# Taber's®

# CYCLOPEDIC MEDICAL DICTIONARY

*Edited by*

CLAYTON L. THOMAS, M.D., M.P.H.

Director Emeritus of Medical Affairs
Tambrands Inc.

*Managing Editor*
Elizabeth J. Egan

*Dictionary Editor*
Dena Ramras Vardara

*Assistant Dictionary Editor*
Anne-Adele Wight

*Online / Production Editors*
Nancee A. Morelli
Marianne Fithian

*Copy Editor*
Ann Houska

*Dictionary Illustrator*
Beth Anne Willert, M.S.

EDITION

18

ILLUSTRATED IN FULL COLOR

# Taber's®

# CYCLOPEDIC MEDICAL DICTIONARY

F. A. DAVIS COMPANY

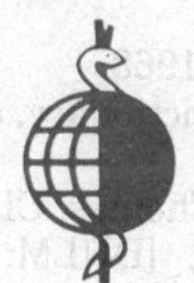

PHILADELPHIA

PRINTED IN THE UNITED STATES OF AMERICA

Last digit indicates print number 10 9 8 7 6 5 4 3 2 1

NOTE: As new scientific information becomes available through basic and clinical research, recommended treatments and drug therapies undergo changes. The author and publisher have done everything possible to make Taber's accurate, up to date, and in accord with accepted standards at the time of publication. The author, editors, and publisher are not responsible for errors or omissions or for consequences from application of the book, and make no warranty, expressed or implied, in regard to the contents of the book. Any practice described in this book should be applied by the reader in accordance with professional standards of care used in regard to the unique circumstances that may apply in each situation. The reader is advised always to check product information (package inserts) for changes and new information regarding dose and contraindications before administering any drug. Caution is especially urged when using new or infrequently ordered drugs.

**Library of Congress Cataloging in Publication Data**

Taber, Clarence Wilbur, 1870–1968
Taber's Cyclopedic Medical Dictionary, edition 18.

Medicine—Dictionaries I. Thomas, Clayton L., 1921– . II. Title. III. Title: Cyclopedic medical dictionary. [DNLM: 1. Dictionaries, Medical. W 13 T113d]
1997 610′.3′21 62-8364
ISSN 1065-1357
ISBN 0-8036-0194-8
ISBN 0-8036-0193-x (indexed)
ISBN 0-8036-0195-6 (deluxe)

# DISTRIBUTORS

**United States of America**
**F. A. DAVIS COMPANY**
1915 Arch St.
Philadelphia, PA 19103

*Atlanta, Georgia*
**J. A. MAJORS COMPANY**
4004 Tradeport Blvd.
P.O. Box 82686, 30354

*Boston, Massachusetts*
**LOGIN BROTHERS NEW ENGLAND**
2 Keith Way
Hingham, MA 02043

**RITTENHOUSE BOOK DISTRIBUTORS, INC.**
Sterling Road
South Lancaster, MA 01561

*Chicago, Illinois*
**LOGIN BROTHERS BOOK COMPANY, INC.**
1436 West Randolph St. 60607

*Cleveland, Ohio*
**LOGIN BROTHERS OHIO**
1550 Enterprise Parkway
Twinsburg, OH 44087

*Dallas, Texas*
**J. A. MAJORS COMPANY**
1851 Diplomat Drive, 75381-9074

*Houston, Texas*
**J. A. MAJORS COMPANY**
9464 Kirby Drive, 77054

*Los Angeles, California*
**J. A. MAJORS COMPANY — CALIFORNIA**
1220 West Walnut St.
Compton, CA 90220

*New York, New York*
**LOGIN BROTHERS NEW JERSEY**
4 Sperry Rd.
Fairfield, NJ 07006

*Philadelphia, Pennsylvania*
**RITTENHOUSE BOOK DISTRIBUTORS, INC.**
511 Feheley Drive
King of Prussia, PA 19406

*St. Louis, Missouri*

**MATTHEWS BOOK COMPANY**
11559 Rock Island Court
Maryland Heights, MO 63043

## Canada

**LOGIN BROTHERS CANADA**
324 Saulteaux Crescent
Winnipeg, Manitoba R3J 3T2

## Europe

**WAVERLY EUROPE, LTD.**
Broadway House
2–6 Fulham Broadway
London SW6 1AA
England

## Australia & New Zealand

**MACLENNAN AND PETTY, PTY. LTD.**
Unit 4/809 Botany Rd.
Rosebery, NSW 2018
Australia

## Mexico & Central America

**LIBRERIA INTERNACIONAL, S. A. DE C.V.**
Av. Sonora 206
Col. Hipodromo
06100 Mexico, D.F.

## Brazil

**ERNESTO REICHMANN, DISTRIBUIDORA DE LIVROS**
Rua Coronel Marques, 335
Tatuape
Sao Paolo—SP 03440-0000
Brazil

## Panama & South America

**INTER-BOOK MARKETING SERVICE**
Rua das Palmeiras, 32-Apt. 701
22270 Rio De Janeiro
Brazil

## India

**JAYPEE BROTHERS MEDICAL PUBLISHERS**
G/16 EMCA House
23/23 B Ansari Rd.
Darya Ganj, New Delhi 110 002
India

## Southeast Asia

**WILLIAMS & WILKINS ASIA-PACIFIC LTD.**
Room 808, Metroplaza Tower 2
223 Hing Fong Rd.
New Territories
Hong Kong

# CONTENTS

# PUBLISHER'S FOREWORD

During the past half century and 17 previous editions, *Taber's Cyclopedic Medical Dictionary* has earned a reputation as the most comprehensive and authoritative reference available for current health science terminology. As the leader in nursing and allied health dictionaries, *Taber's* is the standard against which other dictionaries are measured. At F. A. Davis Company we pride ourselves on that distinction, and the 18th edition of *Taber's* continues that proud tradition.

More than any previous version of this dictionary, the 18th edition reflects our commitment to serve the students and clinicians in the nursing and allied health professions by maintaining the highest standards of editorial excellence. We are especially gratified by the loyalty that the nursing and allied health educators in our audience have shown toward *Taber's* edition after edition. We have welcomed their compliments and, more importantly, listened to their suggestions on how to improve this dictionary.

The 18th edition marks a breakthrough—a coming of age—for *Taber's,* as evidenced by the addition of full-color illustrations and photographs for the first time and by a substantial increase in the total number of images. This edition contains almost three times as many images as the previous edition, most of them in full color and all of them carefully selected (by a team of expert consultants) for relevance to associated entries. Color has also been used to highlight significant elements in the text, making it easier to locate Nursing Implications sections, Caution statements, tables, and cross-references to illustrations and the Nursing Diagnoses Appendix.

Adding the full color spectrum to the overall design of *Taber's* has heightened its visual appeal, but that was not our primary consideration. Our goals were first, to ensure that each illustration was informative and helped to enhance understanding of the related entry, and second, to ensure that current vocabulary entries (which are the essence of any dictionary) were not sacrificed in the process of adding images. Nor did the compactness and portability of the dictionary suffer for this innovation. We avoided the prospect of too much bulk by changing the trim size only slightly (which added less than an inch to the page length).

The primary mission of any dictionary is to define the vocabulary of the language it seeks to explain. In an era of fast-paced communication and technological change in the health sciences, it is essential that students and professionals have a reliable reference tool if they are to communicate effectively within and across health care disciplines. *Taber's* greatest strength continues to be the comprehensiveness of the vocabulary it offers—55,000 entries, a feature unmatched by any other nursing and allied health dictionary. More than 2100 new terms reflecting the latest advances in health care appear in this edition, and virtually every entry in this dictionary has been reviewed for accuracy and clarity. Many of them are encyclopedic entries, offering detailed explanations of important concepts. In addition, there are 65 new and revised tables of easy-to-access, useful information.

*Taber's* extensive set of appendices, a complete resource in themselves, have been fully revised. The Universal Precautions Appendix offers the latest CDC Isolation Precautions (1996) and the OSHA Bloodborne Pathogens Standard. Nursing diagnoses have been updated through the 12th NANDA Conference, and almost 300 diseases/disorders and 124 nursing diagnoses are fully cross-referenced to this appendix from the Vocabulary section of the book. The Interpreter has been expanded and revised to help clinicians communicate with Spanish- and French-speaking patients, and the Medical Emergencies Appendix (including Poisons and Poisonings) has been completely rewritten to reflect the latest thinking. Three new appendices have been added: a glossary of computer terms, a compendium of health care organizations, and a list of professional degrees and titles in the health sciences.

The task of revising a reference book such as *Taber's* is a massive undertaking requiring skill, dedication, and attention to detail on the part of many people. We are indebted primarily to our medical editor, Clayton L. Thomas, M.D., and to Valerie Scanlon, PhD., and a team of consultants from every major nursing and allied health discipline for their expertise in determining the content of the vocabulary entries, in selecting meaningful illustrations to strengthen those entries, and in updating the appendices. Their patience and good humor throughout this long process kept us on an even keel. We also thank Owen Traynor, M.D., Janet Traynor, PharmD., Glenn Morocco, PhD., John C. Lewis, EdD., Barbara Lindsey, M.S., and Margaret Caprara, M.A., for editorial contributions that made this edition even stronger.

Finally, our gratitude goes to everyone who has consulted *Taber's* and taken the time to contact us and let us know what you like or what you would like us to consider for the next edition. We proudly offer the 18th edition of *Taber's Cyclopedic Medical Dictionary* and welcome your comments and suggestions once again.

**Robert H. Craven, Jr.**
**F. A. Davis Company**

# INTRODUCTION TO EDITION 18

From the inception of this dictionary in the 1940s, all concerned with *Taber's* have devoted their efforts to producing an accurate, up-to-date health care resource that would serve any intelligent reader, but especially nurses and allied health professionals. *Taber's* is also invaluable to those in other professions, such as law, who require a reliable source of medical information. The present edition continues this effort by being the most useful dictionary available to the audiences we have traditionally served.

The explosion of information in general and particularly in biological and medical sciences continues. More than 2100 new terms have been added to this edition. Examples are: *airway pressure release ventilation, antibiotic resistance, Canadian Occupational Performance Measure, clinical pathway, functional outcome, hantavirus pulmonary syndrome, Minimum Data Set, monoclonal antibody therapy, nursing protocol,* and *plyometrics*. New appendices include the Computer Glossary, Health Care Resource Organizations, and Professional Designations and Titles in the Health Sciences. As mentioned in the Publisher's Foreword, existing appendices have been updated and their content expanded. The use of hundreds of high-quality four-color illustrations in addition to the excellent two-color illustrations of Beth Anne Willert further enhances the value of this dictionary.

The accuracy of a medical dictionary depends on the editor's ability to stay abreast of the medical and scientific changes that dictate the need to add new words and to delete terms and concepts that are no longer valid or useful. This can be accomplished through constant alertness to the medical literature as well as the spoken words that herald advances in the biological sciences. To do this without comprehensive medical libraries and electronically accessed data banks would be virtually impossible. The Countway Library at the Harvard Medical School Baystate Medical Center Health Sciences Library in Springfield, Massachusetts, and the National Library of Medicine in Bethesda, Maryland, and their staffs are of invaluable assistance in obtaining reference materials.

The several consultants in numerous disciplines important to the nursing, medical, and allied health fields have provided excellent materials and suggestions concerning this edition of *Taber's*. Those individuals are listed on the next page. I appreciate the quality and quantity of their assistance.

I acknowledge also *The Barnhart Dictionary Companion* (published by Springer-Verlag, New York, Inc.) and the *Dictionary of the Rheumatic Diseases* (American College of Rheumatology, Glossary Committee), from which several entries were derived.

An editor's efforts would amount to very little without the excellent leadership and managerial skill provided for F. A. Davis Company by the team of Robert H. and Rob Craven and those directly involved in bringing the book to completion—that is, Elizabeth J. Egan, Dena Ramras Vardara, Anne-Adele Wight, and Nancee Morelli.

Most important of all, my wife, Peggy, provides the support and inspiration for all my efforts, which enabled me to edit this volume.

**Clayton Lay Thomas, M.D., M.P.H.**

# CONSULTANTS

Tonia Dandry Aiken, RN, BSN, JD
Richard J. Barry, MLS
Joea E. Bierchen, RN, EdD
Carroll Conner Bouman, RN, PhD
Virginia Burggraf, RN, C, MSN
Charles Christiansen, EdD, OTR, FAOTA
Marilynn E. Doenges, RN, BSN, MA, CS
Jacqueline Fawcett, PhD, FAAN
Lucien R. Greif, BSME
Barbara Gylys, MEd, CMA-A
Diane B. Hamilton, RN, PhD
Brenda Walters Holloway, RN, MSN, CFNP
Donna Ignatavicius, MS, RNC
Glen Johnson, MD
Terence C. Karselis, MS, MT (ASCP)
Jeanette G. Kernicki, RN, PhD
Carolyn B. Kisner, MS, PT
Susan S. Lampe, RN, MS
Gregg Margolis, MS, NREMT-P
Judith E. Meissner, RN, BSN, MSN
Mary Frances Moorhouse, RN, CRRN, CLNC
Stanley M. Pearson, MSEd, RRT, C-CPT
Betty Reynard, RDH, EdD
Janet Ross Kerr, RN, PhD
Valerie C. Scanlon, PhD
Lydia D. Schafer, BA, PhD
Martha N. Surline, MS
Darlene Travis, BS, RT(R)(T)(CV), ARRT
Morris E. Weaver, PhD
Robert L. Wilkins, MA, RRT

(Material supplied by the consultants has been reviewed and edited by Clayton L. Thomas, MD, MPH, Editor, with whom final responsibility rests for the accuracy of the content.)

# Taber's Feature Finder

MAIN ENTRY

ILLUSTRATION CROSS REFERENCE

**abduction** (ăb-dŭk´shŭn) **1.** Lateral movement of the limbs away from the median plane of the body, or lateral bending of the head or trunk. SEE: illus. **2.** Movement of the digits away from the axial line of a limb. **3.** Outward rotation of the eyes.

**acetaminophen** (ă-sĕt″ă-mĭn´ō-fĕn) A synthetic drug with antipyretic and analgesic effects similar to those of aspirin, but without anti-inflammatory or antirheumatic effects.

CAUTION

Caution: Acute overdose may cause fatal hepatic necrosis.

ABBREVIATION

**ADC** *anodal duration contraction; axiodistocervical*

PRONUNCIATION

ETYMOLOGY

**addict** (ăd´ĭkt) [L. *addictus,* given over] One physically or psychologically, or both, dependent on a substance, esp. alcohol or drugs.

BIOGRAPHICAL INFORMATION

SYNONYM

SYMPTOMS

ETIOLOGY

TREATMENT

CROSS REFERENCE

PROGNOSIS

NURSING IMPLICATIONS

NURSING DIAGNOSES CROSS REFERENCE

**Addison's disease** [Thomas Addison, Brit. physician, 1793-1860] Disease resulting from deficiency in the secretion of adrenocortical hormones. SYN: *adrenocortical hypofunction; chronic hypoadrenocorticism.*

SYMPTOMS: Increased pigmentation of skin and mucous membranes, irregular patches of vitiligo, black freckles over head and neck, weakness, fatigability, hypotension, nausea, vomiting, anorexia, weight loss, and sometimes hypoglycemia.

ETIOLOGY: Progressive destruction of the adrenal gland whether due to an infectious disease, such as tuberculosis, or infiltration by neoplastic tissue or hemorrhage into the gland.

TREATMENT: Adrenocortical hormone therapy is dramatic in its effect and must be given promptly in adrenal crisis in order to prevent death. SEE: *adrenal crisis.*

PROGNOSIS: If untreated, the disease will continue a chronic course with progressive but usually relatively slow deterioration; in some patients the deterioration may be rapid. Patients treated properly have an excellent prognosis.

NURSING IMPLICATIONS: Acute adrenal crisis: The patient is monitored for dehydration, hypotension, hypoglycemia, hyperkalemia, petechial hemorrhages, somnolent state, and profound hypovolemic shock. SEE: Nursing Diagnoses Appendix.

PLURAL

ADJECTIVAL FORM

SUBENTRY

**adenoma** (ăd″ĕ-nō´mă) *pl.* **adenomata** [″+ *oma*, tumor] A neoplasm of glandular epithelium. **adenomatous** (-nō´mă-tŭs),*adj.*

***chromophobe a.*** Tumor of the pituitary gland composed of cells that do not stain readily. It may cause pituitary deficiency or diabetes insipidus.

***follicular a.*** Adenoma of the thyroid.

Not an actual page.

# FEATURES AND THEIR USE

This section describes the major features found in *Taber's* and provides information that may help you use the dictionary more efficiently. The Feature Finder, on page xii, is a graphic representation of many of the features described below.

1. **Vocabulary:** The extensive vocabulary defined in *Taber's* has been updated to meet the ongoing needs of students, educators, and clinicians in the health sciences. The medical editor and the nursing and allied health consultants have researched and written new entries, revised existing entries, and deleted obsolete ones, reflecting the many changes in health care technology, clinical practice, and patient care. American, rather than British, spellings are preferred.
2. **Entry format:** *Taber's* entries are organized according to a main entry–subentry format, which makes it easier—especially for students—to find and compare medical terms that share a common element or classification. All single-word terms (e.g., **cell**) are main entries, and most compound, or multiple-word, terms (e.g., **stem cell**) are subentries under the main entry (or headword)—in this case, **cell.** However, some compound terms (e.g., eponyms, such as **Parkinson's disease,** and the names of individuals and organizations) are listed as main entries. An especially important compound term may be listed as both a main entry and a subentry, with one of the terms serving as a cross-reference to the other. All main entries are printed in bold type; subentries are indented under the main entry and are printed in bold italic type. All entries are listed and defined in the singular whenever possible.
3. **Alphabetization:**

   ***Main entries*** are alphabetized letter by letter, regardless of spaces or hyphens that occur between the words; a comma marks the end of a main entry for alphabetical purposes (e.g., **skin, tenting of** precedes **skin cancer**). In eponyms the **'s** is ignored in alphabetizing (e.g., **Albini's nodules** precedes **albinism**).

   ***Subentries*** are listed in straight-ahead order following the same letter-by-letter alphabetization used for main entries; a comma marks the end of a subentry for alphabetical purposes. The headword is abbreviated in all subentries (such as ***premature l.*** under **labor** or ***emergency medical t.*** under **technician**).
4. **Eponyms:** Included as main entries are the names of individuals who were the first to discover, describe, or popularize a concept, a microorganism, a disease, a syndrome, or an anatomical structure. A brief biography appears in brackets after the pronunciation. Biographical information includes the person's medical designation, the country in which the person was born or worked, and the date of birth and death if known.

5. **Definitions:** The text that occurs before the first period in an entry constitutes the definition for that entry. Many entries are written in encyclopedic style, offering a comprehensive understanding of the disease, condition, or concept defined. See "Encyclopedic entries" for further information.

6. **Pronunciations:** Most main entries are spelled phonetically. Pronunciations, which appear in parentheses after the boldface main entry, are given as simply as possible with most long and short vowels marked diacritically and secondary accents indicated. *Diacritics* are marks over or under vowels. Only two diacritics are used in *Taber's:* the macron ¯ showing the long sound of vowels, as the a in rate, e in rebirth, i in isle, o in over, and u in unite; and the breve ˘ showing the short sound of vowels, as the a in apple, e in ever, i in it, o in not, and u in cut. *Accents* are marks used to indicate stress upon certain syllables. A single accent ′ is called a primary accent. A double accent ″ is called a secondary accent; it indicates less stress upon a syllable than that given by a primary accent. This difference in stress can be seen in the word an″es-the′si-a.

7. **Singular/Plural forms:** When the spelling of an entry's singular or plural form is a nonstandard formation (e.g., **villus** *pl.* **villi,** or **viscera** *sing.* **viscus**), the spelling of the singular or plural form appears in boldface after the pronunciation for the main entry. Nonstandard singular and plural forms appear as entries themselves at their normal alphabetical positions.

8. **Etymologies:** An etymology indicates the origin and historical development of a term. For most medical terms the origin is Latin or Greek. An etymology is given for most main entries and appears in brackets following the pronunciation.

9. **Abbreviations:** Standard abbreviations for entries are included with the definition and also are listed alphabetically throughout the text. Additional abbreviations used for charting and prescription writing are listed in the Appendices. A list of nonmedical abbreviations used in text appears on page xxiv.

10. **Encyclopedic entries:** Detailed, comprehensive information is included with entries that require additional coverage because of their importance or complexity. Often this information is organized into several subsections, each with its own subheading. The most frequently used subheadings are Nursing Implications, Symptoms, Etiology, Treatment, and Caution. Other subheadings that may appear in text include Contraindications, Differential Diagnosis, Examination, Function, Incompatibility, Indications, Pathology, Physiology, and Therapy.

11. **Illustrations:** This edition of *Taber's* includes 560 color illustrations. More than 375 of those are new, four-color illustrations, and the balance are two-color line drawings. The illustrations were carefully chosen to complement the text of the entries with which they are associated. Each illustration is cross-referenced from its associated entry. A complete list of illustrations begins on page xvi.

12. **Tables:** This edition contains 65 color-screened tables located appropriately throughout the Vocabulary section. A list of tables appears on page xxii.

13. **Adjectives:** The adjectival forms of many noun main entries appear at the end of the definition of the noun form or, if the entry is long, at the

end of the first paragraph. Pronunciations for most of the adjectival forms are included. Many common adjectives appear as main entries themselves.

14. **Italics and boldface:** Synonyms and cross references are italicized, as are the Latin names for biological materials, including botanical and zoological specimens, and anatomical structures. The terms for which an abbreviation stands are italicized, as are some foreign words. Boldface type is used for all main entries and subentries, plural or singular forms, adjectival forms, and headings used in tables.
15. **Caution statements:** This notation is used to draw particular attention to clinically important information. The information is of more than routine interest and should be considered when delivering health care. These statements are further emphasized by colored rules above and below the text.
16. **Synonyms:** Synonyms are listed at the end of the entry or, in encyclopedic entries, at the end of the first paragraph. The abbreviation SYN: precedes the synonymous term(s). Terms listed as synonyms have their own entries in the Vocabulary, which generally carry a cross-reference to the entry at which the definition appears.
17. **Cross-references:** Illustrations, tables, appendices, or other relevant vocabulary entries may be given as cross-references. These are indicated by SEE: followed by the name(s) of the appropriate element(s) in italics. Cross-references to the Nursing Diagnoses Appendix are highlighted in color at the end of the entry as SEE: *Nursing Diagnoses Appendix*. Entries at which an illustration appears carry the color-highlighted SEE: illus.
18. **Appendices:** The Appendices contain detailed information that could be organized or presented more easily in that format than the one used in the body of the book. They also include long tables that would interfere with finding entries in the Vocabulary section. This edition features several new appendices: Computer Glossary, Health Care Resource Organizations (in the United States and Canada), and Professional Designations and Titles in the Health Sciences. Among the revised appendices are Nursing Diagnoses, Universal Precautions, Conceptual Models and Theories of Nursing, The Interpreter in Three Languages, Medical Emergencies, and Nutrition.
19. **Nursing Diagnoses Appendix:** This appendix has been updated through the 12th NANDA (North American Nursing Diagnosis Association) conference. It is divided into several sections, including two lists of NANDA's nursing diagnoses organized into Doenges & Moorhouse's Diagnostic Divisions and Gordon's Functional Health Patterns; an at-a-glance look at the most recent diagnoses approved by NANDA; nursing diagnoses commonly associated with almost 300 diseases/disorders (cross-referenced from the body of the dictionary); and a complete description of all NANDA-approved diagnoses through the 12th conference (in 1996) in alphabetical order. Included are the diagnostic division, definition, related factors, and defining characteristics for each nursing diagnosis. See the *Quick View of Contents* on page 2327 for further explanation.

# LIST OF ILLUSTRATIONS

Illustrations are listed according to the main entry or subentry they accompany. Information in parentheses indicates the source of the illustration; a list of sources appears at the end of the list. Wherever possible, a figure will appear on the same page as the entry it illustrates; however, when there is no space on that page for the illustration, it will appear on the preceding or following page.

---

* WB Saunders Company, Philadelphia, PA; with permission.
† Listen, Look, and Learn, vol. 3. Chicago, IL. ASCP Press © 1973; with permission.
‡ TW Diggs, D Sturm, A Bell: Morphology of Human Blood Cells, Abbott Laboratories, Abbott Park, IL, 1985; with permission.
§ BK Hyun, MD; with permission.
¶ The Upjohn Company, Kalamazoo, MI; with permission.

# ILLUSTRATION SOURCES

Harmening, DM: Clinical Hematology and Fundamentals of Hemostasis. FA Davis, Philadelphia, 1992.
Kern, ME: Medical Mycology: A Self-Instructional Text, ed 2. FA Davis, Philadelphia, 1996.
Leventhal, R, and Cheadle, R: Medical Parasitology: A Self-Instructional Text, ed 4. FA Davis, Philadelphia, 1995.
Mazziotta, JC, and Gilman, S: Brain Imaging: Principles and Applications. FA Davis, Philadelphia, 1992.
Reeves, JRT, and Mailbach, H: Clinical Dermatology Illustrated: A Regional Approach. FA Davis, Philadelphia, 1991.
Sacher, RA, and McPherson, RA: Widmann's Clinical Interpretation of Laboratory Tests, ed 10. FA Davis, Philadelphia, 1991.
Scanlon, VC, and Sanders, T: Essentials of Anatomy and Physiology, ed 2. FA Davis, Philadelphia, 1995.
Strasinger, SK: Urinalysis and Body Fluids, ed 3. FA Davis, Philadelphia, 1994.

# LIST OF TABLES

# ABBREVIATIONS USED IN TEXT*

| | | | |
|---|---|---|---|
| ABBR | abbreviation | i.e. | id est (that is) |
| Amerind | American Indian | L. | Latin |
| approx. | approximately | LL. | Late Latin |
| AS | Anglo-Saxon | MD. | Middle Dutch |
| at. no. | atomic number | ME. | Middle English |
| at. wt. | atomic weight | Med. L. | Medieval Latin |
| Brit. | British | NL | New Latin |
| C | centigrade | O.Fr. | Old French |
| CNS | central nervous system | pert. | pertaining |
| e.g. | exempli gratia (for example) | pl. | plural |
| | | rel. | related; relating |
| esp. | especially | sing. | singular |
| F | Fahrenheit | Sp. | Spanish |
| Fr. | French | sp. gr. | specific gravity |
| fr. | from | SYMB | symbol |
| Ger. | German | SYN | synonym |
| Gr. | Greek | | |

* Medical and charting abbreviations appear in the Appendix. Additional abbreviations are listed in the Units of Measurement Appendix and the Medical Abbreviations Appendix.

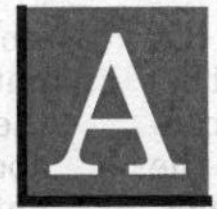

*α* Alpha, the first letter of the Greek alphabet.

**Å** *angstrom unit.*

**$A_2$** *aortic second sound.*

**a** *accommodation; ampere; anode; anterior; aqua; area; artery.*

**ā** [L.] *ante,* before.

**a-, an-** [Gr., not] Prefix meaning *without, away from, not* (a- is usually used before a consonant; an- is usually used before a vowel).

**A.A., a.a.** *achievement age; Alcoholics Anonymous; amino acid; arteriae.*

**aa** [Gr. *ana,* of each] Prescription notation meaning *the stated amount of each of the substances is to be used in compounding the prescription.*

**AAA** *American Ambulance Association.*

**A.A.A.** *American Academy of Allergists; American Association of Anatomists.*

**A.A.A.S.** *American Association for the Advancement of Science.*

**A.A.C.N.** *American Association of Critical-Care Nurses; American Association of Colleges of Nursing.*

**A.A.F.P.** *American Academy of Family Physicians.*

**AAHN** *American Association for the History of Nursing.*

**AAL** *anterior axillary line.*

**A.A.M.A.** *American Association of Medical Assistants.*

**A.A.M.I.** *Association for the Advancement of Medical Instrumentation*

**AAMS** *Association of Air Medical Services.*

**AAMT** *American Association for Medical Transcription.*

**A.A.N.** *American Academy of Nursing.*

**A.A.N.A.** *American Association of Nurse Anesthetists.*

**A.A.N.N.** *American Association of Neuroscience Nurses.*

**A.A.O.H.N.** *American Association of Occupational Health Nurses.*

**A.A.O.S.** *American Academy of Orthopedic Surgeons.*

**A.A.P.** *American Academy of Pediatrics; American Association of Pathologists.*

**A.A.P.A.** *American Academy of Physician Assistants.*

**AAPMR** *American Academy of Physical Medicine and Rehabilitation.*

**A.A.R.C.** *American Association for Respiratory Care.*

**AARP** *American Association of Retired Persons.*

**AAS** *atomic absorption spectroscopy.*

**AASECT** *American Association of Sex Educators, Counselors, and Therapists.*

**ab** *antibody.*

**ab-** [L. *ab,* from] Prefix meaning *from, away from, negative, absent.*

**Abadie's sign** (ă-bă-dēz′) **1.** [Charles A. Abadie, Fr. ophthalmologist, 1842–1932] In exophthalmic goiter, spasm of the levator palpebrae superioris. **2.** [Jean Abadie, Fr. neurologist, 1873–1946] In tabes dorsalis, insensibility to pressure over the Achilles tendon.

**A band** A dark-staining area in the center of a sarcomere in skeletal or cardiac muscle, composed of overlapping myosin and actin filaments. SYN: *anisotropic disk.*

**abandonment** A premature termination of the professional treatment relationship by the health care provider without adequate notice or the patient's consent.

**abaptiston** (ă″băp-tĭs′tŏn) [Gr. *abaptistos,* not dipped] Trephine that cannot slip and injure the brain.

**abarognosis** (ăb″ăr-ŏg-nō′sĭs) [Gr. *a-,* not, + *baros,* weight, + *gnosis,* knowledge] Loss of ability to sense weight. SEE: *baragnosis.*

**abarthrosis** (ăb-ăr-thrō′sĭs) [L. *ab,* from, + Gr. *arthron,* joint, + *osis,* condition] A movable joint or point at which bones move freely against each other. SYN: *diarthrosis.*

**abarticular** [″+ *articulus,* joint] At a distance from a joint.

**abarticulation 1.** Dislocation of a joint. **2.** Diarthrosis. SYN: *abarthrosis.*

**abasia** (ă-bā′zē-ă) [Gr. *a-,* not, + *basis,* step] **1.** Motor incoordination in walking. **2.** Inability to walk due to impairment of coordination. **abasic, abatic** *adj.*

***a.-astasia*** Lack of motor coordination with inability to stand or walk. SYN: *astasia-abasia.*

***a. atactica*** Uncertain movements in walking.

***paralytic a.*** Abasia in which the leg muscles are paralyzed.

***paroxysmal trepidant a.*** Abasia caused by trembling and sudden stiffening of legs on standing, making walking impossible. It may be related to hysteria.

**abate** (ă-bāt′) [L. *ab,* from, + *battere,* to beat] **1.** To lessen or decrease. **2.** To cease or cause to cease.

**abatement** (ă-bāt′mĕnt) Decrease in severity of pain or symptoms.

**abaxial, abaxile** (ăb-ăk′sē-al, -sĭl) [L. *ab,* from, + *axis,* axis] **1.** Not within the axis of a body or part. **2.** At the opposite end of the axis of a part.

**Abbott's method** [Edville G. Abbott, U.S. orthopedic surgeon, 1871–1938] Treatment of scoliosis by a series of plaster jackets.

**ABC** *antigen-binding capacity; airway, breathing, circulation* (mnemonic for assessing status of emergency patients).

**abdomen** (ăb-dō′mĕn, ăb′dō-mĕn) [L., belly] The portion of the trunk located between the pelvis and the thorax. It contains the stomach, lower part of the esophagus, small and large intestines, liver, gallbladder, spleen, pancreas, and bladder. A serous membrane, the peritoneum, lines this cavity, but not all of the organs in the abdomen are covered by this membrane. SEE: *abdominal quadrants* for illus.

INSPECTION: Visual examination of the abdomen is best done while the patient is supine with the knees slightly bent. In a healthy person the abdomen is oval shaped, with elevations and depressions corresponding to abdominal muscles, umbilicus, and to some degree the forms of underlying viscera. Relative to chest size, it is larger in children than in adults; it is more rotund and broader inferiorly in males than in females.

Disease can alter the shape of the abdomen. A general, symmetrical enlargement may result from ascites; a partial and irregular enlargement may result from tumors, hypertrophy of organs such as the liver or spleen, or intestinal distention caused by gas. Retraction of the abdomen may occur in extreme emaciation and in several forms of cerebral disease, esp. tubercular meningitis of children.

The respiratory movements of the abdominal walls are related to movements of the thorax and are often increased when the latter are arrested and vice versa; thus, abdominal movements are increased in pleurisy, pneumonia, and pericarditis, but are decreased or wholly suspended in peritonitis and disease-caused abdominal pain.

The superficial abdominal veins are sometimes visibly enlarged, indicating an obstruction of blood flow in either the portal system (as in cirrhosis) or the inferior vena cava.

AUSCULTATION: Listening to sounds produced in abdominal organs provides useful diagnostic information. Absent or diminished sounds may indicate paralytic ileus or peritonitis. High-pitched tinkling sounds are associated with intestinal obstruction. Bruits may indicate an abdominal aortic aneurysm. During pregnancy, auscultation enables identification and evaluation of the fetal heart rate and vascular sounds from the placenta.

PERCUSSION: The patient should be placed in the same position as for palpation, and percussion should for the most part be mediate. In exploring the abdomen by percussion, the finger should first be placed immediately below the xiphoid cartilage, pressed firmly down, and carried along the median line toward the pubes, striking it all the way and alternating between forcible and gentle. The different tones of the stomach, colon, and small intestines will be distinctly heard. Percussion should then be made laterally, alternately to one side, then the other, until the whole surface is percussed. A large abdominal aneurysm gives dullness or flatness over it unless a distended intestine lies above it.

PALPATION: The abdomen may be palpated with fingertips, the whole hand, or both hands; pressure may be slight or forceful, continuous or intermittent. To obtain the greatest amount of information, the patient should be supine with the head slightly raised and knees bent. The head is supported in order to relax the abdominal wall. It is sometimes necessary to place the patient in a standing position or leaning forward.

Palpation is helpful in detecting the size, consistency, and position of viscera, the existence of tumors and swellings, and whether the tumors change position with respiration or are movable. It is necessary to ascertain whether tenderness exists in any portion of the abdominal cavity, whether pain is increased or relieved by firm pressure, and whether pain is accentuated by sudden release of firm pressure (i.e., rebound tenderness).

Impulse, if one exists, is systolic and expansive, although when situated high there may be a slight diastolic movement also. A thrill is rarely perceptible. A tumor's surface is usually round and smooth but may be nodular. Effusion of blood into surrounding tissues may produce lobulations.

***acute a.*** An abnormal condition of the abdomen in which there is a sudden, abrupt onset of severe pain. It requires immediate evaluation and diagnosis, as it may indicate a need for immediate surgical intervention. SYN: *surgical a.*

***pendulous a.*** A condition in which the excessively relaxed anterior wall of the abdomen hangs down over the pubis.

***scaphoid a.*** A condition in which the anterior wall is hollowed, presenting a sunken appearance as in emaciation.

***surgical a.*** Acute a.

**abdomin-** SEE: *abdomino-*.

**abdominal** (ăb-dŏm′ĭ-năl) Pert. to the abdomen.

**abdominal cavity** The cavity within the abdomen. It is lined with a serous membrane, the peritoneum, and contains the following organs: stomach with the lower portion of the esophagus, small and large intestines (except sigmoid colon and rectum), liver, gallbladder, spleen, pancreas, adrenal glands, kidneys, and ureters. It is continuous with the pelvic cavity; the two constitute the abdominopelvic cavity. SEE: *abdominal quadrants* for illus.

**abdominal crisis** Severe pain in the abdominal area. It usually refers to pain that occurs during sickle cell anemia crisis or that results from syphilis.

**abdominal decompression** A technique used in obstetrics to facilitate childbirth.

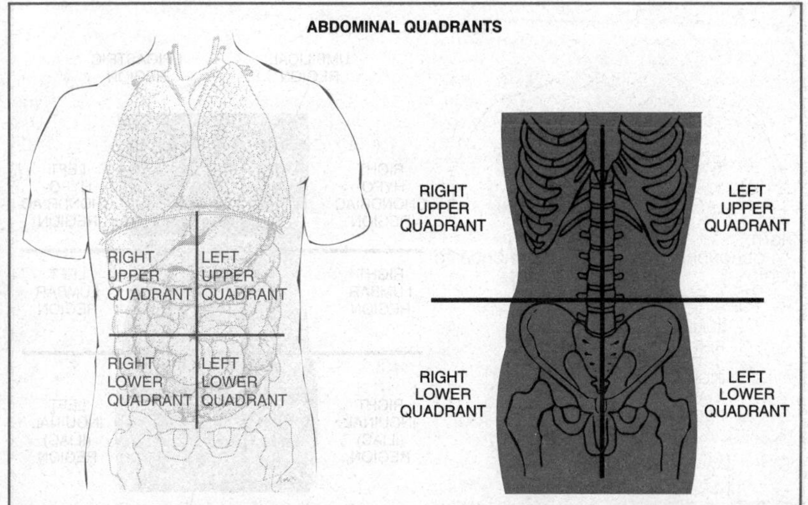


The abdominal area is surrounded by an airtight chamber in which pressure may be intermittently decreased below atmospheric pressure. During labor pains, the pressure is decreased and the uterus is permitted to work more efficiently because the abdominal muscles are elevated away from the uterus.

**abdominalgia** (ăb-dŏm-ĭn-ăl′jē-ă) [L. *abdomen,* belly, + Gr. *algos,* pain] Pain in the abdomen.

**abdominal inguinal ring** The internal opening of the inguinal canal, bounded inferiorly by the inguinal ligament, medially by the inferior epigastric vessels, and above and laterally by the lower free border of the transversus abdominis muscle. SEE: *abdominal rings; canal, inguinal; hernia; ring, abdominal inguinal.*

**abdominal muscles** The group of four muscles that make up the abdominal wall, consisting of: 1. the external oblique (the most superficial of the four), whose fibers are directed downward and medially from the lower ribs to the linea alba and pelvis; 2. the internal oblique, whose fibers are directed upward and medially from the iliac crest and lumbodorsal fascia to the lower ribs; 3. the rectus abdominis, a vertically oriented muscle from the crest of the pubis to the cartilages of the fifth, sixth, and seventh ribs and xiphoid process; and 4. the transversus abdominis, whose fibers are oriented transversely. These muscles participate in a variety of functions, including flexion, side bending and rotation of the trunk, stabilization of the trunk in the upright posture, the expiratory phase of respiration, coughing, and Valsalva's maneuver.

**abdominal quadrants** Four parts or divisions of the abdomen determined by drawing imaginary vertical and horizontal lines through the umbilicus. The quadrants and their contents are:

*Right upper quadrant (RUQ):* right lobe of liver, gallbladder, part of transverse colon, part of pylorus, hepatic flexure, right kidney, and duodenum; *Right lower q. (RLQ):* cecum, ascending colon, small intestine, appendix, bladder if distended, right ureter, right spermatic duct in the male; right ovary and right tube, and uterus if enlarged, in the female; *Left upper q. (LUQ):* left lobe of liver, stomach, transverse colon, splenic flexure, pancreas, left kidney, and spleen; *Left lower q. (LLQ):* small intestine, left ureter, sigmoid flexure, descending colon, bladder if distended, left spermatic duct in the male; left ovary and left tube, and uterus if enlarged, in the female. SEE: illus.

**abdominal reflexes** Contraction of the muscles of the abdominal wall on stimulation of the overlying skin. Absence of these reflexes indicates damage to the pyramidal tract.

**abdominal regions** The abdomen and its external surface, divided into nine regions by four imaginary planes: two horizontal, one at the level of the ninth costal cartilage (or the lowest point of the costal arch) and the other at the level of the highest point of the iliac crest; two vertical, through the centers of the inguinal ligaments (or through the nipples or through the centers of the clavicles) or curved and coinciding with the lateral borders of the two abdominal rectus muscles. SEE: illus.

**abdominal rescue** Emergency cesarean delivery of a fetus jeopardized during labor or failed vaginal birth. Indications for surgical intervention include fetal distress associated with dystocia, arrested descent, abruptio placentae, or umbilical cord prolapse.

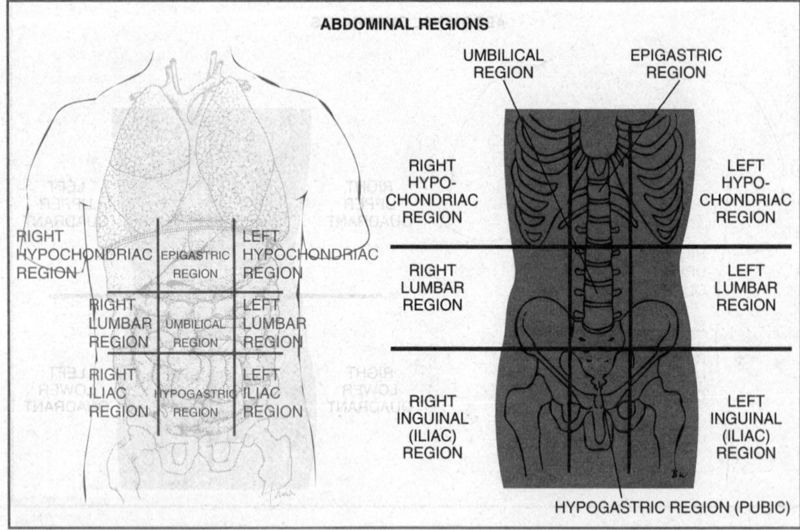


**abdominal rings** The apertures in the abdominal wall. *External:* an interval in the aponeurosis of the external oblique muscle, just above and to the outer side of the crest of the pubic bone. *Triangular:* about 1 in. (2.5 cm) from base to apex and ½ in. (1.3 cm) transversely; provides passage for the spermatic cord in the male and the round ligament in the female. *Internal* or *deep:* situated in the transversalis fascia, midway between the anterior superior spine of the ilium and the symphysis pubis, ½ in. (1.3 cm) above Poupart's ligament; oval form, larger in the male; surrounds spermatic cord in the male and round ligament in the female.

**abdomino-, abdomin-** (ăb-dŏm′ĭ-nō) Combining form meaning *abdomen.*

**abdominocardiac reflex** (ăb-dŏm″ĭ-nō-kăr′dē-ăk) A change in heart rate, usually a slowing, resulting from mechanical stimulation of abdominal viscera.

**abdominocentesis** (ăb-dŏm″ĭ-nō-sĕn-tē′sĭs) [L. *abdomen,* belly, + Gr. *kentesis,* puncture] Puncture of the abdomen with an instrument for withdrawal of fluid from the abdominal cavity. SYN: *abdominal paracentesis.*

**abdominocyesis** (ăb-dŏm″ĭn-ō-sī-ēs′ĭs) SEE: *pregnancy, abdominal.*

**abdominocystic** [″ + Gr. *kystis,* bladder] Pert. to the abdomen and bladder.

**abdominodiaphragmatic breathing** A controlled breathing pattern using reciprocal action of the abdominal muscles for expiration and the diaphragm for inspiration; used to maintain control during exertion or to regain control in dyspnea.

**abdominogenital** (ăb-dŏm″ĭ-nō-jĕn′ĭ-tăl) Pert. to the abdomen and genital organs.

**abdominohysterectomy** [L. *abdomen,* belly, + Gr. *hystera,* womb, + *ektome,* excision] Removal of the uterus through abdominal incision.

**abdominohysterotomy** (ăb-dŏm″ĭ-nō-hĭs-tĕr-ŏt′ō-mē) [″ + ″ + *tome,* incision] Incision of the uterus through a surgical opening in the abdomen.

**abdominoperineal** Pert. to the abdomen and perineal area.

**abdominoplasty** Plastic surgery on the abdomen.

**abdominoscopy** (ăb-dŏm″ĭ-nŏs′kō-pē) [L. *abdomen,* belly, + Gr. *skopein,* to examine] Examination of the abdominal cavity and its contents by use of an endoscope. SEE: *laparoscopy; peritoneoscopy.*

**abdominoscrotal** [″ + *scrotum,* bag] Pert. to the abdomen and scrotum.

**abdominoscrotal muscle** Cremaster.

**abdominothoracic** (ăb-dŏm″ĭ-nō-thō-ră′sĭk) [L. *abdomen,* belly, + Gr. *thorax,* chest] Pert. to the abdomen and thorax.

**abdominothoracic arch** The costal arch; the anterior and lateral boundary between the line dividing the thorax and the abdomen.

**abdominouterotomy** (ăb-dŏm″ĭ-nō-ū-tĕr-ŏt′ō-mē) [L. *abdomen,* belly, + *uterus,* womb, + Gr. *tome,* incision] Abdominohysterotomy.

**abdominovaginal** (ăb-dŏm″ĭ-nō-văj′ĭ-năl) [″ + *vagina,* sheath] Pert. to the abdomen and vagina.

**abdominovesical** (ăb-dŏm″ĭ-nō-vĕs′ĭ-kăl) [″ + *vesica,* bladder] Pert. to the abdomen and urinary bladder.

**abducens** (ăb-dū′sĕnz) [L., drawing away] Pert. to drawing away from the midline of the body.

***a. labiorum*** The muscle that elevates the angle of the mouth. SYN: *caninus muscle; levator anguli oris muscle.* SEE: *Muscles Appendix.*

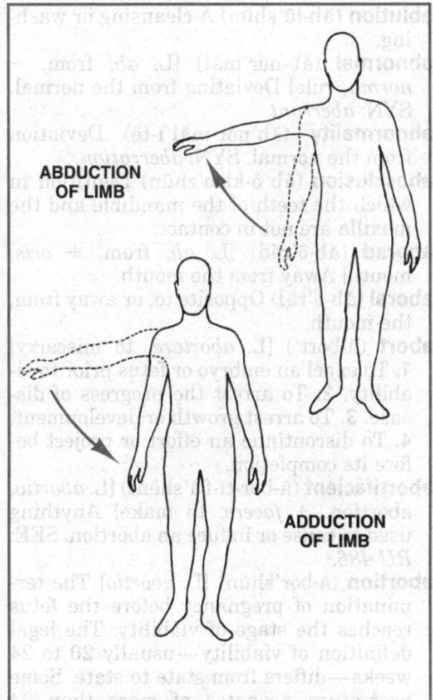


***a. oculi*** Musculus rectus lateralis bulbi.

**abducens muscle** Rectus lateralis muscle of the eye; it moves the eyeball outward.

**abducens nerve** The sixth cranial nerve; it innervates the rectus lateralis muscle of the eye. SEE: *cranial nerves.*

**abducent** (ăb-dū′sĕnt) [L. *abducens,* drawing away] **1.** Abducting; leading away. **2.** Abducens.

**abducent nerve** Abducens nerve.

**abduct** (ăb-dŭkt′) [L. *abductus,* led away] To draw away from the median plane of the body or one of its parts.

**abduction** (ăb-dŭk′shŭn) **1.** Lateral movement of the limbs away from the median plane of the body, or lateral bending of the head or trunk. SEE: illus. **2.** Movement of the digits away from the axial line of a limb. **3.** Outward rotation of the eyes.

**abductor** (ăb-dŭk′tor) A muscle that on contraction draws a part away from the median plane of the body or the axial line of an extremity. Opposite of adductor. SEE: *Muscles Appendix.*

**abenteric** (ăb-ĕn-tĕr′ĭk) [L. *ab,* from, + Gr. *enteron,* intestine] Rel. to or involving organs located outside the intestines.

**Abernethy's fascia** (ăb′ĕr-nē″thē) [John Abernethy, Brit. surgeon, 1764–1831] A layer of areolar tissue separating the external iliac artery from the iliac fascia over the psoas muscle.

**aberrant** (ăb-ĕr′ănt) [L. *ab,* from, + *errare,* to wander] Deviating from the normal. SYN: *abnormal.*

**aberrant conduction** In the electrical conduction system of the heart, the condition of the electrical stimulus traveling via an abnormal pathway. This is diagnosed by examination of the electrocardiogram.

**aberratio** (ăb-ĕr-ā′shē-ō) [L.] Aberration.

***a. testis*** Location of a testis in a position away from the path of normal descent.

**aberration** (ăb-ĕr-ā′shŭn) [L. *ab,* from, + *errare,* to wander] **1.** Deviation from the normal. **2.** Imperfect refraction of light rays.

***chromatic a.*** Unequal refraction of different wavelengths of light through a lens, producing a colored image.

***chromosomal a.*** An abnormality in chromosomes regarding number (aneuploidy, polyploidy) or chromosomal material (translocation, deletion, duplication).

***dioptric a.*** Spherical a.

***lateral a.*** Deviation of a ray from the focus measured on a line perpendicular to the axis.

***longitudinal a.*** Deviation of a ray from the direction parallel to the optic axis.

***spherical a.*** Aberration or distortion of an image due to rays entering the peripheral portion of a spherical mirror or lens being refracted differently from those closer to the center. Thus the peripheral rays are focused on the optical axis at a different point from the central rays.

**abetalipoproteinemia** (ā-bā″tă-lĭp″ō-prō″tēn-ē′mē-ă) [Gr. *a-,* not, + *beta* + *lipos,* fat, + *protos,* first, + *haima,* blood] An inherited disorder marked by an absence of beta lipoproteins in the blood and low levels of cholesterol, fatty acids, and chylomicrons. The red blood cells have a thorny or spiked appearance (i.e., acanthocytosis). It is most often seen in Ashkenazi Jews. Symptoms include retinal macular degeneration and chronic progressive neurological deficits, which usually begin in childhood. Affected infants develop steatorrhea and growth retardation. Later clinical manifestations include ataxia; by adolescence, many patients are unable to walk. Vitamin E may be helpful in arresting the progression of neurological aspects. SYN: *Bassen-Kornzweig syndrome.* SEE: *acanthocyte* for illus.

**abevacuation** (ăb-ē-văk″ū-ā′shŭn) [L. *ab,* from, + *evacuare,* to empty] Abnormal evacuation, either excessive or deficient.

**abeyance** (ă-bā′ăns) [O. Fr.] A temporary suspension of activity, sensation, or pain.

**ABG** *arterial blood gas.*

**ability** An individual's performance capability for a given task, based on genetic makeup and learning.

***cognitive a.*** The ability of the brain to process, retrieve, and store information. Impaired cognitive ability is common in patients with dementia, drug impairment, intoxication, or head injury.

***functional a.*** The ability to perform activities of daily living, including bathing, dressing, and other essential, independent daily activities such as shopping and housework. Many functional assessment tools are available to quantify functional ability. SEE: *activities of daily living.*

***verbal a.*** The ablility to use words, spoken or written, to communicate.

**abiogenesis** (ăb-ē-ō-jĕn′ĕ-sĭs) [Gr. *a-*, not, + *bios,* life, + *genesis,* generation, birth] Spontaneous generation of life; theoretical production of living organisms from nonliving matter. **abiogenetic, abiogenous** (-jĕ-nĕt′ĭk, ăb-ē-ŏj′ĭ-nŭs), *adj.*

**abiosis** (ăb-ē-ō′sĭs) [Gr. *a-*, not, + *bios,* life, + *osis,* condition] Absence of life. **abiotic,** *adj.*

**abiotrophy** (ăb-ē-ŏt′rō-fē) [″ + ″ + *trophe,* nourishment] Premature loss of vitality or degeneration of tissues and cells with consequent loss of endurance and resistance.

**ablactation** (ăb-lăk-tā′shŭn) [L. *ab,* from, + *lactatio,* suckling] **1.** The cessation of milk secretion. **2.** Weaning.

**ablate** (ăb-lāt′) [L. *ablatus,* taken away] To remove.

**ablatio** (ăb-lā′shē-ō) [L., carrying away] Ablation, removal, detachment.

***a. placentae*** Abruptio placentae. SEE: *placenta.*

***a. retinae*** Detachment of the retina. SEE: *retina.*

**ablation** (ăb-lā′shŭn) [L. *ab,* from, + *latus,* carried] Removal of a part, pathway, or function by surgery, chemical destruction, electrocautery, or radiofrequency.

***endometrial a.*** Removal or destruction of the whole thickness of the endometrium and some superficial myometrium. The purpose is to remove all of the endometrial glandular material. This is done to treat benign disturbances of menstrual bleeding in women who do not wish to preserve fertility. Ablation may be done by use of a transcervically placed laser or a thermal balloon system. In the latter method, a balloon is introduced into the endometrial cavity. The balloon is filled with a dextrose and water solution and the solution heated to the appropriate temperature. The temperature and time kept in place are carefully monitored.

***radiofrequency a.*** Ablation in which an electrode delivers a low-voltage, high-frequency current to cauterize and destroy abnormal tissues. An intracardiac catheter-electrode has been used effectively to correct cardiac dysrhythmias. Destruction of electrical conduction pathways in the heart by removing the abnormal conducting tissues has been used to treat Wolff-Parkinson-White syndrome, atrioventricular reentrant tachycardia, and other cardiac arrhythmias.

**ablepharia** (ăb-lĕ-fā′rē-ă) [Gr. *a-*, not, + *blepharon,* eyelid] Congenital absence of or reduction in the size of the eyelids. **ablepharous** (ă-blĕf′ă-rŭs), *adj.*

**ablepsia** (ă-blĕp′sē-ă) [Gr. *a-*, not, + *blepein,* to see] Blindness.

**ablution** (ăb-lū′shŭn) A cleansing or washing.

**abnormal** (ăb-nor′măl) [L. *ab,* from, + *norma,* rule] Deviating from the normal. SYN: *aberrant.*

**abnormality** (ăb″nor-măl′ĭ-tē) Deviation from the normal. SYN: *aberration.*

**abocclusion** (ăb″ō-kloo′zhŭn) Dentition in which the teeth of the mandible and the maxilla are not in contact.

**aborad** (ăb-ō′răd) [L. *ab,* from, + *oris,* mouth] Away from the mouth.

**aboral** (ăb-ō′răl) Opposite to, or away from, the mouth.

**abort** (ă-bort′) [L. *abortare,* to miscarry] **1.** To expel an embryo or fetus prior to viability. **2.** To arrest the progress of disease. **3.** To arrest growth or development. **4.** To discontinue an effort or project before its completion.

**abortifacient** (ă-bor-tĭ-fā′shĕnt) [L. *abortio,* abortion, + *facere,* to make] Anything used to cause or induce an abortion. SEE: *RU 486.*

**abortion** (ă-bor′shŭn) [L. *abortio*] The termination of pregnancy before the fetus reaches the stage of viability. The legal definition of viability—usually 20 to 24 weeks—differs from state to state. Some premature neonates of more than 24 weeks or 500 g are viable. Symptoms of abortion include abdominal cramps and bleeding from the vagina, sometimes with clots and bits of tissue.

ETIOLOGY: Among the most common causes are faulty development of the embryo, abnormalities of the placenta, endocrine disturbances, acute infectious diseases, severe trauma, and shock. Other causes include problems related to the uterus, genetic factors, immunologic factors, and use of certain drugs.

NURSING IMPLICATIONS: Assessment includes monitoring vital signs, fluid balance, and abortion status and progress. Historical data must include duration of pregnancy; Rh status; and time of onset, type, and intensity of abortion symptoms. Character and amount of vaginal bleeding are noted, and any passed tissue (embryonic or fetal) is preserved for laboratory examination. The patient is evaluated for shock, sepsis, and disseminated intravascular coagulation.

The patient's knowledge of her condition and any misconceptions are determined, and appropriate written and verbal information is provided. The nurse assesses the patient's psychological status and remains with her as much as possible to help allay anxiety, is aware of the patient's coping mechanisms, and is alert for responses such as grief, anger, guilt, sadness, depression, relief, or happiness.

If an elective abortion or surgical completion of the abortion is needed, the procedure and expected sensations are explained, and general preoperative and postoperative care are provided. If the patient is Rh negative and Coombs negative (not isoimmune), and if the pregnancy exceeded 8 weeks' gestation, Rho(D) is administered as prescribed within 72 hr of the abortion. Prescribed fluids, oxytocics, antibiotics, and transfusions are administered as required.

After abortion, the patient is instructed to report excessive bleeding, pain, inflammation, or fever and to avoid intercourse, tampon use, and douching until after the follow-up examination in 2 weeks.

***complete a.*** An abortion in which the complete products of conception have been expelled.

***elective a.*** Voluntary termination of a pregnancy for other than medical reasons. The procedure may be recommended when the mother's mental or physical state would be endangered by continuation of the pregnancy or when the fetus has a condition incompatible with life. It may also be performed at the mother's request.

***habitual a.*** Three or more consecutive spontaneous abortions.

***imminent a.*** Impending abortion characterized by bleeding and colicky pains that increase. The cervix is usually effaced and patulous.

***incomplete a.*** An abortion in which part of the products of conception has been retained in the uterus.

***induced a.*** The intentional termination of a pregnancy by means of dilating the cervix and evacuating the uterus. Methods used during the first trimester include cervical dilation and surgical, suction, or vacuum curettage (D&C). In the second trimester, hypertonic saline may be instilled into the uterus or intrauterine and systemic prostaglandins may be used to generate labor and expulsion of the products of conception. SEE: *curettage, uterine; RU 486.*

***inevitable a.*** An abortion that cannot be halted.

***infected a.*** Abortion accompanied by infection of retained material with resultant febrile reaction.

***missed a.*** Abortion in which the fetus has died before completion of the 20th week of gestation but the products of conception are retained in the uterus for 8 weeks or longer.

***septic a.*** Abortion in which there is an infection of the products of conception and the endometrial lining of the uterus.

***spontaneous a.*** Abortion occurring without apparent cause. SYN: *miscarriage.* SEE: *Nursing Diagnoses Appendix.*

***therapeutic a.*** Abortion performed when the pregnancy endangers the mother's mental or physical health or when the fetus has a known condition incompatible with life.

***threatened a.*** The appearance of signs and symptoms of possible loss of the fetus. Vaginal bleeding with or without intermittent pain is usually the first sign. If the fetus is still alive and attachment to the uterus has not been interrupted, the pregnancy may continue. Absolute bedrest and sedation are recommended, with avoidance of coitus, douches, stress, or cathartics.

***tubal a.*** **1.** A spontaneous abortion in which the fetus has been expelled through the distal end of the uterine tube. **2.** The escape of the products of conception into the peritoneal cavity by way of the uterine tube.

**abortionist** (ă-bor′shŭn-ĭst) One who performs an abortion.

**abortive** (ă-bor′tĭv) [L. *abortivus*] **1.** Preventing the completion of something. **2.** Abortifacient; that which prevents the normal continuation of pregnancy.

**abortus** (ă-bor′tŭs) [L.] A fetus born before 20 weeks' gestation or weighing less than 500 g.

**aboulia** SEE: *abulia.*

**ABP** *arterial blood pressure.*

**abrachia** (ă-brā′kē-ă) [Gr. *a-*, not, + *brachium,* arm] Congenital absence of arms.

**abrachiocephalia** (ă-brā″kē-ō-sĕ-fā′lē-ă) [″ + ″ + *kephale,* head] Congenital absence of arms and head.

**abradant** (ă-brād′ĕnt) An abrasive.

**abrade** (ă-brād′) [L. *ab,* from, + *radere,* to scrape] **1.** To chafe. **2.** To roughen or remove by friction.

**abrasion** (ă-brā′zhŭn) [″ + *radere,* to scrape] **1.** A scraping away of skin or mucous membrane as a result of injury or by mechanical means, as in dermabrasion for cosmetic purposes. SEE: *avulsion; bruise.* **2.** The wearing away of the substance of a tooth. It usually results from mastication, but may be done by mechanical or chemical means.

**abrasive** **1.** Producing abrasion. **2.** That which abrades.

**abreaction** (ăb″rē-ăk′shŭn) [L. *ab,* from, + *re,* again, + *actus,* acting] In psychoanalysis, the release of emotion by consciously recalling or acting out a painful experience that had been forgotten or repressed. The painful or consciously intolerable experience may become bearable as a result of the insight gained during this process. The method used to bring about abreaction is called catharsis.

**abruptio** (ă-brŭp′shē-ō) [L. *abruptus*] A tearing away from.

***a. placentae*** Premature detachment of a normally situated placenta after the 20th week of gestation. SYN: *ablatio placentae.* SEE: *placenta.*

SYMPTOMS: The symptoms include hemorrhage, concealed or evident, or a combination of both; constant pain, accompanied by a tetanic contraction if a large portion or all of the placenta separates; rhythmic uterine contractions as in labor; increased fetal movements and changes in heart rate until the fetus dies;

anemia.

ETIOLOGY: The cause is unknown. The condition may be associated with toxemia.

PATHOLOGY: Extravasation of blood occurs between the placenta and the uterine wall, occasionally between muscle fibers of the uterus. SEE: *Couvelaire uterus.*

TREATMENT: In mild cases, bedrest is advised. In severe cases, shock must first be treated. A soft and partially dilated cervix is an indication for immediate artificial rupture of membranes followed by natural or artificial induction of labor. If the fetus is alive and the mother's cervix is firm and not dilated, cesarean section is the treatment of choice. If the uterus fails to contract after cesarean section, an immediate hysterectomy is usually necessary.

NURSING IMPLICATIONS: The nurse monitors the patient's vital signs, fundal height, uterine contractions or tetany, and fetal baseline data, including fetal heart rate and rhythm changes, position, and degree of engagement. Vaginal blood loss is determined by weighing perineal pads and tampons and by recording the character and amount of blood loss. The known pre-use weight of each pad or tampon is subtracted from its weight after use. Prescribed IV fluids and medications are administered through a large-bore catheter. A central venous pressure line may be placed to provide access to the venous circulation, and an indwelling catheter is inserted to monitor urinary output and fluid balance. Noninvasive measures are taken to increase comfort, and a calm atmosphere and reassurance are provided. The patient and family are prepared for labor induction, vaginal delivery, or cesarean birth as appropriate. The possibility of neonatal death should be tactfully mentioned; the neonate's survival depends primarily on gestational age, blood loss, and associated hypertensive disorders. SEE: *Nursing Diagnoses Appendix.*

**abscess** (ăb′sĕs) [L. *abscessus,* a going away] A localized collection of pus in any body part that results from invasion of a pyogenic (pus-forming) bacterium. *Staphylococcus aureus* is a common cause. Pus is made up of dead white blood cells, bacteria, tissue debris, and proteins from the immune response to the bacteria. The abscess is surrounded by a membrane of variable strength created by macrophages, fibrin, and granulation tissue. Abscesses can disrupt function in adjacent tissues and can be life threatening if the swelling interferes with breathing or vital organ function. SEE: *inflammation; pus; suppuration; Universal Precautions Appendix.*

***acute a.*** An abscess associated with significant inflammation, producing intense heat, redness, swelling, and throbbing pain. The tissue over the abscess becomes elevated, soft, and eventually unstable (fluctuant) and discolored as the abscess comes to a head (points). An abscess can rupture spontaneously or be drained via an incision. If it is left untreated, the pathogens may spread to adjacent tissues or to other parts of the body via the bloodstream. Appearance of or increase in fever may indicate systemic spread.

***alveolar a.*** Abscess about the root of a tooth in the alveolar cavity. It is usually the result of necrosis and infection of dental pulp following dental caries. SYN: *apical a.* (2); *root a.*

***amebic a.*** An abscess caused by *Entamoeba histolytica.* SYN: *endamebic a.*

***anorectal a.*** Abscess in the ischiorectal fossa. SYN: *ischiorectal a.*

***apical a.*** **1.** Abscess at the apex of a lung. **2.** Abscess at the extremity of the root of a tooth. SYN: *alveolar a.; root a.*

***appendiceal a., appendicular a.*** Pus formation around an inflamed vermiform appendix.

***axillary a.*** Abscess or multiple abscesses in the axilla.

***Bartholin a.*** Abscess of Bartholin's gland.

***bicameral a.*** Abscess with two pockets.

***bile duct a.*** Abscess of the bile duct. SYN: *cholangitic a.*

***biliary a.*** Abscess of the gallbladder.

***bone a.*** Brodie's a.

***brain a.*** An intracranial abscess involving the brain or its membranes. It is seldom primary but usually occurs secondary to infections of the middle ear, nasal sinuses, face, or skull or from contamination from penetrating wounds or skull fractures. It may also have a metastatic origin arising from septic foci in the lungs (bronchiectasis, empyema, lung abscess), in bone (osteomyelitis), or in the heart (endocarditis). Infection of nerve tissue by the invading organism results in necrosis and liquefaction of the tissue, with edema of surrounding tissues. Brain abscesses may be acute, subacute, or chronic. Their clinical manifestations depend on the part of the brain involved, the size of the abscess, the virulence of the infecting organism, and other factors. SYN: *cerebral a.; intracranial a.* SEE: *Nursing Diagnoses Appendix.*

SYMPTOMS: Symptoms include a severe and persistent headache usually localized over infected area, fever, vomiting, vertigo, malaise, and sometimes irritability and other mental symptoms.

TREATMENT: The usual treatment is chemotherapy. Surgical intervention may be required.

***breast a.*** Mammary a.

***Brodie's a.*** Suppuration of the articular end of a bone, esp. the tibia. SYN: *bone a.*

***bursal a.*** Abscess in a bursa.

***canalicular a.*** Breast abscess that discharges into the milk ducts.

***caseous a.*** Abscess in which the pus has a cheesy appearance.

***cerebral a.*** Brain a.

***cholangitic a.*** Bile duct a.

***chronic a.*** Abscess with pus but without signs of inflammation. It usually develops slowly as a result of liquefaction of tuberculous tissue. It may occur anywhere in or on the body but occurs more frequently in the spine, hips, genitourinary tract, and lymph glands. Symptoms may be very mild. Pain when present is caused by pressure on surrounding parts; tenderness is often absent. Chronic septic changes accompanied by afternoon fever may occur. Amyloid disease may develop if the abscess persists for a prolonged period. SYN: *cold a.*

***circumtonsillar a.*** Peritonsillar a.

***cold a.*** Chronic a.

***collar-button a.'s*** Two pus-containing cavities, one larger than the other, connected by a narrow channel.

***dental a.*** Abscess beside a tooth, usually near the root.

***dentoalveolar a.*** Abscess in the alveolar process surrounding the root of a tooth.

***diffuse a.*** A collection of pus not circumscribed by a well-defined capsule.

***dry a.*** Abscess that disappears without pointing or breaking.

***embolic a.*** Abscess due to movement of infectious material from the site of an infection to another site.

***emphysematous a.*** Abscess containing air or gas. SYN: *tympanitic a.*

***endamebic a., entamebic a.*** Amebic a.

***epidural a.*** Extradural a.

***extradural a.*** Abscess on the dura mater. SYN: *epidural a.*

***fecal a.*** Abscess containing feces. SYN: *stercoral a.*

***filarial a.*** Abscess caused by filaria.

***follicular a.*** Abscess in a follicle.

***fungal a.*** Abscess caused by a fungus.

***gas a.*** An emphysematous abscess; one containing gas due to presence of gas-forming organisms such as *Clostridium perfringens*.

***gingival a.*** Abscess of the gum.

***helminthic a.*** Worm a.

***hemorrhagic a.*** Abscess containing blood.

***hepatic a.*** Abscess of the liver, esp. an amebic abscess. SYN: *liver a.*

***hot a.*** Acute a.

***hypostatic a.*** Wandering a.

***idiopathic a.*** Abscess due to an unknown cause.

***iliac a.*** Abscess in the iliac region.

***iliopsoas a.*** An abscess in the psoas and iliacus muscles.

***intracranial a.*** Brain a.

***intradural a.*** Abscess within the layers of the dura mater.

***ischiorectal a.*** Anorectal a.

***kidney a.*** Abscess or multiple abscesses of the renal cortex. SYN: *renal a.*

***lacrimal a.*** Suppuration of a lacrimal gland or in a lacrimal duct.

***lateral a., lateral alveolar a.*** Abscess in periodontal tissue.

***liver a.*** Hepatic a.

***lumbar a.*** Abscess in the lumbar region.

***lung a.*** Pulmonary a.

***lymphatic a.*** Abscess of a lymph node.

***mammary a.*** Abscess in the female breast, esp. one involving the glandular tissue. It usually occurs during lactation or weaning. SYN: *breast a.*

***mastoid a.*** Suppuration of the mastoid portion of the temporal bone.

***metastatic a.*** Secondary abscess at a distance from the focus of infection.

***miliary a.'s*** Multiple small embolic abscesses.

***milk a.*** Mammary abscess during lactation.

***mycotic a.*** Abscess caused by fungi.

***nocardial a.*** Abscess caused by *Nocardia.*

***orbital a.*** Suppuration in the orbit.

***palatal a.*** Abscess in a maxillary tooth, erupting toward the palate.

***palmar a.*** Purulent effusion into the tissues of the palm of the hand.

***pancreatic a.*** Abscess of pancreatic tissue, usually as a complication of acute pancreatitis or abdominal surgery.

***parafrenal a.*** Abscess on the side of the frenulum of the penis. It usually involves Tyson's gland.

***parametric a., parametritic a.*** Abscess between the folds of the broad ligaments of the uterus.

***paranephric a., paranephritic a.*** Abscess in the tissues around the kidney.

***parapancreatic a.*** Abscess in the tissues adjacent to the pancreas.

***parietal a.*** Periodontal abscess arising in the periodontal tissue other than the orifice through which the vascular supply enters the dental pulp.

***parotid a.*** Abscess of the parotid gland.

***pelvic a.*** Abscess of the pelvic peritoneum, esp. in Douglas' pouch.

***perianal a.*** Abscess of the skin around the anus.

***periapical a.*** An abscess at the apex of a dental root resulting from a variety of causes. Differential diagnosis may classify it further as an acute periapical abscess, a chronic periapical abscess, a periapical granuloma, or a radicular cyst.

***pericemental a.*** Alveolar abscess not involving the apex of a tooth.

***pericoronal a.*** Abscess around the crown of an unerupted molar tooth.

***peridental a.*** Abscess of periodontal tissue.

***perinephric a.*** Abscess in tissue around the kidney.

***periodontal a.*** A localized area of acute or chronic inflammation with pus formation found in the gingiva, periodontal pockets, or periodontal ligament.

***peripleuritic a.*** Abscess in the tissue

surrounding the parietal pleura.

***periproctic a.*** Abscess in the areolar tissue about the anus.

***peritoneal a.*** Abscess within the peritoneal cavity usually following peritonitis.

***peritonsillar a.*** Abscess of the tissue around the tonsillar capsule. SYN: *circumtonsillar a.*

***periureteral a.*** Abscess in the area around a ureter.

***periurethral a.*** Abscess in tissue surrounding the urethra.

***perivesical a.*** Abscess in tissue around the urinary bladder.

***pneumococcic a.*** Abscess due to infection with pneumococci.

***prelacrimal a.*** Abscess of the lacrimal bone producing a swelling at the inner canthus of the eye.

***premammary a.*** Subcutaneous or subareolar abscess of the mammary gland.

***prostatic a.*** Abscess within the prostate gland.

***protozoal a.*** Abscess caused by a protozoon.

***psoas a.*** Abscess with pus descending in the sheath of the psoas muscle due to vertebral disease, usually of tuberculous origin.

***pulmonary a.*** Abscess of the lungs; suppuration of lung tissue with one or more localized areas of necrosis, resulting in pulmonary cavitation. SYN: *lung a.; empyema.*

***pulp a.*** **1.** A cavity discharging pus formed in the pulp of a tooth. **2.** Abscess of the tissues of the pulp of a finger.

***pyemic a.*** A metastatic abscess, usually multiple, due to pyogenic organisms.

***rectal a.*** Abscess in the rectum.

***renal a.*** Kidney a.

***retrocecal a.*** An abscess located behind the cecum.

***retromammary a.*** Abscess between the mammary gland and the chest wall.

***retroperitoneal a.*** Abscess located between the peritoneum and the posterior abdominal wall.

***retropharyngeal a.*** Abscess of the lymph nodes in the walls of the pharynx. It sometimes simulates diphtheritic pharyngitis.

***retrovesical a.*** Abscess behind the bladder.

***root a.*** Apical a. (2).

***sacrococcygeal a.*** Abscess over the sacrum and coccyx.

***septicemic a.*** Abscess resulting from septicemia.

***spermatic a.*** Abscess of the seminiferous tubules.

***spinal a.*** Abscess due to necrosis of a vertebra.

***splenic a.*** Abscess of the spleen.

***stercoral a., stercoraceous a.*** Fecal a.

***sterile a.*** Abscess from which microorganisms cannot be cultivated.

***stitch a.*** Abscess formed about a stitch or suture.

***streptococcal a.*** Abscess caused by streptococci.

***subaponeurotic a.*** Abscess beneath an aponeurosis or fascia.

***subarachnoid a.*** Abscess of the midlayer of the covering of the brain and spinal cord.

***subareolar a.*** Abscess underneath the areola of the mammary gland, sometimes draining through the nipple.

***subdiaphragmatic a.*** Abscess beneath the diaphragm. SYN: *subphrenic a.*

***subdural a.*** Abscess beneath the dura of the brain or spinal cord.

***subfascial a.*** Abscess beneath the fascia.

***subgaleal a.*** Abscess beneath the galea aponeurotica (i.e., the epicranial aponeurosis).

***subpectoral a.*** Abscess beneath the pectoral muscles.

***subperiosteal a.*** Bone abscess below the periosteum.

***subperitoneal a.*** Abscess between the parietal peritoneum and the abdominal wall.

***subphrenic a.*** Subdiaphragmatic a.

***subscapular a.*** Abscess between the serratus anterior and the posterior thoracic wall.

***subungual a.*** Abscess beneath the fingernail. It may follow injury from a pin, needle, or splinter.

***sudoriparous a.*** Abscess of a sweat gland.

***suprahepatic a.*** Abscess in the suspensory ligament between the liver and the diaphragm.

***syphilitic a.*** Abscess occurring in the tertiary stage of syphilis, esp. in bone.

***thecal a.*** Abscess in a tendon sheath.

***thymus a.*** Abscess of the thymus.

***tonsillar a.*** Acute suppurative tonsillitis.

***tooth a.*** Alveolar a.

***tropical a.*** Amebic abscess of the liver.

***tuberculous a.*** Chronic a.

***tubo-ovarian a.*** Abscess involving both the fallopian tube and the ovary.

***tympanitic a.*** Emphysematous a.

***tympanocervical a.*** Abscess arising in the tympanum and extending to the neck.

***tympanomastoid a.*** A combined abscess of the tympanum and mastoid.

***urethral a.*** Abscess in the urethra.

***urinary a.*** Abscess caused by escape of urine into the tissues.

***urinous a.*** Abscess that contains pus and urine.

***verminous a.*** Worm a.

***wandering a.*** Abscess at a distance from the focus of disease with pus along fascial sheaths of muscles. SYN: *hypostatic a.*

***warm a.*** Acute a.

***worm a.*** An abscess caused by or containing insect larvae, worms, or other animal parasites. SYN: *helminthic a.; ver-*

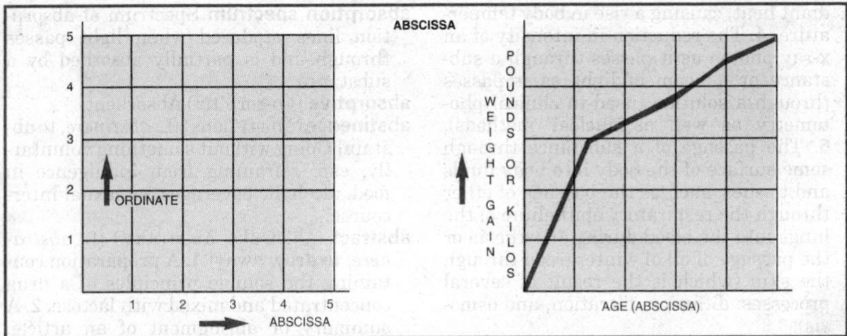


*minous a.*

**abscissa** (ăb-sĭs′ă) [L. *abscindere,* to cut off] The horizontal line, or x-axis, in a graph of a two-dimensional coordinate system wherein horizontal and perpendicular lines are crossed in order to provide a frame of reference. The ordinate is the vertical line, or y-axis. SEE: illus.

**abscission** (ăb-sĭ′zhŭn) [L. *abscindere,* to cut off] Removal by excision.

**abscopal** (ăb-skō′păl) Concerning the effect of radiation on tissues at some distance from the actual radiation site or target.

**absence** (ăb′sĕnz) **1.** Brief temporary loss of consciousness, as may occur in petit mal epilepsy. SYN: *absentia epileptica.* **2.** Lack of development of a structure.

**absence seizure** Seizure in which there is a sudden lapse of consciousness for 2 to 10 sec. There is usually a blank facial expression that may be accompanied by movements such as repeated eye-blinking or lip-smacking. There is no convulsion or fall. The patient resumes activity as if the seizure had not occurred. The seizure may be induced by voluntary hyperventilation for 2 to 3 min. This type of attack is characteristic of petit mal epilepsy.

Nursing Implications: The time, duration, patient's expression, and any repetitive movements occurring during the seizure are observed and documented, as is the patient's postseizure response. Prescribed medications are administered and evaluated for desired effects and adverse reactions. Support, reassurance, and education regarding the condition as well as drug actions and side effects are provided to the patient and family, and they are encouraged to discuss their feelings and concerns and to ask questions.

**absentia epileptica** (ăb-sĕn′shē-ă) [L., absence] Momentary loss of consciousness. There is no convulsion but there may be transient stereotyped muscle movement. SEE: *absence seizure; epilepsy.*

**abs. feb.** [L.] *absente febre,* in the absence of fever.

**Absidia** (ăb-sĭd′ē-ă) Genus of pathogenic fungi of the order Phycomycetes and the family Mucoraceae.

**absinthe, absinth** (ăb′sĭnth) [L. *absinthium,* wormwood] A liquor containing oil of wormwood, anise, and other herbs. It is highly toxic, esp. to the nervous system.

**absinthism** (ăb′sĭn-thĭzm) Deterioration of the nerve centers following excessive use of absinthe.

**absolute** Unrestricted, complete.

**absolute alcohol** Ethyl alcohol with not more than 1% of water by weight.

**absolute scale** Temperature scale in which zero is at the point of absolute zero. SYN: *Kelvin scale.*

**absolute temperature** Temperature measured on the absolute scale.

**absolute zero** The lowest possible temperature, −273.15°C or −459.67°F; equal to zero on the absolute scale.

**absorb** (ăb-sorb′) [L. *absorbere,* to suck in] To take in, suck up, or imbibe. SEE: *absorption; adsorb; adsorption.*

**absorbance** (ăb-sor′băns) The ability of a material or tissue to absorb radiation.

**absorbefacient** (ăb-sor″bĕ-fā′shĕnt) [L. *absorbere,* to suck in, + *facere,* to make] **1.** Causing absorption. **2.** An agent that causes absorption.

**absorbent** (ăb-sor′bĕnt) **1.** A substance that absorbs. **2.** Having the power to absorb.

**absorptiometer** (ăb-sorp″shē-ŏm′ĕ-tĕr) [L. *absorptio,* absorption, + Gr. *metron,* measure] **1.** An instrument that measures the thickness of a layer of liquid, drawn by capillary attraction, between glass plates. **2.** An instrument that measures the absorption of gas by a liquid.

**absorptiometry** A radiographic technique for measuring the dissipation of x-ray energy as the beam goes through tissue.

***dual beam a.*** A radiographic technique to measure tissue density by measuring the amount of absorbed radiation. One use is to detect bone loss in the spine and hips.

***dual photon a.*** Use of two sources of radiation of different energies to measure the density of a material, esp. bone. SEE: *bone densitometry.*

**absorption** (ăb-sorp′shŭn) [L. *absorptio*] **1.** The taking up of liquids by solids, or of gases by solids or liquids. **2.** The taking up of light or of its rays by black or colored rays. **3.** The taking up by the body of radiant heat, causing a rise in body temperature. **4.** The reduction in intensity of an x-ray photon as it passes through a substance or a beam of light as it passes through a solution (used in clinical photometry as well as nuclear methods). **5.** The passage of a substance through some surface of the body into body fluids and tissues, such as the passage of ether through the respiratory epithelium of the lungs into the blood during anesthesia or the passage of oil of wintergreen through the skin (which is the result of several processes: diffusion, filtration, and osmosis).

***colon a.*** The normal absorption of water (important in the conservation of body fluids) and products of bacterial action, esp. in the ascending colon. Some nutrients and drugs are absorbed by the lower bowel. In humans, cellulose is not digested or absorbed but passes from the body as unchanged residue. SEE: *fiber.*

***cutaneous a.*** Absorption through the skin. SYN: *percutaneous a.*

***external a.*** Absorption of material by the skin and mucous membrane.

***mouth a.*** Oral absorption of material. Some substances, but no nutrients, can be absorbed from the mouth; some drugs, esp. alkaloids, can be absorbed through the oral mucosa.

***parenteral a.*** Absorption from a site other than the gastrointestinal tract.

***pathological a.*** Absorption of a substance normally excreted (e.g., urine) or of a product of disease processes (e.g., pus) into the blood or lymph.

***percutaneous a.*** Cutaneous a.

***protein a.*** In the digestive process, hydrolyzation of proteins to their constituent amino acids in the walls of the intestines. They are transported via the portal vein to the liver and then into the general circulation and to the tissues. Each tissue synthesizes its own form of protein from the amino acids received from the blood.

***small intestine a.*** Absorption of digestive products that occurs in the small intestine, esp. the ileum. Products of digestion absorbed from the gastrointestinal tract pass into either blood or lymph. The mesenteric veins unite to form the portal vein and carry such blood to the liver; the mesenteric lymphatics are called lacteals because, during absorption of a fatty meal, the lymph they contain (called chyle) looks milky. The lacteals empty into the cisterna chyli and are joined by lymphatics from other parts of the body; the mixed lymph travels through the thoracic duct to the subclavian vein, where it empties into the bloodstream.

***stomach a.*** Absorption of water, alcohol, and some salts through the gastric mucosa.

**absorption lines** In spectroscopy, dark lines of the solar spectrum. SYN: *Fraunhofer's lines.*

**absorption spectrum** Spectrum of absorption lines produced when light passes through and is partially absorbed by a substance.

**absorptive** (ăb-sorp′tĭv) Absorbent.

**abstinence** (ăb′stĭ-nĕns) [L. *abstinere,* to abstain] Going without something voluntarily, esp. refraining from indulgence in food, alcoholic beverages, or sexual intercourse.

**abstract** (ăb′străkt, ăb-străkt′) [L. *abstrahere,* to draw away] **1.** A preparation containing the soluble principles of a drug concentrated and mixed with lactose. **2.** A summary or abridgment of an article, book, or address.

***discharge a.*** A summary of a patient's record from a health care facility that is prepared after the time of discharge.

**abstraction** (ăb-străk′shŭn) **1.** Removal or separation of a constituent from a mixture or compound. **2.** Distraction of the mind; inattention or absent-mindedness. **3.** The process whereby thoughts and ideas are generalized and dissociated from particular concrete instances or material objects.

**abterminal** (ăb-tĕr′mĭ-năl) [L. *ab,* from, + *terminus,* end] Away from an end and toward the center, said of electric currents in muscles.

**abulia** (ă-bū′lē-ă) [Gr. *a-,* not, + *boule,* will] **1.** Absence of or inability to exercise willpower (or initiative) or to make decisions. **2.** Syndrome of slow reaction, lack of spontaneity, and brief spoken responses. It may be part of the clinical picture that accompanies infarction of a cerebellar vessel.

**abuse** (ă-būs′) [L. *abusus,* using up] Misuse; excessive or improper use.

***domestic a.*** The mistreatment or injury of individuals in a domestic setting. Forms include physical violence, such as striking or forcibly restraining a family member; passive abuse, such as withholding access to resources needed to maintain health; psychological or emotional abuse, such as demeaning, devaluing, intimidating, or instilling fear by threat of physical harm or abandonment; and economic abuse by imposing financial dependency.

***elder a.*** Emotional, physical, or sexual injury, or financial exploitation, of an elder. It may be due to positive action or omission by those responsible for the care of the elder. Elders may also be exploited by individuals and "philanthropic" organizations.

***sexual a.*** SEE: *sexual abuse.*

***spouse a.*** Emotional, physical, or sexual mistreatment of one's spouse.

***substance a.*** An imprecise term for abuse of drugs, alcohol, or other substances that alter mood or behavior. SEE: *Nursing Diagnoses Appendix.*

**abutment** (ă-bŭt′mĕnt) [Fr. *abouter,* to place end to end] The tooth to which a partial denture is anchored.

**ABVD** *adriamycin, bleomycin, vinblastine,* and *dacarbazine,* a combination of chemotherapy drugs.

**A.C.** *acromioclavicular; adrenal cortex; air conduction; alternating current; anodal closure; atriocarotid; auriculocarotid; axiocervical.*

**Ac** Symbol for the element actinium.

**a.c.** L. *ante cibum,* before meals.

**acacia** (ă-kā′shē-ă) Gum arabic. A dried gummy exudation from the tree *Acacia senegal.* It is used as a suspending agent in pharmaceutical products.

**acalculia** (ă-kăl-kū′lē-ă) [Gr. *a-,* not, + L. *calculare,* to reckon] A learning or speech disorder characterized by the inability to perform simple arithmetic operations.

**acampsia** (ă-kămp′sē-ă) [″ + *kamptein,* to bend] Inflexibility of a limb; rigidity; ankylosis.

**acantha** [Gr. *akantha,* thorn] **1.** The spine. **2.** A vertebral spinous process.

**acanthamebiasis** (ă-kăn″thă-mē-bī′ă-sĭs) A rare disease of the brain and meninges caused by free-living amebae. The organisms invade the nasal mucosa of persons swimming in fresh water, the natural habitat of *Acanthamoeba* and *Naegleria fowleri.* The organisms invade the central nervous system through the olfactory foramina. The symptoms begin after an incubation period of 2 to 15 days and are those of acute meningitis. Debilitated or immunocompromised persons are esp. susceptible. Diagnosis is made by finding the amebae in the spinal fluid. Treatment is virtually ineffective and most patients die within a week of onset. Swimming pools adequately treated with chlorine are not a source of the amebae. SEE: *meningoencephalitis, primary amebic.*

**acanthesthesia** (ă-kăn″thĕs-thē′zē-ă) [Gr. *akantha,* thorn, + *aisthesis,* sensation] A sensation as of a pinprick; a form of paresthesia.

**Acanthia lectularia** (ă-kăn′thē-ă lĕk-tū-lă′rē-ă) Cimex lectularius

**acanthiomeatal line** An imaginary line through the acanthion and external auditory meatus.

**acanthion** [Gr. *akanthion,* little thorn] The tip of the anterior nasal spine.

**acantho-** [Gr. *akantha,* thorn] Combining form meaning *thorn, spine.*

**Acanthocephala** (ă-kăn″thō-sĕf′ă-lă) [″ + *kephale,* head] A class of wormlike entozoa related to the Platyhelminthes, including a few species parasitic in humans.

**acanthocephaliasis** (ă-kăn″thō-sĕf-ă-lī′ă-sĭs) An infestation with Acanthocephala.

**Acanthocheilonema perstans** (ă-kăn″thō-kī″lō-nē′mă pĕr′stăns) *Dipetalonema perstans.* A species of filaria that infects wild or domestic animals and occasionally humans. In humans, the adult worm migrates to the subcutaneous tissue and produces a nodule. Rarely, the adult worm may be seen beneath the conjunctiva.

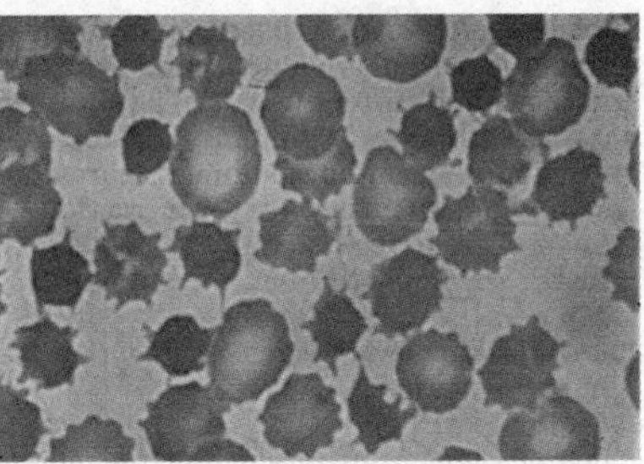

**ACANTHOCYTES** IN PATIENT WITH ABETALIPOPROTEINEMIA (×640)

**acanthocyte** (ă-kăn′thō-sīt″) [Gr. *akantha,* thorn, + *kytos,* cell] An abnormal erythrocyte that in wet preparations has protoplasmic projections so that the cell appears to be covered with thorns. SEE: illus.; *abetalipoproteinemia.*

**acanthocytosis** (ă-kăn″thō-sī-tō′sĭs) [″ + ″ + *osis,* condition] Acanthocytes in the blood.

**acanthoid** (ă-kăn′thoyd) [″ + *eidos,* form, shape] Thorny; spiny; of a spinous nature.

**acanthokeratodermia** (ă-kăn″thō-kĕr″ă-tō-dĕr′mē-ă) [″ + *keras,* horn, + *derma,* skin] Hypertrophy of the horny portion of the skin of the palms of the hands and soles of the feet, and thickening of the nails.

**acantholysis** (ă-kăn-thŏl′ĭ-sĭs) [″ + *lysis,* dissolution] Any disease of the skin accompanied by degeneration of the cohesive elements of the cells of the outer or horny layer of the skin.

***a. bullosa*** Obsolete term for epidermolysis bullosa.

**acanthoma** (ăk″ăn-thō′mă) [″ + *oma,* tumor] A benign tumor of the skin. It was previously used to denote skin cancer.

***a. adenoides cysticum*** A cystic tumor, often familial, occurring on the chest and face and in the axillary regions. The tumor contains tissues resembling sweat glands and hair follicles. SYN: *epithelioma adenoides cysticum.*

**acanthopelvis, acanthopelyx** (ă-kăn″thō-pĕl′vĭs, -pĕl′ĭks) [″ + *pelyx,* pelvis] A prominent and sharp pubic spine on a rachitic pelvis.

**acanthosis** (ăk″ăn-thō′sĭs) [″ + *osis,* condition] Increased thickness of the prickle cell layer of the skin. **acanthotic** (ăk″ăn-thŏt′ĭk), *adj.*

***a. nigricans*** A rare, chronic, inflammatory disease of the skin in adults that is marked by symmetrically distributed hard and soft papillary growths accompanied by hyperpigmentation and hyperkeratosis; it is sometimes associated with cancer of an internal organ. SYN: *keratosis nigricans.*

**acapnia** (ă-kăp′nē-ă) [Gr. *akapnos,* smokeless] Literally, the absence of carbon dioxide, but the term is used to indicate less than the normal amount of carbon dioxide in blood and tissues (e.g., after voluntary overbreathing). Symptoms include depressed respiration, giddiness, paresthesia, cramps, involuntary contraction of fingers, and occasionally convulsions. SEE: *hyperventilation.* **acapnial** (ă-căp′nē-ăl), *adj.*

**acarbia** (ă-kăr′bē-ă) Decrease of bicarbonate in the blood.

**acardia** (ă-kăr′dē-ă) [Gr. *a-*, not, + *kardia,* heart] Congenital absence of the heart. **acardiac** (ă-kăr′dē-ăk), *adj.*

**acardiacus** (ă-kăr-dī′ă-kŭs) A parasitic twin without a heart, therefore using the circulation of its twin. SYN: *acardius.*

**acardiotrophia** (ă-kăr″dē-ŏ-trō′fĕ-a) [Gr. *a-*, not, + *kardia,* heart + *trophe,* nutrition] Atrophy of the heart.

**acardius** Acardiacus.

**acariasis** (ăk″ă-rī′ă-sĭs) [L. *acarus,* mite, + Gr. *-iasis,* condition] Any disease caused by a mite or acarid. SYN: *acarinosis; acaridiasis.*

***demodectic a.*** Infection of hair follicles with *Demodex folliculorum.*

***sarcoptic a.*** Infestation with a burrowing mite, *Sarcoptes scabiei,* which deposits its eggs in the burrows. SEE: *scabies.*

**acaricide** (ă-kăr′ĭ-sīd) [″ + *caedere,* to kill] **1.** An agent that destroys acarids. **2.** Destroying a member of the order Acarina.

**acarid, acaridan** (ăk′ă-rĭd, ă-kăr′ĭ-dăn) [L. *acarus,* mite] A tick or mite of the order Acarina.

**Acaridae** A family of mites that irritate the skin. SEE: *itch, grain; itch, grocer's.*

**acaridiasis** (ă-kăr″ĭ-dī′ă-sĭs) [″ + Gr. *-iasis,* condition] Acariasis.

**Acarina** (ăk″ă-rī′nă) An order of the class Arachnida that includes a large number of species of minute animals known as mites or ticks. Most are ectoparasites, with infestation causing local dermatitis with pruritus and sometimes systemic reactions. They are vectors of a number of diseases. SEE: *Ixodidae; Lyme disease; Sarcoptidae; scabies; tick.*

**acarinosis** (ă-kăr″ĭ-nō′sĭs) [L. *acarus,* mite, + Gr. *osis,* condition] Acariasis.

**acaro-** (ăk-ăro) [L. *acarus,* mite] A combining form meaing mite.

**acarodermatitis** (ăk″ă-rō-dĕr″mă-tī′tĭs) [″ + Gr. *derma,* skin, + *itis,* inflammation] Skin inflammation caused by a mite.

**acaroid** (ăk′ă-royd) [″ + Gr. *eidos,* form, shape] Resembling a mite.

**acarology** (ăk″ă-rŏl′ō-jē) [″ + Gr. *logos,* word, reason] The study of mites and ticks.

**acarophobia** (ăk″ăr-ō-fō′bē-ă) [″ + Gr. *phobos,* fear] Abnormal fear of small objects such as pins, needles, worms, mites, and other small insects.

**Acarus** (ăk′ăr-ŭs) [L., mite] A genus of mites.

***A. folliculorum*** Demodex folliculorum.

***A. scabiei*** *Sarcoptes scabiei.* SEE: *scabies; Sarcoptidae.*

**acarus** [L.] Any mite or tick.

**acaryote** (ă-kăr′ē-ōt) [Gr. *a-*, not, + *karyon,* nucleus] Without a nucleus. SEE: *eukaryote; prokaryote.*

**acatalasemia** Acatalasia.

**acatalasia** (ă″kăt-ă-lā′zē-ă) A rare inherited disease in which there is an absence of the enzyme catalase. The gingival and oral tissues are particularly susceptible to bacterial invasion with subsequent gangrenous changes and alveolar bone destruction. SYN: *acatalasemia.*

**acataphasia** (ă-kăt″ă-fā′zē-ă) [″ + *kataphasis,* affirmation] **1.** Inability to verbalize thoughts coherently. This condition is due to a cerebral lesion. **2.** A form of disordered speech in which statements are incorrectly formulated; individuals may use words that sound like the ones they mean to use but are not appropriate to their thoughts, or they may use totally inappropriate expressions.

**acatastasia** (ă-kăt-ăs-tā′zē-ă) [Gr. *akatastasis,* disorder] Irregularity; deviation from the normal.

**acathexis** (ă″kă-thĕks′ĭs) [Gr. *a-*, not, + *kathexis,* retention] In psychoanalysis, a lack of emotion toward something that is unconsciously important to the individual.

**acathisia** (ă″kă-thĭz′ē-ă) [″+ *kathisis,* sitting] Inability to sit down because the thought of doing so causes severe anxiety. The patient is restless, has an urgent need to move, and complains of muscular quivering. This symptom may appear as a complication of therapy with antipsychotic drugs such as phenothiazines or reserpine. If the condition is due to drugs, the medicine should be decreased or eliminated. Also spelled *akathisia.*

**acaudal, acaudate** (ā-kaw′dăl, -dāt) [″ + L. *cauda,* tail] Having no tail.

**ACC** *anodal closure contraction.*

**acc** *accommodation.*

**accelerated idioventricular rhythm** ABBR: AIVR. An abnormal ectopic cardiac rhythm originating in the ventricular conducting system. This may or may not occur intermittently and is usually 60 to 100 beats per minute.

**acceleration** (ăk-sĕl″ĕr-ā′shŭn) [L. *accelerans,* hastening] **1.** An increase in the speed of an action or function, such as pulse or respiration. **2.** The rate of change in velocity for a given unit of time.

***angular a.*** Rate of change in velocity per unit of time during circular movement.

***central a.*** Centripetal a.

***centripetal a.*** Rate of change in velocity per unit of time while on a circular or curved course. SYN: *central a.*

***fetal heart rate a.*** **1.** The increase in heart rate associated with fetal movement. It may be a criterion for a reactive nonstress test. **2.** A reassuring sign during labor that the fetus is not experiencing intrauterine hypoxemia.

***linear a.*** Rate of change in velocity per unit of time while on a straight course.

***negative a.*** Decrease in the rate of change in velocity per unit of time.

***positive a.*** Increase in the rate of change in velocity per unit of time.

***standard a. of free fall*** The rate of change in velocity of a freely falling body as it is acted on by gravity to travel to the earth. It is 9.81 m (or 32.17 ft)/sec$^2$.

**acceleration injury** Head injury caused when the head remains stationary and is hit by a moving object, such as a batter being hit in the head by a baseball.

**acceleration-deceleration injury** An injury caused when the body abruptly comes to a stop and the internal organs collide with the inside of the body.

**accelerator** (ăk-sĕl′ĕr-ā″tor) **1.** Anything that increases action or function. **2.** In chemistry, a catalyst. **3.** A device that speeds up charged particles to high energy levels to produce x-radiation and neutrons.

**accelerometer** An instrument that detects a change in the velocity of the object to which it is attached. The device may be designed to record the changes and indicate the direction(s) of the acceleration.

**acceptance** According to Dr. Elisabeth Kübler-Ross, the fifth and final stage of dying. Individuals who reach this stage (not all do) come to terms with impending death and await the end with quiet expectation.

**acceptor** (ăk-sĕp′tor) [L. *accipere,* to accept] A compound that unites with a substance freed by another compound, called a donor.

***hydrogen a.*** A substance that combines with hydrogen and is reduced when a substrate is oxidized by an enzyme.

***oxygen a.*** A substance that combines with oxygen and is oxidized when a substrate is reduced by an enzyme.

**access, medical** SEE: *medical access.*

**accessorius** (ăk″sĕs-ō′rē-ŭs) [L., supplementary] Accessory or supplementary, as in certain muscles, glands, and nerves.

**accessory** (ăk-sĕs′ō-rē) Auxiliary; assisting. This term is applied to a lesser structure that resembles in structure and function a similar organ, as the accessory pancreatic duct (of Santorini) or accessory suprarenal glands.

**accessory motion** Motion that accompanies active motion and is necessary for normal motion, but cannot be isolated voluntarily. This includes joint play as well as motion in related joints, such as upward rotation of the scapula during abduction of the arm. It is also called *accessory movement.*

**accessory muscles of respiration** In labored breathing, the use of muscles other than the diaphragm and intercostals. The sternocleidomastoid, spinal, neck, and abdominal muscles, and even the platysma, may be used. Their use is a sign of an abnormal or labored breathing pattern.

**accessory nerve** Motor nerve made up of a cranial and a spinal part that supplies the trapezius and sternomastoid muscles and the pharynx. The accessory portion joins the vagus to supply motor fibers to the pharynx, larynx, and heart (inhibitory). SYN: *spinal accessory nerve.* SEE: *cranial nerve* for illus.

**accident** (ăk′sĭ-dĕnt) [L. *accidens,* happening] **1.** An unforeseen occurrence of an unfortunate nature; a mishap. **2.** An unexpected complicating event in the course of a disease or following surgery. **accidental** (-dĕn′tăl), *adj.*

***cerebrovascular a.*** ABBR: CVA. A sudden, unexpected interference in brain function resulting from a vascular disturbance such as a cerebral hemorrhage, occlusion of a vessel by a thrombus or embolus, vasospasm, or vasodilation. SYN: *apoplexy; stroke.*

***radiation a.*** Undesired contact or excessive exposure to ionizing radiation.

**accident-prone** Said of persons having an unusually high rate of accidents. The validity of this concept is questionable.

**accipiter** (ăk-sĭp′ĭ-tĕr) [L., a hawk] A nose bandage with clawlike ends that spread over the face.

**ACCl** *anodal closure clonus.*

**acclimation, acclimatization** (ăk-lĭ-mā′shŭn, ă-klī″mă-tĭ-zā′shŭn) [Fr. *acclimater,* acclimate] The act of becoming accustomed to a different environment.

**acclimatize** (ăk-klī′mă-tīz) To become accustomed to a different environment.

**accommodation** (ă-kŏm″ō-dā′shŭn) [L. *accommodare,* to suit] ABBR: a; acc. **1.** Adjustment or adaptation. **2.** In ophthalmology, a phenomenon noted in receptors in which continued stimulation fails to elicit a sensation or response. **3.** The adjustment of the eye for various distances whereby it is able to focus the image of an object on the retina by changing the curvature of the lens. In accommodation for near vision, the ciliary muscle contracts, causing increased rounding of the lens, the pupil contracts, and the optic axes converge. These three actions constitute the accommodation reflex. The ability of the eye to accommodate decreases with age. **4.** In the learning theory of Jean Piaget, the process through which a person's schema of understanding incorporates new experiences that do not fit existing ways of understanding the world. SEE: illus.; *adaptation.*

***absolute a.*** Accommodation of one eye independently of the other.

***amplitude of a.*** The difference in the refractive power of the eye when accommodating for near and far vision. It is measured in diopters (D) and normally diminishes progressively from childhood to old age. It is approx. 16 D at age 12, 6.5 D at age 30, and 1 D at age 50. SEE: *diopter.*

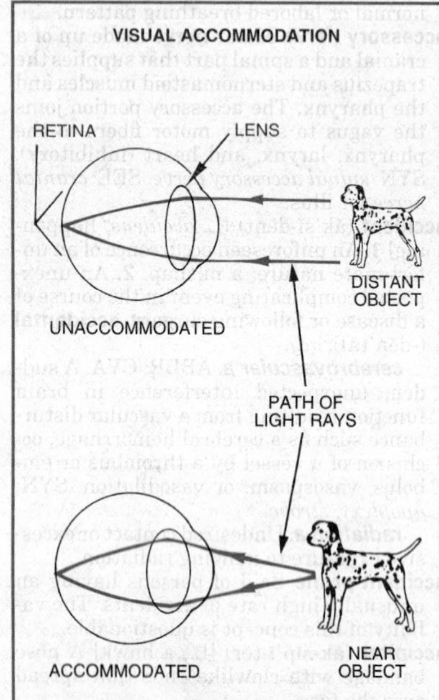


***binocular a.*** Coordinated accommodation of both eyes jointly.

***excessive a.*** Greater-than-needed accommodation of the eye.

***mechanism a.*** Method by which curvature of the eye lens is changed in order to focus close objects on the retina.

***negative a.*** Relaxation of the ciliary muscle to adjust for distant vision.

***positive a.*** Contraction of the ciliary muscle to adjust for near vision.

***range of a.*** Distance of vision from its closest to its most remote points.

***reasonable a.*** An employer's responsibility to provide necessary structural changes, reassignment, equipment modification, devices, training materials, interpreters, and other adjustments that are reasonable for disabled employees.

***relative a.*** The extent to which accommodation is possible for any specific state of convergence of the eyes.

***spasm of a.*** A spasm of the ciliary muscle, usually the result of excessive strain from overuse; it is common in myopia.

***subnormal a.*** Insufficient accommodation.

**accommodation reflex** Contraction of the ciliary muscle resulting in rounding of the lens, contraction of the pupil, and convergence of the eyes in accommodation for near vision. SYN: *near reflex.*

**accommodative iridoplegia** (ă-kŏm′ō-dā″tĭv ĭr″ĭ-dō-plē′jē-ă) Noncontraction of the pupils during accommodation.

**accoucheur, accoucheuse** (ă-koo-shŭr′, ă-koo-shĕz′) [Fr.] An obstetrician or midwife.

**accountability** Responsibility of health care professionals for the actions and judgments involved in patient care.

**ACCP** *American College of Chest Physicians.*

**accreditation** The voluntary process of recognizing that a facility or institution has met established standards. In the U.S. there are two types of educational accreditation, institutional and specialized. The former recognizes the institution for having facilities, policies, and procedures that meet accepted standards. The latter recognizes specific programs of study within institutions for having met established standards.

**Accredited Record Technician** ABBR: A.R.T. A person who, as a result of training and experience, is competent to process, maintain in a secure place, compile, and report information in a patient's medical record. This is done according to rules set by the health care facility to comply with medical, administrative, ethical, legal, and accreditation considerations.

**accrementition** (ăk″rĕ-mĕn-tĭsh′ŭn) [L. *accrescere,* to increase] Growth of tissues by addition of similar tissue.

**accretio** (ă-krē′shē-ō) [L.] Adhesion of parts normally separate from each other.

***a. cordis*** Condition in which fibrous bands extend from the external pericardium to surrounding structures, resulting in angulation and torsion of the heart.

**accretion** (ă-krē′shŭn) [L. *accrescere,* accrue] **1.** An increase by external addition; accumulation. **2.** The growing together of parts naturally separate. **3.** Accumulation of foreign matter in a cavity.

**acculturation** The process by which a member of one culture assumes the values, attitudes, and behavior of a second culture in order to become an accepted member of that culture.

**accuracy 1.** The ratio of the error of measurement to the true value. **2.** State of being free of error.

**Accutane** SEE: *retinoic acid.*

**ACD** *absolute cardiac dullness.*

**ACD sol** Citric acid, trisodium citrate, dextrose solution; an anticoagulant used in collecting blood for transfusions.

**ACE** *angiotensin-converting enzyme.*

**Ace bandage** Trade name for an elastic bandage made of woven material.

**acedia** (ă-sē′dē-ă) [Gr. *a-,* not, + *kedos,* care] Mental state of indifference, insensibility, lack of energy or emotion. SYN: *apathy.*

**acellular** Not containing cells.

**acenesthesia** (ă-sĕn″ĕs-thē′zē-ă) [Gr. *a-,* not, + *koinos,* common, + *aisthesis,* sensation] Absence of a feeling of well-being. It occurs in disorders such as hypochondriasis and neurasthenia.

**acentric** (ă-sĕn′trĭk) [″ + L. *centrum,* center] Not central; peripheral.

**A.C.E.P.** *American College of Emergency*

*Physicians.*

**acephalia, acephalism** (ă-sĕ-fā′lē-ă, ă-sĕf′ă-lĭzm) [Gr. *a-*, not, + *kephale,* head] Congenital absence of the head.

**acephalobrachia** (ă-sĕf″ă-lō-brā′kē-ă) [″ + ″ + *brachion,* arm] Congenital absence of the head and arms.

**acephalocardia** (ă-sĕf″ă-lō-kăr′dē-ă) [″ + ″ + *kardia,* heart] Congenital absence of the head and heart.

**acephalochiria** (ă-sĕf″ă-lō-kī′rē-ă) [″ + ″ + *cheir,* hand] Congenital absence of the head and hands.

**acephalocyst** (ă-sĕf′ă-lō-sĭst) [″ + ″ + *kystis,* bag] A sterile hydatid cyst.

**acephalogastria** (ă-sĕf″ă-lō-găs′trē-ă) [″ + ″ + *gaster,* stomach] Congenital absence of the head, chest, and upper abdomen.

**acephalopodia** (ă-sĕf″ă-lō-pō′dē-ă) [″ + ″ + *pous,* foot] Congenital absence of the head and feet.

**acephalorhachia** (ă-sĕf″ă-lō-rā′kē-ă) [″ + ″ + *rhachis,* spine] Congenital absence of the head and vertebral column.

**acephalostomia** (ă-sĕf″ă-lō-stō′mē-ă) [″ + ″ + *stoma,* mouth] Congenital absence of the head; however, an opening resembling a mouth is present on the superior portion of the body.

**acephalothoracia** (ă-sĕf″ă-lō-thō-rā′sē-ă) [″ + ″ + *thorax,* chest] Congenital absence of the head and chest.

**acephalus** (ă-sĕf′ă-lŭs) A fetus lacking a head.

**acervulus** (ă-sĕr′vū-lŭs) [L.] Sandy, gritty, sabulous.

***a. cerebri*** Gritty matter filling the follicle of the pineal gland. SYN: *brain sand.*

**acetabular** (ăs″ĕ-tăb′ū-lăr) Pert. to the acetabulum.

**acetabulectomy** (ăs″ĕ-tăb″ū-lĕk′tō-mē) [L. *acetabulum,* a little saucer for vinegar, + Gr. *ektome,* excision] Surgical removal of the acetabulum.

**acetabuloplasty** (ăs″ĕ-tăb′ū-lō-plăs″tē) [″ + Gr. *plassein,* to form] Surgical repair and reconstruction of the acetabulum.

**acetabulum** (ăs″ĕ-tăb′ū-lŭm) [L., a little saucer for vinegar] The cavity or depression on the lateral surface of the innominate bone (hip bone) that provides the socket into which the head of the femur fits. SEE: illus.

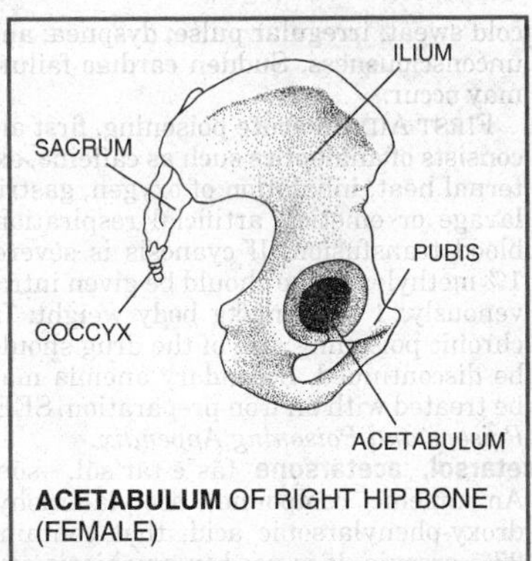

**ACETABULUM** OF RIGHT HIP BONE (FEMALE)

**acetal** (ăs′ĕ-tăl) Chemical combination of an aldehyde with alcohol.

**acetaldehyde** (ăs″ĕt-ăl′dĕ-hīd″) $CH_3CHO$. An intermediate in yeast fermentation and alcohol metabolism. SYN: *acetic aldehyde.*

**acetamide** (ăs″ĕt-ăm′ĭd) $CH_3CONH_2$. Acetic acid amide, used in industry for synthesis of chemicals and as a solvent.

**acetaminophen** (ă-sĕt″ă-mĭn′ō-fĕn) A synthetic drug with antipyretic and analgesic effects similar to those of aspirin, but without anti-inflammatory or antirheumatic effects. It is used for patients who are aspirin-sensitive. Tylenol is a trade name for acetaminophen.

Caution: Acute overdose may cause fatal hepatic necrosis.

**acetaminophen poisoning** Toxicity caused by an overdose of acetaminophen. In therapeutic doses this drug is virtually nontoxic. In oral doses of more than 140 mg/kg in adults, toxicity may occur. Doses of 10 to 25 g or more in adults may be fatal. An estimate of the amount ingested may be determined from the plasma concentration. Values obtained 4 hr after ingestion of more than 140 mg/kg will be associated with minimal hepatic toxicity in children or adults.

SYMPTOMS: The symptoms are nausea, vomiting, drowsiness, pallor, shock, sweating, and liver tenderness. Within 24 to 48 hr these signs subside and evidence of liver damage appears, such as jaundice, liver tenderness, confusion, blood clotting abnormalities, and abnormal liver enzyme tests (aspartate amino transferase, AST; alanine amino transferase, ALT).

TREATMENT: Gastric lavage should be done immediately (the airway must be protected). This is most effective if done within 4 hr of ingestion of the drug. A specific antidote, *N*-acetylcysteine, is given orally within 8 to 10 hr after ingestion in an initial dose of 140 mg/kg and then in 70 mg/kg doses every 4 hr for 17 doses. SEE: *Poisons and Poisoning Appendix.*

**acetanilid** (ăs″ĕ-tăn′ĭ-lĭd) A white powder or crystalline substance obtained by interaction of glacial acetic acid and aniline.

ACTION/USES: Acetanilid has analgesic, antipyretic, and anti-inflammatory effects. Acute or chronic poisoning may develop due to prolonged administration or drug idiosyncrasy. Because of its toxicity, it is rarely used.

**acetanilid poisoning** Toxicity caused by acetanilid ingestion. Symptoms are cyanosis due to formation of methemoglobin;

cold sweat; irregular pulse; dyspnea; and unconsciousness. Sudden cardiac failure may occur.

FIRST AID: In acute poisoning, first aid consists of analeptics such as caffeine, external heat, inhalation of oxygen, gastric lavage or emetics, artificial respiration, blood transfusion. If cyanosis is severe, 1% methylene blue should be given intravenously, 1 to 2 mg/kg body weight. In chronic poisoning, use of the drug should be discontinued. Secondary anemia may be treated with an iron preparation. SEE: *Poisons and Poisoning Appendix.*

**acetarsol, acetarsone** (ăs″ĕ-tăr′sŏl, -sōn) An arsenic compound, acetylaminohydroxy-phenylarsonic acid, that contains 27% arsenic. It is used in amebiasis and *Trichomonas vaginalis* infections.

**acetate** (ăs′ĕ-tāt) A salt of acetic acid.

**acetazolamide** (ăs″ĕt-ă-zŏl′ă-mīd) A drug that inhibits the enzyme carbonic anhydrase. At one time it was used as a diuretic, but more effective drugs are now available. It has been used to treat epilepsy and to reduce intraocular pressure in managing glaucoma. Trade name is Diamox.

**acetic** (ă-sē′tĭk) [L. *acetum,* vinegar] Pert. to vinegar; sour.

**acetic aldehyde** Acetaldehyde.

**acetify** (ă-sĕt′ĭ-fī) [L. *acetum,* vinegar, + *fieri,* to become] To produce acetic fermentation or vinegar.

**Acetobacter** (ă-sĕ″tō-băk′tĕr) [L. *acetum,* vinegar, + Gr. *bakterion,* little rod] A genus of nonpathogenic bacteria of the family Pseudomonadaceae.

***A. aceti*** Species of *Acetobacter* that transforms wine or cider into vinegar. This produces a stringy substance in the liquid, called mother of vinegar.

**acetohexamide** (ăs″ĕ-tō-hĕks′ă-mīd) An orally administered hypoglycemic agent used to treat non–insulin-dependent diabetes mellitus.

**acetoin** (ă-sĕt′ō-ĭn) The substance formed when glucose is fermented by *Enterobacter aerogenes.*

**acetone** (ăs′ĕ-tōn) $C_3H_6O$. Dimethyl ketone, a colorless, volatile, flammable liquid used as a solvent. It has a sweet, fruity, ethereal odor and is found in the blood and urine in diabetes, in other metabolic disorders, and after lengthy fasting. It is produced when fats are not properly oxidized due to inability to oxidize glucose in the blood. SEE: *ketone; ketonuria; ketosis; test, acetone.*

***a. in urine, test for*** **1.** A specially treated paper or stick is wetted with urine. If acetone is present, the paper will turn a certain color. These test papers or sticks are commercially available. **2.** To 5 ml of urine are added a few crystals of ammonium sulfate (which are then dissolved) and a small crystal of sodium nitroprusside. The mixture is shaken a little. Then it is covered with a layer (about 2 ml) of strong ammonia. The presence of acetone is indicated by a purple ring between the layers of liquid. A commercially available tablet is also used for this test.

**acetone body** Ketone body.

**acetonemia** (ăs″ĕ-tō-nē′mē-ă) [*acetone* + Gr. *haima,* blood] Large amounts of acetone in the blood. The symptoms are abnormal excitement, gradual depression, and acidosis.

**acetonitrile** (ăs″ĕ-tō-nī′trĭl) $CH_3CN$. Methyl cyanide, an ingredient of some commercially available nail care products. When ingested, it produces a toxic reaction similar to cyanide poisoning. The onset is delayed 9 to 12 hr or more. It is also found in the urine of cigarette smokers. Treatment for poisoning is the same as for cyanide poisoning. SEE: *cotinine; cyanide poisoning.*

**acetonuria** (ăs″ĕ-tō-nū′rē-ă) [*acetone* + Gr. *ouron,* urine] Ketonuria.

**acetophenazine maleate** (ăs″ĕ-tō-fĕn′ă-zēn măl′ē-āt) An antipsychotic drug of the phenothiazine group. Trade name is Tindal.

**acetophenetidin** (ăs″ĕ-tō-fĕ-nĕt′ĭ-dĭn) Former name for phenacetin.

**acetous** (ăs′ĕ-tŭs) [L. *acetum,* vinegar] **1.** Pert. to vinegar. **2.** Sour in taste.

**acetum** (ă-sē′tŭm) *pl.* **aceta** [L.] **1.** Vinegar. **2.** A drug dissolved in a weak vinegar solution.

**acetyl** (ăs′ĕ-tĭl, ă-sēt′ĭl) [″ + Gr. *hyle,* matter] $CH_3CO$, the univalent radical.

***a. CoA*** Acetylcoenzyme A.

**acetylation** (ă-sĕt″ĭ-lā′shŭn) The introduction of one or more acetyl groups into an organic compound.

**acetylcholine** (ăs″ĕ-tĭl-kō′lēn) ABBR: ACh. An ester of choline that is the neurotransmitter at neuromuscular junctions in the parasympathetic nervous system and sympathetic preganglionic fibers (cholinergic fibers) and at some synapses in the central nervous system. It is inactivated by the enzyme cholinesterase. SEE: *cholinergic fibers.*

***a. chloride*** A salt solution of acetylcholine used in irrigation of the iris to produce contraction of the pupil after cataract surgery. The sterile solution is instilled in the anterior chamber of the eye before suturing. Trade name is Miochol.

**acetylcholinesterase** (ăs″ĕ-tĭl-kō″lĭn-ĕs′tĕr-ās) ABBR: AChE. An enzyme that stops the action of acetylcholine. It is present in various body tissues, including muscles, nerve cells, and red blood cells.

**acetylcoenzyme A** A condensation product of coenzyme A and acetic acid.

**acetylcysteine** (ăs″ĕ-tĭl-sĭs′tē-ĭn) A chemical substance that, when nebulized and inhaled, liquefies mucus and pus. It is also used in the treatment of acetaminophen poisoning. Trade name is Mucomyst. SEE: *acetaminophen poisoning.*

**acetylene** (ă-sĕt′ĭ-lēn) $C_2H_2$. A colorless explosive gas with a garlic-like odor.
**acetylsalicylic acid** (ă-sē″tĭl-săl″ĭ-sĭl′ĭk) Aspirin.
**acetylsalicylic acid poisoning** SEE: *aspirin poisoning.*
**acetyltransferase** (ăs″ĕ-tĭl-trăns′fĕr-ās) Enzyme that is effective in the transfer of an acetyl group from one compound to another.
**ACH** *adrenocortical hormone.*
**ACh** *acetylcholine.*
**achalasia** (ăk″ă-lā′zē-ă) [Gr. *a-,* not, + *chalasis,* relaxation] Failure to relax; said of muscles, such as sphincters, the normal function of which is a persistent contraction with periods of relaxation. SEE: *Nursing Diagnoses Appendix.*
***a. of the cardia*** Failure of the cardiac sphincter to relax, restricting the passage of food to the stomach. In advanced cases, dysphagia is marked and dilation of the esophagus may occur. SYN: *cardiospasm.*
***pelvirectal a.*** Congenital absence of ganglion cells in the distal large bowel, resulting in failure of the colon to relax.
***sphincteral a.*** Failure of the intestinal sphincters to relax.
**AChE** *acetylcholinesterase.*
**ache** (āk) [AS. *acan*] **1.** Pain that is persistent rather than sudden or spasmodic. It may be dull or severe. **2.** To suffer persistent pain.
**acheilia** (ă-kī′lē-ă) [Gr. *a-,* not, + *cheilos,* lip] Congenital absence of one or both lips.
**acheiria** (ă-kī′rē-ă) [″ + *cheir,* hand] **1.** Congenital absence of one or both hands. **2.** A loss of sensation in one or both hands. This may result from temporary or permanent injury or malfunction of the sensory mechanism, or it may occur in hysteria. **3.** Inability to determine to which side of the body a stimulus has been applied. SYN: *achiria.*
**acheiropodia** (ă-kī″rō-pō′dē-ă) [″ + ″ + *pous,* foot] Congenital absence of the hands and feet.
**Achilles jerk** (ă-kĭl′ēz) [Achilles, hero of the *Iliad,* whose vulnerable spot was his heel] Achilles tendon reflex.
**Achilles tendon** The tendon of the gastrocnemius and soleus muscles of the leg. SYN: *calcaneal tendon.*
**Achilles tendon reflex** Plantar flexion, also called extension of the ankle, resulting from contraction of the calf muscles after a sharp blow to the Achilles tendon. The variations and their significance correspond closely to those of the knee jerk. It is exaggerated in upper motor neuron disease and diminished or absent in lower motor neuron disease. Since the character of the response is influenced by the metabolic rate, attempts have been made to use this reflex as an index of thyroid function. The value of such use is controversial.
**achillobursitis** (ă-kĭl″ō-bŭr-sī′tĭs) [*Achilles* + L. *bursa,* a pouch, + Gr. *itis,* inflammation] Inflammation of the bursa lying over the Achilles tendon. SYN: *Albert's disease.*
**achillodynia** (ă-kĭl″ō-dĭn′ē-ă) [″ + Gr. *odyne,* pain] Pain caused by inflammation between the Achilles tendon and bursa.
**achillorrhaphy** (ă-kĭl-or′ă-fē) [″ + Gr. *rhaphe,* seam, ridge] Suture of the Achilles tendon.
**achillotenotomy** (ă-kĭl″ō-tĕn-ŏt′ō-mē) [″ + Gr. *tenon,* tendon, + *tome,* incision] Achillotomy.
**achillotomy** (ă-kĭl-ŏt′ō-mē) [″ + *tome,* incision] Division of the Achilles tendon. SYN: *achillotenotomy.*
**achiria** (ă-kī′rē-ă) [Gr. *a-,* not, + *cheir,* hand] Acheiria.
**achlorhydria** (ă″klor-hī′drē-ă) [″ + *chloros,* green, + *hydor,* water] Absence of free hydrochloric acid in the stomach; may be associated with gastric carcinoma, gastric ulcer, pernicious anemia, adrenal insufficiency, or chronic gastritis. SEE: *achylia.*
***histamine-proved a.*** Absence of free acid in gastric secretion even after subcutaneous injection of histamine hydrochloride.
**achloropsia** (ă-klō-rŏp′sē-ă) [″ + *chloros,* green, + *opsis,* vision] Color blindness in which green cannot be distinguished. SYN: *deuteranopia.*
**acholuria** (ă-kō-lū′rē-ă) [″ + *chole,* bile, + *ouron,* urine] Absence of bile pigments in urine in some forms of jaundice.
**achondrogenesis** (ă-kŏn″drō-jĕn′ĕ-sĭs) [Gr. *a-,* not, + *chondros,* cartilage, + *genesis,* generation, birth] Failure of bone to grow, esp. the bones of the extremities.
**achondroplasia** (ă-kŏn″drō-plā′sē-ă) [″ + ″ + *plasis,* a molding] Defect in the formation of cartilage at the epiphyses of long bones, producing a form of dwarfism; sometimes seen in rickets. SYN: *chondrodystrophy.*
**achroma** (ă-krō′mă) [″ + *chroma,* color] An absence of color or normal pigmentation as in leukoderma, albinism, and vitiligo.
**achromasia** (ăk″rō-mā′zē-ă) [Gr. *achromatos,* without color] **1.** Absence of normal pigmentation of the skin as in albinism, vitiligo, or leukoderma. **2.** Pallor. **3.** Inability of cells or tissues to be stained.
**achromate** (ă-krō′māt) [Gr. *a-,* not, + *chroma,* color] A person who is colorblind.
**achromatic** (ăk″rō-măt′ĭk) [Gr. *achromatos,* without color] **1.** Colorless. **2.** Not dispersing light into constituent components. **3.** Not containing chromatin. **4.** Difficult to stain, with reference to cells and tissues.
**achromatic lens** Lens that transmits light without separating the spectral colors.
**achromatin** (ă-krō′mă-tĭn) The weakly staining substance of a cell nucleus.
**achromatism** (ă-krō′mă-tĭzm″) [Gr. *a-,* not, + *chroma,* color, + *-ismos,* condition] Colorlessness.
**achromatocyte** (ăk″rō-măt′ō-sīt) [Gr. *achro-*

*matos,* without color, + *kytos,* cell] Achromocyte.

**achromatolysis** (ă-krō″mă-tŏl′ĭ-sĭs) [″ + *lysis,* dissolution] Dissolution of cell achromatin.

**achromatophil** (ă″krō-măt′ō-fĭl) [″ + *philos,* love] A cell or tissue not stainable in the usual manner. SYN: *achromophil.*

**achromatopsia** (ă-krō″mă-tŏp′sē-ă) [″ + *opsis,* vision] Complete color blindness.

**achromatosis** (ă-krō″mă-tō′sĭs) [″ + *osis,* condition] The condition of being without natural pigmentation. SEE: *achroma.*

**achromatous** (ă-krō′mă-tŭs) Without color.

**achromaturia** (ă-krō″mă-tū′rē-ă) [Gr. *achromatos,* without color, + *ouron,* urine] Colorless or nearly colorless urine.

**achromia** (ă-krō′mē-ă) [Gr. *a-,* not, + *chroma,* color] **1.** Absence of color; pallor. **2.** Achromatosis. **3.** Condition in which erythrocytes have large central pale areas; hypochromia.

***congenital a.*** Albinism.

**achromic** (ă-krō′mĭk) Lacking color.

**Achromobacter** A genus of gram-negative bacilli that may inhabit the lower gastrointestinal tract; may cause nosocomial infections.

**achromocyte** (ă-krō′mō-sīt) [Gr. *a-,* not, + *chroma,* color + *kytos,* cell] In a blood smear, a large, pale, crescent-shaped cell produced from fragile red cells as the bloodfilm preparation is being made. SYN: *achromatocyte; crescent body; selenoid cell.*

**achromophil** (ă-krō′mō-fĭl) [″ + ″ + *philos,* love] Achromatophil.

**achromotrichia** (ă-krō″mō-trĭk′ē-ă) [″ + ″ + *trichia,* condition of the hair] Lack of color or graying of the hair. SYN: *canities.*

***nutritional a.*** Grayness of the hair due to dietary deficiency.

**Achromycin** (ăk″rō-mī′sĭn) Trade name for tetracycline, an antibiotic effective in the treatment of many bacterial infections.

**achroodextrin** (ăk″rō-ō-dĕks′trĭn) [Gr. *achroos,* colorless, + *dextrin*] One of the varieties of dextrin resulting from hydrolysis of starch.

**achylia** (ă-kī′lē-ă) [Gr. *a-,* not, + *chylos,* juice] Absence of chyle or other digestive ferments. SYN: *achylosis.*

***a. gastrica*** Complete absence or marked decrease in the amount of gastric juice. SEE: *achlorhydria.*

***a. pancreatica*** Absence or deficiency of pancreatic secretion; usually a sign of chronic pancreatitis.

**achylosis** (ă″kī-lō′sĭs) Achylia.

**achylous** (ă-kī′lŭs) [Gr. *achylos,* without chyle] **1.** Lacking in any kind of digestive secretion. **2.** Without chyle.

**acicular** (ă-sĭk′ū-lăr) [L. *aciculus,* little needle] Needle-shaped.

**acid** [L. *acidum,* acid] **1.** Any substance that liberates hydrogen ions (protons) in solution; a hydrogen ion donor. An acid reacts with a metal to form a salt, neutralizes bases, and turns litmus paper red. SEE: *alkali; base; indicator; pH.* **2.** A sour substance. **3.** Slang term for LSD.

***acetic a.*** $CH_3COOH$. Substance that gives sour taste to vinegar; also used as a reagent and as a caustic. Diluted acetic acid contains 6% pure acetic acid by weight. Glacial acetic acid contains at least 99.5% acetic acid by weight.

***acetoacetic a.*** $CH_3COCH_2COOH$. A ketone body formed when fats are incompletely oxidized; appears in urine in abnormal amounts in starvation and in inadequately treated diabetes. SYN: *acetylacetic a.*

***acetylacetic a.*** Acetoacetic a.

***acetylsalicylic a.*** Aspirin.

***adenylic a.*** Adenosine monophosphate.

***amino a.*** SEE: *amino acid.*

***aminoacetic a.*** $NH_2CH_2COOH$, a nonessential amino acid. SYN: *glycine.*

***aminobenzoic a.*** Para-aminobenzoic a.

***aminocaproic a.*** A hemostatic drug; a specific antidote for an overdose of a fibrinolytic agent. Trade name is Amicar.

***aminoglutaric a.*** Glutamic a.

***aminosalicylic a.*** Para-aminosalicylic a.

***aminosuccinic a.*** Aspartic a.

***arachidonic a.*** SEE: *arachidonic acid.*

***ascorbic a.*** $C_6H_8O_6$. Vitamin C, a vitamin that occurs naturally in fresh fruits, esp. citrus, and vegetables, and can also be synthesized. It is essential in maintenance of collagen formation, osteoid tissue of bones, and formation and maintenance of dentin. This essential vitamin is used as a dietary supplement and in the prevention and treatment of scurvy. Scurvy develops after approx. 3 mo. of ascorbic acid deficiency in the diet. The usefulness of large daily doses (1 to 5 g or more a day) of this vitamin in preventing or treating the common cold in otherwise healthy persons has not been established although it may decrease the severity of symptoms. Continuous treatment with large doses can cause kidney stones. SYN: *antiscorbutic vitamin; vitamin C.*

***aspartic a.*** $COOH \cdot CH(NH_2) \cdot CH_2 \cdot COOH$. A nonessential amino acid; a product of pancreatic digestion. SYN: *aminosuccinic a.*

***barbituric a.*** $C_4H_4N_2O_3$. A crystalline compound from which phenobarbital and other barbiturates are derived. SYN: *malonylurea.*

***benzoic a.*** $C_7H_6O_2$. A white crystalline material having a slight odor; used in keratolytic ointments and as a food preservative. Saccharin is a derivative of this acid.

***bile a.*** Any one of the complex acids that occur as salts in bile (e.g., cholic, glycocholic, and taurocholic acids). They give bile its foamy character, are important in the digestion of fats in the intestine, and are reabsorbed from the intestine to be used again by the liver.

***boric a.*** $H_3BO_3$. A white crystalline substance that in water forms a very weak acid solution poisonous to plants and animals. It is soluble in water, alcohol, and glycerin. SEE: *boric acid.*

Caution: Because of its toxicity, boric acid should be used rarely. It is particularly dangerous because it can be accidentally swallowed by children or used in food because of its resemblance to sugar.

***butyric a.*** $C_3H_7COOH$. An acid having a rancid odor; found in cheese, rancid butter, cod liver oil, and perspiration.

***carbolic a.*** Phenol.

***carbonic a.*** $H_2CO_3$. An acid formed when carbon dioxide is dissolved in water.

***carboxylic a.*** Any acid containing the group COOH. The simplest examples are formic and acetic acids.

***cholic a.*** An acid formed in the liver by hydrolysis of other bile acids; important in digestion.

***citric a.*** $C_6H_8O_7$. An acid found in citrus fruits or prepared synthetically in the form of colorless crystals or white crystalline powder, which is soluble in water, ether, and alcohol. The hydrous form is used as a flavoring agent. SEE: *vitamin C.*

***deoxyribonucleic a.*** ABBR: DNA. The nucleic acid that is the hereditary material of the chromosome of cells. SEE: *deoxyribonucleic acid.*

***desoxyribonucleic a.*** Former spelling of deoxyribonucleic acid.

***eicosapenteanoic a.*** ABBR: EPA. One of a group of fatty acids containing 20 carbons and five double bonds that are prevalent in fish oils. SEE: *acids, omega-3 fatty.*

***ethylenediaminetetra-acetic a.*** ABBR: EDTA. A chelating agent that, in the form of its calcium or sodium salts, is used to remove substances such as lead and digitalis from the body. SEE: *chelation.*

***fatty a.*** A carboxylic acid that can be combined with glycerol to form fats; the simplest members of the series are formic and acetic; most typical are stearic and palmitic. A saturated fatty acid has single bonds in its carbon chain, with the general formula $C_nH_{2n}O_2$. An unsaturated fatty acid has one or more double or triple bonds in its carbon chain. In human nutrition, it is believed that decreasing the intake of saturated fatty acids will lower the cholesterol content of the blood.

***folic a.*** $C_{19}H_{19}N_7O_6$. A member of the vitamin B complex; found naturally in green plant tissue, liver, and yeast. When produced synthetically, it is identical with pteroylglutamic acid. Therapeutic use during pregnancy may help to prevent birth defects of the spinal column and spinal cord, such as spina bifida.

Caution: Folic acid should not be used in the treatment of pernicious anemia because it does not protect patients against the development of changes in the central nervous system that accompany this type of anemia.

***formic a.*** HCOOH. The first and strongest member of the monobasic fatty acid series. It occurs naturally in certain animal secretions and in muscle, but it may also be prepared synthetically. It is one of the irritants present in the sting of insects such as bees and ants.

***formiminoglutamic a.*** $C_6N_2O_4H_{10}$. An intermediate product in the metabolism of histidine. Its increase in the urine after administration of histidine in patients with folic acid deficiency is the basis for the FIGLU excretion test.

***gallic a.*** $C_6H_2(OH)_3COOH$. A colorless crystalline acid. It occurs naturally as an excrescence on the twigs of trees, esp. oaks, as a reaction to the deposition of gall wasp eggs. It is used as a skin astringent and in the manufacture of writing inks and dyes.

***glucuronic a.*** $CHO(CHOH)_4COOH$. An oxidation product of glucose that is present in the urine. Toxic products (such as salicylic acid, menthol, and phenol) that have entered the body through the intestinal tract are detoxified in the liver by conjugation with glucuronic acid.

***glutamic a.*** $COOH \cdot (CH_2)_2 \cdot CH(NH_2) \cdot COOH$. A nonessential amino acid formed during protein metabolism. SYN: *aminoglutaric a.*

***glyceric a.*** $CH_2OH \cdot CHOH \cdot COOH$. An intermediate product of the oxidation of fats.

***glycocholic a.*** $C_{26}H_{43}NO_6$. A bile acid yielding glycine and cholic acid on hydrolysis.

***homogentisic a.*** An intermediate product of tyrosine catabolism; found in the urine in alkaptonuria. SYN: *alkapton.*

***hyaluronic a.*** An acid mucopolysaccharide found in the ground substance of connective tissue that acts as a binding and protective agent. It is also found in the synovial fluid and vitreous and aqueous humors.

***hydriodic a.*** HI. In solution, it is used in various forms of chemical analyses. SYN: *hydrogen iodide.*

***hydrochloric a.*** HCl. An inorganic acid that is normally present in gastric juice. It destroys fermenting bacteria that might cause intestinal tract disturbances. Five to 10 ml of a 10% solution of hydrochloric acid in 125 to 250 ml of water is used in treating hypoacidity or achlorhydria.

Caution: When so used, it must be diluted accurately and sipped through a drinking straw. This will prevent the acid from damaging the teeth.

***hydrocyanic a.*** HCN. A colorless, extremely poisonous, highly volatile liquid that occurs naturally in plants but can be produced synthetically. It has many industrial uses: electroplating, fumigation, and production of dyes, pigments, synthetic fibers, and plastic. Exposure of humans to 200 to 500 parts of hydrocyanic acid per 1,000,000 parts of air for 30 min is fatal. It acts by preventing cellular respiration. SYN: *hydrogen cyanide.* SEE: *cyanide* in *Poisons and Poisoning Appendix.*

***hydroxy a.*** An acid containing one or more hydroxyl (OH) groups in addition to the carboxyl (COOH) group (e.g., lactic acid, $CH_3COHCOOH$).

***hydroxybutyric a.*** An acid present in the urine, esp. in diabetes, when fatty acid conversion to ketones increases.

***hypochlorous a.*** An acid, HClO, used as a disinfectant and bleaching agent. It is usually used in the form of one of its salts.

***imino a.*** An acid formed as a result of oxidation of amino acids in the body.

***inorganic a.*** An acid containing no carbon atoms.

***keto a.*** Any organic acid containing the ketone CO (carbonyl radical).

***lactic a.*** A mixture of lactic acid, $C_3H_6O_3$, and lactic acid lactate, $C_6H_{10}O_5$, equal to at least 85% but not more than 90% lactic acid, by weight. It occurs in sour milk from fermentation of lactose, and it is formed in muscles during the anaerobic cell respiration that occurs during strenuous exercise. It is also formed during anaerobic muscle activity when glucose cannot be changed to pyruvic acid in glycolysis. It contributes to muscle fatigue. Lactic acid milk (buttermilk or acidophilus milk) helps to prevent the growth of putrefactive bacteria in the large intestine.

***linoleic a.*** $C_{18}H_{32}O_2$. An unsaturated fatty acid, a dietary essential. It was first isolated from linseed oil but is also found in corn oil. It is required for the synthesis of prostaglandins.

***linolenic a.*** $C_{18}H_{30}O_2$. An unsaturated fatty acid, a dietary essential.

***lysergic a.*** $C_{16}H_{16}N_2O_2$. A crystalline substance derived from ergot. Its derivative, lysergic acid diethylamide (LSD), is a potent hallucinogen. SEE: *LSD.*

***malic a.*** $C_4H_6O_5$. Substance found in certain sour fruits such as apples and apricots and active in the aerobic metabolism of carbohydrates.

***malonic a.*** $C_3H_4O_4$. A dibasic acid formed by the oxidation of malic acid and active in the tricarboxylic acid cycle in carbohydrate metabolism. Its inhibition of succinic dehydrogenase is the classic example of competitive inhibition. Malonic acid is found in beets.

***mandelic a.*** $C_8H_8O_3$. A colorless hydroxy acid. Its salt is used in urinary tract infections.

***monounsaturated fatty a.*** A fatty acid containing one double bond between carbon atoms. This type is found in olive oil. It is thought to lower low-density lipoprotein levels without affecting high-density lipoprotein levels. It is the predominant fat in what has been called the Mediterranean diet. SEE: *Mediterranean diet.*

***nicotinic a.*** $C_6H_5NO_2$. A member of the vitamin B complex; used for the prevention and treatment of pellagra. It occurs naturally in liver, yeast, milk, cheese, and cereals. SYN: *niacin.*

***nitric a.*** $HNO_3$. A strong corrosive acid prepared from sulfuric acid and a nitrate. It is used in the manufacture of explosives and dyes and as a coagulant in testing urine for albumin (Heller's test).

***nucleic a.*** Any one of a group of high-molecular-weight substances found in the cells of all living things. They have a complex chemical structure formed of sugars (pentoses), phosphoric acid, and nitrogen bases (purines and pyrimidines). Most important are ribonucleic acid and deoxyribonucleic acid.

***oleic a.*** $C_{18}H_{34}O_2$. An unsaturated fatty acid found in most organic fats and oils.

***omega-3 (ω3) fatty a.'s*** A group of fatty acids found in the oils of some saltwater fish. They have been used to attempt to reduce levels of very-low-density lipoproteins and chylomicrons in plasma.

***omega-6 (ω6) fatty a.'s*** Fatty acids, such as linoleic and arachidonic, thought to influence cardiovascular and growth function when balanced with omega-3 fatty acids in eicosanoid production.

***organic a.*** An acid containing the carboxyl radical, COOH. Acetic acid, formic acid, lactic acid, and all fatty acids are organic.

***orotic a.*** Uracil-6-carboxylic acid. It is a precursor in the formation of pyrimidine nucleotides.

***oxalic a.*** $C_2H_2O_4$. The simplest dibasic organic acid. Its potassium or calcium salt occurs naturally in rhubarb, wood sorrel, and many other plants. It is the strongest organic acid and is poisonous. When properly diluted, it removes ink or rust stains from cloth. It is used also as a reagent.

***palmitic a.*** $C_{16}H_{32}O_2$. A saturated fatty acid occurring as esters in most natural fats and oils.

***pantothenic a.*** $C_9H_{17}NO_5$. One of the B-complex vitamins.

***para-aminobenzoic a.*** ABBR: PABA. $NH_2C_6H_4COOH$. A B-complex vitamin used as a dietary supplement, an antirickettsial drug, a reagent, and a sunscreening agent. It should not be used in persons known to be sensitive to sulfonamides. It inhibits the bacteriostatic action of sulfonamides, so all but topical use is contraindicated during sulfonamide therapy. SYN: *aminobenzoic a.*

***para-aminosalicylic a.*** ABBR: PAS. $C_7H_7NO_3$. An antituberculosis drug, the effectiveness of which is greatly enhanced when it is combined with streptomycin and isoniazid; a white and practically odorless powder that darkens when exposed to air or light. It is believed to delay development of bacterial resistance. SYN: *aminosalicylic a.*

***pentanoic a.*** Valeric a.

***perchloric a.*** $HClO_4$. A colorless unstable liquid compound; the highest oxygen acid of chlorine.

***phenylglycolic a.*** Mandelic a.

***phosphoric a.*** An acid formed by oxidation of phosphorus, used as an alkaloidal reagent. The phosphoric acids are orthophosphoric acid, $H_3PO_4$; pyrophosphoric acid, $H_4P_2O_7$; metaphosphoric acid, $HPO_3$; and hypophosphoric acid, $H_4P_2O_6$. The salts of these acids are phosphates. Orthophosphoric acid, a tribasic acid, is used as a 30% to 50% solution to etch enamel of teeth in preparation for bonding of resin dental restorations.

***phosphorous a.*** An oxygen acid of phosphorus. The phosphorous acids are orthophosphorous acid, $H_2(HPO_3)$; pyrophosphorous acid, $H_4P_2O_5$; metaphosphorous acid, $HPO_2$; and hypophosphorous acid, $H(H_2PO_2)$. The salts of these acids are phosphites.

***picric a.*** $C_6H_2(NO_2)_3OH$. A yellow crystalline substance that precipitates proteins; used as a dye and a reagent. SYN: *trinitrophenol.*

***pyruvic a.*** $CH_3CO \cdot COOH$. An organic acid that plays an important role in the Krebs cycle. It is an intermediate product in the metabolism of carbohydrates, fats, and amino acids. Its quantity in the blood and tissues increases in thiamine deficiency because thiamine is essential for its oxidation.

***ribonucleic a.*** ABBR: RNA. A nucleic acid that regulates protein synthesis in cells. SEE: *ribonucleic acid.*

***salicylic a.*** $C_7H_6O_3$. White crystalline powder used as a local antiseptic or keratolytic agent.

***saturated fatty a.*** Fatty acid in which the carbon atoms are linked to other carbon atoms by single bonds. SEE: *fatty a.; unsaturated fatty a.*

***silicic a.*** An acid containing silica, as $H_2SiO_3$, $H_2SiO_4$, or $H_2SiO_6$. When silicic acid is precipitated, silica gel is obtained.

***stearic a.*** $C_{18}H_{36}O_2$. A monobasic fatty acid occurring naturally in plants and animals; used in the manufacture of soap and pharmaceutical products such as glycerin suppositories.

***succinic a.*** $COOH(CH_2)_2COOH$. An intermediate in carbohydrate metabolism.

***sulfonic a.*** An organic compound of the general formula $SO_2OH$ derived from sulfuric acid by replacement of a hydrogen atom.

***sulfosalicylic a.*** A crystalline acid soluble in water or alcohol; used as a reagent for precipitating proteins, as in testing for albumin in urine.

***sulfuric a.*** $H_2SO_4$. A colorless, corrosive, heavy liquid prepared from sulfur; used in the production of a great number of industrial products. It is rarely used in medicine.

***sulfurous a.*** $H_2SO_3$. An inorganic acid. It is a powerful chemical reducing agent that is used commercially, esp. for its bleaching properties.

***tannic a.*** A glucoside prepared from oak galls and sumac that yields gallic acid and glucose on hydrolysis. SYN: *tannin.*

***tartaric a.*** $C_4H_6O_6$. Substance obtained from byproducts of wine fermentation; widely used in industry in manufacture of carbonated drinks, flavored gelatins, dyes, and metals; also used as a reagent.

***taurocholic a.*** A bile acid that yields cholic acid and taurine on hydrolysis.

***trichloroacetic a.*** $C_2HCl_3O_2$. A caustic crystalline substance.

***unsaturated fatty a.*** Organic acid in which some of the carbon atoms are linked to other carbon atoms by double bonds, thus containing less than the maximum possible number of hydrogen atoms; for example, unsaturated oleic and linoleic acids as compared with the saturated stearic acid. SEE: *fatty a.; saturated fatty a.*

***uric a.*** $C_5H_4N_4O_3$. An important organic constituent of normal urine; usually occurs in form of salts (urates).

***valeric a.*** $C_5H_{10}O_2$. An oily liquid of the fatty acid series, existing in four isomeric forms and having a distinctly disagreeable odor. SYN: *pentanoic a.*

**acidaminuria** (ăs″ĭd-ăm″ĭ-nū′rē-ă) [L. *acidum,* acid, + *amine* + Gr. *ouron,* urine] An excess of amino acids in urine. SYN: *hyperacidaminuria.*

**acid-base balance** The mechanisms by which the acidity and alkalinity of body fluids are kept in a state of equilibrium so that the pH of arterial blood is maintained at approx. 7.35 to 7.45. This is accomplished by the action of buffer systems of the blood and the regulatory (homeostatic) functions of the respiratory and urinary systems. Disturbances in acid-base balance result in acidosis, or alkalosis. SEE: *pH.*

**acidemia** (ăs-ĭ-dē′mē-ă) [L. *acidum,* acid, + Gr. *haima,* blood] A decrease in the arterial blood pH below 7.35 due to an uncompensated reduction in circulating alkaline substances. The hydrogen ion concentration of the blood increases, as reflected by a lowering of serum pH values. SEE: *acid-base balance; acidity; acidosis.*

**acid fallout** Acid rain.

**acid-fast** Not decolorized easily by acids after staining; pert. to bacteria that after staining are decolorized by a mixture of acid and alcohol. The acid-fast bacteria retain the red dyes, but the surrounding tissues are decolorized. In clinical medicine, an example of this type of organism is *Mycobacterium tuberculosis.*

**acidifiable** (ă-sĭd′ĭ-fī″ă-bl) [L. *acidum,* acid, + *fieri,* to be made, + *habilis,* able] Capable of being transformed to produce an acid reaction.

**acidification** (ă-sĭd″ĭ-fĭ-kā′shŭn) [″ + *factus,* made] Conversion into an acid.

**acidifier** (ă-sĭd′ĭ-fī″ĕr) [″ + *fieri,* to be made] A substance that causes acidity.

**acidify 1.** To make a substance acid. **2.** To become acid.

**acidity** (ă-sĭd′ĭ-tē) **1.** The quality of possessing hydrogen ions (protons). SEE: *acid; hydrogen ion; pH.* **2.** Sourness.

***a. of the stomach*** Sourness due to fermentation of food in the stomach or oversecretion of acid.

***titratable a.*** The amount of hydrogen ion excreted in the urine in a dihydrogen form.

**acidophil(e)** (ă-sĭd′ō-fĭl, -fīl) [″ + Gr. *philos,* love] **1.** Acidophilic. **2.** An acid-staining cell of the anterior pituitary. **3.** A bacterial organism that grows well in an acid medium.

**acidophilic** (ă-sĭd″ō-fĭl′ĭk) **1.** Having affinity for acid or pert. to certain tissues and cell granules. **2.** Pert. to a cell capable of being stained by acid dyes.

**acidophilus milk** (ăs″ĭ-dŏf′ĭ-lŭs) Milk fermented by *Lactobacillus acidophilus* cultures. SEE: *milk.*

**acidoresistant** (ăs″ĭ-dō-rĕ-zĭs′tănt) Acid-resisting; said about bacteria.

**acidosis** (ăs″ĭ-dō′sĭs) [L. *acidum,* acid, + Gr. *osis,* condition] An actual or relative increase in the acidity of blood due to an accumulation of acids (as in diabetic acidosis or renal disease) or an excessive loss of bicarbonate (as in renal disease). The hydrogen ion concentration of the fluid is increased, lowering the pH. SEE: *acid-base balance; acidemia; buffer; pH.* **acidotic** (ăs″ĭ-dŏt′ĭk), *adj.*

***carbon dioxide a.*** Acidosis resulting from carbon dioxide retention, as in drowning or decreased respiration.

***compensated a.*** Acidosis in which the pH of body fluids has returned to normal. Compensatory mechanisms maintain the normal ratio of bicarbonate to carbonic acid (approx. 20 : 1) in blood plasma, even though the bicarbonate level is decreased or the carbon dioxide level is elevated.

***diabetic a.*** Acidosis caused by an accumulation of ketone bodies, in advanced stages of uncontrolled diabetes mellitus. SEE: *coma, diabetic.*

***hypercapnic a.*** Respiratory a.

***hyperchloremic a.*** Acidosis in which there is an abnormally high level of chloride in the blood serum.

***lactic a.*** An accumulation of lactic acid in the blood, whatever the cause. Lactic acid is produced faster than normal when there is inadequate oxygenation of skeletal muscle and other tissues. Thus, any disease that leads to tissue hypoxia, exercise, hyperventilation, or some drugs (e.g., oral hypoglycemic agents) may cause this condition. In general, when blood pH is less than 7.35 and lactate is greater than 5 to 6 mmol/L (5 to 6 mEq/L), lactic acidosis is present.

***metabolic a.*** Acidosis resulting from increase in acids other than carbonic acid. Possible causes are excessive ingestion of acids or acid salts, ketosis, severe dehydration, diarrhea, vomiting, renal disease, and impaired liver function.

NURSING IMPLICATIONS: A history is obtained, focusing on the patient's urine output, fluid intake, dietary habits (including recent fasting), associated disorders (such as diabetes mellitus and kidney or liver dysfunction), and the use of medications (including aspirin) and alcohol. The nurse monitors arterial blood gas values, serum potassium level, and fluid balance. The patient is assessed for lethargy, drowsiness, and headache, and for diminished muscle tone and deep tendon reflexes. The patient is also evaluated for hyperventilation, cardiac dysrhythmias, muscle weakness, and flaccidity, and for gastrointestinal distress such as nausea, vomiting, diarrhea, and abdominal pain. Prescribed intravenous fluids, medications such as sodium bicarbonate or insulin, and other therapies such as oxygen or mechanical ventilation are administered. The patient is positioned to promote chest expansion and repositioned frequently. Frequent oral hygiene with sodium bicarbonate rinses will neutralize mouth acids and a water-soluble lubricant will prevent lip dryness. A safe environment with minimal stimulation is provided, and preparations should be available if seizures occur. Both patient and family are given verbal and written information about managing related disease processes and prescribed medications. SEE: *Nursing Diagnoses Appendix.*

***renal a.*** Acidosis due to impaired kidney function. The acidosis is induced by excessive loss of bicarbonate or inability to excrete phosphoric and sulfuric acids.

***respiratory a.*** Acidosis caused by retention of carbon dioxide due to pulmonary insufficiency.

NURSING IMPLICATIONS: Arterial blood gas values and serum potassium level are monitored. Level of consciousness as it pertains to depression of the central nervous system is determined by assessing for headache, restlessness, irritability, somnolence, disorientation, and blurred vision. The patient is also evaluated for diaphoresis, a fine or flapping tremor (asterixis), depressed reflexes, and cardiac dysrhythmias. Vital signs and ventilatory effort are monitored, and ventilatory difficulties such as dyspnea or hypoventilation are documented. The nurse prepares the patient for and assists with inhalation therapy or mechanical ventilation to decrease carbon dioxide levels. Prescribed intravenous fluids are given to maintain hydration. The patient is oriented as often as necessary, and information and reassurance are given to allay the patient's and family's fears and concerns. Prescribed therapies for associated hypoxemia and underlying conditions are provided, responses evaluated, and related patient education is given.

**acid poisoning** Ingestion of a toxic acid. SEE: *acids* in *Poisons and Poisoning* in *Appendix.*

FIRST AID: Dilute with large volumes of water. Give oral milk, egg white, magnesium oxide, milk of magnesia, lime water, or aluminum hydroxide gel. Avoid carbonates as neutralizers because, in the presence of strong acids, they will react to produce carbon dioxide gas. This may cause distention and rupture of the stomach. Give demulcents and morphine for pain.

---

Caution: The use of emetics and stomach tubes is dangerous.

---

**acid-proof** Acid-fast.

**acid rain** Rain that, in passing through the atmosphere, is contaminated with acid substances, esp. sulfur dioxide and nitrogen oxide. These pollutants are oxidized in the atmosphere to sulfuric acid and nitric acid. Rainwater is considered abnormally acid if the pH is below 5.6. Values as low as pH 2.4 were recorded in Scotland in 1974. Severe harmful effects on aquatic and plant life have been reported in the U.S., Canada, Scandinavia, and western Europe. SYN: *acid fallout.*

**acid-reflux disorder** Any one of a variety of conditions produced when the acid contents of the stomach enter the esophagus. Transient relaxation of the lower esophageal sphincter or the presence of a hiatal hernia may permit the reflux. Symptoms include dysphagia as well as a burning substernal sensation radiating up to the neck. Antacids provide temporary relief. Other treatment measures include elevating the head of the bed and taking medications to prevent stomach acid secretion or to stimulate esophageal contractions. When medical therapy is ineffective or not desired by the patient, surgery should be considered. If the condition is not treated or treatment is ineffective, the result may be esophagitis, acid laryngitis, or pulmonary disease. SEE: *acid-reflux test.*

**acid-reflux test** Test for reflux of acid into the esophagus from the stomach. An electrode for detecting the pH is placed in the stomach and a reading is taken; then the electrode is withdrawn until it is in the esophagus. Normally, the pH will become more alkaline (i.e., rise) as the electrode is moved from the stomach into the esophagus. If there is acid reflux, the pH will be acid in both the stomach and esophagus.

**acid salt** Salt formed when only a part of the hydrogen of an acid is replaced by a metal.

**acidulate** [L. *acidulus,* slightly acid] To make somewhat sour or acid.

**acidulous** (ă-sĭd′ū-lŭs) Slightly sour or acid.

**acidum** (ăs′ĭ-dŭm) [L.] Acid.

**aciduria** (ăs-ĭd-ū′rē-ă) [L. *acidum,* acid, + Gr. *ouron,* urine] The condition of excessive acid in the urine.

***orotic a.*** An inherited disorder of pyrimidine metabolism in which orotic acid accumulates in the body. Clinically, children fail to grow and have megaloblastic anemia and leukopenia. The disease responds to administration of uridine or cytidine.

**aciduric** (ăs″ĭ-dū′rĭk) [″ + *durare,* to endure] Capable of growing in an acid medium, but preferring a slightly alkaline one.

**acinar** (ăs′ĭ-năr) [L. *acinus,* grape] Pert. to an acinus.

**Acinetobacter** (ăs″ĭ-nĕt″ō-băk′tĕr) [Gr. *akinetos,* immovable, + *bakterion,* rod] A genus of microorganisms widely distributed in nature that are usually nonpathogenic. *Acinetobacter lwoffi* was previously known as *Mima polymorpha,* and *Acinetobacter anitratus* was previously known as *Herellea vaginicula.*

**acini** (ăs′ĭ-nī) Pl. of acinus.

**aciniform** (ă-sĭn′ĭ-form) [L. *acinus,* grape, + *forma,* shape] Resembling grapes. SYN: *acinous.*

**acinitis** (ăs″ĭ-nī′tĭs) [″ + Gr. *itis,* inflammation] Inflammation of glandular acini.

**acinose** (ăs′ĭ-nōs) [L. *acinosus,* grapelike] Composed of acini.

**acinous** (ăs′ĭ-nŭs) Pert. to glands resembling a bunch of grapes, such as acini and alveolar glands. SYN: *aciniform.*

**acinus** (ăs′ĭ-nŭs) *pl.* **acini** [L., grape] **1.** The smallest division of a gland; a group of secretory cells surrounding a cavity. **2.** The terminal respiratory gas exchange unit of the lung, composed of airways and alveoli distal to a terminal bronchiole.

**A.C. joint.** *acromioclavicular joint.*

**ackee** (ă′kē) Akee.

**acladiosis** (ăk-lăd″ē-ō′sĭs) An ulcerative skin disease believed to be caused by fungi of the genus *Acladium.*

**aclasis, aclasia** (ăk′lă-sĭs, ă-klā′zē-ă) [Gr. *a-,* not, + *klasis,* a breaking away] Abnormal tissue arising from and continuous with a normal structure, as in chondrodysplasia.

***diaphyseal a.*** Imperfect formation of cancellous bone in cartilage between diaphysis and epiphysis.

**acleistocardia** (ă-klĭs″tō-kăr′dē-ă) [Gr. *akleistos,* not closed, + *kardia,* heart] Patent foramen ovale of the heart.

**ACLS** *Advanced Cardiac Life Support.*

**acme** (ăk′mē) [Gr. *akme,* point] **1.** The highest point; peak. **2.** The time of greatest intensity of a symptom or disease process.

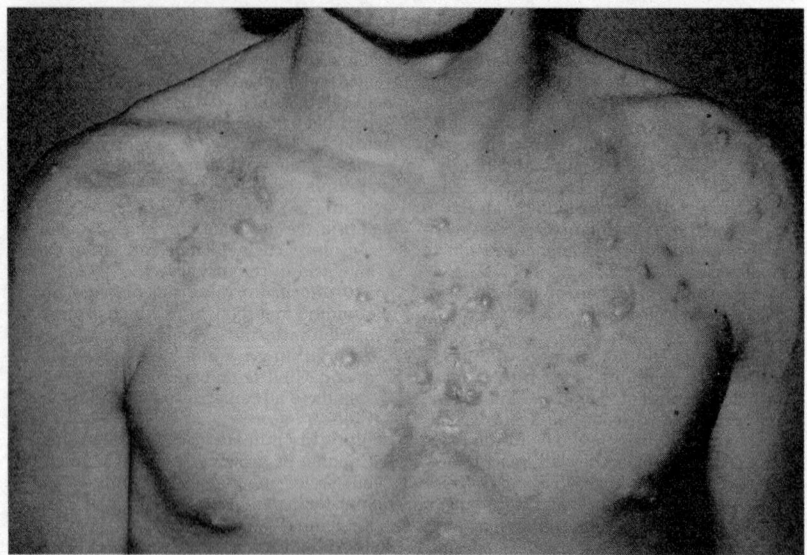

CYSTIC ACNE OF UPPER TRUNK

**3.** The segment of uterine labor contraction during which muscle tension is greatest.

**acne** (ăk′nē) [Gr. *akme,* point] **1.** An inflammatory disease of the sebaceous glands and hair follicles of the skin characterized by comedones, papules, and pustules; usually associated with seborrhea. Cysts and nodules may develop and scarring is common. **2.** Acne vulgaris.

***a. atrophica*** Acne with residual pitting and scarring.

***bromide a.*** Characteristic acne caused by bromide.

***a. ciliaris*** Acne that affects the edges of the eyelids.

***a. conglobata*** Acne vulgaris with abscesses, cysts, and sinuses that leave scars.

***cystic a.*** Acne with cysts containing keratin and sebum. SEE: illus.

TREATMENT: Isotretinoin, a vitamin A derivative, has been effective in treating this condition. For Caution concerning its use, SEE: *isotretinoin*.

***a. fulminans*** A rare type of acne in teenage boys, marked by inflamed, tender, ulcerative, and crusting lesions of the upper trunk and face. It has a sudden onset and is accompanied by fever, leukocytosis, and an elevated sedimentation rate. About half of the cases have inflammation of several joints.

***halogen a.*** Acne due to exposure to halogens such as bromine, chlorine, or iodine.

***a. indurata*** Acne vulgaris with chronic, discolored, indurated surfaces.

***keloid a.*** Infection about the hair follicles at the back of the neck, causing scars and thickening of the skin.

***a. keratosa*** Acne vulgaris in which suppurating nodules crust over to form horny plugs. These occur at the corners of the mouth.

***a. neonatorum*** Acne in the newborn.

***a. papulosa*** Acne characterized by formation of papules with very little inflammation. SEE: illus.

***petroleum a.*** Acne that may occur in those who work with petroleum and oils.

***a. pustulosa*** Acne with pustule formation and subsequent deep scars.

***a. rosacea*** Rosacea.

***steroid a.*** Acne caused by systemic or topical use of corticosteroid drugs.

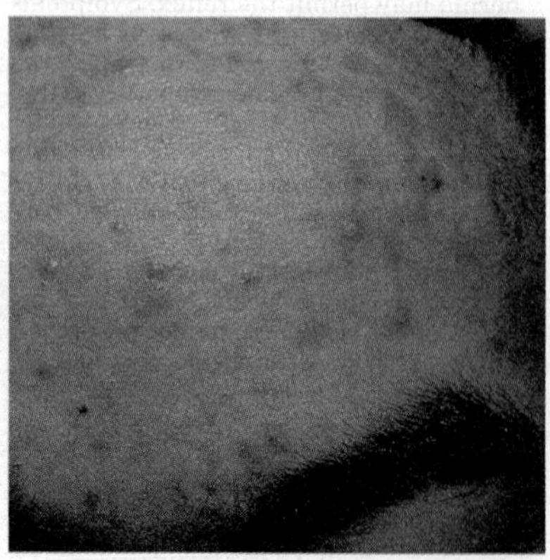

ACNE PAPULOSA

***summer a.*** Acne that appears only in hot, humid weather or that is much worse in such weather. Although the exact cause is unknown, the condition is not caused by increased exposure to the sun's rays.

***tropical a.*** Severe acne caused by or aggravated by living in a hot, humid climate. The skin of the thorax, back, and legs is most commonly affected.

***a. urticaria*** An acneiform eruption of itching wheals.

***a. varioliformis*** Vesiculopustular folliculitis that occurs mostly on the temples and frontal margins of the scalp but may be seen on the chest, back, or nose.

***a. vulgaris*** Common acne.

SYMPTOMS: Acne vulgaris is marked by either papules about comedones with black centers (pustules) or hypertrophied nodules caused by overgrowth of connective tissue. In the indurative type, the lesions are deep-seated and cause scarring. The face, neck, and shoulders are common sites. Acne may be obstinate and recurrent.

ETIOLOGY: The cause is unknown, but predisposing factors include hereditary tendencies and disturbances in the androgen-estrogen balance. Acne begins at puberty, when the increased secretion of androgen in both males and females increases the size and activity of the pilosebaceous glands. Specific inciting factors may include food allergies, endocrine disorders, therapy with adrenal corticosteroid hormones, and psychogenic factors. Vitamin deficiencies, ingestion of halogens, and contact with chemicals such as tar and chlorinated hydrocarbons may be specific causative factors. The fact that bacteria are important once the disease is present is indicated by the successful results following antibiotic therapy. The lesions may become worse in women and girls before the menstrual period.

TREATMENT: Before treatment, patients should consult a dermatologist to ensure that the skin condition is acne. Rashes resembling acne can be caused by cosmetics or other skin irritants. Treatment may be local or systemic. Topical cleansing and peeling (keratolytic) agents and tetracycline may be used, but tetracycline should not be used during the last two trimesters of pregnancy, and not prior to age 12 to prevent tooth discoloration. Topical application of vitamin A acid is effective. Severe cystic acne responds well to orally administered isotretinoin, but because this drug is teratogenic, it cannot be used in women of childbearing age unless they are not sexually active or effective contraceptive use is guaranteed. Comedones should be extracted carefully and cysts and pustules incised and drained. Conditions known to cause exacerbations should be avoided.

NURSING IMPLICATIONS: The patient is instructed to wash the skin thoroughly but gently, avoiding intense scrubbing and skin abrasion; to keep hands away from the face and other sites of lesions; to limit the use of cosmetics; and to observe for, recognize, and avoid or modify predisposing factors that may cause exacerbations. The need to reduce sun exposure is explained, and the patient is advised to use a sunscreen agent when vitamin A acid or tetracycline is prescribed. Information is provided to fill knowledge gaps or correct misconceptions, and emotional support and understanding are offered, particularly if the patient is an adolescent.

**acnegenic** (ăk″nē-jĕn′ĭk) [Gr. *akme,* point, + *gennan,* to produce] Causing acne.

**acneiform** (ăk-nē′ĭ-form) [″ + L. *forma,* shape] Resembling acne; also spelled *acneform.*

**acnemia** (ăk-nē′mē-ă) [Gr. *a-,* not, + *kneme,* lower leg] Wasting of the calves of the legs.

**A.C.N.M.** *American College of Nurse Midwives.*

**A.C.O.G.** *American College of Obstetricians and Gynecologists.*

**aconite** (ăk′ō-nīt) [Gr. *akoniton*] The dried tuberous root of *Aconitum,* esp. *A. napellus* (monkshood) and *A. lycoctonum* (wolfsbane); a poisonous and very powerful alkaloid. Its action, which is due to the presence of two very potent alkaloids, was well known to the ancients. Aconite is believed to have been used as an arrow poison early in Chinese history and perhaps also by the inhabitants of ancient Gaul. Aconite is no longer used but is of historical interest.

**aconitine** (ă-kŏn′ĭ-tĭn) The active ingredient in aconite.

**acorea** (ă-kō-rē′ă) [Gr. *a-,* not, + *kore,* pupil] Absence of the pupil of the eye.

**acoria** (ă-kō′rē-ă) [″ + *koros,* satiety] Lacking in satisfaction after eating but not from hunger.

**acormus** (ă-kor′mŭs) [″ + *kormos,* trunk] **1.** Lack of a trunk. **2.** A fetal abnormality consisting of a head and extremities without a trunk.

**ACOTE** *Accreditation Council for Occupational Therapy Education.*

**acousia** (ă-koo′zē-ă) [Gr. *akousis,* hearing] The hearing faculty. SYN: *acusis.*

**acousmatamnesia** [″ + *amnesia,* forgetfulness] Inability to recall and identify sounds.

**acoustic** (ă-koos′tĭk) [Gr. *akoustikos*] Pert. to sound or to the sense of hearing.

**acoustic center** The hearing center in the brain; located in the temporal lobe of the cerebrum.

**acoustic meatus** The opening to the external or internal auditory canal.

**acoustic nerve** A nerve consisting of two separate parts: the vestibular and cochlear nerves, with superficial origin at the junction of the pons and medulla.

PHYSIOLOGY: The acoustic nerve controls the special senses of hearing and equilibrium. The vestibular and cochlear nerves consist of special somatic afferent fibers. Cells of origin of the vestibular nerve are bipolar and lie in the vestibular ganglion, peripheral branches terminating in receptors of semicircular ducts, saccule, and utricle. Cells of origin of the cochlear nerve are bipolar and lie in the spiral ganglion, peripheral branches terminating in the spiral organ of Corti. The two nerves become joined, enter the internal acoustic meatus with the facial nerve, and then separate. SYN: *auditory nerve; eighth cranial nerve; vestibulocochlear nerve.*

**acousticophobia** (ă-koos″tĭ-kō-fō′bē-ă) [Gr. *akoustos,* heard, + *phobos,* fear] Abnormal fear of loud sounds.

**acoustic reflectometry** Diagnostic technique for the detection of middle ear effusion. It measures the level of sound transmitted and reflected from the middle ear to a microphone located in a probe tip placed against the ear canal opening and directed toward the tympanic membrane.

**acoustic reflex threshold** A test to measure the intensity of a sound at which the stapedial muscle of the inner ear contracts. The test can be used to determine the presence of cochlear pathology and, therefore, is used in differentiating conductive from sensorineural hearing loss.

**acoustics** (ă-koos′tĭks) The science of sound, its production, transmission, and effects.

**acoustic trauma** Injury to hearing by noise, esp. loud noise.

**A.C.P.** *American College of Physicians; American College of Pathologists.*

**acquired** (ă-kwīrd′) [L. *acquirere,* to get] Not hereditary or innate.

**acquired immunodeficiency syndrome** SEE: *AIDS.*

**acquisitus** (ă-kwĭs′ĭ-tŭs) [L.] Acquired.

**A.C.R.** *American College of Radiology.*

**acral** (ăk′răl) [Gr. *akron,* extremity] Pert. to extremities.

**acrania** (ă-krā′nē-ă) [Gr. *a-,* not, + *kranion,* skull] Partial or complete congenital absence of the cranium.

**acrid** (ăk′rĭd) [L. *acer,* sharp] Burning, bitter, irritating.

**acridine** (ăk′rĭ-dĭn) A coal tar hydrocarbon from which certain dyes are prepared.

**acrimony** (ăk′rĭ-mō″nē) Quality of being pungent, acrid, irritating.

**acritical** (ă-krĭt′ĭ-kăl) [Gr. *a-,* not, + *kritikos,* critical] Not marked by a crisis.

**ACRM** *American Congress of Rehabilitation Medicine.*

**acro-** (ăk′rō) [Gr. *akron,* extremity] Combining form meaning *extremity, top, extreme point.*

**acroagnosis** (ăk″rō-ăg-nō′sĭs) [″ + *gnosis,* knowledge] Absence of feeling of one's limb.

**acroanesthesia** (ăk″rō-ăn-ĕs-thē′zē-ă) [″ + *an-,* not, + *aisthesis,* sensation] Lack of sensation in one or more of the extremities.

**acroasphyxia** (ăk″rō-ăs-fĭk′sē-ă) [″ + *asphyxia,* pulse stoppage] Cold, pale condition of hands and feet; symptom of Raynaud's disease.

**acroblast** (ăk′rō-blăst) [″ + *blastos,* germ] A part of the Golgi apparatus in the spermatid from which the acrosome arises.

**acrobrachycephaly** (ăk″rō-brăk″ĭ-sĕf′ă-lē) [″ + *brachys,* short, + *kephale,* head] The condition of having an abnormally short head in the anterior-posterior diameter due to fusion of the coronal suture.

**acrocentric** (ăk″rō-sĕn′trĭk) [Gr. *akron,* extremity + L. *centrum,* center] Pert. to a chromosome in which the centromere is located near one end. At metaphase it has the appearance of a wishbone.

**acrocephalia** (ăk″rō-sĕf-ā′lē-ă) [″ + *kephale,* head] Acrocephaly.

**acrocephalosyndactylia, acrocephalosyndactyly** (ăk″rō-sĕf″ă-lō-sĭn-dăk-tĭl′ē-ă, -sĭn-dăk′tĭl-ē) [″ + ″ + *syn,* together, + *daktylos,* a finger] A congenital condition marked by a peaked head and webbed fingers and toes. SYN: *Apert's syndrome.*

**acrocephaly** (ăk″rō-sĕf′ă-lē) [″ + *kephale,* head] The condition of having a malformed cranial vault with a high or peaked appearance and a vertical index above 77. It is caused by premature closure of the coronal, sagittal, and lambdoidal sutures. SYN: *acrocephalia; oxycephaly.* **acrocephalic** (-sĕ-făl′ĭk), *adj.*

**acrochordon** (ăk″rō-kor′dŏn) [″ + *chorde,* cord] A small outgrowth of epidermal and dermal tissue; a pedunculated, smooth or irregular, flesh-colored, benign tumor that occurs most often on the eyelids, neck, and axillae, but may be seen almost anywhere on the skin. Except for being unsightly, it is harmless, unless it becomes twisted on its pedicle. SYN: *fibroepithelial polyp; skin tag.*

**acrocontracture** (ăk″rō-kŏn-trăkt′ūr) [″ + L. *contrahere,* to draw together] Contracture of the hands or feet.

**acrocyanosis** (ăk″rō-sī-ă-nō′sĭs) [″ + *kyanosis,* dark-blue color] Cyanosis of the extremities. Acrocyanosis of the hands and feet may be normal in a newborn within the first hour after birth. During the transitional period, hemodynamic changes in the pattern of blood flow through the newborn's heart and pulmonary circulation limit flow to peripheral vessels in the extremities.

ETIOLOGY: The condition is caused by vasomotor disturbances. It is seen in catatonia and hysteria.

**acrodermatitis** (ăk″rō-dĕr-mă-tī′tĭs) [″ + *derma,* skin, + *itis,* inflammation] Dermatitis of the extremities.

***a. chronica atrophicans*** Dermatitis of the hands and feet that progresses slowly upward on the affected limbs.

***a. continua*** An obstinate eczematous eruption confined to the extremities.

***a. enteropathica*** Rare disease in children aged 3 weeks to 18 months that may be fatal if untreated. The genetically determined cause is malabsorption of zinc. Onset is insidious with failure to thrive, diarrhea, loss of hair, and development of vesiculobullous lesions, particularly around body orifices.

TREATMENT: Zinc sulfate given orally will abolish all clinical manifestations of the disease within a few days.

***a. hiemalis*** Dermatitis that occurs in winter and affects the extremities. It tends to disappear spontaneously.

***a. perstans*** A. continua.

**acrodermatosis** (ăk″rō-dĕr″mă-tō′sĭs) [Gr. *akron,* extremity, + *derma,* skin, + *osis,* condition] Any skin disease that affects the hands and feet.

**acrodolichomelia** (ăk″rō-dŏl″ĭ-kō-mē′lē-ă) [″ + *dolichos,* long, + *melos,* limb] A condition in which the hands and feet are abnormally long.

**acrodynia** (ăk″rō-dĭn′ē-ă) [″ + *odyne,* pain] A disease of infants and young children caused by chronic mercury poisoning. It has a prolonged clinical course with various grades of severity. The child is listless, irritable, and no longer interested in play. The rash has several variations. Initially, the tips of the fingers and toes become pink; the hands and feet become pink but color shades off at the wrists and ankles. As the disease progresses, the skin of the extremities desquamates, there are profuse sweating and pruritus, and pain is excruciating in the hands and feet. Neurological symptoms with neuritis and mental apathy develop. SYN: *pink disease.*

TREATMENT: Treatment consists of removing the source of the mercury, administering dimercaprol (BAL) antidote, and providing supportive therapy.

**acrodysesthesia** (ăk″rō-dĭs″ĕs-thē′zē-ă) [″ + *dys,* bad, + *aisthesis,* sensation] Dysesthesia in the arms and legs.

**acroesthesia** (ăk″rō-ĕs-thē′zē-ă) [″ + *aisthesis,* sensation] **1.** Abnormal sensitivity of the extremities. **2.** Pain in the extremities.

**acrogeria** (ăk″rō-jĕr′ē-ă) [″ + *geron,* old man] A condition in which the skin of the hands and feet shows signs of premature aging.

**acrognosis** (ăk″rŏg-nō′sĭs) [″ + *gnosis,* knowledge] Sensory perception of limbs.

**acrohyperhidrosis** (ăk″rō-hī″pĕr-hī-drō′sĭs) [″ + *hyper,* excessive, + *hidrosis,* sweating] Excessive perspiration of the hands and feet.

**acrohypothermy** (ăk″rō-hī″pō-thĕr′mē) [″ + *hypo,* below, + *therme,* heat] Abnormal coldness of the extremities.

**acrokeratosis verruciformis** (ăk″rō-kĕr″ă-tō′sĭs vĕ-roo′sĭ-for″mĭs) [″ + *keras,* horn, + *osis,* condition; L. *verruca,* wart, + *forma,* form] Hereditary disease of the skin characterized by warty growths on the extremities, principally on the backs of the hands and on the feet.

**acrokinesia** (ăk″rō-kĭn-ē′sē-ă) [″ + *kinesis,* movement] Excessive motion of the extremities.

**acromacria** (ăk″rō-măk′rē-ă) [Gr. *akron,* extremity, + *makros,* long] Abnormal length of the fingers. SYN: *arachnodactyly.* SEE: *Marfan's syndrome.*

**acromastitis** (ăk″rō-măs-tī′tĭs) [″ + *mastos,* breast, + *itis,* inflammation] Inflammation of the nipple. SYN: *thelitis.*

**acromegaly** (ăk″rō-mĕg′ă-lē) [″ + *megas,* big] A chronic disease of middle-aged persons marked by elongation and enlargement of bones of the extremities and certain head bones, esp. the frontal bone and jaws, with enlargement of the nose and lips and thickening of the soft tissues of the face. It is often associated with somnolence, moodiness, and decreased libido. SYN: *Marie's disease.*

SYMPTOMS: Onset of the disease is so gradual that neither the patients nor their associates notice it. Early complaints include muscular pains, headache, and sweating. Facial features are enlarged, and mandible and malar bones become prominent with protrusion of orbital ridge. Teeth become widely separated; hands and feet gradually enlarge. About one fourth of the patients will develop diabetes. As the disease progresses, muscular weakness becomes a serious feature, and visual impairment may progress to blindness.

ETIOLOGY: The condition is caused by hyperfunction of the eosinophilic cells of the anterior lobe of the pituitary, resulting in excess production of growth hormone. SEE: *somatostatin.*

TREATMENT: The dopamine agonist bromocriptine may be used with either radiation therapy or surgical removal of the pituitary gland.

**acromelalgia** (ăk″rō-mĕl-ăl′jē-ă) [Gr. *akron,* extremity, + *melos,* limb, + *algos,* pain] Erythromelalgia.

**acromelic** (ăk″rō-mĕl′ĭk) [″ + *melos,* limb] Pert. to the end of the extremities.

**acrometagenesis** (ăk″rō-mĕt″ă-jĕn′ĕ-sĭs) [″ + *meta,* beyond, + *genesis,* generation, birth] Abnormal growth of the extremities.

**acromial** (ăk-rō′mē-ăl) [″ + *omos,* shoulder] Rel. to the acromion.

**acromial angle** The angle at the edge of the spine of the scapula where it ascends to become the acromion.

**acromial process** Acromion.

**acromial reflex** Forearm flexion with internal rotation of the hand as a result of a quick blow to the acromion; elicited in hyperkinetic states.

**acromicria** (ăk″rō-mĭk′rē-ă) [Gr. *akron,* extremity, + *mikros,* small] Congenital shortness or smallness of the extremities and face.

**acromioclavicular joint** (ă-krō″mē-ŏ-klă-vĭk′ū-lăr) [″ + *omos,* shoulder, + L. *clavicula,* small key] ABBR: AC joint. An arthrodial joint between the acromion and the acromial end of the clavicle.

**acromiocoracoid** (ă-krō″mē-ŏ-kor′ă-koyd) [″ + ″ + *korax,* crow, + *eidos,* form, shape] Pert. to the acromion and coracoid process.

**acromiohumeral** (ăk-rō″mē-ŏ-hū′mĕr-ăl) [″ + ″ + L. *humerus,* shoulder] Pert. to the acromion and humerus.

**acromion** (ă-krō′mē-ŏn) [Gr. *akron,* extremity, + *omos,* shoulder] The lateral triangular projection of the spine of the scapula that forms the point of the shoulder and articulates with the clavicle. SYN: *acromial process.* SEE: *acromioclavicular joint.*

**acromioplasty** The surgical removal of the distal inferior acromion process of the scapula to relieve impingement of soft tissues in the subacromial space. This is usually performed with release of the coracoacromial ligament, arthroscopically or through open incision.

**acromioscapular** (ă-krō″mē-ŏ-skăp′ū-lăr) [″ + ″ + L. *scapula,* shoulder blade] Pert. to the acromion and scapula.

**acromiothoracic** (ă-krō″mē-ŏ-thō-răs′ĭk) [″ + ″ + *thorax,* chest] Pert. to the acromion and thorax.

**acromphalus** (ăk-rŏm′făl-ŭs) [″ + *omphalos,* umbilicus] **1.** Center of the navel. **2.** Projection of the umbilicus, as in the beginning of an umbilical hernia.

**acromyotonia, acromyotonus** (ăk″rō-mī-ō-tō′nē-ă, -ŏt′ō-nŭs) [″ + *mys,* muscle, + *tonos,* tension] Myotonia of the extremities, causing spasmodic deformity.

**acroneurosis** (ăk″rō-nū-rō′sĭs) [Gr. *akron,* extremity, + *neuron,* nerve, + *osis,* condition] Nervous disorder in the extremities.

**acro-osteolysis** (ăk″rō-ŏs″tē-ŏl′ĭ-sĭs) [Gr. *akron,* extremity, + *osteon,* bone, + *lysis,* dissolution] **1.** A familial disease causing dissolution of the tips of the bones in the extremities of young children. There is no history of trauma, and spontaneous amputation does not occur. The etiology is unknown. **2.** An occupational disease seen in workers who come in contact with vinyl chloride polymerization processes. It is marked by Raynaud's phenomenon, scleroderma-like skin changes, and radiological evidence of bone destruction of the distal phalanges of the hands. Recovery follows removal from exposure. SEE: *Raynaud's disease.*

**acropachyderma** (ăk″rō-păk″ē-dĕr′mă) [″ + ″ + *derma,* skin] Clubbing of the fingers, deformed long bones, and thickening of the skin of the scalp, face, and extremities.

**acroparalysis** (ăk″rō-pă-răl′ĭ-sĭs) [″ + *paralyein,* to disable] Paralysis of one or more extremities.

**acroparesthesia** (ăk″rō-păr-ĕs-thē′zē-ă) [″ + *para,* abnormal, + *aisthesis,* sensation] Sensation of prickling, tingling, or numbness in the extremities.

**acropathology** (ăk″rō-pă-thŏl′ō-jē) [″ + *pathos,* disease, suffering, + *logos,* word, reason] Pathology of disease of the extremities.

**acrophobia** (ăk-rō-fō′bē-ă) [″ + *phobos,* fear] Morbid fear of high places. SYN: *hypsophobia.*

**acroposthitis** (ăk″rō-pŏs-thī′tĭs) [Gr. *akroposthis,* prepuce, + *itis,* inflammation] Inflammation of the prepuce of the penis. SYN: *posthitis.*

**acropustulosis, infantile** Cyclical eruption of pustules on the soles and feet of infants 2 to 10 months of age. The pustules become vesicopapular, crust over, and heal in 7 to 10 days. A new crop appears in 2 to 3 weeks and they also heal. Periodic outbreaks occur for about 2 years and then stop. The cause is unknown; symptomatic therapy is all that is required.

**acroscleroderma** (ăk″rō-sklĕr-ō-dĕr′mă) [Gr. *akron,* extremity, + *scleros,* hard, + *derma,* skin] Hard, thickened skin condition of toes and fingers. SYN: *sclerodactylia.*

**acrosclerosis** (ăk″rō-sklĕr-ō′sĭs) [″ + ″ + *osis,* condition] A scleroderma of the upper extremities, sometimes extending to the neck and face, that usually follows Raynaud's disease.

**acrosome** (ăk′rō-sōm) [″ + *soma,* body] A specialized lysosome on the head of a sperm cell that contains enzymes to digest the membrane of an egg cell. SEE: *spermatozoon* for illus.

**acroteric** (ăk″rō-tĕr′ĭk) [Gr. *akroterion,* summit] Pert. to the outermost parts of the extremities, as the tips of the fingers.

**acrotism** (ăk′rō-tĭzm) [Gr. *a-,* not, + *krotos,* striking, + *-ismos,* condition] Imperceptibility of the pulse.

**acrotrophoneurosis** (ăk″rō-trŏf″ō-nū-rō′sĭs) [Gr. *akron,* extremity, + *trophe,* nourishment, + *neuron,* nerve, + *osis,* condition] Trophoneurosis of the extremities with trophic, neuritic, and vascular changes. It is usually caused by prolonged immersion in water.

**acrylamide** (ă-krĭl′ă-mīd) $C_3H_5NO$. The amide of acrylic acid.

**acrylate** (ăk′rĭ-lāt) A salt or ester of acrylic acid.

**acrylic acid** (ă-krĭl′ĭk) $CH_2$:CH·COOH. A colorless corrosive liquid used in making acrylic polymers and resins.

**acrylic resin** General term for various polymers of acrylic acid and their esters. Some of these compounds are used medically as components of contact lenses and dental materials.

**acrylonitrile** (ăk″rĭ-lō-nī′trĭl) $C_3H_3N$. A toxic compound used in making plastics. SYN: *vinyl cyanide.*

**A.C.S., ACS** *American Cancer Society; American Chemical Society; American College of Surgeons; acute confusional state; anodal closing sound.*

**A.C.S.M.** *American College of Sports Medicine.*

**act** (ăkt) **1.** To accomplish a function. **2.** The accomplishment of a function.

***compulsive a.*** The repetitive, ritualistic performance of an act. This may be done despite the individual's attempts to resist the act.

***impulsive a.*** Sudden action caused by an abnormal impulse or desire.

**ACTH** *adrenocorticotropic hormone,* a pituitary hormone that stimulates the cortex of the adrenal glands to produce adrenal cortical hormones. SEE: *cortisone.*

**actin** (ăk'tĭn) One of the contractile proteins that make up the sarcomeres of muscle tissue. During contraction, the actin filaments are pulled toward the center of the sarcomere by the action of myosin filaments, and the sarcomere shortens.

**acting out** Expressing oneself through actions rather than speech.

***neurotic a.o.*** **1.** A form of transference, in which tension is relieved when one responds to a situation as if it were the same situation that originally gave rise to the tension; a displacement of behavioral response from one situation to another. **2.** In psychoanalysis, a form of displacement, in which the patient relives memories rather than expressing them verbally.

**actinic** (ăk-tĭn'ĭk) [Gr. *aktis,* ray] **1.** Pert. to radiant energy, such as x-rays, ultraviolet light, and sunlight, esp. the photochemical effects. **2.** Pert. to the ability of radiant energy to produce chemical changes.

**actinic burns** Burns caused by ultraviolet or sun rays. Treatment is the same as for dry heat burns. SEE: *burn.*

**actinic dermatitis** Inflammation and erythema of the skin caused by exposure to radiation.

**actinism** (ăk'tĭn-ĭzm) The property of radiant energy that produces chemical changes, as in photography or heliotherapy.

**actinium** (ăk-tĭn'ē-ŭm) [Gr. *aktis,* ray] SYMB: Ac. A radioactive element; atomic weight 227; atomic number 89.

**actino-** (ăk'tĭ-nō) [Gr. *aktis,* ray] Combining form indicating a relationship to a ray or referring to some forms of radiation.

**Actinobacillus** (ăk"tĭ-nō-bă-sĭl'lŭs) Small gram-negative coccobacilli that affect domestic animals mostly; however, *Actinobacillus actinomycetemcomitans* has been implicated in endocarditis in humans.

**actinodermatitis** (ăk"tĭn-ō-dĕr-mă-tī'tĭs) [" + *derma,* skin, + *itis,* inflammation] Dermatitis caused by exposure to radiation.

**actinogenic** (ăk"tĭn-ō-jĕ'nĭk) Radiogenic.

**Actinomyces** (ăk"tĭn-ō-mī'sēz) [" + *mykes,* fungus] A genus of bacteria of the family Actinomycetaceae that contain gram-positive staining filaments. These bacteria cause various diseases in humans and animals.

***A. antibioticus*** A species of *Actinomyces* from which the antibiotic actinomycin is obtained.

***A. bovis*** A species of *Actinomyces* that causes actinomycosis in cattle.

***A. israelii*** A species of *Actinomyces* that causes actinomycosis in humans. One clinical form is called lumpy jaw due to the characteristic appearance of the swollen jaw produced by the infection. Prolonged therapy with very large doses of penicillin G is required.

**Actinomycetales** (ăk"tĭ-nō-mī"sĕ-tā'lēz) An order of bacteria that includes the families Mycobacteriaceae, Actinomycetaceae, Actinoplanaceae, Dermatophilaceae, Micromonosporaceae, Nocardiaceae, and Streptomycetaceae.

**actinomycete** (ăk"tĭ-nō-mī'sēt) Any bacterium of the order Actinomycetales. **actinomycetic** (-mī-sēt'ĭk), *adj.*

**actinomycetin** (ăk"tĭn-ō-mī-sēt'ĭn) A lytic substance obtained from *Actinomyces;* it destroys some gram-positive and gram-negative organisms.

**actinomycin A** (ăk"tĭn-ō-mī'sĭn) A highly toxic antibiotic obtained from *Actinomyces antibioticus* that is effective against gram-positive organisms. This orange-colored heat-stable antibiotic is soluble in alcohol and ether.

**actinomycin B** An antibiotic similar to actinomycin A but not soluble in alcohol. Because of its toxicity, it is not used clinically.

**Actinomycin D** Trade name for dactinomycin.

**actinomycoma** (ăk"tĭ-nō-mī-kō'ma) [Gr. *aktis,* ray, + *mykes,* fungus, + *oma,* tumor] A tumor produced by actinomycosis.

**actinomycosis** (ăk"tĭn-ō-mī-kō'sĭs) [" + " + *osis,* condition] A noncontagious bacterial disease in animals and humans. Infection may be of the cervicofacial, thoracic, or abdominal regions, or it may be generalized. **actinomycotic** (-kŏt'ĭk), *adj.*

SYMPTOMS: Slow-growing granulomas form and later break down, discharging viscid pus containing minute yellowish (sulfur) granules.

ETIOLOGY: Causative organisms are *Actinomyces bovis* in cattle and *Actinomyces israelii* (which is normally present in the mouth) in humans. SEE: *nocardiosis.*

TREATMENT: Prolonged administration of penicillin is usually effective. Tetracyclines are the second choice. Surgical incision and drainage of accessible lesions is helpful when combined with chemotherapy.

**actinon** (ăk'tĭn-ŏn) [Gr. *aktis,* ray] A radioactive isotope of actinium.

**actinoneuritis** (ăk"tĭn-ō-nū-rī'tĭs) [" + *neuron,* nerve, + *itis,* inflammation] Inflammation of a nerve or nerves resulting from exposure to radium or x-rays.

**actinophytosis** (ăk"tĭ-nō-fī-tō'sĭs) [" + *phyton,* plant, + *osis,* condition] Infection due to *Actinomyces.*

**actinotherapy** (ăk″tĭn-ō-thĕr′ă-pē) [″ + *therapeia,* treatment] Treatment of disease by rays of light, esp. actinic or photochemically active rays, or by x-rays or radium.

**action** (ăk′shŭn) [L. *actio*] Performance of a function or process; in pathology, a morbid process.

***antagonistic a.*** The ability of a drug or muscle to oppose or resist the action or effect of another drug or muscle; opposite of synergistic action.

***bacteriocidal a.*** Action that kills bacteria.

***bacteriostatic a.*** Action that stops or prevents the growth of bacteria without killing them.

***ball-valve a.*** Intermittent obstruction of a passageway or opening so that the flow of fluid or air is prevented from moving in the normal direction and at the usual rate.

***calorigenic a.*** Heat produced by the metabolism of food.

***capillary a.*** The movement of fluid to a certain level in a small-diameter tube.

***cumulative a.*** Sudden increased action of a drug after several doses have been given.

***drug a.*** SEE: *drug action.*

***reflex a.*** Involuntary movement produced by sensory nerve stimulation.

***sparing a.*** The effect of a nonessential nutrient in the diet such that it decreases the requirement for an essential nutrient. For example, protein is esp. important for tissue growth and development in children. If protein intake is sufficient but caloric intake is inadequate, a protein deficiency will develop. In this situation, the addition of sufficient carbohydrates to the diet is said to spare the protein.

***specific a.*** The particular action of a drug on another substance or on an organism or part of that organism.

***specific dynamic a.*** Stimulation of the metabolic rate by ingestion of certain foods, esp. proteins.

***synergistic a.*** The ability of a drug or muscle to aid or enhance the action or effect of another drug or muscle; opposite of antagonistic action.

***thermogenic a.*** Action of a food, drug, or physical agent to cause a rise in output of body heat.

***trigger a.*** The initiation of activity, physiological or pathological, that may have no relation to the action that started it.

**action of arrest** The action of decreasing or slowing the function of an organ or cell or a chemical reaction.

**action potential** SEE: under *potential.*

**activate** (ăk′tĭ-vāt) To make active.

**activated partial thromboplastin time** ABBR: APTT. The time required for a fibrin clot to form after the activating factor, calcium, and a phospholipid have been added to the blood sample. The normal value ranges from 16 to 40 sec. A prolonged time indicates a clotting factor deficiency or any one of several diseases or medications.

**activation** The process that stimulates resting, or nonfunctional, white blood cells to assume their role in the immune response. The process involves recognition of an antigen or a response to cytokines. SEE: *antigen processing; cytokine; immune response.*

**activator** (ăk′tĭ-vā″tor) **1.** A substance in the body that converts an inactive substance into an active agent, such as the conversion of pepsinogen into pepsin by hydrogen ions. **2.** Any substance that specifically induces an activity, such as an inductor or organizer in embryonic development or a trophic hormone. **3.** A removable orthodontic appliance that transmits force passively from muscles to the teeth and alveolar process in contact with it. Also called *myofunctional appliance.*

**active plate activator** A removable orthodontic appliance equipped to provide the force for tooth movement. It may be used continuously or intermittently.

**active principle** The chemical substance in a pharmaceutical preparation that is responsible for the therapeutic effects of the medicine. SEE: *drug action.*

**active range of motion** ABBR: AROM. The range of movement of a joint that a patient performs without assistance.

**active transport** The process by which a cell membrane moves molecules against a concentration or electrochemical gradient. This requires metabolic work. An example is the very low concentration of potassium ions in extracellular fluid. Other ions actively transported are sodium, calcium, hydrogen, iron, chloride, iodide, and urate. Several sugars and the amino acids are actively transported.

**activins** A family of polypeptide growth factors which help regulate various biological functions, esp. fertility. SEE: *inhibin.*

**activities of daily living** ABBR: ADL. Tasks that enable individuals to meet basic needs. Examples include eating, toileting, dressing, hygiene, food preparation, laundry, housecleaning, using the telephone, using public transportation, and shopping.

NURSING IMPLICATIONS: The nurse assesses the patient's ability to perform ADL, assists or arranges assistance as needed, and evaluates the patient's response to these interventions. SEE: table.

**activities of daily living, index of** An assessment tool developed by American gerontologist S. Katz and his colleagues. It assesses self-maintenance in the elderly and focuses on the unaided performance of six basic personal care activities: eating, toileting, dressing, bathing, transferring, and continence.

**activity** (ăk-tĭv′ĭ-tē) The production of energy or motion; the state of being active. The word *activity* describes various con-

### Activities of Daily Living and Factors Affecting Them

| Category | Activities | Affecting Factors |
|---|---|---|
| Personal care | Climbing stairs, moving into and out of chair or bed, feeding self, opening containers, dressing, using toilet, maintaining hygiene, taking medication | Altered mobility, physical or emotional illness, elimination problems |
| Family responsibilities | Shopping, cooking, doing laundry, cleaning, caring for yard, caring for family and pets, managing money | Altered mobility, heavy work schedule, insomnia, physical or emotional illness |
| Work or school | Fulfilling work responsibilities or school assignments, getting to and from work or school | Altered mobility, stress, heavy family demands, job dissatisfaction, difficulties in school, physical or emotional illness |
| Recreation | Pursuing hobbies and interests, exercising, reading, watching television | Altered mobility, physical or emotional illness |
| Socialization | Using the telephone, traveling, visiting family and friends, joining group activities, expressing sexuality | Altered mobility, physical or emotional illness, relocation |

ditions: enzyme activity describes the rate of influence of an enzyme on a particular system; extravehicular activity indicates the actions of space travelers while outside a space vehicle; radiation activity indicates the energy produced by a source of radiation.

***graded a.*** In occupational therapy, a principle of therapeutic intervention in which tasks are classified and presented gradually according to the individual's level of function and the challenge or degree of skill (physical, social, or cognitive) required by the task.

***optical a.*** In chemistry, the rotation of the plane of polarized light when the light passes through a chemical solution. Measurement of this property, called polarimetry, is useful in the determination of optically active substances such as dextrose. Sugars are classified according to this criterion. Optical activity of a substance in solution can be detected by placing it between polarizing and analyzing prisms.

***pulseless electrical a.*** ABBR: PEA. A clinical condition in which the patient's heart is beating, as shown on the electrocardiogram, but the pulse cannot be felt or palpated.

***purposeful a.*** The goal-directed use of time, energy, or attention that involves the active participation of the doer. Purposeful activity by humans often involves a social environment (others), a physical environment (objects, tools, and materials), and a process, which often culminates in a product.

**activity analysis** The process used by occupational therapists to determine the social, symbolic, physical, cognitive, and developmental characteristics of a task or activity and thus its therapeutic potential. Typical characteristics of interest include safety, cost, gradability, required space, tools or supplies, complexity, and social or cultural significance.

**activity intolerance** Inadequate mental or physical energy to accomplish daily activities. Risk factors include debilitating physical conditions such as anemia, obesity, musculoskeletal disorders, neurological deficits (such as those following stroke), severe heart disease, chronic pulmonary disease, metabolic disorders, and prolonged sedentary lifestyle. SEE: *Nursing Diagnoses Appendix.*

**activity intolerance, risk for** A state in which an individual is at risk of experiencing insufficient physiologic or psychologic energy to endure or complete required or desired daily activities. SEE: *Nursing Diagnoses Appendix.*

**activity theory** A social theory of aging that stresses a continuation of role performances and asserts that the more active older persons are, the higher their life satisfaction and morale. According to this theory, older individuals find substitutes for former roles that they may have had to relinquish.

**actomyosin** (ăk″tō-mī′ō-sĭn) The combination of actin and myosin in a muscle. On muscle stimulation, these substances shorten without changing their volume and thus cause contraction of the muscle.

**actual** (ăk′chū-ăl) [L. *actus,* doing] Real, existent.

**actual cautery** Cautery acting by heat and not chemically.

**actuator** (ăk′chū-ā-tŏr) A component of a mechanical or electronic device that initiates a given action.

**acufilopressure** (ăk″ū-fī′lō-prĕsh″ŭr) [L. *acus,* needle, + *filum,* thread, + *pressura,* pressure] Acupressure increased by a ligature.

**acuity** (ă-kū′ĭ-tē) [L. *acuere,* to sharpen] Clearness, sharpness.

***visual a.*** Sharpness of vision.

**acuminate** (ă-kū′mĭn-āt) [L. *acuminatus,* sharpened] Conical or pointed.

**acupressure** (ăk′ū-prĕsh″ŭr) [L. *acus,* needle, + *pressura,* pressure] Compression of blood vessels by means of needles in surrounding tissues.

**acupressure forceps** Spring-handled forceps for compressing blood vessels.

**acupressure needles** Elastic needles for compressing blood vessels.

**acupuncture** (ăk′ū-pŭngk″chūr) [L. *acus,* needle, + *punctura,* puncture] Technique for treating certain painful conditions and for producing regional anesthesia by passing long thin needles through the skin to specific points. The free ends of the needles are twirled or in some cases used to conduct a weak electric current. Anesthesia sufficient to permit abdominal, thoracic, and head and neck surgery has been produced by the use of acupuncture alone. The patient is fully conscious during the surgery. Acupuncture has been known in the Far East for centuries but received little attention in Western cultures until the early 1970s.

---

Caution: It is important that the acupuncturist use sterile or disposable needles and that care be taken to prevent puncturing adjacent organs.

---

**acusis** SEE: *presbycusis.*

**acusticus** (ă-kū′stĭ-kŭs) [Gr. *akoustikos,* hearing] Acoustic nerve.

**acute** (ă-kūt′) [L. *acutus,* sharp] **1.** Sharp, severe. **2.** Having rapid onset, severe symptoms, and a short course; not chronic.

**acute care** Health care delivered to patients experiencing acute illness or trauma. Acute care generally occurs in a hospital or emergency room and is generally short-term care rather than long-term, or chronic, care.

**acute confusional states** SEE: *confusional states, acute.*

**acute mountain sickness** ABBR: AMS. Following a recent gain in altitude, the development of a headache, gastrointestinal symptoms such as anorexia, nausea, or vomiting, and fatigue, lassitude or weakness. This condition may occur in aviators and mountain climbers. SEE: *edema, high-altitude pulmonary.*

**acute necrotizing ulcerative gingivitis** ABBR: ANUG. Trench mouth.

**acute phase reaction** The release of physiologically active proteins by the liver into the blood in response to interleukin-6 or other cytokines that participate in the destruction of pathogens and promote healing during inflammation. SYN: *acute phase response.* SEE: *cytokine; inflammation; interleukin-6; protein, acute phase.*

**acute respiratory distress syndrome** ABBR: ARDS. Respiratory insufficiency marked by progressive hypoxemia, due to severe inflammatory damage causing abnormal permeability of the alveolar-capillary membrane. The alveoli fill with fluid, which interferes with gas exchange. SEE: *disseminated intravascular coagulation; sepsis; systemic inflammatory response syndrome; Nursing Diagnoses Appendix.*

SYMPTOMS: Dyspnea and tachypnea are followed by a progressive hypoxemia that, despite oxygen therapy, is the hallmark of ARDS. Fluffy infiltrates appear on chest radiographs.

ETIOLOGY: Acute respiratory distress syndrome may result from direct trauma to the lungs (e.g., near drowning, aspiration of gastric acids, severe lung infection) or systemic disorders such as shock, septicemia, disseminated intravascular coagulation, cardiopulmonary bypass, and reaction to multiple blood transfusions. Widespread damage to the alveolar-capillary membranes is initiated through the aggregation and activity of neutrophils and macrophages and the activation of complement. Cytokines, oxygen free radicals, and other inflammatory mediators damage the walls of capillaries and alveoli, producing diffuse inflammatory interstitial and alveolar edema, fibrin exudates, and hyaline membranes that block oxygen delivery to the blood.

TREATMENT: Endotracheal intubation and the use of mechanical ventilators are required along with high concentrations of oxygen, prevention or treatment of pneumonia, and drugs to maintain blood pressure and organ perfusion. Fluid restriction and a diuretic may be used to reduce pulmonary edema. The patient should be carefully monitored for hypoxia-induced cardiac arrhythmias, oxygen toxicity, renal failure, thrombocytopenia, sepsis, and disseminated intravascular coagulation.

PROGNOSIS: Mortality is high, approx. 60% to 70% depending on the amount of lung tissue involved and the ability to maintain adequate oxygen flow to vital organs. After resolution of the inflammation, the damaged lung tissue becomes fibrotic and can cause chronic restrictive lung disease. Prolonged use of more than 50% oxygen increases the risk of residual lung damage.

NURSING IMPLICATIONS: To avert ARDS, respiratory status is monitored in at-risk patients. Recognizing and treating early signs and symptoms can be crucial to a patient's survival. Ventilatory rate, depth, and rhythm are monitored and subtle changes noted; the patient is also observed for chest wall retractions on inspiration, use of accessory breathing muscles, and dyspnea. Sputum volume and character, esp. frothiness, are noted. The patient's consciousness level, cardiac rate and rhythm, blood pressure, arterial blood gas (ABG) values, serum electrolyte levels, and chest radiograph results are monitored. Fluid balance is closely watched by measuring intravenous (IV) fluid intake and urinary output, central venous pressure, and pulmonary artery wedge pressure; by weighing the patient daily; and by assessing for peripheral edema. A patent airway is maintained, and oxygen therapy with continuous positive airway pressure or mechanical ventilation with positive end-expiratory pressure (PEEP) is provided as prescribed. Routine management of a mechanically ventilated patient includes monitoring breath sounds, chest wall movement, vital signs and comfort, and ventilator settings and function; suctioning the endotracheal tube and oropharynx; and assessing changes in pulse oximetry and ABG values. Any changes in hemodynamic status and cardiac output (decreased because PEEP increases intrathoracic pressure) are noted by closely observing central line pressure and volume readouts, blood pressure, urine output, mental status, and peripheral pulses. The nurse administers inotropic drugs as prescribed if cardiac output falls. Hemoglobin levels and oxygen saturation values are also closely monitored, as packed red blood cell transfusion may be required if hemoglobin is inadequate for oxygen delivery. The nurse observes for signs and symptoms of barotrauma such as subcutaneous emphysema, pneumothorax, and pneumomediastinum (air leaks resulting from alveolar rupture caused by high airway pressures). If pressure control ventilation is used, analgesia, sedation, and paralysis (with pancuronium) are provided as prescribed; the patient's response is monitored with a peripheral nerve stimulator. Because the paralyzed patient cannot blink, moisturizing eye drops are instilled every few hours. The nurse administers enteral and parenteral nutrition, and prescribed IV fluids to maintain fluid volume. Nursing measures are used to prevent problems of immobility. Strict asepsis is observed in dressing changes, suctioning, handwashing, and oral care. The patient is routinely assessed for fever, sputum color changes, and elevated WBC count. Response to therapy is evaluated and adverse reactions are noted. The nurse encourages the family to talk to the patient even though he or she cannot respond verbally.

**acute respiratory failure** SEE: *respiratory failure, acute.*

**acute tubular necrosis** ABBR: ATN. Acute damage to the renal tubules; usually due to ischemia associated with shock. SEE: *renal failure, acute.*

**acute urethral syndrome** Syndrome experienced by women, marked by acute dysuria, urinary frequency, and lack of significant bacteriuria (i.e., less than $10^{-5}$ organisms per milliliter of urine); pyuria may or may not be present. The cause is unknown, but it is important to determine whether a specific bacterial infection of the bladder or vagina is present and to treat appropriately.

NURSING IMPLICATIONS: A history of the illness, including events that cause an increase or a decrease in symptoms, is obtained. The degree and nature of the patient's pain, its location and possible radiation, and its frequency and duration are ascertained. The patient is instructed in the procedure for collecting a clean-catch, midstream urine specimen and prepared for vaginal examination. If a bladder or vaginal bacterial infection is diagnosed, prescribed treatment measures are explained and demonstrated.

**acyanoblepsia** (ă-sī″ă-nō-blĕp′sē-ă) [Gr. *a-*, not, + *kyanos,* blue, + *blepsis,* vision] Inability to discern blue colors. Also called *acyanopsia.*

**acyanotic** (ă-sī″ă-nŏt′ĭk) [″ + *kyanos,* blue] Pert. to the absence of cyanosis.

**acyclic** (ă-sī′klĭk) **1.** Without a cycle. **2.** In chemistry, aliphatic.

**acyclovir** (ā-sī′klō-vĭr) An antiviral drug approved for use in herpes simplex infections of the genitals and herpes infections of the skin of immunocompromised patients. Trade name is Zovirax.

**acyl** (ăs′ĭl) In organic chemistry, the radical derived from an organic acid when the hydroxyl group (OH) is removed.

**acylation** (ăs″ĭ-lā′shŭn) Incorporation of an acid radical into a chemical.

**acystia** (ă-sĭs′tē-ă) [Gr. *a-*, not, + *kystis,* bladder] Congenital absence of the bladder.

**acystinervia, acystineuria** (ă-sĭs″tĭ-nĕr′vē-ă, -nū′rē-ă) [″ + ″ + *neuron,* nerve] Defective nerve supply to or paralysis of the bladder.

**AD** *anodal duration; average deviation.*

**ad** [L., to] In prescription writing, an indication that a substance should be added to the formulation up to a specified volume.

**ad-** [L., to] Prefix indicating *adherence, increase, toward,* as in adduct.

**-ad** [L., to] Suffix meaning *toward* or *in the direction of,* as in cephalad.

**a.d.** [L.] *auris dextra,* right ear.

**A.D.A.** *American Dental Association; American Diabetes Association; American Dietetic Association; Americans with Disabilities Act.*

**A.D.A.A.** *American Dental Assistants Association.*

**adactylia, adactylism, adactyly** (ă″dăk-tĭl′ē-ă, ā-dăk′tĭ-lĭzm, -lē) [Gr. *a-*, not, + *daktylos,* finger] Congenital absence of digits of the hand or foot.

**adamantine** (ăd″ă-măn′tĭn) [Gr. *adamantinos*] Very hard; said of enamel of teeth.

**adamantinoma** (ăd″ă-măn″tĭ-nō′mă) [″ + *oma,* tumor] A tumor of the jaw, esp. of the lower one, that arises from enamel-forming cells and may be partly cystic, partly solid. It may be benign or of low-grade malignancy. SYN: *ameloblastoma.*

**adamantoblast** (ăd″ă-măn′tō-blăst) [Gr. *adamas,* hard surface, + *blastos,* germ] An enamel-forming cell present only during tooth formation. SYN: *ameloblast.*

**adamantoblastoma** (ăd″ă-măn″tō-blăs-tō′mă) [″ + ″ + *oma,* tumor] Overgrowth of an adamantoblast.

**adamantoma** (ăd″ă-măn-tō′mă) [Gr. *adamas,* hard surface, + *oma,* tumor] Adamantinoma.

**Adam's apple** The laryngeal prominence formed by the two laminae of the thyroid cartilage. SYN: *pomum adami; prominentia laryngea.*

**Adams-Stokes syndrome** SEE: *Stokes-Adams syndrome.*

**adaptation** (ăd″ăp-tā′shŭn) [L. *adaptare,* to adjust] **1.** Adjustment of an organism to a change in internal or external conditions or circumstances. **2.** Adjustment of the eye to various intensities of light, accomplished by changing the size of the pupil and accompanied by chemical changes occurring in the rods. **3.** In psychology, a change in quality, intensity, or distinctness of a sensation that occurs after continuous stimulation of constant intensity. **4.** In dentistry, the proper fitting of dentures or bands to the teeth, or closeness of a filling to walls of a cavity.

***chromatic a.*** A change in hue or saturation, or both, resulting from pre-exposure to light of other wavelengths.

***color a.*** The fading of intensity of color perception after prolonged visual stimulation.

***dark a.*** Adjustment of the eyes for vision in dim light. SYN: *scotopia.*

***light a.*** Adjustment of the eyes for vision in bright light. SYN: *photopia.*

***retinal a.*** Adjustment of the rods and cones of the retina to ambient light.

**Adaptation Model** SEE: *Nursing Theory Appendix.*

**adapted clothing** Garments designed with special features, such as Velcro closures, to allow disabled people to dress themselves.

**adapter** (ă-dăp′tĕr) **1.** Device for joining one part of an apparatus to another part. **2.** Device to facilitate connecting electrical supply cords to different receptacles. **3.** Device for adapting one type of electrical supply source to the specific requirements of an instrument.

**adaptive capacity, intracranial, decreased** A clinical state in which intracranial fluid dynamic mechanisms that normally compensate for increases in intracranial volumes are compromised, resulting in repeated disproportionate increases in intracranial pressure in response to a variety of noxious and nonnoxious stimuli. SEE: *Nursing Diagnoses Appendix.*

**adaptive device** Device designed to help disabled people perform life tasks independently.

**adaptometer** A device for determining the time required for retinal adaptation.

**adaxial** (ăd-ăk′sē-ăl) [L. *ad,* toward, + *axis,* axis] Toward the main axis; opposite of abaxial.

**ADC** *anodal duration contraction; axiodistocervical.*

**add** Prescription abbreviation meaning *let there be added.*

**adde** (ăd′ē) [L.] *Add,* used as a direction in writing prescriptions.

**addict** (ăd′ĭkt) [L. *addictus,* given over] One physically or psychologically, or both, dependent on a substance, esp. alcohol or drugs.

**addiction** (ă-dĭk′shŭn) Involvement, for a variety of reasons, in one of several forms of repetitive behavior. Gambling, eating disorders, and reckless driving might be loosely referred to as addiction, but the term is best reserved to indicate dependence on narcotics, drugs of abuse, alcohol, and tobacco.

**Addis count method** (ăd′ĭs) [Thomas Addis, Scot.-born U.S. physician, 1881–1949] Method for counting the sediment (casts and cells) in a 12-hr urine sample.

**Addison's disease** [Thomas Addison, Brit. physician, 1793–1860] Disease resulting from deficiency in the secretion of adrenocortical hormones.

SYMPTOMS: The symptoms are increased pigmentation of skin and mucous membranes, irregular patches of vitiligo, black freckles over the head and neck, weakness, fatigability, hypotension, nausea, vomiting, diarrhea, abdominal discomfort, anorexia, weight loss, and sometimes hypoglycemia. Dehydration, hyponatremia, hyperkalemia, and profound hypovolemic shock may also occur. The patient may experience headache, mental confusion, and lassitude.

ETIOLOGY: The disease is caused by progressive destruction of the adrenal gland because of an infectious disease, such as tuberculosis, or infiltration by neoplastic tissue or hemorrhage into the gland.

TREATMENT: Adrenocortical hormone

therapy is dramatic in its effect and in adrenal crisis must be given promptly to prevent death. The patient should carry an emergency kit of 100 mg of intramuscular hydrocortisone in case oral medication cannot be taken, and both patient and family are taught how to give the injection. The patient should wear or carry a medical identification tag indicating the disease and therapy. SEE: *adrenal crisis.*

PROGNOSIS: If untreated, the disease will continue a chronic course with progressive but usually relatively slow deterioration; in some patients the deterioration may be rapid. Patients treated properly have an excellent prognosis.

NURSING IMPLICATIONS: Patients with primary or secondary adrenocortical insufficiency experiencing physical or emotional stress are assessed for this life-threatening emergency, as are patients who have had adrenal or pituitary surgery, sudden adrenal hemorrhage, or pituitary destruction. Death may occur due to circulatory collapse. The nurse monitors the patient every ½ to 4 hr as necessary, assessing for hypotension, tachycardia, fluid balance (including daily weight and urine output, measured hourly if necessary), and electrolyte and blood glucose levels. Prescribed adrenocortical steroids, with sodium and fluid replacement, are administered. The patient is protected from stressors such as infection, noise, and light and temperature changes. Extra time for rest and relaxation is planned.

*For chronic maintenance therapy:* Both patient and family are taught about the need for lifelong replacement therapy and medical supervision. The nurse instructs the patient regarding self-administration of steroid therapy (two thirds in A.M. and one third in P.M., with antacids or meals to minimize gastric irritation), and about stressful situations or conditions that require a temporary increase in dosage. Symptoms of overdosage and underdosage, and the course of action if either occurs, are explained. The patient is instructed to increase fluid and salt replacement if perspiring and to follow a diet high in sodium, carbohydrates, and protein, with small, frequent meals if hypoglycemia or anorexia occurs. Measures to help prevent infection include getting adequate rest, avoiding fatigue, eating a balanced diet, and avoiding people with infections. The nurse encourages verbalization of feelings and concerns and helps the patient to develop coping strategies. The patient is referred for further mental health or stress management counseling if warranted. SEE: *Medic Alert; Nursing Diagnoses Appendix.*

**addisonism** (ăd′ĭ-sŭn-ĭzm″) Symptom complex resembling Addison's disease but not caused by disease of the adrenal glands; may be seen in pulmonary tuberculosis. There is abnormal skin pigmentation with debility.

**Addison's planes** Imaginary planes that divide the abdomen into nine regions to aid in the location of internal structures. SEE: *abdominal regions.*

**addition** (ă-dĭ′shŭn) In chemistry, a reaction in which two substances unite without loss of atoms or valence.

**additive** (ăd′ĭ-tĭv) In pharmacology, the effect that one drug or substance contributes to the action of another drug or substance. SEE: *synergism.*

***food a.*** Substance added to food to maintain or impart a certain consistency, to improve or maintain nutritive value, to enhance palatability or flavor, to produce a light texture, or to control pH. Food additives are used to help bread rise during baking, to keep bread mold-free, to color margarine, to prevent discoloration of some fruits, and to prevent fats and oils from becoming rancid. The U.S. Food and Drug Administration regulates the use of food additives.

**adducent** (ă-dū′sĕnt) [L. *adducere,* to bring toward] Causing adduction.

**adduct** (ă-dŭkt′) [L. *adductus,* brought toward] To draw toward the main axis of the body or a limb.

**adduction** (ă-dŭk′shŭn) Movement of a limb or eye toward the median plane of the body or, in the case of digits, toward the axial line of a limb. SEE: *abduction* for illus.

***convergent-stimulus a.*** Convergence of the eyes when the gaze is fixed on an object at the near point of vision.

**adductor** (ă-dŭk′tor) A muscle that draws toward the medial line of the body or to a common center.

**adductor reflex** Contraction of the adductor muscles of the thigh on applying pressure to, or tapping, the medial surface of the thigh or knee.

**adelomorphous** (ă-dĕl″ō-mor′fŭs) [Gr. *adelos,* not seen, + *morphe,* shape] Having undefined form, as in the central cells of the gastric glands.

**aden-** SEE: *adeno-.*

**adenalgia** (ăd″ĕn-ăl′jē-ă) [Gr. *aden,* gland, + *algos,* pain] Pain in a gland. SYN: *adenodynia.*

**adenase** (ăd′ĕ-nāz) [″ + *-ase,* enzyme] Enzyme secreted by the pancreas, spleen, and liver that converts adenine into hypoxanthine. SEE: *enzyme.*

**adendric, adendritic** (ă-dĕn′drĭk, ă″dĕn-drĭt′ĭk) [Gr. *a-,* not, + *dendrites,* rel. to a tree] Without dendrites, as in certain cells in the spinal ganglia.

**adenectomy** (ăd″ĕn-ĕk′tō-mē) [Gr. *aden,* gland, + *ektome,* excision] Excision of a gland.

**adenectopia** (ăd″ĕ-nĕk-tō′pē-ă) [″ + ″ + *topos,* place] Malposition of a gland; a gland in a position that is other than its normal position.

**adenia** (ă-dē′nē-ă) Chronic inflammation and enlargement of a lymph gland.

**adeniform** (ă-dĕn′ĭ-form) [Gr. *aden,* gland, + L. *forma,* shape] Glandlike in form.

**adenine** (ăd′ĕ-nīn) $C_5H_5N_5$. A purine base that is part of DNA and RNA; in DNA it is paired with thymine.

**adenitis** (ăd″ĕ-nī′tĭs) [Gr. *aden,* gland, + *itis,* inflammation] Inflammation of lymph nodes or a gland.

**adenization** (ăd″ĕ-nĭ-zā′shŭn) Abnormal change into a glandlike structure.

**adeno-, aden-** [Gr. *aden,* gland] Combining form meaning *gland.*

**adenoacanthoma** (ăd″ĕ-nō-ăk″ăn-thō′mă) [″ + *akantha,* thorn, + *oma,* tumor] Adenocarcinoma in which some cells have undergone squamous metaplasia.

**adenoameloblastoma** (ăd″ĕ-nō-ă-mēl″ō-blăs-tō′mă) [″ + O. Fr. *amel,* enamel, + Gr. *blastos,* germ, + *oma,* tumor] Benign tumor of the jaw, originating from ameloblast cells of forming teeth; an odontogenic tumor.

**adenoblast** (ăd′ĕ-nō-blăst) [″ + *blastos,* germ] **1.** Embryonic cells that produce glandular tissue. **2.** Any tissue that produces secretory or glandular activity.

**adenocarcinoma** (ăd″ĕ-nō-kăr″sĭn-ō′mă) [″ + *karkinos,* crab, + *oma,* tumor] A malignant adenoma arising from a glandular organ.

***acinar a.*** Adenocarcinoma in which the cells are in the shape of alveoli. SYN: *alveolar a.*

***alveolar a.*** Acinar a.

**adenocele** (ăd′ĕ-nō-sēl″) [″ + *kele,* tumor, swelling] **1.** A cystic tumor arising from a gland. **2.** A tumor of glandular structure.

**adenocellulitis** (ăd″ĕ-nō-sĕl″ū-lī′tĭs) [″+ L. *cella,* small chamber, + Gr. *itis,* inflammation] Inflammation of a gland and adjacent cellular tissue.

**adenocyst** (ăd′ĕ-nō-sĭst″) [″ + *kystis,* sac] A cystic tumor arising from a gland.

**adenocystoma** (ăd″ĕ-nō-sĭs-tō′mă) [″ + *kystis,* sac, + *oma,* tumor] Cystic adenoma.

**adenodynia** (ăd″ĕ-nō-dĭn′ē-ă) [″ + *odyne,* pain] Pain in a gland. SYN: *adenalgia.*

**adenoepithelioma** (ăd″ĕ-nō-ĕp″ĭ-thēl-ē-ō′mă) [″ + *epi,* on, + *thele,* nipple, + *oma,* tumor] A tumor consisting of glandular and epithelial elements.

**adenofibroma** (ăd″ĕ-nō-fī-brō′mă) [″ + L. *fibra,* fiber, + Gr. *oma,* tumor] A tumor of fibrous and glandular tissue (connective tissue); frequently found in the uterus or breast.

**adenofibrosis** (ăd″ĕ-nō-fī-brō′sĭs) [″ + ″ + Gr. *osis,* condition] Degeneration of a tumor that contains fibrous connective tissue.

**adenogenous** (ăd″ĕ-nŏj′ĕ-nŭs) [″ + *gennan,* to produce] Originating in glandular tissue.

**adenohypophysis** (ăd″ĕ-nō-hī-pŏf′ĭ-sĭs) [″ + *hypo,* under, + *phyein,* to grow] The anterior lobe of the pituitary gland.

**adenoid** (ăd′ĕ-noyd) [″ + Gr. *eidos,* form, shape] Lymphoid; having the appearance of a gland.

**adenoidectomy** (ăd″ĕ-noyd-ĕk′tō-mē) [″ + ″ + *ektome,* excision] Excision of the adenoids. SEE: *tonsillectomy; Nursing Diagnoses Appendix.*

NURSING IMPLICATIONS: Vital signs are monitored, and the patient is observed for signs of shock. The mouth and pharynx are checked for bleeding, large clot formation, or oozing; the patient is observed for frequent swallowing, which indicates bleeding or large clot formation. Clots should be prevented from obstructing the oropharynx. The patient is placed in either a prone position with the head turned to the side or in a lateral recumbent position to promote drainage. When the operative wound has healed sufficiently, the oral intake of cool (not hot or iced) fluids and soft foods is encouraged. The patient is also advised not to gargle until the surgical site has healed.

*Young patients:* The nurse reassures the child concerning care routines and procedures, provides emotional support, and encourages parental presence. The child is evaluated for vomiting of partially digested swallowed blood, and is monitored for ability to swallow fluids.

**adenoid hypertrophy** Enlargement of the pharyngeal tonsil. It occurs commonly in children and may be congenital or result from infection of Waldeyer's ring.

**adenoiditis** (ăd″ĕ-noyd-ī′tĭs) [Gr. *aden,* gland, + *eidos,* form, + *itis,* inflammation] Inflammation of adenoid tissue.

**adenoids** (ăd′ĕ-noyds) Lymphatic tissue forming a prominence on the wall of the pharyngeal recess of the nasopharynx. SEE: *pharyngeal tonsil.*

**adenoid tissue** SEE: *tissue, adenoid.*

**adenolipoma** (ăd″ĕ-nō-lĭp-ō′mă) [Gr. *aden,* gland, + *lipos,* fat, + *oma,* tumor] A benign tumor having glandular characteristics but composed of fat.

**adenolymphocele** (ăd″ĕ-nō-lĭm′fō-sēl) [″ + ″ + Gr. *kele,* tumor, swelling] Cystic dilatation of a lymph node from obstruction.

**adenolymphoma** (ăd″ĕ-nō-lĭm-fō′mă) [″ + ″ + Gr. *oma,* tumor] A lymph gland adenoma.

**adenoma** (ăd″ĕ-nō′mă) *pl.* **adenomata** [″ + *oma,* tumor] A neoplasm of glandular epithelium. **adenomatous** (-nō′mă-tŭs), *adj.*

***acidophil(ic) a.*** Tumor of the pituitary gland in which cells stain with acid dyes. It causes acromegaly and gigantism. SYN: *eosinophil(ic) adenoma.*

***basophil(ic) a.*** Tumor of the pituitary gland in which cells stain with basic dyes. It causes Cushing's syndrome.

***chromophobe a.*** Tumor of the pituitary gland composed of cells that do not stain readily. It may cause pituitary deficiency or diabetes insipidus.

***eosinophil(ic) a.*** Acidophil(ic) a.

***fibroid a.*** Fibroadenoma.

***follicular a.*** Adenoma of the thyroid.

***Hürthle cell a.*** Tumor of the thyroid that contains mostly eosinophil-staining cells. These are called Hürthle cells and are usually benign.

***islet a.*** Nonmalignant neoplasm of the pancreas sometimes containing beta cells. It may be the cause of hypoglycemia. SYN: *insuloma; langerhansian adenoma.*

***malignant a.*** Adenocarcinoma.

***papillary a.*** Adenoma in which the alveoli of the adenoma are filled with fluid.

***pituitary a.*** Adenoma of the pituitary gland.

***sebaceous a.*** Enlarged sebaceous glands, esp. of the face.

***a. sebaceum*** Benign, usually solitary growth that develops on the face from the epithelium of sebaceous glands.

***villous a.*** Large polyp of the mucosal surface of the large intestine.

**adenomatome** (ăd″ĕ-nō′mă-tōm) [″ + *oma,* tumor, + *tome,* incision] An instrument for removing adenoids.

**adenomatosis** (ăd″ĕ-nō-mă-tō′sĭs) [″ + *oma,* tumor, + *osis,* condition] The condition of multiple glandular tissue overgrowths.

**adenomere** (ăd′ĕ-nō-mēr″) [″ + *meros,* part] The functional part of a gland.

**adenomyoma** (ăd″ĕ-nō-mī-ō′mă) [″ + *mys,* muscle, + *oma,* tumor] Tumor containing glandular and smooth muscular tissue.

**adenomyometritis** (ăd″ĕ-nō-mī″ō-mĕ-trī′tĭs) [″ + ″ + *metra,* womb, + *itis,* inflammation] A hyperplastic condition of the uterus caused by pelvic inflammation; it grossly resembles an adenomyoma.

**adenomyosarcoma** (ăd″ĕ-nō-mī″ō-săr-kō′mă) [″ + ″ + *sarx,* flesh, + *oma,* tumor] Adenosarcoma that includes muscle tissue.

**adenomyosis** (ăd″ĕ-nō-mī-ō′sĭs) [″ + *mys,* muscle, + *osis,* condition] Benign invasive growth of the endometrium into the muscular layer of the uterus. SEE: *endometriosis* for illus.

**adenopathy** (ăd-ĕ-nŏp′ă-thē) [″ + *pathos,* disease, suffering] Swelling and morbid change in lymph nodes; glandular disease.

**adenopharyngitis** (ăd″ĕ-nō-făr″ĭn-jī′tĭs) [″ + *pharynx,* throat, + *itis,* inflammation] Inflammation of tonsils and pharyngeal mucous membrane.

**adenophthalmia** (ăd″ĕ-nŏf-thăl′mē-ă) [″ + *ophthalmos,* eye] Inflammation of the meibomian gland.

**adenosarcoma** (ăd″ĕ-nō-săr-kō′mă) [″ + *sarx,* flesh, + *oma,* tumor] A tumor with adenomatous and sarcomatous characteristics.

**adenosclerosis** (ăd″ĕ-nō-sklĕ-rō′sĭs) [″ + *sklerosis,* hardening] Glandular hardening.

**adenose** (ăd′ĕ-nōs) Glandlike.

**adenosine** (ă-dĕn′ō-sēn) A nucleotide containing adenine and ribose.

***a. 3′,5′-cyclic monophosphate*** ABBR: AMP. A cyclic form of adenosine. Its synthesis from adenosine triphosphate (ATP) is stimulated by an enzyme, adenylate cyclase (also called cyclic AMP synthetase). Adenosine 3′,5′-cyclic monophosphate is important in a wide variety of metabolic responses to cell stimuli.

***a. deaminase conjugated with polyethylene glycol*** ABBR: PEG-ADA. A cytoplasmic enzyme used to treat severe combined immunodeficiency disease (SCID) due to adenosine deaminase deficiency. Trade name is Adagen. SEE: *severe combined immunodeficiency disease.*

***a. diphosphate, a. 5′-diphosphate*** ABBR: ADP. A compound of adenosine containing two phosphoric acid groups. This substance is produced during muscle contraction. It is reformed when the muscle relaxes.

***a. monophosphate, a. 5′-monophosphate*** ABBR: AMP; 5′-AMP. Substance formed by condensation of adenosine and phosphoric acid. It is one of the hydrolytic products of nucleic acids and is present in muscle, red blood cells, yeast, and other nuclear material. SYN: *adenylic acid.*

***a. triphosphatase*** ABBR: ATPase. Enzyme that splits adenosine triphosphate to yield phosphate and energy.

***a. triphosphate*** ABBR: ATP. A compound of adenosine containing three phosphoric acid groups. This substance is present in all cells, but particularly in muscle cells. When it is split by enzyme action, energy is produced. The energy of the muscle is stored in this compound.

**adenosis** (ăd″ĕ-nō′sĭs) [Gr. *aden,* gland, + *osis,* condition] Any disease of a gland, esp. a lymphatic gland.

**adenotome** (ăd′ĕ-nō-tōm) [″ + *tome,* incision] Device for excising a gland, esp. the adenoid glands.

**adenotonsillectomy** (ăd″ĕ-nō-tŏn″sĭl-lĕk′tō-mē) [″ + L. *tonsilla,* almond, + Gr. *ektome,* excision] Surgical removal of the tonsils and adenoids.

**adenous** (ăd′ĕ-nŭs) Like a gland.

**adenovirus** (ăd′ĕ-nō-vī′rŭs) One of a group of closely related viruses that can cause infections of the upper respiratory tract. A large number have been isolated. SEE: illus.

**adenyl** (ăd′ĕ-nĭl) The radical $C_5H_4N_5$;

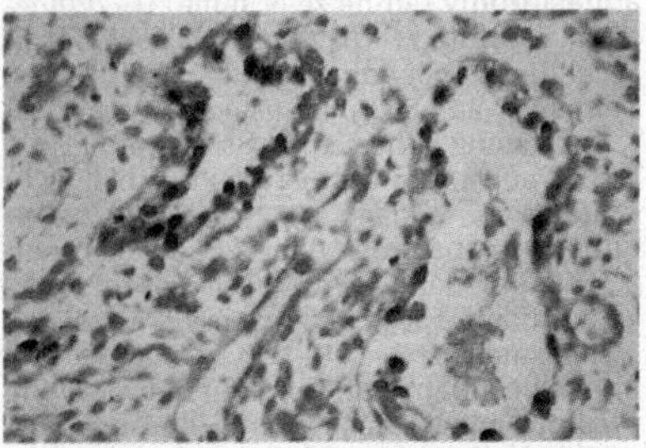

**ADENOVIRUS** INCLUSIONS (STAINED BLUE-BLACK) IN THE CELLS LINING A BRONCHIOLE

present in adenine.

***a. cyclase*** An enzyme that catalyzes the production of cyclic AMP (adenosine 3′,5′-cyclic monophosphate) from ATP (adenosine triphosphate). It is present on most cell surfaces.

**adenylate cyclase** (ă-dĕn′ĭ-lāt sī′klās) An enzyme important in the synthesis of cyclic AMP (adenosine 3′,5′-cyclic monophosphate) from adenosine triphosphate. SYN: *cyclic AMP synthetase.*

**adenylic acid** Adenosine monophosphate.

**adermia** (ă-dĕr′mē-ă) [Gr. *a-,* not, + *derma,* skin] Congenital or acquired defect of or lack of skin.

**adermogenesis** (ă-dĕr″mō-jĕn′ĕ-sĭs) [″ + ″ + *genesis,* generation, birth] Imperfect development of skin.

**ADH** *antidiuretic hormone* (vasopressin).

**A.D.H.A.** *American Dental Hygienists' Association.*

**adherence, bacterial** (ăd-hēr′ĕns) The ability of bacteria to adhere to specific receptors that are present on some cells but not on others. If bacteria normally present in the intestinal tract did not have this ability, they would be washed out of the intestines.

**adherent** (ăd-hē′rĕnt) [L. *adhaerere,* to stick to] Attached to, as of two surfaces.

**adhesin** In conjugation of some bacteria, a protein on the cell surface that causes aggregation of cells.

**adhesio** (ăd-hē′zē-ō) [L. *adhaesio,* stuck to] Adhesion.

**adhesion** (ăd-hē′zhŭn) [L. *adhaesio,* stuck to] **1.** A holding together or uniting of two surfaces or parts, as in wound healing. **2.** A fibrous band holding parts together that are normally separated. **3.** An attraction to another substance: thus, molecules or blood platelets adhere to each other or to dissimilar materials.

***abdominal a.*** Adhesion in the abdominal cavity, usually involving the intestines; caused by inflammation or trauma. If adhesions cause great pain or intestinal obstruction, they are treated surgically.

***pericardial a.*** Adhesion of the pericardial sac. If extensive, adhesions may lead to restriction of the normal movement of the heart. SEE: *pericarditis.*

**adhesiotomy** (ăd-hē″zē-ŏt′ō-mē) [L. *adhaesio,* stuck to, + Gr. *tome,* incision] Surgical division of adhesions.

**adhesive** (ăd-hē′sĭv) [L. *adhaesio,* stuck to] **1.** Causing adhesion. **2.** Sticky; adhering. **3.** A substance that causes two bodies to adhere.

**adhesive capsulitis** Adherence of folds in an articular (joint) capsule, preventing normal joint play and causing restricted movement.

**adhesive inflammation** Inflammation of the serous membrane, making adhesions possible by formation of fibrin.

**adhesive tape** A fabric, film, or paper, one side of which is coated with an adhesive so that it remains in place when applied to the skin. In general, there are two types of backings for the adhesive material: occlusive and nonocclusive. The former prevents air from going through the backing and the latter does not. The occlusive type increases the possibility of skin irritation, so it is rarely used. SEE: *plaster, adhesive.*

NURSING IMPLICATIONS: To prevent skin damage, adhesive tape should be removed by carefully peeling back the tape following the direction of hair growth while the skin is held taut behind the tape removal edge. The skin should be checked for irritation. If the adhesive material has irritated the skin, solvents should not be used to assist in removal. Because some patients are allergic to certain adhesive agents, information about this type of allergy should be gathered as part of the history when tape use is anticipated, any signs of new allergy noted, and an alternative bandage used.

**adiadochokinesia, adiadochokinesis** (ă-dī″ă-dō″kō-kĭ-nē′sē-ă, -nē′sĭs) [Gr. *a-,* not, + *diadochas,* successive, + *kinesis,* movement] **1.** Inability to make rapid alternating movements. **2.** In neurology, rapid antagonistic movements that cannot be carried out smoothly; seen in cerebellar disease.

**adiaphoresis** (ă-dī″ă-fō-rē′sĭs) [″ + *diaphorein,* to perspire] Deficiency or absence of sweat.

**adiastole** (ă″dī-ăs′tō-lē) [″ + *diastole,* dilatation] Imperceptibility of diastole.

**Adie's syndrome** (ā′dēz) [William John Adie, Brit. neurologist, 1886–1935] A syndrome marked by a tonic pupil that responds slowly or not at all to light, with impaired accommodation and slow constriction and relaxation in the change from near to distant vision. The affected pupil is frequently larger than the normal pupil. Loss of certain deep tendon reflexes may also be present, but there are no other signs of central nervous system disease. SEE: *pupil, tonic.*

**adip-** SEE: *adipo-.*

**adipectomy** (ăd″ĭ-pĕk′tō-mē) [L. *adeps,* fat, + Gr. *ektome,* excision] Excision of fat or adipose tissue, usually a large quantity. SEE: *liposuction.*

**adipic** (ă-dĭp′ĭk) Rel. to adipose tissue.

**adipo-, adip-** [L. *adeps,* fat] Combining form meaning fat. See also *lipo-, steato-.*

**adipocele** (ăd′ĭ-pō-sēl″) [L. *adeps,* fat, + Gr. *kele,* tumor] A hernia that contains fat or fatty tissue. SYN: *lipocele.*

**adipocellular** (ăd″ĭ-pō-sĕl′ū-lăr) Containing fat and cellular tissue.

**adipocere** (ăd′ĭ-pō-sēr″) [L. *adeps,* fat, + *cera,* wax] A brown, waxlike substance composed of fatty acids and calcium soaps. It is formed in animal tissues that have been buried in a moist place.

**adipocyte** SEE: *cell, fat.*

**adipofibroma** [″ + *fibra,* fiber, + Gr. *oma,* tumor] A fibroma and adipoma.

**adipogenous, adipogenic** (ăd″ĭ-pŏj′ĕn-ŭs,

-pō-jĕn′ĭk) [″ + Gr. *gennan,* to produce] Inducing the formation of fat.

**adipoid** (ăd′ĭ-poyd) [L. *adeps,* fat, + Gr. *eidos,* form, shape] Fatlike; lipoid.

**adipokinesis** (ăd″ĭ-pō-kĭ-nē′sĭs) [″ + Gr. *kinesis,* movement] **1.** Metabolism of fat with production of free fatty acids. **2.** Mobilization and metabolism of body fat.

**adipokinetic action** The action of substances to promote formation of free fatty acids from body fat stores.

**adiponecrosis** (ăd″ĭ-pō-nĕ-krō′sĭs) [″ + Gr. *nekrosis,* state of death] Necrosis affecting fatty tissue.

**adipose** [L. *adiposus,* fatty] Fatty; pert. to fat.

**adiposis** (ăd″ĭ-pō′sĭs) [L. *adeps,* fat, + Gr. *osis,* condition] Abnormal accumulation of fat in the body. SYN: *corpulence; liposis; obesity.*

***a. cerebralis*** Obesity due to intracranial disease, esp. of the pituitary.

***a. dolorosa*** Scattered areas of painful cutaneous nodules or fat accumulations in menopausal women. SYN: *Dercum's disease.*

***a. hepatica*** Fatty degeneration or infiltration of the liver.

**adipositis** (ăd″ĭ-pō-sī′tĭs) [L. *adiposus,* fatty, + Gr. *itis,* inflammation] Infiltration of an inflammatory nature in and beneath subcutaneous adipose tissue.

**adiposity** (ăd″ĭ-pŏs′ĭ-tē) Excessive fat in the body. SYN: *adiposis; corpulence; obesity.*

**adiposogenital dystrophy** (ăd″ĭ-pō″sō-jĕn′ĭ-tăl dĭs′trō-fē) [L. *adiposus,* fatty, + *genitalis,* genital, + Gr. *dys,* bad, disordered, + *trophe,* nourishment] Combination of adiposity, impaired development of genital organs, and altered secondary sex characteristics. This syndrome is caused by a disturbance of function or a tumor of the hypothalamus and pituitary gland. SYN: *Fröhlich's syndrome.*

**adiposuria** (ăd″ĭ-pō-sū′rē-ă) [″ + Gr. *ouron,* urine] Fat in the urine. SYN: *lipuria.*

**adipsia, adipsy** (ă-dĭp′sē-ă, -sē) [Gr. *a-,* not, + *dipsa,* thirst] Absence of thirst.

**aditus** (ăd′ĭ-tŭs) [L.] An approach; an entrance.

***a. ad antrum*** The recess of the tympanic cavity that leads from the epitympanic recess to the tympanic antrum.

***a. ad aquaeductum cerebri*** The entrance to the sylvian aqueduct, situated at the lower posterior angle of the third ventricle of the brain.

***a. laryngis*** Upper aperture of the larynx.

**adjunct** (ăd′jŭnkt) An addition to the principal procedure or course of therapy.

**adjuster** A device for holding together the ends of the wire forming a suture.

**adjustment** [L. *adjuxtare,* to bring together] **1.** Adaptation to a different environment; a person's relation to his or her environment and inner self. **2.** A change made to improve function or condition. **3.** A modification made to a tooth or a dental prosthesis to enhance fit, function, or patient acceptance. SEE: *occlusal adjustment.*

**adjustment disorder** A maladaptive reaction to an identifiable psychological or social stress that occurs within 3 months of the onset of the stressful situation. The reaction is characterized by impaired function or symptoms in excess of what would be considered normal for that stress. The symptoms are expected to remit when the stress ceases; if the stress continues, a new level of adaptation is achieved.

**adjustment, impaired** The state in which the individual is unable to modify his/her lifestyle or behavior in a manner consistent with a change in health status. SEE: *Nursing Diagnoses Appendix.*

**adjuvant** (ăd′jū-vănt) [L. *adjuvans,* aiding] **1.** That which assists, esp. a drug added to a prescription to hasten or increase the action of a principal ingredient. **2.** In immunology, a variety of substances, including inorganic gels such as alum, aluminum hydroxide, and aluminum phosphate, that increase the antigenic response.

***Freund's complete a.*** A water-in-oil emulsion in which an antigen solution is emulsified in mineral oil with killed mycobacteria to enhance antigenicity. The intense inflammatory response produced by this emulsion makes it unsuitable for use in humans.

***Freund's incomplete a.*** A water-in-oil emulsion in which an antigen solution without mycobacteria is emulsified in mineral oil. On injection, this mixture induces a strong persistent antibody formation.

**adjuvant therapy** In cancer therapy, the use of another form of treatment in addition to the primary therapy. For example, chemotherapy may be the primary treatment and radiation therapy may be an adjuvant therapy.

**ADL** *activities of daily living.*

**Adler, Alfred** Austrian psychiatrist (1870–1937) who founded the school of individual psychology. SEE: *psychology, individual.*

**ad lib** [L. *ad libitum*] Prescription abbreviation meaning *as desired.*

**Administration on Aging** ABBR: AoA. An agency of the U.S. Department of Health and Human Services that conducts research in the field of aging and assists federal, state, and local agencies in planning and developing programs for the aged. It is responsible for implementing the Older Americans Act of 1965.

**A.D.N.** *Associate Degree in Nursing.*

**ad nauseam** (ăd naw′sē-ăm) [L.] Of such degree or extent as to produce nausea.

**adneural** (ăd-nū′răl) [L. *ad,* to, + Gr. *neuron,* nerve] Near or toward a nerve.

**adnexa** (ăd-nĕk′să) [L.] Accessory parts of a structure.

***dental a.*** Tissues surrounding the tooth

(i.e., periodontal ligament and alveolar bone proper).

***a. oculi*** Lacrimal gland.

***a. uteri*** Ovaries and fallopian tubes.

**adnexal** (ăd-nĕk'săl) Adjacent or appending.

**adnexal pain** SEE: *pain, adnexal.*

**adnexitis** (ăd"nĕk-sī'tĭs) [L. *adnexa,* appendages, + Gr. *itis,* inflammation] Inflammation of the adnexa uteri.

**adolescence** (ăd"ō-lĕs'ĕns) [L. *adolescens*] The period from the beginning of puberty until maturity. Because the onset of puberty and maturity is a gradual process and varies among individuals, it is not practical to set exact age or chronological limits in defining the adolescent period.

**adolescent** (ăd"ō-lĕs'ĕnt) **1.** Pert. to adolescence. **2.** A young man or woman not fully grown.

**adolescent turmoil** In psychoanalytic theory, the belief that adolescence is invariably accompanied by turmoil. This is no longer thought to be inevitable, or even the usual case.

**adoption** (ă-dŏp'shŭn) [L. *ad,* to, + *optare,* to choose] Assumption of responsibility for the care of a child by a person or persons who are not the natural parents. This usually requires a legal procedure.

**adoral** (ăd-ō'răl) [" + *os,* mouth] Toward or near the mouth.

**ADP** *adenosine diphosphate.*

**adrenal** (ăd-rē'năl) [L. *ad,* to, + *ren,* kidney] Originally used to indicate nearness to the kidney; now used in reference to the adrenal gland or its secretions.

**adrenal crisis** Acute adrenocortical insufficiency. SEE: *Addison's disease; Waterhouse-Friderichsen syndrome.*

---

Caution: Death will result from circulatory collapse unless the condition is treated promptly and vigorously with corticosteroid therapy. The cause may be a hemorrhage into the adrenal cortex as a result of infection or it may occur at birth, resulting from trauma. In the adult, headache, lassitude, confusion, restlessness, vomiting, and shock progressing to death occur if the cortex is destroyed. Relative adrenal insufficiency can occur for 2 to 3 months after discontinuation of adrenocortical hormone therapy. Sudden stress, such as surgery or trauma, can produce a subacute form of adrenal crisis in these patients.

---

**adrenalectomy** (ăd-rē"năl-ĕk'tō-mē) [L. *ad,* to, + *ren,* kidney, + Gr. *ektome,* excision] Excision of one or both adrenal glands.

NURSING IMPLICATIONS: Vital signs, central venous pressure, and urine output are monitored frequently. Signs and symptoms of hypocorticism are assessed hourly for the first 24 hr and reported to the surgeon immediately. Additional IV glucocorticoids are given as prescribed. The patient is monitored for early indications of shock or infection, and for alterations in blood glucose and electrolyte levels. To counteract shock, IV fluids and vasopressors are administered as prescribed, and the patient's response is evaluated every 3 to 5 min. Increased steroids to meet metabolic demands are needed if a stress such as infection occurs; aseptic technique is used for dressing changes. Corticosteroids and other medications, including analgesics, are given as prescribed, and the patient's response evaluated. The room is kept cool and the patient's clothing and bedding changed often if he or she perspires profusely (a side effect of surgery on the adrenal gland). The abdomen is assessed for distention and return of bowel sounds. Physical and psychological stresses are kept to a minimum. Medications may be discontinued in a few months to a year after unilateral adrenalectomy, but lifelong replacement therapy will be needed after bilateral adrenalectomy. The patient must be taught to recognize the signs of adrenal insufficiency, that sudden withdrawal of steroids can precipitate adrenal crisis, and that continued medical follow-up will be needed so that steroid dosage can be adjusted during stress or illness. Steroids should be taken in a two-thirds A.M. and one-third P.M. dosing pattern to mimic diurnal adrenal activity, with meals or antacids to minimize gastric irritation. Adverse reactions to steroids (e.g., weight gain, acne, headaches, fatigue, and increased urinary frequency) are explained. SEE: *Nursing Diagnoses Appendix.*

**adrenal gland** A triangular body covering the superior surface of each kidney. SYN: *suprarenal gland.* SEE: illus.

EMBRYOLOGY: The adrenal gland is essentially a double organ composed of an outer cortex and an inner medulla. The cortex arises in the embryo from a region of the mesoderm that also gives rise to the gonads, or sex organs. The medulla arises from ectoderm, which also gives rise to the sympathetic nervous system.

ANATOMY: The gland is enclosed in a tough connective tissue capsule from which trabeculae extend into the cortex. The cortex consists of cells arranged into three zones: the outer zona glomerulosa, the middle zona fasciculata, and the inner zona reticularis. The cells are arranged in a cordlike fashion. The medulla consists of chromaffin cells arranged in groups or anastomosing cords. The two adrenal glands are situated retroperitoneally, each embedded in perirenal fat above its respective kidney. In an adult, the average weight of an adrenal gland is 5 g, and the range is 4 to 14 g. It is usually heavier in men than in women.

PHYSIOLOGY: The adrenal medulla synthesizes and stores three catecholamines: dopamine, norepinephrine, and

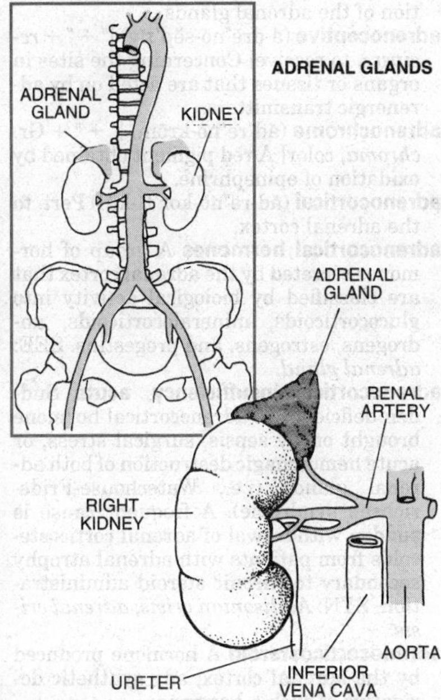


epinephrine. Dopamine's chief effects are dilation of systemic arteries, increased cardiac output, and increased flow of blood to the kidneys. The primary action of norepinephrine is to constrict the arterioles and venules, resulting in increased resistance to blood flow, elevated blood pressure, and slowing of the heart. Epinephrine constricts vessels in the skin and splanchnic area, dilates vessels in skeletal muscle, increases heart activity, dilates the bronchi by relaxing bronchial musculature, increases the glucose level in the blood by stimulating the production of glucose from glycogen in the liver, increases the amount of fatty acid in the blood, and diminishes activity of the gastrointestinal system. The three catecholamines are also produced in other parts of the body.

The adrenal medulla is controlled by the sympathetic nervous system and functions in conjunction with it. It is intimately related to adjustments of the body in response to stress and emotional changes. Anticipatory states tend to bring about the release of norepinephrine. More intense emotional reactions, esp. those in response to extreme stress, tend to increase the secretion of both norepinephrine and epinephrine; epinephrine is important in mobilizing the physiological changes that occur in the "fight or flight" response to emergency situations.

The cortex secretes a group of hormones that vary in quantity and quality. They are all synthesized from cholesterol and contain the basic steroid nucleus perhydrocyclopentanophenanthrene. These compounds are grouped according to their chemical structure and biological activity as follows: glucocorticoids (cortisol, corticosterone), which act principally on carbohydrate metabolism; mineralocorticoids (aldosterone, dehydroepiandrosterone), which affect metabolism of the electrolytes sodium and potassium; androgens (17-ketosteroids), estrogens (estradiol), and progestins (progesterone), all three of which are important in the physiology of reproduction. There is considerable overlap in the biological activity of many of these compounds. SEE: *steroid*.

Almost all body systems are influenced by the action of adrenocortical hormones. Cortisol and cortisone are important in carbohydrate, water, muscle, bone, central nervous system, gastrointestinal, cardiovascular, and hematological metabolism. They are also important anti-inflammatory agents. The principal long-term effect of cortisone and cortisol is catabolic.

The 17-ketosteroids act principally as androgenic and anabolic agents. Aldosterone's principal action is to control sodium and potassium levels in the blood.

PATHOLOGY: In the medulla, increased secretion of catecholamines occurs when a pheochromocytoma develops. In this condition, the patient develops hypertension, excessive sweating, paroxysmal attacks of blanching or flushing of the skin, tachycardia, headache, anorexia, weight loss, personality changes, signs of increased metabolism, constipation, and postural hypotension. Diagnosis may be confirmed by determining the level of catecholamines or their metabolic end products in the urine. SEE: *pheochromocytoma*.

Excess secretion of cortical hormones in the cortex may result in a variety of syndromes, depending on which hormone or group of hormones is increased. If cortisol is increased, the signs of Cushing's syndrome result: obesity with striae and redistribution of fat to produce a "buffalo hump" and "moon face," muscle wasting, osteoporosis, decreased glucose tolerance, atherosclerosis, and systolic hypertension. If the androgens are increased, male sex characteristics are accentuated; in women, this results in voice change, hirsutism, clitoral enlargement, and pronounced muscular development. Baldness and acne will develop in either sex with this condition. It is called adrenogenital syndrome.

When aldosterone is elevated, hypertension, low serum potassium, elevated serum sodium, increased urine volume, and, rarely, edema will be present. This is called primary aldosteronism. SEE: *primary aldosteronism*.

Adrenocortical deficiency may be acute

or chronic. The chronic form is called Addison's disease and is marked by anemia, sluggishness, weakness, weight loss, hypotension, sometimes hypoglycemia, nausea, vomiting, diarrhea, abnormal skin pigmentation, and mental changes. The acute form is called adrenal crisis. Adrenal crisis due to hemorrhage into the adrenal gland caused by meningococcal infection is called the Waterhouse-Friderichsen syndrome.

**adrenal hyperplasia, congenital** ABBR: CAH. An inherited disorder marked by congenital deficiency or absence of one or more enzymes essential to the production of adrenal cortical hormones. It is transmitted as an autosomal recessive trait, most often in Ashkenazi Jews and Mediterranean peoples. The enzyme involved most commonly is 21-hydroxylase (21-OHD). The inability to synthesize mineralocorticoids or glucocorticoids results in an overproduction of adrenal androgens. A severe deficiency or absence of 21-OHD also affects aldosterone synthesis. Symptoms of CAH include ambiguous genitalia or pseudohermaphroditism in infant girls. In other forms of CAH, decreased secretion of corticosterones and increased production of ACTH may cause a variety of clinical changes. Newborns who have salt-losing CAH develop vomiting, fluid and electrolyte imbalances (hyponatremia, hypokalemia), and hypotension within 2 weeks of birth. Treatment consists of hormonal therapy and surgery to correct genital abnormalities.

**Adrenalin** (ă-drĕn′ă-lĭn) Trade name for epinephrine.

**adrenaline** (ă-drĕn′ă-lēn) British designation for epinephrine.

**adrenalinemia** (ă-drĕn″ă-lĭn-ē′mē-ă) [L. *ad,* to, + *ren,* kidney, + Gr. *haima,* blood] Epinephrine in the blood.

**adrenalinuria** (ă-drĕn″ă-lĭn-ū′rē-ă) [″ + ″ + Gr. *ouron,* urine] Epinephrine in the urine.

**adrenarche** (ăd″rĕn-ăr′kē) [″ + ″ + Gr. *arche,* beginning] Changes that occur at puberty as a result of increased secretion of adrenocortical hormones. SEE: *menarche; pubarche.*

**adrenergic** (ăd-rĕn-ĕr′jĭk) [″ + ″ + Gr. *ergon,* work] Relating to nerve fibers that release norepinephrine or epinephrine at synapses. SEE: *sympathomimetic.*

**adrenergic agonist** Any one of a group of therapeutic agents that mimic or stimulate the sympathetic nervous system in different ways depending on the formulation of each drug.

**adrenergic neuron-blocking agents** Substances that inhibit transmission of sympathetic nerve stimuli regardless of whether alpha- or beta-adrenergic receptors are involved. SEE: *alpha-adrenergic receptor; beta-adrenergic receptor.*

**adrenitis** (ăd″rē-nī′tĭs) [L. *ad,* to, + *ren,* kidney, + Gr. *itis,* inflammation] Inflammation of the adrenal glands.

**adrenoceptive** (ă-drē″nō-sĕp′tĭv) [″ + ″ + *recipere,* to receive] Concerning the sites in organs or tissues that are acted on by adrenergic transmitters.

**adrenochrome** (ăd″rē′nō-krōm) [″ + ″ + Gr. *chroma,* color] A red pigment obtained by oxidation of epinephrine.

**adrenocortical** (ăd-rē″nō-kor′tĭ-kăl) Pert. to the adrenal cortex.

**adrenocortical hormones** A group of hormones secreted by the adrenal cortex that are classified by biological activity into glucocorticoids, mineralocorticoids, androgens, estrogens, and progestins. SEE: *adrenal gland.*

**adrenocortical insufficiency, acute** Sudden deficiency of adrenocortical hormone brought on by sepsis, surgical stress, or acute hemorrhagic destruction of both adrenal glands (i.e., Waterhouse-Friderichsen syndrome). A frequent cause is sudden withdrawal of adrenal corticosteroids from patients with adrenal atrophy secondary to chronic steroid administration. SYN: *Addisonian crisis; adrenal crisis.*

**adrenocorticosteroid** A hormone produced by the adrenal cortex; any synthetic derivative of such a hormone.

**adrenocorticotropic** (ăd-rē″nō-kor″tĭ-kō-trŏp′ĭk) [L. *ad,* to, + *ren,* kidney, + *cortex,* bark, + Gr. *tropikos,* turning] Having a stimulating effect on the adrenal cortex.

**adrenocorticotropic hormone** ABBR: ACTH. A hormone secreted by the anterior lobe of the pituitary. It is essential to the growth, development, and continued function of the adrenal cortex. SYN: *corticotropin.*

**adrenocorticotropin** (ăd-rē″nō-kor″tĭ-kō-trŏp′ĭn) Adrenocorticotropic hormone.

**adrenogenital** (ăd-rē-nō-jĕn′ĭ-tăl) [L. *ad,* to, + *ren,* kidney, + *genitalis,* genital] Pert. to the adrenal glands and the genitalia.

**adrenogenital syndrome** Condition caused by excess secretion of androgenic hormones by the adrenal gland or by excess medication with male hormones. In congenital forms, the female infant may be considered erroneously to be male and the male child will have accelerated growth and penile enlargement. In acquired forms, masculine secondary sex characteristics appear in girls, and there is precocious puberty in boys.

**adrenogenous** (ăd″rĕn-ŏj′ĕ-nŭs) [L. *ad,* to, + *ren,* kidney, + Gr. *gennan,* to produce] Originating in or produced by the adrenal gland.

**adrenoleukodystrophy** (ă-drē″nō-loo″kō-dĭs′trō-fē) [″ + ″ + Gr. *leukos,* white, + *dys,* bad, + *trephein,* to nourish] A hereditary disease of children, transmitted as a sex-linked recessive trait. There is an abnormality of the white matter of the brain and atrophy of the adrenal glands. The mental and physical deterioration progresses to dementia, aphasia, apraxia, dysarthria, and blindness. There is no treatment, except symptomatic.

**adrenolytic** (ăd″rēn-ō-lĭt′ĭk) [L. *ad,* to, + *ren,* kidney, + Gr. *lysis,* dissolution] Preventing or inhibiting the activity of adrenergic nerves; interfering with the response of epinephrine.

**adrenomegaly** (ăd-rēn″ō-mĕg′ă-lē) [″ + ″ + Gr. *megas,* large] Enlarged adrenal gland(s).

**adrenomimetic** (ă-drē″nō-mĭ-mĕt′ĭk) [″ + ″ + Gr. *mimetikos,* imitating] Sympathicomimetic.

**adrenopathy** (ăd″rĕn-ŏp′ă-thē) [″ + ″ + Gr. *pathos,* disease, suffering] Any disease of the adrenal glands.

**adrenosterone** (ăd″rĕ-nŏs′tĕ-rōn) An androgenic hormone secreted by the adrenal cortex.

**adrenotoxin** (ăd-rē″nō-tŏk′sĭn) [″ + ″ + *Gr. toxikon,* poison] A substance toxic to the adrenal glands.

**adrenotropic** (ăd-rē″nō-trŏp′ĭk) [″ + ″ + Gr. *tropikos,* turning] Nourishing or stimulating to the adrenal glands, with reference esp. to hormones that stimulate adrenal gland function.

**Adriamycin** Trade name of doxorubicin, an antibiotic, antineoplastic drug.

**ADS** *antidiuretic substance.*

**Adson's maneuver** [Alfred W. Adson, U.S. neurosurgeon, 1887–1951] A test for thoracic outlet syndrome. The patient's arm is moved back into extension and external rotation with the elbow extended and forearm supinated. The radial pulse is palpated while the patient is asked to tuck the chin, side bend the head toward the opposite side, and rotate the chin toward the side of the extended arm. The patient is then asked to inhale. A positive sign of numbness or tingling in the hand or diminished pulse indicates the brachial plexus or blood vessels are compromised at the site of the scalene muscle.

**adsorb** Attachment of a substance to the surface of another material. SEE: *absorb; absorption.*

**adsorbate** (ăd-sor′bāt) Anything that is adsorbed.

**adsorbent** (ăd-sor′bĕnt) **1.** Pert. to adsorption. **2.** A substance that leads readily to adsorption, such as activated charcoal or magnesia.

**adsorption** (ăd-sorp′shŭn) [L. *ad,* to, + *sorbere,* to suck in] Adhesion by a gas or liquid to the surface of a solid.

**adsternal** (ăd-stĕr′năl) [″ + Gr. *sternon,* chest] Near or toward the sternum.

**adterminal** (ăd-tĕr′mĭ-năl) [″ + *terminus,* boundary] Toward the extremity of any structure, such as the end of a nerve or muscle.

**adtorsion** (ăd-tor′shŭn) [″ + *torsio,* twisted] Convergent squint; inward rotation of both eyes.

**adult** (ă-dŭlt′) [L. *adultus,* grown up] The fully grown and mature organism.

**adulteration** (ă-dŭl″tĕr-ā′shŭn) [L. *adulterare,* to pollute] The addition or substitution of an impure, weaker, cheaper, or possibly toxic substance in a formulation or product.

**adult foster care** ABBR: AFC. Long-term care for elderly individuals in an adult foster care facility. Typically, such a facility resembles a residence rather than a nursing home and may have fewer regulations than a nursing home.

**adult onset $G_{M2}$ gangliosidosis** A slowly progressing disease caused by the gradual accumulation of the GM ganglioside in neurons due to defective hexosaminidase (Hex A). It is found among Ashkenazi Jews and manifests itself with symptoms of psychosis or dementia. It may be referred to as adult-onset Tay-Sachs disease.

**adult respiratory distress syndrome** SEE: *acute respiratory distress syndrome.*

**advance** (ăd-văns′) [Fr. *avancer,* to set forth] To carry out the surgical procedure of advancement.

**advanced cardiac life support** ABBR: ACLS. A procedure that includes basic life support (BLS), plus the use of adjunctive equipment to support ventilation, establishment of an IV fluid line, drug administration, cardiac monitoring, defibrillation, control of cardiac arrhythmias, and postresuscitation care. ACLS requires the supervision of a physician in person at the scene of the emergency, direct communication with one, or an alternative method of communication previously defined by the physician, such as standing orders. Patients in whom field resuscitation (i.e., prehospital ACLS) fails are usually rushed to a local emergency department where resuscitation attempts are continued, though few of these patients survive. SEE: *basic life support; cardiopulmonary resuscitation; emergency cardiac care.*

**advance directive** A legal document prepared when an individual is alive, competent, and able to make decisions. It provides guidance to the health care team if the person is no longer capable of making decisions. SEE: *living will; power of attorney, durable, for health care.*

**advancement** (ăd-văns′mĕnt) [Fr. *avancer,* to set forth] An operation to remedy strabismus; the ocular muscle is severed and then attached at a point farther from its origin.

***capsular a.*** Attachment of the capsule of Tenon in front of its normal position.

**adventitia** (ăd″vĕn-tĭsh′ē-ă) [L. *adventicius,* coming from abroad] The outermost covering of a structure or organ, such as the tunica adventitia or outer coat of an artery.

**adventitious** (ăd″vĕn-tĭsh′ŭs) **1.** Acquired; accidental. **2.** Arising sporadically. **3.** Pert. to adventitia.

**adventitious breath sounds** Abnormal breath sounds heard when listening to the chest as the person breathes. These may be rhonchi (wheezes), crackles (rales), or pleural friction rubs. They do not include sounds produced by muscular activity in the chest wall or friction of the stethoscope on the chest.

**adverse reaction** In pharmacology and therapeutics, an undesired side effect or toxicity caused by the administration of drugs. Onset may be sudden or take days to develop. Early detection by use of laboratory tests is sometimes possible in the case of drugs that might adversely affect the blood-forming organs, liver, or kidneys. It is important for health care personnel to be aware that a patient may develop an adverse reaction to a drug. SYN: *drug interaction; drug reaction.*

**advocacy** (ăd′vō-kă-sē) In health care, pleading or representation of the needs of the patient.

**adynamia** (ăd″ĭ-nā′mē-ă) [Gr. *a-*, not, + *dynamis,* strength] Weakness or loss of strength, esp. due to muscular or cerebellar disease. SYN: *asthenia; debility.* **adynamic** (-năm′ĭk, ā-dī-năm′ĭk), *adj.*

**adynamic ileus** Intestinal obstruction resulting from lack of intestinal motility. This causes abdominal distention and interferes with postsurgical recovery, esp. from abdominal surgery.

NURSING IMPLICATIONS: The entire abdomen is auscultated for bowel sounds and assessed for distention by inspection, measurement of abdominal girth, and percussion for tympanic note every 4 to 8 hr as necessary. Nausea and vomiting, lack of passage of flatus, increases in girth, and changes in bowel sounds are documented and reported. If the ileus is still present after 24 to 48 hr, the patient is prepared for diagnostic tests such as abdominal radiographs and for treatment procedures such as insertion of a nasogastric (NG) or intestinal (Cantor) tube for decompression. Prescribed medications, such as gastrointestinal stimulants or cholinergics, are given and the patient is warned that intestinal cramping and diarrhea may result. The NG tube is kept open, the amount and character of drainage are recorded, and ambulation is encouraged to stimulate bowel activity. The nurse evaluates desired therapeutic effects, checking frequently for return of bowel sounds and, if neostigmine (a cholinergic) is prescribed, for adverse cardiovascular effects such as bradycardia and hypotension.

**A.E.** *above elbow;* term refers to the site of amputation of an upper extremity.

**Aedes** (ă-ē′dēs) [Gr. *aedes,* unpleasant] A genus of mosquitoes belonging to the family Culicidae. Many species are troublesome pests and some transmit disease.

***A. aegypti*** A species of *Aedes* that transmits yellow fever and dengue.

***A. triseriatus*** A species that transmits Jamestown Canyon virus or La Crosse virus, either of which can cause encephalitis.

**aer-** (ĕr) [Gr. *aer,* air] Combining form indicating relationship to gas or air.

**aerated** (ĕr′ā″tĕd) Containing air or gas.

**aeration** (ĕr″ā′shŭn) **1.** Act of airing. **2.** Process whereby carbon dioxide is exchanged for oxygen in blood in the lungs. **3.** Saturating or charging a fluid with gases.

**aero-, aer-** (ĕr′ō) Combining form indicating relationship to air or gas.

**aerobe** (ĕr′ōb) *pl.* **aerobes** [″ + *bios,* life] A microorganism that is able to live and grow in the presence of oxygen.

***facultative a.*** A microorganism that prefers an environment devoid of oxygen but has adapted so that it can live and grow in the presence of oxygen.

***obligate a.*** A microorganism that can live and grow only in the presence of oxygen.

**aerobic** (ĕr-ō′bĭk) **1.** Living only in the presence of oxygen. **2.** Concerning an organism living only in the presence of oxygen.

**aerobic exercise** Exercise during which oxygen is metabolized to produce energy. Aerobic exercise is required for sustained periods of hard work and vigorous athletic activity. SEE: *anaerobic exercise.*

**aerobic training** Exercise training for the purpose of attaining aerobic conditioning. No formula can be universally applied, but a general guideline is that aerobic conditioning will be obtained by normal, healthy persons who exercise three to five times a week for 20 to 30 min each time and at an intensity that produces a heart rate of 220 minus the age of the individual.

**aerobiosis** (ĕr″ō-bī-ō′sĭs) [Gr. *aer,* air, + *biosis,* mode of living] Living in an atmosphere containing oxygen.

**aerocele** (ĕr′ō-sēl) [″ + *kele,* tumor, swelling] Distention of a cavity with gas.

**aerocoly** (ĕr″ŏk′ō-lē) [″ + *kolon,* colon] Distention of the colon with gas.

**aerocystoscopy** (ĕr″ō-sĭs-tŏs′kō-pē) [″ + *kystis,* bladder, + *skopein,* to examine] Examination with a cystoscope of the bladder distended by air.

**aerodontalgia** (ĕr″ō-dŏnt-ăl′jē-ă) [″ + *odous,* tooth, + *algos,* pain] Pain in the teeth resulting from a change in atmospheric pressure.

**aerodontia** (ĕr″ō-dŏn′shē-ă) Branch of dentistry concerned with the effect of changes in atmospheric pressure on the teeth.

**aerodynamics** (ĕr″ō-dī-năm′ĭks) [Gr. *aer,* air, + *dynamis,* force] The science of air or gases in motion.

**aeroembolism** (ĕr″ō-ĕm′bō-lĭzm) [″ + *embolos,* plug, + *-ismos,* condition] A condition in which nitrogen bubbles form in body fluids and tissues during rapid ascent to high altitudes; can also occur in skin diving or in hyperbaric oxygen therapy if return to sea level atmospheric pressure is too rapid. SEE: *bends; caisson disease.*

SYMPTOMS: Symptoms include boring, gnawing pain in the joints, itching of skin and eyelids, unconsciousness, convulsions, and paralysis. Symptoms are relieved by recompression (i.e., return to lower altitudes or placement of the patient in a hyperbaric pressure chamber). Even though oxygen by mask may be available, ascents above 25,000 ft should be avoided except in planes with pressurized cabins.

**aerogenesis** (ĕr″ō-jĕn′ĕ-sĭs) [″ + *genesis,* generation, birth] Formation of gas. **aerogenic, aerogenous** (ĕr″ō-jĕn′ĭk, -ŏj′ĕn-ŭs), *adj.*

**aerometer** (ĕr-ŏm′ĕ-tĕr) [Gr. *aer,* air, + *metron,* measure] A device for measuring gas density.

**Aeromonas** (ĕr″ō-mō′năs) A genus of bacteria found in natural water sources and soil. It is a gram-negative, non-spore-forming, motile bacillus. Aeromonads are commonly pathogenic for cold-blooded marine animals. Their importance in serious human diseases has been increasing, esp. in immunocompromised hosts. As opportunistic infections, *Aeromonas* infections may occur in otherwise healthy hosts.

***A. hydrophilia*** A type of *Aeromonas* that is pathogenic for humans; it is sensitive to chloramphenicol, trimethoprim-sulfamethoxazole, and some quinolones.

**aero-otitis** Otitis resulting from pressure changes when auditory tubes are obstructed. It occurs commonly in aviators and divers. SYN: *barotitis.*

**aeroparotitis** Swelling of one or both parotid glands due to introduction of air into the glands. This may occur in those who play wind instruments; it also occurs in nose blowing and Valsalva's maneuver if done too vigorously.

**aeroperitoneum, aeroperitonia** (ĕr″ō-pĕr″ĭ-tō-nē′ŭm, -tō′nē-ă) [″ + *peritonaion,* peritoneum] Distention of the peritoneal cavity caused by gas.

**aerophagia, aerophagy** (ĕr″ō-fā′jē-ă, ĕr″ŏf′ă-jē) [″ + *phagein,* to eat] Swallowing of air.

**aerophilic, aerophilous** (ĕr″ō-fĭl′ĭk, -of′ĭ-lŭs) [″ + *philein,* to love] Requiring air for growth and development. SYN: *aerobic.*

**aerophobia** (ĕr-ō-fō′bē-ă) [″ + *phobos,* fear] Morbid fear of a draft or of fresh air.

**aerophyte** (ĕr′-ō-fīt) [″ + *phyton,* plant] A plant or vegetative organism that derives its sustenance from air.

**aerosinusitis** (ĕr″ō-sī″nŭs-ī′tĭs) [″ + L. *sinus,* a hollow, + Gr. *itis,* inflammation] Chronic inflammation of nasal sinuses due to changes in atmospheric pressure.

**aerosol** (ĕr′ō-sŏl) [″ + L. *solutio,* solution] A colloidal solution dispensed as a mist.

**aerosolization** (ĕr″ō-sŏl″ĭ-zā′shŭn) Production of an aerosol.

**aerosol therapy** The inhalation of aerosolized medicines, such as corticosteroids or mucolytic agents, in the treatment of pulmonary conditions such as asthma, bronchitis, and emphysema. SEE: *inhalation therapy.*

**Aerosporin** (ĕr″ō-spō′rin) Trade name for polymyxin B sulfate. SEE: *polymyxin.*

**aerotherapy** (ĕr″ō-thĕr′ă-pē) [″ + *therapeia,* treatment] The use of air in the treatment of disease, using changes in composition and density. SEE: *hyperbaric oxygen.*

**aerothermotherapy** (ĕr″ō-thĕr″mō-thĕr′ă-pē) [″ + *thermos,* heat, + *therapeia,* treatment] Therapeutic use of hot air.

**aerotitis** (ĕr-ō-tī′tĭs) [″ + *ot-,* ear, + *itis,* inflammation] Inflammation of the ear, esp. the middle ear, due to failure of the eustachian tube to remain open during sudden changes in barometric pressure, as may occur during flying, diving, or working in a pressure chamber. SYN: *barotitis.*

**aerotropism** (ĕr-ŏt′rō-pĭzm) [″ + *trope,* a turn, + *-ismos,* condition] The tendency of organisms, esp. bacteria and protozoa, to move toward air (positive aerotropism) or away from it (negative aerotropism).

**aerourethroscope** (ĕr-ō-ū″rē′thrō-skōp″) [″ + *ourethra,* urethra, + *skopein,* to examine] An apparatus for visual examination of the urethra after dilatation by air.

**aerourethroscopy** (ĕr″ō-ū″rē-thrŏs′kō-pē) Visual examination of the urethra when distended with air.

**Aesculapius** (ĕs″kū-lā′pē-ŭs) The Roman name for the god of medicine; son of Apollo and the nymph Coronis.

***staff of A.*** A rod or crude stick with a snake wound around it, used to signify the art of healing and adopted as the emblem of some medical organizations (e.g., American Medical Association). Snakes were sacred to Aesculapius because they were believed to have the power to renew their youth by shedding their old skin and growing a new one. SEE: *caduceus.*

**aesthetics** (ĕs-thĕt′ĭks) [Gr. *aisthesis,* sensation] The philosophy or the theory of beauty and the fine arts. These concepts are esp. important in dental restorations and in plastic and cosmetic surgery. Also spelled *esthetics.*

***dental a.*** The application of aesthetics to natural or artificial teeth or restorations, usually with regard to form and color.

**afebrile** (ā-fĕb′rĭl) [Gr. *a-,* not, + L. *febris,* fever] Without fever.

**affect** (ăf′fĕkt) [L. *affectus,* exerting influence on] In psychology, the emotional reaction associated with an experience. SEE: *mood.*

***blunted a.*** Greatly diminished emotional response to a situation or condition.

***flat a.*** Virtual absence of emotional response to a situation or condition.

**affection** (ă-fĕk′shŭn) **1.** Love, feeling. **2.** Physical or mental disease.

**affective** (ă-fĕk′tĭv) Pert. to an emotion or mental state.

**affective disorder** A disorder marked by a disturbance of mood accompanied by a full or partial manic or depressive syndrome that is not caused by any other physical or mental disorder. SEE: *Nursing Diagnoses Appendix.*

**afferent** (ăf′ĕr-ĕnt) [L. *ad,* to, + *ferre,* to bear] Carrying impulses toward a center, as when a sensory nerve carries a message toward the brain; also said of certain veins and lymphatics; opposite of efferent.

**afferent loop syndrome** A group of gastrointestinal symptoms that occur in some patients who have had partial gastric resection with gastrojejunostomy. The condition is caused by partial obstruction of an incompletely draining afferent intestinal loop. In some cases there is bacterial overgrowth in the afferent loop. Symptoms include abdominal bloating, nausea, vomiting, and pain after eating.

**afferent nerve** SEE: *nerve, afferent.*

**affidavit** A voluntary written or printed statement of facts that is confirmed by the person's oath or affirmation.

**affiliation** (ă-fĭl-ē-ā′shŭn) [L. *affiliare,* to take to oneself as a son] **1.** Membership in a larger organization. **2.** Association. In nursing education, the administrative association of two hospitals or schools of nursing. This enables nurses to obtain specialized training and experience that might not otherwise be available to them.

**affinity** (ă-fĭn′ĭ-tē) [L. *affinis,* neighboring] Attraction.

***chemical a.*** Force causing certain atoms to combine with others to form molecules. SEE: *chemoreceptor.*

***elective a.*** Force causing a substance to elect one substance rather than another with which to unite.

**A fiber** A heavily medullated, fast-conducting nerve fiber.

**afibrinogenemia** (ă-fī″brĭn-ō-jĕ-nē′mē-ă) [Gr. *a-,* not, + L. *fibra,* fiber, + Gr. *gennan,* to produce, + *haima,* blood] A rare blood disease marked by an absence or decrease of fibrinogen in the blood plasma so that the blood is incoagulable; may be congenital or acquired. (The term *hypofibrinogenemia* more accurately describes the disease process.) The acquired type is due to one of several causes that can reduce the plasma concentration of fibrinogen. This has been observed in severe trauma and burns, following extensive surgery, in obstetric complications of abruptio placentae or retention of a dead fetus, in neoplastic disease, in hepatic cirrhosis, in leukemia, in sarcoidosis, and in polycythemia vera. The clinical picture may develop suddenly. Administration of whole fresh blood and fibrinogen may prevent death from hemorrhage.

**aflatoxicosis** (ăf′lă-tŏk″sĭ-kō′sĭs) Poisoning caused by ingestion of peanuts or peanut products contaminated with *Aspergillus flavus* or other *Aspergillus* strains that produce aflatoxin. Farm animals and humans are susceptible to this toxicosis. SYN: *x-disease.*

**aflatoxin** (ăf′lă-tŏk′sĭn) A toxin produced by some strains of *Aspergillus flavus* and *A. parasiticus* that causes cancer in laboratory animals. It may be present in peanuts and other seeds contaminated with *Aspergillus* molds.

Caution: It is not practical to try to remove aflatoxin from contaminated foods in order to make them edible.

**AFO** *ankle-foot orthosis.*

**AFP** *alpha-fetoprotein.*

**afteraction** Continued reaction for some time after the stimulus ceases, esp. in nerve centers. In the sensory centers this action gives rise to aftersensations.

**afterbirth** The placenta and membranes expelled from the uterus after the birth of a child.

**aftercare 1.** Care of a convalescent after conclusion of treatment in a hospital or mental institution. **2.** A continuing program of rehabilitation designed to reinforce the effects of therapy and to help patients adjust to their environment.

**aftercataract 1.** Secondary cataract. **2.** An opacity of the lens capsule that develops after cataract removal.

**aftercurrent** Current produced in a tissue after electrical stimulation has ceased.

**afterdamp** A gaseous mixture formed by the explosion of methane and air in a mine; contains a large percentage of carbon dioxide, nitrogen, and carbon monoxide.

**afterdischarge** The discharge of impulses from a reflex center after stimulation of the receptor has ceased. It results in prolongation of the response.

**aftereffect** A response occurring some time after the original stimulus or condition has produced its primary effect.

**afterhearing** Perception of sound after the stimulus producing it has ceased to act.

**afterimage** Image that persists subjectively after cessation of the stimulus. If colors are the same as those of the object, it is called positive; it is called negative if complementary colors are seen. In the former case, the image is seen in its natural bright colors without any alteration; in the latter, the bright parts become dark, while dark parts are light.

***negative a.*** Afterimage in which the colors and light intensity are reversed.

***positive a.*** Afterimage in which the colors and light intensity are unchanged.

**afterimpression** Aftersensation.

**afterload** In cardiac physiology, the stress or tension that develops in the ventricular wall during systole. SEE: *preload.*

**afterloading** In brachytherapy, the insertion of the radioactive source after the placement of the applicator has been confirmed. Insertion is usually done in the patient's room.

**aftermovement** Persistent and spontaneous contraction of a muscle after a strong contraction against resistance has ceased. This is easily seen when a person forcibly pushes an arm against a wall while standing with the frontal plane perpendicular to the wall. When this is stopped and the person moves away from the wall, the arm abducts involuntarily and is elevated by the deltoid muscle. SYN: *Kohnstamm's phenomenon.*

**afterpains** Uterine cramps caused by contraction of the uterus and commonly seen in multiparas during the first few days after childbirth. The pains, which are more severe during nursing, rarely last longer than 48 hr postpartum.

TREATMENT: Analgesics provide relief, but aspirin should not be given if there is a bleeding tendency. The sooner an analgesic is given, the less is needed.

**afterperception** Perception of a sensation after cessation of the stimulus.

**afterpotential wave** The wave produced after the action potential wave passes along a nerve. On the recording of the electrical activity, it will be either a negative or positive wave smaller than the main spike.

**afterpressure** A feeling of pressure that remains for a few seconds after removal of a weight or other pressure.

**aftersensation** A sensation that persists after the stimulus causing it has ceased.

**aftertaste** Persistence of gustatory sensations after cessation of the stimulus.

**aftertreatment** Secondary treatment or that which follows the primary treatment regimen. SEE: *aftercare.*

**aftervision** Afterimage.

**Ag** [L. *argentum*] Symbol for the element silver.

**AGA** *appropriate for gestational age.*

**against medical advice** ABBR: AMA. Term used in reference to a patient's decision to discontinue treatment or hospitalization even though the patient was advised by competent professional personnel to continue.

**agamic** (ă-găm'ĭk) [Gr. *a-*, not, + *gamos*, marriage] **1.** Reproducing asexually. **2.** Asexual.

**agammaglobulinemia** (ă-găm″ă-glŏb″ū-lĭn-ē'mē-ă) [″ + *gamma globulin* + Gr. *haima*, blood] A broad term pert. to disorders marked by an almost complete lack of immunoglobulins or antibodies. The cause is abnormal B lymphocyte function. Unless the patient receives a successful bone marrow transplantation, death from infection occurs.

**agamogenesis** (ăg″ă-mō-jĕn'ĕ-sĭs) [″ + *gamos*, marriage, + *genesis*, generation, birth] **1.** Asexual reproduction. **2.** Parthenogenesis.

**agar** (ā'găr, ăg'ăr) [Malay, gelatin] **1.** A dried mucilaginous product obtained from certain species of algae, esp. of the genus *Gelidium.* Because it is unaffected by bacterial enzymes, it is widely used as a solidifying agent for bacterial culture media; it is also used as a laxative because of its great increase in bulk on absorption of water. **2.** A culture medium containing agar.

**agar-agar** Agar.

**agaric** (ă-găr'ĭk) [Gr. *agarikon*, a sort of fungus] A mushroom, esp. species of the genus *Agaricus.*

**agastria** (ă-găs'trē-ă) [Gr. *a-*, not, + *gaster*, stomach] Absence of the stomach. **agastric** (ă-găst'rĭk), *adj.*

**AgCl** Symbol for silver chloride.

**age** [Fr. *age*, L. *aetas*] **1.** The time from birth to the present for a living individual as measured in units of time. **2.** A particular period of life (e.g., middle age or old age). **3.** To grow old. **4.** In psychology, the degree of development of an individual expressed in terms of the age of an average individual of comparable development or accomplishment.

***achievement a.*** ABBR: A.A. The age of a person with regard to level of acquired learning; determined by a proficiency test and expressed in terms of the chronological age of the average person showing the same level of attainment.

***anatomical a.*** An estimate of age as judged by the stage of development or deterioration of the body or tissue as compared with persons or tissues of known age.

***biological a.*** One's present position in regard to the probability of survival. Determination of biological age requires assessment and measurment of the functional capacities of the life-limiting organ system (e.g., the cardiovascular system).

***bone a.*** An estimate of biological age based on radiological studies of the developmental stage of ossification centers of the long bones of the extremities. SEE: *epiphysis.*

***chronological a.*** ABBR: C.A. Age as determined by years since birth.

***conceptional a.*** The estimated gestational age as referenced from the actual time of conception. It is usually considered to be at least 14 days after the first day of the last menstrual period. SYN: *ovulation a.*

***developmental a.*** An index of maturation expressed in months or years, which represents a value obtained by comparing performance with scaled norms for a particular age group. SEE: *age, achievement.*

***emotional a.*** Judgment of age with respect to the stage of emotional development.

***functional a.*** Age defined in terms of physical or functional capacity; frequently applied to the elderly.

***gestational a.*** The age of an embryo or fetus as timed from the date of onset of the last menstrual period.

***menarcheal a.*** Elapsed time expressed in years from menarche.

***mental a.*** ABBR: M.A. The age of a person with regard to mental ability, determined by a series of mental tests devised by Binet and expressed in terms of the chronological age of the average person showing the same level of attainment.

***ovulation a.*** Conceptional a.

***physiological a.*** Age as determined by functional ability as compared with persons of the same chronological age.

**age of consent** The age at which a minor may legally engage in voluntary sexual intercourse or no longer require parental consent for marriage. It varies among states, but is usually between ages 13 and 18.

**aged** (ājd', ā'jĕd) **1.** To have grown older or more mature. **2.** Persons who have grown old. SEE: *aging.*

**ageism** (āj'ĭzm) [Robert Butler, U.S. physician, who coined the term in 1968] Discrimination against aged persons.

**Agency for Health Care Policy and Research** ABBR: AHCPR. An office of the U.S. department of Health and Human Services dedicated to enhancing the quality, appropriateness, and effectiveness of health care services and access to those services in the U.S. Its concerns include scientific research, the promotion of improvements in clinical practice, and the organization, financing, and delivery of health care services.

**agenesia, agenesis** (ă"jĕn-ē'sē-ă, ă-jĕn'ĕ-sis) [Gr. *a-,* not, + *genesis,* generation, birth] **1.** Failure of an organ or part to develop or grow. **2.** Lack of potency.

**agenitalism** (ă-jĕn'ĭ-tăl-ĭzm) [" + L. *genitalis,* genital, + Gr. *-ismos,* condition] Absence of genitals.

**agent** (ā'jĕnt) [L. *agere,* to do] Something that causes an effect; thus, bacteria that cause disease are said to be agents of the specific diseases they cause. A medicine is considered a therapeutic agent.

***chelating a.*** A drug, such as calcium disodium edetate, that is used to chelate substances, esp. toxic chemicals in the body.

***fixing a.*** SEE: *clearing agent.*

***sclerosing a.*** A substance used to cause sclerosis, esp. of the lining of a vein. SEE: *varicose veins.*

***surface-active a.*** Surfactant.

***wetting a.*** In radiographic film processing, a solution used after washing to reduce surface tension and accelerate water flow from the film. This process speeds drying.

**Agent Orange** A defoliant that U.S. military forces used extensively in the Vietnam War. It contained the toxic chemical dioxin as an unwanted and undesired contaminant. SEE: *dioxin.*

**agerasia** (ā-jĕr-ā'sē-ă) [Gr. *a-,* not, + *geras,* old age] Healthy, vigorous old age; youthful appearance of an old person.

**age-specific** Pert. to data, esp. in vital statistics and epidemiology, that are related to age.

**ageusia, ageustia** (ă-gū'sē-ă, ă-goos'tē-ă) [Gr. *a-,* not + *geusis,* taste] Absence, partial loss, or impairment of the sense of taste. SEE: *dysgeusia; hypergeusia; hypogeusia.*

ETIOLOGY: Ageusia may be caused by disease of the chorda tympani or of the gustatory fibers, excessive use of condiments, the effect of certain drugs, aging, or lesions involving sensory pathways or taste centers in the brain.

***central a.*** Ageusia due to a cerebral lesion.

***conduction a.*** Ageusia due to a lesion involving sensory nerves of taste.

***peripheral a.*** Ageusia due to a disorder of taste buds of the mucous membrane of tongue.

**agglomerate** (ă-glŏm'ĕ-rāt) [L. *ad,* to, + *glomerare,* to wind into a ball] To congregate; to form a mass.

**agglutinable** (ă-gloo'tĭ-nă-bl) [L. *agglutinans,* gluing] Capable of agglutination.

**agglutinant** (ă-gloo'tĭ-nănt) **1.** Substance causing adhesion. **2.** Causing union by adhesion, as in the healing of a wound. **3.** An antibody produced in the body in response to stimulation by an antigen (agglutinogen). SYN: *agglutinin.*

**agglutination** (ă-gloo"tĭ-nā'shŭn) **1.** A type of antigen-antibody reaction in which a solid antigen clumps together with a soluble antibody. It requires a cell with antigenic markers close to the surface, available for interaction with the antibody. The term often refers to laboratory tests and to transfusion reactions in which antibodies attach the antigens on red blood cells of a different blood type, causing the cells to clump together. **2.** Adhesion of surfaces of a wound.

***direct a.*** A test for the presence of a specific antibody performed by mixing a dilute antiserum with the antigen it is specific for (e.g., if clumping occurs when type A red blood cells are mixed with serum, the serum contains anti-A immunoglobulins).

***passive a.*** A test for the presence of a specific antibody in which inert particles or cells with no foreign antigenic markers are coated with a known soluble antigen and mixed with serum. If agglutination occurs, an antibody to the antigen is present in the blood. Frequently, red blood cells are used as the carriers after they are washed to remove any known antibodies.

***platelet a.*** Clumping of platelets in response to immunological reactions.

**agglutinative** (ă-gloo'tĭ-nā"tĭv) Causing or capable of causing agglutination.

**agglutinin** (ă-gloo'tĭ-nĭn) [L. *agglutinans,* gluing] An antibody present in the blood that attaches to an antigen on red blood cells, causing them to agglutinate or clump together; used primarily in reference to laboratory tests of agglutination. Agglutinins cause transfusion reactions when blood from a different group is given. These antibodies are present at birth and require no exposure to an antigen to be created, since they are genetically determined.

***anti-Rh a.*** An antibody produced in human plasma but sometimes produced in Rh-negative mothers bearing an Rh-positive fetus or in Rh-negative individuals who have received one or more transfusions of Rh-positive blood.

***cold a.*** A red blood cell agglutinin that acts only at low temperatures (0° to 20°C). It is found in the serum of patients with atypical pneumonia and in certain blood diseases.

**agglutinogen** (ă-gloo-tĭn′ō-jĕn) [L. *agglutinans,* gluing, + Gr. *gennan,* to produce] The specific antigen that stimulates the recognition of an agglutinin, or antibody; used primarily in reference to laboratory testing for antibodies against specific blood types. SEE: *blood groups.* **agglutinogenic, agglutogenic** (ă-gloo″tĭ-nō-jen′ĭk, ă-gloo″tō-jĕn′ĭk), *adj.*

***A and B a.'s*** Antigenic substances discovered by Karl Landsteiner in 1901 that are found on the membranes of red blood cells in humans and that react with the alpha (anti-A) and beta (anti-B) isoagglutinins in mismatched blood. The red corpuscles may contain A or B, both A and B, or neither A nor B agglutinogens. The four resulting blood groups are A, B, AB, and O, respectively. Blood groups are inherited according to Mendel's laws.

***M and N a.'s*** Antigenic substances found on the membranes of red blood cells in humans. Anti-M and anti-N agglutinins are rarely found in normal serum. The red blood cells may contain M or N, or both M and N agglutinogens, resulting in blood types M, N, or MN, respectively.

***Rh a.*** A specific substance called the Rh factor, which is found on the membranes of the red blood cells. It was discovered in 1940 by Landsteiner and Wiener, who prepared anti-Rh serum by injecting red cells from Rhesus monkeys into rabbits or other animals. They found that the red cells of 85% of people of the Caucasian race will be agglutinated when in contact with anti-Rh serum. These people are called Rh-positive. The remaining 15%, whose red cells are not agglutinated by anti-Rh serum, are termed Rh-negative. More than 25 blood factors are known to belong to the Rh system. Their importance in blood typing and blood type incompatibility between mother and fetus makes this blood group system second in importance only to the ABO group.

**agglutinophilic** (ă-gloo″tĭn-ō-fĭl′ĭk) [″ + Gr. *philos,* fond] Readily agglutinating.

**aggregate** (ăg′rĕ-gāt) [L. *aggregatus,* collect] **1.** Total substances making up a mass. **2.** To cluster or come together.

**aggregation** (ăg″rĕ-gā′shŭn) A clustering or coming together of substances.

***cell a.*** Clumping together of blood cells, esp. platelets or red cells.

***familial a.*** A cluster of the same disease in closely related families.

**aggression** (ă-grĕsh′ŭn) [L. *aggredi,* to approach with hostility] **1.** A forceful physical, verbal, or symbolic action. It may be appropriate and self-protective, indicating healthy self-assertiveness, or it may be inappropriate. The behavior may be directed outward toward the environment or inward toward the self. **2.** Activity performed in a forceful manner.

**aging** (āj′ĭng) Growing old, maturing; not replacing enough cells to maintain complete function; progressive changes related to the passage of time. There is no precise method for determining the rate or degree of aging. In a study of 1500 persons aged 100 years or more, the following were determined: longevity is not inheritable; sexual activity is both good and feasible for the aged; the strain of child rearing does not shorten life; the older person's offspring need not love him or her; and one should work hard all during life, however long. Proper care and hygiene usually prolong life and reduce the risk of disability.

The physiological changes occurring with age (diminished neurotransmitters, circulatory capacity, sensory acuity, and perception) affect the brain. These changes do not indicate a loss of cognitive function. There is evidence of slower reaction time and information processing, but the majority of functioning and intelligence remains intact and sufficient.

Emotional trauma and multiple losses occurring in older age often lead to a diminished investment in life, causing professionals to misdiagnose cognitive dysfunction. The stress of demanding situations often contributes to what appears to be an organic disorder. Validation by a team of specialists is important in the diagnosis and treatment of any disorder affecting older persons. SEE: *Alzheimer's disease; dementia.*

**agitated depression** Depression accompanied by restlessness and increased psychomotor activity.

**agitation** (ăj″ĭ-tā′shŭn) [L. *agitare,* to drive] **1.** Excessive restlessness, increased mental and physical activity, esp. the latter. **2.** Tremor. **3.** Severe motor restlessness, usually nonpurposeful, associated with anxiety. **4.** Shaking of a container so that the contents are rapidly moved and mixed.

**agitographia** (ăj″ĭ-tō-grăf′ē-ă) [″ + Gr. *graphein,* to write] Writing with excessive rapidity, with unconscious omission of words and syllables.

**agitophasia** (ăj″ĭ-tō-fā′zē-ă) [″ + Gr. *phasis,* speech] Excessive rapidity of speech, with slurring, omission, and distortion of sounds.

**aglaucopsia, aglaukopsia** (ă″glaw-kŏp′sē-ă) [Gr. *a-,* not, + *glaukos,* green, + *opsis,* vision] Green blindness; color blindness in which there is a defect in the perception of green. SEE: *color blindness.*

**aglossia** (ă-glŏs′ē-ă) [″ + *glossa,* tongue] Congenital absence of the tongue.

**aglossostomia** (ă″glŏs-ō-stō′mē-ă) [″ + ″ + *stoma,* mouth] Congenital absence of the tongue and mouth opening.

**aglutition** (ă-gloo-tĭsh′ŭn) [″+ L. *glutire,* to swallow] Difficulty in swallowing or inability to swallow.

**aglycemia** (ă″glī-sē′mē-ă) [″ + *glykys,* sweet, + *haima,* blood] Lack of sugar in the blood.

**aglycon, aglycone** The substance attached to the chemical structure of digitalis glycosides. It is responsible for the cardiotonic activity of those agents.

**aglycosuric** (ă-glī″kō-sū′rĭk) [″ + ″ + *ouron,* urine] Free from glycosuria.

**agminate(d)** (ăg′mĭ-nāt) [L. *agmen,* a crowd] Aggregated; grouped in clusters.

**agminated follicle** Aggregation of a solitary follicle or a group of lymph nodes, principally in the lower portion of the small intestine. SYN: *Peyer's patch.*

**agnathia** (ăg-nā′thē-ă) [Gr. *a-,* not, + *gnathos,* jaw] Absence of the lower jaw.

**agnea** (ăg′nē-ă) [″ + *gnosis,* knowledge] Inability to recognize objects.

**$AgNO_3$** Symbol for silver nitrate.

**agnogenic** (ăg-nō-jĕn′ĭk) [″ + *gnosis,* knowledge, + *gennan,* to produce] Of unknown origin or etiology.

**agnosia** (ăg-nō′zē-ă) [″ + *gnosis,* knowledge] Loss of comprehension of auditory, visual, or other sensations although the sensory sphere is intact.

***auditory a.*** Mental inability to interpret sounds.

***finger a.*** Inability to identify fingers of one's own hands or of others.

***optic a.*** Mental inability to interpret images that are seen.

***tactile a.*** Inability to distinguish objects by sense of touch.

***time a.*** Unawareness of the sequence and duration of events.

***unilateral spatial a.*** Unilateral visual inattention.

***visual object a.*** SEE: *visual object agnosia.*

**-agogue** (ă-gŏg) [Gr. *agogos,* leading, inducing] Suffix meaning *producer* or *leader.*

**agonad, agonadal** (ă-gō′năd, ă-gŏn′ă-dăl) [Gr. *a-,* not, + *gone,* seed] Lacking gonads.

**agonal** (ăg′ō-năl) [Gr. *agon,* a contest] Rel. to death or agony (e.g., agonal changes in tissue that occur after death).

**agonist** (ăg′ŏn-ĭst) **1.** The muscle directly engaged in contraction as distinguished from muscles that have to relax at the same time; thus, in bending the elbow, the biceps brachii is the agonist and the triceps the antagonist. **2.** In pharmacology, a drug that binds to the receptor and stimulates the receptor's function. Drugs that mimic the body's own regulatory function are called agonists.

**agony** (ăg′ō-nē) **1.** Extreme mental or physical suffering. **2.** Death struggle.

**agoraphobia** (ăg″ō-ră-fō′bē-ă) [Gr. *agora,* marketplace, + *phobos,* fear] Overwhelming symptoms of anxiety, often leading to a panic attack. The attack may occur in a variety of everyday situations (e.g., standing in line, eating in public, in crowds of people, on bridges or in tunnels; while driving) in which a person may be unable to escape or get help and may be embarrassed. Panic attack symptoms often include rapid heartbeat, chest pain, difficulty breathing, gastrointestinal distress, faintness, dizziness, weakness, sweating, fear of losing control or going crazy, and fear of dying or impending doom. People with these symptoms often avoid phobic situations, even to the point of staying at home for their entire lives.

**-agra** [Gr. *agra,* a seizure] Suffix indicating sudden severe pain.

**agranulocyte** (ă-grăn′ū-lō-sīt) [Gr. *a-,* not, + L. *granulum,* granule, + Gr. *kytos,* cell] A nongranular leukocyte.

**agranulocytosis** (ă-grăn″ū-lō-sī-tō′sĭs) [″ + ″ + ″ + *osis,* condition] An acute disease marked by a deficit or absolute lack of granulocytic white blood cells (neutrophils, basophils, and eosinophils). SYN: *granulocytopenia.* **agranulocytic** (-sĭt′ĭk), *adj.*

**agranuloplastic** (ă-grăn″ū-lō-plăs′tĭk) [″ + L. *granulum,* granule, + Gr. *plastikos,* formative] Unable to form granular cells.

**agranulosis** (ă-grăn″ū-lō′sĭs) Agranulocytosis.

**agraphesthesia** Inability to recognize letters or numbers drawn by the examiner on skin. Patients' eyes are closed if this is done on skin visible to them. SEE: *graphesthesia.*

**agraphia** (ă-grăf′ē-ă) [Gr. *a-,* not, + *graphein,* to write] Loss of the ability to write. SYN: *logagraphia.* SEE: *aphasia, motor.*

***absolute a.*** Complete inability to write.

***acoustic a.*** Inability to write words that are heard.

***amnemonic a.*** Inability to write sentences, although letters or words can be written.

***cerebral a.*** Inability to express thoughts in writing.

***motor a.*** Inability to write due to muscular incoordination.

***optic a.*** Inability to copy words.

***verbal a.*** Inability to write words although letters can be written.

**agrypnocoma** (ă-grĭp″nō-kō′mă) [Gr. *agrypnos,* sleepless, + *koma,* a deep sleep] Coma in which the individual is partially awake as if in an extreme lethargic state; may be associated with muttering, delirium, and lack of sleep.

**agrypnotic** (ă″grĭp-nŏt′ĭk) **1.** Afflicted with insomnia. **2.** Causing wakefulness.

**agyria** (ă-jī′rē-ă) [Gr. *a-,* not, + *gyros,* circle] Incompletely developed convolutions of the cerebral cortex. **agyric** (-rĭk), *adj.*

**ah** *hypermetropic astigmatism.*

**A.H.A.** *American Heart Association; American Hospital Association.*

**A.H.C.P.R.** *Agency for Health Care Policy and Research.*

**AHF** *antihemophilic factor,* coagulation factor VIII. SEE: *coagulation factor.*

**AHG** *antihemophilic globulin,* coagulation factor VIII. SEE: *coagulation factor.*

**AHIMA** *American Health Information Management Association.*

**Ahlfeld's sign** (ăl'fĕlts) [Friedrich Ahlfeld, Ger. obstetrician, 1843–1929] Irregular uterine contractions after the third month of pregnancy. It is a presumptive sign of pregnancy.

**A.I.** *aortic insufficiency; artificial insemination; artificial intelligence; axioincisal.*

**aichmophobia** (āk″mō-fō′bē-ă) [Gr. *aichme,* point, + *phobos,* fear] Morbid fear of being touched by pointed objects or fingers.

**A.I.D.** *Agency for International Development; artificial insemination by donor* (heterologous insemination).

**aid** (ād) Assistance provided to a person, esp. one who is sick, injured, or troubled. SEE: *first aid.*

***hearing a.*** SEE: *hearing aid.*

***robotic a.*** A mechanical device guided remotely by a person with a disability to assist with or enable daily living tasks.

**AIDS** *Acquired Immunodeficiency Syndrome.* The combination of specific clinical conditions and CD4+ T lymphocyte counts designated by the Centers for Disease Control and Prevention (CDC) as the final stage of infection by the human immunodeficiency virus (HIV). Approx. 70% of HIV-infected individuals develop AIDS within 10 years. Although there is no evidence that persons infected with AIDS have been cured, some of those infected have survived for a number of years and many of those survivors are asymptomatic.

Information about AIDS may be obtained in the U.S. by calling 1-800-342-AIDS, and in Canada (Ontario) by calling 1-800-668-AIDS.

ETIOLOGY: Two human immunodeficiency viruses, HIV-1 and HIV-2, have been identified. Both cause AIDS, but infection with HIV-2 has been primarily limited to Africa and Europe. Infection results when a glycoprotein on the surface of the virus binds to the CD4 receptors found on T lymphocytes, monocytes, macrophages, follicle dendritic cells in lymph nodes, and certain central and peripheral nerve cells, causing their destruction and a progressive loss of immune function. HIV is a retrovirus that uses an enzyme called reverse transcriptase to convert its viral RNA to viral DNA, using the host cell DNA to do so. The viral DNA then becomes incorporated into the host cell DNA. The change in DNA prevents the cell from functioning normally; it can only create more virus. Eventually, the cell ruptures, releasing more HIV into the bloodstream. The role of other sexually transmitted diseases in increasing the rate of immune depression by HIV is still unclear.

SYMPTOMS: The progress of HIV infection can be roughly divided into five stages, with the recognition that these stages can vary depending on characteristics such as age, sex, race, and country. Exposure to HIV is followed by an asymptomatic incubation period of several weeks during which the virus replicates. The first signs of acute infection are vague: fever, malaise, rash, arthralgias, and lymphadenopathy. Although the infection could be detected by blood analysis for HIV antibodies at this time, individuals rarely seek care because these signs are nebulous and insignificant. Following this acute stage, there is a prolonged asymptomatic phase (5 to 10 years); only a steady drop in CD4+ T lymphocytes indicates progression of the infection. The virus is believed to lie sequestered in the lymph nodes, spleen, and liver. Generalized lymphadenopathy is seen frequently and has become part of the latest CDC classification system.

When the virus has destroyed a sufficient number of CD4+ T lymphocytes and other white blood cells, patients become symptomatic, reporting low-grade fevers, night sweats, chronic diarrhea, and peripheral neuropathy. Vaginal and oral ulcers from *Candida albicans* and shingles from reactivation of varicella zoster virus are common. This phase lasts for approx. 3 years before the AIDS is diagnosed. AIDS is marked by opportunistic infections caused by organisms that would be eliminated in people with healthy immune systems. Organisms responsible for common opportunistic infection include *Candida albicans, Cryptosporidium, Pneumocystis carinii,* and *Toxoplasma gondii.* SEE: table.

DIAGNOSIS: The presence of antibodies to HIV in the blood is a sign of HIV infection. These antibodies do not destroy the virus, they simply serve as markers of infection. Clinical signs and symptoms and laboratory tests confirm it. The Western blot test is the most sensitive laboratory test for HIV antibodies; enzyme-linked immunosorbent assays (ELISA) are used more often, however, because they are less costly and require less time. Positive ELISA tests are validated by the Western blot test. The absolute CD4+ T lymphocyte count and beta-2 microglobulin levels are used, along with clinical signs, to measure the progress of the disease. In 1992, the CDC reported a revised system for categorizing HIV infection and the clinical conditions that constitute AIDS. A CD4+ T-cell count of less than 200/mm$^3$ and the presence of any one of 25 clinical conditions are now used to diagnose AIDS.

**Clinical Conditions and Opportunistic Infections Indicating AIDS**

| | |
|---|---|
| *Candida* infections (candidiasis) of the trachea, bronchi, or lungs | Kaposi's sarcoma |
| Candidiasis of the esophagus | Lymphoma, Burkitt's |
| Cervical cancer, invasive | Lymphoma, immunoblastic |
| *Coccidioides immitis:* Extrapulmonary infections or disseminated | Lymphoma, primary brain |
| *Cryptococcus neoformans:* Infections outside the lung | *Mycobacterium avium* complex or *M. kansasii:* Extrapulmonary infections or disseminated |
| *Cryptosporidium:* Chronic infections of the gastrointestinal tract* | *Mycobacterium tuberculosis:* Pulmonary or extrapulmonary infections |
| Cytomegalovirus: Infections other than liver, spleen, or lymph nodes | *Mycobacterium,* other species: Extrapulmonary infections or disseminated |
| Cytomegalovirus retinitis with loss of vision | *Pneumocystis carinii:* Pneumonia |
| Herpes simplex: Chronic oral ulcers, bronchitis, pneumonitis, or esophagitis | Pneumonia, recurrent |
| *Histoplasma capsulatum:* Infections outside of lung or disseminated | Progressive multifocal leukoencephalopathy |
| HIV-related encephalopathy | *Salmonella:* Septicemia, recurrent |
| Isosporiasis, chronic intestinal | *Toxoplasma:* Brain infections |
| | Wasting syndrome of HIV |

SOURCE: CDC:MMWR 41 (RR-17):2-3, 15, 1992.
* Chronic—more than 1 month's duration

Babies born to HIV-positive mothers are tested for HIV antibodies at birth, and at 1, 3, and 6 months. If their serum is positive but they have no clinical signs, they are considered to have "indeterminate" infection. Positive ELISA results at 15 or 18 months confirm infection. Children have a more rapid onset of the same clinical signs and symptoms displayed by adults plus failure to thrive.

MODE OF TRANSMISSION: HIV infection is spread by bodily secretions of the infected person coming in contact with the recipient's blood through a break in the skin or mucous membranes. Throughout the world, vaginal sexual intercourse, contaminated blood transfusions, needles or other invasive instruments, and transfer from mother to fetus or infant during pregnancy, delivery, or breastfeeding are the most common means of transmission. In the U.S., all blood is screened for HIV antibodies to reduce the risk to those receiving transfusions. Individuals engaging in unsafe sexual behaviors and those abusing intravenous drugs are at greatest risk. As long as they follow universal precautions, health care providers are not at increased risk. Research data indicate that the risk of HIV infection after a stick with a contaminated needle is 0.3%; the risk of seroconversion after mucous membranes are splashed with contaminated blood is 0.09%. The virus cannot survive outside the body (i.e., on counters or other flat surfaces). SEE: *sharps*; *Universal Precautions Appendix*.

PREVENTION: The public should be educated about HIV infection and condom use and safer sex techniques should be encouraged, esp. among teenagers and young adults. The benefits of limiting the number of sexual partners should be stressed. Intravenous drug users should be educated about the hazards of sharing needles and simple methods of disinfecting needles; those with HIV should be taught and encouraged to avoid infecting others. Pregnant women at risk should obtain testing because use of zidovudine during pregnancy reduces the incidence of HIV infection in infants. Maternal-infant transmission of HIV may be reduced if zidovudine is given to the mother before and during delivery and to the infant for 6 weeks after delivery. Long-term follow-up of children born to infected mothers is needed. SEE: *condom, instructions for use; safe sex*.

TREATMENT: The development of effective treatments for AIDS has been relatively slow in contrast to the rapid increase in knowledge about its pathophysiology over the last 10 years. Drugs approved by the U.S. Food and Drug Administration (FDA) include zidovudine (AZT); didanosine (ddI); zalcitabine (ddC); and stavudine (d4T). Combination therapy is more effective than use of a single drug.

The strict safety criteria established by the FDA for new drugs have been the subject of controversy. AIDS activist groups and others have argued that experimental drugs should be made available to volunteers more quickly. As a result, some drugs that have shown promising experimental results are available to a limited number of patients under "compassionate use" protocols.

Evidence supporting the benefits of nonpharmacological therapies remains inconclusive. No drug has been discovered that prevents or cures HIV infection. However, several researchers are working to develop a safe, effective vaccine against AIDS; at least one will be used in phase 2 studies involving large numbers of volunteers.

PROGNOSIS: Despite an increased understanding of the ways in which HIV destroys the immune system, only limited progress has been made in extending the lives of those with AIDS. Life expectancy remains about 10 to 15 years after initial infection.

NURSING IMPLICATIONS: Universal precautions for blood and other body fluids are strictly observed. The nurse teaches the patient about transmission of infectious agents through infected blood or other body fluids and reviews measures to prevent transmission. The patient is assessed for palpable lymph nodes in two or more extrainguinal sites, a sign of lymphadenopathy; and for behavioral, cognitive, or motor changes associated with progressive dementia. Prescribed drug therapy is administered, and the patient is taught to identify and report adverse effects. The patient is encouraged to maintain as much physical activity as is tolerable, allowing time for both exercise and rest. Supportive care is provided for fatigue, anorexia, and fever. Meticulous skin care, with protection from diarrhea and excoriation, is provided, esp. for the debilitated patient. The patient's mouth is rinsed with 0.9% sodium chloride or bicarbonate mouthwash before and after meals; glycerin swabs should be avoided because they dry mucous membranes. Caloric intake is recorded, and the need for small, frequent meals, nutritional supplements, or parenteral nutrition is assessed. Fluid status is monitored and adequate intake ensured. The nurse assists the patient to obtain social service support and funds for housing, food, and medication and for inpatient, outpatient, and hospice care. SEE: *Nursing Diagnoses Appendix*.

***perinatal A.*** AIDS in an infant born to an HIV-positive mother and acquiring the disorder during the perinatal period. The risk of perinatal infection is 25% to 35%. Most infected infants die within the first 18 months of life. Uninfected infants may exhibit positive antibody titers for as long as 15 months after birth due to the presence of maternal antibodies.

SYMPTOMS: Frequent diarrhea, weight loss, enlarged liver, spleen, and lymph nodes, susceptibility to infections, and developmental delays are indications of this disease.

NURSING IMPLICATIONS: The nurse maintains universal precautions and monitors status indicators closely. The infant is bathed as soon as possible after birth; invasive procedures are avoided until after the bath. The nurse demonstrates and explains to parents assessment techniques, such as taking the infant's temperature using an otic or pacifier thermometer for accuracy; health maintenance actions, such as careful skin care for diapered areas; and infection control procedures, such as disinfection of items contaminated with blood or excreta with a 1 : 10 solution of household bleach. The need for follow-up surveillance is emphasized.

**AIDS-dementia complex** ABBR: ADC. Encephalopathy caused by direct infection of brain tissue by the human immunodeficiency virus (HIV). The exact mechanism of infection is not known. The condition is classified as early or late by the type of clinical signs and symptoms. Early infection of the central nervous system is marked by memory loss, decreased ability to concentrate, a general slowing of cognitive processes, personality changes, hyperactive reflexes, difficulty in walking and performing other voluntary muscle movements, and tremor. Late infection is marked by severe cognitive changes, particularly confusion, changes in behavior, and sometimes psychoses. Seizures and significant muscle weakness also may be present. Children tend to have more pronounced central nervous system HIV infections than adults. Drugs that block central nervous system infection are under investigation. SYN: *HIV encephalopathy*.

**AIDS peripheral neuropathies** Direct infection of peripheral nerves by the human immunodeficiency virus (HIV) resulting in sensory and motor changes due to destruction of axons or their myelin covering. Acute or chronic inflammatory myelin damage may be the first sign of peripheral nerve involvement. Patients display gradual or abrupt onset of motor weakness and diminished or absent reflexes. Diagnostic biopsies of peripheral nerves show inflammatory changes and loss of myelin. Distal sensory neuropathy occurs in 20% to 50% of patients during the early symptomatic phase of HIV infection; bilateral foot and ankle pain, particularly on the soles of the feet, is occasionally accompanied by paresthesia. Degeneration of nerve axons seen on nerve biopsy is diagnostic. SEE: *AIDS; Guillain-Barré syndrome; polyneuropathy, chronic inflammatory demyelinating*.

**AIDS-related complex** ABBR: ARC. The progressive appearance of symptoms during the symptomatic stage of human immunodeficiency virus (HIV) infection before the development of AIDS. These clinical signs include fatigue, intermittent fevers, weight loss greater than 10%, chronic or persistent intermittent diarrhea, night sweats, diminished delayed hypersensitivity (skin test) response to common allergens, presence of HIV antibodies in blood, and decreased CD4+ T-lymphocyte count.. The term is not used extensively. SEE: *AIDS*.

**A.I.H.** *artificial insemination by husband*

(homologous insemination).

**ailment** A mild illness.

**ailurophobia** (ă-lū″rō-fō′bē-ă) [Gr. *ailouros,* cat, + *phobos,* fear] Morbid fear of cats.

**ainhum** (ān′hŭm) [East African, to saw] A fissured constriction around a digit; the cause is unknown. Due to the constriction, the digit will eventually require amputation. The fourth or fifth toe is usually affected and less commonly other digits of the feet or hands. It occurs primarily in dark-skinned races. There is no specific treatment.

**air** (ār) [Gr. *aer,* air] The invisible, tasteless, odorless mixture of gases surrounding the Earth. Clean air at sea level comprises approx. 78% nitrogen and 21% oxygen by volume. The remaining constituents are water vapor, carbon dioxide, and traces of ammonia, argon, helium, neon, krypton, xenon, and other rare gases.

***alveolar a.*** Air in the alveoli; that involved in the pulmonary exchange of gases between air and the blood. Its content is determined by sampling the last portion of a maximal expiration.

***complemental a.*** The volume of air that can be inspired over and above the tidal air by deepest possible inspiration. SYN: *inspiratory reserve volume.*

***dead space a.*** The volume of air that fills the respiratory passageways and is not available for exchange of gases with the blood.

***functional residual a.*** The volume of air in the lungs at the end of a normal expiration. It is the sum of supplemental air and residual air.

***liquid a.*** Air liquefied by great pressure. It produces intense cold on evaporation.

***mechanical dead space a.*** Dead space air provided by artificial means, as with mechanical ventilation or the addition of plastic tubing to a ventilator circuit.

***minimal a.*** The small volume of air trapped in the alveoli when lungs collapse with the thorax open; it is impossible to expel, even if the lung is removed.

***reserve a.*** Supplemental a.

***residual a.*** Air remaining in the lungs after the fullest possible expiration; about 1500 cc in the adult.

***supplemental a.*** The volume of air that can be expired after a normal expiration by fullest possible expiration; about 1600 cc in the adult. SYN: *expiratory reserve volume.*

***tidal a.*** The volume of air that flows in and out of the lungs with each normal respiration; average for a man is about 500 cc.

**air bed 1.** Large inflated cushion used as a mattress. **2.** Air-fluidized bed.

**air bronchogram sign** Radiographic appearance of an air-filled bronchus as it passes through an area of increased anatomic density as in pulmonary edema and pneumonia.

**air cell** Air vesicle.

**air conduction** The conduction of sound to the inner ear via the pathway provided by the air in the ear canal.

**air curtain** A current of air directed around a patient to block the air that would normally circulate around and contaminate the patient; used in isolating patients from dustborne bacteria or allergens. SEE: *laminar air flow.*

**air embolism** [L. *embolismus*] Obstruction of a blood vessel by an air bubble.

SYMPTOMS: Symptoms include sudden onset of dyspnea, unequal breath sounds, hypotension, weak pulse, elevated central venous pressure, cyanosis, sharp chest pains, hemoptysis, a churning murmur over the precordium, and decreasing level of consciousness.

ETIOLOGY: Air may enter a vessel postoperatively, during change of an intravenous set on a central line or by injection into a central line port or rupture of a central line balloon, during an intravenous injection if the syringe is not properly filled, or from intravenous tubing if fluid is permitted to flow through tubing from which air has not been evacuated. NOTE: A very small amount of air in the tubing or syringe will not cause symptoms.

NURSING IMPLICATIONS: When an air embolism is suspected in the venous circulation (moving toward the heart), the patient should immediately be turned to the left side with head down to trap air in the right side of the heart and kept in this position for 20 to 30 min to allow the air to dissolve and disperse through the pulmonary artery. The IV should be stopped if air is still in the line and the air evacuated through the port nearest the patient; otherwise the rate of fluid flow should be slowed to keep the vein open. Oxygen should be administered, and the physician notified.

*Prevention:* All air should be purged from the tubing of all IV lines before hookup and when solution bags or bottles are changed; air elimination filters should be used close to the patient; infusion devices with air detection capability should be used, as well as locking tubing, locking connection devices, or taped connections. For central lines, to increase peripheral resistance and prevent air from entering the superior vena cava, the patient should be instructed to perform Valsalva's maneuver as the stylet is removed from the catheter, during attachment of the IV tubing, and when adapters or caps are changed on ports.

**air evacuation** Transport of patients from one location to another by specially equipped helicopters or other aircraft. Indications for air transport include severe trauma, burns, and other conditions requiring immediate skilled care and treatment.

**air flow, laminar** SEE: *laminar air flow.*

**air-fluidized bed** SEE: *bed, air-fluidized.*

**air gap principle** A procedure used to decrease the amount of scattered radiation reaching the radiographic film by increasing the object-film distance.

**air hunger** Shortness of breath marked by rapid, labored breathing. SEE: *dyspnea*.

**air medical services** SEE: *air medical transportation*.

**air medical transportation** Air transportation of patients from a primary treatment area to a regional medical center or emergency hospital. SEE: *air evacuation*.

**airplane splint** An appliance usually used on ambulatory patients in the treatment of fractures of the humerus. It takes its name from the elevated (abducted) position in which it holds the arm suspended in air.

**air sac** Air vesicle.

**airsickness** A form of motion sickness marked by giddiness, nausea, vomiting, headache, and often extreme drowsiness that occurs during air flight. Motion sickness can be controlled by medicines such as transdermal scopolamine. Even for those who are not prone to motion sickness, air travel may not be advisable if certain medical conditions exist. Expansion of gas at cabin pressure may be a problem to those who have had recent abdominal surgery. Persons with blocked sinuses or eustachian tubes should not fly until the condition has cleared up. Patients with a recent history of myocardial infarction should not travel without their physicians' approval. Persons with impaired pulmonary function may need supplemental oxygen, depending on their functional capacity. Those with an intestinal ostomy may need a larger bag because of gas expansion. Those who have had recent surgery involving the inner ear should not travel by air if there is any difficulty with equalizing air pressure between ambient air and the middle ear. If the jaws have been wired as part of the treatment for a jaw fracture, wire cutters must be carried in case motion sickness causes vomiting. Pregnant women will need their physicians' permission to travel during the last several weeks of their pregnancy and immediately after delivery. Diabetics who use insulin will need a supply of it. Patients with infectious disease spread by the airborne route will not be allowed to fly. SEE: *seasickness*.

**air splint** Splint used for immobilizing fractured or injured extremities. It is usually an inflatable cylinder, open at both ends, that becomes rigid when inflated, thus preventing the part confined in the cylinder from moving.

**air swallowing** Voluntary or involuntary swallowing of air. It occurs involuntarily in infants as a result of improper feeding. In adults it occurs in neurasthenia and hysteria and in those on a fluid diet. SYN: *aerophagia*.

**air syringe** A syringe on a dental unit to deliver compressed air through a fine nozzle to clear or dry an area or to evacuate debris from an operative field.

---

Caution: Use of high pressure may injure the tissues.

---

**air vesicle** Pulmonary alveolus; one of the terminal saccules of an alveolar duct where gases are exchanged in respiration.

**airway 1.** A natural passageway for air to and from the lungs. **2.** A device used to prevent or correct an obstructed respiratory passage, esp. during anesthesia and cardiopulmonary resuscitation. Maintaining the airway is, obviously, essential to the life of the patient. In an emergency situation, esp. when the patient is unconscious or has a bilateral fracture of the lower jaw, there is a good possibility that the tongue will close the oropharyngeal airway. Methods for opening the airway are described in the entries for cardiopulmonary resuscitation; chin-lift airway technique, head tilt; jaw-thrust technique, and tracheostomy. SEE: illus.; *jaw-thrust*.

---

Caution: If a patient is unconscious or has an injury to the head and upper neck, one should assume there is spinal injury. To move the patient could cause paralysis by transection of the spinal cord.

---

***esophageal gastric tube a.*** ABBR: EGTA. An esophageal airway with a 37 cm–long, large-bore tube attached to a mask that makes an airtight seal with the patient's face. A balloon at the distal end of the tube is inflated following insertion into the esophagus. This improves ventilation and eliminates the possibility of regurgitation. The EGTA has an opening at the distal end of the tube for decompression of the stomach. SYN: *esophageal obturator a.*

***esophageal obturator a.*** ABBR: EOA. Esophageal gastric tube a.

***laryngeal mask a.*** ABBR: LMA. A device shaped like a miniature mask used in inhalation anesthesia. It is inserted blindly into the hypopharynx and forms a seal around the glottic opening to the larynx. Because laryngoscopy is not necessary in order to properly position the mask, establishing an airway is facilitated even when used by persons with no prior experience in resuscitation. Anesthetic gases may be administered through the device.

---

Caution: Guidelines concerning the risk of aspiration should be followed.

---

***nasopharyngeal a.*** A device used to es-

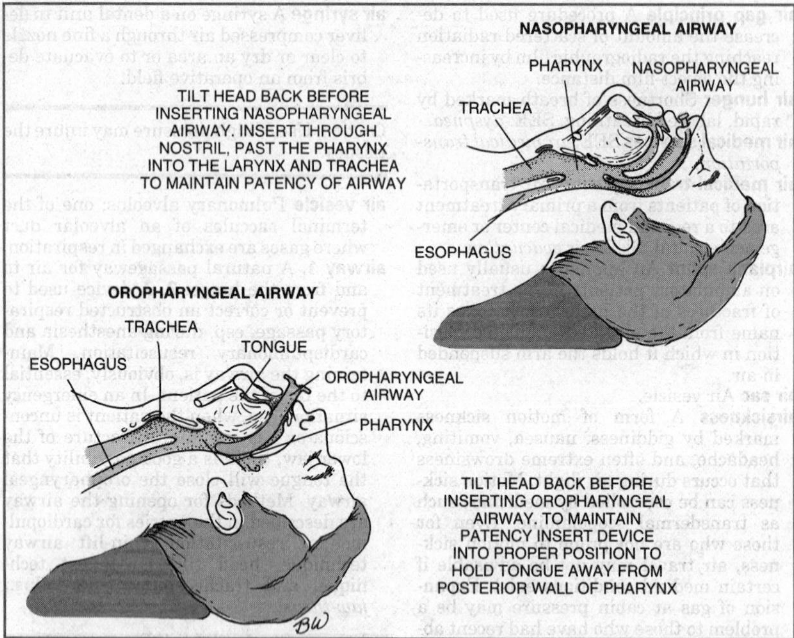


tablish an airway in a patient by placement of a small, soft, flexible tube through the nasal passage into the nasopharynx. The length of the tube should equal the distance from the nose to the ear lobe. It has a flange on the end remaining outside the nose to keep it from sliding into the pharynx. SEE: *Universal Precautions Appendix.*

***oropharyngeal a.*** A curved device used to establish an airway in a patient by displacing the tongue from the posterior wall of the oropharynx. The device should be equal in length to the distance from the corner of the mouth to the ear lobe. It has a flange on the end remaining outside the mouth to keep it from sliding into the pharynx. This device should be reserved for unconscious patients, as it stimulates the gag response in conscious patients. SEE: *cardiopulmonary resuscitation; Universal Precautions Appendix.*

---

Caution: The head of an unconscious patient should not be moved. To do so could cause paralysis.

---

**airway clearance, ineffective** A state in which an individual is unable to clear secretions or obstructions from the respiratory tract to maintain airway patency. SEE: *Nursing Diagnoses Appendix.*

**A.K.** *above knee;* term used to refer to the site of amputation of a lower extremity.

**akaryocyte** (ă-kăr′ē-ō-sīt″) [Gr. *a-*, not, + *karyon,* kernel, + *kytos,* cell] A cell without a nucleus (e.g., an erythrocyte).

**akaryote** (ă-kăr′ē-ōt) [″ + *karyon,* kernel] Akaryocyte.

**akatamathesia** (ă-kăt″ă-mă-thē′zē-ă) [″ + *katamathesis,* understanding] The mental condition of being unable to understand.

**akathisia** (ăk″ă-thĭ′zē-ă) [″ + *kathisis,* sitting] Acathisia.

**akee** (ăk′ē, ă-kē′) [Liberian] The tropical tree *Blighia sapida*. Ingestion of the unripe fruit can cause severe hypoglycemia. Also spelled *ackee.*

**akinesia** (ă″kĭ-nē′zē-ă) [Gr. *a-*, not, + *kinesis,* movement] Complete or partial loss of muscle movement; also spelled *acinesia.* **akinetic** (-nĕt′ĭk), *adj.*

***a. algera*** Akinesia with intense pain caused by voluntary movement.

**Al** Symbol for the element aluminum (British: aluminium).

**-al** [L.] **1.** Suffix meaning *relating to,* as in abdominal, intestinal. **2.** In chemistry, suffix indicating an aldehyde.

**ala** (ā′lă) *pl.* **alae** [L., wing] **1.** An expanded or winglike structure or appendage. **2.** Axilla.

***a. auris*** Protruding portion of the external ear. SYN: *auricle; pinna.*

***a. cerebelli*** Winglike projection of the central lobule of the cerebellum. SYN: *a. lobuli centralis.*

***a. cinerea*** Gray triangular prominence on the floor of the fourth ventricle. The autonomic fibers of the vagus nerve arise from the cells of the nucleus of this area. SYN: *triangle of the vagus nerve; tri-*

*gonum nervi vagi.*

***a. cristae galli*** Small projection on each side of the crista galli of the ethmoid bone.

***a. lobuli centralis*** A. cerebelli.

***a. major ossis sphenoidalis*** Greater wing of the sphenoid bone.

***a. minor ossis sphenoidalis*** Lesser wing of the sphenoid bone.

***a. nasi*** Wing of the nose; broad portion forming the lateral wall of each nostril.

***a. of ethmoid*** Small projection on each side of the ethmoid bone.

***a. of ilium*** Broad, upper portion of the iliac bone.

***a. of sacrum*** Broad projection on each side of the base of the sacrum.

***a. vomeris*** Wing of the vomer; projection on each side of the superior border of the vomer.

**alacrima** (ā-lăk′rĭ-mă) [Gr. *a-*, not, + L. *lacrima,* tear] Deficiency of or absence of tears. SYN: *dry eye.* SEE: *Sjögren's syndrome.*

**Alagille syndrome** [Daniel Alagille, Fr. physician, b. 1925] Arteriohepatic dysplasia with bile duct hypoplasia or paucity.

**alalia** (ă-lā′lē-ă) [″ + *lalein,* to talk] Inability to speak due to defect or paralysis of the vocal organs; aphasia.The cause is organic brain disease or psychoneurosis.

**alanine** (ăl′ă-nēn) $C_3H_7NO_2$. A naturally occurring amino acid considered nonessential in human nutrition.

**alanine aminotransferase** ABBR: ALT. An intracellular enzyme involved in amino acid and carbohydrate metabolism. It is present in high concentrations in muscle, liver, and brain. An increased level of this enzyme in the blood indicates necrosis or disease in these tissues. Formerly called serum glutamic pyruvic transaminase (SGPT) or glutamic-pyruvic transaminase.

**Al-Anon** A nonprofit organization that provides group support for the family and close friends of alcoholics. SEE: *Alcoholics Anonymous.*

**alar** (ā′lăr) [L. *ala,* wing] **1.** Pert. to or like a wing. **2.** Axillary.

**ALARA** *as low as reasonably achievable.*

**alar artery** Branch of the angular artery that supplies the tissues of the ala nasi.

**alar cartilage** Cartilage forming the broad lateral wall of each nostril.

**Alateen** A nonprofit organization that provides support for children of alcoholics. SEE: *Alcoholics Anonymous.*

**alba** [L. *albus,* white] **1.** White. **2.** White substance of the brain.

**albedo** (ăl-bē′dō) [L.] Whiteness. Reflection of light from a surface.

***a. retinae*** Reflections associated with retinal edema.

***a. unguium*** White semilunar area near the nail root. SYN: *lunula.*

**Albers-Schönberg disease** (ăl-bārs-shĕrn′bārg) [Heinrich Ernst Albers-Schönberg, Ger. roentgenologist, 1865–1921] Hereditary condition marked by excessive calcification of bones causing spontaneous fractures and marblelike appearance. SYN: *marble bone; osteopetrosis.*

**Albert's disease** [Eduard Albert, Austrian surgeon, 1841–1900] Inflammation of the bursae lying over the Achilles tendon. SYN: *achillobursitis.*

**albicans** [L.] White; whitish.

***corpus a.*** A mass of fibrous tissue that replaces the regressing corpus luteum following rupture of the graafian follicle. It forms a white scar that gradually decreases in size and eventually disappears.

**Albini's nodules** (ăl-bē′nēz) [Giuseppe Albini, It. physiologist, 1830–1911] Minute nodules on the margins of the mitral and tricuspid valves of the heart; sometimes seen in newborns.

**albinism** (ăl′bĭn-ĭzm) [L. *albus,* white, + Gr. *-ismos,* condition] Genetic, nonpathological, partial or total absence of pigment in skin, hair, and eyes. It is often accompanied by astigmatism, photophobia, and nystagmus because the choroid is not sufficiently protected from light as a result of lack of pigment.

**albino** (ăl-bī′nō) A person afflicted with albinism.

**albinuria** (ăl″bĭ-nū′rē-ă) [L. *albus,* white, + Gr. *ouron,* urine] Passing of white or colorless urine of low specific gravity. SYN: *achromaturia.*

**Albright's disease** [Fuller Albright, U.S. physician, 1900–1969] Polyostotic fibrous dysplasia accompanied by café au lait macules and endocrine disorders, esp. precocious puberty in girls. The patient is fracture prone, and deformity and shortening of bones may develop. SEE: *dysplasia, polyostotic fibrous.*

**albuginea** (ăl-bū-jĭn′ē-ă) [L. from *albus,* white] A layer of firm white fibrous tissue forming the investment of an organ or part, as of the eye, testicle, ovary, or spleen. SYN: *tunica albuginea.*

***a. corporum cavernosorum*** A strong, very elastic, white fibrous coat, forming a sheath common to both corpora cavernosa of the penis.

***a. oculi*** The sclera, or fibrous connective tissue outer layer of the eyeball.

***a. ovarii*** The layer of firm fibrous tissue lying beneath the epithelial ovarian covering.

***a. testis*** The thick, unyielding layer of white fibrous tissue lying under the tunica vaginalis.

**albugineotomy** (ăl″bū-jĭn″ē-ŏt′ō-mē) [*albuginea* + Gr. *tome,* incision] Incision of tunica albuginea, esp. of the testis.

**albugineous** (ăl″bū-jĭn′ē-ŭs) Pert. to or resembling the tunica albuginea.

**albuginitis** (ăl″bū-jĭn-ī′tĭs) [″ + Gr. *itis,* inflammation] Inflammation of the tunica albuginea.

**albumen** (ăl-bū′mĕn) [L.] Albumin.

**albumin** (ăl-bū′mĭn) [L. *albumen,* white of egg] One of a group of simple proteins widely distributed in plant and animal tissues; it is found in the blood as serum albumin, in milk as lactalbumin, and in the white of egg as ovalbumin. In the blood, albumin acts as a carrier molecule and helps to maintain blood volume and blood pressure. In humans, the principal function of albumin is to provide colloid osmotic pressure, preventing plasma loss from the capillaries. Albumin, like all the plasma proteins, can act as a source for rapid replacement of tissue proteins. It is soluble in cold water; when coagulated by heat it is no longer dissolved by cold or hot water. In the stomach, coagulated albumins are made soluble by peptase, being changed at the same time into albumoses and peptones. In general, albumins from animal sources are of higher quality than those from vegetable sources because animal proteins contain greater quantities of essential amino acids. SEE: *albumose; amino acid; peptone.*

***blood a.*** Serum a.

***circulating a.*** Albumin present in body fluids.

***egg a.*** Ovalbumin.

***human a.*** A sterile solution of serum albumin obtained from healthy blood donors. It is administered intravenously to restore blood volume.

***serum a.*** The main protein found in the blood. SYN: *blood a.*

***urinary a.*** Albumin in urine.

***vegetable a.*** Albumin in, or derived from, plant tissue.

**albuminate** (ăl-bū′mĭ-nāt) The compound formed when albumin combines with an acid or alkali (base).

**albuminaturia** (ăl-bū″mĭ-nă-tū′rē-ă) [L. *albumen,* white of egg, + Gr. *ouron,* urine] Presence of albuminates in urine.

**albuminiferous** (ăl-bū″mĭn-ĭf′ĕ-rŭs) [″ + *ferre,* to bear] Producing albumin.

**albuminimeter** (ăl-bū″mĭn-ĭm′ĕ-tĕr) [″ + Gr. *metron,* measure] Instrument for measuring the amount of albumin in urine.

**albuminiparous** (ăl-bū″mĭn-ĭp′ă-rŭs) [″ + *parere,* to bring forth, to bear] Yielding albumin.

**albuminocholia** (ăl-bū″mĭ-nō-kō′lē-ă) [″ + Gr. *chole,* bile] Albumin in the bile.

**albuminogenous** (ăl-bū″mĭn-ŏj′ĕ-nŭs) [″ + Gr. *gennan,* to produce] Producing albumin.

**albuminoid** (ăl-bū′mĭ-noyd″) [″ + Gr. *eidos,* form, shape] **1.** Resembling albumin. **2.** A protein.

**albuminolysis** (ăl-bū″mĭn-ŏl′ĭ-sĭs) [″ + Gr. *lysis,* dissolution] Proteolysis; decomposition of protein.

**albuminoreaction** (ăl-bū″mĭ-nō-rē-ăk′shŭn) [″ + *re,* again, + *agere,* to act] The presence (positive reaction) or absence (negative reaction) of albumin in the sputum. A positive reaction indicates an inflammation of the lungs.

**albuminorrhea** (ăl-bū″mĭ-nō-rē′ă) [″ + Gr. *rhoia,* flow] The presence of albumin in urine. SYN: *albuminuria.*

**albuminose** (ăl-bū′mĭn-ōs) Albuminous.

**albuminosis** (ăl-bū″mĭ-nō′sĭs) [″ + Gr. *osis,* condition] An abnormal increase of albumin in blood plasma.

**albuminous** (ăl-bū′mĭ-nŭs) Pert. to, resembling, or containing albumin.

**albumin test** Any chemical test for the presence of albumin.

The most common type of albumin found in urine is serum albumin. Before testing, certain precautions must be observed: The urine specimen must be fresh. It must also be clear; the safest way to ensure this is to filter it through special filter paper. Because many conditions can cause albuminuria, the test results require careful interpretation. Quantitative methods are also available.

There are many tests for albumin, but the usual ones are:

*Acetic acid test:* The top in. (2.5 cm) of a test tube filled with urine is heated over a Bunsen burner. A cloudiness will occur, which may be due to phosphate or albumin. Then 2 to 3 drops of acetic acid are added. If the cloud disappears, it is due to phosphates; if it becomes intensified, albumin is present.

*Heller's test:* About ½ in. (1.3 cm) of concentrated nitric acid is poured into a test tube and overlaid carefully with the urine, using a pipette. If an opaque line appears at the junction of the fluids, albumin is present. The line may take a few minutes to develop.

*Paper strip or tablet tests:* There are several tests based on the principle that certain chemicals impregnated in paper or in tablet form will change color when exposed to protein-containing urine. In general these tests are fast and reliable.

*Sulfosalicylic acid test:* In a test tube, 10 to 20 drops of sulfosalicylic acid are added to urine. Albumin is shown as a white, cloudy precipitate. This may be carried out as a ring test, as in Heller's test.

**albuminuretic** [L. *albumen,* white of egg, + Gr. *ouretikos,* causing urine to flow] Pert. to or causing albuminuria.

**albuminuria** (ăl-bū-mĭ-nū′rē-ă) [″ + Gr. *ouron,* urine] The presence of readily detectable amounts of serum protein, esp. serum albumin but also serum globulin and others, in the urine. Albuminuria is a common sign of renal impairment (nephrotic syndrome and other kidney disorders); it also occurs in febrile states, malignant hypertension, and congestive heart failure. However, its presence is not always a sign of disease, since it may be found in healthy people after vigorous exercise. SYN: *proteinuria.* SEE: *nephritis; nephrosis.* **albuminuric** (-nū′rĭk), *adj.*

***cyclic a.*** Presence of small amounts of albumin in the urine at regular diurnal intervals, esp. in childhood and adolescence.

***digestive a.*** Albuminuria following ingestion of certain foods.

***extrarenal a., accidental a.*** Albuminuria due to contamination of urine with pus, chyle, or blood.

***functional a.*** Intermittent or temporary albuminuria not associated with a pathological condition. SYN: *physiological a.*

***intrinsic a.*** Albuminuria resulting from intrinsic renal disease. SYN: *true a.*

***orthostatic a.*** Postural a.

***pathological a.*** Albuminuria caused by a disease.

***physiological a.*** Functional a.

***postural a.*** Transient albuminuria in normal individuals who have been erect for a long period. SYN: *orthostatic a.*

***renal a.*** Albuminuria caused by defective renal function, esp. of the glomeruli.

***toxic a.*** Albuminuria caused by internal or external toxins.

***true a.*** Intrinsic a.

**albuminuric retinitis** (ăl″bū-mĭ-nū′rĭk rĕt″ĭ-nī′tĭs) Inflammation of the retina associated with chronic kidney disease and marked by a hazy retina, blurred disk margin, distention of retinal arteries, retinal hemorrhages, and white patches in the fundus, esp. the stellate figure at the macula. SEE: *retinitis.*

**albumoscope** (ăl-bū′mō-skōp) [L. *albumen,* white of egg, + Gr. *skopein,* to examine] An instrument for determining the presence of albumin in the urine.

**albus** [L.] White.

**Albuterol** Bronchodilator administered by inhalation or tablet.

**Alcaligenes** (ăl″kă-lĭj′ĭ-nēz) A genus of rod-shaped, gram-negative bacteria found in the intestinal tract of humans, in dairy products, and in soil.

***A. faecalis*** A species of bacteria normally found in the intestinal tract of humans. It has been associated with septicemia and epidemics of urinary tract infections.

**Alcock's canal** [Benjamin Alcock, Irish anatomist, b. 1801] Pudendal canal; space in the external fascia of the ischiorectal fossa, above the tuberosity of the ischium, through which the internal pudendal artery, veins, and nerve pass.

**alcohol** (ăl′kō-hŏl) [Arabic *al-koh'l,* something subtle] **1.** A class of organic compounds that are hydroxyl derivatives of hydrocarbons. **2.** Ethyl alcohol ($C_2H_5OH$), a colorless, volatile, flammable liquid. Its molecular weight is 46.07; its boiling point is 78.5°C. It is present in fermented or distilled liquors and is obtained, in its pure form, from grain by fermentation and fractionation distillation. SYN: *ethanol; grain a.*

ACTION/USES: Taken in excessive amounts, alcohol acts as a depressant to the nervous system. Because it arrests the growth of putrefactive bacteria, it is useful in preserving biological specimens and in some patent medicines. It is also used in preparing essences, tinctures, and extracts; in the manufacture of ether, ethylene, and other industrial products; as a rubbing compound; and as an antiseptic in 70% solution. SEE: *alcoholism; fetal alcohol syndrome.*

***absolute a.*** A solution that contains 99% alcohol and not more than 1% by weight of water.

***cetyl a.*** A white insoluble solid substance, $C_{16}H_{34}O$, used in the manufacture of ointments.

***dehydrated a.*** Alcohol containing not less than 99.2% by weight of ethyl alcohol. This corresponds to 99.5% by volume of ethyl alcohol.

***denatured a.*** Alcohol rendered unfit for use as a beverage or medicine by the addition of toxic ingredients; used commercially as a solvent.

***diluted a.*** Alcohol containing not less than 41% and not more than 42% by weight of ethyl alcohol; used as a solvent. SYN: *diluted ethanol.*

***ethyl a.*** Ordinary or grain alcohol. SEE: *alcohol* (2).

***grain a.*** Ethyl a. SEE: *alcohol* (2).

***isopropyl a.*** $C_3H_8O$. A clear flammable liquid similar to ethyl alcohol and propyl alcohol; used in medical preparations for external use, antifreeze, cosmetics, and solvents. SEE: *Poisons and Poisoning Appendix.*

---

Caution: Isopropyl alcohol is toxic when taken internally.

---

***methyl a.*** $CH_4O$. A colorless, volatile, flammable liquid obtained from distillation of wood. Even though its physical properties are similar to those of ethyl alcohol, it is not fit for human consumption. Ingestion of methyl alcohol can lead to blindness and death. It is used as a solvent, for fuel, as an additive for denaturing ethyl alcohol, as an antifreeze agent, and in the preparation of formaldehyde. SYN: *carbinol; methanol; wood alcohol.* SEE: *methyl alcohol in Poisons and Poisoning Appendix.*

***pathological reaction to a.*** An exceedingly severe reaction to ingestion of alcohol, esp. to small amounts. It is manifested by irrational violent behavior followed by exhaustion, sleep, and loss of recall of the event. The patient may not be intoxicated. The etiology is unknown but is associated with hypoglycemia, exhaustion, and stress. SEE: *alcoholism.*

***rubbing a.*** SEE: *rubbing alcohol.*

***wood a.*** Methyl a.

**Alcohol, Drug Abuse, and Mental Health Administration** ABBR: ADAMHA. A U.S. government agency that is part of the National Institutes of Health within the Department of Health and Human Services. The agency administers grant programs supporting research, training, and service programs in alcoholism, drug abuse, and mental health.

**alcoholic** (ăl-kō-hŏl′ĭk) [L. *alcoholicus*] **1.** Pert. to alcohol. **2.** One afflicted with alcoholism.

**alcoholic blackout** An episode of forgetting all or part of what occurred during or following a period of alcohol intake.

**alcoholic fermentation** The conversion of carbohydrates to alcohol through the action of yeast.

**alcoholic psychosis** Severe mental disorder caused by alcoholism. Included are pathological intoxication, delirium tremens, Korsakoff's psychosis, and acute hallucinosis. SEE: *alcoholism, acute; delirium tremens; hallucinosis, acute alcoholic; intoxication; Korsakoff's syndrome.*

**Alcoholics Anonymous** ABBR: A.A. An organization consisting of alcoholics who are trying to help themselves and others abstain from alcohol by offering encouragement and discussing experiences, problems, feelings, techniques, and so on. The organization has groups in most U.S. cities; local chapters are listed in the telephone directory. SEE: *Al-Anon; Alateen.*

**alcoholism** (ăl′kō-hŏl-ĭzm) [Arabic *al-koh'l,* something subtle, + Gr. *-ismos,* condition] A chronic progressive, sometimes fatal disease marked by chronic excessive intake of and dependence on alcoholic drinks.

Abuse of alcohol is a major health threat in the U.S. It is much more widely used than any of the illegal drugs. Chronic alcoholism and alcohol-related disorders, accidents, violence, and injuries can be physically, psychologically, and economically devastating to patients and their families. SEE: *Alcoholics Anonymous.*

Alcoholism has been defined as having the following characteristics:

1. "Chronic and progressive"—physical, emotional, and social changes that develop are cumulative and progress as drinking continues.
2. "Tolerance"—brain adaptation to the presence of high concentrations of alcohol.
3. "Physical dependency"—withdrawal symptoms occur from decreasing or ceasing consumption of alcohol.
4. The person with alcoholism cannot consistently predict on any drinking occasion the duration of the episode or the quantity that will be consumed.
5. Pathologic organ changes can be found in almost any organ, but most often involve the liver, brain, peripheral nervous system, and the gastrointestinal tract.
6. The drinking pattern is generally continuous but may be intermittent, with periods of abstinence between drinking episodes.
7. Social, emotional, and behavioral symptoms and consequences of alcoholism result from the effect of alcohol on the function of the brain. The degree to which these symptoms and signs are considered deviant will depend upon the cultural norms of the society or group in which the person lives.

(Definition prepared by the National Council on Alcoholism/American Medical Society on Alcoholism, Committee on Definitions.)

DETECTION: Alcohol concentration in the blood can be measured. In addition, alcohol in the body can be detected by analyzing exhaled air. This provides an estimate of whether the individual has sufficient concentration of blood alcohol to interfere with his or her ability carry out a demanding function such as driving an automobile or piloting an airplane.

ETIOLOGY: The cause of alcoholism is unknown. Psychological, physiological, and sociological factors play an important part. The exhilaration factor is often the cause of intoxication in nonalcoholic individuals. Alcoholism is an illness and should be so treated. Although it is accepted that there is a genetic factor in the development of alcoholism, the precise genetic mechanism has not been determined.

TREATMENT: Naltrexone, an opioid antagonist, has been approved for treating alcoholism.

***acute a.*** Acute intoxication with temporary mental disturbances and muscular incoordination.

Caution: When stupor or coma is observed in a patient suspected of being intoxicated by alcohol, other causes, such as intracranial disease or insulin shock, should also be considered. Acute alcoholism can cause death.

SYMPTOMS: There may be motor instability (staggering gait, blurred or double vision, impaired reflex action), reduced mental function, increased pulse rate, decreased blood pressure, dilated pupils, flushing of skin, and drowsiness or stupor.

TREATMENT: Alcohol-induced coma is a medical emergency and requires vigorous therapy. Intravenous fluids, intubation to prevent aspiration of vomitus, and oxygen inhalation may be required.

***chronic a.*** Pathological state from habitual use of alcohol in toxic amounts. SEE: *intoxication.*

SYMPTOMS: The symptoms include malnutrition, vitamin deficiency, alcoholic cirrhosis of liver, gastritis, pancreatitis, and neurological disorders such as tremulousness, hallucinosis, seizures, delirium tremens, and coma. Prolonged, excessive ingestion of alcohol is toxic to the cells of the liver. This may lead to cirrhosis and death. Alcoholism is, in some urban areas, the third most frequent cause of death in persons between the ages of 25 and 65. The effect of alcohol on the liver is independent of poor diet. Alcohol ingestion during pregnancy may cause congenital defects.

TREATMENT: Treatment involves withdrawal of alcohol, tranquilizing drugs, adequate nutrition and rest, correction of vitamin deficiency, and psychotherapy. SEE: *Alcoholics Anonymous; alcohol withdrawal syndrome; delirium tremens.*

**alcoholuria** (ăl″kō-hŏl-ū′rē-ă) [″ + Gr. *ouron,* urine] The presence of alcohol in urine.

**alcohol withdrawal syndrome** The signs and symptoms produced when an individual with a high tolerance to alcohol suddenly decreases the amount of intake of alcohol. Symptoms include tremors or shaking of the hands; increased pulse, respiration, and temperature; anxiety, panic, hallucinations, and confusion. SEE: *alcoholism, chronic; delirium tremens.*

**aldehyde** (ăl′dĕ-hīd) [*al*cohol *dehyd*rogenatum] **1.** Oxidation product of a primary alcohol; it has the characteristic group—CHO. **2.** Acetaldehyde, $CH_3CHO$; an intermediate in yeast fermentation and alcohol metabolism.

**Alder-Reilly anomaly** [Albert von Alder, Ger. physician, b. 1888; William Anthony Reilly, U.S. pediatrician, b. 1901] Large dark leukocyte granules that stain lilac. They consist of mucopolysaccharide deposits and are indicative of mucopolysaccharidosis.

**aldolase** (ăl′dō-lās) An enzyme present in skeletal and heart muscle and the liver; important in converting glycogen into lactic acid. Its serum level is increased in certain muscle diseases and in viral hepatitis.

**aldopentose** (ăl″dō-pĕn′tōs) A five-carbon sugar with the aldehyde group, —CHO, at the end. Arabinose is an aldopentose.

**aldose** A carbohydrate of the aldehyde group (—CHO).

**aldosterone** (ăl-dŏs′tĕr-ōn, ăl″dō-stēr′ōn) The most biologically active mineralocorticoid hormone secreted by the adrenal cortex. Aldosterone increases sodium reabsorption by the kidneys, thereby indirectly regulating blood levels of potassium, chloride, and bicarbonate, as well as pH, blood volume, and blood pressure. SEE: *adrenal gland.*

**aldosteronism** (ăl″dŏ-stĕr′ōn-ĭzm″) A condition in which the blood contains abnormally high levels of aldosterone. This causes sodium retention, urinary loss of potassium, and alkalosis. The patient develops episodes of tetany, weakness, paralysis, hypertension, cardiac irregularity, polyuria, and polydipsia. SYN: *hyperaldosteronism.*

***primary a.*** Aldosteronism due to disorders of the adrenal gland. SYN: *Conn's syndrome.* SEE: *Nursing Diagnoses Appendix.*

***secondary a.*** Aldosteronism due to extra-adrenal disorders.

**aldrin** (ăl′drĭn) A derivative of chlorinated naphthalene used as an insecticide. SEE: *dieldrin in Poisons and Poisoning Appendix.*

**alemmal** (ă-lĕm′ăl) [Gr. *a-,* not, + *lemma,* husk] Without a neurilemma, as in a nerve fiber.

**Aleppo boil** Cutaneous leishmaniasis, caused by infection with the parasite *Leishmania tropica* and marked by one or multiple ulcerations of the skin. SYN: *Delhi boil; Oriental sore.*

**aleukemia** (ă-loo-kē′mē-ă) [″ + *leukos,* white, + *haima,* blood] A deficiency of leukocytes in the blood; the existence of leukopenia or aleukocytosis.

**aleukemic leukemia** SEE: *leukemia, acute myelogenous.*

**aleukocytosis** (ă-loo″kō-sī-tō′sĭs) [Gr. *a-,* not, + *leukos,* white, + *kytos,* cell, + *osis,* condition] Absence or extreme decrease of leukocytes in the blood.

**aleurone** (ăl-oo′rōn) [Gr. *aleuron,* flour] The protein granules present in the outer layer of the endosperm of cereal grain.

**Alexander-Adams operation** [William Alexander, Brit. surgeon, 1844–1919; James A. Adams, Scot. gynecologist, 1857–1930] Surgery in which the round ligaments of the uterus are shortened and their ends sutured to the exterior abdominal ring; used in treating uterine displacement.

**alexia** [Gr. *a-,* not, + *lexis,* word] Inability to read, or word blindness, caused by a lesion of the central nervous system.

***motor a.*** Inability to read aloud while remaining able to understand what is written or printed.

***musical a.*** Inability to read music. It may be sensory, optic, or visual, but not motor.

***optic a., visual a.*** Inability to understand what is written or printed.

**alexithymia** A clinical feature common in post-traumatic stress disorder (PTSD) characterized by the inability to identify and articulate feelings. Often feelings are reported to the health care worker in the form of physical symptoms. Patients suffering from chemical dependency and somatoform disorders may also display alexithymia.

**ALG** *antilymphocyte globulin.* SEE: *globulin, antilymphocyte.*

**algae** (ăl′jē) [L. *alga,* seaweed] Plants belonging to the subphylum Algae of the phylum Thallophyta, the lowest division of the plant kingdom. They are nonparasitic plants without roots, stems, or leaves; they contain chlorophyll and vary in size from microscopic forms to massive seaweeds. They live in fresh or salt water and in moist places. Some serve as a source of food. Examples are kelp and Irish moss.

***blue-green a.*** Algae that grow in brackish water. Preparations of blue-green algae for medical use are not approved for sale in the U.S.
**algefacient** Refrigerant.
**algesia** (ăl-jē′zē-ă) [Gr. *algesis,* sense of pain] Supersensitivity to pain; a form of hyperesthesia. SYN: *algesthesia.* **algesic, algetic** (ăl-jēz′ĭk, ăl-jĕt′ĭk), *adj.*
**algesthesia** (ăl″jĕs-thē′zē-ă) [Gr. *algos,* pain, + *aisthesis,* sensation] **1.** Perception of pain. **2.** Algesia.
**-algia** (ăl′jē-ă) [Gr.] Suffix meaning *pain.*
**algicide** (ăl′jĭ-sīd) [L. *alga,* seaweed, + *caedere,* to kill] A substance that kills algae.
**algid** (ăl′jĭd) [L. *algidus,* cold] Cold; chilly.
**algid stage** Cold and cyanotic skin that occurs in cholera and some other diseases.
**alginate** (ăl′jĭ-nāt) Any salt of alginic acid. It is derived from kelp, a type of seaweed, and is used as a thickener in foods and as a pharmaceutical aid. In dentistry, this irreversible hydrocolloid is used as a material for taking impressions.
**alginic acid** SEE: *acid, alginic.*
**algiomotor** (ăl″jē-ŏ-mō′tor) [Gr. *algos,* pain, + L. *motor,* a mover] Causing painful contraction of muscles, particularly pain during peristalsis. SYN: *algiomuscular.*
**algiomuscular** (ăl″jē-ŏ-mŭs′kū-lăr) [″ + L. *musculus,* muscle] Algiomotor.
**alglucerase** A drug prepared from human placental tissue. It is used in treating type I Gaucher's disease.
**algolagnia** (ăl″gō-lăg′nē-ă) [Gr. *algos,* pain, + *lagneia,* lust] Sexual satisfaction derived by experiencing pain or by inflicting pain on others.
***active a.*** Sadism.
***passive a.*** Masochism.
**algolagnist** (ăl-gō-lăg′nĭst) One who practices algolagnia.
**algometer** [″ + *metron,* measure] An instrument for measuring the degree of sensitivity to pain.
**algophobia** (ăl″gō-fō′bē-ă) [Gr. *algos,* pain, + *phobos,* fear] Morbid fear of pain.
**algorithm** (ăl′gŏ-rĭthm) A formula or set of rules for solving a particular problem. In medicine, a set of steps used in diagnosing and treating a disease. Appropriate use of algorithms in medicine may lead to more efficient and accurate patient care as well as reduced costs.
**Alice in Wonderland syndrome** [Alice, from Lewis Carroll's *Alice in Wonderland*] Perceptual distortions of space and size. This may be a symptom of neurological involvement in infectious mononucleosis, and may be caused by hallucinogenic drugs.
**alicyclic** (ăl-ĭ-sī′klĭk) Having properties of both aliphatic (open-chain) and cyclic (closed-chain) compounds.
**alienate** (āl′yĕn-āt) To isolate, estrange, or dissociate.
**alienation** (āl″yĕn-ā′shŭn) [L. *alienare,* to make strange] Isolation, estrangement, or dissociation, esp. from society.
**aliform** (ăl′ĭ-form) [L. *ala,* wing, + *forma,* shape] Wing-shaped.
**aliform process** Wing of the sphenoid bone.
**alignment** (ă-līn′mĕnt) [Fr. *aligner,* to put in a straight line] **1.** The act of arranging in a straight line. **2.** The state of being arranged in a straight line. **3.** In orthopedics, the placing of portions of a fractured bone into correct anatomical position. **4.** In dentistry, bringing teeth into correct position. **5.** In radiography, the positioning of the body part in correct relation to the radiographic film and x-ray tube to enable proper visualization.
**aliment** (ăl′ĭ-mĕnt) [L. *alimentum,* nourishment] Nutriment; food.
**alimentary** (ăl″ĭ-mĕn′tăr-ē) [L. *alimentum,* nourishment] Pert. to food or nutrition, or the digestive tract.
**alimentary canal, alimentary tract** The digestive tube from the mouth to the anus, including the mouth or buccal cavity, pharynx, esophagus, stomach, and small and large intestines. Drugs administered orally are absorbed in the stomach or intestine, transported via the portal vein and through the liver before entering the general circulation; or they may be absorbed into the lacteals and enter the bloodstream by way of the thoracic duct of the lymphatic system. SEE: *digestive system* for illus.
**alimentary duct** The thoracic duct of the lymphatic system.
**alimentation** (ăl″ĭ-mĕn-tā′shŭn) The process of nourishing the body, including mastication, swallowing, digestion, absorption, and assimilation. SEE: *hyperalimentation; hypoalimentation; total parenteral nutrition.*
***artificial a.*** Feeding, usually intravenous or by a nasal tube passed into the stomach, of a patient unable to take nourishment normally. SEE: *total parenteral nutrition.*
***forced a.*** **1.** Feeding of a patient unwilling to eat. **2.** Forcing of a person to eat a greater quantity than desired.
***rectal a.*** Feeding by means of nutrient enemas.
**alimentotherapy** (ăl″ĭ-mĕn″tō-thĕr′ă-pē) [L. *alimentum,* nourishment, + Gr. *therapeia,* treatment] Treatment of disease by dietary regulation. SYN: *dietotherapy.* SEE: *dietetics.*
**alinasal** [L. *ala,* wing, + *nasus,* nose] Pert. to the alae nasi, or wings of the nose.
**alinement** (ă-līn′mĕnt) [Fr. *aligner,* to put in a straight line] Alignment.
**aliphatic** (ăl″ĭ-făt′ĭk) [Gr. *aleiphar, aleiphatos,* fat, oil] Belonging to that series of organic chemical compounds characterized by open chains of carbon atoms rather than by rings.
**aliquot** (ăl′ĭ-kwŏt) [L. *alius,* other, + *quot,* how many] A portion obtained by dividing the whole into equal parts without a remainder; a portion that represents a known quantitative relationship to the

whole or to other portions.

**alisphenoid** (ăl-ĭ-sfē′noyd) [L. *ala,* wing, + Gr. *sphen,* wedge, + *eidos,* form, shape] Pert. to the greater wing of the sphenoid bone.

**alizarin** (ă-lĭz′ă-rĭn) [Arabic *ala sara,* extract] A red dye obtained from coal tar or madder.

**alkalemia** (ăl″kă-lē′mē-ă) [Arabic *al-qaliy,* ashes of salt wort, + Gr. *haima,* blood] An increase in the arterial blood pH above 7.45 due to a decrease in the hydrogen ion concentration or an increase in hydroxyl ions. The blood is normally slightly alkaline (pH 7.35 to 7.45).

**alkali** (ăl′kă-lī) *pl.* **alkalis, alkalies** [Arabic *al-qaliy,* ashes of salt wort] A strong base, esp. the metallic hydroxides. Alkalies combine with acids to form salts, combine with fatty acids to form soap, neutralize acids, and turn litmus paper blue. SEE: *acid; base; pH; words beginning with alkal-.*

***corrosive a.*** A strongly corrosive metallic hydroxide most commonly of sodium, ammonium, and potassium, as well as carbonates. Because of their great combining power with water and their action on the fatty tissues, they cause rapid and deep destruction. They have a tendency to gelatinize tissue, turning it a somewhat grayish color and forming a soapy, slippery surface, accompanied by pain and burning. SEE: *corrosion; corrosive poisoning.*

**alkalimetry** (ăl″kă-lĭm′ĕ-trē) Measurement of the alkalinity of a mixture.

**alkaline** (ăl′kă-lĭn) Pert. to or having the reactions of an alkali.

**alkaline phosphatase** SEE: *phosphatase, alkaline.*

**alkaline reserve** The amount of base in the blood, principally bicarbonates, available for neutralization of fixed acids (acetoacetate, β-hydroxybutyrate, and lactate). A fall in alkaline reserve is called acidosis; a rise, alkalosis. Normally, the carbon dioxide combining power of the venous plasma is 21 to 30 mEq/L and the carbon dioxide content of whole blood is 20 to 25 mEq/L.

**alkaline salts** SEE: *hydrogen sulfide in Poisons and Poisoning Appendix.*

**alkaline tide** An increase in alkaline reserve and occasional occurrence of alkaline urine during gastric digestion.

**alkalinity** (ăl″kă-lĭn′ĭ-tē) The state of being alkaline. SEE: *hydrogen ion.*

**alkalinize** (ăl′kă-lĭn-īz″) To make alkaline. SYN: *alkalize.*

**alkalinuria** (ăl″kă-lĭn-ū′rē-ă) [*alkali* + Gr. *ouron,* urine] Alkaline urine.

**alkali poisoning** Ingestion of an alkali.

FIRST AID: Large amounts of water are given by mouth. Mild stimulants are administered to prevent shock. Tracheostomy is performed if necessary. If the esophagus is known to be injured, corticosteroid therapy and a broad-spectrum antibiotic should be used.

TREATMENT: Morphine is useful to allay pain. Rest, heat, quiet, and adequate fluid intake are imperative.

---

Caution: Emetics, strong acids, and lavage should be avoided.

---

**alkali reserve** SEE: *alkaline reserve.*

**alkalization** (ă″kă-lĭ-zā′shŭn) The process of making something alkaline.

**alkalize** (ăl′kă-līz) To make alkaline. SYN: *alkalinize.*

**alkaloid** (ăl′kă-loyd) [*alkali* + Gr. *eidos,* form, shape] One of a group of organic alkaline substances (such as morphine or nicotine) obtained from plants. Alkaloids react with acids to form salts that are used for medical purposes.

**alkalosis** (ăl″kă-lō′sĭs) [″ + Gr. *osis,* condition] An actual or relative increase in blood alkalinity due to an accumulation of alkalies or reduction of acids. SEE: *acid-base balance.* **alkalotic** (-lŏt′ĭk), *adj.*

***altitude a.*** Alkalosis resulting from exposure to decreased oxygen content of air at high altitudes. This causes respiratory alkalosis. SEE: *respiratory alkalosis.*

***compensated a.*** Alkalosis in which the pH of body fluids has been returned to normal. Compensatory mechanisms maintain the normal ratio of bicarbonate to carbonic acid (approx. 20 : 1) even though the bicarbonate level is increased.

***hypochloremic a.*** Metabolic alkalosis due to loss of chloride; produced by severe vomiting.

***hypokalemic a.*** Metabolic alkalosis due to excess loss of potassium; may be caused by diuretic therapy.

***metabolic a.*** Alkalosis in which plasma bicarbonate is increased and there is a proportionate rise in the plasma concentration of carbon dioxide. This is usually the result of increased loss of acid from the stomach or kidney, potassium depletion accompanying diuretic therapy, excessive alkali intake, or continued severe adrenal gland hyperactivity. SEE: *acid-base balance.*

SYMPTOMS: There are no specific signs or symptoms, but if the alkalosis is severe, there may be apathy, confusion, stupor, and tetany as evidenced by a positive Chvostek's sign.

TREATMENT: Therapy for the primary disorder is essential. Saline solution should be administered intravenously and, in patients with hypokalemia due to diuretic therapy, potassium. Only rarely will it be necessary to administer acidifying agents IV.

NURSING IMPLICATIONS: Arterial blood gas values, serum potassium level, and fluid balance are monitored. The patient is assessed for anorexia, nausea and vomiting, tremors, muscle hypertonicity, muscle cramps, tetany, Chvostek's sign, seizures, mental confusion progressing to stupor and coma, cardiac dysrhythmias due to hypokalemia, and compensatory hypoventilation with resulting hypoxia. Prescribed oxygen, oral or IV fluids, sodium chloride or ammonium chloride, and potassium chloride if hypokalemia is a factor, along with therapy prescribed to correct the cause, are administered. Seizure precautions are observed; a safe environment and reorientation as needed are provided for the patient with altered thought processes. The patient's response to therapy is evaluated, and the patient is taught about the dangers of excess sodium bicarbonate intake if that is a factor. The ulcer patient is taught to recognize signs of milk-alkali syndrome, including anorexia, weakness, lethargy, and a distaste for milk. If potassium-wasting diuretics or potassium chloride supplements are prescribed, the nurse ascertains that the patient understands the regimen's purpose, dosage, and possible adverse effects.

***respiratory a.*** Alkalosis with an acute reduction of plasma bicarbonate with a proportionate reduction in plasma carbon dioxide.

SYMPTOMS: Patients may develop paresthesias; hyperventilation; dry oral mucosa; numbness or tingling of the nose, circumoral area, or extremities; muscle twitching; tetany and hyperreflexia; lightheadedness; inability to concentrate; and mental confusion leading to lethargy and coma.

ETIOLOGY: Causes include hyperventilation due to hypoxia, anxiety, fever, salicylate intoxication, exercise, or excessive mechanical assist to breathing, as could occur in a respirator.

TREATMENT: Therapy is given for the underlying cause. The immediate treatment for acute hyperventilation, esp. in the type induced by anxiety, is to increase carbon dioxide by having the patient rebreathe into a paper bag. A simpler method is to have the patient breathe with one nostril closed off and the mouth closed.

NURSING IMPLICATIONS: Patients experiencing risk factors (e.g., pain, fear, anxiety, hysteria) are identified and preventive measures taken, such as having the hyperventilating patient breathe with mouth and one nostril closed into cupped hands or a paper bag. Hyperventilation is prevented or corrected in patients receiving mechanical ventilation by adjusting deadspace or minute volume. Arterial blood gas values, vital signs, and neurological status are monitored. In severe cases the nurse monitors serum potassium level for hypokalemia and cardiac status for dysrhythmias. Prescribed therapy is administered to treat the cause. The nurse provides reassurance and maintains a calm, quiet environment during periods of extreme stress and anxiety. The patient is helped to identify stressors and to learn coping mechanisms and anxiety-reducing techniques, such as guided imagery, controlled breathing, or meditation.

**alkalotherapy** (ăl″kă-lō-thĕr′ă-pē) [*alkali* + Gr. *therapeia,* treatment] Therapeutic use of alkalies.

**alkapton(e)** (ăl-kăp′tōn) [″ + Gr. *hapto,* to bind to] Homogentisic acid; a yellowish-red substance sometimes occurring in urine as the result of the incomplete oxidation of tyrosine and phenylalanine.

**alkaptonuria** (ăl″kăp-tō-nū′rē-ă) [*alkapton* + Gr. *ouron,* urine] A rare inherited disorder marked by the excretion of large amounts of homogentisic acid in the urine, a result of incomplete metabolism of the amino acids tyrosine and phenylalanine. Presence of the acid is indicated by the darkening of urine on standing or when alkalinated and the dark staining of diapers or other linen. SEE: *ochronosis.*

**alkene** (ăl′kēn) A bivalent aliphatic hydrocarbon containing one double bond.

**Alkeran** Trade name for melphalan, an alkylating antineoplastic agent.

**alkyl** (ăl′kĭl) A hydrocarbon molecule from which one atom of hydrogen is absent. The resulting substances are called alkyl groups or alkyl radicals.

**alkylate** (ăl′kĭ-lāt) To provide therapy involving the use of an alkylating agent.

**alkylating agent** A substance that introduces an alkyl radical into a compound in place of a hydrogen atom. Because these substances have the ability to interfere with cell metabolism and growth, they are used in treating certain types of malignancies.

**alkylation** (ăl″kĭ-lā′shŭn) A chemical process in which an alkyl radical replaces a hydrogen atom.

**ALL** *acute lymphocytic leukemia.*

**all-** [Gr. *allos,* other] SEE: *allo-.*

**allachesthesia** (ăl″ă-kĕs-thē′zē-ă) [Gr. *allache,* elsewhere, + *aisthesis,* sensation] Perception of tactile sensation as being remote from the actual point of stimulation.

**allantochorion** (ă-lăn″tō-kō′rē-ŏn) Fusion of the allantois and chorion into one structure.

**allantoic** (ăl″ăn-tō′ĭk) Pert. to the allantois.

**allantoid** [Gr. *allantos,* sausage, + *eidos,* form, shape] **1.** Sausage-shaped. **2.** Pert. to the allantois.

**allantoin** (ă-lăn′tō-ĭn) $C_4H_6N_4O_3$. A white crystalline substance in allantoic and amniotic fluids and the end product of purine metabolism in mammals other than primates. It is produced synthetically by the oxidation of uric acid. At one time allantoin was used to promote wound healing.

**allantoinuria** (ă-lăn″tō-ĭn-ū′rē-ă) [*allantoin* + Gr. *ouron,* urine] Allantoin in the urine.

**allantois** (ă-lăn′tō-ĭs) [Gr. *allantos,* sausage, + *eidos,* form, shape] An elongated bladder developing from the hindgut of the fetus in mammals, birds, and reptiles. In mammals, it contributes to the development of the umbilicus and placenta. In birds and reptiles, it provides for the exchange of gases through the shell.

**allayed** (ă-lād′) Mitigated.

**allele** (ă-lēl′, ă-lĕl′) [Gr. *allelon,* of one another] One of two or more different genes containing specific inheritable characteristics that occupy corresponding positions (loci) on paired chromosomes. A pair of alleles is usually indicated by a capital letter for the dominant and a lowercase letter for the recessive. An individual with a pair of identical alleles, either dominant or recessive, is said to be homozygous for this gene. The union of a dominant gene and its recessive allele produces a heterozygous individual for that characteristic. Some traits may have multiple alleles, that is, more than two possibilities, but an individual has only two of those alleles (e.g., the genes for blood type, A, B, and O, are at the same position on the chromosome pair, but an individual has only two of these genes, which may be the same or different). SYN: *allelic gene; allelomorph.* **allelic** (ă-lĕl′ĭk), *adj.*

***histocompatibility a.*** One of many different forms of the histocompatibility gene. Each allele creates specific cell surface antigenic markers on cells. SEE: *histocompatibility antigens.*

**allelic gene** Allele.

**allelomorph** (ă-lē′lō-morf, ă-lĕl′ō-morf) [″ + *morphe,* form] Allele.

**allelotaxis** (ă-lē″lō-tăk′sĭs) [″ + *taxis,* order] Development of a part from several embryonic structures.

**Allen Cognitive Level Test** A standardized method of assessing information processing based on a theory that postulates six levels of cognitive function. It is used widely by occupational therapists.

**Allen-Doisy test** (ăl′ĕn-doy′sē) [Edgar V. Allen, U.S. endocrinologist, 1892–1943; Edward A. Doisy, U.S. biochemist and physiologist, b. 1893] A test used to determine estrogen content. A spayed mouse is injected with the material being tested. The appearance of cornified cells on a vaginal smear constitutes a positive reaction.

**Allen-Doisy unit** The smallest amount of estrogen that will produce a characteristic change (appearance of cornified cells) in the vaginal epithelium of a spayed mouse. SYN: *mouse unit.*

**Allen test** A test to evaluate patency of the radial and ulnar arteries in the hand. The patient elevates the hand and repetitively makes a fist while the examiner places digital occlusive pressure over the radial and ulner arteries at the wrist. Alternately, the digital pressure is released and the pale palm regains color as circulation returns. A positive Allen test occurs when patency is not demonstrated or the palm does not regain color.

**allergen** (ăl′ĕr-jĕn) [Gr. *allos,* other, + *ergon,* work, + *gennan,* to produce] Any substance that causes manifestations of allergy. It may or may not be a protein or an antigen. Among common allergens are inhalants (dusts, pollens, fungi, smoke, perfumes, odors of plastics), foods (wheat, eggs, milk, chocolate, strawberries), drugs (aspirin, antibiotics, serums), infectious agents (bacteria, viruses, fungi, animal parasites), contactants (chemicals, animals, plants, metals), and physical agents (heat, cold, light, pressure, radiations). SEE: *allergy; antigen; irritation; sensitization.*

**allergenic** (ăl″ĕr-jĕn′ĭk) Producing allergy.

**allergic** (ă-lĕr′jĭk) Pert. to, sensitive to, or caused by an allergen.

**allergist** A physician who specializes in diagnosing and treating allergies.

**allergy** (ăl′ĕr-jē) [Gr. *allos,* other, + *ergon,* work] An acquired, abnormal immune response to a substance (allergen) that does not normally cause a reaction. Sensitization, or an initial exposure to the allergen, is required; subsequent contact with the allergen then results in a broad range of inflammatory responses. Allergic conditions include eczema, allergic rhinitis or coryza, hay fever, bronchial asthma, urticaria (hives), and food allergy. Allergens may be introduced by contact, ingestion (e.g., food), inhalation (e.g., pollen), or injection (e.g., drugs). The hypersensitivity immune reactions of allergies are primarily governed by antibodies, but T cells may also be involved. SEE: *skin test.*

TYPES: *Type I* (immediate) reactions are local or systemic anaphylaxis (extremely rapid) inflammatory responses to allergens mediated by immunoglobulin E (IgE). Local responses include urticaria (hives, allergic rhinitis), asthma, and angioedema. Systemic anaphylaxis is life threatening. The allergen reaches the bloodstream, triggering a massive release of chemical mediators that produce severe bronchial obstruction, vasodilation, and increased vascular permeability, which can cause laryngeal or pulmonary edema and shock.

*Type II* (cytotoxic) reactions are antigen-antibody reactions mediated by IgG and IgM that cause transfusion reactions and many drug reactions. These reactions cause lysis of blood cells (erythrocytes, leukocytes, and platelets) due to the release of complement.

*Type III* (immune complex) reactions occur when IgG or IgM antibodies attach to antigens, creating complexes that circulate in the blood. The complexes cause damage when they adhere to the walls of blood vessels, thus initiating inflammation. Serum sickness, marked by fever, joint and muscle pain, lymphadenopathy, and urticaria, is a type III reaction that can occur in sensitized people who receive penicillins, sulfonamides, or antitoxins developed from animals (e.g., for tetanus, snake venom, or rabies).

*Type IV* (cell mediated) reactions are mediated by sensitized T lymphocytes, not antibodies. Contact dermatitis, one type IV reaction, involves many common allergens, including rubber used in elastic materials, poison ivy, chromium in leather, and nickel used in costume jewelry. These combine with skin proteins, altering the normal self-antigens so that new, foreign antigens are created. Contact dermatitis is marked by acute erythema, edema, itching, and scaling. Delayed hypersensitivity reactions (type IV reactions) are used as a clinical tool in skin tests for sensitivity. In a test, a small amount of an agent is placed on the skin; if the individual is sensitized to the substance and has a competent immune system, an inflammatory reaction will occur. At the end of the test, the site of application is compared with a site exposed to a nonsensitizing substance such as a saline solution.

SYMPTOMS: The symptoms consist of local or systemic inflammatory responses marked by redness, edema, and heat. Respiratory symptoms include wheezing, coughing, sneezing, and nasal congestion. Increased blood eosinophil levels (eosinophilia) are common.

ETIOLOGY: An allergy is caused by an inherited or acquired sensitivity over time to a foreign antigen. The number of exposures needed to produce enough antibodies to cause an allergic response varies. An allergy may occur the second time a person is exposed to a particular allergen or may not occur until years later when repeated exposures have produced sufficient antibodies or sensitized T cells.

TREATMENT: Delayed hypersensitivity demonstrated by skin testing is often used to determine those allergens to which the patient reacts. Many allergens can be eliminated from the environment (e.g., foods, animals). Antihistamines or corticosteroids may be prescribed to reduce symptoms. Desensitization may be used to promote tolerance of allergens if allergic responses significantly interfere with lifestyle or are life threatening. The patient should wear or carry a medical identification device indicating known allergens and usual treatment.

NURSING IMPLICATIONS: A history is obtained to determine any past allergic reactions. The patient receiving blood or blood products is closely observed for the initial 20 min during and after administration of drugs not previously received. Drugs such as epinephrine, diphenhydramine, and corticosteroids should be readily available for treatment of systemic anaphylaxis, which is life threatening. SEE: *anaphylactic shock.* Once the initial emergency has subsided, the nurse administers medications prescribed for long-term management (such as SC or longer-acting epinephrine, corticosteroids, and diphenhydramine), and inhaled bronchodilators or IV aminophylline (over 20 min) for bronchospasm. Patients are taught how to identify and avoid common allergens and identify an allergic reaction. If a patient needs drugs for treatment of systemic anaphylaxis at home, both patient and family are instructed in their use.

***atopic a.*** An inherited allergy.

***contact a.*** Hypersensitivity reaction following direct contact with an allergen.

***drug a.*** Hypersensitivity to a drug.

***food a.*** SEE: *food allergies.*

**allesthesia** (ăl″ĕs-thē′sē-ă) [″ + *aisthesis,* sensation] Perception of stimulus in the limb opposite the one stimulated. SYN: *allochesthesia; allochiria.*

**alleviate** To lessen the effect of.

**alliaceous** (ăl″ē-ā′shŭs) [L. *allium,* garlic, + *-aceus,* of a specific kind] Tasting like garlic or onions.

**allied health professional** An individual who has received special training in an allied health field, such as clinical laboratory science, radiology, emergency medical services, physical therapy, respiratory therapy, medical assisting, athletic training, dental hygiene, or occupational therapy.

**alliesthesia** (ăl″ē-ĕs-thē′sē-ă) [Gr. *allios,* changed, + *aisthesis,* sensation] The perception of an external stimulus as pleasant or unpleasant depending upon internal stimuli. A particular stimulus may be perceived as pleasant at one time and unpleasant at another.

**alliteration** (ă-lĭt″ĕr-ā′shŭn) [L. *ad,* to, + *litera,* letter] A speech disorder in which words beginning with the same consonant sound are used to excess.

**allo-, all-** [Gr. *allos,* other] Combining form indicating *divergence, difference from,* or *opposition to the normal.*

**alloantigen** (ăl″lō-ăn′tĭ-jĕn) [″ + *anti,* against, + *gennan,* to produce] Isoantigen.

**allochesthesia** (ăl″ō-kĕs-thē′zē-ă) [Gr. *allache,* elsewhere, + *aisthesis,* sensation] Allesthesia.

**allochezia, allochetia** (ăl″ō-kē′zē-ă, ăl″ō-kē′shē-ă) [Gr. *allos,* other, + *chezein,* to defecate] The excretion of feces through an abnormal opening.

**allochiria, allocheiria** (ăl″ō-kī′rē-ă) [″ + *cheir,* hand] Allesthesia.

**allochroism** (ăl-ōk′rō-ĭzm, ăl″ō-krō′ĭzm) [″ + *chroa,* color, + *-ismos,* condition] A change in color.

**allochromasia** (ăl″ō-krō-mā′sē-ă) A change in the color of hair or skin.

**allocinesia** (ăl″ō-sĭn-ē′sē-ă) [Gr. *allos,* other, + *kinesis,* movement] Movement on the side of the body opposite the one the patient was asked to move. SEE: *allokinesis.*

**allodiploidy** (ăl″ō-dĭp′loy-dē) [″ + *diploe,*

fold, + *eidos,* form, shape] Possession of two sets of chromosomes, each from a different species. A hybrid is allodiploid.

**allodynia** (ăl″ō-dĭn′ē-ă) The condition in which an ordinarily painless stimulus, once perceived, is experienced as being painful.

**alloeroticism, alloerotism** (ăl″ō-ē-rŏt′ĭ-sĭzm, -ĕr′ō-tĭzm) [″ + *Eros,* god of love] Sexual urges stimulated by and directed toward another person. Opposite of autoerotism.

**alloesthesia** Allesthesia.

**allogeneic, allogenic** (ăl″ō-jĕ-nē′ĭk, ăl″ō-jĕn′ĭk) Having a different genetic constitution but belonging to the same species. SEE: *isogeneic.*

**allograft** (ăl′ō-grăft) [″ + L. *graphium,* grafting knife] Transplant tissue obtained from the same species. The tissues that survive best are cornea, bone, artery, and cartilage. SYN: *homograft.* SEE: *autograft; heterograft.*

**alloimmune** (ăl″ō-ĭm-ūn′) [″ + L. *immunis,* safe] Characterized by immunity to allogeneic antigens.

**allokinesis** (ăl″ō-kĭ-nē′sĭs) [″ + *kinesis,* movement] Passive or reflex movement; involuntary movement. **allokinetic** (-kĭ-nĕt′ĭk), *adj.*

**allolalia** (ăl″ō-lā′lē-ă) [″ + *lalia,* talk] **1.** A speech defect or impairment, esp. due to a brain lesion. **2.** A type of dysphasia in which words are spoken unintentionally or inappropriate words are substituted for appropriate ones.

**allomerism** (ă-lŏm′ĕr-ĭzm) [″ + *meros,* part, + *-ismos,* condition] A change in chemical constitution without a change in form. SEE: *allomorphism.*

**allomorphism** (ăl″ō-mor′fĭzm) [″ + *morphe,* form, + *-ismos,* condition] A change in form without a change in chemical constitution. SEE: *allomerism.*

**allopath** (ăl′ō-păth) One who practices allopathy.

**allopathy** (ăl″ŏp′ă-thē) [Gr. *allos,* other, + *pathos,* disease, suffering] **1.** A system of treating disease by inducing a pathological reaction that is antagonistic to the disease being treated. **2.** A term erroneously used for the regular practice of medicine to differentiate it from homeopathy.

**allophasis** (ăl-ŏf′ă-sĭs) [Gr. *allos,* other, + *phasis,* speech] Incoherent speech.

**alloplasia** (ăl″ō-plā′zē-ă) [″ + *plasis,* a molding] The development of tissue at a location where that type of tissue would not normally occur. SYN: *heteroplasia.*

**alloplasty** (ăl′ō-plăs-tē) [″ + *plasis,* a molding] **1.** Plastic surgery using inert material. **2.** In psychiatry, adaptation by altering the external environment rather than changing oneself. SEE: *autoplasty.*

**alloploidy** (ăl″ō-ploy′dē) [″ + *ploos,* fold, + *eidos,* form, shape] The state of having two or more sets of chromosomes derived from different ancestral species.

**allopolyploidy** (ăl″ō-pŏl′ē-ploy-dē) [″ + *polys,* many, + *ploos,* fold, + *eidos,* form, shape] The state of having more than two sets of chromosomes derived from different ancestral species.

**allopsychic** (ăl-ō-sī′kĭk) [″ + *psyche,* mind] Pert. to mental processes in relation to the external environment.

**allopurinol** (ăl″ō-pū′rĭn-ŏl) A drug that inhibits the enzyme xanthine oxidase. Because its action causes a reduction in both serum and urine levels of uric acid, allopurinol is used in the treatment of gout and of renal calculi caused by uric acid.

Allergic response to this drug has been reported. Trade name is Zyloprim.

**all-or-none law 1.** In response to a stimulus, the heart either contracts to its greatest extent or does not contract at all. **2.** In response to a stimulus, a skeletal muscle cell contracts completely or not at all. **3.** In response to a stimulus, a neuron generates an impulse at a characteristic velocity or none at all.

**allostery** (ăl-ō-stĕrĭ′) [Gr. *allos,* other + *stereos,* shape] In bacteria, alteration of a regulatory site on a protein that changes its shape and activity. This change is important in altering the way the organism responds to its molecular environment.

**allotherm** (ăl′ō-thĕrm) [″ + *therme,* heat] An animal whose body temperature varies according to the temperature of the environment. SYN: *poikilotherm.* SEE: *homotherm.*

**allotransplantation** (ăl″ō-trăns″plăn-tā′shŭn) [″ + L. *trans,* through, + *plantare,* to plant] Grafting or transplantation of tissue from one individual into another of the same species. SYN: *homeotransplantation.*

**allotriogeustia** (ă-lŏt″rē-ō-jūst′ē-ă, -gū′stē-ă) [Gr. *allotrios,* strange, + *geusis,* taste] Perverted appetite or sense of taste. SEE: *parageusia.*

**allotriophagy** (ă-lŏt″rē-ŏf′ă-jē) [″ + *phagein,* to eat] A perversion of appetite with ingestion of material not suitable as food, such as starch, clay, ashes, or plaster. SYN: *pica.*

**allotriosmia** Incorrect identification of odors. SYN: *heterosmia.*

**allotropic** (ăl″ō-trŏp′ĭk) [Gr. *allos,* other, + *tropos,* direction] **1.** Pert. to the existence of an element in two or more distinct forms with different physical properties. **2.** Altered by digestion so as to be changed in its nutritive value. **3.** Indicating one who is concerned with the welfare and interests of others (i.e., not self-centered).

**allotropism, allotropy** (ă-lŏt′rō-pĭzm, -pē) [″ + *trope,* a turn, + *-ismos,* condition] The existence of an element in two or more distinct forms with different physical properties.

**allotype** Any one of the genetic variants of protein that occur in a single species. The serum from a person with one form of allotype could be antigenic to another person.

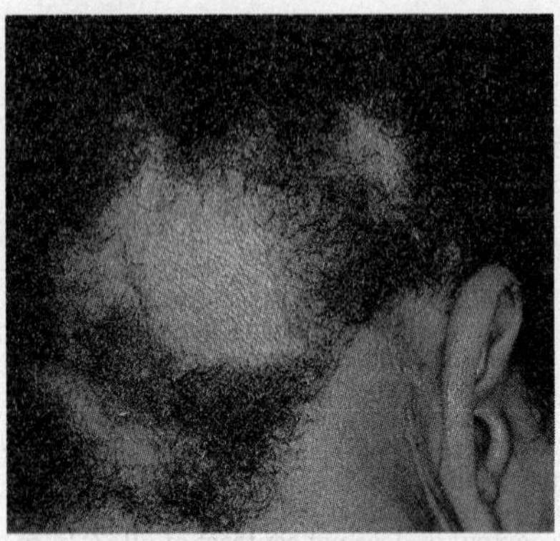

ALOPECIA AREATA

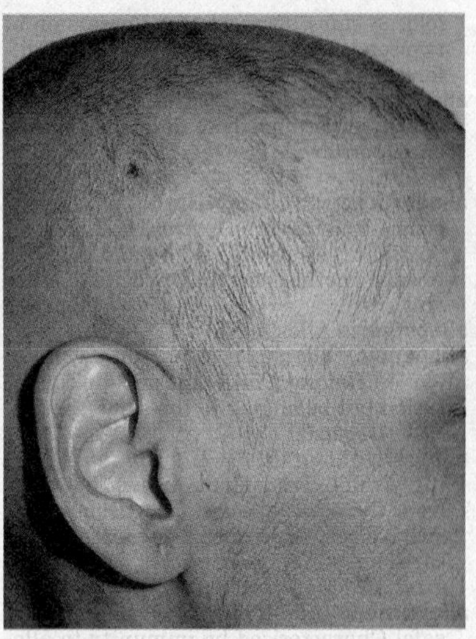

ALOPECIA CAPITIS TOTALIS

**alloxan** (ăl-ŏk′săn) [*all*antoin + *oxa*lic] $C_2H_2N_2O_4$. An oxidation product of uric acid. In laboratory animals, it causes diabetes by destroying the islet cells of the pancreas.

**alloy** (ăl′oy, ă-loy′) [Fr. *aloyer,* to combine] A metallic substance (e.g., brass) resulting from the fusion or mixture of two or more metals; also, a substance (e.g., steel) formed from the fusion or mixture of a metal and a nonmetal. In dentistry, this often contains silver, copper, tin, and mercury and is called an amalgam.

**allyl** (ăl′ĭl) [L. *allium,* garlic, + Gr. *hyle,* matter] $C_3H_5$. A univalent unsaturated radical found in garlic and mustard.

**Alma-Ata Declaration** A declaration made in 1978 at the Conference on Primary Health Care in Alma-Ata, Russia. It stated that primary health care is the key to attaining health for all by the year 2000. Defined as essential to this were eight elements: education, food supply, safe water, maternal and child health including family planning, immunization, prevention and control of endemic diseases, appropriate treatment of common diseases and injuries, and provision of essential drugs.

**ALOC** *altered level of consciousness.*

**alochia** (ă-lō′kē-ă) [Gr. *a-,* not, + *lokhos,* pert. to childbirth] Absence of lochia, the vaginal discharge following childbirth.

**aloe** (ăl′ō) The dried juice of one of several species of plants of the genus *Aloe.*

**alogia** Inability to speak.

**aloin** (ăl′ō-ĭn) A yellow crystalline substance obtained from aloe.

**alopecia** (al″ō-pē′shē-ă) [Gr. *alopekia,* fox mange] Absence or loss of hair, esp. of the head.

ETIOLOGY: Alopecia may result from serious illness, drugs, endocrine disorders, certain forms of dermatitis, hereditary factors, radiation, or physiological changes as a part of the aging process.

TREATMENT: The treatment for dermatitis seborrheica should be followed if present. Scalp baldness may be treated by surgical transplantation of hair follicles from another part of the body to the scalp.

***a. areata*** Loss of hair in sharply defined patches usually involving the scalp or beard. SEE: illus.

***a. capitis totalis*** Complete absence of hair of the scalp. SEE: illus.

***cicatricial a.*** Loss of hair due to formation of scar tissue.

***a. congenitalis*** Baldness due to absence of hair bulbs at birth.

***a. follicularis*** Baldness due to inflammation of the hair follicles of the scalp.

***a. liminaris*** Loss of hair along the hairline, both front and back, of the scalp.

***male pattern a.*** Typical hair loss pattern of males in which the alopecia begins in the frontal area and proceeds until only a horseshoe area of hair remains in the back and temples. This loss is dependent on the presence of the androgenic hormone testosterone.

***a. medicamentosa*** Loss of hair due to administration of certain medicines, esp. those containing cytotoxic agents. SEE: *scalp tourniquet.*

***a. pityroides*** Loss of both scalp and body hair accompanied by desquamation of branlike scales.

***a. prematura*** Premature baldness.

***a. symptomatica*** Loss of hair after prolonged fevers or during the course of a disease; may result from systemic or psychogenic factors.

***a. totalis*** A. capitis totalis.

***a. toxica*** Loss of hair thought to be due to toxins of infectious disease.

***a. universalis*** Loss of hair from the entire body.

**alpha** (ăl′fă) The first letter of the Greek alphabet, $\alpha$. In chemistry, it denotes the first in a series of isomeric compounds or the position adjacent to a carboxyl group.

**alpha-adrenergic blocking agent** A substance that interferes with the transmission of stimuli through pathways that normally allow sympathetic nervous excitatory stimuli to be effective. SEE: *beta-adrenergic blocking agent.*

**alpha-adrenergic receptor** A site in autonomic nerve pathways at which excitatory responses occur when adrenergic agents such as norepinephrine and epinephrine are released. SEE: *beta-adrenergic receptor.*

**alpha-1 antitrypsin** An inhibitor of trypsin that may be deficient in patients who have emphysema.

**alpha-D-galactosidase enzyme** An enzyme, derived from *Aspergillus niger,* used in treating intestinal gas or bloating. SEE: *flatus.*

**alpha-fetoprotein** ABBR: AFP. An antigen present in the human fetus and in certain pathological conditions in the adult. The maternal serum level can be evaluated at 16 to 18 weeks of pregnancy to detect fetal abnormalities. Elevated levels indicate the possibility that neural tube defects (principally anencephaly or spina bifida) are present in the fetus. Decreased levels may indicate an increased risk of having a baby with Down syndrome. If an abnormal level of AFP is found, further tests such as ultrasound or amniocentesis will need to be done. Elevated serum levels are found in adults with certain hepatic carcinomas or chemical injuries. Test results may be abnormal in persons with diabetes, multiple pregnancies, or obesity.

**alpha-globulin** One of the serum globulins. SEE: *globulin, serum.*

**alpha particles, alpha rays** Radioactive, positively charged particles, two protons and two neutrons, ejected at high speeds in certain atomic disintegrations.

**alpha-rhythm** In electroencephalography, rhythmic oscillations in electric potential occurring at an average rate of 10/sec. SYN: *alpha-wave.*

**alpha-tocopherol** Vitamin E.

**alpha-wave** Alpha-rhythm.

**Alport's syndrome** [Arthur Cecil Alport, S. African physician, 1880–1959] Congenital glomerulonephritis associated with deafness and a decrease in large thrombocytes. Occasionally there are eye abnormalities such as cataract. There is no specific treatment for this disease, but renal dialysis or kidney transplantation may be beneficial. SEE: *macrothrombocyte.*

**ALS** *amyotrophic lateral sclerosis.*

**ALT** *alanine aminotransferase.*

**alternans** (awl-tĕr′nănz) [L. *alternare,* to alternate] Alternating.

***pulsus a.*** Regular heart rhythm in which strong beats alternate with weak ones.

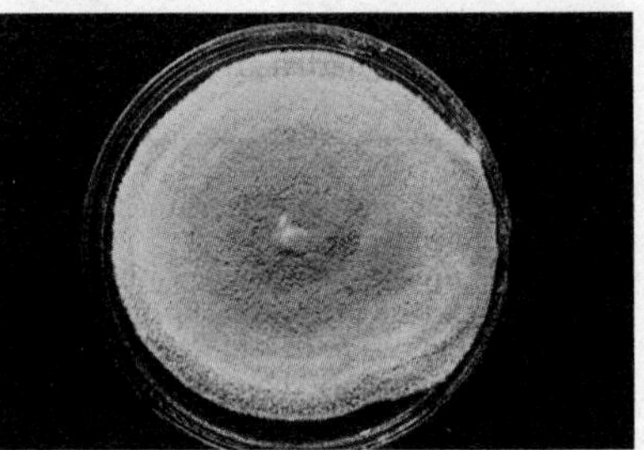

ALTERNARIA IN CULTURE

**Alternaria** (awl″tĕr-nā′rē-ă) A genus of fungi of the Dematiaceae family. The fungus can cause pneumonitis and may cause wound or skin infections in immunocompromised patients. It has been implicated as the cause of pulmonary disease in wood pulp workers. SEE: illus.

**alternating current** ABBR: A.C. An electric current that reverses direction at regular intervals. SEE: *direct current.*

**alternative medicine** Approaches to medical diagnosis and therapy that have not been developed by use of generally accepted scientific methods. Forms of alternative medicine include acupressure, acupuncture, aroma therapy, ayurveda, biofeedback, Christian Science, faith healing, guided imagery, herbal medicine, holistic medicine, homeopathy, hypnosis, macrobiotics, manipulative medicine, massage therapy, naturopathy, ozone therapy, reflexotherapy, relaxation response, Rolfing, shiatsu, and yoga. This is not to say that, were these methods subjected to scientific study, all of them would be found to be ineffective.

The interest of the American public in alternative approaches to health maintenance, the treatment of illness, and the restoration of health has increased over the last several decades. Individuals seeking medical care from either conventional or unconventional practitioners should be advised to inform the caregiver about all behaviors and therapies in recent or current use. In addition, the psychosomatic "placebo" effect and the natural history of the particular disease must be considered in evaluating the efficacy of alternative therapies. In 1992, the Office of Alternative Medicine was established at the National Institutes of Health to investigate the scientific merits of alternative medicine. SEE: *remedy, herbal.*

---

Caution: Individuals who choose to use herbal preparations should be aware that few, if any, of those products are subjected to formulation specifications and manufacturing controls. In their absence the consumer has no assurance of their purity or cleanliness. Furthermore, the possible interaction of pharmacological agents with nutritional and/or herbal preparations must be considered.

**alternator** An electrical generator that produces alternating current.

**alt. hor.** L. *alternis horis,* every other hour.

**altitude sickness** Symptoms produced by decreased oxygen in the environment. The symptoms may come on abruptly, as when an airplane ascends quickly to high altitude, or slowly, as in mountain climbing. The deficiency of oxygen causes headache, shortness of breath, malaise, decreased ability to concentrate, lack of judgment, lightheadedness, fainting and, if severe, death. The initial symptom may be euphoria so that the individual is unaware of the cause of the difficulty. Adaptation to living at high altitudes is best done over a period of weeks and months. SYN: *mountain sickness.* SEE: *bends; altitude hypoxia.*

**altretamine** A drug used for treating persistent or recurrent ovarian cancer.

**altricious** (ăl-trĭsh′ŭs) [L. *altrix,* nourisher] **1.** Slow in developing. **2.** Requiring long-term nursing care.

**alum** (ăl′ŭm) [L. *alumen*] **1.** A double sulfate of aluminum and potassium or aluminum and ammonia; used as an astringent and styptic. **2.** Any of a group of double sulfates of a trivalent metal and a univalent metal.

*ammonia a.* Aluminum ammonia sulfate.

*potassium a.* Aluminum potassium sulfate.

**aluminosis** (ă-loo″mĭn-ō′sĭs) [″ + Gr. *osis,* condition of] Chronic inflammation of the lungs in alum workers due to alum particles in inspired air.

**aluminum** SYMB: Al. A silver-whitish metal used to filter low-energy radiation out of the x-ray beam; atomic weight 26.9815, atomic number 13.

*a. acetate* A salt formed by the reaction between aluminum sulfate and lead acetate. Its aqueous solution (Burow's solution) is used as a local astringent.

*a. ammonia sulfate* An astringent. SYN: *ammonia alum.*

*a. chloride* A chemical substance used as an astringent and antiperspirant.

*a. hydroxide gel* A white viscous suspension containing aluminum hydroxide and hydrated aluminum oxide; an antacid esp. useful in treatment of peptic ulcer.

*a. phosphate gel* An aqueous suspension of aluminum phosphate used as an astringent and antacid.

*a. potassium sulfate* An astringent and styptic. SYN: *potassium alum.*

*a. sulfate* A chemical substance used topically as an antiperspirant.

**alveoalgia** [L. *alveolus,* small cavity, + Gr. *algos,* pain] Pain in the socket of a tooth. SEE: *socket, dry.*

**alveobronchiolitis, alveobronchitis** (ăl″vē-ō-brŏng″kē-ō-lī′tĭs, -brŏng-kī′tĭs) [L. *alveolus,* small hollow or cavity, + Gr. *bronchos,* windpipe, + *itis,* inflammation] Inflammation of the bronchioles and pulmonary alveoli; bronchopneumonia.

**alveolalgia** (ăl″vē-ŏ-lăl′jē-ă) [″ + Gr. *algos,* pain] Pain in the alveolus of a tooth.

**alveolar** (ăl-vē′ō-lăr) Pert. to an alveolus.

**alveolar air** Air in the pulmonary alveoli; that involved in the pulmonary exchange of gases. Its content is determined by sampling the last portion of a maximal expiration.

**alveolar bone** Alveolar process.

**alveolar-capillary block** Impaired ability of gases to pass through the pulmonary alveolar-capillary membrane.

**alveolar duct** A branch of a respiratory bronchiole that leads to the alveoli of the lungs. SEE: *alveolus* for illus.

**alveolar process** The part of the mandible and maxilla containing the tooth sockets. SYN: *alveolar bone.*

**alveolar proteinosis** Pulmonary alveolar proteinosis.

**alveolate** (ăl-vē′ō-lāt) Honeycombed; pitted.

**alveolectomy** (ăl″vē-ŏ-lĕk′tō-mē) [L. *alveolus,* small hollow or cavity, + Gr. *ektome,* excision] Surgical removal of all or part of the alveolar process of the mandible or maxilla; usually performed in treatment of neoplasms.

**alveoli** (ăl-vē′ō-lī) [L.] Pl. of alveolus.

*a. dentales* Tooth sockets.

*a. pulmonis* Air cells of the lungs.

**alveolitis** (ăl″vē-ŏ-lī′tĭs) [″ + Gr. *itis,* inflammation] Inflammation of the alveoli.

*allergic a.* Inflammation of the bronchial tree, interstitial tissue, and alveoli of the lung caused by a hypersensitivity reaction to an inhaled antigen. With repeated exposure, large numbers of macrophages, the primary white blood cell in the lungs, clump together to form granulomas, which produce granulomatous and fibrotic tissue in the lung. Inhaled allergens are most often bacteria or fungi found in grains, fertilizer, grasses, and compost. Farmer's lung and bagassosis are two common names for forms of allergic alveolitis. SYN: *hypersensitivity pneumonitis.*

**alveoloclasia** (ăl-vē″ō-lō-klā′sē-ă) [″ + Gr. *klasis,* fracture] Destruction of a tooth socket.

**alveolodental** (ăl-vē″ō-lō-dĕn′tăl) [″ + *dens,* tooth] Pert. to the alveolus of the tooth and to the tooth itself.

**alveololingual** (ăl-vē″lō-lĭng′gwăl) [″ + *lingua,* tongue] Concerning the alveolar process and tongue.

**alveoloplasty** (ăl-vē″ō-lō-plăs′tē) [″ + Gr. *plassein,* to form] Reconstruction of the alveolus by use of plastic surgery.

**alveolotomy** (ăl″vē-ŏ-lŏt′ō-mē) [″ + Gr. *tome,* incision] Surgical incision of the alveolus of a tooth.

**alveolus** (ăl-vē′ō-lŭs) *pl.* **alveoli** [L., small

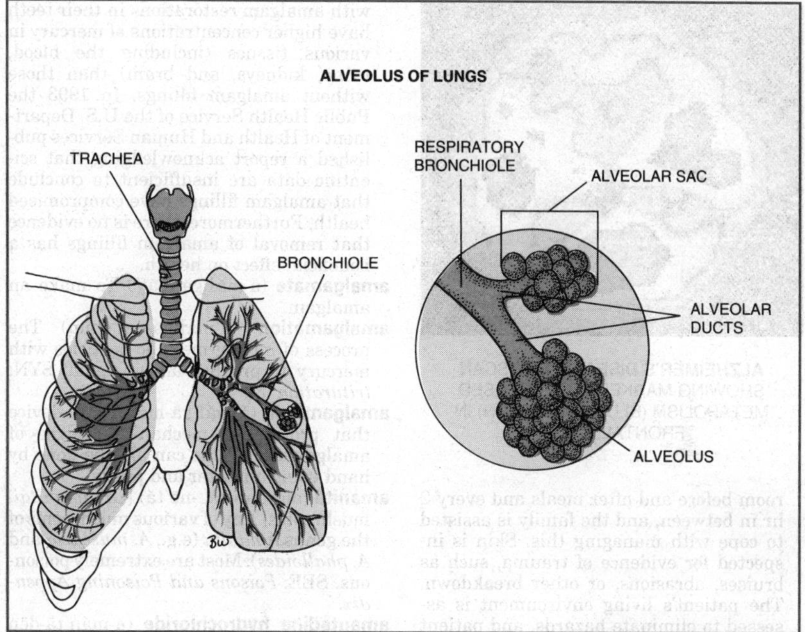


hollow or cavity] **1.** A small hollow. **2.** The socket of a tooth. **3.** An air sac of the lungs. SEE: illus.; *canals of Lambert; pores of Kohn.* **4.** One of the honeycombed depressions of the gastric mucous membrane. **5.** A follicle of a racemose gland.

***a. dentalis*** Tooth socket.

***pulmonary a.*** One of the terminal saccules of an alveolar duct where gases are exchanged in respiration. SYN: *air vesicle.*

**alveus** (ăl'vē-ŭs) [L.] A channel or groove.

***a. hippocampi*** A layer of white matter covering the ventricular surface of the hippocampus.

**alymphia** (ă-lĭm'fē-ă) [Gr. *a-*, not, + L. *lympha,* lymph] Complete or partial deficiency of lymph.

**alymphocytosis** (ă-lĭm″fō-sī-tō'sĭs) [″ + ″ + Gr. *kytos,* cell, + *osis,* condition] Decreased number or absence of lymphocytes in the blood.

**alymphoplasia** (ă″lĭm-fō-plā'zē-ă) [″ + ″ + Gr. *plasis,* a developing] Failure of lymphatic tissue to develop.

***thymic a.*** A sometimes fatal disorder in which the thymus fails to develop, causing a deficiency of gamma globulin. There is a deficiency of lymph tissue throughout the body.

**Alzheimer's disease** (ălts'hī-mĕrz) [Alois Alzheimer, Ger. neurologist, 1864–1915] A chronic, progressive disorder that accounts for more than 50% of all dementias. The most common form occurs in people older than 65, but the presenile form can begin between ages 40 and 60. Characteristic pathological changes in the brain are plaques and neuronal tangles. The disease begins with mild memory loss, which then progresses to deterioration of intellectual functions, personality changes, and speech and language problems. In the terminal stage, patients depend on others for activities of daily living and may have seizures, hallucinations, delusions, paranoia, or depression. Death results from complications of immobility. The course may take 10 to 15 years or more. The exact cause is unknown. The diagnosis is usually made by ruling out other causes of cognitive dysfunction. SEE: illus.; *dementia, senile; tomography, positron emission* for illus.; *Nursing Diagnoses Appendix.*

NURSING IMPLICATIONS: The patient's need for assistance with activities of daily living is assessed. Self-care, exercise, and other activities are encouraged to the fullest extent possible. If sleep disturbances occur, the patient should rest between daytime activities, but sleeping during daytime hours is discouraged. Neurological function, including mental and emotional states and motor capabilities, is monitored for further deterioration. Vital signs and respiratory status are assessed for signs and symptoms of pneumonia and other infections. The patient is evaluated for indications of gastrointestinal or urinary problems (anorexia, dysphagia, and urinary or fecal incontinence), and fluid and food intake is monitored to detect imbalances. The patient is taken to the bath-

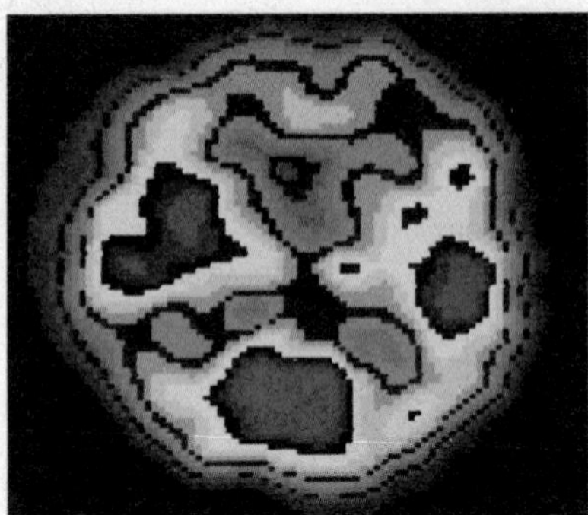

ALZHEIMER'S DISEASE: PET SCAN SHOWING MARKEDLY DECREASED METABOLISM (BLUE AND GREEN) IN FRONTAL LOBES

room before and after meals and every 2 hr in between, and the family is assisted to cope with managing this. Skin is inspected for evidence of trauma, such as bruises, abrasions, or other breakdown. The patient's living environment is assessed to eliminate hazards, and patient activity is monitored to prevent falls, burns, and other injuries. Expectations should not exceed the patient's ability to perform tasks. Because the patient may misperceive the environment, the nurse should speak softly and calmly and allow sufficient time for answers given the patient's slowed thought processes and impaired ability to communicate verbally. The caregiver's ability to manage the patient at home is evaluated, and referral is made to available local resources such as counseling, support groups, and respite care as indicated.

**Am 1.** *mixed astigmatism.* **2.** *ametropia.* **3.** Symbol for the element americium.

**A.M.A.** *American Medical Association.*

**AMA** *against medical advice.*

**amaas** (ă'măs) A mild form of smallpox. SYN: *variola minor.*

**amacrine** (ăm'ă-krĭn) [Gr. *a-*, not, + *makros,* long, + *is, inos,* fiber] Lacking a long process.

**amacrine cell** A modified nerve cell in the retina that has short branches (dendrites) but no long process (axon). SEE: *neuron.*

**amalgam** (ă-măl'găm) [Gr. *malagma,* soft mass] Any alloy containing mercury.

***dental a.*** A dental restorative material made by mixing approx. equal parts of elemental liquid mercury (43% to 54%) and an alloy powder (57% to 46%) composed of silver, tin, copper, and sometimes smaller amounts of zinc, palladium, or indium. It has been used for more than 150 years in dental restorations; only gold has been used longer for this purpose. It is known that a fraction of the mercury in amalgam is absorbed by the body and that people with amalgam restorations in their teeth have higher concentrations of mercury in various tissues (including the blood, urine, kidneys, and brain) than those without amalgam fillings. In 1993 the Public Health Service of the U.S. Department of Health and Human Services published a report acknowledging that scientific data are insufficient to conclude that amalgam fillings have compromised health. Furthermore, there is no evidence that removal of amalgam fillings has a beneficial effect on health.

**amalgamate** (ă-măl'gă-māt") To make an amalgam.

**amalgamation** (ă-măl"gă-mā'shŭn) The process of mixing metallic particles with mercury to produce an amalgam. SYN: *trituration* (3).

**amalgamator** (ă-măl'gă-mā"tor) A device that provides a mechanical means of amalgamation. This can also be done by hand using a mortar and pestle.

**amanita** (ăm"ă-nī'tă, -nē'tă) [Gr. *amanitai,* mushrooms] Any of various mushrooms of the genus *Amanita* (e.g., *A. muscaria* and *A. phalloides*). Most are extremely poisonous. SEE: *Poisons and Poisoning Appendix.*

**amantadine hydrochloride** (ă-măn'tă-dēn hī"drō-klor'īd) An antiviral agent originally used for prophylaxis against certain strains of the influenza virus. Trade name is Symmetrel.

**amastia** (ă-măs'tē-ă) [" + *mastos,* breast] Absence of breast tissue. SYN: *amazia.*

**amaurosis** (ăm"aw-rō'sĭs) [Gr., darkening] Complete loss of vision, esp. that in which there is no apparent pathological condition of the eye. **amaurotic** (ăm-aw-rŏt'ĭk), *adj.*

***albuminuric a.*** Amaurosis caused by kidney disease.

***congenital a.*** Amaurosis present at birth.

***diabetic a.*** Amaurosis associated with diabetes.

***epileptoid a.*** Sudden blindness following an epileptic seizure and lasting up to 2 weeks.

***a. fugax*** Temporary loss of vision in one eye due to insufficient flow of blood to the retina; may last for up to 10 min. The blindness is complete, but it may be limited to a sector of the field of vision. Attacks can be single or multiple. Some patients have hundreds or even thousands of episodes. The prognosis for recovery is good; in a few cases, retinal infarction occurs. SYN: *blindness, transient.*

***lead a.*** Amaurosis caused by lead poisoning.

***a. partialis fugax*** Sudden transitory blindness with symptoms similar to those of migraine: nausea; vomiting; dizziness; and disturbances of vision.

***reflex a.*** Amaurosis due to reflex action caused by irritation of a remote part.

***saburral a.*** Amaurosis in conjunction

with acute gastritis.

***toxic a.*** Amaurosis from optic neuritis caused by toxins that may be endogenous (as in diabetes) or exogenous (as in alcohol or tobacco).

***uremic a.*** Amaurosis caused by acute renal failure.

**amaxophobia** [Gr. *amaxa,* a carriage, + *phobos,* fear] Fear of riding in a vehicle.

**amazia** (ă-mā′zē-ă) [Gr. *a-,* not, + *mazos,* breast] Amastia.

**ambergris** An amorphous gray material formed in the intestinal tract of the sperm whale. It is vomited and usually found floating in the ocean. It is valuable because it is in demand for use in perfume production.

**ambi-** [L. *ambi-,* on both sides] Prefix indicating *both, both sides, around,* or *about.*

**ambidextrous** (ăm″bĭ-dĕk′strŭs) [″ + *dexter,* right] Having the ability to work effectively with either hand.

**ambient** (ăm′bē-ĕnt) [L. *ambiens,* going around] Surrounding.

**ambient noise** The total noise from all sources in a given environment.

**ambiguous** [L. *ambiguus,* to be uncertain] To have several meanings or interpretations. In anatomy, being difficult to classify.

**ambilateral** (ăm″bĭ-lăt′ĕr-ăl) [L. *ambi-,* on both sides, + *latus,* side] Pert. to both sides.

**ambilevous** (ăm-bĭ-lē′vŭs) [″ + *laevus,* left-handed] Awkward in the use of either hand. SYN: *ambisinister.*

**ambiopia** (ăm″bē-ō′pē-ă) [″ + Gr. *ops,* eye] Double vision. SYN: *diplopia.*

**ambisexual** (ăm″bĭ-sĕks′ū-ăl) [″ + *sexus,* sex] Pert. to both sexes. SEE: *bisexual.*

**ambisinister** (ăm″bĭ-sĭn′ĭs-tĕr) [″+ *sinister,* left] Ambilevous.

**ambitendency** (ăm″bĭ-tĕn′dĕn-sē) [″ + *tendere,* to stretch] Ambivalence of the will. SEE: *ambivalence.*

**ambivalence** (ăm-bĭv′ă-lĕns) [″ + *valentia,* strength] Coexistence of contradictory feelings about an object, person, or idea. **ambivalent** (ăm-bĭv′ă-lĕnt), *adj.*

**ambivert** (ăm′bĭ-vĕrt) [″ + *vertere,* to turn] An individual whose personality type falls between introversion and extroversion, possessing some tendencies of each.

**amblyacousia** (ăm″blē-ă-koo′sē-ă) [Gr. *amblys,* dull, + *akousis,* hearing] Dullness of hearing.

**amblychromasia** (ăm″blē-krō-mā′sē-ă) [″ + *chroma,* color] The state in which the cell nucleus stains faintly.

**amblychromatic** (ăm″blē-krō-măt′ĭk) Staining faintly.

**amblyopia** (ăm″blē-ō′pē-ă) [″ + *ops,* eye] Reduction or dimness of vision, esp. that in which there is no apparent pathologic condition of the eye. **amblyopic** (-ō′ĭk), *adj.*

***crossed a.*** Amblyopia of one eye with hemianesthesia of the opposite side of the face. SYN: *a. cruciata.*

***a. cruciata*** Crossed a.

***deprivation a.*** Amblyopia resulting from nonuse of the eye. It is usually secondary to an organic problem such as cataract or ptosis.

***a. ex anopsia*** Amblyopia resulting from disuse. It usually occurs in one eye and is associated with convergent squint or very poor visual acuity.

***reflex a.*** Amblyopia due to irritation of the peripheral area.

***strabismic a.*** Amblyopia secondary to malalignment of the eyes. In this condition, the brain suppresses the visual image from the deviating eye to prevent double vision. Strabismic amblyopia accounts for about 50% of childhood amblyopia.

***toxic a.*** Amblyopia due to the effect of alcohol, tobacco, lead, drugs, or other toxic substances.

***uremic a.*** Dimness or loss of vision during a uremic attack.

**amblyoscope** (ăm′blē-ŏ-skōp″) [″ + ″ + *skopein,* to examine] An instrument for measuring binocular vision. It is used to stimulate vision in an amblyopic eye.

**ambon** (ăm′bŏn) [Gr., edge of a dish] The elevated ring of fibrocartilage around the edge of a bone socket.

**ambos** (ăm′bōs) [Ger.] Incus or anvil bone of the middle ear.

**Ambu bag** (ăm′bū) Proprietary name for a bag used to assist in providing artificial ventilation of the lungs. SEE: *bag-valve-mask resuscitator* for illus.

**ambulance** [L. *ambulare,* to move about] A vehicle for transporting the sick and injured that is equipped and staffed to provide medical care during transit.

**ambulant, ambulatory** (ăm′bū-lănt, -lă-tō″rē) Able to walk; not confined to bed.

**Ambu simulator** Proprietary name for a manikin used in teaching the technique of cardiopulmonary resuscitation.

**Amcill** Trade name for ampicillin.

**ameba** (ă-mē′ba) *pl.* **amebas, amebae** [Gr. *amoibe,* change] A minute, one-celled protozoan of the genus *Amoeba,* found in soil and water. It constantly changes shape by sending out fingerlike processes of protoplasm (pseudopodia), through which it moves about and obtains nourishment. It possesses an outer translucent substance called the ectoplasm; the inner substance, endoplasm, is denser and contains a nucleus. It feeds by surrounding its food and enclosing it in the so-called food vacuole. Oxygen is absorbed from the surrounding water, and carbon dioxide is eliminated through the plasma membrane. Reproduction is by binary fission, in which the nucleus divides by mitosis. Some species of *Entamoeba* are parasitic in humans. **amebic** (ă-mē′bĭk), *adj.*

**amebapore** A pore-forming protein released on a cell membrane by *Entamoeba histolytica.* This forms large pores in the target cell membrane (i.e., the cell the ameba is attacking).

**amebiasis** (am″ĕ-bī′ă-sĭs) [″ + *-iasis,* state] Infection with amebas, esp. *Entamoeba histolytica.* SEE: *amebapore.*

SYMPTOMS: Many patients are asymptomatic. The disease is generally marked by dysentery with diarrhea, weakness, and prostration. Nausea, vomiting, and pain may be present. One serious complication is amebic hepatitis.

ETIOLOGY: *Entamoeba histolytica* is acquired by ingesting food or drink containing encysted forms.

DIAGNOSIS: The diagnosis is by detection of cysts or trophozoites of *E. histolytica* in stools.

PATHOLOGY: Small abscesses form and, later, ulcers of the mucous membrane of the colon, sometimes resulting in perforation. Liver abscesses may result from amebas being carried to the liver via the portal vein.

TREATMENT: In acute amebiasis, metronidazole (Flagyl) is used. Chloroquine and metronidazole are useful in liver abscess. Metronidazole should not be prescribed for pregnant patients. Repeated treatment at intervals for up to 3 months is necessary to ensure that the amebas have been eliminated.

For treatment of asymptomatic carriers of cysts, either iodoquinol or diloxanide furoate is suitable. These are available from the Drug Service, Centers for Disease Control and Prevention, Atlanta, GA 30333; telephone (404) 639-3670.

***hepatic a.*** Infection of the liver by *Entamoeba histolytica,* resulting in hepatitis and abscess formation; usually a sequel to amebic dysentery.

**amebic carrier state** State in which an individual harbors a form of pathogenic ameba but has no clinical signs of the disease.

**amebic dysentery** Infection with *Entamoeba histolytica.* SEE: *amebiasis.*

**amebic hepatitis** Amebic abscess of the liver.

**amebicide, amebacide** (ă-mē′bĭ-sīd) [Gr. *amoibe,* change, + L. *caedere,* to kill] An agent that kills amebas.

**amebiform** (ă-mē′bĭ-form) [″ + L. *forma,* shape] Shaped like an ameba.

**amebocyte** (ă-mē′bō-sīt″) [″ + *kytos,* cell] A cell showing ameboid movements.

**ameboid** (ă-mē′boyd) [″ + *eidos,* form, shape] Resembling an ameba.

**ameboidism** (ă-mē′boyd-ĭzm) **1.** Amebalike movements. **2.** Denoting a condition shown by certain nerve cells.

**ameboid movement** Cellular movement much like that of an ameba. A protoplasmic pseudopod extends, and then the remaining cell contents flow into the pseudopod, which swells gradually. This type of movement allows cells such as leukocytes to move through very small openings. SEE: *diapedesis.*

**ameboma** (ăm″ē-bō′mă) [″ + *oma,* tumor] A tumor composed of inflammatory tissue caused by amebiasis.

**ameburia** (ăm″ĕ-bū′rē-ă) [Gr. *amoibe,* change, + *ouron,* urine] The presence of amebas in the urine.

**amelanotic** (ă″mĕl-ă-nŏt′ĭk) Lacking melanin; unpigmented.

**amelia** (ă-mē′lē-ă) [Gr. *a-,* not, + *melos,* limb] Congenital absence of one or more limbs. SEE: *phocomelia.*

**amelification** (ă-mĕl″ĭ-fĭ-kā′shŭn) [O. Fr. *amel,* enamel, + L. *facere,* to make] Formation of dental enamel by ameloblasts.

**amelioration** (ă-mēl″yō-rā′shŭn) [L. *ad,* to, + *melior,* better] Improvement; moderation of a condition.

**ameloblast** (ă-mĕl′ō-blăst) [O. Fr. *amel,* enamel, + Gr. *blastos,* germ] A cell from which tooth enamel is formed.

**ameloblastoma** (ă-mĕl″ō-blăs-tō′mă) [″ + ″ + *oma,* tumor] A tumor of the jaw, esp. the lower one, arising from enamel-forming cells and having low-grade malignancy. It may be partly cystic and partly solid and may become large. SYN: *adamantinoma.*

**amelodentinal** [O. Fr. *amel,* enamel, + L. *dens, dent-,* tooth] Pert. to both enamel and dentin.

**amelogenesis** (ăm″ĕ-lō-jĕn′ĕ-sĭs) [″ + Gr. *genesis,* generation, birth] The formation of dental enamel.

**amelus** (ăm′ĕ-lŭs) [Gr. *a-,* not, + *melos,* limb] An individual with congenitally absent arms and legs.

**amenorrhea** (ă-mĕn″ō-rē′ă) [″ + ″ + *rhoia,* flow] The absence or suppression of menstruation. It occurs normally before puberty, after menopause, and during pregnancy and lactation. SYN: *amenia.* SEE: *oligomenorrhea.*

ETIOLOGY: The most common causes of abnormal amenorrhea are congenital abnormalities of the reproductive tract; metabolic disorders (obesity, malnutrition, diabetes); systemic diseases (syphilis, tuberculosis, nephritis); emotional disorders (excitement, anorexia nervosa); endocrine disorders, esp. those involving the ovaries and the pituitary, thyroid, and adrenal glands; and hormonal imbalance of estrogen, progesterone, or follicle-stimulating hormones.

TREATMENT: The underlying cause should be determined and corrected. If hormone deficiencies exist, substitutional therapy is recommended.

NURSING IMPLICATIONS: The patient is assessed for other symptoms and encouraged to seek medical attention if absence of menses is not related to pregnancy, menopause, or hormonal therapy. This symptom could have a variety of causes, and a thorough medical evaluation is crucial to identify the exact cause.

**amenorrheic** (-rē′ĭk), *adj.*

***dietary a.*** Cessation of menstruation due to voluntary or involuntary (as in starvation) dietary restriction.

***emotional a.*** Amenorrhea resulting

from shock, fright, or hysteria.

***exercise a.*** A form of stress amenorrhea seen in those whose intense exercise program involves running approx. 100 miles (161 km) or more each week, or the equivalent rate and extent of energy output in other sports. Not all of those who participate in high-level-intensity sports will experience amenorrhea.

***hyperprolactinemic a.*** Amenorrhea due to an excessive secretion of prolactin by the pituitary. SEE: *prolactin.*

***hypothalamic a.*** Amenorrhea due to malfunction of the hypothalamus.

***lactational a.*** Amenorrhea during lactation. Fertility has been shown to be greatly reduced in women who breastfeed for 6 to 12 months.

***pathological a.*** Amenorrhea due to organic disease.

***physiological a.*** Amenorrhea during prepuberty, pregnancy, lactation, and the postmenopausal period. It is not related to organic disease.

***postpartum a.*** Amenorrhea following childbirth that may last for only a month or two and thus would be within normal limits; or it may be permanent and thus abnormal. SEE: *Sheehan's syndrome.*

***primary a.*** Delay of menarche beyond age 18.

***secondary a.*** Cessation of menses in a woman who has previously menstruated.

***stress a.*** Cessation of menstruation due to mental or physical stress. Women in prisoner-of-war camps have experienced this type of amenorrhea. Some athletes who train intensively become amenorrheic. It may be related to hormonal changes caused by stress or to the concomitant alteration in the ratio of muscle to fat as training intensity increases.

**amentia** (ă-mĕn'shē-ă) [L. *ab,* from, + *mens,* mind] **1.** Congenital mental deficiency; mental retardation. **2.** Mental disorder characterized by confusion, disorientation, and occasionally stupor. SEE: *dementia.*

***nevoid a.*** Sturge-Weber syndrome; a congenital syndrome marked by port-wine nevi along trigeminal nerve distribution, angiomas of the leptomeninges and choroid, intracranial calcifications, mental retardation, epileptic seizures, and glaucoma.

***phenylpyruvic a.*** Mental retardation due to phenylketonuria.

**Americaine** Trade name for benzocaine.

**American Academy of Nursing**. An organization formed by the American Nurses' Association. Membership in this honorary association indicates that the person selected has contributed significantly to nursing. A member is titled Fellow of the American Academy of Nursing, abbreviated F.A.A.N.

**American Association for Respiratory Care** ABBR: AARC. The primary professional association for respiratory care practitioners in the U.S.

**American Association of Retired Persons** ABBR: AARP. The largest voluntary association of older people (retired or not) in the U.S., with a membership of almost 30 million. Its goal is to improve every aspect of living for those aged 50 years or over. The group works with Congress and state legislatures to represent the interests of older people.

**American College of Toxicology** The current name of the American Board of Medical Toxicology.

**American Federation for Aging Research** ABBR: AFAR. An association of physicians, scientists, and other individuals involved or interested in research on aging and associated diseases. Its purpose is to encourage and fund research on aging.

**American Geriatrics Society** ABBR: AGS. An association of health care professionals interested in the problems of the elderly. It enourages and promotes the study of geriatrics and stresses the importance of medical research in the field of aging.

**American Medical Records Association** ABBR: AMRA. A professional organization of individuals trained in health information management, including patient records, particularly in medical care facilities.

**American Nurses Association** ABBR: A.N.A. The only full-service professional organization representing the 2.2 million registered nurses in the U.S. It comprises 53 State Nurses Associations. The organization fosters high standards of nursing practice, promotes the economic and general welfare of nurses in the work environment, projects a realistic, positive view of nursing, and lobbies Congress and regulatory agencies about health care issues affecting nurses and the public. SEE: *Code for Nurses..*

**American Nurses Association Network** ABBR: ANA*NET. A wide-area computer network linking the 53 constituent State Nurses Associations with the national headquarters. It provides databases pert. to workplace and practice issues, and various databases and services related to nursing practice. Future plans include subscriber service for all nurses, nursing organizations, and nursing schools.

**American Occupational Therapy Association** ABBR: AOTA. A national professional organization concerned with establishing and enforcing standards of practice for occupational therapists.

**American Occupational Therapy Certification Board** ABBR: A.O.T.C.B. An independent agency recognized to certify the eligibility to practice of occupational therapists and occupational therapy assistants.

**American Red Cross** A branch of the international philanthropic organization Red Cross Society. It provides emergency aid during civil disasters such as floods and earthquakes, offers humanitarian services for armed forces personnel and their families, and operates centers for collecting and processing blood and blood products.

**American Sign Language** ABBR: ASL. A nonverbal method of communicating by deaf or speech-impaired people in which the hands and fingers are used to indicate words and concepts.

**American Standard Association rating** ABBR: ASA rating. A measure of photographic film speed, created by the American Standard Association.

**Americans with Disabilities Act** ABBR: ADA. Legislation passed by the U.S. Congress in 1990 to ensure the rights of persons with disabilities. It provides enforceable standards to ensure access and prohibit discrimination in employment, public services, transportation, public accommodation, communications, and other areas. Also called *Public Law 101-336*.

**americium** (ăm-ĕr-ĭsh′ē-ŭm) SYMB: Am. A metallic radioactive element, atomic number 95. The atomic weight of the longest-lived isotope is 243.

**Ames test** [Bruce Nathan Ames, U.S. biochemist, b. 1928] A laboratory test of the mutagenicity of chemicals. Special strains of organisms are incubated with the test chemical and their growth is an indicator of the mutagenicity of the substance. Most chemicals that test positive are carcinogens. Use of the test has helped reduce the use of mammals for tests of mutagenicity.

**ametria** (ă-mē′trē-ă) [Gr. *a-*, not, + *metra*, uterus] Congenital absence of the uterus.

**ametrometer** (ăm″ĕ-trŏm′ĕ-tĕr) [*ametropia* + Gr. *metron*, measure] An instrument for measuring the degree of ametropia.

**ametropia** (ă″mĕ-trō′pē-ă) [Gr. *ametros*, disproportionate, + *ops*, eye] Imperfect refractive powers of the eye in which the principal focus does not lie on the retina, as in hyperopia, myopia, or astigmatism. **ametropic**, *adj.*

**AMI** *acute myocardial infarction.*

**amicrobic** (ă″mī-krō′bĭk) [Gr. *a-*, not, + *mikros*, small, + *bios*, life] **1.** Lacking microbes. **2.** Not caused by microbes.

**amidase** (ăm′ĭ-dās) A deamidizing enzyme; one that catalyzes the hydrolysis of amides.

**amide** (ăm′ĭd) Any organic substance that contains the monovalent radical $—CONH_2$. It is usually formed by replacing the hydroxyl (—OH) group of the —COOH by the $—NH_2$ group.

**amido-** A prefix signifying the presence of the radical bond $CONH_2$.

**amidulin** (ă-mĭd′ū-lĭn) [Fr. *amidon*, starch] Soluble starch.

**amikacin sulfate** An aminoglycoside antibiotic. Trade name is Amikin.

**amimia** (ă-mĭm′ē-ă) [Gr. *a-*, not, + *mimos*, mimic] Loss of power to express ideas by signs or gestures.

***amnesic a.*** Amimia in which signs and gestures can be made but their meaning is not remembered.

**amine** (ă-mēn′, ăm′ĭn) Any one of a group of nitrogen-containing organic compounds that are formed when one or more of the hydrogens of ammonia have been replaced by one or more hydrocarbon radicals.

**amino-** (ă-mē′nō, ăm′ĭ-nō) Prefix denoting the presence of an amino group ($NH_2$).

**aminoacetic acid** (ăm″ĭn-ō-ă-sē′tĭk) $NH_2$-$CH_2COOH$. A nonessential amino acid. SYN: *glycine.*

**amino acid** One of a large group of organic compounds marked by the presence of both an amino group ($NH_2$) and a carboxyl (COOH) group. Amino acids are the building blocks of proteins and are the end products of protein digestion or hydrolysis.

Approx. 80 amino acids are found in nature, but only 20 are necessary for human metabolism or growth. Of these, some can be produced by the liver; the rest—called essential amino acids—must be supplied by food. These are histidine, isoleucine, leucine, lysine, methionine, cysteine, phenylalanine, tyrosine, threonine, tryptophan, and valine. The nonessential amino acids are alanine, aspartic acid, arginine, citrulline, glutamic acid, glycine, hydroxyglutamic acid, hydroxyproline, norleucine, proline, and serine. Oral preparations of amino acids may be used as dietary supplements.

Arginine, while nonessential for the adult, cannot be formed quickly enough to supply the demand in infants and thus is classed as essential in early life.

Some proteins contain all the essential amino acids and are called complete proteins. Examples are milk, cheese, eggs, and meat. Proteins that do not contain all the essential amino acids are called incomplete proteins. Examples are vegetables and grains. Amino acids pass unchanged through the intestinal wall into the blood, then through the portal vein to the liver and into the general circulation, from which they are absorbed by the tissues according to the specific amino acid needed by that tissue to make its own protein. Amino acids if not otherwise metabolized may be converted into urea. SEE: illus.; *deaminization; digestion; protein.*

***branched-chain a.a.*** ABBR: BCAA. The essential amino acids, leucine, isoleucine, and valine. "Branched-chain" refers to their chemical structure. Therapeutically, they are valuable because they bypass the liver and are available for cellular uptake from the circulation. Parenteral administration, alone or mixed with other amino acids, is thought to be beneficial whenever catabolism due to physiological stress occurs. The skeletal muscle can use these amino acids for energy.

**EXAMPLES OF AMINO ACIDS**

| SERINE | TYROSINE | GLYCINE |
|---|---|---|
| H H<br>H—N—C—C(=O)OH | H H<br>H—N—C—C(=O)OH | H H<br>H—N—C—C(=O)OH |
| $CH_2$<br>OH | $CH_2$<br>(benzene ring)<br>OH | H |
| **ASPARTIC ACID** | **ARGININE** | **HISTIDINE** |
| H H<br>H—N—C—C(=O)OH | H H<br>H—N—C—C(=O)OH | H H<br>H—N—C—C(=O)OH |
| $CH_2$<br>C<br>HO O | $CH_2$<br>$CH_2$<br>$CH_2$<br>NH<br>C=NH<br>$H_2N$ | $CH_2$<br>C=CH<br>HN N<br>HC |

***conditionally dispensable a.a.*** An amino acid that becomes essential when a specific clinical condition is present.

***essential a.a.*** In human nutrition, an amino acid that is required for growth and development and cannot be produced by the body. It must be obtained from food.

***nonessential a.a.*** An amino acid that can be produced by the body and is not required in the diet.

***semi-essential a.a.*** An amino acid of which an adequate amount must be consumed in the diet to prevent the use of essential amino acids to synthesize it. An example is tyrosine. Without adequate dietary intake, the essential amino acid, phenylalanine, is used to make tyrosine.

**aminoacidemia** (ă-mē″nō-, ăm″ĭ-nō-ăs″ĭ-dē′mē-ă) [*amino acid* + Gr. *haima,* blood] Excess of amino acids in the blood.

**amino acid group** The $NH_2$ group that characterizes the amines.

**aminoacidopathies** (ăm″ĭ-nō-ăs″ĭ-dŏp′ă-thēz) [″ + Gr. *pathos,* disease, suffering] Various disorders of amino acid metabolism, of which there are nearly 100, including cystinuria, alkaptonuria, and albinism.

**aminoaciduria** (ă-mē″nō-, ăm″ĭ-nō-ăs″ĭ-dū′rē-ă) [″ + Gr. *ouron,* urine] Excess amino acids in the urine.

**aminobenzene** (ă-mē″nō-, ăm″ĭ-nō-bĕn′zēn) $C_6H_7N$. The simplest aromatic amine, an oily liquid derived from benzene; used in the manufacture of medical and industrial dyes. SYN: *phenylamine.*

**aminobenzoic acid** $NH_2C_6H_4COOH$. A drug used as a topical ultraviolet screening agent. SYN: *para-aminobenzoic acid.*

**aminocaproic acid** SEE: *acid, aminocaproic.*

**aminoglutethimide** (ăm″ĭ-nō-gloo-tĕth′ĭ-mīd) A chemical that interferes with the production of adrenocortical hormone. It has been used to decrease the hypersecretion of cortisol by adrenal tumors and to treat cancer of the adrenal gland and breast cancer that is sensitive to adrenal hormone stimulation.

**aminoglycoside** A chemical compound that is present in a number of antibiotics, some of which are derived from microorganisms and others are produced synthetically.

**aminohippuric acid, sodium** The sodium salt of aminohippuric acid. It is given intravenously to test renal blood flow and the excretory capacity of the renal tubules.

**aminolysis** (ăm″ĭ-nŏl′ĭ-sĭs) [*amine* + Gr. *lysis,* dissolution] Metabolic transformation of amino-containing compounds by removal of the amino group.

**aminometradine** (ăm″ĭ-nō-mĕt′ră-dēn) A nonmercurial diuretic given orally.

**aminophylline** (ăm-ĭ-nŏf′ĭ-lĭn, ăm″ĭ-nō-fĭl′ĭn) $C_{16}H_{24}N_{10}O_4$. A mixture of theophylline and ethylenediamine used esp. to treat acute asthma that has not responded to epinephrine. It is also used as a stimulant to the respiratory center and heart muscle and as a diuretic. SYN: *theophylline ethylenediamine.*

**aminophylline poisoning** SEE: *Poisons and*

*Poisoning Appendix.*

**aminopterin** (ăm-ĭ-nŏp′tĕr-ĭn) A folic acid antagonist used to treat acute leukemia.

**aminopurine** (ăm″ĭ-nō-pū′rĭn) An oxidation product of purine; includes adenine and guanine. SEE: *methyl purine; oxypurine.*

**aminopyrine** (ăm″ĭn-ō-pī′rĭn) An antipyretic and analgesic drug. It is not approved for use in the U.S.

---

Caution: Because this drug may cause fatal agranulocytosis, it should not be used.

---

**aminosalicylic acid** SEE: *acid, aminosalicylic.*

**aminuria** (ăm-ĭ-nū′rē-ă) [*amine* + Gr. *ouron,* urine] Presence of amines in urine.

**amitosis** (ăm″ĭ-tō′sĭs) [Gr. *a-*, not, + *mitos,* a thread, + *osis,* condition] Direct cell division; simple division of the nucleus and cell without the changes in the nucleus that characterize mitosis. **amitotic** (-tŏt′ik), *adj.*

**amitryptyline hydrochloride** (ăm″ĭ-trĭp′tĭ-lēn) An antidepressant administered orally or intramuscularly.

**AML** *acanthiomeatal line; acute myelocytic leukemia.*

**ammeter** (ăm′mĕ-tĕr) [*ampere* + Gr. *metron,* measure] An instrument, calibrated in amperes, that measures the quantity (number of electrons) in an electric current. SEE: *milliammeter.*

**ammoaciduria** (ăm″ō-ăs″ĭ-dū′rē-ă) [*ammonia* + *amino acid* + Gr. *ouron,* urine] An abnormal amount of ammonia and amino acids in the urine.

**ammonia** (ă-mō′nē-ă) [*Ammo,* Egyptian deity near whose temple it was originally obtained] $NH_3$. An alkaline gas formed by decomposition of nitrogen-containing substances such as proteins and amino acids. Ammonia is converted into urea in the liver. It is related to many poisonous substances but also to the proteins and many useful chemicals. Dissolved in water, it neutralizes acids and turns litmus paper blue.

***aromatic spirit of a.*** A pungent solution of approx. 4% ammonium carbonate in 70% alcohol flavored with lemon, lavender, and myristica oil. It is used to elicit reflex stimulation of respiration and as "smelling salts" to stimulate people who have fainted.

***blood a.*** SEE: *ammoniemia.*

**ammoniacal** (ăm″ō-nī′ă-kăl) Having the characteristics of or pert. to ammonia.

**ammonia intoxication** SEE: *ammonia toxicity.*

**ammonia solution, diluted** A solution containing approx. 10 g of ammonia per 100 ml of water.

**ammonia solution, strong** A solution containing approx. 28% ammonia in water.

**ammoniated** (ă-mō′nē-āt′d) Containing ammonia.

**ammonia toxicity** Poisoning caused by an excess of ammonia. Ammonia is produced in the intestinal tract by bacterial action. After absorption it is transported to the liver, where it is converted to the less toxic urea. In diseases such as cirrhosis of the liver, the ammonia absorbed may be shunted past the liver. This results in an accumulation of ammonia in the blood (ammoniemia). The resulting developments, including alterations in consciousness, neurological changes, abnormal electroencephalogram, and a flapping tremor (asterixis), are due at least in part to ammonia toxicity. SEE: *hepatic coma; Poisons and Poisoning Appendix.*

TREATMENT: Treatment is aimed at preventing production and absorption of ammonia in the intestinal tract. Enemas and antibiotics such as neomycin are used to prevent growth of the bacteria that produce ammonia in the intestinal tract. Dietary protein should be limited.

**ammonia water** $NH_4OH$. Ammonium hydroxide.

**ammoniemia** (a-mō″nĭ-ē′mē-ă) [*ammonia* + Gr. *haima,* blood] Excessive ammonia in the blood. Normally only faint traces of ammonia are found in the blood. Increased amounts are due to a pathological condition such as impaired liver function. Also spelled *ammonemia*. SEE: *ammonia toxicity.*

**ammonium** (ă-mō′nē-ŭm) A radical, $NH_4^+$, that forms salts analogous to those of alkaline metals.

***a. alum*** Aluminum ammonium sulfate, an astringent. SEE: *alum.*

***a. carbonate*** A compound used in preparing aromatic ammonia spirit; $(NH_4)_2CO_3$.

***a. chloride*** A compound used as an expectorant and as an acidifier in treating acid-base balance; $NH_4Cl$.

***a. hydroxide*** A solution of ammonia in water, used as a household cleaner and a refrigerant; $NH_4OH$. SEE: *ammonia in Poisons and Poisoning Appendix.*

***a. thiosulfate*** The chemical in fixing solution that removes unexposed silver bromide crystals from radiographic film during the development process.

**ammoniuria** (ă-mō″nē-ū′rē-ă) [″ + Gr. *ouron,* urine] Excessive ammonia in the urine.

**amnesia** (ăm-nē′zē-ă) [Gr.] A loss of memory. The term is often applied to episodes during which patients forget their identity, although they may conduct themselves properly enough, and following which no memory of the period persists. Such episodes are often hysterical and sometimes epileptic, while trauma, senility, alcoholism, and other organic reaction types account for a smaller number. **amnesiac, amnesic, amnestic** (-nē′zē-ăk, -nē′sĭk, nĕs′tĭk), *adj.*

***anterograde a.*** Amnesia for events that occurred after a precipitating event or medication.

Caution: This type of short-term memory loss may be induced in people who use benzodiazepine drugs (e.g., triazolam, lorazepam, or fluazepam) after drinking alcohol.

***auditory a.*** Loss of memory for the meanings of sounds or spoken words. SYN: *auditory aphasia; word deafness.*

***dissociative a.*** Inability to recall important personal information, usually of a traumatic or stressful nature, that is too extensive to be explained by ordinary forgetfulness. This was formerly called psychogenic amnesia.

***lacunar a.*** Loss of memory for isolated events.

***posttraumatic a.*** ABBR: PTA. A state of agitation, confusion, and memory loss that the patient with traumatic brain injury (TBI) enters soon after the injury or on awakening from coma. Edema, hemorrhage, contusions, shearing of axons, and metabolic disturbances impair the brain's ability to process information accurately, resulting in unusual behaviors that often are difficult to manage. Trauma patients with normal brain scans may have a mild TBI and display some of the symptoms of PTA. Posttraumatic amnesia can last for months but usually resolves within a few weeks. During PTA, the patient moves from a cognitive level of internal confusion to a level of confusion about the environment. SEE: *Rancho Los Amigos Guide to Cognitive Levels.*

SYMPTOMS: Symptoms include restlessness, moaning or crying out, uninhibited behavior (often sexual or angry), hallucinations (often paranoid), lack of continuous memory, story fabrication to replace memory (confabulation), combative behavior, confused language, disorientation, repetition of movements or thoughts (perseveration), and sleep disturbances. Deficits in attention and memory may persist, and communication and other cognitive weaknesses may become more apparent, such as difficulty with problem solving, reasoning, organizing thoughts, sequencing, word finding, and carrying out planned motor movements (as in activities of daily living).

NURSING IMPLICATIONS: The nurse assesses the patient for symptoms of PTA. The patient is continually reoriented by keeping a large calendar and clock within sight; each interaction with the patient begins with a repetition of who is in attendance, why the attendant is present, and what activity is planned; and the patient is kept safe and comfortable and is allowed as much freedom of movement as possible. At a cognitive level of internal confusion, the patient does not understand what is happening and becomes agitated. The nurse limits agitation and confusion by speaking softly in simple phrases, using gestures as necessary, allowing time for the patient to respond, and avoiding towering over the patient. The nurse requests regular visits from family, prepares them for the patient's appearance and behavior, and encourages their participation in activities of daily living. The patient may respond best to the person he or she cares about most. Stimulation is limited, and frequent rest periods are scheduled. Equipment designed for agitated patients is used; wrist restraints are avoided if possible. Urinary catheters may increase agitation due to physical discomfort (incontinence briefs can be used during the training period of a toileting program). The patient's swallowing function is evaluated as soon as possible to avoid feeding tubes, but swallowing precautions are observed. A list of stimulations that increase or decrease the patient's agitation is posted for the use of everyone in contact with the patient. Distance is maintained during aggressive outbursts; the aggression is waited out and a soft speaking voice is used. The nurse should not invade the patient's personal space without warning (e.g., should let the patient know when genitals are to be washed), and should approach the patient from the front and place items in positions where they can best be seen. Hallucinations or confabulation are not encouraged, and the patient's attention is redirected when he or she becomes argumentative. As the patient progresses, the nurse recognizes that self-awareness will be limited and variable, and watches closely for impulsive movement that can jeopardize the patient. Others are warned that the patient cannot monitor behavior, and that words and actions will occur without awareness or forethought. All possible independence and self-care are encouraged. The patient is engaged in short activities with a motor component. The nurse should attempt to modify one behavior at a time if the patient displays several that interfere with treatment. To promote abstract reasoning, humor should be used if the patient understands it. A consistent daily schedule continues to be used and the patient is taught to use compensatory cues (a watch or written activity schedule) to aid memory. The patient is also assessed for posttraumatic headache, which is treated with prescribed nonnarcotic analgesics.

***psychogenic a.*** Dissociative a.

***retrograde a.*** Amnesia for events that occurred before the precipitating trauma.

***selective a.*** Inability to remember events that occurred at the same time as other experiences that are recalled.

***tactile a.*** Inability to distinguish objects by sense of touch. SYN: *astereognosis.*

***transient global a.*** Short-term memory loss that occurs in otherwise healthy people; remote memory is retained. Onset is usually sudden and may last for a few hours. Recovery is usually rapid.

***traumatic a.*** Amnesia caused by sudden physical injury.

***visual a.*** Inability to remember the appearance of objects or to be cognizant of printed words.

**amnesiac, amnesic** A person who has amnesia.

**amniocentesis** (ăm″nē-ō-sĕn-tē′sĭs) [Gr. *amnion,* lamb, + *kentesis,* puncture] Transabdominal puncture of the amniotic sac under ultasound guidance using a needle and syringe in order to remove amniotic fluid. The sample obtained is studied chemically and cytologically to detect genetic and biochemical disorders and maternal-fetal blood incompatibility and, later in the pregnancy, to determine fetal maturity. The procedure also allows for transfusion of the fetus with platelets or blood and instillation of drugs for treating the fetus.

This procedure is usually performed no earlier than at 14 weeks' gestation. It is important that the analysis be done by experts in chemistry, cytogenetics, and cell culture. Cell cultures may require 30 days, and if the test has to be repeated, the time required may be insufficient to allow corrective action. SEE: illus.

Caution: The procedure can cause abortion or trauma to the fetus.

NURSING IMPLICATIONS: The nurse reviews the patient's knowledge about the procedure and sensations that may be experienced, and obtains a signed consent form. The amniocentesis equipment is assembled; amber-colored test tubes are used (or clear test tubes are covered with aluminum foil) to shield the fluid from light, which could break down bilirubin. Baseline vital signs and fetal heart rate are obtained, and the fundus is palpated for fetal position and fetal and uterine activity for 30 min before, during, and 30 min after the procedure. The patient is assessed for light-headedness, nausea, and diaphoresis as well as for anxiety, pain, and labor onset. During the procedure, the nurse provides emotional support. After the procedure, the patient is positioned on her left side and is instructed to report unusual fetal hyperactivity or hypoactivity, clear or bloody vaginal drainage, uterine contractions, abdominal pain, or fever and chills, any of which is indicative of complications. SEE: *chorionic villus sampling*; *fetal monitoring in utero.*

**amniochorial, amniochorionic** (ăm″nē-ō-kō′rē-ăl, -kō-rē-ŏn′ĭk) Relating to both the amnion and chorion.

**amniogenesis** (ăm″nē-ō-jĕn′ĕ-sĭs) [″ + *genesis,* generation, birth] Formation of the amnion.

**amniography** [″ + *graphein,* to write] Radiography of the fetus for abnormalities after injection of a water-soluble contrast medium into the amniotic sac. This examination has been replaced with ultrasonography of the fetus.

**amnioinfusion** (ăm″nē-ō-ĭn-fū′zhŭn) The intrauterine instillation of warm normal saline to reduce the risk of cord compression in women with oligohydramnios. Complications may include uterine overdistention and increased uterine resting tone. Hypertonic saline, hypertonic urea, or prostaglandin $F_{2\alpha}$ solutions have been injected to induce late abortion.

**amnion** (ăm′nē-ŏn) [Gr. *amnion,* lamb] The innermost fetal membrane; a thin, transparent sac that holds the fetus suspended in the liquor amnii, or amniotic fluid. The amnion grows rapidly at the expense of the extraembryonic coelom, and by the end of the third month it fuses with the chorion, forming the amniochorionic sac. Commonly called the bag of waters. SEE: *oligohydramnios.* **amniotic** (-ŏt′ĭk), *adj.*

***a. nodosum*** Rounded or oval opaque elevations 1 to 6 mm in diameter in the placenta that are seen in the part of the amnion in contact with the chorionic plate and near the insertion of the cord into the placenta. They are present in approx. 60% of pregnancies.

**amnionitis** (ăm″nē-ō-nī′tĭs) [″ + *itis,* inflammation] Inflammation of the amnion.

**amniorrhea** (ăm″nē-or-rē′ă) [″ + *rhoia,* flow] Escape of the amniotic fluid.

**amniorrhexis** Rupture of the amnion.

**amnioscope** (ăm′nē-ŏ-skōp) [Gr. *amnion,* lamb, + *skopein,* to examine] Optical device for examining the amniotic cavity.

***suction a.*** Amnioscope that allows suction to be applied so that it is held in place against the fetal scalp. This permits evacuation of the amniotic fluid from the area pressing against the scalp, leaving a clear field for sampling blood from that site.

**amnioscopy** Direct visual examination of the fetus through an optical device inserted into the amniotic cavity via the abdominal wall.

**amniote** (ăm′nē-ōt) Any animal or group belonging to the Amniota, a major group of vertebrates, the members of which develop an amnion. Included are reptiles, birds, and mammals.

**amniotic band disruption sequence syndrome** A collection of fetal malformations associated with multiple fibrous strands of amnion that appear to develop or entangle fetal parts in utero. This leads to structural malformations and deformations and disruption of function. Defects associated with this condition include limb defects and amputations; abnormal dermal ridge patterns; simian creases; clubbed feet; craniofacial defects, including cleft lip and palate; and visceral defects such as gastroschisis and omphalocele. Failure to understand the cause of this condition can lead to misdiagnosis

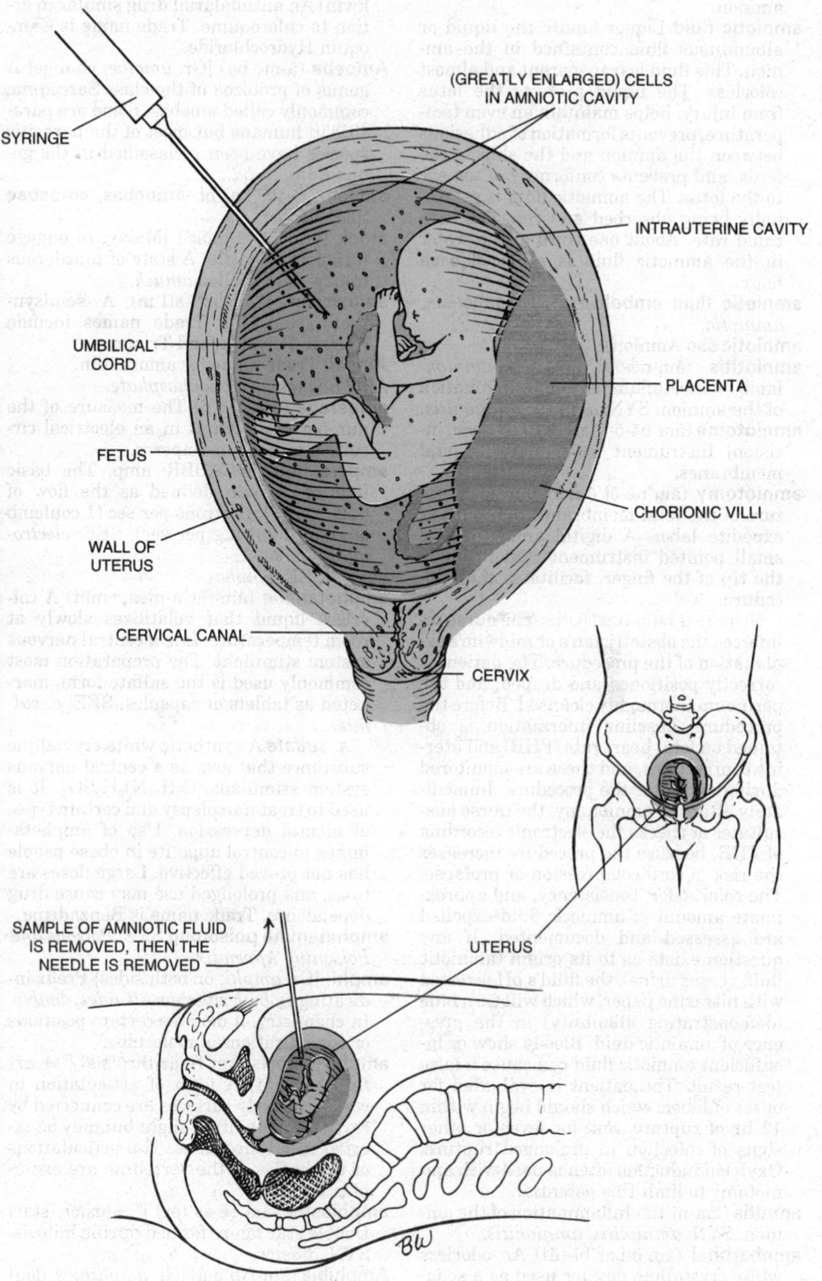
AMNIOCENTESIS
SYRINGE
(GREATLY ENLARGED) CELLS
IN AMNIOTIC CAVITY
INTRAUTERINE CAVITY
UMBILICAL
CORD
PLACENTA
FETUS
CHORIONIC VILLI
WALL OF
UTERUS
CERVICAL CANAL
CERVIX
SAMPLE OF AMNIOTIC FLUID
IS REMOVED, THEN THE
NEEDLE IS REMOVED
UTERUS
BW

and inappropriate family and genetic counseling. SEE: *multiple malformation syndrome.*

**amniotic cavity** The fluid-filled cavity of the amnion.

**amniotic fluid** Liquor amnii; the liquid or albuminous fluid contained in the amnion. This fluid is transparent and almost colorless. The liquid protects the fetus from injury, helps maintain an even temperature, prevents formation of adhesions between the amnion and the skin of the fetus, and prevents conformity of the sac to the fetus. The amniotic fluid is continually being absorbed and renewed at a rapid rate. About one third of the water in the amniotic fluid is replaced each hour.

**amniotic fluid embolism** SEE: *embolism, amniotic.*

**amniotic sac** Amnion.

**amniotitis** (ăm-nē-ŏ-tī'tĭs) [Gr. *amnion,* lamb, + *itis,* inflammation] Inflammation of the amnion. SYN: *amnitis; amnionitis.*

**amniotome** (ăm'nē-ŏ-tōm) [" + Gr. *tome,* incision] Instrument for puncturing fetal membranes.

**amniotomy** (ăm"nē-ŏt'ō-mē) Surgical rupture of the fetal membranes to induce or expedite labor. A digital amniotome, a small pointed instrument that fits over the tip of the finger, facilitates this procedure.

NURSING IMPLICATIONS: The nurse reinforces the obstetrician's or midwife's explanation of the procedure. The patient is correctly positioned and draped, and the perineum thoroughly cleansed. Before the procedure, baseline information is obtained on fetal heart rate (FHR) and uterine contractions, and these are monitored during and after the procedure. Immediately after the amniotomy, the nurse auscultates or checks the electronic recording of FHR, because the procedure increases the risk of cord compression or prolapse. The color, odor, consistency, and approximate amount of amniotic fluid expelled are assessed and documented. If any question exists as to its origin (amniotic fluid versus urine), the fluid's pH is tested with nitrazine paper, which will turn blue (demonstrating alkalinity) in the presence of amniotic fluid. Bloody show or insufficient amniotic fluid can cause a false test result. The patient is evaluated for onset of labor, which should begin within 12 hr of rupture, and for fever or other signs of infection in prolonged rupture. Oxytocin induction often is used with amniotomy to limit this potential.

**amnitis** (ăm-nī'tĭs) Inflammation of the amnion. SYN: *amniotitis; amnionitis.*

**amobarbital** (ăm"ō-bar'bĭ-tăl) An odorless white crystalline powder used as a sedative; $C_{11}H_{18}N_2O_3$.

***a. sodium*** An odorless white granular powder used as a sedative; $C_{11}H_{17}N_2NaO_3$. It is absorbed and inactivated rapidly in the liver.

**A-mode (amplitude modulation) display** SEE: *ultrasound, A-mode.*

**amodiaquine hydrochloride** (ăm"ŏ-dī'ă-kwĭn) An antimalarial drug similar in action to chloroquine. Trade name is Camoquin Hydrochloride.

**Amoeba** (ă-mē'ba) [Gr. *amoibe,* change] A genus of protozoa of the class Sarcodina; commonly called amebas. Some are parasitic in humans but most of the parasitic species have been reclassified in the genus *Entamoeba..*

**amoeba** (ă-mē'ba) *pl.* **amoebas, amoebae** SEE: *ameba.*

**amok** (ă-mŏk', ă-mŭk') [Malay, to engage furiously in battle] A state of murderous frenzy. Also spelled *amuck.*

**amoxicillin** (ă-mŏks"ĭ-sĭl'ĭn) A semisynthetic penicillin. Trade names include Amoxil, Polymox, and Trimox.

**Amoxil** Trade name for amoxicillin.

**AMP** *adenosine monophosphate.*

**amperage** (ăm-pēr'ĭj) The measure of the number of electrons in an electrical circuit, expressed in amperes.

**ampere** (ăm'pēr) ABBR: amp. The basic unit of current, defined as the flow of $6.25 \times 10^{-18}$ electrons per sec (1 coulomb of charge flowing per sec). SEE: *electromotive force.*

**amph-** SEE: *ampho-.*

**amphetamine** (ăm-fĕt'ă-mēn, -mĭn) A colorless liquid that volatilizes slowly at room temperature. It is a central nervous system stimulant. The preparation most commonly used is the sulfate form, marketed as tablets or capsules. SEE: *a. sulfate.*

***a. sulfate*** A synthetic white crystalline substance that acts as a central nervous system stimulant; $C_9H_{13}N)_2H_2SO_4$. It is used to treat narcolepsy and certain types of mental depression. Use of amphetamines to control appetite in obese people has not proved effective. Large doses are toxic, and prolonged use may cause drug dependence. Trade name is Benzadrine.

**amphetamine poisoning** SEE: *Poisons and Poisoning Appendix.*

**amphi-** [Gr. *amphi,* on both sides] Prefix indicating *on both sides, on all sides, double.* In chemistry, it denotes certain positions or configurations of molecules.

**amphiarthrosis** (ăm"fē-ăr-thrō'sĭs) [" + *arthrosis,* joint] A form of articulation in which the body surfaces are connected by cartilage; mobility is slight but may be exerted in all directions. The articulations of the bodies of the vertebrae are examples.

**amphiaster** (ăm"fē-ăs'tĕr) [" + *aster,* star] Double star figure formed during mitosis. SYN: *diaster.*

**Amphibia** (ăm-fĭb'ē-ă) [Gr. *amphibios,* double life] A class of cold-blooded animals that live on land and in water; includes salamanders, frogs, and toads. They breathe through gills during their aquatic larval stage but through lungs in their adult stage. SEE: *metamorphosis*.

**amphibious** (ăm-fĭb'ē-ŭs) Able to live both on land and in water.

**amphiblastula** (ăm"fē-blăs'tū-lă) [Gr. *amphi,* on both sides, + *blastula,* little sprout] A form of blastula in which the blastomeres are of unequal size; seen in sponges.

**amphichroic, amphichromatic** (ăm"fē-krō'ĭk, -krō-măt'ĭk) [" + *chroma,* color] **1.** Turning red litmus paper blue, and blue litmus paper red. **2.** Reacting as both an acid and an alkali. **3.** Capable of exhibiting two colors.

**amphicyte** SEE: *cell, satellite.*

**amphidiarthrosis** (ăm"fē-dī-ăr-thrō'sĭs) [" + *diarthrosis,* articulation] An articulation with amphiarthrosis and diarthrosis, such as that of the lower jaw.

**amphitheater** (ăm"fĭ-thē'ă-tĕr) [" + *theatron,* theater] An operating room with tiers of seats around it for students and other observers.

**amphitrichate, amphitrichous** (ăm-fĭt'rĭ-kāt, -kŭs) [" + *thrichos,* hair] Having a flagellum or flagella at both ends, said of microorganisms.

**ampho-, amph-** [Gr. *ampho,* both] Prefix indicating *both, both sides, on all sides,* or *double.*

**amphocyte** (ăm'fō-sīt) [" + *kytos,* cell] A cell that stains with either acid or basic stains.

**amphodiplopia** (ăm-fō-dĭ-plō'pē-ă) [" + *diploos,* double, + *ops,* vision] Double vision in each eye. SYN: *amphoterodiplopia.*

**Amphojel** (ăm'fō-jĕl) A trade name for aluminum hydroxide gel.

**ampholyte** (ăm'fō-līt) [" + *electrolyte*] A substance that acts as a base or an acid, depending on the pH of the solution into which it is introduced.

**amphoric** (ăm-for'ĭk) [L. *amphoricus*] Pert. to a sound such as that caused by blowing across the mouth of a bottle; a resonance; a cavernous sound on percussion of a pulmonary cavity.

**amphoricity** (ăm"for-ĭs'ĭ-tē) The condition of producing amphoric sounds.

**amphoriloquy** (ăm"for-ĭl'ō-kwē) [L. *amphora,* jar, + *loqui,* to speak] The presence of amphoric sounds in speaking.

**amphorophony** (ăm"for-ŏf'ō-nē) [Gr. *amphoreus,* jar, + *phone,* voice] Amphoric voice sound.

**amphoteric, amphoterous** (ăm-fō-tĕr'ĭk, ăm-fŏt'ĕr-ŭs) [Gr. *amphoteros,* both] Being able to react as both an acid and a base.

**amphoteric compound** A compound that reacts as both an acid and a base.

**amphotericin B** (ăm"fō-tĕr'ĭ-sĭn) An antibiotic agent obtained from a strain of *Streptomyces nodosus.* It is used in treatment of deep-seated mycotic infections. The drug usually is administered parenterally. Trade name is Fungizone.

**amphoteric reaction** Reaction in which a compound reacts as both an acid and a base.

**amphoterism** (ăm-fō'tĕr-ĭzm) State of reacting as both an acid and a base.

**amphoterodiplopia** (ăm-fŏt"ĕr-ō-dĭ-plō'pē-ă) [" + *diploos,* double, + *ops,* vision] Double vision in each eye. SYN: *amphodiplopia.*

**ampicillin** (ămp"ĭ-sĭl'ĭn) A semisynthetic penicillin; a broad-spectrum antibiotic. Trade names include Amcill, Omnipen, Polycillin, and Principen.

***a. sodium*** Monosodium salt of ampicillin. Trade names include Omnipen-N and Principen/N.

**amplification** (ăm"plĭ-fĭ-kā'shŭn) [L. *amplificatio,* making larger] Enlargement, magnification, expansion.

**amplifier** (ăm'plĭ-fī"ĕr) **1.** That which enlarges, extends, increases, or makes more powerful. **2.** In electronics, a device for increasing the electric current or signal.

**amplitude** (ăm'plĭ-tūd) [L. *amplitudo*] **1.** Amount, extent, size, abundance, or fullness. **2.** In physics, the extent of movement, as of a pendulum or sound wave. The maximum displacement of a particle, as that of a string vibrating, as measured from the mean to the extreme. **3.** Magnitude of an action potential. **4.** In radiography, the extent of tube travel during tomography.

**amplitude modulation** Modification of the amplitude, esp. of a current used for muscle stimulation.

**ampule** (ăm'pūl) [Fr. *ampoule*] A small glass container that can be sealed and its contents sterilized. This is a French invention for containing hypodermic solutions.

**ampulla** (ăm-pŭl'lă) *pl.* **ampullae** [L., little jar] Saclike dilatation of a canal or duct.

***a. ductus deferentis*** An irregular and nodular dilatation of the vas deferens just before its junction with the excretory duct of the seminal vesicle.

***hepatopancreatic a.*** The entry of the common bile duct and main pancreatic duct into the duodenum. SYN: *a. of Vater; papilla of Vater.*

***a. of lacrimal duct*** Slight dilatation of the lacrimal duct medial to the punctum.

***a. of rectum*** Slight dilatation of the rectum proper just before continuing as the anal canal. Also called *infraperitoneal portion of rectum proper.*

***a. of semicircular canal*** A dilatation at the end of the semicircular canal that houses an ampulla of a semicircular duct.

***a. of semicircular ducts*** Dilatation of semicircular ducts near their junction with the utricle. In their walls are the cristae ampullares.

***a. of uterine tube*** The dilated distal end of a uterine tube terminating in a funnel-like infundibulum.

***a. of vas deferens*** A. ductus deferentis.

***a. of Vater*** Hepatopancreatic a.

**ampullitis** (ăm"pŭl-lī'tĭs) [" + Gr. *itis,* inflammation] Inflammation of any ampulla, esp. of the ductus deferens.

**ampullula** (ăm-pŭl'ū-lă) [dim. of L. *ampulla*] A small dilatation, esp. of a lymph or blood vessel.

**amputation** (ăm"pū-tā'shŭn) [L. *amputare,* to cut around] Removal, usually by surgery, of a limb, part, or organ.

NURSING IMPLICATIONS: In the immediate postoperative period, vital signs are assessed, the dressing is observed for bleeding at least every 2 hr, drain patency is checked, and the amount and character of drainage are documented. Limb circulation is ascertained by checking proximal pulses, skin color, and temperature. Postoperative pain is managed by oral and injected medicine. To prevent contracture formation, the patient is encouraged to ambulate, change position, rest in proper body alignment with the residual limb in extension rather than in flexion, do range-of-motion exercises (esp. extension), and do muscle-strengthening exercises as soon as these are prescribed postoperatively. Residual limb-conditioning exercises and correct residual limb bandaging (applying even, moderate pressure to mold the residual limb into a cone shape that allows a good prosthesis fit) assist limb shrinkage. The residual limb may initially have a rigid plaster dressing; nursing care for this type of cast is the same as for any plaster cast. The patient is instructed to wash the residual limb daily with mild soap and water, rinse it well, and dry it gently; to massage the limb; to examine the entire limb daily, using a mirror to visualize hidden areas; and to report symptoms such as swelling, redness, excessive drainage, increased pain, and residual limb skin changes (rashes, blisters, or abrasions). The patient is taught how to bandage the residual limb or, when it is dry, to apply a residual limb shrinker (a custom-fitted elastic stocking that fits over the residual limb) and is advised against applying body oil or lotion because it can interfere with proper fit of a prosthesis. The need for constant bandaging until edema subsides and the prosthesis is properly fitted and the use of a residual limb sock and proper prosthesis care are explained. The patient is encouraged to verbalize anger and frustration, to cope with grief, self-image, and lifestyle adjustments, and to deal with phantom limb sensation (itching, numbness, or pain "felt" in the area of amputation even though the limb is no longer there) if this occurs. The patient may require referral to a local support group or for further psychological counseling. SEE: *Nursing Diagnoses Appendix.*

***congenital a.*** Amputation of parts of the fetus in utero, formerly believed to be caused by constricting bands but now believed to be a developmental defect.

***double-flap a.*** Amputation in which two flaps of soft tissue are formed to cover the end of the bone.

***a. in contiguity*** Amputation at a joint.

***a. in continuity*** Amputation at a site other than a joint.

***primary a.*** Amputation performed before inflammation sets in.

***secondary a.*** Amputation performed during suppuration.

***spontaneous a.*** Nonsurgical separation of an extremity or digit. SEE: *ainhum.*

***traumatic a.*** The sudden amputation of some part of the body due to an accidental injury.

**amputee** (ăm"pū-tē') One who has had an amputation, esp. of the arm(s) or leg(s).

**Amsler grid** [Marc Amsler, Swiss ophthalmologist, 1891–1968] A grid of lines used in testing for macular degeneration. The grid is observed with each eye separately.

**A.M.T.** *American Medical Technologists.*

**amuck** (ă-mŭk') Amok.

**amusia** (ă-mū'sē-ă) [Gr. *amousos,* unmusical] Music deafness; inability to produce or appreciate musical sounds.

***motor a.*** Inability to produce musical sounds.

***sensory a.*** Music deafness; inability to appreciate musical sounds.

***vocal a.*** Inability to sing.

**Amussat's operation** (ăm'ū-săz) [Jean Z. Amussat, Fr. surgeon, 1796–1856] Surgical formation of an artificial anus, by lumbar colotomy in ascending colon.

**amychophobia** (ă-mī"kō-fō'bē-ă) [Gr. *amyche,* scratch, + *phobos,* fear] Morbid fear of being scratched; fear of the claws of any animal.

**amyelencephaly** (ă-mī"ĕl-ĕn-sĕf'ă-lē) [Gr. *a-,* not, + *myelos,* marrow, + *enkephalos,* brain] Congenital absence of the brain and spinal cord.

**amyelia** (ă-mī-ē'lē-ă) [" + *myelos,* marrow] Congenital absence of the spinal cord.

**amyelinic** (ă-mī"ĕ-lĭn'ĭk) Not possessing a myelin sheath.

**amyelus** (ă-mī'ĕ-lŭs) An individual with congenital absence of the spinal cord.

**amygdala** (ă-mĭg'dă-lă) *pl.* **amygdalae** [L., almond] **1.** A mass of gray matter in the anterior portion of the temporal lobe. It is believed to play an important role in arousal. **2.** Obsolete term for the tonsil.

**amygdalin** (ă-mĭg'dă-lĭn) A bitter-tasting glycoside derived from the pit or other seed parts of several plants, including almonds and apricots. Amygdalin, from which the poisonous hydrocyanic acid can be produced by enzymatic action, is the substance known in the U.S. as Laetrile. Amygdalin has no therapeutic or nutritional value. SEE: *Laetrile.*

**amygdaline** (ă-mĭg'dă-līn, -lĭn) [L. *amygdalinus*] **1.** Pert. to a tonsil. **2.** Pert. to or shaped like an almond. SYN: *amygdaloid.*

**amygdaloid** (ă-mĭg'dă-loyd) [Gr. *amygdale,* almond, + *eidos,* form, shape] Resembling a tonsil or an almond.

**amygdaloid fossa** A depression that contains the tonsil.

**amygdaloid tubercle** A projection from the middle cornu of the lateral ventricle, marking the area of the amygdaloid nucleus.

**amygdalolith** (ă-mĭg′dă-lō-lĭth″) [″ + *lithos,* stone] Stone in a distended crypt of a tonsil.

**amygdalopathy** (ă-mĭg″dă-lŏp′ă-thē) [″ + *pathos,* disease, suffering] Any disease of a tonsil.

**amygdalotome** (ă-mĭg′dă-lō-tōm″) [″ + *tome,* incision] An instrument for excision of a tonsil.

**amyl** (ăm′ĭl) [Gr. *amylon,* starch] $C_5H_{11}$. A hypothetical univalent radical, nonexistent in a free state.

***a. nitrite*** $C_5H_{11}NO_2$. A volatile and highly flammable clear liquid used as a vasodilator, esp. for anginal pain.

**amylaceous** (ăm″ĭ-lā′shē-ŭs) Starchy.

**amylase** (ăm′ĭ-lās) [″ + *-asis,* colloid enzyme] A class of enzymes that split or hydrolyze starch. Those found in animals are called alpha-amylases; those in plants are called beta-amylases. SEE: *antiamylase; enzyme; macroamylase.*

***pancreatic a.*** Amylopsin.

***salivary a.*** Ptyalin.

***vegetable a.*** Diastase.

**amylasuria** (ăm″ĭ-lās-ū′rē-ă) [″+ *ouron,* urine] Increased amount of amylase in the urine; occurs in pancreatitis.

**amylodextrin** [″ + *dexter,* right] Soluble substance produced during the hydrolysis of starch into sugar.

**amylodyspepsia** (ăm″ĭ-lō-dĭs-pĕp′sē-ă) [″ + *dys,* bad, + *pepsis,* digestion] Inability to digest starchy foods.

**amylogenesis** (ăm″ĭ-lō-jĕn′ĕ-sĭs) [″ + *genesis,* generation, birth] The production of starch. **amylogenic** (-jĕn′ĭk), *adj.*

**amyloid** (ăm′ĭ-loyd) [Gr. *amylon,* starch, + *eidos,* form, shape] **1.** Resembling starch; starchlike. **2.** A protein-polysaccharide complex having starchlike characteristics produced and deposited in tissues during certain pathological states. It is a homogeneous, highly refractile substance staining readily with Congo red. It is associated with a variety of chronic diseases, particularly tuberculosis, osteomyelitis, leprosy, Hodgkin's disease, and carcinoma.

**amyloid degeneration** Degeneration of organs or tissues from amyloid deposits, which are waxy and translucent and have a hyaline appearance. The liver, spleen, and kidneys are usually involved, but any tissue may be infiltrated.

**amyloid disease** Amyloidosis.

**amyloid kidney** An enlarged, firm, smooth kidney usually associated with amyloid disease of the spleen or liver.

SYMPTOMS: Symptoms include a pale face and waxy skin that may be edematous. The liver and spleen may also be enlarged and are not tender to pressure. Diarrhea occurs if the intestines are involved. Albumin, hyaline, and waxy casts are found in the urine.

**amyloid nephrosis** A nephrotic syndrome from myeloid degeneration of the kidney.

**amyloidosis** (ăm″ĭ-loy-dō′sĭs) [Gr. *amylon,* starch, + *eidos,* form, shape, + *osis,* condition] A metabolic disorder marked by amyloid deposits in organs and tissue. It is thought to be the result of disordered function of the reticuloendothelial system and abnormal immunoglobulin synthesis. There is no known method of preventing formation of amyloid deposits except to control the primary disease with which it is associated. SYN: *amylosis.*

SYMPTOMS: Symptoms include decreased sensations of pain and temperature and inability to sweat. The patient may experience difficulty in breathing, coughing, lightheadedness with position change, palpitations, delayed blood clotting, abdominal pain, constipation, diarrhea, gastrointestinal bleeding, morning joint stiffness, and fatigue. Raised papules or plaques may be found on or near the face or in the axillary, inguinal, or anal region. Congestive heart failure may be present.

NURSING IMPLICATIONS: The patient is assessed for cardiac, respiratory, renal, gastrointestinal, skin, neurological, and joint dysfunction, depending on the body site involved. A history is obtained of any associated disease or condition.

Airway patency is monitored if the patient's tongue is involved. The patient is observed for signs of congestive heart failure such as jugular vein distention, peripheral edema, crackles, dyspnea, and oliguria. Electrolyte levels and the results of coagulation studies are monitored. Proper nutrition and fluid balance are maintained and taught. Prescribed medications are given to decrease amyloid deposits, relieve pain, and control constipation or diarrhea, and the patient is instructed in their use. Special mouth care, and referral for speech therapy if necessary, are provided for the patient with tongue involvement, and referral for speech therapy may be necessary. Alternative communication methods are also provided for the patient with tongue involvement. Gentle suctioning of oral and respiratory secretions helps to prevent ventilatory compromise. When bedrest is required, the patient is positioned in correct body alignment to improve ventilation and repositioned frequently; range-of-motion exercises help to prevent joint contractures (and muscle atrophy). Slow movements are encouraged when the patient stands, and the temperature of bath water is tested for the patient with sensory impairment.

Use of available support systems is encouraged, and referral for further counseling is made as necessary.

Desired outcomes include the patient's ability to manage the prescribed medication regimen and report adverse developments; to communicate understanding of special dietary needs, consume adequate calories, and maintain body weight; to maintain fluid balance and communicate understanding of fluid and sodium intake limits; to communicate needs and desires without undue frustration, using alternative communication methods when necessary; and to use available resources to maximize communication skills.

***lichen a.*** A form of amyloidosis limited to the skin.

***localized a.*** Amyloidosis in which isolated amyloid tumors are formed.

***primary a.*** Amyloidosis not associated with a chronic disease.

***secondary a.*** Amyloidosis associated with a chronic disease, such as tuberculosis, syphilis, Hodgkin's disease, or rheumatoid arthritis, and with extensive tissue destruction. The spleen, liver, kidneys, and adrenal cortex are most frequently involved.

**amylolysis** (ăm″ĭl-ŏl′ĭ-sĭs) [″ + *lysis,* dissolution] Hydrolysis of starch into sugar in the process of digestion. **amylolytic** (-ō-lĭt′ĭk), *adj.*

**amylopectin** (ăm″ĭl-ō-pĕk′tĭn) The insoluble component of starch. The soluble component is amidin.

**amylophagia** (ăm″ĭ-lō-fā′jē-ă) [″ + *phagein,* to eat] Abnormal craving for starch.

**amylopsin** (ăm″ĭ-lŏp′sĭn) [″ + *opsis,* appearance] An enzyme in pancreatic juice that hydrolyzes starch into achroodextrin and maltose. SYN: *pancreatic amylase.* SEE: *digestion; duodenum; enzyme.*

**amylose** (ăm′ĭ-lōs) [Gr. *amylon,* starch] A group of carbohydrates that includes starch, cellulose, and dextrin.

**amylosuria** (ăm″ĭ-lō-sū′rē-ă) [″ + *ouron,* urine] Amylose in the urine.

**amyluria** [″ + Gr. *ouron,* urine] Starch in the urine.

**amyosthenia** (ă-mī″ŏs-thē′nē-ă) [Gr. *a-,* not, + *mys,* muscle, + *sthenos,* strength] Muscular weakness. SEE: *myasthenia.* **amyosthenic, amyasthenic,** *adj.*

**amyotonia** (ă-mī″ō-tō′nē-ă) [″ + ″ + *tonos,* tone] Deficiency or lack of muscular tone.

***a. congenita*** SEE: *Oppenheim's disease.*

**amyotrophia, amyotrophy** (ă-mī″ō-trō′fē-ă, ă-mī-ŏt′rō-fē) [″ + ″ + *trophe,* nourishment] Muscular atrophy. **amyotrophic** (-trŏf′ĭk), *adj.*

***progressive spinal a.*** Progressive muscular atrophy.

**amyotrophic lateral sclerosis** ABBR: ALS. A syndrome marked by muscular weakness and atrophy with spasticity and hyperreflexia due to degeneration of the motor neurons of the spinal cord, medulla, and cortex. Even though the prognosis is poor, some patients have remained active for 10 to 20 years after the disease was diagnosed. If only cells of motor cranial nuclei in the medulla are involved, the condition is called progressive bulbar palsy. No specific therapy is available but research is ongoing to develop drugs that slow the progress of the disease. Patients often benefit from referral to occupational or physical therapy, or both. Also called *Lou Gehrig's disease.* SYN: *motor neuron disease.* SEE: *Nursing Diagnoses Appendix.*

SYMPTOMS: Symptoms include progressive weakness in the arms, legs, and trunk; and difficulty in talking, chewing, swallowing, and eventually breathing.

ETIOLOGY: The cause is unknown, but the possibility of the illness being associated with a specific genetic defect holds promise of determining the course of the disease. Once this is done, it might be possible to treat the genetic abnormality.

NURSING IMPLICATIONS: Neuromuscular function is monitored to assess the progression of deterioration. Ventilatory status is assessed frequently. The patient is evaluated for respiratory infection, which can be fatal. Nutritional intake and fluid balance are monitored. The skin is inspected regularly for evidence of breakdown.

A rehabilitation program is instituted to help the patient maintain independence. Prescribed medications for symptomatic relief are administered, and the patient is instructed in their use. The patient is encouraged to do active exercise and active range-of-motion exercises on unaffected muscle groups; assistance is provided with stretching exercises. Other assistance is provided according to the patient's muscular capacity. As mobility decreases, skin care is provided, the patient is turned and repositioned frequently, and special low-pressure mattresses and pads are used to prevent skin breakdown. Equipment such as a walker, wheelchair, or special bed is obtained as necessary. Alternative methods of communication are devised for the patient who cannot talk. The nurse helps the patient perform deep-breathing and coughing exercises and uses incentive spirometry, chest physiotherapy, and suctioning as necessary. The patient having trouble swallowing is positioned upright, and soft, semisolid foods are offered, with suctioning equipment available to prevent or treat aspiration. If the patient cannot swallow, nasogastric or gastrostomy tube feedings are provided.

The patient and family are instructed about the signs and symptoms of ALS and about problem management. Referral is made to social and home health care services, hospice care, and available local and national support and information services such as the Amyotrophic Lateral

Sclerosis Association.

Desired outcomes include the patient's and family's ability to express feelings about life changes and future losses; to cope appropriately with grief; to make continual adjustments to the home to allow the patient to be independent as long as possible and perform activities of daily living; to maintain the patient's highest degree of mobility, using assistive devices as necessary; and limited or no evidence of complications due to impaired physical mobility.

**Amytal** Trade name for amobarbital.

**Amytal Sodium** Trade name for amobarbital sodium.

**amyxia** (ă-mĭks′ē-ă) [″ + *myxa,* mucus] Absence or deficiency of mucus.

**amyxorrhea** (ă-mĭks-ō-rē′ă) [″ + ″ + *rhoia,* flow] Lack of normal secretion of mucus.

**An 1.** Symbol for actinon. **2.** *anisometropia.* **3.** *anode.* **4.** *antigen.*

**an-** [Gr.] SEE: *a-.*

**A.N.A.** *American Nurses' Association.*

**ana** (ăn′ă) ABBR: $\overline{aa}$. **1.** Prescription term meaning *so much of each.* **2.** *antinuclear antibody.*

**ana-** Prefix used in words derived from Greek. It indicates *up, against,* or *back.*

**anabolic agent** Testosterone, or a steroid hormone resembling testosterone, which stimulates anabolism (rather than catabolism) in the body. Anabolic steroids have been used, sometimes in large doses, by male and female athletes to improve performance, esp. in events requiring strength. This use has been judged to be illegal by various organizations that supervise sports, including the International Olympic Committee and the U.S. Olympic Committee. SEE: *doping; ergonomic aid.*

---

Caution: Indiscriminate use of anabolic agents is inadvisable because of the undesirable side effects they may produce, particularly in women, in whom hirsutism, masculinization, and clitoral hypertrophy may occur.

---

**anabolism** (ă-năb′ō-lĭzm) [Gr. *anabole,* a building up, + *-ismos,* condition] The building up of the body's substance; the constructive phase of metabolism by which a cell takes from the blood the substance required for repair and growth, building it into a cytoplasm, thus converting a nonliving material into the living cytoplasm of the cell. Anabolism is the opposite of catabolism, the destructive phase of metabolism. **anabolic** (ăn″ă-bŏl′ĭk), *adj.*

**anabolite** (ă-năb′ō-līt″) Any product of anabolism.

**anacamptometer** (ăn″ă-kămp-tŏm′ĕ-tĕr) [Gr. *ana,* up, + *kamptos,* bent, + *metron,* to measure] A device for measuring the intensity of deep reflexes.

**anacatesthesia** (ăn″ă-kăt″ĕs-thē′zē-ă) [″ + ″ + *aisthesis,* sensation] A sensation of hovering.

**anacidity** (ăn″ă-sĭd′ĭ-tē) [Gr. *an-,* not, + L. *acidum,* acid] Abnormal deficiency of acidity, esp. of hydrochloric acid in the gastric juice.

**anaclasis** (ă-năk′lă-sĭs) [Gr. *anaklasis,* reflection] **1.** Refraction or reflection of light. **2.** Refraction of light in the interior of the eye. **3.** Reflex action. **4.** Refraction for therapeutic reasons. **5.** Forcible movement of a joint in order to treat fibrous ankylosis.

**anaclitic** (ăn″ă-klĭt′ĭk) Leaning or depending on. In psychoanalysis, pert. to the dependence of an infant on the mother figure for care.

**anaclitic depression** SEE: *depression, anaclitic.*

**anacrotic** (ăn″ă-krŏt′ĭk) [Gr. *ana,* up, + *krotos,* stroke] **1.** Pert. to the ascending or vertical upstroke of a sphygmogram. **2.** Pert. to a pulse with more than one expansion of the artery. **3.** Pert. to two heartbeats traced on the ascending line of a sphygmogram. SYN: *anadicrotic.* SEE: *pulse.*

**anacrotic pulse** Pulse in which one or more small waves occur on the ascending limb of the tracing of pulse waves, as in aortic stenosis.

**anacrotism** (ă-năk′rō-tĭzm) Existence of a double beat on the ascending line of a sphygmogram. SYN: *anadicrotism.*

**anacusia, anacusis, anakusis** (ăn-ă-kū′sē-ă, -sĭs) [Gr. *an-,* not, + *akouein,* to hear] Total deafness.

**anadicrotism** (ăn-ă-dĭk′rō-tĭzm) [Gr. *ana,* up, + *dikrotos,* double beating] Anacrotism. **anadicrotic** (ăn-ă-dī-krŏt′ĭk), *adj.*

**anadidymus** (ăn″ă-dĭd′ĭ-mŭs) [″ + *didymos,* twin] A developmental abnormality in which the lower extremities of two fetuses are joined together.

**anadipsia** (ăn″ă-dĭp′sē-ă) [Gr. *ana,* intensive, + *dipsa,* thirst] Intense thirst.

**anadrenalism** (ăn″ă-drē′năl-ĭzm) [Gr. *an-,* not, + *adrenal* + Gr. *-ismos,* condition] Failure of the adrenal gland to function.

**anadromous** [Gr. *anadromos,* running upward] Descriptive of fish that migrate from sea water to fresh water.

**anaerobe** (ăn′ĕr-ōb) [Gr. *an-,* not, + *aer,* air, + *bios,* life] A microorganism that can live and grow in the absence of oxygen.

***facultative a.*** An organism that can live and grow with or without oxygen.

***obligatory a.*** An organism that can live and grow only in the absence of oxygen.

**anaerobic** (ăn″ĕr-ō′bĭk) **1.** Pert. to an anaerobe. **2.** Able to live without oxygen.

**anaerobic exercise** Exercise during which the energy needed is provided without use of inspired oxygen. This type of exercise is limited to short bursts of vigorous activity. SEE: *aerobic exercise.*

**anaerobiosis** (ăn″ĕr-ō-bī-ō′sĭs) [″ + *aer,* air, + *bios,* life, + *osis,* condition] **1.** Life in an

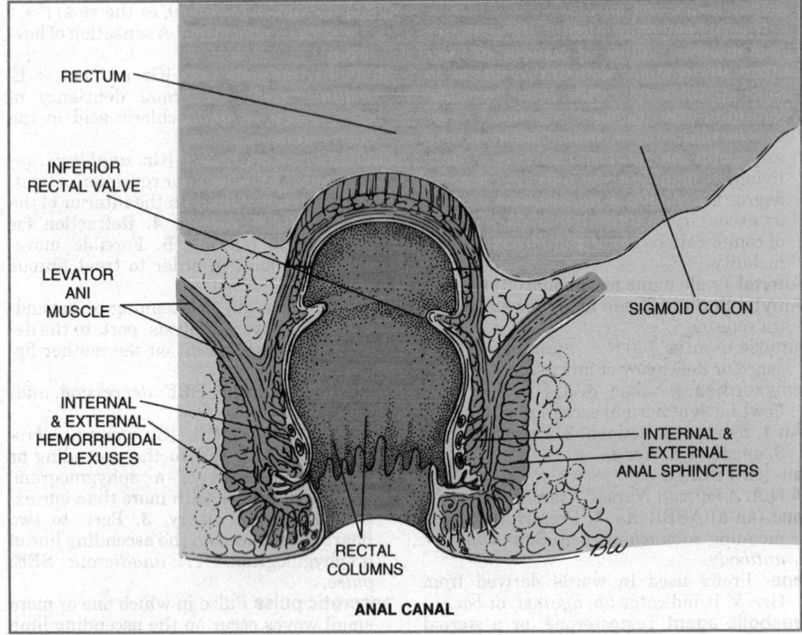


ANAL CANAL

oxygen-free atmosphere. **2.** Functioning of an organ or tissue in the absence of free oxygen.

**anagen** (ăn'ă-jĕn) [Gr. *ana*, up, + *genesis*, generation, birth] The growth stage of hair development. SEE: *catagen; telogen.*

**anakatadidymus** (ăn"ă-kăt"ă-dĭd'ĭ-mŭs) [Gr. *ana*, up, + *kata*, down, + *didymos*, twin] A congenital anomaly in which twins are separated above and below but joined at the trunk.

**anakré** [African, big nose] Goundou.

**anal** (ā'năl) [L. *analis*] Rel. to the anus or outer rectal opening.

**anal canal** The terminal portion of the large intestine, its external aperture being the anus. This includes the internal and external sphincter muscles of the anus. The canal remains closed except during defecation and passage of flatus. It is about 1½ in. (3.8 cm) long. SEE: illus.

**anal continence plug** A disposable device inserted in the anal canal to prevent anorectal incontinence. It is useful in incontinence involving both liquid and solid fecal material. SEE: *anal dynamic graciloplasty.*

**anal dynamic graciloplasty** The construction of a new anal sphincter to treat severe intractable fecal incontinence. The gracilis muscle is moved and reattached around the anal sphincter. A sustained contraction can be stimulated by implanted electrodes, closing the anus.

**analeptic** (ăn"ă-lĕp'tĭk) [Gr. *analeptikos*, restorative] **1.** A drug that stimulates the central nervous system. **2.** A restorative agent.

**anal erotism** Localization of the libido in the anal region. SEE: *anal stage.*

**analgesia** (ăn-ăl-jē'zē-ă) [Gr. *an-*, not, + *algos*, pain] Absence of a normal sense of pain.

***a. algera, a. dolorosa*** Spontaneous pain with loss of sensibility in a part.

***continuous caudal a.*** Analgesia to reduce the pain of childbirth. The anesthetic is injected continuously into the epidural space at the sacral hiatus.

***epidural a.*** A postoperative pain management technique in which narcotics are infused into the peridural space through an indwelling catheter. Administration may be at a continuous basal infusion rate or self-administered within programmed limits.

***infiltration a.*** Anesthesia produced in a local area by injecting an anesthetic agent into the nerve endings.

***paretic a.*** Complete analgesia of an upper limb in conjunction with partial paralysis.

***patient-controlled a.*** ABBR: PCA. A drug administration method that permits the patient to control the rate of drug delivery for the control of pain. It is usually accomplished by the use of an infusion pump. The patient must have complete understanding of the system and be willing to use it. The system should be designed so that the patient will be unable to administer an overdose of the analgesic; also, as with all narcotics, the system has to be designed to prevent its theft.

**analgesic** (ăn″ăl-jē′sĭk) **1.** Relieving pain. **2.** A drug that relieves pain. Analgesic drugs include nonprescription drugs, such as aspirin and other nonsteroidal anti-inflammatory agents, and those classified as controlled substances and available only by prescription. SYN: *analgetic.*

**analgesic nephropathy** SEE: *nephritis, analgesic.*

**analgetic** (ăn″ăl-jĕt′ĭk) Analgesic.

**analgia** (ăn-ăl′jē-ă) [″ + *algos,* pain] State of being without pain.

**anal incontinence** Failure of the anal sphincter to prevent involuntary expulsion of gas, liquid, or solids from the lower bowel.

**analog, analogue** (ăn′ă-lŏg) [Gr. *analogos,* analogy, proportion] **1.** One of two organs in different species that are similar in function but different in structure. **2.** In chemistry, a compound that is structurally similar to another.

**analogous** (ă-năl′ō-gŭs) Similar in function but different in origin or structure.

**analogy** (ă-năl′ō-jē) [Gr. *analogos,* analogy, proportion] **1.** Likeness or similarity between two things that are otherwise unalike. **2.** In biology, similarity in function, but difference in structure or origin; opposite of homology.

**anal personality** In Freudian psychology, a personality disorder marked by excessive orderliness, stinginess, and obstinacy. If carried to an extreme, these qualities lead to the development of obsessive-compulsive behavior.

**anal reflex** Contraction of the anal sphincter following irritation of the skin around the anus. The reflex is lost in lesions of the posterior columns of the cord and is exaggerated in anal fissures.

**anal stage** In Freudian psychology, the second phase of sexual development, from infancy to childhood, in which the libido is concentrated in the anal region. In order of appearance, the phases of sexual development are oral, anal, phallic, and genital.

**anal wink** Contraction of the anal sphincter in response to pinprick stimulus of the perineum.

**analysand** (ăn-ăl′ĭ-zănd) A patient who is being psychoanalyzed.

**analysis** (ă-năl′ĭ-sĭs) *pl.* **analyses** [LL. *ana,* up, back, + Gr. *lysis,* dissolution] **1.** Separation of anything into its constituent parts. **2.** In chemistry, determination of or separation into constituent parts of a substance or compound. **3.** Psychoanalysis. **analytic** (ăn-ă-lĭt′ĭk), *adj.*

***batch a.*** An automated analysis in which all of the samples undergo the same test or test profile.

***chromatographic a.*** Analysis of substances on the basis of color reaction of the constituents as they are differentially absorbed on one of a variety of materials such as filter paper.

***cohort a.*** The tabulation and analysis of morbidity or mortality in relation to the ages of a specific group of people (cohort), identified at a particular period of time and followed as they pass through different ages during part or all of their life span.

***colorimetric a.*** Analysis by adsorption of a compound and the identification of its element by color.

***continuous-flow a.*** Analysis using a type of laboratory instrument that, prior to analyzing specimens, separates them by placing an air bubble between individual specimens as they are injected into a tube. Specimens are then analyzed as they flow along the tube.

***densimetric a.*** Analysis by determination of the specific gravity (density) of a solution and estimation of the amount of solids.

***discrete a.*** An automated methodology in which samples are held in separate containers to be assayed. In a continuous flow system, all samples flow through the same tubing.

***gastric a.*** Analysis of the stomach contents to determine the concentration of free hydrochloric acid and combined (total) acid and the presence of lactic acid, occult blood, pus, and excessive mucus, and the amount and types of bacteria.

***hair a.*** Investigation of the chemical composition of hair. It is used in studying exposure to toxic chemicals in the environment, in poisoning investigations, in nutritional studies, and in monitoring the course of certain diseases. The sample should be obtained from new-growth hair within 5 cm of the scalp to reduce the chance of contamination of the hair by air pollutants.

***qualitative a.*** Determination of the nature of the elements in a substance.

***quantitative a.*** Determination of the quantity of each element in a substance.

***spectrophotometric a.*** Determination of materials in a compound by measuring the amount of light they absorb in the infrared, visible, or ultraviolet region of the spectrum.

***volumetric a.*** Quantitative analysis performed by the measurement of the volume of solutions or liquids.

**analysis of variance** ABBR: ANOVA. A statistical technique for defining and segregating the causes of variability affecting a set of observations. Use of this technique provides a basis for analyzing the effects of various treatments or variables on the subjects or patients being investigated. In an experimental design in which several samples or groups are drawn from the same population, estimates of population variance between samples should differ from each other only by chance. ANOVA provides a method for testing the hypothesis that several random and independent samples are from a common, normal population.

**analyst** (ăn′ă-lĭst) [Fr. *analyse,* analysis] **1.** One who analyzes. **2.** A practitioner of psychoanalysis. SYN: *psychoanalyst.*

**analyte** A substance being analyzed, esp. a chemical analysis.

**analytical balance** A very sensitive scale used in chemical analysis.

**analyze** (ăn′ă-līz) [Fr. *analyse,* analysis] To separate into parts or principles in order to determine the nature of the whole; to examine methodically.

**analyzer** (ăn′ă-lī″zĕr) **1.** A device used to determine the optical rotation produced when polarized light passes through a solution. **2.** An oxygen device used to monitor delivered oxygen concentration by the measurement of partial pressure or concentration. Analyzers are physical, electric, and electrochemical and use paramagnetic, thermal conductive polarographic, and galvanic cells, respectively. **3.** Any device that determines some characteristic of the object, chemical, or action being investigated. There are devices for analyzing a voice; the breath for presence of certain chemicals such as alcohol; images; cells in a solution; and chemicals.

***automated a.*** A chemical instrument system designed to perform assays that were done, and may still be done, manually.

***batch a.*** A discrete automated chemical analyzer in which the instrument system sequentially performs a single test on each of a group of samples.

***continuous flow a.*** An automated chemical analyzer in which the samples and reagents are pumped continuously through a system of modules interconnected by tubing.

***discrete a.*** An automated chemical analyzer in which the instrument performs tests on samples that are kept in "discrete containers," in contrast to a continuous flow analyzer.

***parallel a.*** A discrete automated chemical analyzer that performs a single test on a group of samples at practically the same time (actually, within milliseconds).

***pulse height a.*** ABBR: PHA. A circuit that differentiates between pulses of varying sizes. It is used in scintillation, blood cell, and particle counters.

**anamnesis** (ăn″ăm-nē′sĭs) [Gr. *anamnesis,* recalling] **1.** Recollection; the faculty of remembering. **2.** That which is remembered. **3.** The medical history of a patient. SEE: *catamnesis.*

**anamnestic** (ăn″ăm-nĕs′tĭk) **1.** Pert. to the medical history of a patient. **2.** Assisting the memory.

**anamniotic** [Gr. *an-,* not, + *amnion,* amnion] Without an amnion.

**ANA*NET** *American Nurses Association Network.*

**anangioplasia** (ăn-ăn″jē-ō-plā′sē-ă) [Gr. *an-,* not, + *angeion,* vessel, + *plassein,* to form] Imperfect vascularization of a part. **anangioplastic** (-plăs′tĭk), *adj.*

**anaphase** (ăn′ă-fāz) [″ + *phainein,* to appear] The third stage in meiosis, and mitosis, (between metaphase and telophase) in which there is longitudinal bisection of chromosomes (the chromatids), which separate and move toward their respective poles.

**anaphoresis** (ăn″ă-fō-rē′sĭs) [″ + *phoresis,* bearing] The flow of electropositive particles toward the anode (positive pole) in electrophoresis.

**anaphoria** (ăn″ă-for′ē-ă) [Gr. *ana,* up, + *phorein,* to carry] The tendency of the eyeballs to turn upward. SYN: *anatropia.*

**anaphrodisia** (ăn-ăf″rō-dĭz′ē-ă) [Gr. *an-,* not, + *aphrodisia,* sexual desire] Diminished or absent desire for sex. SEE: *aphrodisiac.*

**anaphrodisiac** (ăn″ăf-rō-dĭz′ē-ăk) **1.** Repressing sexual desire. **2.** An agent that represses sexual desire.

**anaphrodite** (ăn-ăf′rō-dīt) A person with impaired or absent sexual desire.

**anaphylactia** (ăn″ă-fĭ-lăk′shē-ă) [Gr. *ana,* up, + *phylaxis,* protection] Anaphylaxis.

**anaphylactic shock** Systemic anaphylaxis that produces life-threatening changes in circulation and bronchioles consistent with shock. SEE: *allergy; anaphylaxis.*

SYMPTOMS: Symptoms include acute respiratory distress, hypotension, edema, rash, tachycardia, pale cool skin, convulsions, and cyanosis. If no treatment is received, unconsciousness and death may result. Edema can be life-threatening if the larynx is involved, since air flow is obstructed with even minimal swelling.

ETIOLOGY: The condition is the result of a type I allergic or hypersensitivity reaction during which the allergen is absorbed into the blood directly or through the mucosa. The most common agents are radiographic contrast media used in diagnostic studies, and drugs. Chemical mediators released during the reaction cause constriction of the bronchial smooth muscle, vasodilation, and increased vascular permeability.

TREATMENT: Treatment consists of vasopressor agents, esp. epinephrine, antihistamines, and corticosteroids; oxygen; and intravenous fluids given rapidly, if indicated. Epinephrine acts not only as a vasopressor but also to relax smooth muscles in the airway and to increase myocardial contractions. Endotracheal intubation and mechanical ventilation are often necessary. The patient should carry a medical identification device indicating known allergens and usual treatment.

PROGNOSIS: Death may occur if emergency treatment is not given.

NURSING IMPLICATIONS: *Prevention:* A history of past allergic reactions, particularly to drugs, blood, or contrast media, is obtained. The at-risk patient is observed for reaction during and immediately after administration of any of the these agents. At the first sign of life-threatening respiratory distress, the nurse establishes an airway, notifies the appropriate physician, and administers epinephrine, diphenhydramine, corticosteroids, oxygen, and other emergency drugs per protocol or prescription. Drugs should be administered IV if the patient is unconscious or hypotensive, SC or IM if the patient is conscious and normotensive. Airway patency is maintained, and the patient is observed for early signs of laryngeal edema (such as stridor, hoarseness, and dyspnea); endotracheal intubation or tracheostomy, in addition to oxygen therapy, may be required. Cardiopulmonary resuscitation is initiated in cases of respiratory or cardiac arrest. The patient is assessed for hypotension and shock; circulatory volume is maintained with prescribed volume expanders, and blood pressure is stabilized with prescribed vasopressors. Blood pressure, central venous pressure, and urinary output are monitored. Once the initial emergency has subsided, the nurse administers prescribed drugs for long-term management and inhaled bronchodilators or IV aminophylline (over 20 min) for bronchospasm. The patient is taught to identify and avoid common allergens and to recognize an allergic reaction. If a patient is unable to avoid exposure to allergens and requires medication, both patient and family are instructed in its use.

**anaphylactogenesis** (ăn″ă-fĭ-lăk″tō-jĕn′ĕ-sĭs) The process of producing anaphylaxis.

**anaphylactogenic** (ăn″ă-fĭ-lăk″tō-jĕn′ĭk) **1.** Producing anaphylaxis. **2.** The agent producing anaphylactic reactions.

**anaphylatoxin** (ăn″ă-fĭ-lă-tŏk′sĭn) A substance composed of the C3 and C5 components of complement, which cause vasoactive mediators to be released from mast cells, promoting increased vascular permeability and the formation of edema during an anaphylactic reaction.

**anaphylaxis** (ăn″ă-fĭ-lăk′sĭs) [″ + *phylaxis,* protection] A form of type I allergic or hypersensitivity reaction to an allergenic antigen mediated by interactions between factors released by mast cells and immunoglobulin E. These interactions produce the antigen-antibody reaction. SEE: *anaphylactic shock.* **anaphylactic** (-lăk′tĭk), *adj.*

***active a.*** Anaphylaxis resulting from injection of an antigen.

***exercise-induced a.*** Onset of anaphylaxis during exercise. It is more common in women than in men. The cause is unknown. Treatment is the same as for anaphylaxis associated with an allergen.

***local a.*** Local inflammatory reaction following repeated injections of antigenic material; includes allergic rhinitis to animal dander or pollen, hives, and angioneurotic edema in which fluid accumulates in the eyelids, hands, and lips. SYN: *Arthus reaction.*

***passive a.*** Anaphylaxis induced by injection of serum from a sensitized animal into a normal one. After a few hours the latter becomes sensitized.

***passive cutaneous a.*** ABBR: PCA. A laboratory test of antibody levels in which serum from a sensitized individual is injected into the skin. Intravenous injection of an antigen accompanied by Evans blue dye at a later time reacts with the antibodies produced in response to the antigen, creating a wheal and blue spot at the site, indicating local anaphylaxis.

***systemic a.*** Anaphylaxis involving the systemic release of histamine and other chemical mediators, leading to respiratory and vascular changes that can result in life-threatening anaphylactic shock. SEE: *allergy; anaphylactic shock.*

**anaplasia** (ăn″ă-plā′zē-ă) [″ + *plassein,* to form] Loss of cellular differentiation and function, characteristic of most malignancies. **anaplastic** (-plăs′tĭk), *adj.*

**anapnea** (ăn″ăp-nē′ă) [Gr. *anapnein,* to breathe again] **1.** Respiration. **2.** Regaining the breath.

**anapneic** (ăn″ăp-nē′ĭk) Pert. to anapnea or relieving dyspnea.

**anapophysis** (ăn″ă-pŏf′ĭ-sĭs) [Gr. *ana,* back, + *apophysis,* offshoot] An accessory spinal process of a vertebra, esp. a thoracic or lumbar vertebra.

**anarthria** (ăn-ăr′thrē-ă) [Gr. *an-,* not, + *arthron,* joint] Loss of motor power to speak distinctly. It may result from a neural lesion or a muscular defect.

***a. literalis*** Stammering.

**anasarca** (ăn″ă-săr′kă) [Gr. *ana,* through, + *sarkos,* flesh] Severe generalized edema. SYN: *dropsy.* **anasarcous** (-săr′kŭs), *adj.*

**anaspadias** (ăn″ă-spā′dē-ăs) [″ + *spadon,* a rent] Congenital opening of the urethra on the dorsum of the penis; or opening by separation of the labia minora and a fissure of the clitoris. SYN: *epispadias.*

**anastole** (ăn-ăs′tō-lē) [Gr.] Shrinking away or retraction of the edges of a wound.

**anastomose** (ă-năs′tō-mōs) [Gr. *anastomosis,* opening] **1.** To communicate directly or by means of connecting two parts together, esp. nerves or blood vessels. **2.** To make such a connection surgically.

**anastomosis** (ă-năs″tō-mō′sĭs) *pl.* **anastomoses** [Gr., opening] **1.** A natural communication between two vessels; may be direct or by means of connecting channels. **2.** The surgical or pathological connection of two tubular structures. **anastomotic** (-mŏt′ĭk), *adj.*

***antiperistaltic a.*** Anastomosis between two parts of the intestine such that the peristaltic flow in one part is the opposite of that in the other.

***arteriovenous a.*** Anastomosis between an artery and a vein by which the capillary bed is bypassed.

***crucial a.*** An arterial anastomosis on the back of the thigh, formed by the medial femoral circumflex, inferior gluteal, lateral femoral circumflex, and first perforating arteries.

***end-to-end* a.** Anastomosis in which the ends of two structures are joined.

***Galen's* a.** Anastomosis between the superior and inferior laryngeal nerves.

***heterocladic* a.** Anastomosis between branches of different arteries.

***homocladic* a.** Anastomosis between branches of the same artery.

***Hyrtl's* a.** An occasional looplike anastomosis between the right and left hypoglossal nerves in geniohyoid muscle.

***intestinal* a.** Surgical connection of two portions of the intestines. SYN: *enteroenterostomy.*

***isoperistaltic* a.** Anastomosis between two parts of the intestine such that the peristaltic flow in both parts is in the same direction.

***precapillary* a.** Anastomosis between small arteries just before they become capillaries.

***Schmiedel's* a.** Abnormal communications between the vena cava and the portal system.

***side-to-side* a.** Anastomosis between two structures lying or positioned beside each other.

***terminoterminal* a.** Anastomosis between the peripheral end of an artery and the central end of the corresponding vein and between the distal end of the artery and the terminal end of the vein.

***ureterotubal* a.** Anastomosis between the ureter and the fallopian tube.

***ureteroureteral* a.** Anastomosis between two parts of the same ureter.

**anatomic, anatomical** (ăn″ă-tŏm′ĭk, -tŏm′ĭ-kăl) [Gr. *anatome,* dissection] Rel. to the anatomy or structure of an organism.

**anatomical snuffbox** Tabatière anatomique.

**anatomist** (ă-năt′ō-mĭst) A specialist in the field of anatomy.

**anatomy** (ă-năt′ō-mē) [Gr. *anatome,* dissection] **1.** The structure of an organism. **2.** The branch of science dealing with the structure of organisms.

***applied* a.** Application of anatomy to diagnosis and treatment, esp. surgical treatment.

***comparative* a.** Comparison of homologous structures of different animals.

***descriptive* a.** Description of individual parts of the body. SYN: *systematic anatomy.*

***developmental* a.** Embryology of the organism from the time of egg fertilization until adulthood is attained.

***gross* a.** Study of structures able to be seen with the naked eye. SYN: *macroscopic a.*

***macroscopic* a.** Gross a.

***microscopic* a.** Study of structure by use of a microscope. SYN: *histology.*

***morbid* a.** Pathological a.

***pathological* a.** Study of the structure of abnormal, diseased, or injured tissue. SYN: *morbid a.*

***radiological* a.** Anatomical investigation based on the radiological appearance of tissues and organs. SYN: *x-ray a.*

***surface* a.** Study of form and markings of the surface of the body, esp. as they relate to underlying tissues and organs.

***systematic* a.** Descriptive a.

***topographic* a.** Study of the structure and form of a portion of the body with particular emphasis on the relationships of the parts to each other.

***x-ray* a.** Radiological a.

**anatoxin** (ăn″ă-tŏks′ĭn) [Gr. *ana,* backward, + *toxikon,* poison] A toxin that has been treated to destroy its toxicity but is still capable of inducing antibody formation on injection. SYN: *toxoid.* **anatoxic** (-tŏks′ĭk), *adj.*

**anatricrotism** (ăn″ă-trĭk′rō-tĭzm) [Gr. *ana,* up, + *tresis,* three, + *krotos,* stroke] The existence of three beats on the ascending line of a sphygmogram. **anatricrotic** (-trī-krŏt′ĭk), *adj.*

**anatripsis** (ăn″ă-trĭp′sĭs) [″ + *tripsis,* friction] Therapeutic use of rubbing or friction massage.

**anatriptic** (ăn″ă-trĭp′tĭk) [″ + *tripsis,* friction] **1.** Pert to anatripsis. **2.** An agent applied by rubbing.

**anatropia** (ăn″ă-trō′pē-ă) [″+ *trope,* a turning] Tendency of eyeballs to turn upward. SYN: *anaphoria.*

**anaxon(e)** (ăn-ăk′sŏn) [Gr. *an-,* not, + *axon,* axis] A nerve cell, as of the retina, having no axon.

**ANC** *absolute neutrophil count.*

**A.N.C.** *Army Nurse Corps.*

**AnCC** *anodal closure contraction.*

**anchor** (ăng′ker) [Gr. *ankyra,* anchor] A metal implant placed within the alveolar bone to provide retention for a tooth crown, bridge, or denture anchorage.

**anchorage** (āng′kĕr-ĭj) **1.** Surgical fixation, as of prolapsed abdominal organs. **2.** The part to which anything is fixed, as a tooth to which a bridge is fastened.

**ancillary** (ăn′sĭl-lār″ē) [L. *ancillaris,* handmaid] **1.** Subordinate, secondary. **2.** Auxiliary, supplementary.

**anconad** (ăn′kō-năd) [Gr. *ankon,* elbow, + L. *ad,* to] Toward the elbow.

**anconagra** (ăn″kŏn-ăg′ră) [″ + *agra,* a seizure] Gout of the elbow.

**anconal, anconeal** (ăn′kō-năl, ăn-kō′nē-ăl) Pert. to the elbow.

**anconal fossa, anconeal fossa** Fossa olecrani; the hollow on the distal end of the humerus, in which the olecranon rests when the elbow is extended.

**anconeus** (ăn-kō′nē-ŭs) [Gr. *ankon,* elbow] The short extensor muscle of the forearm, located on the back of the elbow. It arises from the back portion of the lateral epicondyle of the humerus, and its fibers insert on the side of the olecranon and upper fourth of shaft of ulna. It extends the forearm and abducts the ulna in pronation of the wrist.

**anconitis** (ăn″kō-nī′tĭs) [″ + *itis,* inflammation] Inflammation of the elbow joint.

**ancrod** An enzyme purified from the venom of a Malayan pit viper and used as an anticoagulant.

**Ancylostoma** (ăn″sĭl-ŏs′tō-mă) [Gr. *ankylos,* crooked, + *stoma,* mouth] A genus of nematodes of the family Ancylostomatidae whose members are intestinal parasites and include the hookworms.

***A. braziliense*** Species of hookworm that infests dogs and cats and may cause cutaneous larva migrans in humans. SEE: *larva migrans, cutaneous.*

***A. caninum*** Species of hookworm that infests dogs and cats and may cause cutaneous larva migrans in humans. SEE: *larva migrans, cutaneous.*

***A. duodenale*** Species of hookworm that commonly infests humans, causing ancylostomiasis; widely found in temperate regions. SEE: *Necator americanus.*

**Ancylostomatidae** (ăn″sĭ-lŏs″tō-măt′ĭ-dē) A family of nematodes belonging to the suborder Strongylata. It includes the genera *Ancylostoma* and *Necator,* common hookworms of humans.

**ancylostomiasis** (ăn″sĭ-lŏs-tō-mī′ă-sĭs) [Gr. *ankylos,* crooked, + *stoma,* mouth, + *-iasis,* condition] Hookworm infestation, esp. *Ancylostoma duodenale* or *Necator americanus.* The disease is common in tropical and semitropical areas where the effects of climate and poor sanitation bring the larvae—found in infected feces—in contact with bare skin, usually of the foot. SYN: *hookworm disease.*

When the hookworm eggs hatch, the larvae enter through the host's skin, causing inflammation, itching, and sometimes allergic reactions. They pass from the skin to the venous circulation, where they migrate to the lungs and respiratory tree. If larvae are numerous, they may cause eosinophilic pneumonia. They travel up the bronchi and are finally swallowed, thus gaining entry to the intestinal tract. Larvae mature in the intestines, where they attach to the mucous membrane and suck blood from the host. The adults secrete an anticoagulant, which causes additional bleeding; the loss of blood leads to anemia. Nausea, colicky pains, and diarrhea may also result. In children, normal mental and physical growth is retarded. If the condition is untreated, adult worms may live in the intestinal tract for as long as 30 years. However, most individuals lose the infection within 2 years.

TREATMENT: In severe cases it may be necessary to treat the severe anemia prior to ridding the patient of the parasites. Mebendazole and pyrantel pamoate are the drugs of choice for *Necator* and *Ancylostoma* infections. The latter has the advantage of single-dose administration. A nutritional supplement with iron will be needed when anemia is severe. In some severe cases in children, blood transfusion may be needed.

**ancyroid** (ăn′sĭ-royd) [Gr. *ankyra,* anchor, + *eidos,* form, shape] Shaped like the fluke of an anchor.

**Andernach's ossicles** (ŏn′dĕr-nŏks) [Johann Winther von Andernach, Ger. physician, 1487–1574] Ossa suturarum; small bones found in cranial sutures. SYN: *wormian bones; sutural bone.*

**Andersen's disease** [Dorothy H. Andersen, U.S. pediatrician, 1901–1963] Glycogen storage disease, type IV. SEE: *glycogen storage disease.*

**andro-** [Gr. *andros,* man] Combining form meaning *man, male,* or *masculine.*

**androgalactozemia** (ăn″drō-găl-ăk″tō-zē′mē-ă) [″ + *gala,* milk, + *zemia,* loss] Oozing of milk from a man's breast.

**androgen** (ăn′drō-jĕn) [Gr. *andros,* man, + *gennan,* to produce] A substance producing or stimulating the development of male characteristics (masculinization), such as the hormones testosterone and androsterone.

**androgenic** (ăn″drō-jĕn′ĭk) Causing masculinization. SYN: *andromimetic.*

**androgyne** (ăn′drō-jīn) [″ + *gyne,* woman] A female pseudohermaphrodite. SYN: *androgynus.*

**androgynoid** (ăn-drŏj′ĭ-noyd) [″ + ″ + *eidos,* form, shape] A person possessing female gonads (ovaries) but secondary sex characteristics of a male (a female pseudohermaphrodite). Term is less commonly used for a person possessing male gonads (testes) but secondary sex characteristics of a female (a male pseudohermaphrodite).

**androgynous** (ăn-drŏj′ĭ-nŭs) [″ + *gyne,* woman] **1.** Resembling or pert. to an androgynoid. **2.** Without definite sexual characteristics.

**androgynus** (ăn-drŏj′ĭ-nŭs) A female pseudohermaphrodite. SYN: *androgyne.*

**android** (ăn′droyd) [″ + *eidos,* form, shape] Resembling a male; manlike.

**andromimetic** (ăn″drō-mĭ-mĕt′ĭk) [″ + *mimetikos,* imitative] Androgenic.

**andromorphous** (ăn″drō-mor′fŭs) [″ + *morphe,* form] Resembling a male in physical structure and appearance.

**androphobia** (ăn″drō-fō′bē-ă) [″ + *phobos,* fear] Morbid fear of the male sex.

**androstane** (ăn′drō-stān) $C_{19}H_{32}$. A steroid hydrocarbon that is the precursor of androgenic hormones.

**androsterone** (ăn″drō-stēr′ōn, ăn-drŏs′tĕr-ōn) $C_{19}H_{30}O_2$. An androgenic steroid found in the urine. It is a metabolite of testosterone and androstenedione. It has been synthesized. As one of the androgens (male sex hormones), androsterone contributes to the characteristic changes of growth and development of the genitals and axillary and pubic hair, deepening of the voice, and development of the sweat glands in the male.

**-ane** In chemistry, a suffix indicating a saturated hydrocarbon.

**anecdotal evidence** (ăn″ĭk-dōt′l) [Gr. *an,*

not, + *ekdotos,* given out] Information that is subjective or not subject to objective verification.

**anecdotal records** Notes used in nursing education to document observed incidents of a student's clinical behavior related to attainment of clinical learning objectives. Such anecdotal notes have been upheld in court as documented evidence for failing a student; the notes have not been treated as hearsay evidence.

**anechoic room** A room in which the boundaries are made so that all sound produced in the room is absorbed (i.e., not reflected).

**Anectine** Trade name for succinylcholine chloride.

**Anel's operation** (ă-nĕlz′) [Dominique Anel, Fr. surgeon, 1679–1725] Ligation of an artery immediately above and on the proximal side of an aneurysm.

**anemia** (ă-nē′mē-ă) [Gr. *an-,* not, + *haima,* blood] A reduction in the number of circulating red blood cells per cubic millimeter, the amount of hemoglobin per 100 ml, or the volume of packed red cells per 100 ml of blood. It exists when hemoglobin content is less than that required to provide the oxygen demands of the body. Because variables such as lifestyle, residential altitude, age, and sex can influence red cell and hemoglobin concentration, it is not possible to state that anemia exists when the hemoglobin content is lower than a specific value. If the onset of anemia is slow, the body may adjust so well that there will be no functional impairment even though the hemoglobin may be less than 6 g/100 ml of blood.

Anemia is not a disease; it is a symptom of various diseases. Anemia is classified on the basis of mean corpuscular volume as microcytic (<80), normocytic (80–94), and macrocytic (>94); on the basis of mean corpuscular hemoglobin as hypochromic (<27), normochromic (27–32), and hyperchromic (>32); and on the basis of etiological factors.

SYMPTOMS: Symptoms include pallor of the skin, nailbeds of the fingers, and mucous membranes, weakness, vertigo, headache, sore tongue, drowsiness, general malaise, dyspnea, tachycardia, palpitation, angina pectoris, gastrointestinal disturbances, amenorrhea, loss of libido, and slight fever.

ETIOLOGY: Anemia may result from excessive blood loss due to acute or chronic hemorrhage, from excessive blood cell destruction as occurs in hemolytic diseases and hypersplenism, or from decreased blood cell formation that may result from defective nucleoprotein synthesis (as in pernicious and other macrocytic anemias), iron deficiency in the diet, inhibition of bone marrow (as in certain toxic states), loss of bone marrow, or bone marrow failure.

TREATMENT: Treatment of anemia must be specific for the cause.

*Anemia due to excessive blood loss:* For acute blood loss, immediate measures should be taken to stop the bleeding, to restore blood volume by transfusion, and to combat shock. Chronic blood loss usually produces iron-deficiency anemia.

*Anemia due to excessive blood cell destruction:* The specific hemolytic disorder should be treated.

*Anemia due to decreased blood cell formation:* For deficiency states, use replacement therapy to combat the specific deficiency (e.g., iron, vitamin $B_{12}$, folic acid, ascorbic acid). For bone marrow disorders: if anemia is due to a toxic state, removal of the toxic agent may result in spontaneous recovery.

NURSING IMPLICATIONS: The patient is evaluated for signs and symptoms, and the results of laboratory studies are reviewed for evidence of inadequate erythropoiesis or premature erythrocyte destruction. The nurse schedules or carries out prescribed diagnostic studies. *Rest:* The patient is evaluated for fatigue; care and activities are planned and regular rest periods are scheduled. *Mouth care:* The patient's mouth is inspected daily for glossitis, mouth lesions, or ulcers. The sponge stick is recommended for oral care, and alkaline mouthwashes are suggested if mouth ulcers are present. A dental consultation may be required. *Diet:* The patient is encouraged to eat small portions at frequent intervals. Mouth care is provided before meals. The nurse or a nutritionist provides counseling based on type of anemia. *Medications:* The nurse teaches the patient about medication actions, desired effects, adverse reactions, and correct dosing and administration. *Patient education:* The cause of the anemia and the rationale for prescribed treatment are explained to the patient and family. Teaching should cover the prescribed rest and activity regimen, diet, prevention of infection including the need for frequent temperature checks, and the continuing need for periodic blood testing and medical evaluation. SEE: *Nursing Diagnoses Appendix.*

***achlorhydric a.*** A hypochromic, microcytic anemia associated with a lack of free hydrochloric acid in gastric juice.

***aplastic a.*** Anemia caused by deficient red cell production due to bone marrow disorders. SEE: illus.; *marrow* for illus. of normal marrow.

ETIOLOGY: Idiopathic cases range from 40% to 70% and are most common in adolescents and young adults. Exposure to chemical and antineoplastic agents and ionizing radiation can result in aplastic anemia and chronic renal failure; and infiltration of the bone marrow by cells that are not normally present there can interfere with normal blood production. Examples are metastatic carcinoma, miliary

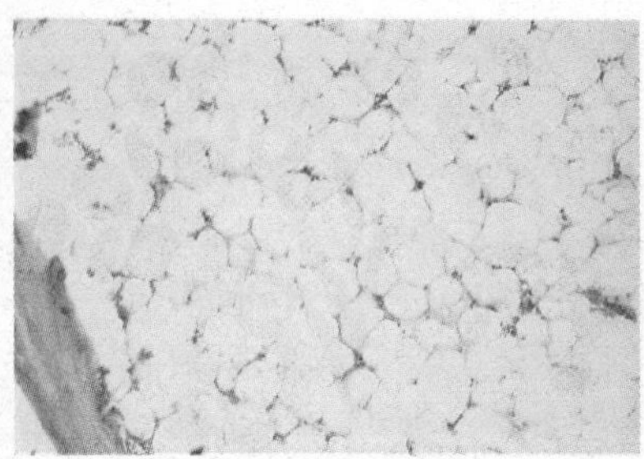

HYPOCELLULAR BONE MARROW OF
**APLASTIC ANEMIA**

tuberculosis. A congenital form has been described.

TREATMENT: Most patients can be treated effectively with bone marrow transplantation or immunosuppressive drugs.

NURSING IMPLICATIONS: The nurse ensures that the patient and family understand the cause and treatment of the illness. Measures to prevent infection are explained, and the importance of adequate rest emphasized. In the acute phase, the nurse carries out prescribed treatment, explains the side effects of drugs and transfusions, and ensures a restful environment. If the patient's platelet count is low (less than 20,000/cu mm), the following steps are taken to prevent hemorrhage: avoiding parenteral injections, suggesting the use of an electric razor, humidifying oxygen to prevent dry mucous membranes, and promoting regular bowel movements with stool softeners and dietary measures. Pressure is applied to all venipuncture sites until bleeding has stopped, and bleeding is detected early by checking for occult blood in urine and stools and by assessing the skin for petechiae and ecchymoses. Universal precautions and careful handwashing (and protective isolation if necessary) are used, a diet high in vitamins and protein is provided, and meticulous oral and perianal care are provided. The patient is assessed for life-threatening hemorrhage, infection, adverse effects of drug therapy, or blood transfusion reactions. Throat, urine, and blood cultures are done regularly. SEE: *protective isolation.*

***autoimmune hemolytic a.*** ABBR: AIHA. Anemia caused by antibodies produced by the patient's own immune system. They are classified by the thermal properties of the anti–red-cell antibody involved. Drug-induced hemolytic anemias are clinically indistinguishable from AIHA and for that reason are classified with this disorder.

***congenital hemolytic a.*** An inherited chronic disease marked by hemolysis of blood cells, jaundice, and splenomegaly. SYN: *icterus, hemolytic; jaundice, hemolytic.*

***Cooley's a.*** Erythroblastic a.

***deficiency a.*** Condition resulting from lack of an essential ingredient, such as iron or vitamins, in the diet or the inability of the intestine to absorb them. SYN: *nutritional a.*

***erythroblastic a.*** Anemia resulting from inheritance of a recessive trait responsible for interference with hemoglobin synthesis. SYN: *Cooley's a.; thalassemia major.*

***folic acid deficiency a.*** Anemia resulting from a deficiency of folic acid.

NURSING IMPLICATIONS: Fluid and electrolyte balance is monitored, particularly in the patient with severe diarrhea. The patient can obtain daily folic acid requirements by including an item from each food group in every meal; a list of foods rich in folic acid (green leafy vegetables, asparagus, broccoli, liver, organ meats, milk, eggs, yeast, wheat germ, kidney beans, beef, potatoes, dried peas and beans, whole-grain cereals, nuts, bananas, cantaloupe, lemons, and strawberries) is provided. The rationale for replacement therapy is explained, and the patient is advised not to stop treatment just because he or she feels better.

***hemolytic a.*** Anemia resulting from hemolysis of red blood cells; may be congenital or may be caused by the effects of toxic agents or by severe pre-eclampsia. SEE: *hemolytic uremic syndrome.*

***hyperchromic a.*** Anemia in which mean corpuscular hemoglobin concentration (MCHC) is greater than normal. The red blood cells are darker staining than normal.

***hypochromic a.*** Anemia in which hemoglobin is deficient and mean corpuscular hemoglobin concentration is less than normal.

***hypoplastic a.*** Term that has been used to describe aplastic anemia. If anemia due to failure of formation of red blood cells is meant, pure red blood cell aplasia is the term of choice.

***iron-deficiency a.*** Anemia resulting from a greater demand on the stored iron than can be supplied. The red blood cell count may be normal, but there will be insufficient hemoglobin. Erythrocytes will be pale (hypochromia) and have abnormal shapes (poikilocytosis). Iron-deficiency anemia is probably the most common chronic disease of humankind. It is estimated that at least 18,000,000 people in the U.S. are iron deficient. SEE: illus.; *koilonychia.*

ETIOLOGY: The condition is caused by inadequate iron intake, malabsorption of iron, chronic blood loss, pregnancy and lactation, intravascular hemolysis, or a combination of these factors.

TREATMENT: Treatment consists of oral ferrous sulfate or ferrous gluconate

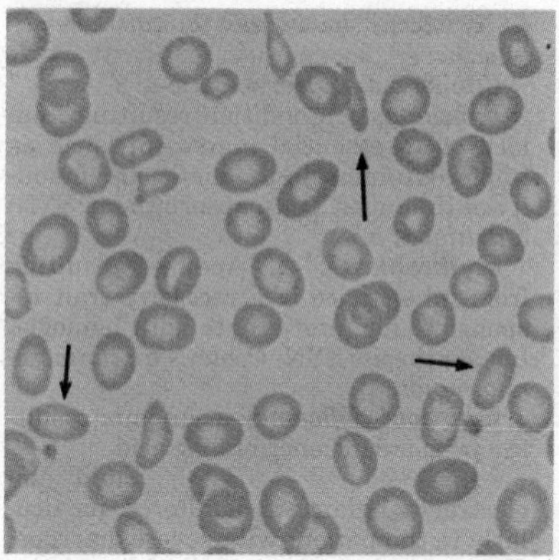

**IRON-DEFICIENCY ANEMIA**

HYPOCHROMIA AND POIKILOCYTOSIS, WITH OVALOCYTES (ARROWS) (×640)

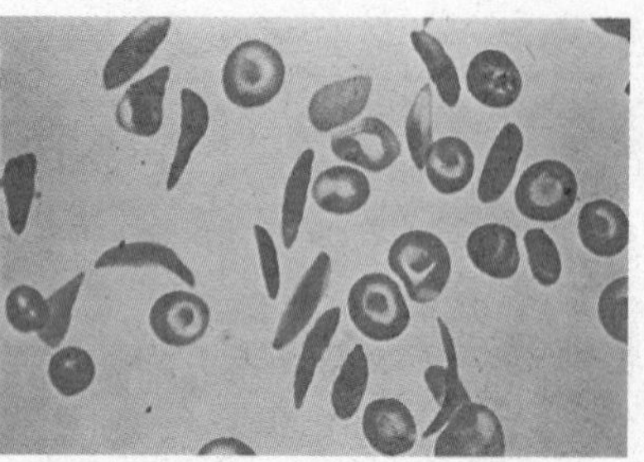

**SICKLE CELL ANEMIA** (×600)

and a well-balanced diet.

***macrocytic a.*** Anemia marked by abnormally large erythrocytes.

***Mediterranean a.*** SEE: *thalassemia.*

***megaloblastic a.*** Anemia in which megaloblasts are found in the blood.

***microcytic a.*** Anemia marked by abnormally small red blood cells.

***milk a.*** In a young child, iron-deficiency anemia caused by consistent consumption of milk in amounts greater than 1 qt daily. This excessive milk intake displaces iron-rich foods in the diet.

***normochromic a.*** Anemia in which the red blood cells contain the normal amount of hemoglobin.

***normocytic a.*** Anemia in which the size and hemoglobin content of red blood cells remain normal.

***nutritional a.*** Deficiency a.

***pernicious a.*** A chronic, macrocytic anemia marked by achlorhydria. It occurs most often in 40- to 80-year-old northern Europeans of fair skin, but has been reported in other races and ethnic groups. It is rare in blacks and Asians.

SYMPTOMS: Symptoms include weakness, sore tongue, paresthesias (tingling and numbness) of extremities, and gastrointestinal symptoms such as diarrhea, nausea, vomiting, and pain; in severe anemia, there may be signs of cardiac failure.

ETIOLOGY: Pernicious anemia is thought to be an autoimmune disease. The parietal cells of the stomach lining fail to secrete enough intrinsic factor to ensure intestinal absorption of vitamin $B_{12}$, the extrinsic factor. This is due to atrophy of the glandular mucosa of the fundus of the stomach and is associated with absence of hydrochloric acid.

TREATMENT: Intramuscular injection of vitamin $B_{12}$ is given.

***physiological a. of pregnancy*** SEE: *pseudoanemia of pregnancy.*

***pure red cell aplasia a.*** Anemia due to decreased production of red cells.

***runner's a.*** Mild hemolysis with hematuria, hemoglobinemia, and hemoglobinuria produced by strenuous exercise including running. Blood may be lost in the feces, presumably due to transient ischemia of the gut during vigorous exercise.

***septic a.*** Anemia due to severe infection.

***sickle cell a.*** An inherited disorder transmitted as an autosomal recessive trait that causes an abnormality of the globin genes in hemoglobin. The frequency of the genetic defect responsible for this chronic anemia disorder is highest among African-American, native African, and Mediterranean populations. SEE: illus.; *Nursing Diagnoses Appendix.*

ETIOLOGY: When both parental genes carry the same defect, the person is homozygous for hemoglobin S, that is, HbSS, and manifests the disorder. When exposed to a decrease in oxygen, hemoglobin S becomes viscous. This causes the red cells to become crescent-shaped (sickling), rigid, sticky, and fragile. When they clump together, circulation through the capillaries is impeded, causing obstruction, tissue hypoxia, and further sickling. In infants younger than 5 months old, high levels of fetal hemoglobin inhibit the reaction of the hemoglobin S molecule to decreased oxygen.

SYMPTOMS: The shortened lifespan of the abnormal red cells (10 to 20 days) results in a chronic anemia; pallor, weakness, and fatigue are common. Jaundice may result from the hemolysis of red cells. Crisis may occur as a result of sickling, thrombi formation, vascular occlusion, tissue hypoxia, and infarction. SEE: *sickle cell crisis.*

TREATMENT: Supportive therapy includes supplemental iron and blood transfusion. Administration of hydroxyurea stimulates the production of hemoglobin S and decreases the need for blood transfusions and painful crises. Prophylactic daily doses of penicillin have demon-

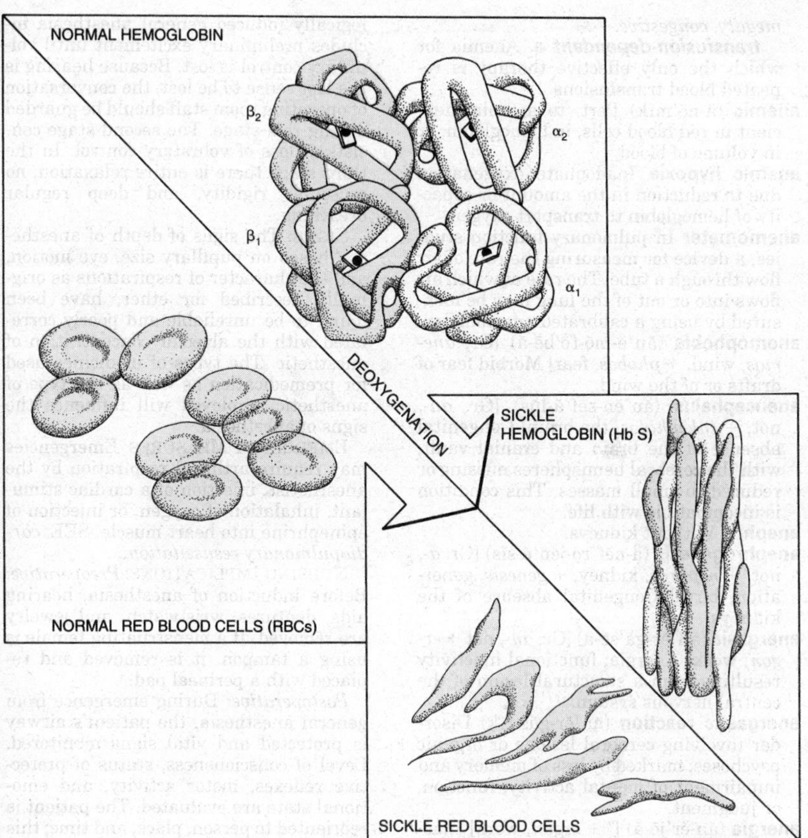


SICKLE CELL ANEMIA

STRUCTURE OF HEMOGLOBIN A AND HEMOGLOBIN S AND THEIR EFFECT ON ERYTHROCYTES

strated effectiveness in reducing the incidence of acute bacterial infections in children. Supportive therapy includes supplemental iron and transfusions.

NURSING IMPLICATIONS: Sickle cell crisis should be suspected in the sickle cell patient with pale lips, tongue, palms, or nailbeds; lethargy; listlessness; difficulty awakening; irritability; severe pain; or temperature over 104°F (37.8°C) lasting at least 2 days. During a crisis, warm compresses are applied to the painful areas, and the patient is covered with a blanket. (Cold compresses aggravate the condition.) Prescribed analgesic-antipyretics such as aspirin or acetaminophen are given. Bedrest is encouraged, with the patient in a sitting position. Dehydration and severe pain are the two chief reasons for hospitalization; the patient should increase fluid intake to prevent dehydration that may result from impaired urine-concentrating ability. During remission, the patient can prevent exacerbations by avoiding tight clothing that restricts circulation; strenuous exercise; vasoconstricting drugs; cold temperatures; and unpressurized aircraft, high altitudes, and other hypoxia-provoking conditions. Parents are warned against being overprotective. The child must avoid strenuous exercise and body-contact sports but can still enjoy most activities. Parents are referred for genetic counseling regarding risks to future children, and screening of family members is recommended to determine heterozygote carriers. Both parents and patients are referred to community-based support groups; parents may also require psychological counseling to cope with guilt feelings.

***splenic a.*** Enlargement of the spleen due to portal or splenic hypertension with accompanying anemia, leukopenia, thrombocytopenia, and gastric hemorrhage. SYN: *Banti's syndrome; spleno-*

*megaly, congestive.*

***transfusion-dependent a.*** Anemia for which the only effective therapy is repeated blood transfusions.

**anemic** (ă-nē′mĭk) Pert. to anemia; deficient in red blood cells, in hemoglobin, or in volume of blood.

**anemic hypoxia** Inadequate oxygenation due to reduction in the amount or capacity of hemoglobin to transport oxygen.

**anemometer** In pulmonary function studies, a device for measuring the rate of air flow through a tube. The rate at which air flows into or out of the lung may be measured by using a calibrated anemometer.

**anemophobia** (ăn″ĕ-mō-fō′bē-ă) [Gr. *anemos,* wind, + *phobos,* fear] Morbid fear of drafts or of the wind.

**anencephalus** (ăn″ĕn-sĕf′ă-lŭs) [Gr. *an-,* not, + *enkephalos,* the brain] Congenital absence of the brain and cranial vault, with the cerebral hemispheres missing or reduced to small masses. This condition is incompatible with life.

**anephric** Without kidneys.

**anephrogenesis** (ă-nĕf″rō-jĕn′ĕ-sĭs) [Gr. *a-,* not, + *nephros,* kidney, + *genesis,* generation, birth] Congenital absence of the kidneys.

**anergasia** (ăn″ĕr-gā′sē-ă) [Gr. *an-,* not + *ergon,* work] Anergia; functional inactivity resulting from a structural lesion of the central nervous system.

**anergastic reaction** (ăn″ĕr-găs′tĭk) Disorder involving cerebral lesions or organic psychoses; marked by loss of memory and impairment of mental activity, function, or judgment.

**anergia** (ăn-ĕr′jē-ă) [″ + *ergon,* work] Inactivity; lack of energy.

**anergic stupor** Acute phase of dementia.

**anergy** (ăn′ĕr-jē) **1.** Impaired or absent ability to react to common antigens administered through skin testing. **2.** Lack of energy. **anergic** (ăn-ĕr′jĭk), *adj.*

**aneroid** (ăn′ĕr-ŏyd) [Gr. *a-,* not, + *neron,* water, + *eidos,* form, shape] Operating without fluid, such as an aneroid barometer that uses atmospheric pressure instead of a liquid such as mercury.

**anerythroplasia** (ăn″ĕ-rĭth″rō-plā′zē-ă) [Gr. *an-,* not, + *erythros,* red, + *plasis,* a molding] Absence of red blood cell formation in the bone marrow. **anerythroplastic** (-plăs′tĭk), *adj.*

**anerythropsia** (ăn″ĕ-rĭ-thrŏp′sē-ă) [″ + ″ + *opsis,* vision] Inability to distinguish clearly the color red.

**anesthecinesia, anesthekinesia** (ăn-ĕs-thē″sĭn-ē′zē-ă, -kĭ-nē′zē-ă) [″ + *aisthesis,* sensation, + *kinesis,* movement] Sensory and motor paralysis.

**anesthesia** (ăn″ĕs-thē′zē-ă) [″ + *aisthesis,* sensation] Partial or complete loss of sensation, with or without loss of consciousness, as a result of disease, injury, or administration of an anesthetic agent, usually by injection or inhalation.

STAGES: The first stage of pharmacologically induced general anesthesia includes preliminary excitement until voluntary control is lost. Because hearing is the last sense to be lost, the conversation of operating room staff should be guarded during this stage. The second stage consists of loss of voluntary control. In the third stage there is entire relaxation, no muscular rigidity, and deep regular breathing.

SIGNS: The signs of depth of anesthesia, based on pupillary size, eye motion, and the character of respirations as originally described for ether, have been found to be unreliable and poorly correlated with the alveolar concentration of anesthetic. The types of medicines used for premedication as well as the type of anesthetic employed will influence the signs of anesthesia.

EMERGENCY MEASURES: Emergencies may require artificial respiration by the anesthetist, injection of a cardiac stimulant, inhalation of oxygen, or injection of epinephrine into heart muscle. SEE: *cardiopulmonary resuscitation.*

NURSING IMPLICATIONS: *Preoperative:* Before induction of anesthesia, hearing aids, dentures, wristwatch, and jewelry are removed. If a menstruating female is using a tampon, it is removed and replaced with a perineal pad.

*Postoperative:* During emergence from general anesthesia, the patient's airway is protected and vital signs monitored. Level of consciousness, status of protective reflexes, motor activity, and emotional state are evaluated. The patient is reoriented to person, place, and time; this information is repeated as often as necessary. For patients who have received ketamine, a quiet area with minimal stimulation is provided. Before nerve block anesthesia, the nurse establishes an intravenous infusion to ensure hydration. The patient is protected with side rails and other safety measures, and the anesthetized body part protected from prolonged pressure. For regional anesthesia, the nurse assesses sympathetic blockade by monitoring sensory response along with vital signs (the block will wear off from head to toe). In obstetrics, maternal hypotension results in diminished placental perfusion and potential fetal compromise. Outcomes indicating returned sympathetic innervation include stable vital signs and temperature, ability to vasoconstrict, perianal pinprick sensations ("anal wink"), plantar flexion of the foot against resistance, and ability to sense whether the great toe is flexed or extended. The nurse ensures that the patient with postanesthesia headache remains flat in bed, administers prescribed analgesics, provides comfort measures and abdominal support, assists with position changes, and offers fluids to increase hydration.

***audio a.*** Anesthesia produced by sound;

used by dentists to inhibit pain perception.

***basal a.*** A level of unconsciousness that is just above the level of complete surgical anesthesia. The patient does not respond to verbal stimuli but does react to noxious stimuli, such as a pinprick. Basal anesthesia is useful in combination with local or regional anesthesia, making the patient unaware of the surgical experience.

***block a.*** A regional anesthetic injected into a nerve (intraneural) or immediately around it (paraneural). SYN: *conduction a.; neural a.*

***bulbar a.*** Anesthesia produced by a lesion of the pons.

***caudal a.*** Anesthesia produced by insertion of a needle into sacrococcygeal notch and injection of a local anesthetic into the epidural space.

***central a.*** Pathological anesthesia due to a lesion of the central nervous system.

***closed a.*** Inhalation anesthesia technique in which the gases are rebreathed. This requires appropriate treatment of the exhaled gas in order to absorb the expired carbon dioxide and to replenish the oxygen and the anesthetic.

***conduction a.*** Block a.

***crossed a.*** Anesthesia of the side opposite to the site of the lesion.

***dissociative a.*** A type of anesthesia marked by catalepsy, amnesia, and marked analgesia. The patient experiences a strong feeling of dissociation from the environment.

***a. dolorosa*** Pain in an anesthetized zone, as in thalamic lesions.

***electric a.*** Anesthesia induced by the use of an electric current.

***endotracheal a.*** Anesthesia in which gases are administered via a tube inserted into the trachea.

***epidural a.*** Anesthesia produced by injection of a local anesthetic into the peridural space of the spinal cord. SYN: *peridural a.*

***general a.*** Anesthesia that is complete and affects the entire body with loss of consciousness when the anesthetic acts on the brain. This type of anesthesia is usually accomplished following administration of inhalation or intravenous anesthetics. It is commonly used for surgical procedures.

***Gwathmey's a.*** Anesthesia induced by injection of an olive oil and ether solution into the rectum.

***hypotensive a.*** Anesthesia during which the blood pressure is lowered.

***hypothermic a.*** General anesthesia during which the body temperature is lowered.

***hysterical a.*** Bodily anesthesia occurring in hysteria.

***ice a.*** Refrigeration a.

***infiltration a.*** Local anesthesia produced by injection of the local anesthetic solution directly into the tissues, such as injection of procaine solution into the gums for dental procedures.

***inhalation a.*** General anesthesia produced by the inhalation of vapor or gaseous anesthetics such as ether, nitrous oxide, and methoxyflurane.

***insufflation a.*** Instillation of gaseous anesthetics into the inhaled air.

***intratracheal a.*** Anesthesia administered through a catheter passed to the level of the trachea.

***local a.*** Anesthesia affecting a local area only, the anesthetic acting upon nerves or nerve tracts. Local anesthesia to allow placement of a needle in the skin, as in a hypodermic injection, can be produced by applying an ice cube to the site for 10 to 30 sec just prior to the needle stick. This affords anesthesia for a few seconds. A longer period of anesthesia—2 to 5 min—is produced by subcutaneous injection of bacteriostatic saline solution with benzyl alcohol. It allows enough time for surgical removal of skin tags, warts, and non-melanotic moles. SEE: *block anesthesia; infiltration anesthesia.*

***mixed a.*** General anesthesia produced by more than one drug, such as nitrous oxide gas for induction followed by ether for maintenance of anesthesia.

***neural a.*** Block a.

***neuroleptic a.*** General anesthesia produced by a neuroleptic agent such as droperidol, a narcotic analgesic, and nitrous oxide.

***open a.*** Application, usually by dropping, of a volatile anesthetic agent onto gauze held over the nose and mouth.

***peridural a.*** Epidural a.

***peripheral a.*** Local anesthesia produced when a nerve is blocked with an appropriate agent.

***primary a.*** The first stage of anesthesia, before unconsciousness.

***pudendal a.*** A type of local anesthesia used in obstetrics. The pudendal nerve on each side, near the spinous process of the ischium, is blocked.

***rectal a.*** General anesthesia produced by introduction of an anesthetic agent into the rectum, used esp. in labor.

***refrigeration a.*** Anesthesia induced by lowering the temperature of a body part to near freezing either by spraying it with ethyl chloride or by immersing it in a container of finely cracked ice.

***regional a.*** Nerve or field blocking, causing insensibility over a particular area. SEE: *block anesthesia; infiltration anesthesia.*

***saddle block a.*** A type of anesthesia produced by introducing the anesthetic agent into the fourth lumbar interspace. This anesthetizes the perineum and the buttocks area.

***segmental a.*** Anesthesia due to a pathological or surgically induced lesion of a nerve root.

***sexual a.*** Absence of sexual desire.

***spinal a.*** **1.** Anesthesia resulting from disease or injury to conduction pathways of the spinal cord. **2.** Anesthesia produced by injection of anesthetic into the subarachnoid space of the spinal cord.

***splanchnic a.*** Anesthesia produced by injection of an anesthetic into the splanchnic ganglion.

***surgical a.*** Depth of anesthesia at which relaxation of muscles and loss of sensation and consciousness are adequate for the performance of surgery.

***tactile a.*** Loss of sense of touch.

***topical a.*** Local anesthesia induced by application of an anesthetic directly to the surface of the area to be anesthetized.

***traumatic a.*** Loss of sensation resulting from nerve injury.

***twilight a.*** State of light anesthesia. SEE: *twilight sleep.*

**anesthesiologist** (ăn″ĕs-thē″zē-ŏl′ō-jĭst) A physician specializing in anesthesiology.

**anesthesiology** (ăn″ĕs-thē″zē-ŏl′ō-jē) [″ + ″ + *logos,* word, reason] The science of anesthesia.

**anesthetic** (ăn″ĕs-thĕt′ĭk) **1.** Pert. to or producing anesthesia. **2.** An agent that produces anesthesia; subdivided into general and local, according to its action. SEE: *anesthesia.*

**anesthetist** (ă-nĕs′thĕ-tĭst) One who administers anesthetics, esp. for general anesthesia; may be an anesthesiologist or specially trained nurse.

**anesthetization** (ă-nĕs″thĕ-tĭ-zā′shŭn) Induction of anesthesia.

**anesthetize** (ă-nĕs′thĕ-tīz) To induce anesthesia.

**anetoderma** (ăn″ĕt-ō-dĕr′mă) [Gr. *anetos,* relaxed, + *derma,* skin] Localized laxity of the skin with protruding, saclike areas. These lesions are due to loss of normal skin elasticity. They may be excised. SYN: *macular atrophy.*

**aneuploidy** (ăn″ū-ploy′dē) [Gr. *an-,* not, + *eu,* well, + *ploos,* fold, + *eidos,* form, shape] Condition of having an abnormal number of chromosomes for the species indicated. **aneuploid** (ăn′ū-ployd), *adj.*

**aneurysm** (ăn′ū-rĭzm) [Gr. *aneurysma,* a widening] Localized abnormal dilatation of a blood vessel, usually an artery; due to a congenital defect or weakness in the wall of the vessel. SEE: illus.

ETIOLOGY: In the aorta, arteriosclerosis accompanied by hypertension is a cause, as is syphilis. Bacterial or mycotic infection and trauma are common causes of aneurysms in peripheral arteries. **aneurysmal** (ăn″ū-rĭz′măl), *adj.*

***abdominal aortic a.*** A localized dilatation (saccular, fusiform, or dissecting) of the wall of the abdominal aorta (the portion of the descending aorta that passes from the aortic hiatus of the diaphragm into the abdomen, descending ventral to the vertebral column, and ending at the fourth lumbar vertebra where it divides into the two common iliac arteries). It is

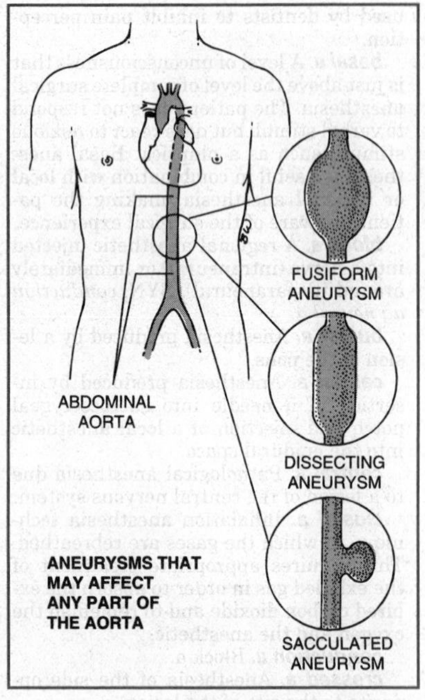


generally found to involve the renal arteries and frequently the iliac arteries. Occasionally the dilatation can extend upward through the diaphragm.

SYMPTOMS: Symptoms, when present, include generalized abdominal pain, low back pain unaffected by movement, sensations of gastric or abdominal fullness, sudden lumbar or abdominal pain radiating to the flank and groin, a pulsating mass in the periumbilical area, and a systolic bruit over the aorta.

TREATMENT: If untreated, most abdominal aneurysms will continue to enlarge and will rupture. Surgical repair is recommended for all aneurysms 6 cm or greater in size but smaller ones also can rupture. If an aneurysm is tender and known to be enlarging rapidly (no matter what its size), surgery is essential. Surgical therapy consists of replacing the aneurysmal segment with a synthetic fabric graft. Immediate surgery is indicated for ruptured aortic abdominal aneurysm.

NURSING IMPLICATIONS: Vital signs are monitored, esp. blood pressure, every 4 hr or more frequently, depending on the severity of the patient's condition. Blood pressure may be much lower in the legs than in the arms. Renal function is assessed by monitoring blood urea nitrogen, creatinine, and electrolyte levels and by measuring fluid intake and output. Complete blood count is monitored for evidence of blood loss. In acute situations, arterial blood gas values and cardiac rhythm are monitored, and a pulmonary artery line is inserted to monitor blood pressure. The patient is observed for signs of rupture, which may be fatal; these include acute blood loss and shock; increasing pulse and respiratory rates; cool, clammy skin; restlessness; and decreased sensorium. Palpation of the abdomen for a mass is avoided if abdominal aortic aneurysm has been diagnosed or is suspected, because deep palpation may precipitate rupture.

Prescribed medications are administered, and the patient is instructed in their use. In acute situations, admission to the intensive care unit is arranged, a blood sample obtained for typing and crossmatching, and a large-bore (14G) venous catheter inserted to facilitate blood replacement. The patient is prepared for, and informed about, elective surgery if indicated or emergency surgery if rupture occurs.

Desired outcomes include the patient's ability to express anxiety; to use support systems and perform stress reduction techniques to assist with coping; demonstrated abatement of physical signs of anxiety; avoidance of activities that increase the risk of rupture; understanding of, and cooperation with, the prescribed treatment regimen; ability to identify indications of rupture and to institute emergency measures; maintenance of normal fluid and blood volume in acute situations; recovery from elective or emergency surgery with no complications.

***aortic a.*** An aneurysm affecting any part of the aorta. Symptoms include dyspnea, cough, sputum, dysphagia, congestion of the head and neck, and inequality in the right and left radial pulses. The condition produces pressure on the trachea, esophagus, veins, or nerves and is treated with surgery.

***arteriovenous a.*** An aneurysm of congenital or traumatic origin in which the artery and vein become connected by a saccule. Symptoms include pain, expansive pulsation, and bruits.

***atherosclerotic a.*** Aneurysm due to degeneration or weakening of the arterial wall caused by atherosclerosis.

***berry a.*** A small saccular congenital aneurysm of a cerebral vessel. It communicates with the vessel by a small opening. Rupture of this type of aneurysm may cause bleeding severe enough to be fatal.

***cerebral a.*** Aneurysm of a blood vessel in the brain.

***cirsoid a.*** A dilatation of a network of vessels commonly occurring on the scalp. The mass may form a pulsating subcutaneous tumor. SYN: *racemose a.*

***compound a.*** Aneurysm in which some of the layers of the vessel are ruptured and others dilated.

***dissecting a.*** Aneurysm in which the blood makes its way between the layers of a blood vessel wall, separating them; a result of necrosis of the medial portion of the arterial wall. SEE: *aneurysm* for illus.

***fusiform a.*** Aneurysm in which all the walls of a blood vessel dilate more or less equally, creating a tubular swelling. SEE: *aneurysm* for illus.

***mycotic a.*** Aneurysm due to bacterial infection.

***racemose a.*** Cirsoid a.

***sacculated a.*** Aneurysm in which there is weakness on one side of the vessel; usually due to trauma. It is attached to the artery by a narrow neck. SEE: *aneurysm* for illus.

***varicose a.*** Aneurysm forming a blood-filled sac between an artery and a vein.

***venous a.*** Aneurysm of a vein.

**aneurysmectomy** (ăn″ū-rĭz-mĕk′tō-mē) [″ + *ektome,* excision] Surgical removal of the sac of an aneurysm.

**aneurysmoplasty** (ăn″ū-rĭz′mō-plăs″tē) [″ + *plassein,* to form] Surgical repair of an aneurysm.

**aneurysmorrhaphy** (ăn″ū-rĭz-mor′ă-fē) [″ + *rhaphe,* seam, ridge] Surgical closure of the sac of an aneurysm.

**aneurysmotomy** (ăn″ū-rĭz-mŏt′ō-mē) [″ + *tome,* incision] Incision of the sac of an aneurysm, allowing it to heal by granulation.

**A.N.F.** *American Nurses' Foundation.*

**angel dust** Phencyclidine hydrochloride.

**angel's trumpet** [*Datura ruaveolens*] A flowering shrub native to the southeastern U.S. Portions of the plant are used for hallucinogenic effects. The flowers are made into a stew or tea, and the leaves are eaten. The flowers contain large quantities of the alkaloids atropine, hyoscyamine, and hyoscine. Ingestion of the plant produces intense thirst, visual disturbances, flushing, central nervous system hyperexcitability, sensory flooding, and a delirious incoherent state. This is followed by hyperthermia, tachycardia, hypertension, visual hallucinations, disturbed consciousness, clonus, and subsequent convulsions. If the condition is untreated, death may occur.

TREATMENT: Treatment consists of gastric lavage, followed by 1 to 4 mg of intravenous physostigmine sulfate. This dosage should reverse the acute delirious state in 1 to 2 hr, but it may need to be repeated several times.

**angel's wing** Posterior projection of the scapula; usually caused by paralysis of the serratus anterior muscle. SYN: *winged scapula.*

**Angelucci's syndrome** (ăn″jĕ-loo′chēz) [Arnaldo Angelucci, It. ophthalmologist, 1854–1934] Great excitability, palpitation, and vasomotor disturbance associated with vernal conjunctivitis.

**anger** (ăng′er) [L. *angere,* anguish] The basic emotion of extreme displeasure or exasperation in reaction to a person, a situation, or an object. Anger is instrumental in mobilizing and enhancing our ability to respond to adverse situations; for that reason, it may be essential to survival in some situations. It has been suggested that anger may be a reaction to dying and that a patient's anger may be directed to friends or family and to those responsible for his or her medical care.

**angi-** (ăn′jē) [Gr. *angeion,* vessel] SEE: *angio-*.

**angiasthenia** (ăn″jē-ăs-thē′nē-ă) [″ + *a-*, not, + *sthenos,* strength] Loss of vascular tone.

**angiectomy** (ăn″jē-ĕk′tō-mē) [″ + *ektome,* excision] Excision or resection of a blood vessel.

**angiectopia** (ăn″jē-ĕk′tō′pē-ă) [″ + *ektopos,* out of place] Displacement of a vessel.

**angiemphraxis** (ăn″jē-ĕm-frăk′sĭs) [″ + *emphraxis,* stoppage] Obstruction of a vessel.

**angiitis** (ăn″jē-ī′tĭs) [″ + *itis,* inflammation] Inflammation of a blood or lymph vessel. SYN: *vasculitis.*

**angina** (ăn-jī′nă, ăn′jĭ-nă) [L. *angina,* quinsy, from *angere,* to choke] **1.** Angina pectoris. **2.** Acute sore throat. **anginal** (ăn′jĭ-nal), *adj.*

***a. decubitus*** Attacks of angina pectoris occurring while an individual is in a recumbent position.

***a. of effort*** Angina pectoris with onset during exercise. SYN: *exertion a.*

***exertion a.*** A. of effort.

***intestinal a.*** Abdominal pain caused by insufficient blood supply to the intestines; usually occurs after eating.

***Ludwig's a.*** Submaxillary cellulitis; a deep infection of the tissues of the floor of the mouth.

***a. pectoris*** Severe pain around the heart caused by a relative deficiency of oxygen supply to the heart muscle. It occurs most often after increased activity, exercise, or a stressful event. Pain or numbness typically radiates to the left shoulder and down the left arm and may also radiate to the back or jaw. SEE: illus.

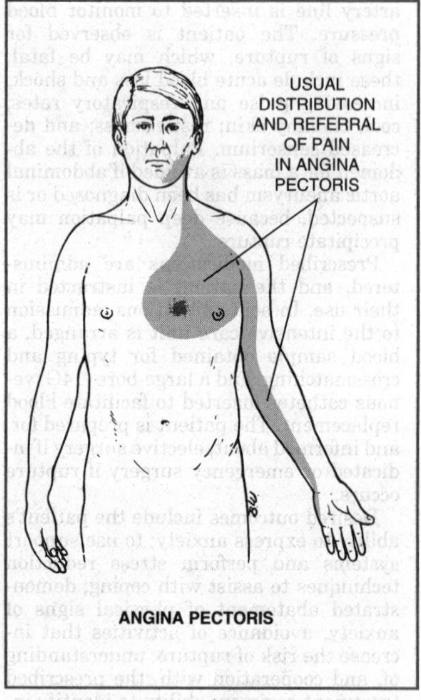

ANGINA PECTORIS

SYMPTOMS: Symptoms include steady, severe pain in the region of the heart; great anxiety, fear, and fixation of the body; and a pale, ashen, or livid face. Dyspnea may be present; the pulse is variable and is usually quick and tense. Blood pressure is raised during an attack. Cardiac arrhythmia may be present. Attacks usually last less than 30 min and are relieved by rest or medication.

TREATMENT: During an attack, treatment consists of inhalation of amyl nitrite or use of nitroglycerin sublingually. Nitroglycerin may be administered by using transdermal patches. Beta-blocking drugs (e.g., propanolol) are effective in treating angina but their side effects may make them undesirable. Calcium channel blockers, such as nifedipine, verapamil, or diltiazem, are used in treating angina. The patient should avoid excitement and get plenty of rest.

PROGNOSIS: The prognosis may be grave. Attacks may be intermittent, and with proper rest and care, recovery is possible. SEE: *myocardial ischemia; percutaneous transluminal coronary angioplasty.*

NURSING IMPLICATIONS: The pattern of pain, including time of onset, location and radiation, intensity, quality, duration, and precipitating circumstances, is monitored and documented. Cardiopulmonary status is evaluated for evidence of tachypnea, dyspnea, diaphoresis, pulmonary crackles, bradycardia or tachycardia, altered pulse strength, the appearance of a systolic third or fourth heart sound or mid- to late-systolic murmurs over the apex on auscultation, pallor, hypotension or hypertension, gastrointestinal distress, and increased need to void. The electrocardiogram is monitored for ST-segment elevation or depression, T-wave inversion, and cardiac arrhythmias. Prescribed medication and oxygen are administered and the patient's response noted. The nurse remains with the patient and provides emotional support throughout the episode. The patient is taught how to use the prescribed form of nitroglycerin for anginal attacks and about the importance of seeking medical attention if prescribed dosing does not provide relief. The patient is also taught about prescribed beta-adrenergic or calcium channel blockers, and cardiac catheterization and surgical interventions are discussed to ensure the patient's understanding of these procedures should they become necessary. SEE: *Nursing Diagnoses Appendix.*

***Prinzmetal's a.*** Variant a.

***silent a.*** Angina that causes no pain. Approx. 10% to 20% of patients with diabetes mellitus and coronary artery disease have silent angina; a similar percentage of patients with acute myocardial infarctions have silent infarctions (i.e., infarctions that cause no pain).

***stable a.*** Angina that occurs with exercise and is predictable; usually promptly relieved by rest or nitroglycerin.

***unstable a.*** Angina that has changed to a more frequent and more severe form. It can occur during rest and may be an indication of impending myocardial infarction. Unstable angina should be treated as a medical emergency and the patient hospitalized without delay.

***variant a.*** Angina occurring during rest. It is not preceded by exercise or an increase in heart rate. These patients have normal exercise potential when the angina is not present. This type of angina is caused by coronary artery spasm. SYN: *Prinzmetal's a.*

***Vincent's a.*** SEE: *Vincent's angina.*

**anginoid** (ăn′jĭ-noyd) [″ + Gr. *eidos,* form, shape] Resembling angina, esp. angina pectoris.

**anginophobia** (ăn″jĭ-nō-fō′bē-ă) [″ + Gr. *phobos,* fear] Morbid fear of an attack of angina pectoris.

**anginose, anginous** (ăn′jĭ-nōs, -nŭs) [L. *angina,* quinsy] Pert. to or resembling angina.

**angio-, angi-** (ăn′jē-ō) [Gr. *angeion,* vessel] Combining form denoting *lymph* or *blood vessels.*

**angioataxia** (ăn″jē-ō-ă-tăk′sē-ă) [″ + *ataktos,* out of order] Variability in arterial tonus.

**angioblast** (ăn′jē-ō-blăst) [″ + *blastos,* germ] **1.** The earliest tissue arising from the mesenchymal cells of the embryo, from which blood vessels develop. **2.** A cell that participates in vessel formation.

**angioblastoma** (ăn″jē-ō-blăs-tō′mă) [″ + ″ + *oma,* tumor] A tumor of particular blood vessels of the brain or of the meninges of the brain.

**angiocardiogram** (ăn″jē-ō-kăr′dē-ō-grăm) [″ + *kardia,* heart, + *gramma,* something written] The image of the heart and great blood vessels obtained by angiocardiography.

**angiocardiography** (ăn″jē-ō-kăr″dē-ŏg′ră-fē) [″ + ″ + *graphein,* to write] Serial imaging, usually cineradiography, of the heart and great blood vessles after intravascular or intracardiac injection of a water-soluble contrast medium.

**angiocardiopathy** (ăn″jē-ō-kăr″dē-ŏp′ă-thē) [″ + ″ + *pathos,* disease, suffering] Disease of the blood vessels of the heart.

**angiocarditis** (ăn″jē-ō-kăr-dī′tĭs) [″ + ″ + *itis,* inflammation] Inflammation of the heart and large blood vessels.

**angiocavernous** (ăn″jē-ō-kăv′ĕr-nŭs) [″ + L. *caverna,* cavern] Rel. to angioma cavernosum.

**angiocholecystitis** (ăn″jē-ō-kō″lĕ-sĭs-tī′tĭs) [″ + *chole,* bile, + *kystis,* bladder, + *itis,* inflammation] Inflammation of the gallbladder and bile vessels.

**angiocholitis** (ăn″jē-ō-kō-lī′tĭs) [″ + ″ + *itis,* inflammation] Inflammation of the biliary vessels. SYN: *cholangitis.*

**angiodysplasia** (ăn″jē-ō-dĭs-plā′zē-ă) Recurrent gastrointestinal bleeding due to vascular ectasis in the mucosa of the intestine, usually the cecum. Lesions increase with advancing age and accompany various bleeding syndromes, from chronic anemia and occult blood in stools to hematochezia.

**angioedema** (ăn″jē-ō-ĕ-dē′mă) [″ + *oidema,* swelling] A condition marked by development of urticaria and edematous areas of skin, mucous membranes, or viscera. It is usually benign when limited to the skin. The reaction may be dependent on immunoglobulin E and may be associated with atopic diathesis, specific antigen sensitivity to foods, drugs, stings, or molds; or it may be a physical reaction of the skin to cold, light, pressure, or exercise. The condition may also be complement mediated as in hereditary angioedema, necrotizing vasculitis, or serum sickness reactions to blood products. SYN: *angioneurotic edema.*

TREATMENT: Antihistamines and sympathomimetic agents are used for symptomatic relief. If the disease is related to complement, attenuated androgens or epsilon-aminocaproic acid can prevent or treat attacks, respectively.

**angioendothelioma** (ăn″jē-ō-ĕn″dō-thē″lē-ō′mă) *pl.* **angioendotheliomas, -mata** [″ + *endon,* within, + *thele,* nipple, + *oma,* tumor] A tumor consisting of endothelial cells, commonly occurring as single or multiple tumors of bone.

**angiofibroma** (ăn″jē-ō-fī-brō′mă) *pl.* **angiofibromas, -mata** [″ + L. *fibra,* fiber, + Gr. *oma,* tumor] A tumor consisting of fibrous tissue.

**angiogenesis** (ăn″jē-ō-jĕn′ĕ-sĭs) [″ + *genesis,* generation, birth] Development of blood vessels. **angiogenic** (-jĕn′ĭk), *adj.*

**angiogenic factors** A group of polypeptides that act in one of two ways: (1) to stimulate vascular endothelial cells to move or divide or (2) to act indirectly by mobilizing host cells, such as macrophages, to release endothelial growth factors. These factors are found in tumors in which new vessels are being formed and in normal tissues in which new vessels are not being formed. The importance of these factors in both tumors and other pathological conditions is unclear.

**angioglioma** (ăn″jē-ō-glī-ō′mă) [Gr. *angeion,* vessel, + *glia,* glue, + *oma,* tumor] A mixed angioma and glioma.

**angiogram** (ăn′jē-ō-grăm) [″ + *gramma,* something written] A radiographic record of the size, shape, and location of the heart and blood vessels after introduction of a radiopaque contrast medium. A catheter is usually inserted into a peripheral vessel and guided to the affected area by use of the Seldinger technique. The recording can be either serial film or digital imaging. The function may be therapeutic as well as diagnostic.

***aortic a.*** Angiogram of the aorta; used in diagnosing aneurysms or tumors that contact and deform the aorta.

***cardiac a.*** Angiogram of the heart; used to determine the size and shape of the cavities of the heart and the condition of the valves.

***cerebral a.*** Angiogram of blood vessels of the brain.

**angiograph** (ăn′jē-ō-grăf″) [″ + *graphein,* to write] A variety of sphygmograph.

**angiography** (ăn″jē-ŏg′ră-fē) **1.** A description of blood vessels and lymphatics. **2.** Diagnostic or therapeutic radiography of the heart and blood vessels using a radiopaque contrast medium. Types include magnetic resonance imaging, interventional radiology, and computed tomography. **3.** Recording of arterial pulse movements by use of a sphygmograph.

***aortic a.*** Angiography of the aorta and its branches.

***cardiac a.*** Angiography of the heart and coronary arteries.

***cerebral a.*** Angiography of the vascular system of the brain.

***coronary a.*** Angiography of the coronary vessels of the heart. This can provide useful information about the adequacy of blood supply to the myocardium.

***digital subtraction a.*** Use of a computer technique to investigate arterial blood circulation. A reference image is obtained by fluoroscopy. Then a contrast medium is injected intravenously. Another film is produced from the fluoroscopic image, and then the computer technique "subtracts" the image produced by surrounding tissues. The third image is an enhanced view of the arteries.

***pulmonary a.*** Angiography of the pulmonary vessels.

***selective a.*** Angiography in which a catheter is introduced directly into the vessel to be visualized.

**angiohyalinosis** (ăn″jē-ō-hī-″ă-lĭn-ō′sĭs) [Gr. *angeion,* vessel, + *hyalos,* glass, + *osis,* condition] Hyaline degeneration of blood vessel walls.

**angiohypertonia** (ăn″jē-ō-hī″pĕr-tō′nē-ă) [″ + *hyper,* over, + *tonos,* act of stretching, tension] Spasm of blood vessels, esp. arteries. SYN: *angiospasm; vasospasm.* SEE: *hypertension.*

**angiohypotonia** (ăn″jē-ō-hī″pō-tō′nē-ă) [″ + *hypo,* under, + *tonos,* act of stretching, tension] Angioparalysis; angioparesis; vascular dilatation. SEE: *hypotension.*

**angioid** (ăn′jē-oyd) [″ + *eidos,* form, shape] Resembling a blood vessel.

**angioid streaks** Dark, wavy, anastomosing striae lying beneath retinal vessels.

**angiokeratoma** (ăn″jē-ō-kĕr″ă-tō′mă) [″ + *keras,* horn, + *oma,* tumor] A skin disorder occurring chiefly on the feet and legs, marked by formation of telangiectases or warty growths accompanied by thickening of the epidermis along the course of dilated capillaries.

**angiokinetic** (ăn″jē-ō-kĭ-nĕt′ĭk) [″ + *kinesis,* movement] Pert. to constriction and dilation of blood vessels. SYN: *vasomotor.*

**angioleukitis** (ăn″jē-ō-loo-kī′tĭs) [″ + *leukos,* white, + *itis,* inflammation] Inflammation of lymphatics.

**angiolipoma** (ăn′jē-ō-lĭp-ō′mă) [″ + *lipos,* fat, + *oma,* tumor] A mixed angioma and lipoma.

**angiolith** (ăn′jē-ō-lĭth) [″ + *lithos,* stone] Calcareous deposit in the wall of a blood vessel.

**angiology** (ăn″jē-ŏl′ō-jē) [″ + *logos,* word, reason] The study of blood vessels and lymphatics.

**angiolymphitis** (ăn″jē-ō-lĭm-fī′tĭs) [″ + L. *lympha,* lymph, + *itis,* inflammation] Inflammation of the lymphatics. SYN: *lymphangitis.*

**angiolysis** (ăn″jē-ŏl′ĭ-sĭs) [″ + *lysis,* dissolution] Obliteration of blood vessels, as in the umbilical cord when it is tied just after birth.

**angioma** (ăn″jē-ō′mă) [″ + *oma,* tumor] A form of tumor, usually benign, consisting principally of blood vessels (hemangioma) or lymph vessels (lymphangioma). It is considered to be remnants of fetal tissue misplaced or undergoing disordered development. SEE: *choristoma; epithelioma; hamartoma; nevus.* **angiomatous** (-ō′mă-tŭs), *adj.*

***capillary a.*** Congenital, superficial hemangioma appearing as an irregularly shaped, red discoloration of otherwise normal skin; due to overgrowth of capillaries. SYN: *a. simplex.*

***a. cavernosum*** Congenital hemangioma appearing as an elevated dark-red benign tumor, ranging in size from a few millimeters to several centimeters. It may pulsate. It commonly involves the subcutaneous or submucous tissue and consists of blood-filled vascular spaces. Small ones may disappear without therapy.

***senile a.*** Hemangioma common in older people due to weakening of capillary walls; consists of a compressible mass of blood vessels. SYN: *spot, ruby.*

***serpiginous a.*** A skin disorder marked by the appearance of small red vascular dots arranged in rings; due to proliferation of capillaries.

***a. simplex*** Capillary a.

***spider a.*** SEE: *spider nevus.*

***stellate a.*** Hemangioma in which numerous telangiectatic vessels radiate from a central point; commonly associated with liver disease, hypertension, and pregnancy. SYN: *spider nevus.*

***telangiectatic a.*** Angioma composed of abnormally dilated blood vessels.

***a. venosum racemosum*** Swelling associated with severe varicosities of superficial veins.

**angiomalacia** (ăn″jē-ō-mă-lā′sē-ă) [Gr. *angeion,* vessel, + *malakia,* softness] Softening of blood vessel walls.

**angiomatosis** (ăn″jē-ō-mă-tō′sĭs) [″ + *oma,* tumor, + *osis,* condition] Condition of having multiple angiomas.

***bacillary a.*** An infectious disease causing proliferation of small blood vessels in the skin and visceral organs of patients with human immunodeficiency virus (HIV) infection and in others with compromised immune systems. The causative organism, *Bartonella quintana* (formerly *Rochalimaea quintana*), can be cultured from the blood. Treatment consists of oral antibiotics such as erythromycin, tetracycline, minocycline, or clarithromycin. SYN: *epithelioid angiomatosis.* SEE: *cat scratch disease; trench fever.*

**angiomegaly** (ăn″jē-ō-mĕg′ă-lē) [″ + *megas,* large] Enlargement of blood vessels, esp. in the eyelid.

**angiomyocardiac** (ăn″jē-ō-mī″ō-kăr′dē-ăk) [″ + *mys,* muscle, + *kardia,* heart] Pert. to blood vessels and cardiac muscle.

**angiomyolipoma** (ăn″jē-ō-mī″ō-lĭ-pō′mă) [″ + ″ + *lipos,* fat, + *oma,* tumor] A benign tumor containing vascular, fatty, and muscular tissue.

**angiomyoma** (ăn″jē-ō-mī-ō′mă) [″ + ″ + *oma,* tumor] A tumor composed of blood vessels and muscle tissue. SYN: *myoma telangiectodes.*

**angiomyoneuroma** (ăn″jē-ō-mī″ō-nū-rō′mă) [″ + ″ + *neuron,* nerve, + *oma,* tumor] A painful, benign tumor of the arteriovenous anastomoses of the skin. SYN: *glomangioma.*

**angiomyosarcoma** (ăn″jē-ō-mī″ō-săr-kō′mă) [″ + ″ + *sarx,* flesh, + *oma,* tumor] A tumor composed of blood vessels, muscle tissue, and connective tissue.

**angioneurectomy** (ăn″jē-ō-nū-rĕk′tō-mē) [″ + *neuron,* nerve, + *ektome,* excision] Excision of vessels and nerves.

**angioneuromyoma** Angiomyoneuroma.

**angioneurotic edema** Angioedema.

**angioneurotomy** (ăn″jē-ō-nū-rŏt′ō-mē) [″ + ″ + *tome,* incision] Cutting of vessels and nerves.

**angionoma** (ăn″jē-ō-nō′mă) [Gr. *angeion,* vessel, + *nome,* ulcer] Ulceration of a vessel.

**angioparalysis** (ăn″jē-ō-pă-răl′ĭ-sĭs) [″ + *paralyein,* loosen, dissolve] Vasomotor relaxation of blood vessel tone.

**angiopathology** (ăn″jē-ō-pă-thŏl′ō-jē) [″ + *pathos,* disease, suffering, + *logos,* word, reason] Morbid changes in diseases of the blood vessels.

**angiopathy** (ăn-jē-ŏp′ă-thē) Any disease of blood or lymph vessels. SYN: *angiosis.*

**angiophacomatosis, angiophakomatosis** (ăn″jē-ō-făk″ō-mă-tō′sis) [″ + *phakos,* lens, + *oma,* tumor, + *osis,* condition] Hippel's disease.

**angioplasty** (ăn′jē-ō-plăs″tē) [″ + *plassein,* to form] Alteration of a blood vessel, either surgically or by dilating the vessel using a balloon inside the lumen. SEE: illus.; *percutaneous transluminal coronary a.*

***laser coronary a.*** The use of laser energy to vaporize an atherosclerotic plaque in a diseased coronary vessel. SEE: *percutaneous transluminal coronary a.*

***percutaneous transluminal coronary a.*** ABBR: PTCA. A method of treating localized coronary artery narrowing. A special double-lumen catheter is designed so that a cylindrical balloon surrounds a portion of it. After the catheter is inserted transcutaneously in the artery, inflation of the balloon with pressure between 45 and 150 p.s.i. dilates the narrowed vessel. This technique may be used on narrowed arteries other than the coronaries. SEE: *laser coronary a.*

NURSING IMPLICATIONS: *Preoperative:* The cardiologist's explanation of the procedure is reinforced, the patient is encouraged to verbalize feelings and concerns, and misconceptions are clarified. The nurse prepares the patient physically for the procedure according to the surgeon's orders. Baseline data needed for comparison with postoperative assessment data are gathered.

*Postoperative:* Vital signs, cardiac rate and rhythm, and neurovascular status distal to the catheter insertion site are monitored. A Doppler stethoscope should be used if peripheral pulses are difficult to palpate. The catheter site is inspected periodically for hematoma formation, ecchymosis, or hemorrhage, and the dressing is marked and physician notified of any rapid progression. If bleeding occurs, direct pressure is applied to the catheter site. The patient should keep the leg straight and limit head elevation to no more than 15 degrees to prevent hip flexion and potential catheter migration. The patient is assessed for chest pain, which may indicate vasospasm or reocclusion of the ballooned vessel. Intravenous fluids are administered as prescribed at least 100 ml/hr to promote excretion of contrast medium and the patient is assessed for signs and symptoms of fluid overload (dyspnea, pulmonary crackles, distended neck veins, tachycardia, bounding pulse, hypertension, gallop rhythms). Pharmacological therapy is continued as prescribed (I.V. nitroglycerin, heparin). The nurse explains catheter removal to the patient and assists the physician by applying direct pressure to the insertion site for 30 min and then pressure dressing. Vital signs continue to be monitored until nurse is certain that no occult hemor-

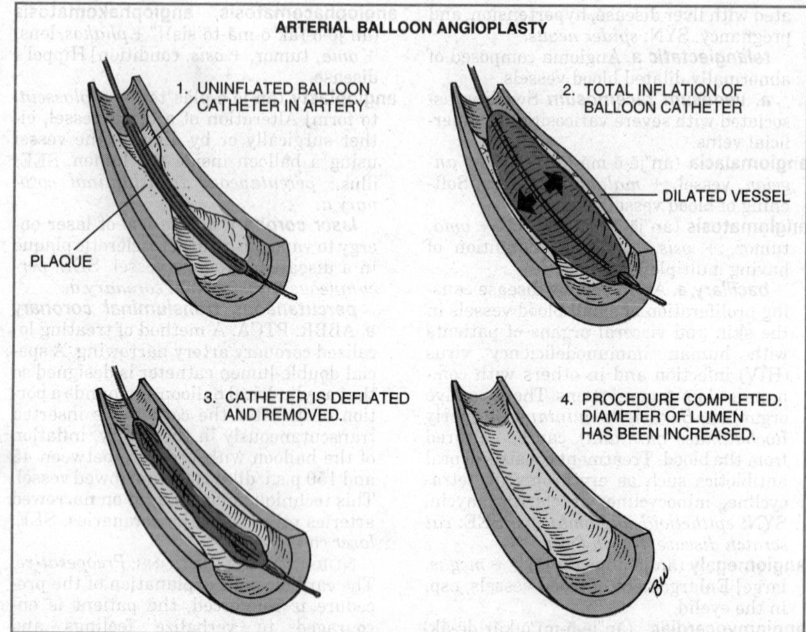


rhage is occurring. Discharge instructions are provided to the patient and family regarding scheduled return visit with cardiologist, follow-up exercise, thallium stress testing or angiography, and any exercise prescriptions or activity restrictions (usually patients can walk 24 hr after procedure and return to work in 2 weeks). The importance of continuing the drug regimen and the drug's desired effects and potential adverse reactions are reinforced.

***rescue a.*** The use of angioplasty to open coronary arteries that remain occluded after intravenous thrombolytic therapy for acute myocardial infarction.

**angiopoiesis** (ăn″jē-ō-poy-ē′sĭs) [″ + *poiein,* to make] The formation of blood vessels. **angiopoietic** (-poy-ĕt′ĭk), *adj.*

**angiopressure** (ăn′jē-ō-prĕsh″ŭr) Pressure applied to a blood vessel to arrest hemorrhage.

**angiorrhaphy** (ăn″jē-or′ă-fē) [″ + *rhaphe,* seam, ridge] Suture of a vessel, esp. a blood vessel.

**angiorrhexis** (ăn″jē-or-ĕk′sĭs) [″ + *rhexis,* rupture] Rupture of a vessel, esp. a blood vessel.

**angiosarcoma** (ăn″jē-ō-săr-kō′mă) [″ + *sarx,* flesh, + *oma,* tumor] Malignant neoplasm originating from blood vessels. SYN: *hemangiosarcoma.*

**angiosclerosis** (ăn″jē-ō-sklĕ-rō′sĭs) [″ + *sklerosis,* hardening] Hardening of the walls of the vascular system.

**angioscotoma** (ăn″jē-ō-skō-tō′mă) [″ + *skotoma,* darkness] The defect produced in the visual field by the shadows of the retinal blood vessels.

**angiosis** (ăn″jē-ō′sĭs) [Gr. *angeion,* vessel, + *osis,* condition] Any disease of blood vessels or lymph vessels. SYN: *angiopathy.*

**angiospasm** (ăn′jē-ō-spăzm) [″ + *spasmos,* a convulsion] Spasmodic contraction of blood vessels; may cause cramping of muscles or intermittent claudication. **angiospastic** (ăn″jē-ō-spăs′tĭk), *adj.*

**angiostenosis** (ăn″jē-ō-stĕ-nō′sĭs) [″ + *stenoein,* to make narrow, + *osis,* condition] Narrowing of a vessel, esp. a blood vessel.

**angiosteosis** (ăn″jē-ŏs″tē-ō′sĭs) [″ + *osteon,* bone, + *osis,* condition] Calcification of a vessel.

**angiostomy** (ăn″jē-ŏs′tō-mē) [″ + *stoma,* mouth] An operation that makes an artificial fistulous opening into a blood vessel.

**angiostrophy** (ăn″jē-ŏs′trō-fē) [″ + *strophe,* twist] The twisting of the cut end of a blood vessel to arrest bleeding.

**angiotelectasis** (ăn″jē-ō-tĕl-ĕk′tă-sĭs) [″ + *telos,* end, + *ektasis,* stretching out] Dilatation of terminal arterioles.

**angiotensin** (ăn″jē-ō-tĕn′sĭn) A vasopressor substance produced when renin is released from the kidney. Renin is formed by the juxtaglomerular apparatus of the kidney. SEE: *apparatus, juxtaglomerular.*

***a. I*** Physiologically inactive form of angiotensin; precursor of angiotensin II.

***a. II*** Physiologically active form of angiotensin; a powerful vasopressor and stimulator of aldosterone production and secretion.

***a. amide*** A vasoconstricting compound

of angiotensin.

**angiotensin-converting enzyme** ABBR: ACE. An enzyme essential for conversion of angiotensin I to angiotensin II.

**angiotensin-converting enzyme inhibitor** Any of the therapeutic agents that inhibit conversion of angiotensin I to angiotensin II. The result is vasodilation and increased renal blood flow. These agents are used in treating hypertension, heart failure, and myocardial infarction.

**angiotensinogen** (ăn″jē-ō-tĕn-sĭn′ō-jĕn) A serum globulin fraction formed in the liver; converted to angiotensin as a result of hydrolysis by renin.

**angiotitis** (ăn″jē-ō-tī′tĭs) [″ + *otos,* ear, + *itis,* inflammation] Inflammation of the blood vessels of the ear.

**angiotome** (ăn′jē-ō-tōm″) [Gr. *angeion,* vessel, + *tome,* incision] Any segment of the embryonic vascular system.

**angiotomy** (ăn″jē-ŏt″ō-mē) Sectioning of blood vessels.

**angiotonic** (ăn″jē-ō-tŏn′ĭk) [″ + *tonos,* tension] Increasing arterial tension.

**angiotribe** [″ + Gr. *tribein,* to crush] A forceps designed for application of a strong, crushing force to a tissue containing an artery. This is done to control hemorrhage.

**angiotrophic** (ăn″jē-ō-trŏf′ĭk) [″ + *trophe,* nourishment] Pert. to nutrition of blood vessels or lymph vessels.

**angle** (ăng′gl) [L. *angulus*] **1.** The figure or space outlined by the diverging of two lines from a common point or by the meeting of two planes. **2.** A projecting or sharp corner.

***acromial a.*** The angle formed by the junction of the lateral and posterior borders of the acromion.

***acute a.*** An angle less than 90°.

***alpha a.*** The angle formed by intersection of the visual line with the optic axis.

***alveolar a.*** The angle between the horizontal plane and a line drawn through the base of the nasal spine and the middle point of the alveolus of the upper jaw.

***biorbital a.*** The angle formed by the meeting of the axes of the orbits.

***cardiophrenic a.*** The medial, inferior corner of the pulmonary cavity bordered by the heart and diaphragm.

***carrying a.*** The angle made at the elbow by extending the long axis of the forearm and the upper arm. This obtuse angle is more pronounced in women than in men.

***caudal a.*** In radiology, angulation of the central ray toward the patient's feet.

***cavity a.*** The angle formed by two or more walls of a cavity preparation in restorative dentistry.

***cephalic a.*** In radiology, angulation of the central ray toward the patient's head.

***cephalometric a.*** The angle formed by intersecting anthropometric lines used in studies of the skull and for diagnosis of orthodontic problems.

***cerebellopontine a.*** The angle formed by the junction of the cerebellum and the pons. SYN: *pontine a.*

***costal a.*** The meeting point of the lower border of the false ribs with the axis of the sternum.

***costophrenic a.*** The lateral, inferior corner of the pulmonary cavity bordered by the ribs and diaphragm.

***costovertebral a.*** The angle formed on each side of the trunk by the junction of the last rib with the lumbar vertebrae.

***craniofacial a.*** The angle formed by the basifacial and basicranial axes at the midpoint of the sphenoethmoidal suture.

***facial a.*** The angle made by lines from the nasal spine and external auditory meatus meeting between the upper middle incisor teeth.

***flat a.*** The angle between two lines that join at an angle of almost 180°.

***gamma a.*** The angle between the line of vision and the optic axis.

***gonial a.*** A. of jaw.

***metafacial a.*** The angle between the base of the skull and the pterygoid process.

***obtuse a.*** An angle greater than 90°.

***occipital a.*** The angle formed at the opisthion by the intersection of lines from the basion and from the lower border of the orbit.

***a. of convergence*** The angle between the visual axis and the median line when an object is looked at.

***a. of incidence*** The angle between a ray striking a surface and a line drawn perpendicular to the surface at the point of incidence.

***a. of iris*** The angle between the cornea and iris at the periphery of the anterior chamber of the eye.

***a. of jaw*** The angle formed by the junction of the posterior edge of the ramus of the mandible and the lower surface of the body of the mandible. SYN: *gonial a.; a. of mandible.*

***a. of mandible*** A. of jaw.

***ophryospinal a.*** The angle formed at the anterior nasal spine by the intersection of lines drawn from the auricular point and the glabella.

***parietal a.*** The angle formed by the meeting of a line drawn tangent to the maximum curve of the zygomatic arch and a line drawn tangent to the end of the maximum frontal diameter of the skull. If these lines are parallel, the angle is zero; if they diverge, a negative angle is formed.

***pontine a.*** Cerebellopontine a.

***pubic a.*** The angle formed by the junction of the rami of the pubes.

***right a.*** An angle of 90°.

***sphenoid a.*** The angle formed at the top of the sella turcica by the intersection of lines drawn from the nasal point and the tip of the rostrum of the sphenoid.

***sternal a.*** The angle formed by the junction of the manubrium and the body of the sternum.

***a. of Treitz*** Sharp curve at the duodenojejunal junction.

***venous a.*** The angle formed by the junction of the internal jugular and subclavian veins.

***visual a.*** The angle formed by lines drawn from the nodal point of the eye to the edges of the object viewed.

**Angle's classification** SEE: *malocclusion.*

**angor** (ăng'gor) [L., strangling] Violent distress, as in angina pectoris.

**angor animi** (ăng'gor ăn'ĭ-mē) [" + L. *animus,* soul] The feeling that one is dying, as may occur in connection with angina pectoris.

**angstrom unit** (ŏng'strŭm) [Anders J. Ångström, Swedish physicist, 1814–1874] ABBR: A. SYMB: Å. U. An internationally adopted unit of length equal to $10^{-10}$ m, or 0.1 nm; used esp. to measure radiation wavelengths.

**angular** (ăng'gū-lăr) [L.] Having corners or angles.

**angular artery** The artery at the inner canthus of the eye; the facial artery.

**angulation** (ăng"ū-lā'shŭn) **1.** Abnormal formation of angles by tubular structures such as the intestines, blood vessels, or ureter. **2.** In radiology, the direction of the primary beam in relation to the film and the object being imaged.

**anhedonia** (ăn"hē-dō'nē-ă) [Gr. *an-,* not, + *hedone,* pleasure] Lack of pleasure in acts that are normally pleasurable. SEE: *hedonism.* **anhedonic** (-dŏn'ĭk), *adj.*

**anhidrosis** (ăn"hī-drō'sĭs) [" + *hidros,* sweat] Diminished or complete absence of secretion of sweat. It may be generalized or localized, temporary or permanent, disease related or congenital. SYN: *anidrosis.*

TREATMENT: Treatment consists of therapy for the cause or accompanying conditions. The patient should wear soft, nonirritating clothing and use bland, soothing skin ointments and lubricants. Air conditioning provides comfort in most instances.

**anhidrotic** (ăn"hī-drŏt'ĭk) **1.** Inhibiting or preventing perspiration. **2.** An agent that inhibits or prevents perspiration. SYN: *anidrotic; antihidrotic; antiperspirant; antisudorific.*

**anhydrase** (ăn"hī'drās) [" + *hydor,* water, + *-ase,* enzyme] An enzyme that promotes the removal of water from a chemical compound.

**anhydration** (ăn-hī'drā'shŭn) [" + *hydor,* water] Removal of water from a substance. SYN: *dehydration.*

**anhydride** (ăn-hī'drīd) [Gr. *an-,* not, + *hydor,* water] A compound formed by removal of water from a substance, esp. from an acid.

**anhydrochloric** (ăn-hī-drō-klō'rĭk) [" + " + *chloros,* green] Lacking hydrochloric acid.

**anhydrous** (ăn-hī'drŭs) [" + *hydor,* water] Lacking water.

**anianthinopsy** (ăn-ē-ăn'thĭn-ŏp"sē) [" + *ianthinos,* violet, + *opsis,* vision] Inability to recognize violet or purple.

**anicteric** (ăn"ĭk-tĕr'ĭk) [" + *ikteros,* jaundice] Without jaundice.

**anidrosis** (ăn-ĭ-drō'sĭs) Anhidrosis.

**anidrotic** (ăn-ĭ-drŏt'ĭk) Anhidrotic.

**aniline** (ăn'ĭ-lĭn) [Arabic *an-nil,* the indigo plant] $C_6H_7N$. The simplest aromatic amine, an oily liquid derived from benzene; used in the manufacture of medical and industrial dyes. Aniline has antipyretic action but is too toxic to use as a medicine. SYN: *aminobenzene; phenylamine.*

**aniline poisoning** SEE: *Poisons and Poisoning Appendix.*

**anilingus** [L. *anus* + *lingere,* to lick] Oral stimulation of the anus by use of the tongue or lips. SEE: *cunnilingus.*

**anilism** (ăn'ĭl-ĭzm) [Arabic *an-nil,* the indigo plant, + Gr. *-ismos,* condition] Chronic aniline poisoning. Symptoms include cardiac block, weakness, intermittent pulse, vertigo, muscular depression, and cyanosis. SEE: *aniline in Poisons and Poisoning Appendix.*

**anima** (ăn'ĭ-mă) [L., soul] **1.** Soul. **2.** According to Carl Jung, an individual's inner self as distinguished from the external personality (persona). **3.** Jung's term for the feminine inner personality present in men. SEE: *animus.*

**animal** (ăn'ĭ-măl) [L. *animalis,* living] **1.** A living organism that requires oxygen and organic foods, is incapable of photosynthesis, has limited growth, and is capable of voluntary movement and sensation. **2.** Any animal other than humans. **3.** Pert. to or from an animal. **4.** A person who is beastlike.

***cold-blooded a.*** An animal whose body temperature varies according to the temperature of the environment. SYN: *allotherm; poikilotherm.*

***control a.*** In medical research involving the use of animals, an animal that is not treated, but is housed and cared for under the same conditions as the treated animal(s). SEE: *control* (2).

***warm-blooded a.*** An animal whose body temperature remains constant regardless of the temperature of the environment. SYN: *homotherm.*

**animation** (ăn-ĭ-mā'shŭn) [L. *animus,* soul] State of being alive or active.

***suspended a.*** Temporary cessation of vital functions with loss of consciousness; state of apparent death.

**animatism** (ăn'ĭ-mă-tĭzm) The belief that everything in nature, animate and inanimate, contains a spirit or soul.

**animi agitatio** (ăn'ĭ-mē ă-jĭ-tā'shē-ō) [" + *agitare,* to turn over] Mental agitation.

**animism** (ăn'ĭ-mĭzm) Attribution of spiritual qualities and mental capabilities to inanimate objects.

**animus** [L., breath, mind, soul] **1.** An animating or energizing motive or intention. **2.** A feeling of bitter hostility; a grudge.

3. According to Carl Jung, the masculine inner personality present in women. SEE: *anima*.

**anion** (ăn′ī-ŏn) [Gr. *ana*, up, + *ion*, going] An ion carrying a negative charge; the opposite of cation. An anion is attracted by, and travels to, the anode (positive pole). Examples are acid radicals and corresponding radicals of their salts. SEE: *electrolyte; ion*. **anionic** (ăn″ī-ŏn′ĭk), *adj*.

**anion channel** Channels in red blood cells that cross the cell membrane. Chloride ions ($Cl^-$) and bicarbonate ions ($HCO_3^-$) are exchanged via these channels.

**anion exchange** SEE: *resin, ion-exchange*.

**anion gap** The difference between the measured cations sodium ($Na^+$) and potassium ($K^+$) and the measured anions chloride ($Cl^-$) and bicarbonate ($HCO_3^-$). In accordance with the principle of electroneutrality, in any body fluid the number of net positive charges contributed by cations must equal the number of net negative charges contributed by anions. The result of an imbalance in the 1 : 1 ratio of cations to anions is known as an anion gap. The difference will be the unmeasured anions that are present; these include sulfates, phosphates, proteins, ketones, and other organic acids. In general, an anion gap of 8 to 18 mmol/L is considered normal. A value greater than 25 mmol/L strongly suggests metabolic acidosis.

**anionic detergent** A natural or synthetic chemical substance with disinfectant properties due to the presence of an active, negatively charged chemical group.

**aniridia** (ăn″ī-rĭd′ē-ă) [Gr. *an-*, not, + *iris*, rainbow, iris] Congenital absence of all or part of the iris. SYN: *irideremia*.

**anisakiasis** (ăn″ĭs-să-kī′ă-sĭs) Disease of the gastrointestinal tract accompanied by intestinal colic, fever, and abscesses; caused by eating uncooked fish containing larval nematodes of the family Anisakidae.

**aniseikonia** (ăn-ĭs-ī-kō′nē-ă) [Gr. *anisos*, unequal, + *eikon*, image] A condition in which the size and shape of the ocular image of one eye differ from those of the other. SYN: *anisoiconia*.

**anismus** Excessive contraction of the external sphincter of the rectum.

**aniso-** (ăn-ī′sō) [Gr. *anisos*, unequal] Combining form meaning *unequal, asymmetrical*, or *dissimilar*.

**anisoaccommodation** (ăn-ī″sō-ă-kŏm″mō-dā′shŭn) [″ + L. *accommodare*, to suit] Difference in the ability of the eyes to accommodate. SEE: *accommodation*.

**anisochromatic** (ăn-ī″sō-krō-măt′ĭk) [″ + *chroma*, color] Not of uniform color.

**anisocoria** (ăn-ī″sō-kō′rē-ă) [″ + *kore*, pupil] Inequality of the size of the pupils; may be congenital or associated with aneurysms, head trauma, diseases of the nervous system, brain lesion, paresis, or locomotor ataxia.

**anisocytosis** (ăn-ī″sō-sī-tō′sĭs) [″ + *kytos*, cell, + *osis*, condition] Condition in which there is excessive inequality in the size of cells, esp. erythrocytes. SEE: illus.

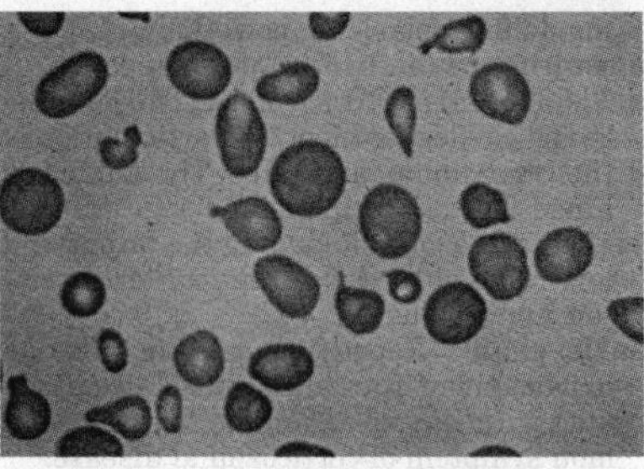

ANISOCYTOSIS IN SEVERE PERNICIOUS ANEMIA

**anisogamy** (ăn″ī-sŏg′ă-mē) [″ + *gamos*, marriage] Sexual fusion of two gametes of different form and size.

**anisognathous** (ăn″ī-sŏg′nă-thŭs) [″ + *gnathos*, jaw] Having an upper jaw wider than the lower one.

**anisoiconia** (ăn-ī″sō-ī-kō′nē-ă) [″ + *eikon*, image] Aniseikonia.

**anisokaryosis** (ăn-ī″sō-kăr″ē-ō′sĭs) [″ + *karyon*, nucleus, + *osis*, condition] Unequal size of the cell nuclei.

**anisomastia** (ăn-ī-sō-măs′tē-ă) [″ + *mastos*, breast] Condition in which the breasts are markedly unequal in size.

**anisomelia** (ăn-ī″sō-mē′lē-ă) [″ + *melos*, limb] Condition in which paired limbs are noticeably unequal.

**anisometrope** (ăn-ī″sō-mĕt′rōp) [Gr. *anisos*, unequal, + *metron*, measure, + *ops*, vision] One afflicted with anisometropia.

**anisometropia** (ăn-ī″sō-mĕ-trō′pē-ă) Condition in which the refractive power of the eyes is unequal. **anisometropic** (-trŏp′ĭk), *adj*.

**anisonormocytosis** (ăn-ī″sō-nor″mō-sī-tō′sĭs) [″ + L. *norma*, rule, + Gr. *kytos*, cell, + *osis*, condition] Condition in which the total number of leukocytes is normal but the proportion of different types is abnormal.

**anisophoria** (ăn″ī-sō-fō′rē-ă) [″ + *phoros*, bearing] Eye muscle imbalance so that the horizontal visual plane of one eye is different from that of the other.

**anisopia** (ăn″ī-sō′pē-ă) [″ + *ops*, vision] Condition in which the visual power of the eyes is unequal.

**anisosthenic** (ăn-ī″sŏs-thĕn′ĭk) [″ + *sthenos*, strength] Of unequal strength; used of paired muscles.

**anisotonic** (ăn-ī″sō-tŏn′ĭk) [″ + *tonos*, act of stretching, tension] Pert. to a solution not isotonic as compared with another.

**anisotropal** (ăn″ī-sŏt′rō-păl) [″ + *tropos*, a turning] **1.** Not equal in every direction. **2.** Unequal in power of refraction. SYN: *anisotropous*.

**anisotropic** (ăn-ī″sō-trŏp′ĭk) **1.** Having different optical properties in different directions, as with certain crystals. **2.** Having double polarizing power.

**anisotropous** (ăn-ī-sŏt′rō-pŭs) Anisotropal.

**ankle** (ăng′kl) [AS. *ancleow*] **1.** The joint between the leg and foot; the articulation of the tibia, fibula, and talus. The ankle is a hinge joint. **2.** In popular usage, the region of this joint, including the tarsus and lower end of the leg. SEE: *foot* for illus.

**ankle bone** Talus.

**ankle clonus** Repetitive extension-flexion movement of the ankle muscles, associated with increased muscle tonus; a common symptom of corticospinal disease.

NURSING IMPLICATIONS: The patient's foot is maintained at a right angle to the horizontal plane of the body, usually with a foot splint. When the splint is removed, dorsiflexion of the foot should be avoided to prevent ankle movement, clonus, or spasm. The nurse demonstrates and teaches correct movement of the involved joint, which should be slow and even, with the extremity supported on the palms rather than grasped; exercise should be performed when the joint is warm and relaxed.

***a.c. reflex*** A reflex elicited by quick, vigorous dorsiflexion of the foot while the knee is held in a flexed position, resulting in repeated clonic movement of the foot as long as it is maintained in dorsiflexion. In women with pregnancy-induced hypertension, this reflects hyperirritability of the central nervous system and increased risk for eclamptic convulsions.

**ankle-foot orthosis** ABBR: AFO. Any of a class of splints for the foot, commonly made of lightweight thermoplastic splinting material, which are fitted to provide stability and prevent deformities.

**ankle jerk** Extension of the foot produced by contraction of the calf muscles after a brisk tap to the Achilles tendon.

**ankle joint** Ankle.

**ankylo-, ankyl-** (ăng′kĭ-lō) [Gr. *ankylos,* crooked] Combining form meaning *crooked, bent,* or *a fusion or growing together of parts.*

**ankyloblepharon** (ăng″kĭ-lō-blĕf′ăr-ŏn) [″ + *blepharon,* eyelid] Blepharosynechia.

**ankylochilia** (ăng″kĭ-lō-kī′lē-a) [″ + *cheilos,* lip] Adhesion of the upper and lower lips.

**ankylodactylia** (ăng-kĭ-lō-dăk-tĭl′ē-a) [″ + *daktylos,* finger] Adhesion of two or more fingers or toes.

**ankyloglossia** (ăng″kĭ-lō-glŏs′sē-ă) [″ + *glossa,* tongue] Abnormal shortness of the frenulum of the tongue. SYN: *lingua frenata; tongue-tie.*

**ankylopoietic** (ăng″kĭ-lō-poy-ĕt′ĭk) [Gr. *ankyle,* stiff joint, + *poiein,* to form] **1.** Indicating the presence of ankylosis. **2.** Causing ankylosis.

**ankyloproctia** (ăng″kĭ-lō-prŏk′shē-ă) [Gr. *ankylos,* crooked, + *proktos,* anus] Stricture or imperforation of the anus.

**ankylosed 1.** Fixed; stiffened; held by adhesions. **2.** Affected with ankylosis.

**ankylosis** (ăng″kĭ-lō′sĭs) [Gr. *ankyle,* stiff joint, + *osis,* condition] Immobility of a joint. The condition may be congenital (sometimes hereditary), or it may be the result of disease, trauma, surgery, or contractures resulting from immobility.

NURSING IMPLICATIONS: Immobility-induced contractures that can result in ankylosis are prevented by putting joints through their normal range of motion passively whenever they cannot be exercised actively. If a nonsurgical ankylosis is present, the joint is maintained in a functional position, splints are used for patients with spastic muscles, passive range-of-motion exercises to affected joints are initiated, and physical therapy or orthopedic intervention may be appropriate. If an ankylosis is surgically created, the joint is immobilized until the bone has healed (usually in 6 to 12 weeks), and correct body alignment is maintained.

***artificial a.*** The surgical fixation of a joint.

***bony a.*** The abnormal union of the bones of a joint. SYN: *True a.*

***dental a.*** A condition marked by the loss of tooth movement due to the fusion of the root cementum with the adjacent alveolar bone.

***extracapsular a.*** Ankylosis caused by rigidity of parts outside a joint.

***false a.*** Fibrous a.

***fibrous a.*** Ankylosis due to the formation of fibrous bands within a joint. SYN: *false a; ligamentous a.*

***intracapsular a.*** Ankylosis due to undue rigidity of structures within a joint.

***ligamentous a.*** Fibrous a.

***true a.*** Bony a.

**Ankylostoma** (ăng″kĭ-lŏs′tō-mă) Ancylostoma.

**ankylostomiasis** (ăng″kĭ-lō-stō-mī′ă-sĭs) Ancylostomiasis.

**ankylotia** (ăng″kĭ-lō′shē-ă) [Gr. *ankylos,* crooked, + *ot-,* ear] Stricture or imperforation of the external auditory meatus of the ear.

**ankylotome** (ăng′kĭl-ō-tōm, ăng-kĭl′ō-tōm) [″ + *tome,* incision] An instrument for cutting the frenulum of the tongue in tongue-tie.

**ankylurethria** (ăng″kĭl-ū-rē′thrē-ă) [″ + *ourethra,* urethra] Stricture or imperforation of the urethra.

**anlage** (ŏn′lŏ-jhă) [Ger., a laying on] The first accumulation of cells in an embryo; the beginning of an organized tissue, organ, or part. SYN: *primordium.*

**A.N.N.A.** *American Nephrology Nurses' Association.*

**anneal** (an-nēl′) [AS. *anaelan,* to burn] To soften a material, such as glass, metal, or wax, by heating and cooling to remove internal stresses and to make it more easily adapted or swaged, as in preparation of materials for restorative dentistry.

**annectant, annectent** (ă-nĕk′tĕnt) [L. *annectens,* tying or binding to] Linking; connecting.

**Annelida** (ă-nĕl′ĭ-dă) The phylum that includes earthworms, leeches, and other segmented worms. Some annelids serve as intermediate hosts for parasitic worms.

**annexa** (ă-nĕks′ă) [L. *annectere,* to tie or bind to] Accessory parts of a structure. SYN: *adnexa.*

**annexitis** (ă-nĕks-ī′tĭs) [″ + Gr. *itis,* inflammation] Inflammation of the adnexa uteri. SYN: *adnexitis.*

**annular** (ăn′ū-lăr) [L. *annulus,* ring] Circular; ring-shaped (e.g., annular ligament of the elbow).

**annulorrhaphy** (ăn″ū-lor′ă-fē) [″ + Gr. *rhaphe,* seam, ridge] Closure of a hernial ring by suture.

**annulus** (ăn′ū-lŭs) *pl.* **annuli** [L.] A ring-shaped structure; a ring. Also spelled *anulus.*

**anococcygeal** (ā″nō-kŏk-sĭ′jē-al) [L. *anus,* anus, + Gr. *kokkyx,* coccyx] Rel. to both the anus and coccyx.

**anococcygeal body** The muscle and fibrous tissue lying between the coccyx and the anus.

**anococcygeal ligament** A band of fibrous tissue joining the tip of the coccyx with the external sphincter ani.

**anodal closure contraction** ABBR: ACC. Contraction of the muscles at the anode on closure of the circuit.

**anodal opening contraction** Contraction of the muscles at the anode when the electrical circuit is open.

**anode** (ăn′ōd) [Gr. *ana,* up, + *hodos,* way] The positive pole of an electrical source. In radiography, the target of the x-ray tube. SEE: *cathode.* **anodal** (ăn-ō′dăl), *adj.*

**anodmia** (ăn-ŏd′mē-ă) [Gr. *an-,* not, + *odme,* stench] Anosmia.

**anodontia** (ăn″ō-dŏn′shē-ă) [″ + *odous,* tooth] Absence of teeth. SYN: *edentia.*

**anodyne** (ăn′ō-dīn) [″ + *odyne,* pain] A drug that relieves pain. SYN: *analgesic.*

**anodynia** (ăn″ō-dĭn′ē-ă) Cessation or absence of pain.

**anogenital** Concerning the anal and genital areas.

**anomaloscope** (ă-nŏm′ă-lō-skōp″) [Gr. *anomalos,* irregular, + *skopein,* to examine] A device for detecting color blindness.

**anomalous** (ă-nŏm′ă-lŭs) [Gr. *anomalos,* uneven] Irregular; deviating from or contrary to normal.

**anomaly** (ă-nŏm′ă-lē) [Gr. *anomalia,* irregularity] Deviation from normal.

***congenital a.*** Intrauterine development of an organ or structure that is abnormal in form, structure, or position. SYN: *birth defect.*

**anomia** (ă-nō′mē-ă) [Gr. *a-,* not, + *onoma,* name] Inability to remember names of objects.

**anomie** (ăn′ŏ-mē) [Fr. from Gr. *anomia,* lawlessness] A term coined by the French sociologist Emile Durkheim (1858–1917) to indicate a condition similar to alienation. The individual feels there has been a disintegration of his or her norms and values. Durkheim felt such individuals were prone to take their lives because of the anxiety, isolation, and alienation that they experience.

**anonychia** (ăn-ō-nĭk′ē-ă) [Gr. *an-,* not, + *onyx,* nail] Absence of the nails.

**anoperineal** (ā″nō-pĕr-ĭ-nē′ăl) Rel. to both the anus and perineum.

**Anopheles** (ă-nŏf′ĕ-lēz) [Gr. *anopheles,* harmful, useless] A genus of mosquitoes belonging to the family Culicidae, order Diptera. It is a vector of *Plasmodium,* the causative agent of malaria, and may be involved in transmitting the causative agent of dengue, filariasis, and possibly other diseases. Of the almost 100 species of Anopheles, only a few are capable of transmitting the causative organism of malaria. SEE: *malaria.*

**anophoria** Hyperphoria.

**anophthalmia** (ăn-ŏf-thăl′mē-ă) [Gr. *an-,* not, + *ophthalmos,* eye] Congenital absence of one or both eyes. SYN: *anopia* (1).

**anopia** (an-ō′pē-ă) [″ + *ops,* eye] **1.** Anophthalmia. **2.** Anophoria.

**anoplasty** (ā′nō-plăs″tē) [L. *anus,* anus, + Gr. *plassein,* to form] Plastic surgery of the anus.

**Anoplura** (an-ō-ploo′ră) [Gr. *anoplos,* unarmed, + *oura,* tail] An order of insects composed of the sucking lice. SEE: *louse; pediculosis.*

**anopsia** (ăn-ŏp′sē-ă) [Gr. *an-,* not, + *opsis,* sight] **1.** Hyperphoria. **2.** Inability to use the vision, as occurs in strabismus, cataract, or refractive errors or in those confined in the dark.

**anorchia** Anorchism.

**anorchidism, anorchism** (ăn-or′kĭ-dĭzm″, ăn-or′kĭzm) [″ + *orchis,* testicle, + *-ismos,* condition] Congenital absence of one or both testes. SYN: *anorchia.*

**anorectal** (ā-nō-rĕk′tăl) Pert. to both the anus and rectum.

**anorectic, anorectous** (ăn-ō-rĕk′tĭc, -tŭs) [Gr. *anorektos,* without appetite for] Having no appetite.

**anorexia** (ăn-ō-rĕk′sē-ă) [Gr. *an-,* not, + *orexis,* appetite] Loss of appetite. Anorexia is seen in depression, malaise, commencement of fevers and illnesses, disorders of the alimentary tract (esp. the stomach), and alcoholism and drug addiction (esp. cocaine). Many medicines and medical procedures have the undesired side effect of causing malaise with concurrent anorexia.

NURSING IMPLICATIONS: Oral hygiene is provided before and after eating. The patient's food preferences are determined, and only preferred foods are offered. Small, frequent meals or smaller meals with between-meal and bedtime nutritional snacks are provided. The patient area is kept free of odors, and a quiet atmosphere is provided for meals. Family and friends are encouraged to bring favorite home-cooked meals and to join the patient for meals. Mealtime conversation should converge on pleasant topics and should not address the patient's food intake. Actual intake is documented, indicating food types, amounts eaten, and approximate caloric and nutrient intake.

***a. nervosa*** An eating disorder marked by excessive fasting; occurs most commonly in females between the ages of 12 and 21 but may occur in older women and men.

Diagnosis is made by the following criteria: Intense fear of becoming obese. This does not diminish as weight loss progresses. The patient claims to feel fat even when emaciated. A loss of 25% of original weight may occur. No known physical illness accounts for the weight loss. There is a refusal to maintain body weight over a minimal normal weight for age and height.

Psychiatric therapy in a hospital is usually required if the patient refuses to eat. The patient may need to be fed parenterally. SEE: *bulimia; Nursing Diagnoses Appendix.*

NURSING IMPLICATIONS: The nurse monitors the patient's vital signs and electrolyte balance; daily fluid intake and output; food types, amounts, and approximate nutrient intake; and laboratory values. The patient is weighed daily or weekly weights as prescribed. As necessary, the patient's body orifices, underarm area, and hair are checked for hidden weight before weighing. Small, frequent meals and nutritionally complete fluids are provided; the latter may be accepted more readily. If tube feeding or parenteral nutrition is required, the procedure is explained to the patient and family. Edema or bloating, if present, is also explained, and the nurse reassures the patient of its temporary nature. The patient's activities are strictly monitored as a precaution against vomiting, catharsis, or excessive exercise. The nurse explains that improved nutrition can correct abnormal laboratory findings, and avoids arguments about food or related subjects. The patient is encouraged to recognize and express feelings; assertive behavior is supported. Assistance is offered to the family and close friends in dealing with their feelings about the patient and the patient's behavior, and they are instructed not to discuss food or weight with the patient. The patient and family are encouraged to seek professional counseling, and are referred to local and national support and information organizations. Stable weight and eating patterns, the ability to express feelings, and the establishment of healthier patient-family relationships are good indicators of successful intervention.

**anorexigenic** (ăn″ō-rĕk″sĭ-jĕn′ĭk) [″ + ″ + *gennan,* to produce] Causing loss of appetite.

**anorgasmic** One who does not or cannot experience orgasm.

**anorgasmy** (ăn-or-găz′mē) [″ + *orgasmos,* swelling] Failure to reach orgasm during sexual intercourse or masturbation.

**anorthopia** (ăn″or-thō′pē-ă) [″ + ″ + *ops,* eye] **1.** Vision in which straight lines do not appear straight; symmetry and parallelism not properly perceived. **2.** Strabismus.

**anoscope** (ā′nō-skōp) [L. *anus,* anus, + Gr. *skopein,* to examine] Speculum for examining the anus and lower rectum.

**anosigmoidoscopy** (ā″nō-sĭg″moy-dŏs′kō-pē) [″ + Gr. *sigmoeides,* shaped like Greek S, + *skopein,* to examine] Direct visual examination of the anus, rectum, and colon by use of an endoscope.

**anosmatic** (ăn-ŏz-măt′ĭk) [Gr. *an-,* not, + *osme,* smell] Lacking the sense of smell.

**anosmia** (ăn-ŏz′mē-ă) Loss of the sense of smell. SYN: *anodmia.*

**anosmic, anosmous** (ăn-ŏz′mĭk, -mŭs) **1.** Lacking the sense of smell. **2.** Odorless.

**anosognosia** (ăn-ō-sŏg-nō′zē-ă) [″ + ″ + *gnosis,* knowledge] The apparent denial or unawareness of one's own neurological defect.

***visual a.*** A neurological syndrome in which patients who cannot see deny that they are blind. An excuse such as "I lost my glasses" may be offered. The lesion is in the visual association areas of the cortex of the brain. SYN: *Anton's syndrome.*

**anosphrasia** (ăn-ŏs-frā′zē-ă) [Gr. *an-,* not, + *osphresis,* smell] Absence of or imperfect sense of smell.

**anospinal** (ā″nō-spī′năl) [L. *anus* + *spina,* thorn] Pert. to the anus and spinal cord or to the center in the spinal cord that controls the contraction of the anal sphincter.

**anostosis** (ăn-ŏs-tō′sĭs) [Gr. *an-,* not, + *osteon,* bone, + *osis,* condition] A defective formation or development of bone; failure to ossify.

**anotia** (ăn-ō′shē-ă) [″ + *ours,* ear] Congenital malformation with absence of the ears.

**anotropia** (ăn″ō-trō′pē-ă) [Gr. *ana,* up, + *trope,* a turning] Tendency of the eyes to turn upward and away from the visual axis.

**ANOVA** Term used in statistics for *an*alysis *o*f *va*riance. SEE: *analysis of variance.*

**anovaginal** (ā″nō-văj′ĭ-năl) Pert. to the anus and vagina.

**anovarism** (ăn-ō′văr-ĭzm) [Gr. *an-,* not, + LL. *ovarium,* ovary, + Gr. *-ismos,* condition] Absence of ovaries.

**anovesical** (ā″nō-vĕs′ĭ-kl) [L. *anus,* anus, + *vesica,* bladder] Rel. to both the anus and urinary bladder.

**anovular, anovulatory** (ăn-ŏv′ū-lăr, ăn-ŏv′ū-lă-tō″rē) [Gr. *an-,* not, + LL. *ovarium,* ovary] Not accompanied by production of and discharge of an ovum.

**anovular cycle** Menstrual cycle in which ovulation is absent.

**anoxemia** (ăn-ŏk-sē′mē-ă) [″ + *oxygen* + Gr.

*haima,* blood] Insufficient oxygenation of the blood. SEE: *hypoxemia; respiration.*

**anoxia** (ăn-ŏk′sē-ă) [″ + *oxygen*] Absence of oxygen. This term is often used incorrectly to indicate hypoxia. **anoxic** (ăn-ŏks′ĭk), *adj.*

**ANP** *advanced nurse practitioner.*

**ANS** *autonomic nervous system.*

**ansa** (ăn′să) *pl.* **ansae** [L., a handle] In anatomy, any structure in the form of a loop or arc.

***a. cervicalis*** A nerve loop in the neck formed by fibers from the first three cervical nerves. Formerly called *ansa hypoglossi.*

***a. hypoglossi*** A. cervicalis.

***a. lenticularis*** Tortuous fiber tract from the globus pallidus, extending around the internal capsule, to the ventral thalamic nucleus.

***a. nervorum spinalium*** Connecting loops of nerve fibers between the anterior spinal nerves.

***a. peduncularis*** Complex fiber tract from the anterior temporal lobe, extending around the internal capsule to the mediodorsal thalamic nucleus.

***a. sacralis*** Nerve loop connecting the sympathetic trunk with the coccygeal ganglion.

***a. subclavia*** Nerve loop that passes anterior and inferior to the subclavian artery, connecting the middle and inferior cervical sympathetic ganglia.

**anserine bursitis** SEE: *bursitis, anserine.*

**ANSER system** A group of questionnaires for evaluating developmental dysfunction in children.

**A.N.S.I.** *American National Standards Institute.*

**ansiform** (ăn′sĭ-form) [L. *ansa,* a handle, + *forma,* shape] Shaped like a loop.

**ant-** SEE: *anti-.*

**ant** Small social insect of the order Hymenoptera and family Formicidae, distributed worldwide. Ants live in highly organized colonies whose members specialize in performing specific tasks. Because some ants secrete formic acid their bite can be painful.

**Antabuse** (ăn′tă-būs″) Proprietary name for disulfiram; administered orally in treatment of alcoholism. Drinking alcohol after taking this drug causes severe reactions, including nausea and vomiting, and may endanger the life of the patient. SEE: *Poisons and Poisoning Appendix.*

**antacid** (ănt-ăs′ĭd) [Gr. *anti,* against, + L. *acidum,* acid] An agent that neutralizes acidity, esp. in the stomach and duodenum. Examples are aluminum hydroxide and magnesium oxide.

**antagonism** (ăn-tăg′ō-nĭzm″) [Gr. *antagonizesthai,* to struggle against] Mutual opposition or contrary action, as between muscles or medicines.

***microbial a.*** The inhibition of one bacterial organism by another. This is a function of the normal bacterial flora and is one of the most important host defenses against microbial pathogens. SEE: *opportunistic infections.*

**antagonist** (ăn-tăg′ō-nĭst) That which counteracts the action of something else, such as a muscle or drug; opposite of synergist.

***dental a.*** The tooth in the opposite arch with which a tooth occludes in function.

***drug a.*** A drug that prevents receptor stimulation. An antagonist drug has an affinity for a cell receptor and, by binding to it, the cell is prevented from responding.

***muscular a.*** A muscle that opposes the action of the prime mover and produces a smooth movement by balancing the opposite forces.

***narcotic a.*** A drug that prevents or reverses the action of a narcotic. SEE: *nalorphine hydrochloride.*

**antalkaline** (ănt-ăl′kă-līn, -lĭn) [″ + *alkaline*] An agent that neutralizes alkalinity.

**antaphrodisiac** (ănt″ăf-rō-dĭz′ē-ăk) [″ + *aphrodisiakos,* sexual] An agent that depresses sexual desire. SYN: *anaphrodisiac.*

**antasthenic** (ănt″ăs-thĕn′ĭk) [″ + *astheneia,* weakness] **1.** Relieving weakness; strengthening, invigorating. **2.** An agent that relieves weakness or strengthens.

**antasthmatic** (ănt″ăz-măt′ĭk) [″ + Gr. *asthma,* panting] **1.** Preventing or relieving asthma. **2.** An agent that prevents or relieves an asthma attack.

**antatrophic** (ănt″ă-trō′fĭk) [″ + *atrophia,* atrophy] Preventing or curing atrophy.

**antazoline phosphate** (ăn-tăz′ō-lēn) An antihistamine used in dilute solution to treat allergic conjunctivitis. A component of the trade name preparation Vasocon-A.

**ante-** [L.] Prefix meaning *before.*

**antebrachium** (ăn″tē-brā′kē-ŭm) [L. *ante,* before, + *brachium,* arm] The forearm. **antebrachial** (-ăl), *adj.*

**antecardium** (ăn″tē-kăr′dē-ŭm) [″ + Gr. *kardia,* heart] The area on the anterior surface of the body overlying the heart and the lower part of the thorax; also spelled *anticardium.* SYN: *precordia; precordium.*

**antecedent** (ăn″tē-sē′dĕnt) [L. *antecedere,* to precede] Something that comes before something else; a precursor.

***plasma thromboplastin a.*** ABBR: PTA. Blood coagulation factor XI. SYN: *Christmas factor.* SEE: *coagulation factors.*

**ante cibum** (ăn′tē sē′bŭm) [L.] ABBR: a.c. Used in prescription writing to indicate *before meals.*

**antecubital** (ăn″tē-kū′bĭ-tăl) [″ + *cubitum,* elbow] In front of the elbow; at the bend of the elbow.

**antecubital fossa** Triangular area lying anterior to and below the elbow, bounded medially by the pronator teres and laterally by the brachioradialis muscles. SYN: *cubital fossa.*

**antecurvature** (ăn″tē-kŭr′vă-tūr″) [″ + *curvatura,* bend] Bending forward abnormally. SYN: *anteflexion.*

**antefebrile** (an″tē-fē′brĭl, -fē′brīl, -fĕb′rĭl) [L. *ante,* before, + *febris,* fever] Before the development of fever. SYN: *antepyretic.*

**anteflect** (ăn′tē-flĕkt) [″ + *flectere,* to bend] To bend or cause to bend forward.

**anteflexion** (ăn″tē-flĕk′shŭn) The abnormal bending forward of part of an organ, esp. of the uterus at its body and neck. SEE: *anteversion.*

**antegrade** (ăn′tē-grād) Moving forward or in the same direction as the flow.

**antelocation** (ăn″tē-lō-kā′shŭn) [″ + *locare,* to place] Forward displacement of an organ.

**antemortem** (ăn′tē-mor′tĕm) [L.] Before death.

**antemortem statement** Declaration made by an individual immediately preceding death. SYN: *deathbed statement.*

**antenatal** (ăn″tē-nā′tăl) [″ + *natus,* born] Before birth. SYN: *prenatal.*

**antenatal diagnosis** Prenatal diagnosis.

**antenatal surgery** Surgical procedure done on the fetus prior to delivery. This type of surgery is done only at certain medical centers. SEE: *amnioscopy; embryoscopy.*

**antepartal, ante partum** (ăn″tē-păr′tăl, -tŭm) [L.] Before the onset of labor, used with reference to the mother.

**antepyretic** (ăn″tē-pī-rĕt′ik) [L. *ante,* before, + Gr. *pyretos,* fever] Before the development of fever. SYN: *antefebrile.*

**anterior** [L.] Before or in front of; in anatomical nomenclature, refers to the ventral or abdominal side of the body.

**anterior chamber** The front of the aqueous cavity of the eye, between the cornea and the iris. SEE: *eye.*

**anterior drawer test, anterior drawer sign**

KNEE: A test for anterior cruciate ligament rupture. It is positive if anterior glide of the tibia is increased.

ANKLE: A test for stability of the anterior talofibular ligament of the ankle. It is positive if movement is increased as the examiner grasps the heel with one hand and the distal tibia with the other and draws the heel forward.

**anterior horn cell** A somatic motor neuron with its cell body in the ventral (anterior) horn of the gray matter of the spinal cord, and an axon that innervates skeletal muscle.

**antero-** [L.] Prefix denoting *anterior, front, before.*

**anteroexternal** (ăn″tĕr-ō-ĕks-tĕr′năl) [L. *antero,* anterior, + *externus,* outside] In anatomy, located to the front and laterally.

**anterograde** [″ + *gradior,* to step] Moving frontward.

**anteroinferior** [″ + *inferior,* below] In front and below.

**anterointernal** (ăn″tĕr-ō-ĭn-tĕr′năl) [″ + *internus,* within] In anatomy, located to the front and to the inner side.

**anterolateral** [″ + *latus,* side] In front and to one side.

**anteromedial** [″ + *medius,* middle] In front and toward the center.

**anteroposterior** [″ + *posterior,* rear] Passing from front to rear.

**anterosuperior** [″ + *superior,* above] In front and above.

**anteversion** (ăn″tē-vĕr′zhŭn) [″ + *vertere,* to turn] **1.** A tipping forward of an organ as a whole, without bending. SEE: *anteflexion.* **2.** Excessive anterior angulation of the neck of the femur (i.e., femoral neck anteversion), leading to excessive internal rotation of the femur. The normal value for femoral neck anteversion is approx. 15°. Any increase in this anterior angulation is called femoral anteversion.

**anteverted** (ăn″tē-vĕrt′ĕd) Tipped forward.

**anthelix** (ănt′hē-lĭks, ăn′thē-lĭks) [Gr. *anti,* against, + *helix,* coil] Antihelix.

**anthelmintic, anthelminthic** (ănt″hĕl-mĭn′tĭk, -thĭk) [″ + *helmins,* worm] An agent that destroys parasitic intestinal worms. SYN: *helminthagogue; vermicide.*

**Anthemis** (ăn′thĕm-ĭs) **1.** A genus of aromatic flowering plants. **2.** Chamomile; dried blossoms of *Anthemis nobilis;* a bitter tonic and antispasmodic.

**anthemorrhagic** (ănt″hĕm-ō-răj′ĭk) [″ + *haima,* blood, + *rhegnynai,* to burst forth] Antihemorrhagic.

**anthocyanin** (ăn″thō-sī′ă-nĭn) [Gr. *anthos,* flower, + *kyanos,* a blue substance] Any one of a group of reddish-purple pigments occurring in flowers.

**Anthomyia** (ăn″thō-mī′yă) [″ + *myia,* fly] A genus of fly of the order Diptera, related to the housefly. Larvae sometimes infest humans.

***A. canicularis*** A small black housefly, whose larvae may infest the human intestine after accidental ingestion, often resulting in gastrointestinal disturbances.

**anthophobia** (ăn″thō-fō′bē-ă) [″ + *phobos,* fear] Morbid dislike or fear of flowers.

**anthracene** (ăn′thră-sēn) $C_{14}H_{10}$. A hydrocarbon obtained from distilling coal tar; used in manufacturing dyes.

**anthracoid** (an′thră-koyd) [″+ *eidos,* form, shape] Resembling or pert. to anthrax.

**anthracosilicosis** (ăn″thră-kō-sĭl″ĭ-kō′sĭs) [″ + L. *silex,* flint, + Gr. *osis,* condition] A form of pneumoconiosis in which carbon and silica deposits accumulate in the lungs due to coal dust inhalation. SYN: *coal worker's pneumoconiosis.* SEE: *anthracosis; silicosis.*

**anthracosis** (ăn-thră-kō′sĭs) [″ + *osis,* condition] Accumulation of carbon deposits in the lungs due to inhalation of smoke or coal dust. SYN: *black lung.*

**anthralin** (ăn′thră-lĭn) A synthetic hydrocarbon used in ointment form for treating various skin diseases, including fungal infections and eczema. Trade names are Anthra-Derm and DrithoCreme HP.

**anthrax** (ăn′thrăks) [Gr., coal, carbuncle] Acute, infectious disease caused by *Bacillus anthracis,* usually attacking cattle, sheep, horses, and goats. Humans contract it from contact with animal hair, hides, or waste. Workers who handle wools and hides, and manufacture brushes are commonly affected. Immunization with a cell-free vaccine is recommended for persons handling potentially contaminated industrial raw materials.

SYMPTOMS: The disease may attack the lungs (wool-sorter's disease) or the loose connective tissue, giving rise to malignant edema, necrosis of mediastinal lymph nodes, and pleural effusion. This is followed by respiratory distress, cyanosis, shock, and coma. More commonly anthrax occurs in the form of a pustule called an anthrax boil or malignant pustule. This cutaneous form will exhibit redness, vesiculation and induration with central ulceration, and development of a black eschar. Rarely, the disease may occur in the intestinal tract. If untreated, anthrax may be fatal.

TREATMENT: Treatment consists of penicillin or tetracycline. Erythromycin is also effective.

NURSING IMPLICATIONS: The nurse provides health supervision to at-risk employees, along with prompt medical care of all lesions. The nurse also supervises terminal disinfection of textile mills contaminated with *B. anthracis*, using vaporized formaldehyde or other recommended treatment, and reports all cases of anthrax to local health authorities. Isolation procedures (mask, gown, gloves, handwashing, and incineration of contaminated materials) are maintained to protect against drainage and secretions for the duration of illness in both inhalation and cutaneous anthrax. For patients with inhalation anthrax, vital signs are monitored and respiratory support is provided. For patients with cutaneous anthrax, lesions are kept clean and covered with sterile dressings. Prescribed antibiotics are administered. Frequent oral hygiene and skin care are provided. Oral fluid intake and frequent small, nutritious meals are encouraged. Appropriate nursing measures and prescribed medical therapies are instituted to control hyperpyrexia. SEE: *Universal Precautions Appendix.*

**anthropo-** [Gr. *anthropos,* man] Combining form denoting *relationship to human beings or human life.*

**anthropobiology** (ăn″thrō-pō-bī-ŏl′ō-jē) [″ + *bios,* life, + *logos,* word, reason] Study of the biology of humans and the great apes.

**anthropoid** (ăn′thrō-poyd) [″ + *eidos,* form, shape] **1.** Resembling humans. **2.** An ape.

**anthropological baseline** An imaginary line that passes from the lower border of the orbit to the superior margin of the external auditory meatus.

**anthropology** (ăn″thrō-pŏl′ō-jē) [″ + *logos,* word, reason] The scientific study of humans. It includes the investigation of human origin and the development of the physical, cultural, religious, and social attributes.

***physical a.*** The branch of anthropology concerned with physical measurement of human beings (as living subjects or skeletal remains).

**anthropometer** (ăn″thrō-pŏm′ĕ-tĕr) [″ + *metron,* measure] A device for measuring the human body and its parts.

**anthropometry** (ăn-thrō-pŏm′ĕt-rē) The science of measuring the human body, including craniometry, osteometry, skin fold evaluation for subcutaneous fat estimation, and height and weight measurements; usually performed by an anthropologist. **anthropometric** (-pō-mĕt′rĭk), *adj.*

**anthropomorphism** (ăn″thrō-pō-mor′fĭzm) [″ + *morphe,* form, + *-ismos,* condition] Attributing human qualities to nonhuman organisms or objects.

**anthropophilic** (ăn″thrō-pō-fĭl′ĭk) [″ + *philein,* to love] Preferring humans, said of parasites that prefer a human host to an animal.

**anthropozoonosis** (ăn″thrō-pō-zō″ō-nō′sĭs) [″ + *zoon,* animal, + *nosis,* disease] An infectious disease acquired by humans from vertebrate hosts of the causative agents. Examples are rabies and trichinosis.

**anti-, ant-** [Gr.] Prefix meaning *against, opposing, counteracting.*

**antiadrenergic** (ăn″tē-ă-drĕn-ĕr′jĭk) [Gr. *anti,* against, + L. *ad,* to, + *ren,* kidney, + Gr. *ergon,* work] Preventing or counteracting adrenergic action.

**antiagglutinin** (ăn″tē-ă-gloo′tĭ-nĭn) A specific antibody opposing the action of an agglutinin.

**antiaggregant, platelet** A medicine, such as aspirin, that interferes with the aggregation or clumping of platelets.

**antiamebic** (ăn″tē-ă-mē′bĭk) [″ + *amoibe,* change] A medicine used to prevent or treat amebiasis.

**antianaphylaxis** (ăn″tē-ăn-ă-fĭ-lăks′ĭs) [″ + *ana,* away from, + *phylaxis,* protection] Prevention of anaphylaxis; usually attained by administering repeated doses of the sensitizing substance in an amount too small to cause an anaphylactic reaction. SYN: *desensitization.*

**antiandrogen** (ăn″tē-ăn′drō-jĕn) [″ + *androgen*] A substance that inhibits or prevents the action of an androgen.

**antianemic** (ăn″tē-ă-nē′mĭk) Preventing or curing anemia.

**antiantibody** (ăn″tē-ăn′tĭ-bŏd-ē) [″ + *antibody*] An antibody specific for, and produced in response to the administration of, another antibody.

**antiantitoxin** (ăn″tē-ăn″tĭ-tŏk′sin) [″ + *antitoxin*] An antibody, produced in response to the administration of an antitoxin, that counteracts the effect of the antitoxin.

**antiarrhythmic** (ăn″tē-ă-rĭth′mĭk) [″ + *a-,* not, + *rhythmos,* rhythm] A drug or physical force that acts to control or prevent cardiac arrhythmias.

**antiarthritic** (ăn″tē-ăr-thrĭt′ĭk) [″ + *arthritikos,* gouty] Relieving arthritis.

**antibacterial** (ăn″tĭ-băk-tē′rē-ăl) **1.** Destroying or stopping the growth of bacteria. **2.** An agent that destroys or stops the growth of bacteria.

**antibiosis** (an″tĭ-bī-ō′sĭs) [″ + *bios,* life] An association or relationship between two organisms in which one is harmful to the other.

**antibiotic** (ăn″tĭ-bī-ŏt′ĭk) **1.** Destructive to life. **2.** Pert. to antibiosis. **3.** A natural or synthetic substance that destroys microorganisms or inhibits their growth. Antibiotics are used extensively to treat infectious diseases in plants, animals, and humans. SEE: *antimicrobial drugs* for table.

***bactericidal a.*** An antibiotic that kills microorganisms.

***bacteriostatic a.*** An antibiotic that inhibits the growth of microorganisms.

***broad-spectrum a.*** An antibiotic that is effective against a wide variety of microorganisms.

***narrow-spectrum a.*** An antibiotic that is effective against only a few kinds of microorganisms.

**antibiotic-impregnated polymethacrylate beads** Vehicles for delivering high-concentration antibiotic therapy to a specific area. The antibiotic-impregnated beads are implanted in open wounds with loss of tissue substance, such as open fractures.

**antibiotic resistant** Having the ability to resist the action of antibiotics.

**antibody** (ăn′tĭ-bŏd″ē) Any of the complex glycoproteins produced by B lymphocytes in response to the presence of an antigen. A single antibody molecule consists of four polypeptide chains, two light chains and two heavy chains, all of which are joined by disulfide bonds. The heavy chains form the compliment binding site, and the light and heavy chains form the antigen binding site. Antibodies, all of which are immunoglobulins, may combine with specific antigens to destroy or control them, providing protection against most common infections. Almost all antibodies except natural antibodies (e.g., antibodies to different blood types) are created by B cells linking with a foreign antigen on the surface of an invading organism. SYN: *immunoglobulin.* SEE: illus.; *antigen; autoantibody; cytokines; immunoglobulin.*

Antibodies neutralize or destroy antigens in several ways. They can initiate lysis of the antigen by activating the complement system, neutralizing toxins released by bacteria, opsonizing the antigen or forming a complex to stimulate phagocytosis, promoting antigen clumping (agglutination), or preventing the antigen from adhering to host cells.

***antireceptor a.*** An antibody that acts against the receptor on a cell rather than on the cell itself.

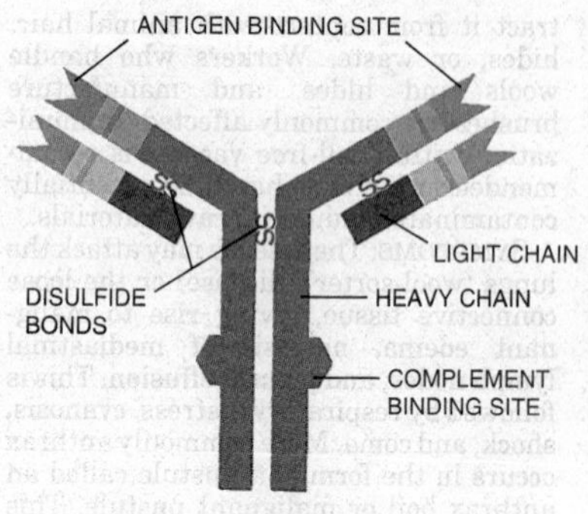


ANTIBODY

SCHEMATIC STRUCTURE OF AN IgG ANTIBODY

***blocking a.*** An antibody that combines with an antigen and specifically blocks its ability to produce sensitizing reactions.

***cross-reacting a.*** An antibody that reacts with antigens functionally similar to its specific antigen.

***cytotoxic a.*** An antibody that lyses cells by binding to a cellular antigen and activating complement or killer cells.

***fluorescent a.*** Antibody reaction made visible by incorporating a fluorescent dye into the antigen-antibody reaction and examining the specimen with a microscope equipped for fluorescent microscopy.

***immune a.*** An antibody produced by immunization or as a result of transfusion of incompatible blood.

***maternal a.*** An antibody produced by the mother and transferred to the fetus in utero.

***monoclonal a.*** SEE: *hybridoma; monoclonal antibodies.*

***natural a.*** An antibody present in a person without known exposure to the specific antigen, such as an anti-A antibody in a person with B blood type; may be the result of unknown accidental exposure.

***protective a.*** An antibody produced in response to an infectious disease. SEE: *immunity.*

**antibody combining site** The particular area on an antibody molecule to which part of an antigen links, creating an antigen-antibody reaction. SEE: *antibody; antigen; antigenic determinant.*

**antibody therapy** The use of antibodies to treat patients with immunodeficiency. This is done by using parenteral immune globulin.

**antibrachium** (ăn″tĭ-brā′kē-ŭm) Antebrachium; the forearm.

**antibromic** (ăn″tĭ-brō′mĭk) [Gr. *anti,* against, + *bromos,* smell] **1.** Deodorizing. **2.** A deodorant.

**anti-burn scar garment** A carefully fitted garment of material with calibrated stretch characteristics worn to provide uniform pressure over burn graft sites in order to reduce scarring during healing.

**anticarcinogenic 1.** Tending to delay or prevent tumor formation. **2.** A substance or action that prevents or delays tumor formation.

**anticariogenic** A substance or action that interferes with the development of dental caries.

**anticarious** (ăn″tĭ-kā′rē-ŭs) [″ + *caries,* decay] Preventing decay of teeth.

**anticholagogue** (ăn″tĭ-kŏl′ă-gŏg) [Gr. *anti,* against, + *chole,* bile, + *agein,* to lead forth] Medicine used to decrease secretion of bile.

**anticholinergic** (ăn″tĭ-kō″lĭn-ĕr′jĭk) **1.** Impeding the impulses of cholinergic, esp. parasympathetic, nerve fibers. **2.** An agent that blocks parasympathetic nerve impulses. The side effects, which include dry mouth and blurred vision, are seen in phenothiazine and tricyclic antidepressant drug therapy. SYN: *parasympatholytic.*

**anticholinesterase** (ăn″tĭ-kō-lĭn-ĕs′tĕr-ās) A substance that opposes the action of cholinesterase.

**anticipate** (ăn-tĭs′ĭ-pāt) [L. *ante,* before, + *capere,* to take] **1.** To occur prior to the usual time of onset of a particular illness or disease, said of an event, sign, or symptom. **2.** In nursing and medicine, to prepare for other than the routine or fully expected.

**anticipatory grief** Mental anguish caused by the impending loss of a body part, a function, or a loved one.

**anticipatory guidance** Information concerning normal expectations of an age group or disease entity in order to provide support for coping with problems before they arise.

**anticlinal** (ăn″tĭ-klī′năl) [Gr. *anti,* against, + *klinein,* to incline] Inclined in opposite directions.

**anticoagulant** (ăn″tĭ-kō-ăg′ū-lănt) [″ + L. *coagulans,* forming clots] **1.** Delaying or preventing blood coagulation. **2.** An agent that prevents or delays blood coagulation. Anticoagulants used for storing whole blood include anticoagulant citrate dextrose solution, anticoagulant citrate phosphate dextrose solution, anticoagulant heparin solution, and anticoagulant sodium citrate solution.

***warfarin sodium a.*** SEE: *warfarin sodium.*

**anticoagulant therapy** The use of drugs that interfere with blood coagulation to prevent disorders, such as pulmonary embolism and stroke, that result from vascular thrombosis. Thrombus formation is associated with narrowing of and injury to atherosclerotic blood vessels, venous stasis, and hypercoagulability. Risk factors include dehydration, pregnancy, varicose veins, heart valve disease, congestive heart failure, cardiac irregularities, and thrombophlebitis. The normal rate of blood flow can be slowed also in a variety of conditions associated with prolonged inactivity such as paralysis, or recovery from major surgical procedures. SEE: *heparin; thrombosis; warfarin sodium.*

---

Caution: Anticoagulant therapy increases the risk of internal bleeding.

---

**anticodon** (ăn″tĭ-kō′dŏn) A triplet (codon) of bases on tRNA (transfer RNA) that complements the corresponding codon on mRNA (messenger RNA), which ensures the proper sequence of amino acids in the protein being synthesized.

**anticonvulsant** (ăn″tĭ-kŏn-vŭl′sănt) [″ + L. *convulsio,* pulling together] **1.** Preventing or relieving convulsions. **2.** An agent that prevents or relieves convulsions.

**anticytotoxin** Something that opposes the action of a cytotoxin. SEE: *cytotoxin.*

**antidepressant** (ăn″tĭ-dē-prĕs′sănt) Any medicine or other mode of therapy that acts to prevent, cure, or alleviate mental depression.

***tricyclic and tetracyclic a.'s*** A class of antidepressant agents whose chemical structure has three fused rings. These drugs block the reuptake of norepinephrine and serotonin at the nerve endings. They are used frequently in elderly patients.

**antidiabetic** (ăn″tĭ-dī″ă-bĕt′ĭk) **1.** Preventing or relieving diabetes. **2.** An agent that prevents or relieves diabetes.

**antidiarrheal** (ăn″tĭ-dī-ă-rē′ăl) A substance used to prevent or treat diarrhea.

**antidiuretic** (ăn″tĭ-dī-ū-rĕt′ĭk) [″+ *dia,* intensive, + *ouresis,* urination] **1.** Lessening urine secretion. **2.** A drug that decreases urine secretion.

**antidotal** (ăn″tĭ-dō′tăl) Acting as or pert. to an antidote.

**antidote** (ăn′tĭ-dōt) [Gr. *antidoton,* given against] A substance that neutralizes poisons or their effects.

***chemical a.*** An antidote that reacts with the poison to produce a harmless chemical compound. For example, table salt precipitates silver nitrate and forms the much less toxic silver chloride. Chemical antidotes should be used sparingly and, after their use, should be removed from the stomach by gastric lavage because they may produce serious results if allowed to remain there.

***mechanical a.*** An antidote that prevents absorption of the poison. Examples are fats, oils, milk (casein coagulum), whites of eggs, finely divided charcoal, fuller's earth, and mineral oil. (Fats and oils are not to be used in treating phosphorus, camphor, aspidium, and cantharides poisonings.)

***physiologic a.*** An antidote that produces physiological effects opposite to the effects of the poison; e.g., sedatives are given for convulsants and stimulants are given for hypnotics. These should not be given without a physician's definite instructions.

***universal a.*** An antidote that is effective against many poisons (there is no known antidote that is literally universal). The mixture consists of two parts activated charcoal, one part tannic acid, and one part magnesium oxide. (The charcoal absorbs; the tannic acid precipitates metals, alkaloids, and some glucosides; and the magnesium oxide neutralizes acids.) Give orally by dissolving 5 tsp (approx. 25 ml) of the mixture in 4 oz (120 ml) of warm water. After the patient has swallowed the antidote, the stomach contents should then be removed by gastric lavage within a few minutes. Treatment may be repeated.

Caution: Gastric lavage should not be used in patients who have ingested caustics. The stomach or esophagus may be ruptured by introduction of the tube.

**antidromic** (ăn″tĭ-drŏm′ĭk) [Gr. *anti,* against, + *dromos,* running] Denoting nerve impulses traveling in the opposite direction from normal.

**antiemetic** (ăn″tĭ-ē-mĕt′ĭk) [″ + *emetikos,* inclined to vomit] **1.** Preventing or relieving nausea and vomiting. **2.** An agent that prevents or relieves nausea and vomiting.

**antienzyme** (an″tĭ-ĕn′zīm) A substance that opposes the action of an enzyme.

**antiepileptic** (ăn″tĭ-ĕp″ĭ-lĕp′tĭk) **1.** Opposing epilepsy. **2.** Any procedure or therapy that combats epilepsy.

**antiestrogen** (ăn″tĭ-ĕs′trō-jĕn) A substance that blocks or modifies the action of estrogen.

**antifebrile** (ăn″tĭ-fē′brĭl, -fē′brĭl, -fĕb′rĭl) [″ + L. *febris,* fever] **1.** Reducing fever. **2.** An agent that reduces fever. SYN: *antipyretic.*

**antifibrinolysin** (ăn″tĭ-fī″brĭ-nŏl′ĭ-sĭn) [″ + L. *fibra,* fiber, + Gr. *lysis,* dissolution] A substance that counteracts fibrinolysis.

**antifungal** (ăn″tĭ-fŭng′găl) **1.** Destroying or inhibiting the growth of fungi. **2.** An agent that destroys or inhibits the growth of fungi.

**antigalactic** (ăn″tĭ-gă-lăk′tĭk) **1.** Preventing or diminishing the secretion of milk. **2.** An agent that prevents or diminishes the secretion of milk.

**antigen** (ăn′tĭ-jĕn) [Gr. *anti,* against, + *gennan,* to produce] A protein or oligosaccharide marker on the surface of cells that identifies the cell as *self* or *non-self;* identifies the type of cell, e.g., skin, kidney; stimulates the production of antibodies, by B lymphocytes that will neutralize or destroy the cell if necessary; and stimulates cytotoxic responses by granulocytes, monocytes, and lymphocytes.

Antigens on the body's own cells are called autoantigens. Antigens on all other cells are called foreign antigens. Matching certain types of tissue antigens is essential for the success of an organ transplant. Inflammation occurs when neutrophils, monocytes, and macrophages encounter an antigen from any source during bodily injury. The antigen may be foreign or may be an autoantigen that has been damaged and, therefore, appears to be foreign. Reactions to antigens by T and B cells are part of the specific immune response. SEE: *autoantigen; cytokines; histocompatibility antigens.*

***allogeneic a.*** An antigen that occurs in some individuals of the same species. Examples are the human blood group antigens.

***alpha-fetoprotein a.*** SEE: *alpha-fetoprotein.*

***carcinoembryonic a.*** ABBR: CEA. One of a class of antigens normally present in the fetus. Originally isolated from colon tumors, they were thought erroneously to be specific for those tumors. If the previously elevated CEA level returns to normal after surgery, removal of the colonic tumor is thought to be complete.

***CD a.'s*** Cell surface molecules (markers) present on cells. They are designated CD1, CD2, and so on. This system of designating CD antigens has been accepted by international convention. The markers may be identified by specific monoclonal antibodies and used to designate cell populations.

***CD4 a.*** A cell surface molecule present on T cells. It is the receptor for the human immunodeficiency virus associated with AIDS.

***class I a.*** One of the major histocompatibility molecules present on almost all cells except human red blood cells. These antigens are important in rejecting grafts and transplanted organs.

***class II a.*** One of the major histocompatibility molecules present on immunocompetent cells.

***cross-reacting a.*** An antigen having the ability to react with more than one specific antibody.

***H a.*** A flagellar protein present on the surface of some enteric bacilli such as *Escherichia coli.* The antigen is important in classifying these bacilli.

***histocompatibility locus a.*** SEE: *histocompatibility locus antigen.*

***human leukocyte a.*** Histocompatibility locus a.

***H-Y a.*** A histocompatibility antigen located on the cell membrane. It has a primary role in determining the sexual differentiation of the male embryo.

***K a.*** A capsular antigen present on the surface of some enteric bacilli. The antigen is important in classifying these bacilli.

***O a.*** A surface antigen of some enteric bacilli. The antigen is important in classifying these bacilli.

***oncofetal a.*** An antigen normally expressed in the fetus that may reappear in the adult in association with certain tumors. Examples include alpha-fetoprotein and carcinoembryonic antigens.

***prostate-specific a.*** ABBR: PSA. A marker for cancer of the prostate, found in the blood. It is excreted by both benign and malignant prostate tumors, but cancerous prostate cells secrete it at much higher levels. Prostate-specific antigen is used as a diagnostic tool with blood levels and digital examination if possible. SEE: *prostate cancer.*

***soluble a.*** An antigen present in a liquid (aqueous) substance.

***specific a.*** The property of mature B and T lymphocytes that enables them to respond to specific foreign antigens entering the body. Antigen specificity requires mature B and T cells that have been previously exposed to the antigen and, therefore, are able to recognize it again and respond by neutralizing or destroying it. The exact process by which B lymphocytes become capable of recognizing and responding to antigens is unknown. Development of antigen specificity by T cells requires macrophage processing, of the antigen for recognition.

***T-dependent a.*** An antigen that can stimulate an antibody response only in the presence of helper T cells.

***tumor-specific a.*** An antigen produced by certain tumors. It appears on the tumor cells but not on normal cells derived from the same tissue.

**antigen-antibody reaction** The combination of an antigen with its specific antibody. It may result in agglutination, precipitation, neutralization, complement fixation, or increased susceptibility to phagocytosis. The antigen-antibody reaction forms the basis for B-cell–mediated immunity.

**antigen binding site** SEE: *antibody combining site.*

**antigenic** (ăn-tĭ-jĕn′ĭk) Capable of causing the production of an antibody.

**antigenic determinant** The specific area of an antigen that binds with an antibody combining site and determines the specificity of the antigen-antibody reaction. SEE: *antigen.*

***epitope a.d.*** The simplest form of an antigenic determinant within a complex antigenic marker. The epitope links with a paratope, one area of an antibody combining site.

**antigenic drift** A change in the protein marker or antigen on an organism. As a result, the body's previous immune response to the organism must change. This is often seen in the influenza virus, since it changes its antigenic makeup from year to year.

**antigenicity** The condition of being able to produce an immune response to an antibody.

**antigen-presenting cell** ABBR: APC. A cell that breaks down antigens and displays their fragments on surface receptors next to major histocompatibility complex molecules. This presentation is necessary for some T lymphocytes that are unable to recognize soluble antigens. Macrophages are the primary antigen-presenting cells, but B cells and dendritic cells also can act as APCs. SEE: *cell, T; macrophage processing.*

**antigen processing** The series of events that occur when an antigen is recognized by the immune system as foreign, culminating in the production of a specific antibody or cytotoxic cell response. SEE: *antigen; macrophage processing; self.*

**antiglobulin** (ăn″tĭ-glŏb′ū-lĭn) A substance that opposes the action of globulin.

**antiglobulin test** A test for the presence of antibodies against the Rh factor on red blood cells. Antiglobulin antiserum produced in rabbits is mixed with serum containing Rh-positive red blood cells. If anti-Rh antibodies have coated the red cells, the cells will agglutinate or clump together. SYN: *Coombs' test.*

**antigoitrogenic** (ăn″tĭ-goy″trō-jĕn′ĭk) [″ + L. *guttur,* throat, + Gr. *gennan,* to produce] Preventing the formation of a goiter.

**anti-G suit** [″ + *G,* gravity] A garment designed to produce uniform pressure on the lower extremities and abdomen. Normally the suit is used by aviators to help prevent pooling of blood in the lower half of the body during certain flight maneuvers. The garment has also been used in treating severe forms of postural hypotension. The suit's usefulness in treating shock is questionable.

Caution: This garment is contraindicated in congestive heart failure, cardiogenic shock, and penetrating chest trauma.

**antihelix** (ăn″tĭ-hē′lĭks) [″ + Gr. *helix,* coil] The inner curved ridge of the external ear parallel to the helix. SYN: *anthelix.*

**antihemolysin** (ăn″tĭ-hĕ-mŏl′ĭ-sĭn) A substance that opposes the action of hemolysin.

**antihemophilic factor** ABBR: AHF. Blood coagulation factor VIII. Trade names are Hemofil M and Profilate. SEE: *coagulation factor.*

**antihemorrhagic** (ăn″tĭ-hĕm-ō-răj′ĭk) [″ + *haima,* blood, + *rhegnynai,* to burst forth] **1.** Preventing or arresting hemorrhage. **2.** An agent that prevents or arrests hemorrhage.

**antihidrotic** (ăn″tĭ-hī-drŏt′ĭk) [″ + *hidrotikos,* sweating] **1.** Preventing or decreasing perspiration. **2.** An agent that prevents or decreases perspiration. SYN: *anhidrotic; antiperspirant; antisudorific.*

**antihistamine** (ăn″tĭ-hĭs′tă-mēn, -mĭn) A

drug that opposes the action of histamine. Many of the first antihistamines were noted for their side effects of drowsiness and dry mouth. Antihistamines that have fewer side effects are now available. Examples are terfenadine (short acting) and astemizole (long acting). Trade names are Seldane and Hismanal, respectively. SEE: *histamine.*

**antihistamine poisoning** SEE: *Poisons and Poisoning Appendix.*

**antihistaminic** (ăn″tĭ-hĭs″tă-mĭn′ĭk) **1.** Opposing the action of histamine. **2.** An agent that opposes the action of histamine.

**antihormone** A substance that interferes with the action of a hormone.

**antihypercholesterolemic** (ăn″tĭ-hī″pĕr-kō-lĕs″tĕr-ŏl-ē′mĭk) [″ + *hyper,* above, + *chole,* bile, + *stereos,* solid, + *haima,* blood] **1.** Preventing or controlling elevation of the serum cholesterol level. **2.** An agent that prevents or controls elevation of the serum cholesterol level.

**antihypertensive** (ăn″tĭ-hī″pĕr-tĕn′sĭv) [″ + ″ + L. *tensio,* tension] **1.** Preventing or controlling high blood pressure. **2.** An agent that prevents or controls high blood pressure.

**antihypnotic** (ăn″tĭ-hĭp-nŏt′ĭk) **1.** Preventing or inhibiting sleep. **2.** An agent that prevents or inhibits sleep.

**anti-icteric** (ăn″tĭ-ĭk-tĕr′ĭk) [″ + *ikteros,* jaundice] **1.** Preventing or relieving jaundice. **2.** An agent that prevents or relieves jaundice.

**anti-inflammatory** (ăn″tĭ-ĭn-flăm′ă-tō-rē) **1.** Counteracting inflammation. **2.** An agent that counteracts inflammation.

**antiketogenesis** (ăn″tĭ-kē-tō-jĕn′ĕ-sĭs) [″ + *ketone* + Gr. *gennan,* to produce] The prevention or inhibition of formation of ketone bodies. In starvation, diabetes, and certain other conditions, production of ketones is increased, but they accumulate in the blood because cells do not use them as rapidly as they would carbohydrate energy sources. Increased carbohydrate intake will help to prevent or treat this. Carbohydrates are therefore antiketogenic. In ketonemia due to diabetes, both insulin and carbohydrates are needed to allow carbohydrate metabolism to proceed at a rate that would control ketone formation. **antiketogenetic, antiketogenic** (-jĕ-nĕt′ik, -jĕn′ĭk), *adj.*

**antilactase** (ăn″tĭ-lăk′tās) [″ + *lac,* milk, + *-ase,* enzyme] A substance that opposes the action of lactase.

**antilipemic** (ăn″tĭ-lī-pē′mĭk) **1.** Preventing or counteracting the accumulation of fatty substances in the blood. **2.** An agent that prevents or counteracts the accumulation of fatty substances in the blood.

**Antilirium** Trade name for physostigmine salicylate.

**antilithic** (ăn″tĭ-lĭth′ĭk) [″ + *lithos,* stone] **1.** Preventing or relieving calculi. **2.** An agent that prevents or relieves calculi.

**antilymphocyte serum** (ăn″tĭ-lĭm″fō-sīt′) ABBR: ALS. Serum, developed in animals, containing antibodies directed against lymphocytes that promotes some degree of immunosuppression when injected into a patient. The antibodies do not affect the activities of other white blood cells. Antilymphocyte serum is used to reduce rejection of transplanted organs or other tissue such as skin grafts. It may cause excessive immunosuppression. SEE: *monoclonal antibody.*

**antilysin** (ăn-tĭ-lī′sĭn) Antibody that opposes the action of lysin.

**antilysis** (ăn-tĭ-lī′sĭs) [″ + *lysis,* dissolution] Prevention or inhibition of lysis due to the action of antilysin. **antilytic** (-lĭt′ĭk), *adj.*

**antilyssic** (ăn-tĭ-lĭs′ĭk) [″ + *lyssa,* frenzy] Preventing or curing rabies.

**antimalarial** (ăn″tĭ-mă-lā′rē-ăl) **1.** Preventing or relieving malaria. **2.** An agent that prevents or relieves malaria.

**antimere** (ăn′tĭ-mēr) [″ + *meros,* a part] One of corresponding parts of the body on opposite sides of the long axis.

**antimetabolite** (ăn″tĭ-mĕ-tăb′ō-līt) **1.** A substance that opposes the action of or replaces a metabolite and is structurally similar to it. It is believed that certain antibiotics are effective because they act as antimetabolites. **2.** A class of antineoplastic drugs used to treat cancer. Antimetabolites are structurally similar to vitamins, coenzymes, or other substances essential for growth and division of normal and neoplastic cells. These drugs are most effective against rapidly growing tumors. A drug-induced block of DNA synthesis occurs when the cells take in the antimetabolite rather than the necessary nutrient or enzyme.

**antimetropia** (ăn″tĭ-mĕ-trō′pē-ă) [″ + *metron,* measure, + *ops,* eye] An ocular disorder in which each eye has a different error of refraction (e.g., one eye may be hyperopic; the other, myopic).

**antimicrobial** (ăn″tĭ-mī-krō′bē-ăl) **1.** Destructive to or preventing the development of microorganisms. **2.** An agent that destroys or prevents the development of microorganisms.

**antimicrobial drug** A chemical substance that either kills microorganisms or prevents their growth.

**antimicrobic** (ăn″tĭ-mī-krō′bĭk) [″ + *mikros,* small, + *bios,* life] Antimicrobial.

**Antiminth** Trade name for pyrantel pamoate.

**antimitotic** (ăn″tĭ-mī-tŏt′ĭk) Interfering with or preventing mitosis.

**antimonial** (ăn″tĭ-mō′nē-ăl) Pert. to or containing antimony.

**antimony** (ăn′tĭ-mō″nē) SYMB: Sb. Stibium; a crystalline metallic element, atomic weight 121.75, atomic number 51. Its compounds are used in alloys and medicines and may form poisons.

**antimony poisoning** Toxicity caused by ingestion of antimony. Symptoms include an acrid metallic taste; cardiac depression; sweating and vomiting about 30 min after ingestion. In large doses, it causes irritation of the lining of the alimentary tract, resembling arsenic poisoning.

FIRST AID: Vomiting caused by the poison may be sufficient, or gastric lavage with 1% sodium bicarbonate solution may be needed. British antilewisite (BAL) is effective, esp. if the poisoning is due to a trivalent form such as tartar emetic. Otherwise, it should be treated symptomatically. SEE: *arsenic* in *Poisons and Poisoning Appendix.*

**antimuscarinic** Opposing the action of muscarine or agents that act like muscarinics. Atropine and scopolamine are antimuscarinic drugs.

**antimycotic** (ăn″tĭ-mī-kŏt′ĭk) [Gr. *anti,* against, + *mykes,* fungus] Inhibiting or preventing the growth of fungi.

**antinarcotic** (ăn″tĭ-năr-kŏt′ĭk) [″ + *narkotikos,* benumbing] **1.** Opposing the action of a narcotic. **2.** An agent that opposes the action of a narcotic.

**antinatriuresis** (ăn″tĭ-nā″trĭ-ū-rē′sĭs) [″ + L. *natrium,* sodium, + Gr. *ouresis,* making water] Decreasing the excretion of sodium in the urine.

**antinauseant** (ăn″tĭ-naw′sē-ănt) **1.** Preventing or relieving nausea. **2.** An agent that prevents or relieves nausea.

**antineoplastic** (ăn″tĭ-nē″ō-plăs′tĭk) **1.** Preventing the development, growth, or proliferation of malignant cells. **2.** An agent that prevents the development, growth, or proliferation of malignant cells.

**antinephritic** (ăn″tĭ-nĕ-frĭt′ĭk) **1.** Preventing or relieving inflammation of the kidneys. **2.** An agent that prevents or relieves inflammation of the kidneys.

**antineuralgic** (ăn″tĭ-nū-răl′jĭk) [″ + *neuron,* nerve, + *algos,* pain] **1.** Relieving neuralgia. **2.** An agent that relieves neuralgia.

**antineuritic** (ăn″tĭ-nū-rĭt′ĭk) **1.** Preventing or relieving inflammation of a nerve. **2.** An agent that prevents or relieves inflammation of a nerve.

**antinuclear** (ăn″tĭ-nū′klē-ăr) Having an affinity for or reacting with the nucleus of a cell.

**antinuclear antibodies** ABBR: ANA. A group of antibodies that react against normal components of the cell nucleus. These antibodies are present in a variety of immunologic diseases, including systemic lupus erythematosus, progressive systemic sclerosis, Sjögren's syndrome, scleroderma, polymyositis, and dermatomyositis, and in persons taking hydralazine, procainamide, or isoniazid. In addition, ANA is present in some normal individuals.

**antiodontalgic** (ăn″tē-ō″dŏn-tăl′jĭk) [″ + *odous,* tooth, + *algos,* pain] **1.** Relieving toothache. **2.** An agent that relieves toothache.

**anti-oncogene** A gene that inhibits or prevents the growth of tumor cells. SEE: *oncogene.*

**antiovulatory** (ăn″tē-ŏv′ū-lă-tō″rē) Inhibiting or preventing ovulation.

**antioxidant** (ăn″tē-ŏk′sĭ-dănt) An agent that prevents or inhibits oxidation. Antioxidants are naturally occurring or synthetic substances that help protect cells from the damaging effects of oxygen free radicals, highly reactive compounds created during normal cell metabolism. Antioxidants (such as the enzymes superoxidase dismutase and peroxidases and vitamins A, C, and E) scavenge oxygen free radicals. Superoxide dismutase and other cellular enzymes convert the very destructive hydroxyl radicals into hydrogen peroxide and then into water and harmless oxygen before they can damage important cell and mitochondrial membranes, destroy cellular proteins or enzymes, and even cause DNA mutations. Assisting the cell's enzyme protectors are the antioxidant vitamins E and C and beta-carotene, a precursor of vitamin A. These vitamins absorb or attach to the free radicals, preventing them from attacking normal tissues. In some circumstances, excessive production of oxygen free radicals overwhelms the available oxidants, causing DNA mutation that can lead to cancer. Radiation therapy, tissue infarction, and aging contribute to this dangerous process.

Current antioxidant therapy consists mainly of oral vitamins and food additives. However, drugs with antioxidant activity are under investigation to prevent cancer, to slow aging, and to limit the spread of tissue infarctions. In the future, these drugs may be administered by intravenous push during such crises as myocardial infarction or evolving stroke.

**antiparalytic** (ăn″tĭ-păr-ă-lĭt′ĭk) Relieving paralysis.

**antiparkinsonian** **1.** Pert. to any effective therapy for parkinsonism. **2.** An agent effective against parkinsonism.

**antiparasitic** (ăn″tĭ-păr-ă-sĭt′ĭk) **1.** Destructive to parasites. **2.** An agent that destroys parasites.

**antipathy** (ăn-tĭp′ă-thē) **1.** Feeling of strong aversion. **2.** Antagonism. **antipathic** (ăn″tĭ-păth′ĭk), *adj.*

**antipedicular** (ăn″tĭ-pĕ-dĭk′ū-lăr) Effective against pediculosis, said of a medicine or procedure.

**antiperistalsis** (ăn″tĭ-pĕr″ĭ-stăl′sĭs) [″ + *peri,* around, + *stalsis,* constriction] Reversed peristalsis; a wave of contraction in the gastrointestinal tract moving toward the oral end. In the duodenum it is associated with vomiting; in the ascending colon it occurs normally. SEE: *peristalsis.* **antiperistaltic** (-stăl′tĭk), *adj.*

**antiperspirant** (ăn″tĭ-pĕr′spĭ-rănt) **1.** Inhibiting perspiration. **2.** A substance that inhibits perspiration. SYN: *anhidrotic; antihidrotic; antisudorific.*

**antiphagocytic** (ăn″tĭ-făg-ō-sĭt′ĭk) Preventing or inhibiting phagocytosis.

**antiplastic** (ăn″tĭ-plăs′tĭk) [″ + *plassein,* to form] **1.** Preventing or inhibiting wound healing. **2.** An agent that prevents or inhibits wound healing by preventing formation of granulation tissue.

**antiplatelet** (ăn″tĭ-plāt′lĕt) **1.** Destructive to platelets. **2.** An agent that destroys platelets.

**antipodal** (ăn-tĭp′ō-dăl) [Gr. *antipous,* with feet opposite] Located at opposite positions.

**antiprostaglandin** (ăn″tĭ-prŏs″tă-glăn′dĭn) A drug that interferes with prostaglandin activity. Such drugs are used in treating arthritis and dysmenorrhea.

**antiprostatitis** (ăn″tĭ-prŏs″tă-tī′tĭs) Inflammation of Cowper's gland.

**antiprotease** (ăn″tĭ-prō′tē-ās) A substance that interferes with proteolysis.

**antiprotozoal** (ăn″tĭ-prō″tō-zō′ăl) Destructive to protozoa.

**antipruritic** (ăn″tĭ-proo-rĭt′ĭk) **1.** Preventing or relieving itching. **2.** An agent that prevents or relieves itching.

**antipsoriatic** (ăn″tĭ-sō″rē-ăt′ĭk) [Gr. *anti,* against, + *psora,* itch] **1.** Preventing or relieving psoriasis. **2.** An agent that prevents or relieves psoriasis.

**antipyresis** (ăn″tĭ-pī-rē′sĭs) [″ + *pyretos,* fever] Use of antipyretics.

**antipyretic** (ăn-tĭ-pī-rĕt′ĭk) **1.** Reducing fever. **2.** An agent that reduces fever. SYN: *antifebrile.*

**antipyrotic** (ăn″tĭ-pī-rŏt′ĭk) [″ + *pyrotikos,* burning] **1.** Promoting the healing of burns. **2.** An agent that promotes the healing of burns.

**antirachitic** (ăn″tĭ-ră-kĭt′ĭk) [″ + *rachitis,* rickets] **1.** Helping to cure rickets. **2.** An agent for treating rickets.

**antiretroviral drug** Any one of several drugs used in treating patients with human immunodeficiency virus (HIV) infection.

**antirheumatic** (ăn″tĭ-roo-măt′ĭk) **1.** Preventing or relieving rheumatism. **2.** An agent that prevents or relieves rheumatism.

**antiscabietic** (ăn″tĭ-skā″bē-ĕt′ĭk) [Gr. *anti,* against, + L. *scabies,* itch] **1.** Preventing or relieving scabies. **2.** An agent that prevents or relieves scabies.

**antiscorbutic** (ăn″tĭ-skor-bū′tĭk) [″ + L. *scorbutus,* scurvy] **1.** Preventing or relieving scurvy. **2.** An agent that prevents or relieves scurvy.

**antiseborrheic** (ăn″tĭ-sĕb″ō-rē′ĭk) **1.** Counteracting or effectively treating seborrhea. **2.** An agent that counteracts or relieves seborrhea.

**antisecretory** (ăn″tĭ-sē-krē′tō-rē) **1.** Inhibiting secretion of a gland or organ. **2.** An agent that inhibits secretion of a gland or organ.

**antiself** The reaction of antibodies or lymphocytes with antigens present in the host.

**antisense compounds** Manufactured compounds that are being investigated for the possibility that they may alter disease processes by blocking the production of harmful proteins by diseased cells. These molecules seek out and impede the functioning of a diseased cell's messenger RNA (i.e., a "sense" strand). Without this intervention, the RNA would carry basic directions for the production of disease-causing proteins. If this method proves effective, it will be an important procedure for treating a number of diseases.

**antisepsis** (ăn″tĭ-sĕp′sĭs) [″ + *sepsis,* putrefaction] The prevention of sepsis by preventing or inhibiting the growth of causative microorganisms.

**antiseptic** (ăn″tĭ-sĕp′tĭk) **1.** Rel. to antisepsis. **2.** An agent capable of producing antisepsis.

Chemically, antiseptics may be inorganic, such as the mercury preparations, or organic, such as carbolic acid (phenol). Oxidizing disinfectants liberate oxygen when in contact with pus or organic substances. When in use they should be washed away and replaced frequently to help remove pus, blood, and other substances. Different types of bacteria are sensitive to different antiseptics. SEE: *disinfectant.*

**antiserum** (ăn″tĭ-sē′rŭm) A serum that contains antibodies for a specific antigen. It may be of human or animal origin. SYN: *immune serum.*

***monovalent a.*** Antiserum containing antibodies specific for one antigen.

***polyvalent a.*** Antiserum containing antibodies specific for more than one antigen.

**antishock garment** A special garment that can be placed quickly on a patient in hypovolemic shock. The device contains inflatable compartments that, when filled with air, compress the lower extremities and abdominal area. This compression helps to prevent pooling of blood and fluids in the tissues. The value of this garment in treating shock is questionable. Also known as MAST *(military antishock trousers).*

---

Caution: This garment is contraindicated in congestive heart failure, cardiogenic shock, and penetrating chest trauma.

---

Nursing Implications: Inflatable compartments are filled to appropriate pressure from the bottom up, and inflation is maintained until venous access and fluid resuscitation are initiated. Compartments are then deflated from top to bottom; blood pressure and pulse are monitored frequently for evidence of hypotension. SEE: *anti-G suit.*

**antisialagogue** (ăn″tĭ-sī-ăl′ă-gŏg) [Gr. *anti,* against, + *sialon,* saliva, + *agogos,* drawing forth] An agent, such as atropine, that lessens or prevents production of saliva.

**antisialic** (ăn″tĭ-sī-ăl′ĭk) **1.** Inhibiting the

secretion of saliva. **2.** An agent that inhibits the secretion of saliva.

**antisocial** (ăn″tĭ-sō′shăl) Pert. to a person whose outlook and actions are socially negative and whose behavior is repeatedly in conflict with what society perceives as the norm. SEE: *asocial.*

**antispasmodic** [″ + *spasmos,* convulsion] **1.** Preventing or relieving spasm. **2.** An agent that prevents or relieves spasm. SEE: *spasm.*

**antistaphylococcic** (ăn″tĭ-stăf″ĭ-lō-kŏk′sĭk) [Gr. *anti,* against, + *staphyle,* bunch of grapes, + *cocci,* bacteria] Destructive to staphylococci.

**antistreptococcic** (ăn″tĭ-strĕp″tō-kŏk′sĭk) Destructive to streptococci.

**antistreptolysin** (ăn″tĭ-strĕp-tŏl′ĭ-sĭn) Antibody that opposes the action of streptolysin, a hemolysin produced by streptococci.

**antisudorific** (ăn″tĭ-soo″dor-ĭf′ĭk) Antiperspirant.

**antisyphilitic** (ăn″tĭ-sĭf″ĭ-lĭt′ĭk) [″ + L. *syphiliticus,* pert. to syphilis] **1.** Curing or relieving syphilis. **2.** An agent that cures or relieves syphilis.

**antithenar** (ăn-tĭth′ĕn-ăr) [″ + *thenar,* palm] The eminence on the ulnar side of the palm, formed by the muscles of the little finger. SYN: *hypothenar eminence.*

**antithrombin** Any agent that prevents the action of thrombin.

***a. III*** A plasma protein that inactivates thrombin and inhibits coagulation factors IX, X, XI, and XII, preventing abnormal clotting.

**antithrombotic** (ăn″tĭ-thrŏm-bŏt′ĭk) Interfering with or preventing thrombosis or blood coagulation.

**antithyroid** (ăn″tĭ-thī′royd) [″ + *thyreoeides,* thyroid] **1.** Preventing or inhibiting the functioning of the thyroid gland. **2.** An agent that prevents or inhibits the functioning of the thyroid gland.

**antitoxic serum** Serum that contains antitoxin.

**antitoxigen** (ăn″tĭ-tŏk′sĭ-jĕn) [″ + ″ + *gennan,* to produce] Antitoxinogen.

**antitoxin** (ăn″tĭ-tŏk′sĭn) An antibody produced in response to and capable of neutralizing a specific biologic toxin such as those that cause diphtheria, gas-gangrene, or tetanus. Antitoxins are used for prophylactic and therapeutic purposes. SEE: *antivenin.* **antitoxic** (-tŏk′sĭk), *adj.*

**antitoxinogen** (ăn″tĭ-tŏk-sĭn′ō-jĕn) [Gr. *anti,* against, + *toxikon,* poison, + *gennan,* to produce] An antigen that stimulates production of antitoxin. SYN: *antitoxigen.*

**antitragicus** (ăn″tĭ-trăj′ĭ-kŭs) A small muscle in the pinna of the ear.

**antitragus** (ăn″tĭ-trā′gŭs) [″ + L. *tragus,* goat] A projection on the ear of the cartilage of the auricle in front of the tail of the helix, posterior to the tragus.

**antitrichomonal** **1.** Resistant to or lethal to trichomonads. **2.** A medicine effective in treating trichomonal infections.

**antitrismus** (ăn″tĭ-trĭs′mŭs) [″ + *trismos,* grinding] A condition in which the mouth cannot close because of tonic spasm. SEE: *trismus.*

**antitrypsin** (ăn″tĭ-trĭp′sĭn) A substance that inhibits the action of trypsin.

***alpha 1- a.*** A low-molecular-weight glycoprotein that inhibits proteolytic enzymes. Deficiency of this enzyme in the serum is associated with early-onset emphysema in some patients and liver disease in others. There is no specific therapy, but liver transplant may be of benefit in those with liver disease.

**antitryptic** (ăn″tĭ-trĭp′tĭk) Inhibiting the action of trypsin.

**antituberculotic** (ăn″tĭ-too-bĕr′kū-lŏt″ĭk) Inhibiting the spread or progress of tuberculosis in the body.

**antitussive** (ăn″tĭ-tŭs′ĭv) [Gr. *anti,* against, + L. *tussis,* cough] **1.** Preventing or relieving coughing. **2.** An agent that prevents or relieves coughing.

***centrally acting a.*** An agent that depresses medullary centers, suppressing the cough reflex.

**antivenene** (ăn″tĭ-vĕn′ēn) Antivenin.

**antivenereal** (ăn″tĭ-vĕ-nē′rē-ăl) Preventing or curing venereal diseases.

**antivenin** (ăn″tĭ-vĕn′ĭn) A serum that contains antitoxin specific for an animal or insect venom. Antivenin is prepared from immunized animal sera and is used in the treatment of poisoning by animal or insect venom. SYN: *antivenene.*

***black widow spider a.*** Antitoxic serum obtained from horses immunized against the venom of the black widow spider *(Latrodectus mactans)* and used specifically to treat bites of the black widow spider. The serum is available from Merck Sharp & Dohme, West Point, PA 19486.

***(Crotalidae) polyvalent a.*** Anti-snakebite serum obtained from serum of horses immunized against venom of four types of pit vipers: *Crotalus atrox, C. adamanteus, C. terrificus,* and *Bothrops atrox* (family Crotalidae). The serum is used specifically to treat bites of these snakes.

**antivenomous** (ăn″tĭ-vĕn′ŏ-mŭs) Opposing the action of venom.

**Antivert** Trade name for meclizine hydrochloride.

**antiviral** (ăn″tĭ-vī′răl) Opposing the action of a virus.

**antiviral resistance** The developed resistance of a virus to specific antiviral therapy.

**antivitamin** A vitamin antagonist; a substance that makes a vitamin ineffective.

**antivivisection** (ăn″tĭ-vĭv″ĭ-sĕk′shŭn) Opposition to the use of live animals in experimentation. SEE: *vivisection.*

**antixerotic** (ăn″tĭ-zē-rŏt′ĭk) [″ + *xerosis,* dryness] Preventing dryness of the skin.

**antizymotic** (ăn″tĭ-zī-mŏt′ĭk) [″ + *zymosis,* fermentation] An agent that prevents or arrests fermentation (e.g., alcohol or salicylic acid).

**Anton's syndrome** [Gabriel Anton, Ger. psychiatrist, 1858–1933] SEE: *anosognosia, visual.*

**antr-, antro-** [L. *antrum,* cavity] Combining form denoting *relationship to an antrum.*

**antra** (ăn′tră) [L.] Pl. of antrum.

**antrectomy** (ăn-trĕk′tō-mē) [L. *antrum,* cavity, + Gr. *ektome,* excision] Excision of the walls of an antrum.

**antritis** (ăn″trī′tĭs) [″ + Gr. *itis,* inflammation] Inflammation of an antrum, esp. the maxillary sinus.

**antroatticotomy** (ăn″trō-ăt″ĭ-kŏt′ō-mē) [″ + *atticus,* attic, + Gr. *tome,* incision] Operation to open the maxillary sinus and the attic of the tympanum.

**antrobuccal** (ăn″trō-bŭk′ăl) [″ + *bucca,* cheek] Concerning the maxillary sinus and the cheek.

**antrocele** (ăn′trō-sēl) [″ + Gr. *kele,* tumor, swelling] Fluid accumulation in a cyst in the maxillary sinus.

**antroduodenectomy** (ăn″trō-dū″ō-dĕ-nĕk′tō-mē) [″ + *duodeni,* twelve, + Gr. *ektome,* excision] Surgical removal of the pyloric antrum and the upper portion of the duodenum.

**antronasal** (ăn″trō-nā′zăl) [″ + *nasalis,* nasal] Rel. to the maxillary sinus and nasal fossa.

**antroscope** (ăn′trō-skōp) [″ + Gr. *skopein,* to examine] An instrument for visual examination of a cavity, esp. the maxillary sinus.

**antrostomy** (ăn-trŏs′tō-mē) [″ + Gr. *stoma,* mouth] Operation to form an opening in an antrum.

**antrotomy** (ăn″trŏt′ō-mē) Cutting through an antral wall.

**antrotympanic** (ăn″trō-tĭm-păn′ĭk) [L. *antrum,* cavity, + Gr. *tympanon,* drum] Rel. to the mastoid antrum and the tympanic cavity.

**antrotympanitis** (ăn″trō-tĭm″păn-ī′tĭs) [″ + ″ + *itis,* inflammation] Chronic inflammation of the tympanic cavity and mastoid antrum.

**antrum** (ăn′trŭm) *pl.* **antra** [L., cavity] Any nearly closed cavity or chamber, esp. in a bone. **antral** (-trăl), *adj.*

***a. auris*** External acoustic meatus.

***a. cardiacum*** The thoracic portion of the esophagus, functionally the superior portion of the stomach.

***duodenal a.*** The duodenal cap; a dilatation of the duodenum near the pylorus. It is seen during digestion.

***gastric a.*** Distal non–acid-secreting segment of the stomach or pyloric gland region that produces the hormone gastrin.

***a. of Highmore*** Maxillary a.

***mastoid a., mastoideum a.*** A cavity in the mastoid portion of the temporal bone. SYN: *tympanic a.*

***maxillary a.*** The maxillary sinus; a cavity in the maxillary bone communicating with the middle meatus of the nasal cavity. SYN: *a. of Highmore.*

***puncture of the a.*** Puncture of the maxillary sinus by insertion of a trocar through the sinus wall in order to drain fluid. The instrument is inserted near the floor of the nose, approx. 1½ in. (3.8 cm) from the nasal opening. SYN: *antrotomy.*

NURSING IMPLICATIONS: The antrum is irrigated with the prescribed solution (often warm normal saline solution) according to protocol. The character and volume of the returned solution and the patient's response to treatment are carefully monitored and documented. Ice packs are applied as prescribed for edema and pain; these are replaced by warm compresses as healing progresses. The nurse assesses for chills, fever, nausea, vomiting, facial or periorbital edema, visual disturbances, and personality changes, which indicate the development of complications.

***pyloric a., pyloricum a.*** A bulge in the pyloric portion of the stomach along the greater curvature on distention.

***tympanic a., tympanicum a.*** Mastoid a.

**ANTU** Alpha-naphthylthiourea, a powerful rat poison.

**Antuitrin S** Trade name for human chorionic gonadotropin.

**Anturane** Trade name for sulfinpyrazone.

**anuclear** (ă-nū′klē-ăr) Lacking a nucleus, said of erythrocytes.

**ANUG** *acute necrotizing ulcerative gingivitis.* SEE: *trench mouth.*

**anulus** (ăn′ū-lŭs) *pl.* **anuli** [L.] A ring-shaped structure; a ring. Also spelled *annulus.*

***a. abdominalis*** A. inguinalis profundus.

***a. femoralis*** Femoral ring; the abdominal opening of the femoral canal.

***a. fibrosus*** The outer portion of the intervertebral disk, consisting of concentric rings of collagen fibers (lamellae) oriented in varying directions and designed to withstand tensile and compressive loads on the spine as it transmits weight.

***a. inguinalis profundus*** Deep inguinal ring; the opening in the fascia transversalis for the ductus deferens in the male and the round ligament in the female. SYN: *a. abdominalis.*

***a. inguinalis superficialis*** Superficial inguinal ring; the opening in the external oblique muscle for the ductus deferens in the male and the round ligament in the female.

***a. tympanicus*** Tympanic ring; the part of the temporal bone forming a ring at the inner end of the external auditory canal.

***a. umbilicalis*** An opening in the abdominal wall of a fetus through which the umbilical vessels pass.

***a. urethralis*** Elevated muscular ring surrounding the opening of the bladder into the urethra. SYN: *bladder sphincter.*

**anuresis** (ăn-ū-rē′sĭs) [Gr. *an-,* not, + *ouresis,* urination] Absence of urination. SEE: *anuria.* **anuretic** (-rĕt′ĭk), *adj.*

**anuria** (ăn-ū′rē-ă) [″ + *ouron,* urine] Absence of urine formation. SEE: *anuresis.* **anuric,** *adj.*

**anus** (ā′nŭs) [L.] The outlet of the rectum lying in the fold between the buttocks.

***artificial a.*** An opening into the bowel formed by colostomy.

***imperforate a.*** Condition in which the anus is closed.

***vulvovaginal a.*** Congenital anomaly in a female in which the anus is imperforate but there is an opening from the rectum to the vagina.

**anvil** (ăn′vĭl) [AS. *anfilt*] A common name for the incus, the second of the three bones in the middle ear. SYN: *incus.* SEE: *ear* for illus.

**anxiety** (āng-zī′ĕ-tē) A vague feeling of apprehension, worry, uneasiness, or dread, the source of which is often nonspecific or unknown to the individual. Anxiety is the normal reaction to anything that threatens one's body, lifestyle, values, or loved ones. A certain amount of anxiety is normal and stimulates the individual to purposeful action. Excess anxiety interferes with efficient functioning of the individual. SEE: *neurosis, anxiety; Nursing Diagnoses Appendix.*

NURSING IMPLICATIONS: The nurse evaluates the patient's level of anxiety and documents related behaviors and physical characteristics, such as sympathetic nervous system arousal and effects on the patient's perceptual field and ability to learn and solve problems. Coping and defense mechanisms, avoidance behaviors, and surrounding circumstances are also assessed. The presence of a calm, caring nurse in a quiet, controlled atmosphere can prevent progression of the patient's anxiety and even reduce it by lessening feelings of isolation and instability. Patients with lower anxiety are assisted to identify and eliminate stressors, if possible. Appropriate outlets are provided for excess energy. The nurse establishes a trusting relationship, encouraging the patient to express feelings and concerns. False reassurance is never offered. Nursing care for patients with higher anxiety is focused on reducing environmental and other stimuli. Clear, simple validating statements are used to communicate with the patient and are repeated as often as necessary, and reality is reinforced if distortion is evident. The nurse attends to the patient's physical needs and encourages activity to help the patient discharge excess energy and relieve stress.

***free-floating a.*** Anxiety unrelated to an identifiable condition, situation, or cause.

**anxiety attack** An imprecise term for sudden onset of anxiety, sometimes accompanied by a sense of imminent danger or impending doom and an urge to escape. SEE: *panic attack.*

**anxiety disorder** Any of a group of mental conditions that include panic disorder with or without agoraphobia, agoraphobia without panic disorder, simple (specific) phobia, social phobia, obsessive-compulsive disorder, posttraumatic stress disorder, acute stress disorder, generalized anxiety disorder, anxiety caused by a general medical condition, and substance-induced anxiety disorder. The symptoms vary widely but interfere significantly with normal functioning. SEE: *Nursing Diagnoses Appendix.*

***generalized a.d.*** Excessive anxiety and worry predominating for at least 6 mo. Restlessness, easy fatiguability, difficulty in concentrating, irritability, muscle tension, and disturbed sleep may be present. Adults with this disorder often worry about everyday, routine circumstances such as job responsibilities, finances, the health of family members, misfortune to their children, or minor matters such as being late or completing household chores. Frequently they experience cold, clammy hands; dry mouth; sweating; nausea or diarrhea; urinary frequency; trouble swallowing or a "lump in the throat"; an exaggerated startle response; or depressive symptoms. The intensity, duration, or frequency of the anxiety and worry is far out of proportion to the actual likelihood or impact of the feared event.

**anxiolytic** (ăng″zī-ō-lĭt′ĭk) [L. *anxietas,* anxiety, + Gr. *lysis,* dissolution] **1.** Counteracting or relieving anxiety. **2.** A drug that relieves anxiety.

**A.O.A.** *Alpha Omega Alpha,* an honorary medical fraternity in the U.S.; *American Osteopathic Association.*

**AoA** *Administration on Aging.*

**A.O.C.** *anodal opening contraction.*

**A.O.R.N.** *Association of Operating Room Nurses.*

**aorta** (ā-or′tă) *pl.* **aortas, aortae** [L. from Gr. *aorte*] The main trunk of the arterial system of the body.

The aorta is about 3 cm in diameter at its origin in the upper surface of the left ventricle. It passes upward as the ascending aorta, turns backward and to the left (arch of the aorta) at about the level of the fourth thoracic vertebra, and then passes downward as the descending aorta, which is divided into the thoracic and abdominal aorta. The latter terminates at its division into the two common iliac arteries. At the junction of the aorta and the left ventricle is the aortic semilunar valve, which contains three cusps. This valve opens when the ventricle contracts and is closed by the backup of blood when the ventricle relaxes. SEE: illus.

The divisions of the aorta are as follows:

*Ascending aorta* (two branches): Two coronary arteries (right and left) provide blood supply to the myocardium.

*Aortic arch* (three branches): The brachiocephalic artery divides into the right subclavian artery, which provides blood to the right arm and other areas, and right common carotid artery, which

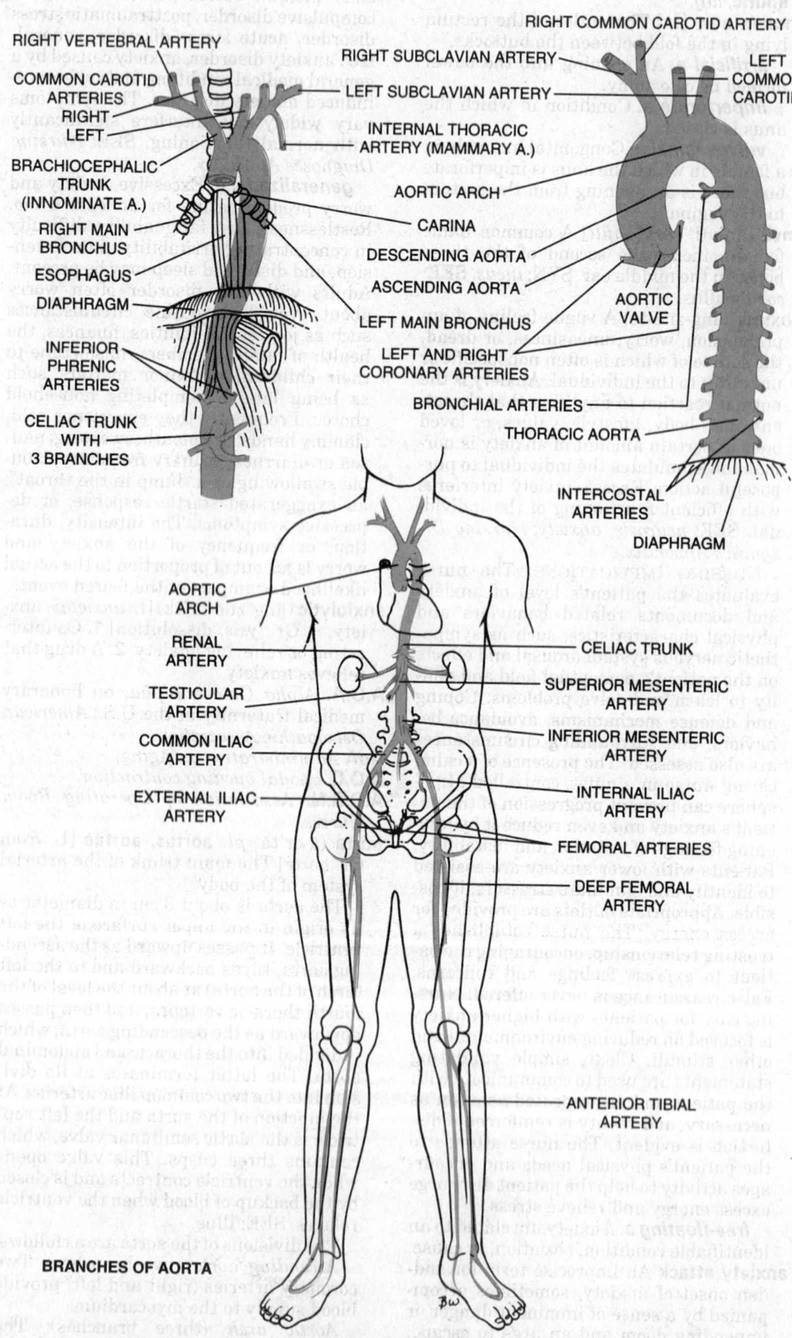


BRANCHES OF AORTA

supplies the right side of the head and neck. The left common carotid artery supplies the left side of the head and neck. The left subclavian artery provides blood for the left arm and portion of the thoracic area.

*Thoracic aorta:* Two or more bronchial arteries provide blood for bronchi. Esophageal arteries provide blood to the esophagus. Pericardial arteries supply the pericardium. Nine pairs of intercostal arteries supply blood for intercostal areas. Mediastinal branches supply lymph glands and the posterior mediastinum. Superior phrenic arteries supply the diaphragm.

*Abdominal aorta:* The celiac artery supplies the stomach, liver, and spleen. The superior mesenteric artery supplies all of the small intestine except the superior portion of the duodenum. The inferior mesenteric artery supplies all of the colon and rectum except the right half of the transverse colon. The middle suprarenal branches supply the adrenal (suprarenal) glands. The renal arteries supply the kidneys, ureters, and adrenals. The testicular arteries supply the testicles and ureter. The ovarian arteries (which correspond to internal spermatic arteries of the male) supply the ovaries, part of the ureters, and the uterine tubes. The inferior phrenic arteries supply the diaphragm and esophagus. The lumbar arteries supply the lumbar and psoas muscles and part of the abdominal wall musculature. The middle sacral artery supplies the sacrum and coccyx. The right and left common iliac arteries supply the lower pelvic and abdominal areas and the lower extremities. **aortal, aortic** (ā-or′tăl, -tĭk), *adj.*

**aortalgia** (ā″or-tăl′jē-ă) [L. from Gr. *aorte,* aorta, + *algos,* pain] Pain in the aortic area.

**aortarctia** (ā″or-tărk′shē-ă) [″ + L. *arctare,* to narrow] Aortic narrowing. SEE: *coarctation.*

**aortectasia** (ā″or-tĕk-tā′zē-ă) [″ + *ek,* out, + *tasis,* a stretching] Dilatation of the aorta.

**aortectomy** (ā″or-tĕk′tō-mē) [″ + *ektome,* excision] Excision of part of the aorta.

**aortic** (ā-or′tĭk) Pert. to the aorta.

***a. balloon pump*** SEE: *phase-shift balloon pumping.*

***a. bodies*** Chemoreceptors located in the wall of the aortic arch. They detect changes in oxygen concentration in the blood and generate nerve impulses to the medulla to increase or decrease respiration and peripheral vasoconstriction in order to restore normal oxygen concentration.

***a. insufficiency*** A. regurgitation.

***a. murmur*** An abnormal, soft sound heard on auscultation; may be due to obstruction or regurgitation. It is a symptom of aortic valvular disease. SEE: *Auscultation* under *heart.*

***a. opening*** A path through the diaphragm for the aorta.

***a. regurgitation*** Leakage of the blood from the aorta through the aortic valve back into the left ventricle after the ventricular contraction is completed. It is caused by diseases of the heart or aortic valves with defects or weakness of the heart muscle. SYN: *a. insufficiency.*

SYMPTOMS: Symptoms include an uncomfortable awareness of the heartbeat, especially when lying down; palpitations accompanied by a pounding in the head; dyspnea on exertion or paroxysmal nocturnal dyspnea with diaphoresis, orthopnea, and cough; fatigue and syncope with exertion or emotion; and anginal chest pain unrelieved by sublingual nitroglycerin. Heartbeats may seem to jar the entire body and the head may bob with each systole. Inspection of arterial pulses shows a rapidly rising pulse that collapses suddenly as arterial pressure falls late in systole (water-hammer pulse). The patient's nailbeds may appear to pulsate, and if pressure is applied at the nail tip, the nail root alternately flushes and pales (Quincke's sign). The chest may show a visible apical impulse, and the ankles may show edema and ascites associated with left ventricular failure. Peripheral pulses may rise and collapse rapidly (pulsus biferiens) and pulse irregularities may be present.

NURSING IMPLICATIONS: A history of related cardiac illnesses and symptoms is obtained. Fever and other signs of infection are noted. Vital signs, weight, and fluid intake and output are monitored for indications of fluid overload. Activity tolerance and degree of fatigue are assessed regularly, and the patient is taught to intersperse periods of activity with rest. If bedrest is required, its importance is explained, assistance is offered as necessary, and a bedside commode is provided because it requires less cardiac effort than the use of a bedpan. The patient is encouraged to express concerns about activity restrictions and is reassured of their temporary nature. The patient is placed in an upright position to relieve dyspnea if necessary, and prescribed oxygen is administered to prevent tissue hypoxia. When sitting in a chair, the patient should keep the legs elevated to improve venous return. The diet should consist of foods that the patient enjoys, but prescribed dietary restrictions must be maintained. The patient receives appropriate instruction regarding prescribed medications.

Desired outcomes include adequate cardiopulmonary tissue perfusion and cardiac output, reduced fatigue with exertion, and ability to manage the treatment regimen.

***a. septal defect*** A congenital abnormality in which there is a communication between the ascending aorta and the pulmonary artery, requiring surgery to correct.

***a. stenosis*** Narrowing of the aorta or its orifice due to lesions of the wall with scar formation. It is caused by infection, as in rheumatic fever, or by embryonic anomalies. Hypertrophy of the heart is a common result. SYN: *aortostenosis*. SEE: *Nursing Diagnoses Appendix*.

SYMPTOMS: Symptoms include dyspnea on exertion, fatigue, exertional syncope, angina, and palpitations. Orthopnea and paroxysmal nocturnal dyspnea are due to left ventricular failure. Peripheral edema may be present. Palpation detects diminished carotid pulses and pulsus alternans, displacement of the apical impulse, and a systolic thrill at the base of the heart, at the jugular notch, and along the carotid arteries.

NURSING IMPLICATIONS: The nurse obtains a history of related cardiac disorders. Cardiopulmonary function is assessed regularly by monitoring vital signs and weight, intake, and output for signs of fluid overload. The patient is monitored for chest pain, which may indicate cardiac ischemia, and the electrocardiogram evaluated for ischemic changes. Activity tolerance and fatigue are assessed.

After cardiac catheterization, the insertion site is checked according to protocol (often every 15 min for 6 hr) for signs of bleeding; the patient is assessed for chest pain, and vital signs, heart rhythm, and peripheral pulses distal to the insertion site are monitored. Problems are reported to the cardiologist.

Desired outcomes include adequate cardiopulmonary tissue perfusion and cardiac output, reduced fatigue with exertion, absence of fluid volume excess, and ability to manage the treatment regimen.

***a. valve*** The valve between the left ventricle and the ascending aorta that prevents regurgitation of blood back into the left ventricle. It is composed of three segments, each of which is called a semilunar cusp. The valve is open during ventricular systole and closed during diastole.

**aortitis** (ā-or-tī'tĭs) [L. from Gr. *aorte,* aorta, + *itis,* inflammation] Inflammation of the aorta. This condition is associated with syphilis and other diseases in which vascular changes have taken place. It is a common cause of aortic aneurysm. Symptoms include possible cough, cyanosis, dyspnea, cardiac asthmatic attacks, and hemoptysis.

**aortoclasia** (ā″or-tō-klā'zē-ă) [″ + *klasis,* a breaking] Aortic rupture.

**aortocoronary** (ā-or″tō-kor'ŏ-nā-rē) Pert. to both the aorta and the coronary arteries.

**aortocoronary bypass** Coronary artery bypass surgery.

**aortogram** (ā-or'tō-grăm″) [″ + *gramma,* something written] An image of the aorta obtained through radiography, computed tomography, or magnetic resonance imaging, usually after the injection of a contrast agent.

**aortography** (ā″or-tog'ră-fē) [L. from Gr. *aorte,* aorta, + *graphein,* to write] Radiography of the aorta after injection of a contrast medium. **aortographic** (-grăf'ĭk), *adj.*

***retrograde a.*** Aortography by injection of a contrast medium into the aorta via one of its branches, and thus against the direction of the blood flow.

***translumbar a.*** Aortography by injection of a contrast medium into the abdominal aorta through a needle inserted into the lumbar area near the level of the 12th rib.

**aortoiliac** (ā-or″tō-ĭl'ē-ăk) Pert. to both the aorta and the iliac arteries.

**aortolith** (ā-or'tō-lĭth) [″ + *lithos,* stone] Calcareous deposit in the aortic wall.

**aortomalacia** (ā-or″tō-mă-lā'shē-ă) [″ + *malakia,* softness] Softening of the walls of the aorta.

**aortoplasty** (ā-or″tō-plăs″tē) Surgical repair of the aorta.

**aortorrhaphy** (ā″or-tor'ă-fē) [″ + *rhaphe,* seam, ridge] Suture of the aorta.

**aortosclerosis** (ā-or″tō-sklĕr-ō'sĭs) [″ + *skleros,* hard] Aortic sclerosis.

**aortostenosis** (ā-or″tō-stĕ-nō'sĭs) Aortic stenosis.

**aortotomy** (ā″or-tŏt'ō-mē) [″ + *tome,* incision] Incision of the aorta.

**AOS** *anodal opening sound.*

**A.O.S.S.M.** *American Orthopedic Society for Sports Medicine.*

**A.O.T.A.** *American Occupational Therapy Association.*

**A.O.T.F.** *American Occupational Therapy Foundation.*

**A.P.** *anteroposterior.*

**A.P.A.** *American Pharmaceutical Association; American Physiotherapy Association; American Podiatry Association; American Psychiatric Association; American Psychological Association.*

**APACHE II** Acronym for *Acute Physiology and Chronic Health Evaluation,* a severity of disease classification system.

**apallesthesia** (ă-păl″ĕs-thē'zē-ă) [″ + *pallein,* to tremble, + *aisthesis,* sensation] Inability to sense vibrations. SEE: *pallesthesia.*

**apancreatic** (ă-păn″krē-ăt'ĭk) **1.** Caused by absence of the pancreas. **2.** Pert. to noninvolvement of the pancreas.

**aparalytic** (ă-păr″ă-lĭt'ĭk) [Gr. *a-,* not, + *paralyein,* to loosen] Marked by lack of paralysis.

**aparathyrosis** (ă-păr″ă-thī-rō'sĭs) [″ + *para,* near, + *thyreos,* an oblong shield, + *osis,* condition] Parathyroid deficiency.

**apareunia** (ă″păr-ū'nē-ă) [″ + *pareunos,* lying with] Inability to accomplish sexual intercourse. SEE: *dyspareunia.*

**aparthrosis** (ăp″ăr-thrō'sĭs) [Gr. *apo,* from, + *arthron,* joint, + *osis,* condition] **1.** A joint that moves freely in any direction, such as the shoulder joint. SYN: *diarthrosis.* **2.** Dislocation of a joint.

**apathetic** (ăp″ă-thĕt′ĭk) [″ + *pathos,* disease, suffering] Indifferent; without interest. SYN: *apathic.*

**apathic** (ă-păth′ĭk) Apathetic.

**apathism** (ăp′ă-thĭzm) [″ + *pathos,* disease, suffering, + *-ismos,* condition] Slowness to react to stimuli; opposite of erethism.

**apathy** (ăp′ă-thē) [Gr. *apatheia*] Indifference; insensibility; lack of emotion. SYN: *acedia.*

**apatite** (ăp′ă-tīt″) [Ger. *Apatit,* "the deceptive stone"] A mineral containing calcium and phosphate ions and a univalent anion in a specific ratio; the major constituent of teeth and bones.

**APC** *absolute phagocyte count.*

**A.P.C.** *aspirin, phenacetin,* and *caffeine,* common ingredients in various headache and cold tablets. Phenacetin is no longer considered suitable for use in any form.

**APE** *anterior pituitary extract.*

**apellous** (ă-pĕl′ŭs) [Gr. *a-,* not, + L. *pellis,* skin] **1.** Lacking skin. **2.** Lacking foreskin; circumcised.

**apepsia** (ă-pĕp′sē-ă) [Gr. *a-,* not, + *pepsis,* digesting] Cessation of digestion.

**apepsinia** (ă″pĕp-sĭn′ē-ă) Absence of pepsin in the gastric juice.

**aperient** (ă-pĕr′ē-ĕnt) [L. *aperiens,* opening] **1.** Having a mild laxative effect. **2.** A mild laxative.

**aperiodic** Occurring other than periodically.

**aperistalsis** (ă″pĕr-ĭ-stăl′sĭs) [Gr. *a-,* not, + *peri,* around, + *stalsis,* constriction] Absence of peristalsis.

**apéritif** (ă-pĕr″ĭ-tēf′) [L. *aperire,* to open] An alcoholic beverage, such as wine, taken before a meal to stimulate the appetite.

**aperitive** (ă-pĕr′ĭ-tĭv) **1.** Stimulating the appetite. **2.** Aperient.

**Apert's syndrome** (ă-pārz′) [Eugene Apert, Fr. pediatrician, 1868–1940] A congenital condition marked by a peaked head and webbed fingers and toes. Oral manifestations include cleft palate or uvula, a prognathic mandible, and maxillary hypoplasia, resulting in extreme malocclusion.

**apertura** (ăp″ĕr-tū′ră) *pl.* **aperturae** [L.] An opening.

**aperture** (ăp′ĕr-chūr″) An orifice or opening, esp. to anatomical or bony spaces or canals.

**apex** (ā′pĕks) *pl.* **apexes, apices** [L., tip] The pointed extremity of a conical structure. **apical** (ăp′ĭ-kal, ā′pĭ-kal), *adj.*

***a. of the lung*** The superior, subclavicular portion of the lung.

***root a.*** The end of the root of a tooth.

**apex beat** In systole, the movement of the apex of the left ventricle against the chest wall. It is felt in the fifth left intercostal space, approx. 3 ½ in. (8.9 cm) from the middle of the sternum, about 1 in. (2.5 cm) within a line drawn down from the middle of the clavicle parallel with the sternum (the mammary line). Generally it may be detected by inspection or palpation; when these fail, it may be localized by auscultation. As a rule, the patient should be examined in an erect or sitting position while breathing quietly. If the patient is lying down, the apex beat may be detected 1 in. (2.5 cm) or more higher. When the body is inclined to the left, the beat may be detected inside or outside the mammary line. During forced inspiration, it may become imperceptible or be found below its usual place. During forced expiration, the beat becomes more forcible and may be found above its usual place.

ABNORMALITIES: A weak apex beat may be noted in healthy persons at rest and in heart failure, pericardial effusion, emphysema, shock, or collapse.

Changes in the force and extent of the apex beat may be increased by hypertrophy of the heart, exercise, drugs, reflex irritation, excitement, or disease (such as exophthalmic goiter).

Deformity of the chest may cause displacement in any direction. Displacement to the left may result from hypertrophy and dilatation of the heart (down and to the left); pneumothorax (on the right); pericardial effusion (up and to the left); chronic diseases of the left lung and pleura associated with retraction, as fibroid tuberculosis and pleural adhesions; abdominal tumors and effusions (up and to the left); or pressure of a pleural effusion on the right side (up and to the left).

Displacement to the right may be caused by chronic disease of the right lung or pleura associated with retraction; pneumothorax on the left; or pressure of a pleural effusion on the left side.

Displacement downward may result from hypertrophy and dilatation of the heart, chiefly the left ventricle; pressure of solid growths in the upper mediastinum; an aneurysm of the aortic arch; or enlargement of the liver, causing traction through the central tendon of the diaphragm.

Precordial prominence may result from deformity, enlargement of the heart, or pericardial effusions.

**apexcardiogram** A graphic record of chest wall movements produced by the apex beat.

**apexigraph, apexograph** (ā-pĕks′ĭ-grăf, -ō-grăf) [L. *apex,* tip, + Gr. *graphein,* to write] An instrument for determining the location and size of the apex of a tooth root.

**apex murmur** Murmur over the apex of the heart.

**Apgar score** [Virginia Apgar, U.S. anesthesiologist, 1909–1974] A system for evaluating an infant's physical condition at birth. The infant's heart rate, respiration, muscle tone, response to stimuli, and color are rated at 1 min, and again at 5 min, after birth. Each factor is scored 0, 1, or 2; the maximum total score is 10. *Interpretation of scores:* 7 to 10, good to ex-

**Apgar Score**

| Sign | Score 0 | Score 1 | Score 2 |
|---|---|---|---|
| Heart rate | Absent | Slow (less than 100) | Greater than 100 |
| Respiratory effort | Absent | Slow, irregular | Good; crying |
| Muscle tone | Limp | Some flexion of extremities | Active motion |
| Reflex irritability | No response | Grimace | Cough or sneeze |
| Color* | Blue, pale | Body pink; extremities blue | Completely pink |

* Skin color or its absence may not be a reliable guide in nonwhites, although melanin is less apparent at birth than later.

cellent; 4 to 6, fair; less than 4, poor condition. A low score at 1 min is a sign of perinatal asphyxia and the need for immediate assisted ventilation. Infants with scores below 7 at 5 min should be assessed again in 5 more min; scores less than 6 at any time may indicate need for resuscitation. In depressed infants, a more accurate determination of the degree of fetal hypoxia may be obtained by direct measures of umbilical cord oxygen, carbon dioxide partial pressure, and pH. SEE: table; *biophysical profile.*

**A.P.H.A.** *American Public Health Association.*

**aphacia, aphakia** (ă-fā′sē-ă, -kē-ă) [″ + *phakos,* lentil] Absence of the crystalline lens of the eye. **aphacic, aphakic** (ă-fā′sĭk, -kĭk), *adj.*

**aphagia** (ă-fā′jē-ă) [Gr. *a-,* not, + *phagein,* to eat] Inability to swallow.

**aphalangia** (ă″fă-lăn′jē-ă) [″ + *phalanx,* closely knit row] Absence of fingers or toes.

**aphanisis** (ă-făn′ĭ-sĭs) [Gr. *aphaneia,* disappearance] Fear or apprehension that sexual potency will be lost.

**aphasia** (ă-fā′zē-ă) [Gr. *a-,* not, + *phasis,* speaking] Absence or impairment of the ability to communicate through speech, writing, or signs because of brain dysfunction. It is considered complete or total when both sensory and motor areas are involved. **aphasic** (-zĭk), *adj.* SEE: *alalia.*

***amnesic a.*** Anomic a.

***anomic a.*** Inability to name objects; loss of memory for words.

***auditory a.*** Inability to understand spoken words. SYN: *word deafness.*

***Broca's a.*** Motor a.

***conduction a.*** Aphasia due to a lesion of the conduction path between the motor and speech centers.

***fluent a.*** Aphasia in which words are easily spoken but those used are incorrect and may be unrelated to the content of the other words spoken.

***gibberish a.*** Utterance of meaningless phrases.

***global a.*** Total aphasia involving failure of all forms of communication.

***jargon a.*** Communication that results in the use of jargon or disconnected words.

***mixed a.*** Combined sensory and motor aphasia.

***motor a.*** Aphasia in which patients know what they want to say but cannot say it; inability to coordinate the muscles controlling speech. It may be complete or partial. Broca's area is disordered or diseased.

***nominal a.*** Inability to name objects.

***optic a.*** Inability to name an object recognized by sight without the aid of sound, taste, or touch; a form of agnosia.

***semantic a.*** Inability to understand the meaning of words.

***sensory a.*** Inability to understand spoken words if the auditory word center is involved (auditory aphasia) or written words if the visual word center is affected (visual aphasia). If both centers are involved, the patient will not understand spoken or written words.

***syntactic a.*** Loss of the ability to use proper grammatical construction.

***traumatic a.*** Aphasia caused by head injury.

***visual a.*** Inability to understand the written word. SYN: *word blindness.*

***Wernicke's a.*** An injury to Wernicke's area in the temporal lobe of the dominant hemisphere of the brain, resulting in an inability to comprehend the spoken or written word. Visual and auditory pathways are unaffected; however, patients are unable to differentiate between words and interpret their meaning. Although patients speak fluently, they are unable to function socially because their ability to communicate effectively is impaired by a disordered speech pattern called paraphasia (i.e., inserting inappropriate syllables into words or substituting one word for another). They also may be unable to repeat spoken words.

**aphasiac** (ă-fā′zē-ăk) An individual affected with aphasia.

**aphasic** (ă-fā″zĭk) **1.** Pert. to aphasia. **2.** An individual affected with aphasia.

**aphasiologist** (ă-fā″zē-ŏl′ō-jĭst) [Gr. *a-,* not, + *phasis,* speaking, + *logos,* word, reason] A person who studies the pathology of language and the production of speech and written language.

**aphemia** (ă-fē′mē-ă) [″ + *pheme,* speech]

**1.** Loss of the power to speak. SYN: *motor aphasia.* **2.** Loss of the power to speak distinctly. SYN: *anarthria.*

**aphephobia** (af″ĕ-fō′bē-ă) [Gr. *haphe,* touch, + *phobos,* fear] Morbid fear of being touched.

**apheresis, therapeutic** (ă-fĕr′ē-sĭs) [Gr. *aphairesis,* separation] Removal of unwanted or pathological components from a patient's blood by means of a continuous-flow separator; the process is similar to hemodialysis, as detoxified blood is returned to the patient. The removal of cellular material is termed cytapheresis; leukapheresis describes the removal of leukocytes only. Plasmapheresis, also called plasma exchange, involves removal of noncellular materials. Therapeutic apharesis has been used to treat blood hyperviscosity, cold agglutinin hemolytic anemia, posttransfusion purpura, thrombotic thrombocytopenic purpura, myasthenia gravis, sickle cell anemia, Guillain-Barré syndrome, familial hypercholesterolemia, and certain drug overdoses.

**aphonia** (ă-fō′nē-ă) [Gr. *a-,* not, + *phone,* voice] Loss of speech sounds from the larynx, as may occur in chronic laryngitis. It is not caused by a brain lesion. The condition may be caused by disease of the vocal cords, paralysis of the laryngeal nerves, or pressure on the recurrent laryngeal nerve; or it may be functional due to hysteria or psychiatric causes.

***hysterical a.*** Aphonia due to hysteria. There is no organic defect.

***a. paranoica*** Obstinate silence in the mentally ill.

***spastic a.*** Aphonia resulting from spasm of the vocal muscles, esp. that initiated by efforts to speak.

**aphonogelia** (ă-fō″nō-jē′lē-ă) [″ + *phone,* voice, + *gelos,* laughter] Inability to laugh out loud.

**aphose** (ăf′ōz) [″ + *phos,* light] A subjective visual perception of darkness or of a shadow.

**aphrasia** (ă-frā′zē-ă) [″ + *phrasis,* speech] Inability to speak or understand phrases.

**aphrodisiac** (ăf″rō-dĭz′ē-ăk) **1.** Stimulating sexual desire. **2.** A drug, food, environment, or other agent that arouses sexual desire.

**aphtha** (ăf′thah) *pl.* **aphthae** [Gr. *aphtha,* small ulcer] A small ulcer on a mucous membrane of the mouth, as in thrush. **aphthic** (-thik), *adj.*

***Bednar's a.'s*** SEE: *Bednar's aphthae.*

***cachectic a.*** A lesion formed beneath the tongue and accompanied by severe constitutional symptoms.

**aphthoid** (ăf′thoyd) Resembling aphthae.

**aphthongia** (ăf-thŏn′jē-ă) [Gr. *a-,* not, + *phthongos,* voice] Inability to speak due to spasm of muscles controlling speech.

**aphthosis** (ăf-thō′sĭs) [Gr. *aphtha,* small ulcer, + *osis,* condition] Any condition characterized by aphthae.

**aphthous** (ăf′thŭs) [Gr. *aphtha,* small ulcer] Pert. to, or characterized by, aphthae.

**aphthous ulcer** An oral lesion caused by recurrent stomatitis. It is usually less than 0.5 cm in diameter. If it persists for longer than 2 weeks, it should be biopsied in order to rule out cancer. SYN: *aphthous stomatitis; canker sore.*

ETIOLOGY: The cause is unknown, but an autoimmune basis is suspected. Fever, mental stress, or exposure to certain foods may precede these lesions.

TREATMENT: Application of topical tetracycline several times a day relieves pain and shortens healing time. Application of a topical anesthetic or a protective paste, such as Orabase, provides symptomatic relief and makes it possible to eat without pain.

**apical** (ăp′ĭ-kal, ā′pĭ-kal) [L. *apex,* tip] Pert. to the apex of a structure.

**apical heave** In children, visible heaving of the chest over the apex of the heart. This indicates left ventricular hypertrophy. SEE: *substernal thrust.*

**apicectomy** (ăp″ĭ-sĕk′tō-mē) [L. *apex,* tip, + Gr. *ektome,* excision] Excision of the apex of the petrous portion of the temporal bone.

**apices** (ā′pĭ-sēz, ăp′ĭ-sēz) [L.] Pl. of apex.

**apicitis** (ăp-ĭ-sī′tĭs) [L. *apices,* tips, + Gr. *itis,* inflammation] Inflammation of an apex, esp. that of a lung or tooth root.

**apicoectomy** (ăp-ĭ-kō-ĕk′tō-mē) [L. *apex,* tip, + Gr. *ektome,* excision] Excision of the apex of the root of a tooth.

**apicolocator** (ă″pĭ-kō-lō′kā-tor) [″ + *locare,* to place] An instrument for locating the apex of the root of a tooth.

**apicolysis** (ăp″ĭ-kŏl′ĭ-sĭs) [″ + Gr. *lysis,* dissolution] Artificial collapse of the apex of a lung by creation of an opening through the anterior chest wall.

NURSING IMPLICATIONS: The patient's understanding of the procedure is determined and misinformation corrected. At the same time, the nurse evaluates the patient for symptoms of anxiety and provides emotional support. During and after the procedure, the patient is assessed for symptoms of tension pneumothorax (increased pulse and respirations, cyanosis, and marked dyspnea, along with severe sharp pain, tympanic resonance to percussion, and absent breath sounds on auscultation of the affected side) and for symptoms of a mediastinal shift (cyanosis, severe dyspnea, distended neck veins, increased pulse and respiratory rate, and excessive, uncontrollable coughing). After the procedure, the patient is positioned as prescribed, usually on the affected side.

**Apicomplexa** A phylum of the kingdom Protista (formerly a division of protozoa called *Sporozoa*; named for a complex of cell organelles (apical microtubule complex) at the apex of the sporozoite form that can penetrate host cells. It includes the medically important genera *Plasmo-*

*dium, Toxoplasma, Cryptosporidium*, and *Isospora*.

**apicostomy** (āp″ĭ-kŏs′tō-mē) [L. *apex*, tip, + Gr. *stoma*, mouth] Surgical removal of the mucoperiosteum and bone in order to expose the apex of the root of a tooth.

**apicotomy** (ăp″ĭ-kŏt′ō-mē) [L. *apex*, tip, + Gr. *tome*, incision] Incision of an apical structure.

**apinealism** (ă-pĭn′ē-ăl-ĭzm) [Gr. *a-*, not, + L. *pinea*, pine cone, + Gr. *-ismos*, condition] Absence of the pineal gland.

**apiphobia** [L. *apis*, bee, + phobia] Unrealistic fear of bees.

**A.P.L.** Trade name for chorionic gonadotropin, human.

**aplanatic** (ă″plă-năt′ĭk) [Gr. *a-*, not, + *planetos*, wandering] Free from or correcting spherical aberration.

**aplasia** (ă-plā′zē-ă) [″ + *plasis*, a developing] Failure of an organ or tissue to develop normally. **aplastic** (ă-plăs′tĭk), *adj.*

***a. axialis extracorticalis congenita*** Congenital defect of the axon formation on the surface of the cerebral cortex.

***a. cutis congenita*** Defective development of a localized area of the skin, usually on the scalp. The area is usually covered by a thin, translucent membrane.

**aplastic crisis, transient** ABBR: TAC. A serious complication of infection with human parvovirus B-19 infection in patients with chronic hemolytic anemia such as sickle cell disease. This virus causes erythema infectiosum. SEE: *erythema infectiosum*.

**Apley's scratch test** A test to functionally assess range of motion of the shoulders. The patient reaches over the head with one hand and behind the back with the other hand and is then asked to scratch the back. This is a quick method of testing abduction and lateral rotation of one shoulder and adduction and medial rotation of the other shoulder.

**A.P.M.A.** *American Podiatric Medical Association*. Formerly called the American Podiatry Association.

**apnea** (ăp-nē′ă) [″ + *pnoe*, breathing] Temporary cessation of breathing. Apnea may result from reduction in stimuli to the respiratory center (as in overbreathing, in which carbon dioxide content of the blood is reduced), from failure of the respiratory center to discharge impulses (as in voluntary breath-holding), or from Cheyne-Stokes respiration. SEE: *apnea monitoring; Cheyne-Stokes respiration; sleep apnea* under *sleep, disorders of; sudden infant death syndrome*.

It is a serious symptom, esp. in conditions such as arteriosclerosis, meningitis, coma, heart and kidney diseases, and concussion of the brain. Sometimes Cheyne-Stokes respiration is noticed in healthy children and in the aged during profound sleep.

***a. of prematurity*** ABBR: AOP. A condition of the immature newborn marked by repeated episodes of apnea lasting longer than 20 sec. It is thought to be related to neurological immaturity, pharyngeal obstruction, or both. Increased frequency of apneic episodes is directly related to the degree of prematurity. Apneic episodes may result in bradycardia, hypoxia, respiratory acidosis, and death.

TREATMENT: Methylxanthines such as theophylline are helpful.

NURSING IMPLICATIONS: Care should include maintenance of a neutral thermal environment, avoidance of prolonged oral feedings, use of tactile stimulation early in the apneic episode, and ventilatory support as needed. The infant is maintained on cardiac and respiratory monitoring devices. Before discharge, parents are taught cardiopulmonary resuscitation, use of monitoring equipment, and how to recognize signs of medication toxicity.

***sleep a.*** Suspension of breathing during sleep. SEE: *sleep apnea*.

**apnea alarm mattress** A mattress that is designed to sound an alarm when the infant lying on it ceases to breathe. SEE: *apnea monitoring; sudden infant death syndrome*.

**apnea monitoring** Monitoring the respiratory movements, esp. of infants. This may be done by use of an apnea alarm mattress, or devices to measure the infant's thoracic and abdominal movements and heart rate. SEE: *sudden infant death syndrome*.

**apneic oxygenation** The supplying of oxygen to the upper airway of patients who are not breathing.

**apneumatic** (ăp″nū-măt′ĭk) [Gr. *a-*, not, + *pneuma*, air] **1.** Free of air, as in a collapsed lung. **2.** Pert. to a procedure done in the absence of air.

**apneumatosis** (ăp″nū-mă-tō′sĭs) [″ + ″ + *osis*, condition] Noninflation of air cells of the lung; congenital atelectasis.

**apneumia** (ăp-nū′mē-ă) [″ + *pneumon*, lung] Congenital absence of the lungs.

**apneusis** (ăp-nū′sĭs) Abnormal respiration marked by sustained inspiratory effort; caused by surgical removal of the upper portion of the pons.

**apo-** (ăp′ō) [Gr. *apo*, from] Combining form meaning *separated from* or *derived from*.

**apo(a)** Abbreviation for apolipoprotein(a).

**apocamnosis** (ăp″ō-kăm-nō′sĭs) [Gr. *apokamnein*, to grow weary] Weariness; easily induced fatigue.

**apochromatic** (ăp″ō-krō-măt′ĭk) Free from spherical and chromatic aberrations.

**apocrine** (ăp′ō-krēn, -krīn, -krĭn) [Gr. *apo*, from, + *krinein*, to separate] Denoting secretory cells that contribute part of their protoplasm to the material secreted. SEE: *eccrine; holocrine; merocrine*.

**apocrine sweat glands** Sweat glands located in the axillae and pubic region that open into hair follicles rather than directly onto the surface of the skin as do eccrine sweat glands. They appear after puberty and are better developed in women than in men. The characteristic odor of perspiration is produced by the action of bacteria on the material secreted by the apocrine sweat glands. SEE: *sweat glands.*

**apodal** (ă-pō′dăl) [Gr. *a-*, not, + *pous*, foot] Lacking feet.

**apodia** (ă-pō′dē-ă) [Gr. *a-*, not, + *pous*, foot] Congenital absence of one or both feet.

**apoenzyme** (ăp-ō-ĕn′zīm) The protein portion of an enzyme. SEE: *holoenzyme; prosthetic group.*

**apoferritin** (ăp″ō-fĕr′ĭ-tĭn) A protein that combines with iron to form ferritin. In the body, it is always bound to iron.

**apogee** (ăp′ō-jē) [Gr. *apo*, from, + *gaia*, earth] The climax or period of greatest severity of a disease.

**apolar** (ă-pō′lăr) [Gr. *a-*, not, + *polos*, pole] Without poles or processes. Some nerve cells are apolar.

**apolipoprotein** The nonlipid protein portion of a lipoprotein. The apolipoproteins are classified according to function into five major groups—B100, A-I, A-II, B, and E—with subclasses in some groups. Apolipoproteins bind to specific enzymes on cell membranes and transport the lipoproteins to their sites of metabolism. SEE: *lipoprotein.*

**apomorphine** (ăp″ō-mor′fĕn) [Gr. *apo*, from, + *morphine*] A morphine derivative prepared by removal of one molecule of water from the morphine molecule.

***a. hydrochloride*** A grayish white powder that becomes green on exposure to water or air. An emetic, apomorphine hydrochloride may be valuable in cases of poisoning when gastric lavage cannot be employed. In small doses it may be used as an expectorant.

**aponeurology** (ăp″ō-nū-rŏl′ō-jē) [″ + *neuron*, nerve, tendon, + *logos*, word, reason] The branch of anatomy dealing with aponeuroses.

**aponeurorrhaphy** (ăp″ō-nū-ror′ă-fē) [″+ ″ + *rhaphe*, seam, ridge] Suture of an aponeurosis.

**aponeurosis** (ăp″ō-nū-rō′sĭs) *pl.* **aponeuroses** [″ + *neuron*, nerve, tendon] A flat fibrous sheet of connective tissue that attaches muscle to bone or other tissues; may sometimes serve as a fascia. **aponeurotic** (-rŏt′ĭk), *adj.*

***epicranial a.*** Fibrous membrane connecting the occipital and frontal muscles. SYN: *galea aponeurotica.*

***lingual a.*** Connective tissue sheet of the tongue to which lingual muscles attach.

***palatine a.*** Connective tissue sheet of the soft palate to which palatal muscles attach.

***pharyngeal a.*** Sheet of connective tissue lying between the mucosal and muscular layers of the pharyngeal wall. SYN: *pharyngobasilar fascia.*

***plantar a.*** Sheet of connective tissue investing the muscles of the sole of the foot. SYN: *plantar fascia.*

**aponeurositis** (ăp″ō-nū-rō-sī′tĭs) [″ + ″ + *itis*, inflammation] Inflammation of an aponeurosis.

**aponeurotome** (ăp″ō-nū′rō-tōm) [″ + ″ + *tome*, incision] Surgical instrument for cutting an aponeurosis.

**aponeurotomy** (ăp″ō-nū-rŏt′ō-mē) Incision of an aponeurosis.

**apophysis** (ă-pŏf′ĭ-sĭs) *pl.* **apophyses** [Gr. *apophysis*, off-shoot] A projection, esp. from a bone (e.g. a tubercle); an outgrowth without an independent center of ossification. **apophyseal, apophysial** (ăp″ō-fĭz′ē-ăl), *adj.*

***basilar a.*** Basilar process of the occipital bone.

***a. of Ingrassia*** Smaller wing of the sphenoid bone.

***lenticular a.*** Lenticular process of the incus, which articulates with the stapes.

***a. of Rau, a. raviana*** Anterior process of the malleus.

***temporal a.*** Mastoid process of the temporal bone.

***vertebral a.*** Superior and inferior articular process of the vertebral arches.

**apophysitis** (ă-pŏf″ĭ-sī′tĭs) [Gr. *apo*, from, + *physis*, growth, + *itis*, inflammation] Inflammation of an apophysis.

**apoplectic** (ăp″ō-plĕk′tĭk) [Gr. *apoplektikos*, crippled by stroke] Pert. to apoplexy.

**apoplectiform** (ăp″ō-plĕk′tĭ-form) [Gr. *apoplexia*, stroke, + L. *forma*, form] Resembling apoplexy. SYN: *apoplectoid.*

**apoplectoid** (ăp″ō-plĕk′toyd) [″ + *eidos*, form, shape] Apoplectiform.

**apoplexia** (ăp″ō-plĕk′sē-ă) [Gr. *apoplessein*, to cripple by a stroke] Apoplexy.

***a. uteri*** Sudden hemorrhage from the uterus.

**apoplexy** (ăp′ō-plĕk″sē) [Gr. *apoplessein*, to cripple by a stroke] **1.** Copious effusion of blood into an organ, as in abdominal apoplexy or pulmonary apoplexy. **2.** Sudden loss of consciousness followed by paralysis caused by hemorrhage into brain; formation of an embolus or thrombus that occludes an artery; or rupture of an extracerebral artery causing subarachnoid hemorrhage. SYN: *cerebrovascular accident; stroke.*

SYMPTOMS: Onset is acute, with unconsciousness, stertorous respiration due to paralysis of part of the soft palate, and expiration puffing out the cheeks and mouth. The pupils are sometimes unequal, the larger one being on the side of the hemorrhage. Paralysis usually involves one side of the body, with eyeballs turned away from the affected side; the skin is covered with clammy sweat, and the surface temperature of the skin is often subnormal; speech may be disordered or impossible. Onset is more gradual in the case of a thrombosis.

FIRST AID: In the hospital or at home, the patient, if conscious, should be kept quiet and sitting up or lying down with head and shoulders elevated. This will help to prevent aspiration of saliva. Clothing should be loosened, esp. around the neck. Stimulants should not be given. Cooling applications should be used on the head and neck.

PROGNOSIS: Prognosis depends on symptoms, but is often poor.

**apoptosis** (ă-pŏp-tō′sĭs, ă-pō-tō′sĭs) [Gr. *apo,* from, + *ptosis,* a dropping] **1.** Disintegration of cells into membrane-bound particles that are then phagocytosed by other cells. The process may be important in limiting growth of tumors. **2.** Programmed death of cells.

**aporepressor** (ăp″ō-rē-prĕs′or) A protein, the synthesis of which is directed by a regulator gene, that functions only when bound with specific low-molecular-weight compounds called corepressors.

**aposia** (ă-pō′zē-ă) [Gr. *a-,* not, + *posis,* drink] Absence of thirst. SYN: *adipsia.*

**apotemnophilia** (ăp″ō-tĕm″nō-fēl′ē-ă) [Gr. *apo,* away, + *temnein,* to cut, + *philein,* to love] A form of paraphilia characterized by the individual requesting amputation of an extremity for erotic reasons.

**apothecaries' weights and measures** An outdated and obsolete system of weights and measures formerly used by physicians and pharmacists; based on 480 grains to 1 oz and 12 oz to 1 lb. It has been replaced by the metric system. SEE: *Weights and Measures Appendix.*

**apothecary** (ă-pŏth′ĕ-kā-rē) [Gr. *apotheke,* storing place] A druggist or pharmacist. In England and Ireland, one licensed by the Society of Apothecaries of London or the Apothecaries' Hall of Ireland as an authorized physician and dispenser of drugs.

**apothem, apotheme** (ăp′ō-thĕm, -thēm) [Gr. *apo,* from, + *thema,* deposit] The brown precipitate that appears when vegetable decoctions or infusions are exposed to the air or are boiled a long time.

**apotripsis** (ăp″ō-trĭp′sĭs) [Gr. *apotribein,* to abrade] Removal of a corneal scar or opacity.

**apparatus** (ăp″ă-rā′tŭs, -răt′ŭs) [L. *apparare,* to prepare] **1.** A number of parts that act together to perform a special function. **2.** A group of structures or organs that work together to perform a common function. **3.** A mechanical device or appliance used in operations and experiments.

***acoustic a.*** Auditory apparatus; the anatomical structures essential for hearing.

***attachment a.*** The cementum, periodontal ligament, and alveolar bone at the attachment of a tooth.

***biliary a.*** Structures concerned with secretion and excretion of bile; includes liver, gallbladder, and hepatic, cystic, and common bile ducts.

***dental a.*** The tooth and its supporting tissues.

***Golgi a.*** SEE: *Golgi apparatus.*

***juxtaglomerular a.*** The juxtaglomerular cells of the afferent arteriole and the macula densa of the distal tubule. This structure initiates the renin-angiotensin mechanism to elevate blood pressure and increase sodium retention.

***kite a.*** An apparatus for the reeducation of weak muscles and for assistance in overcoming contractures of the forearm, wrist, and fingers.

***lacrimal a.*** SEE: *lacrimal apparatus.*

***masticatory a.*** The teeth, jaws, muscles of mastication, and the temporomandibular joints; used for chewing.

***respiratory a.*** The respiratory system.

***sound-conducting a.*** Those parts of the acoustic apparatus that transmit sound.

***urogenital a.*** The genitourinary system.

***vocal a.*** The organs that produce sounds and speech.

**apparent** [L. *apparens,* appearing] **1.** Obvious and easily seen; not disguised or hidden. **2.** Appearing to the senses to be obvious and clear based on evidence that, with greater knowledge or closer examination, may or may not be valid.

**appearance** The visible presentation of an object.

**appendage** (ă-pĕn′dĭj) Anything attached or appended to a larger or major part, as a tail or a limb. SEE: *appendix.*

***atrial a.*** A small muscular pouch attached to each atrium of the heart.

***auricular a.*** Atrial a.

***a.'s of the eye*** The eyelid, eyelashes, eyebrow, lacrimal apparatus, and conjunctiva.

***a.'s of the fetus*** The amnion, chorion, and umbilical cord.

***a.'s of the skin*** The nails, hair, sebaceous and sweat glands.

***uterine a.*** The ovaries, fallopian tubes, and uterine ligaments.

**appendectomy** (ăp″ĕn-dĕk′tō-mē) [″ + Gr. *ektome,* excision] Surgical removal of the vermiform appendix.

***incidental a.*** Removal of the appendix during another surgical procedure in the abdominal cavity.

**appendical, appendiceal** (ă-pĕn′dĭ-kăl, ăp-ĕn-dĭs′ē-ăl) Pert. to an appendix.

**appendicectasis** (ă-pĕn″dĭ-sĕk′tă-sĭs) [L. *appendere,* hang to, + Gr. *ektasis,* a stretching] Dilatation of the vermiform appendix.

**appendicectomy** (ă-pĕn″dĭ-sĕk′tō-mē) Appendectomy.

**appendicitis** (ă-pĕn″dĭ-sī′tĭs) [L. *appendere,* hang to, + Gr. *itis,* inflammation] Inflammation of the vermiform appendix. It generally occurs in the young, most often between ages 15 and 25, rarely before age 5 or after age 50. It is more common in males than in females. The disease may be acute, subacute, or chronic. When this diagnosis is considered in a woman, it must be differentiated from pain associated with ovulation (mittelschmerz), ruptured ectopic pregnancy, torsion of the ovary, and pelvic inflammatory disease. SEE: *Nursing Diagnoses Appendix*.

TREATMENT: Surgery is usually required. From 10% to 30% of appendices removed will be normal.

***acute a.*** Appendicitis marked by abdominal pain, usually severe throughout the abdomen, followed by nausea and vomiting. Symptoms include localization of pain in the right lower quadrant of the abdomen with tenderness and rigidity over the right rectus muscle or McBurney's point; a fever that usually rises within several hours, 99° to 101°F (37.2° to 38.3°C); a pulse that increases with temperature; the patient lying in a supine position with the right lower extremity frequently flexed to relieve muscle tension; leukocytosis present shortly after onset. In mild cases symptoms begin to subside on the second day. A well-defined abscess usually develops 24 to 72 hr after the onset of symptoms and may be palpable in the right ileocecal region.

NURSING IMPLICATIONS: *Preoperative:* The patient is assessed for signs and symptoms of appendicitis, such as elevated temperature; nausea or vomiting; onset, location, quality, and intensity of pain; rebound tenderness; constipation or diarrhea; and an elevated white blood cell count. The patient is positioned for comfort and prepared physically and emotionally for surgery.

---

Caution: To prevent possible rupture of an inflamed appendix, cathartics or enemas should not be used, nor should heating pads, for a patient with suspected appendicitis.

---

*Postoperative:* The nurse monitors and documents vital signs, the status of bowel sounds, abdominal flatus, lung sounds, and intake and output, including prescribed intravenous fluids. The patient is positioned comfortably (Fowler's position in the case of a ruptured appendix or peritonitis). Prescribed analgesics and noninvasive nursing measures are provided to ensure comfort. Position changes, deep breathing and coughing, and early ambulation are encouraged. The patient's ability to urinate is ascertained and documented. If required, antibiotics are administered as prescribed. The dressing is inspected for any bleeding or drainage and the findings documented. The patient is prepared for return to home, work, and other activities.

***chronic a.*** Appendicitis that may follow an acute attack, leaving adhesions or a cicatricial narrowing of the lumen of the appendix. Symptoms include gastric indigestion, frequently simulating a gastric ulcer, duodenal ulcer, or gallbladder disease. Tenderness is manifested in the right lower abdomen. Surgery is required.

***gangrenous a.*** Appendicitis in which inflammation is extreme, blood vessels are blocked in the mesentery, circulation to the appendix is cut off, and diffuse peritonitis ensues.

**appendicoenterostomy** (ă-pĕn″dĭk-ō-ĕn″tĕr-ŏs′tō-mē) [L. *appendere,* hang to, + Gr. *enteron,* intestine, + *stoma,* mouth] **1.** Appendicostomy. **2.** The establishment of an anastomosis between the appendix and intestine.

**appendicolysis** (ă-pĕn″dĭ-kŏl′ĭ-sĭs) [″ + Gr. *lysis,* dissolution] Surgery to free the appendix from adhesions. This is done by slitting the serosa at its base.

**appendicopathy** (ă-pĕn″dĭ-kŏp′ă-thē) [″ + Gr. *pathos,* disease, suffering] Any disease of the vermiform appendix.

***a. oxyurica*** A lesion of the appendical mucosa supposedly due to oxyurids (intestinal parasitic worms).

**appendicular** (ăp″ĕn-dĭk′ū-lăr) [L. *appendere,* to hang to] **1.** Pert. to an appendix. SYN: *appendical; appendiceal.* **2.** Pert. to the limbs.

**appendicular skeleton** The bony structure that makes up the shoulder girdle, upper extremities, pelvis, and lower extremities.

**appendix** (ă-pĕn′dĭks) *pl.* **appendixes, appendices** [L.] An appendage, esp. the appendix vermiformis. SYN: *appendage.* SEE: *digestive system and omentum* for illus.

***atrial a.*** A small muscular pouch attached to each atrium of the heart.

***auricular a.*** Atrial a.

***ensiform a.*** Xiphoid a.

***a. epididymidis*** A cystic structure attached to the epididymis, a vestigial remnant of the mesonephric duct.

***a. epiploica*** One of numerous pouches of the peritoneum, filled with fat and attached to the colon.

***a. testis*** A small bladder-like structure at the upper end of the testis, a vestigial remnant of the cephalic portion of the müllerian duct.

***ventricular a.*** SEE: *saccule, laryngeal.*

***a. vermiformis*** A worm-shaped process projecting from the blind end of the cecum and lined with a continuation of the mucous membrane of the cecum. SEE: *vermiform appendix.*

***vesicular a.*** A cystic structure attached to the fimbriated end of the uterine tube. It is a vestigial remnant of the mesonephric duct.

***xiphoid a.*** Xiphoid process. SYN: *ensiform a.*

**apperception** (ăp″ĕr-sĕp′shŭn) [L. *ad,* to, + *percipere,* to perceive] The perception and interpretation of sensory stimuli; awareness of the meaning and significance of a particular sensory stimulus as modified by one's own experiences, knowledge, thoughts, and emotions. **apperceptive** (-tĭv), *adj.*

**appestat** (ăp′ĕ-stăt) [L. *appetitus,* longing

for, + Gr. *states,* stand] The area of the brain (probably in the hypothalamus) that is thought to control appetite and food intake.

**appetite** (ăp′ĕ-tīt) [L. *appetitus,* longing for] A strong desire, esp. for food. Appetite differs from hunger in that the latter is an uncomfortable sensation caused by lack of food, whereas appetite is a pleasant sensation based on previous experience that causes one to seek food for the purpose of tasting and enjoying.

***perverted a.*** Pica.

**appetizer** (ăp′ĕ-tī″zĕr) That which promotes appetite.

**applanation** (ăp″lă-nā′shŭn) [L. *ad,* toward, + *planare,* to flatten] Abnormal flattening, esp. of the corneal surface.

**applanometer** (ăp″lă-nŏm′ĕ-tĕr) [″ + *planum,* plane, + Gr. *metron,* measure] A device for measuring intraocular pressure. SEE: *tonometer.*

**apple packer's epistaxis** Nosebleed due to handling packing trays containing certain dyes.

**apple picker's disease** Bronchitis resulting from a fungicide used on apples.

**apple sorter's disease** Contact dermatitis caused by chemicals used in washing apples.

**appliance** (ă-plī′ăns) **1.** In dentistry, a device to provide or facilitate a particular function, such as artificial dentures or a device used to correct bite. **2.** A device for influencing a specific function (e.g., a cane, crutch, or walker to assist walking or an appliance to discourage thumb sucking). SEE: *prosthesis.*

**applicator** (ăp′lĭ-kā″tor) [L. *applicare,* to attach] A device, usually a slender rod with a pledget of cotton on the end, for making local applications.

**apposition** (ăp″ō-zĭ′shŭn) [L. *ad,* toward, + *ponere,* to place] **1.** Condition of being positioned side by side or fitted together. SYN: *contiguity.* **2.** Addition of one substance to another, as one layer of tissue upon another. **3.** Development by means of accretion, as in the formation of bone or dental cementum.

**approach** (ă-prōch′) The surgical procedure for exposing an organ or tissue.

**approximal** (ă-prŏk′sĭ-măl) [″ + *proximus,* nearest] Contiguous; next to.

**approximate** (ă-prŏk′sĭ-māt) [″ + *proximare,* to come near] To place or bring objects close together.

**apractagnosia** Agnosia marked by the inability to use common instruments or tools whether they are being used on the individual's body or in the environment. This is usually due to a lesion in the parietal area of the brain.

**apraxia** (ă-prăk′sē-ă) [Gr. *a-,* not, + *praxis,* action] **1.** Inability to perform purposive movements although there is no sensory or motor impairment. **2.** Inability to use objects properly. **apraxic** (ă-prăk′sĭk), *adj.*

***akinetic a.*** Inability to carry out spontaneous movements.

***amnesic a.*** Inability to produce a movement on command because the command is forgotten, although the ability to perform the movement is present.

***constructional a.*** Inability to draw or construct two- or three-dimensional forms or figures and impairment in the ability to integrate perception into kinesthetic images.

***developmental a.*** Disorder of motor planning and execution occurring in developing children; thought to be due to central nervous system immaturity.

***dressing a.*** Inability to dress due to patient's deficient knowledge of the spatial relations of his or her body.

***ideational a.*** Misuse of objects due to inability to perceive their correct use. SYN: *sensory a.*

***motor a.*** Inability to perform movements necessary to use objects properly, although the names and purposes of the objects are known and understood.

***sensory a.*** Ideational a.

**Apresoline hydrochloride** Trade name for hydralazine hydrochloride.

**aproctia** (ă-prŏk′shē-ă) [Gr. *a-,* not, + *proktos,* anus] Absence or imperforation of anus.

**apron** (ā′prŏn) [O. Fr. *naperon,* cloth] **1.** Outer garment covering the front of the body for protection of clothing during surgery or certain nursing procedures. **2.** Part of the body resembling an apron.

***Hottentot a.*** SEE: *Hottentot apron.*

***lead a.*** An apron that contains lead but is sufficiently pliable to wear as protection from ionizing radiation. It is used to shield patients and personnel during radiological procedures.

**aprosody** (ă-prŏs′ō-dē) [Gr. *a-,* not, + *prosodia,* voice modulation] Absence of normal variations of pitch, rhythm, and stress in the speech.

**aprosopia** (ăp″rō-sō′pē-ă) [″ + *prosopon,* face] Congenital defect in which part or all of the face is absent.

**aprotes** Chemical substances that are either cations such as sodium, calcium, potassium, and magnesium that carry a positive charge, or anions such as chloride and sulfate that carry a negative charge. These chemicals are unable to donate or accept protons; thus they are not acids, bases, or buffers. SEE: *buffer.*

**aprotinin** A serine protease inhibitor obtained from bovine pancreas. Its action is believed to be inhibition of plasmin and kallikrein. It is used to decrease blood loss and thus transfusion requirements during surgery.

**APRV** *airway pressure release ventilation.*

**APT** *alum-precipitated toxoid.*

**A.P.T.A.** *American Physical Therapy Association.*

**aptitude** (ăp′tĭ-tūd) Inherent ability or skill in learning or performing physical or mental endeavors.

**aptitude test** A mental or physical (or both) test designed to evaluate skill or ability to perform certain tasks or assignments.

**APT test** In infants, a method of differentiating swallowed maternal blood in the stool from gastrointestinal bleeding from the infant. The blood could be swallowed during delivery or from a bleeding nipple fissure. To test: 1. A bloody stool or diaper is rinsed until a pink supernatant is obtained. 2. The supernatant is centrifuged and the top fluid is removed. 3. To 5 parts of the removed solution,1 part of 0.25 normal (1%) sodium hydroxide is added. Within 1 to 2 min, a color reaction takes place. A yellow-brown color indicates the blood originated from the mother; a persistent pink color indicates the blood is from the infant. It is advisable to test control specimens from both the mother and the infant. SYN: *swallowed blood syndrome.*

**aptyalia, aptyalism** (ăp″tē-ā′lē-ă, ă-tī′ă-lĭzm) [″ + *ptyalon,* saliva] Absence of or deficiency in secretion of saliva. The condition may be caused by disease (mumps, typhoid fever), dehydration, drugs, radiation therapy to the salivary glands, old age, obstruction of salivary ducts, or Sjögren's syndrome, in which there is deficient function of lacrimal, salivary, and other glands. SYN: *asialia; dry mouth; xerostomia.*

**APUD cells** *amine precursor uptake and decarboxylation* cells. A class of cells that produce hormones (such as insulin, ACTH, glucagon, and thyroxin) and amines (such as dopamine, serotonin, and histamine). These cells are involved in multiple endocrine neoplasia, types I and II.

**apudoma** [from *APUD cells*] A tumor of APUD cells.

**apulmonism** (ă-pool′mŏn-ĭzm) [Gr. *a-,* not, + L. *pulmo,* lung, + Gr. *-ismos,* condition] Congenital absence of part or all of a lung.

**apus** (ā′pŭs) [″ + *pous,* foot] A person who has apodia, congenital absence of the feet.

**apyknomorphous** (ă-pĭk″nō-mor′fŭs) [″ + *pyknos,* thick, + *morphe,* form] Not pyknomorphous; pert. to a cell that does not stain deeply because its stainable material is not compact.

**apyogenous** (ā-pī-ŏj′ĕn-ŭs) [″ + *pyon,* pus, + *genos,* origin] Not producing pus.

**apyretic** (ā-pī-rĕt′ĭk) [″ + *pyretos,* fever] Without fever. SYN: *afebrile.*

**apyrexia** (ā-pī-rĕks′ē-ă) [″ + *pyrexis,* feverishness] Absence of fever.

**apyrogenetic, apyrogenic** (ā″pī-rō-jĕ-nĕt′ĭk, -jĕn′ĭk) [″ + ″ + *genos,* origin] Not causing fever.

**AQ** *achievement quotient.*

**aq** L. *aqua,* water.

**aqua** (awk′wă) *pl.* **aquae** [L. *aqua*] ABBR: a; aq. Water.

***a. ammonia*** $NH_4OH$. Ammonium hydroxide.

***a. destillata*** Distilled water.

***a. fortis*** Weak nitric acid.

***medicated a.*** An aqueous solution of a volatile substance. It usually contains only a comparatively small percentage of the active drug. Some of these solutions are merely water saturated with a volatile oil. They are used mostly as vehicles to give odor and taste to solutions.

***a. oculi*** The fluid (aqueous humor) of the eye.

***a. pura*** Pure water.

***a. purificata*** Purified water.

***a. regia*** Nitrohydrochloric acid water (20% nitric acid and 80% hydrochloric acid). SYN: *nitromuriatic acid.*

***a. rosea*** Rose water.

***a. sterilisata*** Sterilized water.

***a. tepida*** Lukewarm water.

**Aquamephyton** Trade name for phytonadione (vitamin K).

**aquaphobia** (ăk″wă-fō′bē-ă) [″ + Gr. *phobos,* fear] An abnormal fear of water. SYN: *hydrophobia.*

**Aquaplast** A type of low-temperature thermoplastic splinting material principally used for making upper-extremity orthoses.

**aquapuncture** (ăk″wă-pŭngk′chūr) [″ + *punctura,* puncture] Subcutaneous injection of water, as to produce counterirritation.

**aquatic 1.** Pert. to water. **2.** Inhabiting water.

**aqueduct** (ăk′wĕ-dŭkt″) [″ + *ductus,* duct] Canal or channel. SYN: *aqueductus.*

***cerebral a.*** Canal in the midbrain connecting the third and fourth ventricles. SYN: *aqueductus cerebri.*

***vestibular a.*** Small passage reaching from the vestibule to the posterior surface of the temporal bone's petrous section.

**aqueductus** (ăk″wĕ-dŭk′tŭs) A canal or channel. SYN: *aqueduct.*

***a. cerebri*** Canal in the midbrain connecting the third and fourth ventricles. SYN: *cerebral aqueduct.*

***a. cochleae*** Canal connecting subarachnoid space and the perilymphatic space of the cochlea.

***a. Fallopii*** Canal for facial nerve in the temporal bone.

***a. vestibuli*** Small passage reaching from the vestibule to the posterior surface of the temporal bone's petrous section.

**aqueous** (ā′kwē-ŭs) [L. *aqua,* water] **1.** Of the nature of water; watery. **2.** Aqueous humor.

**aqueous chambers** Anterior and posterior chambers of the eye, which contain the aqueous humor.

**aqueous humor** Transparent liquid contained in the anterior and posterior chambers of the eye; produced by the ciliary processes. It passes from the posterior to the anterior chamber, and then to the venous system through the canal of Schlemm.

**aquiparous** (ăk-wĭp′ă-rŭs) [″ + *parere,* to bring forth, to bear] Producing water.

**AR 1.** *achievement ratio.* **2.** *alarm reaction.*
**Ar** Symbol for the element argon.
**ara-A** Vidarabine.
**arabinose** (ă-răb′ĭ-nōs) Gum sugar, a pentose obtained from plants; sometimes found in urine.
**arabinosuria** (ă-răb″ĭ-nō-sū′rē-ă) [*arabinose* + Gr. *ouron,* urine] Arabinose in the urine.
**Ara-C** Cytarabine, an antineoplastic drug of the antimetabolite class.
**arachidonic acid** (ă-răk″ĭ-dŏn′ĭk) An essential fatty acid, 5,8,11,14-eicosatetraenoic acid, formed from unsaturated acids of plants and present in peanuts. It is a precursor of prostaglandins. An essential fatty acid present in peanuts. It is metabolized in the body via two principal pathways to produce a group of chemicals called eicosanoids. Included in these are prostaglandins, thromboxane, and leukotrienes. Synthesis of prostaglandins and thromboxane is directly inhibited by nonsteroidal anti-inflammatory agents such as salicylates, indomethacin, and ibuprofen. Corticosteroids inhibit formation of arachidonic acid from phospholipases.
**arachnid** (ă-răk′nĭd) A member of the class Arachnida.
**Arachnida** (ă-răk′nĭ-dă) [Gr. *arachne,* spider] A class of the Arthropoda, including the spiders, scorpions, ticks, and mites.
**arachnidism** (ă-răk′nĭd-ĭzm) [″ + *eidos,* form, shape, + *-ismos,* condition of] Systemic poisoning from a spider bite. SYN: *arachnoidism.* SEE: *spider bite.*
**arachnitis** (ă″răk-nī′tĭs) Arachnoiditis.
**arachnodactyly** (ă-răk″nō-dăk′tĭl-ē) [″ + *dactylos,* finger] Spider fingers; a state in which fingers and sometimes toes are abnormally long, slender, and curved. SYN: *acromacria.* SEE: *Marfan's syndrome.*
**arachnoid** (ă-răk′noyd) [″ + *eidos,* form, shape] **1.** Resembling a web. **2.** Arachnoid membrane; arachnoidea.

***cranial a.*** Arachnoidea encephali.

***a. granulation*** A. villus.

***a. membrane*** The thin, delicate, intermediate membranes of the meninges that enclose the brain and spinal cord. It is separated from the pia mater, the inner membrane, by the subarachnoid space and from the dura mater, the outer membrane, by the subdural space. SYN: *arachnoidea.*

***spinal a.*** Arachnoidea spinalis.

***a. villus*** One of numerous small ovoid or villuslike projections of the arachnoid membrane of the brain. They may project into the superior sagittal sinus as arachnoid villi or press against the outer dura and grow into the inner plate of the cranium, forming ovoid depressions. Cerebrospinal fluid is reabsorbed from the cranial subarachnoid space through the arachnoid villi into the blood in the cranial venous sinuses. SYN: *a. granulation; pacchionian body.*

**arachnoidea** (ă-răk-noyd′ē-ă) Arachnoid membrane.

***a. encephali*** The part of the arachnoidea enclosing the brain. SYN: *cranial arachnoid.*

***a. spinalis*** The part of the arachnoidea enclosing the spinal cord. SYN: *spinal arachnoid.*

**arachnoidism** (ă-răk′noyd-ĭzm) Arachnidism.
**arachnoiditis** (ă-răk″noyd-ī′tĭs) [″ + *eidos,* form, shape, + *itis,* inflammation] Inflammation of the arachnoid membrane. SYN: *arachnitis.*
**arachnolysin** (ă-răk-nŏl′ĭ-sĭn) [″ + *lysis,* dissolution] The hemolysin present in spider venom.
**arachnophobia** (ă-răk″nō-fō′bē-ă) [″ + *phobos,* fear] Morbid fear of spiders.
**Aralen hydrochloride** Trade name for chloroquine hydrochloride.
**Aralen phosphate** Trade name for chloroquine phosphate.
**Aran-Duchenne disease** Spinal muscular atrophy.
**Arantius' body, Arantius' nodule** (ăr-ăn′shē-ŭs) *pl.* **Arantii** [Julius Caesar Arantius, It. anatomist and physician, 1530–1589] A small nodule at the center of each of the aortic valve cusps.
**arbor** A structure resembling a tree with branches.
**arborescent** (ăr″bor-ĕs′ĕnt) [L. *arborescere,* to become a tree] Branching; treelike.
**arborization** (ăr″bor-ĭ-zā′shŭn) [L. *arbor,* tree] Ramification; branching, esp. terminal branching of nerve fibers and capillaries. SEE: *nerve.*
**arbor vitae** (ăr′bor vī′tē) [L. *arbor,* tree, + *vita,* life] **1.** A treelike structure; a treelike outline seen in a section of the cerebellum. **2.** A tree or shrub of the genus *Thuja* or *Thujopsis.* **3.** A series of branching ridges within the cervix of the uterus. SYN: *palmate plica.*
**arbovirus** (ăr″bō-vī′rŭs) [*ar*thropod-*bo*rne *virus*] Any of a large group of viruses that multiply in both vertebrates and arthropods such as mosquitoes and ticks. Arboviruses cause diseases such as yellow fever and viral encephalitis. SEE: *arenaviruses; Togaviridae.*
**ARC** *AIDS-related complex.* SEE: *AIDS.*
**arc** (ărk) [L. *arcus,* bow] A curved line; a portion of a circle.

***reflex a.*** The path followed by a nerve impulse to produce a reflex action. The impulse originates in a receptor at the point of stimulation, passes through an afferent neuron or neurons to a reflex center in the brain or spinal cord, and from the center out through efferent neurons to the effector organ, where the response occurs. SEE: illus.

**arcade** (ăr-kād) Any anatomic structure composed of a series of arches.

***Flint's a.*** The arteriovenous anastomoses at the bases of the pyramids of the kidney.

**arcanum** (ăr-kā′nŭm) *pl.* **arcana** [L. *arca-*

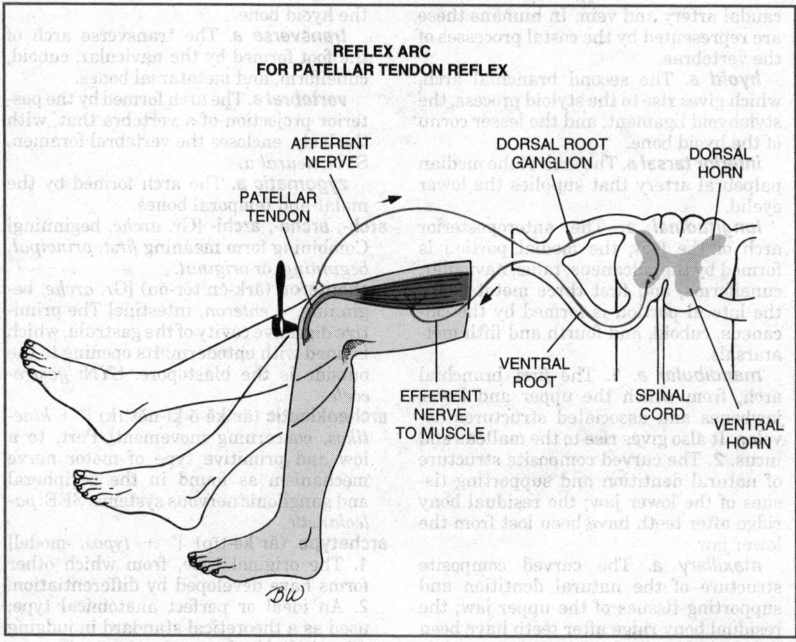


*num,* a secret] Secret remedy.

**arcate** (ăr′kăt) [L. *arcatus,* bow-shaped] Arched; bow-shaped.

**arc eyes** Eye burn caused when welders fail to wear protective eye shields while welding or following extended periods of welding even though protective eye gear was worn. Irrigation of the eyes with copious amounts of sterile saline may be necessary for several hours in addition to pain medication and instillation of anti-inflammatory eye drops and other medications.

**arch** [L. *arcus,* a bow] Any anatomical structure having a curved or bowlike outline. SYN: *arcus.*

***abdominothoracic a.*** The lower boundary of the front of the thorax.

***alveolar a.*** Arch of the alveolar process of either jaw.

***aortic a.*** Proximal curved part of the aorta, at about the level of the fourth thoracic vertebra. The brachiocephalic, left common carotid, and left subclavian arteries arise from the aortic arch.

***aortic a.'s*** A series of six pairs of vessels that develop in the embryo and connect the aortic sac with the dorsal aorta. During the fifth to seventh weeks of gestation, the arches undergo transformation, some persisting as functional vessels, others persisting as rudimentary structures, and some disappearing entirely.

***axillary a.*** An anomalous muscular slip across the axilla, between the pectoralis major and latissimus dorsi muscles. SYN: *Langer's muscle.*

***branchial a.'s*** Five pairs of arched structures that form the lateral and ventral walls of the pharynx of the embryo. The first is the mandibular arch; the second is the hyoid arch; the third, fourth, and fifth arches are transitory. They are partially separated from each other externally by the branchial clefts and internally by the pharyngeal pouches. They are important in the formation of structures of the face and neck. SYN: *pharyngeal a.'s.*

***carotid a.*** The third aortic arch, which provides the common carotid artery.

***costal a.*** Arch formed by the ribs.

***crural a.*** The inguinal ligament, which extends from the anterior superior iliac spine to the pubic tubercle. SYN: *Poupart's ligament.*

***deep crural a.*** A band of fibers arching in front of the sheath of femoral vessels; the downward extension of the transversalis fascia.

***deep palmar a.*** An arch formed in the palm by the communicating branch of the ulnar and the radial artery.

***dental a.*** The arch formed by the alveolar process and teeth in each jaw.

***glossopalatine a.*** The anterior pillar of the fauces; one of two folds of mucous membrane extending from the soft palate to the sides of the tongue.

***hemal a.*** **1.** Arch formed by the body and processes of a vertebra, such as a pair of ribs and the sternum; also the sum of all such arches. **2.** In lower vertebrates, extensions from the lateral areas of the caudal vertebrae that fuse to enclose the caudal artery and vein. In humans these are represented by the costal processes of the vertebrae.

***hyoid a.*** The second branchial arch, which gives rise to the styloid process, the stylohyoid ligament, and the lesser cornu of the hyoid bone.

***inferior tarsal a.*** The arch of the median palpebral artery that supplies the lower eyelid.

***longitudinal a.*** The anteroposterior arch of the foot; the medial portion is formed by the calcaneus, talus, navicular, cuneiforms, and first three metatarsals; the lateral portion is formed by the calcaneus, cuboid, and fourth and fifth metatarsals.

***mandibular a.*** **1.** The first branchial arch, from which the upper and lower jawbones and associated structures develop. It also gives rise to the malleus and incus. **2.** The curved composite structure of natural dentition and supporting tissues of the lower jaw; the residual bony ridge after teeth have been lost from the lower jaw.

***maxillary a.*** The curved composite structure of the natural dentition and supporting tissues of the upper jaw; the residual bony ridge after teeth have been lost from the upper jaw.

***nasal a.*** Arch formed by the nasal bones and by the nasal processes of the maxilla.

***neural a.*** Vertebral a.

***a.'s of Corti*** A series of arches made up of the rods of Corti in the inner ear.

***a.'s of foot*** The instep of the foot formed by the longitudinal arch and the transverse arch.

***palmar a.*** SEE: *deep palmar a.; superficial palmar a.*

***pharyngeal a.'s*** Branchial a.'s.

***pharyngopalatine a.*** The posterior pillar of the fauces; one of two folds of mucous membrane extending from the soft palate to the sides of the pharynx.

***plantar a.*** The arch formed by the external plantar artery and the deep branch of the dorsalis pedis artery.

***pubic a.*** The arch formed by the rami of the ischia.

***pulmonary a.*** The fifth aortic arch on the left side. It becomes the pulmonary artery.

***superciliary a.*** A curved process of the frontal bone lying just above the orbit and subjacent to the eyebrow.

***superficial palmar a.*** An arch in the palm forming the termination of the ulnar artery.

***superior tarsal a.*** The arch of the median palpebral artery that supplies the upper eyelid.

***supraorbital a.*** A bony arch formed by the upper margin of the orbit.

***tarsal a.*** SEE: *inferior tarsal a.; superior tarsal a.*

***thyrohyoid a.*** The third branchial arch, which gives rise to the greater cornu of the hyoid bone.

***transverse a.*** The transverse arch of the foot formed by the navicular, cuboid, cuneiform, and metatarsal bones.

***vertebral a.*** The arch formed by the posterior projection of a vertebra that, with the body, encloses the vertebral foramen. SYN: *neural a.*

***zygomatic a.*** The arch formed by the malar and temporal bones.

**arch-, arche-, archi-** [Gr. *arche,* beginning] Combining form meaning *first, principal, beginning,* or *original.*

**archenteron** (ărk-ĕn'tĕr-ŏn) [Gr. *arche,* beginning, + *enteron,* intestine] The primitive digestive cavity of the gastrula, which is lined with entoderm. Its opening to the outside is the blastopore. SYN: *gastrocoele.*

**archeokinetic** (ăr"kē-ō-kĭ-nĕt'ĭk) [" + *kinetikos,* concerning movement] Pert. to a low and primitive type of motor nerve mechanism as found in the peripheral and ganglionic nervous systems. SEE: *paleokinetic.*

**archetype** (ăr'kĕ-tīp) [" + *typos,* model] **1.** The original type, from which other forms have developed by differentiation. **2.** An ideal or perfect anatomical type; used as a theoretical standard in judging other individuals.

**ARCF** *American Respiratory Care Foundation.*

**archiblast** (ăr'kĭ-blăst) [" + *blastos,* a germ, bud] The outer layer that surrounds the germinal vesicle.

**archiblastic** (ăr"kĭ-blăs'tĭk) Derived from or pert. to the archiblast.

**archiblastoma** (ăr"kĭ-blăs-tō'mă) [" + *blastos,* germ, + *oma,* tumor] A tumor of archiblastic tissue.

**archigaster** (ăr'kĭ-găs"tĕr) [" + *gaster,* belly] The primitive embryonic alimentary canal.

**archinephron** (ăr"kĭ-nĕf'rŏn) Mesonephros.

**archineuron** (ăr-kĭ-nū'rŏn) [" + *neuron,* nerve, tendon] The central cell of the cerebral cortex and all its processes. The nervous impulse transmitted to initiate physiological function originates in the archineuron.

**archipallium** (ăr"kĭ-păl'ē-ŭm) [" + L. *pallium,* a cloak] Olfactory cortex; phylogenetically older than the neopallium.

**archiplasm** (ăr'kĭ-plăzm) [" + LL. *plasma,* form, mold] **1.** The most primitive living substance. **2.** The substance of the fertilized ovum.

**archistome** (ăr'kĭ-stōm) Blastopore.

**architectural barrier** Any limitation in the design of facilities that restricts the access of persons with disabilities and limited mobility, including those using wheelchairs.

**architis** (ăr-kī'tĭs) [Gr. *archos,* anus, + *itis,* inflammation] Inflammation of the anus; proctitis.

**arch width** The measured distance between the canines, bicuspids, and the first molars. These distances establish the shape and size of the dental arch.

**arciform** (ăr′sĭ-form) Arcuate.

**arctation** (ărk-tā′shŭn) [L. *arctatus,* pressing together] Stricture of any canal opening.

**arcuate** (ăr′kū-āt) [L. *arcuatus,* bowed] Bowed; shaped like an arc. SYN: *arciform.*

**arcuation** (ăr-kū-ā′shŭn) A bending; curvature.

**arcus** (ăr′kŭs) *pl.* **arcus** [L. *arcus,* a bow] Arch.

***a. alveolaris mandibulae*** The arch formed by the alveolar process of the body of the mandible.

***a. alveolaris maxillae*** The arch formed by the alveolar process of the maxilla.

***a. dentalis*** Dental arch.

***a. juvenilis*** Opaque ring about the periphery of the cornea similar to arcus senilis but occurring in young individuals; may be due to hypercholesterolemia, corneal irritation or inflammation, or a congenital anomaly.

***a. plantaris*** Plantar arch.

***a. senilis*** Opaque white ring about the periphery of the cornea, seen in aged persons; caused by the deposit of fat granules in the cornea or by hyaline degeneration.

**ARD** *acute respiratory distress.*

**ardor** (ăr′dor) [L., heat] Burning; great heat.

***a. urinae*** A burning sensation during urination.

**ARDS** *acute respiratory distress syndrome.*

**area** (ā′rē-ă) *pl.* **areae, areas** [L. *area,* an open space] **1.** A circumscribed space; one having definite boundaries. **2.** Part of an organ that performs a specialized function.

***acoustic a.*** Vestibular a.

***association a.*** Area of the cerebral cortex that is not sensory or motor, in the usual meaning of those terms. It is thought to be a region in which higher mental processes are mediated.

***auditory a.*** The hearing center of the cerebral cortex; located in the floor of the lateral fissure and surfacing on the dorsal surface of the superior temporal gyrus. It receives auditory fibers from the medial geniculate body.

***body surface a.*** SEE: *body surface area.*

***Broca's a.*** SEE: *Broca's area.*

***Brodmann's a.'s*** SEE: *Brodmann's areas.*

***catchment a.*** a geographical area defining the portion of a population served by a designated medical facility.

***controlled a.*** An area in which a protection officer oversees the occupational exposure of personnel to ionizing radiation. Controlled access, occupancy, and working conditions are necessary for radiation protection.

***Kiesselbach's a.*** SEE: *Kiesselbach's area.*

***macular a.*** Area of the retina that provides central vision.

***mitral a.*** Area over the apex of the heart where mitral valve sounds are heard.

***motor a.*** Posterior part of frontal lobe anterior to the central sulcus, from which impulses for volitional movement arise.

***occipital a.*** The portion of the brain below the occipital bone.

***olfactory a.*** An area in the hippocampal convolution; the anterior portion of the callosal gyrus and the uncus of the brain. This area includes the olfactory bulb, tract, and trigone and is perforated by many blood vessels.

***a. pellucida*** The clear central portion of the area germinativa.

***silent a.*** Any cortical area in the brain that on stimulation produces no detectable motor activity or sensory phenomenon, and in which a lesion may occur without producing detectable motor or sensory abnormalities.

***vestibular a.*** Fundus of the internal auditory meatus. SYN: *acoustic a.*

***uncontrolled a.*** For radiation protection purposes, an area occupied by the general public.

**Area Agency on Aging** ABBR: AAA. An agency that develops, coordinates, and in some cases provides a wide range of community-based services for persons aged 60 and older.

**areata, areatus** (ă″rē-ā′tă, ă″rē-ā′tŭs) Occurring in circumscribed areas or patches.

**areflexia** (ă″rĕ-flĕk′sē-ă) [Gr. *a-,* not, + L. *reflectere,* to bend back] Absence of reflexes.

**arenaceous** (ăr″ĕ-nā′sē-ŭs) [L. *arenaceus,* sandy] Resembling sand or gravel. SYN: *arenoid.*

**arenation** (ă″rĕ-nā′shŭn) [L. *arena,* sand] A sand bath or application of hot sand.

**arenaviridae** Arenaviruses.

**arenaviruses** (ă″rē-nă-vī′rŭs-ĕs) [″ + *virus,* poison] A group of viruses once classed as causing disease by being arthropod borne. This method of transmission is not obligatory. The principal viruses in this group are lymphocytic choriomeningitis virus (LCM virus) and Lassa virus. The LCM virus rarely infects humans, but when it does, the disease is usually a mild form of meningitis. The Lassa virus causes a highly contagious, severe febrile illness and may be fatal. SEE: *Lassa fever.*

**arenoid** (ăr′ĕ-noyd) Arenaceous.

**areola** (ă-rē′ō-lă) *pl.* **areolae, areolas** [L. *areola,* a small space] **1.** A small space or cavity in a tissue. **2.** A circular area of different pigmentation, as around a wheal, around the nipple of the breast, or the part of the iris around the pupil. **areolar** (-lăr), *adj.*

***a. mammae*** The pigmented area surrounding the nipple. SYN: *a. papillaris.*

***a. papillaris*** A. mammae.

***second a.*** A pigmented area surrounding the areola mammae during pregnancy.

***a. umbilicalis*** A pigmented area surrounding the umbilicus.

**areolitis** (ăr″ē-ō-lī′tĭs) [″ + Gr. *itis,* inflammation] Inflammation of a mammary areola.

**arevareva** (ăr-ē″vā-rā′vă) [Tahitian, skin rash] Severe skin disease marked by scales and general debility. Arevareva is thought to be caused by excess use of kava, an intoxicating beverage. Use of kava should be stopped. SEE: *kava.*

**ARF** *acute respiratory failure; acute renal failure.*

**Arfonad** Trade name for trimethaphan camsylate.

**Argasidae** (ăr-găs′ĭ-dī) [Gr. *argeeis,* shining] A family of soft ticks that usually infest birds but may attack humans, causing severe pain and fever.

**argentaffin, argentaffine** (ăr-jĕnt′ă-fĭn) [L. *argentum,* silver, + *affinis,* associated with] Denoting cells that react with silver salts, thus taking a brown or black stain.

**argentaffinoma** (ăr″jĕn-tăf″ĭ-nō′mă) [″ + ″ + Gr. *oma,* tumor] An argentaffin cell tumor that may arise in the intestinal tract, bile ducts, pancreas, bronchus, or ovary. Tumors of this type secrete serotonin and may produce the carcinoid syndrome. SYN: *carcinoid.*

**argentum** (ăr-jĕn′tŭm) [L.] SYMB: Ag. Silver; atomic weight 107.868, atomic number 47.

**arginase** (ăr′jĭ-nās) A liver enzyme that converts arginine into urea and ornithine.

**arginine** (ăr′jĭ-nēn, -nĭn) [L. *argentum,* silver] $C_6H_{14}N_4O_2$. A crystalline basic amino acid obtained from the decomposition of vegetable tissues, protamines, and proteins. It is a guanidine derivative, yielding urea and ornithine on hydrolysis. It may also be produced synthetically. SEE: *amino acid.*

***a. glutamate*** The L(+)—arginine salt of L(+)—glutamic acid. It has been used to treat ammonia intoxication due to severe liver insufficiency.

***a. hydrochloride*** L(+)—arginine salt of hydrochloric acid. It has been used to treat ammonia intoxication due to severe liver insufficiency.

***suberyl a.*** A combination of suberic acid and arginine. It forms a portion of the molecule of various bufotoxins (toad poisons).

**argininosuccinic acid** (ăr″jĭ-nĭ″nō-sŭk-sĭn′ĭk) A compound intermediate in the synthesis of arginine; formed from citrulline and aspartic acid.

**argininosuccinicaciduria** (ăr″jĭn-ĭn-ō-sŭk-sĭn″ĭk-ăs-ĭ-dū′rē-ă) Hereditary metabolic disease caused by excessive excretion, and thus deficiency, of argininosuccinase, an enzyme required to metabolize argininosuccinic acid. Clinical evidence of this defect includes mental retardation, friable tufted hair, convulsions, ataxia, liver disease, and epilepsy.

**argon** (ăr′gŏn) [Gr. *argos,* inactive] SYMB: Ar. An inert gas; atomic weight 39.948, atomic number 18. It composes approx. 1% of the atmosphere.

**Argyll Robertson pupil** (ăr-gīl′ rŏb′ĕrt-sŏn) [Douglas Argyll Robertson, Scottish ophthalmologist, 1837–1909] More properly the name of a symptom often present in paralysis and locomotor ataxia (due to syphilis), in which the light reflex is absent but there is no change in the power of contraction during accommodation. Usually bilateral. SYN: *Robertson's pupil.*

**argyria, argyriasis** (ăr-jĭr′ē-ă, ăr″jĭ-rī′ă-sĭs) [Gr. *argyros,* silver] Bluish discoloration of the skin and mucous membranes as a result of prolonged administration of silver. SYN: *argyrosis.*

**argyric** (ăr-jĭr′ĭk) Pert. to silver.

**Argyrol S S** (ăr′jĭ-rŏl) Trade name for mild silver protein; used as an antiseptic in infections of the eye, nose, and throat and for urethral irrigations.

**argyrophil** (ăr-jī′rō-fĭl) [″ + *philos,* fond] Denoting cells that bind with silver salts, which can then be reduced to produce a brown or black stain.

**argyrosis** (ăr″jĭ-rō′sĭs) Argyria.

**arhinia** Arrhinia.

**arhythmia** Arrhythmia.

**Arias-Stella reaction** [Javier Arias-Stella, Peruvian pathologist, b. 1924] An endometrial gland cell abnormality consisting of hyperchromatic nuclei, which may be present in normal or ectopic pregnancy. It is not a sign of endometrial adenocarcinoma.

**ariboflavinosis** (ă-rī″bō-flā″vĭn-ō′sĭs) [Gr. *a-,* not, + *riboflavin* + Gr. *osis,* condition] Condition arising from a deficiency of riboflavin in the diet. Symptoms include lesions on the lips, stomatitis and, later, fissures in the angles of the mouth, seborrhea around the nose, and vascularization of the cornea. Riboflavin is given orally.

**Aristocort** Trade name for triamcinolone.

**Aristocort Acetonide** Trade name for triamcinolone acetonide.

**Aristocort Forte Parenteral** Trade name for triamcinolone diacetate.

**Aristospan** Trade name for triamcinolone hexacetonide.

**arithmetic mean** In statistics, the number obtained by adding all of the values listed in a group and dividing by the total number of values in the group. SYN: *average.*

**arkyochrome** (ăr′kē-ō-krōm) [Gr. *arkys,* net, + *chroma,* color] A nerve cell in which the stainable substance is arranged in a network.

**arkyostichochrome** (ar″kē-ō-stĭk′ō-krōm) [″ + *stichos,* row, + *chroma,* color] A nerve cell in which the stainable material is arranged both as a network and in parallel lines.

**arm** [AS] **1.** In anatomy, the upper extremity from shoulder to elbow. **2.** In popular usage, the entire upper extremity, from shoulder to hand. SEE: illus.

***bird a.*** Atrophy of the forearm muscles.

***brawny a.*** Hard, swollen arm caused by

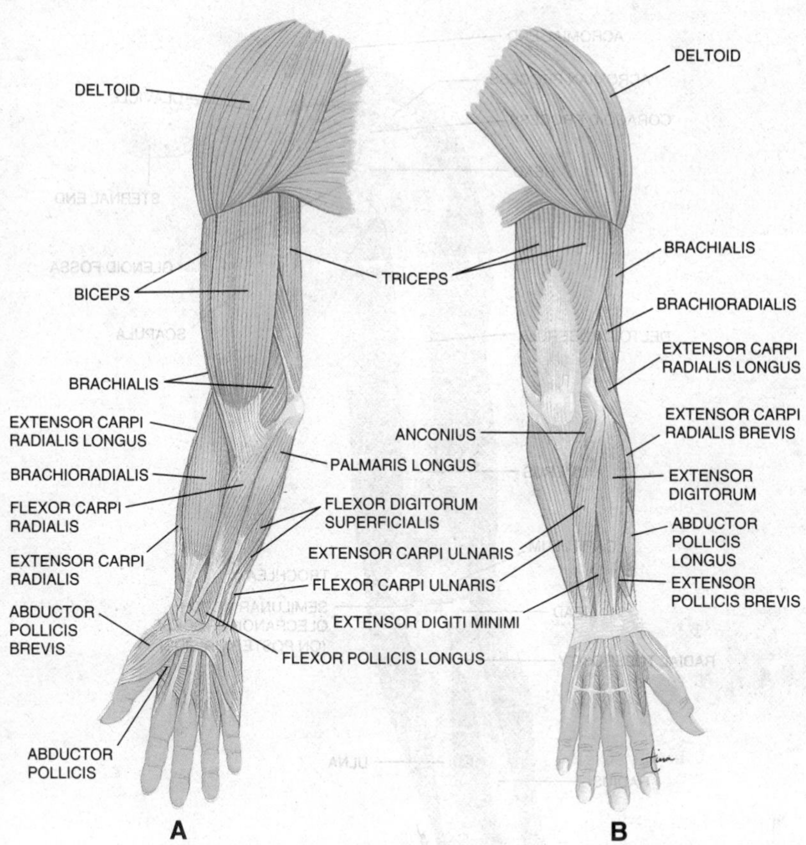


MUSCLES OF THE **ARM (A)** ANTERIOR VIEW, **(B)** POSTERIOR VIEW

lymphedema after mastectomy.

***Saturday-night a.*** A form of paralysis of the brachial plexus, sometimes seen in intoxicated persons. It may be caused by sleeping in a chair, with the arm hanging over the back of the chair while the head rests on the shoulder or arm.

**arm, carrying angle of** The angle between the long axes of the upper and lower arm. This angle is nearly straight in the male and is increased in the female (i.e., in the female the lower part of the arm will deviate away from the body more than is the case in the male). This is a secondary sex characteristic.

**armamentarium** (ăr″mă-mĕn-tā′rē-ŭm) [L. *armamentum,* implement] The total equipment of a physician or institution, such as instruments, drugs, books, and supplies.

**armature** (ăr′mă-tūr) [L. *armatura,* equipment] **1.** In biology, a structure that serves to protect or is used to attack a predator (e.g., a stinger). **2.** A part of an electrical generator, consisting of a coil of insulated wire mounted around a soft iron core.

**arm board 1.** A board placed under and attached to the arm for stabilization during intravenous administration. **2.** A device attached to the sides of a wheelchair to permit support or positioning of the arm, esp. for persons with upper-extremity paralysis.

**armpit** Axilla.

**Arneth, Joseph** (ăr′nāt) German physician, 1873–1955.

***A.'s classification of neutrophils*** A classification of polymorphonuclear neutrophils based on the number of lobes (one to five) in the nucleus, termed stages one to five, respectively.

***A.'s formula*** The normal ratio of various types of polymorphonuclear neutrophils based on the number of lobes (one to five) in the nucleus.

**Arnold, Friedrich** German anatomist, 1803–1890.

***A.'s canal*** Passage in the temporal bone for lesser superficial petrosal nerve.

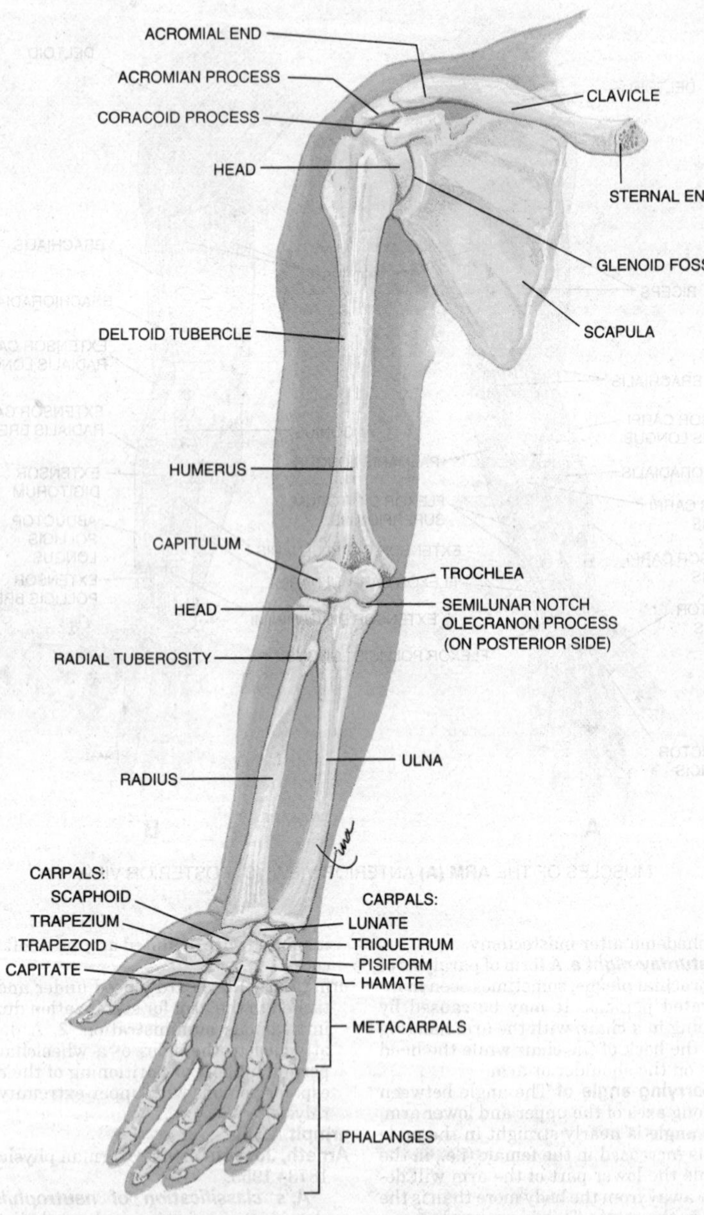


BONES OF THE **ARM** AND SHOULDER GIRDLE

***A.'s ganglion*** Otic ganglion.

***A.'s nerve*** Auricular branch of the vagus nerve. SEE: *cough, reflex.*

**Arnold-Chiari deformity** (ăr′nōlt-kē′ă-rē) [Julius Arnold, Ger. pathologist, 1835–1915; Hans Chiari, Austrian pathologist, 1851–1916] A condition in which the inferior poles of the cerebellar hemispheres and the medulla protrude through the foramen magnum into the spinal canal. It is one of the causes of hydrocephalus and is usually accompanied by spina bifida cystica and meningomyelocele.

**AROM** *active range of motion.*

**aroma** (ă-rō′mă) [Gr. *aroma,* spice] An agreeable odor.

**aromatic** (ăr″ō-măt′ĭk) **1.** Having an agreeable odor. **2.** Denoting an organic chemical compound in which the carbon atoms form closed rings (as in benzene) as distinguished from the aliphatic series, in which the carbon atoms form straight or branched chains.

***a. ammonia spirit*** A solution consisting of 34 g of ammonium carbonate in 1000 ml of diluted ammonia solution, fragrant oils, alcohol, and purified water; used as an antacid and carminative. It acts as a reflex stimulant when its vapor is inhaled.

***a. compounds*** Ring or cyclic compounds related to benzene, many having a fragrant odor.

***a. elixir*** A flavoring agent used in preparing medicines.

**arousal** **1.** Alertness; the state of being prepared to act. **2.** Erotic excitement.

***a. level*** An individual's degree of alertness or responsiveness to stimuli. In testing a newborn's behavior, the level of arousal is important. These levels are deep sleep; sleep with rapid eye movements; drowsy state; a quiet, alert state; an awake and active state; and a state of active, intense crying. The infant is capable of the most responsive and complex interactions with the environment in the quiet and alert states. SEE: *psychomotor and physical development of infant.*

**arrector pili** (ă″rĕk-tō′rēz pĭl-ō′rŭm) *pl.* **arrectores pilorum** [L. *arrectores,* raisers, + *pilus,* hair] One of the involuntary muscle fibers arising in the skin and extending down to connect with the hair follicles on the side toward which the hair slopes. After certain stimuli, including cold or fright, the muscle fibers contract, straighten the follicles, and raise the hairs, resulting in gooseflesh (cutis anserina).

**arrest** (ă-rĕst′) **1.** The condition of being stopped. **2.** To bring to a stop.

***bradyasystolic a.*** The type of cardiac arrest marked by a slow pulse. This can be due to increased vagal stimulation or progressive heart block.

***cardiac a.*** Cessation of the heartbeat. SEE: *cardiopulmonary resuscitation.*

***epiphyseal a.*** Arrest of the growth of long bones.

***pelvic a.*** Condition in which the presenting part of the fetus becomes fixed in the maternal pelvis.

***respiratory a.*** Cessation of spontaneous respirations.

***sinus a.*** Condition in which the sinus node of the heart does not initiate impulses for heartbeat. If this condition persists, it usually requires implantation of a permanent cardiac pacemaker. SEE: *pacemaker, cardiac, artificial.*

**arrhenoblastoma** (ă-rē″nō-blăs-tō′mă) [Gr. *arren,* male, + *blastos,* germ, + *oma,* tumor] An ovarian tumor that secretes male sex hormone, causing secondary male sex characteristics (virilization) in the female.

**arrhinia** (ă-rĭn′ē-ă) [Gr. *a-,* not, + *rhis,* nose] Congenital absence of the nose.

**arrhythmia** (ă-rĭth′mē-ă) [″ + *rhythmos,* rhythm] Irregularity or loss of rhythm, esp. of the heartbeat. SYN: *dysrhythmia.* **arrhythmic** (-mĭk), *adj.*

***cardiac a.*** Irregular heart action caused by physiological or pathological disturbances in the discharge of cardiac impulses from the sinoatrial node or their transmission through conductile tissue of the heart. SEE: *bradycardia; cardioversion; pacemaker, cardiac, artificial; sick sinus syndrome; tachycardia; Nursing Diagnoses Appendix.*

***reperfusion a.*** Cardiac arrhythmia that occurs as the damaged heart is resupplied with blood following angioplasty or thrombolysis.

***sinus a.*** Cardiac irregularity marked by an increased heart rate during inspiration and decrease in heart rate on expiration. This arrhythmia has no clinical significance except in older patients, in which case it may occur in coronary artery disease.

**A.R.R.T.** *American Registry of Radiologic Technologists.*

**arseniasis** (ăr″sē-nī′ă-sĭs) [L. *arsenium,* arsenic, + *-iasis,* condition] Chronic arsenic poisoning. SYN: *arsenicalism.*

**arsenic** (ăr′sĕ-nĭk) [L. *arsenicum*] SYMB: As. A very poisonous, grayish-white metallic element, atomic weight 74.922, atomic number 33, specific gravity 5.73. It is used in the manufacture of dyes and medicines.

Arsenic may be present in soil, water, and air as a common environmental toxicant. Minute traces of arsenic are found in vegetable and animal forms of life and are present in eggs. Many household and garden pesticides contain various forms of arsenic. All of these are toxic if ingested or inhaled in sufficient quantity. An accumulation of arsenic in the body will cause alimentary tract disorders, nausea, vomiting, diarrhea, dehydration, neuritis, and paralysis of the wrist and ankle muscles. SEE: *arsenic poisoning; Poisons and Poisoning Appendix.*

***a. trioxide*** $As_2O_3$. A white powder formerly used internally in a 1% solution. Its toxicity makes it unsafe to use.

**arsenical** (ăr-sĕn′ĭ-kăl) **1.** Pert. to or containing arsenic. **2.** A drug containing arsenic.

**arsenicalism** (ăr-sĕn′ĭ-kăl-ĭzm) [L. *arsenicum,* arsenic, + Gr. *-ismos,* condition of] Chronic arsenic poisoning. SYN: *arseniasis.*

**arsenicophagy** (ăr″sĕn-ĭ-kŏf′ă-jē) [″ + *phagein,* to eat] Habitual eating of arsenic.

**arsenic poisoning** Morbid condition produced by ingestion of arsenic.

SYMPTOMS: In acute poisoning, symptoms may appear in a few minutes; if arsenic was taken with solid food, symptoms may not appear for many hours.

Symptoms include a metallic taste in the mouth, garlic odor on the breath, burning pain throughout the gastrointestinal tract, vomiting, dehydration, shock syndrome, coma, convulsions, paralysis, and death.

FIRST AID: Stomach lavage should be performed with copious amounts of water. If this cannot be done, vomiting should be induced. Dimercaprol (British antilewisite) should be given immediately.

TREATMENT: After first aid, fluid and electrolyte balance is maintained. Morphine is given for pain. Shock and pulmonary edema are treated. Blood transfusion may be required because of hemolysis. SEE: *Poisons and Poisoning Appendix.*

**arsenium** (ăr-sē′nē-ŭm) [L.] Arsenic.

**arsine** (ăr′sĭn) A very poisonous gas used in chemical warfare.

**arsphenamine** (ărs-fĕn′ă-mēn) A light yellow powder containing about 30% arsenic; formerly used in the treatment of syphilis. SYN: *salvarsan.*

**ART** *assisted reproduction technologies.*

**A.R.T.** *Accredited Record Technician.*

**Artane** Trade name for trihexyphenidyl hydrochloride.

**artefact** SEE: *artifact.*

**arterectomy** (ăr″tĕ-rĕk′tō-mē) [Gr. *arteria,* artery, + *ektome,* excision] Excision of an artery or arteries.

**arteri-** SEE: *arterio-.*

**arteria** (ăr″tē′rē-ă) *pl.* **arteriae** Artery.

**arterial** (ăr-tē′rē-ăl) Pert. to one or more arteries.

**arterial bleeding** Bleeding from an artery. The blood is bright red and comes in spurts. The bleeding may be arrested by application of pressure on the proximal side of the vessel (nearest the heart).

**arterial blood gas** ABBR: ABG. Literally, any of the gases present in blood; clinically, the determination of levels of oxygen, $O_2$, and carbon dioxide, $CO_2$, in the blood. ABGs are important in the diagnosis and treatment of disturbances of acid-base balance. Values are usually expressed as the partial pressure of carbon dioxide or oxygen. Several other blood chemistry values are important in managing acid-base disturbances; included are the levels of the bicarbonate ion, $HCO_3$, blood pH, sodium, potassium, and chloride. These data are then used to calculate the anion gap.

**arterial circulation** Movement of blood through the arteries. It is maintained by the pumping of the heart and influenced by the elasticity and extensibility of arterial walls, peripheral resistance in the areas of small arteries, and the quantity of blood in the body. SEE: *circulation.*

**arterial line** A hemodynamic monitoring system consisting of a catheter in an artery connected to pressure tubing, a transducer, and an electronic monitor. It is used to measure systemic blood pressure and to provide ease of access for the drawing of blood for study of gases present. It is considered to be more accurate than conventional methods using venous blood.

**arterial varix** An enlarged and tortuous artery.

**arteriectasis, arteriectasia** (ăr″tĕ-rē-ĕk′tă-sĭs, -ĕk-tā′zē-ă) [″ + *ektasis,* a stretching out] Arterial dilatation.

**arteriectomy** (ăr″tĕ-rē-ĕk′tō-mē) [″ + *ektome,* excision] Surgical removal of part of an artery.

**arterio-, arteri-** [Gr. *arteria,* artery] Combining form indicating *relationship to an artery.*

**arteriocapillary** (ăr-tē″rē-ō-kăp′ĭ-lăr″ē) [″ + L. *capillus,* like hair] Pert. to both arteries and capillaries.

**arteriocapillary fibrosis** Sclerosis of capillaries and arterioles.

**arteriofibrosis** (ăr-tē″rē-ō-fī-brō′sĭs) [″ + L. *fibra,* fiber, + Gr. *osis,* condition] Arteriocapillary fibrosis.

**arteriogram** (ăr″tē-rē-ō-grăm) [″ + *gramma,* something written] A radiograph of an artery after injection of a radiopaque contrast medium, usually directly into the artery or near its origin. SEE: *angiogram.*

**arteriography** (ăr″tē-rē-ŏg′ră-fē) [″ + *graphein,* to write] **1.** A radiographic procedure for obtaining an arteriogram. SEE: *angiography.* **2.** Description of arteries.

**arteriola** (ăr-tē″rē-ō′lă) *pl.* **arteriolae** [L.] A small artery; an arteriole.

***a. macularis inferior*** The inferior macular arteriole, which supplies the macula retinae of the eye.

***a. macularis superior*** The superior macular arteriole, which supplies the macula retinae of the eye.

***a. medialis retinae*** The medial arteriole of the retina.

***a. nasalis retinae inferior*** The inferior nasal arteriole of the retina.

***a. nasalis retinae superior*** The superior nasal arteriole of the retina.

***a. recta*** One of the small arteries of the kidney that supply the renal pyramids.

***a. temporalis retinae inferior*** The inferior temporal artery of the retina.

***a. temporalis retinae superior*** The superior temporal artery of the retina.

**arteriole** (ăr-tē′rē-ōl) *pl.* **arterioles** [L. *arteriola*] A minute artery, esp. one that, at its distal end, leads into a capillary. SYN: *arteriola.* **arteriolar** (ăr-tē-rē-ō′lăr), *adj.*

**arteriolith** (ăr-tē′rē-ō-lĭth) [″ + Gr. *lithos,* stone] An arterial calculus.

**arteriolitis** (ăr-tēr″ē-ō-lī′tĭs) [″ + Gr. *itis,* inflammation] Inflammation of the arteriolar wall.

**arteriolonecrosis** (ăr-tē″rē-ō″lō-nĕ-krō′sĭs) [″ + Gr. *nekros,* corpse, + *osis,* condition] Destruction of an arteriole.

**arteriolosclerosis** (ăr-tē″rē-ō″lō-sklĕ-rō′sĭs) [L. *arteriola,* small artery, + Gr. *sklerosis,* hardening] Thickening of the walls of the arterioles, with loss of elasticity and contractility. **arteriolosclerotic** (-rŏt′ĭk), *adj.*

**arteriomotor** (ăr-tē″rē-ō-mō′tor) [Gr. *arteria,* artery, + L. *movere,* to move] Causing changes in the interior diameter of arteries by dilatation and constriction.

**arteriomyomatosis** (ăr-tē″rē-ō-mī″ō-mă-tō′sĭs) [″ + *mys,* muscle, + *oma,* tumor, + *osis,* condition] Thickening of arterial walls due to overgrowth of muscle fibers.

**arterionecrosis** (ăr-tē″rē-ō-nĕ-krō′sĭs) [″ + *nekros,* corpse, + *osis,* condition] Arterial necrosis.

**arteriopathy** (ăr″tē-rē-ŏp′ă-thē) [″ + *pathos,* disease, suffering] Any disease of the arteries.

**arterioplasty** (ăr-tē″rē-ō-plăs′tē) [″ + *plassein,* to form] Repair or reconstruction of an artery.

**arteriopressor** (ăr-tē″rē-ō-prĕs′or) [″ + L. *pressura,* force] Causing increased arterial blood pressure.

**arteriorrhaphy** (ăr-tē″rē-or′ă-fē) [″ + *rhaphe,* seam, ridge] Arterial suture.

**arteriorrhexis** (ăr-tē″rē-ō-rĕk′sĭs) [″ + *rhexis,* rupture] Rupture of an artery.

**arteriosclerosis** (ăr-tē″rē-ō-sklĕ-rō′sĭs) [″ + *sklerosis,* to harden] A disease of the arterial vessels marked by thickening, hardening, and loss of elasticity in the arterial walls. This results in altered function of tissues and organs. Changes may occur in the intima, media, or both. In the Western world, this condition is the leading cause of death and serious morbidity. The terms *arteriosclerosis* and *atherosclerosis* should not be used interchangeably. Atherosclerosis is a type of arteriosclerosis involving cholesterol deposits and triglycerides.

SYMPTOMS: Symptoms may include intermittent claudication, changes in skin temperature and intensity of pulse, headache, dizziness, or memory defects, depending on the organ system involved. **arteriosclerotic** (-rŏt′ĭk), *adj.*

ETIOLOGY: The cause is unknown. Risk factors include age, familial predisposition, sedentary lifestyle, hypertension, increased blood lipids (particularly cholesterol and triglycerides), obesity, cigarette smoking, diabetes mellitus, inability to cope with stress, family history of early-onset atherosclerosis, and male sex (at ages 35 to 44, the death rate for white men is six times that of white women).

TREATMENT: Treatment includes regular exercise; a diet low in saturated fats; abstaining from use of tobacco; general moderation in all things to reduce or avoid stress; therapy for treatable diseases such as obesity, diabetes, and hypertension if any of these are present.

NURSING IMPLICATIONS: The patient and family are taught about risk factors associated with arteriosclerosis, and the nurse assists the patient to modify these factors. Patients who smoke cigarettes are referred to support services and for nicotine patch replacement or reduction therapy to assist them to stop smoking. Community-based plans and programs to change sedentary activity patterns, reduce stress, control obesity, and decrease saturated fat intake to control triglyceride and cholesterol levels are explored with the patient. The nurse refers the patient for medical treatment to control hypertension and diabetes mellitus and supports the patient's efforts to cooperate with lifestyle and health care changes. Regular exercise of a type and extent appropriate to the patient's health and adequate rest are prescribed. The patient is informed of the need for long-term follow-up care to prevent a wide variety of body system complications.

***a. obliterans*** Arteriosclerosis in which the lumen of the artery is completely occluded.

**arteriospasm** (ăr-tē′rē-ō-spăzm″) [Gr. *arteria,* artery, + *spasmos,* a convulsion] Arterial spasm.

**arteriostenosis** (ăr-tē″rē-ō-stĕ-nō′sĭs) [″ + *stenosis,* act of narrowing] Narrowing of the lumen of an artery; may be temporary or permanent.

**arteriostosis** (ăr-tē″rē-ŏs-tō′sĭs) [″ + *osteon,* bone, + *osis,* condition] Calcification of an artery.

**arteriostrepsis** (ăr-tē″rē-ō-strĕp′sĭs) [″ + *strepsis,* a twisting] Twisting of the divided end of an artery to arrest hemorrhage.

**arteriosympathectomy** (ăr-tē″rē-ō-sĭm″pă-thĕk′tō-mē) [″ + *sympatheia,* suffer with, + *ektome,* excision] Removal of the arterial sheath containing fibers of the sympathetic nerve.

**arteriotomy** (ăr″tē-rē-ŏt′ō-mē) Surgical division or opening of an artery.

**arteriovenous** (ăr-tē″rē-ō-vē′nŭs) [″+ L. *vena,* a vein] ABBR: A-V. Rel. to both arteries and veins.

**arteriovenous access** Use of a shunt to connect an artery to a vein. This may be used in renal dialysis.

**arterioversion** (ăr-tē″rē-ō-vĕr′shŭn) [″ + L. *versio,* a turning] Eversion of an arterial wall to arrest hemorrhage from the open end.

**arteritis** (ăr″tĕ-rī′tĭs) [″ + *itis,* inflammation] Inflammation of an artery. SEE: *endarteritis; polyarteritis.* **arteritic** (-rĭt′ĭk), *adj.*

***a. nodosa*** Widespread inflammation of adventitia of small and medium-sized arteries with impaired function of the involved organs. SYN: *periarteritis nodosa; polyarteritis nodosa.*

***a. obliterans*** Inflammation of the intima of an artery, causing occlusion of the lumen. SYN: *endarteritis obliterans.*

***rheumatic a.*** Inflammation of small arteries as a result of rheumatic fever.

***Takayasu's a.*** SEE: *Takayasu's arteritis.*

***temporal a.*** A relatively common chronic inflammation of large arteries, usually the temporal, occipital, or ophthalmic arteries, accompanied by the presence of giant cells. It causes thickening of the intima, with narrowing and eventual occlusion of the lumen. It occurs in elderly people. Symptoms include headache, tenderness over the affected artery, loss of vision, and facial pain. The cause is unknown, but there is a genetic predisposition. Corticosteroids are administered.

**artery** (ăr'tĕr-ē) *pl.* **arteries** [Gr. *arteria,* windpipe] One of the vessels carrying blood from the heart to the tissues.

There are two divisions, pulmonary and systemic. The pulmonary arteries carry deoxygenated blood from the right ventricle to the lungs. The systemic arteries carry oxygenated blood from the left ventricle to the rest of the body. SEE: illus. (Systemic Arteries); *aorta* and *coronary artery disease* for illus.

ANATOMY: An arterial wall has three layers: the inner or serous layer (tunica intima) is endothelial tissue; the middle or yellow fibrous layer (tunica media) is smooth muscle and elastic connective tissue; and the outer or white fibrous layer (tunica adventitia) is fibrous connective tissue. SEE: illus. (Structure of an Artery); *Arteries Appendix.*

***brachiocephalic a.*** Innominate a.

***celiac a.*** The first branch of the abdominal aorta. Its branches supply the stomach, liver, spleen, duodenum, and pancreas.

***coiled a.*** Spiral a.

***conducting a.*** Elastic a.

***elastic a.*** A large artery in which elastic tissue is predominant in the tunica intima and tunica media. Elastic arteries include the aorta and its larger branches (innominate, common carotid, subclavian, and common iliac), which conduct blood to the muscular arteries. SYN: *conducting a.*

***end a.*** An artery whose branches do not anastomose with those of other arteries (e.g., arteries to the brain and spinal cord). SYN: *terminal a.*

***hyaloid a.*** A fetal artery that supplies nutrition to the lens. It disappears in the later months of gestation.

***innominate a.*** The right artery arising from the arch of the aorta, and dividing into the right subclavian and right common carotid arteries. SYN: *brachiocephalic a.*

***muscular a.*** A medium-sized artery with more smooth muscle than elastic tissue in the tunica media. Muscular arteries include the axillary, brachial, radial, intercostal, splenic, mesenteric, femoral, popliteal, and tibial arteries.

***sheathed a.*** The terminal portion of a pulp artery in the spleen. It has distinctive thickenings in its walls.

***spiral a.*** The coiled terminal branch of a uterine artery. It supplies the superficial two thirds of the endometrium, and in a pregnant uterus it empties into intervillous spaces, supplying blood that bathes the chorionic villi at the placental site. SYN: *coiled a.*

***terminal a.*** End a.

**arthr-** SEE: *arthro-.*

**arthral** (ăr'thrăl) Pert. to a joint.

**arthralgia** (ăr-thrăl'jē-ă) [Gr. *arthron,* joint, + *algos,* pain] Pain in a joint. **arthralgic** (-jĭk), *adj.*

***a. saturnina*** Joint pain resulting from lead poisoning.

**arthrectomy** (ăr-thrĕk'tō-mē) [" + *ektome,* excision] Excision of a joint.

**arthrempyesis, arthroempyesis** Suppuration in a joint.

**arthresthesia** (ăr"thrĕs-thē'zē-ă) [" + *aisthesis,* sensation] Joint sensibility; the perception of articular motions.

**arthritic** (ăr-thrĭt'ĭk) **1.** Pert. to arthritis. **2.** A person afflicted with arthritis.

**arthritis** (ăr-thrī'tĭs) *pl.* **arthritides** [" + *itis,* inflammation] Inflammation of a joint, usually accompanied by pain, swelling, and, frequently, changes in structure. **arthritic** (-thrĭ'tĭk), *adj.*

ETIOLOGY: Arthritis may result from or be associated with infection (gonococcal, tuberculous, pneumococcal); rheumatic fever; ulcerative colitis; trauma; neurogenic disturbances such as tabes dorsalis; degenerative joint disease such as osteoarthritis; metabolic disturbances such as gout; neoplasms such as synovioma; hydrarthrosis; periarticular conditions such as fibromyositis, myositis, or bursitis; and various other conditions such as acromegaly, psoriasis, and Raynaud's disease. Patients often benefit from referral to occupational or physical therapy, or both. SEE: *bursitis; osteoarthritis; rheumatism.*

***acute suppurative a.*** A serious arthritic condition marked by purulent distention of a synovial sac.

***allergic a.*** Arthritis following ingestion of food allergens or occurring in serum sickness.

***bacterial a.*** Inflammation of synovial membranes with purulent effusion into one or more joints. The etiological agent is usually streptococcus or staphyloccus.

***degenerative a.*** Osteoarthritis.

***gonorrheal a.*** Arthritis, usually of the knee joint, caused by gonorrheal infection. During the acute stage, several joints may be affected.

TREATMENT: Penicillin is given parenterally in an appropriate dosage for 10 to 14 days. If the gonococcal organism is resistant to penicillin, an appropriate antibiotic is substituted.

***gouty a.*** Arthritis caused by gout.

***hypertrophic a.*** Osteoarthritis.

***juvenile rheumatoid a.*** A chronic, inflammatory, systemic disease that may cause joint or connective tissue damage and visceral lesions throughout the body. It affects juveniles, with onset prior to age 16. Complete remission occurs in 75% of

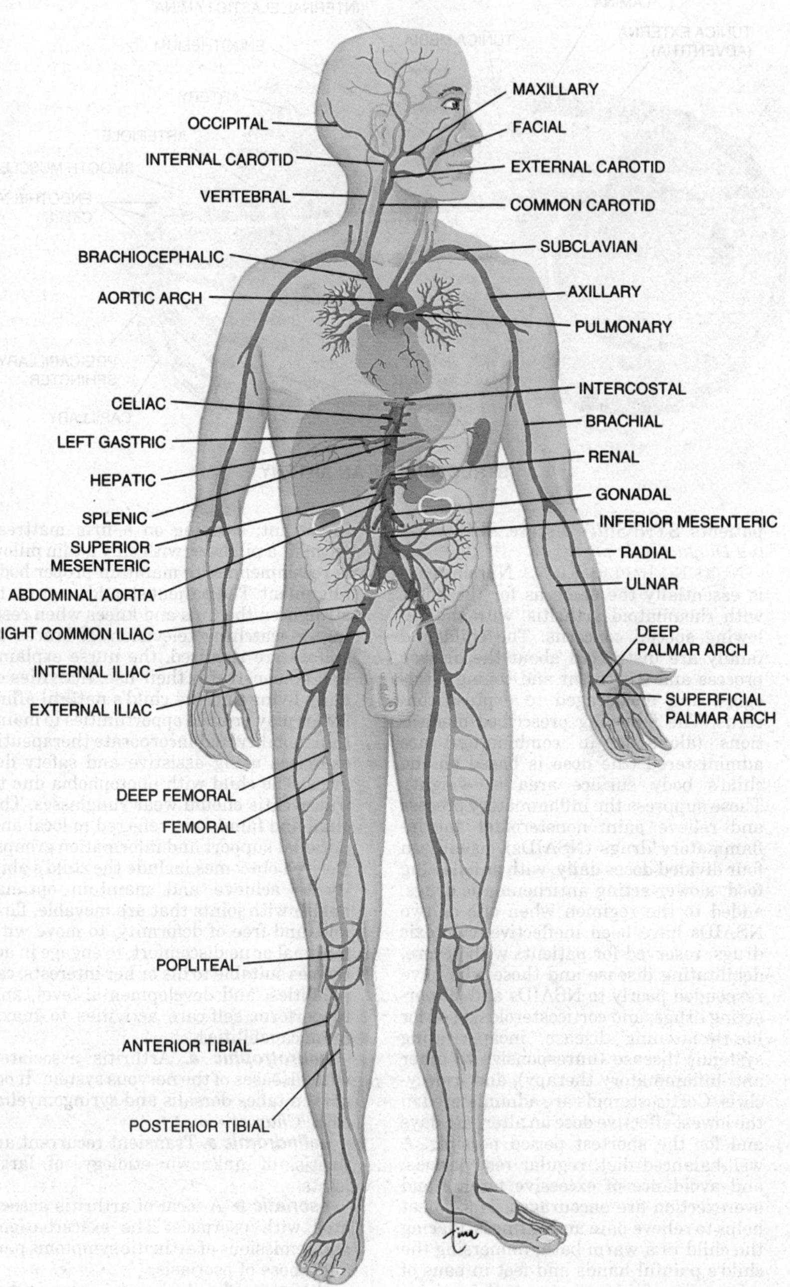


SYSTEMIC ARTERIES

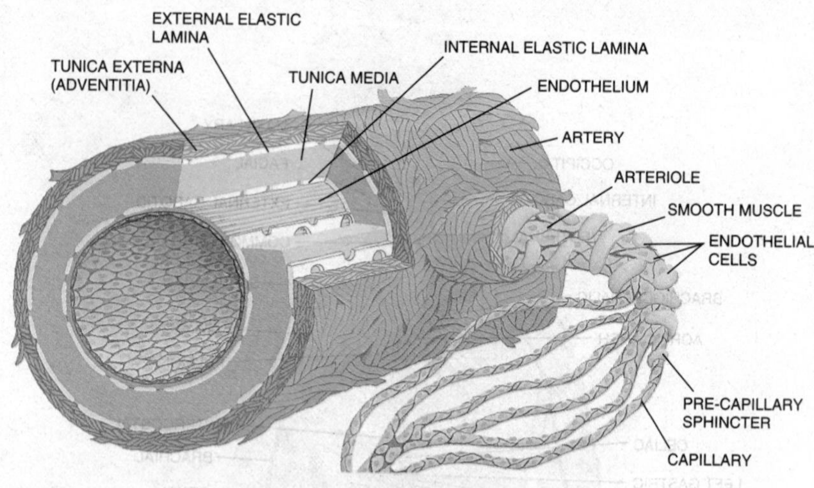


STRUCTURE OF AN ARTERY

patients. SYN: *Still's disease*. SEE: *Nursing Diagnoses Appendix.*

NURSING IMPLICATIONS: Nursing care is essentially the same as for the adult with rheumatoid arthritis, with the following special concerns: The child and family are instructed about the disease process and treatment and coping strategies, and encouraged to express concerns. The following prescribed medications (alone or in combination) are administered (the dose is based on the child's body surface area or weight). These suppress the inflammatory process and relieve pain: nonsteroidal anti-inflammatory drugs (NSAIDs), usually in four divided doses daily, with or following food; slower-acting antirheumatic drugs, added to the regimen when one or two NSAIDs have been ineffective; cytotoxic drugs, reserved for patients with severe, debilitating disease and those who have responded poorly to NSAIDs and slower-acting drugs; and corticosteroids, used for life-threatening disease, incapacitating systemic disease (unresponsive to other anti-inflammatory therapy), and iridocyclitis. Corticosteroids are administered in the lowest effective dose on alternate days and for the shortest period possible. A well-balanced diet, regular rest periods, and avoidance of excessive fatigue and overexertion are encouraged. Moist heat helps to relieve pain and stiffness. Placing the child in a warm bath, immersing the child's painful hands and feet in pans of warm water for 10 min two to three times daily, or using daily whirlpool baths, a paraffin bath, or hot packs provides temporary relief of acute swelling and pain. Swimming is recommended to strengthen muscles and maintain mobility. Good posture and body mechanics are important; sleeping on a firm mattress without a pillow or with only a thin pillow is recommended to maintain proper body alignment. The patient should lie prone to straighten the hips and knees when resting or watching television. If braces or splints are required, the nurse explains and demonstrates their use. Activities of daily living and the child's natural affinity for play provide opportunities to maintain mobility and incorporate therapeutic exercises using assistive and safety devices. The child with photophobia due to iridocyclitis should wear sunglasses. The child and family are referred to local and national support and information groups. Desired outcomes include the child's ability to achieve and maintain optimal health with joints that are movable, flexible, and free of deformity, to move with minimal or no discomfort, to engage in activities suitable to his or her interests, capabilities, and developmental level, and to perform self-care activities to maximum capabilities.

***neurotrophic a.*** Arthritis associated with diseases of the nervous system. It occurs in tabes dorsalis and syringomyelia. SEE: *Charcot's joint.*

***palindromic a.*** Transient recurrent arthritis, of unknown etiology, of large joints.

***psoriatic a.*** A form of arthritis associated with psoriasis. The exacerbations and remissions of arthritic symptoms parallel those of psoriasis.

***rheumatoid a.*** A chronic systemic disease marked by inflammatory changes in joints and related structures that result in crippling deformities. SEE: illus.

ETIOLOGY: The pathological changes in the joints are generally thought to be caused by an autoimmune disease. Envi-

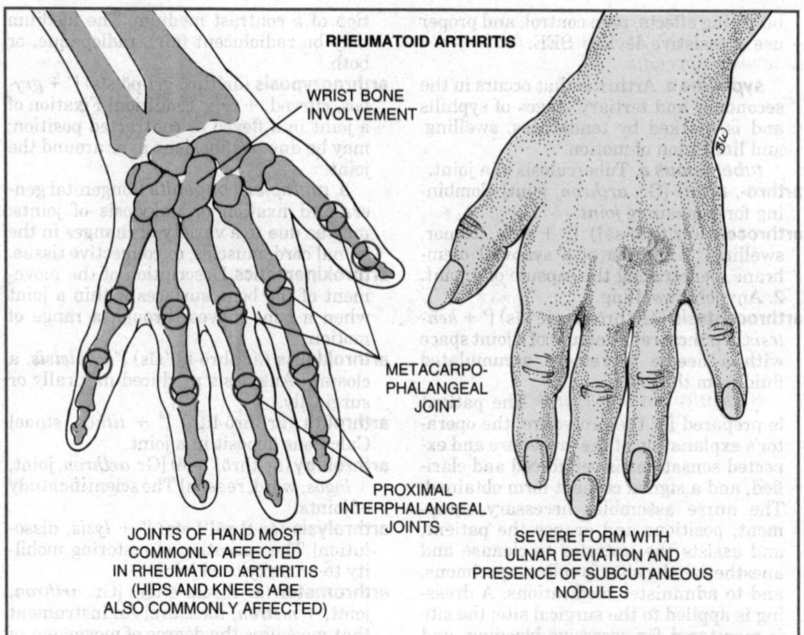


ronmental and familial factors are of doubtful importance. Onset may vary, but it usually occurs in middle age.

TREATMENT: There is no specific therapy. If the condition is severe and painful, bedrest may be required for a short time. Drug therapy usually is initiated with large doses of enteric-coated aspirin, nonsteroidal anti-inflammatory agents and, sometimes, brief use of corticosteroids.

Caution: The continued use of corticosteroids is contraindicated due to the development of serious side effects, and the use of second-line drugs requires regular monitoring for adverse effects.

Exercise and physical therapy are important in maintaining range of motion of the affected joints. Until the inflammatory response has subsided, passive exercise is employed to prevent contractures. When inflammation has subsided, active exercise is used to maintain muscle strength and range of motion. A variety of self-help devices are available for patients with severe limitation of joint movement, enabling these patients to remain self-sufficient. Surgical procedures such as arthroplasty (e.g., total joint replacements) have been effective in treating severe forms of rheumatoid arthritis.

NURSING IMPLICATIONS: All joints are assessed for inflammation, deformities, and contractures, and the patient's ability to perform activities of daily living (ADL) is evaluated. The patient is assessed for fatigue, irritability, and temperature elevation; vital signs are monitored; and weight changes, sensory disturbances, pain (location, quality, severity, inciting and relieving factors), and morning stiffness (esp. duration) are documented. Use of moist heat is encouraged to relieve stiffness and pain. Prescribed anti-inflammatory and analgesic drug therapy is administered and evaluated; the patient is taught about the use of these medications. Inflamed joints are splinted in extension as prescribed to prevent contractures, pressure areas noted, and range of motion is maintained with gentle, passive exercise. Once inflammation has subsided, the nurse instructs the patient about active range-of-motion exercise for specific joints and encourages warm baths or soaks before or during exercise. Cleansing lotions or oils should be used for dry skin. The patient is encouraged to perform ADLs if possible, allowing extra time. Assistive and safety devices may be recommended for some patients. Activities should be paced, sitting and standing alternated, and short rest periods taken. The patient should sleep on a firm mattress, preferably in a supine position. Referral to an occupational therapist may be needed. Both patient and family are referred to local and national support and information groups. Desired outcomes include cooperation with prescribed medication and exercise regimens, ability to perform ADLs, slowed progression of debilitating effects, pain control, and proper use of assistive devices. SEE: *Nursing Diagnoses Appendix.*

***syphilitic a.*** Arthritis that occurs in the secondary and tertiary stages of syphilis and is marked by tenderness, swelling, and limitation of motion.

***tuberculous a.*** Tuberculosis of a joint.

**arthro-, arthr-** [Gr. *arthron,* joint] Combining form meaning *joint.*

**arthrocele** (ăr′thrō-sēl) [″ + *kele,* tumor, swelling] **1.** Hernia of a synovial membrane, penetrating the capsule of a joint. **2.** Any joint swelling.

**arthrocentesis** (ăr″thrō-sĕn-tē′sĭs) [″ + *kentesis,* a puncture] Puncture of a joint space with a needle to remove accumulated fluid from the joint.

NURSING IMPLICATIONS: The patient is prepared for the procedure; the operator's explanation of the procedure and expected sensations is reinforced and clarified, and a signed consent form obtained. The nurse assembles necessary equipment, positions and drapes the patient, and assists the operator to cleanse and anesthetize the site, to collect specimens, and to administer medications. A dressing is applied to the surgical site; the site is monitored for excessive bleeding, and bleeding controlled should it occur. Follow-up care includes elevating the affected limb and applying ice or cold packs to the joint for 24 to 36 hr to decrease pain and swelling; reporting symptoms such as fever and increased joint pain, redness, or swelling; and avoiding overuse of the affected joint for several days.

**arthrochondritis** (ăr″thrō-kŏn-drī′tĭs) [″ + *chondros,* cartilage, + *itis,* inflammation] Inflammation of an articular cartilage.

**arthroclasia** (ăr″thrō-klā′zē-ă) [″ + *klasis,* a breaking] Artificial breaking of adhesions of an ankylosed joint to provide movement.

**arthrodesis** (ăr-thrō-dē′sĭs) [″ + *desis,* binding] The surgical immobilization of a joint; artificial ankylosis.

**arthrodia** (ăr-thrō′dē-ă) [Gr.] A type of synovial joint that permits only simple gliding movement within narrow limits imposed by ligaments.

**arthrodynia** (ăr″thrō-dĭn′ē-ă) [Gr. *arthron,* joint, + *odyne,* pain] Pain in a joint.

**arthrodysplasia** (ăr″thrō-dĭs-plā′zē-ă) [″ + *dys,* bad, + *plassein,* to form] A hereditary condition marked by deformity of various joints.

**arthroendoscopy** (ăr″thrō-ĕn-dŏs′kō-pē) [″ + *endon,* within, + *skopein,* to examine] Inspection of the interior of a joint with an endoscope.

**arthrogram** (ăr′thrō-grăm) [″ + *gramma,* something written] Visualization of a joint by radiographic study after injection of a contrast medium into the joint space.

**arthrography** (ăr-thrŏg′ră-fē) [″ + *graphein,* to write] **1.** Radiography of a joint. **2.** Radiography of a synovial joint after injection of a contrast medium. The medium may be radiolucent (air), radiopaque, or both.

**arthrogryposis** (ăr″thrō-grĭ-pō′sĭs) [″ + *grypos,* curved, + *osis,* condition] Fixation of a joint in a flexed or contracted position; may be due to adhesions in or around the joint.

***a. multiplex congenita*** Congenital generalized fixation or ankylosis of joints; may be due to a variety of changes in the spinal cord, muscles, or connective tissue.

**arthrokinematics** Description of the movement of the bone surfaces within a joint when a bone moves through a range of motion.

**arthrokleisis** (ăr″thrō-klī′sĭs) [″ + *kleisis,* a closure] Ankylosis produced naturally or surgically.

**arthrolith** (ăr′thrō-lĭth) [″ + *lithos,* stone] Calculous deposit in a joint.

**arthrology** (ăr-thrŏl′ō-jē) [Gr. *arthron,* joint, + *logos,* word, reason] The scientific study of joints.

**arthrolysis** (ăr-thrŏl′ĭ-sĭs) [″ + *lysis,* dissolution] The operation of restoring mobility to an ankylosed joint.

**arthrometer** (ăr-thrŏm′ĕ-tĕr) [Gr. *arthron,* joint, + *metron,* measure] An instrument that measures the degree of movement of a joint. SYN: *goniometer.*

**arthroneuralgia** (ăr″thrō-nū-răl′jē-ă) [″ + *neuron,* nerve, + *algos,* pain] Pain in or around a joint.

**arthropathology** (ăr″thrō-pă-thol′ō-jē) [″ + *pathos,* disease, + *logos,* word, reason] The pathology of joint disease.

**arthropathy** (ăr-thrŏp′ă-thē) [″ + *pathos,* disease, suffering] Any joint disease.

***Charcot's a.*** SEE: *Charcot's joint.*

***inflammatory a.*** An inflammatory joint disease; arthritis.

**arthrophyte** (ăr′thrō-fīt) [Gr. *arthron,* joint, + *phyton,* growth] Abnormal growth in a joint cavity.

**arthroplasty** (ăr′thrō-plăs″tē) [″ + *plassein,* to form] Plastic surgery to reshape or reconstruct a diseased joint. This may be done to alleviate pain, to permit normal function, or to correct a developmental or hereditary joint defect. The procedure may require use of an artificial joint.

NURSING IMPLICATIONS: *Preoperative:* The nurse prepares the patient physically and emotionally for the procedure and gathers baseline data.

*Postoperative:* The surgeon may prescribe traction or other immobilization devices, such as splints, pillows, or casts, or a continuous passive motion device. Bedrest is maintained for the prescribed period, and the patient is positioned as prescribed. The affected joint is maintained in proper alignment, immobilization devices are inspected for pressure, and frequent neurovascular and motor checks are performed on the involved extremity distal to the operative site. Prescribed analgesics are administered, and the patient is taught about self-administration. Noninvasive measures are employed to reduce pain and anxiety. Vital signs are monitored for hypovolemic shock due to blood loss, and the patient is assessed for other complications such as thromboembolism, fat embolism, and infection. The nurse re-dresses the incision according to protocol, assessing for local signs of infection. Deep breathing and coughing, frequent position changes, and adequate fluid intake are encouraged. The nurse assists the patient with prescribed exercise and activity, taking appropriate measures to prevent dislocation of the prosthesis, and reinforces prescribed activity restrictions. The patient is taught to report symptoms such as fever, pain, and increased joint stiffness and is referred for home care and outpatient physical therapy. SEE: *Nursing Diagnoses Appendix.*

**arthropneumoradiography** (ăr″thrō-nū″mō-rā-dē-ŏg′ră-fē) [″ + *pneuma,* air, + *radiography*] Radiography of a synovial joint after injection of a radiolucent contrast medium such as air or helium. SEE: *arthrogram.*

**arthropod** (ăr′thrō-pŏd) A member of the phylum Arthropoda.

**Arthropoda** (ăr-thrŏp′ō-dă) [″ + *pous,* foot] A phylum of invertebrate animals marked by bilateral symmetry, a hard, jointed exoskeleton, segmented bodies, and jointed paired appendages. It includes the crustaceans, insects, myriapods, arachnids, and similar forms. It is the largest animal phylum, containing over 700,000 species. Many have medical importance as causative agents of disease, as vectors, or as parasites.

**arthropyosis** (ăr″thrō-pī-ō′sĭs) [″ + *pyosis,* suppuration] Suppuration of a joint.

**arthrosclerosis** [Gr. *arthron,* joint, + *sklerosis,* a hardening] Stiffening or hardening of the joints, esp. in the aged.

**arthroscope** (ăr′thrō-skōp) [″ + *skopein,* to examine] An endoscope for examining the interior of a joint.

**arthroscopy** (ăr-thrŏs′kō-pē) Direct joint visualization by means of an arthroscope.

NURSING IMPLICATIONS: *Preoperative:* The nurse prepares the patient physically and emotionally for the procedure and gathers baseline data. The operative site is prepared according to protocol and type of anesthesia.

*Postoperative:* Vital signs are monitored until stable, and intravenous or oral fluids provided depending on the type of anesthesia used. The surgical dressing is inspected for drainage, and the presence of any drainage devices and their contents are documented. The dressing is reinforced or replaced under strict asepsis according to protocol. Postoperative teaching stresses expected sensations, such as joint soreness and grinding; the application of ice to relieve pain and swelling; analgesic use; activity or ambulation restrictions; weight-bearing exercises; and use of crutches or other assistive devices. The patient is instructed to report any unusual drainage, redness, joint swelling, "mushy" feeling in the joint, severe or persistent pain, or fever, because these may indicate infection, effusion, hemarthrosis, or a synovial cyst. The patient is referred for outpatient follow-up care as necessary. SEE: *Nursing Diagnoses Appendix.*

**arthrosis** (ăr-thrō′sĭs) [″ + *osis,* condition] **1.** Joint. **2.** A joint disorder caused by trophic degeneration.

**arthrospore** (ăr′thrō-spor) [″ + *sporos,* a seed] A bacterial spore formed by segmentation.

**arthrosteitis** (ăr″thrŏs-tē-ī′tĭs) [″ + *osteon,* bone, + *itis,* inflammation] Inflammation of the bony structures of a joint.

**arthrostenosis** (ăr″-thrō-stĕ-nō′sĭs) [″ + *stenos,* narrow] Pathological narrowing of a joint.

**arthrostomy** (ăr-thrŏs′tō-mē) [″ + *stoma,* mouth] The surgical formation of a temporary opening into a joint for drainage purposes.

**arthrosynovitis** (ăr″thrō-sĭn″ō-vī′tĭs) [″ + L. *synovia,* joint fluid, + Gr. *itis,* inflammation] Inflammation of the synovial membrane of a joint.

**arthrotome** (ăr′thrō-tōm) [″ + *tome,* incision] A knife for making incisions into a joint.

**arthrotomy** (ăr-thrŏt′ō-mē) Cutting into a joint.

**arthrous** (ăr′thrŭs) [Gr. *arthron,* joint] Jointed or pert. to a joint.

**arthroxesis** (ăr-thrŏk′sĭ-sĭs) [″ + *xexis,* scraping] Scraping of diseased tissue from a joint.

**Arthus reaction, Arthus phenomenon** (ăr-toos′) [Nicholas Maurice Arthus, Fr. bacteriologist, 1862–1945] A severe local inflammatory reaction that occurs at the site of injection of an antigen in a previously sensitized individual. Arthus reactions are a form of type III hypersensitivity reactions producing an antigen-antibody immune complex and are the cause of occupational pneumonitis or alveolitis in certain individuals.

**articulate** (ăr-tĭk′ū-lāt) [L. *articulatus,* jointed] **1.** To join together as a joint. **2.** In dentistry, to arrange teeth on a denture. **3.** To speak clearly.

**articulatio** (ăr-tĭk″ū-lā′shē-ō) [L.] The site of union or junction of two bones.

**articulation** **1.** The place of union between two or more bones; a joint. It may be immovable (as in synarthrosis), slightly movable (amphiarthrosis), or freely movable (diarthrosis). Cartilage (fibrous connective tissue) lines the opposing surfaces of all joints. **2.** The relative position of the tongue and palate necessary to produce a given sound. **3.** Enunciation of words and sentences. **4.** The movement of articulating surfaces through their available joint play or range of motion, used to determine joint mobility or to treat joint pain. **articular** (ăr-tĭk′ū-lăr), *adj.*

***apophyseal a.*** The joint between the superior and the inferior articulating processes of the vertebrae.

***articulator a.*** The use of a mechanical device to simulate the action of the temporomandibular joint when placing teeth in complete dentures or partial removable dentures so that they articulate properly.

***confluent a.*** Speech in which syllables are run together.

***dental a.*** The contact relationship between upper and lower teeth when moving against each other or into or out of centric position.

***working a.*** The occlusion of teeth on the side toward which the mandible is moved. *Also called* working bite.

**articulator** (ăr-tĭk′ū-lā″tor) In dentistry, a device for maintaining casts of the teeth in a precise and natural relationship.

**articulo mortis** (ăr-tĭk′ū-lō″ mor′tĭs) [L.] At the time of death.

**articulus** (ăr-tĭk′ū-lŭs) [L.] **1.** A knuckle or a joint. **2.** A segment.

**artifact, artefact** (ăr′tĭ-făkt) [L. *ars,* art, + *facere,* to make] **1.** Anything artificially produced. **2.** In histology and radiography, any structure or feature produced by the technique used and not occurring naturally. **3.** In electronics, the appearance of a spurious signal not consistent with results expected from the signal being studied. For example, an electrocardiogram may contain artifacts produced by a defective machine, electrical interference, patient movement, or loose electrodes.

**artificial** (ăr″tĭ-fĭsh′ăl) Not natural; formed in imitation of nature.

**artificial assist** A device used to support a bodily function (e.g., a crutch, an artificial limb, a cardiac pacemaker, or a respirator).

**artificial heart** A device designed to be implanted in a patient to assist the action of the heart or to replace it. Efforts to perfect such a device continue.

**artificial hyperemia** Bringing of blood to the superficial tissues by means of counterirritation, such as may be produced by cupping or acupuncture.

**artificial impregnation** Artificial insemination.

**artificial insemination** ABBR: AI. Mechanical placement of semen containing viable spermatozoa into the vagina.

***donor a.i.*** ABBR: AID. Artificial insemination of a woman with sperm from an anonymous donor. This procedure is generally done in cases in which the husband is sterile. SEE: *Universal Precautions Appendix.*

***husband a.i.*** ABBR: AIH. Use of a husband's sperm to artificially inseminate his wife.

**artificial kidney transplant** The implantation of a device to take over kidney function. Efforts to perfect such a device are experimental.

**artificial pneumothorax** Artificial introduction of air into the pleural cavity. Oxygen, nitrogen, or filtered atmospheric air is used.

**artificial respiration** Maintenance of respiratory movements by artificial means. SEE: *cardiopulmonary resuscitation.*

**artisan's cramp** A muscle spasm induced by prolonged work requiring delicate coordination; most likely to occur in writing, piano playing, sewing, and typing. SEE: *writer's cramp.*

**arum family poisoning** Poisoning caused by ingestion of plants of the genus *Arum* (e.g., dieffenbachia, caladium, and philodendron), which contain poisonous calcium oxalate crystals. Symptoms include irritation, pain, burning, and swelling of the affected areas. The affected area should be washed with water, and ice should be applied. If pain is severe, corticosteroids are of benefit.

**aryepiglottic** (ăr″ē-ĕp″ĭ-glŏt′ĭk) [Gr. *arytaina,* ladle, + *epi,* upon, + *glottis,* back of tongue] Pert. to the arytenoid cartilage and epiglottis.

**aryl-** Prefix denoting a radical derived from an aromatic hydrocarbon.

***a. group*** In chemistry, a radical group of the aromatic or benzene series.

**arytenoid** (ăr″ĭ-tē′noyd) [Gr. *arytaina,* ladle, + *eidos,* form, shape] **1.** Resembling a ladle or pitcher mouth. **2.** Pert. to the arytenoid cartilages or muscles of the larynx. SEE: *larynx* for illus.

**arytenoidectomy** (ăr″ĭ-tē″noyd-ĕk′tō-mē) [″ + ″ + *ektome,* excision] Excision of arytenoid cartilage.

**arytenoiditis** (ăr-ĭt″ĕ-noy-dī′tĭs) [″ + ″ + *itis,* inflammation] Inflammation of arytenoid cartilage or muscles.

**arytenoidopexy** (ăr″ĭ-tĕ-noy′dō-pĕk″sē) [″ + ″ + *pexis,* fixation] Surgical fixation of the arytenoid muscle or cartilage.

**AS** L. *auris sinistra,* left ear; *aortic stenosis.*

**As** **1.** *astigmatic.* **2.** *astigmatism.* **3.** Symbol for the element arsenic.

**ASA** *acetylsalicylic acid.*

**asafetida, asafoetida** (ăs-ă-fĕt′ĭd-ă) [L. *asa,* gum, + *foetida,* smelly] A gum resin, obtained from the roots of *Ferula asafoetida,* with a characteristic strong odor and garlic taste. Although this substance is no longer used in medicine, it has historical interest. In the early 20th century, it was used as a carminative and as an amulet to ward off disease. It is used in Asia as a condiment and food flavoring and as an animal repellent in veterinary medicine.

**ASAHP** *Association of Schools of Allied Health Professions.*

**ASAP** *as soon as possible.* SEE: *stat.*

**asaphia** (ă-săf′ē-ă, ă-sā′fē-ă) [Gr. *asapheia,* obscurity] Inability to speak distinctly.

**asbestiform** (ăs-bĕs′tĭ-form) [Gr. *asbestos,* unquenchable, + L. *forma,* appearance] Having a structure similar to that of asbestos.

**asbestos** (ăs-bĕs′tŏs) [Gr. *asbestos,* unquenchable] A fibrous, incombustible form of magnesium and calcium silicate used to make insulating materials.

**asbestos bodies** A beaded, dumbbell-shaped body formed when a macrophage engulfs asbestos fibers.

**asbestosis** (ăs″bĕ-stō′sĭs) [″ + *osis,* condition] Lung disease, a form of pneumonoconiosis resulting from protracted inhalation of asbestos particles. Exposure to asbestos has been linked with lung cancer, including bronchogenic carcinoma and esp. mesothelioma. The latency period may be 20 years or more.

SYMPTOMS: Symptoms include exertional dyspnea or, with extensive fibrosis, dyspnea at rest. In advanced disease, the patient may complain of a dry cough (productive in smokers), chest pain (often pleuritic), and recurrent respiratory tract infections. Tachypnea, crackles, and clubbing may be present.

NURSING IMPLICATIONS: A history of occupational, family, or neighborhood exposure to asbestos fibers is obtained. The chest is auscultated for tachypnea and crackles in the lung bases, and the fingers inspected for clubbing. The nurse monitors for and documents changes in sputum quality and quantity, restlessness, increased tachypnea, and changes in breath sounds. Complications such as cor pulmonale or pulmonary hypertension are noted.

Prescribed aerosol therapy, inhaled mucolytics, and oxygen are administered, and the patient is instructed in their use. Mechanical ventilation is used if the patient's arterial oxygen level cannot be maintained above 40 mm Hg. Both patient and family are instructed in chest physiotherapy. Frequent small meals of high-calorie, high-protein foods are offered. The patient is weighed two or three times weekly. Adequate fluids are provided to help thin and loosen secretions. Respiratory therapy is scheduled for at least 1 hr before or after meals, and oral hygiene provided after inhaled bronchodilator therapy. Daily activities are recommended, but should be interspersed with rest.

The patient is advised to avoid crowds and persons with known respiratory infections and to obtain influenza and pneumococcal immunizations. Instruction is given in the use and care of required oxygen and aerosol equipment, inhalers, or transtracheal catheters. Patients who smoke cigarettes are referred to smoking cessation programs or for nicotine therapy if necessary.

**ascariasis** (ăs″kă-rī′ă-sĭs) [Gr. *askaris,* pinworm, + *-iasis,* condition of] Condition resulting from infestation by *Ascaris lumbricoides.*

**ascaricide** (ăs-kăr′ĭ-sīd) [″ + L. *cidus,* killing] An agent that kills ascarids. **ascaricidal** (ăs-kăr-ĭ-sī′dăl), *adj.*

**ascarid** (ăs′kă-rĭd) A nematode worm of the family Ascaridae.

**Ascaris** (ăs′kă-rĭs) A genus of nematode worms belonging to the family Ascaridae. They inhabit the intestines of vertebrates.

***A. lumbricoides*** A species of *Ascaris* that lives in the human intestine. Eggs are passed with the feces and require at least 2 weeks' incubation in the soil before they become infective. After being swallowed, the eggs hatch in the intestinal tract and the larvae enter the venous circulation and pass to the lungs. From there they migrate up the respiratory passages, are swallowed, and reach their site of continued residence, the jejunum. In a 1- to 2-year life span, the female is capable of producing 200,000 eggs per day. The eggs are passed with the feces, and a new cycle is started. Children up to the ages of 12 to 14 are likely to be infected. Intestinal obstruction may be a complication in children under 6 years of age. SEE: illus.

TREATMENT: Pyrantel pamoate is the drug of choice. Mebendazole is also effective. No drug is useful during the pulmonary phase of the infection.

**ascaris** *pl.* **ascarides** A worm of the genus *Ascaris.*

**Aschner's phenomenon** (ăsh′nĕrz) [Bernhard Aschner, Austrian gynecologist, 1883–1960] Slowing of the pulse after pressure is applied to the eyeball or the carotid sinus. It may be used to slow the heart during attacks of supraventricular tachycardia or as a diagnostic test for angina pectoris. Slowing of the heart produced by this reflex may relieve anginal pain. Also called *Aschner's reflex* and *sign.* SYN: *oculocardiac reflex.*

**Aschoff, Ludwig** (ăsh′ŏf) German pathologist, 1866–1942.

***A.'s cells*** Large cells with basophilic cytoplasm and a large vesicular nucleus, often multinucleated. They are characteristic of Aschoff's nodules.

***A.'s nodules*** Small nodules composed of cells and leukocytes found in the interstitial tissues of the heart in rheumatic myocarditis.

**asci** (ăs′ī) Pl. of ascus.

**ascia** (ăs′ē-ă, ăs′kē-ă) [L. *ascia,* ax] A form of spiral bandage with each turn overlapping the previous one for a third of its width.

**ascites** (ă-sī′tēz) [Gr. *askitēs* from *askos,* a leather bag] The accumulation of serous fluid in the peritoneal cavity. SEE: *edema.*

ETIOLOGY: Ascites may be caused by interference in venous return as occurs in cardiac disease; obstruction of flow in the vena cava or portal vein; obstruction in lymphatic drainage; disturbance in electrolyte balance as occurs in sodium retention; depletion of plasma proteins; or cirrhosis of the liver.

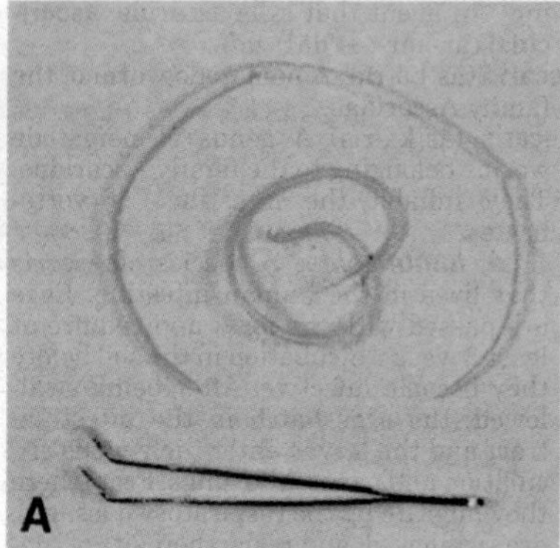



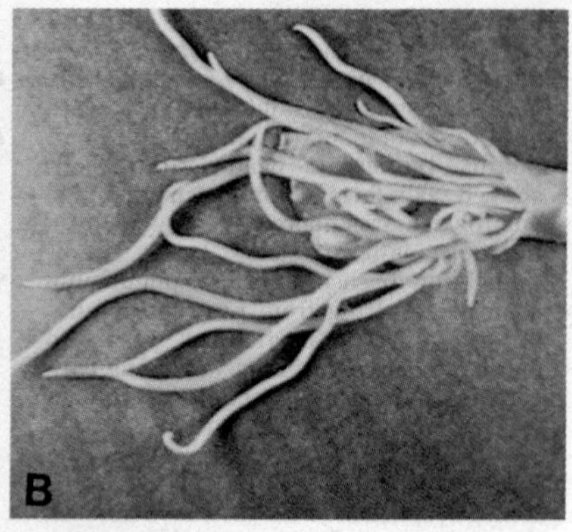



**ASCARIS LUMBRICOIDES**

**(A)** THE SMALLER MALE ENCIRCLED BY THE FEMALE **(B)** OBSTRUCTION OF SMALL INTESTINE BY HEAVY INFESTATION

NURSING IMPLICATIONS: Ventilatory effort, appetite and food intake, fluid intake and output, and weight are assessed. Abdominal girth is measured at the largest point, and the site marked for future measurements. Paracentesis procedure and expected sensations are explained to the patient. The nurse assists the operator to perform the paracentesis: assembling the equipment; preparing the site; monitoring vital signs, weight, and girth; and obtaining serum protein, sodium, and potassium levels before and after the procedure. The nurse also provides emotional and physical support to the patient throughout the procedure. Desired outcomes include eased ventilatory effort, improved appetite, and improved general comfort. **ascitic** (-sĭt′ĭk), *adj.*

***a. chylosus*** Chyle in the ascitic fluid, usually resulting from rupture of the thoracic duct.

**ascitic fluid** Clear and pale straw-colored fluid occurring in ascites. Specific gravity is 1.005 to 1.015.

**A.S.C.L.S.** *American Society for Clinical Laboratory Science,* formerly American Society for Medical Technology.

**Ascoli's reaction** (ăs-kō′lēz) [Alberto Ascoli, It. serologist, 1877–1957] Precipitation test for anthrax; used for detection of anthrax bacilli in animal hides and meat. Also called *Ascoli's test.*

**Ascomycetes** (ăs″kō-mī-sē′tēz) [Gr. *askos,* leather bag, + *mykes,* fungus] The largest class of Eumycetes (or true fungi) of the phylum Thallophyta; the sac fungi, which includes the true yeasts, blue molds, and penicillin. Organisms in this group are characterized by possession of a saclike sporangium (or ascus), in which ascospores are developed.

**ascorbic acid** (ăs-kor′bĭk) [Gr. *a-,* not, + L. *scorbutus,* scurvy] SEE: *acid, ascorbic; vitamin C.*

**ascospore** (ăs′kō-spor) [Gr. *askos,* leather bag, + *sporos,* seed] A spore produced within an ascus or spore sac.

**ascus** (ăs′kŭs) *pl.* **asci** [Gr. *askos,* leather bag] A saclike spore case in which ascospores, typically eight, are formed; characteristic of the Ascomycetes.

**-ase** A suffix used in forming the name of an enzyme. It is added to the name of the substance upon which it acts (e.g., lipase, which acts on lipids).

**asemia** Asymbolia.

**asepsis** (ā-sĕp′sĭs) [Gr. *a-,* not, + *sepesthai,* to decay] A condition free from germs, infection, and any form of life. SEE: *antisepsis; sterilization.* **aseptic** (-tĭk), *adj.*

**aseptic-antiseptic** [Gr. *a-,* not, + *sepsis,* decay, + *anti,* against, + *sepsis,* decay] Both aseptic and antiseptic.

**aseptic technique** A method used in surgery to prevent contamination of the wound and operative site. All instruments used are sterilized, and physicians and nurses wear sterile caps, masks, and gloves. SEE: *Universal Precautions Appendix.*

**Asepto syringe** Trade name for a type of syringe with a bulb top and blunt-tipped end; generally used for aseptic irrigation of wounds.

**asexual** (ā-sĕk′shū-ăl) [″ + L. *sexualis,* having sex] Without sex; nonsexual.

**asexualization** (ā-sĕk″shū-ăl-ĭ-zā′shŭn) Sterilization by ablation of the ovaries or testes.

**ash** (ăsh) [AS. *aesc,* ash] Incombustible powdery residue of a substance that has been incinerated.

**ASHD** *arteriosclerotic heart disease.*

**Asherman's syndrome** [Joseph G. Asherman, Czech. physician, b. 1889] Intrauterine adhesions. These may cause amenorrhea.

**asialia** (ă″sī-ā′lē-ă, ā″sē-ā′lē-ă) [Gr. *a-*, not, + *sialon,* spittle] Absence or deficiency of saliva. SYN: *aptyalism.*

**Asiatic cholera** SEE: *cholera.*

**asiderosis** (ă″sĭd-ĕ-rō′sĭs) [″ + *sideros,* iron, + *osis,* condition] Deficiency of iron reserve in the body.

**ASIS** *anterior superior iliac spine.* Radiographic palpation point on the skin on each side of the front of the pelvis.

**-asis** Suffix meaning *condition, state.*

**ASLO** *antistreptolysin-O.*

**as low as reasonably achievable** ABBR: ALARA. In radiology, a program of radiation protection in which personnel attempt to keep their exposure to ionizing radiation at an absolute minimum.

**asocial** (ā-sō′shĭl) **1.** Withdrawn from society. **2.** Inconsiderate of the needs of others.

**asoma** (ā-sō′mă) [Gr. *a-*, not, + *soma,* body] A deformed fetus with an imperfectly formed trunk and head.

**asonia** (ă-sō′nē-ă) [″ + L. *sonus,* sound] Tone deafness.

**asparaginase** (ăs-păr′ă-jĭn-āz) An antineoplastic agent derived from the bacterium *Escherichia coli.*

**asparagine** (ăs-păr′ă-jĭn) Aminosuccinic acid, a nonessential amino acid.

**Asparagus** (ă-spăr′ă-gŭs) [Gr. *asparagos*] A genus of liliaceous herbs.

**aspartame** (ă-spăr′tām) An artificial sweetener synthesized from two amino acids, aspartic acid and phenylalanine. It is 180 times sweeter than sugar. It is unsuitable for use in cooking because its flavor is changed when heated. Trade names are Equal and NutraSweet.

**aspartate aminotransferase** ABBR: AST. An intracellular enzyme involved in amino acid and carbohydrate metabolism. It is present in high concentrations in muscle, liver, and brain. An increased level of this enzyme in the blood indicates necrosis or disease in these tissues. Formerly called serum glutamic-oxaloacetic transaminase (SGOT) or glutamic-oxaloacetic transaminase.

**aspartic acid** $COOH \cdot CH(NH_2) \cdot CH_2 \cdot COOH$. A nonessential amino acid.

**aspastic** (ă-spăs′tĭk) [Gr. *a-*, not, + *spastikos,* having spasms] Nonspastic.

**aspecific** (ă-spĕ-sĭf′ĭk) Not specific.

**aspect** (ăs′pĕkt) [L. *aspectus,* a view] **1.** The part of a surface facing in any designated direction. **2.** Appearance, looks.

**A.S.P.E.N.** *American Society for Parenteral and Enteral Nutrition.*

**Asperger's disorder** A severe and sustained impairment of social interaction and functioning. In contrast to autism, there are no clinically significant delays in language, cognitive, or developmental age-appropriate skills.

**aspergillin** (ăs″pĕr-jĭl′ĭn) A pigment produced by *Aspergillus niger.*

**aspergillosis** (ăs″pĕr-jĭl-ō′sĭs) [*aspergillus* + Gr. *osis,* condition] *Aspergillus* infection in the tissues or on any mucous surface; marked by inflammatory granulomatous lesions. This condition may develop in the bronchi, lungs, aural canal, or skin, or in the mucous membranes of the eye, nose, or urethra. It may extend through the various viscera, producing mycotic nodules in the lungs, liver, kidney, and other organs. The disease is not transmissible from humans to animals or vice versa. SEE: illus.

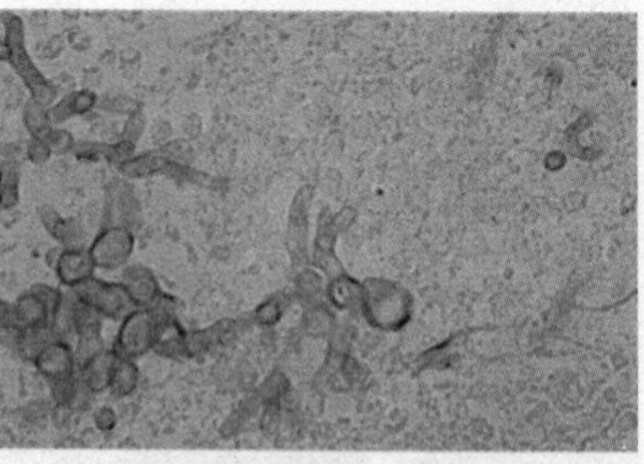

ASPERGILLOSIS OF LUNG

GROWTH OF FUNGUS (PURPLE) FILLS THE ALVEOLI (×450)

TREATMENT: Amphotericin B is administered. At construction sites, application of 8-copper quinolate may control fungal growth on inanimate objects.

***allergic bronchopulmonary a.*** Inflammation of the bronchioles and surrounding interstitial tissue in patients with atopic or inherited asthma exposed to *Aspergillus fumigatus.* The cause is the response of immunoglobulins E and G and their mediators. Permanent fibrotic damage may occur.

***aural a.*** A form of otomycosis caused by *Aspergillus.*

***pulmonary a.*** Lung disease caused by *Aspergillus.*

**Aspergillus** (ăs″pĕr-jĭl′ŭs) [L. *aspergere,* to sprinkle] A genus of Ascomycetes fungi, including several mold species, some of which are pathogenic. The principal pathogen is *Aspergillus fumigatus,* although others (*A. flavus, A. nidulans,* and *A. niger*) may be pathogenic. SEE: *aspergillosis.*

***A. clavatus*** A species found in soil and manure.

***A. concentricus*** A species once thought to be the cause of tinea imbricata ringworm.

***A. flavus*** A mold found on corn, peanuts, and grain.

***A. fumigatus*** The fungus that is the common cause of aspergillosis in humans and birds. It is found in soil and manure.

***A. glaucus*** A bluish mold found on dried fruit.

***A. nidulans*** A species common in soil, causing one form of white mycetoma.

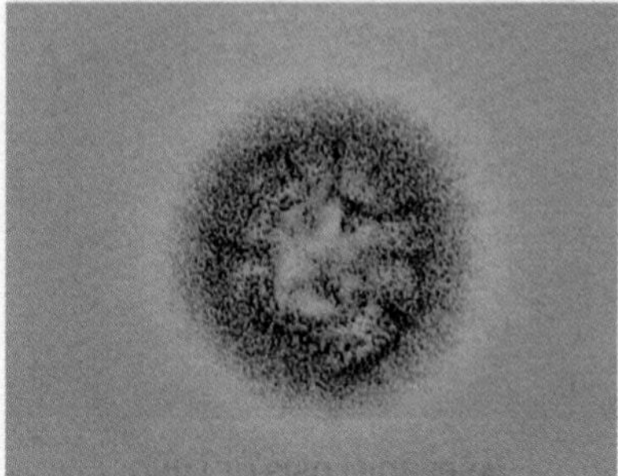

ASPERGILLUS NIGER IN CULTURE

***A. niger*** A pathogenic form with black spores, frequently present in the external auditory meatus. It may cause otomycosis. SEE: illus.

***A. ochraceus*** A species that produces the characteristic odor of brewing coffee.

***A. versicolor*** A species that produces a toxin similar to aflatoxin.

**aspermatogenesis** (ă-spĕr″mă-tō-jĕn′ĕ-sĭs) [″ + ″ + *genesis,* generation, birth] Nonfunction of the sperm-producing system of the testicles.

**aspermia** (ă-spĕr′mē-ă) [″ + *sperma,* seed] Failure to form semen or to ejaculate. **aspermic** (-mĭk), *adj.*

**aspersion** (ăs-pĕr′zhŭn) [L. *aspersio,* sprinkling] Sprinkling an affected part with water; a form of hydrotherapy.

**asphalgesia** (ăs″făl-jē′zē-ă) [Gr. *asphe-,* self, + *algos,* pain] A burning sensation sometimes felt on touching certain articles during hypnosis.

**asphyctic, asphyctous** (ăs-fĭk′tĭk, -tŭs) [Gr. *a-,* not, + *sphyxis,* pulse] **1.** Pert. to, or affected with, asphyxia. **2.** Without pulse.

**asphyxia** (ăs-fĭk′sē-ă) [″ + *sphyxis,* pulse] Condition caused by insufficient intake of oxygen. **asphyxial** (-sē-ăl), *adj.*

SYMPTOMS: In general, symptoms include dyspnea, cyanosis, rapid pulse, impairment of senses, and mental disturbances; in extreme cases, convulsions, unconsciousness, and death.

ETIOLOGY: Extrinsic causes include choking, toxic gases, exhaust gas (principally carbon monoxide), electric shock, drugs, anesthesia, trauma, crushing injuries of the chest, compression of the chest, injury of the respiratory nerves or centers, diminished environmental oxygenation, and drowning.

Intrinsic causes include hemorrhage into the lungs or pleural cavity, foreign bodies in the throat, swelling of the airways, diseases of the airways, ruptured aneurysm or abscess, edema of the lung, cardiac deficiency, tumors such as goiter, and pharyngeal and retropharyngeal abscesses. Other causes include paralysis of the respiratory center or of respiratory muscles, anesthesia, pneumothorax, narcotic drugs, electrocution, and child abuse.

FIRST AID: Artificial respiration should be given.

***autoerotic a.*** SEE: *autoerotic hypoxia.*

***a. carbonica*** Suffocation from inhalation of coal or water gas or of carbon monoxide.

***fetal a.*** Asphyxia occurring in a fetus; results from interference in placental circulation or from premature separation of the placenta, as in abruptio placentae.

***a. livida*** Asphyxia in which the skin is cyanotic from lack of oxygen in the blood.

***local a.*** Asphyxia affecting a limited portion of the body (e.g., fingers, hands, toes, or feet) due to insufficient blood supply; a symptom usually associated with Raynaud's disease.

***a. neonatorum*** Respiratory failure in the newborn.

***a. pallida*** Asphyxia in which difficulty in breathing is accompanied by weak and thready pulse, pale skin, and absence of reflexes.

***sexual a.*** SEE: *autoerotic hypoxia.*

**asphyxiant** (ăs-fĭk′sē-ănt) An agent, esp. any gas, that will produce asphyxia.

**asphyxiate** (ăs-fĭk′sē-āt) To cause asphyxiation or asphyxia.

**asphyxiation** (ăs-fĭk″sē-ā′shŭn) **1.** A state of asphyxia or suffocation. **2.** The act of producing asphyxia.

**asphyxiophilia** Dependence on self-strangulation for production of cerebral hypoxia. This act may intensify enjoyment of orgasm, but if continued too long may result in death. SEE: *asphyxia, sexual.*

**aspidium** (ăs-pĭd′ē-ŭm) [Gr. *aspidion,* little shield] The root and stalk of *Dryopteris filixmas* (male fern) or *D. marginalis* (marginal fern); used medicinally in the form of oleoresin.

***a. oleoresin*** Extract of the male fern; male fern oleoresin; used as an anthelmintic in the treatment of tapeworm infestation of the intestines. Care should be taken that it is not administered with an oil, since absorption may occur.

**aspirate** (ăs′pĭ-rāt) [L. *ad,* to, + *spirare,* to breathe] **1.** To draw in or out by suction. **2.** To make a sound like that of the letter *h.*

**aspiration** (ăs-pĭ-rā′shŭn) **1.** Drawing in or out by suction. Foreign bodies may be aspirated into the nose, throat, or lungs on inspiration. **2.** Withdrawal of fluid from a cavity by suctioning with an aspirator. The purpose of aspiration is to remove fluid or air from an affected area (as in pleural effusion, pneumothorax, ascites, or an abscess) or to obtain specimens (such as blood from a vein or serum from the spinal canal).

EQUIPMENT: Aspiration equipment includes disinfecting solution for the skin; local anesthetic; two aspirating needles with the aspirating apparatus as indicated; a utensil for receiving the fluid and a sterile receptacle for the specimen; sterile sponges, towels, basins; sterile gloves, face masks, and gowns; sterile forceps; surgical dressings as the case may require; a stimulant ordered if the indication arises.

NURSING IMPLICATIONS: Pathological respiratory aspiration is prevented by placing the unconscious patient (or any other patient with defective swallowing or cough protective reflexes) in a head-low position to protect the airway, to prevent silent regurgitation, and to promote evacuation of mucus or vomitus; and by suctioning the nasopharynx as necessary. The nurse assists with the aspiration procedures by assembling necessary equipment, by explaining the procedure and expected sensations to the patient, and by ascertaining that a consent form has been signed. The patient is draped to ensure privacy and warmth as well as emotional comfort. Emotional support is provided throughout the procedure. The nurse also assists the operator in obtaining and processing specimens, carefully observes and documents the type and amount of any drainage or aspirated material, dresses the operative site, and evaluates for desired patient outcomes and for any complications.

**aspiration, risk for** The state in which an individual is at risk for entry of gastric secretions, oropharyngeal sections, [or exogenous food] or fluids into tracheobronchial passages solids due to dysfunction or absence of normal protective mechanisms]. SEE: *Nursing Diagnoses Appendix.*

**aspirator** (ăs′pĭ-rā-tor) An apparatus for evacuating the fluid contents of a cavity. Varieties are piston pump, compressible rubber tube, rubber bulb, and siphon, a trocar and cannula, and hypodermic needle and syringe.

***dental a.*** An aspirator that suctions water, saliva, blood, or tissue debris from the oral cavity.

**aspirin** (ăs′pĕr-ĭn) ABBR: ASA. $C_9H_8O_4$. Acetylsalicylic acid, a nonsteroidal anti-inflammatory drug that is a derivative of salicylic acid. It occurs as white crystals or powder. It is one of the most widely used and prescribed analgesic-antipyretic and anti-inflammatory agents. Because of its ability to bind irreversibly to blood platelets and inhibit platelet aggregration, aspirin in a dose of 80 to 325 mg/day is used prophylactically to prevent coronary artery disease, transient ischemic attacks, and thromboembolic disease of the cerebral vessels. Aspirin causes prolongation of the bleeding time. A single dose of 65 mg approx. doubles the bleeding time of normal persons for a period of 4 to 7 days. This same antiplatelet effect can cause the undesired effects of intestinal bleeding and peptic ulceration.

Caution: Children with viral infections such as varicella or influenza should not be given aspirin because of the possibility of increasing their risk of developing Reye's syndrome.

**aspirin poisoning** Toxicity caused by ingesting an excessive amount of aspirin. In acute poisoning, signs vary with increasing doses from mild lethargy and hyperpnea to coma and convulsions. Sweating, dehydration, hyperpnea, hyperthermia, and restlessness may be present with moderate doses. In chronic poisoning, tinnitus, skin rash, bleeding tendency, weight loss, and mental symptoms may be present. Aspirin poisoning in very young infants may produce very few signs and symptoms other than dehydration or hyperpnea.

TREATMENT: Repeated gastric lavage with activated charcoal is required. Intravenous (IV) fluids are given for dehydration, but must not be overloaded. Enough IV fluids should be given to establish 3 to 4 ml/kg/hr of urine flow. Just as important as IV fluid therapy is alkalinization of urine by administering bicarbonate. The goal is a urine pH of 8 or higher. Also, after urine flow is established, potassium 30 mEq/L of administered fluid should be added. After serum potassium levels reach 5 mEq/L, potassium should be discontinued. If alkalinization of the urine is not accomplished, hemodialysis may be needed. Treat tachycardia with appropriate drug. SEE: *salicylates in Poisons and Poisoning Appendix.*

**asplenia** (ă-splē′nē-ă) [Gr. *a-*, not, + L. *splen*, spleen] Absence of the spleen.

**asplenia syndrome** A developmental disorder that occurs before the fifth week of pregnancy. The vascular structures on the left side, including the spleen, are absent.

**asporogenic** (ăs″pō-rō-jĕn′ĭk) [″ + *sporos*, seed, + *gennan*, to produce] Not reproducing by spores.

**asporous** (ă-spō′rŭs) Having no spores.

**A.S.R.T.** *American Society of Radiologic Technologists.*

**assault** (ă-sawlt′) [L. *assultus*, having assailed] **1.** The threat of unlawful touching of another. **2.** The willful attempt to harm someone. SEE: *battery.*

***sexual a.*** Actual or attempted oral, anal, or vaginal penetration against the victim's will. This includes sexual intercourse and forced entry of the orifices with an object. It may be extended to include grasping of the victim's breasts or genitals. SEE: *rape.*

**assay** (ă-sā′, ăs′ā) [O. Fr. *assai*, trial] The analysis of a substance or mixture to determine its constituents and the relative proportion of each.

***biological a.*** Bioassay.

***intracellular killing a.*** A laboratory test

of bacterial ingestion by phagocytes. Neutrophils or macrophages are placed in a culture with bacteria. After 30 min, the remaining bacteria are killed with an antibiotic and the phagocytes are stained and examined for the number of bacteria they have ingested. This assay is only accurate if the phagocytes have been tested previously for the ability to ingest bacteria. SYN: *neutrophil microbicidal a.*

***neutrophil microbicidal a.*** Intracellular killing a.

**assessment 1.** An appraisal or evaluation of a patient's condition by a physician or nurse, based on clinical and laboratory data, medical history, and the patient's account of symptoms. **2.** The process by which a patient's condition is appraised or evaluated.

***functional a.*** In rehabilitation, the determination of a person's ability to perform everyday tasks and requirements of living. Functional assessment scales vary greatly with respect to the number, type, and scoring of the tasks used to determine performance levels, their degree of standardization, and their predictive validity. SEE: *activities of daily living.*

***nursing a.*** SEE: *nursing assessment.*

**Assessment of Motor and Process Skills** ABBR: AMPS. A performance test of complex tasks required for activities of daily living, used in rehabilitation. It is one of the first of a new generation of functional performance assessments designed to accommodate differences in settings and raters through statistical mechanisms. SEE: *functional assessment.*

**assimilable** (ă-sĭm′ĭ-lă-bl) [L. *ad,* to, + *similare,* to make like] Capable of assimilation.

**assimilate** (ă-sĭm′ĭ-lāt) **1.** To absorb digested food. **2.** In psychology, to absorb newly perceived information into the existing subjective conscious structure.

**assimilation** (ă-sĭm″ĭ-lā′shŭn) **1.** The transformation of food into living tissue; the constructive phase of metabolism (i.e., anabolism). **2.** In psychology, the absorption of newly perceived information into the existing subjective conscious structure.

**assistant** One who aids or supports.

***dental a.*** SEE: *dental assistant.*

***physician a.*** ABBR: PA. A specially trained and (when necessary) licensed individual who performs tasks usually done by physicians and works under the direction of a supervising physician. PA training programs are accredited by the American Medical Association. Nearly all states require PAs to pass the certification examination of the National Commission on Certification of Physician Assistants.

**assisted circulation** Use of a mechanical device to augment or replace the action of the heart in pumping blood.

**assisted death** Help given an individual who wants to die to do so. This may take the form of counseling or actually providing the means and instruments for allowing the person to act to commit suicide. The legal and moral questions concerning such acts, esp. if the assisting person is a physician or someone involved in medical care, are debatable. SEE: *assisted suicide; euthanasia.*

**assisted reproduction technologies** ABBR: ART. Techniques to assist infertile women to conceive and give birth. These include in vitro fertilization with embryonic transfer, zygote intrafallopian transfer for women whose infertility results from tubal factors, and gamete intrafallopian transfer for couples whose infertility stems from semen inadequacy.

**assisted suicide** The rendering of assistance to a person who wants to end his or her life but is not able to do this alone. This may be due to a physical disability or due to lack of knowledge of how to accomplish suicide. Whether or not physicians should become involved in helping patients commit suicide is debatable. Physicians or other medical care personnel who do assist a patient who wishes to take his or her life may be considered in the U.S. legal system to have murdered the patient. However, some state governments have legalized this procedure. SEE: *assisted death; euthanasia.*

**assistor** A ventilation system in which the patient initiates the inspiration cycle.

**associated movements** Synchronous correlation of two or more muscles or muscle groups that, although not essential for the performance of some function, normally accompany it, as the swinging of arms accompanies normal walking. Associated movements are characteristically lost in cerebellar disease.

**association** [L. *ad,* to, + *socius,* companion] **1.** The act of joining or uniting; coordination with another idea or structure; relationship. In psychiatry, association refers in particular to the interrelationship of the conscious and unconscious ideas. **2.** In genetics, the occurrence together of two characteristics at a frequency greater than would be predicted by chance. **3.** In clinical epidemiology, the relationship of the occurrence of two events, without evidence that the event being investigated actually causes the second condition (e.g., malaria occurs in warm climates with proper breeding conditions for certain types of mosquitoes, but those conditions are *associations*). The actual *cause* is the malaria parasite.

***controlled a.*** Induced a.

***free a.*** In psychoanalysis, the uninhibited and uncensored oral expression of ideas as they arise in the patient's mind.

***induced a.*** The idea suggested when the physician gives a stimulus word. SYN: *controlled a.* SEE: *association test.*

**association areas** Areas of the cerebral cortex connected to motor and sensory areas of the same side, to similar areas on the other side, and to other regions of the brain (e.g., the thalamus). They integrate the simpler motor and sensory functions.

**association center** Center controlling associated movements.

**Association for Gerontology in Higher Education** ABBR: AGHE. An agency that promotes the education and training of persons preparing for research or careers in gerontology. It is committed to the development of education, research, and public service, and works to increase public awareness of the needs of gerontological education.

**association neuron** A neuron of the central nervous system that transmits impulses from sensory to motor neurons or to other association neurons. SYN: *interneuron.*

**association of ideas** The linking together in a memory chain of two or more ideas because of their similarity, relationship, or timing.

**association test** Test in which the patient is given a word (stimulus word) and replies immediately with another word (reaction word) suggested by the first. The words chosen and the time taken in responding (association time) may be indicative of the patient's mental condition.

**association time** SEE: *association test.*

**assonance** (ăs′ō-năns) [L. *assonans,* answering with same sound] **1.** Similarity of sounds in words or syllables. **2.** Abnormal tendency to use alliteration.

**assumption of risk** A doctrine of law whereby the plaintiff assumes the risk of medical treatment or procedures and may not recover damages for injuries sustained as a result of the known and described dangers.

**AST** *aspartate aminotransferase.*

**Ast** *astigmatism.*

**astasia** (ă-stā′zē-ă) [Gr. *a-,* not, + *stasis,* stand] Inability to stand or sit erect due to motor incoordination.

**astasia-abrasia** A form of hysterical ataxia, with incoordination and inability to stand or walk although all leg movements can be performed while sitting or lying down.

**astatine** (ăs′tă-tēn, -tīn) [Gr. *astatos,* unstable] SYMB: At. A radioactive element, atomic number 85, atomic weight 210.

**asteatosis** (ăs″tē-ă-tō′sĭs) [Gr. *a-,* not, + *stear,* tallow, + *osis,* condition] Any disease condition in which there is persistent scaling of the skin, suggesting deficiency or absence of sebaceous secretion.

***a. cutis*** A dry, fissured condition of the skin with a deficient sebaceous secretion. The symptomatic form is caused by senility or systemic disorders that give rise to trophic changes in the nervous system. The local form may be caused by frequent contact with irritants. The underlying cause must be removed. Local application of oils and fats offers some relief.

**aster** (ăs′tĕr) [Gr., star] The stellate rays forming around the dividing centrosome during mitosis.

**astereognosis** (ă-stĕr″ē-ŏg-nō′sĭs) [Gr. *a-,* not, + *stereos,* solid, + *gnosis,* knowledge] Inability to recognize objects or forms by touch.

**asterion** (ăs-tē′rē-ŏn) *pl.* **asteria** [Gr., starlike] A craniometric point at the junction of the lambdoid, occipitomastoid, and parietomastoid sutures.

**asterixis** (ăs″tĕr-ĭk′sĭs) [Gr. *a-,* not, + *sterixis,* fixed position] Abnormal muscle tremor consisting of involuntary jerking movements, esp. in the hands, but also seen in the tongue and feet. It may be due to various diseases that interfere with brain metabolism. When due to hepatic coma, asterixis is called liver flap or liver tremor. SYN: *tremor, flapping.* SEE: *alcoholism; hepatic coma.*

**asternal** (ā-stĕr′năl) [″ + *sternon,* chest] **1.** Not connected with the sternum. **2.** Having no sternum.

**asternia** (ă-stĕr′nē-ă) Congenital absence of the sternum.

**asteroid** (ăs′tĕr-oyd) [Gr. *aster,* star, + *eidos,* form, shape] Star-shaped.

**asthenia** (ăs-thē′nē-ă) [Gr. *asthenes,* without strength] Lack or loss of strength; debility; any weakness, but esp. one originating in muscular or cerebellar disease. SYN: *adynamia.*

***neurocirculatory a.*** A psychosomatic disorder marked by mental and physical fatigue, dyspnea, giddiness, precordial pain, and palpitation, esp. on exertion. The cause is unknown but the condition occurs in those under stress. It is common among soldiers in combat. Psychotherapy and removal of the stress situation are needed. SYN: *cardiac neurosis.* SEE: *chronic fatigue syndrome; posttraumatic stress syndrome.*

**asthenic** (ăs-thĕn′ĭk) **1.** Weak; pert. to asthenia. **2.** Pert. to a body habitus marked by a narrow, shallow thorax, a long thoracic cavity, and a short abdominal cavity.

**asthenobiosis** (ăs-thē″nō-bī-ō′sĭs) [Gr. *asthenes,* without strength, + *bios,* life, + *osis,* condition] Condition of reduced biological activity of an animal, resembling hibernation but not related to temperature or humidity.

**asthenocoria** (ăs-thē″nō-kō′rē-ă) [″ + *kore,* pupil] A sluggish pupillary light reflex.

**asthenometer** (ăs″thĕ-nŏm′ĕ-ter) [″ + *metron,* measure] An instrument for determining muscular strength or weakness.

**asthenope** (ăs′thĕ-nōp) [″ + *opsis,* power of sight] An individual who is affected with asthenopia.

**asthenopia** (ăs″thĕ-nō′pē-ă) Weakness or tiring of the eyes accompanied by pain, headache, and dimness of vision. Symptoms include pain in or around the eyes; headache, usually aggravated by use of the eyes for close work; fatigue; vertigo; reflex symptoms such as nausea, twitching of facial muscles, or migraine. **asthe-**

**nopic** (-nŏp′ĭk), *adj.*

***accommodative a.*** Asthenopia due to strain of the ciliary muscles.

***muscular a.*** Asthenopia caused by weakness of the extrinsic ocular muscles.

***nervous a.*** Asthenopia of hysteric or neurasthenic origin.

**asthenospermia** (ăs″thĕ-nō-spĕr′mē-ă) [″ + *sperma,* seed] Loss or reduction of motility of spermatozoa in semen; associated with infertility.

**asthma** (ăz′mă) [Gr., panting] A disease caused by increased responsiveness of the tracheobronchial tree to various stimuli, which results in paroxysmal constriction of the bronchial airways.

Clinically, there is severe dyspnea accompanied by wheezing. The patient may assume a hunched-forward position in an attempt to get more air. Between attacks the patient may be quite comfortable. In some cases the attacks become continuous, a condition called status asthmaticus, and may be fatal. The recurrence and severity of attacks are greatly influenced by secondary factors, including mental or physical fatigue, endocrine changes at various periods in life, emotional situations, and exposure to noxious fumes. There is always an allergic component. Other allergic disorders may coexist.

Asthma attacks have a slow or sudden onset. In slow onset, the patients have time to seek help; however, sudden-onset attacks are marked by rapid development of airway obstruction, and death may occur within minutes. Sudden-onset fatal asthma is considered to have occurred if the patient dies within an hour of onset. As many as 25% of asthma deaths may be attributed to this condition. Patients who have survived such an attack should wear a bracelet describing their disease, with the advice that they immediately be taken to an emergency department. Also, the patient should carry a written emergency treatment plan. This will be useful for emergency department physicians who may not be familiar with this type of asthma and not appreciate that it is potentially life threatening. Patients should always carry injectable epinephrine and use it (unless contraindicated) at the onset of an attack even prior to seeking medical assistance.

No age is exempt, but asthma occurs most frequently in childhood or early adulthood. The leading cause of chronic illness in childhood, asthma is estimated to occur in 5% to 10% of children at some time during their development. Prior to puberty, twice as many boys as girls have asthma; the attack rate is equal in adults. SYN: *chronic desquamating eosinophilic bronchitis; reactive airway disease.*

ETIOLOGY: Asthma may be caused by allergens inhaled from the air (pollen, mold spores, animal dander, or dust). Occasionally food (e.g., eggs, shellfish, or chocolate) or drugs (e.g., aspirin) may precipitate an attack. This type of asthma involves immunoglobulin E (IgE). In some cases asthma develops in people with allergies of unknown etiology. It may be triggered by a respiratory tract infection.

TREATMENT: Indoor inhalants such as house dust, danders, molds, tobacco smoke, and strong odors should be avoided. Acute attacks are managed by inhalation of nebulized beta$_2$ agonists such as terbutaline or albuterol. The more severe the episode, the longer the therapy will need to be maintained. Because the inhaled medications may cause a temporary decrease in oxygen saturation, they should be administered with oxygen. Patients with recurrent, nonacute attacks of asthma are managed by use of cromolyn sodium, which blocks release of histamine from mast cells but requires several weeks to become fully effective. A brief, intense course of oral corticosteroids will hasten remission. Salmeterol, a longer-acting inhaled drug, is also available.

For persistent asthma (status asthmaticus), treatment consists of adrenocortical hormones plus continuous oxygen, intravenous fluids if the patient is dehydrated, and continued bronchodilator therapy. Careful monitoring of blood gases and pH, and electrocardiography are indicated. Sedation is indicated but should be used only if the patient is carefully monitored. Even though adrenocortical hormones may provide dramatic relief, they should be used only as long as is necessary to control the acute attack; prolonged use may cause serious side effects. The use of sedatives and expectorants is sometimes necessary.

In all cases, effort should be made to control the causative factors, including the component of the disease due to emotional disturbance. Elimination of antigen, or countermeasures such as immunization, desensitization, or hyposensitization, are desirable. For asthma due to infection of the respiratory tract, antibiotics should be used to control infection or prevent recurrence. SEE: *bronchoalveolar lavage.*

NURSING IMPLICATIONS: The nurse assesses for ventilatory rate and effort; inspiratory-expiratory ratio; presence, location, and timing of wheezing; use of ancillary muscle groups; presence of retractions; and other symptoms of respiratory fatigue or distress. Vital signs are monitored and mental status is evaluated for evidence of anxiety, irritability, and reduced level of consciousness. Arterial blood gas and oxygen saturation values are monitored according to protocol. The patient is positioned to ease ventilatory effort and facilitate ventilation. Humidified air or oxygen is administered according to prescription. Prescribed medications are given; the patient is evaluated for desired responses and adverse reactions. The nurse remains with and reassures the patient. The patient is assessed for dehydration, and oral fluids are provided in frequent, small amounts, or IV fluids are administered as necessary to help thin inspissated respiratory secretions. Characteristics of the cough and any sputum are documented. When the acute attack has subsided, the patient is taught breathing exercises and the proper use of inhalers. The patient is advised to eat a balanced diet, drink sufficient fluids, avoid excessive fatigue, and avoid contact with persons with upper respiratory infections. The nurse instructs the patient about eliminating allergens or irritants, teaches home measures to prevent or decrease the severity of future attacks, and assists the patient in identifying and reducing stressors associated with the attacks. The patient and family may be referred to community-based programs for further support and information. SEE: *Nursing Diagnoses Appendix.* **asthmatic** (ăz-măt′ĭk), *adj.*

***bronchial a.*** Allergic asthma; a common form of asthma due to hypersensitivity to an allergen.

***cardiac a.*** Paroxysmal nocturnal dyspnea. SEE: *heart failure, congestive.*

***exercise-induced a.*** Asthmatic attacks that occur during exercise. They can usually be prevented by breathing air at body temperature fully saturated with water vapor.

***extrinsic a.*** Asthma due to some environmental factor, usually allergic.

***intrinsic a.*** Asthma assumed to be due to some endogenous cause because no external cause can be found.

**asthmagenic** Producing asthma.

**astigmatism** (ă-stĭg′mă-tĭzm) [Gr. *a-*, not, + *stigma,* point, + *-ismos,* condition of] ABBR: As; Ast. A form of ametropia in which the refraction of a ray of light is spread over a diffuse area rather than sharply focused on the retina. It is due to differences in the curvature in various meridians of the cornea and lens of the eye. The exact cause is unknown. Some types show a familial pattern. **astigmatic** (ăs″tĭg-măt′ĭk), *adj.*

***compound a.*** Astigmatism in which both horizontal and vertical curvatures are involved.

***index a.*** Astigmatism resulting from inequalities in the refractive indices of different parts of the lens.

***mixed a.*** Astigmatism in which one meridian is myopic and the other hyperopic.

***simple a.*** Astigmatism along one meridian only.

**astigmatometer, astigmometer** (ăs″tĭg-mă-tŏm′ĕ-tĕr, -mŏm′ĕ-tĕr) [″ + *stigma,* point, + *metron,* measure] An instrument for measuring astigmatism.

**astigmia** (ă-stĭg′mē-ă) Astigmatism.

**astomatous, astomous** (ăs-tŏm′ă-tŭs, ăs′tō-mŭs) [Gr. *a-*, not, + *stoma,* mouth] Without a mouth or oral aperture; as certain protozoa.

**astomia** (ă-stō′mē-ă) Congenital absence of the mouth.

**astragalectomy** (ăs″trăg-ă-lĕk′tō-mē) [*astragalus* + Gr. *ektome,* excision] Surgical removal of the talus (astragalus).

**astragalus** (ă-străg′ă-lŭs) [Gr. *astragalos,* ball of the ankle joint] Obsolete term for the talus of the ankle. SEE: *talus.*

**astraphobia** (ăs-tră-fō′bē-ă) [Gr. *astrape,* the heavens, + *phobos,* fear] Fear of thunder and lightening.

**astriction** (ă-strĭk′shŭn) Action of an astringent.

**astringent** (ă-strĭn′jĕnt) [L. *astringere,* to bind fast] **1.** Drawing together, constricting, binding. **2.** An agent that has a constricting or binding effect (i.e., one that checks hemorrhages or secretions by coagulation of proteins on a cell surface). The principal astringents are salts of metals such as lead, iron, zinc (ferric chloride, zinc oxide); permanganates; and tannic acid. SEE: *styptic.*

**astro-** [Gr. *astron,* star] Combining form indicating *relationship to a star,* or *star-shaped.*

**astrobiology** Study of extraterrestrial life.

**astroblast** (ăs′trō-blăst) [″+ Gr. *blastos,* germ] A cell that gives rise to an astrocyte. It develops from spongioblasts derived from embryonic neuroepithelium.

**astroblastoma** (ăs″trō-blăs-tō′mă) [″+ ″+ *oma,* tumor] A grade II astrocytoma, composed of cells with abundant cytoplasm and two or three nuclei.

**astrocyte** (ăs′trō-sīt) [″ + *kytos,* cell] Spider cell.

**astrocytoma** (ăs″trō-sī-tō′mă) [″ +″+ *oma,* tumor] Tumor of the brian or spinal cord composed of astrocytes. They are graded according to the prognosis.

***malignant a.*** A tumor of the brainstem, cerebellum, spinal cord, or the white matter of the cerebral hemispheres. Onset is typically in the fifth decade of life. Prognosis after treatment by surgery, radiation, or other means is poor in that few survive more than 2 years.

**astroglia** (ăs-trŏg′lē-ă) [″ + *glia,* glue] Astrocytes making up neuroglial tissue.

**astrokinetic motions** (ăs″trō-kĭ-nĕt′ĭk) [″ + *kinesis,* movement] Pert. to movements of the centrosome.

**astrophobia** (ăs″trō-fō′bē-ă) [″ + *phobos,* fear] Morbid fear of stars and celestial space.

**astrosphere** (ăs′trō-sfēr) [″ + *sphaira,* sphere] A group of fibrils or fine rays that radiate from the centrosome (microcentrum) of a dividing cell. SYN: *aster.*

**astrostatic** (ăs″trŏ-stăt′ĭk) [″ + *statikos,* standing] Pert. to an astrosphere in its resting condition.

**Astroviridae** A recently identified virus family that causes epidemic viral gastroenteritis in adults and children. The incubation period has been estimated to be 3 to 4 days. The outbreaks are self-limiting and in the absence of coexisting pathogens, the intestinal signs and symptoms last 5 days or less. Treatment, if required, is supportive and directed to maintaining hydration and electrolyte balance. SEE: *Caliciviridae.*

**astrovirus** (ăs′trō-vī″rŭs) An adenovirus with worldwide distribution that causes gastroenteritis in children. Clinical symptoms include anorexia, headache, fever, diarrhea, and vomiting.

**ASV** *Anodic stripping voltammetry,* an analytical technique used to assay for blood lead content.

**asyllabia** (ă″sĭl-ā′bē-ă) [Gr. *a-,* not, + *syllabe,* syllable] A form of alexia, in which the patient recognizes letters but cannot form syllables or words.

**asymbolia** (ā-, ă-sĭm-bō′lē-ă) [Gr. *a-,* not, + *symbolon,* a sign] Inability to comprehend words, gestures, or any type of symbol. SYN: *asemia.* SEE: *aphasia.*

**asymmetry** (ă-sĭm′ĕ-trē) [″ + *symmetria,* symmetry] Lack of symmetry. **asymmetric, asymmetrical** (ā-sĭ-mĕ′-trĭk, -trĭ-kăl), *adj.*

**asymphytous** (ă-sĭm′fĭ-tŭs) [″ + *symphysis,* a growing together] Separate or distinct; not grown together.

**asymptomatic** (ā″sĭmp-tō-măt′ĭk) [″ + *symptoma,* occurrence] Without symptoms.

**asynchronism** (ă-sĭn′krō-nĭzm) [″+ *syn,* together, + *chronos,* time, + *-ismos,* condition of] **1.** The failure of events to occur in time with each other as they usually do. **2.** Incoordination. **asynchronous** (-nŭs), *adj.*

**asynclitism** (ă-sĭn′klĭ-tĭzm) [″ + *synklinein,* to lean together, + *-ismos,* condition of] An oblique presentation of the fetal head in labor. SEE: *presentation* for illus.

***anterior a.*** Anterior parietal presentation. SYN: *Naegele's obliquity.*

***posterior a.*** Posterior parietal presentation. SYN: *Litzmann's obliquity.*

**asyndesis** (ă-sĭn′dĕ-sĭs) [Gr. *a-,* not, + *syn,* together, + *desis,* binding] Mental defect in which related thoughts cannot be assembled to form a comprehensive concept.

**asynechia** (ă″sĭ-nĕk′ē-ă) [″ + *synecheia,* continuity] Lack of continuity of structure in an organ or tissue.

**asynergia, asynergy** (ă-sĭn-ĕr′jē-ă, ă-sĭn′ĕr-jē) [″ + Gr. *synergia,* cooperation] Lack of coordination among parts or organs normally acting in unison; in neurology, lack of coordination between muscle groups. Movements are jerky and in sequence instead of being made together. It is seen in cerebellar diseases. **asynergic** (ā-sĭ-nĕr-gĭk), *adj.*

**asynovia** (ă-sĭn-ō′vē-ă) [″ + *syn,* with, + *oon,* egg] Lack or insufficient secretion of synovial fluid of a joint.

**asyntaxia** (ă″sĭn-tăk′sē-ă) [″ + *syntaxis,* orderly arrangement] Failure of the embryo to develop properly.

**asystematic** (ă-sĭs″tĕ-măt′ĭk) [″ + LL. *systema,* arrangement] Not systematic; not limited to one system or set of organs.

**asystole, asystolia** (ă-sĭs′tō-lē, ă″sĭs-tō′lē-ă) [″ + *systole,* contraction] Cardiac standstill; absence of contractions of the heart.

**asystolic cardiac rhythm** A flat (isoelectric) line in an electrocardiographic tracing during cardiac arrest.

**At** Symbol for the element astatine.

**Atabrine Hydrochloride** (ăt′ă-brĭn) Trade name for quinacrine hydrochloride.

**atactiform** (ă-tăk′tĭ-form) [″ + L. *forma,* form] Similar to ataxia.

**ataractic** (ăt″ă-răk′tĭk) [Gr. *ataraktos,* quiet] **1.** Of or pert. to ataraxia. **2.** A tranquilizer.

**Atarax** Trade name for hydroxyzine hydrochloride.

**ataraxia, ataraxy** (ăt″ă-răk′sē-ă, -sē) [Gr. *ataraktos,* quiet] A state of complete mental calm and tranquility, esp. without depression of mental faculties or clouding of consciousness.

**atavism** (ăt′ă-vĭzm) [L. *atavus,* ancestor, + Gr. *-ismos,* condition] The appearance of a characteristic presumed to have been present in some remote ancestor; due to chance recombination of genes or environmental conditions favorable to their expression in the embryo. **atavistic** (ăt-ă-vĭs′tĭk), *adj.*

**ataxia** (ă-tăk′sē-ă) [Gr., lack of order] Defective muscular coordination, esp. that manifested when voluntary muscular movements are attempted. **atactic, ataxic** (ă-tăk′tĭk, -tăk′sĭk), *adj.*

***alcoholic a.*** In chronic alcoholism, ataxia due to a loss of proprioception.

***bulbar a.*** Ataxia due to a lesion in the medulla oblongata or pons.

***cerebellar a.*** Ataxia due to cerebellar disease.

***choreic a.*** Lack of muscular coordination seen in patients with chorea.

***Friedreich's a.*** An inherited degenerative disease with sclerosis of the dorsal and lateral columns of the spinal cord, accompanied by ataxia, speech impairment, lateral curvature of the spinal column, and peculiar swaying and irregular movements, with paralysis of the muscles, esp. of the lower extremities. Onset occurs in childhood or adolescence.

***hysterical a.*** Ataxia of leg muscles due to hysteria.

***locomotor a.*** Tabes dorsalis.

***motor a.*** Inability to perform coordinated muscle movements.

***sensory a.*** Ataxia resulting from interference in conduction of sensory responses, esp. proprioceptive impulses from muscles. The condition becomes aggravated when the eyes are closed. SEE: *Romberg's sign; spinal a.*

***spinal a.*** Ataxia due to spinal cord disease.

***static a.*** Loss of deep sensibility, causing inability to preserve equilibrium in standing.

**ataxiagram** (ă-tăk′sē-ă-grăm) [Gr. *ataxia,* lack of order, + *gramma,* something written] A record or tracing produced by an ataxiagraph.

**ataxiagraph** (ă-tăk′sē-ă-grăf) [″ + *graphein,* to write] Instrument for measuring the degree and direction of swaying in ataxia.

**ataxiameter** (ă-tăk″sē-ăm′ĕ-tĕr) [″ + *metron,* measure] Apparatus measuring ataxia.

**ataxiamnesia** (ă-tăk″sē-ăm-nē′zē-ă) [″ + *amnesia,* forgetfulness] Condition marked by ataxia and amnesia.

**ataxiaphasia** (ă-tăk″sē-ă-fā′zē-ă) [″ + *phasis,* speech] Inability to arrange words into sentences. Also spelled *ataxaphasia.*

**ataxia-telangiectasia** A degenerative brain disease of children, marked by a specific immunological dysfunction and progressive cerebellar degeneration, telangiectasis of the bulbar conjunctiva, and increased tendency to experience malignancy. It is transmitted as an autosomal recessive trait. Death usually occurs in adolescence or early adulthood. Parents should be informed that subsequent children have a 25% risk of having this condition. SYN: *Louis-Bar syndrome.*

**ataxophobia** (ă-tăk″sō-fō′bē-ă) [″ + *phobos,* fear] Fear of disorder or untidiness.

**A.T.B.C.B.** *Architectural and Transportation Barriers Compliance Board,* a federal agency charged with enforcing legislation requiring that federal buildings and transportation facilities be accessible to the disabled.

**ATC** *Athletic trainer, certified.*

**atelectasis** (ăt″ĕ-lĕk′tă-sĭs) [Gr. *ateles,* imperfect, + *ektasis,* expansion] **1.** A condition in which the lungs of a fetus remain partially or totally unexpanded at birth. **2.** A collapsed or airless condition of the lung. It may be caused by obstruction, by hypoventilation as occurs secondary to pain as in fractured ribs and in patients being ventilated with inadequate tidal volumes, mucus plugs or excessive secretions, or by compression from without as by tumors, aneurysms, or enlarged lymph nodes. It sometimes is a complication following abdominal operations. Middle lobe syndrome, a chronic form, results from compression of the middle lobe bronchus by surrounding lymph nodes. SEE: *canals of Lambert; pores of Kohn.*

NURSING IMPLICATIONS: Patients at risk are evaluated for dyspnea, decreased chest wall movement, inspiratory substernal or intercostal retractions, diaphoresis, anxiety, tachycardia, and pleuritic chest pain. Lung fields are percussed for dullness, and the chest is auscultated for decreased breath sounds. Pulse oximetry and arterial blood gas values are monitored for evidence of hypoxemia. Respiratory toilet and incentive spirometry or intermittent positive pressure breathing treatments are provided as prescribed. Atelectasis can be prevented in at-risk patients by encouraging deep breathing and coughing exercises every 1 to 2 hr, by repositioning the patient often, and by administering prescribed analgesics. Adequate fluid intake is encouraged; inspired air is humidified as necessary; and the patient is assisted to mobilize and clear secretions. Intubated or obtunded patients are suctioned as necessary. If the patient is being mechanically ventilated, tidal volume is maintained at 10 to 15 cc/kg of body weight to ensure adequate lung expansion, and the ventilator's sigh mechanism is used three to four times each hour.

***absorption a.*** Lung collapse associated with high alveolar oxygen concentrations.

**atelencephalia** (ăt-ĕl″ĕn-sĕ-fā′lē-ă) [Gr. *ateleia,* incompleteness, + *enkephalos,* brain] Congenital anomaly with imperfect development of the brain. Also spelled *ateloencephalia.*

**atelia** (ă-tē′lē-ă) [Gr. *ateleia,* incompleteness] Imperfect or incomplete development.

**ateliosis** (ă-tē″lē-ō′sĭs) [Gr. *a-,* not, + *teleios,* complete, + *osis,* condition] A form of infantilism due to pituitary insufficiency, in which there is arrested growth but no deformity. The voice and face may resemble those of a child. **ateliotic** (-ŏt′ĭk), *adj.*

**atelo-** (ăt′ĕ-lō) [Gr. *ateles,* imperfect] Combining form meaning *imperfect* or *incomplete.*

**atelocardia** (ăt″ĕ-lō-kăr′dē-ă) [″ + *kardia,* heart] Congenital incomplete development of the heart.

**atelocephaly** (ăt″ĕ-lō-sĕf′ă-lē) [″ + *kephale,* head] Incomplete development of the head.

**atelocheilia** (ăt″ĕ-lō-kī′lē-ă) [″ + *cheilos,* lip] Incomplete development of the lip.

**atelocheiria** (ăt″ĕ-lō-kī′rē-ă) [″ + *cheir,* hand] Incomplete development of the hand.

**ateloglossia** (ăt″ĕ-lō-glŏs′ē-ă) [″ + *glossa,* tongue] Incomplete development of the tongue.

**atelognathia** (ăt″ĕ-lŏg-nā′thē-ă) [″ + *gnathos,* jaw] Incomplete development of the jaw.

**atelomyelia** (ăt″ĕ-lō-mī-ē′lē-ă) [″ + *myelos,* marrow] Incomplete development of the spinal cord.

**atelopodia** (ăt″ĕ-lō-pō′dē-ă) [″ + *pous,* foot] Incomplete development of the foot.

**ateloprosopia** (ăt″ĕ-lō-prō-sō′pē-ă) [″ + *prosopon,* face] Incomplete development of the face.

**atelorhachidia** (ăt″ĕ-lō-ră-kĭd′ē-ă) [″ + *rhachis,* spine] Incomplete development of the spinal cord.

**atelostomia** (ăt″ĕ-lō-stō′mē-ă) [″ + *stoma,* mouth] Incomplete development of the mouth.

**atenolol** (ă-tĕn′ō-lŏl) A beta-blocking agent. Trade name is Tenormin.

**athelia** (ă-thē′lē-ă) [Gr. *a-*, not, + *thele*, nipple] Congenital absence of the nipples.

**atherectomy** An experimental technique for removing atheromatous plaques from arteries. Under direct visualization, intravascular devices are used for removing the atheromas.

**atherogenesis** (ăth″ĕr-ō-jĕn′ĕ-sĭs) [Gr. *athere*, porridge, + *genesis*, generation, birth] Formation of atheromata in the walls of arteries.

**atheroma** (ăth″ĕr-ō′mă) *pl.* **atheromata** [″ + *oma*, tumor] Fatty degeneration or thickening of the walls of the larger arteries occurring in atherosclerosis. SEE: *arteriosclerosis*. **atheromatous** (-ō′mă-tŭs), *adj.*

**atheromatosis** (ăth″ĕr-ō″mă-tō′sĭs) Generalized atheromatous disease of the arteries.

**atheronecrosis** (ăth″ĕr-ō″nĕ-krō′sĭs) [″ + *nekros*, corpse, + *osis*, condition] Necrosis or degeneration accompanying arteriosclerosis.

**atherosclerosis** (ăth″ĕr-ō″sklĕ-rō′sĭs) [″ + Gr. *sklerosis*, hardness] The most common form of arteriosclerosis, marked by cholesterol-lipid-calcium deposits in arterial linings. SEE: *coronary artery disease* for illus.

PATHOLOGY: The initial pathological alterations, called fatty streaks, are visible on the endothelial surface of the aorta and coronary arteries. They are composed of lipid deposition in the macrophages (foam cells) in the intima of these vessels. Whether they progress to advanced lesions depends on hemodynamic forces, such as hypertension, and the plasma levels of atherogenic lipoproteins. Progression of the arteriosclerotic process leads to the next stage, in which fibrous plaques form. They appear first in the abdominal aorta, coronary arteries, and carotid arteries. The changes, beginning in about the third decade of life, appear in men before women; and in women they appear in the aorta before the coronary arteries. In both men and women these changes increase with age. The final stage, termed *complicated lesion*, is a calcified plaque which may be necrotic, contain thrombi, and be ulcerated. As this condition continues the vessel walls weaken, and the intima may rupture and lead to aneurysm of the vessel. An arterial embolus occurs if the plaque breaks off into the lumen of the vessel.

**athetoid** (ăth′ĕ-toyd) [Gr. *athetos*, unfixed, changeable, + *eidos*, form, shape] Resembling or affected with athetosis.

**athetosis** (ăth-ĕ-tō′sĭs) [″ + *osis*, condition] A condition in which slow, irregular, twisting, snakelike movements occur in the upper extremities, esp. in the hands and fingers. These involuntary movements prevent sustaining the body, esp. the extremities, in one position. All four limbs may be affected or the involvement may be unilateral. The symptoms may be due to encephalitis, cerebral palsy, hepatic encephalopathy, drug toxicity, or Huntington's chorea or may be an undesired side effect of prolonged treatment of parkinsonism with levodopa.

There are several types of athetosis. In *athetosis with spasticity*, muscle tone fluctuates between normal and hypertonic; often there is moderate spasticity in the proximal parts and athetosis more distally. Modified primitive spinal reflex patterns are often present. In *athetosis with tonic spasms*, muscle tone fluctuates between hypotonic and hypertonic. Excessive extension or flexion is evident. There are strong postural asymmetry and frequent spinal or hip abnormalities or deformities.

In *choreoathetosis*, muscle tone fluctuates from hypotonic to normal or hypertonic. There are extreme ranges of motion. Deformities are rare, but subluxation of the shoulder and finger joints often occurs. *Pure athetosis* is much rarer than the others. Muscle tone fluctuates between hypotonic and normal. Deformities are rare. Twitches and jerks of muscles or individual muscle fibers are seen, along with slow, writhing, involuntary movements that are more proximal than distal.

NURSING IMPLICATIONS: Muscle tone and joint range of motion are assessed; and joints are inspected for involuntary movements, spasticity, and joint deformities and subluxations. Degree of interference with activities of daily living and self-image is evaluated. Prescribed therapies (based on the etiology) are administered and evaluated for desired effects and adverse reactions. Emotional support and acceptance are provided, and the patient is informed about local and national groups and services offering support and information.

**athlete's foot** A fungal infection of the foot caused by various dermatophytes, esp. *Trichophyton rubrum*, *T. mentagrophytes*, and *Epidermophyton floccosum*, which invade the dead, outer layers of the skin. SYN: *dermatophytosis; tinea pedis*. SEE: illus.; *Nursing Diagnoses Appendix*.

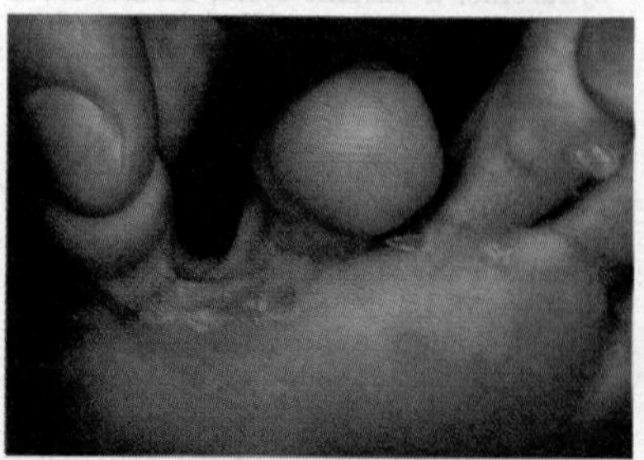

ATHLETE'S FOOT

TREATMENT: Careful attention to hygiene is important. The feet, esp. the skin between the toes, should be carefully dried after bathing. Loose, macerated skin should be gently removed and a bland drying powder applied. Well-ventilated shoes and absorbent socks made of 100% cotton or polypropylene are important treatment adjuncts. In suitable climates, going barefoot is beneficial. Severe cases should be treated with griseofulvin, but most subacute or chronic cases will respond to a fungicidal medication such as 2% miconazole cream, 1% clotrimazole cream or lotion, or Whitfield's tincture (3% salicylic acid, 6% benzoic acid in 70% alcohol).

NURSING IMPLICATIONS: The patient should practice scrupulous foot care, washing the feet daily and drying thoroughly, with special attention to areas between the toes. Prescribed medications (prepared as creams, lotions, or powders) are applied as directed. The importance of keeping the feet as dry as possible and wearing well-ventilated shoes and clean, absorbent socks is stressed.

**athletic trainer** A person who, as a result of training and experience, is capable of working with athletes and their environment to help prevent injuries, advise them concerning appropriate equipment, recognize and evaluate injuries, administer emergency treatment, and determine if specialized medical care is required. The athletic trainer also works with the health care team to rehabilitate those with sports injuries. In many instances, the first member of the health care team an injured athlete encounters is an athletic trainer, who must be able to provide the best possible treatment. In some states, athletic trainers must be licensed to practice. SEE: *training, athletic.*

**athrepsia, athrepsy** (ă-thrĕp'sē-ă, -sē) [Gr. *a-*, not, + *threpsis*, nourishment] Marasmus. **athreptic** (-thrĕp'tĭk), *adj.*

**Athrombin-K** Trade name for warfarin potassium.

**athyroidemia** (ath"ĭ-roy-, ă-thī"roy-dē'mē-ă) [" + " + " + *haima*, blood] Absence of thyroid hormone in the blood.

**athyroidism** (ă-thī'roy-dĭzm) [" + " + " + *-ismos*, condition of] Suppression of thyroid secretions, or absence of the thyroid gland; hypothyroidism.

**atlantad** (ăt-lăn'tăd) Toward the atlas.

**atlantal** (ăt-lăn'tăl) Pert. to the atlas.

**atlantoaxial** (ăt-lăn"tō-ăk'sē-ăl) [Gr. *atlas*, a support, + L. *axis*, a pivot] Pert. to the atlas (first cervical vertebra) and the axis (second cervical vertebra).

**atlantodidymus** (ăt-lăn"tō-dĭd'ĭ-mŭs) [" + *didymus*, twin] Atlodidymus.

**atlanto-occipital** (ăt-lăn"tō-ŏk-sĭp'ĭ-tăl) [" + L. *occipitalis*, occipital] Pert. to the atlas and the occipital bones.

**atlas** (ăt'lăs) [Gr.] The first cervical vertebra by which the spine articulates with the occipital bone of the head; named for Atlas, the Greek god who was supposed to support the world on his shoulders.

**atloaxoid** (ăt"lō-ăk'soyd) [" + L. *axis*, a pivot, + Gr. *eidos*, form, shape] Pert. to the atlas and axis.

**atlodidymus** (ăt-lō-dĭd'ĭ-mŭs) [" + Gr. *didymos*, twin] A malformed fetus with one body and two heads.

**ATLS** *advanced trauma life support.*

**atm** *atmosphere; atmospheric.*

**atmo-** [Gr. *atmos*, vapor or steam] Prefix denoting *steam* or *vapor.*

**atmosphere** (ăt'mŏs-fēr) [" + *sphaira*, sphere] **1.** The gases surrounding the earth. **2.** Climatic condition of a locality. **3.** In physics, the pressure of the air on the earth at mean sea level, approx. 14.7 lb/sq in. (101,325 pascals or 760 torr). **4.** In chemistry, any gaseous medium around a body. **atmospheric** (ăt"mŏs-fēr'ĭk), *adj.*

***standard a.*** The pressure of air at sea level when the temperature is 0°C (32°F). This is equal to 14.7 lb/sq in., or 760 torr, or 101,325 pascals (newtons per square meter).

**ATN** *acute tubular necrosis.*

**ATNR** *asymmetrical tonic neck reflex.*

**atom** (ăt'ŏm) [Gr. *atomos*, indivisible] The smallest part of an element. An atom consists of a nucleus (which contains protons and neutrons) and surrounding electrons. The nucleus is positively charged, and this determines the atomic number of an element. A large number of entities in the atomic nucleus have been identified, and the search for others continues. Dimensions of atoms are of the order of $10^{-8}$ cm. SEE: *atomic theory; electron.* **atomic** (ă-tŏm'ĭk), *adj.*

***tagged a.*** Radioactive tracer.

**atomic number** SEE: *number.*

**atomic theory 1.** The theory that all matter is composed of atoms. **2.** Theories pert. to the structure, properties, and behavior of the atom.

**atomic weight** ABBR: at. wt. The relative weight of an atom as compared with the standard carbon atom isotope with a mass of 12. Therefore, carbon has an at. wt. of 12; oxygen, 16; hydrogen, 1.008; and nitrogen, 14.008.

**atomization** (ăt"ŏm-ĭ-zā'shŭn) Converting a fluid into spray or vapor form. SEE: *nebulizer; vaporizer.*

**atomize** (ăt'ŏm-īz) To convert a liquid to a spray or vapor.

**atomizer** (ăt'ŏm-ī-zĕr) An apparatus for converting a jet of liquid to a spray.

**atonicity** (ăt-ō-nĭs'ĭ-tē) [Gr. *a-*, not, + *tonos*, stretching] State of being atonic or without tone.

**atony** (ăt'ō-nē) [" + *tonos*, stretching] Debility; lack of normal tone or strength. **atonic** (ă-tŏn'ĭk), *adj.*

***gastric a.*** Lack of muscle tone in the stomach and failure to contract normally, causing a delay in movement of food out of the stomach.

**atopen** (ăt′ō-pĕn) [″+ *topos,* place] An allergen that causes atopy.

**atopic** (ă-tŏp′ĭk) **1.** Pert. to atopy. **2.** Displaced; malpositioned.

**atopognosis** (ă-tŏp″ŏg-nō′sĭs) [″ + *topos,* place, + *gnosis,* knowledge] Inability to locate a sensation of touch or feeling.

**atopy** (ăt′ō-pē) [Gr. *atopia,* strangeness] A type I hypersensitivity or allergic reaction for which there is a genetic predisposition. It differs from normal hypersensitivity reactions to allergies that are not genetically determined. The basis for the predisposition lies in the histocompatibility genes. The child of two parents with the atopic allergy has a 75% chance of developing similar symptoms; if one parent is affected, the child has a 50% chance of developing the atopy. Hay fever and asthma are two of the most commonly inherited allergies; contact dermatitis and gastrointestinal reactions may also be inherited. As with all type I hypersensitivity reactions, IgE is the primary antibody involved. SEE: *allergy; immunity; reagin.*

**atoxic** [Gr. *a-,* not, + *toxikon,* poison] Nonpoisonous.

**ATP** *adenosine triphosphate.*

**ATPase** *adenosine triphosphatase.*

**ATPS** *ambient temperature and pressure* (saturated with water vapor).

**atraumatic** (ā″traw-măt′ĭk) [Gr. *a-,* not, + *traumatikos,* relating to injury] Not causing trauma or injury. SEE: *needle, atraumatic.*

**atresia** (ă-trē′zē-ă) [″ + *tresis,* a perforation] Congenital absence or closure of a normal body opening or tubular structure. **atresic, atretic** (-zĭk, -trĕ-tĭk), *adj.*

***anal a., ani a.*** Imperforate anus.

***aortic a.*** Congenital closure of the aortic valvular opening into the aorta.

***biliary a.*** Closure or absence of some or all of the major bile ducts.

***choanal a.*** A congenital occlusion of the passage between the nose and pharynx by a bony or membranous structure.

***duodenal a.*** Congenital closure of a portion of the duodenum.

***esophageal a.*** Congenital failure of the esophageal tube to develop.

***follicular a.*** Normal death of the ovarian follicle following failure of the ovum to be fertilized.

***intestinal a.*** Congenital closure of any part of the intestine.

***mitral a.*** Congenital closure of the mitral valve opening between the left atrium and ventricle.

***prepyloric a.*** Congenital closure of the pyloric end of the stomach.

***pulmonary a.*** Congenital closure of the pulmonary valve between the right ventricle and the pulmonary artery.

***tricuspid a.*** Congenital closure of the tricuspid valve between the right atrium and ventricle.

***urethral a.*** Absence or closure of the urethral orifice or canal.

***vaginal a.*** Congenital closure or absence of the vagina.

**atreto-** (ă-trē′tō) [Gr. *atretos,* imperforate] Prefix signifying *absence of an opening.*

**atria** (ā′trē-ă) Pl. of atrium.

**atrial** (ā′trē-ăl) Pert. to the atrium.

**atrial fibrillation** ABBR: AF. Irregular and rapid discharges from multiple ectopic atrial foci that cause randomized quivering of the atria. There is no real atrial systole to force blood into the ventricles and enhance cardiac output, and no real atrial diastole. Impulses are transmitted through the atrioventricular node at irregular intervals, causing an irregular ventricular response, often very rapid when untreated. The apical impulse varies in strength and some beats are not transmitted to peripheral sites, resulting in a pulse deficit.

Etiology: The condition may occur in normal persons, esp. during stress or exercise, in acute alcoholism, and after surgery. It may be present in persons with cardiopulmonary disease who develop acute hypoxia, increased carbon dioxide (hypercapnia), or metabolic disorders. Persistent atrial fibrillation usually occurs in patients with rheumatic heart disease, mitral valve disease, hypertension, or thyrotoxicosis.

Treatment: In acute AF, therapy is directed to a precipitating factor such as fever, alcoholic intoxication, thyrotoxicosis, pulmonary emboli, congestive heart failure, or pericarditis. If the patient's clinical status is severely compromised, electrical cardioversion is indicated. Anticoagulant therapy should be started 2 weeks before and continued for 2 weeks following cardioversion. In less severe cases and chronic AF, the primary goal is to slow the ventricular rate, using digitalis, calcium channel blockers, or beta-adrenergic blockers. When drug therapy is ineffective or not tolerated by the patient, electrical ablation of the bundle of His may be tried, but this requires implantation of a permanent cardiac pacemaker to guarantee an adequate ventricular rate. An experimental method of reducing ventricular rate during AF is to modify atrioventricular nodal conduction by application of radiofrequency energy to the atrioventricular junction. This is done by using a special transvenous, steerable electrode catheter. SEE: *ablation; atrioventricular reentrant tachycardia.*

Nursing Implications: Apical and radial pulses are assessed simultaneously to evaluate for pulse deficit, and the findings documented. The patient is assessed for evidence of forward cardiac failure (activity intolerance and fatigue) and backward failure (pulmonary congestion, neck vein distention, anorexia, peripheral edema, and weight gain). Energy conservation methods are taught, and frequent rest periods are recommended for optimal physical functioning. Desired actions and adverse effects of the prescribed drug therapy are explained, and the patient is taught how to manage the prescribed dietary sodium restriction. If elective cardioversion is required for symptomatic rapid ventricular rate, the nurse explains the procedure and expected sensations, assists with the procedure, and evaluates outcomes.

**atrial flutter** A cardiac arrhythmia originating in the atrial muscle cells; marked by rapid (approx. 300 times per minute) regular atrial activity and usually regular ventricular response of varying rates.

**atrial natriuretic factor** A peptide secreted by the atrial tissue of the heart in response to an increase in blood pressure. It influences blood pressure, blood volume, and cardiac output. It increases the excretion of sodium and water in urine, thereby lowering blood volume and blood pressure and influencing cardiac output. Its secretion rate depends on glomerular filtration rate and inhibits sodium reabsorption in distal tubules. These actions reduce the workload of the heart. Also called *atrial natriuretic hormone* or *atrial natriuretic peptide*.

**atrial septal defect** A congenital heart defect in which there is an opening between the atria.

**atrichia** (ă-trĭk′ē-ă) [Gr. *a-*, not, + *thrix*, hair] **1.** Absence of hair. **2.** Lack of cilia or flagella.

**atrichosis** (ă-trĭ-kō′sĭs) [″ + ″ + *osis*, condition] Congenital absence of hair.

**atrichous** (ă-trĭk′ŭs) **1.** Without flagella. **2.** Without hair.

**atrionector** (ăt″rē-ō-nĕk′tor) [L. *atrium*, corridor, + *nector*, connector] Sinoatrial node.

**atriopeptin** (āt′rē-ō-pĕp″tĭn) Atrial natriuretic factor.

**atrioseptopexy** (ā″trē-ō-sĕp′tō-pĕk″sē) [″ + *saeptum*, a partition, + Gr. *pexis*, fixation] Plastic surgical repair of an interatrial septal defect.

**atriotome** (ā′trē-ō-tōm) [″ + Gr. *tome*, incision] Instrument used in surgically opening the cardiac atrium.

**atrioventricular** (ā″trē-ō-vĕn-trĭk′ū-lăr) [″ + *ventriculus*, ventricle] Pert. to both the atrium and the ventricle.

**atrioventricular bundle** SEE: *bundle, atrioventricular*.

**atrioventricular junction** SEE: *junction, atrioventricular*.

**atrioventricularis communis** (ā″trē-ō-vĕn-trĭk″ū-lā′rĭs kŏ-mū′nĭs) Persistence of the common atrioventricular canal. In this congenital anomaly of the heart, the division of the common atrioventricular canal in the embryo fails to occur. This causes atrial septal defect and atrioventricular valve incompetence.

**atriplicism** (ă-trĭp′lĭ-sĭzm) Poisoning due to eating one form of spinach, *Atriplex littoralis*.

**atrium** (ā′trē-ŭm) *pl.* **atria** [L., corridor] A chamber or cavity communicating with another structure.

***a. of the ear*** The portion of the tympanic cavity lying below the malleus; the tympanic cavity proper.

***a. of the heart*** The upper chamber of each half of the heart. The right atrium receives deoxygenated, dark red blood from the entire body (except lungs) through the superior and inferior venae cavae and coronary sinus; the left atrium receives oxygenated red blood from the lungs through the pulmonary veins. Blood passes from the atria to the ventricles through the atrioventricular valves. In the embryo, the atrium is a single chamber that lies between the sinus venosus and the ventricle.

***a. of the lungs*** The space at the end of an alveolar duct that opens into the alveoli, or air sacs, of the lungs.

**Atromid-S** Trade name for clofibrate.

**atrophoderma** (ăt″rō-fō-dĕr′mă) [Gr. *a-*, not, + *trophe*, nourishment, + *derma*, skin] Atrophy of the skin.

**atrophy** (ăt′rō-fē) [Gr. *atrophia*] **1.** A wasting; a decrease in size of an organ or tissue. Atrophy may result from death and resorption of cells, diminished cellular proliferation, pressure, ischemia, malnutrition, decreased activity, or hormonal changes. **2.** To undergo or cause atrophy. **atrophic** (ā-trō′fĭk), *adj.*

***acute yellow a.*** Extensive necrosis of liver cells, with jaundice, mental disturbances, and cutaneous hemorrhages; a complication of hepatitis. Early central nervous system symptoms appear before jaundice sets in. Onset is slow. Malaise and some fever are accompanied by nausea with black vomitus.

***brown a.*** Atrophic tissue that is yellowish-brown rather than its normal color. It is seen principally in the heart and liver of the aged. The pigmentation is due to the presence of lipofuscin, the "wear and tear" pigment associated with aging. Its presence in tissue is a sign of injury from free radicals. SEE: *lipofuscin; radical, free*.

***compression a.*** Atrophy due to constant pressure on a part.

***correlated a.*** Wasting of a part following destruction of a correlated part.

***Cruveilhier's a.*** Spinal muscular a.

***disuse a.*** Atrophy, esp. in muscular tissue, due to lack of exercise.

***healed yellow a.*** Postnecrotic cirrhosis of the liver.

***Hoffmann's a.*** SEE: *Werdnig-Hoffmann disease*.

***Landouzy-Déjérine a.*** A hereditary form of progressive muscular dystrophy with onset in childhood or adolescence. It is marked by atrophic changes in the muscles of the shoulder girdle and face, inability to raise the arms above the head, myopathic facies, eyelids that remain partly open in sleep, and inability to whistle or purse the lips. SYN: *dystrophy, Landouzy-Déjérine.*

***macular a.*** Anetoderma.

***muscular a.*** Atrophy of muscle tissue, esp. due to lack of use or denervation.

***myelopathic a.*** Muscular atrophy resulting from a lesion of the spinal cord.

***myotonic a.*** Myotonia congenita.

***a. of disuse*** Atrophy from failure to exercise a part normally.

***optic a.*** Atrophy of the optic disk as a result of degeneration of the second cranial (optic) nerve.

***pathological a.*** Atrophy that results from the effects of disease processes.

***peroneal muscular a.*** Charcot-Marie-Tooth disease.

***physiological a.*** Atrophy caused by the normal aging processes in the body. Examples are atrophy of embryonic structures; atrophy of childhood structures on reaching maturity, as the thymus; atrophy of structures in cyclic phases of activity, as the corpus luteum; atrophy of structures following cessation of functional activity, as the ovary and mammary glands; and atrophy of structures with aging.

***postmenopausal vaginal a.*** SEE: *vaginal atrophy, postmenopausal.*

***progressive muscular a.*** Spinal muscular a.

***spinal muscular a.*** An autosomal recessive hereditary disorder in which motor neurons in the spinal cord die, leading to muscle paralysis. The type 1 form is usually fatal by age 4; the cause of death is respiratory paralysis. Types 2 and 3 are slower to progress. There is no treatment. SYN: *Aran-Duchenne disease; Cruveilhier's a.; Duchenne-Aran disease; progressive muscular a.; progressive muscular dystrophy.*

***Sudeck's a.*** Acute atrophy of a bone at the site of injury; probably due to reflex local vasospasm.

***trophoneurotic a.*** Atrophy due to disease of the nerves or nerve centers supplying the affected muscles.

***unilateral facial a.*** Progressive atrophy of one side of the facial tissues.

**atropine sulfate** (ăt′rō-pēn sŭl′fāt) Salt of an alkaloid obtained from belladonna. A parasympatholytic agent, it counteracts the effects of parasympathetic stimulation. It is administered prior to a general anesthetic to inhibit salivation and secretions of the respiratory tract. The use of relatively nonirritating anesthetics has decreased the need for atropine for that purpose.

**atropine sulfate poisoning** A toxic reaction caused by an overdose of atropine sulfate. SYN: *atropinism; atropism.*

SYMPTOMS: Symptoms include dry mouth, thirst, burning pain in the throat, hyperpyrexia, palpitations, restlessness, excitement, delirium, and dry, hot, and flushed skin.

FIRST AID: Treatment consists of lavage with a slurry of activated charcoal or 1% tannic acid. Pilocarpine will make the patient more comfortable, but barbiturates are required to control excitement. SEE: *Poisons and Poisoning Appendix.*

**atropinism, atropism** (ăt′rō-pĭn-ĭzm, -pĭzm) Atropine sulfate poisoning.

**atropinization** (ăt-rō″pĭn-ĭ-zā′shŭn) Administration of atropine until desired pharmacologic effect is achieved.

**Atropisol** Trade name for atropine sulfate.

**ATS** *American Thoracic Society.*

**attachment** (ă-tăch′mĕnt) **1.** A device or other material affixed to something else. **2.** In dentistry, a plastic or metal device used for retention or stabilization of a dental prosthesis, such as a partial denture. **3.** An enduring psychological bond of affection.

***epithelial a.*** The mechanism by which the surrounding soft tissue is attached to the calcified tooth root.

***parent-newborn a.*** Unconscious incorporation of the infant into the family unit. Characteristic parental claiming behaviors include seeking mutual eye contact with the infant, initiating touch with their fingertips, calling the infant by name, and expressing recognition of physical and behavioral similarities with other family members. Attachment is enhanced or impeded by the infant's responses. SEE: *bonding, mother-infant; engrossment; position, en face.*

**attack** (ă-tăk′) [Fr. *attaquer,* join] **1.** The onset of an illness or symptom, usually dramatic (e.g., a heart attack or an attack of gout). **2.** An assault.

**attendant** A paramedical hospital employee who assists in the care of patients.

**attending** The person having primary responsibility for a patient.

**attention-deficit hyperactivity disorder** ABBR: ADHD. A persistent pattern of inattention and hyperactivity-impulsivity or both, occurring more frequently and severely than is typical in individuals at a comparable level of development. The illness may begin in early childhood, but may not be diagnosed until after the symptoms have been present for many years. The prevalence is estimated to be 3% to 5% in children; data for adults are not available.

SYMPTOMS: The disorder is marked by inattention, hyperactivity, impulsivity, or a combination of these. Signs may be minimal or absent when the person is under strict control or is engaged in esp. interesting or challenging situations. They are more likely to occur in group situations. Although behaviors vary widely, children usually exhibit low frustration levels, marked intolerance for changes in their immediate environments, and failure to respond to discipline. Young children commonly exhibit temper tantrums, excessive large muscle activity, and negativity. Older children frequently display restlessness, carelessness, stubbornness, rapid mood swings, and low self-esteem.

ETIOLOGY: The origin is unknown; however, the disorder may reflect a deficiency in neurochemicals that influence functions of the reticular activating system of the brain.

DIAGNOSIS: The disorder is difficult to diagnose in children under age 5. It is important to distinguish this illness from age-appropriate behaviors in active children, and from disorders such as mental retardation, alteration of mood, anxiety, or personality changes caused by illness or drugs. The criteria determined by the American Psychiatric Association now include specific limits concerning the duration and severity of symptoms of inattention and hyperactivity-impulsivity. The findings must be severe enough to be maladaptive and inconsistent with specified levels of development.

TREATMENT: In both children and adults, the domestic, school, social, and occupational environments are evaluated to determine contributing factors and their relative importance. The drug of choice for use in children is methylphenidate. Dextroamphetamine may used for those who do not tolerate methylphenidate. Pemoline, although weaker, also may be used.

**attention reflex** Change in the size of the pupil when attention is suddenly fixed. SYN: *Piltz's reflex.*

**attenuate** (ă-tĕn'ū-āt) To render thin or make less virulent. In radiology, to make less intense. **attenuated,** *adj.*

**attenuation** (ă-tĕn"ū-ā'shŭn) **1.** Dilution. **2.** The lessening of virulence. Bacteria and viruses are made less virulent by being heated, dried, treated with chemicals, passed through another organism, or cultured under unfavorable conditions. **3.** The decrease in intensity (quantity and quality) of an x-ray beam as it passes through matter. **4.** In acoustics, the reduction in sound intensity of the initial sound source as compared with the sound intensity at a point away from the source. **5.** The reduction of amplitude, magnitude, or strength of an electrical signal. In electronics, it is the opposite of amplification.

**Attenuvax** Trade name for measles virus vaccine, live.

**attic** (ăt'ĭk) [L. *atticus*] The cavity of the middle ear or the portion lying above the tympanic cavity proper. It contains the head of the malleus and the short limb of the incus. SYN: *epitympanic recess.* SEE: *ear; tympanum.*

**attic disease** Chronic suppurative inflammation of the attic of the ear.

**atticitis** (ăt"ĭ-sī'tĭs) [L. *atticus,* attic, + Gr. *itis,* inflammation] Inflammation of the attic of the ear.

**atticoantrotomy** (ăt"ĭ-kō-ăn-trŏt'ō-mē) [" + Gr. *antron,* cave, + *tome,* incision] Surgical opening of the attic and mastoid antrum of the ear.

**atticotomy** (ăt"ĭ-kŏt'ō-mē) [" + Gr. *tome,* incision] Surgical opening of the tympanic attic of the ear.

**attitude** [LL. *aptitudo,* fitness] **1.** Bodily posture or position, esp. the position of the limbs. A particular attitude is often a symptom of disease or abnormal mental state (e.g., the stereotyped position assumed by catatonics or the theatric expression seen in hysteria). **2.** Behavior based on conscious or unconscious mental views developed through cumulative experience.

***crucifixion a.*** Position in which the body is rigid with the arms at right angles to the long axis of the body; seen in catatonia.

***defense a.*** Position automatically assumed to avert pain.

***fetal a.*** Position of the fetus with respect to maternal anatomical landmarks.

***forced a.*** Abnormal position due to disease or contractures.

***frozen a.*** Stiffness of gait, seen in amyotrophic lateral sclerosis.

***stereotyped a.*** Position taken and held for a long period, seen frequently in mental diseases.

**atto** [Danish, *atten,* eighteen] Symbol: a. In SI units, a prefix indicating $10^{-18}$.

**attolens** (ă-tōl'ĕnz) [L.] Raising or lifting up.

**attraction** (ă-trăk'shŭn) [L. *attrahere,* to draw toward] A force that causes particles of matter to be drawn to each other.

***capillary a.*** The force by which liquids rise in fine tubes or through pores of loose material.

***chemical a.*** The tendency of atoms of one element to unite with those of another to form compounds.

***molecular a.*** The tendency of molecules with unlike electrical charges to attract each other. SEE: *adhesion; cohesion.*

**attrahens** To bring toward.

**attribute** [L. *attributus,* character, reputation] A quality or characteristic of animate or inanimate objects (e.g., adaptability is an attribute of living organisms).

**attrition** (ă-trĭsh'ŭn) [L. *attritio,* a rubbing against] **1.** The act of wearing away by friction or rubbing. **2.** Any friction that breaks the skin. **3.** The process of wearing away, as of teeth, in the course of normal use.

**atypia** (ā-tĭp'ē-ă) [Gr. *a-,* not, + *typos,* type] Deviation from a standard or regular type.

**atypical** (ā-tĭp'ĭ-kăl) [" + *typikos,* pert. to type] Deviating from the normal; not conforming to type.

**A.U.** *angstrom unit; aures unitas,* both ears; *auris uterque,* each ear.

**Au** [L. *aurum*] Symbol for the element gold.

**Aub-Dubois table** (awb-dū-boy′) [Joseph C. Aub, U.S. physician, 1890–1973; Eugene F. Dubois, U.S. physician, 1882–1959] Table of normal basal metabolic rates according to age.

**audible** Capable of being heard.

**audible sound** Sound containing frequency components between 15 and 15,000 Hz (cycles per second).

**audile** (aw′dĭl) **1.** Pert. to hearing; auditory. **2.** A person who retains more auditory information than information received through other senses. **3.** In psychoanalysis, one whose mental images are auditory. SEE: *motile; visile.*

**audioanesthesia** (aw″dē-ō-ăn″ĕs-thē′zē-ă) [L. *audire,* to hear, + Gr. *an-,* not, + *aisthesis,* sensation] Anesthesia or analgesia produced by sound; used by dentists to help prevent perception of pain.

**audiogenic** (aw-dē-ō-jĕn′ĭk) [″ + Gr. *genesis,* generation, birth] Originating in sound.

**audiogram** (aw′dē-ō-grăm″) [″ + Gr. *gramma,* something written] A graphic record produced by an audiometer. SEE: illus.

**audiologist** A specialist in audiology.

**audiology** (aw″dē-ŏl′ō-jē) [″ + Gr. *logos,* word, reason] The study of hearing disorders through identification and evaluation of hearing loss, and the rehabilitation of those with hearing loss, esp. that which cannot be improved by medical or surgical means.

**audiometer** (aw″dē-ŏm′ĕ-tĕr) [″ + Gr. *metron,* measure] An instrument for testing hearing.

**audiometry** (aw″dē-ŏm′ĕ-trē) Testing of the hearing sense. SEE: *spondee threshold.*

***averaged electroencephalic a.*** A method of testing the hearing of children who cannot be adequately tested by conventional means. The test is based on the electroencephalogram's being altered by perceived sound without the need for a behavioral response, so the test may be done on an autistic, severely retarded, or hyperkinetic child who is asleep or sedated. SEE: *auditory evoked response.*

***evoked response a.*** Use of computer-aided technique to average the brain's response to latency of auditory stimuli. Auditory brainstem evoked response (ABER) is one form of this type of audiometry. This method is used to test the hearing of individuals, esp. children, who cannot be tested in the usual manner.

***pure tone a.*** Measurement of hearing using pure tones, which are almost completely free of extraneous noise.

***speech a.*** Test of the ability to hear and understand speech. The threshold of detection is measured in decibels.

**audit** In medical care facilities, an official examination of the record of all aspects of patient care. This is done by trained staff who are not usually affiliated with the institution. The purpose of an audit is to compare the quality of care provided with accepted standards.

**audition** (aw-dĭ′shŭn) [L. *auditio,* hearing] Hearing.

***chromatic a.*** Condition in which certain color sensations are aroused by sound stimuli. SYN: *colored a.*

***colored a.*** Chromatic a.

***gustatory a.*** Condition in which certain taste sensations are aroused by sound stimuli.

***mental a.*** Recollection of a sound based on previous auditory impressions.

**audito-oculogyric reflex** (aw″dĭt-ō-ŏk″ū-lō-jī′rĭk) The sudden turning of the head and eyes toward an alarming sound.

**auditory** (aw′dĭ-tō″rē) [L. *auditorius*] Pert. to the sense of hearing.

**auditory bulb** The membranous labyrinth and cochlea.

**auditory canal** One of the two canals associated with the structures of each ear. They are the external auditory canal, leading from the external auditory meatus to the tympanic membrane, length less than 1 in. (2.5 cm); and the internal auditory canal, leading from the structures of the inner ear to the internal auditory meatus and the cranial cavity. Both auditory canals transmit the nerves of hearing and equilibrium.

**auditory epilepsy** Epilepsy triggered by certain sounds. SEE: *epilepsy.*

**auditory evoked response** Response to auditory stimuli as determined by a method independent of the individual's subjective response. The electroencephalogram has been used to record response to sound. By measuring intensity of sound and presence of response, one can test the acuity of hearing of psychiatric patients, persons who are asleep, and children too young to cooperate in a standard hearing test. SEE: *audiometry, averaged electroencephalic.*

**auditory muscles** The tensor tympani and stapedius muscles. SEE: *Muscles Appendix.*

**auditory nerve** The eighth cranial nerve; a sensory nerve with two sets of fibers: cochlear nerve (hearing) and vestibular nerve (equilibrium), the latter having three branches, the superior, inferior, and middle branches. SYN: *vestibulocochlear nerve.*

**auditory placode** The embryonic thickenings of the epithelial layer, which become the inner ear of the embryo.

**auditory reflex** Any reflex produced by stimulation of the auditory nerve, esp. blinking of the eyes at the sudden unexpected production of a sound.

**auditory tube** Eustachian tube.

**Auenbrugger's sign** (ow-ĕn-broog′ĕrz) [Leopold Joseph Auenbrugger, Austrian physician, 1722–1809] Epigastric prominence due to marked pericardial effusion.

**Auerbach's plexus** (ow′ĕr-băks) [Leopold Auerbach, Ger. anatomist, 1828–1897]

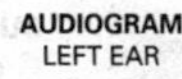


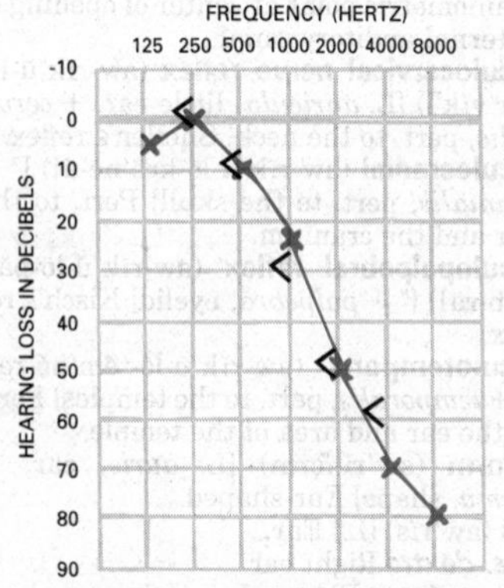


A PRESBYACUSIS. AIR AND BONE CONDUCTION ARE EQUALLY AFFECTED

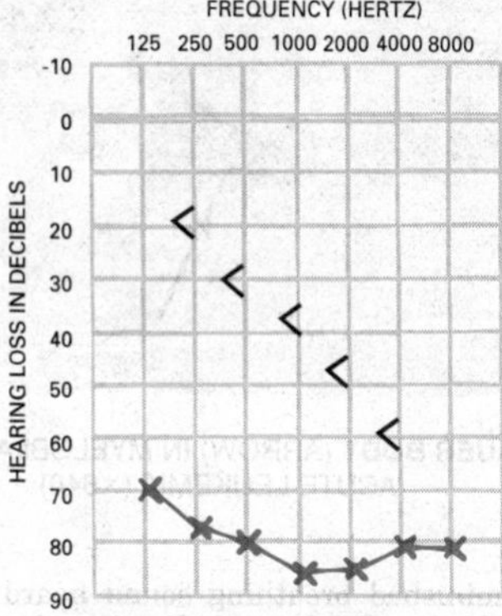


B SEVERE MIXED HEARING LOSS

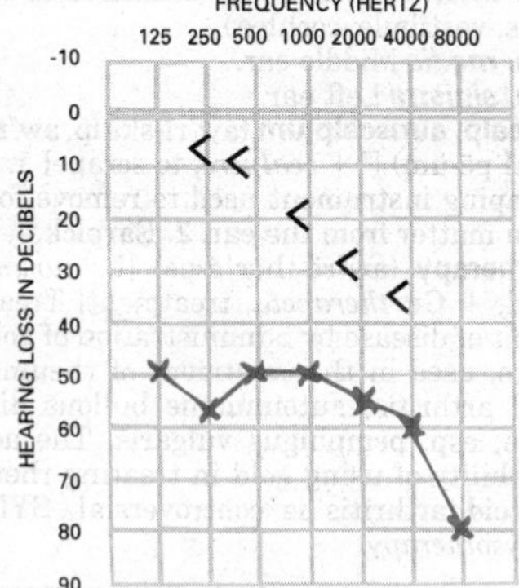


C MODERATELY SEVERE MIXED HEARING LOSS

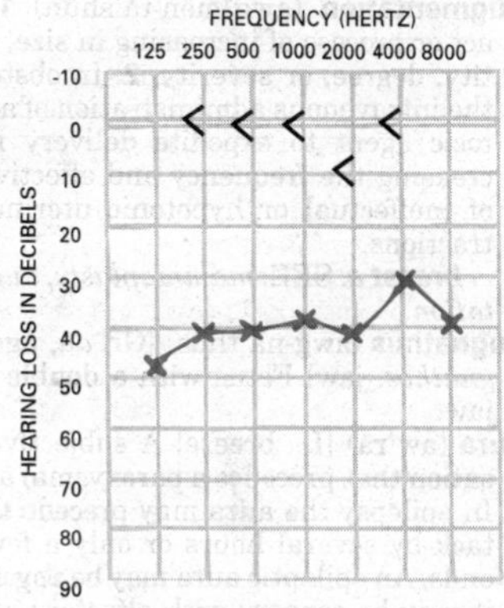


D PURE AIR CONDUCTION LOSS BECAUSE OF UNCOMPLICATED OTOSCLEROSIS

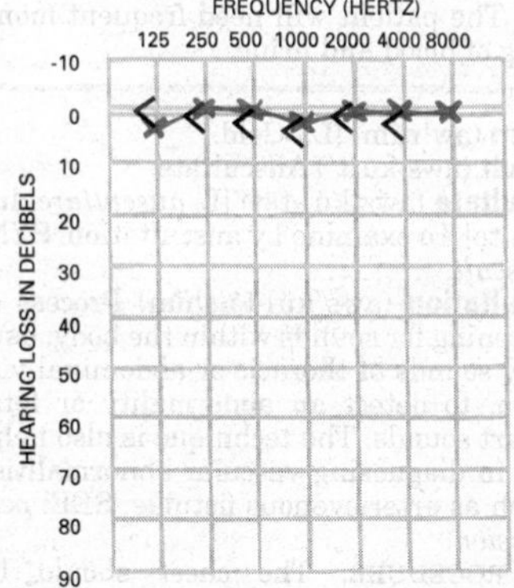


E NORMAL AUDIOGRAM

< LEFT EAR BONE CONDUCTION, RIGHT EAR MASKED

✕ LEFT EAR CONDUCTION

An autonomic nerve plexus between the circular and longitudinal fibers of the muscular layer of the stomach and intestines. SYN: *myenteric plexus.*

**Auer bodies** (ow′ərz) [John Auer, U.S. physician, 1875–1948] Rod-shaped structures, present in the cytoplasm of myeloblasts, myelocytes, and monoblasts, found in leukemia. Also called *Auer rods.* SEE: illus.

**Aufrecht's sign** (owf′rĕkhts) [Emanuel Aufrecht, Ger. physician, 1844–1933] Di-

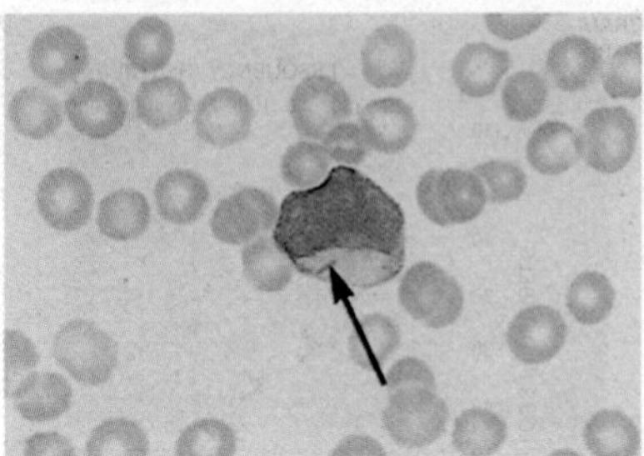

**AUER BODY** (ARROW) IN MYELOBLAST IN ACUTE LEUKEMIA (×640)

minished breathing sound heard above the jugular fossa; indicative of tracheal stenosis.

**augmentation** (awg″mĕn-tā′shŭn) **1.** The act or process of increasing in size, quantity, degree, or severity. **2.** In obstetrics, the intravenous administration of an oxytocic agent to expedite delivery by increasing the frequency and effectiveness of ineffectual or hypotonic uterine contractions.

***breast a.*** SEE: *mammaplasty, augmentation.*

**augnathus** (awg-nā′thŭs) [Gr. *au,* again, + *gnathos,* jaw] Fetus with a double lower jaw.

**aura** (aw′ră) [L., breeze] A subjective sensation that precedes a paroxysmal attack. In epilepsy the aura may precede the attack by several hours or only a few seconds. An epileptic aura may be psychic, or it may be sensory with olfactory, visual, auditory, or taste hallucinations. In migraine the aura immediately precedes the attack and consists of ocular sensory phenomena.

**aural** (aw′răl) [L. *auris,* the ear] **1.** Pert. to the ear. **2.** Pert. to an aura.

**aurantiasis cutis** (aw″răn-tī′ă-sĭs kū′tĭs) [L. *aurantium,* orange, + Gr. *-iasis,* condition of; L. *cutis,* skin] Yellow pigmentation of skin due to ingestion of excessive amounts of food that contain carotene, such as carrots, oranges, and squash. SEE: *carotenemia.*

**Aureomycin** (aw″rē-ŏ-mī′sĭn) Trade name for the antibiotic chlortetracycline hydrochloride.

**auriasis** (aw-rī′ă-sĭs) Chrysiasis.

**auric** (aw′rĭk) [L. *aurum,* gold] Pert. to gold.

**auricle** (aw′rĭ-kl) [L., little ear] **1.** The portion of the external ear not contained within the head; the pinna. **2.** A small conical pouch forming a portion of the right and left atria of the heart. Each projects from the upper anterior portion of each atrium. **3.** An obsolete term for the atrium of the heart.

**auricula** (aw-rĭk′ū-lă) *pl.* **auriculae** Auricle.

**auricular** (aw-rĭk′ū-lăr) Pert. to the auricle of the ear.

**auriculare** (aw-rĭk″ū-lā′rē) *pl.* **auricularia** A craniometric point at center of opening of external auditory canal.

**auriculocervical nerve reflex** (aw-rĭk″ū-lō-sĕr′vĭk′l) [L. *auricula,* little ear, + *cervicalis,* pert. to the neck] Snellen's reflex.

**auriculocranial** (aw-rĭk″ū-lō-krā′nē-ăl) [″ + *cranialis,* pert. to the skull] Pert. to the ear and the cranium.

**auriculopalpebral reflex** (aw-rĭk″ū-lō-păl′pĕb-răl) [″ + *palpebra,* eyelid] Kisch's reflex.

**auriculotemporal** (aw-rĭk″ū-lō-tĕm′pŏ-răl) [″ + *temporalis,* pert. to the temples] Pert. to the ear and area of the temple.

**auriform** (aw′rĭ-form) [L. *auris,* ear, + *forma,* shape] Ear-shaped.

**auris** (aw′rĭs) [L.] Ear.

***a. dextra*** Right ear.

***a. externa*** External ear (pinna and external auditory meatus).

***a. interna*** Internal ear (semicircular canals, vestibule, cochlea).

***a. media*** Middle ear.

***a. sinistra*** Left ear.

**auriscalp, auriscalpium** (aw′rĭ-skălp, aw″rĭ-skăl′pē-ŭm) [″ + *scalpere,* to scrape] **1.** A scraping instrument used to remove foreign matter from the ear. **2.** Earpick.

**aurotherapy** (aw″rō-thĕr′ă-pē) [L. *aurum,* gold, + Gr. *therapeia,* treatment] Treatment of disease by administration of gold salts; used in the treatment of rheumatoid arthritis, autoimmune bullous disease, esp. pemphigus vulgaris. The advisability of using gold in treating rheumatoid arthritis is controversial. SYN: *chrysotherapy.*

---

Caution: Side effects, including toxicity to the kidneys and bone marrow, are significant. The patient will need frequent monitoring of blood and urine.

---

**aurum** (aw′rŭm) [L.] Gold.

**auscult** (aws-kŭlt′) Auscultate.

**auscultate** (aws′kŭl-tāt) [L. *auscultare,* listen to] To examine by auscultation. SYN: *auscult.*

**auscultation** (aws″kŭl-tā′shŭn) Process of listening for sounds within the body, usually sounds of thoracic or abdominal viscera, to detect an abnormality or fetal heart sounds. The technique is also helpful in diagnosing vascular abnormalities such as arteriovenous fistulae. SEE: *percussion.*

PROCEDURE: The chest should be draped with a loose-fitting garment that can easily be moved aside to allow the stethoscope to be placed directly against the skin. If chest hair is thick, it should be moistened to prevent friction sounds, which resemble crackles. Auscultation is performed all over the chest anteriorly and posteriorly, on full inspiration, on full expiration, and after the patient coughs. For a comparison of the two sides, symmetrical parts should be auscultated. The patient should be relaxed. The examiner should be positioned so that his or her vascular sounds cannot be confused with those of the patient.

***immediate a.*** Auscultation in which the ear is applied directly to a bare or thinly covered surface.

***mediate a.*** Auscultation in which sounds are conducted from the surface to the ear through an instrument such as a stethoscope.

**auscultatory** (aws-kŭl'tă-tō"rē) Pert. to auscultation.

**auscultatory percussion** Auscultation at the same time percussion is made.

**Austin Flint murmur** [Austin Flint, U.S. physician, 1812–1886] A presystolic or late diastolic heart murmur best heard at the apex of the heart. It is present in some cases of aortic insufficiency. It is thought to be due to the vibration of the mitral valve caused by the backward-flowing blood from the aorta meeting the blood flowing in from the left atrium.

**Australia antigen, Australian antigen** An antigen present in the sera of patients with hepatitis B, but rarely in patients with other forms of hepatitis. This antigen is also found in normal populations in the Tropics and southeast Asia. It was first isolated in the serum of an Australian aborigine. SYN: *hepatitis B surface antigen.*

**autacoid** (aw'tă-koyd) [Gr. *autos,* self, + *akos,* remedy, + *eidos,* form, shape] **1.** A term originally used by the British physiologists Edward Shäfer and Sharpey-Shafer as a substitute for the word *hormone.* **2.** A term used to describe prostaglandins and related compounds that form rapidly, act, and then decay or are destroyed enzymatically.

**autism** (aw'tĭzm) [Gr. *autos,* self, + *-ismos,* condition] Mental introversion in which the attention or interest is fastened on the patient's own ego; a self-centered mental state from which reality tends to be excluded. SEE: *Nursing Diagnoses Appendix.*

***infantile a.*** A syndrome appearing in childhood with symptoms of self-absorption, inaccessibility, aloneness, inability to relate, highly repetitive play and rage reactions if interrupted, predilection for rhythmical movements, and many language disturbances. The cause is unknown.

**auto-** [Gr. *autos,* self] Combining form meaning *self.*

**autoactivation** (aw"tō-ăk"tĭ-vā'shŭn) [" + L. *agere,* to act] Gland activation by its own secretion.

**autoagglutination** (aw"tō-ă-gloo"tĭ-nā'shŭn) [" + L. *agglutinare,* adhere to] Agglutination, or clumping of red blood cells, in response to an autotransfusion (e.g., the transfusion of a person's own blood that has been removed by phlebotomy or during surgery).

**autoagglutinin** (aw"tō-ă-glū'tĭ-nĭn) A substance present in an individual's blood that agglutinates that person's red blood cells.

**autoamputation** (aw"tō-ăm"pū-tā'shŭn) Spontaneous amputation of a part or limb. SEE: *ainhum.*

**autoanalysis** (aw"tō-ă-năl'ĭ-sĭs) [" + *analyein,* break down] A patient's own analysis of the mental state underlying his or her mental disorder.

**Autoanalyzer** (aw"tō-ăn'ă-līz"ĕr) Trade name of a device for performing analytic tests on a large number of laboratory specimens. The testing is done automatically with the specimens being tested sequentially.

**autoantibody** (aw"tō-ăn'tĭ-bŏd"ē) [" + *anti,* against, + AS *bodig,* body] ABBR: AAb. An antibody, produced by B cells in response to an altered "self" antigen on one type of the body's own cells, that attacks and destroys these cells. Autoantibodies are the basis for autoimmune diseases such as rheumatoid arthritis and diabetes mellitus. Several theories exist as to why autoantibodies are formed. The most commonly accepted theory proposes that a virus or direct trauma damages the antigen, changing its appearance. Consequently, B cells see it as "non-self" or foreign, and antibodies are produced for its destruction. SEE: *antibody; antigen; autoimmunity; immunoglobulin.*

**autoantigen** (aw"tō-ăn'tĭ-jĕn) [" + " + *gennan,* to produce] A substance that stimulates the production of antibodies in the individual from whom it was derived.

**autoantitoxin** (aw"tō-ăn"tĭ-tŏk'sĭn) [" + " + *toxikon,* poison] Antitoxin produced by the body itself.

**autocatalysis** (aw"tō-kă-tăl'ĭ-sĭs) [" + *katalysis,* dissolution] Increase in the rate of a chemical reaction resulting from products that are produced in the reaction acting as catalysts. SEE: *catalyst.*

**autocatharsis** (aw-tō-kă-thăr'sĭs) [" + *katharsis,* a cleansing] A form of psychotherapy in which patients in discussing their own problems gain an insight into their mental difficulties.

**autocatheterization** Catheterization of oneself, esp. urinary catheterization.

**autochthonous** (aw-tŏk'thō-nŭs) [Gr. *autos,* self, + *chthon,* earth] **1.** Found where developed, as in the case of a blood clot or a calculus. **2.** Pert. to a tissue graft to a new site on the same individual.

**autochthonous infection** Infection due to organisms normally present in the patient's body. It may occur when host defenses are compromised, or when resistant flora are introduced into an abnormal site.

**autocinesia, autocinesis** (aw"tō-sĭ-nē'sē-ă, -nē'sĭs) Autokinesis.

**autoclasis** (aw"tŏk'lă-sĭs) [" + *klasis,* a breaking] Destruction of a part from internal causes.

**autoclave** (aw'tō-klāv) [" + L. *clavis,* a key] A device that sterilizes by steam pressure, usually at 250°F (121°C) for a specified length of time. SEE: *sterilization.*

**autocrine factor** A growth factor produced by the cell, probably in response to a virus. This factor is important in the development of malignancies.

**autocrine system** The secretion of a cell that acts to influence only its own growth. SEE: *paracrine.*

**autocystoplasty** (aw"tō-sĭs'tō-plăs"tē) [" + *kystis,* bladder, + *plassein,* to mold] Plastic repair of the bladder with grafts from one's own body.

**autocytolysis** (aw"tō-sī-tŏl'ĭ-sĭs) Self-digestion or self-destruction of cells.

**autodermic** (aw"tō-dĕr'mĭk) [" + *derma,* skin] Pert. to one's own skin, esp. pert. to dermatoplasty with a patient's own skin.

**autodigestion** (aw"tō-dī-jĕs'chŭn) [" + L. *dis,* apart, + *gerere,* to carry] Digestion of tissues by their own secretion, such as digestion of the stomach wall by gastric juice, which occurs in certain stomach disorders.

**autodiploid** (aw"tō-dĭp'loyd) [" + *diploe,* fold, + *eidos,* form, shape] Having two sets of chromosomes; caused by redoubling the chromosomes of the haploid cell.

**autodrainage** (aw"tō-drān'ĭj) [" + AS *dreahnian,* drain] Drainage of a cavity by the fluid passing through a channel in one's own tissues or to the outside of the body.

**autoecholalia** (aw"tō-ĕk-ō-lā'lē-ă) [" + *echo,* echo, + *lalia,* babble] Repetition of the last portion of one's own statements.

**autoecic** (aw-tē'sĭk) [" + *oikos,* house] Pert. to a parasite that spends its entire life cycle in one organism.

**autoerotic hypoxia** A state of cerebral oxygen deprivation resulting from intermittent interruption of blood flow to the brain during masturbation. A mechanism is used to constrict the neck vessels and induce hypoxia. Although difficult to prove, it is thought that hypoxia intensifies perceived pleasure during orgasm. Cases are on record in which the masturbating individual failed to release the constricting device around the neck in time to prevent brain damage or death from hypoxia. SYN: *autoerotic asphyxia; sexual asphyxia.* SEE: *asphyxiophilia.*

**autoeroticism** Autoerotism.

**autoerotism** (aw"tō-ē-rŏt'ĭsm) [Gr. *autos,* self, + *erotikos,* rel. to love] **1.** Self-gratification of the sexual instinct, usually by manual stimulation of erogenous areas, esp. the penis or clitoris. SEE: *asphyxia, sexual; masturbation; urolagnia.* **2.** Self-admiration combined with sexual emotion, such as that obtained from viewing one's naked body or one's genitals. SYN: autoeroticism. **autoerotic** (-ē-rŏt'ĭk), *adj.*

**autoexamination** (aw"tō-ĕg-zăm"ĭ-nā'shŭn) [" + L. *examinare,* to examine] Self-examination. SEE: *breast self-examination.*

**autofundoscope** (aw"tō-fŭn'dō-skōp) [" + L. *fundus,* bottom, + Gr. *skopein,* to examine] Apparatus for autoexamination of retinal vessels of the eye.

**autogenesis** (aw-tō-jĕn'ĕ-sĭs) [" + *genesis,* generation, birth] Self-generation; abiogenesis. **autogenetic** (-jĕ-nĕt'ĭk), *adj.*

**autogenous** (aw-tŏj'ĕ-nŭs) **1.** Self-producing; originating within the body. **2.** Denoting a vaccine from a culture of the patient's own bacteria.

**autograft** (aw'tō-grăft) [" + L. *graphium,* grafting knife] A graft transferred from one part of a patient's body to another.

**autohemagglutination** (aw"tō-hĕm"ă-glū"tĭ-nā'shŭn) Agglutination of one's own red cells.

**autohemic** (aw"tō-hē'mĭk) [" + *haima,* blood] Done with one's own blood.

**autohemolysin** (aw"tō-hē-mŏl'ĭ-sĭn) [" + " + *lysis,* dissolution] An antibody that acts on the corpuscles of the individual in whose blood it is formed.

**autohemolysis** (aw"tō-hē-mŏl'ĭ-sĭs) Hemolysis of one's blood corpuscles by one's own serum.

**autohemotherapy** (aw"tō-hē"mō-thĕr'ă-pē) [" + *haima,* blood, + *therapeia,* treatment] Treatment by withdrawal and injection intramuscularly of one's own blood.

**autohypnosis** (aw"tō-hĭp-nō'sĭs) Self-induced hypnosis.

**autoimmune disease** (aw"tō-ĭm-mūn') [" + L. *immunis,* safe] A disease produced when the body's normal tolerance of its own antigenic markers on cells disappears. Autoantibodies (AAbs) are produced by B lymphocytes and attack normal cells whose surface contains a "self" antigen, or autoantigen (AAg), causing destruction of tissue. Diabetes mellitus, in which AAbs attack the insulin-producing cells of the pancreas, is an autoimmune disease. Others include rheumatoid arthritis, caused by inflammatory changes in the connective tissue of joints, and multiple sclerosis, caused by AAb destruction of the myelin sheath covering nerves. Hemolytic anemia, some forms of glomerulonephritis, myasthenia gravis, chronic thyroiditis, Reiter's syndrome, Graves' disease, and systemic lupus erythematosus are also considered autoimmune diseases. SEE: *autoimmunity.*

**autoimmune theory of aging** A physiological theory of aging, originally proposed by Dr. Ray Walford. Aging occurs because antibodies develop, attack, and destroy the normal cells in the body. According to this theory, defects occur in the body's immune system so that it cannot distinguish itself from foreign structures.

**autoimmunity** (aw"tō-ĭm-mū'nĭ-tē) The body's tolerance of the antigens present on its own cells (i.e., self- or autoantigens). The most current theory of self-tolerance is that developing self-reactive T lymphocytes (those with receptors that react to self-antigens) are destroyed in the thymus by negative selection. Self-reactive T cells that escape destruction in the thymus may become tolerant because they are exposed to thousands of self-antigens as they circulate in the blood.

The loss of self-tolerance is believed to occur when self-antigens are damaged, when they link with a foreign antigen, or when the structure of a self-antigen is very similar to that of a foreign antigen (molecular mimicry). The changes in the appearance of the self-antigen cause T-cell receptors to perceive them as foreign and stimulate B-cell production of autoantibodies that attack self-antigens, producing inflammation and cell destruction. SEE: *antigen; autoantibody; autoimmune disease.*

**autoinfusion** (aw″tō-ĭn-fū′zhŭn) [Gr. *autos,* self, + L. *in,* into, + *fundere,* to pour] Forcing of blood from extremities to the body core by applying Esmarch bandages.

**autoinoculation** (aw″tō-ĭn-ŏk″ū-lā′shŭn) [″ + L. *inoculare,* to ingraft] Inoculation with organisms obtained from one's own body.

**autointoxication** (aw″tō-ĭn-tŏk″sĭ-kā′shŭn) [″ + L. *in,* into, + Gr. *toxikon,* poison] A condition caused by toxic substances produced within the body. SYN: *autotoxemia; autotoxicosis; endogenic toxicosis.*

**autoisolysin** (aw″tō-ī-sŏl′ĭ-sĭn) [″ + *isos,* equal, + *lysis,* dissolution] An antibody that causes dissolution of cells of the individual from which it was obtained and of other individuals of the same species.

**autokeratoplasty** (aw″tō-kĕr′ă-tō-plăs″tē) [″ + *keras,* horn, + *plassein,* to form] Grafting of corneal tissue taken from the patient's other eye.

**autokinesis** (aw″tō-kĭ-nē′sĭs) [″ + *kinesis,* movement] Voluntary movement. SYN: *autocinesia.* **autokinetic** (-nĕt′ĭk), *adj.*

***visual a.*** The illusion that an object in space, esp. at night, moves as one continues to look at it. Thus, an aviator looking at a distant light may perceive that the light has moved even though it is stationary.

**autolesion** (aw′tō-lē″zhŭn) [″ + L. *laedere,* to wound] Self-inflicted injury.

**autologous** (aw-tŏl′ō-gŭs) [″ + *logos,* word, reason] Originating within an individual, esp. a factor present in tissues or fluids.

**autologous blood transfusion** Transfusion of blood donated by the patient before surgery or collected from the patient during surgery. The latter is also called blood salvage. Use of the patient's own blood, rather than blood from a donor, prevents accidental exposure to the AIDS virus and other blood-borne diseases.

**autolysate** (aw-tŏl′ĭ-sāt) [″ + *lysis,* dissolution] Specific product of autolysis.

**autolysis** (aw-tŏl′ĭ-sĭs) **1.** The self-dissolution or self-digestion that occurs in tissues or cells by enzymes in the cells themselves, such as occurs after death and in some pathological conditions. **2.** Hemolysis of blood cells occurring as a result of the action of an animal's own serum or plasma. **autolytic** (aw″tō-lĭt′ĭk), *adj.*

**autolysosomes** The lysosomes that enable digestion of injured portions of the cell in which they are located.

**automatic** [Gr. *automatos,* self-acting] Spontaneous; involuntary.

**automatic implanted ventricular defibrillator** Cardioverter surgically implanted in patients at high risk for sudden cardiac death from ventricular arrhythmias. This device is capable of automatically restoring normal heartbeat.

**automaticity** The unique property of cardiac muscle tissue to contract without nervous stimulation.

**automation, laboratory** The use of clinical laboratory instruments that assay large numbers of samples mechanically.

**automatism** (aw-tŏm′ă-tĭzm) [″ + *-ismos,* condition of] **1.** Automatic actions or behavior without conscious volition or knowledge. The subject, though amnesic, appears normal to an observer, but the real personality is latent during a secondary state or period of automatism, usually a hysterical trance. Such patients are not responsible for their actions and must not be left alone. They may carry out complicated acts and not remember doing so. **2.** The spontaneous activity of cells or tissues, as the movement of cilia or the contraction of smooth muscles in tissues or organs removed from the body.

**autonomic** (aw-tō-nŏm′ĭk) [Gr. *autos,* self, + *nomos,* law] **1.** Self-controlling; functioning independently. **2.** Rel. to the autonomic nervous system.

**autonomic hyperreflexia** A condition commonly seen in patients with injury to the upper spinal cord. It is caused by massive sympathetic discharge of stimuli from the autonomic nervous system. It may be triggered by distention of the bladder or colon, catheterization of or irrigation of the bladder, cystoscopy, or transurethral resection. Symptoms include sudden hypertension, bradycardia, sweating, severe headache, and gooseflesh. Ganglionic blocking agents such as mecamylamine hydrochloride or trimethaphan camsylate are given.

NURSING IMPLICATIONS: The nurse assesses vital signs and symptoms, with the patient seated (to decrease blood pressure), and monitors them until the episode resolves. The urinary bladder is drained by catheterization. The indwelling catheter is checked for kinking or other obstruction and irrigated with no more than 30 ml of sterile normal saline solution if necessary. If the catheter remains obstructed, it is removed and a new catheter inserted immediately. The patient's rectum is checked for impaction; a local anesthetic ointment is used for lubrication and for anesthesia if removal of an impaction is necessary. Any other stimuli that may be triggering the response are also removed. A urine specimen is obtained for culture because infection may be a cause. Prescribed medications to reduce blood pressure are administered, and the patient's response evaluated. A calm atmosphere is created and emotional support offered throughout the episode. The nurse educates the patient about this complication and explains actions to prevent and alleviate it.

**autonomic nervous system** ABBR: ANS. The part of the nervous system that controls involuntary bodily functions. It is inappropriately named because rather than being truly "autonomic," it is intimately responsive to changes in somatic activities. The ANS consists of motor nerves to visceral effectors: smooth muscle, cardiac muscle, glands such as the salivary, gastric, and sweat glands, and the adrenal medullae.

The two divisions of the ANS are the sympathetic or thoracolumbar division and the parasympathetic or craniosacral division. The sympathetic division consists of the paired chains of ganglia on either side of the backbone, their connections (rami communicantes) with the thoracic and lumbar segments of the spinal cord, the splanchnic nerves, and the celiac and mesenteric ganglia in the abdomen and their axons to visceral effectors. The parasympathetic division consists of some fibers of cranial nerves 3, 7, 9, and 10; the fibers of some sacral spinal nerves and ganglia; and short axons near or in the visceral effectors. SEE: illus.

FUNCTION: Sympathetic impulses have the following effects: vasodilation in skeletal muscle and vasoconstriction in the skin and viscera occur; heart rate and force are increased; the bronchioles dilate; the liver changes glycogen to glucose; sweat glands become more active; peristalsis and gastrointestinal secretions decrease; the pupils dilate; the salivary glands secrete small amounts of thick saliva; and the hair stands on end (gooseflesh). The sympathetic division dominates during stressful situations such as anger or fright, and the body responses contribute to fight or flight, with unimportant activities such as digestion markedly slowed. Most sympathetic neurons release the neurotransmitter norepinephrine at the visceral effector.

The parasympathetic division dominates during nonstressful situations, with the following effects: the heart slows to normal, the bronchioles constrict to normal, peristalsis and gastrointestinal secretion increase for normal digestion, the pupils constrict to normal, secretion of thin saliva increases, and the urinary bladder constricts normally. If parasympathetic supply to the bladder is impaired, there will be incomplete emptying and urinary retention. All parasympathetic neurons release the transmitter acetylcholine at the visceral effector. SEE: *nervous system.*

EXAMINATION: The following tests are helpful in evaluating the state of the autonomic nervous system: Blood pressure and body temperature may be measured serially with respect to diurnal variation. Sweating by painting an area of the skin may be tested with iodine and dusting the area with starch; the areas without autonomic function will fail to turn dark. Parasympathetic function may be tested by instilling a 2% solution of methacholine into one conjunctival sac. This produces constriction of the pupil in patients with parasympathetic disorders.

**autonomous** (aw-tŏn'ō-mŭs) Independent of external influences.

**autonomy** (aw-tŏn'ō-mē) [Gr. *autos,* self, + *nomos,* law] Independent functioning.

**auto-PEEP** The inadvertent application of positive end-expiratory pressure to the lungs of a patient receiving mechanical ventilation.

**autophagia, autophagy** (aw"tō-fā'jē-ă, aw-tŏf'ă-jē) [" + *phagein,* to eat] **1.** Biting oneself. **2.** Self-consumption by a cell.

**autophagocytosis** In a cell, the digestion of portions of cell organelles or mitochondria injured or atrophied. This digestive process is essential to the survival of the cell. SEE: *endocytosis; phagocytosis; pinocytosis.*

**autophil** (aw'tō-fĭl) [" + *philein,* to love] A person who has a sensitive autonomic nervous system.

**autophilia** (aw-tō-fĭl'ē-ă) Narcissism; self-love.

**autophobia** (aw"tō-fō'bē-ă) [" + *phobos,* fear] **1.** A psychoneurotic fear of being alone. **2.** Abnormal fear of being egotistical.

**autophony** (aw-tŏf'ō-nē) [" + *phone,* voice] The vibration and echolike reproduction of one's own voice, breath sounds, and murmurs; usually due to diseases of the middle ear and auditory tube.

**autoplasmotherapy** (aw"tō-plăs"mō-thĕr'ă-pē) [" + LL. *plasma,* form, mold, + *therapeia,* treatment] Treatment that consists of injection of the patient's own blood plasma.

**autoplasty** (aw'tō-plăs"tē) Plastic surgery using grafts from the patient's body. **autoplastic** (aw"tō-plăs'tĭk), *adj.*

**autopolyploidy** (aw"tō-pŏl'ē-ploy"dē) [" + *polys,* many, + *ploos,* fold, + *eidos,* form, shape] The condition of having more than two complete sets of chromosomes.

**autoprecipitin** (aw"tō-prē-sĭp'ĭ-tĭn) [Gr. *autos,* self, + L. *praecipitare,* to cast down] Precipitin active against the serum of the animal in which it was formed.

**autopsy** (aw'tŏp-sē) Postmortem examination of the organs and tissues of a body to determine the cause of death or patholog-

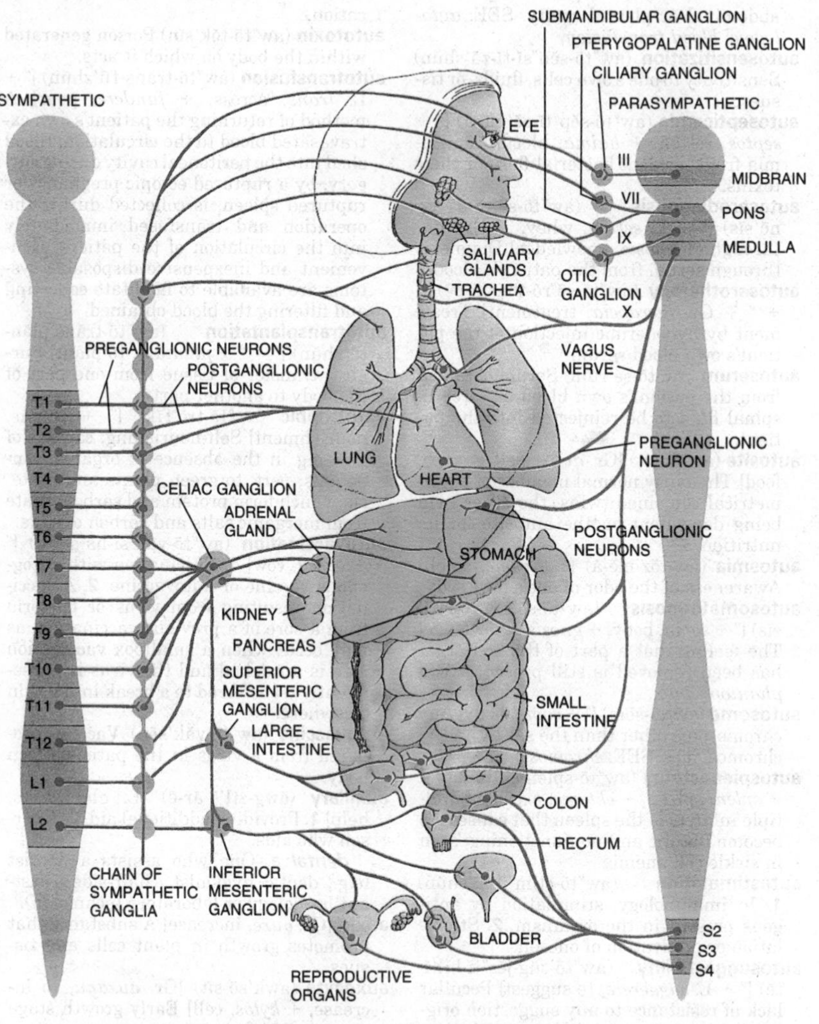


AUTONOMIC NERVOUS SYSTEM

ical conditions. SYN: *necropsy; necroscopy; postmortem examination.*

***psychological a.*** An attempt to determine what, if any, emotional or psychological factors caused or contributed to an individual's suicide.

**autopsychic** (aw″tō-sī′kĭk) [″ + *psyche,* soul] Aware of one's own personality.

**autopsychosis** (aw″tō-sī-kō′sĭs) [″ + *psyche,* soul] Mental disease in which patients' ideas about themselves are disordered.

**autoradiogram** Autoradiograph.

**autoradiograph** (aw″tō-rā′dē-ō-grăf) The radiograph formed by radioactive materials present in the tissue or individual. This is made possible by injecting radiochemicals into the person or tissue and then exposing x-ray film by placing the individual or tissue adjacent to the film. SYN: *autoradiogram; radioautograph.*

**autoradiography** Use of autoradiographs in investigating certain diseases.

**autoregulation** (aw″tō-rĕg″ū-lā′shŭn) Control of an event such as blood flow through a tissue (e.g., cardiac muscle) by alteration of the tissue. If not enough blood is flowing through a tissue, certain changes cause an increase; if the flow is too great, another type of change causes a decrease.

**autoreinfusion** (aw″tō-rē″ĭn-fū′zhŭn) [″ + L. *re,* back, + *in,* into, + *fundere,* to pour] Intravenous injection of patient's blood that has been collected from a site in which bleeding had occurred, such as the abdominal or pleural cavity. SEE: *autologous blood transfusion.*

**autosensitization** (aw″tō-sĕn″sĭ-tĭ-zā′shŭn) Sensitivity to one's own cells, fluids, or tissues.

**autosepticemia** (aw″tō-sĕp″tĭ-sē′mē-ă) [″ + *septos,* rotten, + *haima,* blood] Septicemia from resident bacterial flora or their toxins.

**autoserodiagnosis** (aw″tō-sē″rō-dī-ăg-nō′sĭs) [″ + L. *serum,* whey, + Gr. *dia,* through, + *gnosis,* knowledge] Diagnosis through serum from the patient's blood.

**autoserotherapy** (aw″tō-sē″rō-thĕr′ă-pē) [″ + ″ + Gr. *therapeia,* treatment] Treatment by hypodermic injection of the patient's own blood serum.

**autoserum** (aw″tō-sē′rŭm) Serum obtained from the patient's own blood or cerebrospinal fluid to be reinjected into the patient.

**autosite** (aw′tō-sīt) [Gr. *autos,* self, + *sitos,* food] The fairly normal member of asymmetrical conjoined twins, the other twin being dependent on the autosite for its nutrition.

**autosmia** (aw-tŏz′mē-ă) [″ + *osme,* smell] Awareness of the odor of one's own body.

**autosomatognosis** (aw″tō-sō″mă-tŏg-nō′sĭs) [″ + *soma,* body, + *gnosis,* knowledge] The feeling that a part of the body that has been removed is still present. SEE: *phantom limb.*

**autosome** (aw′tō-sōm) [″ + *soma,* body] Any chromosome other than the sex (X and Y) chromosomes. SEE: *chromosome.*

**autosplenectomy** (aw″tō-splĕn-ĕk′tō-mē) [″ + *splen,* spleen, + *ektome,* excision] Multiple infarcts of the spleen that cause it to become fibrotic and nonfunctioning; seen in sickle cell anemia.

**autostimulation** (aw″tō-stĭm″ū-lā′shŭn) **1.** In immunology, stimulation by antigens present in the organism. **2.** Stimulation or motivation of oneself.

**autosuggestibility** (aw″tō-sŭg-jĕs″tĭ-bĭl′ĭ-tē) [″ + L. *suggerere,* to suggest] Peculiar lack of resistance to any suggestion originating in one's own mind.

**autosuggestion** (aw″tō-sŭg-jĕs′chŭn) The acceptance of an idea or thought arising from within one's own mind, bringing about some physical or mental action or change.

**autotemnous** (aw″tō-tĕm′nŭs) [″ + *temnein,* to divide] Pert. to cells propagating by spontaneous division.

**autotomography** (aw″tō-tō-mŏg′ră-fē) [″ + Gr. *tome,* incision, + *graphein,* to write] Radiographic tomography in which the patient rather than the x-ray tube is moved.

**autotopagnosia** (aw″tō-tŏp-ăg-nō′zē-ă) [″ + *topos,* place, + *a-,* not, + *gnosis,* knowledge] Inability to orient various parts of the body correctly; occurs in lesions of the thalamoparietal pathways of the cortex.

**autotoxemia, autotoxicosis** (aw″tō-tŏk-sē′mē-ă, aw″tō-tŏk″sĭ-kō′sĭs) Autointoxication.

**autotoxin** (aw″tō-tŏk′sĭn) Poison generated within the body on which it acts.

**autotransfusion** (aw″tō-trăns-fū′zhŭn) [″ + L. *trans,* across, + *fundere,* pour] A method of returning the patient's own extravasated blood to the circulation. Blood shed into the peritoneal cavity during surgery, by a ruptured ectopic pregnancy or ruptured spleen, is collected during the operation and transfused immediately into the circulation of the patient. Convenient and inexpensive disposable systems are available to facilitate collecting and filtering the blood obtained.

**autotransplantation** (aw″tō-trăns″plăn-tā′shŭn) [″ + ″ + *plantare,* to plant] Surgical transfer of tissue from one part of the body to another part.

**autotrophic** (aw″tō-trō′fĭk) [″ + *trophe,* nourishment] Self-nourishing; capable of growing in the absence of organic compounds; pert. to green plants and bacteria, which form protein and carbohydrate from inorganic salts and carbon dioxide.

**autovaccination** (aw″tō-văk″sĭ-nā′shŭn) [″ + *vacca,* cow] **1.** Vaccination with autogenous vaccine or autovaccine. **2.** A vaccination resulting from virus or bacteria from a sore of a previous vaccination, as may occur when a smallpox vaccination sore is scratched and the virus is subsequently transferred to a break in the skin elsewhere.

**autovaccine** (aw″tō-văk′sēn) Vaccine prepared from a virus in the patient's own body.

**auxiliary** (ăwg-zĭl′ē-ăr-ē) [L. *auxiliarius,* help] **1.** Providing additional aid. **2.** A person who aids.

***dental a.*** One who assists a dentist (e.g., dental hygienist, chair-side assistant, radiology or laboratory technician).

**auxin** [Gr. *auxe,* increase] A substance that promotes growth in plant cells and tissues.

**auxocyte** (awk′sō-sīt) [Gr. *auxanu,* to increase, + *kytos,* cell] Early growth stage of a spermatocyte, oocyte, or sporocyte.

**auxotroph** (awk′sō-trōf) [″ + *trophe,* nutrition] An auxotrophic organism.

**auxotrophic** (awk-sō-trō′fĭk) Requiring a growth factor that is different from that required by the parent organism.

**A-V 1.** *arteriovenous.* **2.** *atrioventricular.*

**A-V access** *Arteriovenous access.*

**availability** In nutrition, the extent to which a nutrient is present in a form that can be absorbed and used by the body.

**avalanche theory** [Fr. *avaler,* to descend] The theory that nervous impulses are reinforced and thereby become more intense as they travel peripherally.

**avalvular** (ă-văl′vū-lăr) Without valves.

**avascular** (ă-văs′kū-lăr) [Gr. *a-,* not, + L. *vasculum,* little vessel] Lacking in blood vessels or having a poor blood supply, said of tissues such as cartilage.

**avascularization** (ă-văs″kū-lăr-ĭ-zā′shŭn)

Expulsion of blood from tissues, esp. the extremities, as in the use of Esmarch's bandage.

**Avazyme** Trade name for chymotrypsin.

**A-V block** SEE: under *block*.

**A-V bundle** A bundle of fibers of the impulse-conducting system of the heart. From its origin in the atrioventricular node, it enters the interventricular septum, where it divides into two branches whose fibers pass to the right and left ventricles respectively. These fibers become continuous with the Purkinje fibers of the ventricles. SYN: *bundle of His*.

**Avellis' paralysis syndrome** [Georg Avellis, Ger. laryngologist, 1864–1916] Paralysis of half of the soft palate, pharynx, and larynx and loss of pain, heat, and cold sensations on the opposite side.

**Aventyl hydrochloride** Trade name for nortriptyline hydrochloride.

**average** SEE: *arithmetic mean*.

**aversion therapy** A form of behavior in which an undesired stimulus (e.g., drinking alcohol) is presented to the patient at the same time as an unpleasant or painful stimulus. The goal is to have the individual associate the undesired stimulus with the unpleasant one and thus discontinue the former.

**avian** Concerning birds.

**aviation medicine** Aerospace medicine.

**aviation physiology** The branch of physiology that deals with conditions encountered by humans in flying, mountain climbing, or space flight. The conditions studied are hypoxia, extreme temperature and radiation, effects of acceleration and deceleration, weightlessness, motion sickness, enforced inactivity, mental stress, acclimatization, and disturbance of biological rhythm.

**avidin** (ăv'ĭ-dĭn) [L. *avidus*, greedy] A protein isolated from raw egg white. It is thought to be an inhibitor of biotin, thereby causing a deficiency in biotin.

**avidity 1.** Eagerness; a strong attraction for something. **2.** Concerning the ability of antibodies to bind to antigens.

**avirulent** (ă-vĭr'ū-lĕnt) [Gr. *a-* not, + L. *virus*, poison] Without virulence.

**avitaminosis** (ā-vī"tă-mĭ-nō'sĭs) [" + *vitamin* + *osis*, condition] Disease caused by vitamin deficiency. SEE: *vitamin*. **avitaminotic** (-mĭ-nŏt'ĭk), *adj.*

**avivement** (ă-vēv-mŏn') [Fr.] Surgical trimming of wound edges before suturing them.

**Avogadro's law** (ŏv-ō-gŏd'rōs) [Amadeo Avogadro, It. physicist, 1776–1856] Equal volumes of gases at the same pressure and temperature contain equal numbers of molecules.

**Avogadro's number** Number of molecules, $6.0221367 \times 10^{23}$, in one gram-molecular weight of a compound.

**avoidance** (ă-voyd'ăns) The conscious or unconscious effort to escape from situations or events perceived by the individual to be threatening to personal comfort, safety, or well-being.

**avoirdupois measure** (ăv"ĕr-dĕ-poyz') [Fr., to have weight] A system of weighing or measuring articles in which 7000 grains equal 1 lb. SEE: *Weights and Measures Appendix*.

**avulsion** (ă-vŭl'shŭn) [Gr. *a-*, not, + L. *vellere*, to pull] **1.** A tearing away forcibly of a part or structure. If surgical repair is necessary, a sterile dressing may be applied while surgery is awaited. If fingers, toes, feet, or hands are completely avulsed, they may be successfully rejoined to the body if prompt and expert surgical care is available. **2.** The complete separation of a tooth from its alveolus. The term usually refers to dental injuries resulting from acute trauma. SYN: *evulsion*.

***phrenic a.*** Elevation of a side of the diaphragm and semicollapse of the corresponding lung by excision of part of the phrenic nerve.

**awareness, fertility** The identification of the days during a woman's menstrual cycle when her potential for conception is highest. SEE: *basal temperature chart; mucus, cervical; mittelschmerz*.

**A.W.H.O.N.N** *Association of Women's Health, Obstetric, and Neonatal Nurses.* Formerly Nurses' Association of the American College of Obstetrics and Gynecology (NAACOG).

**axanthopsia** (ăk"săn-thŏp'sē-ă) [" + *xanthos*, yellow, + *opsis*, vision] Yellow blindness.

**axenic** (ā-zĕn'ĭk) [" + *xenos*, stranger] Germ free, as pert. to animals, or pure, as pert. to cultures or microorganisms; sterile.

**axial** (ăk'sē-ăl) [L. *axis*, axle] Situated in or pert. to an axis.

**axifugal** (ăks-ĭf'ū-găl) Centrifugal.

**axilemma** (ăk"sĭ-lĕm'ă) [" + Gr. *lemma*, husk] Axolemma.

**axilla** (ăk-sĭl'ă) *pl.* **axillae** [L. *axilla*] The armpit.

**axilla conformer** A splint designed to prevent adduction contractures after severe burns to the axillary region.

**axillary** (ăk'sĭ-lār-ē) Pert. to the axilla.

**axillofemoral bypass graft** (ăk"sĭl-ō-fĕm'or-ăl) The surgical establishment of a connector between the axillary artery and the common femoral arteries. A synthetic artery graft is used and implanted subcutaneously. This technique is used in treating patients with insufficient blood flow to the legs.

**axio-** (ăk'sē-ō) [L. *axis*, axle] Combining form meaning *relating to an axis*; in dentistry, the long axis of the tooth.

**axiobuccal** (ăk"sē-ō-bŭk'kăl) [L. *axis*, axle, + *bucca*, cheek] Concerning the angle formed by the long axis of the tooth and the buccal walls of a cavity of the tooth.

**axioincisal** (ăk"sē-ō-ĭn-sī'zăl) [" + *incisor*, a cutter] Concerning the angle formed by the long axis of the tooth and the incisal

walls of a cavity in the tooth.
**axiolabial** (ăk″sē-ō-lā′bē-ăl) [″ + *labialis*, pert. to the lips] Concerning the angle formed by the long axis of the tooth with the labial walls of a cavity in the tooth.
**axiolingual** (ăk″sē-ō-lĭng′gwăl) [″ + *lingua*, tongue] Concerning the angle formed by the long axis of the tooth and the lingual walls of a cavity in the tooth.
**axiomesial** (ăk″sē-ō-mē′zē-ăl) [″ + Gr. *mesos*, middle] Concerning the angle formed by the long axis of a tooth and the mesial walls of a cavity in the tooth.
**axio-occlusal** (ăk″sē-ō-ŏ-klū′zăl) [″ + *occlusio*, closure] Concerning the angle formed by the long axis of the tooth and the occlusal walls of a cavity in the tooth.
**axioplasm** (ăk′sē-ō-plăzm) [″ + LL. *plasma*, form, mold] Neuroplasm of an axis cylinder.
**axiopulpal** (ăk″sē-ō-pŭl′păl) [″ + *pulpa*, pulp] Concerning the angle formed by the long axis of a tooth and the pulpal walls of a cavity in the tooth.
**axipetal** (ăk-sĭp′ĕt-ăl) Centripetal.
**axis** [L.] **1.** A real or imaginary line that runs through the center of a body or about which a part revolves. **2.** The second cervical vertebra, or epistropheus; it bears the odontoid process (dens), about which the atlas rotates.

***basicranial a.*** Axis connecting the basion and gonion.

***basifacial a.*** Axis from the subnasal point to the gonion.

***binauricular a.*** Axis between the two auricular points.

***cardiac a.*** A graphic representation of the main conduction vector of the heart, determined through measurements of direction and amplitude of the complexes in several leads on a 12-lead electrocardiogram. Normal axis is zero to +90°.

***celiac a.*** Axis between the celiac artery and the abdominal aorta.

***condylar a.*** Axis through the two condyles of the mandible, about which movement takes place when the mouth opens. SYN: *hinge a.; transverse mandibular a.*

***frontal a.*** An imaginary line, running from side to side in the frontal plane, about which the anterior to posterior movement occurs. Also called *coronal axis*.

***hinge a.*** A projected line connecting the condyles of the mandible. When the mandible starts to move, it rotates around this imaginary line. SYN: *mandibular a.*

***mandibular a.*** Hinge a.

***neural a.*** Central nervous system.

***optic a.*** A line that connects the anterior and posterior poles of the eye.

***principal a.*** In optics, a line that passes through the optical center or nodal point of a lens perpendicular to the surface of the lens.

***sagittal a.*** Imaginary line running anterior-posterior, about which frontal plane motion occurs.

***transverse mandibular a.*** Condylar a.

***visual a.*** A line passing from the object of vision directly through the center of the cornea and lens to the fovea.

**axis cylinder** Axon (2).
**axis deviation** An abnormal cardiac axis. Left axis deviation is −1° to −89°. Right axis deviation is 91° to −90°. This condition usually indicates cardiac disease.
**axo-** [Gr. *axon*, axis] Combining form meaning *axis* or *axon*.
**axodendrite** (ăk″sō-dĕn′drīt) [″ + *dendron*, tree] Process given off from a nerve cell axon (not an axis cylinder).
**axofugal** (ăk-sŏf′ū-găl) Axifugal.
**axolemma** (ăk″sō-lĕm′ă) [″ + *lemma*, husk] The cell membrane of an axon. SYN: *axilemma*.
**axolysis** (ăk-sŏl′ĭ-sĭs) [″ + *lysis*, dissolution] Destruction of the axis cylinder of a nerve.
**axometer** (ăk-sŏm′ĕ-tĕr) [″ + *metron*, measure] Measuring device for adjusting eyeglasses so that the lenses are suitable for the optic axes of the eyes.
**axon, axone** (ăk′sŏn, -sōn) [Gr. *axon*, axis] **1.** A process of a neuron that conducts impulses away from the cell body. Typically, it arises from a portion of the cell devoid of Nissl granules, the axon hillock. Axons may possess either or both of two sheaths (myelin sheath and neurilemma) or neither. Axons are usually long and straight, and most end in synapses in the central nervous system or ganglia or in effector organs (e.g., motor neurons). They may give off side branches or collaterals. An axon with its sheath(s) constitutes a nerve fiber. **2.** A nerve cell process that resembles an axon in structure; specifically, the peripheral process of a dorsal root ganglion cell (sensory neuron) that functionally and embryologically is a dendrite, but structurally is indistinguishable from an axon. SYN: *axis cylinder; neuraxon*. SEE: *nerve; neuron*. **axonal** (ăk′sŏn-ăl), *adj.*
**axoneme** (ăk′sōn-nēm) [″ + *nema*, a thread] Axial thread of a chromosome.
**axonometer** (ăk-sō-nŏm′ĕ-tĕr) [″ + *metron*, measure] Device for determining the axis of astigmatism.
**axonotmesis** (ăk″sŏn-ŏt-mē′sĭs) [″ + *tmesis*, incision] Nerve injury that damages the nerve tissue without actually severing the nerve.
**axopetal** (ăk-sŏp′ĕ-tăl) [″ + L. *petere*, to seek] Conducted along an axon toward a cell body of a neuron.
**axoplasm** (ăk′sō-plăzm) [″ + LL. *plasma*, form, mold] The cytoplasm (neuroplasm) of an axon that encloses the neurofibrils.
**axospongium** (ăk-sō-spŏn′jē-ŭm) [″ + *spongos*, sponge] The fine fibrillar network of the axon substance of a nerve cell.
**ayurvedic medicine** (ă″yūr-vă′dĭc) [Sanskrit *ayus*, lifespan, life, + *veda*, knowledge, science] An ancient Hindu medical system. Its goal is to improve health by harmonizing mind and body. It uses herbal

remedies, massage therapy, yoga, and pulse diagnosis. A modern revival of this system is known as Maharishi Ayur-Veda and has been directed by Maharishi Mahesh Yogi.

**azalein** (ă-ză′lē-ĭn) [L. *azalea,* azalea] A red dye.

**azathioprine** (ā″ză-thī′ō-prēn) A cytotoxic chemical substance used for immunosuppression. Trade name is Imuran.

**azidothymidine** Zidovudine.

**azo-** Prefix indicating the presence of —N: N— group in a chemical structure. This group is usually connected at both ends to carbon atoms. SEE: *azo compounds.*

**azo compounds** Organic substances that contain the azo group. An example is azobenzene, $C_6H_5N:NC_6H_5$. They are related to aniline and include important dyes and indicators. SEE: *indicator* for table.

**Azolid** Trade name for phenylbutazone.

**azoospermia** (ă-zō-ō-spĕr′mē-ă) [″ + *zoon,* animal, + *sperma,* seed] Absence of spermatozoa in the semen.

**Azorean disease** (ā-zor′ē-ăn) A form of hereditary ataxia present in Portuguese families whose ancestors lived in the Azores. It is a degenerative disease of the nervous system. Symptoms vary but may include gait ataxia, limitation of eye movements, widespread muscle fasciculations, mild cerebellar tremor, loss of reflexes in lower limbs, and extensor plantar reflex response.

**azotemia** (ăz″ō-tē′mē-ă) [″ + ″ + *haima,* blood] Presence of nitrogenous bodies, esp. urea in increased amounts, in the blood. SEE: *uremia.*

**Azotobacter** (ă-zō″tō-băk′tĕr) Rod-shaped, gram-negative, nonpathogenic soil and water bacteria that fix atmospheric nitrogen; the single genus of the family Azotobacteraceae.

**azoturia** (ăz″ō-tū′rē-ă) [″ + ″ + *ouron,* urine] An increase in nitrogenous compounds, esp. urea, in urine.

**AZT** *Azidothymidine,* the former name for zidovudine.

**Azulfidine** Trade name for sulfasalazine.

**azure lunulae** (ăz′ŭr loo′nū-lē) [O. Fr. *azur,* blue, + L. *lunula,* little moon] Blue discoloration of the base, or lunulae, of the fingernails. It may be seen in patients with hepatolenticular degeneration (Wilson's disease). Blue discoloration of the entire nail may be present in argyria and following therapy with quinacrine hydrochloride.

**azurophil(e)** (ăz-ū′rō-fĭl) [″ + Gr. *philein,* to love] Staining readily with azure dye.

**azurophilia** (ăz″ū-rō-fĭl′ē-ă) Condition in which some blood cells have azurophil granules.

**azygography** (ăz″ĭ-gŏg′ră-fē) [Gr. *a-,* not, + *zygon,* yoke, + *graphein,* to write] Radiography of the azygos veins by the use of an intravenous contrast medium.

**azygos** (ăz′ĭ-gŏs) [″ + *zygon,* yoke] **1.** Occurring singly, not in pairs. **2.** An unpaired anatomical part. **azygos, azygous** (ăz′ĭ-gŭs), *adj.*

**azygos vein** A single vein arising in the abdomen as a branch of the ascending lumbar vein. It passes upward through the aortic hiatus of the diaphragm into the thorax, then along the right side of the vertebral column to the level of the fourth thoracic vertebra, where it turns and enters the superior vena cava. In the thorax, it receives the hemiazygos, accessory azygos, and bronchial veins, as well as the right intercostal and subcostal veins. If the inferior vena cava is obstructed, the azygous vein is the principal vein by which blood can return to the heart.

**azymia** (ă-zī′mē-ă) [″ + *zyme,* ferment] State of being without a ferment or enzyme.

# B

***β*** Beta, second letter of the Greek alphabet. SEE: *beta.*

**B 1.** Symbol for the element boron. **2.** *Bacillus; Balantidium; barometric; base; bath; behavior; buccal.*

**B.A.** *Bachelor of Arts.*

**Ba** Symbol for the element barium.

**Babbitt metal** (băb′ĭt) [Isaac Babbitt, U.S. inventor, 1799–1862] An antifriction alloy of copper, antimony, and tin used occasionally in dentistry.

**Babcock's operation** (băb′kŏks) [William Wayne Babcock, U.S. surgeon, 1872–1963] Extirpation of the saphenous vein; a treatment for varicose veins.

**Babesia** (bă-bē′zē-ă) [Victor Babès] A genus of the family Babesiidae that consists of tick-borne parasites, which invade the red blood cells of cattle, sheep, horses, dogs, and other vertebrate animals. Destruction of the red blood cells results in hemoglobinuria.

***B. bigemina*** The causative organism of Texas fever in cattle.

***B. bovis*** The causative organism of hemoglobinuria and jaundice (red-water fever) in cattle.

**babesiosis** (bă-bē-zē-ō′sĭs) A rare, often severe, and sometimes fatal disease of humans caused by an intraerythrocytic protozoan, *Babesia microti,* and perhaps other *Babesia* species. The disease is transmitted by ticks, and at one time was thought to be limited, in the U.S., to New England. It has since been reported from many other areas. Severe forms are most likely to occur in persons over age 40 and those with a nonfunctioning spleen or no spleen. In rare cases the infection is transmitted by blood transfusion from an asymptomatic carrier. The incubation period may last from weeks to months.

SYMPTOMS: Symptoms include fever, chills, drenching sweats, myalgia, arthralgia, nausea and vomiting, and hemolytic anemia.

DIAGNOSIS: Diagnosis is based on the presence of the parasite in red blood cells and on serologic studies. On the blood smear it may be difficult to differentiate the *Babesia* parasite from *Plasmodium falciparum,* a malarial parasite. Use of the polymerase chain reaction test provides a sensitive method of detecting the associated parasitemia.

TREATMENT: Quinine given orally and clindamycin given intravenously or intramuscularly have been effective. Exchange transfusion may be needed in asplenic patients in whom a large proportion of their red blood cells contain parasites.

**Babinski's reflex** (bă-bĭn′skēz) [Joseph Babinski, Fr. neurologist, 1857–1932] Dorsiflexion of the great toe when the sole of the foot is stimulated. Normally, when the lateral aspect of the sole of the relaxed foot is stroked, the great toe is flexed. If the toe extends instead of flexes and the outer toes spread out, Babinski's reflex is present. It is a normal reflex in infants under the age of 6 months but indicates a lesion of the pyramidal (corticospinal) tract in older individuals. Care must be taken to avoid interpreting voluntary extension of the toe as Babinski's reflex.

**Babinski's sign** Loss of or diminished Achilles tendon reflex in sciatica.

**baby** [ME. *babie*] An infant.

***battered b.*** A baby or child whose body provides evidence of physical abuse such as bruises, cuts, scars, fractures, or abdominal visceral injuries that have occurred at various times in the past. SEE: *battered child syndrome.*

***blue b.*** An infant born with cyanosis, which may be caused by anything that prevents proper oxygenation of the blood, esp. a congenital anomaly that permits blood to go directly from the right to the left side of the heart without going through the lungs. The most common cyanotic congenital heart defects are tetralogy of Fallot, transposition of the great vessels, and hypoplastic left heart syndrome.

***collodion b.*** A newborn covered with a collodion-like layer of desquamated skin; may be due to ichthyosis vulgaris.

**baby bottle syndrome** Decay of primary teeth in older infants and toddlers related to taking a bottle of punch or other sweet liquid to bed and retaining the liquid. This creates massive caries. SYN: *bottle mouth caries; nursing-bottle syndrome.*

**Baby Doe regulations** Federal, state, and hospital policies insuring that handicapped infants will receive life-saving treatment without regard to the quality of life.

**BAC** *blood alcohol concentration.*

**bacciform** (băk′sĭ-form) [″ + *forma,* form] Berry-shaped; coccal.

**Bacid** Trade name for lactobacillus acidophilus.

**Bacillaceae** (băs-ĭ-lā′sē-ē) A family of rod-shaped, usually gram-positive bacteria of the order Eubacteriales that produce endospores and are commonly found in soil. Genera of this family include *Bacillus* and *Clostridium.*

**bacillar, bacillary** (băs′ĭl-ăr, băs′ĭl-ăr-ē) **1.** Pert. to or caused by bacilli. **2.** Rodlike.

**bacillary angiomatosis** An acute infectious disease caused by *Bartonella quintana.* It is characterized by skin lesions that may vary from small papules to pyogenic granulomas or pedunculated masses. These occur anywhere on the skin and may involve mucous membranes. If the lesions ulcerate, they can extend to and destroy underlying bone. In addition, the organisms are disseminated to the liver, spleen, bone marrow, and lymph nodes. In the liver there may be painful, multiple, cystic, blood-filled spaces (peliosis hepatitis). Most patients with this disease are immunocompromised or infected with human immunodeficiency virus (HIV). In the untreated immunocompetent patient, recovery may be prolonged but is usually complete. In the untreated immunocompromised patient, death is the likely outcome. When the organisms are disseminated, treatment for several months with oral doxycycline or oral erythromycin will be of benefit in altering the course of the disease. Culture of the organism provides diagnosis. SEE: *cat scratch disease; trench fever*.

NURSING IMPLICATIONS: Universal precautions should be maintained. The nurse provides emotional support, describes signs and symptoms that should be promptly reported to the primary caregiver, and discusses common side effects of prolonged antibiotic therapy. The necessity of completing prescribed therapy is emphasized.

**bacille Calmette-Guérin** (bă-sēl′) An organism of the strain *Mycobacterium bovis,* rendered avirulent by long-term cultivation on bile-glycero-potato medium and used in BCG vaccine, in prevention of human tuberculosis.

**bacillemia** (băs-ĭ-lē′mē-ă) [L. *bacillus,* rod, + Gr. *haima,* blood] The presence of bacilli in the blood.

**bacilli** (bă-sĭl′ī) Pl. of bacillus.

**bacilliform** (bă-sĭl′ĭ-form) [″ + *forma,* form] Resembling a bacillus in shape.

**bacillophobia** (băs″ĭ-lō-fō′bē-ă) [″ + Gr. *phobos,* fear] Morbid fear of bacilli.

**bacillosis** (băs″ĭ-lō′sĭs) [″ + Gr. *osis,* infection] Infection by bacilli.

**bacilluria** (băs″ĭ-lū′rē-ă) [″ + Gr. *ouron,* urine] Bacilli in the urine. SEE: *clean-catch method.*

**Bacillus** (bă-sĭl′ŭs) [L.] A genus of bacteria of the family Bacillaceae. All species are rod-shaped, sometimes occurring in chains. They are spore-bearing, aerobic, motile or nonmotile; most are gram-positive and nonpathogenic. A well-known species pathogenic to humans is *Bacillus anthracis,* which causes anthrax. SEE: *bacterium.*

**bacillus** *pl.* **bacilli 1.** Any rod-shaped microorganism. **2.** A rod-shaped microorganism belonging to the class Schizomycetes. SEE: *Bacillus; bacterium.*

***acid-fast b.*** A bacillus not readily decolorized by acids or other means when stained.

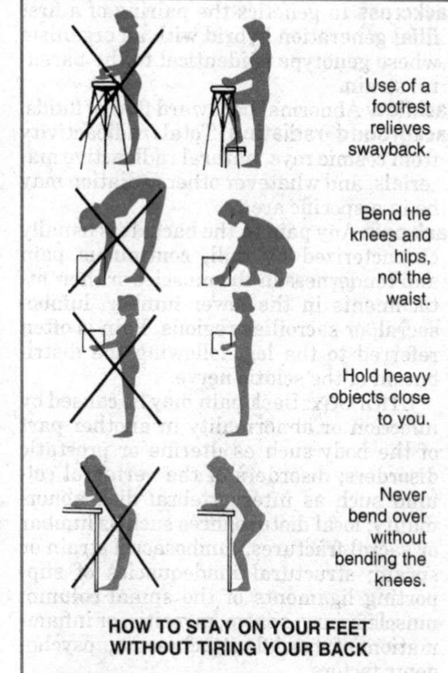


**HOW TO STAY ON YOUR FEET WITHOUT TIRING YOUR BACK**

Adapted from "Your Back and How to Care for It," Copyright 1965, Shering Corporation, Bloomfield, N.J.

**Bacillus species** ABBR: *Bacillus* spp. All of the species of *Bacillus*.

**bacitracin** (băs-ĭ-trā′sĭn) An antibiotic substance obtained from a strain of *Bacillus subtilis.* Its antibacterial actions are similar to those of penicillin, including gram-positive cocci and bacilli and some gram-negative organisms. Because of its toxicity when used parenterally, bacitracin is usually applied topically in ointment form.

***zinc b.*** The zinc salt of bacitracin, used in topical antibacterial ointments.

**back 1.** The dorsum. **2.** The posterior region of the trunk from neck to pelvis.

Misuse of the back is common among those who care for the sick. Therefore, it is important to learn basic concepts in back care. SEE: illus.; *back pain*

**back board** A stiff board placed on a stretcher so that the patient's back is kept flat in spinal injury cases.

***long b.b.*** A long, flat board approx. 6 ft long and 2 ft wide, often made of wood, fiberglass, or plastic, used to immobilize a patient with a potential head injury. This device should be used with a head immobilization device and a cervical collar.

***short b.b.*** A long, flat board, approx. 3 ft long and 2 ft wide, used to immobilize a seated patient with a potential spinal injury. The short back board is often used to remove an injured patient from a vehicle, after which the long back board is used for full immobilization.

**backbone** The vertebral column; spinal column. SEE: *vertebra.*

**backcross** In genetics the pairing of a first filial generation hybrid with an organism whose genotype is identical to the parental strain.

**backflow** Abnormal backward flow of fluids.

**background radiation** Total radioactivity from cosmic rays, natural radioactive materials, and whatever other radiation may be in a specific area.

**back pain** Any pain in the back. It is usually characterized by dull, continuous pain and tenderness in the muscles or their attachments in the lower lumbar, lumbosacral, or sacroiliac regions. Pain is often referred to the leg, following the distribution of the sciatic nerve.

ETIOLOGY: Back pain may be caused by infection or abnormality in another part of the body such as uterine or prostatic disorders; disorders of the vertebral column such as intervertebral disk abnormality; local disturbances such as lumbar or sacral fractures, lumbosacral strain or sprain; structural inadequacies of supporting ligaments of the spinal column; muscle injury, spasm, myositis, or inflammation of fascial attachments; psychogenic factors.

TREATMENT: The specific primary cause must be treated. General treatment includes allowing time for the condition to improve without specific therapy such as surgery. Important in this phase are measures to allay pain and discomfort, such as analgesics (preferably salicylates or other nonsteroidal anti-inflammatory agents), muscle relaxants, heat, or whirlpools. Tender areas or trigger points may be anesthetized by local infiltration with 1% procaine or topical application of ethyl chloride spray. Special measures to relax tense muscles and improve blood flow are helpful. In some cases orthopedic supports and strapping may be needed as well as physical therapy with therapeutic exercises to retrain muscles and balance forces in the pelvis and spine. After an acute attack, several activities are esp. good for the back: brisk walking, bicycling and swimming. All of these involve minimal impact and will not put the back into an awkward position. Psychotherapy may be necessary, esp. when excessive muscle tension results from emotional disturbances.

Most patients will not need surgery, but some conditions, such as herniated disk, persistent pain upon vertebral column rotation, overgrowth of bone that causes narrowing of the spinal canal (lumbar spinal stenosis), and spondylolisthesis, may need surgery.

NURSING IMPLICATIONS: The nurse encourages bedrest in William's position. Local heat is applied as directed. The treatment regimen is explained, implemented, and reinforced. Factors that precipitate symptoms are identified and preventive actions are discussed.

**backrest** An adjustable device that supports the back in bed.

**backscatter** In radiation physics, the deflection of ionizing radiation back more than 90° from interactions with intervening matter.

**back school** A term for educational programs, often sponsored by industry, that emphasize body mechanics and ergonomic principles with the goal of preventing initial or recurring injuries to the spine.

**backup** Anything that serves to replace a function or system that fails.

**bacteremia** (băk-tĕr-ē′mē-ă) [Gr. *bakterion,* rod, + *haima,* blood] Bacteria in the blood. SEE: *sepsis.*

**bacteri** SEE: *bacterio-.*

**bacteria** (băk-tē′rē-ă) [Gr. *bakterion,* rod] Pl. of bacterium. **bacterial** (-ăl), *adj.*

**bacterial adherence** The process of attachment of bacteria to tissue cells. Some bacteria need to adhere to cells in order to colonize a site and cause infection.

**bacterial pathogenesis** SEE: under *pathogenesis.*

**bacterial plasmid** SEE: *plasmid.*

**bacterial resistance** Development of resistance to a drug by an organism previously susceptible to it. This has been manifested by pathogenic organisms (as gonococci, streptococci, staphylococci, and tubercle bacilli) to various chemotherapeutic drugs, and occurs both in vitro and in vivo. It may be due to appearance of resistant mutant strains, development of alternate metabolic pathways by the organisms, decomposition of the drug, or unknown factors. SEE: *antiviral resistance; resistance, antibiotic; transfer factor.*

**bacterial synergism** The interaction of indigenous flora to allow a strain of bacteria to become pathogenic when it would normally be harmless.

**bactericidal** (băk″tĕr-ĭ-sī′dăl) Destructive to or destroying bacteria.

**bactericide** (băk-tĕr′ĭ-sīd) [Gr. *bakterion,* rod, + L. *caedere,* to kill] An agent that destroys bacteria, but not necessarily their spores.

**bactericidin** Anything lethal to bacteria.

**bacteriemia** (băk-tĕr-ē-ē′mē-ă) Bacteremia.

**bacterio-, bacteri-** (băk-tē′rē-ō) Combining form meaning *bacteria.*

**bacterioagglutinin** (băk-tē″rē-ō-ă-gloo′tĭ-nĭn) [″ + L. *agglutinans,* gluing] An antibody in serum that causes agglutination, or clumping, of bacteria in vitro.

**bacteriocidal** (băk″tĕr-ē-ō-sī′dăl) Bactericidal.

**bacteriocin** (băk-tē′rē-ō-sĭn) Protein produced by certain bacteria that exerts a lethal effect on closely related bacteria. In general, bacteriocins are more potent but have a narrower range of activity than antibiotics. SEE: *colicin.*

**bacteriogenic** (băk-tē″rē-ō-jĕn′ĭk) [″ + *gennan,* to produce] **1.** Caused by bacteria.

2. Producing bacteria.

**bacteriohemagglutinin** (băk-tē″rē-ō-hĕm″ă-gloo′tĭ-nĭn) [″ + *haima,* blood, + L. *agglutinans,* gluing] A hemagglutinin formed in the body by bacterial action.

**bacteriohemolysin** (băk-tē″rē-ō-hē-mŏl′ĭ-sĭn) [″ + ″ + *lysis,* dissolution] A hemolysin formed in the body by bacterial action.

**bacteriologic, bacteriological** [″ + *logos,* word, reason] Pert. to bacteriology.

**bacteriologist** An individual trained in the field of bacteriology.

**bacteriology** Scientific study of bacteria.

**bacteriolysin** (băk-tē″rē-ŏl′ĭ-sĭn) [″ + *lysis,* dissolution] A substance, esp. an antibody produced within the body of an animal, that is capable of bringing about the lysis of bacteria.

**bacteriolysis** (băk-tē″rē-ŏl′ĭ-sĭs) The destruction or dissolution of bacteria. **bacteriolytic** (-ō-lĭt′ĭk), *adj.*

**bacteriophage** (băk-tē′rē-ō-fāj″) [Gr. *bakterion,* rod, + *phagein,* to eat] A virus that infects bacteria. Bacteriophages are widely distributed in nature, having been isolated from feces, sewage, and polluted surface waters. They are regarded as bacterial viruses, the phage particle consisting of a head composed of either RNA or DNA and a tail by which it attaches to host cells. SYN: *phage.*

**bacteriophytoma** (băk-tē″rē-ō-fī-tō′mă) [″ + *phyton,* plant, + *oma,* tumor] A tumorlike growth caused by bacteria.

**bacterioprecipitin** (băk-tē″rē-ō-prē-sĭp′ĭ-tĭn) Precipitin produced in the body by the action of bacteria.

**bacterioprotein** (băk-tē″rē-ō-prō′tē-ĭn) Any of the proteins within the cells of bacteria.

**bacteriopsonin** (băk-tē″rē-ŏp′sō-nĭn) An opsonin, acting on bacteria.

**bacteriosis** (băk-tē″rē-ō′sĭs) [″ + *osis,* condition] Any disease caused by bacteria.

**bacteriostasis** (băk-tē″rē-ŏs′tă-sĭs) [″ + *stasis,* standing still] The arrest of bacterial growth.

**bacteriostatic** (băk-tē-rē-ō-stăt′ĭk) Inhibiting or retarding bacterial growth.

**bacteriotoxic** (băk-tē″rē-ō-tŏk′sĭk) **1.** Toxic to bacteria. **2.** Due to bacterial toxins.

**bacteriotoxin** (băk-tē″rē-ō-tŏk′sĭn) [″ + *toxikon,* poison] Toxin specifically produced by or destructive to bacteria.

**bacteriotropin** (băk-tē″rē-ŏt′rō-pĭn) [″ + *tropos,* a turn] An opsonin or a substance that enhances the ability of phagocytes to engulf bacteria.

**bacteristatic** Inhibiting the growth of bacteria. SEE: *bactericidal.*

**bacterium** *pl.* **bacteria** A one-celled organism without a true nucleus or functionally specific components of metabolism that belongs to the kingdom Procaryotae (Monera). The internal cytoplasm is surrounded by a one- or two-layered rigid cell wall composed of phospholipids. Some bacteria also produce a mucoid extracellular capsule for additional protection, particularly from phagocytosis by white blood cells. Bacteria can synthesize DNA, RNA, and other vital proteins and can reproduce independently, but need a host to supply food and a supportive environment. Millions of nonpathogenic bacteria live on the skin and mucous membranes of the human gastrointestinal tract; these are called *normal flora.* Bacteria that cause disease are called *pathogens.* SEE: table.

CHARACTERISTICS: *Shape:* There are three principal forms of bacteria. *Spherical* or *ovoid* bacteria occur as single cells (micrococci) or in pairs (diplococci), clusters (staphylococci), chains (streptococci) or cubical groups (sarcinae). *Rod-shaped* bacteria are called bacilli, more oval ones are called coccobacilli; and those forming a chain are called streptobacilli. *Spiral* bacteria are rigid (spirilla), flexible (spirochetes) or curved (vibrios). SEE: illus.

*Size:* An average rod-shaped bacterium measures about 1 $\mu$m in diameter by 4 $\mu$m in length. They vary considerably in size from less than 0.5 to 1.0 $\mu$m in diameter to 10 to 20 $\mu$m in length in some of the longer spiral forms.

*Reproduction:* Simple cell division is the usual method of reproduction, but some bacteria produce buds or branches that eventually break off. Growth rate is significantly affected by changes in temperature, nutrition, and other factors. Bacilli can form reproductive cells called *spores* whose thick coats are highly resistant to adverse environmental conditions. When a better environment develops, the spores being to grow. Spores are difficult to kill because they are highly resistant to heat, drying, and disinfectant action.

*Colony formation:* A group of bacteria growing in one place is called a colony. A colony is usually composed of the descendants of a single cell. Colonies differ in shape, size, color, texture, type of margin, and other characteristics. Each species of bacteria has a characteristic type of colony formation.

*Mutation:* Most bacteria, like all living organisms, have the ability to adapt their shape or functions when faced with changes in their environment, but there are limits to this ability. They can also mutate to adapt to potentially lethal agents such as antibiotics.

*Motility:* None of the spherical or ovoid cocci are capable of moving, but most bacilli and spiral forms exhibit independent movement. The power of locomotion depends on the possession of one or more flagella, slender whiplike appendages that work like propellers.

*Food and oxygen requirements:* Most bacteria are heterotrophic (require organic material as food). If they feed on living organisms, they are called *parasites*; if they feed on nonliving organic material, they are called *saprophytes.* Bacteria that

## Common Bacterial Infections

| Organism | Type of and/or Site of Infection |
|---|---|
| **Gram-Positive Bacteria** | |
| **Clostridium difficile* | Pseudomembranous colitis |
| †*Staphylococcus aureus* | Pneumonia, cellulitis, boils, toxic shock, postoperative bone/joints, eyes, peritonitis |
| †*Staphylococcus epidermidis* | Postoperative bone/joints, IV line–related phlebitis |
| *Streptococcus pneumoniae* (pneumococcus) | Pneumonia, meningitis, otitis media, sinusitis, septicemia |
| *Streptococcus pyogenes* | Scarlet fever, pharyngitis, impetigo, rheumatic fever, erysipelas |
| *Streptococcus viridans* | Endocarditis |
| **Gram-Negative Bacteria** | |
| *Campylobacter jejuni* | Diarrhea (most common worldwide cause) |
| *Escherichia coli* | Urinary tract, pyelonephritis, septicemia, gastroenteritis, peritonitis |
| *Haemophilus influenzae* | Pneumonia, meningitis, otitis media, epiglottitis |
| *Klebsiella pneumoniae* | Pneumonia, wounds |
| *Legionella pneumophilia* | Pneumonia |
| *Neisseria gonorrhoeae* | Gonorrhea |
| *Neisseria meningitidis* (meningococcus) | Meningitis |
| †*Pseudomonas aeruginosa* | Wounds, urinary tract, pneumonia, IV lines |
| *Salmonella enteritidis* | Gastroenteritis, food poisoning |
| *Salmonella typhi* | Typhoid fever |
| *Shigella dysenteriae* | Dysentery |
| *Vibrio cholerae* | Cholera |

* Anaerobic
† Pyogenic (pus forming)

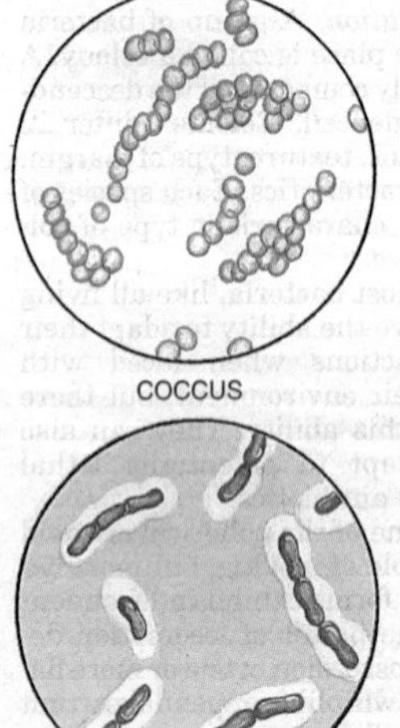

COCCUS

BACTERIAL CAPSULES

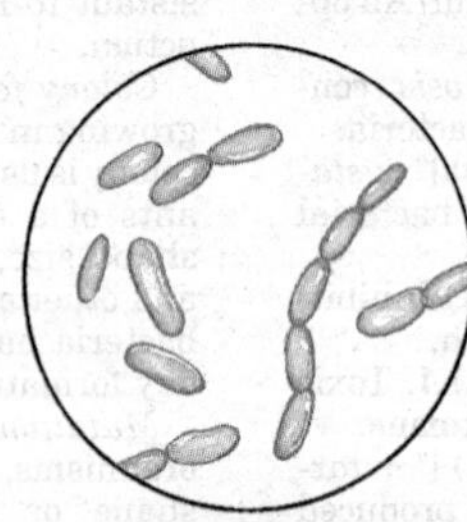

BACILLUS

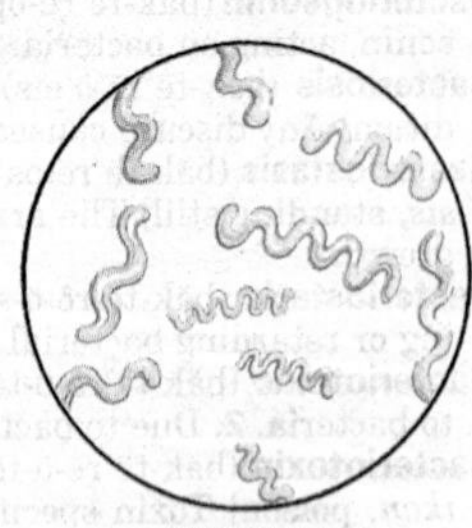

SPIRILLUM

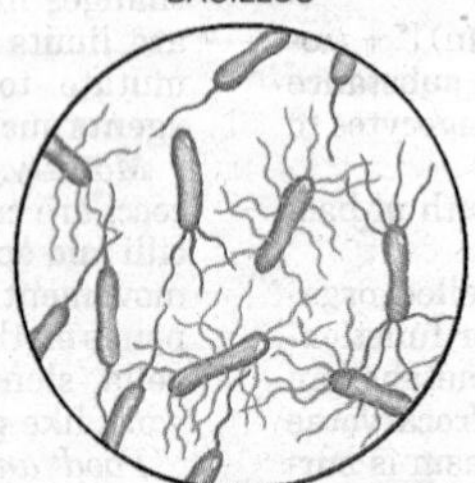

FLAGELLA

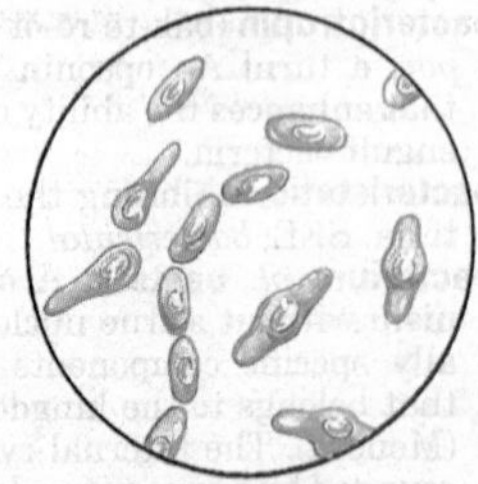

BACTERIAL SPORES

**BACTERIA**

BACTERIAL SHAPES AND SPECIALIZED STRUCTURES (×1000)

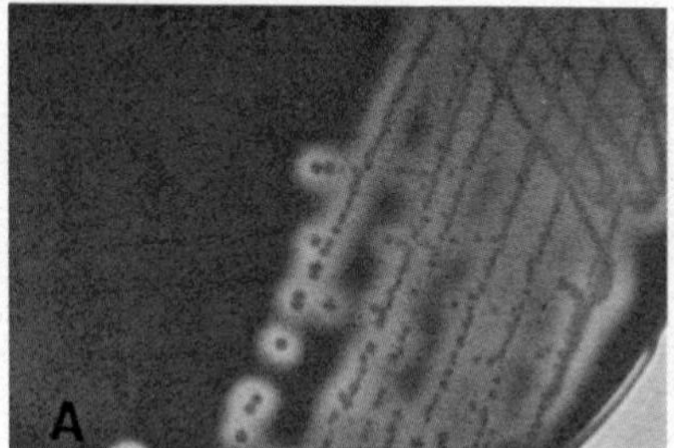


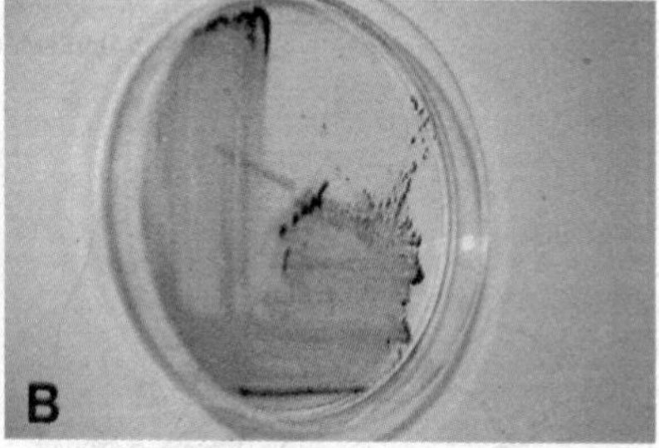


**BACTERIA**

**(A)** GROUP A STREPTOCOCCI; BETA-HEMOLYSIS ON BLOOD AGAR; **(B)** SALMONELLA; $H_2S$ PRODUCTION (BLACK) ON SS AGAR

obtain their energy from inorganic substances, including many of the soil bacteria, are called *autotrophic* (self-nourishing). Most bacteria are also aerobes (require oxygen). Bacteria that do not need oxygen are called *anaerobes*; most bacteria in the gastrointestinal tract are anaerobic. SEE: *infection, opportunistic*

*Temperature requirements:* Although some bacteria live at very low or very high temperatures, the optimum temperature for most pathogens is 98.6°F (37°C).

ACTIVITIES: *Enzyme production:* Bacteria produce enzymes that act on complex food molecules, breaking them down into simpler materials; they are the principal agents of decay and putrefaction. Putrefaction, the decomposition of nitrogenous and other organic materials in the absence of air, produces foul odors. Decay is the gradual decomposition of organic matter exposed to air by bacteria and fungi.

*Toxin production:* Special molecules called *adhesins* bind bacteria to the host cells. Once attached, the bacteria may produce poisonous substances called toxins. There are two types: exotoxins, enzymes that disrupt the cell's function or kill it, and endotoxins, which are parts of the cell walls of gram-negative bacteria and are toxic even after the death of the cell. Endotoxins stimulate production of cytokines that can produce widespread vasodilation and shock. SEE: *endotoxin; sepsis.*

*Miscellaneous:* Some bacteria produce pigments; some produce light, thus appearing luminescent at night. Many chemical substances are produced as a result of bacterial activity, among them acids, gases, alcohol, aldehydes, ammonia, carbohydrates, and indole. Pathogenic forms produce hemolysins, leukocidins, coagulases, and fibrolysins. Soil bacteria play an important role in various phases of the nitrogen cycle (nitrification, nitrogen fixation, and denitrification).

IDENTIFICATION: Several methods are used to identify bacteria in the laboratory: SEE: illus.

*Culture:* Bacteria are grown on various culture media; a visible colony containing millions of cells is visible within several hours. Groups of cells can then be examined under a microscope, usually with Gram's stain. In addition, colonies can be separated and antibiotics applied to assess their sensitivity to different drugs.

*Hanging drop:* Unstained bacteria in a drop of liquid are examined under ordinary or dark-field illumination.

*Gram's stain:* Gram-positive bacteria retain dye, turning purple; gram-negative bacteria can be decolorized by alcohol and colored red by a second dye; acid-fast bacteria retain the dye even when treated with an acid. Bacteria are often described by a combination of their response to Gram's stain and their appearance. For example, "gram-positive staphylococcus" indicates a cluster of oval bacteria that stain purple, whereas gram-negative bacilli are rod-shaped and lose their purple color.

*Immunofluorescence:* Bacteria stained with fluorescein and examined under a microscope equipped with fluorescent light appear yellow-green.

***antibody-coated b.*** **1.** A bacterium coated with an antibody that acts as an opsonin to make the bacterium more susceptible to phagocytosis. **2.** A laboratory test using fluorescein-labeled antibodies to locate antigens with which the antibody links. SEE: *opsonin.*

**bacteriuria** (băk-tē″rē-ū′rē-ă) [Gr. *bakterion,* rod, + *ouron,* urine] The presence of bacteria in the urine.

***significant b.*** Concentration of pathogenic bacteria in the urine of $10^5$ per ml or greater. Concentrations above this level are thought to represent evidence of urinary tract infection, but this is not always the case.

**bacteroid** (băk′tĕr-oyd) [″ + *eidos,* form, shape] **1.** Resembling a bacterium. **2.** A structurally modified bacterium.

**Bacteroides** (băk-tĕr-oyd′ēz) A genus of non-spore-forming, gram-negative, rod-

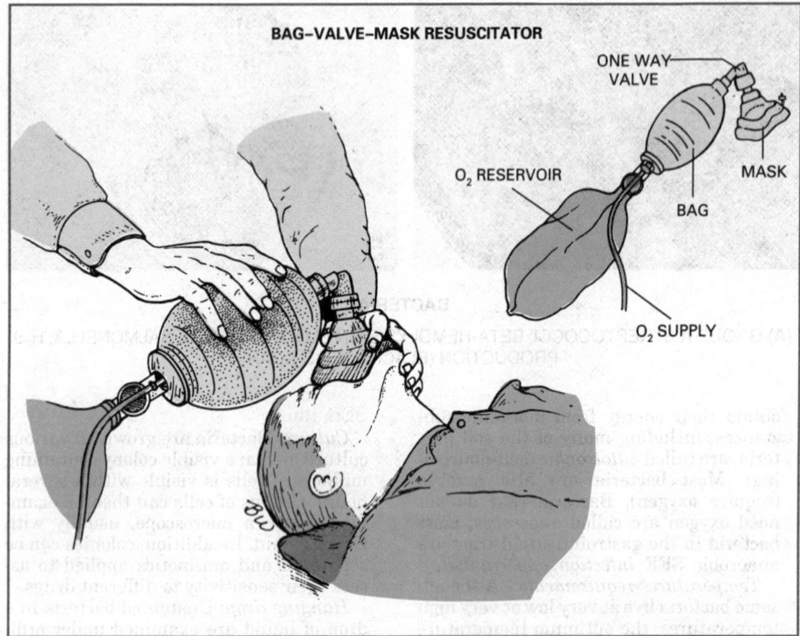


shaped, anaerobic bacteria that occur normally in digestive, respiratory, and genital tracts and are often found in necrotic tissue and in the blood after an infection. Some species are pathogenic and may be implicated in peritonitis and peritoneal abscesses. *Bacteroides* are the most common bacteria in the colon, where they outnumber *Escherichia coli* by at least 100 to 1; the species most commonly encountered is *B. fragilis*.

**bad breath** Offensive odor of the breath. Its origin may be in the mouth or nose, lungs, blood, or digestive tract. Many individuals have bad breath due to drying of the oral mucosa. On awakening, those who snore or sleep with their mouths open may have particularly noticeable bad breath. If bad breath is due to an ingested food, such as onions or garlic, local therapy with a mouthwash will be of no benefit because the odor is present in the blood and is excreted from the lungs. It is caused by respiratory infections such as bronchiectasis or lung abscess, acute necrotizing gingivitis, herpetic gingivostomatitis, periodontal disease, dental caries, cigarette smoking, hepatic failure, or diabetic ketoacidosis. SYN: *halitosis*. SEE: *hepatic coma*.

**baffle** In respiratory care, a component of a nebulizer designed to remove large airborne particles.

**bag** [ME. *bagge*] A sack or pouch.

***colostomy b.*** A watertight receptacle that holds the discharge from a colostomy site.

***Douglas b.*** SEE: *Douglas bag*.

***b. of waters*** Amnion.

***Politzer b.*** SEE: *Politzer bag*.

**bagassosis** (băg-ă-sō′sĭs) [Sp. *bagazo*, husks, + Gr. *osis*, condition] A form of hypersensitivity pneumonitis, due to inhalation of bagasse dust, the moldy, dusty fibrous waste of sugar cane after removal of the sugar-containing sap. The dust contains antigens from thermophilic actinomycetes.

**bag-valve-mask resuscitator** A manually operated resuscitator consisting of a bag reservoir, a one-way flow valve, and a face mask capable of ventilating a nonbreathing patient; commonly known as an Ambu bag. SEE: illus.

**Bailey, Harriet** [U.S. nurse educator, b. 1875] The first nurse educator to write a textbook on psychiatric nursing. *Nursing Mental Diseases* was published by Macmillan in 1920 and was the standard text for psychiatric nursing for two decades.

**baker** [AS. *bacan*, cook by dry heat] Two or more electric lamps mounted in semicircular containers used for applying heat to various parts of the body. They are also called *electric light bakers*.

**Baker's cyst** [William M. Baker, Brit. surgeon, 1839–1896] A synovial cyst (pouch) arising from the synovial lining of the knee. It occurs in the popliteal fossa.

**baker leg** Knock-knee; genu valgum.

**BAL** *British anti-lewisite*.

**balance** (băl′ăns) [L. *bilanx*] **1.** Scale; a device for measuring weight. **2.** A state of equilibrium; condition in which the intake and output of substances such as water and nutrients are approx. equal. SEE: *homeostasis*. **3.** The ability to maintain the center of gravity over the base of support, as in standing balance.

***acid-base b.*** SEE: *acid-base balance*.

***analytical b.*** A very sensitive scale.

***fluid b.*** The balance between intake and excretion of fluids, esp. water, in the body.

***metabolic b.*** Comparison of the intake and excretion of a specific nutrient. The balance may be negative when an excess of the nutrient is excreted or positive when more is taken in than excreted.

***nitrogen b.*** The body state in which intake of nitrogen in protein foods is equal to nitrogen output, principally through loss of nitrogenous substances in the urine and feces.

**balance beam** In occupational and physical therapy, a device used to assess and improve balance and motor coordination; usually consists of a narrow beam elevated several inches from the floor.

**balance board** A device usually consisting of a padded platform mounted on a curved base and commonly used in therapy with children having central nervous system deficits. It is designed to facilitate the development of appropriate equilibrium-related postural reflexes.

**balan-** SEE: *balano-*.

**balanic** (bă-lăn′ĭk) [Gr. *balanos,* glans] Pert. to the glans clitoridis or glans penis.

**balanitis** (băl-ă-nī′tĭs) [″ + *itis,* inflammation] Inflammation of the skin covering the glans penis.

***b. xerotica obliterans*** A pathological condition of the skin of the penis. There are sclerotic and atrophic patches that can cause narrowing of the urinary meatus and phimosis. The cause is thought to be chronic balanoposthitis.

TREATMENT: Treatment is symptomatic and may be of little benefit.

**balano-, balan-** (băl′ă-nō) [Gr. *balanos,* glans] Combining form meaning *glans penis* or *glans clitoridis*.

**balanocele** (băl′ă-nō-sēl″) [″ + *kele,* tumor, swelling] Protrusion of the glans penis through a rupture of the prepuce.

**balanoplasty** (băl′ă-nō-plăs″tē) [″ + *plassein,* to form] Plastic surgery of the glans penis.

**balanoposthitis** (băl″ă-nō-pŏs-thī′tĭs) [″ + *posthe,* prepuce, + *itis,* inflammation] Balanitis.

**balanopreputial** (băl″ă-nō-prē-pū′shē-ăl) Pert. to the glans penis and prepuce.

**balanorrhagia** (băl″ă-nŏ-rā′jē-ă) [″ + *rhegnynai,* burst forth] Balanitis with pus formation.

**balantidial** (băl-ăn-tĭd′ē-ăl) Pert. to *Balantidium,* a genus of protozoa.

**balantidiasis** (băl″ăn-tĭ-dī′ă-sĭs) Infection caused by infestation with *Balantidium coli.*

SYMPTOMS: Symptoms include abdominal pain, diarrhea, vomiting, weakness, and weight loss.

TREATMENT: Treatment consists of tetracyclines, metronidazole, or paromomycin.

**Balantidium** (băl-ăn-tĭd′ē-ŭm) [Gr. *balantidion,* a bag] A genus of ciliated protozoa. A number of species are found in the intestines of both vertebrates and invertebrates.

***B. coli*** A normal parasite of swine and the largest protozoan parasitic of humans. It causes balantidiasis. SEE: illus.

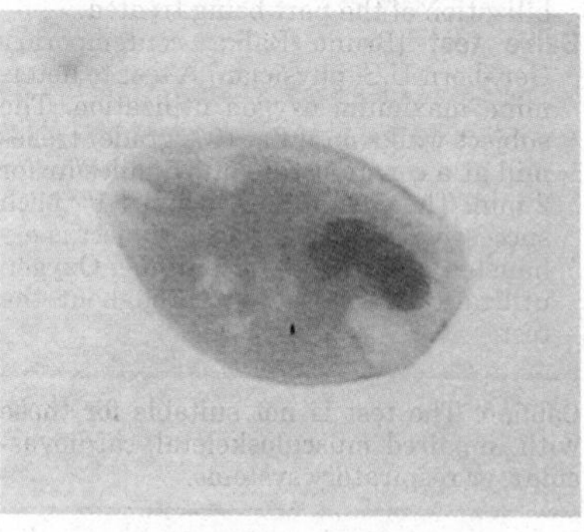


**BALANTIDIUM COLI** (×400)

EDGE OF CELL APPEARS INDISTINCT BECAUSE OF CILIA

**balanus** (băl′ă-nŭs) [Gr. *balanos,* glans] The glans penis or glans clitoridis.

**baldness** [ME. *ballede,* without hair] Lack of or partial loss of hair on the head. SEE: *alopecia*.

***male pattern b.*** Baldness in the male due to influence of the male hormone testosterone. Genetic predisposition is also a factor, and baldness does not usually occur in males having no familial tendency to become bald. The use of minoxidil has helped stimulate growth of hair in some individuals. SEE: illus.

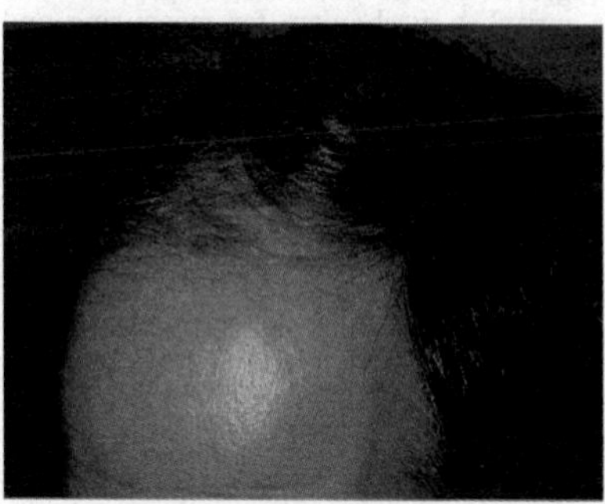

**MALE PATTERN BALDNESS**

**Balint's syndrome** [Rudolph Balint, Hungarian physician, 1874–1929] Inability to scan the peripheral visual field and to grasp an object under visual guidance, and visual inattention; usually due to bilateral occipitoparietal lesions of the brain.

**Balkan frame** A framework that fits over a bed. Suspended from the frame and connected through ropes and pulleys are weights used to produce desired continuous traction while permitting freedom of motion, thus maintaining desired immobilization of the part being treated.

**Balke test** [Bruno Balke, contemporary Ger.-born U.S. physician] A test to determine maximum oxygen utilization. The subject walks on a flat (0% grade) treadmill at a constant rate of 3.5 miles/hr for 2 min. The treadmill is inclined 1% each successive minute until the subject is exhausted and unable to continue. Oxygen utilization is measured throughout the test.

---

Caution: The test is not suitable for those with impaired musculoskeletal, cardiovascular, or respiratory systems.

---

**ball** A spherical object.

***b. of the foot*** The padded portion of the anterior extremity of the sole of the foot.

***b. of the thumb*** The thenar eminence of the thumb.

**ball-and-socket joint** A synovial joint in which one rounded bone head moves within a concavity of another bone. SYN: *enarthrosis.*

**ball bearing feeder** SEE: *mobile arm support.*

**ballism, ballismus** (băl′ĭzm, bă-lĭz′mŭs) [Gr. *ballismos,* jumping about] **1.** A condition marked by the jerking, twisting movements seen in chorea. **2.** An obsolete term for paralysis agitans.

**ballistics** (bă-lĭs′tĭks) [Gr. *ballein,* to throw] The science of the motion and trajectory of bullets, bombs, rockets, and guided missiles.

**ballistocardiograph** (bă-lĭs″tō-kăr′dē-ō-grăf) [″ + *kardia,* heart, + *graphein,* to write] A mechanism for measuring and recording the impact caused by the discharge of blood from the heart at each beat and the resulting recoil. The minute movements of the body with each heartbeat are recorded as they are transmitted to the special platform that supports the subject.

**balloon** [Fr. *ballon,* great ball] **1.** To expand, dilate, or distend, as to expand a cavity by filling it with air or water in a bag. **2.** A flexible, expandable object that can be placed inside a vessel or cavity to expand it or at the end of a catheter to prevent its removal. SEE: *catheter; percutaneous transluminal coronary angioplasty.*

**balloon tamponade, nasal** SEE: *nosebleed* for illus.; *epistaxis.*

**ballottable** (bă-lŏt′ă-bl) Capable of identification by ballottement.

**ballottement** (băl-ŏt-mŏn′) [Fr. *balloter,* to toss about] **1.** A palpatory technique used to detect or examine a floating object in the body, such as an organ. It is used in examining the abdomen esp. when ascites is present. **2.** A diagnostic maneuver in pregnancy. The fetus or a fetal part rebounds when displaced by a light tap of the examining finger through the vagina.

**ball-valve action** Action of a mass, such as a pedunculated cyst or thrombus, moving to open and close the passageway of a tube or chamber and causing intermittent obstruction. A ball-valve thrombus may form in the heart and cause repeated blockage of an opening connecting two chambers of the heart.

**balm** [Gr. *balsamon,* balsam] **1.** A balsam. **2.** A soothing or healing ointment.

***b. of Gilead*** **1.** Mecca balsam from *Commiphora opobalsamum,* probably biblical myrrh. **2.** Balsam fir, source of Canadian balsam. **3.** Poplar bud resin.

**balneology** (băl-nē-ŏl′ō-jē) [L. *balneum,* bath, + Gr. *logos,* word, reason] The science of baths and bathing.

**balneotherapy, balneotherapeutics** (băl″nē-ō-thĕr′ă-pē, -thĕr″ă-pū′tĭks) [″ + Gr. *therapeia,* treatment] The use of baths in treatment of disease.

**balsam** (bawl′săm) [Gr. *balsamon,* balsam] A fragrant, resinous, oily exudate from various trees and plants. It is used in topical preparations to treat irritated skin or mucous membrane.

***b. of Peru*** A dark brown, viscid, resinous liquid obtained from the bark of the tree *Myroxylon perierae* or *M. balsamum.*

**BALT** *bronchus-associated lymphoid tissue.*

**bamboo spine** In ankylosing spondylitis, a spinal column that on a radiograph resembles a bamboo stalk.

**Bancroft's filariasis** [Joseph Bancroft, Brit. physician, 1836–1894] A filarial infection caused by *Wuchereria bancrofti.* SEE: *elephantiasis.*

**band 1.** A cord or tapelike tissue that connects or holds structures together. SEE: *bundle; ligament; tract.* **2.** Any appliance that encircles or binds the body or a limb. **3.** A segment of a myofibril. **4.** A metal strip or seamless band for attaching orthodontic appliances to teeth. **5.** An immature, unsegmented neutrophil in the differential section of a complete blood count. An increase in bands indicates that all mature neutrophils have been released from the bone marrow, usually during severe inflammation or infection, and that the marrow is releasing immature cells.

***H b.*** A narrow band in the center of the A band of a sarcomere; it contains only thick (myosin) filaments and is bisected by the M line. SYN: *Engelmann's disk; H zone.*

***I b.*** In muscle fibers, the light band segment of a sarcomere, containing lateral ends of thin (actin) filaments. There is one to either side of the medial A band. SYN: *isotropic b.*

***iliotibial b.*** A thick, wide fascial layer from the iliac crest along the lateral thigh to the fascia around the lateral aspect of the knee joint. Fibers from the tensor fascia lata and gluteus maximus insert into the proximal band.

***isotropic b.*** I b.

**bandage** [ME. *bande,* a band] **1.** A piece of soft, usually absorbent gauze or other material applied to a limb or other part of the body as a dressing. **2.** To cover by wrapping with a piece of gauze or other material.

Bandages are used to hold dressings in place, apply pressure to a part, immobilize a part, obliterate cavities, support an injured area, and check hemorrhages. Types of bandages include roller, triangular, four-tailed, many-tailed (Scultetus), quadrangular, elastic (elastic knit, rubber, synthetic, or combinations of these), adhesive, elastic adhesive, newer cohesive bandages under various proprietary names, impregnated bandages (plaster of paris, waterglass [silica], starch), and stockinet. Use of a self-adhering, form-fitting roller bandage facilitates bandaging by eliminating the special techniques needed when ordinary gauze roller bandages are used. SEE: illus.; *sling.*

---

Caution: Skin-to-skin contact will, if continued, cause severe skin infection.

---

***abdomen b.*** A single wide cravat or several narrow ones used to hold a dressing in place or to exert a moderate pressure.

***Ace b.*** Trade name for a woven elastic bandage available in various widths and lengths. It provides uniform support, yet permits joint movement without loosening the bandage.

***adhesive b.*** A bandage made of adhesive tape.

***amputation-stump b.*** An elastic bandage applied to an amputation stump to control postoperative edema and to shape the stump. The elastic bandage is applied in a recurrent or figure-of-eight fashion with more pressure applied to the distal, rather than the proximal, portion of the limb.

***ankle b.*** Bandage in which one loop is brought around the sole of foot and the other around the ankle; it is secured in front or on the side.

***axilla b.*** A bandage with a spica-type turn starting under the affected axilla, crossing over the shoulder of the affected side, and making the long loop under the opposite armpit.

***back b.*** Open bandage to the back; applied the same as a chest bandage, the point being placed above the scapula of the injured side.

***Barton b.*** A double figure-of-eight bandage for the lower jaw.

***breast b.*** Suspensory bandage and compress for the breasts.

***butterfly b.*** An adhesive bandage used in place of sutures to hold wound edges together.

***buttocks b.*** T or double-T bandage or open triangular bandage for the buttocks.

***capeline b.*** A bandage applied to the head or shoulder or to a stump like a cap or hood.

***chest b.*** Figure-of-eight (spica), many-tailed (Scultetus), or triangular (open-chest) bandage for the chest.

***circular b.*** A bandage applied in circular turns about a part.

***cohesive b.*** A bandage made of material that sticks to itself but not to other substances; used to bandage fingers and extremities or to build up pads.

***cravat b.*** A triangular bandage folded to form a band around an injured part. This is done by pulling the point over toward the base, folding the base over the point, and then folding again. This makes a bandage wide enough to cover a large knee. Folded a second time, it is suitable for an elbow. Folded a third time, it could be used in making a figure-of-eight bandage for the foot, ankle, hand, wrist, or head. It is an effective bandage in arresting hemorrhages and in retaining splints and dressings. The center of the cravat should be laid against the affected part, the ends of the cravat carried around the limb and tied over the center of the base. When used to retain splints, it should be tied on the outer side of the limb and against the splint, thus preventing the knot from irritating the skin. When used to retain a dressing in the axilla, the center of the cravat should be placed under the arm and the ends carried upward and crossed over the shoulder and tied in the axillary space of the opposite side, thus forming a figure-of-eight. The cravat can also be used as a sling when only a simple support is needed.

In using cravats for ties or splints, care should be taken so that the knots do not pass over and press unduly on the surface of the limb. Knots should be placed where they are easily found and not subject to pressure; the ends should be neatly tucked in. All knots should be square or reef knots.

***cravat elbow b.*** A bandage in which the elbow is bent about 45° and the center of bandage is placed over the point of the elbow. One end is brought around the forearm and the other end around the upper arm; the bandage is pulled tight and tied.

***cravat b. for clenched fist*** A hand bandage to arrest bleeding or to produce pres-

TYPES OF BANDAGES

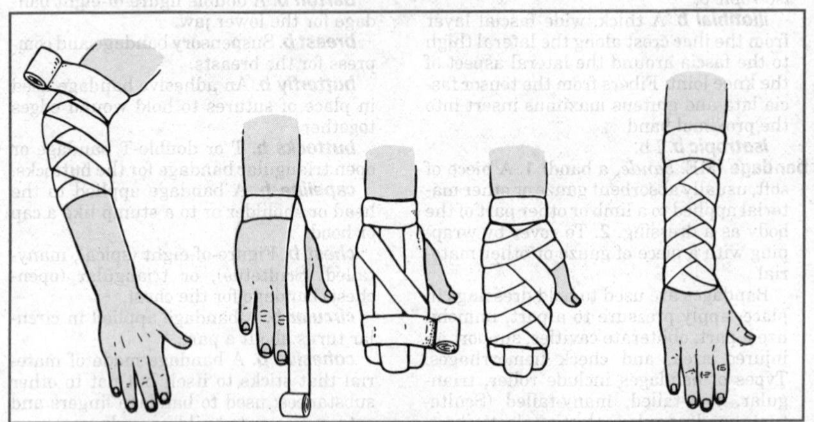

FIGURE-OF-EIGHT RECURRENT SPIRAL REVERSE

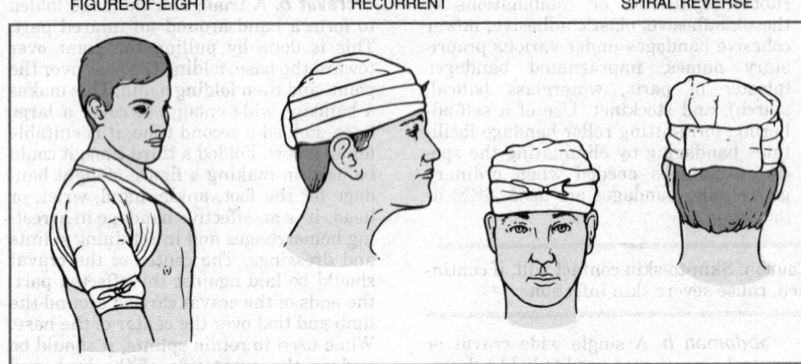

BANDAGE OF SHOULDER RECURRENT B. OF HEAD

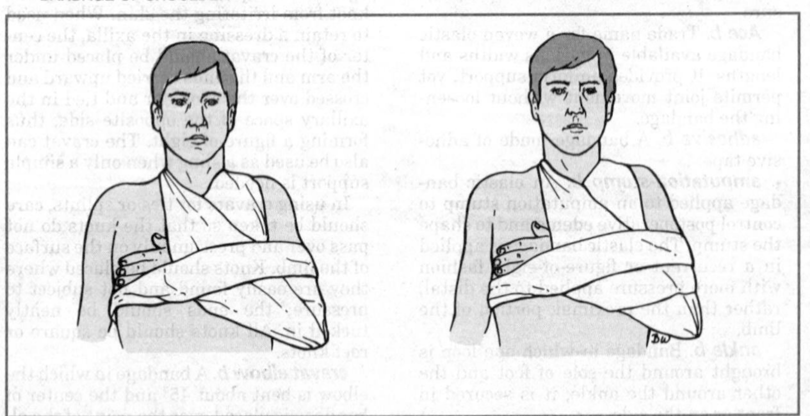

TRIANGULAR BANDAGE OF ELBOW AND ARM

## TYPES OF BANDAGES

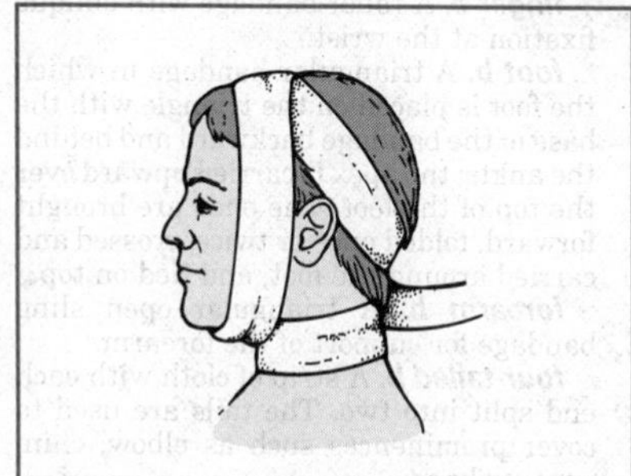
BARTON

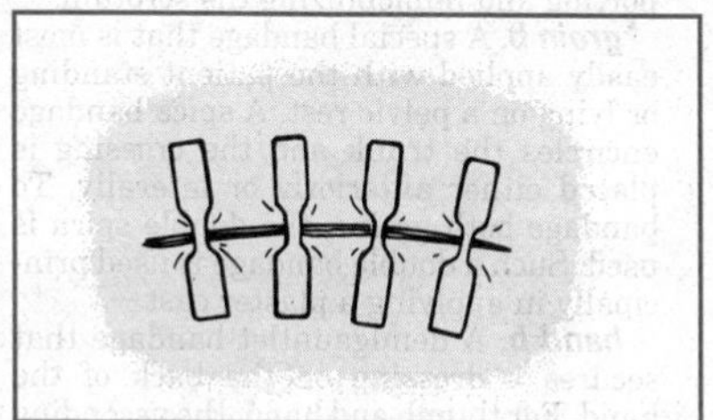
BUTTERFLY STRIPS

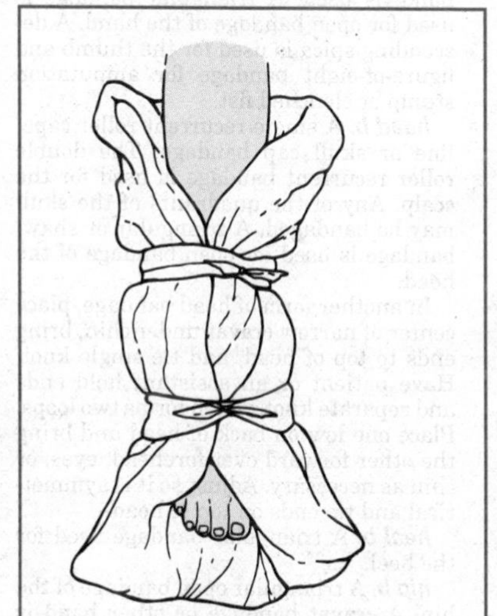
PILLOW SPLINT

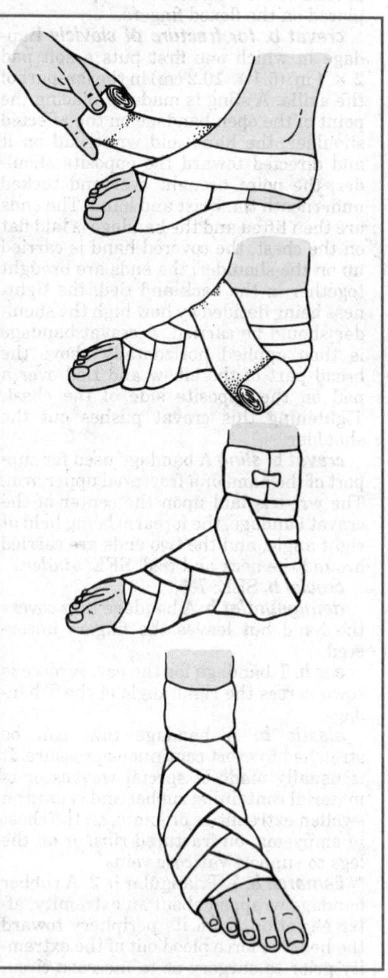
ANKLE STRAPPING

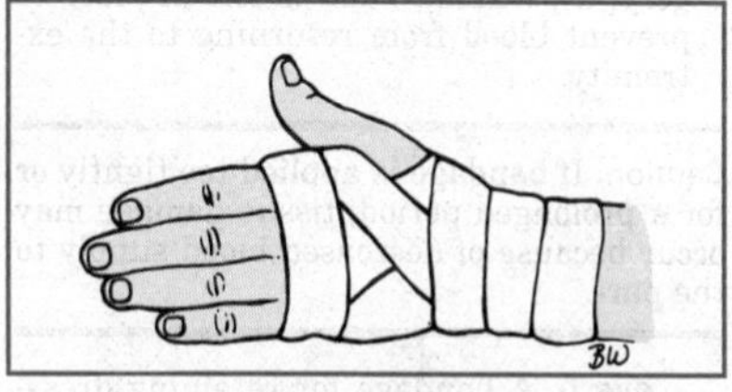

WRIST BANDAGE

sure. The wrist is placed on the center of the cravat, one end is brought around over the fist and back to the starting point, and the same procedure is then repeated with the other end. The two ends are pulled tight, twisted, and carried around the fist again so that pressure is placed on the flexed fingers.

***cravat b. for fracture of clavicle*** Bandage in which one first puts a soft pad 2 × 4 in. (5.1 × 10.2 cm) in the forepart of the axilla. A sling is made by placing the point of the open bandage on the affected shoulder, the hand and wrist laid on it and directed toward the opposite shoulder, the point brought over and tucked underneath the wrist and hand. The ends are then lifted and the bandage is laid flat on the chest, the covered hand is carried up on the shoulder, the ends are brought together in the back and tied, the tightness being decided by how high the shoulder should be carried. A cravat bandage is then applied horizontally above the broad part of the elbow and tied over a pad on the opposite side of the chest. Tightening this cravat pushes out the shoulder.

***cravat b. sling*** A bandage used for support of the hand or a fractured upper arm. The wrist is laid upon the center of the cravat bandage, the forearm being held at right angle, and the two ends are carried around the neck and tied. SEE: *binder*.

***crucial b.*** SEE: *T b.*

***demigauntlet b.*** A bandage that covers the hand but leaves the fingers uncovered.

***ear b.*** T bandage for the ear. A piece is sewn across the right angle of the T bandage.

***elastic b.*** A bandage that can be stretched to exert continuous pressure. It is usually made of special weaves or of material containing rubber and is used on swollen extremities or joints, on the chest in empyema, on fractured ribs, or on the legs to support varicose veins.

***Esmarch b.*** **1.** Triangular b. **2.** A rubber bandage wrapped about an extremity, after elevation, from its periphery toward the heart to force blood out of the extremity prior to surgery or to increase circulating blood. When it is removed for surgery, a proximal band is left in place to prevent blood from returning to the extremity.

Caution: If bandage is applied too tightly or for a prolonged period, tissue damage may occur because of decreased blood supply to the part.

***eye b.*** A bandage for retaining dressings. The simple roller bandage for one eye or the monocle or crossed bandage. The binocular or crossed bandage for both eyes is 2 in. × 6 yd (5.1 cm × 5.49 m).

***figure-of-eight b.*** A bandage in which the turns cross each other like the figure eight; used to retain dressings, to exert pressure for joints (or to leave the joint uncovered), to fix splints for the foot or hand, for the great toe, and for sprains or hemorrhage.

***finger b.*** A roller bandage with oblique fixation at the wrist.

***foot b.*** A triangular bandage in which the foot is placed on the triangle with the base of the bandage backward and behind the ankle; the apex is carried upward over the top of the foot. The ends are brought forward, folded once or twice, crossed and carried around the foot, and tied on top.

***forearm b.*** A triangular open sling bandage for support of the forearm.

***four-tailed b.*** A strip of cloth with each end split into two. The tails are used to cover prominences such as elbow, chin, nose, or knee.

***Fricke's b.*** A special bandage for supporting and immobilizing the scrotum.

***groin b.*** A special bandage that is most easily applied with the patient standing or lying on a pelvic rest. A spica bandage encircles the trunk and the crossing is placed either anteriorly or laterally. To bandage both groins, the double spica is used. Such a double bandage is used principally in applying a plaster cast.

***hand b.*** A demigauntlet bandage that secures a dressing on the back of the hand. For thumb and hand, the ascending spica of the thumb, with spiral of the hand, is used. A triangular bandage is used for open bandage of the hand. A descending spica is used for the thumb and figure-of-eight bandage for amputation stump or clenched fist.

***head b.*** A single recurrent roller capeline or skull cap bandage. The double roller recurrent bandage is used for the scalp. Any of the quadrants of the skull may be bandaged. A triangular or shawl bandage is used for open bandage of the head.

In another form of head bandage, place center of narrow cravat under chin, bring ends to top of head, and tie single knot. Have patient or an assistant hold ends and separate knot, which forms two loops. Place one low on back of head and bring the other forward over forehead, eyes, or chin as necessary. Adjust so it is symmetrical and tie ends on top of head.

***heel b.*** A triangular bandage used for the heel.

***hip b.*** A triangular open bandage of the hip. A cravat bandage or other band is tied around the waist; the point of another bandage is slipped under and rolled or pinned directly above the position of the wound. The base is rolled up and the ends are carried around the thigh, crossed, and tied.

***immovable b.*** A bandage for immobilizing a part.

***impregnated b.*** A wide-meshed bandage used to make molds or immobilize parts of the body. The material is impregnated with a substance such as plaster of paris, which is applied wet and hardens after drying.

***knee b.*** The knee cravat; triangular and the figure-of-eight bandages are used.

***leg b.*** A bandage applied by fixing the initial end by a circular or oblique fixation at the ankle or with a figure-of-eight of the foot and ankle.

***many-tailed b.*** A bandage with split ends used for the trunk and limbs; a piece of roller to which slips are stitched in an imbricated fashion. SEE: *four-tailed b.; Scultetus b.*

***Martin's b.*** A roller bandage of rubber used for exerting pressure on an extremity, as for varicose veins, and for exsanguination, as with an Esmarch bandage.

***neck b.*** *Neck spica:* Bandage 2½ in. × 8 yd (6.4 cm × 7.3 m). *Bandage following thyroid gland surgery:* Roller bandage 2½ in. × 9 yd (6.4 cm × 8.2 m). *Adhesive plaster bandage for thyroidectomy:* Used to hold dressing on wound in place. A small dressing is applied to center of strip and then applied to back of neck. *Special bandage:* A double-loop bandage of the head and neck made by using a figure-of-eight turn.

***oblique b.*** A bandage applied obliquely to a limb, without reverses.

***plaster b.*** A bandage stiffened with a paste of plaster of paris, which sets and becomes very hard.

***pressure b.*** A bandage for applying pressure; usually used to stop hemorrhage.

***protective b.*** A bandage that covers a part or keeps dressings in place.

***quadrangular b.*** A towel or large handkerchief, folded variously and applied as a bandage of head, chest, breast, or abdomen.

***recurrent b.*** A bandage over the end of a stump.

***reversed b.*** A bandage applied to a limb in such a way that the roller is inverted or half twisted at each turn so as to make it fit smoothly and resist slipping off the limb. SEE: *spiral reverse b.*

***roller b.*** A long strip of soft material, usually from ½ to 6 in. (1.3 to 15.2 cm) wide and 2 to 5 yd (1.83 to 4.57 m) long, rolled on its short axis. When rolled from both ends to meet at center, it is called a double-headed roller.

***rubber b.*** A rubber roller bandage used to apply pressure to swollen parts for immobilization.

***Scultetus b.*** A many-tailed bandage; a succession of interlocking, overlapping bands originally used to enclose a rigid support against a fractured extremity but now used without the splint or impregnated as a supporting bandage of the abdomen or lower extremity. SEE: *binder, Scultetus,* for illus.

***shoulder b.*** An open bandage of the shoulder (spica bandage); a shawl bandage of both shoulders and neck.

***spica b.*** A bandage in which a number of figure-of-eight turns are applied, each a little higher or lower, overlapping a portion of each preceding turn so as to give an imbricated appearance. This type of bandage is used to support, to exert pressure, or to retain dressings on the breast, shoulder, limbs, thumb, great toe, and hernia at the groin.

***spiral reverse b.*** A technique of twisting, in its long axis, a roller bandage on itself at intervals during application to make it fit more uniformly. These reverse folds may be necessary every turn or less, depending on the contour of the part being bandaged.

***suspensory b.*** A bandage for supporting any part but esp. the breast or scrotum.

***T b.*** A bandage shaped like the letter T and used for the perineum and, in certain cases, the head.

***tailed b.*** A bandage split at the end.

***toe b.*** A small bandage, about 2 in. (5.1 cm) wide.

***triangular b.*** A 36- to 42-in. (232- to 271-cm) square of material, usually muslin, that is cut diagonally, making two triangular bandages; frequently used in first aid. SYN: *Esmarch bandage* (1). SEE: *triangular bandage* for illus.

***Velpeau b.*** A special immobilizing roller bandage that incorporates the shoulder, arm, and forearm.

**bandage roller** A device for rolling bandages.

**banding** The use of chemicals to stain chromosomes so that the characteristic bands may be visualized.

**Bandl's ring** (băn′d'ls) [Ludwig Bandl, Ger. obstetrician, 1842–1892] Ringlike thickening and indentation at the junction of the upper and lower uterine segments that obstructs delivery of the fetus. SEE: *retraction ring.*

**bandpass, photometric** The wavelength selectivity of a laboratory photometer.

**bandwidth** In electronics the range of frequencies within which performance with respect to some characteristic falls within specified limits.

**bandy leg** Bowleg. SYN: *genu varum.*

**bank** A stored supply of body fluids or tissues for use in another individual (e.g., blood bank, eye bank, kidney bank, tissue bank).

***sperm b.*** A repository for the storage of semen used for artificial insemination. In some banks the specimen is frozen. SEE: *Universal Precautions Appendix.*

**Bankart lesion** An avulsion injury of the capsule and labrum from the glenoid rim of the glenohumeral joint. This lesion is the most common reason for recurrent shoulder dislocations.

**Banthine** Trade name for methantheline bromide, an anticholinergic.

**Banting, Sir Frederick Grant** Canadian scientist, 1891–1941; co-discoverer of insulin, with Charles Herbert Best and John J. R. Macleod in 1922; Nobel laureate 1923.

**Banti's syndrome** (băn'tēz) [Guido Banti, It. physician, 1852–1925] A syndrome combining anemia, splenic enlargement, hemorrhages, and ultimately cirrhosis of the liver; secondary to portal hypertension.

**bar 1.** A metal piece attaching two or more units of a removable dental prosthesis. **2.** A rigid component of a splint or brace. **3.** A section of tissue that connects two similar structures.

***lumbrical b.*** A component of a hand splint that rests on the dorsal surface of the proximal phalanges to prevent hyperextension of the metacarpophalangeal joints.

***median b.*** Contracture or constriction of the vesical neck of the bladder caused by benign hypertrophy or fibrosis of the prostate. It may obstruct the flow of urine from the bladder.

**baragnosis** (băr-ăg-nō'sĭs) [Gr. *baros,* weight, + *a-,* not, + *gnosis,* knowledge] The inability to estimate weights; the opposite of barognosis. It is indicative of a parietal lobe lesion. SYN: *abarognosis.*

**Bárány's caloric test** [Robert Bárány, Austrian physician and physiologist, 1876–1936. Won Nobel Prize in medicine in 1914] Evaluation of vestibular function by irrigation of the ear canal with either warm or cold water. Normally when warm water is used, rotatory nystagmus toward the irrigated ear is observed; with cold water, the normal response is rotatory nystagmus away from the irrigated ear. If vestibular function is impaired, the response may be absent or diminished. If one ear is normal and the other is not, a comparison between the two may be made.

**barber's itch 1.** The formation of papules and pustules on the face due to infection of hair follicles and associated glands by staphylococci. SYN: *folliculitis barbae.* **2.** A dermatomycosis caused by a fungus, *Microsporum lanosum, Trichophyton mentagrophytes, T. violaceum,* or *T. purpureum.* SYN: *tinea barbae.*

**barbiturates** (băr-bĭt'ū-rāts, băr-bĭ-tū'rāts) A group of organic compounds derived from barbituric acid (e.g., Amytal, Pentothal, phenobarbital, and Seconal). These derivatives depress the central nervous system, depress respiration, affect heart rate, and decrease blood pressure and temperature. These drugs can be habit forming. For sedative action, these drugs have been replaced by safer drugs such as benzodiazepines. SEE: *Poisons and Poisoning Appendix.*

**barbotage** (băr-bō-tŏzh') [Fr. *barboter,* to dabble] Repeated injection and withdrawal of fluid, as in gastric lavage, or the administration of an anesthetic into the subarachnoid space by alternate injection of anesthetic and withdrawal of cerebrospinal fluid into the syringe.

**barbula hirci** (băr'bū-lă hĭr'sī) [L. *barbula,* little beard, + *hircus,* goat] **1.** Hairs present on the ears. **2.** Axillary hair.

**bar code** A parallel array of alternately spaced black bars and white spaces representing a coded number, numbers, or letters, depending on the format employed. It is used clinically for patient sample identification.

**barefoot doctor** In the People's Republic of China, one who is trained to administer medical care in areas where there is a shortage of physicians.

**baresthesia** (băr-ĕs-thē'zē-ă) [Gr. *baros,* weight, + *aisthesis,* sensation] Sense of weight or pressure; pressure sense.

**bariatrics** (băr"ē-ă'trĭks) [" + *iatrike,* medical treatment] The branch of medicine that deals with prevention, control, and treatment of obesity.

**baritosis** Pneumoconiosis caused by inhalation of barium dust.

**barium** (bă'rē-ŭm) SYMB: Ba. A soft metallic element of the alkaline earth group; atomic weight 137.373, atomic number 56.

***b. sulfate*** A radiopaque contrast medium used in radiographic studies of the gastrointestinal tract. It should not be used as a water-soluble agent because it is not absorbed by the body. Trade names are Barosperse and Esophotrast.

**barium compounds** Compounds containing barium and suitable diluents or additives. They are used to color fireworks and, in the form of insoluble barium sulfate, to visualize the hollow viscera in roentgenography. Poisoning occasionally occurs when the soluble salts are used accidentally in place of the insoluble sulfate. SEE: *Poisons and Poisoning Appendix.*

**barium enema** The use of barium sulfate solution as an enema to facilitate x-ray and fluoroscopic examination of the colon.

PROCEDURE: Careful preparation of the patient will greatly increase the chances of the test producing useful information. The patient is given the following written instructions with a careful explanation to ensure compliance. 1. A minimum-residue diet must be followed for all meals for 2 days prior to the test. 2. Two nights before the test, 60 ml (2 oz) of milk of magnesia must be taken in 120 ml (4 oz) of water at bedtime. 3. On the day before the test, a clear liquid diet must be taken for all meals. 4. At 5 P.M. on the day before the test, 60 ml (2 oz) of castor oil must be taken. 5. At 10 P.M. on the day before the test, a cleansing enema consisting of 1500 ml (50 oz) of lukewarm water must be given. 6. On the day of the test, only clear liquids are allowed for meals. SEE: *diet, minimum residue.*

***double-contrast b.e.*** A technique of barium enema x-ray study of the large intestine in which air is insufflated into the rectum and colon. This technique is considered more effective in demonstrating pathologic lesions of the large intestine than an ordinary barium enema.

**barium meal** The use of ingested barium sulfate to visualize the outline of the esophagus, stomach, and small intestines during x-ray or fluoroscopic examination. Also called *upper G.I. series.*

PROCEDURE: If the test does not follow a barium enema, the patient should receive nothing by mouth after midnight on the night before the test. No food or liquids should be taken by mouth until the last roentgenogram is taken. If the test is done within a few days after a barium enema examination, it is important to be sure the colon is free of barium, which could interfere with visualization of the stomach and intestines. A cleansing enema and 60 ml (2 oz) of milk of magnesia in 120 ml (4 oz) of water the evening before the test will remove residual barium from the colon.

**barium swallow** Radiographic examination of the esophagus during and after introduction of a contrast medium consisting of barium sulfate. Structural abnormalities of the esophagus and vessels such as esophageal varices may be diagnosed by use of this technique.

**barium test** Nonspecific term for any test involving use of barium sulfate as a radiopaque material for outlining anatomical areas such as the esophagus and other portions of the intestinal tract by use of radiographic or fluoroscopic examinations. SEE: *barium enema; barium meal.*

**Barlow's disease** [Sir Thomas Barlow, Brit. physician, 1845–1945] A deficiency disease due to lack of vitamin C (ascorbic acid). It occurs in both breast-fed and bottle-fed babies—usually between 6 and 12 months of age—who fail to receive adequate supplements of vitamin C. SEE: *scurvy, infantile.*

TREATMENT: Therapy includes vitamin C and adequate daily intake of fruit juices (orange, grapefruit, tomato).

**Barlow's test** An assessment maneuver designed to detect subluxation or dislocation of the hip. The examiner adducts and then extends the legs with his fingers over the heads of the femurs. A dysplastic joint will be felt to dislocate as the femur leaves the acetabulum.

**baro-** [Gr. *baros,* weight] Combining form indicating relationship to *weight* or *pressure.*

**barognosis** (băr-ŏg-nō'sĭs) [" + *gnosis,* knowledge] The ability to estimate weights; the opposite of baragnosis.

**barograph** A device used to measure and record changes in atmospheric pressure.

**baroreceptor** (băr"ō-rē-sĕp'tor) A sensory nerve ending that is stimulated by changes in pressure. Baroreceptors are found in the walls of the atria of the heart, vena cava, aortic arch, and carotid sinus. SYN: *pressoreceptor.*

**baroreflexes** (băr"ō-rē'flĕk-sĕs) [" + L. *reflexus,* bent back] Reflexes mediated or activated through a group of nerves located in various blood vessels in the intrathoracic and cervical areas and in the heart and its great vessels. They are sensitive to mechanical changes produced when the pressure inside the vessel to which they are attached is altered. The response is called a baroreflex. Because the nerve groups are stimulated by mechanical rather than chemical means, they are called mechanoreceptors.

**baroscope** (băr'ō-skōp) [" + *skopein,* to examine] An instrument that registers changes in the density of air.

**barostat** A receptor that is sensitive to changes in pressure and provides feedback stimuli to counteract the changes. Such a feedback system is present in the part of the carotid sinus sensitive to changes in blood pressure.

**barotitis** (băr"ō-tī'tĭs) Aerotitis.

**barotrauma** (băr"ō-traw'mă) [" + *trauma,* wound] Any injury caused by a change in atmospheric pressure between a potentially closed space and the surrounding area. SEE: *aerotitis; barotitis; bends; caisson disease.*

**Barr body** [Murray L. Barr, Canadian anatomist, b. 1908] Sex chromatin mass seen within the nuclei of normal female somatic cells. According to the Lyon hypothesis, one of the two X chromosomes in each somatic cell of the female is genetically inactivated. The Barr body represents the inactivated X chromosome.

**barrel chest** A condition of increased anteroposterior chest diameter caused by increased functional residual capacity due to air trapping from small airway collapse in patients with chronic obstructive pulmonary disease (i.e., chronic bronchitis and emphysema).

**barren** [O. Fr. *barhaine,* unproductive] Sterile; incapable of producing offspring.

**Barrett's esophagus** [Norman R. Barrett, Brit. surgeon, 1903–1979] Inflammation and possibly ulceration of the lower part of the esophagus caused by gatroesophageal reflux or mucosal damage due to chemotherapy. The condition may be complicated by peptic stricture higher in the esophagus and by adenocarcinoma of the inflamed area. SEE: *disorder, acid-reflux.*

**barrier** [O. Fr. *barriere*] An obstacle, impediment, obstruction, boundary, or separation.

***blood-brain b.*** A barrier that exists between circulating blood and the brain, preventing certain damaging substances from reaching brain tissue and cerebrospinal fluid. It consists of either the perivascular glial membrane or the vascular endothelium or both.

***placental b.*** A barrier provided by placental tissues, between the fetal and the maternal circulation. Small substances, excluding blood cells, may cross this barrier.

***primary radiation b.*** A wall or partition that shields the radiology technician from direct exposure to x-rays.

***secondary radiation b.*** A wall or partition that shields against scattering or leakage of x-rays.

**barrier-free design** The planning and arrangement of living environments that emphasizes accessibility by persons with physical disability.

**Barthel index** A widely used functional assessment of activities of daily living. It assesses a person's ability to perform feeding, transfers, personal grooming and hygiene, toileting, walking, negotiating stairs, and controlling bowel and bladder functions.

**Bartholin's abscess** (băr'tō-lĭnz) [Caspar Bartholin, Danish anatomist, 1655–1738] An abscess that develops when Bartholin's glands become occluded in an acute inflammatory process.

**Bartholin's cyst** Cyst commonly formed in chronic inflammation of Bartholin's glands. Carcinoma is rare.

**Bartholin's ducts** Large ducts of the sublingual salivary gland. They parallel Wharton's duct.

**Bartholin's gland** One of two small compound mucous glands located one in each lateral wall of the vestibule of the vagina, near the vaginal opening at the base of the labia majora.

**bartholinitis** (băr″tō-lĭn-ī'tĭs) [*Bartholin* + Gr. *itis,* inflammation] Inflammation of Bartholin's gland.

**Barton, Clara** U.S. nurse, 1821–1912. Founder of the American National Red Cross. She aided the wounded in the Civil War and was a contemporary of Florence Nightingale.

**Bartonella** (băr″tō-nĕl'ă) [A.L. Barton, S. Amer. physician, 1871–1950] A genus of bacteria of the family Bartonellaceae.

***B. bacilliformis*** Motile gram-negative bacillus that causes bartonellosis. SEE: *bartonellosis.*

***B. henselae*** A gram-negative rod of the family Bartonellaceae that, together with *B. quintana,* causes acute and persistent bacteremia and localized tissue infection, which may lead to bacillary angiomatosis, bacillary peliosis, and other inflammatory responses. This infection can occur in immunocompromised and immunocompetent individuals but is seen most frequently in patients with HIV infection. *B. henselae,* previously named *Rochalimaea henselae,* is the causative agent of cat scratch disease. Therapy for bacillary angiomatosis is oral antibiotics. SEE: *angiomatosis, bacillary; disease, cat scratch; peliosis, bacillary.*

***B. quintana*** The organism previously known as *Rochalimaea quintana* or *Rickettsia quintana.* During World War I, it caused trench fever, a debilitating febrile illness, in battlefield troops. Together with *B. henselae,* it may cause bacillary angiomatosis, bacillary peliosis, and other inflammatory responses. Treatment includes oral antibiotics. SEE: *B. henselae; angiomatosis, bacillary; peliosis, bacillary.*

***B. elizabethae*** The organism previously known as *Rochalimaea elizabethae.* It causes an infection that has been identified most often in immunocompromised patients with HIV infection. It has been implicated as a cause of bacteremia and endocarditis.

**bartonellosis** (băr″tō-nĕl-ō'sĭs) [*Bartonella* + Gr. *osis,* condition] A disease caused by infection with *Bartonella bacilliformis,* transmitted by female sandflies *(Phlebotomus).* It occurs in the valleys of the Andes Mountains in Peru, Chile, Bolivia, and Colombia. The first clinical stage is noneruptive and is called Oroya fever, a severe febrile, hemolytic anemia. The second stage, called verruga peruana, is eruptive and is marked by the appearance of small tumors on the skin and mucous membranes. SYN: *Carrion's disease.*

TREATMENT: The causative organism responds to several antibiotics, but ampicillin or chloramphenicol has the advantage of being effective against *Salmonella,* which may be present as a secondary infection.

**Bartter's syndrome** [Frederic Crosby Bartter, U.S. physician, 1914–1983] Hyperplasia of the juxtaglomerular cells of the kidney, hypokalemic alkalosis, and hyperaldosteronism without a rise in blood pressure. It usually occurs in children and may be accompanied by dwarfism. Etiology is unknown. Some patients have responded to therapy with prostaglandin inhibitors.

**Baruch's law** (băr'ooks) [Simon Baruch, Ger.-born U.S. physician, 1840–1921] The theory that water has a sedative effect when its temperature is the same as that of the skin and a stimulating effect when it is below or above the skin temperature.

**bary-** [Gr. *barys,* heavy] Prefix indicating *heavy, dull, hard.*

**baryglossia** (băr-ĭ-glŏs'ē-ă) [Gr. *barys,* heavy, + *glossa,* tongue] Slow, thick utterance of speech.

**barylalia** (băr-ĭ-lā'lē-ă) [″ + *lalia,* speech] Indistinct, husky speech due to imperfect articulation. SYN: *baryphonia* (2).

**baryophobia** The unreasonable fear that one's child will become obese. The allowed diet may be insufficient to support the child's growth and development needs.

**baryphonia** (băr″ĭ-fō'nē-ă) [″ + *phone,* voice] **1.** Heavy, thick quality of the voice. **2.** Barylalia.

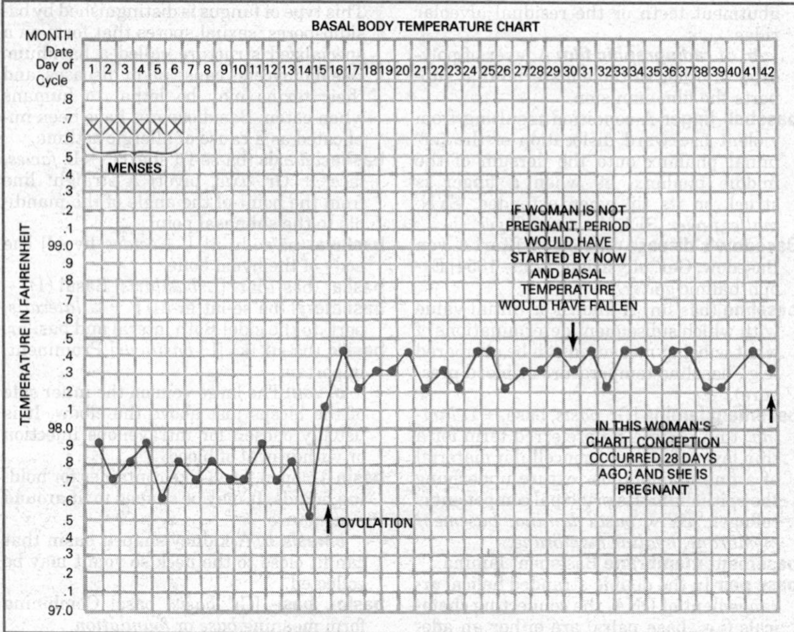


**basad** (bā′săd) [Gr. *basis,* base, + L. *ad,* toward] Toward the base.

**basal** (bā′săl) **1.** Pert. to the base. **2.** Of primary importance.

**basal ganglia** Four masses of gray matter located deep in the cerebral hemispheres—caudate, lentiform, and amygdaloid nuclei and the claustrum. The caudate and lentiform nuclei and the fibers of the internal capsule that separate them constitute the corpus striatum. The function of the basal ganglia is complex. They contribute to some of the subconscious aspects of voluntary movement such as accessory movements and inhibiting tremor. They initiate stimuli for movement but provide essential links in complex motor circuits. Chemical substances that affect basal ganglionic function are acetylcholine, dopamine, gamma-aminobutyric acid (GABA), and serotonin.

**basal lamina** Basement lamina.

**basal metabolic rate** ABBR: BMR. The metabolic rate as measured under so-called basal conditions: 12 hr after eating, after a restful sleep, no exercise or activity preceding test, elimination of emotional excitement, and in a comfortable temperature. It is usually expressed in terms of kilocalories per square meter of body surface per hour. The use of this test is no longer justified due to the availability of better tests of thyroid function. SEE: *thyroid function tests.*

**basal metabolism** The amount of energy needed for maintenance of life when the subject is at digestive, physical, and emotional rest.

**basal ridge** An eminence on the lingual surface of the incisor teeth, esp. the upper ones. It is situated near the gum. SYN: *cingulum* (2).

**basal temperature chart** A daily chart of temperature (usually taken rectally) obtained upon awakening. Some women are able to predict the time of ovulation by carefully analyzing the character and rhythm of the temperature chart. This information and other data can be used to establish that the woman is ovulating. Use of this method to control conception by predicting time of ovulation is unreliable in most cases. SEE: illus.; *conception.*

**base** [Gr. *basis,* base] **1.** The lower part of anything; the supporting part. **2.** The principal substance in a mixture. **3.** Any substance that combines with hydrogen ions (protons); a hydrogen ion acceptor. Strong bases (such as sodium hydroxide, or lye) are corrosive to human tissues. Whether an unknown chemical compound is a base or an acid may be determined by the color produced when it is added to a solution containing an indicator. SYN: *alkali.* SEE: *acid; pH.*

***cavity b., cement b.*** In dentistry, the lining material placed in a cavity preparation, such as zinc phosphate, zinc oxide-eugenol, or calcium hydroxide along with small amounts of other medicinal or adhesive materials.

***denture b.*** That part of the denture made of metal or resin, or both, that supports the artificial teeth and rests on abutment teeth or the residual alveolar ridge.

***b. of radiographic film*** A layer of polyester or other suitable material that supports the film emulsion.

**baseball finger** A condition resulting from violent backward dislocation of the terminal phalanx onto the dorsum of the middle phalanx, as when a finger is struck on its tip when extended. SYN: *mallet finger.* SEE: *hammer finger.*

**Basedow's disease** (băz'ē-dōz) [Karl A. von Basedow, Ger. physician, 1799–1854] Exophthalmic goiter.

**baseline** (bās'līn) A known or initial value with which subsequent determinations of what is being measured can be compared (e.g., baseline temperature or blood pressure).

**basement lamina** [Gr. *basis,* base, + L. *lamina,* thin plate] The preferred term for a thin layer of delicate noncellular material of a fine filamentous texture underlying the epithelium. Its principal component is collagen. SYN: *basal lamina; basement membrane; hyaline membrane.*

**basement membrane** Basement lamina.

**base pair** In the double-stranded helical arrangement of DNA, the connecting chemicals (i.e., base pairs) are either an adenine-thymine pair or a guanine-cytosine pair. These base pairs connect the helical strands of DNA like the steps of a spiral staircase.

**baseplate** (bās'plāt) A temporary, preformed shape made of wax, metal, or acrylic resin that represents the base of a denture; used in assessing the relations of maxillary-mandibular teeth or for placement of artificial teeth in denture preparation.

**basi-** [Gr. *basis,* base] SEE: *basio-.*

**basial** (bā'sē-ăl) [L. *basialis*] Pert. to the basion.

**basiarachnoiditis** (bā″sē-ă-răk″noy-dī'tĭs) [Gr. *basis,* base, + *arachne,* spider, + *eidos,* form, shape, + *itis,* inflammation] Inflammation of the arachnoid membrane at the base of the brain.

**basic 1.** In chemistry, possessing the properties of a base. **2.** Fundamental.

**basicranial axis** (bā″sē-krā'nē-ăl) [″ + *kranion,* skull, + *axis,* pivot] A straight line from the basion to point of angle of mandible.

**basic salt** A compound formed when only part of the hydroxide radicals of a base is replaced by the acid radical of an acid.

**Basic Trauma Life Support** ABBR: BTLS. A continuing education program sponsored by the American College of Emergency Physicians for emergency medical personnel to develop the skills of rapid assessment, treatment, and transportation of the traumatized person.

**Basidiomycetes** (bă-sĭd″ē-ō-mī-sē'tēz) One of the four major classes of true fungi of the division Eumycetes, which includes toadstools, mushrooms, and tree fungi. This type of fungus is distinguished by basidiospores, sexual spores that form on a specialized structure called a basidium. Basidiomycetes cause plant diseases, and their toxins may be lethal to humans when eaten. Basidiospores have been implicated as a cause of allergic asthma.

**basifacial axis** (bā-sē-fā'shăl) [″ + L. *facies,* face, + Gr. *axis,* pivot] A straight line from the point of the angle of the mandible to the subnasal point.

**basihyal** (bā″sē-hī'ăl) [″ + *oeides,* hyoid] The body of the hyoid bone.

**basilar** (băs'ĭ-lăr) [L. *basilaris*] Basal (1).

**basilateral** (bā″sē-lăt'ĕr-ăl) [″ + L. *lateralis,* pert. to the side] Both lateral and basilar.

**basilic** (bă-sĭl'ĭk) [L. *basilicus*] Prominent, important.

***b. vein*** The large vein on the inner side of the biceps just above the elbow. It is usually chosen for intravenous injection or withdrawal of blood.

**basin** An open, bowl-like container for holding liquids. It may be shaped to fit around a structure.

***emesis b.*** A kidney-shaped basin that can fit close to the neck so vomit may be collected.

**basio-, basi-** [Gr. *basis,* base] Combining form meaning *base* or *foundation.*

**basioccipital bone** (bā″sē-ŏk-sĭp'ĭ-tăl) [″ + L. *occiput,* head] The basilar process of the occipital bone.

**basion** (bā'sē-ŏn) The midpoint of the anterior border of the foramen magnum.

**basiphobia** (bā″sē-fō'bē-ă) [Gr. *basis,* a stepping, + *phobos,* fear] Fear of walking.

**basirhinal** (bā-sē-rī'năl) [Gr. *basis,* base, + *rhis,* nose] Pert. to the base of the brain and the nose.

**basis** (bā'sĭs) *pl.* **bases** [L., Gr.] The base of a structure or organ.

**basisphenoid** (bā-sē-sfē'noyd) [Gr. *basis,* base, + *sphen,* wedge, + *eidos,* form, shape] An embryonic bone that becomes the lower portion of the sphenoid bone.

**basket** [ME.] A netlike terminal arborization of an axon (or its collateral) of a basket cell that forms a network about the cell body of a Purkinje cell.

**Basle Nomina Anatomica** ABBR: BNA. An official anatomical nomenclature adopted by the German Anatomical Society in 1895, at Basel, Switzerland. It includes some 4500 terms. Revisions were published until 1955, when the Congress of Anatomists modified the nomenclature and applied the name Nomina Anatomica. SEE: *Nomina Anatomica.*

**basophil(e)** (bā'sō-fĭl, -fīl) [Gr. *basis,* base, + *philein,* to love] **1.** A cell or part of a cell that stains readily with basic dyes such as methylene blue. **2.** A type of cell found in the anterior lobe of the pituitary gland. It produces corticotropin, the substance that stimulates the adrenal cortex to secrete adrenocortical hormone. **3.** One type of granulocytic white blood cell. Basophils make up less than 1% of all leukocytes but are essential to the nonspecific immune response to inflammation because of their important role in releasing histamine and other chemicals that act on blood vessels. SEE: *blood* for illus.

**basophilia** (bā-sō-fĭl'ē-ă) **1.** A pathological condition in which basophilic erythrocytes are found in the blood. **2.** A condition marked by a high number of basophilic leukocytes in the blood.

**basophilic** (bā-sō-fĭl'ĭk) Pert. to the staining characteristics of various cells.

**basophilism** (bā-sŏf'ĭ-lĭzm) A condition marked by an excessive number of basophils in the blood.

***pituitary b.*** Cushing's syndrome.

**basophobia** (bās-ō-fō'bē-ă) [Gr. *basis,* a stepping, + *phobos,* fear] **1.** Abnormal fear of walking. **2.** Emotional inability to stand or walk in the absence of muscle disease.

**Bassen-Kornzweig syndrome** [Frank A. Bassen, U.S. physician, b. 1903; Abraham L. Kornzweig, U.S. physician, b. 1900] Abetalipoproteinemia.

**Bassini's operation** (bă-sē'nēz) [Edoardo Bassini, It. surgeon, 1844–1924] A specific surgical procedure for inguinal hernia.

**bath** [AS. *baeth*] The medium and method of cleansing the body or any part of it, or treating it therapeutically as with air, light, vapor, or water. The temperature of the cleansing bath for a bed patient should be about 95°F (35°C) with a room temperature of 75° to 80°F (23.9° to 26.7°C). SEE: table.

THERAPEUTIC EFFECT: Warm and hot baths and applications soothe both the mind and the body. Thus they tend to calm and relax a nervous, agitated patient. Gradually elevated hot tub and vapor baths relax all the muscles of the body. Hot baths promote vasodilation in the skin, drawing blood from the deeper tissues, and also help to relieve pain and stimulate nerves. Cold baths and applications abstract heat and stimulate reaction, esp. if followed by brisk rubbing of the skin. Cold contracts small blood vessels when applied locally. SEE: *hydrotherapy.*

***air b.*** The therapeutic use of air, warmed or vaporized, on the nude body.

**Bath Temperatures for Treating Hyperthermia or Hyperpyrexia**

| Rectal Temperature | | Water Should Be | |
|---|---|---|---|
| F | C | F | C |
| 103° | 39.4° | 90° | 32.2° |
| 104° | 40° | 86° | 30° |
| 104.5° | 40.3° | 82° | 27.8° |
| 105° | 40.6° | 76° | 24.4° |
| 105.5° | 40.8° | 60°–70° | 15.6°–21.1° |

***alcohol b.*** Application of a diluted alcohol solution to the skin as a stimulant and defervescent.

***alkaline b.*** A bath in which 8 oz (227 g) of sodium bicarbonate or washing soda is added to 30 gal (114 L) of water.

***alum b.*** A bath using alum in washing solution as an astringent.

***antipyretic b.*** A cool water bath (65° to 75°F or 18.3° to 28.9°C). The patient should not be cooled to the point of shivering, as this indicates excessive heat loss.

***aromatic b.*** A bath to which some volatile oil, perfume, or some herb is added.

***astringent b.*** Bathing in liquid containing an astringent.

***bed b.*** A bath for a patient confined to bed.

NURSING IMPLICATIONS: All necessary equipment is assembled, the room temperature adjusted to a comfortable level, and the room checked for drafts. While shielding the patient, the nurse removes the top covers and replaces them with a bath blanket for the patient's physical warmth. The patient's ability to bathe independently is assessed, and the patient is encouraged to do so to the extent possible and permitted. Bath water should be comfortably warm, 110° to 120°F (43.3° to 48.1°C), and the water changed as often as necessary to maintain the desired temperature and to permit thorough rinsing. The entire body, including the perineal area and genitalia, is washed, rinsed, and dried thoroughly, one area at a time. The patient remains covered except for the area being bathed. After the bath, lotion is applied to the skin, a clean gown applied, the bed remade with clean linens, and the patient's hair combed or brushed. Oral hygiene is performed in conjunction with bathing; the nurse helps if the patient requires it. When bathing obese patients, the nurse may facilitate the drying of crevices by using a hand-held hair dryer. Additional hair care (shampoo, dry shampoo, styling) is provided as necessary, following protocols.

***bland b.*** Bath containing substances such as starch, bran, or oatmeal for the relief of skin irritation; an emollient bath.

***brine b.*** Saline b.

***bubble b.*** A bath in which the water contains many small bubbles produced mechanically as by an air pump or chemically by bubble bath preparations.

Caution: Perfumes used in bubble baths are frequently the cause of vaginitis and skin irritation, esp. in children.

***carbon dioxide b.*** An effervescent saline bath consisting of water, salts, and carbon dioxide ($CO_2$). The natural $CO_2$ baths are known as Nauheim baths.

***cold b.*** A bath in water at a temperature below 65°F (18.3°C).

***colloid b.*** Emollient b.

***continuous b.*** A bath administered for an extended period but seldom for longer than several hours. It is used in treating hypothermia or hyperthermia and certain skin diseases.

***contrast b.*** Alternate immersion of hands or feet in hot water (1 min) then cold water (30 sec) for a prescribed length of time to promote circulation. The initial water temperature should be maintained throughout the bath, and the bath should end with immersion in cold water.

***emollient b.*** A bath used for irritation and inflammation of skin and after erysipelas. SYN: *colloid b.* SEE: *glycerin b; oatmeal b; powdered borax b; starch b.*

***foam b.*** A tub bath to which an extract of a saponin-containing vegetable fiber has been added. Oxygen or carbon dioxide is driven through this mixture to create foam.

***foot b.*** Immersion of the feet and legs to a depth of 4 in. (10 cm) above the ankles in water at 98°F (36.7°C).

***full b.*** A bath in which the whole body except the head is immersed in water.

***glycerin b.*** A bath consisting of 10 oz (300 ml) of glycerin added to 30 gal (114 L) water.

***herb b.*** A full bath to which is added a mixture of 1 to 2 lb (454 to 907 g) of herbs such as chamomile, wild thyme, or spearmint tied in a bag and boiled with 1 gal (3.8 L) of water.

***hip b.*** Sitz b.

***hot b.*** A tub bath with the water covering the body to slightly above the nipple level. The temperature is gradually raised from 98°F (36.7°C) to the desired degree, usually to 108°F (42.2°C).

***hot air b.*** Exposure of entire body except head to hot air in a bath cabinet.

***hyperthermal b.*** A bath in which the whole body except the head is immersed in water from 105° to 120°F (40.6° to 48.9°C) for 1 to 2 min.

***kinetotherapeutic b.*** A bath given for underwater exercises of weak or partially paralyzed muscles.

***lukewarm b.*** A bath in which patient's body except head is immersed in water from 94° to 96°F (34.4° to 35.6°C) for 15 to 60 min.

***medicated b.*** A bath to which substances such as bran, oatmeal, starch, sodium bicarbonate, Epsom salts, pine products, tar, sulfur, potassium permanganate, and salt are added.

***milk b.*** A bath taken in milk for emollient purposes.

***mud b.*** The use of mud in order to apply moist heat.

***mustard b.*** A stimulative hot foot bath consisting of a mixture of 1 tablespoon (15 ml) of dry mustard in a quart (946 ml) of hot water added to a pail or large basin filled with water of 100° to 104°F (37.8° to 40°C).

***Nauheim b.*** A bath in which the body is immersed in warm water through which carbon dioxide is bubbled.

***needle b.*** A bath in which water is forcibly sprayed on the body in fine jet streams.

***neutral b.*** A bath in which no circulatory or thermic reaction occurs, temperature 92° to 97°F (33.3° to 36.1°C).

***neutral sitz b.*** Same as sitz bath, except temperature is 92° to 97°F (33.3° to 36.1°C) or for foot bath 104° to 110°F (37.8° to 40°C), duration 15 to 60 min.

***oatmeal b.*** A bath consisting of 2 to 3 lb (907 g to 1.4 kg) oatmeal added to 30 gal (114 L) water.

***oxygen b.*** A bath given by introducing oxygen into the water through a special device that is connected to an oxygen tank.

***paraffin b.*** A bath used to apply topical heat to traumatized or inflamed limbs. The limb is repeatedly immersed in warm paraffin, 104° to 150°F (37.8° to 65.6°C), and quickly withdrawn until it is encased in layers of the material. Paraffin may be applied with a paintbrush for larger joints.

***powdered borax b.*** Bath consisting of ½ lb (227 g) added to 30 gal (114 L) water; 5 oz (150 ml) glycerin may be added.

***saline b.*** Bath given in artificial seawater made by dissolving 8 lb (3.6 kg) of sea salt or a mixture of 7 lb (3.2 kg) of sodium chloride and ½ lb (227 g) of magnesium sulfate in 30 gal (114 L) of water. SYN: *brine b; salt b; seawater b.*

***salt b.*** Saline b.

***sauna b.*** A hot, humid atmosphere created in a small enclosed area by pouring water on heated rocks.

***seawater b.*** Saline b.

***sedative b.*** A prolonged warm bath. A continuous flow of water as well as an air cushion or back rest may be used.

***sheet b.*** A bath given by wrapping the patient in a sheet previously dipped in water 80° to 90°F (26.7° to 32.2°C), and by rubbing the whole body with vigorous strokes on the sheet.

***shower b.*** Water sprayed down upon the body from an overhead source.

***sitz b.*** The immersion of thighs, buttocks, and abdomen below the umbilicus in water. In a hot sitz bath the water is first 92°F (33.3°C) and then elevated to 106°F (41.1°C). SYN: *hip b.*

***sponge b.*** A bath in which patient is not immersed in a tub but washed with a washcloth or sponge.

***starch b.*** A bath consisting of 1 lb (454 g) of starch mixed into cold water, with boiling water added to make a solution of gluelike consistency, then added to 30 gal (114 L) of water.

***stimulating b.*** A bath that increases cutaneous blood flow. SEE: *cold b.; mustard b.; saline b.*

***sun b.*** Exposure of all or part of the nude body to sunlight.

***sweat b.*** A bath given to induce perspiration.

***towel b.*** A bath given by applying towels dipped in water 60° to 70°F (15.6° to 21.1°C) to the arms, legs, and anterior and posterior surfaces of trunk, and then removing the towels and drying the parts.

***whirlpool b.*** A bath consisting of continuous localized jets of water at a temperature of 105° to 120°F (40.6° to 48.9°C) that agitate the water into which the body or a part of it is immersed.

**bathophobia** (băth″ō-fō′bē-ă) [Gr. *bathos,* deep, + *phobos,* fear] Abnormal fear of depths; commonly refers to fear of height or of looking down from a high place.

**bathyanesthesia** (băth-ē-ăn″ĕs-thē′zē-ă) [″ + *an-,* not, + *aisthesis,* sensation] Loss of deep sensibility.

**bathyesthesia** (băth″ē-ĕs-thē′zē-ă) [″ + *aisthesis,* sensation] A consciousness or sensibility of parts of the body beneath the skin.

**bathyhyperesthesia** (băth-ē-hī″pĕr-ĕs-thē′zē-ă) [″ + *hyper,* above, + *aisthesis,* sensation] Excessive sensitivity of muscles and other deep body structures.

**bathyhypesthesia** (băth″ē-hīp″ĕs-thē′zē-ă) [″ + *hypo,* under, + *aisthesis,* sensation] Impairment of sensitivity in muscles and other deep body structures.

**Batten disease** [Frederick E. Batten, English ophthalmologist, 1865–1918] A hereditary disturbance of metabolism that results in blindness and mental retardation. SYN: *Spielmeyer-Vogt disease.* SEE: *sphingolipidosis.*

**battered child syndrome** Physical abuse of a child by an adult, usually a parent or guardian, often under circumstances that make it appear that the injury was accidental. The child may exhibit bruises, scratches, burns, hematomas, or fractures of the long bones, ribs, or skull. Poor skin hygiene and some degree of malnutrition also may be present. SEE: *child abuse; shaken baby syndrome; Nursing Diagnoses Appendix.*

ETIOLOGY: Most parents or guardians of abused children were abused as children themselves.

DIAGNOSIS: The most distinguishing feature is variation in the stages of healing of bone lesions seen in radiographic images, indicating injuries incurred at different times.

PROGNOSIS: Prognosis is variable. The death rate is high, and surviving children often suffer from long-term physical and mental injuries and may become abusive parents. If a child has been abused by parents, it is important to examine the child's siblings because about 20% of them will have signs of physical abuse. That examination should be done without delay to prevent further abuse of children in that home.

**battered woman syndrome** A pattern of repeated physical assault of a woman by her husband or partner. Typically, the pattern begins with verbal abuse and progresses to increasingly violent physical abuse and sometimes death. Estimates indicate that over one million women a year are victims. Shelters for battered women are available in many cities. Frequently, women are afraid to report this type of abuse because they feel trapped in the relationship. Women from any socioeconomic level may be affected.

**battery** [Fr. *battre,* to beat] **1.** A device for generating electric current by chemical action. **2.** A series of tests, procedures, or diagnostic examinations given to or done on a patient. **3.** The unlawful touching of another without consent, justification or excuse. In legal medicine, battery occurs if a medical or surgical procedure is performed without proper consent. SEE: *assault; sexual harassment.*

**Battle sign** [William Henry Battle, Brit. surgeon, 1855–1936] Bogginess of the temporal or postauricular region of the head, which indicates fracture of the basilar area of the skull.

**Baudelocque's diameter** (bōd-lŏks′) [Jean Louis Baudelocque, Sr., Fr. obstetrician, 1746–1810] The distance between the depression beneath the last lumbar vertebra and the margin of the symphysis pubis; the external conjugate diameter of the pelvis. SYN: *Baudelocque's line.*

**Baudelocque's method** In obstetrics, manipulation to convert a fetal face presentation into a vertex presentation.

**Baumé scales** (bō-mā′) [Antoine Baumé, Fr. chemist, 1728–1805] Hydrometer scales for determination of the specific gravity of liquids.

**bay** (bā) An anatomical recess or depression filled with liquid.

**Bayes' theorem** [Thomas Bayes, Brit. mathematician, 1702–1761] A theorem, published posthumously in 1764, concerned with analyzing the probability that a patient may have a certain diagnosis or disease when it is known that the patient has certain attributes such as an abnormal test. It is usually known how frequently that particular attribute is present in the population considered to have the specific disease. Two reasons for applying this theorum are to determine the probability that a positive test result indicates the presence of the disease and the probability that a negative test is found even though the patient actually has the disease.

**Bayley Scales of Infant Development** A standardized battery of tests used to provide information about the developmental status of children aged 2 to 30 months. The battery is designed to indicate motor, mental and behavioral levels based on performance and parental reports.

**Bazin's disease** (bă-zăz′) [Antoine P.E. Bazin, Fr. dermatologist, 1807–1878] A chronic skin disease occurring in young adult females; characterized by hard cutaneous nodules that break down to form necrotic ulcers that leave atrophic scars. The disease is almost invariably preceded by tuberculosis, but the etiological relationship to that disease is debated. SYN: *erythema induratum.*

**BCAA** *branched-chain amino acids.*

**B-cell–mediated immunity** SEE: *immunity, humoral.*

**BCG vaccine** Bacille Calmette-Guérin vaccine, a form of tuberculosis vaccine that consists of a freeze-dried preparation of a live, attenuated strain of *Mycobacterium bovis.* It is used to immunize children against tuberculosis, but its efficacy is questionable. BCG vaccine is indicated in a tuberculin-negative infant who resides in a household in which repeated exposure to untreated or ineffectively treated cases of tuberculosis occurs. It may also be instilled in the bladder to prevent recurrence of bladder tumors. SEE: *bacille Calmette-Guérin.*

**b.d.** L. *bis die,* twice a day.

**Bdellovibrio** [Gr. *bdella,* leech, + *vibrio*] A parasite that invades bacteria by forming a hole in the cell wall. It lives and reproduces inside the cell.

**B.E.** *below elbow,* a term that refers to the site of amputation of an arm; *barium enema.*

**Be** Symbol for the element beryllium.

**beaded** (bēd′ĕd) Referring to disjointed colonies along the inoculation line in a streak or stab culture.

**beads, rachitic** Visible swelling where the ribs join their cartilages, seen in rickets. SYN: *rachitic rosary.*

**beaker** (bē′kĕr) A widemouthed glass vessel for mixing or holding liquids.

**beam 1.** In nuclear medicine and radiology, a group of atomic particles traveling a parallel course. **2.** The part of an analytical balance to which the weighing pans are attached. **3.** A long, slender piece of wood, metal, or plastic resin that serves as a support in some part of a dental appliance.

**beard** The hair on the face and throat.

**bearing down** The expulsive effort of a parturient woman in the second stage of labor. Valsalva's maneuver is used, causing increased pressure against the uterus by increasing intra-abdominal pressure.

**beat** [AS. *beatan,* to strike] A pulsation or throb as in contraction of the heart or the passage of blood through a vessel.

***apex b.*** The impulse of the heartbeat felt by the hand when held over the fifth intercostal space in the left midclavicular line.

***artificially paced b.*** A heartbeat stimulated by an artificial pacemaker.

***capture b.*** A ventricular contraction responding to an impulse from the sinus that reaches the atrioventricular node at a time at which the node is nonrefractory.

***dropped b.*** The absence of a ventricular contraction of the heart.

***ectopic b.*** A heartbeat beginning at a place other than the sinoatrial node.

***escape b.*** A heartbeat that occurs after a prolonged pause, or failure of the sinus node to stimulate the heart to contract.

***forced b.*** Extrasystole brought on by artificial heart stimulation.

***premature b.*** A heartbeat that arises from a site other than the sinus node and occurs early in the cardiac cycle before the expected sinus beat.

**Beau's lines** (bōz) [Joseph Honoré Simon Beau, Fr. physician, 1806–1865] White lines across the fingernails, usually a sign of systemic disease. They may be due to trauma, coronary occlusion, hypercalcemia, or skin disease. The lines are visible until the affected area of the nail has grown out and been trimmed away.

**Bechterew's reflex, Bekhterev's reflex** (bĕk′tĕr-ĕvs) [Vladimir Mikhailovich von Bechterew, Russ. neurologist, 1857–1927] **1.** Contraction of the facial muscles due to irritation of the nasal mucosa. **2.** Dilatation of the pupil on exposure to light. **3.** Contraction of the lower abdominal muscles when the skin on the inner thigh is stroked.

**Beck's triad** Signs seen with pericardial tamponade, consisting of hypotension, distended neck veins, and muffled heart sounds.

**beclomethasone dipropionate** A corticosteroid drug. Trade names are Vancenase and Beclovent inhaler.

**becquerel** (bĕk′rĕl) [Antoine Henri Becquerel, French physicist, 1852–1908] SYMB: Bq. An SI-derived unit of measure of activity of a radionuclide equal to one spontaneous nuclear transition per second. It is equal to $3.7 \times 10^{10}$ curies. SEE: *curie; SI Units Appendix.*

**bed** [AS. *bedd*] **1.** A supporting structure or tissue. **2.** A couch or support for the body during sleep.

***air b.*** A bed inflated with air.

***air-fluidized b.*** A bed consisting of a mattress filled with approx. 100 billion ceramic spheres that are suspended by a continuous flow of warm air at the rate of approx. 40 cu ft/ min. This creates a surface that feels like a liquid, having a specific gravity of 1.3. The patient "floats" on the mattress with only minimal penetration. Because of the even distribution of weight, the bed is particularly useful in treating patients with burns or decubitus ulcers. Nursing care of the patient is simplified because the patient can be moved by fingertip pressure.

***b. blocks*** Blocks of sturdy material, usually wood, placed under the legs of a bed to elevate one end of it. Raising the foot of the bed may be useful in treatment of shock, inguinal hernia, bleeding from the lower limbs, or edema of the lower limbs, vulva, or scrotum. It may also be helpful when weight is used on the lower limbs or when a patient has difficulty with enema retention. Raising the head of the bed may be used to drain the abdomen or pelvis, to treat congestive heart failure, to aid respiration, or to treat bleeding from the head, neck, or upper chest.

***b. board*** A firm board placed beneath a mattress to keep it from sagging. It is used to treat some persons with back difficulties. SEE: *board, back.*

***capillary b.*** A network of capillaries.

***circular b.*** A bed that allows a patient to be turned end-over-end while held between two frames. This permits turning the patients without disturbing them by turning the two frames inside a circular apparatus that holds the ends of the frames. It is useful in treating paralyzed or immobilized patients. SYN: *Circ-O-Lectric bed.*

***float b.*** A bed in which the patient is supported either on a water mattress or on minute ceramic beads with air flowing through them. This type of bed is useful for patients with decubitus ulcers or burns.

***flotation b.*** A bed in which the patient reclines in a hollow, flexible, mattress-shaped device filled with water. This enables equal distribution of pressure on the body. It is used to treat and prevent decubiti.

***fracture b.*** A bed for patients who have fractures.

***Gatch b.*** An adjustable bed that provides elevation of the back and the knees.

***hydrostatic b.*** Water b.

***kinetic b.*** A bed that constantly turns patients side to side through 270°. It is used to prevent the hazards of immobility in patients requiring prolonged bedrest, as in multiple trauma and some neuromuscular diseases. Trademark is Roto-Bed. SEE: *Circ-O-Lectric bed.*

***metabolic b.*** A bed arranged to facilitate collection of feces and urine of a patient so that metabolic studies can be done.

***nail b.*** The skin that lies beneath a nail at the tip of a digit.

***open b.*** A bed available for assignment to a patient.

***recovery b.*** A bed, usually a portable bed or stretcher, prepared to receive a patient immediately after surgery.

***rocking b.*** A device used to create abdominal displacement ventilation in patients with respiratory failure.

***surgical b.*** A bed equipped with a mechanism by which the head or the foot of the bed can be raised or lowered independently of each other.

***tilt b.*** SEE: *table, tilt.*

***water b.*** A water-filled rubber mattress used for prevention of bedsores. SYN: *hydrostatic b.* SEE: *flotation b.*

**bedbug** An insect, *Cimex lectularius* of the family *Cimicidae,* the saliva of which contains an irritating substance that causes a purpuric reaction or an urticarial wheal. The adult bugs are about 4 to 5 mm in length and survive for up to a year without feeding and at low temperature. The female ingests 0.0185 ml of blood each feeding, and the male 0.015 ml. Bedbugs can be a cause of anemia in infants. There is much speculation but no proof that bedbugs transmit diseases to humans, either through bites or infected feces. Treatment for bites consists of application of antipruritic lotions containing phenol, camphor, and menthol. Infestation control is largely a matter of cleanliness. In heavy infestations, an appropriate insecticide should be used to spray furniture, mattresses, floors, baseboards, and walls. The use of wooden frames for beds should be avoided, as this provides a nesting and breeding site for these insects.

**bedfast** Unable or unwilling to leave the bed; bedridden.

**bedlam** [From Hospital of St. Mary of Bethlehem, pronounced Bedlem in Middle English.] **1.** An asylum for the insane. **2.** Any place or situation characterized by a noisy uproar.

**Bednar's aphthae** [Alois Bednar, physician in Vienna, 1816–1888] Infected, traumatic ulcers appearing on the hard palate of infants; usually caused by sucking infected objects.

**bedpan** [AS. *bedd,* bed, + *panna,* flat vessel] A pan-shaped device placed under a bedridden patient for collecting fecal and urinary excreta.

NOTE: In general, because bedpan use is uncomfortable and awkward, it requires more exertion on the patient's part than using a bedside toilet. Patients, esp. those recovering from myocardial infarction, should not be forced to use a bedpan if it is possible for them to use a bedside toilet.

**bedrest 1.** A device for propping up patients in bed. **2.** The confining of a patient to bed for rest.

**bedridden** Unable or unwilling to leave the bed; bedfast.

**bedsore** [AS. *bedd,* bed, + *sare,* open wound] Decubitus ulcer.

**bedwetting** Enuresis.

**BEE** *basal energy expenditure.*

**bee** [AS. *beo,* bee] An insect of the order Hymenoptera and superfamily Apoidea. Included is the common honeybee, *Apis mellifera,* which produces honey and beeswax.

***b. sting*** Injury resulting from bee venom and causing pain, redness, and swelling. The stinger of the honeybee has multiple barbs that usually anchor it in the skin. The stinger, if present, should be removed and the area cooled as quickly and efficiently as possible to prevent the venom from entering the general circulation. To prevent further injection of venom, the stinger should be grasped gently by fingernails or forceps. Fairly strong household ammonia or a baking soda paste can be applied. If pain is severe, an injection of 2% procaine solution may be needed. Antihistamines help to relieve discomfort.

---

Caution: Some individuals are hypersensitive to bee venom and may suffer severe anaphylactic reactions leading to death. In such cases immediate subcutaneous or intravenous administration of epinephrine is indicated.

---

**Beer's law** [August Beer, Ger. physicist, 1825–1863] The basic law, also known as the Beer-Lambert or Bougher-Beer law, that is the foundation for all absorption photometry. It predicts the linear relationship between the absorbance (A) of a solution and its concentration (c). Given as: $A = \epsilon lc$, where A = absorbance, $\epsilon$ = molar absorptivity, l = path distance, and c = concentration.

**Beer's operation** [Georg Joseph Beer, Ger. ophthalmologist, 1763–1821] A flap operation for cataract or artificial pupil.

**beeswax** (bēz'wăks) Yellow wax obtained from the honeycomb of bees. A purified form is used in ointments.

**beeturia** (bēt-ū'rē-ă) Deep red or pink coloration of urine caused by betanin, the pigment in beets. This condition is common in iron-deficient adults and children and can occur after ingestion of even one beet.

**behavior** [ME. *behaven,* to hold oneself in a certain way] **1.** The manner in which one acts; the actions or reactions of individuals under specific circumstances. **2.** Any response elicited from an organism.

***self-consoling b.'s*** The self-quieting actions of infants, such as sucking on their fists and watching mobiles and other moving objects.

***self-injurious b.*** ABBR: SIB. Maladaptive behaviors of various types, sometimes exhibited by persons with mental retardation; they include self-scratching, repeated head banging, and other potentially dangerous acts. The cause is unknown, but one theory is that the behaviors are self-stimulatory.

***type A b.*** A behavior pattern marked by the characteristics of competitiveness, aggressivity, easily aroused hostility, and an overdeveloped sence of urgency. The importance of this type of behavior pattern in coronary artery disease, hypertension, and peptic ulcer may be considerable. The risk of accidents, suicide, and murder is higher in type A individuals.

***type B b.*** A behavior pattern that is best defined by the absence of the factors present in the type A behavior pattern.

**behavioral science** The science concerned with all aspects of behavior.

**behavioral system model** A conceptual model of nursing developed by Dorothy Johnson. The person is regarded as a behavioral system with seven subsystems—attachment, dependency, ingestion, elimination, sexual, aggression, achievement. The goal of nursing is to restore, maintain, or attain behavioral system balance and stability. SEE: *Nursing Theory Appendix.*

**behaviorism** A theory of conduct that regards normal and abnormal behavior as the result of conditioned reflexes quite apart from the concept of will. It does not apply to conditions resulting from organic disease.

**behavior therapy** Various techniques used to change maladaptive behaviors, based on principles of learning theory. Cigarette smoking, eating disorders, and alcohol abuse are commonly treated through behavior therapy, which may include the use of positive reinforcement, aversive conditioning, discrimination, and modeling.

**Behçet's syndrome** (bā'sĕts) [Hulusi Behçet, Turkish dermatologist, 1889–1948] A multisystem, chronic, recurrent disease marked by ulceration of the mouth and genitalia and by iritis, uveitis, arthritis, and thrombophlebitis. The joint pain usually comes later in the history of the disease than the ulcers of the mouth and genitalia. Iritis is often accompanied by conjunctivitis, episcleritis, keratitis, retinal thrombophlebitis, and optic atrophy. The central nervous system, heart, and intestinal tract may be involved. The disease occurs worldwide, but is most common in the eastern Mediterranean area and eastern Asia. In these areas it occurs mostly in young men and is a leading cause of blindness. In the Western world, where the disease is less severe, it affects men twice as frequently as it does women but is not a leading cause of blindness. The period between attacks is irregular, but may be as short as days or as long as years. Needle punctures provoke inflammatory skin lesions and, for that reason, should be avoided.

TREATMENT: Immunosuppressive therapy (e.g., chlorambucil) is helpful. Corticosteroids control serious inflammation until the immunosuppressive agents begin to have an effect. The immunosuppressive agent azathioprine has been found to prevent progression of Behçet's syndrome.

**bejel** (bĕj'ĕl) A nonvenereal form of syphilis endemic in Arab countries; children are especially susceptible.

**bel** (bĕl) SYMB: B. A unit of measurement of the intensity of sound. It is expressed as a logarithm of the ratio of two sounds of acoustic intensity, one of which is fixed or standard; the ratio is expressed in decibels.

**belch** [AS. *baelcan,* to eructate] **1.** To expel

gas from the stomach through the mouth; to eructate. 2. An act of belching; eructation.

**belching** Raising of gas from the stomach and expelling it through the mouth and nose. For belching to occur, there is first an increase in gastric pressure; then the lower esophagus sphincter relaxes to allow equalization of pressure in the stomach and esophagus. Relaxation of the upper esophagus sphincter allows the gas to escape through the pharynx and mouth. SEE: *water brash.*

ETIOLOGY: Belching may be caused by gastric fermentation, air swallowing, or ingestion of carbonated drinks or gas-producing foods.

**belemnoid** (bē-lĕm′noyd) [Gr. *belemnon,* dart, + *eidos,* form, shape] Dart-shaped; styloid.

**Bell, Sir Charles** Scottish physiologist and surgeon, 1774–1842.

***B.'s law, B.-Magendie's law*** The fact that anterior spinal nerve roots contain only motor fibers and posterior roots only sensory fibers.

***B.'s nerve*** Long thoracic nerve; nervus thoracicus longus.

***B.'s palsy*** Unilateral facial paralysis of sudden onset. The patient cannot control salivation or lacrimation and, in severe cases, cannot close the eye on the affected side. Facial expression is distorted. The cause is unknown but is presumed to involve swelling of the seventh (facial) nerve due to immune or viral disease, resulting in ischemia and compression of the nerve at the point where it leaves the bony tissue. Either the right or left side of the face may be affected, and less than 1% of cases will have bilateral involvement. Attacks recur in about 10% of cases.

TREATMENT: The affected eye should be protected by a temporary patch or by methylcellulose drops. Corticosteroids, such as 60 to 80 mg of oral prednisone per day for 1 week (with a smaller dosage the second week), may decrease acute pain.

PROGNOSIS: Partial facial paralysis is usually resolved within several months. The likelihood of complete recovery after total paralysis varies from 20% to 90%.

***B.'s phenomenon*** Rolling of the eyeball upward and outward when an attempt is made to close the eye on the side of the face affected in peripheral facial paralysis.

**belladonna** (bĕl″ă-dŏn′ă) [It., beautiful lady] An anticholinergic derived from *Atropa belladonna,* a poisonous plant with reddish flowers and shiny black berries. Belladonna is the source of various alkaloids (stramonium, hyoscyamus, scopolamine, and atropine) and is used mainly for its sedative and spasmolytic effects on the gastrointestinal tract. All alkaloids derived from belladonna are highly toxic. SEE: *atropine in Poisons and Poisoning Appendix.*

***b. leaf*** Powder from the dried leaf and flowering top of *Atropa belladonna Linné* or *A. belladonna acuminata.* An anticholinergic agent, it is used generally in tincture form though the dry extract in tablet form may be used.

**Bellini's tubule** (bĕ-lē′nēz) [Lorenzo Bellini, It. anatomist, 1643–1704] The straight connecting tubule of the kidney.

**bell-metal resonance** In cases of pneumothorax, a metallic sound heard when a coin placed on the chest wall is struck by another coin.

**Bellocq's cannula** (bĕl-ŏks′) [Jean Jacques Bellocq, Fr. surgeon, 1732–1807] An instrument for drawing in a plug through the nostril and mouth to control epistaxis.

**belly** [AS. *baelg,* bag] **1.** The abdomen or abdominal cavity. **2.** The fleshy, central portion of a muscle.

**bellyache** Colic; gastralgia.

**belly button** Umbilicus; navel.

**belonephobia** (bĕl″ō-nĕ-fō′bē-ă) [Gr. *belone,* needle, + *phobos,* fear] Morbid fear of sharp-pointed objects.

**belonoskiascopy** (bĕl″ō-nō-skī-ăs′kō-pē) [″ + *skia,* shadow, + *skopein,* to examine] Subjective retinoscopy by means of shadows and movements to determine refraction.

**Benadryl** (bĕn′ă-drĭl) Trade name for diphenhydramine hydrochloride, an antihistaminic agent.

**Bence Jones protein** [Henry Bence Jones, Brit. physician, 1814–1873] A protein that occurs in the urine of patients with multiple myeloma and occasionally in patients with other diseases of the reticuloendothelial system. When urine samples are heated to 50° to 60°C, a precipitate forms. It disappears when the urine is boiled and reappears when the urine cools.

**Bender's Visual Motor Gestalt test** [Lauretta Bender, N.Y. psychiatrist, 1897–1987] A test in which the subject copies a series of patterns. The results vary with the type of psychiatric disorder present.

**Bendopa** Trade name for levodopa.

**bendroflumethiazide** (bĕn″drō-floo″mĕ-thī′ă-zīd) A thiazide-type diuretic. Trade name is Naturetin.

**bends** Pain in the limbs and abdomen caused by bubbles of nitrogen in blood and tissues as a result of rapid reduction of atmospheric pressure. This condition may also develop when a person ascends too rapidly after being exposed to increased pressure while deep sea diving. Pressure should be restored by placing the patient in a hyperbaric chamber and slowly returning to ambient pressure. SEE: *caisson disease; decompression illness; hyperbaric chamber.*

**benediction hand** Paralysis in the intrinsic muscles of the hand innervated by the ulnar nerve. This results in marked flexion of the joints of the fourth and fifth digits so that the hand resembles that of the

Pope when he gives a blessing.

**Benedict's solution** (bĕn′ĕ-dĭkts) [Stanley R. Benedict, U.S. chemist, 1844–1936] A solution used to test for the presence of sugar. To 173 g sodium or potassium citrate and 100 g anhydrous sodium carbonate (dissolved in 700 ml water) is added 17.3 g crystalline copper sulfate that has been dissolved in 100 ml of water. Sufficient water is added to the mixture to make 1000 ml. SEE: *Benedict's test.*

**Benedict's test** A test to determine the presence of sugar in the urine by adding 8 drops of clear urine (filtered if necessary) to a test tube containing 5 ml of Benedict's solution. The mixture is boiled from 1 to 2 min, with the test tube agitated during this time, and is then allowed to cool undisturbed. Formation of red, yellow, olive green, or green precipitate indicates presence of sugar.

**Benedikt's syndrome** [Moritz Benedikt, Austrian physician, 1835–1920] Hemiplegia with oculomotor paralysis and clonic spasm or tremor on the opposite side. It is caused by lesions that damage the third nerve and involve the nucleus ruber and corticospinal tract.

**benefit 1.** Something that promotes health. **2.** A term for service stipulations of an insurance policy, esp. a medical policy.

**Benemid** Trade name for probenecid.

**benign** (bē-nīn′) [L. *benignus,* mild] Not recurrent or progressive; nonmalignant.

**benign forgetfulness** A memory defect marked by the inability to immediately recall a name or date. The item, whether recent or remote, is eventually recalled.

**benign positional vertigo** SEE: *vertigo, benign positional.*

**benign prostatic hypertrophy** ABBR: BPH. A nonmalignant enlargement of the prostate due to excessive growth of prostatic tissue. It is the most common benign neoplasm of the aging human male. It is present in 50% of men by age 60; and by age 85, about 90% of men will have microscopic evidence of BPH. One out of every four men in the U.S. will require treatment for the symptoms of BPH by age 80. More than 300,000 surgical procedures for BPH are performed annually in the U.S. SEE: *Nursing Diagnoses Appendix; prostate; prostate cancer; transurethral resection of the prostate.*

SYMPTOMS: Symptoms include nocturia, a sudden desire to urinate that is difficult to delay (urgency), difficulty in initiating urination, urination that starts and stops, diminished force of the urinary stream, and a feeling that the bladder is not completely emptied after urination.

ETIOLOGY: These symptoms are related to the growth of the prostate pressing on the urethra at the point it leaves the bladder. The hypertrophy may eventually be sufficient to prevent passage of urine from the bladder, causing acute urinary retention.

TREATMENT: If the symptoms are not particularly troublesome to the patient, watchful waiting is an option. In those cases, the patient should be periodically monitored in order to reassess the symptoms. Other treatment options include surgical removal of the excess tissue. This is usually done with an instrument passed through the urethra into the prostate. This is called transurethral resection of the prostate. Balloon dilation of the prostatic urethra is also used; however, it is not suitable when there is enlargement of the middle lobe of the prostate. Medicines that may be used to relax smooth muscle of the bladder neck and prostate include alpha-1 blockers such as terazosin. Other medicines known as 5-alpha reductase inhibitors are used to reduce the size of the prostate. Laser therapy, hyperthermia, and cryotherapy have been used to decrease prostate size. Acute urinary retention is treated by draining the bladder by use of a urethral catheter.

**benign senescent forgetfulness** Minor, nonprogressive memory loss that does not interfere with daily living. This generally is a normal age-related cognitive change.

**Bennett double-ring splint** A metal splint that slips on the finger and limits hyperextension of the proximal interphalangeal joint.

**bentonite** (bĕn′tŏn-īt) [Fort Benton, U.S.] A hydrated aluminosilicate that forms a thick, slippery substance when water is added. It is used as a suspending and clarifying agent. It may be heat-sterilized.

**Bentyl** Trade name for dicyclomine hydrochloride.

**benzaldehyde** (bĕn-zăl′dĕ-hīd) A pharmaceutical flavoring agent derived from oil of bitter almond.

**benzalkonium chloride** (bĕnz″ăl-kō′nē-ŭm klō′rīd) An antimicrobial preservative. White or yellowish-white thick gel. Usually has a mild aromatic odor. In aqueous solution it has a bitter taste. Used as a detergent and germicide. Trade names are Zephiran Chloride, Roccal, and Hyamine 3500.

**benzene, benzin, benzine** (bĕn′zēn, bĕn-zēn′, bĕn′zĭn) [*benz*(oin) + Gr. *ene,* suffix used in chemistry to denote unsaturated compound] $C_6H_6$. A volatile liquid that is the simplest member of the aromatic series of hydrocarbons. It is immiscible with water and it dissolves fats. It is used as a solvent and is used in the synthesis of innumerable dyes and drugs. The phenyl radical, $C_6H_6$, will be recognized in the formulae for phenol, dimethylaminoazobenzene (see under *azo compounds*), and benzoic acid. SYN: *benzol.* SEE: *Poisons and Poisoning Appendix.*

**benzestrol** (bĕn-zĕs′trŏl) A synthetic estrogenic substance used orally.

**benzethonium chloride** (bĕn″zĕ-thō′nē-ŭm) A synthetic quaternary ammonium detergent compound used as a disinfectant and antiseptic. It is incompatible with soap. Trade names are Hyamine 1622 and Phemerol Chloride.

**benzidine** (bĕn′zĭ-dĭn) Compound used as a test to determine traces of blood in feces.

Prepare benzidine solution as follows: to a saturated solution of benzidine in glacial acetic acid add an equal volume of 3% hydrogen peroxide and about 1 ml of the suspected material. Appearance of a blue color indicates the presence of blood.

A diet free of iron-containing foods should be followed for at least 48 hr before the test. This clears the intestinal tract of iron-containing foods and helps to prevent a false-positive test for iron.

**benzoate** (bĕn′zō-āt) A salt of benzoic acid.

**benzocaine** (bĕn′zō-kān) Ethyl aminobenzoate, a local anesthetic used topically. Trade name is Americaine.

**benzodiazepine** (bĕn″zō-dī-ăz′ĕ-pēn) Any of a group of chemically similar psychotropic drugs with potent hypnotic and sedative action; used predominantly as antianxiety and sleep-inducing drugs. Side effects of these drugs may or may not be of importance in a patient. They include impairment of psychomotor performance; amnesia; euphoria; dependence; and rebound (i.e., the return of symptoms) transiently worse than before treatment, upon discontinuation of the drug. Treatment with benzodiazepines should not exceed 4 months.

**benzoic acid** $C_7H_6O_2$. A white crystalline material having a slight odor. It is used in keratolytic ointments and in food preservation. Saccharin is a derivative of this acid.

**benzoin** (bĕn′zoyn, -zō-ĭn) [Fr. *benjoin*] A balsamic resin obtained from trees of various species of *Styrax,* esp. *S. benzoin* or *S. paralleloneuris*. It is used as a stimulant expectorant, as an inhalant in laryngitis and bronchitis, and as a protective coating for ulcers. It is also used as a solution applied to the skin to prepare it for application of adhesives, esp. adhesive tape.

**benzol** Benzene.

**benzonatate** (bĕn-zō′nă-tāt) A substance chemically related to procaine; used in anticough preparations. Trade name is Tessalon.

**benzoyl peroxide** A keratolytic agent. Trade name is Benoxyl.

**benzthiazide** (bĕnz-thī′ă-zīd) A diuretic agent.

**benztropine mesylate** (bĕnz′trō-pēn) An antiparasympathomimetic agent usually used with other drugs in treating parkinsonism. Trade name is Cogentin.

**benzyl** The hydrocarbon radical of benzyl alcohol and various other compounds.

***b. benzoate*** An aromatic, clear, colorless oily liquid with a sharp, burning taste. It is used as a topical scabicide. Trade name is Benylate.

**benzylpenicillin procaine** (bĕn″zĭl-pĕn-ĭ-sĭl′ĭn) Penicillin G procaine.

**Bérard's aneurysm** (bā-rărz′) [Auguste Bérard, Fr. surgeon, 1802–1846] An arteriovenous aneurysm in the tissues surrounding the injured vein.

**Béraud's valve** (bā-rōz′) [Bruno J.J. Béraud, Fr. surgeon, 1823–1865] A fold of mucous membrane of the lacrimal sac at the junction of the lacrimal duct. SYN: *Krause's valve*.

**berdache** (bĕr-dăsh′) [Fr.] An individual of a definite sex, male or female, who assumes the status and role of the opposite sex and who is viewed by the community as being of one physiologic sex but as having assumed the status and role of the opposite sex. Transvestism is not synonymous with berdache, nor is homosexual behavior necessarily a component of this condition.

**bereavement** The expected reactions of grief and sadness upon learning of the loss of a loved one. The period of bereavement is associated with increased mortality. It is important for those who care for the bereaved to emphasize human resilience and the power of life rather than the stress that accompanies bereavement.

**beriberi** (bĕr′ē-bĕr′ē) [Singhalese *beri,* weakness] A disease marked by peripheral neurologic, cerebral, and cardiovascular abnormalities and caused by a lack of thiamine. Early deficiency produces fatigue, irritation, poor memory, sleep disturbances, precordial pain, anorexia, abdominal discomfort, and constipation. Beriberi is endemic in Asia, the Philippines, and other islands of the Pacific. SYN: *kakke*.

ETIOLOGY: Deficiency is caused by subsistence on highly polished rice, which has lost all thiamine content through the milling process. Secondary deficiency can arise from decreased absorption, impaired absorption, or impaired utilization of thiamine.

TREATMENT: Treatment consists of oral or parenteral administration of thiamine and establishment of a balanced diet.

**Berkefeld filter** (bĕr′kē-fĕld) [Wilhelm Berkefeld, Ger. manufacturer, 1836–1897] A filter of diatomaceous earth designed to allow virus-size particles to pass through.

**berkelium** (bĕrk′lē-ŭm) [U. of California at Berkeley, where first produced] SYMB: Bk. A transuranium element; atomic weight 247, atomic number 97.

**berloque dermatitis** SEE: *dermatitis, berlock*.

**Bernard's glandular layer** The inner layer of cells lining the acini of the pancreas.

**Bernard-Soulier syndrome** [Jean A. Bernard, Fr. hematologist, b. 1907; Jean-Pierre Soulier, Fr. hematologist, b. 1915] An autosomal recessive bleeding disorder marked by an inherited deficiency of a platelet glycoprotein. The platelets are large. Bleeding results from defective adhesion of platelets to subendothelial collagen and is disproportionate to the reduction in platelets.

**Bernoulli effect** [Jakob Bernoulli, Swiss mathematician, 1654–1705] In pulmonology, the inverse variation in pressure with gas velocity in tubal air flow.

**Bernstein test** [Lionel Bernstein, U.S. physician, b. 1923] Test to reproduce the pain of heartburn. This is done by swallowing a dilute solution (0.1 N) hydrochloric acid. This is compared with infusion of normal saline into the esophagus. The latter does not cause heartburn.

**Bertin, column of** (bĕr'tăn) [Exupère Joseph Bertin, Fr. anatomist, 1712–1781] Any of the renal cortical columns that support the blood vessels in the kidneys and separate the medullary pyramids. Also called *columnae renales.*

**Bertin's ligament** Iliofemoral ligament.

**berylliosis** (bĕr"ĭl-lē-ō'sĭs) [*beryllium* + Gr. *osis,* condition] Beryllium poisoning, usually of the lungs. The beryllium particles cause fibrosis and granulomata at any site, whether inhaled or accidentally introduced into or under the skin.

**beryllium** (bĕ-rĭl'ē-ŭm) [Gr. *beryllos,* beryl] A metallic element, symbol Be, atomic weight 9.0122, atomic number 4, specific gravity 1.848. It is used as a window in some x-ray tubes to produce an unfiltered beam.

**bestiality** (bĕs-tē-ăl'ĭ-tē) [L. *bestia,* beast] The use of animals for the purpose of sexual enjoyment. Animals used include snakes, poultry, and nonhuman mammals. SYN: *zooerasty.*

**beta** (bā'tă) **1.** Second letter of Gr. alphabet, written $\beta$. **2.** In chemistry, a prefix to denote isomeric variety or position in compounds of substituted groups.

**beta-adrenergic agent** A synthetic or natural drug that stimulates beta (sympathetic) receptors.

**beta-adrenergic blocking agent** A substance that interferes with the transmission of stimuli through pathways that normally allow sympathetic nervous inhibiting stimuli to be effective.

These agents are used in treating hypertension, angina, certain cardiac arrhythmias, and postmyocardial infarction. They may also be helpful in preventing migraine and in treating stage fright and benign essential tremor.

**beta-adrenergic receptor** A site in autonomic nerve pathways wherein inhibitory responses occur when adrenergic agents such as norepinephrine and epinephrine are released.

**beta carotene** A carotenoid precursor of vitamin A found in many fresh vegetables and fruits; an antioxidant that minimizes the damage caused by free radicals. The daily human requirement for vitamin A can be met by dietary intake of beta carotene ($\beta$-carotene). Ingestion of large doses of vitamin A either acutely or chronically causes a variety of toxic changes, and $\beta$-carotene does not. For this reason labeling of food products containing large amounts of vitamin A should indicate whether the vitamin A activity is from vitamin A or $\beta$-carotene. Vitamin A activity in foods is expressed as retinol equivalents (RE). One RE equals 6 g of $\beta$-carotene. SEE: *vitamin A; retinol.*

**beta cells 1.** Basophilic cells in the anterior lobe of pituitary that give a positive periodic acid stain reaction. **2.** Insulin-secreting cells of the islets of Langerhans of the pancreas.

**betacism** (bā'tă-sĭzm) [Gr. *beta,* the letter b, + *-ismos,* condition] A speech defect giving the *b* sound to other consonants.

**Betadine** Trade name for povidone-iodine, a topical anti-infective.

**betaine hydrochloride** (bē'tă-ĭn) [L. *beta,* beet] A colorless crystalline substance containing 23% hydrochloric acid. It is obtained from an alkaloid found in the beet and other plants and is used orally as a source of hydrochloric acid in treating hypochlorhydria.

**beta-lactamase resistance** The ability of microorganisms that produce the enzyme beta-lactamase, also called penicillinase, to resist the action of certain types of antibiotics, including some but not all forms of penicillin.

**betamethasone** (bā"tă-mĕth'ă-sōn) A synthetic glucocorticoid that has the pharmaceutical actions of cortisone. Various preparations and dose forms, including an ointment or cream for topical application, are available. Trade name is Celestone.

**beta$_2$ microglobulin** ABBR: $\beta_2$-m. A polypeptide that is one of the class I major histocompatability markers on cell surfaces. Blood levels increase with activation of the immune system and contribute to determining the progress and stage of HIV infection. SEE: *major histocompatability complex.*

**beta particle, beta ray.** A negatively charged particle emitted by radium. It is more penetrating than an alpha ray and is absorbed by 1 mm lead or 0.6 mm platinum. SEE: *electron.*

**beta subunit** Glycoprotein hormones containing two different polypeptide subunits designated $\alpha$ and $\beta$ chains. Analysis of the units of these hormones (e.g., follicle-stimulating, luteinizing, chorionic gonadotropin, and thyrotropin) enables early diagnosis of such conditions as pregnancy and ectopic pregnancy.

**betatron** (bā'tă-trŏn) A circular electron accelerator that produces either high-energy electrons or x-ray photons.

**betazole hydrochloride** (bā'tă-zōl) An isomer of histamine used intramuscularly to stimulate gastric secretion. It is contraindicated in those with atopic allergy. Trade name is Histalog.

**bethanechol chloride** (bĕ-thā'nĕ-kŏl) A cholinergic drug used to treat paralytic ileus and also urinary retention not caused by organic disease. Trade names are Urecholine and Duvoid.

**Bethesda System, The** ABBR: TBS. A system for reporting cervical or vaginal cytologic diagnoses. Use of TBS replaces the numerical designations (Class 1 through 5) of the Papanicolaou smear with descriptive diagnoses of cellular changes. Cellular changes are identified as benign; reactive, such as those due to inflammation, atrophy, radiation, or use of an intrauterine device; or malignant, and includes hormonal evaluation of vaginal smears. Low-grade squamous intraepithelial lesions include what was previously called grade 1 cervical intraepithelial neoplasia (CIN 1) and cellular changes due to human papilloma virus, that is, koilocytosis. High-grade squamous intraepithelial neoplasia includes what was once identified as CIN 2 and CIN 3. SEE: *cervix, cancer of; cervical intraepithelial neoplasia.*

**Betz cells** [Vladimir A. Betz, Russ. anatomist, 1834–1894] A type of giant pyramidal cell in the cortical motor area of the brain. The axons of these cells are included in the pyramidal tract.

**bevel** (bĕv'ĕl) **1.** A surface slanting from the horizontal or vertical. **2.** In dentistry, to produce a slanting surface in the enamel margins of a cavity preparation, named according to the surface resulting.

**bezoar** (bē'zor) [Arabic *bazahr,* protecting against poison] A hard mass of entangled material sometimes found in the stomachs and intestines of animals and humans, such as a hairball (trichobezoar), a hair and vegetable fiberball (trichophytobezoar), or a foodball (phytobezoar).

**BFP** *biologically false positive.*

**Bi** Symbol for the element bismuth.

**bi-** (bī) [L. *bis,* twice] Combining form indicating *two, double, twice.*

**biarticular** (bī"ăr-tĭk'ū-lăr) [" + *articulus,* joint] Pert. to two joints; diarthric (e.g., temporomandibular joints).

**bias** (bī'ŭs) In experimental medicine, statistics, and epidemiology, any effect or interference at any stage of an investigation tending to produce results that depart systematically from the true value. The reasons this may occur include selection bias, response bias, or observer bias.

**bibasic** (bī-bā'sĭk) [" + Gr. *basis,* foundation] Pert. to an acid with two hydrogen atoms replaceable by bases to form salts.

**bibliomania** (bĭb"lē-ō-mā'nē-ă) [Gr. *biblion,* book, + *mania,* madness] An obsession with the collecting of books.

**bibliotherapy** (bĭb"lē-ō-thĕr'ă-pē) [" + *therapeia,* treatment] A nonphysical, psychotherapeutic technique in which the patient is induced to read books. It is used in treating mental illness.

**bibulous** (bĭb'ū-lŭs) [L. *bibulus,* from *bibere,* to drink] Absorbent. SYN: *hydrophilous; hygroscopic.*

**bicameral** (bī-kăm'ĕr-ăl) [L. *bis,* twice, + *camera,* a chamber] Having two cavities or chambers.

**bicapsular** (bī-kăp'sū-lăr) [" + *capsula,* container] Having two capsules.

**bicarbonate** (bī-kăr'bō-nāt) Any salt containing the $HCO_3^-$ (bicarbonate) anion. SEE: *carbonic acid.*

***blood b.*** Bicarbonate in the blood. The amount present is an indicator of the alkali reserve.

***b. of soda*** Sodium bicarbonate, $NaHCO_3$.

**bicellular** (bī-sĕl'ū-lăr) [" + *cellularis,* little cell] **1.** Composed of two cells. **2.** Having two chambers or compartments.

**biceps** (bī'sĕps) [" + *caput,* head] A muscle with two heads.

***b. brachii*** The muscle of the upper arm that flexes the arm and forearm and supinates the hand.

***b. femoris*** One of the hamstring muscles lying on the posterior lateral side of the thigh. It flexes the knee and rotates it outward.

**Bichat, Marie François X** (bē-shă') French physiologist and anatomist, 1771–1802; founder of scientific histology and pathological anatomy.

***B.'s canal*** The subarachnoid canal, which extends from the third ventricle to the middle of Bichat's fissure and carries the veins of Galen.

***B.'s fat ball*** The mass of fat behind the buccinator muscle. SYN: *sucking pad.*

***B.'s fissure*** The horseshoe fissure separating the cerebrum from the cerebellum.

***B.'s ligament*** The lower fasciculus of the posterior sacroiliac ligament.

***B.'s tunic*** Tunica intima.

**bichloride of mercury** (bī-klō'rīd) $HgCl_2$. Corrosive mercuric chloride; a crystalline salt. SEE: *mercuric chloride; mercuric chloride poisoning; mercuric chloride in Poisons and Poisoning Appendix.*

**bicipital** (bī-sĭp'ĭ-tăl) [L. *biceps,* two heads] **1.** Pert. to a biceps muscle. **2.** Having two heads.

**BiCNU** Trade name for carmustine.

**biconcave** (bī-kŏn'kāv) [L. *bis,* twice, + *concavus,* concave] Concave on each side, esp. as a type of lens. SEE: illus.

**biconvex** (bī-kŏn'vĕks) [" + *convexus,* rounded raised surface] Convex on two sides, esp. as a type of lens. SEE: *biconcave* for illus.

**bicornate, bicornis** (bī-kor'nāt, -nĭs) [" + *cornutus,* horned] Having two processes or hornlike projections.

**bicoronal** (bī"kō-rō'năl) [" + Gr. *korone,* crown] Pert. to the two coronas.

**bicorporate** (bī-kor'pŏ-rāt) [" + *corpus,* body] Having two bodies.

**bicuspid** (bī-kŭs'pĭd) [" + *cuspis,* point] Having two cusps or projections or having two cusps or leaflets.

***b. tooth*** A premolar tooth; a permanent

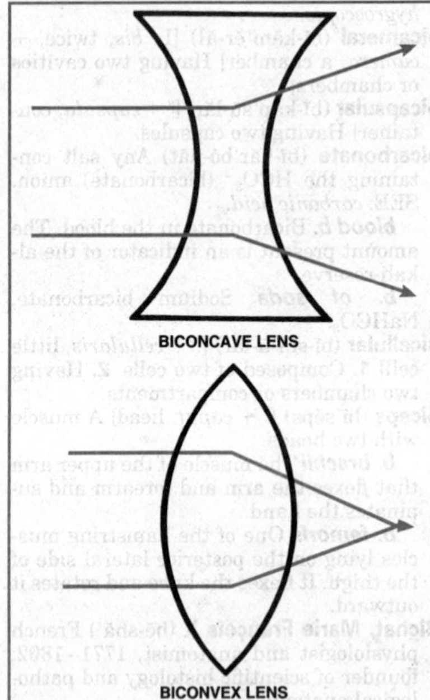


tooth with two cusps on the grinding surface and a flattened root. There are four premolars in each jaw, two on each side between the canines and the molars. SEE: *tooth*.

***b. valve*** The valve between the left atrium and left ventricle of the heart. SYN: *mitral valve*. SEE: *heart*.

**b.i.d.** L. *bis in die*, twice daily.

**bidet** (bē-dā′) [Fr., a small horse] A basin used for cleaning the perineum.

**Bielschowsky disease** (bē″ĕl-shō′skē) [Max Bielschowsky, Ger. neuropathologist, 1869–1940] An early juvenile type of cerebral sphingolipidosis.

**bifacial** (bī-fā′shē-ăl) [″ + *facies*, face] Having similar opposite surfaces.

**bifid** (bī′fĭd) [″ + *findere*, to cleave] Cleft or split into two parts.

***b. spine*** Spina bifida cystica.

***b. tongue*** Cleft tongue.

**bifocal** (bī-fō′kăl) [″ + *focus*, hearth] Having two foci, as in bifocal eyeglasses.

***b. glasses*** SEE: *glasses, bifocal*.

**bifurcate, bifurcated** (bī′fŭr-kāt, bī-fŭr′kāt′d) [″ + *furca*, fork] Having two branches or divisions; forked.

**bifurcation** (bī-fŭr-kā′shŭn) **1.** A separation into two branches; the point of forking. **2.** The anatomical area where roots divide in a multirooted tooth.

**bigemina** (bī-jĕm′ĭ-nă) [L.] Pl. of bigeminum.

**bigeminal** (bī-jĕm′ĭ-năl) [L. *bigeminum*, twin] Double; paired.

***b. pulse*** Pulse in which two beats follow each other in rapid succession, each group of two being separated by a longer pause. The initial beat is considered the normal one and is usually more intense than the second one. Detection of this type of irregular pulse should alert one to look for its cause, which may be one of several forms of heart disease.

**bigeminum** (bī-jĕm′ĭ-nŭm) *pl.* **bigemina** [L.] A bigeminal body.

**bigeminy** (bī-jĕm′ĭ-nē) The condition of occurring in pairs. **bigeminal,** *adj.*

***junctional b.*** Cardiac arrhythmia in which every other beat is a junctional ectopic or premature junctional contraction. SYN: *nodal b.*

***nodal b.*** Junctional b.

***ventricular b.*** Cardiac arrhythmia in which every other beat is a ventricular ectopic or premature ventricular contraction.

**bi-ischial** Concerning both ischial tuberosities.

**bilabe** (bī′lāb) [L. *bis*, twice, + *labium*, lip] A long, thin device equipped with a hinged lower jaw. It is inserted into the bladder via the urethra to remove small calculi from the bladder.

**bilateral** (bī-lăt′ĕr-ăl) [″ + *latus*, side] Pert. to, affecting, or relating to two sides.

***b. carotid body resection*** ABBR: BCBR. A rarely used method of treating carotid sinus syncope. The carotid body is removed bilaterally. SEE: *syncope, carotid sinus*.

***b. symmetry*** The symmetry of paired organs or of an organism whose right and left halves are mirror images of each other or in which a median longitudinal section divides the organism into equivalent right and left halves. SYN: *bilateralism*.

**bilateralism** (bī-lăt′ĕr-ăl-ĭzm) [″ + ″ + Gr. *-ismos*, condition] Bilateral symmetry.

**bilayer** A two-component layer.

***lipid b.*** The outer membrane of most cells includes two layers of lipid molecules. These are arranged so that one part of each molecule is soluble in water and is hydrophilic; the other is water-insoluble and is hydrophobic. The membrane is virtually impermeable to water and water-soluble substances, such as ions, glucose, and urea; but fat-soluble substances, such as oxygen, carbon dioxide, and alcohols, can freely cross it. SEE: *cell* for illus.

**bile** (bīl) [L. *bilis*, bile] A thick, viscid, bitter-tasting fluid secreted by the liver. It passes from the bile duct of the liver into the common bile duct and then into the duodenum as needed. The bile from the liver is straw colored, while that from the gallbladder varies from yellow to brown or green.

Bile also is stored in the gallbladder, where it is concentrated, drawn upon as needed, and discharged into the duodenum. Contraction of the gallbladder is brought about by cholecystokinin-pancreozymin, a hormone produced by the duodenum; its secretion is stimulated by the entrance of fatty foods into the duodenum. Added to water, bile decreases surface tension, giving a foamy solution favoring the emulsification of fats and oils; this action is due to the bile salts, mainly sodium glycocholate and taurocholate.

COMPOSITION: Bile pigments (principally bilirubin, and biliverdin.) are responsible for the variety of colors observed. In addition, bile contains cholesterol, lecithin, mucin, and other organic and inorganic substances.

FUNCTION: Bile's importance as a digestive juice is due to its emulsifying action, which facilitates the digestion of fats in the small intestine by pancreatic lipase. Bile also stimulates peristalsis. Normally the ejection of bile occurs only during duodenal digestion. Bile is both an antiseptic and a purgative. About 800 to 1000 ml/24 hr are secreted in the normal adult. SEE: *gallbladder*.

PATHOLOGY: Interference with the flow of bile produces jaundice, which results in the presence of unabsorbed fats in the feces. In such instances, fats should be restricted in the diet. A restricted flow of bile may also produce gallstones in the gallbladder.

TESTS: There are several methods of testing for bile in the urine.

*Gmelin's test:* A depth of 1 in. (2.5 cm) of concentrated nitric acid is carefully overlaid with the sample of urine. Bile is present when there is a play of colors at the junction of the fluids. This test also can be carried out by pouring some urine onto blotting or filter paper and then placing a drop of concentrated nitric acid on the moist paper. From the spreading edge of the drop of acid, a ring of various colors will develop in which green predominates and forms the outer band.

*Iodine test:* Urine is poured into a test tube to a depth of 1 in. (2.5 cm) and carefully overlaid with dilute tincture of iodine. A bright green ring will appear at the junction of the fluids if bile is present.

***b. acids*** Complex acids, of which cholic, glycocholic, and taurocholic acids are examples, and which occur as salts in bile. They give bile its foamy character, are important in the digestion of fats in the intestine, and are reabsorbed from the intestine to be used again by the liver. This circulation of bile acids is called the enterohepatic circulation. In Hay's test for bile acids, some urine is placed in a watchglass and a little powdered sulfur is sprinkled on the surface. If bile acids are present, the sulfur sinks because of the lowering of the surface tension by the bile salts.

***cystic b.*** Bile stored in the gallbladder. It is concentrated as compared with hepatic bile.

***b. ducts*** Intercellular passages that convey bile from the liver to the hepatic duct, which joins the duct from the gallbladder (cystic duct) to form the common bile duct (ductus choledochus), and which enters the duodenum about 3 in. (7.6 cm) below the pylorus. SEE: illus.

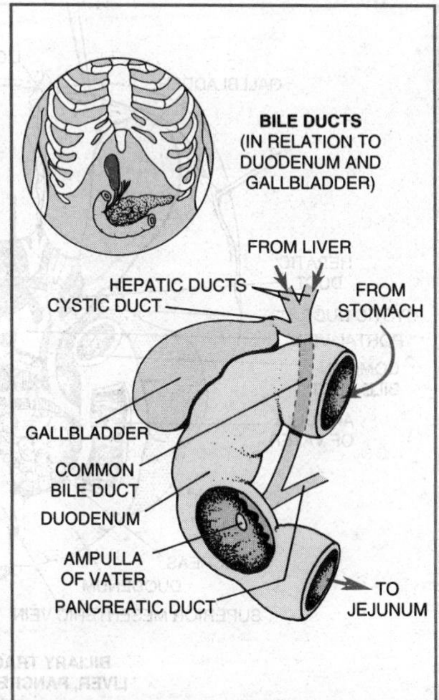


***hepatic b.*** Bile secreted by the liver cells. It is collected in the bile ducts and flows to the gallbladder.

***lithogenic b.*** Bile that favors gallstone production. This may be associated with several conditions; the most important is increased secretion of cholesterol in the bile as occurs with obesity, high-caloric diets, or drugs such as clofibrate.

***b. pigments*** Complex, highly colored substances (e.g., bilirubin and biliverdin) found in bile derived from hemoglobin. They impart brown color to intestinal contents and feces. Van den Bergh's test is used to detect the type of bilirubin in the blood serum.

***b. salts*** Alkali salts of bile sodium glycocholate and sodium taurocholate.

**Bilharzia** (bĭl-hăr′zē-ă) [Theodor Maximilian Bilharz, Ger. helminthologist, 1825–1862] Former name for *Schistosoma*, the human blood fluke. SEE: *Schistosoma*.

**bilharzial, bilharzic** (bĭl-hăr′zē-ăl, -zĭk) Pert. to *Bilharzia* (*Schistosoma*).

**bilharziasis** (bĭl″hăr-zī′ă-sĭs) *Schistosomiasis*. SEE: *Bilharzia*.

**bili-** [L. *bilis*] Combining form meaning *bile*.

**biliary** (bĭl′ē-ār-ē) Pert. to bile.

***b. calculus*** Gallstone.

***b. colic*** Pain caused by the pressure or passing of gallstones.

***b. tract*** The organs and ducts that par-

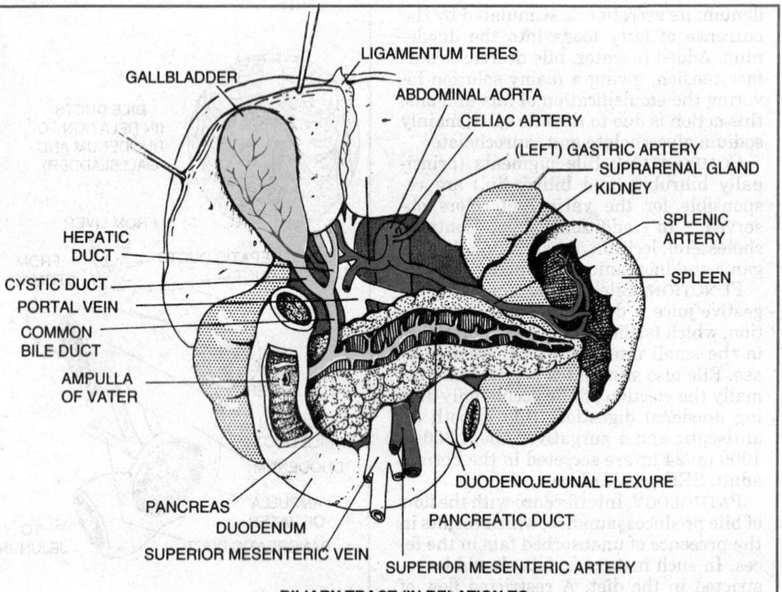

LIGAMENTUM TERES
GALLBLADDER
ABDOMINAL AORTA
CELIAC ARTERY
(LEFT) GASTRIC ARTERY
SUPRARENAL GLAND
KIDNEY
SPLENIC ARTERY
HEPATIC DUCT
SPLEEN
CYSTIC DUCT
PORTAL VEIN
COMMON BILE DUCT
AMPULLA OF VATER
DUODENOJEJUNAL FLEXURE
PANCREAS
PANCREATIC DUCT
DUODENUM
SUPERIOR MESENTERIC VEIN
SUPERIOR MESENTERIC ARTERY

**BILIARY TRACT (IN RELATION TO LIVER, PANCREAS, AND DUODENUM)**

ticipate in the secretion, storage, and delivery of bile into the duodenum. SEE: illus.; *bile ducts; gallbladder; liver.*

**bilicyanin** (bĭl″ĭ-sī′ă-nĭn) [L. *bilis,* bile, + *cyaneus,* blue] A blue or purple pigment, an oxidation product of biliverdin.

**biliflavin** (bĭl″ĭ-flā′vĭn) [″ + *flavus,* yellow] A yellow pigment derived from biliverdin.

**bilifuscin** (bĭl″ĭ-fŭs′ĭn) [″ + *fuscus,* brown] A dark brown pigment from bile and gallstones.

**biligenesis** (bĭl″ĭ-jĕn′ĕ-sĭs) [″ + Gr. *genesis,* generation, birth] The formation of bile.

**biligenetic, biligenic** (bĭl″ĭ-jĕn-ĕt′ĭk, -jĕn′ĭk) [″ + Gr. *gennan,* to produce] Forming bile.

**bilious** (bĭl′yŭs) [L. *bilosus*] **1.** Pert. to bile. **2.** Afflicted with biliousness.

**biliousness** (bĭl′yŭs-nĕs) **1.** A symptom of a disorder of the liver causing constipation, headache, loss of appetite, and vomiting of bile. **2.** An excess of bile.

**bilirubin** (bĭl-ĭ-roo′bĭn) [″ + *ruber,* red] $C_{33}H_{36}O_6N_4$. The orange-colored or yellowish pigment in bile. It is derived from hemoglobin of red blood cells that have completed their life span and are destroyed and ingested by the macrophage system of the liver, spleen, and red bone marrow. When produced elsewhere, it is carried to the liver by the blood. It is changed chemically in the liver and excreted in the bile via the duodenum. As it passes through the intestines, it is converted into urobilinogen by bacterial enzymes, most of it being excreted through the feces. If urobilinogen passes into the circulation, it is excreted through the urine or re-excreted in the bile. The accumulation of bilirubin leads to jaundice in many cases, esp. to physiologic jaundice of the newborn. SEE: illus.

***direct b.*** Bilirubin conjugated by the liver cells to form bilirubin diglucuronide, which is water-soluble.

***indirect b.*** Unconjugated bilirubin that is present in the blood. It is fat-soluble.

**bilirubinate** (bĭl-ĭ-roo′bĭn-āt) A salt of bilirubin.

**bilirubinemia** (bĭl″ĭ-roo-bĭn-ē′mē-ă) [″ + *ruber,* red, + Gr. *haima,* blood] Bilirubin in the blood, usually in excessive amounts. Bilirubin is normally present in the blood in small amounts. However, it

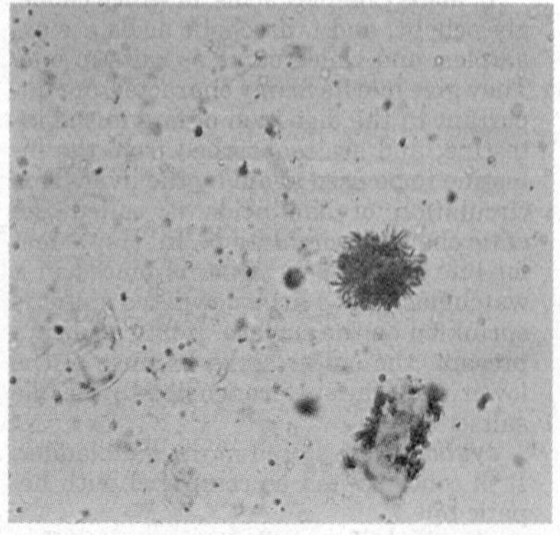

**BILIRUBIN CRYSTALS** (×400)

increases in certain pathological conditions in which there is excessive destruction of red blood cells or interference with bile excretion; the amount is also increased when the liver is diseased or damaged. In a newborn infant with erythroblastosis fetalis and greatly elevated bilirubin, exchange transfusion may be required. Also called *hyperbilirubinemia*.

**bilirubinuria** (bĭl″ĭ-roo-bĭn-ū′rē-ă) [″ + ″ + Gr. *ouron,* urine] Presence of bilirubin in urine.

**biliuria** (bĭl-ĭ-ū′rē-ă) The presence of bile in the urine.

**biliverdin** (bĭl-ĭ-vĕr′dĭn) [″ + *viridis,* green] $C_{33}H_{34}O_6N_4$. A greenish pigment in bile formed by the oxidation of bilirubin.

**billion** [Fr. *bi,* two, + *million,* million] **1.** In the U.S., billion is a number equal to 1 followed by 9 zeros (1,000,000,000) or ($10^9$). **2.** In Europe, billion is a number equal to 1 followed by 12 zeros ($10^{12}$), that is, bi-million, or twice the number of zeros in a million ($10^6$).

**Billroth, Christian A.T.** Austrian surgeon, 1829–1894.

***B. I operation*** Gastroduodenostomy.

***B. II operation*** Gastrojejunostomy.

**bilobate** (bī-lō′bāt) [L. *bis,* twice, + *lobus,* lobe] Having two lobes.

**bilobular** (bī-lŏb′ū-lăr) Having two lobules.

**bilocular** (bī-lŏk′ū-lăr) [″ + *loculus,* cell] **1.** Having two cells. **2.** Divided into compartments.

**bimanual** (bī-măn′ū-ăl) [″ + *manus,* hand] With both hands, as in bimanual palpation.

***b. examination*** SEE: *pelvic examination.*

**bimaxillary** (bī-măk′sĭ-lĕr″ē) [″ + *maxilla,* jawbone] Pert. to or afflicting both jaws.

**bimodal** (bī-mō′dăl) [″ + *modus,* mode] Pert. to a graphic presentation that contains two peaks.

**binary** (bī′nār-ē) [L. *binarius,* of two] **1.** Composed of two elements. **2.** Separating into two branches.

***b. acid*** An acid containing hydrogen and one other element.

***b. code*** SEE: *b. system.*

***b. digit*** One of two digits, usually 0 or 1, used in a binary system of enumeration.

***b. gas*** A toxic gas composed of two ingredients, neither of which is toxic by itself. Used in chemical warfare.

***b. system*** A numbering system particularly well suited to use by computers. All of the information placed into a computer is in binary form, that is, numbers made up of zeros and ones (0's and 1's). In this system each "place" in a binary number represents a power of 2 (i.e., the number of times 2 is to be multiplied by itself).

**binaural** (bĭn-aw′răl) [L. *bis,* twice, + *auris,* ear] Pert. to both ears.

**binauricular** (bĭn″aw-rĭk′ū-lăr) [″ + *auricula,* little ear] Binaural; pert. to both auricles of the ear.

**bind 1.** To fasten, wrap, or encircle with a bandage. **2.** In chemistry and immunology, the uniting or adherence (i.e., bonding) of one molecule or chemical entity to another (e.g., the joining of a toxin to an antitoxin or of a hormone to its receptor on a cell surface).

**binder** (bīnd′ĕr) [AS. *bindan,* to tie up] **1.** A broad bandage most commonly used as an encircling support of the abdomen or chest. SEE: *bandage.* **2.** In dental materials, a substance that holds a mixture of solid particles together.

***abdominal b.*** A wide band fastened snugly about the abdomen for support.

***chest b.*** A broad band that encircles the chest and is used for applying heat, dressings, or pressure and for supporting the breasts. Shoulder straps may be used to keep the binder from slipping.

***double-T b.*** A horizontal band about the waist to which two vertical bands are attached in back, brought around the leg, and again fastened to the horizontal band. The binder holds dressings about the perineum or genitalia, esp. in males.

***obstetrical b.*** A broad bandage that encircles the entire abdomen from ribs to pelvis, affording support.

***Scultetus b.*** (skŭl-tē′tŭs) [Johann Schultes (Scultetus), German surgeon, 1595–1645] A many-tailed binder or bandage, applied around the abdomen so that the ends overlap each other as if they were roof shingles. The binder holds dressings in place and supports abdominal muscles postoperatively. SEE: illus.

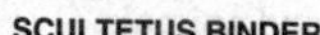


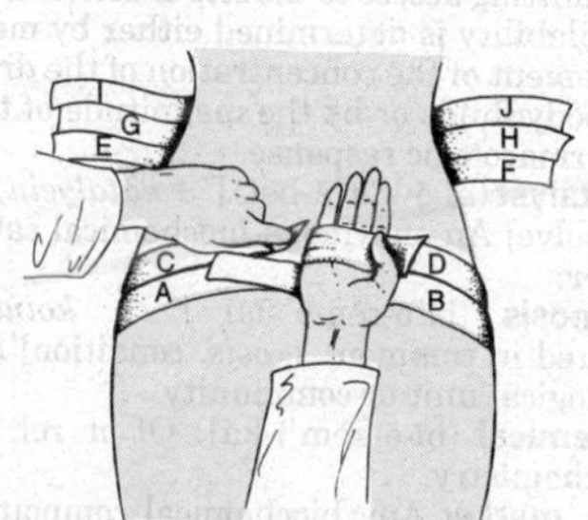


A MULTIPLE-TAIL BINDER APPLIED SEQUENTIALLY STARTING AT THE END SHOWN. EACH TAIL IS PULLED FIRM AND THEN OVERLAPPED BY THE NEXT ONE. THEY MAY BE HELD IN PLACE BY SAFETY PINS OR ADHESIVE TAPE. THIS BINDER IS UNSUITABLE FOR USE ON THE CHEST DUE TO MOVEMENT DURING BREATHING.

***T b.*** Two strips of material fastened together resembling a T, used as a bandage to hold a dressing on the perineum of women.

***towel b.*** A towel that encircles the abdomen or chest and whose ends are pinned together.

**Binder's syndrome** A syndrome related to facial growth, with hypoplasia of the maxillae and nasal bones resulting in a flattened face, elongated nose, and smaller maxillary arch with crowding of the teeth and malocclusions.

**binge eating** An eating disorder marked by rapid consumption of large amounts of food in a short period of time. SEE: *bulimia.*

**binocular** (bĭn-ŏk'ū-lăr) [L. *bis,* twice, + *oculus,* eye] Pert. to both eyes.

***b. vision*** Normal vision involving simultaneous use of both eyes.

**binomial** (bī-nō'mē-ăl) [" + *nomen,* name] In mathematics and statistics, an equation containing two variables.

**binotic** (bĭn-ŏt'ĭk) [" + Gr. *ous,* ear] Pert. to or having two ears.

**binovular** (bĭn-ŏv'ū-lăr) Biovular.

**binuclear, binucleate** (bī-nū'klē-ăr, -āt) [" + *nucleus,* kernel] Having two nuclei.

**bio-** [Gr. *bios,* life] Combining form indicating *relationship to life.*

**bioactive** Affecting living tissues.

**bioassay** (bī"ō-ăs'ā) [" + O. Fr. *asaier,* to try] In pharmacology, the determination of the strength of a drug or substance by comparing its effect on a live animal or an isolated organ preparation with that of a standard preparation.

**bioastronautics** (bī"ō-ăs"trō-naw'tĭks) The study of the effects of space travel on living plants and animals.

**bioavailability** (bī"ō-ă-văl"ă-bĭl'ĭ-tē) The rate and extent to which an active drug or metabolite enters the general circulation, permitting access to the site of action. Bioavailability is determined either by measurement of the concentration of the drug in body fluids or by the magnitude of the pharmacologic response.

**biocatalyst** (bī-ō-kăt'ă-lĭst) [" + *katalyein,* to dissolve] An enzyme; a biochemical catalyzer.

**biocenosis** (bī"ō-sĕn-ō'sĭs) [" + *koinos,* shared in common, + *osis,* condition] An ecological unit or community.

**biochemical** (bī-ō-kĕm'ĭ-kăl) Of or rel. to biochemistry.

***b. marker*** Any biochemical compound such as an antigen, antibody, abnormal enzyme, or hormone that is sufficiently altered in a disease to serve as an aid in diagnosing or in predicting susceptibility to the disease.

**biochemistry** [" + *chemeia,* chemistry] The chemistry of living things; the science of the chemical changes accompanying the vital functions of plants and animals.

**biochemorphology** (bī"ō-kĕ-mor-fŏl'ō-jē) [" + " + *morphe,* shape, + *logos,* word, reason] The science of the relationship between chemical structure and biological action. SEE: *stereochemistry.*

**biocide** (bī'ō-sīd) [" + L. *caedere,* to kill] A substance, esp. a pesticide or an antibiotic, that destroys living organisms.

**bioclimatology** (bī"ō-klī-mă-tŏl'ō-jē) [" + *klima,* climate, + *logos,* word, reason] Study of the relationship of climate to life.

**biocolloid** (bī"ō-kŏl'oyd) [" + *kollodes,* glutinous] A colloid from animal, vegetable, or microbial tissue.

**biocompatibility** The condition of being harmless to living systems.

**biocontainment** In infectious disease laboratories, the process and procedures used to confine harmful microorganisms to the areas in which they are being investigated. The precise regulations vary with the pathogenicity of the organisms. SEE: *biosafety levels.*

**biodegradable** Susceptible to degradation by biological processes, such as bacterial or enzymatic action.

**biodegradation** (bī"ō-dĕg"rĕ-dā'shŭn) The breakdown of organic materials into simple chemicals by biochemical processes. Also called *biological degradation.*

**biodynamics** (bī"ō-dī-năm'ĭks) [Gr. *bios,* life, + *dynamis,* force] The science of the force or energy of living matter.

**bioelectronics** (bī"ō-ē"lĕk-trŏn'ĭks) The study of the transfer of electrons between molecules in biological systems.

**bioenergetics** (bī"ō-ĕn"ĕr-jĕt'ĭks) Study of energy transfer and relationships between all living systems.

**bioengineering** The application of engineering concepts, equipment, skills and techniques to solving medical problems. SEE: *biomedical engineering.*

**bioequivalence** (bī"ō-ĭ-kwĭv'ă-lĕnts) The property of having the same biological effects of that to which a medicine was compared.

**bioequivalent. 1.** Of or relating to bioequivalence. **2.** A bioequivalent drug.

**biofeedback.** A training program designed to develop one's ability to control the autonomic (involuntary) nervous system. After learning the technique, the patient may be able to control heart rate, blood pressure, and skin temperature or to relax certain muscles. The patient learns by using monitoring devices that sound a tone when changes in pulse, blood pressure, brain waves, and muscle contractions occur. Then the patient attempts to reproduce the conditions that caused the desired changes.

**biofilm** A moist film that covers surfaces, esp. those of implanted devices, including catheters. This film consists of bacteria imbedded in a film of an adhesive biopolymer. Bacteria within the film may be protected from the action of antibiotics. The film may be seen with a scanning electron microscope.

**biogenesis** (bī"ō-jĕn'ĕ-sĭs) [" + *genesis,* generation, birth] The accepted theory that life can originate only from pre-existing life and never from nonliving material. **biogenetic** (-jĕ-nĕt′ĭk), *adj.*

**biogenic** (bī-ō-jĕn′ĭk) Produced by living organisms.

***b. amines*** A group of chemical compounds, most of which are important in neurotransmission. Included are norepinephrine, histamine, serotonin, and dopamine.

**biohazard** Anything that is harmful or potentially harmful to humans, other species, or the environment. SEE: *biosafety levels.*

**bioinequivalent** Not being equivalent to that to which a drug is compared.

**bioinstrument** A device placed in the body to record or transmit data from the individual.

**biokinetics** (bī″ō-kĭ-nĕt′ĭks) [″ + *kinetikos,* moving] The study of growth changes and movements in developing organisms.

**biologic** [″ + *logos,* word, reason] Pert. to biology.

***b. fitness*** SEE: *fitness, biologic.*

***b. half-life*** The time required to reduce the concentration of a drug in the blood, plasma, or serum by 50%. This is a measure of the rate of drug distribution and elimination. SEE: *half-life; pharmacokinetics.*

**biological** [″ + *logos,* word, reason] **1.** Pert. to biology. **2.** A medicinal compound (such as a serum, vaccine, antigen, or antitoxin) prepared from living organisms and their products.

***b. armature*** SEE: *armature, biological.*

***b. degradation*** The breakdown of organic materials into simple chemicals by biochemical processes.

***b. mother*** The individual who actually gives birth to a child. This term does not apply to an individual who provided the uterus for the gestation of a fertilized ovum obtained from a donor. SEE: *birth mother; surrogate parenting.*

***b. response modifier*** An agent that intensifies normal immune responses. Examples include interferon, interleukin-2, and monoclonal antibodies. Usually, these agents are used as adjuncts to other pharmacological agents and therapies in the management of selected malignancies, immunodeficiency and autoimmune disorders, and certain viral infections such as hepatitis C.

***b. rhythm*** SEE: *clock, biological.*

***b. warfare*** ABBR: BW. Warfare in which disease-producing microorganisms, toxins, or organic biocides (e.g., anthrax, brucellosis, plague) are deliberately used to destroy, injure, or immobilize livestock, vegetation, or human life. SEE: *chemical warfare.*

**biologist** A specialist in biology.

**biology** (bī-ŏl′ō-jē) [Gr. *bios,* life, + *logos,* word, reason] The science of life and living things.

***molecular b.*** The branch of biology dealing with analysis of the structure and development of biological systems with respect to the chemistry and physics of their molecular constituents.

***radiation b.*** SEE: *radiation biology.*

**bioluminescence** (bī″ō-loo″mĭ-nĕs′ĕns) [″ + L. *lumen,* light] Emission of visible light from living organisms. The best known example is the cold light produced by fireflies. SEE: *luciferase.*

**biolysis** (bī-ŏl′ĭ-sĭs) [″ + *lysis,* dissolution] The chemical decomposition of living tissue by the action of living organisms. **biolytic** (bī-ō-lĭt′ĭk), *adj.*

**biomarker** A signal that serves as a guide or indicator of the state of a living organism. An example of a simple biomarker is body temperature. In a more sophisticated context, hormonal or enzymatic changes in response to toxic substances serve as biomarkers.

**biomass** (bī′ō-măs) [″ + L. *massa,* mass] All of the living organisms in a specified area.

**biome** (bī′ōm) [″ + *oma,* mass] The totality of living organisms in a specified ecological area.

**biomechanics** (bī″ō-mĕ-kăn′ĭks) The application of mechanical forces to living organisms and the investigation of the effects of the interaction of force and the body or system. Includes forces that arise from within and outside the body. SEE: *kinesiology.*

**biomedical** Biological and medical; pert. to application of natural sciences to the study of medicine.

***b. engineer*** A certified design engineer, usually with a Bachelor of Science degree and employed in a hospital or a commercial company to design and/or maintain medical equipment. Also referred to as a *clinical engineer.*

***b. engineering*** Application of the principles and practices of engineering science to biomedical research and health care, as seen in the development of devices such as cardiac pacemakers, hearing aids, and sophisticated artificial limbs and joints.

***b. engineering technologist*** A certified repair specialist usually with an AAS degree usually employed in a hospital or commercial company to repair and maintain medical equipment.

**biomedicalization of aging** The treatment of aging as a biological or medical problem that must be combatted or cured.

**biometeorology** (bī″ō-mē″tē-or-ŏl′ō-jē) [″ + *meteoros,* raised from off the ground, + *logos,* word, reason] Study of the effects of meteorology on all forms of life.

**biometrics** (bī″ō-mĕt′rĭks) The study of the application of mathematics and statistics to the analysis and solution of problems in the fields of biology and other life sciences.

**biometry** (bī-ŏm′ĕ-trē) [″ + *metron,* measure] **1.** The application of statistics to biological science. **2.** The computation of life expectancy.

**biomicroscope** (bī″ō-mī′krŏ-skōp) A microscope used with a slit lamp for viewing segments of the living eye.

**bion** (bī′ŏn) [Gr. *bios,* life] Any living organism.

**bionics** (bī-ŏn′ĭks) The study of biological functions and mechanisms and the application of these findings to the design of machines, esp. computers.

**biophysical profile** A system of estimating current fetal status determined by analysis of five variables via ultrasonography and nonstress testing. Fetal breathing movements, gross body movement, fetal tone, amniotic fluid volume, and fetal heart rate reactivity are compared to specific criteria. Each expected normal finding is rated as 2; each abnormal finding is rated as 0. Scores of 8 to 10 with normal amniotic fluid volume indicate satisfactory fetal status. A score of 6 with normal amniotic fluid volume requires reassessment of a preterm fetus within 24 hours of delivery. Scores below 6 indicate fetal compromise and require prompt delivery. SEE: *Apgar score.*

**biophysics** (bī″ō-fĭz′ĭks) [″ + *physikos,* natural] Application of physical laws to biological processes and functions. **biophysical** (-ĭ-kăl), *adj.*

**biopsy** (bī′ŏp-sē) [″ + *opsis,* vision] The obtaining of a representative tissue sample for microscopic examination, usually to establish a diagnosis. The tissue may be obtained surgically or through a syringe and needle. The procedure can be guided by computed tomography, ultrasonography, magnetic resonance imaging, ultrasound, or radiography.

***aspiration b.*** The removal of tissue by use of a needle and syringe.

***brush b.*** The removal of tissue for investigation by use of a brush.

***cone b.*** The removal of a cone-shaped piece of tissue for examination.

***liver b.*** The removal of tissue from the liver by use of a large-bore needle that permits removal of a core of tissue.

***muscle b.*** The removal of muscle tissue for microscopic examination and chemical analysis.

***needle b.*** The removal of tissue by use of a needle. Usually it is attached to a syringe.

***percutaneous transthoracic needle aspiration b.*** Use of a fluoroscopically guided aspiration needle to obtain a sample of tissue in cases of suspected pulmonary malignancies or unknown lesions. Because of the risk of pneumothorax, the procedure is usually contraindicated in patients receiving mechanical ventilation.

***punch b.*** The removal of a small bit of tissue by use of a hollow punch.

***stereotactic breast b.*** A radiographically guided method of localizing and sampling breast lesions discovered on mammography that indicate possible malignancy. The procedure is comparable in sensitivity to surgical biopsy. The procedure is quicker, easier, and less expensive than the standard surgical biopsy.

**biopsychosocial** Biological, psychological and social; pert. to the application of knowledge from the biological and behavioral sciences to solve human problems.

**biopterin** (bī-ŏp′tĕr-ĭn) The chemical 2-amino-4-hydroxy-6-(1,2-hydroxypropyl) pteridine, important in metabolizing phenylalanine. A deficiency of biopterin is a rare cause of phenylketonuria.

**bioremediation** The conversion of hazardous wastes and pollutants into harmless materials by the action of microorganisms.

**biorhythm** (bī′ō-rĭth″ŭm) [″ + *rhythmos,* rhythm] A cyclic phenomenon (e.g., circadian rhythm, sleep cycle, and menstrual cycle) that occurs with established regularity in living organisms. SEE: *clock, biological.*

**bios** (bī′ŏs) [Gr., life] **1.** Organic life. **2.** A group of substances (including inositol, biotin, and thiamine) necessary for the most favorable growth of some yeasts.

**biosafety levels** ABBR: BSL. A classification system used to indicate the safety precautions required for those investigating microorganisms, especially viruses known to be dangerous or lethal to those exposed to them. There are four BSLs, with BSL-4 requiring the highest level of security.

**bioscience** (bī″ō-sī′ĕns) [Gr. *bios,* life, + L. *scientia,* knowledge] Life science.

**biosensor** [Gr. *bios,* life, + sensor] A device that senses and analyzes biological information. This may be simple temperature, blood pressure, or heart rate or more sophisticated determination of chemicals and enzymes in body fluids. The device may be used in the laboratory or placed within the body.

**biospectrometry** (bī″ō-spĕk-trŏm′ĕ-trē) [″ + L. *spectrum,* image, + Gr. *metron,* measure] Use of a spectroscope to determine the amounts and kinds of substances in tissues.

**biospectroscopy** (bī″ō-spĕk-trŏs′kō-pē) [″ + ″ + Gr. *skopein,* to examine] Examination of tissue by use of a spectroscope.

**biosphere** (bī′ō-sfēr″) [″ + *sphaira,* ball] **1.** The parts of earth's land, water, and atmosphere in which living organisms can exist. **2.** In Arizona an enclosed, supposedly self-contained experimental ecosystem designed to provide environmental insights. The initial 2-year test, begun in 1991, was called Biosphere 1; the second one, Biosphere 2, began in early 1994. The scientific importance of Biosphere studies is being evaluated.

**biostatistics** The application of statistical processes and methods to the analysis of biological data. SEE: *rate, morbidity; vital statistics.*

**biosynthesis** (bī″ō-sĭn′thĕ-sĭs) [″ + *synthesis,* a putting together] The formation of chemical compounds by a living organism.

**biota** (bī-ō′tă) [Gr. *bios,* life] The combined animal and plant life in an area.

**biotaxis, biotaxy** (bī″ō-tăk′sĭs, -sē) [″ + *taxis,* arrangement] **1.** The selecting and arranging activity of living cells. **2.** Systematic classification of living organisms.

**Biot's breathing** (bē-ōz′) [Camille Biot, Fr. physician, b. 1878] Breathing marked by several short breaths followed by long, irregular periods of apnea. It is seen in patients with increased intracranial pressure. SEE: *Cheyne-Stokes respiration.*

**biotechnology** The application of biological systems and organisms to technical and industrial processes. This broad definition includes such ancient endeavors as the use of yeast in preparing bread for baking, and such modern concepts as genetic engineering. SEE: *molecular biology.*

**biotelemetry** (bī″ō-tĕl-ĕm′ĕ-trē) [Gr. *bios,* life, + *tele,* distant, + *metron,* measure] Recording biological events such as temperature, heart rate, ECG, and EEG in subjects remote from the investigator. This is done by transmitting and receiving by telephone or other electronic methods.

**biotics** (bī-ŏt′ĭks) [Gr. *biotikos,* living] The science that deals with the functions of life.

**biotin** (bī′ō-tĭn) A component of the vitamin B complex formerly designated as vitamin H. This heat-sensitive substance, poorly soluble in water, is essential for the metabolism of fat and carbohydrates. It is present in many foods, but liver, kidney, milk, egg yolks, and yeast are particularly rich sources. Deficiencies have been reported in humans and laboratory animals when the diet contains large amounts of raw egg white, which contains avidin, a biotin antagonist that renders the biotin in the diet unavailable. Children with biotin deficiency have retarded mental and physical development, alopecia, impaired immunity, and anemia.

**biotoxin** (bī-ō-tŏk′sĭn) [Gr. *bios,* life, + *toxikon,* poison] A toxin produced by or found in a living organism.

**biotransformation** The chemical alteration that a substance undergoes in the body.

**biotype** (bī′ō-tīp) [″ + *typos,* mark] **1.** Individuals possessing the same genotype. **2.** In microbiology, the former name for biovar. SEE: *biovar.*

**biovar** [*bio*logical *var*iation] In microbiology, a term for variants within a species. These are usually distinguished by certain biochemical or physiological characteristics. SEE: *morphovar; serovar.*

**biovular** (bī-ŏv′ū-lăr) [L. *bis,* twice, + *ovum,* egg] Derived from or pert. to two ova. SYN: *binovular.*

**BiPAP** *bilevel continuous positive airway pressure.*

**bipara** (bĭp′ă-ră) [″ + *parere,* to bring forth, to bear] A woman who has given birth for the second time to an infant or infants, alive or dead, weighing 500 g or more. SYN: *secundipara.*

**biparental** (bī″pă-rĕn′tăl) [″ + *parere,* to bring forth, to bear] Derived from two parents, male and female.

**biparietal** (bī″pă-rī′ĕ-tăl) Concerning the parietal bones or their eminences.

**biparous** (bĭp′ă-rŭs) Producing two ova or offspring at one time.

**biped** (bī′pĕd) [″ + *pes,* foot] An animal with two feet.

**bipenniform** (bī-pĕn′ĭ-form) [″ + *penna,* feather, + *forma,* shape] Muscle fibers that come from each side of a tendon in the manner in which barbs come from the central shaft of a feather.

**biperforate** (bī-pĕr′fō-rāt) [″ + *perforatus,* pierced with holes] Having two openings or perforations.

**biperiden** (bī-pĕr′ĭ-dĕn) An anticholinergic drug used in treating parkinsonism. Trade name is Akineton.

**biphasic** (bī-fāz′ĭk) Consisting of two phases.

**bipolar** (bī-pōl′ăr) [″ + *polus,* a pole] **1.** Having two poles or processes. **2.** Pert. to the use of two poles in electrotherapeutic treatments. The term *biterminal* should be used when referring to an alternating current. **3.** A two-poled nerve cell.

**bipolar disorder** SEE: under *disorder.*

**biramous** (bī-rā′mŭs) [″ + *ramus,* a branch] Possessing two branches.

**bird breeder's lung** Attacks of chills, fever, and cough with shortness of breath in persons closely associated with birds such as pigeons and parakeets. In some patients the onset is slow rather than acute. The symptoms are caused by antigens in the bird's excreta. Symptoms usually subside when exposure to the excrement ceases. SYN: *pigeon breeder's disease.* SEE: *psittacosis.*

**birefractive** (bī″rē-frăk′tĭv) [″ + *refrangere,* to break up] Birefringent.

**birefringence** (bī″rē-frĭn′jĕns) The splitting of a ray of light in two. **birefringent** (-jĕnt), *adj.*

**birth** [Old Norse *burdhr*] The act of being born; passage of a child from the uterus.

***complete b.*** The instant of complete separation of the body of the infant from that of the mother, regardless of whether the cord or placenta is detached.

***cross b.*** Labor in which the fetus lies transversely across the uterus.

***dry b.*** A birth following premature rupture of the fetal membranes.

***live b.*** An infant showing one of the three evidences of life (breathing, heart action, movements of a voluntary muscle) after complete birth. In some countries a live birth is considered not to have occurred if the infant dies during the 24 hr following delivery. Obviously, which of these two definitions is used has considerable effect on various vital statistics concerned with the viability of the fetus at time of delivery.

***multiple b.*** The birth of two or more offspring produced in the same gestation period.

***premature b.*** The birth of a fetus any time between the date of defined viability and 38 weeks' gestation. SYN: *preterm b.* SEE: *prematurity.*

***preterm b.*** Premature b.

**birth canal** The canal through which the fetus passes in birth, comprising the cervix, vagina, and vulva.

**birth center** An alternative nonhospital facility that provides family-oriented maternity care for women judged to be at low risk of experiencing obstetrical complications.

**birth certificate** A legal written record of the birth of a child, as required by U.S. law.

**birth control** Prevention of conception or implantation of the fertilized ovum, or termination of pregnancy. Methods of birth control may be temporary and reversible, or permanent. Temporary methods to avoid conception include physical barriers (e.g., male and female condoms, diaphragm, cervical cap, and vaginal sponge) that are most effective when used in conjunction with chemical barriers, such as spermicidal vaginal suppositories, creams, jellies, or foams. Hormonal methods include oral contraceptive pills and progestin implants to suppress ovulation. Fertility awareness methods, such as rhythm, involve identification of and abstinence during ovulation, graphing basal body temperature and changes in cervical mucus consistency, assist in estimating the day of ovulation. Intrauterine devices (IUD) prevent zygote implantation. Sterilization techniques include male vasectomy and female tubal ligation. Sterilization usually is permanent, but may be reversible. SEE: *abortion; contraceptive; family planning; infanticide; RU 486.*

**birth control pill** A class of medicines taken in pill form to control conception. They contain synthetic forms of estrogen and progesterone or synthetic progesterone alone. SEE: *contraceptive.*

**birth defect** A congenital anomaly. Birth defects are the leading cause of infant mortality in the U.S. and most developed countries. Each year in the U.S. about 150,000 babies are born with serious birth defects. Known causes include human teratogens, chromosomal defects, and single-gene defects. The cause is unknown in about two thirds of the cases.

**birthing chair** A chair designed for use during childbirth. The mother is in a sitting or semireclining position, which facilitates the labor process and is more comfortable than the usual supine position.

**birth injury** Injury sustained by the neonate during the birth process.

**birthmark** Nevus (1).

**birth mother** The biological mother. SEE: *surrogate parenting.*

**birth palsy** Paraplegia or hemiplegia due to birth injury.

**birth parent(s)** The biological parent(s) of a child. SEE: *surrogate parenting.*

**birth rate** The number of live births in 1 year per thousand population.

**birth trauma** Otto Rank's term to describe what he considered the basic source of anxiety in human beings, the birth process. The importance of this concept is controversial.

**birth weight** The weight of the newborn. Normal weight of the newborn is between 5.5 lb (2.5 kg) and 10 lb (4.5 kg). Birth weight is an important index of maturation and chance for survival. Weight of less than 2.5 kg is associated with an increased chance of death in the perinatal period. Medical advances have increased the chance of survival of newborns of 2.0 kg or more.

**birth weight, low** SEE: *low birth weight.*

**bisacodyl** (bĭs-ăk′ō-dĭl; bĭs″ă-kō′dĭl) A cathartic drug that acts by its direct effect on the colon. It may be administered orally or by rectal suppository. Trade names are Dulcolax and Theralax.

**bisacromial** (bĭs″ă-krō′mē-ăl) [L. *bis,* twice, + Gr. *akron,* point, + *omos,* shoulder] Pert. to the two acromial processes.

**bisection** (bī-sĕk′shŭn) [″ + *sectio,* a cutting] Division into two parts by cutting.

**bisexual** (bī-sĕks′ū-ăl) [″ + *sexus,* sex] **1.** Hermaphroditic; having imperfect genitalia of both sexes in one person. **2.** An individual who is sexually attracted to others of either sex. SEE: *heterosexual; homosexual; lesbian.*

**bisferious** (bĭs-fĕr′ē-ŭs) [″ + *ferire,* to beat] Having two beats; dicrotic.

**bisiliac** (bĭs-ĭl′ē-ăk) [″ + *ilium,* ilium] Pert. to the two iliac crests or any corresponding iliac structures.

**bis in die** [L.] ABBR: b.d.; b.i.d. Twice in a day.

**bismuth** (bĭz′mŭth) [Ger. *Wismuth,* white mass] SYMB: Bi. A silvery metallic element; atomic weight 208.980, atomic number 83. Its compounds are used as a protective for inflamed surfaces. Its salts are used as an astringent and as a treatment for diarrhea.

***b. subcarbonate*** An odorless, tasteless powder used as an antacid, astringent, and protective.

INCOMPATIBILITY: Sulfides, acids, acid salts.

***b. subgallate*** A bright yellow powder without odor or taste. It was first used for treatment of skin diseases. General use is the same as for bismuth subnitrate.

***b. subnitrate*** A heavy white odorless powder; used as an astringent, protective, and antiseptic.

INCOMPATIBILITY: Acids, tannins, and

sulfides.

***b. subsalicylate*** ABBR: BSS. BSS has antisecretory and antimicrobial effects in vitro. Its unlabeled use is for prevention of travelers' diarrhea due to enterotoxigenic *Escherichia coli*. It also relieves abdominal cramps. Trade name is Pepto-Bismol.

**bismuth colloids** Several bismuth compounds that are effective in treating peptic ulcers. They act in an acid medium by inhibiting the action of pepsin and reacting with the proteins in the ulcer crater to form a barrier that prevents the diffusion of acid into the area. SEE: *peptic ulcer*.

**bismuth poisoning** Poisoning due to ingestion of bismuth.

SYMPTOMS: Symptoms include metallic taste, foul breath, fever, gastrointestinal irritation, a bluish line at the gum margin, ulcerative process of the gums and mouth, headache, and renal tubular damage.

FIRST AID: The source of bismuth is removed; gastric lavage and high enemas are performed; respiratory support and chelation therapy with BAL are provided.

**bisulfate** (bī-sŭl′fāt) An acid sulfate in which a monovalent metal and a hydrogen ion are combined with the sulfate radical. SEE: *disulfate*.

**bite** (bīt) [AS. *bitan,* to bite] **1.** To cut with the teeth. **2.** An injury in which the body surface is torn by an insect or animal, resulting in abrasions, punctures, or lacerated wounds. There may be evidence of a wound, usually surrounded by a zone of redness and swelling, often accompanied by pain, itching, or throbbing. This type of wound often becomes infected and may contain specific noxious materials such as bacteria, toxins, viruses, or venom. **3.** In dentistry, the angle and manner in which the upper and lower teeth meet.

***balanced b.*** Balanced occlusion of the teeth.

***closed b.*** A bite in which the lower incisors lie behind the upper incisors.

***dog b.*** A lacerated or punctured wound made by the teeth of a dog. The dog should be observed for 10 days to determine the presence of rabies. SEE: *Capnocytophaga canimorsus; rabies*.

TREATMENT: The wound must be cleansed thoroughly. It should be washed vigorously with soap and water for at least 10 min to remove saliva. Flushing with a viricidal agent should be followed with a clear rinse. Unless massive, bleeding should not be stopped because blood flow helps to cleanse the wound. Routine tetanus prophylaxis should be provided and information obtained about the animal, its location, and its owner. These data should be included in a report to public health authorities. Appropriate antirabies therapy must be initiated if the animal is known to have rabies.

***end-to-end b.*** A bite in which the incisors of both jaws meet along the cutting edge when the jaw is closed.

***fire ant b.*** Injury caused by fire ant venom, resulting in local redness and tenderness; the allergic response may be life threatening.

TREATMENT: The area, which may contain multiple bites, should be washed with soap and water. Epinephrine, 0.3 to 0.5 ml of a 1:1000 aqueous solution, should be given subcutaneously every 20 to 30 min. This may be life saving. Use of a tourniquet slows absorption of the venom. Application of ice packs to the area relieves pain. Oxygen, endotracheal intubation, and vasopressors, as well as corticosteroids and antibiotics, may be required.

***flea b.*** SEE: under *flea*.

***human b.*** A lacerated or punctured wound caused by the teeth of a human. The aerobic and anaerobic organisms in the mouth may cause a severe necrotizing lesion.

TREATMENT: The wound should be cleaned thoroughly but not sutured. A moist dressing should be applied and tetanus prophylaxis administered. Both penicillin and a beta-lactamase–resistant penicillin should also be given.

***insect b.*** An injury in which the body surface is torn by an insect, resulting in abrasions, punctures, or lacerated wounds. Insect bites cause more deaths than do snake bites. For more information, see entries for individual insects.

SYMPTOMS: The reaction of a previously sensitized person is a potentially life-threatening medical emergency that requires prompt, effective therapy. Symptoms may include hives, itching and swelling in areas other than the site of the bite, tightness in the chest and difficulty in breathing, hoarse voice, swelling of the tongue, dizziness or hypotension, unconsciousness, and cardiac arrest.

FIRST AID: If the wound is suspected of containing venom, a bandage sufficiently tight to prevent venous return is applied if the bite is on an extremity. The wound is washed with saline solution thoroughly and a dry sterile dressing is applied. Appropriate antitetanus therapy is applied. Treatment for shock may be needed.

Some insect bites contain an acid substance resembling formic acid and consequently are relieved by topically applied alkalies, as ammonia water or baking soda paste. For intense local pain, injection of local anesthetic may be required. Systemic medication may be needed for generalized pain.

Individuals who have had an allergic reaction to an insect bite may benefit from venom immunotherapy. This treatment involves administration of very small amounts of the insect venom over several weeks until immunity develops. Immunity is then maintained by periodic venom boosters.

Persons who have a history of an anaphylactic reaction to insect bites should avoid exposure to insects by wearing protective clothing, gloves, and shoes. Cosmetics, perfumes, and hair sprays should be avoided because they attract some insects, as do brightly colored and white clothing. Because foods and odor attract insects, care should be taken when cooking and eating outdoors.

***mosquito b.*** SEE: under *mosquito*.

***open b.*** A bite in which a space exists between the upper and lower incisors when the mouth is closed.

***snake b.*** SEE: under *snake*.

***spider b.*** SEE: under *spider*.

***stork b.*** Colloquial term for telangiectasia.

***tick b.*** SEE: under *tick*.

**bitelock** A device used in dentistry for retaining bite rims outside the mouth in the same position as they were inside the mouth.

**bitemporal** (bī-tĕm′pō-răl) [L. *bis*, twice, + *temporalis*, pert. to a temple] Pert. to both temples or temporal bones.

**biteplate** (bīt′plāt) A dental device used to correct or diagnose malocclusion. It is worn in the palate, usually on a temporary basis.

**bitewing radiograph** A type of radiograph that shows the crowns and upper third of the roots of upper and lower teeth. It is made by using a dental film with a tab (bitewing) or placement device that holds the film in place when the jaws are closed on the tab. The purpose is to detect proximal caries and the interdental bone. SYN: *interproximal radiograph*.

**Bitot's spots** (bē′tōz) [Pierre A. Bitot, Fr. physician, 1822–1888] Triangular shiny gray spots on the conjunctiva seen in vitamin A deficiency.

**bitrochanteric** (bī″trō-kăn-tĕr′ĭk) Concerning both greater trochanters of the two femurs.

**bitter** (bĭt′ĕr) [AS. *biter*, strong] Having a disagreeable taste.

**bituminosis** (bī-tū″mĭ-nō′sĭs) A form of pneumoconiosis from dust of soft coal.

**biuret** (bī′ū-rĕt) [L. *bis*, twice, + *urea*] A crystalline decomposition derivative of urea.

**biuret test** A method for measuring protein in the serum. The presence of biuret can be detected by the addition of sodium hydroxide and copper sulfate solutions to the sample. A rose to violet color indicates the presence of protein, and a pink and finally blue color indicates the presence of urea.

**bivalent** (bī-vā′lĕnt) [″ + *valens*, powerful] **1.** Divalent. **2.** In cytology, a structure consisting of two paired homologous chromosomes, each split into two sister chromatids during meiosis.

**biventer** (bī-vĕn′tĕr) [″ + *venter*, belly] A muscle with two bellies.

**biventral** (bī-vĕn′trăl) Digastric.

**bizygomatic** (bī″zī-gō-măt′ĭk) Concerning the most prominent point on each of the two zygomatic arches.

**Bjerrum's screen** (byĕr′oomz) [Jannik P. Bjerrum, Danish ophthalmologist, 1827–1892] A 1-m square planar surface viewed from a distance of 1 m and consisting of a large square of black cloth with a central mark for fixation. It is used to plot the physiological blind spot, the central and paracentral scotomata, and other visual field defects. SYN: *tangent screen*.

**Bjerrum's sign** A sickle- or comet-shaped blind spot usually found in the central zone of the visual field; seen in glaucoma.

**B.K.** *below knee*, a term used to refer to the site of amputation of a lower extremity.

**Bk** Symbol for the element berkelium.

**black** (blăk) [AS. *blaec*] **1.** Devoid of color or reflecting no light. **2.** Marked by dark pigmentation.

**blackdamp** An atmosphere formed by the slow absorption of oxygen and the release of carbon dioxide by the coal in a mine.

**black death** SEE: *plague*.

**black eye** Bruising, discoloration, and swelling of the eyelid and tissue around the eye due to trauma.

TREATMENT: Application of ice packs during the first 24 hr will inhibit swelling. Hot compresses after the first day may aid absorption of the fluids that produce discoloration. Topically applied leeches have been used to extract the pigment from the traumatized area. SEE: *leech*.

**blackhead** An open comedo. SEE: *comedo*.

**black lung** Lay term for the chronic lung disease or pneumoconiosis found in coal miners. SYN: *coal worker's pneumoconiosis*.

**blackout 1.** Sudden loss of consciousness. This may occur while coughing, following nocturnal urination, or while swallowing in patients who have esophageal disease. SEE: *postural hypotension*. **2.** Temporary loss of consciousness. In aviators, temporary or transient loss of vision or consciousness is usually due to loss of blood supply to the brain. This is caused by the centrifugal force experienced in high-speed aircraft maneuvers that produce positive gravitational forces. SEE: *alcoholic blackout; red-out*.

**blackwater fever** Hemoglobinuria following chronic falciparum malaria infection.

SYMPTOMS: Symptoms include sudden onset, fever, tender and enlarged liver and spleen, dark urine, epigastric pain, vomiting, jaundice, and sudden shock.

**bladder** (blăd′dĕr) [AS. *blaedre*] A membranous sac or receptacle for a secretion, as the gallbladder; commonly used to designate the urinary bladder. SEE: *bladder, urinary; genitourinary system*.

***atony of b.*** Inability to urinate due to lack of muscle tone. It is frequently seen after traumatic deliveries or after the use

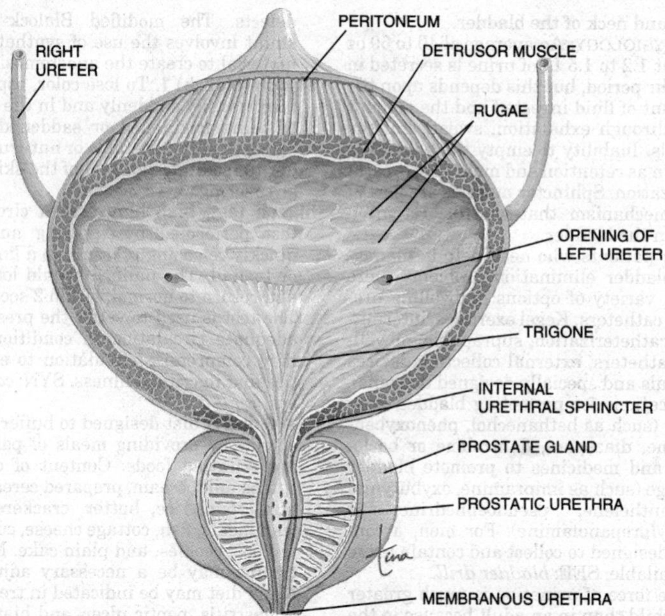


**URINARY BLADDER,** MALE, FRONTAL SECTION

of epidural anesthesia.

***autonomous b.*** A bladder in which there is interruption in both the afferent and efferent limbs of the reflex arcs. Bladder sensation is absent; dribbling is constant; residual urine amount is large.

***exstrophy of b.*** Congenital eversion of the urinary bladder. The abdominal wall fails to close and the inside of the bladder may protrude through the abdominal wall.

***hypertonic b.*** **1.** A bladder with excessive muscle tone. **2.** Increased muscular activity of the bladder.

***irritable b.*** Bladder condition marked by increased frequency of contraction with an associated desire to urinate.

***motor paralytic b.*** A neurogenic bladder caused by defective nerve supply to the bladder. In the acute form urination is not possible. In the chronic form there is difficulty in urinating, which may lead to recurrent urinary tract infections.

***nervous b.*** A condition marked by the repeated desire to urinate, but doing so fails to empty the bladder.

***neurogenic b.*** Any dysfunction of the urinary bladder caused by lesions of the central nervous system or nerves supplying the bladder.

***spastic b.*** Neurogenic bladder due to complete transection of the spinal cord above the sacral segments.

***urinary b.*** A muscular, membranous, distensible reservoir that holds urine situated in the pelvic cavity. It receives urine from the kidneys through the ureters and discharges it from the body through the urethra. SYN: *vesica urinaria.* SEE: illus.; *urinary system.*

ANATOMY: The bladder is situated in the anterior inferior portion of the pelvic cavity. In the female it lies in front of the anterior wall of the vagina and the uterus; in the male it lies in front of the rectum. The lower portion of the bladder, continuous with the urethra, is called the neck; its upper tip, connected with the umbilicus by the median umbilical ligament, is called the apex. The region between the two openings of the two ureters and the urethra is the trigone. The wall of the bladder consists of an inner mucous layer of transitional epithelium, a coat of smooth muscle (the outer layer comprising the detrusor urinae), and a fibrous layer. On its free superior surface is a layer of peritoneum. The bladder is supported by numerous ligaments; it is supplied with blood by the superior, middle, and inferior vesical arteries and numerous veins and lymphatics; and it is innervated with nerves derived from the third and fourth sacral nerve by way of the hypogastric plexus.

The bladder has a normal storage capacity of 500 ml (about 34 oz) or more. In disease states it may be greatly distended. A frequent cause of distention of the bladder in elderly men is interference with urination due to hypertrophy of the prostate gland, which surrounds the urethra and neck of the bladder.

PHYSIOLOGY: An average of 40 to 50 oz (about 1.2 to 1.5 L) of urine is secreted in a 24-hr period, but this depends upon the amount of fluid ingested and the amount lost through exhalation, sweat, and the bowels. Inability to empty the bladder is known as retention and may require catheterization. Sphincter muscles are part of the mechanism that controls retention within the bladder.

For patients who need help in managing bladder elimination problems there are a variety of options: indwelling urethral catheters, Kegel exercises, intermittent catheterization, suprapubic indwelling catheters, external collecting devices (urinals and specially designed bedpans), medications for promoting bladder emptying (such as bethanechol, phenoxybenzamine, diazepam, dantrolene or baclofen), and medicines to promote bladder storage (such as imipramine, oxybutynin, propanthelene, pseudoephedrine, or phenylpropanolamine). For men, a condom designed to collect and contain urine is available. SEE: *bladder drill.*

The force of urination is much greater in a child than in an adult because in the child the bladder is more an abdominal organ than a pelvic one. The child's abdominal muscles help to expel the urine.

EXAMINATION: *Palpation:* The bladder cannot be palpated when empty. When full it appears as a tumor in the suprapubic region that is smooth and oval on palpation.

*Percussion:* When it is distended with urine, the rounded superior margin is easily made out by observing the tympanic sound of the intestines on one hand and dull sound of the bladder on the other.

**bladder drill** A technique used to treat stress urinary incontinence in women in which the patient charts the number of urinations, the intervals between urination, and the volume of urine passed. She also notes the degree and frequency of incontinence. The intervals between urinations are gradually increased. Also called *bladder training.*

**bladder worm** Cysticercus.

**Blalock-Hanlon procedure** [Alfred Blalock, U.S. surgeon, 1899–1965; C. Rollins Hanlon, U.S. surgeon, b. 1915] The surgical creation of an atrial septal defect or enlargement of the foramen ovale in an infant with transposition of the great arteries. This procedure helps to improve oxygenation until total repair is undertaken.

**Blalock-Taussig shunt** [Alfred Blalock, U.S. surgeon; 1899–1965; Helen B. Taussig, U.S. pediatrician; 1898–1986] ABBR: B-T shunt. An anastomosis of a subclavian artery to the pulmonary artery on the same side. This procedure increases blood flow to the lungs in children with cardiac defects. The modified Blalock-Taussig shunt involves the use of synthetic graft material to create the anastomosis.

**blanch** (blănch) **1.** To lose color, esp. of the face, usually suddenly and in the context of being frightened or saddened. **2.** To briefly scald a vegetable or nut-fruit in order to facilitate removal of the skin, peel, or covering. **3.** To bleach.

**blanch test, blanching test** A circulation test performed by applying and then quickly releasing pressure to a fingernail or toenail. The nailbed should lose color and return to normal within 2 sec or less. The test is used to verify the presence of adequate circulation in conditions that may compromise circulation to extremities and in critical illness. SYN: *capillary nail refill test.*

**bland diet** A diet designed to buffer gastric acidity by providing meals of palatable, nonirritating foods. Content of diet includes milk, cream, prepared cereals, gelatin, soup, rice, butter, crackers, eggs, lean meats, fish, cottage cheese, custards, tapioca, cookies, and plain cake. Multivitamins may be a necessary adjunct. A bland diet may be indicated in treatment of gastritis, peptic ulcer, and hiatal hernia.

**Blandin's glands** (blŏn-dănz′) [Philippe F. Blandin, Fr. surgeon, 1798–1849] Small glands situated deep on each side of the frenulum of the tongue near the apex. SYN: *Nuhn's glands.*

**blast** [AS. *bloest,* a puff of wind] A violent movement of air such as accompanies the explosion of a shell or bomb; a violent sound, as the blast of a horn.

**blast-** [Gr. *blastos,* germ] Combining form indicating *germ, bud, embryonic state of development.*

**-blast** [Gr. *blastos,* germ] Combining form used as a suffix indicating *an embryonic state of development.*

**blast** A cell that produces something (e.g., osteoblast, fibroblast).

**blastema** (blăs-tē′mă) [Gr. *blastema,* sprout] The immature material from which cells and tissues are formed.

**blastid** (blăs′tĭd) [Gr. *blastos,* germ] The clear space marking the site of the organizing nucleus in the impregnated ovum.

**blastocele, blastocoele** (blăs′tō-sēl) [″ + *koilos,* hollow] The cavity in the blastula of the developing embryo.

**blastochyle** (blăs′tō-kīl) [″ + *chylos,* juice] Fluid contained in the blastocele.

**blastocyst** (blăs′tō-sĭst) [″ + *kystis,* bag] In mammalian embryo development, the stage that follows the morula. It consists of an outer layer of trophoblast, which is attached to an inner cell mass. The enclosed cavity is the blastocele. The whole is called blastodermic vesicle or blastocyst. At this stage, implantation in the endometrium (lining of the uterus) occurs. SYN: *blastodermic vesicle.*

**blastocyte** (blăs′tō-sīt) [″ + *kytos,* cell] An

undifferentiated embryonic cell.

**blastocytoma** (blăs-tō-sī-tō'mă) [" + " + *oma,* tumor] Blastoma.

**blastoderm** (blăs'tō-dĕrm) [" + *derma,* skin] A disk of cells (germinal disk or blastodisk) that develops on the surface of the yolk in an avian or reptilian egg from which the embryo develops; also, in mammalian embryos a disk of cells lying between the yolk sac and the amniotic cavity from which the embryo develops. From the blastoderm, the three germ layers (ectoderm, mesoderm, and endoderm) arise.

**blastodermic vesicle** Blastocyst.

**blastodisk** (blăs'tō-dĭsk) [" + *diskos,* disk] A flat disk of embryonic cells on the surface of the yolk of the ovum. It forms from the blastomeres.

**blastogenesis** (blăs"tō-jĕn'ĕ-sĭs) [" + *genesis,* generation, birth] **1.** Multiplication by budding. **2.** Transmission of characteristics by the germ plasm.

**blastokinin** (blăs"tō-kī'nĭn) A globulin found in the uterine lumen of some mammals near the time of blastocyst implantation.

**blastolysis** (blăs-tŏl'ĭ-sĭs) [" + *lysis,* dissolution] Lysis or destruction of a germ cell or a blastoderm.

**blastoma** (blăs-tō'mă) *pl.* **blastomata** [" + *oma,* tumor] A neoplasm composed of immature, undifferentiated cells derived from the blastema of an organ or tissue. SYN: *blastocytoma.*

**blastomere** (blăs'tō-mēr) [" + *meros,* a part] One of the cells resulting from the cleavage of a fertilized ovum.

**blastomerotomy** (blăs"tō-mēr-ŏt'ō-mē) [" + " + *tome,* incision] Destruction of blastomeres.

**Blastomyces** (blăst-ō-mī'sēz) [Gr. *blastos,* germ, + *mykes,* fungus] A genus of yeastlike budding fungi pathogenic to humans. At room temperature the genus grows as a mycelial (fungal) form and at body temperature as a yeastlike form.

***B. brasiliensis*** The fungus that causes South American blastomycosis. This organism and disease are also called *Paracoccidioides brasiliensis* and paracoccidioidomycosis, respectively.

***B. dermatitidis*** The fungus that causes North American blastomycosis, a rare fungal infection in humans. SEE: illus.

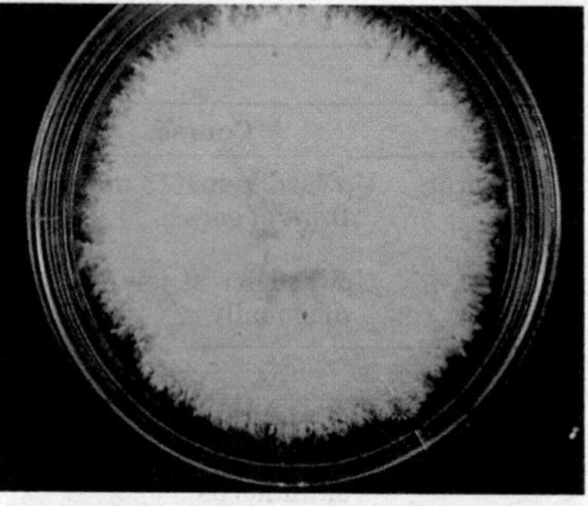

BLASTOMYCES DERMATITIDIS IN CULTURE; FUNGAL FORM AT ROOM TEMPERATURE

**blastomycete** (blăs"tō-mī'sēt) Any organism of the genus *Blastomyces.*

**blastomycosis** (blăs"tō-mī-kō'sĭs) [" + *mykes,* fungus, + *osis,* condition] Infection caused by inhalation of the conidia of *Blastomyces dermatitidis.* This rare fungal infection may produce inflammatory lesions of the skin (cutaneous form) or lungs or a generalized invasion of the skin, lungs, bones, central nervous system, kidneys, liver, and spleen. SYN: *North American b.; Gilchrist's disease.*

TREATMENT: Treatment consists of amphotericin B or ketoconazole.

***North American b.*** Blastomycosis.

***South American b.*** Paracoccidiodomycosis.

**blastopore** (blăs'tō-por) [" + *poros,* passageway] In the embryo of mammals, the small opening into the archenteron made by invagination of the blastula.

**blastospore** (blăs'tō-spor) [" + *sporos,* seed] A spore formed by budding from a hypha, as in yeast.

**blastula** (blăs'tū-lă) *pl.* **blastulae** [L.] An early stage in the development of an ovum, consisting of a hollow sphere of cells enclosing a cavity, the blastocele. In large-yolked eggs, the blastocele is reduced to a narrow slit. In mammalian development, the blastocyst corresponds to the blastula of lower forms.

**Blatta** (blăt'ă) [L.] A genus of insects (that includes the cockroaches) of the order Orthoptera.

***B. germanica*** The German cockroach or croton bug.

***B. orientalis*** The Oriental cockroach, also known as the black beetle, a common European house pest.

**bleaching** Use of an oxidizing chemical to remove stain or discoloration from a tooth.

**bleaching powder** Chlorinated lime or calcium hypochlorite.

**bleb** (blĕb) An irregularly shaped elevation of the epidermis; a blister or a bulla. Blebs may vary in size from less than 1 cm to as much as 5 to 10 cm; they may contain serous, seropurulent, or bloody fluid. Blebs are a primary skin lesion that may occur in dermatitis herpetiformis, pemphigus, and syphilis. SEE: *bulla.*

**bleeder** [AS. *bledan,* to bleed] **1.** One whose ability to coagulate blood is either deficient or absent, so that small cuts and injuries lead to prolonged bleeding. SEE: *hemophilia.* **2.** A small artery that has been cut or torn.

**bleeding** [AS. *bledan,* to bleed] **1.** Emitting blood, as from an injured vessel. **2.** The process of emitting blood, as a hemorrhage or the operation of letting blood.

**Control of Arterial Bleeding**

| Artery | Course | Bone Involved | Spot to Apply Pressure |
|---|---|---|---|
| *For Wounds of the Face* | | | |
| Temporal | Upward ½ in. (13 mm) in front of ear | Temporal bone | Against bony prominence immediately in front of ear or on temple |
| Facial | Upward across jaw diagonally | Lower part of lower maxilla | 1 in. (2.5 cm) in front of angle of lower jaw |
| *For Wounds of the Upper Extremity* | | | |
| Axillary | Downward across outer side of armpit to inside of humerus | Head of humerus | High up in armpit against upper part of humerus |
| Brachial | Along inner side of humerus under edge of biceps muscle | Shaft of humerus | Against shaft of humerus by pulling aside and gripping biceps, pressing tips of fingers deep down against bone |
| *For Wounds of the Lower Extremity* | | | |
| Femoral | Down thigh from pelvis to knee from a point midway between iliac spine and symphysis pubis to inner side of end of femur at knee joint | Brim of pelvis | Against brim of pelvis, midway between iliac spine and symphysis pubis |
| Femoral | | Shaft of femur | High up on inner side of thigh, about 3 in. (7.6 cm) below brim of pelvis, over line given in direction of knee |
| Posterior tibial | Downward to foot in hollow just behind prominence of inner ankle | Inner side of tibia, low down above ankle | For wounds in sole of foot, against tibia in center of hollow behind inner ankle |

Normally, when blood plasma is exposed to air, it changes to allow fibrin to form. This entangles the corpuscles and forms a blood clot. SEE: *coagulation, blood; coagulation factors; hemorrhage*.

***arterial b.*** Bleeding in spurts of bright red blood.

FIRST AID: Arterial bleeding may be controlled by applying pressure with the fingers at the nearest pressure point between it and the heart. The artery is located and digital pressure is applied above it until bleeding stops or until the artery is ligated. A tourniquet should not be used. SEE: table.

***breakthrough b.*** Intermenstrual spotting or bleeding experienced by some women who are taking oral contraceptives.

***dysfunctional uterine b.*** ABBR: DUB. A diagnosis of exclusion in which there is abnormal bleeding from the uterus not caused by tumor, inflammation or pregnancy. These causes of bleeding must be ruled out before DUB may be diagnosed. The condition may occur with ovulatory cycles, but most often occurs with anovulation. It is common in women with polycystic ovary syndrome. Endometrial hyperplasia followed by sloughing of the endometrium may occur in women with repeated anovulatory cycles.

ETIOLOGY: The absence of the luteal progesterone phase interferes with normal endometrial preparation for implantation or menstruation. Prolonged constant levels of estrogen stimulate uneven endometrial hypertrophy so that some areas slough and bleed before others, causing intermittent bleeding.

***internal b.*** Hemorrhage from an internal organ or site, esp. the gastrointestinal tract.

***menstrual b.*** SEE: *menstruation*.

***occult b.*** Inapparent bleeding, esp. that which occurs into the intestines and can be detected only by chemical tests of the feces.

***venous b.*** A continuous flow of dark red blood.

FIRST AID: Venous bleeding may be controlled by firm, continuous pressure applied directly to the bleeding site. If bleeding is from an area over soft tissues, a large, compact bandage should be held firmly against the site.

---

Caution: A tourniquet should not be used. If the bleeding is over a bony area, as in the case of a ruptured varicose vein of the leg, a coin held firmly against the vein will provide immediate control of the blood loss. The patient should be taken to a physician as soon as possible.

---

**bleeding time** The time required for blood to stop flowing from a small wound or pinprick. This test is done using one of several techniques. Depending on the method used, the time may vary from 1 to 3 min (Duke method) or from 1 to 9 min (Ivy method). The Duke method consists of timing the cessation of bleeding after the ear lobe has received a standardized puncture. The Ivy method is done in a similar manner following puncture of the skin of the forearm. The validity of this test to predict clinically significant bleeding has been questioned.

**blenn-** SEE: *blenno-*.

**blennadenitis** (blĕn″ăd-ĕ-nī′tĭs) [″ + *aden,* gland, + *itis,* inflammation] Inflammation of the mucous glands.

**blennemesis** (blĕn-ĕm′ĕ-sĭs) [″ + *emesis,* vomiting] Vomiting of mucus.

**blenno-, blenn-** [Gr. *blennos,* mucus] Combining form meaning *mucus.*

**blennogenic, blennogenous** (blĕn″ō-jĕn′ĭk, blĕn-ŏj′ĕ-nŭs) [″ + *gennan,* to produce] Secreting mucus.

**blennoid** (blĕn′oyd) [″ + *eidos,* form, shape] Like mucus; mucoid.

**blennophthalmia** (blĕn″ŏf-thăl′mē-ă) [″ + *ophthalmos,* eye] **1.** Catarrhal conjunctivitis. **2.** Gonorrheal ophthalmia.

**blennorrhagia** (blĕn″ō-rā′jē-ă) [″ + *rhegnynai,* to break forth] Blennorrhea.

**blennorrhea** (blĕn″ō-rē′ă) [Gr. *blennos,* mucus, + *rhoia,* flow] Any discharge from mucous membranes. SYN: *blennorrhagia.*

***inclusion b.*** B. neonatorum.

***b. neonatorum*** Inflammation of the conjunctiva in newborns. It is caused by *Chlamydia trachomatis,* a special group of bacteria that forms cytoplasmic inclusion bodies in the epithelial cells. SYN: *inclusion b.*

**blennothorax** (blĕn″ō-thō′răks) [″ + *thorax,* chest] The accumulation of mucus in the bronchial tubes or alveoli.

**blennuria** (blĕn-ū′rē-ă) [″ + *ouron,* urine] The presence of mucus in the urine.

**Blenoxane** Trade name for bleomycin sulfate.

**bleomycin** (blē-ō-mī′sĭn) Any one of a group of antitumor agents produced by *Streptomyces verticillus.*

***sterile sulfate b.*** Bleomycin used in treating various carcinomas of the skin, head, neck, and lungs, as well as testicular tumors. Trade name is Blenoxane.

**blephar-** SEE: *blepharo-*.

**blepharadenitis** (blĕf″ăr-ăd-ĕ-nī′tĭs) [Gr. *blepharon,* eyelid, + *aden,* gland, + *itis,* inflammation] Inflammation of the meibomian glands.

**blepharal** (blĕf′ăr-ăl) Pert. to an eyelid.

**blepharectomy** (blĕf″ă-rĕk′tō-mē) [″ + *ektome,* excision] Surgical excision of all or part of an eyelid.

**blepharedema** (blĕf″ăr-ĕ-dē′mă) [″ + *oidema,* swelling] Edema of the eyelids, causing swelling and a baggy appearance.

**blepharism** [″ + *-ismos,* condition] Twitching or blinking of the eyelids. SEE: *blepharospasm.*

**blepharitis** (blĕf″ăr-ī′tĭs) [″ + *itis,* inflammation] Ulcerative or nonulcerative inflammation of the hair follicles and glands along the edges of the eyelids.

SYMPTOMS: The eyelids become red, tender, and sore with sticky exudate and scales on the edges; the eyelids may become inverted; there may be watering of the eyes and loss of eyelashes. Styes and meibomian cysts are associated with the condition.

ETIOLOGY: The ulcerative type is usually caused by infection with staphylococci. The cause of the nonulcerative type is often unknown; it may be due to allergy or exposure to dust, smoke, or irritating chemicals.

NURSING IMPLICATIONS: The patient's scalp, eyebrows, and eyelids should be kept clean; and patient hand contact with the eyes should be avoided. The nurse demonstrates the proper technique for bathing the eyelids with warm saline solution and for applying warm compresses to remove any drainage or crusts. The nurse instructs the patient to wash the hands first, then the eyelids, before applying the prescribed antibiotic ointment, which is applied to the lid margins in a narrow ribbon, beginning at the inner and working toward the outer canthus of the eye. The ointment container should not touch the lid or eye surface. The procedure ends with handwashing, and the patient's or caregiver's ability to perform eye care as instructed is evaluated.

***b. angularis*** Blepharitis in which the medial angle of the eye is involved with blocking of openings of lacrimal ducts.

***b. ciliaris*** Inflammation affecting the ciliary margins of the eyelids. SYN: *b. marginalis.*

***b. marginalis*** B. ciliaris.

***b. parasitica*** Blepharitis caused by parasites such as mites or lice.

***seborrheic b.*** A nonulcerative form of blepharitis in which waxy scales form on the eyelids. It is usually associated with seborrheic dermatitis of the surrounding skin.

***b. squamosa*** Chronic blepharitis with scaling.

***b. ulcerosa*** Blepharitis with ulceration.

**blepharo-, blephar-** [Gr. *blepharon,* eyelid]

Combining form meaning *eyelid.*

**blepharoadenitis** SEE: *blepharadenitis.*

**blepharoadenoma** (blĕf″ăr-ō-ăd-ĕ-nō′mă) [″ + ″ + *oma,* tumor] A glandular tumor of the eyelid.

**blepharoatheroma** (blĕf″ăr-ō-ăth″ĕ-rō′mă) [″ + *athere,* thick fluid, + *oma,* tumor] A sebaceous cyst of the eyelid.

**blepharochalasis** (blĕf″ăr-ō-kăl′ă-sĭs) [″ + *chalasis,* relaxation] Hypertrophy of the skin of the upper eyelid due to loss of elasticity following edematous swellings as in recurrent angioneurotic edema of the lids. The skin may droop over the edge of the eyelid when the eyes are open.

**blepharoclonus** (blĕf″ă-rŏk′lō-nŭs) [″ + *klonos,* tumult] Clonic spasm of the muscles that close the eyelids (orbicularis oculi).

**blepharoconjunctivitis** (blĕf″ă-rō-kŏn-jŭnk″tĭ-vī′tĭs) [″ + L. *conjungere,* to join together, + Gr. *itis,* inflammation] Inflammation of the eyelids and conjunctiva.

**blepharodiastasis** (blĕf-ă-rō-dī-ăs′tă-sĭs) [″ + *diastasis,* separation] Excessive separation of the eyelids, causing the eyes to open wide.

**blepharoncus** (blĕf″ă-rŏn′kŭs) [″ + *onkos,* tumor] A tumor of the eyelid.

**blepharopachynsis** (blĕf″ă-rō-pă-kĭn′sĭs) [″ + *pachynsis,* thickening] Abnormal thickening of the eyelid.

**blepharophimosis** (blĕf″ă-rō-fī-mō′sĭs) [″+ *phimosis,* narrowing] Blepharostenosis.

**blepharoplast** (blĕf′ă-rō-plăst) A minute mass of chromatin in a cell, forming the base of a flagellum. Morphologically it is identical to a centriole. SYN: *basal body.*

**blepharoplasty** (blĕf′ă-rō-plăs″tē) Plastic surgery upon the eyelid.

**blepharoplegia** (blĕf″ă-rō-plē′jē-ă) [Gr. *blepharon,* eyelid, + *plege,* a stroke] Paralysis of an eyelid.

**blepharoptosis** (blĕf″ă-rō-tō′sĭs) [″ + *ptosis,* a dropping] Drooping of the upper eyelid.

**blepharopyorrhea** (blĕf″ă-rō-pī-ō-rē′ă) [″+ *pyon,* pus, + *rhoia,* flow] Purulent discharge from the eyelid.

**blepharorrhaphy** (blĕf″ă-ror′ă-fē) [″ + *rhaphe,* seam, ridge] Tarsorrhaphy.

**blepharorrhea** (blĕf″ă-rō-rē′ă) [″ + *rhoia,* flow] Discharge from the eyelid.

**blepharospasm** (blĕf′ă-rō-spăsm) [″ + *spasmos,* a convulsion] A twitching or spasmodic contraction of the orbicularis oculi muscle due to habit spasm, eyestrain, or nervous irritability. SEE: *Marcus-Gunn syndrome.*

***essential b.*** Blepharospasm of unknown cause. It may be so severe as to be debilitating. Surgery has helped some patients. Botulinum toxin A injected into the muscles that control the spasm has been of benefit. This treatment will need to be repeated after 2 to 3 months.

**blepharosphincterectomy** (blĕf″ă-rō-sfĭnk″tĕr-ĕk′tō-mē) [″ + *sphinkter,* a constrictor, + *ektome,* excision] Excision of part of the orbicularis palpebrarum to relieve pressure of the eyelid on the cornea.

**blepharostat** (blĕf′ă-rō-stăt) [″ + *histanai,* cause to stand] A device for separating the eyelids during an operation.

**blepharostenosis** (blĕf″ă-rō-stĕn-ō′sĭs) [″ + *stenosis,* act of narrowing] Narrowing of the palpebral slit due to an inability to open the eye normally. SYN: *blepharophimosis.*

**blepharosynechia** (blĕf″ă-rō-sĭ-nē′kē-ă) [″ + *synecheia,* a holding together] Adhesion of the edges of the upper eyelid to the lower one. SYN: *ankyloblepharon.*

**blepharotomy** (blĕf-ă-rŏt′ō-mē) [″ + *tome,* incision] Surgical incision of the eyelid.

**Bleuler, Eugen** [1857–1939] Swiss psychiatrist known for studies on schizophrenia.

**blind** [AS.] **1.** Without sight. **2.** In medical research, pert. to a situation in which one group of patients receives a form of therapy, a second group receives another form or a placebo, and a third group (the control group) remains untreated but is followed in the same manner as the other group(s). In such studies, it is the practice that physicians treating and following the patients do not know which groups received which therapy. The treating physicians are said to be "blinded." The study is designed this way to prevent the treating physicians from being influenced (i.e., biased, in their judgment of the efficacy of the therapy or of the placebo effects).

**blind loop syndrome** A condition caused by intraluminal growth of bacteria in the upper portion of the small intestine. Conditions associated with this syndrome are anatomical lesions that lead to stasis of such as diverticula or surgically created blind loops; diseases associated with motor function of the small intestine; and any condition that decreases gastric acid secretion. This leads to malabsorption. The syndrome is diagnosed by the clinical signs and symptoms of malabsorption and the use of breath tests for detecting overgrowth of bacteria in the intestine.

TREATMENT: Antimicrobial therapy and nutritional support are needed. Tetracyclines may be ineffective due to bacterial resistance.

**blindness** Inability to see. The leading causes of blindness in the U.S. are cataracts, glaucoma, and age-related macular degeneration.

A variety of free services are available for the blind and physically handicapped. Talking Book Topics published bimonthly in large-print, cassette, and disc formats is distributed free to blind and physically handicapped individuals who participate in the Library of Congress free reading program. It lists recorded books and magazines available though a national network of cooperating libraries and provides news of developments and activities in library services. Subscription requests may be sent to Talking Books Topics, CMLS,

P.O. Box 9150, Melbourne, FL 32902-9150.

***amnesic color b.*** An inability to remember the names of colors.

***color b.*** SEE: *color blindness.*

***cortical b.*** Blindness due to lesions in the left and right occipital lobes of the brain. The eyes are still able to move and the pupillary light reflexes remain, but the blindness is as if the optic nerves had been severed. The usual cause is occlusion of the posterior cerebral arteries. Transitory cortical blindness may follow head injury.

***day b.*** An inability to see in daylight; hemeralopia.

***eclipse b.*** Blindness due to burning the macula while viewing an eclipse without using protective lenses. Looking directly at the sun anytime can damage the eyes. SYN: *solar b.*

***hysterical b.*** Partial or total blindness associated with attacks of hysteria and occurring in the absence of any organic defect.

***legal b.*** A degree of loss of visual acuity that prevents a person from performing work requiring eyesight. In the U.S. this is defined as corrected visual acuity of 20/200 or less, or a visual field of 20° or less in the better eye. In the U.S. in 1978 there were an estimated 498,000 blind people. It is estimated there are 20 to 40 million blind people worldwide.

***letter b.*** An inability to understand the meaning of letters; a form of aphasia.

***night b.*** An inability to see at night; nyctalopia.

***object b.*** A disorder in which the brain fails to recognize things even though the eyes are functioning normally. SEE: *apraxia.*

***psychic b.*** Sight without recognition due to a brain lesion.

***river b.*** SEE: *onchocerciasis.*

***snow b.*** Blindness, usually temporary, resulting from the glare of sunlight on snow. It may result in photophobia and conjunctivitis, the latter resulting from effects of ultraviolet radiation.

***solar b.*** Eclipse b.

***transient b.*** Temporary blindness in one or both eyes. The onset is usually sudden. It may be caused in both eyes by any condition that temporarily interferes with maintenance of blood pressure in the ophthalmic arteries, such as migraine; carotid artery insufficiency; temporal arteritis; retinal artery spasm caused by hypertensive encephalopathy; uremia; or eclampsia; optic neuritis; glaucoma; and hysteria. SYN: *amaurosis fugax.*

***word b.*** An inability to understand written or printed words.

**blind spot 1.** Physiological scotoma situated 15° to the outside of the visual fixation point; the point where the optic nerve enters the eye (optic disk), a region devoid of rods and cones. **2.** In psychiatry, the inability of an individual to have insight into his or her own personality.

**blink** To open and close the eye involuntarily; to wink rapidly, esp. in response to being surprised or startled or in response to an object closely approaching the eye without warning.

**blink reflex** Automatic closing of the eyes in response to a sudden movement of an object toward the eyes.

**blister** [MD. *bluyster,* a swelling] **1.** A collection of fluid below or within the epidermis. **2.** To form a blister.

TREATMENT: The area should be cleansed with mild soap and a protective dressing applied. Unless a blister is painful or interferes with function due to its size, it should not be punctured. If puncturing is needed, it should be done aseptically, with the skin left in place. A sterile pressure bandage should be applied. After about 2 days, debridement may be necessary. SEE: *Universal Precautions Appendix.*

---

Caution: If infection develops, treatment is the same as for any other wound, including tetanus prophylaxis or booster as required.

---

***blood b.*** A small subcutaneous or intracutaneous extravasation of blood due to the rupture of blood vessels.

TREATMENT: A firm dressing should be applied with moderate pressure to prevent extravasation and hasten absorption. In some cases it is desirable to puncture aseptically and aspirate.

***fever b.*** Herpes simplex of the lip.

***fly b.*** A blister produced by application of cantharides to the skin.

**bloated** (blōt′ĕd) [AS. *blout*] Swollen or distended beyond normal size as by serum, water, or gas.

**bloating** Abdominal distress of distention caused by abnormal intestinal motility and not by excess gas. Therapy for this troublesome symptom is rarely effective.

**block** [MD. *blok,* trunk of a tree] **1.** An obstruction or stoppage. **2.** A method of regional anesthesia used to stop the passage of sensory impulses in a nerve, a nerve trunk, the dorsal root of a spinal nerve, or the spinal cord, thus depriving a patient of sensation in the area involved. SEE: *anesthesia.* **3.** To obstruct any passageway or opening.

***air b.*** Leakage of air from the respiratory passageways and its accumulation in connective tissues of the lungs, forming an obstruction to the normal flow of air.

***atrioventricular b.*** A condition in which the depolarization impulse is delayed or blocked at the atrioventricular (A-V) node or a more distal site, as in the A-V bundle or bundle branches. A-V block can be partial or complete. There are several degrees of A-V block. *First-degree* block is due to prolonged A-V conduction; electrocardiograms show a characteristic prolonged PR interval. *Second-degree* blocks are intermittent (i.e., some, but not all, A-V impulses are transmitted to the ventricles). *Third degree* block, also known as complete A-V block, is present when no atrial impulses are conducted to the ventricles; it is clinically indistinguishable from bilateral bundle branch block.

***A-V b.*** Atrioventricular b.

***bite b.*** **1.** A wedge of sturdy material used to maintain space between the two jaws. **2.** A film holder held between the teeth for stable retention of the film packet during dental radiology.

***ear b.*** Blockage of the auditory tube to the middle ear. It may result from trauma, infection, or an accumulation of cerumen.

***epidural b.*** SEE: *anesthesia, epidural.*

***field b.*** Regional anesthesia in which a limited operative area is walled off by an anesthetic.

***heart b.*** SEE: *heart block.*

***mandibular b.*** Regional anesthesia of the lower face and mandibular tissues by infiltration of the mandibular division of the trigeminal nerve.

***maxillary b.*** Second division b.

***nerve b.*** The induction of regional anesthesia by preventing sensory nerve impulses from reaching the centers of consciousness. This is usually done on a temporary basis, by using chemical or electrical means. In the former case, it is accomplished by injecting an anesthetic solution, such as procaine, around the nerve but at some distance, or by anesthetizing nerve endings in the region itself (infiltration).

***neuromuscular b.*** A disturbance in the transmission of impulses from a motor endplate to a muscle. It may be caused by an excess or deficiency of acetylcholine or by drugs that simulate such action.

***paravertebral b.*** Infiltration of the stellate ganglion with a local anesthetic.

***saddle b.*** SEE: under *anesthesia.*

***second division b.*** Regional anesthesia of the upper face and maxillary tissues by infiltration of the maxillary division of the trigeminal nerve. SYN: *maxillary b.*

***sinoatrial b.*** Heart block in which there is interference in the passage of impulses between the sinus node and the atria.

***spinal b.*** Blockage in the flow of cerebrospinal fluid within the spinal canal.

***ventricular b.*** Interference in the flow of cerebrospinal fluid between the ventricles or from the ventricles through the foramina to the subarachnoid space.

**blockade** (blŏk-ād′) Prevention of the action of something, such as a drug or a body function.

***adrenergic b.*** Inhibition of responses to adrenergic sympathetic nerve impulses and to agents such as epinephrine.

***cholinergic b.*** Inhibition of cholinergic nerve stimuli or cholinergic agents.

***lymphatic b.*** A local defense mechanism in which minute bits of material, such as fibrinous exudate from injured tissue, enter local lymphatic vessels, obstructing them and preventing foreign substances, esp. bacteria, from passing through them.

**blocker** A drug that prevents the normal action of a system or cell receptor.

**blocking 1.** Obstructing. **2.** In psychoanalysis, a sudden break in free association as a defense against unpleasant ideas.

**blocking factors** Substances present in the serum of tumor-bearing animals that are capable of blocking the ability of immune lymphocytes to kill tumor cells.

**blood** [AS. *blod*] The cell-containing fluid that circulates through the heart, arteries, veins, and capillaries, carrying nourishment, electrolytes, hormones, vitamins, antibodies, heat, and oxygen to the tissues and taking away waste matter and carbon dioxide. SEE: *erythropoietin.*

CHARACTERISTICS: Blood has a distinctive, somewhat metallic, odor. Arterial blood is bright red or scarlet and usually pulsates if the artery has been cut. Venous blood is dark red or crimson and flows steadily from a cut vein.

COMPOSITION: Human blood is 52% to 62% plasma and 38% to 48% cells. The plasma is mostly water and transports many materials. The cells are the erythrocytes (red cells), leukocytes (white cells), and thrombocytes (platelets). The leukocytes comprise neutrophils, eosinophils, basophils, lymphocytes, and monocytes. SEE: illus.; *buffy coat; plasma; serum.*

An adult weighing 70 kg has a blood volume of about 5 L or 70 ml/kg of body weight. Blood constitutes approx. 7% to 8% of the body weight. The pH of the blood is from 7.35 to 7.45. The specific gravity of blood varies from 1.048 to 1.066, the corpuscles being heavier and plasma lighter than this. Blood is of slightly higher specific gravity in men than in women. Specific gravity is higher after exercise and at night. SEE: *blood count; corpuscle; plasma; platelet.*

FUNCTION: In passing through the lungs the blood gives up carbon dioxide and absorbs oxygen; after leaving the heart, it is carried to the tissues as arterial blood and then returned to the heart in the venous system. It moves in the aorta at an average speed of 30 cm/sec, and it makes the circuit of the vascular system in about 20 sec. Red blood cells carry oxygen; white blood cells participate in the immune response to infection; platelets are important in blood clotting. The plasma transports nutrients, waste products, hormones, carbon dioxide, and other substances, and contributes to fluid-electrolyte balance and thermal regulation.

FORMATION: Red blood cells are pro-

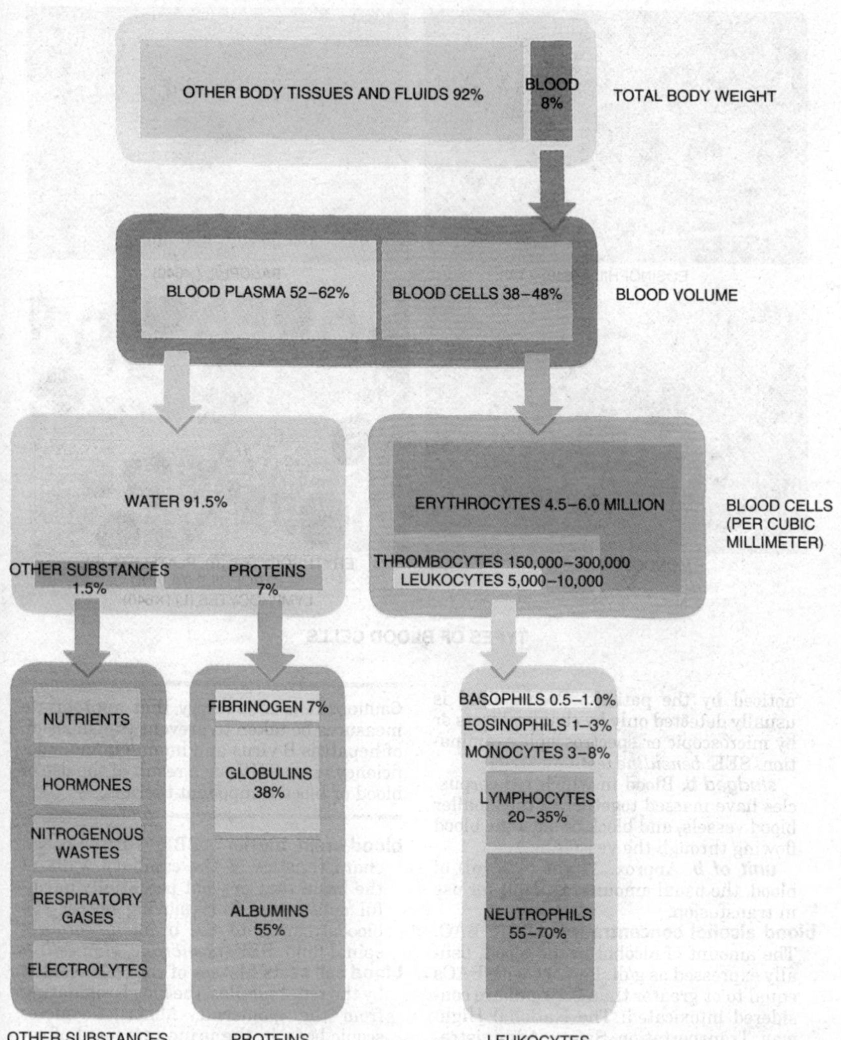


**BLOOD COMPOSITION**

COMPONENTS OF BLOOD AND RELATIONSHIP OF BLOOD TO OTHER BODY TISSUES

duced at the rate of approx. 2,400,000 each second. Since each red blood cell lives for approx. 120 days, the number of red cells remains at a level concentration.

***arteriolized b.*** Blood that has been exposed to oxygen in the lung.

***clotting of b.*** SEE: *coagulation, blood.*

***cord b.*** The blood present in the umbilical vessels connecting the placenta with the fetus.

***defibrinated b.*** Whole blood from which fibrin was separated during the clotting process. If whole blood is stirred, the stringy elastic fibrin comes out on the stirrer; the fibrin can be washed until white. The remaining thick red blood, called defibrinated blood, can no longer clot. If it is centrifuged, a clear liquid called serum appears in the upper half of the centrifuged tube; serum differs from plasma chiefly in that it does not contain fibrinogen (the precursor of fibrin). The corpuscles are in the lower part of the tube. SEE: *buffy coat.*

***occult b.*** Blood that is present in such small quantities that it is not apparent to the eye. Blood may be present in feces but of such color and consistency as to be un-

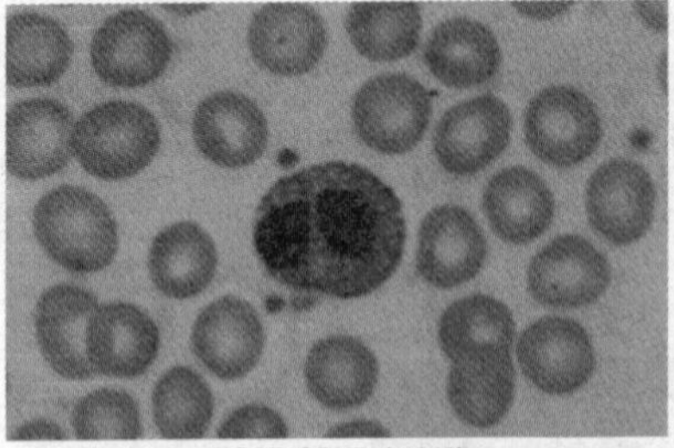
EOSINOPHIL (×640)

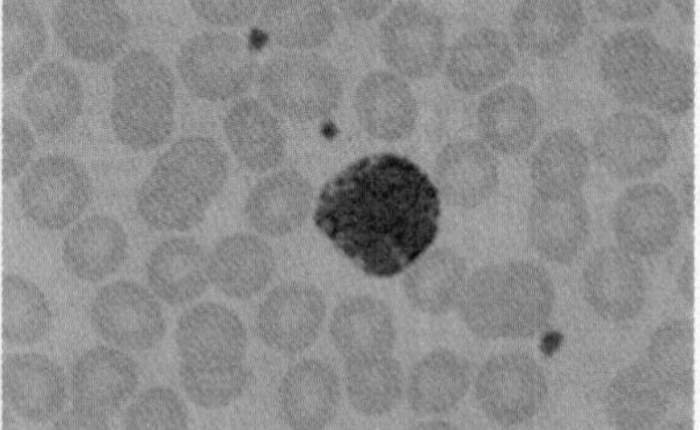
BASOPHIL (×640)

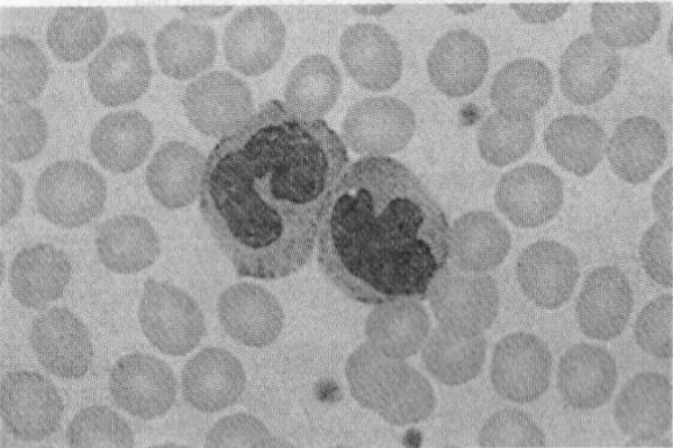
MONOCYTES (×640)

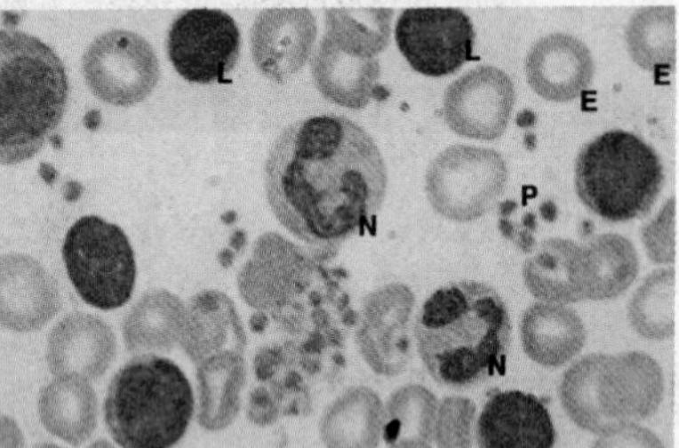

ERYTHROCYTES (E), PLATELETS (P), NEUTROPHILS (N), AND LYMPHOCYTES (L) (×640)

**TYPES OF BLOOD CELLS**

noticed by the patient. Occult blood is usually detected only by chemical tests or by microscopic or spectroscopic examination. SEE: *benzidine test.*

***sludged b.*** Blood in which red corpuscles have massed together in the smaller blood vessels, and block or slow the blood flowing through the vessels.

***unit of b.*** Approx. 1 pint (473 ml) of blood, the usual amount available for use in transfusion.

**blood alcohol concentration** ABBR: BAC. The amount of alcohol in the blood, usually expressed as g/dl. Persons with BACs equal to or greater than 0.10 g/dl are considered intoxicated. The National Highway Transportation Safety Administration considers a fatal crash to be alcohol-related if the individual—driver or pedestrian—has a BAC equal to or greater than 0.01 g/dl. In the U.S., injuries from motor vehicle crashes are the leading cause of death in people aged 6 to 33 years.

**blood bank** A place in which whole blood and certain derived components are processed, typed, and stored until needed for transfusion. Blood is mixed with adenine-supplemented citrate phosphate dextrose and is stored at 4°C (39°F). Heparin may be used as a preservative. Banked blood should be used as soon as possible because the longer it is stored, the fewer red blood cells survive in usable form. Ninety percent of the red cells survive up to 14 days of storage, but only 70% remain after 24 days.

Caution: It is mandatory that appropriate measures be taken to prevent transmission of hepatitis B virus and human immunodeficiency virus (HIV) as a result of the use of blood or blood component therapy.

**blood-brain barrier** ABBR: BBB. Special characteristics of the capillary walls of the brain that prevent potentially harmful substances from moving out of the bloodstream into the brain or cerebrospinal fluid. SEE: *membrane, glial cell.*

**blood cell casts** Masses of red cells molded by the renal tubules, the blood originating from the glomeruli. Abnormal microscopic body in the urine composed of coagulated serum covered with red blood cells.

**blood clot** A coagulated mass of blood. SEE: *coagulation, blood.*

**blood coagulation** SEE: *coagulation, blood.*

**blood component therapy** Transfusion of one or more of the components of whole blood. The blood components may have been taken from the patient previously (autologous transfusion) or donated by someone else (homologous transfusion). Except in the case of acute hemorrhage, the transfusion of whole blood is rarely needed. Use of a component rather than whole blood permits several patients to benefit from a single blood donation. Components used in clinical medicine include packed red blood cells; leukocyte-poor red blood cells; frozen glycerolized red blood cells (RBCs); thawed deglycerolized

RBCs; washed RBCs; whole blood; heparinized whole blood; granulocytes; platelets; plasma and plasma fractions. The latter include antihemophilic factor (factor VIII), prothrombin complex (factors VII, IX, and X), gamma globulin, and albumin. SEE: *blood transfusion; Universal Precautions Appendix.*

---

Caution: It is mandatory that appropriate measures be taken to prevent transmission of hepatitis B virus and human immunodeficiency virus (HIV) as a result of the use of blood or blood component therapy.

---

**blood corpuscle** Blood cell.

**blood count** The number of red corpuscles and leukocytes per microliter (μl) of whole blood. Normally, the number of erythrocytes in men averages 5 million/μl; in women, 4.5 million/μl. Prolonged exposure to high altitude increases the number. Leukocytes average 5000 to 10,000/μl. Platelets range from 140,000 to 400,000/μl by direct counting method. A special chamber is filled with blood and the cells are visualized under the microscope and then counted. The type of fluid used to dilute the blood depends upon whether the white or red cells are to be counted. Hemoglobin and hematocrit are determined from samples of whole blood.

***differential b.c.*** The number and type of white blood cells as determined by microscopic examination of a thin layer of blood on a glass slide after it has been suitably stained to show the morphology of the various cells. The number and variety of white cells in a sample of a given size are obtained. Also, even though the red cells are not counted by this method, their shape, size, and color can be evaluated. Some blood diseases and inflammatory conditions may be recognized in this way. In a differential count, the varieties of the leukocytes and their percentages normally should be: neutrophils (segmented), 40% to 60%; eosinophils, 1% to 3%; basophils, 0.5% to 1%; lymphocytes, 20% to 40%; monocytes, 4% to 8%.

**blood crossmatching** The process of mixing a sample of the donor's red blood cells with the recipient's serum (major crossmatching), and mixing a sample of the recipient's blood with the donor's serum (minor crossmatching). It is done before transfusion to determine compatibility of blood.

**blood donation, preoperative** The preoperative collection of blood from a patient for the purpose of reinfusing it at the time of elective surgery. SEE: *blood salvage.*

**blood donor** One who gives blood to be used for transfusion.

**blood doping** SEE: *doping, blood; erythrocyte reinfusion.*

**blood gas analysis** Chemical analysis of the blood for the concentration of oxygen and carbon dioxide. This may be done on arterial or venous blood; the specimen may be obtained from an arm vein or, by way of a catheter, from a peripheral vein to the heart. The blood sample is usually collected in a heparinized vacuum tube with care being taken to ensure that the specimen is not exposed to air. SEE: *blood gases.*

**blood gases** The oxygen utilized and carbon dioxide produced during metabolic processes. Levels of these gases vary in response to certain disease conditions. Analysis of the blood for these gases is important in helping to evaluate the extent of the deviation of acids and bases from the normal. Before appropriate therapy can be instituted, information obtained from those values is analyzed with respect to other laboratory results and the clinical condition. SEE: *acidosis; alkalosis.*

**blood group** A genetically determined system of antigens located on the surface of the erythrocyte. There are a number of human blood group systems; each system is determined by a series of two or more genes that are allelic or closely linked on a single autosomal chromosome. The ABO system (discovered in 1901 by Karl Landsteiner) is of prime importance in blood transfusions. The Rhesus (Rh) system is esp. important in obstetrics. There are about 30 Rh antigens. SEE: illus.; *Rh factor.*

The population can be phenotypically divided into four ABO blood groups: A, B, AB, and O. Individuals in the A group have the A antigen on the surface of their red cells; B group has the B antigen on red cells; AB group has A and B antigens on red cells; and O group has neither A nor B antigens on red cells. The individuals in each group have in their sera the corresponding antibody agglutinin to the red cell antigens that they lack. Thus, a group A person has in the blood serum the anti-B antibody; group B has anti-A antibodies; group AB has no antibodies for A and B; and group O individuals have anti-A and anti-B antibodies in their sera.

Blood group factors are important in clinical medicine because of the interaction of the antigens on cells with their agglutinin(s) in the serum.

For example, destruction of red cells transfused from either a group A or group B donor to a group O recipient—the anti-A and anti-B agglutinins in the recipient's serum would react with the A or B antigens on the donor's red cells.

Analysis of blood groups is important in identification of bloodstains for medicolegal purposes, in genetic and anthropological studies, and in the past in determination of the probability of fatherhood in paternity suits.

**bloodless** Without blood.

**bloodletting** Removal of blood from the

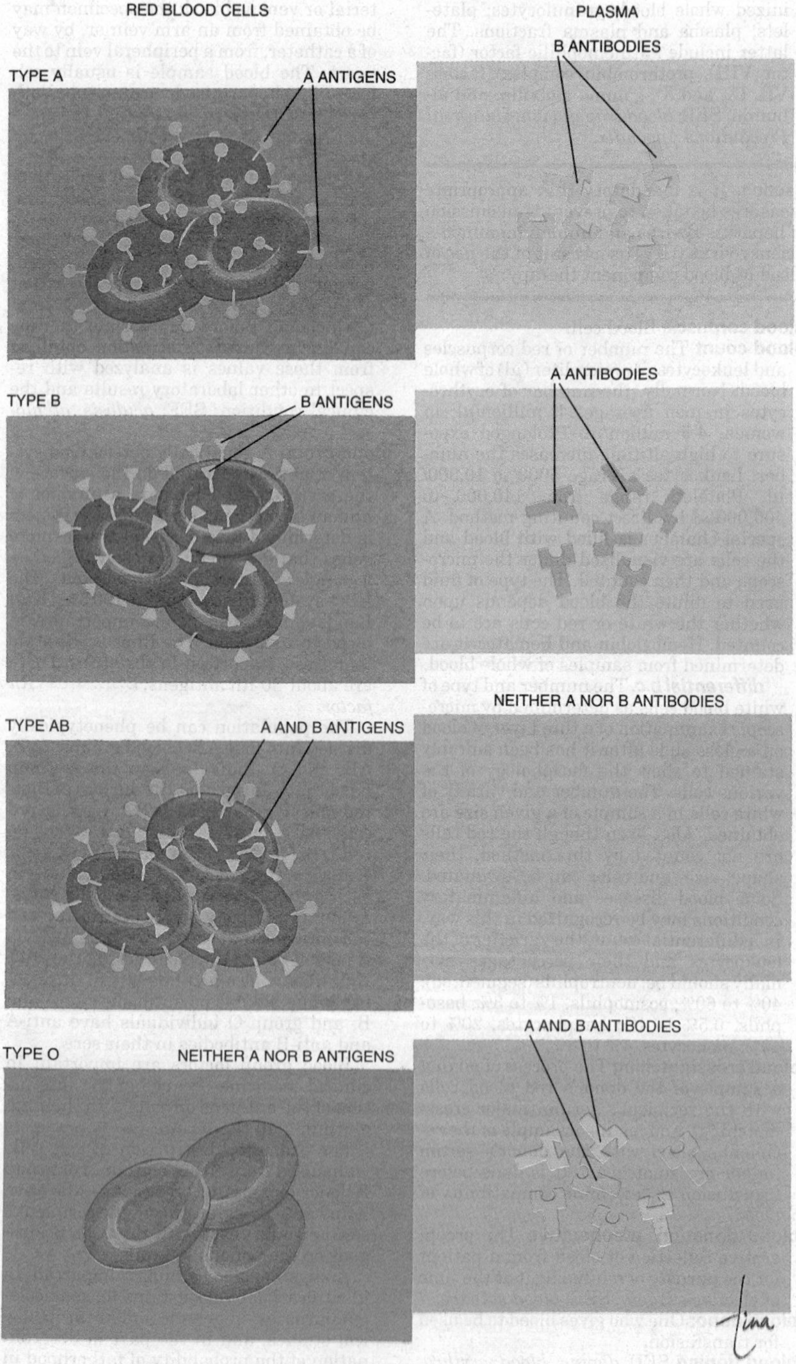

RED BLOOD CELLS

PLASMA

TYPE A

A ANTIGENS

B ANTIBODIES

TYPE B

B ANTIGENS

A ANTIBODIES

TYPE AB

A AND B ANTIGENS

NEITHER A NOR B ANTIBODIES

TYPE O

NEITHER A NOR B ANTIGENS

A AND B ANTIBODIES

ABO BLOOD TYPES

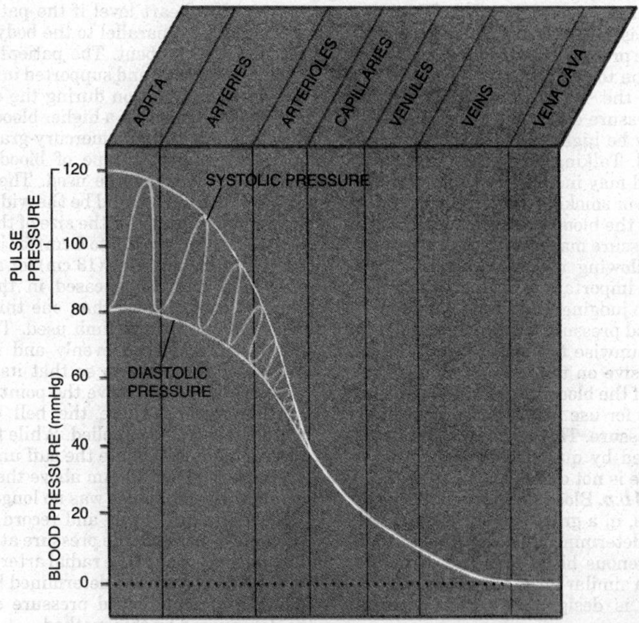


SYSTEMIC **BLOOD PRESSURE** CHANGES THROUGH THE VASCULAR SYSTEM; SYSTOLIC AND DIASTOLIC PRESSURES MERGE AS BLOOD ENTERS CAPILLARIES

body as a therapeutic measure, usually by venipuncture. This technique is used in treating hemochromatosis, polycythemia vera, and in infants born with elevated hematocrits.

**blood level** The concentration of anything, esp. a drug, in the plasma, serum, or blood.

**blood patch** SEE: *postlumbar puncture headache.*

**blood platelet** A small cell fragment in circulating blood, averaging about 3 microns in diameter. Platelets tend to agglutinate into small clusters in shed blood. They originate from giant bone marrow cells (megakaryocytes). Ten substances associated with or derived from platelets are involved in blood coagulation. Only three of these 10 factors, platelet factors 2, 3, and 4, are unique to platelets. Platelets promote hemostasis by adhering to damaged vascular surfaces. There they begin a complex process to participate in blood coagulation.

The normal number of platelets in circulating blood in adults ranges from 140,000 to 440,000 ($\mu$l) with an average of 250,000$\mu$l. There is no difference in blood platelet counts in men and women. Reduction below normal is called thrombocytopenia. In certain forms of hemophilia, blood platelets are abnormally stable and fail to release thrombokinase, thus increasing coagulation time. SEE: *coagulation, blood.*

**blood poisoning** An outdated term for septicemia.

**blood pressure** The tension exerted by blood against the arterial walls. Determining factors include ventricular contraction, arteriolar and capillary resistance, elasticity of the arterial walls, and blood volume and viscosity. SEE: *chronic low blood pressure; normal blood pressure.*

The blood pressure reaches its highest values in the left ventricle during systole. It decreases in the arterial system as the distance from the heart increases, and is lower in capillaries than in arteries. The systolic arterial blood pressure rises during activity or excitement and falls during sleep. In the normal, relaxed, sitting adult, it may be as low as 100 or as high as 140 mm Hg. SEE: illus.

The following findings in adults are considered abnormal: systolic pressure persistently above 140; diastolic pressure persistently above 90. When either the systolic pressure is 160 or more or the diastolic pressure is 115 or above, the elevation is considered severe. Blood pressure varies with age, sex, altitude, muscular development, and states of mental and physical stress and fatigue. Usually it is lower in women than in men, low in childhood, and higher in the elderly.

There are a variety of conditions and factors which can lead to an erroneous blood pressure being recorded. When the pressure is taken in a clinic or by a physician the pressure may be temporarily elevated due to the patient's anxiety. This is called the "white coat effect." If the blood pressure cuff is too small the pressure may be higher than if a larger cuff was used. Talking while the pressure is measured may increase the value; drinking coffee or smoking a cigarette just prior to taking the blood pressure may raise it; blood pressure may be reduced for several hours following vigorous exercise. It is therefore important to evaluate these factors when judging whether or not the person's blood pressure is within normal limits. It is unwise to judge a person to be hypertensive on the basis of a single recording of the blood pressure. Devices are available for use in the home to monitor blood pressure. This technique is reliable when used by qualified persons. Use of the device is not difficult.

***central b.p.*** Blood pressure in the heart chambers, in a great vein, or close to the heart. If determined in a vein, it is termed central venous blood pressure; if in the aorta or a similar large artery close to the heart, it is designated central arterial blood pressure.

***chronic low b.p.*** A condition in which the systolic blood pressure is consistently less than 100 mm Hg. In the absence of associated disease, low blood pressure is often a predictor of longevity and continued health. SEE: *hypotension; hypotension, orthostatic.*

***diastolic b.p.*** Blood pressure when the ventricles are relaxed; systemic pressure is normally 60 to 85 mm Hg. It is dependent primarily upon the elasticity of the arteries and peripheral resistance, which in turn is dependent upon the diameter of the arterioles.

***direct measurement of b.p.*** Determination of the blood pressure in one of several arteries. It is done by placing a sterile needle or small catheter inside an artery and having the blood pressure transmitted through that system to a suitable recorder. As the blood pressure fluctuates, the changes are recorded graphically.

***high b.p.*** Blood pressure that is above the normal range. The person making this diagnostic judgment must consider the person's age, body build, previous blood pressure, and state of mental and physical health at the time the blood pressure is measured. Generally it is inadvisable to declare that a person has elevated blood pressure if the opinion is based on one blood pressure measurement. SYN: *hypertension.*

***indirect measurement of b.p.*** A simple external method for measuring blood pressure.

*Palpation method:* The same arm, usually the right, should be used each time the pressure is measured. The arm should be raised to heart level if the patient is sitting, or kept parallel to the body if the patient is recumbent. The patient's arm should be relaxed and supported in a resting position. Exertion during the examination could result in a higher blood pressure reading. Either a mercury-gravity or aneroid-manometer type of blood pressure apparatus may be used. The blood compression cuff should be the width and length appropriate for the size of the subject's arm: narrow (2.5 to 6 cm) for infants and children and wide (13 cm) for adults. The inflatable bag encased in the cuff should be 20% wider than one third the circumference of the limb used. The deflated cuff is placed evenly and snugly around the upper arm so that its lower edge is about 1 in. above the point of the brachial artery where the bell of the stethoscope will be applied. While feeling the radial pulse, inflate the cuff until the pressure is about 30 mm above the point where the radial pulse was no longer felt. Deflate the cuff slowly and record as accurately as possible the pressure at which the pulse returns to the radial artery. Systolic blood pressure is determined by this method; diastolic blood pressure cannot be determined by this method.

*Auscultatory method:* Begin as above. After inflating the cuff until the pressure is about 30 mm above the point where the radial pulse disappears, place the bell of the stethoscope over the brachial artery just below the blood pressure cuff. Then deflate the cuff slowly, about 2 to 3 mm Hg per heartbeat. The first sound heard from the artery is recorded as the systolic pressure. The point at which sounds are no longer heard is recorded as the diastolic pressure. For convenience the blood pressure is recorded as figures separated by a slash. The systolic value is recorded first.

Sounds heard over the brachial artery change in quality at some point prior to the point the sounds disappear. Some physicians consider this the diastolic pressure. This value should be noted when recording the blood pressure by placing it between the systolic pressure and the pressure noted when the sound disappears. Thus, 120/90/80 indicates a systolic pressure of 120 with a first diastolic sound change at a pressure of 90 and a final diastolic pressure of 80. The latter pressure is the point of disappearance of all sounds from the artery. When the values are so recorded, the physician may use either of the last two figures as the diastolic pressure. When the change in sound and the disappearance of all sound coincide, the result should be written as follows: 120/80/80.

***mean b.p.*** Half of the sum of systolic and diastolic values (for a normal person in good health, about 100 mm Hg).

***negative b.p.*** Blood pressure that is

less than atmospheric pressure, as in the great veins near the heart.

***normal b.p.*** In healthy young persons, a blood pressure reading of 100 to 140 mm Hg systolic and 60 to 90 mm Hg diastolic. Loss of resilience in the vascular tree and physiological changes of age must be considered when levels above 140 systolic or above 90 diastolic are obtained in apparently healthy older persons.

***systolic b.p.*** Blood pressure during contraction of the ventricles; systemic pressure is normally 90 to 135 mm Hg.

**blood pressure monitor** A device that automatically obtains and usually records the blood pressure at certain intervals, using the direct or indirect method of determining pressure. In some models, an alarm or light signal is activated if the pressure rises or falls to an abnormal level.

**blood pressure monitoring, ambulatory** Use of a portable device worn by the patient that automatically inflates and deflates a blood pressure cuff and records the blood pressure. The machine may be programmed to obtain readings at frequent intervals.

**blood salvage** During or following surgery, collection of blood from a patient's operative site. The blood is then reinfused in the patient. Some patients whose religious beliefs prohibit transfusion of allogeneic blood will permit reinfusion of their own blood. SEE: *autologous blood transfusion.*

**bloodshot** Local congestion of the smaller blood vessels of a part, as when the vessels of the conjunctiva are dilated and visible.

**blood shunting** A condition in which blood, by going through an abnormal pathway or bypass, does not travel its normal route. It may occur when an arteriovenous fistula forms or in congenital anomalies of the heart in which the blood passes from the right atrium or ventricle directly to the left atrium or ventricle respectively, through a defect in the wall (septum) that normally separates the atria and ventricles.

**blood smear** A drop of blood spread thin on a slide for examination.

*Procedure:*

1. The slide must be grease-free. It is cleaned with alcohol, rinsed in warm water, and wiped clean with a lint-free towel or lens paper.
2. A small drop of blood is placed on the slide; the end of another slide (spreader slide) is placed against the first slide at a 45° angle and pulled back against the drop of blood so that the drop spreads between the point of contact of the two slides. Then the spreader slide is pushed forward against the first slide; the blood will form an even, thin smear.
3. The slide is dried by waving it in the air; the slide should not be heated.
4. The blood smear is covered with Wright's stain and allowed to stand 2 min.
5. An equal amount of distilled water or buffer solution is added and mixed uniformly. It is allowed to stand 5 min.
6. The stain is gently washed off and the slide is allowed to dry.
7. If a permanent slide is desired, balsam or methacrylate and a glass cover slip are applied.

*Stain:* A common method is to cover the blood smear with Wright's stain. Allow to stand 2 min. Add an equal amount of distilled water or buffer solution, mixing uniformly. Let stand 5 min. Gently wash off stain. Allow to dry. If permanent slide is desired, apply balsam or methacrylate and apply a glass cover slip.

**bloodstream** The blood that flows through the circulatory system of an organism.

**blood sugar** Glucose in the blood, normally 60 to 100 mg/100 ml of blood. It rises after a meal to as much as 150 mg/100 ml of blood but this may vary. SEE: *glucose.*

**blood test** A test to determine the chemical, physical, or serological characteristics of the blood or some portion of it.

**blood thinner** A popular but erroneous name for an anticoagulant.

**blood transfusion** The replacement of blood or one of its components. Effective and safe transfusion therapy requires a thorough understanding of the clinical condition being treated. This is essential to determine whether a transfusion of whole blood or one of the blood components is indicated. Also it is contraindicated to add an extra load on the circulation of a patient whose cardiovascular system is already severely compromised. Most patients require blood components rather than whole blood. SEE: *autologous blood transfusion; blood component therapy; transfusion, exchange; transfusion reactions; Universal Precautions Appendix.* In general, a patient who receives only a single unit of blood is in no more need of a blood transfusion than the donor. Nevertheless, administration of a single unit may be indicated in elderly surgical patients with coronary disease and in patients who have an acute blood loss of several units but are stabilized by use of one unit. Also, if at surgery or during bleeding from the intestinal tract, a single unit controls the bleeding, then a single unit is justified. Nevertheless, it is important to remember that each blood transfusion has the potential of being infected with HIV or hepatitis B virus, or other blood-borne pathogens.

NURSING IMPLICATIONS: The nurse identifies the patient from both the hospital identification band and blood bank band. Two health-care professionals (one the administering nurse) verify the patient's ABO and Rh blood type and its compatibility with the unit of blood or packed cells to be administered, as well as the unit's expiration date and time. Outdated blood is not used but returned to the blood bank for disposal. The blood or blood product is retrieved from the blood bank refrigerator immediately before administration, because blood should not be stored in other than approved refrigerators and cannot be returned to blood bank storage if the unit's temperature exceeds 50°F (10°C), a change that will occur within approx. 30 min of removal from storage. Before the transfusion is started, the patient's vital signs (including temperature) are checked and documented. The nurse visually inspects the blood for clots or discoloration and then administers the transfusion through an approved line containing a blood filter, preferably piggybacked through physiological saline solution on a Y-type blood administration set. No other IV solutions or drugs may be infused with blood (unless specifically prescribed) because of potential incompatibility. In the first 15 min, the blood flow rate is slowed to limit intake to no more than 50 ml. The nurse remains with the patient during this time and instructs the patient to report any adverse reactions, such as back or chest pain, hypotension, fever, increase in temperature of more than 1.8°F (1°C), chills, pain at the infusion site, tachycardia, tachypnea, wheezing, cyanosis, urticaria, or rashes. If any of these occurs, the transfusion is stopped immediately, the vein is kept open with physiological saline solution, and the patient's physician and the blood bank are notified. If incompatibility is suspected, the nurse returns the blood and set to the blood bank, obtains samples of the patient's blood and urine for laboratory analysis, and records the data from the unit. If no symptoms occur in the first 15 min and vital signs remain stable, the transfusion rate is increased to complete the tranfusion within the prescribed time, or (if necessary) the transfusion is administered as fast as the patient's overall condition permits. Once the transfusion begins, the nurse administers the blood within a maximum of 4 hr to maintain biological effectiveness and limit the risk of bacterial growth. (If the patient's condition does not permit transfusing the prescribed amount within this time frame, the nurse arranges to have the blood bank split the unit and properly store the second portion.) The patient's vital signs and response are monitored every 30 min throughout the transfusion and 30 min afterward; stated precautions are observed and indications of volume overload (distended neck veins, bounding pulse, hypertension, dyspnea) are assessed for. Blood should not be administered through a central line unless an approved in-line warming device is used. A warmer also should be used whenever multiple transfusions place the patient at risk for hypothermia, which can lead to dysrhythmias and cardiac arrest.

***autologous b.t.*** SEE: *autologous blood transfusion.*

**blood typing** The method used to determine various factors when blood is tested according to blood group systems such as ABO, MN, or Rh-Hr.

**blood urea nitrogen** ABBR: BUN. Nitrogen in the blood in the form of urea, the metabolic product of the breakdown of amino acids used for energy production. The normal concentration is 8 to 18 mg/dl. The level of urea in the blood provides a rough estimate of kidney function. An increase in the blood urea nitrogen level usually indicates decreased renal function. SEE: *creatinine.*

**blood vessels** The veins, arteries, and capillaries.

**blood warmer** A device for warming banked blood to body temperature before it is transfused.

**bloody sweat** Hemathidrosis.

**bloody weeping** Hemorrhage from the conjunctiva.

**blotch** A blemish, spot, or area of discoloration on the skin.

**blotting method** A technique for analyzing a tiny portion of the primary structure of genomic material (DNA or RNA).

***Northern b.m.*** A blot analysis technique for analyzing a small portion of RNA.

***Southern b.m.*** A blot analysis technique used in molecular genetics to analyze a small portion of DNA.

***Western b.m.*** A technique for analyzing protein antigens. SYN: *immunoblotting.*

**blowfly** One of the flies belonging to the family Calliphoridae. Most blowflies are scavengers. Their larvae live in decaying flesh or meat, although occasionally they may live in decaying or suppurating tissue. However, one species, the screwworm fly, *Callitroga hominivorax,* attacks living tissue, laying its eggs in the nostrils or open wounds of its domestic animal or human host, giving rise to myiasis. SEE: *Calliphora vomitoria; myiasis.*

**blowpipe** A tube through which a gas or current of air is passed under pressure and directed upon a flame to concentrate and intensify the heat.

**BLS** *basic life support.*

**blue** [O. Fr. *bleu*] **1.** A primary color of the spectrum; sky color; azure. **2.** Cyanotic.

**blue baby** SEE: *baby, blue.*

**bluebottle fly** A fly of the family Calliphoridae. It breeds in dung or the flesh of dead animals.

**Blue Cross** A nonprofit medical care insurer in the U.S. The insurance is mostly for hospital services. SEE: *Blue Shield.*

**Blue Shield** A nonprofit medical care insurer in the U.S. The insurance is for that part of medical care provided by health care professionals. SEE: *Blue Cross.*

**Blumberg's sign** (blŭm'bĕrgs) [Jacob Moritz Blumberg, Ger. surgeon and gynecologist, 1873–1955] The occurrence of a sharp acute pain when the examiner presses his or her hand over McBurney's point and then releases the hand pressure suddenly. This sign is indicative of peritonitis. SYN: *rebound tenderness.*

**Blumenbach's clivus** (bloo'mĕn-bawks) [Johann F. Blumenbach, Ger. physiologist and anthropologist, 1752–1840] The sloping part of the sphenoid bone behind the posterior clinoid processes.

**blush** [AS. *blyscan,* to be red] Redness of the face and neck due to vasodilation caused by emotion or heat. Blushing may also be associated with certain diseases, including carcinoid syndrome, pheochromocytoma, and Zollinger-Ellison syndrome.

**B lymphocyte** B cell.

**B.M.A.** *British Medical Association.*

**B.M.E** *Biomedical Engineer.*

**B.M.E.T** *Biomedical Engineering Technologist.*

**B-mode (brightness mode) display** In ultrasonography, imaging dots on the screen indicate echoes. The brighter the dot relative to the background, the greater the strength of the echo.

**B.M.R.** *basal metabolic rate.*

**B.M.S.** *Bachelor of Medical Science.*

**BMT** *bone marrow transplant.*

**BNA** *Basle Nomina Anatomica.*

**board 1.** A long, flat piece of a substance such as wood or firm plastic. SEE: *bed board.* **2.** A corporate or governmental body, such as a board of directors or board of health.

**board certification** In medicine, a process that ensures that an individual has met standards beyond those of admission to licensure and has passed specialty examinations in the field. The various medical professional organizations establish their own standards and administer their own board certification examinations. Individuals successfully completing all requirements are called Fellows, such as Fellow of the American College of Surgeons (F.A.C.S.) or Fellow of the American College of Physicians (F.A.C.P.). Board certification may be required by a hospital for admission to the medical staff or for determination of a staff member's rank (e.g., general staff, associate staff, or full attending status).

**board eligible** In medicine, a designation that signifies that a physician has completed all of the requirements for admission to the medical specialty board certification examination but has not taken and passed the examination.

**boarder baby** An infant kept in a hospital nursery until status permits discharge to family care or transfer to another agency for maintenance or adoption.

**Boas' point** (bō'ăz) [Ismar I. Boas, Ger. physician, 1858–1938] A tender spot left of the 12th dorsal vertebra in patients with gastric ulcer.

**Bochdalek's ganglion** (bŏk'dăl-ĕks) [Victor Bochdalek, Czech. anatomist, 1801–1883] A ganglion of the plexus of the dental nerve in the maxilla above the canine tooth.

**Bodo** (bō'dō) A genus of nonpathogenic, flagellate protozoa of the family Bodonidae often found in stale feces or urine and sometimes in the urinary bladder.

**body** [AS. *bodig*] **1.** The physical part of the human as distinguished from mind and spirit. SYN: *soma* (1). **2.** Trunk (1). **3.** The principal mass of any structure. **4.** The largest or most important part of any organ.

EXAMINATION: The nude body is examined and both sides are compared. Physical examination is made by inspection, palpation, manipulation, mensuration, auscultation, and use of the sense of smell. It should also include observation of the body as the person walks and goes through the various ranges of motion of the trunk, neck, and extremities. Chemical and microscopic examination may be made of the blood, sputum, feces, urine, cerebrospinal fluids, and other bodily fluids. Radiological studies also may be used.

***acetone b.*** Ketone b.

***amygdaloid b.*** An almond-shaped mass of gray matter in the lateral wall and roof of the third ventricle of the brain.

***aortic b.*** One of two small bodies located in the arch of the aorta and containing the endings of the aortic nerve.

***asbestosis b.*** One of the minute bodies formed by the deposition of various salts and minerals around an asbestos particle. These may be found in the sputum, lung, or feces.

***Aschoff b.'s*** Microscopic foci of fibrinoid degeneration and granulomatous inflammation found in the interstitial tissues of the heart in rheumatic fever.

***Barr b.*** SEE: *Barr body.*

***basal b.*** A small granule usually present at the base of a flagellum or cilium in protozoa. SYN: *basal granule; blepharoplast.*

***carotid b.*** A sensory structure at the bifurcation of the common carotid artery that contains chemoreceptors and pressoreceptors. SYN: *carotid gland.*

***chromaffin b.*** One of a number of bodies composed principally of chromaffin cells, arranged serially along both sides of the dorsal aorta and in the kidney, liver, and gonads. They are ectodermal in origin, having the same origin as cells of the sympathetic ganglia. SYN: *paraganglion.*

***ciliary b.*** A structure directly behind the iris of the eye. It secretes the aqueous humor and contains the ciliary muscle that changes the shape, and thus the refractive power, of the lens by tightening and relaxing the tension on the lens zonule. SEE: *eye* for illus.

***coccygeal b.*** An arteriovenous anastomosis at the tip of the coccyx formed by the middle sacral artery. SYN: *glomus coccygeum.*

***Donovan b.'s*** The common name for *Calymmatobacterium granulomatis,* which causes granuloma inguinale.

***foreign b.*** SEE: *foreign body.*

***Heinz b.*** SEE: *Heinz body.*

***Hensen's b.*** A modified Golgi net found in the hair cells of the organ of Corti.

***hyaline b.*** A homogeneous substance resulting from colloid degeneration; found in degenerated cells. SEE: *degeneration, hyaline.*

***inclusion b.*** A nonliving substance in the protoplasm of cells, as seen in diseases caused by viral infections.

***ketone b.*** One of a number of substances that increase in the blood as a result of faulty carbohydrate metabolism. Among them are $\beta$-hydroxybutyric acid, acetoacetic acid, and acetone. They increase in persons with untreated or inadequately controlled diabetes mellitus and are the primary cause of acidosis. They may also occur in other metabolic disturbances. SYN: *acetone b.*

***lateral geniculate b.*** One of two bodies forming elevations on the lateral portion of the posterior part of the thalamus. Each is the termination of afferent fibers from the retina, which it receives through the optic nerves and tracts.

***Leishman-Donovan b.'s*** Small bodies found in the spleen and liver of victims of kala-azar or dum-dum fever; now known as *Leishmania donovani,* the causative organism of the disease. They are found both within and outside living cells and in circulating blood.

***malpighian b.*** **1.** A renal corpuscle consisting of a glomerulus enclosed in Bowman's capsule. **2.** A lymph nodule found in the spleen.

***mammillary b.*** A rounded body of gray matter found in the diencephalon. It forms a rounded eminence projecting into the anterior portion of the interpeduncular fossa, and its nucleus constitutes an important relay station for olfactory impulses.

***medial geniculate b.*** One of two bodies lying in the posterior part of the dorsal thalamus. Each receives fibers from the acoustic center of the medulla and the inferior colliculus through the brachium.

***medullary b.*** The deeper white matter of the cerebellum enclosed within the cortex.

***Negri b.'s*** SEE: *Negri bodies.*

***Nissl b.'s*** SEE: *Nissl bodies.*

***olivary b.*** A rounded mass in the anterolateral portion of the medulla oblongata. It consists of a convoluted sheet of gray matter enclosing white matter. SYN: *oliva.*

***pacchionian b.*** SEE: *arachnoid villus.*

***perineal b.*** A mass of tissue that separates the anus from the vestibule and the lower part of the vagina. SEE: *perineum* for illus.

***pineal b.*** SEE: *gland, pineal.*

***pituitary b.*** Pituitary gland.

***polar b.*** A small cell produced in oogenesis resulting from the divisions of the primary and secondary oocytes.

***postbranchial b.*** One of two bodies that develop from the posterior wall of the fourth pharyngeal pouch and become incorporated into the thyroid glands. SYN: *ultimobranchial b.*

***psammoma b.*** A laminated calcareous body seen in certain types of tumors and sometimes associated with chronic inflammation.

***quadrigeminal b.'s*** Four rounded projections from the roof of the midbrain. SEE: *colliculus inferior; colliculus superior.*

***restiform b.*** One of the inferior cerebellar peduncles of the brain, found along the lateral border of the fourth ventricle. These two bands of fibers, principally ascending, connect the medulla oblongata with the cerebellum.

***striate b.*** The corpus striatum, composed of the cordate and lenticular nucleoli of the brain.

***trachoma b.*** A mass of cells present as an inclusion body in the conjunctival epithelial cells of individuals with trachoma.

***ultimobranchial b.*** Postbranchial b.

***vertebral b.*** A short column of bone forming the weight-supporting portion of a vertebra. From its dorsolateral surfaces project the roots of the arch of a vertebra.

***vitreous b.*** A jellylike substance within the eye that fills the space between the lens and the retina. It is colorless, structureless, and transparent. Nevertheless, it may contain minute particles called floaters.

***wolffian b.*** Mesonephros.

**body composition** Quantitation of the various components of the body, esp. of the fat, water, protein, and bone. Determination of the specific gravity of the body is done to estimate the percentage of fat. This may be calculated by various methods, including underwater weighing, which determines the density of the individual; use of radioactive potassium, $^{40}K$; measuring the total body water by dilution of tritium; and use of various anthropometric measurements such as height, weight, and skin fold thickness at various sites. None of these methods is free of the potential for error. Underwater weighing is useful but may provide misleading information when used in analyzing body composition of highly trained athletes. The obese person has a lower body density than does the lean person, because the specific gravity of fat tissue is less than that of muscle tissue. The fat content for young men will vary from about 5% to 27% and for women from about 18% to 35%.

**body fluid** A fluid found in one of the fluid compartments of the body. The principal fluid compartments are intracellular and extracellular. A much smaller segment, the transcellular, includes fluid in the tracheobronchial tree, the gastrointestinal tract, and the bladder; cerebrospinal fluid; and the aqueous humor of the eye. The chemical composition of fluids in the various compartments is carefully regulated. In a normal 154 lb (70 kg) adult human male, 60% of total body weight (i.e., 42 L) is water; a similar female is 55% water (39 L). SEE: *acid-base balance; fluid replacement; fluid balance.*

**body image 1.** The subjective image or picture people have of their physical appearance based on their own observations and the reaction of others. **2.** The conscious and unconscious perception of one's body at any particular time.

**body image disturbance** Disruption in the way one perceives one's body image. SEE: *Nursing Diagnoses Appendix.*

**body language** The unconscious use of posture, gestures, or other nonverbal expression in communication. SEE: *kinesics.*

**body mass index** ABBR: BMI. An index for estimating obesity, obtained by dividing weight in kilograms by height in meters squared. Age is an important factor in interpreting these values because a high level in a young person is more likely to indicate obesity than in an old one. In adult males, a BMI greater than 27.8 $kg/m^2$ indicates obesity; in females, 27.3 $kg/m^2$. For adult males, being underweight is specified as a BMI less than 20.7 $kg/m^2$; for females, 19.1 $kg/m^2$.

**body mechanics** Application of kinesiology to use of the body in daily life activities and to the prevention and correction of problems related to posture and lifting.

**body odor** An unpleasant smell emanating from the human body. It may be derived from sweat gland secretions, urine, feces, expiration, saliva, breasts, skin, and sex organs. The major sources are the eccrine and apocrine sweat glands. Sebaceous gland secretions from the skin contribute to these odors. Eating garlic or onions or taking certain drugs may add to the odors produced by sweat glands, but the major sources of body sweat odor are the volatile fatty acids, steroids, and amines emitted by apocrine glands. Bacteria and fungi in and around these glands can intensify the odors. The secretions increase at puberty and decrease after menopause, are enhanced by stress, and are partially genetically controlled. SEE: *halitosis.*

**body packer syndrome** Drug overdose as a result of the ingestion of multiple small packages, usually containing drugs of abuse (esp. cocaine), to transport them illegally. Inadvertent overdose may occur if the packages rupture.

**body rocking** Rhythmic, purposeless body movement seen in individuals, whether adults or infants, who are bored, lonely, mentally subnormal, or disturbed. It is also seen in some blind children.

**body section radiography** Tomography.

**body snatching** Robbing a grave of its body, which was done in the past to obtain bodies for anatomical study in medical schools.

**body surface area** The surface area of the body expressed in square meters. Body surface area is an important measure in calculating pediatric dosages, in managing burn patients, and in determining radiation doses. Nomograms for accurately determining body surface area are available for both pediatric and adult patients. SEE: illus.; *burn; rule of nines.*

**body temperature, altered, risk for** The state in which the individual is at risk for failure to maintain body temperature within normal range. SEE: *Nursing Diagnoses Appendix.*

**body type** Classification of the human body according to muscle and fat distribution. SEE: *ectomorph; endomorph; mesomorph; somatotype.*

**Boeck's sarcoid** (běks) [Caesar P.M. Boeck, Norwegian dermatologist, 1845–1917] Former name for sarcoidosis.

**Boerhaave syndrome** (boor'hă-vě) [Hermann Boerhaave, Dutch physician, 1668–1738] Complete, spontaneous rupture of the esophagus usually associated with violent retching or vomiting. SEE: *Mallory-Weiss syndrome.*

**Bohr effect** [Niels Bohr, Danish physicist, 1855–1911] The effect of an acid environment on hemoglobin; hydrogen ions alter the structure of hemoglobin and increase the release of oxygen. It is esp. important in active tissues producing carbon dioxide and lactic acid.

**boil** [AS. *byl,* a swelling] An acute circumscribed inflammation of the subcutaneous layers of the skin or of a gland or hair follicle. The deeper tissue inflammation is so severe that blood clots in the vessels and forms a core. This is the cause of the acuteness of the pain; the core is ultimately expelled or reabsorbed. Boils are most commonly due to a localized infection with staphylococci. SYN: *furuncle.*

TREATMENT: The affected area should be protected from irritation, the skin should be kept scrupulously clean, and injury or trauma to the involved region should be avoided. Moist heat can be applied intermittently. Bedrest may be necessary in severe cases. After lesions are fluctuant, surgical incision and drainage are advisable. The area around draining abscesses should be protected by an antibiotic ointment to prevent new lesions on surrounding areas. If lesions are large and located on the face, an appropriate antibiotic should be used systematically

## Nomogram for the Assessment of Body Surface Area*

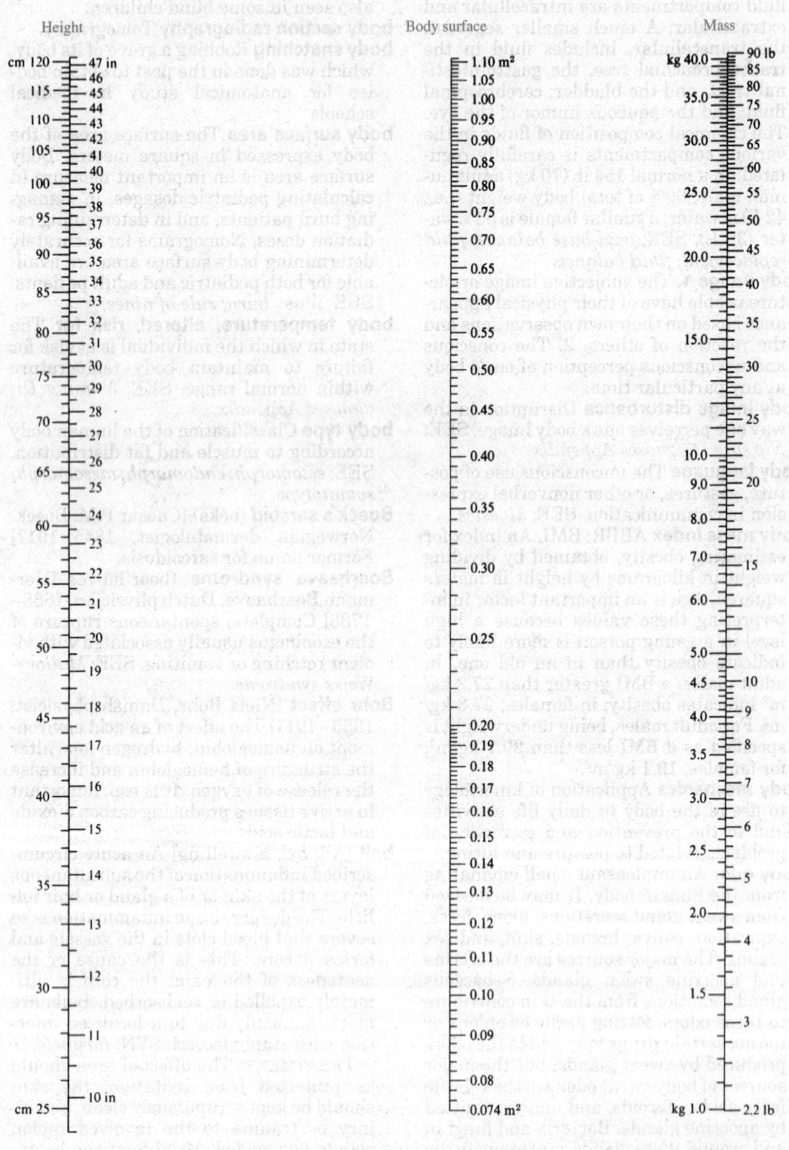


**Source: Lentner, C (ed): Geigy Scientific Tables, ed 8. Ciba Geigy, Basle, Switzerland, 1981.**

***The body surface area is given by the point of intersection with the middle scale of a straight line joining height and weight.**

## Nomogram for the Assessment of Body Surface Area* *(Continued)*

**Height**

cm 200, 195, 190, 185, 180, 175, 170, 165, 160, 155, 150, 145, 140, 135, 130, 125, 120, 115, 110, 105, cm 100

79 in, 78, 77, 76, 75, 74, 73, 72, 71, 70, 69, 68, 67, 66, 65, 64, 63, 62, 61, 60, 59, 58, 57, 56, 55, 54, 53, 52, 51, 50, 49, 48, 47, 46, 45, 44, 43, 42, 41, 40, 39 in

**Body surface**

2.80 m², 2.70, 2.60, 2.50, 2.40, 2.30, 2.20, 2.10, 2.00, 1.95, 1.90, 1.85, 1.80, 1.75, 1.70, 1.65, 1.60, 1.55, 1.50, 1.45, 1.40, 1.35, 1.30, 1.25, 1.20, 1.15, 1.10, 1.05, 1.00, 0.95, 0.90, 0.86 m²

**Mass**

kg 150, 145, 140, 135, 130, 125, 120, 115, 110, 105, 100, 95, 90, 85, 80, 75, 70, 65, 60, 55, 50, 45, 40, 35, kg 30

330 lb, 320, 310, 300, 290, 280, 270, 260, 250, 240, 230, 220, 210, 200, 190, 180, 170, 160, 150, 140, 130, 120, 110, 105, 100, 95, 90, 85, 80, 75, 70, 66 lb

***The body surface area is given by the point of intersection with the middle scale of a straight line joining height and weight.**

to prevent possible complications such as meningitis or septicemia.

**boiling** Process of vaporizing a liquid. Boiling water destroys most microorganisms (but may not kill spores and some viruses); toughens and hardens albumin in eggs; toughens (i.e., denatures) fibrin and dissolves tissues in meat; bursts starch granules; and softens cellulose in cereals and vegetables.

**boiling point** The temperature at which a liquid boils. The boiling point of a liquid varies according to the chemicals present in it. Under ordinary conditions water boils at 212°F (100°C) at sea level. To kill most vegetative forms of microorganisms, water should be boiled for 30 min. Aeration (pouring from one vessel to another) will overcome the flat taste of boiled water.

**bolometer** (bō-lŏm′ĕ-tĕr) [Gr. *bole,* a ray, + *metron,* measure] An instrument for measuring small amounts of radiated heat.

**bolus** (bō′lŭs) [L., from Gr. *bolos,* a lump] **1.** A mass of masticated food ready to be swallowed. **2.** A rounded preparation of medicine for oral ingestion. **3.** A concentrated mass of a diagnostic substance given rapidly intravenously, such as an opaque contrast medium, or an intravenous medication. **4.** In radiology, a tissue-equivalent material placed on the surface of the body to minimize the effects of an irregularly shaped body surface. The dose at the skin surface tends to increase, minimizing the skin-sparing effect of megavoltage radiation.

***alimentary b.*** A mass of masticated food in the esophagus that is ready to be passed into the stomach.

**bombesin** (bŏm′bĕ-sĭn) A neuropeptide present in the gut and brain tissue of humans. It is also present in increased concentrations in cell cultures of small-cell carcinomas of the lung.

**bond** A force that binds ions or atoms together. It is represented by a line drawn from one molecule or atom to another as in H—O—H.

***hydrogen b.*** The chemical linkage of hydrogen to other chemicals, esp. nitrogen and oxygen.

**bonding 1.** In dentistry, using an adhesive or cement to hold a covering to a stained or damaged tooth or to secure orthodontic appliances to the teeth. **2.** Development of a strong emotional attachment between individuals (e.g., a mother and child) after frequent or prolonged close contact.

***mother-infant b.*** The emotional and physical attachment between infant and mother that is initiated in the first hour or two after normal delivery of a baby who has not been dulled by anesthetic agents or drugs. It is believed that the stronger this bond, the greater the chances of a mentally healthy infant-mother relationship in both the short- and long-term periods after childbirth. For that reason, the initial contact between mother and infant should be in the delivery room and the contact should continue for as long as possible in the first hours after birth.

**bone** [AS. *ban,* bone] **1.** Osseous tissue, a specialized form of dense connective tissue consisting of bone cells (osteocytes) embedded in a matrix of calcified intercellular substance. SEE: illus. (Bone). **2.** Individual unit of the skeleton. Bones provide shape and support for the body of a vertebrate. They also serve as storage sites for mineral salts, and bone marrow provides a site for the formation of blood cells. Bone consists of about 50% water and 50% solid matter, the solids being chiefly calcium carbonate and calcium phosphate. They surround and protect some vital organs, and give points of attachment for the muscles, serving as levers and making movement possible. The outer surface of a bone is compact bone, and the inner more porous portion is cancellous (spongy) bone. The shafts of long bones are made of compact bone that surrounds a marrow canal. Compact bone is made of haversian systems, which are precise arrangements of osteocytes, blood vessels, and lymphatics within the bony matrix. All of these contribute to the maintenance and repair of bone. The periosteum is the fibrous connective tissue membrane that covers a bone. It has blood vessels that enter the bone, and it provides a site of attachment for tendons and ligaments. According to their shape, bones are classified as flat, irregular, long, or short. In the elderly, esp. women, osteoporosis may develop, a condition in which bones become brittle and break easily. SEE: illus. (Relationship of Bones to Thoracic, Abdominal, and Pelvic Areas); *skeleton* for names of principal bones.

***alveolar b.*** The bony tissue or process of the maxilla or mandible that supports the teeth.

***ankle b.*** Talus.

***breast b.*** Sternum.

***brittle b.*** A bone that is abbnormally fragile.

***cancellous b.*** A spongy bone in which the matrix forms connecting bars and plates, partially enclosing many intercommunicating spaces filled with bone marrow. SYN: *spongy b.*

***cartilage b.*** A bone formed by endochondral ossification developing from the primary centers of bone formation. SYN: *endochondral b.*

***cavalry b.*** Rider's b.

***compact b.*** The hard, dense bone made of haversian systems that forms the surface layer of all bones and the shafts of long bones, in contrast to spongy bone that forms the bulk of the short, flat, and irregular bones and the ends of long bones.

***cotyloid b.*** A bone that forms a part of

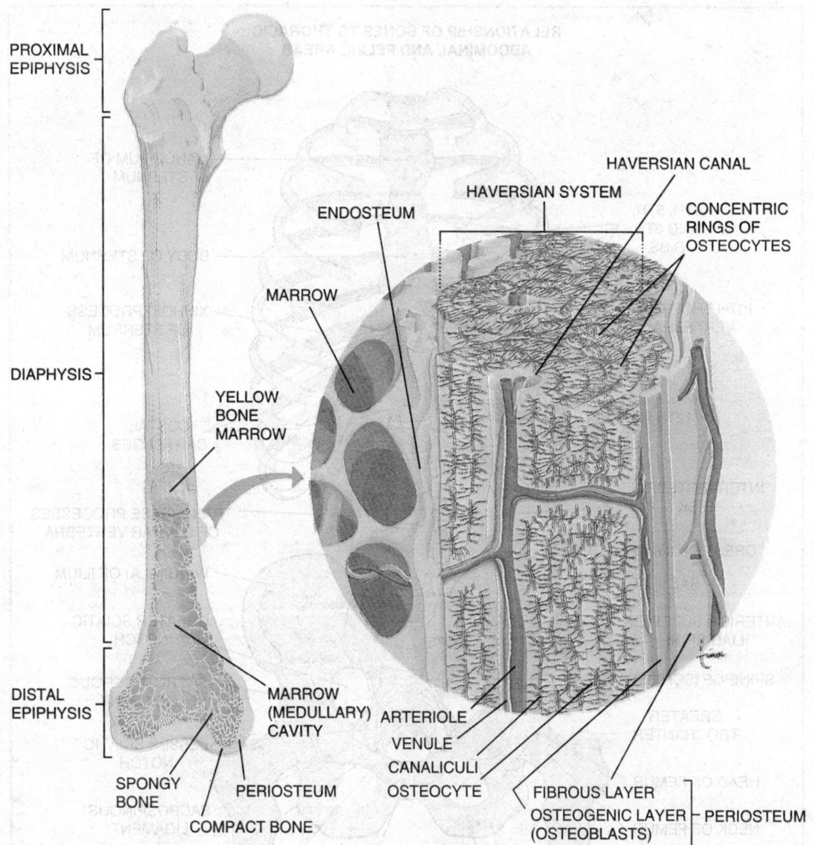


**BONE TISSUE**

**(A)** FEMUR WITH DISTAL END SECTIONED; **(B)** COMPACT BONE WITH HAVERSIAN SYSTEMS

the medial portion of the acetabulum during fetal development. It subsequently fuses with the pubis.

***cranial b.*** A bone of the skull or brain case.

***cuboid b.*** The outer bone of the instep bones of the foot that articulates posteriorly with the calcaneus and anteriorly with the fourth and fifth metatarsals.

***cuneiform b.*** One of the bones of the internal, middle, and external tarsus.

***dermal b.*** Membrane b.

***endochondral b.*** Cartilage b.

***hip b.*** Innominate b.

***incisive b.*** The part of maxilla bearing the incisor teeth.

***innominate b.*** The hip bone or os coxae, composed of the ilium, ischium, and pubis. It is united with the sacrum and coccyx by ligaments to form the pelvis. SYN: *pelvic b.*

***interparietal b.*** The squamous portion of the occipital bone.

***interradicular b.*** The alveolar bone between the roots of multirooted teeth.

***intramembraneous b.*** A bone formed directly from a condensation of mesenchyme, which differentiates into osteoblasts. It forms layers of bone without any cartilage model and includes the bones of the face and cranium.

***ivory b.*** Marble b.

***lacrimal b.*** The bone at the medial side of the orbital cavity.

***marble b.*** An abnormally calcified bone with a spotted appearance on a radiograph. SYN: *ivory b.* SEE: *Albers-Schönberg disease; osteopetrosis.*

***membrane b.*** Bone that is formed within fibrous connective tissue in the embryo (e.g., most of the skull bones). SYN: *dermal b.*

***mosaic b.*** Bone appearing as small pieces fitted together, characteristic of Paget's disease.

***pelvic b.*** Innominate b.

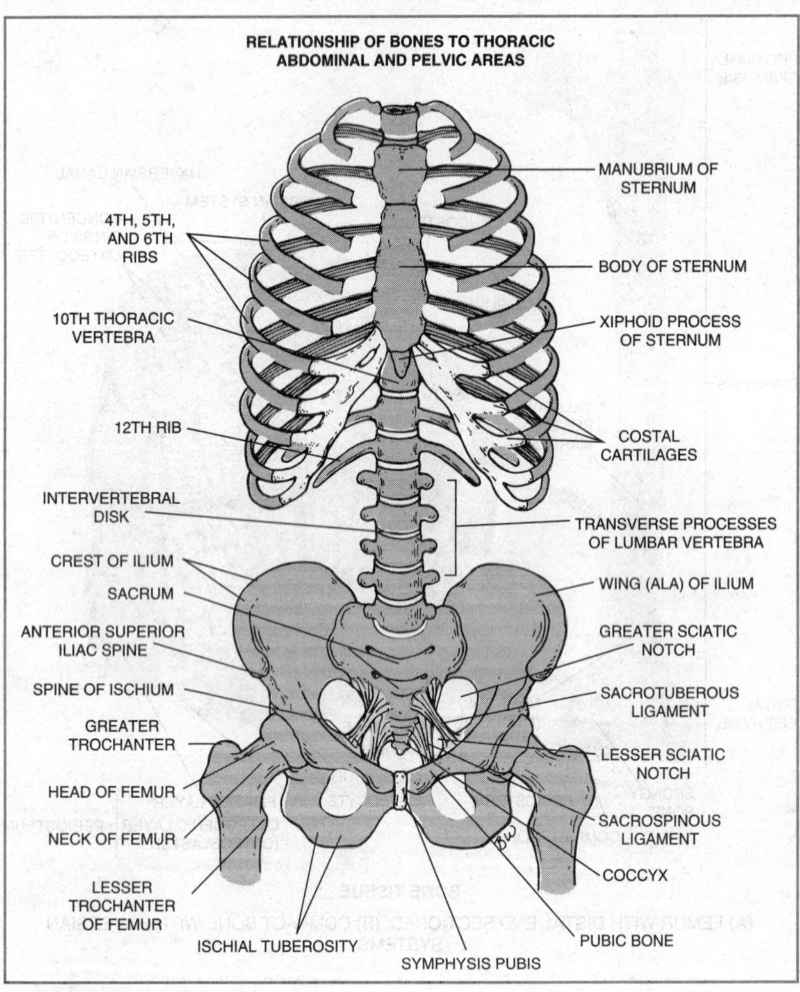


***perichondral b., perichondrial b.*** Bone formed beneath the perichondrium.

***periosteal b.*** Bone formed by osteoblasts of the periosteum.

***ping pong b.*** A thin shell of osseous tissue covering a giant-cell sarcoma in a bone.

***replacement b.*** Any bone that develops within cartilage.

***rider's b.*** Ossification of the distal end of the adductor muscles of the thigh, as may be seen in horseback riders. SYN: *calvary b.*

***sesamoid b.*** A type of short bone occurring in the hands and feet and embedded in tendons or joint capsules.

***spongy b.*** Cancellous b.

***sutural b.*** Wormian b.

***thigh b.*** Femur.

***wormian b.*** A small, irregularly shaped bone often found in the sutures of the cranium. SYN: *sutural b.*

***woven b.*** Embryonic or rapidly growing bone characterized microscopically by a prominent fibrous matrix.

**bone age** In children, an estimate of biological age based on radiological studies of the stage of development of the ossification centers of the wrist bones and long bones of the extremities. SEE: *epiphysis.*

**bone cell** A nucleated cell occupying a separate lacuna of bone. SEE: *osteoblast; osteoclast; osteocyte.*

**bone cyst** A cystic bone tumor.

**bone densitometry** A method of determining the density of bone by use of radiographic techniques. The use of dual photon absorptiometry will provide density data of the axial skeleton with a precision of 97% to 98%. It is used in testing for degree of osteoporosis. SEE: *absorptiometry, dual photon.*

**bone fracture, nonunion** SEE: *nonunion.*

**bone fracture, nonunion, electrical stimulation for** A noninvasive method of stimulating a nonunion bone fracture to heal. The electrical stimulation is applied to the skin over the area of the fracture. SEE: *nonunion.*

**bonelet** An ossicle.

**bone marrow** The soft organic material that fills the cavities of the bone. SEE: *marrow.*

**bone marrow transplantation** ABBR: BMT. Transplantation of bone marrow from one individual to another. It is used in treating aplastic anemia, thalassemia and sickle cell anemia, and immunodeficiency disorders. Some diseases can be treated with either allogeneic or autologous BMT (e.g., acute leukemia, chronic myelogenous leukemia, non-Hodgkin's lymphoma, Hodgkin's disease, and testicular cancer).

***autologous b.m.t.*** ABBR: ABMT. The harvest, cryopreservation, and reinfusion of a patient's own bone marrow, a procedure that may be used in post-treatment marrow hypoplasia following cancer therapy. After the red bone marrow is removed from the patient, it may be purged of malignant cells and then returned to the patient. Cells are purged by using monoclonal antibodies to bind the unwanted cells, by using chemotherapy to kill cancer cells, and by using magnetic microspheres to bind to the unwanted cells and separate them by use of a magnetic field. Purging cells by use of these methods is experimental and is not used in the majority of patients undergoing autologous transplantation. SEE: *immunomagnetic technique; magnetic microspheres.*

**bone paste** A mixture of a calcium compound, phosphoric acid, and sodium phosphate in a solution. The material hardens in 10 min and becomes as strong as bone in 12 hr. It is applied directly to the gaps left by broken or injured bones. It has been used successfully in some countries and is being investigated for use in the U.S.

**bone remodeling** The process in which bone is resorbed and new bone formed at the same site. This process keeps the bone tissue in dynamic equilibrium.

**bone scan** The use of short half-life radiopharmaceutical agents to visualize bones. This is esp. useful in delineating osteomyelitis and metastases to the bone.

**bone wax** The nontoxic, biocompatible wax used during surgery to plug bleeding cavities in cranial bones or other bones to control bleeding.

**Bonine** (bō′nēn) Trade name for meclizine hydrochloride.

**bony** Resembling or of the nature of bone. SYN: *osseous.*

**booster** (boo′stĕr) An additional dose of an immunizing agent to increase the protection afforded by the original series of injections. The booster is given some months or years after the initial immunization.

**boot** A special shoe or bandage for covering the foot, ankle, and lower leg.

**borate** (bō′rāt) Any basic salt of boric acid. SEE: *Poisons and Poisoning Appendix.*

**borated** Mixed with borax.

**borax** (bor′ăks) [L., from Arabic, from Persian *burah*] Sodium borate, used as a detergent, a water softener, and a weak antiseptic.

**borborygmus** (bor″bō-rĭg′mŭs) *pl.* **borborygmi** [Gr. *borborygmos,* rumbling in the bowels] A gurgling, splashing sound normally heard over the large intestine; it is caused by passage of gas through the liquid contents of the intestine. Its absence may indicate paralytic ileus or obstruction of the bowels due to torsion, volvulus, or strangulated hernia.

**border** (bor′dĕr) The outer part or edge; boundary.

***brush b.*** The microvilli on the free surface of the cells lining the small intestine and the proximal convoluted portion of the renal tubules. Microvilli are folds of the cell membrane and greatly increase the surface area for absorption.

***vermilion b.*** The red boundary of the lips that represents the highly vascular, hyalinized, keratinized epithelial covering between the outer skin and the moist oral mucosa of the mouth.

**borderline** An incomplete state, as in a borderline diagnosis, in a patient who has some of the requirements for a definite diagnosis but not enough for certainty; a condition judged numerically (e.g., high blood pressure in which the value is close to a hypertensive level but not at a level to be clearly a case of hypertension).

**borderline personality disorder** SEE: *personality, borderline.*

**Bordetella** (bor″dĕ-tĕl′lă) [Jules Bordet, Belg. physician, bacteriologist, and physiologist, 1870–1961] A genus of hemolytic gram-negative coccobacilli of the family Brucellaceae. Some species are parasitic and pathogenic in warm-blooded animals, including humans.

***B. pertussis*** The causative agent of whooping cough; formerly called *Haemophilus pertussis.* SEE: *pertussis.*

**bore** The internal diameter of a tube.

**boredom** A feeling of tiredness or depression because of lack of activity or challenging, meaningful stimuli. SEE: *apathy.*

**boric acid** $H_3BO_3$. An odorless white crystalline powder that contains boron and is obtained by condensation and evaporation from certain mineral salts. It is used as a mild antiseptic solution, esp. for the eyes, mouth, and bladder.

**boric acid poisoning** Poisoning as the result of taking boric acid internally.

SYMPTOMS: Symptoms include nausea,

vomiting, diarrhea, convulsions, central nervous system depression, livid skin rash, and shock.

TREATMENT: Ipecac should be administered to induce vomiting and the stomach should be washed out. A saline cathartic and large volumes of water should be given. Dialysis may be required if poisoning is severe. SEE: *Poisons and Poisoning Appendix.*

**borism** The symptoms caused by the internal use of borax or boron compounds. These include dry skin, eruptions, and gastric disturbances.

**Bornholm disease** (born′hōm) [named for the Danish island Bornholm] An epidemic disease caused by coxsackie B virus and marked by sudden onset of chest pain and fever. SYN: *epidemic myositis; epidemic pleurodynia.*

**boron** [*bor*ax + carb*on*] SYMB: B. A nonmetallic element found only as a compound such as boric acid or borax; atomic weight 10.81, atomic number 5.

**Borrelia** (bor-rē′lē-ă) A genus of spirochetes, some of which are causative agents for relapsing fevers and Lyme disease in humans. Though classed as bacteria, spirochetes differ in physical appearance from most bacteria in that they have a spiral shape.

***B. burgdorferi*** The causative agent of Lyme disease.

***B. duttonii*** The causative agent for tick-borne relapsing fever in Central and South America.

***B. recurrentis*** The causative agent of louse-borne relapsing fever.

**borreliosis** Any of several arthropod-borne diseases caused by spirochetes of the genus *Borrelia.*

**boss** [O. Fr. *boce,* a swelling] A round circumscribed swelling or growth (e.g., a tumor) that becomes large enough to produce swelling.

**bosselated** (bŏs′ĕ-lāt-ĕd) Marked by numerous bosses.

**bossing** Prominence of the forehead.

**Boston arm** A myoelectric prosthesis for above-the-elbow amputations. The elbow is powered by a small battery-driven motor, activated in proportion to the strength of contraction detected in the control muscle. SYN: *Boston elbow; Liberty Mutual elbow.*

**Boston brace** A low-profile plastic thoracolumbosacral orthosis (spinal jacket) with no metal suprastructure, used to treat mild to moderate lower thoracic and lumbar scoliosis.

**Boston elbow** Boston arm.

**Botallo's duct** (bō-tăl′ōz) [Leonardo Botallo, It. anatomist, 1530–1600] Ductus arteriosus.

**botany** (bŏt′n-ē) [Gr. *botanikos,* pert. to plants] The study of plants; a division of biology.

**botfly** (bŏt′flī) *pl.* **botflies** An insect that belongs to the family Oestridae of the order Diptera and is parasitic to mammals, esp. horses and sheep. Human infestation is rare.

**botryoid** (bŏt′rē-oyd) [Gr. *botrys,* bunch of grapes, + *eidos,* form, shape] Resembling a bunch of grapes. SYN: *staphyline.*

**botuliform** (bŏt-ū′lĭ-form) [L. *botulus,* sausage, + *forma,* shape] Shaped like a sausage.

**botulin** (bŏt′chū-lĭn) The neurotoxin responsible for botulism. It is not destroyed by the action of gastric or intestinal secretions.

**botulinic acid** A toxin found in putrid sausage.

**botulism** (bŏt′ū-lĭzm) [″ + Gr. *-ismos,* condition] A severe form of food poisoning from food containing the botulinus toxins A, B, C, D, E, F, and G, produced by *Clostridium botulinum* bacteria, which are found in soil and in the intestinal tract of domestic animals. Botulism in humans is usually associated with development of the bacteria under anaerobic conditions in raw, improperly canned or otherwise preserved foods, esp. meats (as ham and sausage) and nonacid vegetables (as string beans). The toxin is a neurotoxin that blocks the release of acetylcholine at neuromuscular junctions and in much of the autonomic nervous system. It is thermolabile, losing its toxic properties when exposed to temperature of 80°C (176°F) for 30 min or boiling at 100°C (212°F) for 10 min. In the absence of acetylcholine, skeletal muscles become paralyzed; this is usually first apparent in the muscles of the eyes and those for speaking and swallowing. In fatal cases, the respiratory muscles have become paralyzed. The fatality rate in the U.S. is 20% to 35%.

SYMPTOMS: The symptoms of botulism are fatigue, weakness, dizziness, blurred or double vision, dry mouth, sore throat, and headache; digestive complaints, such as nausea, vomiting, diarrhea, and abdominal pain, may or may not be present. Without treatment, these symptoms progress to dyspnea, muscle weakness, and paralysis in the extremities or trunk.

TREATMENT: It is important to administer trivalent (ABE) antitoxin as soon as the condition is suspected (even if laboratory results are not yet available) and before the onset of neurological symptoms. The antitoxin is available from the state or local health department or the Bacterial Diseases Division, Centers for Disease Control and Prevention, Atlanta, GA 30333, (404) 639–3670 during the day or (404) 639–2888 at night. SEE: *Poisons and Poisoning Appendix.*

NURSING IMPLICATIONS: If ingestion of contaminated food is suspected, the nurse obtains a careful history of food intake for the preceding few days and determines whether relatives or others around the patient have eaten the same food or shown similar symptoms. If the patient ate the suspected food within the past several hours, vomiting is induced and gastric lavage begun; a high enema is administered to purge unabsorbed toxins from the GI tract. (Family members and other persons around the patient who have eaten the same food should receive the same treatment, even if asymptomatic.)

If clinical signs of botulism appear, the patient is admitted to the intensive care unit. Cardiopulmonary and hemodynamic function are monitored, vital capacity assessed frequently, and reduced inspiratory effort, or respiratory distress documented and reported. Arterial blood gases are monitored, and mechanical ventilation is instituted and maintained if required. Neurological status, including bilateral motor status, is evaluated and abnormalities are documented and reported. Before administering botulism antitoxin, a history of the patient's allergies, esp. to horses, is obtained, and a skin test performed. With epinephrine 1 : 1000 and emergency airway equipment nearby, prescribed botulism antitoxin is administered and the patient observed for anaphylaxis or other hypersensitivity reactions, including serum sickness. The patient's cough and gag reflexes are checked, and fluid intake and output monitored. If the patient has swallowing difficulties or an impaired cough or gag reflex, suctioning is performed, and nasogastric feeding, IV fluid, or total parenteral nutrition administered as prescribed. Deep-breathing exercises are encouraged, the patient is repositioned frequently, proper body alignment is maintained, and assistance with range-of-motion exercises is provided. If the patient has difficulty speaking, other communication methods are provided, and reassurance is given that this symptom will pass. Both patient and family are informed about the course of the disease and its sometimes fatal outcome.

***infant b.*** An infectious form of botulism first recognized in 1976. Most cases occur in infants younger than 1 year who have ingested botulism spores. The infant's protective colon flora is not yet established, and the spores germinate into active bacteria that produce the neurotoxin. Treatment entails supportive care.

SYMPTOMS: The symptoms include constipation, lethargy, listlessness, poor feeding, ptosis, loss of head control, difficulty in swallowing, hypotonia, generalized weakness, and respiratory insufficiency. The disease may be mild or severe.

***wound b.*** Botulism acquired when spores of the bacteria contaminate an anaerobic wound, germinate, and produce the neurotoxin.

**Bouchard's nodes** Bony enlargements or nodules, located at the proximal interphalangeal joints, that result from osteoarthritis or degenerative joint disease.

**Bouchut's respiration** (boo-shooz') [Jean A.E. Bouchut, Fr. physician, 1818–1891] Respiration in which expiration is longer than inspiration, as seen in children with bronchopneumonia and asthma.

**Bouchut's tubes** A set of tubes used for intubation of the larynx.

**bougie** (boo'zhē) [Fr. *bougie,* candle] A slender, flexible instrument for exploring and dilating tubal organs, esp. the male urethra.

**bouillon** (boo-, bool-yŏn') [Fr.] A clear broth made from meat. It may be used as a culture medium for bacteria.

**Bouin's fluid** (boo-ēnz') [Paul Bouin, Fr. anatomist, 1870–1962] A fixative for embryological and histological tissue. It consists of formaldehyde, glacial acetic acid, trinitrophenol (picric acid), and water.

**bound 1.** In chemistry, the holding in combination of one molecule by another. SEE: *bind* (2). **2.** Contained, not free.

**bouquet** (boo-kā') [Fr., nosegay] A cluster or bunch of structures, esp. blood vessels.

**Bourdon gauge** A low-pressure flow metering device.

**boutonnière** (boo-tŏn-yār') [Fr., buttonhole] **1.** Incision through the perineum behind an impervious stricture. **2.** A buttonhole-like opening in a membrane.

**boutonnière deformity** Contracture of hand musculature marked by proximal interphalangeal joint flexion and distal interphalangeal joint hyperextension.

**boutons terminaux** (boo-tŏn' tĕr-mĭ-nō') [Fr., terminal buttons] The bulblike expansions at the tips of axons that come into synaptic contact with the cell bodies of other neurons.

**bovine** (bō'vīn) [L. *bovinus*] Pert. to cattle.

**bovine somatotropin A** A growth hormone used to increase milk production in cows.

**bowel** [O. Fr. *boel,* intestine] Intestine.

**bowel incontinence** A state in which an individual experiences a change in normal bowel habits characterized by involuntary passage of stool. SEE: *Nursing Diagnoses Appendix.*

**bowel movement** Evacuation of feces. The number of bowel movements varies in normal individuals, some having a movement after each meal, others one in the morning and one at night, and still others only one in several days. Thus, to say that the healthy person must have at least one bowel movement a day in order to maintain health is unreasonable and not based on factual evidence. SYN: *defecation.*

---

Caution: A persistent change in bowel habits should be investigated thoroughly because it may be a sign of a malignant growth in the gastrointestinal tract.

---

NURSING IMPLICATIONS: A history is obtained of the patient's usual bowel habits, and any change documented. The patient is questioned and the stool is inspected for color, shape, odor, consistency, and other characteristics, as well as the presence of any unusual coatings or contents (mucus, blood, fat, parasites). Privacy is provided for the patient when using a bed pan, toilet, or bedside commode. The nurse ventilates the area or uses a deodorant spray after the bowel movement to limit the patient's embarrassment and to reduce the discomfort of others sharing the area. (Burning several matches in the area will help to remove malodors.) The patient is taught the use of diet and activity to help prevent constipation, and the rationale for testing the stool for occult blood, if this is required, is explained.

**bowel sounds** The normal sounds associated with movement of the intestinal contents through the lower alimentary tract. Auscultation of the abdomen for bowel sounds may provide valuable diagnostic information. Absent or diminished sounds may indicate paralytic ileus or peritonitis. High pitched tinkling sounds are associated with intestinal obstruction.

**bowel training** A program for assisting adult patients to reestablish regular bowel habits. Patients with chronic constipation, colostomies, or spinal cord injuries affecting the muscles involved in defecation may benefit from bowel training. Assessments include determining the etiology and duration of the bowel problem (e.g., a patient complaining of chronic constipation also should be queried regarding the usual normal pattern and the use of enemas, suppositories, or laxatives to promote bowel evacuation). Interventions include dietary changes, supervised training to elicit evacuation at convenient times, biofeedback, and psychotherapy.

NURSING IMPLICATIONS: The patient is encouraged to increase the dietary intake of fresh fruits and vegetables, and whole grains, and to drink 3000 ml of fluid each day. The nurse emphasizes the need to heed normal evacuatory urges, discourages the use of laxatives, and explains the actions of stool softeners. The nurse explains the advantages of generating evacuation 30 min after meals to enlist normal peristaltic action and demonstrates digital anal stimulation or insertion of suppository, if indicated.

**bowleg** (bō'lĕg) A bending outward of the leg. SYN: *bandy leg; genu varum.*

**Bowman's capsule** (bō'măns) [Sir William Bowman, Brit. physician, 1816–1892] Part of the renal corpuscle. It consists of a visceral layer closely applied to the glomerulus and an outer parietal layer. It functions as a filter in the formation of urine. SEE: *kidney* for illus.

**Bowman's glands** The olfactory glands, or branched tubuloalveolar glands located in the lamina propria of the olfactory membrane. Mucus from these glands keeps the olfactory surface moist.

**Bowman's membrane** The thin homogeneous membrane separating the corneal epithelium from the corneal substance. SYN: *anterior elastic lamina.*

**boxing** In dentistry, the building up of vertical walls, usually in wax, around an impression to produce the desired size and form of the base of the cast and to preserve certain landmarks of the impression.

**box-note** In emphysema, a hollow sound heard on percussion.

**Boyden chamber** A chamber used to measure chemotaxis. Cells are placed on one side of a membrane and chemotactic material on the other. The number of cells migrating to the filter quantitates the chemotactic effect.

**Boyer's bursa** (bwă-yāz') [Baron Alexis de Boyer, Fr. surgeon, 1757–1833] A bursa anterior to the thyrohyoid membrane.

**Boyer's cyst** A painless and gradual enlargement of the subhyoid bursa.

**Boyle's law** [Robert Boyle, Brit. physicist, 1627–1691] A law stating that at a constant temperature, the volume of a gas varies inversely with the pressure. SEE: *Charles' law; Gay-Lussac's law.*

**Bozeman-Fritsch catheter** (bōz'măn-frĭtch) [Nathan Bozeman, U.S. surgeon, 1825–1905; Heinrich Fritsch, Ger. gynecologist, 1844–1915] A double-lumen uterine catheter with several openings at tip.

**B.P.** *blood pressure; British Pharmacopoeia.*

**b.p.** *boiling point.*

**BPD** *biparietal diameter; bronchopulmonary dysplasia.*

**BPH** *benign prostatic hypertrophy.*

**Bq** *becquerel.*

**Br 1.** *Brucella.* **2.** Symbol for the element bromine.

**brace** (brās) *pl.* **braces 1.** Any of a variety of devices used in orthopedics for holding joints or limbs in place. **2.** A colloquial term for temporary dental prostheses used to align or reposition teeth.

**brachial** (brā'kē-ăl) [L. *brachialis*] Pert. to the arm.

**brachial artery** The main artery of the arm; a continuation of the axillary artery on the inside of the arm. SEE: illus.

**brachialgia** (brā″kē-ăl'jē-ă) [L. *brachialis,* brachial, + Gr. *algos,* pain] Intense pain in the arm.

**brachialis** (brā″kē-ăl'ĭs) [L. *brachialis,* brachial] A muscle of the arm lying immediately under the biceps brachii.

**brachial plexus** A network of the last four cervical and the first thoracic spinal nerves supplying the arm, forearm, and hand. SEE: *Nerve Plexuses Appendix.*

**brachial veins** The veins that accompany the brachial artery.

**brachiocephalic** (brā″kē-ō-sĕ-făl'ĭk) [L. *brachium,* arm, + Gr. *kephale,* head] Pert. to the arm and head.

**brachiocrural** (brā″kē-ō-kroo'răl) [″ + *crur-*

*alis*, pert. to the leg] Pert. to the arm and thigh.

**brachiocubital** (brā″kē-ō-kū′bĭ-tăl) [″ + *cubitus*, forearm] Pert. to the arm and forearm.

**brachiocyllosis** (brā″kē-ō-sĭl-ō′sĭs) [″ + Gr. *kyllosis*, a crooking] Abnormal curvature of the arm.

**brachioradialis** (brā″kē-ō-rā″dē-ă′lĭs) [″ + *radialis*, radius] A muscle lying on the lateral side of the forearm. SEE: *Muscles Appendix*.

BRACHIAL ARTERY

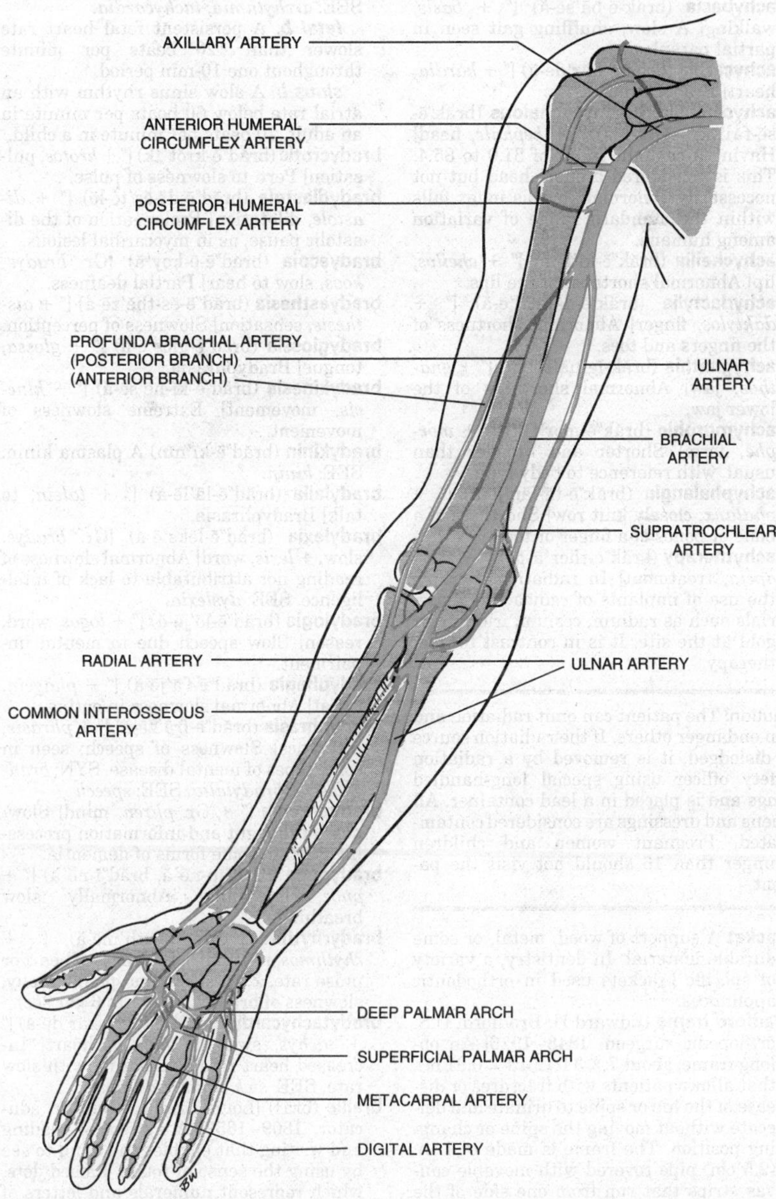


RIGHT ANTERIOR ARM

**brachium** (brā′kē-ŭm) *pl.* **brachia** [L., arm, from Gr. *brakhion,* shorter, hence "upper arm" as opposed to longer forearm] **1.** The upper arm from shoulder to elbow. **2.** Anatomical structure resembling an arm.

***b. conjunctivum*** Superior cerebellar peduncle.

***b. pontis*** Middle cerebellar peduncle.

**brachy-** [Gr. *brachys,* short] Combining form meaning *short.*

**brachybasia** (brăk-ē-bā′sē-ă) [″ + *basis,* walking] A slow, shuffling gait seen in partial paraplegia.

**brachycardia** (brăk-ē-kăr′dē-ă) [″ + *kardia,* heart] Bradycardia.

**brachycephalic, brachycephalous** (brăk″ē-sĕ-făl′ĭk, -sĕf′ă-lŭs) [″ + *kephale,* head] Having a cephalic index of 81.0 to 85.4. This is considered a short head but not necessarily abnormal, as this index falls within the standard range of variation among humans.

**brachycheilia** (brăk″ē-kī′lē-ă) [″ + *cheilos,* lip] Abnormal shortness of the lips.

**brachydactylia** (brăk″ē-dăk-tĭl′ē-ă) [″ + *daktylos,* finger] Abnormal shortness of the fingers and toes.

**brachygnathia** (brăk-ĭg-nā′thē-ă) [″ + *gnathos,* jaw] Abnormal shortness of the lower jaw.

**brachymorphic** (brăk″ē-mor′fĭk) [″ + *morphe,* form] Shorter and broader than usual, with reference to body type.

**brachyphalangia** (brăk″ē-fă-lăn′jē-ă) [″ + *phalanx,* closely knit row] Shortness of a bone or bones of a finger or toe.

**brachytherapy** (brăk″ē-thĕr′ă-pē) [″ + *therapeia,* treatment] In radiation therapy, the use of implants of radioactive materials such as radium, cesium, iridium, or gold at the site. It is in contrast to teletherapy.

Caution: The patient can emit radiation and can endanger others. If the radiation source is dislodged, it is removed by a radiation safety officer using special long-handled tongs and is placed in a lead container. All linens and dressings are considered contaminated. Pregnant women and children younger than 16 should not visit the patient.

**bracket** A support of wood, metal, or some durable material. In dentistry, a variety of specific brackets used in orthodontic appliances.

**Bradford frame** [Edward H. Bradford, U.S. orthopedic surgeon, 1848–1926] An oblong frame, about 7 × 3 ft (2.13 × 0.91 m), that allows patients with fractures or disease of the hip or spine to urinate and defecate without moving the spine or changing position. The frame is made of 1 in. (2.5 cm) pipe covered with movable canvas strips that run from one side of the frame to the other.

**brady-** [Gr. *bradys,* slow] Combining form meaning *slow.*

**bradyacusia** (brăd″ē-ă-koo′sē-ă) [″ + *akouein,* to hear] An abnormally diminished hearing acuity.

**bradyarrhythmia** (brăd″ē-ă-rĭth′mē-ă) [″ + *a-,* not, + *rhythmos,* rhythm] A slow and irregular heart rate.

**bradycardia** (brăd″ē-kăr′dē-ă) [″ + *kardia,* heart] A slow heartbeat characterized by a pulse rate below 60 beats per minute. SEE: *arrhythmia; tachycardia.*

***fetal b.*** A persistent fetal heart rate slower than 120 beats per minute throughout one 10-min period.

***sinus b.*** A slow sinus rhythm with an atrial rate below 60 beats per minute in an adult, 70 beats per minute in a child.

**bradycrotic** (brăd″ē-krŏt′ĭk) [″ + *krotos,* pulsation] Pert. to slowness of pulse.

**bradydiastole** (brăd″ē-dī-ăs′tō-lē) [″ + *diastole,* dilatation] Prolongation of the diastolic pause, as in myocardial lesions.

**bradyecoia** (brăd″ē-ē-koy′ă) [Gr. *bradyekoos,* slow to hear] Partial deafness.

**bradyesthesia** (brăd″ē-ĕs-thē′zē-ă) [″ + *aisthesis,* sensation] Slowness of perception.

**bradyglossia** (brăd″ē-glŏs′ē-ă) [″ + *glossa,* tongue] Bradyphrasia.

**bradykinesia** (brăd″ē-kī-nē′sē-ă) [″ + *kinesis,* movement] Extreme slowness of movement.

**bradykinin** (brăd″ē-kī′nĭn) A plasma kinin. SEE: *kinin.*

**bradylalia** (brăd″ē-lā′lē-ă) [″ + *lalein,* to talk] Bradyphrasia.

**bradylexia** (brăd″ē-lĕks′ē-ă) [Gr. *bradys,* slow, + *lexis,* word] Abnormal slowness of reading not attributable to lack of intelligence. SEE: *dyslexia.*

**bradylogia** (brăd″ē-lō′jē-ă) [″ + *logos,* word, reason] Slow speech due to mental impairment.

**bradyphagia** (brăd″ē-fā′jē-ă) [″ + *phagein,* to eat] Abnormal slowness in eating.

**bradyphrasia** (brăd″ē-frā′zē-ă) [″ + *phrasis,* utterance] Slowness of speech; seen in some types of mental disease. SYN: *bradyglossia; bradylalia.* SEE: *speech.*

**bradyphrenia** [″ + Gr. *phren,* mind] Slowness of thought and information processing, seen in some forms of dementia.

**bradypnea** (brăd″ĭp-nē′ă, brăd″ī-nē′ă) [″ + *pnoe,* breathing] Abnormally slow breathing.

**bradyrhythmia** (brăd″ē-rĭth′mē-ă) [″ + *rhythmos,* rhythm] **1.** Slowness of heart or pulse rate. **2.** In electroencephalography, slowness of brain waves (1 to 6 per sec).

**bradytachycardia** (brăd″ē-tăk″ē-kăr′dē-ă) [″ + *tachys,* swift, + *kardia,* heart] Increased heart rate alternating with slow rate. SEE: *sick sinus syndrome.*

**braille** (brāl) [Louis Braille, blind Fr. educator, 1809–1852] A system of reading and writing that enables the blind to see by using the sense of touch. Raised dots, which represent numerals and letters of the alphabet, can be identified by the fingers. SEE: *Optacon II.*

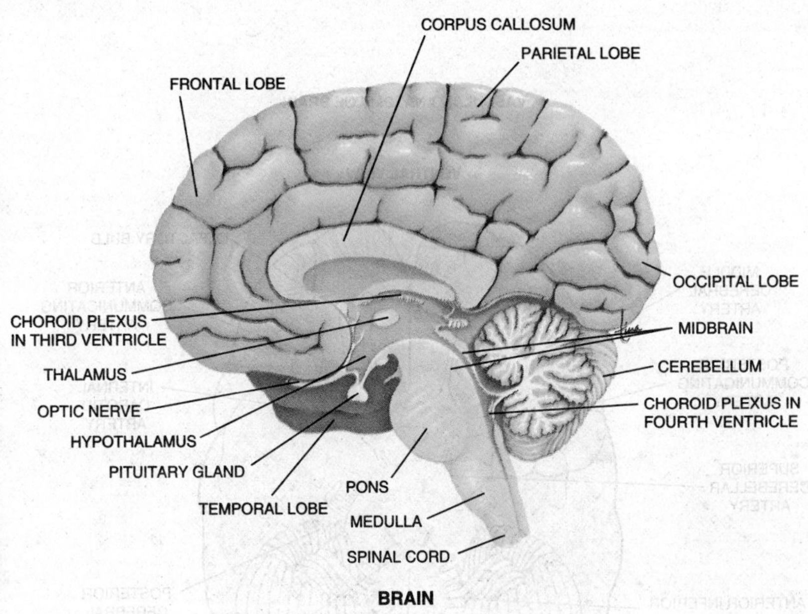


**BRAIN**

MIDSAGITTAL SECTION OF BRAIN AS SEEN FROM LEFT

**brain** (brān) [AS. *braegen*] A large soft mass of nerve tissue contained within the cranium; the cranial portion of the central nervous system. SYN: *encephalon.*

ANATOMY: The brain is composed of neurons (nerve cells) and neuroglia or supporting cells. The brain consists of gray and white matter. Gray matter is composed mainly of neuron cell bodies and is concentrated in the cerebral cortex and the nuclei and basal ganglia. White matter is composed of neuron processes, which form tracts connecting parts of the brain with each other and with the spinal cord.

The brain consists of three major parts: the cerebrum, cerebellum, and brainstem (medulla, pons, and midbrain). The weight of the brain and spinal cord is about 1350 to 1400 g, of which 2% is the cord. The cerebrum represents about 85% of the weight of the brain. *Lobes:* Frontal, parietal, occipital, temporal, insular. *Glands:* Pituitary, pineal. *Membranes:* Meninges—dura mater (external), arachnoid (middle), and pia mater (internal). *Nerves:* Cranial. SEE: illus. (Brain); *cranial nerve* for illus.; *Cranial Nerves Appendix*

*Subdivisions* of the brain are (1) diencephalon, including the epithalamus, thalamus, and hypothalamus (optic chiasma, tuber cinereum, and maxillary bodies); (2) myelencephalon, including the corpora quadrigemina, tegmentum, crura cerebri, and the medulla oblongata; (3) metencephalon, including the cerebellum and pons; (4) telencephalon, including the rhinencephalon, corpora striata, and cerebrum (cerebral cortex).

*Ventricles:* The cavities of the brain are the first and second lateral ventricles, which lie in the cerebral hemispheres, the third ventricle of the diencephalon, and the fourth ventricle posterior to the medulla and pons. The first and second communicate with the third by the interventricular foramina, the third with the fourth by the cerebral aqueduct (of Sylvius), the fourth with the subarachnoid spaces by the two foramina of Luschka and the foramen of Magendie. The ventricles are filled with cerebrospinal fluid, which is formed by the choroid plexuses in the walls and roofs of the ventricles. SEE: illus. (Vascular Anatomy of Brain).

PHYSIOLOGY: The brain is the primary center for regulating and coordinating body activities. Sensory impulses are received through afferent nerves and register as sensations, the basis for perception. It is the seat of consciousness, thought, memory, reason, judgment, and emotion. Motor impulses are discharged through efferent nerves to muscles and glands initiating activities. Through reflex centers automatic control of body activities is maintained. The most important reflex centers are the cardiac, vasomotor, and respiratory centers, which regulate circulation and respiration. SEE: *central nervous system; spinal cord.*

**brain attack** SEE: *stroke.*

**VASCULAR ANATOMY OF BRAIN**

**VENTRAL VIEW**

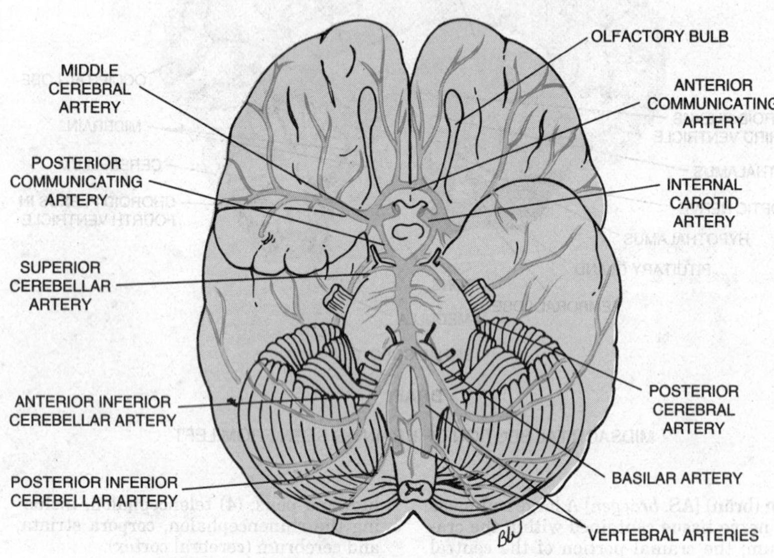


**LATERAL VIEW** **MEDIAL VIEW**

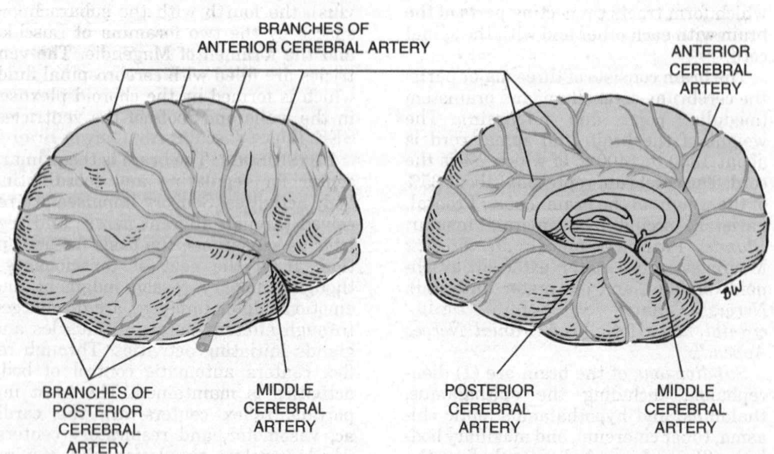

**brain death** The cessation of brain function. The criteria for concluding that the brain has died include lack of response to stimuli, lack of all reflexes, absent respirations, and an isoelectric electroencephalogram that for at least 30 min will not change in response to sound or pain stimuli. Before making this diagnosis, two physicians, including one experienced in caring for severely brain-damaged patients, should review the medical records. It is inadvisable for physicians associated with transplantion procedures to participate in the review. The patient may be kept alive by life-support devices, but death is the inevitable outcome.

---

Caution: Some drugs (e.g., barbiturates, methaqualone, diazepam, mecloqualone, meprobamate, trichloroethylene can produce short periods of isoelectric encephalograms. Hypothermia must be excluded as the cause of apparent brain death.

---

**brain edema** Swelling of the brain due to an increase in its water content. It is caused by a variety of conditions but the mechanisms are several, including increased permeability of brain capillary endothelial cells; swelling of brain cells associated with hypoxia or water intoxication; and interstitial edema resulting from obstructive hydrocephalus. SYN: *brain swelling*.

**brain fever** Meningitis.

**brain graft** An experimental technique in which brain cells are transplanted into the brain.

**Brain's reflex** [Walter Russell Brain, Brit. physician, 1895–1966] Extension of the flexed arm when the quadrupedal posture is assumed.

**brain sand** Corpora arenacea.

**brain scan** The use of radioactive isotopes injected into the circulation to detect abnormalities in the structure and function of the brain.

**brainstem** The stemlike part of the brain that connects the cerebral hemispheres with the spinal cord. It comprises the medulla oblongata, the pons, and the midbrain.

**brainstem auditory evoked potential** ABBR: BAEP. The study of brain (ECG) waves during sound stimuli. It is used to determine the threshold of sound required to produce a brainstem response. This provides an objective measure of hearing acuity. SEE: *auditory evoked response; evoked response; somatosensory evoked responses; visual evoked responses*.

**brain swelling** Brain edema.

**brain tumor** An inexact term to describe any intracranial mass—neoplastic, cystic, inflammatory (abscess), or syphilitic. Treatment includes surgery, radiation, and chemotherapy. Immunologic therapy, hyperthermia, and laser photoactivation have been investigated, but none has proved clinically useful. SEE: *neoplasm; tumor; Nursing Diagnoses Appendix*.

SYMPTOMS: The general symptoms are caused by an increase in intracranial pressure, such as headache, vomiting (without nausea), and changes in the retina such as choked disk seen on ophthalmoscopic examination. Mental changes (esp. dullness), epileptiform convulsions, and giddiness may be present. History and cranial radiography are esp. valuable.

In general, neoplasms of the brain do not metastasize to other parts of the body. They contain almost no blood vessels and may produce pain or other sensations. The most malignant ones in childhood are gliomas.

**brainwashing** Intense psychological indoctrination, usually political, for the purpose of displacing the individual's previous thoughts and attitudes with those selected by the regime or person inflicting the indoctrination.

**bran** The outer coating or husk of cereal grains, such as wheat or oats, produced as a by-product of milling these grains. Because some of the cellulose in bran is indigestible, it may be used to add bulk to the diet, helping to prevent or treat constipation. SEE: *fiber, dietary*.

**branch** In anatomy, a subdivision arising from a main or larger portion, esp. of an artery, vein, nerve, or lymphatic vessel.

**branchial** (brăng′kē-ăl) [L. *branchia*, gills] Pert. to or resembling gills of a fish or a homologous structure in higher animals.

**branchiogenic, branchiogenous** (brăng″kē-ō-jĕn′ĭk, brăng″kē-ŏj′ĕ-nŭs) [L. *branchia*, gills, + Gr. *gennan*, to produce] Having origin in a branchial cleft.

**branchioma** (brăng″kē-ō′mă) [″ + Gr. *oma*, tumor] A tumor derived from the branchial epithelium.

**branchiomeric** (brăng″kē-ō-mĕr′ĭk) [″ + Gr. *meros*, part] Pert. to the branchial arches.

**Brandt-Andrews maneuver** A technique for expressing the placenta from the uterus during the third stage of labor. One hand puts gentle traction on the cord while the other presses the anterior surface of the uterus backward. SEE: *Credé's method*.

**brash** A burning sensation in the stomach sometimes accompanied by belching of sour fluid. SYN: *heartburn; pyrosis*.

***water b.*** Reflex salivary hypersecretion in response to peptic esophagitis.

**brass chills** SEE: *metal fume fever*.

**brass poisoning** Poisoning due to the inhalation of fumes of zinc and zinc oxide, causing destruction of tissue in the respiratory passage. It is rarely fatal. Symptoms include dryness and burning in respiratory tract, coughing, headache, and chills. Treatment is symptomatic. Inhalations of humidified air make the patient more comfortable.

**brawny induration** Pathological hardening and thickening of tissues, usually due to inflammation.

**Braxton Hicks contractions** [John Braxton Hicks, Brit. gynecologist, 1823–1897] Intermittent painless uterine contractions that may occur every 10 to 20 min. They occur after the third month of pregnancy. These contractions are not true labor pains but are often interpreted as such. They are not present in every pregnancy. SYN: *Hicks sign*.

**Brazelton Neonatal Assessment Scale** [T. Berry Brazelton, American pediatrician, b. 1918] A scale for evaluating the behavior and responses of the newborn infant. It is based on four dimensions: interaction with the environment; motor processes, including motor responses, general activity level, and reflexes; control of physiologic state as determined by reaction to a distinct stimulus such as a rattle, bell, light, or a pinprick; and response to stress as judged by tremulousness, startle reaction, and change in skin coloration. The test has been used as late as 1 week after birth to demonstrate alteration in an infant's behavior due to drugs administered to the mother while the infant was in utero.

**break 1.** In orthopedics, a fracture. **2.** To interrupt the continuity in a tissue or electric circuit or the channel of flow or communication.

**breakage, chromosomal** The breaking of a chromosome. When this occurs, the two fragments may rejoin or a fragment may rejoin another broken chromosome. Unrepaired chromosome breaks may be associated with Fanconi's anemia or ataxia-telangiectasia.

**breakbone fever** An acute febrile disease marked by sudden onset, with headache, fever, prostration, joint and muscle pain, lymphadenopathy, and a rash that appears simultaneously with a second temperature rise after an afebrile period. The causative agent is a group B arbovirus. SYN: *dengue*.

**breakdown, nervous** SEE: *nervous breakdown*.

**breast** [AS. *breost*] **1.** The upper anterior aspect of the chest. **2.** The mammary gland, a compound alveolar gland consisting of 15 to 20 lobes of glandular tissue separated from each other by interlobular septa. Each lobe is drained by a lactiferous duct that opens on the tip of the nipple. The mammary gland secretes milk used for nourishment of the infant. SEE: illus.; *lactiferous glands; milk*.

DEVELOPMENT: During puberty, estrogens from the ovary stimulate growth and development of the duct system. During pregnancy, progesterone secreted by the corpus luteum and placenta acts synergistically with estrogens to bring the alveoli to complete development. Following parturition, prolactin (luteotrophin) in conjunction with adrenal corticoids initiates lactation, and oxytocin from the posterior pituitary induces ejection of milk. Sucking or milking reflexly stimulates both milk secretion and discharge of milk.

CHANGES IN PREGNANCY: During the first 6 to 12 weeks, there are fullness and tenderness, erectile tissues develop in the nipples, nodules are felt, pigment is deposited around the nipple (primary areola) (in blondes the areolae and nipples become darker pink and in brunettes they become dark brown and in some cases even black), and a few drops of fluid may be squeezed out. During the next 16 to 20 weeks, the secondary areola shows small whitish spots in pigmentation due to hypertrophy of the sebaceous glands (glands of Montgomery).

***chicken b.*** A deformity in which the sternum projects anteriorly; caused by rickets or obstructed respiration in childhood. SYN: *pigeon b.*

***ductal carcinoma in situ of the b.*** ABBR: DCIS. A cluster of abnormal cells in the milk ducts. In their early development they are not life-threatening. If left untreated, as many as 50% of patients with DCIS will develop invasive cancer. Because these cells grow in the ducts they develop without forming a palpable mass. Thus, in their early stage they are diagnosed through the use of mammography. SEE: *breast cancer; mammography*.

***pigeon b.*** Chicken b.

***b. self-examination*** ABBR: BSE. A technique that enables a woman to detect changes in her breasts. The accompanying illustration explains the specific steps to be followed. The examination should be done each month soon after the menstrual period ends, as normal physiological changes that may confuse results occur in the premenstrual period. This method of self-examination is useful in the early detection of breast cancer, but is not as accurate as mammography. SEE: illus.; *mammography*.

**breast cancer** A malignant neoplasm of the breast. Breast cancer is the leading cause of death in women between the ages of 30 and 50, and is second only to heart disease as a cause of death in women over 50. Approx. one woman in 10 will develop breast cancer in her lifetime. About 1000 men develop breast cancer each year. The gene BRCA1, believed to indicate susceptibility to cancer of the breast and ovary, has been isolated. SEE: illus.

DIAGNOSIS: About 90% of the cases of breast masses are discovered by breast self-examination (BSE) or accidentally by the patient. The remainder are detected by physical examination by a health professional or by screening techniques, such as mammography. Positive diagnosis can be made only by obtaining tissue for microscopic examination. SEE: *breast, self-examination of; double reading; mammography*.

The American Cancer Society recom-

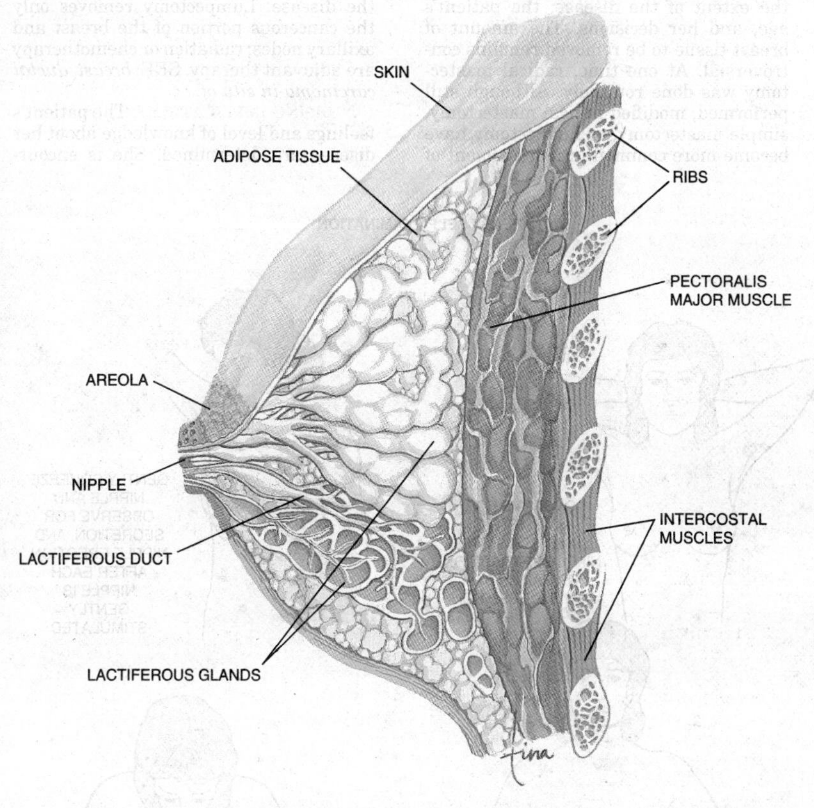


**BREAST**

MAMMARY GLAND IN MIDSAGITTAL SECTION

mends that all women perform BSE monthly. In addition, women 20 to 40 years of age should be examined by a clinician every 3 years. In the 40 to 49 age group, mammography is recommended every 1 to 2 years, and clinical breast examination every year; women 50 years of age and older should have clinical breast examination and mammography annually.

NOTE: BSE is a useful procedure and should not be neglected, but mammography should also be performed because it can detect a much smaller suspicious lesion than can be felt by use of BSE.

RISK FACTORS: It is estimated that in the U.S. 75% of breast cancer cases occur in women with no known high-risk factors. The risk of developing breast cancer increases with age. Persons born in northern Europe and North America have higher rates of breast cancer than those born in other countries. The more full-term pregnancies a woman has had may decrease her risk of breast cancer after about age 45, but increases her risk for developing it at an earlier age. The data are not conclusive but in general the longer the total period of lactation after childbirth, the less risk there is of developing breast cancer.

Risk factors in order of importance include: having a mother who had bilateral breast cancer diagnosed prior to menopause; having a close relative who developed breast cancer but was menopausal; being over age 50 and nulliparous or having a first pregnancy after age 30; a history of chronic breast disease, esp. epithelial hyperplasia; exposure to ionizing radiation of more than 0.5 Gy (50 rad) during adolescence; and obesity. Early menarche, late menopause, and menstrual cycle irregularity also increase the chances of breast cancer development. Artificial menopause prior to age 35 and childbearing prior to age 18 provide some protection from breast cancer. SEE: *menopause*.

TREATMENT: The type of treatment, whether surgical, chemotherapeutic, or a combination of the two, is determined by the extent of the disease, the patient's age, and her decisions. The amount of breast tissue to be removed remains controversial. At one time, radical mastectomy was done routinely. Although still performed, modified radical mastectomy, simple mastectomy, or lumpectomy have become more common in management of the disease. Lumpectomy removes only the cancerous portion of the breast and axillary nodes; radiation or chemotherapy are adjuvant therapy. SEE: *breast, ductal carcinoma in situ of.*

NURSING IMPLICATIONS: The patient's feelings and level of knowledge about her disease are determined. She is encour-

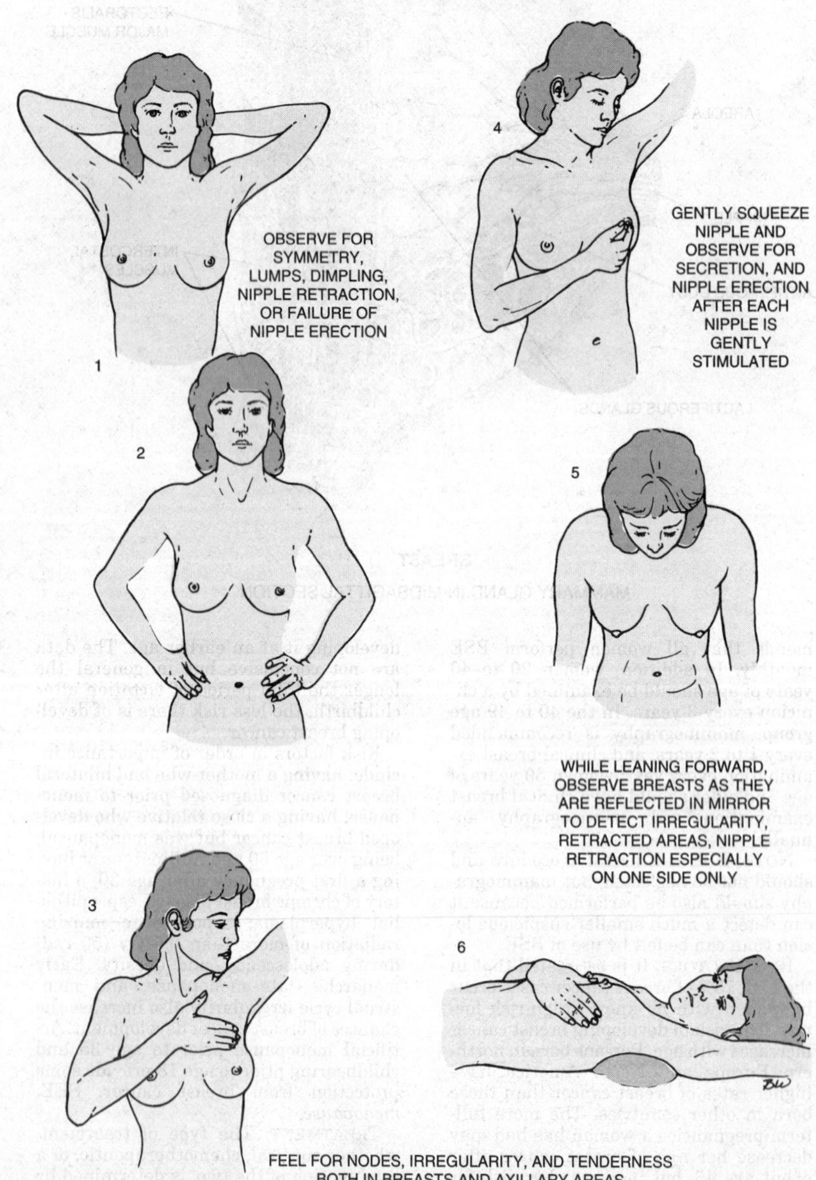

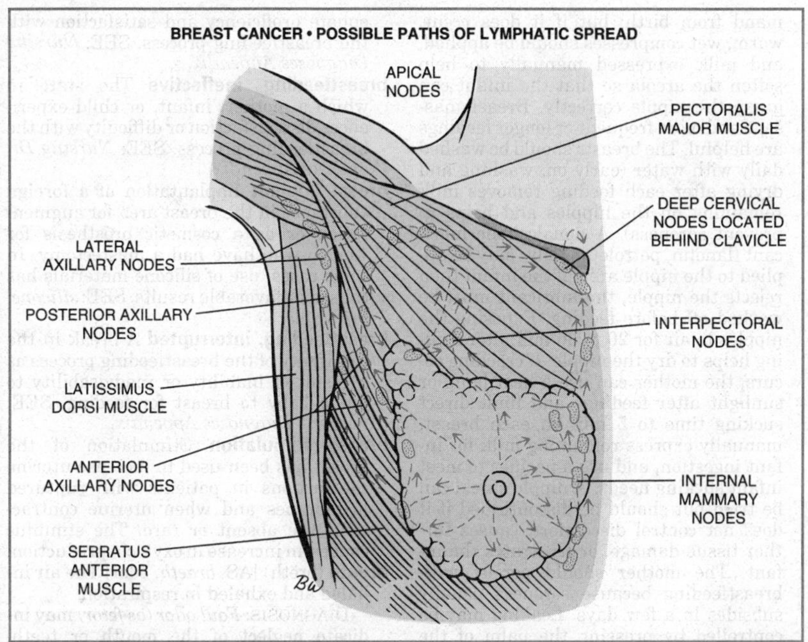


aged to express fears and concerns, and the nurse stays with her during periods of anxiety or anguish. If surgery is planned, the procedure, postoperative care, and expected outcomes are explained.

Prescribed chemotherapy is administered, and the patient is monitored for adverse reactions, such as nausea, vomiting, anorexia, stomatitis, GI ulceration, leukopenia, thrombocytopenia, and bleeding, so that they can be managed early. Weight and nutrition status are evaluated. Skin is inspected for redness, irritation, or breakdown if radiation therapy is prescribed. Prescribed analgesics are administered, and noninvasive nursing measures to relieve pain are instituted and taught to the patient. Comfort measures are used to promote relaxation and rest and to relieve anxiety. If immobility develops late in the disease, careful repositioning, excellent skin care, respiratory toilet, and low-pressure mattresses are used to prevent complications (skin breakdown, respiratory problems, pathological fractures). The patient's and family's coping abilities are evaluated, and referral for counseling and support services may be necessary.

**breastfeeding** The act of providing milk to a newborn or infant from the mother's breasts. Mature mother's milk and its precursor, colostrum, are considered to be the most balanced foods available for normal newborns and infants. Breast milk is sterile, easily digested, nonallergenic, and transmits maternal antibodies that protect against many infections and illness. In addition, the baby's suckling causes release of oxytocin, a pituitary hormone that stimulates uterine contractions and promotes the return of the uterus to a normal nongravid size and state. Breastfeeding may engender and strengthen early bonding. Frequency and duration of nursing may vary. Initially, newborns may nurse for only a few min on each breast, and demand-feed on an average of every 1 to 3 hr. Time spent in nursing gradually increases, and the demand intervals stabilize. The time for weaning is a personal decision; however, many women choose to breastfeed until solid foods are introduced and well-accepted by the infant.

Nursing Implications: Gentle massage during the third trimester will prepare the nipples and areolar areas for nursing. During nursing, the nipple and surrounding tissue should be positioned well back in the infant's mouth, because sucking on the end of the nipple may cause soreness, erosion, and cracking. If the nipple appears retracted, the mother is taught to roll it gently between her fingers until it becomes erect.

The infant will begin nursing for several minutes on alternating breasts. The time that the infant spends breastfeeding is gradually increased according to nipple tolerance. When lactation is well established, the infant takes 10 to 15 min to empty each breast. Engorgement may be prevented by nursing the infant on demand from birth; but if it does occur, warm, wet compresses should be applied, and milk expressed manually to help soften the areola so that the infant can grasp the nipple correctly. Breast massage and more frequent or longer feedings are helpful. The breasts should be washed daily with water (early on, washing and drying after each feeding removes milk remaining on the nipples and helps to prevent soreness). A nonalcoholic lubricant (lanolin, petroleum jelly) may be applied to the nipple area; if the infant then rejects the nipple, the lubricant must be washed off before feeding. Exposing the nipples to air for 20 to 30 min after feeding helps to dry the nipple. If cracking occurs, the mother can use a heat lamp or sunlight after feedings and limit direct sucking time to 5 min on each breast, manually express remaining milk for infant ingestion, and use a pacifier to meet infant sucking needs. A nipple shield can be tried but should be discontinued if it does not control discomfort, causes further tissue damage, or frustrates the infant. The mother should persist with breastfeeding because soreness usually subsides in a few days. Leaking may be controlled by pressing the palm of the hand firmly over the nipple or by crossing the arms firmly across the breasts. The mother should wear a well-fitted brassiere that supports the breasts in an upward and inward position. The cups may be lined with soft pads of disposable material or folded soft-flannel or cotton fabric to absorb released milk, but the nurse advises the mother to avoid plastic liners because they retain moisture, which softens and macerates the nipple. The nurse refers the mother to local nursing mothers' groups for practical and emotional support and for further information.

*Lactation suppression:* If the mother chooses not to breast-feed, she is instructed in traditional (nonpharmacological) therapies to relieve postpartum breast engorgement and suppress lactation. These include wearing a tight-fitting brassiere, applying ice packs, and avoiding local stimulation of the breast. Level of discomfort is assessed, and mild analgesics (such as acetaminophen or aspirin) are administered for relief of pain and discomfort. Some women prefer to gently express a small amount of milk manually if breasts are painfully engorged, although this may delay lactation suppression. Breast engorgement usually resolves within a few days, and lactation ceases in 1 to 2 weeks when treated nonpharmacologically, with no risk of adverse reactions. (Up to 40% of patients who take drugs prescribed to suppress lactation begin lactating again after completion of the usual 14-day medication regimen.)

**breastfeeding, effective** The state in which a mother-infant dyad/family exhibits adequate proficiency and satisfaction with the breastfeeding process. SEE: *Nursing Diagnoses Appendix.*

**breastfeeding, ineffective** The state in which a mother, infant, or child experiences dissatisfaction or difficulty with the breastfeeding process. SEE: *Nursing Diagnoses Appendix.*

**breast implant** Implantation of a foreign substance in the breast area for augmentation or as a cosmetic prosthesis for women who have had a mastectomy. In some cases, use of silicone materials has caused unfavorable results. SEE: *silicone, injectable.*

**breastfeeding, interrupted** A break in the continuity of the breastfeeding process as a result of inability or inadvisability to put a baby to breast for feeding. SEE: *Nursing Diagnoses Appendix.*

**breast stimulation** Stimulation of the breast has been used to increase uterine contractions in patients with ruptured membranes and when uterine contractions are absent or rare. The stimulus causes an increase in oxytocin production.

**breath** (brĕth) [AS. *braeth,* odor] The air inhaled and exhaled in respiration.

DIAGNOSIS: *Foul odor (os fetor)* may indicate neglect of the mouth or teeth, improper diet, constipation, breathing through the mouth, lack of exercise, or the use of drugs, alcohol, or tobacco. It also depends upon the food ingested and may indicate stomatitis, necrosis of the jaw, caries of the teeth, tonsillitis, diphtheria, gangrene and abscess of the lungs, fetid bronchitis, bronchiectasis, pyothorax, diabetes, kidney disease, or other disorders. Mouthwashes and gargles are ineffective in removing the odor if it is due to systemic causes or ingestion of food such as garlic. *Urinous odor* indicates uremia. *Sweet odor* (like ripe apples) occurs in diabetes mellitus, esp. during coma. This sweet odor is due to the excretion of acetone in the breath. This condition develops quickly in infants and children who have gone several hours without food. SEE: *breath tests.*

*Rattling and shortness of breath* indicates edema and the presence of fluids in the air passages. *Sighing breath* (air hunger) occurs with bleeding into the lung. Therefore be alert to the development of this symptom following abdominal surgery and in typhoid fever.

***liver b.*** The characteristic odor of the breath that accompanies severe liver disease. It has been described as "mousy."

***uremic b.*** The "fishy" or ammoniacal breath odor characteristic of individuals with uremia.

**Breathalyzer** (brĕth′ă-lī-zĕr) Trade name for an apparatus used to analyze the specific content of expired air. It may be used to test for the presence of alcohol in expired air to determine whether a person is legally intoxicated.

**breath-holding** The voluntary or involuntary stopping of breathing may be seen in children who use this to attempt to control the behavior of their parents.

**breath-holding attacks** A benign condition that always has its onset with crying. The young child stops breathing and becomes cyanotic, the limbs become rigid and extended, and consciousness may be lost. This is followed by the body becoming limp, resumption of respirations and, after a few seconds, full alertness. This pattern of behavior usually disappears spontaneously prior to school age.

**breathing** The act of inhaling and exhaling air. SEE: *chest; respiration.*

***apneuistic b.*** An abnormal breathing pattern marked by prolonged inspiratory pauses. This is usually associated with brainstem injuries.

***asthmatic b.*** Harsh breathing with a prolonged wheezing expiration heard all over the chest.

***ataxic b.*** An irregular, uncoordinated breathing pattern common in infants.

***bronchial b.*** Harsh breathing with a tubular quality. It is heard when consolidated lung tissue is present.

***Cheyne-Stokes b.*** SEE: *Cheyne-Stokes respiration.*

***continuous positive-pressure b.*** A method of mechanically assisted pulmonary ventilation. A device administers air or oxygen to the lungs under a continuous pressure that never returns to zero. SYN: *continuous positive-pressure ventilation.*

***diaphragmatic b.*** A rehabilitative retraining technique is which patients can learn to control breathing with the least possible effort by using the muscles of the diaphragm.

***frog b.*** A respiratory pattern in which the air in the mouth and pharynx is forced into the lungs by gulping and swallowing it. This may be observed in patients whose respiratory muscles are weak or paralyzed.

***inspiratory resistive b.*** Inspiration with an added workload to increase the strength and endurance of the inspiratory muscles.

***intermittent positive-pressure b.*** ABBR: IPPB. A mechanical method for assisting pulmonary ventilation employing a device that administers air or oxygen for the inflation of the lungs under positive pressure. Exhalation is usually passive. SYN: *intermittent positive-pressure ventilation.*

***Kussmaul b.*** SEE: *Kussmaul's breathing.*

***periodic b.*** An irregular respiratory pattern marked by alternating periods of rapid and slow respirations and by apneic periods lasting 15 sec or less. This breathing pattern is considered normal in newborns.

***pursed-lip b.*** An expiratory maneuver to alter flow rate and prevent bronchial collapse.

***shallow b.*** The type of breathing present in acute pulmonary disease. It is noted in the old and feeble, in those with thick chest walls, and in those with pneumonia, atelectasis, pleural effusion, incipient tuberculosis, fractured ribs, pleurodynia, early pleurisy, and pulmonary edema.

***vesicular b.*** Normal breathing. SEE: *eupnea.*

**breathing pattern, ineffective** The state in which the rate, depth, timing, rhythm or chest/abdominal wall excursion during inspiration, expiration or both does not maintain optimum ventilation for the individual. SEE: *Nursing Diagnoses Appendix.*

**breathlessness** The feeling of being short of breath. This may be normal, as during and immediately after vigorous and prolonged exercise. In other cases, it is a symptom of an abnormality such as acute asthma, congestive heart failure, hyperventilation syndrome, or acute anxiety attack. The feeling of breathlesssness is thought to be caused, at least in some cases, by an increase in the concentration of carbon dioxide in the blood.

**breath test** A test that may be used to detect a specific substance in the breath to help explain metabolic changes. Certain breath tests are used to detect evidence of bacterial overgrowth in the intestines and to investigate intestinal malabsorption.

**breath test for lactase deficiency** The measurement of hydrogen in the breath after ingestion of 50 g of lactase. SEE: *lactase deficiency syndrome.*

**breech** [AS. *brec,* buttocks] The nates, or buttocks.

**breech presentation** SEE: *presentation, breech.*

**bregma** (brĕg′mă) *pl.* **bregmata** [Gr., front of head] The point on the skull where the coronal and sagittal sutures join. The anterior fontanel in the fetus and young infant. **bregmatic** (-măt′ĭk), *adj.*

**bregmocardiac reflex** (brĕg″mō-kăr′dē-ăk) [Gr. *bregma,* front of head, + *kardia,* heart] A reduced heart rate following pressure on the posterior fontanel.

**Brenner's tumor** [Fritz Brenner, Ger. pathologist, 1877–1969] A benign fibroepithelioma of the ovary.

**Breokinase** Trade name for urokinase.

**brevicollis** (brĕv″ĭ-kŏl′ĭs) [L. *brevis,* short, + *collum,* neck] Shortness of the neck.

**brevilineal** (brĕv-ĭ-lĭn′ē-ăl) [L. *brevis,* short, + *linea,* line] Having a body build that is shorter and broader than usual. SYN: *brachymorphic.*

**Brevital Sodium** Trade name for methohexital sodium.

**Bricanyl** Trade name for terbutaline sulfate.

**bridge** (brĭj) [AS. *brycg*] **1.** A narrow band of tissue. **2.** A dental appliance that replaces missing teeth and is attached to adjacent teeth for support. SYN: *fixed partial den-*

*ture.*

***b. of nose*** The upper part of the external nose formed by the junction of the nasal bones.

**bridgework** (brĭj'work) A partial denture held in place by attachments other than clasps.

***fixed b.*** A partial plate held by crowns or inlays cemented to the natural teeth.

***removable b.*** A partial plate held by clasps that permit its removal.

**bridle** (brī'dl) In anatomy, a frenum.

**Bright's disease** [Richard Bright, Brit. physician, 1789–1858] A vague and obsolete term for kidney disease. It usually refers to nonsuppurative inflammatory or degenerative kidney disease marked by proteinuria and hematuria and sometimes by edema, hypertension, and nitrogen retention. SEE: *nephritis.*

**brightness gain** The increase in the intensity of a fluoroscopic image by use of an image intensifier.

**brim 1.** An edge or margin. **2.** The brim of the pelvis; the superior aperture of the lesser or true pelvis; the inlet. It is formed by the iliopectineal line of the innominate bone and the sacral promontory. It is oval-shaped in the female, heart-shaped in the male.

**Briquet's syndrome** [Paul Briquet, Fr. physician, 1796–1881] A personality disorder in which alcoholism and somatization disorder occur.

**Brissaud's reflex** (brĭs-sōz') [Edouard Brissaud, Fr. physician, 1852–1909] Contraction of the tensor fasciae latae muscle when the sole of the foot is stroked or tickled; a component of the extensor plantar response.

**British antilewisite** ABBR: BAL. Trade name for dimercaprol, a compound used as an antidote in poisoning due to heavy metals such as arsenic, gold, and mercury.

**British Pharmacopoeia** ABBR: B.P. The standard reference on drugs and their preparations used in Great Britain.

**British thermal unit** ABBR: BTU. The amount of heat needed to raise the temperature of 1 lb of water from 39°F to 40°F. One BTU is equal to 252 calories or 1055 joules.

**brittle diabetes** Previous name for insulin-dependent diabetes.

**broach** (brōch) [ME. *broche,* pointed rod] **1.** A dental instrument used for enlarging a root canal or removing the pulp. **2.** A technique used for preparing the intramedullary canal of a bone by using a cutting device. This is done in preparation for a prosthetic replacement.

**Broadbent's sign** [Sir William Henry Broadbent, Brit. physician, 1835–1907] A visible retraction of the left side and back in the region of the 11th and 12th ribs synchronous with the cardiac systole in adhesive pericarditis.

**Broca's area** (brō'kăs) [Pierre Paul Broca, Fr. anatomist, anthropologist, neurologist, and surgeon, 1824–1880] The area of the left hemisphere of the brain at the posterior end of the inferior frontal gyrus. It contains the motor speech area and controls movements of tongue, lips, and vocal cords. Loss of speech may follow hemorrhage into this area. SYN: *motor speech area; speech center.* SEE: *aphasia, motor.*

**Brodie's abscess** [Sir Benjamin Collins Brodie, Brit. surgeon, 1783–1862] An abscess of the head of a bone, esp. the tibia.

SYMPTOMS: There may be aching pain in the affected area, followed by slight swelling and tenderness on movement. The symptoms are similar to those of osteomyelitis but are less acute.

ETIOLOGY: It is usually of tubercular origin or from subacute staphylococcal infection.

**Brodmann's areas** [Korbinian Brodmann, Ger. neurologist, 1868–1918] The division of the cerebral cortex into 47 areas. This was originally done on the basis of cytoarchitectural characteristics, but the areas are now classified according to their functions.

**brom-, bromo-** [Gr. *bromos,* stench] Combining form indicating the presence of bromine.

**bromelain** (brō'mĕ-lān) A proteolytic enzyme present in the pineapple plant.

**bromide** (brō'mīd) [Gr. *bromos,* stench] A binary compound of bromine combined with an element or a radical. It is a central nervous system depressant, and overdosage can cause serious mental disturbance.

**bromide poisoning** Poisoning due to an overdose of bromide.

SYMPTOMS: Symptoms include vomiting; abdominal pain; respiratory and eye irritation if inhaled; corrosion of the mouth and intestinal tract if swallowed; cyanosis; tachycardia; and shock.

FIRST AID: If bromide is inhaled, oxygen is administered, respiratory support provided, and pulmonary edema treated. If bromide is swallowed, emesis should be induced with ipecac, gastric lavage should be performed, and shock should be treated. SEE: *Poisons and Poisoning Appendix.*

**bromidrosiphobia** (brō"mĭ-drō-sĭ-fō'bē-ă) [" + *hidros,* sweat, + *phobos,* fear] An abnormal fear of personal odors, accompanied by hallucinations.

**bromidrosis, bromhidrosis** (brō"mĭ-drō'sĭs) Sweat that is fetid or offensive due to bacterial decomposition. It occurs mostly on the feet, in the groin, and under the arms.

NURSING IMPLICATIONS: The axillae, groin, and feet should be cleansed daily with soap and water, rinsing well and drying thoroughly. Deodorant preparations should be used; and clothing and shoes changed, aired, and cleaned frequently. SYN: *kakidrosis.*

**bromine** (brō′mēn, -mĭn) [Gr. *bromos,* stench] SYMB: Br. A liquid nonmetallic element obtained from natural brines from wells and sea water; atomic weight 79.904, atomic number 35. Its compounds are used in medicine and photography. SEE: *bromide.*

**bromism, brominism** (brō′mĭzm, brō′mĭn-ĭzm) [″ + *-ismos,* condition] Poisoning that results from prolonged use of bromides. SEE: *bromides in Poisons and Poisoning Appendix.*

**bromocriptine mesylate** (brō″mō-krĭp′tēn) An ergot derivative that suppresses secretion of prolactin. It has been used to stimulate ovulation in the galactorrhea-amenorrhea syndrome. It is used to treat acromegaly and is of limited usefulness in treating parkinsonism. Trade name is Parlodel.

**bromoderma** (brō″mō-dĕr′mă) [″ + *derma,* skin] An acnelike eruption due to allergic sensitivity to bromides.

**bromodiphenhydramine hydrochloride** (brō″mō-dī″fĕn-hī′dră-mēn) An antihistamine. It also has sedative properties. Trade name is Ambodryl Hydrochloride.

**bromoiodism** (brō″mō-ī′ō-dĭzm) [″ + *ioeides,* violet colored, + *-ismos,* condition] Poisoning from bromine and iodine or their compounds.

**bromomenorrhea** (brō″mō-mĕn-ō-rē′ă) [″ + *men,* month, + *rhoia,* flow] Menstrual discharge marked by an offensive odor.

**brompheniramine maleate** (brōm″fĕn-ĭr′ă-mēn) An antihistamine. Trade name is Dimetane.

**Brompton's cocktail** [Brompton Chest Hospital, England] A mixture of cocaine, morphine, and antiemetics used to alleviate pain and induce euphoria, esp. in patients with cancer.

**bromsulphalein** ABBR: BSP. Trade name for sulfobromophthalein sodium, a dye used for testing liver function in nonjaundiced patients.

**bronch-** SEE: *broncho-.*

**bronchi-** SEE: *broncho-.*

**bronchi** (brŏng′kī) *sing.,* **bronchus** [L.] The two main branches leading from the trachea to the lungs, providing a passageway for air. The trachea divides opposite the third thoracic vertebra into the right and left main bronchi. The point of division, called the carina tracheae, is the site where foreign bodies too large to enter either bronchus would rest after passing through the trachea. The right bronchus is shorter and more vertical than the left one. After entering the lung each bronchus divides further and terminates in bronchioles. SEE: *bronchus* for illus.

***foreign bodies in b.*** The presence of any foreign material in the bronchi may cause various diseases, large objects leading to collapse of the lung. Beans, nuts, or seeds may cause pneumonia, bronchitis, or lung abscess. Foreign bodies usually are aspirated into the right bronchus because it has a less acute angle compared with the left.

SYMPTOMS: Choking and gagging occur immediately. Later, symptoms of bronchitis, atelectasis, pneumonia, or lung abscess may develop. Small metal bodies may produce no symptoms.

TREATMENT: A bronchoscope may be used to remove the object.

PROGNOSIS: Prognosis is good if the object is removed before complications occur. The outlook is better in cases involving metal objects than in those involving vegetable matter.

**bronchial** (brŏng′kē-ăl) Pert. to the bronchi or bronchioles.

**bronchial breath sounds** SEE: under *sound.*

**bronchial crisis** A paroxysm of coughing in persons with locomotor ataxia due to syphilis.

**bronchial tree** The bronchi and bronchial tubes.

**bronchial tube** One of the smaller divisions of the bronchi.

**bronchial washing** Irrigation of one or both bronchi to collect cells for cytologic study or to help cleanse the bronchi.

**bronchiectasis** (brŏng″kē-ĕk′tă-sĭs) [″ + *ektasis,* dilatation] Chronic dilatation of a bronchus or bronchi, with a secondary infection that usually involves the lower portion of the lung. Dilatation may be in an isolated segment or spread throughout the bronchi.

SYMPTOMS: Symptoms include coughing, dyspnea, and expectoration of foul secretion, esp. in the morning or when the individual changes position. When allowed to stand, the sputum separates into three layers: a bottom layer that is thick and contains pus cells; a middle layer of greenish fluid; and an upper layer of froth.

ETIOLOGY: The condition may be acquired or congenital and may occur in one or both lungs. Acquired bronchiectasis usually occurs secondary to an obstruction or an infection such as bronchopneumonia, chronic bronchitis, tuberculosis, or whooping cough.

TREATMENT: Therapy consists of antibiotics, prophylaxis, and postural drainage. Resection of affected areas may be done in selected patients. Aerosols may be useful for bronchodilation if bronchospasm is present. SEE: *postural drainage.*

NURSING IMPLICATIONS: The patient is assessed for the presence or increased severity of respiratory distress. Ventilatory rate, pattern, and effort are observed, breath sounds are ausculated, and sputum is inspected for changes indicating a worsening condition or development of a respiratory infection. Gas exchange is evaluated by monitoring arterial blood gas values, and oxygen is administered according to protocol or as prescribed. The patient is observed for complications, such as right ventricular failure or cor pulmonale. The patient should increase oral fluid intake and be shown how to use a humidifier or vaporizer to help thin inspissated secretions. The patient is also taught to breathe deeply and cough effectively. Chest physiotherapy is most effective and least disruptive if carried out in the morning, ½ hr before meals, and at bedtime. The nurse suctions the oropharynx if the patient is unable to clear the airway and teaches the patient and family how to do this. The need for frequent oral hygiene to remove foul-smelling secretions and to help prevent anorexia is explained. The patient is taught to dispose of secretions, to cleanse items contaminated by secretions, and to wash hands thoroughly to avoid spreading infections. A well-balanced high-calorie, high-protein diet (in small, frequent meals) is encouraged to promote tissue healing and prevent fatigue. Periods of activity and rest should be alternated, and activity should be pursued in a warm, comfortable environment. Air pollutants and people with upper respiratory infections should be avoided. If the patient smokes, referral may be needed for a smoking cessation program or nicotine patch therapy. Prescribed medications, such as antibiotics, bronchodilators, and expectorants, are given and both patient and family instructed in their use, action, and side effects. The patient is advised not to take over-the-counter drugs without the physician's approval. Supportive care is provided to help the patient adjust to the lifestyle changes that irreversible lung damage requires. If surgery is scheduled, the nurse prepares the patient physically and emotionally, provides preoperative and postoperative teaching and care, and monitors the patient's status to prevent complications.

***saccular b.*** Dilated bronchi that are of saccular or irregular shape. The proximal third to fourth branches of the bronchi are severely dilated and end blindly with extensive collapse.

***varicose b.*** Dilated bronchi that resemble varicose veins; irregular dilatation and constriction as seen in cystic fibrosis.

**bronchiloquy** (brŏng-kĭl′ō-kwē) [″ + L. *loqui,* to speak] Unusual vocal resonance over a bronchus covered with consolidated lung tissue.

**bronchiocele** (brŏng′kē-ō-sēl) [″ + *kele,* tumor, swelling] Circumscribed dilatation of a bronchus.

**bronchiogenic** (brŏng″kē-ō-jĕn′ĭk) [″ + *gennan,* to produce] Having origin in the bronchi.

**bronchiole** (brŏng′kē-ōl) *pl.* **bronchioles** [L. *bronchiolus,* air passage] One of the smaller subdivisions of the bronchial tubes.

***respiratory b.*** The last division of the bronchial tree. Respiratory bronchioles are branches of terminal bronchioles and continue to the alveolar ducts, which lead to the alveoli.

***terminal b.*** The next-to-last subdivision of a bronchiole, leading to the respiratory bronchioles.

**bronchiolectasis** (brŏng″kē-ō-lĕk′tă-sĭs) [″ + Gr. *ektasis,* dilatation] Dilatation of the bronchioles; capillary bronchiectasis.

**bronchiolitis** (brŏng″kē-ō-lī′tĭs) [″ + Gr. *itis,* inflammation] Inflammation of the bronchioles.

***b. exudativa*** Bronchiolitis with fibrinous exudation and grayish sputum; often associated with asthma.

***b. obliterans*** Bronchiolitis in which the bronchioles and, occasionally, some of the smaller bronchi are partly or completely obliterated by nodular masses that contain granulation and fibrotic tissue.

**bronchiolus** (brŏng-kē′ō-lŭs) *pl.* **bronchioli** [L.] Bronchiole.

**bronchiospasm** (brŏng′kē-ō-spăzm) [Gr. *bronchos,* windpipe, + *spasmos,* a convulsion] Spasmodic contraction of the bronchial airways.

**bronchiostenosis** (brŏng″kē-ō-stĕn-ō′sĭs) [″ + *stenosis,* act of narrowing] Narrowing of the bronchial tubes.

**bronchitis** (brŏng-kī′tĭs) [″ + *itis,* inflammation] Inflammation of the mucous membrane of the bronchial airways. SEE: *Nursing Diagnoses Appendix.*

ETIOLOGY: Bronchitis is caused by infectious agents such as viruses, esp. influenza, or pyogenic organisms such as various species of *Streptococcus, Pneumococcus, Staphylococcus,* and *Haemophilus.* Infection is often preceded by the common cold. Predisposing factors are exposure, chilling, fatigue, and malnutrition. Acute bronchial irritation may also be caused by various physical and chemical agents such as dusts and fumes. Allergic factors may be important.

NOTE: Although the pathway of air to the bronchi and lungs is capable of warming inspired cold air, there are limits beyond which this system fails. Therefore, it is inadvisable to sleep in an area that is extremely cold or to exercise vigorously in extremely cold air without wearing a face mask so that the heat produced from exhalation will be available to the inspired air.

NURSING IMPLICATIONS: A history is obtained documenting tobacco use, including type, duration, and frequency, and a pack-year history is calculated. The nurse assesses for other known respiratory irritants and allergens, exertional or worsening dyspnea, and productive cough. The patient is evaluated for changes in baseline respiratory function such as use of accessory muscles in breathing, pedal edema, neck vein distention, tachypnea, prolonged expiratory time, and altered breath sounds such as wheezes and gurgles. The color and characteristics of sputum are documented, and the patient is observed for signs of respiratory infection. Diagnostic testing such as pulmonary function testing, arterial blood gas analysis, and sputum culture are explained, including expected sensations. Prescribed bronchodilators, oxygen therapy, chest physiotherapy and respiratory toilet, nebulizer treatments, inhaled corticosteroids, and diuretics (if necessary for edema) are administered, the response is documented, and the patient is instructed in their use. Daily activities are interspersed with rest periods to conserve energy and to prevent fatigue. Adequate fluids (at least 3 L per day unless otherwise restricted) are needed to loosen secretions, and fluid intake is monitored. Weight and nutritional status are monitored, and a high-calorie, protein-rich diet is offered in small, frequent meals. The patient should avoid exposure to cold air, crowds, individuals with known respiratory infections, and known allergens and respiratory irritants. Patients needing help to quit smoking are referred to smoking cessation programs and for nicotone patch therapy. The nurse encourages both patient and family to express concerns about the illness, and answers their questions, offers emotional support, and refers them to any needed support services. Both patient and family should be encouraged to participate in care decisions.

***acute b.*** Bronchitis that has a short, severe course and is marked by chilliness, malaise, soreness and constriction behind the sternum, coughing, and a slight fever of 100° to 102°F (37.8° to 38.9°C). At first the cough may be dry and painful, but later it produces mucopurulent expectoration that becomes free as inflammation subsides.

TREATMENT: Treatment consists of bedrest, increased fluid intake, an antipyretic and analgesic, antibiotics, and steam inhalations.

***asthmatic b.*** Bronchitis that aggravates an existing asthma.

***chronic b.*** Bronchitis marked by increased mucus secretion by the tracheobronchial tree. The productive cough is usually present for at least 3 months of 2 consecutive years. The diagnosis can be made only if bronchopulmonary diseases such as bronchiectasis, tuberculosis, and tumor have been excluded. The predominant pathological change is hypertrophy and hyperplasia of the mucus-secreting glands of the trachea, bronchi, and bronchioles.

TREATMENT: It is important to have the patient who smokes stop smoking. Change of climate and occupation may be indicated but may be impossible due to social and economic circumstances. If infection is present, appropriate antibiotics should be administered.

***plastic b.*** Bronchitis marked by violent cough and paroxysms of dyspnea in which casts of the bronchial tubes are expectorated.

***putrid b.*** A chronic form of bronchitis with foul-smelling sputum.

***vegetal b.*** Bronchitis resulting from lodging of foods of vegetable origin in the bronchus.

**bronchium** (brŏng′kē-ŭm) *pl.* **bronchia** [Gr. *bronchos*] One of the subdivisions of the bronchus. It is smaller than a bronchus and larger than a bronchiole.

**broncho-, bronch-, bronchi-** [Gr. *bronchos,* windpipe] Combining form meaning *airway.*

**bronchoalveolar** (brŏn″kō-ăl-vē′ō-lăr) [″ + *alveolus,* small hollow] Concerning the bronchi and alveoli.

**bronchoalveolar lavage** The removal of secretions, cells, and protein from the lower respiratory tract by insertion of sterile saline solution into the lung through a fiberoptic bronchoscope. The fluid is usually used to treat cystic fibrosis, pulmonary alveolar proteinosis, and severe asthma with bronchial obstruction due to mucus plugging and to obtain materials for diagnostic purposes.

**bronchoblennorrhea** (brŏng″kō-blĕn″ō-rē′ă) [″ + *blennos,* mucus, + *rhoia,* flow] Chronic bronchitis in which sputum is copious and thin.

**bronchocele** (brŏng′kō-sēl) [″ + *kele,* tumor, swelling] A localized dilatation of a bronchus.

**bronchoconstriction** (brŏng″kō-kŏn-strĭk′shŭn) [″ + L. *constringere,* to draw together] Constriction of the bronchial tubes.

**bronchodilatation** (brŏng″kō-dĭl-ă-tā′shŭn) [″ + L. *dilatare,* to open] Dilatation of a bronchus.

**bronchodilator** A drug that expands the bronchial tubes by relaxing bronchial muscle. There are three classes of bronchodilators: $\beta_2$ adrenergic-receptor agonists, methylxanthines, and anticholinergic agents. The $\beta_2$ adrenergic-receptor agonists produce the greatest bronchodilation in patients with bronchial asthma. They are also preferred for relief of acute symptoms and for prevention of exercise-induced bronchospasm. Long-acting inhaled $\beta_2$ adrenergic-receptor agonists are available.

**bronchoedema** (brŏng″kō-ĕ-dē′mă) [″+ *oidema,* swelling] Edematous swelling of the mucosa of the bronchial tubes, reducing the size of air passageways and inducing dyspnea.

**bronchoesophageal** (brŏng″kō-ĕ-sŏf″ă-jē′ăl) [″ + *oisophagos,* esophagus] Concerning the bronchus and the esophagus.

**bronchofiberscope** (brŏng″kō-fī′bĕr-skōp) [″ + L. *fibra,* fiber, + Gr. *skopein,* to examine] A fiberoptic endoscope for visual examination of the bronchi.

**bronchogenic** (brŏng-kō-jĕn′ĭk) [″ + *gen-*

*nan,* to produce] Having origin in a bronchus.

**bronchogram** (brŏng′kō-grăm) [″ + *gramma,* something written] Previously used term for a radiograph of the lung obtained during bronchography.

**bronchography** (brŏng-kŏg′ră-fē) [″ + *graphein,* to write] Radiography of the tracheobronchial tree after instillation of an oil-based contrast medium. This examination has been replaced by bronchoscopy and computed tomography.

**broncholith** (brŏng′kō-lĭth) [″ + *lithos,* stone] A calculus in a bronchus.

**broncholithiasis** (brŏng″kō-lĭth-ī′ă-sĭs) [″ + *lithos,* stone, + *-iasis,* state] Bronchial inflammation or obstruction caused by calculi in the bronchi.

**bronchomotor** (brŏng″kō-mō′tor) [″ + L. *motus,* moving] Causing dilation or constriction of the bronchi.

**bronchomycosis** (brŏng″kō-mī-kō′sĭs) [″ + *mykes,* fungus, + *osis,* condition] Any fungal infection of the bronchi or bronchial tubes, usually caused by fungi of the genus *Candida.*

**bronchopathy** (brŏng-kŏp′ă-thē) [″ + *pathos,* disease, suffering] Any pathological condition involving the bronchi or bronchioles.

**bronchophony** (brŏng-kŏf′ō-nē) [″ + *phone,* voice] An abnormal increase in tone or clarity in vocal resonance.

**bronchoplasty** (brŏng′kō-plăs″tē) [″ + *plassein,* to form] Surgical repair of a bronchial defect.

**bronchopleural** (brŏng″kō-ploor′ăl) [″ + *pleura,* side, rib] Pert. to the bronchi and the pleural cavity.

**bronchopneumonia** (brŏng″kō-nū-mō′nē-ă) [″+ *pneumonia,* lung inflammation] Inflammation of the terminal bronchioles and alveoli. SEE: *pneumonia.*

SYMPTOMS: Symptoms include cough and expectoration; short, shallow respiration (50 to 75 breaths per minute). Cyanosis may ensue. The nostrils dilate with each inspiration, and in children the temperature reaches 103° to 105°F (39.4° to 40.6°C). Before death, the temperature may go as high as 108°F (42.2°C), with a pulse of 140, and may last 2 to 3 weeks. Improvement may be followed by increased severity as new patches form.

In the elderly, many of these symptoms are absent. There is a slight cough with little sputum, and a fever of 100° to 101°F (37.8° to 38.3°C) may be evident. Weakness, sore throat, chills, and chest pain may be present. The elderly and bedridden are esp. susceptible to bronchopneumonia.

ETIOLOGY: Bronchopneumonia may be caused by Group A hemolytic streptococcus, *Klebsiella pneumoniae, Francisella tularensis,* or various types of pneumococci or staphylococci. It may also be caused by other pathogenic bacteria, viruses, rickettsias, and fungi.

TREATMENT: Patients will require bedrest, increased intake of fluids, analgesics for pain, antibiotics, a soft diet, oxygen for cyanosis, and treatment for shock if it occurs.

PROGNOSIS: Early treatment (during the first 3 days) improves the patient's chances of recovery. The prognosis is more favorable for those under 50, less favorable for the very young and the elderly. The use of antibiotics has greatly reduced mortality from this disease.

COMPLICATIONS: Lung abscess, atelectasis, empyema, pericarditis, and paralytic ileus are possible complications.

NURSING IMPLICATIONS: The patient is monitored for changes in respiratory status. The lungs are percussed for dullness, and the chest is auscultated for decreased breath sounds, crackles, gurgles, or wheezes, and decreased vocal fremitus at regular intervals as indicated by the patient's condition. A patent airway is maintained, and lung expansion and aeration are promoted through frequent repositioning. The patient is encouraged to breathe deeply and cough 8 to 10 times per hour, and to use incentive spirometry if prescribed. Arterial blood gas values are monitored and supplemental oxygen is administered as prescribed if the $PaO_2$ falls below a specified level (often 55 to 60 mm Hg). If intubation or mechanical ventilation becomes necessary, the nurse explains the procedure, assists with and monitors the therapy, provides emotional support, and (as necessary) suctions the patient using aseptic technique to remove secretions. The character and amount of sputum or secretions are documented, the patient is taught to dispose of secretions hygienically in the proper receptacle, and specimens are collected as required. Prescribed antibiotic therapy, analgesics, antipyretics, and IV fluid and electrolyte replacement are administered, and desired effects and adverse reactions are evaluated. Patients are advised to complete the entire course of prescribed antibiotics or other medication even if they feel better, but to avoid using antibiotics indiscriminately for minor infections, because upper-airway colonization with antibiotic-resistant organisms may result. An annual influenza vaccination and a one-time pneumococcal pneumonia vaccination are recommended for high-risk patients. A high-calorie, high-protein soft diet is provided in small, frequent meals to prevent fatigue and decrease the potential for abdominal distention. Oral feedings are supplemented with nasogastric or parenteral nutrition if necessary. A calm, quiet environment with frequent rest periods is provided.Respiratory irritants, esp. cigarette smoke, and individuals with respiratory infections should be avoided. SEE: *Nursing Diagnoses Appendix.*

**bronchopulmonary** (brŏng″kō-pŭl′mō-nă-rē) [Gr. *bronchos,* windpipe, + L. *pulmonarius,* pert. to lung] Pert. to the bronchi and lungs.

**bronchopulmonary lavage** Irrigation of the bronchi and bronchioles to remove tenacious secretions.

**bronchorrhagia** (brŏng″kor-ā′jē-ă) [″ + *rhegnynai,* to break forth] A bronchial hemorrhage.

**bronchorrhaphy** (brŏng-kor′ă-fē) [″ + *rhaphe,* seam, ridge] The suturing of a bronchial wound.

**bronchorrhea** (brŏng-kō-rē′ă) [″ + *rhoia,* flow] An abnormal, sometimes offensive secretion from the bronchial mucous membrane.

**bronchorrhoncus** (brŏng″kor-ŏn′kŭs) [″ + *rhonchos,* snore] A bronchial crackle.

**bronchoscope** (brŏng′kō-skōp) [″ + *skopein,* to examine] An endoscope designed to pass through the trachea for visual inspection of the tracheobronchial tree. The device also allows passage of an instrument to remove tissue for biopsy or a foreign body from the tracheobronchial tree.

**bronchoscopy** (brŏng-kŏs′kō-pē) Examination of the bronchi through a bronchoscope.

**bronchosinusitis** (brŏng″kō-sī″nŭs-ī′tĭs) [″ + L. *sinus,* a hollow, + Gr. *itis,* inflammation] Infection of a bronchus and a sinus at the same time.

**bronchospasm** (brŏng′kō-spăzm) [″ + *spasmos,* a convulsion] An abnormal narrowing with partial obstruction of the lumen of the bronchi due to spasm of the peribronchial smooth muscle. Clinically this is accompanied by coughing and wheezing. Bronchospasm occurs in asthma and bronchitis. Treatment includes active bronchodilators and corticosteroids. SEE: *asthma.*

**bronchospirometer** (brŏng″kō-spĭ-rŏm′ĕ-tĕr) [″ + L. *spirare,* to breathe, + Gr. *metron,* measure] An instrument for determining the volume of air inspired from one lung and for collecting air for analysis.

**bronchostaxis** (brŏng″kō-stăk′sĭs) [″ + *staxis,* dripping] Hemorrhage from the walls of a bronchus.

**bronchostenosis** (brŏng″kō-stĕn-ō′sĭs) [″ + *stenosis,* act of narrowing] Stenosis of a bronchus.

**bronchostomy** (brŏng-kŏs′tō-mē) [″ + *stoma,* mouth] The surgical formation of an opening into a bronchus.

**bronchotomy** (brŏng-kŏt′ō-mē) [″ + *tome,* incision] Surgical incision of a bronchus, the larynx, or the trachea.

**bronchotracheal** (brŏng″kō-trā′kē-ăl) [″ + *trachea,* rough] Pert. to the bronchi and trachea.

**bronchovesicular** (brŏng″kō-vĕ-sĭk′ū-lăr) [″ + L. *vesicula,* a tiny bladder] Pert. to bronchial tubes and alveoli with special reference to sounds intermediate between bronchial or tracheal sounds and alveolar sounds.

***b. breath sounds*** SEE: under *sound.*

**bronchus** (brŏng′kŭs) *pl.* **bronchi** [Gr. *bronchos,* windpipe] One of the two large branches of the trachea. The trachea proper terminates at the level of the fourth thoracic vertebra. SEE: illus.; *bronchi.*

**Bronkaid Mist** Trade name for epinephrine.

**Bronkephrine** Trade name for ethylnorepinephrine hydrochloride.

**Bronkosol** Trade name for isoetharine.

**brontophobia** (brŏn″tō-fō′bē-ă) [Gr. *bronte,* thunder, + *phobos,* fear] An abnormal fear of thunder.

**bronzed skin** A condition seen in chronic adrenocortical insufficiency (Addison's disease). It is also seen in hemochromatosis, some cases of diabetes mellitus, and cirrhosis of the liver.

**brood capsule** A cystlike body that develops within a hydatid cyst of *Echinococcus granulosus.*

**brood** To worry or ponder anxiously.

**broth** [ME.] **1.** A nutrient drink made from meat (e.g., bouillon) usually served hot. **2.** A liquid medium made from meat, used in making bacterial culture media.

**brow** The forehead.

**brown baby syndrome** The dark grayish brown skin color seen in infants undergoing extensive phototherapy for hyperbilirubinemia. The condition may last for months but is not known to produce permanent harm.

**brownian movement** (brow′nē-ăn) [Robert Brown, Brit. botanist, 1773–1858] The oscillatory movement of particles resulting from chance bombardment by molecules moving at high velocities.

**Brown-Séquard's syndrome** (brown′sā-kărz′) [Charles E. Brown-Séquard, Fr. physician, 1817–1894] Hemisection of the spinal cord with the following neurological changes: paralysis on the same side as the lesion, loss of position and vibratory sense, and ataxia; loss of pain and temperature sensitivity on the side opposite the lesion.

**Brucella** (broo-sĕl′ă) [Sir David Bruce, Brit. physician and bacteriologist, 1855–1931] A genus of nonmotile, aerobic, gram-negative coccobacilli that are pathogenic to humans and cause undulant fever and abortion in cattle, hogs, and goats. SEE: *brucellosis.*

**brucella** *pl.* **brucellae, brucellas** Any bacterium of the genus *Brucella.* **brucellar** (broo-sĕl′ĕr), *adj.*

**brucellin** (broo-sĕl′ĭn) An extract of a suspension of any species of *Brucella.* Injected intradermally, it may help in diagnosing brucellosis.

**brucellosis** (broo″sĕl-ō′sĭs) [*Brucella* + Gr. *osis,* condition] A widespread infectious febrile disease affecting principally cattle, swine, and goats, and sometimes other animals and humans. It is caused by bacteria of several *Brucella* species. *B. meli-*

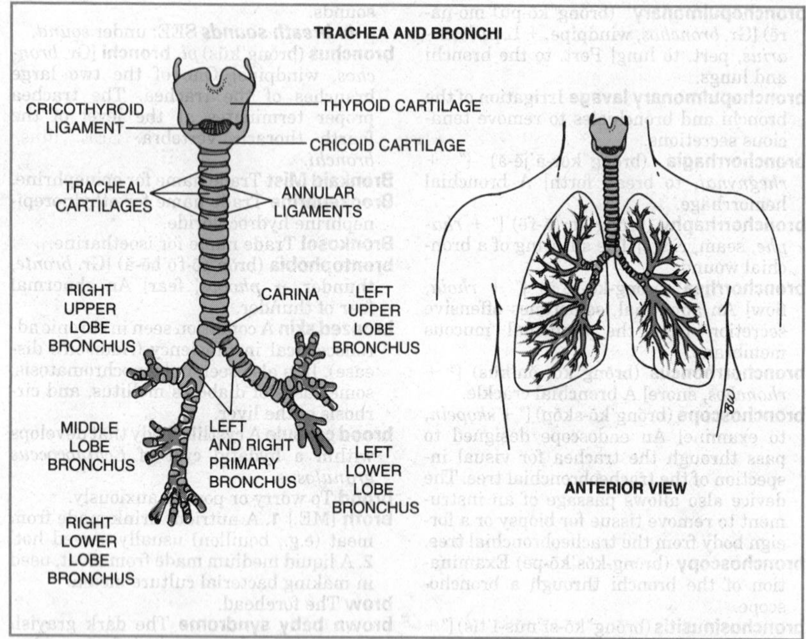


*tensis* and *B. suis* cause brucellosis in goats and swine, respectively, and *B. abortus* causes contagious abortion in cattle, dogs, and other domestic animals. The organisms are intracellular parasites. In humans it is called brucellosis or Malta fever and is caused by any of the three species.

TREATMENT: In adult humans, treatment consists of combined tetracycline for 4 to 6 weeks and streptomycin for the first 2 weeks of the tetracycline therapy. Doxycycline is also effective. In children, tetracycline may cause staining of developing teeth.

**Bruch's membrane** (brooks) [Karl W.L. Bruch, Ger. anatomist, 1819–1884] A glassy membrane of the uvea of the eye, lying between the choroid membrane and the pigmented epithelium of the retina. SYN: *lamina basalis choroideae; vitreous lamella.*

**Bruck's disease** (brooks) [Alfred Bruck, Ger. physician, b. 1865] A rare disease marked by muscle atrophy and skeletal disorders such as multiple fractures and ankyloses.

**Brudzinski sign** [Józef Brudzinski, Polish physician, 1874–1917] Flexion of the hips when the neck is flexed from a supine position. It occurs in children with meningitis. SEE: *Kernig's sign; meningitis.*

**Bruininks-Oseretsky Test of Motor Proficiency** ABBR: BOTMP. A standardized test of gross and fine motor performance for children from 4 to 14 years of age.

**bruise** (brooz) [O. Fr. *bruiser,* to break] An injury with diffuse effusion into subcutaneous tissue and in which skin is discolored but not broken. SYN: *contusion.*

***b. of head, chest, and abdomen*** A bruise that may be associated with internal injuries. SEE: *ecchymosis.*

SYMPTOMS: Symptoms include pain, swelling, tenderness, and discoloration.

NURSING IMPLICATIONS: Historical data are collected regarding the exact cause and location of the injury. The nurse inspects the bruised area and documents the location, color, size, discomfort, and other pertinent characteristics. The patient is assessed for other injuries dependent on the specific location and severity of the original injury. Related skin abrasions are cleansed thoroughly. Neurological status is monitored hourly or as needed for any patient with a suspected head injury.

***stone b.*** Bruise of the bottom of the foot, usually seen in children who walk barefoot on stones.

**bruissement** (broo-ēs-mŏn′) [Fr., droning noise] A purring sound heard upon auscultation.

**bruit** (brwē, broot′) [Fr., noise] An adventitious sound of venous or arterial origin heard on auscultation.

***carotid b.*** SEE: *carotid bruit.*

***placental b.*** A purring or blowing noise originating in the pregnant uterus due to fetal circulation of blood. It is synchronous with the maternal pulse.

**Brunner's glands** (brŭn′ĕrz) [Johann C. Brunner, Swiss anatomist, 1653–1727] Compound glands of the duodenum and upper jejunum that are similar to the pyloric glands of the stomach. They are embedded in the submucous tissue and lined with columnar epithelium. They secrete a clear, alkaline mucinous solution. SYN: *duodenal glands.*

**Brushfield spots** [T. Brushfield, Brit. physician, 1858–1937] Gray or pale yellow spots sometimes present at the periphery of the iris of children with Down syndrome.

**brushing 1.** A technique of tactile stimulation using small, electrically rotated brushes over selected dermatomes to elicit muscular responses in the rehabilitation of persons with central nervous system damage. **2.** Cleaning with a brush, as in toothbrushing.

**bruxism** (brŭk′sĭzm) [Gr. *brychein,* to grind the teeth, + *-ismos,* condition] The grinding of the teeth, esp. in children, during sleep. If untreated, it can damage teeth and the temporomandibular joint. In severe cases the teeth are worn down due to attrition.

ETIOLOGY: Psychological stress or abnormalities of tooth occlusion are the principal causes.

TREATMENT: If the condition is due to psychological causes, tension, anxiety, and stress should be reduced. The teeth should be treated for caries, malocclusion, or periodontal disease. Occlusal guards for the teeth may be of benefit.

**Bryant's traction** [Sir Thomas Bryant, Brit. surgeon, 1828–1914] Traction applied to the lower legs with the force pulling vertically. It is used esp. in treating fractures of the femur in children.

**B.S.** *Bachelor of Science; Bachelor of Surgery.*

**BSE** *breast self-examination.*

**B.S.N** *Bachelor of Science in Nursing.* The individual who earns this degree may apply to take the registered nurse (R.N.) licensing examination.

**BSP** *Bromsulphalein.*

**BTE work simulator** [Trademark, Baltimore Therapeutic Equipment Company] A mechanical device with interchangeable handles that simulates the work demands of many jobs and can objectively measure the work output of the user. This device is widely used in rehabilitation settings where injured workers are trained for return to employment.

**BTPS** *body temperature and pressure* (saturated with water vapor).

**BTU** *British thermal unit.*

**bubo** (boo′bō) *pl.* **buboes** [Gr. *boubon,* groin, swollen gland] An inflamed, swollen, or enlarged lymph node often exhibiting suppuration, occurring commonly after infective disease due to absorption of infective material. The nodes most commonly affected are those of the groin and axilla.

***axillary b.*** A bubo in the armpit.

***indolent b.*** A bubo in which suppuration does not occur.

***inguinal b.*** A bubo in the region of the groin.

***venereal b.*** A bubo resulting from a venereal disease. SEE: *lymphogranuloma venereum.*

**bubonadenitis** (boo-bŏn-ăd-ĕ-nī′tĭs) [″ + *aden,* gland, + *itis,* inflammation] Inflammation of an inguinal gland.

**bubonic plague** [″ + L. *plaga,* stroke, wound] An acute, infectious disease associated with a high fatality rate; called the black death in the Middle Ages. SEE: *plague.*

ETIOLOGY: Bubonic plague is caused by *Yersinia pestis,* which is usually present in infected rats and ground squirrels, and is transmitted to humans by the bite of the rat flea. It is marked by enlarged lymph glands and severe toxic symptoms, accompanied by intense adenitis or pneumonia.

**bucca** (bŭk′ă) *pl.* **buccae** [L., cheek] The cheek.

**buccal** (bŭk′ăl) Relating to the cheek or mouth.

***b. fat pad*** An encapsulated mass of fat lying superficial to the buccinator muscle. It is well developed in infants and is thought to aid in the act of sucking. SYN: *sucking pad.*

**buccinatolabialis** (bŭk″sĭn-ā-tō-lā″bē-ă′lĭs) [L. *buccinator,* trumpeter, + *labialis,* pert. to the lips] The buccinator and orbicularis oris considered as a single muscle.

**buccinator** (bŭk′sĭn-ā-tor) The muscle of the cheek. SEE: *Muscles Appendix.*

**bucco-** [L. *bucca,* mouth] Combining form meaning *cheek.*

**buccoaxiocervical** (bŭk″kō-ăk″sē-ō-sĕr′vĭ-kăl) The angle formed by the intersection of the buccal, axial, and cervical walls of a cavity in a tooth.

**buccocervical** (bŭk″kō-sĕr′vĭ-kăl) Concerning the buccal surface and cervical margin of a tooth.

**buccodistal** (bŭk″kō-dĭs′tăl) Concerning the buccal and distal surfaces of a tooth.

**buccogingival** (bŭk″kō-jĭn′jĭ-văl) Concerning the buccal and gingival surfaces of a tooth.

**buccolabial** (bŭk″kō-lā′bē-ăl) Concerning the buccal and labial surfaces of a tooth.

**buccolingual** (bŭk″kō-lĭng′gwăl) Concerning the buccal and lingual surfaces of a tooth.

**buccomesial** (bŭk″kō-mē′zē-ăl) Concerning the buccal and mesial surfaces of a tooth.

**bucco-occlusal** (bŭk″kō-ŏ-kloo′săl) Concerning the buccal and occlusal surfaces of a tooth.

**buccopharyngeal** (bŭk″kō-fă-rĭn′jē-ăl) Concerning the mouth and pharynx.

**buccopulpal** (bŭk″kō-pŭl′păl) Concerning the buccal and pulpal surfaces of a tooth.

**buccoversion** (bŭk″kō-vĕr′zhŭn) [L. *bucca,* cheek, + *versio,* turning] A tooth that twists in a buccal direction.

**buccula** (bŭk′ū-lă) [L., a little cheek] A fold of fatty tissue under the chin. SYN: *double chin.*

**Buck's extension** [Gurdon Buck, U.S. surgeon, 1807–1877] SEE: *extension.*

**Bucky diaphragm** [Gustav P. Bucky, Ger.-born U.S. radiologist, 1880–1963] A specialized film holder with a moving grid located immediately beneath the radiographic table or upright apparatus. It decreases the effects of scatter and secondary radiation during a radiographic exposure.

**Bucky factor** A measure of the amount of radiation absorbed by the Bucky diaphragm. This indicates the amount by which to increase the technical factors when a grid is being used.

**buclizine hydrochloride** (bū′klĭ-zēn) An antihistamine used to treat motion sickness.

**bud** [ME. *budde,* to swell] **1.** In anatomy, a small structure resembling a bud of a plant. **2.** In embryology, a small protuberance or outgrowth that is the anlage or primordium of an organ or structure.

***taste b.*** An ovoid body embedded in the stratified epithelium of the tongue and also found sparingly on the epiglottis and soft palate. Buds contain the sensory receptors for taste. SEE: *taste cells.*

***tooth b.*** The earliest evidence of tooth development. SEE: *enamel organ.*

**Budd-Chiari syndrome** SEE: *thrombosis, hepatic vein.*

**budding** A method of asexual reproduction in which a budlike process grows from the side or end of the parent and develops into a new organism, which in some cases remains attached and in others separates and lives an independent existence. Budding is common in lower animals (e.g., sponges and coelenterates) and plants (e.g., yeasts and molds).

**Buerger's disease** (bŭr′gĕrz) [Leo Buerger, U.S. physician, 1879–1943] A chronic, recurring, inflammatory, vascular occlusive disease, chiefly of the peripheral arteries and veins of the extremities. The disease is seen most commonly in males 20 to 40 years of age who smoke cigarettes. SYN: *thromboangiitis obliterans.*

SYMPTOMS: Symptoms include paresthesia of the foot or pain confined to one toe, easy fatiguability, and leg cramps. The legs fatigue quickly, esp. during walking. Ulceration or moist gangrene may set in; amputation may be necessary.

TREATMENT: Absolute and continued abstinence from tobacco in all forms is extremely important. The patient should avoid excessive use of the affected limb, exposure to temperature extremes, use of drugs that diminish the blood supply to extremities, trauma, and fungus infections. If gangrene, pain, or ulceration is present, complete bedrest is advised; if these are absent, patient should walk for 30 min twice daily. For arterial spasm, blocking of the sympathetic nervous system by injection of various drugs or by sympathectomy may be done.

NURSING IMPLICATIONS: The history should document occurrences of painful, intermittent claudication of the instep, which is aggravated by exercise and relieved by rest; the patient's walking ability (distance, time, and rest required); the patient's foot response to exposure to cold temperatures (initially cold, numb, and cyanotic; later reddened, hot, and tingling); and any involvement of the hands, such as digital ischemia, trophic nail changes, painful fingertip ulcerations, or gangrene. Peripheral pulses are palpated, and absent or diminished radial, ulnar, or tibial pulses documented. Feet and legs are inspected for superficial vein thrombophlebitis, muscle atrophy, peripheral ulcerations, and gangrene, which occur late in the disease. Soft padding is used to protect the feet; they are washed gently with a mild soap and tepid water, rinsed thoroughly, and patted dry with a soft towel. The patient is instructed in this and advised to inspect tissues for injury such as cuts, abrasions, and signs of skin breakdown (redness or soreness) and to report all injuries to the physician for treatment. The patient is advised to avoid wearing tight or restrictive clothing, sitting or standing in one position for long periods, and walking barefoot; also, shoes and stockings should be carefully fitted, but stockings should not be tight enough to hinder venous return from the legs. Extremities must be protected from temperature extremes, esp. cold. The patient is taught Buerger's postural exercises if prescribed. The nurse administers prescribed medications, evaluates the patient's response, explains desired and adverse reactions, and cautions the patient to avoid use of over-the-counter drugs without the attending physician's approval. The patient who smokes is referred to a smoking cessation program, but nicotine patch therapy would not be prescribed given the patient's associated hypersensitivity to nicotine. Both patient and family should receive emotional support and psychological counseling if necessary to help them cope with this chronic disease. For the patient with ulcers and gangrene, bedrest is prescribed, and a padded footboard or cradle used to prevent pressure from bed linens. If amputation has been done, rehabilitative needs are considered, esp. regarding changes in body image, and the patient is referred for physical and occupational therapy and for social services as appropriate. SEE: *exercise, Buerger's postural.*

**buffalo hump** A deposit of fat in the lower midcervical and upper thoracic area of the back. It is usually caused by excessive adrenocortical hormone production or therapy.

**buffer** (bŭf′ĕr) [ME. *buffe,* to deaden shock

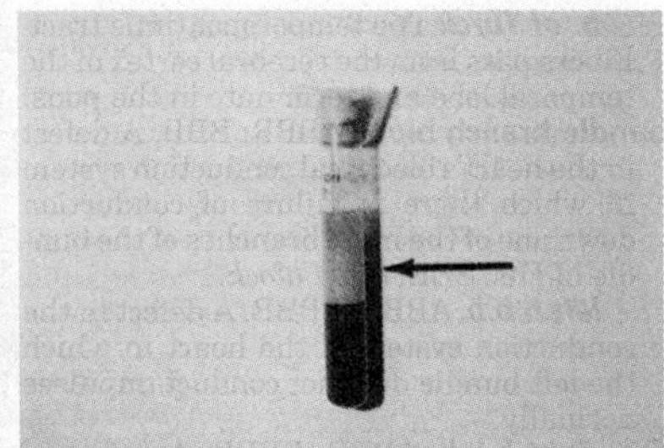

**BUFFY COAT** (ARROW) IN LEUKEMIA

of] **1.** A substance, esp. a salt of the blood, tending to preserve original hydrogen-ion concentration of its solution, upon adding an acid or base. **2.** A substance tending to offset reaction of an agent administered in conjunction with it.

***blood b.*** A buffer present in the blood. The principal buffers are carbonic acid, carbonates and bicarbonates, monobasic and dibasic phosphates, and proteins. Hemoglobin is an important protein buffer.

**buffy coat** A light stratum of blood seen when the blood is centrifuged or allowed to stand in a test tube. The red blood cells settle to the bottom and, between the plasma and the red blood cells, a light-colored layer contains mostly white blood cells. Platelets are at the top of this coat; the next layers, in order, are lymphocytes and monocytes; granulocytes; and reticulocytes. With normal blood, the buffy coat is barely visible; with leukemia, it is much larger. SEE: illus.

**bufotoxin** [L. *bufo,* toad, + Gr. *toxikon,* poison] A general term for any toxin present in the skin of a toad.

**bug** A term applied loosely to any small insect or arthropod, esp. of the order Hemiptera, that has sucking mouth parts, incomplete metamorphosis, and two pairs of wings, the fore pair being half membranous. SEE: *bedbug; chigger.*

***assassin b.*** A member of the family Reduviidae. Many are predaceous; others are blood-sucking. *Panstrongylus, Triatoma,* and *Rhodnius* are vectors of trypanosome diseases (Chagas' disease) in humans. SEE: *trypanosomiasis.*

***kissing b.*** Several species of the family Reduviidae. *Melanolestes picipes* is the common kissing bug, or black corsair.

***red b.*** Chigger.

**buggery** Sodomy.

**bulb** [L. *bulbus,* bulbous root; Gr. *bolbos*] Any rounded or globular structure.

***aortic b.*** The dilated portion of the truncus arteriosus in the embryo that gives rise to the roots of the aorta and pulmonary arteries.

***duodenal b.*** The upper duodenal area just beyond the pylorus.

***hair b.*** The expanded portion at the lower end of the hair root. The growth of a hair results from the proliferation of cells of the hair bulb.

***b. of the eye*** Eyeball.

***b. of the urethra*** The posterior portion of the corpus spongiosum found between the two crura of the penis.

***b. of the vestibule*** Bulbus vestibuli.

***olfactory b.*** An anterior enlargement of the olfactory tract.

***terminal b. of Krause*** An encapsulated sensory nerve ending similar in structure to the corpuscles of Pacini. SYN: *corpuscle of Golgi-Mazzoni.*

**bulbar** Pert. to or shaped like a bulb.

**bulbiform** (bŭl′bĭ-form) [″ + *forma,* shape] Shaped like a bulb.

**bulbitis** (bŭl-bī′tĭs) [″ + Gr. *itis,* inflammation] Inflammation of the urethra in its bulbous portion.

**bulbocavernosus** (bŭl″bō-kăv″ĕr-nō′sŭs) [″ + *cavernosus,* hollow] A muscle ensheathing the bulb of the penis in the male or covering the bulbus vestibuli in the female. It is also called *ejaculator urinae* or *accelerator urinae* in males and *sphincter vaginae* in females.

**bulbocavernosus reflex** Contraction of bulbocavernosus muscle on percussing the dorsum of the penis.

**bulboid** (bŭl′boyd) [″ + Gr. *eidos,* form, shape] Shaped like a bulb.

**bulbomimic reflex** (bŭl″bō-mĭm′ĭk) [″ + Gr. *mimikos,* imitator] In coma, contraction of facial muscles following pressure on the eyeball. SYN: *facial reflex; Mondonesi's reflex.*

**bulbonuclear** (bŭl″bō-nū′klē-ăr) [″ + *nucleus,* kernel] Pert. to the nuclei in the medulla oblongata.

**bulbospongiosus** (bŭl″bō-spŏn″jē-ō′sŭs) One of the three voluntary muscles of the penis. It acts to empty the canal of the urethra after urination and to assist in erection of the corpus cavernosum urethrae. The anterior fibers contribute to penile erection by contracting to compress the deep dorsal vein of the penis.

**bulbospongiosus reflex** Contraction of bulbospongiosus muscle on percussing the dorsum of the penis.

**bulbourethral gland** (bŭl″bō-ū-rē′thrăl) [″ + Gr. *ourethra,* urethra] Either of two small glands, one on each side of the prostate gland, each with a duct about 1 in. (2.5 cm) long, terminating in the wall of the urethra. They secrete a viscid fluid forming part of the seminal fluid. These round bodies are yellow and correspond to the Bartholin glands in the female. SYN: *Cowper's glands.* SEE: *prostate; urethra.*

**bulbous** (bŭl′bŭs) [L. *bulbus*] Bulb-shaped; swollen; terminating in an enlargement.

**bulbus** [L.; Gr. *bolbos*] Bulb.

***b. corpus spongiosum*** Bulb of the urethra. A bulbous swelling of the corpus spongiosum penis at the base of the penis.

***b. vestibuli*** Either of two oval masses of erectile tissue lying beneath the vestibule

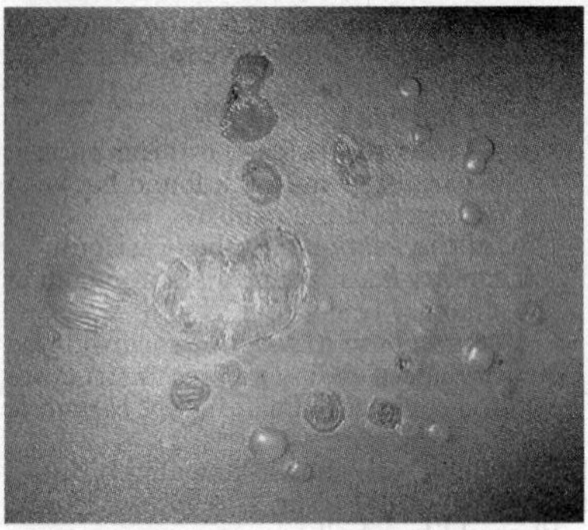

BULLAE OF IMPETIGO

and resting on the urogenital diaphragm. In the female they are homologous to the bulbus spongiosum of the penis.

**bulimia** (bū-lĭm'ē-ă) [L.] Excessive and insatiable appetite. **bulimic** (-ĭk), *adj.*

***b. nervosa*** A disorder marked by recurrent episodes of binge eating, self-induced vomiting and diarrhea, excessive exercise, strict dieting or fasting, and an exaggerated concern about body shape and weight. SEE: *anorexia nervosa.*

**bulk** In nutrition, a substance that absorbs water in the intestinal tract. The increased mass (i.e., bulk) helps to stimulate peristalsis. Bulk materials are used to treat constipation.

**bulla** (bŭl'lă) *pl.* **bullae** [L., a bubble] A large blister or skin vesicle filled with fluid; a bleb. SEE: illus.

***b. ethmoidalis*** A rounded projection into the middle meatus of the nose underneath the middle turbinated bone, formed by an anterior ethmoid cell.

***b. ossea*** The dilated portion of the bony external meatus of the ear. SEE: *pompholyx.*

**bullous** (bŭl'ŭs) [L. *bulla,* bubble] Having the nature of a bulla.

**BUN** *blood urea nitrogen.*

**bundle** A group of fibers. SYN: *fasciculus; fasciola.*

***Arnold's b.*** The frontopontile tract. It passes from the cerebral cortex of the frontal lobe through the internal capsule and cerebral peduncle to the pons.

***atrioventricular b.*** A bundle of fibers of the impulse-conducting system of the heart. From its origin in the atrioventricular node, it enters the interventricular septum, where it divides into two branches whose fibers pass to the right and left ventricles respectively, the fibers of each trunk becoming continuous with the Purkinje fibers of the ventricles. SYN: *A-V bundle; bundle of His.* SEE: *heart block.*

***A-V b.*** Atrioventricular b.

***b. of His*** Atrioventricular b.

***b. of Kent*** SEE: *Kent's bundles.*

***b. of Türck*** The temporopontinus tract. Fibers pass from the cerebral cortex of the temporal lobe and terminate in the pons.

**bundle branch block** ABBR: BBB. A defect in the heart's electrical conduction system in which there is failure of conduction down one of the main branches of the bundle of His. SEE: *heart block.*

***left b.b.b.*** ABBR: LBBB. A defect in the conduction system of the heart in which the left bundle does not conduct impulses normally.

***right b.b.b.*** ABBR: RBBB. A defect in the conductive system of the heart in which the right bundle does not conduct impulses normally.

**bundling** A mandatory system of drug distribution involving monitoring and reporting side effects to the U.S. Food and Drug Administration.

**bunion** (bŭn'yŭn) Inflammation and thickening of the bursa of the joint of the great toe, usually associated with marked enlargement of the joint and lateral displacement of the toe.

ETIOLOGY: Bunions may be caused by heredity, degenerative bone or joint diseases such as arthritis, or tight-fitting shoes and high heels that force toes together and displace weight onto the forefoot.

**Bunnell block** An orthotic device used after surgical repair of flexor tendon hand injuries. It prevents flexion at joints proximal to the one being exercised during the rehabilitation regimen.

**Bunsen burner** (bŭn'sĕn) [Robert W. E. von Bunsen, Ger. chemist, 1811–1899] A gas burner in which air holes at the bottom of the tube can be closed or opened. If the holes are closed, the flame burns yellow and gives light but a relatively small amount of heat. If the air intake is adjusted, a blue flame is produced. This is the hottest, most efficient, smokeless flame that can be produced by the burner.

**Bunyaviridae** (bŭn"yă-vĭr'ĭ-dē) A family of viruses that includes a large group of arthropod-borne viruses. Diseases caused by these viruses include certain types of encephalitis, some types of hemorrhagic fevers, phlebotomus fever, and Rift Valley fever.

**buphthalmia, buphthalmos** (būf-thăl'mē-ă, -mōs) [Gr. *bous,* ox, + *ophthalmos,* eye] Infantile glaucoma resulting in uniform enlargement of the eye, particularly the cornea. The disease may stop spontaneously or continue until it produces blindness. SEE: *glaucoma; hydrophthalmos.*

**burp 1.** To belch. **2.** To hold a baby against the chest and pat it on the back to induce belching.

**bur, burr** (bŭr) A device that rotates at high speed and is designed and held in a special tool to enable a dentist to cut by grinding the tooth, bone, or previous restorations.

**Burdach's tract** (boor'dăks) [Karl F. Burdach, Ger. physiologist, 1776–1847] Continuation of the dorsolateral column of the spinal cord into the medulla oblongata. SYN: *fasciculus cuneatus*.

**buret, burette** (bū-rět′) [Fr.] **1.** A special hollow glass tube usually with a stopcock at the lower end. It is used in chemical analysis to measure the amount of liquid reagent used. **2.** A calibrated chamber used to ensure accurate measurement of small amounts of intravenous fluid and to prevent fluid infusion overload. The chamber is usually connected to a larger container of fluid.

**Burkitt's lymphoma** [Denis P. Burkitt, Ugandan physician, b. 1911] A highly undifferentiated lymphoblastic lymphoma that involves sites other than the lymph nodes and reticuloendothelial system. It is rare in the U.S. but common in Central Africa, where the distribution suggests that environmental and climatic factors, such as insect vectors, are determinants. There is a strong association of this disease with the Epstein-Barr virus.

**Bureau of Medical Devices** ABBR: BMD. A branch of the U.S. Food and Drug Administration that regulates medical devices.

**burn** [AS. *baernan,* to burn] Tissue injury resulting from excessive exposure to thermal, chemical, electrical, or radioactive agents. The effects vary according to the type, duration, and intensity of the agent and the part of the body involved. The effects may be local, resulting in cell injury or death, or both local and systemic, involving primary shock (which occurs immediately after the injury and is rarely fatal) or secondary shock (which develops insidiously following severe burns and is often fatal). Burns are usually classified as:

*First degree* (minimal depth in skin): Superficial burns. Damage is limited to the outer layer of the epidermis; characterized by erythema, hyperemia, tenderness, and pain. There is no vesiculation.

*Second degree* (superficial to deep partial thickness of skin): Burns in which damage extends through the epidermis and into the dermis but not of sufficient extent to interfere with regeneration of the epidermis. If secondary infection results, the damage from a second-degree burn may be equivalent to that of a third degree. Vesicles are usually present.

*Third degree* (full thickness of skin including tissue beneath skin): Burns in which both epidermis and dermis are destroyed with damage extending into underlying tissues. Tissues may be charred or coagulated. SEE: illus.

COMPLICATIONS: Sloughing, gangrene, erysipelas, nephritis, pneumonia, or intestinal disturbances are possible complications. Sudden attacks of rigor, vomiting, rise of temperature, and convulsions are all suspicious symptoms. A superficial burn covering a large part of the body is more serious than a small, deep one, unless important nerves and blood vessels are involved. If two thirds of the skin is involved, death may be expected, even in a burn of the first degree. Shock and infection must always be anticipated regardless of the degree of burn.

PRECAUTIONS: A person in burning clothing should never be allowed to run. The individual should lie down and roll. A rug, blanket, or anything within reach can be used to smother the flames. Care must be taken so that the individual does not inhale the smoke. The clothing should be cut off carefully so that the skin is not pulled away. Blisters should not be opened, as this increases the chance for infection. All burned patients must receive appropriate tetanus prophylaxis.

NOTE: In severe, widespread burns, the patient must be transferred to a burn center as soon as is practical.

TREATMENT: The principal points in the initial care of burn patients include immediate evaluation of respiratory system for evidence of respiratory distress or smoke inhalation injury; cardiovascular status; percent of body burned and depth of burns; evaluation of other injuries. Immediate therapy of respiratory distress should be instituted by use of endotracheal intervention and mechanical ventilation with positive end-expiratory pressure and supplemental oxygen. Necessary volume resuscitation with Ringer's lactate solution is calculated as 4 ml/kg of body weight for each percent of body surface area burned. Half of this amount is administered during the first 8 hr after the burn. A nasogastric tube is inserted for gastric decompression and a Foley catheter is inserted to monitor urinary output. A stress ulcer (Curling's) may develop in the stomach. SEE: *ulcer, Curling's*.

*Emergency Wound Care:* Burned areas should be cleaned and old devitalized tissues gently removed with aseptic techniques; a topical antimicrobial agent should be applied to all second and third degree burns; burns should be covered with a closed dressing; the patient should be kept warm. If there are circumferential third-degree burns of extremities, decompressive escharotomies may be needed. Ice or cold dressings should not be used because of the risk of hypothermia. Diagnosis of the organism causing infection of the burn sites or systemic infection should be treated by appropriate antibiotic therapy and surgical excision of necrotic tissue. The use of artificial skin may be helpful in immediately closing the wound and in improving the quality of the resulting skin cover. Nutritional therapy should be instituted without delay.

NURSING IMPLICATIONS: *Emergency care:* The nurse establishes a patent airway, flushes chemical contact areas,

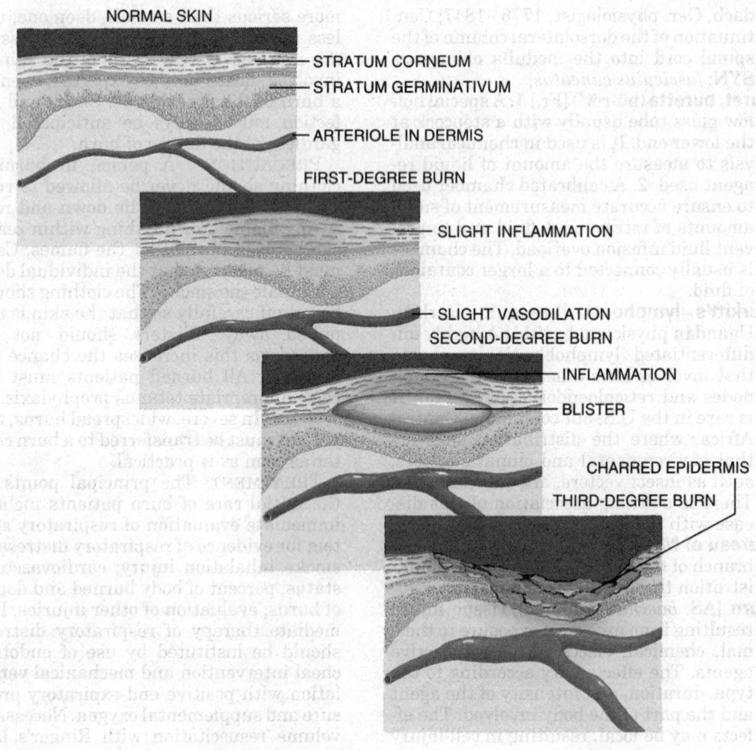


BURNS

starts an IV line, and stops the burning process by applying cool, saline-soaked towels (cold and ice are avoided to prevent hypothermia and further thermal damage). Constricting apparel (such as rings, collars, and belts) and easily separated clothing are removed, and adherent clothing soaked thoroughly to aid removal. The burn wound is covered (with sterile dressings if available) to prevent fluid and heat loss, pain, and shock. Bleeding is controlled, shock symptoms assessed for, and the extent of burn injury determined by using the rule of nines (or more accurate body surface area charts if available). If necessary, transportation to a burn center is arranged, and injured limbs are splinted to prevent further tissue damage.

*Stage 1* (injury onset to full resuscitation): The nurse maintains a patent airway and adequate ventilation and oxygenation, monitors arterial blood gas and oxygen saturation values, assesses for inhalation injury and respiratory distress (singed nasal hairs, mucosal damage, voice changes, coughing, wheezing, soot in the nose or mouth, and darkened sputum), and initiates intubation and mechanical ventilation if required. Soaked adherent clothing and initial dressings are carefully removed, and the depth and extent of burns determined. The patient is weighed at least once a day. Fluid replacement therapy is begun to manage fluid shift to tissue spaces, fluid loss, and shock; the specific infusion rate varies according to the patient's urine output. A central line is inserted as required. Vital signs are checked frequently as determined by the patient's ongoing status; urine output is determined hourly; a urine specimen for myoglobinuria and hemoglobinuria is obtained; and fluid balance and serum electrolyte levels are monitored closely. Using universal precautions and aseptic technique, the nurse debrides or assists with debridement of devitalized tissue, taking care not to disturb blisters, and dresses the burn wound with an antimicrobial agent and a nonadhesive bulky dressing. Prescribed tetanus prophylaxis, antibiotic therapy, and analgesics (the latter usually IV in small increments) are administered and the response is evaluated. The nurse explains all procedures and provides noninvasive pain relief measures and emotional support. Gastrointestinal function is assessed, and gastric dilatation and ileus are prevented or managed with nasogastric drainage. Any concomitant injuries are evaluated and treated.

*Stage 2* (beginning of diuresis to wound closure): The nurse monitors fluid balance, electrolyte status, and replacement therapy, assesses respiratory status for pulmonary edema, explains wound debridement procedures, administers premedication, and provides support before, during, and after such procedures. Nursing care of the wound consists of cleansing, debriding, and assessing for slough; assisting with escharotomies and graft application and care; and preventing and treating infection. Enteral (parenteral if the GI system is nonfunctional) nutrition is provided to meet hypermetabolic needs. The patient's mental and emotional status and pain are assessed, and prescribed invasive and noninvasive measures instituted. Continued emotional support is offered to help the patient to cope with altered body image or lifestyle concerns. General nursing measures are used to prevent complications related to immobility, such as contractures, loss of muscle mass, pneumonia, and venous thrombosis. The patient is also assessed for other complications, such as GI bleeding or sepsis, and these are reported to the physician.

*Stage 3* Rehabilitation (major wound closure to return to optimal physical and psychological function): Interventions to heal remaining wounds and to protect healed wounds are continued. Individually fitted elastic garments are applied to prevent hypertrophic scar formation, and joints are exercised to promote full range of motion. The nurse encourages the patient to increase activity tolerance, obtain adequate rest, strive for physical and emotional independence, and resume vocational and social functioning. Referrals for occupational therapy, psychological counseling, support groups, or social services are often necessary. Reconstructive and cosmetic surgery may be required. Support groups and services are available to assist the patient with life adjustments. SEE: *Nursing Diagnoses Appendix.*

***acid b.*** A burn caused by exposure to corrosive acids such as sulfuric, hydrochloric, and nitric.

FIRST AID: The burn area should be washed with large volumes of water and dilute alkalies such as baking soda (sodium bicarbonate) paste, soap solution dressing, or chalk paste should be applied, followed by a bland oil or ointment.

***alkali b.*** A burn caused by caustic alkalies such as lye, caustic potash (potassium hydroxide), and caustic soda (sodium hydroxide), and marked by a painful lesion of the skin often associated with gelatinization of tissue.

FIRST AID: The burn is washed with large volumes of water and dressed with bland ointments.

***brush b.*** A combined burn and abrasion resulting from friction.

TREATMENT: Loose dirt is carefully brushed away and the area is cleansed with soap and water. An antiseptic solution or ointment is applied and covered with a dressing. Tetanus toxoid or antitoxin is given if required.

***chemical b.*** Injuries due to the action of corrosive or irritating chemicals such as acid or alkali. Burns from chemical acids or alkalies should be treated by flushing the surface with water, thereby removing all traces of the chemical. Irrigation should not be delayed because sterile water or saline is unavailable, even for eye burns. The nearest available supply of clean water should be used. An acid usually counteracts an alkali, so weak vinegar (an acid) or weak ammonia (an alkali) is safe. A carbolic acid burn is almost always counteracted by alcohol. Oil should never be used because it promotes the absorption of acid. If lime gets into the eye, the eye should be flushed with water, followed by normal saline solution irrigation.

***electric b.*** A burn caused by exposure to electricity. The extent of destruction is likely to be much greater than that evidenced by initial inspection.

***fireworks b.*** Injury from fireworks; usually a burn, often with embedded foreign bodies and a high incidence of infection and tetanus, which should be prevented by meticulous care of injury and use of antitetanus serum.

***flash b.*** A burn resulting from an explosive blast such as occurs from ignition of highly inflammable fluids, or in war from a high-explosive shell or a nuclear blast.

***gunpowder b.*** A burn resulting from exploding gunpowder. It is often followed by tetanus, which should be prevented by administration of antitetanus serum and meticulous care of injury area.

***inhalation b.*** A burn caused by inhalation of flames or very hot gases. This type of burn is suspected in all patients with facial burns or with singed nose hairs or elevated carboxyhemoglobin greater than 5 in arterial blood gases. A major complication is airway obstruction from edema of the air passages. SYN: *respiratory b.*

TREATMENT: The usual treatment is early intubation and ventilatory management with high oxygen levels and positive end-expiratory pressure or constant positive airway pressure.

***b. of eye*** A burn of the eyeball due to contact with chemical, thermal, electrical, or radioactive agents.

FIRST AID: The eye should be washed immediately with the nearest available supply of water, even if it is not sterile.

Irrigation may need to be continued for hours if burn is due to lye.

***radiation b.*** A burn resulting from overexposure to radiant energy as from x-rays, radium emanations, sunlight, or nuclear blast.

***respiratory b.*** Inhalation b.

***thermal b.*** A burn resulting from contact with fire, hot objects, or fluids.

***x-ray b.*** SEE: *radiation burn.*

**burner** A traction injury to the brachial plexus that occurs in contact sports. The burner (also called a *stinger*) is a sharp burning sensation that radiates down the arm as the head and neck are forcefully deviated and the ipsilateral shoulder is depressed, causing traction to the brachial plexus. Weakness and numbness follow the burning sensation but are usually transient.

**Burnett's syndrome** [Charles Hoyt Burnett, U.S. physician, 1913–1967] Milk-alkali syndrome.

**burning foot syndrome** A sensation of burning on the sole of the foot. It occurs in certain vitamin deficiencies and in patients with chronic renal failure, due to build-up of toxic waste products.

**burning mouth syndrome** A burning sensation in one or several parts of the mouth. It occurs in the elderly and is generally related to menopausal, psychological, or psychopathological factors. Identified causes are denture irritation, yeast infection, decreased salivary production, systemic factors such as nutritional and estrogen deficiencies, and sensory neuropathies. It is also called *oral dysesthesia*. Treatment consists of therapy for the causative condition.

**burnish** (bĕr′nĭsh) To condense or polish a metal surface with a smooth metal instrument.

**burnisher** (bĕr′nĭsh-ĕr) An instrument with a blade or nib for smoothing the margins of a dental restoration.

**burnout 1.** Rendering unserviceable by excessive heat. **2.** A condition resulting from chronic job stress. It is characterized by physical and emotional exhaustion and sometimes physical illness. Frustration from a perceived inability to end the stresses and problems associated with this lack of power in the job contribute to the individual's loss of concern for patients or good job performance. Nurses are esp. prone to burnout, particularly those working in highly stressful conditions.

***inlay b.*** Wax b.

***radiographic b.*** Loss of radiographic detail by excessive exposure.

***wax b.*** Removal of an invested wax pattern from a mold by heating, thereby preparing the mold for casting metal. SYN: *inlay burnout.*

**Burow's solution** [Karl August von Burow, Ger. surgeon, 1809–1874] A solution of aluminum acetate; used in dermatology as a drying agent for weeping skin lesions.

**burr** SEE: *bur.*

**burrow** (bŭr′rō) A tunnel made in the skin by the itch mite, *Sarcoptes scabiei,* or any of several parasitic worms. SEE: *creeping eruption; cutaneous larva migrans.*

**burrowing** The formation of a subcutaneous tunnel made by a parasite or of a fistula or sinus containing pus.

**bursa** (bŭr′să) *pl.* **bursae** [Gr., a leather sack] **1.** A padlike sac or cavity found in connective tissue usually in the vicinity of joints. It is lined with synovial membrane and contains a fluid (synovia), that reduces friction between tendon and bone, tendon and ligament, or between other structures where friction is likely to occur. **2.** A blind sac or cavity.

***Achilles b.*** A bursa located between the tendon of Achilles and the calcaneus.

***adventitious b.*** A bursa not usually present but developing in response to friction or pressure.

***olecranon b.*** A bursa at the elbow joint lying between olecranon process and the skin.

***omental b.*** The lesser peritoneal cavity; the cavity of the great omentum. It communicates with the greater or true peritoneal cavity via the vestibule and epiploic foramen.

***patellar b.*** One of several bursae located in the region of the patella; includes the suprapatellar, infrapatellar, and prepatellar bursae. Some communicate with the cavity of the knee joint.

***pharyngeal b.*** A small, median, blind sac found in lower portion of the pharyngeal tonsil.

***subacromial b.*** The large bursa lying between the acromion and coracoacromial ligament above and the insertion of the supraspinatus muscle below. It is also known as subdeltoid bursa.

**bursae** (bŭr′sē) Pl. of bursa.

**bursal** (bŭr′săl) Pert. to a bursa.

**bursalis** (bŭr-săl′ĭs) [L., pert. to a bursa] Obturator internus muscle.

**bursectomy** (bŭr-sĕk′tō-mē) [Gr. *bursa,* a leather sack, + *ektome,* excision] Excision of a bursa.

**bursitis** (bŭr-sī′tĭs) [″ + *itis,* inflammation] Inflammation of a bursa, esp. those located between bony prominences and muscle or tendon, as the shoulder and knee. Common forms include painful shoulder, miner's or tennis elbow, housemaid's knee (prepatellar bursitis), and bunion. SEE: *Nursing Diagnoses Appendix.*

TREATMENT: Therapy includes rest and immobilization of the affected part during the acute stage. Active mobilization as soon as acute symptoms subside will help to prevent adhesions. Analgesics, heat, and diathermy are helpful. Injection of local anesthetics or cortisone into bursa may be required. In chronic bursitis, surgical removal of calcification may be necessary.

NURSING IMPLICATIONS: Rest is prescribed and movement of the affected part is restricted during the acute phase if pain and limited range of joint motion are present. If pain and loss of function are severe and do not improve with rest, the patient is referred for medical evaluation; physical therapy may also be needed.

***anserine b.*** Inflammation of the sartorius bursa located over the medial side of the tibia just below the knee. This causes pain upon climbing stairs.

**bursolith** (bŭr′sō-lĭth) [″ + *lithos,* stone] A calculus formed in a bursa.

**bursopathy** (bŭr-sŏp′ă-thē) [″ + *pathos,* disease, suffering] Any pathological condition of a bursa.

**bursotomy** (bŭr-sŏt′ō-mē) [″ + *tome,* incision] Incision of a bursa.

**bursula** (bŭr′sū-lă) [L., little sack] A small bursa.

***b. testium*** The scrotum.

**Burton's line** (bŭr′tŏns) [Henry Burton, Brit. physician, 1799–1849] A blue line along the margin of the gingiva visible in chronic lead poisoning.

**Buschke's scleredema** [Abraham Buschke, Ger. dermatologist, 1868–1943] Generalized nonpitting edema that begins on the head or neck and spreads to the body. This lasts a year or less and leaves no sequelae. The cause is unknown. SYN: *scleredema adultorum.*

**bush tea disease** Veno-occlusive disease of the liver due to ingesting of pyrrolidizine alkaloids present in some herbal teas.

**buspirone hydrochloride** An antianxiety agent that is neither a benzodiazepine nor a barbiturate. It has minimal central nervous system depressant actions, produces minimal sedation, and does not enhance the depressant effects of alcohol and other central nervous system depressants. The drug is used in treating short-term anxiety.

**busulfan** (bū-sŭl′făn) An antineoplastic agent used in treating chronic granulocytic leukemia. Trade name is Myleran.

**butacaine sulfate** (bū′tă-kān) A topical local anesthetic. Trade name is Butyn.

**butamben** (bū-tăm′bĕn) An anesthetic agent that is used topically. It is poorly and slowly absorbed and thus does not cause systemic toxicity. Trade name is Butesin.

**butane** (bū′tān) $C_4H_{10}$. A gaseous, inflammable hydrocarbon derived from petroleum.

**Butazolidin** (bū″tă-zŏl′ĭ-dĭn) Trade name for phenylbutazone, used in treatment of acute rheumatic disease. It has a potent anti-inflammatory action.

**Butisol sodium** (bū′tĭ-sŏl sō′dē-ŭm) Trade name for butabarbital sodium, a sedative and hypnotic.

**butt** [ME. *butte,* end] To join the ends of two objects together.

**butterfly 1.** Anything shaped like a butterfly. **2.** An adhesive bandage used in place of sutures to hold wound edges together.

**buttocks** (bŭt′ŭks) [AS. *buttuc,* end] The external prominences posterior to the hips; formed by the gluteal muscles and underlying structures. SYN: *nates.*

**button** (bŭt′n) An anatomical or pathological structure that resembles a button.

**button aid** An adaptive aid permitting button closure by persons with the functional use of only one extremity.

**buttonhole** A straight cut through the wall of a cavity.

**butylene** (bū′tĭ-lēn) A hydrocarbon gas, $C_4H_8$.

**butyraceous** (bū″tĭ-rā′shŭs) [L. *butyrum,* butter] Containing or resembling butter.

**butyrate** (bū′tĭ-rāt) A salt of butyric acid.

**butyric acid** (bū-tĭr′ĭk) [L. *butyrum,* butter] $C_3H_7COOH$. A fatty acid derived from butter but rare in most fats. It is a viscid liquid with a rancid odor; it is used in disinfectants, emulsifying agents, and pharmaceuticals.

**butyrin** (bū′tĭr-ĭn) A soft, yellow semiliquid fat that is present in butter.

**butyroid** (bū′tĭ-royd) [″ + Gr. *eidos,* form, shape] Having the appearance or consistency of butter.

**butyrometer** (bū″tĭ-rŏm′ĕ-tĕr) [″ + Gr. *metron,* measure] A device for estimating the amount of butterfat in milk.

**butyrophenone** (bū″tĭ-rō-fē′nōn) A class of chemicals, some of which are useful in treating mental disorders. One, haloperidol, is particularly useful in treating Tourette's syndrome.

**Byler's disease** An inherited disorder in which infants develop cholestatic jaundice and, gradually, cirrhosis. A high incidence of retinitis pigmentosa is associated with this disease, and mental retardation is frequently seen in the children. Death from liver disease occurs by adolescence.

**bypass** A means of circumvention; a shunt. It is surgically possible to install an alternate route for the blood to bypass an obstruction if a main or vital artery such as the abdominal aorta or a coronary artery becomes obstructed. The various procedures are named according to the arteries involved (e.g., coronary artery, aortoiliac, or femoropopliteal bypasses). The heart itself may be bypassed by providing an extracorporeal device to pump blood while a surgical procedure is being done on the heart. SEE: illus.

***ileal b.*** A surgical procedure for decreasing absorption of nutrients from the small intestine by anastomosing one portion of the upper small intestine to another portion some distance farther along the intestine. This method is used in treating obesity.

**byssinosis** (bĭs″ĭ-nō′sĭs) [Gr. *byssos,* cotton, + *osis,* condition] Pneumonoconiosis of cotton, flax, and hemp workers. It is char-

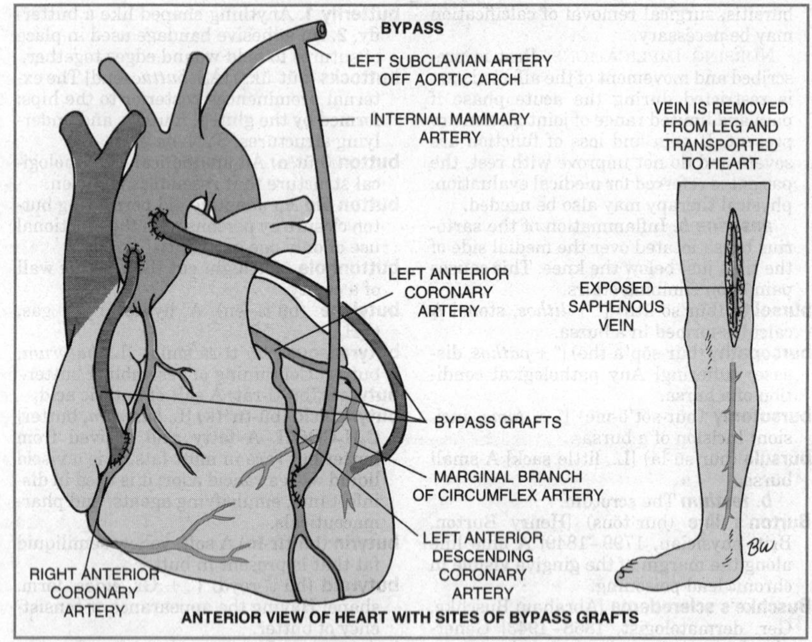

ANTERIOR VIEW OF HEART WITH SITES OF BYPASS GRAFTS

acterized by wheezing and tightness in the chest. Byssinosis is caused by the inhalation of dust and foreign materials contained therein, including bacteria, mold, and fungi. The disease does not occur in textile workers who work with cotton after it is bleached. Symptoms are usually more pronounced at the beginning of each work week than later on. SEE: *Monday chest tightness; pneumoconiosis.*

**byssocausis** (bĭs″ō-kaw′sĭs) [″ + *kausis,* burning] Moxibustion.

# C

**C 1.** Symbol for the element carbon. **2.** *Celsius*; *centigrade*; *cervical vertebra* (C1 to C7); *kilocalorie* (large calorie).

**$^{14}$C** Carbon-14.

**c** *calorie*; *centum* (a hundred); *circa* (about); *clonus; closure; compound; congius* (gallon).

**c̄** [L.] *cum*, with.

**CA 125** An antigen produced by tissues derived from coelomic epithelium. It is associated with various epithelial cancers, including ovarian cancer. It may be used experimentally to assess response to treatment in women with known ovarian cancer.

**Ca 1.** Symbol for the element calcium. **2.** *cathode*.

**CAAHEP** *Commission on Accreditation for Allied Health Educational Programs.*

**CABG** *coronary artery bypass graft.*

**Cabot's rings** (kăb'ŏts) [Richard C. Cabot, U.S. physician, 1868–1939] Blue-staining threadlike inclusions of unknown origin, found in the red blood cells in severe anemia. They may appear as rings, figures-of-eight, or twisted. They seem to be parts of the nucleus, with histones and iron but no DNA. SEE: illus.

**cac-, caci-** [Gr. *kakos,* bad] SEE: *caco-*.

**$CaC_2$** Calcium carbide.

**cacao** (kă-kā'ō, kă-kaw'ō) [Mex.-Sp. from Nahuatl *cacahuatl,* cacao beans] **1.** The seed of *Theobroma cacao* used to prepare cacao butter (theobroma oil), chocolate, and cocoa. **2.** A reddish to brown powder prepared from the roasted ripe seeds of *Theobroma cacao* (family Sterculiaceae), having a chocolate odor and taste. It is used as a syrup base, as a flavoring for certain medications, and in beverages and confections.

**cachectin** (kă-kĕk'-tĭn) Tumor necrosis factor alpha.

**cachexia** (kă-kĕks'ē-ă) [Gr. *kakos,* bad, + *hexis,* condition] A state of ill health, malnutrition, and wasting. It may occur in many chronic diseases, certain malignancies, and advanced pulmonary tuberculosis. **cachectic** (-kĕk'tĭk), *adj.*

Nursing Implications: Activities should be interspersed with frequent rest periods, and the patient's response to activity monitored to prevent fatigue. Oral hygiene is provided before and after eating. Small, frequent meals of high-calorie, high-nutrient, concentrated soft foods are offered along with fluids to reduce the effort required in eating. The patient is repositioned frequently to promote ventilatory excursions, to mobilize secretions, and to prevent skin breakdown. The skin is inspected for breakdown, and tissues are protected from pressure with flotation pads or mattresses and other assistive devices. When moved, the patient is handled gently and the joints are supported to prevent pain and pathological fractures. Assisted passive or active range-of-motion exercises are provided to maintain joint mobility. Elimination is monitored to prevent retention of urine or stools, and the patient is assisted with toileting. If incontinence occurs, steps are taken to protect skin integrity and to preserve the patient's self-esteem. Assistance is offered to the patient and family in coping with feelings about change in body image, illness state, and approaching death.

***cancerous c.*** Cachexia caused by cancer.

***c. hypophysiopriva*** Symptoms resulting from total loss of function of the pituitary gland.

***malarial c.*** Cachexia due to chronic malaria.

***pituitary c.*** A group of symptoms caused by atrophy of the pituitary gland, including emaciation, premature aging, genital atrophy with loss of secondary sex characteristics, and lowering of the basal metabolic rate. SYN: *Simmonds' disease.*

**cachinnation** (kăk-ĭ-nā'shŭn) [L. *cachinnare,* to laugh aloud] Excessive, inappropriate, loud laughter. It may be associated with schizophrenia.

**$CaCl_2$** Calcium chloride.

**caco-, caci-, cac-** [Gr. *kakos,* bad] Combining form denoting *bad* or *ill.*

**$CaCO_3$** Calcium carbonate.

**$CaC_2O_4$** Calcium oxalate.

**cacodylate** (kăk'ō-dĭl-āt) A salt of cacodylic acid.

**cacogeusia** (kăk"ō-gū'sē-ă) [" + *geusis,* taste] An unpleasant taste in the mouth.

**cacosmia** (kă-kŏz'mē-ă) [" + *osme,* smell] **1.** An unpleasant odor. **2.** Subjective perception of a disagreeable odor. SYN: *kakosmia.* SEE: *hallucination, olfactory; parosmia.*

**cacumen** (kăk-ū'mĕn) *pl.* **cacumina** [L. *cacumen,* summit] **1.** The anterior portion of the superior vermis of the cerebellum. SYN: *culmen.* **2.** The top or apex of a plant.

**CAD** *coronary artery disease; computer-assisted design; computer-aided dispatch.*

**cadaver** (kă-dăv'ĕr) *pl.* **cadavera** [L. *cadere,* to fall, die] A dead body, a corpse; usually applied to a body used for dissection.

**cadaveric** (kă-dăv'ĕr-ĭk) Pert. to a dead body.

**cadaverous** (kă-dăv'ĕr-ŭs) Resembling, esp. having the color or appearance of, a corpse.

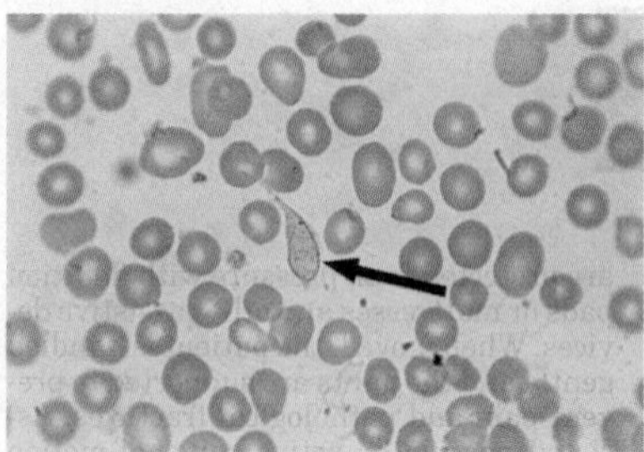

CABOT'S RING (ARROW) IN PERNICIOUS ANEMIA (ORIG. MAG. ×640)

**cadmiosis** (kăd-mē-ō'sĭs) A form of pneumoconiosis caused by inhalation of and tissue reaction to cadmium dust.

**cadmium** (kăd'mē-ŭm) [Gr. *kadmia,* earth] SYMB: Cd. A soft bluish-white metal present in zinc ores; atomic number 48, atomic weight 112.40, specific gravity 8.65. It is used industrially in electroplating and in atomic reactors. Its salts are poisonous. SEE: *Poisons and Poisoning Appendix.*

**caduceus** (kă-dū'sē-ŭs) [L., a herald's wand] In mythology, the wand or staff that belonged to Apollo and was given to Hermes, or Mercury. It consists of two serpents entwined around a staff, surmounted by two wings, and is used as the medical insignia of certain groups such as the U.S. Army Medical Corps. Although the caduceus is sometimes used to symbolize the medical profession, the staff of Aesculapius is usually considered the more appropriate symbol.

**caecum** Cecum.

**caelotherapy** (sē″lō-thĕr'ă-pē) [L. *caelum,* heaven, + Gr. *therapeia,* treatment] Therapy using religion or religious symbols.

**café au lait macules** Pale brown areas of increased melanin in the skin. The sites are usually 0.8 to 8 in. (2 to 20 cm) in diameter with irregular borders. They appear in infancy and tend to disappear with age. These macules are common and can occasionally be markers for systemic disease including neurofibromatosis.

**Cafergot** Trade name for a combination of caffeine and ergotamine tartrate.

**caffeine** (kăf'ēn, kă-fēn') $C_8H_{10}N_4O_2$. An alkaloid present in coffee, chocolate, tea, many cola drinks, cocoa, and some over-the-counter medicines. The amount of caffeine in these beverages varies from 110 to 150 mg in 6 oz (180 ml) of coffee, from 2 to 5 mg in decaffeinated coffee, and from 20 to 46 mg in 5 oz (150 ml) of tea. The caffeine in cola drinks ranges from 30 to 60 mg in a 360-ml (12-oz) serving.

The pharmacological action of caffeine includes stimulation of the central nervous system and of gastric acid and pepsin secretion, elevation of free fatty acids in plasma, diuresis, basal metabolic rate increase, total sleep time decrease, and possible blood glucose level increase. Caffeine is considered an ergogenic aid in athletics because it tends to enhance endurance and improves reaction time. The possibility that normal consumption of caffeine is a risk factor for cardiovascular disease, birth defects, breast disease, or cancer has been investigated but definitive supporting evidence is lacking. SEE: *caffeine intoxication; caffeine withdrawal.*

***c. and sodium benzoate*** A mixture of equal parts of caffeine and sodium benzoate. It is used as a central nervous system stimulant.

***c. and sodium salicylate*** A mixture of caffeine with sodium salicylate, containing about 52% caffeine. It combines the actions of caffeine and salicylate. SEE: *salicylate, sodium.*

***citrate c.*** A mixture of equal parts of caffeine and citric acid; used as a central nervous system stimulant.

**caffeine intoxication** The reaction that follows the ingestion of excessive caffeine, usually more than 250 mg. At least five of the following side effects are experienced: restlessness, nervousness, excitement, insomnia, flushed face, gastrointestinal disturbance, muscle twitching, diuresis, rambling flow of thought and speech, tachycardia or arrhythmia, periods of inexhaustibility, and psychomotor agitation. Other physical or mental disorders such as anxiety disorder must be ruled out. SYN: *caffeinism.*

**caffeine withdrawal** Abrupt cessation of long-term intake of caffeine resulting in headache within 12 to 24 hr and one or more of the following symptoms: marked fatigue, drowsiness, anxiety or depression, nausea or vomiting. This condition has been noted in patients instructed to discontinue caffeine intake for a few hours before and after surgery. Preoperative management of persons at risk of developing these withdrawal signs should include either gradual withdrawal beginning several days prior to surgery or, if possible, continuation of caffeine intake preoperatively and postoperatively. SEE: *caffeine; coffee; tea.*

**caffeinism** (kăf'ēn-ĭzm) Caffeine intoxication.

**Caffey, John** (kăf'fē) U.S. pediatrician, 1895–1966.

***C.'s disease*** Infantile cortical hyperostosis.

**cage, Faraday** A room or space entirely enclosed within a wire mesh to prevent electromagnetic interference with electronic devices.

**cage, thoracic** The soft tissue and bones enclosing the thorax.

**CAH** congenital adrenal hyperplasia.

**CAI** computer-assisted instruction.

**cainotophobia** (kī-nō″tō-fō'bē-ă) [Gr. *kainotes,* novelty, + *phobos,* fear] Cenotophobia.

**caked breast** Accumulation of milk in the secreting ducts of the breast following delivery. SEE: *breast.*

**Cal** large *calorie.*

**cal** small *calorie.*

**calamine** (kăl'ă-mīn) A pink powder, containing zinc oxide with a small amount of ferric oxide. It is used externally in various skin conditions as a protective and astringent, an ointment, or a lotion.

**calamus scriptorius** [L.] The inferior portion of the floor of the fourth ventricle of the brain. It is shaped like a pen and lies between the restiform bodies.

**calcaneoapophysitis** (kăl-kā'nē-ō-ă-pŏf"ĕ-zī'tĭs) [L. *calcaneus,* heel, + Gr. *apophysis,* offshoot, + *itis,* inflammation] Pain and inflammation of the posterior portion of the calcaneus at the place of insertion of the Achilles tendon.

**calcaneocuboid** (kăl-kā"nē-ō-kū'boyd) [" + Gr. *kubos,* cube, + *eidos,* form, shape] Pert. to the calcaneus and cuboid bone.

**calcaneodynia** (kăl-kā"nē-ō-dĭn'ē-ă) [" + Gr. *odyne,* pain] Pain in the heel.

**calcaneofibular** (kăl-kā"nē-ō-fĭb'ū-lăr) [" + *fibula,* pin] Pert. to the calcaneus and fibula.

**calcaneonavicular** (kăl-kā"nē-ō-nă-vĭk'ū-lăr) [" + *navicula,* boat] Pert. to the calcaneus and navicular bone.

**calcaneoscaphoid** (kăl-kā"nē-ō-skā'foyd) [" + Gr. *skaphe,* skiff, + *eidos,* form, shape] Pert. to the calcaneus and scaphoid bone.

**calcaneotibial** (kăl-kā"nē-ō-tĭb'ē-ăl) [" + *tibia,* shinbone] Pert. to the calcaneus and tibia.

**calcaneum** (kăl-kā'nē-ŭm) *pl.* **calcanea** [L. *calcaneus,* heel] Calcaneus.

**calcaneus** (kăl-kā'nē-ŭs) *pl.* **calcanei** [L.] The heel bone, or os calcis. It articulates with the cuboid bone and with the talus. SEE: *leg* for illus. **calcaneal, calcanean** (-kā'nē-ăl, -ăn), *adj.*

**calcanodynia** (kăl"kăn-ō-dĭn'ē-ă) [" + Gr. *odyne,* pain] Pain in the heel when standing or walking; calcaneodynia.

**calcar** (kăl'kăr) [L., a spur] A spurlike process.

***c. avis*** Hippocampus minor.

***c. femorale*** A bony spur that strengthens the femoral neck.

***c. pedis*** The heel.

**calcareous** (kăl-kā'rē-ŭs) [L. *calcarius,* of lime] Having the nature of lime; chalky.

**calcarine** (kăl'kăr-ĭn) [L. *calcar,* spur] Spur-shaped.

**calcariuria** (kăl-kăr"ē-ū'rē-ă) [L. *calcarius,* of lime, + Gr. *ouron,* urine] The presence of calcium lime salts in the urine.

**calcemia** (kăl-sē'mē-ă) [L. *calx,* lime, + Gr. *haima,* blood] Hypercalcemia.

**calcic** (kăl'sĭk) [L. *calcarius*] Pert. to calcium or lime.

**calcicosis** (kăl"sĭ-kō'sĭs) [L. *calx,* lime, + Gr. *osis,* infection] Pneumoconiosis caused by inhaling dust from limestone (marble).

**calciferol** (kăl-sĭf'ĕr-ŏl) Vitamin $D_2$. A synthetic vitamin D. It has the most vitamin D activity of those substances derived from ergosterol. It is used for prophylaxis and treatment of vitamin D deficiency, rickets, and hypocalcemic tetany. SYN: *ergocalciferol.*

**calciferous** (kăl-sĭf'ĕr-ŭs) [" + *ferre,* to carry] Containing calcium, chalk, or lime.

**calcific** (kăl-sĭf'ĭk) [" + *facere,* to make] Forming or composed of lime.

**calcification** (kăl"sĭ-fĭ-kā'shŭn) The process in which organic tissue becomes hardened by the deposition of lime salts in the tissues.

***arterial c.*** Calcium deposition in the arterial walls.

***dystrophic c.*** A necrotic process in which calcium salts and other minerals attach to cellular debris that is not promptly destroyed and reabsorbed.

***metastatic c.*** Calcification of soft tissue with transference of calcium from bone, as in osteomalacia and disease of the parathyroid glands.

***Mönckeberg's c.*** Calcium deposition in the media of arteries.

**calcific tendinitis** Calcium deposition in a chronically inflamed tendon, esp. a tendon of the shoulder.

**calcigerous** (kăl-sĭj'ĕr-ŭs) [" + *gerere,* to bear] Containing calcium or lime salts.

**Calcimar** Trade name for calcitonin.

**calcination** (kăl"sĭ-nā'shŭn) [L. *calcinare,* to char] Drying by roasting to produce a powder.

**calcine** (kăl'sĭn) **1.** To expel water and volatile materials by heating to a high temperature. Lime is formed from limestone in this way by the removal of carbon dioxide. **2.** A powder produced by roasting.

**calcinosis** (kăl"sĭ-nō'sĭs) [L. *calx,* lime, + Gr. *osis,* condition] A condition marked by abnormal deposition of lime salts in tissues.

***c. circumscripta*** Subcutaneous calcification.

**calcipenia** (kăl"sĭ-pē'nē-ă) [" + Gr. *penia,* poverty] Calcium deficiency in body tissues and fluids.

**calcipexis, calcipexy** (kăl"sĭ-pĕk'sĭs, -pĕk'sē) [" + Gr. *pexis,* fixation] Fixation of calcium in body tissues. **calcipectic** (-pĕk'tĭk), *adj.*

**calciphylaxis** (kăl"sĭ-fĭ-lăk'sĭs) [" + Gr. *phylaxis,* protection] A state of induced tissue sensitivity marked by calcification of tissue when challenged by an appropriate stimulus.

**calciprivia** (kăl"sĭ-prĭv'ē-ă) [" + *privus,* without] Deficiency or absence of calcium.

**calcitonin** (kăl"sĭ-tō'nĭn) A hormone produced by the human thyroid gland that is important for maintaining a dense, strong bone matrix and regulating the blood calcium level. SEE: illus.

**calcitriol** A metabolite of vitamin D that promotes the absorption of calcium and phosphate in the intestines and their deposition in bone tissue.

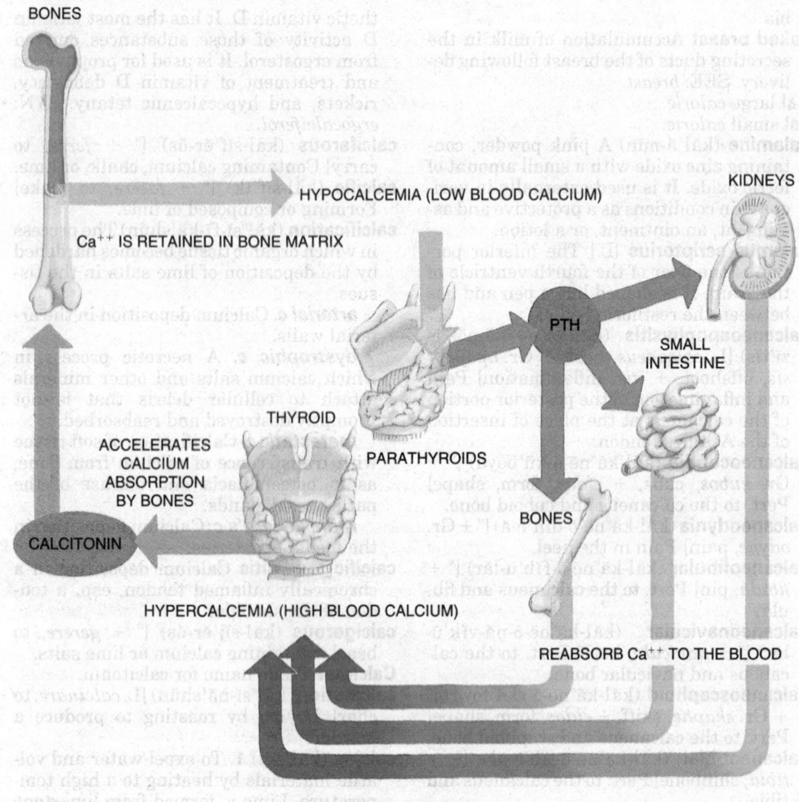


COMPLEMENTARY FUNCTIONS OF CALCITONIN AND PARATHYROID HORMONE

**calcium** (kăl′sē-ŭm) [L. *calx,* lime] SYMB: Ca. A silver-white metallic element; atomic number 20, atomic weight 40.08. It is a major component of limestone. Lime, CaO, is its oxide. Calcium phosphate constitutes 75% of body ash and about 85% of mineral matter in bones.

FUNCTION: Calcium must be carried by the blood in solution to be available for bone growth and metabolism. Unless certain activating substances, such as vitamin D, are present, increased calcium intake does not affect the tissues or blood calcium. The parathyroid gland secretions are a factor in calcium use, making it possible for the blood to carry dissolved calcium. Although some foods may influence calcium absorption, none of these is believed to be important in persons whose intake of calcium is typical for the diet of individuals living in the U.S.

Calcium is very important to blood coagulation, enzyme activation, and acid-base balance; it gives firmness and rigidity to bones and teeth; and it is essential for lactation, the function of nerves and muscles, including the myocardium, and maintenance of membrane permeability.

Calcium is taken into the body as a constituent of various foods. Although much of it may prove insoluble and escape absorption, some of it passes through the intestine into the blood, where it can be measured by chemical tests. Its serum level is normally 8.5 to 10.5 mg/dl. Low blood calcium causes tetany with muscular twitching, spasms, and convulsions. Blood deprived of its calcium will not clot. Calcium is essential for the curdling of milk.

Calcium is deposited in the bones but can be mobilized again to keep the blood level constant when there is a period of insufficient intake. At any given time the body of an adult contains about 700 g of calcium phosphate; of this, 120 g is the element calcium. Ordinarily an adult takes in 0.8 g of calcium per day. During pregnancy, 1.3 g of calcium a day is required.

SOURCES: Excellent calcium sources include milk, yogurt, cheese, and ice cream. Good sources include canned salmon and sardines, broccoli, tofu, rhubarb, almonds, figs, and turnip greens.

DEFICIENCY: Symptoms are brittle bones, poor development of bones and teeth, osteoporosis, dental caries, rickets, tetany, heart atony, hyperirritability, and excessive bleeding. Laboratory error and variation may cause inaccurate or inconsistent values in evaluating the calcium level. SEE: *osteoporosis; Recommended Daily Dietary Allowances Appendix.*

EXCESS: Signs and symptoms are cardiac arrhythmia, including cardiac arrest, decreased respirations, lethargy progressing to coma, profound muscle weakness, renal calculi, anorexia, nausea, and constipation. The treatment is with diuretics and calcium-reducing agents.

***c. carbonate, precipitated*** $CaCO_3$. Precipitated chalk, a fine, white, tasteless, and odorless powder. It is used as an antacid and as an antidote to corrosive acid poisoning.

***c. chloride*** $CaCl_2 \cdot 2H_2O$. A deliquescent salt occurring as translucent crystals but used in solution, having a sharp saline taste. It is used to raise the calcium content of the blood in disorders resulting from lack of sufficient calcium, such as in hypocalcemic tetany. It is used in solution and administered intravenously. It is incompatible with ephedrine.

***c. cyclamate*** An artificial sweetening agent. SEE: *cyclamate.*

***c. disodium edetate*** A substance used to bind certain metallic ions in the body. It is used in treating poisoning caused by those metals.

***c. gluconate*** A granular or white powder without odor or taste. Its actions and uses are the same as those of calcium chloride, but calcium gluconate is more pleasant to taste and nonirritating when administered orally or intramuscularly in a 10% solution.

***c. glycerophosphate*** The calcium salt of glycerophosphoric acid. It is used as a dietary supplement and in formulating drugs.

***c. hydroxide*** $Ca(OH)_2$. A white powder used in preparing calcium hydroxide solution, which is used as an astringent applied to the skin and mucous membranes. In solution it is called lime water. It is used in dentistry as cavity liner or a pulp-capping material under a layer of zinc phosphate. It induces tertiary dentin formation for bridging or root closure, but may be related to a chronic pulpitis and pulp necrosis after pulp capping. SYN: *slaked lime.*

***c. lactate*** A white, odorless, and nearly tasteless powder, less irritating than calcium chloride. It is used orally or parenterally as an alternative to calcium gluconate.

***c. levulinate*** A soluble white powder used when intravenous administration of calcium is required.

***c. mandelate*** The calcium salt of mandelic acid. It is used in treating urinary tract infections.

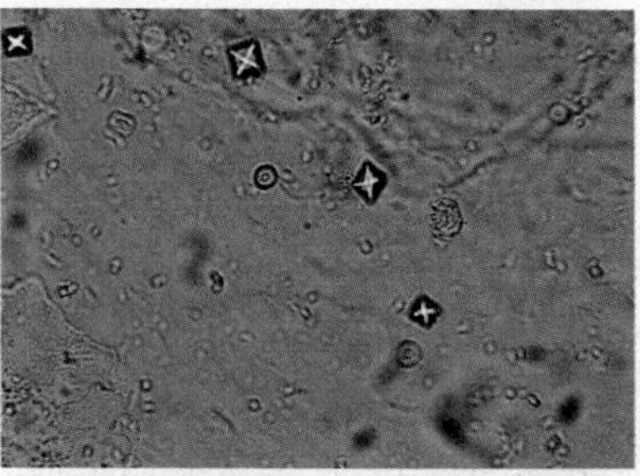

**CALCIUM OXALATE** CRYSTALS IN URINE (ORIG. MAG. ×400)

***c. oxalate*** A calcium-containing substance present in urine in crystalline form. It is a constituent of some renal calculi. SEE: illus.

***c. oxide*** A corrosive and easily pulverized mineral occurring as a hard white or grayish-white mass. It is used as a germicide and disinfectant.

***c. pantothenate*** One of the B complex vitamins. SEE: *vitamin B complex.*

***c. phosphate, precipitated*** A white, amorphous powder used as an antacid in treating gastric hyperacidity.

***c. saccharin*** An artificial sweetening agent. SEE: *saccharin.*

***c. sulfate*** A white powder that absorbs water. It is used in making plaster of paris.

***total serum c.*** The sum of the diffusible and nondiffusible calcium in the blood serum.

***c. tungstate*** A fluorescent material used for radiological imaging. It is used in intensifying screens.

**calcium-45 ($^{45}$Ca)** A radioactive isotope of calcium. It has a half-life of 164 days.

**calcium channel blocker** Any of a group of drugs that slow the influx of calcium ions into muscle cells, resulting in decreased arterial resistance and decreased myocardial oxygen demand. These drugs are used in treating angina, hypertension, and supraventricular tachycardia, but may cause hypotension. Therefore it is important to monitor blood pressure during the initial treatment period. These drugs have not been shown to provide protection against coronary artery disease.

**Calcium Disodium Versenate** Trade name for edetate calcium disodium.

**calciuria** (kăl″sē-ū′rē-ă) [″ + Gr. *ouron,* urine] Calcium in the urine.

**calcospherite** (kăl″kō-sfē′rīt) [″ + Gr. *sphaira,* sphere] One of many small calcareous bodies found in tumors, nervous tissue, the thyroid, and the prostate.

**calculogenesis** (kăl″kū-lō-jĕn′ĕ-sĭs) [″ + Gr. *genesis,* generation, birth] The formation of calculi.

**calculous** (kăl′kū-lŭs) Like a calculus.

**calculus** (kăl′kū-lŭs) *pl.* **calculi** [L., pebble] Any abnormal concretion, commonly called a stone, within the animal body. A calculus is usually composed of mineral salts. These pathological concretions can occur in the kidneys, ureters, bladder, or urethra, and are usually formed of crystalline urinary salts held together by viscid organic matter. SEE: *gallstone; kidney stone.*

ETIOLOGY: Calculi can be caused by abnormal function of the parathyroid glands, disordered uric acid metabolism as in gout, or excessive intake of milk and alkali. The cause of most kidney stones is unknown.

***biliary c.*** Cholelith; gallstone. It is usually composed of cholesterol, some with bile pigments, such as bilirubin, or calcium deposits. SEE: *gallbladder.*

***dental c.*** Calcified deposits on teeth and located on subgingival, supragingival, or occlusal surfaces. SEE: *dental plaque; tartar.*

***hemic c.*** A calculus formed from coagulated blood.

***pancreatic c.*** A calculus in the pancreas, formed of calcium carbonate with other salts and inorganic materials.

***renal c.*** A calculus in the kidney that may block urine flow. If the ureter is blocked by the stone, there is sudden, severe, and paroxysmal renal colic with chills, fever, hematuria, and frequency of urination. The prognosis is serious if the condition is allowed to continue untreated. SYN: *nephrolith.*

TREATMENT: Pain relief should be a priority, as should forcing fluids unless passage is completely blocked by the calculus. Smooth muscle relaxants help in passing the stone and relieving pain. If the stone is preventing urine flow or continues to grow and cause infection, surgery must be performed. Alternatively, the stone may be disintegrated ultrasonically. SEE: *extracorporeal shock-wave lithotriptor; kidney stone removal, laser treatment for.*

***salivary c.*** A calculus in the salivary duct. It usually affects the duct of the submandibular gland. The calculus obstructs the flow of saliva, causing severe pain and swelling of the gland, esp. during eating. Surgical removal of the stone is the treatment.

***urinary c.*** A calculus in any part of the urinary system. SEE: *renal c.; Nursing Diagnoses Appendix.*

***vesical c.*** A calculus in the bladder, marked by increased frequency of urination, pain, and diurnal hematuria increased by exercise.

TREATMENT: An analgesic and antispasmodic should be used if necessary, and fluid intake should be adequate. Special urological, ultrasonic, or surgical procedures should be performed if the stone is large or impacted. These stones are usually small enough to pass through the urethra. SEE: *extracorporeal shock-wave lithotriptor.*

**calefacient** (kăl″ĕ-fā′shĕnt) [L. *calere,* to be warm, + *facere,* to make] Conveying a sense of warmth when applied to a part of the body; something that conveys such a sense.

**calf** (kăf) [AS. *cealf*] The fleshy muscular back part of the leg below the knee, formed by the gastrocnemius and soleus muscles.

**caliber** (kăl′ĭ-bĕr) [Fr. *calibre,* diameter of bore of gun] The diameter of any orifice, canal, or tube.

**calibration** (kăl-ĭ-brā′shŭn) **1.** Determination of the accuracy of an instrument by comparing the measurement or other information provided with that of a known standard or an instrument known to be accurate. **2.** Measuring of size, esp. the diameter of vessels or the caliber of an orifice.

***c. of instruments*** A procedure in which the electrical circuitry of an electronic device is brought into alignment.

**calibrator** (kăl′ĭ-brā-tor) An instrument for measuring the inside diameter of tubes or orifices.

**caliceal** (kăl″ĭ-sē′ăl) [Gr. *kalyx,* cup of a flower] Pert. to a calix.

**calicectasis** (kăl″ĭ-sĕk′tă-sĭs) [″ + *ektasis,* dilatation] Dilatation of the renal calyx. SYN: *caliectasis.*

**calices** Pl. of calix.

**Caliciviridae** (kăl-ĭ-sē-vĭ′rĭ-dā) [L. *chalice, calyx,* "cuplike" appearance of viral particles under electron microscopy] A virus family that was previously classed as a genus in the family of picornaviruses. SEE: *Astroviridae; Calicivirus.*

**Calicivirus** (kăl-ĭs′ĭ-vī″rŭs) A genus of the family Caliciviridae that causes epidemic viral gastroenteritis in adults and children. Genera are classed in accordance with the geographic areas in which they have been identified. SEE: *Norwalk agent.*

**caliculus** (kă-lĭk′ū-lŭs) [L., small cup] A cup-shaped structure.

***c. gustatorius*** A taste bud.

***c. ophthalmicus*** The optic cup.

**caliectasis** (kăl″ē-ĕk′tă-sĭs) [Gr. *kalyx,* cup of a flower, + *ektasis,* dilatation] Dilatation of the renal calyx. SYN: *calicectasis.*

**californium** (kăl″ĭ-for′nē-ŭm) [Named for California, the state and university where it was first discovered in 1950] SYMB: Cf. A chemical element prepared by bombardment of curium with alpha particles; atomic weight 251, atomic number 98. It has properties similar to dysprosium.

**caligo** (kă-lī′gō) [L., darkness] Dimness of vision.

**caliper(s)** (kăl′ĭ-pĕr) [Fr. *calibre,* diameter of bore of gun] An instrument for measuring diameters of solids, such as those of the chest or pelvis.

**calisthenics** (kăl″ĭs-thĕn′ĭks) [Gr. *kalos,* beautiful, + *sthenos,* strength] An exercise program that emphasizes development of gracefulness, suppleness, and range of motion and the strength required for such movement.

**Calliphora vomitoria** (kă-lĭf′ĕr-ă) The common blowfly, whose larvae sometimes cause myiasis disorders.

**callomania** (kăl″ō-mā′nē-ă) [Gr. *kalos,* beautiful, + *mania,* madness] **1.** Belief in one's own beauty, a delusion of the insane. **2.** Unrealistic attraction to something only because of its beauty.

**callosal** (kă-lō′săl) [L. *callus,* hardened skin] Pert. to the corpus callosum.

**callosity, callositas** (kă-lŏs′ĭ-tē, -ĭ-tăs) [L. *callosus,* hard] A circumscribed thickening and hypertrophy of the horny layer of the skin. It may be oval or elongated, gray or brown, slightly elevated, with a smooth burnished surface. It appears on the flexor surfaces of hands and feet and is caused by friction, pressure, or other irritation. SYN: *callus.*

TREATMENT: Salicylic acid or careful shaving will remove the callosity temporarily. Removal is made permanent only by elimination of the cause.

**callosomarginal** (kă-lō″sō-măr′jĭ-năl) [L. *callus,* hardened skin, + *margo,* margin] Pert. to the corpus callosum and marginal gyrus; marking the sulcus between them.

**callosum** (kă-lō′sŭm) [L. *callosus,* hard] The great commissure of the brain between the cerebral hemispheres. SYN: *corpus callosum.*

**callous** (kăl′ŭs) Hard; like a callus.

**callus** (kăl′ŭs) [L., hardened skin] **1.** Callosity. **2.** The osseous material woven between the ends of a fractured bone that is ultimately replaced by true bone in the healing process. SEE: *porosis.*

***definitive c.*** The exudate, found between two ends of a fractured bone, that develops into true bone.

***provisional c.*** A temporary deposit between the ends of a fractured bone that is reabsorbed when true bone develops.

**calmative** (kă′-, kăl′mă-tĭv) **1.** Sedative; soothing. **2.** An agent that acts as a sedative.

**calmodulins** Intracellular proteins that combine with calcium and activate a variety of cellular processes.

**calomel** (kăl′ō-mĕl) [Gr. *kalos,* beautiful, + *melas,* black] Mercurous chloride.

**calor** (kā′lor) [L., heat] **1.** Heat. **2.** The heat of fever. It is one of the five classic signs of inflammation, the others being redness (rubor), swelling (tumor), pain (dolor), and loss of function (functio laesa).

**Calori's bursa** (kăl-ō′rēz) [Luigi Calori, It. anatomist, 1807–1896] The bursa found between the arch of the aorta and the trachea.

**caloric** (kă-lor′ĭk) [L. *calor,* heat] Relating to heat or to a calorie.

**caloric test** A procedure used to assess vestibular function in patients who complain of dizziness or exhibit standing balance disturbances or unexplained sensorineural hearing loss. With the patient supine, each ear canal is irrigated with warm (44°C) water for 30 sec, followed by irrigation with cold (30°C) water. Warm water elicits rotatory nystagmus to the side being irrigated; cold water produces the opposite reaction (i.e., nystagmus to the opposite side). SYN: *oculovestibular test; Bárány's test.*

**calorie** (kăl′ō-rē) [L. *calor,* heat] A unit of heat. A calorie may be equated to work or to other units of heat measurement. Small calories are converted to joules by multiplying by 4.1855. SEE: table.

***gram c.*** Small c.

***kilogram c.*** Large c.; one thousand calories.

***large c.*** ABBR: C, Cal, or kcal. The amount of heat needed to change the temperature of 1 kg of water from 14.5°C to 15.5°C. It is commonly used in metabolic studies and in reference to human nutrition. It is always capitalized to distinguish it from a small calorie. SYN: *kilogram c.; kilocalorie.*

***small c.*** ABBR: c, cal. The amount of heat needed to change the temperature of 1 g of water 1°C. SYN: *gram c.; microcalorie.*

**calorifacient** (kă-lor″ĭ-fā′shĕnt) [L. *calor,* heat, + *faciens,* making] Producing heat.

**calorific** (kăl″ō-rĭf′ĭk) Producing heat.

**calorigenic** (kă-lor″ĭ-jĕn′ĭk) [″ + Gr. *gennan,* to produce] Pert. to the production of heat or energy.

**calorimeter** (kăl″ō-rĭm′ĕ-tĕr) [″ + Gr. *metron,* measure] An instrument for determining the amount of heat exchanged in a chemical reaction or by the animal body under specific conditions.

***bomb c.*** An apparatus for determinating potential food energy. Heat produced in combustion is measured by the amount of heat absorbed by a known quantity of water in which the calorimeter is immersed.

***respiration c.*** An apparatus for measuring heat produced from exchange of respiratory gases.

**calorimetry** (kăl″ō-rĭm′ĕ-trē) The determination of heat loss or gain.

**calvaria** (kăl-vā′rē-ă) [L., skull] The domelike superior portion of the cranium, composed of the superior portions of the frontal, parietal, and occipital bones. SYN: *skullcap.*

**Calvé-Perthes disease** (kăl-vā′pĕr′tās) [Jacques Calvé, Fr. orthopedist, 1875–1954; Georg C. Perthes, Ger. surgeon, 1869–1927] A disorder marked by aseptic necrosis of the epiphysis of the head of the femur.

**calx** (kălks) [L.] **1.** Lime. **2.** The heel.

***c. chlorinata*** Chlorinated lime. It is used as a deodorant and disinfectant.

**calyces** Pl. of calyx.

## Recommended Daily Caloric and Protein Allowances*†

Designed for the Maintenance of Good Nutrition of Practically All Healthy People in the U.S.

| | Age (yr) | Weight‡ kg | Weight‡ lb | Height‡ cm | Height‡ in. | Protein (g) | Average Energy Allowance (kcal)§ |
|---|---|---|---|---|---|---|---|
| Infants | 0.0–0.5 | 6 | 13 | 60 | 24 | 13 | 650 |
| | 0.5–1.0 | 9 | 20 | 71 | 28 | 14 | 850 |
| Children | 1–3 | 13 | 29 | 90 | 35 | 16 | 1300 |
| | 4–6 | 20 | 44 | 112 | 44 | 24 | 1800 |
| | 7–10 | 28 | 62 | 132 | 52 | 28 | 2000 |
| Males | 11–14 | 45 | 99 | 157 | 62 | 45 | 2500 |
| | 15–18 | 66 | 145 | 176 | 69 | 59 | 3000 |
| | 19–24 | 72 | 160 | 177 | 70 | 58 | 2900 |
| | 25–50 | 79 | 174 | 176 | 70 | 63 | 2900 |
| | 51+ | 77 | 170 | 173 | 68 | 63 | 2300 |
| Females | 11–14 | 46 | 101 | 157 | 62 | 46 | 2200 |
| | 15–18 | 55 | 120 | 163 | 64 | 44 | 2200 |
| | 19–24 | 58 | 128 | 164 | 65 | 46 | 2200 |
| | 25–50 | 63 | 138 | 163 | 64 | 50 | 2200 |
| | 51+ | 65 | 143 | 160 | 63 | 50 | 1900 |
| Pregnant | 1st trimester | | | | | 60 | +0 |
| | 2nd trimester | | | | | 60 | +300 |
| | 3rd trimester | | | | | 60 | +300 |
| Lactating | 1st 6 months | | | | | 65 | +500 |
| | 2nd 6 months | | | | | 62 | +500 |

SOURCE: Adapted with permission from Recommended Daily Allowances, ed. 10, copyright 1989 by the National Academy of Sciences, National Research Council, Washington, D.C. Revised 1990.

* For complete table, SEE: *Appendix*.

† The allowances, expressed as average daily intakes over time, are intended to provide for individual variations among most normal persons as they live in the U.S. under usual environmental stresses. Diets should be based on a variety of common foods in order to provide other nutrients for which human requirements have been less well defined.

‡ Weights and heights of Reference Adults are actual medians for the U.S. population of the designated age. The use of these figures does not imply that the height-to-weight ratios are ideal.

§ Kilojoules (kJ) = 4.1855 × kcal.

**calyciform** (kă-lĭs′ĭ-form) [Gr. *kalyx,* cup of a flower, + L. *forma,* shape] Cup-shaped.

**Calymmatobacterium granulomatis** (kă-lĭm″mă-tō-băk-tē′rē-ŭm) The organism, a gram-negative bacillus, that causes granuloma inguinale. The presence of Donovan bodies in lesions is diagnostic.

**calyx** (kā′lĭx) *pl.* **calyces** [Gr. *kalyx,* cup of a flower] **1.** Any cuplike organ or cavity. **2.** A cuplike extension of the renal pelvis that encloses the papilla of a renal pyramid; urine from the papillary duct is emptied into it.

**camera** (kăm′ĕr-ă) [Gr. *kamara,* vault] In anatomy, a chamber or cavity.

***c. anterior bulbi*** The anterior chamber of the eye between the cornea and the iris.

***c. posterior bulbi*** The posterior chamber of the eye between the iris and the lens.

**camomile** The flowering heads of the plant *Anthemis nobilis*. Used in bitters to improve appetite and digestion. SYN: *chamomile.*

**Camoquin Hydrochloride** Trade name for amodiaquine hydrochloride.

**cAMP** *cyclic adenosine monophosphate.*

**camphor** (kăm′for) [Malay, *kapur,* chalk] A gum obtained from an evergreen tree native to China and Japan. Topically, as a 0.1% preparation, it is used as an antipruritic.

**camphorated** Combined with or containing camphor.

**camphorated oil** Liniment containing camphor.

**camphor poisoning** SEE: *Poisons and Poisoning Appendix.*

**campimeter** (kămp-ĭm′ĕ-tĕr) [L. *campus,* field, + Gr. *metron,* measure] A device for measuring the field of vision.

**campimetry** (kămp-ĭm′ĕ-trē) Perimetry (2).

**campospasm** Camptocormia.

**camptocormia** (kămp″tō-kor′mē-ă) [Gr. *kamptos,* bent, + *kormos,* trunk] A deformity marked by habitual forward flexion of the trunk when the individual is erect. SYN: *camptospasm.*

**camptodactylia** (kămp″tō-dăk-tĭl′ē-ă) [″ + *dactylos,* finger] Permanent flexion of the fingers or toes.

**camptomelic dwarfism** A condition in which infants have craniofacial anomalies, defects of the ribs, and scapular hypoplasia. The cause is unknown, and death usually occurs in the neonatal period.

**camptospasm** (kămp′tō-spăzm) [″ + *spasmos,* spasm] Camptocormia.

**Campylobacter** (kăm′pĭ-lō-băk′tĕr) [Gr. *kampylos,* curved, + *bakterion,* little rod] A genus of gram-negative, spirally curved, rod-shaped bacteria of the family Spirillaceae that are motile and non–spore-forming. One or both ends of the cell have a single polar flagellum.

***C. fetus*** A species with several subspecies that can cause disease in both humans and animals.

***C. jejuni*** A subspecies of *C. fetus* formerly called *Vibrio fetus.* It can cause an acute enteric disease characterized by diarrhea, abdominal pain, malaise, fever, nausea, and vomiting. The disease is usually self-limiting. Treatment consists of fluid and electrolyte replacement and administration of the antibiotic to which the organism is sensitive.

**Canadian Nurses' Association** ABBR: CNA. The official national organization for professional nurses from the 10 provinces of Canada and the Northwest Territories. All services provided by the organization are offered in English and French.

**Canadian Nurses' Association Testing Service** ABBR: CNATS. An organization affiliated with the Canadian Nurses' Association that is responsible for administering the nursing licensure examination to graduates of approved nursing schools. Successful completion of the examination qualifies the candidate as a registered nurse. The examination is analogous to the National Council Licensure Examination (NCLEX) in the U.S.

**Canadian Occupational Performance Measure** ABBR: COPM. An outcome measure designed for use by occupational therapists to assess self-care, productivity, and leisure. The patient identifies problems in daily function that are then measured on the basis of performance and client satisfaction.

**canal** (kă-năl′) [L. *canalis,* channel] A narrow tube, channel, or passageway. SEE: *duct; foramen; groove; space.*

***adductor c.*** A triangular space lying beneath the sartorius muscle and between the adductor longus and vastus medialis muscles. It extends from the apex of the femoral triangle to the popliteal space and transmits the femoral vessels and the saphenous nerve. Also called *Hunter's canal.*

***Alcock's c.*** Canalis pudendalis; a canal on the pelvic surface of the obturator internus muscle formed by the obturator fascia. It transmits the pudendal vessels and nerve. SYN: *pudendal c.*

***alimentary c.*** The digestive tract from the mouth through the anus.

***alveolar c.*** Canalis alveolaris; one of several canals in the maxilla that transmit the posterior superior alveolar blood vessels and nerves to the upper teeth. SYN: *dental c.; maxillary c.*

***anal c.*** Canalis analis; the terminal portion of the rectum opening at the anus.

***auditory c.*** SEE: *external auditory c.; internal auditory c.*

***birth c.*** The parturient canal; the passageway through which the fetus passes during delivery; specifically, the cervix, vagina, and vulva.

***bony semicircular c.*** One of several canals located in the bony labyrinth of the internal ear and enclosing the three semicircular ducts (superior, posterior, and lateral) that open into the vestibule. They are enclosed within the petrous portion of the temporal bone.

***carotid c.*** Canalis caroticus; a canal in the petrous portion of the temporal bone that transmits the interior carotid artery and the interior carotid plexus of sympathetic nerves.

***central c. of bone*** **1.** Canalis centralis; a small canal in the center of the spinal cord extending from the fourth ventricle to the conus medullaris. It contains cerebrospinal fluid. **2.** The haversian canal of an osteon in bone.

***cervical c.*** Canalis cervicis uteri; a canal in the cervix of the uterus extending from the internal to the external os.

***cochlear spiral c.*** Canalis spiralis cochleae; a part of the bony labyrinth of the ear. A spiral tube about 30 mm long makes two and three quarters turns about a central bony axis, the modiolus. It contains the scala tympani, scala vestibuli, and cochlear duct. SYN: *spiral c. of the cochlea.*

***condylar c.*** Canalis condylaris; a canal in the occipital bone for passage of the emissary vein from the transverse sinus. It opens anterior to the occipital condyle.

***craniopharyngeal c.*** A canal in the fetal sphenoid bone that contains the stalk of Rathke's pouch.

***dental c.*** Alveolar c.

***ethmoidal c.*** One of two grooves running transversely across the lateral mass of the ethmoid bone to the cribriform plate and lying between the ethmoid and frontal bones. The anterior ethmoidal canal transmits the anterior ethmoidal vessels and the nasociliary nerve; the posterior ethmoidal canal transmits the posterior ethmoidal vessels and nerve.

***external auditory c.*** The external auditory meatus, which transmits sound waves.

***facial c.*** Canalis facialis; a canal in the internal acoustic meatus of the temporal bone that transmits the facial nerve.

***femoral c.*** Canalis femoralis; the medial division of the femoral sheath. It is a short compartment about 1.5 cm long, lying behind the inguinal ligament. It contains some lymphatic vessels and a lymph node.

***gastric c.*** A longitudinal groove on the inner surface of the stomach following the lesser curvature. It extends from the esophagus to the pylorus.

***haversian c.*** **1.** One of many minute canals found in compact bone that contain blood and lymph vessels, nerves, and sometimes marrow, each surrounded by lamellae of bone constituting a haversian system. SEE: *bone*. **2.** A canal in osseous tissue that carries a neurovascular bundle to the teeth, seen most often in periapical radiographs of the mandible. SYN: *interdental c.*

***hyaloid c.*** Canalis hyaloideus; a canal in the vitreous body of the eye extending from the optic papilla to the central posterior surface of the lens. It serves as a lymph channel. In the fetus the canal contains the hyaloid artery. This normally disappears 6 weeks before birth.

***hypoglossal c.*** Canalis hypoglossi; a canal in the occipital bone that transmits the hypoglossal nerve and a branch of the posterior meningeal artery.

***incisive c.*** Canalis incisivus; a short canal in the maxillary bone leading from the incisive fossa in the roof of the mouth to the floor of the nasal cavity. It transmits the nasopalatine nerve and the branches of the greater palatine arteries to the nasal fossa.

***inferior alveolar c.*** Mandibular c.

***infraorbital c.*** Canalis infraorbitalis; a canal in the maxilla lying in the floor of the orbit that transmits the infraorbital nerve and artery. It terminates anteriorly at the infraorbital foramen.

***interdental c.*** Haversian c. (2).

***internal auditory c.*** The canal in the petrous portion of the temporal bone that transmits the acoustic and facial nerves and the acoustic artery.

***intestinal c.*** The alimentary canal from the stomach to the anus.

***lacrimal c.*** The lacrimal duct.

***mandibular c.*** Canalis mandibulae; a canal in the mandible that transmits the inferior alveolar blood vessels and nerve to the teeth. SYN: *inferior alveolar c.*

***maxillary c.*** Alveolar c.

***medullary c.*** The marrow cavity of long bones.

***membranous semicircular c.*** A semicircular duct. SEE: *duct, semicircular.*

***nasolacrimal c.*** The canal lying between the lacrimal bone and the inferior nasal conchae. It contains the nasolacrimal duct.

***nutrient c.*** An opening on the surface of compact bone through which blood vessels gain access to the medullary cavity of long bones.

***obturator c.*** An opening in the obturator membrane of the hip bone that transmits the obturator vessels and nerve.

***c. of Lambert*** One of several bronchioalveolar communications in the lung. These may help to prevent atelectasis. SEE: *pores of Kohn.*

***optic c.*** The foramen through which the optic nerve passes.

***pharyngeal c.*** A canal between the sphenoid and palatine bones that transmits branches of the sphenopalatine vessels.

***portal c.*** The connective tissue (a continuation of Glisson's capsule) and its contained vessels (interlobular branches of the hepatic artery, portal vein, and bile duct and lymphatic vessel) located between adjoining liver lobules.

***pterygoid c.*** Canalis pterygoideus; a canal of the sphenoid bone transmitting the pterygoid vessels, artery, and nerve.

***pterygopalatine c.*** Canalis palatinus major; a canal between the maxillary and palatine bones that transmits the descending palatine nerves and artery.

***pudendal c.*** Alcock's c.

***pulp c.*** The central cavity of a tooth, filled with pulp. It contains blood vessels and sensory nerve endings.

***root c.*** **1.** The passageway in the root of a tooth through which the nerve and blood vessels pass. **2.** Colloquially, the procedure for preserving a tooth by removing its diseased pulp cavity.

***sacral c.*** Canalis sacralis; a cavity within the sacrum. It is a continuation of the vertebral canal.

***Schlemm's c.*** The space or series of spaces at the junction of the sclera and the cornea of the eye into which aqueous humor is drained from the anterior chamber through the pectinate villi.

***semicircular c.*** SEE: *bony semicircular c.; membranous semicircular c.*

***spinal c.*** Vertebral c.

***spiral c. of the cochlea*** Cochlear spiral c.

***spiral c. of the modiolus*** Canalis spiralis modioli; a series of irregular spaces that follow the course of the attached margin of the osseous spiral lamina to the modiolus. They transmit filaments of the cochlear nerve and blood vessels. The spiral ganglion lies in the spiral canal.

***uterine c.*** The cavity of the uterus.

***uterocervical c.*** The cavity of the cervix of the uterus.

***uterovaginal c.*** The combined cavities of the uterus and vagina.

***vaginal c.*** The cavity of the vagina.

***vertebral c.*** Canalis vertebralis, the cavity formed by the foramina of the vertebral column. It contains the spinal cord and its meninges.

***Volkmann's c.'s*** Small canals found in bone through which blood vessels pass from the periosteum. They connect with the blood vessels of haversian canals or the marrow cavity.

**canaliculus** (kăn″ă-lĭk′ū-lŭs) *pl.* **canaliculi** [L. *canalicularis*] A small channel or canal. In bone or cementum, radiating out from lacunae and anastomosing with canaliculi of neighboring lacunae. **canalicular** (-lĭk′ū-lăr), *adj.*

**canalis** (kă-nā′lĭs) *pl.* **canales** [L., channel] Canal.

**canalization** (kăn″ăl-ī-zā′shŭn) Formation of channels in tissue.

**canavanine** (kă-năv′ă-nĭn) An amino acid originally isolated from soybean meal. It prevents growth of some bacteria.

**Canavan's disease** An autosomal recessive disorder of infants, marked by spongy white matter with Alzheimer's type II cells. Also called *Canavan–van Bogaert–Bertrand disease.*

**cancellated** (kăn′sĕ-lāt″ĕd) [L. *cancellus,* lattice] Reticulated; said of a lattice-like structure.

**cancelli** (kăn-sĕl′ī) Pl. of cancellus.

**cancellous** (kăn′sĕl-ŭs) Having a reticular or latticework structure, as the spongy tissue of bone.

**cancellus** (kăn-sĕl′ŭs) *pl.* **cancelli** [L.] An osseous plate composing cancellous bone; any structure arranged as a lattice.

**cancer** (kăn′sĕr) [G. *karkinos,* crab] An imprecise term used to describe an estimated 200 different kinds of malignant neoplasms, marked by uncontrolled growth and the spread of abnormal cells. Cancers may be lethal by invading adjacent normal tissues or by spread (metastasis) to sites distant from the place of origin. Cancers that arise in epithelial tissues are called carcinomas; from mesenchymal tissues, sarcomas. Leukemias are also considered malignant growths. SYN: *neoplasia; malignancy.*

Four attributes differentiate cancer cells from normal cells: 1. *Clonality:* Cancer cells originate from genetic changes in a single cell, which then multiplies to form a clone of malignant cells. 2. *Autonomy:* Cancerous growth is not controlled or regulated by the normal biochemical and physical forces present in the body. 3. *Anaplasia:* The abnormally growing cells do not develop into normal cells similar to the one from which the clone arose. 4. *Metastasis:* Cancer cells are able to grow in parts of the body other than their site of origin. The process by which normal cells develop into cancer cells is called malignant transformation.

Cancer is the second leading cause of death in the U.S. In the last 40 years in the U.S., the cancer death rate has declined in women and increased in men. SEE: illus. (Cancer Statistics).

SYMPTOMS: There are seven warning signs of cancer, which may be remembered by the mnemonic CAUTION. *C*hange in bowel or bladder habits; *A* sore that does not heal; *U*nusual bleeding or discharge; *T*hickening or lump in breast or elsewhere; *I*ndigestion or difficulty in swallowing; *O*bvious change in a wart or mole; *N*agging cough or hoarseness. If any one of these signs is observed, it should be brought to a physician's attention without delay.

ETIOLOGY: Unregulated, disorganized proliferation of cell growth may be stimulated by various chemicals, viruses, and physical agents such as ionizing radiation and ultraviolet light. Ironically, cytotoxic agents used to treat cancer may cause it. Several agents are specific carcinogens, notably the chemicals contained in tobacco products. Other lifestyle factors such as dietary high-fat and low-fiber intake may be important contributors to the development of cancer in humans. Familial predisposition to certain types of cancers has been evidenced. A family history of some malignancies, for example breast cancer, may be a risk factor.

DIAGNOSIS: Depending on the site, diagnosis is made by various means, the most important being biopsy, use of devices to visualize hollow organs, radiography including computed tomography (CT), mammography, ultrasound, cytology such as the Papanicolaou test, and palpation for lumps. Although some of these techniques and devices may demonstrate an increase in the size or change in the shape of an organ, such alteration may be due to either a benign or a malignant growth. SEE: illus. (Cancer).

The most effective screening tests to detect cancers in the symptomless stage are those for cancer of the uterine cervix, breast, and prostate. Tests for cancer of the ovary, lung, and colon are being researched.

Metastatic cancer in which it is not possible to determine the site of the primary malignancy frequently involves adenocarcinoma, melanoma, lymphoma, sarcoma, or squamous carcinoma. Even though the prognosis is poor for patients with these types of malignancies, the response may be improved when the cell type is specifically identified.

Various cancer staging systems exist to help delineate the extent and prognosis of tumors. An example of one of these is the tumor, node, metastasis (TNM) system. Numbers are added to each category to indicate the degree of dissemination. SEE: table; *cancer staging.*

TREATMENT: Surgery, chemotherapy, hormone therapy, radium, and radiotherapy are all recognized effective methods for treating patients with cancer. Application of the proper method or combination of methods is necessary for effective therapy. Therefore, early diagnosis is the most important factor.

Because the pain associated with cancer is frequently undertreated in both adults and children, the U.S. Department

**1996 ESTIMATED CANCER INCIDENCE BY SITE AND SEX**

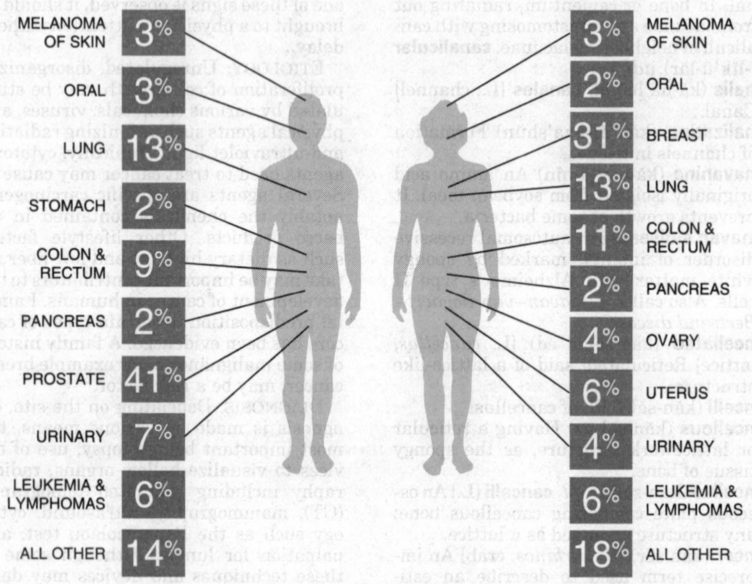


Excluding basal and squamous cell skin cancers and in situ carcinoma except bladder.

**1996 ESTIMATED CANCER DEATHS BY SITE AND SEX**

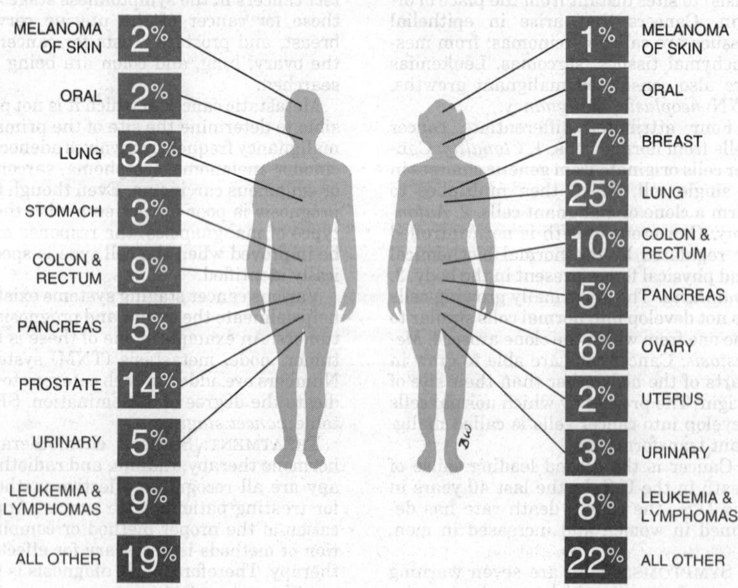


Cancer Statistics, 1995, American Cancer Society, New York, N.Y.

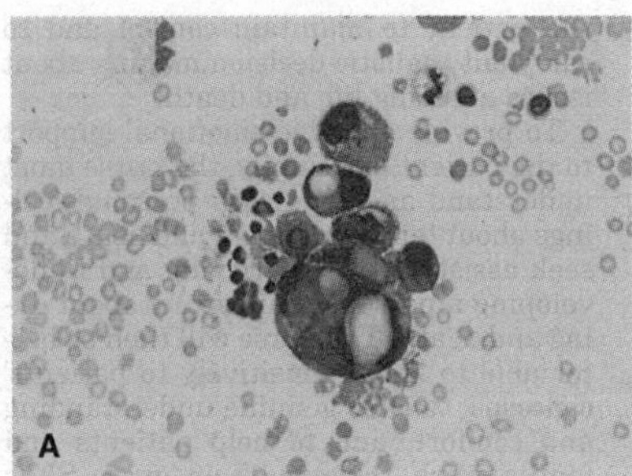


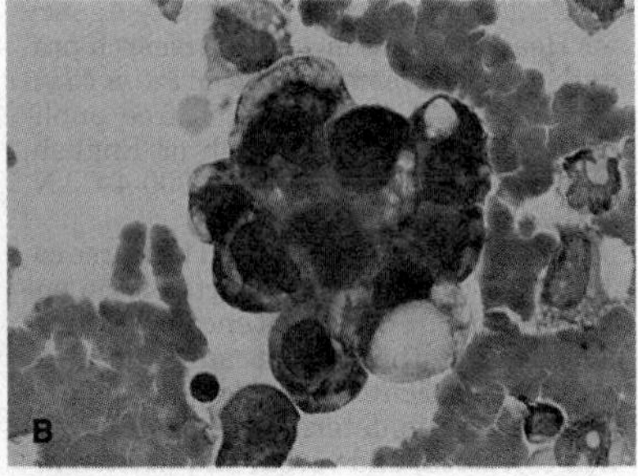


**CANCER**

COLON **(A)** AND OVARIAN **(B)** CANCER CELLS IN PERITONEAL FLUID (ORIG. MAG. ×500)

## American Cancer Society Recommendations for Early Detection of Cancer in Asymptomatic People

| Test or Examination | To Detect | Who | Frequency |
|---|---|---|---|
| Sigmoidoscopy, preferably flexible | Colorectal cancer | Everyone 50 and over | Every 3–5 years |
| Fecal occult blood test | Colorectal cancer | Everyone 50 and over | Every year |
| Digital rectal examination* | Rectal cancer | Everyone 40 and over | Every year |
| | Prostate cancer | Men 50 and over | Every year |
| Prostate-specific antigen test* | Prostate cancer | Men 50 and over | Every year |
| Pap test | Cervical cancer | All women who are or have been sexually active or have reached 18 should have annual Pap test and pelvic examination. After three or more consecutive normal, satisfactory annual examinations, the Pap test may be performed less frequently at the discretion of the physician. | |
| Pelvic examination | Reproductive system cancers in women | Women 18–40 | Every 1–3 years with Pap test |
| | | Women over 40 | Every year |
| Endometrial tissue sample | Uterine cancer | Women at high risk† | At menopause and thereafter at the physician's discretion |
| Breast self-examination | Breast cancer | Women 20 and over | Every month |
| Breast clinical examination | Breast cancer | Women 20–40 | Every 3 years |
| | | Women over 40 | Every year |
| Mammography‡ | Breast cancer | Women 40–49 | Every 1–2 years |
| | | Women 50 and over | Every year |
| Health counseling and cancer checkup | Cancer of thyroid, testes, ovaries, lymph nodes, mouth, and skin | Everyone over 20 | Every 3 years |
| | | Everyone over 40 | Every year |

SOURCE: American Cancer Society; adapted with permission.

* If either test is abnormal, further evaluation for prostate cancer should be considered.

† History of infertility, obesity, failure to ovulate, abnormal uterine bleeding, or unopposed estrogen or tamoxifen therapy.

‡ Screening mammography should begin by age 40.

of Health and Human Services' Agency for Health Care Policy and Research produced *Management of Cancer Pain: Clinical Practice Guideline*. This free publication, available in Spanish or English, may be obtained by calling 1-800-4-CANCER.

NURSING IMPLICATIONS: The nurse coordinates collaborative efforts of the entire health-care team and encourages participation of the patient and family in care. The patient's knowledge of the disease process is determined, misinformation corrected, and verbal and written information supplied about the disease, its progression, its treatment, and expected outcomes. The patient's and family's positive coping mechanisms are identified and supported, and verbalization of feelings and fears, particularly with regard to changes in body image, pain and suffering, and dying and death, is encouraged.

Assistance is provided with personal hygiene and physical care. Physical care is directed at the maintenance of fluid and electrolyte balance and proper nutrition. Nutrition is a special concern because tumors compete with normal tissues for nutrients and grow at their expense and because the disease or treatments can cause anorexia, altered taste sensations, mouth ulcerations, vomiting, diarrhea, and draining fistulas. Nutritional support includes assessing the patient's status and problems, experimenting to find foods that the patient can tolerate, avoiding highly aromatic foods, and offering frequent small meals of high-calorie, high-nutrient soft foods along with fluids to limit fatigue and to encourage overall intake. Elimination is maintained by administering stool softeners as necessary if analgesic drugs result in constipation.

Using careful, gentle handling techniques, the nurse assists with range of motion exercises, encourages ambulation when possible, and turns and repositions the patient frequently to decrease the deleterious multisystemic effects of immobilization. Comfort is achieved through correct body alignment, noninvasive measures such as guided imagery and cutaneous stimulation, and prescribed pharmacological measures, preferably administered on a regular schedule to prevent pain, with additional dosing to relieve breakthrough pain. The nurse also strives to decrease the patient's fears of helplessness and loss of control; provides hope for remission or long-term survival, but avoids giving false hope; and provides the patient with realistic reassurance about pain control, comfort, and rest.

Hospice care if needed is discussed with the patient and family. The nurse encourages family members to assume an active role in the patient's care, fosters communication between patient and family and other health-care providers, and assists the patient to maintain control and to carry out realistic decision making about issues affecting life and death.

To provide effective emotional support to the patient and family, the nurse must understand and cope with personal feelings about terminal illness and death and seek assistance with grieving and in developing a personal philosophy about dying and death. The nurse will then be better able to listen sensitively to patients' concerns, to offer genuine understanding and comfort, and to help patients and family work through their grief. SEE: *Nursing Diagnoses Appendix*.

***bone c.*** A malignancy of bone tissue. Primary bone tumors are rare in adults; they are seen more often in children and adolescents. Secondary or metastatic bone tumors are far more common. Tumors arising in other areas of the body which metastasize to the bones most often spread to areas such as the spine and pelvis.

***chimney sweeps' c.*** Cancer of the skin of the scrotum due to chronic irritation by coal soot.

***hard c.*** A cylindrical cancer composed of fibrous tissue. SYN: *scirrhous c.*

***lip c.*** An epithelioma of the lower lip usually seen in men or smokers.

***lung c.*** Cancer that may appear in the trachea, air sacs, and other lung tubes. It may appear as an ulcer in the windpipe, as a nodule or small flattened lump, or on the surface blocking air tubes. It may extend into the lymphatics and blood vessels. The majority of lung cancers are caused by carcinogens inhaled via cigarette smoking. The relative risk of developing lung cancer is increased by about 13 times by active smoking and about 1.5 times by long time exposure to cigarettes (passive smoking).

***ovarian c.*** Any malignant growth in an ovary. About 85% to 90% of ovarian cancers arise from the surface epithelium of the ovary. More women die of epithelial ovarian cancer than of all other gynecologic cancers combined. SEE: *inhibin*.

***scirrhous c.*** Hard c.

**cancer cell** A cell present in a neoplasm and differentiated from normal tissue cells because of its degree of anaplasia, irregularity of shape, indistinct outline, nuclear size, changes in the structure of the nucleus and cytoplasm, increased number of mitoses, and ability to metastasize.

**cancer, chemoprevention of** The use of certain foods and drugs to prevent the progression of preneoplastic and some neoplastic conditions. This topic is the object of extensive investigation.

**cancer cluster** The occurrence of a rare type of cancer in a small geographical area and in much greater number than could be expected through chance alone.

**cancer grading and staging** The standardized procedure for expressing cancer cell differentiation, called grading, and the extent of dissemination of the cancer, called staging. This procedure is very helpful in comparing the results of various forms of therapy. Cancer is graded on the differentiation of the tumor cells and the number of mitoses present. These are thought to be correlated with the ability of the tumor to grow and spread. Some cancers are graded I to IV, the latter being the most anaplastic and having the least resemblance to normal tissue.

Cancers are staged according to size, amount of local spread (metastases), and whether or not blood-borne metastasis has occurred. There are two major staging systems. The TNM judges the size of primary tumor (T), evidence of regional extension, or nodes (N), and evidence of metastases (M). Another system classifies cancers as Stage 0 to IV according to the size of the tumor and its spread.

It is not possible to determine the site of the primary malignancy for some metastatic cancers. The most frequent cell types are adenocarcinoma, melanoma, lymphoma, sarcoma, and squamous carcinoma. Even though the prognosis is poor for these patients, the response may be improved when the cell type is specifically identified.

**cancericidal** (kăn″sĕr-ĭ-sī′dăl) [L. *cancer,* crab, + *cidus,* killing] Lethal to malignant cells.

**cancerigenic** (kăn″sĕr-ĭ-jĕn′ĭk) [″ + Gr. *gennan,* to produce] Carcinogenic.

**Cancer Information Service** A program sponsored by the National Cancer Institute that provides cancer information to patients and their families, health professionals, and the general public. Information may be obtained by calling the toll-free number 1-800-4-CANCER (1-800-422-6237).

**cancerogenic** (kăn″sĕr-ō-jĕn′ĭk) [″ + Gr. *gennan,* to produce] Carcinogenic.

**cancerophobia** [″ + Gr. *phobos,* fear] Unreasonable fear of cancer.

**cancerous** (kăn′sĕr-ŭs) Pert. to malignant growth.

**cancer screening** A program to detect cancer in its symptomless stage. Because the number of lives lost to cancer is so great, it has been the object of intense investigation for effective screening tests. Effective screening tests for cancers of the breast, uterine cervix, and prostate are available. Evaluation of screening tests includes determining the chance that the test will be negative when the patient does indeed have the disease (false negative) and the reverse when the test is positive but cancer is not present (false positive). SEE: *breast self-examination; CA 125; mammography; Papanicolaou test; prostate-specific antigen.*

**cancra** (kăng′kră) Pl. of cancrum.

**cancroid** (kăng′kroyd) [″ + Gr. *eidos,* form, shape] **1.** Like a cancer. **2.** A type of keloid. **3.** Epithelioma.

**cancrum** (kăng′krŭm) *pl.* **cancra** [L. *cancer,* crab, creeping ulcer] A rapidly spreading ulcer.

***c. nasi*** A gangrenous inflammation of the nasal membranes.

***c. oris*** Trench mouth.

***c. pudendi*** Ulceration of the vulva.

**candela** (kăn-dĕl′ă) [L. *candela,* candle] SYMB: cd. The SI base unit of luminous intensity.

**candicidin** (kăn″dĭ-sī′dĭn) An antibiotic produced by certain species of *Streptomyces.*

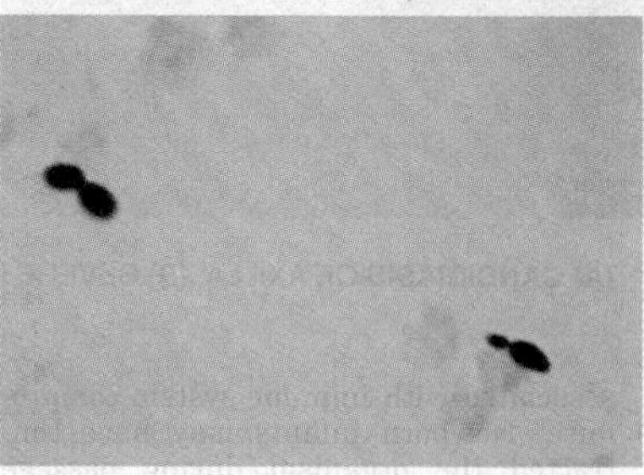

GRAM STAIN OF **CANDIDA** VAGINITIS

**Candida** (kăn′dĭ-dă) [L. *candidus,* glowing white] A genus of yeasts that develop a pseudomycelium and reproduce by budding. *Candida* (formerly *Monilia*) species are part of the normal flora of the mouth, skin, intestinal tract, and vagina. SEE: illus.

***C. albicans*** A small, oval budding fungus that is the primary etiological organism of moniliasis (candidiasis). It was formerly called *Monilia albicans.* SEE: illus.

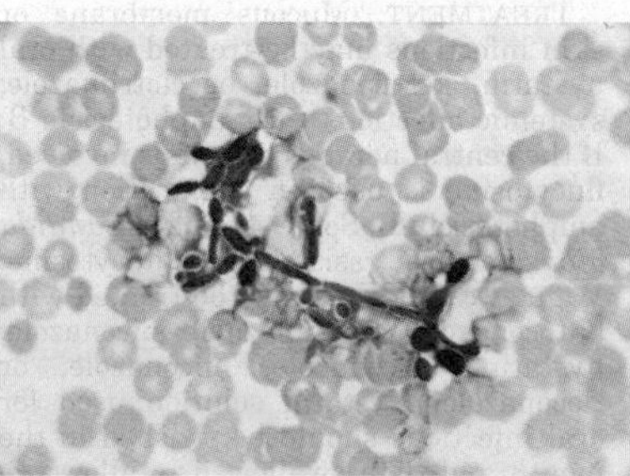

**CANDIDA ALBICANS** (PURPLE) IN BLOOD (ORIG. MAG. ×640)

**candidemia** The presence of yeast cells from the genus *Candida* in the blood.

**candidiasis** (kăn″dĭ-dī′ă-sĭs) Infection of the skin or mucous membrane with any species of *Candida,* but chiefly *Candida albicans.* It is usually localized in the skin, nails, mouth, vagina, vulva, bronchi, or lungs, but may invade the bloodstream. It occurs commonly as a secondary infection

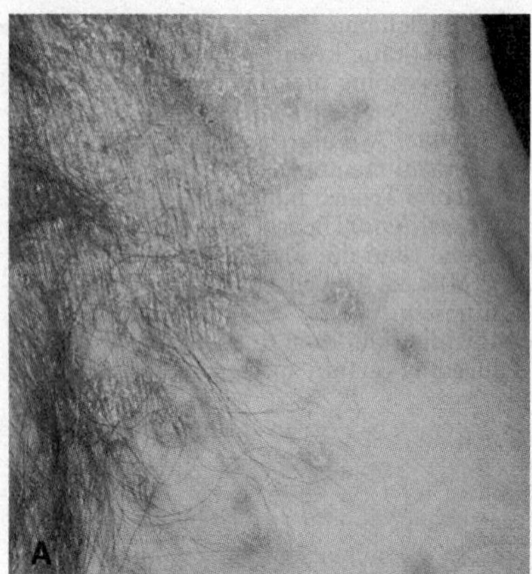

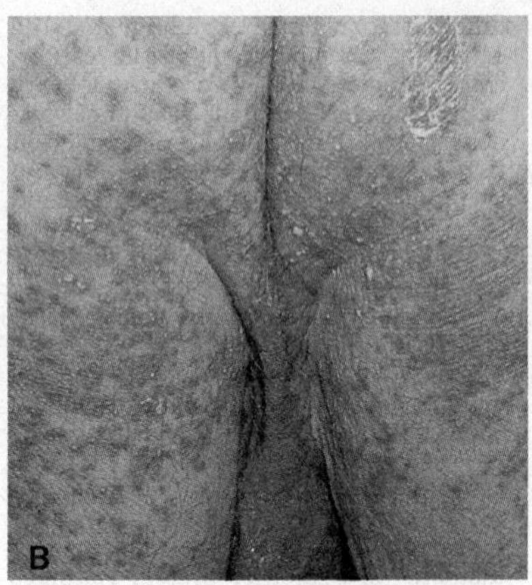

**(A) CANDIDIASIS** OF AXILLA, **(B)** SEVERE INFECTION IN DIABETIC (SKIN OF BUTTOCKS)

associated with immune system compromise. Newborn infants may have contracted the organism during passage through the birth canal. SEE: illus.; *thrush*.

SYMPTOMS: Oral lesions consist of painless, discrete white plaques that adhere on the oral and pharyngeal mucosa, including the tongue. Skin lesions are red and macerated, and usually occur in intertriginous areas. Other sites include the nails (paronychia), penis (balanitis), and anus (pruritis ani). Invasive systemic infections may be present in any organ, including the brain, heart, kidneys, and eyes. The symptoms produced in systemic infections depend on the extent of the infection and the organs affected.

TREATMENT: Mucous membrane or skin infections may be treated with oral nystatin, ketoconazole, or clotrimazole; systemic infections with amphotericin B. If the central nervous system is involved, flucytosine is used in conjunction with amphotericin B. Some strains of *Candida albicans* are resistant to flucytosine. Vaginal candidiasis may be treated with butoconazole, clotrimazole, miconazole, nystatin, terconazole, miconazole, or tioconazole. Nystatin solution used for oral infections should be swished in the mouth and then swallowed to allow the medicine to contact the mucosa being treated. Nystatin is not absorbed from the gastrointestinal tract. Pregnant patients should consult their physician before taking or applying these drugs.

NURSING IMPLICATIONS: Universal precautions are observed in assessing or caring for the patient. The patient is observed for a scaly, erythematous, papular skin rash, possibly covered with exudate and erupting in breast folds, between fingers, and at the axillae, groin, and umbilicus. Red, swollen, darkened nailbeds, occasionally with purulent discharge, and sometimes with nail separation from the nailbed, accompany this rash. Cream-colored or bluish-white lacelike pseudomembranous patches appear on the patient's mucous membranes; these patches reveal bloody engorgement when scraped. The patient also complains of a burning sensation in the mouth and throat and a white or yellow vaginal discharge accompanied by pruritus. The infection may progress to systemic involvement as evidenced by symptoms of myalgia, arthralgia, chills with a high and spiking fever, and prostration. Additional signs and symptoms will depend on the particular organ system(s) infected.

In a patient with systemic infection, vital signs are closely monitored. The patient is instructed about prescribed drug therapy, including procedures for "swish and swallow" of oral antifungals or application of vaginal medication. A nonirritating mouthwash and a soft toothbrush or sponge toothette are provided to loosen tenacious secretions without causing irritation. A topical anesthetic is prescribed to relieve mouth discomfort, and a soft diet is recommended for the patient experiencing severe dysphagia. An antifungal powder as prescribed or dry padding is applied to intertriginous areas of obese patients to prevent irritation and candidal growth.

Supportive care is provided for the patient with a systemic infection, including premedication with aspirin, antihistamines, or antiemetics to help reduce adverse reactions if the patient is prescribed amphotericin B systemically. A woman in her third trimester of pregnancy should be examined and treated for vaginitis to protect her infant from being infected during passage through the birth canal. The patient with dyspareunia is counseled that sexual impairment should resolve as the infection subsides, but to complete the full course of medication as prescribed. Although the sexual partners of infected patients usually will not need treatment, partners of patients with recurrent vaginal infections should be examined and treated to prevent reinfection of the patient.

**candle** (kăn'dl) [L. *candela*] A solid mass of combustible material such as tallow or wax in which a wick is imbedded. When the wick is lighted, the wax burns slowly to produce heat and light. Candles are used in bacteriology, where they are placed lighted in an airtight jar and allowed to extinguish themselves. This process produces an atmosphere containing approx. 10% carbon dioxide. This carbon dioxide concentration is required for culturing certain organisms, particularly *Neisseria gonorrhoeae.*

**cane** (kān) A slender stick held in the hand and used for support during walking.

**canine** (kā'nīn) [L. *caninus,* dog] **1.** Pert. to a dog. **2.** A canine tooth; any of the four teeth, also known as the eyeteeth (upper and lower), between the incisors and molars. SEE: *dentition* for illus.

**canities** (kăn-ĭsh'ē-ēz) [L., gray hair] Congenital (rare) or acquired whiteness of the hair. The acquired form may develop rapidly or slowly and be partial or complete. SYN: *achromatrichia.*

***c. unguium*** Gray or white streaks in the nails. SYN: *leukonychia.*

**canker sore** (kăng'kĕr) [L. *cancer,* crab, creeping ulcer] Ulceration of the mouth and lips. SEE: *aphthous ulcer.*

**cannabis** (kăn'ă-bĭs) [Gr. *kannabis,* hemp] Marijuana.

**cannibalism** The human consumption of human flesh. SEE: *kuru.*

**cannula** (kăn'ū-lă) [L., a small reed] A tube or sheath enclosing a trocar; the tube allowing the escape of fluid after withdrawal of the trocar from the body.

***nasal c.*** Tubing used to deliver oxygen at levels from 1 to 6 L/min. It extends approx. 1 cm into each naris and is connected to a common tube, which is then connected to the oxygen source. It is used in situations such as cardiac disease, in which a low-flow, small-percentage oxygen therapy is desirable. The exact percentage of oxygen delivered to the patient varies with respiratory rate and other factors.

**cannulate** (kăn'ū-lāt) To introduce a cannula through a passageway.

**cannulation of large veins** The technique of providing access to venous circulation by placing a flexible cannula in one of the large veins, usually the femoral or subclavian. The cannula is used to provide hyperalimentation or fluid replacement to patients in shock. When the subclavian vein is used, pneumothorax is a possible complication.

**cantharides** (kăn-thăr'ĭ-dēz) *sing.,* **cantharis** [Gr. *kantharis,* beetle, + *eidos,* form, shape] Dried insects of the species *Cantharis vesicatoria;* poisonous if taken internally in large doses. It was formerly used externally as a counterirritant and vesicant, and internally for its supposed aphrodisiac effect. It is no longer used. SYN: *Spanish fly.* **cantharidal** (-thăr'ĭ-dăl), *adj.*

**Cantharis** (kăn'thă-rĭs) A genus of beetles, *C. vesicatoria,* known as Spanish fly. SEE: *cantharides.*

**canthectomy** (kăn-thĕk'tō-mē) [Gr. *kanthos,* angle, + *ektome,* excision] Excision of a canthus.

**canthi** (kăn'thī) Pl. of canthus.

**canthitis** (kăn-thī'tĭs) [" + *itis,* inflammation] Inflammation of a canthus.

**cantholysis** (kăn-thŏl'ĭ-sĭs) [" + *lysis,* dissolution] Incision of an optic canthus of an eye to widen the palpebral slit.

**canthoplasty** (kăn'thō-plăs"tē) [" + *plassein,* to form] **1.** Plastic surgery of an optic canthus. **2.** Enlargement of the palpebral fissure by division of the external canthus.

**canthorrhaphy** (kăn-thor'ă-fē) [" + *rhaphe,* seam, ridge] Suturing of a canthus.

**canthotomy** (kăn-thŏt'ō-mē) [" + *tome,* incision] Surgical division of a canthus.

**canthus** (kăn'thŭs) *pl.* **canthi** [Gr. *kanthos,* angle] The angle at either end of the slit between the eyelids; the external canthus (commissura palpebrarum lateralis) and the internal canthus (commissura palpebrarum medialis). **canthal** (-thăl), *adj.*

**Cantil** Trade name for mepenzolate bromide.

**CaO** Calcium oxide.

**$CaO_2$** The content of oxygen in arterial blood.

**$Ca(OH)_2$** Calcium hydroxide.

**C.A.O.T.** *Canadian Association of Occupational Therapists.*

**cap** (kăp) [LL. *cappa,* hood] **1.** A covering. SYN: *tegmentum.* **2.** The first part of the duodenum. SYN: *pyloric cap.* **3.** The protective covering of a developing tooth. **4.** The artificial covering of a tooth, used for cosmetic reasons. SEE: *enamel organ.* **5.** [L.] *capiat,* let (the patient) take.

***cradle c.*** Seborrhea of the scalp seen in infants.

***knee c.*** Patella.

**capacitance** (kă-păs'ĭ-tăns) [L. *capacitas,* holding] **1.** The ability to store an electrical charge. **2.** The ratio of the charge transferred between a pair of conductors to the potential difference between the conductors.

**capacitation** (kă-păs"ĭ-tā'shŭn) The process occurring in the female reproductive tract that enables sperm to fertilize ova.

**capacitor** (kă-păs'ĭ-tor) An electronic device for storing electric charges.

**capacity** **1.** The potential ability to contain; the potential power to do something. **2.** Cubic content. **3.** The ability to perform mentally. **4.** The measure of the electrical output of a generator.

***timed vital c.*** A test of vital capacity of the lungs expressed with respect to the volume of air that can be quickly and forcibly breathed out in a certain amount of time. SEE: *FEV*$_1$.

***total lung c.*** ABBR: TLC. The volume of air left in the lungs after a maximal inspiration. This amount is important in evaluating the ability of the lung to exchange oxygen and carbon dioxide. SEE: *pulmonary function test; vital c.; volume, residual.*

***vital c.*** The volume of air that can be exhaled from the lungs after a maximal inspiration. This amount is important in evaluating the ability of the lung to exchange oxygen and carbon dioxide. SEE: *pulmonary function test; total lung c.; volume, residual.*

**CAPD** *continuous ambulatory peritoneal dialysis.*

**Capdepont-Hodge syndrome** Dentinogenesis imperfecta.

**capeline** (kăp′ĕ-lĭn) [Fr., a hat] A bandage used for the head or for the stump of an amputated limb.

**Capgras' syndrome** [Jean Marie Joseph Capgras, Fr. psychiatrist, 1873–1950] The patient's delusion that a close relative or friend has been replaced by an impostor.

**capillarectasia** (kăp″ĭ-lăr″ĕk-tā′sē-ă) [L. *capillaris,* hairlike, + Gr. *ektasis,* dilatation] Distention of capillary vessels.

**Capillaria** (kăp″ĭ-lăr′ē-ă) A genus of parasitic nematodes.

***C. philippinensis*** A species of roundworm discovered in the Philippines. It causes severe diarrhea, malabsorption, and enteric protein loss in humans; mortality is high.

**capillariasis** (kăp″ĭ-lă-rī′ă-sĭs) [*Capillaria* + Gr. *-iasis,* condition] A disease, first described in 1968, caused by infestation of the small bowel with the roundworm *Capillaria philippinensis.* It was reported from northern Luzon in the Philippine Islands. Treatment is with thiabendazole.

**capillaritis** (kăp″ĭ-lăr-ī′tĭs) [″ + Gr. *itis,* inflammation] Telangiitis.

**capillarity** (kăp″ĭ-lăr′ĭ-tē) A surface tension effect shown by the elevation or depression of a liquid at the point of contact with a solid, as in capillary tubes. SYN: *capillary attraction.*

**capillaropathy** (kăp″ĭ-lăr-ŏp′ă-thē) [″ + Gr. *pathos,* disease] A capillary disorder or disease.

**capillaroscopy** (kăp″ĭ-lăr-ŏs′kō-pē) [″ + Gr. *skopein,* to examine] Examination of capillaries for diagnostic purposes.

**capillary** (kăp′ĭ-lăr″ē) *pl.* **capillaries** [L. *capillaris,* hairlike] **1.** Any of the minute blood vessels, averaging 0.008 mm in diameter, that connect the ends of the smallest arteries (arterioles) with the beginnings of the smallest veins (venules). **2.** Pert. to a hair; hairlike.

***arterial c.*** One of the very small vessels that are the terminal branches of the arterioles or metarterioles.

***bile c.*** One of the intercellular biliary passageways that convey bile from liver cells to the interlobular bile ducts. SYN: *bile canaliculus.*

***blood c.*** One of the minute blood vessels that convey blood from the arterioles to the venules and form an anastomosing network that brings the blood into intimate relationship with the tissue cells. Its wall consists of a single layer of squamous cells (endothelium) through which oxygen diffuses to the tissue and products of metabolic activity enter the bloodstream. Blood capillaries average about 8 $\mu$m in diameter.

***venous c.*** One of the minute vessels that convey blood from a capillary network into the small veins (venules).

**capillary attraction** Capillarity.

**capillary nail refill test** Blanch test.

**capillary permeability** The ability of substances to diffuse through capillary walls into tissue spaces. It is influenced by hypoxia, adrenocortical hormone, and the concentration of calcium ions in the blood.

**capillus** (kă-pĭl′ŭs) *pl.* **capilli** [L., a hair] **1.** A hair, esp. of the head. **2.** A filament. **3.** A hair's breadth.

**capital** (căp′ĭ-tăl) [L. *capitalis*] Pert. to the head.

**capital punishment** Sentencing a criminal to death and carrying out the sentence via a legal method such as hanging, electrocution, or lethal injection.

**capitate** (kăp′ĭ-tāt) [L. *caput,* head] Head-shaped; having a rounded extremity.

**capitation fee** (kăp″ĭ-tā′shŭn) The amount paid a physician annually from each patient in a medical group plan.

**capitatum** (kăp″ĭ-tā′tŭm) Os capitatum; the third bone in the distal row of the carpus (i.e., the wrist). SYN: *os magnum.*

**capitellum** (kăp″ĭ-tĕl′ŭm) [L., small head] The round eminence at the lower end of the humerus articulating with the radius; the radial head of the humerus. SYN: *capitulum humeri.*

**capitula** [L.] Pl. of capitulum.

**capitular** (kă-pĭt′ū-lăr) Pert. to a capitulum.

**capitulum** (kă-pĭt′ū-lŭm, -pĭch′ŭ-lŭm) *pl.* **capitula** [L., small head] A small, rounded articular end of a bone.

***c. fibulae*** The proximal extremity or head of the fibula. It articulates with the tibia.

***c. humeri*** Capitellum.

***c. mallei*** In the middle ear, the head (the large rounded extremity) of the malleus. It carries the facet for the incus.

***c. stapedis*** The head of the stapes. It articulates with the lenticular process of the incus of the middle ear.

**Caplan's syndrome** [Anthony Caplan, Brit. physician, 1907–1976] Rheumatoid arthritis and pneumoconiosis with progressive massive fibrosis of the lung in coal workers. SYN: *pneumoconiosis*.

**Capnocytophaga** A genus of gram-negative, facultative, anaerobic bacteria that may be isolated from the oral cavity of humans and canines and are associated with serious systemic infections, esp. in asplenic patients.

***C. canimorsus*** A species associated with infections from dog bites. The resulting illness may be mild or life threatening. Alcoholics, splenectomized individuals, and those taking corticosteroids are esp. susceptible, but the illness can be fatal even in previously healthy people. Treatment consists of penicillin; it may be given prophylactically to asplenic patients following a dog bite.

**capnography** Continuous recording of the carbon dioxide level in expired air in mechanically ventilated patients.

**capnophilic** (kăp-nō-fĭl′ĭk) [Gr. *kapnos*, smoke, + *philein*, to love] Pert. to bacteria that grow best in an atmosphere containing carbon dioxide.

**capotement** (kă-pōt-mŏn′) [Fr.] A splashing sound that may be heard when the dilated stomach contains air and fluid.

**Capoten** Trade name for captopril.

**capping** (kăp′ĭng) **1.** Placing a protective substance over the exposed pulp of a tooth. **2.** Placing an artificial crown on a tooth for cosmetic purposes. **3.** In immunology, the aggregation of living B lymphocytes that have reacted with fluorescein-labeled anti-immune globulin cells to form a polar cap.

**capsicum** (kăp′sĭ-kŭm) The fruit of pepper plants, of which there are more than 200 varieties, including jalapeno and tabasco. The amount of chemicals in some peppers makes them too hot to eat. Even in amounts comfortable to ingest, peppers cause mucosal changes in the stomach that are consistent with irritation. In large doses, they can cause acute gastroenteritis.

**capsid** (kăp′sĭd) The protein covering around the central core of a virus. The capsid, which develops from protein units called protomers, protects the nucleic acid in the core of the virus from the destructive enzymes in biological fluids and promotes attachment of the virus to susceptible cells.

**capsitis** (kăp-sī′tĭs) [L. *capsa*, box, + Gr. *itis*, inflammation] Capsulitis of the crystalline lens of the eye.

**capsomer** (kăp′sō-mĕr) [″ + Gr. *meros*, part] Short ribbons of protein that make up a portion of the capsid of a virus.

**capsula** [L., little box] A sheath or continuous enclosure around an organ or structure.

***c. articularis*** The capsule of a joint.

***c. bulbi*** Tenon's capsule.

***c. fibrosa perivascularis*** Glisson's capsule.

***c. glomeruli*** Bowman's capsule.

***c. lentis*** The crystalline lens capsule of the eye.

**capsulae** (căp′sū-lē) [L.] Pl. of capsula.

**capsular** Pert. to a capsule.

**capsulation** Enclosure in a capsule.

**capsule** [L. *capsula*, little box] **1.** Capsula. **2.** A special container made of gelatin, sized for a single dose of a drug. The enclosure prevents the patient from tasting the drug.

***articular c.*** A two-layered sleeve or covering for a synovial joint. The inner layer is synovial and the outer is fibrous.

***auditory c.*** The embryonic cartilaginous capsule that encloses the developing ear.

***bacterial c.*** The membrane that surrounds some bacterial cells, offering protection against phagocytosis and allowing evasion of host defense mechanisms.

***Bowman's c.*** The glomerular capsule of the kidneys. SYN: *glomerular c.*

***cartilage c.*** The layer of matrix that forms the innermost portion of the wall of a lacuna enclosing a single cell or a group of cartilage cells. It is basophilic.

***Glisson's c.*** An outer capsule of fibrous tissue that covers the liver, its ducts, and its vessels. SYN: *capsula fibrosa perivascularis.*

***glomerular c.*** Bowman's capsule.

***joint c.*** The sleevelike membrane that encloses the ends of bones in a diarthrodial joint. It consists of an outer fibrous layer and an inner synovial layer and contains synovial fluid.

***c. of the kidney*** The fat-containing connective tissue surrounding the kidney.

***lens c.*** A transparent, structureless membrane that surrounds and encloses the lens of the eye.

***nasal c.*** The cartilaginous capsule that develops in the embryonic skull to enclose the nasal cavity.

***optic c.*** The cartilaginous capsule that develops in the embryonic skull to enclose the eye.

***otic c.*** The cartilaginous capsule that develops in the embryonic skull to enclose the ear.

***c. of Tenon*** The thin fibrous sac enveloping the eyeball, forming a socket in which it rotates.

***renal c.*** The fibrous capsule surrounding the kidney.

***suprarenal c.*** A tough connective tissue capsule that encloses the adrenal gland.

***temporomandibular joint c.*** The fibrous covering of the synovial joint between the skull and mandible on each side of the head.

**capsulectomy** (kăp″sū-lĕk′tō-mē) [L. *capsula*, little box, + Gr. *ektome*, excision] Surgical removal of a capsule.

**capsulitis** (kăp″sū-lī′tĭs) [″ + Gr. *itis*, inflammation] Inflammation of a capsule.

**capsulociliary** (kăp″sū-lō-sĭl′ē-ĕr-ē) [″ + *ciliaris*, pert. to the eyelashes] Pert. to the lens capsule and the ciliary structures of the eye.

**capsulolenticular** (kăp″sū-lō-lĕn-tĭk′ū-lăr) [″ + *lenticularis,* pert. to a lens] Pert. to the capsule of the eye and the lens.

**capsuloplasty** (kăp′sū-lō-plăs″tē) [″ + Gr. *plassein,* to mold] Plastic surgery of a capsule, esp. a joint capsule.

**capsulorrhaphy** (kăp″sū-lor′ă-fē) [″ + Gr. *rhaphe,* seam, ridge] Suture of a joint capsule or of a tear in a capsule.

**capsulotome** (kăp′sū-lō-tōm″) [″ + Gr. *tome,* incision] An instrument for incising the capsule of the crystalline lens.

**capsulotomy** (kăp″sū-lŏt′ō-mē) Cutting of a capsule of the lens or a joint.

***laser c.*** The use of a laser to make a hole in the capsule surrounding the lens of the eye to let light pass. Extracapsular removal of a cataract allows the capsule surrounding the lens to remain in the eye; however, if the capsule becomes cloudy, laser capsulotomy is needed.

**captopril** A drug that blocks the conversion of angiotensin I to angiotensin II. It is used in diagnosing renovascular hypertension that can be alleviated by surgery. In addition, it is useful in lowering the blood pressure of most patients with hypertension, in treating congestive heart failure, and in treating the vascular and renal crises that may occur in scleroderma. Trade name is Capoten.

**capture** In atomic physics, the joining of an elementary particle such as an electron or neutron with the atomic nucleus.

***ventricular c.*** The normal response of the ventricle of the heart to the electrical impulse from the electrical conducting system.

**caput** (kā′pŭt, kăp′ŭt) *pl.* **capita** [L.] **1.** The head. **2.** The chief extremity of an organ.

***c. medusae*** A plexus of dilated veins about the umbilicus seen in one form of cirrhosis of the liver (Cruveilhier-Baumgarten syndrome) and indicating portal vein obstruction. It may be seen in newborns.

***c. succedaneum*** Diffuse edema of the fetal scalp that crosses the suture lines. Head compression against the cervix impedes venous return, forcing serum into the interstitial tissues. The swelling reabsorbs within 1 to 3 days.

**Carafate** Trade name for sucralfate.

**carbachol** (kăr′bă-kŏl) A drug with action similar to that of acetylcholine. It is used intraocularly to produce miosis during eye surgery and topically to lower intraocular pressure in glaucoma.

**carbamazepine** (kăr-bă-măz′ĕ-pēn) A drug used for treatment of trigeminal neuralgia and temporal lobe epilepsy. It is used in psychiatry as a mood stabilizer in bipolar affective disorder. Trade name is Tegretol.

**carbamide** (kăr′bă-mīd, kăr-băm′ĭd) $CO(NH)_2$. Urea in an anhydrous, sterile powder form.

**carbaminohemoglobin** (kăr-băm″ĭ-nō-hē″mō-glō′bĭn) A chemical combination of carbon dioxide and hemoglobin.

**carbenicillin indanyl sodium** (kăr″bĕn-ĭ-sĭl′ĭn) A semisynthetic antibiotic of the penicillin group. Trade name is Geocillin.

**carbidopa** (kăr″bĭ-dō′pă) A drug used with levodopa in treating parkinsonism.

**carbinoxamine maleate** (kăr″bĭn-ŏk′să-mēn) An antihistamine and decongestant.

**carbohydrase** (kăr″bō-hī′drās) One of a group of enzymes (such as amylase and lactase) that hydrolyze carbohydrates.

**carbohydrate** (kăr″bō-hī′drāt) [L. *carbo,* carbon, + Gr. *hydor,* water] One of a group of chemical substances, including sugars, glycogen, starches, dextrins, and celluloses, that contain only carbon, oxygen, and hydrogen. Usually the ratio of hydrogen to oxygen is 2 : 1. Glucose and its polymers (including starch and cellulose) are estimated to be the most abundant organic chemical compounds on earth, surpassing in quantity even the great stores of fuel hydrocarbons beneath the earth's crust. Carbohydrates are one of the six classes of nutrients needed by the body (the others are proteins, fats, minerals, vitamins, and water).

Green plants use the sun's energy to combine carbon dioxide and water to form carbohydrates. Most plant carbohydrates (celluloses) are unavailable for direct metabolism by vertebrates. However, the bacteria present in the intestinal tracts of some vertebrates break down cellulose to molecules that can be absorbed. The human intestinal tract lacks the enzyme that splits cellulose into sugar molecules, but humans do split starch into maltose by means of their salivary and pancreatic amylase enzymes.

CLASSIFICATION: Carbohydrates are grouped according to the number of carbon atoms they contain and how many of the basic types are combined into larger molecules. The most common simple sugars, monosaccharides, contain five or six carbon atoms and are called pentoses and hexoses, respectively. Two monosaccharides linked together are called a disaccharide. A series (chain) of monosaccharides or disaccharides is called a polysaccharide. Ribose and deoxyribose are the most important pentoses; glucose, fructose, and galactose are the most important hexoses in human metabolism. The disaccharide sugars in the diet are maltose (2 D-glucose molecules), sucrose or cane sugar (glucose and fructose), and lactose or milk sugar (D-glucose and D-galactose). These sugars are split and eventually converted to glucose by enzyme action. The two important polysaccharides are starch and glycogen; the latter is called animal starch. The basic monosaccharide building block for both of these large polymers is glucose. Dietary starch and glycogen are metabolized first to glucose and then to carbon dioxide and water

**Classification of Important Carbohydrates**

| Classification | Examples | Some Properties |
|---|---|---|
| Monosaccharides $C_6H_{12}O_6$ | Glucose | Crystalline, sweet, very soluble, readily absorbed |
| Pentoses $C_5H_{10}O_5$ or $C_5H_{10}O_4$ | Ribose<br>Deoxyribose | Part of nucleic acid, RNA<br>Part of nucleic acid, DNA |
| Disaccharides $(C_6H_{10}O_5)_2 \cdot H_2O$ or $C_{12}H_{22}O_{11}$ hydrolyzed to simple sugars | Sucrose<br>Lactose<br>Maltose | Crystalline, sweet, soluble, digestible<br>Present in milk |
| Polysaccharides $(C_6H_{10}O_5)_n$ composed of many molecules of simple sugars. (Since polysaccharides can be composed of various numbers of monosaccharides and disaccharides, *n* refers to an unknown number of these groups.) | Starch<br>Dextrin<br>Cellulose<br>Glycogen | Amorphous, little or no flavor, less soluble. Vary in solubility and digestibility. |

in humans. SEE: table (Classification of Important Carbohydrates).

FUNCTION: Carbohydrates are a basic source of energy. They are stored in the body as glycogen in virtually all tissues, but principally in the liver and muscles. Carbohydrates can be mobilized from those sites, making these stores an important source of reserve energy.

DIGESTION AND ABSORPTION: Cooked but not raw starch is broken down to disaccharide by salivary amylase. Both cooked and raw starches are split in the small intestine by pancreatic amylase. Disaccharides cannot be absorbed until they have been split into monosaccharides by the enzymes present in the brush border of cells lining the intestinal tract. Glucose and galactose are the actively absorbed sugars. Fructose is absorbed by diffusion. SEE: table (Digestion of Carbohydrates).

METABOLISM: Although very complex at the molecular level, carbohydrate metabolism can be explained as follows. Carbohydrates are absorbed as glucose, galactose, or fructose. Fructose and galactose are converted to glucose by the liver and are then available for energy production, or they may be stored after conversion to glycogen. The glycogen is available for metabolism to glucose whenever reserve energy is needed. SEE: *muscle metabolism.*

SOURCES: Carbohydrates are present in food in digestible and indigestible forms. The digestible type are an important source of energy. Those that cannot be used, usually some form of cellulose, are beneficial in adding bulk to the diet. Whole grains, vegetables, legumes (peas and beans), tubers (potatoes), fruits, honey, and refined sugar are excellent sources of carbohydrate. Calories derived from sugar and candy have been termed "empty" calories because these foods lack essential amino acids, vitamins, and minerals. SEE: *fiber, dietary.*

NUTRITION: Carbohydrates contain 4.1 kcal/g and are esp. useful as a source of energy. As indicated, however, some forms are virtually devoid of dietary essentials other than calories.

**carbohydrate loading** Dietary manipulation to enhance the amount of glycogen stored in muscle tissue. This technique is used by athletes before high-intensity en-

**Digestion of Carbohydrates**

| Enzyme | Produced in | Carbohydrates Digested | End Product |
|---|---|---|---|
| Sucrase (invertase) | Small intestine | Sucrose | Glucose and fructose |
| Maltases | Small intestine and mucosal cells of small intestine | Maltose | Two D-glucose |
| Lactase | Small intestine | Lactose | D-glucose and D-galactose |
| Salivary amylase | Saliva (mouth) | Cooked starch, glycogen, and dextrins | Maltose |
| Pancreatic amylase | Pancreas | Raw and cooked starch and glycogen | Maltose |

durance events such as a marathon foot race. Phase I is begun 7 days before competition. It depletes glycogen from specific muscles used in the event by exercise to exhaustion in the sport for which the athlete is preparing. The glycogen exhaustion is maintained by a high-fat, high-protein diet for 3 days. It is important to include 100 g of carbohydrate to prevent ketosis. Phase II consists of a high-carbohydrate diet of at least 1000 to 2000 kcal for 3 days. This is called the supersaturation phase because the goal is to enhance glycogen storage. Glycogen synthesis is facilitated by the extended period of depletion in phase I. Carbohydrates used should be complex ones (as in grain-derived foods such as bread and pasta) rather than simple carbohydrates (as in candy and soft drinks). Phase III begins on the day of the event. Any type of food may be eaten up to 4 to 6 hr before competition. Food eaten from that time up to the time of competition is a matter of individual preference.

**carbolize** (kăr′bŏl-īz) To mix with or add carbolic acid.

**carbon** [L. *carbo,* carbon] SYMB: C. The nonmetallic element that is the characteristic constituent of organic compounds; atomic weight 12.0111, atomic number 6.

Carbon occurs in two pure forms, diamond and graphite, and in impure form in charcoal, coke, and soot. Its compounds are constituents of all living tissue. Carbon combines with hydrogen, nitrogen, and oxygen to form the basis of all organic matter. Organic carbon compounds provide energy in foods.

***impregnated c.*** An electrode having a carbon shell with a core of various metals or salts of metals for use in a carbon arc lamp.

**carbon-14** SYMB: $^{14}C$. A radioactive isotope of carbon with a half-life of 5600 years. It is used as a tracer in metabolic studies and in archeology to date materials containing carbon.

**carbonate** (kăr′bŏn-āt) [L. *carbo,* carbon] Any salt of carbonic acid.

***c. of soda*** Sodium carbonate used commercially in crude form, such as washing soda. The free alkali present is irritating and in strong concentrations has the effect of sodium hydroxide.

**carbon dioxide** SYMB: $CO_2$. A colorless gas that is heavier than air and is produced in the combustion or decomposition of carbon or its compounds. It is the final metabolic product of carbon compounds present in food. The body eliminates $CO_2$ through the lungs, in urine, and in perspiration. It is also given off by decomposition of vegetable and animal matter and is formed by alcoholic fermentation as in rising bread. Green plants absorb it directly from the air and use it in photosynthesis. Approx. 1 sq m of leaf surface can absorb the $CO_2$ from 2500 L of air in 1 hr. An acre of trees uses an estimated 4½ tons (4082 kg) of $CO_2$ a year. Commercially, $CO_2$ gas is used in carbonated drinks and the solid form is used to make dry ice.

***c.d. combining power*** The amount of carbon dioxide that the blood serum can hold in chemical combination. $CO_2$ in aqueous solution forms carbonic acid; the amount of this acid that the blood serum can take up is a measure of its reserve power to prevent acidosis. The normal amount is 50 to 70 ml/dl of blood (usually expressed as 50 to 70 vol%). Values below 50 indicate acidosis; above 70, alkalosis.

***c.d. inhalation*** Inspiration of oxygen and carbon dioxide. It is used as an accessory during artificial respiration and as a continuation of resuscitation after the return of spontaneous breathing. It is also used to stimulate respiration in patients with pulmonary diseases.

***c.d. poisoning*** Toxicity from carbon dioxide inhalation. In small quantities (up to about 5%) in inspired air, $CO_2$ stimulates respiration in humans; in greater quantities it produces an uncomfortable degree of mental activity with confusion. Although not toxic in low concentrations, $CO_2$ can cause death by suffocation. Poisoning is rarely fatal unless exposure occurs in a closed space.

SYMPTOMS: Symptoms include extremely deep breathing, a sensation of pressure in the head, ringing in the ears, an acid taste in the mouth, and a slight burning in the nose. Within a short time, respiration almost ceases and the patient becomes unconscious.

TREATMENT: The patient should be removed to fresh air and given artificial respiration and oxygen inhalation.

***c.d. solid therapy*** Solid carbon dioxide ($CO_2$ snow) used for therapeutic refrigeration. Solid $CO_2$ has a temperature of −80°C. Its application to the skin for 1 to 2 sec causes superficial frostbite; 4 to 5 sec, a blister; 10 to 15 sec, superficial necrosis; and 15 to 45 sec, ulceration. It is used mostly for removal of certain nevi and warts, occasionally for telangiectasia.

**carbonemia** (kăr″bō-nē′mē-ă) [L. *carbo,* carbon, + Gr. *haima,* blood] An excess accumulation of carbonic acid in the blood.

**carbonic** Pert. to carbon.

***c. acid*** $H_2CO_3$. Acid resulting from a mixture of carbon dioxide and water.

***c. anhydrase*** An enzyme that catalyzes union of water and carbon dioxide to form carbonic acid, or performs the reverse action. It is present in red blood cells.

**carbonize** (kăr′bŏn-īz) To char or convert into charcoal.

**carbon monoxide** SYMB: CO. A poisonous gas resulting from the inefficient and incomplete combustion of coal. Colorless, tasteless, and odorless, it cannot be detected by the senses. Carbon monoxide is distributed widely because of imperfect

**Toxic Symptoms of Carbon Monoxide**

| Carbon Monoxide Concentration | | |
|---|---|---|
| **Percent in Air** | **Parts Per Million** | **Response** |
| 0.005 | 50 | No apparent toxic symptoms. |
| 0.01 | 100 | Can be tolerated for several hr without symptoms. |
| 0.02 | 200 | Possible mild frontal headache in 2–3 hr. |
| 0.08 | 800 | Headache, dizziness, and nausea in 45 min; collapse and possible unconsciousness in 2 hr. |
| 0.16 | 1600 | Headache, dizziness, and nausea in 20 min; collapse and possible death in 2 hr. |
| 0.32 | 3200 | Headache and dizziness in 5–10 min; unconsciousness and possible death in 10–15 min. |
| 0.64 | 6400 | Headache and dizziness in 1–2 min; possible death in 10–15 min. |
| 1.28 | 12,800 | Immediate unconsciousness; possible death in 1–3 min. |

SOURCE: Adapted from Hamilton, A and Hardy, H: Industrial Technology, ed 3. Publishing Sciences Group, Littleton, MA, 1974.

combustion and oxidation and is found in illuminating gas, in the exhaust gas from the internal combustion engines in most motor-powered vehicles, and in sewers, cellars, and mines.

***c.m. poisoning*** Toxicity that results from inhalation of small amounts of carbon monoxide over a long period or from large amounts inhaled for a short time. For example, riding in a closed automobile or parking in an automobile in an enclosed space with the motor running may cause death from inhalation of these noxious fumes, which may come from leaking exhausts and exhaust heaters. Another cause of death is the operation of a gasoline motor in an enclosed area such as a closed garage or basement. Carbon monoxide poisoning results from a chemical combination of this gas with the hemoglobin of the blood, preventing blood from carrying oxygen to the tissues. Because this combination is relatively stable, patients may need prolonged periods of oxygen administration in addition to artificial respiration. The affinity of carbon monoxide for hemoglobin is more than 200 times as great as that of oxygen. Therefore exposure to carbon monoxide causes a marked reduction in the ability of the blood to transport oxygen. SEE: *Poisons and Poisoning Appendix*.

SYMPTOMS: The symptoms of carbon monoxide poisoning are somewhat variable. Respiration is deep and difficult. Carboxyhemoglobin (COHb), the substance formed when carbon monoxide combines with hemoglobin, is cherry red. The tissues and skin of individuals with carbon monoxide poisoning and a carboxyhemoglobin level of 30% or greater are much pinker than normal. Their appearance has been described as "cherry red." The pulse may be slowed initially but soon increases. There may be pounding of the heart, dizziness is frequent, and muscular function may be so weakened that the individual is unable to stand. There may be ringing in the ears, throbbing in the temples, headache, faintness and nausea, and dilated pupils. A patient who is breathing when found usually recovers when brought into fresh air and given stimulants. SEE: table.

TREATMENT: The person should be removed immediately from exposure to carbon monoxide. Using a tight-fitting mask, 100% oxygen is given, under pressure (hyperbaric) if possible. Artificial respiration should be used if indicated. The patient should be kept absolutely quiet and immobile to reduce the body's oxygen requirements. If cerebral edema develops, 50 ml of 50% glucose and 1 mg/kg of prednisone are given intravenously every 4 hr as needed. If hypotension is present it should be corrected; cardiac function is monitored and altered function treated as indicated. A sedative such as diazepam may be needed if the patient becomes excited during recovery.

COMPLICATIONS: When such patients recover, they often have some nervous system involvement including various types of paralysis, blindness, interference with sensation, muscular spasms, or twitchings for an indefinite period. Most of these complications disappear in time, but occasionally they remain permanently.

**carbon tetrachloride** (tĕt″ră-klō′rīd) SYMB: $CCl_4$. A clear, colorless liquid, not flammable, with an ethereal odor like that of chloroform. Although having narcotic and anesthetic properties resembling chloroform, it is too toxic to be suitable as an anesthetic or for any medical use. Inhalation of a small quantity can produce death by means of acute atrophy of the liver and kidney.

***c.t. poisoning*** Toxic effects due to prolonged inhalation of carbon tetrachloride. Symptoms are irritation of the eyes, nose, and throat, headache, confusion, central nervous system depression, ventricular fibrillation, visual disturbances, nausea, and anorexia.

FIRST AID: Clothes contaminated with carbon tetrachloride are removed. Oxygen inhalation and artificial respiration, and lavage with saline solution, are given. Saline cathartic should be left in the stomach. SEE: *Poisons and Poisoning Appendix.*

**carbonuria** (kăr″bō-nū′rē-ă) [L. *carbo,* carbon, + Gr. *ouron,* urine] The presence or excretion of carbon compounds in the urine.

**carbonyl** (kăr′bŏn-ĭl) [″ + Gr. *hyle,* matter] The divalent radical carbon monoxide, characteristic of aldehydes and ketones.

**carboplatin** A cytotoxic, platinum-containing drug used in treating ovarian cancer. SEE: *cisplatin.*

**carboxyhemoglobin** (kăr-bŏk″sē-hē″mō-glō′bĭn) [″ + Gr. *oxys,* acid, + *haima,* blood, + L. *globus,* sphere] A compound formed by carbon monoxide and hemoglobin in carbon monoxide poisoning.

**carboxyhemoglobinemia** The presence of carboxyhemoglobin in the blood. SEE: *carbon monoxide poisoning.*

**carboxyl** (kăr-bŏk′sĭl) The characteristic group (COOH) of organic carboxylic acids, such as formic acid (HCOOH) and acetic acid ($CH_2COOH$).

**carboxylase** (kăr-bŏk′sĭ-lās) An enzyme that catalyzes the removal of the carboxyl group (COOH) from amino acids. Found in brewer's yeast, it catalyzes the decarboxylation of pyruvic acid by producing acetaldehyde and carbon dioxide. In the body, this process requires the presence of vitamin $B_1$ (thiamine), which acts as a coenzyme.

**carboxylation** In chemistry, the replacement of hydrogen by a carboxyl (—COOH) molecule.

**carboxylic acid** One of a group of organic acids that contain the carboxyl (—COOH) group.

**carboxylmethylcellulose sodium** A chemical used as a pharmaceutical aid and a food additive.

**carbuncle, carbunculus** (kăr′bŭng″k′l, kăr-bŭng′kū-lŭs) [L. *carbunculus,* small glowing ember] A circumscribed inflammation of the skin and deeper tissues that terminates in a slough and suppuration and is accompanied by marked constitutional symptoms. **carbuncular** (-bŭng′kū-lăr), *adj.*

SYMPTOMS: The lesion is marked by a painful node, at first covered by tight reddened skin that later becomes thin and perforates, discharging pus through several openings. Fever, leukocytosis, and sometimes prostration may accompany the lesion. The most common sites are the nape of the neck, the upper back, and the buttocks.

ETIOLOGY: Staphylococci are the causative agents. Predisposing factors are the same as in a furuncle. Persons with diabetes are particularly susceptible.

TREATMENT: Antibiotics given systemically are usually effective. Incision and drainage may be performed when the lesion is about to point (come to a head). The area should be covered with warm compresses to promote blood supply.

NURSING IMPLICATIONS: Universal precautions are observed in assessing or caring for the patient. Sterile technique is used in re-dressing the lesion, and dressings are changed frequently to facilitate drainage and promote healing. All contaminated equipment is disinfected, and soiled dressings are disposed of correctly. Both patient and family are instructed to avoid contact with wound drainage and to prevent spread of infection by thorough handwashing, disinfecting contaminated linens and equipment, and disposing of dressings in an impermeable, sealable bag. SEE: *Universal Precautions Appendix.*

**carbunculosis** (kăr-bŭng″kū-lō′sĭs) [″ + Gr. *osis,* condition] The appearance of several carbuncles in succession.

**carbutamide** (kăr-bū′tă-mīd) An oral hypoglycemic agent.

**carcass** (kăr′kăs) A dead body; usually applied to nonhuman bodies.

**carcinogen** (kăr′sĭn-, kăr-sĭn′ō-jĕn) Any substance or agent that produces cancer or increases the risk of developing cancer in humans or lower animals.

***chemical c.*** Any chemical substance capable of causing cancer.

**carcinogenesis** (kăr″sĭ-nō-jĕn′ĕ-sĭs) [Gr. *karkinos,* crab, + *genesis,* generation, birth] The production or origin of cancer.

**carcinogenic** (kăr″sĭ-nō-jĕn′ĭk) Producing cancer.

**carcinoid** (kăr′sĭ-noid) [″ + *eidos,* form, shape] A tumor derived from the argentaffin cells in the intestinal tract, bile ducts, pancreas, bronchus, or ovary. It secretes serotonin (5-hydroxytryptamine) and other vasoactive substances.

**carcinoid syndrome** A condition produced by metastatic carcinoid tumors that secrete excessive amounts of serotonin. Serotonin is metabolized to 5-hydroxyindoleacetic acid (5-HIAA).

SYMPTOMS: One or more of the following may occur: brief episodes of flushing, esp. of the face and neck, tachycardia, facial and periorbital edema, hypotension, intermittent abdominal pain with diarrhea, valvular heart lesions, weight loss, hypoproteinemia, and signs of pellagra. The latter symptom reflects the ability of tryptophan to partially compensate for a niacin deficiency. In the syndrome, however, tryptophan is used to synthesize serotonin and is not available for that function.

DIAGNOSIS: The diagnosis is based on clinical presentation and greatly increased excretion of 5-HIAA in urine. Some foods, including bananas, pineapples, tomatoes, walnuts, avocados, and certain drugs, can cause an increased level of this chemical.

TREATMENT: Surgery, except in the case of an isolated tumor, is not indicated. A high-protein diet with nicotinamide supplement is used to prevent pellagra. A serotonin antagonist is given to control diarrhea and malabsorption. Somatostatin and its analogues have been effective in inhibiting flushing and diarrhea and reversing hypotension.

**carcinolysis** (kăr″sĭ-nŏl′ĭ-sĭs) [Gr. *karkinos,* crab, + *lysis,* dissolution] Destruction of carcinoma cells. **carcinolytic** (-nō-lĭt′ĭk), *adj.*

**carcinoma** (kăr″sĭ-nō′mă) [″ + *oma,* tumor] A new growth or malignant tumor that occurs in epithelial tissue. These neoplasms tend to infiltrate and produce metastases. It may affect almost any organ or part of the body and spread by direct extension, through lymphatics, or through the bloodstream. The etiology is unknown. SYN: *cancer.*

***alveolar cell c.*** A type of lung carcinoma.

***basal cell c.*** A skin malignancy that rarely metastasizes. Typically it begins as a small, shiny papule that is difficult to distinguish from discrete dermatitis. The lesion enlarges to form a whitish border around a central depression or ulcer that may bleed. When the lesion reaches this stage, it is often called a rodent ulcer. After biopsy, the removal method used is determined by the size, location, and appearance of the lesion. SEE: illus.

***bronchogenic c.*** A malignant lung tumor that originates in the bronchi and is usually associated with cigarette smoking. The most common bronchogenic tumors are squamous cell or epidermoid tumors. Oat cell and adenocarcinoma are the next most common tumors.

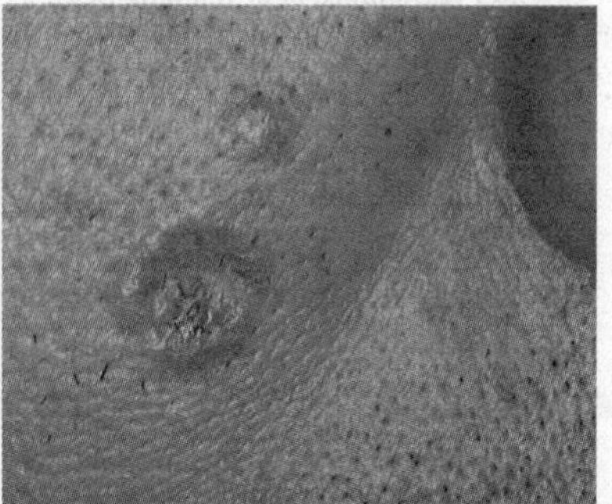

EARLY BASAL CELL CARCINOMA

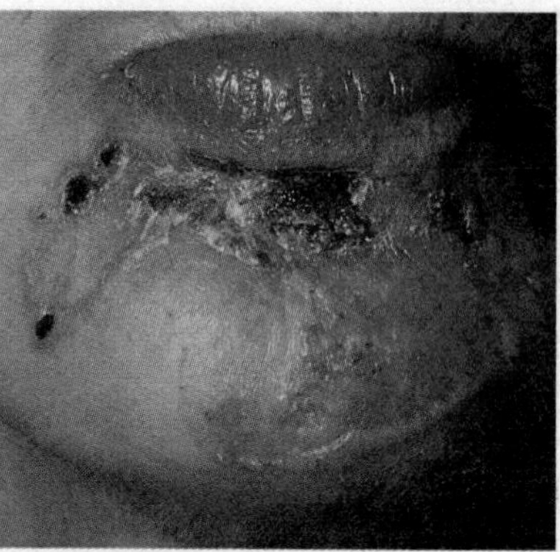

NEGLECTED BASAL CELL CARCINOMA

TREATMENT: Surgery is the most effective treatment. More than one half of the tumors are advanced and inoperable when diagnosed. The prognosis for patients with bronchogenic carcinoma is very poor, with the 5-year survival rate less than 10%.

***chorionic c.*** Choriocarcinoma.

***embryonal c.*** Malignant teratoma.

***epidermoid c.*** A tumor on a surface, such as the skin. It is usually one of two types: a wartlike growth, slow growing and mildly malignant; or a flat, rapidly infiltrating neoplasm.

***giant cell c.*** Carcinoma marked by the presence of unusually large cells.

***glandular c.*** Adenocarcinoma.

***c. in situ*** ABBR: CIS. Malignant cell changes in the epithelial tissue that do not extend beyond the basement membrane.

***medullary c.*** Carcinoma that is soft because of the predominance of cells and in which there is little fibrous tissue.

***melanotic c.*** Carcinoma containing melanin.

***mucinous c.*** Carcinoma in which the glandular tissue secretes mucin.

***oat cell c.*** A poorly differentiated tumor of the bronchus that contains small oat-shaped cells.

***scirrhous c.*** Hard cancer.

***squamous cell c.*** Epidermoid carcinoma that develops primarily from squamous cells. SEE: illus.

**carcinomatophobia** (kăr″sĭ-nō″mă-tō-fō′bē-ă) [Gr. *karkinos,* crab, + *oma,* tumor, + *phobos,* fear] Morbid fear of cancer.

**carcinomatosis** (kăr″sĭ-nō″mă-tō′sĭs) [″ + ″ + *osis,* condition] Widespread dissemination of carcinoma in the body. SYN: *car-*

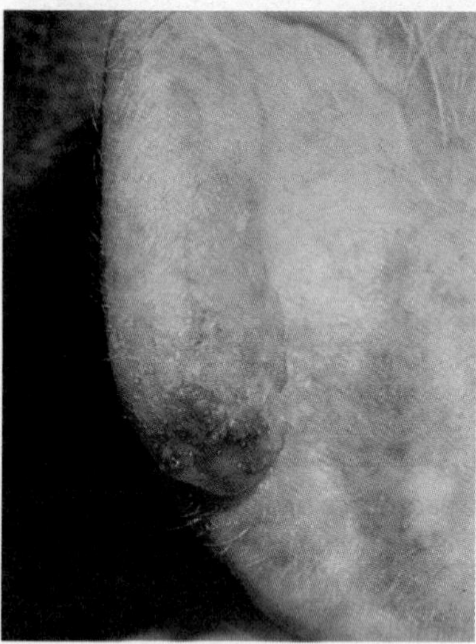

EARLY SQUAMOUS CELL CARCINOMA ON EAR

*cinosis.*

**carcinophilia** (kăr″sĭ-nō-fĭl′ē-ă) [″ + *philos,* love] An affinity for cancer cells.

**carcinosarcoma** (kăr″sĭ-nō-săr-kō′mă) [″ + *sarx,* flesh, + *oma,* tumor] A malignant tumor containing the elements of both carcinoma and sarcoma.

***embryonal c.*** A malignant germ-cell tumor derived from embryonic cells.

**carcinosis** (kăr″sĭ-nō′sĭs) [″ + *osis,* condition] Carcinomatosis.

**cardamom, cardamon** [Gr. *kardamomon*] The dried ripe fruit of an herb, *Elettaria repens* or *E. cardamomum.* It is used as an aromatic and carminative.

**Cardarelli's sign** (kăr″dă-rĕl′lēz) [Antonio Cardarelli, It. physician, 1831–1926] Pulsating movement of the trachea to one side. It may be present with aortic aneurysm.

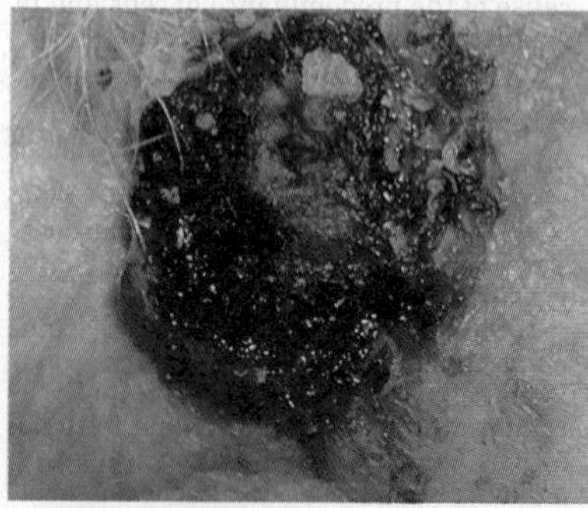

NEGLECTED SQUAMOUS CELL CARCINOMA OF FACE

**cardi-** SEE: *cardio-.*

**cardia** (kăr′dē-ă) [Gr. *kardia,* heart] The upper orifice of the stomach connecting with the esophagus.

**cardiac** (kăr′dē-ăk) [L. *cardiacus*] **1.** Pert. to the heart. **2.** Pert. to the cardia.

**cardiac arrest** Sudden cessation of functional circulation. The care of a patient suffering from a cardiac arrest begins with institution of basic life support measures as soon as possible. This intervention may be carried out by physicians, nurses, paramedical personnel, or trained lay persons. Thereafter, advanced life support measures are begun as soon as possible followed by postresuscitation care. The long-term management of patients after survival of cardiac arrest occurring out of hospital is guided by diagnosis of the disease process associated with the arrest. The overall rate of survival in the 2-year period following out-of-hospital cardiac arrest is about 40%. SEE: *cardiopulmonary resuscitation.*

***sudden c.a.*** ABBR: SCA. Sudden death due to cardiac causes rather than to trauma. The event begins with an abrupt loss of consciousness within 1 hr of the onset of acute symptoms. SCA occurs most commonly in individuals with known preexisting heart disease, but in whom the time and mode of death were unexpected. SEE: *cardiopulmonary resuscitation* for illus.; *advanced cardiac life support; cardiac arrest; cardiovascular collapse.*

ETIOLOGY: Cessation of cardiac function is most often associated with ventricular fibrillation. Almost any structural abnormality of the heart, such as coronary artery disease, myocarditis, cardiac hypertrophy, valvular heart disease, or disease of the electrical conducting system, can cause sudden cardiac failure. Other conditions that may contribute to SCA are cardiotoxic agents such as drugs of abuse or digitalis intoxication. The most important risk factors for SCD are age, hypertension, left ventricular hypertrophy, cigarette smoking, elevated serum cholesterol levels, and obesity. The more risk factors an individual has, the greater the chance of developing SCA.

PREVENTION: Therapy is directed to reduction or control of the risk factors. Because the majority of SCA cases occur in persons with few, if any, of the risk factors, better methods for identifying and controlling the unpredictable components are needed.

**cardiac catheterization** Percutaneous intravascular insertion of a catheter into any chamber of the heart or great vessels for diagnosis, assessment of abnormalities, interventional treatment, and evaluation of the effects of pathology on the heart and great vessels. Diagnostic tests include radiography, blood sampling, and measurement of pressure and cardiac output.

NURSING IMPLICATIONS: *Precatheterization:* The nurse prepares the patient physically and emotionally by explaining the procedure and expected sensations. The patient's vital signs, including the presence and intensity of peripheral pulses, are assessed to establish a baseline measure. Anxiety and activity levels are documented, as well as the presence and pattern of any chest pain. Any known allergies, particularly to shellfish or iodine (suggestive of sensitivity to radiopaque dye), are also documented, and the cardiologist is alerted to these allergies or any changes in the patient's condition. The groin is shaved and cleansed, and the patient is informed that an oral or intravenous mild sedative (rather than general anesthesia) will probably be given before or during the procedure, so that he or she is able to cough and breathe deeply as instructed during testing. A radiopaque contrast medium is injected into the arteries and nitroglycerin may be administered to aid visualization. After the injection, the patient may feel light-headed, warm, or nauseated for a few moments. The patient will have to lie on the back for several hours after the procedure and should report chest pain immediately both during and after the procedure.

*During catheterization:* The nurse assists with the procedure according to protocol by monitoring cardiac pressures and rhythm and the results of hemodynamic studies. Patient comfort and safety are assured; and changes in emotional status, level of consciousness, and verbal and nonverbal responses are assessed to determine the patient's response to the procedure and need for reassurance or medication to prevent vasovagal reactions or coronary artery spasm. Any complications, such as cardiac dysrhythmias or allergic reaction to the contrast medium, are also evaluated and reported.

*Postcatheterization:* The nurse provides emotional support to the patient and answers questions. Cardiac rhythm and vital signs (including apical pulse and temperature) are monitored until stable according to protocol (usually every 15 min for the first 1 to 2 hr) or more frequently as the patient's condition requires. The blood pressure should not be checked in any limb used for catheter insertion. As bleeding poses the most serious risk, the dressing is inspected frequently for signs of bleeding, and the patient is instructed to report any increase in dressing tightness (which may indicate hematoma formation). Pressure is applied over the entry site and the extremity is maintained in extension according to protocol (pressure dressing, sandbag; 3 to 8 hr). The patient is cautioned to avoid flexion or hyperextension of the affected limb for another 12 to 24 hr depending on protocol.

Neurovascular status of the involved extremity distal to the insertion site is monitored for changes, which may indicate arterial thrombosis (the most frequent complication), embolus, or another complication requiring immediate attention. The head of the bed is elevated no more than 30 degrees, and the patient is confined to bedrest according to protocol, usually 2 to 3 hr for a brachial site or 6 hr for a femoral site, or until fluid balance is restored (angiographic contrast medium may cause osmotic diuresis). The patient may complain of urinary urgency immediately after the procedure. Fluids are given orally to flush out the dense radiopaque contrast medium, and urine output is monitored, esp. in patients with impaired renal function. The patient is assessed for complications such as pericardial tamponade, myocardial infarction, pulmonary embolism, stroke, congestive heart failure, cardiac dysrhythmia, infection, and thrombophlebitis. The patient's preoperative medication regimen is resumed as prescribed (or revised). Postprocedural pain is managed and any unusually severe pain at the catheter insertion site or involved extremity or any chest discomfort is documented and reported.

The patient will need to be driven home, and a responsible adult should be in attendance until the next morning. Both patient and family are provided with written discharge instructions explaining the need to report any of the following symptoms to the physician: bleeding or swelling at the entry site; increased tenderness; redness; drainage or pain at the entry site; fever; and any changes in color, temperature, or sensation in the involved extremity. The patient may take acetaminophen or other nonaspirin analgesic every 3 to 4 hr as needed for pain. The entry site should be covered with an adhesive bandage for 24 hr or until stitches, if present, are removed (usually within 6 days). The patient usually is permitted to shower the day after the procedure and to take a tub bath 48 hr after the procedure (if no sutures are present). Strenuous activity should be avoided for 24 hr after the procedure. The patient is scheduled for a follow-up appointment. SEE: *Nursing Diagnoses Appendix.*

**cardiac compensation** The ability of the heart to compensate for impaired valvular functioning through its reserve power.

**cardiac failure** A condition resulting from the heart's inability to pump sufficient blood to meet the body's needs. SEE: *heart failure.*

**cardiac hypertrophy** SEE: *hypertrophy, heart.*

**cardiac insufficiency** Inadequate cardiac output due to failure of the heart to function properly, as in valvular deficiency.

**cardiac massage** SEE: *cardiopulmonary resuscitation.*

**cardiac output** The amount of blood discharged from the left or right ventricle per minute. For an average adult at rest, cardiac output is approx. 3.0 L per sq m of body surface area each minute. Cardiac output is determined by multiplying the stroke volume by the heart rate. SYN: *minute volume.*

**cardiac output, decreased** A state in which the blood pumped by the heart is inadequate to meet the metabolic demands of the body. (NOTE: In a hypermetabolic state, although cardiac output may be within normal range, it may still be inadequate to meet the needs of the body's tissues. Cardiac output and tissue perfusion are interrelated, although there are differences. When cardiac output is decreased, tissue perfusion problems will develop; however, tissue perfusion problems can exist without decreased cardiac output.) SEE: *Nursing Diagnoses Appendix.*

**cardiac plexus** Plexus cardiacus; the nerve plexus at the base of the heart made up of branches of the vagus nerves and sympathetic trunks. Afferent nerves from this plexus provide the nerve supply to the heart.

**cardiac reflex** An involuntary response consisting of a change in cardiac rate. Stimulation of sensory nerve endings in the wall of the carotid sinus by increased arterial blood pressure reflexively slows the heart (Marey's law). Stimulation of vagus fibers in the right side of the heart by increased venous return reflexively increases the heart rate (Bainbridge's reflex).

**cardiac reserve** The capacity of the heart to increase cardiac output and raise blood pressure above basal pressure to meet body requirements.

**cardiac surgery** SEE: *Nursing Diagnoses Appendix.*

**cardiac troponin I** A protein that is a highly sensitive and specific indicator of myocardial infarction.

**cardiac troponin T** ABBR: cTnT. A muscle protein, not normally present in blood, that can be detected in the blood following myocardial injury. Assay of this material in the blood can provide a rapid test for myocardial infarction. Bedside detection methods are available.

**cardialgia** (kăr″dē-ăl′jē-ă) [Gr. *kardia,* heart, + *algos,* pain] Pain at the pit of the stomach or region of the heart, usually occurring in paroxysms.

**cardiaortic** (kăr″dē-ā-or′tĭk) [″ + *aorte,* aorta] Pert. to the heart and aorta.

**cardiasthenia** (kăr″dē-ăs-thē′nē-ă) [″ + *astheneia,* weakness] A type of neurasthenia with predominance of cardiac symptoms.

**cardiasthma** (kăr″dē-ăz′mă) [″ + *asthma,* panting] Dyspnea due to heart disease.

**cardiectasia, cardiectasis** (kăr″dē-ĕk-tā′sē-ă, -ĕk′tă-sĭs) [″ + *ektasis,* dilatation] Dilatation of the heart.

**cardiectomy** (kăr″dē-ĕk′tō-mē) [″ + *ektome,* excision] Excision of the cardiac end of the stomach.

**cardinal** [LL. *cardinalis,* important] Of primary importance, as in the cardinal symptoms: temperature, pulse, and respiration.

**cardio-, cardi-** [Gr. *kardia,* heart] Combining form meaning *heart.*

**cardioaccelerator** (kăr″dē-ō-ăk-sĕl′ĕr-ā-tor) [″ + L. *accelerare,* to hasten] Something that increases the rate of the heartbeat.

**cardioactive** (kăr″dē-ō-ăk′tĭv) [″ + L. *activus,* acting] Acting on the heart.

**cardioangiography** (kăr″dē-ō-ăn″jē-ŏg′ră-fē) [″ + *angeion,* vessel, + *graphein,* to write] Angiocardiography.

**cardioangiology** (kăr″dē-ō-ăn″jē-ŏl′ō-jē) [″ + ″ + *logos,* word, reason] The science of the heart and blood vessels.

**cardioaortic** (kăr″dē-ō-ā-or′tĭk) [″ + *aorte,* aorta] Pert. to the heart and the aorta.

**cardiocele** (kăr′dē-ō-sēl) [″ + *kele,* tumor, swelling] A herniation or protrusion of the heart through an opening in the diaphragm or through a wound.

**cardiocentesis** Cardiopuncture.

**cardiochalasia** (kăr″dē-ō-kă-lā′zē-ă) [″ + *chalasis,* relaxation] Relaxation of the muscles of the cardiac sphincter of the stomach.

**cardiocirrhosis** (kăr″dē-ō-sĭr-rō′sĭs) [″ + *kirrhos,* orange-yellow, + *osis,* condition] Cirrhosis of the liver with heart disease.

**cardiodiaphragmatic** (kăr″dē-ō-dī″ă-frăg-măt′ĭk) Concerning the heart and the diaphragm.

**cardiodilator** (kăr″dē-ō-dī′lā-tor) [″ + L. *dilatare,* to enlarge] A device for dilating the cardia of the gastroesophageal junction.

**cardiodynamics** (kăr″dē-ō-dī-năm′ĭks) The science of the forces involved in propulsion of blood from the heart to the tissues and back to the heart.

**cardiodynia** (kăr″dē-ō-dĭn′ē-ă) [Gr. *kardia,* heart, + *odyne,* pain] Pain in the region of the heart.

**cardioesophageal** Pert. to the junction of the esophagus and the stomach.

**cardioesophageal reflux** SEE: *gastroesophageal reflux.*

**cardiogenesis** (kăr″dē-ō-jĕn′ĕ-sĭs) [″ + *genesis,* generation, birth] Formation and growth of the embryonic heart.

**cardiogenic** (kăr″dē-ō-jĕn′ĭk) [″ + *gennan,* to produce] Originating in the heart.

**cardiogram** (kăr′dē-ō-grăm″) [″ + *gramma,* something written] A graph of the electrical activity of the heart muscle, made with an electrocardiograph machine. SYN: *electrocardiogram.*

**cardiograph** (kăr′dē-ō-grăf″) [″ + *graphein,* to write] A device for registering the electrical activity of the heart muscle.

**cardiography** (kăr″dē-ŏg′ră-fē) The recording and study of the electrical activity of the heart. **cardiographic** (-ō-grăf′ĭk), *adj.*

**cardiohepatic** (kăr″dē-ō-hĕ-păt′ĭk) [″ + *he-*

*patos,* liver] Pert. to the heart and liver.

**cardiohepatomegaly** (kăr″dē-ō-hĕp″ă-tō-mĕg′ă-lē) [″ + ″ + *megas,* large] Enlargement of the heart and liver.

**cardioinhibitory** (kăr″dē-ō-ĭn-hĭb′ĭ-tō-rē) [″ + L. *inhibere,* to check] Inhibiting the action of the heart.

**cardiokinetic** (kăr″dē-ō-kĭ-nĕt′ĭk) [″ + *kinesis,* movement] Pert. to the action of the heart.

**cardiokymography** ABBR: CKG. The radiographic method of recording the outline of the heart as it beats. Its usefulness in clinical medicine has not been shown.

**cardiolipin** (kăr″dē-ō-lĭp′ĭn) [″ + *lipos,* fat] Previously used term for diphosphatidylglycerol.

**cardiolith** (kăr′dē-ō-lĭth″) [″ + *lithos,* stone] A concretion or calculus in the heart.

**cardiologist** (kăr-dē-ŏl′ō-jĭst) [″ + *logos,* word, reason] A physician specializing in treatment of heart disease.

**cardiology** (kăr-dē-ŏl′ō-jē) The study of the physiology and pathology of the heart.

***nuclear c.*** A noninvasive method for studying cardiovascular disease by use of nuclear imaging techniques. These tests are usually done while the individual is exercising. Coronary artery disease can be investigated as can damage to the myocardium following coronary infarction. The size and function of the ventricles can be evaluated using these techniques.

**cardiolysin** (kăr″dē-ŏl′ĭ-sĭn) [″ + *lysis,* dissolution] An antibody acting destructively on the heart muscle.

**cardiolysis** (kăr-dē-ŏl′ĭ-sĭs) An operation that separates adhesions constricting the heart in adhesive mediastinopericarditis. It involves resection of the ribs and sternum over the pericardium.

**cardiomalacia** (kăr″dē-ō-mă-lā′shē-ă) [Gr. *kardia,* heart, + *malakia,* softening] Softening of the heart muscle.

**cardiomegaly** (kăr″dē-ō-mĕg′ă-lē) [″ + *megas,* large] Enlargement of the heart.

**cardiomotility** (kăr″dē-ō-mō-tĭl′ĭ-tē) [″ + L. *motilis,* moving] The ability of the heart to move.

**cardiomyoliposis** (kăr″dē-ō-mī″ō-lĭp-ō′sĭs) [″ + *mys,* muscle, + *lipos,* fat, + *osis,* condition] Fatty degeneration of the heart.

**cardiomyopathy** (kăr″dē-ō-mī-ŏp′ă-thē) [″ + ″ + *pathos,* disease, suffering] ABBR: CMP. Disease of the myocardium, esp. that caused by primary disease of the heart muscle. SEE: *myocarditis.*

***alcoholic c.*** Disease of the heart muscle due to alcohol consumption.

***congestive c.*** Myocardial disease associated with enlargement of the left ventricle of the heart and congestive heart failure.

***constrictive c.*** Restrictive c.

***hypertrophic c.*** A common heart muscle disorder marked by asymptomatic hypertrophy of the interventricular septum. The disorder may be present in newborns. In some patients the disease is transmitted genetically. Its cause is unknown.

SYMPTOMS: The patient exhibits congestive heart failure, dyspnea, fatigue, chest pain similar to angina, dizziness, and syncope. In addition, the electrocardiogram readings are usually abnormal, as are those of the chest radiograph and echocardiogram. Many children with the disease are asymptomatic except for having a heart murmur. The disease may have a long, benign course or may result in sudden death during exercise.

TREATMENT: Symptomatic treatment of dyspnea and chest pain is needed. Calcium entry blockers, particularly verapamil, are given. Cardioversion is required for arrhythmias. Surgery may be indicated in patients who do not respond to conservative therapy.

NURSING IMPLICATIONS: The patient's cardiopulmonary status and vital signs, intake and output, and weight are monitored regularly. The patient is evaluated for signs and symptoms of complications such as pulmonary hypertension or heart failure. Prescribed medications (beta-blockers, calcium channel blockers) are administered and evaluated for desired effects and any adverse reactions.

Propranolol therapy may cause depression, and both patient and family are encouraged to notify the primary health-care provider if such symptoms occur. If propranolol is to be discontinued, the patient should be advised not to stop the drug abruptly, but rather to taper it slowly, because abrupt discontinuance of propranolol may cause rebound effects, resulting in myocardial infarction or sudden death. Any physician who might care for the patient should be informed not to prescribe nitroglycerin, digitalis glycosides, or diuretics without consulting with the patient's cardiologist, because these drugs can worsen the obstructive process and result in reduced left ventricular function and congestive heart failure.

A nutritious diet is provided, and sodium and fluid intake is restricted as prescribed. Activities of daily living and treatments are interspersed with periods of rest, and personal care is provided as needed to prevent fatigue. If the patient is restricted to bedrest, active or passive range-of-motion exercises will prevent muscle atrophy (or at least maintain joint mobility); these exercises are taught to both patient and family.

Because therapeutic restrictions and an uncertain prognosis usually result in profound anxiety and depression, emotional support is offered and the patient is encouraged to express feelings and concerns. Flexible visiting hours are permitted, with care taken to balance the patient's need for family and diversion against the need for rest. If hospitalization is prolonged (whether in an acute care or supportive care environment), permission may be obtained for the patient to spend occasional days at home. Assistance is provided to the patient and family to identify and use effective coping strategies.

Before any dental work, surgery, or other invasive procedure, the patient will need antibiotic prophylaxis to prevent subacute bacterial endocarditis. Because syncope or sudden death may follow usually well-tolerated exercise, the patient is warned against strenuous physical activity, such as running, and a medically supervised cardiac rehabilitation exercise program is recommended instead. The family is also advised to learn cardiopulmonary resuscitation.

***idiopathic dilated c.*** ABBR: IDC. An uncommon disease of the heart muscle of unknown cause. The possibility that factors such as viruses, cytotoxic insults, or immune abnormalities can cause this condition is unproven. There does seem to be a genetic predisposition to IDC. The first change in the heart is dilatation of both ventricles; the most common initial clinical sign of IDC is heart failure. The course of the disease is difficult to describe because asymptomatic cardiomegaly may be present for months or years. Once patients become symptomatic, the prognosis is poor.

TREATMENT: General supportive therapy includes rest, weight control, abstinence from tobacco, and moderate exercise at a level that does not cause symptoms. A salt-restricted diet is mandatory in patients with congestive heart disease symptoms. Therapy includes the use of vasodilators when there is left ventricular dysfunction. Anticoagulants are important to prevent thrombus formation. Antiarrhythmic therapy may be indicated; use of digitalis is controversial. IDC is a principal indication for cardiac transplant.

***c. of overload*** Cardiomyopathy in which enlarged cardiac myocytes fail to function efficiently. Because cardiac myocytes are not able to divide, they can respond to cardiac overload by increasing in size but not in number. When the overload is chronic, the life span of myocytes is shortened and myocardial ability is decreased. This process eventually leads to heart failure.

***primary c.*** Cardiomyopathy in which the origin (i.e., cause) is unknown.

***restrictive c.*** A disease of the heart muscle associated with lack of flexibility of the ventricular walls. SYN: *constrictive c.* SEE: *pericarditis.*

***secondary c.*** Any cardiomyopathy in which the cause is either known or associated with a well-defined systemic disease. Included are cardiomyopathies associated with inflammation, toxic chemicals, metabolic abnormalities, and inherited muscle disorders.

**cardiomyopexy** (kăr″dē-ō-mī′ō-pĕk″sē) [″ + ″ + *pexis,* fixation] Surgical fixation of a vascular tissue such as pectoral muscle to the cardiac muscle and pericardium to improve blood supply to the myocardium.

**cardiomyoplasty** Surgical implantation of skeletal muscle to either supplement or replace myocardial muscle.

**cardiomyotomy** Surgical therapy for achalasia. The muscles surrounding the cardioesophageal junction are cut, while the underlying mucous membrane is left intact.

**cardionecrosis** (kăr″dē-ō-nĕ-krō′sĭs) [″ + *nekros,* dead, + *osis,* condition] Death of heart tissue.

**cardionecteur, cardionector** (kăr″dē-ō-nĕk′tĕr) [″ + L. *nektor,* joiner] The conduction system of the heart. It includes the sinoatrial node, which transmits impulses to the atrioventricular node, which in turn transmits impulses to the bundle of His, which transmits impulses to the bundle branches and Purkinje fibers to produce ventricular contraction.

**cardionephric** (kăr″dē-ō-nĕf′rĭk) [″ + *nephros,* kidney] Pert. to the heart and kidney.

**cardioneural** (kăr″dē-ō-nū′răl) [″ + *neuron,* nerve] Pert. to nervous control of the heart.

**cardioneurosis** (kăr″dē-ō-nū-rō′sĭs) [″ + ″ + *osis,* condition] Functional neurosis with cardiac symptoms.

**cardiopathy** (kăr″dē-ŏp′ă-thē) [″ + *pathos,* disease, suffering] Any disease of the heart.

**cardiopericarditis** (kăr″dē-ō-pĕr″ĭ-kăr-dī′tĭs) [″ + *peri,* around, + *kardia,* heart, + *itis,* inflammation] Inflammation of the myocardium and pericardium.

**cardiophobia** (kăr″dē-ō-fō′bē-ă) [″ + *phobos,* fear] Morbid fear of heart disease.

**cardioplasty** (kăr″dē-ō-plăs′tē) [″ + *plassein,* to form] An operation on the cardiac sphincter of the stomach to relieve cardiospasm.

**cardioplegia** (kăr″dē-ō-plē′jē-ă) [″ + *plege,* stroke] Intentional, temporary arrest of cardiac function by means of hypothermia, medication, or electrical stimuli to reduce the need of the myocardium for oxygen. This is done during surgery requiring cardiopulmonary bypass.

**cardiopneumograph** (kăr″dē-ō-nū′mō-grăf) [″ + ″ + *graphein,* to write] A device for recording the motion of the heart and lungs.

**cardioptosis** (kăr″dē-ŏp-tō′sĭs) [″ + *ptosis,* a dropping] Prolapse of the heart.

**cardiopulmonary** (kăr″dē-ō-pŭl′mō-nĕr-ē) [″ + L. *pulmo,* lung] Pert. to the heart and lungs.

**cardiopulmonary arrest** Sudden cessation of functional ventilation and circulation. SEE: *cardiopulmonary resuscitation.*

**cardiopulmonary resuscitation** ABBR: CPR. The process of ventilating and circulating blood for a patient in cardiopulmonary arrest, usually by combining mouth-to-mouth ventilation with external chest compressions. The victim is then carefully placed in a supine position on a firm, flat surface. The rescuer should ensure that the head is not elevated and that the arms are alongside the body. While kneeling at the level of the victim's shoulder, the rescuer should *open an airway*. The head is tilted back and the chin lifted up unless spinal injury is present or suspected. In that case, the spine is moved as little as possible by using the jaw-thrust technique for opening the airway. This prevents the tongue and epiglottis from obstructing the airway. If liquid or solid material is visible in the mouth, it is removed. If dentures are present and interfere with resuscitation, they are removed too. Next, *breathing* is assessed by listening for breath signs while maintaining an open airway, and watching for rise and fall of the chest. If this does not happen, the victim is breathless. This assessment should require no more than 3 to 5 sec.

The goal of CPR is to provide oxygen quickly to the lungs, brain, heart, and other vital organs until appropriate, definitive medical treatment can restore normal heart and pulmonary function. Rescue breathing is begun using the mouth-to-mouth technique. The rescuer gently pinches the victim's nose closed, using the hand on the victim's forehead to prevent air from escaping through the nose while the lung is being inflated. The rescuer takes a deep breath and seals his or her lips around the outside of the victim's mouth, creating an airtight seal, and then gives two full breaths, each taking 1 to 1½ sec. The rescuer inhales air between each ventilation and makes certain that the victim's chest rises. Using too much air too swiftly may increase pharyngeal pressure and allow air to enter the stomach. If signs of adequate ventilation (rising chest and palpable escape of air during exhalation) are not present, the head is repositioned and rescue breathing repeated. If this does not result in ventilation, the Heimlich maneuver is performed to clear the airway of a foreign body.

---

Caution: To prevent transmission of disease from the victim to the rescuer, a bag-valve-mask or other suitable device should be used in place of mouth-to-mouth technique.

---

Next, *circulation* is assessed by checking the pulse in the carotid artery. This is done in 5 to 10 sec by locating the groove between the trachea and the strap muscles of the neck. Pressure on this area should be gentle to avoid compressing the artery. If a pulse is present but there is no breathing, rescue breathing should be initiated at a rate of one per 5 sec (12 per min). If there is no pulse, the diagnosis of cardiac arrest is confirmed and external chest compression is begun after the initial two breaths. This consists of serial, rhythmic applications of pressure over the lower half of the sternum. To reduce the chance of rib fracture, the heels of the hands must be properly placed over the middle of the sternum, just above the notch where the ribs meet the sternum in the middle of the lower part of the chest. The fingers may be either extended or interlaced, but must not be pressed against the lateral chest wall. Proper compression is accomplished by locking the elbows in position. The rescuer's arms extend straight up from the victim's chest, with the shoulders directly over the hands. This forces the thrust of each external chest compression straight down on the sternum. The chest is depressed 1.5 to 2.0 in. (3.8 to 5.0 cm) for a normal-sized adult. For a child, the chest is depressed 1.0 to 1.5 in. (2.8 to 3.8 cm); for an infant, 0.5 to 1.0 in. (1.3 to 2.54 cm). The chest compression pressure is released completely to allow blood to flow into the heart. The chest should return to its normal position after each compression. Pressure should be released for the amount of time required for compression. This is necessary to allow the administered air to leave the lungs. The compression rate should be between 80 and 100 per min if possible for an adult or child, and at least 100 per min for an infant.

While these maneuvers are being continued, it is imperative to try to activate the emergency medical system (EMS), but CPR should not be interrupted for more than 7 sec. This is done by calling or having someone call the local emergency telephone number, 911, if available. The person contacting the EMS should provide full details concerning the location of the emergency, the telephone number from which the call is being made, the nature of the emergency, the number of persons who need help, and the type of aid being given. Lay persons being instructed in CPR should use the one-rescuer technique. If trained professionals arrive at the scene, they will proceed with two-rescuer CPR and advanced cardiac life support as appropriate for the situation. In two-rescuer CPR, one rescuer does ventilation while the second rescuer does external chest compressions at the same rate as for one-person CPR. When the compressor becomes fatigued, the rescuers exchange positions. It is important to monitor the victim's condition to assess the effectiveness of the rescue effort. This is done by checking the pulse during chest compression. To determine whether spontaneous breathing has returned, chest compression is stopped for 5 sec at about the end of the first minute and every few minutes thereafter. SEE: illus.; table; *ad-*

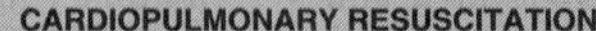

CARDIOPULMONARY RESUSCITATION

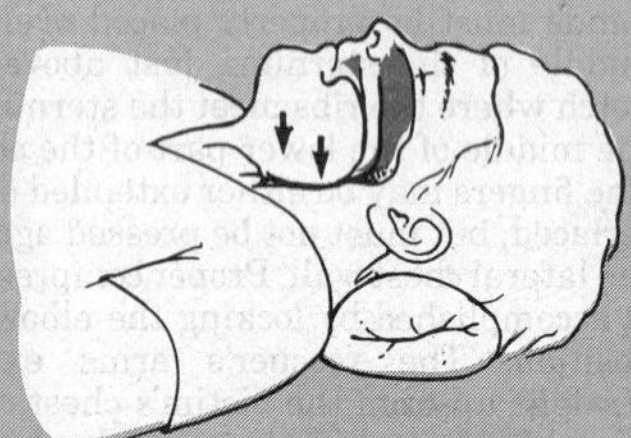

ARROWS INDICATE RELAXED TONGUE OCCLUDING AIRWAY

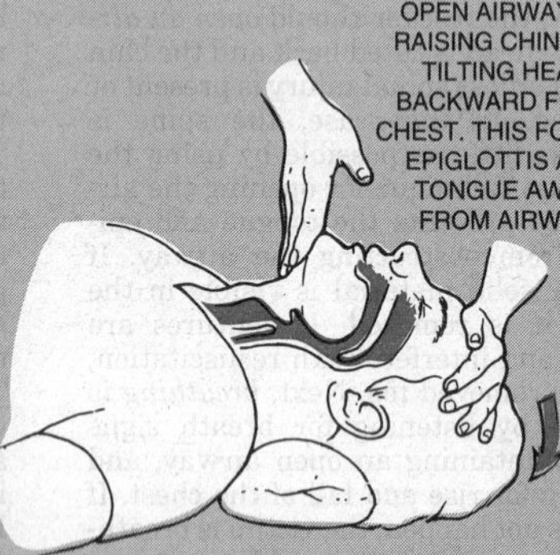

OPEN AIRWAY BY RAISING CHIN AND TILTING HEAD BACKWARD FROM CHEST. THIS FORCES EPIGLOTTIS AND TONGUE AWAY FROM AIRWAY

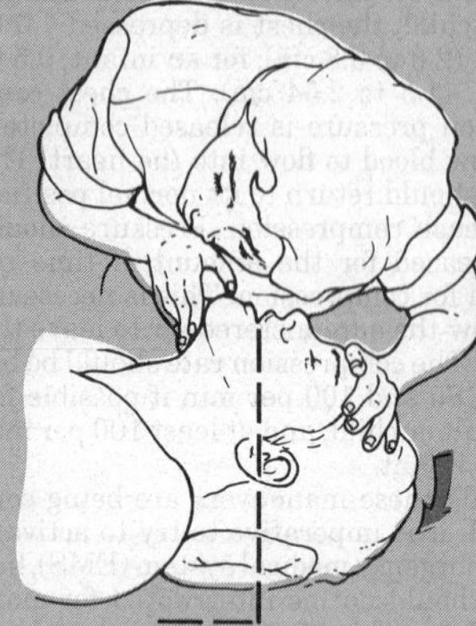

MAINTAIN HEAD TILT AND CHIN RAISED. LISTEN FOR BREATH, OR IT CAN BE FELT

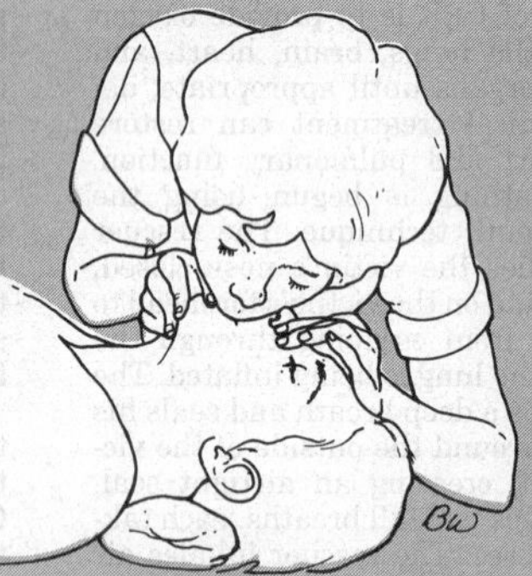

MAINTAIN HEAD TILT, CHIN RAISED POSITION. INFLATE LUNGS WHILE HOLDING NOSE CLOSED

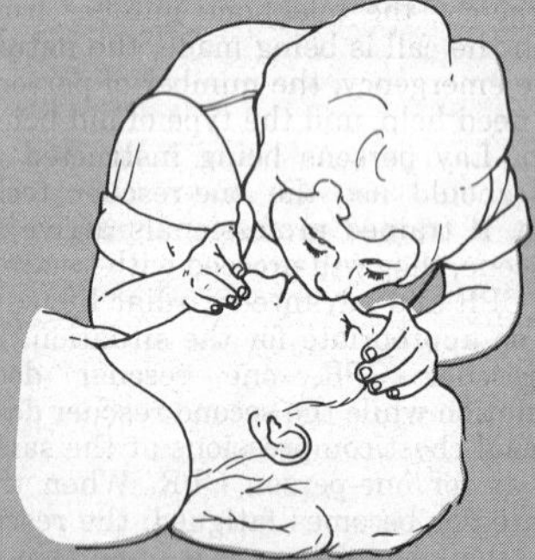

IF MOUTH IS HELD CLOSED LUNGS MAY BE INFLATED BY BLOWING THROUGH PATIENT'S NOSE

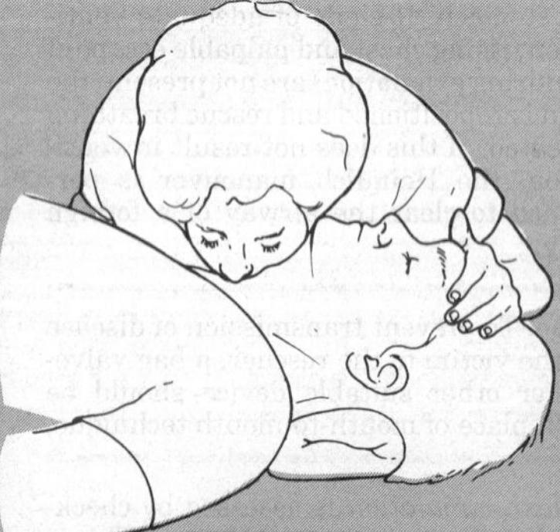

IF TRACHEOSTOMY IS PRESENT INFLATE LUNGS BY BLOWING THROUGH STOMA

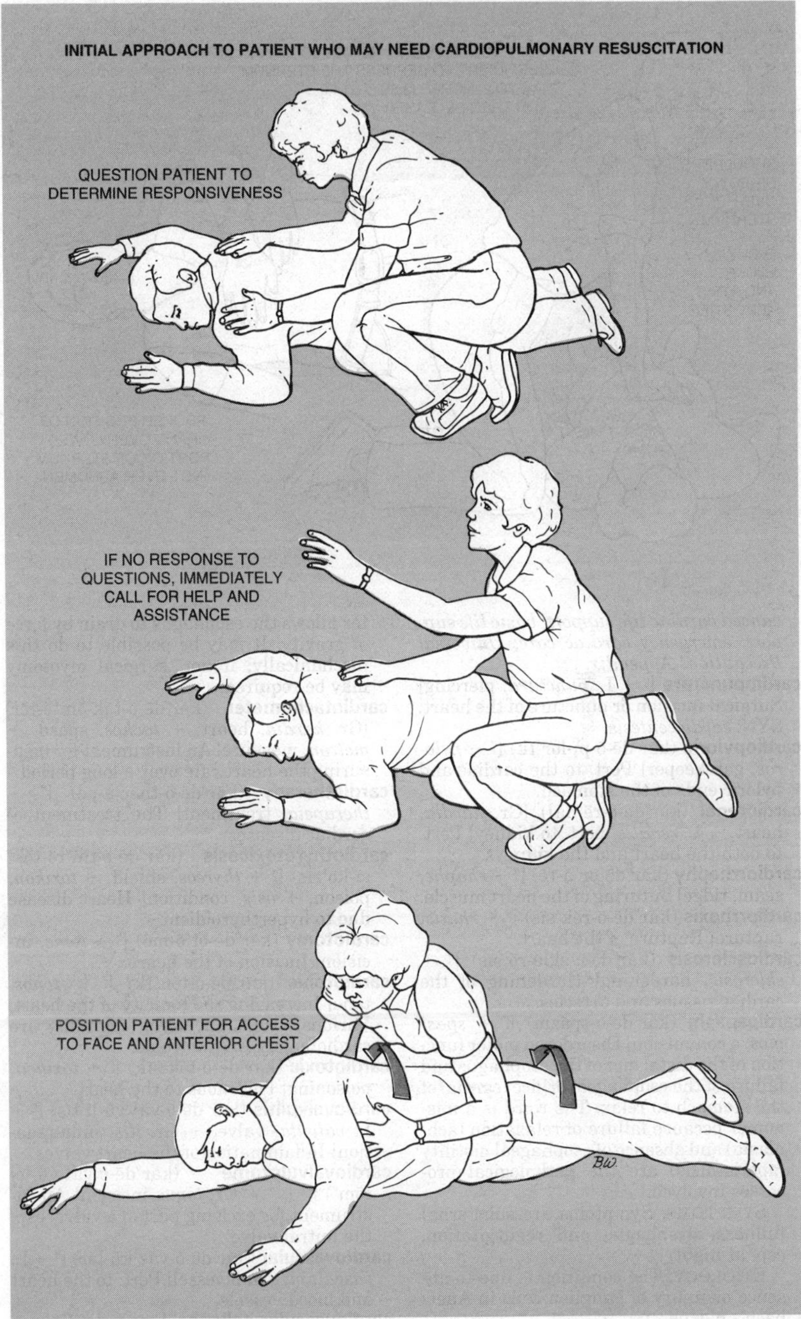
INITIAL APPROACH TO PATIENT WHO MAY NEED CARDIOPULMONARY RESUSCITATION
QUESTION PATIENT TO DETERMINE RESPONSIVENESS
IF NO RESPONSE TO QUESTIONS, IMMEDIATELY CALL FOR HELP AND ASSISTANCE
POSITION PATIENT FOR ACCESS TO FACE AND ANTERIOR CHEST
BW.

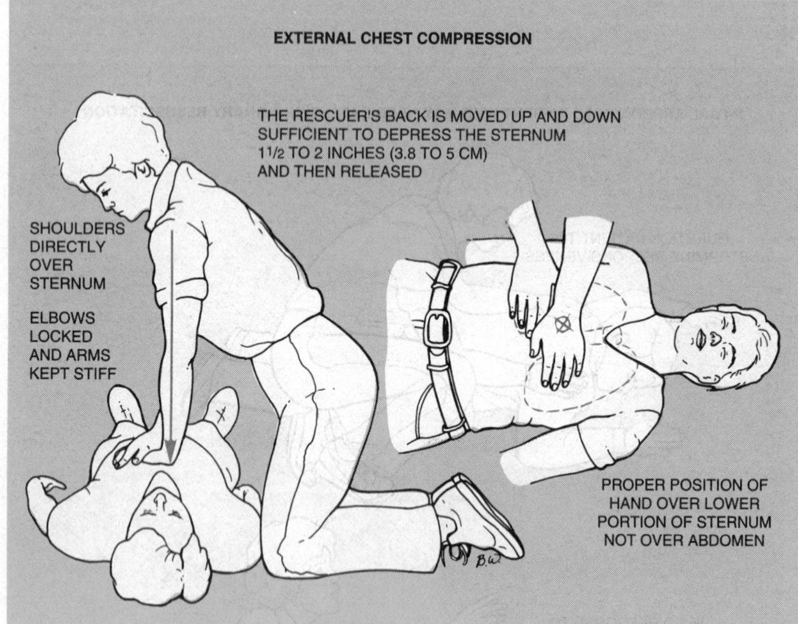


*vanced cardiac life support; basic life support; emergency cardiac care; Universal Precautions Appendix.*

**cardiopuncture** [″ + L. *punctura,* piercing] Surgical incision or puncture of the heart. SYN: *cardiocentesis.*

**cardiopyloric** (kăr″dē-ō-pī-lor′ĭk) [″ + *pyloros,* gatekeeper] Pert. to the cardiac and pyloric ends of the stomach.

**cardiorenal** (kăr″dē-ō-rē′năl) [Gr. *kardia,* heart, + L. *renalis,* pert. to kidney] Pert. to both the heart and the kidneys.

**cardiorrhaphy** (kăr″dē-or′ă-fē) [″ + *rhaphe,* seam, ridge] Suturing of the heart muscle.

**cardiorrhexis** (kăr″dē-ō-rĕk′sĭs) [″ + *rhexis,* rupture] Rupture of the heart.

**cardiosclerosis** (kăr″dē-ō-sklĕ-rō′sĭs) [″ + *sklerosis,* hardening] Hardening of the cardiac tissues and arteries.

**cardiospasm** (kăr′dē-ō-spăzm) [″ + *spasmos,* a convulsion] Disordered motor function of the distal end of the esophagus and failure of the esophageal orifice (cardia) of the stomach to relax. The word is a misnomer because failure of relaxation (achalasia) and absence of esophageal motility (aperistalsis) are the pathological processes involved.

SYMPTOMS: Symptoms are substernal fullness, dysphagia, and regurgitation, esp. at night.

ETIOLOGY: The condition is due to absence or injury of ganglion cells in Auerbach's plexus.

TREATMENT: Bland semisolid foods warmed to body temperature are of some help. Dilatation of the esophageal sphincter allows the esophagus to drain by force of gravity. It may be possible to do this mechanically; if not, surgical myotomy may be required.

**cardiotachometer** (kăr″dē-ō-tăk-ŏm′ĕ-tĕr) [Gr. *kardia,* heart, + *tachos,* speed, + *metron,* measure] An instrument for measuring the heart rate over a long period.

**cardiotherapy** (kăr″dē-ō-thĕr′ă-pē) [″ + *therapeia,* treatment] The treatment of cardiac diseases.

**cardiothyrotoxicosis** (kăr″dē-ō-thī″rō-tŏk″sĭ-kō′sĭs) [″ + *thyreos,* shield, + *toxikon,* poison, + *osis,* condition] Heart disease due to hyperthyroidism.

**cardiotomy** (kăr″dē-ŏt′ō-mē) [″ + *tome,* incision] Incision of the heart.

**cardiotonic** (kăr″dē-ō-tŏn′ĭk) [″ + *tonos,* tone] Increasing the tonicity of the heart. Various drugs, including digitalis, are cardiotonic. SEE: *inotropic.*

**cardiotoxic** (kăr″dē-ō-tŏk′sĭk) [″ + *toxikon,* poisoning] Poisonous to the heart.

**cardiovalvulitis** (kăr″dē-ō-văl″vū-lī′tĭs) [″ + L. *valvula,* valve, + Gr. *itis,* inflammation] Inflammation of the heart valves.

**cardiovalvulotome** (kăr″dē-ō-văl′vū-lō-tōm″) [″ + ″ + Gr. *tome,* incision] An instrument for excising part of a valve, esp. the mitral valve.

**cardiovascular** (kăr″dē-ō-văs′kū-lăr) [″ + L. *vasculum,* small vessel] Pert. to the heart and blood vessels.

**cardiovascular collapse** A nonspecific condition associated with sudden loss of effective blood flow to the tissue, which may be caused by vasovagal syncope or pos-

**Basic Cardiac Life Support Guidelines**

| Former Guidelines | Present Guidelines | Rationale |
|---|---|---|
| **Training of rescuers** | | |
| One- and two-person CPR | Lay rescuers: One-person CPR only. If present, second lay rescuer should call for professional help. If first rescuer tires, second may provide relief.<br>Professional rescuers (nurses, physicians, emergency medical technicians): Both one- and two-person CPR | One-person CPR improves performance and retention of skills. Two-person CPR may be confusing and has not been used often.<br>Two-person CPR: Less fatiguing; performance may be extended over longer time periods. |
| **Opening airway (establishing breathlessness)** | | |
| Head tilt/chin lift and jaw thrust | Lay rescuers: Head tilt/chin lift only<br>Professional rescuers: Both head tilt/chin lift and jaw thrust | Head tilt/chin lift is safe, effective, simple, and easy to learn. Although effective, jaw thrust is tiring and technically difficult. |
| **After establishing breathlessness (victim over 1 year of age)** | | |
| Four quick "staircase" breaths | Two slow breaths of 1.5–2 sec each. After delivering first breath, pause to inhale before delivering second. | Slower breaths prevent air entrapment between breaths. Decreased air pressure minimizes risk of opening the esophagus and creating gastric distention with possible regurgitation and aspiration. Pause allows rescuer to increase lung volume, enabling more oxygen delivery to lungs. |
| **After establishing breathlessness (infant victim)** | | |
| Four quick, full puffs of air | Same as above (two slow breaths of 1.5–2 sec each; pause between breaths) | Same as above |
| **After establishing complete airway obstruction** | | |
| Four back blows and four abdominal thrusts (Heimlich maneuver) | The abdominal thrust is the only recommended technique for removal of a foreign body causing airway obstruction in victims over 1 year of age. The chest thrust remains the approved technique for obese persons and women in late pregnancy.<br>Due to risk of abdominal injury, the combination of chest thrusts and back blows remains accepted protocol in infant victims under 1 year of age. | Exclusive use of abdominal thrusts is more effective and safer than back blows alone or back blows in combination with abdominal thrusts. |

*Table continued on following page*

**Basic Cardiac Life Support Guidelines** (Continued)

| Former Guidelines | Present Guidelines | Rationale |
|---|---|---|
| **Near-drowning victims** | | |
| No clear guidelines available. Instruction usually in rescue breathing or CPR. Some emphasis on clearing lower airway of water before initiation of CPR. | Start rescue breathing as soon as possible. Perform abdominal thrusts only if a foreign object appears to be obstructing the airway or if victim does not respond to mouth-to-mouth ventilation. If necessary, start CPR after abdominal thrusts have been performed. | The necessity of clearing lower airway of aspirated water has not been proved. Attempts to remove water from airway by nonsuctioning techniques are unnecessary and may be dangerous by causing ejection of gastric contents and subsequent aspiration. |
| **After establishing lack of pulse (infant victim)** | | |
| Compress victim's sternum at nipple line with two or three fingers. | Compress victim's sternum one fingerwidth below nipple line with two or three fingers. | Recent studies demonstrate that an infant's heart lies lower in the chest (in relation to external landmarks) than previously believed. |
| **External chest compression, one-person CPR** | | |
| 60–80 external chest compressions per min | 80–100 external chest compressions per min | Rapid chest compressions increase blood flow from the heart. Increase in intrathoracic pressure promotes blood flow from the thoracic cavity to the brain and heart. |
| **Delivering breaths, two-person CPR** | | |
| One breath on the upstroke of every fifth chest compression, no pause in chest compressions | One breath of 1–1.5 sec *during a pause* after every fifth chest compression. Pause may be shorter. | Slower breaths minimize risk of gastric distention, regurgitation, and aspiration. |

tural hypotension. These may revert spontaneously. SEE: *cardiac arrest; cardiac arrest, sudden.*

**cardiovascular reflex 1.** A sympathetic increase in heart rate when increased pressure in, or distention of, great veins occurs. **2.** Reflex vasoconstriction resulting from reduced venous pressure.

**cardioversion** (kăr′dē-ō-vĕr″zhŭn) [″ + L. *versio,* a turning] Synchronized electric shock used to terminate cardiac arrhythmias. Unlike defibrillation, which is an unsynchronized shock, cardioversion is timed to avoid the T wave of the cardiac cycle. A conscious patient may require sedation before the procedure.

Caution: Cardioversion should not be used in sinus tachycardia or arrhythmias (other than ventricular fibrillation) caused by digitalis toxicity. It should be used only in emergency situations when potassium administration and other measures have failed. The cardioverter may induce lethal ventricular fibrillation unresponsive to further electric shocks.

Nursing Implications: The procedure and expected sensations are explained to the patient, the physician's explanation of complications and risks is reinforced and clarified, and emotional support is provided throughout the procedure. The patient's medication history is reviewed, and cardiac glycoside use is reported to the physician, along with the patient's potassium level. Emergency equipment (crash cart) is available nearby. The patient's vital signs are checked, an intravenous infusion started, and the patient hooked up to the ECG monitor. Chest electrodes are placed to facilitate recording of tall R waves without interfering with paddle placement, and a 12-lead ECG is obtained. The patient is placed in a supine position, and adequate ventilation is ensured while oxygen is temporarily stopped. A sedative is provided as prescribed unless the patient is profoundly hypotensive.The defibrillator leads are attached to the patient, and the oscilloscope and recorder are turned on to document the cardioversion and postprocedure rhythm. Then the synchronization control is turned on and the recording checked to ensure that each R wave is marked, or the gain is turned up to create taller R waves and the recording checked to ensure that each R wave is marked. The control is set to the energy level prescribed by the physician or by protocol. The paddles are prepared, and the charge button is pushed until the display indicates that the desired energy level has been achieved. The paddles are then placed firmly on the patient's chest (as for defibrillation), and the operator shouts "all clear" and verifies that no one is in contact with the patient or the bed. The operator holds the discharge button down until the paddles discharge; a slight delay can be expected for electrical synchronization with the patient's R wave. After discharge, the operator removes the paddles from the chest and evaluates the ECG to determine whether cardioversion was successful. If the arrhythmia was not corrected, the procedure is repeated using a higher-energy setting.

After successful cardioversion, the nurse monitors the posttreatment rhythm and position of the ST segment; vital signs are also monitored every 15 min for an hour (or according to protocol) until baseline levels are reached. The skin is inspected for burns, and the patient is assessed for respiratory problems and hypotension.

**cardioverter** (kăr′dē-ō-vĕr″tĕr) A device used to administer electric shocks to the heart when electrodes are placed on the chest wall. It is useful in emergency treatment of cardiac arrhythmias such as ventricular tachycardia. Changing the arrhythmia to normal sinus rhythm is called cardioversion.

***automatic implantable c.*** An implantable device for detecting and terminating ventricular tachycardia or fibrillation.

**carditis** (kăr-dī′tĭs) [″ + *itis,* inflammation] Inflammation of the layers of the wall of the heart. It usually involves two of the following: pericardium, myocardium, or endocardium.

***Coxsackie c.*** Carditis or pericarditis that may occur in infections with enteroviruses of the Coxsackie groups, and also with echovirus groups.

***rheumatic c.*** Carditis occurring in conjunction with rheumatic fever.

**care, adult day** ABBR: ADC. A licensed agency where chronically ill, disabled, or cognitively impaired persons can stay during the day under health care supervision. Most people who attend adult day care are elderly and need some assistance with care. They are able to participate in structured activities programs and to ambulate with or without an assistive device. Most day care centers operate 5 days a week for 8 to 12 hr a day.

**care, cluster** A system of home care for the elderly that allows the needs of many clients who live in proximity to be met by a team of workers.

**care, family-centered** In obstetrics, a philosophy of maternal and child care that emphasizes the family as the unit of care.

**care, home health** The provision of equipment and services to patients in their homes to restore and maintain the individual's maximal levels of comfort, function, and health.

**care, intensive** Care of critically ill patients.

**care, long-term** A range of care services from health to social services for individuals with chronic physical or mental impairments, or both, to maintain continuity from one discipline or institution to another. The goal is to maintain an optimal level of functioning and ensure use of the patient's potential. SEE: *Nursing Diagnoses Appendix.*

**care, medical** The use of medical skill to benefit a patient.

**care, mouth** Personal and bedside care of the oral cavity including the gingivae, teeth, lips, epithelial covering of the mucosa, pharynx, and tongue. When ill, persons who would normally be able to provide their own oral hygiene may require assistance in maintaining a healthy oral environment. The intensity and frequency of care is dictated by patient comfort; the severity of the illness; potential or existing irritation or inflammation secondary to trauma or therapy; and the patient's state of consciousness, level of cooperation, and ability to provide self-care. SEE: *stomatitis.*

**care, personal** Self-care (2).

**care, primary medical** The medical care of a person at the initial time and place the patient presents. This service is usually provided in a physician's office, an outpatient clinic, or the emergency department of a hospital.

**care, respiratory** The evaluation, treatment, and rehabilitation of patients with cardiopulmonary disease by respiratory therapy professionals working under a physician's supervision.

**care, respite** Provision of short-term care to older persons in the community to allow caregivers a temporary relief from their responsibilities. This service also may be available for persons who care for severely disabled children. Respite care is similar to adult day care, but organized activities or services are not available. The care may be provided either in the patient's home, a church, community center, or in the caregiver's home. The cost for this service is usually minimal and may be free.

**care, secondary medical** Medical care of a patient by a physician acting as a consultant. The provider of primary medical care usually refers the patient for this level of care.

**care, tertiary medical** Medical care of a patient in a facility staffed and equipped to administer comprehensive care. In the usual situation, this level of care is provided in a large hospital to which the patient has been referred or transferred.

**caregiver** One who provides care to a dependent or partially dependent patient. In an acute care setting, the caregiver is most often a professional; however, in the home care situation, this person is often a family member. Care of caregivers is a focus of nurses, social workers, and other health care providers who manage chronic patients. Generally, caregivers need emotional support and comfort owing to the extreme stress of their lives. SEE: *caregiver burden.*

**caregiver burden** The perception of stress and fatigue caused by the sustained effort required in caring for persons with chronic illness or other conditions with special needs for care.

**caregiver role strain** A caregiver's felt difficulty in performing the family caregiver role. SEE: *Nursing Diagnoses Appendix.*

**caregiver role strain, risk for** The vulnerability of the caregiver for felt difficulty in performing the family caregiver role. SEE: *Nursing Diagnoses Appendix.*

**Caregiver Stress Inventory** ABBR: CSI. A 50-item scale specific to professionals caring for patients with Alzheimer's disease. It is divided into three subscales measuring stress related to the patient's verbal and physical behavior, the patient's mental, emotional, and social behavior, and the resources, knowledge, and abilities of the staff.

**C.A.R.F.** *Commission on Accreditation of Rehabilitation Facilities.*

**caries** (kār′ēz, kār′ĭ-ēz) [L., rottenness] Gradual decay and disintegration of soft or bony tissue or of a tooth. If the decay progresses, the surrounding tissue becomes inflamed and an abscess forms (e.g., chronic abscess, tuberculosis, and bacterial invasion of teeth). In caries, the bone disintegrates by pieces, whereas in necrosis, large masses of bone are involved. **carious** (-rē-ŭs), *adj.*

***arrested c.*** Apparent lack of progress in a carious lesion between dental examinations.

***bottle mouth c.*** Extensive caries and discoloration of the teeth observed in children from 19 months to 4 years of age who have had prolonged bottle feedings.

***cervical c.*** Caries involving the neck of the tooth, slightly above or below the junction between the root cementum and the enamel crown.

***classification of c.*** G.V. Black's classification of dental caries according to the part of the tooth involved: class I, occlusal; class II, interproximal, commonly at the dentinoenamel junction of bicuspids and molars; class III, interproximal surfaces not involving incisal surfaces; class IV, interproximal but involving an incisal surface; class V, the faciocervical area.

***dental c.*** Tooth decay; progressive decalcification of the enamel and dentin of a tooth. The causes are not fully known, but minimizing intake of dietary refined carbohydrates and good dental hygiene prevent growth of bacteria that contribute to the development of caries. Proper brushing of the teeth is effective in preventing and removing dental plaque in all areas except those between the teeth and deep fissures. Use of dental floss or tape removes plaque from between adjacent tooth surfaces; deep pits and fissures may be sealed by the application of resins. The sealant may need to be replaced periodically. Early detection and dental restorations offer the best form of control once caries has formed. Topical application of fluoride promotes resistance to dental caries if applied during tooth formation. Dental caries is less likely to develop if appropriate amounts of fluoride are ingested while the teeth are developing. It is important that excess fluoride not be ingested because greater amounts than required (about 1 mg/day) cause mottling of the teeth. Fluoride in the diet does not obviate the need for topical application of fluoride to the teeth. SEE: illus.; *plaque, dental.*

***incipient c.*** One of the two distinct stages in the development of a carious dental lesion. The first stage is the incipient lesion, marked by the appearance of a white spot. Microscopic pores course through the enamel to the subsurface demineralization, where the main body of the lesion is located.

***necrotic c.*** A disease in which masses of bone lie in a suppurating cavity.

***pit and fissure c.*** Caries in the pits and fissures of tooth enamel.

***radiation c.*** Dental caries that develops as a side effect of treatment of malignancies of the oral cavity with ionizing radiation.

***rampant c.*** A sudden onset of widespread caries that affects most of the teeth and penetrates quickly to the dental pulp.

***recurrent c.*** Dental caries that develops at the small imperfections between the tooth surface and a restoration, caused by plaque at the imperfections. SYN: *secondary c.*

***root c.*** Caries on the root of a tooth. The root is more susceptible to decay than the rest of the tooth due to the lack of an enamel covering, difficulty in maintaining a clean root surface, and the lack of effective preventive therapies.

***secondary c.*** Recurrent c.

***c. sicca*** Dry caries of the bone.

***spinal c.*** Pott's disease.

**carina** (kă-rī′nă) *pl.* **carinae** [L., keel of a

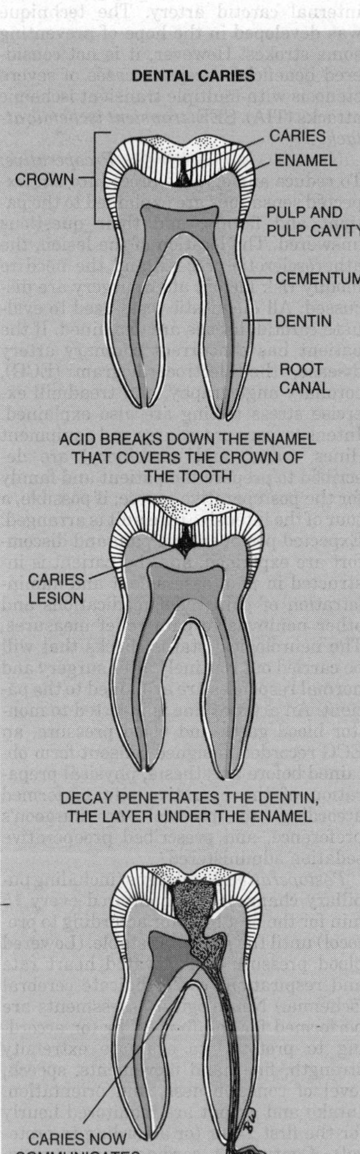


boat] A structure with a projecting central ridge.

*c. nasi* The olfactory nasal sulcus.

*c. tracheae* The ridge at the lower end of the trachea separating the openings of the two bronchi.

*c. urethralis* The ridge extending posteriorly from the urethral orifice and continuous with the anterior column of the vagina.

**carinate** (kăr′ĭ-nāt) [L. *carina,* keel of a boat] Keel-shaped; having a conspicuous central ridge.

**caring behaviors** The actions or responses of providing patient services.

NURSING IMPLICATIONS: The following are the 10 highest-ranked caring behaviors, derived from nursing literature, then selected by nurses as evident in caring situations with patients: attentive listening, comforting, honesty, patience, responsibility, providing information so the patient can make an informed decision, touch, sensitivity, respect, calling the patient by name.

**cariogenesis** (kār″ē-ō-jĕn′ĕ-sĭs) [L. *caries,* rottenness, + Gr. *genesis,* generation, birth] The formation of caries. SEE: *caries, dental.*

**cariogenic** (kā″rē-ō-jĕn′ĭk) [″ + Gr. *gennan,* to produce] Conducive to caries formation.

**carious** (kā′rē-ŭs) **1.** Affected with or pert. to caries. **2.** Having pits or perforations.

**carisoprodol** (kăr″ī-sō-prō′dŏl) A drug that relaxes muscles by acting on the central nervous system.

**carminative** (kăr-mĭn′ă-tĭv) [L. *carminativus,* cleanse] An agent that helps to prevent gas formation in the gastrointestinal tract.

**carmustine (BCNU)** An antineoplastic drug. Trade name is BiCNU.

**carnal** (kăr′năl) [L. *carnalis,* flesh] Pert. to the desires and appetites of the flesh; sensual.

**carneous** (kăr′nē-ŭs) [L. *carneus,* fleshy] Fleshy.

**carnitine** (kăr′nĭ-tĭn) A chemical, $\gamma$-trimethylamine-$\beta$-hydroxybutyrate, important in metabolizing palmitic and stearic acids. It has been used therapeutically in treating myopathy due to carnitine deficiency.

**carnivore** (kăr′nĭ-vor) An animal that eats primarily meat, particularly an animal of the order Carnivora, which includes cats, dogs, and bears.

**carnivorous** (kăr-nĭv′ō-rŭs) [L. *carnivorus*] Flesh-eating.

**carnophobia** (kăr″nō-fō′bē-ă) [″ + Gr. *phobos,* fear] An abnormal aversion to meat.

**carnose** (kăr′nōs) Having the consistency of or resembling flesh.

**carnosine** (kăr′nō-sĭn) A chemical, $\beta$-alanylhistidine, present in muscle. Its function is unknown.

**carnosity** (kăr-nŏs′ĭ-tē) [L. *carnositas,* fleshiness] An excrescence resembling flesh; a fleshy growth.

**carotenase** (kăr-ŏt'ĕ-nās) [Gr. *karoton,* carrot] An enzyme that converts carotene into vitamin A. SYN: *carotinase.*

**carotene** (kăr'ō-tēn) [Gr. *karoton*] A yellow crystalline pigment present in various plant and animal tissues. It is abundant in yellow vegetables (carrots, squash, corn). It exists in several forms and is the precursor of vitamin A. It is stored in and converted to vitamin A in the liver.

Retinol is the form of vitamin A found in mammals. One retinol equivalent is equal to 6 μg of beta-carotene. Beta-carotene is safer than vitamin A because the latter has much greater toxic potential in large doses.

**carotenemia** (kăr"ō-tĕ-nē'mē-ă) [" + *haima,* blood] Carotene in the blood, marked by yellowing of the skin (pseudojaundice). It can be distinguished from true jaundice by the lack of yellow discoloration of the conjunctivae in carotenemia. It is a benign condition.

**carotenoid** (kă-rŏt'ĕ-noyd) [" + *eidos,* form, shape] **1.** One of a group of pigments (e.g., carotene) ranging in color from light yellow to red, widely distributed in plants and animals. The best known is beta carotene present in carrots, but others are lycopene in tomatoes and lutein in spinach. The carotenoids are antioxidants and they are thought to be important in helping to prevent various diseases including age-related macular degeneration. The possibility that some carotenoids may be of benefit in treating cancer is being investigated. **2.** Resembling carotene.

**carotic** (kă-rŏt'ĭk) [Gr. *karos,* deep sleep] **1.** Carotid. **2.** Resembling stupor; stupefying.

**caroticotympanic** (kă-rŏt"ĭ-kō-tĭm-păn'ĭk) Pert. to the carotid canal and the tympanic cavity (the middle ear).

**carotid** (kă-rŏt'ĭd) [Gr. *karos,* deep sleep] **1.** Pert. to the right and left common carotid arteries, which comprise the principal blood supply to the head and neck. The left arises directly from the aorta and the right from the brachiocephalic artery. Each of these two arteries divides to form external and internal carotid arteries. **2.** Pert. to any carotid part, such as the carotid sinus.

**carotid body** A flat structure at the bifurcation of the common carotid artery. It contains cells that respond to changes in oxygen concentration in the blood and to changes in blood pressure.

**carotid bruit** A murmur heard in the cervical area that does not disappear with venous compression, is maximal over the carotid bifurcation, and is not due to transmitted cardiac murmurs. The presence of asymptomatic carotid bruits increases with advanced age but is not associated with increased risk for stroke in elderly patients. Carotid bruits may spontaneously disappear without sequelae.

**carotid endarterectomy** A surgical technique for removing intra-arterial obstructions of the lower cervical portion of the internal carotid artery. The technique was developed in the hope of preventing some strokes. However, it is not considered beneficial except in cases of severe stenosis with multiple transient ischemic attacks (TIA). SEE: *transient ischemic attack.*

NURSING IMPLICATIONS: *Preoperative:* To reduce anxiety, the procedure and expected sensations are explained to the patient and family, and their questions answered. The location of the lesion, the atherosclerotic process, and the need to modify risk factors after surgery are discussed. All diagnostic tests used to evaluate carotid disease are explained. If the patient has concurrent coronary artery disease, the electrocardiogram (ECG), coronary angiography, and treadmill exercise stress testing are also explained. Intensive care procedures and equipment (lines, tubes, and machinery) are described to prepare the patient and family for the postoperative course; if possible, a tour of the intensive care unit is arranged. Expected postoperative pain and discomfort are explained, and the patient is instructed in pain assessment and administration of pain relief medications and other noninvasive pain relief measures. The neurological status checks that will be carried out routinely after surgery and normal responses are explained to the patient. An arterial line is inserted to monitor blood gases and blood pressure, an ECG recorded, a signed consent form obtained before anesthesia, physical preparation of the operative site performed according to protocol or surgeon's preference, and prescribed preoperative sedation administered.

*Postoperative:* Vital signs (including pupillary changes) are monitored every 15 min for the first hour (or according to protocol) until the patient is stable. (Lowered blood pressure and elevated heart rate and respirations could indicate cerebral ischemia.) Neurological assessments are performed for the first 24 hr (or according to protocol) to evaluate extremity strength, fine hand movements, speech, level of consciousness, and orientation. Intake and output are monitored hourly for the first 24 hr (or according to protocol). Continuous cardiac and hemodynamic monitoring is performed for the first 24 hr (or according to protocol), and an ECG is obtained if the patient has chest pain or arrhythmias. Prescribed analgesic medication is administered, and other noninvasive pain relief measures are offered.

Surgical wound care is provided and taught to the patient and family, and the signs and symptoms of infection to be reported to the surgeon (redness, swelling, or drainage from the incision, fever, or sore throat) are reviewed. Patients who smoke cigarettes are encouraged to stop and may be referred to a smoking cessation program or for nicotine patch therapy if appropriate. Modification of risk factors such high lipid levels or excessive weight is also advised. Prescribed medications are administered, and the patient is instructed in their use and adverse reactions to report to the physician.

The patient who has had a cerebrovascular accident and needs follow-up care is referred to a rehabilitation or home health care agency. Instruction is given in the management of postsurgical neurological, sensory, or motor deficits, and the importance of regular checkups explained. The surgeon or neurologist should be contacted immediately if any new neurological symptoms occur. The patient should wear or carry a medical identification tag to alert others to the condition and treatments in case of an emergency.

**carotid siphon** The S-shaped terminal portion of the internal carotid artery. It is the origin of most of the arteries to the brain.

**carotidynia, carotodynia** (kăr-ŏt″ĭ-dĭn′ē-ă) [″ + *odyne,* pain] Pain in the face, neck, or jaw. It may be produced in persons with atypical facial neuralgia by pressure on the common carotid artery. The pain is dull and referred to the same side to which pressure was applied. Treatment is with analgesics.

**carotinase** Carotenase.

**carotinemia** Carotenemia.

**carpal** [Gr. *karpalis*] Pert. to the carpus or wrist.

**carpal boss** A bony growth on the dorsal surface of the third metacarpocarpal joint.

**carpale** (kăr-pā′lē) [Gr. *karpos*] Any wrist bone.

**carpal spasm** Involuntary contraction of the muscles of the hand. SEE: *tetany*.

**carpal tunnel** The canal in the wrist bounded by osteofibrous material through which the flexor tendons and the median nerve pass.

**carpal tunnel syndrome** Pain or numbness that affects some part of the median nerve distribution of the hand (the palmar side of the thumb, the index finger, the radial half of the ring finger, and the radial half of the palm) and may radiate into the arm. There may be a history of cumulative trauma to the wrist, for example, in carpenters, rowers, or those who regularly use vibrating tools or machinery. SEE: *repetitive motion injury*.

TREATMENT: The patient should rest the extremity, avoiding anything that aggravates the symptoms. This may require intermittent splinting of the wrist to relieve tension on the median nerve. The patient's job requirements should be analyzed and recommendations provided for modified tools or a change in job assignment. The patient is taught how to avoid tension on the median nerve. Corticosteroids are injected under the actual tunnel but not the median nerve. Surgery is required in most cases. However, cortisone injection into the painful site or use of nonsteroidal anti-inflammatory drugs may eliminate the symptoms.

NURSING IMPLICATIONS: Medical evaluation is encouraged to determine the severity and underlying cause of the problem. The patient is evaluated for symptoms, degree of immobility, and changes that may have occurred over time. The patient's ability to make a fist is assessed, and the fingernails are inspected for atrophy and for surrounding dry, shiny skin. The transverse carpal ligament over the median nerve is lightly percussed to elicit pain, burning, numbness, or tingling in the hands and fingers (Tinel's sign). The patient is instructed to flex the wrists for 30 sec, and the hands and fingers are assessed for pain and numbness. The prescribed analgesic drug is administered, the patient's response evaluated, and the patient instructed in the drug's use, including the need to take it with food or antacids if stomach upset or irritation occurs. The patient should use the hands for self-care as much as immobility and pain allow. If a splint is prescribed to relieve symptoms, the patient is taught how to apply it without making it too tight, and how to remove it and perform gentle range-of-motion exercises daily.

Lifestyle changes needed to help minimize symptoms are demonstrated and explained to the patient. Occupational counseling is suggested if the syndrome necessitates a change in jobs.

If surgery (carpal tunnel release) is required, the nurse prepares the patient by explaining the procedure and expected sensations. Postoperatively, neurovascular status in the affected extremity is carefully assessed, and the patient is encouraged to keep the hand elevated to reduce swelling and discomfort. Prescribed wrist and finger exercises should be performed daily to improve circulation and to enhance muscle tone; these exercises can be performed in warm water if they are painful (wearing a surgical glove if dressings are still in place). Lifting anything weighing more than a few ounces should be avoided. The patient should report severe, persistent pain or tenderness, which may point to tenosynovitis or hematoma formation. The incision should be kept clean and dry, and dressings changed daily until the incision has healed completely. Dressings should also be checked for bleeding; any unusual bleeding or drainage should be reported. The patient is encouraged to express any concerns, and support is offered. SEE: *Nursing Diagnoses Appendix*.

**carpectomy** (kăr-pĕk'tō-mē) [" + *ektome,* excision] Excision of the carpus or a portion of it.

**carphology, carphologia** (kăr-fō-lō'jē-ă, -fŏl'ō-jē) [Gr. *karphos,* dry twig, + *legein,* to pluck] Involuntary picking at bedclothes, seen esp. in febrile or exhaustive delirium of the low muttering type. This is a grave symptom in cases of extreme exhaustion or approaching death. SYN: *floccillation.*

**carpo-** [Gr. *karpos*] Combining form for carpus.

**carpometacarpal** [" + *meta,* beyond, + *karpos,* wrist] Pert. to both the carpus and the metacarpus.

**carpopedal** (kăr"pō-pĕd'ăl) [" + L. *ped,* foot] Pert. to both the wrist and the foot.

**carpoptosis** (kăr"pŏp-tō'sĭs) [" + *ptosis,* a falling] Wrist drop.

**carpus** (kăr'pŭs) [L.] The eight bones of the wrist joint. SEE: *skeleton; wrist drop.*

**carrageen, carragheen** (kăr'ă-gēn) Irish moss; dried red alga, *Chondrus crispus,* from which the substance carrageenan, or carragheenan, is obtained. It is used as a demulcent and thickening agent in medicines and foods. SYN: *Irish moss.*

**Carrel-Dakin treatment** (kăr-ĕl'dā'kĭn) [Alexis Carrel, Fr.-U.S. surgeon, 1873–1944; Henry D. Dakin, U.S. chemist, 1880–1952] A method of wound irrigation first used in 1915. The wound is intermittently irrigated with Dakin's solution.

**carrier** [O. Fr. *carier,* to bear] **1.** A person who harbors a specific pathogenic organism, has no discernible symptoms or signs of the disease, and is potentially capable of spreading the organism to others. **2.** Something that carries anything, as an insect that passively carries infectious organisms. **3.** A substance that, when combined with another substance (transport substance), can pass through cell membranes as occurs in active transport mechanisms. SEE: *fomes; isolation; microorganism; vector; Universal Precautions Appendix; disease, communicable* for table. **4.** A heterozygote; one who carries a recessive gene together with its normal allele. **5.** An instrument or apparatus for transporting something; in dentistry, an amalgam carrier.

CLASSIFICATION: *Infection by animal carriers:* Some microorganisms may be carried from animals to humans by direct contact, indirect transfer, or intermediary hosts.

*Airborne infection:* Pathogenic organisms in the respiratory tract, discharged from the mouth or nose, may be airborne and may settle on food, clothing, walls, and floors. If they are of the type that resists drying for a long period, they may remain virulent until transmitted to another person. Coughing, sneezing, and expectorating may be responsible for droplet infection.

*Contact infection:* This is caused by transmission from person to person as in kissing, or coming in contact with persons who have communicable diseases or with utensils handled by such persons.

*Food-borne infection:* Bacteria may be transported by food. Root and salad vegetables may carry bacteria from the soil or from manure used as fertilizer. Cooking provides safeguards by destroying microorganisms on food.

*Human carriers:* Some parasites may live in or on the bodies of persons who themselves do not suffer from the parasites but may carry them to others. Carriers may be asymptomatic contact carriers (who never show symptoms), incubationary carriers (in whom the infection is starting but has not completed the incubation period), and convalescent carriers (who have recovered but still harbor the organism causing their disease).

*Insect vectors:* An insect may act as a physical carrier, such as the tick that may transmit the organism causing Rocky Mountain spotted fever, or an active intermediate host, such as the Anopheles mosquito, which transmits malaria.

*Prenatal infection:* This is caused by infection of the fetus from the mother's bloodstream or from contiguity with the maternal membranes.

*Soil-borne infection:* Soil-borne, spore-forming organisms commonly enter the body through wounds as in tetanus and gas gangrene.

*Water-borne infection:* Organisms producing typhoid, dysentery, cholera, and amebic infections may be carried through a water supply or in public swimming pools. These organisms may pass into the water from the feces of an infected person and be communicated to others.

***active c.*** One who harbors a pathogenic organism for a considerable period after recovery from disease caused by it.

***convalescent c.*** One who harbors an infective organism during recovery from the disease caused by the organism.

***genetic c.*** One whose chromosomes contain a pathological mutant gene that may be transmitted to offspring. In some cases, such as Tay-Sachs disease, this can be detected prenatally by a laboratory test done on amniotic fluid.

***healthy c.*** One who harbors an infectious organism but does not succumb to the disease. SYN: *passive c.*

***incubatory c.*** One who harbors and spreads an infectious organism during the incubation period of a disease.

***intermittent c.*** One who is capable of spreading infectious organisms at intervals.

***passive c.*** Healthy c.

**carrier-free** (kăr'ē-ĕr-frē) Not attached to a carrier; said of radioactive isotopes.

**Carrion's disease** (kăr-ē-ōnz') [Daniel A. Carrion, 1850–1885, a Peruvian student who died after voluntarily injecting himself with a disease] Bartonellosis.

**cartilage** (kăr′tĭ-lĭj) [L. *cartilago,* gristle] A specialized type of dense connective tissue consisting of cells embedded in a ground substance or matrix. The matrix is firm and compact and can withstand considerable pressure or tension. Cartilage is bluish-white or gray and is semiopaque; it has no nerve or blood supply of its own. The cells lie in cavities called lacunae. They may be single or in groups of two, three, or four.

Cartilage forms a part of the skeleton in adults. It also occurs in the costal cartilages of the ribs, in the nasal septum, in the external ear and lining the eustachian tube, in the wall of the larynx, in the trachea and bronchi, between vertebral bodies, and covering the articular surfaces of bones. It forms the major portion of the embryonic skeleton, providing a model in which most bones develop.

***articular c.*** The thin layer of smooth, elastic cartilage located on the joint surfaces of a bone, as in a synovial joint.

***costal c.*** A cartilage that connects the end of a true rib with the sternum or the end of a false rib with the costal cartilage above.

***cricoid c.*** The lowermost cartilage of the larynx; shaped like a signet ring, the broad portion or lamina being posterior, the anterior portion forming the arch. SEE: *larynx* for illus.

***cuneiform c.*** One of two small pieces of yellow elastic cartilage that lie in the aryepiglottic fold of the larynx immediately anterior to the arytenoid cartilage.

***fibrous c.*** Fibrocartilage.

***hyaline c.*** A bluish-white, glassy, translucent cartilage. The matrix appears homogeneous although it contains collagenous fibers forming a fine network. The walls of the lacunae stain intensely with basic dyes. Hyaline cartilage is flexible and slightly elastic. Its surface is covered by the perichondrium except on articular surfaces. It is found in articular cartilage, costal cartilages, the nasal septum, the larynx, and the trachea.

***repair of c. defects*** The experimental treatment of full-thickness knee cartilage defects by culturing cartilage cells from the patient and then implanting them in cartilage tears. The cells are covered with a thin patch of bone tissue.

***semilunar c.*** One of two crescentic cartilages (medial and lateral) of the knee joint between the femur and tibia.

***thyroid c.*** The largest cartilage of the larynx, a shield-shaped cartilage that forms the prominence known as the Adam's apple.

***yellow c.*** A network of yellow elastic fibers that holds cartilage cells and pervades intercellular substance. It is found in the epiglottis, the external ear, and the auditory tube. It strengthens these and maintains their shape.

**cartilaginification** (kăr″tĭ-lă-jĭn″ĭ-fĭ-kā′shŭn) [″ + *facere,* to make] Cartilage formation or chondrification; the development of cartilage from undifferentiated tissue.

**cartilaginoid** (kăr″tĭ-lăj′ĭ-noyd) [″ + Gr. *eidos,* form, shape] Resembling cartilage.

**cartilaginous** (kăr″tĭ-lăj′ĭ-nŭs) Pert. to or consisting of cartilage.

**cartilago** (kăr″tĭ-lă′gō) *pl.* **cartilagines** [L.] Cartilage.

**caruncle** (kăr′ŭng-kl) [L. *caruncula,* small flesh] A small fleshy growth.

***lacrimal c.*** Caruncula lacrimalis; a small reddish elevation found on the conjunctiva near the inner canthus, at the medial angle of the eye.

***sublingual c.*** A protuberance on each side of the frenulum of the tongue, containing the openings of the ducts from the submandibular and sublingual salivary glands.

***urethral c.*** A small, red, papillary growth that is highly vascular and is sometimes found in the urinary meatus in females. It is characterized by pain on urination and is very sensitive to friction.

**caruncula** (kăr-ŭng′kū-lă) *pl.* **carunculae** [L.] Caruncle.

***c. hymenales*** Small irregular nodules representing remains of the hymen.

**Carvallo's sign** [J. M. Rivero-Carvallo, contemporary Mexican physician] An increase in intensity of the presystolic murmur heard in patients with tricuspid stenosis during inspiration, and its decrease during expiration. This is best demonstrated with the patient in an erect position.

**carver** A knife or other instrument used to fashion or shape an object. In dentistry, it is used with artificial teeth or dental restorations.

***amalgam c.*** A small, sharp instrument of varying shape used to carve or contour amalgam for interdental occlusion.

***wax c.*** A blunt instrument of varying shape to heat and carve or shape wax patterns.

**cary-, caryo-** [Gr. *karyon,* nucleus] Combining form meaning *nucleus.* SEE: *kary-, karyo-.*

**Casal necklace** [Gaspar Casal, Sp. physician, 1691–1759] Bilaterally symmetrical lesions of the neck that represent a portion of the skin's involvement in pellagra. The lesions begin as erythemas and progress to vesiculation and crusting.

**cascade** (kăs-kād′) The continuation of a process through a series of steps, each step initiating the next, until the final step is reached. The action may or may not become amplified as each step progresses.

**cascara sagrada** (kăs-kăr′ă să-gră′dă) The dried bark of *Rhamnus purshiana,* a small tree grown on the western U.S. coast and in parts of South America. It is the main ingredient in aromatic cascara sagrada fluid extract, a cathartic.

**case** [L. *casus,* happening] **1.** An occurrence of disease; incorrectly used to refer to a patient. **2.** An enclosing structure.

**caseate** (kā′sē-āt) [L. *caseus,* cheese] To undergo cheesy degeneration, as in certain necroses.

**caseation** (kā″sē-ā′shŭn) **1.** The process in which necrotic tissue is converted into a granular amorphous mass resembling cheese. **2.** The precipitation of casein during coagulation of milk.

**case control** In epidemiology, a study in which index cases are matched with comparison cases to discover risk factors or exposure.

**casefinding** An active attempt to identify persons who have disease.

**case history** The complete medical, family, social, and psychiatric history of a patient up to the time of admission for the present illness.

**casein** (kā′sē-ĭn) [L. *caseus,* cheese] The principal protein in milk. It is present in milk curds. It supplies all of the amino acids necessary for growth and development. When coagulated by rennin or acid, it becomes one of the principal ingredients of cheese. SEE: *caseinogen.*

**caseinogen** (kā-sē-ĭn′ō-jĕn) [″ + Gr. *gennan,* to produce] The principal protein, from which casein is derived, in milk. It is the substance in solution, and casein is the result of its precipitation. Its conversion into casein is the essential process in the curdling of milk.

**case law** Opinions or decisions made by the courts.

**case management** An individualized approach to obtaining needed services for a patient by using a case manager to link the patient to direct service providers. It is a particularly valuable approach to meeting the service needs of the homebound elderly.

***hospital c.m.*** A system of patient care delivery in which a case manager, typically a registered nurse, coordinates interdisciplinary care for a group of patients. The advantages are improved quality, continuity of care, and decreased hospital costs.

**caseous** (kā′sē-ŭs) **1.** Resembling cheese. **2.** Pert. to transformation of tissues into a cheesy mass.

**$CaSO_4$** Calcium sulfate.

**cassava** A group of perennial herbs of the genus *Manihot.* The plant is one of the most efficient converters of solar energy to carbohydrate. The root of *M. esculenta* provides an excellent source of starch and can thrive in poor, dry, acid soils. To be suitable for eating, the root is processed by one of several methods to remove or control the amount of cyanide present. Tapioca is made from cassava.

**cassette** (kă-sĕt′) [Fr., little box] A flat, lightproof box with an intensifying screen, for holding x-ray film; a case for film or magnetic tape.

**cassette, screen-type** A film holder usually made of metal, with the exposure side usually made of a material with a low atomic number such as aluminum or magnesium.

**cast** [ME. *casten,* to carry] **1.** In dentistry, a positive copy of jaw tissues over which denture bases may be made. **2.** To make an accurate metallic reproduction of a wax pattern of a dental appliance, tooth crown, or inlay cavity preparation. **3.** Pliable or fibrous material shed in various pathological conditions; the product of effusion. It is molded to the shape of the part in which it has been accumulated. Casts are classified as bronchial, intestinal, nasal, esophageal, renal, tracheal, urethral, and vaginal; constituents are classified as bloody, fatty, fibrinous, granular, hyaline, mucous, and waxy. **4.** A solid mold of a part, usually applied in situ for immobilization as in fractures, dislocations, and other severe injuries. It is usually made of plaster of paris, sodium silicate, starch, or dextrin that is rubbed into crinoline, then soaked in water, carefully applied to the immobilized part, and allowed to harden. Synthetic materials, such as fiberglass, are also used, esp. for non–weight-bearing parts of the body. SEE: illus.

NURSING IMPLICATIONS: Neurovascular status distal to the cast is monitored; and any deterioration in circulation and in sensory or motor abilities, such as paresthesias, paralysis, diminished pulses, pallor, coldness, or pain, is documented and reported. Pain or burning under the cast, including the region involved, is also documented and reported. The cast is bivalved or removed to relieve pressure. Objects should not be placed inside a cast to relieve itching, but relief often can be obtained by applying cold (a well-sealed ice bag) to the cast over the area that itches, or by scratching the opposite extremity in the same area. The patient is instructed in cast care and and ways to protect the cast from damage; prescribed exercises or activity limitations; and use of any assistive devices such as slings, crutches, or walker. SEE: *Nursing Diagnoses Appendix.*

***body c.*** A cast used to immobilize the spine. It may extend from the thorax to the groin.

***bronchial c.*** A cast seen in the sputum of patients with asthma and some patients with bronchitis.

***broomstick c.*** A type of cast used following skin traction for Legg's disease (Legg-Calvé-Perthes disease). A bar is used between upper femoral casts to maintain abduction. SEE: *Legg's disease.*

***epithelial c.*** An aggregation of renal epithelium with cells filled with granules or fat droplets. It is seen in acute nephritis. SEE: illus.

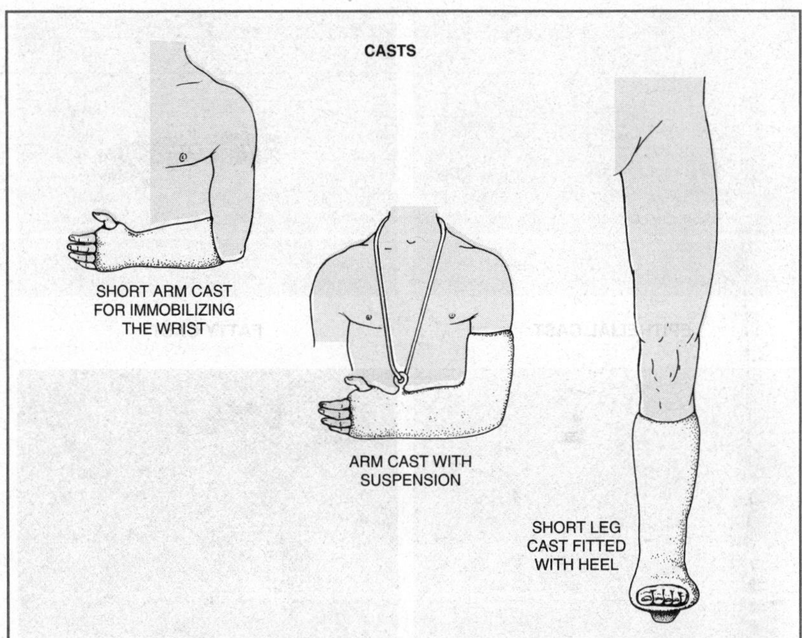


***fatty c.*** Any cast made up of fat globules. SEE: illus.

***fibrinous c.*** A yellow-brown cast seen in acute nephritis.

***granular c.*** A dark urinary cast of a granular substance, usually a degenerative form of a hyaline or waxy cast.

***hyaline c.*** The most common form of cast found in the urine, transparent, pale, and having homogeneous rounded ends. Its presence indicates nephropathy. SEE: illus.

***light c.*** A cast used in orthopedics, made of a lightweight material that is usually applied and then hardened by treating with the heat from a light.

***red blood cell c.*** A urinary cast composed principally of red blood cells. SEE: illus.

***urinary c.*** A cast, found in the urine, formed from protein precipitates in the renal tubules. SEE: *mucoprotein, Tamm-Horsfell.*

***uterine c.*** A cast from the uterus passed in exfoliative endometritis or membranous dysmenorrhea.

***waxy c.*** A light yellowish, well-defined urinary cast with a tendency to split transversely, found in some cases of amyloid degeneration and advanced nephritis. SEE: illus.

***white blood cell c.*** A leukocyte cast found in urine in suppuration of the kidney. SEE: illus.

**Castellani's paint** (kăs-tĕl-ăn′ēz) [Aldo Castellani, It. physician, 1878–1971] Paint used to disinfect skin and to treat fungus infections of the skin. Its components are phenol, resorcinol, basic fuchsin, boric acid, and acetone.

**casting** The forming of an object in a mold.

**Castle's intrinsic factor** [William Bosworth Castle, U.S. physician and educator, 1897–1990] A substance secreted by the stomach, essential for the absorption of cyanocobalamin (vitamin $B_{12}$; extrinsic factor). Absence of the intrinsic factor causes pernicious anemia.

**castor oil** A fixed oil expressed from the seed of the plant *Ricinus communis.* It is used externally as an emollient and internally as a cathartic. In the digestive tract it is hydrolyzed to ricinoleic acid, which acts as an irritant type of laxative.

**castrate** (kăs′trāt) [L. *castrare,* to prune] **1.** To remove the testicles or ovaries. SEE: *spay.* **2.** One who has been castrated.

**castrated** Rendered incapable of reproduction by removal of the testicles or ovaries.

**castration** (kăs-trā′shŭn) **1.** Excision of the testicles or ovaries. **2.** Destruction or inactivation of the gonads.

***female c.*** Removal of the ovaries. SYN: *oophorectomy; spaying.*

***male c.*** Removal of the testes. SYN: *orchiectomy.*

***parasitic c.*** Destruction of the gonads by parasitic organisms early in life. It may result from direct infestation of the gonad or indirectly from effects of infestation in other parts of the body.

**castration anxiety, castration complex** Anxiety about the possibility of injury to or loss of the testicles or ovaries.

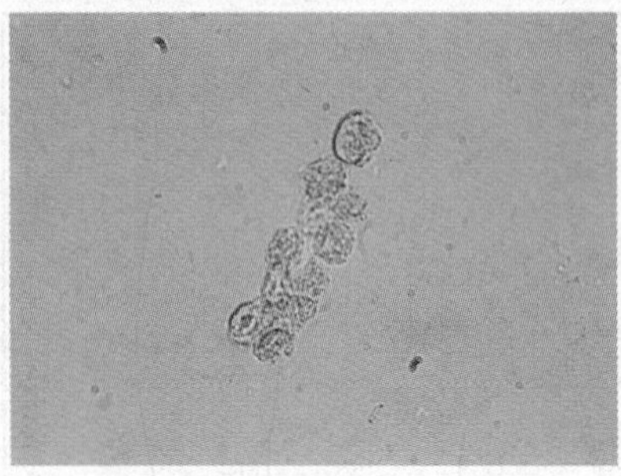

EPITHELIAL CAST

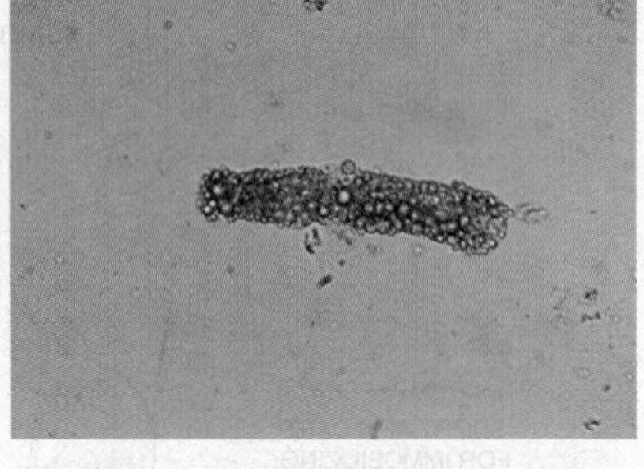

FATTY CAST

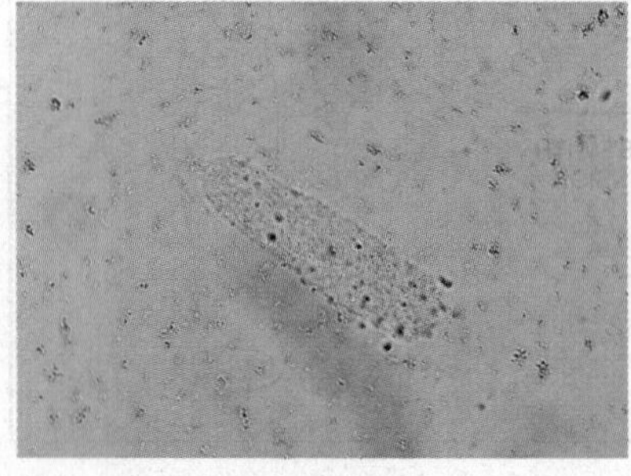

HYALINE CAST

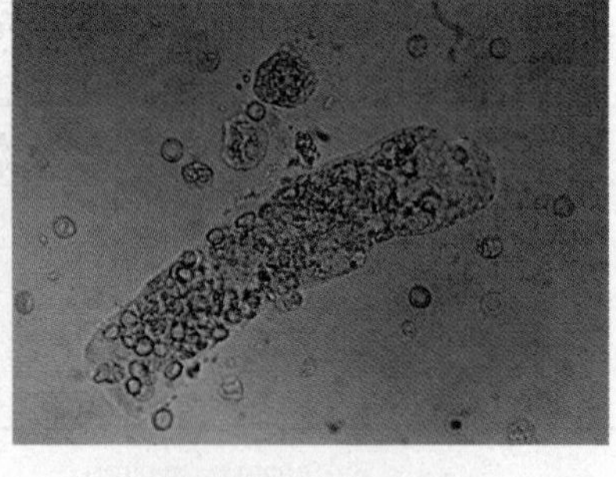

RED BLOOD CELL CAST

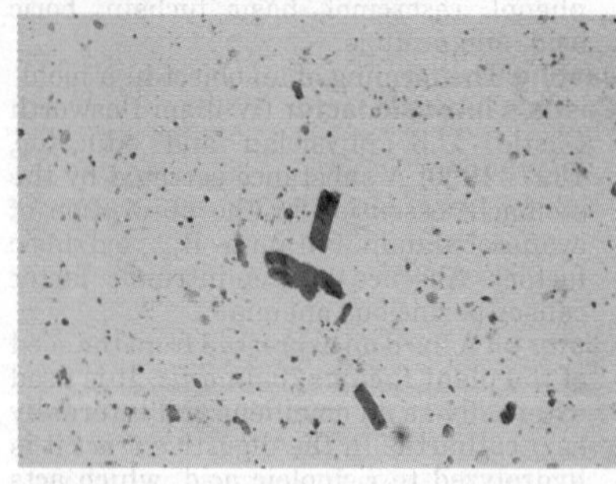

WAXY CAST

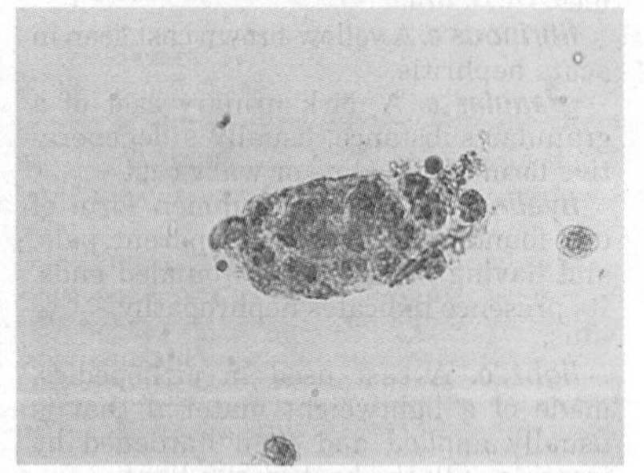

WHITE BLOOD CELL CAST

**URINARY CASTS** (ORIG. MAG. ×400)

**casualty** (kăz′ū-ăl-tē) [L. *casualis,* accidental] **1.** An accident causing injury or death. **2.** A person injured or killed in an accident. **3.** A military person captured, missing, injured, or killed.

**casuistics** (kăz-ū-ĭs′tĭks) [L. *casus,* chance] **1.** Analysis of clinical case records to establish the general characteristics of a disease. **2.** In moral questions, the determination of right and wrong by application of ethical principles to a particular case.

**cata-** [Gr. *kata,* down] Prefix indicating *down, downward, destructive,* or *against.*

**catabasis** (kă-tăb′ă-sĭs) [Gr. *kata,* down, + *basis,* going] The decline of a disease.

**catabatic** (kăt-ă-băt′ĭk) Pert. to catabasis.

**catabolin** (kă-tăb′ō-lĭn) Catabolite.

**catabolism** (kă-tăb′ō-lĭzm) [Gr. *katabole,* a casting down, + *-ismos,* condition] The destructive phase of metabolism; the opposite of anabolism. Catabolism includes all the processes in which complex substances are converted into simpler ones, usually with the release of energy. SEE: *anabolism; metabolism.* **catabolic** (kăt″ă-bŏl′ĭk), *adj.*

**catabolite** (kă-tăb′ō-līt) Any product of catabolism. SYN: *catabolin.*

**catacrotic** (kăt″ă-krŏt′ĭk) [″ + *krotos,* beat] Indicating the downstroke of pulse tracing interrupted by an upstroke.

**catacrotism** (kă-tăk′rō-tĭzm) [″ + ″ + *-ismos,* condition] A pulse with one or more secondary expansions of the artery following the main beat.

**catadicrotic** (kăt″ă-dī-krŏt′ĭk) [″ + *dis,* twice, + *krotos,* beat] Manifesting one or more secondary expansions of a pulse on the descending limb of the tracing.

**catadicrotism** (kăt″ă-dī′krō-tĭzm) [″ + ″ + ″ + *-ismos,* condition] Two minor expansions following the main beat of an artery.

**catagen** (kăt′ă-jĕn) [″ + *gennan,* to produce] The intermediate phase of the hair-growth cycle, between the growth or anagen stage and the resting or telogen phase.

**catagenesis** (kăt″ă-jĕn′ĕ-sĭs) [″ + *genesis,* generation, birth] Retrogression or involution.

**catalase** (kăt′ă-lās) An enzyme present in almost all cells that catalyzes the decomposition of hydrogen peroxide to water and oxygen.

**catalepsy** (kăt′ă-lĕp″sē) [Gr. *kata,* down, + *lepsis,* seizure] A condition seen in psychotic patients in which generalized diminished responsiveness usually is marked by a trancelike state. Physicians and nurses should keep in mind that although the patient is in a trance, conversations may be heard. Therefore, one's actions toward and talk about such patients should be the same as if they were fully conscious. **cataleptic** (kăt″ă-lĕp′tĭk), *adj.*

**cataleptoid** (kăt″ă-lĕp′toyd) [″ + ″+ *eidos,* form, shape] Resembling or simulating catalepsy.

**catalysis** (kă-tăl′ĭ-sĭs) [Gr. *katalysis,* dissolution] The speeding of a chemical reaction by a catalyst. **catalytic** (kăt-ăl-ĭt′ĭk), *adj.*

**catalyst** (kăt′ă-lĭst) A substance that speeds the rate of a chemical reaction without being permanently altered in the reaction. Catalysts are effective in small quantities and are not used up in the reaction (i.e., they can be recovered unchanged). All enzymes are catalysts; the human body has thousands of enzymes, each specific for a particular reaction. For example, pepsin catalyzes the hydrolysis of protein; amylase catalyzes the hydrolysis of starch; transaminases catalyze the transfer of an amino group from one molecule to another. SYN: *catalyzer.*

**catalyze** (kăt′ă-līz) [Gr. *katalysis,* dissolution] To cause catalysis.

**catalyzer** (kăt′ă-lī-zĕr) A catalyst.

**catamenia** (kăt-ă-mē′nē-ă) [Gr. *kata,* according to, + *men,* month] Menstruation. **catamenial** (-ăl), *adj.*

**catamnesis** (kăt-ăm-nē′sĭs) [Gr. *kata,* down, + *mneme,* memory] A patient's medical history after treatment; the follow-up history. SEE: *anamnesis.*

**cataphasia** (kăt-ă-fā′zē-ă) [″ + *phasis,* speech] A speech disorder causing an involuntary repetition of the same word.

**cataphoresis** (kăt″ă-fō-rē′sĭs) [Gr. *kata,* down, + *phoresis,* being carried] Transmission of electronegative ions or drugs into the body tissues or through a membrane by use of an electric current.

**cataphoria** (kăt″ă-fō′rē-ă) [″ + *pherein,* to bear] The tendency of visual axes to incline below the horizontal plane.

**cataphoric** Pert. to cataphora or cataphoresis.

**cataplectic** (kăt-ă-plĕk′tĭk) [″ + *plexis,* stroke] Pert. to cataplexy.

**cataplexy, cataplexia** (kăt′ă-plĕks-ē, kăt-ă-plĕk′sē-ă) A sudden, brief loss of muscle control brought on by strong emotion or emotional response, such as a hearty laugh, excitement, surprise, or anger. Although this may cause collapse, the patient remains fully conscious. The episode lasts from a few seconds to as long as several minutes. The condition may be less severe with age. About 70% of patients with narcolepsy, also have cataplexy. Imipramine hydrochloride is beneficial in treating this disorder.

**Catapres** Trade name for clonidine hydrochloride.

**cataract** (kăt′ă-răkt) [L. *cataracta,* waterfall] Opacity of the lens of the eye, its capsule, or both. Varieties are capsular, polar, lamellar, nuclear, cortical, morgagnian, congenital, infantile, traumatic, diabetic, and senile. An estimated 1.25 million people worldwide are blinded by cataracts each year. SEE: illus.

STAGES: The stages of cataracts are as follows: the incipient stage (spoke-shaped opacities, cloudlike opacities, opacity of the cortex or nucleus); the swelling or immature stage (swollen lens, shallow anterior chamber); the mature stage in which the lens has become completely opaque; and the hypermature stage (lens becoming either solid and shrunken or soft and liquid). SEE: *cataract, mature.*

SYMPTOMS: At first, vision is distorted, particularly during night driving or in very bright light, due to light sensitivity (photophobia). As the cataract progresses, severe visual impairment develops.

ETIOLOGY: The common form is a result of aging. Other forms may be congenital or caused by infection, injury, exposure to radiation, or adrenocortical hormones taken for long periods. Cataracts may also occur as a complication of diabetes. Premature cataract development has been linked to cigarette smoking.

TREATMENT: Surgical removal of the lens is required unless associated inflammation is present. In the past, this procedure required an incision large enough to permit extraction of the lens and implantation of an artificial lens. Now the procedure can be done through a very small (3 mm) incision in the cornea. Ultrasound is used to fragment the cataract, which can then be removed through the incision. The replacement lens is folded

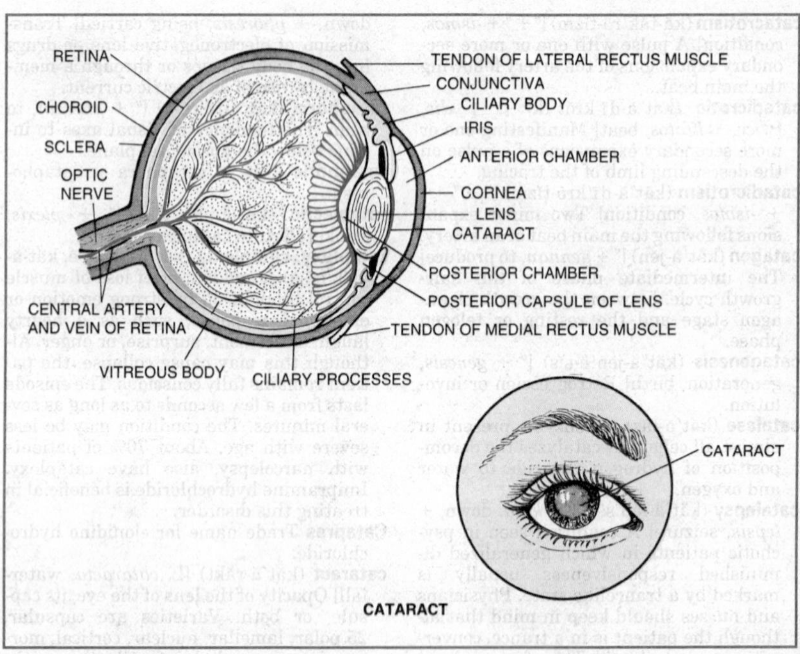


CATARACT

and inserted through the small incision. Because the operation is done on an outpatient basis using topical anesthesia, the patient is able to recover at home. SEE: *lens, intraocular; phacoemulsification.*

NURSING IMPLICATIONS: *Preoperative:* The procedure is explained to the patient. An antiseptic facial scrub is performed. Mydriatic and cycloplegic eye drops are instilled to dilate the pupil, and osmotic diuretics are given to reduce intraocular pressure. Antibiotics, a sedative, and a local anesthetic are provided.

*Postoperative:* The nurse orients the patient to the surroundings and speaks with him or her at frequent intervals to decrease the effects of sensory deprivation. Any severe pain, which may signify an increase in intraocular pressure or hemorrhage; increased drainage; bleeding; or fever, are assessed, documented, and reported. Prescribed antiemetics are administered, and the patient is instructed about use of prescribed analgesics. An eye patch and shield are required temporarily to prevent injury and infection; these coverings will result in temporary loss of peripheral vision on the operative side. The patient will need help when getting up from bed and should sleep on the unaffected side to reduce intraocular pressure. Safety measures, such as using up-and-down head movements to judge distance and turning the head fully toward the operative side to view objects in that area, help to protect the patient from injury due to decreased peripheral vision. Both patient and family are taught how to change an eye patch, to inspect the eye for redness or watering and to report these conditions as well as any photophobia or sudden visual changes, to instill eye drops as prescribed, and to maintain the eye patch and shield as directed (usually for several weeks, esp. during sleep).

Activities that raise intraocular pressure, including heavy lifting, bending from the waist, straining during defecation, or vigorous coughing and sneezing, should be avoided. Strenuous activity should also be avoided for 6 to 10 weeks or as directed by the ophthalmologist. Keeping follow-up appointments is important. Dark glasses should be worn to counteract glare. If the patient will be wearing contact lenses, proper insertion, removal, and care are explained, as is the need to visit the ophthalmologist routinely for removal, cleaning, and reinsertion of extended-wear lenses. SEE: *Nursing Diagnoses Appendix.*

***capsular c.*** A cataract occurring in the capsule.

***hypermature c.*** Overripe c.

***immature c.*** An early cataract, too poorly developed to require therapy.

***lenticular c.*** A cataract occurring in the lens.

***mature c.*** Sufficiently dense changes in the anterior cortex of the lens to prevent the examiner from viewing the posterior portion of the lens and the posterior portion of the eye, that is, the entire lens is opaque and ophthalmoscopic examination of the eye past the lens is not possible.

***morgagnian c.*** SEE: *Morgagni's cataract.*

***nuclear c.*** A cataract in which the central portion of the lens is opacified.

***overripe c.*** A cataract in which the lens solidifies and shrinks. This stage follows the mature stage. SYN: *hypermature c.*

***radiation c.*** A cataract caused by exposure to radiation, esp. from sunlight.

***ripe c.*** A mature cataract.

***senile c.*** A cataract occurring in an elderly person.

**cataractogenic** (kăt″ă-răk″tō-jĕn′ĭk) [L. *cataracta,* waterfall, + Gr. *gennan,* to produce] Causing or forming cataracts.

**catarrh** (kă-tăr′) [Gr. *katarrhein,* to flow down] Term formerly applied to inflammation of mucous membranes, esp. of the head and throat. **catarrhal** (-ăl), *adj.*

***dry c.*** Severe spells of coughing with little or no expectoration. It is generally seen in the elderly in association with emphysema or asthma.

**catatonia** (kăt-ă-tō′nē-ă) [″ + *tonos,* tension] **1.** A phase of schizophrenia in which the patient is unresponsive, marked by the tendency to assume and remain in a fixed posture and the inability to move or talk. **2.** Stupor. **catatonic** (-tŏ′nĭk), *adj.*

**catatricrotic** (kăt″ă-trī-krŏt′ĭk) [″ + *treis,* three, + *krotos,* beat] Manifesting a third impulse in the descending stroke of the sphygmogram of the pulse.

**catatricrotism** (kăt″ă-trī′krō-tĭzm) A condition in which the pulse shows a third impulse in the descending stroke of a pulse tracing.

**catatropia** (kăt″ă-trō′pē-ă) [″ + *tropos,* turning] A condition in which both eyes are turned downward.

**cat-cry syndrome** SEE: *syndrome, cri du chat.*

**catecholamine** (kăt″ĕ-kōl′ă-mēn) One of two biologically active amines, epinephrine and norepinephrine, derived from the amino acid tyrosine. They have a marked effect on the nervous and cardiovascular systems, metabolic rate, temperature, and smooth muscle. SEE: *serotonin.*

**catelectrotonus** (kăt″ē-lĕk-trŏt′ō-nŭs) [″ + *elektron,* amber, + *tonos,* tension] The increased excitability produced in a nerve or muscle in the region near the cathode during the passage of an electric current.

**catenating** (kăt′ĕn-āt″ĭng) [L. *catena,* chain] **1.** Pert. to a disease that is linked with another. **2.** Forming a series of symptoms.

**catenation** Concatenation.

**catenoid** (kăt′ĕ-noyd) [″ + Gr. *eidos,* form, shape] Chainlike; pert. to protozoan colonies whose individuals are joined end to end.

**catgut** Sheep intestine twisted for use as an absorbable ligature.

***chromic c.*** Catgut treated with chromium trioxide. This enhances the strength of the suture material.

**catharsis** (kă-thăr′sĭs) [Gr. *katharsis,* purification] **1.** Purgative action of the bowels. **2.** The Freudian method of freeing the mind by recalling from the patient's memory the events or experiences that were the original causes of a psychoneurosis. SEE: *abreaction.*

**cathartic** (kă-thăr′tĭk) [Gr. *kathartikos,* purging] An active purgative, producing bowel movements (e.g., cascara sagrada, castor oil). SEE: *purgative.*

**cathepsin-D** (kă-thĕp′sĭn) An estrogen-induced lysomal protease, the level of which in the blood may be a predictor of breast cancer recurrence in patients whose lymph nodes show no evidence of metastasis.

**catheter** (kăth′ĕ-tĕr) [Gr. *katheter,* something inserted] A tube passed through the body for evacuating fluids or injecting them into body cavities. It may be made of elastic, elastic web, rubber, glass, metal, or plastic. SEE: illus.

***arterial c.*** A catheter inserted into an artery to measure pressure, remove blood, inject medication or radiographic contrast media, or perform an interventional radiological procedure.

***balloon c.*** A double-lumened catheter surrounded by a balloon. The balloon may be expanded by injecting air, saline, or contrast medium.

***cardiac c.*** A long, fine catheter specially designed for passage through the lumen of a blood vessel into the chambers of the heart. SEE: *cardiac catheterization.*

***central c.*** A catheter inserted into a central vein or artery for diagnostic or therapeutic purposes or both.

***central venous c.*** A catheter inserted into the superior vena cava to permit intermittent or continuous monitoring of central venous pressure and to facilitate obtaining blood samples for chemical analysis. SEE: illus.

***condom c.*** A specially designed condom that includes a catheter attached to the end. The catheter carries urine to a collecting bag. Its use prevents men with uri-

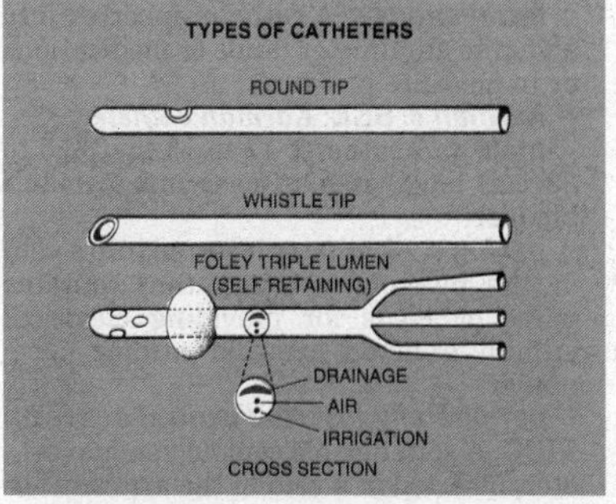

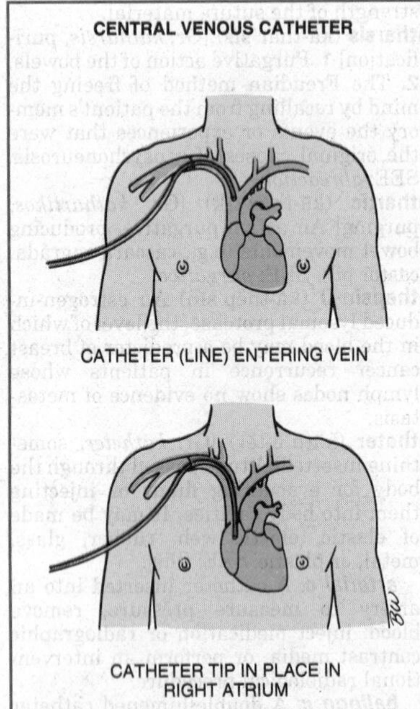


nary incontinence from soiling clothes or bed linens.

---

Caution: Continual use of this device may excoriate the skin of the penis.

---

***double-channel c.*** A catheter providing for inflow and outflow.

***elbowed c.*** Prostatic c.

***eustachian c.*** A catheter passed into the eustachian tube through the nasal passages.

***female c.*** A catheter about 5 in. (12.7 cm) long, used to pass into a woman's bladder.

***Foley c.*** SEE: *Foley catheter*.

***indwelling c.*** Any catheter that is allowed to remain in place in a vein, artery, or body cavity.

***intra-aortic c.*** SEE: *intra-aortic balloon counterpulsation*.

***intravenous c.*** A catheter inserted into a vein to administer fluids or medications or to measure pressure.

***Karman c.*** SEE: *Karman catheter*.

***male c.*** A catheter 12 to 13 in. (30.5 to 33 cm) long, used to pass into a man's bladder.

***pacing c.*** A catheter inserted into a vein or the pulmonary artery that contains wires or leads for providing electrical stimuli from an external cardiac pacemaker.

***peripherally inserted central c.*** ABBR: PICC. A soft, flexible central venous catheter, inserted in a vein in the arm and advanced until the tip is positioned in the axillary, subclavian, or bracheocephalic vein. It may also be advanced into the superior vena cava. A PICC is commonly used for prolonged antibiotic therapy, total parenteral nutrition, or continuous opioid infusion.

***pharyngeal suction c.*** A rigid tube used to suction the pharynx during direct visualization. SYN: *Yankauer suction c.*

***prostatic c.*** A catheter, 15 to 16 in. (38 to 40.6 cm) long, with a short elbowed tip designed to pass prostatic obstruction. SYN: *elbowed c.*

***pulmonary artery c.*** A catheter inserted into the pulmonary artery to measure pulmonary artery pressures, pulmonary capillary wedge pressure, and cardiac output.

***self-retaining c.*** A bladder catheter designed to remain in place (e.g., a Foley catheter).

***suprapubic c.*** A urinary catheter used for closed drainage. It is inserted through the skin, about 2.5 cm above the symphysis pubis, into the distended bladder. This is usually done under general anesthesia. If it is to remain in place, it is sutured to the abdominal skin.

***Swan-Ganz c.*** SEE: *Swan-Ganz catheter*.

***Tenckhoff peritoneal c.*** SEE: *Tenckhoff peritoneal catheter*.

***triple-lumen c.*** A central catheter containing three separate channels or passageways.

***tunneled central venous c.*** An intravenous catheter inserted into the subclavian or internal jugular vein and then advanced into the right atrium or superior vena cava. The proximal end is tunneled subcutaneously from the insertion site and brought out through the skin at an exit site below the nipple line. Commonly used tunneled catheters include the Hickman and Broviac catheters.

***vertebrated c.*** A catheter in sections to be fitted together so that it is flexible.

***winged c.*** A catheter with little flaps at each side of the beak to help retain it in the bladder.

***Yankauer suction c.*** SEE: *Yankauer suction catheter*.

**catheterization** (kăth″ĕ-tĕr-ĭ-zā′shŭn) [Gr. *katheterismos*] Use or passage of a catheter.

***cardiac c.*** SEE: *cardiac catheterization*.

***urinary bladder c.*** Introduction of a catheter through the urethra into the bladder for withdrawal of urine.

Both men and women may be instructed in the technique of clean intermittent self-catheterization. The method is similar to the clean-catch method, except that a catheter is used. Patients need instruction in understanding their own anatomy and physiology, ensuring that the catheter is clean, and washing and storing it after use. Self-catheterization must be done three or four times each day. It allows patients to be free of indwelling catheters and may permit return to normal activities of daily living. SEE: illus.

NURSING IMPLICATIONS: The procedure is explained to the patient. The necessary equipment is assembled, the patient properly positioned and draped, the site prepared, and the catheter inserted. Sterile technique is maintained throughout these procedures, and the indwelling catheter is connected to a closed drainage system prior to insertion. The tube is secured to the patient's leg, the drainage tubing is looped on the bed, and the tubing leading to the collection bag is straightened to facilitate gravity drainage. The collection bag is suspended above the floor. The drainage tube is prevented from touching a surface when the collection bag is emptied; the spout is wiped with an alcohol swab before being refastened to the bag. The meatal area should be cleansed daily. The patient's ability to void and remain continent is periodically evaluated and catheterization is discontinued when this is possible. Results of the procedure, including the character and volume of urine drained and the patient's response, are observed and documented. SEE: *urinary tract infection.*

*Female:* The patient should be in the dorsal recumbent position on a firm mattress or examining table to enhance visualization of the urinary meatus. Alternately, the lithotomy position, with buttocks at the edge of the examining table and feet in stirrups, may be used. For female patients with difficulties involving hip and knee movements, the Sims' or left lateral position may be more comfortable and allow for better visualization. Pillows may be placed under the head and shoulders to relax the abdominal muscles.

*Male:* The patient should be in a supine position with legs extended. After the procedure, care should be taken to return the prepuce to its normal position to prevent any subsequent swelling.

**catheterize** (kăth′ĕ-tĕr-īz) To pass or introduce a catheter into a part. Term usually refers to bladder catheterization.

**cathexis** (kă-thĕk′sĭs) [Gr. *kathexis,* retention] The emotional or mental energy used in concentrating on an object or idea.

**cathode** (kăth′ōd) [Gr. *kathodos,* downward path] ABBR: ca. **1.** The negative electrode from which electrons are emitted; the opposite of the anode or positive pole. **2.** In a vacuum tube, the electrode that serves as the source of the electron stream. **cathodal** (-ăl), *adj.*

**cathodic** (kă-thŏd′ĭk) **1.** Pert. to a cathode. **2.** Proceeding outwardly or efferently as applied to a nerve impulse.

**cation** (kăt′ī-ŏn) [Gr. *kation,* descending] An ion with a positive electric charge; opposite of anion. It is attracted by and travels to the cathode (negative pole). SEE: *ion.*

CATHETERIZATION OF URINARY BLADDER

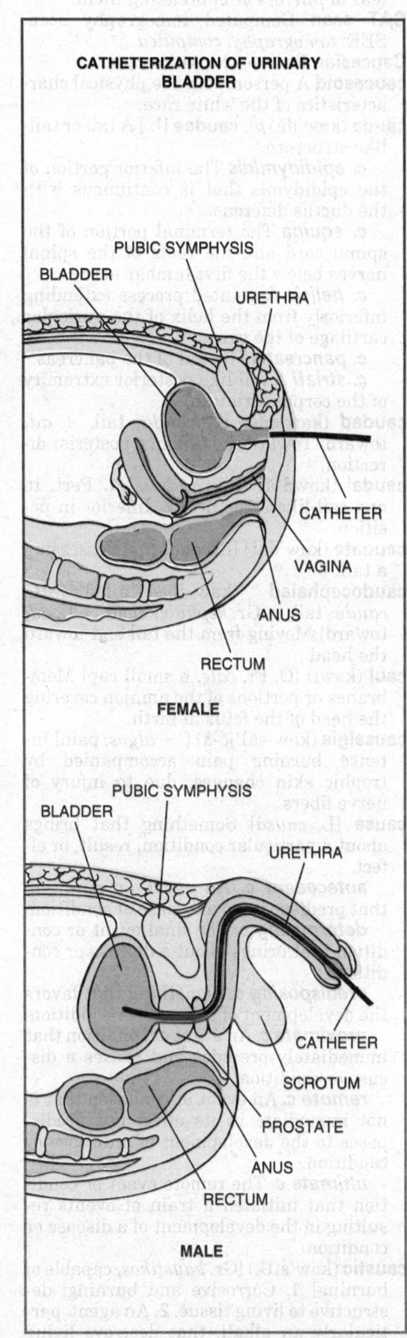

**catoptrophobia** (kăt″ŏp-trō-fō′bē-ă) [Gr. *katoptron,* mirror, + *phobos,* fear] A morbid fear of mirrors or of breaking them.

**CAT scan** Computed tomography scan. SEE: *tomography, computed.*

**Caucasian** Pert. to the white race.

**caucasoid** A person with the physical characteristics of the white race.

**cauda** (kaw′dă) *pl.* **caudae** [L.] A tail or tail-like structure.

***c. epididymidis*** The inferior portion of the epididymis that is continuous with the ductus deferens.

***c. equina*** The terminal portion of the spinal cord and the roots of the spinal nerves below the first lumbar nerve.

***c. helicis*** A pointed process extending inferiorly from the helix of the auricular cartilage of the ear.

***c. pancreatis*** The tail of the pancreas.

***c. striati*** A tail-like posterior extremity of the corpus striatum.

**caudad** (kaw′dăd) [L. *cauda,* tail, + *ad,* toward] Toward the tail; in a posterior direction.

**caudal** (kawd′ăl) [L. *caudalis*] **1.** Pert. to any tail-like structure. **2.** Inferior in position.

**caudate** (kaw′dāt) [L. *caudatus*] Possessing a tail.

**caudocephalad** (kaw-dō-sĕf′ă-lăd) [L. *cauda,* tail, + Gr. *kephale,* head, + L. *ad,* toward] Moving from the tail end toward the head.

**caul** (kawl) [O. Fr. *cale,* a small cap] Membranes or portions of the amnion covering the head of the fetus at birth.

**causalgia** (kaw-săl′jē-ă) [″ + *algos,* pain] Intense burning pain accompanied by trophic skin changes, due to injury of nerve fibers.

**cause** [L. *causa*] Something that brings about a particular condition, result, or effect.

***antecedent c.*** An event or condition that predisposes to a disease or condition.

***determining c.*** The final event or condition that brings about a disease or condition.

***predisposing c.*** Something that favors the development of a disease or condition.

***proximate c.*** An event or condition that immediately precedes and causes a disease or condition.

***remote c.*** An event or condition that is not immediate in its effect but predisposes to the development of a disease or condition.

***ultimate c.*** The remote event or condition that initiated a train of events resulting in the development of a disease or condition.

**caustic** (kaw′stĭk) [Gr. *kaustikos,* capable of burning] **1.** Corrosive and burning; destructive to living tissue. **2.** An agent, particularly an alkali, that destroys living tissue (e.g., silver nitrate, potassium hydroxide, nitric acid). SEE: *poisoning; Poisons and Poisoning Appendix.*

**cauterant** (kaw′tĕr-ănt) [Gr. *kauter,* a burner] **1.** Cauterizing. **2.** A cauterizing agent.

**cauterization** (kaw″tĕr-ī-zā′shŭn) [Gr. *kauteriazein,* to burn] Destruction of tissue with a caustic, an electric current, a hot iron, or by freezing.

***chemical c.*** Cauterization by the use of chemical agents, esp. caustic substances.

***electrical c.*** Electrocautery.

**cauterize** (kaw′tĕr-īz) To burn with a cautery, or to apply one.

**cautery** (kaw′tĕr-ē) [Gr. *kauter,* a burner] A device used to destroy tissue by electricity, freezing, heat, or corrosive chemicals. It is used in potentially infected wounds and to destroy excess granulation tissue. Thermocautery consists of a red-hot or white-hot object, usually a piece of wire or pointed metallic instrument, heated in a flame or with electricity (electrocautery, galvanocautery).

**cava** (kā′vă) **1.** A hollow area or a body cavity. **2.** The vena cava.

**caval** (kā′văl) Pert. to the vena cava.

**caveola** (kăv-ē-ō′lă) *pl.* **caveolae** A small pit or depression formed on the cell surface during pinocytosis.

**cavernitis** (kăv″ĕr-nī′tĭs) [L. *caverna,* hollow, + Gr. *itis,* inflammation] Inflammation of the corpus cavernosum of the penis.

**cavernoma** (kăv″ĕr-nō′mă) [″ + Gr. *oma,* tumor] A cavernous angioma. SEE: *angioma; hemangioma.*

**cavernositis** (kăv″ĕr-nō-sī′tĭs) [″ + Gr. *itis,* inflammation] Inflammation of the corpus cavernosum.

**cavernous** (kăv′ĕr-nŭs) [L. *caverna,* a hollow] Containing hollow spaces.

**cavitary** (kăv′ĭ-tā″rē) Pert. to a cavity.

**cavitation** [L. *cavitas,* hollow] Formation of a cavity. This process may be normal, as in the formation of the amnion in human development, or pathological, as in the development of cavities in lung tissue in pulmonary tuberculosis.

**cavitis** (kā-vī′tĭs) [″ + Gr. *itis,* inflammation] Inflammation of a vena cava.

**cavity** (kăv′ĭ-tē) [L. *cavitas,* hollow] A hollow space, such as a body organ or the hole in a tooth produced by caries.

***abdominal c.*** The ventral cavity between the diaphragm and pelvis that contains all the abdominal organs.

***alveolar c.*** A tooth socket.

***amniotic c.*** The fluid-filled cavity around the developing embryo.

***articular c.*** The synovial cavity of a joint.

***body c.*** Either of the two major body cavities, one containing the viscera of the trunk, abdomen, and pelvic areas (ventral), and the other composed of the cranial and spinal cavities (dorsal). SYN: *coelom.* SEE: illus.

***buccal c.*** Oral c.

***cotyloid c.*** The acetabulum (1).

***cranial c.*** The cavity of the skull, which

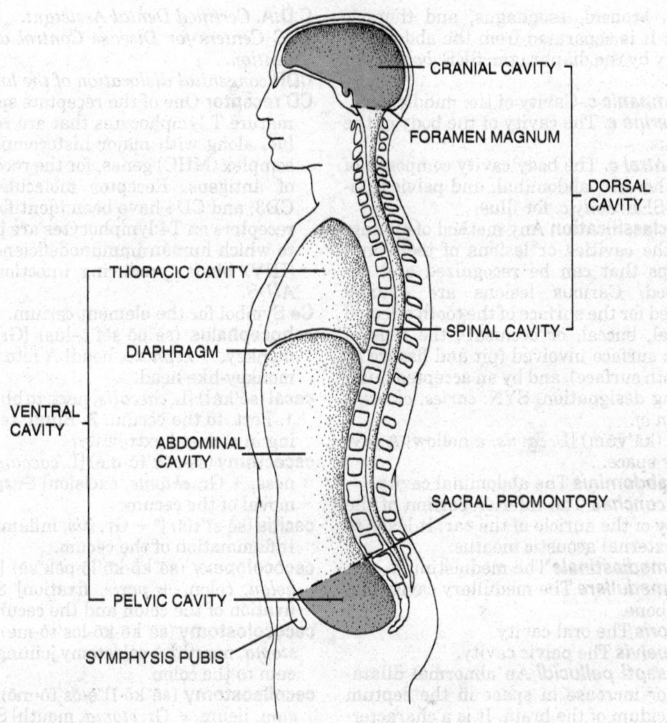


CAVITIES OF THE BODY

contains the brain.

***dental c.*** A hole in a tooth caused by dental caries.

***dorsal c.*** The body cavity composed of the cranial and spinal cavities. SEE: *body c.* for illus.

***glenoid c.*** A shallow concavity on the lateral surface of the head of the scapula that receives the head of the humerus.

***joint c.*** The articular cavity or space enclosed by the synovial membrane and articular cartilages. It contains synovial fluid.

***lesser peritoneal c.*** The omental bursa.

***oral c.*** The cavity of the mouth. It includes the vestibule and oral cavity proper. SYN: *buccal c.*

***pelvic c.*** The cavity of the pelvis. It includes the major pelvic cavity, which lies between the iliac fossa and above the iliopectineal lines, and the minor pelvic cavity, which lies below the iliopectineal lines or the inlet of the pelvis.

***pericardial c.*** The potential space between the epicardium (visceral pericardium) and the parietal pericardium. SEE: *friction rub, pericardial; pericarditis.*

***peritoneal c.*** The potential space between the parietal peritoneum, which lines the abdominal wall, and the visceral peritoneum, which forms the surface layer of the visceral organs. It contains serous fluid.

***pleural c.*** The potential space between the parietal pleura that lines the thoracic cavity and the visceral pleura that covers the lungs. It contains serous fluid that prevents friction.

***pulp c.*** The cavity in a tooth containing the dental pulp and nerve termination.

***Rosenmüller's c.*** The cavity on either side of the openings of the eustachian tube.

***serous c.*** The space between two layers of serous membrane (e.g., the pleural, pericardial, and peritoneal cavities).

***spinal c.*** The cavity that contains the spinal cord. SEE: *body c.* for illus.

***splanchnic c.*** One of the cavities of the body, such as the cranial, thoracic, and abdominal cavities, that contain important organs.

***thoracic c.*** The space lying above the diaphragm and enclosed within the walls of the thorax; the space occupied by the thoracic viscera. It includes the pleural cavities occupied by the lungs and the mediastinum, the space between the lungs (which is occupied by the heart, lying within the pericardium), the thoracic aorta, pulmonary artery and veins, vena cava, thymus gland, lymph nodes, trachea, bronchi, esophagus, and thoracic duct. It is separated from the abdominal cavity by the diaphragm. SEE: *body c.* for illus.

***tympanic c.*** Cavity of the middle ear.

***uterine c.*** The cavity of the body of the uterus.

***ventral c.*** The body cavity composed of the thoracic, abdominal, and pelvic cavities. SEE: *body c.* for illus.

**cavity classification** Any method of arranging the cavities or lesions of teeth into groups that can be recognized and described. Carious lesions are usually named for the surface of the tooth affected (labial, buccal, or occlusal), the type of tooth surface involved (pit and fissure or smooth surface), and by an accepted numbering designation. SYN: *caries, classification of.*

**cavum** (kā'vŭm) [L. *cavus,* a hollow] A cavity or space.

***c. abdominis*** The abdominal cavity.

***c. conchae*** The inferior portion of the cavity of the auricle of the ear. It leads to the external acoustic meatus.

***c. mediastinale*** The mediastinum.

***c. medullare*** The medullary cavity of a long bone.

***c. oris*** The oral cavity.

***c. pelvis*** The pelvic cavity.

***c. septi pellucidi*** An abnormal dilatation or increase in space in the septum pellucidum of the brain. It is a characteristic pathological change in boxers who have experienced many blows to the head.

***c. trigeminale*** The space between the two layers of the dura mater of the brain in which the trigeminal ganglion is located. SYN: *Meckel's space.*

***c. tympani*** The cavity of the middle ear.

***c. uteri*** The cavity of the uterus.

**cavus** (kā'vŭs) [L., hollow] Talipes arcuatus.

**cayenne pepper** (kī-ĕn', kā-ĕn') Capsicum.

**C bar** The curved part of a hand splint that maintains the thumb web space.

**CBC** *complete blood count.*

**C.C.** *chief complaint; Commission Certified.*

**cc** *cubic centimeter.*

**$CCl_3$·CHO** Chloral.

**$CCl_4$** Carbon tetrachloride.

**CCNU** Code name for a chemotherapeutic agent used in treating certain neoplastic conditions; also called *lomustine.*

**CCPD** *continuous cycling peritoneal dialysis.*

**CCRN** Registered trademark indicating certification by the American Association of Critical-Care Nurses Certification Corporation.

**C.C.U.** *coronary care unit.*

**Cd** Symbol for the element cadmium.

**CD** *cluster of differentiation.*

**CD4** A protein on the surface of cells that normally helps the body's immune system combat disease. Human immunodeficiency virus (HIV) attaches itself to the protein to attack white blood cells, causing a failure of host defense. SEE: *AIDS.*

**C.D.A.** *Certified Dental Assistant.*

**CDC** *Centers for Disease Control and Prevention.*

**CDH** *congenital dislocation of the hip.*

**CD receptor** One of the receptors specific to mature T lymphocytes that are responsible, along with major histocompatibility complex (MHC) genes, for the recognition of antigens. Receptor molecules CD2, CD3, and CD4 have been identified. CD4 receptors on T4 lymphocytes are the sites to which human immunodeficiency virus (HIV) binds, producing infection. SEE: *AIDS.*

**Ce** Symbol for the element cerium.

**cebocephalus** (sē″bō-sĕf'ă-lŭs) [Gr. *kebos,* monkey, + *kephale,* head] A fetus with a monkey-like head.

**cecal** (sē'kăl) [L. *caecalis,* pert. to blindness] **1.** Pert. to the cecum. **2.** Blind, terminating in a closed extremity.

**cecectomy** (sē-sĕk'tō-mē) [L. *caecum,* blindness, + Gr. *ektome,* excision] Surgical removal of the cecum.

**cecitis** (sē-sī'tĭs) [″ + Gr. *itis,* inflammation] Inflammation of the cecum.

**cecocolopexy** (sē″kō-kō'lō-pĕk″sē) [″ + Gr. *kolon,* colon, + *pexis,* fixation] Surgical fixation of the colon and the cecum.

**cecocolostomy** (sē″kō-kō-lŏs'tō-mē) [″ + ″ + *stoma,* mouth] A colostomy joining the cecum to the colon.

**cecoileostomy** (sē″kō-ĭl″ē-ŏs'tō-mē) [″ + *ileum,* ileum, + Gr. *stoma,* mouth] Surgical formation of an anastomosis between the cecum and the ileum.

**Cecon** Trade name for ascorbic acid.

**cecopexy** (sē'kō-pĕk″sē) [″ + Gr. *pexis,* fixation] Surgical fixation of the cecum to the abdominal wall.

**cecoplication** (sē″kō-plĭ-kā'shŭn) [″ + *plica,* fold] The reduction of a dilated cecum by making a fold in its wall.

**cecoptosis** (sē″kŏp-tō'sĭs) [″ + Gr. *ptosis,* a dropping] Falling displacement of the cecum.

**cecosigmoidostomy** (sē″kō-sĭg″moyd-ŏs'tō-mē) [″ + Gr. *sigmoeides,* shaped like Gr. letter Σ (sigma), + *stoma,* mouth] A surgical connection between the cecum and the sigmoid.

**cecostomy** (sē-kŏs'tō-mē) [″ + Gr. *stoma,* mouth] Surgical formation of an artificial opening into the cecum.

**cecotomy** (sē-kŏt'ō-mē) [″ + Gr. *tome,* incision] An incision into the cecum.

**cecum, caecum** (sē'kŭm) [L. *caecum,* blindness] A blind pouch or cul-de-sac that forms the first portion of the large intestine, located below the entrance of the ileum at the ileocecal valve. It averages about 6 cm in length and 7.5 cm in width. At its lower end is the vermiform appendix.

**Cedilanid-D** Trade name for deslanoside.

**Cefadyl** Trade name for cephapirin sodium.

**cefamandole nafate** An antibacterial drug. Trade name is Mandol.

**cefoxitin sodium** An antibacterial drug.

**cel-** SEE: *celo-*.

**-cele** [Gr. *kele,* tumor, swelling; *koilia,* cavity] Suffix indicating *swelling, hernia,* or *tumor.*

**Celestone** Trade name for betamethasone.

**celiac** (sē′lē-ăk) [Gr. *koilia,* belly] Pert. to the abdominal cavity.

***c. sprue*** SEE: *sprue, celiac.*

**celiectomy** (sē″lē-ĕk′tō-mē) [″ + *ektome,* excision] **1.** Surgical removal of an abdominal organ. **2.** Excision of the celiac branches of the vagus nerve.

**celiocentesis** (sē″lē-ō-sĕn-tē′sĭs) [″ + *kentesis,* puncture] Puncture of the abdomen.

**celiocolpotomy** (sē″lē-ō-kōl-pŏt′ō-mē) [″ + *kolpos,* vagina, + *tome,* incision] A surgical incision of the vagina through the abdominal wall.

**celioenterotomy** (sē″lē-ō-ĕn″tĕr-ŏt′ō-mē) [″ + *enteron,* intestine, + *tome,* incision] An incision in the abdominal wall to gain access to the intestines.

**celiogastrostomy** (sē″lē-ō-găs-trŏs′tō-mē) [″ + *gaster,* stomach, + *stoma,* mouth] Laparogastrostomy.

**celiogastrotomy** (sē″lē-ō-găs-trŏt′ō-mē) [Gr. *koilia,* belly, + *gaster,* stomach, + *tome,* incision] Laparogastrotomy.

**celiohysterectomy** (sē″lē-ō-hĭs-tĕr-ĕk′tō-mē) [″ + *hystera,* uterus, + *ektome,* excision] Removal of the uterus through the abdomen.

**celiohysterotomy** (sē″lē-ō-hĭs″tĕr-ŏt′ō-mē) [″ + ″ + *tome,* incision] An incision into the uterus through the abdominal wall.

**celioma** (sē-lē-ō′mă) [″ + *oma,* tumor] An abdominal tumor.

**celiomyomectomy** (sē″lē-ō-mī″ō-mĕk′tō-mē) [″ + ″ + *oma,* tumor, + *ektome,* excision] Cutting of muscular tissue via an abdominal incision.

**celiomyomotomy** (sē″lē-ō-mī″ō-mŏt′ō-mē) [″ + ″ + ″ + *tome,* incision] Incision of the abdominal muscles.

**celiomyositis** (sē″lē-ō-mī″ō-sī′tĭs) [″ + ″ + *itis,* inflammation] Inflammation of the abdominal muscles.

**celioparacentesis** (sē″lē-ō-păr″ă-sĕn-tē′sĭs) [″ + *para,* beside, + *kentesis,* puncture] Needle puncture of the abdomen for tapping or drainage.

**celiopathy** (sē″lē-ŏp′ă-thē) [″ + *pathos,* disease, suffering] Any disease of the abdomen.

**celiorrhaphy** (sē″lē-or′ă-fē) [″ + *rhaphe,* seam, ridge] Laparorrhaphy.

**celiosalpingectomy** (sē″lē-ō-săl″pĭn-jĕk′tō-mē) [″ + *salpinx,* tube, + *ektome,* excision] Removal of the fallopian tubes through an abdominal incision.

**celioscope** (sē′lē-ō-skōp) [″ + *skopein,* to examine] An endoscope for visual examination of a body cavity.

**celioscopy** (sē″lē-ŏs′kō-pē) Examination of a body cavity through a celioscope.

**celiotomy** (sē″lē-ŏt′ō-mē) [″ + *tome,* incision] Surgical incision into the abdominal cavity.

***vaginal c.*** Incision into the abdomen through the vagina.

**cell** [L. *cella,* a chamber] **1.** A small enclosed or partly enclosed cavity such as an air cell. **2.** A mass of protoplasm containing a nucleus or nuclear material; the structural unit of all animals and plants. Cells and their products make up all the tissues of the body. Cells carry out all the body's functional activities, and their structure and form are closely correlated with their functions. Cells arise only from pre-existing cells; new cells arise by cell division. Growth and development result from the increase in numbers of cells and their differentiation into different types of tissues. Specialized germ cells, the spermatozoa and ova, contain in their nuclei the genes for hereditary characteristics.

STRUCTURE: When a typical cell is fixed and stained, it exhibits a centrally located nucleus surrounded by cytoplasm. The nucleus contains the chromosomes, which are made of DNA and protein. It also possesses a nuclear membrane that encloses clear karyoplasm. One or more densely staining bodies, the nucleoli, are usually present. The cell membrane is made of phospholipids, protein, and cholesterol; it forms the outer boundary of the cells and selectively allows substances to enter or leave the cell. The functional and structural elements, called organelles, within the cell include ribosomes, endoplasmic reticulum, mitochondria, Golgi apparatus, centrioles, lipid droplets, and glycogen granules. SEE: illus.

CELL DIVISION: *Meiosis* is the type of cell division in which two successive divisions of the germ cell nuclei produce cells that contain half the number of chromosomes present in somatic cells. In *mitosis,* the other type of cell division, each daughter cell contains the same number of chromosomes as the parent cell. SEE: *meiosis* and *mitosis* for illus.

***accessory c.*** A monocyte or macrophage; refers to the immune response. SEE: *antigen-presenting cell; macrophage.*

***acidophil c.*** A cell with an affinity for staining with acid dyes.

***acinar c.*** A cell present in the acinus of an acinous gland (e.g., of the pancreas).

***adipose c.*** Fat c.

***adventitial c.*** A macrophage along a blood vessel, together with perivascular undifferentiated cells associated with it.

***alpha c.*** A cell of the anterior lobe of the pituitary and the pancreas. In the latter, these cells are the source of glucagon.

***alveolar c., type I*** One of the thin, flat cells that form the epithelium of the alveoli.

***alveolar c., type II*** An epithelial cell of the alveoli of the lungs that secretes pulmonary surfactant.

***ameloblast c.*** The type of cell that produces the enamel rods of the tooth crown.

***argentaffin c.*** A cell found in the epi-

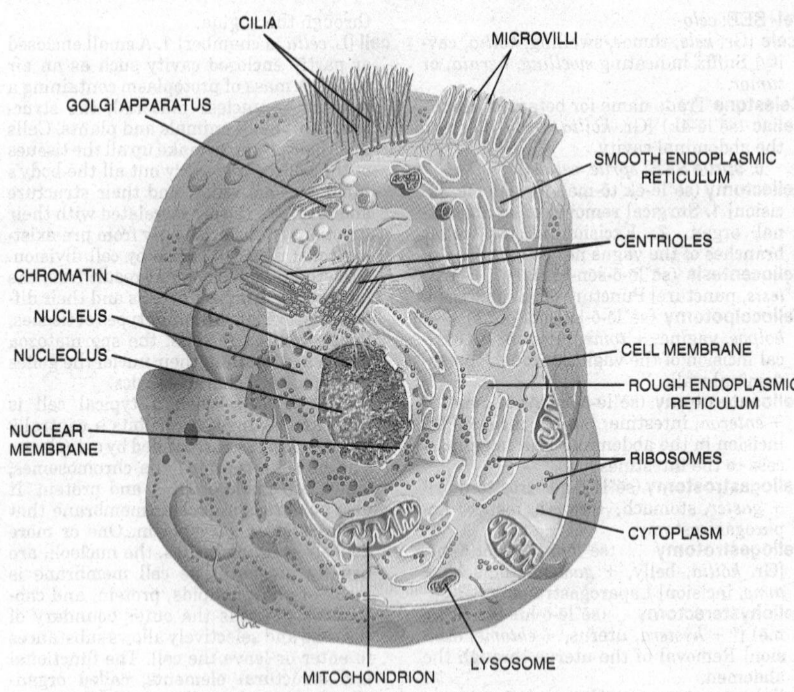


GENERALIZED HUMAN CELL AND ORGANELLES

thelium of the digestive tract (stomach, intestine, appendix). The cytoplasm of these cells contains granules that stain selectively with silver.

***B c.*** A lymphoid stem cell from the bone marrow that migrates to, and becomes a mature antigen-specific cell in, the spleen and lymph nodes. The spleen contains many immature B cells, which, because of the large amount of blood passing through the spleen, become exposed to new antigens and differentiate into functional cells. Each mature B cell can be stimulated by a specific antigen entering the body. After a B cell comes in contact with an antigen, it changes into a plasma cell or a memory cell. Plasma cells produce antibodies that destroy the invading cell. Memory cells are available to produce antibodies quickly if the same antigen reappears. All B cells are antigen specific and respond to only one foreign protein. The antigen-antibody reaction is part of the specific immune response. It is the basis for vaccination and plays a major role in defense against infection from common organisms. SYN: *B lymphocyte.* SEE: *B c.; plasma c.; antibody; antigen; cytokine; immunoglobulin; vaccination.*

***band c.*** The developing leukocyte at a stage at which the nucleus is not segmented.

***basal c.*** A type of cell in the deepest layer of the epidermis.

***basket c.*** **1.** A branching basal or myoepithelial cell of the salivary and other glands. **2.** A type of cell in the cerebellar cortex in which Purkinje cells rest.

***basophil c.*** A cell with an affinity for staining with basic dyes.

***beta c.*** **1.** One of the insulin-secreting cells of the pancreas that constitute the bulk of the islets of Langerhans. **2.** A basophil cell of the anterior lobe of the pituitary.

***Betz c.*** SEE: *Betz cell.*

***bipolar c.*** A neuron with two processes, an axon and a dendrite. It is found in the retina of the eye and in the cochlear and vestibular ganglia of the acoustic nerve.

***blast c.*** A newly formed cell of any type. Large numbers of blast cells in the peripheral blood indicate that the bone marrow is producing a high level of the particular cell (e.g., lymphoblast [lymphocyte], monoblast [monocyte]).

***blood c.*** Any type of nucleated or nonnucleated cell normally found in the blood or blood-forming tissues. SEE: *blood* for illus.

***burr c.*** An erythrocyte with 10 to 30 spicules distributed over the surface of the cell, as seen in heart disease, stomach cancer, kidney disease, and dehydration. SEE: illus.

***capsule c.*** Satellite c.

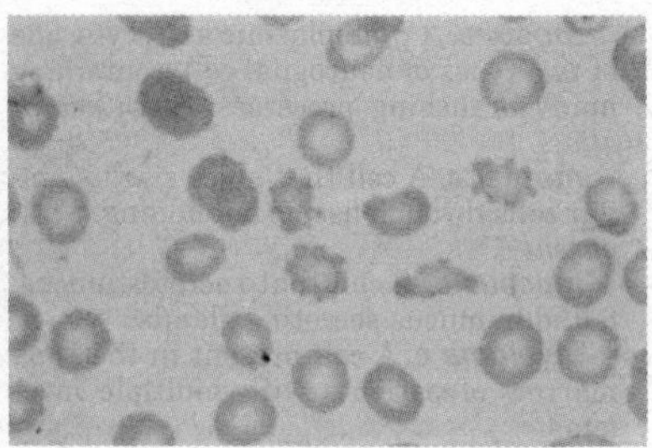

BURR CELLS

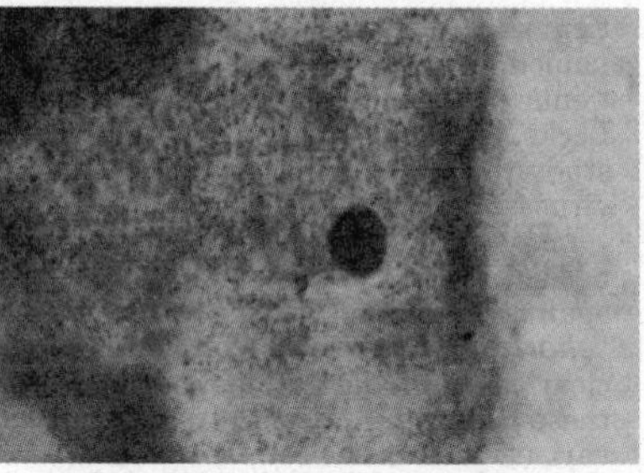

CLUE CELL (ORIG. MAG. ×400)

***castration c.*** An enlarged and vacuolated basophil cell seen in the pituitary in gonadal insufficiency or following castration.

***cementoblast c.*** One of the cells that produce the cementum layer, which covers the tooth root and provides attachment for the supporting periodontal ligament.

***cementocyte c.*** One of the cells trapped within cementum that maintain cementum as a living calcified tissue by their metabolic activity.

***centroacinar c.*** A duct cell of the pancreas more or less invaginated into the lumen of an acinus.

***chalice c.*** Goblet c.

***chief c.*** **1.** One of the cells of the parathyroid gland that secrete the parathyroid hormone. **2.** One of the secretory cells that line the gastric glands and secrete pepsin or its precursor. **3.** A chromophobe cell of the pituitary.

***chromaffin c.*** An epinephrine-containing cell of the adrenal medulla whose granules stain brown when cells are stained with a fluid containing potassium bichromate.

***cleavage c.*** A cell that results from mitosis or splitting of the fertilized ovum; a blastomere.

***clue c.*** A type of vaginal epithelial cell coated with coccobacillary organisms. The cells, which apppear granular, are seen in bacterial vaginosis. SEE: illus.

***columnar c.*** An epithelial cell with height greater than its width.

***cone c.*** A cell in the retina whose scleral end forms a cone that serves as a light receptor. Vision in bright light, color vision, and acute vision depend on the function of the cones. SEE: *rod c.*

***cuboid c.*** A cell with height about equal to width and depth.

***cytotoxic T c.*** A CD8+ T lymphocyte that can destroy microorganisms directly. SEE: *T c.*

***daughter c.*** Any cell formed from the division of a mother cell.

***delta c.*** A cell of the islets of Langerhans of the pancreas that secretes somatostatin.

***endothelial c.*** One of the flat cells that form the lining of the blood and lymph vessels.

***ependymal c.*** One of the cells of the developing neural tube that give rise to the ependyma. They originate from spongioblasts derived from the neural epithelium.

***epithelial c.*** One of the cells forming the epithelial surfaces of membranes and skin. SEE: *tissue, epithelial.*

***ethmoidal c.*** One of several cavities that honeycomb the lateral masses of the ethmoid bone, forming a part of the paranasal air sinuses. SYN: *ethmoid sinus.*

***fat c.*** A cell that stores fat. SYN: *adipose c.; adipocyte; lipocyte.*

***foam c.*** A cell that contains vacuoles; a lipid-filled macrophage.

***ganglion c.*** **1.** Any neuron whose cell body is located within a ganglion. **2.** A neuron of the retina of the eye whose cell body lies in the ganglion cell layer. The axons of ganglion cells form the fibers of the optic nerve.

***germ c.*** A cell whose function is to reproduce the organism. It usually has a single set of chromosomes (haploid). Germ cells are called ova in females and spermatozoa in males.

***giant c.*** **1.** A large cell, often with many nuclei, found in bone marrow. They are thought to produce blood platelets. SYN: *megakaryocyte.* **2.** Any large cell, containing one or multiple nuclei.

***glia c.*** Neuroglia c.

***goblet c.*** An epithelial cell, containing a large globule of mucin, giving it the appearance of a goblet. SYN: *chalice c.*

***Golgi c.*** SEE: *Golgi cell.*

***granule c.*** A small neuron of the cerebrum or the cerebellum that contains granules.

***gustatory c.*** A neuroepithelial cell or taste cell of a taste bud.

***hair c.*** An epithelial cell possessing fine nonmotile cilia found in the maculae and the organ of Corti of the membranous labyrinth of the inner ear. These cells are receptors for the senses of position and hearing.

***HeLa c.*** A cell from a strain that has been continuously cultured from a patient's carcinoma of the cervix. It is named for the first two letters of the patient's first and last names, Henrietta Lacks. The cultured cells are used to study the growth of other cells including viruses.

**helper T c.** A type of T lymphocyte needed for the production of antibodies against certain antigens.

**horizontal c.** A neuron of the inner nuclear layer of the retina. The axons of these cells run horizontally and connect various parts of the retina.

**Hürthle c.** SEE: *Hürthle cell.*

**hybridoma c.** SEE: *hybridoma.*

**hyperchromatic c.** All or part of a cell that contains more than the normal number of chromosomes and hence stains more densely.

**interstitial c.** One of the many cells found in connective tissue of the ovary and the seminiferous tubules of the testes, accounting for their internal secretion.

**islet c.** A cell of the islets of Langerhans of the pancreas.

**juvenile c.** The early developmental form of a white blood cell.

**juxtaglomerular c.** A modified smooth muscle cell in the wall of the afferent arteriole leading to a glomerulus of the kidney. This type of cell secretes renin when blood pressure decreases to activate the renin-angiotensin mechanism, which elevates blood pressure and increases sodium retention.

**killer c.** SEE: *T c.*

**killer T c.** SEE: *T c.*

**Kupffer c.** SEE: *Kupffer cell.*

**L.E. c.** SEE: *L.E. cell.*

**Leydig's c.** SEE: *Leydig's cell.*

**littoral c.** A macrophage found in the sinuses of lymphatic tissue.

**lutein c.** A cell of the corpus luteum of the ovary that contains fatty yellowish granules. Granulose lutein cells are hypertophied follicle cells; these lutein (paralutein) cells develop from the theca interna.

**lymph c.** Lymphocyte.

**lymphokine-activated killer c.** ABBR: LAK cell. A cytotoxic lymphoid cell activated by interleukin-2 (IL-2) that acts against malignant tumor cells.

**mast c.** A cell found in connective tissue of vertebrates that contains heparin and histamine.

**mastoid c.** One of the air spaces in the mastoid process of the temporal bone.

**memory c.** A cell derived from B or T lymphocytes that can quickly recognize a foreign antigen to which the body has been previously exposed. These cells stimulate antibody production by plasma cells or initiate other immune responses. SEE: *B c.; lymphocyte.*

**microglia c.** A neuroglial cell of mesodermal origin present in the brain and spinal cord and capable of phagocytosis.

**mossy c.** A protoplasmic astrocyte; one of two types of neuroglial cell, containing many branching processes. SEE: *neuroglia.*

**mother c.** A cell that gives rise to similar cells through fission or budding. SYN: *parent c.*

**mucous c.** A cell that secretes mucus; found in mucus-secreting glands.

**myeloma c.** A cell present in the bone marrow of patients with multiple myeloma.

**myoepithelial c.** A spindle-shaped or branched contractile epithelial cell found between glandular cells and basement membrane of sweat, mammary, and salivary glands.

**natural killer c.** ABBR: NK cell. A large granular lymphocyte that bonds to cells and lyses them by releasing cytotoxins. These cells are known to be effective against cells infected with viruses and some types of tumor cells. The are proliferated by gamma interferon, interleukin-2, antibodies, retinoic acid, and prostaglandin-E.

**nerve c.** A special cell of nerves that has processes extending from the cell body. One process, the axon, transmits nerve impulses; the other, the dendrite, receives impulses and transmits them to the cell body.

**neuroglia c.** A nonnerve cell of the supporting tissue of the central nervous system and the retina of the eye. This type includes astrocytes, oligodendrocytes, and microglia. SYN: *glia c.*

**Niemann-Pick c.** SEE: *Niemann-Pick cell.*

**null c.** A white blood cell that is a lymphocyte but does not have the characteristics of either a T cell or a B cell.

**odontoblast c.** A cell that produces dentin and is responsible for the sensitivity of and metabolism of dentin in the tooth.

**olfactory c.** A special cell of the olfactory mucosa that has a combined neuroepithelial function.

**osteoblast c.** A mesodermal cell that produces the bone matrix and forms bone layer by layer on its surface.

**osteocyte c.** A type of cell trapped within bone matrix that maintains bone as a living tissue by its metabolic activity.

**oxyntic c.** A parietal cell of the stomach. In humans, hydrochloric acid is formed in these cells.

**parent c.** Mother c.

**phalangeal c.** One of the cells supporting the hair cells of the organ of Corti. These cells form several rows of outer phalangeal cells (Deiters' cells) and a single row of inner phalangeal cells.

**pigment c.** Any cell that normally contains pigment granules.

**plasma c.** A cell derived from B lymphocytes that has been sensitized to a specific foreign antigen and produces antibodies to that particular antigen. It may be found in the blood or in tissue fluid. SYN: *plasmacyte.*

***prickle c.*** A cell possessing spinelike protoplasmic processes that connect with similar processes of adjoining cells. These are found in the stratum spinosum (Malphighian layer) of the epidermis of keratinized epithelium.

***primordial c.*** One of the original germ cells that in the embryo migrate to the gonadal ridge, where they form all of the germ cells.

***Purkinje c.*** SEE: *Purkinje cell.*

***pus c.*** A leukocyte present in pus. Cells of this type are often degenerated or necrotic.

***pyramidal c.*** A nerve cell of the cerebral cortex.

***red c.*** The erythrocyte of the blood. Its principal purpose is to transport oxygen to the cells of the body. The hemoglobin that the red cell contains is oxygenated in the lungs, and the oxygen contained in the arterial system is released to the tissues throughout the body.

***Renshaw c.*** SEE: *Renshaw cell.*

***reticular c.*** **1.** An undifferentiated cell of the spleen, bone marrow, or lymphatic tissue that can develop into one of several types of connective tissue cells or into a macrophage. **2.** A cell of reticular connective tissue. SEE: *reticular tissue.*

***reticuloendothelial c.*** A macrophage or phagocytic cell.

***Rieder c.*** SEE: *Rieder cell.*

***rod c.*** A cell in the retina of the eye whose scleral end is long and narrow, forming a rod that acts as a sensory element. Rods are stimulated by dim light. SEE: *cone c.*

***rosette c.*** A cell that composes the nuclear material surrounded by phagocytes. These cells occur frequently in blood in which L.E. cells are present. Rosette cells are not diagnostic of lupus erythematosus. SEE: *L.E. c.; rosette, E.*

***Rouget c.*** SEE: *Rouget cell.*

***satellite c.*** **1.** One of the flat epithelium-like cells forming the inner portion of a double-layered capsule that covers a neuron. **2.** One of the neuroglia cells enclosing the cell bodies of sensory neurons in spinal ganglia. SYN: *capsule c.*

***segmented c.*** A segmented neutrophil (i.e., one with a nucleus of two or more lobes connected by slender filaments).

***sensory c.*** A cell that when stimulated gives rise to nerve impulses that are conveyed to the central nervous system.

***septal c.*** A type II alveolar cell that secretes pulmonary surfactant; it is attached to or in the septa of the lungs.

***Sertoli c.*** SEE: *Sertoli cell.*

***sickle c.*** An abnormal erythrocyte shaped like a sickle. SEE: *anemia, sickle cell.*

***signet-ring c.*** A vacuolated cell with the nucleus off center. Mucus-secreting adenocarcinomas usually contain these cells.

***somatic c.*** A cell that is not a germ cell. Somatic cells have two sets of chromosomes (diploid) and are represented by cells of many different shapes and functions.

***spider c.*** Astrocyte.

***squamous c.*** A flat, scalelike epithelial cell.

***stellate c.*** A star-shaped cell with processes extending from it.

***stellate reticuloendothelial c.*** A star-shaped, fixed macrophage found in the sinusoids of the liver and in some nerve tissue. SYN: *Kupffer's cell.* SEE: *reticuloendothelial system.*

***stem c.*** **1.** A cell capable of both differentiation and self-renewal. **2.** In transplantation, a hematopoietic cell in bone marrow, umbilical cord blood, and peripheral blood, capable of reconstituting lethally damaged bone marrow (i.e., after myeloablative conditioning chemoradiotherapy) to restore lymphohematopoietic function.

***Sternberg-Reed c.*** SEE: *Reed-Sternberg cell.*

***stipple c.*** A red blood cell that contains small basophilic-staining dots. It is seen in lead poisoning, malaria, severe anemia, and leukemia.

***suppressor T c.*** A previously used term for a type of lymphocyte that inhibits CD4+ and B cell activity. Because no specific CD markers have been identified for these cells, it is unclear whether they exist as a separate group.

***sympathicotrophic c.*** One of the large epithelial cells that occur in groups in the hilus of the ovary. They are thought to be chromaffin cells.

***sympathochromaffin c.*** A chromaffin cell of ectodermal origin present in the fetal adrenal gland. Sympathetic and medullary cells originate from these cells.

***T c.*** A lymphoid cell from the bone marrow that migrates to the thymus gland, where it develops into a mature differentiated lymphocyte that circulates between blood and lymph. Immature T cells are called thymocytes. Mature T cells are "antigen specific," meaning that each one responds to only one antigen. T cells are identified by surface protein markers called clusters of differentiation (CD). All T cells have the CD3 marker; additional markers differentiate different T subsets. CD4+/CD8− helper T cells serve primarily as regulators, secreting lymphokines that influence the activities of other immune cells during inflammation and T-cell–mediated immunity. CD4+ cells also secrete gamma interferon, one of the strongest stimulators of macrophage activity. CD8+/CD4− T cells are effector cells that directly lyse (kill) organisms. Natural killer cells were originally believed to be a subset of T cells, but are now recognized as being a third type of lymphocyte. SYN: *killer c.; killer T c.* SEE: *B c.; plasma c.; antigen; immune response; immunity; lymphocyte; macrophage processing; rejection; surveillance, immunological; T-cell receptors.*

T cells cannot recognize foreign antigens without the help of macrophage processing. However, once the macrophage has helped them identify an antigen as "non-self," T cells dominate the specific immune response directing macrophages, B cells, and other T cells in the body's defense. T cells also play a major role in graft rejection, some hypersensitivity reactions, and recognition and destruction of tumor cells because of the unique antigens these cells carry.

Subpopulations of T lymphocytes include T4 (CD4) or helper cells, which are the major regulatory cells. These cells secrete interleukin-2, which stimulates the activity of B cells and other T lymphocytes. They also secrete gamma interferon, which inhibits viruses. T4 cells are the primary cells attacked by the human immunodeficiency virus (HIV) in AIDS. T8 (CD8) or suppressor cells stop the specific immune response after several days and create memory cells. At least two classes of T lymphocytes, cytotoxic T cells and natural killer cells, kill other cells directly.

***target c.*** An erythrocyte with a rounded central area surrounded by a lightly stained clear ring, which in turn is surrounded by a dense ring of peripheral protoplasm. It is present in certain blood disorders.

***tart c.*** A phagocyte that has ingested the unaltered nuclei of cells. These nuclei can be observed unchanged within the phagocytic cell.

***taste c.*** A cell of a taste bud.

***totipotent c.*** An undifferentiated embryonic cell that has the potential to develop into any type of cell.

***Touton giant c.*** SEE: *Touton cell.*

***Türk's irritation c.*** SEE: *Türk's irritation cell.*

***Tzanck c.*** SEE: *Tzanck cell.*

***undifferentiated c.*** A cell resembling an embryonic cell in that it has not demonstrated a change into a mature cell of any type.

***visual c.*** A rod c. or cone c. of the retina.

***wandering c.*** A macrophage capable of ameboid movement.

***white c.*** Any of the leukocytes of the blood.

***zymogenic c.*** Any of the chief cells or enzyme-producing cells of the gastric glands.

**cell bank** A facility for keeping cells frozen at extremely low temperatures. These cells are used for investigating hereditary diseases, human aging, and cancer. Collections of banked cells are kept by the National Institutes of Health (the Human Genetic Mutant Cell Repository and the Aging Cell Repository) and at the Cornell Institute for Medical Research.

**cell counter, electronic** An electronic instrument used to count blood cells, employing either an electrical resistance or an optical gating technique. SEE: *flow cytometry.*

**cell culture** The growth of cells in vitro for experimental purposes. The cells proliferate but do not organize into tissue.

**cell cycle** The series of events that occur during the growth and development of a cell. SEE: *meiosis* and *mitosis* for illus.

**cell division** The fission of a cell. SEE: *meiosis* and *mitosis* for illus.

**cell-free** Pertaining to fluids or tissues that contain no cells or in which all the cells have been disintegrated by laboratory treatment.

**cell growth cycle** The order of physical and biochemical events that occur during the growth of cells. In tissue culture studies, the cyclic changes are divided into specific periods or phases: the DNA synthesis or S period, the $G_2$ period or gap, the M or mitotic period, and the $G_1$ period.

**cell kill** In antineoplastic therapy, the number of malignant tumor cells destroyed by a treatment.

**cell kinetics** The study of cells and their growth and division. Study of these factors has led to understanding of cancer cells and has been useful in developing chemotherapeutic methods.

**cell mass** In embryology, the mass of cells that develops into an organ or structure.

**cell membrane** SEE: under *membrane.*

**cellobiose** (sĕl″ō-bī′ōs) A disaccharide resulting from the hydrolysis of cellulose.

**cellophane** (sĕl′ō-fān) A thin, transparent, waterproof sheet of cellulose acetate. It is used as a dialysis membrane.

**cell organelle** Any of the structures in the cytoplasm of a cell. These include mitochondria, endoplasmic reticulum, Golgi complex, ribosomes, lysosomes, and centriole. SEE: *cell* for illus.

**cell receptor** SEE: *receptor.*

**cell sorting** A technique used to separate cells with a surface antigen from those without it. SEE: *flow cytometry.*

**cellucidal** (sĕl″ū-sī′dăl) [L. *cella,* a chamber, + *caedere,* to kill] Destructive to cells.

**cellula** (sĕl′ū-lă) *pl.* **cellulae** [L., little cell] **1.** A minute cell. **2.** A small compartment.

**cellular** (sĕl′ū-lăr) Pertaining to, composed of, or derived from cells.

**cellular immunity** T-cell–mediated immune functions requiring cell interactions (e.g., graft rejection, or destruction of infected cells).

**cellulase** (sĕl′ū-lās) An enzyme that converts cellulose to cellobiose. It is present in some microorganisms and marine life.

**cellulifugal** (sĕl″ū-lĭf′ū-găl) [″ + *fugere,* to flee] Extending or moving away from a cell.

**cellulipetal** (sĕl″ū-lĭp′ĭ-tăl) [″ + *petere,* to seek] Extending or moving toward a cell.

**cellulite** A nontechnical term for subcutaneous deposits of fat, especially in the buttocks, legs, and thighs.

**cellulitis** (sĕl-ū-lī'tĭs) [" + Gr. *itis,* inflammation] Inflammation of cellular or connective tissue, spreading as in erysipelas. An infection in or close to the skin is usually localized by the body defense mechanisms. However, if inflammation spreads through the tissue, the process is called cellulitis.

***pelvic c.*** Parametritis.

**cellulofibrous** (sĕl"ū-lō-fī'brŭs) [" + *fibra,* fiber] Both cellular and fibrous.

**cellulose** (sĕl'ū-lōs) [L. *cellula,* little cell] A polysaccharide that forms plant fiber; a fibrous form of carbohydrate, $(C_6H_{10}O_5)_n$, constituting the supporting framework of most plants. It is composed of many glucose units. When ingested, it stimulates peristalsis and aids in intestinal elimination. When ingested by humans, cellulose provides no nutrient value because it is not chemically changed or absorbed in digestion; it remains a polysaccharide.

Some foods that contain cellulose are apples, apricots, asparagus, beans, beets, bran flakes, broccoli, cabbage, celery, mushrooms, oatmeal, onions, oranges, parsnips, prunes, spinach, turnips, wheat flakes, whole grains, and whole wheat bread. SEE: *fiber, dietary.*

***c. acetate*** A support medium commonly used in electrophoresis. Normally it is white. When treated with a clearing agent of methanol and acetic acid, it becomes transparent, allowing the sample bands to be visualized.

***carboxymethyl sodium c.*** ABBR: CMC. A hydrophilic cellulose derivative used as a bulk-forming laxative. It is also used as a food additive to thicken various types of prepared foods.

***oxidized c.*** Cellulose that has been oxidized and is made to resemble cotton or gauze. It is used to arrest bleeding by direct application to the site of hemorrhage.

**cellulotoxic** (sĕl"ū-lō-tŏk'sĭk) [" + Gr. *toxikon,* poison] **1.** Poisonous to cells. **2.** Caused by cell toxins.

**cell wall** A wall made of cellulose and other materials that encloses a plant cell in a rigid framework. Plant cells have both cell membranes and cell walls. Plant cell walls cannot be digested by humans. SEE: *cellulose.*

**celo-, cel-** **1.** [Gr. *kele,* tumor, swelling] Combining form meaning *tumor* or *hernia.* **2.** [Gr. *koilia,* cavity] Combining form meaning *cavity.*

**celom, celoma** (sē'lŏm, sē-lō'mă) [Gr. *koiloma,* a hollow] The coelom.

**celoschisis** (sē-lŏs'kĭ-sĭs) [Gr. *koilia,* cavity, + *schisis,* fissure] A congenital fissure of the abdominal wall.

**celoscope** (sē'lō-skōp) [" + *skopein,* to examine] A device for visual examination of a body cavity.

**celosomia** (sē-lō-sō'mē-ă) [" + *soma,* body] A congenital fissure of the sternum with herniation of the fetal viscera.

**Celsius scale** (sĕl'sē-ŭs) [Anders Celsius, Swedish astronomer, 1701–1744] A temperature scale on which the boiling point of water is 100° and the freezing point is 0°. This is the official scientific name of the temperature scale, also called the centigrade scale. SEE: *Fahrenheit scale* for table; *thermometer* for table; *Conversion Factors Appendix.*

**cement** (sē-mĕnt') **1.** Any material that hardens into a firm mass when prepared appropriately. **2.** To cause two objects to stick together, as in using an adhesive to join a gold inlay to the cavity of a tooth and to insulate the pulp from metallic fillings. **3.** The material used to make one substance adhere to another.

**cementicle** (sē-mĕn'tĭ-kl) The small calcified area in the periodontal membrane of the root of a tooth.

**cementitis** (sē"mĕn-tī'tĭs) [L. *cementum,* cement, + Gr. *itis,* inflammation] Inflammation of the dental cementum.

**cementoblast** (sē-mĕn'tō-blăst) [" + Gr. *blastos,* germ] A cell of the inner layer of the dental sac of a developing tooth. It deposits cementum on the dentin of the root.

**cementoclasia** (sē-mĕn"tō-klā'sē-ă) [" + Gr. *klasis,* breaking] Decay of the cementum of a tooth root.

**cementoclast** (sē-mĕn'tō-klăst) A very large multinucleated cell associated with the removal of cementum during root resorption, more correctly called an odontoclast.

**cementogenesis** (sē-mĕn"tō-jĕn'ĕ-sĭs) [" + Gr. *genesis,* generation] The development of cementum on the root dentin of a tooth.

**cementoid** (sē"mĕn'toyd) [" + Gr. *eidos,* form, shape] The noncalcified matrix of cementum.

**cementoma** (sē"mĕn-tō'mă) [" + Gr. *oma,* tumor] A benign fibrous connective tissue growth containing small masses of cementum, usually found in the periodontal ligament near the apex of the tooth.

**cementum** (sē-mĕn'tŭm) [L.] The thin layer of calcified tissue formed by cementoblasts which covers the tooth root. In it are embedded the collagenous fibers of the periodontal ligament, which are also attached to the surrounding alveolar bone proper, thereby supporting the tooth. Also called *substantia ossea dentis.*

**CEN** *certified emergency nurse.*

**Cenolate** Trade name for ascorbic acid.

**cenosite** (sĕn'ō-, sē'nō-sīt) [Gr. *koinos,* common, + *sitos,* food] A parasitic microorganism that can live without a host.

**cenotophobia** (sĕn"ō-, sē"nō-tō-fō'bē-ă) [Gr. *kainotes,* novelty, + *phobos,* fear] Pathological aversion to new things and new ideas. SYN: *cainotophobia.*

**cenotype** (sē'nō-, sĕn'ō-tīp) [" + *typos,* a type] An original type; term used in ontogeny and cytology.

**censor** (sĕn'sĕr) [L. *censor,* judge] In psychoanalysis, a psychic inhibition that prevents abhorrent unconscious thoughts or impulses from being expressed objectively in any form recognized at the conscious level.

**census** In hospital management, the number of patients in the hospital.

**centenarian** A person over the age of 100.

**center** (sĕn′tĕr) [L. *centrum,* center] **1.** The middle point of a body. **2.** A group of nerve cells within the central nervous system that controls a specific activity or function. **3.** A facility specializing in a particular service.

***apneustic c.*** A respiratory center in the pons that may prolong inhalation.

***auditory c.*** The center for hearing in the anterior gyri of the transverse temporal gyri. SEE: *area, auditory.*

***autonomic c.*** The center in the brain or spinal cord that regulates any of the activities under the control of the autonomic nervous system. Most cortical centers are located in the hypothalamus, medulla oblongata, and spinal cord.

***Broca's c.*** SEE: *Broca's area.*

***burn c.*** A hospital-based health care facility staffed with specialists essential to the comprehensive care of burn patients.

***cardioaccelerator c.*** The center in the medulla oblongata that gives rise to impulses that speed up the heart rate. Impulses reach the heart by way of sympathetic fibers.

***cardioinhibitory c.*** The center in the medulla oblongata containing neurons whose axons, parasympathetic fibers, pass by way of the vagus nerves to the heart. Impulses from this center cause the heart rate to slow down.

***chondrification c.*** The center of cartilage formation.

***ciliospinal c.*** The center in the spinal cord that produces sympathetic impulses that dilate the pupils of the eyes.

***community health c.*** A health care facility for treatment of ambulatory patients. SYN: *neighborhood health c.*

***defecation c.*** Either of two centers, a medullary center located in the medulla oblongata and a spinal center located in the second to fourth sacral segments of the spinal cord. The anospinal centers control the sphincter reflexes for defecation.

***deglutition c.*** The center in the medulla oblongata on the floor of the fourth ventricle that controls swallowing.

***epiotic c.*** The ossification center of the mastoid process.

***feeding c.*** An area in the ventrolateral nucleus of the hypothalamus that originates signals to the cerebral cortex that stimulate eating. SEE: *satiety c.; weight, set point.*

***germinal c.*** The area in lymph node tissue that responds in a specific manner to antigenic stimulation.

***gustatory c.*** The cerebral center that controls taste. SYN: *taste c; taste area.*

***heat-regulating c.*** One of two centers, a heat loss and a heat production center, located in the hypothalamus. They regulate body temperature.

***higher c.*** **1.** The center in the cerebrum from which impulses based on conscious sensations, wishes, or desires are initiated. **2.** A center in any portion of the brain, in contrast to one in the spinal cord.

***independent living c.*** A facility in the community that coordinates services for the disabled, including counseling, training, rehabilitation, assistance with devices, and respite care.

***lower c.*** A center in the brainstem or spinal cord.

***medullary c.*** The area in the brainstem that regulates respiratory activity.

***micturition c.*** A center that controls the reflexes of the urinary bladder. These are located in the second to fourth and fourth to sixth sacral segments of the cord. Higher centers are present in the medulla oblongata, hypothalamus, and cerebrum.

***motor cortical c.*** An area in the frontal lobe in which impulses for voluntary movements originate.

***neighborhood health c.*** Community health c.

***nerve c.*** One of many centers in cerebrospinal or ganglionic systems originating or controlling certain functions.

***ossification c.*** The spot in bones where ossification begins.

***pneumotaxic c.*** The center in the pons that rhythmically inhibits inspiration.

***psychocortical c.*** One of the centers of the cerebral cortex concerned with voluntary muscular movements.

***reflex c.*** A region within the brain or spinal cord where connections (synapses) are made between afferent and efferent neurons of a reflex arc.

***respiratory c.*** The region in the medulla oblongata that controls respiratory movements. It consists of inspiratory and expiratory centers.

***satiety c.*** An area in the ventromedial hypothalamus that modulates the stimulus to eat by sending inhibitory impulses to the feeding center. Blood glucose and insulin level influence its activity. SEE: *feeding c.; weight, set point.*

***senior c.*** A community building or meeting room where elderly persons congregate for services and activities that reflect their interests, enhance their dignity, support their independence, and encourage their involvement with the community.

***speech c.*** Broca's area.

***suicide prevention c.*** A health care facility dedicated to preventing suicide by counseling and crisis intervention.

***taste c.*** Gustatory c.

***temperature c.*** Thermoregulatory c.

***thermoregulatory c.*** One of the temperature-regulating centers in the hypothalamus. SYN: *temperature c.*

***vasoconstrictor c.*** The center in the medulla oblongata that brings about the constriction of blood vessels.

***vasodilator c.*** The center in the medulla oblongata that brings about the dilation of blood vessels.

***vasomotor c.*** The center that controls the diameter of blood vessels; the vasoconstrictor and vasodilator centers.

***visual c.*** A center in the occipital lobes of the cerebrum that receives visual information transmitted from the retina.

***Wernicke's c.*** SEE: *Wernicke's center.*

***word c.*** The area in the dominant hemisphere of the brain that recognizes and perceives spoken or written words.

**Centers for Disease Control and Prevention** ABBR: CDC. A division of the U.S. Public Health Service in Atlanta, Georgia, that investigates and controls various diseases, especially those that have epidemic potential. The agency is also responsible for national programs to improve laboratory conditions and encourage health and safety in the workplace. Telephone number is (404) 639-3311. SEE: *Health Care Resources Appendix.*

**centesis** (sĕn-tē′sĭs) [Gr. *kentesis,* puncture] Puncture of a cavity.

**centigrade** (sĕn′tĭ-grād) [L. *centum,* a hundred, + *gradus,* a step] ABBR: C. **1.** Having 100 degrees. **2.** Pertaining to a thermometer divided into 100°. The boiling point of water is 100° and the freezing point is 0°. SEE: *Celsius scale; thermometer.*

**centigram** (sĕn′tĭ-grăm) [″ + Gr. *gramma,* a small weight] One hundredth of a gram. SEE: *metric system; Weights and Measures Appendix.*

**centiliter** (sĕn′tĭ-lē-tĕr) [″ + Gr. *litra,* measure of wt.] One hundredth of a liter. SEE: *metric system.*

**centimeter** (sĕn′tĭ-mē-tĕr) [″ + Gr. *metron,* measure] ABBR: cm. One hundredth of a meter. To convert centimeters to inches, multiply by 0.3937. To convert inches to centimeters, multiply by 2.54. SEE: *metric system.*

**centimorgan** ABBR: cM. One hundreth of a morgan; a measure of genetic distance that indicates the likelihood of crossover of two loci on a gene.

**centinormal** (sĕn″tĭ-nor′măl) [″ + *norma,* rule] One hundredth of the normal, as the strength of a solution.

**centipede** (sĕn′tĭ-pēd″) [″ + *pes,* foot] An arthropod of the subclass Chilopoda distinguished by an elongated flattened body of many segments, each with a pair of jointed legs. The first pair of appendages are hooklike claws bearing openings of ducts from poison glands. The bites of large tropical centipedes may cause severe local and sometimes general symptoms, but they are rarely fatal.

**centipoise** (sĕn′tĭ-poyz) A unit of viscosity, one hundredth of a poise. SEE: *poise.*

**centrad** (sĕn′trăd) [Gr. *kentron,* center, + L. *ad,* toward] Toward the center.

**central** (sĕn′trăl) **1.** Situated at or pertaining to a center. **2.** Principal or controlling.

**central core disease** A rare form of benign familial polymyopathy marked by hypotonia, delay in walking, and muscle weakness that does not progress. When the muscle fibers are stained in certain ways and studied microscopically, a central area does not stain.

**central intravenous line** SEE: *catheter, central venous; central line.*

**central line** A venous access device inserted into and kept in the vein. It maintains a route for administering fluids and medicines, or for gaining access to the heart to obtain information about pressures in the venous circulation. Keeping the line open permits later venous access when the veins might be collapsed and difficult to enter. SEE: *catheter, central venous.*

**central nervous system** ABBR: CNS. The brain and spinal cord. SEE: *brain* and *cranial nerve* for illus.; *autonomic nervous system; nerve; neuron; parasympathetic nervous system; sympathetic nervous system.*

COMPOSITION: Nerve tissue that forms the brain and spinal cord consists of gray and white matter. Gray matter is made of the cell bodies of neurons, and white matter is made of the axons and dendrites of these neurons. White matter transmits impulses within the CNS.

**central venous pressure** ABBR: CVP. The pressure within the superior vena cava. It reflects the pressure under which the blood is returned to the right atrium. The normal range is between 5 and 10 cm $H_2O$. A high CVP indicates circulatory overload (as in congestive heart failure), whereas a low CVP indicates reduced blood volume (as in hemorrhage or fluid loss). CVP can be estimated by examining the cervical veins or the dorsal veins of the hand if the neck and hand are at the level of the heart. Those veins are well filled if CVP is normal or high, and tend to collapse if it is low.

**centration** The ability of the preschool child to focus or center attention on only one aspect or characteristic of a situation at a time. It was first described by Piaget.

**centre** Center.

**centriciput** (sĕn-trĭs′ĭ-pŭt) [″ + L. *caput,* head] The central part of the upper surface of the skull between the occiput and sinciput.

**centrifugal** (sĕn-trĭf′ū-găl) [″ + L. *fugere,* to flee] Receding from the center. SYN: *axifugal.* SEE: *centrifuge.*

**centrifuge** (sĕn′trĭ-fūj) A device that spins test tubes at high speeds. Centrifugal force causes the heavy particles in the liquid to settle to the bottom of the tubes and the lighter liquid to go to the top. When unclotted blood is centrifuged, the plasma goes to the top and the heavy red cells go to the bottom of the tube. The white blood cells are heavier than the plasma but lighter than the red blood cells. Therefore they form a thin layer between the red blood cells and the plasma. SEE: *buffy coat.*

***human c.*** A device that accommodates a human subject being rotated while suspended from a long arm. It is used to investigate the ability of subjects to withstand positive gravitational forces.

**centrilobular** (sĕn″trĭ-lŏb′ū-lăr) Pertaining to the center of a lobule.

**centriole** (sĕn′trē-ōl) A minute organelle consisting of a hollow cylinder closed at one end and open at the other, found in the cell center or attraction sphere of a cell. Before mitosis it divides, forming two daughter centrioles (diplosomes). During mitosis the centrioles migrate to opposite poles of the cell, and each forms the center of the aster to which the spindle fibers are attached. SEE: *mitosis.*

**centripetal** (sĕn-trĭp′ĕ-tăl) [″ + L. *petere,* to seek] Directed toward the axis. SYN: *axipetal.*

**centrocyte** (sĕn′trō-sīt) [″ + *kytos,* cell] A cell with single and double hematoxylin-stainable granules of varying size in its protoplasm.

**centrodesmus** (sĕn-trō-dĕz′mŭs) [Gr. *kentron,* center, + *desmos,* a band] The matter connecting the two centrosomes in a nucleus during mitosis.

**centrolecithal** (sĕn″trō-lĕs′ĭ-thăl) [″ + *lekithos,* yoke] Pertaining to an egg, especially an ovum, with the yolk centrally located.

**centromere** (sĕn′trō-mēr) [″ + *meros,* part] A constricted region of a chromosome, a specific sequence of about 200 nucleotides that connects the chromatids during cell division. Attached to this DNA is a protein disk called a kinetochore, which attaches the pair of chromatids to a spindle fiber.

**centrosclerosis** (sĕn″trō-sklĕ-rō′sĭs) [″ + *sklerosis,* a hardening] Filling of the bone marrow space with bone tissue.

**centrosome** (sĕn′trō-sōm) [″ + *soma,* body] A region of the cytoplasm of a cell usually lying near the nucleus, containing in its center one or two centrioles, the diplosomes. SEE: *mitosis.*

**centrosphere** (sĕn′trō-sfēr) [″ + *sphaira,* sphere] The cytoplasm of the centrosome.

**centrostaltic** (sĕn″trō-stăl′tĭk) [″ + *stellein,* send forth] Pert. to a center of motion.

**centrum** (sĕn′trŭm) *pl.* **centra** [L.] **1.** Any center, esp. an anatomical one. **2.** The body of a vertebra.

***c. semiovale*** The mass of white matter at the center of each cerebral hemisphere.

***c. tendineum*** The central tendon of the diaphragm.

**cepacia** SEE: *Pseudomonas cepacia.*

**cephalad** (sĕf′ă-lăd) [Gr. *kephale,* head, + L. *ad,* toward] Toward the head.

**cephalalgia** (sĕf-ă-lăl′jē-ă) [″ + *algos,* pain] Headache. SYN: *cephalodynia.* **cephalalgic** (-jĭk), *adj.*

**cephalea** (sĕf-ă-lē′ă) [Gr. *kephale,* head] Cephalalgia.

**cephaledema** (sĕf″ăl-ĕ-dē′mă) [″ + *oidema,* swelling] Edema of the head, esp. of the brain.

**cephalexin** (sĕf″ă-lĕk′sĭn) An analogue of the antibiotic cephalosporin. It is effective against gram-positive and gram-negative organisms.

**cephalhematocele** (sĕf″ăl-hē-măt′ō-sēl) [″ + *haima,* blood, + *kele,* tumor] A bloody tumor communicating with the dural sinuses.

**cephalhematoma** (sĕf″ăl-hē″mă-tō′mă) [″ + ″ + *oma,* tumor] A mass composed of clotted blood, located between the periosteum and the skull of a newborn. The swelling is confined between suture lines and usually is unilateral. The cause is rupture of periosteal bridging veins due to pressure and friction during labor and delivery, resulting in the collection of clotted blood between the periosteum and the fetal skull. The swelling reabsorbs gradually within a few weeks of birth.

**cephalic** (sĕ-făl′ĭk) [L. *cephalicus*] **1.** Cranial. **2.** Superior in position.

**cephalic index** An arbitrary measure of cranial capacity, derived by dividing the maximal length of the head into the value of the maximal breadth multiplied by 100.

**cephalocele** (sĕf′ă-lō-sēl) [″ + *kele,* hernia] Protrusion of the brain from the cranial cavity.

**cephalocentesis** (sĕf″ă-lō-sĕn-tē′sĭs) [″ + *kentesis,* puncture] Surgical puncture of the cranium.

**cephalodynia** (sĕf″ă-lō-dĭn′ē-ă) [″ + *odyne,* pain] Headache.

**cephalogyric** (sĕf″ă-lō-jī′rĭk) [″ + *gyros,* a turn] Pert. to rotation of the head.

**cephalohemometer** (sĕf″ă-lō-hē-mŏm′ĕ-tĕr) [″ + *haima,* blood, + *metron,* measure] An instrument for determining changes in intracranial blood pressure.

**cephalomenia** (sĕf″ă-lō-mē′nē-ă) [″ + *men,* month] Vicarious menstruation from the nose or head.

**cephalomeningitis** (sĕf″ă-lō-mĕn″ĭn-jī′tĭs) [″ + *meninx,* membrane, + *itis,* inflammation] Inflammation of the cerebral meninges.

**cephalometer** (sĕf-ă-lŏm′ĕ-tĕr) [″ + *metron,* measure] **1.** A device for measuring the head. **2.** In radiology, a device that maintains the head in a certain position for radiographic examination and measurement.

**cephalometry** (sĕf″ă-lŏm′ĕ-trē) Measurement of the head of a living person by using certain bony points directly, or by tracing radiographs made using well-established planes for linear and angular measurements. This technique is used in dentistry to assess growth and to determine orthodontic or prosthetic treatment plans.

**cephalomotor** (sĕf″ă-lō-mō′tor) [Gr. *kephale,* head, + L. *motus,* motion] Pert. to movements of the head.

**cephalonia** (sĕf″ă-lō′nē-ă) A condition marked by mental retardation and enlargement of the head.

**cephalopathy** (sĕf″ă-lŏp′ă-thē) [″ + *pathos,* disease, suffering] Any disease of the head or brain.

**cephalopelvic** (sĕf″ă-lō-pĕl′vĭk) Pert. to the relationship between the measurements of the fetal head and the diameters of the maternal pelvis, esp. to the size of the pelvic outlet through which the fetal head will pass during delivery.

**cephaloplegia** (sĕf″ă-lō-plē′jē-ă) [″ + *plege,* stroke] Paralysis of head or neck muscles or both.

**cephalorhachidian** (sĕf″ă-lō-ră-kĭd′ē-ăn) [″ + *rhachis,* spine] Pert. to the head and spine.

**cephaloridine** (sĕf″ă-lor′ĭ-dēn) An analogue of the antibiotic cephalosporin C.

**cephalosporin** (sĕf″ă-lō-spor′ĭn) General term for a group of antibiotic derivatives of cephalosporin C, which is obtained from the fungus *Cephalosporium.*

**Cephalosporium** A genus of imperfect fungi that inhabit soil. Cephalosporins are derived from them.

**cephalothin sodium** (sĕf′ă-lō-thĭn″) A semisynthetic analogue of the antibiotic cephalosporin C. Trade name is Keflin.

**cephalothoracic** (sĕf″ă-lō-thō-răs′ĭk) [″ + *thorakos,* chest] Pert. to the head and thorax.

**cephalothoracopagus** (sĕf″ă-lō-thō″ră-kŏp′ă-gŭs) [″ + ″ + *pagos,* thing fixed] A double fetus joined at the head and thorax.

**cephalotome** (sĕf′ă-lō-tōm) [″ + *tome,* incision] An instrument for cutting the head of the fetus to facilitate delivery.

**cephalotomy** (sĕf-ă-lŏt′ō-mē) Cutting the fetal head to facilitate delivery.

**cephapirin sodium** (sĕf-ă-pī′rĭn) An antibiotic similar to cephalothin. Trade name is Cefadyl.

**Cephulac** Trade name for lactulose.

**ceptor** (sĕp′tor) [L. *receptor,* receiver] Receptor (2).

***chemical c.*** A ceptor that initiates chemical reactions in the body.

***contact c.*** A ceptor that receives stimuli contributed by direct physical contact.

***distance c.*** A ceptor that perceives stimuli remote from the immediate environment.

**cera** (sē′ră) [L.] Wax (1).

***c. alba*** White wax.

***c. flava*** Yellow wax.

**ceramics, dental** [Gr. *keramos,* potter's clay] The use of porcelain or porcelain-type materials in dental work.

**ceramide** (sĕr′ă-mīd) A class of lipids that do not contain glycerol. They are derived from a sphingosine. Glycosphingolipids and sphingomyelins are derived from ceramides.

***c. oligosaccharides*** A class of glycosphingolipids.

**ceramodontia** (sē-răm″ō-dŏn′sheē-ă) [Gr. *keramos,* potter's clay, + *odous,* tooth] Dental ceramics.

**cerate ceratum** (sē′rāt) [L. *ceratum*] A medicinal formulation for topical use containing wax. It can be spread easily with a spatula on muslin or similar material at ordinary temperature, but is not soft enough to liquefy and run when applied to the skin. It is rarely prescribed.

**ceratocele** (sĕr′ă-tō-sēl) [Gr. *keras,* horn, + *kele,* hernia] Keratocele.

**ceratotome** (sĕ-răt′ō-tōm) [″ + *tome,* incision] A knife for division of the cornea.

**cercaria** (sĕr-kā′rē-ă) *pl.* **cercariae** [Gr. *kerkos,* tail] A free-swimming stage in the development of a fluke or trematode. Cercariae develop within sporocysts or rediae that parasitize snails or bivalve mollusks. They emerge from the mollusk and either enter their final host directly or encyst in an intermediate host that is ingested by the final host. In the latter case, the encysted tailless form is known as a metacercaria. SEE: *fluke; trematode.*

**cercaricide** An agent that is lethal to cercaria.

**cerclage** (sār-klōzh′) [Fr., hooping] Encircling tissues with a ligature, wire, or loop.

***cervical c.*** The use of ligatures around the cervix uteri to treat cervical incompetence during pregnancy. This helps to prevent spontaneous abortion.

**Cercomonas** (sĕr-kŏm′ō-năs) [Gr. *kerkos,* tail, + *monas,* unit] A genus of free-living flagellate protozoa. It may be present in stale specimens of feces or urine. It is not pathogenic.

**cercomoniasis** (sĕr″kō-mō-nī′ă-sĭs) Infestation with *Cercomonas intestinalis.*

**cercus** (sĕr′kŭs) *pl.* **cerci** [L., tail] A hairlike structure.

**cerea flexibilitas** (sē′rē-ă flĕk″sĭ-bĭl′ĭ-tăs) [L. *cera,* wax, + *flexibilitas,* flexibility] A cataleptic state in which limbs retain any position in which they are placed. It is characteristic of catatonic patients. SEE: *catalepsy.*

**cereal** [L. *cerealis,* of grain] An edible seed or grain. All cereals are similar in composition. Carbohydrates are the principal nutrient present and protein is next. Cereals contain 70% to 80% carbohydrate in the form of starch, and 8% to 15% protein. Vitamin B complex is abundant in wheat germ. Many cereals are high in fiber.

**cerebellifugal** (sĕr″ĕ-bĕl-ĭ-fū′găl) [L. *cerebellum,* little brain, + *fugere,* to flee] Extending or proceeding from the cerebellum.

**cerebellipetal** (sĕr″ĕ-bĕl-lĭp′ĭ-tăl) [″ + *petere,* to seek] Extending toward the cerebellum.

**cerebellitis** (sĕr″ĕ-bĕl-ī′tĭs) [″ + Gr. *itis,* inflammation] Inflammation of the cerebellum.

**cerebellospinal** (sĕr″ĕ-bĕl-ō-spī′năl) [″ +

*spina,* thorn] Pert. to the cerebellum and spinal cord.

**cerebellum** (sĕr-ĕ-bĕl′ŭm) [L., little brain] The portion of the brain forming the largest segment of the rhombencephalon. It lies dorsal to the pons and medulla oblongata, overhanging the latter. It consists of two lateral cerebellar hemispheres and a narrow medial portion, the vermis. It is connected to the brainstem by three pairs of fiber bundles, the inferior, middle, and superior peduncles. The cerebellum is involved in synergic control of skeletal muscles and plays an important role in the coordination of voluntary muscular movements. It receives afferent impulses and discharges efferent impulses but is not a reflex center in the usual sense; however, it may reinforce some reflexes and inhibit others.

Although the cerebellum does not initiate movements, it interrelates with many brainstem structures in executing various movements, including maintaining proper posture and balance; walking and running; fine voluntary movements as required in writing, dressing, eating, and playing musical instruments; and smooth tracking movements of the eyes. The cerebellum controls the property of movements, such as speed, acceleration, and trajectory. **cerebellar** (-ăr), *adj.*

**cerebral dominance** In 90% to 95% of human beings the left cerebral hemisphere is functionally dominant, and those persons are right-handed. This preference of one hand over the other may be more nearly complete in some than others. Speech and handedness are interrelated. In those who are right-handed, speech impairment is almost always related to a lesion in the left cerebral hemisphere. Aphasia rarely occurs in right-handed persons as a result of a right cerebral lesion. In 60% of left-handed individuals with aphasia owing to a cerebral lesion, the left side is affected. In some left-handed patients, it is possible that language function is controlled partially by both the left and right cerebal hemispheres. SEE: *stroke.*

**cerebral hemorrhage** The result of rupture of a sclerosed or diseased blood vessel in the brain. It is often associated with high blood pressure.

**cerebral palsy** ABBR: CP. An "umbrella" term for a group of nonprogressive, but often changing, motor impairment syndromes secondary to lesions or anomalies of the brain arising in the early stages of its development. CP is a symptom complex rather than a specific disease. For the vast majority of children born at term in whom CP later develops, the disorder cannot reasonably be ascribed to birth injury or hypoxic-ischemic insults during delivery. CP rarely occurs without associated defects such as mental retardation (60% of cases) or epilepsy (50% of cases).

Risk factors have been divided into three groups: those occurring prior to pregnancy, such as an unusually short interval (less than 3 months) or unusually long interval since the previous pregnancy; those occuring during pregnancy, including physical malformations, twin gestation, abnormal fetal presentation, fetal growth retardation, or maternal hypothyroidism; and perinatal factors such as prematurity, premature separation of the placenta, or newborn encephalopathy. Of infants with one or more of these risk factors, 95% do not have CP.

The disorder is classified by the extremities involved and the type of neurological dysfunction, such as spastic, hypotonic, dystonic, athetotic, or a combination of these. It is not possible to diagnose CP in the neonatal period, and early clinical diagnosis is complicated by the changing pattern of the disease in the first year of life.

TREATMENT: Therapy is directed to maximizing function and preventing secondary handicaps. Essential to the outcome of patients with CP is establishing good hand function, which will help compensate for other motor deficits. SEE: *Nursing Diagnoses Appendix.*

**cerebral palsy feeder** A mechanical device operated by simple gross movements; designed to permit independent eating by persons with severe motor control difficulties.

**cerebration** (sĕr″ĕ-brā′shŭn) [L. *cerebratio,* brain activity] Mental activity; thinking.

**cerebrifugal** (sĕr″ĕ-brĭf′ū-găl) [L. *cerebrum,* brain, + *fugere,* to flee] Away from the brain; pert. to efferent nerve fibers.

**cerebripetal** (sĕr″ĕ-brĭp′ĕ-tăl) [″ + *petere,* to seek] Proceeding toward the cerebrum; pert. to afferent nerve fibers or impulses.

**cerebroid** (sĕr′ē-broyd) [″ + Gr. *eidos,* form, shape] Resembling brain tissue.

**cerebromedullary** Cerebrospinal.

**cerebromeningitis** (sĕr″ĕ-brō-mĕn″ĭn-jī′tĭs) [″ + Gr. *meninx,* membrane, + *itis,* inflammation] Inflammation of the cerebrum and its membranes.

**cerebropathy** (sĕr-ĕ-brŏp′ă-thē) [″ + *pathos,* disease, suffering] Any disease of the brain, esp. the cerebrum.

**cerebrophysiology** (sĕr″ĕ-brō-fĭz-ē-ŏl′ō-jē) [″ + Gr. *physis,* nature, + *logos,* word, reason] The physiology of the brain.

**cerebropontile** (sĕr″ĕ-brō-pŏn′tĭl) [″ + *pons,* bridge] Pert. to the cerebrum and pons varolii.

**cerebrosclerosis** (sĕr″ĕ-brō″sklĕ-rō′sĭs) [″ + Gr. *sklerosis,* hardening] Hardening of the brain, esp. of the cerebrum.

**cerebroside** (sĕr′ĕ-brō-sīd″) A lipid or fatty substance present in nerve and other tissues.

**cerebrosidosis** (sĕr″ĕ-brō″sī-dō′sĭs) A form of lipoidosis with kerasin in the fatty cells. SEE: *Gaucher's disease.*

**cerebrospinal** (sĕr″ĕ-brō-spī′năl) [″ + *spina,*

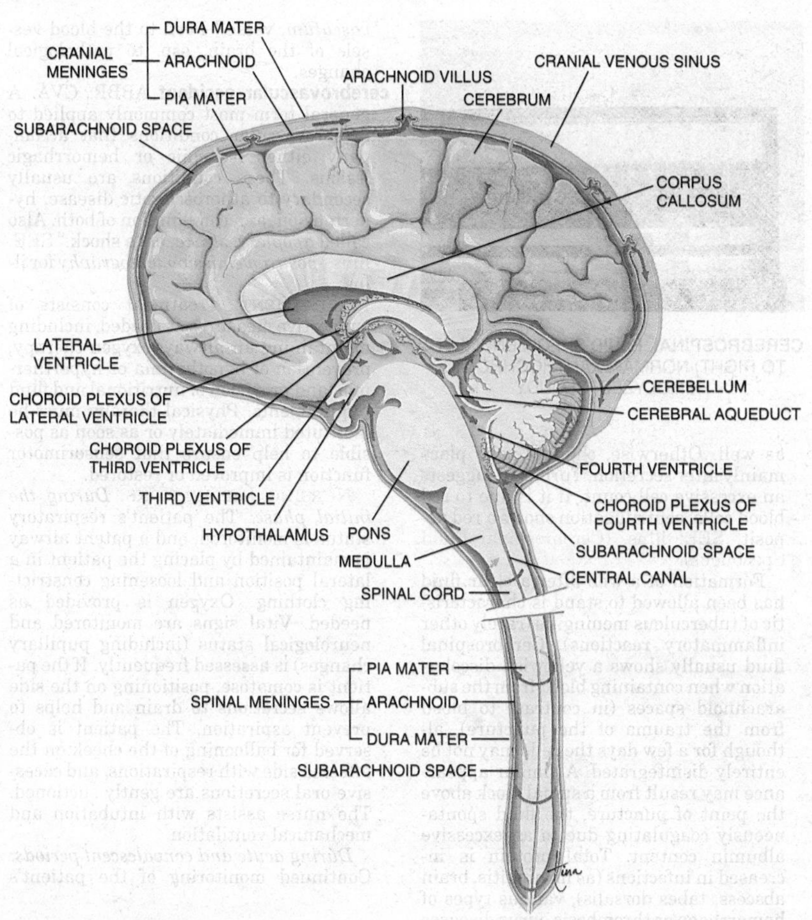


FORMATION, CIRCULATION, AND REABSORPTION OF **CEREBROSPINAL FLUID**

thorn] Pert. to the brain and spinal cord, as the cerebrospinal axis.

**cerebrospinal axis** The central nervous system.

**cerebrospinal fluid** ABBR: CSF. A water cushion protecting the brain and spinal cord from physical impact. Shrinkage or expansion of the cranial contents is usually balanced quickly by an increase or a decrease in the amount of this fluid. SEE: *blood-brain barrier; lumbar puncture.*

FORMATION: The fluid is formed by the choroid plexuses of the lateral and third ventricles. That of the lateral ventricles passes through the foramen of Monro to the third ventricle, and through the aqueduct of Sylvius to the fourth ventricle. There it may escape through the central foramen of Magendie or the lateral foramen of Luschke into the cisterna magna, and so over the brain and cord surfaces, occupying the subarachnoid spaces. It is reabsorbed through the arachnoid villi into the blood in the cranial venous sinuses, and through the perineural lymph spaces of both the brain and the cord. SEE: illus. (Formation, Circulation, and Reabsorption of Cerebrospinal Fluid).

CHARACTERISTICS: The fluid is watery, clear, and colorless. Normally the initial pressure of spinal fluid in a recumbent adult, as determined by spinal puncture, is equivalent to 70 to 180 mm of water. The amount in normal adults is 100 to 140 ml. Its specific gravity ranges from 1.003 to 1.008. The total cell count in adults is 0 to 10/ml, and in children, 0 to 20/ml (cells should be counted at once). Its total protein is 20 to 45 mg/dl; the total glucose is 0 to 75 mg/dl. Its concentration and alkaline reserve are similar to those of blood. It does not clot on standing. Although the choroid plexuses can reflect certain blood constituents (e.g., iodides), changes in blood sugar, chloride, and urea manifest themselves quickly in the fluid

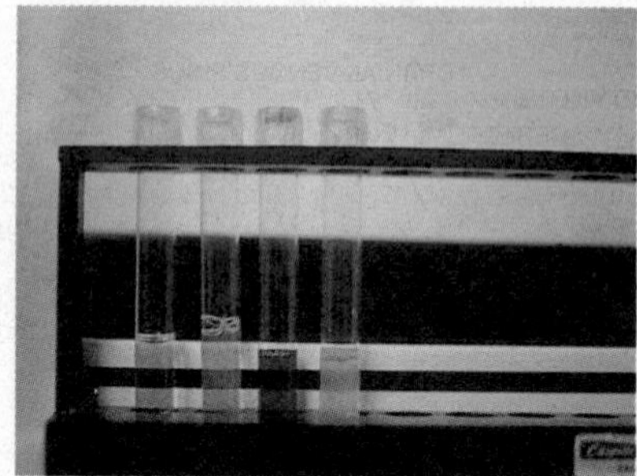

**CEREBROSPINAL FLUID** SPECIMENS: (LEFT TO RIGHT) NORMAL, XANTHOCHROMIC, HEMOLYZED, CLOUDY

as well. Otherwise, changes take place mainly after secretion. Turbidity suggests an excessive cell count. If it is due to red blood cells, centrifugation shows a red deposit. SEE: illus. (Cerebrospinal Fluid Specimens).

Formation of a web after a clear fluid has been allowed to stand is characteristic of tuberculous meningitis (rarely other inflammatory reactions). Cerebrospinal fluid usually shows a yellowish discoloration when containing blood from the subarachnoid spaces (in contrast to blood from the trauma of the puncture), although for a few days the cells may not be entirely disintegrated. A similar appearance may result from a spinal block above the point of puncture, the fluid spontaneously coagulating due to an excessive albumin content. Total protein is increased in infections (as meningitis, brain abscess, tabes dorsalis), various types of hemorrhage or thrombosis, virus diseases (as encephalitis, anterior poliomyelitis, lymphocytic meningitis), and conditions such as chronic alcoholism. Cell count increases esp. in tuberculous meningitis, epidemic encephalitis, lymphocytic choriomeningitis, poliomyelitis (several days after onset), syphilis of the central nervous system, and certain types of tumors of the spinal cord or brain.

**cerebrospinal ganglia** Sensory ganglia on the roots of cranial and spinal nerves.

**cerebrospinal nerves** Cranial nerves and spinal nerves.

**cerebrospinal puncture** A puncture for the collection of cerebrospinal fluid or the injection of contrast media or medications. Puncture sites include the spaces around the spinal cord (lumbar puncture), the cisterna magna (cisternal puncture), or open fontanelles in infants (ventricular puncture).

**cerebrotomy** (sĕr″ĕ-brŏt′ō-mē) [L. *cerebrum,* brain, + Gr. *tome,* incision] **1.** Incision of the brain to evacuate an abscess. **2.** Dissection of the brain.

**cerebrovascular** (sĕr″ĕ-brō-văs′kū-lăr) [″ + *vasculum,* vessel] Pert. to the blood vessels of the brain, esp. to pathological changes.

**cerebrovascular accident** ABBR: CVA. A general term most commonly applied to cerebrovascular conditions that accompany either ischemic or hemorrhagic lesions. These conditions are usually secondary to atherosclerotic disease, hypertension, or a combination of both. Also called *apoplexy*, *stroke*, or "a shock." SEE: illus.; *positron emission tomography* for illus.

TREATMENT: Treatment consists of supportive measures as needed, including maintaining an airway, oxygen therapy, prevention of hypothermia or hyperthermia, and provision of nutritional and fluid requirements. Physical therapy must be instituted immediately or as soon as possible to help ensure that sensorimotor function is improved or restored.

NURSING IMPLICATIONS: *During the initial phase:* The patient's respiratory status is monitored, and a patent airway is maintained by placing the patient in a lateral position and loosening constricting clothing. Oxygen is provided as needed. Vital signs are monitored and neurological status (including pupillary changes) is assessed frequently. If the patient is comatose, positioning on the side allows secretions to drain and helps to prevent aspiration. The patient is observed for ballooning of the cheek on the affected side with respirations, and excessive oral secretions are gently suctioned. The nurse assists with intubation and mechanical ventilation.

*During acute and convalescent periods:* Continued monitoring of the patient's

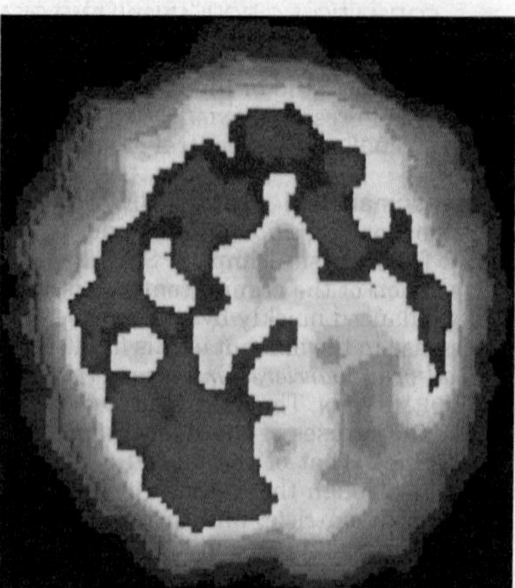

**CEREBROVASCULAR ACCIDENT**
PET SCAN OF BRAIN SHOWING INFARCTION IN TEMPORAL LOBE (GREEN)

neurological status is performed. Respiratory status is assessed by auscultating for adventitious sounds, and the patient is encouraged to breathe deeply to prevent respiratory complications. Fluid and electrolyte balance are monitored and maintained; oral fluids are provided as patient's condition permits, or intravenous fluids are administered as prescribed. The urinal or bedpan is offered to the conscious patient every 2 hr; and urinary catheterization is used only when necessary for the unconscious patient because it may result in urinary tract infection. Bladder function is assessed, bladder training initiated, and the incontinent patient kept clean and dry.

To ensure adequate nutrition, gag reflex and swallowing ability are assessed before small meals of semisolid foods and thickened liquids are offered, and the patient is positioned upright with the head slightly forward for meals. The patient is also assessed for visual field deficits, dysphagia, and one-sided facial weakness, which can interfere with eating; the patient with facial weakness is encouraged to chew on the unaffected side. Enteral nutrition via a feeding tube is provided if the patient is unable to eat, or parenteral nutrition, if the gastrointestinal system is nonfunctional. Oral care is provided.

The daily elimination pattern is assessed, and the patient is advised to avoid straining at stool. Dietary modifications such as increased fiber and fluid and stool softeners are provided, and laxatives or enemas are used if needed. Bowel training is initiated by encouraging defecation at the usual time in as natural a position and setting as possible; suppositories are used to stimulate the bowel if necessary.

Eye secretions are removed with approved irrigation solutions, artificial tears are applied to prevent drying, and the eye is patched closed if the patient is unable to close the eyelid.

The patient is maintained in correct body alignment; trochanter rolls are used to prevent external hip rotation, pillow supports to prevent hip dislocation, pillow supports or slings to prevent shoulder subluxation, and right-angle splints to prevent footdrop. The patient is repositioned frequently, but positioning on the affected side for more than short periods is avoided. Skin is inspected and pressure areas are massaged and cushioned. Distal parts of extremities are positioned higher than proximal areas to encourage venous return. Passive or active-assisted range of motion exercises to both the affected and unaffected sides are performed to maintain joint mobility. The patient is encouraged to exercise joints as ability permits, using the unaffected side to exercise the affected side.

The nurse collaborates in obtaining assistive appliances to help in performing activities of daily living. The nurse sets up a simple method for the aphasic patient to communicate basic needs and documents this system for use by other caregivers; speaks slowly, quietly, and calmly; and uses gestures to aid understanding. All communication attempts by the patient are encouraged, and the speech therapist's prescribed treatment plan is followed. The unresponsive patient can hear; therefore, nothing should be said in this patient's presence that should not be heard.

The family needs assistance to understand and deal with the patient's emotions. A plan of care is established to promote the patient's physical, intellectual, and communicative abilities and to help the patient regain lost functions to facilitate independence. Both patient and family are instructed about the prescribed drug regimen, management of the plan of care at home, safety measures, and modification of risk factors to decrease the potential for another CVA. As necessary, referrals are made to home health care agencies and support services. SEE: *Nursing Diagnoses Appendix.*

**cerebrum** (sĕr′ĕ-brŭm, sĕr-ē′brŭm) [L.] The largest part of the brain, consisting of two hemispheres separated by a deep longitudinal fissure. The hemispheres are united by three commissures—the corpus callosum and the anterior and posterior hippocampal commissures. The surface of each hemisphere is thrown into numerous folds or convolutions called gyri, which are separated by furrows called fissures or sulci.

EMBRYOLOGY: The cerebrum develops from the telencephalon, the most anterior portion of the prosencephalon or forebrain.

ANATOMY: Each cerebral hemisphere consists of three primary portions—the rhinencephalon or olfactory lobe, the corpus striatum, and the pallium or cerebral cortex. The cortex is a layer of gray matter that forms the surface of each hemisphere. The part in the rhinencephalon (phylogenetically the oldest) is called the archipallium; the larger nonolfactory cortex is called the neopallium. The cerebrum contains two cavities, the lateral ventricles (right and left) and the rostral portion of the third ventricle. The white matter of each hemisphere consists of three kinds of myelinated fibers: commissural fibers, which pass from one hemisphere to the other; projection fibers, which convey impulses to and from the cortex; and association fibers, which connect various parts of the cortex within one hemisphere.

*Lobes:* The principal lobes are the frontal, parietal, occipital, and temporal lobes and the central (the insula or island of Reil). *Basal ganglia:* Masses of gray matter are deeply embedded within each

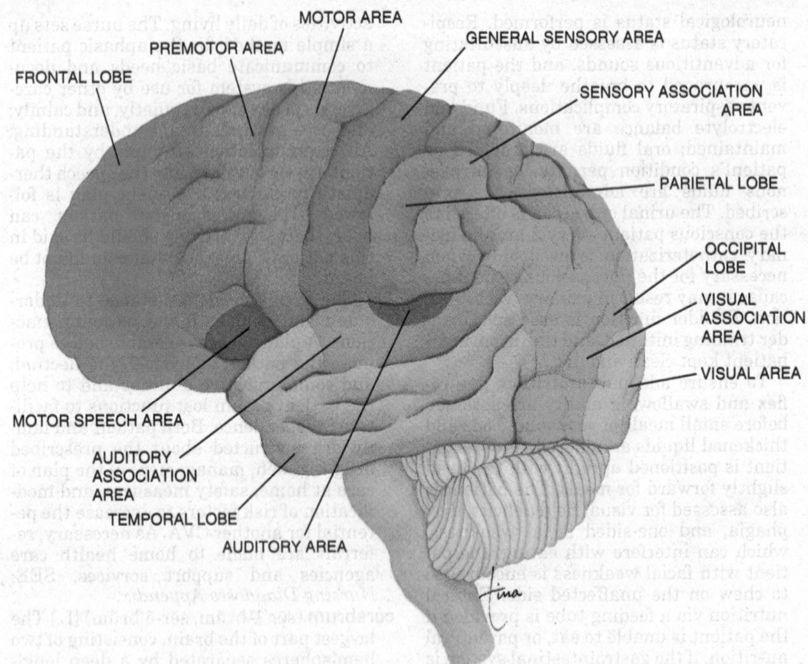


CEREBRUM (LEFT HEMISPHERE)

hemisphere. They are the caudate, lentiform, and amygdaloid nuclei and the claustrum. *Fissures and sulci:* These include the lateral cerebral fissure (of Sylvius), the central sulcus (of Rolando), the parieto-occipital fissure, the calcarine fissure, the cingulate sulcus, the collateral fissure, the sulcus circularis, and the longitudinal cerebral fissure. *Gyri:* These include the superior, middle, and inferior frontal gyri, the anterior and posterior central gyri, the superior, middle, and inferior temporal gyri, and the cingulate, lingual, fusiform, and hippocampal gyri.

PHYSIOLOGY: The cerebrum is concerned with sensations (the interpretation of sensory impulses) and all voluntary muscular activities. It is the seat of consciousness and the center of the higher mental faculties such as memory, learning, reasoning, judgment, intelligence, and the emotions. SEE: illus.

On the basis of function, several areas have been identified and located. Motor areas in the frontal lobes initiate all voluntary movement of skeletal muscles. Sensory areas in the parietal lobes are for taste and cutaneous senses, those in the temporal lobes are for hearing and smell, and those in the occipital lobes are for vision. Association areas are concerned with integration, analysis, learning, and memory.

**cerium** (sē′rē-ŭm) [L.] SYMB: Ce. A metallic element obtained from the rare earths; atomic weight 140.12, atomic number 58.

**ceroid** (sē′royd) A fatty pigment present in various tissues.

**ceroma** (sē-rō′mă) [L. *cera*, wax, + Gr. *oma*, tumor] A waxy tumor that has undergone amyloid degeneration.

**ceroplasty** (sē′rō-plăs″tē) [″ + Gr. *plassein*, to mold] The manufacture of anatomical models and pathological specimens in wax.

**certifiable** (sĕr″tĭ-fī′ă-b′l) **1.** Pert. to infectious diseases that must be reported or registered with the health authorities. **2.** In forensic medicine, a term applied to a mentally incompetent individual who requires the care of a guardian or institution.

**certification** (sĕr″tĭ-fĭ-kā′shŭn) **1.** A legal document prepared by an official body that indicates a person or institution has met certain standards, or that a person has completed a prescribed course of instruction or training. **2.** The completion of a form indicating the cause of death. **3.** The legal process of declaring a person insane or mentally incompetent on the basis of medical evidence. SEE: *commitment.*

**certified emergency nurse** ABBR: CEN. A nurse who has passed the examination administered by the Board of Certification of Emergency Nursing. To maintain certification as a CEN, a nurse must pass the examination every 4 years.

**certify** [L. *certus,* certain, + *facio,* to make] **1.** To make a declaration concerning the sanity of an individual. **2.** To report certain specified diseases to public health authorities.

**ceruloplasmin** (sĕ-roo″lō-plăz′mĭn) A blue glycoprotein to which most of the copper in the blood is attached. It is decreased in Wilson's disease.

**cerumen** (sĕ-roo′mĕn) [L. *cera,* wax] A substance secreted by glands at the outer third of the ear canal. Usually cerumen does not accumulate in the ear canal, but it may clog the channel in some persons. In this case, the cerumen may become impacted and must be physically removed, not by irrigation of the canal but by use of a curette. Soft cerumen is easily removed by gentle syringe instillation of plain water in the canal. SYN: *earwax.* **ceruminal, ceruminous** (-mĭ-năl, -mĭ-nŭs), *adj.*

**ceruminolysis** (sĕ-roo″mĭ-nŏl′ĭ-sĭs) The dissolution or disintegration of cerumen in the external ear canal.

**ceruminolytic agent** (sĕ-roo″mĭ-nō-lĭt′ĭk) An agent that dissolves cerumen in the external ear canal. Obstruction of the ear canal with cerumen can cause itching, pain, and temporary conductive hearing loss. The first approach to treatment should be removal of the obstruction manually with a blunt curette or loop or by irrigation. Cerumen solvents are not always recommended because they often do not eliminate the problem and frequently cause maceration of skin of the canal and allergic reactions.

**ceruminosis** (sĕ-roo″mĭ-nō′sĭs) [″ + Gr. *osis,* condition] Excessive secretion of cerumen.

**ceruminous gland** One of the modified sweat glands in the skin lining the external auditory canal that secrete cerumen.

**cervic-** SEE: *cervico-.*

**cervical** (sĕr′vĭ-kăl) [L. *cervicalis*] **1.** Pert. to or in the region of the neck. **2.** Pert. to the cervix of an organ, as the cervix uteri.

**cervical cap** A device made of a flexible material that is shaped to provide a covering for the uterine cervix. It is used to prevent conception.

**cervical intraepithelial neoplasia** ABBR: CIN. Dysplasia of the basal layers of the squamous epithelium of the uterine cervix. This may progress to involve deeper layers of the epithelium. Grades 1, 2, and 3 represent increasing progression of the pathological process. Grade 3 (CIN 3) represents carcinoma in situ. CIN 3 is also classed stage 0 of cancer of the cervix. SEE: *Bethesda system; cervix, cancer of.*

**cervical nerve** A nerve in the first eight pairs of spinal nerves. SEE: *skeleton; spinal nerve.*

**cervical plexus** A network formed by the first four cervical spinal nerves. It innervates parts of the face, neck, shoulder, and chest, and gives rise to the phrenic nerve to the diaphragm. SEE: *Nerve Plexus Appendix.*

**cervical rib syndrome** Pain and paresthesias in the the hand, neck, shoulder, or arms, usually due to compression of the brachial plexus of nerves by an accessory cervical rib. SEE: *scalenus syndrome.*

**cervical ripening** The process of physical softening and dilation of the uterine cervix in preparation for childbirth. Normally this occurs naturally, but in postterm pregnancies it may be necessary to use mechanical dilators or drugs. Placement of laminaria or prostaglandin $E_2$ gel in the vagina or cervical canal promotes cervical ripening and onset of labor.

NURSING IMPLICATIONS: The nurse assesses fetal status by monitoring the heart rate for 30 min before gel insertion and for approx. 1 hr after the procedure. The mother is assessed for uterine contractions and signs of hyperstimulation, nausea, or vomiting. If hyperstimulation occurs, the nurse removes the gel and notifies the primary health care provider.

**cervical spondylosis** Degenerative arthritis (osteoarthritis) of the cervical vertebrae and related tissues. If severe, it may cause pressure on nerve roots with subsequent pain or paresthesia in the arms.

**cervical vertebra** One of the first seven bones of the spinal column. SEE: *skeleton.*

**cervicectomy** (sĕr″vĭ-sĕk′tō-mē) [L. *cervix,* neck, + Gr. *ektome,* excision] Surgical removal of the cervix uteri.

**cervices** Pl. of cervix.

**cervicitis** (sĕr-vĭ-sī′tĭs) [″ + Gr. *itis,* inflammation] Inflammation of the cervix uteri.

**cervico-, cervic-** (sĕr′vĭ-kō) [L. *cervix*] Combining form pert. to the neck or to the neck of an organ.

**cervicobrachial** (sĕr″vĭ-kō-brā′kē-ăl) [″ + Gr. *brachion,* arm] Pert. to the neck and arm.

**cervicocolpitis** (sĕr″vĭ-kō-kŏl-pī′tĭs) [″ + Gr. *kolpos,* vagina, + *itis,* inflammation] Inflammation of the cervix uteri and vagina.

**cervicodynia** (sĕr″vĭ-kō-dĭn′ē-ă) [″ + Gr. *odyne,* pain] A pain or cramp of the neck; cervical neuralgia.

**cervicofacial** (sĕr″vĭ-kō-fā′shē-ăl) [″ + *facies,* face] Pert. to the neck and face.

**cervicography** Photographic study of the uterine cervix.

**cervicovaginitis** (sĕr″vĭ-kō-văj″ĭ-nī′tĭs) [″ + *vagina,* sheath, + Gr. *itis,* inflammation] Inflammation of the cervix uteri and the vagina.

**cervicovesical** (sĕr″vĭ-kō-vĕs′ĭ-kăl) [″ + *vesica,* bladder] Pert. to the cervix uteri and bladder.

**cervix** (sĕr′vĭks) *pl.* **cervices** [L.] The neck or a part of an organ resembling a neck. SEE: words beginning with *cervico-.*

***cancer of c.*** A malignant neoplasm of the cervix of the uterus (cervix uteri). Annually, it causes 5% of the cancer deaths in women. It may occur at any age, beginning at puberty. The mortality increases with age. Symptoms are absent except in advanced cases. Periodic Papanicolaou tests, beginning after the individual becomes sexually active, and colposcopy constitute the diagnostic procedures. The disease begins insidiously and may progress slowly or rapidly through the earliest change, dysplasia of the squamous epithelium of the cervix, through the various grades of cervical intraepithelial neoplasm (CIN), to carcinoma in situ, to the five stages of carcinoma of the cervix (stages 0 through IV). The treatment consists of radiation, surgery, or cytotoxic agents. SEE: *Bethesda system; cervical intraepithelial neoplasia; colposcopy; loop electrode excision procedure; Papanicolaou test.*

ETIOLOGY: A precise cause is unknown, but the risk factors include early age at first intercourse, multiple sexual partners, and promiscuous male sexual partners, esp. those whose previous partners had cervical cancer. It is suspected that an oncogenic factor, probably a virus, is transmitted sexually. The human papilloma virus is thought to be an important factor.

In the past, it was thought that cervical cancer did not occur in celibate women, such as nuns. There is little evidence to support this. Therefore, when a celibate woman has symptoms suggesting cervical cancer, that diagnosis should be considered.

***c. uteri*** The neck of the uterus; the lower part from the internal os outward to the external os. It is rounded and conical, and a portion protrudes into the vagina. It is about 1 in. (2.5 cm) long and is penetrated by the cervical canal, through which the fetus and menstrual flow escape. It may be torn in childbirth, esp. in a primigravida.

Deeper tears may occur in manual dilatation and use of forceps; breech presentation also may be a cause. Laceration may be single, bilateral, stellate, or incomplete. Tears are repaired by suturing to prevent hemorrhage and later complications.

***c. vesicae*** Neck of the bladder.

**c.e.s.** *central excitatory state.*

**cesarean birth** Cesarean section.

**cesarean hysterectomy** (sē-sār'ē-ăn) [L. *caesarea,* cut] Cesarean section immediately followed by hysterectomy.

**cesarean section** Delivery of the fetus by means of incision into the uterus. Operative approaches and techniques vary. A horizontal incision through the lower uterine segment is most common; the classic vertical midline incision may be used in times of profound fetal distress. Elective cesarean section is indicated for known cephalopelvic disproportion, malpresentations, and active herpes infection. The most common reason for emergency cesarean delivery is fetal distress. Many women can experience successful vaginal birth with a later pregnancy.

NURSING IMPLICATIONS: *Preoperative:* The procedure is explained to the patient and her partner. The partner should be included in the experience if possible. Baseline measures of maternal vital signs and fetal heart rate are obtained; maternal and fetal status is monitored until delivery according to protocol. Laboratory data, ultrasound results, or the results of other studies are available to the obstetrical team. The operative area is shaved according to protocol, and an indwelling urinary catheter inserted as prescribed. An intravenous infusion with a large-bore catheter is started, and oral food and fluid are restricted according to protocol and as time permits. Two units of blood are crossmatched and available. The patient is premedicated to reduce anxiety and discomfort.

*Postoperative:* On recovery from general anesthesia, or as soon as possible thereafter, the mother is allowed to see, hold, and touch her newborn. Vital signs are monitored and a patent airway is established. The dressing and perineal pad are assessed for bleeding (often every 15 min times 4, then every 30 min times 4, then every hour times 4, and finally every 4 hr for 24 hr, or as prescribed for the specific patient). The fundus is gently palpated for firmness without touching the incision, and intravenous oxytocin is administered as prescribed. If general anesthesia is used, routine postoperative care and positioning are provided; if regional anesthesia is used, the anesthesia level is assessed until sensation has completely returned. Intake and output are monitored, and any evidence of blood-tinged urine is documented and reported. Cold is applied to the incision to control pain and swelling if prescribed, analgesics are administered, and noninvasive pain-relief measures are instituted. The mother is assisted to turn from side to side and encouraged to breathe deeply, cough, and use incentive spirometry to improve ventilation and to mobilize secretions. When bowel sounds have returned, oral fluids and food are encouraged and bowel and bladder activity are monitored.

The patient is assisted with early ambulation and urged to visit her newborn in the nursery if the neonate is not healthy enough to be brought to her bedside. Usual postpartal instruction is provided regarding fundus, lochia, and perineal care; breast and nipple care; and infant care. Instruction is also given on incision care and the need to report any hemorrhage, chest or leg pain (possible thrombosis), dyspnea, separation of the wound's edges, or signs of infection, such as fever, difficult urination, or flank pain. Any activity restrictions after discharge are discussed with both patient and partner. SEE: *Nursing Diagnoses Appendix.*

***cervical c.s.*** Surgical removal of the fetus, placenta, and membranes through an incision in the portion of the uterus just above the cervix.

***classic c.s.*** Surgical removal of the fetus, placenta, and membranes through an incision in the abdominal and uterine walls.

***extraperitoneal c.s.*** Surgical removal of the fetus, placenta, and membranes through an incision into the lowest portion of the anterior aspect of the uterus. This approach does not entail entering the peritoneal cavity.

***low transverse c.s.*** Surgical removal of the fetus, placenta, and membranes through a transverse incision into the lower uterine segment. Use of this incision is associated with a decreased incidence of maternal and fetal mortality and morbidity in future pregnancies.

***postmortem c.s.*** Surgical removal of the fetus from the uterus immediately after maternal death.

**cesium** (sē′zē-ŭm) [L. *caesius,* sky blue] SYMB: Cs. A metallic element; atomic weight 132.905, atomic number 55. It has several isotopes. The radioactive isotope $^{137}$Cs, which has a half-life of 30 years, is used therapeutically for irradiation of cancerous tissue.

**cesspool** Colloquial term for *septic tank.*

**Cestan-Chenais syndrome** (sĕs-tăn′shĕn-ā′) [Raymond Cestan, Fr. neurologist, 1872–1934; Louis J. Chenais, Fr. physician, 1872–1950] A neurological disorder produced by a lesion of the pontobulbar area of the brain.

**Cestoda** (sĕs-tōd′ă) [Gr. *kestos,* girdle] A subclass of the class Cestoidea, phylum Platyhelminthes, which includes the tapeworms, having a scolex and a chain of segments (proglottids) (e.g., Taenia, intestinal parasites of humans and other vertebrates).

**cestode** (sĕs′tōd) [″ + *eidos,* form, shape] A tapeworm; a member of the Cestoda family. **cestoid** (-toyd), *adj.*

**cestodiasis** (sĕs″tō-dī′ă-sĭs) [″ + ″ + *-iasis,* condition] Infestation with tapeworms. SEE: *Cestoda.*

**Cestoidea** (sĕs-toy′dē-ă) A class of flatworms of the phylum Platyhelminthes; it includes the tapeworms.

**Cetamide** Trade name for sulfacetamide sodium.

**cetyl alcohol** A white insoluble solid substance, $C_{16}H_{34}O$, used in the manufacture of ointments.

**cetylpyridinium chloride** An anti-infective agent used topically and as a preservative in the manufacture of drugs.

**CF** *Christmas factor; citrovorum factor.*

**Cf** Symbol for the element californium.

**C.F.T.** *complement fixation test.*

**cGMP** *cyclic guanosine monophosphate.*

**C.G.S.** *centimeter-gram-second,* a name given to a system of units for length, weight, and time.

**$CH_4$** Methane; marsh gas.

**$C_2H_2$** Acetylene.

**$C_2H_4$** Ethylene.

**$C_6H_6$** Benzene.

**Chaddock's reflex** (chăd′ŏks) [Charles G. Chaddock, U.S. neurologist, 1861–1936] **1.** Extension of the great toe when the outer edge of the dorsum of the foot is stroked. It is present in disease of the corticospinal tract. **2.** Flexion of the wrist and fanning of the fingers when the tendon of the palmaris longus muscle is pressed.

**Chadwick's sign** [James R. Chadwick, U.S. gynecologist, 1844–1905] A deep blue-violet color of the cervix and vagina caused by increased vascularity; a presumptive sign of pregnancy that becomes evident around the fourth week of gestation.

**chafe** (chāf) [O. Fr. *chaufer,* to warm] To injure by rubbing or friction.

**chafing** (chāf′ĭng) A superficial inflammation that develops when skin is subjected to friction from clothing or adjacent skin. This may occur at the axilla, groin, or anal region, between digits of hands and feet, or at the neck or wrists. Erythema, maceration, and sometimes fissuring occur. Bacterial or mycotic infection may result secondarily.

**Chagas' disease** (chăg′ăs) [Carlos Chagas, Braz. physician, 1879–1934] South American trypanosomiasis.

**chagoma** An erythematous swelling following the bite of the parasite that transmits trypanosomiasis. SEE: *trypanosomiasis, South American.*

**chain** (chān) [O. Fr. *chaine,* chain] **1.** A related series of events or things. **2.** In bacteriology, bacterial organisms strung together. **3.** In chemistry, the linkage of atoms in a straight line or in a circle or ring. The ring or straight-line structures may have side chains branching off from the main compound.

***electron transport c.*** SEE: *system, cytochrome transport.*

***food c.*** SEE: *food chain.*

***heavy c.'s*** The large polypeptide chains of antibodies. SEE: *heavy chain disease.*

***kinematic c.*** A series of bones connected by joints. Movement of one segment influences other parts of the chain.

***light c.'s*** the small polypeptide chains of antibodies.

**chaining** (chān′ĭng) A behavioral therapy process whereby reinforcement is given for behaviors related to established behavior. Also called *chained reinforcement.*

**chain of custody** In legal medicine, the procedure for ensuring that material obtained for diagnosis has been taken from the named patient, is properly labeled, and has not been tampered with en route to the laboratory.

**chain of survival concept** In emergency cardiac care, the concept that more people could survive cardiac arrest when a particular sequence of events occurs as rapidly as possible. This sequence is (1) early access, (2) early CPR, (3) early defibrillation, (4) early advanced life support. Each of these interventions is regarded as a link in a chain, and weakness in any link lessens the chance of survival. SEE: *cardiopulmonary resuscitation.*

**chair, birthing** SEE: *birthing chair.*

**chalasia** (kă-lā′zē-ă) [Gr. *chalasis,* relaxation] Relaxation of sphincters.

**chalazion** (kă-lā′zē-ŏn) *pl.* **chalazia, chalazions** [Gr. *khalaza,* hailstone] A small, hard tumor analogous to a sebaceous cyst developing on the eyelids, formed by distention of a meibomian gland with secretion. SYN: *meibomian cyst.* SEE: *steatoma.*

**chalicosis** (kăl-ĭ-kō′sĭs) [Gr. *chalix,* limestone, + *osis,* condition] Pneumonoconiosis associated with the inhalation of dust produced by stone cutting.

**chalinoplasty** (kăl′ĭ-nō-plăs″tē) [Gr. *chalinos,* corner of mouth, + *plassein,* to mold] Plastic surgery of the mouth and lips, esp. of the corners of the mouth.

**challenge** (chăl′ĕnj) In immunology, administration of a specific antigen to an individual known to be sensitive to that antigen in order to produce an immune response.

**chalone** (kăl′ōn) [Gr. *chalan,* to relax] A protein that inhibits mitosis in the tissue in which it is produced.

**chamber** (chām′bĕr) [Gr. *kamara,* vault] A compartment or closed space.

***altitude c.*** Low-pressure c.

***anterior c.*** The space between the cornea and iris of the eye. SEE: *posterior c.*

***aqueous c.*** The anterior and posterior chambers of the eye, containing the aqueous humor.

***hyperbaric c.*** An airtight enclosure strong enough to withstand high internal pressure. It is used to expose animals, humans, or an entire surgical team to increased air pressure. SYN: *pressure c.* SEE: *hyperbaric oxygen therapy.*

***ionization c.*** A device used to measure radiation by equating ion production in a gas chamber with the intensity of an electrical charge.

***low-pressure c.*** An enclosure designed to simulate high altitudes by exposing humans or animals to low atmospheric pressure. Such studies are essential for simulated flights into the atmosphere and space. SYN: *altitude c.*

***posterior c.*** In the eye, the space behind the iris and in front of the vitreous body. It is occupied by the lens, its zonules, and the aqueous humor. SEE: *anterior c.; eye* for illus.

***pressure c.*** Hyperbaric c.

***pulp c.*** The part of the pulp cavity contained within the crown of the tooth. It is continuous with the root canals.

***vitreous c.*** The cavity behind the lens in the eye that contains the vitreous humor.

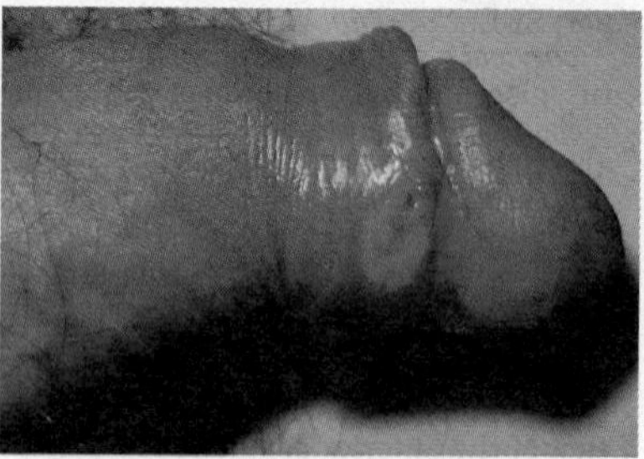

TYPICAL **CHANCRE** OF PRIMARY SYPHILIS

**chamomile; camomile** (kăm′ĕ-mīl) [Gr. *khamaemelon,* earth apple] The flowers of the *Anthemis;* they yield a bluish volatile oil and a bitter infusion.

**chancre** (shăng′kĕr) [Fr., ulcer] A hard, syphilitic primary ulcer, the first sign of syphilis, appearing approx. 2 to 3 weeks after infection. SEE: illus.; *syphilis.* **chancrous** (-krŭs), *adj.*

SYMPTOMS: The ulcer begins as a painless erosion or papule that ulcerates superficially. It occurs generally singly, but sometimes may be multiple. It has a scooped-out appearance due to level or sloping edges that are adherent, and a shining red or raw floor. Induration is persistent, and there is a slightly purulent secretion. The ulcer heals without leaving a scar. It may appear at almost any site including the mouth, penis, urethra, hand, toe, eyelid, conjunctiva, vagina, or cervix. SYN: *hard c.; hunterian c.; true c.*

---

Caution: During the chancre stage, the condition is highly contagious and the chancre itself contains many spirochetes. Discovery of these organisms in the chancre is the basis for the positive dark-field test for syphilis. However, syphilis may occur without a chancre developing.

---

***hard c.*** Chancre.

***hunterian c.*** Chancre.

***simple c.*** Chancroid.

***soft c.*** Chancroid.

***true c.*** Chancre.

**chancroid** (shăng′kroyd) [″ + Gr. *eidos,* form, shape] A highly infectious nonsyphilitic venereal ulcer. It is caused by *Haemophilus ducreyi* (also called Ducrey's bacillus), a gram-negative bacillus. Incubation is approx. 3 to 5 days. Treatment is with ceftriaxone or erythromycin. SYN: *simple chancre; soft chancre.*

SYMPTOMS: A chancroid begins with multiple pustules or ulcers having abrupt edges, a rough floor, yellow exudate, and purulent secretion. It is sensitive and inflamed. It heals rapidly, leaving a scar. Chancroids may affect the penis, urethra, vulva, or anus. Multiple lesions may develop by autoinoculation. Types include transient, phagedenic, giant, and serpiginous.

**change, fatty** Any abnormal accumulation of fat within parenchymal cells. It may occur in the heart or other organs. When seen in the liver, it usually is a result of excessive and prolonged alcohol intake.

**change of life** Menopause; the climacteric.

**channel** [L. *canalis,* a waterpipe] **1.** A conduit, groove, or passageway through which various materials may flow. **2.** In cell biology, a passageway in the cell membrane through which materials may pass. The passageway is open or closed, depending on the molecular interaction between the material and the opening.

**chapped** (chăpt) [ME. *chappen*] Inflamed, roughened, fissured, as from exposure to cold.

**character** (kăr′ăk-tĕr) **1.** A person's pattern of thought and action, esp. regarding moral choices. Character differs from personality, although in psychiatry the terms are often used interchangeably. **2.** The feature of an organism or individual that results from the expression of genetic information inherited from the parents.

***acquired c.*** A trait or quality that was not inherited but is the result of environmental influence.

***anal c.*** A term sometimes used to describe an individual with obsessive-compulsive personality disorder.

***dominant c.*** In genetics, a trait that is expressed although it was present in only one gene.

***primary sex c.*** An inherited trait directly concerned with the reproductive tract.

***recessive c.*** In genetics, a trait that is not expressed unless it was present in the genes received from both parents.

***secondary sex c.*** A trait peculiar to a specific sex but not concerned with the reproductive tract. Voice quality, facial hair, and body fat distribution are examples.

***sex-conditioned c.*** A genetic trait carried by both sexes but expressed or inhibited by the sex of the individual.

***sex-limited c.*** A trait present in only one sex even though the gene responsible is present in both sexes.

***sex-linked c.*** A trait for which the gene is present on one of the sex chromosomes.

**characteristic** (kăr″ăk-tĕr-ĭs′tĭk) **1.** A trait or character that is typical of an organism or individual. **2.** In logarithmic expressions, the number to the left of the decimal point, as distinguished from the mantissa, which is the number to the right of the decimal point.

**characterize** To mark, identify, or describe the attributes of something. This helps to distinguish an individual or material from other examples of similar individuals or materials.

**charcoal** (chăr′kōl) [ME. *charcole*] Activated charcoal; very fine powder prepared from soft charred wood.

ACTION/USES: In treating persons who have ingested poisons, activated charcoal is given orally as a suspension in water, using 8 ml of diluent per gram of charcoal. This may be given to infants by using a nippled bottle. The dose is 1 to 2 g/kg of body weight. Superactivated charcoal is two to three times more effective than activated charcoal. Charcoal should be administered as soon as possible after intake of the toxin. It is contraindicated in patients who have ingested corrosive chemicals. Ionized chemicals such as acids, alkalis and salts of cyanide, iron, and lithium are not well absorbed by charcoal.

***superactivated c.*** A type of charcoal used in treating poisoning. It is several more times as effective as activated charcoal. Trade name is SuperChar.

**Charcot's joint** (shăr-kōz′) [Jean M. Charcot, Fr. neurologist, 1825–1893] A type of diseased joint, marked by hypermobility, associated with tabes dorsalis, syringomyelia, or other conditions involving spinal cord disease or injury. Bone decalcification occurs on the joint surfaces, accompanied by bony overgrowth about the margins. Pain is usually absent, although there are exceptions. Deformity and instability of the joint are characteristic.

**Charcot-Bouchard aneurysm** [Charcot; Charles Jaques Bouchard, Fr. physician, 1837–1986] A microaneurysm in a small artery of the brain resulting from vascular wall injury with segmental weakening and dilation leading to rupture. This type of aneuryusm is caused by hypertension.

**Charcot-Leyden crystal** (shăr-kō′lī′dĕn) [Charcot; Ernest V. von Leyden, Ger. physician, 1832–1910] A type of colorless, hexagonal, double-pointed, often needlelike crystals found in the sputum in asthma and bronchial bronchitis or in the feces in ulceration of the intestine, esp. amebiasis.

**Charcot-Marie-Tooth disease** [Charcot; Pierre Marie, Fr. neurologist, 1853–1940; Howard Henry Tooth, Brit. physician, 1856–1925] A form of progressive neural atrophy of muscles supplied by the peroneal nerves. The disease has hereditary tendencies and is marked by progressive weakness of the distal muscles of the arms and feet. The muscles atrophy, reflexes are lost, foot drop develops, and cutaneous sensations are lost. The disease usually develops in childhood but may occur in adults. It is more common in males. Its cause is unknown. SYN: *atrophy, peroneal muscular.*

**Charcot's triad** The combination of nystagmus, intention tremor, and scanning speech. It is frequently associated with multiple sclerosis.

**charge 1.** In electricity, the amount of electrical force present. **2.** To add electrical energy to a battery. **3.** The cost to the patient of a medical service or hospitalization.

***customary and reasonable c.*** The usual cost of a specific service to a patient. The term is used in the medical insurance industry to determine the amount the provider will be reimbursed for the service or procedure. Under Medicare, this is the lowest customary charge by a physician for a service, or the prevailing charge of other area physicians for the same service.

**charlatan** (shăr′lă-tăn) [It. *ciarlatano*] A pretender to special knowledge or ability, as in medicine. SYN: *quack.*

**charlatanry** (shăr′lă-tăn-rē) Undue pretension to knowledge or skill that is not possessed.

**Charles' law** (shărl) [Jacques A. C. Charles, Fr. physicist, 1746–1823] At constant pressure, a given amount of gas expands its volume in direct proportion to the absolute temperature. SYN: *Gay-Lussac's law.* SEE: *Boyle's law.*

**charleyhorse** A colloquial term for pain and tenderness in the fibromuscular tissue of the thighs, usually caused by muscle strain or tear. The condition is marked by sudden onset and aggravation on movement. Relief can be obtained from rest, local applications of cold, gentle massage, and nonsteroidal anti-inflammatory drugs.

**chart** [L. *charta,* paper] **1.** A form or sheet of paper used to record the course of a patient's illness. It includes records of temperature, pulse, respiratory rate, blood pressure, urinary and fecal output, and doctors' and nurses' notes. **2.** To record on a graph the sequence of events such as vital signs. SEE: *charting.* **3.** The complete clinical record of a patient, including physical and psychosocial state of health as well as results of diagnostic tests. Plans for meeting the needs of the patient are also included. SEE: *problem-oriented medical record.* **4.** To record the clinical, radiographic, and forensic findings of the teeth and surrounding tissues.

***dental c.*** A diagram of the teeth on which clinical and radiographic findings can be recorded. These often include existing restorations, decayed surfaces, missing teeth, and periodontal conditions.

**charta** (kăr′tă) [L.] A preparation intended principally for external application, made either by saturating paper with medicinal substances or by applying the latter to the surface of the paper by adding adhesive liquid.

**charting** The process of making a tabulated record of a patient's progress during an illness; keeping a clinical record of information about the patient and his or her treatment. The physician needs detailed information about the patient that the nurse or others may contribute through observation and contact. These notes and flowsheet entries, containing details of the patient's reactions, assessments, and progress, aid the physician, nurse, and other health professionals in planning, implementing, and evaluating patient care. Almost any member of the professional health-care team may be responsible for providing and recording information concerning the patient's therapy, course, and progress. Verbal reports are not sufficient; they take time and may be misunderstood. SEE: *Abbreviations Appendix; nursing process; problem-oriented medical record.*

NOTE: Charting procedures may differ among health care institutions, so it is important to use the system specified. Written documentation is considered legal evidence. It must be recorded promptly and be dated, clear, concise, and legible. Authorized abbreviations should be used. Mistakes should be corrected by noting the mistaken entry and correction. If an entry is made late, it should follow the most recent entry in the chart and include the date and time at which it was made. Slang should not be used.

GENERAL RECORDS: *Blood pressure:* This is usually recorded on the sheet with the temperature, pulse, and respiration records. *Diet:* The percentage of intake for each meal and type of diet consumed are recorded. If calorie count is needed, the type and amount of each food and liquid taken are recorded. If the patient is on intake and output record, the amount of each liquid consumed is documented. The following should be included: amount of liquids taken (not "Water p.r.n."); hours of giving; type of diet (full, light, soft, liquid, special); and appetite. *Discharge or death:* This must include the date and hour of discharge or death and the name of the person who ordered the discharge or pronounced the patient dead.

*Fluids:* The hours of giving, kind, and amount of fluids should be recorded. *Heat:* This should include the names of the person who ordered heat applied to an unconscious patient and the person who executed the order, the period for which heat was applied, and the method used. *Infant feeding:* The formula should be charted the first time; afterward, the amount given, and if regurgitated, the approximate amount. *Laboratory:* This record includes the date and time, the type of specimen, the person who took the specimen, the person who ordered the specimen (not necessary for a routine urine specimen on admission), and the method by which the specimen was sent to the laboratory. SEE: *chain of custody.*

*Dressings:* This chart should include change of dressings on wounds and amount and character of drainage (including "Specimen Saved" if this has been done), the hour, the person who changed the dressing, the removal of stitches or drains, and the patient's reaction if pained or shocked by the dressing. *Drugs:* Any unfavorable reaction from drugs or treatments should be recorded, as should the time when the drugs or treatments are administered. All medicines, treatments, preparation, and so on should be charted by the nurse who administers them whether or not the nurse is in charge of the patient. The name of the medicine, the dosage, the route of administration, and the frequency should be confined to the prescribed column. When soluble salts or medicines are dispensed in liquid form, the actual dose administered should be stated rather than the amount of solution. Any unusual therapeutic action or idiosyncrasy resulting from a drug should be recorded.

*Nursing care:* The nurse should chart the date and time, assessments, special treatments, activity, ambulation, evaluation of care, independent interventions, and medications. *Surgery:* Documentation includes the procedure; preparation, including medications; the time of going to and leaving surgery; the time of admission and discharge from the postanesthesia care unit (PACU) or critical care unit; the time of readmission or initial admission to the patient's room; the condition, tubes, lines, monitors, and assessment on return to the room; and frequent assessment during the first few hours after surgery. PACU and critical care unit staff members record treatment and condition while the patient is in their care. NOTE: If a patient dies, it is important to record the precise time and identify the person who declared the patient to be dead. It is also important to state the basis for the declaration of death.

*Personal care:* Baths, personal hygiene, and the patient's reactions to these should be recorded. For women, this includes menstruation and the type of menstrual protection used. *Physician:* The physician's visit is recorded. This includes the physician's orders and the time they are written and carried out. *Physical therapy:* The hour of going for treatment, the hour of return, and the condition of the patient should be charted. *Postoperative:* Changing of the patient's position should be recorded under "Remarks." Passive and active exercise should be charted. *Specimens:* The taking of specimens of blood, exudates, transudates, and so on, for examination is recorded. The result is shown by the pathologist's report. *Surgical preparations:* The signature of the nurse who does surgical preparations should appear after "Preliminary preparation of field of operation." The same rule is observed for narcotics.

*Symptoms:* An accurate description of all symptoms (i.e., character of pulse and respiration, mental state, description of pain, and any discharge) should be given. The remarks should be appropriate and accurate. Both subjective and objective symptoms should be recorded. *Time:* Everything relating to the patient's progress should be charted as it occurs. All statements on charts must include the hour they were written. The first line of the sheet should include the day, date of admission, whether the patient walked in or was admitted by ambulance, and the patient's condition. Four-hour graphic charts are kept for all surgical patients the first 3 days (usually at 8, 12, and 4, around the clock), for all obstetrical patients, and for all patients whose temperature is above normal. The temperature, pulse, and respirations of all other patients are charted according to the requirements of the institution.

*Treatments:* The hour of treatment, the nature of the treatment, by whom it was given, and the patient's reaction are recorded. *Radiograph:* The chart includes the hour, the use of the radiology room or a portable machine at the bedside, the time of return from the radiology room (if applicable) and the patient's condition.

*Visits of clergy:* The hour, the name of the visitor, and the rite performed are charted.

*Miscellaneous:* Any sudden or marked change in the patient's condition is charted, as well as notification of the patient's relatives and clergy. Charts provided for specific purposes include temperature, pulse, and respiration charts; an anesthesia chart, generally kept by the anesthetist; a blood-pressure chart, used in conditions likely to affect the blood pressure; intake and output charts, used in all patients with fluid and electrolyte imbalance; and laboratory records, usually filed with the patient's chart. If any laboratory records have not been filed with the chart, their existence should be noted on the clinical chart at the time made and also on the final page of the chart.

PHYSICAL SYMPTOMS: *Appetite:* This may include remarks such as "Good" or "Poor" and special likes or dislikes. *Convulsions:* The type, duration, and whether consciousness was lost should be recorded; fecal or urinary incontinence should also be charted. The record should note whether the patient was injured during the convulsion or the accompanying fall, and whether any aura was experienced. *Defecation:* (see Excretions; Feces; Urine in this entry). *Diaphoresis* (perspiration): The chart should state whether this was slight, moderate, or profuse. *Emesis:* The amount, color, odor, and consistency of the vomitus and the manner of ejection are recorded (see Vomiting in this entry.)

*Enemas:* Unusual appearances, distention before or after, and results should be described fully. Any expulsion of flatus with the return of the enema is included. The type of solution, strength, temperature, and amount, as well as any douches and irrigations, are noted.

*Excretions:* Time, character, and other facts are included. *Feces:* Enema or natural movement, amount, consistency, color, abnormal odor, and abnormal constituents are recorded. The record should show whether defecation was accompanied by pain or tenesmus.

*General appearance:* The patient's color, posture, mood, mental state, and any rash should be documented. *Hemorrhages and discharges:* These should be described and any unusual specimens saved for examination. *Nausea:* The chart should note whether this was accompanied by vomiting, and whether it followed certain foods, drugs, or treatments. *Nerves:* All symptoms of nervousness or excitability must be charted. *Pain:* This includes location, time of onset, character (e.g., sharp, dull, burning, grinding, throbbing), duration (constant or intermittent, and if intermittent, how long), and intervals.

*Pathological conditions:* Vomiting, convulsions: The time of onset, duration, severity, and general appearance of the patient before, during, and after the attack should be recorded. It is important to record any localization of the convulsive motion and whether or not the patient was incontinent; and if the patient fell, whether any injury was sustained and what treatment was provided. Temperature, pulse, and respiration (TPR), and what was done to relieve the condition, should be noted immediately after. The cause should be explained if known. *Pulse:* This includes rate (beats per minute), character (e.g., full, bounding, weak, thready, faint), and rhythm (e.g., regular, irregular, intermittent). *Respiration:* This includes rate per minute, character (e.g., deep, shallow, difficult, easy, labored, quiet, stertorous, Cheyne-Stokes), and rhythm (e.g., regular, irregular, gasping).

*Sleep:* Hours of sleeping during both day and night are charted. If an accurate estimate is impossible, an approximation should be made and noted as such. The times and amount of sleep are noted, as are sleepwalking, nightmares, or talking in sleep. *Temperature:* The chart should indicate whether this was taken by mouth, rectum, or axilla, the degree, any following chill, and any treatment. If the temperature is high and the patient does not appear to have a corresponding fever, the temperature should be taken again with the nurse at the bedside to make sure the patient is not placing the thermometer against some hot object.

*Temperature, pulse, and respiration:* These should be charted as ordered. They are recorded before the patient goes to the operating room, and the pulse, respiration, and general condition are recorded on return from the operating room. *Unconsciousness or coma:* Time of onset, conditions associated with or that caused onset, appearance of the patient while in coma, medicines or treatment given while in coma, and duration are charted. *Unusual conditions:* These include appearance of blood, twitching, convulsions, fecal or urinary incontinence, coma, drowsiness, lethargy, and unconsciousness.

*Urine:* The chart should note the time of voiding, amount, color and appearance, and whether the urine was voided or obtained through a catheter. The time of beginning a 24-hr specimen collection is noted; when the bladder is emptied for that purpose, the specimen is sent to a laboratory for qualitative testing. The chart should note time of completion of collecting a 24-hr specimen; the amount should be noted on the chart and laboratory label. Specimens should be sent to the laboratory for all patients remaining in the hospital overnight. A check mark may be used in the urine column when the patient urinates or defecates. At all other times the amount of urine is to be charted every 12 hr. The nurse should record any urination accompanied by pain or burning, any abnormal appearance, and the time the specimen was sent to the laboratory.

*Vomiting:* The cause; forcible or projectile ejection; vomitus amount, color, odor, consistency, and any unusual constituents are recorded.

MENTAL SYMPTOMS: The record should document the mood, esp. sudden change; delirium; depression; ability to follow directions; teaching and learning ability; and presence and specific description of psychotic symptoms, such as hallucinations or delusions.

*Visitors:* Reaction to visitors and mood change after visitors depart are noted. This is esp. important in depressed and psychiatric patients.

***dental c.*** Recording on a chart the clinical findings in the mouth. Each tooth is examined and the gingival sulcus probed. Restorations and missing teeth are noted, as are periodontal pocket depth and the conditions of all soft tissues.

**chartula** (kăr'tū-lă) [L., small piece of paper] A paper folded to form a receptacle containing a dose of medicine.

**chasma** (kăz'mă) [Gr., a cleft] An opening, gap, or wide cleft.

**chaude-pisse** (shōd-pēs') [Fr.] A burning sensation during urination, esp. in acute gonorrhea.

**chaulmoogra oil** (chŏl-moo'grŭ, chŏl-mŏ'grŭ) [Bengali *caulmugra*] A vegetable oil used to treat leprosy and some dermatoses. Although generally replaced by sulfones in treatment of leprosy, chaulmoogra oil is still used in endemic areas because of its availability and low cost. Also spelled *chaulmugra* or *chaulmaugra*.

**Chaussier's areola** (shō-sē-āz') [François Chaussier, Fr. physician, 1746–1828] Indurated tissue around the lesion of a malignant pustule.

**CHB** *complete heart block.*

**Ch.B.** *Bachelor of Surgery;* used mostly in the United Kingdom.

**CHD** *congenital hip dislocation; congenital heart disease; coronary heart disease.*

**check** [O. Fr. *eschec*] **1.** To slow down or arrest the course of a condition. **2.** To verify.

**check bite** A sheet of hard wax used to make an impression of teeth to check articulation.

**check-up** General term for a visit to a physician for a physical examination.

**Chédiak-Higashi syndrome** (shē'dē-ăk-hē-gă'shē) [M. Chédiak and O. Higashi, contemporary French and Japanese physicians, respectively] A lethal metabolic disorder, inherited as an autosomal recessive trait, in which neutrophils contain peroxidase-positive inclusion bodies. Partial albinism, photophobia, and pale optic fundi are clinical features. Children usually die by the 5 to 10 years of age of a lymphoma-like disease.

**cheek** [AS. *ceace*] **1.** The side of the face forming the lateral wall of the mouth below the eye. SYN: *bucca.* **2.** The buttock.

**cheekbone** The malar bone; os zygomaticum; the zygomatic bone.

**cheek retractor** A device that encloses the cheek at the angle of the mouth for proper exposure of the operating field.

**cheil-** SEE: *cheilo-.*

**cheilectomy** (kī-lĕk'tō-mē) [Gr. *cheilos,* lip, + *ektome,* excision] **1.** Surgical removal of abnormal bone around a joint to facilitate joint mobility. **2.** Surgical removal of a lip.

**cheilectropion** (kī"lĕk-trō'pē-ŏn) [" + *ektrope,* a turning aside] Eversion of the lip.

**cheilitis** (kī-lī'tĭs) [" + *itis,* inflammation] Inflammation of the lip.

***angular c.*** An inflammation of the corners of the mouth occurring in elderly persons. The cause is bacterial infection of the skin. Erythema and painful fissures are present. This condition usually occurs in edentulous patients. SYN: *perlèche.*

***solar c.*** Skin changes including papules and plaques that occur on sun-exposed areas of the lips.

***c. venenata*** Dermatitis of the lips resulting from chemical irritants in lipsticks, lip cream, and various other materials.

**cheilo-, cheil-** Combining form meaning *lip.* SEE: *chilo-.*

**cheilognathopalatoschisis** (kī"lō-nā"thō-păl-ă-tŏs'kĭ-sĭs) [" + *gnathos,* jaw, + L. *palatum,* palate, + Gr. *schisis,* a splitting] A developmental anomaly in which there is a cleft in the hard and soft palate, upper jaw, and lip.

**cheilophagia** (kī"lō-fā'jē-ă) [" + *phagein,* to eat] The habit of biting one's own lip.

**cheiloplasty** (kī'lō-plăs"tē) [" + *plassein,* to form] Plastic surgery on the lips.

**cheilorrhaphy** (kī-lor'ă-fē) [" + *rhaphe,* seam, ridge] Surgical repair of a cleft lip.

**cheiloschisis** (kī-lŏs'kĭ-sĭs) [" + *schisis,* a splitting] A cleft lip.

**cheilosis** (kī-lō'sĭs) [" + *osis,* condition] A morbid condition in which the lips become reddened and develop fissures at the angles. It is seen frequently in deficiency of vitamin B complex, esp. riboflavin.

**cheilostomatoplasty** (kī"lō-stō-măt'ō-plăs"tē) [" + *stoma,* mouth, + *plassein,* to form] Plastic surgery and restoration of the mouth.

**cheilotomy, chilotomy** (kī-lŏt'ō-mē) [" + *tome,* incision] Excision of part of the lip.

**cheirognostic, chirognostic** (kī"rŏg-nŏs'tĭk) [Gr. *cheir,* hand, + *gnostikos,* knowing] Able to distinguish the left from the right side of the body; able to perceive which side of the body is being stimulated.

**cheirology** (kī-rŏl'ō-jē) [" + *logos,* word, reason] Dactylology.

**cheirospasm** (kī'rō-spăsm) [" + Gr. *spasmos,* a convulsion] Writer's cramp; a spasm of the muscles of the hand.

**chelate** (kē'lāt) [Gr. *chele,* claw] **1.** In chemistry, to combine with a ring structure as a claw would grasp an object; used of the ion of a metal. **2.** In toxicology, to use a compound to enclose or grasp a toxic substance and make it nonactive and therefore nontoxic.

**chelation** (kē-lā'shŭn) [Gr. *chele,* claw] The combining of metallic ions with certain heterocyclic ring structures so that the ion is held by chemical bonds from each participating ring. When this structure is diagrammed, it appears that the metallic ion is being held by a claw. Calcium disodium edetate, is a chelating agent.

**cheloid** (kē'loyd) [Gr. *kele,* tumor, swelling, + *eidos,* form, shape] Keloid.

**chemabrasion** (kēm-ă-brā'shŭn) The use of a chemical to destroy superficial layers of skin. This technique may be used to treat scars, tattoos, or abnormal pigmentation. SYN: *chemexfoliation.*

**chemexfoliation** (kēm'ĕks-fō'lē-ā"shŭn) Chemabrasion.

**CHEMFET** *chemically sensitive field effect transistor.*

**chemical** [Gr. *chemeia,* chemistry] Pert. to chemistry.

**Chemical Abstract Service** ABBR: CAS. A branch of the American Chemical Society that maintains a registry of chemicals, active ingredients used in drugs, and food additives. Each chemical is assigned a permanent CAS number through which current data can be traced.

**chemical barriers** **1.** The chemical characteristics of certain areas of the body that oppose colonization by microorganisms. Examples are the acidic properties of the stomach mucosa and urinary bladder, which effectively prevent invasion by pathogenic microorganisms. **2.** A contraceptive cream, foam, jelly, or suppository that contains chemical spermicides.

**chemical change** A process in which a substance breaks up or combines with other substances to make new substances with new properties or characteristics. For example, oxygen and hydrogen combine to form water. Sodium (a metal) and chlorine (a gas) combine to form sodium chloride, or common salt. Glucose ($C_6H_{10}O_5$) is metabolized to carbon dioxide ($CO_2$) and water ($H_2O$). Oxygen combines with hemoglobin to form oxyhemoglobin when the hemoglobin in the blood comes into contact with the oxygen in the air contained in the alveoli of the lungs. The arterial blood containing oxyhemoglobin is bright scarlet; the venous blood containing reduced hemoglobin is dark red.

**chemical compound** **1.** A substance consisting of two or more chemical elements, in specific proportions and in chemical combination, for which a chemical formula can be written. Examples include water ($H_2O$) and salt (NaCl). **2.** A substance that can be separated chemically into simpler substances.

**chemical disaster** The accidental release of large amounts of chemicals. The effects suffered by people in the area are determined by the toxicity of the chemical, its speed in spreading, its composition (liquid, solid, or gaseous), and the spill site, esp. its proximity to a water supply or buildings. The major effect may be due to the chemical itself or to a resulting fire or explosion. In general, the medical care facilities of any area probably could not care for hundreds or thousands of casualties. SEE: *chemical warfare.*

**chemical element** SEE: *element.*

**chemically sensitive field effect transistor** ABBR: CHEMFET. A specialized chemical sensor found in some clinical laboratory instruments.

**chemical reflex** Chemoreflex.

**chemical warfare** The tactics and technique of conducting warfare by using toxic chemical agents. The chemicals include nerve gases; agents that cause temporary blindness, paralysis, hallucinations, or deafness; eye and lung irritants; blistering agents, including mustard gas; defoliants; and herbicides. SEE: *biological warfare.*

**chemiluminescence, chemoluminescence** (kĕm″ĭ-loo″mĭ-nĕs′ĕns, kĕm″ō-loo″mĭ-nĕs′ĕns) Cold light or light resulting from a chemical reaction and without heat production. Certain bacteria, fungi, and fireflies produce this type of light. SEE: *luciferase.*

**chemist** (kĕm′ĭst) Someone who is trained in chemistry.

**chemistry** [Gr. *chemeia,* chemistry] The science dealing with the molecular and atomic structure of matter and the composition of substances—their formation, decomposition, and various transformations.

***analytical c.*** Chemistry concerned with the detection of chemical substances (qualitative analysis) or the determination of the amounts of substances (quantitative analysis) in a compound.

***biological c.*** Biochemistry.

***general c.*** The study of the entire field of chemistry with emphasis on fundamental concepts or laws.

***inorganic c.*** The chemistry of compounds not containing carbon.

***nuclear c.*** Radiochemistry; the study of changes that take place within the nucleus of an atom, esp. when the nucleus is bombarded by electrons, neutrons, or other subatomic particles.

***organic c.*** The branch of chemistry dealing with substances that contain carbon compounds.

***pathological c.*** The study of chemical changes induced by disease processes (e.g., changes in the chemistry of organs and tissues, blood, secretions, or excretions.

***pharmaceutical c.*** The chemistry of medicines, their composition, synthesis, analysis, storage, and actions.

***physical c.*** Theoretical chemistry; the chemistry concerned with fundamental laws underlying chemical changes and the mathematical expression of these laws.

***physiological c.*** The study of the chemistry of living matter and the changes occurring in the metabolic activities of plants and animals.

**chemocautery** (kĕm″ō-kaw′tĕr-ē) [Gr. *chemeia,* chemistry, + *kauterion,* branding iron] Cauterization by chemical agents.

**chemoceptor** (kĕm′ō-sĕp-tĕr) Chemoreceptor.

**chemocoagulation** (kē″mō-kō-ăg″ū-lā′shŭn) [″ + L. *coaglutio,* coagulation] Coagulation caused by chemical agents.

**chemodectoma** (kē″mō-dĕk-tō′mă) [″ + *dektikos,* receptive, + *oma,* tumor] A tumor of the chemoreceptor system. SEE: *paraganglioma.*

**chemokine** Any cytokine that causes chemotaxis, attracting neutrophils, monocytes, and T lymphocytes to assist in destroying an invading microorganism. SEE: *cytokine; inflammation.*

**chemokinesis** The accelerated random locomotion of cells, usually in response to chemical stimuli.

**chemoluminescence** Chemiluminescence.

**chemolysis** (kē-mŏl′ĭ-sĭs) [″ + *lysis,* dissolution] Destruction by chemical action.

**chemonucleolysis** (kēm″ō-nū-klē-ŏl′ĭ-sĭs) A method of dissolving a herniated nucleus pulposus, by injecting the enzyme chymopapain into it. This procedure is controversial and is contraindicated for patients with a herniated lumbar disk in which the nucleus pulposis protrudes through the annulus.

**chemopallidectomy** (kē″mō-păl″ĭ-dĕk′tō-mē) [″ + L. *pallidum,* globus pallidus, + Gr. *ektome,* excision] Destruction of a portion of the globus pallidus of the brain by use of a chemical.

**chemoprophylaxis** (kē″mō-prō″fĭ-lăk′sĭs) The use of a drug or chemical to prevent a disease (e.g., the taking of an appropriate medicine to prevent malaria).

**chemopsychiatry** (kē″mō-sī-kī′ă-trē) The use of drugs in treating psychiatric illnesses.

**chemoreceptor** (kē″mō-rē-sĕp′tor) [″ + L. *recipere,* to receive] A sense organ or sensory nerve ending (as in a taste bud) that is stimulated by and reacts to certain chemical stimuli and that is located outside the central nervous system. Chemoreceptors are found in the large arteries of the thorax and neck (carotid and aortic bodies), the taste buds, and the olfactory cells of the nose. SYN: *chemoceptor.* SEE: *carotid body; taste bud.*

**chemoreflex** (kē″mō-rē′flĕks) [″ + L. *reflectere,* to bend back] Any involuntary response initiated by a chemical stimulus. SYN: *chemical reflex.*

**chemoresistance** (kē″mō-rē-zĭs′tăns) The specific resistance of a body cell or microorganism to the effect of a drug.

**chemosensitive** (kē″mō-sĕn′sĭ-tĭv) Reacting to the action of a chemical or a change in chemical composition.

**chemosensory** (kē″mō-sĕn′sō-rē) Pert. to the sensory detection of a chemical, esp. by odor.

**chemoserotherapy** (kē″mō-sē″rō-thĕr′ă-pē) The combined use of a drug and serum in treating disease.

**chemosis** (kē-mō′sĭs) [Gr. *cheme,* cockleshell, + *osis,* condition] Edema of the conjunctiva around the cornea. **chemotic** (-mŏt′ĭk), *adj.*

**chemosterilant** (kē″mō-stĕr′ĭ-lănt) **1.** A chemical that kills microorganisms. **2.** A chemical that causes sterility, usually of the male, in organisms such as insects.

**chemosurgery** Destruction of tissue by the use of chemical compounds.

**chemosynthesis** (kē″mō-sĭn′thĕ-sĭs) The formation of a chemical compound from other chemicals or agents. In biological systems, this involves metabolism.

**chemotactic** (kē″mō-tăk′tĭk) Pert. to chemotaxis.

**chemotaxin** A substance released by bacteria, injured tissue, and white blood cells that stimulates the movement of neutrophils and other white blood cells to the injured area. Complement factors 3a (C3a) and 5a (C5a), cytokines, leukotrienes, prostaglandins, and fragments of fibrin and collagen are common chemotaxins. SEE: *inflammation.*

**chemotaxis** (kē″mō-tăk′sĭs) [Gr. *chemeia,* chemistry, + *taxis,* arrangement] The movement of additional white blood cells to an area of inflammation in response to the release of chemical mediators by neutrophils, monocytes, and injured tissue. SYN: *chemotropism.*

**chemothalamectomy** (kē″mō-thăl-ă-mĕk′tō-mē) Chemical destruction of a part of the thalamus.

**chemotherapy** (kē″mō-thĕr′ă-pē) [″ + *therapeia,* treatment] In the treatment of disease, the application of chemical reagents that have a specific and toxic effect on the disease-causing microorganism. SEE: *Nursing Diagnoses Appendix.*

***combination c.*** In antineoplastic drug therapy, the use of two or more drugs to treat disease.

***peritoneal c.*** Intraperitoneal injection of antineoplastic drugs.

**chemotropism** (kē-mŏt′rō-pĭzm) [″ + *tropos,* a turning] The ability or impulse to progress or turn in a certain direction due to the influence of certain chemical stimuli, as the root of a plant toward its food supply.

**chenodeoxycholic acid** A drug given orally to dissolve cholesterol gallstones. SEE: *gallstone.*

**cherophobia** (kē″rō-fō′bē-ă) [Gr. *chairein,* to rejoice, + *phobos,* fear] Morbid fear of and aversion to gaiety.

**cherubism** (chĕr′ū-bĭzm) Cherubic appearance of the face of a child due to infiltration of the jaw, esp. the mandible, with masses of vascular fibrous tissue containing giant cells.

**chest** [AS. *cest,* a box] The thorax.

MENSURATION: The object of measuring the chest is to determine the comparative bulk of the two sides and the amount of expansion and retraction accompanying inspiration and expiration on both sides. The points of measurement are between the spinous processes in back and the median line in front on the level of the sixth costosternal articulation. The right side is from ½ in. to 1 in. (1.3 to 2.5 cm) larger than the left. When a pleural cavity is distended with air or fluid, the measurement of the affected side may exceed that of the healthy side by 2 or 3 in. (5.6 to 7.6 cm); after removal of the fluid, the measurement of the affected side may diminish in correct proportion to the healthy one. In unilateral emphysema, the total difference between the fullest inspiration and fullest expiration on the affected side barely exceeds 1/16 in. (1.6 mm), whereas the other side may show a difference of 2 or 3 in. (5.6 to 7.6 cm).

PALPATION: This detects any thoracic tenderness, edema, friction fremitus, or crackles. Edema of the chest walls is shown by pitting when pressure is applied with a finger. This may be observed in empyema and certain types of heart failure.

The friction sound of pleurisy and harsh, sonorous crackles can sometimes be detected by palpation. Thoracic tenderness is observed in pleurisy, pneumonia associated with pleurisy, pleurodynia, intercostal neuralgia (confined to certain spots), fracture of the ribs, and contusion and inflammation of the pleural surfaces.

PERCUSSION: The finger being used as a pleximeter is placed firmly against the chest and preferably parallel to the ribs. The plexor finger strikes the finger on the chest perpendicularly, the forearm is fixed, and no more force is used than can be obtained from a gentle swing of the wrist. All parts of the chest are percussed anteriorly and posteriorly during both inspiration and expiration. In comparing sides, it is essential to percuss corresponding parts.

*Normal resonance:* On the right side, pulmonary resonance extends from ½ in. to 1 in. (1.3 to 2.5 cm) above the clavicle, downward to the upper border of the sixth rib in front, and to a line drawn through the 10th spinous process posteriorly. On the left side, pulmonary resonance extends from ½ in. to 1 in. (1.3 to 2.5 cm) above the clavicle downward within the mammary line to the 10th rib, and posteriorly to a line drawn through the 10th spinous process.

*Cracked pot sound:* Modified tympany can be simulated by percussing over the cheek when the mouth is partially open. It may be heard normally over the chest of a crying infant. In the adult it usually indicates a cavity that has a free communication with a bronchus. It is best detected by keeping the ear near the open mouth of the patient while percussing.

*Dullness or flatness:* This is recognized in tuberculous conditions, consolidation of the lung, pleural effusions of all kinds, lung collapse, lung congestion and edema, enlargement of the liver or spleen (at the base), and neoplastic lung growths. It is important to determine the extent of diaphragm movement. For this, the patient holds his or her breath in deep inspiration while sitting. Then the examiner quickly percusses the chest on both sides posteriorly to find and mark the lowest point of pulmonary resonance. This is repeated while the patient holds the breath following complete expiration. On both sides of the chest, the top and bottom marks should be from ¾ to 2½ in. (2 to 6 cm) apart. The top line on the right is usually 1 to 2 cm higher than the left owing to the presence of the liver below the right side of the diaphragm. Diseases that interfere with aeration of the lungs or that paralyze the diaphragm alter the normal movement of the diaphragm.

*Hyperresonance:* This is observed in pneumothorax, lung collapse, tuberculous or bronchiectatic cavities, emphysema, lowered pulmonary tension in the initial stage of pneumonia and above a pleural effusion (Skoda's resonance), and flatulent distention of the stomach or colon frequently observed over the left base.

*Tympanitic note:* This hollow drumlike sound resembles that normally obtained by percussing the larynx or empty stomach. The conditions mentioned under Hyperresonance in this entry can also produce tympany.

*Pitch:* This depends largely on the volume of air and the tension of the cavity walls, and on the size of the opening that communicates with the cavity. The less air, the greater the tension; the smaller the opening, the higher the pitch. In beginning tuberculous consolidation, the note over the affected apex is higher pitched. Normally the note over the right apex is higher pitched than that over the left.

***emphysematous c.*** The chest characteristic of advanced emphysema. The thorax is short and round, the anteroposterior diameter is often as long as the transverse diameter, the ribs are horizontal, and the angle formed by divergence of the costal margin from the sternum is very obtuse or obliterated. This type of chest is often termed barrel-shaped.

***flail c.*** A condition of the chest wall due to multiple fractures of the rib cage in which it moves paradoxically (i.e., in with inspiration and out during expiration).

***flat c.*** A deformity of the chest in which the anteroposterior diameter is short, the thorax long and flat, and the ribs oblique. The scapula is prominent; the spaces above and below the clavicles are depressed. The angle formed by divergence of the costal margins from the sternum is very acute.

***funnel c.*** Pectus excavatum.

***pigeon c.*** A condition in which the sides of the chest are considerably flattened and the sternum is prominent. The sternal ends of the ribs are enlarged or beaded; this characteristic has produced the term "rachitic rosary." Often there is a circular construction of the thorax at the level of the xiphoid cartilage. The condition is due to obstruction of infantile respiration or to rickets.

**chest physical therapy, chest physiotherapy** ABBR: CPT, Chest P.T. A type of pulmonary care intervention usually incorporating postural drainage, cough facilitation, breathing exercises, and total body conditioning and used for loosening and removing lung secretions. It involves percussion (clapping) and vibration over the affected areas of the lungs, followed by postural drainage to remove secretions. Auscultation of breath sounds is done before and after the procedure. SYN: *pulmonary rehabilitation.*

**chest prominences and depressions** An unnatural prominence or depression often observed over the lower part of the sternum and generally congenital. The sternal depression has been called "funnel breast" or "shoemaker's breast" (because it may result from pressure of tools). The correct term is pectus excavatum.

A unilateral or local depression may be caused by consolidation, cavity, or pleurisy with fibrous adhesions.

A unilateral or local prominence may be due to pleurisy with effusion; pneumothorax, hydrothorax, or hemothorax; aneurysm or tumor; compensatory emphysema resulting from impairment of the opposite lung; cardiac enlargement (left side); or enlargement of abdominal organs, esp. the liver and spleen.

**chest P.T.** chest physical therapy.

**chest regions** The anterior, posterior, and lateral chest areas. Anterior divisions (right and left) are the clavicular, infraclavicular, and supraclavicular, the mammary and inframammary, and the upper and lower sternal. Posterior divisions (right and left) are the scapular, infrascapular, interscapular, and suprascapular. Lateral divisions are the axillary and infra-axillary.

**chest thump** A sharp blow to the chest in the precordial area. This is done to attempt restoration of normal heartbeat in patients with cardiac arrest or ventricular tachycardia.

**Cheyne-Stokes respiration** (chān′stōks′) [John Cheyne, Scot. physician, 1777–1836; William Stokes, Irish physician, 1804–1878] A common and bizarre breathing pattern marked by a period of apnea lasting 10 to 60 sec, followed by gradually increasing depth and frequency of respirations. It accompanies frontal lobe depression and diencephalic dysfunction. This condition may be present as a normal finding in children. SEE: *respiration* for illus.

**CHF** *congestive heart failure.*

**Chiari's deformity** SEE: *Arnold-Chiari deformity.*

**Chiari-Frommel syndrome** (kē-ăr′ē-frŏm′mĕl) [Hans Chiari, Austrian pathologist, 1851–1916; Richard Julius Ernst Frommel, Ger. gynecologist, 1854–1912] Persistent lactation and amenorrhea following childbirth, caused by continued prolactin secretion and decreased gonadotropin production. A pituitary adenoma may be present.

**chiasm, chiasma** (kī′ăzm, kī-ăz′mă) [Gr. *khiasma,* cross] A crossing or decussation.

***optic c.*** An X-shaped crossing of the optic nerve fibers in the brain. Past this point, the fibers travel in optic tracts. Fibers that originate in the outer half of the retina end on the same side of the brain; those from the inner half cross over.

**chickenpox** Varicella.

**chiggers** (chĭg′ĕrs) Redbugs; the six-legged larvae of mites of the family Trombiculidae, order Acarina of the class Arachnida. They are parasitic on insects, various vertebrates, and humans. The most common species attacking humans in North America is *Trombicula alfreddugesi.* Eggs are laid on the ground and hatch in about 12 days, after which the mites attach to a host at the first opportunity. They attach themselves to the skin surface and inject a salivary secretion that dissolves the surrounding tissue, producing a wheal with intense itching and severe dermatitis. The tubular structure or stylostome that develops is used in ingesting the semidigested tissue debris. The mites do not feed on blood. The irritation is the result of sensitization to the injected saliva. To prevent being infested when exposed, one should wear clothes that completely cover the skin and are tight at the neck and arms, and stuff pant legs into high-topped shoes. Certain chemical compounds such as diethyltoluamide repel chiggers. SEE: *Tunga.*

TREATMENT: Proprietary preparations are available that asphyxiate the mite when applied to the affected area. One of these, Kwell, contains hexachlorohexane. Benzyl benzoate ointment and gamma benzene hexachloride are also effective.

**chigoe infestation** Infestation of a parasite of dogs, pigs, and barefooted humans by the flea *Tunga penetrans.* In humans the usual sites of invasion are the spaces between the toes, where the burrowing female swells and causes a painful open sore.

TREATMENT: The gravid flea is removed with a sterile needle. The site is treated with tincture of iodine, which is toxic to the remaining fleas and eggs.

**chil-** SEE: *chilo-.*

**chilblain** (chĭl′blān) [AS. *cele,* cold, + *blegen,* to puff] A form of cold injury marked by localized erythema and sometimes blistering. The affected area itches, may be painful, and may progress to crusted ulcerations. The cause is thought to be prolonged constriction of arterioles in reaction to exposure to cold and dampness. SYN: *pernio.*

NURSING IMPLICATIONS: The patient is evaluated for circulatory insufficiency. Susceptible areas need to be protected from cold exposure.

**child** [AS. *cild,* child] Any human between infancy and puberty. SEE: *pediatrics.*

**child abuse** Emotional, physical, or sexual injury to a child. It may be seen after instances of severe disruption in the process of parental attachment. It may be due to either a positive action or an omission on the part of those responsible for the care of the child. In domestic situations in which a child is abused, it is important to examine other children and infants living in the same home because about 20% will have signs of physical abuse. That examination should be done without delay to attempt to prevent further child abuse in that home. An infant or child must never be allowed to remain in the hostile environment where the abuse occurred; such a situation might be disastrous for the child. SEE: *battered child syndrome; shaken baby syndrome.*

DIAGNOSIS: Caregivers should carefully note signs of current and previous physical violence, such as bruises, abrasions, burns, fractures, or deformities related to untreated old fractures. Genital or perianal bruises or bleeding suggests sexual abuse. Signs of malnutrition, dehydration, dirty skin, or poor hygiene are indicators of parental neglect. In addition, the examiner should note the child's behaviors; parental behaviors, reactions, and comments, and parent-child interactions. The child's behaviors should be compared with established developmentally appropriate norms.

NURSING IMPLICATIONS: The nature, frequency, and extent of physical abuse are determined. The child's neurological status is assessed. Vital signs are monitored, and all parts of the child's body are inspected and palpated for signs of injury, such as burns, scalds, bruises, scratches, hematomas, and long bone fractures. The child is also assessed for indications of neglect, such as poor skin hygiene and malnutrition. The child's memory of the abuse and of the person or people involved is carefully and gently explored. The child and accompanying adult are encouraged to voice feelings and concerns, and realistic reassurance and support are provided. Statements made by any adult accompanying the child are documented, and the speaker's identity and relationship to the child are noted. Institutional policy and state law should be followed in reporting the abuse.

A nonpunitive, noncritical approach is assumed in dealing with the parents to prevent them from feeling rejected and further abusing their children. The nurse must work through personal feelings of anger or disgust at the parental behavior. Appropriate physical care and assistance in meeting developmental needs through sensory stimulation and education are provided.

If the child is to return to the parents, the nurse supports the parents' positive coping efforts and parenting skills by acknowledging parental strengths, by encouraging participation in care, and by demonstrating positive care behaviors. Parents are referred to local self-help groups and day-care services and for psychological counseling as available and appropriate. The goal of nursing care is to provide the abused child with a safe, secure environment to promote physical and psychosocial growth and development.

**childbearing** The act of carrying and being delivered of a child.

***delayed c.*** SEE: *elderly primigravida.*

**childbed** The period during and immediately following parturition. SYN: *puerperium.*

**childbed fever** Puerperal sepsis.

**childbirth** The process of giving birth to a child. SYN: *labor; parturition.*

***natural c.*** The delivery of a fetus without the use of analgesics, sedatives, or anesthesia. Contemporary natural childbirth is termed "natural" because it was the only approach to childbirth before the development of modern obstetrical techniques. The woman, and often her partner, go through a training period beginning months before the actual delivery. This training is called psychoprophylactic preparation for childbirth. More recently, natural childbirth has come to include a more noninterventionist approach, with less reliance on technology and more reliance on emotional support during labor and delivery, as appropriate. SEE: *Lamaze technique or method; psychoprophylactic childbirth.*

***prepared c.*** Childbirth in which the mother, and often also the father, of the baby has been educated about childbirth, anesthesia, and analgesia during labor. The mother may choose to have natural childbirth or to receive medications or regional anesthesia. SEE: *natural c.; Lamaze technique or method; psychoprophylactic preparation for childbirth.*

**child neglect** Failure by those responsible for caring for a child to provide for the child's nutritional, emotional, and physical needs.

**childproof** Designed to be harmless to children; used esp. of medicine containers that children cannot open.

**chilectropion** Cheilectropion.

**chilitis** Cheilitis.

**chill** (chĭl) [AS. *cele*, cold] An attack of shivering, accompanied by the sensation of coldness and skin pallor, produced by involuntary contraction of many muscle groups. It may be caused by a disturbance in the temperature-regulating centers of the hypothalamus. Chills accompany various diseases, esp. malaria and pneumococcal pneumonia, and may be coarse or fine, diffuse, or trembling.

SYMPTOMS: A real chill is ushered in by a sensation of extreme cold, shivering, teeth chattering, and in extreme cases, a marked tremor of the entire body followed by a rapidly rising temperature.

ETIOLOGY: Chills are caused by infections or diseases (e.g., malaria, pneumococcal pneumonia, bacteremia), parasites in the blood, bacterial vaccines, and transfusion reactions. Postoperative chills or chills in the puerperium indicate infection.

NURSING IMPLICATIONS: The patient's temperature is checked, and the patient questioned about related symptoms. The patient is covered with a warm blanket and placed in a warm (not hot) environment to increase comfort. Warm drinks are offered when the patient is able to tolerate them or when they are permitted by the physician. Baseline vital signs are obtained and the patient is assessed for signs of septic shock. The duration and severity of the chill are documented. The patient's temperature and other vital signs are rechecked 20 to 30 min after the chill has subsided.

***nervous c.*** A tremor accompanied by a chilly sensation but not by fever. It may follow severe pain or extreme nervousness. It usually passes quickly and seldom is serious.

**chilo-, chil-** [Gr. *cheilos,* lip] Combining form meaning *lip.*

**Chilomastix mesnili** (kī″lō-măs′tĭks mĕs-nĭl′ē) A species of Mastigophora, a protozoon that is considered a presumptive parasite in the intestines. SEE: illus.

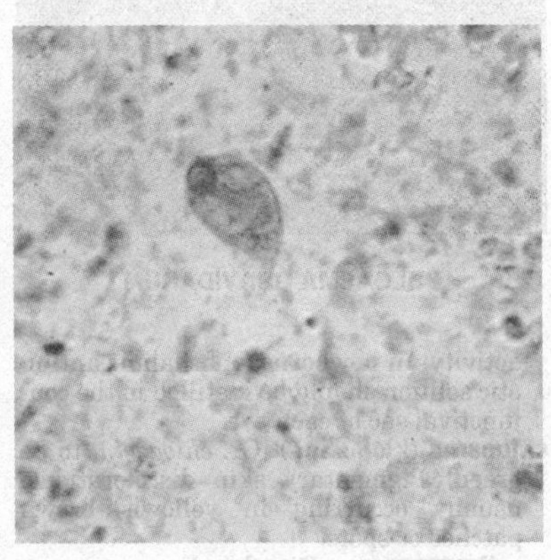


CHILOMASTIX MESNILI IN FECAL DEBRIS (ORIG. MAG. ×1000)

**chimera** (kī-mē′ră) In human biology, a double-egg twin whose blood and blast cells have been mixed in embryo with those of the other twin. Therefore, although each twin originally had a different blood group, each now has a mixed group.

**chimpanzee** (chĭm-păn′zē) An intelligent ape native to parts of Africa. It is used in experimental medicine because of its similarity to humans.

**chin** [AS. *cin,* chin] The point of the lower jaw; the region below the lower lip. SYN: *mentum.*

**China clay** Kaolin.

**Chinese restaurant syndrome** A group of transient symptoms that some persons report after eating at restaurants that add monosodium glutamate (MSG) to some of their recipes. The syndrome may be a valid clinical condition, but it has not been proven that MSG is the cause.

**chin jerk** A reflex contraction of the muscles of mastication when the jaw is suddenly depressed.

**chin-lift airway technique, head-tilt** A method of opening the airway of an unconscious patient by elevating his or her chin and tilting the head. This provides the maximum opening, esp. in an unconscious patient whose tongue is blocking the airway. SEE: *airway; bag-valve-mask resuscitator; cardiopulmonary resuscitation; Universal Precautions Appendix.*

Caution: This technique is not to be used in patients with neck or spinal injuries.

The fingertips are used to bring the patient's chin forward and support the lower jaw. This maneuver also tilts the patient's head. The maneuver can be completed by applying gentle pressure to the patient's forehead with the other hand. The patient's mouth must be kept open; however, the thumb must not be used for this purpose.

**chiragra** (kī-răg′ră) [Gr. *cheir,* hand, + *agra,* seizure] Pain in the hand.

**chiralgia** (kī-răl′jē-ă) [″ + *algos,* pain] Nontraumatic or neuralgic pain in the hand.

***c. paresthetica*** Numbness and pain in the hand, esp. in the region supplied by the radial nerve.

**chirokinesthesia** (kī″rō-kĭn″ĕs-thē′zē-ă) [″ + *kinesis,* movement, + *aisthesis,* sensation] A subjective sensation of hand motions.

**chiromegaly** (kī″rō-mĕg′ă-lē) [″ + *megas,* large] Enlargement of the hands, wrists, or ankles.

**chiroplasty** (kī′rō-plăs″tē) [″ + *plassein,* to form] Plastic surgery on the hand.

**chiropodist** (kī-rŏp′ō-dĭst, kĭ-) [″ + *pous,* foot] An obsolete term for podiatrist. SEE: *podiatrist.*

**chiropody** (kĭ-rŏp′ō-dē) Obsolete term for treatment of foot disorders. SEE: *podiatry.*

**chiropractic** (kī″rō-prăk′tĭk) [Gr. *cheir,* hand, + *prattein,* to do] A system of health care based on the premise that the relationship between structure and function in the human body is a significant health factor and that such relationships between the spinal column and the nervous system are important because the normal transmission and expression of nerve energy are essential to the restoration and maintenance of health. (Adapted from a definition supplied by the American Chiropractic Association.)

**chiropractor** A person certified and licensed to provide chiropractic care.

**chirospasm** (kī′rō-spăzm) [″ + *spasmos,* spasm] A spasm of the hand muscles; writer's cramp.

**chisel** (chĭs′l) A beveled-edge steel cutting instrument used in dentistry and orthopedics.

**chi-square** (kī-skwār) A statistical test to determine the correlation between the number of actual occurrences and the expected occurrences. The symbol for chi-square is $\chi^2$.

**chitin** (kī′tĭn) [Gr. *chiton,* tunic] A white, horny substance in the outer covering of the body of invertebrates such as crabs. It also occurs in some fungi. **chitinous** (-nŭs), *adj.*

**Chlamydia** (klă-mĭd'ē-ă) [Gr. *chlamys,* cloak] A single genus of intracellular parasites with three recognized species: *C. psittaci*, *C. trachomatis*, and *C. pneumoniae*. The organisms are characterized as bacteria because of the composition of their cell walls and their growth by binary division; but they grow only intracellularly. These species cause a variety of diseases.

***C. pneumoniae*** A species of chlamydia that is an important cause of pneumonia, bronchitis, and sinusitis. It is believed to be transmitted from person to person by respiratory tract secretions, but this has not been proven. It is more common in the elderly and is uncommon in persons less than 20 years of age. In closed populations, it is spread slowly. Most cases of respiratory infection are mild and rarely require hospitalization. Treatment consists of daily tetracycline or erythromycin for 14 days.

***C. psittaci*** A species of chlamydia that is common in birds and animals, thus pet owners, pet shop employees, poultry farmers, and workers in meat processing plants are at risk of developing psittacosis. After an incubation period of 5 to 15 days, nonspecific symptoms similar to a viral illness with malaise and fever may develop. Or the illness may resemble infectious mononucleosis with fever, pharyngitis, hepatosplenomegaly, and adenopathy. The severity may vary from mild or inapparent to a fatal systemic disease. In patients who are untreated, the fatality rate is approximately 20%. Treatment consists of administration of tetracycline or doxycycline for 10 to 21 days. SEE: *ornithosis.*

***C. trachomatis*** An organism that causes a great variety of diseases, including genital infections in men and women. The specific diseases caused by *C. trachomatis* include 35% to 50% of cases of nonspecific urethritis, neonatal inclusion conjunctivitis, lymphogranuloma venereum, pneumonia, and trachoma.

In industrialized countries *C. trachomatis* is the most common sexually transmitted pathogen, causing an estimated 3 million new infections annually. Men with chlamydial infection experience urethritis and penile discharge. Women experience urethral or vaginal discharge, painful or frequent urination, lower abdominal pain, or acute pelvic inflammatory disease, which may result in infertility. A test for chlamydia-specific monoclonal antibodies establishes the diagnosis. A pregnant woman with a chlamydial infection can transmit the disease to her infant during birth.

Contact with infected persons should be avoided or condoms used during sexual activity. In newborns, ophthalmic antibiotic solition should be instilled in the conjunctival sac of each eye.

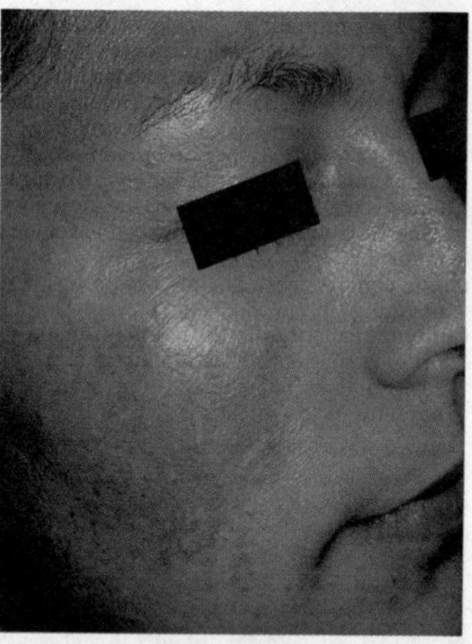

CHLOASMA GRAVIDARUM

**chloasma** (klō-ăz'mă) [Gr. *chloazein,* to be green] Pigmentary skin discolorations, usually occurring in yellowish-brown patches or spots.

SYMPTOMS: Discolored areas are rounded or oval with ill-defined margins. They are light yellow to black. In those due to external factors, pigmentation develops only at the site of irritation or beyond it.

***c. gravidarum*** Brownish pigmentation of the face, often occurring in pregnancy. It usually disappears after delivery. It is also seen in some women who take progestational oral contraceptives. SYN: *mask of pregnancy*. SEE: illus.

***c. hepaticum*** Liver spot. SEE: *lentigines* for illus.

***idiopathic c.*** Chloasma caused by external agents such as sun, heat, mechanical means, and x-rays.

***c. traumaticum*** Skin discoloration following trauma.

**chloracne** (klor-ăk'nē) A generalized acneiform dermatitis that may occur in persons exposed to chemicals containing chlorine.

**chloral** (klō'răl) [Gr. *chloras,* green] **1.** An oily liquid having a bitter taste. **2.** Chloral hydrate.

**chloral hydrate** Colorless, transparent crystals having an aromatic, slightly acrid odor and a caustic, faintly bitter taste; soluble in alcohol and water. Trade names are Noctec and SK-Chloral Hydrate.

ACTION/USES: Chloral hydrate is used as a sedative and hypnotic. It is most commonly used to induce sleep because it allows an almost normal sleep pattern in most patients.

**chloral hydrate poisoning** Toxicity caused by excessive ingestion of chloral hydrate. The drug depresses and eventually paralyzes the central nervous system and may cause liver toxicity. There may be nausea and vomiting due to gastric irritation. The pulse is feeble and respirations are shallow and irregular. Lassitude, weakness, dizziness, and sleep occur.

FIRST AID: An airway must be maintained and a cuffed endotracheal tube used if necessary. Assisted respiration may be required. Emesis should be induced. If this is not accomplished, a slurry of activated charcoal is administered and removed by suction through the same tube used to instill the charcoal. The patient should be placed in a Trendelenburg position and given intravenous glucose. If the overdose was administered by enema, an activated charcoal cleansing enema should be given. SEE: *Poisons and Poisoning Appendix*.

**chlorambucil** (klō-răm′bū-sĭl) A cytotoxic agent used in treating chronic lymphocytic leukemia, Hodgkin's disease, and certain lymphomas. Trade name is Leukeran.

**chloramine T** A strong antiseptic used to irrigate wounds and as a disinfectant in dentistry.

**chloramphenicol** (klō″răm-fĕn′ĭ-kōl) An antibiotic originally isolated from *Streptomyces venezuelae* that is now made synthetically. It is a broad-spectrum agent and is esp. useful in typhoid fever (for which it is the antibiotic of choice), other infections caused by *Salmonellae*, and rickettsial infections. SEE: *gray syndrome of the newborn*.

---

Caution: Chloramphenicol may cause certain blood disorders, esp. in newborns; consequently it should not be used indiscriminately or for minor infections. If it is used for prolonged periods, careful blood checks should be made. One should read the literature that comes with each package of this medicine before choosing it over another antibiotic.

---

**chlorate** (klō′rāt) A salt of chloric acid. SEE: *potassium chlorate; Poisons and Poisoning Appendix*.

**chlordane** (klor′dān) A poisonous substance used as an insecticide. SEE: *Poisons and Poisoning Appendix*.

**chlordiazepoxide hydrochloride** (klor″dī-ăz″ĕ-pŏk′sīd) A benzodiazepine derivative used in treating anxiety and alcohol withdrawal syndrome and as a premedication in anesthesia.

**chloremia** (klō-rē′mē-ă) [Gr. *chloros*, green, + *haima*, blood] Increased chloride in the blood.

**chlorhexidine gluconate** (klor-hĕk′sĭ-dēn) A topical anti-infective agent. Trade name is Hibiclens.

**chlorhydria** (klor-hī′drē-ă) [″ + *hydor*, water] An excess of hydrochloric acid in the stomach.

**chloride** (klō′rīd) [Gr. *chloros*, green] A binary compound of chlorine; a salt of hydrochloric acid. Blood serum contains 100 to 110 mEq/L (350 to 390 mg/dl) of chloride ions. Chloride levels are elevated in nephritis, eclampsia, anemia, and cardiac disease; decreased in fevers, diabetes, and pneumonia.

FUNCTION: Chloride is the major extracellular anion and contributes to osmotic pressure and the movement of water between fluid compartments. Chlorine is found combined with sodium in the blood. It exerts some influence on metabolism, helps to maintain osmotic pressure, and helps to regulate and stimulate muscular action. The body fluids contain 0.85% salt concentration. The inorganic salts keep proteins of the blood, milk, and other secretions in solution. Chlorine is present in the hydrochloric acid of the gastric juice. It aids digestion, activates enzymes, and is essential to normal gastric secretion.

**chloridemia** (klō″rĭ-dē′mē-ă) [″ + *haima*, blood] Chlorides in the blood.

**chloride poisoning** SEE: *barium salts, absorbable, in Poisons and Poisoning Appendix*.

**chloridimeter** (klor-ĭ-dim′ĕ-tur) An instrument for determining the amount of chloride in a body fluid.

**chloriduria** (klō″rĭ-dū′rē-ă) [″ + *ouron*, urine] Excess of chlorides in the urine.

**chlorinated** (klō′rĭn-ā-tĕd) Impregnated with chlorine.

**chlorinated lime** Calcium hypochlorite and calcium chloride; widely used in solution as a bleach and as an antiseptic. It was the first agent used for disinfecting birth attendants' hands to prevent iatrogenic "childbed fever." SEE: *Semmelweiss, Ignaz Phillip*.

**chlorination** (klō″rĭ-nā′shŭn) Treatment of water by adding chlorine and its compounds to kill bacteria. For effective disinfection, a concentration of 0.5 to 1 part chlorine per million parts water is necessary.

**chlorine** (klō′rēn) [Gr. *chloros*, green] SYMB: Cl. A highly irritating, very poisonous gas; atomic weight 35.453, atomic number 17. It is destructive to the mucous membranes of the respiratory passages, and excessive inhalation may cause death. Chlorine is an active bleaching agent and germicide, owing to its oxidizing powers. It is used extensively to disinfect water supplies and treat sewage.

**chlorite** (klō′rīt) A salt of chlorous acid; used as a disinfectant and bleaching agent.

**chlorobutanol** (klō-rō-bū′tă-nōl) Colorless crystals with camphor odor and taste. It is used as an antiseptic and local anesthetic in dentistry, and as a preservative in many pharmaceuticals. SYN: *chlorbu-*

*tanol; chlorbutol.*

INCOMPATIBILITY: Chlorobutanol is decomposed by alkalies and should not be mixed with borax or carbonates. It is soluble in ether, chloroform, and volatile oils.

**chloroform** (klō′rō-form) [Gr. *chloros,* green, + L. *forma,* form] $CHCl_3$. A heavy, clear, colorless liquid with a strong etherlike odor, formed by the action of chlorinated lime on methyl alcohol. At one time chloroform was administered by inhalation to produce anesthesia, but this use is obsolete.

**chloroformism** (klō′rō-form″ĭzm) The habit of inhaling chloroform for pleasure.

**chloroleukemia** (klō″rō-loo-kē′mē-ă) [″ + *leukos,* white, + *haima,* blood] Leukemia with chlorosis.

**chloroma** (klō-rō′mă) [″ + *oma,* growth] A greenish sarcoma of the periosteum of the cranial bones; green cancer.

**Chloromycetin** (klō″rō-mī-sē′tĭn) Trade name for chloramphenicol.

**chloropenia** (klō″rō-pē′nē-ă) Hypochloremia. **chloropenic** (-nĭk), *adj.*

**chlorophane** (klō′rō-fān) [″ + *phainein,* to show] A green-yellow pigment in the retina.

**chlorophenothane** (klō″rō-fĕn′ō-thān) An insecticide, better known as DDT, that is effective but should not be used because of its toxicity to various animals.

**chlorophyll, chlorophyl** (klō′rō-fĭl) [″ + *phyllon,* leaf] The green pigment in plants that accomplishes photosynthesis. In this process, carbon dioxide and water are combined to form glucose and oxygen according to the following equation: $6\,CO_2 + 6\,H_2O + \text{light} \rightarrow C_6H_{12}O_6 + 6\,O_2$. Thus, the primary energy source for our planet is the sunlight absorbed by chlorophyll. Four forms of chlorophyll (a, b, c, and d) occur in nature. Magnesium is an important component of chlorophyll and an important dietary source of this mineral.

**chloropia, chloropsia** (klō-rō′pē-ă, klō-rŏp′sē-ă) [″ + *opsis,* vision] A sign of digitalis toxicity in which viewed objects appear green.

**chloroplast, chloroplastid** (klō′rō-plăst, klō″rō-plăs′tĭd) [″ + *plastos,* formed] A small green cell organelle found in the leaves and some stems of plants. Chloroplasts are the sites of photosynthesis. They possess a stroma and contain four pigments: chlorophyll a, chlorophyll b, carotene, and xanthophyll.

**chloroprivic** (klō″rō-prĭv′ĭk) [″ + L. *privare,* to deprive of] Lacking in or caused by loss of chlorides.

**chloroprocaine hydrochloride** (klō″rō-prō′kān) A local anesthetic more potent and less toxic than procaine. Trade name is Nesacaine.

**chloroquine hydrochloride** (klō′rō-kwĭn) $C_{18}H_{26}ClN_3 \cdot 2HCl$. A white crystalline powder used for its antimicrobial action, esp. in the treatment of malaria. It is useful also in amebic dysentery complicated by liver abscess and in lupus erythematosus. Trade name is Aralen Hydrochloride.

**chlorosis** (klō-rō′sĭs) [″ + *osis,* condition] A form of iron-deficiency anemia. SEE: *anemia, iron-deficiency.* **chlorotic** (-rŏt′ĭk), *adj.*

**chlorothiazide sodium** (klō″rō-thī′ă-zīd) An effective diuretic that is administered orally. Trade name is Sodium Diuril.

**chlorotrianisene** (klō″rō-trī-ăn′ĭ-sēn) $C_{23}H_{21}ClO_3$. A synthetic estrogen that is about one eighth as potent as diethylstilbestrol. It is little used because it accumulates in fat tissue. Trade name is TACE.

**chlorpheniramine maleate** (klor″fĕn-ĭr′ă-mēn) An antihistamine that may be used orally or by injection. It is available under several trade names, including Chlor-Trimeton and Teldrin.

**chlorpromazine** (klor-prō′mă-zēn) A tranquilizing agent used primarily in its hydrochloride form in major and minor psychotic states. Trade name for chlorpromazine hydrochloride is Thorazine.

**chlorpromazine poisoning** SEE: *Poisons and Poisoning Appendix.*

**chlorpropamide** (klor-prō′pă-mīd) An oral hypoglycemic agent of the sulfonylurea class. Trade name is Diabinese.

---

Caution: This drug should be used only in patients with non–insulin-independent diabetes who, if weight reduction and dietary control fail, cannot be treated with diet alone and who are unwilling or unable to take insulin.

---

**chlorprothixene** (klor-prō-thĭks′ēn) A drug used in treating mental illness. Trade name is Taractan.

**chlortetracycline hydrochloride** (klor″tĕt-rā-sī′klēn) A golden-colored, broad-spectrum antibiotic isolated from a strain of *Streptomyces aureofaciens.* It inhibits growth of or destroys some strains of streptococci, staphylococci, pneumococci, rickettsiae. Trade name is Aureomycin.

**chlorthalidone** (klor-thăl′ĭ-dōn) An effective diuretic. Trade name is Hygroton.

**Chlor-Trimeton** Trade name for chlorpheniramine maleate.

**chlorzoxazone** (klor-zŏk′să-zōn) A muscle relaxant.

**Ch.M.** *chirurgiae magister,* Master of Surgery.

**choana** (kō′ă-nă) *pl.* **choanae** [Gr. *choane,* funnel] A funnel-shaped opening, esp. of the posterior nares; one of the communicating passageways between the nasal fossae and the pharynx.

**choanoid** (kō′ăn-oyd) [″ + *eidos,* form, shape] Shaped like a funnel.

**choke** [ME. *choken*] To prevent respiration by compressing or obstructing the larynx or trachea.

**chokes** Respiratory symptoms such as substernal distress, paroxysmal cough, tachypnea, or asphyxia. These may occur in decompression illness, esp. in cases of aeroembolism resulting from exposure to pressure lower than atmospheric. SEE: *disease, caisson.*

**choke-saver** Commercial name for a curved tweezer-like forceps, usually made of plastic, for inserting into the throat of a person who is choking. The device is used to grasp and remove the food from the obstructed airway. SEE: *Heimlich maneuver.*

**choking** [ME. *choken,* to suffocate] Obstruction within a respiratory passage or constriction about the neck, interfering with breathing and circulation of blood to the brain. It may also result from spasm of the larynx induced by an irritating gas. The symptoms of choking include purple face, protruding eyes, arms thrown about, coughing, constriction and injury of the neck, cyanosis, dizziness, and unconsciousness. SEE: *choking on food; Heimlich maneuver.*

**choking on food** Choking caused by inadvertent inhalation of inadequately chewed food. Most commonly involved is a piece of meat or other solid food. The usual result is panic accompanied by inability to speak, cyanosis, and fainting. Lay persons in the vicinity may assume the patient is having a heart attack.

EMERGENCY MEASURES: For complete airway obstruction, evidenced by inability to speak, one should reach into the throat using the fingers or curved forceps, dislodge the obstruction, and remove it. It may be possible to forcibly eject the food by quickly and forcibly compressing the abdomen and lower chest (the Heimlich maneuver). This maneuver consists of (1) wrapping the arms around the victim's waist from behind; (2) making a fist with one hand and placing it against the victim's abdomen between the navel and rib cage; (3) clasping the fist with the free hand and pressing in with a quick, forceful upward thrust. This produces sudden air pressure on the object. The maneuver may be repeated several times if necessary. If an object is lodged in the throat and breathing is possible, interference should be limited until professional aid is available. Emergency cricothyroidotomy may be needed. SEE: *Heimlich maneuver.*

**cholagogue** (kō'lă-gŏg) [Gr. *chole,* bile, + *agein,* to lead forth] An agent that increases the flow of bile into the intestine (i.e., a choleretic or cholecystagogue).

**cholangiectasis** (kō-lăn"jē-ĕk'tă-sĭs) [" + *angeion,* vessel, + *ektasis,* dilatation] Dilation of the bile ducts.

**cholangiocarcinoma** (kō-lăn"jē-ō-kăr"sĭ-nō'mă) [" + " + *karkinos,* crab, + *oma,* tumor] Carcinoma of the bile ducts.

**cholangioenterostomy** (kō-lăn"jē-ō-ĕn"tĕr-ŏs'tō-mē) [" + " + *enteron,* intestine, + *stoma,* mouth] Surgical formation of a passage between a bile duct and the intestine.

**cholangiogastrostomy** (kō-lăn"jē-ō-găs-trŏs'tō-mē) [" + " + *gaster,* stomach, + *stoma,* mouth] Surgical formation of a passage between a bile duct and the stomach.

**cholangiography** (kō-lăn"jē-ŏg'ră-fē) [" + " + *graphein,* to write] Radiography of the bile ducts.

***percutaneous transhepatic c.*** ABBR: PTC. Direct percutaneous puncture of an intrahepatic duct by a needle inserted through the eighth or ninth intercostal space into the center of the liver. Radiopaque material is injected into the dilated intrahepatic biliary tree. The procedure is useful in determining the cause of jaundice. SEE: *endoscopic retrograde cholangiopancreatography; jaundice.*

**cholangiole** (kō-lăn'jē-ōl) [" + " + *ole,* dim. suffix] The small terminal portion of the bile duct.

**cholangiolitis** (kō-lăn"jē-ō-lī'tĭs) [" + " + " + Gr. *itis,* inflammation] Inflammation of the bile ducts, occurring in various forms of hepatitis.

**cholangioma** (kō-lăn-jē-ō'mă) [" + *angeion,* vessel, + *oma,* tumor] A tumor of the bile ducts.

**cholangiostomy** (kō"lăn-jē-ŏs'tō-mē) [" + " + *stoma,* mouth] Surgical formation of a fistula into the gallbladder.

**cholangiotomy** (kō"lăn-jē-ŏt'ō-mē) [" + " + *tome,* incision] Incision of an intrahepatic bile duct for removal of gallstones.

**cholangitis** (kō"lăn-jī'tĭs) [" + *angeion,* vessel, + *itis,* inflammation] Inflammation of the bile ducts.

***primary sclerosing c.*** A chronic liver disease of unknown origin marked by inflammation and obliteration of the intrahepatic and extrahepatic bile ducts. The disease progresses silently and steadily and in most patients leads to cirrhosis, portal hypertension, and liver failure. Seventy percent of patients are men and the mean age at diagnosis is 39. The only effective treatment is liver transplantation. This disease is the fourth leading indication for liver transplantation in adults.

**cholanopoiesis** (kō"lă-nō-poy-ē'sĭs) [Gr. *chole,* bile, + *ano,* upward, + *poiesis,* making] Synthesis of cholic acid in the liver.

**cholate** (kō'lāt) Any salt or ester of cholic acid.

**cholecalciferol** (ko"lē-kăl-sĭf'ĕr-ŏl) Vitamin $D_3$; an antirachitic, oil-soluble vitamin occurring as white, odorless crystals.

**cholecystagogue** (kō"lē-sĭs'tă-gŏg) [" + " + *agogos,* leader] A drug or action that empties the gallbladder.

**cholecystalgia** (kō"lē-sĭs-tăl'jē-ă) [" + " + *algos,* pain] Biliary colic.

**cholecystangiography** (kō"lē-sĭs"tăn-jē-ŏg'ră-fē) [" + " + *angeion,* vessel, + *graph-*

*ein,* to write] Radiographic examination of the gallbladder and bile ducts after injection of a contrast medium.

**cholecystectasia** (kō″lē-sĭs-tĕk-tā′zē-ă) [″ + ″ + *ektasis,* dilatation] Dilatation of the gallbladder.

**cholecystectomy** (kō″lē-sĭs-tĕk′tō-mē) [″ + ″ + *ektome,* excision] Excision of the gallbladder by abdominal incision or laparoscopy.

NURSING IMPLICATIONS: *Preoperative:* The patient is prepared physically and emotionally for the procedure, and any expected intubation or catheterization is explained in advance.

*Postoperative:* Vital signs are monitored every 2 to 4 hr or as necessary, and dressings inspected frequently and redressed as necessary. The patient is assessed for pain and for gastrointestinal and urinary function; analgesics and antiemetics are provided as needed, and voiding is encouraged. Fluid and electrolyte balance is monitored, and prescribed replacement therapy administered. Respiratory status is assessed every 2 to 4 hr, and the patient is encouraged to breathe deeply and to perform incentive spirometry if prescribed. The nurse assists the patient to splint the abdomen for coughing and helps with early ambulation. Peripheral circulation is evaluated and venous return promoted with leg exercises and elastic stockings or pneumatic leg dressings as prescribed.

If a laparoscopic approach is used, the patient is discharged the day of or the day after surgery. Clear liquids are offered after recovery from general anesthesia, and a normal diet is resumed within a few days. If an abdominal approach is used, the patient is placed in the semi-Fowler position, a nasogastric (NG) tube attached to low intermittent suction, and the volume and characteristics of drainage from the NG tube and any abdominal drains are documented. If a T-tube is in place, the position and patency of the tube and drainage bag are assessed; the bag is situated level with the abdomen to prevent excess drainage; and the volume and characteristics of drainage, which may be bloody or blood-tinged bile for the first few hours after surgery, are documented. Skin care is provided around the tube insertion site.

The patient is assessed for bowel sounds; when they are present, the NG tube is removed as directed and oral intake, beginning with clear liquids, is initiated. The T-tube usually is clamped for an hour before and after each meal to allow bile to travel to the intestine. Signs and symptoms of postcholecystectomy syndrome (fever, abdominal pain, and skin and scleral jaundice) and other complications involving obstructed bile drainage are reported; urine and stool samples are collected for analysis of bile content should any such complications occur.

Discharge teaching for the patient and family focuses on wound care; T-tube care if appropriate (the T-tube may remain in place up to 2 weeks); the need to report any signs of biliary obstruction (fever, jaundice, pruritus, pain, dark urine, and clay-colored stools); the importance of daily exercise such as walking; avoidance of heavy lifting or straining for the prescribed period; and any restrictions on motor vehicle operation. Although diet is not restricted, the patient may be more comfortable avoiding excessive intake of fats and gas-forming foods for 4 to 6 weeks. Arrangements for home health care may be necessary. SEE: *Nursing Diagnoses Appendix.*

***laparoscopic laser c.*** Removal of the gallbladder using the laser technique. This procedure is not attempted for patients with severe acute cholecystitis, a palpable gallbladder, or evidence of a stone in the common bile duct. The procedure was previously called endoscopic laser cholecystectomy.

**cholecystenterorrhaphy** (kō″lē-sĭs-tĕn″tĕr-or′ă-fē) [″ + ″ + *enteron,* intestine, + *rhaphe,* seam, ridge] Suture of the gallbladder to the intestinal wall.

**cholecystenterostomy** (kō″lē-sĭs-tĕn″tĕr-ŏs′tō-mē) [″ + ″ + *enteron,* intestine, + *stoma,* mouth] Surgical formation of a passage between the gallbladder and the small intestine.

**cholecystic** (kō″lē-sĭs′tĭk) Pert. to the gallbladder.

**cholecystitis** (kō″lē-sĭs-tī′tĭs) [Gr. *chole,* bile, + *kystis,* bladder, + *itis,* inflammation] Inflammation of the gallbladder.

SYMPTOMS: In acute cholecystitis there is fever, gradually developing or sudden pain in the upper abdomen, nausea, vomiting, and visible but mild jaundice in about 20% of patients. Frequently pain is referred to the back or the right shoulder. Approx. 10% of patients do not have pain.

ETIOLOGY: Acute cholecystitis is caused by chemical irritation due to obstruction of the cystic duct preventing the outflow of bile from the gallbladder. However, not all patients with gallstones experience cholecystitis.

TREATMENT: In acute cholecystitis, cholecystectomy is required. If this is not possible, the gallbladder should be drained (cholecystostomy) and cholecystectomy should be performed at a later date.

NURSING IMPLICATIONS: The patient is assessed for biliary colic, which is characterized by a sudden onset of severe steady or aching midepigastric or right upper quadrant pain that may radiate to the back shoulder area, often following eating a fatty or large meal after fasting. The patient is evaluated for evidence of nausea, vomiting, flatulence, food intolerance, fever or chills, increased pulse and respiratory rate, pallor, diaphoresis, and exhaustion. A history of earlier attacks, which may have been milder or more vague, is obtained. In chronic cases, the skin and sclera are inspected for jaundice, the urine for dark coloration, and stools for clay coloration. The abdomen is auscultated for bowel sounds, which may be absent, and lightly palpated for tenderness over the gallbladder area, which increases on inspiration. During an acute attack, the vital signs and fluid balance are monitored, oral intake is withheld, prescribed antiemetics are administered as necessary, and intravenous fluid and electrolyte therapy is maintained as prescribed. Patient comfort is ensured, and prescribed narcotic analgesics and anticholinergics are administered to relieve pain.

The condition is managed nonsurgically with a low-fat diet offered in small, frequent meals to help prevent biliary colic attacks. Obese patients are advised to lose weight. Fat-soluble vitamins (A, D, E, and K) are replaced and bile salts administered as prescribed. Diagnostic tests including pretest instructions and aftercare are explained; the surgeon's explanation of any prescribed surgical interventions, including possible complications, is reinforced; and the patient is prepared physically and emotionally for such procedures.

**cholecystnephrostomy** (kō″lē-sĭst″nē-frŏs′tō-mē) [″ + *kystis,* bladder, + *nephros,* kidney, + *stoma,* mouth] Surgical formation of a passage between the gallbladder and the renal pelvis.

**cholecystocolostomy** (kō″lē-sĭs″tō-kō-lŏs′tō-mē) [″ + ″ + *kolon,* colon, + *stoma,* mouth] Surgical formation of a passage between the gallbladder and the colon.

**cholecystocolotomy** (kō″lē-sĭs″tō-kō-lŏt′ō-mē) [″ + ″ + ″ + *tome,* incision] A surgical incision into the gallbladder and colon.

**cholecystoduodenostomy** (kō″lē-sĭs″tō-dū″ō-dē-nŏs′tō-mē) [″ + ″ + L. *duodeni,* twelve, + Gr. *stoma,* mouth] Surgical formation of a passage between the gallbladder and the duodenum.

**cholecystogastrostomy** (kō″lē-sĭs″tō-găs-trŏs′tō-mē [″ + ″ + *gaster,* belly, + *stoma,* mouth]. Surgical formation of a passage between the gallbladder and the stomach.

**cholecystogram** (kō″lē-sĭs′tō-grăm) [″ + ″ + *gramma,* something written] A radiograph of the gallbladder.

**cholecystography** (kō″lē-sĭs-tŏg′ră-fē) [″ + ″ + *graphein,* to write] Radiography of the gallbladder.

**cholecystoileostomy** (kō″lē-sĭs″tō-ĭl-ē-ŏs′tō-mē) [″ + *kystis,* bladder, + L. *ileum,* + Gr. *stoma,* mouth] Surgical formation of a passage between the gallbladder and the ileum.

**cholecystojejunostomy** (kō″lē-sĭs″tō-jĕ-jū-nŏs′tō-mē) [″ + ″ + L. *jejunum,* empty, + Gr. *stoma,* mouth] Surgical formation of a passage between the gallbladder and the jejunum.

**cholecystokinin** A hormone secreted into the blood by the mucosa of the upper small intestine. It stimulates gallbladder contraction and secretion of pancreatic enzymes. SEE: *Zollinger-Ellison syndrome.*

**cholecystolithiasis** (kō″lē-sĭs″tō-lĭ-thī′ă-sĭs) [″ + ″ + *lithos,* stone, + *-iasis,* condition] Gallstones in the gallbladder.

**cholecystolithotripsy** (kō″lē-sĭs″tō-lĭth′ō-trĭp″sē) [″ + ″ + ″ + *tripsis,* a rubbing] Crushing of a gallstone in the unopened gallbladder with an extracorporeal shock-wave lithotriptor.

**cholecystomy** (kō″lē-sĭs′tō-mē) [Gr. *chole,* bile, + *kystis,* bladder, + *tome,* incision] Cholecystotomy.

**cholecystopathy** (kō″lē-sĭs-tŏp′ă-thē) [″ + ″ + *pathos,* disease, suffering] Any gallbladder disorder.

**cholecystopexy** (kō″lē-sĭs′tō-pĕk″sē) [″ + ″ + *pexis,* fixation] Suturing of the gallbladder to the abdominal wall.

**cholecystoptosis** (kō″lē-sĭs-tŏp-tō′sĭs) [″ + ″ + *ptosis,* a dropping] Downward displacement of the gallbladder.

**cholecystorrhaphy** (kō″lē-sĭs-tor′ă-fē) [″ + *kystis,* bladder, + *rhaphe,* seam, ridge] Suturing of the gallbladder.

**cholecystostomy** (kō″lē-sĭs-tŏs′tō-mē) [″ + ″ + *stoma,* mouth] Surgical formation of an opening into the gallbladder through the abdominal wall.

**cholecystotomy** (kō″lē-sĭs-tŏt′ō-mē) [″ + ″ + *tome,* incision] Incision of the gallbladder through the abdominal wall for removal of gallstones.

**choledochal** (kō-lē-dŏk′ăl) [″ + *dochos,* receptacle] Pert. to the common bile duct.

**choledochectasia** (kō-lĕd″ō-kĕk-tā′zē-ă) [″ + ″ + *ektasis,* distention] Distention of the common bile duct.

**choledochectomy** (kō-lĕd″ō-kĕk′tō-mē) [″ + ″ + *ektome,* excision] Excision of a portion of the common bile duct.

**choledochitis** (kō″lē-dō-kī′tĭs) [″ + ″ + *itis,* inflammation] Inflammation of the common bile duct.

**choledochoduodenostomy** (kō-lĕd″ō-kō-dū-ō-dē-nŏs′tō-mē) [″ + ″ + L. *duodeni,* twelve, + Gr. *stoma,* mouth] Surgical formation of a passage between the common bile duct and the duodenum.

**choledochoenterostomy** (kō-lĕd″ō-kō-ĕn-tĕr-ŏs′tō-mē) [″ + ″ + *enteron,* intestine, + *stoma,* mouth] Surgical formation of a passage between the common bile duct and the intestine.

**choledochography** (kō-lĕd″ō-kŏg′ră-fē) [″ + *dochos,* receptacle, + *graphein,* to write] Radiography of the bile duct following administration of a radiopaque contrast medium.

**choledochojejunostomy** (kō-lĕd″ō-kō-jĕ-jū-nŏs′tō-mē) [″ + ″ + L. *jejunum,* empty, + Gr. *stoma,* mouth] Surgical joining of the common bile duct to the jejunum of the small intestine.

**choledocholith** (kō-lĕd′ŏ-kō-lĭth″) [″ + ″ + *lithos,* stone] A calculus, or stone, in the common bile duct.

**choledocholithiasis** (kō-lĕd″ō-kō-lĭ-thī′ă-sĭs) [″ + ″ + *lithos,* stone, + *-iasis,* condition] Calculi in the common bile duct.

**choledocholithotomy** (kō-lĕd″ō-kō-lĭth-ŏt′ō-mē) [″ + ″ + ″ + *tome,* incision] Removal of a gallstone through an incision of the bile duct.

**choledocholithotripsy** (kō-lĕd′ō-kō-lĭth″ō-trĭp-sē) [″ + ″ + ″ + *tripsis,* a crushing] Crushing of a gallstone in the common bile duct.

**choledochoplasty** (kō-lĕd′ō-kō-plăs″tē) [Gr. *chole,* bile, + *dochos,* receptacle, + *plassein,* to form] Surgical repair of the common bile duct.

**choledochorrhaphy** (kō-lĕd″ō-kor′ă-fē) [″ + ″ + *rhaphe,* seam, ridge] Suturing of the severed ends of the common bile duct.

**choledochostomy** (kō-lĕd″ō-kŏs′tō-mē) [″ + ″ + *stoma,* mouth] Surgical formation of a passage into the common bile duct through the abdominal wall.

**choledochotomy** (kō″lĕd-ō-kŏt′ō-mē) [″ + ″ + *tome,* incision] Surgical incision of the common bile duct.

**cholelithiasis** (kō″lē-lĭ-thī′ă-sĭs) [″ + ″ + *-iasis,* condition] The formation or presence of calculi, or bilestones, in the gallbladder or common duct. The stones may or may not cause symptoms. SYN: *gallstone.* SEE: *Nursing Diagnoses Appendix.*

SYMPTOMS: The condition is marked by digestive disturbances, heaviness in the right hypochondrium, and tenderness on pressure over the gallbladder. Gallstone colic is present when a stone obstructs the bile duct. Pain may radiate to the back and right shoulder. Colic is usually manifest when the stomach is empty. Jaundice is present if the flow of bile is obstructed. Pain may be associated with vomiting and sweating. If distended, the gallbladder is palpable.

TREATMENT: Cholecystectomy is the usual treatment. Cholecystostomy is required in very poor-risk patients. Lithotripsy has been used to disintegrate stones so that they are small enough to pass.

**cholelithic** (kō″lē-lĭth′ĭk) Pert. to or caused by biliary calculus.

**cholelithotomy** (kō″lē-lĭ-thŏt′ō-mē) [″ + *lithos,* stone, + *tome,* incision] Removal of gallstones through a surgical incision.

**cholelithotripsy, cholelithotrity** (kō″lē-lĭth′ō-trĭp-sē, kō″lē-lĭ-thŏt′rĭ-tē) [″ + ″ + *tripsis,* a crushing] Crushing of a biliary calculus.

**cholemesis** (kō-lĕm′ĕ-sĭs) [″ + *emein,* to vomit] Bile in the vomitus.

**choleperitoneum** (kō″lē-pĕr″ĭ-tō-nē′ŭm) [″ + *peri,* around, + *teinein,* to stretch] Bile in the peritoneum.

**cholera** (kŏl′ĕr-ă) [L. *cholera,* bilious diarrhea] An acute infection involving the entire small intestine, marked by profuse watery diarrhea and vomiting. This produces severe loss of fluids and electrolytes, muscular cramps, oliguria, dehydration, and collapse. The incubation period is from a few hours to 4 or 5 days. SYN: *Asiatic cholera.*

SYMPTOMS: Four stages are usually described as follows:

*Invasion:* At the conclusion of the incubation period, malaise, headache, diarrhea, anorexia, and slight fever are present. These may last a few days and then subside. This is termed the cholerine stage. Sometimes this stage is missing entirely.

*Evacuation:* Purging, violent vomiting, and muscular cramps characterize this stage. Stools are loose, copious, and watery, and the flecks of mucus present a typical rice-water appearance. Sometimes there are particles of blood and mucus. Vomiting is severe and persistent; the material expelled may also resemble rice water. Muscular cramps commonly start in the extremities; they involve the calves of the legs and later the arms, hands, feet, and trunk. Thirst is unquenchable, and hiccough sometimes develops. Signs of physical depression soon terminate in collapse. This stage seldom lasts longer than 2 to 12 hr.

*Collapse:* At this stage, circulation is almost completely arrested. The eyes are sunken, the cheeks are hollow, the nose is pinched, the skin is dry and wrinkled, the body surface is cold and covered with clammy sweat, and the breath is cool. The temperature in the axilla is 85° to 95°F (29.4° to 35°C), whereas in the rectum it may be 103°F (39.4°C) or more. Respirations are quickened, the pulse is weak, and the systolic blood pressure is decreased. Urine output is diminished or absent; diarrhea and cramps may continue. The mind usually is clear until shortly before death, when coma develops. This stage lasts from few hours to 1 or 2 days and usually ends in death. The cause of death is dehydration and electrolyte imbalance.

*Reaction:* Sometimes, even when death seems imminent, the surface temperature begins to rise, vomiting ceases, bowel evacuations become less frequent and more feculent, and convalescence follows. Complete recovery may take from 1 to 2 weeks. Occasionally, typhoid symptoms set in, the temperature goes to 106° to 107°F (41.1° to 41.7°C), and the outcome is fatal. Sometimes in this stage, an erythemal or urticarial eruption appears, particularly on the extremities. Such eruptions have no known significance.

ETIOLOGY: The causative organism, *Vibrio cholerae,* is a short, curved, motile gram-negative rod producing a potent enterotoxin, a mucolytic enzyme that causes increased secretion of chloride, bicarbonate, and water into the small intestine. Transmission is through water, milk, or other foods contaminated with excreta of patients or carriers.

TREATMENT: Fluid and electrolytes must be replaced vigorously by intravenous administration of a 2-to-1 mixture of normal saline and ⅙ molar sodium lactate. If the patient is in shock, 100 ml/kg of body weight is given; less is given if shock is not present. The fluid should be given rapidly until blood pressure returns to normal. Children require additional potassium. Fluids also should be given *ad lib* by mouth. Tetracycline given early in the disease is effective in killing the causative organism. Hypoglycemia is a reversible life-threatening complication of cholera, esp. in small children. It is treated by intravenous infusion of 3 to 4 ml/kg of 25% glucose as a bolus, then adding glucose to the infusion to provide 10 ml/kg/hr.

PROPHYLAXIS: Cholera vaccine is relatively ineffective. If traveling in an area where cholera exists, one should not drink unboiled or untreated water, not add ice to beverages, avoid raw or partially cooked fish or shellfish, avoid uncooked vegetables or fruits one has not peeled oneself, not assume bottled water is safe, and swim only in chlorinated swimming pools. Medical attention should be sought immediately if diarrhea or a febrile illness develops.

***c. sicca*** A fulminating variety of cholera that occurs without vomiting or diarrhea.

**choleresis** (kŏl-ĕr-ē′sĭs, kō-lĕr′ĕ-sĭs) [Gr. *chole,* bile, + *hairesis,* removal] The secretion of bile by the liver.

**choleretic** (kŏl-ĕr-ĕt′ĭk) **1.** Stimulating excretion of bile by the liver. **2.** Any agent that increases excretion of bile by the liver.

**choleric** (kŏl′ĕr-ĭk) Irritable; quick-tempered without apparent cause.

**choleriform** (kŏl-ĕr′ĭ-form) [L. *cholera,* + *forma,* shape] Resembling cholera.

**choleroid** (kŏl′ĕr-oyd) [″ + Gr. *eidos,* form, shape] Resembling cholera.

**cholerophobia** (kŏl″ĕr-ō-fō′bē-ă) [″ + Gr. *phobos,* fear] A morbid fear of acquiring cholera.

**cholestasia** (kō″lē-stā′zē-ă) [Gr. *chole,* bile, + *stasis,* stoppage] Cholestasis. **cholestatic** (-stă′tĭk), *adj.*

**cholestasis** Arrest of the flow of bile. This may be due to intrahepatic causes, obstruction of the bile duct by gallstones, or any process that blocks the bile duct (e.g., cancer). SYN: *cholestasia.*

**cholesteatoma** (kō″lē-stē″ă-tō′mă) [″ + *steatos,* fat, + *oma,* tumor] An epithelial pocket or cystlike sac filled with keratin debris. It can occur in the meninges, central nervous system, and skull bones, but is most common in the middle ear and mastoid area. The cyst, which is filled with a combination of epithelial cells and cholesterol, most commonly enlarges to occlude the middle ear. Enzymes formed within the sac cause erosion of adjacent bones, including the ossicles, and destroy them. Cholesteatomas are classified as congenital, primary acquired, and secondary acquired.

**cholesteremia, cholesterolemia** (kō-lĕs″tĕ-rē′mē-ă, kō-lĕs″tĕr-ŏl-ē′mē-ă) [″ + *stereos,* solid, + *haima,* blood] Hypercholesterolemia.

**cholesterol** (kō-lĕs′tĕr-ŏl) [″ + *stereos,* solid] $C_{27}H_{45}OH$. A monohydric alcohol; a sterol widely distributed in animal tissues and occurring in the egg yolks, various oils, fats, the nerve tissue of the brain and spinal cord, the liver, the kidneys, and the adrenal glands. It can be synthesized in the liver and is a normal constituent of bile. It is the principal constituent of most gallstones. It is important in metabolism, serving as a precursor of various steroid hormones (e.g., sex hormones, adrenal corticoids). SEE: illus.

In most individuals, an elevated blood level of cholesterol constitutes an increased risk of developing coronary heart disease (CHD). Scientific evidence has established that lowering definitely elevated blood cholesterol (specifically, blood levels of low-density lipoprotein cholesterol) reduces the risk of heart attacks due to CHD. Risk categories and recommended actions are included in the accompanying table. SEE: table.

Cholesterol levels may be decreased by several factors, including diet (e.g., decreased total dietary fat; decreased percentage of dietary fat derived from cholesterol and saturated fats), avoiding smoking, and avoiding anabolic steroids. Drugs used to control cholesterol include lovastatin, niacin, gemfibrozil, clofibrate, probucol, and bile-acid resins (cholestyramine, colestipol).

Devices have been designed for testing cholesterol at home. In one method, a drop of blood is placed onto a test strip and the resulting color is compared with a color guide. These tests measure total

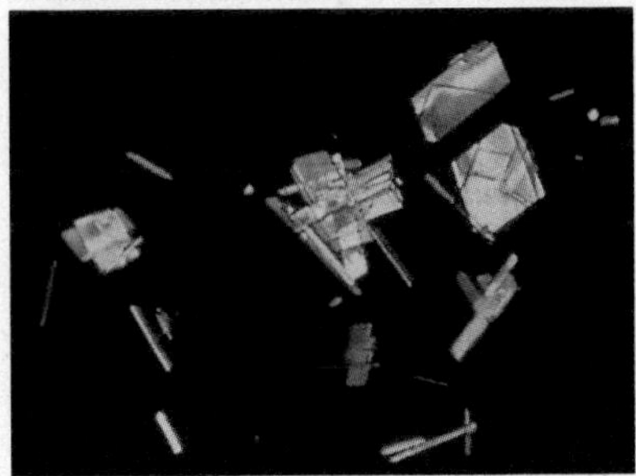

CHOLESTEROL CRYSTALS, POLARIZED
(ORIG. MAG. ×400)

**Cholesterol Risk Categories and Recommendations**

| Total Cholesterol Level | Recommendation |
|---|---|
| **Desirable level** Less than 200 mg/dl | Recheck cholesterol level every 5 years. |
| **Borderline high** 200–239 mg/dl | Dietary control of cholesterol. Recheck cholesterol level annually. |
| **Borderline high with risk factors** Family history of premature coronary artery disease; cigarette smoking; hypertension; low level of high-density lipoprotein; diabetes; history of stroke; severe obesity. | For men with one risk factor, women with two risk factors, or anyone with coronary artery disease, determine level of low-density lipoprotein and initiate stringent dietary program for lowering cholesterol; further treatment with drugs if necessary. |
| **High** 240 mg/dl or higher | Same as above. |

cholesterol only. SEE: *coronary artery disease*; *heart disease, ischemic*.

***high-density lipoprotein c.*** SEE: under *lipoprotein*.

***low-density lipoprotein c.*** SEE: under *lipoprotein*.

***total c.*** The sum of low- and high-density lipoproteins.

**cholesterolosis** The abnormal accumulation of cholesterol in tissues.

**cholestyramine resin** (kō″lĕ-stī′ră-mĭn) An ion-exchange resin used to treat itching associated with jaundice. It acts by lowering the level of bile acids in the serum. Trade name is Questran.

**choleverdin** SEE: *biliverdin*.

**cholic acid** (kō′lĭk) The sodium salt of conjugated taurocholic or glycocholic acid.

**choline** (kō′lĭn, -lēn) [Gr. *chole*, bile] $C_5H_{15}NO_2$. An amine, widely distributed in plant and animal tissues. It is a constituent of lecithin and other phospholipids. It is essential in normal fat and carbohydrate metabolism. A deficiency leads to lipoidosis of the liver. Choline is also involved in protein metabolism, serving as a methylating agent, and is a precursor of acetylcholine.

**cholinergic** (kō″lĭn-ĕr′jĭk) [″ + *ergon*, work] **1.** Liberating acetylcholine; used of nerve endings. **2.** An agent that produces the effect of acetylcholine.

**cholinergic blocking agent** A substance that blocks the action of acetylcholine at nerve cell receptors.

**cholinesterase** (kō″lĭn-ĕs′tĕr-ās) Any enzyme that catalyzes the hydrolysis of choline esters, such as acetylcholinesterase, which catalyzes the breakdown of acetylcholine to acetic acid and choline. Cholinesterases are inhibited by physostigmine (eserine).

**cholinoceptive** (kō″lĭn-ō-sĕp′tĭv) [″ + L. *receptor*, receiver] Pert. to sites on cells that are acted on by cholinergic transmitters.

**cholinolytic** (kō″lĭn-ō-lĭt′ĭk) [″ + *lysis*, dissolution] A drug or chemical that blocks the action of acetylcholine.

**cholinomimetic** (kō″lĭ-nō-mī-mĕt′ĭk) [″ + *mimetikos*, imitating] Acting in the same way as acetylcholine.

**chologenic** (kō″lō-jĕn′ĭk) [″ + *gennan*, to produce] Promoting or stimulating bile production.

**cholelith** (kŏl′ō-lĭth) [″ + *lithos*, stone] A gallstone; a biliary calculus.

**chololithiasis** (kŏl″ō-lĭth-ī′ăs-ĭs) [″ + ″ + *-iasis*, state] Cholelithiasis.

**cholorrhea** (kŏl″ō-rē′ă) [″ + *rhoia*, flow] Excessive secretion of bile.

**chondral** (kŏn′drăl) [Gr. *chondros*, cartilage] Pert. to cartilage.

**chondralgia** (kŏn-drăl′jē-ă) [″ + *algos*, pain] Pain in or around a cartilage.

**chondralloplasia** (kŏn″drăl-ō-plā′zē-ă) [″ + *allos*, other, + *plassein*, to form] Cartilage in abnormal places.

**chondrectomy** (kŏn-drĕk′tō-mē) [″ + *ektome*, excision] Surgical excision of a cartilage.

**chondric** (kŏn′drĭk) [Gr. *chondros*, cartilage] Pert. to cartilage.

**chondrification** (kŏn-drĭ-fĭ-kā′shŭn) [″ + L. *facere*, to make] Conversion into cartilage.

**chondrigen, chondrogen** (kŏn′drĭ-jĕn) [″ + *gennan*, to produce] The basal substance of cartilage and corneal tissue, which turns into chondrin on boiling.

**chondrin** (kŏn′drĭn) [Gr. *chondros*, cartilage] Gelatin-like matter obtained by boiling cartilage.

**chondritis** (kŏn-drī′tĭs) [″ + *itis*, inflammation] Inflammation of cartilage.

**chondroadenoma** (kŏn″drō-ăd-ē-nō′mă) [″ + *aden*, gland, + *oma*, tumor] Cartilaginous tissue in an adenoma.

**chondroangioma** (kŏn″drō-ăn-jē-ō′ma) [″ + *angeion*, vessel, + *oma*, tumor] Cartilaginous elements in an angioma.

**chondroblast** (kŏn′drō-blăst) [″ + *blastos*, germ] A cell that forms cartilage. SYN: *chondroplast*.

**chondroblastoma** (kŏn″drō-blăs-tō′mă) [″ + ″ + *oma*, tumor] A benign neoplasm in which the cells resemble cartilage cells and the tumor appears to be cartilage.

**chondrocalcinosis** (kŏn″drō-kăl″sĭn-ō′sĭs) [″ + L. *calx,* lime, + Gr. *osis,* condition] Pseudogout; chronic recurrent arthritis clinically similar to gout. The crystals found in the synovial fluid are calcium pyrophosphate dihydrate and not urate crystals. The most commonly involved joint is the knee.

**chondroclast** (kŏn′drō-klăst) [″ + *klastos,* broken into bits] A giant cell involved in the absorption of cartilage.

**chondrocostal** (kŏn″drō-kŏs′tăl) [″ + L. *costa,* rib] Pert. to the ribs and costal cartilages.

**chondrocranium** (kŏn-drō-krā′nē-ŭm) [″ + *kranion,* head] The cartilaginous embryonic cranium before ossification.

**chondrocyte** (kŏn′drō-sīt) [″ + *kytos,* cell] A cartilage cell.

**chondrodermatitis nodularis chronica helicis** Growth of nodules on the helix of the ear.

**chondrodynia** (kŏn″drō-dĭn′ē-ă) [″ + *odyne,* pain] Pain in or about a cartilage.

**chondrodysplasia** (kŏn″drō-dĭs-plā′zē-ă) [″ + Gr. *dys,* + *plasis,* a molding] A disease, usually hereditary, resulting in disordered growth. It is marked by multiple exostoses of growth of the epiphyses, esp. of the long bones, metacarpals, and phalanges. SYN: *dyschondroplasia.*

**chondrodystrophy** (kŏn″drō-dĭs′trō-fē) [″ + ″ + *trophe,* nourishment] Achondroplasia.

**chondroendothelioma** (kŏn″drō-ĕn″dō-thē″lē-ō′mă) [″ + *endon,* within, + *thele,* nipple, + *oma,* tumor] An endothelioma that contains cartilage.

**chondroepiphysitis** (kŏn″drō-ĕp″ĭ-fĭz-ī′tĭs) [″ + *epiphysis,* a growing on, + *itis,* inflammation] Inflammation of the epiphyseal portion of the bone and the attached cartilage.

**chondrofibroma** (kŏn″drō-fī-brō′mă) [″ + L. *fibra,* fiber, + Gr. *oma,* tumor] A mixed tumor with elements of chondroma and fibroma.

**chondrogenesis** (kŏn″drō-jĕn′ĕ-sĭs) [″ + *genesis,* generation, birth] Formation of cartilage. **chondrogenic** (-jĕn′ĭk), *adj.*

**chondroid** (kŏn′droyd) [″ + *eidos,* form, shape] Resembling cartilage; cartilaginous.

**chondroitin** (kŏn-drō′ĭ-tĭn) A substance present in connective tissue, including the cornea and cartilage.

**chondrolipoma** (kŏn-drō-lĭp-ō′mă) [″ + *lipos,* fat, + *oma,* tumor] A tumor made of cartilaginous and fatty tissue.

**chondrology** (kŏn-drŏl′ō-jē) [″ + *logos,* word, reason] The scientific study of cartilage.

**chondrolysis** (kŏn-drŏl′ĭ-sĭs) [″ + *lysis,* dissolution] The breaking down and absorption of cartilage.

**chondroma** (kŏn-drō′mă) [″ + *oma,* tumor] A slow-growing, painless cartilaginous tumor. It may occur wherever there is cartilage. **chondromatous** (-ă-tŭs), *adj.*

**chondromalacia** (kŏn-drō-măl-ā′shē-ă) [″ + *malakia,* softness] Softening of the articular cartilage, usually involving the patella.

**chondromatosis** (kŏn″drō-mă-tō′sĭs) [″ + *oma,* tumor, + *osis,* condition] Formation of multiple chondromas of the hands and feet.

**chondromucin** (kŏn″drō-mū′sĭn) Chondromucoid.

**chondromucoid** (kŏn″drō-mū′koyd) [″ + L. *mucus,* mucus, + Gr. *eidos,* form, shape] A basophilic glycoprotein present in the interstitial substance of cartilage. SYN: *chondromucin.*

**chondromucoprotein** (kŏn″drō-mū″kō-prō′tē-ĭn) [″ + ″ + *protos,* first] The ground substance (the fluid or solid material) that occupies the space between the cells and fibers of cartilage.

**chondromyoma** (kŏn″drō-mī-ō′mă) [″ + *mys,* muscle, + *oma,* tumor] A combined myoma and cartilaginous neoplasm.

**chondromyxoma** (kŏn″drō-mĭks-ō′mă) [″ + *myxa,* mucus, + *oma,* tumor] A chondroma with myxomatous elements.

**chondromyxosarcoma** (kŏn-drō-mĭk″sō-săr-kō′mă) [″ + ″ + *sarx,* flesh, + *oma,* tumor] A cartilaginous and sarcomatous tumor.

**chondro-osseus** (kŏn″drō-ŏs′ē-ŭs) [″ + L. *osseus,* bony] Composed of cartilage and bone.

**chondro-osteodystrophy** (kŏn″drō-ŏs″tē-ō-dĭs′trō-fē) [″ + *osteon,* bone, + *dys,* bad, + *trophe,* nourishment] Developmental deformity of the epiphyses. This produces dwarfism, kyphosis, and pigeon breast.

**chondropathology** (kŏn″drō-pă-thŏl′ō-jē) [Gr. *chondros,* cartilage, + *pathos,* disease, + *logos,* word, reason] The pathology of cartilage disease.

**chondropathy** (kŏn-drŏp′ă-thē) Any disease of cartilage.

**chondroplasia** (kŏn″drō-plā′zē-ă) [″ + *plassein,* to mold] The formation of cartilage.

**chondroplast** (kŏn′drō-plăst) Chondroblast.

**chondroplasty** (kŏn′drō-plăs″tē) [″ + *plassein,* to mold] Plastic or reparative surgery on cartilage.

**chondroporosis** (kŏn″drō-pō-rō′sĭs) [″ + *poros,* passage] The porous condition of pathological or normal cartilage during ossification.

**chondroprotein** (kŏn-drō-prō′tē-ĭn) [″ + *protos,* first] Any of a group of glucoproteins found in cartilage, tendons, and connective tissue.

**chondrosarcoma** (kŏn-drō-săr-kō′mă) [″ + *sarx,* flesh, + *oma,* tumor] A cartilaginous sarcoma.

**chondrosin** (kŏn′drō-sĭn) Material produced when chondroitin sulfate is hydrolyzed.

**chondrosis** (kŏn-drō′sĭs) [″ + *osis,* condition] The development of cartilage.

**chondrosternal** (kŏn″drō-stĕr′năl) [″ + *sternon,* chest] Pert. to sternal cartilage.

**chondrosternoplasty** (kŏn″drō-stĕr′nō-plăs″tē) [″ + ″ + *plassein,* to mold] Surgical correction of a deformed sternum.

**chondrotome** (kŏn′drō-tōm) [″ + *tome,* incision] A device for cutting cartilage.

**chondrotomy** (kŏn-drŏt′ō-mē) Dissection or surgical division of cartilage.

**chondroxiphoid** (kŏn″drō-zĭ′foyd) [″ + *xiphos,* sword, + *eidos,* form, shape] Pert. to the sternum and the xiphoid process.

**Chondrus** [L., cartilage] A genus of red algae that includes *Chondrus crispus,* the source of carrageenan, a mucilaginous substance used as an emulsifying agent. Chondrus is commonly called Irish moss or carrageen.

**choosing death** Deciding to die. In particular, an individual may choose to withdraw from chronic kidney dialysis with no medical reason for withdrawing. In one study, stopping dialysis in this situation was three times more common in patients treated at home than in those treated at dialysis centers. SEE: *death; death with dignity; do not attempt resuscitation; suicide.*

**Chopart's amputation** (shō-părz′) [François Chopart, Fr. surgeon, 1743–1795] Disarticulation at the midtarsal joint.

**chorda** (kor′dă) *pl.* **chordae** [Gr. *chorde,* cord] A cord or tendon.

***c. dorsalis*** The notochord.

***c. gubernaculum*** An embryonic structure forming a part of the gubernaculum testis in males and the round ligament in females.

***c. obliqua*** The oblique ligament, an oblique cord that connects the shafts of the radius and ulna. It extends from the lateral side of the tubercle of the ulna to a point just below the radial tuberosity.

***c. tendinea*** One of several small tendinous cords that connect the free edges of the atrioventricular valves to the papillary muscles and prevent inversion of these valves during ventricular systole.

***c. tympani*** A branch of the facial nerve that leaves the cranium through the stylomastoid foramen, traverses the tympanic cavity, and joins a branch of the lingual nerve. Efferent fibers innervate the submandibular and sublingual glands; afferent fibers convey taste impulses from the anterior two thirds of the tongue.

***c. umbilicalis*** The umbilical cord connecting the fetus and placenta.

***c. vocalis*** The vocal folds of the larynx.

***c. willisii*** One of several fibrous cords across the superior longitudinal sinus of the brain.

**chordal** (kor′dăl) Pert. to a chorda, esp. the notochord.

**Chordata** (kor-dā′tă) [LL., notochord] A phylum of the animal kingdom including all animals that have a notochord during their development (i.e., all vertebrates).

**chordee** (kor-dē′) [Fr., corded] Painful downward curvature of the penis during erection. It occurs in congenital anomaly (hypospadia) or in urethral infection such as gonorrhea. SEE: *Peyronie's disease.*

**chorditis** (kor-dī′tĭs) [Gr. *chorde,* cord, + *itis,* inflammation] Inflammation of the spermatic or vocal cord.

***c. nodosa*** The formation of small whitish nodules on one or both vocal cords in individuals who misuse the voice. Hoarseness and an inability of singers to produce the desired sounds characterize this condition. It is treated by resting the voice. Surgical removal of the nodules is necessary if they do not respond to conservative therapy. SYN: *singer's node.*

**chordoma** (kor-dō′mă) [″ + *oma,* tumor] A rare type of tumor that occurs at any place along the vertebral column. It is composed of embryonic nerve tissue and vacuolated physaliform cells. The neoplasm may cause death because of its surgical inaccessibility and the damage caused by the expanding tissue.

**chordotomy** (kor-dŏt′ō-mē) Cordotomy.

**chorea** (kō-rē′ă) [Gr. *choreia,* dance] A nervous condition marked by involuntary muscular twitching of the limbs or facial muscles. **choreal** (kō-rē′al, kō′rē-ăl), *adj.*

***acute c.*** Sydenham's chorea.

***Bergeron's c.*** Electric c.

***chronic c.*** Huntington's c.

***electric c.*** A rare form of chorea marked by sudden involuntary contraction of a muscle group. This causes violent movements as if the patient had been stimulated by an electric current. SYN: *Bergeron's c.; Dubini's disease.*

***epidemic c.*** Dancing mania; uncontrolled dancing. It was manifested in the 14th century in Europe. SYN: *dancing mania.*

***c. gravidarum*** A form of Sydenham's chorea seen in some pregnant women, usually in those who have had chorea before, esp. in their first pregnancy. SEE: *Sydenham's chorea.*

***Henoch's c.*** A form of progressive electric chorea.

***hereditary c.*** Huntington's c.

***Huntington's c.*** SEE: *Huntington's chorea.*

***hyoscine c.*** Movements simulating chorea and sometimes accompanied by delirium, seen in acute scopolamine intoxication.

***hysteric c.*** A form of hysteria with choreiform movements.

***mimetic c.*** Chorea caused by imitative movements.

***c. minor*** Sydenham's chorea.

***posthemiplegic c.*** Chorea affecting partially paralyzed muscles subsequent to a hemiplegic attack.

***senile c.*** A mild, usually benign disorder of the elderly marked by chorea-like movements but not associated with mental disorder.

**choreiform** (kō-rē′ĭ-form) [Gr. *choreia,* dance, + L. *forma,* form] Of the nature of chorea.

**choreoathetoid** (kō″rē-ō-ăth′ĕ-toyd) [″ +

*athetos,* not fixed, + *eidos,* form, shape] Pert. to choreoathetosis.

**choreoathetosis** (kō″rē-ō-ăth″ĕ-tō′sĭs) [″ + ″ + *osis,* condition] A type of athetosis frequently seen in cerebral palsy, marked by extreme range of motion, jerky involuntary movements that are more proximal than distal, and muscle tone fluctuating from hypotonia to hypertonia.

**chorioadenoma** (kō″rē-ō-ăd″ĕn-ō′mă) [Gr. *chorion,* outer membrane enclosing an embryo, + *aden,* gland, + *oma,* tumor] An adenoma of the chorion.

***c. destruens*** A type of hydatidiform mole in which the chorionic villi penetrate the myometrium.

**chorioallantois** (kō″rē-ō-ă-lăn′tō-ĭs) In embryology, the membrane formed by the union of the chorion and allantois. In the human embryo, this develops into the placenta.

**chorioamnionitis** (kō″rē-ō-ăm″nē-ō-nī′tĭs) [″ + *amnion,* lamb, + *itis,* inflammation] Inflammation of the membranes that cover the fetus.

**chorioangioma** (kō″rē-ō-ăn-jē-ō′mă) [″ + *angeion,* vessel, + *oma,* tumor] A vascular tumor of the chorion.

**choriocapillaris** (kō″rē-ō-kăp-ĭl-lā′rĭs) [Gr. *choroeides,* resembling a membrane, + L. *capillaris,* hairlike] The capillary layer of choroid.

**choriocarcinoma** (kō″rē-ō-kăr″sĭ-nō′mă) [Gr. *chorion,* + *karkinoma,* cancer] An extremely rare, very malignant neoplasm, usually of the uterus but sometimes at the site of an ectopic pregnancy. Although the actual cause is unknown, it may occur following a hydatid mole, a normal pregnancy, or an abortion. This cancer may respond dramatically to methotrexate combined with actinomycin. Complete remissions for over 10 years have been observed. SYN: *chorioepithelioma; chorionepithelioma.*

**choriocele** (kō′rē-ō-sēl) [Gr. *choroeides,* resembling a membrane, + *kele,* tumor, swelling] A protrusion of the choroid coat of the eye through a defective sclera.

**chorioepithelioma** (kō″rē-ō-ĕp″ĭ-thē″lē-ō′mă) Choriocarcinoma.

**choriogenesis** (kō″rē-ō-jĕn′ĕ-sĭs) [Gr. *chorion,* chorion, + *genesis,* generation, birth] Formation of the chorion.

**chorioid** (kō′rē-oyd) Choroid.

**choriomeningitis** (kō″rē-ō-mĕn″ĭn-jī′tĭs) [″ + *meninx,* membrane, + *itis,* inflammation] Cerebral meningitis with cellular infiltration of the meninges.

***lymphocytic c.*** An acute viral disease of the central nervous system marked by flu-like symptoms (fever, malaise, headache) sometimes followed by acute septic meningitis.

**chorion** (kō′rē-ŏn) [Gr.] An extraembryonic membrane that, in early development, forms the outer wall of the blastocyst. It is formed from the trophoblast and its inner lining of mesoderm. From it develop the chorionic villi, which establish an intimate connection with the endometrium, giving rise to the placenta. SEE: *embryo, placenta,* and *umbilical cord* for illus.; *trophoblast.* **chorionic** (kō-rē-ŏn′ĭk), *adj.*

***c. frondosum*** The outer surface of the chorion. Its villi contact the decidua basalis. This is the placental portion of the chorion.

***c. laeve*** The smooth, nonvillous portion of the chorion.

**chorionepithelioma** (kō″rē-ŏn-ĕp″ĭ-thē″lē-ō′mă) [″ + *epi,* on, + *thele,* nipple, + *oma,* tumor] Choriocarcinoma.

**chorionic plate** In the placenta, the portion of the chorion attached to the uterus.

**chorionic villi** The vascular projections from the chorion.

**chorionic villus sampling** ABBR: CVS. The procedure for obtaining a sample of the chorionic villi. In one method, a catheter is inserted into the cervix and the outer portion of the membranes surrounding the fetus. Microscopic and chemical examination of the sample is useful in prenatal evaluation of the chromosomal, enzymatic, and DNA status of the fetus. CVS should not be done before 10 weeks' gestation. The chance of having a successful pregnancy outcome is less after CVS than after amniocentesis. In addition, the accuracy of data obtained from CVS is lower than that obtained from amniocentesis.

**chorionitis** (kō″rē-ŏn-ī′tĭs) [″ + *itis,* inflammation] Inflammation of the chorion. SYN: *choroidoretinitis; retinochoroiditis.*

**chorioretinal** (kō″rē-ō-rĕt′ĭ-năl) Pert. to the choroid and retina. SYN: *retinochoroid.*

**chorioretinitis** (kō″rē-ō-rĕt″ĭn-ī′tĭs) [Gr. *chorioeides,* skinlike, + L. *rete,* network, + Gr. *itis,* inflammation] Inflammation of the choroid and retina.

**chorista** (kō-rĭs′tă) [Gr. *choristos,* separated] An error of development in which tissues grow in a displaced position. These tissues are histologically normal.

**choristoma** (kō-rĭs-tō′mă) [″ + *oma,* tumor] A neoplasm due to overdevelopment of embryonic rudiments in sites where the tissues are not normally found.

**choroid** (kō′royd) [Gr. *chorioeides,* skinlike] The dark blue vascular layer of the eye between the sclera and retina, extending from the ora serrata to the optic nerve. It consists of blood vessels united by connective tissue containing pigmented cells and contains five layers: the suprachoroid, the layer of large vessels, the layer of medium-sized vessels, the layer of capillaries, and the lamina vitrea (a homogeneous membrane next to the pigmentary layer of the retina). It is a part of the uvea or vascular tunic of the eye. SYN: *chorioid.*

**choroideremia** (kō-roy-dĕr-ē′mē-ă) [″ + *eremia,* destitution] A hereditary primary choroidal degeneration transmitted as an X-linked trait. In males, the earliest symptom is night blindness followed by constricted visual field and eventual blindness. In females, the condition is nonprogressive and vision is usually normal.

**choroiditis** (kō″royd-ī′tĭs) [″ + *itis,* inflammation] Inflammation of the choroid.

***anterior c.*** Choroiditis in which outlets of exudation are at the choroidal periphery.

***areolar c.*** Choroiditis in which inflammation spreads from around the macula lutea.

***central c.*** Choroiditis in which exudation is limited to the macula.

***diffuse c.*** Choroiditis in which the fundus is covered with spots.

***exudative c.*** Choroiditis in which the choroid is covered with patches of inflammation.

***metastatic c.*** Choroiditis due to embolism.

***suppurative c.*** Choroiditis in which suppuration occurs.

***Tay's c.*** A familial condition marked by degeneration of the choroid, esp. in the region about the macula lutea. It occurs in aged persons.

**choroidocyclitis** (kō-roy″dō-sĭk-lī′tĭs) [Gr. *chorioeides,* skinlike, + *kyklos,* a circle, + *itis,* inflammation] Inflammation of the choroid coat and ciliary processes.

**choroidoiritis** (kō-royd″ō-ī-rī′tĭs) [″ + *iris,* iris, + *itis,* inflammation] Inflammation of the choroid coat and iris.

**choroidopathy** (kō″roy-dŏp′ă-thē) [″ + *pathos,* disease, suffering] Any disease of the choroid.

**choroidoretinitis** (kō-royd″ō-rĕt″ĭn-ī′tĭs) [″ + L. *rete,* network, + Gr. *itis,* inflammation] Chorioretinitis.

**Christian Science** A system of religious teaching based on Christian Scientists' interpretation of Scripture, founded in 1866 by Mary Baker Eddy. The system emphasizes full healing of disease by mental and spiritual means because a major belief is that cause and effect are mental.

**Christian-Weber disease** SEE: *Weber-Christian disease.*

**Christmas disease** [*Christmas,* family name of the first patient with the disease who was studied] A form of hemophilia in males resulting from plasma thromboplastin component (PTC or Factor IX) deficiency. It is transmitted as an X-linked trait. SYN: *hemophilia B.*

**Christmas factor** ABBR: CF. Plasma thromboplastin component (PTC); a thromboplastin activator present in blood plasma.

**chromaffin** (krō-măf′ĭn) [Gr. *chroma,* color, + L. *affinis,* having affinity for] **1.** Staining readily with chromium salts. **2.** Denoting the pigmented cells forming the medulla of the adrenal glands and the paraganglia. SYN: *chromaphil.*

**chromaffinoma** (krō″măf-ĭ-nō′mă) [″ + ″ + Gr. *oma,* tumor] A chromaffin cell tumor. SYN: *paraganglioma.*

**chromaffinopathy** (krō″măf-ĭn-ŏp′ă-thē) [″ + ″ + Gr. *pathos,* disease] Any disease of chromaffin tissue.

**chromaffin reaction** The turning brown of cytoplasmic granules containing epinephrine when subjected to stains containing chromium salts. Such granules stain green with ferric chloride, yellow with iodine, and brown with osmic acid.

**chromaffin system** The mass of tissue forming the paraganglia and medulla of the suprarenal glands. It secretes adrenalin and stains readily with chromium salts. Similar tissue is found in the organs of Zuckerkandl and in the liver, testes, ovary, and heart. SEE: *adrenal gland.*

**chromaphil** (krō′mă-fĭl) [″ + *philein,* to love] Chromaffin.

**chromate** (krō′māt) [Gr. *chromatos,* color] A salt of chromic acid. SEE: *potassium chromate.*

**chromatic** (krō-măt′ĭk) Pert. to color.

**chromatid** (krō′mă-tĭd) One of the two potential chromosomes formed by DNA replication of each chromosome before mitosis and meiosis. They are joined together at the centromere and separate at the end of metaphase; then the new chromosomes migrate to opposite poles of the cell at anaphase.

**chromatin** (krō′mă-tĭn) [Gr. *chroma,* color] The deeply staining genetic material present in the nucleus of a cell that is not dividing. It is the largely uncoiled chromosomes, made of DNA and protein.

***sex c.*** SEE: *Barr body.*

**chromatin-negative** Lacking the sex chromatin; characteristic of nuclei in cells of normal male humans. SEE: *Barr body.*

**chromatinolysis** (krō″mă-tĭn-ŏl′ĭ-sĭs) [″ + *lysis,* dissolution] **1.** Destruction of chromatin. **2.** The emptying of a cell, bacterial or other, by lysis.

**chromatinorrhexis** (krō″mă-tĭn-or-rĕk′sĭs) [″ + *rhexis,* rupture] Splitting of chromatin.

**chromatin-positive** Having the sex chromatin (the Barr body); characteristic of nuclei in cells of normal females.

**chromatism** (krō′mă-tĭzm) [″ + *-ismos,* condition] **1.** Unnatural pigmentation. **2.** A chromatic aberration.

**chromatogenous** (krō″mă-tŏj′ĕn-ŭs) [″ + *gennan,* to produce] Causing pigmentation or color.

**chromatogram** (krō-măt′ō-grăm) [″ + *gramma,* something written] A record produced by chromatography.

**chromatography** (krō″mă-tŏg′ră-fē) [″ + *graphein,* to write] The separation of two or more chemical compounds in solution by their removal from the solution at different rates. This is done by percolating them down a column of a powdered absorbent or passing them across the surface of an absorbent paper.

***adsorption c.*** Chromatography accomplished by applying the test material to one end of a sheet or column containing a solid. As the material moves, the various constituents adhere to the surface of the particles of the solid at different distances from the starting point according to their chemical characteristics.

***column c.*** A form of adsorption chromatography in which the adsorptive material is packed into a column.

***gas c.*** An analytical technique in which a sample is separated into its component parts between a gaseous mobile phase and a chemically active stationary phase.

***gas-liquid c.*** ABBR: GLC. Chromatography in which a gas moves over a liquid, and chemical substances are separated on the liquid by their different adsorption rates.

***high-performance liquid c.*** ABBR: HPLC. Application of high pressure to liquid chromatography technique to increase separation speed and enhance resolution.

***paper c.*** Chromatography in which paper strips are used as the porous solid medium.

***partition c.*** Chromatography in which substances in solution are separated by being exposed to two immiscible solvents. The immobile solvent is located between the spaces of an inert material such as starch, cellulose, or silica. The substances move with the mobile solvent as it passes down the column at a rate governed by their partition coefficient.

***thin layer c.*** ABBR: TLC. Chromatography involving the differential adsorption of substances as they pass through a thin layer or sheet of cellulose or some other inert compound.

**chromatoid** (krō′mă-toyd) [Gr. *chroma,* color, + *eidos,* form, shape] Staining in the same manner as chromatin.

**chromatokinesis** (krō″mă-tō-kī-nē′sĭs) [″ + *kinesis,* movement] The movement of chromatin during the division of a cell.

**chromatolysis** (krō″mă-tŏl′ĭ-sĭs) [″ + *lysis,* dissolution] The dissolution of chromophil substance (Nissl bodies) in neurons in certain pathological conditions, or following injury to the cell body or axon. SYN: *chromolysis; karyolysis.*

**chromatometer** (krō-mă-tŏm′ĕt-ĕr) [″ + *metron,* measure] A scale of colors for testing color perception.

**chromatophil, chromatophilic** (krō′mă-tō-fĭl″, krō″mă-tō-fĭl′ĭk) [″ + *philein,* to love] Staining easily.

**chromatophore** (krō-măt′ō-for) [″ + *phoros,* bearing] A pigment-bearing cell.

**chromatopsia** (krō″mă-tŏp′sē-ă) [″ + *opsis,* vision] Abnormally colored vision.

**chromatoptometry** (krō″măt-ŏp-tŏm′ĕ-trē) [″ + *optos,* visible, + *metron,* measure] Measurement of color perception.

**chromatosis** (krō″mă-tō′sĭs) [″ + *osis,* condition] **1.** Pigmentation. **2.** The pathological deposition of pigment in any part of the body where it is not normally present, or excessive deposition where it is normally present.

**chromaturia** (krō-mă-tū′rē-ă) [″ + *ouron,* urine] Abnormal color of the urine.

**chromesthesia** (krō″mĕs-thē′zē-ă) [″ + *aisthesis,* sensation] The association of color sensations with words, taste, smell, or sounds.

**chromidrosis, chromhidrosis** (krō″mĭd-rō′sĭs) [″ + *hidros,* sweat] Excretion of colored sweat. Red sweat may be caused by an exudation of blood into the sweat glands or by color-producing microorganisms in those glands. This disorder is treated by relief of the underlying condition.

SYMPTOMS: Colored sweat may be localized in the eyelids, breasts, axillae, and genitocrural regions, and occasionally on the hands and limbs. It may be grayish, bluish, violaceous, brownish, or reddish; it collects on skin, giving a greasy, powdery appearance to parts.

ETIOLOGY: Colored sweat may be due to ingestion or absorption of certain substances, such as pigment-producing bacteria. It may also be caused by certain metabolic disorders.

**chromium** (krō′mē-ŭm) [L., color] SYMB: Cr. A very hard, metallic element; atomic weight 51.996, atomic number 24. It is an essential trace element required for normal glucose metabolism.

**chromium-51** A radioactive isotope of chromium. The half-life is 27.7 days. Red blood cells are labeled with this isotope in order to study their length of life in the body.

**chromium poisoning** Toxicity caused by excess chromium. It is marked by a disagreeable taste in the mouth, pain, diarrhea, collapse, and cramping. If it is fatal, death is due to uremia.

TREATMENT: Chalk, magnesia, and other weak alkalies are given to neutralize the acid effects of chromium. The stomach is washed out. Cathartics and analgesics are given for pain.

**chromoblast** (krō′mō-blăst) [Gr. *chroma,* color, + *blastos,* germ] An embryonic cell that becomes a pigment cell.

**chromocenter** (krō′mō-sĕn″tĕr) [″ + *kentros,* middle] Karyosome.

**chromocyte** (krō′mō-sīt) [″ + *kytos,* cell] Any colored cell.

**chromodacryorrhea** (krō″mō-dăk″rē-ō-rē′ă) [″ + *dacryon,* tear, + *rhoia,* flow] A flow of blood-stained tears.

**chromogen** (krō′mō-jĕn) [″ + *gennan,* to produce] Any chemical that may be changed into a colored material.

**chromogenesis** (krō″mō-jĕn′ĕ-sĭs) [″ + *genesis,* generation, birth] Production of pigment.

**chromolipoid** (krō″mō-lĭp′oyd) [″ + *lipos,* fat, + *eidos,* form, shape] Lipochrome.

**chromolysis** (krō-mŏl′ĭ-sĭs) Chromatolysis.

**chromomere** (krō′mō-mēr) [Gr. *chroma,* color, + *meros,* part] One of a series of chromatin granules found in a chromosome.

**chromomycosis** (krō″mō-mī-kō′sĭs) [″ + *myxa,* mucus, + *osis,* condition] A chronic fungal skin infection marked by itching and warty plaques on the skin and subcutaneous swellings of the feet, legs, and other exposed areas. Various fungi have been implicated, including *Phialophora verrucosa, P. pedrosoi, P. compacta,* and *Cladosporium carrionii.* Some of these are also called *Fonsecaea pedrosoi* and *F. compacta.*

**chromopexic, chromopectic** (krō″mō-pĕk′sĭk, -pĕk′tĭk) [″ + *pexis,* fixation] Pert. to fixation of coloring matter, as the liver function in forming bilirubin.

**chromophane** (krō′mō-fān) [″ + *phainein,* to show] Retinal pigment.

**chromophil(e)** (krō′mō-fĭl, -fīl) [″ + *philein,* to love] **1.** Any structure that stains easily. **2.** One of two types of cells present in the pars distalis of the pituitary gland. It is considered a secretory cell.

**chromophilic, chromophilous** (krō-mō-fĭl′ĭk, krō-mŏf′ĭl-ŭs) Staining readily.

**chromophobe** (krō′mō-fōb) [″ + *phobos,* fear] Any cell or tissue that stains either poorly or not at all. A type of cell found in the pars distalis of the pituitary gland.

**chromophobia** (krō″mō-fō′bē-ă) The condition of staining poorly. **chromophobic** (-bĭk), *adj.*

**chromophore** (krō′mō-for) [″ + *pherein,* to bear] Any chemical that displays color when present in a cell that has been prepared properly. **chromophoric** (-for′ĭk), *adj.*

**chromophose** (krō′mō-fōz) [″ + *phos,* light] A subjective sensation of a spot of color in the eye.

**chromoprotein** (krō″mō-prō′tē-ĭn) [″ + *protos,* first] One of a group of conjugated proteins consisting of a protein combined with hematin or another colored, metal-containing, prosthetic group (e.g., hemoglobin, hemocyanin, chlorophyll, flavoproteins, cytochromes).

**chromosomal map** SEE: *gene map.*

**chromosome** (krō′mō-sōm) [Gr. *chroma,* color, + *soma,* body] A linear thread made of DNA (and proteins in eukaryotic cells) in the nucleus of a cell. Chromosomes stain deeply with basic dyes and are esp. conspicuous during mitosis. The DNA is the genetic code of the cell; specific sequences of DNA nucleotides are the genes for the cell's particular proteins (the DNA in a cell contains all the genes for the organism, but only those needed for a particular cell will be active). The normal number of chromosomes, the diploid number, is constant for each species. For humans, the diploid number is 46 (23 pairs in all somatic cells). In the formation of the gametes (ovum and spermatozoon), the number is reduced to one half (haploid number); that is, the ovum and sperm each contain 23, or one of each pair. Of these, 22 are autosomes and one is the sex chromosome (X or Y). At fertilization, the chromosomes from the sperm unite with the chromosomes from the ovum. This random union determines the sex of the embryo. The female sex chromosome from the ovum always contributes an X to the embryo. The male sex chromosome may contribute an X or a Y to join with the chromosome derived from the ovum. Thus the embryo may have an XX pair of sex chromosomes, which will produce a girl, or an XY pair, which will produce a boy. SEE: illus.; *Barr body; gene; heredity; karyotype.*

***accessory c.*** An unpaired sex chromosome. SEE: *sex chromosome.*

***banded c.*** A chromosome specially stained to delineate bands of various width on its regions or loci. This technique facilitates analysis and investigation.

***bivalent c.*** A double chromosome resulting from the conjugation of two homologous chromosomes in synapsis, which occurs during the first meiotic division.

***giant c.*** Any of the extremely large chromosomes found in the salivary glands and other organs and tissues of insects.

***homologous c.*** One of a pair of chromosomes that contain genes for the same traits; one is maternal in origin, the other paternal.

***Philadelphia c., Ph¹ c.*** An abnormal chromosome 22 in which there is translocation of the distal portion of its long arm to chromosome 9. It is found in leukocyte cultures of many patients with chronic myelocytic leukemia. The Philadelphia chromosome was the first chromosomal change found to be characteristic of a human disease.

***sex c.*** One of two chromosomes, the X and Y chromosomes, that determine sex in humans and that carry the genes for sex-linked characteristics.

***somatic c.*** An autosome.

***X c.*** One of the sex chromosomes; women have two (XX) present in all somatic cells, and men have one (XY). Characteristics transmitted on the X chromosome are said to be X-linked or sex-linked.

***Y c.*** The male-determining member of a pair of human chromosomes (XY) present in the somatic cells of all male humans.

**chromotherapy** (krō″mō-thĕr′ă-pē) [Gr. *chroma,* color, + *therapeia,* treatment] The use of colored light in the treatment of disease.

**chromotrichia** (krō″mō-trĭk′ē-ă) [″ + *thrix,* hair] Coloration of the hair.

**chromotropic** (krō″mō-trŏp′ĭk) [″ + *tropikos,* turning] **1.** Being attracted to color. **2.** Attracting color.

**chronaxie** (krō′năk-sē) [Gr. *chronos,* time, + *axia,* value] A number expressing the sensitivity of a nerve to electrical stimulation. It is the minimum duration, in mil-

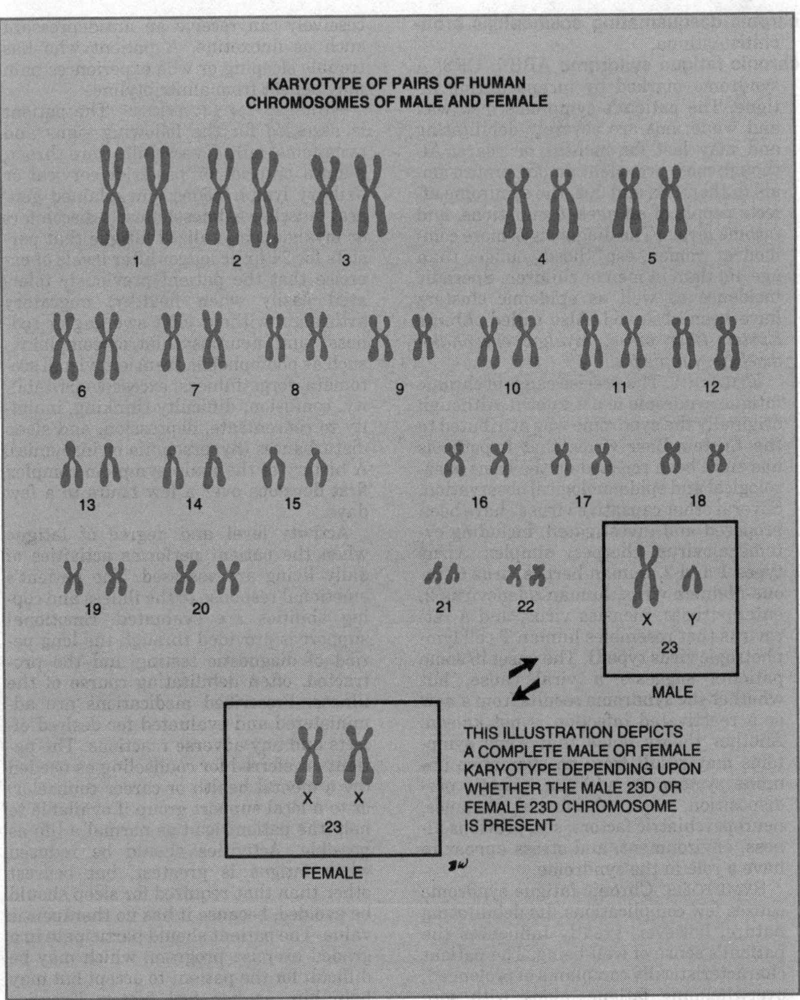


liseconds, during which a current of prescribed strength must pass through a motor nerve to cause contraction in the associated muscle. The strength of direct current (rheobasic voltage) that will just suffice if given an indefinite time is first determined, and exactly double this strength is used for the final determinations.

**chronic** [Gr. *chronos,* time] **1.** Of long duration. **2.** Denoting a disease showing little change or of slow progression; the opposite of acute.

**chronic airflow limitation** ABBR: CAL. Newer term for chronic lung disease. SEE: *chronic obstructive pulmonary disease.*

**chronically neurologically impaired** ABBR: CNI. Having a general level of intellectual function that is significantly below average and exists concurrently with deficits in adaptive behavior. These behavioral changes must have been manifested during the developmental period. This condition is often referred to as mental retardation, but the concept is broader. Chronologically neurologically impaired persons are often grouped epidemiologically with persons who have other developmental disabilities including chronic epilepsy, autism, and cerebral palsy.

**chronic bacterial prostatitis** ABBR: CBP. Inflammation of the prostate due to long-standing bacterial infection. Clinical symptoms of fever, pain, and dysuria may be relatively mild as compared with acute infection. Therapy depends on the causative organism and in addition to antibiotics may involve treatment of prostatic hypertrophy.

**chronic desquamating eosinophilic bronchitis** Asthma.

**chronic fatigue syndrome** ABBR: CFS. A syndrome marked by incapacitating fatigue. The patient's symptoms may wax and wane, but are severely debilitating and may last for months or years. Although most prevalent among professionals in their 20s and 30s, the syndrome affects people of all ages, occupations, and income levels. The diagnosis is more common in women, esp. those younger than age 45, than in men or children. Sporadic incidence as well as epidemic clusters have been observed. Also called *chronic Epstein-Barr virus, myalgic encephalomyelitis, yuppie flu*.

ETIOLOGY: The precise cause of chronic fatigue syndrome is not known. Although originally the syndrome was attributed to the Epstein-Barr virus, that hypothesis has since been rejected on the basis of serological and epidemiological observation. Several other causative viruses have been proposed and investigated, including cytomegalovirus, herpes simplex virus types 1 and 2, human herpes virus 6, Inoue-Melnick virus, human adenovirus 2, enteroviruses, measles virus, and a retrovirus that resembles human T-cell lymphotropic virus type II. The onset in some patients suggests a viral cause, but whether the syndrome results from a new or a reactivated infection is not known. Another theory holds that some symptoms may result from an overactive immune system. In addition, genetic predisposition, age, hormonal balance, neuropsychiatric factors, sex, previous illness, environment, and stress appear to have a role in the syndrome.

SYMPTOMS: Chronic fatigue syndrome causes few complications. Its debilitating nature, however, greatly influences the patient's sense of well-being. The patient characteristically complains of prolonged, overwhelming fatigue, along with sore throat, myalgia, and cognitive dysfunction. No definitive test exists for this disorder. Diagnostic studies should include tests to rule out other similar clinical pictures.

TREATMENT: Polyribonucleotide, an investigational antiviral agent and immunomodulator, is in clinical trials as a treatment for this disorder. Acyclovir, intravenous immune globulin, and intramuscular magnesium sulfate also have been studied, but acyclovir has been found no better than a placebo. The role of immune globulin remains unclear after two clinical trials that yielded contradictory results. Intramuscular magnesium sulfate can improve the patient's energy and emotional state and relieve pain. Treatment focuses on supportive care. The patient with myalgia or arthralgia can benefit from nonsteroidal anti-inflammatory drugs. A patient who sleeps excessively can receive an antidepressant such as fluoxetine. A patient who has trouble sleeping or who experiences pain may benefit from amitriptyline.

NURSING IMPLICATIONS: The patient is assessed for the following signs and symptoms: mild fever; chills; sore throat; painful anterior or posterior cervical or axillary lymph nodes; unexplained general muscle weakness; muscle discomfort or myalgia; generalized fatigue that persists for 24 hr or longer after levels of exercise that the patient previously tolerated easily when healthy; migratory arthralgia without joint swelling or redness; and neuropsychiatric complaints such as photophobia, transient visual scotomata, forgetfulness, excessive irritability, confusion, difficulty thinking, inability to concentrate, depression, and sleep disturbances (hypersomnia or insomnia). A history of the main symptom complex first develops over a few hours to a few days.

Activity level and degree of fatigue when the patient performs activities of daily living are assessed. The patient's emotional response to the illness and coping abilities are evaluated. Emotional support is provided through the long period of diagnostic testing and the protracted, often debilitating course of the illness. Prescribed medications are administered and evaluated for desired effects and any adverse reactions. The patient is referred for counseling as needed (by a mental health or career counselor) or to a local support group if available to help the patient lead as normal a life as possible. Activities should be reduced when fatigue is greatest, but bedrest other than that required for sleep should be avoided, because it has no therapeutic value. The patient should participate in a graded exercise program, which may be difficult for the patient to accept but may help him or her feel better. Exercise should be carried out for short periods and slowly increased to avoid increasing fatigue.

Desired outcomes include maintenance of normal muscle mass and strength and joint range of motion; expression of a willingness to maximize activity as tolerated; performance of self-care activities as tolerated; identification and incorporation of activities that modify fatigue into daily routine; restoration of a normal energy level; verbalization of feelings related to self-esteem; and steps to achieve a higher level of physical and emotional wellness.

**chronic granulomatous disease** A congenital disease marked by polymorphonuclear leukocytes that are able to ingest but not kill certain bacteria. It occurs mostly in children. Twenty percent of reported cases are in girls. Evidence for X-linked (i.e., sex-linked) inheritance is present in most boys but not girls with the disease. Female carriers rarely experience severe bacterial infections. Death is due to chronic and recurrent infections. SEE: *nitroblue tetrazolium test.*

TREATMENT: There is no specific therapy. Prolonged antibiotic therapy helps prevent infection. Bone marrow transplantation has been tried experimentally.

**chronicity** (krŏn-ĭs′ĭt-ē) The condition of being long lasting or of showing little or slow progress.

**chronic obstructive pulmonary disease** ABBR: COPD. A disease process that decreases the ability of the lungs to perform ventilation. Diagnostic criteria include a history of persistent dyspnea on exertion, with or without chronic cough, and less than half of normal predicted maximum breathing capacity. Diseases that cause this condition are chronic bronchitis, pulmonary emphysema, chronic asthma, and chronic bronchiolitis. Also called *chronic obstructive lung disease.* SEE: *emphysema; Nursing Diagnoses Appendix.*

**chrono-** [Gr. *chronos,* time] Combining form indicating a relationship to time or timing.

**chronobiology** (krŏn″ō-bī-ŏl′ō-jē) [Gr. *chronos,* time, + *bios,* life, + *logos,* word, reason] The study of the timing characteristics of life processes to describe the factors that influence biological rhythms; the influence of biological rhythms on life processes. SEE: *circadian; clock, biological.*

**chronognosis** (krŏn″ŏg-nō′sĭs) [″ + *gnosis,* knowledge] The subjective realization of the passage of time.

**chronograph** (krŏn′ō-grăf) [″ + *graphein,* to write] A device for recording intervals of time.

**chronological** (krŏn″ō-lŏj′ĭ-kăl) [″ + *logos,* word, reason] Occurring in natural sequence according to time.

**chronopharmacology** A method used in pharmacokinetics to describe the diurnal changes in plasma drug concentrations.

**chronophobia** Fear of time or its perceived duration, esp. in prisoners.

**chronotaraxis** (krō-nō-tăr-ăk′sĭs) [″ + *taraxis,* without order] Inability to orient oneself with respect to time.

**chronotropic** (krŏn″ō-trŏp′ĭk) [″ + *tropikos,* turning] Influencing the rate of occurrence of an event, such as the heartbeat. SEE: *inotropic.*

**chronotropism** [″ + ″ + *-ismos,* condition] Interference with periodic events such as the heartbeat.

***negative c.*** Deceleration of the rate of an event such as the heartbeat.

***positive c.*** Acceleration of the rate of an event such as the heartbeat.

**chrysarobin** (krĭs″ă-rō′bĭn) [Gr. *chrysos,* gold, + Brazilian *araraba,* bark] A mixture of neutral principles obtained from goa powder, which is deposited in the wood of Araroba, a leguminous tree of South America. It is used topically as an ointment for treatment of certain skin disorders.

**chrysiasis** (krĭ-sī′ă-sĭs) **1.** Gray patches of skin discoloration after therapeutic administration of gold. **2.** Deposition of gold in tissues. SYN: *auriasis.*

**chrysoderma** (krĭs″ō-dĕr′mă) [″ + *derma,* skin] Discoloration of the skin due to deposition of gold.

**chrysotherapy** (krĭs″ō-thĕr′ă-pē) [″ + *therapeia,* treatment] The medical use of gold compounds. They are still used in treating rheumatoid arthritis.

**Chvostek's sign** (vōs′tĕks) [Franz Chvostek, Austrian surgeon, 1835–1884] A spasm of the facial muscles following a tap on one side of the face over the facial nerve; seen in tetany.

**chylangioma** (kī″lăn-jē-ō′mă) [Gr. *chylos,* juice, + *angeion,* vessel, + *oma,* tumor] A tumor of the intestinal lymph vessels containing chyle.

**chyle** (kīl) [Gr. *chylos,* juice] The milklike, alkaline contents of the lacteals and lymphatic vessels of the intestine, consisting of digestive products and principally absorbed fats. It is carried by the lymphatic vessels to the cisterna chyli, then through the thoracic duct to the left subclavian vein, where it enters the bloodstream. A large amount forms in 24 hr.

**chylemia** (kī-lē′mē-ă) [″ + *haima,* blood] Chyle in the peripheral circulation.

**chylifacient, chylifactive** (kī″lĭ-fā′shĕnt, kī-lĭ-făk′tĭv) [″ + L. *facere,* to make] Forming chyle.

**chylifaction, chylification** (kī-lĭ-făk′shŭn, kī-lĭ-fĭ-kā′shŭn) Chylopoiesis.

**chyliferous** (kī-lĭf′ĕr-ŭs) [″ + L. *ferre,* to carry] Carrying chyle.

**chyliform** (kī′lĭ-form) [″ + L. *forma,* shape] Resembling chyle.

**chylocele** (kī′lō-sēl) [″ + *kele,* tumor, swelling] Distention of the tunica vaginalis testis with chyle.

**chyloderma** (kī″lō-dĕr′mă) [″ + *derma,* skin] Lymph accumulated in the enlarged lymphatic vessels and thickened skin of the scrotum. SYN: *elephantiasis, scrotal.*

**chylomediastinum** (kī″lō-mē″dē-ăs-tī′nŭm) [″ + L. *mediastinum,* median] Chyle in the mediastinum.

**chylomicron** (kī″lō-mī′krŏn) [″ + *mikros,* small] A lipoprotein molecule formed in the small intestine from digested fats for transport of fats to other tissues.

**chylopericardium** (kī″lō-pĕr″ĭ-kăr′dē-ŭm) [″ + L. *peri,* around, + Gr. *kardia,* heart] Chyle in the pericardium.

**chyloperitoneum** (kī″lō-pĕr″ĭ-tō-nē′ŭm) [″ + *peritonaion,* peritoneum] Chyle in the peritoneal cavity.

**chylopneumothorax** (kī″lō-nū″mō-thō′răks) [″ + *pneumon,* air, + *thorax,* chest] Chyle and air in the pleural space.

**chylopoiesis** (kī″lō-poy-ē′sĭs) [″ + *poiesis,* production] Formation of chyle and its absorption by lacteals in the intestines. SYN: *chylifaction; chylification.*

**chylorrhea** (kī″lō-rē′ă) [Gr. *chylos,* juice, + *rhoia,* flow] Escape of chyle resulting from rupture of the thoracic duct.
**chylothorax** [″ + *thorax,* chest] Chyle in the pleural cavities.
**chylous** (kī′lŭs) Pert. to or of the nature of chyle.
**chyluria** (kī-lū′rē-ă) [″ + *ouron,* urine] The presence of chyle in the urine, giving it a milky appearance. SYN: *galacturia.*
**chymase** (kī′mās) An enzyme in gastric juice that accelerates the action of the pancreatic enzymes.
**chyme** (kīm) [Gr. *chymos,* juice] The mixture of partly digested food and digestive secretions found in the stomach and small intestine during digestion of a meal. It is a varicolored, thick, nearly liquid mass.
**chymopapain** (kī-mō-pă′pā-ĭn) An enzyme related to papain.
**chymosin** (kī′mō-sĭn) [Gr. *chymos,* juice] An enzyme that curdles milk; present in the gastric juice of young ruminants. It is the preferred term for rennin owing to possible confusion with renin.
**chymotrypsin** (kī″mō-trĭp′sĭn) [″ + *tryein,* to rub, + *pepsis,* digestion] A digestive enzyme produced by the pancreas and functioning in the small intestine that, with trypsin, hydrolyzes proteins to peptones or further. It is secreted by the pancreas. Trade names are Avazyme and Enzeon.
**C.I.** *chemotherapeutic index* (parasitology); *color index.*
**Ci** *curie.*
**cib** Abbreviation for L. *cibus,* food.
**cibophobia** (sī″bō-fō′bē-ă) [L. *cibus,* food, + Gr. *phobos,* fear] A morbid aversion to or fear of food.
**cicatricotomy** (sĭk″ă-trĭk-ŏt′ō-mē) [″ + Gr. *tome,* incision] Incision of a cicatrix or scar.
**cicatrix** (sĭk′ă-trĭks, sĭk-ā′trĭks) [L.] A scar left by a healed wound. Lack of color is due to an absence of pigmentation. Cicatricial tissue is less elastic than normal tissue, so it usually appears contracted. **cicatricial**(-trĭsh′ăl), *adj.* SEE: *keloid.*
**cicatrizant** (sĭk-ăt′rĭ-zănt) [L. *cicatrix,* scar] Favoring or causing cicatrization; an agent that aids in scar formation.
**cicatrization** (sĭk″ă-trĭ-zā′shŭn) Healing by scar formation. SEE: *intention.*
**cicatrize** (sĭk′ă-trīz) To heal by scar tissue.
**cicutism** (sĭk′ū-tĭzm) Poisoning resulting from ingestion of *Cicuta maculata* or *C. virosa,* water hemlock.
**Cieszynski's rule** A geometric theorem stating that two triangles are equal if they share one complete side and have two equal angles. In dental radiography, the theorem is applied in the bisecting angle technique to guide film placement and angulation of the central beam of the x-ray. The resulting image on the radiograph is the same length as the projected object. SEE: *technique, bisecting angle.*
**ciguatera poisoning** (sē″gwă-tā′ră) [Sp. Amer. from W. Indies *cigua,* sea snail] A

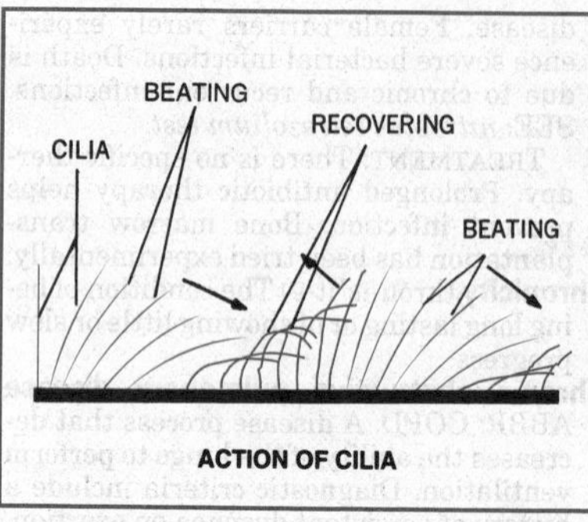

ACTION OF CILIA

form of fish poisoning caused by eating fish normally considered safe to eat, such as sea bass, grouper, or snapper. The fish become toxic after ingesting certain dinoflagellates, marine plankton that are the source of toxin. Clinically there is tingling about the lips, tongue, and throat with nausea, vomiting, diarrhea, weakness, and numbness. There is no specific therapy but treatment of respiratory paralysis may be required. Intravenous mannitol has been reported to be effective. Gastric lavage is indicated if vomiting has not occurred. Mortality is less than 10%.
**ciguatoxin** (sē″gwă-tŏk′sĭn) The toxic substance that causes ciguatera poisoning. The structure is unknown, but the toxin interferes with nerve impulse transmission.
**cilia** (sĭl′ē-ă) *sing.,* **cilium** [L. eyelid] **1.** Eyelashes. **2.** Threadlike projections from the free surface of certain epithelial cells such as those lining the trachea, bronchi, and some reproductive ducts (e.g., the fallopian tubes). They propel or sweep materials, such as mucus or dust, across a surface, such as the respiratory tract. SEE: illus.

***immotile c. syndrome*** A group of inherited conditions characterized by immotility of the cilia (or in the case of sperm the flagellum) of the respiratory tract epithelium, sperm, and other cells. Sperm flagella and respiratory tract cilia lack the protein dynein, essential to cilia movement. SYN: *Kartagener's syndrome.*
**ciliariscope** (sĭl″ē-ă′rĭ-skōp) [L. *ciliaris,* pert. to eyelid, + Gr. *skopein,* to examine] An instrument for examining the ciliary region of the eye.
**ciliarotomy** (sĭl″ē-ă-rŏt′ō-mē) [″ + Gr. *tome,* incision] Surgical section of the ciliary zone in glaucoma.
**ciliary** (sĭl′ē-ĕr″ē) [L. *ciliaris,* pert. to eyelid] Pertaining to any hairlike processes, esp. the eyelashes, and to eye structures such as the ciliary body.
**ciliary apparatus** A ciliary body.
**ciliary artery** Any of the branches of the ophthalmic artery that supply the choroid layer.

**ciliary glands** SEE: *Moll's glands.*

**ciliary muscle** The smooth muscle forming a part of the ciliary body of the eye. Contraction pulls the choroid forward, lessening tension on the fibers of the zonula (suspensory ligament) and allowing the lens, which is elastic, to become more spherical. Accommodation for near vision is accomplished by this process.

**ciliary nerve, long** One of the two or three branches of the nasal nerves supplying the ciliary muscle, iris, and cornea.

**ciliary nerve, short** One of the several branches of the ciliary ganglion supplying the ciliary muscle, iris, and tunics of the eyeball.

**Ciliata** (sĭl″ē-ā′tă) Formerly a class of protozoa characterized by locomotion by cilia. Now called Ciliophora, a phylum of the kingdom Protista.

**ciliate** (sĭl′ē-āt) [L. *cilia,* eyelids] Ciliated.

**ciliated** (sĭl′ē-ā-tĕd) Possessing cilia.

**ciliated epithelium** Epithelium with hairlike processes on the surface that wave actively only in one direction. This type is present in the respiratory tract and fallopian tubes.

**ciliectomy** (sĭl″ē-ĕk′tō-mē) [″ + Gr. *ektome,* excision] Excision of a portion of the ciliary body or ciliary border of the eyelid.

**ciliogenesis** (sĭl″ē-ō-jĕn′ĕ-sĭs) Formation of cilia.

**Ciliophora** A phylum of the kingdom Protista that includes unicellular and colonial forms possessing cilia for locomotion. Some are free living and others are parasitic species such as *Balantidium coli.*

**ciliospinal** (sĭl″ē-ō-spī′năl) [″ + *spinalis,* pert. to a spine] Pert. to the ciliary body and spinal cord.

**ciliostatic** (sĭl″ē-ō-stăt′ĭk) [″ + Gr. *statos,* placed] Interfering with or preventing movement of the cilia.

**ciliotomy** (sĭl″ē-ŏt′ō-mē) [″ + Gr. *tome,* incision] Surgical cutting of the ciliary nerve.

**ciliotoxicity** The action of anything that interferes with ciliary motion.

**cilium** (sĭl′ē-ŭm) [L.] Sing. of cilia.

**cillosis** (sĭl-ō′sĭs) [L.] Spasmodic twitching of the eyelid.

**cimbia** (sĭm′bē-ă) [L.] A slender band of white fibers crossing the ventral surface of a cerebral peduncle.

**cimetidine** A histamine $H_2$ receptor antagonist that represents a new class of pharmacological agents. It inhibits gastric secretions and is indicated for treatment of gastric and duodenal ulcers. Trade name is Tagamet. SEE: *peptic ulcer.*

**Cimex lectularius** (sī′mĕks lĕk-tū-lā′rē-ŭs) The bedbug. An insect belonging to the order Hemiptera. SYN: *Acanthia lectularia.* SEE: *bedbug.*

**cimicosis** (sĭm″ĭ-kō′sĭs) Itching due to the bite of a bedbug.

**CIN** *cervical intraepithelial neoplasia.*

**CINAHL** *Cumulative Index to Nursing and Allied Health Literature,* an index of literature related to nursing and allied health. The index is available in electronic form from 1982 on.

**CINAHL-CD** A computer-accessible index to nursing and allied health literature. SEE: *CINAHL.*

**cinchona** (sĭn-kō′nă, -chō′nă) [Sp. *cinchon,* Countess of Cinchon] The dried bark of the tree cinchona, the source of quinine. SEE: *quinine.*

**cinchonism** (sĭn′kŏn-ĭzm) [″ + Gr. *-ismos,* condition] Poisoning from cinchona or its alkaloids. SYN: *quininism.*

**cinclisis** (sĭn′klĭ-sĭs) [Gr. *kinklisis,* a wagging] Swift spasmodic movement of any part of the body.

**cine-** [Gr. *kinesis,* movement] Combining form indicating a relationship to movement.

**cineangiocardiography** (sĭn″ē-ăn″jē-ō-kăr″dē-ŏg′ră-fē) [Gr. *kinesis,* movement, + *angeion,* vessel, + *kardia,* heart, + *graphein,* to write] Cinefluorographic 35-mm imaging of the heart chambers or coronary vessels after injection of a radiopaque contrast medium. SEE: *cardiac catheterization.*

***radionuclide c.*** The use of a scintillation camera to record and project the image of a radioisotope as it travels through the heart and great vessels.

**cinecystourethrogram** (sĭn-ĕ-sĭs″tō-ū-rē′thrō-grăm) A radiographic motion picture record of the urinary bladder and urethra when they have been filled with and are eliminating a radiopaque contrast medium.

**cinefluorography** (sĭn″ĕ-floo″or-ŏg′ră-fē) The production of moving images during image-intensified fluoroscopy.

**cinematics** (sĭn″ĕ-măt′ĭks) [Gr. *kinema,* motion] The science of motion; kinematics.

**cinematoradiography** (sĭn″ĕ-măt-ō-rā″dē-ŏg′ră-fē) [″ + L. *radius,* ray, + Gr. *graphein,* to write] Radiography of an organ in motion.

**cinemicrography** (sĭn″ĕ-mī-krŏg′ră-fē) [Gr. *kinesis,* movement, + *mikros,* small, + *graphein,* to write] A motion picture record of an object seen through a microscope.

**cineplastics** (sĭn″ĕ-plăs′tĭks) [″ + *plassein,* to form] The arrangement of muscles and tendons in a stump after amputation so that it is possible to impart motion and direction to an artificial limb.

**cineradiography** (sĭn″ĕ-rā″dē-ŏg′ră-fē) [″ + L. *radius,* ray, + Gr. *graphein,* to write] A motion picture record of images produced during fluoroscopic examination.

**cinerea** (sĭn-ē′rē-ă) [L. *cinereus,* ashen-hued] Gray matter of the brain or spinal cord. **cinereal** (-ăl), *adj.*

**cineurography** (sĭn″ĕ-ū-rŏg′ră-fē) [″ + *ouron,* urine, + *graphein,* to write] The use of cineradiography to obtain motion pictures of the urinary tract.

**cingulotomy** (sĭn′gū-lŏt″ō-mē) [L. *cingulum,* girdle, + Gr. *tome,* incision] Surgical excision of the anterior half of the cingulate gyrus of the brain. It may be done to alleviate intractable pain.

**cingulum** (sĭn′gū-lŭm) *pl.* **cingula** [L., girdle] **1.** A band of association fibers in the cingulate gyrus extending from the anterior perforated substance posteriorly to the hippocampal gyrus. **2.** A convexity on the cervical third of the lingual aspect of incisors and canines. SYN: *basal ridge.*

**cinnamic acid** A white insoluble powder derived from cinnamon. It is used as a flavoring agent in cooking and in the preparation of perfumes and medicines.

**cinnamon** A volatile oil derived from the bark of *Cinnamomum zeylanicum.* It is used as a flavoring agent in cooking and in preparing pharmaceutical products.

**circa** (sĭr′kă) [L.] ABBR: c. About; used before dates or figures that are approximate.

**circadian** (sĭr″kă-dē′ăn, sĭr-kā′dē-ăn) [L. *circa,* about, + *dies,* day] Pert. to events that occur at approx. 24-hr intervals, such as certain physiological phenomena. SEE: *desynchronosis; night work, maladaption to.*

**circinate** (sĕr′sĭ-nāt) [L. *circinatus,* made round] Circular.

**circle** [L. *circulus,* a little ring] Any ring-shaped structure.

***c. of diffusion*** One or more circles on the projection plane of an image not in focus of the lens of the eye.

***c. of Willis*** SEE: *Willis' circle.*

**Circ-O-Lectric bed** A bed that allows the patient's position to be changed from supine to prone by rotating the bed through 180° by electromechanical rotation.

**circuit** (sĕr′kĭt) [L. *circuire,* to go around] **1.** The course or path of an electric current. **2.** The path followed by a fluid circulating in a system of tubes or cavities. **3.** The path followed by nerve impulses in a reflex arc from sensory receptor to effector organ.

***ventilator c.*** The external or internal pneumatic delivery component of a mechanical ventilator.

**circular** [L. *circularis*] **1.** Shaped like a circle. **2.** Recurrent.

**circulation** [L. *circulatio*] Movement in a regular or circular course.

***bile salt c.*** Circulation of the sodium glycocholate and taurocholate found in hepatic bile. They pass with the bile into the duodenum and then into the intestine, where they are absorbed along with the fats.

***blood c.*** Circulation in which the blood leaving the left ventricle enters the aorta, from which it is pumped into the various large arteries. It reaches the coronary arteries of the heart itself and the arteries of the head, body wall, abdominal viscera, and extremities. It passes through the various capillary systems into the veins, which have two collecting systems: (1) Most veins empty their blood into the superior and inferior venae cavae. (2) The veins from the stomach, pancreas, spleen, and intestine unite to form the portal vein, which runs to the liver. In the liver, it breaks up into a new capillary system, which drains through the hepatic veins into the vena cava inferior. The combined blood of the venae cavae and the coronary veins enters the right atrium, passes through the right ventricle, and is forced out into the pulmonary artery. The pulmonary capillary system drains through the pulmonary veins into the left atrium and thence into the left ventricle.

***collateral c.*** Circulation established through an anastomosis between two vessels supplying or draining two adjacent vascular areas. This enables blood to bypass an obstruction in the larger vessel that supplies or drains both areas, or enables blood to flow to or from a tissue when the principal vessel involved is obstructed.

***coronary c.*** Circulation through the muscular tissue of the heart. Blood leaves the aorta through the right and left coronary arteries, which supply the myocardium. Blood passes through capillaries and is collected in veins, most of which empty into the coronary sinus, which opens into the right atrium. A few of the small veins open directly into the atria and ventricles. SEE: illus.

***enterohepatic c.*** Circulation in which substances excreted by the liver pass into the intestines where some are absorbed into the bloodstream and returned to the liver and re-excreted. Bile and bile salts follow this pathway.

***extracorporeal c.*** Circulation of blood outside the body. This may be through an artificial kidney or a heart-lung device.

***fetal c.*** Circulation through the fetus. Blood, oxygenated in the placenta, passes through the umbilical vein and ductus venosus to the inferior vena cava and thence to the right atrium of the fetus. From there it may follow one of two courses—through the foramen ovale to the left atrium and then through the aorta to the tissues; or through the right ventricle, pulmonary artery, and ductus arteriosus to the aorta and then to the tissues. In either case the blood bypasses the lungs, which do not function before birth. Blood is returned to the placenta through the umbilical arteries, which are continuations of the hypogastric arteries. At birth or shortly after, the ductus arteriosus and the foramen ovale close, establishing normal circulation. Failure of either to occur may produce a blue baby. SEE: *fetal circulation* for illus.; *ductus arteriosus, patent.*

***lymph c.*** The flow of lymph from the tissues into the lymphatic collecting system. Lymph is formed from the tissue fluid that fills the tissue spaces of the body. It is collected into lymph capillaries, which carry the lymph to the larger lymph vessels. These converge to form one of two main trunks, the right lymphatic duct and the thoracic duct. The right lymphatic duct drains the right side of the head, neck, and trunk and the right upper extremity; the thoracic duct drains the rest of the body. The thoracic duct originates at the cisterna chyli, which receives the lymphatics from the abdominal organs. It courses upward through the diaphragm and thorax and empties into the left subclavian artery near its junction with the left interior jugular vein. The right lymphatic duct empties into the right subclavian vein. Along the course of lymph vessels are lymph nodes, which remove bacteria and other foreign materi-

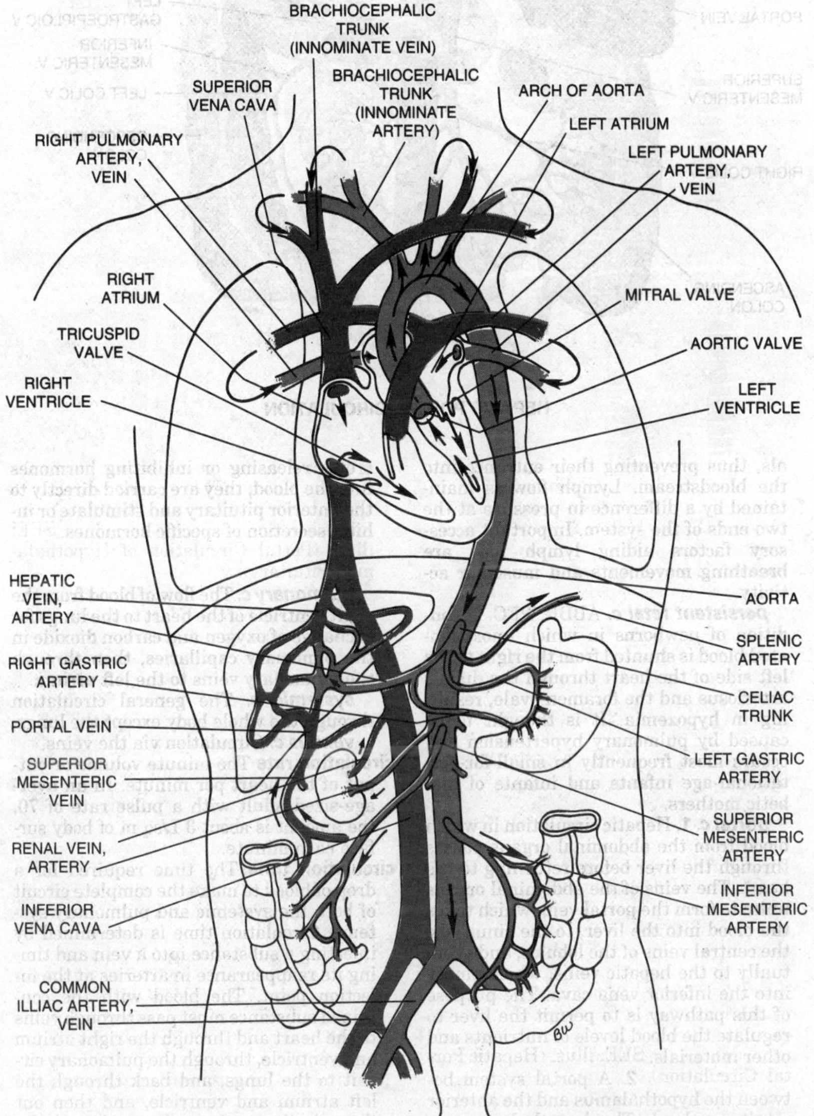

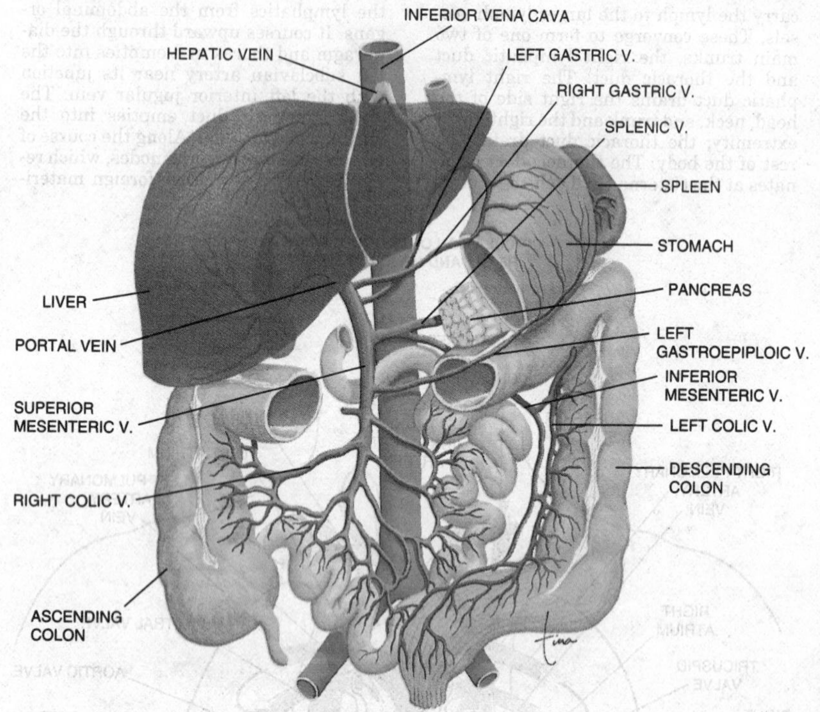


**HEPATIC PORTAL CIRCULATION**

als, thus preventing their entrance into the bloodstream. Lymph flow is maintained by a difference in pressure at the two ends of the system. Important accessory factors aiding lymph flow are breathing movements and muscular activity.

***persistent fetal c.*** ABBR: PFC. A condition of newborns in which unoxygenated blood is shunted from the right to the left side of the heart through the ductus arteriosus and the foramen ovale, resulting in hypoxemia. It is thought to be caused by pulmonary hypertension and occurs most frequently in small-for-gestational-age infants and infants of diabetic mothers.

***portal c.*** **1.** Hepatic circulation in which blood from the abdominal organs passes through the liver before returning to the heart. The veins of the abdominal organs unite to form the portal vein, which takes the blood into the liver, to the sinusoids, the central veins of the lobules, and eventually to the hepatic veins, which empty into the inferior vena cava. The purpose of this pathway is to permit the liver to regulate the blood levels of nutrients and other materials. SEE: illus. (Hepatic Portal Circulation). **2.** A portal system between the hypothalamus and the anterior pituitary gland. The hypothalamus secretes releasing or inhibiting hormones into the blood; they are carried directly to the anterior pituitary and stimulate or inhibit secretion of specific hormones. SEE: illus. (Portal Circulation of Hypothalamus-Pituitary).

***pulmonary c.*** The flow of blood from the right ventricle of the heart to the lungs for exchange of oxygen and carbon dioxide in the pumonary capillaries, then through the pulmonary veins to the left atrium.

***systemic c.*** The general circulation through the whole body except the lungs.

***venous c.*** Circulation via the veins.

**circulation rate** The minute volume or output of the heart per minute. In an average-sized adult with a pulse rate of 70, the amount is about 3 L/sq m of body surface each minute.

**circulation time** The time required for a drop of blood to make the complete circuit of both the systemic and pulmonary systems. Circulation time is determined by injecting a substance into a vein and timing its reappearance in arteries at the injection point. The blood with the contained substance must pass through veins to the heart and through the right atrium and ventricle, through the pulmonary circuit to the lungs, and back through the left atrium and ventricle, and then out through the aorta and arteries to the

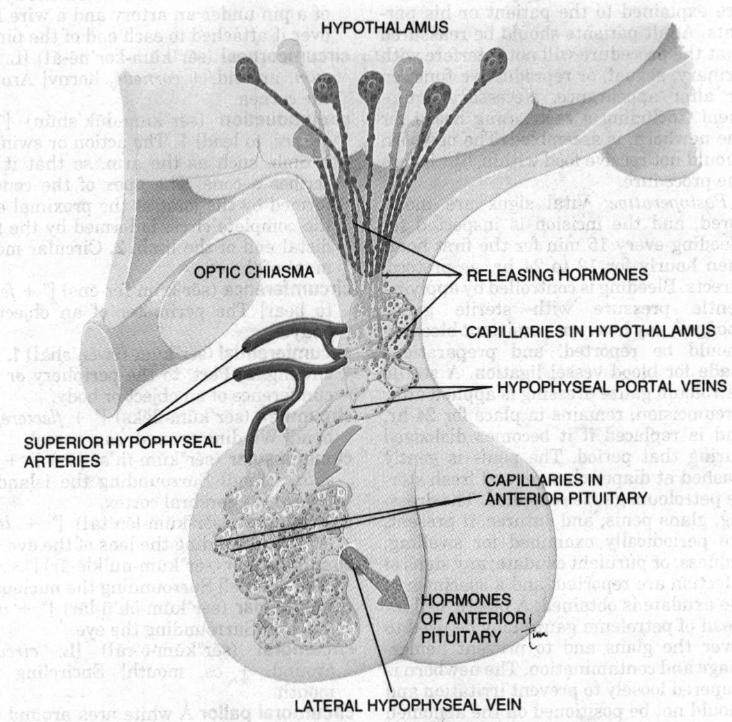

PORTAL CIRCULATION OF HYPOTHALAMUS-PITUITARY

place of detection. Dyes such as fluorescein and methylene blue and substances such as potassium ferrocyanide and histamine have been used as tracers. Average circulation time is 18 to 24 sec.

Circulation time is reduced in anemia and hyperthyroidism and is increased in hypertension, myxedema, and cardiac failure. Circulation time may also be measured by injecting into a vein a substance that can be tasted when it is transported to the tongue. The normal circulation time from an arm vein to the tongue is 10 to 16 sec. In the aorta, the blood flows at a speed of approx. 30 cm/sec.

**circulatory** Pert. to circulation.

**circulatory failure** Failure of the cardiovascular system to provide body tissues with enough blood for proper functioning. It may be caused by cardiac failure or peripheral circulatory failure, as occurs in shock, in which there is general peripheral vasodilation with "pooling" of blood in the expanded vascular space, resulting in decreased venous return.

**circulatory overload** Increased blood volume, usually caused by transfusions that increase the venous pressure, esp. in patients with heart disease. This can result in heart failure, pulmonary edema, and cyanosis.

**circulatory system** The cardiovascular system, consisting of the heart and blood vessels (arteries, arterioles, capillaries, venules, veins, and sinuses) and the lymphatic system. SEE: *abdominal examination; apex beat; blood; chest; heart; lung; pulsation; pulse.*

INSPECTION: Inspection detects any abnormal centers of pulsation; the apex beat and its position, force, and extent; and any unnatural prominence over the precordial region.

**circulus** (sĕr′kū-lŭs) [L.] A circle.

**circum-** [L.] Prefix meaning *around.*

**circumanal** Around the anus.

**circumarticular** (sĕr″kŭm-ăr-tĭk′ū-lăr) [L. *circum,* around, + *articulus,* small joint] Surrounding a joint. SYN: *periarthric; periarticular.*

**circumcision** (sĕr″kŭm-sĭ′zhŭn) [L. *circumcisio,* a cutting around] Surgical removal of the end of the prepuce of the penis. Circumcision is usually performed at the request of the parents. There are very few medical indications for this procedure. Uncircumcised males exhibit a higher incidence of syphilis, gonorrhea, and penile malignancies.

NURSING IMPLICATIONS: *Preoperative:*

The procedure and expected sensations are explained to the patient or his parents. Adult patients should be reassured that the procedure will not interfere with urinary, sexual, or reproductive function or alter appearance. Necessary equipment, including a restraining board for the newborn, is assembled. The newborn should not receive food within 1 hr before the procedure.

*Postoperative:* Vital signs are monitored, and the incision is inspected for bleeding every 15 min for the first hour, then hourly for 12 to 24 hr, as protocol directs. Bleeding is controlled by applying gentle pressure with sterile gauze sponges; any heavy or persistent bleeding should be reported, and preparations made for blood vessel ligation. A sterile petroleum gauze dressing is applied after circumcision, remains in place for 24 hr, and is replaced if it becomes dislodged during that period. The penis is gently washed at diaper change, and fresh sterile petroleum gauze reapplied. The dressing, glans penis, and sutures, if present, are periodically examined for swelling, redness, or purulent exudate; any signs of infection are reported, and a specimen of the exudate is obtained. A plastic bell instead of petroleum gauze may be used to cover the glans and to prevent hemorrhage and contamination. The newborn is diapered loosely to prevent irritation and should not be positioned on the abdomen for the first few hours after the procedure.

For the older patient, analgesics are provided, and a topical anesthetic ointment or spray is applied as needed. If prescribed, a sedative is provided to help prevent nocturnal penile tumescence and resulting pressure on the suture line. The patient is encouraged to void within 6 hr after the procedure. Either patient or family is instructed how to keep the area clean and how to change and apply dressings. They are also instructed to watch for and report renewed bleeding or signs of infection. Adult patients can resume normal sexual activity as soon as healing is complete, usually within a week or so, and use of prescribed analgesics is recommended to relieve discomfort during intercourse.

***female c.*** Partial or complete removal of the clitoris, a procedure widespread in Africa and in certain groups in the Middle and Far East. The surgery is usually performed before puberty. The untoward results include infection, scarring that may prevent sexual intercourse, and death from excessive bleeding or postoperative shock owing to lack of proper medical care. SYN: *female genital mutilation.* SEE: *infibulation.*

***ritual c.*** The religious rite performed by the Jews and Muslims at the time of removal of the prepuce.

**circumclusion** (sĕr″kŭm-klū′zhŭn) [L. *circumcludere,* to shut in] Occlusion by use of a pin under an artery and a wire loop over it attached to each end of the pin.

**circumcorneal** (sĕr″kŭm-kor′nē-ăl) [L. *circum,* around, + *corneus,* horny] Around the cornea.

**circumduction** (sĕr″kŭm-dŭk′shŭn) [″ + *ducere,* to lead] **1.** The action or swing of a limb, such as the arm, so that it describes a cone. The apex of the cone is formed by the joint at the proximal end; the complete circle is formed by the free distal end of the limb. **2.** Circular movement of the eye.

**circumference** (sĕr-kŭm′fĕr-ĕns) [″ + *ferre,* to bear] The perimeter of an object or body.

**circumferential** (sĕr″kŭm-fĕr-ĕn′shăl) **1.** Encircling. **2.** Pert. to the periphery or circumference of an object or body.

**circumflex** (sĕr′kŭm-flĕks) [″ + *flectere,* to bend] Winding around, as a vessel.

**circuminsular** (sĕr″kŭm-ĭn′sū-lăr) [″ + *insula,* island] Surrounding the island of Reil in the cerebral cortex.

**circumlental** (sĕr″kŭm-lĕn′tăl) [″ + *lens,* lens] Surrounding the lens of the eye.

**circumnuclear** (sĕr″kŭm-nū′klē-ăr) [″ + *nucleus,* kernel] Surrounding the nucleus.

**circumocular** (sĕr″kŭm-ŏk′ū-lăr) [″ + *oculus,* eye] Surrounding the eye.

**circumoral** (sĕr″kŭm-ō′răl) [L. *circum,* around, + *os,* mouth] Encircling the mouth.

**circumoral pallor** A white area around the mouth contrasting vividly with the color of the face, seen esp. in scarlet fever.

**circumorbital** (sĕr″kŭm-or′bĭt-ăl) [″ + *orbita,* orbit] Around an orbit.

**circumpolarization** (sĕr″kŭm-pō″lăr-ĭ-zā′shŭn) [″+ *polaris,* polar] The rotation of a ray of polarized light.

**circumrenal** (sĕr″kŭm-rē′năl) [″+ *renalis,* pert. to kidney] Surrounding or partly surrounding the kidney.

**circumscribed** (sĕr′kŭm-skrībd) [″ + *scribere,* to write] Limited in space by something drawn around or confining an area.

**circumstantiality** (sĕr″kŭm-stăn″shē-ăl′ĭ-tē) [L. *circum,* around, + *stare,* to stand] Disturbance of the associative thought and speech processes in which the patient digresses into unnecessary details and inappropriate thoughts before communicating the central idea. It is observed in schizophrenia, obsessional disturbances, and certain cases of dementia.

**circumvallate** (sĕr″kŭm-văl′āt) [″ + *vallare,* to wall] Surrounded by a wall or raised structure.

**circumvascular** (sĕr″kŭm-văs′kū-lăr) [″ + *vasculum,* vessel] Perivascular; around a blood vessel.

**cirrhosis** (sĭ-rō′sĭs) [Gr. *kirrhos,* orange yellow, + *osis,* condition] A chronic disease of the liver marked by formation of dense perilobular connective tissue, degenerative changes in the parenchymal cells, structural alteration of the cords of liver lobules, fatty and cellular infiltration, and sometimes development of areas of regeneration. In addition to the clinical signs and symptoms inherent in the cause of the cirrhosis, those caused by it are due to loss of functioning liver cells and increased resistance to blood flow through the liver (portal hypertension). When severe enough, cirrhosis leads to ammonia toxicity. Therapy depends on the cause and severity of the disease. SEE: *coma, hepatic; esophageal varix; liver; liver flap.*

SYMPTOMS: Symptoms include anorexia, chronic dyspepsia, indigestion, nausea and vomiting, constipation or diarrhea, and dull aching abdominal pain; bleeding tendencies such as easy bruising, frequent nosebleeds, and bleeding gums; hemorrhage from esophageal varices; "mousy" breath, pruritus, extreme skin dryness, poor tissue turgor, abnormal pigmentation, telangiectasis, spider angiomas, palmar erythema, distended abdominal blood vessels, umbilical hernia, thigh and leg edema, ascites, and jaundice. Indications of progressive hepatic encephalopathy are lethargy, behavioral or personality changes, slurred speech, asterixis (i.e., "liver flap"), peripheral neuritis, paranoia, hallucinations, mental dullness, and coma. Limited thoracic expansion due to hepatomegaly or ascites and endocrine changes such as menstrual irregularities, testicular atrophy, gynecomastia, and loss of chest and axillary hair may also be present.

ETIOLOGY: Cirrhosis may be due to various factors such as nutritional deficiency (lack of proteins, choline, or methionine), poisons (including alcohol, carbon tetrachloride, and phosphorus), or previous inflammation caused by a virus or bacterium.

NURSING IMPLICATIONS: Daily weights are obtained, fluid and electrolyte balance is monitored, and abdominal girth is measured. The ankles, sacrum, and scrotum are also assessed for dependent edema. The stools are inspected for color, amount, and consistency. Stools and vomitus are tested for occult blood. Surface bleeding sites are monitored frequently, and direct pressure is applied to the site if bleeding occurs. The patient is observed for indications of internal bleeding, such as anxiety, epigastric fullness, weakness, and restlessness; and vital signs are monitored as appropriate. Dependent areas are exercised and elevated, and pruritus-associated skin breakdown is prevented by eliminating soaps and by using lubricating oils and lotions for bathing. The patient is frequently repositioned. The patient should avoid straining at stool and should use stool softeners as necessary and prescribed. Violent sneezing and nose blowing should also be avoided. A soft toothbrush or sponge stick and an electric razor are used. Aspirin or aspirin products and other over-the-counter medications should not be taken without the physician's knowledge. Alcohol or products containing alcohol are prohibited.

Both patient and family may require referral to alcohol cessation and related support groups. Prescribed therapies, including sodium and fluid restriction, dietary modifications, supplemental vitamin therapy, antiemetics, and diuretics, are administered. The patient's response to prescribed therapies is assessed, and the patient is instructed in their use and any adverse reactions. A regimen of moderate exercise alternating with periods of rest is prescribed; energy conservation measures are explained; small, frequent, nutritious meals are recommended; and exposure to infections should be avoided. Appropriate safety measures are instituted, esp. if the patient demonstrates hepatic encephalopathy, and the patient is frequently reoriented to time and place. Albumin is administered and paracentesis performed, if prescribed, to control ascites, and the patient is physically and psychologically prepared for required medical and surgical procedures. SEE: *Nursing Diagnoses Appendix.*

***alcoholic c.*** Cirrhosis occurring in persons who are chronic alcoholics. Approx. 20% of chronic alcoholics develop cirrhosis.

***atrophic c.*** Cirrhosis in which the liver is decreased in size.

***biliary c.*** Cirrhosis marked by prolonged jaundice due to chronic retention of bile and inflammation of bile ducts. SEE: *obstructive biliary c.; primary biliary c.*

***cardiac c.*** Congestive cirrhosis resulting from passive congestion of the liver due to congestive heart failure.

***fatty c.*** Cirrhosis with fatty infiltration of the liver cells.

***hypertrophic c.*** Cirrhosis in which connective tissue hyperplasia causes the liver to be greatly enlarged.

***infantile c.*** Cirrhosis occurring in childhood as a result of protein malnutrition. SEE: *kwashiorkor.*

***metabolic c.*** Cirrhosis resulting from metabolic disease such as hemochromatosis, glycogen storage disease, or Wilson's disease.

***obstructive biliary c.*** Cirrhosis resulting from obstruction of the common duct by a stone or tumor.

***primary biliary c.*** A rare, progressive form of cirrhosis marked by liver enlargement, jaundice, and pruritus.

***syphilitic c.*** Cirrhosis occurring in tertiary syphilis, in which gummas form in the liver and cause coarse lobulation on healing.

***toxic c.*** Cirrhosis resulting from toxic substances as in poisoning by carbon tetrachloride or phosphorus.

***zooparasitic c.*** Cirrhosis resulting from infestation with animal parasites, esp. blood flukes of the genus *Schistosoma* or liver flukes, *Clonorchis sinensis*.

**cirrhotic** (sĭ-rŏt′ĭk) Pert. to or affected with cirrhosis.

**cirsectomy** (sĕr-sĕk′tō-mē) [Gr. *kirsos,* varix, + *ektome,* excision] Excision of a portion of a varicose vein.

**cirsoid** (sĕr′soyd) Varicose.

**cirsomphalos** (sĕr-sŏm′fă-lŏs) [″ + *omphalos,* navel] Varicose veins around the navel.

**cirsotome** (sĕr′sō-tōm) [″ + *tome,* incision] An instrument for cutting varicose veins.

**cirsotomy** (sĕr-sŏt′ō-mē) Incision of a varicose vein.

**C.I.S.** *central inhibitory state.*

**cis** (sĭs) [L., on the same side] In organic chemistry, a form of isomerism in which similar atoms or radicals are on the same side. In genetics, a prefix meaning the location of two or more genes on the same chromosome of a homologous pair.

**cisplatin** (sĭs′plă-tĭn) An antineoplastic chemical used in treating testicular tumors and ovarian cancer. The nephrotoxicity of the drug may be almost eliminated by ensuring a diuresis of 150 ml/hr when it is administered.

**cis-retinal** The form of retinal combined with a glycoprotein opsin (rhodopsin in rods) during darkness. Light striking the retina changes it to *trans*-retinal and begins the generation of a nerve impulse.

**cistern** (sĭs′tĕrn) A reservoir for storing fluid.

**cisterna** [L.] A reservoir or cavity.

***c. chyli*** A dilated sac; the origin of the thoracic duct. Into it empty the intestinal, two lumbar, and two descending lymphatic trunks. SYN: *receptaculum chyli.*

***c. subarachnoidalis*** A wide space in the cranial cavity between the arachnoid and the pia mater. It contains cerebrospinal fluid.

**cisternal** (sĭs-tĕr′năl) Concerning a cavity filled with fluid.

**cisternography** Radiography of the basal cistern of the brain after the injection of a contrast medium into the subarachnoid space.

**cisvestitism** (sĭs-vĕs′tĭ-tĭzm) [L. *cis,* on the same side, + *vestitus,* dressed, + Gr. *-ismos,* condition] Wearing of clothes appropriate to one's sex but suitable for a calling or profession other than one's own. An example would be a civilian who dresses in a uniform of the armed services.

**Citelli's syndrome** (chē-tĕl′ēz) [Salvatore Citelli, It. laryngologist, 1875–1947] Insomnia or drowsiness, and lack of concentration associated with intelligence disorders, seen in children with infected adenoids or sphenoid sinusitis.

**citrate** (sĭt′rāt, sī′trāt) A compound of citric acid and a base.

**citrated** (sĭt′rāt-ĕd) Combined or mixed with citric acid or a citrate.

**citrate solution** A solution used to prevent clotting of the blood. Its use permits whole blood to be stored in a refrigerator until it is needed for transfusion.

**citric acid cycle** The Krebs cycle.

**citronella** (sĭt″rŏn-ĕl′ă) A volatile oil obtained from *Cymbopogon citratus,* or lemongrass, that contains geraniol and citronellal. It is used in perfumes and as an insect repellent.

**citrovorum factor** Folic acid.

**citrulline** (sĭt-rŭl′lĭn) An amino acid, $C_6H_{13}N_3O_3$, formed from ornithine. It is found in watermelons.

**citrullinemia** (sĭt-rŭl″lĭ-nē′mē-ă) A type of aminoaciduria accompanied by increased amounts of citrulline in the blood, urine, and spinal fluid. Clinical findings include ammonia intoxication, liver disease, vomiting, mental retardation, convulsions, and failure to thrive.

**Cl** **1.** Symbol for the element chlorine. **2.** *chloride; clavicle; Clostridium.*

**cladosporiosis** (klăd″ō-spō-rē-ō′sĭs) [Gr. *klados,* branch, + *sporos,* seed, + *osis,* condition] A general term for an infection, usually of the central nervous system, caused by the fungus *Cladosporium.*

**Cladosporium** A genus of fungi. The condition tinea nigra is caused by either *C. werneckii* or *C. mansonii.* SEE: illus.

**clairvoyance** (klār-voy′ăns) [Fr.] The alleged ability to be aware of events that occur at a distance without receiving any sensory information concerning those events.

**clamp** (klămp) [MD. *klampe,* metal clasp] A device used in surgery to grasp, join, compress, or support an organ, tissue, or vessel.

***rubber dam c.*** An attachment that fits on the cervical part of the tooth for retention of a rubber dam. SEE: *rubber dam.*

**clang** [L. *clangere,* to peal] **1.** A loud, metallic sound. **2.** In psychiatry, clang association is speech directed by the sound of words, as in combining words that rhyme, rather than using appropriate ones.

**clap** A colloquial term for gonorrhea.

**clapotage, clapotement** (klă″pō-tăzh′, klă-

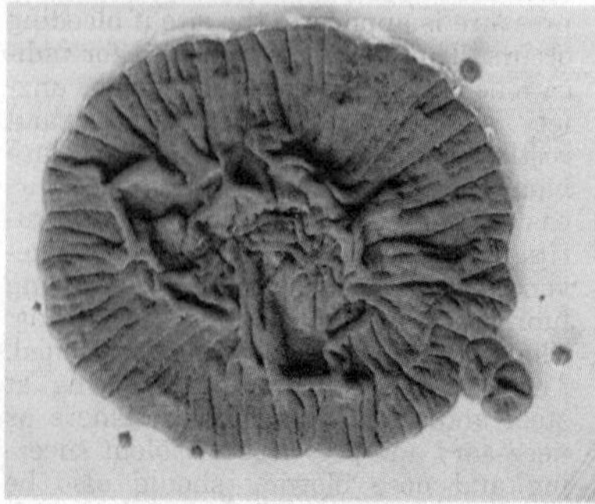

CLADOSPORIUM IN CULTURE

pŏt-maw') [Fr.] Any splashing sound in succussion of a dilated stomach.

**clapping** (klăp'ĭng) Percussion of the chest to loosen secretions; also called *cupping* or *tapping*. The hand is held in a cupped position.

**Clapton's lines** Green lines on the dental margin of the gums in copper poisoning.

**Clara cell** [Max Clara, Austrian anatomist, b. 1899] One of the secreting cells in the surface epithelium of the bronchioles. These cells, along with goblet cells, provide secretions for the respiratory tract. The secretion is a mucus-poor protein that coats the epithelium.

**clarificant** (klăr-ĭf'ĭk-ănt) [L. *clarus,* clear, + *facere,* to make] Any agent that clears turbidity from a liquid.

**clarification** (klăr"ĭ-fĭ-kā'shŭn) **1.** The removal of turbidity from a solution. **2.** In psychiatry, a technique used to help a patient recognize inconsistencies in his or her statements.

**Clark electrode** Oxygen electrode.

**Clark's rule** A method of calculating pediatric drug dosages. The weight of the child in pounds is multiplied by the adult dose and the result is divided by 150. SEE: *dosage.*

**Clarke, Jacob A.L.** British anatomist, 1817–1880.

***C.'s body*** One of the alveolar sarcomatous intranuclear bodies of the breast.

***C.'s column*** The dorsal nucleus of the spinal cord.

**Clarke-Hadfield syndrome** [Cecil Clarke, 20th-century Brit. physician; Geoffrey John Hadfield, Brit. pathologist, 1899–1968] Infantilism caused by pancreatic insufficiency. A child suffering from this syndrome is underweight and fails to grow.

**clasmatodendrosis** (klăz-măt"ō-dĕn-drō'sĭs) [Gr. *klasma,* fragment, + *dendron,* tree, + *osis,* condition] Breaking up of astrocytic protoplasmic expansions.

**clasmatosis** (klăz"mă-tō'sĭs) [" + *osis,* condition] Crumbling into small bits; fragmentation, as of cells.

**clasp** (klăsp) A device for holding objects or tissues together. In dentistry, a type of wire or metal retainer or attachment used to stabilize dentures or prosthetic devices in the mouth.

**clasp-knife phenomenon** Increased muscle resistance to passive movement of a joint followed by a sudden release of the muscle; commonly seen in patients with spasticity.

**class** [L. *classis,* division] **1.** In biology, a taxonomic group of clearly defined organisms classified below a phylum and above an order. **2.** In statistics, a group of variables that fall within certain value limits.

**classification** (klăs"sĭ-fĭ-kā'shŭn) The orderly separation of a group of similar organisms, animals, or individuals into classes according to traits or characteristics common to each class or group.

***Dukes c.*** A system of classifying the extent of spread of adenocarcinoma of the colon or rectum.

**classification of living organisms** A systematic method of assigning organisms to various groups. Living organisms are classified into five kingdoms: Monera (Prokaryota), Protista, Fungi, Plantae, and Animalia. Within a kingdom, the subdivisions usually are phylum, class, order, family, genus, and species. The genus and species names are referred to as binomial nomenclature, with the larger (genus) category first and the precise species name second. SEE: *taxonomy.*

**class restriction** The requirement of certain T lymphocytes for the presence of either class I or class II major histocompatibility complex markers on antigen-presenting cells. These markers enable the T cells to recognize and respond to foreign antigens. CD4+ T cells require class II antigens and CD8+ T cells require class I antigens. Class restriction is a type of clonal restriction. SEE: *cell, antigen-presenting; clonal restriction.*

**clastic** (klăs'tĭk) [Gr. *klastos,* broken] Causing division into parts.

**clastogenic** (klăs'tō-jĕn"ĭc) [" + *gennan,* to produce] Capable of breaking chromosomes (e.g., able to cause chromosomal abnormalities).

**clastothrix** (klăs'tō-thrĭks) [" + *thrix,* hair] Trichorrhexis nodosa.

**Claude's syndrome** (klawdz) [Henri Claude, Fr. psychiatrist, 1869–1945] Paralysis of the third cranial nerve, contralateral ataxia, and tremor; caused by a lesion in the red nucleus of the brain.

**claudication** (klaw-dĭ-kā'shŭn) [L. *claudicare,* to limp] Lameness.

***intermittent c.*** A severe pain in the calf muscles that occurs during walking but subsides with rest. It results from inadequate blood supply, which may be due to arterial spasm, atherosclerosis, arteriosclerosis obliterans, or an occlusion of an artery to the limb. This symptom, which occurs more frequently in men than women, has been reported in 1.8% of the population under 60 years of age, in 3.7% of those 60 to 70 years of age, and in 5.2% of those over 70 years of age. Prognosis is favorable because the condition stabilizes or improves in most patients. Therefore, conservative therapy is advisable. Walking for exercise is helpful in increasing the distance that the patient can walk without experiencing symptoms.

***venous c.*** Claudication resulting from inadequate venous drainage.

**Claudius' cell** (klaw'dē-ŭs) [Friedrich Claudius, Austrian anatomist, 1822–1869] One of the large columnar cells external to the organ of Corti.

**Claudius' fossa** A small depression on either side of the posterior part of the pelvis; each contains an ovary.

**claustrophilia** (klaws-trō-fĭl′ē-ă) [L. *claustrum,* a barrier, + Gr. *philein,* to love] Dread of being in an open space; a morbid desire to be shut in with doors and windows closed.

**claustrophobia** (klaws-trō-fō′bē-ă) [″ + Gr. *phobos,* fear] Fear of being confined in any space, as in a locked room.

**claustrum** (klŏs′trŭm) [L.] **1.** A barrier. **2.** The thin layer of gray matter separating the external capsule of the brain from the island of Reil.

**clava** (klā′vă) *pl.* **clavae** [L., club] An elevation on the dorsal surface of the medulla oblongata caused by the underlying nucleus gracilis, the superior extremity of the fasciculus gracilis.

**clavate** (klā′vāt) Club-shaped.

**clavicle** (klăv′ĭ-k′l) [L. *clavicula,* little key] A bone curved like the letter *f* that articulates with the sternum and the scapula. SYN: *collar bone.*

***dislocation of c.*** Traumatic displacement of either end of the clavicle.

TREATMENT: The procedure is done by an emergency care physician or an orthopedist. The knee is placed against the spine and the shoulders are drawn back. A clavicle bandage is applied with the pad on the dislocated end of the bone.

***fracture of c.*** Symptoms include swelling, pain, and protuberance with a sharp depression over the injured bone. The patient holds the immobile arm by supporting it at the elbow.

TREATMENT: This procedure is done by an emergency care physician or an orthopedist. An assistant draws the patient's arms and shoulders backward. The shoulders are raised and supported upward, backward, and outward. The position is maintained by a clavicle strap or a figure-of-eight wrap between the shoulders and over the back.

FIRST AID: A ball of cloth or one or two handkerchiefs are tightly rolled and placed under the armpit. An arm sling is applied and the elbow bandaged to the side, with the hand and forearm extending across the chest. Alternatively, the patient may lie on his or her back on the floor with a rolled-up blanket under the shoulders until medical aid arrives. This position keeps the shoulders back and prevents the broken ends of the bone from rubbing.

**clavicotomy** (klăv″ĭ-kŏt′ō-mē) [″ + Gr. *tome,* incision] Surgical division of the clavicle.

**clavicular** (klă-vĭk′ū-lăr) Pert. to the clavicle.

**clavus** (klā′vŭs) [L., nail] A corn or callosity.

***c. hystericus*** A sharp pain in the head described as feeling like a nail being driven into the head.

**clawfoot** A deformity of the foot marked by an excessively high longitudinal arch, usually accompanied by dorsal contracture of the toes.

**clawhand** A hand marked by hyperextension of the proximal phalanges of the digits and extreme flexion of the middle and distal phalanges. Usually it is caused by injury to the ulnar and median nerves. SYN: *main en griffe.*

**claw toe** Hammertoe.

**Clayton gas** Sulfur dioxide; used to fumigate ships.

**clean-catch method** A procedure for obtaining a urine specimen that exposes the culture sample to minimal contamination. For females, the labia are held apart and the periurethral area is cleaned with a mild soap or antibacterial solution, rinsed with copious amounts of plain water, and dried from front to back with a dry gauze pad. The urine is then passed and the specimen collected in a sterile container. It is important that the labia be held apart and that the urine flow directly into the container without touching the skin. If possible, the sample should be obtained after the urine flow is well established (i.e., a midstream specimen). For males, the urethral meatus is cleaned and the midstream specimen is collected in a sterile container. If the male is uncircumcised, the foreskin is retracted before the penis is cleaned.

**cleaning, ultrasonic** The use of high-frequency vibrations to clean instruments.

**clean room** A controlled environment facility in which all incoming air passes through a filter capable of removing 99.97% of all particles 0.3 $\mu$m and larger. The temperature, pressure, and humidity in the room are controlled. Clean rooms are used in research and in controlling infections, esp. for persons who may not have normally functioning immune systems (e.g., individuals who have been treated with immunosuppressive drugs in preparation for organ transplantation).

In very rare instances a child is born without the ability to develop an immune system. Such children are kept in a clean room while waiting for specific therapy such as bone marrow transplantation. Alternatively, these children may be kept in a suit that isolates them completely from physical contact with the environment but allows them to be mobile. The suit, sometimes called a "space bubble," is attached to filtering devices that screen the air supplied to the child.

**clearance** The elimination of a substance from the blood plasma by the kidneys. SEE: *renal clearance test.*

**clearing agent** **1.** A substance that increases the transparency of tissues prepared for microscopic examination. **2.** In radiographic film processing, the active agent in the fixer that clears undeveloped silver bromide crystals from the film. The most common agent is ammonium thiosulfate. SYN: *fixing agent.*

**cleavage** (klē′vĕj) [AS. *cleofian,* to cleave] **1.** Splitting a complex molecule into two or more simpler ones. **2.** Division of a fertilized egg into many smaller cells or blastomeres. SYN: *segmentation.* SEE: *blastomere; embryo.*

**cleft** (klĕft) [ME. *clift,* crevice] **1.** A fissure or elongated opening. **2.** Divided or split.

***alveolar c.*** An anomaly resulting from lack of fusion between the medial nasal process and the maxillary process. A cleft maxillary alveolar process is usually associated with a cleft lip and palate or both.

***branchial c.*** An opening between the branchial arches of an embryo. In lower vertebrates it becomes a gill cleft.

***facial c.*** An anomaly resulting from failure of the facial processes of the embryo to fuse. Common types are oblique facial cleft, an open nasolacrimal furrow extending from the eye to the lower portion of the nose that is sometimes continuous with a cleft in the upper lip, and transverse facial cleft, which extends laterally from the angle of the mouth.

***synaptic c.*** The synapse of a neuromuscular junction (between the axon terminal of a motor neuron and the sarcolemma of a muscle fiber). Impulse transmission is accomplished by a neurotransmitter.

**cleft cheek** Transverse facial cleft.

**cleft hand** A bipartite hand resulting from failure of a digit and its corresponding metacarpal to develop.

**cleft lip** A vertical cleft or clefts in the upper lip. This congenital condition, resulting from the faulty fusion of the median nasal process and the lateral maxillary processes, is usually unilateral and on the left side, but may be bilateral. It may involve either the lip or the upper jaw, or both, and often accompanies cleft palate. Nongenetic factors may also be responsible for causing this condition. The incidence of cleft lip is from one in 600 to one in 1250 births. SYN: *harelip.*

**cleft palate** A congenital fissure in the roof of the mouth forming a communicating passageway between mouth and nasal cavities. It may be unilateral or bilateral and complete or incomplete.

***incomplete c.*** A cleft involving only a part of the hard or soft palate.

**cleido-, cleid-** (klī′dō) [L. *clavis,* key] Combining form pert. to the clavicle.

**cleidocostal** (klī″dō-kŏs′tăl) [″ + *costa,* rib] Pertaining to the clavicle and ribs.

**cleidorrhexis** (klī″dō-rĕk′sĭs) [″ + Gr. *rhexis,* rupture] Fracture or bending of the clavicles of the fetus for delivery.

**cleidotomy** (klī-dŏt′ō-mē) [″ + Gr. *tome,* incision] Division of a fetal clavicle to facilitate delivery.

**clemastine fumarate** (klĕm′ăs-tēn) An antihistamine drug.

**clenching** (klĕnch′ĭng) With the teeth in contact, forcible, repeated contraction of the jaw muscles. This causes pulsating, bilateral contractions of the temporalis and pterygomasseteric muscles. It may be done consciously, subconsciously while awake, or during sleep. SEE: *bruxism.*

**cleptomania** (klĕp″tō-mā′nē-ă) Kleptomania.

**click** (klĭk) **1.** An abrupt, brief sound heard in listening to the heart sounds. **2.** Any brief sound but esp. one heard during a joint movement. **3.** In dentistry, a noise associated with temporomandibular joint movement, sometimes accompanied by pain or joint dysfunction.

**clidinium bromide** (klĭ-dĭn′ē-ŭm) A drug used in treating peptic ulcers and other conditions in which it is desirable to inhibit the action of the parasympathetic nervous system. Trade name is Quarzan.

**client** The patient of a health care professional.

**climacteric** (klī-măk′tĕr-ĭk, klī-măk-tĕr′ĭk) [Gr. *klimakter,* a rung of a ladder] The period that marks the cessation of a woman's reproductive ability (female climacteric or menopause); a corresponding period of lessened sexual activity in a man (male climacteric).

**climatology, medical** [Gr. *klima,* sloping surface of the earth, + *logos,* word, reason] The branch of meteorology that includes the study of climate and its relationship to disease. SEE: *bioclimatology.*

**climatotherapy** (klī″măt-ō-thĕr′ăp-ē) [″ + *therapeia,* treatment] Treatment of disease by having the patient move to a more favorable climate.

**climax** (klī′măks) [Gr. *klimax,* ladder] **1.** The period of greatest intensity. **2.** The sexual orgasm.

**clindamycin hydrochloride** (klĭn″dă-mī′sĭn) An antibiotic effective against gram-positive cocci. It was once thought to have the side effect of causing colitis. It is now believed that the colitis that may develop during therapy with clindamycin is due to resistant strains of *Clostridium difficile.*

**clinic** (klĭn′ĭk) [Gr. *klinikos,* pert. to a bed] **1.** Medical and dental instruction in which patients are observed directly, symptoms noted, and treatments discussed. **2.** A center for physical examination and treatment of ambulant patients who are not hospitalized. **3.** A center where preliminary diagnosis is made and treatment given, as an x-ray clinic, a dental clinic, or a child-guidance clinic.

***walk-in c.*** A general medical care clinic that is open to those who walk in without having made an appointment.

**clinical 1.** Founded on actual observation and treatment of patients as distinguished from data or facts obtained from other sources. **2.** Pert. to a clinic.

**clinical ecology** A form of medical practice based on two concepts: that a broad range of environmental chemicals and foods can cause an illness in which an unlimited variety of symptoms occur without objective physical findings, pathological abnormalities, or specific abnormal test results; and that the immune system is functionally depressed by many environmental chemicals. Environmental illness, a disease related to the mentioned environmental factors, has also been known by other names, such as environmentally induced disease, chemical hypersensitivity syndrome, multiple chemical sensitivities, chemically induced immune dysregulation, 20th-century disease, total allergy syndrome, ecological illness, and food and chemical sensitivity.

**clinical judgment** The exercise of the clinician's experience and knowledge in diagnosing and treating illness and disease. SEE: *decision analysis.*

**clinical pathway** A method being used in health care settings as a way of organizing, evaluating, and limiting variations in patient care. This method integrates the components of the nursing care plan into one comprehensive plan that addresses the needs and services provided to the whole patient. Development of a clinical pathway usually begins with establishment of a multidisciplinary steering committee that examines agency data to determine which diagnostic-related groups (DRG) will have pathways. Most agencies are developing paths for diagnoses that are of large volume and high cost (often related to the use of technologies), involve multiple specialties, and require the patient to be cared for on different units.

The most typical content found in a clinical pathway includes consultations and assessments, tests and treatments, nutrition and medications, activity and safety, and teaching and discharge planning. Clinical pathways address timelines, actions, and outcomes, and ensure that essential components of care are provided on time, every time. Many agencies use clinical pathways as a primary documentation tool, including prewritten physicians' orders and a space for other team members to merely sign off if the identified action or patient outcome has been established.

Agencies using clinical pathways report the following advantages: reduced length of stay for patients in given DRGs; greater accountability for patient care; greater patient and family satisfaction; enhanced staff and physician satisfaction and communication; an improved and integrated process for care delivery; minimal prejudices and elitism between departments; lower patient charges and costs; and 20% to 40% less time spent on documentation.

**clinical thermometer** A glass or electronic instrument that measures body temperature. The glass nondisposable type may be disinfected by first cleansing with cotton and soap solution, using a rotary motion down toward the bulb end. This removes adherent mucus, which coagulates in some disinfectants, thereby retaining organisms. It should be rinsed thoroughly in tepid, not hot, water, submerged in 70% alcohol for 10 min, and rinsed before use. SEE: *thermometer.*

**clinical trial** A carefully designed and executed investigation of the effects of a drug administered to human subjects. The goal is to define the clinical efficacy and pharmacological effects (toxicity, side effects, incompatibilities, or interactions). The U.S. government requires strict testing of all new drugs before their approval for use as therapeutic agents. SEE: *randomization.*

**clinician** (klĭn-ĭsh′ăn) [Gr. *klinikos,* pert. to a bed] A health professional with expertise in clinical practice as distinguished from one specializing in research.

**clinicopathological** (klĭn″ĭ-kō-pă″thō-lŏj′ĭk-ăl) Concerning the clinical and pathological manifestations of a disease.

**clinicopathological conference** ABBR: CPC. A teaching conference in which clinical findings are presented to a physician previously unfamiliar with a case, who then attempts to diagnose the disease that would explain the clinical findings. The exact diagnosis is then presented by the pathologist, who has either examined the tissue removed at surgery or has performed the autopsy. SEE: *medical grand rounds.*

**clinocephaly** (klī″nō-sĕf′ă-lē) [Gr. *klinein,* to bend, + *kephale,* head] Congenital flatness or saddle shape of the top of the head, caused by bilateral premature closure of the sphenoparietal sutures.

**clinodactyly** (klī″nō-dăk′tĭ-lē) [″ + *daktylos,* finger] Hypoplasia of the middle phalanx of one or more of the fingers resulting in these fingers curving inward. This condition occurs in Down syndrome.

**clinoid** (klī′noyd) [Gr. *kline,* bed, + *eidos,* form, shape] Shaped like a bed.

**clinometer** (klī-nŏm′ĕ-tĕr) [Gr. *klinein,* to slope, + *metron,* measure] An instrument for estimating torsional deviation of the eyes; used to measure ocular muscle paralysis. SYN: *clinoscope.*

**clinoscope** (klī′nō-skōp) Clinometer.

**clip** A metallic instrument for holding tissue or other material together.

**clithrophobia** (klĭth″rō-fō′bē-ă) [Gr. *kleithria,* keyhole, + *phobos,* fear] A morbid fear of being locked in.

**clition** (klĭt′ē-ŏn) [Gr. *kleitys,* slope] A craniometric point in the center of the highest part of the clivus on the sphenoid bone.

**clitoridectomy** (klī″tō-rĭd-ĕk′tō-mē) [Gr. *kleitoris,* clitoris, + *ektome,* excision] Excision of the clitoris.

**clitoriditis** (klī″tō-rĭd-ī′tĭs) Clitoritis.

**clitoridotomy** (klī″tō-rĭd-ŏt′ō-mē) [″ + *tome,* incision] Incision of the clitoris; female circumcision.

**clitoris** (klī′tō-rĭs, klĭt′ō-rĭs) [Gr. *kleitoris*] One of the structures of the female genitalia; a small erectile body located beneath the anterior labial commissure and partially hidden by the anterior portion of the labia minora. It is homologous to the penis.

STRUCTURE: It consists of three parts: a body, two crura, and a glans. The body, about 1 in. (2.5 cm) long, consists of two fused corpora cavernosa. It extends from the pubic arch above to the glans below. The two crura are continuations of the corpora cavernosa and attach them to the inferior rami of the pubic bones. They are covered by the ischiocavernosus muscles. The glans, which forms the free distal end, is a small rounded tubercle composed of erectile tissue. It is highly sensitive. The glans is usually covered by a hoodlike prepuce, and its ventral surface is attached to the frenulum of the labia.

**clitorism** (klī'tō-rĭzm) **1.** The counterpart of priapism; a long-continued, painful condition with recurring erection of the clitoris. **2.** Enlargement of the clitoris.

**clitoritis** (klī"tō-rī'tĭs) Inflammation of the clitoris. SYN: *clitoriditis.*

**clitoromegaly** (klī"tō-rō-mĕg'ă-lē) [" + *megas,* large] Enlargement of the clitoris. This may be caused by an endocrine disease, or by use of anabolic steroids by female athletes.

**clivus** (klī'vŭs) [L., a slope] A surface that slopes, as the sphenoid bone.

***c. blumenbachii*** The slope at the base of the skull.

**clo** A unit for thermal insulation of clothing; the amount of insulation necessary to maintain comfort in a sitting-resting subject in a normally ventilated room (air movement at the rate of 10 cm/sec) at a temperature of 70°F (21°C) with relative humidity of less than 50%.

**cloaca** (klō-ā'kă) [L. *cloaca,* a sewer] **1.** A cavity lined with endoderm at the posterior end of the body that serves as a common passageway for urinary, digestive, and reproductive ducts. It exists in adult birds, reptiles, and amphibia, and in the embryos of all vertebrates. **2.** An opening in the sheath covering necrosed bone.

**clobetasol propionate** A high-potency topical corticosteroid; used for short-term treatment to cortisone-responsive dermatoses.

**clock** [LL. *clocca*] A device for measuring time.

***biological c.*** An internal system in organisms that influences behavior in a rhythmic manner. Functions such as growth, feeding, secretion of hormones, the rate of drug action, the wake-sleep cycle, the menstrual cycle, and reproduction coincide with certain external events such as day and night, the tides, and the seasons. Biological clocks appear to be set by environmental conditions in some animals, but if these animals are isolated from their environment they continue to function according to the usual rhythm. A gradual change in environment does produce a gradual change in the timing of the biological clock. SEE: *night work, maladaptation to.*

**clofazimine** (klō-fă'zĭ-mēn) A drug used in treating patients with leprosy whose disease is caused by sulfone-resistant bacteria.

**clofibrate** (klō-fī'brāt) A drug used to reduce plasma concentration of lipids; used in treating hyperlipoproteinemias III, IV, and V. Trade name is Atromid-S.

**Clomid** Trade name for clomiphene citrate.

**clomiphene citrate** (klō'mĭ-fēn) A nonsteroidal agent used to stimulate ovulation in women who have potentially functioning pituitary and ovarian systems. Women treated with this medicine who become pregnant have an increased incidence of multiple births. Trade name is Clomid.

**clonal** (klōn'ăl) Pert. to a clone.

**clonal restriction** The occurrence of the same characteristics as the parent cell in all clones (offspring) of one B or T lymphocyte. For example, surface receptors are identical, so clones react to the same group of specific antigens as the parent cell does.

**clonazepam** (klō-năz'ĕ-păm) An anticonvulsant drug.

**clone** (klōn) [Gr. *klon,* a cutting used for propagation] **1.** In microbiology, the asexual progeny of a single cell. **2.** A group of plants propagated from one seedling or stock. Members of the group are identical but do not reproduce from seed. **3.** In tissue cultures or in the body, a group of cells descended from a single cell. The term commonly refers to the multiple offspring of single T or B lymphocytes that have identical surface receptors or immunoglobulins, and to the offspring of malignant white blood cells. **4.** In immunology, a group of lymphocytes that develop from a sensitized lymphocyte; they are all capable of responding to a specific foreign antigen.

**clonic** (klŏn'ĭk) [Gr. *klonos,* turmoil] Pert. to clonus; alternately contracting and relaxing the muscles.

**clonicity** (klŏn-ĭs'ĭ-tē) The condition of being clonic.

**clonicotonic** (klŏn"ĭ-kō-tŏn'ĭk) [Gr. *klonos,* turmoil, + *tonikos,* tonic] Both clonic and tonic, as some forms of muscular spasm.

**clonidine hydrochloride** (klō'nĭ-dēn) An antihypertensive drug. Trade name is Catapres.

**clonorchiasis** (klō"nor-kī'ă-sĭs) A disease of the Orient caused by the Chinese liver fluke, *Clonorchis sinensis,* which infects the bile ducts of humans. Infection is caused by eating uncooked freshwater fish containing encysted larvae. Early symptoms are loss of appetite and diarrhea; later there may be signs of cirrhosis of the liver. The disease may be prevented by cooking fish thoroughly, or by freezing it at −10°C (14°F) for a minimum of 5 days. The disease rarely causes death, but it may last for 30 years. Treatment with Praziquantel is effective.

**Clonorchis sinensis** (klō-nor'kĭs sī-nĕn'sĭs)

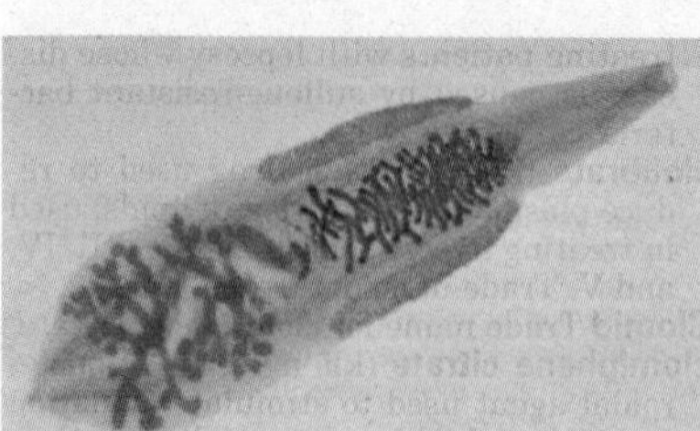

CLONORCHIS SINENSIS (ORIG. MAG. ×4)

The trematode fluke, Chinese liver fluke. It is an important cause of disease, esp. in the Orient. SEE: illus.; *clonorchiasis*.

**clonospasm** (klŏn′ō-spăzm) [″ + *spasmos*, spasm] Rapid alternation of muscular contraction and relaxation. The rate is much slower than a tremor. In upper motor neuron paralysis, sharp flexion of the ankle often produces ankle clonus.

**clonus** (klō′nŭs) Spasmodic alternation of muscular contractions between antagonistic muscle groups caused by a hyperactive stretch reflex from an upper motor neuron lesion. Usually, sustained pressure or stretch of one of the muscles inhibits the reflex.

**Cloquet's canal** (klō-kāz′) [Jules Germain Cloquet, Fr. surgeon, 1790–1883] An irregular passage (hyaloid) through the center of the vitreous body in the fetus.

**closed-packed position** The joint position in which there is maximum congruency of the articular surfaces and the ligaments and joint capsule usually are taut. This is the opposite of the maximum loose-packed position.

**Clostridium** (klō-strĭd′ē-ŭm) [Gr. *kloster*, spindle] A genus of bacteria belonging to the family Bacillaceae. These anaerobic, spore-forming rods are widely distributed in nature, with more than 250 species recognized. They are common in the soil and in the intestinal tract of humans and animals and are frequently found in wound infections. In humans several species are pathogenic, being the primary causative agents of gas gangrene.

***C. botulinum*** A species of soil bacteria that may grow in improperly processed food or in wounds under anaerobic conditions; it produces the neurotoxin that causes botulism.

***C. chauvoei*** The organism causing blackleg or symptomatic anthrax in cattle.

***C. difficile*** A species that causes pseudomembranous colitis. An antibiotic that diminishes the normal colon flora may permit this species to overgrow and cause necrosis of the intestinal mucosa.

***C. histolyticum*** A proteolytic organism found in feces and soil, isolated from necrotic war wounds and found in some cases of gas gangrene.

***C. novyi*** A species found in many cases of gas gangrene.

***C. perfringens*** The most common causative agent of gas gangrene. SYN: *C. welchii; gas bacillus*.

***C. septicum*** A species found in cases of gangrene in humans, as well as in cattle, hogs, and other domestic animals.

***C. sporogenes*** A species frequently associated with other organisms in mixed gangrenous infections.

***C. tetani*** The causative organism of tetanus or lockjaw. It produces a powerful exotoxin, one portion of which affects nerve tissue and the other of which is hemolytic. SEE: *tetanus*.

***C. welchii*** C. perfringens.

**closure** (klō′shŭr) **1.** Shutting or bringing together as in suturing together the edges of a laceration wound. **2.** In psychotherapy, the resolution of an issue that was a topic in therapy and a cause of distress for the patient.

**clot** (klŏt) [AS. *clott*, lump] **1.** A thrombus; a coagulum, as of blood or lymph. SEE: *coagulation, blood; coagulation factor; thrombosis*. **2.** To coagulate.

***agony c.*** A clot formed in the heart when death follows prolonged heart failure.

***antemortem c.*** A clot formed in the heart or its cavities before death.

***blood c.*** A coagulation formed of blood.

***chicken fat c.*** A yellow blood clot appearing to contain no erythrocytes.

***currant jelly c.*** A soft red postmortem blood clot found in the heart and vessels.

***distal c.*** A clot formed in a vessel on the distal side of a ligature.

***external c.*** A clot formed outside a blood vessel.

***heart c.*** A clot within the heart.

***internal c.*** A clot formed by coagulation of blood within a vessel.

***laminated c.*** A clot formed in a succession of layers filling an aneurysm.

***muscle c.*** A clot formed in muscle tissue.

***passive c.*** A clot formed in the sac of an aneurysm.

***plastic c.*** A clot formed from the intima of an artery at the point of ligation.

***postmortem c.*** A clot formed in the heart or in a blood vessel after death.

***proximal c.*** A clot formed on the proximal side of a ligature.

***stratified c.*** A clot consisting of layers of different colors.

**clothes louse** SEE: *Pediculus humanus corporis*.

**clothing** [AS. *clath*, cloth] Wearing apparel; used both functionally and decoratively. From the medical standpoint, clothes conserve heat or protect the body (e.g., gloves, sunhelmets, and shoes). Air spaces in a fabric and its texture, rather than the material alone, conserve heat. In matted woolen fabrics, the air spaces are destroyed and insulation is lost. Wool and silk absorb more moisture than other fabrics, but silk loses it more readily. Cotton and linen come next, but linen loses moisture more quickly than cotton. Knitted fabrics absorb and dry more readily than woven fabrics of the same material. The temperature inside an individual's hat may vary from 13° to 20°F (7° to 11°C) warmer than the outside temperature. Body heat is increased when moisture from wet garments cannot escape. SEE: *clo; hypothermia.*

**clotrimazole** (klō-trĭm′ă-zōl) An antifungal drug that is also used in treating vulvovaginal candidiasis. Intravaginal use occasionally causes burning, redness, and itching in the patient, her sex partner, or both. Trade names are Gyne-Lotrimin, Mycelex G, and Lotrimin.

**clotting** The formation of a jelly-like substance from blood shed at the site of an injury to a blood vessel. This action usually halts blood flow from the wound. SEE: *coagulation, blood.*

**clouding of consciousness** A state of mental confusion marked by insufficiency of perception and impaired attention and resulting in disorientation to time and place, amnesia, and altered reaction time or disordered reactions. It occurs when the brain receives insufficient oxygen, and in delerium due to a toxic or febrile condition. SEE: *consciousness.*

**cloven spine** Congenital defect of spinal canal walls caused by lack of union between laminae of the vertebrae. SYN: *spina bifida cystica.*

**clove oil** [L. *clavus,* a nail or spike] A volatile oil distilled from the dried flower buds of the clove tree, *Eugenia caryophyllus.* It is used as an antiseptic and an aromatic and is applied directly to relieve pain in teeth.

**clownism** (klown′ĭzm) Grotesque actions and attitudes, esp. in certain hysterical states or in epilepsy.

**cloxacillin sodium** (klŏks″ă-sĭl′ĭn) A penicillinase-resistant antibiotic.

**clozapine** A drug approved for use in treating schizophrenic patients who have not responded to standard antipsychotic drugs. This drug is less likely to produce restlessness or muscle stiffness than standard drugs. In about 8% of cases, the drug must be discontinued because of the development of side effects such as grand mal seizures, sedation, orthostatic hypotension, leukopenia, or agranulocytosis.

**clubbing** (klŭb′ĭng) A condition that affects the fingers and toes in many diseases of varying etiologies. The most outstanding feature of clubbing is a lateral and longitudinal curvature of the nails accompanied by soft-tissue enlargement, presenting a bulbous, shiny appearance. It is most commonly found in lung diseases, infective endocarditis, steatorrhea, and occasionally as a familial condition not associated with pathology. SEE: illus.

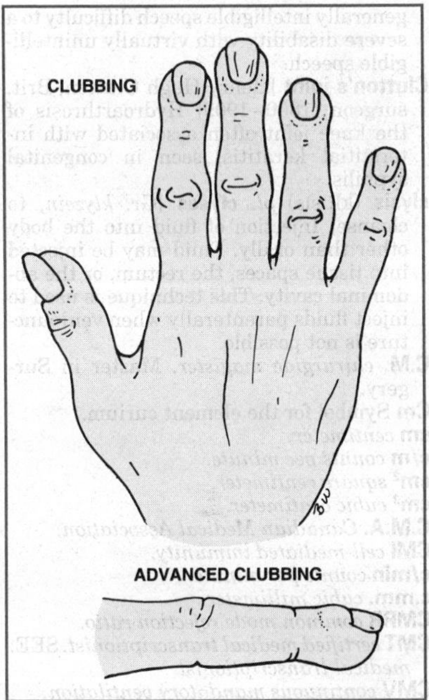


**clubfoot** Talipes equinovarus.

**clubhand** Talipomanus.

**clump** (klŭmp) [AS. *clympre,* a lump] **1.** A mass of bacteria in solution; may be caused by an agglutination reaction. **2.** To gather together.

**clumping** Agglutination.

**cluster** A closely grouped series of events or cases of a disease or other health-related phenomenon with well-defined distribution patterns, in relation to time or place or both.

***c. of differentiation*** ABBR: CD. A group of protein markers on the surface of a white blood cell. These markers are used to classify immune cell types and establish international nomenclature standards. Although found on many blood cells and some nonblood cells, they are used most often to refer to lymphocytes. Markers for CD3 are found on all mature T cells in association with T-cell antigen receptors; CD2 and CD7 markers are found on immature T cells. Markers for CD4 are found on all T helper cells, macrophages, and some B cells. Markers for CD8 identify cytotoxic T cells, which are essential to the defense against viral infections. Each marker has a specific function in the cell, such as passing a signal from the T-cell receptor to the cytoplasm. SEE: *cell, T.*

**cluttering** (klŭt′ĕr-ĭng) A form of speech difficulty marked by excessive speed and irregular rhythm, often with condensation of sounds and collapsing of words. It may range in severity from an annoying but generally intelligible speech difficulty to a severe disability with virtually unintelligible speech.

**Clutton's joint** [Henry Hugh Clutton, Brit. surgeon, 1850–1909] Hydroarthrosis of the knee joint often associated with interstitial keratitis, seen in congenital syphilis.

**clysis** (klī'sĭs) *pl.* **clyses** [Gr. *klyzein,* to cleanse] Injection of fluid into the body other than orally. Fluid may be injected into tissue spaces, the rectum, or the abdominal cavity. This technique is used to inject fluids parenterally when venipuncture is not possible.

**C.M.** *chirurgiae magister,* Master in Surgery.

**Cm** Symbol for the element curium.

**cm** *centimeter.*

**c/m** *counts per minute.*

**cm²** *square centimeter.*

**cm³** *cubic centimeter.*

**C.M.A.** *Canadian Medical Association.*

**CMI** *cell-mediated immunity.*

**c/min** *counts per minute.*

**c.mm.** *cubic millimeter.*

**CMRR** *common mode rejection ratio.*

**CMT** *certified medical transcriptionist.* SEE: *medical transcriptionist.*

**CMV** *continuous mandatory ventilation.*

**CN** *cyanogen.*

**C.N.A.** *Canadian Nurses' Association.*

**C.N.M.** *certified nurse-midwife.*

**CNS** *central nervous system; clinical nurse specialist.*

**CO** Formula for carbon monoxide; *cardiac output.*

**$CO_2$** Formula for carbon dioxide.

**$CO_2$ therapy** **1.** Therapeutic application of low temperatures with solid carbon dioxide. SEE: *cryotherapy; hypothermia* (2). **2.** Inhalation of carbon dioxide to stimulate breathing.

**Co** Symbol for the element cobalt.

**Co1** *coccygeal spinal nerve.*

**CoA** *coenzyme A.*

**coacervate** (kō-ăs'ĕr-vāt) [L. *coacervatus,* heaped up] The formation of an aggregate in a solution that is about to emulsify or in an emulsion that is demulsifying.

**coadaptation** (kō"ăd-ăp-tā'shŭn) Mutual adaptation of two independent organisms, organs, or persons.

**coagglutination** (kō"ă-gloo"tĭn-ā'shŭn) [L. *coagulare,* to curdle] Clumping by an antigen and the homologous antibody of the corpuscles of another organism.

**coagula** (kō-ăg'ū-lă) [L.] Pl. of coagulum.

**coagulability** (kō-ăg"ū-lă-bĭl'ĭ-tē) The capacity to form clots, esp. blood clots.

**coagulable** (kō-ăg'ū-lă-b'l) Capable of clotting; likely to clot.

**coagulant** (kō-ăg'ū-lănt) [L. *coagulans,* congealing] **1.** Something that causes a fluid to coagulate. **2.** Causing coagulation.

**coagulase** (kō-ăg'ū-lāz) [L. *coagulum,* blood clot] Any enzyme, such as thrombin, that causes coagulation.

**coagulate** (kō-ăg'ū-lāt) [L. *coagulare,* to congeal] To solidify; to change from a fluid state to a semisolid mass.

**coagulated** Clotted or curdled.

**coagulated protein** One of the derived (insoluble) proteins, resulting from the action of alcohol on protein, or heat on protein solutions.

**coagulation, blood** (kō-ăg"ū-lā'shŭn) [L. *coagulatio,* clotting] The process of clumping together of blood cells to form a clot. This may occur in vitro, intravascularly, or when a laceration of the skin allows the escape of blood from an artery, vein, or capillary. Coagulation of blood may occur in two pathways, depending on the beginning of the process.

*Extrinsic:* The extrinsic pathway (in an abbreviated outline form) requires the blood to be exposed to a subendothelial tissue factor originating outside the blood. This factor begins a complex pathway involving thromboplastin, factor VII, and calcium; binding to factor X, causing its conversion to factor Xa; and the resulting conversion of prothrombin to thrombin to fibrinogen and eventually fibrin.

*Intrinsic:* The intrinsic pathway (in abbreviated outline form) occurs when blood is drawn without contamination by tissue factor. This clotting pathway does not require an additive. It is triggered when the blood is exposed to a foreign surface and factor XII is activated. Factor XII may also be activated through limited cleavage by kallikrein. This process is accelerated by high-molecular-weight kininogen (HMWK). This leads to formation of factor XII, a process that produces more HMWK to accelerate kallikrein production. The process continues and factors XI and IX, and HMWK, in concert with calcium, generate factor Xa. The clotting cascade then continues as in the extrinsic pathway, and prothrombin is converted to thrombin, which acts on fibrinogen to produce fibrin. SEE: illus.

**coagulation factor** One of the various factors involved in the coagulation process. The generally accepted terms for the factors and their Roman numeral designations are as follows:

*Factor I,* fibrinogen; *Factor II,* prothrombin; *Factor III,* tissue factor; *Factor IV,* calcium ions; *Factor V,* proaccelerin (an unstable protein substance also called labile factor); *Factor VII,* proconvertin or serum prothrombin conversion accelerator; *Factor VIII,* antihemophilic factor; *Factor IX,* Christmas factor; *Factor X,* Stuart-Prower factor; *Factor XI,* plasma thromboplastin antecedent (PTA); *Factor XII,* Hageman or glass factor; *Factor XIII,* fibrin-stabilizing factor (FSF); prekallikrein, also called *Fletcher factor;* and HMWK, also called *Fitzgerald, Falujenc,* or *Williams factor,* or *contact activation cofactor.* Factor VI, once called *accelerin,* is no longer used.

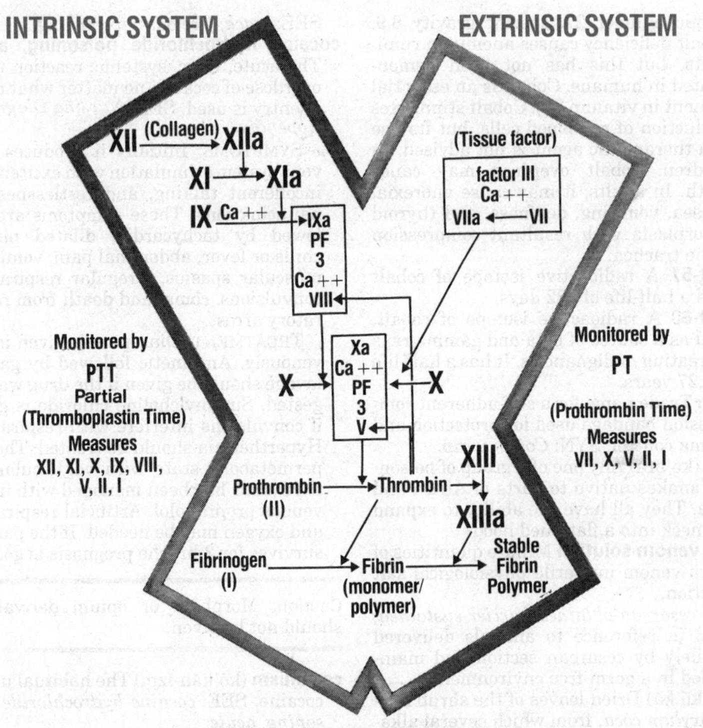


CASCADE THEORY OF COAGULATION

**coagulation time** The time required for a small amount of blood to clot. This can be determined by collecting blood in a small test tube and noting elapsed time from the moment blood is shed to the time it coagulates, or by collecting blood in a small capillary tube and breaking off small pieces of the tube at 30-sec intervals. Coagulation is indicated by the appearance of fine threads of fibrin between the broken ends of the tube. Normal time, using the capillary tube method, is 6 to 17 min.

**coagulopathy** (kō-ăg″ū-lŏp′ă-thē) [″ + Gr. *pathos,* disease, suffering] A defect in blood-clotting mechanisms. SEE: *coagulation, blood.*

*consumption c.* Disseminated intravascular clotting.

**coalesce** (kō-ăl-ĕs′) [L. *coalescere*] To fuse; to run or grow together.

**coalescence** (kō-ă-lĕs′ĕns) The fusion or growing together of two or more body parts.

**coal worker's pneumoconiosis** ABBR: CWP. A form of pneumoconiosis in which carbon and silica accumulate in the lungs as a result of breathing coal dust. SYN: *black lung.*

**coapt** (kō′ăpt) [L. *coaptare,* to fit together] To bring together, as in suturing a laceration.

**coaptation** (kō″ăp-tā′shŭn) [L. *coaptare,* to fit together] The adjustment of separate parts to each other, as the edges of fractures.

**coarctate** (kō-ărk′tāt) [L. *coarctare,* to tighten] To press together; pressed together.

**coarctation** (kō″ărk-tā′shŭn) **1.** Compression of the walls of a vessel. **2.** Shriveling. **3.** A stricture.

*c. of aorta* A localized malformation resulting in narrowing of the aorta.

**coarctotomy** (kō″ărk-tŏt′ō-mē) [″ + Gr. *tome,* incision] Cutting or dividing of a stricture.

**coat** [L. *cotta,* a tunic] A covering or a layer in the wall of a tubular structure, as the inner coat (tunica intima), middle coat (tunica media), or outer coat (tunica adventitia) of an artery.

**Coats' disease** [George Coats, Brit. ophthalmologist, 1876–1915] The development of large white masses deep in the blood vessels of the retina. This term is now used to describe at least six separate retinal disorders.

**cobalamin** (kō-băl′ă-mĭn) A chemical that contains cobalt and is contained in all of the several $B_{12}$ vitamins. SEE: *cyanocobalamin.*

**cobalt** (kō′bălt) SYMB: Co. A gray, hard, ductile metal; atomic weight 59.933, atomic number 27, specific gravity 8.9. Cobalt deficiency causes anemia in ruminants, but this has not been demonstrated in humans. Cobalt is an essential element in vitamin $B_{12}$. Cobalt stimulates production of red blood cells, but its use as a therapeutic agent is not advised. In children, cobalt overdose may cause death. In adults, it may cause anorexia, nausea, vomiting, deafness, and thyroid hyperplasia with resultant compression of the trachea.

**cobalt-57** A radioactive isotope of cobalt with a half-life of 272 days.

**cobalt-60** A radioactive isotope of cobalt, used as a source of beta and gamma rays in treating malignancies. It has a half-life of 5.27 years.

**Coban** Trade name for a self-adherent compression bandage used for protection and edema control. SYN: *Coban wrap.*

**cobra** (kō′bră) Any one of a group of poisonous snakes native to parts of Africa and Asia. They all have the ability to expand the neck into a flattened hood.

**cobra venom solution** Minute quantities of cobra venom in sterile physiological salt solution.

**COBS** *cesarean-obtained barrier-sustained;* used in reference to animals delivered sterilely by cesarean section and maintained in a germ-free environment.

**coca** (kō′kă) Dried leaves of the shrub *Erythroxylum coca,* from which several alkaloids including cocaine are obtained.

**cocaine baby** An infant exposed to cocaine in utero through maternal use of the drug. Cocaine abuse during pregnancy has been correlated with birth defects, intrauterine growth retardation, and perinatal loss related to premature separation of the placenta, preterm labor and delivery, low birth weight, and sudden infant death syndrome. It is known that cocaine crosses the placenta and enters the fetal circulation. In addition, use of cocaine by the father at the time of conception may have a negative effect on sperm quality.

Follow-up studies suggest that children who were cocaine babies have short attention spans and learning disorders.

SYMPTOMS: Newborns may exhibit signs of drug withdrawal, tachycardia, hyperirritability, muscle rigidity and seizures, and feeding problems. Hyperirritability causes negative responses to common parental claiming behaviors and interferes with bonding.

**cocaine hydrochloride** (kō-kān′, kō′kān) The hydrochloride of an alkaloid obtained from the shrub *Erythroxylum coca,* native to Bolivia and Peru and cultivated extensively in South America. Cocaine is classed as a drug of abuse when used for nonmedical purposes. "Street" names for cocaine include snow, coke, crack, lady, flake, gold dust, green gold, blow, and toot. Medically it is used as a topical anesthetic applied to mucous membranes. SEE: *crack; free base; freebasing.*

**cocaine hydrochloride poisoning, acute** The acute, toxic, systemic reaction to an overdose of cocaine, no matter what route of entry is used. SEE: *Nursing Diagnoses Appendix.*

SYMPTOMS: Initially it produces nervous system stimulation with excitement, incoherent talking, and restlessness or hallucinations. These symptoms are followed by tachycardia, dilated pupils, chills or fever, abdominal pain, vomiting, muscular spasms, irregular respiration, convulsions, coma, and death from respiratory arrest.

TREATMENT: Diazepam is given intravenously. An emetic followed by gastric lavage should be given if the drug was ingested. Succinylcholine chloride is given if convulsions interfere with respiration. Hyperthermia should be treated. The hypermetabolic state with ventricular arrhythmias has been managed with intravenous propranolol. Artificial respiration and oxygen may be needed. If the patient survives for 3 hr, the prognosis is good.

---

Caution: Morphine or opium derivatives should not be given.

---

**cocainism** (kō′kān-ĭzm) The habitual use of cocaine. SEE: *cocaine hydrochloride poisoning, acute.*

**cocainization** (kō″kān-ĭ-zā′shŭn) The use of cocaine to induce analgesia.

**cocainomania** (kō″kān-ō-mā′nē-ă) An intense desire for cocaine and its effects.

**cocarboxylase** (kō″kăr-bŏk′sĭ-lās) Thiamine pyrophosphate.

**cocarcinogen** (kō-kăr′sĭ-nō-jĕn″) A chemical or environmental factor that enhances the action of a carcinogen, the end result being the development of a malignancy.

**coccal** (kŏk′ăl) Pert. to or caused by cocci.

**cocci** (kŏk′sī) Pl. of coccus.

**Coccidia** (kŏk-sĭd′ē-ă) [Gr. *kokkos,* berry] A subclass of the phylum Apicomplexa (apical microtubule complex) of the kingdom Protista. All are intracellular parasites usually infecting epithelial cells of the intestine and associated glands. They are principally parasites of lower animals and cause great economic loss owing to their toxic effect on domestic and game animals. Only one species, *Isospora hominis,* infects humans. The geographical area of infestation is largely confined to Asia.

**coccidian** (kŏk-sĭd′ē-ăn) **1.** Pert. to Coccidia. **2.** Any member of the order Coccidia.

**Coccidioides** A genus of fungi with only one species, *Coccidioides immitis,* that is pathogenic for humans. SEE: illus.; *coccidioidomycosis.*

**coccidioidin** (kŏk″sĭd-ē-oy′dĭn) An antigenic substance prepared from *Coccidioides immitis.* It is used as a skin test in diagnosing coccidioidomycosis.

**coccidioidomycosis** (kŏk-sĭd″ĭ-oyd-ō-mī-

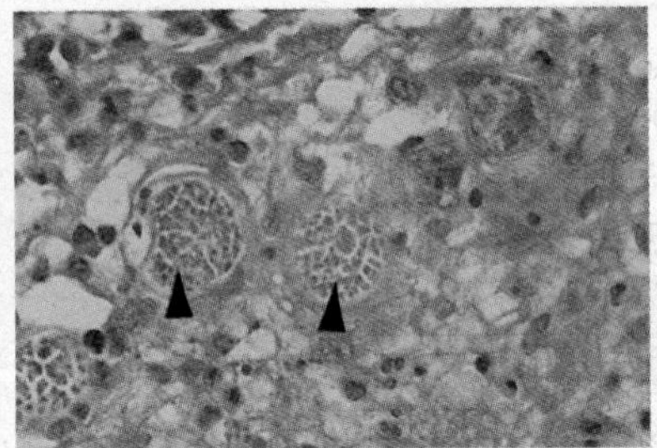

**COCCIDIOIDES IMMITIS SPHERULES (ARROWS)** (ORIG. MAG. ×450)

kō'sĭs) [" + *eidos,* form, shape, + *mykes,* fungus, + *osis,* condition] A coccidioidal granuloma caused by a pathogenic fungus, *Coccidioides immitis.* It exists in two forms: primary coccidioidomycosis, an acute self-limiting disease involving only the respiratory organs, and progressive coccidioidomycosis, a chronic, diffuse granulomatous disease involving almost any part of the body. SYN: *desert fever; granuloma, coccidioidal; valley fever.* SEE: *Nursing Diagnoses Appendix.*

TREATMENT: Most patients with primary infection recover without therapy. Patients with disseminated disease require prolonged chemotherapy. Amphotericin B is administered for 1 to 3 months. Meningitis due to *Coccidioides immitis* is treated with amphotericin B injected directly into the cerebrospinal fluid.

PROGNOSIS: For the primary type, the prognosis is favorable. For the progressive type, the prognosis is grave because the disease is often fatal.

**coccidiosis** (kŏk-sĭd-ē-ō'sĭs) [" + *osis,* condition] A pathogenic condition resulting from infestation with coccidia. SEE: *Coccidia.*

**coccobacilli** (kŏk"ō-bă-sĭl'ī) Bacilli that are short, thick, and somewhat ovoid. SEE: *bacterium* for illus.

**coccobacteria** (kŏk"ō-băk-tē'rē-ă) **1.** Spherical-shaped bacteria. **2.** Any kind of cocci.

**coccogenous** (kŏk-ŏj'ĕn-ŭs) [Gr. *kokkos,* berry, + *gennan,* to produce] Produced by cocci.

**coccoid** (kŏk'oyd) [" + *eidos,* form, shape] Resembling a micrococcus.

**coccus** (kŏk'ŭs) *pl.* **cocci** [Gr. *kokkos,* berry] A bacterial type that is spherical or ovoid. When cocci appear singly, they are designated micrococci; in pairs, diplococci; in clusters like bunches of grapes, staphylococci; in chains, streptococci; in cubical packets of eight, sarcinae. Many are pathogenic, causing such diseases as septic sore throat, erysipelas, scarlet fever, rheumatic fever, pneumonia, gonorrhea, meningitis, and puerperal fever. SEE: *bacterium.*

**coccyalgia, coccydynia** (kŏk"sē-ăl'jē-ă, kŏk"sē-dĭn'ē-ă) [Gr. *kokkyx,* coccyx, + *algos,* pain; " + *odyne,* pain] Pain in the coccyx. SYN: *coccygodynia.*

**coccygeal** (kŏk-sĭj'ē-ăl) Pert. to or in the region of the coccyx.

**coccygeal body** A small arteriovenous anastomosis at the level of the coccyx. It is associated with the median sacral artery.

**coccygeal nerve** The lowest of the spinal nerves; one of the pair of nerves arising from the coccygeal section of the spinal cord and entering the pudendal plexus.

**coccygectomy** (kŏk"sĭ-jĕk'tō-mē) [" + *ektome,* excision] Excision of the coccyx.

**coccygeus** (kŏk-sĭj'ē-ŭs) Pert. to the coccyx.

**coccygodynia** (kŏk-sĭ-gō-dĭn'ē-ă) [" + *odyne,* pain] Coccyalgia; coccydynia.

**coccyx** (kŏk'sĭks) [Gr. *kokkyx,* coccyx] A small bone at the base of the spinal column in humans, formed by four fused rudimentary vertebrae. It is usually ankylosed and articulated with the sacrum above.

**cochineal** (kŏch'ĭn-ēl) [L. *coccinus,* scarlet] A dried female insect, *Coccus cacti,* previously used as a dye.

**cochlea** (kŏk'lē-ă) [Gr. *kokhlos,* land snail] A winding cone-shaped tube forming a portion of the inner ear. It contains the organ of Corti, the receptor for hearing.

The cochlea is coiled, resembling a snail shell, winding two and three quarters turns about a central bony axis, the modiolus. Projecting outward from the modiolus, a thin bony plate, the spinal lamina, partially divides the cochlear canal into an upper passageway, the scala vestibuli, and a lower one, the scala tympani. Between the two scalae is the cochlear duct, in the floor of which lies the spiral organ (organ of Corti). The base of the cochlea adjoins the vestibule. At the cupola or tip, the two scalae are joined at the helicotrema. SEE: illus. **cochlear** (-ăr), *adj.*

**cochleariform** (kŏk"lē-ăr'ĭ-form) [" + L. *forma,* shape] Spoon-shaped.

**cochlear implant** An experimental electrical device that receives sound and transmits the resulting signal to electrodes implanted in the cochlea. That signal stimulates the cochlea and the subject is able to perceive sound. Eventually the ability to understand speech should be possible through use of this device.

**cochlear nerve** The division of the vestibulocochlear nerve (eighth cranial nerve) that supplies the cochlea. SEE: *vestibulocochlear nerve.*

**cochleitis** (kŏk"lē-ī'tĭs) [Gr. *kokhlos,* land snail, + *itis,* inflammation] Inflammation of the cochlea.

**cochleo-orbicular reflex** SEE: *cochleopalpebral reflex.*

**cochleopalpebral reflex** (kŏk"lē-ō-păl'pĕ-brăl) Contraction of the orbicularis palpebrarum muscle resulting from a sudden

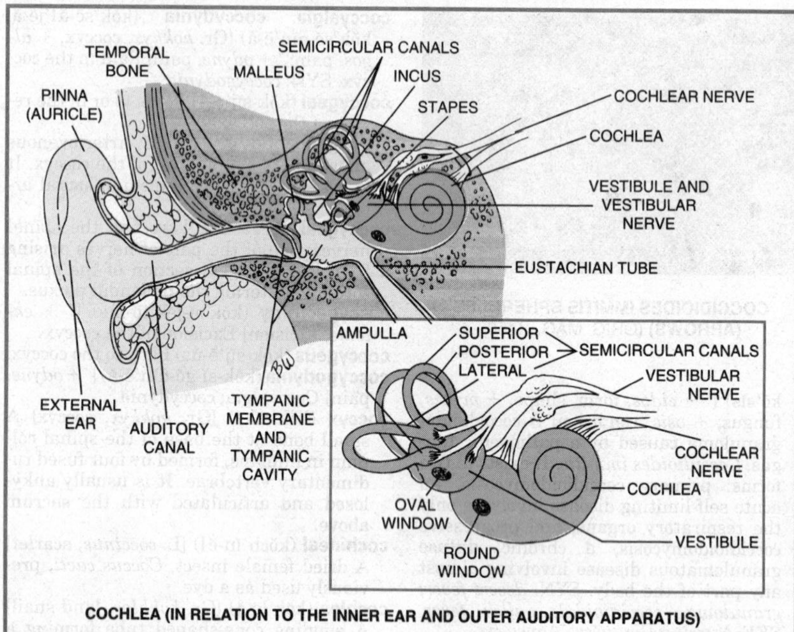

COCHLEA (IN RELATION TO THE INNER EAR AND OUTER AUDITORY APPARATUS)

noise produced near the ear. SYN: *cochleo-orbicular reflex.*

**cochleovestibular** (kŏk″lē-ō-vĕs-tĭb′ū-lăr) [″ + L. *vestibulum,* vestibule] Pert. to the cochlea and vestibule of the ear.

**cockroach** [Sp. *cucaracha*] *Blatta orientalis,* a common insect of the order Orthoptera that infests homes and food handling and food storage places. These swift-running, omnivorous insects average about 2 cm in length, but may be much larger and may have wings. Through their dual contact with filth and food, they may mechanically transmit bacteria, protozoan cysts, and helminth ova. Common genera are *Blatta, Blatella,* and *Periplaneta.*

**cocktail** (kŏk′tāl) Any beverage containing several ingredients.

***lytic c.*** A mixture of analgesic and phenothiazine derivatives used in anesthesia as a premedication. The term originated in France.

**cock-up splint** A static splint designed to maintain the wrist in either extension or dorsal flexion.

**cock-up toe** A toe deformity with dorsiflexion of the metatarsophalangeal joint and flexion of the interphalangeal and distal interphalangeal joints. SEE: *claw toe; hammertoe.*

**cocoa butter** Theobroma oil; the fat obtained from the roasted seed of *Theobroma cacao.* It is used as a base in suppositories and as a topical skin lubricant.

**coconsciousness** (kō-kŏn′shŭs-nĕs) A conscious state of which we are unaware because it is not in the focus of attention but is at the fringe of consciousness.

**cocontraction** (kō″kŏn-trăk′shŭn) A condition in which muscles around a joint or the spinal column contract simultaneously to provide stability.

**coconut "water"** [Sp. and Port. *coco,* coconut, + Eng. *nut*] The liquid obtained from an unripe coconut. The composition of the "water" varies with the species of coconut, maturation of the fruit, and location in which it was grown. Because the fluid is poor in sodium, chloride, and bicarbonate, and rich in potassium, calcium, and magnesium as compared with recommended oral rehydration solution (ORS), it is unsuitable for use in treating acute diarrhea.

**code** (kōd) **1.** A collection of rules and regulations or specifications. **2.** A set of symbols that communicate information or conceal it from people not familiar with the true meaning of the symbols. **3.** A form of coded message used in transmitting information in a hospital, esp. when the information is broadcast over a public address system (e.g., "code blue" or "code 9" could indicate a particular type of emergency to an emergency care team). SEE: *code cart; code drug.* **4.** A system of symbols that represents information contained in a computer data bank.

***genetic c.*** The sequence of bases in the DNA of living cells that provides the instructions for the synthesis of polypeptides and proteins from amino acids. These instructions are contained in 64 nucleotide triplet sequences, called codons,

61 of which specify the 20 amino acids present in proteins and 3 of which halt the addition of amino acids to a polypeptide being synthesized. These three triplets are called *termination codons*. The genetic code is the same in all living things, except that in some viruses and fungi, it is contained in RNA rather than DNA.

***pacemaker c.*** A code of three to five letters to describe pacemaker type and function. The first letter indicates the chamber(s) paced: V for ventricle pacing, A for atrial pacing, and D for dual chamber (i.e., both atrial and ventricular) pacing. The second letter indicates the chamber from which electrical activity is sensed (i.e., A for atrium, V for ventricle, or D for dual sensing). Other notations indicate the response to a sensed electrical signal, that is, none, inhibition, triggering of pacing, and dual response that may inhibit or trigger pacing in the atrium or ventricle or both.

***triplet c.*** In DNA or mRNA, the sequence of three nucleotides that is the code for a particular amino acid. The triplet sequence controls the amino acid sequence during protein synthesis.

**code cart** A container or cart that can easily and quickly be moved to a patient who has suddenly developed a life-threatening emergency. Supplies should always be replenished and arranged so that the most frequently used first-line drugs and equipment are readily available. Powered equipment, such as a defibrillator, is tested as often as necessary to be certain it is functioning properly. SEE: *basic life support; code* (3).

**code drug** A drug needed for the emergency care of patients, esp. those with sudden onset of life-threatening cardiopulmonary conditions. Included are drugs and equipment required for treating shock, cardiac arrhythmias, and cardiac standstill. SEE: *basic life support; code (3); code cart.*

**Code of Ethics for Physical Therapists** A code of ethics that sets forth ethical principles for the physical therapy profession. According to its preamble, members of this profession are responsible for maintaining and promoting ethical practice. This code of ethics, adopted by the American Physical Therapy Association, is binding on physical therapists who are members of the Association.

Principle 1. Physical therapists respect the rights and dignity of all individuals.

Principle 2. Physical therapists comply with the laws and regulations governing the practice of physical therapy.

Principle 3. Physical therapists accept responsibility for the exercise of sound judgment.

**Code for Nurses** A statement by the American Nurses Association to guide nurses in their legal and ethical practice.

1. The nurse provides services with respect for human dignity and the uniqueness of the client, unrestricted by considerations of social or economic status, personal attributes, or the nature of health problems.
2. The nurse safeguards the client's right to privacy by judiciously protecting information of a confidential nature.
3. The nurse acts to safeguard the client and the public when health care and safety are affected by the incompetent, unethical, or illegal practice of any person.
4. The nurse assumes responsibility and accountability for individual nursing judgments and actions.
5. The nurse maintains competence in nursing.
6. The nurse exercises informed judgment and uses individual competence and qualifications as criteria in seeking consultation, accepting responsibilities, and delegating nursing activities to others.
7. The nurse participates in activities that contribute to the ongoing development of the profession's body of knowledge.
8. The nurse participates in the profession's efforts to implement and improve standards of nursing.
9. The nurse participates in the profession's efforts to establish and maintain conditions of employment conducive to high quality nursing care.
10. The nurse participates in the profession's effort to protect the public from misinformation and misrepresentation and to maintain the integrity of nursing.
11. The nurse collaborates with members of the health professions and other citizens in promoting community and national efforts to meet the health needs of the public.

[From Code for Nurses with Interpretive Statements, Kansas City, MO, American Nurses' Association, 1985]

**codeine** (kō′dēn) [Gr. *kodeia*, poppyhead] An alkaloid obtained from opium, or synthetically from morphine as methylmorphine. It is used as an analgesic or a hypnotic sedative; its effects resemble those of morphine. It is used for its effectiveness in suppressing coughs.

***c. phosphate*** The phosphate of the alkaloid codeine; used because of its free solubility in water.

***c. sulfate*** The sulfate of the alkaloid codeine. It has the same uses as codeine.

**codeine poisoning** Poisoning due to an acute overdose of codeine.

SYMPTOMS: The most serious effects are depression of the central nervous system, including the centers that control respiration and heart rate. A sufficiently high dose may be fatal.

TREATMENT: Emetics should not be

given. Treatment is similar to the treatment for morphine poisoning. SEE: *morphine in Poisons and Poisoning Appendix.*

**codependency** The acute and chronic stress of living in close association with a dependent person. The individual's dependency or addiction may relate to drugs, alcohol, gambling, eating, or sexual activity. Whether or not the codependent person reinforces the dependent person's addiction is a matter of individual consideration, and generalities may be misleading.

**cod liver oil** A fixed oil obtained from fresh codfish livers. The official oil is standardized for its vitamin A and D content.

ACTION/USES: Cod liver oil was widely used in cases of nutritional deficiency to supply vitamins A and D, esp. for prophylaxis of rickets in infants. It is rarely used now because more efficient and more palatable agents are available.

INCOMPATIBILITY: Light and air both cause the oil to become rancid.

**codon** (kō′dŏn) A sequence of three bases in a strand of DNA or mRNA (messenger RNA) that is the genetic code for a specific amino acid.

**Codroxomin** Trade name for hydroxocobalamin.

**coefficient** (kō″ĕ-fĭsh′ĕnt) [L. *co-*, together, + *efficere,* to produce] **1.** In chemistry, a numeral put before a chemical formula or compound to indicate the number of molecules of that substance taking part in the chemical reaction. **2.** An expression of a ratio between two different quantities, or the effect produced by varying certain factors.

***activity c.*** **1.** A factor used in potentiometry to describe the activity of free ions in solution. **2.** A vitamin deficiency factor that describes the enhancement of enzyme activity after saturation with a vitamin.

***diffusion c.*** The number of milliliters of gas at 1 atmosphere of pressure that will diffuse a distance of 1 $\mu$m over 1 sq cm/min.

***c. of absorption*** The volume of gas absorbed by a unit volume of a liquid at 0°C and a pressure of 760 mm Hg.

***c. of elastic expansion*** The volumetric expression in cubic centimeters of a compressed gas cylinder under hydrostatic test conditions.

**Coelenterata** (sē-lĕn″tĕr-ā′tă) [Gr. *koilos,* hollow, + *enteron,* intestine] A phylum of invertebrates that includes corals, hydras, jellyfish, and sea anemones. Contact with some species can result in sting injuries. SEE: *bite; sting.*

**coelom** (sē′lŏm) [Gr. *koiloma,* a cavity] The cavity in an embryo between the split layers of lateral mesoderm. In mammals it develops into the pleural, peritoneal, and pericardial cavities. SYN: *body cavity.*

***extraembryonic c.*** In humans, the cavity in the developing blastocyst that lies between the mesoderm of the chorion and the mesoderm covering the amniotic cavity and yolk sac.

**coenocyte** (sē′nō-sīt, sĕn′ō-sīt) [Gr. *koinos,* common, + *kytos,* cell] A multinucleated mass of protoplasm; a mass of protoplasm in which there are no cell membranes between the nuclei. SYN: *syncytium.*

**coenzyme** (kō-ĕn′zīm) [L. *co-*, together, + Gr. *en,* in, + *zyme,* leaven] An enzyme activator; a diffusible, heat-stable substance of low molecular weight that, when combined with an inactive protein called apoenzyme, forms an active compound or a complete enzyme called a holoenzyme (e.g., adenylic acid, riboflavin, and coenzymes I and II).

**coenzyme A** A derivative of pantothenic acid, important as a carrier molecule for acetyl groups in many reactions including the Krebs cycle and the oxidation of fatty acids.

**coetaneous** (kō″ē-tā′nē-ŭs) [″ + *aetas,* age] Having the same age or date.

**coexcitation** (kō-ĕk-sī-tā′shŭn) [″ + *excitare,* to arouse] Simultaneous excitation of two parts or bodies.

**cofactor** (kō′făk-tor) A factor acting in conjunction with another. In general, the cofactor must be present for the other factor to be active.

**coffee** The beverage made from the seed of trees of the genus *Coffea,* called coffee beans. Coffee has a 2500-year history of use. For the last several decades, the possibility that its use causes harm has been investigated. Complicating these studies is the fact that roasted coffee contains more than 700 volatile and nonvolatile compounds. The investigations have not produced evidence that normal consumption of caffeine is a risk factor for cardiovascular disease, birth defects, breast disease, or cancer. SEE: *caffeine; caffeine withdrawal; tea.*

**Cogan's syndrome** (kō′găns) [David G. Cogan, U.S. ophthalmologist, b. 1908] Interstitial keratitis associated with tinnitus, vertigo, and usually deafness.

**cognition** (kŏg-nĭsh′ŭn) [L. *cognoscere,* to know] Awareness with perception, reasoning, judgment, intuition, and memory; the mental process by which knowledge is acquired. A patient with normally functioning mental processes would have insight into his or her illness. **cognitive** (kŏg′nĭ-tĭv), *adj.*

**cogwheel rigidity** The condition that occurs when tremor coexists with rigidity as in Parkinson's syndrome. In this condition, manually manipulated body parts may take on the feel of a cogwheel. This can occur also as an extrapyramidal side effect of antipsychotic drug therapy.

**coherent** (kō-hĕr′ĕnt) [L. *cohaerere,* to stick together] **1.** Sticking together, as parts of bodies or fluids. **2.** Consistent; making a logical whole.

**cohesion** (kō-hē′zhŭn) The property of adhering.

**cohesive** (kō-hē′sĭv) Adhesive; sticky.

**Cohnheim's areas** (kōn′hīmz) [Julius Friedrich Cohnheim, Ger. pathologist, 1839–1884] One of the irregular groups of fibrils seen in a cross section of a striated muscle fiber.

**Cohnheim's theory** The theory that tumors result from embryonal cells not used for fetal development.

**cohort** A population component born during a particular period and traced through life as it enters successive time and age periods. SEE: *analysis, cohort.*

**cohort study** In epidemiology, a method of investigation using a cohort studied prospectively or retrospectively.

**coil** (koyl) **1.** A continuous material such as tubing, rope, or a spring arranged in a spiral, loop, or circle. **2.** Popular term for a type of intrauterine contraceptive device.

**coilonychia** (koy″lō-nĭk′ē-ă) [Gr. *koilos,* hollow, + *onyx,* nail] Koilonychia; dystrophy of the fingernails in which they are thin and concave with raised edges. This condition is sometimes associated with iron-deficiency anemia.

**coin counting** A sliding movement of the tips of the thumb and index finger over each other. This may occur in Parkinson's disease.

**coinfection** The simultaneous infection of an organism or individual cells by two different pathological microorganisms.

**coitarche** Age at first sexual intercourse.

**coition** (kō-ĭsh′ŭn) [L. *coire,* to come together] Coitus.

**coitophobia** (kō″ĭ-tō-fō′bē-ă) [″ + Gr. *phobos,* fear] Morbid fear of sexual intercourse.

**coitus** (kō′ĭ-tŭs) Sexual intercourse between a man and a woman by insertion of the penis into the vagina. SYN: *coition; copulation; sexual intercourse.* **coital** (-tăl), *adj.*

***c. à la vache*** Coitus from behind with the woman in the knee-chest position.

***c. interruptus*** Coitus with withdrawal of the penis from the vagina before seminal emission occurs. This is not an effective method of contraception.

***c. reservatus*** Coitus with intentional suppression of ejaculation.

***c. Saxonius*** Coitus with manual pressure of the urethra at the underside of the penis or in the perineum to block the emission of semen at ejaculation; also called the squeeze technique. The woman may do this to prevent her partner's premature ejaculation.

**col** (kŏl) The nonkeratinized, depressed gingival tissue that lies between adjacent teeth; it extends labiolingually between the interdental papillae below the interproximal contact of the teeth.

**Cola** (kō′lă) [W. African *kola*] A genus of tropical trees that produce the kola nut. A kola nut extract is used in pharmaceutical preparations and as a main ingredient in some carbonated beverages.

**Colace** Trade name for docusate sodium.

**colation** (kō-lā′shŭn) [L. *colare,* to strain] Straining, filtering.

**colchicine** (kŏl′chĭ-sĭn) Medicine used in treating an acute attack of gout. Because the drug stimulates the smooth muscles, diarrhea may be an undesired side effect.

**COLD** *chronic obstructive lung disease.* SEE: *chronic obstructive pulmonary disease.*

**cold** [AS. *ceald,* cold] **1.** A general term for coryza or inflammation of the respiratory mucous membranes known as the common cold. **2.** Lacking heat or warmth; having a low temperature; the opposite of heat.

***chest c.*** SEE: *bronchitis.*

***common c.*** An acute catarrhal inflammation of any or all parts of the respiratory tract from the nasal mucosa to the nasal sinuses, throat, larynx, trachea, and bronchi; also called acute coryza. The contagious period begins prior to the onset of symptoms; and the spread is usually by nasal secretions. The incubation period is from 12 to 72 hr. Children develop immunity to each virus on exposure, thus they have more colds than adults. Although the common cold does not cause death, its economic importance is vast because it is the greatest cause of absenteeism in industry and schools.

SYMPTOMS: The common cold is marked by congestion of the nasal mucosa with partial or complete occlusion of the nostrils and a continuous watery discharge with more or less continuous sniffling and blowing of the nose. Also present may be sneezing, lacrimation, irritated nasopharynx, chilliness, and malaise. Fever in adults is rare; if fever is present, influenza or another cause of the infection must be suspected. Symptoms are usually resolved within 2 to 10 days. Persons with chronic diseases such as diabetes or heart or lung diseases should consult a physician when they have a cold, esp. if it is severe, accompanied by fever, or lasts more than 10 days.

ETIOLOGY: Colds may be due to any one of many viruses including rhinoviruses, coxsackieviruses, and coronaviruses.

TREATMENT: Treatment is mainly for the relief of symptoms. Nasal congestion, lacrimation, or sneezing may be treated with over-the-counter (OTC) preparations that are taken orally or sprayed on the nasal mucosa. Spray-type nasal decongestants should not be used for more than 3 days. Longer use may cause rebound reaction, which worsens the congestion. OTC medications are available for treating cough and headache. Analgesics are useful to relieve aching. Preparations containing codeine usually relieve a cough but should not be used when the cough is productive. There is no evidence that high doses of vitamin C are of benefit in treating the common cold; however, some studies have shown a reduced period of disability in persons who took as much as 8 g of vitamin C on the first day of the disease. There is no effective vaccine. Antibiotics are of use only if there is secondary bacterial infection.

CONTAGIOUSNESS: The virus may be present in the nasal secretions for a week or longer after the onset of symptoms.

**cold agglutinin disease** Term applied to a group of disorders marked by hemolytic anemia, obstruction of the microcirculation, or both. It is caused by agglutination of red blood cells by cold agglutinin. In some people this is caused by a transient infectious disease; in others, the cause is idiopathic. The latter occurs mostly in women over 50 years of age.

**cold cream** A water-in-oil emulsion ointment base used on the skin.

**cold-damp** Foggy vapor in a mine charged with carbon dioxide.

**cold pack** Wrapping of a patient or an area in towels dipped in cold water before application. A more effective method is to place crushed ice in a small plastic bag with a small amount of water. Application of cold by this method does not cause frostbite in healthy adults. Cold packs applied to ankle injuries in the first 36 hr have reduced recovery time as compared with early heat treatment. Cold packs are usually used to reduce fever, pain, swelling, or inflammation.

**cold pressor test** A test that measures blood pressure response to the immersion of one hand in ice water. An excessive increase in pressure may indicate a latent hypertensive state.

**coldspray** An aerosol coolant used to lower the temperature quickly and thus harden thermoplastic splinting material during fitting or molding.

**cold stress** SEE: *hypothermia.*

**colectomy** (kō-lĕk′tō-mē) [Gr. *kolon,* colon, + *ektome,* excision] Excision of part or all of the colon.

**coleocystitis** (kō″lē-ō-sĭs-tī′tĭs) Colpocystitis.

**coleoptosis** (kō″lē-ŏp-tō′sĭs) [″ + *ptosis,* a dropping] Prolapse of the wall of the vagina.

**coleotomy** (kō″lē-ŏt′ō-mē) Colpotomy.

**colestipol hydrochloride** (kō-lĕs′tĭ-pōl) An ion-exchange resin similar in action to cholestyramine.

**colibacillemia** (kō″lĭ-băs-ĭl-lē′mē-ă) [Gr. *kolon,* colon, + L. *bacillus,* little rod, + Gr. *haima,* blood] Colon bacillus (*Escherichia coli*) in the blood.

**colibacillosis** (kō″lĭ-băs-ĭ-lō′sĭs) [″ + ″ + Gr. *osis,* condition] Infection with the colon bacillus (*Escherichia coli*).

**colibacilluria** (kō-lĭ-băs-ĭl-ū′rē-ă) [″ + ″ + Gr. *ouron,* urine] Presence of the colon bacillus (*Escherichia coli*) in the urine.

**colibacillus** (kō″lĭ-bă-sĭl′ŭs) [″ + L. *bacillus,* little rod] The colon bacillus, *Escherichia coli.*

**colic** (kŏl′ĭk) [Gr. *kolikos,* pert. to the colon] **1.** Spasm in any hollow or tubular soft organ accompanied by pain. **2.** Pert. to the colon. SEE: *cholecystalgia; tormina.*

***biliary c.*** Colic in bile ducts usually associated with a gallstone.

***infantile c.*** Colic occurring in infants, principally during the first few months.

***intestinal c.*** Colic in which pain may occur throughout the abdomen.

***lead c.*** Severe abdominal colic associated with lead poisoning. A lead line may be found on the gums and basic stippling in the red blood cells.

***menstrual c.*** Dysmenorrhea.

***renal c.*** Pain in the region of one of the kidneys and toward the thigh. The pain radiates from the kidney region around and over the abdomen into the groin. This condition may be associated with the passage of renal calculi.

***uterine c.*** Severe abdominal pain arising in the uterus, usually during the menstrual period. SEE: *dysmenorrhea.*

**colica** (kŏl′ĭ-kă) [L.] Colic.

**colicin** (kŏl′ĭ-sĭn) A bacteriocin produced by some strains of *Escherichia coli* that is lethal to other *E. coli.* Since its discovery in 1925, approx. 20 colicins have been described, some produced by bacteria other than *E. coli.* All colicins are now called bacteriocins.

**colicky** (kŏl′ĭk-ē) Concerning colic or affected by it.

**colicolitis** (kō″lĭ-kō-lī′tĭs) [Gr. *kolon,* colon, + *kolon,* colon, + *itis,* inflammation] Colitis due to *Escherichia coli.*

**colicoplegia** (kō″lĭ-kō-plē′jē-ă) [″ + *plege,* stroke] Colic and paralysis due to lead poisoning.

**colicystitis** (kō″lĭ-sĭs-tī′tĭs) [″ + *kystis,* bladder, + *itis,* inflammation] Inflammation of the bladder resulting from *Escherichia coli* infection.

**colicystopyelitis** (kō-lĭ-sĭs″tō-pī″ĕ-lī′tĭs) [″ + ″ + *pyelos,* pelvis, + *itis,* inflammation] *Escherichia coli* inflammation of the bladder and renal pelvis.

**coliform** (kō′lĭ-form) [″ + L. *forma,* form] **1.** Sieve form; cribriform. **2.** A general term applied to some species of the family Enterobacteriaceae, including *Escherichia coli, Enterobacter,* and *Klebsiella* species. Their presence in water, esp. that of *E. coli,* is presumptive evidence of fecal contamination.

**colinephritis** (kō″lĭ-nē-frī′tĭs) [″ + *nephros,* kidney, + *itis,* inflammation] Nephritis caused by the colon bacillus, *Escherichia coli.*

**coliplication** (kō″lĭ-plĭ-kā′shŭn) [″ + L. *plica,* fold] Operation for correcting a dilated colon.

**colipuncture** (kō′lĭ-pŭnk″chūr) Colocentesis.

**colisepsis** [″ + *sepsis,* putrefaction] Infection caused by *Escherichia coli.*

**colistimethate sodium, sterile** (kō-lĭs″tĭ-mĕth′āt) A form of colistin, suitable for use intramuscularly or intravenously.

**colistin sulfate** (kō-lĭs′tĭn) Polymyxin E; an

antibiotic effective against some gram-negative bacteria, esp. *Pseudomonas* organisms, that are resistant to other antibiotics. Trade name is Coly-Mycin S.

**colitis** (kō-lī'tĭs) [" + *itis*, inflammation] Inflammation of the colon. SEE: *irritable bowel syndrome.*

***amebic c.*** Amebiasis.

***antibiotic-associated c.*** Antibiotic-induced diarrhea. SEE: *colitis, pseudomembranous.*

***pseudomembranous c.*** Colitis associated with antibiotic therapy. This is usually due to a toxin produced by *Clostridium difficile* and is marked by formation of a pseudomembrane on the mucosa of the colon. The symptoms—diarrhea with gross blood and mucus, abdominal cramps, fever, and leukocytosis—usually begin 4 to 10 days after the start of antibiotic therapy. The disease is treated by discontinuation of the antibiotic and institution of therapy with either oral vancomycin or metronidazole.

***radiation c.*** Colitis due to damage of the bowel by radiation therapy. The symptoms are those of an inflamed bowel: pain, cramps, diarrhea, and rectal bleeding. Malabsorption may develop as a result of permanent injury to the mucosa.

***ulcerative c.*** Ulceration of the mucosa of the colon. SEE: *disease, inflammatory bowel; Nursing Diagnoses Appendix.*

SYMPTOMS: The passage of offensive watery stools with mucus and pus; abdominal pain, tenderness, or colic; and intermittent or irregular fever are characteristic. Hemorrhage and perforation may occur. SEE: *irritable bowel syndrome.*

**colla** (kŏl'lă) Pl. of collum.

**collagen** (kŏl'ă-jĕn) [Gr. *kolla*, glue, + *gennan*, to produce] A strong, fibrous insoluble protein found in connective tissue, including the dermis, tendons, ligaments, deep fascia, bone, and cartilage. Collagen is the protein typical of dental tissues (except enamel), forming the matrix of dentin, cementum, and alveolar bone proper. Collagen fibers also form the periodontal ligament, which attaches the teeth to their bony sockets.

**collagenase** (kŏl-lăj'ĕ-nās) [" + " + *-ase*, enzyme] An enzyme that induces changes in collagen to cause its degradation.

**collagenic** (kŏl"ă-jĕn'ĭk) Producing or containing collagen.

**collagenoblast** (kŏl-lăj'ĕ-nō-blăst) [" + " + *blastos*, germ] A fibroblast-derived cell that produces collagen when mature.

**collagenolysis** (kŏl"ă-jĕn-ŏl'ĭ-sĭs) [" + " + *lysis*, dissolution] The degradation or destruction of collagen.

**collagenosis** (kŏl-lăj"ĕ-nō'sĭs) [" + " + *osis*, condition] A connective tissue disease.

**collapse** [L. *collapsus*, fallen to pieces] **1.** An abnormal retraction of the walls of an organ. **2.** A sudden exhaustion, prostration, or weakness due to decreased circulation of the blood.

SYMPTOMS: The symptoms are similar to those of hemorrhage. The peripheral arteries are depleted of blood, and the veins are congested, esp. in the splanchnic region. Other symptoms include apathy, extreme pallor, cold, clammy perspiration, a thin, rapid pulse, fall of blood pressure, and unconsciousness.

NURSING IMPLICATIONS: A patent airway is maintained, and the patient's head is lowered and the lower extremities are elevated slightly to enhance venous return. Vital signs and level of consciousness are assessed for signs of shock or aspiration of vomitus; prescribed intravenous fluid therapy is administered; and the patient is kept warm, but not hot. The nurse remains with the patient and briefly and calmly orients the patient to surroundings and explains procedures to provide reassurance of appropriate care.

***circulatory c.*** Shock.

***c. of lung*** An airless state of all or part of a lung. This is normal in the fetus. It is artificially induced by pneumothorax, thoracoplasty, or avulsion of the phrenic nerve. It may occur spontaneously owing to rupture of a bleb on the pleural surface of the lung.

**collapsing** Falling into extreme and sudden prostration resembling shock.

**collapsotherapy** (kŏ-lăp"sō-thĕr'ă-pē) [L. *collapsus*, fallen to pieces, + Gr. *therapeia*, treatment] Treatment of pulmonary disorders by unilateral pneumothorax and immobilization of the affected lung.

**collar** (kŏl'ăr) [L. *collum*, neck] **1.** A band worn around the neck. **2.** A structure or marking formed like a neckband.

***cervical c.*** A rigid or soft collar used to limit neck movement in patients with suspected or confirmed cervical injuries. SYN: *extrication c.; orthosis.*

***extrication c.*** Cervical c.

***c. of Venus*** Syphilitic leukoderma.

***rigid cervical c.*** A firm collar appled to a traumatized patient to prevent neck movement.

**collar bone** Clavicle.

**collateral** (kŏ-lăt'ĕr-ăl) [L. *con*, together, + *lateralis*, pert. to a side] **1.** Accompanying, side by side, as in a small side branch of a blood vessel or nerve. **2.** Subordinate or accessory.

**collateral ligament** SEE: under *ligament.*

**collateral trigone** The angle between the diverging inferior and posterior horns of the lateral ventricle.

**collecting tubule** One of the small ducts that receive urine from several renal tubules, which join together to provide a passage for the urine to larger straight collecting tubules (papillary ducts of Bellini) that open into the pelvis of the kidney. SEE: *kidney* for illus.

**Colles, Abraham** Irish surgeon, 1773–1843.

***C.'s fascia*** The inner layer of the superficial fascia of the perineum.

***C.'s fracture*** A transverse fracture of

the distal end of the radius (just above the wrist) with displacement of the hand backward and outward.

NURSING IMPLICATIONS: A history of the injury is obtained, and the patient is assessed for pain, swelling, mobility, and any deformity of the distal forearm. The areas above and below the fracture site are inspected for color changes and palpated for pulses, temperature, and the presence of sensation. The extremity is temporarily immobilized with a splint, and cold is applied according to protocol to reduce pain and limit swelling. The patient is scheduled for radiography, all procedures are explained, and noninvasive pain relief measures are instituted to reduce discomfort. The nurse assists with closed reduction and casting if carried out in the emergency department or refers the patient to an orthopedic surgeon for treatment and follow-up care.

**colliculectomy** (kŏl-lĭk″ū-lĕk′tō-mē) [L. *colliculus,* mound, + Gr. *ektome,* excision] Removal of the colliculus seminalis.

**colliculitis** (kŏl-lĭk″ū-lī′tĭs) [″ + Gr. *itis,* inflammation] Inflammation of the colliculus seminalis.

**colliculus** (kŏl-lĭk′ū-lŭs) *pl.* **colliculi** [L.] A little eminence.

***c. bulbi, c. bulbi intermedius*** Erectile tissue encircling the male urethra at the entrance to the bulb.

***c. cervicalis*** The crest on the posterior wall of the female urethra.

***c. inferior*** One of two elevations forming the lower portion of the corpora quadrigemina of the midbrain.

***c. seminalis*** An oval enlargement on the crista urethralis, an elevation in the floor of the prostatic portion of the urethra. On its sides are the openings of the ejaculatory ducts and numerous ducts of the prostate gland. SYN: *c. urethralis.*

***c. superior*** One of two elevations forming the upper portion of the corpora quadrigemina of the midbrain.

***c. urethralis*** C. seminalis.

**collimation** (kŏl″ĭ-mā′shŭn) [L. *collineare,* to align] **1.** The process of making parallel. **2.** In radiography, the process of limiting the scatter and extent of the x-ray beam to the part being radiographed.

**collimator** (kŏl′ĭ-mā″tur) [L. *collineare,* to align, direct, aim] A radiographic device used to limit the scatter and extent of the x-ray beam.

**colliquation** (kŏl″ĭ-kwā′shŭn) [L. *con,* together, + *liquare,* to melt] **1.** Abnormal discharge of a body fluid. **2.** Softening of tissues to liquefaction. **3.** Wasting.

**colliquative** (kŏ-lĭk′wă-tĭv) Pert. to a liquid and excessive discharge, as a colliquative diarrhea.

**collodion** (kō-lō′dē-ŏn) [Gr. *kollodes,* resembling glue] A preparation containing pyroxylin, a preparation of cellulose nitrate, dissolved thoroughly in ether and alcohol. It is a viscous liquid with an etheric odor and is highly flammable. When applied, it dries to form a strong, thin, transparent film that is useful in sealing the edge of a dressing, esp. on the scalp.

***flexible c.*** A collodion preparation containing camphor and castor oil. It is more elastic than collodion.

***salicylic acid c.*** A flexible collodion with salicylic acid; used as a keratolytic agent.

**colloid** (kŏl′oyd) [Gr. *kollodes,* glutinous] **1.** A gluelike substance such as a protein or starch whose particles (molecules or aggregates of molecules), when dispersed as much as possible in a solvent, remain uniformly distributed and do not form a true solution. **2.** The size of a microscopic colloid; particles ranging from $10^{-9}$ to $10^{-11}$ meters (1 to 100 nm). **3.** A homogenous gelatinous substance found within the follicles of the thyroid gland and containing the thyroid hormones. **colloidal** (-loyd′ăl), *adj.*

***thyroid c.*** A semifluid, jelly-like substance filling the follicles of the thyroid gland. It contains the thyroid hormones.

**colloid chemistry** The application of chemistry to systems and substances, and the problems of emulsions, mists, foams, and suspensions.

**colloidin** (kŏl-loy′dĭn) A jelly-like substance seen in colloid degeneration.

**colloidoclasia** (kŏl-oyd″ō-klā′sē-ă) [″ + *klasis,* fracture] An alteration in the equilibrium of body colloids producing anaphylactic shock. It results from the entrance into the bloodstream of unaltered colloids such as proteins.

**colloidopexy** (kŏl-oyd′ō-pĕk″sē) [″ + *pexis,* fixation] Fixation of colloids during metabolism.

**colloid suspension** A mixture with suspended particles whose forms change with the forces acting on them, such as milk or fat.

**colloma** (kŏ-lō′mă) [Gr. *kolla,* glue, + *oma,* tumor] A colloid degeneration of a cancer.

**collopexia** (kŏl″ō-pĕk′sē-ă) [L. *collum,* neck, + Gr. *pexis,* fixation] Fixation of the cervix uteri.

**collum** (kŏl′lŭm) *pl.* **colla** [L.] **1.** The necklike part of an organ. **2.** The neck.

**collyrium** (kō-lĭr′ē-ŭm) [Gr. *kollyrion,* eye salve] An eyewash or lotion for the eye.

**coloboma** (kŏl″ō-bō′mă) [Gr. *koloboma,* a mutilation] A lesion or defect of the eye, usually a fissure or cleft of the iris, ciliary body, or choroid. It may be congenital, pathological, or surgical. Sometimes the eyelid is involved.

**colocecostomy** (kō″lō-sē-kŏs′tō-mē) [Gr. *kolon,* colon, + L. *caecum,* blindness, + Gr. *stoma,* mouth] Surgical joining of the colon to the cecum of the small intestine.

**colocentesis** (kō″lō-sĕn-tē′sĭs) [″ + *kentesis,* puncture] Surgical puncture of the colon to relieve distention. SYN: *colipuncture; colopuncture.*

**colocolostomy** (kō″lō-kō-lŏs′tō-mē) [″ + *kolon,* colon, + *stoma,* mouth] The surgical formation of a passage between two portions of the colon.

**colocutaneous** (kō″lō-kū-tā′nē-ŭs) [″ + L. *cutis,* skin] **1.** Pert. to the colon and the skin. **2.** Pert. to a pathological or surgical connection between the colon and the skin. SEE: *colostomy.*

**coloenteritis** (kŏ″lō-ĕn″tĕr-ī′tĭs) [Gr. *kolon,* colon, + *enteron,* intestine, + *itis,* inflammation] Inflammation of the mucous membrane of the small and large intestines.

**colofixation** (kō″lō-fĭk-sā′shŭn) Suspension of the colon in treatment of ptosis.

**Cologel** Trade name for methylcellulose.

**colon** [L.; Gr. *kolon*] The large intestine from the end of the ileum to the anal canal that surrounds the anus, about 59 in. (1.5 m) long; divided into the ascending, the transverse, the descending, and the sigmoid or pelvic colon. Beginning at the cecum, the first part of the large intestine (ascending colon) passes upward to the right colic or hepatic flexure, where it turns as the transverse colon passing ventral to the liver and stomach. On reaching the spleen, it turns downward (left colic or splenic flexure) and continues as the descending colon to the brim of the pelvis, where it is continuous with the sigmoid colon and extends to the rectum. SEE: illus.

FUNCTION: *Mechanical:* The colon mixes the intestinal contents. *Chemical:* No digestive enzymes are secreted by the colon. The products of bacterial action that are absorbed into the bloodstream are carried by the portal circulation to the liver before they enter the general circulation. More water is absorbed in the colon than in the small intestine. Body fluids are conserved in this way, and despite the large volumes of secretions added to the food during its progress through the alimentary canal, the contents of the colon are gradually dehydrated until they assume the consistency of normal feces or even become quite hard. SEE: *absorption, colon*; *defecation.* **colonic** (kō-lŏn′ĭk), *adj.*

***bacteria of c.*** The bacteria present in the colon. Several conditions, such as use of antibiotics, corticosteroids, or dieting, may alter the normal flora. In addition, the type and number of bacteria in the colon may be influenced by genetic factors. Although *Escherichia coli* is the most important bacterium that normally inhabits the colon, it is not the most common, being outnumbered by the gram-negative anaerobic *Bacteroides* bacilli by at least 100 to 1. Whatever digestion takes place in the colon results from bacterial action. A large number of fermentative bacteria are found in the middle portion of the colon. Putrefying bacteria, found in the lower part of the colon, may produce toxic products, such as indole and skatole; however, if absorbed, such products undergo detoxification in the liver.

***irritable c.*** The most frequently seen gastrointestinal disease. Women are three times more likely to have this disease than men. Both the small and large intestines are involved in this syndrome

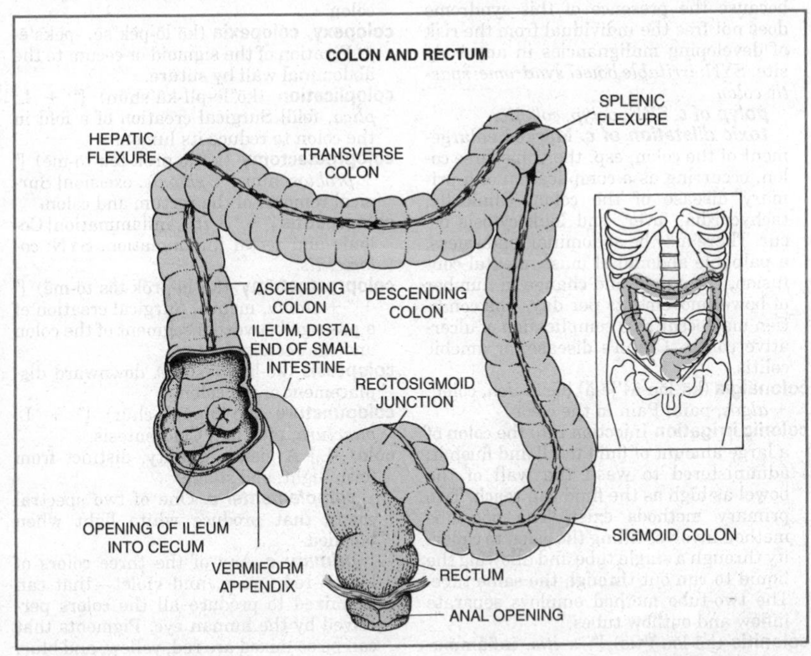

of disordered motility accompanied by pain, including cramping, usually in the lower abdomen, and constipation alternating with diarrhea. The pain is usually relieved by the passage of either small-diameter stools of varying consistency or gas and mucus. The symptoms, which may be chronic or recurring at intervals, are usually triggered by anxiety-producing periods of stress from social, family, or occupational problems. The cause is unknown, but the disease is related to the patient's reaction to stress, which induces changes in the motility pattern of the intestinal tract. Typically, patients have little insight into their disease and regard their altered bowel habits and stool size as being the cause of their discomfort. The disease subsides as the stress is relieved.

TREATMENT: A careful history, physical examination, and special studies of the gastrointestinal tract are required to assure the patient and physician that no organic disease is present. The patient is then treated for chronic anxiety neurosis. It is essential to reassure the patient that the disease will not cause chronic colitis or colon cancer. The use of laxatives for constipation and antispasmodics such as tincture of belladonna for abdominal cramps may be helpful but may prevent the patient from learning to recognize the importance of the gastrointestinal signs and symptoms.

NOTE: Although the disease does not cause malignancy of the gastrointestinal tract, it is important to review the patient periodically for such pathological changes because the presence of this syndrome does not free the individual from the risk of developing malignancies in any body site. SYN: *irritable bowel syndrome; spastic colon.*

***polyp of c.*** SEE: *polyp, colonic.*

***toxic dilatation of c.*** Marked enlargement of the colon, esp. the transverse colon, occurring as a complication of a primary disease of the colon. Clinically, tachycardia, fever, and leukocytosis occur. There may be abdominal tenderness, a palpable abdominal mass, mental confusion, cramping, and change in number of bowel movements per day. The condition may occur as a complication of ulcerative colitis, Crohn's disease, or amebic colitis.

**colonalgia** (kō″lŏn-ăl′jē-ă) [Gr. *kolon,* colon, + *algos,* pain] Pain in the colon.

**colonic irrigation** Injection into the colon of a large amount of fluid to fill and flush it; administered to wash the wall of the bowel as high as the fluid can reach. Two primary methods exist. The one-tube method involves filling the colon to capacity through a single tube and allowing the liquid to run out through the same tube. The two-tube method employs separate inflow and outflow tubes.

**colonitis** (kō-lŏn-ī′tĭs) [″ + *itis,* inflammation] Colitis.

**colonization** (kŏl″ŏ-nĭ-zā′shŭn) **1.** The process of a group of organisms, esp. bacteria, living together. **2.** Innidiation.

**colonopathy** (kō″lō-nŏp′ă-thē) [Gr. *kolon,* colon, + *pathos,* disease] Any disease of the colon.

**colonopexy** (kō-lŏn′ō-pĕk″sē) [″ + *pexis,* fixation] Surgical attachment of part of the colon to the abdominal wall.

**colonorrhagia** (kō″lŏn-ō-rā′jē-ă) [″ + *rhegnynai,* to burst forth] Hemorrhage from the colon.

**colonorrhea** (kō″lŏn-ō-rē′ă) [″ + *rhoia,* flow] **1.** Colitis. **2.** Discharge of watery fluid from the colon.

**colonoscope** (kō-lŏn′ō-skōp) [″ + *skopein,* to examine] An instrument for examining the colon. SEE: *sigmoidoscope.*

**colonoscopy** (kō″lŏn-ŏs′kō-pē) Examination of the upper portion of the rectum with an elongated speculum or a colonoscope.

**colony** (kŏl′ō-nē) [L. *colonia*] A growth of microorganisms in a culture; usually considered to have grown from a single organism.

**colony-stimulating factor–1** ABBR: CSF-1. A protein in human serum that promotes monocyte differentiation. SEE: *granulocyte-macrophage colony-stimulating factor.*

**colopexostomy** (kō″lō-pĕks-ŏs′tō-mē) [Gr. *kolon,* colon, + *pexis,* fixation, + *stoma,* mouth] Resection of the colon and fixation to the abdominal wall to establish an artificial anus.

**colopexotomy** (kō″lō-pĕks-ŏt′ō-mē) [″ + ″ + *tome,* incision] Incision and fixation of the colon.

**colopexy, colopexia** (kō′lō-pĕk″sē, -pĕks′ē-ă) Fixation of the sigmoid or cecum to the abdominal wall by suture.

**coloplication** (kō″lō-plĭ-kā′shŭn) [″ + L. *plica,* fold] Surgical creation of a fold in the colon to reduce its lumen.

**coloproctectomy** (kō″lō-prŏk-tĕk′tō-mē) [″ + *proktos,* anus, + *ektome,* excision] Surgical removal of the rectum and colon.

**coloproctitis** [″ + ″ + *itis,* inflammation] Colonic and rectal inflammation. SYN: *colorectitis.*

**coloproctostomy** (kō″lō-prŏk-tŏs′tō-mē) [″ + ″ + *stoma,* mouth] Surgical creation of a passage between a segment of the colon and the rectum.

**coloptosis** (kō-lŏp-tō′sĭs) A downward displacement of the colon.

**colopuncture** (kō′lō-pŭnk-chūr) [″ + L. *punctura,* piercing] Colocentesis.

**color** [L.] A visible quality, distinct from form, light, and shade.

***complemental c.*** One of two spectral colors that produce white light when blended.

***primary c.*** Any of the three colors of light—red, green, and violet—that can be mixed to produce all the colors perceived by the human eye. Pigments that can be so mixed are red, yellow, and blue.

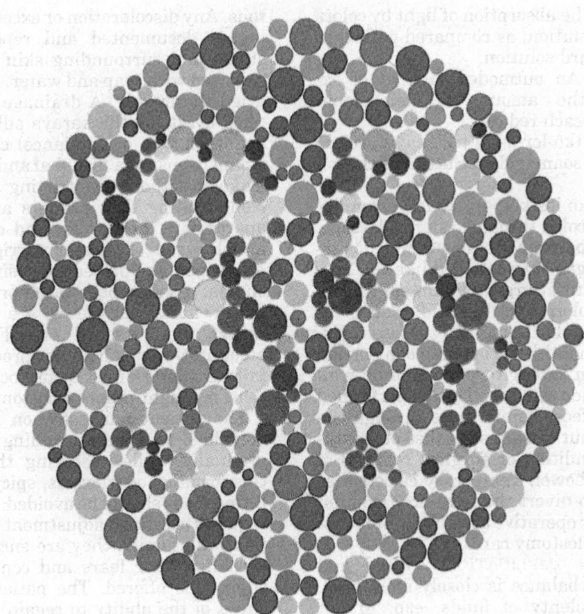

PATTERN USED TO DETECT **COLOR BLINDNESS**

**color additives** Any dye, pigment, or substance that can impart color when added or applied to a food, drug, or cosmetic. Use of color additives in the U.S. is regulated by the Food and Drug Administration (FDA). Food Drug and Cosmetic (FD&C) colors certified for food use are FD&C Blue No. 1, No. 2, and No. 3; Green No. 3; Red No. 3 and No. 40; and Yellow No. 5 and No. 6.

**color blindness** A genetically determined condition in which color perception is defective or absent. Color vision is based on perception of red, green, and blue (termed the first, second, and third color factors, respectively). If there is a defect in the perception of one of these colors, a color will be perceived as if it were composed only of the other two colors. A person may suffer from red, green, or blue blindness. Color blindness in which all colors are perceived as gray is termed *monochromasia*. SEE: illus.

**color deficiency** A preferred term for color blindness, the inability to identify one or more of the primary colors. Children may become unduly alarmed by hearing the words "color blindness"; therefore, "color deficiency," which is technically correct, is preferred.

**colorectal carcinoma** A malignant neoplasm of the colon or rectum, of which an estimated 55,000 persons in the U.S. die annually. It is the second most common cause of death from cancer in the U.S.

SYMPTOMS: Symptoms are nonspecific and include change in the usual pattern of bowel habits, esp. in patients over 40 years of age; recent onset of constipation, diarrhea, or tenesmus in an older patient; bright red or dark blood in the stool; and hypochromic microcytic anemia.

DIAGNOSIS: Diagnosis is based on findings from the digital rectal examination, anoscopy, proctosigmoidoscopy, colonoscopy, barium enema examination, and biopsy of suspicious lesions and polyps.

TREATMENT: Surgical resection is the treatment for this disease. Then a combination of levamisole hydrochloride and fluorouracil is given if the cancer has metastasized to regional lymph nodes.

**colorectitis** (kō″lō-rĕk-tī′tĭs) Coloproctitis.

**colorectostomy** (kō″lō-rĕk-tŏs′tō-mē) [″ + ″ + Gr. *stoma*, mouth] Surgical formation of a passage between the colon and rectum.

**colorectum** (kōl″ō-rĕk′tŭm) The colon and rectum.

**color gustation** A sense of color aroused by stimulation of taste receptors.

**color hearing** A sense of color caused by a sound.

**colorimeter** (kŭl″or-ĭm′ĕ-tĕr) [L. *color*, color, + Gr. *metron*, measure] An instrument for measuring the intensity of color in a substance or fluid, esp. one for determining the amount of hemoglobin in the blood.

**colorimetry** A photometric technique that

measures the absorption of light by colors in a test solution, as compared with that in a standard solution.

**color index** An outmoded method of expressing the amount of hemoglobin present in each red cell.

**colorrhaphy** (kō-lor′ă-fē) [Gr. *kolon,* colon, + *rhaphe,* seam, ridge] Suture of the colon.

**coloscopy** (kō-lŏs′kō-pē) Visual examination of the colon through a sigmoidoscope.

**colosigmoidostomy** (kō″lō-sĭg″moy-dŏs′tō-mē) [″ + *sigmoeides,* shaped like Gr. Σ, + *stoma,* mouth] Surgical joining of the descending colon to the sigmoid colon.

**colostomy** (kō-lŏs′tō-mē) [Gr. *kolon,* colon, + *stoma,* mouth] The opening of a portion of the colon through the abdominal wall to its outside surface. This is performed when the feces cannot pass through the colon and out the anus because of a pathological condition or surgical removal of the distal bowel. Temporary colostomies are done to divert the fecal flow from an inflamed or operative area. SEE: illus.; *ostomy* for colostomy care.

NURSING IMPLICATIONS: Fluid and electrolyte balance is closely monitored. Drinking plenty of fluids, esp. in hot weather, is recommended; fruit juices and bouillon are particularly beneficial because of their potassium content. Alcohol should be avoided. Persistent diarrhea should be reported. The stoma and surrounding skin are inspected for irritation and excoriation; the stoma should be smooth, cherry red, and slightly edematous. Any discoloration or excessive swelling is documented and reported. The stoma and surrounding skin are gently cleansed with soap and water, rinsed, and dried thoroughly. A drainage bag is applied by fitting the karaya adhesive ring (or other type of appliance) close to the stoma to ensure a firm seal and to prevent leakage without constricting the stoma. Nonirritating skin barriers are used as appropriate. Stool color and consistency are observed. If colostomy irrigations are prescribed, the procedure is similar to an enema: a soft rubber catheter is used to instill fluid, and feces are evacuated rather than washed out. Fluid type, amount, timing, and other procedural details are determined by protocol. The patient is taught proper colostomy care.

The patient must stay on a low-fiber diet for 6 to 8 weeks, adding new foods gradually while observing their effect. Gas-forming, odoriferous, spicy, and irritating foods should be avoided. Colostomy requires a difficult adjustment by both patient and family; they are encouraged to verbalize their fears and concerns, and support is offered. The patient is reassured of the ability to regain continence with dietary control and bowel retraining. Both patient and partner are encouraged to discuss their feelings and concerns about body image changes and about resumption of sexual relations, and they should be assured that the appliance will not dislodge if empty. Food and fluids should be avoided a few hours before sex-

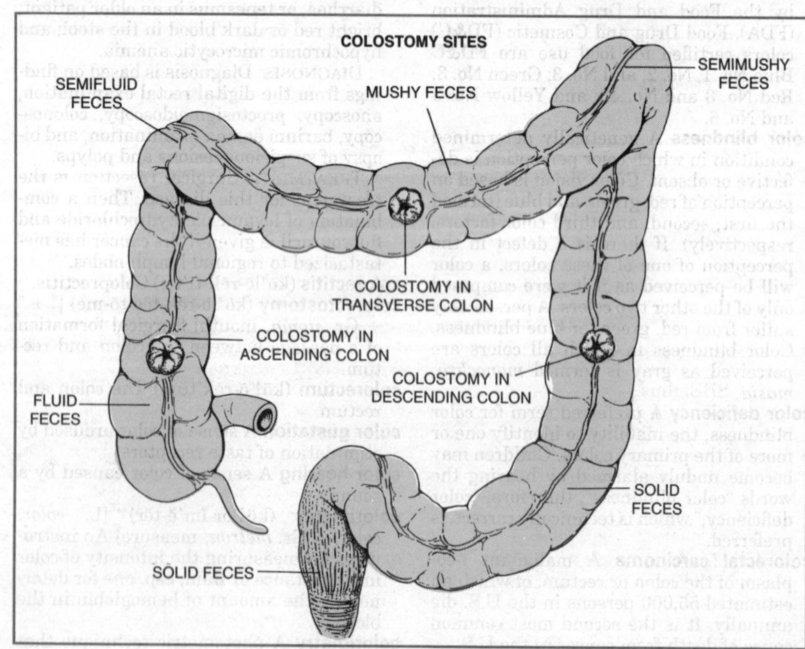

ual activity. Depression is not uncommon after ostomy surgery, and psychological counseling is recommended if depression persists. The patient and family are referred to available support groups. SEE: *Nursing Diagnoses Appendix.*

***double-barrel c.*** A temporary colostomy with two openings into the colon: one distal and one proximal. Elimination occurs through the proximal stoma, allowing the distal length of the colon to rest and heal as in colitis. When healing is complete, the two ends are rejoined and returned to the peritoneal cavity, and normal function resumes.

***terminal c.*** A colostomy in which the proximal cut end of the colon is formed into a stoma and the distal colon is either resected or closed.

***wet c.*** **1.** A colostomy in the right side of the colon or in the ileum. The drainage from this type of colostomy is liquid. **2.** A colostomy in the left side of the colon distal to the point where the ureters have been anastomosed to it. Thus the urine and fecal material are excreted through the same stoma.

**colostrorrhea** (kō-lŏs″trō-rē′ă) [L. *colostrum,* + Gr. *rhoia,* flow] Abnormal secretion of colostrum.

**colostrum** [L.] Breast fluid that may be secreted from the second trimester of pregnancy onward but that is most evident in the first 2 to 3 days after birth and before the onset of true lactation. This thin yellowish fluid contains a great number of proteins and calories in addition to immune globulins.

**colotomy** (kō-lŏt′ō-mē) [Gr. *kolon,* colon, + *tome,* incision] Incision of the colon.

**colovaginal** (kō″lō-văj′ĭ-năl) Concerning the colon and vagina or communication between the two.

**colovesical** (kō″lō-vĕs′ĭ-kăl) Concerning the colon and the urinary bladder or communication between the two.

**colpalgia** (kŏl-păl′jē-ă) [Gr. *kolpos,* vagina, + *algos,* pain] Vaginal pain.

**colpectomy** (kŏl-pĕk′tō-mē) [″ + *ektome,* excision] Surgical removal of the vagina.

**colpeurysis** (kŏl-pū′rĭs-ĭs) Surgical dilatation of the vagina.

**colpitis** SEE: *vaginitis* (2).

***c. macularis*** Small erythematous lesions on the squamous epithelium of the upper vagina and cervix. The lesions are seen best by use of colposcopy, and have the appearance of "strawberry spots." These spots have a high positive predictive value for women with trichomoniasis. SEE: *Trichomonas vaginalis.*

**colpocele** (kŏl′pō-sēl) [″ + *kele,* tumor, swelling] A hernia into the vagina.

**colpoceliotomy** (kŏl″pō-sē″lē-ŏt′ō-mē) [″ + *koilia,* belly, + *tome,* incision] An incision into the abdomen through the vagina. SEE: *culdoscopy.*

**colpocleisis** (kŏl″pō-klī′sĭs) [″ + *kleisis,* a closure] Surgical occlusion of the vagina.

**colpocystitis** (kŏl″pō-sĭs-tī′tĭs) [″ + *kystis,* bladder, + *itis,* inflammation] Inflammation of the vagina and bladder. SYN: *coleocystitis.*

**colpocystocele** (kŏl″-pō-sĭs′tō-sēl) [″ + *kystis,* bladder, + *kele,* tumor, swelling] Prolapse of the bladder into the vagina.

**colpocystoplasty** (kŏl″pō-sĭs′tō-plăs″tē) [″ + ″ + *plassein,* to form] Surgical repair of a vesicovaginal fistula.

**colpocystotomy** (kŏl″pō-sĭs-tŏt′ō-mē) [″ + ″ + *tome,* incision] An incision into the bladder through the vagina.

NURSING IMPLICATIONS: Fluid balance is monitored and documented. The patient is carefully assessed for bladder distention, and the retention catheter is inspected for patency and character of drainage. If irrigation is required, a three-way catheter, which permits continuous or intermittent irrigation as prescribed, should be used. Sterility of irrigation fluid and equipment is maintained to help prevent nosocomial infections.

**colpohyperplasia** (kŏl″pō-hī-pĕr-plā′zē-ă) [″ + *hyper,* over, + *plasis,* a forming] Excessive growth of the mucous membrane of the vagina.

***c. cystica*** Infectious inflammation of the vaginal walls marked by the production of small blebs.

**colpomicroscope** (kŏl″pō-mī′krō-skōp) [″ + *mikros,* small, + *skopein,* to view] An optical device for viewing under very high–power magnification of the vaginal mucosa and the cervix.

**colpomyomectomy** (kŏl″pō-mī″ō-mĕk′tō-mē) [″ + *mys,* muscle, + *oma,* tumor, + *ektome,* excision] Removal of a fibroid tumor of the uterus through the vagina.

**colpomyomotomy** (kŏl″pō-mī″ō-mŏt′ō-mē) [″ + ″ + ″ + *tome,* incision] Incision of the uterus through the vagina for removal of a tumor.

**colpoperineoplasty** (kŏl″pō-pĕr″ĭn-ē′ō-plăs″tē) [″ + *perinaion,* perineum, + *plassein,* to form] Plastic surgery on the vagina and perineum.

**colpoperineorrhaphy** (kŏl″pō-pĕr″ĭn-ē-or′ră-fē) [″ + ″ + *rhaphe,* seam, ridge] Surgical repair of perineal tears in the vagina.

**colpopexy** (kŏl′pō-pĕk″sē) [″ + *pexis,* fixation] Suture of a relaxed and prolapsed vagina to the abdominal wall.

**colpoplasty** (kŏl′pō-plăs″tē) [″ + *plassein,* to form] Plastic surgery of the vagina.

**colpoptosis** (kŏl″pŏp-tō′sĭs) [″ + *ptosis,* a dropping] Prolapse of the vagina.

**colporrhaphy** (kŏl-por′ă-fē) [″ + *rhaphe,* seam, ridge] Suture of the vagina.

**colporrhexis** (kŏl″pō-rĕk′sĭs) [″ + *rhexis,* rupture] Laceration or rupture of the vaginal walls.

**colposcope** (kŏl′pō-skōp) [″ + *skopein,* to examine] An instrument used to examine the tissues of the vagina and cervix through a magnifying lens.

**colposcopy** (kŏl-pŏs′kō-pē) The examination of vaginal and cervical tissues by means of a colposcope. Colposcopy is used to select sites of abnormal epithelium for biopsy in patients with abnormal Pap smears. It is helpful in defining tumor extension, for evaluating benign lesions, and in postpubertal vaginal examination of diethylstilbestrol-exposed daughters.

**colpostat** (kŏl'pō-stăt) [" + *statikos,* standing] A device for holding an instrument, such as a radium applicator, in place in the vagina.

**colpostenosis** (kŏl"pō-stĕn-ō'sĭs) [" + *stenosis,* narrowing] Stenosis or narrowing of the vagina.

**colpotomy** (kŏl-pŏt'ō-mē) [" + *tome,* incision] An incision into the wall of the vagina. SYN: *coleotomy.*

**colpoureterotomy** (kŏl"pō-ū-rē"tĕr-ŏt'ō-mē) [" + " + *tome,* incision] Incision of the ureter through the vagina.

**columbium** Former name for the element niobium.

**columella** (kŏl"ū-mĕl'lă) [L., small column] **1.** A little column. **2.** In microbiology or mycology, the portion of the sporangiophore on which the spores are borne.

***c. cochleae*** The modiolus of the cochlea.

***c. nasi*** The anterior part of the septum of the nose.

**column** (kŏl'ŭm) [L. *columna,* pillar] A cylindrical supporting structure.

***anal c.*** Vertical folds in the anal canal. SYN: *rectal c.*

***anterior c.*** The anterior portion of the gray matter on each side of the spinal cord; in reference to white matter, the posterior funiculus.

***c. of Burdach*** The fasciculus cuneatus.

***Clarke's c.*** A group of large cells in the medial portion of the base of the posterior gray column of the spinal cord.

***fornix c.*** A column of the fornix; two arched bands of fibers that form its anterior portion. The fibers lead to the mammillary body.

***gray c.*** Gray matter in the anterior and posterior horns of the spinal cord.

***lateral c.*** **1.** A column in the lateral portion of the gray matter of the spinal cord. It contains cell bodies of preganglionic neurons of the sympathetic nervous system. **2.** The lateral funiculus or the white matter between roots of spinal nerves.

***c. of Goll*** The fasciculus gracilis.

***c. of Gowers*** The tract of ascending fibers anterior to the direct cerebellar column and on the lateral surface of the spinal cord.

***c. of Morgagni*** One of several vertical ridges in the mucous membrane at the junction of the anus and rectum.

***posterior c.*** **1.** The posterior horn of the gray matter of the spinal cord. It consists of an expanded portion or caput connected by a narrower cervix to the main portion of the gray matter. **2.** The posterior funiculus of the white matter.

***rectal c.*** Anal c.

***renal c.*** A column of Bertin, cortical material of the kidney that extends centrally, separating the pyramids.

***spinal c.*** Vertebral c.

***vertebral c.*** The portion of the axial skeleton consisting of vertebrae (7 cervical, 12 thoracic, 5 lumbar, the sacrum, and the coccyx) joined together by intervertebral disks and fibrous tissue. It forms the main supporting axis of the body, encloses and protects the spinal cord, and attaches the appendicular skeleton and muscles for moving the various body parts. SYN: *spinal c.*

**columna** (kō-lŭm'nă) *pl.* **columnae** [L.] A column or pillar.

***c. carnea*** The trabecula carnea cordis.

***c. nasi*** The nasal septum.

***c. rugarum vaginae*** The folds of mucous membrane of the vagina that are arranged in a columnar fashion.

**columnar layer** SEE: *layer, columnar.*

**Coly-Mycin M** Trade name for colistimethate sodium.

**Coly-Mycin S Oral** Trade name for colistin sulfate.

**coma** (kō'mă) [Gr. *koma,* a deep sleep] An abnormal deep stupor occurring as a result of illness or injury. The patient cannot be aroused by external stimuli. More than 50% of cases are caused by trauma to the head or circulatory accidents in the brain due to hypertension, arteriosclerosis, thrombosis, tumor, abscess formation, or insufficient blood flow to the brain. Other frequent causes of coma are acute systemic infection of the brain or meninges; acute infection and bacterial intoxication as in fevers, botulism, and other infectious diseases; effects of drugs (alcohol, atropine, barbiturates, chloral, hyoscine, paraldehyde, and phenols); trauma as in accidents, hemorrhage, or electrocution; gases or fumes such as carbon dioxide or carbon monoxide; extreme temperature; and neurosis as in malingering. SEE: *Glasgow Coma Scale.*

TREATMENT: Treatment is symptomatic until evidence shows the need for definitive therapy. Basic life support measures should be instituted.

FIRST AID: First aid should be instituted cautiously. The patient should not be moved except to position the head to help clear the airway. Sudden movement of the patient by unskilled persons may be dangerous. The shirt collar should be loosened.

---

Caution: If there is a question of whether the coma is due to an overdose of insulin or to diabetes mellitus, it is safe to give glucose intravenously. Administration of insulin might be disastrous.

---

The urine should be examined for albumin, sugar, narcotics, and acetone. In uremic coma, diuresis should be stimulated. In coma due to hysteria, the patient requires careful nursing care and observation but no specific therapy other than maintaining the airway.

NURSING IMPLICATIONS: A patent airway is maintained. Neurological status is monitored with the Glasgow Coma Scale. Frequency of assessment depends on protocol and the patient's stability. Findings are documented, and evidence of clinical deterioration is reported.

Fluid and electrolyte balance is monitored and maintained; gastrointestinal and urinary functions are assessed; care for the indwelling urinary catheter, intravenous line, and nasogastric or PEG feeding tube is provided, as well as adequate enteral or parenteral nutrition; and bowel elimination is maintained with stool softeners, suppositories, or enemas as prescribed. Ventilatory status is assessed by auscultating for adventitious lung sounds, and adequate ventilation and oxygenation are determined by arterial blood gas or oxygen saturation values. The nurse assists with intubation and provides mechanical ventilation. The patient is repositioned to improve aeration of lung bases, and drainage of secretions is encouraged. The oropharynx (and endotracheal tube) is suctioned gently but briefly as necessary, considering concerns for increased intracranial pressure. The corneas are protected from ulceration by applying artificial tears to moisturize the eyes and by patching the eyes closed if the patient is unable to close them. Skin status is assessed and a plan instituted to prevent or manage pressure areas; passive range-of-motion exercises are provided; the patient is repositioned frequently; distal extremities are supported and elevated to prevent dependent edema; and appropriate supportive devices are used to prevent external hip rotation, flexion and extension, contractures, and footdrop.

Verbal and gentle touch stimulation are provided; the patient is assessed for orientation to person, time, place, and activities; and nothing is said in the patient's presence that the patient should not hear, because the unresponsive patient is still aware of surroundings and can hear what is said. Emotional support is offered family members to help them interact appropriately with the patient and reinforce their decisions about care. SEE: *shock*.

***alcoholic c.*** A coma due to ingestion of alcohol.

***apoplectic c.*** A coma due to an intracranial vascular accident (so-called shock or stroke). One side of the body and one or more extremities may be paralyzed. Initially fever is not present. One pupil may be larger than the other. Coma usually indicates increased intracranial pressure. SEE: *apoplexy; stroke.*

***barbiturate c.*** A coma caused by ingestion or injection of barbiturates. It is used clinically in the treatment of elevated intracranial pressure.

NURSING IMPLICATIONS: The patient usually requires intubation and mechanical ventilation. Ventilatory status and oxygenation are monitored, adequate ventilation is maintained, and pulmonary toilet is provided. Septic technique is used for all procedures to prevent nosocomial respiratory infections.

***diabetic c.*** A coma occurring in diabetes mellitus, caused by lack of insulin, which produces metabolic changes with excess production of acetone bodies and metabolic acidosis. Paralysis is not present. SEE: *diabetes mellitus; Nursing Diagnoses Appendix.*

SYMPTOMS: Symptoms include sweet-smelling (acetone odor) breath and hyperglycemia.

TREATMENT: The correct use of insulin has prevented diabetic coma to a large extent, but an insulin overdose may induce hypoglycemic coma. Therefore, insulin should not be given until the diagnosis of diabetic coma is made. Urine should be examined hourly for dextrose; if it is sugar free, more dextrose must be given.

***hepatic c.*** SEE: *hepatic coma.*

***hyperglycemic, hyperosmolar, nonketotic c.*** ABBR: HHNC. A coma in which the patient has a relative insulin deficiency and resulting hyperglycemia, but enough insulin to prevent fatty acid breakdown. The condition occurs most often in non–insulin-dependent diabetes and involves hyperosmolarity of extracellular fluids and subsequent intracellular dehydration. It is often precipitated by physical stress or administration of hyperosmolar solutions.

***hypoglycemic c.*** Unconsciousness due to a decreased level of blood glucose. This may be caused by a disease of the pancreas, an overdose of insulin, or starvation.

***irreversible c.*** A coma from which the patient cannot recover. SYN: *brain death.*

***Kussmaul's c.*** The coma, acidosis, and deep breathing seen in diabetic coma.

***uremic c.*** A coma due to disturbed kidney metabolism. This causes autointoxication through the retention of metabolic end products that would normally be excreted by the kidneys. Interference with the acid-base balance develops.

SYMPTOMS: In general, respirations are stertorous and the face is livid. The skin is dry and may be covered with "uremic frost," a collection of urea excreted in the sweat. The pulse is forceful and rapid, and the blood pressure is elevated. The sphincters may be relaxed. Urine is scanty and contains albumin and many casts; the breath has a urinous odor. Complete urinary retention may occur.

***vigil c.*** A coma in which the patient's

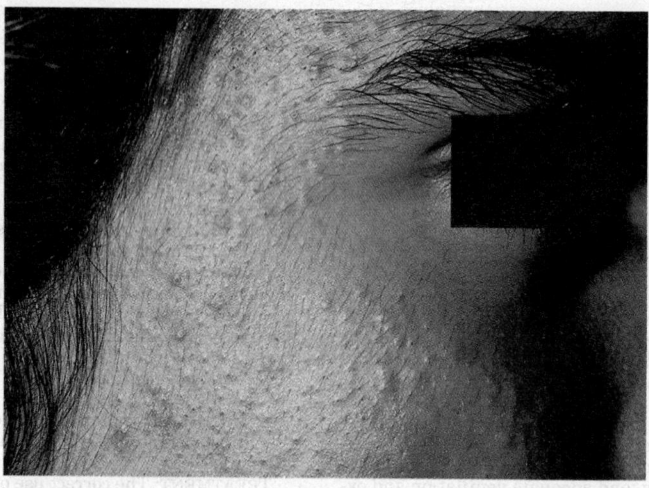

COMEDOS

eyes are open wide in a vacant stare and the face is expressionless, although the patient is unconscious. This may occur in typhus or typhoid fever, or in organic brain syndrome associated with systemic infection.

**coma scale** SEE: *Glasgow Coma Scale.*

**comatose** (kō′mă-tōs) In a coma.

**combustion** (kŏm-bŭst′yŭn) **1.** Burning. **2.** In metabolism, the oxidation of food with production of heat.

**comedo** (kŏm′ē-dō) *pl.* **comedones, comedos** [L. *comedere,* to eat up] The typical small skin lesion of acne vulgaris. One, a closed form, is called a whitehead. It consists of a papule from which the contents are not easily expressed. When inflamed these lesions form pustules and nodules. The open form of comedo, called a blackhead, is rarely inflamed. It has a dilated opening from which the oily debris is easily expressed. Both forms are usually located on the face, but the chest and back may be involved. The condition may be chronic and is frequently associated with seborrheic dermatitis or acne. It usually occurs during adolescence. SEE: illus.; *acne vulgaris.*

**comes** (kō′mēz) *pl.* **comites** [L., companion] A blood vessel that accompanies a nerve or another blood vessel.

**comma tract of Schultze** The fasciculus interfascicularis, a tract of descending fibers located between the fasciculus cuneatus and fasciculus gracilis in the posterior funiculus of the spinal cord.

**commensal** (kŏ-mĕn′săl) [L. *com-,* together, + *mensa,* table] One of two organisms that live in different species in an intimate, nonparasitic relationship. SEE: *symbiosis.*

**commensalism** (kŏ-mĕn′săl-ĭzm″) The symbiotic relationship of two organisms of different species in which neither is harmful to the other and one gains some benefit such as protection or nourishment (e.g., nonpathogenic bacteria in the human intestine).

**comminute** (kŏm′ĭ-nūt) [L. *com-,* together, + *minuere,* to crumble] To break into pieces.

**comminution** (kŏm″ĭ-nū′shŭn) [L. *comminutio,* crumbling] The reduction of a solid body to varying sizes by grating, pulverizing, slicing, granulating, and other processes.

**commissura** (kŏm″mĭ-sū′ră) [L.] *pl.* **commissurae** A commissure.

**commissure** (kŏm′ĭ-shūr) [L. *commissura,* a joining together] **1.** A transverse band of nerve fibers passing over the midline in the central nervous system. **2.** The meeting of two structures, as the lips, eyelids, or labia, across the midline or dividing space. **commissural** (kŏm-mĭs′ū-răl), *adj.*

***anterior cerebral c.*** The band of white fibers that passes through the lamina terminalis, connecting the two cerebral hemispheres.

***anterior gray c.*** The commissure in the spinal cord that lies in front of the central canal.

***anterior white c.*** The commissure in the spinal cord that lies in front of the central canal and the anterior gray commissure.

***c. of fornix*** Hippocampal c.

***hippocampal c.*** A thin sheet of fibers passing transversely under the posterior portion of the corpus callosum. They connect the medial margins of the crura of the fornix. SYN: *c. of fornix.*

***posterior c. of brain*** The commissure just above the midbrain containing fibers that connect the superior colliculi.

***posterior c. of spinal cord*** The gray

commissure connecting the halves of the spinal cord, lying behind the central canal.

**commissurorrhaphy** (kŏm"ĭ-shūr-or'ă-fē) [" + Gr. *rhaphe,* seam, ridge] The surgical joining of the parts of a commissure to decrease the size of the opening.

**commissurotomy** (kŏm"ĭ-shūr-ŏt'ō-mē) [" + Gr. *tome,* incision] Surgical incision of any commissure; used in treating mitral stenosis to increase the size of the mitral orifice. This is done by incising the adhesions that cause the leaves of the valve to stick together. Commissurotomy may also be used in treating certain psychiatric conditions by incising the anterior commissure of the brain.

**commitment** (kŏ-mĭt'mĕnt) The legal procedure for hospitalization of a patient who may not be competent to make that decision or who does not choose to be hospitalized. It is usually done in connection with mental illness, but may be used to hospitalize patients with certain contagious diseases. SEE: *certification.*

**committee, patient care advisory** A multidisciplinary group of individuals who advise health-care agencies facing ethical dilemmas. This committee ususally comprises health-care professionals, clergy, legal counsel, and administrative personnel. Also called *institutional ethics committee.* SEE: *institutional review board.*

**commode** A receptacle suitable for use as a toilet.

***bedside c.*** A bedside toilet that enables a patient to sit comfortably while using it. For many patients using a bedside commode is less stressful than using a bedpan.

**communicable disease** A disease that may be transmitted directly or indirectly from one individual to another. SEE: table; *Universal Precautions Appendix.*

**communicans** (kŏ-mū'nĕ-kănz) [L. *communicare,* to connect with] One of several communicating nerves or arteries.

**communication board** A small, flat surface on which pictures can be placed. It is used to communicate with patients who are unable to voice the names of objects but can point to them.

**communication, impaired verbal** The state in which an individual experiences a decreased or absent ability to use or to understand language in human interaction. SEE: *Nursing Diagnoses Appendix.*

**communication, nonverbal** In interpersonal relationships, the use of communication techniques that do not involve words. A grimace, shrug, silence, smile, wink, raised eyebrows, avoidance, turning away, or even fighting are examples of nonverbal communication.

**communication board** Any of a variety of devices with letters or words that permit communication by patients with impaired physical and verbal ability.

**communicator** An electronic device that permits persons with impaired verbal and physical ability to communicate through graphic or symbolic light-emitting diode (LED) displays, printed messages, or synthetic speech.

**community coping, enhanced, potential for** A pattern of community activities for adaptation and problem solving that is satisfactory for meeting the demands or needs of the community but can be improved for management of current and future problems/stressors. SEE: *Nursing Diagnoses Appendix.*

**community coping, ineffective** A pattern of community activities for adaptation and problem solving that is unsatisfactory for meeting the demands or needs of the community. SEE: *Nursing Diagnoses Appendix.*

**community medicine** SEE: *medicine, community.*

**Comolli's sign** (kō-mōl'lēz) [Antonio Comolli, It. pathologist, b. 1879] A triangular swelling corresponding to the outline of the fractured scapula.

**comorbid disease** A disease coexisting with the primary disease (e.g., the primary disease could be cancer and the comorbid disease emphysema).

**compact** [L. *compactus,* joined together] Closely and tightly packed together; solid.

**compaction** (kŏm-păk'shŭn) **1.** Simultaneous engagement of the presenting parts of twins in the pelvis so that labor cannot progress. **2.** In dentistry, the act or process of joining or packing together powdered gold, mat gold, or gold foil in a prepared cavity in a tooth.

**comparative negligence** In forensic medicine, negligence of the plaintiff and defendant measured in terms of percentages. Damages awarded are decreased in proportion to the plaintiff's amount of negligence provided it is less than that of the defendant.

**compartment syndrome** Any condition in which a structure such as a nerve or tendon is being constricted in a space (e.g., carpal tunnel syndrome). The sheath or tendon may be enlarged due to disease or inflammation and no longer able to move freely in the compartment. The condition may also be present inside a cast when edema causes increased pressure on the limb immobilized.

Nursing Implications: The patient at risk is assessed for deep, throbbing pain out of proportion to the original problem; pain that is not relieved by analgesic drugs; pain that occurs in response to passive flexion or extension of the digits; decreased mobility of the digits; and paresthesias. The painful extremity is elevated, and pertinent findings are documented and reported immediately to the physician. Constricting dressings or casts are removed while the injured limb is supported. The patient is prepared for surgical decompression (fasciotomy) if symp-

## Method of Transmission of Some Common Communicable Diseases

| Disease | How Agent Leaves the Bodies of the Sick | How Organisms May Be Transmitted | Method of Entry into the Body |
|---|---|---|---|
| Acquired immunodeficiency syndrome (AIDS) | Blood, semen, or other body fluids, including breast milk | Sexual contact<br>Contact with blood or mucous membranes or by way of contaminated syringes<br>Placental transmission | Reproductive tract<br>Contact with blood<br>Placental transmission<br>Breastfeeding |
| Cholera | Feces | Water or food contaminated with feces | Mouth to intestine |
| Diphtheria | Sputum and discharges from nose and throat<br>Skin lesions (rare) | Droplet infection from patient coughing | Through mouth or nose to throat |
| Gonococcal disease | Lesions<br>Discharges from infected mucous membranes | Sexual activity<br>Hands of infected persons soiled with their own discharges | Reproductive tract or any mucous membrane |
| Hepatitis A, viral | Feces | Food or water contaminated with feces | Mouth to intestine |
| Hepatitis B, viral and delta hepatitis | Blood and serum-derived fluids, including semen and vaginal fluids | Contact with blood and body fluids | Exposure to body fluids including during sexual activity<br>Contact with blood |
| Hepatitis C | Blood and other body fluids | Parenteral drug use<br>Laboratory exposure to blood<br>Health care workers exposed to blood (i.e., dentists and their assistants, and clinical and laboratory staff) | Infected blood<br>Contaminated needles |
| Hookworm | Feces | Cutaneous contact with soil polluted with feces<br>Eggs in feces hatch in sandy soil | Larvae enter through skin (esp. of feet), migrate through the body, and settle in small intestine |
| Influenza | As in pneumonia | Respiratory droplets or objects contaminated with discharges | As in pneumonia |
| Leprosy | Cutaneous or mucosal lesions that contain bacilli<br>Respiratory droplets | Cutaneous contact or nasal discharges of untreated patients | Nose or broken skin |
| Measles (rubeola) | As in streptococcal pharyngitis | As in streptococcal pharyngitis | As in streptococcal pharyngitis |
| Meningitis, meningococcal | Discharges from nose and throat | Respiratory droplets | Mouth and nose |

*Table continued on following page*

**Method of Transmission of Some Common Communicable Diseases**
(Continued)

| Disease | How Agent Leaves the Bodies of the Sick | How Organisms May Be Transmitted | Method of Entry into the Body |
|---|---|---|---|
| Mumps | Discharges from infected glands and mouth | Respiratory droplets and saliva | Mouth and nose |
| Ophthalmia neonatorum (gonococcal infection of eyes of newborn) | Vaginal secretions of infected mother | Contact with infected areas of vagina of infected mother during birth | Directly on conjunctiva |
| Pertussis | Discharges from respiratory tract | Respiratory droplets | Mouth and nose |
| Pneumonia | Sputum and discharges from nose and throat | Respiratory droplets | Through mouth and nose to lungs |
| Poliomyelitis | Discharges from nose and throat, and via feces | Respiratory droplets<br>Contaminated water | Through mouth and nose |
| Rubella | As in streptococcal pharyngitis | As in streptococcal pharyngitis | As in streptococcal pharyngitis |
| Streptococcal pharyngitis | Discharges from nose and throat | Respiratory droplets | Through mouth and nose |
| Syphilis | Lesions<br>Blood<br>Transfer through placenta to fetus | Kissing or sexual intercourse<br>Contaminated needles and syringes | Directly into blood and tissues through breaks in skin or membrane<br>Contaminated needles and syringes |
| Trachoma | Discharges from infected eyes | Cutaneous contact<br>Hands, towels, handkerchiefs | Directly on conjunctiva |
| Tuberculosis, bovine | | Milk from infected cow | Mouth to intestine |
| Tuberculosis, human | Sputum<br>Lesions<br>Feces | Droplet infection from person coughing with mouth uncovered<br>Sputum from mouth to fingers, thence to food and other things | Through nose to lungs or intestines<br>From intestines via lymph channels to lymph vessels and to tissues |
| Typhoid fever | Feces and urine | Food or water contaminated with feces, or urine from patients | Through mouth via infected food or water and thence to intestinal tract |

toms are not resolved within 30 min.

**compassionate use** The administration of investigational drugs to a patient in a special circumstance in which it is felt that the drug may be life saving or effective when no other therapy would be. The procedure requires the treating physician to contact either the Food and Drug Administration or the drug manufacturer to obtain permission for use in a specific case.

**compatibility** [L. *compati*, to sympathize with] **1.** The suitability to be mixed or taken together without unfavorable results, as drugs. **2.** The ability of two individuals or groups to live together without undue strife or tension.

**compatible** In pharmacology, pert. to the ability to combine two medicines without interfering with their action.

**Compazine** Trade name for prochlorperazine maleate.

**compensating** Making up for a deficiency.

**compensation** [L. *cum,* with, + *pensare,* to weigh] **1.** Making up for a defect, as cardiac circulation competent to meet demands regardless of valvular defect. **2.** In psychoanalysis, a psychic mechanism best described by an example. An individual handicapped by a physical deformity or variation or by a character defect may escape the consciousness of the defect by accomplishment resulting from compensatory ambition. More simply, a short person may strut or an incompetent one brag. Sublimation, is often similar, but varies by substituting a higher social goal to gratify the infrasocial drive by replacement rather than mere camouflaging. **3.** Restitution by payment to a person injured, esp. in the work place. **compensatory,** *adj.*

***failure of c.*** The inability of the heart muscle to cope with the required cardiac output. It indicates a diseased heart muscle. This is caused by a myocardial disorder, back pressure due to mitral regurgitation, mitral or aortic stenosis, or aortic regurgitation.

**competence** (kŏm′pĕ-tĕns) **1.** In psychiatry, being able to manage one's affairs, and by inference, being sane; usually stated as mental competence. **2.** Performance in a manner that satisfies the demands of a situation; interaction effectively with the environment.

**competition** (kŏm″pĕ-tĭsh′ŭn) The simultaneous attempt of similar substances to attach to a receptor site of a cell membrane.

**complaint** (kŏm-plānt′) **1.** Verbal or other communication of the principal reason the patient is seeking medical assistance. **2.** An initial pleading or document that commences a legal action, states grounds for such an action, names the parties to the lawsuit, and demands relief for injuries and damages suffered.

***chief c.*** The symptom or group of symptoms that represents the primary reason for a patient's seeking health care.

**complement** (kŏm′plĕ-mĕnt) [L. *complere,* to complete] A group of proteins in the blood that play a vital role in the body's immune defenses through a cascade of interations. Components of complement are labeled C1 through C9. C3 and C5 are the most important of these. Complement acts by directly lysing (killing) organisms; by opsonizing an antigen, thus stimulating phagocytosis; and by stimulating inflammation and the B-cell–mediated immune response. All complement proteins lie inactive in the blood until activated by either the classic or the alternative pathways.

A deficiency or abnormality in complement is an autosomal recessive trait. The lack of C3 increases susceptibility to common bacterial infections, whereas deficits in C5 through C9 are usually associated with increased incidence of autoimmune diseases, particularly systemic lupus erythematosus and glomerulonephritis. Lack of C1 causes hereditary angioedema of the extremities and gastrointestinal tract. The lack of any of the more than 25 proteins involved in the complement system may affect the body's defenses adversely.

**complemental, complementary** Supplying something that is lacking in another system or entity.

**complementarity** In individual and group interactions, the extent to which emotional requirements are met.

**complement fixation** A common blood assay used to determine if antigen-antibody reactions have occurred. Complement that combines with the antigen-antibody complex becomes inactive and is unable to lyse (kill) red blood cells in vitro. The degree of complement fixation is determined by the number of red blood cells destroyed, which indicates the amount of free complement not bound to the antigen-antibody complexes. Complement fixation can measure the severity of an infection because it helps indicate the extent and effectiveness of antigen-antibody reactions occurring in the body.

**complex** [L. *complexus,* woven together] **1.** All the ideas, feelings, and sensations connected with a subject. **2.** Intricate. **3.** An atrial or ventricular systole as it appears on an electrocardiograph tracing. **4.** A subconscious idea (or group of ideas) that has become associated with a repressed wish or emotional experience and that may influence behavior, although the person may not realize the connection with the repressed thoughts or actions. **5.** In Freudian theory, a grouping of ideas with an emotional background. These may be harmless, and the individual may be fully aware of them (e.g., an artist sees every object with a view to a possible picture and is said to have established a complex for art). Often, however, the complex is aroused by some painful emotional reaction such as fright or excessive grief that, instead of being allowed a natural outlet, becomes unconsciously repressed and later manifests itself in some abnormality of mind or behavior. According to Freud, the best method of determining the complex is through psychoanalysis. SEE: *Electra complex; Jocasta complex; Oedipus complex.*

***castration c.*** A morbid fear of being castrated.

***Ghon c.*** The primary lesion in tuberculosis, consisting of the affected area of the lung and a corresponding lymph node. These usually heal and become calcified. If the calcium surrounding the lesion is later dissolved, the contained tubercle bacilli are free to spread throughout the body. SEE: *tuberculosis, miliary.*

***Golgi c.*** An organelle present in most

cells but larger in secretory cells. Enclosed are vacuoles, sacs, and secretory material. This complex is vital to the cell's function. SEE: *Golgi apparatus; organelle* for illus.

***inferiority c.*** The condition of having low self-esteem; a mid–20th-century term stemming from Freudian therapy.

***membrane attack c.*** The combination of complement factors C5 through C9 that directly attack and kill the cell membranes of microorganisms during the terminal attack phase of the complement cascade. SEE: *complement, inflammation.*

***nodal premature c.*** ABBR: NPC. Ectopic cardiac beat originating in the atrioventricular node.

***superiority c.*** Exaggerated conviction of one's own superiority; the pretense of being superior to compensate for a real or imagined inferiority.

**complexion** (kŏm-plĕk′shŭn) The color and appearance of the facial skin.

**complexus** (kŏm-plĕk′sŭs) [L.] Semispinalis capitis muscle. SEE: under *muscle.*

**compliance** (kŏm-plī′ăns) **1.** The property of altering size and shape in response to application of force, weight, or release from force. The lung and thoracic cage of a child may have a high degree of compliance as compared with that of an elderly person. SEE: *elastance.* **2.** The extent to which a patient's behavior coincides with medical advice. Compliance may be estimated by carefully questioning the patient and family members, evaluating the degree of clinical response to therapy, the presence or absence of side effects from drugs, measuring serum drug levels or testing for excretion of the drug in the urine, and counting remaining pills.

***dynamic c.*** A measure of the ease of lung inflation with positive pressure.

***effective c.*** Patient compliance during positive-pressure breathing using a tidal volume corrected for compressed volume divided by static pressure.

***frequency-dependent c.*** A condition in which pulmonary compliance decreases with rapid breathing; used to identify small airway disease.

***pulmonary c.*** A measure of the force required to distend the lungs.

***static c.*** A volume-to-pressure measurement of lung distensibility with exhalation against a closed system, taken under conditions of no airflow.

***tubing c.*** The loss of ventilator tubing compression or volume to dead space in the tube. It is calculated by closing the ventilator circuit and measuring the volume under pressurization.

**complication** [L. *cum,* with, + *plicare,* to fold] An added difficulty; a complex state; a disease or accident superimposed on another without being specifically related, yet affecting or modifying the prognosis of the original disease (e.g., pneumonia is a complication of measles and is the cause of many deaths from that disease).

**component** A constituent part.

**component blood therapy** SEE: *blood component therapy.*

**compos mentis** (kŏm″pŭs mĕn′tĭs) [L.] Of sound mind; sane. SEE: *non compos mentis.*

**compound** [L. *componere,* to place together] **1.** A substance composed of two or more units or parts combined in definite proportions by weight and having specific properties of its own. Compounds are formed by all living organisms and are of two types, organic and inorganic. **2.** Made up of more than one part.

***dental c.*** A nonelastic molding or impression material used in dentistry that softens when heated and solidifies without chemical change when cooled (i.e., a thermoplastic material).

***inorganic c.*** One of many compounds that, in general, contain no carbon.

***organic c.*** A compound containing carbon. Such compounds include carbohydrates, proteins, and fats.

**compound astigmatism** Myopia of both the vertical and horizontal meridians.

**comprehend** To understand something.

**Comprehensive Occupational Assessment and Training System** ABBR: C.O.A.T.S. A pretreatment test battery used to determine interests and abilities that may be used in the rehabilitation regimen of persons with disabilities.

**compress** [L. *compressus,* squeezed together] **1.** (kŏm′prĕs) A cloth, wet or dry, folded and applied firmly to a body part. **2.** (kŏm-prĕs′) To press together into a smaller space. **3.** To close by squeezing together, as a wound.

***cold c.*** A soft, absorbent cloth, several layers thick, dipped in cold water, slightly wrung out, and applied to the part being treated. To maintain constant temperature, the compress is frequently renewed, or an ice bag or rubber coil through which ice water is circulating is placed on it. The duration of the application is usually 30 to 60 min.

***hot c.*** A soft, absorbent cloth folded into several layers, dipped in hot water 107° to 115°F (41.7° to 46.1°C), barely wrung out, and placed on the part to be treated. It is covered with a piece of flannel large enough to overlap the linen slightly. The temperature is maintained at a constant level by renewing the compress or by applying a rubber coil through which hot water 107° to 115°F (41.7° to 46.1°C) is circulated.

***wet c.*** Two or more folds of soft cloth wrung out of water at prescribed temperatures and covered with flannel.

**compression** (kŏm-prĕsh′ŭn) [L. *compressio,* a compression] A squeezing together; the condition of being pressed together.

***cerebral c.*** Pressure on the brain produced by increased intracranial fluids, embolism, thrombosis, tumors, and skull fractures. This is more serious than a concussion.

SYMPTOMS: The condition is marked by deep unconsciousness, full, bounding pulse, deep, stertorous, slow respirations, flushed face, high blood pressure, and varying pupil size. Fever may develop, and there may be retention or incontinence of urine and feces. Danger signals include coma, Cheyne-Stokes respiration, fever, and a quickened pulse. SEE: *Glasgow Coma Scale*.

NURSING IMPLICATIONS: The patient is closely assessed for signs and symptoms of increased intracranial pressure, respiratory distress, convulsions, bleeding from the ears or nose, or drainage of cerebrospinal fluid from the ears or nose (which most probably indicates a fracture). Neurological status is monitored for any alterations in level of consciousness, pupillary signs, ocular movements, verbal response, sensory and motor function (including voluntary and involuntary movements), or behavioral and mental capabilities; and vital signs are assessed, esp. respiratory patterns. Any signs of deterioration are documented and reported. Seizure precautions are maintained. SEE: *coma*.

***digital c.*** Compression of blood vessels with the fingers to stop hemorrhage.

***myelitis c.*** Compression due to pressure on the spinal cord, often caused by a tumor.

**compression glove** Any type of glove made of stretch material so that pressure is maintained against the fingers and hands. This helps to reduce edema.

**compressor** **1.** An instrument or device that applies a compressive force, as in compaction of gold. **2.** A muscle that compresses a part, as the compressor hemispherium bulbi, which compresses the bulb of the urethra.

***air c.*** A machine that compresses air into storage tanks for use in air syringes, air turbine handpieces, and other air-driven tools.

**compromised host** A person who lacks resistance to infection owing to a deficiency in any of the host defenses. SEE: *AIDS; host defense mechanisms; immunocompromised*.

**Compton scattering** An interaction between x-rays and matter in which the incoming photon ejects a loosely bound outer-shell electron. The resulting change in the direction of the x-ray photon causes scatter, increasing the dose and degrading the radiographic image. Most interactions between x-rays and matter are of this type, esp. at high energies.

**compulsion** (kŏm-pŭl′shŭn) [L. *compulsio*, compulsion] A repetitive stereotyped act performed to relieve fear connected with obsession. It is dictated by the subconscious against the person's wishes and, if denied, causes uneasiness. **compulsive** (-sĭv), *adj*.

**compulsory** (kŏm-pŭl′sor-ē) Compelling action against one's will.

**CON** *certificate of need*.

**con-** [L.] Prefix meaning *together* or *with*. SEE: *syn-*.

**con-A** *concanavalin-A*.

**conarium** (kō-nā′rē-ŭm) [L.] The pineal body of the brain.

**conation** (kō-nā′shŭn) [L. *conatio*, an attempt] The initiative, impulse, and drive to act, arising from inside oneself. All of these may be diminished in cerebral diseases, esp. those involving the medial orbital parts of the frontal lobes. SEE: *abulia*.

**concanavalin-A** (kŏn″kā-năv′ĭ-lĭn) ABBR: con-A. A mitogen, protein from the jack bean used to stimulate proliferation of T lymphocytes. SEE: *mitogen*.

**concatenation** (kŏn-kăt″ĭ-nā′shŭn) [L. *con*, together, + *catena*, chain] A group of events or effects acting in concert or occurring at the same time.

**Concato's disease** (kŏn-kŏ′tōs) [Luigi M. Concato, It. physician, 1825–1882] Polyserositis.

**concave** (kŏn′kāv, kŏn-kāv′) [″ + *cavus*, hollow] Having a spherically depressed or hollow surface.

**concavity** (kŏn-kăv′ĭ-tē) A surface with curved, bowl-like sides.

**concavoconcave** (kŏn-kā″vō-kŏn′kāv) [″ + *cavus*, hollow, + *con*, with, + *cavus*, hollow] Concave on opposing sides.

**concavoconvex** (kŏn-kā″vō-kŏn′vĕks) [″ + ″ + *convexus*, vaulted] Concave on one side and convex on the opposite surface. SEE: *convex*.

**conceive** (kŏn-sēv′) [L. *concipere*, to take to oneself] **1.** To become pregnant. **2.** To form a mental image or to bring into mind; to form an idea.

**concentration** (kŏn-sĕn-trā′shŭn) [L. *con*, together with, + *centrum*, center] **1.** Fixation of the mind on one subject to the exclusion of all other thoughts. **2.** An increase in the strength of a fluid by evaporation. **3.** The amount of a substance in a mixture or solution expressed as a percentage of weight or volume.

***hydrogen ion c.*** $H^+$, the relative proportion of hydrogen ions in a solution, the factor responsible for the acidic properties of a solution. SEE: *pH*.

***mean corpuscular hemoglobin c.*** ABBR: MCHC. The average concentration of hemoglobin in a given volume (usually 100 ml) of packed red blood cells, obtained by multiplying the number of grams of hemoglobin in the unit volume by 100 and dividing by the hematocrit.

***minimum inhibitory c.*** ABBR: MIC. In bacteriology, the minimum antibiotic concentration needed to cause a 99% reduction in colony-forming units on a culture medium.

**concentric** (kŏn-sĕn′trĭk) [″+ *centrum*, center] Having a common center.

**concept** (kŏn′sĕpt) [L. *conceptum,* something understood] An idea.
**conception** (kŏn-sĕp′shŭn) **1.** The mental process of forming an idea. **2.** The union of the male sperm and female ovum; fertilization. With a 28-day cycle, menstruation normally lasts 5 days, followed by a period of repair and proliferation of the uterine lining (endometrium) for about 1 week. In general, ovulation occurs about 12 to 14 days before the beginning of the next menstrual period. Therefore, sexual intercourse during the middle of the menstrual cycle is most likely to result in conception. During this period, the ovum is discharged from the follicle and moves through the fallopian tube to the uterus. If fertilization does not occur during this time, the ovum disintegrates.

However, the menstrual cycle is one of the most variable events known in human biology. It is therefore difficult, and often impossible, to predict the optimum time of conception (or the reverse) by attempting to calculate ovulation from the time of the last menstrual period. Also, sperm survival time in the female reproductive tract is variable. SEE: *basal temperature chart; contraception.*
**conceptual models in nursing** SEE: *Nursing Theory Appendix.*
**conceptus** (kŏn-sĕp′tŭs) The products of conception.
**concha** (kŏng′kă) *pl.* **conchae** [Gr. *konche,* shell] **1.** The outer ear or the pinna. **2.** One of the three nasal conchae. SEE: *nasal concha.*

***c. auriculae*** A concavity on the median surface of the auricle of the ear, divided by a ridge into the upper cymba conchae and a lower cavum conchae. The latter leads to the external auditory meatus.

***c. bullosa*** A distention of the turbinate bone due to cyst formation.

***nasal c.*** One of the three scroll-like bones that project medially from the lateral wall of the nasal cavity; a turbinate bone. The superior and middle conchae are processes of the lateral mass of the ethmoid bone; the inferior concha is a facial bone. Each overlies a meatus.

***c. sphenoidalis*** In a fetal skull, one of the two curved plates located on the anterior portion of the body of the sphenoid bone and forming part of the roof of the nasal cavity.
**conchoidal** (kŏng-koy′dăl) [″ + *eidos,* form, shape] Shell-shaped.
**conchoscope** (kŏng′kō-skōp) [″ + *skopein,* to examine] An instrument for examining the nasal cavity.
**conchotome** (kŏng′kō-tōm) [″ + *tome,* incision] A device for excising the middle turbinate bone.
**concoction** (kŏn-kŏk′shŭn) [L. *con,* with, + *coquere,* to cook] A mixture of two medicinal substances, usually done with the aid of heat.
**concomitant** (kŏn-kŏm′ĭ-tănt) [″ + *comes,* companion] Accessory; taking place at the same time.
**concordance** (kŏn-kor′dăns) In twins, the equal representation of a genetic trait in each.
**concrement** (kŏn′krē-mĕnt) [L. *concrementum*] A concretion as of protein and other substances. If infiltrated with calcium salts, it is termed a calculus.
**concrescence** (kŏn-krĕs′ĕns) [L. *con,* with, + *crescere,* to grow] The union of separate parts; coalescence, esp. the attachment of a tooth to an adjacent one by deposition of cementum to the roots.
**concrete** (kŏn′krēt, kŏn-krēt′) [L. *concretus,* solid] Condensed, hardened, or solidified.
**concretio cordis** (kŏn-krē′shē-ō kor′dĭs) Obliteration of the pericardial space caused by chronic constrictive pericarditis.
**concretion** (kŏn-krē′shŭn) [″ + *crescere,* to grow] A calculus.
**concussion** (kŏn-kŭsh′ŭn) [L. *concussus,* shaken violently] **1.** An injury resulting from impact with an object. **2.** Partial or complete loss of function, as that resulting from a blow or fall.

***c. of brain*** Cerebral concussion; a common result of a blow to the head or fall on the end of the spine with sufficient force to be transmitted upward. This usually causes unconsciousness, either temporary or prolonged. Return of consciousness may be gradual. The patient may suddenly draw up the knees and vomit. SEE: *Nursing Diagnoses Appendix.*

SYMPTOMS: These vary with location and extent of injury, ranging from transient dizziness to various paralyses or unconsciousness, unequal pupils, and shock. If there are no complications, the patient regains consciousness in a short time. There may be a reactive period, accompanied by vomiting, temperature 99° to 100°F (37.2° to 37.8°C), rapid pulse, flushed face, restlessness, headache, and cerebral irritation, lasting for 12 to 24 hr.

FIRST AID: The patient is kept lying down quietly with the head and shoulders slightly elevated. Stimulants should not be given; sedatives are generally contraindicated. Transportation should be delayed if possible. Cool applications to the head and neck are soothing. One should reassure the patient if he or she is conscious and maintain a suitable temperature. Any adverse symptoms, such as bleeding, or alteration in pupil size or reaction, should be reported at once. SEE: *coma; Glasgow Coma Scale; transportation of the injured.*

---

Caution: Morphine should not be given.

---

***c. of labyrinth*** Deafness resulting from a blow to the head or ear.

***spinal c.*** Loss of function in the spinal cord resulting from a blow or severe jarring.

**condensation** (kŏn″dĕn-sā′shŭn) [L, *con*, with, + *densare*, to make thick] **1.** Making more dense or compact. **2.** Changing of a liquid to a solid or a gas to a liquid. **3.** In psychoanalysis, the union of ideas to form a new mental pattern. **4.** In chemistry, a type of reaction in which two or more molecules of the same substance react with each other and form a new and heavier substance with different chemical properties. **5.** A mechanical process used in dentistry to remove excess mercury from amalgam or to form a dense gold foil restoration. It improves the physical properties of the material used and forces it to adapt more closely to the cavity preparation.

**condenser** (kŏn-dĕn′sĕr) **1.** A device for solidifying vapors and liquids. **2.** An instrument or tool used to compact and condense restorative materials in dental cavity preparations; also called a plugger.

***electrical c.*** A device for storing electricity by using two conducting surfaces and a nonconductor.

***substage c.*** The part of the lens system of a microscope that supplies the illumination critical to the resolving power of the instrument; also called an Abbé condenser.

**condiment** (kŏn′dĭ-mĕnt) [L. *condire*, to pickle] An appetizing ingredient added to food.

CLASSIFICATION: *Aromatic:* vanilla, cinnamon, cloves, chervil, parsley, bay leaf. *Acrid or peppery:* pepper, ginger, tabasco, all-spice. *Alliaceous or allylic:* onion, mustard, horseradish. *Acid:* vinegar, capers, gherkins, citron. *Animal origin:* caviar, anchovies. *Miscellaneous:* salt, sugar, truffles.

In general, with the exception of sugar, condiments have little nutritional value. They are appetizers, stimulating the secretion of saliva and intestinal juices.

**condition 1.** A state of health; physical, esp. athletic, fitness. **2.** To train a person or animal to respond in a predictable way to a stimulus.

**conditioning** (kŏn-dĭsh′ŭn-ĭng) **1.** Improving the physical capability of a person by an exercise program. **2.** In psychology, the use of a special and different stimulus in conjunction with a familiar one. After a sufficient period in which the two stimuli have been presented simultaneously, the special stimulus alone will cause the response that could originally be produced only by the familiar stimulus. The late Russian physiologist Ivan Pavlov used dogs to demonstrate that the strange stimulus, ringing of a bell, could cause the animal to salivate if the test was done after a period of *conditioning* during which the bell and the familiar stimulus, food, were presented simultaneously. SYN: *classical conditioning.*

***aversive c.*** SEE: *aversion therapy.*

***operant c.*** The learning of a particular action or type of behavior followed by a reward. This technique was publicized by the Harvard psychologist B.F. Skinner, who trained animals to activate (by pecking, in the case of a pigeon, or pressing a bar, in the case of a rat) an apparatus that released a pellet of food.

**condom** (kŏn′dŭm) [L. *condus*, a receptacle] A thin, flexible sheath made of rubber (latex) or the cecum of a sheep and worn over the penis during sexual intercourse to prevent sperm from entering the vagina and to help prevent sexually transmitted disease. A supply of condoms should be kept at hand, ideally in a cool, dry place, so that one is easily available for use at every intercourse. Condoms cannot be reused. They should not be tested by inflating or stretching. They must be handled gently and kept away from water-insoluble oily substances and sharp objects. For maximum effectiveness, the condom should be put on before genital contact takes place. Either the man or the woman may put the condom in place, but long fingernails can damage it. A man who is reluctant to use a condom may be more receptive to the idea if his partner puts it on for him. The condom must be placed with the rolled portion out so that it will unroll properly. It is unrolled on the erect penis, leaving a space at the end to accommodate the ejaculate. If desired, the outside of the condom may be lubricated using contraceptive jelly or another water-soluble lubricant. Use of oil-based lubricants, however, may damage the condom. After ejaculation, the condom must not become dislodged until the penis is withdrawn. Its rim should be held firmly against the base of the penis during withdrawal. The condom should be checked for tears before it is thrown away. If it has torn, a contraceptive suppository, jelly, or foam should be inserted into the vagina immediately. SEE: *AIDS; contraception; sexually transmitted disease.*

---

Caution: Only a water-based lubricant such as K-Y Jelly should be used with a condom. Oil-based products begin to deteriorate latex in less than 1 min.

---

***female c.*** An intravaginal device, similar to the male condom, that is designed to prevent unwanted pregnancy and sexually transmitted diseases. It consists of a soft loose-fitting polyurethane sheath closed at one end. A flexible polyurethane ring is inside the closed end and another is at the open end. The inner ring is used for insertion, covering the cervix the way a contraceptive diaphragm does and also anchoring and positioning the condom well inside the vagina. During use the external ring remains outside the vagina and covers the area around the vaginal opening. This prevents contact between the labia and the base of the penis. The female condom is prelubricated and additional lubrication is provided in the package. It is designed for one-time use. As a contraceptive, it is as effective as other barrier methods.

**conductance** (kŏn-dŭk′tăns) [L. *conducere,* to lead] The conducting ability of a body or a circuit for electricity. The best conductor is one that offers the least resistance such as gold, silver, or copper. When expressed as a numerical value, conductance is the reciprocal of resistance. The unit is the ohm.

***airway c.*** ABBR: G. The amount of airflow divided by the amount of pressure that produces it; a measure of the ability of the respiratory airways to maintain airflow.

**conduction** (kŏn-dŭk′shŭn) **1.** The process whereby a state of excitation affects adjacent portions of a tissue or cell, so that the disturbance is transmitted to remote points. Conduction occurs not only in the fibers of the nervous system but also in muscle fibers. **2.** The transfer of electrons, ions, heat, or sound waves through a conductor or conducting medium.

***bone c.*** Sound conduction through the cranial bones.

**conductivity** (kŏn″dŭk-tĭv′ĭ-tē) The specific electric conducting ability of a substance. Conductivity is the reciprocal of unit resistance or resistivity. The unit is the ohm/cm. Specific conductivity is sometimes expressed as a percentage. In such cases, it is given as a percentage of the conductivity of pure copper under certain standard conditions.

**conductor** (kŏn-dŭk′tor) **1.** A medium that transmits a force, a signal, or electricity. **2.** A guide directing a surgical knife or probe.

**conduit** (kŏn′doo-ĭt) An aqueduct; a channel, esp. one constructed surgically.

***ileal c.*** A method of diverting the urinary flow by transplanting the ureter into a prepared and isolated segment of the ileum, which is sutured closed on one end. The other end is connected to an opening in the abdominal wall. Urine is collected there in a special receptacle.

**condylar** (kŏn′dĭ-lăr) [Gr. *kondylos,* knuckle] Pert. to a condyle.

**condylarthrosis** (kŏn″dĭl-ăr-thrō′sĭs) [″ + *arthrosis,* a joint] A form of diarthrosis; an ovoid head in an elliptical cavity.

**condyle** (kŏn′dīl) *pl.* **condyles** [Gr. *kondylos,* knuckle] A rounded protuberance at the end of a bone forming an articulation.

**condylectomy** (kŏn″dĭ-lĕk′tō-mē) [″ + *ektome,* excision] Excision of a condyle.

**condylion** (kŏn-dĭl′ē-ŏn) [Gr. *kondylion,* knob] A point on either the lateral or the medial surface of the mandibular condyle.

**condyloid** (kŏn′dĭ-loyd) [Gr. *kondylos,* knuckle, + *eidos,* form, shape] Pert. to or resembling a condyle.

**condyloma** (kŏn″dĭ-lō′mă) [Gr. *kondyloma,* wart] A wartlike skin growth, usually on the external genitalia or near the anus.

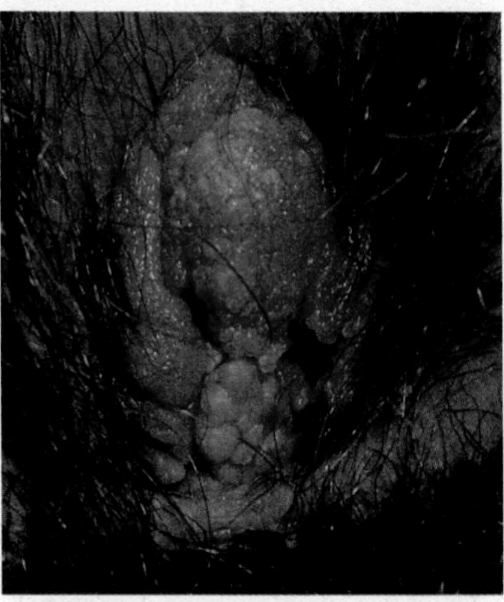

**CONDYLOMA ACUMINATUM** (PERIANAL WARTS)

***c. acuminatum*** An ordinary wart in the genital and perianal areas. It is caused by various types of human papilloma virus and may be spread by physical contact with an area containing a wart. The spread of a wart from one labium to the other by auto-inoculation is possible. The virus that causes the wart is usually transmitted sexually. SYN: *genital wart.* SEE: illus.

TREATMENT: Podophyllum applied locally, cryosurgery, electrocautery, and laser surgery are some methods of treatment. Also, intralesional injection of interferon alfa is effective in treating some patients in whom other forms of therapy failed.

***c. latum*** A mucous patch, characteristic of syphilis, on the vulva or anus. It is flat and coated with gray exudate and has a delimited area. SYN: *moist papule.*

**condylomatous** (kŏn″dĭ-lō′mă-tŭs) Pert. to a condyloma.

**condylotomy** (kŏn″dĭ-lŏt′ō-mē) [Gr. *kondylos,* knuckle, + *tome,* incision] Division of a condyle without its removal.

**condylus** (kŏn′dĭ-lŭs) *pl.* **condyli** Condyle.

**cone** ( kōn) [Gr. *konos,* cone] **1.** A solid or hollow three-dimensional figure with a circular base and sides sloping up to a point. **2.** In the outer layer of the retina (the layer adjacent to the choroid), one of the flask-shaped cells that are stimulated by the wavelengths of light of different colors. The cones are essential for color discrimination. SYN: *retinal c.; cone cell.* SEE: *retina* for illus.; *rod; rod cell.* **3.** A hollow, tapered, cylindrical device used in upper-extremity exercise to improve grasp, coordination, and range of motion. **4.** A device on a dental radiography machine that indicates the direction of the central beam and helps to establish the desired source-to-film distance.

***c. of light*** One of the triangular areas of reflected light on the membrana tympani extending downward from the umbo.

***ocular c.*** A cone of light in the eye with the point on the retina.

***retinal c.*** One of the specialized cone-shaped cells of the retina. These cells, along with the retinal rods, are light sensitive. The cones receive color stimuli. SYN: *cone* (2).

**cone cutting** Failure to cover or expose the whole area of a radiograph with the useful beam. The film is only partially exposed.

**cone shell poisoning** A toxic reaction to the neurotoxin delivered by the pointed, hollow teeth of the marine animal contained in the cone shell. Intense local pain, swelling, and numbness may last several days. In severe poisoning, muscular incoordination and weakness can progress to respiratory paralysis. Although death can occur, recovery within 24 hr is the usual outcome. There is no specific therapy, but supportive measures including artificial respiration and supplemental oxygen may be needed.

**conexus** (kŏ-nĕk′sŭs) [L.] A connecting structure.

**confabulation** (kŏn-făb″ū-lā′shŭn) [L. *confabulari,* to talk together] A behavioral reaction to memory loss in which the patient fills in memory gaps with inappropriate words.

**confectio, confection** (kŏn-fĕk′shē-ō, -shŭn) [L. *conficere,* to prepare] A sugar-like soft solid in which one or more medicinal substances are incorporated so that they can be administered agreeably and preserved conveniently. This is not often prescribed and is not official.

**confidentiality** Information the health care team obtains from or about a patient (e.g., laboratory data, psychiatric history, sexual preference) that is considered to be privileged and cannot be disclosed to a third party without the patient's consent. In some instances when the information is important to public health, it may be illegal not to disclose the data.

**configuration** (kŏn-fĭg″ū-rā′shŭn) **1.** The shape and appearance of something. **2.** In chemistry, the position of atoms in a molecule.

***activity c.*** An assessment approach used by occupational therapists to determine an individual's usual use of time during a typical week. The technique is designed to elicit the person's perceptions of the nature of daily activities and satisfaction with them.

**confinement** (kŏn-fīn′mĕnt) [O. Fr. *confiner,* to restrain in a place] The period of childbirth.

**conflict** (kŏn′flĭkt) [L. *confligere,* to contend] **1.** The opposing action of incompatible substances. **2.** In psychiatry, the conscious or unconscious struggle between two opposing desires or courses of action; applied to a state in which social goals dictate behavior contrary to more primitive (often subconscious) desires.

**confluence of sinuses** The union of the sagittal and transverse sinuses.

**confluent** (kŏn′floo-ĕnt) [L. *confluere,* to run together] Running together, as when pustules merge.

**conformation** (kŏn″for-mā′shŭn) The form or shape of a part, body, material, or molecule.

**confrontation** (kŏn″frŭn-tā′shŭn) [L. *con,* together with, + *frons,* face] **1.** The examination of two patients together, one with a disease and the other from whom the disease was supposedly contracted. **2.** A method of determining the extent of visual fields in which that of the patient is compared with that of the examiner. **3.** In psychiatry, a feedback procedure in which a patient's behavior and apparent feelings are presented to facilitate better understanding of his or her actions.

**confusion** (kŏn-fū′zhŭn) Not being aware of or oriented to time, place, or self.

***acute c.*** The abrupt onset of a cluster of global, transient changes and disturbances in attention, cognition, psychomotor activity level of consciousness, and/or sleep/wake cycle. SEE: *Nursing Diagnoses Appendix.*

***chronic c.*** An irreversible, long-standing, and/or progressive deterioration of intellect and personality characterized by a decreased ability to interpret environmental stimulli, a decreased capacity for intellectual thought processes, and manifested by disturbances of memory, orientation, and behavior. SEE: *Nursing Diagnoses Appendix.*

***mental c.*** An abnormal mental state in which the individual experiences reduced mental functions, attentiveness, alertness, and ability to comprehend the immediate situation.

**confusional state, acute** A condition seen frequently in hospitalized patients of any age, but particularly in geriatric patients with dementia. Clinical manifestations are clouding of consciousness, memory impairment, impaired cognitive function, impaired perception, and emotional disturbances. Psychomotor activity is depressed, but repetitive, stereotyped activity such as plucking at bedclothes or tossing from side to side may be seen. Primary neurological disease must be distinguished from confusion due to systemic disease or toxic causes.

TREATMENT: It is helpful to reassure the patient and have a relative or friend stay with him or her. Agitated patients may require sedation with a long-acting tranquilizer or short-term sedation for diagnostic procedures. If present, hypoxia, hypoglycemia, hyperthermia, or dehydration should be corrected. The primary disease should be treated and an adequate diet provided.

**congener** (kŏn′jĕn-ĕr) [L. *con,* together, + *genus,* race] **1.** Two or more muscles with the same function. **2.** Something that resembles something else in structure, function, or origin. In the production of alcoholic beverages by fermentation, chemical substances termed congeners are also produced. These chemicals, more than 100 of which are known, impart aroma and flavor to the alcoholic compound. The precise role of these congeners in producing toxic effects is unknown.

**congenital** (kŏn-jĕn′ĭ-tăl) [L. *congenitus,* born together] Present at birth.

**congested** (kŏn-jĕs′tĕd) [L. *congerere,* to heap together] Containing an abnormal amount of blood or tissue fluid.

**congestion** (kŏn-jĕs′chŭn) An excessive amount of blood or tissue fluid in an organ or in tissue. **congestive** (-tĭv), *adj.*

***active c.*** Congestion resulting from increased blood flow to a part or from dilatation of blood vessels.

***passive c.*** Hyperemia resulting from interference with blood flow from capillaries into venules. It may also result from myocardial insufficiency.

***pulmonary c.*** The accumulation of an abnormal amount of blood in the pulmonary vascular bed. It usually occurs in association with heart failure.

**conglobate** (kŏn′glō-bāt) [L. *con,* together, + *globare,* to make round] In one mass, as lymph glands.

**conglobation** (kŏn″glō-bā′shŭn) An aggregation of particles in a rounded mass.

**conglomerate** (kŏn-glŏm′ĕr-āt) [″ + *glomerare,* to heap] **1.** An aggregation in one mass. **2.** Clustered; heaped together.

**conglutinant** (kŏn-gloo′tĭ-nănt) Promoting adhesion, as of the edges of a wound.

**congregate housing** Housing for the elderly that provides individual living units for tenants who range from independence to the institutional level of dependence.

**coniasis** (kō-nī′ă-sĭs) [Gr. *konis,* dust, + *-iasis,* condition] Dustlike calculi in gallbladder and bile ducts.

**conidia** (kō-nĭd′ē-ă) *sing.,* **conidium** Asexual spores of fungi.

**conidiophore** (kŏn-ĭd′ē-ō-for) [″ + *phoros,* bearing] The stalk supporting conidia.

**coniofibrosis** (kō″nē-ō-fī-brō′sĭs) [Gr. *konis,* dust, + L. *fibra,* fiber, + Gr. *osis,* condition] Pneumoconiosis produced by dust such as that from asbestos or silica. This causes fibrosis to develop in the lung.

**coniology** (kō-nē-ŏl′ŏ-jē) [″ + *logos,* study of] The study of dust and its effects.

**coniosis** (kō″nē-ō′sĭs) [″ + *osis,* condition] Any condition caused by inhalation of dust.

**coniosporosis** (kō″nē-ō-spō-rō′sĭs) [″ + *sporos,* seed, + *osis,* condition] A hypersensitivity reaction consisting of asthma and pneumonitis caused by breathing the spores of *Cryptostroma corticale* or *Coniosporium corticale.* These fungi grow under the bark of some types of trees. Workers who strip the bark from these trees may develop this condition.

**coniotomy** (kō″nē-ŏt′ō-mē) [Gr. *konos,* cone, + *tome,* incision] Cricothyrotomy.

**conization** (kŏn″ĭ-zā′shŭn) [Gr. *konos,* cone] Excision of a cone of tissue, as the mucous membrane of the cervix.

**conjugata** (kŏn″jū-gā′tă) Conjugate (2).

***c. diagonalis*** Diagonal conjugate.

***c. vera*** True conjugate.

**conjugate** (kŏn′jū-gāt) **1.** Paired or joined. **2.** An important diameter of the pelvis, measured from the center of the promontory of the sacrum to the back of the symphysis pubis. In obstetrics, the diagonal conjugate is measured and the true conjugate is estimated. SYN: *conjugata.* SEE: *diagonal c.*

***diagonal c.*** The distance between the sacral promontory and the lower inner surface of the symphysis pubis, usually more than 4.52 in. (11.5 cm). SYN: *conjugata diagonalis.*

***c. diameter*** Conjugate (2).

***external c.*** The diameter measured (with calipers) from the spine of the last lumbar vertebra to the front of the pubes; it is normally about 8 in. (20.3 cm).

***obstetrical c.*** The distance between the sacral promontory and a point slightly below the upper inner margin of the symphysis pubis; the shortest diameter to which the fetal head must accommodate to descend successfully through the pelvic inlet.

***true c.*** In obstetrics, the distance between the midline superior point of the sacrum and the upper margin of the symphysis pubis. It is the anteroposterior diameter of the pelvic inlet, estimated by subtracting 1.5 to 2 cm from the measurement of the diagonal conjugate. SYN: *conjugata vera.*

**conjugation** (kŏn″jū-gā′shŭn) **1.** A coupling together. **2.** In biology, the union of two unicellular organisms accompanied by an interchange of nuclear material as in *Paramecium.*

**conjunctiva** (kŏn″jŭnk-tī′vă, kŏn-jŭnk′tĭ-vă) [L. *conjungere,* to join together] The mucous membrane that lines the eyelids and is reflected onto the eyeball.

DIVISIONS: The palpebral conjunctiva covers the undersurface of the eyelids. The bulbar conjunctiva coats the anterior portion of the eyeball. The fornix conjunctiva is the transition portion forming a fold between the lid and the globe.

INSPECTION: The palpebral and ocular portions should be examined. Color, degree of moisture, presence of foreign bodies or petechial hemorrhages, and inflammation should be observed.

PATHOLOGY: Conjunctival pathology includes trachoma, pannus, and discoloration. Yellowish discoloration is seen in jaundice and pale conjunctivae are seen in anemias. Note: The skin of a person with hypercarotinemia is yellow, but the conjunctivae are not.

**conjunctival reflex** Closure of eyelids when the conjunctiva is touched or threatened.

**conjunctivitis** (kŏn-jŭnk″tĭ-vī′tĭs) [″ + Gr. *itis,* inflammation] Inflammation of the conjunctiva. Treatment is directed against the specific type of infection.

***actinic c.*** Conjunctivitis resulting from exposure to ultraviolet (actinic) radiations.

***acute contagious c.*** Pinkeye.

***acute hemorrhagic c.*** A contagious viral eye infection marked by rapid onset of pain. It progresses to swollen eyelids, hyperemia of the conjunctiva, and later subconjunctival hemorrhage. The disease, which is self-limiting and for which there is no specific therapy, usually affects both eyes. Several viral agents can cause this disease. Included are enterovirus 70, echovirus 7, and a variant of coxsackievirus A24.

***angular c. of Morax-Axenfeld*** Conjunctivitis affecting the inner angle of the conjunctivae.

***catarrhal c.*** Conjunctivitis due to causes such as foreign bodies, bacteria, or irritation from heat, cold, or chemicals.

***chlamydial c.*** Conjunctivitis caused by *Chlamydia trachomatis.* In newborns, this type of conjunctivitis is encountered more frequently than ophthalmia neonatorum caused by gonococci. Prophylaxis for chlamydial conjunctivitis is 1% silver nitrate. If the disease develops, tetracycline or sulfonamides are used.

***follicular c.*** A type of conjunctivitis characterized by pinkish round bodies in the retrotarsal fold.

***gonorrheal c.*** A severe, acute form of purulent conjunctivitis caused by the gonococcus *Neisseria gonorrhoeae.* SEE: *ophthalmia neonatorum.*

***granular c.*** Acute contagious inflammatory conjunctivitis with granular elevations on the lids that ulcerate and cicatrize.

***inclusion c.*** An acute purulent inflammation of the conjunctivae caused by *Chlamydia trachomatis.* The newborn is infected as it passes through the mother's genital tract. Adults may be infected while swimming or by a sex partner.

***membranous c.*** Acute conjunctivitis marked by a false membrane with or without infiltration.

***c. of newborn*** Ophthalmia neonatorum.

***phlyctenular c.*** An allergenic form of conjunctivitis common in children and marked by nodules that may ulcerate.

***purulent c.*** A form of conjunctivitis caused by organisms producing purulence, esp. gonococci.

***vernal c.*** Conjunctivitis beginning in the spring; probably due to allergy.

**conjunctivoma** (kŏn-jŭnk″tĭ-vō′mă) [L. *conjungere,* to join together, + Gr. *oma,* tumor] A tumor of the conjunctiva.

**conjunctivoplasty** (kŏn″jŭnk-tī′vō-plăs″tē) [″ + Gr. *plassein,* to form] Removal of part of the cornea and replacement with flaps from the conjunctiva.

**connective** [L. *connectere,* to bind together] Connecting or binding together.

**Conn's syndrome** [J. W. Conn, U.S. physician, b. 1907] Primary hyperaldosteronism. The symptoms and clinical condition include muscle weakness, polyuria, hypertension, hypokalemia, and alkalosis associated with an abnormally high rate of aldosterone secretion by the adrenal cortex. SEE: *Nursing Diagnoses Appendix.*

**conoid** (kō′noyd) [Gr. *konos,* cone, + *eidos,* form, shape] Resembling a cone; conical.

**conoid tubercle** An eminence on the inferior surface of the clavicle to which the conoid ligament is attached.

**consanguinity** (kŏn″săn-gwĭn′ĭ-tē) [L. *consanguinitas,* kinship] Relationship by blood (i.e., descent from a common ancestor).

**conscience** (kon′shŭntz) One's inner sense of what is right, wrong, or fair, esp. regarding relations with people or society. This sense can inhibit or reinforce the individual's actions and thoughts. SEE: *superego.*

**conscious** (kŏn′shŭs) [L. *conscius,* aware] Being aware and having perception; awake. SEE: *coma.*

**consciousness** A state of awareness, implying that the individual is oriented to time, place, and person (i.e., knows approx. the date, the nature of the environment, his or her name, and other pertinent personal data). Consciousness combines memories and the comprehension of external reality, as well as the person's emotional status and goals. It is, then, a significant part of what is described as "personality" in its largest sense.

Consciousness varies in intensity and extent from minute to minute. In crises, vivid ideational association may lead to exaggerated awareness. In states of relaxed contentment it lessens, and disappears completely in sleep. This differs from the pathological condition of coma, in which the patient cannot be aroused.

In so-called pathological sleep (i.e., encephalitis lethargica) and in stupor, though aroused, the patient is unable to postpone again lapsing into dullness. Up to a point, however, normal sleep can be adequately combatted by the demands of reality. Stupor is produced largely by the factors resulting in coma; the personality is relatively intact but "hazy." However, a real personality change manifests itself in certain conditions. Clouding of consciousness may simulate the dullness but usually not the other characteristics of stupor. On the contrary, such patients may seem alert.

Altered consciousness and attention, and impaired orientation and recent memory, are characteristic of delirium. A quiet delirium may not reveal itself easily, even in certain states of automatism in which one finds evidence of the "real personality." There is little to arouse suspicion on casual examination, yet total absence of memory may indicate major abnormalities.

In somnambulistic (i.e., sleepwalking) states, experiences may register but cannot be recalled after return to a normal state. In contrast, consciousness may seem to be present in so-called "coma vigil" because the eyes are open and the expression may be alert. SEE: *levels of consciousness.*

***clouding of c.*** A phase of delirium in which the patient's consciousness is cloudy or not clear.

Clouding of consciousness may be diagnosed from the appearance of a patient in catatonic stupor, and it may be difficult to realize that the patient is quite lucid and that experiences are being registered accurately and can be recalled later. In true clouding, stimuli usually fail to register.

***cosmic c.*** The inner reaches of consciousness in which knowledge or facts are recognized independently of physical influence.

***disintegration of c.*** Disorganization of the personality; the cause of most mental disorders not resulting from organic conditions. It is produced by the contents of the unconscious gradually disrupting the conscious.

***levels of c.*** States of awareness; may vary from alert wakefulness to coma. It is important to use a standardized system of description rather than vague terms such as semiconscious, semicomatose, or semistuporous.

*Alert wakefulness:* The patient perceives the environment clearly and responds quickly and appropriately to visual, auditory, and other sensory stimuli.

*Drowsiness:* The patient does not perceive the environment fully and responds to stimuli appropriately but slowly and with delay. He or she may be roused by verbal stimuli but may ignore some of them. The patient is capable of verbal response unless aphasia, aphonia, or anarthria is present. Lethargy and obtundation also describe the drowsy state.

*Stupor:* The patient is aroused by intense stimuli only. Loud noise may elicit a nonspecific reaction. Motor response and reflex reactions are usually preserved unless the patient is paralyzed.

*Coma:* The patient does not perceive the environment and intense stimuli produce a rudimentary response if any. The presence of reflex reactions depends on the location of the lesion(s) in the nervous system.

**consensual** (kŏn-sĕn′shū-ăl) [L. *consensus,* agreement] Pert. to reflex stimulation of one part or side produced by excitation of another part or the opposite side.

**consensual light reflex** The reaction of both pupils that occurs when one eye is exposed to a greater intensity of light than the other. SEE: *reflex, pupillary.*

**consensual reflex** SEE: *reflex, crossed.*

**consent** The granting of permission by the patient for another person to perform an act (e.g., permission for a surgical or therapeutic procedure or experiment to be performed by a physician, dentist, or other health-care professional).

***implied c.*** Consent implied in certain actions by the patient, as when he or she enters the dental office and sits in a dental chair. This implies consent to examination, diagnosis, and consultation.

***informed c.*** The consent given by a person after receipt of the following information: the nature and purpose of the proposed procedure or treatment, the expected outcome and the likelihood of success, the risks, and the alternatives to the procedure and supporting information regarding these and the effect of no treatment or procedure, including the effect on the prognosis and the material risks associated with no treatment. Also included are instructions concerning what should be done if the procedure turns out to be harmful or unsuccessful, and who will pay for additional medical expenses incurred as a result of an unsuccessful procedure. Informed consent promotes individual autonomy, protects patients, avoids duress, encourages introspection by health care professionals, and involves the public in promoting autonomy and controlling biomedical research. SEE: *institutional review board.*

**consenting adult** A mature individual who consents to participate in social or sexual activity that is or formerly was regarded as abnormal (e.g., sadomasochistic sexual activity or homosexual acts).

**conservative** (kŏn-sĕr′vă-tĭv) [L. *conservare,* to preserve] Pert. to the use of a simple rather than a radical method of medical or surgical therapy.

**conservation** A cognitive principle, first described by Piaget, indicating that a certain quantity remains constant despite the transformation of shape. Children develop conservation ability for number, length, liquid amount, solid amount, space, weight, and volume.

**conservation model** A conceptual model of nursing developed by Myra Levine. The person is viewed as a holistic being who adapts to environmental challenges. In this model the goal of nursing is to promote wholeness through conservation of energy, structural integrity, personal integrity, and social integrity. SEE: *Nursing Theory Appendix.*

**conservatorship** The most restrictive way

in which someone's person and property can be legally managed by another. The term does not refer to imprisonment or confinement in a psychiatric facility. This is called *guardianship* in some states.

**consolidation** (kŏn-sŏl-ĭ-dā'shŭn) [L. *consolidare,* to make firm] The process of becoming solid, esp. in connection with the lungs. Solidification of the lungs is caused by pathological engorgement of the lung tissues as occurs in acute pneumonia.

**constant** (kŏn'stănt) [L. *constans,* standing together] **1.** Unchanging. **2.** A condition, fact, or situation that does not change.

**constellation** (kŏn″stĕl-lā'shŭn) [L. *con,* together, + *stella,* star] A group, set, or configuration of objects, individuals, or conditions.

**constipation** (kŏn″stĭ-pā'shŭn) [L. *constipare,* to press together] A state in which an individual experiences a change in normal bowel habits characterized by a decrease in frequency and/or passage of hard, dry stools; difficult defecation; sluggish action of the bowels. SEE: *Nursing Diagnoses Appendix.*

ETIOLOGY: Predisposing factors include a lack of regular bowel habits from childhood, worry, anxiety, fear, and a sedentary life. Direct factors include failure to establish definite and regular times for bowel movements, improper diet, intestinal obstruction, tumors, excessive laxative use, weakness of intestinal musculature (atony) or excessive tonicity (spasticity), use of certain drugs, and anal lesions. It is also a concomitant in some types of insanity.

NOTE: It is virtually impossible to state how frequently the bowels should move in order to be classed as "normal." In healthy individuals such frequency can vary, ranging from two to three bowel movements per day to two per week.

---

Caution: A change in frequency of bowel movements may be a sign of serious intestinal or colonic disease (e.g., a malignancy). A change in bowel habits should be discussed with a physician.

---

TREATMENT: Consumption of plenty of fresh vegetables, fruits, milk, and an abundance of water is effective in treating constipation. One should also try to establish regular bowel, eating, and exercise habits.

***atonic c.*** Constipation due to weakness of the muscles of the colon and rectum.

***colonic c.*** The state in which an individual's pattern of elimination is characterized by hard, dry stools which results from a delay in passage of food residue. SEE: *Nursing Diagnoses Appendix.*

***obstructive c.*** Constipation due to an obstruction in the intestines, possibly requiring surgery. The preoperative diet should contain low-residue and no gas-forming foods.

***perceived c.*** The state in which an individual makes a self-diagnosis of constipation and ensures a daily bowel movement through use of laxatives, enemas, and suppositories. SEE: *Nursing Diagnoses Appendix.*

***spastic c.*** Constipation due to excessive tonicity of the intestinal wall, esp. the colon.

**constitution** (kŏn-stĭ-tŭ'shŭn) [L. *constituere,* to establish] The physical makeup and functional habits of the body. **constitutional** (-ăl), *adj.*

**constriction** [L. *con,* together, + *stringere,* to draw] **1.** The binding or squeezing of a part. **2.** The narrowing of a vessel or opening (e.g., blood vessels or the pupil of the eye).

**constrictor 1.** Something that binds or restricts a part. **2.** A muscle that constricts a vessel, opening, or passageway, as the constrictors of the faucial isthmus and pharynx and the circular fibers of the iris, intestine, and blood vessels.

**consultant** [L. *consultare,* to counsel] A health care worker, such as a nurse, physician, dentist, pharmacist, or psychologist, who acts in an advisory capacity.

**consultation** For a specific patient, diagnosis and proposed treatment by two or more health care workers at one time.

**consummation** The first act of sexual intercourse after marriage.

**consumption** (kŏn-sŭmp'shŭn) [L. *consumere,* to waste away] **1.** Tuberculosis. **2.** Wasting. **3.** The using up of anything.

**consumption-coagulopathy** Disseminated intravascular coagulation.

**consumptive** Pert. to or afflicted with tuberculosis.

**contact** [L. *con,* with, + *tangere,* to touch] **1.** Mutual touching or apposition of two bodies. **2.** One who has been recently exposed to a contagious disease.

***complete c.*** The contact that occurs when the entire proximal surface of a tooth touches the entire surface of an adjoining tooth, proximally.

***defective occlusal c.*** Interceptive occlusal c.

***direct c.*** Transmission of a communicable disease from the host to a healthy person by way of body fluids, such as respiratory droplets, blood, and semen; cutaneous contact; or placental transmission.

***indirect c.*** Transmission of a communicable disease in which the pathogen is carried by some medium between the host and the healthy person. This may be contaminated food or water or an arthropod vector.

***interceptive occlusal c.*** Tooth contact that can divert the mandible from a normal to an abnormal path of motion. SYN: *defective occlusal c.*

***intercuspal c.*** Contact between the cusps of opening teeth.

***occlusal c.*** The normal contact between teeth when the maxilla and mandible are brought together in habitual or centric occlusion.

***proximal c., proximate c.*** Touching of teeth on their adjacent surfaces.

**contactant** (kŏn-tăk′tănt) A substance that produces an allergic or sensitivity response when it contacts the skin directly.

**contact lens** SEE: under *lens*.

**contact surface** A proximal tooth surface.

**contagion** (kŏn-tā′jŭn) [L. *contingere,* to touch] **1.** A contagious disease. **2.** Any virus or other microorganism that causes a contagious disease. SEE: *virulent; virus.*

**contagious** (kŏn-tā′jŭs) A disease that is easily transmitted from host to host by casual cutaneous contact or respiratory droplets.

**contagious pustular dermatitis** A cutaneous disease of sheep and goats transmitted to humans by direct contact. The lesion on humans is usually solitary and on the hands, arms, or face. This maculopapular area may progress to a pustule up to 3 cm in diameter and may last 3 to 6 weeks. The etiological agent is *Parapoxvirus,* which is a genus of poxvirus. There is no specific treatment. SYN: *orf.*

**contagium** (kŏn-tā′jē-ŭm) [L.] The agent causing infection or contagion.

**container** (kŏn-tā′nĕr) A receptacle for storing a medical specimen or supplies. Use of sterile disposable containers for collecting specimens is recommended, since contamination of the container may alter the results of the specimen analysis and therefore interfere with the diagnosis. SEE: *Universal Precautions Appendix.*

**contaminant** (kŏn-tăm′ĭ-nănt) A substance or organism that causes contamination.

**contaminate** (kŏn-tăm′ĭ-nāt) [L. *contaminare,* to render impure] **1.** To soil, stain, or pollute. **2.** To render unfit for use through introduction of a harmful or injurious substance. **3.** To make impure or unclean. **4.** To deposit a radioactive substance in any place where it is not supposed to be.

**contamination 1.** The act of contaminating, esp. the introduction of disease germs or infectious material into or on normally clean or sterile objects, spaces, or surfaces. **2.** In psychiatry, the fusion and condensation of words so that they run together when spoken.

***radiation c.*** Radiation in or on a place where it is not wanted.

**contiguity** (kŏn″tĭ-gū′ĭ-tē) [L. *contiguus,* touching] Contact or close association.

***law of c.*** The law stating that if two ideas occur in association, they are likely to be repeated.

***solution of c.*** The dislocation or displacement of two normally contiguous parts.

**continence** (kŏn′tĭ-nĕns) [L. *continere,* to hold together] Self-restraint, used esp. in reference to refraining from sexual intercourse, and to the ability to control urination and defecation. SEE: *incontinence.*

**continent** (kŏn′tĭ-nĕnt) **1.** Able to control urination and defecation. **2.** Not engaging in sexual intercourse. SEE: *continence.*

**continuing care community** A type of combined health housing and social care insurance for older persons. The person signs a contract, paying an entrance fee and a monthly service charge. The contract remains in effect as long as the person lives.

**continuing education** The enhancement or expansion of an individual's knowledge or skills by further schooling. Postgraduate courses may be required for continued certification in a practice such as medicine or nursing.

**continuity** (kŏn″tĭ-nū′ĭ-tē) [L. *continuus,* continued] The condition of being unbroken, uninterrupted, or intimately united.

**continuous passive motion** ABBR: CPM. The use of a mechanical apparatus to provide continuous movement through specific ranges of motion at selected joints. This is used following surgery to reduce complications and promote recovery.

**continuous spectrum 1.** An unbroken series of wavelengths, either visible or invisible. **2.** An unbroken range of radiations of different wavelengths in any portion of the invisible spectrum.

**continuous subcutaneous insulin infusion** ABBR: CSII. SEE: *insulin pump.*

**continuum of care** A range of services available to elderly people in the community. They include supportive, rehabilitative, preventive, and social services and meet various levels of need or impairment.

**contour** (kŏn′toor) [It. *contornare,* to go around] **1.** The outline or surface configuration of a part. **2.** To shape or form a surface, as in carving dental restorations to approximate the conditions of the original tooth surface.

***gingival c.*** The normal arching appearance of the gingiva along the cervical part of the teeth and rounding off toward the attached gingiva.

***gingival denture c.*** The form of the denture base or other materials around the cervical parts of artificial teeth.

**contoured** (kŏn′toord) Having an irregular, undulating surface resembling a relief map; said of bacterial colonies.

**contra-** [L.] Prefix indicating *opposite* or *against.*

**contra-aperture** [L. *contra,* against, + *apertura,* opening] A second opening made in an abscess.

**contraception** (kŏn″tră-sĕp′shŭn) [″ + *conceptio,* a conceiving] The prevention of conception.

***postcoital c.*** ABBR: PCC. The prevention of conception in the immediate postcoital period. These methods include diethylstilbestrol and RU 486.

**contraceptive** (kŏn″tră-sĕp′tĭv) Any process, device, or method that prevents con-

## Contraceptive Use by Women, 15 to 44 Years Old: 1995

Based on Samples of the Female Population of the United States

| Contraceptive Status and Method | All Women[1] | Age: 15–24 Years | Age: 25–34 Years | Age: 35–44 Years | Race: White | Race: Black | Race: Hispanic |
|---|---|---|---|---|---|---|---|
| All women (1,000) | 58,381 | 17,637 | 21,728 | 19,016 | 42,968 | 7,510 | 5,500 |
| **Percent Distribution** | | | | | | | |
| Sterile | 32.1 | 3.8 | 26.4 | 64.6 | 32.9 | 34.0 | 27.5 |
| Surgically sterile | 30.2 | 3.1 | 24.8 | 61.1 | 31.2 | 31.4 | 23.9 |
| Noncontraceptively sterile[2] | 5.2 | 0.3 | 2.7 | 12.5 | 5.4 | 6.5 | 3.2 |
| Contraceptively sterile[3] | 25.0 | 2.8 | 22.1 | 48.6 | 25.8 | 24.9 | 20.7 |
| Nonsurgically sterile[4] | 1.9 | 0.7 | 1.6 | 3.5 | 1.7 | 2.6 | 3.6 |
| Pregnant, postpartum | 5.4 | 7.0 | 7.9 | 1.2 | 5.2 | 5.5 | 7.7 |
| Seeking pregnancy | 4.0 | 1.8 | 7.6 | 2.0 | 3.7 | 4.7 | 5.1 |
| Other nonusers | 24.2 | 46.4 | 17.1 | 12.0 | 23.6 | 22.1 | 28.3 |
| Never had intercourse | 9.4 | 26.4 | 2.8 | 1.3 | 8.7 | 7.0 | 16.4 |
| No intercourse in last month | 7.0 | 7.7 | 7.1 | 6.4 | 7.2 | 7.5 | 5.1 |
| Had intercourse in last month | 7.8 | 12.3 | 7.2 | 4.3 | 7.7 | 7.6 | 6.8 |
| Nonsurgical contraceptors | 34.3 | 41.2 | 41.3 | 20.1 | 34.6 | 33.8 | 31.7 |
| Pill | 16.9 | 23.9 | 22.0 | 4.7 | 17.3 | 16.7 | 16.4 |
| IUD | 0.8 | 0.2 | 0.4 | 1.8 | 0.8 | 0.8 | 1.0 |
| Diaphragm | 1.7 | 0.2 | 2.3 | 2.4 | 1.8 | 1.0 | 0.8 |
| Condom | 10.5 | 13.9 | 11.0 | 6.7 | 10.3 | 11.4 | 8.9 |
| Periodic abstinence | 1.6 | 1.0 | 2.0 | 1.6 | 1.6 | 0.7 | 1.9 |
| Natural family planning | 0.2 | 0.1 | 0.4 | 0.2 | 0.2 | — | — |
| Withdrawal | 0.6 | 0.6 | 0.6 | 0.5 | 0.6 | 0.4 | 0.4 |
| Other methods[5] | 2.3 | 1.4 | 3.0 | 2.4 | 2.2 | 2.8 | 2.3 |

SOURCE: Adapted from U.S. National Center for Health Statistics. *Advance Data from Vital and Health Statistics.*

— Represents or rounds to zero. [1] Includes other races, not shown separately. [2] Persons who had sterilizing operation and who gave as one reason that they had medical problems with their reproductive organs. [3] Includes all other sterilization operations, and sterilization of the husband or current partner. [4] Persons sterile from illness, accident, or congenital conditions. [5] Douche, suppository, and less frequently used methods.

ception. Categories of contraceptives include steroids; chemical; physical or barrier; combinations of physical or barrier and chemical; "natural"; abstinence; and permanent surgical procedures. SEE: table; *abortion; RU 486*.

STEROIDS: Oral contraceptives, colloquially termed "the pill," consist of chemicals that are quite similar to natural hormones (estrogen or progesterone). They act by preventing ovulation. When taken according to instructions, these pills are almost 100% effective. Long-acting contraceptives including the implanted levonorgestrel are available. Diethylstilbestrol is used as a "morning-after" contraceptive, esp. in cases of rape or incest. SEE: *Norplant*.

CHEMICAL: Spermicides in the form of foam, cream, jelly, spermicide-impregnated sponge, or suppositories are placed in the vagina before intercourse. They may be used alone or in combination with a barrier contraceptive. They act by killing the sperm. Douching after intercourse is not effective enough to be considered a method of contraception.

PHYSICAL OR BARRIER: Intrauterine contraceptive devices (IUD) are plastic or metal objects placed inside the uterus. They are thought to prevent the fertilized egg from attaching itself to the lining of the uterus. Their effectiveness is only slightly lower than that of oral contraceptives. Diaphragms are made of a dome-shaped piece of rubber with a flexible spring circling the edge. They are available in various sizes and are inserted into the vagina so as to cover the cervix. A diaphragm must be used in conjunction with a chemical spermicide, which is used before positioning the diaphragm. A specially fitted cervical cap is also available as a barrier-type contraceptive. A sponge impregnated with a contraceptive cream or jelly is available. It is placed in the vagina up to several hours prior to intercourse. The male partner can use a condom, a flexible tube-shaped barrier placed over the erect penis so that the ejaculate is contained in the tube and is not deposited in the vagina. Made of rubber or animal membranes, condoms are available in both dry and wet-lubricated forms and in various colors. Used properly, the condom is a reliable means of contraception. It is more effective if combined with a chemical spermicide. Condoms also help prevent transmission of diseases by sexual intercourse by providing a physical barrier. SEE: *condom*.

NATURAL: These methods involve abstaining from intercourse for a specified number of days before, during, and after ovulation. The rhythm method is based on calculating the fertile period by the use of a calendar, on which the supposed infertile days are marked. In practice, this method has a high rate of failure. Other methods include determining ovulation by keeping a basal temperature chart and judging the time of ovulation by observing cyclical changes in the cervical mucus. SEE: *basal temperature chart*. Sophisticated home-diagnostic tests for the hormonal changes present at ovulation are available. Withdrawal, the removal of the penis from the vagina just before ejaculation, is subject to a high failure rate because sperm may be contained in the preejaculatory fluid from the penis.

PERMANENT: *For women:* Tubal ligation involves surgical division of the fallopian tubes and ligation of the cut ends. This procedure does not interfere with the subsequent enjoyment of sexual intercourse. This form of sterilization is effective but virtually irreversible. *For men:* Vasectomy consists of cutting the vas deferens and ligating each end so that the sperm can no longer travel from the testicle to the urethra. The procedure must be done bilaterally and the ejaculate tested for several months postoperatively to make certain sperm are not present. Until two successive tests reveal absence of sperm, the method should not be regarded as having succeeded. Attempts to reverse this surgical procedure have succeeded in only a small percentage of cases. Vasectomy does not interfere with the normal enjoyment of sexual intercourse.

**contract** (kŏn-trăkt′) [L. *contrahere,* to draw together] **1.** To draw together, reduce in size, or shorten. **2.** To acquire through infection, as to contract a disease.

**contractile** (kŏn-trăk′tĭl) Able to contract or shorten.

**contractility** (kŏn-trăk-tĭl′ĭ-tē) **1.** Having the ability to contract or shorten. **2.** In cardiac physiology, the force with which left ventricular ejection occurs. It is independent of the effects of preload or afterload.

**contraction** (kŏn-trăk′shŭn) A shortening or tightening, as of a muscle; a shrinking or a reduction in size.

***Braxton Hicks c.*** SEE: *Braxton Hicks sign*.

***carpopedal c.*** A contraction of the flexor muscles of the hands and feet due to tetany hypocalcemia or hyperventilation.

***hourglass c.*** An excessive, irregular contraction of an organ at its center. SEE: *ectasia*.

***idiomuscular c.*** Motion produced by degenerated muscles without nerve stimulus.

***isoinertial muscle c.*** Shortening and increased tension in a muscle against a constant load or resistance.

***isometric c.*** A muscular contraction in which the muscle increases tension but does not change its length; also called a *static muscle contraction*.

***isotonic c.*** A muscular contraction in which the muscle maintains constant tension by changing its length during the action.

***tetanic c.*** **1.** Continuous muscular contraction. **2.** A sudden, strong, sustained uterine contraction that jeopardizes maternal and fetal status. It may occur during oxytocin induction or stimulation of labor and can cause profound fetal distress, premature placental separation, or uterine rupture.

***tonic c.*** Spasmodic contraction of a muscle for an extended period.

**contraction stress test** ABBR: CST. SEE: *oxytocin challenge test*.

**contracture** (kŏn-trăk′chūr) [L. *contractura*] Fibrosis of connective tissue in skin, fascia, muscle, or a joint capsule that prevents normal mobility of the related tissue or joint.

***Dupuytren's c.*** SEE: *Dupuytren's contracture*.

***fibrotic c.*** Contraction of a muscle in which the muscle tissue has been replaced by fibrous tissue because of injury.

***functional c.*** Contraction of a muscle that decreases during anesthesia or sleep.

***myostatic c.*** Adaptive shortening of muscle, usually caused by immobilization and without tissue pathology.

***physiological c.*** A temporary condition in which tension and shortening of a muscle are maintained for a considerable time although there is no tetanus. It may be induced by heat, drug action, or acids.

***pseudomyostatic c.*** Apparent permanent contraction of a muscle due to a central nervous system lesion, resulting in loss of range of motion and resistance of the muscle to stretch.

***Volkmann's c.*** Pronation and flexion of the hand, with atrophy of the forearm muscles, resulting from circulatory impairment due to pressure from a cast, constricting dressings, or injury to the radial artery. This can be prevented by alertness to signs of cold, pallor, cyanosis, pain, and swelling of the part below the injury or constriction and removal of the cause.

**contrafissura** (kŏn″tră-fĭ-shū′ră) [L. *contra,* against, + *fissura,* fissure] A skull fracture at a point opposite where the blow was received. SEE: *contrecoup injury.*

**contraindication** (kŏn″tră-ĭn-dĭ-kā′shŭn) [″ + *indicare,* to point out] Any symptom or circumstance indicating the inappropriateness of an otherwise advisable treatment.

**contralateral** (kŏn″tră-lăt′ĕr-ăl) [″ + *latus,* side] Originating in or affecting the opposite side of the body, as opposed to homolateral and ipsilateral.

**contralateral reflex 1.** Passive flexion of one part following flexion of another. **2.** Passive flexion of one leg, causing similar movement of opposite leg.

**contrast** (kŏn′trăst) The difference between adjacent densities on a radiograph. This is controlled by the energy of the beam and influenced by the characteristics of the part radiographed, production of scatter radiation, type of film and screen combination, and processing.

**contrast medium** In radiology, the use of a foreign substance to provide a difference in density (contrast) so that the tissue or organ can be better visualized. The substance can be radiopaque and positive (e.g., barium sulfate, tri-iodinated media) or radiolucent and negative (e.g., air). When swallowed, barium sulfate is more dense than the intestinal tract and creates enough contrast to successfully image the organ.

***high-osmolarity c.m.*** ABBR: HOCM. A water-soluble contrast medium with high osmolarity. These agents increase the probability of an adverse reaction and are generally ionic.

***low-osmolarity c.m.*** ABBR: LOCM. A water-soluble contrast medium with low osmolarity. These agents produce fewer undesired effects after intravascular administration than do high-osmolarity contrast media. They are generally nonionic, with the exception of Hexabrix (an ionic dimer).

***nonionic c.m.*** A water-soluble contrast medium whose base molecules dissociate into cations and anions in solution. These agents tend to have low osmolarity and decreased patient adverse reactions, but they are expensive.

***tri-iodinated c.m.*** A derivative of tri-iodobenzoic acid that is the base for water-soluble contrast media. It contains three atoms of iodine per molecule.

**contrast spray** A method of stimulating blood circulation by having the patient sit on the side of a bathtub and spraying the feet and legs with warm water for 1 min and cold water for 1 min. This is done for 10 min twice daily.

**contravolitional** (kŏn″tră-vō-lĭ′shŭn-ăl) [L. *contra,* against, + *velle,* to wish] In opposition to or without the will; involuntary.

**contrecoup** (kŏn-tr-koo′) An injury to parts of the brain located on the side opposite that of the primary injury, as when a blow to the back of the head forces the frontal and temporal lobes against the irregular bones of the anterior portion of the cranial vault.

**contributory negligence** In forensic medicine, the concept that the plaintiff's negligence in combination with the defendant's negligence is the cause of the plaintiff's injuries or damages.

**control** (kŏn-trōl′) [L. *contra,* against, + *rotulus,* little wheel] **1.** To regulate or maintain. **2.** A standard against which observations or conclusions may be checked to establish their validity, as a control animal (e.g., one that has not been exposed to the treatment or condition being studied in the other animals). **3.** In clinical investigations, the matching of cases and controls with as many major variables as appear to be important in the particular study. This leaves the suspected factor open for study in the two groups.

***automatic exposure c.*** ABBR: AEC. In radiology, an ionization chamber or solid-state device that terminates the radiation exposure at a preset level. SYN: *phototimer.*

***motor c.*** The ability to voluntarily execute planned, coordinated movement. SEE: *learning, motor.*

**controlled substance act** The Comprehensive Drug Abuse Prevention and Control Act; a law enacted in 1971 to control the distribution and use of all depressant and stimulant drugs and other drugs of abuse or potential abuse as may be designated by the Drug Enforcement Administration of the Department of Justice.

The act specifies record keeping by the pharmacist, the format for prescription writing, and the limit on the amount of a drug that can be legally dispensed. This limit and whether refills are allowed varies with the nature of the drug. Centrally acting drugs such as narcotics, stimulants, and certain sedatives are divided into five classes called schedules I through V. Schedule I drugs are experimental. Prescriptions for schedule II drugs may not be refilled. Prescriptions for schedule III and IV drugs may be refilled up to five times within 6 months of the time the initial prescription was written. Schedule V drugs are restricted only to the extent that all nonscheduled prescription drugs are regulated.

Controlled substances are labeled with a large "C" followed by the Roman numeral designation. Alternatively the Roman numeral is within the large "C."

**contrude** (kŏn-trood′) [L. *con,* with, + *trudere,* to thrust] To crowd together, as the teeth.

**contrusion** (kŏn-troo′zhŭn) **1.** Abnormal lingual curve or line of the dental arch. **2.** Having the teeth crowded.

**contuse** (kŏn-tooz′) [L. *contundere,* to bruise] To bruise.

**contusion** (kŏn-too′zhŭn) An injury in which the skin is not broken; a bruise. Pain, swelling, and discoloration are characteristic.

FIRST AID: Cold applications are needed first, followed by application of a firm bandage to prevent swelling. Twenty-four to 48 hr later, application of heat is desirable, followed by gentle massage.

**conus** (kō′nŭs) [Gr. *konos*] **1.** A cone. **2.** A posterior staphyloma of a myopic eye.

***c. arteriosus*** The upper rounded anterior angle of the right cardiac ventricle, where the pulmonary artery arises.

***c. medullaris*** The conical portion of the lower spinal cord.

**convalescence** (kŏn″văl-ĕs′ĕns) [L. *convalescere,* to become strong] The period of recovery after the termination of a disease or an operation.

**convalescent 1.** Getting well. **2.** One who is recovering from a disease or operation.

**convalescent diet** A diet suitable for the condition from which the patient is recovering. SEE: *soft diet.*

**convection** (kŏn-vĕk′shŭn) [L. *convehere,* to convey] **1.** Heat transference by means of currents in liquids or gases. **2.** Loss of body heat by means of transfer to the surrounding cooler air.

**convergence** (kŏn-vĕr′jĕns) [L. *con,* with, + *vergere,* to incline] **1.** The moving of two or more objects toward the same point. **2.** In reflex activity, the coming together of several axons or afferent fibers on one or a few motor neurons; the condition in which impulses from several sensory receptors converge on the same motor center, resulting in a limited and specific response. **3.** The directing of visual lines to a nearby point.

**convergent** (kŏn-vĕr′jĕnt) Tending toward a common point.

**conversion** (kŏn-vĕr′zhŭn) [L. *convertere,* to turn round] **1.** The change from one condition to another. **2.** In obstetrics, a change in position of a fetus in the uterus by the physician to facilitate delivery. SEE: *version.*

**conversion disorder** A mental disorder marked by symptoms or deficits affecting voluntary motor or sensory function that suggest a neurological or other general medical condition. Psychological factors are associated with and precede the condition. Symptoms include loss of sense of touch, double vision, blindness, deafness, paralysis, and hallucinations. Individuals with conversion symptoms show "la belle indifference" or relative lack of concern. The symptoms are not intentionally produced or feigned. The diagnosis cannot be established if the condition can be explained by the effects of medication or a neurological or other general medical condition. SYN: *conversion hysteria.*

**conversion symptom** The unconscious change of an anxiety-producing state to a somatic symptom. In hysteria the manifestation may be imagined pain or disability. SEE: *somatoform disorder.*

**convex** (kŏn′vĕks, kŏn-vĕks′) [L. *convexus,* vaulted, arched] Curved evenly; resembling the segment of a sphere.

**convexoconcave** (kŏn-vĕk″sō-kŏn′kāv, -kŏn-kāv′) Concavoconvex.

**convexoconvex** [″ + *convexus,* arched] Convex on two opposite faces.

**convolute, convoluted** (kŏn′vō-loot; -loot′ ĕd) [L. *convolvere,* to roll together] Rolled, as a scroll.

**convolution** (kŏn″vō-loo′shŭn) [L. *convolvere,* to roll together] **1.** A turn, fold, or coil of anything that is convoluted. **2.** In anatomy, a gyrus, one of the many folds on the surface of the cerebral hemispheres. They are separated by grooves (sulci or fissures). SEE: *gyrus.*

***angular c.*** A gyrus forming the posterior portion of the inferior parietal lobule.

***annectant c.*** One of the four gyri connecting the convolutions on the upper surface of the occipital lobe with the parietal and temporosphenoidal lobes.

***anterior choroid c.*** Gyrus choroides.

***anterior orbital c.*** The convolution that lies in front of the orbital sulcus.

***Arnold's c.*** One of the gyri posteriores inferiores.

***ascending frontal c.*** The convolution forming the anterior boundary of Rolando's fissure.

***ascending parietal c.*** The convolution parallel to the ascending frontal convolution, separated from it by Rolando's fissure, except at the extremities, where they are generally united.

***Broca's c.*** Broca's area.

***callosal c.*** Gyrus cinguli.

***cerebral c.*** One of the convolutions of the cerebrum.

***c. of corpus callosum*** Gyrus fornicatus.

***cuneate c.*** Gyral isthmus.

***dentate c.*** A small, notched gyrus, rudimentary in humans, situated in the dentate fissure.

***exterior olfactory c.*** One of the small projections forming the outer boundary of the olfactory grooves.

***hippocampal c.*** Uncinate gyrus.

***inferior frontal c.*** The lower and outer part of the frontal lobe.

***inferior occipital c.*** A small convolution lying between the middle and inferior occipital fissures.

***insular c.*** One of a group of small convolutions forming the island of Reil, entirely concealed by the operculum.

***intestinal c.*** A coil of the intestines.

***marginal c.*** The convolution beginning in front of the locus perforatus anterior and bounding the longitudinal fissure on the mesial aspect of the hemisphere.

***middle frontal c.*** Second frontal c.

***middle occipital c.*** The convolution between the first and third occipital convolutions.

***middle temporosphenoidal c.*** A small gyrus continuous with the middle occipital or angular gyrus.

***occipitotemporal c.*** One of two small convolutions on the lower surface of the temporosphenoidal lobe.

***olfactory c.*** Olfactory lobe.

***orbital c.*** One of the small gyri on the orbital surface of the frontal lobe.

***parietal c.*** The ascending parietal or the superior parietal convolution.

***posterior orbital c.*** A small convolution on the posterior and outer side of the orbital sulcus, and continuous with the inferior frontal convolution.

***second frontal c.*** A convolution on the frontal lobes, lying posteriorly between the superior and inferior frontal sulci. SYN: *middle frontal c.*

***superior frontal c.*** A convolution that bounds the great longitudinal fissure, originating behind the upper end of the ascending frontal convolution.

***superior occipital c.*** The uppermost of the three convolutions on the superior surface of the occipital lobe.

***superior parietal c.*** The portion of the parietal lobe limited anteriorly by the upper part of Rolando's fissure, posteriorly by the exterior parieto-occipital fissure, and inferiorly by the intraparietal sulcus.

***superior temporosphenoidal c.*** The uppermost of three convolutions forming the temporosphenoidal lobe. It is just below and parallel to the sylvian fissure.

***supramarginal c.*** The anterior portion of the interior parietal lobule behind the inferior extremity of the intraparietal sulcus, below which it joins the ascending parietal convolution.

***c. of the sylvian fissure*** The convolution that bounds the fissure of Sylvius.

***transverse orbital c.*** The gyrus occupying the posterior portion of the inferior surface of the frontal lobe, at the anterior extremity of the fissure of Sylvius.

***uncinate c.*** The convolution extending from near the posterior extremity of the occipital lobe to the apex of the temporosphenoidal lobe.

**convulsant** (kŏn-vŭl′sănt) [L. *convellere,* to pull together] **1.** An agent that produces a convulsion. **2.** Causing the onset of a convulsion.

**convulsion** (kŏn-vŭl′shŭn) Paroxysms of involuntary muscular contractions and relaxations.

NOTE: It is important for the person who observes the convulsion to record on the chart the following: time of onset, duration, whether the convulsion started in a certain area of the body or became generalized from the start, type of contractions, whether the patient became incontinent, whether the patient's breath had an abnormal odor, and whether the convulsion caused the patient to be injured or strike the head during the convulsion. This information, in addition to its medicolegal importance, is valuable in diagnosis and in caring for the patient.

ETIOLOGY: General causes are epilepsy, eclampsia, meningitis, heat cramps, brain lesions, tetanus, uremia, and poisoning from camphor, cyanide compounds, and strychnine. In children, the cause is often fever. Other causes include rickets, syphilis, malnutrition, malaria, acute infectious disease, or toxemia of pregnancy.

TREATMENT: Febrile convulsions in children are usually controlled by phenobarbital with or without aspirin as an antipyretic. In adults, the cause must first be found. The patient should be prevented from self-injury. A firm pad between the teeth prevents biting the tongue or cheeks. If fever is present, a tepid or cool bath may be helpful. Sedatives or anesthesia may be ordered by the physician. Aftercare includes rest in bed, absolute quiet, and careful diagnosis without undue disturbance to the patient. SEE: *febrile convulsion.*

***clonic c.*** A convulsion with intermittent contractions, the muscles being alternately contracted and relaxed.

***febrile c.*** SEE: *febrile convulsion.*

***hysterical c.*** A convulsion caused by hysteria.

***mimetic c.*** A facial muscle spasm.

***puerperal c.*** An eclamptic convulsion in a pregnant or puerperal woman.

***salaam c.*** A nodding spasm.

***tonic c.*** Convulsion in which the contractions are maintained for a time, as in tetany.

***toxic c.*** Convulsion caused by the action of a toxin on the nervous system.

***uremic c.*** Convulsion caused by uremia.

**convulsive** (kŏn-vŭl′sĭv) Pert. to convulsions.

**convulsive reflex** Incoordinate contraction of muscles in a convulsive manner.

**cooking** [L. *coquere,* to cook] The process of heating foods to prepare them for eating. Cooking makes most foods more palatable and easier to chew, improves their digestibility, and destroys or inactivates harmful organisms or toxins that may be present. Cooking releases the aromatic substances and extractives that contribute odors and taste to foods. These odors help to stimulate the appetite.

---

Caution: Not all toxic substances are inactivated by heat. Most microorganisms and parasites are destroyed in the ordinary process of cooking, but some require a higher degree of heat and longer cooking to effect this result. Pork must be cooked completely throughout to kill the encysted larvae of *Trichinella.*

---

ACTION: *Protein:* Soluble proteins become coagulated. *Soluble substances:* These, including heat-labile vitamins, are often inactivated by boiling, and even mineral substances and starches, although insoluble to a certain extent, may be altered in this process. *Starch:* The starch granules swell and are changed from insoluble (raw) starch to soluble starch capable of being converted into sugar during digestion and of being assimilated in the system.

**Cooley's anemia** [Thomas Cooley, U.S. pediatrician, 1871–1945] Thalassemia major.

**Coombs' test** [R. R. A. Coombs, Brit. immunologist, b. 1921] A postnatal test of a sample of umbilical cord blood for maternal antibodies against the fetal blood type. An absence of agglutination signifies a normal negative finding and qualifies Rh-negative mothers for administration of RhoGam to protect a subsequent pregnancy.

**Cooper's ligaments** [Sir Astley Paston Cooper, Eng. surgeon, 1768–1841] Supportive fibrous structures throughout the breast that partially sheathe the lobes shaping the breast. These ligaments affect the image of the glandular tissue on a mammogram.

**coordination** (kō-or″dĭn-ā′shŭn) [L. *co-*, same, + *ordinare,* to arrange] The working together of various muscles to produce a certain movement. More generally, it is the working together of different body systems in a given process, as the coordination between the systems of glands and involuntary muscles in digestion.

**COPD** *chronic obstructive pulmonary disease.*

**cope** (kōp) [ME. *caupen,* to contend with] **1.** To deal effectively with and handle stresses. **2.** The upper half of a flask used in casting. **3.** In dentistry, the cavity side of a denture flask.

**coping** Use of resourcefulness and ability to deal with the stress of daily life and unusual challenges posed by chronic disease, disability, and pain.

***defensive c.*** The state in which an individual repeatedly projects falsely positive self-evaluation based on a self-protective pattern which defends against underlying perceived threats to positive self-regard. SEE: *Nursing Diagnoses Appendix.*

***ineffective individual c.*** Impairment of adaptive behaviors and abilities of a person in meeting life's demands and roles. SEE: *Nursing Diagnoses Appendix.*

***c. mechanism*** A conscious or physical effort to manage anxiety or a stressful situation.

***c. skills*** The characteristics or behavior patterns of a person that enhance adaptation. Coping skills include a stable value or religious belief system, problem solving, social skills, health-energy, and commitment to a social network.

**copodyskinesia** (kō″pō-dĭs″kĭn-ē′sē-ă) [Gr. *kopos,* fatigue, + *dys,* difficult, + *kinesis,* motion] Fatigue of or difficulty in moving a group of muscles used in working. If disproportionate to the amount of work done, it is called occupational neurosis. SEE: *chronic fatigue syndrome; cramp, writer's.*

**copolymer** (kō-pŏl′ĭ-mĕr) A polymer composed of two different kinds of monomers.

**copper** [L. *cuprum*] SYMB: Cu. A metal, small quantities of which are used by the body, with atomic weight 63.54, atomic number 29, and specific gravity 8.96. Its salts are irritant poisons. Symptoms of deficiency include anemia, weakness, impaired respiration and growth, and poor use of iron. SEE: *Wilson's disease; Poisons and Poisoning Appendix.*

FUNCTION: The total body content of copper is 100 to 150 mg; the amount normally ingested each day is less than 2 mg. It is found in many vegetable and animal tissues. Copper is an essential component of several enzymes, including those for hemoglobin synthesis and cell respiration. It is stored in the liver and excess is excreted in bile or by the kidneys.

**copperas** (kŏp′ĕr-ăs) $FeSO_4 \cdot 7H_2O$. Pale blue-green crystals of ferrous sulfate, used as a disinfectant and deodorizer. SYN: *ferrous sulfate.*

**copperhead** A poisonous snake, *Agkistrodon contortrix,* common in the southern U.S. SEE: *snake bite; snake, poisonous.*

**copper sulfate** $CuSO_4 \cdot 5H_2O$. Deep-blue shiny crystals or granular powder. It is used as an astringent in proper dilution and also as an algicide.

**copper sulfate poisoning** The systemic response to ingestion of toxic amounts of copper sulfate.

SYMPTOMS: Toxicity from copper sulfate, marked by a disagreeable coppery metallic taste with tightness in the throat, nausea and vomiting, thirst, abdominal pains, cramps, and suppression of urine.

FIRST AID: Emesis should be initiated and the stomach washed out. Penicillamine or dimercaprol should be given. The caregiver should monitor vital signs, treat shock, administer oxygen if needed, control convulsions, and maintain electrolyte balance. One should be alert to possible renal and hepatic failure. SEE: *Poisons and Poisoning Appendix.*

**copremesis** (kŏp-rĕm′ĕ-sĭs) [Gr. *kopros,* dung, + *emesis,* vomiting] The vomiting of fecal material.

**coproantibody** (kŏp″rō-ăn′tĭ-bŏd″ē) Any one of a group of antibodies to various bacteria in the feces. They are of the IgA type. Their ability to protect the host has not been shown.

**coprolagnia** (kŏp″rō-lăg′nē-ă) [″ + *lagneia,* lust] An erotic satisfaction at the sight or odor of excreta.

**coprolalia** (kŏp″rō-lā′lē-ă) [″ + *lalia,* babble] The use of vulgar, obscene, or sacrilegious language, seen in schizophrenia and Tourette's syndrome.

**coprolith** (kŏp′rō-lĭth) [″ + *lithos,* stone] Hard, inspissated feces.

**coprology** (kŏp-rŏl′ō-jē) [″ + *logos,* word, reason] Scientific study of the feces. SYN: *scatology* (1).

**coprophagy** (kŏp-rŏf′ă-jē) [″ + *phagein,* to eat] The eating of excrement. SYN: *scatophagy.*

**coprophilia** (kŏp″rō-fĭl′ē-ă) [″ + *philein,* to love] Abnormal interest in feces; a perversion in adults.

**coprophilic** A term applied to organisms that normally live in fecal material.

**coprophobia** (kŏp″rō-fō′bē-ă) [″ + *phobos,* fear] Abnormal fear of defecation and feces.

**coproporphyria** (kŏp″rō-por-fĭr′ē-ă) [″ + *porphyra,* purple] An inherited form of porphyria in which an excess amount of coproporphyrin is excreted in the feces.

**coproporphyrin** (kŏp″rō-por′fĭr-ĭn) A porphyrin present in urine and feces. Coproporphyrins I and II are normally present in minute and equal amounts, but quantities are altered in certain diseases such as poliomyelitis and in infectious hepatitis and lead poisoning.

**coproporphyrinuria** (kŏp″rō-por″fĭr-ĭn-ū′rē-ă) Excess coproporphyrin in the urine.

**coprozoa** (kŏp″rō-zō′ă) [″ + *zoon,* animal] Protozoa in the fecal matter outside of the intestine.

**copula** (kŏp′ū-lă) [L., link] **1.** Any connecting part. **2.** A median elevation on the floor of the embryonic pharynx that is the future root of the tongue; copula linguae.

**copulation** (kŏp″ū-lā′shŭn) [L. *copulatio*] Sexual intercourse. SYN: *coition; coitus.*

**cor** (kor) [L.] The heart.

***c. pulmonale*** SEE: *cor pulmonale.*

**coracoacromial** (kor″ă-kō-ă-krō′mē-ăl) [Gr. *korax,* raven, + *akron,* point, + *omos,* shoulder] Pert. to the acromial and coracoid processes.

**coracoid** (kor′ă-koyd) [″ + *eidos,* form, shape] Shaped like a crow's beak.

**cord** [Gr. *khorde*] **1.** A stringlike structure. **2.** The umbilical cord. **3.** A firm elongated structure consistent with a thrombosed vein, esp. in the extremities, where it may be detected by palpation.

***nuchal c.*** The umbilical cord wrapped around the neck of the fetus in utero.

***spermatic c.*** The cord by which the testis is connected to the abdominal inguinal ring. It surrounds the ductus deferens, blood vessels, lymphatics, and nerves supplying the testis and epididymis. These are enclosed in the cremasteric fascia, which forms an investing sheath.

***spinal c.*** The portion of the central nervous system contained in the spinal canal. The center of the cord is gray matter in the shape of the letter H; it consists of the cell bodies and dendrites of motor neurons and interneurons. The white matter is arranged in tracts outside the gray matter. It consists of myelinated axons that transmit impulses to and from the brain, or between levels of the gray matter of the spinal cord, or that will leave the cord and become peripheral nerves. The cord is the pathway for sensory impulses to the brain and motor impulses from the brain. It also serves as a reflex center for many reflex acts. SYN: *medulla spinalis.*

***umbilical c.*** The cord that connects the circulatory system of the fetus to the placenta.

***vocal c.*** One of two thin, reedlike folds of tissue within the larynx that vibrate with the passage of air between them, producing sounds that are the basis of speech.

**cordal** (kor′dăl) Pert. to a cord (e.g., a spinal or vocal cord).

**cordate** (kor′dāt) [L. *cor,* heart] Shaped like a heart.

**cord bladder** Distention of the bladder without discomfort. Symptoms include a tendency to void frequently and dribbling after urination. The condition is caused by a lesion affecting the posterior roots of the spinal column at the level of bladder innervation above the sacrum.

**cordectomy** (kor-dĕk′tō-mē) [Gr. *khorde,* cord, + *ektome,* excision] Surgical removal of a cord.

**cordiform** (kor′dĭ-form) [L. *cor,* heart, + *forma,* shape] Shaped like a heart.

**corditis** (kor-dī′tĭs) Funiculitis.

**cordocentesis** A technique for obtaining a blood sample from the umbilical cord while the fetus is in utero.

**cordopexy** (kor′dō-pĕk″sē) [″ + *pexis,* fixation] Surgical fixation of anatomical cords, esp. the vocal cords.

**cordotomy** (kor-dŏt′ō-mē) [″ + *tome,* incision] Spinal cord section of lateral pathways to relieve pain. SYN: *chordotomy.*

**Cordran** Trade name for flurandrenolide.

**core** (kor) The center of a structure.

**coreclisis** (kor″ē-klī′sĭs) [Gr. *kore,* pupil of the eye, + *kleisis,* closure] Occlusion of the pupil.

**corectasia, corectasis** (kor-ĕk-tā′zē-ă, -ĕk′tă-sĭs) [″ + *ektasis,* dilatation] Dilatation of the pupil of the eye resulting from disease.

**corectome** (kō-rĕk′tōm) Iridectome.

**corectomy** (kō-rĕk′tō-mē) Iridectomy.

**corectopia** (kor-ĕk-tō′pē-ă) [″ + *ek,* out of, + *topos,* place] A condition in which the pupil is to one side of the center of the iris.

**coredialysis** (kō″rē-dī-ăl′ĭ-sĭs) [″ + *dia,* through, + *lysis,* dissolution] Separation of the outer border of the iris from its ciliary attachment.

**corelysis** (kor-ĕl′ĭ-sĭs) [″ + *lysis,* dissolution]

Obliteration of the pupil caused by adhesions of the iris to the cornea.

**coremorphosis** (kor″ē-mor-fō′sĭs) [″ + *morphe,* form, + *osis,* condition] Establishment of an artificial pupil.

**coreometer** (kō″rē-ŏm′ĕ-tĕr) [″ + *metron,* measure] An instrument for measuring the pupil.

**coreometry** (kō″rē-ŏm′ĕ-trē) Measurement of the pupil.

**coreoplasty** (kō′rē-ō-plăs″tē) [″ + *plassein,* to form] Any operation for forming an artificial pupil.

**corepressor** (kō″rē-prĕs′sor) The substance capable of activating the repressor produced by a regulator gene.

**corestenoma** (kor″ē-stĕn-ō′mă) [″ + *stenoma,* contraction] Narrowing of the pupil.

***c. congenitum*** Partial congenital obliteration of the pupil by outgrowths from the iris that form a partial gridlike covering over the pupil.

**core temperature** The body's temperature in deep structures such as the liver or heart, as opposed to peripheral areas such as the mouth or axilla.

**coretomedialysis** (kor″ĕt-ō-mē-dē-ăl′ĭ-sĭs) [″ + *tome,* incision, + *dialysis, dia,* through, + *lysis,* dissolution] Making of an artificial pupil through the iris.

**coretomy** (kō-rĕt′ō-mē) Iridotomy.

**CORF** *comprehensive outpatient rehabilitation facility* .

**Cori cycle** (kō′rē) [Carl Ferdinand Cori, Czech.-born U.S. physician and biochemist, 1896–1984; Gerty T. Cori, Czech.-born U.S. biochemist, 1896–1957] The cycle in carbohydrate metabolism in which muscle glycogen breaks down, forms lactic acid, which enters the bloodstream, and is converted to liver glycogen. Liver glycogen then breaks down into glucose, which is carried to muscles, where it is reconverted to muscle glycogen.

**corium** (kō′rē-ŭm) *pl.* **coria** [L., skin] Dermis. SYN: *cutis vera.* SEE: *skin* for illus.

**corm** (korm) [Gr. *kormos,* a trimmed tree trunk] A short, bulb-shaped underground stem of a plant such as the colchicum.

**corn** [L. *cornu,* horn] A horny induration and thickening of the skin that may be hard or soft according to location. Pressure, friction, or both from ill-fitting shoes cause this condition. SYN: *clavus; heloma.*

SYMPTOMS: Hard corns on exposed surfaces have a horny, conical core extending down into the derma, causing pain and irritation. Soft corns that occur between the toes are kept soft by moisture and maceration. This may lead to inflammation beneath the corn. Infection with pyogenic organisms results in suppuration.

TREATMENT: Properly fitting shoes of soft leather and proper shape should be worn. Spongelike materials that absorb energy and thus prevent friction are available for lining shoes or bandaging the area of the foot being abraded. Local application of a keratolytic agent is effective for removal of the corn. Corn pads are used to relieve pressure. The services of a podiatrist may be necessary. Patients with diabetes or a circulatory condition who have corns need special care to prevent foot infections.

**cornea** (kor′nē-ă) [L. *corneus,* horny] The transparent anterior portion of the fibrous outer layer of the eyeball composing about one sixth of its surface. Its curvature is greater than that of the remainder of the bulb; therefore, it is able to function as an important refractive medium. It is continuous at its periphery with the sclera, the "white" of the eye. It is composed of five layers: an epithelial layer, Bowman's membrane (anterior limiting membrane), the substantia propria corneae, Descemets' membrane, and a layer of endothelium. SEE: *geographic ulceration of cornea.* **corneal** (-ăl), *adj.*

**corneal impression test** In diagnosing rabies, the staining of material obtained from the corneas of patients suspected of having the disease. The rabies virus may be seen in the stained material.

**corneal reflex** Closure of eyelids resulting from direct corneal irritation.

**corneal transplant** The implantation of a cornea from a healthy donor eye. This is the most common organ transplantation procedure in the U.S. There are two major types of procedures. Lamellar keratoplasty, or split-thickness technique, involves removing a portion of the anterior host cornea and attaching a partial thickness of the donor cornea. Penetrating keratoplasty, or full-thickness transplantation, involves complete removal of the patient's cornea and replacement with the donor cornea.

Transmission of donor disease to the recipient is rare, but rabies, Creutzfeldt-Jakob disease, and hepatitis B have been acquired by graft recipients. The technique is more likely to be successful when histocompatibility matching of donor and recipient is as close as possible. The success rate is more than 90% at 1 year. SEE: *keratoplasty.*

NURSING IMPLICATIONS: *Preoperative:* The surgical transplant procedure is explained, including duration (1 hr), the need to remain still throughout the procedure, and expected sensations. Healing is slow, and vision may not be completely restored until the sutures are removed, which may take as long as a year. Any straining or jerking movements should be avoided to prevent external and intraocular pressure. Prescribed osmotic agents are administered orally to reduce intraocular pressure, and a preoperative sedative is given.

*Postoperative:* Evidence of any sudden, sharp, or excessive pain; bloody, purulent, or clear viscous drainage; or fever is reported immediately. Prescribed corticosteroid eye drops or topical antibiotics are administered to prevent inflammation and graft rejection, and prescribed analgesics are provided as necessary. A calm, restful environment is provided, and the patient is instructed to lie on the back or on the unaffected side, with the head of the bed flat or slightly elevated according to protocol. Rapid head movements, hard coughing or sneezing, or any other activities that could increase intraocular pressure should be avoided, and the patient should not squint or rub the eyes. Assistance is provided with standing or walking until the patient adjusts to vision changes, and personal items should be within the patient's field of vision.

Both patient and family are taught to recognize signs of graft rejection such as inflammation, cloudiness, drainage, and pain at the graft site and to report such signs immediately. Graft rejection may occur years after surgery; consequently, the graft must be assessed daily for the rest of the patient's life. The patient is encouraged to verbalize feelings of anxiety and concerns about graft rejection, and is helped to develop effective coping behaviors to deal with these feelings and concerns. Photophobia is a common adverse reaction, but it will gradually decrease as healing progresses; patients are advised to wear dark glasses in bright light. The patient is taught how to correctly instill prescribed eye drops and should wear an eye shield when sleeping.

**corneitis** (kor″nē-ī′tĭs) [L. *corneus,* horny, + Gr. *itis,* inflammation] Keratitis.

**Cornelia de Lange's syndrome** De Lange's syndrome.

**Cornell Medical Index** A lengthy, all-inclusive, self-administered history form developed at Cornell University Medical School.

**corneoblepharon** (kor″nē-ō-blĕf′ă-rŏn) [″ + Gr. *blepharon,* eyelid] Adhesion of the eyelid to the cornea.

**corneomandibular reflex** (kor″nē-ō-măn-dĭb′ū-lăr) Deflexion of the mandible toward opposite side when the cornea is irritated while the mouth is open and relaxed.

**corneosclera** (kor″nē-ō-sklē′ră) [L. *corneus,* horny, + *skleros,* hard] The cornea and sclera, constituting the tunica fibrosa or fibrous coat of the eye.

**corneous** (kor′nē-ŭs) [L. *corneus*] Horny (1); hornlike.

**corneum** (kor′nē-ŭm) [L., horny] Stratum corneum.

**corniculate** (kor-nĭk′ū-lāt) Containing small horn-shaped projections.

**corniculum** (kor-nĭk′ū-lŭm) [L., little horn] A small hornlike process.

**cornification** (kor″nĭ-fĭ-kā′shŭn) Keratinization.

**cornified** (kor′nĭ-fīd) Changed into horny tissue.

**cornu** (kor′nū) *pl.* **cornua** [L., horn] Any projection like a horn. **cornual** (-ăl), *adj.*

***c. ammonis*** The hippocampus major of the brain.

***c. anterius*** The anterior horn of the lateral ventricle.

***c. coccygeum*** One of the two upward-projecting processes that articulate with the sacrum.

***c. cutaneum*** A hornlike excrescence on the skin.

***c. of the hyoid*** The greater or the lesser horn of the hyoid bone.

***c. inferius*** The inferior horn of the lateral ventricle of the brain.

***c. posterius*** The posterior horn of the lateral ventricle.

***c. of the sacrum*** The two small processes projecting inferiorly on either side of the sacral hiatus leading into the sacral canal.

**cornua** (kor′nū-ă) Pl. of cornu.

**corona** (kŏ-rō′nă) [Gr. *korone,* crown] Any structure resembling a crown. **coronal** (-năl), *adj.*

***c. capitis*** The crown of the head.

***c. ciliaris*** The circular figure on the inner surface of the ciliary body.

***c. dentis*** The crown of a tooth.

***c. glandis*** The posterior border of the glans penis.

***c. radiata*** **1.** The ascending and descending fibers of the internal capsule that extend in all directions to the cerebral cortex above the corpus callosum. Many of the fibers arise in the thalamus. **2.** A thin mass of follicle cells that adhere firmly to the zona pellucida of the human ovum following ovulation.

***c. veneris*** Syphilitic blotches on the forehead that parallel the hairline.

**coronary** (kor′ō-nă-rē) [L. *coronarius,* pert. to a crown or circle] Encircling, as the blood vessels that supply blood directly to the heart muscle; loosely used to refer to the heart and to coronary artery disease. Coronary pain is usually dull and heavy and may radiate to the arm, jaw, or back. Typically, the patient describes the pain as being viselike or producing a feeling of compression or squeezing of the chest.

**coronary artery** **1.** One of a pair of arteries that supply blood to the myocardium of the heart. They arise within the right and left aortic sinuses at the base of the aorta. Decreased flow of blood through these arteries induces attacks of angina pectoris. SEE: illus. **2.** The cervical branch of the uterine artery.

**coronary artery bypass surgery** Surgical establishment of a shunt that permits blood to travel from the aorta to a branch of the coronary artery at a point past an obstruction. It is used in treating coronary artery disease.

NURSING IMPLICATIONS: *Preoperative:* The procedure, and the equipment and procedures used in the postanesthesia and intensive care units, are explained, and if possible, a tour of the facilities is

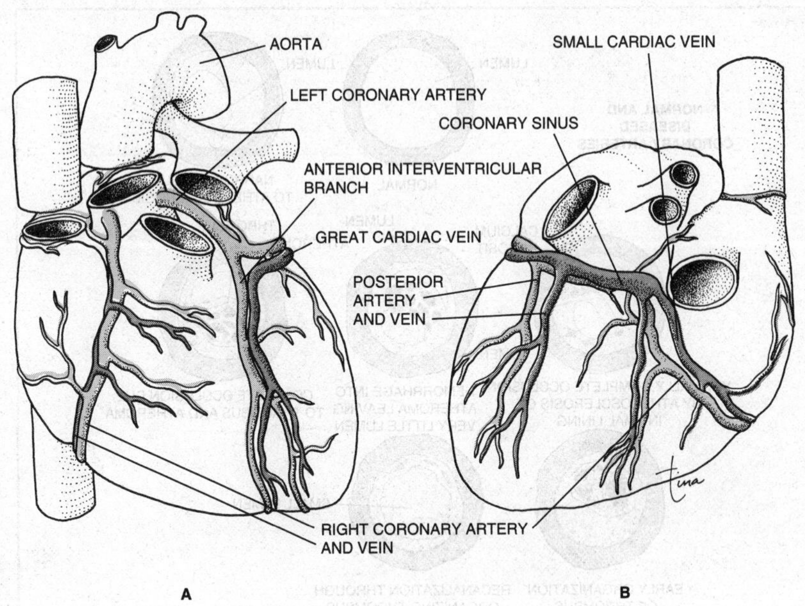


**CORONARY ARTERIES: (A)** ANTERIOR, **(B)** POSTERIOR

arranged. The nurse assists with insertion of arterial and central lines and initiates cardiac monitoring just before surgery.

*Postoperative:* Initially after surgery, the patient will have a breathing tube; will be mechanically ventilated and connected to a cardiac monitor; and will have a nasogastric tube, a chest tube and drainage system, an indwelling urinary catheter, arterial and venous lines, epicardial pacing wires, and a pulmonary artery catheter.

Signs of hemodynamic compromise, such as severe hypotension, decreased cardiac output, and shock, are monitored, and vital signs are obtained and documented every 5 to 15 min or according to protocol until the patient's condition stabilizes. Disturbances in heart rate or rhythm are monitored, and any serious abnormalities documented and reported. Preparations are made to initiate or assist with epicardial pacing, cardioversion, or defibrillation as necessary. Pulmonary artery, central venous, and left arterial pressures are monitored, and arterial pressure is maintained within prescribed guidelines (usually between 110 and 70 mm Hg). Peripheral pulses, capillary refill time, and skin temperature and color are assessed frequently, and the chest is auscultated for changes in heart sounds; any abnormalities are documented and reported to the surgeon. Tissue oxygenation is monitored by assessing breath sounds, chest excursion, symmetry of chest expansion, and arterial blood gas (ABG) values; ventilator settings are adjusted as needed. Fluid intake and output and electrolyte levels are assessed for imbalances. Chest tube drainage is maintained at the prescribed negative pressure (usually −10 to −40 cm $H_2O$), and chest tubes are inspected for patency. The patient is assessed for hemorrhage, excessive drainage (>200 ml/hr), and sudden decrease or cessation of drainage. Prescribed analgesics and other medications are administered.

Throughout the recovery period, the patient is evaluated for indications of cerebrovascular accident, pulmonary embolism, and impaired renal perfusion. After the patient is weaned from the ventilator and extubated, chest physiotherapy and incentive spirometry are instituted, and the patient is encouraged to breathe deeply and cough and assisted to change position frequently. Assistance is also provided with range-of-motion exercises and with active leg movement and gluteal and quadriceps setting exercises.

Before discharge, the patient is instructed to report any signs of infection (fever; sore throat; redness, swelling, or drainage from the leg or chest incisions) or possible arterial reocclusion (angina, dizziness, rapid or irregular pulse, or increasing fatigue or prolonged recovery time following activity or exercise). Postpericardiotomy syndrome, characterized by fever, muscle and joint pain, weakness,

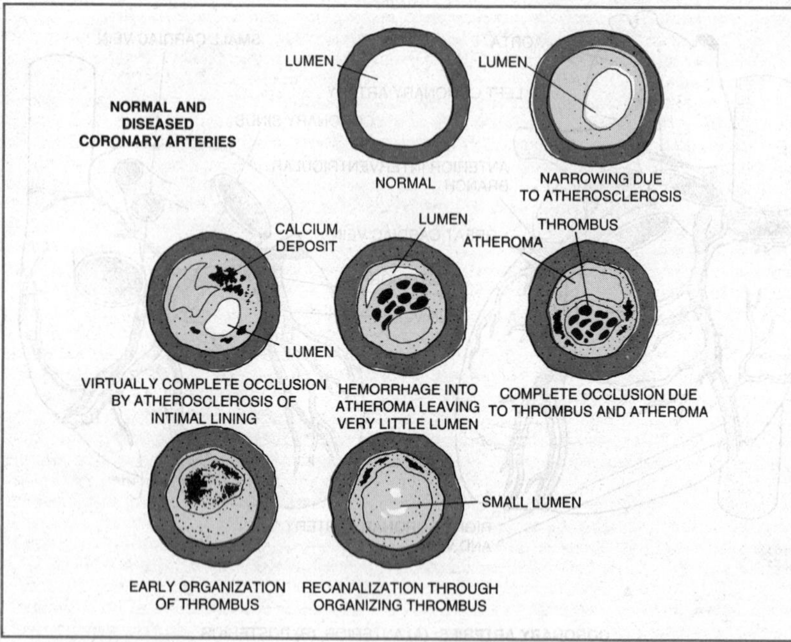


or chest discomfort, often develops after open heart surgery. Postoperative depression may also develop up to weeks after discharge; both patient and family are reassured that this is normal and usually passes quickly. The patient is advised to observe any sodium, cholesterol, fat, or calorie restrictions, because this diet can help reduce the risk of recurrent arterial occlusion. The patient needs to maintain a balance between activity and rest and should schedule a short afternoon rest period and plan to get 8 hours' sleep nightly. Frequent rest should also follow any tiring activity, participation in the prescribed cardiac rehabilitative exercise program is recommended, and any activity restrictions (avoiding lifting heavy objects, driving a car, or doing strenuous work until specific permission is granted) are reinforced. Appropriate reassurance is offered that the patient can climb stairs, engage in sexual activity, take baths or shower, and do light chores. The patient is referred to local information and support groups or organizations, such as the Mended Hearts Club and the American Heart Association. SEE: *Nursing Diagnoses Appendix.*

**coronary artery disease** ABBR: CAD. Narrowing of the coronary arteries sufficient to prevent adequate blood supply to the myocardium. Either basal oxygen needs are unmet or the oxygen supply is insufficient to meet any increased demand, as in work. The narrowing is usually caused by atherosclerosis; any other factor that limits blood flow through the coronary arteries may also be involved. Narrowing may progress to the point where the heart muscle is damaged due to lack of blood supply. The plasma concentrations of fibrinogen, von Willebrand factor antigen, and tissue plasminogen activator antigen are independent predictors of subsequent myocardial infarction or sudden death from coronary artery disease. SEE: illus.; *angina pectoris; cholesterol; heart disease, ischemic; lipoprotein; percutaneous transluminal coronary angioplasty; thrombosis, coronary.*

NURSING IMPLICATIONS: During anginal episodes, blood pressure and heart rate are monitored, a long rhythm strip is run from the patient's heart monitor or a 12-lead electrocardiogram (ECG) is obtained as directed by the physician or according to protocol, and the patient's description of the pain (severity, location, quality, radiation, precipitating factors), its duration, accompanying symptoms, and amount of medication required for pain relief are recorded. Prescribed nitroglycerin should be available for immediate use, and the patient is instructed to call for or use the medication whenever he or she feels chest, arm, or neck pain.

The patient is prepared for cardiac catheterization; the procedure and expected sensations are explained, and a signed consent form obtained. To counter the diuretic effect of the contrast medium, intravenous flow rate and potassium dosage are increased as prescribed (periodically checking the patient's potassium level), and oral fluids are offered in increased amount when the patient is able to tolerate them.

After cardiac catheterization, the catheter insertion site is monitored for bleeding and distal pulses are evaluated. Recurrent anginal symptoms after percutaneous transluminal coronary angioplasty or rotational ablation may signify recurrent obstruction. The catheterization findings and the planned course of treatment are reviewed with the patient and family.

The patient is prepared for surgery if indicated or is taught about the drug, diet, and exercise regimen prescribed. Nursing assistance is provided to help the patient to identify which activities precipitate episodes of pain and to identify and select more effective coping mechanisms to deal with stress. As necessary, the patient is referred to a prescribed cardiac rehabilitation program, smoking cessation program, or a local support group.

**coronary artery spasm** Intermittent constriction of the large coronary arteries. This may lead to angina pectoris in various conditions and is not necessarily associated with exertion (e.g., Prinzmetal's angina).

**coronary artherectomy** The technique of removing obstructions in the coronary artery. This is done by use of a cutting instrument inserted through a cardiac catheter. The same approach has been used experimentally to introduce a laser device into the coronary arteries for removal of plaques.

**coronary blood flow** Quantitation of the amount of blood flowing to the coronary arteries. This may be done by one of several techniques including indicator dilution or use of radioisotopes.

**coronary care unit** A specially equipped area of a hospital providing intensive nursing and medical care for patients who have acute coronary thrombosis.

**coronary occlusion** Coronary thrombosis.

**coronary plexus** A network of autonomic nerve fibers that lies close to the base of the heart.

**coronary sinus** The vessel cavity or passage that receives the cardiac veins from the heart. It opens into the right atrium. SEE: *coronary artery* for illus.

**coronary thrombosis** Occlusion of one or more of the coronary arteries.

**coronavirus** (kor″ō-nă-vī′rŭs-ĕs) [L. *corona,* crown, + *virus,* poison] One of a group of viruses, morphologically similar, ether sensitive, and containing RNA, that are responsible for some but not all common colds. They are so named because their microscopic appearance is that of a virus particle surrounded by a crown.

**coroner** (kor′ŏ-nĕr) [L. *corona,* crown] An official (originally, English crown officer) who investigates and holds inquests concerning people dead from unknown or violent causes. The coroner may or may not be a physician, depending on the law in each state.

**coronoid** (kor′ō-noyd) [Gr. *korone,* something curved, kind of crown, + *eidos,* form, shape] Shaped like a crown.

**coronoidectomy** (kor″ō-noy-dĕk′tō-mē) [″ + ″ + *ektome,* excision] Excision of the coronoid process of the mandible.

**coroparelcysis** (kor″ō-păr-ĕl′sĭ-sĭs) [Gr. *kore,* pupil, + *parelkein,* to draw aside] Surgical moving of the pupil to one side so that it no longer lies under a scar but under a transparent area.

**coroscopy** (kō-rŏs′kō-pē) [″ + *skopein,* to examine] Shadow test to determine refractive error of an eye. SYN: *retinoscopy; skiascopy.*

**corotomy** (kō-rŏt′ō-mē) Iridotomy.

**corpora** (kor′pō-ră) Pl. of corpus.

***c. arantii*** Tubercles found in the center of the semilunar valves of the heart.

***c. arenacea*** Psammoma bodies found in the pineal body. SYN: *brain sand.*

***c. olivaria*** Two oval masses behind the pyramids of the medulla oblongata.

***c. para-aortica*** Aortic bodies.

***c. quadrigemina*** The superior portion of the midbrain consisting of two pairs of rounded bodies, the superior and inferior colliculi.

**corporeal** (kor-pō′rē-ăl) Having a physical body.

**corpse** (korps) [L. *corpus,* body] The dead human body.

**corpsman** (kor′măn) An enlisted person in the U.S. Armed Forces who works as a member of the medical team. During duty in the armed forces he or she receives training and experience in one or more health-related fields. In wartime, a corpsman may be assigned as the only medically trained person to a field unit or a small ship. SYN: *medic; medical corpsman.*

**corpulence** (kor′pū-lĕns) [L. *corpulentia*] Obesity. **corpulent** (-lĕnt), *adj.*

**cor pulmonale** Hypertrophy or failure of the right ventricle resulting from disorders of the lungs, pulmonary vessels, or chest wall. Living for an extended period at a high altitude also may cause this condition.

NURSING IMPLICATIONS: The patient is assessed for exacerbation of related signs and symptoms. Symptoms include chronic productive cough, exertional dyspnea, wheezing respirations, fatigue, weakness, drowsiness, and alterations in level of consciousness. Dependent edema is present, and the neck veins are distended. The pulse is weak and rapid with a gallop rhythm and tricuspid insufficiency. Sometimes an early right ventricular murmur or a systolic pulmonary ejection sound may be heard. The liver is enlarged and tender, and hepatojugular reflux is present.

Serum potassium levels are monitored closely if diuretics are prescribed, signs of digitalis toxicity (anorexia, nausea, vomiting, yellow haloes seen around objects) noted, and cardiac arrhythmias monitored. Periodically, arterial blood gas levels are measured, and signs of respiratory failure are noted. Prescribed medications are administered and evaluated for desired effects and any adverse reactions. A nutritious diet (limiting carbohydrates if the patient is a carbon dioxide retainer) is provided in frequent small meals to limit fatigue. Fluid retention is prevented by limiting the patient's intake as prescribed (usually 1 to 2 L daily) and by providing a low-sodium diet. The rationale for fluid restriction is explained, because those patients with chronic obstructive pulmonary disease would previously have been encouraged to increase fluid intake to help loosen and thin secretions. Frequent position changes are encouraged and meticulous respiratory care is provided, including prescribed oxygen therapy and breathing exercises or chest physiotherapy. Assistance is provided to help the patient rinse the mouth after respiratory therapies.

Care activities are paced and rest periods provided. The patient is encouraged to verbalize fears and concerns about the illness, and the nurse remains with the patient during times of stress or anxiety. The patient is encouraged to identify actions and care measures that promote comfort and relaxation and to participate in care decisions. The importance of avoiding respiratory infections and of reporting signs of infection immediately (increased sputum production, changes in sputum color, increased coughing or wheezing, fever, chest pain, and tightness in the chest) is stressed. Immunizations against influenza and pneumococcal pneumonia are recommended. Use of over-the-counter medications should be avoided unless the health care provider is consulted first. If the patient needs supplemental oxygen or suctioning at home, referral is made to a social service agency for assistance in obtaining the necessary equipment, and correct procedures are taught for equipment use. As appropriate, the patient is referred to smoking cessation programs or for nicotine patch therapy and to local support groups.

**corpus** (kor′pŭs) *pl.* **corpora** [L., body] The principal part of any organ; any mass or body.

***c. albicans*** A mass of fibrous tissue that replaces the regressing corpus luteum following rupture of the graafian follicle. It forms a white scar that gradually decreases and eventually disappears.

***c. amygdaloideum*** Almond-shaped gray matter in the lateral wall and roof of the third ventricle of the brain.

***c. amylaceum*** A mass having an irregular laminated structure like a starch grain; found in the prostate, meninges, lungs, and other organs in various pathologies. SYN: *colloid corpuscle.*

***c. annulare*** Pons varolii.

***c. callosum*** The great commissure of the brain that connects the cerebral hemispheres.

***c. cavernosum*** Any erectile tissue, esp. the erectile bodies of the penis, clitoris, male or female urethra, bulb of the vestibule, or nasal conchae.

***c. cavernosum penis*** One of the two columns of erectile tissue on the dorsum of the penis.

***c. cerebellum*** One of the two lateral portions of the cerebellum exclusive of the central flocculonodular node.

***c. ciliare*** Ciliary body.

***c. dentatum*** The gray layer in the white substance of the cerebellum. SYN: *c. rhomboidale.*

***c. fimbriatum*** The white layer edging the lower cornu of the lateral ventricle.

***c. flavum*** A waxy body seen in the central nervous system.

***c. fornicis*** The body of the fornix.

***c. geniculatum*** The medial or lateral geniculate body; a mass of gray matter lying in the thalamus.

***c. hemorrhagicum*** A blood clot formed in the cavity left by rupture of the graafian follicle.

***c. highmorianum*** Mediastinum testis.

***c. interpedunculare*** The gray matter between the peduncles in front of the pons varolii.

***c. luteum*** The small yellow endocrine structure that develops within a ruptured ovarian follicle and secretes progesterone and estrogen. SEE: *ovary* for illus.

***c. Luysii*** C. subthalamicum.

***c. mammillare*** Mamillary body.

***c. restiforme*** Restiform body.

***c. rhomboidale*** C. dentatum.

***c. spongiosum*** Erectile tissue surrounding the male urethra.

***c. striatum*** A structure in the cerebral hemispheres consisting of two basal ganglia (the caudate and lentiform nuclei) and the fibers of the internal capsule that separate them.

***c. subthalamicum*** The subthalamic nucleus, lying in the ventral thalamus. SYN: *c. Luysii.*

***c. trapezoideum*** Trapezoid body.

***c. uteri*** The main body of the uterus, located above the cervix.

***c. vitreum*** The vitreous part of the eye.

***c. wolffianum*** Wolffian body.

**corpuscle** (kor′pŭs-ĕl) [L. *corpusculum,* little body] **1.** Any small rounded body. **2.** An encapsulated sensory nerve ending. **3.** Old term for a blood cell. SEE: *erythrocyte; leukocyte.* **corpuscular** (kor-pŭs′kū-lăr), *adj.*

***axile c., axis c.*** The center of a tactile corpuscle.

***blood c.*** An erythrocyte or leukocyte.

***bone c.*** A bone cell.

***cancroid c.*** The characteristic nodule in cutaneous epithelioma.

***cartilage c.*** A cell characteristic of cartilage.

***chromophil c.*** Nissl body.

***chyle c.*** A corpuscle seen in chyle.

***colloid c.*** Corpus amylaceum.

***colostrum c.*** A cell containing phagocytosed fat globules, present in milk secreted the first few days after parturition; also called *colostrum body*.

***corneal c.*** A type of connective tissue corpuscle found in the fibrous tissue of the cornea.

***Drysdale's c.*** SEE: *Drysdale's corpuscle.*

***genital c.*** An encapsulated sensory nerve ending resembling a pacinian corpuscle that is found in the skin of the external genitalia and nipple.

***ghost c.*** Achromatocyte.

***Gierke's c.*** Hassall's c.

***Golgi-Mazzoni c.*** A tactile corpuscle in the skin of the fingertips.

***Hassall's c.*** A corpuscle in the thymus gland. SYN: *Gierke's c.*

***Krause's c.*** One of the sensory encapsulated nerve endings in the mucosa of the genitalia, mouth, nose, and eyes.

***lymph c.*** A lymphocyte.

***malpighian c.*** **1.** Renal c. **2.** A malpighian body of the spleen.

***Mazzoni's c.*** A nerve ending resembling a Krause corpuscle.

***Meissner's c.*** SEE: *Meissner's corpuscle.*

***milk c.*** A fat-filled globule present in milk. It represents the distal end of a mammary gland cell broken off in apocrine secretion.

***pacinian c.*** A large, ovoid, sensory end organ consisting of concentric layers or lamellae of connective tissue surrounding a nerve ending. Pacinian corpuscles are present in the dermis, tendons, intermuscular septa, connective tissue membranes, and sometimes internal organs, and function as proprioceptive and deep pressure receptors.

***phantom c.*** Achromatocyte.

***Purkinje's c.*** SEE: *Purkinje cell.*

***red c.*** Erythrocyte.

***renal c.*** A glomerulus and the capsule (Bowman's capsule) that surrounds it. It is located at the proximal end of a renal tubule. SYN: *malpighian c.* (1).

***reticulated c.*** An erythrocyte that shows filamentous reticulations when properly stained.

***splenic c.*** A nodule of lymphatic tissue in the spleen.

***tactile c.*** A sensory end organ that responds to touch, as Meissner's corpuscle. They are located in the dermal papillae just beneath the epidermis and are most numerous on the fingertips, toes, soles, palms, lips, nipples, and tip of the tongue.

***terminal c.*** A nerve ending.

***white c.*** Leukocyte.

**corpuscular** (kor-pŭs′kū-lăr) Pert. to corpuscles.

**correction** The altering of a condition that is abnormal or malfunctioning.

**corrective** (kŏ-rĕk′tĭv) [L. *corrigere,* to correct] **1.** A drug that modifies the action of another. **2.** Pert. to such a drug.

**correlation** (kor″ĕ-lā′shŭn) [L. *com-,* together, + *relatio,* relation] **1.** The processes by which the various activities of the body, esp. nervous impulses, occur in proper relation to each other. **2.** In statistics, the degree to which one variable increases or decreases with respect to another variable. A variable can have a positive or negative correlation with another variable. The positive correlation is greatest when the coefficient of correlation is + 1.0, the negative correlation is greatest when the coefficient is − 1.0, and the correlation is least when the value is zero.

**correspondence** The act or condition of corresponding (i.e., occurring in proper relationship to other phenomena).

***retinal c.*** A condition occurring in normal vision in which the images formed on the maculae or other points of both retinas are mentally blended and seen as a single image.

**corresponding** Agreeing with, matching, or fitting.

**Corrigan's pulse** (kor′ĭ-găns) [Sir Dominic J. Corrigan, Ir. physician, 1802–1880] Waterhammer pulse.

**corroborating** (kŏr-ŏb′ō-rā-tĭng) Confirming or supporting with evidence.

**corrosion** (kŏ-rō′zhŭn) [L *corrodere,* to corrode] The slow disintegration or wearing away of something by a destructive agent.

**corrosive** (kŏ-rō′sĭv) Producing corrosion.

**corrugator** (kor′ū-gā″tor) [L. *con,* together, + *rugare,* to wrinkle] A muscle that lies above the orbit, arises medially from the frontal bone, and has its insertion on the skin of the medial half of the eyebrows. It draws the brow medially and inferiorly.

**Cortenema** Trade name for hydrocortisone retention enema.

**cortex** (kor′tĕks) *pl.* **cortices** [L., rind] **1.** The outer layer of an organ as distinguished from the inner medulla, as in the adrenal gland, kidney, ovary, lymph node, thymus, and cerebrum and cerebellum. **2.** The outer layer of a structure, as a hair or the lens of the eye. **3.** The outer superficial portion of the stem or root of a plant.

***adrenal c.*** The outer layer of the adrenal gland, which secretes mineralocorticoids, androgens, and glucocorticoids.

***cerebellar c.*** The surface layer of the cerebellum consisting of three layers: the outer or molecular, the middle, and the inner or granular. Purkinje's cells are present in the middle layer.

***cerebral c.*** The thin, convoluted surface layer of gray matter of the cerebral hemispheres, consisting principally of cell bodies of neurons arranged in five layers. There are also numerous fibers.

***interpretive c.*** The temporal cortex, where memories of the past may be evoked by electrical stimulation.

***olfactory c.*** The portion of the cerebral cortex concerned with the sense of smell. It includes the pyriform lobe and the hippocampal formation.

***renal c.*** SEE: *kidney.*

**Corti, Alfonso Giacomo Gaspare** (kor′tē) Italian anatomist, 1822–1876.

***canal of C.*** A triangular-shaped canal extending the entire length of the organ of Corti. Its walls are formed by the external and internal pillar cells.

***C.'s membrane*** A delicate gelatinous film that covers the cochlear duct of the inner ear. SEE: *organ of C.*

***organ of C.*** An elongated spiral structure running the entire length of the cochlea in the floor of the cochlear duct and resting on the basilar membrane. It is the end organ of hearing and contains hair cells, supporting cells, and neuroepithelial receptors stimulated by sound waves. SYN: *organum spirale; spiral organ of Corti.* SEE: illus.; *C.'s membrane; Claudius' cells; ear.*

**cortical** (kor′tĭ-kăl) Pert. to a cortex.

**corticate** (kor′tĭ-kāt) Possessing a cortex or bark.

**corticectomy** (kor″tĭ-sĕk′tō-mē) [″ + Gr. *ektome,* excision] Surgical removal of a portion of the cerebral cortex.

**cortices** (kor′tĭ-sēz) Pl. of cortex.

**corticifugal** (kor″tĭ-sĭf′ū-găl) [L. *cortex,* rind, + *fugere,* to flee] Conducting impulses away from the outer surface, or cortex; particularly denoting axons of the pyramidal cells of the cerebral cortex. SYN: *corticoefferent.*

**corticipetal** (kor″tĭ-sĭp′ĕ-tăl) [″ + *petere,* to seek] Conducting impulses toward the outer surface, or cortex; particularly denoting thalamic radiation fibers conveying impulses to sensory areas of the cerebral cortex. SYN: *corticoafferent.*

**corticoadrenal** (kor″tĭ-kō-ăd-rē′năl) [″ + *ad,* toward, + *ren,* kidney] Pert. to the cortex of the adrenal gland.

**corticoafferent** (kor″tĭ-kō-ăf′fĕr-ĕnt) [″ + *adferre,* to bear to] Corticipetal.

**corticobulbar** (kor″tĭ-kō-bŭl′băr) [″ + *bulbus,* bulb] Pert. to the cerebral cortex and upper portion of the brainstem, as the corticobulbar tract.

**corticoefferent** (kor″tĭ-kō-ĕf′-ĕr-ĕnt) [″+ *effere,* to bring out of] Corticifugal.

**corticoid** (kor′tĭ-koyd) [″+ Gr. *eidos,* form, shape] Corticosteroid.

**corticopeduncular** (kor″tĭ-kō-pē-dŭng′kū-lăr) [″ + *pedunculus,* little foot] Pert. to the cerebral cortex and cerebral peduncles.

**corticopleuritis** (kor″tĭ-kō-ploo-rī′tĭs) [″ + Gr. *pleura,* rib, + *itis,* inflammation] Inflammation of the outer parts of the pleura.

**corticopontine** (kor″tĭ-kō-pŏn′tīn) [″ + *pons,* bridge] Pert. to or connecting the cerebral cortex and the pons.

**corticospinal tract** (kor″tĭ-kō-spī′năl) [″ + *spina,* thorn] One of three descending tracts (lateral, ventral, ventrolateral) of the spinal cord. It consists of fibers arising from giant pyramidal cells of Betz present in the motor area of the cerebral cortex. SYN: *pyramidal tract.*

**corticosteroid** (kor″tĭ-kō-stēr′oyd) Any of several hormonal steroid substances secreted by the cortex of the adrenal gland. They are classified according to their biological activity as glucocorticoids, mineralocorticoids, and androgens. Adrenal corticosteroids do not initiate cellular and enzymatic activity but permit many biochemical reactions to proceed at optimal rates. SYN: *corticoid.*

**corticosterone** (kor″tĭ-kŏs′tĕ-rōn) A hormone of the adrenal cortex that influences carbohydrate, potassium, and sodium metabolism. It is essential for normal absorption of glucose, the formation of glycogen in the liver and tissues, and the normal use stof carbohydrates by the tissues. SEE: *adrenocorticotropic hormone.*

**corticothalamic** (kor″tĭ-kō-thă-lăm′ĭk) [″ + Gr. *thalamos,* chamber] Concerning or connecting the cerebral cortex and the thalamus of the brain.

**corticotropic, corticotrophic** (kor″tĭ-kō-trŏp′ĭk, -trŏf′ĭk) [″ + Gr. *trophe,* nourishment; ″ + Gr. *trope,* a turn] Pert. to corticotropin.

**corticotropin, corticotrophin** (kor″tĭ-kō-trō′pĭn, -trō′fĭn) The adrenocorticotropic factor or principle in the anterior lobe of the pituitary gland. It stimulates the adrenal cortex to secrete steroid hormones. Trade name is Acthar Gel; trade name for corticotropin zinc hydroxide is Cortrophin Zinc ACTH. SYN: *ACTH.*

**corticotropin production, ectopic** The production of corticotropin by nonendocrine tissue. This is usually but not always associated with a cancer such as a small-cell cancer of the lung. In some cases, the production site may not be found. SEE: *dexamethasone suppression test.*

**cortin** (kor′tĭn) [L. *cortex,* rind] An extract of the cortex of the adrenal gland; contains a mixture of the active steroid agents such as corticosterone.

**cortisol** (kor′tĭ-sŏl) A glucocortical hormone of the adrenal cortex, usually referred to pharmaceutically as hydrocortisone. It is closely related to cortisone in its physiological effects.

**cortisone** (kor′tĭ-sōn) A hormone isolated from the cortex of the adrenal gland and also prepared synthetically. It is closely related to cortisol and is largely inactive in humans until it is converted to cortisol. It is important for its regulatory action in metabolism of fats, carbohydrates, sodium, potassium, and proteins, and is also

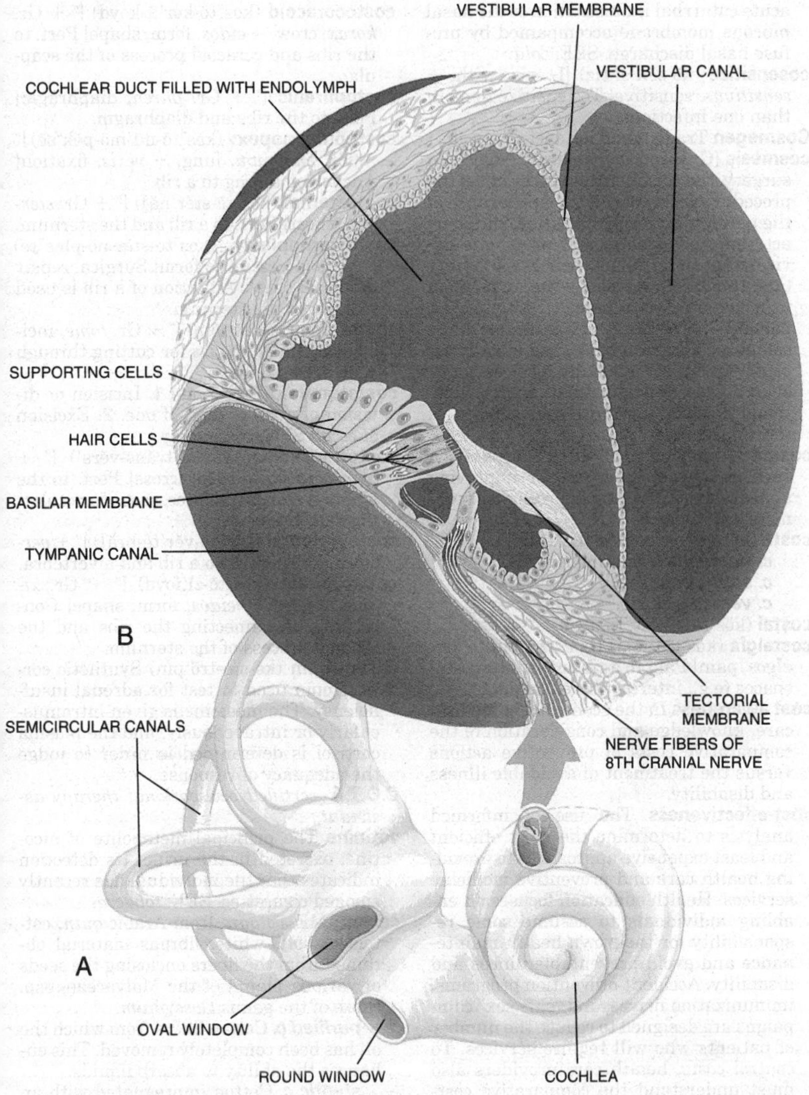


**ORGAN OF CORTI (A)** INNER EAR STRUCTURE, **(B)** ORGAN OF CORTI WITHIN THE COCHLEA

used as an anti-inflammatory agent.

**coruscation** (kŏ-rŭs-kā′shŭn) [L. *coruscare,* to glitter] The subjective sensation of flashes of light before the eyes. SEE: *Moore's lightning streaks*.

**Corynebacterium** (kō-rī″nē-băk-tē′rē-ŭm) [Gr. *coryne,* a club, + *bacterion,* a small rod] A genus of the family Corynebacteriaceae. The bacteria are rod shaped, gram positive, and nonmotile. Although many of the species are pathogens in domestic animals, birds, reptiles, and plants, the most important is the species *C. diphtheriae,* pathogenic in humans.

***C. diphtheriae*** The causative agent of diphtheria in humans. SYN: *Klebs-Loeffler bacillus.* SEE: *diphtheria*.

***C. parvum*** An organism used as part of a nonspecific immunotherapy regimen (investigational) in the treatment of lung cancer.

***C. vaginale*** An organism that may cause vaginitis, also known as *Haemophilus vaginalis*. The currently accepted name is *Gardnerella vaginalis*.

**coryza** (kŏ-rī′ză) [Gr. *koryza,* catarrh] An

acute catarrhal inflammation of the nasal mucous membrane accompanied by profuse nasal discharge. SEE: *cold*.

**cosensitize** (kō-sĕn′sĭ-tīz) [L. *con*, with, + *sensitivus*, sensitive] To sensitize to more than one infection.

**Cosmegen** Trade name for dactinomycin.

**cosmesis** [G. *kosmesus*, an arranging] **1.** In surgery, the consideration of the effect the procedure will have on the appearance of the patient. **2.** In rehabilitation, the characteristic of orthotic and prosthetic devices that determines their acceptability (and thus their successful use) in relation to a person's body image. For example, persons with hand amputations may sometimes prefer a more cosmetically acceptable but functionally useless glove over a less appealing but highly functional artificial limb with a stainless steel terminal device.

**cosmetic** (kŏz-mĕt′ĭk) **1.** A preparation such as powder or cream for improving appearance. **2.** Serving to preserve or promote appearance.

**costa** (kŏs′tă) *pl.* **costae** [L.] Rib.

***c. fluctuans*** A floating rib.

***c. spuria*** A false rib.

***c. vera*** A true rib.

**costal** (kŏs′tăl) Pert. to a rib.

**costalgia** (kŏs-tăl′jē-ă) [L. *costa*, rib, + Gr. *algos*, pain] Pain in a rib or the intercostal spaces (e.g., intercostal neuralgia).

**cost awareness** In the economics of medical care, knowledge and consideration of the comparative costs of preventive actions versus the treatment of avoidable illness and disability.

**cost-effectiveness** The use of informed analysis to determine the most efficient and least expensive approaches to providing health care and preventive medicine services. Health education focuses on enabling individuals to assume some responsibility for their own health maintenance and avoid preventable illness and disability. Accident prevention programs, immunization drives, and "safe sex" campaigns are designed to reduce the number of patients who will require services. To control costs, health care providers also must understand the comparative cost-benefit value of procedures and medicines. SEE: *preventive medicine; preventive nursing*. **cost-effective,** *adj.*

**costectomy** (kŏs-tĕk′tō-mē) [″ + Gr. *ektome*, excision] Surgical excision or resection of a rib.

**Costen's syndrome** [James B. Costen, U.S. otolaryngologist, 1895–1961] Temporomandibular joint syndrome.

**costocervical** (kŏs″tō-sĕr′vĭ-kăl) Concerning the ribs and neck.

**costochondral** (kŏs″tō-kŏn′drăl) [L. *costa*, rib, + Gr. *chondros*, cartilage] Pert. to a rib and its cartilage.

**costoclavicular** (kŏs″tō-klă-vĭk′ū-lăr) [″ + *clavicula*, a little key] Pert. to the ribs and clavicle.

**costocoracoid** (kŏs″tō-kor′ă-koyd) [″ + Gr. *korax*, crow, + *eidos*, form, shape] Pert. to the ribs and coracoid process of the scapula.

**costophrenic** [″ + Gr. *phren*, diaphragm] Pert. to the ribs and diaphragm.

**costopneumopexy** (kŏs″tō-nū′mō-pĕk″sē) [″ + Gr. *pneumon*, lung, + *pexis*, fixation] Anchoring a lung to a rib.

**costosternal** (kŏs″tō-stĕr′năl) [″ + Gr. *sternon*, chest] Pert. to a rib and the sternum.

**costosternoplasty** (kŏs″tō-stĕr′nō-plăs″tē) [″ + ″ + *plassein*, to form] Surgical repair of funnel chest. A portion of a rib is used to support the sternum.

**costotome** (kŏs′tō-tōm) [″ + Gr. *tome*, incision] Knife or shears for cutting through a rib or cartilage.

**costotomy** (kŏs-tŏt′ō-mē) **1.** Incision or division of a rib or part of one. **2.** Excision of a rib. SYN: *costectomy*.

**costotransverse** (kŏs″tō-trăns-vĕrs′) [″ + *transvertere*, to turn across] Pert. to the ribs and transverse processes of articulating vertebrae.

**costovertebral** (kŏs″tō-vĕr′tĕ-brăl) [″ + *vertebra*, joint] Pert. to a rib and a vertebra.

**costoxiphoid** (kŏs″tō-zĭ′foyd) [″ + Gr. *xiphos*, sword, + *eidos*, form, shape] Concerning or connecting the ribs and the xiphoid process of the sternum.

**cosyntropin** (kō-sĭn-trō′pĭn) Synthetic corticotropin used to test for adrenal insufficiency. The medicine is given intramuscularly or intravenously, and the plasma cortisol is determined in order to judge the adequacy of response.

**C.O.T.A.** *certified occupational therapy assistant.*

**cotinine** The principal metabolite of nicotine; excreted in the urine. Its detection indicates that the individual has recently smoked cigarettes. SEE: *tobacco*.

**cotton** [ME. *cotoun*, from Arabic *qutn*, cotton] A soft, white, fibrous material obtained from the fibers enclosing the seeds of various plants of the Malvaceae, esp. those of the genus *Gossypium*.

***purified c.*** Cotton fibers from which the oil has been completely removed. This enhances the ability to absorb liquids.

***styptic c.*** Cotton impregnated with an astringent.

**cotton-wool spot** The appearance of the retina in certain conditions, including hypertension and other diseases.

**co-twin** (kō-twĭn) Either one of twins.

**cotyledon** (kŏt″ĭ-lē′dŏn) [Gr. *kotyledon*, hollow of a cup] **1.** A mass of villi on the chorionic surface of the placenta. **2.** Any of the rounded portions into which the placenta's uterine surface is divided. **3.** The seed leaf of a plant embryo.

**cotyloid** (kŏt′ĭ-loyd) [Gr. *kotyloeides*, cup-shaped] Shaped like a cup.

**cough** (kawf) [ME. *coughen*] A forceful and sometimes violent expiratory effort preceded by a preliminary inspiration. The glottis is partially closed, the accessory muscles of expiration are brought into action, and the air is noisily expelled.

There is no one course of therapy for a cough, as it may be due to a variety of conditions. Each disease is evaluated and treated accordingly. It is usually inadvisable to suppress completely coughs due to inflammation of the respiratory tract. This is particularly true if sputum is produced as a result of coughing. SEE: *expectoration.*

***aneurysmal c.*** A cough that is brassy and clanging, heard in patients suffering from an aneurysm.

***asthmatic c.*** A cough that is more like an attack of dyspnea.

***brassy c.*** A cough heard in patients who have pressure on the left recurrent laryngeal nerve, as in aortic aneurysm.

***bronchial c.*** A cough heard in patients with bronchiectasis or bronchitis. It may be provoked by a change of posture, as when getting up in the morning, and produces frothy, mucous sputum that is copious, dirty gray, and has a fetid odor. The cough is hacking and irritating in the earlier stages; in later stages it is looser and easier.

***diphtherial c.*** A cough heard in laryngeal diphtheria. It is noisy and brassy, and breathing is stridulous.

***dry c.*** A cough unaccompanied by sputum production.

***ear c.*** A reflex cough induced by irritation in the ear that stimulates Arnold's nerve (ramus auricularis nervi vagi).

***hacking c.*** A series of repeated efforts, as occurs in the early stages of pulmonary tuberculosis.

***harsh c.*** A metallic cough occurring in laryngitis.

***moist c.*** A loose cough accompanied by production of mucus or exudate.

***paroxysmal c.*** A cough occurring in whooping cough and bronchiectasis.

***productive c.*** A cough in which mucus or an exudate is expectorated.

***pulmonary c.*** A cough that is hard and painful, seen in pneumonia. It is hacking and irritating in the early stages of tuberculosis; in later stages, it is frequent and paroxysmal. SEE: *sputum.*

***reflex c.*** A cough due to irritation from the middle ear, pharynx, stomach, or intestine. It may occur singly or coupled, or may be hacking. Stimulation of Arnold's nerve of the ear can cause this type of cough.

***whooping c.*** **1.** Pertussis. **2.** The paroxysmal cough ending in a whooping inspiration that occurs in pertussis.

**coulomb** (koo'lŏm, -lōm) [Charles A. de Coulomb, Fr. physicist, 1736–1806] ABBR: C. A unit of electrical quantity; the quantity of electricity that flows across a surface when a steady current of 1 ampere flows for 1 sec.

**coumarin anticoagulant** One of a group of natural and synthetic compounds that antagonize the biosynthesis of vitamin K–dependent coagulation factors in the liver. SEE: *dicumarol; warfarin sodium.*

**counseling** The providing of advice and guidance to a patient by a health professional.

**count** The computation obtained by determining the number of units of the object being counted per unit of volume or, in the case of radiation, counts per unit of time. Types of counts include bacteria count, various blood cell counts, platelet count, reticulocyte count, differential count of white blood cells, emissions from radioactive substances, and parasite count.

***absolute neutrophil c.*** ABBR: ANC. The actual number of neutrophils in a cubic millimeter of blood. The approximate normal range is 3000 to 6000 cells/mm$^3$. This figure is used to measure bone marrow production of blood cells before and after cancer chemotherapy. Generally, chemotherapy is not given unless the patient's ANC is greater than 1000. Patients with an ANC of less than 500 cells/mm$^3$ are at high risk for infection and require protective isolation measures. SEE: *neutrophil.*

***absolute phagocyte c.*** ABBR: APC. The number of phagocytes (neutrophils and monocytes-macrophages) in a cubic millimeter of blood. The APC is the sum of the neutrophils ("segs" and "bands"), monocytes, and macrophages times one hundredth of the white blood cell count. This figure is used to measure bone marrow production of these cells before and after cancer chemotherapy. SEE: *absolute neutrophil c.; blood count.*

**counter** (kown'tĕr) A device for counting anything.

***colony c.*** An apparatus for counting bacterial colonies in a culture plate.

***Coulter c.*** A device for automatically counting the blood cells.

***impedance c.*** A blood cell counter that employs the impedance method of cell counting. The principle is based on the fact that cell membranes "impede" the flow of direct electrical current. When cells suspended in an electrolyte are passed through an aperture, each cell creates an impedance that produces a change in electrical current. The magnitude of the current is proportional to the cell volume.

***particle c.*** An electronic device for counting and differentiating cells, platelets, and small particles according to their volume.

***scintillation c.*** A device for detecting and counting radiation. Flashes of light are produced when radiation is detected.

**counteract** (kown"tĕr-ăkt') To act against or in opposition to.

**counteraction** (kown"tĕr-ăk'shŭn) The action of a drug or chemical agent having an action opposing that of another agent.

**countercurrent exchanger** The exchange of

chemicals between two countercurrent streams separated by a membrane. This permits the fluid leaving one side of the membrane to be similar to the composition of the fluid entering the other end of the other stream.

**counterextension** (kown″tĕr-ĕks-tĕn′shŭn) [L. *contra,* against, + *extendere,* to extend] Back pull or resistance to extension on a limb.

**counterimmunoelectrophoresis** (kown″tĕr-ĭm″ū-nō-ē-lĕk″trō-fō-rē′sĭs) [″ + *immunis,* safe, + Gr. *elektron,* amber, + *phoresis,* bearing] The process in which antigens and antibodies are placed in separate wells and an electric current is passed through the diffusion medium. Antigens migrate to the anode and antibodies to the cathode. If the antigen and antibody correspond to each other, they will precipitate and form a precipitin band or line upon meeting in the diffusion medium.

**counterincision** (kown″tĕr-ĭn-sĭzh′ŭn) [″ + *incisio,* incision] A second incision made to promote drainage or relieve the stress on a wound as it is sutured.

**counterirritant** (kown″tĕr-ĭr′ĭ-tănt) [″ + *irritare,* to excite] An agent such as mustard plaster that is applied locally to produce inflammatory reaction for the purpose of affecting some other part, usually adjacent to or underlying the surface irritated. Three degrees of irritation are produced by the following classes of agents: 1. rubefacients, which redden the skin; 2. vesicants, which produce a blister or vesicle; and 3. escharotics, which form an eschar or slough or cause death of tissue. SEE: *acupuncture; escharotic; moxibustion; plaster, mustard.*

**counterirritation** (kown″tĕr-ĭr″ĭ-tā′shŭn) Superficial irritation that relieves some other irritation of deeper structures.

**counteropening** (kown″tĕr-ō′pĕn-ĭng) [L. *contra,* against, + AS. *open,* open] A second opening, as in an abscess that is not draining satisfactorily from the first incision.

**counterpressure instrument** An instrument that provides counterretraction to offset that exerted by the exit of a needle.

**counterpulsation, intra-aortic balloon** ABBR: IABC. The use of a balloon attached to a catheter inserted through the femoral artery into the descending thoracic aorta for producing alternating inflation and deflation during diastole and systole, respectively. This permits lowering resistance to aortic blood flow during systole and increasing resistance during diastole. The result is to decrease the work of the heart and to increase flow of blood to the coronary arteries. The inflation of the balloon is accomplished by using helium. This technique is rarely used.

**counterresistance** A term rooted in Freudian psychoanalysis that refers to resistance by a psychotherapist that corresponds to the patient's resistance to closeness and change of life patterns. Examples include coming late to sessions, avoiding certain subjects, and fascination with the patient. Three types are countertransferance, characterological resistance, and cultural resistance.

**countershock** The application of an electric current to the heart directly or indirectly in order to alter a disturbance in cardiac rhythm.

**counterstain** (kown′tĕr-stān) Application of a different stain to tissues that have already been prepared for microscopic examination by having been stained. The added stain helps to contrast the tissues originally stained.

**countertraction** (kown″tĕr-trăk′shŭn) The application of traction so the force opposes the traction already established; used in reducing fractures.

**countertransference** (kown″tĕr-trăns-fĕr′ĕns) In psychoanalytic theory, the development by the analyst of an emotional (i.e., transference) relationship with the patient. In this situation, the therapist may lose objectivity.

**coup** SEE: *contrecoup.*

**coup de soleil** (kū-dă-sŏ-lā′) [Fr.] Sunstroke.

**couple 1.** To join together. **2.** To have sexual intercourse.

**coupling** (kŭp′lĭng) In cardiology, the regular occurrence of premature systole just after a normal systolic beat.

**Courvoisier's law** (koor-vwă′zē-āz) [Ludwig Georg Courvoisier, Swiss surgeon, 1843–1918] A law pert. to dilatation of the gallbladder. Disease processes that cause sudden blockage of the common bile duct (e.g., a stone) do not usually cause dilatation of the gallbladder. When the duct is obstructed slowly, as would be the case in infiltration of tissue around the duct (as in cancer), dilatation of the gallbladder is usually present.

**couvade** (koo-văd′) The custom in some primitive cultures of the father remaining in bed as if ill during the time the mother is confined for childbirth. In other cultures, expectant fathers may experience psychosomatic pregnancy-simulating symptoms of nausea, fatigue, and backache.

**Couvelaire uterus** [Alexandre Couvelaire, French obstetrician, 1873–1948] The condition in which, in abruptio placentae, blood is extravasated into the uterine musculature. This acute condition may be associated with disseminated intravascular coagulation, and hysterectomy may be required.

**covalence** (kō-vāl′ĕns) The sharing of electrons between two atoms, which bonds the atoms. **covalent** (-ĕnt), *adj.*

**covariance** (kō-vā′rē-ăns) In statistics, the expected value of the product of the deviations of corresponding values of two variables from their respective means.

**covariant** (kō-vā′rē-ănt) In mathematics, pert. to variation of one variable with another so that a specified relationship is unchanged.

**cover** To provide protection, esp. in the sense of assisting the body to protect against something that would normally not require such protection. For example, the adrenal gland is normally capable of responding to stress by increasing the secretion of adrenocortical hormones. However, if a patient has received adrenocortical hormones for some time and then discontinues them, the adrenal will for a certain period be unable to respond adequately to stress such as surgery or trauma. In that case, replacement hormone therapy will be needed until the stress is over. Thus the patient would be covered by receiving adrenocortical hormones in the period of stress.

**cover glass, cover slip** A thin glass disk to cover a tissue or bacterial specimen to be examined microscopically.

**Cowden's disease, Cowden's syndrome** [Cowden, family name of first patient described] Multiple hamartoma.

**Cowling's rule** A method for calculation of pediatric drug dosages in which the age of the child at the next birthday is divided by 24. However, the most safe and accurate methods of pediatric dosage calculation include the weight and body surface area or both of the patient. SEE: *Clark's rule; Young's rule.*

**Cowper's glands** [William Cowper, Brit. anatomist, 1666–1709] Bulbourethral glands.

**cowperitis** (kow″pĕr-ī′tĭs) [*Cowper* + Gr. *itis,* inflammation] Inflammation of Cowper's glands.

**cowpox** (kow′poks) Vaccinia.

**coxa** (kŏk′să) *pl.* **coxae** [L.] Hip or hip joint.

***c. plana*** Legg's disease.

***c. valga*** A deformity produced when the angle of the head of the femur with the shaft is increased above 120°; as opposed to coxa vara.

***c. vara*** A deformity produced when the angle made by the head of the femur with the shaft is decreased below 120°. In coxa vara it may be 80° to 90°. Coxa vara occurs in rickets or may result from bone injury.

**coxalgia** (kŏk-săl′jē-ă) [L. *coxa,* hip, + Gr. *algos,* pain] Pain in the hip.

**coxarthrosis** (kŏks″ărth-rō′sĭs) [″ + Gr. *arthron,* joint, + *osis,* condition] Arthrosis of the hip joint.

**Coxiella** (kŏk″sē-ĕl′lă) [Harold Rae Cox, U.S. bacteriologist, b. 1907] A genus of bacteria of the order Rickettsiales.

***C. burnetii*** Causative organism of Q fever.

**coxitis** (kŏk-sī′tĭs) [L. *coxa,* hip, + Gr. *itis,* inflammation] Inflammation of the hip joint.

**coxodynia** (kŏk″sō-dĭn′ē-ă) [″ + Gr. *odyne,* pain] Pain in the hip joint.

**coxofemoral** (kŏk″sō-fĕm′ŏ-răl) [″ + *femur,* thigh] Pert. to the hip and femur.

**coxotuberculosis** (kŏk″sō-tū-bĕr″kū-lō′sĭs) [″ + *tuberculum,* a little swelling, + *osis,* diseased condition] Tuberculosis of the hip joint.

**coxsackievirus** (kŏk-săk′ē-vī″rŭs) Any of a group of viruses, the first of which was isolated in 1948 from two children in Coxsackie, New York. There are 23 group A and 6 group B coxsackieviruses. Most coxsackievirus infections in humans are mild, but the viruses do produce a variety of illnesses including aseptic meningitis, herpangina, epidemic pleurodynia, epidemic hemorrhagic conjunctivitis, acute upper respiratory infection, and myocarditis of the newborn. It is also possible that coxsackie infection during the first trimester of pregnancy is causally related to increased incidence of congenital heart lesions in newborns. SEE: *picornaviruses.*

**cozymase** (kō-zī′mās) ABBR: NAD. Nicotinamide-adenine dinucleotide.

**C.P.** *candle power; cerebral palsy; chemically pure.*

**C.P.A.** *Canadian Physiotherapy Association.*

**CPAP** *continuous positive air pressure.*

**CPFT** *Certified Pulmonary Function Technician.*

**CPK** *creatine phosphokinase.*

**c.p.m.** *counts per minute.*

**CPPV** *continuous positive pressure ventilation.*

**CPR** *cardiopulmonary resuscitation.*

**C.P.S.** *cycles per second.*

**CPT** *chest physical therapy.*

**CR** *conditioned reflex; complement receptor.*

**C.R.** *crown-rump; central ray.*

**Cr** Symbol for the element chromium.

**crab louse** *Phthirus inguinalis* and *Phthirus pubis;* the louse that infests the pubic region and other hairy areas of the body. SEE: *pediculosis.*

**crack** Street name for an almost pure form of cocaine. It is prepared from an aqueous solution of cocaine hydrochloride to which ammonia (with or without baking soda) has been added. This causes the alkaloidal form of cocaine to be precipitated. Because crack is not destroyed by heating, it may be smoked. The effects of crack are very brief compared with those of ingested or injected cocaine. SEE: *cocaine hydrochloride poisoning, acute.*

**crack baby** An infant exposed to crack cocaine in utero owing to the mother's use of the drug during the pregnancy. SEE: *cocaine baby.*

**cracking joint** The sound produced by forcible movement of a joint by contracting the muscles that contract or extend a joint, esp. the metacarpophalangeal joints. This is probably caused by the sudden creation of negative pressure in the joint space to produce a temporary vacuum. SEE: *crepitation.*

**crackle** An adventitious lung sound heard on auscultation of the chest, produced by air passing over retained airway secretions or the sudden opening of collapsed airways. It may be heard on inspiration or expiration. A crackle is a discontinuous adventitious lung sound as opposed to a wheeze, which is continuous. Crackles are described as fine or coarse. SYN: *rales*. SEE: *sounds, adventitious lung*.

***coarse c.'s*** Louder, rather long, low-pitched lung sounds. Coarse inspiratory and expiratory crackles indicate excessive airway secretion.

***fine c.'s*** Soft, very short, high-pitched lung sounds. Fine, late-inspiratory crackles are often heard in pulmonary fibrosis and acute pulmonary edema.

**cradle** [AS. *cradel*] A light-weight frame placed over part of the bed and patient to provide protection of an injured or burned part or to contain either heat or cold.

**cradle cap** Seborrheic dermatitis of the newborn, usually appearing on the scalp, face, and head. Thick, yellowish, crusted lesions develop on the scalp, and scaling, papules, or fissuring appear behind the ears and on the face. SEE: *seborrhea*.

TREATMENT: The head is cleansed with a mild shampoo daily. Corticosteroid cream is applied to the affected area twice daily.

**cramp** [ME. *crampe*] **1.** A pain, usually sudden and intermittent, of almost any area of the body, esp. abdominal and pelvic viscera. SEE: *dysmenorrhea*. **2.** A painful, involuntary skeletal muscle contraction. SEE: *heat c.; muscle c.; writer's c; systremma*.

TREATMENT: Therapy depends on the cramp's cause and location. In muscular cramps, the muscle is extended and compressed, and heat and massage are applied.

***heat c.*** Painful muscle contraction occurring in persons who have performed hard muscular work in high environmental heat, sweated profusely, and replaced their fluid losses with water. The usual muscles affected are those used during work (i.e., the hand, arm, or leg muscles). The cramps may come on during work or up to 18 hr after completing a work shift.

***menstrual c.'s*** An abdominal cramp associated with menstruation. SEE: *dysmenorrhea*.

***muscle c.*** A painful, involuntary skeletal muscle contraction. This occurs at rest, mostly at night, is asymmetrical, and usually affects the gastrocnemius muscle and small muscles of the foot. Persons with cirrhosis, with well-developed muscles, or in the last months of pregnancy may experience this type of cramp. Ordinary muscle cramps are not due to fluid or electrolyte abnormality. These cramps begin when a muscle already in its most shortened position involuntarily contracts.

TREATMENT: Passive stretching of the involved muscle and active contraction of the antagonists will relieve an established cramp. Quinine, methocarbamol, or chloroquine may help to relieve muscle cramps.

***occupational c.*** A form of focal dystonia in which agonist and antagonist muscles contract at the same time. This can occur in writers, pianists, typists, and almost any occupation; and they are not considered to have an emotional basis.

TREATMENT: Rest from the specific task and administration of anticholinergics and benzodiazepine may provide temporary relief. Injection of botulinum toxin into the most active muscle has also been of help.

***pianists' c.*** Spasm, or occupational neurosis, of muscles of fingers and forearms from piano playing.

***writer's c.*** A cramp affecting muscles of the thumb and two adjacent fingers after prolonged writing.

**crani-** SEE: *cranio-*.

**cranial** (krā'nē-ăl) [L. *cranialis*] Pert. to the cranium.

**cranial nerve** One of the twelve pairs of nerves originating in the brain. In addition to these cranial nerves, there is a small combined efferent and afferent nerve that goes from the olfactory area of the brain to the nasal septum. This nerve, which is thought by some anatomists to be the first cranial nerve, is called the terminal nerve. SEE: illus.

DIAGNOSIS: Lesions of the cranial nerves give rise to the following alteration(s) (lesions are described as if one of each pair of nerves were diseased): *First* (olfactory): Loss or disturbance of the sense of smell. *Second* (optic): Blindness of various types, depending on the exact location of the lesion. *Third* (oculomotor): Ptosis (drooping) of the eyelid, deviation of the eyeball outward, dilatation of the pupil, double vision. *Fourth* (trochlear): Rotation of the eyeball upward and outward, double vision. *Fifth* (trigeminal): Sensory root: Pain or loss of sensation in the face, forehead, temple, and eye. Motor root: Deviation of the jaw toward the paralyzed side, difficulty in chewing. *Sixth* (abducens): Deviation of the eye outward, double vision. *Seventh* (facial): Paralysis of all the muscles on one side of the face; inability to wrinkle the forehead, to close the eye, to whistle; deviation of the mouth toward the sound side. *Eighth* (vestibulocochlear): Deafness or ringing in the ears; dizziness; nausea and vomiting; reeling. *Ninth* (glossopharyngeal): Disturbance of taste; difficulty in swallowing. *Tenth* (vagus): Disease of the vagus nerve is usually limited to one or more of its divisions. Paralysis of the main trunk on one side causes hoarseness and difficulty in swallowing and talking. The commonest disease of the vagus is of its left recurrent branch, which causes hoarseness as its principal manifestation. *Eleventh* (spinal accessory): Drooping of the shoulder; inability to rotate the head away from the affected side. *Twelfth* (hypoglos-

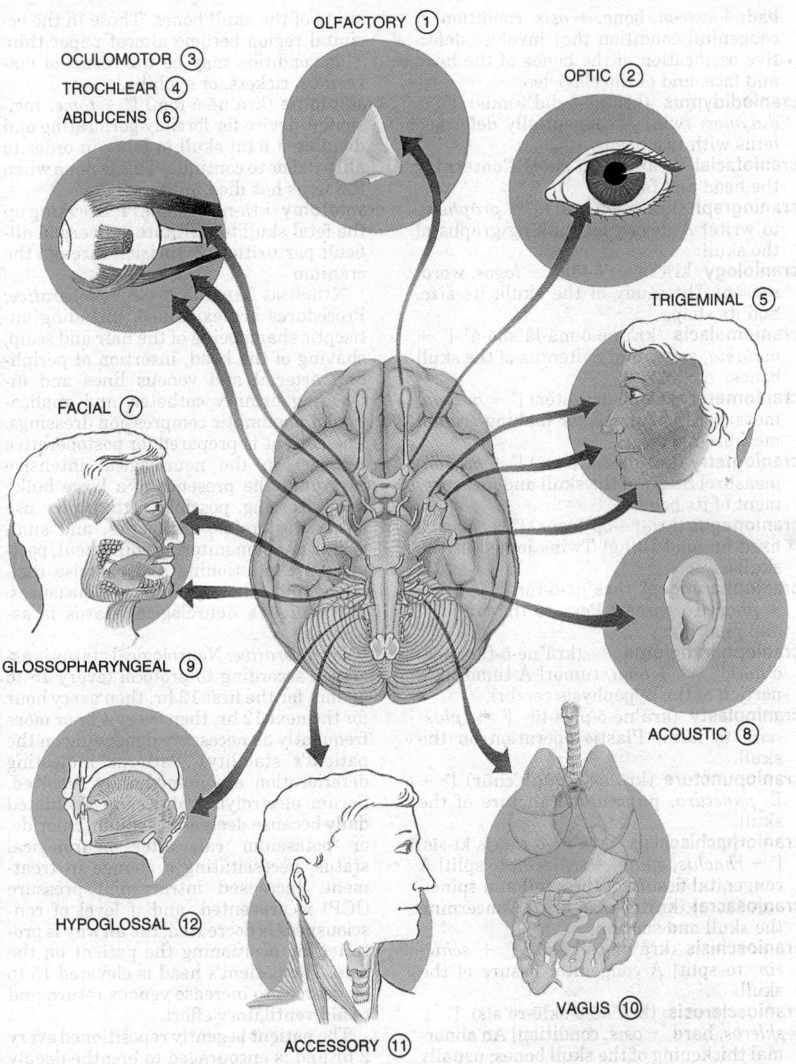

CRANIAL NERVES AND THEIR DISTRIBUTIONS

sal): Paralysis of one side of the tongue; deviation of the tongue toward the paralyzed side; thick speech.

**craniectomy** (krā-nē-ĕk′tō-mē) [Gr. *kranion,* skull, + *ektome,* excision] Opening of the skull and removal of a portion of it.

**cranio-, crani-** [Gr. *kranion,* L. *cranium,* skull] Combining form meaning *skull* or *cranium.*

**cranioacromial** (krā″nē-ō-ă-krō′mē-ăl) [Gr. *kranion,* skull, + *akron,* extremity] Relating to the cranium and the acromion.

**craniocaudal** (krā″nē-ō-kawd′ăl) [″ + L. *cauda,* tail] Direction from head to foot.

**craniocele** (krā′nē-ō-sēl) [″ + *kele,* tumor, swelling] Protrusion of the brain from the skull. SEE: *encephalocele.*

**craniocerebral** (krā″nē-ō-sĕr-ē′brăl) [″+ L. *cerebrum,* brain] Relating to the skull and brain.

**cranioclasis** (krā″nē-ŏk′lă-sĭs) [″ + *klasis,* fracture] Crushing of the fetal head to permit delivery.

**cranioclast** (krā′nē-ō-klăst) [″ + *klastos,* broken] An instrument for crushing the fetal skull to facilitate delivery.

**cranioclasty** (krā′nē-ō-klăs″tē) Crushing of the fetal head in dystocia.

**craniocleidodysostosis** (krā″nē-ō-klī″dō-dĭs-ŏs-tō′sĭs) [″ + *kleis,* clavicle, + *dys,* bad, + *osteon,* bone, + *osis,* condition] A congenital condition that involves defective ossification of the bones of the head and face, and of the clavicles.

**craniodidymus** (krā″nē-ō-dĭd′ĭ-mŭs) [″ + *didymos,* twin] A congenitally deformed fetus with two heads.

**craniofacial** (krā″nē-ō-fā′shăl) Concerning the head and face.

**craniograph** (krā-′nē-ō-grăf) [″ + *graphein,* to write] A device for making graphs of the skull.

**craniology** (krā″nē-ŏl′ō-jē) [″ + *logos,* word, reason] The study of the skull, its size, and its shape.

**craniomalacia** (krā-nē-ō-mă-lā′shē-ă) [″ + *malakia,* softening] Softening of the skull bones.

**craniometer** (krā-nē-ŏm′ĕ-tĕr) [″ + *metron,* measure] Instrument for making cranial measurements.

**craniometry** (krā-nē-ŏm′ĕ-trē) [″ + *metron,* measure] Study of the skull and measurement of its bones.

**craniopagus** (krā-nē-ŏp′ă-gŭs) [″ + *pagos,* a fixed or solid thing] Twins joined at the skulls.

**craniopharyngeal** (krā″nē-ō-făr-ĭn′jē-ăl) [″ + *pharynx,* throat] Pert. to the cranium and pharynx.

**craniopharyngioma** (krā″nē-ō-făr-ĭn-jē-ō′mă) [″ + ″ + *oma,* tumor] A tumor of a portion of the hypophysis cerebri.

**cranioplasty** (krā′nē-ō-plăs-tē) [″ + *plassein,* to form] Plastic operation on the skull.

**craniopuncture** (krā′nē-ō-pŭnk″chūr) [″ + L. *punctura,* puncture] Puncture of the skull.

**craniorhachischisis** (krā″nē-ō-ră-kĭs′kĭ-sĭs) [″ + *rhachis,* spine, + *schizein,* to split] A congenital fissure of the skull and spine.

**craniosacral** (krā″nē-ō-sā′krăl) Concerning the skull and sacrum.

**cranioschisis** (krā″nē-ŏs′kĭ-sĭs) [″ + *schizein,* to split] A congenital fissure of the skull.

**craniosclerosis** (krā″nē-ō-sklē-rō′sĭs) [″ + *skleros,* hard, + *osis,* condition] An abnormal thickening of the skull bones; usually associated with rickets.

**cranioscopy** (krā″nē-ŏs′kō-pē) [″ + *skopein,* to examine] Examination of the intracranial structures using endoscopy.

**craniospinal** (krā′nē-ō-spī′năl) Concerning the skull and spine.

**craniostenosis** (krā″nē-ō-stē-nō′sĭs) [″ + *stenosis,* act of narrowing] A contracted skull caused by premature closure of the cranial sutures.

**craniostosis** (krā-nē-ŏs-tō′sĭs) [″ + *osteon,* bone, + *osis,* condition] Congenital ossification of the cranial sutures.

**craniosynostosis** (krā″nē-ō-sĭn″ŏs-tō′sĭs) [″ + *syn,* together, + *osteon,* bone, + *osis,* condition] Premature closure of the skull sutures.

**craniotabes** (krā″nē-ō-tā′bēz) [″ + L. *tabes,* a wasting] In infancy, an abnormal softening of the skull bones. Those in the occipital region become almost paper thin. This condition may be the result of marasmus, rickets, or syphilis.

**craniotome** (krā′nē-ō-tōm) [″ + *tome,* incision] A device for forcibly perforating and dividing a fetal skull in labor in order to allow labor to continue. This is done when the fetus has died in utero.

**craniotomy** (krā-nē-ŏt′ō-mē) **1.** Breaking up the fetal skull to facilitate delivery in difficult parturition. **2.** Incision through the cranium.

NURSING IMPLICATIONS: *Preoperative:* Procedures are explained, including antiseptic shampooing of the hair and scalp, shaving of the head, insertion of peripheral arterial and venous lines and indwelling urinary catheter, and application of pneumatic compression dressings. The patient is prepared for postoperative recovery in the neurological intensive care unit: the presence of a large bulky head dressing, possibly with drains; use of corticosteroids, antibiotics, and analgesics; use of monitoring equipment; postoperative positioning and exercise regimens; and other specific care measures. The patient's neurological status is assessed.

*Postoperative:* Neurological status is assessed according to protocol (every 15 to 30 min for the first 12 hr, then every hour for the next 12 hr, then every 4 hr or more frequently as necessary depending on the patient's stability). Patterns indicating deterioration are immediately reported. Serum electrolyte values are evaluated daily because decreased sodium, chloride, or potassium can alter neurological status, necessitating a change in treatment. Increased intracranial pressure (ICP) is prevented, and if level of consciousness is decreased, the airway is protected by positioning the patient on the side. The patient's head is elevated 15 to 30 degrees to increase venous return and to aid ventilatory effort.

The patient is gently repositioned every 2 hr and is encouraged to breathe deeply and cough without straining, and the airway is gently suctioned if necessary. Fluid is restricted as prescribed or according to protocol to minimize cerebral edema and prevent increased ICP and seizures. Wound care is provided as appropriate; dressings are assessed for increased tightness (indicative of swelling); and closed drainage systems are checked for patency and for volume and characteristics of any drainage. Excessive bloody drainage, possibly indicating cerebral hemorrhage, and any clear or yellow drainage, indicating a cerebrospinal fluid leak, is reported to the surgeon. The patient is observed for signs of wound infection.

Prescribed stool softeners are also administered to prevent increased ICP from straining during defecation. Before discharge, the patient and family are taught to perform wound care; to assess the incision regularly for redness, warmth, or tenderness; and to report such findings to the neurosurgeon. If self-conscious about appearance, the patient can wear a wig, hat, or scarf until the hair grows back and can apply a lanolin-based lotion to the scalp (but not to the incision line) to keep it supple and to decrease itching as the hair grows. Prescribed medications, such as anticonvulsants, should be continued after discharge.

**craniotonoscopy** (krā″nē-ō-tō-nŏs′kō-pē) [″ + *tonos,* tone, + *skopein,* to examine] Auscultatory percussion of the cranium.

**craniotrypesis** (krā″nē-ō-trĭ-pē′sis) [″ + Gr. *trypesis,* a boring] The introduction of trephine or burr holes into the cranial bones.

**craniotympanic** (krā″nē-ō-tĭm-păn′ĭk) [″ + *tympanon,* kettle-drum] Pert. to the skull and middle ear.

**cranium** (krā′nē-ŭm) *pl.* **crania** [L.] The portion of the skull that encloses the brain, consisting of single frontal, occipital, sphenoid, and ethmoid bones and the paired temporal and parietal bones. SEE: *skeleton.*

**crapulous** (L. *crapula,* excessive drinking]. Relating to the effects of excessive drinking and eating; relating to intoxication.

**crash cart** A specially equipped cart for transporting the materials needed to the bedside or other location for administration of life-saving medicines or procedures to acutely ill patients. These conditions have usually arisen suddenly as in the case of life-threatening cardiac arrhythmias, septic or other kinds of shock, acute pulmonary edema, cardiac arrest, or life-threatening trauma.

**crater** (krā′tĕr) A circular depression with an elevated area at the periphery.

**crateriform** (krā-tĕr′ĭ-form) [Gr. *krater,* bowl, + L. *forma,* shape] In bacteriology, relating to colonies that are saucer shaped, crater-like, or goblet shaped.

**Crawford Small Parts Dexterity Test** A performance test that uses the manipulation of small tools under standardized conditions to measure fine motor skills and eye-hand coordination.

**crazing** Minute fissures on the surface of natural or artificial teeth.

**crazy bone** Funny bone.

**C-reactive protein** A globulin that, in the presence of calcium ions, precipitates the C substance of pneumococcal cells. C-reactive protein is an abnormal protein detectable in blood only during the active phase of certain acute illnesses, esp. rheumatic fever.

**cream** The fat portion of milk. When untreated milk is allowed to stand undisturbed, the cream rises to the top of the container. Approx. 90% of the calories in cream come from fat.

**cream of tartar** Potassium bitartrate.

**crease** (krēs) [ME. *crest,* crest] A line produced by a fold.

***gluteofemoral c.*** The crease that bounds the inferior border of the buttocks.

***inframammary c.*** The attachment of the inferior breast to the chest wall; the location of the film during craniocaudal filming of the breast.

**creatinase** (krē-ăt′ĭn-ās) [Gr. *kreas,* flesh, + *-ase,* enzyme] An enzyme that decomposes creatinine.

**creatine** (krē′ă-tĭn) [Gr. *kreas,* flesh] $C_4H_9O_2N_3$. A colorless, crystalline substance that can be isolated from various animal organs and body fluids. It combines readily with phosphate to form phosphocreatine (creatine phosphate), which serves as a source of high-energy phosphate released in the anaerobic phase of muscle contraction. Creatine may be present in a greater quantity in the urine of women than in that of men. Creatine excretion is increased in pregnancy and decreased in hypothyroidism.

**creatine kinase** An enzyme present in skeletal muscle (CK-MM), cardiac muscle (CK-MB), and the brain (CK-BB). It catalyzes the reversible transfer of high-energy phosphate between creatine and phosphocreatine and between adenosine diphosphate (ADP) and adenosine triphosphate (ATP). The serum level is increased 10 to 25 times the normal level in the first few hours after myocardial infarction and returns to normal within 2 to 4 days. Serum levels are also increased in progressive muscular dystrophy and following trauma to skeletal muscle. They are not elevated in liver disease or pulmonary infarction.

**creatinemia** (krē″ă-tĭn-ē′mē-ă) [″ + *haima,* blood] An excess of creatine in circulating blood.

**creatinine** (krē-ăt′ĭn-ĭn) [Gr. *kreas,* flesh] $C_4H_7ON_3$. The decomposition product of the metabolism of phosphocreatine, a source of energy for muscle contraction. Increased quantities of it are found in advanced stages of renal disease. It is a normal, alkaline constituent of urine and blood. The normal serum creatinine value is less than 1.2 mg/dL. About 0.02 g/kg of body weight is excreted by the kidneys per day. SEE: *blood urea nitrogen.*

**creatinine phosphokinase** Improper term for creatine kinase.

**creatinuria** (krē-ă″tĭn-ū′rē-ă) [″ + *ouron,* urine] Excess concentration of creatinine in urine.

**creatorrhea** (krē″ă-tō-rē′ă) [″ + *rhoia,* flow] The presence of undigested muscle fibers in the feces, seen in some cases of pancreatic disease.

**credentialing** (krē-dĕn′shăl-ĭng) Recognition by licensure and certification that an individual has met certain criteria.

**Credé's method** (krā-dāz′) [Karl S.F. Credé, Ger. gynecologist, 1819–1892] **1.** The means whereby the placenta is expelled by downward pressure on the uterus through the abdominal wall with the thumb on the posterior surface of the fundus uteri and the flat of the hand on the anterior surface, the pressure being applied in the direction of the birth canal. This may cause inversion of the uterus if done improperly. **2.** For treatment of the eyes of the newborn, the use of 1% silver nitrate solution instilled into the eyes immediately after birth for the prevention of ophthalmia neonatorum (gonorrheal ophthalmia). **3.** For emptying a flaccid bladder, the method of applying pressure over the symphysis pubis to expel the urine periodically. This technique is sometimes used therapeutically to initiate voiding in bladder retention for persons with paralysis following spinal cord injury (neurogenic bladder).

**cremains** [contraction of *cre*mated *re*mains] That which remains after the body has been prepared for burial by cremation.

**cremaster** (krē-măs'tĕr) [L., to suspend] One of the fascia-like muscles suspending and enveloping the testicles and spermatic cord. **cremasteric** (-ĭk), *adj.*

**cremate** (krē'māt) [L. *crematio,* a burning] To dispose of the body of a dead person by burning. The ashes may or may not be buried.

**crematorium** (krē"mă-tō'rē-ŭm) [L.] A place for the burning of corpses.

**crenate** (krē'nāt) [L. *crenatus*] Notched or scalloped, as crenated condition of blood corpuscles.

**crenation** (krē-nā'shŭn) The conversion of normally round red corpuscles into shrunken, knobbed, starry forms, as when blood is mixed with salt solution of 5% strength. SEE: *plasmolysis.*

**crenocyte** (krē'nō-sīt) Crenated red blood cell.

**creosote** (krē'ō-sōt) [Gr. *kreas,* flesh, + *sozein,* to preserve] A mixture of phenols obtained from the destructive distillation of coal or wood. This toxic substance has been used as a disinfectant and as a preserver of wood. Because creosote is a potent carcinogen, contact with it should be avoided by wearing protective garments, gloves, and masks.

**crepitant** (krĕp'ĭ-tănt) [L. *crepitare*] Crackling; having or making a crackling sound.

**crepitation** (krĕp-ĭ-tā'shŭn) **1.** A crackling sound heard in certain diseases, as the crackle heard in pneumonia. **2.** A grating sound heard on movement of ends of a broken bone. **3.** A clicking or crackling sound often heard in movements of joints, such as the temporomandibular, elbow, or patellofemoral joints, due to roughness and irregularities in the articulating surfaces. SEE: *temporomandibular joint syndrome.*

**crepuscular** (krē-pŭs'kū-lăr) [L. *crepusculum,* twilight] Pert. to twilight; used to describe twilight mental state.

**crescent** (krĕs'ĕnt) [L. *crescens*] Shaped like a sickle or the new moon.

***articular c.*** A crescent-shaped cartilage present in certain joints, as the menisci of the knee joint.

***c. body*** Achromocyte.

***myopic c.*** A grayish patch in the fundus of the eye caused by atrophy of the choroid.

***c. of Giannuzzi*** A crescent-shaped group of serous cells lying at the base of or along the side of a mucous alveolus of a salivary gland.

**crescentic** (krĕs-ĕn'tĭk) Sickle-shaped.

**Crescormon** Trade name for somatropin.

**cresol** (krē'sŏl) Yellow-brown liquid obtained from coal tar and containing not more than 5% of phenol, used as a disinfectant in a 1% to 5% solution for articles or areas that do not come in direct contact with food.

**cresomania, croesomania** (krē"sō-mā'nē-ă) [Croesus, wealthy king of Lydia, 6th century B.C.] Delusion of possessing great wealth.

**crest** [L. *crista,* crest] A ridge or an elongated prominence, esp. one on a bone.

***alveolar c.*** The most coronal portion of the bone surrounding the tooth; the continuous upper ridge of bone of the alveolar process, which is usually the first bone lost as a result of periodontal disease.

***iliac c.*** The anatomical landmark for the superior margin of the pelvis, located between the anterior superior and posterior superior iliac spines.

***intertrochanteric c.*** On the posterior femoral shaft, the ridge of bone extending from the greater to the lesser trochanter. SYN: *intertrochanteric line.*

**CREST syndrome** The presence of *c*alcinosis, *R*aynaud's phenomenon, *e*sophageal dysfunction, *s*clerodactyly, and *t*elangiectasia, indicative of scleroderma. SYN: *progressive systemic sclerosis.*

**cretin** (krē'tĭn) [Fr.] One afflicted with congenital myxedema owing to lack of thyroid secretion; characterized by lack of growth and mental development. The patient rarely if ever exceeds the mental age of 10. The skin is rough and dry and the hair coarse, dry, and brittle. Teeth erupt slowly and are of poor quality and irregularly placed. The tongue is large and apt to protrude from the mouth. The individuals drool saliva constantly. A child with cretinism is characteristically potbellied, swaybacked, and prone to umbilical hernia. **cretinous,** *adj.* (-ŭs) SEE: *cretinism.*

**cretinism** (krē'tĭn-ĭzm) [" + Gr. *-ismos,* condition] A congenital condition caused by a lack of thyroid secretion, characterized by arrested physical and mental development, myxedema, dystrophy of the bones and soft parts, and lowered basal metabolism. The treatment consists of administration of appropriate thyroid preparation. The acquired form of this disease is referred to as myxedema.

**cretinoid** (krē'tĭ-noyd) [" + Gr. *eidos,* form, shape] Having the symptoms of cretinism, or resembling a cretin, owing to a congenital condition.

**Creutzfeldt-Jakob disease** [Hans Gerhard Creutzfeldt, 1855–1964; Alfons Maria Jakob, 1884–1931, German psychiatrists] ABBR: CJD. A central nervous system disease that causes presenile dementia, myoclonus, and distinctive electroencephalographic changes. The causative organism is assumed to be a prion. Creutzfeldt-Jakob disease has developed in the recipient of a cornea from a donor with the disease, and in a few recipients of human growth hormone. There is no treatment, and the disease is fatal. SEE: *Universal Precautions Appendix.*

Caution: The causative agent of CJD is extremely resistant to most sterilization procedures; thus, the same precautions as used for AIDS should be exercised when handling body fluids and tissues from patients with CJD.

**crevice** (krĕv'ĭs) [Fr. *crever,* to break] A small fissure or crack.

***gingival c.*** The fissure produced by the marginal gingiva with the tooth surface.

**crevicular** (krĕv-ĭk'ū-lăr) Pert. to the gingival crevice.

**CRF** *corticotropin-releasing factor.*

**crib** (krĭb) [AS. *cribbe,* manger] **1.** A framework around a denture or a natural tooth to serve as a brace or supporting structure. **2.** A small bed with long legs and high sides for an infant or young child.

**crib death** SEE: *sudden infant death syndrome.*

**cribrate** (krĭb'rāt) [L. *cribratus*] Profusely pitted or perforated like a sieve.

**cribration** (krĭb-rā'shŭn) The state of being perforated.

**cribriform** (krĭb'rĭ-form) [L. *cribrum,* a sieve, + *forma,* form] Sievelike.

**crick** A muscle spasm or cramp, esp. in the neck.

**cricoarytenoid** (krī"kō-ă-rĭt'ĕn-oyd) [Gr. *krikos,* ring, + *arytaina,* pitcher, + *eidos,* form, shape] Extending between the cricoid and arytenoid cartilages.

**cricoid** (krī'koyd) [" + *eidos,* form, shape] Shaped like a signet ring.

**cricoidectomy** (krī"koyd-ĕk'tō-mē) [" + " + *ektome,* excision] Excision of the cricoid cartilage.

**cricoidynia** (krī-koy-dĭn'ē-ă) [" + " + *odyne,* pain] Pain in the cricoid cartilage.

**cricopharyngeal** (krī"kō-făr-ĭn'jē-ăl) [" + *pharynx,* throat] Pert. to the cricoid cartilage and pharynx.

**cricothyroid** (krī-kō-thī'royd) [" + *thyreos,* shield, + *eidos,* form, shape] Pert. to the thyroid and cricoid cartilages.

**cricothyrotomy** (krī"kō-thī-rŏt'ō-mē) [" + " + *tome,* incision] Division of the cricoid and thyroid cartilages. SYN: *coniotomy.*

**cricotomy** (krī-kŏt'ō-mē) [" + *tome,* incision] Division of the cricoid cartilage.

**cricotracheotomy** (krī"kō-trā"kē-ŏt'ō-mē) [" + *tracheia,* windpipe, + *tome,* incision] Division of the cricoid cartilage and upper trachea in closure of the glottis.

**Crigler-Najjar syndrome** (krēg'lĕr-nă'hār) [John Fielding Crigler, U.S. physician, b. 1919; Victor A. Najjar, U.S. physician, b. 1914] A familial form of congenital hyperbilirubinemia associated with brain damage and resembling kernicterus. The syndrome is caused by an enzyme deficiency in the liver and faulty bilirubin conjugation. It is transmitted as an autosomal recessive trait; death usually occurs within 15 months after birth.

**crinogenic** (krĭn"ō-jĕn'ĭk) [Gr. *krinein,* to secrete, + *gennan,* to produce] Producing or stimulating secretion.

**crisis** (krī'sĭs) *pl.* **crises** [Gr. *krisis,* turning point] **1.** The turning point of a disease; a very critical period often marked by a long sleep and profuse perspiration. **2.** The term used for the sudden descent of a high temperature to normal or below; generally occurs within 24 hr. **3.** Sharp paroxysms of pain occurring over the course of a few days in certain diseases. **4.** In counseling, an unstable period in a person's life characterized by inability to adapt to a change resulting from a precipitating event.

***abdominal c.*** A general term for severe abdominal pain due to many possible causes.

***addisonian c.*** Acute failure of the adrenal gland.

***celiac c.*** The rapid onset of malnutrition in celiac disease with severe watery diarrhea, vomiting, dehydration, and acidosis. Vigorous antibiotic and nutritional therapy is required.

***Dietl's c.*** A sudden, severe attack of gastric pain, chills, fever, nausea, and general collapse. In cases of floating kidney, the ureter becomes kinked and urine is obstructed, producing symptoms of renal colic.

***salt-losing c.*** Acute vomiting, dehydration, hypotension, and sudden death as a result of acute loss of sodium; may be caused by adrenal hyperplasia, salt-losing nephritis, or gastrointestinal disease.

***sickle cell c.*** Severe abdominal pain due to sickle cell anemia.

***tabetic c.*** Abdominal pain due to tabes dorsalis in patients with syphilis.

***thyroid c.*** Thyroid storm.

***true c.*** Temperature drop accompanied by a fall in the pulse rate.

**crisis intervention** Problem-solving activity intended to correct or prevent the continuation of a crisis, as in poison control centers or suicide prevention services. Usually these activities are mediated through telephone services operated by professional or paraprofessional workers in the medical and social fields.

**crista** (krĭs′tă) *pl.* **cristae** [L.] **1.** A crest or ridge. **2.** A projection, sometimes branched, of the inner wall of a mitochondrion into its fluid-filled cavity.

***c. ampullaris*** A localized thickening of the membrane lining the ampullae of the semicircular canals; it is covered with neuroepithelium containing hair cells that are stimulated by movement of the head.

***c. galli*** A ridge on the ethmoid bone to which the falx cerebri is attached.

***c. lacrimalis posterior*** A vertical ridge on the lateral surface of the lacrimal bone.

***c. spiralis*** A ridge on the spiral lamina of the cochlea.

**criterion** (krī-tē′rē-ŏn) *pl.* **criteria** [Gr. *kriterion,* a means for judging] A standard or attribute for judging a condition or establishing a diagnosis.

**critical** (krĭt′ĭ-kăl) [Gr. *kritikos,* critical] **1.** Pert. to a crisis. **2.** Dangerous.

**critical care unit** SEE: *intensive care unit.*

**critical period** **1.** The phase of the life cycle during which cells are responsive to certain regulators. **2.** The time during gestation when important organ systems are being formed and the fetus is most vulnerable to environmental factors that may cause deformities.

**CRNA** *certified registered nurse anesthetist.*

**Crohn's disease** (krōnz) [Burrill B. Crohn, U.S. gastroenterologist, 1884–1983] Regional ileitis. SEE: *disease, inflammatory bowel; Nursing Diagnoses Appendix.*

**cromolyn sodium** (krō′mŏ-lĭn) A prophylactic mast cell stabilizer used as an antiasthmatic. Trade name is Intal as a powder inhalant and Gastrocrom as oral capsules. It is also used in an ophthalmic solution to treat allergic conjunctivitis.

**Crookes' dark space** [Sir William Crookes, Brit. physicist, 1832–1919] The nonluminous region enveloping the outline of the cathode in a discharge tube. SEE: *cathode.*

**Crookes' tube** An early form of vacuum discharge tube used for the study of cathode rays.

**Crosby capsule** [William Holmes Crosby, Jr., U.S. physician, b. 1914] A device attached to a flexible tube that is introduced into the gastrointestinal tract per os. It is designed so that a sample of tissue may be obtained from the mucosal surface with which it is in contact. The capsule is then removed and the tissue examined for evidence of pathological changes.

**cross** [L. *crux*] **1.** Any structure or figure in the shape of a cross. **2.** In genetics, the mating or the offspring of the mating of two individuals of different strains, varieties, or species.

**crossbirth** Presentation of the fetus in which the long axis of the fetus is at right angles to that of the mother and requires version. Also called *transverse lie.*

**cross bite** A form of dental malocclusion in the buccolingual direction.

**crossbreeding** Mating of individuals of different breeds or strains.

**cross-bridge** In the sarcomere of a muscle cell, the portion of the myosin filaments that pulls the actin filaments toward the center of a sarcomere during contraction.

**cross-cultural** Concerning the physiological and social differences and similarities of two or more cultures.

**cross-dress** To dress in clothing appropriate for one of the opposite sex.

**crossed** Passing from one side to the other, as the crossed corticospinal tract, in which nerve fibers cross from one side of the medulla to the other.

**crossed finger airway technique** A method used to open an unconscious patient's mouth by placing the thumb and index finger on opposite rows of teeth and spreading the jaw open.

**cross education** Contralateral facilitation or changes resulting from exercise.

**cross-eye** Manifest inward deviation of the visual axis of one eye toward that of the other eye when looking at an object. SYN: *esotropia.* SEE: *squint; strabismus.*

**cross-fertilization** Fusion of male and female gametes from different individuals.

**crossing over** In genetics, the mutual interchange of blocks of genes between two homologous chromosomes. It occurs during synapsis in meiosis. In this process, there is no gain or loss of genetic material, but a recombination does occur.

**crossmatching** A test to establish blood compatibility before transfusion. SEE: *blood group.*

**crossover** The result of the reciprocal exchange of genetic material between chromosomes.

**cross-training** **1.** A cost-containment measure whereby instruction and experience are provided to enable health care workers to perform procedures and provide services previously limited to other members of the health team. **2.** In physical fitness training, the use of one or more sports to train for another. For example, training in both cycling and running strengthens all of the leg muscle groups and makes them less vulnerable to injury.

**Crotalus** (krŏt′ă-lŭs) [Gr. *krotalon,* rattle] A genus of snakes that includes most rattlesnakes; all are highly poisonous.

**crotamiton** (krō″tă-mī′tŏn) An effective scabicide. Trade name for a preparation of which crotamiton is a component is Eurax.

**crotaphion** (krō-tăf′ē-ŏn) [Gr. *krotaphos,* the temple] The tip of the greater wing of the sphenoid bone.

**crotonism** (krō′tŏn-ĭzm) Poisoning from croton oil.

**croton oil** (krō′tŏn) [Gr. *kroton,* castor oil plant seed] Oleum tiglii; a fixed oil expressed from the seed of the croton plant, *Croton tiglium.*

ACTION: A drastic cathartic, it is used externally as a rubefacient. Because this substance is toxic, it is no longer used.

**croup** (croop) An acute viral disease of childhood, marked by a resonant barking cough, suffocative and difficult breathing, and laryngeal spasm. Because of respiratory distress, the child is hypoxic. Blood gas may show increased carbon dioxide content.

TREATMENT: Supportive measures include rest and supervised hydration. Humidification by use of mist reduces the viscosity of tracheobronchial secretions, but humidification of the bronchi requires use of an ultrasonic nebulizer with a mask or in an oxygen tent. Hospitalization may be needed. Intubation may be necessary if hypoxemia persists. Antibiotics are rarely needed because the viruses involved do not predispose to secondary bacterial infections.

NURSING IMPLICATIONS: A quiet, calm environment is maintained, all procedures are explained, and support and reassurance are provided to the child and family to reduce fear and anxiety. Intubation is performed if necessary. Ventilation and heart rate are monitored, and a high-humidity atmosphere, with cool moisture to help control fever, if present, is provided, but the child is kept dry to prevent chilling. Prescribed antipyretics and sponge baths are provided for fever. If the child becomes dehydrated, prescribed intravenous rehydration is administered. Sore throat is relieved with water-based ices (fruit sherbets, iced popsicles), and thicker fluids are avoided if the child is producing thick mucus or has difficulty in swallowing. Humidified cool air is provided at home, and symptoms of croup can be relieved by having the child breathe the warm moist air generated by running hot water in the shower or sink in a closed bathroom. SEE: *Nursing Diagnoses Appendix.*

***diphtheritic c.*** Laryngeal diphtheria.

***membranous c.*** Inflammation of the larynx with exudation forming a false membrane. SYN: *croupous laryngitis.* SEE: *carpopedal spasm; Nursing Diagnoses Appendix.*

SYMPTOMS: Symptoms include those of laryngitis; loss of voice; noisy, difficult, and stridulous breathing; weak, rapid pulse; livid skin; and moderate fever.

ETIOLOGY: Several viruses may cause this disease. These include parainfluenza, respiratory syncytial virus, and various influenza viruses.

TREATMENT: The air should be humidified by whatever means is available such as vaporizers or steam. Antibiotics are indicated only if there is secondary bacterial infection; corticosteroids are of no benefit. If hypoxia is present, inhalation of 40% concentration of well-humidified oxygen is indicated. This is best accomplished by use of a face mask. SEE: *steam tent.*

PROGNOSIS: The prognosis is grave, unless tracheostomy has been performed. The illness usually subsides in 3 to 4 days.

***spasmodic c.*** Recurrent attacks of croup.

**croupous** (kroo'pŭs) Pert. to croup or having a fibrinous exudation.

**Crouzon's disease** (kroo-zŏnz') [Octave Crouzon, Fr. neurologist, 1874–1938] A congenital disease characterized by hypertelorism (widely spaced eyes), craniofacial dysostosis, exophthalmos, optic atrophy, and divergent squint.

**crowing** (krō'ĭng) A noisy, harsh sound on inspiration.

**crown** [L. *corona,* wreath] The top or highest part of an organ, tooth, or other structure, as the top of the head; the corona.

***anatomical c.*** The part of a tooth extending from the cementoenamel junction to the occlusal surface or the incisal edge.

***clinical c.*** The portion of the natural tooth that is exposed in the mouth, from the gingiva to the occlusal plane or the incisal edge.

***dental c.*** SEE: *crownwork.*

**crowning** [L. *corona,* wreath] The stage in delivery when the fetal head presents at the vulva. It occurs when the largest diameter of the infant's head comes through the vulvar opening.

**crown-rump** ABBR: CR. The axis for measurement of a fetus.

**crownwork** An artificial surface for a tooth.

**CRP** *C-reactive protein.*

**CRT** *cathode-ray tube.*

**CRTT** *certified respiratory therapy technician.*

**crucial** (kroo'shăl) [L. *crucialis*] **1.** Cross-shaped. **2.** Decisive; of supreme importance; critical.

**cruciate** (kroo'shē-āt) Cross-shaped, as in the cruciate ligaments of the knee.

**crucible** (kroo'sĭ-b'l) [L. *crucibulum*] A dish or container for substances that are being melted, burned, or dehydrated while exposed to high temperatures.

**cruciform** (kroo'sĭ-form) [L. *crux,* cross, + *forma,* shape] Shaped like a cross.

**crude** (krood) [L. *crudus,* raw] Raw, unrefined, or in a natural state.

**crura** (kroo'ră) *sing.* **crus** [L., legs] A pair of elongated masses or diverging bands, resembling legs.

***c. cerebelli*** Cerebellar peduncles.

***c. cerebri*** A pair of bands joining the cerebrum to the medulla and pons.

***c. of diaphragm*** Two pillars connecting the spinal column and diaphragm.

***c. of the fornix*** Arches made by division of the fornicate extremities.

**crural** (kroo'răl) [L. *cruralis*] Pert. to the leg or thigh; femoral.

***c. hernia*** Femoral hernia.

***c. nerve*** Femoral nerve. SEE: *Nerves Appendix.*

***c. palsy*** Paralysis of the nerves of the legs (e.g., 12th thoracic, first to fifth lumbar, and first to third sacral spinal nerves).

**crus** (krŭs) *pl.* **crura** [L.] **1.** The leg. **2.** Any structure resembling the leg.

***c. cerebri*** Either of the two peduncles connecting the cerebrum with the pons.

**crush syndrome** The result of prolonged, continuous pressure on large muscles (e.g., the legs or arms). As a result of the trauma, the muscle tissue disintegrates. Once the pressure is released and circulation is restored, myoglobin, potassium, and phosphorus leak into the circulation. If left untreated, hypovolemic shock and hyperkalemia are followed by acute renal failure. This condition, also known as traumatic rhabdomyolysis, is associated with a high rate of morbidity and mortality. SEE: *renal failure, acute; reperfusion; rhabdomyolysis.*

**crust** [L. *crusta*] **1.** A scab; a secondary lesion. Dry serous or seropurulent brown, yellow, red, or green exudations may appear. Crusts are seen in eczema, seborrhea, syphilis, impetigo, favus, and ringworm of the scalp. **2.** An outer covering or coat.

**crusta** [L.] Crust.

**crutch** [AS. *crycc*] A device for aiding a paralyzed, weak, or injured person in walking. It is usually a long staff with a padded crescent-shaped portion at the top for placing under the armpit. A great variety of crutches and devices that serve the same purpose are available. These include the axillary (most common); various forms of walkers that provide a mobile stable platform that the patient holds onto while walking; the forearm crutch or lofstrand crutch, which provides points of contact between the hand and forearm; the shelf crutch, an adapted forearm crutch that permits a person unable to bear weight on the hands to use a crutch; and a three- or four-legged cane for a person with poor balance who needs mild support. It is important that the patient be instructed in the proper use of a crutch, because nerve lesions can result from improper use.

NURSING IMPLICATIONS: Depending on activity restrictions, the patient is taught appropriate gaits for crutch walking, including negotiating stairs and moving safely through doorways. The patient should not lean on the crutches to transfer from a standing to sitting position. The patient's safety and dexterity while on crutches are evaluated, and use of a walker is recommended if safety is a concern.

**Crutchfield tongs** [William Gayle Crutchfield, U.S. surgeon, 1900–1972] Device for inserting into each side of the skull. Traction is then applied parallel to the long axis of the cervical spine by applying traction to the device.

**Cruveilhier-Baumgarten syndrome** (kroo-văl-yā'bŏm'găr-tĕn) [Jean Cruveilhier, Fr. pathologist, 1791–1874; Paul Clemens von Baumgarten, Ger. pathologist, 1848–1928] Cirrhosis of the liver caused by patency of the umbilical or paraumbilical veins and the resultant collateral circulation. It is associated with prominent periumbilical veins, portal hypertension, liver atrophy, and splenomegaly.

**cry-** SEE: *cryo-*.

**cry** (krī) The production of inarticulate sounds, with or without weeping, which may be sudden, loud, or quiet as in a sob. These sounds are made in response to a variety of stimuli: fright, fear, pain, apprehension, sadness, glee, or joy. They may occur during nightmares. SEE: *cry reflex.*

***cephalic c.*** A sudden shrill cry by an infant that may be indicative of cerebral disease.

***epileptic c.*** A sudden, loud cry that may accompany the onset of an epileptic seizure.

***hydrocephalic c.*** An involuntary night cry by a child with acute tuberculous meningitis or acute-onset hydrocephalus.

***night c.*** Any sudden outcry at night. It may be caused by onset of acute joint pain.

**cryalgesia** (krī-ăl-jē'zē-ă) [Gr. *kryos,* cold, + *algos,* pain] Pain from the application of cold.

**cryanesthesia** (krī-ăn-ĕs-thē'zē-ă) [" + *an-,* not, + *aisthesis,* sensation] Loss of sense of cold.

**cryesthesia** (krī-ĕs-thē'zē-ă) [" + *aisthesis,* sensation] Sensitivity to the cold.

**cry for help** An action by an individual who is potentially suicidal or severely depressed to inform others of his or her distress. This may be done by leaving cryptic messages or making telephone calls that are later interpreted to mean that the individual was asking for help more or less covertly.

**crymodynia** (krī"mō-dĭn'ē-ă) [Gr. *krymos,* frost, + *odyne,* pain] Pain from cold, esp. rheumatic pain aggravated by cold or damp weather.

**crymophilic** (krī"mō-fĭl'ĭk) [" + *philein,* to love] Cryophilic.

**crymotherapy** (krī"mō-thĕr'ă-pē) [" + *therapeia,* treatment] Cryotherapy.

**cryo-, cry-** [Gr. *krymos,* cold] Combining form concerning cold. SEE: *psychro-*.

**cryoanesthesia** SEE: *anesthesia, refrigeration.*

**cryobank** (krī'ō-bănk) A facility for storage of biological tissues at very low temperatures.

**cryobiology** (krī"ō-bī-ŏl'ō-jē) [" + *bios,* life, + *logos,* word, reason] The study of the effect of cold on biological systems.

**cryocautery** (krī"ō-kaw'tĕr-ē) [" + *kauter,* a burner] A device for application of cold sufficient to kill tissue.

**cryoextraction** (krī"ō-ĕks-trăk'shŭn) The use of a cooling probe introduced into the lens of the eye to produce an ice ball limited to the lens. The ice ball, which includes the lens, is then removed. This is used in treating cataracts.

**cryofibrinogen** (krī″ō-fī-brĭn′ō-jĕn) An abnormal fibrinogen that precipitates when cooled and dissolves when reheated to body temperature.

**cryogen** (krī′ō-jĕn) [″ + *gennan,* to produce] A substance that produces low temperatures.

**cryogenic** (krī″ō-jĕn′ĭk) Producing or pert. to low temperatures.

**cryoglobulin** (krī″ō-glŏb′ū-lĭn) [″ + L. *globulus,* globule] An abnormal protein, globulin, that precipitates when cooled and dissolves when reheated to body temperature.

**cryoglobulinemia** (krī″ō-glŏb″ū-lĭn-ē′mē-ă) [″ + ″ + Gr. *haima,* blood] The presence in the blood of an abnormal protein that forms gels at low temperatures. It is found in association with pathological conditions such as multiple myeloma, leukemia, and certain forms of pneumonia.

**cryohypophysectomy** (krī″ō-hī″pō-fĭz-ĕk′tō-mē) [Gr. *kryos,* cold, + *hypo,* under, + *physis,* growth, + *ektome,* excision] Destruction of the hypophysis by the use of cold.

**cryolesion 1.** The cooling of an area in order to injure or destroy it. This is done for therapeutic reasons. **2.** A lesion produced by exposure to cold (e.g., frostbite).

**cryophilic** (krī″ō-fĭl′ĭk) [″ + *philein,* to love] Showing preference for cold, as in psychrophilic bacteria. SYN: *crymophilic; psychrophilic.*

**cryoprecipitate** (krī″ō-prē-sĭp′ĭ-tāt) The precipitate formed when serum from patients with rheumatoid arthritis, glomerulonephritis, systemic lupus erythematosus, and other chronic diseases in which immune complexes are pathogenic is stored at 4°C. The joint fluid from rheumatoid arthritis patients also forms a precipitate when so stored.

**cryopreservation** Preservation of biological materials, such as tissue, sperm, fluids, blood, or plasma at very low temperatures. This enables the tissue to be used in another individual at a later time, as it remains viable after thawing. The technique is used to preserve human semen for artificial insemination.

**cryoprobe** (krī′ō-prōb) A device for applying cold to a tissue. Liquid nitrogen is the coolant frequently used. SEE: *cryoextraction.*

**cryoprotectant** A drug that permits cells to survive freezing and thawing.

**cryoprotective** (krī″ō-prō-tĕk′tĭv) Pert. to a chemical that protects cells from the effect of cold.

**cryoprotein** (krī″ō-prō′tē-ĭn) Any protein that precipitates when cooled below body temperature. SEE: *cryofibrinogen; cryoglobulin.*

**cryostat** (krī′ō-stăt) A device for maintaining very low temperatures.

**cryosurgery** (krī″ō-sĕr′jĕr-ē) [″ + ME. *surgerie,* surgery] The technique of exposing tissues to extreme cold in order to produce well-demarcated areas of cell injury and destruction. The tissue is usually cooled to below −20°C. It is used in treating malignant tumors, to control pain, to produce lesions in the brain, and to control bleeding. The cold is usually produced by use of a probe through which liquid nitrogen circulates.

**cryothalamotomy** (krī″ō-thăl″ă-mŏt′ō-mē) [″ + L. *thalamus,* inner chamber, + Gr. *tome,* incision] The destruction of a portion of the brain by cooling the end of a slender probe placed in the thalamus, usually done by circulating liquid nitrogen through the hollow stylus. This was formerly used to treat parkinsonism.

**cryotherapy** (krī-ō-thĕr′ă-pē) [″ + *therapeia,* treatment] The therapeutic use of cold.

**cryotolerant** (krī″ō-tŏl′ĕr-ănt) [″ + L. *tolerare,* to bear] Able to tolerate very low temperatures.

**crypt** (krĭpt) [Gr. *kryptos,* hidden] **1.** A small sac or cavity extending into an epithelial surface. **2.** A tubular gland, esp. one of the intestine.

***anal c.*** One of a number of small indentations lying immediately behind the junction of the anal skin and rectal mucosa.

***dental c.*** A space in the bony jaw occupied by a developing tooth.

***c. of iris*** An irregular excavation on the anterior surface of the iris near the pupillary and ciliary margins.

***c. of Lieberkühn*** A tubular gland of the intestine that secretes intestinal juice. Its wall is composed of columnar epithelium containing argentaffin cells and, at the base of the gland, cells of Paneth. They open between bases of the villi.

***synoviparous c.*** A saclike extension of the synovial cavity into the capsule of a joint. Sometimes these crypts become blind sacs.

***tonsillar c.*** A deep invagination of the surface-stratified epithelium into substance of the lingual or palatine tonsils. It is surrounded by lymph nodules and may be branched.

**cryptanamnesia** (krĭpt″ăn-ăm-nē′zē-ă) [″ + *an-,* not, + *amnesia,* forgetfulness] Cryptomnesia.

**cryptectomy** (krĭp-tĕk′tō-mē) [″ + *ektome,* excision] Excision of a crypt.

**cryptesthesia** (krĭp-tĕs-thē′zē-ă) [″ + *aisthesis,* sensation] Subconscious awareness of facts or occurrences other than through the senses or through rational thinking, such as intuition or clairvoyance.

**cryptic** (krĭp′tĭk) [Gr. *kryptikos,* hidden] **1.** Having a hidden meaning; occult. **2.** Tending to hide or disguise.

**cryptitis** (krĭp-tī′tĭs) [Gr. *kryptos,* hidden, + *itis,* inflammation] Inflammation of a crypt or follicle, esp. an anal crypt.

**cryptocephalus** (krĭp″tō-sĕf′ă-lŭs) [″ + *kephale,* head] A congenital deformity in

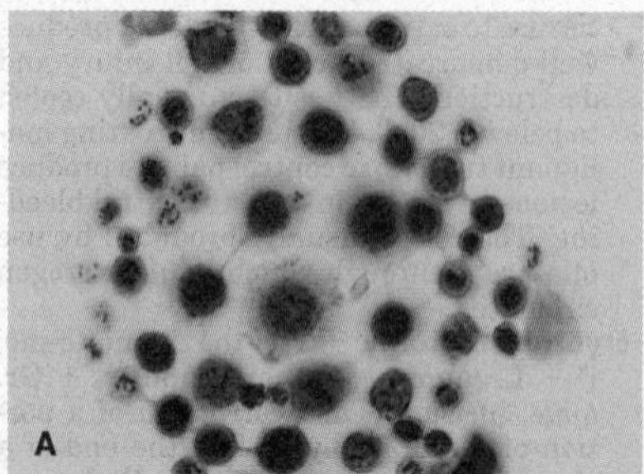


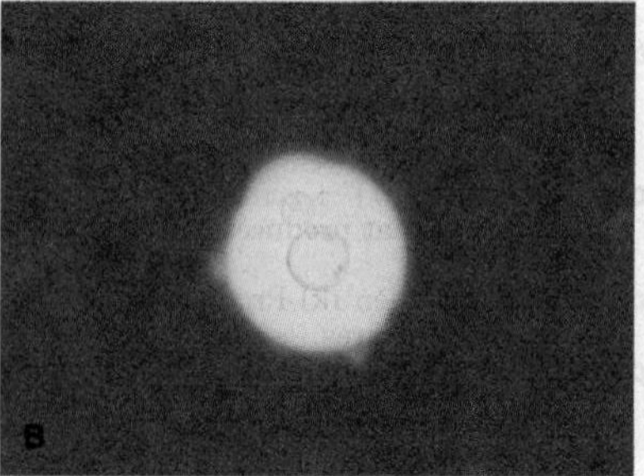


**CRYPTOCOCCUS NEOFORMANS** IN **(A)** CEREBROSPINAL FLUID (ORIG. MAG. ×1000) AND **(B)** INDIA INK PREPARATION SHOWING LARGE CAPSULE (ORIG. MAG. ×400)

which the head is inapparent.

**cryptococcosis** (krĭp″tō-kŏk-ō′sĭs) [″ + *kokkos,* berry, + *osis,* condition] A systemic fungus infection that may involve any organ of the body, lungs, or skin, but having a marked predilection for the brain and its meninges. SYN: *torulosis.*

SYMPTOMS: Single or multiple abscesses develop. In the cerebral type headache, dizziness, vertigo, and stiffness of neck muscles are present; in the final stages, coma and respiratory failure occur. This condition is often mistaken for brain tumor.

ETIOLOGY: Cryptococcosis is caused by *Cryptococcus neoformans (Torula histolytica),* a fungus.

TREATMENT: Amphotericin B may be beneficial.

PROGNOSIS: The prognosis is poor; the cerebral and meningeal forms are usually fatal.

**Cryptococcus** (krĭp″tō-kŏk′ŭs) A genus of pathogenic yeastlike fungi. The former term was *Torula.*

***C. neoformans*** A species that is the causative agent of cryptococcus. SEE: illus.

**cryptodidymus** (krĭp-tō-dĭd′ĭ-mŭs) [″ + *didymos,* twin] A congenital anomaly in which one fetus is concealed within another.

**cryptogenic** (krĭp″tō-jĕn′ĭk) [″ + *gennan,* to produce] Of unknown or indeterminate origin.

**cryptolith** (krĭp′tō-lĭth) [″ + *lithos,* stone] A concretion in a glandular follicle.

**cryptomenorrhea** (krĭp″tō-mĕn″ō-rē′ă) [″ + *men,* month, + *rhoia,* flow] Monthly subjective symptoms of menses without flow of blood; may be caused by an imperforate hymen.

**cryptomerorachischisis** (krĭp″tō-mē″rō-ră-kĭs′kĭ-sĭs) [″ + *meros,* part, + *rhachis,* spine, + *schisis,* a splitting] Spina bifida occulta without a tumor but with bony deficiency.

**cryptomnesia** (krĭp-tŏm-nē′zē-ă) [″ + *mnesis,* memory] Subconscious memory. SYN: *cryptanamnesia.*

**cryptophthalmus** (krĭp″tŏf-thăl′mŭs) [″ + *ophthalmos,* eye] Complete congenital adhesion of the eyelid to the globe of the eye.

**cryptoplasmic** (krĭp″tō-plăz′mĭk) [″ + LL. *plasma,* form, mold] Having existence in a concealed form.

**cryptorchid, cryptorchis** (krĭpt-or′kĭd, -or′kĭs) [″ + *orchis,* testis] An individual in whom either or both testicles have not descended into the scrotum. SEE: *monorchid.*

**cryptorchidectomy** (krĭpt″or-kĭ-dĕk′tō-mē) [″ + ″ + *ektome,* excision] Operation for correction of an undescended testicle.

**cryptorchidism, cryptorchism** (krĭpt-or′kĭd-ĭzm, -kĭzm) [″ + *orchis,* testis, + *-ismos,* condition] Failure of the testicles to descend into the scrotum.

**cryptoscope** (krĭp′tō-skōp) [″ + *skopein,* to examine] Fluoroscope.

**cryptosporidiosis** A diarrheal disease caused by protozoa of the genus *Cryptosporidium.* It was first described in humans in 1976. *C. parvum* is the most common species in human infections. Travelers to endemic areas have an increased chance of becoming infested with this organism. The typical infection, in immunocompetent individuals, causes explosive diarrhea and abdominal cramps following an incubation period of 4 to 14 days; these usually last for 5 to 11 days but may continue for a month. In immunocompromised patients, the disease often causes death. This disease is commonly seen in patients with AIDS and in immunocompromised cancer and organ transplant patients. In immunocompetent patients, no effective specific therapy exists, and the disease is self-limiting. In the immunocompromised patient, the only effective therapy is reversal of the immunological defect. SEE: *Universal Precautions Appendix*

When the organism contaminates public water supplies hundreds of thousands of those drinking that water may develop diarrhea. A frequent source of the contamination is surface water from livestock grazing areas. Resistant to chlorine,

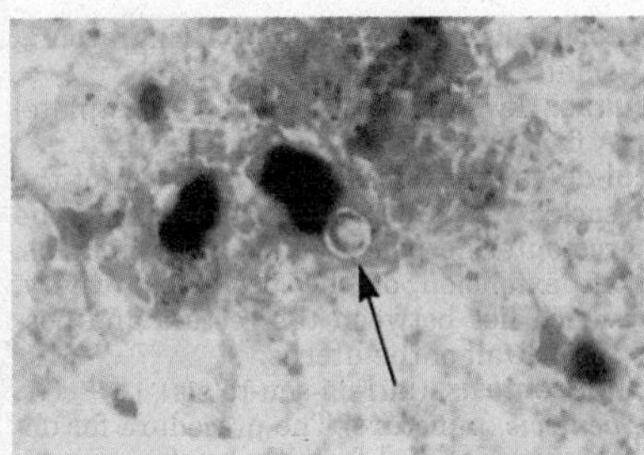

CRYPTOSPORIDIUM IN STOOL SPECIMEN (ORIG. MAG. ×500)

cryptosporidial cysts are incompletely removed by standard water-filtration systems. The least expensive method of killing the organism in water is to boil the water for 1 min. Some types of bottled water come from above-ground sources and are likely to contain cryptosporidia. Water filters effective against the organism are labeled "absolute 1 micron" or "National Sanitation Foundation (NSF) certified for Standard 53 cyst removal."

---

Caution: Stools from these patients are highly infectious. Standard techniques must be used in handling and disposing of them.

---

**Cryptosporidium** A genus of protozoa in the kingdom Protista classed as a coccidian parasite. It is an important cause of diarrhea, esp. in immunocompromised patients, but may cause large outbreaks in the general population when it contaminates supplies of drinking water. SEE: illus.; *cryptosporidiosis.*

**cryptoxanthin** (krĭp″tō-zăn′thĭn) A substance present in a variety of foods (e.g., eggs and corn) that can be converted to vitamin A in the body.

**cry reflex 1.** The normal ability of an infant to cry; not usually present in premature infants. **2.** The spontaneous crying by infants during sleep. It may be caused by a painful joint disease.

**crystal** (krĭs′tăl) [Gr. *krystallos,* ice] A solid body in which the atoms are arranged in a definite symmetrical pattern, with faces lying at definite angles to each other as crystals formed from salts or water.

***apatite c.*** In dentistry, the hydroxyapatite crystal typical of calcified tissues; a complex of calcium phosphate and other elements, present in bone and in the cementum, dentin, and enamel layers of teeth. The most dense crystalline pattern is found in enamel, the hardest tissue of the body.

***Charcot-Leyden c.*** A protein-containing crystal found in diseased tissues wherein eosinophils are being destroyed. It is present in sputum from asthma patients, leukemic bloods, and pleural effusions containing large numbers of eosinophils.

***Charcot-Neumann c.*** A spermin crystal found in semen and some animal tissues.

***Charcot-Robin c.*** A type of crystal formed in the blood in leukemia.

***c. of hemin*** A yellowish or brown crystal that appears when dried blood or hemoglobin is heated, after adding a few drops of acetic acid and salt. The presence of this crystal, the hydrochloride of heme, is a delicate and reliable test for blood.

***liquid c.*** A substance that alters its color or changes from opaque to transparent when subjected to changes in temperature, electric current, pressure, or electromagnetic waves, or when impurities are present. Liquid crystals have been used to detect temperature fluctuation in infants, and may be divided into two general classes: cholestric, which change color, and nematic, which can change back and forth from transparent to opaque.

***spermin c.*** A crystal composed of spermine phosphate and seen in prostatic fluid on addition of a drop of ammonium phosphate solution.

**crystallin** (krĭs′tăl-ĭn) Globulin of the crystalline lens.

**crystalline** (krĭs′tă-līn) Resembling crystal.

***c. deposits*** An acid group including the urates, oxalates, carbonates, and sulfates. The alkaline group includes the phosphates and cholesterin ammonium urate.

**crystallization** (krĭs″tă-lī-zā′shŭn) [Gr. *krystallos,* ice] The formation of crystals.

**crystallography** (krĭs″tă-lŏg′ră-fē) [″ + *graphein,* to write] The study of crystals; useful in investigating renal calculi.

**crystalloid** [″ + *eidos,* form, shape] **1.** Like a crystal. **2.** A substance capable of crystallization, which in solution can be diffused through animal membranes; the opposite of colloid.

**crystalloiditis** (krĭs″tăl-oyd-ī′tĭs) [″ + ″ + *itis,* inflammation] Inflammation of the crystalline lens.

**crystallophobia** [Gr. *krystallos,* ice, + *phobos,* fear] An abnormal fear of glass or objects made of glass.

**crystalluria** (krĭs-tă-lū′rē-ă) [″ + *ouron,* urine] The appearance of crystals in the urine. It may occur following the administration of sulfonamides. This condition can be prevented by administration of adequate amounts of alkali.

**Crystodigin** Trade name for digitoxin.

**CS** *cesarean section.*

**Cs** Symbol for the element cesium.

**c-section** *cesarean section.*

**CSF** *cerebrospinal fluid.*

**CST** *Certified Surgical Technologist.*

**C substance** A complex carbohydrate present in the cell wall of pneumococcal cells. SEE: *C-reactive protein.*

**CT** *computed tomography.*

**C.T.D.** *connective tissue disease.*

**Ctenocephalides** (tĕn-ō-sĕf-ăl'ĭ-dēz) [Gr. *ktenodes,* like a cockle, + *kephale,* head] A genus of fleas belonging to the order Siphonaptera. Common species are *Ct. canis* and *Ct. felis,* the dog flea and cat flea, respectively. The adults feed on their hosts, whereas the larvae live on dried blood and feces of adult fleas. Adults may attack humans and other animals. They serve as intermediate host of the dog tapeworm, *Dipylidium caninum,* and may transmit other helminth and protozoan infections.

**c-terminal** In chemical nomenclature, the alpha carboxyl group of the last amino acid.

**CTZ** *chemoreceptor trigger zone.*

**Cu** [L. *cuprum*] Symbol for the element copper.

**cubic measure** A unit or a system of units used to measure volume or capacity as distinguished from liquid measure. SEE: *Weights and Measures Appendix.*

**cubital** (kū'bĭ-tăl) [L. *cubitum,* elbow] Pert. to the ulna or to the forearm.

**cubital fossa** Antecubital fossa.

**cubitus** (kū'bĭ-tŭs) [L] Elbow; forearm; ulna.

***c. valgus*** A deformity of the arm in which the forearm deviates laterally; may be congenital or caused by injury or disease. In women, slight cubitus valgus is normal and is one of the secondary sex characteristics.

***c. varus*** A deformity of the arm in which the forearm deviates medially.

**cuboid** (kū'boyd) [Gr. *kubos,* cube, + *eidos,* form, shape] Like a cube.

**cu cm** *cubic centimeter.*

**cucurbit** (kū-kĕr'bĭt) [L. *cucurbita,* gourd] Cupping glass. SEE: *cupping.*

**cue** In psychology, a stimulus or set of stimuli that results in action or attempted action.

**cuff** (kŭf) [ME. *cuffe,* glove] An anatomical structure encircling a part.

***attached gingival c.*** Attachment or junctional epithelium attached to the calcified root of the tooth apical to the gingival sulcus.

***gingival c.*** The most coronal portion of the gingiva around the tooth.

***rotator c.*** A musculotendinous structure consisting of supraspinatus, infraspinatus, teres minor, and subscapularis tendons blending with the shoulder joint capsule. The muscles, which surround the glenohumeral joint below the superficial musculature, stabilize and control the head of the humerus in all arm motions, function with the deltoid to abduct the arm, and rotate the humerus. Weakness in the cuff muscles may lead to impingement syndromes and tendinitis; tears in the cuff may lead to subluxations; and continued irritation may lead to immobilization of the shoulder.

**cuffing** (kŭf'ĭng) A collection of inflammatory cells in the shape of a ring around small blood vessels.

**cuirass** (kwē-răs') [Fr. *cuirasse,* breastplate] A firm bandage around the chest.

**cul-de-sac** (kŭl"dĭ-săk') [Fr., bottom of the sack] **1.** A blind pouch or cavity. **2.** The rectouterine pouch or pouch of Douglas, an extension of the peritoneal cavity, which lies between the rectum and posterior wall of the uterus.

**culdocentesis** (kŭl"dō-sĕn-tē'sĭs) [" + Gr. *kentesis,* puncture] The procedure for obtaining material from the posterior vaginal cul-de-sac by aspiration or surgical incision through the vaginal wall, performed for therapeutic or diagnostic reasons.

**culdoscope** (kŭl'dō-skōp) An endoscope used in performing a culdoscopic examination.

**culdoscopy** (kŭl-dŏs'kō-pē) Examination of the viscera of the female pelvic cavity after introduction of an endoscope through the wall of the posterior fornix of the vagina.

**-cule, -cle** [L.] Suffix indicating little, as molecule, corpuscle.

**Culex** (kū'lĕks) [L., gnat] A genus of small to medium-sized mosquitoes of cosmopolitan distribution. Some species are vectors of disease organisms.

***C. pipiens*** The common house mosquito; serves as a vector of *Wuchereria bancrofti,* the causative agent of filariasis.

***C. quinquefasciatus*** Mosquito common in the tropics and subtropics; the most important intermediate host of *Wuchereria bancrofti.*

**Culicidae** (kū-lĭs'ĭ-dē) A family of insects belonging to the order Diptera; includes the mosquitoes.

**culicide** (kū'lĭ-sīd) [L. *culex,* gnat, + *caedere,* to kill] An agent that destroys gnats and mosquitoes.

**Cullen's sign** (kŭl'ĕnz) [Thomas Stephen Cullen, U.S. gynecologist, 1868–1953] Bluish discoloration of the periumbilical skin caused by intraperitoneal hemorrhage. This may be caused by ruptured ectopic pregnancy or acute pancreatitis.

**culling** The process of removal of abnormal or damaged blood cells from the circulation by the spleen. SEE: *pitting; spleen.*

**culmen** (kŭl'mĕn) *pl.* **culmina** [L., summit] **1.** The top or summit of a thing. **2.** The most prominent part of the vermis superior of the cerebellum, located near its anterior extremity.

**cult** [L. *cultus,* care] A group of people with an obsessive commitment to an ideal or principle or to an individual personifying that ideal.

**cultivation** (kŭl"tĭ-vā'shŭn) [L. *cultivare,* to cultivate] The propagation of living organisms, esp. growing microorganisms in an artificial medium.

**cultural** (kŭl'tū-răl) [L. *cultura,* tillage] Pert. to cultures of microorganisms.

**cultural formulation** A systematic review of

a person's cultural background and the role of culture in the manifestation of symptoms and dysfunction. It includes the cultural identity of the individual, cultural explanations of the illness, cultural factors related to the environment and individual functioning, cultural elements of the clinician-patient relationship, and a general discussion of how cultural considerations may influence the diagnosis and treatment of a psychiatric illness.

**culture** (kŭl'tūr) **1.** The propagation of microorganisms or of living tissue cells in special media that are conducive to their growth. **2.** The part of the environment made by humans; symbols, ideas, values, traditions, institutions, and technology of humanity.

***blood c.*** A bacterial culture used in the diagnosis of specific infectious diseases. This test consists of withdrawing blood from a vein under sterile precautions, placing it in or on suitable culture media, and determining whether or not bacteria grow in the media. If organisms do grow, they are identified by bacteriological methods. Multiple blood cultures may be needed to isolate an organism.

***cell c.*** An in vitro growth of cells.

***contaminated c.*** Culture in which bacteria from a foreign source have infiltrated the original bacteria being grown.

***continuous flow c.*** A bacterial culture in which a fresh flow of culture media is maintained. This allows the bacteria to maintain their growth rate.

***gelatin c.*** A culture of bacteria on a gelatin medium.

***hanging block c.*** A thin slice of agar seeded on its surface with bacteria and then inverted on a cover slip and sealed in the concavity of a hollow glass slide.

***hanging drop c.*** A culture accomplished by inoculating the bacterium into a drop of culture medium on a cover glass and mounting it upside down over the depression on a concave slide.

***negative c.*** A culture made from suspected matter that fails to reveal the suspected organism.

***positive c.*** A culture that reveals the suspected organism.

***pure c.*** A culture of a single form of microorganism uncontaminated by other organisms.

***c. shock*** The emotional trauma of being exposed to the culture, mores, and customs of a culture that is vastly different from the one to which one has been accustomed.

***slant c.*** A culture in which the medium is placed in a tube that is slanted to allow greater surface for growth of the inoculum of bacteria.

***stab c.*** A bacterial culture made by thrusting into the culture medium a point inoculated with the matter under examination.

***stock c.*** A permanent culture from which transfers may be made.

***streak c.*** The spreading of the bacteria inoculum by drawing a wire containing the inoculum across the surface of the medium.

***tissue c.*** A culture in which tissue cells are grown in artificial nutrient media.

***type c.*** A culture of standard strains of bacteria that are maintained in a suitable storage area. These permit bacteriologists to compare known strains with unknown or partially identified strains.

**cu mm** *cubic millimeter.*

**cumulative** (kū'mū-lă-tĭv) [L. *cumulus,* a heap] Increasing in effect by successive additions; the total is usually greater than the sum of all the additions.

**cumulative drug action** The action of small but repeated doses of drugs that are not immediately eliminated from the body. For example, preparations containing lead, silver, and mercury tend to accumulate in the system and can produce symptoms of poisoning.

**Cumulative Index to Nursing and Allied Health Literature** SEE: *CINAHL.*

**cumulus** (kū'mū-lŭs) [L., a little mound] A small elevation; a heap of cells.

***c. oophorus*** A solid mass of follicular cells that surrounds the developing ovarian follicle. It projects into the antrum of the graafian follicle. SYN: *discus proligerus.*

**cuneate** (kū'nē-āt) [L. *cuneus,* wedge] Wedge-shaped.

**cuneiform** (kū-nē'ĭ-form) [" + *forma,* shape] Wedge-shaped.

**cuneo-** (kū'nē-ō) [L. *cuneus,* wedge] Combining form rel. to a wedge.

**cuneocuboid** (kū"nē-ō-kū'boyd) [" + Gr. *kubos,* cube, + *eidos,* form, shape] Pert. to cuboid and cuneiform bones.

**cuneohysterectomy** (kū"nē-ō-hĭs"tĕr-ĕk'tō-mē) [" + Gr. *hystera,* womb, + *ektome,* excision] Excision of a wedge of tissue from the posterior surface of the cervix uteri to correct abnormal anteflexion.

**cuneus** (kū'nē-ŭs) *pl.* **cunei** [L., wedge] A wedge-shaped lobule of the brain on the mesial surface of the occipital lobe.

**cuniculus** (kū-nĭk'ū-lŭs) *pl.* **cuniculi** [L., an underground passage] A burrow in the epidermis made by the itch mite.

**cunnilinguist** (kŭn-ĭ-lĭn'gwĭst) [L. *cunnus,* pudenda, + *lingua,* tongue] One who practices cunnilingus.

**cunnilingus** (kŭn-ĭ-lĭn'gŭs) Sexual activity in which the mouth and tongue are used to stimulate the female genitalia. SEE: *fellatio.*

**cunnus** (kŭn'ŭs) [L.] The vulva; pudenda.

**cup** [LL. *cuppa,* drinking vessel] **1.** Small drinking vessel. **2.** A cupping glass. SEE: *cupping.* **3.** An athletic supporter (jockey strap) reinforced with a piece of firm material to cover the male genitalia; worn to protect the penis and testicles during vigorous and contact sports. **4.** Either of the two cup-shaped halves of a brassiere that fit over a breast. **5.** A method of producing counterirritation. SEE: *cupping.*

***favus c.*** A cup-shaped crust that develops in certain fungus infections. SEE: *favus.*

***glaucomatous c.*** A depression in the optic disk occurring in late stages of glaucoma.

***optic c.*** In the embryo, a double-layered cuplike structure connected to the diencephalon by a tubular optic stalk. It gives rise to the sensory and pigmented layers of the retina.

***physiological c.*** A slight concavity in the center of the optic disk.

**cup arthroplasty of hip** Surgical technique for remodeling the femoral head and acetabulum and then covering the head with a metal cup. It is rarely used in treating arthritis of the hip. Total hip replacement is usually the procedure of choice in the elderly as well as in young adults on a selective basis.

**Cupid's bow** The normal bow-shape of the upper lip of the mouth.

**cupola, cupula** (kū′pō-lă, -pū-lă) [L. *cupula,* little tub] **1.** The little dome at the apex of the cochlea and spiral canal of the ear. **2.** The portion of costal pleura that extends superiorly into the root of the neck. It is dome shaped and accommodates the apex of the lung.

**cupping** Application to the skin of a glass vessel, from which air has been exhausted by heat, or of a special suction apparatus in order to draw blood to the surface. This is done to produce counterirritation. SEE: *leech; moxibustion.*

**cupric** (kū′prĭk) Concerning divalent copper, $Cu^{++}$, in solution.

***c. sulfate*** Copper sulfate.

**cuprous** (kū′prŭs) Concerning monovalent copper, $Cu^{+}$, in a compound.

**cuprum** (kū′prŭm) [L.] ABBR: Cu. Copper.

**cupruresis** (kū″proo-rē′sĭs) [L. *cuprum,* copper, + Gr. *ouresis,* to void urine] Excretion of copper in the urine.

**cupulolithiasis** (kū″pū-lō-lĭth-ī′ă-sis) [L. dim. of *cupa,* a tub, + Gr. *lithos,* stone, + *iasis,* state or condition of] A disease of calculi in the cupula of the posterior semicircular canal of the middle ear. The condition may be associated with positional vertigo.

**curare** (kū-, koo-răr′ē) [phonetic equivalent of a South American Indian name for extracts of plants used as arrow poisons] One of several different resinous substances obtained from extracts of South American trees including species of chondrodendron. The pharmacologically active ingredient of curare used medically is the alkaloid D-tubocurarine. This drug is used to facilitate skeletal muscle relaxation during anesthesia. SEE: *tubocurarine chloride.*

**curarization** (kū″răr-ī-zā′shŭn) A condition following introduction of a purified form of curare, characterized by heavy eyelids, nystagmus, husky voice, weak jaw and throat muscles, and inability to raise the head, arms, and legs. It is used to lessen severity of convulsions produced by pentylenetetrazol and electric shock therapy and relaxation of muscles as in tetanus.

**curative** (kū′ră-tĭv) [L. *curare,* to take care of] Having healing or remedial properties.

**curb cut** An area in which a sidewalk has been modified or designed to eliminate the vertical curb. By providing a gradual slope to the street at this point, an environmental obstacle has been removed, thus improving access for persons with wheelchairs, who have difficulty walking, or for persons pushing wheeled vehicles.

**curd** [ME] Milk coagulum, composed mainly of casein.

**cure** [L. *cura,* care] **1.** Course of treatment to restore health. **2.** Restoration to health.

**curet, curette** (kū-rĕt′) [Fr. *curette,* a cleanser] **1.** A spoon-shaped scraping instrument for removing foreign matter from a cavity. **2.** In dentistry, one of a variety of sharp instruments used to remove calculus and to smooth tooth roots or to remove soft tissues from a periodontal pocket or extraction site.

**curettage** (kū″rĕ-tăzh′) [Fr.] **1.** Scraping of a cavity. SYN: *curettement.* **2.** The use of a curet in removal of necrotic tissue from around the tooth, dental granulomata, or cysts and tissue fragments or debris from the bony socket after tooth extraction; also called débridement.

***periapical c.*** Use of a curet to remove pathological tissues from around the apex of the tooth root.

***suction c.*** Vacuum aspiration.

***uterine c.*** Scraping with a curet to remove the contents of the uterus, as is done following inevitable or incomplete abortion; to produce abortion; to obtain specimens for use in diagnosis; and to remove growths, such as polyps.

NURSING IMPLICATIONS: *Preoperative:* The physician's explanation of the procedure is reinforced and clarified, any questions are answered, and expected sensations are described. Physical preparation of the patient is completed according to protocol, and the patient is placed in the lithotomy position. Asepsis is maintained throughout the procedure.

*Postoperative:* Vital signs are monitored until stable, and the patient is monitored until she is able to tolerate liquids by mouth and to urinate without difficulty. A perineal pad count is performed to determine the extent of uterine bleeding, and excessive bleeding is documented and reported to the physician. Prescribed analgesics are administered to relieve pain and discomfort. Before discharge, the patient is instructed to report profuse bleeding immediately; to report any bleeding lasting longer than 10 days; to avoid use of tampons, diaphragms, and douches; and to report signs of infections such as fever or foul-smelling vaginal discharge. Gradual resumption of usual activities is encouraged as long as they do not result in vaginal bleeding.

**curettement** (kū-rĕt′mĕnt) [Fr.] Curettage.

**Curie** (kūr′ē, kū-rē′) **1.** Marie, the Polish-born Fr. chemist, 1867–1934, who discovered the radioactivity of thorium, who discovered polonium and radium, and who isolated radium from pitchblende. She was awarded the Nobel Prize in physics in 1903 with her husband, and in chemistry in 1911. **2.** Pierre, Fr. chemist, 1859–1906, who, with his wife, was awarded the Nobel Prize in 1903.

**curie** [Marie Curie] ABBR: Ci. The standard unit of quantity of radon, being the amount in equilibrium with 1 g of radium element. This quantity decays at the rate of $3.7 \times 10^{10}$ disintegrations per second.

**curietherapy** (kū″rē-thĕr′ă-pē) [″ + Gr. *therapeia,* treatment] Radium therapy.

**curium** (kū′rē-ŭm) [Pierre and Marie Curie] SYMB: Cm. An artificially made element of the actinide series; atomic weight of the longest-lived isotope, 247, atomic number 96. The half-life of the most stable isotope is 16 million years.

**Curling's ulcer** (kŭr′lĭngz) [Thomas Curling, Brit. physician, 1811–1888] An acute peptic ulcer that sometimes follows acute stress (e.g., a severe burn); a form of stress ulcer.

**current** [L. *currere,* to run] A flow, as of water or the transference of electrical impulses.

***alternating c.*** A current that periodically flows in opposite directions; may be either sinusoidal or nonsinusoidal. The alternating current wave usually used therapeutically is the sinusoidal.

***direct c.*** A current that flows in one direction only. When used medically it is called the galvanic current.

**curriculum** (kŭ-rĭk′ū-lŭm) [L.] A course of study in a special field or covering a specific time.

**Curschmann's spirals** (koorsh′mănz) [Heinrich Curschmann, Ger. physician, 1846–1910] Coiled spirals of mucus occasionally seen in sputum of asthma patients. SEE: *sputum.*

**curse** (kĕrs) **1.** To attempt to inflict injury by appeal to a malevolent supernatural power. **2.** Injury assumed to have been inflicted by a malevolent supernatural power. **3.** To use foul, offensive language.

**curvature** [L. *curvatura,* a slope] A normal or abnormal bending or sloping away; a curve.

***angular c.*** A sharp bending of the vertebral column.

***c. of spine*** One of four normal curves or flexures of the vertebral column as seen in profile: cervical, thoracic, lumbar, and sacral. Abnormal curvatures may occur as a result of maldevelopment or disease processes. SEE: *kyphosis; lordosis; scoliosis.*

**curve** [L. *curvus*] A bend.

***characteristic c.*** Sensitometric c.

***dye-dilution c.*** A graph of the disappearance rate of a known amount of injected dye from the circulation; used to measure cardiac function.

***epidemic c.*** A chart or graph in which the number of new cases is plotted for each time interval selected.

***Hurter and Driffield c.*** ABBR: H and D curve. Sensitometric c.

***learning c.*** A graph of the effect of learning or practice on the performance of an intellectual or physical task.

***normal c.*** In statistics, the theoretical frequency of a set of data. It is usually a bell-shaped curve. SYN: *normal distribution.*

***c. of Carus*** An arc corresponding to the pelvic axis.

***sensitometric c.*** In radiographic film analysis, the curve derived by graphing the exposure to the film versus the film density. Analysis yields information about the contrast, speed, latitude, and maximum and minimum densities of the film or film-screen system. SYN: *characteristic c.; Hurter and Driffield c.*

***c. of Spee*** A curve established by viewing the occlusal alignment of teeth, beginning with the tip of the lower canine and extending back along the buccal cusps of the natural premolar and molar teeth to the ramus of the mandible.

**curvilinear** Concerning or pert. to a curved line.

**Cushing, Harvey** (koosh′ĭng) U.S. surgeon, 1869–1939.

***C.'s disease*** C.'s syndrome.

***C.'s syndrome*** A syndrome resulting from hypersecretion of the adrenal cortex in which there is excessive production of glucocorticoids. It may be caused by a tumor of the adrenal gland or excess stimulation of that gland as a result of hyperfunction of the anterior pituitary. Prolonged administration of large doses of adrenocortical hormones will also cause this syndrome. Symptoms are protein loss, adiposity, fatigue and weakness, osteoporosis, amenorrhea, impotence, capillary fragility, edema, excessive hair growth, diabetes mellitus, skin discoloration and turgidity (plethora), and purplish striae of skin. SEE: *dexamethasone suppression test.*

NURSING IMPLICATIONS: When prolonged administration of therapeutic, as opposed to replacement, doses of adrenocortical hormones is required, the patient is monitored for development of adverse reactions. A diet high in protein and potassium but low in calories, carbohydrates, and sodium is provided. Protective measures to prevent infection are instituted and taught to the patient. The patient is assisted to adjust to changes in body image and strength. Realistic reassurance and emotional support are provided, and the patient is encouraged to verbalize feelings about losses and to develop positive coping strategies. Intermittent rest periods are recommended, and assistance is provided with mobility, esp. with movements requiring arm-shoulder strength. Safety measures are instituted to prevent falls. Corticosteriods should be given in the smallest possible maintenance dose, usually every other day, and the dose should gradually be decreased after an increase during an exacerbation. If the corticosteroids are being used for a chronic respiratory disorder, inhaled therapy can provide the desired therapeutic effect better than oral medication while reducing side effects. SEE: *Nursing Diagnoses Appendix.*

**Cushing response** A reflex due to cerebral ischemia that causes an increase in systemic blood pressure. This maintains cerebral perfusion during increased intracranial pressure.

**cushingoid** (koosh′ĭng-oyd) Resembling Cushing's syndrome.

**cushion** In anatomy, a mass of connective tissue, usually adipose, that acts to prevent undue pressure on underlying tissues or structures.

***wheelchair c.*** A padded surface for wheelchair seats designed to prevent pressure sores. There are several static varieties, including air-filled, polyurethane foam, and flotation, the latter filled with water or gel. Dynamic surfaces, which require an external power source, protect pressure points by alternating high and low air pressures through a system of valves and pumps. SYN: *pressure relief device.*

**cusp** (kŭsp) [L. *cuspis,* point] **1.** A rounded or cone-shaped point on the crown of a tooth. **2.** One of the leaflike divisions or parts of the valves of the heart. SEE: *bicuspid valve; semilunar cusps; tricuspid valve.*

***Carabelli's c.*** An accessory cusp found on the upper molars.

**cuspid** (kŭs′pĭd) The canine teeth. SEE: *dentition* for illus.

**cuspidate** (kŭs′pĭ-dāt) [L. *cuspidatus*] Having cusps.

**custom** A generally accepted practice or behavior by a particular group of people or a social group.

**cut 1.** Separating or dividing of tissues by use of a sharp surgical instrument such as a scalpel. **2.** To dilute a substance in order to decrease the concentration of the active ingredient.

**cutaneous** (kū-tā′nē-ŭs) [L. *cutis,* skin] Pert. to the skin. SYN: *dermal; integumentary.*

**cutaneous nerves** Nerves that provide sensory pathways for stimuli to the skin. SEE: illus.; *Nerves Appendix.*

**cutaneous respiration** The transpiration of gases through the skin.

**cutdown** (kŭt′down) A surgical procedure for locating a vein or artery to permit intravenous or intra-arterial administration of fluids or drugs; required in patients with vascular collapse caused by shock or other conditions.

**cuticle** (kū′tĭ-k′l) [L. *cuticula,* little skin] A layer of solid or semisolid substance that covers the free surface of a layer of epithelial cells. It may be horny or chitinous, and sometimes is calcified. Examples include the enamel cuticle of a tooth and the capsule of the lens of the eye.

***acquired c.*** A layer of salivary products, bacteria, and food debris on the surface of the teeth; not a true cuticle. SYN: *pellicle.*

***attachment c.*** Dental c.

***dental c.*** The glycosaminoglycans layer produced by attachment epithelium on the cementum of the tooth root. It is continuous with and identical in origin and function to enamel cuticle, which is present on the enamel crown. SYN: *attachment c.*

***enamel c.*** The thin, calcified layer that covers the enamel crown of the tooth prior to eruption. Remnants that persist after decalcification of the tooth for microscopy are called Nasmyth's membrane. SYN: *cuticula dentis.*

**cuticula** (kū-tĭk′ū-lă) [L.] Cuticle.

***c. dentis*** A skinlike membrane that may cover the teeth after they have erupted and usually is lost in ordinary mastication of food. The membrane is easily removed by a dentist. SYN: *enamel cuticle; Nasmyth's membrane.*

**cuticularization** (kū-tĭk″ū-lăr-ī-zā′shŭn) Growth of skin over a sore or wound.

**cutin** (kū′tĭn) [L. *cutis,* skin] A wax that combines with cellulose to form the cuticle of plants.

**cutireaction** (kū″tē-rē-ăk′shŭn) An inflammatory or irritative reaction appearing on the skin; skin reaction.

***von Pirquet's c.*** The reaction of the skin after inoculation with tuberculosis toxins.

**cutis** (kū′tĭs) [L.] The skin; consisting of the epidermis and the corium (dermis), and resting on the subcutaneous tissue.

***c. anserina*** Piloerection.

***c. aurantiasis*** Yellow discoloration of the skin resulting from ingesting excessive quantities of vegetables, such as carrots, containing carotenoid pigments. SEE: *carotenemia.*

***c. hyperelastica*** Ehlers-Danlos syndrome.

***c. laxa*** A rare inherited condition in which there is loss of elastic fibers of the skin. The skin becomes so loose it hangs and sags. Pulmonary emphysema, intestinal diverticula, and hernias also may be present. There are at least three inheritable patterns of this disease. There is no known treatment. SYN: *c. pendula.*

***c. marmorata*** Transitory purplish discoloration of skin on exposure to cold.

***c. pendula*** C. laxa.

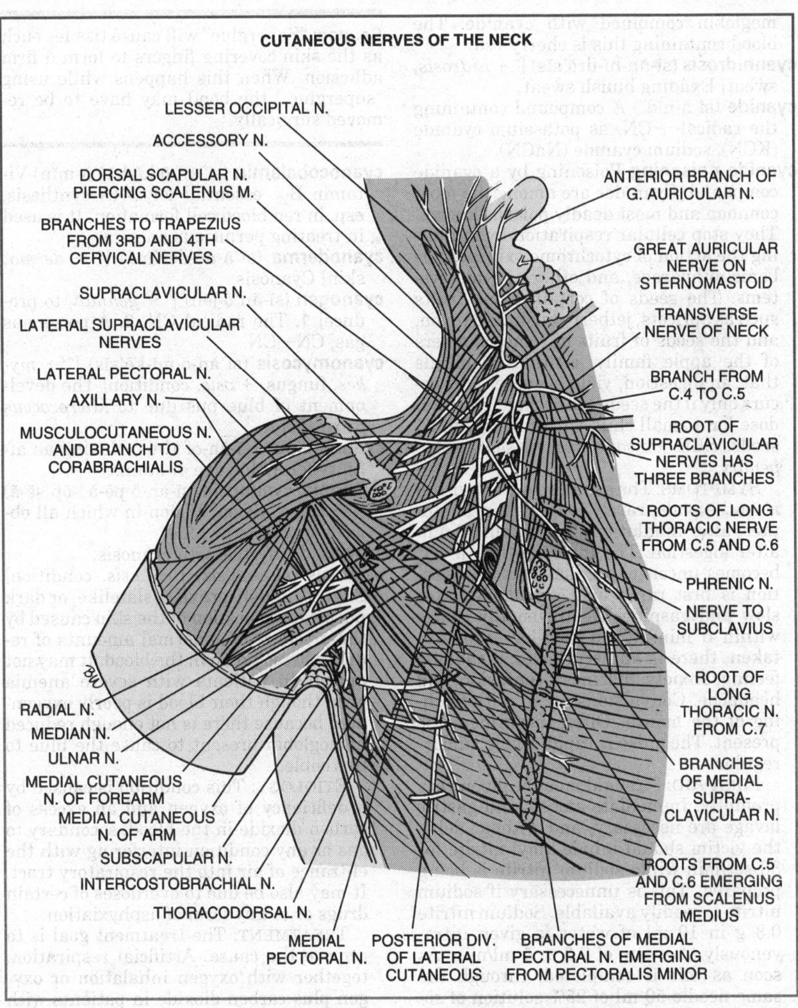


***c. vera*** Dermis.

***c. verticis gyrata*** Convoluted scalp folds 1 to 2 cm thick. The appearance of those with this condition is that the scalp is too big for the head. It may develop any time from birth to adolescence and is more common in males. The skin cannot be flattened by traction.

**cutization** (kū-tĭ-zā′shŭn) Skinlike condition of a mucous membrane as a result of continued exposure.

**cut throat** Laceration of the throat. The seriousness of the injury depends on the angle of thrust of the cutting object, the location of the injury, and the amount of tissue damage.

First Aid: A physician must be sent for. The patient should lie down, head and shoulders raised. (If there is bleeding into the airway, the patient should be positioned so blood flows away from the pharynx. This may require a head-low position.) If the trachea is severed, it should be kept open and free of clots. Bleeding points should be compressed with sterile cloths. Such patients should be reassured, their lips kept moist, and should not be left for an instant. Artificial respiration should be given if necessary.

**cuvette** (kŭv-ĕt′) [Fr. *cuve,* a tub] A small transparent glass or plastic container, esp. one used to hold liquids to be examined photometrically.

**CVA** *cerebrovascular accident.*

**CVP** *central venous pressure.*

**cyan-** SEE: *cyano-.*

**cyanephidrosis** (sī″ăn-ĕf″ĭ-drō′sĭs) [Gr. *kyanos,* dark blue, + *ephidrosis,* sweating] Bluish sweat.

**cyanhemoglobin** (sī″ăn-hē″mō-glō′bĭn) Hemoglobin combined with cyanide. The blood containing this is cherry-red.

**cyanhidrosis** (sī-ăn-hī-drō′sĭs) [″ + *hidrosis,* sweat] Exuding bluish sweat.

**cyanide** (sī′ă-nīd″) A compound containing the radical —CN, as potassium cyanide (KCN), sodium cyanide (NaCN).

**cyanide poisoning** Poisoning by a cyanide compound. Cyanides are among the most common and most deadly poisons known. They stop cellular respiration by inhibiting the action of cytochrome oxidase, carbonic anhydrase, and other enzyme systems. The seeds of certain stone fruits such as apricots, jetberry bush, and toyon, and the seeds of fruits of some members of the apple family, contain chemicals that, on digestion, yield cyanide. This occurs only if the seeds are broken. The fatal dose for a small child varies from 5 to 25 seeds. SEE: *Poisons and Poisoning Appendix.*

SYMPTOMS: The symptoms start within a few seconds, rarely longer than 2 minutes, after inhalation, and within 30 min after ingestion. The patient utters a cry, becomes unconscious, and falls. Respiration is first rapid and convulsive, later slow and gasping. Death usually comes within 5 min. When smaller doses are taken, there is an acrid taste, a choking feeling, anxiety, dizziness, confusion, and headache. Convulsions occur, with frothing of the mouth. Often incontinence is present. The pulse is rapid, feeble, and irregular.

FIRST AID: First aid must be given very promptly. Immediate emesis and gastric lavage are necessary, and without delay the victim should inhale amyl nitrite for 30 sec/min while sodium nitrite is being prepared. This is unnecessary if sodium nitrite is readily available. Sodium nitrite 0.3 g in 10 ml of water is given intravenously at a rate of 2.5 to 5 ml/min. As soon as this is completed, through the same needle 50 ml of 25% solution of sodium thiosulfate is given. Immediate artificial respiration with 100% oxygen is required also. In 1 hr, half doses of the medicines listed here should be given. Hyperbaric oxygen therapy should be used if immediately available. External heat is applied and epinephrine given for collapse. The patient should be kept in a recumbent position. An alternative antidote, hydroxocobalamin-thiosulfate mixture, is used outside the U.S. It is given in doses of 4 to 10 g.

**cyanmethemoglobin** (sī″ăn-mĕt″hē-mō-glō′bĭn) Combination of cyanide and methemoglobin.

**cyano-, cyan-** [Gr. *kyanos,* dark blue] Combining form meaning *blue.*

**cyanoacrylate adhesives** Monomers of *N*-alkyl cyanoacrylate that have been used as a tissue adhesive. This use is limited by the toxicity of the glue. Commercially available versions are called “superglue.”

Caution: “Superglue” will cause tissues such as the skin covering fingers to form a firm adhesion. When this happens while using “superglue,” the bond may have to be removed surgically.

**cyanocobalamin** (sī″ăn-ō-kō-băl′ă-mĭn) Vitamin $B_{12}$, essential for DNA synthesis, esp. in red blood cell formation. It is used in treating pernicious anemia.

**cyanoderma** (sī″ă-nō-dĕr′mă) [″ + *derma,* skin] Cyanosis.

**cyanogen** (sī-ăn′ō-jĕn) [″ + *gennan,* to produce] **1.** The radical CN. **2.** A poisonous gas, CN—CN.

**cyanomycosis** (sī″ăn-ō-mī-kō′sĭs) [″ + *mykes,* fungus, + *osis,* condition] The development of blue pus due to *Micrococcus pyocyaneus.*

**cyanophilous** (sī-ăn-ŏf′ĭl-ŭs) Having an affinity for a blue dye or stain.

**cyanopia, cyanopsia** (sī-ăn-ō′pē-ă, -ŏp′sē-ă) [″ + *opsis,* vision] Vision in which all objects appear to be blue.

**cyanosed** Affected with cyanosis.

**cyanosis** (sī-ă-nō′sĭs) [″ + *osis,* condition] Slightly bluish, grayish, slatelike, or dark purple discoloration of the skin caused by the presence of abnormal amounts of reduced hemoglobin in the blood. It may not appear in patients with severe anemia even though their blood is poorly oxygenated because there is not enough reduced hemoglobin present to cause the blue to be visible.

ETIOLOGY: This condition is caused by a deficiency of oxygen and an excess of carbon dioxide in the blood, secondary to gas or any condition interfering with the entrance of air into the respiratory tract. It may also be due to overdoses of certain drugs or to any form of asphyxiation.

TREATMENT: The treatment goal is to remove the cause. Artificial respiration, together with oxygen inhalation or oxygen plus carbon dioxide in patients with chronic lung disease, is necessary. Stimulants, heat, and massage are valuable adjuncts. SEE: *asphyxia; unconsciousness.*

***circumoral c.*** Cyanosis of the area surrounding the mouth, an indication of hypoxia.

***congenital c.*** Cyanosis usually associated with stenosis of the pulmonary orifice, an imperfect ventricular septum, or a patent foramen ovale or ductus arteriosus. SEE: *tetralogy of Fallot.*

***delayed c.*** Tardive c.

***enterogenous c.*** Cyanosis induced by intestinal absorption of toxins or by certain drugs. SEE: *methemoglobinemia.*

***c. retinae*** Bluish appearance of the retina seen in congenital heart disease, polycythemia, and in certain poisonings, such as dinitrobenzol.

***tardive c.*** Cyanosis caused by congenital heart disease and appearing only after cardiac failure. SYN: *delayed c.*

**cyanotic** (sī-ăn-ŏt′ĭk) Of the nature of, affected with, or pert. to cyanosis.

**cyanuria** (sī″ă-nū′rē-ă) The voiding of blue urine.

**cybernetics** (sī″bĕr-nĕt′ĭks) [Gr. *kybernetes,* helmsman] The science of control and communication in biological, electronic, and mechanical systems. This includes analysis of feedback mechanisms that serve to govern or modify the actions of various systems.

**cyberphilia** (sī″bĕr-fĭl′ē-ă) [″ + *philein,* to love] Fascination with the use of machines, esp. computers, their use, and programming them.

**cyberphobia** (sī″bĕr-fō′bē-ă) [″ + *phobos,* fear] Tension, anxiety, and stress in persons required to work with a computer.

**cycad** (sī′kăd) A variety of plants including *Cycas revoluta* and *C. circinalis,* from which cycasin has been isolated.

**cycasin** (sī′kă-sĭn) A toxic substance present in cycad plants. The chemical may be important in inducing cancer in some lower animals.

**cycl-** SEE: *cyclo-*.

**cyclamate** (sī′klă-māt) A salt of cyclamic acid that is used as a nonnutritive artificial sweetener. It is about 30 times as sweet as sugar. Its general use has been restricted because of its toxic effect on lower animals.

**cyclarthrosis** (sī-klăr-thrō′sĭs) [Gr. *kyklos,* circle, + *arthron,* joint, + *osis,* condition] A lateral ginglymus or pivot joint, which makes rotation possible.

**cycle** (sī′kl) [Gr. *kyklos,* circle] A series of movements or events; a sequence usually recurring at regular intervals.

***cardiac c.*** The period from the beginning of one heartbeat to the beginning of the succeeding beat, including the *systole,* the contraction of the atria and ventricles that propels the blood, and the *diastole,* the period during which the cavities are being refilled with blood. The atria contract immediately before the ventricles. The ordinary cycle lasts 0.8 sec with the heart beating approx. 60 to 85 times a minute in the adult at rest. The atrial systole lasts 0.1 sec; the ventricular systole 0.3 sec, and the diastole 0.4 sec; although the heart seems to be working continuously, it actually rests for a good portion of each cardiac cycle. SEE: illus.

***gastric c.*** The progression of peristaltic waves over the stomach wall.

***genesial c.*** **1.** The period from puberty to menopause. **2.** The period of sexual maturity.

***glycolytic c.*** The successive steps by which glucose is broken down in living tissue.

***life c.*** All of the developmental history of an organism whether in a free-living condition or in a host (e.g., as a parasite that experiences part of its cycle inside another organism).

***menstrual c.*** A series of periodically recurring changes in the hormonal status of women and in the endometrium of the uterus, culminating in menstruation. SEE: *menstruation*.

**cyclectomy** (sī-klĕk′tō-mē) [Gr. *kyklos,* circle, + *ektome,* excision] **1.** Excision of part of the ciliary body or muscle. **2.** Excision of the ciliary border of the eyelids.

**cycles per second** ABBR: cps. SEE: *hertz.*

**cyclic** (sī′klĭk) Periodic; occurring in cycles.

**cyclic AMP** Adenosine 3′,5′-cyclic monophosphate.

**cyclic AMP synthetase** Adenylate cyclase.

**cyclicotomy** (sĭk″lĭ-kŏt′ō-mē) [″ + *tome,* incision] Cutting of the ciliary muscle.

**cyclins** A group of proteins important in regulating mitosis.

**cyclitis** (sĭk-lī′tĭs) [″ + *itis,* inflammation] An inflammation of the ciliary body of the eye.

SYMPTOMS: The patient exhibits tenderness in the ciliary region, swelling of the upper lid, circumcorneal injection, deposits on Descemet's membrane, reduced or hazy vision, and increased or decreased intraocular tension. Pain in or about the eye is present, which is worse at night and on pressure. Its course is rapid and progressively unfavorable. Complications include iritis, choroiditis, scleritis, and glaucoma.

TREATMENT: Local treatment involves administration of atropine, application of heat, and protection from light. General treatment includes salicylates, induced diaphoresis, and rest. The underlying cause should be treated if possible.

***plastic c.*** Ciliary body inflammation accompanied by inflammation of the entire uveal tract, giving rise to a fibrinous exudate in the anterior chamber and vitreous.

***purulent c.*** Suppurative inflammation of the ciliary body and iris.

***serous c.*** Simple inflammation of the ciliary body without iritis.

**cyclizine hydrochloride** An antihistamine used in treating and preventing motion sickness. Trade name is Marezine.

**cyclo-, cycl-** [Gr. *kyklos,* circle] **1.** Combining form meaning *circular* or pert. to a cycle. **2.** Combining form meaning pert. to the ciliary body of the eye.

**cycloceratitis** (sī″klō-sĕr″ă-tī′tĭs) Cyclokeratitis.

**cyclochoroiditis** (sī″klō-kō″royd-ī′tĭs) [″ + *chorioeides,* skinlike, + *itis,* inflammation] Inflammation of the ciliary body and choroid coat of the eye.

**cyclodialysis** (sī″klō-dī-ăl′ĭ-sĭs) [″ + *dialysis,* dissolution] An operation performed in certain types of glaucoma to produce communication between the anterior chamber and suprachoroidal space for the escape of aqueous humor.

**cycloid** (sī′kloyd) [″ + *eidos,* form, shape] **1.** Resembling a circle. **2.** Denoting a ring of atoms. **3.** Extreme variations of mood

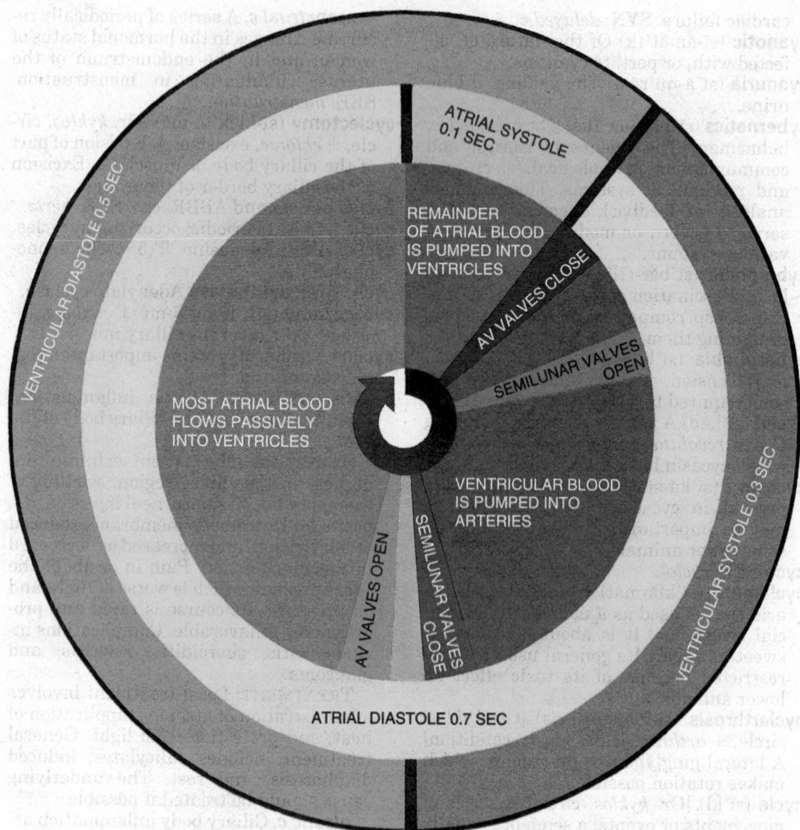


CARIDAC CYCLE; ONE HEARTBEAT, PULSE 75. THE OUTER CIRCLE REPRESENTS THE VENTRICLES, THE MIDDLE CIRCLE THE ATRIA, AND THE INNER CIRCLE THE MOVEMENT OF BLOOD AND ITS EFFECT ON THE HEART VALVES

from elation to melancholia.

**cyclokeratitis** (sī″klō-kĕr-ă-tī′tĭs) [″ + *keras,* cornea, + *itis,* inflammation] Inflammation of the cornea and ciliary body. SYN: *cycloceratitis.*

**cyclopentolate hydrochloride** (sī″klō-pĕn′tō-lāt) A moderately long-acting drug used as a cycloplegic and mydriatic. Trade name is Cyclogyl.

**cyclophoria** (sī″klō-fō′rē-ă) [″ + *phoros,* bearing] Deviation of the eye around its anteroposterior axis due to weakness of the oblique muscles. SYN: *periphoria.*

**cyclophosphamide** (sī″klō-fŏs′fă-mīd) An effective antineoplastic agent that has also been used as an immunosuppressive agent in organ transplantation. Trade name is Cytoxan.

**cyclopia** (sī-klō′pē-ă) [Gr. *kyklos,* circle, + *ops,* eye] The condition of being a cyclops.

**cycloplegia** (sī″klō-plē′jē-ă) [″ + *plege,* a stroke] Paralysis of the ciliary muscle. This can be an anticholinergic side effect of antipsychotic or antidepressant medications.

**cycloplegic** (sī″klō-plē′jĭk) Producing cycloplegia.

**cyclopropane** (sī″klō-prō′pān) $C_3H_6$. An anesthetic agent that is colorless and slightly heavier than air and has a characteristic odor. Administered with 70% to 95% oxygen, it produces unconsciousness in 1 to 2 min. Fire and explosion must be guarded against.

**cyclops** (sī′klŏps) A fetal malformation in which there is only one eye. SYN: *monoculus* (2).

**cycloserine** (sī″klō-sĕr′ĕn) A broad-spectrum antibiotic that has been used in combination with other drugs in treating tuberculosis. It is contraindicated in patients with epilepsy and in those with depression or anxiety. Trade name is Seromycin.

**cyclosis** (sī-klō′sĭs) [Gr. *kyklosis,* circulation] A streaming movement of protoplasm, as is seen in certain plant and animal cells.

**cyclosporine** (sī′klō-spor-een) An immunosuppressive drug useful in suppressing rejection phenomena in organ transplant recipients.

**cyclothiazide** (sī″klō-thī′ă-zīd) A diuretic of the benzothiazide group. The drug also lowers blood pressure in hypertensive patients. Trade name is Anhydron.

**cyclotomy** (sī-klŏt′ō-mē) [″ + *tome,* incision] Surgical incision of the ciliary muscle of the eye.

**cyclotron** (sī′klō-trŏn) A particle accelerator in which the particle is rotated between magnets, gaining speed with each rotation.

**cyclotropia** (sī″klō-trō′pē-ă) Permanent cyclophoria.

**cyesis** (sī-ē′sĭs) [Gr. *kyesis*] Pregnancy.

**cylicotomy** (sĭl″ĭ-kŏt′ō-mē) [Gr. *kylix,* cup, + *tome,* incision] Cutting of the ciliary muscle.

**cylinder** (sĭl′ĭn-dĕr) [Gr. *kylindros*] A hollow, tube-shaped body.

***crossed c.'s*** Two cylindrical lenses at right angles to each other; used in diagnosing astigmatism.

***extension c.*** A hollow tube attached to the end of the collimator apparatus of an x-ray tube. It limits the size of the beam, decreasing scatter radiation and increasing detail.

***gas c.*** A high-pressure, nonreactive, seamless tempered steel container for compressed medical, therapeutic, or diagnostic gas.

***urinary c.'s*** Cylindrically shaped casts in the urine.

**cylindroadenoma** (sĭ-lĭn″drō-ăd″ē-nō′mă) [Gr. *kylindros,* cylinder, + *aden,* gland, + *oma,* tumor] An adenoma containing cylindrical masses of hyaline material.

**cylindroid** (sĭl-ĭn′droyd) [″ + *eidos,* form, shape] **1.** Cylinder-shaped. **2.** A mucous, spurious cast in urine; recognized by its twists and turns, varying markedly in diameter in different places, most frequently pointed at the ends and frequently crossing an entire field. It does not usually have cellular intrusions.

**cylindroma** (sĭl″ĭn-drō′mă) [″ + *oma,* tumor] A malignant tumor containing a collection of cells forming cylinders.

**cylindruria** (sĭl″ĭn-drū′rē-ă) [″ + *ouron,* urine] The presence of cylindroids in the urine.

**cymbocephalic** (sĭm″bō-sĕ-făl′ĭk) [Gr. *kymbe,* boat, + *kephale,* head] Having a boat-shaped head.

**cynanthropy** (sĭn-ăn′thrō-pē) [Gr. *kyon,* dog, + *anthropos,* man] Insanity in which the patient behaves like a dog.

**cynic spasm** [Gr. *kynikos,* doglike] Spasm of the facial muscles causing a grin or snarl like a dog. SYN: *risus sardonicus.*

**cynophobia** (sī″nō-fō′bē-ă) [″ + *phobos,* fear] **1.** Unreasonable fear of dogs. **2.** Morbid fear of rabies. SYN: *lyssophobia* (2).

**cypridophobia** (sĭp″rĭ-dō-fō′bē-ă) [Gr. *Kypris,* Venus, + *phobos,* fear] **1.** Morbid fear of venereal disease. **2.** Abnormal fear of the sexual act. **3.** False belief of having a venereal disease.

**cypriphobia** (sĭp-rĭ-fō′bē-ă) Morbid aversion to and fear of coitus.

**cyproheptadine hydrochloride** (sī″prō-hĕp′tă-dēn) An antiallergy drug that is also used in postgastrectomy dumping syndrome.

**cyrtosis** (sĭr-tō′sĭs) [″ + *osis,* condition] Any abnormal curvature of the spine. SEE: *kyphosis.*

**cyst-** SEE: *cysto-.*

**cyst** (sĭst) [Gr. *kystis,* bladder, sac] **1.** A closed sac or pouch, with a definite wall, that contains fluid, semifluid, or solid material. It is usually an abnormal structure resulting from developmental anomalies, obstruction of ducts, or parasitic infection. **2.** In biology, a structure formed by and enclosing certain organisms, in which they become inactive, as the cyst of certain protozoans or of the metacercariae of flukes.

***adventitious c.*** A cyst formed around a foreign body.

***alveolar c.*** Dilation and rupture of pulmonary alveoli to form air cysts.

***apical c.*** A cyst near the apex of the tooth root.

***blood c.*** Hematoma.

***blue dome c.*** A cyst close to the surface of the breast. The blue color is caused by bleeding into the cyst.

***branchial c.*** Cervical c.

***cervical c.*** A closed epithelial sac derived from a branchial groove of its corresponding pharyngeal pouch. SYN: *branchial c.*

***chocolate c.*** An ovarian cyst with darkly pigmented gelatinous contents.

***colloid c.*** A cyst with gelatinous contents.

***congenital c.*** A cyst present at birth resulting from abnormal development, as a dermoid cyst, imperfect closure of a structure as in spina bifida cystica, or nonclosure of embryonic clefts, ducts, or tubules, such as cervical cysts.

***daughter c.*** A cyst growing out of the walls of another cyst.

***dental c.*** A cyst that forms from any of the odontogenic tissues.

***dentigerous c.*** A fluid-filled cyst usually surrounding the crown of an unerupted tooth; often involves incomplete enamel formation. SYN: *eruption c.; follicular c.; follicular odontoma.* SEE: *dermoid c.*

***dermoid c.*** A cyst containing elements of hair, teeth, or skin. It occurs commonly in the ovary or testes and contains derivatives of all three germ layers.

***distention c.*** A cyst formed in a natural enclosed cavity, as a follicular cyst of the ovary.

***echinococcus c.*** Hydatid c.

***epidermal c.*** **1.** A cyst that forms in the skin due to the blockage of a pillosebaceous follicle. **2.** A cyst that contains epidermis.

***eruption c.*** Dentigerous c.

***extravasation c.*** A cyst arising from hemorrhage into tissues.

***exudation c.*** A cyst caused by trapping of an exudate in a closed area.

***follicular c.*** A cyst arising from a follicle, as a follicular cyst of the thyroid gland, the ovary, or a forming tooth. SYN: *dentigerous c.*

***Gartner's c.*** A cyst developing from a vestigial mesonephric duct (Gartner's duct) in a female.

***hydatid c.*** A cyst formed by the growth of the larval form of *Echinococcus granulosus,* usually in the liver. SYN: *echinococcus c.*

***implantation c.*** A cyst resulting from displacement of portions of the epidermis as may occur in injuries.

***intraligamentary c.*** A cystic formation between the layers of the broad ligament.

***involutional c.*** A cyst occurring in the normal involution of an organ or structure, as in the mammary gland.

***keratin c.*** A cyst containing keratin.

***meibomian c.*** Chalazion.

***meniscus c.*** A fluid-filled cyst often associated with a degenerative horizontal meniscal tear, more frequently seen in the lateral meniscus of the knee. This ganglion-like cyst is a palpable mass at the joint line of the knee and can be visualized by arthrography and magnetic resonance imaging.

***morgagnian c.*** A cystlike remnant of the müllerian duct that is attached to the fallopian tube.

***mother c.*** A hydatid cyst enveloping smaller ones.

***mucous c.*** A retention cyst composed of mucus.

***nabothian c.*** SEE: *nabothian cyst.*

***odontogenic c.*** A cyst associated with the teeth, such as a dentigerous or radicular cyst.

***ovarian c.*** A cyst in the ovary. SEE: *ovary.*

***parasitic c.*** A cyst enclosing the larval form of certain parasites, as the cysticercus or hydatid of tapeworms or the larva of certain nematodes (i.e., *Trichinella.*)

***parovarian c.*** A cyst of the parovarium.

***pilar c.*** An epithelial cyst with a wall that resembles the follicular epithelium. It is filled with a homogeneous mixture of keratin and lipid. SYN: *trichilemma c.*

***pilonidal c.*** A cyst in the sacrococcygeal region, usually at the upper end of the intergluteal cleft. It is due to a developmental defect that permits epithelial tissue to be trapped below the skin. This type of cyst may become symptomatic in early adulthood when an infected draining sinus forms. SYN: *pilonidal sinus.*

***porencephalic c.*** An anomalous cavity of the brain that communicates with the ventricular system.

***proliferative c.*** A cyst lined with epithelium that proliferates, forming projections that extend into the cavity of the cyst.

***radicular c.*** A granulomatous cyst located alongside the root of a tooth.

***retention c.*** A cyst retaining the secretion of a gland, as in a mucous or sebaceous cyst.

***sebaceous c.*** A cyst of a sebaceous gland.

***seminal c.*** A cyst of the epididymis, ductus deferens, or other sperm-carrying ducts that contain semen.

***suprasellar c.*** A cyst of the hypophyseal stalk just above the floor of the sella turcica. Its wall is frequently calcified or ossified.

***trichilemma c.*** Pilar c.

***tubo-ovarian c.*** An ovarian cyst that ruptures into the lumen of an adherent uterine tube.

***unilocular c.*** A cyst containing only one cavity.

***vaginal c.*** A cyst in the vagina.

***vitelline c.*** A congenital cyst of the gastrointestinal canal. Lined with ciliated epithelium, it is the remains of the omphalomesenteric duct.

**cystadenocarcinoma** (sĭs-tăd″ē-nō-kăr″sĭ-nō′mă) [Gr. *kystis,* bladder, + *aden,* gland, + *karkinos,* crab, + *oma,* tumor] A glandular malignancy that forms cysts as it grows.

**cystadenoma** (sĭst″ăd-ĕn-ō′mă) [″ + ″ + *oma,* tumor] An adenoma containing cysts; cystoma blended with adenoma.

***pseudomucinous c.*** A cyst filled with a thick, viscid fluid and lined with tall epithelial cells.

***serous c.*** A cyst filled with a clear serous fluid and lined with cuboidal epithelial cells.

**cystalgia** (sĭs-tăl′jē-ă) [″ + *algos,* pain] Pain in the bladder. SYN: *cystodynia.*

**cystathionine** (sĭs″tă-thī′ō-nīn) An intermediate compound in the metabolism of methionine to cysteine.

**cystathioninuria** (sĭs″tă-thī″ō-nī-nū′rē-ă) A hereditary disease caused by a deficiency of the enzyme important in metabolizing cystathionine, resulting in mental retardation, thrombocytopenia, and acidosis.

**cystectasy** (sĭs-tĕk′tă-sē) [″ + *ektasis,* dilatation] **1.** An operation for extracting calculus from the bladder by dividing the membranous portion of the urethra and then dilating the neck of the bladder. **2.** Dilatation of the bladder.

**cystectomy** (sĭs-tĕk′tō-mē) [″ + *ektome,* excision] **1.** Removal of a cyst. **2.** Excision of the cystic duct and the gallbladder, or just the cystic duct. **3.** Excision of the urinary bladder or a part of it.

**cysteic acid** Acid produced by the oxidation of cysteine. Further oxidation produces taurine.

**cysteine hydrochloride** (sĭs′tē-ĭn, sĭs-tē′ĭn) An amino acid, $C_3H_7NO_2S \cdot HCl \cdot H_2O$, containing sulfur and found in many proteins. It is valuable as a source of sulfur in metabolism.

**cystelcosis** (sĭs″tĕl-kō′sĭs) [″ + *helkosis,* ulceration] Ulceration of the urinary bladder.

**cystic** (sĭs′tĭk) [Gr. *kystis,* bladder] **1.** Of or pert. to a cyst. **2.** Pert. to the gallbladder. **3.** Pert. to the urinary bladder.

**cysticercoid** (sĭs″tĭ-sĕr′koyd) [″ + *kerkos,* tail, + *eidos,* form, shape] The larval encysted form of a tapeworm. It differs from a cysticercus in having a much reduced bladder.

**cysticercosis** (sĭs″tĭ-sĕr-kō′sĭs) [″ + ″ + *osis,* condition] Infestation with cysticerci (plural of cysticercus). This occurs when ingested *Taenia solium* larvae from uncooked pork burrow through the intestinal wall and are carried to other tissues. They may encyst in the heart, eye, muscles, or brain. In the brain, they may cause a wide variety of neurological symptoms. A patient history of eating habits (undercooked pork or other meats) may be helpful in establishing the diagnosis.

**cysticercus** (sĭs″tĭ-sĕr′kŭs) *pl.* **cysticerci** The encysted larval form of a tapeworm, consisting of a rounded cyst or bladder into which the scolex is invaginated. SYN: *bladder worm.*

***c. cellulosae*** The bladder worm that is the larva of the pork tapeworm, *Taenia solium.*

**cystic fibrosis** ABBR: CF. A single-gene defect manifesting in multiple body systems as chronic obstructive pulmonary disease, pancreatic exocrine deficiency, urogenital dysfunction, and abnormally high electrolyte concentration in the sweat. The name is derived from the characteristic histologic changes in the pancreas. CF usually begins in infancy and is the major cause of severe chronic lung disease in children. The etiology and primary defect of cystic fibrosis are unknown. In the U.S., CF occurs in 1 in 2500 white live births and 1 in 17,000 black live births. Also called *fibrocystic disease of pancreas.* SYN: *mucoviscidosis.*

SYMPTOMS: A great variety of clinical manifestations may be present, including nasal polyposis; bronchiectasis; bronchitis; pneumonia; respiratory failure; gallbladder diseases; intussusception; meconium ileus; salt depletion; pancreatic exocrine deficiency causing intestinal malabsorption of fats, proteins, and, to a lesser extent, carbohydrates; pancreatitis; peptic ulcer; rectal prolapse; diabetes; nutritional deficiencies; arthritis; absent vas deferens with consequent aspermia and absence of fructose in the ejaculate; failure to thrive; and delayed puberty.

TREATMENT: Therapy must be individualized, carefully monitored, and continued throughout the life span. High doses of ibuprofen taken consistently for years slows the progression of the disease without serious adverse effects. Pulmonary disease is controlled with antibiotics. It is essential that secretions be cleaned from the airway by intermittent aerosol therapy with a mixture of phenylephrine, propylene glycol, and saline. A mucolytic agent such as *N*-acetylcysteine may be helpful, as well as postural drainage, mist inhalation, and bronchodilator therapy. Bronchoalveolar lavage has been of use in some patients. In addition, bronchial drainage may be improved by use of aerosolized recombinant human DNase (rhDNase). Use of a Flutter device for airway mucus clearance is considerably more effective in increasing sputum expectoration than traditional postural drainage and clapping the chest. Lung transplantation may also be used to treat CF. SEE: *bronchoalveolar lavage; Flutter device.*

PROGNOSIS: Median cumulative survival is approximately 30 years, with males surviving much longer than females for unknown reasons.

NURSING IMPLICATIONS: Both patient and family are taught to perform pulmonary chest physiotherapy followed by deep breathing and coughing to help mobilize secretions. Fluid intake is encouraged to thin inspissated secretions. Humidified air, with intermittent positive-pressure breathing therapy if prescribed, is provided; and prescribed pancreatic enzyme replacement is administered with meals and snacks. Dornase alpha is also administered by nebulizer as prescribed. A DNA enzyme produced by recombinant gene therapy, the drug is used to reduce the frequency of respiratory infections, to decrease sputum viscosity, and to improve pulmonary functioning in patients with this condition.

The patient should take precautions to prevent respiratory infections, and should learn to recognize and report signs and symptoms, and to initiate prescribed antibiotic prophylaxis promptly. A well-balanced high-calorie, high-protein diet is recommended, including replacement of fat-soluble vitamins if laboratory analysis indicates any deficiencies. Aerobic exercise and physical activity within permitted limits are encouraged; breathing exercises should be performed during activity to improve ventilatory capacity and activity tolerance. The child is encouraged in age-appropriate developmental tasks, and acceptable activities are substituted for those in which the child is unable to participate.

The nurse involves the child in care by offering valid choices and encouraging decision making. The family is encouraged to discuss their feelings and concerns. Genetic testing is explained. Realistic reassurance is offered regarding expectations after an exacerbation, and emotional support is provided to help both patient and family work through feelings of anticipatory grief. Referral is made to available local chapters of support groups such as the Cystic Fibrosis Foundation. SEE: *Nursing Diagnoses Appendix.*

**cysticotomy** (sĭs″tĭ-kŏt′ō-mē) [″ + *tome,* incision] Incision of cystic bile duct. SYN: *choledochotomy.*

**cystiform** (sĭs′tĭ-form) [″ + L. *forma,* form] Having the form of a cyst.

**cystigerous** (sĭs-tĭj′ĕr-ŭs) [″ + L. *gerere,* to bear] Containing cysts.

**cystine** (sĭs′tēn) [Gr. *kystis,* bladder] $C_6H_{12}N_2S_2O_4$. A sulfur-containing amino acid, produced by the action of acids on proteins that contain this compound. It is an important source of sulfur in metabolism.

**cystinemia** (sĭs″tĭ-nē′mē-ă) [*cystine* + Gr. *haima,* blood] The presence of cystine in blood.

**cystinosis** (sĭs′tĭ-nō′sĭs) [″ + Gr. *osis,* condition] An inherited disease of cystine metabolism resulting in abnormal deposition of cystine in body tissues. The cause is disordered proximal renal tubular function. Clinically, failure to grow is accompanied by the development of rickets, corneal opacities, acidosis, and deposition of cystine in tissues. SYN: *cystine storage disease.*

**cystinuria** (sĭs″tĭ-nū′rē-ă) [″ + *ouron,* urine] **1.** The presence of cystine in urine. **2.** A hereditary metabolic disorder characterized by excretion of large amounts of cystine, lysine, arginine, and ornithine in the urine. It results in the development of recurrent urinary calculi.

**cystitis** (sĭs-tī′tĭs) [Gr. *kystis,* bladder, + *itis,* inflammation] Inflammation of the bladder usually occurring secondary to ascending urinary tract infections. Associated organs (kidney, prostate, urethra) may be involved. This condition may be acute or chronic. SEE: *Nursing Diagnoses Appendix.*

SYMPTOMS: Frequent painful urination characterizes acute cystitis. Chronic cystitis occurs secondary to some other lesion with possibly pyuria as the only symptom.

TREATMENT: Antibiotics are useful in treating the infection, but more definitive therapy is required if the basic cause is a renal calculus or a structural defect in the urinary tract such as obstruction.

NURSING IMPLICATIONS: The patient is assessed for pain, burning, urinary frequency, bladder spasms, chills, and fever, and the urinary bladder is palpated and percussed for distention. Volume and frequency of urinary output are monitored, and urine is inspected for cloudiness and gross hematuria. A clean-catch specimen is sent to the laboratory for urinalysis and culture and sensitivity tests. Oral fluid intake is encouraged to dilute urine and to decrease pain on voiding. Heat is applied to the lower abdomen to decrease bladder spasms. Prescribed urinary antiseptics, analgesics, and antibiotics are administered and evaluated for therapeutic effectiveness and any adverse reactions. The patient is warned that prescribed urinary antiseptics such as phenazopyridine hydrochloride (Pyridium) will color the urine reddish orange and may stain fabric. The importance of follow-up urinalysis and culture testing to ensure that the cause of cystitis has been eliminated, and is not just quiescent, is emphasized.

***interstitial c.*** A chronically irritable and painful inflammatory bladder condition of unknown etiology that is poorly understood and for which there is no agreed upon definition. Most commonly, the disease is seen in women 30 to 70 years of age. The disease is not life-threatening, but the pain can make a patient's life intolerable. Hunner's ulcer of the bladder is thought to have the same pathological basis as this disease and, if present, confirms the diagnosis. The most common symptoms are urinary frequency, nocturia, and suprapubic pain on bladder filling. There is no curative therapy but hydraulic distention of the bladder and intravesical installation of dimethyl sulfoxide have been used. If these fail, the tricyclic antidepressant amitriptyline has been beneficial. Transcutaneous electrical nerve stimulation and intravesical heparin instillation have also been used.

**cystitome** (sĭs′tĭ-tōm) [″ + *tome,* incision] Instrument for incision into the sac of the crystalline lens.

**cystitomy** (sĭs-tĭt′ō-mē) **1.** Surgical incision of a cavity. **2.** Incision of the capsule of the crystalline lens. **3.** Incision into the gallbladder. SYN: *cholecystotomy.*

**cysto-, cyst-** [Gr. *kystis,* bladder] Combining form denoting a relationship to the urinary bladder or a cyst.

**cystoadenoma** (sĭs″tō-ăd″ĕ-nō′mă) [″ + *aden,* gland, + *oma,* tumor] A tumor containing cystic and adenomatous elements.

**cystocele** (sĭs′tō-sēl) [″ + *kele,* tumor, swelling] A bladder hernia that protrudes into the vagina. Injury to the vesicovaginal fascia during delivery may allow the bladder to pouch into the vagina, causing a cystocele. It may cause urinary frequency, urgency, and dysuria. SYN: *vesicocele.*

**cystocolostomy** (sĭs″tō-kō-lŏs′tō-mē) [″ + *kolon,* colon, + *stoma,* mouth] Formation of communication between the gallbladder and colon.

**cystodiaphanoscopy** (sĭs″tō-dī″ă-făn-ŏs′kō-pē) [″ + *dia,* through, + *phanein,* to shine, + *skopein,* to examine] Transillumination of the abdomen by an electric light in the bladder.

**cystodynia** (sĭs″tō-dĭn′ē-ă) [″ + *odyne,* pain] Cystalgia.

**cystoelytroplasty** (sĭs″tō-ē-lĭt′rō-plăs-tē) [″ + *elytron,* sheath, + *plassein,* to form] Repair of a vesicovaginal fistula.

**cystoepiplocele** (sĭs″tō-ē-pĭp′lō-sēl) [″ + *epiploon,* omentum, + *kele,* tumor, swelling]

Herniation of a portion of the bladder and the omentum.

**cystoepithelioma** (sĭs″tō-ĕp″ĭ-thē″lē-ō′mă) [″ + *epi,* upon, + *thele,* nipple, + *oma,* tumor] Epithelioma in the stage of cystic degeneration.

**cystofibroma** (sĭs″tō-fī-brō′mă) [″ + L. *fibra,* fiber, + Gr. *oma,* tumor] Fibrous tumor containing cysts.

**cystogastrostomy** (sĭs″tō-găs-trŏs′tō-mē) [″ + *gaster,* stomach, + *stoma,* mouth] Joining an adjacent cyst, usually of the pancreas, to the stomach.

**cystogram** (sĭs′tō-grăm) [″ + *gramma,* something written] A radiograph of the bladder.

**cystography** (sĭs-tŏg′ră-fē) [″ + *graphein,* to write] Radiography of any cyst into which a contrast medium has been instilled, esp. the bladder.

**cystoid** (sĭs′toyd) [″ + *eidos,* form, shape] Resembling a cyst.

**cystojejunostomy** (sĭs″tō-jē-jū-nŏs′tō-mē) [″ + L. *jejunum,* empty, + Gr. *stoma,* mouth] Joining of an adjacent cyst to the jejunum.

**cystolith** (sĭs′tō-lĭth) [″ + *lithos,* stone] A vesical calculus.

**cystolithectomy** (sĭs-tō-lĭ-thĕk′tō-mē) [″ + *lithos,* stone, + *ektome,* excision] Excision of a stone from the bladder.

**cystolithiasis** (sĭs-tō-lĭ-thī′ă-sĭs) [Gr. *kystis,* bladder, + *lithos,* stone, + *-iasis,* condition] Formation of calculi in the bladder.

**cystolithic** (sĭs″tō-lĭth′ĭk) Pert. to a vesical calculus.

**cystolutein** (sĭs″tō-loo′tē-ĭn) [″ + L. *luteus,* yellow] Yellow pigment found in some ovarian cysts.

**cystoma** (sĭs-tō′mă) *pl.* **cystomata, cystomas** [″ + *oma,* tumor] A cystic tumor; a growth containing cysts.

**cystometer** (sĭs-tŏm′ĕ-tĕr) [″ + *metron,* measure] A device for estimating the capacity of the bladder and pressure changes in it during micturition.

**cystometrography** (sĭs″tō-mĕ-trŏg′ră-fē) [″ + ″ + *graphein,* to write] A graphic record of the pressure in the bladder at varying stages of filling.

**cystomorphous** (sĭs″tō-mor′fŭs) [″ + *morphe,* form] Cystlike; cystoid.

**cystopexy** (sĭs′tō-pĕk″sē) [″ + *pexis,* fixation] Surgical fixation of the bladder to the wall of the abdomen.

**cystoplasty** (sĭs′tō-plăs″tē) [″ + *plassein,* to form] Plastic operation on the bladder.

**cystoplegia** (sĭs″tō-plē′jē-ă) [″ + *plege,* stroke] Paralysis of the bladder.

**cystoproctostomy** (sĭs″tō-prŏk-tŏs′tō-mē) [″ + *proktos,* rectum, + *stoma,* mouth] Surgical formation of a connection between the urinary bladder and the rectum.

**cystoptosia, cystoptosis** (sĭs″tŏp-tō′sē-ă, -sĭs) [″ + *ptosis,* a dropping] Prolapse into the urethra of the vesical mucous membrane.

**cystoradiography** (sĭs″tō-rā″dē-ŏg′ră-fē) [″ + L. *radius,* ray, + Gr. *graphein,* to write] Radiography of the gallbladder or urinary bladder.

**cystorrhaphy** (sĭst-or′ă-fē) [″ + *rhaphe,* seam, ridge] Surgical suture of the bladder.

**cystorrhea** (sĭs″tō-rē′ă) [″ + *rhoia,* flow] A discharge of mucus from the urinary bladder.

**cystorrhexis** [″ + *rhexis,* rupture] Rupture of the bladder.

**cystosarcoma** (sĭs″tō-săr-kō′mă) [″ + *sarx,* flesh, + *oma,* tumor] A sarcoma containing cysts or cystic formations.

**cystoscope** (sĭst′ō-skōp) [″ + *skopein,* to examine] An instrument for interior examination of bladder and ureter. It is introduced through the urethra into the bladder.

**cystoscopy** (sĭs-tŏs′kō-pē) [″ + *skopein,* to examine] Examination of the bladder with a cystoscope.

**cystospasm** (sĭs′tō-spăzm) [Gr. *kystis,* bladder, + *spasmos,* a convulsion] A spasmodic contraction of the urinary bladder.

**cystostomy** (sĭs-tŏs′tō-mē) [″ + *stoma,* mouth] Surgical incision into the bladder.

**cystotome** (sĭs′tō-tōm) [″ + *tome,* incision] An instrument for incision of the bladder.

**cystotomy** (sĭs-tŏt′ō-mē) [″ + *tome,* incision] Incision of the bladder.

***suprapubic c.*** Surgical opening of the bladder from just above the symphysis pubis.

**cystotrachelotomy** (sĭs″tō-trā″kē-lŏt′ō-mē) [″ + *trachelos,* neck, + *tome,* incision] Incision into the neck of the bladder.

**cystoureteritis** (sĭs″tō-ū-rē″tĕr-ī′tĭs) [″ + *oureter,* ureter, + *itis,* inflammation] Inflammation of the ureter and urinary bladder.

**cystoureterogram** (sĭs″tō-ū-rē′tĕr-ō-grăm) [″ + ″ + *gramma,* something written] A radiograph of the bladder and ureter obtained after instillation of a contrast medium.

**cystourethritis** (sĭs″tō-ū″rē-thrī′tĭs) [″ + *ourethra,* urethra, + *itis,* inflammation] Inflammation of the urinary bladder and urethra.

**cystourethrocele** (sĭs″tō-ū-rē′thrō-sēl) [″ + ″ + *kele,* tumor, swelling] Prolapse of the bladder and urethra of the female.

**cystourethrography** (sĭs″tō-ū-rē-thrŏg′ră-fē) [″ + ″ + *graphein,* to write] Radiography of the bladder and urethra by use of a radiopaque contrast medium.

***chain c.*** Radiography in which a sterile beaded radiopaque chain is introduced into the bladder by means of a special catheter so that one end of the chain is in the bladder and the other extends outside via the urethra. This examination is useful in demonstrating anatomical relationships, esp. in women with persistent urinary incontinence.

***voiding c.*** Cystourethrography done before, during, and after voiding.

**cystourethropexy, retropubic** A general term for a surgical procedure for correction of stress urinary incontinence.

**cystourethroscope** (sĭs″tō-ū-rē′thrō-skōp) [″ + *ourethra,* urethra, + *skopein,* to examine] A device for examining the posterior urethra and urinary bladder.

**cystovesiculography** (sĭs″tō-vĕ-sĭk-ū-lŏg′ră-fē) Radiography of the bladder and seminal vesicles after instillation of a contrast medium.

**cyt-** SEE: *cyto-.*

**cytarabine** (sī-tăr′ă-bēn) A drug originally developed as an antileukemic agent and now used in treating herpesvirus hominis infections that cause either keratitis or encephalitis. Trade name is Cytosar-U. SYN: *cytosine arabinoside; ara-C.* SEE: *ara-A.*

**-cyte** (sīt) [Gr. *kytos,* cell] Suffix denoting cell.

**cytidine** (sī′tĭ-dĭn) A nucleoside that is one of the four main riboside components of ribonucleic acid. It consists of a cytosine and D-ribose.

**cyto-, cyt-** [Gr. *kytos,* cell] Combining form meaning *cell.*

**cytoanalyzer** (sī″tō-ăn″ă-lī′zĕr) A device for detecting malignant cells in microscopic preparations or in fluids. The technique has not been perfected.

**cytoarchitectonic** (sī″tō-ărk″ĭ-tĕk-tŏn′ĭk) [″ + *architektonike,* architecture] Pert. to structure and arrangement of cells.

**cytobiology** (sī″tō-bī-ŏl′ō-jē) [″ + *bios,* life, + *logos,* word, reason] Biology of cells.

**cytobiotaxis** (sī″tō-bī-ō-tăk′sĭs) [″ + ″ + *taxis,* arrangement] The influence of living cells on other living cells. SYN: *cytoclesis.*

**cytoblast** (sī′tō-blăst) [″ + *blastos,* germ] A cell nucleus. SEE: *cyton.*

**cytocentrum** (sī″tō-sĕn′trŭm) [″ + *kentron,* center] A minute body in the cytoplasm of a cell close to the nucleus. SYN: *centrosome.* SEE: *sphere, attraction.*

**cytochalasin B** (sī″tō-kăl′ă-sĭn) A substance that destroys the contractile microfilaments in cells. This fragments cells and permits the fragments to be investigated.

**cytochemistry** (sī″tō-kĕm′ĭs-trē) The chemistry of the living cell.

**cytochrome** (sī′tō-krōm) [″ + *chroma,* color] An iron-containing protein found in the mitochondria of eukaryotic cells; they are given letter names (a, b, c). The cytochrome transport system (electron transport chain) is the last stage in aerobic cell respiration. SEE: *c. oxidase; c. P450; chain, electron transport.*

***c. oxidase*** An enzyme complex of two cytochromes and two copper atoms found in the mitochondria of eukaryotic cells; part of the electron transport chain, the last stage of aerobic cell respiration. It transfers electrons to oxygen which then combines with hydrogen to form metabolic water. SEE: *chain, electron transport.*

***c. P450*** A group of enzymes, called hemethiolate protein P450, present in every type of cell in the body except red blood cells and skeletal muscle cells. They are important in metabolizing substances normally present in the body such as steroids, fat-soluble vitamins, fatty acids, prostaglandins, and alkaloids. The P450 enzymes also detoxify a great number of environmental pollutants such as carcinogens present in tobacco smoke and charcoal-broiled meat, polychlorinated biphenyls, and dioxin. Specialized types of cytochrome P450 are involved in the synthesis of nitric oxide.

**cytochylema** (sī″tō-kī-lē′mă) [Gr. *kytos,* cell, + *chylos,* juice] Hyaloplasm.

**cytocidal** (sī″tō-sī′dăl) [″ + L. *caedere,* to kill] Lethal to cells.

**cytocide** (sī′tō-sīd) An agent that kills cells.

**cytoclasis** (sī″tŏk′lă-sĭs) [″ + *klasis,* destruction] Destruction of cells.

**cytoclastic** [″ + *klasis,* destruction] Destructive to cells.

**cytoclesis** (sī″tō-klē′sĭs) [″ + *klesis,* a call] Cytobiotaxis.

**cytodendrite** (sī″tō-dĕn′drīt) [″ + *dendron,* tree] A dendrite given off from the body of a nerve cell.

**cytodiagnosis** (sī″tō-dī″ăg-nō′sĭs) [″ + *dia,* through, + *gignoskein,* to know] Diagnosis of pathogenic conditions by the study of cells present in exudates, fluids, and so forth.

**cytodieresis** (sī″tō-dī-ĕr′ē-sĭs) [″ + *diairesis,* division] Cytokinesis.

**cytodistal** (sī″tō-dĭs′tăl) [″ + *distare,* to be distant] Pert. to a neoplasm remote from the cell of origin.

**cytogenesis** (sī″tō-jĕn′ĕs-ĭs) [″ + *genesis,* generation, birth] Origin and development of the cell.

**cytogenetics** (sī″tō-jĕ-nĕt′ĭks) The study of cytology in relation to genetics, esp. the study of chromosomal behavior in mitosis and meiosis. Modern cytogenetics has led to the identification of chromosomes as bearers of the genes and deoxyribonucleic acid (DNA) as the key molecule of the gene. The diagnosis of fetal abnormalities can be made as early as 11 to 14 weeks of gestation by using cytogenetic technique applied to cells from the amniotic fluid or placenta. SEE: *amniocentesis; chorionic villus sampling.*

**cytogenic** (sī-tō-jĕn′ĭk) [″ + *gennan,* to produce] Producing cells or promoting the production of cells.

**cytogenous** (si-tŏj′ĕn-ŭs) [″ + *gennan,* to produce] Producing cells.

**cytogeny** (sī-tŏj′ĕ-nē) [″ + *genesis,* generation, birth] The formation and development of the cell.

**cytogerontology** The study of cell aging developed by Leonard Hayflick.

**cytoglycopenia** (sī″tō-glī-kō-pē′nē-ă) [″ + *glykys,* sweet, + *penia,* poverty] Deficient glucose of blood cells; also called cytoglucopenia.

**cytohistogenesis** (sī″tō-hĭs″tō-jĕn′ĕ-sĭs) [″ + *histos,* web, + *genesis,* generation, birth] The structural development of cells.

**cytohyaloplasm** (sī″tō-hī′ăl-ō-plăzm) [″ + *hyalos,* glass, + LL. *plasma,* form, mold] Hyaloplasm.

**cytoid** (sī′toyd) [″ + *eidos,* form, shape] Resembling a cell.

**cytoinhibition** (sī″tō-ĭn″hĭ-bĭsh′ŭn) [″ + L. *inhibere,* to restrain] Phagocytic cell action that prevents the destruction of ingested bacteria by the cell.

**cytokine** One of more than 100 distinct proteins produced primarily by white blood cells. They provide signals to regulate immunological aspects of cell growth and function during both inflammation and specific immune response. Each cytokine is secreted by a specific cell in response to a specific stimulus. Cytokines produced by monocytes or macrophages and lymphocytes are called monokines and lymphokines, respectively. Cytokines include the interleukins, interferons, tumor necrosis factors, erythropoietin, and colony-stimulating factors. They act by changing the cells that produce them (autocrine effect), and altering other cells close to them (paracrine effect); a few affect cells systemically (endocrine effect). SEE: *granulocyte-macrophage colony-stimulating factor; immune response; inflammation; interferon; interleukin; macrophage; tumor necrosis factor.*

**cytokinesis** (sī″tō-kĭ-nē′sĭs) [″ + *kinesis,* movement] The separation of the cytoplasm into two parts, which occurs in the latter stages of mitosis or cell division. SYN: *cytodieresis.*

**cytologist** A person trained in cytology.

**cytology** (sī-tŏl′ō-jē) [″ + *logos,* word, reason] The science that deals with the formation, structure, and function of cells.

**cytolymph** (sī′tō-lĭmf) [″ + L. *lympha,* lymph] Hyaloplasm.

**cytolysin** (sī-tŏl′ĭ-sĭn) [″ + *lysis,* dissolution] An antibody that causes disintegration of cells.

**cytolysis** (sī-tŏl′ĭ-sĭs) Dissolution or destruction of living cells. Hemolysis is used in the case of red blood corpuscles, and bacteriolysis for bacteria.

**cytomegalic inclusion disease** A disease, esp. of the neonatal period, caused by cytomegalovirus (CMV) and characterized by variable severity ranging from an asymptomatic infection with no sequelae to a disease with fever, hepatosplenomegaly, microcephaly, and, in neonates, mental or motor retardation and perhaps death. About four out of five persons over age 35 have been infected with CMV, usually during childhood or early adulthood. In most, the disease is so mild that it is overlooked; however, CMV can be devastating to a fetus or to an immunosuppressed individual. The disease can occur congenitally, postnatally, or later in life. The virus can produce a latent infection that may be subsequently activated by pregnancy, multiple blood transfusions, or immunosuppression therapy. There is no specific therapy. SEE: *ganciclovir; Nursing Diagnoses Appendix.*

NURSING IMPLICATIONS: An immunosuppressed patient is assessed for a history of mild, nonspecific clinical symptoms, such as fatigue, myalgia, and headache, although the patient may have no symptoms. The patient is also assessed for extensive organ involvement, for a nonproductive cough, dyspnea, and hypoxia (CMV pneumonia); for explosive, watery diarrhea (CMV colitis); for gastrointestinal bleeding (CMV ulcerative disease); and for blurred vision and scotoma, progressing to blindness in one or both eyes (CMV retinitis). Fever is a common finding.

The immunosuppressed patient with CMV mononucleosis may demonstrate 3 or more weeks of irregular high fever as the only symptom. Depending on the systems involved, tachypnea, shortness of breath, cyanosis, and nonproductive coughing (respiratory) or jaundice and spider angiomas (liver involvement) may be noted on inspection. In all CMV patients, palpation reveals splenomegaly and hepatomegaly.

Vital signs, esp. temperature, and intake and output are monitored and documented. The patient is assessed for signs of opportunistic infections. If the patient has splenomegaly, the patient is evaluated for signs of rupture and protected from excess activity and injury. If the patient has respiratory involvement, respiratory status is watched closely. If the patient has diarrhea, the number and characteristics of stools and signs and symptoms of fluid, electrolyte, and acid-base imbalances are noted.

Universal precautions should be instituted before contact is made with the patient's blood or other body fluids. Secretion precautions are esp. important for the infant known to be shedding CMV. Patients with CMV are urged to wash their hands thoroughly to help prevent contagion.

Prescribed medications such as ganciclovir or acyclovir, or foscarnet, along with medications prescribed to reduce symptoms, are administered and evaluated for desired effects and any adverse reactions. Nutritious meals are offered, and fluids increased to replace those lost if diarrhea is present. For the patient with respiratory involvement, oxygen is administered and assistance with ventilation is provided, as necessary, by positioning the patient in a semi-Fowler or sitting position. For the patient with impaired vision, a safe environment encourages optimal independence is provided, and both patient and family are instructed in providing this type of environment at home. These patients are also referred to community resources as appropriate.

Emotional support and counseling are provided to the parents of a child with severe CMV infection; assistance is provided to help them to find support systems and coordination of referrals to other health-care professionals.

Female health care workers trying to become pregnant should be advised to have CMV titers drawn to identify their risk of contracting the infection. (A Centers for Disease Control and Prevention study showed that 50% of pregnant women exposed to CMV also had fetal exposure, with 20% of the fetuses contracting the infection.) Immunosuppressed or pregnant patients are warned to avoid contact with any person who has confirmed or suspected CMV infection. The immunosuppressed patient who is CMV seronegative should wear or carry a medical identification tag with this information and should relay this information to any caregiver to prevent the possibility of receiving CMV-positive blood products.

**cytomegalovirus** (sī″tō-mĕg″ă-lō-vī′rŭs) A widely distributed species-specific herpesvirus; in humans, it inhabits the salivary glands and causes cytomegalic inclusion disease. A mother with a latent infection may transmit the virus to her fetus either transplacentally or at the time of birth. The virus may also be transmitted by blood transfusion. Although it is usually not harmful to those with functional immune systems, it may cause a fatal pneumonia in immunocompromised patients. Cytomegalovirus may infect the retinas and cause blindness in AIDS patients.

**cytometaplasia** (sī″tō-mĕt″ă-plā′zē-ă) [Gr. *kytos,* cell, + *metaplasis,* change] Change in form or function of cells.

**cytometer** (sī-tŏm′ĕ-ter) [″ + *metron,* measure] An instrument for counting and measuring cells.

***flow c.*** A device for measuring thousands of cells as they are forced one at a time through a focused light beam, usually a laser. Cells studied by this device need to be in an evenly dispersed suspension.

**cytometry** (sī-tŏm′ĕ-trē) The counting and measuring of cells.

***flow c.*** A sophisticated technique for analyzing individual cells passing through a detector system. In one method, the cells are tagged with a monoclonal antibody carrying a fluorescent label. They pass through the detector at about 10,000 cells per second. Flow cytometry has many clinical and research applications. These include analysis of cell size, structure, and viability; examination of DNA and RNA in the cells; determination of pH in the cells; and chromosome analysis. Flow cytometry is also used to determine the percentages of cells in various stages of development in a population, making it possible to estimate the extent or controllability of a malignant tumor. Monitoring the number of populations of T cells, B cells, and T helper and suppressor cells, and using that information to calculate the helper : suppressor ratio, assists in determining the patient's immune status. Flow cytometry has been used in monitoring survival of transplanted organs and tissues such as bone marrow. SEE: *cell sorting.*

**cytomicrosome** (sī-tō-mī′krō-sōm) [″ + *mikros,* small, + *soma,* body] One of the minute granules in the protoplasm (cytoplasm) of the cell.

**cytomitome** (sī″tō-mī′tōm) [″ + *mitos,* thread] Any part of the network of the cytoplasm.

**cytomorphology** (sī″tō-mor-fŏl′ō-jē) [″ + *morphe,* form, + *logos,* word, reason] The study of the structure of cells.

**cytomorphosis** (sī″tō-mor-fō′sĭs) [″ + ″ + *osis,* condition] The cellular transformations that a cell undergoes during its life.

**cyton** (sī′tŏn) [Gr. *kytos,* cell] **1.** A cell. **2.** The body of a nerve cell. SYN: *perikaryon.*

**cytopathic** (sī″tō-păth′ĭk) [″ + *pathos,* disease] **1.** Concerning pathological changes in a cell. **2.** Concerning the ability of an agent, esp. a virus, to injure or destroy a cell.

**cytopathogenic effect** (sī″tō-păth″ō-jĕn′ĭk) [″ + *pathos,* disease, + *gennan,* to produce] In tissue culture, the morphological changes seen in the cultured cells owing to the effect of some pathogenic agent such as a virus.

**cytopathology** (sī″tō-păth-ŏl′ō-jē) [″ + ″ + *logos,* word, reason] The study of the cellular changes in disease.

**cytopenia** [″ + *penia,* lack] Diminution of cellular elements in blood or other tissues.

**cytophagocytosis** (sī″tō-făg″ō-sī-tō′sĭs) [″ + *phagein,* to eat, + *kytos,* cell, + *osis,* condition] Cytophagy.

**cytophagy** (sī-tŏf′ă-jē) The destruction of other cells by phagocytes. SYN: *cytophagocytosis.*

**cytophotometry** SEE: *cytometry, flow.*

**cytophylaxis** (sī″tō-fī-lăk′sĭs) [″ + *phylaxis,* protection] The protection of cells against lysis.

**cytophyletic** (sī″tō-fī-lĕt′ĭk) [″ + *phyle,* tribe] Pert. to the genealogy of cells.

**cytophysics** (sī″tō-fĭz′ĭks) [″ + *physike,* (study of) nature] The physics of cellular activity.

**cytophysiology** (sī″tō-fĭz-ē-ŏl′ō-jē) [″ + *physis,* nature, + *logos,* word, reason] Physiology of the cell.

**cytoplasm** (sī′tō-plăzm) [″ + LL. *plasma,* form, mold, from Gr. *plassein,* to mold, spread out] The protoplasm of a cell outside the nucleus. SEE: *cell.*

**cytoplast** (sī′tō-plăst) The cytoplasm of a cell body as distinguished from the contents of the nucleus.

**cytoproximal** (sī″tō-prŏk′sĭ-măl) [″ + L. *proximus,* nearest] Pert. to the portion of an axon nearest to the cell body from which it originates.

**cytoreticulum** (sī″tō-rĕ-tĭk′ū-lŭm) [″ + L. *reticulum,* network] The fibrillar network supporting fluid of protoplasm.

**cytorrhyctes** (sī″tō-rĭk′tēz) [″ + *oryssein,* to dig] Inclusion bodies in cells. Composed of virus elementary bodies, they were once thought to be of protozoal origin.

**cytoscopy** (sī-tŏs′kō-pē) [″ + *skopein,* to examine] Microscopic examination of cells for purposes of diagnosis.

**cytosine** (sī′tō-sĭn) $C_4H_5N_3O$. A pyrimidine base that is part of DNA and RNA. In DNA it is paired with guanine.

***c. arabinoside*** Cytarabine.

**cytoskeleton** (sī″tō-skĕl′ĕ-tŏn) The internal structural framework of a cell consisting of three types of filaments: microfilaments, microtubules, and intermediate filaments. These form a dynamic framework for maintaining cell shape and allowing rapid changes in the three-dimensional structure of the cell.

**cytosol** (sī′tō-sŏl) Hyaloplasm.

**cytosome** (sī′tō-sōm) [″ + *soma,* body] The portion of a cell exclusive of the nucleus.

**cytostasis** (sī-tŏs′tă-sĭs) [Gr. *kytos,* cell, + *stasis,* standing still] Stasis of white blood corpuscles, as in the early stage of inflammation.

**cytostatic** (sī″tŏ-stăt′ĭk) [″ + *stasis,* standing still] Preventing the growth and proliferation of cells.

**cytotactic** (sī″tō-tăk′tĭk) Pert. to cytotaxia.

**cytotaxia, cytotaxis** (sī-tō-tăk′sē-ă, -sĭs) [″ + *taxis,* arrangement] Attraction or repulsion of cells for each other.

**cytotechnologist** A medical laboratory technologist who works under the supervision of a pathologist to examine cells in order to diagnose cancer or other diseases.

**cytotechnology** Microscopic examination of cells to identify abnormalities.

**cytotherapy** [″ + *therapeia,* treatment] **1.** Treatment by use of glandular extracts; organotherapy. **2.** Use of cytotoxic or cytolytic substances or serums in treating disease.

**cytothesis** (sī-tŏth′ĕ-sĭs) [″ + *thesis,* a placing] Restoration or repair of injured cells.

**cytotoxic** (sī″tō-tŏks′ĭk) Destructive to cells.

**cytotoxic agent** A chemical that destroys cells or prevents their multiplication. This group of compounds was developed for use in cancer chemotherapy. The ideal agent for such use should destroy the fast-growing cancer cells without injuring the normal cells of the body.

**cytotoxin** (sī″tō-tŏk′sĭn) [″ + *toxikon,* poison] An antibody or toxin that attacks the cells of particular organs. SEE: *endotoxin; erythrotoxin; exotoxin; leukocidin; lysis; neurotoxin.*

**cytotrophoblast** (sī″tō-trō′fō-blăst) [″ + *trophe,* nourishment, + *blastos,* germ] The thin inner layer of the trophoblast composed of cuboidal cells, the outer layer being the syntrophoblast. SYN: *Langhans' layer.*

**cytotropic** (sī″tō-trŏp′ĭk, -trōp′ĭk) [″ + *trope,* a turn] Having an affinity for cells.

**cytotropism** (sī-tŏt′rō-pĭzm) [″ + *trope,* a turn, + *-ismos,* condition] The movement of cells toward or away from a stimulus such as drugs, viruses, bacteria, or physical conditions such as heat or cold.

**Cytoxan** (sī-tŏk′săn) Trade name for cyclophosphamide.

**cytozoic** (sī″tō-zō′ĭk) [″ + *zoon,* animal] Living within or attached to a cell, as certain protozoa.

**cytozoon** (sī-tō-zō′ŏn) A protozoon that lives as an intracellular parasite.

**cyturia** (sī-tū′rē-ă) [Gr. *kytos,* cell, + *ouron,* urine] The presence of any kind of cells in the urine.

**Czermak's spaces** (chār′măks) [Johann Czermak, Ger. physiologist, 1828–1873] The interglobular spaces in dentin caused by failure of calcification. SYN: *space, interglobular.*

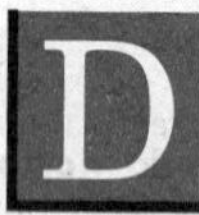

**Δ, δ** Upper- and lower-case delta, respectively, for the fourth letter of the Greek alphabet.

**D 1**. L. *da,* give; *date; daughter; deciduous;* L. *detur,* let it be given; *died; diopter; divorced; doctor.* **2.** Symbol for the element deuterium.

**D-** In biochemistry, a prefix indicating the structure of certain organic compounds with asymmetric carbon atoms. If a carbon atom is attached to four different substituent groups that can be arranged in two ways and represent nonsuperimposable mirror images, it is classed as asymmetrical. The name of such a compound is preceded by D. When there are only three dissimilar groups around the carbon atom, only one configuration in space is possible. The carbon atom is classed as symmetrical (or chiral), and the name is preceded by L.

In other chemical nomenclature, a lower-case *d-* or *l-* indicates the rotational direction of a polarized light shined through a solution of the compound. When the plane of the light is rotated to the right (i.e., is dextrorotatory), the compound's name is preceded by *d-*. When the light is rotated to the left (i.e., is levorotatory), the name is preceded by *l-*.

If a D compound that has an asymmetrical carbon can also rotate light and is dextrorotatory, its name is preceded by D(+); if levorotatory, D(−). If the asymmetrical carbon is of the L form and is dextrorotatory, its name is prefixed by L(+); if it is levorotatory, the name is preceded by L(−).

**d** *density;* L. *dexter* or *dextro,* right; L. *dies,* day; *distal; dorsal; duration.*

**2,4-D** Herbicide, 2,4-dichlorophenoxyacetic acid, that acts by stimulating broad-leaf plants to grow. It is toxic to humans and animals.

**D/A** *digital to analog.*

**Da** Symbol for dalton.

**daboia, daboya** (dă-boy′ă) Russell's viper, a large poisonous snake of India, Burma, and Thailand. Its venom is used to enhance the action of certain blood coagulation factors.

**dacarbazine** (dă-kăr′bă-zēn) An alkylating agent used in treating neoplasms including malignant melanoma and Hodgkin's disease.

**dacryadenalgia** (dăk″rē-ăd-ĕn-ăl′jē-ă) [Gr. *dakryon,* tear, + *aden,* gland, + *algos,* pain] Pain in a lacrimal gland. SYN: *dacryoadenalgia.*

**dacryadenitis** (dăk″rē-ăd-ĕ-nī′tĭs) [″ + ″ + *itis,* inflammation] Inflammation of a lacrimal gland.

**dacryadenoscirrhus** (dăk″rē-ăd″ĕn-ō-skĭr′us) [″ + ″+ *skirrhos,* hardening] Induration of a lacrimal gland.

**dacryagogatresia** (dăk″rē-ă-gŏg″ă-trē′sē-ă) [Gr. *dakryon,* tear, + *agogos,* leading, + *a-,* not, + *tresis,* perforate] Occlusion of a tear duct.

**dacryagogue** (dăk′rē-ă-gŏg) An agent that stimulates the secretion of tears.

**dacrycystalgia** (dăk″rē-sĭs-tăl′jē-ă) [″ + *kystis,* cyst, + *algos,* pain] Pain in a lacrimal sac. SYN: *dacryocystalgia.*

**dacryelcosis** (dăk″rē-ĕl-kō′sĭs) [″ + *helkosis,* ulceration] Ulceration of the lacrimal apparatus.

**dacryoadenalgia** (dăk″rē-ō-ăd″ĕn-ăl′jē-ă) [″ + *aden,* gland, + *algos,* pain] Pain in a lacrimal gland. SYN: *dacryadenalgia.*

**dacryoadenectomy** (dăk″rē-ō-ăd″ĕ-nĕk′tō-mē) [″ + ″ + *ektome,* excision] Surgical removal of a lacrimal gland.

**dacryoadenitis** (dăk″rē-ō-ăd″ĕn-ī′tĭs) [″ + ″ + *itis,* inflammation] Inflammation of a lacrimal gland. It is rare, seen as a complication in epidemic parotitis (mumps involving the lacrimal gland), and present in Mikulicz's disease. It may be acute or chronic.

**dacryoblennorrhea** (dăk″rē-ō-blĕn″ō-rē′ă) [″ + *blenna,* mucus, + *rhoia,* flow] Discharge of mucus from a lacrimal sac, and chronic inflammation of the sac.

**dacryocele** (dăk′rē-ō-sēl) [″ + *kele,* tumor, swelling] Protrusion of a lacrimal sac.

**dacryocyst** (dăk′rē-ō-sĭst) [″ + *kystis,* cyst] Lacrimal sac.

**dacryocystalgia** (dăk″rē-ō-sĭs-tăl′jē-ă) [″ + ″ + *algos,* pain] Pain in a lacrimal sac. SYN: *dacrycystalgia.*

**dacryocystectomy** (dăk″rē-ō-sĭs-tĕk′tō-mē) [″ + *kystis,* cyst, + *ektome,* excision] Excision of membranes of the lacrimal sac.

**dacryocystitis** (dăk″rē-ō-sĭs-tī′tĭs) [″ + ″ + *itis,* inflammation] Inflammation of a lacrimal sac involving mucous membrane of the sac with submucous membrane, which later extends to connective tissue, surrounding it with resulting cellulitis. It is usually secondary to prolonged obstruction of a nasolacrimal duct.

SYMPTOMS: The symptoms are profuse tearing (epiphora); redness and swelling in the area of a lacrimal sac, which may also extend to the lids and conjunctiva; pain, esp. on pressure over the sac; and overflow of tears.

TREATMENT: Hot compresses should be applied to the area. Appropriate topical and systemic antibiotic therapy depend on the organisms isolated from the inflamed area. The physician should incise and drain the sac if it is fluctuant; attempt to restore permeability of the duct with a probe when acute symptoms have subsided; and in chronic cases, extirpate the sac or perform an intranasal operation (dacryocystorhinostomy).

**dacryocystoblennorrhea** (dăk″rē-ō-sĭs″tō-blĕn-ō-rē′ă) [″ + ″ + *blenna,* mucus, + *rhoia,* flow] Chronic inflammation of and discharge from a lacrimal sac.

**dacryocystocele** (dăk″rē-ō-sĭs′tō-sēl) [Gr. *dakryon,* tear, + *kystis,* cyst, + *kele,* tumor, swelling] A herniated protrusion of a lacrimal sac.

**dacryocystography** (dăk″rē-ō-sĭs-tŏg′ră-fē) [″+ ″ + *graphein,* to write] Radiographic examination of the nasolacrimal drainage system after introduction of a contrast agent.

**dacryocystoptosis** (dăk″rē-ō-sĭs-tŏp-tō′sĭs) [″ + ″ + *ptosis,* a dropping] Prolapse of a lacrimal sac.

**dacryocystorhinostenosis** (dăk″rē-ō-sĭs″tō-rī-nō-stĕ-nō′sĭs) [″ + ″ + *rhis,* nose, + *stenosis,* act of narrowing] Narrowing or obliteration of the canal connecting a lacrimal sac with the nasal cavity. Patency is tested by placing a weak sugar solution in the conjunctival space. If the duct is patent, the patient will report a sweet taste in the mouth.

**dacryocystorhinostomy** (dăk″rē-ō-sĭs″tō-rī-nŏs′tō-mē) [″ + ″ + ″ + *stoma,* mouth] Surgical connecting of the lumen of a lacrimal sac with the nasal cavity.

**dacryocystorhinotomy** (dăk″rē-ō-sĭs″tō-rī-nŏt′ō-mē) [″ + ″ + ″+ *tome,* incision] Surgical probing of the duct leading from a lacrimal sac into the nose.

**dacryocystosyringotomy** (dăk″rē-ō-sĭs″tō-sĭr″ĭn-gŏt′ō-mē) [″ + *kystis,* cyst, + *syrinx,* tube, + *tome,* incision] A surgically created opening between a lacrimal sac and the nasal cavity.

**dacryocystotome** (dăk″rē-ō-sĭs′tō-tōm) [″ + ″ + *tome,* incision] A device for incision of a lacrimal sac.

**dacryocystotomy** (dăk″rē-ō-sĭs-tŏt′ō-mē) Incision of a lacrimal sac.

**dacryogenic** Promoting the shedding of tears.

**dacryohelcosis** (dăk″rē-ō-hĕl-kō′sĭs) [″ + *helcosis,* ulceration] Ulceration of a lacrimal sac or duct.

**dacryohemorrhea** (dăk″rē-ō-hĕm″ō-rē′ă) [″ + *haima,* blood, + *rhoia,* flow] Discharge of bloody tears.

**dacryolithiasis** (dăk″rē-ō-lĭ-thī′ă-sĭs) [″+ *lithiasis,* formation of stones] Presence of stones or calculi in the lacrimal apparatus.

**dacryoma** (dăk″rē-ō′mă) [″+ *oma,* tumor] **1.** A lacrimal tumor. **2.** A tumorlike swelling due to obstruction of the lacrimal duct.

**dacryon** (dăk′rē-ŏn) [Gr. *dakryon*] The lacrimal juncture point of the lacrimal, frontal, and upper maxillary bones.

**dacryopyorrhea** (dăk″rē-ō-pī″ō-rē′ă) [″ + *pyon,* pus, + *rhoia,* discharge] Discharge of pus from a lacrimal duct.

**dacryopyosis** [″ + *pyosis,* suppuration] Suppuration in a lacrimal sac or duct.

**dacryorrhea** (dăk″rē-ō-rē′ă) [″ + *rhoia,* flow] Excessive flow of tears.

**dacryosolenitis** (dăk″rē-ō-sō-lĕn-ī′tĭs) [″ + *solen,* duct, + *itis,* inflammation] Inflammation of a lacrimal or nasal duct.

**dacryostenosis** (dăk″rē-ō-stĕn-ō′sĭs) [″ + *stenosis,* act of narrowing] Obstruction or narrowing of a lacrimal or nasal duct.

**dacryosyrinx** (dăk″rē-ō-sī′rĭnks) [″ + *syrinx,* tube] A lacrimal fistula.

**dactinomycin** An antibiotic of the actinomycin complex used as an antineoplastic agent.

**dactyl** (dăk′tĭl) [Gr. *daktylos,* finger] A finger or toe; a digit of the hand or foot.

**dactyledema** (dăk″tĭl-ĕ-dē′mă) [″+ *oidema,* swelling] Edema of the fingers or toes.

**dactylion** Adhesions between or union of fingers or toes.

**dactylitis** [″ + *itis,* inflammation] Chronic inflammation of finger and toe bones in very young children, usually of tuberculous or syphilitic origin.

***sickle cell d.*** Painful swelling of the feet and hands during the first several years of life in children with sickle cell anemia.

**dactylogryposis** (dăk″tĭ-lō-grĭ-pō′sĭs) [″ + *gryposis,* curve] Permanent contraction of the fingers.

**dactylolysis** (dăk″tĭ-lŏl′ĭ-sĭs) [″ + *lysis,* dissolution] Spontaneous dropping off of fingers or toes, seen in leprosy and ainhum and sometimes produced in utero when a hair firmly wrapped around a digit causes amputation.

**dactylomegaly** (dăk″tĭ-lō-mĕg′ă-lē) [″ + *megas,* large] Abnormally large size of fingers and toes. SEE: *acromegaly.*

**dactylospasm** (dăk′tĭ-lō-spăzm) [″ + *spasmos,* a convulsion] Cramp of a finger or toe.

**dactylus** (dăk′tĭ-lŭs) [Gr. *daktylos*] A digit.

**dairy food substitute** A food resembling an existing dairy food in taste and appearance but differing in composition from the dairy food for which it is substituted.

**Dakin's solution** (dā′kĭns) [Henry D. Dakin, U.S. chemist, 1880–1952] A very neutral solution of sodium hypochlorite and boric acid. It was developed during World War I and is still used for cleansing wounds.

**Dale reaction** [Sir Henry H. Dale, 1875–1968, Brit. scientist and Nobel prize winner in 1936] A test result that demonstrates the ability of muscle tissues from an anaphylactic organism to contract on re-exposure to the antigen. Either guinea pig uterine muscle or intestine is used. The test is very specific, as unrelated antigens will not cause the sensitized muscle to contract. SYN: *Schultz reaction.*

**dalton** (dawl′tŏn) ABBR: Da. An arbitrary unit of mass equal to 1/12 the mass of carbon 12 or $1.657 \times 10^{-24}$ g.

**Dalton-Henry law** When a mixture of gases is in equilibrium with a liquid, each gas will dissolve in the liquid in proportion to its partial pressure in the gas.

**Dalton's law** [John Dalton, Brit. chemist, 1766–1844] A law that states that, in a mixture of gases, the total pressure is equal to the sum of the partial pressures of each gas.

**dam** A thin sheet of rubber used in dentistry and surgery to isolate a part from the surrounding tissues and fluids.

**damp 1.** Moist, humid. **2.** A noxious gas in a mine.

**damping** Steady diminution of the amplitude of successive vibrations, as of an electric wave or current.

**danazol** (dă'nă-zōl) A drug that suppresses the action of the anterior pituitary. It is used in treating endometriosis.

**dancing disease** In Europe during the Middle Ages, an epidemic dancing mania supposed to have been caused by the bite of the tarantula. SEE: *tarantism.*

**dancing mania** Epidemic chorea.

**D and C** *dilatation and curettage.*

**D and E** *dilation and evacuation* of the uterus. SEE: *dilation and curettage.*

**dander** (dăn'dĕr) Small scales from the hair or feathers of animals that may cause allergy in sensitive individuals.

**dandruff** Normal exfoliation of the epidermis of the scalp in the form of dry white scales. Several over-the-counter products, including salicylic acid, pyrithione zinc, sulfur, selenium sulfide, and coal tar, are approved for treating this condition.

**dandy fever** Dengue; an acute, epidemic, febrile disease occurring in tropical areas.

**Dandy-Walker syndrome** (dăn'dē-wawk'ĕr) [Walter E. Dandy, U.S. neurosurgeon, 1886–1946; Arthur E. Walker, U.S. surgeon, b. 1907] Congenital hydrocephalus caused by blockage of the foramina of Magendie and Luschka, through which the cerebrospinal fluid passes.

**Dane particle** [David S. Dane, contemporary Brit. virologist] A type of viral particle present in the serum of patients with hepatitis B. Dane particles contain DNA and are infectious.

**dantrolene sodium** (dăn'trō-lēn) A muscle relaxant used to relieve spasticity.

**Danysz phenomenon** [Jean Danysz, Polish-born pathologist in France, 1860–1928] A phenomenon that illustrates the reversibility of precipitation of antibody and antigen complexes. When a specified amount of diphtheria toxin is added all at once to an antitoxin serum, the mixture is nontoxic; but when the same quantity of toxin is added in portions at about 30-min intervals, the mixture is toxic.

**dapsone** (dăp'sōn) An antibacterial sulfone that was once the drug of choice for treatment of all forms of leprosy and is also used in the treatment of dermatitis herpetiformis. Frequent blood studies must be performed on patients receiving this drug for prolonged periods, as hemolysis, leukopenia, and methemoglobinemia can occur.

**Darier, Ferdinand Jean** (dăr-ē-ā') French dermatologist, 1856–1938.

***D.'s disease*** A rare hereditary condition characterized by verrucous papular growths that coalesce into plaques of various sizes on the scalp, face, neck, trunk, and axillae. SYN: *keratosis follicularis.*

***D.'s sign*** The skin change produced when the skin lesion in urticaria pigmentosa is rubbed briskly. The area usually begins to itch and becomes raised and surrounded by erythema. SEE: *mastocytosis; urticaria pigmentosa.*

**Darling's disease** (dăr'lĭngz) [Samuel Taylor Darling, U.S. pathologist, 1872–1925] Histoplasmosis.

**dartoid** (dăr'toyd) [Gr. *dartos,* skinned, + *eidos,* form, shape] Resembling the tunica dartos in its slow, involuntary contractions.

**dartos** [Gr.] The muscular, contractile tissue beneath the skin of the scrotum. SYN: *tunica dartos.*

**dartos muliebris** A veil-like smooth muscle just under the skin of the labia majora.

**dartos muscle reflex** Wormlike contraction of the dartos muscle following sudden cold application to the perineum.

**dartrous** [Gr. *dartos,* skinned] Of the nature of herpes; herpetic.

**darwinian ear** [Charles Robert Darwin, Brit. naturalist, 1809–1882]. An exaggeration of the darwinian tubercle.

**darwinian tubercle** [Charles Robert Darwin] A blunt point projecting from the upper part of the helix of the ear.

**darwinism** (dăr'wĭ-nĭzm) The theory of biological evolution through natural selection.

**Datura** (dā-tū'ră) A genus of plants, one member of which, *Datura stramonium,* contains constituents of hyoscyamine and scopolamine, which have anticholinergic properties.

**daughter** (daw'tĕr) **1.** The product of the decay of a radioactive element. **2.** A product of cell division, as a daughter cell or daughter nucleus. **3.** One's female child.

**daughter, DES** The daughter of a mother who received diethylstilbestrol (DES) during pregnancy. SEE: *DES syndrome; diethylstilbestrol.*

**daunorubicin hydrochloride** An antineoplastic drug used in treating acute leukemia.

**Davidsohn's sign** [Hermann Davidsohn, Ger. physician, 1842–1911] Lessening or absence of the pupillary light reflex when an electric light is held in the closed mouth. It indicates the presence of a tumor or fluid in the maxillary sinus.

**DAWN** *Drug Abuse Warning Network.*

**dawn phenomenon** A marked increase in insulin requirements between 6 A.M. and 9 A.M. as compared with the midnight to 6 A.M. period. The increased dose of insulin required during this period is in contrast to the Somogyi phenomenon, which is managed by decreasing insulin during the critical period. Dawn phenomenon may occur in persons with diabetes mellitus of either type and in some normal persons. SEE: *diabetes mellitus.*

**day blindness** Inability to see well in a bright light.

**day care center** A place for the care of preschool children both of whose parents are employed or for some other reason are unable to care for their child during normal working hours.

***adult d.c.c.*** A center for day care of adult patients. These centers provide supervised social, recreational, and health-related activities, usually in a group setting. The centers permit caregivers a respite and enable them to continue to work during the day.

**daydream** Mental musing or fantasy while awake.

**dazzle** Dimming of vision due to intense stimulus of very bright light. SEE: *glare.*

**dB, db** *decibel.*

**D.C.** *Doctor of Chiropractic; direct current.*

**d/c** *discontinue.*

**DCIS** *ductal carcinoma in situ.*

**DDD pacing** SEE: *pacemaker, cardiac, artificial.*

**D.D.S.** *Doctor of Dental Surgery.* SEE: *D.M.D.*

**DDT** Dichlorodiphenyltrichloroethane, now called chlorophenothane; a powerful insecticide effective against a wide variety of insects, esp. the flea, fly, louse, mosquito, bedbug, cockroach, Japanese beetle, and European corn borer. However, many species develop resistant populations, and birds and fish that feed on affected insects suffer toxic effects. In 1972, the U.S. banned DDT except for essential public health use and a few minor uses to protect crops for which there were no effective alternatives.

When ingested orally, it may cause acute poisoning. Symptoms are vomiting, numbness and partial paralysis of limbs, anorexia, tremors, and depression, resulting in death. SEE: *Poisons and Poisoning Appendix.*

**de-** [L. *de,* from] Prefix indicating *down* or *from.*

**deacidification** [″ + *acidus,* sour, + *facere,* to make] Neutralization of acidity.

**deactivation** [″ + *activus,* acting] The process of becoming or making inactive.

**dead** [AS. *dead*] Without life or life processes. SEE: *death.*

**deadman switch** A switch or control that requires continuous pressure by the operator.

**deadspace** The portion of the tidal volume not participating in gas exchange.

***alveolar d.*** The volume of gas in alveoli that are ventilated but not perfused with capillary blood.

***anatomical d.*** In pulmonary physiology, the air in the mouth, nose, pharynx, larynx, trachea, and bronchial tree at the end of inhalation. This is termed dead space because the air does not reach the alveoli and is not involved in gas exchange. One purpose of this space is to permit warming of very cold inhaled air before it comes in contact with the alveoli.

***mechanical d.*** The volume of gas exhaled into a tubing system and rebreathed on the subsequent breath.

***physiological d.*** The sum of anatomical and alveolar deadspace.

**dead tooth** A nonvital tooth by clinical standards, having had the pulp removed by endodontic treatment. The term is a poor choice because, if the periodontal tissues are healthy, the tooth will continue to function without symptoms.

**deaf** [AS. *deaf*] **1.** Partially or completely lacking the sense of hearing. **2.** Unwilling to listen; heedless.

**deafferentation** (dē-ăf″ĕr-ĕn-tā′shŭn) Cutting off of the afferent nerve supply. SEE: *denervation.*

**deaf-mute** A person who is unable to hear or speak.

**deaf-mutism** The state of being both deaf and unable to speak.

**deafness** [AS.] Complete or partial loss of the ability to hear. Some forms of conduction deafness may be remedied by a fenestration operation or stapes mobilization. SEE: *American Sign Language; otosclerosis.*

ETIOLOGY: Deafness may occur from several causes, such as injury or disease of the part of the cortex controlling the center for hearing; disease of the middle ear or the eighth cranial nerve; toxic effects of certain drugs; hysteria without any abnormality of the ear or brain; injury of the ear from loud noises such as the firing of a gun at close range, or prolonged and repetitive exposure to loud noise, whether in the workplace or in connection with a hobby done in a noisy environment.

NURSING IMPLICATIONS: Patients can prevent damage to hearing from excessively loud noises by wearing sound-muffling ear plugs or muffs when exposed to loud noise from any source, esp. industrial noise, and by recognizing that loud music can be as detrimental to hearing as the noise of a jackhammer. Patients should avoid cleaning inside the ears or putting sharp objects in the ears. Many antibiotics and chemotherapeutic drugs are ototoxic, and hearing should be evaluated continually when such drugs are used.

When interacting with a person with a hearing deficit, the nurse should make his or her presence known to the patient by sight or gentle touch before beginning to speak. If possible, background noise should be decreased or the patient removed from a noisy area before the nurse speaks. The nurse's face should be illuminated to facilitate the patient's visualization of the lips and expressions. The nurse faces directly to the patient's face or toward the ear with the best hearing and does not turn away while speaking. To facilitate lip reading, short words and simple sentences should be used and spoken clearly and distinctly in a normal tone and speed. Exaggerated mouthing of words or loud tones should be avoided. Placing a stethoscope in the patient's ears and speaking into the bell helps to cut out extraneous sounds and to direct words into the patient's ears. If the patient is literate, sign language or finger spelling may be used to communicate. Written information should be presented clearly and in large letters, esp. if the patient has poor visual acuity.

***acoustic trauma d.*** Impaired hearing due to repeated exposure to loud noise.

***aviator's d.*** A temporary or permanent nerve deafness found in some aviators. It is caused by prolonged exposure to loud noise.

***bass d.*** Inability to hear low-frequency tones.

***central d.*** Deafness resulting from lesions of the auditory tracts of the brain or the auditory centers of the cerebral cortex.

***cerebral d.*** Deafness due to a brain lesion.

***ceruminous d.*** Deafness due to plugs of cerumen (ear wax) blocking the ear canal.

***conduction d.*** Deafness resulting from any condition that prevents sound waves from being transmitted to the auditory receptors. It may result from wax obstructing the external auditory meatus, inflammation of the middle ear, ankylosis of the ear bones, or fixation of the footplate of the stirrup. SEE: *otosclerosis; Rinne test; Weber test.*

***cortical d.*** Deafness due to disease of the cortical centers without a lesion.

***high-frequency d.*** Inability to hear high-frequency sounds.

***hysterical d.*** Deafness that comes and goes in a hysterical patient.

***nerve d.*** Deafness due to a lesion of the auditory nerve or central neural pathways.

***occupational d.*** Deafness caused by working in places where noise levels are quite high. Persons working in such an environment should wear protective devices.

***ototoxic d.*** Hearing loss due to the toxic effect of certain chemicals or medicines on the eighth cranial nerve.

***perceptive d.*** Deafness resulting from lesions involving sensory receptors of the cochlea or fibers of the acoustic nerve, or a combination of these.

***psychic d.*** A condition in which auditory sensations are perceived but not comprehended.

***sensorineural d.*** Deafness due to defective function of the cochlea or acoustic nerve.

***tone d.*** Inability to distinguish musical sounds.

***word d.*** A form of aphasia in which sounds are heard but interpretation of the words is impossible.

**deamidase** (dē-ăm′ĭ-dās) An enzyme that splits amides to form carboxylic acid and ammonia.

**deamidization** (dē-ăm″ĭ-dĭ-zā′shŭn) The removal of an amide group by hydrolysis.

**deaminase** An enzyme that causes the removal of an amino group from organic compounds.

**deamination** Deaminization.

**deaminization** Loss of the $NH_2$ radical from amino compounds. Alanine can be deaminized to give ammonia and pyruvic acid: $CH_3CH(NH_2)COOH + OCH_3CO \cdot COOH + NH_3$. Deaminization may be simple, oxidative, or hydrolytic. Oxidizing enzymes are called deaminizing enzymes when the oxidation is accompanied by splitting off of amino groups. Deaminization is the first step in the use of amino acids in cell respiration; the $NH_2$ is converted to urea.

**dearterialization** (dē″ăr′tēr″ē-ăl-ī-zā′shŭn) [L. *de,* from, + Gr. *arteria,* artery] Changing of arterial into venous blood; deoxygenation.

**dearticulation** (dē″ăr-tĭk″ū-lā′shŭn) Dislocation of a joint.

**death** [AS. *death*] Permanent cessation of all vital functions; the loss of brainstem and spinal reflexes and flat electroencephalograms over at least 24 hr. The following definitions of death have also been considered: (1) Total irreversible cessation of cerebral function, spontaneous function of the respiratory system, and spontaneous function of the circulatory system. (2) Final and irreversible cessation of perceptible heartbeat and respiration. If any heartbeat or respiration can be perceived, with or without mechanical or electric aids, and regardless of how the heartbeat and respiration have been maintained, death has not occurred.

Conditions such as cardiac standstill or complete lack of renal function no longer means certain death. The use of cardiac pacemakers, artificial hearts and kidneys, heart transplants, and kidney transplants has made this definition of death untenable. SEE: *life.*

SIGNS: The principal sign of death is cessation of the heart's action. Other indications are absence of reflexes, cessation of electric activity in the brain as determined by electroencephalogram, manifestations of rigor mortis, and a mottled discoloration of the body, esp. over all parts where there is pressure. In case of an emergency, the usual symptoms of death often are found to be unreliable. Attempts at resuscitation should continue indefinitely. No harm can be caused by attempting to resuscitate a person who seems to be deceased; successes are numerous.

*Determining time lapse since death occurred:* The rectal temperature should be taken. In general the body loses 1°F each hour following death. Of course, the rate of heat loss varies with temperature of the surrounding air, water, or snow.

*Emotional aspects of dying:* Patients and their families rely on physicians to provide technical expertise when illness occurs. In addition, when the patient is dying, the patient and the family require emotional and physical support. The dying patient who is conscious needs to be touched and assured that the physician is providing all necessary care. SEE: *advance directive; choosing death; death investigation; "death with dignity"; donor card; do not attempt resuscitation; euthanasia; living will.*

NURSING IMPLICATIONS: Legal procedures and insitutional protocols should be followed concerning requests for organ donation. Appropriate health care professionals are notified of the patient's and family's wishes regarding organ donation. The time of cessation of respirations and heartbeat is documented, and the physician or other legally authorized health care professional is notified and requested to certify death. The family is notified according to insitutional policy, and emotional support is provided. Auxiliary equipment is removed, but the hospital identification bracelet is left in place. The body is cleansed, clean dressings are applied as necessary, and the rectum is packed with absorbent material to prevent drainage. The patient is placed in a supine position with the limbs extended and the head slightly elevated. Dentures are inserted, if appropriate, the mouth and eyes closed, and the body covered to the chin with a sheet.

The patient's belongings are collected and documented. Witnesses should be present, esp. if personal items have great sentimental or monetary value. The family is encouraged to visit, touch, and hold the patient's body as desired. In some situations (e.g., neonatal death, accidental death) and according to protocol, a photograph of the deceased is obtained to assist the family in grieving and remembering their loved one. The nurse and a family member sign for and remove the patient's belongings.

After the family has gone, the nurse prepares the body for the morgue by applying a chin strap, wrist and ankle protection and restraint, and shroud. Body tags, imprinted with the patient's identification plate or card information (name, identification number, room and bed number, attending physician), along with the date and time of death, are tied to the patient's foot or wrist as well as to the outside of the shroud. The body is then transported to the morgue and placed in a refrigerated unit according to protocol.

***biological d.*** Death due directly to natural causes.

***black d.*** Former name for bubonic plague.

***brain d.*** SEE: *brain death.*

***crib d.*** Sudden infant death syndrome.

***fetal d.*** Death of a fetus in utero.

***functional d.*** Central nervous system death with vital functions being artificially supported.

***good d.*** Death in which the rights of the individual have been respected, and during which the dying person was made as comfortable as possible and was in the company of persons he or she knew and loved. SEE: *advance directive; donor card; hospice; living will.*

***local d.*** Gangrene or necrosis of a part.

***man-made d.*** Death due to something other than natural causes (e.g., murder, war, political violence).

***molecular d.*** Death of cell life.

***sudden d.*** SEE: *sudden death.*

**deathbed statement** A declaration made at the time immediately preceding death. Such a statement, if made with the consciousness and belief that death is impending and in the presence of a witness, is legally considered as binding as a statement made under oath. SYN: *antemortem statement.*

**death investigation** The customary investigation of a violent, suspicious, or unexpected death, or of a death unattended by a physician. The investigation is, by law, done by an officially appointed person. The investigation system includes medical examiners, coroners, and combined medical examiner and coroner. The system used varies from state to state. SEE: *coroner; medical examiner.*

**death rate** The number of deaths occurring per 1000 of the population in a given area within a specified time. SYN: *mortality.*

**death rattle** A sound heard in the throat of a dying person, caused by the accumulation of mucus in the throat due to absence of the cough reflex. The breath moving through the mucus makes the "rattle" sound.

**death with dignity** Death that is allowed to occur in accordance with the wishes of a patient who might remain comatose for life. To prevent artificial prolongation of life, a patient, or the family if the patient is unconscious, may sign this statement: "I request that I be allowed to die and not be kept alive by artificial means or heroic measures. I ask also that drugs be mercifully administered to me to alleviate terminal suffering even if they may hasten the moment of death." SEE: *advance directive; assisted suicide; do not attempt resuscitation; "no code" orders.*

**debilitant** [L. *debilis,* weak] **1.** A remedy used to reduce excitement. **2.** Something that weakens.

**debilitate** To produce weakness or debility.

**debility** Weakness or lack of strength.

**débouchement** (dā-boosh-mŏn′) [Fr.] An opening or emptying into another part.

**Debove's membrane** (dĕ-bōvz′) [Georges Maurice Debove, Fr. physician, 1845–1920] A layer of connective tissue cells between the epithelium and basement tissue of respiratory and intestinal epithelia.

**débride** (dā-brēd′) [Fr.] To perform the action of debridement.

**débridement** (dā-brēd-mŏn′) [Fr.] The removal of foreign material and dead or damaged tissue, esp. in a wound.

***canal d., root canal d.*** The removal of organic and inorganic debris from a dental root canal by mechanical or chemical methods. This procedure is done in preparation for sealing the canal to prevent further decay of the tooth.

***enzymatic d.*** Use of proteolytic enzymes to remove dead tissue from a wound. The enzymes do not attack viable tissues.

***epithelial d.*** The removal of the entire epithelial lining or attachment epithelium from a periodontal pocket. SEE: *curettage.*

**debris** (dĕ-brē′) [Fr., remains] The remains of broken-down or damaged cells or tissue.

**debrisoquin** (dĕb-rĭs′ō-kwĭn) An antihypertensive medicine not generally available in the U.S.

**debt** (dĕt) Deficit.

***oxygen d.*** After strenuous (i.e., anaerobic) physical activity, the oxygen required (in addition to that required in the resting, or recovery, period) to oxidize the excess lactic acid produced and to replenish the depleted stores of adenosine triphosphate and phosphocreatine.

**debulking** The surgical procedure of removing a portion of a neoplasm when complete excision is not possible.

**deca-, dec-** [Gr. *deka*] Prefix indicating *ten.*

**decagram** (dĕk′ă″grăm) [Gr. *deka,* ten, + *gramma,* small weight] A weight of 10 g.

**decalcification** (dē″kăl-sĭ-fĭ-kā′shŭn) [L. *de,* from, + *calx,* lime, + *facere,* to make] The removal or withdrawal of calcium salts from bone or teeth.

**decalcify 1.** To soften bone through removal of calcium or its salts by acids. **2.** To remove the mineral content from bones or teeth so that sections can be cut and stained for microscopic examination.

**decaliter** (dĕk′ă-lē″tĕr) [Gr. *deka,* ten, + Fr. *litre,* liter] A measure of 10 L, equivalent to 10,000 ml, or about 10.57 qt. SEE: *deciliter.*

**decameter** (dĕk′ă-mē-tĕr) [Gr. *deka,* ten, + *metron,* measure] A measure of 10 m; 393.71 in.

**decannulation** (dē-kăn″nū-lā′shŭn) The removal of a cannula.

**decanormal** (dĕk″ă-nor′măl) [″ + L. *norma,* rule] Pert. to a solution 10 times as strong as one normal solution. It contains 10 gram-equivalent weights of the substance per liter. SEE: *normal.*

**decant** (dē-kănt′) [L. *de,* from, + *canthus,* rim of a vessel] To pour off liquid so the sediment remains in the bottom of the container.

**decantation** Gentle pouring off of a liquid so the sediment remains.

**decapitation** (dē-kăp″ĭ-tā′shŭn) [″ + *caput,* head] **1.** Separation of the head from the body; beheading. **2.** Separation of the head from the shaft of a bone.

**decapsulation** [″ + *capsula,* little box] Removal of a capsule of an organ.

**decarboxylase** (dē″kăr-bŏk′sĭ-lās) An enzyme that catalyzes the release of carbon dioxide from compounds such as amino acids.

**decarboxylation** (dē″kăr-bŏks-ĭ-lā′shŭn) A chemical reaction whereby the carboxyl group, —COOH, is removed from an organic compound.

**decarboxylization** (dē″kăr-bŏks-ĭ-lĭ-zā′shŭn) Decarboxylation.

**decavitamin capsule** (dĕk″ă-vī′tă-mĭn) A vitamin preparation that contains vitamins A, D, and C, calcium pantothenate, folic acid, niacinamide, pyridoxine hydrochloride (vitamin $B_6$), riboflavin, thiamine hydrochloride (vitamin $B_1$), a suitable form of alpha-tocopherol (vitamin E), and cyanocobalamin (vitamin $B_{12}$).

**decay** (dē-kā′) [″ + *cadere,* to fall, die] **1.** Gradual loss of vigor with physical and mental deterioration as in aging. SEE: *senility.* **2.** To waste away. **3.** Decomposition of organic matter by the action of microorganisms. SEE: *caries; cementoclasia.* **4.** Disintegration of radioactive substances.

***radioactive d.*** The continual loss of energy by radioactive substances. Disintegration of the nucleus by the emission of alpha, beta, or gamma rays eventually results in the complete loss of radioactivity. The time required for some materials to become stable may be minutes and, for others, thousands of years. SEE: *half-life.*

***tooth d.*** Caries.

**deceleration** (dē-sĕl″ĕ-rā′shŭn) **1.** A decrease in velocity. **2.** A fall in the baseline fetal heart rate as recorded by the fetal monitor.

*Early deceleration* coincides with contraction acme and reflects the fetal vagal response to head compression during uterine contractions. Normal baseline variability is evident throughout the interval between uterine contractions. *Late deceleration* occurs after contraction acme and reflects insufficient blood flow through the intervillous spaces of the placenta. *Variable deceleration* does not occur at any consistent point during contractions. The monitor record also exhibits different degrees and shapes. Variable deceleration indicates interference with blood flow through the umbilical vessels caused by cord compression.

**deceleration injury** A head injury in which the moving head hits a stationary object, such as a dancer hitting a wall.

**decerebrate** (dē-sĕr′ĕ-brāt) [″ + *cerebrum*, brain] **1.** To eliminate cerebral function by decerebration. **2.** A person or animal who has been subjected to decerebration.

**decerebrate posture** The posture of an individual with decerebrate rigidity. The extremities are stiff and extended, and the head is retracted.

**decerebration** (dē-sĕr-ĕ-brā′shŭn) Removal of the brain or cutting of the spinal cord at the level of the brainstem. SEE: *pithing.*

**dechlorination, dechloridation** [″ + Gr. *chloros*, green] Reduction in the amount of chlorides in the body by reduction of or withdrawal of salt in the diet.

**deci-** [L. *decimus*, tenth] Prefix indicating *one tenth.*

**decibel** (dĕs′ĭ-bĕl) [L. *decimus*, tenth, + *bel*, unit of sound] The unit for expressing logarithmically the pressure or power (and thus degree of intensity or loudness) of sound.

**decidophobia** [*decide* + Gr. *phobos*, fear] Fear of making a decision; an unofficial term.

**decidua** (dē-sĭd′ū-ă) [L. *deciduus*, falling off] The endometrium or lining of the uterus during pregnancy, and the tissue around the ectopically located fertilized ovum, e.g., in the fallopian tube or peritoneal cavity. The gland structures of the endometrium and the interstitial cells undergo marked hypertrophy. The decidua divides itself into an outer compact layer and an inner spongy layer. **decidual** (-ăl), *adj.*

***d. basalis*** The part of the decidua that unites with the chorion to form the placenta. SYN: *d. serotina.*

***d. capsularis*** The part of the decidua that surrounds the chorionic sac.

***d. menstrualis*** The layer of the uterine endometrium that is shed during menstruation.

***d. parietalis*** The endometrium during pregnancy except at the site of the implanted blastocyst.

***d. serotina*** D. basalis.

**deciduation** (dē-sĭd″ū-ā′shŭn) The loss of the decidua during menstruation.

**deciduitis** (dē-sĭd″ū-ī′tĭs) [″ + Gr. *itis*, inflammation] Inflammation of the decidua.

**deciduoma** (dē-sĭd″ū-ō′mă) [″ + Gr. *oma*, tumor] A uterine tumor containing decidual tissue, thought to arise from portions of decidua retained within the uterus following an abortion.

***benign d.*** During pregnancy, the normal invasion of the uterine musculature by the syncytium, which disappears after the gestation is completed.

***Loeb's d.*** Decidual tissue produced within the uteri of experimental animals as a result of mechanical or hormonal stimulation.

***malignant d.*** A uterine tumor consisting of syncytial and Langhans' cells, which tend to invade the general system by way of the bloodstream. Specific therapy with methotrexate may cause a complete remission. SYN: *choriocarcinoma; chorioepithelioma.*

ETIOLOGY: This tumor may arise following a full-term pregnancy, an ectopic pregnancy, an abortion, a miscarriage, and particularly a vesicular mole.

DIAGNOSIS: The diagnosis may be made by histological study, aided by the symptoms and the pregnancy test, the results of which remain strongly positive during the presence of this type of tumor.

TREATMENT: Chemotherapy with dactinomycin or the folic acid antagonist methotrexate should be administered.

**deciduosarcoma** [″ + Gr. *sarx*, flesh, + *oma*, tumor] A tumor of the chorion. SYN: *choriocarcinoma; chorioepithelioma.*

**deciduous** (dē-sĭd′ū-ŭs) [L. *deciduus*] Falling off; subject to being shed.

**deciduous teeth** An old term for the primary dentition, which begins to appear at about 6 months of age and proceeds until the last teeth are replaced by permanent teeth in the 12th or 13th year. SEE: *dentition.*

**decigram** (dĕs′ĭ-grăm) [L. *decimus*, tenth, + Gr. *gramma*, small weight] One tenth of a gram.

**deciliter** (dĕs′ĭ-lē-tĕr) [″ + Fr. *litre*] ABBR: dL. A unit of volume in the SI system of measurement that is equal to 0.1 L or 100 ml.

**decimeter** (dĕs′ĭ-mē″tĕr) [″ + Gr. *metron*, measure] One tenth of a meter.

**decinormal** (dĕs″ĭ-nor′măl) [″ + *norma*, rule] Having one tenth the strength of a normal solution. SEE: *normal.*

**decipara** (dĕ-sĭp′ă-ră) [″ + *parere*, to bring forth, to bear] A woman who has given birth for the tenth time to an infant or infants, alive or dead, weighing 500 g or more.

**decisional conflict** The state of uncertainty about course of action to be taken when choice among competing actions involves risk, loss, or challenge to personal life values. SEE: *Nursing Diagnoses Appendix.*

**decision analysis** A logically consistent approach to making a decision when its consequences cannot be foretold with certainty. The uncertainties in medical practice are due to many factors including biological variation and the inadequacy of the clinical data available for an individual patient. There are three steps in this process: the outcome, or consequences, of each option is described schematically by the use of a decision tree; probability is used to quantify the uncertainties inherent in each option; and each possible outcome is designated by a number that measures the patient's preference for that outcome as compared with the others. After the last step is completed, each outcome is assigned a "utility" value in which 1.0 indicates a perfect outcome and 0 is the worst possibility. Use of decision analysis will probably become increasingly important in helping all members of the health care team and the patient make logical choices concerning management of illness.

**decision making** The process of using all of the available information about a patient and arriving at a decision concerning the therapeutic plan.

**decision tree** A graphical analysis of the decisions or choices available to the physician in deciding a course of treatment. Included in the graph are the probabilities of all of the events that may result from each decision. SEE: *decision analysis*.

**Declaration of Geneva** A statement adopted in 1948 by the Second General Assembly of the World Medical Association. Some medical schools use it at graduation exercises.

"At the time of being admitted as Member of the Medical Profession I solemnly pledge myself to consecrate my life to the service of humanity. I will give to my teachers the respect and gratitude which is their due; I will practice my profession with conscience and dignity. The health of my patient will be my first consideration; I will respect the secrets which are confided in me; I will maintain by all the means in my power, the honor and the noble traditions of the medical profession; my colleagues will be my brothers; I will not permit considerations of religion, nationality, race, party politics or social standing to intervene between my duty and my patient; I will maintain the utmost respect for human life, from the time of conception; even under threat, I will not use my medical knowledge contrary to the laws of humanity. I make these promises solemnly, freely and upon my honor." SEE: *Hippocratic oath; Nightingale Pledge; Prayer of Maimonides*.

**Declaration of Hawaii** Ethical guidelines laid down by the General Assembly of the World Psychiatric Association for psychiatrists all over the world. These guidelines were unanimously adopted by the association in 1976.

(1) The aim of psychiatry is to promote health and personal autonomy and growth. To the best of his or her ability, consistent with accepted scientific and ethical principles, the psychiatrist shall serve the best interests of the patient and be also concerned for the common good and a just allocation of health resources.

To fulfill these aims requires continuous research and continual education of health care personnel, patients, and the public.

(2) Every patient must be offered the best therapy available and be treated with the solicitude and respect due to the dignity of all human beings and to their autonomy over their own lives and health.

The psychiatrist is responsible for treatment given by the staff members and owes them qualified supervision and education. Whenever there is a need, or whenever a reasonable request is forthcoming from the patient, the psychiatrist should seek the help or the opinion of a more experienced colleague.

(3) A therapeutic relationship between patient and psychiatrist is founded on mutual agreement. It requires trust, confidentiality, openness, cooperation, and mutual responsibility. Such a relationship may not be possible to establish with some severely ill patients. In that case, as in the treatment of children, contact should be established with a person close to the patient and acceptable to him or her.

If and when a relationship is established for purposes other than therapeutic, such as in forensic psychiatry, its nature must be thoroughly explained to the person concerned.

(4) The psychiatrist should inform the patient of the nature of the condition, of the proposed diagnostic and therapeutic procedures, including possible alternatives, and of the prognosis. This information must be offered in a considerate way and the patient be given the opportunity to choose between appropriate and available methods.

(5) No procedure must be performed or treatment given against or independent of a patient's own will, unless the patient lacks capacity to express his or her own wishes or, owing to psychiatric illness, cannot see what is in his or her best interest or, for the same reason, is a severe threat to others.

In these cases compulsory treatment may or should be given, provided that it is done in the patient's best interests and over a reasonable period of time, a retroactive informed consent can be presumed, and, whenever possible, consent has been obtained from someone close to the patient.

(6) As soon as the above conditions for compulsory treatment no longer apply the patient must be released, unless he or she voluntarily consents to further treatment.

Whenever there is compulsory treatment or detention there must be an independent and neutral body of appeal for regular inquiry into these cases. Every patient must be informed of its existence and be permitted to appeal to it, personally or through a representative, without interference by the hospital staff or by anyone else.

(7) The psychiatrist must never use the possibilities of the profession for maltreatment of individuals or groups, and should be concerned never to let inappropriate personal desires, feelings, or prejudices interfere with the treatment.

The psychiatrist must not participate in compulsory psychiatric treatment in the absence of psychiatric illness. If the patient or some third party demands actions contrary to scientific or ethical principles the psychiatrist must refuse to cooperate. When, for any reason, either the wishes or the best interests of the patient cannot be promoted he or she must be so informed.

(8) Whatever the psychiatrist has been told by the patient, or has noted during examination or treatment, must be kept confidential unless the patient releases the psychiatrist from professional secrecy, or else vital common values or the patient's best interest makes disclosure imperative. In these cases, however, the patient must be immediately informed of the breach of secrecy.

(9) To increase and propagate psychiatric knowledge and skill requires participation of the patients. Informed consent must, however, be obtained before presenting a patient to a class and, if possible, also when a case history is published, and all reasonable measures be taken to preserve the anonymity and to safeguard the personal reputation of the subject.

In clinical research, as in therapy, every subject must be offered the best available treatment. His or her participation must be voluntary, after full information has been given of the aims, procedures, risks, and inconveniences of the project, and there must always be a reasonable relationship between calculated risks or inconveniences and the benefit of the study.

For children and other patients who cannot themselves give informed consent this should be obtained from someone close to them.

(10) Every patient or research subject is free to withdraw for any reason at any time from any voluntary treatment and from any teaching or research program in which he or she participates. This withdrawal, as well as any refusal to enter a program, must never influence the psychiatrist's efforts to help the patient or subject.

The psychiatrist should stop all therapeutic, teaching, or research programs that may evolve contrary to the principles of this Declaration. SEE: *Declaration of Geneva; Hippocratic oath; Nightingale Pledge; Prayer of Maimonides.*

**declination** (dĕk″lĭ-nā′shŭn) Cyclophoria.

**declinator** (dĕk′lĭn-ā″tor) [L. *declinare,* to turn aside] An instrument used during trephining for holding apart the dura mater.

**decline** (dē-klīn′) **1.** Progressive decrease. **2.** The declining period of a disease.

**declivis cerebelli** (dē-klīv′ĭs sĕr-ĕ-bĕl′ī) [L.] The sloping posterior portion of the monticulus of the superior vermis of the cerebellum.

**decoction** (dē-kŏk′shŭn) [L. *de,* down, + *coquere,* to boil] A liquid medicinal preparation made by boiling vegetable substances with water. When the strength and method of preparation are not otherwise specified, it is made by boiling five parts of the coarsely comminuted drug for 15 min with enough water to make 100 parts. There are no official decoctions.

**decoloration** (dē-kŭl″or-ā′shŭn) Loss or removal of color or pigment.

**decompensation** [L. *de,* from, + *compensare,* to make good again] **1.** Failure of the heart to maintain adequate circulation. **2.** In psychology, failure of defense system mechanisms such as occurs in relapses of mental patients.

**decomposition** (dē-kŏm-pō-zĭsh′ŭn) [″ + *componere,* to put together] **1.** The putrefactive process; decay. **2.** Reducing a compound body to its simpler constituents. SEE: *biodegradation; fermentation; resolution.*

***double d.*** A chemical change in which the molecules of two interacting compounds exchange a portion of their constituents.

***hydrolytic d.*** A chemical change in substances due to addition of a molecule of water.

***simple d.*** A chemical change by which a molecule of a single compound breaks into its simpler constituents or substitutes the entire molecule of another body for one of these constituents.

**decompress 1.** To pass from a state of stress to tranquillity. **2.** To relieve pressure, esp. that produced by air or gas.

**decompression** [″ + *compressio,* a squeezing together] **1.** The removal of pressure, as from gas in the intestinal tract. SEE: *Wangensteen tube.* **2.** The slow reduction or removal of pressure on deep-sea divers and caisson workers to prevent development of nitrogen bubbles in the tissue spaces. SEE: *caisson disease.*

***explosive d.*** In aviators or divers, decompression resulting from an extremely rapid rate of change to a much lesser pressure. This may occur if a high-altitude aircraft suddenly loses its cabin pressurization or if a diver ascends rapidly. Either of these causes violent expansion of body gases. SEE: *bends.*

**decompression illness** A condition that develops in divers subjected to rapid reduction of air pressure after coming to the surface following exposure to compressed air. The cause is nitrogen bubbles in the tissue spaces. The condition may occur when an individual participates in underwater sports and flies in an aircraft shortly afterward. It may also occur when an aviator suddenly ascends to high altitudes without taking measures to clear the body of nitrogen. SYN: *caisson disease.* SEE: *bends; hyperbaric chamber.*

TREATMENT: The person is placed in a pressure chamber. The pressure in the chamber is then increased to the level that relieves the patient's symptoms and then decreased very slowly until the pressure inside the chamber is equal to outside pressure.

**deconditioning** A loss of physical fitness due to failure to maintain an optimal level of physical training. Inactivity for any reason may lead to deconditioning. For example, astronauts exposed to weightlessness for prolonged periods become deconditioned.

**decongestant** **1.** Reducing congestion or swelling. **2.** An agent that reduces congestion, esp. nasal.

**decontamination** The use of physical, chemical, or other means to remove, inactivate, or destroy harmful microorganisms or poisonous or radioactive chemicals from persons, spaces, surfaces, or objects.

**decorticate posture** The characteristic posture of a patient with a lesion at or above the upper brainstem. The patient is rigidly still with arms flexed, fists clenched, and legs extended.

**decortication** [″ + *cortex,* bark] Removal of the surface layer of an organ or structure, as removal of a portion of the cortex of the brain from the underlying white portion.

***pulmonary d.*** Removal of the pleura of the lung or a portion of the surface lung tissue.

***renal d.*** Removal of the capsule of the kidney.

**decrement** (dĕk′rĕ-mĕnt) [L. *decrementum,* decrease] **1.** The period in the course of a febrile disease when the fever subsides. **2.** A reduction in the response of the nervous system to repeated stimulation. **3.** A decrease in the quantity or force of an entity. **4.** The portion of each uterine contraction between acme and baseline. The downslope is recorded by the fetal monitor.

**decrepitate** (dē-krĕp′ĭ-tāt) [L. *decrepitare,* to crackle] To cause decrepitation.

**decrepitation** A crackling noise.

**decrepitude** (dē-krĕp′ĭ-tūd) A state of general feebleness and decline that sometimes accompanies old age; weakness; infirmity.

**decrudescence** (dē-kroo-dĕs′ĕns) A decrease in the severity of disease symptoms.

**decubation** (dē-kū-bā′shŭn) [L. *de,* down, + *cumbere,* to lie] **1.** The act of lying down. **2.** The recovery stage of an infectious disease.

**decubitus** (dē-kū′bĭ-tŭs) [L., a lying down] **1.** A bedsore. **decubital** (-tăl), *adj.* **2.** A patient's position in bed.

***acute d.*** A severe, sometimes fatal bedsore that can occur on the affected side in hemiplegia.

***Andral's d.*** Lying on the sound side during the early stages of pleurisy.

***dorsal d.*** Lying on the back.

***lateral d.*** Lying on the side.

***ventral d.*** Lying on the stomach.

**decubitus projection** A radiographic procedure, using the decubitus positions and the central ray of the x-ray beam placed horizontally, that aids in the demonstration of air-fluid levels.

**decubitus ulcer** An ulcer, initially of the skin, due to prolonged pressure, usually in a person who is lying down. However, pressure ulcers or sores may occur at any site (e.g., on the buttocks of patients confined to wheelchairs). The most common sites are over bony prominences (i.e., the sacrum, heels, trochanter, lateral malleoli, and ischial areas). The combination of pressure, shearing forces, friction, and moisture lead to the death of tissue due to the lack of blood supply. If not treated vigorously, the ulcer will progress from a simple erosion to complete involvement of the deep layers of the skin and may eventually extend to the underlying muscle and bone tissue. SYN: *bedsore; pressure sore.*

The most important principle is to prevent the continuous pressure that causes the ulcer.

The size of a decubitus ulcer may be determined by covering the area with a transparent film that adheres to the ulcer and touches the surrounding skin. Sterile isotonic saline is then injected under the film until the film is level with the surrounding skin. The amount of fluid required is recorded. Repetition of this procedure at intervals provides an index of the healing progress or lack of it.

NURSING IMPLICATIONS: In at-risk patients, decubiti can be prevented by inspecting the skin regularly for redness and signs of breakdown, documenting findings, and instituting any preventive measures or treatment. Reddened areas should not be massaged because this can damage ischemic deep layers of tissue. The skin is thoroughly cleansed, rinsed, and dried, and emollients are gently applied by minimizing the force and friction used, esp. over bony prominences. The patient is repositioned every 1 to 2 hr with a turning sheet or pad and by lifting rather than sliding to relieve pressure. Raising the head higher than 30 degrees except for short periods should be avoided to decrease shearing forces. Range-of-motion exercises are provided, early ambulation is encouraged, and nutritious high-protein meals are offered. Low-pressure mattresses and special beds are kept in proper working order. Doughnut-type cushions should not be used because they decrease blood flow to tissues resting in the center of the doughnut.

Ulcers are cleansed and debrided, and other therapeutic measures are instituted according to institutional protocol or prescription. Topical agents include absorbable gelatin sponges, karaya gum patches, antiseptic irrigations, air-permeable occlusive clear dressings that allow aspiration of collected fluid, supportive adhesive-backed foam padding, surgical debridement, proteolytic enzyme debriding agents, and absorptive dextranomer beads. Continuity of care is probably more important than the agent used; the nurse's main efforts are directed at relieving pressure and preventing further damage.

**decussate** (dē-kŭs′āt) [L. *decussare,* to make an X] **1.** To cross, or crossed, as in the form of an X. **2.** Interlacing or crossing of parts.

**decussation 1.** A crossing of structures in form of an X. **2.** A place of crossing. SYN: *chiasma.*

***d. of pyramids*** Crossing of fibers of pyramids of the medulla oblongata from one pyramid to the other.

***optic d.*** Crossing of fibers of the optic nerves; the optic chiasma.

**dedifferentiation 1.** The return of parts to a homogeneous state. **2.** The process by which mature differentiated cells or tissues become sites of origin for immature elements of the same type, as in some cancers.

**deduction** (dē-dŭk′shŭn) Reasoning from the general to the particular.

**de-efferented state** Locked-in syndrome.

**deep** [AS. *deop*] Below the surface.

**deep tendon reflex** A reflex within the body, or fractional stretch reflex; opposed to a superficial or skin reflex. In obstetrics, deep tendon reflexes are used to assess central nervous system irritability in women with pregnancy-induced hypertension. Hyperreflexia indicates increased risk of eclamptic seizures.

**deer fly** A biting fly, *Chrysops discalis,* that transmits the causative organism of deer fly fever, a form of tularemia.

**deer fly fever** Tularemia.

**DEF** *decayed, extracted, filled.*

**defamation** In law, an intentional wrong that occurs when a person communicates to a third party information that injures or harms the reputation of another. Oral defamation is slander. Written defamation is libel.

**defatted** [L. *de,* from, + AS. *faelt,* to fatten] Freed from or deprived of fat.

**defecalgesiophobia** (dĕf″ĕ-kăl″jē-sē-ō-fō′bē-ă) [L. *defaecare,* to remove dregs, + Gr. *algesis,* sense of pain, + *phobos,* fear] Fear of defecating because of pain.

**defecation** (dĕf-ĕ-kā′shŭn) [L. *defaecare,* to remove dregs] Evacuation of the bowels. The bulk of the feces depends on the amount and composition of food ingested. One does not, however, have to eat to have bowel movements. A large quantity of cellular material is desquamated from the epithelial lining of the intestinal tract each day. The food residues, reaching the rectum, cause the urge to defecate. The sensation is related to periodic increase of pressure within the rectum and contracture of its musculature. The expulsion of a fecal mass is accompanied by coordinated action of the following mechanisms: involuntary contraction of the circular muscle of the rectum behind the bowel mass followed by contraction of the longitudinal muscle; relaxation of the internal (involuntary) and external (voluntary) sphincter ani; voluntary closure of the glottis, fixation of the chest, and contraction of the abdominal muscles, causing an increase in intra-abdominal pressure. SEE: *constipation; feces; stool.*

**defecation syncope** Syncope occurring during or immediately after defecation. It may be associated with disease of the gastrointestinal tract, the cardiovascular or cerebrovascular systems, or orthostatic hypotension. In many cases the potential cause is not discovered.

**defecography** (dĕ″fē-kŏ′grăfē) Radiography of the anorectal region after instillation of a barium paste into the rectum. The defecation process is imaged by direct filming or video recording.

**defect** (dē′fĕkt) A flaw or imperfection.

***alcohol-related birth d.*** A congenital abnormality that reflects the teratogenic effects of alcohol on developing fetal structures. The most common abnormalities involve the heart, eyes, kidneys, and skeleton. These defects are caused by maternal alcohol abuse during pregnancy. SEE: *effects, fetal alcohol; fetal alcohol syndrome.*

***congenital d.*** An imperfection present at birth.

***congenital heart d.*** A structural abnormality of the heart and great blood vessels that occurs during intrauterine development. Abnormalities are commonly classified by the presence or absence of cyanosis. Acyanotic abnormalities include atrial and ventricular septal defects, coarctation of the aorta, and patent ductus arteriosus. Cyanotic defects include tetralogy of Fallot, transposition of the great vessels, and hypoplastic left heart syndrome.

***filling d.*** An interruption of the contour of the inner surface of the stomach or intestine revealed by radiography. It may be due to a benign obstruction or a malignancy.

***luteal phase d.*** A deficiency in either the amount or the duration of postovulatory progesterone secretion by the corpus luteum. Insufficient hormonal stimulation results in inadequate preparation of the endometrium for successful implantation and support of the growing embryo. This rare condition is associated with infertility or habitual spontaneous first-trimester abortion. SEE: *menstrual cycle.*

***septal d.*** A defect in one or more of the septa between the heart chambers.

**defective** [L. *defectus,* a failure] **1.** Not perfect. **2.** A person deficient in one or more physical, mental, or moral powers.

**defendant** In law, the person or party charged in a lawsuit or legal action seeking damages or other legal relief. SEE: *plaintiff.*

**defense** [L. *defendere,* to repel] **1.** Resistance to disease. **2.** Protective action against harm or injury.

**defense mechanism** **1.** Any reaction, whether general or cellular, that protects against something harmful, as in immune reactions. Any defense mechanism occurring in excess can be pathological. **2.** In psychoanalysis, a method of unconscious behavior (such as compensation, denial, or projection) used to resolve or conceal conflicts or anxieties.

**defense reflex** Retraction or tension in defense against an action or threatened action.

**defensin** [term coined by Robert I. Lehrer, U.S. physician, b. 1938] Antimicrobial peptide present in leukocytes from several species including humans. Defensins are active against bacteria, fungi, and enveloped viruses in vitro. They may contribute to host defenses against susceptible organisms.

**defensive** Defending; protecting from injury.

**defensive medicine** Medicine practiced as if each patient were planning a malpractice suit. This is done by ordering an inordinate number of laboratory and test procedures.

**deferens** (dĕf′ĕr-ĕnz) [L. *deferens,* carrying away] Deferent.

**deferent** (dĕf′ĕr-ĕnt) Conveying something away from or downward. SEE: *afferent; efferent.*

**deferentectomy** (dĕf-ĕr-ĕn-tĕk′tō-mē) [″ + Gr. *ektome,* excision] Cutting of a ductus deferens.

**deferential** (dĕf-ĕr-ĕn′shăl) [L. *deferre,* to bring to] Pert. to or accompanying the ductus deferens.

**deferentitis** (dĕf″ĕr-ĕn-tī′tĭs) [″ + Gr. *itis,* inflammation] Inflammation of the ductus deferens.

**deferoxamine mesylate** (dē-fĕr-ŏks′ă-mēn) A drug with a very high affinity for iron. It is used parenterally to reduce the iron stored in the body in patients with hemochromatosis, acute iron poisoning, or abnormal storage of iron due to multiple blood transfusions.

**defervescence** [L. *defervescere,* to become calm] The period that marks the subsidence of fever to normal temperature.

**defibrillation** Stopping fibrillation of the heart through the use of drugs or by physical means. SEE: *electric d.; cardioversion.*

***electric d.*** Defibrillation done by using an electric device that applies countershocks to the heart through electrodes placed on the chest wall. The purpose of this countershock is to allow the heart's normal pacemaker to take over. The electric "dose" required for defibrillation is less for lightweight persons than for larger ones. SEE: *cardioversion; cardioverter; pacemaker, cardiac, artificial.*

**defibrillator** (dē-fĭb″rĭ-lā′tor) An electric device that produces defibrillation of the heart. It may be used externally or in the form of an automatic implanted cardioverter defibrillator. The latter is used in patients who have had a life-threatening ventricular tachyarrhythmia or cardiac arrest and in whom drug therapy is unsuitable. SEE: *cardioversion.*

***automatic implanted cardioverter d.*** ABBR: AICD. A defibrillator surgically implanted in patients at high risk for sudden cardiac (arrhythmia-induced) death. This machine automatically detects and treats life-threatening arrhythmias.

***fully automatic d.*** A defibrillator that performs all functions by computer (analyzes rhythm, selects an energy level, charges the machine, and shocks the patient). The operator applies adhesive paddles and turns the machine on.

***implantable cardioverter d.*** SEE: *pacemaker, artificial cardiac.*

***manual d.*** A defibrillator that requires the operator to assess the need for defibrillation (electrocardiogram and condition), select an energy level, charge the machine, and deliver shock.

***semi-automatic d.*** A defibrillator that assesses rhythm and gives voice prompts to the operator concerning the patient's condition, the energy level, charging, and shocking the patient.

**defibrination, defibrinization** [L. *de,* from, + *fibra,* fiber] The process of removing fibrin, usually from blood. SEE: *coagulation, blood.*

**deficiency** (dē-fĭsh′ĕn-sē) [L. *deficere,* to lack] A lack; less than the normal amount.

**deficiency disease** A condition due to lack of a substance essential in body metabolism. The deficiency may be due to inadequate intake, digestion, absorption, or use of foods, minerals, water, or vitamins. It may also be due to excess loss through excretion or to an intestinal parasite such as hookworm or tapeworm. Deficiency diseases include night blindness and keratomalacia (caused by lack of vitamin A); beriberi and polyneuritis (lack of thiamine); pellagra (lack of niacin); scurvy (lack of vitamin C); rickets and osteomalacia (lack of vitamin D); pernicious anemia (lack of gastric intrinsic factor and vitamin $B_{12}$).

**deficit** (dĕf′ĭ-sĭt) A deficiency (e.g., a muscular or mental deficit).

***reversible ischemic neurological d.*** ABBR: RIND. A transient focal neurological dysfunction resulting from a decrease in cerebral blood flow. Symptoms typically last longer than 24 hr but less than 1 week.

**defined medium** SEE: *medium, defined.*

**definition** [L. *definire,* to limit] **1.** The precise determination of limits, esp. of a disease process. **2.** The detail with which images are recorded on radiographic film or screens.

**definitive** Clear and final; without question.

**deflection** (dē-flĕk′shŭn) A turning away from a previous or usual course.

**defloration** (dĕf″lō-rā′shŭn) [L. *de*, from, + *flos, flor-*, flower] Rupture of the hymen during coitus, by accident, surgically, or through vaginal examination. Not many women have a hymen that is of such size or consistency as to require its surgical rupture. SEE: *hymen; virginity*.

**deflorescence** Disappearance of an eruption of the skin.

**defluvium** (dē-floo′vē-ŭm) [L.] The process of falling out.

**deformability** (dē-form″ă-bĭl′ĭ-tē) Capability of being deformed.

**deformation** [L. *de*, from, + *forma*, form] **1.** The act of deforming. **2.** A disfiguration.

**deformity** Alteration in the natural form of a part or organ; distortion of any part or general disfigurement of the body. It may be acquired or congenital. If present after injury, deformity usually implies the presence of fracture, dislocation, or both. It may be due to extensive swelling, extravasation of blood, or rupture of muscles.

***anterior d.*** Abnormal anterior convexity of the spine. SYN: *lordosis*.

***gunstock d.*** A deformity in which the forearm, when extended, makes an angle with the arm because of displacement of the axis of the extended arm. It is caused by a condylar fracture at the elbow.

***Madelung's d.*** SEE: *Madelung's deformity*.

***seal fin d.*** Lateral deviation of the fingers in rheumatoid arthritis.

***silverfork d.*** The peculiar deformity seen in Colles' fracture of the forearm. SYN: *Velpeau's d.* SEE: *Colles' fracture*.

***Sprengel's d.*** Congenital upward displacement of the scapula.

***Velpeau's d.*** Silverfork d.

***Volkmann's d.*** Congenital tibiotarsal dislocation.

**defundation** [″ + *fundus*, base] Excision of the uterine fundus.

**defurfuration** (dē″fĕr-fū-rā′shŭn) [″ + *furfur*, bran] Shedding of epidermis in scales; branny desquamation. It may occur in various skin conditions, including seborrheic dermatitis (dandruff), psoriasis, ichthyosis, and eczema.

**deg** *degeneration; degree*.

**deganglionate** (dē-găn′glē-ŏn-āt″) [″ + Gr. *ganglion*, knot] To deprive of ganglia.

**degenerate** [L. *degenerare*, to fall from one's ancestral quality] **1.** To deteriorate. **2.** Characterized by deterioration.

**degeneration** [L. *degeneratio*] Deterioration or impairment of an organ or part in the structure of cells and the substances of which they are a component; opposed to regeneration. **degenerative,** *adj.*

***ascending d.*** Nerve fiber degeneration progressing to the center from the periphery.

***calcareous d.*** Infiltration of lime salts into tissues.

***caseous d.*** Cheesy alteration of tissues seen in tuberculosis.

***cloudy swelling d.*** A condition in which protein substances in cells become cloudy, the cells increasing in size with minute droplets of protein substances. It may occur in any inflamed tissue.

***colloid d.*** Mucoid degeneration seen in the protoplasm of epithelial cells.

***congenital macular d.*** Congenital degeneration of the macula of the eye.

***cystic d.*** Cyst formation accompanying degeneration.

***descending d.*** Nerve fiber degeneration progressing toward the periphery from the original lesion.

***fatty d.*** Deposition of abnormal amounts of fat in the cytoplasm of cells, or replacement or infiltration of tissues by fat cells.

***fibroid d.*** Change of membranous tissue into fibrous tissue.

***gray d.*** Degeneration in white nerve tissue due to chronic inflammation, causing it to turn gray.

***hepatolenticular d.*** Wilson's disease.

***hyaline d.*** A form of degeneration in which the tissues assume a homogeneous and glassy appearance. It is caused by hyaline deposits replacing musculoelastic elements of blood vessels with a firm, transparent substance that causes loss of elasticity. It is responsible for hardening of the arteries and is often followed by calcification or deposit of lime salts in dead tissue. Calcification also may result in concretions. SYN: *vitreous d.; Zenker's d.*

***hydropic d.*** Pathological change in cells marked by the appearance of water droplets in the cytoplasm.

***lipoidal d.*** Deposition of fat droplets in cells.

***macular d.*** SEE: *macular degeneration*.

***mucoid d.*** Deposition of mucus in the connective tissues. SYN: *myxomatous d.*

***mucous d.*** Deposition of mucus or mucoid substance in the connective tissue of organs or in epithelial cells.

***myxomatous d.*** Mucoid d.

***Nissl d.*** Nerve cell degeneration after division of the axon.

***pigmentary d.*** Degeneration in which affected cells develop an abnormal color.

***polypoid d.*** Formation of polyp-like growths on mucous membrane.

***secondary d.*** Wallerian d.

***senile d.*** The bodily and mental changes of the aged.

***senile macular d.*** ABBR: SMD. Degeneration of the retina that may begin and increase as a person ages.

***spongy d.*** Familial demyelination of the deep layers of the cerebral cortex. The affected area has a spongy appearance. Symptoms include mental retardation, enlarged head, muscular flaccidity, and blindness. Death usually occurs before 18 months of age.

***subacute combined d. of spinal cord*** Degeneration of the posterior and lateral columns of the spinal column. Clinically, paresthesia, sensory ataxia, and sometimes spastic paraplegia are present. The disease is the result of pernicious anemia.

***vitreous d.*** Hyaline d.

***wallerian d.*** Nerve fiber degeneration after separation from its nutritive center. SYN: *secondary d.*

***Zenker's d.*** Hyaline d.

**deglutition** (dē″gloo-tĭsh′ŭn) The act of swallowing.

**deglutitive** Pert. to deglutition.

**degradation** (dĕg″rĕ-dā′shŭn) [LL. *degradare,* to go down a step] Physical, metabolic, or chemical change to a less complex form. Foods are physically degraded during chewing, and then chemically degraded from complete compounds, such as proteins and starches, to amino acids and sugars, respectively. SEE: *biodegradation.*

**degranulation** Loss of granules, esp. in a phagocytic cell.

**degree** (dĕ-grē′) **1.** A unit of measurement on a scale. **2.** A unit of angular measure. **3.** A stage of severity of a disease. **4.** Evidence of academic attainment granted by the institution in which the individual studied.

**degrees of freedom** ABBR: d.f. In statistics, in defining the properties of a sample, the number of independent observations in a quantity. For example, if a sample contains a total of 10 children who are being classified by hair color (brown, black, or blond) and it is known that four of the children have blond hair, then there are two degrees of freedom. If, at the beginning of the investigation, the hair color of all the subjects is unknown, there are three degrees of freedom.

**degustation** (dē″gŭs-tā′shŭn) [L. *degustatio*] The sense of taste; the function or act of tasting.

**dehiscence** (dē-hĭs′ĕns) [L. *dehiscere,* to gape] **1.** A bursting open, as of a graafian follicle or a wound, esp. a surgical abdominal wound. **2.** In dentistry, an isolated area in which the tooth root is denuded of bone from the margin nearly to the apex. It occurs more often in anterior than posterior teeth, and more on the vestibular than the oral surface.

NURSING IMPLICATIONS: Dehiscence can be prevented by assessing nutritional status and risk factors such as obesity or malnourishment before surgery; by ensuring proper nutrition; and by providing support for the wound during coughing and movements that strain the incision. If dehiscence occurs, the surgeon is notified immediately, and the wound is covered with a sterile dressing or towel moistened with warm sterile physiological saline solution. The covering may need to be held in place by hand to keep abdominal tissues from "spilling" into the bed until a restraining bandage can be applied. The patient should flex the knees slightly to decrease tension on the abdominal muscles. The patient is kept calm and quiet, is reassured that measures are being taken to care for the wound, and is prepared physically and emotionally for surgery to close the wound. SEE: *Nursing Diagnoses Appendix.*

**dehumanization** (dē-hū″măn-ĭ-zā′shŭn) [L. *de,* from, + *humanus,* human] Loss of human qualities, as occurs in persons who are psychotic or in previously normal individuals subjected to torture or mental stress imposed by others, as could occur in prisoners.

**dehumidifier** (dē″hū-mĭd′ĭ-fī″ĕr) A device for removing moisture from the air.

**dehydrate** [L. *de,* from, + Gr. *hydor,* water] **1.** In chemistry, to deprive of, lose, or become free of water. **2.** To lose or be deprived of water from the body or tissues. **3.** To become dry.

**dehydration** (dē″hī-drā′shŭn) **1.** Removal of water from a substance. **2.** A condition, resulting from excessive loss of body fluid, that occurs when fluid output exceeds fluid intake. It may result from deprivation or excessive loss of fluid, reduction in total quantity of electrolytes, or injection of hypertonic solutions. SEE: *skin, tenting of; Nursing Diagnoses Appendix.*

**dehydroandrosterone** (dē-hī″drō-ăn-drō-stēr′ōn, -drŏs′tĕr-ōn) A previously used name for dehydroepiandrosterone.

**dehydrocholesterol** (dē-hī″drō-kō-lĕs′tĕr-ōl) A sterol found in the skin and other tissues that forms vitamin D after activation by irradiation.

**dehydrocholic acid** A bile salt that stimulates production of bile from the liver.

**dehydrocorticosterone** (dē-hī″drō-kor-tĭ-kōs′tĕr-ōn) 11-dehydrocorticosterone (Kendall's compound A). $C_{21}H_{28}O_4$. A physiologically active steroid isolated from the adrenal cortex. It is important in water and salt metabolism. SEE: *adrenal gland.*

**dehydroepiandrosterone** (dē-hī″drō-ĕp″ē-ăn-drŏs′tĕr-ōn) An androgenic substance, $C_{19}H_{28}O_2$, present in urine. It has about one fifth the potency of androsterone. The level of this hormone in plasma decreases with age.

**dehydrogenase** (dē-hī-drŏj′ĕ-nās) An enzyme that catalyzes the oxidation of a specific substance, causing it to give up its hydrogen.

***alcohol d.*** An enzyme that catabolizes ethyl alcohol (ethanol) in the liver. When ethanol is consumed in relatively large amounts, it is instead catabolized by the microsomal ethanol oxidizing system, also in the liver. SEE: *system, microsomal ethanol oxidizing.*

**dehydrogenate** (dē-hī″drŏj′ĕn-āt) To remove hydrogen from a chemical compound.

**dehydroisoandrosterone** (dĕ-hī″drō-ī″sō-ăn-drŏs′tĕr-ōn) A 17-ketosteroid excreted in normal male urine. It possesses androgenic activity.

**deinstitutionalization** A planned program for placing hospitalized psychiatric patients in the community by way of halfway houses, residential hotels, group homes, and boarding houses.

**deionization** (dē-ī″ŏn-ī-zā′shŭn) Removal of ions from a substance, producing a substance free of minerals.

**Deiters' cells** (dī′tĕrz) [Otto F. C. Deiters, Ger. anatomist, 1834–1863] **1.** Supporting cells in the organ of Corti. **2.** Neuroglia cells.

**Deiters' nucleus** Collection of cells behind the acoustic nucleus.

**Deiters' process** Axis cylinder process or neuraxon.

**déjà entendu** (dā′zhă ŏn-tŏn-doo′) [Fr., already heard] **1.** Recognition of something previously understood. **2.** The illusion that what one is hearing was heard previously.

**déjà vu** (dā′zhă voo) [Fr., already seen] The illusion that something seen or some situation being experienced for the first time has been previously seen or experienced.

**dejecta** (dē-jĕk′tă) [L. *dejectio*, injection] Feces; intestinal waste.

**dejection, dejecture** (dē-jĕk′shŭn, -tūr) **1.** A cast-down feeling or mental depression. **2.** Defecation or act of defecation.

**Déjérine, Joseph Jules** (dā″zhĕr-ēn′) French neurologist, 1849–1917.

***D.'s disease*** Interstitial neuritis of infants.

***D.'s syndrome*** A condition in which deep sensation is depressed but tactile sense is normal, caused by a lesion of the long root fibers of the posterior spinal column.

**Déjérine-Sottas disease** Progressive and hypertrophic interstitial neuritis of infants. It progresses slowly; the life span may be normal.

**dekaliter** A unit of volume in the SI system of measurement that is equal to 10 L. SEE: *decaliter; deciliter.*

**delacrimation** (dē-lăk″rĭ-mā′shŭn) [L. *de*, from, + *lacrima*, tear] Excessive flow of tears. SEE: *epiphora.*

**delamination** [″ + *lamina*, plate] Division into layers, esp. that of a blastoderm into two layers—epiblast and hypoblast.

**de Lange's syndrome** [Cornelia de Lange, Dutch pediatrician, 1871–1950] A congenital disorder marked by mental retardation, a small round head, thin lips, downward curve of the mouth, small feet, short stature, failure to thrive, and generalized hirsutism. Mental retardation is present and autism may develop. The cause is unknown. SYN: *Cornelia de Lange's syndrome.*

**delead** (dē-lĕd) To remove lead from the body or a tissue. SEE: *chelate.*

**deleterious** (dĕl″ĕ-tē′rē-ŭs) [Gr. *deleterios*] Harmful.

**deletion** (dē-lē′shŭn) In cytogenetics, the loss of a portion of a chromosome.

**Delhi boil** Aleppo boil.

**delicate** Having a fine, fragile structure.

**delimitation** [L. *de*, from, + *limitare*, to limit] Determination of limits of an area or organ in diagnosis.

**delinquent** (dē-lĭn′kwĕnt) **1.** Someone, esp. a juvenile, whose behavior is criminal or antisocial. **2.** Of a criminal or antisocial nature.

**deliquescence** (dĕl″ĭ-kwĕs′ĕns) The process of becoming liquefied or moist by absorbing of water from the air. Ordinary table salt has this property. **deliquescent,** *adj.*

**délire de toucher** (dā-lēr′ dŭ too-shā′) [Fr.] An abnormal desire to touch or feel things.

**deliriant, delirifacient** (dē-lĭr′ē-ănt, dē-lĭr″ĭ-fā′shĭ-ĕnt) [L. *delirare*, to be deranged] An agent that produces delirium (e.g., atropine or hyoscine).

**delirium** (dē-lĭr′ē-ŭm) [L.] A state of mental confusion and excitement marked by disorientation for time and place, usually with illusions and hallucinations. The mind wanders, speech is incoherent, and the patient is in a state of continual aimless physical activity. There are many forms of delirium, depending on the cause, which may be fever, shock, exhaustion, anxiety, or drug overdose.

***acute d.*** Delirium developing suddenly and speedily, resulting in recovery or death.

***alcoholic d.*** D. tremens.

***chronic d.*** Delirium of chronic psychoses without febrile characteristics.

***d. cordis*** Atrial fibrillation.

***d. epilepticum*** Delirium following an epileptic attack or appearing instead of an attack.

***febrile d.*** Delirium occurring with fever.

***lingual d.*** Delirium in which meaningless sounds are muttered constantly.

***d. of negation*** Delirium in which the patient thinks body parts are missing.

***d. of persecution*** Delirium in which the patient feels persecuted by surrounding persons.

***partial d.*** Delirium acting on only a portion of the mental faculties, causing only some of the patient's actions to be unreasonable.

***senile d.*** An intermittent or permanent state of disorientation, hallucinations, confusion, and wandering that may come on abruptly in old age or may be associated with senile dementia.

***toxic d.*** Delirium produced by a toxin.

***traumatic d.*** Delirium following injury or shock.

***d. tremens*** ABBR: DTs. A dramatic complication of alcoholism. The onset may follow a period of abstinence after a prolonged drinking spree, or it may occur in the chronic alcoholic who has been admitted to the hospital for an unrelated illness. Its onset is usually sudden and initially may present with any of the following: restlessness, irritability, confusion, tremulousness, insomnia, and, in about 30% of cases, generalized convulsions. This somewhat benign clinical onset progresses to visual, auditory, and tactile hallucinations, incessant and incoherent talking, disorientation, tremors, and jerky, restless movements. Signs of overactivity of the autonomic nervous system, with dilated pupils, fever, tachycardia, and profuse sweating, are present. Of these patients, 5% to 15% die depending on the presence of pre-existing illness. In most cases, recovery occurs within 3 to 5 days. The patient may fall into a deep sleep and awaken with little or no memory of the illness. SYN: *alcoholic d.; acute alcohol withdrawal*. SEE: *alcoholism; alcohol withdrawal syndrome*.

TREATMENT: Because the illness is potentially fatal and treatment is controversial, it is important that the patient be hospitalized. This is particularly true for those who have a history of previous attacks.

NURSING IMPLICATIONS: The patient and those around him or her are protected from harm while prescribed treatment is carried out to relieve withdrawal symptoms. The patient's mental status, cardiopulmonary and hepatic function, and vital signs, including body temperature, are monitored in anticipation of complicating hyperthermia or circulatory collapse. Prescribed drug and fluid therapy, titrated to the patient's symptoms and blood pressure response, are administered; and the patient's need for anticonvulsant drugs is evaluated, and such drugs given as prescribed. A calm, nonstressful, evenly illuminated environment is provided to reduce visual hallucinations. The patient is called by name, surroundings are validated frequently to orient the patient to reality, and all procedures are explained. The patient is observed closely and left alone as little as possible. Physical restraints should be reserved for patients who are combative or who have attempted to injure themselves. Patience, tact, understanding, and support are imperative throughout the acute withdrawal period. Once the acute withdrawal has subsided, the patient is advised of the need for further treatment and supportive counseling. SEE: *Nursing Diagnoses Appendix*.

---

Caution: This syndrome is a true medical emergency that should be treated aggressively due to the possibility of death. Also, it is important to be certain there is not a coexisting condition such as head trauma with concussion, or an acute infectious disease, or that the signs and symptoms are not due to some toxic substance other than ethanol.

---

**deliver** [L. *deliberare*, to free completely] **1.** To aid in childbirth. **2.** To remove or extract, as a tumor from a cystic enclosure or a cataract.

**delivery** Expulsion of a child with the placenta and membranes from the mother at birth. SEE: *labor*.

***abdominal d.*** Delivery of a child by cesarean section.

***breech d.*** Delivery of the fetus that presents in the breech position (i.e., the buttocks are the first part of the body to be delivered). Also called *breech extraction*. SEE: *presentation, breech*.

***forceps d.*** Delivery of a child by application of forceps to the fetal head. These may be applied prior to head engagement. This method is called *high forceps delivery;* if the forceps are applied after the head is visible, *low forceps delivery;* or, if they are applied after engagement but prior to the head becoming visible, *midforceps delivery*.

***postmortem d.*** Delivery of the child by either the abdominal or vaginal route after death of the mother.

***precipitous d.*** Swift progression of the second stage of labor, marked by rapid descent and expulsion of the fetus.

NURSING IMPLICATIONS: The patient should be monitored carefully. A multipara needs more careful monitoring than a primipara. Nevertheless, the condition may occur in a primipara. The nurse should heed the patient's statements that delivery is imminent and perform vaginal examination.

During preparation for delivery, the head does not need to be visible in a multipara if she is having frequent hard contractions, particularly if she is bearing down. A physician should see her immediately. In a primipara it is usually fairly safe to wait until a small portion of the head is seen at the vaginal orifice during a contraction before preparing for delivery. The primipara or multipara who has received an analgesic should be monitored because precipitation can occur with little or no warning. This involves watching for perineal bulging during the contractions by viewing the vulva, and not taking it for granted that because the patient is fairly quiet she is not progressing in labor.

***premature d.*** Preterm d.

***preterm d.*** Delivery of a fetus before full term. SYN: *premature d.*

***spontaneous d.*** Delivery of an infant without external aid.

***vaginal d.*** Delivery of an infant through the birth canal.

**dellen** (dĕl′ĕn) A depression or thinning in the corneal surface of the eye. It may be due to swelling of adjacent tissue from wearing contact lenses or degenerative changes.

**delomorphous cell** A granular cell that stains easily. It is found next to the basement membrane in the stomach and the glands in the cardiac region.

**delousing** (dē-lows′ĭng) [L. *de,* from, + AS. *lus,* louse] Ridding the body of lice. SEE: *louse.*

**delta** **1.** Δ or δ, respectively, the uppercase and lowercase symbols for the fourth letter of the Greek alphabet. **2.** A triangular space. **3.** Change in value or amount of something being measured or monitored.

**deltacortisone** (dĕl″tă-kor′tĭ-sōn) Prednisone, a steroid hormone with glucocorticoid activity.

**delta fornicis** (dĕl′tă for′nĭ-sĭs) [L.] A triangular surface on the lower side of the fornix.

**delta hepatitis virus** ABBR: HDV. SEE: *hepatitis D.*

**deltoid** [Gr. *delta,* letter d, + *eidos,* form, shape] Shaped like the uppercase form of the Greek letter delta (Δ); triangular.

**deltoid ligament** The internal lateral ligament of the ankle joint.

**deltoid muscle** The musculus deltoideus, which covers the shoulder prominence.

**deltoid ridge** The ridge on the humerus where the deltoid muscle is attached.

**delusion** (dē-loo′zhŭn) [L. *deludere,* to cheat] A false belief brought about without appropriate external stimulation and inconsistent with the individual's own knowledge and experience. It is seen most often in psychoses, in which patients cannot separate delusion from reality. It differs from hallucination, in that the latter involves the false excitation of one or more senses. The most serious delusions are those that cause patients to harm others or themselves (e.g., fear of being poisoned may cause the patient to refuse food). Delusions may lead to suicide or self-injury. False beliefs might include being persecuted or being guilty of an unpardonable sin.

***d. of control*** A delusion that one's thoughts and actions are under the control of an external force.

***depressive d.*** A delusion causing a saddened state.

***expansive d.*** An unreasonable conviction of one's own power, importance, or wealth, accompanied by a feeling of wellbeing, seen in manic patients. These beliefs are not consistent with reality. SEE: *megalomania.*

***fixed d.*** A delusion that remains unaltered.

***d. of grandeur*** A false sense of possessing wealth or power. SYN: *megalomania.*

***d. of negation*** Nihilistic d.

***nihilistic d.*** A delusion that everything has ceased to exist. SYN: *d. of negation.*

***d. of persecution*** A delusion in which patients believe everyone around them is against them.

***reference d.*** A delusion that causes the patient to read an unintended meaning into the acts or words of others; often the interpretation is of slight or ridicule.

***systematized d.*** A logical correlation with false reasoning and deduction.

***unsystematized d.*** A delusion with no correlation between ideas and actual circumstances.

**delusional** Pert. to a delusion.

**demand** **1.** A need for something. **2.** A legal obligation asserted in courts, such as a payment of a debt or monetary award for injuries suffered by the plaintiff and allegedly caused by the defendant.

***biological oxygen d.*** The amount of oxygen required for a biological reaction, esp. the oxygen required to oxidize materials in natural water supplies, such as rivers or lakes. SEE: *eutrophication.*

**demand valve manually cycled resuscitator** A resuscitator using high-flow oxygen, which is cycled by pushing a button and watching the chest rise. It can be used during cardiopulmonary resuscitation efforts, but the high oxygen pressure may result in gastric distention and barotrauma.

**demarcation** (dē″măr-kā′shŭn) [L. *demarcare,* to limit] A limit or boundary.

**demasculinization** Loss of male sexual characteristics. This may be caused by lack of the male hormone or by the action of certain drugs.

**demecarium bromide** (dĕm″ē-kā′rē-ŭm) An anticholinesterase agent used in treating glaucoma.

**demeclocycline hydrochloride** (dĕm″ĕ-klō-sī′klēn) A tetracycline-type antibiotic.

**demented** Of unsound mind.

**dementia** (dē-mĕn′shē-ă) [L. *dementare,* to make insane] A broad term that refers to cognitive deficit, including memory impairment. There are many causes. The current classifications include dementia of Alzheimer's disease; vascular dementia; AIDS dementia; dementia due to head trauma; dementia due to Parkinson's, Huntington's, or Creutzfeldt-Jakob disese; and demential induced by substance abuse.

SYMPTOMS: The onset of primary dementia may be slow, over months or years. Memory deficits, impaired abstract thinking, poor judgment, and clouding of consciousness and orientation are not present until the terminal stages; depression, agitation, sleeplessness, and paranoid ideation may be present. Patients become dependent for activities of daily living and typically die from complications of immobility in the terminal stage.

ETIOLOGY: The cause may be primary as with Alzheimer's disease; or secondary as with brain tumors, fever, or severe medical or surgical disease.

TREATMENT: The treatment is symptomatic therapy for primary dementia and appropriate specific therapy for the reversible causes.

***alcoholic d.*** Dementia in the terminal portion of the chronic alcoholic state.

***apoplectic d.*** Dementia due to cerebral hemorrhage or tumor.

***dialysis d.*** SEE: *dialysis dementia.*

***epileptic d.*** Dementia seen in some cases of long-term epilepsy.

***multi-infarct d.*** Dementia resulting from damage to the cerebral blood vessels, marked by facial presentation of aphasia, apraxia, and alexia. The onset occurs in middle age after an episode of hypertension or stroke.

***d. paralytica*** A form of neurosyphilis marked by a sudden onset with irritability and deterioration of memory and concentration. Behavior deteriorates and emotional instability develops. Neurasthenia, depression, and delusions of grandeur with lack of insight may be present.

***postfebrile d.*** Dementia following a severe febrile illness.

***presenile d.*** Dementia beginning in middle age, usually resulting from cerebral arteriosclerosis. The symptoms are apathy, loss of memory, and disturbances of speech and gait. SEE: *Nursing Diagnoses Appendix.*

***primary d.*** Dementia associated with Alzheimer's disease.

***d. pugilistica*** Punchdrunk.

***senile d.*** Dementia occurring in the aged. It is marked by progressive mental deterioration with loss of memory, esp. for recent events, with occasional intercurrent attacks of excitement.

***senile d. of the Alzheimer's type*** ABBR: SDAT. Alzheimer's disease.

***syphilitic d.*** Dementia caused by a lesion of syphilis.

***toxic d.*** Dementia due to excessive use of a drug or drugs toxic to the central nervous system.

**Demerol** (dĕm′ĕr-ŏl) Trade name for meperidine hydrochloride, a white, odorless, crystalline compound, soluble in water, having a neutral reaction and an analgesic effect similar to that of morphine.

---

Caution: Continued use will lead to addiction.

---

**demi-** [L. *dimidius,* half] Prefix indicating *half.*

**demibain** (dĕm′ĭ-băn) [Fr., half bath] Half a bath; a sitz bath.

**demifacet** In the thoracic spine, a notch on the superior and inferior aspects of the posterior vertebral bodies that articulates with the head of the rib. It occurs in all vertbrae except the superior first and the 10th, 11th, and 12th.

**demilune** (dĕm′ĭ-loon) [L. *dimidius,* half, + *luna,* moon] A crescent-shaped group of serous cells that form a caplike structure over a mucous alveolus. They are present in mixed glands, esp. the submandibular gland.

**demineralization** [L. *de,* from, + *minare,* to mine] Loss of mineral salts, esp. from the bones. SEE: *decalcification.*

**demise** (dĕ-mīz′) [L. *dimittere,* to dismiss] Death.

**demodectic** (dĕm-ō-dĕk′tĭk) Concerning or caused by the mite *Demodex.*

**Demodex** [Gr. *demos,* fat, + *dex,* worm] A genus of mites and ticks of the class Arachnida and order Acarina.

***D. folliculorum*** The hair follicle or face mite; an almost microscopic elongated wormlike organism that infests hair follicles and sebaceous glands of various mammals, including humans.

**demography** (dē-mŏg′ră-fē) [Gr. *demos,* people, + *graphein,* to write] The statistical and quantitative study of characteristics of human populations. Size, growth, density, age and sex distribution, and vital statistics are included in the data collected.

**demoniac 1.** Concerning or resembling a demon. **2.** Frenzied, as if possessed by demons or evil spirits.

**demorphinization** (dē-mor″fĭn-ĭ-zā′shŭn) Gradual decrease in the dose of morphine being used by one addicted to that drug.

**demotivate** To cause loss of incentive or motivation.

**Demours' membrane** (dē-mūr′) [Pierre Demours, Fr. ophthalmologist, 1702–1795] A fine membrane between the endothelial layer of the cornea and the substantia propria. SYN: *Descemet's membrane.*

**demucosation** (dē″mū-kō-sā′shŭn) [L. *demucosatio*] Removal of mucosa from any part of body.

**demulcent** [L. *demulcens,* stroking softly] An oily or mucilaginous agent used to soothe or soften an irritated surface, esp. mucous membranes. SEE: *emollient.*

**de Musset's sign** SEE: *Musset's sign.*

**demyelinate** (dē-mī′ĕ-lĭ-nāt) [″ + Gr. *myelos,* marrow] To remove the myelin sheath of nerve tissue.

**demyelinating** An inflammatory process of nerves that destroys normal, healthy myelin.

**demyelination** Destruction or removal of the myelin sheath of nerve tissue, seen in Guillain-Barré syndrome.

**denaturation** (dē-nā″chŭr-ā′shŭn) Addition of a substance to alcohol that makes it toxic and unfit for human consumption but usually does not interfere with its use for other purposes.

**denatured** [″ + *natura,* nature] Having the usual nature, as of a substance, altered, as when the addition of methanol to alcohol renders it unfit for consumption.

**denatured protein** A protein that has been treated to remove some of its physical and chemical properties. For example, cooking egg white denatures the albumin.

**dendraxon** (dĕn-drăk′sŏn) [Gr. *dendron,* tree, + *axon,* axle] A terminal filament of the neuraxon of a nerve cell.

**dendric** (dĕn′drĭk) Pert. to or possessing a

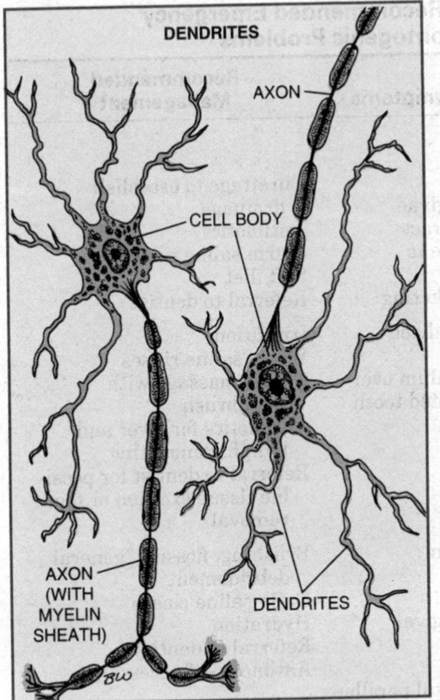


dendron.

**dendriform** (děn′drĭ-form) [″ + L. *forma*, shape] Branching or treelike.

**dendrite** (děn′drīt) [Gr. *dendrites*, pert. to a tree] A branched protoplasmic process of a neuron that conducts impulses to the cell body. There are usually several to a cell. They form synaptic connections with other neurons. SYN: *dendron; neurodendrite*. SEE: illus.

***extracapsular d.*** A dendrite of a neuron of autonomic ganglia that pierces the capsule surrounding the cell and extends for a considerable distance from the cell body.

***intracapsular d.*** A dendrite of a neuron of autonomic ganglia that branches beneath the capsule, forming a network about the cell body.

**dendritic** Treelike.

**dendritic calculus** A renal stone molded in the form of the pelvis and calyces.

**dendroid** (děn′droyd) [″ + *eidos*, form, shape] **1.** Dendriform; dendritic; pert. to dendrites. **2.** Arborescent; treelike.

**dendron** (děn′drŏn) [Gr., tree] A dendrite; a protoplasmic branch from a nerve cell. SYN: *neurodendrite*.

**dendrophagocytosis** (děn″drō-făg-ō-sī-tō′sĭs) [Gr. *dendron*, tree, + *phagein*, to eat, + *kytos*, cell, + *osis*, condition] Absorption of portions of astrocytes by microglia cells.

**denervation** [L. *de*, from, + Gr. *neuron*, nerve] **1.** Excision, incision, or blocking of a nerve supply. **2.** A condition in which the afferent and efferent nerves are cut. SEE: *deafferentation*.

**dengue** (dāng′gā, -gĕ) [Sp.] An acute febrile disease marked by sudden onset, with headache, fever, prostration, joint and muscle pain, lymphadenopathy, and a rash that appears simultaneously with a second temperature rise following an afebrile period. SYN: *breakbone fever; dengue fever*.

SYMPTOMS: Symptoms include two fever periods with intermissions; eruptions similar to those of measles; and severe pain in muscles and joints.

ETIOLOGY: Dengue is caused by Group B arbovirus transmitted by mosquitoes. The incubation period is 3 to 15 days, usually 5 to 6 days.

TREATMENT: There is no specific treatment. Analgesic and sedative agents should be used, but aspirin should be avoided because of the potential for bleeding or the development of Reye's syndrome. Prophylaxis consists of mosquito control.

**denial** (dĕ-nī′ăl) **1.** Refusal to admit the reality, or to acknowledge the presence or existence, of something; keeping of anxiety-producing realities from conscious awareness. This is a defense mechanism. **2.** In medical care reimbursement, the decision by the patient's insurer that part or all of the medical care administered was not justified. The result of the denial is that the insurer refuses to pay for all or a portion of the medical costs incurred.

***ineffective d.*** The state of a conscious or unconscious attempt to disavow the knowledge or meaning of an event to reduce anxiety/fear to the detriment of health. SEE: *Nursing Diagnoses Appendix*.

**denial and isolation** According to Elisabeth Kübler-Ross, the initial emotional reactions to being told of impending death. Individuals refuse to accept the diagnosis and seek additional professional opinions in the hope that the predicted outcome is erroneous. When these efforts are in vain, the patient feels isolated and abandoned. SEE: *acceptance*.

**denitrify** To remove nitrogen from something.

**denitrogenation** In aerospace medicine, the removal of nitrogen from the body of a person preparing to fly in an environment in which the barometric pressure will be much lower than at sea level. Prior to the flight, the person breathes 100% oxygen for a variable length of time, depending on the anticipated degree of reduced barometric pressure. SYN: *preoxygenation*. SEE: *bends; decompression illness*.

**Dennie's line** [Charles Clayton Dennie, U.S. dermatologist, 1883–1971] An extra fold of skin below the lower eyelid. It may be present in patients with atopic dermatitis.

**dens** (dĕnz) *pl.* **dentes** [L.] **1.** A tooth. SEE: *dentition* for illus. **2.** The odontoid process of the axis, which serves as a pivot for the rotation of the atlas.

## Signs and Symptoms and Recommended Emergency Management of Odontogenic Problems

| Condition | Signs and Symptoms | Recommended Management |
|---|---|---|
| **Acute periodontal disease** | | |
| Acute periodontal abscess | Localized pain<br>Swelling of gingivae<br>Possible sinus tract<br>Lack of response to percussion<br>Periodontal pocketing | Curettage to establish drainage<br>Antibiotics<br>Warm saline rinses<br>Soft diet<br>Referral to dentist |
| Pericoronitis | Pain and generalized soreness<br>Inflamed operculum over partially erupted tooth | Irrigation<br>Warm saline rinses<br>Gentle massage with toothbrush<br>Antibiotics for fever and lymphadenopathy<br>Referral to dentist for possible tissue excision or tooth removal |
| Acute necrotizing ulcerative gingivitis | Generalized pain<br>Bleeding gums<br>Fetid odor<br>Generalized gingival inflammation<br>Necrotic tissue<br>Loss of interdental papillae | Brushing, flossing, general debridement<br>Daily saline rinses<br>Hydration<br>Referral to dentist<br>Antibiotics if necessary |
| Acute primary herpetic gingivostomatitis (highly infectious) | Gingival ulceration<br>Fever<br>Punctate lesions of gingivae and possibly dorsum of tongue, buccal mucosa, floor of mouth, lips<br>Malaise<br>Headache<br>Irritability<br>Lymphadenopathy | Rest<br>Diluted mouthwashes<br>Increased fluid intake<br>Soft diet<br>Topical analgesics<br>Referral to dentist |
| **Pulpitis and periapical problems** | | |
| Reversible pulpitis | Sharp, transient pain response to cold stimuli<br>Recent dental restoration | Analgesics<br>Avoidance of thermal stimuli<br>Referral to dentist |
| Irreversible pulpitis | Spontaneous pain<br>Persistent pain response to thermal stimuli | Referral to dentist for removal of pulp or extraction of tooth |
| Periapical inflammation | Acute pain on percussion | Examination for lymph node involvement, intraoral and extraoral swelling, fever<br>Analgesics<br>Referral to dentist |
| Periapical abscess | Tooth sensitive to touch<br>Tooth mobile<br>Fever<br>Swelling | Thorough systemic examination<br>Incision and drainage<br>Antibiotics<br>Analgesics<br>Warm water rinses<br>Referral to dentist |
| **Posttreatment complications** | | |
| Alveolar osteitis (dry socket) | Throbbing pain 2–4 days after extraction | Irrigation of extraction site<br>Sedative dressing (eugenol) |

**Signs and Symptoms and Recommended Emergency Management of Odontogenic Problems** (Continued)

| Condition | Signs and Symptoms | Recommended Management |
|---|---|---|
| | | Analgesics<br>Gauze packs, bone wax, or gelatin sponge to control hemorrhage<br>Referral to dentist |
| Tooth sensitivity | Thermal sensitivity<br>Pain on closing mouth<br>Imbalance when teeth contact | Referral to dentist |

SOURCE: Adapted from Comer, RW, et al: Dental emergencies. Postgrad Med 85:63, Feb. 1989.

***d. bicuspidus*** D. premolaris.

***d. caninus*** A canine tooth.

***d. deciduus*** A milk tooth, or first tooth.

***d. incisivus*** An incisor tooth.

***d. in dente*** A dental anomaly in which the radiograph of a tooth shows the outline of a second dental structure inside it. Outwardly, on inspection, the visible tooth is normal. SYN: *d. invaginatus.*

***d. invaginatus*** D. in dente.

***d. molaris*** A molar tooth, or grinder.

***d. permanens*** One of the 32 permanent teeth.

***d. premolaris*** A premolar tooth. SYN: *d. bicuspidus.*

***d. serotinus*** A wisdom tooth (third molar).

**densitometer** (dĕn″sĭ-tŏm′ĕ-tĕr) **1.** An instrument that measures bacterial growth and the effect on it of antiseptics and bacteriophages. **2.** In radiology, an instrument that measures the optical density of a radiograph.

**densitometry** (dĕn″sĭ-tŏm′ĕ-trē) **1.** The determination of the density of a substance (e.g., bone). **2.** The determination of the amount of ionizing radiation to which a person has been exposed.

**density** [L. *densitas,* thickness] **1.** The relative weight of a substance compared with a reference standard. SEE: *specific gravity.* **2.** The quality of being dense. **3.** The degree of blackness on a radiograph or the relationship between the light given and the light passing through a radiograph.

**dent-** SEE: *dento-.*

**dental** Pert. to the teeth.

**dental assistant** One who assists in the care and treatment of dental patients. The responsibilities vary according to the needs of the dentist, the training and capability of the individual, and the state regulations of duties.

**dental caries** SEE: under *caries.*

**dental chart** A diagram of the mouth on which clinical and radiographic findings can be recorded. It often includes restorations, decayed surfaces, missing teeth, and periodontal conditions.

**dental consonant** A consonant pronounced with the tongue at or near the front upper teeth. The term is used in speech therapy.

**dental curve** The curve or bow of the line of the teeth. Its different portions are described as follows: *alignment curve,* the line passing through the center of the teeth from the middle line through the last molar; *buccal curve,* the curve extending from the cuspid to the third molar; *compensating curve,* the occlusal line of the bicuspids and molars; *labial curve,* the curve extending from cuspid to cuspid.

**dental disk** A thin circular piece of paper, cloth, or other substance charged with abrasive powder for cutting or polishing teeth and fillings.

**dental dysfunction** Malfunctioning of the parts of the dental structure.

**dental emergency** An acute condition affecting the teeth, such as inflammation of the soft tissues surrounding teeth or post-treatment complications of dental surgery. It is best treated by a dentist. Nevertheless, the primary care physician and other health care professionals must be familiar with these emergency conditions and their management. SEE: table.

**dental engine** A machine operated by foot power or by an electric or water motor to give a swift rotary motion to drills, burs, and burnishers.

**dental engineering** Use of the principles of engineering in dentistry.

**dental floss** Waxed or unwaxed thread or tape used for cleaning, removing plaque between the teeth, and testing for defects in the teeth.

**dental formula** A brief method of expressing the dentition of mammals in which the numbers of the teeth are given in the form of a fraction, each portion representing one quadrant; the numbers of the upper teeth form the numerator, and those of the lower teeth the denominator.

The first number listed represents the incisors; the second, the canines; the third, the premolars; and the fourth, the molars. The dental formula of the upper and lower right half of the mouth in humans is:

$$\frac{2-1-2-3 \text{ (right upper jaw)}}{2-1-2-3 \text{ (right lower jaw)}}$$

**dental geriatrics** The scientific study and treatment of dental conditions of the aged.

**dentalgia** (dĕn-tăl′jē-ă) [L. *dens,* tooth, + Gr. *algos,* pain] Toothache.

**dental handpiece** An instrument designed to hold the rotary instruments used in dentistry to remove tooth structure or to smooth and polish restorative materials; it may be powered by foot pedal, electric motor, air, or water turbines.

**dental hygienist** A licensed allied health professional who by training and practice is skilled in performing preventive dental services such as cleaning teeth (dental prophylaxis), and in promoting dental health by instructing persons in how to care for their teeth. A dental hygienist may or may not work under the supervision of a dentist.

**dental index** A system of numbers for indicating comparative size of the teeth.

**dental instrument** A variety of steel instruments with points or cutting surfaces at either or both ends, which can be sharpened, sterilized, and used in the special procedures of dentistry.

**dental material** Any of several types of colloids, plastics, resins, and metal alloys used in dentistry to take impressions, restore teeth, or duplicate dentition.

**dental plaque** A gummy mass of microorganisms that grows on the crowns and spreads along the roots of teeth. It usually is too small to be seen and is both colorless and transparent. Dental plaque can calcify and is the forerunner of dental caries and periodontal disease. Preventive measures include proper daily self-care of the teeth, careful use of dental floss, and periodic prophylaxis by a dentist or dental hygienist. SEE *calculus; caries; periodontitis; pyorrhea alveolaris.*

**dental prosthesis** An artificial part used in the mouth to replace missing structural tissue or teeth. SYN: *denture.*

**dental pulp** The embryonic connective tissue that occupies the central space within the tooth and its roots. It is vascular and well innervated.

**dental sealant** Plastic film applied to the chewing surface of a tooth to seal pits and grooves where food and bacteria can be trapped; it is used to reduce the occurrence of dental caries. Dental sealants are used in addition to fluorides and other preventive measures.

**dental tape** Waxed or unwaxed thin tape used for cleaning and removing plaque from between the teeth.

**dental trephination** Surgical creation of a drainage tract, with a bur or sharp instrument, in the soft tissue or bone overlying a tooth root apex. This is usually done to permit drainage of an apical abscess. SYN: *apicostomy.*

**dentate** (dĕn′tāt) [L. *dentatus,* toothed] Notched; having short triangular divisions at the margin; toothed.

**dentes** [L.] Teeth; pl. of dens.

**denti-** SEE: *dento-.*

**dentia** (dĕn′shē-ă) [L.] Eruption of teeth.

***d. praecox*** Premature eruption of teeth.

***d. tarda*** Delayed eruption of teeth.

**dentibuccal** (dĕn-tĭ-bŭk′l) [L. *dens,* tooth, + *bucca,* cheek] Pert. to both the cheek and the teeth.

**denticle** (dĕn′tĭ-kl) [L. *denticulus,* little tooth] **1.** A small toothlike projection. **2.** A calcified structure within the pulp of the tooth. SYN: *pulp stone.*

**denticulate** [L. *denticulatus,* small-toothed] Finely toothed or serrated.

**denticulate body** The corpus dentatum of the cerebellum.

**dentification** [L. *dens,* tooth, + *facere,* to make] Conversion into dental structure.

**dentiform** [″ + *forma,* shape] Toothlike.

**dentifrice** (dĕn′tĭ-frĭs) [″ + *fricare,* to rub] A paste, liquid, gel, or powder for cleaning teeth. A dentifrice may be cosmetic or therapeutic. Cosmetic dentifrices must clean and polish; therapeutic dentifrices must reduce some disease process in the oral cavity. Each dentifrice generally contains an abrasive, water, humectants, a foaming agent, a binder, a flavoring agent, a sweetener, a therapeutic agent, a coloring material, and a preservative.

**dentigerous** (dĕn-tĭj′ĕr-ŭs) [″ + *gerere,* to bear] Having or containing teeth.

**dentilabial** (dĕn-tĭ-lā′bē-ăl) [″ + *labium,* lip] Pert. to both the teeth and the lips.

**dentilingual** (dĕn-tĭ-lĭn′gwăl) [″ + *lingua,* tongue] Pert. to both the teeth and the tongue.

**dentin** (dĕn′tĭn) [L. *dens,* tooth] The calcified part of the tooth surrounding the pulp chamber, covered by enamel in the crown and cementum in the root area. It is called primary, secondary, or reparative according to its location inside the tooth and its relative sensitivity.

***interglobular d.*** Dentin that contains spaces or hypomineralized areas between mineralized globules or calcospherites.

**dentinal** Pert. to dentin.

**dentinitis** [″ + Gr. *itis,* inflammation] Inflammation of dentin.

**dentinoclast** (dĕn′tĭn-ō-clăst) [″ + Gr. *clastos,* broken] A multinucleate cell indistinguishable from an osteoclast. It is involved with resorption of dentin. The same cells probably resorbed cementum before contacting dentin and would be better called odontoclasts. SEE: *osteoclast.*

**dentinogenesis** (dĕn″tĭn-ō-jĕn′ĕ-sĭs) [″ + *genesis,* generation, birth] Formation of dentin in the development of a tooth.

***d. imperfecta*** Hereditary aplasia or hypoplasia of the enamel and dentin of a

DENTITION

CHILD

ERUPTION OF DECIDUOUS (MILK) TEETH

| UPPER | ERUPTION |
|---|---|
| CENTRAL INCISOR | 5–7 MO |
| LATERAL INCISOR | 7–10 MO |
| (CUSPID) CANINE | 16–20 MO |
| FIRST MOLAR | 10–16 MO |
| SECOND MOLAR | 20–30 MO |
| **LOWER** | |
| SECOND MOLAR | 20–30 MO |
| FIRST MOLAR | 10–16 MO |
| (CUSPID) CANINE | 16–20 MO |
| LATERAL INCISOR | 8–11 MO |
| CENTRAL INCISOR | 6–8 MO |

ADULT

ERUPTION OF PERMANENT TEETH

| UPPER | COMPLETED BY |
|---|---|
| CENTRAL INCISOR | 9–10 YR |
| LATERAL INCISOR | 10–11 YR |
| (CUSPID) CANINE | 12–15 YR |
| FIRST PREMOLAR (BICUSPID) | 12–13 YR |
| SECOND PREMOLAR (BICUSPID) | 12–14 YR |
| FIRST MOLAR | 6–7 YR |
| SECOND MOLAR | 14–16 YR |
| THIRD MOLAR | 18–25 YR |
| **LOWER** | |
| THIRD MOLAR | 18–25 YR |
| SECOND MOLAR | 13–16 YR |
| SECOND PREMOLAR (BICUSPID) | 13–14 YR |
| FIRST PREMOLAR (BICUSPID) | 12–15 YR |
| FIRST MOLAR | 6–7 YR |
| (CUSPID) CANINE | 10–13 YR |
| LATERAL INCISOR | 9–10 YR |
| CENTRAL INCISOR | 8–9 YR |

tooth, resulting in missphapen blue or brown teeth.

**dentinoid** [″ + Gr. *eidos,* form, shape] **1.** Resembling dentin. **2.** The noncalcified matrix of dentin, similar to the noncalcified matrix of bone, which is called osteoid. SYN: *dentoidin; predentin.*

**dentinoma** [″ + Gr. *oma,* tumor] A tumor composed of tissues from which the teeth originate, consisting mainly of dentin.

**dentinosteoid** (dĕn″tĭn-ŏs′tē-oyd) [″ + Gr. *osteon,* bone, + *eidos,* form, shape] A tumor composed of dentin and bone.

**dentist** [L. *dens,* tooth] An authorized practitioner of dentistry.

**dentistry 1.** The branch of medicine dealing with the care of the teeth and associated structures of the oral cavity. It is concerned with the prevention, diagnosis, and treatment of diseases of the teeth and gums. **2.** The art or profession of a dentist. SYN: *dentology; odontology.*

***d. for children*** Pedodontia.

***esthetic d.*** Repair and restoration or replacement of carious or broken teeth.

***forensic d.*** The area of dentistry particularly related to jurisprudence; usually, the identification of unknown persons by the details of their dentition and tooth restorations.

Whereas forensic medicine often is used to establish the time and cause of death, forensic dentistry may be used to establish identity on the basis of dental records only.

***four-handed d.*** Extensive use of a chairside dental assistant to facilitate and enhance the productivity of the dentist.

***geriatric d.*** The area of dentistry devoted to the dental health care of the aged.

***hospital d.*** The practice of dentistry in a hospital where the dentist is an integral part of the comprehensive health care team.

***operative d.*** The branch of dentistry dealing with restorative dental surgery.

***preventive d.*** That phase of dentistry concerned with the maintenance of the normal masticatory apparatus by teaching good oral hygiene and dietary practice, and preserving dental health by early restorative procedures.

***prosthodontic d.*** The replacement of defective or missing teeth with artificial appliances such as bridges, crowns, and dentures.

***public health d.*** The area of dentistry that seeks to improve the dental health of communities by epidemiological studies, research in preventive methods, and better distribution, management, and use of dental skills.

**dentition** [L. *dentitio*] The type, number, and arrangement of teeth in the dental arch. SEE: illus.; *teeth* for illus.

***diphyodont d.*** Two sets of teeth (i.e., primary and permanent, as in many mammals and humans).

***heterodont d.*** A set of teeth of various shapes which may serve different functions (e.g., incisors, canines, and molars).

***mixed d.*** A set of both primary and permanent teeth, as in humans between 6 and 13 years of age. SYN: *transitional dentition.*

***monophyodont d.*** A single set of teeth.

***permanent d.*** The 32 permanent teeth, which begin to erupt at about 6 years of age in humans. These are completed by the 16th year with the exception of third molars, which appear between the 18th and 25th years. The incisors are followed by the bicuspids (premolars) and the canines; then the second molars are followed by the third molars. In some individuals the third molars, although present beneath the gingiva, do not erupt. The appearance of the first molars is highly variable, but in some instances they may be the first permanent teeth to appear. SEE: *teeth.*

***polyphyodont d.*** Several successive sets of teeth developing during a lifetime.

***primary d.*** The 20 primary or deciduous teeth in humans. In general, the order of eruption is two lower central incisors, 6 to 8 months; two upper central incisors, 5 to 7 months; two lower lateral incisors, 8 to 11 months; two upper lateral incisors, 7 to 10 months; four canines (cuspids), lower and upper, 16 to 20 months; four first molars, lower and upper, 10 to 16 months; four second molars, upper and lower, 20 to 30 months.

**dento-, denti-, dent-** Combining form concerning teeth.

**dentoalveolar** (dĕn″tō-ăl-vē′ō-lăr) [L. *dens,* tooth, + *alveolus,* small hollow] Pert. to the alveolus of a tooth and the tooth itself.

**dentoalveolitis** (dĕn″to-ăl″vē-ō-lī′tĭs) [″ + ″ + Gr. *itis,* inflammation] A purulent inflammation of the tooth socket linings characterized by loose teeth and shrinkage of the gum.

**dentofacial** (dĕn″tō-fā′shăl) Concerning the teeth and face.

**dentoid** [″ + Gr. *eidos,* form, shape] Dentiform; odontoid; tooth-shaped.

**dentoidin** The organic ground substance of dentin. SYN: *dentinoid; predentin.*

**dentolegal** Concerning dentistry and legal matters.

**dentulous** (dĕn′tū-lŭs) Having one's natural teeth. SEE: *edentulous.*

**denture** (dĕn′chūr) A partial or complete set of artificial teeth set in appropriate plastic materials to substitute for the natural dentition and related tissues. SYN: *dental prosthesis.*

NURSING IMPLICATIONS: Proper denture care involves cleansing the dentures after each meal by gently brushing them with warm water and by scrubbing them with only moderate pressure. Cleansing solutions and mixtures accepted by the American Dental Association are ammonia water 28% (2 ml in 30 ml water); trisodium phosphate (0.6 g in 30 ml water); sodium hypochlorite, or bleach, (2 ml in 120 ml water). Dentures should be properly fitted in the patient's mouth; when stored outside the mouth, they should be placed in a well-identified, opaque, closed container. Dentures are stored wet or dry according to their particular composition and according to instructions by the dentist. Dentures are removed from comatose or moribund patients as well as from patients undergoing surgery

***fixed partial d.*** A dental restoration of one or more missing teeth that is cemented to prepared natural teeth.

***full d.*** A dental appliance that replaces all of the teeth in both jaws.

***immediate d.*** A complete set of artificial teeth inserted immediately after removal (extraction) of natural teeth.

***implant d.*** An artificial denture placed in and supported by bone. The denture may be implanted at the site of a previously removed natural tooth. SEE: *implant, dental* for illus.

***partial d.*** A dental appliance replacing less than the full number of teeth in either jaw.

**denturism** A movement among dental technicians to be permitted to provide dentures legally to the public without the supervision of a dentist. SEE: *denturist.*

**denturist** A person licensed in some states to fabricate and fit dentures. This person is not a dentist or a dental technician.

**denucleated** (dē-nū′klē-āt″ĕd) [L. *de,* from, + *nucleus,* kernel] Deprived of a nucleus.

**denudation** [L. *denudare,* to lay bare] Removal of a protecting layer or covering through surgery, pathological change, or trauma.

**Denver classification** A system for classifying chromosomes based on the size and position of the centromere. SEE: *chromosome.*

**Denver Developmental Screening Test** ABBR: DDST. A widely used screening test to detect problems in the development of very young children.

**deodorant** (dē-ō′dor-ănt) [″ + *odorare,* to perfume] An agent that masks or absorbs foul odors. SEE: *odor.*

**deodorize** (dē-ō′dor-īz) [″ + *odor,* odor] To remove foul odor.

**deodorizer** (dē-ō′dor-īz-ĕr) Something that deodorizes.

**deontology** (dē″ŏn-tŏl′ō-jē) [Gr. *deonta,* needful, + *logos,* word, reason] The theory or study of moral obligations and commitments (e.g., medical ethics). SEE: *ethics.*

**deorsum** (dē-or′sŭm) [L.] Downward.

***d. vergens*** Turning downward.

**deorsumduction** (dē-or″sŭm-dŭk′shŭn) [L. *deorsum,* downsard, + *ducere,* to lead] A downward turn.

**deorsumversion** (dē-or″sŭm-vĕr′zhŭn) [″ + *vertere,* to turn] A downward turning or movement of the eyes.

**deossification** (dē-ŏs″ĭ-fĭ-kā′shŭn) [L. *de,* from, + *os,* bone, + *facere,* to make] Loss or removal of mineral matter from bone or osseous tissue.

**deoxidation** The process of depriving a chemical compound of oxygen.

**deoxidizer** (dē-ŏk′sĭ-dī-zĕr) An agent that removes oxygen.

**deoxycholic acid** (dē-ŏk″sē-kō′lĭk) $C_{24}H_{40}O_4$. A crystalline acid found in bile.

**deoxycorticosterone** (dē-ŏk″sē-kor″tē-kŏs′tĕr-ōn) A hormone from the adrenal gland. It acts principally on salt and water metabolism.

**deoxygenation** (dē-ŏk″sĭ-jĕn-ā′shŭn) Removal of oxygen from a chemical compound or tissue.

**deoxyhemoglobin** Chemically reduced (deoxygenated) hemoglobin.

**deoxyribonuclease** (dē-ŏk″sē-rī″bō-nū′klē-ās) ABBR: DNase. An enzyme that hydrolyzes and thus depolymerizes deoxyribonucleic acid (DNA).

**deoxyribonucleic acid** (dē-ŏk″sē-rī″bō-nū-klē′ĭk) ABBR: DNA. A complex nucleic acid of high molecular weight consisting of deoxyribose, phosphoric acid, and four bases (two purines, adenine and guanine, and two pyrimidines, thymine and cytosine). These are arranged as two long chains that twist around each other to form a double helix joined by bonds between the complementary components. Nucleic acid, present in chromosomes of the nuclei of cells, is the chemical basis of heredity and the carrier of genetic information for all organisms except the RNA viruses. Formerly spelled desoxyribonucleic acid. SEE: *chromosome; gene; ribonucleic acid; virus; Watson-Crick helix.*

**deoxyribonucleoprotein** (dē-ŏk″sē-rī″bō-nū″klē-ō-prō′tē-ĭn) One of a class of conjugated proteins that contain deoxyribonucleic acid.

**deoxyribonucleoside** (dē-ŏk″sē-rī″bō-nū′klē-ō-sīd) One of a class of nucleotide in which the pentose is 2-deoxyribose.

**deoxyribose** (dē-ŏk″sē-rī′bōs) A pentose sugar that is part of DNA.

**Department of Health and Human Services** ABBR: HHS. The U.S. Government agency that administers federal health programs, including the Federal Drug Administration and the Centers for Disease Control and Prevention. Its previous name was Department of Health, Education, and Welfare.

**dependence** (dē-pĕn′dĕns) [L. *dependere,* to hang down] **1.** A form of behavior that suggests inability to make decisions. **2.** A psychic craving for a drug that may or may not be accompanied by physiological dependency. **3.** A state of reliance on another. SEE: *habituation; withdrawal.*

**dependent care** The practice of caring for persons who cannot meet their own needs. Included would be elderly parents and other relatives, as well as children. SEE: *dumping* (2).

**depersonalization disorder** The belief that one's own reality is temporarily lost or altered. The patient feels estranged or unreal and may feel that the extremities have changed size. A feeling of being automated or as if in a dream may be present. The onset is usually rapid, and it usually occurs in adolescence or under extreme stress, fatigue, or anxiety.

**depersonalize** To make impersonal; to deprive of personality or individuality.

**dephosphorylation** (dē-fŏs″for-ī-lā′shŭn) [L. *de,* from, + *phosphorylation*] Removal of a phosphate group from a compound.

**depigmentation** (dē″pĭg-mĕn-tā′shŭn) **1.** The pathological loss of normal pigment as in vitiligo. **2.** Removal of pigment, esp. from the skin, by chemical or physical means.

**depilate** (dĕp′ĭl-āt) [L. *depilare,* to deprive of hair] To remove hair.

**depilation** (dĕp″ĭl-ā′shŭn) The process of hair removal. SEE: *epilation.*

**depilatory** An agent used to remove hair.

**depilatory technique** One of several temporary procedures to remove hair from the body, including shaving the area, plucking a few unsightly hairs, chemical means, or wax treatment. If chemical depilation is used, care must be taken to avoid skin irritation. The wax treatment involves application of molten wax, which is allowed to cool; then, when the wax is pulled away, the hair comes with it. Permanent depilation is accomplished by electrolysis of each hair follicle. This time-consuming process is done by an electrologist trained in the technique. SEE: *electrolysis; hirsutism.*

**deplete** (dē-plēt′) [L. *depletus,* emptied] To empty; to produce depletion.

**depletion** (dē-plē′shŭn) Removal of substances such as blood, fluids, iron, fat, or protein from the body.

**depolarization** (dē-pō″lăr-ĭ-zā′shŭn) [″ + *polus,* pole] A reversal of charges at a cell membrane; an electrical change in an excitable cell in which the inside of the cell becomes positive (less negative) in relation to the outside. This is the opposite of polarization and is caused by a rapid inflow of sodium ions. SEE: illus.

**depolymerization** (dē-pŏl″ĭ-mĕr-ī-zā′shŭn) The breakdown or splitting of polymers into their basic building blocks or monomers. The glucose monomer may be polymerized to form the large glycogen polymer and then broken down (i.e., depolymerized) to form glucose.

**deposit** (dē-pŏz′ĭt) [L. *depositus,* having put aside] **1.** A sediment; a precipitate (1). **2.** Matter collected in any part of an organism.

***calcareous d.*** A deposit of calcified material, as in calculus on teeth.

***tooth d.*** Soft or hard material deposited on the surface of a tooth. Also called *plaque* or *calculus.*

**deposition** In law, an oral interrogation about the subject at issue. The party or witness is under oath and the interrogation is recorded word for word by a judi-

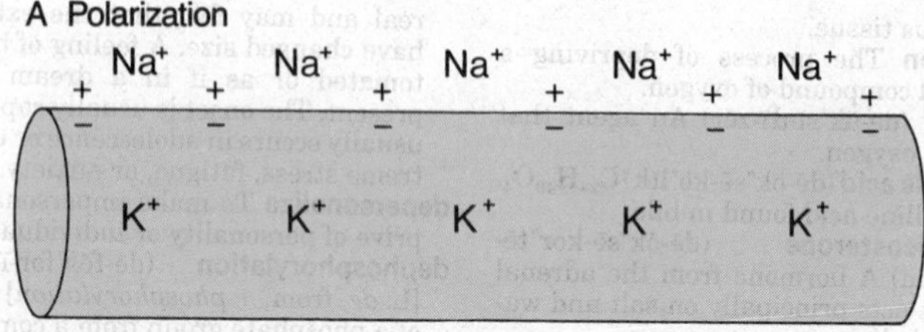


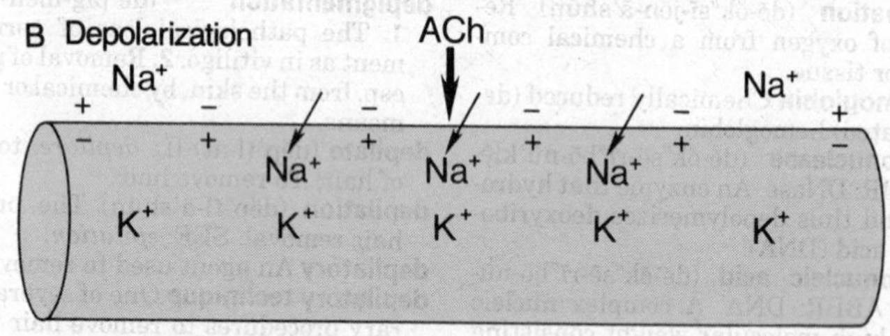


C Repolarization
K+ K+ K+
Na+ Na+ Na+ Na+ Na+
K+ K+

ELECTRICAL CHARGES AND ION CONCENTRATIONS AT THE CELL MEMBRANE. **(A)** POLARIZATION, **(B) DEPOLARIZATION, (C)** REPOLARIZATION

cial officer such as a court reporter.

***diffusion d.*** The accumulation of aerosol particles on a surface due to their random bombardment by gas molecules.

**depot** (dē′pō, dĕp′ō) [Fr. *depot,* fr. L. *depositum*] A place of storage, esp. in the body, such as a fat depot.

**depravation** (dĕp″ră-vā′shŭn) [L. *depravare,* completely destroyed] A pathological deterioration of function or secretion.

**depressant** [L. *depressus,* pressed down] An agent that decreases the level of a body function or nerve activity (e.g., a sedative medicine).

***cardiac d.*** An agent that decreases heart rate and contractility.

***cerebral d.*** An agent that lessens brain activity, making the patient dull and less active. Large doses may produce sleep.

***motor d.*** An agent that lessens contractions of involuntary muscles.

***respiratory d.*** An agent that lessens frequency and depth of breathing.

**depressed** (dĕ-prĕst′) **1.** Below the normal level, as when fragments of bone are forced below their normal level and that of surrounding portions of bone. **2.** Low in spirits; dejected. **3.** Having a decreased level of function. SEE: *depression.*

**depression** (dē-prĕsh′ŭn) [L. *depressio,* a pressing down] **1.** A hollow or lowered region. **2.** The lowering of a part, such as the mandible. **3.** The decrease of a vital function such as respiration. **4.** A mental disorder marked by altered mood. An estimated 3% to 5% of the world's population experiences depression on any given date. There is loss of interest in all usually pleasurable outlets such as food, sex, work, friends, hobbies, or entertainment. Diagnostic criteria include the presence of altered mood nearly every day, markedly diminished interest or pleasure in most or all activities, and three or more of the following: (1) Poor appetite or significant weight loss, or increased weight gain. (2) Insomnia or hypersomnia. (3) Psychomotor agitation or retardation. (4) Feelings of hopelessness. (5) Loss of energy, or fatigue. (6) Feelings of worthlessness, self-reproach, or excessive or inappropriate guilt. (7) Complaints or evidence of a diminished ability to think or concentrate. (8) Recurrent thoughts of death, suicidal ideation, a wish to be dead, or attempted suicide.

TREATMENT: Therapy must be individualized because the various types of depression have different underlying causes. Thus, to attempt to treat all persons suffering depression with the same medication would be ill advised. Psychotherapy, electroconvulsive therapy, or both may be helpful. SEE: *depression, situational; electroconvulsive therapy; grief reaction; suicide.*

---

Caution: Depressed persons may attempt suicide and should not be left alone, esp. if hospitalized.

---

NURSING IMPLICATIONS: The patient is assessed for feelings of worthlessness or self-reproach, inappropriate guilt, concern with death, and attempts at self-injury. Level of activity and socialization are evaluated. Adequate nutrition and fluids are provided, and the patient is fed if necessary. Dietary interventions and increased physical activity are recommended to manage constipation; assistance with grooming and other activities of daily living may be required. A structured routine, including noncompetitive activities, is provided to build the patient's self-confidence and to encourage interaction. The nurse demonstrates warmth and interest in the patient and maintains an optimistic attitude while guarding against excessive cheerfulness. Support is gradually reduced as the patient demonstrates an increasing ability to resume self-care. Prescribed drug therapies are administered and evaluated.

If electroconvulsive therapy (ECT) is required, the patient is informed that a series of treatments may be needed. Before each ECT session, the prescribed sedative is administered, and a nasal or oral airway inserted. Vital signs are monitored, and the nurse offers support by talking calmly or by gentle touch. After ECT, mental status and response to therapy are evaluated. The patient may be drowsy and experience transient amnesia but should become alert and oriented within 30 min. The period of disorientation lengthens after subsequent treatments. SEE: *Nursing Diagnoses Appendix.*

***anaclitic d.*** Depression in infants separated from their mothers between the first months and 1 year of age. These infants have been cared for in a suitable physical situation, but without the love, affection, and nurturing usually present in the mother-child relationship. They may have severe disturbances in health and in motor, language, and social development. They may die. Symptoms include crying, panic behavior, and increased motor activity at first. Later, the infants manifest dejection, apathy, staring into space, and silent crying.

***bipolar d.*** Depression in which both dejection and elation are alternately present.

***endogenous d.*** Melancholia.

***postpartum d.*** Depression, occurring in a new mother, in which the signs and symptoms do not dissipate within several weeks following delivery, or strong feelings of dejection and anger begin 1 to 2 months after childbirth. The symptoms are tearfulness, despondency, a feeling of hopelessness, inadequacy, inability to cope with infant care, mood swings, extreme anxiety over the infant, guilt of not loving the infant enough, irritability, fatigue, loss of normal interests, and insomnia. This depression occurs in about 3% of women and may occur in other family members, including the father. SEE: *postpartum blues.*

***situational d., reactive d.*** Depression that is usually self-limiting, following a serious event such as a death in the family, the loss of a job, or a personal financial catastrophe. The disorder is longer lasting and more marked than the normal reaction.

***unipolar d.*** Depression characterized by mental shifts from a normal baseline to a depressed state.

**depressive disorder** SEE: *Nursing Diagnoses Appendix.*

**depressomotor** (dē-prĕs′ō-mō″tor) [″ + *motor,* mover] Having the ability to diminish muscular movements by lessening the impulses for motion sent from the brain or spinal cord; said of drugs.

**depressor** [L.] An instrument for drawing down a body part.

***tongue d.*** A device used to draw down and displace the tongue to facilitate visual examination of the throat.

**depressor fiber** A muscle that depresses or draws down a body part.

**depressor nerve** A nerve whose stimulation lessens or inhibits the activity of an organ or tissue.

**depressor reflex** A reflex that results in slowed muscle activity, as in the heart rate.

**deprivation** (dĕp″rĭ-vā′shŭn) [L. *de,* from, + *privare,* to remove] Loss or absence of a necessary part or function.

***emotional d.*** Isolation of an individual, esp. an infant, from normal emotional stimuli. In infants, this produces impairment of mental and physical development.

***sensory d.*** Absence of the usual sensory stimuli, including noise, light, and human contact, or masking of noise by a continuous dull sound. Persons exposed partially or completely to such an environment include astronauts, patients in artificial respirators, and patients with temporary loss of a sense (i.e., through bandaging of both eyes). Prolonged exposure to lack of sensory stimuli may cause hallucinations and other signs and symptoms of mental disorder.

***sleep d., effects of*** SEE: *sleep depriva-*

*tion, effects of.*

**deprogram** To free an individual from some mentally harmful cult, religion, or political brainwashing program.

**depth** [ME. *depthe*] Richness; intensity; the quality of being deep.

**depth dose** The actual amount of radiation exposure at a specific point below the surface of the body.

**depth perception** The perception of spatial relationships; three-dimensional perception.

**depth psychology** The psychology of unconscious behavior, as opposed to psychology of conscious behavior.

**depulization** (dē-pū l″ĭ-zā′shŭn) [L. *de*, from, + *pulex*, flea] Destruction of fleas, including those that carry the plague bacillus.

**depurant** (dĕp′ū-rănt) [L. *depurare*, to purify] **1.** A medicine that helps to purify by promoting the removal of waste material from the body. **2.** Any agent that removes waste material.

**depuration** The process of freeing from impurities. **depurative,** *adj.*

**depurator** An agent that purifies.

**de Quervain's disease** Tenosynovitis due to relative narrowness of the tendon sheath of the abductor pollicis longus and the extensor pollicis brevis.

**deradelphus** (dĕr-ă-dĕl′fŭs) [Gr. *dere*, neck, + *adelphos*, brother] A pair of malformed twins, fused above the thorax and having one head, but separated below the chest as two bodies.

**deradenoncus** (dĕr″ăd-ĕn-ŏnk′ŭs) [″ + *onkos*, bulk, mass] A swelling or tumor of a neck gland.

**derangement** (dē-rānj′mĕnt) [Fr. *deranger*, unbalance] **1.** Lack of order or organization, esp. as compared with the previous condition; confusion. **2.** A defect in the annulus fibrosus of the intervertebral disk allowing the nucleus pulposus to herniate.

**Dercum's disease** (dĕr′kŭms) [Francis X. Dercum, U.S. neurologist, 1856–1931] Scattered areas of painful cutaneous nodules or fat accumulations in menopausal women. SYN: *adiposis dolorosa.*

**derealization** A sense that reality has changed; a sense of detachment from one's surroundings.

**dereism** (dē′rē-ĭzm) [L. *de*, from, + *res*, thing] In psychiatry, activity and thought based on fantasy and wishes rather than logic or reason; overexercise of the imagination to the extent of ignoring reality, as seen in daydreaming. SEE: *autism.* **dereistic** (dē-rē-ĭst′ik), *adj.*

**derencephalus** (dĕr″ĕn-sĕf′ă-lŭs) [Gr. *dere*, neck, + *enkephalos*, brain] A congenitally deformed fetus with a rudimentary skull and bifid cervical vertebrae.

**derivation** (dĕr″ĭ-vā′shŭn) [L. *derivare*, to draw off] The source or origin of a substance.

**derivative** (dĕ-rĭv′ă-tĭv) **1.** Something that is not original or fundamental. **2.** Something derived from another body or substance. **3.** Something that produces derivation. **4.** In embryology, anything that develops from a preceding structure, as the derivatives of the germ layers.

**derm-** SEE: *dermato-*.

**derm, derma** [Gr. *derma*, skin] The cutis vera, or true skin. **dermal,** *adj.*

**dermabrasion** (dĕrm′ă-brā″zhŭn) [″ + L. *abrasio*, wearing away] A surgical procedure for removal of acne scars, nevi, tattoos, or fine wrinkles on the skin by using sandpaper or mechanical methods on the frozen epidermis. The procedure is dangerous and should not be used indiscriminately. SEE: *chemical peel of skin; planing.*

**Dermacentor** (dĕr″mă-sĕn′tor) A genus of ticks belonging to the order Acarina, family Ixodidae.

***D. andersoni*** The wood tick, a species of ticks that is parasitic on humans or other mammals during some part of its life cycle. It may transmit causative agents of Rocky Mountain spotted fever, scrub typhus, tularemia, tick paralysis, brucellosis, Q fever, and several forms of viral encephalomyelitis.

***D. variabilis*** A species of ticks similar to *D. andersoni.* In the central and eastern U.S., it is the main vector for Rocky Mountain spotted fever. It is parasitic to dogs, horses, cattle, rabbits, and humans.

**dermad** [Gr. *derma*, skin, + L. *ad*, toward] Toward the skin; externally.

**dermalgia** (dĕr-măl′jē-ă) [″ + *algos*, pain] Pain localized in the skin.

**dermamyiasis** (dĕr-mă-mī-ī′ă-sĭs) [″ + *myia*, fly, + *-iasis*, condition] A skin disease caused by invasion of larvae of dipterous insects. SEE: *myiasis.*

**dermat-** SEE: *dermato-*.

**dermatalgia** (dĕr″mă-tăl′jē-ă) [Gr. *dermatos*, skin, + *algos*, pain] A paresthesia with localized pain in the skin. SYN: *dermalgia.*

**dermatatrophia** (dĕrm″ăt-ă-trō′fē-ă) [″ + *atrophia*, atrophy] Atrophy of the skin.

**dermatitides** Pl. of dermatitis.

**dermatitis** (dĕr″mă-tī′tĭs) [Gr. *dermatos*, skin, + *itis*, inflammation] Inflammation of skin evidenced by itching, redness, and various skin lesions.

ETIOLOGY: Dermatitis may be due to one of several causes: systemic disease; skin irritants such as poison ivy, corrosives, acids, and alkalies; or hypersusceptibility to conditions that would not normally cause skin irritation.

TREATMENT: The primary cause should be removed if the condition is due to a systemic effect. If it is due to a local agent, the irritant should be removed by washing with soap and water.

NURSING IMPLICATIONS: Patients should avoid harsh soaps, known irritants, temperature extremes, emotional stress, and other potential precipitants. Local measures (tepid sponge baths, cool

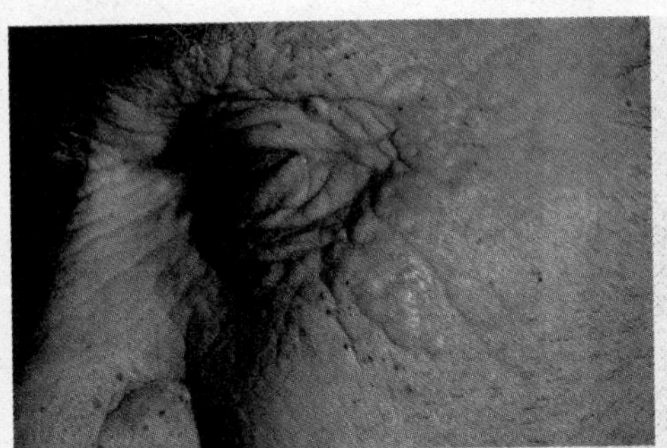

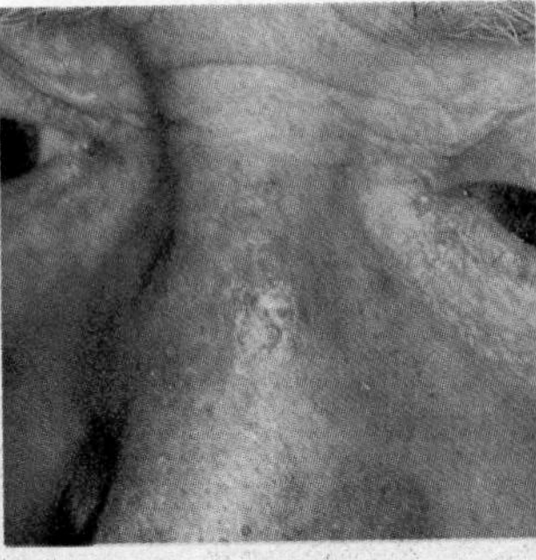

**ACTINIC DERMATITIS: (A)** ERYTHEMA AND WRINKLING, **(B)** SOLAR KERATOSIS AND TELANGIECTASIA

compresses) are used to relieve inflammation and pruritus. Prescribed drug therapy is administered and evaluated for desired effects and adverse reactions. The patient is instructed in the application of prescribed topical medications and warned about drowsiness produced by systemic antihistamines and about the serious side effects of systemic corticosteroids. The nurse encourages the patient to express feelings about the condition and avoids showing distaste when caring for the patient's lesions.

***actinic d.*** Reaction of the skin to sunlight or other sources of photochemical activity such as x-rays or ultraviolet light. SEE: illus.

***allergic d.*** Inflammation believed to be due to an allergy. SEE: *allergen*; *allergy*.

***atopic d.*** Dermatitis of unknown etiology marked by itching and scratching in an individual with inherently irritable skin. There may be allergic, hereditary, or psychological components. The disease rarely occurs before 2 months of age and may occur initially quite late in life. In about 70% of all cases there is a family history of the disease. About 3% of all infants have atopic dermatitis. The symptoms are made worse by contact with wool, climatic changes, and excessive exposure to soap, water, and oils. The skin lesions in infants consist of swollen papules that itch and become exudative and crusty from scratching. Secondary infection and lymphadenopathy are common. About half of the infantile cases clear up by 18 months of age. The lesions in children and adults are similar to those of infancy but lichenification is present. SEE: illus.

TREATMENT: The patient should avoid soaps and ointments. Bathing is kept to a minimum, but bath oils may help to prevent drying of the skin. Clothing should be soft textured and should not contain wool. Fingernails should be kept short to decrease damage from scratching. Antihistamines may help to reduce itching at night. Heavy exercise should be avoided because it induces perspiration. The patient should use a nonlipid softening lotion followed by a cortisone or hydrocortisone lotion in a propylene glycol base twice daily. Oral antibiotics may be needed for a brief period to control secondary infection.

***berlock d., berloque d.*** A type of phytophotodermatitis with postinflammatory hyperpigmentation at the site of application of perfumes or colognes containing oil of bergamot.

***d. calorica*** Inflammation due to heat, as in sunburn, or cold.

***cercarial d.*** Dermatitis resulting from infestation with the cercaria of blood flukes belonging to the genus *Schistosoma*. SYN: *schistosome d.; swimmer's itch*.

***contact d.*** Inflammation and irritation of the skin due to contact with an irritating substance. It is usually due to a combination of reduced ability of the skin to resist injury and exposure to a material in strong concentration such as soap or a chemical. Some individuals are sensitive to such apparently innocuous compounds as perfumes and deodorants. SYN: *d. venenata* (1). SEE: illus.

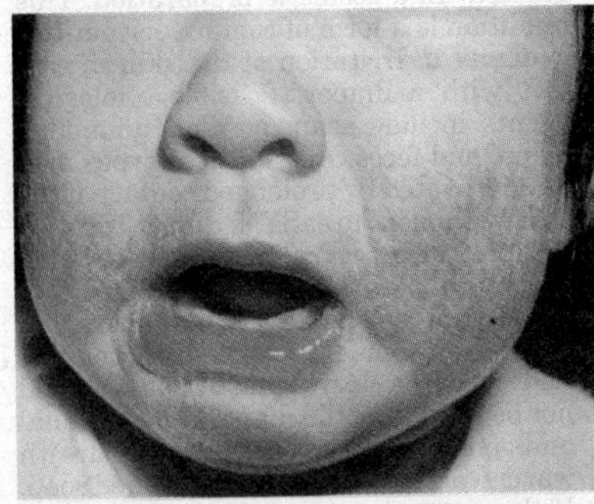

**ATOPIC DERMATITIS**

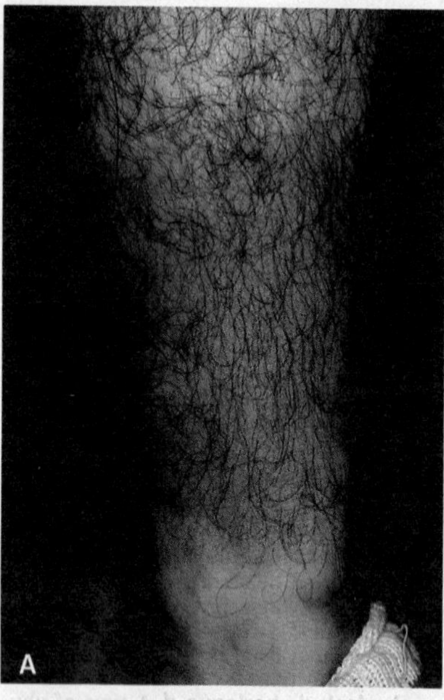


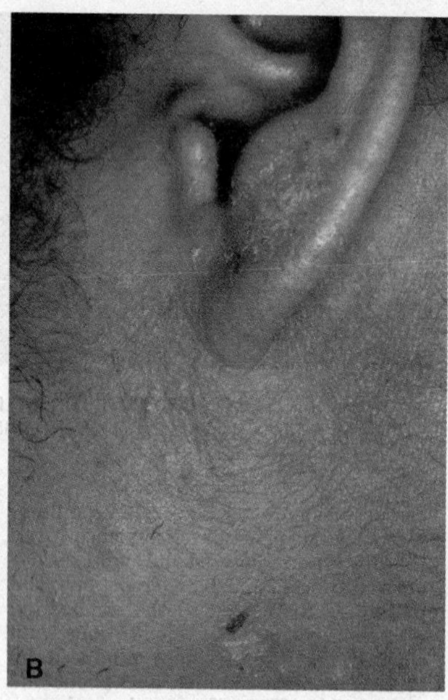


**CONTACT DERMATITIS: (A)** ALLERGY TO ELASTIC IN SOCKS, **(B)** ALLERGY TO NICKEL IN EARRING

SYMPTOMS: Symptoms vary from simple hyperemia to gangrene and sloughing. Most eruptions are erythematous and limited to the part touched by the irritant. They become papular, vesicular, or pustular with burning or itching.

ETIOLOGY: The causes are drugs, acids, alkalies, and plants (poison ivy, oak, or sumac). The inflammation runs an acute course with recurrence on re-exposure to the sensitizing agent.

TREATMENT: Local drying solutions such as aluminum acetate should be applied. Calamine lotion is helpful in drying the lesions and controlling itching. In severe cases, topical and systemic cortisone may be needed.

***cosmetic d.*** Dermatitis caused by an ingredient in a cosmetic preparation. This condition is a form of contact dermatitis.

***diaper d.*** Irritation of the skin in contact with a diaper. Possible etiological agents include soap, powder, ammonia, urine, and feces. Any of these types may be aggravated by prolonged contact of the skin with moisture. SYN: *diaper rash.*

TREATMENT: Treatment is symptomatic. Diapers should be changed frequently; if washable cloth diapers are used, they should be washed thoroughly and rinsed. Occlusive plastic pants should not be used over the diaper. The perianal and genital areas should be washed with warm water and mild, nonperfumed soap. If these measures and the application of a bland protective agent (e.g., zinc oxide paste) do not promote healing, a small amount of 0.5% to 1% topical hydrocortisone cream should be applied to the area after each diaper change. This should be repeated for several days.

***exfoliative d.*** An erythematous condition in which scaling follows the erythema. In addition to the increased loss of exfoliated skin, there is systemic involvement with lymphadenopathy in 60% of cases and hepatomegaly in about 30%, fever without other signs of infection, anemia in 65%, eosinophilia in 30%, and hypothermia in some cases. Although the cause of idiopathic exfoliative dermatitis is unknown, the condition is secondary to or associated with many other disease processes of the skin (atopic dermatitis, contact dermatitis, mycosis fungoides, psoriasis), systemic diseases (Hodgkin's disease, lymphomas, leukemias, certain cancers), and toxic chemicals and drugs (antibiotics, arsenic, mercury, aspirin, codeine, BAL, gold, iodine, quinidine).

When the skin involvement is extensive the patient may become depressed because of the cosmetic changes.

TREATMENT: If the cause can be determined it should be removed or treated appropriately. The idiopathic type is treated with corticosteroids, emollients, and antihistamines for pruritis.

---

Caution: Corticosteroids are not indicated if this condition is a manifestation of psoriasis.

***factitial d.*** A skin irritation or injury that is self-inflicted.

***d. herpetiformis*** A chronic inflammatory disease characterized by erythematous, papular, vesicular, bullous, or pustular lesions with a tendency to grouping and with intense itching and burning.

SYMPTOMS: The lesions develop suddenly and spread peripherally. The disease is variable and erratic, and an attack may be prolonged for weeks or months. Secondary infection may follow trauma to the inflamed areas.

ETIOLOGY: The direct cause is unknown. The condition occurs mostly in men; no age is exempt. Some patients have associated asymptomatic gluten-sensitive enteropathy. In those persons the HLA-B8 antigen may be present.

TREATMENT: Oral dapsone provides substantial relief of symptoms in a few days. Sulfapyridine also may be used.

***d. hiemalis*** Dermatitis occurring in cold weather.

***d. infectiosa eczematoides*** A pustular eruption during or following a pyogenic disease.

***d. medicamentosa*** A skin eruption due to ingested or applied medicines. Treatment consists of discontinuing use of the causative agent. SEE: *idiosyncracy*.

SYMPTOMS: With the exception of those caused by bromine and iodine, the eruption is not characteristic and may resemble almost any skin condition or disease.

ETIOLOGY: The cause is an idiosyncrasy or sensitization to the drug in question. Cosmetics, arsenic, iodides, bromides, phenobarbital, and antibiotics are some of the offending agents.

***d. multiformis*** A form of dermatitis with pustular lesions.

***d. papillaris capillitii*** Formation on the scalp and neck of surface elevations interspersed with pustules and ending in scarlike elevations resembling keloids.

***photoallergic contact d.*** Inflammation of the skin due to substances made allergenic by the effect of ultraviolet or visible light. SEE: *photoallergy*.

***poison ivy d.*** Dermatitis resulting from irritation or sensitization of the skin by urushiol, the toxic resin of the poison ivy plant. There is no absolute immunity, although susceptibility varies greatly, even in the same individual.

Persons sensitive to poison ivy may also react to contact with other plants such as the mango rind and cashew oil. These plants contain chemicals that cross-react with the *Rhus* sap present in poison ivy.

SYMPTOMS: An interval of time elapses between skin contact with the poison and first appearance of symptoms, varying from a few hours to several days and depending on the sensitivity of the patient and the condition of the skin. Moderate itching or a burning sensation is soon followed by small blisters; later manifestations vary. Blisters usually rupture and are followed by oozing of serum and subsequent crusting.

PREVENTION: Certain substances, including organoclay compounds, have been useful in preventing poison ivy dermatitis. They are sprayed on the skin, where they serve as a barrier to prevent the irritating agent, urushiol, from bonding with the skin. Organoclay compounds are present in some antiperspirants. Shoes and clothes as well as the hair of cats and dogs can carry the toxic resin to those who handle them.

TREATMENT: In mild dermatitis, a lotion to relieve itching is usually sufficient. In severe dermatitis, cool, wet dressings or compresses, potassium permanganate baths, and perhaps a course of intramuscular or oral corticosteroid therapy will be required. Sedation is also necessary in some cases.

Application of moderately hot water to nonblistered areas for 2 or 3 min may provide symptomatic relief from itching and burning. The comfort produced is dramatic and may last several hours.

NURSING IMPLICATIONS: Prevention is important in both persons with known sensitivity and those with no previous contact with or reaction to it. Patient teaching focuses on helping the patient to recognize the plant, to avoid contact with it, and to wear long-sleeved shirts and long pants in wooded areas. If contact occurs, the patient should wash with soap and water immediately to remove the toxic oil, apply antipruritic lotion (e.g., calamine) or a cool wet dressing of aluminum acetate (Borrow's) solution or Epsom salts, and cover skin with plastic wrap to retain moisture.

***primary d.*** Dermatitis that is a direct rather than an allergic response.

***radiation d.*** Dermatitis due to radiation exposure.

***rhus d.*** Contact dermatitis caused by substances present in certain plants. SEE: *poison ivy dermatitis; Toxicodendron*.

***schistosome d.*** Cercarial d.

***d. seborrheica*** An acute or subacute inflammatory skin disease of unknown cause, beginning on the scalp and characterized by rounded, irregular, or circinate lesions covered with yellow or brown-gray greasy scales. SYN: *alopecia furfuracea; pityriasis capitis; seborrhea corporis; seborrhea sicca*. SEE: *Nursing Diagnoses Appendix*.

SYMPTOMS: On the scalp, it may be dry with abundant grayish branny scales, or oozing and crusted, constituting eczema capitis, and may spread to the forehead and postauricular regions. The forehead shows scaly and infiltrated lesions with dark red bases, some itching, and localized loss of hair. The eyebrows and eyelashes show dry, dirty white scales with itching. On nasolabial folds or the vermilion border of the lips, there is inflammation with itching. On the sternal region, the lesions are greasy to the touch. Eruptions may appear in interscapular, axillary, and genitocrural regions also.

TREATMENT: When the condition is limited to the scalp, frequent shampooing and use of mild keratolytic agents is indicated. Selenium-containing shampoos have been helpful. Generalized seborrheic dermatitis requires careful attention including scrupulous skin hygiene, keeping the skin as dry as possible, and using dusting powders. Topical and systemic cortisone preparations may be required.

***stasis d.*** Eczema of the legs with edema, pigmentation, and sometimes chronic inflammation. It is usually due to impaired circulation. SEE: illus.

***d. venenata*** **1.** Contact d. **2.** Any inflammation caused by local action of various animal, vegetable, or mineral substances contacting the surface of the skin.

***d. verrucosa*** A chronic fungal infection of the skin characterized by the formation of wartlike nodules. These may enlarge and form papillomatous structures that sometimes ulcerate. SYN: *chromoblastomycosis*.

ETIOLOGY: This condition may be due to one of several fungi including *Hormodendrum pedrosoi* or *Phialophora verrucosa*.

***x-ray d.*** Skin inflammation due to effects of x-rays.

**dermato-, dermat-, derm-** Combining form meaning *skin*.

**dermatoautoplasty** (dĕr″mă-tō-aw′tō-plăs″tē) [Gr. *dermatos*, skin, + *autos*, self, + *plassein*, to form] Grafting of skin taken from some portion of the patient's own body.

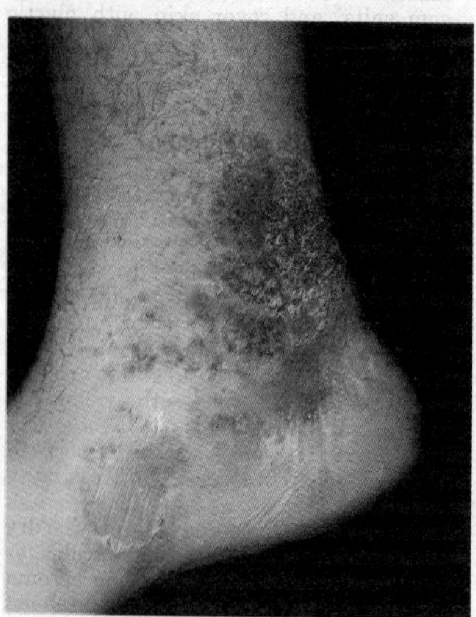

STASIS DERMATITIS

**Dermatobia** (dĕr″mă-tō′bē-ă) [″ + *bios*, life] A genus of botflies belonging to the order Diptera of the family Oestridae.

***D. hominis*** A species of botflies, found in parts of tropical America, whose larvae infest humans and cattle. The eggs are transported by mosquitoes.

**dermatobiasis** (dĕr″mă-tō-bī′ă-sĭs) Infestation by the larvae of *Dermatobia hominis*, the eggs of which are carried to the skin by mosquitoes. The larvae then hatch and bore into the skin while the mosquito feeds. Marblelike boils form at the site of infestation.

**dermatocele** (dĕr′mă-tō-sēl″) [″ + *kele*, tumor, swelling] A tendency of hypertrophied skin and subcutaneous tissue to hang loosely in folds. SYN: *dermatolysis*.

***d. lipomatosa*** A pedunculated lipoma with cystic degeneration.

**dermatocelidosis** (dĕr″mă-tō-sĕl″ĭ-dō′sĭs) [″ + *kelis*, spot, + *osis*, condition] A macular eruption; a freckle. SYN: *dermatokelidosis*.

**dermatocellulitis** (dĕr″mă-tō-sĕl″ū-lī′tĭs) [″ + L. *cellula*, little cell, + Gr. *itis*, inflammation] Inflammation of subcutaneous connective tissue.

**dermatoconiosis** (dĕr″mă-tō-kō″nē-ō′sĭs) [″ + *konia*, dust] Any irritation of the skin caused by dust, esp. one due to occupational exposure.

**dermatocyst** (dĕr′mă-tō-sĭst) [″ + *kystis*, cyst] A skin cyst.

**dermatofibroma** [″ + L. *fibra*, fiber, + Gr. *oma*, tumor] A nonmalignant skin fibroma. SEE: *dimple sign*.

**dermatofibrosarcoma** (dĕr″mă-tō-fī″brō-săr-kō′mă) [″ + ″ + Gr. *sarx*, flesh, + *oma*, tumor] Fibrosarcoma of the skin.

**dermatogen** (dĕr-măt′ō-jĕn) [″ + *gennan*, to produce] Antigen from a skin disease.

**dermatogenous** (dĕr″mă-tŏj′ĕn-ŭs) Producing skin or skin disease.

**dermatoglyphics** (dĕr″mă-tō-glĭf′ĭks) [″ + *glyphe*, a carving] Study of the surface markings of the skin, esp. those of hands and feet, used in identification and genetic studies. SEE: *fingerprint* for illus.

**dermatographism** A form of physical allergy in which a pale raised wheal with red flare on each side is produced when the skin is scratched by using a blunt object.

**dermatoheliosis** Sun-induced degenerative changes in the skin. Included are wrinkling, atrophy, hypermelanotic and hypomelanotic macules, telangiectasia, yellow papules and plaques, keratoses, and degeneration of elastic tissue. This condition can be prevented by avoiding exposure to the sun or by using topically applied effective sunscreens.

**dermatoheteroplasty** (dĕr″mă-tō-hĕt′ĕr-ō-plăs″tē) [″ + *heteros*, other, + *plassein*, to mold] Skin grafting from a member of a different species.

**dermatokelidosis** (dĕr″mă-tō-kĕl″ĭ-dō′sĭs) Dermatocelidosis.

**dermatologist** (dĕr″mă-tŏl′ō-jĭst) [Gr. *dermatos,* skin, + *logos,* word, reason] A physician who specializes in treating diseases of the skin.

**dermatology** (dĕr″mă-tŏl′ō-jē) The science of the skin and its diseases.

**dermatolysis** (dĕr″mă-tŏl′ĭ-sĭs) [″ + *lysis,* dissolution] A tendency of hypertrophied skin and subcutaneous tissue to hang in folds; loose skin. SYN: *cutis laxa; cutis pendula; pachydermatocele* (1).

**dermatoma** (dĕr″mă-tō′mă) [″ + *oma,* tumor] A circumscribed thickening of skin.

**dermatome** (dĕr′mă-tōm) [Gr. *derma,* skin, + *tome,* incision] **1.** An instrument for incising the skin or cutting thin slices for skin transplantation. **2.** A delineated area of skin innervated by a spinal cord segment. Each cord segment has a representative skin area. SEE: illus. **3.** The lateral portion of the somite of an embryo, where the dermis of the skin originates; the cutis plate.

**dermatomere** (dĕr′mă-tō-mēr) [Gr. *dermatos,* skin, + *meros,* part] A segment of embryonic integument.

**dermatomucosomyositis** (dĕr″mă-tō-mū-kō″sō-mī-ō-sī′tĭs) [″ + L. *mucosa,* mucous membrane, + Gr. *mys,* muscle, + *itis,* inflammation] An inflammation involving the mucosa and muscles.

**dermatomycosis** (dĕr″mă-tō-mī-kō′sĭs) *pl.* **dermatomycoses** [″ + *mykes,* fungus, + *osis,* condition] A skin infection caused by certain fungi of the genera *Trichophyton, Epidermophyton,* and *Microsporum.* SYN: *tinea.*

**dermatomyoma** [″ + *mys,* muscle, + *oma,* tumor] Myoma of the skin.

**dermatomyositis** (dĕr″mă-tō-mī″ō-sī′tĭs) [″ + ″ + *itis,* inflammation] A disease of connective tissue. It may be acute, subacute, or chronic. The etiology is unknown. Characteristics are edema, dermatitis, and inflammation of the muscles.

SYMPTOMS: Symptoms include fever, malaise, general weakness, and weakness of the pelvic and shoulder girdle muscles; skin and mucosal lesions are often present. About one third of patients have dysphagia.

TREATMENT: The treatment is symptomatic and includes bedrest, physical therapy, and salicylates. Adrenocortical steroids are helpful in most cases. Cytotoxic drugs such as azathioprine, cyclophosphamide, and methotrexate may be beneficial in patients who do not respond to adrenocortical steroids.

NURSING IMPLICATIONS: The patient's level of discomfort, muscle weakness, and joint range of motion are assessed and documented daily. The patient's face, neck, upper back, chest, nailbeds, eyelids, and interphalangeal joints are evaluated for rashes, and any findings documented. Frequent assistance is provided to help the patient reposition in correct body alignment; appropriate supportive devices and graduated exercises are used to prevent and treat muscle atrophy and joint contractures. Warm baths, moist heat, and massage are provided to relieve stiffness, and prescribed analgesics are administered. Oral lesions are irrigated with warm saline solution as necessary. Tepid sponge baths and compresses are used to relieve pruritus and to prevent scratching; antihistamines are also administered as prescribed. Self-care activities, with assistance if necessary, are encouraged and paced according to response. Prescribed corticosteroid or cytotoxic drugs are administered, and the patient's response is evaluated.

Both patient and family are educated about the disease process, treatment expectations, and possible adverse reactions to corticosteroid and cytotoxic drugs. Good nutrition and a low-sodium diet are recommended to prevent fluid retention. The patient is reassured that steroid-induced weight gain will diminish when the drug can be reduced or discontinued. The patient is encouraged to express feelings, fears, and concerns about the illness; realistic support and encouragement are provided.

**dermatopathia** [″ + *pathos,* disease, suffering] Any skin disease.

**dermatopathology** [″ + ″ + *logos,* word, reason] The study of skin diseases.

**dermatopathy** Any skin disease. SYN: *dermatopathia.*

**dermatophiliasis** (dĕr″mă-tō-fĭ-lī′ă-sĭs) **1.** Infestation with *Tunga penetrans,* a pathogenic actinomycete. **2.** Dermatophilosis.

**dermatophilosis** (dĕr″mă-tō-fī-lō′sĭs) An actinomycotic infection that occurs in certain hooved animals and rarely in humans. SYN: *dermatophiliasis.*

**dermatophobia** [″ + *phobos,* fear] Abnormal fear of having a skin disease.

**dermatophyte** (dĕr′mă-tō-fīt) [″ + *phyton,* plant] A fungal parasite that grows in or on the skin. Dermatophytes rarely penetrate deeper than the epidermis or its appendages—hair and nails. They cause such skin diseases as favus, tinea, ringworm, and eczema. Important dermatophytes include the genera *Microsporum, Trichophyton,* and *Epidermophyton.*

**dermatophytid** (dĕr″mă-tŏf′ĭ-tĭd) A toxic rash or eruption occurring in dermatomycosis.

**dermatophytosis** (dĕr″mă-tō-fī-tō′sĭs) [″ + *phyton,* plant, + *osis,* condition] A fungus infection of the skin of the hands and feet, esp. between the toes. SYN: *athlete's foot; ringworm; tinea pedis.*

**dermatoplastic** [″ + *plassein,* to form] Pert. to skin grafting.

**dermatoplasty** (dĕr′mă-tō-plăs″tē) Trans-

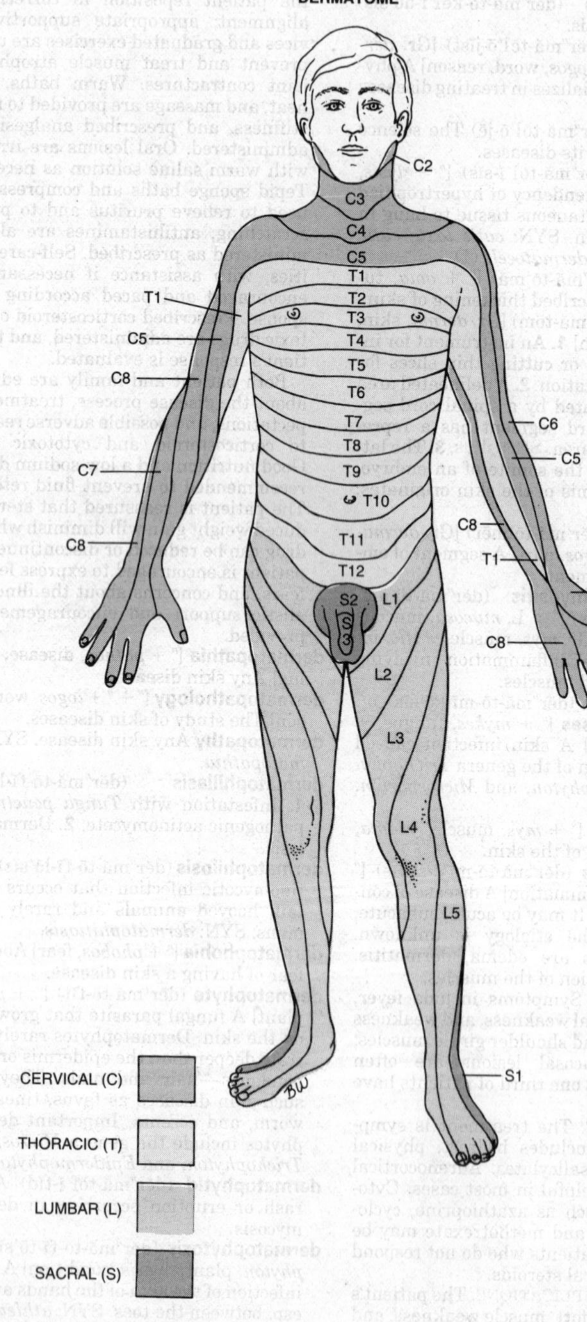
DERMATOME
C2
C3
C4
C5
T1
T2
T3
T1
C5
T4
T5
C8
T6
T7
C6
T8
C5
C7
T9
T10
C8
T11
C8
T1
T12
C6
S2
L1
S3
C8
C7
L2
L3
L4
L5
S1
BW
CERVICAL (C)
THORACIC (T)
LUMBAR (L)
SACRAL (S)

plantion of living skin to cover cutaneous defects caused by injury, operation, or disease.

NURSING IMPLICATIONS: Nursing measures are directed toward protecting the graft site from dislodgement, trauma, or infection and toward promoting healing of the donor site. Signs of infection such as fever and pain are monitored, and assistance is offered to help the patient to cope with altered mobility. Any discomfort is assessed, and pain relief provided as indicated. Nutritious meals are provided to aid healing.

**dermatorrhexis** [" + *rhexis,* rupture] Rupture of the skin and capillaries in the skin.

**dermatosclerosis** (dĕr"mă-tō-sklĕr-ō'sĭs) [" + *sklerosis,* hardening] Infiltration of the skin with fibrous material.

**dermatosis** (dĕr"mă-tō'sĭs) *pl.* **dermatoses** [" + *osis,* condition] Any disease of the skin in which inflammation is not necessarily a feature; not a synonym for dermatitis.

***d. papulosa nigra*** An eruption consisting of many tiny tumors, or milia, on the skin of the face. The greatest incidence is among blacks.

***progressive pigmentary d.*** A slowly progressive eruption of reddish papules principally on the legs.

**dermatosome** (dĕr'mă-tō-sōm) [" + *soma,* body] A section of the equatorial plate in mitosis.

**dermatotherapy** [" + *therapeia,* treatment] Treatment of skin disease.

**dermatotome** (dĕr'mă-tō-tōm") [" + *tome,* incision] **1.** One of the fetal skin segments. **2.** A knife for incising the skin or small lesions. SYN: *dermatome* (1).

**dermatotropic** (dĕr"mă-tō-trŏp'ĭk) [" + *trope,* a turning] Acting preferentially on the skin.

**dermatozoon** [" + *zoon,* animal] An animal parasite of the skin.

**dermatozoonosis** (dĕr"mă-tō-zō"ō-nō'sĭs) [" + " + *nosos,* disease] Any skin disease caused by an animal parasite.

**dermic** (dĕr'mĭk) [Gr. *derma,* skin] Pert. to the skin.

**dermis** (dĕr'mĭs) [L.] The layer of the skin lying immediately under the epidermis; the true skin. It consists of two layers, papillary and reticular. The corium dermis is composed of fibrous connective tissue made of collagen and elastin, and contains numerous capillaries, lymphatics, and nerve endings. In it are hair follicles and their smooth muscle fibers, sebaceous glands and sweat glands, and their ducts. SYN: *corium; cutis vera.*

**dermoblast** [Gr. *derma,* skin, + *blastos,* germ] Part of the mesoblastic layer, developing into the corium.

**dermographia, dermography** A form of urticaria due to allergy.

**dermoid** (dĕr'moyd) [" + *eidos,* form, shape] **1.** Resembling the skin. **2.** A dermoid cyst.

**dermoid cyst 1.** An ovarian teratoma. **2.** A nonmalignant cystic tumor containing elements derived from the ectoderm, such as hair, teeth, or skin. These tumors occur frequently in the ovary but may develop in other organs such as the lungs.

**dermoidectomy** (dĕr"moyd-ĕk'tō-mē) [" + " + *ektome,* excision] Excision of a dermoid cyst.

**dermolipoma** (dĕr"mō-lĭ-pō'mă) **1.** A growth of yellow fatty tissue beneath the bulbar conjunctiva. **2.** A lipoma of the skin.

**dermomycosis** (dĕr"mō-mī-kō'sĭs) [" + *mykes,* fungus, + *osis,* condition] A skin disease produced by a fungus; dermatomycosis. SYN: *tinea.*

**dermonosology** (dĕr"mō-nō-sŏl'ō-jē) [" + *nosos,* disease, + *logos,* word, reason] The science of classification of skin diseases.

**dermoskeleton** [" + *skeleton*] The apparent external covering of the body; the hair, nails, and teeth in humans. SYN: *exoskeleton.*

**dermosynovitis** (dĕr"mō-sĭn-ō-vī'tĭs) [" + L. *synovia,* joint fluid, + Gr. *itis,* inflammation] Inflammation of the skin overlying an inflamed bursa or tendon.

**dermovascular** (dĕr"mō-văs'kū-lăr) [" + *vas,* vessel] Concerning the skin and its blood vessels.

**derodidymus** (dĕr"ō-dĭd'ĭ-mŭs) [Gr. *dere,* neck, + *didymos,* double] A malformed fetus with two necks and heads but a single body and normal limbs. SYN: *dicephalus.*

**DES** *diethylstilbestrol.*

**desalination** Partial or complete removal of salts from a substance, as from seawater or brackish water, so that it is suitable for agricultural or household purposes but not for drinking.

**desaturation** [L. *de,* from, + *saturare,* to fill] A process whereby a saturated organic compound is converted into an unsaturated one, as when stearic acid, $C_{18}H_{36}O_2$, is changed into oleic acid, $C_{18}H_{34}O_2$. The product has different physical and chemical properties after this transformation. SEE: *saturated hydrocarbon.*

**Desault's apparatus** (dĕ-sōz') [Pierre J. Desault, Fr. surgeon, 1744–1795] A bandage used for fracture of the clavicle. SEE: *bandage.*

**descemetitis** (dĕs"ĕ-mĕ-tī'tĭs) Inflammation of Descemet's membrane on the corneal posterior surface.

**descemetocele** (dĕs"ĕ-mĕt'ō-sēl) A protrusion of Descemet's membrane.

**Descemet's membrane** (dĕs-ĕ-māz') [Jean Descemet, Fr. anatomist, 1732–1810] A fine membrane between the endothelial layer of the cornea and the substantia propria. SYN: *vitreous membrane.*

**descendens** (dē-sĕn'dĕns) [L. *de,* from, + *scendere,* to climb] Descending; a descending structure.

***d. hypoglossi*** A branch of the hypoglossal nerve occurring at the point at which the nerve curves around the occipital artery, which passes down obliquely across (sometimes within) the sheath of the carotid vessels to form a loop just below the middle of the neck with branches of the second and third cervical nerves.

**descensus** (dē-sĕn′sŭs) [L.] The process of falling; descent.

***d. testis*** The normal passage of the testicle from the abdominal cavity down into the scrotum. This occurs during the last few months of fetal life. SYN: *migration of testicle.*

***d. uteri*** SEE: *uterus, prolapse of.*

***d. ventriculi*** Downward displacement of the stomach. SYN: *gastroptosis.*

**desensitization** **1.** Treatment of an allergy by repeated injections of a dilute solution containing the allergen. The concentration is too weak to cause symptoms, but slowly promotes tolerance of the antigen by the immune system. It increases the levels of immunoglobulin G, which blocks immunoglobulin E from binding to mast cells and initiating the release of the chemical mediators of inflammation. Although not always successful, densensitization is still commonly used, particularly for patients whose allergic response to an antigen is systemic anaphylaxis. SEE: *allergy; anaphylaxis; tolerance.* **2.** In psychiatry, the alleviation of an emotionally upsetting life situation.

Nursing Implications: The patient is closely monitored for signs of anaphylaxis for at least 20 min after each injection of dilute antigen. Emergency drug therapy is maintained nearby for immediate treatment of anaphylaxis. Prescribed antihistamine therapy is provided to relieve lesser allergic symptoms (urticaria, pruritus, wheezing).

***phobic d.*** A method of treating phobias in which the patient is taught to relax while slowly re-entering the phobic situation, first in imagination and then in real life. Anxiety and fear are kept to a minimum at all times. SEE: *implosion flooding.*

***systematic d.*** A form of behavior therapy, used particularly for phobias, in which the patient is gradually exposed to anxiety-producing stimuli until they no longer produce anxiety. SEE: *implosion flooding.*

**desensitize** [L. *de,* from, + *sentire,* to perceive] **1.** To deprive of or lessen sensitivity by nerve section or blocking. **2.** To abate anaphylactic sensitivity by administration of the specific antigen in low dosage.

**desert fever, desert rheumatism** Coccidioidomycosis.

**desexualize** (dē-sĕks′ū-ăl-īz) [″ + *sexus,* sex] To castrate; to remove sexual traits.

**desferrioxamine** (dĕs-fĕr′ē-ŏks′ă-mēn) Deferoxamine mesylate.

**desiccant** (dĕs′ĭ-kănt) Causing desiccation or dryness.

**desiccate** (dĕs′ĭ-kāt) [L. *desiccare,* to dry up] To dry.

**desiccation** (dĕs″ĭ-kā′shŭn) The process of drying up. SEE: *electrodesiccation.*

**desipramine hydrochloride** (dĕs-ĭp′ră-mēn) An antidepressant.

**deslanoside** (dĕs-lăn′ō-sīd) A cardiac glycoside, obtained from digitalis leaf, that has the same action as lanatoside C.

**desmectasia, desmectasis** (dĕs-mĕk-tā′zē-ă, -ĕk′tă-sĭs) [Gr. *desmos,* band, + *ektasis,* dilatation] Stretching of a ligament.

**desmepithelium** (dĕs-mĕp-ĭ-thē′lē-ŭm) [″ + *epi,* upon, + *thele,* nipple] The epithelial lining of vessels and synovial cavities.

**desmitis** (dĕs-mī′tĭs) [″ + *itis,* inflammation] Inflammation of a ligament.

**desmo-** [Gr. *desmos,* band] Combining form indicating a band or ligament.

**desmocranium** (dĕs″mō-krā′nē-ŭm) [″ + L. *cranium*] In the embryo, the earliest form of the skull.

**desmocyte** (dĕs′mō-sīt) [″ + *kytos,* cell] A supporting tissue cell. SYN: *fibroblast; fibrocyte.*

**desmocytoma** (dĕs″mō-sī-tō′mă) [″ + ″ + *oma,* tumor] A tumor formed of desmocytes; a sarcoma.

**desmogenous** (dĕs-mŏj′ĕ-nŭs) [″ + *gennan,* to produce] Originating in connective tissue.

**desmography** (dĕs-mŏg′ră-fē) [″ + *graphein,* to write] A description of or treatise on ligaments.

**desmoid** (dĕs′moyd) [″ + *eidos,* form, shape] **1.** Tendonlike; fibroid (1). **2.** A very tough and firm fibroma.

**desmology** (dĕs-mŏl′ō-jē) [″ + *logos,* word, reason] The science of tendons and ligaments.

**desmoma** [″ + *oma,* tumor] A tumor of the connective tissue.

**desmoneoplasm** (dĕs″mō-nē′ō-plăzm) [″ + *neos,* new, + LL. *plasma,* form, mold] A newly developed connective tissue tumor.

**desmopathy** (dĕs-mŏp′ă-thē) [″ + *pathos,* disease, suffering] Any disease affecting ligaments.

**desmoplasia** (dĕs-mō-plā′zē-ă) [″ + Gr. *plassein,* to form] An abnormal tendency to form fibrous tissue or adhesive bands.

**desmoplastic** [″ + *plassein,* to form] Causing or forming adhesions.

**desmopressin acetate** A synthetic antidiuretic, a vasopressin analogue, with greater antidiuretic activity but less pressor activity than vasopressin. Used intranasally, this medicine has been very beneficial in treating primary nocturnal enuresis.

**desmopyknosis** (dĕs″mō-pĭk-nō′sĭs) [″ + *pyknosis,* condensation] A surgical procedure for shortening round ligaments by attaching them by loops to the anterior uterine wall.

**desmorrhexis** (dĕs-mō-rĕk′sĭs) [″ + *rhexis,* rupture] Rupture of a ligament.

**desmosis** (dĕs-mō′sĭs) [″+ *osis,* condition] Any disease of the connective tissue.

**desmosome** (dĕs′mō-sōm) [″ + *soma,* body] A structure binding adjacent epithelial cells.

**desmotomy** (dĕs-mŏt′ō-mē) [″ + *tome,* incision] Dissection of a ligament.

**desoximetasone** (dĕs-ŏk″sē-mĕt′ă-sōn) A corticosteroid used topically.

**desoxy-** Prefix meaning deoxidized or a reduced form of.

**desoxycorticosterone** (dĕs-ŏk″sē-kor-tĭ-kŏs′tĕr-ōn) An active steroid hormone produced by the adrenal cortex. It plays an important role in the regulation of water and salt metabolism.

***d. acetate*** An acetate ester of desoxycorticosterone and the form in which the hormone is usually administered in its therapeutic use. It may be injected intramuscularly or used buccally.

**desoxyribonucleic acid** (dĕs″ŏk-sē-rī″bō-nū′klē-ĭk) The former spelling for deoxyribonucleic acid.

**despair** The eighth stage in Erikson's developmental theory; the opposite of ego integrity. The individual experiences sorrow over past life events and dismay over a foreshortened life.

**desquamate** (dĕs′kwă-māt) [L. *desquamare,* to remove scales] To shed or scale off the surface epithelium.

**desquamation** (dĕs″kwă-mā′shŭn) **1.** Shedding of the epidermis. **2.** The peeling skin characteristic of postmature infants.

***furfuraceous d.*** Shedding of branlike scales.

**desquamative** (dĕs-kwŏm′ă-tĭv) Of the nature of desquamation, or pert. to or causing it. SYN: *keratolytic.*

**DES syndrome** The occurrence of neoplasms and malformation of the vagina in young women whose mothers received diethylstilbestrol early in their pregnancy.

**destructive** [L. *destructus,* destroyed] Causing ruin or destruction; the opposite of constructive.

**destructive lesion** A pathological change such as an infection, tumor, or injury that causes the death of tissue or an organ.

**desulfhydrase** (dē″sŭlf-hī′drās) An enzyme that cleaves cysteine into hydrogen sulfide, ammonia, and pyruvic acid.

**desynchronosis** (dē-sĭn″krō-nō′sĭs) [″ + Gr. *synkhronos,* same time] An upset of the internal biological clock, caused by the difference between the time at a person's present location and the time to which the person is accustomed. This condition occurs in persons traveling across several time zones in a short period. The lay term for this condition is "jet lag."

**DET** *diethyltryptamine.*

**det** L. *detur,* let it be given.

**detachment** [O. Fr. *destachier,* to unfasten] The process of separation.

**detail** In radiology, the sharpness with which an image is presented on a radiograph.

**detector** [L. *detectus,* uncovered] A device for determining the presence of something.

***flame ionization d.*** ABBR: FID. A device used in gas chromatography in which a sample burned in a flame changes the conductivity between two electrodes.

***lie d.*** A polygraph.

***optical d.*** The sensor in a typical colorimeter or photometer that senses the light transmitted by the sample.

***radiation d.*** An instrument used to detect the presence of radiation. SEE: *dosimeter.*

**detergent** [L. *detergere,* to cleanse] **1.** Something that purges or cleanses; cleansing. **2.** A cleaning or wetting agent prepared synthetically from any of several chemicals. These are classed as anionic if they have a negative electric charge or cationic if they have a positive charge. SEE: *soap.*

**deterioration** [L. *deteriorare,* to deteriorate] Retrogression; said of impairment of mental or physical functions.

**determinant** (dē-tĕr′mĭ-nănt) [L. *determinare,* to limit] That which determines the character of something.

**determination** [L. *determinatus,* limiting] The establishing of the nature or precise identity of a substance, organism, or event.

**determinism** (dē-tĕr′mĭn-ĭzm) [″ + Gr. *-ismos,* condition] The theory that all human action is the result of predetermined and inevitable physical, psychological, or environmental conditions that are uninfluenced by the will of the individual.

**detersive** [L. *detergere,* to cleanse] Detergent (1).

**detortion, detorsion** (dē-tor′shŭn) **1.** Surgical therapy for torsion of a testicle, ureter, or volvulus of the bowel. **2.** Correction of any bodily curvature or deformity.

**detoxification** [″ + ″ + L. *facere,* to make] **1.** Reduction of the toxic properties of a poisonous substance. SEE: *biotransformation.* **2.** The process of removing the physiological effects of a drug or substance from an addicted individual.

**detoxify** (dē-tŏk′sĭ-fī) **1.** To remove the toxic quality of a substance. **2.** To treat a toxic overdose of any medicine, but esp. of the toxic state produced by drug abuse or acute alcoholism.

**detrition** (dē-trĭsh′ŭn) [L. *detritus,* to rub away] The wearing away of a part, esp. through friction, as of the teeth. SEE: *bruxism.*

**detritus** (dĭ-trī′tŭs) [L., to rub away] Any broken-down, degenerative, or carious matter produced by disintegration.

**detrusor urinae** (dē-trū′sor ū-rī′nē) [L.] The external longitudinal layer of the muscular coat of the bladder.

**detumescence** (dē″tū-mĕs′ĕns) [L. *de,* down, + *tumescere,* to swell] **1.** Subsidence of a swelling. **2.** Subsidence of the swelling of erectile tissue of the genital organs (penis or clitoris) following erection.

**deuter-** SEE: *deutero-.*

**deuteranomalopia** (doo″tĕr-ă-nŏm″ă-lō′pē-ă) [″ + *anomalos,* irregular, + *ops,* eye] Partial color blindness in which the primary colors are perceived but green is poorly appreciated.

**deuteranopia, deuteranopsia** (dū″tĕr-ăn-ō′pē-ă, -ŏp′sē-ă) [″ + *anopia*, blindness] Green blindness; color blindness in which there is a defect in the perception of green. SEE: *color blindness*.

**deuterate** (dū′tĕr-āt) To combine with deuterium.

**deuterium** (dū-tē′rē-ŭm) [Gr. *deuteros*, second] SYMB: $H^2$ or D. The mass two isotope of hydrogen, sometimes called heavy hydrogen.

***d. oxide*** An isotope of water in which hydrogen has been displaced by its isotope, deuterium. Its properties differ from ordinary water in that it has a higher freezing and boiling point and is incapable of supporting life. SYN: *heavy water*.

**deutero-, deuter-, deuto-** [Gr. *deuteros*, second] Prefix indicating *second* or *secondary*.

**deuteron** (dū′tĕr-ŏn) SYMB: d. The nucleus of deuterium or heavy hydrogen.

**deuteroplasm** [″ + LL. *plasma*, form, mold] The reserve food supply in the yolk or ovum.

**deuto-** SEE: *deutero-*.

**deutoscolex** (dū″tō-skō′lĕks) [″ + *skolex*, worm] A secondary daughter cyst that develops on the inner wall of a hydatid cyst.

**devascularization** (dē-văs″kū-lăr-ĭ-ză′shŭn) [″ + *vascularis*, pert. to a vessel] **1.** Loss or draining of blood from a body part. **2.** A decrease in the blood supply to a body part.

**developer** In radiology and photography, the solution used to make the latent image visible on the radiographic film.

**development** [O. Fr. *desveloper*, to unwrap] Growth to full size or maturity, as in the progress of an egg to the adult state. SEE: *growth*.

***cognitive d.*** The sequential acquisition of the ability to learn, reason, and analyze that begins in infancy and progresses as the individual matures.

***psychomotor and physical d. of infant*** SEE: *psychomotor and physical development of infant*.

**developmental** Pert. to development.

**developmental milestone** A skill regarded as having special importance in the development of infants and toddlers and usually associated with a particular age range (e.g., sitting, crawling, walking).

**deviance** [L. *deviare*, to turn aside] A variation from the accepted norm.

**deviant** Something (or someone) that is variant when compared with the norm or an accepted standard.

***sex d.*** One whose sexual behavior is considered to be abnormal or socially unacceptable. SEE: *paraphilia*.

**deviant behavior** Any action considered to be abnormal.

**deviate** (dē′vē-āt″) [L. *deviare*, to turn aside] **1.** To move steadily away from a designated norm. **2.** An individual whose behavior, esp. sexual behavior, is so far removed from societal norms that it is classed as socially, morally, or legally unacceptable.

**deviation** (dē-vē-ā′shŭn) **1.** A departure from the normal. **2.** To alter course or direction.

***axis d.*** A change in the direction of the major electrical axis of the heart as determined by the electrocardiogram.

***conjugate d.*** Deviation of the eyes to the same side.

***minimum d.*** The smallest deviation that a prism can produce.

***standard d.*** ABBR: SD. In statistics, the measure of variability from the central tendency of any frequency curve. It is the square root of the variance.

**device** (dĭ-vīs′) [O. Fr. *devis*, contrivance] An apparatus, machine, or shaped object constructed to perform a specific function.

***abduction d.*** A trapezoid-shaped pillow, wedge, or splint placed between the legs to prevent adduction. It is commonly used postoperatively for patients having total hip replacement or open reduction or internal fixation of the hip.

***adapted seating d.*** ABBR: ASD. A device that provides proper positioning for persons with limited motor control. These include seating inserts, wheelchairs, and postural support systems designed to prevent deformities and enhance function. SYN: *seating system*.

***adaptive d.*** Any equipment or device used to aid disabled or handicapped individuals to perform daily tasks. SYN: *assistive d.*

***assistive d.*** Adaptive d.

***head immobilization d.*** A device that attaches to a long back board and holds the patient's head in neutral alignment. Also called *cervical immobilization device*. SEE: *back board, long*.

***input d.*** In assistive technology, the apparatus that activates an electronic device. This can be a manual switch, a remote control, or a joystick. SEE: *switch*.

***Kendrick extrication d.*** SEE: *Kendrick extrication device*.

***pointing d.*** A type of input device for sending commands to a microcomputer. Moving the device results in movement of a cursor on the monitor or computer screen. Pointing devices range from the conventional desktop mouse, trackball, and touch-sensitive screens to infrared and ultrasound pointers mounted on the head. SYN: *input d.* SEE: *pointer, light; switch*.

***position-indicating d.*** ABBR: PID. A device used to guide the direction of the x-ray beam during the exposure of dental radiographs. These devices improve and standardize dental radiographic imaging and reduce the patient's risk of radiation exposure.

***positive beam limiting d.*** A collimator that automatically adjusts the size of the radiation field to match the size of the imaging device. Also called *automatic colli-*

*mator.*

***pressure relief d.*** Wheelchair cushion.

***telecommunication d. for the deaf*** A device that allows hearing-impaired people to use the telephone even if they cannot comprehend speech. A keyboard and display screen are used on each end of the transmission.

**devil's grip** Epidemic pleurodynia.

**deviometer** (dē″vē-ŏm′ĕ-tĕr) [L. *de,* from, + *via,* way, + Gr. *metron,* measure] A machine for estimating degrees of strabismus.

**devitalization** [″ + *vita,* life] **1.** Destruction or loss of vitality. **2.** Anesthetizing of the sensitive pulp of a tooth; known as killing the nerve.

**dew point** Temperature at which dew begins to form as the moisture in the air condenses.

**dexamethasone** (dĕk″să-mĕth′ă-sōn) A synthetic glucocorticoid drug.

**dexamethasone suppression test** A test performed by administering dexamethasone to determine the effect on cortisol production. This is done as part of the diagnostic investigation for Cushing's syndrome. Normally this test causes a decrease in cortisol production, but in a patient with Cushing's syndrome, suppression is minimal. The test may be positive in patients with ectopic corticotropin production. SEE: *corticotropin production, ectopic; Cushing's syndrome.*

**dexbrompheniramine maleate** (dĕks″brŏm-fĕn-ĭr′ă-mēn) An antihistamine.

**dexchlorpheniramine maleate** (dĕks″klor-fĕn-ĭr′ă-mēn) An antihistamine.

**dexter** (dĕks′tĕr) [L.] On the right side. SEE: *sinister.*

**dexterity** Skill in using the hands, usually requiring both fine and gross motor coordination.

**dextrad** (dĕks′trăd) [L. *dexter,* right, + *ad,* toward] **1.** Toward the right side. **2.** A right-handed person.

**dextral** (dĕks′trăl) Pert. to the right side.

**dextrality** (dĕks-trăl′ĭ-tē) Right-handedness. SEE: *sinistrality.*

**dextran** (dĕks′trăn) [L. *dexter,* right] A polysaccharide produced by the action of *Leuconostoc mesenteroides* on sucrose. It is available in various molecular weights and is used as a plasma volume expander.

**dextranomer beads** A cross-linked network of dextran prepared in the form of beads. Because this compound has great ability to absorb moisture, it has been used in helping to debride wounds. SEE: *decubitus ulcer.*

**dextrase** (dĕks′trās) An enzyme that splits dextrose and converts it into lactic acid.

**dextraural** (dĕks-traw′răl) [L. *dexter,* right, + *auris,* ear] Hearing better with the right ear.

**dextrin** (dĕks′trĭn) [L. *dexter,* right] A yellow-white powder that forms mucilaginous solutions in water and can be prepared by the action of heat or acid on starch. It is a carbohydrate of the formula $(C_6H_{10}O_5)_{11}$. In digestion, it is a soluble or gummy matter into which starch is converted by diastase; it is the result of the first chemical change in the digestion of starch.

**dextro-** [L. *dexter,* right] Combining form meaning *to the right.*

**dextroamphetamine sulfate** (dĕks″trō-ăm-fĕt′ă-mēn sŭl′fāt) A compound related to amphetamine sulfate (i.e., an isomer of amphetamine); sometimes written D-amphetamine sulfate or dextroamphetamine sulfate. It is used as a central nervous system stimulant in the treatment of mild depression. The drug is of benefit in treating abnormally hyperactive children, but concomitant psychotherapy and parent counseling are essential. Continued use of this drug in children depresses their growth; thus growth should be carefully monitored. The drug is used in the treatment of obesity but should not be used long term or in children under age 12 years. Prolonged use can cause psychological dependence. The "street" name is "speed."

**dextrocardia** (dĕks″trō-kăr′dē-ă) [″ + Gr. *kardia,* heart] The condition of having the heart on the right side of the body.

**dextrocular** (dĕks-trŏk′ū-lăr) [″ + *oculus,* eye] Having a stronger right eye than left.

**dextrocularity** (dĕks″trŏk-ū-lăr′ĭ-tē) The condition of having the right eye stronger than the left.

**dextroduction** [″ + *ducere,* to lead] Movement of the visual axis to the right.

**dextrogastria** [″ + Gr. *gaster,* belly] The condition of having the stomach on the right side of the body.

**dextromanual** [″ + *manus,* hand] Right-handed.

**dextromethorphan** (dĕk″strō-mĕth′or-făn) A cough suppressant. A great number of cough medicines include this drug in their formula.

**dextropedal** (dĕks-trŏp′ĕ-dăl) [″ + *pes, ped-,* foot] Having greater dexterity in using the right leg than the left.

**dextrophobia** [″ + Gr. *phobos,* fear] Abnormal aversion to objects on the right side of the body.

**dextroposition** (dĕks″trō-pō-zĭsh′ŭn) Displacement to the right.

**dextropropoxyphene** (dĕk″strō-prō-pŏk′sē-fēn) Propoxyphene, an analgesic that can cause addiction and may be fatal in an overdose.

**dextrorotatory** (dĕks″trō-rō′tă-tor-ē) [″ + *rotare,* to turn] Causing to turn to the right, applied esp. to substances that turn polarized rays of light to the right.

**dextrose** (dĕks′trōs) $C_6H_{12}O_6$. Glucose, a simple sugar of the monosaccharose group; a crystalline solid that can be made by the action of acids on starches. It is very soluble in water, is an important constituent of corn syrup and honey, and is an example of one kind of carbohydrate.

It is the most important of the monosaccharide group. Its presence in the urine in large amounts is usually a result of diabetes. However, this may be associated with brain injuries, cirrhosis of the liver, normal pregnancies, and the administration of epinephrine or thyroxine. It is formed in the digestive tract by the action of enzymes on carbohydrates. It occurs naturally in plants and in the body fluids of animals.

**dextrose and sodium chloride injection** A sterile solution of dextrose, salt, and water for use intravenously. It contains no antimicrobial agents.

**dextrosinistral** (dĕks″trō-sĭn′ĭs-trăl) [L. *dexter,* right, + *sinister,* left] From right to left.

**dextrosuria** (dĕks-trō-sū′rē-ă) Dextrose in the urine.

**dextrothyroxine sodium** (dĕks″trō-thī-rŏk′sĭn) A thyroxine-like drug used in treating type II hyperlipoproteinemia.

**dextrotropic, dextrotropous** (dĕks″trō-trŏp′ĭk, -trō′pŭs) [″ + Gr. *tropos,* a turning] Turning to the right.

**dextroversion** [″ + *vertere,* to turn] Turned or location toward the right.

**DFP** *di-isopropyl fluorophosphate.* SEE: *isoflurophate.*

**dg** *decigram.*

**dhobie itch** (dō′bē) [Hindi, laundryboy] Tropical name for form of tinea cruris more intense than that observed in temperate zones.

**di-** [Gr. *dis,* twice] Prefix indicating *twice, double,* or *two.*

**diabetes** (dī″ă-bē′tēz) [Gr. *diabetes,* passing through] A general term for diseases marked by excessive urination; usually refers to diabetes mellitus. SEE: *Nursing Diagnoses Appendix.*

***brittle d.*** A term applied previously to insulin-dependent diabetes in which the disorder was controlled for varying periods of time before patients experienced persistent problems maintaining a normal concentration of glucose in the blood. Frequent episodes of hypoglycemia followed by hyperglycemia required constant adjustment of dietary intake and insulin dosage. Causes of this condition include inadequate absorption of insulin due to lipodystrophy, the effects of concurrent therapeutic or over-the-counter medications, insulin resistance related to pregnancy, inadequate preparation or administration of insulin, Somogyi phenomenon (chronic insulin overdosage), and persistent physiological or psychological stress. SEE: *insulin-dependent d. mellitus.*

***bronze d.*** Hemochromatosis.

***chemical d.*** A stage of diabetes mellitus in which the various tests for altered glucose metabolism other than the fasting blood glucose level are abnormal, but there are no obvious clinical signs or symptoms of diabetes.

***endocrine d.*** Diabetes mellitus associated with certain diseases of the pituitary, thyroid, or adrenal glands.

***gestational d.*** Diabetes mellitus that first manifests clinically during pregnancy as a result of hormonal changes. It usually subsides after delivery.

***iatrogenic d.*** Diabetes mellitus brought on by administration of drugs such as corticosteroids, certain diuretics, or birth control pills.

***d. insipidus*** Polyuria and polydipsia caused by inadequate secretion of antidiuretic hormone from the hypothalamus or its release by the posterior pituitary gland.

SYMPTOMS: Urine output of 5 to 10 L/24 hr is common. The specific gravity is usually 1.001 to 1.005, and urine is free of glucose (sugar) and albumin. Symptoms include thirst, weakness, and dry skin.

ETIOLOGY: In almost half of all cases the cause is unknown. Trauma to the head that damages the pituitary, or a tumor in that area, causes the remainder of cases.

TREATMENT: The causative factor should be eradicated if it is known. When not due to specific injury of the pituitary, the disease is easily controlled by vasopressin replacement therapy. This may be given by injection or nasal spray.

PROGNOSIS: The disease is generally chronic and not life-threatening if properly treated.

NURSING IMPLICATIONS: Fluid balance is monitored. Fluid intake and output, urine specific gravity, and weight are assessed for evidence of dehydration and hypovolemic hypotension. Serum electrolyte and blood urea nitrogen levels are monitored. If the patient is receiving chlorpropamide, laboratory values are reviewed for evidence of hypoglycemia and hyponatremia, and the patient is assessed for signs of hypoglycemia. Safety measures are instituted if the patient complains of dizziness or weakness. If the patient is receiving chlorpropamide, adequate caloric intake is provided and orange juice or other carbohydrates are available to treat hypoglycemia.

The patient is instructed in nasal insufflation of vasopressin and administration of subcutaneous or intramuscular hormones. The length of the therapy and the importance of taking medications as prescribed and not discontinuing them abruptly are stressed. Meticulous skin and oral care are provided; use of a soft toothbrush is recommended, and petroleum jelly is applied to lips and an emollient lotion to the skin to reduce dryness. Adequate fluid intake should be maintained during the day but fluids should be limited in the evening to prevent nocturia.

Both patient and family are taught to identify signs of dehydration and to report signs of severe dehydration and impend-

**Comparison of Diabetic Ketoacidosis and Hypoglycemia**

| | Diabetic Ketoacidosis | Hypoglycemia |
|---|---|---|
| Onset | Gradual | Often sudden |
| History | Often acute infection in a diabetic or insufficient insulin intake<br>Previous history of diabetes may be absent | Recent insulin injection, inadequate meal, or excessive exercise after insulin |
| Musculoskeletal | Muscle wasting or weight loss | Weakness<br>Tremor<br>Muscle twitching |
| Gastrointestinal | Abdominal pains or cramps, sometimes acute<br>Nausea and vomiting | Nausea and vomiting |
| Central nervous system | Headache<br>Double or blurred vision<br>Irritability | Convulsions<br>Coma |
| Cardiovascular | Rapid, feeble pulse<br>Decrease in blood pressure<br>Flushed, dry skin | Pallor<br>Diaphoresis<br>Decrease in pulse rate followed by increase<br>Decrease in blood pressure followed by increase<br>Palpitations |
| Respiratory | Air hunger<br>Acetone odor of breath<br>Dyspnea | Air hunger<br>Increased respiratory rate |
| Laboratory values | Elevated blood glucose (>200 mg/dl)<br>Glucose and acetone in urine | Subnormal blood glucose (20–50 mg/dl)<br>Absence of glucose and acetone in urine unless bladder is full |

ing hypovolemia. The patient is taught to measure intake and output, monitor weight daily, and use a hydrometer to measure urine specific gravity. The patient should wear or carry a medical identification tag and keep a supply of medication with him or her at all times.

***insulin-dependent d. mellitus*** ABBR: IDDM. Diabetes mellitus that usually has its onset before the age of 25 years, in which the essential abnormality is related to absolute insulin deficiency. This form usually is quite difficult to regulate. SYN: *brittle d.; juvenile-onset d.; type I d.* SEE: table.

***juvenile-onset d.*** Insulin-dependent d. mellitus.

***latent d.*** Diabetes mellitus that manifests itself during times of stress such as pregnancy, infectious disease, obesity, or trauma. Previous to the stress, no clinical or laboratory findings of diabetes are present. There is a very strong chance that such individuals will eventually develop overt diabetes mellitus.

***d. mellitus*** A chronic disorder of carbohydrate metabolism, marked by hyperglycemia and glycosuria and resulting from inadequate production or use of insulin. Persons fulfilling these conditions are not a homogeneous group. Diabetes mellitus is classified according to two syndromes: Type I, or insulin-dependent diabetes mellitus (IDDM) and type II, or non–insulin-dependent diabetes mellitus (NIDDM). In type I, the patient secretes no insulin. In the past, this form of diabetes was called juvenile-onset, ketotic, or brittle diabetes. In type II, insulin is produced, but exogenous insulin is needed to control hyperglycemia. Older terms for this form of diabetes were maturity-onset, nonketotic, or stable diabetes. Type II diabetes occurs much more frequently than type I and is most common in individuals over 40 years of age. SEE: table; *insulin-dependent d. mellitus; non–insulin-dependent d. mellitus; dawn phenomenon; insulin; insulin pump; insulin resistance; polyneuropathy, diabetic; Somogyi phenomenon.*

SYMPTOMS: Principal symptoms are elevated blood glucose (hyperglycemia), glucose in urine (glycosuria), excessive urine production (polyuria), excessive thirst (polydipsia), increase in food intake (polyphagia), and itching, frequently about the genitals. Urine specific gravity is 1.020 to 1.040; glucose is excessive; urine contains diacetic acid, beta-hydroxybutyric acid, and acetone when the disease process is advanced. Fasting blood

## Comparison of Type I Insulin-Dependent Diabetes Mellitus and Type II Non–Insulin-Dependent Diabetes Mellitus

| | Type I | Type II |
|---|---|---|
| Age at onset | Usually under 30 | Usually over 40 |
| Type of onset | Abrupt | Gradual |
| Body weight | Normal | Obese—80% |
| HLA association | Positive | Negative |
| Insulin in blood | Little to none | Some usually present |
| Islet cell antibodies | Present at onset | Absent |
| Prevalence | 0.2%–0.3% | 2%–4% |
| Symptoms | Polyuria, polydipsia, polyphagia, weight loss, ketoacidosis | Polyuria, polydipsia, pruritis, peripheral neuropathy |
| Control | Insulin and diet | Diet (sometimes diet only), hypoglycemic agents, sometimes insulin |
| Vascular and neural changes | Eventually develop | Will usually develop |
| Stability of condition | Fluctuates, difficult to control | Fairly stable, usually easy to control |

glucose is raised above normal range of 90 to 120 mg/dl of blood; boils, carbuncles, and vascular changes may be present. Loss of weight, emaciation, weakness, and debility are present. When severe diabetes is allowed to progress without proper treatment, coma ensues with weakness and sweet (acetone) odor of breath. The process includes nausea, headache, vomiting, dyspnea, sense of intoxication, delirium, and deep coma resulting in death.

ETIOLOGY: Insulin-dependent diabetes mellitus, type I, is now generally accepted to be an autoimmune disease triggered by a nonspecific viral infection that inflames the beta cells of the pancreas. The most common such infections are caused by cytomegalovirus, rubella virus, mumps virus, or influenza virus. Although the exact mechanism is unclear, the inflammatory process seems to stimulate the beta cells to produce slightly abnormal class II histocompatibility locus antigens (HLA). Lymphocytes recognize these antigens as "non-self" and therefore destroy them, releasing more beta cell proteins that can make additional HLA and stimulating an ongoing immune response that eventually destroys all the beta cells producing insulin. The HLAs in the pancreas are determined genetically. Because most patients with IDDM have HLA-DR3, HLA-DR4, or both, the tendency to develop an autoimmune response and subsequent IDDM is considered hereditary. IDDM may occur at any age but is usually diagnosed before age 30 years.

COMPLICATIONS: Diabetic acidosis can occur due to excessive production of ketone bodies. Other complications include low resistance to infections, esp. those involving extremities; ulceration of lower extremities; an increased incidence of toxemia in pregnancy; cardiovascular and renal disorders; and disturbances in electrolyte balance.

Diabetic persons are prone to developing retinopathy, glaucoma, and various types of neuropathy. Eye involvement is common, and 0.2% of diabetics become blind each year. This complication is much less frequent in the insulin-dependent than the non–insulin-dependent type. The retinal changes may be nonproliferative with retinal ischemia and areas of infarction. In the proliferative type, new vessels are formed in the retina and may lead to retinal detachment. These new vessels are destroyed by the use of photocoagulation; this helps to prevent further deterioration of vision.

Diabetic neuropathy is estimated to occur in 40% of patients in whom diabetes has been present 25 years. It may affect a single peripheral nerve, the autonomic nervous sytem, or the cranial nerves.

Cardiovascular disease is the major cause of death in diabetics. In addition, peripheral vascular disease may lead to ischemia and gangrene of the lower limbs. One or more amputations may be required.

TREATMENT: Careful study of patients with IDDM confirms that intensive therapy, sometimes referred to as "tight control," is more effective than conventional therapy in preventing the progression of serious microvascular complications such as nephropathy and retinopathy. Intensive therapy consists of three or more doses of insulin injected daily or administered by infusion pump, frequent self-monitoring of blood glucose levels, and changes in therapy as a result of weekly telephone contacts with the health care team. Some negative aspects of this intensive care program for patients with IDDM are a three times more frequent occurrence of severe hypoglycemia, and weight gain that is greater than in those who receive conventional therapy. Participation in an intensive therapy program requires a highly motivated patient who must be frequently monitored by the health care team.

Conventional treatment consists of diet, insulin, exercise, and hygienic measures. At first the patient should be placed on a well-balanced diet adequate in all basic essentials: carbohydrates, proteins, fats, vitamins, minerals, and fluids. Many patients may require no further measures. Control of diabetes is much more difficult in an obese person. Obese persons with diabetes should be placed on a diet that will enable them to lose weight. Blood glucose determinations may be necessary at frequent intervals. Glucose levels in the urine may be monitored by the patient or family as often as necessary. In addition, kits are available to help patients monitor blood glucose levels at home. Long-term blood glucose regulation may be objectively assessed by determining the glycosylated hemoglobin (hemoglobin $A_{1c}$) in blood. SEE: *hemoglobin $A_{1c}$*.

When a patient is given an adequate diet and glucose still appears in the urine, use of insulin may be necessary. Its use is not required in every case and may be dangerous if it is not properly administered and monitored. Oral hypoglycemic agents have controlled mild cases of diabetes. They have been used with success mostly in middle-aged and older patients who still have some beta cell function.

*Diet:* A balanced diet of approx. 1000 to 1200 kcal may be prescribed. The diet is modified according to the weight of the patient. It should be increased promptly if levels of blood glucose are brought within normal limits. The age, weight, and type of work or physical activity in which the patient is engaged are important in the planning of a diet. Standardized diets have been created in which the necessary proportions of carbohydrates, proteins, and fats are outlined. The diets vary from 1200 to 3000 kcal. Frequent feedings (five to six each day) rather than the standard three meals are preferred. The older the patient, as a rule, the smaller the proportion of fat in the diet. SEE: *exchange list*.

*Exercise:* Physical exercise is important in helping to improve glucose metabolism. Thus, a regular exercise program should be encouraged. The individual with diabetes should not be excluded from any athletic endeavor at any level. Initially, high-level physical activity will necessitate careful management of insulin intake and monitoring of glucose levels in the blood.

PROGNOSIS: Diabetes is a chronic, incurable disease, but symptoms can be ameliorated and life prolonged by proper therapy. The isolation and eventual production of insulin in 1922 by Canadian physicians Banting and Best made it possible to allow persons with the disease to lead a normal life.

NURSING IMPLICATIONS: Acute complications of diabetic therapy are monitored, esp. hypoglycemia and insulin shock, vagueness, slow cerebration, dizziness, weakness, pallor, tachycardia, diaphoresis, seizures, and coma. Signs and symptoms of hyperglycemic complications are also monitored. These include diabetic ketoacidosis, acetone breath, weak and rapid pulse, and Kussmaul's respirations; or hyperglycemic, hyperosmolar, nonketotic syndrome or coma, characterized by polyuria, thirst, neurological abnormalities, and stupor.

Vital signs, weight, fluid intake, urine output, and caloric intake are accurately documented. Serum glucose and urine acetone levels are evaluated. The effects of diabetes on other body systems, such as cerebrovascular, coronary artery, and peripheral vascular impairment; visual impairment; and peripheral and autonomic nervous system impairment are assessed. The patient is observed for signs and symptoms of diabetic neuropathy, such as numbness or pain in the hands and feet, decreased vibratory sense, footdrop, and neurogenic bladder. The urine is checked for urinary tract and vaginal infections and for protein, an early indication of nephropathy.

Insulin or oral hypoglycemic agents are administered as prescribed and their action and use explained. With help from a dietician, a diet is planned based on the recommended amount of calories, protein, carbohydrates, and fats. The patient is taught how to choose food exchanges and how to read food container labels. A steady, consistent level of daily exercise is prescribed, and participation in a supervised exercise program is recommended.

Hypoglycemic reactions are promptly treated by giving carbohydrates (oral orange juice, hard candy, honey, or any sugar-containing food); as necessary, SC or IM glucagon or IV dextrose (if the patient is not conscious) is administered. Hyperglycemic crises are treated initially with prescribed intravenous fluids and insulin, and later, with potassium replacement based on laboratory values.

Skin care, esp. to the feet and legs, are provided, and the patient is instructed in these techniques. All injuries, cuts, and blisters should be treated promptly; and constricting hose, slippers, shoes, and bed linens, and walking barefoot, should be avoided. The patient is referred to a podiatrist for ongoing foot care and is warned that decreased sensation can mask injuries. Regular ophthalmological examinations are recommended for early detection of diabetic retinopathy.

The patient is educated about diabetes, its possible complications and their management, and the importance of strict adherence to the prescribed therapy. Emotional support and a realistic assessment of the patient's condition are offered; this assessment stresses that with proper treatment, the patient can have a near-normal lifestyle and life expectancy. Assistance is offered to help the patient to develop positive coping strategies. The patient and family may be referred for counseling and to local and national support and information groups. SEE: *Nursing Diagnoses Appendix.*

***non–insulin-dependent d. mellitus*** ABBR: NIDDM. A group of forms of diabetes mellitus that occur predominantly in adults. The insulin produced is sufficient to prevent ketoacidosis but insufficient to meet the total needs of the body. This form of diabetes in nonobese patients can usually be controlled by diet and oral hypoglycemic agents, such as sulfonylurea drugs or metformin, a nonsulfonylurea drug. Occasionally insulin therapy is required. In obese patients the condition can be controlled by avoidance of overfeeding. SYN: *maturity-onset d.; type II d.* SEE: *insulin-dependent d. mellitus* for table.

***pancreatic d.*** Diabetes associated with disease of the pancreas.

***phlorhizin d.*** Glycosuria caused by administration of phlorhizin.

***renal d.*** Renal glycosuria; this condition is marked by a low renal threshold for glucose. Glucose tolerance is normal and diabetic symptoms are lacking.

***true d.*** D. mellitus.

***type I d.*** Insulin-dependent d. mellitus.

***type II d.*** Non–insulin-dependent d. mellitus.

**diabetic** (dī-ă-bĕt′ĭk) Pert. to diabetes.

**diabetic acidosis** SEE: *acidosis, diabetic.*

**diabetic center** An area in the floor of the fourth ventricle of the brain.

**diabetic coma** Loss of consciousness due to severe diabetes mellitus that has not been treated or to treatment that has not been adequately regulated. SEE: *coma, diabetic.*

**diabetic ear** Otitis media diabetica.

**diabetic ketoacidosis** SEE: *Nursing Diagnoses Appendix.*

**diabetic polyneuropathy** SEE: *polyneuropathy, diabetic.*

**diabetic tabes** Diabetes with neuritic pains in the leg and loss of the patellar tendon reflex.

**diabetogenic** (dī″ă-bĕt″ō-jĕn′ĭk) [″ + *gennan,* to produce] Causing diabetes.

**diabetogenous** (dī″ă-bē-tŏj′ĕn-ŭs) Caused by diabetes.

**diacele** (dī′ă-sēl) [Gr. *dia,* between, + *koilia,* a hollow] The third ventricle of the brain.

**diacetate** (dī-ăs′ĕ-tāt) A salt of diacetic acid.

**diacetemia** (dī-ăs″ĕ-tē′mē-ă) The presence of diacetic acid in the blood.

**diacetic acid** (dī″ă-sĕt′ĭk) Acetoacetic acid, found in acidosis and in the urine of diabetic persons. Like acetone, it is found in serious diabetes and in any condition that produces starvation and excessive fat metabolism, such as persistent vomiting.

**diacetonuria, diaceturia** (dī-ăs″ĕ-tō-nū′rē-ă, dī-ăs″ĕ-tū′rē-ă) Diacetic acid in urine.

**diacetylmorphine** (dī″ă-sē″tĭl-mor′fēn) Heroin.

**diacidic** (dī-ăs′ĭd-ĭk) [Gr. *dis,* twice, + L. *acidus,* soured] Containing two acidic hydrogen ions.

**diaclasis** (dī-ă-klā′sĭs) [Gr. *dia,* through, + *klan,* to break] A surgical procedure in which a bone is intentionally fractured. SYN: *osteoclasia.*

**diaclast** (dī′ă-klăst) [″ + *klan,* to break] A device for perforating the fetal skull.

**diacrinous** (dī-ăk′rĭn-ŭs) [Gr. *diakrinein,* to separate] Pert. to cells that secrete outwardly rather than into the vascular system. SYN: *exocrine.*

**diaderm** [Gr. *dia,* through, + *derma,* skin] A blastoderm composed of ectoderm and entoderm, and containing between them the segmentation cavity.

**diadochokinesia** (dī-ăd″ō-kō-kĭn-ē′zē-ă) [Gr. *diadokos,* succeeding, + *kinesis,* movement] The ability to make antagonistic movements, such as pronation and supination of the hands in quick succession. SEE: *disdiadochokinesia.*

**diagnose** (dī′ăg-nōs) [Gr. *diagignoskein,* to discern] To determine the cause and nature of a pathological condition; to recognize a disease.

**diagnosis** (dī″ăg-nō′sĭs) *pl.* **diagnoses** **1.** The term denoting the disease or syndrome a person has or is believed to have. **2.** The use of scientific and skillful methods to establish the cause and nature of a person's illness. This is done by evaluating the history of the disease process, the signs and symptoms, and the laboratory data, and by special tests such as radiography and electrocardiography. The value of establishing a diagnosis is to provide a logical basis for treatment and prognosis.

***antenatal d.*** Diagnostic procedures to determine the health status of a fetus including amniocentesis, cell culture, biochemical studies, amnioscopy, nonstress test, oxytocin challenge test, biophysical profile, amniography, ultrasound, and chorionic villus biopsy.

***clinical d.*** Identification of a disease by

history, laboratory studies, and symptoms. Most diseases have a symptom or symptoms in common with other diseases.

***cytological d.*** Identification of a disease based on cells present in body tissues or exudates.

***differential d.*** Identification of a disease by comparison of the symptoms of two or more similar diseases.

***d. by exclusion*** Identification of a disease by eliminating other possibilities.

***medical d.*** The entire process of identifying the cause of the patient's illness or discomfort. The method of determination depends on several factors including the type of illness or injury present. For example, the diagnosis of a simple and superficial skin laceration of the lower leg is much less involved than that of a scalp laceration. In the latter, the depth of the wound is of utmost importance in determining the number of layers of the scalp to be sutured. Also, the diagnosis of an obscure infectious disease or an unexplained fever involves clinical skills and sophisticated laboratory investigations that would not be required when diagnosing a simple cold or influenza. *Medical diagnosis* is to be differentiated from *nursing diagnosis.*

***nursing d.*** SEE: *nursing diagnosis.*

***oral d.*** SEE: *oral diagnosis.*

***pathological d.*** Identification of an illness based on structural lesions.

***physical d.*** Identification of an illness by external examination only.

***radiographic d.*** Identification of an illness by the interpretation of radiographic findings.

***serological d.*** Identification of an illness through a serological test such as that for syphilis or typhoid.

**diagnosis-related group** ABBR: DRG. A system designed to standardize prospective payment for medical care. The reimbursement for treating all individuals within the same DRG is the same, regardless of actual cost to the health care facility. The facility may earn a profit if the patient's hospitalization is shorter than the specified average length of stay in that category of illness.

**diagnostic** Pert. to a diagnosis.

**Diagnostic and Statistical Manual of Mental Disorders (Fourth Edition)** ABBR: DSM IV. The standard nomenclature of emotional illness used by all health care practitioners. DSM IV, published by the American Psychiatric Association, was introduced in 1994.

**diagnostician** (dī″ăg-nŏs-tĭsh′ŭn) [Gr. *diagignoskein,* to discern] One skilled in diagnosis.

**diakinesis** (dī″ă-kĭ-nē′sĭs) [Gr. *dia,* through, + *kinesis,* motion] In cell division, the final stage in the prophase of meiosis. At this time the homologous chromosomes shorten and thicken.

**dial** (dī′ăl) [L. *dialis,* daily, fr. *dies,* day] A graduated circular face, similar to a clock face, on which some measurement is indicated by a pointer that moves as the entity being measured (pressure, temperature, or heat) changes.

***astigmatic d.*** A circular dial with black lines of uniform width drawn as if they were connecting opposing numbers on the face of a clock. It is used in testing for astigmatism.

**dialy-** [Gr. *dia,* through, + *lysis,* dissolution] Prefix denoting *separation.*

**dialysance** (dī″ă-lī′săns) In renal dialysis, the minute rate of net exchange of a substance between blood and dialysis fluid per unit of blood-bath concentration gradient.

**dialysate** (dī-ăl′ĭ-sāt) **1.** A liquid that has been dialyzed. **2.** In renal failure, the fluid used to remove or deliver compounds or electrolytes that the failing kidney cannot excrete or retain in the proper concentrations.

**dialysis** (dī-ăl′ĭ-sĭs) [Gr. *dia,* through, + *lysis,* dissolution] **1.** The passage of a solute through a membrane. **2.** The process of diffusing blood across a semipermeable membrane to remove toxic materials and to maintain fluid, electrolyte, and acid-base balance in cases of impaired kidney function or absence of the kidneys. SEE: *hemodialysis; Nursing Diagnoses Appendix.*

***continuous ambulatory peritoneal d.*** ABBR: CAPD. A type of maintenance dialysis that uses an implanted peritoneal catheter. Fluid is drained into and from the peritoneal cavity by gravity. CAPD is an alternative to chronic hemodialysis and is considerably less expensive.

***continuous cyclic peritoneal d.*** ABBR: CCPD. Dialysis performed every night with fluid remaining in the peritoneal cavity until the next night.

***intermittent peritoneal d.*** ABBR: IPD. Dialysis using automated equipment, often performed overnight. The fluid is drained from the peritoneal cavity at the end of the treatment.

***peritoneal d.*** Dialysis in which the lining of the peritoneal cavity is used as the dialyzing membrane. Dialyzing fluid introduced into the peritoneal cavity is left there for 1 or 2 hr and is then removed. The procedure may be repeated as often as is indicated. Care must be taken to prevent the development of peritonitis. This is done by using strict sterile technique.

This dialysis technique is used to remove toxic substances from the body by perfusing specific warm sterile chemical solutions through the peritoneal cavity. It is used in treating renal failure and in certain types of poisoning. Some of the drugs and chemicals that may be so removed are salicylates, barbiturates, meprobamate, amphetamines, bromide, methanol, boric acid, sulfonamide, and various antibiotics.

This technique, using chilled, sterile isotonic saline, has been used in treating heatstroke. SEE: *Nursing Diagnoses Appendix.*

Caution: Peritoneal dialysis may be dangerous and may cause death if not done with adequate supervision of body fluid and electrolyte balance.

NURSING IMPLICATIONS: Strict aseptic technique is maintained throughout the procedure. The patient is observed for signs of peritonitis, pain, respiratory difficulty, and low blood pressure. Many persons can ably perform the procedure at home using equipment designed for home use. The nurse ensures that the patient understands the procedure and its rationale, care of the peritoneal catheter, and symptoms of infection; can change medication schedule before and after dialysis; and can adjust lifestyle to provide a balance of adequate rest and activity.

***renal d.*** Dialysis of blood to remove liquid and chemicals that the kidneys would normally remove.

**dialysis acidosis** Metabolic acidosis due to prolonged hemodialysis in which the pH of the dialysis bath has been inadvertently reduced by the action of contaminating bacteria.

**dialysis dementia** A neurological disturbance seen in patients who have been on dialysis for several years. There are speech difficulties, myoclonus, dementia, seizures, and eventually death. The pathological mechanism is unknown.

**dialysis disequilibrium** A disturbance in which nausea, vomiting, drowsiness, headache, and seizures occur shortly after the patient begins hemodialysis or peritoneal dialysis. The cause is related to the rapid pH changes in the blood and the decrease in the osmolarity of the extracellular fluid. The urea in the brain is higher than in the serum.

**dialytic** Belonging to or resembling the process of dialysis.

**dialyzable** (dī-ă-līz'ă-b'l) Capable of receiving dialysis.

**dialyze** (dī'ă-līz) To perform a dialysis or to undergo one.

**dialyzer** (dī'ă-līz"ĕr) [Gr. *dia,* through, + *lysis,* dissolution] The apparatus used in performing dialysis.

**diameter** (dī-ăm'ĕ-tĕr) [" + *metron,* a measure] The distance from any point on the periphery of a surface, body, or space to the opposite point.

***anteroposterior d. of pelvic cavity*** The distance between the middle of the symphysis pubis and the upper border of the third sacral vertebra (about 13.5 cm in women).

***anteroposterior d. of pelvic inlet*** The distance from the posterior surface of the symphysis pubis to the promontory of the sacrum (about 11 cm in women). SYN: *conjugata vera; true conjugate d. of pelvic inlet.*

***anteroposterior d. of pelvic outlet*** The distance between the tip of the coccyx and the lower edge of the symphysis pubis.

***bigonial d.*** The distance between the two gonia. The gonion is the anthropometric point at the most inferior, posterior, and lateral points on the angle of the mandible.

***biparietal d.*** The transverse distance between the parietal eminences on each side of the head (about 9.25 cm).

***bitemporal d.*** The distance between the temporal bones (about 8 cm).

***bitrochanteric d.*** The distance between the highest points of the greater trochanters.

***bizygomatic d.*** The greatest transverse distance between the most prominent points of the zygomatic arches.

***buccolingual d.*** The measurement of a tooth from the buccal to the lingual surface.

***cervicobregmatic d.*** The distance between the anterior fontanel and the junction of the neck with the floor of the mouth.

***diagonal conjugate d. of pelvis*** The distance from the upper part of the symphysis pubis to the most distant part of the brim of the pelvis.

***external conjugate d.*** The anteroposterior diameter of the pelvic inlet measured externally; the distance from the skin over the upper part of the symphysis pubis to the skin over a point corresponding to the sacral promontory. SYN: *Baudelocque's diameter.*

***frontomental d.*** The distance from the top of the forehead to the point of the chin.

***interspinous d.*** The distance between the two anterior superior spines of the ilia.

***intertuberous d.*** The distance between the ischial tuberosities. Most commonly, this measure of the female pelvic outlet is greater than 9 cm, allowing the exit of an average-sized term fetus.

***labiolingual d.*** The measurement of an anterior tooth from the labial to the lingual surface.

***mentobregmatic d.*** The distance from the chin to the middle of the anterior fontanel.

***mesiodistal d.*** The measurement of a tooth from the ventral or mesial surface to the distal or dorsal surface.

***obstetrical d. of pelvic inlet*** The shortest distance between the sacrum and the symphysis pubis. This diameter is shorter than the true conjugate. SYN: *obstetrical conjugate.*

***occipitofrontal d.*** The distance from the posterior fontanel to the root of the nose.

***occipitomental d.*** The greatest distance between the most prominent portion of the occiput and the point of the chin (about 13.5 cm).

***d. of pelvis*** Any diameter of the pelvis found by measuring a straight line between any two points. *Anteroposterior:* the distance between the sacrovertebral angle and the symphysis pubis. *Biischial:* the distance between the ischial spines. *Conjugata diagonalis:* the distance between the sacrovertebral angle and the symphysis pubis. *Conjugata vera:* the true conjugate between the sacrovertebral angle and the middle of the posterior aspect of the symphysis pubis (about 1.5 cm less than the diagonal conjugate). *Intercristal:* the distance between the crests of the ilia. *Interspinous:* the distance between the spines of the ilium. *Intertrochanteric:* the distance between the greater trochanters when the hips are extended and the legs are held together. *Obstetrical conjugate:* the distance between the promontory of the sacrum and the upper edge of the symphysis pubis. SEE: *pelvis.*

***true conjugate d. of pelvic inlet*** Anteroposterior d. of pelvic inlet.

**diamid(e)** (dī-ăm′ĭd, -īd) [L. *di,* two, + *amide*] A compound that contains two amine groups. The term is sometimes used incorrectly to indicate a diamine or hydrazine.

**diamidine** (dī-ăm′ĭ-dēn) Any chemical compound that contains two amidine, C(NH)$NH_2$, groups.

**diamine** (dī-ăm′ĭn, -ēn) A chemical compound with two amino, —$NH_2$, groups.

**diaminuria** (dī-ăm″ĭ-nū′rē-ă) Presence of diamines in the urine.

**diapause** (dī′ă-pawz) [Gr. *dia,* through, + *pausis,* pause] The state of metabolic inactivity that some plants, seeds, eggs, and insect forms assume to survive adverse conditions such as winter.

**diapedesis** (dī″ă-pĕd-ē′sĭs) [″ + *pedan,* to leap] The movement of white blood cells and other cells out of small arterioles, venules, and capillaries as part of the inflammatory response. The cells move through gaps between cells in the vessel walls. SEE: *inflammation.*

**diaper rash, diaper dermatitis** SEE: *rash, diaper.*

**diaphane** (dī′ă-fān) [Gr. *dia,* through, + *phainein,* to appear] A very small electric light used in transillumination.

**diaphanography** Transillumination of the breast.

**diaphanometer** (dī″ă-făn-ŏm′ĕ-tĕr) [″ + ″ + *metron,* measure] A device for estimating the amount of solids in a fluid by its transparency.

**diaphanometry** (dī″ă-făn-ŏm′ĕ-trē) Determination of the translucency of a fluid (e.g., urine).

**diaphanoscope** (dī-ă-făn′ō-skōp) [″ + *phainein,* to appear, + *skopein,* to examine] A device for transillumination of body cavities.

**diaphanoscopy** (dī″ă-făn-ŏs′kō-pē) Examination using the diaphanoscope; transillumination.

**diaphemetric** (dī″ă-fĕ-mĕt′rĭk) [″ + *haphe,* touch, + *metron,* measure] Pert. to the degree of tactile sensibility.

**diaphorase** (dī-ăf′ō-rās) The flavoprotein catalyst of the reoxidation of nicotinamide-adenine dinucleotide (NAD) or nicotinamide-adenine dinucleotide phosphate (NADP) by the mitochondrial electron transport chain.

**diaphoresis** (dī″ă-fō-rē′sĭs) [″ + *pherein,* to carry] Profuse sweating.

**diaphoretic** (dī″ă-fō-rĕt′ĭk) [″ + *pherein,* to carry] **1.** A sudorific, or an agent that increases perspiration. **2.** A patient who is sweating profusely.

**diaphragm** (dī′ă-frăm) [Gr. *diaphragma,* a partition] **1.** A thin membrane such as one used for dialysis. **2.** In microscopy, an apparatus located beneath the opening in the stage and permitting regulation of the amount of light passing through the object. **3.** A rubber or plastic cup that fits over the cervix uteri and is used for contraceptive purposes. SEE: illus. (Contraceptive Diaphragm). **4.** The dome-shaped skeletal muscle separating the abdomen from the thoracic cavity with its convexity upward. It contracts with each inspiration, flattening out downward, permitting the bases of the lungs to descend. It relaxes with each expiration, elevating itself and restoring the inverted basin

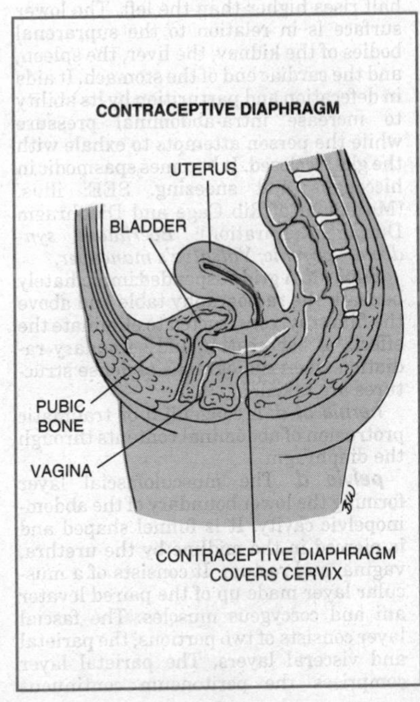

CONTRACEPTIVE DIAPHRAGM

MOVEMENT OF RIB CAGE AND DIAPHRAGM DURING RESPIRATION

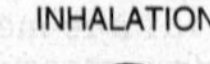


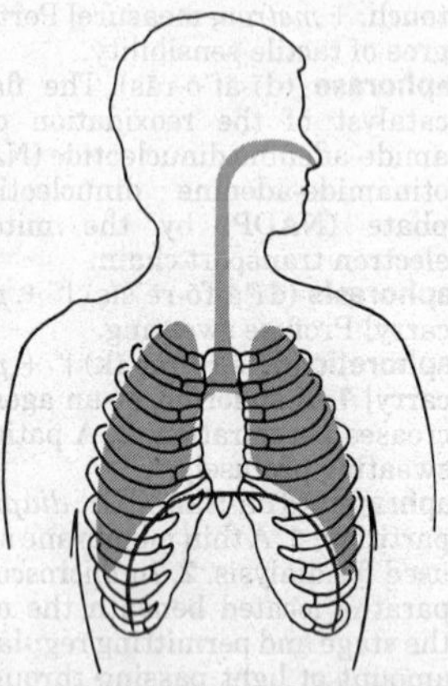

EXHALATION

THE DIAPHRAGM HAS CONTRACTED AND DESCENDED AND THE RIB CAGE HAS BEEN PULLED UP AND OUT TO EXPAND THE LUNGS

THE DIAPHRAGM HAS ASCENDED (RELAXED) AND THE RIB CAGE HAS MOVED DOWN AND IN TO COMPRESS THE LUNGS

shape. The deeper the inspiration, the lower it descends; the greater the expiration, the higher it rises.

Its origin is at a level with the sixth ribs or intercostal spaces anteriorly and the 11th or 12th ribs posteriorly. The right half rises higher than the left. The lower surface is in relation to the suprarenal bodies of the kidney, the liver, the spleen, and the cardiac end of the stomach. It aids in defecation and parturition by its ability to increase intra-abdominal pressure while the person attempts to exhale with the glottis closed. It becomes spasmodic in hiccoughs and sneezing. SEE: illus. (Movement of Rib Cage and Diaphragm During Respiration); *Boerhaave syndrome; phrenic; Valsalva's maneuver.*

***Bucky d.*** A grid suspended immediately beneath the radiography table and above the film tray, constructed to eliminate the effects of backscatter and secondary radiation when radiographs of dense structures are taken.

***hernia of d.*** A congenital or traumatic protrusion of abdominal contents through the diaphragm.

***pelvic d.*** The musculofascial layer forming the lower boundary of the abdominopelvic cavity. It is funnel shaped and is pierced in the midline by the urethra, vagina, and rectum. It consists of a muscular layer made up of the paired levator ani and coccygeus muscles. The fascial layer consists of two portions, the parietal and visceral layers. The parietal layer comprises the peritoneum continuous with the connective tissue sheaths of the psoas and iliac muscles. The visceral layer is split from the parietal layer at the white line passing downward and inward to form the upper sheath of the levator ani muscles; the anterior part of this layer unites the bladder with the posterior wall of the pubes. The middle portion splits into three parts: the vesical layer, investing the bladder and urethra; the rectovaginal layer, forming the rectovaginal septum; and the rectal layer, investing the rectum. The posterior part is the base of the broad ligament, where it sheaths the uterine arteries and supports the cervix.

***urogenital d.*** The urogenital trigone, or triangular ligament. A musculofascial sheath that lies between the ischiopubic rami, it is superficial to the pelvic diaphragm. In males it surrounds the membranous urethra; in females, the vagina.

**diaphragmatic** Pert. to the diaphragm.

**diaphragmatocele** (dī″ă-frăg-măt′ō-sēl) [″ + *kele*, tumor, swelling] A hernia of the diaphragm.

**diaphragmitis** (dī″ă-frăg-mī′tĭs) [″ + *itis*, inflammation] Inflammation of the diaphragm.

**diaphyseal** (dī″ă-fĭz′ē-ăl) [Gr. *diaphysis*, a growing through] Part of or affecting the shaft of a long bone.

**diaphysectomy** [″ + *ektome*, excision] Removal of part of the shaft of a long bone.

**diaphysis** (dī-ăf′ĭ-sĭs) The shaft or middle part of a long cylindrical bone. SEE: *apophysis; epiphysis.*

**diaphysitis** (dī″ă-fĭ-zī′tĭs) [Gr. *diaphysis*, a

growing through, + *itis,* inflammation] Inflammation of the shaft of a long bone.

**diaplexus** [Gr. *dia,* through, + L. *plexus,* braid] The choroid plexus of the third ventricle.

**diapophysis** (dī-ă-pŏf′ĭ-sĭs) [″ + *apophysis,* outgrowth] The upper articular surface of the transverse process of a vertebra.

**diarrhea** (dī-ă-rē′ă) [″ + *rhein,* to flow] A state in which an individual experiences a change in normal bowel habits characterized by the frequent passage of loose, fluid, unformed stools. It is a common symptom of gastrointestinal disturbances. SEE: *cholera; epidemic viral gastroenteropathy; oral rehydration therapy; Nursing Diagnoses Appendix.*

ETIOLOGY: Diarrhea can be due to diet, inflammation or irritation of the intestinal mucosa, gastrointestinal infections, certain drugs, and psychogenic factors.

NURSING IMPLICATIONS: The patient is assessed for signs and symptoms of dehydration. Indications of metabolic acidosis, such as headache, lethargy, decreasing level of consciousness, and compensatory hyperventilation also require assessment. The frequency, consistency, color, and volume of stools are monitored, and bowel sounds auscultated for changes from normal patterns. Fluid balance, intake and output, and daily weights are also monitored. Prescribed oral or intravenous fluid and electrolyte and nutrient replacements are administered, and the patient's response is evaluated. The anal area is assessed for skin excoriation and gently but thoroughly washed and rinsed after each bowel movement, and protective ointment is applied. Universal precautions are observed for these interventions. Antidiarrheal medications are administered as prescribed. The spread of infectious diarrhea is prevented by practicing and teaching thorough handwashing and hygiene measures, by correctly handling and refrigerating foods at risk for bacterial contamination, and by reporting unusual numbers of diarrheal cases to appropriate public health authorities.

***acute d.*** Diarrhea marked by sudden onset.

TREATMENT: Strong tea, whey, rice milk, arrowroot, and blackberry brandy are all therapeutic. Adsorbents, such as aluminum hydroxide and bismuth subsalicylate (Pepto-Bismol), are useful. The return to an ordinary diet should be gradual. Basically, these are home remedies that act as demulcents or astringents for the irritated intestinal mucosa. They are often effective, but severe cases of diarrhea may require additional therapy. Specific therapy depends on the cause of the diarrhea. Also, in severe cases, fluid and electrolyte replacement therapy may be needed. Agents that reduce intestinal activity, such as antispasmodics and paregoric, may provide distinct symptomatic relief.

***antibiotic-associated d.*** Mild to moderate diarrhea in individuals taking oral antibiotics. The antibiotics destroy the normal flora in the gastrointestinal tract.

***dysenteric d.*** Diarrhea due to dysentery, characterized by mucus or bloody stools.

***emotional d.*** Diarrhea caused by emotional stress.

***epidemic d. in the newborn*** Contagious diarrhea in a newborn caused by pathogenic strains of *Escherichia coli,* occurring in epidemics in hospitals.

***factitious d.*** Self-induced diarrhea. This can be accomplished, for example, by self-medication with laxatives. SEE: *Munchausen syndrome.*

***fatty d.*** Diarrhea with stools containing undigested fat particles.

***infantile d.*** Diarrhea in children under 2 years of age.

SYMPTOMS: Dry skin, high temperature, thirst, pains, and increased frequency and amount of stools with change of color and consistency are all symptoms of diarrhea.

TREATMENT: Each year the deaths of thousands of children with diarrhea are prevented by the use of oral rehydration solutions consisting of clean (i.e., potable) water, salt, potassium, bicarbonate, and glucose. SEE: *oral rehydration solution.*

***lienteric d.*** Watery stools with undigested food particles.

***membranous d.*** Diarrhea with pieces of intestinal mucosa.

***mucous d.*** Diarrhea with mucus.

***osmotic d.*** Diarrhea caused by the retention of osmotically active solutes in the small intestine. This causes fluid to be drawn into the intestinal lumen. The retained fluid is more than the colon can resorb. The solute may be the result of maldigestion, malabsorbed nutrient, or drugs.

***purulent d.*** Diarrhea with pus, a result of intestinal ulceration.

***secretory d.*** Diarrhea in which there is a large volume of fecal output caused by abnormalities of the movement of fluid and electrolytes into the intestinal lumen. This can be caused by hormonal abnormalities present in disorders such as carcinoid syndrome, Zollinger-Ellison syndrome, certain types of pancreatic adenomas, and medullary carcinomas of the thyroid.

***simple d.*** Diarrhea in which stools contain only normal excreta.

***summer d.*** Diarrhea occurring in children during summer heat.

***travelers' d.*** ABBR: TD. Diarrhea experienced by travelers. The cause of some cases is enteropathogenic strains of *E. coli.* When travelers go from an area in which organisms that commonly cause diarrhea are endemic to an area of low risk of exposure to contamination, from 2% to 4% will develop mild diarrhea. In travelers who go from low-risk areas to high-risk areas, as many as 40% will experience diarrhea, and 20% of those will be confined to bed for 1 to 2 days. There is no completely effective method of prophylaxis. Nevertheless, it is important to avoid eating uncooked food or drinking beverages that could be contaminated. In general, the disease is self-limiting and usually lasts for 3 to 4 days. Symptomatic therapy for tenesmus, fluid loss, vomiting, and malaise is indicated. If diarrhea persists without signs of severe systemic disease such as blood in the stools, the use of paregoric, loperamide (trade name: Imodium), or diphenoxylate is beneficial. The latter two are the drugs of choice for symptomatic treatment of TD. Diphenoxylate with atropine (trade name: Lomotil) is contraindicated in children under 2 years of age. Bismuth subsalicylate taken as tablets or in its liquid form of Pepto-Bismol helps to decrease the severity of the symptoms. If there is blood in the stools, an appropriate antibiotic such as ciprofloxacin, norfloxacin, or ofloxacin is appropriate. If diarrhea continues for more than a day, the traveler can prepare an oral rehydration solution of 1 qt of safe drinking water, 6 level tsp of sugar, and 1 level tsp of salt.

PREVENTION: The ingestion of contaminated food and water, including ice, should be avoided, along with uncooked vegetables and food containing raw or undercooked eggs (e.g., mayonnaise and some desserts, sauces, and salads). Unpasteurized milk and cream may be used in ice cream, which should be avoided. Fish and shellfish may contain biotoxins even when well cooked; local residents can provide valuable advice concerning this. Unpasteurized milk should be boiled before drinking. Pepto-Bismol can be effective in preventing TD. Persons taking Pepto-Bismol should not take other salicylates at the same time. Two antimicrobials, doxycycline or trimethoprim-sulfamethoxazole, may be taken prophylactically and will greatly reduce the attack rate of TD, but like all drugs, their benefit must be weighed against the development of potentially serious side effects. Resistance to trimethoprim-sulfamethaxole has become common.

**diarthric** (dī-ăr′thrĭk) [Gr. *dis,* two, + *arthron,* joint] Pert. to two or more joints.

**diarthrosis** [Gr., a movable articulation] An articulation in which opposing bones move freely (e.g., a hinge joint or a pivot joint).

**diarticular** [Gr. *dis,* two, + L. *articulus,* joint] Pert. to two joints; specifically, the temporomandibular joints, where the mandible articulates in two places with the skull.

**diascope** (dī′ă-skōp) [Gr. *dia,* through, + *skopein,* to examine] A glass plate held against the skin for examining superficial lesions. Erythematous lesions will show the compressed capillary bed, but a hemorrhagic area will not blanch when the glass is pressed against the skin.

**diastalsis** (dī-ă-stăl′sĭs) [″+ *stalsis,* contraction] A wave of inhibition before a downward contraction in the intestine. The process is similar to peristalsis.

**diastaltic 1.** Pert. to diastalsis. **2.** Denoting reflex action.

**diastase** (dī′ăs-tās) [Gr. *diastasis,* a separation] A specific enzyme or ferment in plant cells, such as sprouting grains and malt, that converts starch into sugar.

**diastasis** (dī-ăs′tă-sĭs) [Gr.] **1.** In surgery, injury to a bone involving separation of an epiphysis. **2.** In cardiac physiology, the last part of diastole. It follows the period of most rapid diastolic filling of the ventricles, consists of a period of retarded inflow of blood from atria into ventricles, lasts (in humans under average conditions) about 0.2 sec, and is immediately followed by atrial systole.

***d. recti*** A separation of the two halves of the rectus abdominis muscles in the midline at the linea alba.This condition is benign when it occurs in pregnant women.

**diastema** (dī″ă-stē′mă) *pl.* **diastemata** [Gr. *diastema,* an interval or space] **1.** A fissure. **2.** A space between two adjacent teeth.

**diastematocrania** (dī″ă-stĕm″ă-tō-krā′nē-ă) [″ + *kranion,* cranium] A congenital sagittal fissure of the skull.

**diastematomyelia** (dī″ă-stĕm″ă-tō-mī-ē′lē-ă) [″ + *myelos,* marrow] A congenital fissure of the spinal cord, frequently associated with spina bifida cystica.

**diastematopyelia** (dī″ă-stĕm″ă-tō-pī-ē′lē-ă) [″ + *pyelos,* pelvis] A congenital median slit of the pelvis.

**diaster** [Gr. *dis,* two, + *aster,* star] A double star figure formed during mitosis. SYN: *amphiaster.*

**diastole** (dī-ăs′tō-lē) [Gr. *diastellein,* to expand] The normal period in the heart cycle during which the muscle fibers lengthen, the heart dilates, and the cavities fill with blood; diastole of the atria occurs before that of the ventricles. Roughly, the period of relaxation alternating with systole or contraction. SEE: *blood pressure; heart; murmur; pulse; systole.*

**diastolic** (dī-ăs-tŏl′ĭk) Pert. to diastole.

**diastolic pressure** ABBR: DP. The period of least pressure in the arterial vascular system.

***augmented d.p.*** An increase in diastolic pressure, usually by an artificial device, such as an intra-aortic balloon pump. SEE: *counterpulsation, intra-aortic balloon.*

**diataxia** [Gr. *dis,* two, + *ataxia,* lack of order] Bilateral ataxia.

**diatela, diatele** (dī-ă-tē′lă, -tēl′) [Gr. *dia,* between, + L. *tela,* web] The membranous roof of the third ventricle.

**diaterma** [″ + *terma,* end] A portion of the floor of the third ventricle.

**diathermal** (dī″ă-thĕr′măl) [Gr. *dia,* through, + *therme,* heat] Able to absorb heat rays.

**diathermic** Of the nature of diathermy or of its results.

**diathermy** (dī′ă-thĕr″mē) [Gr. *dia,* through, + *therme,* heat] The therapeutic use of a high-frequency current to generate heat within some part of the body. The frequency is greater than the maximum frequency for neuromuscular response and ranges from several hundred thousand to millions of cycles per second. It is used to increase blood flow to specific areas. It should not be used in the acute stage of recovery from trauma.

***medical d.*** The generation of heat within the body by the application of high-frequency oscillatory current for warming, but not damaging, tissues.

***short-wave d.*** Diathermy using wavelengths of 3 to 30 m.

***surgical d.*** Diathermy of high frequency for electrocoagulation or cauterization.

**diathesis** (dī-ăth′ĕ-sĭs) [Gr. *diatithenai,* to dispose] A constitutional predisposition to certain disease conditions.

**diathetic** Pert. to diathesis.

**diatom** (dī′ă-tŏm) [Gr. *diatemnein,* to cut through] One of a group of unicellular microscopic algae. They possess a siliceous or calcium-containing cell wall.

**diatomaceous earth** (dī″ă-tō-mā′shus) A substance composed of diatoms. SEE: *diatom.*

**diatomic 1.** Containing two atoms; said of molecules. **2.** Bivalent.

**diatrizoate meglumine** (dī″ă-trī-zō′āt) A high-osmolarity, water-soluble ionic contrast medium with the cation consisting of meglumine during ionic dissociation. It is used intra-arterially to visualize the arteries and veins of the heart and brain, great vessels such as the aorta, and the kidneys and bladder.

**diatrizoate sodium** A high-osmolarity, water-soluble contrast medium with the cation consisting of sodium during ionic dissociation. It is used to visualize various hollow body organs such as the kidney, bladder, uterus, and fallopian tubes.

**diaxon, diaxone** [Gr. *dis,* two, + *axon,* axis] A neuron having two axons.

**diazepam** (dī-ăz′ĕ-păm) An antianxiety and sedative drug used extensively in the U.S. It is effective in treating status epilepticus, acute cocaine poisoning, and a variety of anxiety disorders.

**diazo-** A prefix used in chemistry to indicate that a compound contains the —N=N— group.

**diazo reaction** A deep red color in urine, produced by the action of *p*-diazobenzenesulfonic acid and ammonia on aromatic substances found in the urine in certain conditions.

**diazotize** (dī-ăz′ō-tīz) In chemistry, to convert $NH_2$ groups into diazo, —N=N—, groups.

**diazoxide** (dī-ăz-ŏk′sīd) A drug used to lower blood pressure in acute hypertension emergencies, and to treat hypoglycemia due to hyperinsulinism.

**dibasic** (dī-bā′sĭk) [″ + *basis,* base] Capable of neutralizing or accepting two hydrogen ions.

**diblastula** (dī-blăs′tū-lă) [″ + *blastos,* sprout] A blastula containing the ectoderm and entoderm.

**Dibothriocephalus** (dī-bŏth″rē-ō-sĕf′ăl-ŭs) Former name for the genus *Diphyllobothrium.*

**dibucaine hydrochloride** A local anesthetic similar to cocaine in action when applied topically and similar to procaine and cocaine when injected.

**DIC** *disseminated intravascular coagulation.*

**dicalcic, dicalcium** (dī-kăl′sĭk) [″ + L. *calx,* lime] Containing two atoms of calcium.

**dicalcium phosphate** (dī-kăl′sē-ŭm fŏs′fāt) Dibasic calcium phosphate. It is used as a source of calcium to supplement the diet.

**dicentric** (dī-sĕn′trĭk) Having two centers or two centromeres.

**dicephalus** (dī-sĕf′ă-lŭs) [″ + *kephale,* head] A congenitally deformed fetus with two heads.

**2,4-dichlorophenoxyacetic acid** ABBR: 2,4-D. A toxic substance previously used as a weed killer. SEE: *Poisons and Poisoning Appendix.*

**dichlorphenamide** (dī″klor-fĕn′ă-mīd) A carbonic anhydrase inhibitor used in treating glaucoma.

**dichorionic** (dī″kō-rē-ŏn′ĭk) Having two chorions. This may occur in two-egg (dizygotic) twins.

**dichotomy, dichotomization** (dī-kŏt′ō-mē, dī-kŏt″ō-mī-zā′shŭn) [Gr. *dicha,* twofold, + *tome,* incision] **1.** Bifurcation of a vein. **2.** Cutting or dividing into two parts.

**dichroic** (dī-krō′ĭk) Pert. to dichroism.

**dichroic mirror** An optical device used in some spectrophotometers to split a beam of light into reference and sample beams.

**dichroism** (dī′krō-ĭzm) [Gr. *dis,* two, + *chroa,* color] The property of appearing to be one color by direct light and another by transmitted light.

**dichromate** (dī-krō′māt) A chemical that contains the $Cr_2O_7$ group.

**dichromatic** Able to see only two colors.

**dichromatism** (dī-krō′mă-tĭzm) The ability to distinguish only two primary colors. SYN: *dichromatopsia.*

**dichromatopsia** (dī″krō-mă-tŏp′sē-ă) [″ + *chroma,* color, + *opsis,* sight] Dichromatism.

**dichromic 1.** Containing two atoms of chromium. **2.** Seeing only two colors.

**dichromophil** [″ + *chroma,* color, + *philein,* to love] Double staining with both acid and basic dyes.

**dichromophilism** (dī″krō-mŏf′ĭl-ĭzm) [″ + ″ + ″ + *-ismos,* condition] The capacity for double staining.

**Dick method** [George F. Dick, 1881–1967, and Gladys H. Dick, 1881–1963, U.S. bacteriologists] A toxin-antitoxin injection for the prevention of scarlet fever.

**Dick test** A test for susceptibility or immunity to scarlet fever. The erythrogenic toxin from *Streptococcus* is injected intracutaneously. In a negative reaction, some slight inflammatory changes may occur due to irritation by proteins in administered fluid. Somewhat similar to the Schick test for diphtheria, the Dick test ascertains a person's susceptibility to scarlet fever by the injection of a standardized toxin of the beta-hemolytic streptococcus. A positive (susceptible) reaction in the form of erythema appears in about 12 to 24 hr. Patients convalescing from scarlet fever invariably have a negative reaction. SEE: *Schick test.*

**dicloxacillin sodium** (dī-klŏks″ă-sĭl′ĭn) A semisynthetic penicillin useful in treating penicillinase-resistant staphylococci.

**dicoelous** (dī-sē′lŭs) [″ + *koilos,* hollow] **1.** Concave or hollowed out on two sides. **2.** Containing two cavities.

**dicophane** (dī′kō-fān) A powerful insecticide now rarely used because of its toxicity. SYN: *chlorophenothane; DDT.*

**dicoria** (dī-kō′rē-ă) [″ + *kore,* pupil] A double pupil in each eye.

**dicoumarol** (dī-koo′mă-rŏl) Dicumarol.

**dicrotic** (dī-krŏt′ĭk) [Gr. *dikrotos,* beating double] Having one heartbeat for two arterial pulsations; relating to a double pulse.

**dicrotic notch** In a pulse tracing, a notch on the descending limb.

**dicrotic wave** A positive wave following the dicrotic notch.

**dicrotism** (dī′krŏt-ĭzm) [″ + *-ismos,* condition] The state of being dicrotic.

**dictyoma, diktyoma** (dĭk″tē-ō′mă) [Gr. *diktyon,* net, + *oma,* tumor] A tumor of the ciliary epithelium.

**dictyosome** (dĭk′tē-ō-sōm) [″ + *soma,* body] A cytoplasmic body similar to the Golgi apparatus. It is thought to be a dispersed element of the Golgi apparatus.

**dicumarol** (dī-koo′mă-rŏl) A drug that acts in the liver to impair the synthesis of six vitamin K–dependent coagulation factors including prothrombin. It is used in the prophylaxis and treatment of intravascular clotting, and in postoperative thrombophlebitis, pulmonary embolism, acute peripheral embolism and thrombosis, and recurrent idiopathic thrombophlebitis. It is used also in management of acute coronary thrombosis. Frequently it is given as an adjunct to heparin. The dose is determined by periodically testing the prothrombin time. If heparin is being given, it is important that 3 to 4 hr elapse between the last dose of heparin and the time the blood is drawn for the prothrombin test. SYN: *dicoumarol.*

CONTRAINDICATIONS: Contraindications are subacute bacterial endocarditis; recent brain, spinal, or eye surgery; purpura and blood disorders; gastrointestinal bleeding; vitamin K deficiency; and absence of prothrombin determination. The drug is excreted in breast milk. Thus, breast-fed infants whose mothers are receiving dicumarol should be carefully observed for bleeding tendency. If the drug causes hemorrhaging, it should be stopped immediately and vitamin K should be given intravenously; whole fresh blood may be needed. SEE: *anticoagulant; heparin; tissue plasminogen activator; vitamin K.*

**dicyclic** (dī-sī′klĭk) **1.** Having or concerning two cycles. **2.** In chemistry, containing two cyclic ring structures.

**dicyclomine hydrochloride** (dī-sī′klō-mēn) An anticholinergic drug used as an antispasmodic.

**didactic** (dī-dăk′tĭk) [Gr. *didaktikos*] Concerning medical instruction by lectures and use of texts as opposed to clinical or bedside teaching.

**didactylism** (dī-dăk′tĭ-lĭzm) [Gr. *dis,* two, + *daktylos,* finger] The congenital condition of having only two digits on a hand or foot.

**didanosine** ABBR: DDI. A drug used in treating AIDS.

**didelphic** (dī-dĕl′fĭk) [″ + *delphys,* uterus] Having or pert. to a double uterus.

**didymalgia, didymodynia** (dĭd-ĭ-măl′jē-ă, dĭd″ĭ-mō-dĭn′ē-ă) [Gr. *didymos,* twin, + *algos,* pain] Pain in a testicle.

**didymitis** (dĭd-ĭ-mī′tĭs) [″ + *itis,* inflammation] Inflammation of a testicle. SYN: *orchitis.*

**didymus** (dĭd′ĭ-mŭs) [Gr. *didymos,* twin] **1.** A twin. **2.** A congenital abnormality involving joined twins. **3.** A testicle.

**die 1.** To cease living. **2.** In dentistry, a positive duplicate made from an impression of a tooth.

**dieldrin** (dī-ĕl′drĭn) A chlorinated hydrocarbon used as an insecticide. It is toxic to humans and marine and terrestrial animals. SEE: *Poisons and Poisoning Appendix.*

**dielectric** [Gr. *dia,* through, + *elektron,* amber] Insulating by offering great resistance to the passage of electricity by conduction.

**diencephalon** (dī″ĕn-sĕf′ă-lŏn) [Gr. *dis,* two, + *enkephalos,* brain] The second portion of the brain, or that lying between the telencephalon and mesencephalon. It includes the epithalamus, thalamus, metathalamus, and hypothalamus. SYN: *interbrain; thalamencephalon.*

**dienestrol** (dī″ēn-ĕs′trŏl) A nonsteroid, synthetic estrogen used for estrogen therapy.

**Dientamoeba** (dī″ĕn-tă-mē′bă) A genus of parasitic protozoa marked by possession of two similar nuclei.

***D. fragilis*** A species of parasitic ameba

inhabiting the intestine of humans. Persons infected may have diarrhea with blood or mucus, abdominal pain, and anal pruritus. This organism has been found inside the eggs of pinworms, and the eggs are thought to serve as the vector.

**dieresis** (dī-ĕr′ĕ-sĭs) [Gr. *diairesis,* a division] **1.** Breaking up or dispersion of things normally joined, as by an ulcer. **2.** Mechanical separation of parts by surgical means.

**dieretic** Pert. to dieresis; dissolvable or separable.

**diet** [ Gr. *diaita,* way of living] **1.** Liquid and solid food substances regularly consumed in the course of normal living. **2.** A prescribed allowance of food adapted for a particular state of health or disease, as a diet prescribed for use by a diabetic. **3.** To eat or drink sparingly in accordance with prescribed rules. SEE: *energy expenditure, basal.*

***acid-ash d.*** A diet designed to acidify the urine. It contains acidic foods such as meat, fish, eggs, and cereals and is lacking in fruits, vegetables, cheese, and milk.

***alkali-ash d.*** A diet designed to produce an alkaline urine. It contains foods such as fruits, vegetables, and milk and is lacking in meat, fish, eggs, and cereals.

***balanced d.*** A diet adequate in energy-providing substances (carbohydrates and fats), tissue-building compounds (proteins), inorganic chemicals (water and mineral salts), agents that regulate or catalyze metabolic processes (vitamins), and substances for certain physiological processes, such as bulk for promoting peristaltic movements of the digestive tract.

***gluten-free d.*** SEE: *gluten-free diet.*

***high-calorie d.*** A diet that contains more calories than normally required for an individual's metabolic and energy needs. The diet should include three meals plus between-meal feedings, avoiding fermentable and bulky foods. A high-calorie diet may be used to prevent weight loss in wasting diseases, in high basal metabolism, and after a long illness; in deficiency caused by anorexia, poverty, and poor dietary habits; and during lactation (when an extra 1000 and 1200 kcal each day are indicated).

***high-cellulose d.*** High-residue d.

***high-residue d.*** A diet that contains considerable amounts of substances such as fiber or cellulose, which the human body is unable to metabolize and absorb. This diet is particularly useful in treating constipation and may be beneficial also in preventing certain diseases of the gastrointestinal tract. Lay persons may refer to a high-residue diet as one containing a lot of roughage. SYN: *high-cellulose d.* SEE: *fiber.*

***ketogenic d.*** A diet that produces acetone or ketone bodies, or mild acidosis.

***light d.*** A diet consisting of all foods allowed in a soft diet, plus whole-grain cereals, easily digested raw fruits, and vegetables. Foods are not pureed or ground. This diet is used as an intermediate regimen for patients who do not require a soft diet but are not yet able to resume a full diet.

***liquid d.*** A diet for persons unable to tolerate solid food or for patients whose gastrointestinal tract must be free of solid matter. This type of diet may contain coffee with hot milk, tea, water, milk in all forms, milk and cream mixtures, cocoa, strained cream soups, fruit juices, meat juices, beef tea, clear broths, gruels, strained meat soups, and eggnogs.

***low-protein d.*** A diet that contains a limited amount of protein. The principal sources of food energy are fats and carbohydrates. This diet is used in treating severe liver disease and hepatic coma.

***low-salt d.*** A diet in which no salt is allowed on the patient's tray and no salty foods are served. This diet is used in treating hypertension and congestive heart failure.

***macrobiotic d.*** A diet consisting of unprocessed foods, vegetables, beans, whole grains, and some fish and fruits.

***Mediterranean d.*** Dietary recommendations developed by Harvard University and the World Health Organization for the prevention of cardiovascular disease. The daily use of wine and olive oil are the main factors in which it differs from the recommendations of the U.S. Department of Agriculture in the Food Guide Pyramid. The fat content is higher than that recommended by the American Heart Association. SEE: *Food Guide Pyramid.*

***minimum residue d.*** A diet used for short periods to ensure a minimum of solid material in the intestinal tract. Foods allowed include one glass of milk per day, clear fluids and juices, lean meat, noodles, and refined cereals.

***National Cholesterol Education Program d.*** A two-step approach designed to lower blood cholesterol in adults, children, and adolescents. It is similar to the "Prudent Diet," designed by the American Heart Association.

***National Renal d.*** A diet designed by the American Dietetic Association (ADA) and the National Kidney Foundation for the treatment of kidney disease. It consists of six food planning systems based on the ADA Exchange Lists. The incidence of diabetes and the use of peritoneal dialysis and hemodialysis are considered.

***"Prudent d."*** A diet designed by the American Heart Association for protection against and treatment of cardiovascular disease. A multistep approach decreases fat, cholesterol, and protein. This diet is similar to those created by the National Cholesterol Education Program.

***purine-restricted d.*** A diet that limits purine and fats and encourages fluid intake; used to control the excessive levels of uric acid caused by gout. SEE: *purine* for table.

***soft d.*** A diet consisting of soft but otherwise normal foods for individuals who find it difficult to chew or swallow.

***very low calorie d.*** A commercially available diet in which caloric intake may be from 400 to 800 kcal/day. The very low calorie diet is usually in the form of a powdered supplement that is taken 3 to 5 times a day with large amounts of water. This type of diet can be effective, but the long-range efficacy in maintaining the weight loss may be discouraging.

***weight reduction d.*** A diet that reduces the caloric content sufficiently to cause weight loss. Normal metabolism must be preserved, and bulk, mineral, protein, vitamin, and water requirements must be met. During weight loss, intake should be 600 to 1500 kcal below maintenance levels for the individual's weight. SEE: *obesity*.

***yo-yo d.*** A popular term to describe a dietary practice resulting in alternating cycles of losing and regaining weight. The demonstration of successful weight loss should be emphasized to motivate the patient to commit to lifelong changes in behaviors related to diet and physical activity. Concerns about the possible ill effects of weight cycling should not prevent persons from attempting to control their body weight. SYN: *weight cycling*.

**dietary** (dī′ĕ-tā″rē) **1.** Pert. to diet. **2.** A system of dieting. **3.** A regulated food allowance.

**dietary guidelines for Americans** Seven recommendations from the U.S. Department of Agriculture and the U.S. Department of Health and Human Services for planning and eating a healthy diet. They are as follows:

Eat a variety of foods.
Maintain healthy weight.
Choose a diet low in fat, saturated fat, and cholesterol.
Choose a diet with plenty of vegetables, fruits, and grain products.
Use sugars only in moderation.
Use salt and sodium only in moderation.
If you drink alcoholic beverages, do so in moderation. SEE: *Food Guide Pyramid*.

**dietetic** (dī″ĕ-tĕ′tĭk) **1.** Pert. to diet or its regulation. **2.** Food specially prepared for restrictive diets.

**dietetics** [Gr. *diaitetikos*] The science of applying nutritional data to the regulation of the diet of healthy and sick individuals. Some fundamental principles and facts of this science are summarized here. SEE: *energy expenditure, basal; Recommended Daily Dietary Allowances Appendix*.

CONSERVATION OF ENERGY: To produce metabolic balance, the number of calories consumed must equal the energy required for basic metabolic needs plus additional energy output resulting from muscular work and added heat losses. Thus a person whose basal rate is 1000 kcal per 24 hr may do work and lose heat during the day, adding about 1500 kcal to the energy output; he or she must, therefore, obtain 2500 kcal.

One g of fat yields approx. 9 kcal. One g of carbohydrate or protein yields about 4 kcal.

NOTE: To convert kilocalories to kilojoules, multiply them by 4.1855.

CONSERVATION OF MATTER: Everything that leaves the body, whether exhaled as carbon dioxide and water or excreted as urea and minerals, must be replaced by food. Thus, a person excreting 10 g of nitrogen daily must receive the same in his or her diet, for the element can be neither created nor destroyed. This metabolic balance may be monitored by careful chemical analysis of all that is eaten and excreted.

**diethylcarbamazine citrate** (dī-ĕth″ĭl-kăr-băm′ă-zēn) A medicine used in treating filarial infections.

**diethylpropion hydrochloride** (dī-ĕth″ĭl-prō′pē-ŏn) An adrenergic drug with actions similar to those of the amphetamines.

**diethylstilbestrol** (dī-ĕth″ĭl-stĭl″bĕs′trŏl) ABBR: DES. A synthetic preparation possessing estrogenic properties. It is several times more potent than natural estrogens and may be given orally. It is used therapeutically in the treatment of menopausal disturbances and other disorders due to estrogen deficiencies. SEE: *DES daughter; DES syndrome*.

---

Caution: Diethylstilbestrol should not be administered during pregnancy. Such use has been found to be related to subsequent vaginal malignancies in the daughters of mothers who were given it.

---

This drug was once used extensively during pregnancy to treat threatened and habitual abortion. An estimated 5 million to 10 million Americans received DES during pregnancy or were exposed to the drug in utero. Those who were exposed to DES in utero were found to be at risk of developing reproductive tract abnormalities such as clear-cell cervicovaginal cancer in women and reproductive tract abnormalities in men. These findings were reported in 1970; the use of the drug during pregnancy was subsequently banned in the U.S. in 1971 and in Europe in 1978. Women who took the drug are now known as DES mothers and their daughters and sons are known as DES daughters and DES sons, respectively.

**diethyltoluamide** (dī-ĕth″ĭl-tŏl-ū′ă-mīd) ABBR: DEET. An effective insect repellant, esp. for repelling arthropods.

**diethyltryptamine** (dī-ĕth″ĭl-trĭp′tă-mĭn) A hallucinogenic agent that at low doses has effects similar to those of LSD.

**dietitian, dietician** (dī-ĕ-tĭsh′ăn) [Gr. *diaita,* way of living] An individual whose training and experience are in the area of nutrition, and who has the ability to apply that information to the dietary needs of the healthy and sick.

***registered d.*** ABBR: RD. A specialist in dietetics who has met the requirements for certification stipulated by the American Dietetic Association.

**Dietl's crisis** (dē′t′ls) [Joseph Dietl, Pol. physician, 1804–1878] Renal colic resulting from kinking and partial obstruction of the ureter, accompanied by pain and scanty bloodstained urine.

**dietotherapy** (dī″ĕ-tō-thĕr′ă-pē) Use of the sciences of dietetics and nutrition in treating disease.

**Dieulafoy's triad** (dyū-lă-fwăhz′) [Georges Dieulafoy, Fr. physician, 1839–1911] Tenderness, muscular contraction, and skin hyperesthesia at McBurney's point in acute appendicitis.

**differential** (dĭf″ĕr-ĕn′shăl) [L. *differre,* to carry apart] Marked by or relating to differences.

**differential amplifier** An amplifier used to increase the difference between two signals, one of which is usually a reference.

**differential blood count** The determination of the number of each variety of leukocyte in 1 μl of blood. SEE: *blood count, differential.*

**differential diagnosis** SEE: *diagnosis, differential.*

**differentiation 1.** In embryology, the aquiring of individual characteristics. This occurs in progressive diversification of cells of the developing pre-embryo and embryo. **2.** The distinguishing of one disease from another. **3.** In psychiatry, the integration of emotional and intellectual functions in an individual.

***lymphocyte d.*** The process by which immature lymphocytes are stimulated to become functional T and B cells able to recognize and respond to antigens.

**diffraction** (dĭ-frăk′shŭn) [L. *diffringere,* to break to pieces] The change occurring in light when it passes through crystals, prisms, or parallel bars in a grating, in which the rays are deflected and thus appear to be turned aside. This produces dark or colored bands or lines. The term is also applied to similar phenomena in sound.

**diffraction grating** The device in a spectrophotometer that disperses white light into the colors of the spectrum. This is done to isolate wavelengths.

**diffusate** (dĭf′ū-sāt) [L. *dis,* apart, + *fundere,* to pour] In the process of dialysis, the portion of a liquid that passes through a membrane and that contains crystalloid matter in solution. SYN: *dialysate.*

**diffuse** (dĭ-fūs′) Spreading, scattered, spread.

**diffusible** (dĭ-fūz′ĭ-bl) Capable of being diffused.

**diffusing capacity** The ability of gas to cross the alveolar-capillary membrane in the lung. This may be measured by using the rate of movement of a single breath of inhaled 0.3% carbon monoxide across the alveolar-capillary membrane.

**diffusion** (dĭ-fū′zhŭn) [″ + *fundere,* to pour] **1.** The tendency of molecules of a substance (gaseous, liquid, or solid) to move from a region of high concentration to one of lower concentration. **2.** Absorption of a liquid, such as the absorption by cells of water from lymph when the percentage of salt is less in the lymph than in the cells. When the percentage is greater in the lymph, water is withdrawn from the cells. SEE: *osmosis.* **3.** A process whereby various gases interpenetrate and become mixed through the incessant motion of their molecules. Similarly, if aqueous solutions of different materials stand in contact, mixing occurs on standing even if the solutions are separated by thin membranes. SEE: illus.

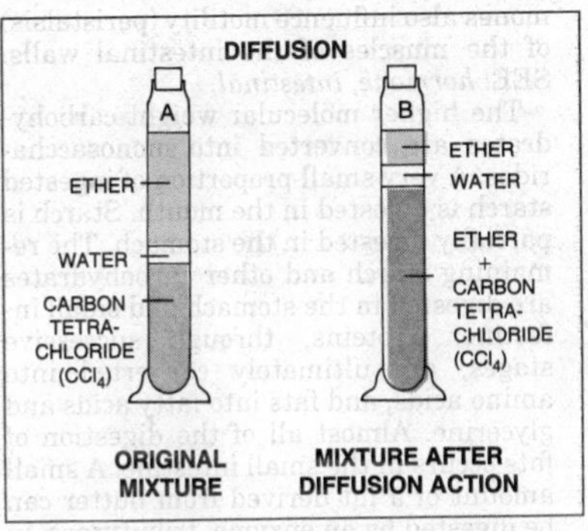


***facilitated d.*** Diffusion of a substance such as glucose through a membrane by way of membrane proteins that act as carrier molecules.

**digastric** (dī-găs′trĭk) [Gr. *dis,* twice, + *gaster,* belly] Having two bellies; said of certain muscles.

**Digenetica** (dī-jĕ-nĕt′ĭ-kă) An order of parasitic flatworms belonging to the class Trematoda. It reproduces asexually, lives usually in molluscs, and alternates with a sexual generation living in vertebrates as their final host. It includes all four groups of flukes parasitic in humans. SEE: *fluke.*

**digest** [L. *dis,* apart, + *gerere,* to carry] **1.** To undergo the process involved in changing food from a solid physical form to a soft, moisturized mass broken down in the intestinal tract by chemicals, bacteria, and enzymes. SEE: *metabolism.* **2.** To make a condensation of a subject.

**digestant 1.** An agent that digests food or

aids in digestion, such as pepsin or pancreatin. **2.** A preparation made from the digestive glands or lining membrane of the stomach, classified according to the foods it digests, such as carbohydrate or protein.

**digestible** Capable of being digested.

**digestion** [L. *digestio,* a taking apart] The process by which food is broken down mechanically and chemically in the gastrointestinal tract and converted into absorbable forms. Salt, the simplest sugars (such as glucose), cystalloids in general, and water can be absorbed unchanged, but starches, fats, and proteins generally are not absorbable until they have been split into smaller molecules. Even the sugar sucrose (a disaccharide) must first be split into two simple hexoses, glucose and fructose, to be absorbed. The chemical actions are chiefly hydrolytic; they are caused by various enzymes, each of which acts in an acid, alkaline, or neutral juice according to its properties. In addition, hormones released by the gastrointestinal mucosa facilitate the digestive process by targeting specific tissues to release acid, enzymes, or emulsifiers. These hormones also influence motility (peristalsis) of the muscles of the intestinal walls. SEE: *hormone, intestinal.*

The higher molecular weight carbohydrates are converted into monosaccharides. A very small proportion of ingested starch is digested in the mouth. Starch is partially digested in the stomach. The remaining starch and other carbohydrates are digested in the stomach and small intestine. Proteins, through successive stages, are ultimately converted into amino acids, and fats into fatty acids and glycerine. Almost all of the digestion of fats occurs in the small intestine. A small amount of a fat derived from butter can be digested by an enzyme, tributyrase, in the stomach. In the stomach the soluble casein of milk is converted into insoluble paracasein, causing it to coagulate or clot. This is caused by the enzyme pepsin. This digestive process does not occur in the absence of gastric acid. Proteins are also digested by the action of enzymes secreted into the small intestine from the pancreas, and by enzymes present in the epithelial cells of the small intestine. The enzyme lipase is able to act on emulsified fats. For instance, it liberates butyric acid from the fats in milk. This chemical causes the characteristic odor of vomitus. The chemical actions are facilitated by the churning wavelike motions (i.e., peristalsis) of the stomach walls. When the chyme is ready to leave the stomach, the pylorus opens from time to time and the chyme is quickly propelled into the duodenum. SEE: tables.

***artificial d.*** Digestion outside the living organism by a ferment.

***duodenal d.*** The chyme, which is usually acid as it comes from the stomach, is made alkaline and the fats it contains are emulsified by the action of bile. Enzymes adapted to these new conditions are supplied by pancreatic juice, which enters the duodenum by two ducts, and intestinal juice, which comes from small glands in the wall of the intestine itself. The hydrolysis of starches, fats, and proteins is carried to its physiological completion here and in the remainder of the small intestine.

***extracellular d.*** Digestion occurring outside the body of the cell.

***gastric d.*** The portion of the digestive process taking place in the stomach.

***intestinal d.*** In the intestines, the continuation of hydrolytic processes and the active absorption of food products. From the ileum, the food residues pass in a nearly liquid state through a small opening into the ascending colon. A sphincter muscle prevents backflow. True digestive processes in the colon are slight, but there are normally bacterial action (the products of which are mostly absorbed) and reabsorption of water. The remaining substances, now colored by pigments that entered with bile and changed to a firm consistency by the loss of water, pass on through the transverse colon, the descending colon, and the sigmoid colon. The rectum is usually empty until peristalsis propels feces in, stimulating the defecation reflex; contraction of the anal sphincters may prevent defecation. SEE: *absorption.*

***intracellular d.*** The metabolic processes within cells.

***oral d.*** The portion of the digestive process taking place in the mouth. It includes the physical process of chewing food and the chemical process of starch splitting by the enzyme ptyalin, present in the saliva.

***pancreatic d.*** The portion of digestive process influenced by pancreatic juice.

***salivary d.*** SEE: *salivary digestion.*

**digestive** (dī-jĕs′tĭv) Pert. to digestion.

**digestive juice** One of several secretions that aid in processes of digestion.

**digestive system** All the organs and glands associated with ingestion and digestion of food; the tract from the mouth to the anus. SEE: illus.

**digit** (dĭj′ĭt) *pl.* **digits** [L. *digitus,* finger] A finger or toe. **digital** (-ĭ-tăl), *adj.*

**digital amniotome** A small apparatus that fits over the tip of the index finger. A small knifelike projection at the end of the device is used to puncture the bag of waters before delivery of the fetus. This usually expedites progression of labor.

**digitalis** (dĭj″ĭ-tăl′ĭs) [L. *digitus,* finger] Foxglove. The dried leaves of *Digitalis purpurea* used in powdered form in tablets or capsules. Cardiotonic glycosides, esp. digitoxin and digoxin, are obtained from various species of the digitalis plant. SEE: *Poisons and Poisoning Appendix.*

**Action of Digestive Enzymes on Foods**

| Food Component | Enzyme | Secretion | Site of Action |
|---|---|---|---|
| Proteins | Pepsin | Gastric juice, acid | Stomach |
| | Trypsin | Pancreatic juice, alkaline | Small intestine |
| Fats | Lipase | Gastric juice | Stomach |
| | | Pancreatic juice | Small intestine |
| Carbohydrates | Salivary amylase | Saliva, alkaline | Mouth |
| | Pancreatic amylase | Pancreatic juice | Small intestine |
| | Sucrase, maltase, lactase | Intestinal juice | Small intestine |

ACTION/USES: Digitalis glycosides increase the force of myocardial contraction, increase the refractory period of the atrioventricular node, and to a lesser degree affect the sinoatrial node. Digitalis increases cardiac output by increasing the contractility of cardiac muscle. Digitalis is indicated in congestive heart failure, and its use causes diuresis and general amelioration of this condition. It is usually necessary to continue the drug after the heart failure is controlled. Digitalis is also used in atrial fibrillation and flutter and in paroxysmal atrial tachycardia.

CONTRAINDICATIONS: Digitalis is not indicated in sinus tachycardia or premature systoles in the absence of heart failure. Its use in shock caused by infections is of no benefit and may be harmful. It should not be used in ventricular fibrillation or if the patient is allergic to digitalis.

PRECAUTIONS: Potassium depletion, which may accompany diuresis, sensitizes the myocardium to digitalis and may permit toxicity to develop with what would otherwise be the usual dose. Patients with acute myocardial infarction, severe pulmonary disease, or far-advanced heart failure may be more sensitive to digitalis and thus prone to develop arrhythmia. Calcium affects the heart in a manner similar to that of digitalis; its use in a digitalized patient may produce serious arrhythmias. In myxedema, digitalis requirements are decreased because the excretion rate of the drug is decreased. Patients with incomplete atrioventricular block, esp. those with Stokes-Adams attacks, may develop complete heart block if given digitalis. Because renal insufficiency delays the excretion of digitalis, the dose must be adjusted accordingly in those patients.

**digitalis poisoning** Toxicity that may develop acutely or chronically from the cumulative effect of digitalis. Patients on digitalis therapy must know how to take their pulse and be aware of the signs and symptoms of heart block or other adverse effects. They should also include potassium-containing foods in their daily diet. SEE: *Nursing Diagnoses Appendix.*

SYMPTOMS: Symptoms include digestive disturbances such as nausea and vomiting, irregular pulse, diarrhea, and yellow vision. Frequently a severe headache is present. Cardiac irregularities are

**Action of Digestive Secretions on Proteins, Fats, and Carbohydrates**

| Secretion | Proteins | Fats | Carbohydrates |
|---|---|---|---|
| Saliva | | | Cooked starch into maltose |
| Gastric juice | Curdles milk<br>Proteins into polypeptides | | |
| Pancreatic juice | Polypeptides to peptides | Fats to fatty acids and glycerol | Raw and cooked starch into maltose |
| Bile | | Emulsifies fats | |
| Intestinal juice | Completes the change of peptones into amino acids | | Completes the change of all sugars into the simplest form. NOTE: Disaccharides are hydrolyzed to monosaccharides in the mucosal cells lining the small intestine. |

common, esp. slowing of the heart, ventricular extrasystoles, or partial heart block.

FIRST AID: The stomach must be evacuated and digitalis and diuretics discontinued. Because these patients are usually chronically ill, special care is necessary in their management. Serious cases of poisoning should be treated with digoxin immune Fab (ovine).

**digitalization** (dĭj″ĭ-tăl-ĭ-zā′shŭn) Subjection of an organism to the action of digitalis.

**digital radiography** Radiography using computerized imaging instead of conventional film or screen imaging.

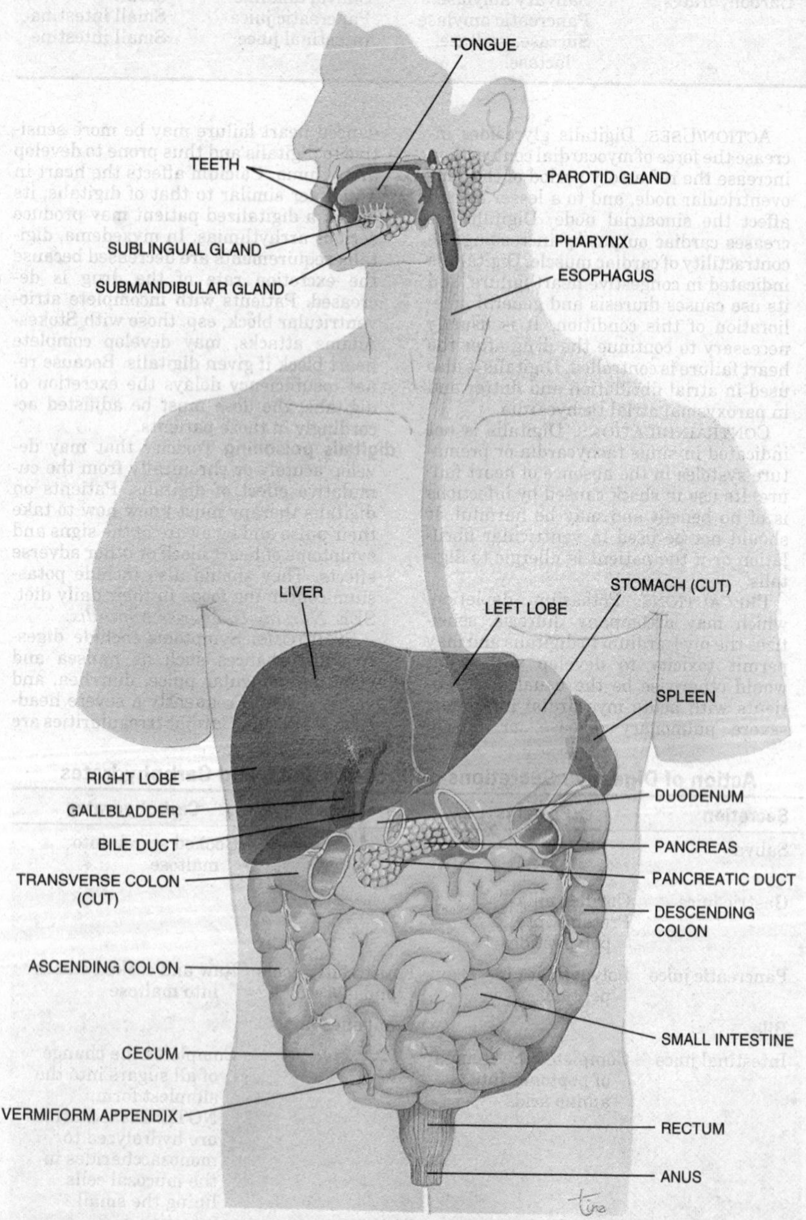


THE DIGESTIVE SYSTEM (WITH SPLEEN SHOWN)

**digital reflex** Sudden flexion of the terminal phalanx of a finger or thumb when the nail is suddenly tapped.

**digital subtraction angiography** SEE: *angiography, digital subtraction.*

**digitate** [L. *digitus,* finger] Having finger-like impressions or processes.

**digitation** (dĭj-ĭ-tā'shŭn) A finger-like process.

**digiti** (dĭj'ĭ-tī) Pl. of digitus.

**digitiform** (dĭj'ĭ-tĭ-form) Similar to a finger.

**digitoxin** (dĭj-ĭ-tŏk'sĭn) A cardiotoxic glycoside obtained from various species of the digitalis plant and used as a heart stimulant, administered orally or parenterally. SEE: *digitalis.*

**digit span test** A test of immediate memory. The patient is asked to repeat a string of numerals spoken by the examiner. The string is made progressively longer in order to determine the numerals that can be recalled. Normally six or seven numbers could be repeated. SEE: *memory; object span test; temporal-sequential organization.*

**digitus** [L] A finger or toe.

**diglossia** (dī-glŏs'ē-ă) [Gr. *dis,* double, + *glossa,* tongue] The condition of having a double tongue.

**diglyceride** (dī-glĭs'ĕr-īd) A glyceride combined with two fatty acid molecules. SEE: *triglyceride.*

**dignathus** (dĭg-nā'thŭs) [" + *gnathos,* jaw] Having two jaws due to a congenital deformity.

**digoxin** (dĭ-jŏk'sĭn) A cardiotonic glycoside obtained from *Digitalis lanata* and used as a heart stimulant, administered orally or parenterally.

**digoxin immune Fab (ovine) for injection** A biological substance for use in treating severe overdose of digoxin or digitoxin. This fragment antigen binding (Fab) substance combines with molecules of digoxin or digitoxin, which are then excreted by the kidneys.

**dihydric** (dī-hī'drĭk) A compound containing two hydrogen atoms.

**dihydrocodeinone bitartrate** (dī-hī"drō-kō'dē-ĭ-nōn) An opioid analgesic used in combination with certain other drugs.

**dihydroergotamine mesylate** (dī-hī"drō-ĕr-gŏt'ă-mēn) A vasoconstrictor used in treating migraine.

**dihydrosphingosine** $CH_3—[CH_2]_{14}—CHOH—CH(NH_2)—CH_2OH$. A long-chain amino alcohol present in sphingolipids, also known as sphinganine. SEE: *sphingolipid; sphingosine.*

**dihydrotachysterol** (dī-hī"drō-tăk-ĭs'tĕr-ŏl) A hydrogenated tachysterol; a steroid obtained by irradiation of ergosterol. It aids the absorption of calcium from the digestive tract in hypoparathyroidism.

**dihydroxyaluminum aminoacetate** (dī"hī-drŏk"sē-ă-lū'mĭ-nŭm) An antacid used in treating gastric hyperacidity.

**dihydroxyaluminum sodium carbonate** A gastric antacid preparation.

**dihydroxycholecalciferol** (dī"hī-drŏk"sē-kō"lē-kăl-sĭf'ĕ-rŏl) A group of compounds considered to be hormones because of their ability to influence absorption and metabolism of calcium. One of these, calcitriol, is thought to be the active form of vitamin D.

**3,4-dihydroxyphenylalanine** (dī-hī-drŏk"sē-fĕn"ĭl-ăl'ă-nēn) Dopa.

**di-iodohydroxyquin** (dī"ī-ō"dō-hī-drŏk'sē-kwĭn) The previously used name for iodoquinol.

**diktyoma** Dictyoma.

**dilaceration** (dī"lăs-ĕr-ā'shŭn) [L. *dilacerare,* to tear apart] **1.** A tearing apart, as of a cataract. SEE: *discission.* **2.** Bending of the root of a tooth due to injury during development.

**Dilantin** (dī-lăn'tĭn) Trade name for phenytoin sodium, previously termed diphenylhydantoin sodium. A derivative of glyceryl urea, it is an anticonvulsant used esp. in the treatment of epilepsy.

**dilatant** (dī-lā'tănt) [L. *dilatare,* to enlarge] Anything that causes dilation.

**dilatation** (dĭl-ă-tā'shŭn) **1.** Expansion of an organ or vessel. **2.** Expansion of an orifice with a dilator.

***digital d.*** Dilatation of an opening or a cavity by use of the fingers.

***heart d.*** Abnormal increase in the size of the cavities of the heart, a common result of valvular disease or hypertension.

***stomach d.*** A condition in which the stomach is extremely distended. Acute dilatation of the stomach or acute gastromesenteric ileus may occur as a postoperative or postpartum condition and usually results from obstruction of the duodenum.

**dilation 1.** Expansion of an orifice with a dilator. **2.** Expansion of an organ, orifice, or vessel. SYN: *dilatation.*

**dilation and curettage** ABBR: D and C. A surgical procedure that expands the cervical canal of the uterus (dilation) so that the surface lining of the uterine wall can be scraped (curettage). SEE: *Nursing Diagnoses Appendix.*

**dilation and evacuation** ABBR: D and E. During the second trimester, removal of the products of conception by suction curettage and use of forceps.

**dilator** (dī-lā'tor) [L. *dilatare,* to expand] An instrument for dilating muscles or for stretching cavities or openings.

***Barnes' d.*** A rubber bag filled with fluid for dilation of the cervix uteri.

***Bossi's d.*** A multiple-pronged instrument that dilates by separation of its prongs. It is used for dilation of the cervix uteri.

***Goodell's d.*** An instrument similar to the Bossi dilator except that it has three prongs.

***gynecological d.*** An instrument for dilating the cervix uteri.

***Hegar's d.*** Graduated metal sounds that are inserted into the cervical canal and cause a graded dilation.

***tent d.*** A small cone made of seaweed, sponge, or tree roots that is inserted into the uterine canal dry and, on absorbing moisture, expands to cause a slow dilation. SEE: *Laminaria digitata.*

***vaginal d.*** A glass, plastic, or metal device for dilating the vagina.

**Dilaudid** Trade name for hydromorphone hydrochloride.

**dildo, dildoe** An artificial penis-shaped device used intravaginally to produce sexual pleasure.

**dilemma, ethical** A situation that requires an individual to choose between two equally unfavorable alternatives.

**diluent** (dĭl′ū-ĕnt) [L. *diluere,* to wash away] An agent that dilutes the substance or solution to which it is added.

**dilution** (dī-loo′shŭn) **1.** The process of attenuating or weakening a substance. **2.** A diluted substance. SEE: *adulteration.*

**dimenhydrinate** (dī″mĕn-hī′drĭn-āt) A drug used to prevent or treat motion sickness and to control nausea, vomiting, and dizziness in other conditions.

**dimension, vertical** A vertical measurement of the face; used in dentisty for growth studies and for reference in denture placement.

**dimer** (dī′mĕr) **1.** In chemistry, esp. polymer chemistry, a combination of two identical molecules to form a single compound. **2.** In virology, a capsomer containing two subunits.

**dimercaprol** (dī-mĕr-kăp′rōl) $C_3H_8OS_2$. A compound, 2,3-dimercaptopropanol, used as an antidote in poisoning from heavy metals such as arsenic, gold, and mercury. It is a colorless liquid with a disagreeable odor. Mixed with benzyl benzoate and oil, it is administered intramuscularly.

**Dimetane** Trade name for brompheniramine maleate.

**dimethicone** (dī-mĕth′ĭ-kōn) A silicone oil used to protect the skin against water-soluble irritants.

**dimethindene maleate** (dī″mĕth-ĭn′dēn) An antihistamine.

**dimethylamine** (dī-mĕth″ĭl-ăm′ĭn) A malodorous product of decaying materials that contain proteins.

***p*-dimethylaminoazobenzene** (dī-mĕth″ĭl-ăm″ĭ-nō-ăz″ō-bĕn′zēn) A carcinogenic dye, butter yellow.

**dimethyl phthalate** (dī-mĕth″ĭl thăl′āt) An insect repellent.

**dimethyl sulfoxide** (dī-mĕth′ĭl sŭlf-ŏks′īd) ABBR: DMSO. A penetrating solvent used to hasten absorption of medicines through the skin. First used in veterinary medicine, it has been proposed for use in sports medicine but has not been approved in the U.S. for use in humans.

**dimethyltryptamine** (dī-mĕth″ĭl-trĭp′tă-mēn) An agent that in low doses has hallucinogenic action similar to that of LSD.

**dimetria** (dī-mē′trē-ă) [Gr. *dis,* double, + *metra,* uterus] A double uterus.

**dimorphous** (dī-mor′fŭs) [″ + *morphe,* form] Occurring in two different forms.

**dimple** A small depression in the skin, esp. of the cheek or chin.

**dimple sign** A sign used to differentiate a benign lesion, dermatofibroma, from nodular melanoma, which it may mimic. On application of lateral pressure with the thumb and index finger, the dermatofibroma dimples or becomes indented; melanomas, melanocytic nevi, and normal skin protrude above the initial plane.

**dimpling** The formation of slight depressions in the flesh due to retraction of the subcutaneous tissue. It occurs in certain carcinomas, such as cancer of the breast. SEE: *peau d'orange.*

**2,4-dinitrophenol** (dī-nī″trō-fē′nōl) An isomeric compound formerly used in making dyes. It is very toxic and is used only as a reagent. SEE: *Poisons and Poisoning Appendix.*

**Dinoflagellata** (dī″nō-flăj″ĕ-lā′tă) [″ + *flagellum,* whip] A phylum of the kingdom Protista; photosynthetic unicellular organisms that are part of the phytoplankton in fresh and ocean water. Some marine species bloom explosively in what are called "red tides"; shellfish that feed on the dinoflagellates are toxic to humans (paralytic shellfish poisoning). Another species produces ciguatera toxin, which is poisonous to fish and to humans who consume such fish.

**dinoprostone** (dī′nō-prŏs-tōn) A drug that causes uterine contractions and may be used to induce abortion during the very early stage of pregnancy. Also called prostaglandin $E_2$.

**dinucleotide** (dī-nū′klē-ō-tīd) The product of cleaving a polynucleotide.

**Dioctophyma** (dī-ŏk″tō-fī′mă) A genus of roundworms found in dogs but rarely in humans.

**dioctyl calcium sulfosuccinate** (dī-ŏk′tĭl) A stool softener. The name was previously used for docusate calcium.

**dioctyl sodium sulfosuccinate** Previously used name for docusate sodium.

**Diodrast** (dī′ō-drăst) Trade name for iodopyracet, a radiopaque medium used in radiographic studies, esp. of the urinary tract.

**Diogenes syndrome** [Diogenes, Gr. philosopher, 4th century B.C.] A lack of interest in personal cleanliness or cleanliness of the home, usually occurring in elderly individuals who live alone. These people are usually undernourished, but not necessarily from poverty; this condition occurs in all socioeconomic circumstances.

**diopter** (dī-ŏp′-tĕr, dī′ŏp-) [Gr. *dia,* through, + *optos,* visible] The refractive power of a lens; the reciprocal of the focal length expressed in meters. It is used as a unit of measurement in refraction. **dioptric** (-ŏp′trĭk), *adj.*

**dioptometer** (dī″ŏp-tŏm′ĕ-tĕr) [″ + ″ + *met-*

*ron,* measure] A device for measuring ocular refraction.

**dioptometry** (dī″ŏp-tŏm′ĕ-trē) The determination of refraction and accommodation of the eye.

**dioptrics** (dī-ŏp′trĭks) The science of light refraction.

**diovulatory** (dī-ŏv′ū-lă-tō″rē) Producing two ova in the same ovarian cycle.

**dioxide** (dī-ŏk′sīd) [Gr. *dis,* two, + *oxys,* sharp] A compound having two oxygen atoms per molecule.

**dioxin** 2,3,7,8-tetrachlorodibenzo-*p*-dioxin (TCDD). This chemical is important because of its being an unwanted and undesirable contaminant in widely used herbicides and preservatives. There are more than 75 different isomers of dioxin. Exposure to dioxin can produce chloracne, liver injury, peripheral neuropathy, central nervous system changes, and psychiatric difficulties. The possibility that dioxin causes cancer in humans is being investigated. At low concentrations, dioxin, which is carcinogenic in animals, is one of the most toxic substances to which workers in the industrial and agricultural environment can be exposed. SEE: *Agent Orange; pentachlorophenol; 2,4,5-trichlorophenoxyacetic acid.*

**dioxybenzone** (dī-ŏks″ĭ-bĕn′zōn) A chemical that protects skin from the sun.

**dipalmityl lecithin** ABBR: DPL. A major constituent of pulmonary surfactant.

**dipeptid(e)** (dī-pĕp′tĭd, -tīd) [″ + *peptein,* to digest] A derived protein obtained by hydrolysis of proteins or condensation of amino acids.

**dipeptidase** (dī-pĕp′tĭ-dās) An enzyme that catalyzes the hydrolysis of dipeptides to amino acids.

**Dipetalonema perstans** (dī-pĕt″ă-lō-nē′mă) A species of filariae that infests wild or domestic animals and occasionally humans. In humans, the adult worm migrates to the subcutaneous tissue and produces a nodule. Rarely, the adult worm may be seen beneath the conjunctiva.

**diphallus** (dī-făl′ŭs) [″ + *phallos,* penis] A condition in which there is either complete or incomplete doubling of the penis or clitoris.

**diphasic** (dī-fā′zĭk) [″ + *phasis,* a phase] Having two phases.

**diphenhydramine hydrochloride** (dī″fĕn-hī′dră-mēn hī-drō-klō′rīd) An antihistamine.

**diphenoxylate hydrochloride** (dī″fĕn-ŏk′sĭ-lāt) A smooth muscle relaxant used in combination with atropine in treating diarrhea.

**diphenylhydantoin sodium** (dī-fĕn″ĭl-hī-dăn′tō-ĭn) An anticonvulsant used esp. in the treatment of epilepsy. Its official name is phenytoin. Trade name is Dilantin.

**diphonia** (dī-fō′nē-ă) [Gr. *dis,* two, + *phone,* voice] Simultaneous production of two different voice tones. SYN: *diplophonia.*

**diphosphatidylglycerol** An extract of beef hearts that contains phosphorylated polysaccharide esters of fatty acids. It is used in certain tests for syphilis.

**2,3-diphosphoglycerate** ABBR: 2,3-DPG. An organic phosphate in red blood cells that alters the affinity of hemoglobin for oxygen. Blood cells stored in a blood bank lose 2,3-diphosphoglycerate, but once they are infused, the substance is resynthesized or reactivated.

**diphtheria** (dĭf-thē′rē-ă) [Gr. *diphthera,* membrane] A rare acute infectious disease marked by the formation of a false membrane on any mucous surface and occasionally on the skin. It is usually accompanied by severe prostration. **diphterial** (-thē′rē-ăl), *adj.*

SYMPTOMS: The onset is gradual. Slight headache and malaise are usually present. Temperatures reach 100° to 101°F (37.8° to 38.3°C), and sore throat is present with yellow-white or gray pseudomembrane adherent to tonsils or pharyngeal walls. The membrane can form a cast of the pharynx and tracheobronchial tree. The cast may dislodge and be aspirated. This is a common cause of death. Cervical adenitis may develop early in severe types. In nasal diphtheria, fever is a much more evident symptom. Adenitis often is severe, with a serous, sometimes blood-tinged discharge from the nostrils. A strong, fetid breath odor is common. Myocarditis and late neuritis are often present.

ETIOLOGY: The causative organism is *Corynebacterium diphtheriae,* a gram-positive nonmotile, non–spore-forming, club-shaped bacillus. In stained smears, the bacilli are usually arranged at sharp angles to each other. The disease is rare under 1 year of age. The vast majority of cases occur before 10 years of age, but older children and adults are not exempt. Both sexes are equally susceptible. Transmission is through direct contact with a human carrier, or as a result of exposure through contact with articles that have been contaminated by the patient with diphtheria.

INCUBATION: The incubation period is 2 to 5 days and occasionally longer.

DIFFERENTIAL DIAGNOSIS: Similar symptoms may be due to tonsillitis, scarlet fever, acute pharyngitis, streptococcus sore throat, peritonsillar abscess, infectious mononucleosis, Vincent's angina, acute moniliasis, and staphylococcus infections in the respiratory tract following chemotherapy. Examination of a smear from the infected area is advisable; cultures should be obtained in every instance to confirm the diagnosis. In the laryngeal type of diphtheria, edema of the glottis, foreign bodies, and retropharyngeal abscess must be considered.

ACTIVE IMMUNIZATION: Not all individuals are susceptible to diphtheria, and this factor may be determined by means of the Schick test. Therefore, it is advisable to use this test in adults before administering either toxin-antitoxin or toxoid. Routine immunization should begin at 3 months of age, diphtheria toxoid being administered in combination with pertussis vaccine and tetanus toxoid; this is then followed by booster doses. Diphtheria toxoid, following a subcutaneous test for hypersensitivity, is used for immunization of adults. Many adults are susceptible to diphtheria. Therefore, all older children and adults who have not been immunized should receive primary immunization series of diphtheria toxoid (DT) in two doses administered 4 to 8 weeks apart followed by a third dose 6 to 12 months later. For older children and adults who have been previously immunized, a booster dose of DT should be given every 10 years throughout life.

GENERAL MEASURES: Strict bedrest is needed during the acute and convalescent stages of the disease. In cases with myocardial involvement, prolonged rest in bed is extremely important.

TREATMENT: Patients should be hospitalized in an intensive care unit without delay and diphtheria antitoxin administered intravenously even before culture results are known.

---

Caution: The skin test for sensitivity to the toxin must precede administration of the antitoxin.

---

The dose of antitoxin given is governed by the location and duration of the disease. If the patient is sensitive to antitoxin, desensitization will be required. Specific antimicrobial therapy is needed to eradicate the organisms, but it cannot substitute for the antitoxin. Erythromycin, penicillin G procaine, or ampicillin is effective. To determine that the organism has been eliminated, three consecutive negative cultures must be obtained after completion of antibiotic therapy.

Surgical interference is sometimes a necessity in laryngeal diphtheria. Intubation is always to be preferred to tracheotomy, if an experienced operator is available, and hospitalization is provided so that any attention can be given within a moment's notice.

Symptomatic patients should be kept in isolation until two cultures are negative for the organism. These should be taken 24 and 48 hr after the patient discontinues antibiotics.

PROGNOSIS: The prognosis is favorable when antitoxin is administered in sufficient amounts within 3 days from the time of onset. If it is given on the first day, death hardly ever occurs. In laryngeal diphtheria, intubation or, rarely, tracheotomy may be necessary as well as an adequate dose of diphtheria antitoxin. Age is an important factor, with death more frequent in very young or very old patients than in the intermediate age group. When therapy is not given promptly, the incidence of nerve damage is high. If the patient survives, the myocarditis and neuritis will completely resolve.

NURSING IMPLICATIONS: The patient is monitored for anaphylaxis after prescribed antitoxin or antibiotics are administered, and for thrombophlebitis if erythromycin has been given. Respiratory status is assessed for ventilatory effort, use of accessory muscles, nasal flaring, stridor, cyanosis, and alterations in level of consciousness and oxygen saturation. The skin is inspected in the patient with cutaneous diphtheria. Neuromuscular function is monitored for weakness, paralysis, or sensory changes, and such findings are documented and reported immediately. Necessary culture specimens are obtained. Humidified oxygen is administered as prescribed, and the head of the bed is elevated. Prescribed drug therapies are administered.

Before diphtheria antitoxin is given, eye and skin test results are reviewed to determine the patient's sensitivity. Desensitization should be attempted if test results indicate sensitivity to diphtheria antitoxin. If test results are normal, antitoxin usually is given before laboratory confirmation of the diagnosis, because mortality increases when drug administration is delayed.

Frequent small feedings of liquids and soft foods are offered in cases of mild to moderate dysphagia. The prescribed parenteral fluids are given to a patient who cannot swallow. The patient is suctioned as needed to prevent aspiration. Strict infection and isolation precautions are maintained. Nasopharyngeal secretions are disposed of correctly until two consecutive negative nasopharyngeal cultures have been obtained at least 1 week after drug therapy stops. The need for follow-up testing is explained, and the patient is prepared for a prolonged convalescence. A rehabilitation program is initiated if any paralysis has occurred.

The family is educated about diphtheria, and nonimmunized members are advised to receive diphtheria toxoid appropriate to age, and to complete the proper series of diphtheria immunizations. All parents are advised to immunize their children. All cases of diphtheria must be reported to local public health authorities, and others who have been exposed followed up as appropriate. If the patient sustains paralysis, a rehabilitation program is initiated to restore normal functioning.

***cutaneous d.*** Diphtheritic lesions of the skin, usually limited to the site of infec-

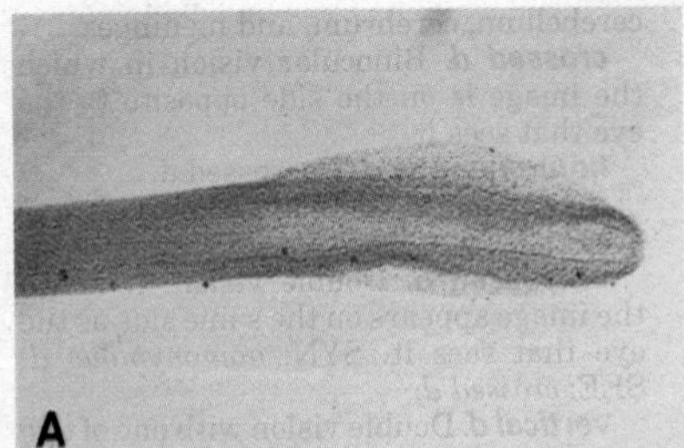


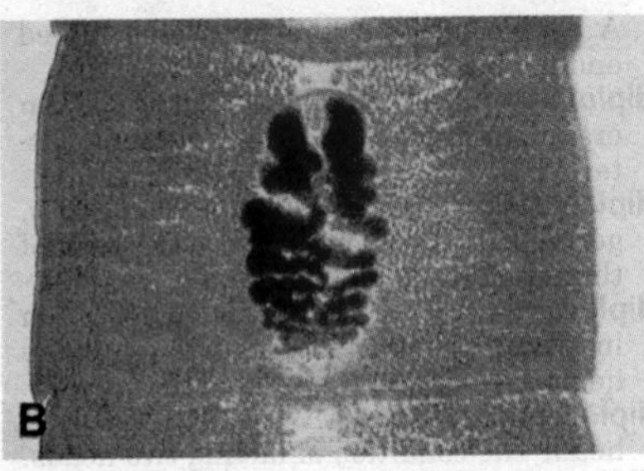


**DIPHYLLOBOTHRIUM LATUM**

**(A)** SCOLEX WITH GROOVED SUCKERS (ORIG. MAG. ×5), **(B)** PROGLOTTID (ORIG. MAG. ×10)

tion.

***laryngeal d.*** A complication of diphtheria caused by extension of the membrane from the pharynx with gradual occlusion of the airway. The signs are restlessness, use of accessory respiration muscles, and development of cyanosis. If this condition is not remedied effectively, death results.

***surgical d.*** Diphtheritic membrane formation on wounds.

**diphtheria antitoxin** The antitoxin used in treating diphtheria.

**diphtheria toxin** The potent exotoxin of *Corynebacterium diphtheriae.* It affects all the cells in the body; however, cells of the heart, nerves, and kidneys are most often damaged.

**diphtheria toxin for Schick test** The toxin used for determining immunity to diphtheria. SEE: *Schick test.*

**diphtheria toxoid** The immunizing agent for diphtheria.

**diphtheroid** (dĭf′thĕ-royd) [″ + *eidos,* form, shape] **1.** Resembling diphtheria or the bacteria that cause diphtheria. **2.** A false membrane or pseudomembrane not due to the diphtheria bacillus.

**diphthongia** (dĭf-thŏn′jē-ă) [Gr. *dis,* two, + *phtongos,* voice] The simultaneous utterance of two vocal sounds of different pitch in pathological conditions of the larynx.

**Diphyllobothrium** (dī-fĭl″ō-bŏth′rē-ŭm) [″ + *phyllon,* leaf, + *bothrion,* pit] A genus of tapeworm belonging to the order Pseudophyllidea and marked by possession of a scolex with two slitlike grooves or bothria. Formerly called *Dibothriocephalus.*

***D. cordatum*** The heart-shaped tapeworm, a small species infesting dogs and seals in Greenland, formerly known as *D. mansoni.* The plerocercoids are occasionally found in humans.

***D. erinacei*** A species infesting dogs, cats, and other carnivores. Larval stages are occasionally found in humans.

***D. latum*** The broad or fish tapeworm. The adult lives in the intestine of fish-eating mammals, including humans. The largest tapeworm infesting humans, it may reach a length of 50 to 60 ft or 15.2 to 18.3 m (average 20 ft or 6.1 m). The eggs develop into ciliated larvae called coracidia. These are eaten by certain species of copepod, of which each becomes an oncosphere, which develops into a procercoid. Further development occurs in a fish, where it develops into a wormlike plerocercoid or sparganum larva. Infection of the final host occurs after the host eats raw or improperly cooked fish. Infection can be prevented by thoroughly cooking all freshwater fish, or by keeping the fish frozen at −10°C (14°F) for 48 hr prior to eating. SEE: illus.

SYMPTOMS: Pathological effects are abdominal pain, loss of weight, digestive disorders, progressive weakness, and a severe type of anemia that is clinically identical with pernicious anemia because the worm absorbs ingested vitamin $B_{12}$.

TREATMENT: Niclosamide or praziquantel is indicated. The therapy may need to be repeated if examination of the stools indicates presence of infection after 3 months of treatment.

**diphyodont** (dĭf′ē-ō-dŏnt) [″ + *phyein,* to produce, + *odous,* tooth] Having two sets of teeth, a primary and a permanent set, as in humans.

**diplacusis** (dĭp″lă-kū′sĭs) [″ + *akousis,* hearing] A disturbed perception of pitch in which two tones are heard for every sound produced.

**diplegia** (dī-plē′jē-ă) [Gr. *dis,* twice, + *plege,* a stroke] **1.** Paralysis of similar parts on both sides of the body. **2.** In cerebral palsy, excessive stiffness usually in all limbs, but greater stiffness in the legs than in the arms. **diplegic** (-jĭk), *adj.*

***infantile d.*** Birth palsy.

***spastic d.*** Congenital spastic stiffness of the limbs.

**diplo-** Combining form meaning *double* or *twin.*

**diploalbuminuria** (dĭp″lō-ăl-bū″mĭn-ū′rē-ă) [Gr. *diplous,* double, + L. *albumen,* white of egg, + Gr. *ouron,* urine] The coexistence of physiological and pathological albuminuria.

**diplobacillus** [″ + L. *bacillus,* a little stick]

A double bacillus, the two being linked end to end.

**diplobacterium** [″ + *bakterion,* little rod] An organism made up of two adherent bacteria.

**diploblastic** (dĭp″lō-blăs′tĭk) [″ + *blastos,* germ] Having two germ layers, used of the ectoderm and endoderm.

**diplocardia** [″ + *kardia,* heart] A condition in which the two lateral halves of the heart are partially separated by a groove.

**diplocephaly** (dĭp″lō-sĕf′ă-lē) [″ + *kephale,* head] The condition of having two heads.

**diplococcemia** (dĭp″lō-kŏk-sē′mē-ă) [″ + *kokkos,* berry, + *haima,* blood] The presence of diplococci in the blood.

**diplococci** (dĭp″lō-kŏk′sē, -kŏk′ī) Pl. of diplococcus. SEE: *bacterium* for illus.

**Diplococcus** (dĭp-lō-kŏk′ŭs) [″ + *kokkus,* berry] A genus of bacterium belonging to the family Lactobacillaceae. They are gram-positive organisms occurring in pairs.

***D. pneumoniae*** SEE: *Streptococcus pneumoniae.*

**diplococcus** (dĭp″lō-kŏk′ŭs) *pl.* **diplococci** Any of various spherical bacteria appearing in pairs, esp. of the genus *Neisseria.* SEE: *Neisseria* for illus.

**diplocoria** (dĭp″lō-kō′rē-ă) [″ + *kore,* pupil] A double pupil in the eye.

**diploë** (dĭp′lō-ē) [Gr. *diploē,* fold] Spongy bone containing red bone marrow between the two layers of compact bone of the skull bones. **diploetic** (-lō-e′tĭc), *adj.*

**diplogenesis** [Gr. *diplous,* double, + *genesis,* generation, birth] The condition of having two parts or producing two substances; the production of a double fetus or the doubling of some fetal parts.

**diploid** (dĭp′loyd) [″ + *eidos,* form, shape] Having two sets of chromosomes; said of somatic cells, which contain twice the number of chromosomes present in the egg or sperm. SEE: *chromosome; meiosis; mitosis.*

**diplokaryon** (dĭp″lō-kăr′ē-ŏn) [″ + *karyon,* nucleus] A nucleus containing twice the diploid number of chromosomes.

**diplomyelia** (dĭp″lō-mī-ē′lē-ă) [″ + *myelos,* marrow] A condition in certain types of spina bifida in which the spinal cord appears to be doubled due to a lengthwise fissure.

**diploneural** [″ + *neuron,* nerve] Having two nerves from different origins, as certain muscles.

**diplopagus** (dĭp-lŏp′ă-gŭs) [″ + *pagos,* a thing fixed] Conjoined and sharing some organs, used of twins with this condition.

**diplophonia** (dĭp-lō-fō′nē-ă) [″ + *phone,* voice] Simultaneous production of two different voice tones. SYN: *diphonia.*

**diplopia** (dĭp-lō′pē-ă) [″ + *ope,* sight] Double vision, which may be monocular.

***binocular d.*** Double vision occurring when both eyes are used but not in focus. It is seen in disease of the eyeballs, cranial nerve disease, and disease of the cerebellum, cerebrum, and meninges.

***crossed d.*** Binocular vision in which the image is on the side opposite to the eye that sees it.

***homonymous d.*** Uncrossed d.

***monocular d.*** Double vision with one eye.

***uncrossed d.*** Double vision in which the image appears on the same side as the eye that sees it. SYN: *homonymous d.* SEE: *crossed d.*

***vertical d.*** Double vision with one of two images higher than the other.

**diploscope** [″ + *skopein,* to examine] A device for studying binocular vision.

**diplosomatia, diplosomia** (dĭp″lō-sō-mā′shē-ă, dip″lō-sō′mē-ă) [″ + *soma,* body] A condition in which twins are joined at one or more points.

**diplotene** (dĭp′lō-tēn) In cell division, the stage of the first meiotic prophase. The homologous pairs of chromatids begin to separate.

**dipole** (dī′pōl) A molecule in which each end has an equal but opposite charge. The intensity of the charge is given by its dielectric moment or constant.

**dipping 1.** Palpation of the liver by a quick depressive movement of the fingers while the hand is held flat on the abdomen. **2.** Immersion of an object in a solution, esp. applied to the dipping of cattle or dogs for tick control.

**diprosopus** (dĭp-rō-sōp′ŭs) [Gr. *dis,* twice, + *prosopon,* face] A malformed fetus with a double face.

**dipsophobia** (dĭp-sō-fō′bē-ă) [″ + *phobos,* fear] Morbid fear of drinking.

**dipsosis** (dĭp-sō′sĭs) [″+ *osis,* condition] Abnormal thirst.

**dipstick** (dĭp′stĭk) A chemical-impregnated paper strip used for analysis of body fluids, principally urine.

**Diptera** (dĭp′tĕr-ă) [Gr. *dipteros,* having two wings] An order of insects characterized by sucking or piercing mouth parts, one pair of wings, and complete metamorphosis. It includes the flies, gnats, midges, and mosquitoes. It contains many species involved in the transmission of pathogenic organisms, such as malaria.

**dipterous** (dĭp′tĕr-ŭs) Having two wings; characteristic of the order Diptera.

**dipygus** (dī-pī′gŭs) [Gr. *dis,* two, + *pyge,* rump] Having a double pelvis; said of a congenitally deformed fetus.

**dipylidiasis** (dĭp″ĭ-lĭ-dī′ă-sĭs) Infestation with the tapeworm *Dipylidium caninum.*

**Dipylidium** (dĭp″ĭ-lĭd′ē-ŭm) [Gr. *dipylos,* having two entrances] A genus of tapeworms belonging to the family Dipylidiae that infests dogs and cats.

***D. caninum*** A common parasite of dogs and cats. Occasionally, human infestation may occur through the accidental ingestion of lice or fleas, which serve as the intermediate host.

**directionality** The ability to perceive one's position in relation to the environment;

the sense of direction. Problems with directionality are frequently found in children with learning disabilities or suspected minimal brain dysfunction.

**direct light reflex** Prompt contraction of the sphincter of the iris when light entering through the pupil strikes the retina.

**directly observed therapy** ABBR: DOT. Oral administration of a drug(s) to a patient and observing to ensure the drug is swallowed. DOT is of particular importance in treating infectious diseases in which development of drug-resistant microorganisms is more likely to occur if the drug is not taken as prescribed.

**director** A grooved device for guiding a knife in surgery.

**direct reflex** A reflex in which response occurs on same side as the stimulus.

**dirigomotor** (dĭr″ĭ-gō-mō′tor) [L. *dirigere,* to direct, + *motor,* mover] Controlling or directing muscular activity.

**Dirofilaria** (dī″rō-fĭ-lā′rē-ă) A genus of filariae.

***D. immitis*** Heartworm, a species of filariae that occurs in dogs, but may infest humans.

**dis-** **1.** [L. *dis,* apart] Prefix indicating *free of, undone from.* **2.** [Gr. *dis,* twice] Prefix meaning *double* or *twice.*

**disability** (dĭs″ă-bĭl′ĭ-tē) Any physical or mental impairment that limits a major activity. It may be partial or complete. SEE: *handicap.*

***developmental d.*** A condition due to congenital abnormality, trauma, deprivation, or disease that interrupts or delays the sequence and rate of normal growth, development, and maturation.

***excess d.*** The discrepancy that exists when a person's functional limitations are greater than those warranted by the objective degree of impairment. Often excess disability is created by attitudes and policies that create barriers to a disabled person's full participation.

***learning d.*** An inability or defect in the ability to learn. It occurs in children and is manifested by difficulty in learning basic skills such as writing, reading, and mathematics.

**disability analysis** The attempt to determine the relative importance of life events that might contribute to disability. For example, persons with chronic respiratory difficulty may have had long-term exposure to coal dust, asbestos, certain chemicals, and cigarettes. Determining the relationship of occupational or other exposures to the development of chronic illness is difficult. Similarly, persons who have been exposed to a noisy work and recreational environment will be difficult to evaluate with respect to the impact of each these factors on hearing.

**disaccharidase** (dī-săk′ă-rĭ-dās) A group of enzymes that split disaccharides into monosaccharides.

**disaccharide** (dī-săk′ĭ-rĭd) [Gr. *dis,* twice, + *sakkharon,* sugar] A carbohydrate composed of two monosaccharides. SEE: *carbohydrate.*

**disarticulation** [L. *dis,* apart, + *articulus,* joint] Amputation through a joint.

**disassimilation** [″ + *ad,* to, + *similare,* to make like] The conversion of assimilated material into less complex compounds for energy production.

**disaster** [″ + L. *astrum,* star, ill-starred] A natural or man-made occurrence such as a flood, tornado, earthquake, forest fire, bridge or building collapse, nuclear reactor accident, war, explosion, terrorist attack or bombing, or train wreck. The need for emergency evacuation and medical services is increased during and following a disaster. It is essential that hospitals and community services have a plan for the expeditious mobilization and use of their services at such times.

**disaster planning** A comprehensive plan of action to cope with a sudden, unexpected event such as a flood, fire, famine, terrorist attack or bombing, nuclear bomb attack, oil spill, earthquake, explosion, electric power failure, poison gas attack, aircraft accident, or contamination of the water supply. The plan may be for a community, state, or nation. Involved will be a plan for mobilizing all available emergency sources and to do this in a minimum of time. Frequent disaster planning drills are essential to being adequately prepared for an actual disaster.

**disc** SEE: *disk.*

**discharge** (dĭs-chărj′, dĭs′chărj) [ME. *dischargen,* to discharge] **1.** To release from care; done by a physician, other medical care worker, or a medical care facility. **2.** The escape (esp. by violence) of pent-up or accumulated energy or of explosive material. **3.** The flowing away of a secretion or excretion of pus, feces, urine, and so forth. **4.** The material thus ejected.

***cerebrocortical d.*** The violent action of an injured or malfunctioning portion of the cerebral cortex that gives rise to an epileptic paroxysm.

***convective d.*** The discharge from a high-potential source in the form of electrical energy passing through the air to the patient.

***disruptive d.*** The passage of current through an insulating medium due to the breakdown of the medium under electrostatic stress.

***lochial d.*** Uterine excretion following childbirth. SEE: *lochia.*

**discharge summary** A summary of the hospital or clinic record of a patient. It is prepared after the time of discharge.

**discharging** The emission of or the flowing out of material, as the discharge of pus from a lesion; excretion.

**discharging lesion** A lesion of a nerve center in the brain that suddenly discharges motor impulses.

**discission** (dĭs-sĭzh′ŭn) [L. *dis,* apart, +

*scindere*, to cut] Rupture of the capsule of the crystalline lens in cataract surgery.

**disclosing agent** A diagnostic aid used in dentistry to reveal areas of the teeth that are not being cleaned adequately. The dye, erythrosine sodium, is applied to the teeth in a 2% solution or by a tablet that is chewed by the patient.

**discoblastic** [" + *blastos*, germ] Meroblastic.

**discoblastula** (dĭs″kō-blăs′tū-lă) A modified blastula found in highly telolecithal eggs, as in birds in which the blastomeres form a cellular cap (germinal disk or blastoderm) that is separated from the yolk by a space, the blastocele.

**discogenic** (dĭs″kō-jĕn′ĭk) [" + *gennan*, to produce] Caused by an intervertebral disk.

**discography** (dĭs-kŏg′ră-fē) Use of a contrast medium injected into the intervertebral disk so that it can be examined radiographically.

**discoid** Like a disk.

**disconnection syndrome** Disturbance of the visual and language functions of the central nervous system due to interruption of the connections between two cerebral hemispheres in the corpus callosum, occlusion of the anterior cerebral artery, or interruption of the connections between different parts of one hemisphere. These disorders also may be produced by tumors or hypoxia. They can manifest in several ways including the inability, when blindfolded, to match an object held in one hand with that in the other; the inability to execute a command with the right hand but not the left; if blindfolded, the ability to correctly name objects held in the right hand but not those in the left; and the inability to understand spoken language while being able to speak normally. SEE: *neglect*.

**discoplacenta** [Gr. *diskos*, quoit, + *plakous*, a flat cake] A disklike placenta.

**discordance** (dĭs-kor′dăns) In genetics, the expression of a trait in only one of a twin pair. SEE: *concordance*.

**discovery** The stage in a lawsuit in which all information, facts, and circumstances surrounding the allegations are "discovered" by the plaintiff and defendant. Techniques include interrogatories, requests for production of documents and items, admissions of facts, records of physical and mental examinations, and depositions.

**discrete** (dĭs-krēt′) [L. *discretus*, separated] Separate; said of certain eruptions on the skin. SEE: *confluent*.

**discrimination** [L. *discriminare*, to divide] **1.** The process of distinguishing or differentiating. **2.** Unequal and unfair treatment or denial of privileges without reasonable cause. Federal statutes prohibit discrimination based on age, sex, sexual preference, religion, race, and disability.

***figure-ground d.*** The ability to see the outline of an object as distinct from visually competing background stimuli. This ability is often impaired following central nervous system damage.

***one-point d.*** The ability to locate specifically a point of pressure on the surface of the skin.

***tonal d.*** The ability to distinguish one tone from another. This is dependent on the integrity of the transverse fibers of the basilar membrane of the organ of Corti.

***two-point d.*** The ability to localize two points of pressure on the surface of the skin and to identify them as discrete sensations. SYN: *tactile discrimination*. SEE: *two-point discrimination test*.

**discus** [Gr. *diskos*, quoit] A disk.

***d. articularis*** An interarticular fibrocartilage; an articular disk.

***d. proligerus*** Cumulus oophorus.

**disdiaclast** (dĭs-dī′ă-klăst) [Gr. *dis*, twice, + *diaklan*, to break through] A doubly refracting element in the tissues of striated muscles.

**disdiadochokinesia** (dĭs-dī″ă-dō″kō-kĭ-nē′zē-ă) [L. *dis*, apart, + Gr. *diadochos*, succeeding, + *kinesis*, movement] The inability to make finely coordinated antagonistic movements, as when quickly supinating and pronating the hand. SEE: *diadochokinesia*.

**disease** (dĭ-zēz′) [Fr. *des*, from, + *aise*, ease] Literally the lack of ease; a pathological condition of the body that presents a group of clinical signs, symptoms, and laboratory findings peculiar to it and setting the condition apart as an abnormal entity differing from other normal or pathological condition. SYN: *dyscrasia*. SEE: *health; syndrome*.

The concept of disease may include illness or suffering not necessarily arising from pathological changes in the body. There is a major distinction between disease and illness in that disease is usually tangible and may even be measured, whereas illness is highly individual and personal, as with pain, suffering, and distress. A person may have a serious disease such as hypertension but no feeling of pain or suffering, and thus no illness. Conversely, a person may be extremely ill, as with hysteria or mental illness, but have no evidence of disease as measured by pathological changes in the body.

***acute d.*** A disease having a rapid onset and relatively short duration.

***anticipated d.*** A disease that may be predicted to occur in individuals with a certain genetic, physical, or environmental predisposition.

***autoimmune d.*** A disease produced when the body's normal tolerance of the antigens on its own cells (i.e., self-antigens or autoantigens [AAgs]) disappears. Current theories are that the loss of self-tolerance is the result of damage to AAgs by microorganisms, a strong similarity in appearance between the AAg and a foreign antigen, or a foreign antigen linking with an AAg. T cells identify the altered AAg as foreign and stimulate B cells to produce autoantibodies (AAbs) that produce inflammation and damage. Researchers have found links between AAb production and the inheritance of certain histocompatibility antigens, indicating that genetic susceptibility is probably a component in autoimmune diseases. Other unknown factors within the immune system may prevent it from stopping the abnormal inflammatory process once it has begun.

Many diseases are based on AAb-AAg reactions. Systemic lupus erythematosus is an unusual autoimmune disease in that multiple tissues are affected; most disorders are limited to a single tissue. The damage to cardiac valves in rheumatic fever occurs because AAgs on the valves are similar in structure to antigens on Group A beta-hemolytic streptococci. Insulin-dependent diabetes mellitus is caused by AAb destruction of the islets of Langerhans, rheumatoid arthritis is caused by inflammatory changes in the connective tissue of joints, and multiple sclerosis is caused by AAb destruction of the myelin sheath covering nerves. Hemolytic anemia, some forms of glomerulonephritis, myasthenia gravis, chronic thyroiditis, Reiter's syndrome, and Graves' disease also are considered to be autoimmune diseases. SEE: *antigen; autoantibody; autoantigen; histocompatability locus antigens; inflammation.*

***caisson d.*** A condition that develops in divers subjected to rapid reduction of air pressure after coming to the surface following exposure to compressed air. The cause is nitrogen bubbles in the tissue spaces and small blood vessels. Symptoms appear when a diver is exposed to a depth of at least 30 ft (9.1 m) long enough for the tissues to be saturated with nitrogen, and then ascends to the surface rapidly; or when an aviator ascends rapidly in an unpressurized aircraft from sea level to at least 18,000 ft (5486 m). SYN: *decompression illness.*

SYMPTOMS: Symptoms include deep boring, usually constant joint pain; itching or burning skin; burning sensation in the lungs and coughing; and various neurological signs.

TREATMENT: Recompression and then slow decompression is performed in a special hyperbaric chamber. SEE: *bends.*

***cat scratch d.*** A febrile disease characterized by lymphadenitis, thought to be transmitted by cats. A distinctive manifestation of this disease is the oculoglandular syndrome, which follows primary inoculation of the conjunctiva or eyelid. Regional lymphadenopathy develops within about 2 weeks, but may take as long as 2 months. Fever, malaise, headache, and anorexia accompany the lymphadenopathy. The causative organism is *Bartonella henselae* (formerly *Rochalimaea*), a gram-negative rod that in cats usually produces asymptomatic infection. Diagnosis is based on clinical findings combined with the history of cat contact and positive results from a cat scratch antigen skin test. Currently, antibiotics are not recommended because of minimal response. Aminoglycoside therapy, quinolone therapy, or both may be indicated for severe, disseminated disease. Hot compresses are used to promote drainage of the pustule. The prognosis is usually excellent; rare complications are encephalitis and endocarditis. SEE: *angiomatosis, bacillary; Nursing Diagnoses Appendix.*

***celiac d.*** SEE: *sprue, celiac.*

***chronic d.*** A disease having a slow onset and lasting for a long period of time.

***chronic granulomatous d.*** ABBR: CGD. An X-linked congenital disease of phagocytes (neutrophils and macrophages) marked by defects in the respiratory burst (the metabolic process by which these cells kill bacteria after ingesting them). Patients are usually diagnosed by 2 years of age. Life expectancy is limited and depends on the success of early treatment and the degree of damage to organs, particularly the liver and lungs. Most patients die within 20 years.

SYMPTOMS: Symptoms include chronic and acute infections of the skin, liver, lymph nodes, intestinal tract, and bone, often involving bacteria or other microorganisms that usually do not cause infections such as *Staphylococcus epidermidis, Pseudomonas, Escherichia coli, Candida,* and *Aspergillus*. SEE: *phagocytosis.*

TREATMENT: High doses of antibiotics, usually an aminoglycoside and penicillin, are administered until blood cultures reveal the pathogenic organism. Antifungal agents such as fluconazole or amphotericin B are used if fungi are involved. Usually, 6 weeks of antibiotic therapy is required. Experimental treatments include the use of gamma interferon and bone marrow transplantation.

***communicable d.*** A disease in which the causative organism is transmissible from one person to another either directly or indirectly through a carrier or vector.

***complicating d.*** A disease that occurs during the course of another disease.

***congenital d.*** A disease that is present at birth. It may be due to hereditary factors, prenatal infection, injury, or the effect of a drug the mother took during pregnancy.

***connective tissue d.*** ABBR: CTD. A group of diseases that affect connective tissue, including muscle, cartilage, tendons, vessels, skin, and ligaments. CTDs may be acute but are usually chronic. They may be localized or systemic.

***contagious d.*** An infectious disease readily transmitted from one person to another.

***cystine storage d.*** An inherited disease of cystine metabolism resulting in abnormal deposition of cystine in body tissues. The cause is disordered proximal renal tubular function. Clinically, the child fails to grow and develops rickets, corneal opacities, and acidosis. SYN: *cystinosis.*

***deficiency d.*** A disease resulting from inadequate intake or absorption of essential dietary factors such as vitamins or minerals.

***degenerative d.*** A disease resulting from deterioration of tissues and organs, characteristic of old age.

***degenerative joint d.*** Osteoarthritis.

***demyelinating d.*** A disturbance of nerve cells due to destruction of their myelin sheaths.

***endemic d.*** A disease that is present more or less continuously, or recurs frequently, in a community.

***epidemic d.*** A disease that attacks a large number of individuals in a community at the same time.

***epizootic d.*** An epidemic that affects animals of a particular area, usually in a short period of time.

***extrapyramidal d.*** Any of several degenerative diseases of the nervous system that involve the extrapyramidal system and the basal ganglion of the brain. Symptoms include tremors, chorea, athetosis, and dystonia. Parkinsonism is a form of extrapyramidal disease.

***familial d.*** A disease that occurs in several members of the same family.

***fibrocystic d. of the breast*** A nonspecific diagnosis for a condition marked by palpable lumps in the breasts, usually associated with pain and tenderness, that fluctuate with the menstrual cycle and become progressively worse until menopause. At least 50% of women of reproductive age have palpably irregular breasts caused by this condition. SYN: *chronic cystic mastitis*. SEE: *breast self-examination of.*

Women with fibrocystic breast disease have a two to five times greater risk of developing breast cancer. Some women with this disease have atypical hyperplasia in the lesion. If these patients also have a family history of breast cancer, their risk of developing breast cancer is greatly increased. They should have a breast examination every 6 months and mammography once a year.

NURSING IMPLICATIONS: Teach patient importance of monthly breast self-examination, mapping known lumps (round, movable and well-delineated), also examination by a health professional and mammography annually or earlier as prescribed. Teach the patient that knowing the contours (feel, texture) of her breasts will make it possible for her to detect any changes, often sooner or more accurately than the health care provider who examines her infrequently. Discuss use of fine-needle aspiration for diagnosis and treatment, encouraging patient to verbalize feelings and concerns. Wearing a well-fitted, supportive brassiere both day and night can help reduce discomfort, as can application of ice packs intermittently to tender areas and treatment with aspirin or nonsteroidal anti-inflammatory drugs available over the counter. In severe cases, hormone therapy may be prescribed. Nurse should caution patient that relief may not be noted for 4 to 6 months, and should assess for annoying and upsetting side effects such as weight gain, amenorrhea, and masculinization. Provide emotional support for patient, who may have a heightened awareness of and fear about developing breast cancer.

***fibrocystic d. of the pancreas*** Cystic fibrosis.

***fifth d.*** Erythema infectiosum, so named because it is the fifth most common rash-producing illness in children. SEE: *erythema infectiosum.*

***focal d.*** A disease located at a specific and distinct area such as the tonsils, adenoids, or a boil.

***foot and mouth d.*** A viral disease of cattle and horses that is rarely transmitted to humans.

SYMPTOMS: In humans, symptoms include fever, headache, and malaise with dryness and burning sensation of the mouth. Vesicles develop on the lips, tongue, mouth, palms, and soles.

TREATMENT: Therapy is symptomatic. Full recovery occurs in 2 to 3 weeks.

***functional d.*** A disease in which no anatomical changes can be observed to account for the symptoms present.

***glycogen storage d.*** SEE: *glycogen storage disease.*

***heavy chain d.*** A group of diseases involving serum immunoglobulins. The globulins contain heavy chain subunits. If immunoglobulin A is affected, abdominal lymphoma and malabsorption occur. If immunoglobulin D is involved, a clinical picture similar to multiple myeloma is present. If immunoglobulin G is affected, there are lymphadenopathy, weakness, weight loss, and repeated bacterial infections. If immunoglobulin M is involved, the lymphadenopathy affects the abdominal lymph nodes, the liver, and the spleen. Bence Jones proteinuria is present.

***hemolytic d. of the newborn*** Erythroblastosis fetalis.

***hemorrhagic d. of the newborn*** A bleeding tendency in newborns characterized by melena, purpura, and prothrombin deficiency. The disease is self-limiting.

***hereditary d.*** A disease due to genetic factors transmitted from parent to offspring.

***hookworm d.*** SEE: *ancylostomiasis;*

*Necator americanus.*

***hydatid d.*** The disease produced by the cysts of the larval stage of the tapeworm *Echinococcus.* SYN: *echinococcosis.* SEE: *hydatid.*

***hypokinetic d.*** Physical and mental illness produced by lack of or insufficient exercise.

***iatrogenic d.*** A disease caused by medical or surgical intervention. The implication is that the disease would not have occurred if the individual had not sought medical care.

***idiopathic d.*** A disease for which no causative factor can be recognized.

***infectious d.*** Any disease caused by growth of pathogenic microorganisms in the body. It is not necessarily contagious. SEE: *quarantine; incubation* for table.

***inflammatory bowel d.*** ABBR: IBD. The term for a number of chronic inflammatory diseases of the gastrointestinal tract. The names previously used include irritable bowel syndrome, Crohn's disease, ulcerative colitis, and regional ileitis or enteritis. There are no specific features or diagnostic tests for this illness; thus, it is established by exclusion.

Chronic IBD is divided into ulcerative colitis and Crohn's disease. The major clinical symptoms of ulcerative colitis are bloody diarrhea and abdominal pain. In severe cases, there may be acute bowel cramps, dehydration, anemia, fever, and weight loss. The physical findings may include tenderness along the colon. In severe cases, signs of arthritis and liver disease also may be present. A major complication of severe ulcerative colitis is toxic megacolon.

In Crohn's disease, the clinical signs and symptoms are similar to those of ulcerative colitis except fatigability is more common in Crohn's disease, and a palpable mass in the colon area may be present. Complications of Crohn's disease include intestinal obstruction, fistula formation between bowel segments, and intestinal perforation.

TREATMENT: The therapy for ulcerative colitis and Crohn's disease is similar, and in both conditions, treatment will depend on the severity. The objectives are to control the inflammation and to replace fluid and nutritional losses. If bleeding is severe and chronic, blood transfusion may be needed. In ulcerative colitis, control of diarrhea by the use of codeine and antispasmodics must be done carefully to prevent colonic dilatation and toxic megacolon. Anti-inflammatory agents such as glucocorticoids and sulfasalazine are used. Intravenous cyclosporine is effective in patients with corticosteroid-resistant ulcerative colitis. Toxic megacolon manifests by segmental dilatation of the large intestine with areas of ulceration and thinning of the intestinal wall to the point that perforation may occur. This condition requires immediate intensive therapy with IV fluids, electrolyte replacement, nasogastric suction, and blood transfusion. Glucocorticoids are given IV, and broad-spectrum antibiotics are administered after stool cultures have been obtained. If the patient does not stabilize within 24 to 48 hr and intestinal perforation is a possibility, emergency colectomy is done. The mortality rate after perforation is almost 50%

Therapy of Crohn's disease is similar to ulcerative colitis, except in the latter use of glucocorticoids may mask signs of intestinal perforation or fistula formation. When the colon and small intestine are involved, the nutritional problems are more severe than with colonic involvement alone. Once the disease is in remission glucocorticoids should be discontinued gradually.

***intercurrent d.*** A disease occurring during the course of another, unrelated disease.

***iron storage d.*** Hemochromatosis.

***kinky hair d.*** A congenital syndrome caused by an autosomal recessive gene, consisting of short, sparse, often poorly pigmented, kinky hair and physical and mental retardation. The disease is due to a metabolic defect that causes an abnormality in the fatty acid composition of the gray matter of the brain. Death follows progressive severe degenerative changes in the central nervous system.

***lysosomal storage d.*** A disease caused by deficiency of specific lysosomal enzymes that normally degrade glycoproteins, glycolipids, or mucopolysaccharides. Thus, the substances that cannot be catabolized accumulate in lysosomes. Specific enzymes account for specific storage diseases. Included in this group are Gaucher's, Hurler's, Tay-Sachs, Niemann-Pick, Fabry's, Morquio's, Scheie's, and Maroteaux-Lamy diseases.

***malignant d.*** **1.** Cancer. **2.** A disease, including but not limited to cancer, in which the progress is extremely rapid and generally threatening or resulting in death within a short time.

***Mediterranean d.*** Thalassemia.

***metabolic d.*** A disease due to abnormality of the body chemistry. The abnormality may be due to underproduction of a needed substance, such as insulin in diabetes, or overproduction, such as thyroid hormone in thyrotoxicosis.

***mixed connective tissue d.*** ABBR: MCTD. A rare disease that combines the signs and symptoms of certain connective tissue diseases including lupus erythematosus, scleroderma, and polymyositis. The cause is unknown.

***motor neuron d.*** One of several diseases of the motor neurons: progressive muscular atrophy, progressive bulbar palsy, and amyotrophic lateral sclerosis. These diseases are marked by degeneration of anterior horn cells of the spinal cord, the motor cranial nerve nuclei, and the corticospinal tracts. They occur principally in men. In the U.S., amyotrophic lateral sclerosis is commonly known as Lou Gehrig's disease. Gehrig was a well-known athlete whose baseball career and life ended prematurely as a result of this disease.

***occupational* d.** A disease resulting from factors associated with the occupation in which the patient is engaged.

***organic* d.** A disease resulting from recognizable anatomical changes in an organ or tissue of the body.

***pandemic* d.** An extremely widespread epidemic disease involving the populations of several countries.

***parasitic* d.** A disease resulting from the growth and development of parasitic organisms (plants or animals) in or on the body.

***periodontal* d.** SEE: *periodontitis*.

***polycystic kidney* d.** A hereditary disorder in which cysts form in the kidneys, eventually destroying kidney tissue and function. The autosomal recessive form usually appears in early childhood; the autosomal dominant form usually develops later in life. The only treatments are dialysis and kidney transplant.

***psychosomatic* d.** A physical illness caused or exacerbated by psychological factors. Conditions in the general category of psychosomatic disorders are obesity, tension headache, some types of asthma, neurodermatitis, peptic ulcer, some attacks of angina pectoris, and frequency of urination.

NOTE: It is not possible for a human being to be consciously sick without some interplay between the emotions and the bodily functions.

***pulmonary veno-occlusive* d.** A rare condition marked by extensive occlusion of the small and medium-sized veins of the lung by loose, sparsely cellular, fibrous tissue. Some larger veins may be involved. This disease produces severe pulmonary venous hypertension.

***reactive airway* d.** Asthma.

***restrictive lung* d.** Any chest disease that results in a reduced lung volume.

***secondary* d.** A disease caused by another disease, as when obesity causes diseases of the joints and muscles of the lower limbs due to the increased trauma of transporting and supporting the added weight.

***self-limited* d.** A disease that eventually goes away even if untreated.

***storage* d.** A disorder involving abnormal deposition of a substance in body tissues. SEE: *glycogen storage disease; Wilson's disease.*

***subacute* d.** A disease in which symptoms are less pronounced but more prolonged than in an acute disease; this type is intermediate between acute and chronic disease.

***systemic* d.** A generalized disease rather than a localized or focal one.

***thyrotoxic heart* d.** A disease due to increased activity of the thyroid gland, marked by cardiac enlargement, atrial fibrillation, and heart failure. SEE: *thyrotoxicosis*.

***trophoblastic* d.** ABBR: TD. Any neoplasm of trophoblastic origin. SEE: *chorioadenoma destruens; choriocarcinoma; hydatiform mole.*

***venereal* d.** ABBR: VD. A disease usually acquired through sexual relations. It includes acquired immunodeficiency syndrome (AIDS), syphilis, gonorrhea, granuloma inguinale, herpes genitalis, *Chlamydia trachomatis* infections, trichomoniasis, anogenital warts, scabies, pediculosis pubis, enteric infections due to anal-oral contacts, lymphogranuloma venereum, and chancroid. SEE: *sexually transmitted disease.*

**disease burden** The total effect of a disease or diseases on an individual as well as society. Knowledge concerning this is important, particularly in attempting to plan prevention programs and in evaluating the success or failure of intervention. However, without a rational system for measuring disease burden, the concept is of little value. In 1993 the disease-adjusted life-year (DALY) concept was described in a publication from the World Bank. It is based on the quantitation not only of mortality but also of suffering and loss of health. Data obtained using the DALY concept will permit establishing the priority for treating specific diseases and conditions. The goal would be to allot research and treatment resources according to where they would have the best chance to make a difference in alleviating suffering and prevention of death from specific illnesses.

**disengagement** [Fr.] **1.** The emergence of the fetal head from within the maternal pelvis. **2.** Any withdrawal from participation in customary social activity. **3.** In psychiatry, autonomous functioning with little or no emotional attachment and a distorted sense of independence.

**disentanglement** A rescue technique used to free a trapped victim that involves removing the wreckage from around the patient (rather than removing the patient from the wreckage). For example, freeing a person trapped in a crushed car often requires the car to be pried apart with heavy rescue tools capable of cutting through metal.

**disequilibrium** (dĭs-ē″kwĭ-lĭb′rē-ŭm) [L. *dis*, apart, + *aequus*, equal, + *libra*, balance] An unequal and unstable equilibrium.

**disequilibrium syndrome** A complication of renal dialysis in which symptoms of nervous irritability, agitation, muscle cramps, headache, nausea, drowsiness, convulsions, and intracranial hypertension occur in the third or fourth hour of dialysis and persist for several hours.

Symptoms may occur as late as 8 to 48 hours following dialysis. Approx. 70% of patients will experience headaches; 5% to 10% of patients will develop other symptoms.

ETIOLOGY: The rapidly diminishing levels of urea in the blood cause an acute shift of the intracellular water in the brain, cerebral edema, and increased intracranial pressure.

**disharmony** Lack of harmony; discord.

**disinfect** (dĭs-ĭn-fĕkt′) [″ + *inficere,* to corrupt] To free from infection by physical or chemical means.

**disinfectant** A substance that prevents infection by killing bacteria. Most disinfectants are used on equipment or surfaces rather than in or on the body. Common disinfectants are halogens: chlorine, iodine; salts of heavy metals: mercuric chloride (bichloride of mercury), silver nitrate; boric acid; chloride of lime; organic compounds: formaldehyde, alcohol 70%, iodoform, organic acids, phenol (carbolic acid), cresols, benzoic and salicylic acids and their sodium salts; and miscellaneous substances: thymol, hydrogen peroxide, potassium permanganate, ethylene oxide. The term is usually applied to a chemical or physical agent that kills vegetative forms of microorganisms.

**disinfection** The application of a disinfectant to materials and surfaces to destroy pathogenic microorganisms.

***d. of blankets and woolens*** The use of chemicals to disinfect blankets and woolens before washing. Blankets and woolens may be soaked for 2 hr in a 5% carbolic acid solution and then washed and rinsed thoroughly. Cotton goods may be treated in the same way or boiled before washing. Materials that might be harmed by conventional methods of disinfection may be treated in a chamber with ethylene oxide gas.

***concurrent d.*** Prompt disinfection and suitable disposal of infected excreta during the entire course of a disease.

***d. of excreta*** Excreta should be soaked in a 5% carbolic acid solution for 1 hr before disposal. All infected excreta should be burned. Sputum may be treated as excreta if impossible to burn.

***d. of field of operation*** Disinfection of the area of the body where surgery is to be performed. The area of disinfection should be extensive. Thus, in operations on large scalp wounds and in all operations on the skull and its contents, the entire scalp must be shaved and disinfected.

In operations on the breast, the axilla and half of the chest must be prepared. If glands of the neck are involved, the entire neck must be included in the field of operation.

In amputation of the foot and lower third of the leg, the disinfection must extend as far as the knee, and in all higher amputations it should include the whole limb and corresponding side of the pelvis.

In all abdominal operations below the umbilicus, the pubic area must be shaved and the surface disinfection must include the whole anterior surface and both sides as far as the breasts.

In operations on the stomach, liver, and bile ducts, the field extends from the pubic area to the breasts. A general warm bath with liberal use of tincture of green soap should precede disinfection of the field of operation in all abdominal and pelvic operations, including hernia and varicocele.

In operations on parts of the body difficult to disinfect such as the scalp, palm of the hand, and sole of the foot, it is advisable to scrub with warm water and tincture of green soap and then rinse. A seventy-percent ethyl alcohol solution, povidone-iodine, benzalkonium chloride, or any other suitable disinfectant should be used. Seventy-percent ethyl alcohol is useful in hand and surface disinfection.

---

Caution: The mucous membranes are active, absorbing surfaces, and therefore solutions of carbolic acid, mercuric bichloride, and other potent antiseptics may not be used in these areas. The use of any of these agents in the vagina, uterus, or rectum frequently has resulted in serious poisoning and in some instances death.

---

In operations in the oral cavity, such as excision of the superior or inferior maxilla and amputation of the tongue, the use of a disinfecting solution is preceded by thorough cleansing of the teeth and swabbing of the mucous membrane with hydrogen peroxide.

In operations on the rectum, the usual procedure consists of shaving the perianal area and giving cleansing enemas.

Vaginal disinfection is preceded by shaving and disinfection of the external genitals. After a thorough cleansing with warm water and tincture of green soap, a douche of warm water with a suitable disinfectant is recommended.

Catheterization should always be preceded by disinfection of the meatus with green soap solution and thorough rinsing of the area with sterile water.

The external ear canal should be mechanically cleansed of wax, dirt, or blood clots, and then carefully disinfected by a low-pressure stream of warm hydrogen peroxide, until it is absolutely clean. This should not be done if the eardrum has been ruptured or if there is doubt of its integrity.

***terminal d.*** Disinfection of the room and infected materials at the end of the infectious stage of a disease.

**disinfestation** (dĭs″ĭn-fĕs-tā′shŭn) [L. *dis,*

apart, + *infestare,* to strike at] The process of killing infesting insects or parasites.

**disinhibition** (dĭs″ĭn-hĭ-bĭsh′ŭn) **1.** Abolition or countering of inhibition. **2.** In psychiatry, freedom to act in accordance with one's drives with a decrease in social or cultural constraint.

**disinsertion** Detachment of the retina at its periphery. SYN: *retinodialysis.*

**disintegration** [″ + *integer,* entire] **1.** The product of catabolism; the falling apart of the constituents of a substance. **2.** Disorganization of the psyche.

**disjoint** To disarticulate or to separate bones from their natural positions in a joint.

**disjunction** (dĭs-jŭnk′shŭn) Separation of the homolgous pairs of chromosomes during anaphase of the first meiotic division.

**disk** [Gr. *diskos,* a disk] A flat, round, platelike structure. SYN: *disc.*

***anisotropic d.*** SEE: *band, A.*

***articular d.*** The biconcave oval disk of fibrous connective tissue that separates the two joint cavities of the temporomandibular joint on each side.

***choked d.*** A swollen optic disk due to inflammation or edema. SYN: *papilledema.*

***dental d.*** A thin circular paper or other substance carrying polishing or cutting materials; it is driven by a dental engine and used in a variety of procedures with natural or artificial teeth.

***embryonic d.*** An oval disk of cells in the blastocyst of a mammal from which the embryo proper develops. Its lower layer, the endoderm, forms the roof of the yolk sac. Its upper layer, the ectoderm, forms the floor of the amniotic cavity. The primitive streak develops on the upper surface of the disk.

***epiphyseal d.*** A disk of cartilage at the junction of the diaphysis and epiphyses of growing long bones. Cartilage synthesis provides for growth in length; eventually the cartilage is replaced by bone.

***germinal d.*** A disk of cells on the surface of the yolk of a teloblastic egg from which the embryo develops. SYN: *proligerous d.; blastoderm.*

***herniated intervertebral d.*** A rupture or herniation of the nucleus pulposus, esp. between the lumbar vertebrae. It usually causes pain on the affected side. SYN: *slipped d.* SEE: *herniation of nucleus pulposus* for illus.

***intercalated d.*** A modification of the cell membrane of adjacent cardiac muscle cells; it contains intercellular junctions for electrical and mechanical linkage of contiguous cells.

***intervertebral d.*** The fibrocartilaginous tissue uniting the vertebral bodies. The outer portion is the anulus fibrosus; the inner portion is the nucleus pulposus.

***M d.*** M line.

***Merkel's d.*** The tiny expanded end of a sensory nerve fiber found in the epidermis and in the epithelial root sheath of a hair. SYN: *tactile d.*

***optic d.*** The area of the retina where the optic nerve enters it. SEE: *blind spot.*

***proligerous d.*** Germinal d.

***slipped d.*** Lay term for herniated intervertebral d.

***tactile d.*** Merkel's d.

***Z d.*** Z line.

**diskectomy** (dĭs-kĕk′tō-mē) Surgical removal of a herniated intervertebral disk.

**diskiform** (dĭs′kĭ-form) Shaped like a dish or disk.

**diskitis** (dĭsk-ī′tĭs) [Gr. *diskos,* disk, + *itis,* inflammation] Inflammation of a disk, esp. an interarticular cartilage. SYN: *meniscitis.*

**dislocation** [L. *dis,* apart, + *locare,* to place] The displacement of any part, esp. the temporary displacement of a bone from its normal position in a joint.

***closed d.*** Simple d.

***complete d.*** A dislocation that separates the surfaces of a joint completely.

***complicated d.*** A dislocation associated with other major injuries.

***compound d.*** A dislocation in which the joint communicates with the external air.

***condylar d.*** In the jaw, a displacement of the mandibular condyle in front of the condylar eminence. It is often caused by keeping the mouth wide open for an extended time, as in dental treatment that involves a rubber dam. SEE: *subluxation.*

***congenital d.*** A dislocation existing from or before birth.

***consecutive d.*** A dislocation in which the luxated bone has changed position since its first displacement.

***divergent d.*** A dislocation in which the ulna and radius are displaced separately.

***d. fracture*** A fracture near a dislocated joint.

***habitual d.*** A dislocation that often recurs after replacement.

***incomplete d.*** A subluxation (1); a slight displacement.

***mandibular d.*** SEE: *subluxation.*

***metacarpophalangeal joint d.*** The dislocation of a finger. It is usually complicated by an interposition of tendons or other structures. When reduced, it tends to slip out immediately. In many instances, manipulation of this region only makes subsequent reduction more difficult; therefore, the disturbed area should be immobilized with well-placed padded splints on the hand and wrist. The patient should be sent to a physician promptly.

***Monteggia's d.*** A dislocation of the hip joint in which the head of the femur is near the anterosuperior spine of the ilium.

***Nélaton's d.*** Dislocation of the ankle in which the talus is forced up between the end of the tibia and the fibula.

***old d.*** A dislocation in which no reduction has been accomplished even after many days, weeks, or months.

***partial d.*** Incomplete d.

***pathological d.*** A dislocation resulting from paralysis or disease of the joint or supporting tissues.

***primitive d.*** A dislocation in which the bones remain as originally displaced.

***recent d.*** A dislocation seen shortly after it occurred.

***simple d.*** A dislocation in which the joint is not penetrated by a wound.

***slipped d.*** SEE: *herniated disk*.

***subastragalar d.*** Separation of the calcaneum and the scaphoid from the talus.

***traumatic d.*** Dislocation due to injury or violence.

**dismember** To remove an extremity or a portion of it.

**dismutase** (dĭs-mū′tās) An enzyme that acts on two molecules of the same substance. One of these is oxidized and the other reduced; two new compounds are thus produced.

***superoxide d.*** An enzyme present in aerobic but not in strictly anaerobic bacteria. It destroys the poisonous, highly reactive free-radical form of $O_2$, superoxide ($O_2^-$), formed by flavoenzymes. Thus, aerobic bacteria are protected from the lethal effect of superoxide by the action of this enzyme.

**disocclusion** Loss of contact between opposing teeth.

**disomus** (dī-sō′mŭs) [Gr. *dis*, twice, + *soma*, body] A malformed fetus with a double trunk.

**disopyramide phosphate** (dī-sō-pēr′ă-mīd) A drug used in treating cardiac arrhythmias. Trade name is Norpace.

**disorder** A pathologic condition of the mind or body. SEE: *disease*.

***acute stress d.*** A disorder characterized by severe anxiety, dissociative symptoms, and depersonalization. Symptoms occur within 1 month of exposure to an extremely traumatic stressor and persist for at least 2 days.

***amnestic d.'s*** A group of disorders marked by memory disturbance that is due either to the direct physiological effects of a general medical condition or to the persistent effects of a drug, toxin, or similar substance. Affected patients are unable to recall previously learned information or past events, and social or occupational functioning is significantly impaired.

***bipolar d.*** A disorder marked by manic or manic and depressive episodes. Bipolar disorders are divided into four categories: bipolar I, bipolar II, cyclothymia, and nonspecified disorders. There are six separate disorders within the bipolar I category. Mania is the essential feature of bipolar I, whereas bipolar II is marked by recurrent moods of both mania and depression. SEE: *Nursing Diagnoses Appendix*.

TREATMENT: The usual medication is lithium carbonate. If the patient is concerned about the side effects of lithium, valproate and carbamazepine may be tried.

***body dysmorphic d.*** ABBR: BDD. A preoccupation with one or more imagined defects in appearance.

***breathing-related d.*** A sleep disturbance due to a sleep-related breathing condition such as obstructive sleep apnea. Excessive sleepiness is the most common presenting complaint because of frequent arousals during night sleep as the person attempts to breathe normally. The person may fall asleep while talking, eating, or driving. Electrocardiographic abnormalities, elevated pulmonary and systolic arterial pressure, cardiac arrhythmias, and oxyhemoglobin desaturation may be associated laboratory findings. The disorder occurs in both sexes and often has a chronic course.

***character d.*** A personality disorder manifested by a chronic, habitual, maladaptive pattern of reaction that is relatively inflexible, limits the optimal use of potentialities, and often provokes the responses from the environment that the individual wants to avoid.

***childhood disintegrative d.*** A personality disorder of children marked by regression in many areas of functioning after at least 2 yr of normal development. Individuals exhibit social, communicative, and behavioral characteristics similar to those of autistic disorder. Also called *Heller's syndrome*, *dementia infantalis*, or *disintegrative psychosis*.

***d. factitious*** A disorder that is not real, genuine, or natural. The symptoms, physical and psychological, are produced by the individual and are under voluntary control. These symptoms and the behavior are used to pursue a goal (i.e., to assume the role of patient and to stay in a hospital). This is attained by various means, such as taking anticoagulants and feigning right lower quadrant pain with nausea and vomiting, dizziness, fainting, fever of unknown origin, and massive hemoptysis. Mental symptoms may include memory loss, hallucinations, and uncooperativeness. These patients have a severe personality disturbance. SEE: *malinger; Munchausen syndrome*.

***functional d.*** SEE: *illness, functional*.

***gender identity d.*** A disorder marked by a strong cross-gender identification and a persistent discomfort with the biologically assigned sex. Generally, adults with the disorder are preoccupied with the wish to live as a member of the other sex; this often impairs the social, occupational, or other types of functioning. SEE: *Nursing Diagnoses Appendix*.

***habit d.*** A tension-discharging phenomenon such as head banging, body rocking, thumb sucking, nail biting, hair pulling, tics, or teeth grinding, usually beginning in childhood. The habit's importance depends upon its etiology and persistence. Almost all children will demonstrate one or more of these disorders during their development, but if it does not interfere with function it should be of no concern.

***impulse-control d.*** A disorder marked by failure to resist impulses, drives, or temptations that cause harm. Impulse-control disorders include kleptomania, pyromania, pathological gambling, trichotillomania, and intermittent explosive disorder.

***inhalant-induced d.*** A disorder caused by the use and overuse of inhalants. Abuse may lead to anxiety, psychosis, dementia, liver disease, and peripheral nervous system damage.

***intermittent explosive d.*** A personality disorder marked by episodes of impulsive aggressiveness that are out of proportion to precipitating events. In contrast to amok, a culture-specific, one-time outburst, intermittent explosive disorder is a pattern of behavior. It results in serious assaults or destruction of property.

***late luteal phase dysphoric d.*** SEE: *premenstrual dysphoric disorder.*

***learning d.*** A disorder of academic functioning such as reading, mathematics, or written expression. These disorders are marked by difficulties in learning far greater than would be expected for the person's age and measured intelligence. Formerly called *learning disability*.

***mental d.*** An imprecise term for a clinically significant behavioral or psychological syndrome or pattern typically associated with either a distressing symptom or impaired function. It is important to remember that different individuals described as having the same mental disorder are not alike in the way they react to their illness and how they need to be treated.

***pain d.*** A mental disorder in which pain is the predominant symptom, is of such severity to warrant clinical attention, and interferes with function. Psychological factors are important in the onset, severity, exacerbation, or maintenance of the pain. The condition is not intentionally produced or feigned.

***phonological d.*** A disorder in which the individual does not use speech sounds that are appropriate for age and dialect. The disorder may involve production, use, organization, or omission of sounds.

***substance dependence d.*** An addictive disorder caused by drug use. It is marked by a cluster of behavioral and physiological symptoms that indicate continual use of the substance despite significant related problems. The term includes a variety of substances but excludes caffeine. Patients develop a tolerance for the substance and require progressively greater amounts to elicit the effects desired. In addition, patients experience physical and psychological signs and symptoms of withdrawal if the agent is not used. SEE: *substance-induced d.; substance-related d.; substance abuse.*

***substance-induced d.*** A disorder related to drug use but excluding drug dependency. Substance-induced disorders include intoxication, withdrawal, and other substance-induced mental disorders such as delirium and psychosis. SEE: *substance dependence d.; substance-related d.; substance abuse.*

***substance-related d.*** Any disorder related to drug abuse or the effects of medication. Substances include alcohol, amphetamines, cannabis, cocaine, hallucinogens, inhalants, nicotine, opioids, phencyclidine (PCP), sedatives, hypnotics, and anxiolytics. SEE: *substance dependence d.; substance-induced d.; substance abuse.*

**disorganization** [L. *dis,* apart, + Gr. *organon,* a unified organ] Alteration in an organic part, causing it to lose most or all of its distinctive characteristics.

**disorganized infant behavior** Alteration in integration and modulation of the physiological and behavioral systems of functioning (i.e., autonomic, motor, state, organizational, self-regulatory, and attentional-interactional systems). SEE: *Nursing Diagnoses Appendix.*

**disorganized infant behavior, risk for** Risk for alteration in integration and modulation of the physiological and behavioral systems of functioning (i.e., autonomic, motor, state, organizational, self-regulatory, and attentional-interactional systems). SEE: *Nursing Diagnoses Appendix.*

**disorientation** (dĭs″ō-rē-ĕn-tā′shŭn) [″ + *oriens,* arising] Inability to estimate direction or location, or to be cognizant of time or of persons.

***spatial d.*** In aerospace medicine, a term used to describe a variety of incidents occurring in flight, when the pilot fails to sense correctly the position, motion, or attitude of the aircraft or himself or herself within the coordinate system provided by the surface of the earth and gravitation.

**disparate** [L. *disparitas,* unequal] Dissimilar, not equally paired.

**dispensary** [L. *dispensare,* to give out] A clinic or similar place for obtaining medical care.

**dispensatory** (dĭs-pĕn′să-tō-rē) [L. *dispensatorium*] A publication, in book form, of the description and composition of medicines.

**dispense** (dĭs-pĕns′) To prepare or deliver medicines.

**dispersate** (dĭs′pŭr-sāt) A suspension of finely divided particles in a liquid.

**disperse** (dĭs-pĕrs′) [L. *dis,* apart, + *spargere,* to scatter] **1.** To scatter, esp. applied to light rays. **2.** To dissipate or cause to disappear, as a tumor or the particles of a colloidal system.

**dispersion** (dĭs-pĕr′zhŭn) **1.** The act of dispersing. **2.** That which is dispersed.

***coarse d.*** Mechanical suspension.

***colloidal d.*** A mixture containing colloid particles that fail to settle out and are held in suspension. They are common in animal and plant tissues; the protoplasm of cells is an example. Particles of colloidal dispersions are too large to pass through cell membranes. Such dispersions usually appear cloudy.

***molecular d.*** A true solution.

**dispersoid** A colloid with very finely divided particles.

**dispersonalization** (dĭs-pĕr″sŏn-ăl-ī-zā′shŭn) A mental state in which the individual denies the existence of his or her personality or parts of the body.

**displacement** [Fr. *deplacer,* to lay aside] **1.** Removal from the normal or usual position or place. **2.** Addition to a fluid of another more dense, causing the first fluid to be dispersed. **3.** Transference of emotion from the original idea with which it was associated to a different idea, thus allowing the patient to avoid acknowledging the original source.

**disposition** [L. *disponere,* to arrange] **1.** A natural tendency or aptitude exhibited by an individual or group. It may be manifested by acquiring a certain disease, presumably due to hereditary factors. **2.** The sum of a person's behavior as determined by his or her mood. SEE: *diathesis.*

**disproportion** (dĭs″prō-por′shŭn) A size different from that considered to be normal.

***cephalopelvic d.*** ABBR: CPD. Disparity between the dimensions of the fetal head and those of the maternal pelvis. When the fetal head is larger than the pelvic diameters through which it must pass, or when the head is extended as in a face or brow presentation and cannot rotate to accommodate to the size and shape of the birth canal, fetal descent and delivery are not possible.

**disruptive behavior disorder** SEE: *Nursing Diagnoses Appendix.*

**dissect** (dĭ-sĕkt′, dī-sĕkt′) [L. *dissecare,* to cut up] To separate tissues and parts of a cadaver for anatomical study.

**dissection** (dĭ-, dī-sĕk′shŭn) In surgical procedures, the cutting of parts for separation and study.

***blunt d.*** In surgical procedures, separation of tissues by use of a blunt instrument. This provides minimal damage to the part being dissected.

***sharp d.*** In surgical procedures, gaining access to tissues by incising them with some sort of sharp instrument such as a scalpel.

**dissemble** To mislead, to give a false impression, or to conceal the truth.

**disseminated** [L. *dis,* apart, + *seminare,* to sow] Scattered or distributed over a considerable area, esp. applied to disease organisms; scattered throughout an organ or the body.

**disseminated intravascular coagulation** ABBR: DIC. A pathological form of coagulation that is diffuse rather than localized, as would be the case in normal coagulation. The process damages rather than protects the area involved, and several clotting factors are consumed to such extent that generalized bleeding may occur. Various conditions have been associated with DIC including septic shock; acute intravascular hemolysis; acute viral, rickettsial, or protozoal infection; abruptio placentae; septic abortion; surgical procedures; heatstroke; certain poisonous snake bites; severe head injury; malignancy; retained dead fetus; liver disease; and systemic lupus erythematosis. SEE: *acute respiratory distress syndrome; sepsis; serine protease inhibitor; systemic inflammatory response syndrome; Nursing Diagnoses Appendix.*

SYMPTOMS: Symptoms of DIC include bleeding from surgical or invasive procedure sites and bleeding gums, cutaneous oozing, petechiae, ecchymoses, and hematomas. The patient may also experience nausea and vomiting; severe muscle, back, and abdominal pain; chest pain; hemoptysis; epistaxis; seizures; and oliguria. Peripheral pulses and blood pressure may be decreased; the patient may demonstrate confusion or other changes in mental status. SEE: illus.

TREATMENT: The primary illness must be treated. Heparin should be administered; adults should receive fibrinolytic inhibitors. The latter may be dangerous if the thrombotic process has not been previously treated with heparin. Transfusion should be initiated to re-establish normal hemostatic potential if the thrombosis is blocked by heparin.

NURSING IMPLICATIONS: In acute DIC, intake and output are monitored hourly, esp. when blood products are given, and the patient is observed for transfusion reactions and fluid overload. The blood pressure cuff is used infrequently to avoid triggering subcutaneous bleeding. Any emesis or drainage should undergo a hematest, and dressings and linens should

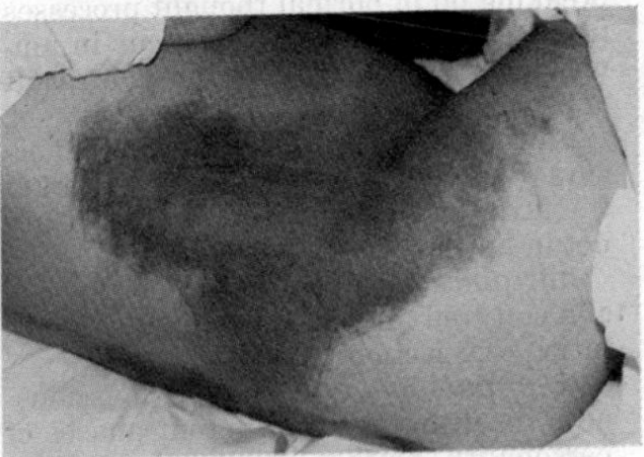

**DISSEMINATED INTRAVASCULAR COAGULATION**

WIDESPREAD CUTANEOUS HEMORRHAGE

be weighed to measure the amount of blood lost. Daily weights are obtained, particularly in cases of renal involvement. The patient is checked for evidence of gastrointestinal and genitourinary bleeding; all urine and stool specimens are tested for occult blood. The patient is observed closely for signs of shock, and the abdominal girth measured every 2 to 4 hr if intra-abdominal bleeding is suspected.

The results of serial blood studies, such as hemoglobin and hematocrit and coagulation studies, are monitored. All venipuncture sites are checked frequently for bleeding. Analgesics are given as prescribed, as well as heparin therapy if prescribed (the latter is controversial). The patient is repositioned every 2 hr, and meticulous skin care is provided. Prescribed oxygen therapy is administered. Areas at risk can be washed gently with hydrogen peroxide and water to remove crusted blood. Pressure, cold compresses, and topical hemostatic agents are applied to control bleeding. Parenteral injections are avoided and venipunctures limited whenever possible; pressure should be applied to an injection site for at least 10 min after removal of a needle or intravenous catheter. The patient is protected from injury by enforcing complete bedrest during bleeding episodes and by padding the bed rails if the patient is at risk for agitation. Frequent rest periods are provided.

The disorder, the patient's progress, and treatment options and posttreatment appearance are explained and the patient and family are encouraged to express their feelings and concerns and are referred for further counseling or support as needed.

**dissipation** (dĭs-ĭ-pā'shŭn) [L. *dissipare,* to scatter] **1.** Dispersion of matter. **2.** The act of living a wasteful and dissolute life, esp. drinking alcoholic beverages to excess.

**dissociation** (dĭs-sō″sē-ā'shŭn) [L. *dis,* apart, + *sociatio,* union] **1.** Separation, as the separation by heat of a complex compound into simpler molecules. **2.** The ability to move one body segment independently of another. **3.** In psychiatry, the breaking off of normal thought processes from consciousness, as can occur in amnesia, conversion reaction, or as a result of psychoactive drugs. SEE: *hysteria.*

***atrioventricular d.*** Dissociation that occurs when the independent pacemakers of the atria and ventricles of the heart are not in harmony.

***microbic d.*** A change in the morphology of a cultured microbial colony due to mutation or selection.

***d. of personality*** A split in consciousness resulting in two different phases of personality, neither being aware of the words, acts, and feelings of the other. SEE: *dual personality; multiple personality; vigilambulism.*

***psychological d.*** A disunion of mind of which the person is not aware (e.g., dual personality, fugue, somnambulism, selective amnesia).

**dissociative disorder** SEE: *Nursing Diagnoses Appendix.*

**dissolution** [L. *dissolvere,* to dissolve] **1.** Death. **2.** A pathological resolution or breaking up of the integrity of an anatomical entity.

**dissolve** (dĭ-zŏlv') [L. *dissolvere,* to dissolve] To cause absorption of a solid in and by a liquid.

**dissonance** (dĭs'ō-năns) **1.** Discord or disagreement. **2.** Unpleasant sounds, particularly musical ones.

***cognitive d.*** Incongruity of thought, philosophy, or action.

**distad** (dĭs'tăd) [L. *distare,* to be distant] Away from the center.

**distal** (dĭs'tăl) [L. *distare,* to be distant] **1.** Farthest from the center, from a medial line, or from the trunk; opposed to proximal. **2.** In dentistry, the tooth surface farthest from the midline of the arch.

**distance** The space between two objects.

***focal d.*** The distance from the optical center of a lens to the focal point.

***focal-film d.*** The distance between the focal target of an x-ray and the film.

***interocclusal d.*** The distance between the occlusal surfaces of opposed teeth when the mandible is at rest.

***interocular d.*** The distance between the eyes. SEE: *hypertelorism.*

***interpupillary d.*** The distance between the centers of the pupils of the eyes.

***object-film d.*** ABBR: OFD. In radiography, the distance between the anatomical structure to be imaged and the radiographic film.

***source-skin d.*** The distance from a radioactive source to the skin of the patient.

***source-to-image receptor d.*** The distance from the source of radiation to the imaging device.

***target-skin d.*** ABBR: TSD. The distance at which it is safe to deliver an appropriately timed exposure of ionizing radiation for treatment or diagnosis.

**distemper** (dĭs-tĕm'pĕr) In veterinary medicine, one of several virus infections of animals.

**distend** [L. *distendere,* to stretch out] **1.** To stretch out. **2.** To become inflated.

**distensibility** (dĭs-tĕn″sĭ-bĭl'ĭ-tē) The ability to become distended.

**distention** The state of being distended.

**distichiasis** (dĭs″tĭ-kī'ă-sĭs) [Gr. *distichia,* a double row] A condition in which there are two rows of eyelashes, one or both being directed inward toward the eye.

**distill** (dĭs-tĭl') [L. *destillare,* to drop from] To vaporize by heat and condense and collect the volatilized products.

**distillate** (dĭs'tĭl-āt, dĭs-tĭl'āt) That which has been derived from the distillation process.

**distillation** Condensation of a vapor that has been obtained from a liquid heated to the volatilization point, as the condensation of steam from boiling water. Distillation is used to purify water and for other purposes. Distilled water should be stored in covered containers because it readily takes up impurities from the atmosphere.

***destructive d.*** The process of decomposing complex organic compounds by heat in the absence of air and condensing the vapor of the liquid products.

***dry d.*** Distillation of solids without added liquids.

***fractional d.*** Separation of liquids based on the difference in their boiling points.

**distobuccal** (dĭs″tō-bŭk′ăl) [L. *distare,* to be distant, + *bucca,* cheek] Pert. to the distal and buccal walls of bicuspid and molar teeth; also pert. to the distal or buccal walls of a cavity preparation.

**distoclusion** (dĭs″tō-kloo′zhŭn) A condition in which the lower teeth meet the upper teeth behind the normal position.

**distogingival** (dĭs″tō-jĭn′jĭ-văl) [″ + *gingiva,* gum] Pert. to the distal and gingival walls of a cavity being prepared for restoration.

**distolabial** (dĭs″tō-lā′bē-ăl) [″ + *labialis,* lips] Pert. to the distal and labial surfaces of a tooth.

**distolingual** (dĭs″tō-lĭng′gwăl) [″ + *lingua,* tongue] Pert. to the distal and lingual surfaces of a tooth.

**distome** A fluke with two suckers, an oral and a ventral sucker, or acetabulum.

**distomia** (dī-stō′mē-ă) [Gr. *dis,* two, + *stoma,* mouth] A congenital deformation producing a fetus with two mouths.

**disto-occlusal** (dĭs″tō-ŏ-kloo′zăl) Concerning the distal and occlusal surfaces of a tooth or the distal and occlusal walls of a cavity preparation.

**distortion** [L. *distortio,* twist, writhe] **1.** A twisting or bending out of regular shape. **2.** A writhing or twisting movement as of the muscles of the face. **3.** A deformity in which the part or structure is altered in shape. **4.** In ophthalmology, visual perception of an image that does not provide a true picture, due to astigmatism or to retinal abnormalities. **5.** In psychiatry, the process of modifying unconscious mental elements so that they can enter consciousness without being censored. **6.** In radiology, the difference in size and shape of a radiographic image as compared with the actual part examined. **7.** Variation in the amplitude or frequency of a signal that may be caused by overdriving the amplifier in the circuit.

**distractibility 1.** A condition of mental wandering in which the thoughts are attracted by extraneous conditions or influenced by a dissociation of consciousness. **2.** Inability to focus one's attention.

**distraction** (dĭs-trăk′shŭn) [L. *dis,* apart, + *tractio,* a drawing] **1.** A state of mental confusion or derangement. **2.** Separation of joint surfaces by extension without injury or dislocation of the parts. **3.** A joint mobilization technique causing separation of opposing joint surfaces. It is used to inhibit pain, move synovial fluid, or stretch a tight joint capsule.

**distraught** (dĭs-trawt′) [L. *distrahere,* to perplex] In doubt, deeply troubled, and having conflicting thoughts. The patient may be frantic and may need to be continuously occupied.

**distress** (dĭs-trĕs′) [L. *distringere,* to draw apart] Physical or mental pain or suffering.

***fetal d.*** SEE: *fetal distress.*

**distribution** [L. *dis,* apart, + *tribuere,* to allot] **1.** The dividing and spreading of anything, esp. blood vessels and nerves, to tissues. **2.** The presence of entities, such as hair, fat, or nutrients, at various sites or in particular patterns throughout the body. **3.** In demography or statistics, the location pattern of particular individuals who are ill, or of events.

***frequency d.*** In statistics, the grouping of data by rate of occurrence at arbitrarily determined values although the variable may vary continuously (e.g., disease occurrences could be grouped by weeks, months, or years rather than by the precise day of occurrence).

***gaussian d.*** Normal d.

***normal d.*** In statistics, the smooth, bell-shaped, hypothetical curve made by a frequency distribution diagram in which the occurrences are plotted on the vertical axis (ordinate), and the values of the variable are plotted on the horizontal axis (abscissa). SYN: *bell-shaped curve; gaussian curve.*

**districhiasis** (dĭs-trĭk-ī′ă-sĭs) [Gr. *dis,* double, + *thrix,* hair] A condition in which two hairs grow from the same hair follicle.

**disturbance 1.** Interruption of the normal sequence of continuity. **2.** A departure from the considered norm.

***emotional d.*** Mental disorder.

**disulfate** (dī-sŭl′fāt) A compound containing two sulfate radicals. SEE: *bisulfate.*

**disulfiram** (dī-sŭl′fĭ-răm) A drug administered orally to treat alcoholism. Alcohol is acted on by alcohol dehydrogenase to produce the toxic substance acetaldehyde. The toxic effect of disulfiram is due to the prevention of the further degradation of acetaldehyde. Trade name is Antabuse.

---

Caution: The reaction to use of alcohol while this drug is being administered may cause severe reactions such as respiratory depression, shock, acute congestive heart failure, myocardial infarction, unconsciousness, convulsions, and sudden death.

---

**disulfiram poisoning** SEE: *Antabuse in Poisons and Poisoning Appendix.*

**disuse syndrome, risk for** A state in which an individual is at risk for deterioration of body systems as the result of prescribed or unavoidable musculoskeletal inactivity. SEE: *Nursing Diagnoses Appendix.*

**dithiazanine iodide** (dī″thī-ăz′ă-nēn) An anthelmintic.

**Dittrich's plugs** (dĭt′rĭks) [Franz Dittrich, Ger. pathologist, 1815–1859] Small particles in fetid sputum composed of pus, detritus, bacteria, and fat globules.

**diurese** (dī″ū-rēs′) To cause diuresis.

**diuresis** (dī″ū-rē′sĭs) [Gr. *diourein,* to urinate] Secretion and passage of large amounts of urine. This condition occurs in diabetes mellitus. It can be an early sign of chronic interstitial nephritis. It may also be due to hysteria, fear and anxiety, ingestion of large amounts of liquid, diabetes insipidus, recent childbirth, or the action of drugs that can cause diuresis. Cold applications have a diuretic action by contracting superficial vessels and raising blood pressure. SEE: *diuretic.*

***postpartum* d.** Diuresis due to the rapid decline in estrogen levels shortly after childbirth. This causes excretion of the large amount of fluid retained in the extravascular tissue during pregnancy. The daily urine output may exceed 3 L.

**diuretic** (dī″ū-rĕt′ĭk) **1.** Increasing urine secretion. SEE: *diuresis.* **2.** An agent that increases urine secretion. Diuretics act in two ways: by increasing glomerular filtration or by decreasing reabsorption from the tubules. An increase in blood flow in the renal vessels increases urine formation by raising glomerular filtration pressure.

**diurnal** [L. *dies,* day] **1.** Daily. **2.** Happening in the daytime or pert. to it. SEE: *circadian; clock, biological; desynchronosis; nocturnal.*

**divagation** (dī-vă-gā′shŭn) [L. *divagatus,* to wander off] **1.** Wandering astray. **2.** Rambling or incoherent speech.

**divalent** (dī-vā′lĕnt) In a molecule, having an electric charge of two. SYN: *bivalent.*

**divergence** (dī-vĕr′jĕns) [L. *divergere,* to turn aside] Separation from a common center, especially that of the eyes.

**divergent** Radiating in different directions.

**diversional activity deficit** The state in which an individual experiences a decreased stimulation from or interest or engagement in recreational or leisure activities (because of internal/external factors that may or may not be beyond the individual's control). SEE: *Nursing Diagnoses Appendix.*

**diver's paralysis** An occupational disease due to returning too suddenly to normal atmosphere after working under high air pressure. SYN: *bends; caisson disease.*

**diverticulectomy** (dī″vĕr-tĭk″ū-lĕk′tō-mē) [″ + Gr. *ektome,* excision] Surgical removal of a diverticulum.

**diverticulitis** (dī″vĕr-tĭk″ū-lī′tĭs) [″ + Gr. *itis,* inflammation] Inflammation of a diverticulum or diverticula in the intestinal tract, esp. in the colon, causing stagnation of feces in little distended sacs of the colon (diverticula) and pain. SEE: *Nursing Diagnoses Appendix.*

Nursing Implications: During an acute episode, prescribed treatment with fluid and electrolyte replacement, antibiotic, antispasmodic, analgesic, and stool softener therapy, and nasogastric suction if required is initiated. The patient is then observed for increasing or decreasing distress and for any adverse reactions to the therapy. Stools are inspected for color and consistency, and the frequency of bowel movements is noted. The patient is assessed for fever, increasing abdominal pain, blood in the stools, and leukocytosis. Rest is prescribed, and the patient is instructed not to lift, strain, bend, cough, or perform other actions that increase intra-abdominal pressure.

Patients with chronic diverticulitis (diverticulosis) are educated about the disease and its symptoms. A well-balanced diet that provides dietary roughage in the form of fruit, vegetable, and cereal fiber, but that is nonirritating to the bowel, is recommended; and fluid intake should be increased to 2 to 3 L daily (unless otherwise restricted). Constipation and straining at stool should be avoided, and the patient is advised relieve constipation with stool softeners and bulk cathartics, taken with plenty of water. The importance of regular medical evaluation is emphasized.

***acute* d.** Diverticulitis in which the symptoms are similar to those of appendicitis: inflammation of the peritoneum, formation of an abscess, and finally, gangrene accompanied by perforation may ensue.

***chronic* d.** Diverticulitis marked by worsening constipation, mucus in the stools, and griping abdominal pains at intervals. The walls of the bowels may thicken, which may produce chronic intestinal obstruction.

**diverticulosis** (dī″vĕr-tĭk″ū-lō′sĭs) [″ + Gr. *osis,* condition] Diverticula in the colon without inflammation or symptoms. Only a small percentage of persons with diverticulosis develop diverticulitis.

**diverticulum** (dī″vĕr-tĭk′ū-lŭm) *pl.* **diverticula** [L. *devertere,* to turn aside] A sac or pouch in the walls of a canal or organ. SEE: illus.

***d. of the colon*** An outpocketing of the colon. These may be asymptomatic until they become inflamed.

***d. of the duodenum*** A diverticulum commonly located near the entrance of the common bile or pancreatic duct.

***false* d.** A diverticulum without a muscular coat in the wall or pouch. This type of diverticulum is acquired.

***gastric* d.** A pulsion-type diverticulum usually on the lesser curvature of the esophagogastric junction.

***d. of the jejunum*** A diverticulum usually marked by severe pain in the upper abdomen, followed occasionally by a massive hemorrhage from the intestine.

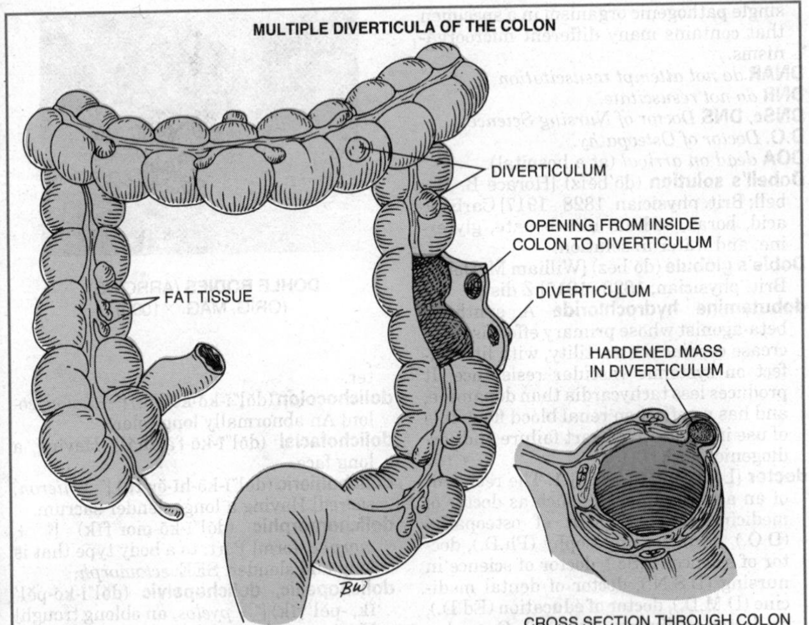


***Meckel's d.*** SEE: *Meckel's diverticulum.*

***d. of the stomach*** A diverticulum of the stomach wall.

***true d.*** A diverticulum involving all the coats of muscle in the pouch wall. It is usually congenital.

***Zenker's d.*** SEE: *Zenker's diverticulum.*

**diving reflex** A complex cardiovascular reflex produced by submersion of the face and nose of animals, including humans, in water. It constricts blood flow except to the brain, decreases cardiac output and rate, and produces stable or slightly increased arterial blood pressure. The reflex enables aquatic animals to remain submerged for long periods because it reduces their oxygen requirements. In humans, it has been used to treat paroxysmal atrial tachycardia.

**divulsion** (dĭ-vŭl′shŭn) [L. *dis*, apart, + *vellere*, to pluck] A forcible pulling apart.

**divulsor** (dĭ-vŭl′sor) [L. *dis*, apart, + *vellere*, to pluck] A device for dilatation of a part, esp. the urethra.

***pterygium d.*** An instrument for separating the corneal portion of the pterygium.

***tendon d.*** A device for separating a tendon from the surrounding tissue.

**Dix, Dorothea Lynde** A Massachusetts schoolteacher (1802–1887) who crusaded for prison reform and for care of the mentally ill. She was responsible for founding many hospitals in the U.S., Canada, and several other countries. During the Civil War, she organized the nursing service of the Union armies.

**dizziness** [AS. *dysig*, foolish] A sensation of lightheadness, whirling, or a tendency to fall. SYN: *giddiness*. SEE: *vertigo*.

**DKA** *diabetic ketoacidosis*.

**dl** *deciliter*.

**DM** *diabetes mellitus*.

**D.M.D.** *Doctor of Dental Medicine*.

**DMF index** The total number of decayed, missing, and filled teeth.

**DMSO** *dimethyl sulfoxide*.

**DMT** *dimethyltryptamine*.

**DNA** *deoxyribonucleic acid*.

**DNA fingerprint** A distinctive pattern of bands formed by repeating sequences of base pairs of satellite DNA. These patterns are different in every individual. The technique of identifying the pattern, known as DNA fingerprinting, can be helpful in establishing the origin of tissues and body fluids and is used in forensic medicine.

**DNA probe** A single-strand DNA fragment used to detect the complementary fragment. DNA probes are used widely in bacteriology. Recombinant DNA techniques are used to isolate, reproduce, and label a portion of the genetic material, DNA, from the nucleus of a microorganism that is specific for it. This fragment can be added to a specimen containing the organisms. The specimen and known DNA are treated so that the DNA strands from the organisms in the specimen are separated into single strands. The DNA from the specimen rejoins (is annealed to) the known labeled DNA and is thereby labeled. This permits the identification of a single pathogenic organism in a specimen that contains many different microorganisms.

**DNAR** *do not attempt resuscitation.*

**DNR** *do not resuscitate.*

**DNSc, DNS** *Doctor of Nursing Science.*

**D.O.** *Doctor of Osteopathy.*

**DOA** *dead on arrival* (at a hospital).

**Dobell's solution** (dō'bĕlz) [Horace B. Dobell, Brit. physician, 1828–1917] Carbolic acid, borax, sodium bicarbonate, glycerine, and water in solution.

**Dobie's globule** (dō'bēz) [William M. Dobie, Brit. physician, 1828–1915] Z disk.

**dobutamine hydrochloride** A synthetic beta-agonist whose primary effect is to increase cardiac contractility, with little effect on systemic vascular resistance. It produces less tachycardia than dopamine, and has no effect on renal blood flow. It is of use in congestive heart failure and cardiogenic shock.

**doctor** [L. *docere,* to teach] **1.** The recipient of an advanced degree, such as doctor of medicine (M.D.), doctor of osteopathy (D.O.), doctor of philosophy (Ph.D.), doctor of science (D.Sc.), doctor of science in nursing (D.S.N.), doctor of dental medicine (D.M.D.), doctor of education (Ed.D.), or doctor of divinity (D.D.). **2.** One who, after graduating from a medical, veterinary, or dental school, successfully passes an examination and is licensed by a state government to practice medicine, veterinary medicine, or dentistry. SEE: *optometry; osteopathy.*Because of the great variety of doctoral degrees, the use of the word doctor is sometimes confusing. This may be remedied by using the word physician when writing or speaking of those who possess an M.D. or D.O. (doctor of osteopathy) degree.

***barefoot d.*** A practitioner of traditional or native medicine in the People's Republic of China. These individuals have not attended a medical school.

**doctrine** (dŏk'trĭn) A system of principles taught or advocated.

**docusate calcium** (dŏk'ū-sāt) A stool softener.

**docusate sodium** A stool softener.

**dogmatic** Pert. to the expression of opinions in an uncompromising, arrogant manner.

**Döhle bodies** (dē'lēz) [Paul Döhle, Ger. pathologist, 1855–1928] A leukocyte inclusion in the periphery of a neutrophil. It is composed of liquefied endoplasmic reticulum and is frequently accompanied by toxic granulations. Döhle bodies are present in association with burns, severe or systemic infections, exposure to cytotoxic agents, uncomplicated pregnancy, trauma, and neoplastic diseases. SEE: illus.

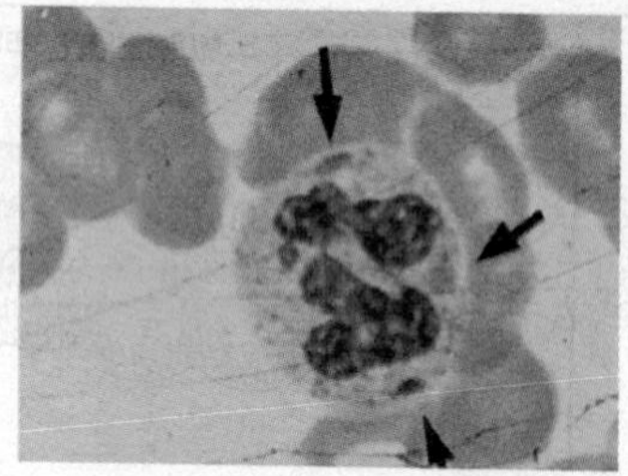

**DOHLE BODIES** (ARROWS), (ORIG. MAG. ×1000)

**dol** Symbol for degree of pain intensity registered on the dolorimeter.

**dolichocephalic** (dŏl″ĭ-kō-sĭ-făl'ĭk) [Gr. *dolichos,* long, + *kephale,* head] Having a skull with a long anteroposterior diameter.

**dolichocolon** (dŏl″ĭ-kō-kō'lŏn) [″ + *kolon,* colon] An abnormally long colon.

**dolichofacial** (dŏl″ĭ-kō-fā'shăl) Having a long face.

**dolichohieric** (dŏl″ĭ-kō-hī-ĕr'ĭk) [″ + *hieron,* sacred] Having a long, slender sacrum.

**dolichomorphic** (dŏl″ĭ-kō-mor'fĭk) [″ + *morphe,* form] Pert. to a body type that is long and slender. SEE: *ectomorph.*

**dolichopellic, dolichopelvic** (dŏl″ĭ-kō-pĕl'ĭk, -pĕl'vĭk) [″ + *pyelos,* an oblong trough] Having an abnormally long or narrow pelvis.

**dolichosigmoid** (dŏl″ĭ-kō-sĭg'moyd) [″ + *sigmoeides,* sigmoid] Having an abnormally long sigmoid flexure of the colon.

**dolichuranic** (dŏl″ĭk-ū-răn'ĭk) [″ + *ouranos,* palate] Having a long alveolar arch of the maxilla.

**doll's eye movement** Oculocephalic reflex. SYN: *doll's head maneuver.*

**doll's head maneuver** A test of eye movement in comatose patients. The head is quickly rotated from one side to the other. Normally the eyes deviate together to the side opposite the direction of head rotation. If this response is absent, there may be damage to the brainstem or oculomotor nerves. SEE: *coma.*

**dolor** (dō'lor) *pl.* **dolores** [L.] Pain. This is one of the principal indications of inflammation. The others are rubor (redness), tumor (swelling), functio laesa (loss of function), and calor (heat).

**dolorimeter** (dō″lor-ĭm'ĭ-tĕr) [″ + Gr. *metron,* measure] A device for measuring degrees of pain.

**dolorogenic** [″ + Gr. *gennan,* to produce] Causing pain.

**domain** In immunology, the portion of a protein, such as an immunoglobulin, that has a functional role independent of the remainder of the protein.

**domatophobia** (dō-măt-ō-fō'bē-ă) [Gr. *doma,* house, + *phobos,* fear] Abnormal aversion to being in a house; a form of claustrophobia.

**domiciliary** (dŏm″ĭ-sĭl'ē-ār″ē) [L. *domus,* house] Pert. to or carried on in a house.

**domiciliary care facility** A home providing mainly custodial and personal care for persons who do not require medical or nursing supervision, but may need assistance with activities of daily living because of a physical or mental disability. This may also be referred to as a sheltered living environment. SEE: *adult foster care.*

**dominance** [L. *dominans,* ruling] **1.** A genetic pattern of inheritance in which one of an allelic pair of genes has the capacity to suppress the expression of the other so that the first prevails in the heterozygote. **2.** Often, the preferred hand or side of the body, as in right-hand dominance. **3.** In psychiatry, the tendency to be commanding or controlling of others.

***ocular d.*** The use of one eye by choice for particular tasks such as aiming a gun. This may or may not be related to right-hand or left-hand dominance.

**dominant** In genetics, concerning a trait or characteristic that is expressed in the offspring although it is carried on only one of the homologous chromosomes. SEE: *recessive.*

**domoic acid** An excitotoxin reported to have contaminated mussels.

**Donath-Landsteiner phenomenon** (dō′năth-lănd′stī-nĕr) [Julius Donath, Austrian physician, 1870–1950; Karl L. Landsteiner, Austrian-born U.S. biologist, 1868–1943] A test for paroxysmal hemoglobinuria. Blood from the patient is cooled to 5°C, and a cold hemolysin in the plasma combines with the red blood cells if the patient has the disease. On warming, the sensitized red cells are hemolyzed by the complement normally present.

**donation, organ** Donation of organs for transplantation in human beings. The success rate of transplantation procedures has led to a great demand for organ donation. Donating an organ does not disfigure the body of the deceased. The family of the donor is not responsible for the expense of providing the organ or tissue. The major religious organizations support organ and tissue donation. SEE: *donor card; transplantation.*

**donee** (dō-nē′) [L. *donare,* to give] One who receives something, such as a blood transfusion, from a donor.

**Don Juan** [After the legendary, promiscuous Spanish nobleman, Don Juan de Tenorio] A man whose sexual promiscuity arises from insecurity concerning his masculinity or latent and unconscious homosexual preference.

**Donnan's equilibrium** (dŏn′ănz) [Frederick G. Donnan, Brit. chemist, 1871–1956] A condition in which an equilibrium is established between two solutions separated by a semipermeable membrane so that the sum of the anions and cations on one side is equal to that on the other side.

**Donohue's syndrome** SEE: *leprechaunism.*

**donor 1.** A person who furnishes blood, tissue, or an organ to be used in another person. **2.** In chemistry, a compound that frees part of itself to unite with another compound called an acceptor.

***universal d.*** A person whose blood is of group O and is therefore usually compatible with most other blood types. In actual practice this compatibility rarely occurs because of the many factors besides the major blood antigens (A, B, AB) that determine compatibility.

**donor card** A document used by a person who wishes to make an anatomical gift, at the time of his or her death, of an organ or other body part needed for transplantation. SEE: illus.; *transplantation.*

**do not attempt resuscitation** ABBR: DNAR. An order somewhat more precise than "do not resuscitate" (DNR). DNR implies that, if a resuscitation attempt is made, the patient can be revived. DNAR indicates that resuscitation efforts should not be attempted regardless of their expected outcome. SEE: *do not resuscitate.*

**do not resuscitate** ABBR: DNR. An order stating that a patient should not be revived. It may be written by a physician at the patient's request. If the patient is not competent or is unable to make such a decision, the family, legal guardian, or health care proxy may request and give consent for such an order to be written on the patient's chart and followed by the health care providers. The hospital or physician should have policies regarding time limits and reordering. SEE: *do not attempt resuscitation.*

**Donovan body** [Charles Donovan, Ir. physician, 1863–1951] The common name for the causative organism, *Calymmatobacterium granulomatis,* of granuloma inguinale.

**donovanosis** SEE: *granuloma inguinale.*

**dopa** A chemical substance, 3,4-dihydroxyphenylalanine, produced by the oxidation of tyrosine to tyrosinase. It is a precursor of catecholamines and melanin.

**dopamine hydrochloride** (dō′pă-mēn) **1.** A catecholamine synthesized by the adrenal gland. It is the immediate precursor in the synthesis of norepinephrine. Dopamine is used to treat hypotension unrelated to hypovolemia (which should be treated with transfusions, intravenous fluids, and surgery). It has different actions at various doses. Low doses (2 to 5 μg/kg/min) cause increased renal and mesenteric blood flow. Intermediate doses (5 to 15 μg/kg/min) increase cardiac contractility, which increases cardiac output, blood pressure, and perfusion pressure. High doses (above 15 μg/kg/min) cause generalized vasoconstriction by activating alpha-adrenergic receptors. It is also used in the treatment of shock. **2.** A catecholamine neurotransmitter, or brain messenger, implicated in some forms of psychosis and abnormal movement disorders.

---

Caution: This drug should not be adminis-

# UNIFORM DONOR CARD

OF__________________________________________

Print or type name of donor

In the hope that I may help others, I hereby make this anatomical gift, if medically acceptable, to take effect upon my death. The words and marks below indicate my desires.

I give: (a) _____ any needed organs or parts

(b) _____ only the following organs or parts

__________________________________________

Specify the organ(s) or part(s)

for the purposes of transplantation, therapy, medical research or education;

(c) _____ my body for anatomical study if needed.

Limitations or special wishes, if any:____________________________

Signed by the donor and the following two witnesses in the presence of each other:

____________________ ____________________

Signature of Donor — Date of Birth of Donor

____________________ ____________________

Date Signed — City & State

____________________ ____________________

Witness — Witness

This is a legal document under the Uniform Anatomical Gift Act or similar laws.

tered by intravenous push. The intravenous line should be monitored frequently to make certain there is no extravasation. Other drugs should not be administered in the same intravenous line. Use is discontinued gradually. When dopamine is used in life-threatening states of shock, blood pressure and renal function must be monitored carefully.

**dopaminergic** (dō″pă-mĕn-ĕr′jĭk) **1.** Caused by dopamine. **2.** Concerning tissues that are influenced by dopamine.

**dopa-oxidase** (dō″pă-ŏk′sĭ-dās) An enzyme in some epithelial cells that converts dopa to melanin.

**dope** An imprecise slang term used to describe almost any drug of abuse. SEE: *doping; doping, blood.*

**doping** In athletic medicine, use of a drug or blood product by an athlete to improve performance. The existence of a drug that safely accomplishes this has not been demonstrated. The administration of anabolic hormones to women causes signs of masculinization, including facial hair growth, deepening of the voice, and clitoromegaly.

***blood d.*** The practice by athletes of storing several units of their own blood and having it transfused to themselves a day or two before competition. The safety and effectiveness of this practice is questionable, and it is unapproved by sports governing bodies.

**Doppler echocardiography** A sensitive, noninvasive technique for determining the blood flow velocity in different locations in the heart. It is an adaptation of ultrasound technology. This same method can be used in determining the uterine artery blood flow velocity during pregnancy. SEE: *echocardiography*.

**Doppler effect** (dŏp′lĕr) [Johann Christian Doppler, Austrian scientist, 1803–1853] The variation of the apparent frequency of waves, such as sound waves, with change in distance between the source and the receiver. The frequency seems to increase as the distance decreases and to decrease as the distance increases.

**Doppler measurement of blood pressure and fetal heart rate** Use of Doppler sound waves to determine systolic blood pressure, as well as to determine the fetal heart rate.

**doraphobia** (dō″ră-fō′bē-ă) [Gr. *dora*, hide, + *phobos*, fear] Abnormal aversion to touching the hair or fur of animals.

**Dorello's canal** [Primo Dorello, It. anatomist, 1872–1963] A bony canal in the tip of the temporal bone enclosing the abducens nerve.

**Dorendorf's sign** [Hans Dorendorf, Ger. physician, b. 1866] A filling or fullness of the supraclavicular groove in an aneurysm of the aortic arch.

**dormancy 1.** The condition of greatly reduced metabolic activity that permits long-term survival and possible reactivation. The term refers to bacterial endospores, protozoan cysts, larval stages of some worm parasites, and viruses such as herpesviruses. **2.** The state in which a disease or disease process is no longer active. **dormant,** *adj.*

**dornase** (dor′nās) Short for deoxyribonuclease.

***pancreatic d.*** Dornase prepared from beef pancreas, used to loosen thick pulmonary secretions.

**dors-** SEE: *dorso-*.

**dorsabdominal** [L. *dorsum*, back, + *abdomen*, belly] Pert. to the back and abdomen.

**dorsad** [″ + *ad*, toward] Toward the back.

**dorsal** [L. *dorsum*, back] **1.** Pert. to the back. **2.** Indicating a position toward a rear part; opposed to ventral.

**dorsal cord stimulation** A procedure for relieving pain by electric stimulation of the spinal cord through electrodes sutured to the posterior spinal cord.

**dorsalgia** (dōr-săl′jē-ă) [″ + Gr. *algos*, pain] Pain in the back. SYN: *notalgia*.

**dorsalis** (dor-sā′lĭs) [L.] Dorsal (i.e., pert. to the back).

**dorsal nerve** A branch of spinal nerves that pass dorsally to innervate skin, muscle, and bone near the vertebral column; also called a *dorsal ramus* or *posterior branch*.

**dorsal reflex** Irritation of the skin over the erector spinae muscles, causing contraction of muscles of the back.

**dorsal rigid posture** A position in which both legs (or the right leg only) are drawn up. It is observed in peritonitis, meningitis, ascites, and tympanites. The right leg is drawn up in appendicitis, pelvic inflammation, renal calculus in the right ureter, psoas abscess, and peritonitis on the right side.

**dorsal slit** A surgical method of making the foreskin of the penis easily retractable. The foreskin is cut in the dorsal midline but not far enough to extend into the mucous membrane next to the glans.

**dorsi-** SEE: *dorso-*.

**dorsiduct** [L. *dorsum*, back, + *ducere*, to lead] To draw toward the back or backward.

**dorsiduction** Drawing toward the back.

**dorsiflect** (dor′sĭ-flĕkt) [″ + *flectere*, to bend] To bend backward.

**dorsiflexion** Movement of a part at a joint to bend the part toward the dorsum, or posterior aspect of the body. Thus, dorsiflexion of the foot indicates movement backward, in which the foot moves toward its top, or dorsum; the opposite of plantar flexion. Dorsiflexion of the toes indicates a movement of the toes away from the sole of the foot. When the hand is extended, or bent backward at the wrist, it is dorsiflexed; this is the opposite of palmar flexion, or volar flexion of the wrist.

**dorsimesal** (dor″sĭ-mĕs′ăl) In the direction of the dorsimeson.

**dorsimeson** (dor-sĭ-mĕs′ŏn) [″ + Gr. *meson*, middle] The median plane of the back.

**dorsispinal** (dor″sĭ-spī′năl) [″ + *spina*, thorn] Pert. to the back and spine.

**dorso-, dorsi-, dors-** Combining form indicating *back*.

**dorsocephalad** (dor″sō-sĕf′ă-lăd) [″ + Gr. *kephale*, head, + L. *ad*, toward] Situated toward the back of the head.

**dorsodynia** (dor″sō-dĭn′ē-ă) [″ + Gr. *odyne*, pain] Pain in the muscles of the upper part of the back.

**dorsolateral** (dor″sō-lăt′ĕr-ăl) Pert. to the back and side.

**dorsolumbar** Pert. to the lower thoracic and upper lumbar (loin) area of the back.

**dorsoplantar** (dor″sō-plăn′tăr) [″ + *planta*, sole of the foot] From the top to the bottom of the foot.

**dorsosacral** [″ + *sacrum*, sacred bone] Pert. to the lower back.

**dorsoventral** (dor″sō-vĕn′trăl) Concerning the back and frontal surfaces of the body.

**dorsum** [L.] The back or posterior surface of a part; in the foot, the top of the foot.

**dosage** [Gr. *dosis*, a giving] The determination of the amount, frequency, and number of doses of medication or radiation for a patient.

***d. calculation for children*** Specialized determination of dosage allowing for smaller size. There is no absolutely reliable formula for calculating the dosage of a medicine an infant or child should receive. Several rules for calculating a child's dosage have been used in the past, but those that use body surface area are most accurate. SEE: *body surface area*.

**dose** (dōs) [Gr. *dosis*, a giving] The amount of medicine or radiation to be administered at one time.

***absorbed d.*** SEE: under *radiation.*

***air d.*** The intensity of radiation measured in air at the target.

***bolus d.*** An amount of medicine given intravenously at a controlled but rapid rate.

***booster d.*** SEE: *booster.*

***cumulative d.*** **1.** The total dose resulting from repeated exposure to radiation, either to one site or to the whole body. **2.** The amount of a drug present in the body after repeated doses.

***curative d.*** The dose required to cure an illness or disease.

***divided d.*** Fractional portions administered at short intervals.

***equianalgesic d.*** A dose of one form of analgesic drug equivalent in pain-relieving potential to another analgesic. In pain control, this equivalence permits substitution of one analgesic to avoid undesired side effects from another.

***erythema d.*** The smallest amount of radiation that will produce erythema within 2 weeks following treatment. SYN: *threshold d.*

***fatal d.*** A dose that kills. SEE: *median lethal d.*

***infective d.*** The amount of an infectious organism, esp. a bacterium or virus, that will cause disease.

***maintenance d.*** The dose required to maintain the desired effect.

***maximum d.*** The largest dose that is safe to administer.

***maximum permissible d.*** ABBR: MPD. The highest dose of radiation allowed to a person exposed over 1 year. Lower MPDs exist for the general public than for occupationally exposed individuals.

***mean marrow d.*** ABBR: MMD. An estimated measure of average exposure to the entire active bone marrow by ionizing radiation. The percentage of active bone marrow in the useful beam is multiplied by the average absorbed dose.

***median curative d.*** A dose that cures half of the persons treated.

***median infective d.*** An infective dose that causes disease in half of the susceptible subjects given that dose.

***median lethal d.*** ABBR: $LD_{50}$. The amount of a substance, bacterium, or toxin that will kill 50% of the animals exposed to it. SEE: *minimum lethal d.*

***minimum d.*** The smallest effective dose.

***minimum lethal d.*** The smallest amount of a substance capable of producing death. SEE: *median lethal d.*

***primary d.*** The initial, large dose given to provide a high blood level without delay.

***skin d.*** A radiation dose to the skin including secondary radiation from backscatter.

***therapeutic d.*** The dose required to produce the desired effect.

***threshold d.*** Erythema d.

***tissue tolerance d.*** The largest dose, esp. of radiation, that will not harm tissues.

***tolerance d.*** The dose of a drug or physical agent such as radiation that can be received without harm. This dose will vary between individuals.

***toxic d.*** A dose that causes signs and symptoms of drug toxicity.

**dose response curve** A graph that charts the effect of a specific dose of drug, chemical, or ionizing radiation. In radiology, also called *survival curve.*

**dosimeter** (dō-sĭm′ĭ-tĕr) [″ + *metron,* measure] A device for measuring x-ray output.

**dosimetric** (dō″sĭ-mĕt′rĭk) Pert. to dosimetry.

**dosimetry** (dō-sĭm′ĕ-trē) [″ + *metron,* measure] Measurement of doses.

**DOT** *directly observed therapy.*

**dotage** [ME. *doten,* to be silly] Senility; the feeblemindedness of very old age.

**double** (dŭb′l) [L. *duplus,* twofold] Being twofold; combining two qualities.

**double-blind technique** A method of scientific investigation in which neither the subject nor the investigator knows what treatment, if any, the subject is receiving. At the completion of the experiment, the "code" is broken and data are analyzed with respect to the various treatments used. This method attempts to eliminate observer and subject bias. SEE: *open-label study.*

**double chin** Buccula.

**double personality** A split in consciousness, neither personality being aware of the actions and words of the other. SEE: *multiple personality.*

**double reading** Evaluation of the results of a test, especially a mammogram, by two individuals. SEE: *mammography.*

**double touch** Exploration with a finger in one cavity and the thumb in another.

**double uterus** Dihysteria. SYN: *uterus didelphys.*

**double vision** Two images of an object seen at the same time. SYN: *diplopia.*

**doubling time** The time required to double in size, as in the growth of a malignant tumor.

**douche** (doosh) [Fr.] A current of vapor or a stream of hot or cold water directed against a part. A douche may be plain water or a medicated solution. It may be for personal hygiene or treatment of a local condition.

***air d.*** An air current directed onto the body for therapeutic purposes, usually directed to the tympanum for opening the eustachian tube.

***astringent d.*** A douche containing substances such as alum or zinc sulfate for shrinking the mucous membrane.

***circular d.*** A needle spray or application of water to the body through horizontal needle-sized jets. Several small rows of sprays project the water from four directions simultaneously.

***cleansing d.*** An external or perineal douche for cleansing genitalia following defecation or after operations such as hemorrhoidectomy, curettage, rectal surgery, circumcision, or perineorrhaphy. A mild antiseptic or disinfectant solution, 98° to 104°F (36.7° to 40°C), is poured or sprayed over the parts, followed by gentle drying and inspection for cleanliness.

***deodorizing d.*** A douche used to deodorize the vagina and vaginal secretions when they have an offensive odor.

***high d.*** A douche in which the bag is at least 4 ft (1.2 m) above the hips of the patient.

***jet d.*** A douche applied to the body in a solid stream from the douche hose.

***medicated d.*** A douche containing a medicinal substance for the treatment of local conditions.

***nasal d.*** An injection of fluid into the nostril with fluid escaping through the nasopharynx out of the mouth. The patient should keep the mouth open and the glottis closed to prevent fluid from entering the throat and bronchus, and should not blow his or her nose during the treatment. The force of the douche must be moderate. The container should not be suspended more than 6 in. (9.2 cm) above the patient. An atomized spray works more quickly.

***neutral d.*** A douche given at the average surface temperature of the body (i.e., 90° to 97°F [32.2° to 36.1°C]).

***perineal d.*** A spray projected upward from a bidet, placed just above the floor; the patient sits on the seat and receives the douche on the perineum.

***vaginal d.*** A douche of the vagina used for deodorant, antiseptic, stimulating, or hemostatic purposes. The temperature of the solutions varies: for an antiseptic or deodorant douche, 105° to 112°F (40.6° to 44.4°C); for a stimulating or hemostatic douche, 118° to 120°F (47.8° to 48.9°C). The solution should flow slowly with little pressure, the container being elevated up to 2 ft (61 cm) above the patient's pelvis. The quantity generally is 2 to 3 qt (2 or 3 L) of solution unless otherwise ordered.

NOTE: The vagina, like many other areas of the body, can cleanse itself. Thus there is very little reason for a normal, healthy woman to use a vaginal douche. Douching can upset the balance of the vaginal flora and change the vaginal pH, thus predisposing the woman to vaginitis. There is no evidence that a postcoital vaginal douche is effective as a contraceptive.

In at least one investigation, vaginal douching has been shown to be a risk factor for pelvic inflammatory disease (PID). The more frequently the subjects douched, the more likely they were to have PID.

**Douglas bag** [Claude G. Douglas, Brit. physiologist, 1882–1963] A container, usually a bag made of flexible material, for collecting expired air. It is used in investigating respiratory function and physiology.

**Douglas' cul-de-sac, Douglas' pouch** [James Douglas, Scot. anatomist, 1675–1742] The peritoneal space or pouch that lies behind uterus and in front of rectum.

**Douglas' fold** The arcuate line of the sheath of the rectus abdominis muscle.

**douglasitis** (dŭg-lăs-ī′tĭs) Inflammation of Douglas' cul-de-sac.

**dowager's hump** Cervical lordosis with dorsal kyphosis due to slow, painless loss of bone (i.e., osteoporosis). This may occur at any age but is seen most commonly in elderly women. SEE: *buffalo hump.*

**dowel** [ME. *dowle,* peg] A metal pin for fastening an artificial crown to a tooth root.

**down 1.** Lanugo, the fine hairs of the skin of the newborn. **2.** The fine soft feathers of the young of some birds; and the small feathers underneath the large feathers of adult birds, particularly waterfowl. It is used in clothing to protect from the cold.

**downregulate** To inhibit or suppress the normal response of an organ or system (e.g., the immune system or the central nervous system). SEE: *immunocompromised.*

**Down syndrome** [J. Langdon Down, Brit. physician, 1828–1896] A variety of congenital moderate-to-severe mental retardation. It is marked by a sloping forehead, small ear canals, gray or very light yellow spots at the periphery of the iris (Brushfield's spots), short broad hands with a single palmar crease (simian crease), a flat nose or absent bridge, low-set ears, and generally dwarfed physique. SYN: *trisomy 21.* SEE: *amniocentesis; Nursing Diagnoses Appendix.*

Women at high risk of giving birth to a child with Down syndrome are those over 40; those who have had a previous child with the syndrome; and those who themselves have Down syndrome (pregnancy is rare in this condition). In addition, there is a high risk of having a child with Down syndrome when there is parental mosaicism with a 21 trisomic cell population.

Down syndrome may be diagnosed antenatally by several techniques.

ETIOLOGY: Patients with Down syndrome have an extra chromosome, usually number 21 or 22.

**doxapram hydrochloride** (dŏk′să-prăm) A respiratory stimulant.

**doxorubicin hydrochloride** (dŏk″sō-rū′bĭ-sĭn) An antineoplastic antibiotic agent.

**doxycycline** (dŏk″sē-sī′klēn) A broad-spectrum antibiotic of the tetracycline group.

**doxylamine succinate** (dŏk-sĭl′ă-mēn) An antihistamine.

**Doyère's eminence** (dwă-yārz′) [Louis Doyère, Fr. physiologist, 1811–1863] An elevation where a nerve filament enters a muscle.

**D.P.** *Doctor of Pharmacy.*

**2,3-D.P.G.** *2,3-diphosphoglycerate.*

**D.P.H.** *Diploma in Public Health.*

**D.P.M.** *Doctor of Podiatric Medicine.*

**DR** *reaction of degeneration.*

**Dr.** *Doctor.*

**dr** *drachm; dram.*

**drachm** Dram.

**dracontiasis** (drăk″ŏn-tī′ă-sĭs) [Gr. *drakontion,* little dragon] Dracunculiasis.

**dracunculiasis** (dră-kŭng″kū-lī′ă-sĭs) Infestation with the nematode *Dracunculus medinensis.*

**dracunculosis** (dră-kŭng″kū-lō′sĭs) Dracunculiasis.

**Dracunculus** (dră-kŭng′kū-lŭs) A genus of parasitic nematodes.

***D. medinensis*** The guinea worm or "fiery serpent." This species of nematode is a common human parasite, esp. in Africa and India. Infection of humans occurs when water containing infected crustacea of the genus *Cyclops* is swallowed. The larvae are liberated in the stomach or duodenum, then migrate through the viscera and become adults. The adult female, after mating, burrows under the skin of the leg. Larvae are discharged into the environment through the ulcer caused by the worm, esp. when the legs are in water. The infection may be prevented by boiling suspect water, treating it with chlorine, or filtering it to remove the infected *Cyclops.*

TREATMENT: The head of the adult worm can be seen in the ulcer. Slow traction on the worm will remove it. This is done by making a small incision, grasping the front end of the worm, and winding it around a small object. The winding is increased each day until the worm is removed. It is important not to break the worm. Use of thiabendazole or metranidazole has no effect on the worms themselves but produces resolution of the skin inflammation in several days. Unerupted worms may be removed surgically under local anesthesia. SEE: illus.

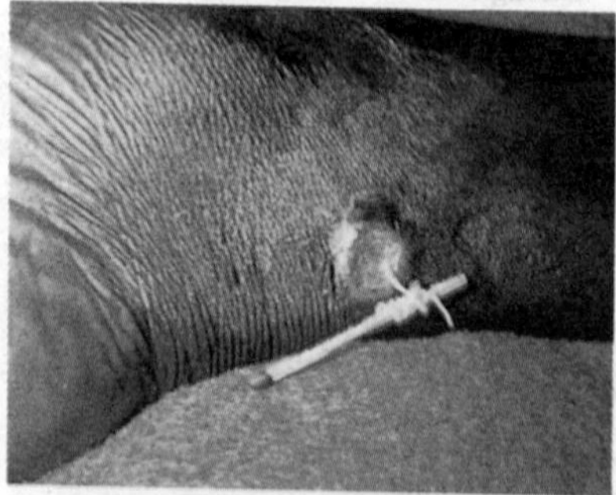

**DRACUNCULUS MEDINENSIS**
GUINEA WORM BEING REMOVED FROM ULCER

**draft, draught** A dose of liquid medicine intended to be taken all at once.

**drain** (drān) [AS. *dreahnian,* to draw off] **1.** An exit or tube for discharge of a morbid matter. **2.** To draw off a fluid.

***capillary d.*** A drawing off by capillary attraction.

***cigarette d.*** A drain made by covering a small strip of gauze with rubber.

***Mikulicz's d.*** SEE: *Mikulicz's drain.*

***nonabsorbable d.*** A drain made from horsehair, gauze, rubber, glass, or metal. Types are abdominal, antrum, perineal, and suprapubic.

***Penrose d.*** A cigarette drain made with a piece of small rubber tubing through which gauze has been pulled.

**drainage** (drān′ĭj) The free flow or withdrawal of fluids from a wound or cavity, such as pus from a cavity or wound. SEE: *autodrainage; drain.*

***capillary d.*** Drainage by means of capillary attraction.

***chest d.*** Placement of a drainage tube in the chest cavity, usually in the pleural space. The tube is used to drain air, fluid, or blood from the pleural space so the compressed and collapsed lung can expand. The tube is connected to a system that produces suction. This helps to remove the material from the pleural space and also prevents air from being sucked into the space.

***closed d.*** Drainage of a wound or body space so that the air is excluded.

***closed sterile d.*** A sterile tube draining a body site, such as the abdominal cavity or pleural space, that is designed to prevent the entry of air and bacteria into the tubing or the area being drained.

***negative pressure d.*** Drainage in which negative pressure is maintained in the tube. It is used in treating pneumothorax and in certain types of drains or catheters in the intestinal tract. SYN: *suction d.*

***open d.*** Drainage of a wound or body cavity so that does not exclude air from the area of the cavity.

***postural d.*** Drainage for the nasal area, bronchi, and sinuses. The patient is placed so that gravity will allow drainage. SEE: *postural drainage* for illus.

***suction d.*** Negative pressure d.

***tidal d.*** A method, controlled mechanically, of filling the bladder with solution by gravity and periodically emptying the bladder by siphonage. It is usually used when the patient lacks bladder control as in injuries or lesions of the spinal cord.

***Wangensteen d.*** SEE: *Wangensteen tube.*

**drainage tube** A device for allowing escape of pus, serum, blood, or other fluids from a wound or abscess.

**drained weight** The actual weight of food that has been allowed to drain to remove the liquids in which it has been prepared.

**dram** (drăm) [Gr. *drachme,* a Gr. unit of weight] ABBR: dr. SYMB: ʒ. A unit of weight in the apothecaries' system. SYN: *drachm.*

**Dramamine** (drăm'ă-mēn) Trade name for dimenhydrinate, the chlorotheophylline salt of the antihistaminic agent diphenhydramine. Dramamine has a depressant effect on hyperstimulated labyrinthine function and is used to treat or prevent nausea, vomiting, vertigo, and motion sickness.

**dramatism** [Gr. *drama,* acting, + *-ismos,* condition] Dramatic behavior and lofty speech seen in psychological disturbances.

**drapetomania** (drăp"ĕt-ō-mā'nē-ă) [Gr. *drapetes,* runaway, + *mania,* madness] An insane impulse to wander from home.

**drastic** [Gr. *drastikos,* effective] **1.** Acting strongly. **2.** A very active cathartic, usually producing many explosive bowel movements accompanied by pain and tenesmus. The use of this type of cathartic is not advisable.

**draught** (drăft) [ME. *draught,* a pulling] **1.** A drink. **2.** Liquid drawn into the mouth. **3.** A breeze produced by wind or a fan. **4.** Draft.

**Draw-a-Person test** A widely used projective assessment that is assumed to reveal information about a patient's body image or self-concept. SYN: *Machover test.*

**drawer sign, drawer test** A sign diagnostic of rupture of the cruciate ligament(s) of the knee. The knee is flexed to 90 degrees with the foot stabilized on the examination table. The examiner applies an anterior, then a posterior, force against the upper tibia, perpendicular to the long axis of the leg. An increased glide, anterior or posterior, of the tibia is caused by rupture of the anterior or posterior cruciate ligament, respectively. This is sometimes called the "draw sign."

**draw sheet** Historically, the term designating a long roll or bolt of muslin that was stretched across the width of the bed with the free end initially placed under the patient's buttocks. When this became soiled, it was drawn from under the patient and rolled up on the opposite side of the cot or bed, allowing the patient to lie on a clean section of the roll of muslin.

The draw sheet is used to protect the bottom sheet and mattress from drainage and soilage and is easier to change, for both the patient and nurse, than the entire bed. When a draw sheet is folded and placed under a patient to use for lifting and turning, it is called a lift sheet. In many hospitals, draw sheets have been replaced by paper and plastic pads that resemble disposable diapers.

**DRE** *digital rectal examination.*

**dream** [AS. *dream,* joy] The occurrence of ideas, emotions, and sensations during sleep. Some dreams may be recalled on awakening; others may not be. SEE: *REM; sleep; sleep disorder; wet dream.*

Interpretation of the meaning of dreams has been of interest to the laity as well as psychoanalysts, not to mention the person who recalls having the dream. The idea that a dream conceals a meaning buried deep in the subconscious is controversial. A dream may reveal more than it conceals. Any idea, emotion, or wish may be the subject of a dream. Less controversial are the research results correlating changes in the electroencephalogram and rapid eye movements (REM) during sleep with dream activity. Under experimental conditions, it has been possible to communicate with the person who is dreaming. Some lower animals (i.e., cats and dogs) dream. There is no evidence that two people asleep together have the same dream simultaneously.

**drench** A dose of medicine that is administered to an animal by pouring into its mouth.

**drepanocyte** (drĕp'ă-nō-sīt) [Gr. *drepane,* sickle, + *kytos,* cell] Crescent or sickle cell.

**drepanocytemia** (drĕp"ă-nō-sī-tē'mē-ă) [" + " + *haima,* blood] Sickle cell anemia.

**drepanocytic** (drĕp"ă-nō-sĭt'ĭk) Pert. to or resembling a sickle cell.

**dressing** [O. Fr. *dresser,* to prepare] A covering, protective or supportive, for diseased or injured parts.

NURSING IMPLICATIONS: The procedure and expected sensations are explained, patient privacy is ensured, and necessary equipment assembled. Strict aseptic technique is followed during dressing changes; dressings are properly disposed of, and hands are washed before and after the procedure. The wound or incision and dressing are assessed for the presence and character of any drainage and the findings are documented. The condition of the wound or suture line is also checked, and the presence of erythema or edema is noted. Instruction in wound assessment and dressing change techniques is provided.

***absorbent d.*** A dressing consisting of gauze, sterilized gauze, or absorbent cotton.

***antiseptic d.*** A dressing consisting of gauze permeated with an antiseptic solution.

***clear transparent covering d.*** Transparent synthetic d.

***dry d.*** A dressing consisting of dry gauze, absorbent cotton, or other dry material.

***hot moist d.*** A dressing that most commonly uses a normal saline solution no hotter than the bare forearm of the nurse can tolerate. The sterile towel is unfolded, and the gauze dressing is dropped into it. Then the center of the towel is immersed in solution and wrung out by turning the dry ends in opposite directions. The dressing is applied with sterile forceps directly to the wound. Sometimes a dry sterile towel is used over it to keep the dressing in place. Heat is best maintained by infrared lamp.

Caution: Care must be taken not to burn the patient.

***hydrocolloid d.*** A flexible dressing made of an adhesive, gumlike (hydrocolloid) material such as karaya or pectin covered with a water-resistant film. The dressing keeps the wound surface moist, but, because it excludes air, it may promote anaerobic bacterial growth. It should not be used on wounds that are, or are suspected to be, infected. The directions that come with the dressing should be followed.

***nonadherent d.*** A dressing that has little or no tendency to adhere to dried secretions from the wound.

***occlusive d.*** A dressing that seals a wound completely to prevent infection from outside and to prevent inner moisture from escaping through the dressing.

***pressure d.*** A dressing used to apply pressure to the wound. It may be used following skin grafting.

***protective d.*** A dressing applied for the purpose of preventing injury or infection to the treated part.

***self-adhering roller d.*** A rolled gauze strip made of a material that adheres to one side of the gauze. It comes in various widths.

***transparent synthetic d.*** A dressing usually made of a plastic material with the skin-contact side coated with a hypoallergenic adhesive. SYN: *clear transparent covering d.*

***universal d.*** A large flat bandage that may be folded several times to make a relatively large dressing or folded several more times to make a smaller and thicker dressing. This process can be continued until the unit is suitable for use as a cervical collar. The bandage is easily made and stored. SEE: illus.

***water d.*** A dressing consisting of gauze, cotton, or similar material that is kept wet by the application of sterilized water.

***wet-to-dry d.*** A dressing consisting of gauze moistened by sterile saline applied directly to the wound and covered with dry gauze pads and a bandage. It is used to prevent gauze from adhering to the wound.

**dressing stick** An adaptive device designed to permit independent dressing by persons with limited motion. SYN: *dressing wand.*

**Dressler's syndrome** [William Dressler, U.S. physician, 1890-1960] Postmyocardial infarction syndrome.

**DRG** *diagnosis-related group.*

**drift** Movement due to an external force, often in an aimless fashion.

***genetic d.*** The chance variation of genetic frequency, seen most often in a small population.

***mesial d.*** Movement of teeth in the arch in a mesial or ventral direction due to occlusal forces and interproximal wear of teeth.

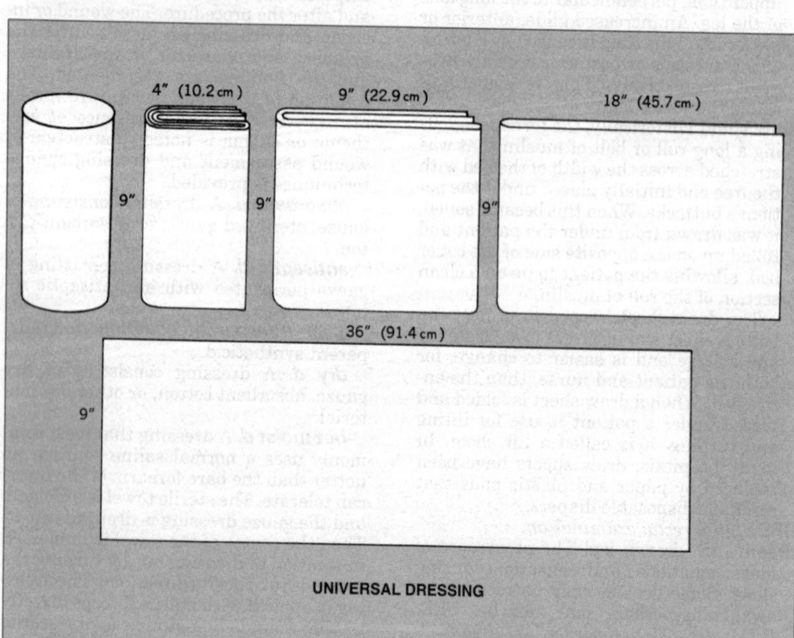


UNIVERSAL DRESSING

**drill** A device for rotating a sharp and shaped cutting instrument, used for preparing teeth for restoration and in orthopedics. SEE: *bur*.

**Drinker respirator** [Philip Drinker, U.S. engineer in industrial hygiene, 1894–1972] An apparatus in which alternating positive and negative air pressure on the patient's thoracic area produces artificial respiration by allowing the air in the otherwise immobile lung to be alternately filled with air and emptied. This device is commonly called an *iron lung*.

**drip** [ME. *drippen,* to drip] **1.** To fall in drops. **2.** To instill a liquid slowly, drop by drop.

***intravenous d.*** Slow injection of a solution into a vein a drop at a time.

***Murphy d.*** Slow rectal instillation of a fluid drop by drop.

***nasal d.*** A method of administering fluid slowly to dehydrated babies by means of a catheter with one end placed through the nose into the esophagus.

***postnasal d.*** A condition due to chronic sinusitis in which a discharge flows from the postnasal region into the pharynx.

**drive** (drīv) [AS. *drifan*] The force or impulse to act.

**drive control** One of various devices and adapted equipment, including hand or foot controls, for modifying a motor vehicle for use by persons with physical disability.

**dromomania** (drō″mō-mā′nē-ă) [Gr. *dromos,* a running, + *mania,* madness] An insane impulse to wander.

**dromostanolone propionate** (drō″mō-stăn′ō-lōn) An antineoplastic drug.

**dromotropic** [″ + *tropikos,* a turning] Affecting the conductivity of nerve or muscle fibers. SEE: *inotropic*.

**dronabinol** The principal psychoactive substance present in Cannabis sativa (marijuana). The trade name is Marinol. SEE: *marijuana*.

**drop** [AS. *dropa*] **1.** A minute spherical mass of liquid. **2.** Failure of a part to maintain its normal position, usually due to paralysis or injury.

***culture d.*** A bacterial culture in a drop of culture medium.

***foot d.*** A condition in which the toes drag and the foot hangs, caused by paralysis of the anterior tibial muscles.

***hanging d.*** Application of a drop of solution to a small glass coverslip. This is then inverted over a glass slide with a depression in it. The contents of the suspended solution can be examined microscopically.

***knock-out d.'s*** The mythical nonlethal dose (i.e., a few drops) of a substance such as chloral hydrate that is erroneously thought to cause immediate unconsciousness if given orally or mixed with an alcoholic beverage. Movies have perpetrated and perpetuated this myth.

***nose d.'s*** Medication instilled in or sprayed into the nasal cavity.

***wrist d.*** Paralysis of extensor muscles causing the hand to hang down from the forearm.

**drop attack** A condition of unknown origin marked by falling, often without warning, with loss of consciousness or dizziness. Patients are usually elderly and female. The sudden fall is usually forward and occurs while walking or standing. The attacks may occur several times over a period of weeks and then do not recur. The only treatment necessary is therapy for trauma caused by the fall. SEE: *stroke; transient ischemic attack*.

**droperidol** (drō-pĕr′ĭ-dŏl) A drug used for premedication for surgery. It is neuroleptic, sedative, and tranquilizing.

**droplet** A very small drop.

**droplet infection** Invasion of a pathogenic agent conveyed by particles, as when carried in a spray from the nose or mouth. This is the usual mode of transmission for the common cold.

**dropper** A tube, usually narrowed at one end, for dispensing drops of liquid. If water is so dispensed, about 20 drops equals 1 ml. SEE: *medicine dropper*.

***medicine d.*** According to *USP XXII,* a tube made of glass or other suitable transparent material that generally is fitted with a collapsible bulb and, while varying in capacity, is constricted at the delivery end to a round opening having an external diameter of 3 mm. When held vertically, it delivers water in drops each weighing between 45 mg and 55 mg.

In using a medicine dropper, one should keep in mind that few medicinal liquids have the same surface and flow characteristics as water, and therefore the size of drops may vary considerably from one preparation to another.

When accurate dosing is important, one should use a dropper that has been calibrated for and supplied with the preparation. The volume error incurred in measuring any liquid by means of a calibrated dropper should not exceed 15% under normal use conditions.

**dropsy** (drŏp′sē) [Gr. *hydor,* water] An obsolete term for generalized edema.

**Drosophila** (drō-sŏf′ĭ-lă) A genus of flies belonging to the order Diptera. Includes the common fruit flies.

***D. melanogaster*** A genus of fruit flies used extensively in the study of genetics. The development of the chromosome theory of heredity was largely the outcome of research on this species.

**drowning** [ME. *dr(o)unen,* to drown] Asphyxiation due to immersion in liquid. It may also result from a spasm of the glottis that allows neither air nor water to pass into the lungs (dry drowning). An acute asphyxial reaction to ingested water or liquid followed by laryngeal relaxation and flooding of the respiratory tract with water is another mechanism of drowning

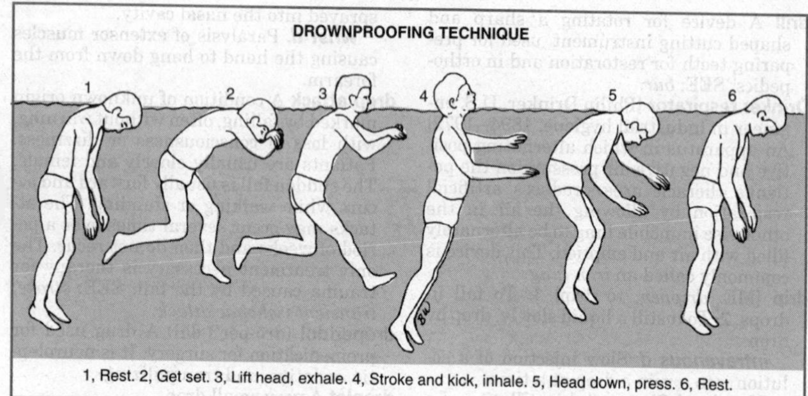

1, Rest. 2, Get set. 3, Lift head, exhale. 4, Stroke and kick, inhale. 5, Head down, press. 6, Rest.

(wet drowning). Drowning can occasionally result from vagally induced cardiac arrest after immersion in extremely cold water.

NOTE: Delayed death due to hypoxia can occur 15 min to 3 days after immersion. It is imperative that resuscitated patients be kept in the hospital for observation until this possibility can be excluded or treated if it occurs.

SYMPTOMS: The symptoms of drowning include unconsciousness, cessation of respiration, and cyanosis, depending on the duration of submersion. Due to action of the epiglottis, there is very little, if any, water in the lung.

FIRST AID: Immediate efforts to aerate the victim's lungs are essential, but this will be futile if the airway is not clear. Abdominal thrust maneuver should not be used routinely but reserved for when the airway is obstructed with a foreign body or when the victim fails to respond to mouth-to-mouth ventilation. An abdominal thrust may lead to regurgitation and pulmonary aspiration of gastric contents. Air may be administered artificially by any means available including mouth-to-mouth resuscitation. Cardiac resuscitation may be required.

It is important to examine for head or neck injuries, esp. if the patient was diving into water where it was possible to strike a submerged object. If there is damage to the head, neck, or vertebral column, it is important to keep the neck in a neutral position. SEE: *cardiopulmonary resuscitation; drownproofing*.

NOTE: Prolonged immersion does not necessarily mean that resuscitation will result in brain damage. This is true esp. if the individual has been immersed in very cold water. SEE: *diving reflex*.

**drownproofing** A method of staying afloat by using a minimum amount of energy. It may be kept up for hours even by nonswimmers, whereas only the most fit and expert could swim for more than 30 min. Details of the drownproofing technique may be obtained from local chapters of the American Red Cross. SEE: illus.

TECHNIQUE: 1. *Rest:* The person takes a deep breath and sinks vertically beneath the surface, relaxes the arms and legs, keeps the chin down, and allows the fingertips to brush against the knees. The neck is relaxed and the back of the head is above the surface. 2. *Get set:* The arms are raised gently to a crossed position with the back of the wrists touching the forehead. At the same time, the person steps forward with one leg and backward with the other. 3. *Lift head, exhale:* With the arms and legs in the previous position, the head is raised quickly but smoothly to the vertical position and the person exhales through the nose. 4. *Stroke and kick, inhale:* To support the head above the surface while inhaling through the mouth, the arms sweep gently outward and downward and both feet step downward. 5. *Head down, press:* As the person drops beneath the surface, the head goes down and the arms and hands press downward to arrest descent. 6. *Rest:* It is important to relax completely as in the first step for 6 to 10 sec.

**drowsiness** The state of almost falling asleep.

***daytime d.*** Drowsiness occurring during the day rather than just before normal bedtime. The cause may be inadequate sleep the preceding night; however, it may also be associated with anxiety, ill health, or side effects of either prescribed drugs or drugs of abuse. The condition is not equivalent to narcolepsy.

**Dr.P.H.** *Doctor of Public Health.*

**drug** [O. Fr. *drogue,* chemical material] Any substance that, when taken into a living organism, may modify one or more of its functions.

***"brake" d.*** A popular term for a hormonal agent that prevents excessive growth in children.

***"designer" d.*** [Term coined by Gary

Henderson, contemporary pharmacologist] An illicitly produced drug of abuse such as methamphetamine, fentanyl and its analogues, and phencyclidine hydrochloride (PCP). In several attempts to produce these drugs, toxic chemicals have been made. Also, the compounds are not standardized with respect to potency, so deaths from overdose may occur.

***generic d.*** SEE: *generic drug.*

***look-alike d.*** One of a group of solid dosage forms of drugs that mimic various prescription drugs by size, shape, color, and markings. Some of these may be controlled drugs.

***neuromuscular blocking d.*** A type of drug used during the administration of anesthesia to allow surgical access to body cavities, in particular the abdomen and thorax, by preventing voluntary or reflex muscle movement. These drugs are also used to facilitate compliance in critically ill patients undergoing intensive therapy such as mechanical ventilation.

***nonprescription d.*** Over-the-counter medication.

***recreational d.*** A drug used for enjoyment rather than for a medical purpose.

***scheduled d.*** SEE: *controlled substance act.*

***street d.*** A drug obtained illegally. Usually it is a drug of abuse.

**drug abuse** The use or overuse, usually by self-administration, of any drug in a manner that deviates from the prescribed pattern.

Health care workers, many of whom have easy access to narcotics, are at high risk of abusing analgesics. Increased awareness of this problem has led hospitals to establish special programs for identifying these individuals, esp. physicians, nurses, and pharmacists, in order to provide support and education in an attempt to control the problem and prevent loss of license.

**Drug Abuse Warning Network** ABBR: DAWN. A system for obtaining statistical data concerning admission to a sample of emergency treatment facilities for drug abuse.

**drug action** The function of a drug in various body systems.

*Local:* When the drug is applied locally or directly to a tissue or organ, it may combine with the cells' albumin to form an albuminate. This action may be (1) astringent when the drug cannot act because the albuminate does not dissolve, (2) corrosive when the drug is strong enough to destroy cells, or (3) irritating when too much of the drug combines with cells and impairs them.

*General, or systemic:* This type of action occurs when the drug enters the bloodstream by absorption or direct injection, affecting tissues and organs not near the site of entry. Systemic action may be (1) specific, when it cures a certain disease; (2) substitutive or replenishing, when it supplies substances deficient in the body; (3) physical, when some cell constituents are dissolved by the action of the drug in the bloodstream; (4) chemical, when the drug or some of its principles combine with the constituents of cells or organs to form a new chemical combination; (5) active by osmosis, caused by dilution of salt (also acids, sugars, and alkalies) in the stomach or intestines by fluid withdrawn from the blood and tissues; or by diffusion, when water is absorbed by cells from the lymph; (6) selective, when action is produced by drugs that affect only certain tissues or organs; (7) synergistic, when one drug increases the action of another; (8) antagonistic, when one drug counteracts another; (9) physiological, when the drug exerts a potentially beneficial effect similar to that which the body normally produces; (10) therapeutic, when the effect is to treat or repair diseased organs or tissues; (11) side active, creating an undesired effect; (12) empiric, producing results not proved by clinical or laboratory tests to be effective; or (13) toxicological, having a toxic or undesired effect, generally the result of overdose or long-term usage.

*Cumulative:* Some drugs are slowly excreted or absorbed so that with repeated doses an accumulation in the body produces a toxic effect. Such drugs should not be administered continuously.

*Incompatible:* Undesired side effects occur when some drugs are administered together. This may be due to the antagonistic action of one drug to others, or to a physical interaction of the drugs that inactivates one of them (e.g., precipitation of some drugs mixed in intravenous fluids).

**drug addiction** A condition caused by excessive or continued use of habit-forming drugs. Illicit drugs may or may not contain the kind and amount of drug the user thought was purchased. For this reason, a user may have a serious reaction (even death) to the unknown substance present in the material.

SYMPTOMS: The symptom pattern may change according to the drug used. In general there may be a change in personality, dulled or lost appetite, disturbance in normal sleep rhythm, and weight loss. The addict may be dull, sleepy, and uncoordinated in movement, having the appearance of intoxication. The eyes are often tearing and bloodshot; a watery fluid at times may drip from the nose. If intramuscular or intravenous injection has been used, there may be scars and hardening and swelling of the arm tissues. Hepatitis, AIDS, or both may occur when narcotic addicts use dirty needles and syringes to administer drugs to themselves or fellow addicts. SEE: *AIDS; hepatitis.*

**drug administration** *Acids:* When administered orally, acids should be given well diluted through a glass tube or by stomach tube because they are corrosive to the enamel and dentin of the teeth. They should be given with much water, and the drinking tube should be placed well back in the mouth to prevent the fluid coming in contact with the teeth before passing into the throat. Diluted hydrochloric acid is one preparation that should always be given using this technique.

*Habit-forming drugs:* These drugs should be given as ordered by the physician.

*Horse serum:* When injections containing it are administered, information should be obtained as to whether the patient has ever received vaccine containing horse serum and what reaction there was at that time. If the patient is allergic to horse serum, a sensitivity test should always be done by injecting hypodermically a few drops of the greatly diluted material containing horse serum. Reaction occurs within a short time. A small spot appears at the site of the injection if the patient is allergic. The physician will provide instructions for desensitizing a person allergic to horse serum.

*Insulin:* When insulin is administered, it should be given hypodermically or intravenously according to the instructions of the attending physician. The type of insulin, dosage, and dosing frequency vary greatly with each patient. SEE: *insulin pump.*

*Laxatives:* These are best given in the evening because they usually take 6 to 8 hr to produce an effect. Saline purgatives are usually given well diluted on an empty stomach in the morning. Other purgatives usually are given as ordered and needed.

*Mouthwash:* Stock solutions used for mouthwash should be diluted by half or more before being given to the patient. Only enough for the immediate mouth washing should be given to the patient at a particular time.

*Oxygen:* The most commonly used method for administration of oxygen consists of inserting a catheter into one or both nostrils. Oxygen may also be given from a tank by means of a mask over the patient's nose and mouth, or the patient may be placed in an oxygen tent, chamber, or room. The last two methods are not only expensive and less effective than use of a mask or nasal catheters but are also extremely dangerous and must be used cautiously because of the fire hazard. Oxygen given by catheter should be hydrated by bubbling through water before passage into the nose. Dry oxygen in high concentration for a prolonged period will cause severe irritation of the nasal and respiratory mucosa.

*Saline purgatives:* These should always be given to the patient when the stomach is empty, preferably in the morning.

*Sleeping pills:* All such preparations should be given from 30 min to 1 hr before sleep is desired. All procedures should be finished before the drug is given so that nothing disturbs the patient after the drug is administered.

*Vaccines:* If vaccines are alum precipitated or alumina absorbed, the preferred route of administration is intramuscular.

**drug delivery, new methods of** Several methods of drug delivery have been used experimentally. Included are chemical modification of a drug to enable it to penetrate membranes such as the blood-brain barrier; incorporation of microparticles in colloidal carriers made of proteins, carbohydrates, lipids, or synthetic polymers; controlled-release systems that permit a drug to be delivered for very long periods; and transdermal controlled-release systems (e.g., those currently in use for administration of scopolamine or nitroglycerin). In addition to the use of various carriers for drugs, cell transplantation could be used to provide therapeutic agents, and the possibility of inserting genes into cells to produce desired effects is being explored. SEE: *liposome.*

**drug dependence** A psychic (and sometimes physical) state resulting from interaction of a living organism and a drug. Characteristic behavioral and other responses include a compulsion to take the drug on a continuous or periodic basis to experience its psychic effects or to avoid the discomfort of its absence. Tolerance may be present, and a person may be dependent on more than one drug.

**drug eruption** Dermatitis medicamentosa.

**drug-fast** Resistant, as in bacteria, to the action of a drug or drugs.

**drug fever** Fever caused by the administration of a drug or drugs. Almost any drug can produce this undesired side effect.

**druggist** (drŭg′ĭst) A pharmacist.

**drug handling** It is important to carefully read the label or other printed instruction issued with medicine. The ordered doses (quantities) should be measured accurately and never estimated. A measuring glass or spoon marked in milliliters, ounces, or both should be used. In giving a dose of medicine, it is necessary to know to whom it has to be given, what has to be given, when it has to be given, and the prescribed amount. If medicine is to be taken orally, the patient should be observed until he or she has actually swallowed it.

NOTE: The cover must never be left off the container because a necessary property may evaporate, the drug may become dangerously concentrated, or it may absorb moisture from the air and become difficult to handle or dilute. The drug storage compartment must be kept locked.

**drug interaction** The combined effect of

**Comparison of Toxic and Allergic Drug Reactions***

| | Toxic | Allergic |
|---|---|---|
| Incidence | May occur with any drug | Occurs infrequently |
| Dosage | Usually high | Therapeutic |
| Reaction time | May occur with first dose, or may be due to cumulative effect | Usually only upon re-exposure, but some drugs cross-react with chemicals of similar structure |
| Symptoms | May be similar to pharmacological action of drug | Not related to pharmacological action of drug |
| Associated disorders | None | Asthma, hay fever |

* Differences may be indistinct. Shock from drug overdose may be no different from allergic shock.

drugs taken concurrently. The result may be antagonism or synergism, and consequently may be lethal in some cases. It is important for the patient, physician, and nurse to be aware of the potential interaction of drugs that are prescribed as well as those that the patient may be self-administering.

Many patients, esp. the elderly, may take several medicines each day. The chances of developing an undesired drug interaction increases rapidly with the number of drugs used. It is estimated that if eight or more medications are being used, there is a 100% chance of interaction.

**drug overdose** Literally, any excess dose of a drug, but in our present culture, a self-administered, potentially lethal dose of a drug of abuse. The individual's action may be inadvertent—the dose is an accustomed one but the potency of the "street drug" is much greater than expected. When such a dose results in coma or death, the person is said to have OD'd (i.e., overdosed). SEE: *Nursing Diagnoses Appendix.*

**drug product problem reporting program** A program managed by the U.S. Pharmacopeial Convention, Inc., that informs the product manufacturer, the labeler, and the Food and Drug Administration (FDA) of potential health hazards and defective drug products. The reports may be submitted by any health professional.

**drug rash** Dermatitis produced in some patients by application or ingestion of drugs. Drug rashes are usually not specific for certain drugs. Therefore the following should be used only as a rough guide.

*Antibiotics:* erythema. *Antipyrine:* papular, erythematous rash, sometimes accompanied by edema and much irritation. *Arsenic:* papular or erythematous rash, sometimes urticarial. Prolonged use may produce pigmentation of skin. *Belladonna:* erythematous rash, usually accompanied by intense itching. *Bromides:* usually a rash similar to acne vulgaris; sometimes erythema. *Chloral:* papular erythema. *Iodides:* usually papular erythema, sometimes with acnelike pustules. *Phenolphthalein:* macular rash, sometimes purpuric. *Quinine:* very irritable erythema or urticaria. *Salicylate:* erythematous rash, possibly morbilliform.

**drug reaction** Adverse and undesired reaction to a substance taken for its pharmacological effects. An estimated 15% of hospitalized patients develop toxic or allergic drug reactions. SEE: table.

**drug receptor** A part of a cell that interacts with a drug or drugs. The proteins contained in cells in the form of enzymes are the most important class of drug receptors. Chemotherapeutic agents used in treating malignancies react with nucleic acid receptors. Some anesthetic agents react with lipid receptors on the cell membrane.

**drug screen** A clinical laboratory procedure that checks a comatose patient's blood or urine sample for presence of certain drugs such as barbiturates and amphetamines. Also called a *tox screen.*

**drug testing, mandated** The enforced testing of individuals for evidence of drug use or abuse. Certain U.S. governmental regulatory agencies have instituted programs for testing employees in industries important to public safety such as ground and air transportation. To date, the programs have not mandated testing for alcohol abuse.

**drum** The membrane of the tympanic cavity; the tympanum or cavity of the middle ear.

**drunkenness** [AS. *drinean,* to drink] Alcoholic intoxication. In legal medicine, intoxication or being "under the influence" of alcohol is defined according to the concentration of alcohol in the blood or exhaled air. The precise concentration used to define legal intoxication varies among states. Clinically, a blood level of 0.3% to 0.4% of ethyl alcohol is classed as marked intoxication. A level of 0.4% to 0.5% is consistent with alcoholic stupor, and a level over 0.5% is sufficient to cause alcoholic coma.

**drusen** (droo'zĕn) [Ger. *Druse,* weathered ore] Small, hyaline, globular pathological growths on the optic papilla or on Descemet's membrane.

**dry eye** Insufficient lubrication in the eye and abnormal lack of moisture in the conjunctiva. This condition produces pain and discomfort in the eyes. Dry eye may occur in any disorder that scars the cornea (e.g., erythema multiforme, trachoma, or corneal burns), Sjögren's syndrome, lagophthalmos, Riley-Day syndrome, absence of one or both of the lacrimal glands, paralysis of the facial or trigeminal nerves, medication with atropine, deep anesthesia, and debilitating diseases. Suitably prepared water-soluble polymers are effective in treating this condition.

**dry ice** Solidified carbon dioxide used for commercial refrigeration. It is also used in the form of a pencil-shaped block for treating certain skin lesions, such as warts, by freezing. The temperature of solid carbon dioxide is −78.5°C. For this reason it is extremely important to use thick cloth gloves when handling it. Momentary skin contact with dry ice can cause severe frostbite and blisters.

**dry measure** A measure of volume for dry commodities. SEE: *Weights and Measures Appendix.*

**dry mouth** Decrease or lack of saliva. This condition may be due to the action of drugs such as anorectics, anticholinergics, antidepressants, antihistamines, diuretics, nicotine, caffeine, hypnotics, or sedatives. Radiation therapy in the area of the salivary glands may destroy those glands. SYN: *xerostomia.* SEE: *Sjögren's syndrome; saliva, artificial.*

TREATMENT: Pilocarpine may help. If saliva is completely absent, saliva substitutes are beneficial. Dry mouth due to dehydration is ameliorated by fluid intake.

**Drysdale's corpuscle** (drīz'dālz) [Thomas M. Drysdale, U.S. gynecologist, 1831–1904] A type of nonnucleated granular cell found in the fluid of certain ovarian cysts.

**DSA** *digital subtraction angiography.*

**DSM IV** *Diagnostic and Statistical Manual of Mental Disorders (Fourth Edition).*

**DT's** *delirium tremens.*

**dualism** (dū'ă-lĭzm) [L. *duo,* two, + Gr. *-ismos,* condition] **1.** The condition of being double or twofold. **2.** The theory that human beings consists of two entities, mind and matter, that are independent of each other. **3.** The theory that various blood cells arise from two types of stem cells: myeloblasts, giving rise to the myeloid elements, and lymphoblasts, giving rise to the lymphoid elements.

**duazomycin** (dū-ăz″ō-mī'sĭn) An antineoplastic agent.

**DUB** *dysfunctional uterine bleeding.*

**Dubini's disease** (dū-bē'nēz) [Angelo Dubini, It. physician, 1813–1902] Rapid rhythmic contractions of a group or groups of muscles. SYN: *electric chorea; spasmus Dubini.*

**Dubin-Johnson syndrome** [Isadore Nathan Dubin, U.S. pathologist, 1913–1980; Frank B. Johnson, U.S. pathologist, b. 1919] An inherited defect of bile metabolism that causes retention of conjugated bilirubin in hepatic cells. The patient is asymptomatic except for mild intermittent jaundice. No treatment is required.

**duboisine** (dū-bŏy'sēn) An alkaloid derivative of the plant *Duboisia myoporoides.* It is a form of hyoscyamine used as a mydriatic.

**Dubowitz tool, Dubowitz score** [Lilly and Victor Dubowitz, contemporary South African physicians] A method of estimating the gestational age of an infant based on 21 strictly defined physical and neurological signs. This method provides the correct gestational age ±2 weeks in 95% of infants.

**Duchenne, Guillaume B. A.** (dū-shĕn') A French neurologist, 1806–1875.

***D.'s disease*** Degeneration of the posterior roots and column of the spinal cord and of the brainstem. It is marked by attacks of pain, progressive ataxia, loss of reflexes, functional disorders of the bladder, larynx, and gastrointestinal system, and impotence. This disorder develops in conjunction with syphilis and most frequently affects middle-aged men. SYN: *tabes dorsalis.*

***D.'s muscular dystrophy*** Pseudohypertrophic muscular dystrophy marked by weakness and pseudohypertrophy of the affected muscles. It is caused by mutation of the gene responsible for producing the protein dystrophin. The disease begins in childhood, is progressive, and affects the shoulder and pelvic girdle muscles. The disease, mostly of males, is transmitted as a sex-linked recessive trait. Most patients die before age 20. SEE: *Nursing Diagnoses Appendix.*

***D.'s paralysis*** Bulbar paralysis.

**Duchenne-Aran disease** (dū-shĕn'ăr-ăn') [Duchenne; Francois Amilcar Aran, Fr. physician, 1817–1861] Spinal muscular atrophy.

**Duchenne-Erb paralysis** (dū-shĕn'ayrb) [Duchenne; Wilhelm Heinrich Erb, Ger. neurologist, 1840–1921] Paralysis of muscles supplied by nerves from the upper brachial plexus.

**duct** [L. *ducere,* to lead] **1.** A narrow tubular vessel or channel, esp. one that conveys secretions from a gland. **2.** A narrow enclosed channel containing a fluid (e.g., the semicircular duct of the ear).

***accessory pancreatic d.*** A duct of the pancreas leading into the pancreatic duct or the duodenum near the mouth of the common bile duct. SYN: *d. of Santorini.*

***alveolar d.*** A branch of a respiratory bronchiole that leads to the alveolar sacs of the lungs.

***Bartholin's d.*** The major duct of the sublingual gland.

***biliary d.*** A canal that carries bile. The intrahepatic ducts include the bile canaliculi and interlobular ducts; the extrahepatic ducts include the hepatic, cystic, and common bile ducts. SYN: *bile duct.*

***cochlear d.*** Canal of the cochlea.

***common bile d.*** The duct that carries bile and pancreatic juice to the duodenum. It is formed by the union of the cystic duct of the gallbladder and the hepatic duct of the liver and is joined by the main pancreatic duct. SYN: *ductus choledochus.* SEE: *biliary tract* for illus.

***cystic d.*** The secretory duct of the gallbladder. It unites with the hepatic duct from the liver to form the common bile duct. SEE: *biliary tract* for illus.

***efferent d.*** One of a group of 12 to 14 small tubes that constitute the efferent ducts of the testis. They lie within the epididymis and connect the rete testis with the ductus epididymidis. Their coiled portions constitute the lobuli epididymidis.

***ejaculatory d.*** The duct that conveys semen from the vas deferens and seminal vesicle to the urethra.

***endolymphatic d.*** In the embryo, a tubular projection of the otocyst ending in a blind extremity, the endolymphatic sac. In the adult, it connects the endolymphatic sac with the utricle and saccule of the inner ear.

***d. of the epoophoron*** Gartner's d.

***excretory d.*** Any duct that conveys a waste product from an organ, such as the collecting duct of the renal tubule.

***Gartner's d.*** The caudal part of the mesonephric duct, extending from the parovarium through the broad ligament into the vagina. SYN: *d. of the epoophoron.*

***hepatic d.*** A duct that receives bile from the right or left lobe of the liver and carries it to the common bile duct. SYN: *ductus hepaticus dexter; ductus hepaticus sinister.*

***intercalated d.*** One of several short, narrow ducts that lie between the secretory ducts and the terminal alveoli in the parotid and submandibular glands and in the pancreas.

***interlobular d.*** A duct passing between lobules within a gland (e.g., one of the ducts carrying bile).

***lacrimal d.*** One of two short ducts, inferior and superior, that convey tears from the lacrimal lake to the lacrimal sac. Their openings are on the margins of the upper and lower eyelids. SYN: *lacrimal canal.*

***lactiferous d.*** One of 15 to 20 ducts that drain the lobes of the mammary gland. Each opens in a slight depression in the tip of the nipple. SYN: *milk d.*

***lymphatic d.*** One of two main ducts conveying lymph to the bloodstream: the left lymphatic (thoracic) and the right lymphatic duct, which drains lymph from the right side of the body above the diaphragm. It discharges into the right subclavian vein. It is smaller than the left lymphatic duct. SEE: *thoracic d.; lymphatic system* for illus.

***mesonephric d.*** Embryonic duct that connects the mesonephros with the cloaca. In males it develops into the reproductive ducts (the duct of the epididymis, deferent duct, seminal vesicle, and ejaculatory duct). In females it develops into the duct of the epoophoron, a rudimentary structure. SYN: *wolffian d.*

***milk d.*** Lactiferous d.

***müllerian d.*** One of the bilateral ducts in the embryo that form the uterus, vagina, and fallopian tubes. SYN: *Müller's duct.*

***nasolacrimal d.*** A duct that conveys tears from the lacrimal sac to the nasal cavity. It opens beneath the inferior nasal concha.

***omphalomesenteric d.*** Vitelline d.

***pancreatic d.*** A duct that conveys pancreatic juice to the duodenum. SYN: *d. of Wirsung.*

***papillary d.*** Any of the large collecting tubules of the kidney.

***paramesonephric d.*** The genital canal in the embryo. In females it develops into the oviducts, uterus, and vagina; in males it degenerates to form the appendix testis.

***paraurethral d.*** Skene's d.

***parotid d.*** A duct through which secretions from the parotid gland enter the oral cavity. The duct is approx. 2 in. (5.1 cm) long. It extends from the anterior border of the parotid gland, crossing the masseter muscle and piercing the buccinator muscle, and then runs between the buccinator muscle and the mucous membrane. It opens into the mouth opposite the second upper molar. The transverse facial artery is above the duct, and the buccal branch of the seventh cranial nerve is below. Stenosis of the duct causes pain and swelling in the parotid gland. SYN: *Stensen's d.*

***prostatic d.*** One of about 20 ducts that discharge prostatic secretion into the urethra. SYN: *ductus prostatici.*

***d. of Rivinus*** One of 5 to 15 ducts (the minor sublingual ducts) that drain the posterior portion of the sublingual gland.

***salivary d.*** Any of the ducts that drain a salivary gland.

***d. of Santorini*** Accessory pancreatic d.

***secretory d.*** Any of the smaller canals of a gland.

***segmental d.*** One of a pair of embryonic tubes located between the visceral and parietal layers of the mesoblast on each side of the body.

***semicircular d.*** One of three membranous tubes forming a part of the membranous labyrinth of the inner ear. They lie within the semicircular canals and bear corresponding names: anterior, posterior, and lateral.

***seminal d.*** Any of the ducts that convey semen, specifically the ductus deferens and the ejaculatory duct.

***Skene's d.*** One of the two slender ducts of Skene's glands that open on either side of the urethral orifice in women. SYN: *paraurethral d.*

***spermatic d.*** The secretory duct of the testicle that later joins the duct of the seminal vesicle to become the ejaculatory duct. SYN: *ductus deferens; testicular d.; vas deferens.*

***Stensen's d.*** Parotid d.

***striated d.*** One of a class of ducts contained within the lobules of glands, esp. salivary glands, that contain radially appearing striations within the cells, denoting the presence of mitochondria.

***sublingual d.*** Any of the secretory ducts of the sublingual gland. SEE: *Bartholin's d.*

***submandibular d.*** A duct of the submandibular gland. It opens on a papilla at the side of the frenulum of the tongue. SYN: *Wharton's d.*

***tear d.*** A duct that conveys tears. These include secretory ducts of lacrimal glands, and lacrimal and nasolacrimal ducts.

***testicular d.*** Spermatic d.

***thoracic d.*** The duct that drains the left side of the body above the diaphragm and all of the body below the diaphragm, and discharges into the left subclavian vein. SYN: *lymphatic d.*

***umbilical d.*** Vitelline d.

***utriculosaccular d.*** A narrow tube emanating from the utricle, connecting it to the saccule, and opening into the endolymphatic duct of the inner ear.

***vitelline d.*** The narrow duct that, in the embryo, connects the yolk sac (umbilical vesicle) with the intestine. SYN: *omphalomesenteric d.; umbilical d.; yolk stalk.*

***Wharton's d.*** Submandibular d.

***d. of Wirsung*** Pancreatic d.

***wolffian d.*** Mesonephric d.

**duct ectasia** An inflammatory condition of the lactiferous ducts of the breast. There is nipple discharge, nipple inversion, and periareolar sepsis. This may occur at any age following menarche. The condition resembles carcinoma of the breast.

ETIOLOGY: The cause is unknown, but in some cases may be associated with hyperprolactinemia due to a pituitary tumor.

TREATMENT: Duct ectasia is treated with surgical drainage of the abscess and antibiotics.

**ductal carcinoma in situ of breast** SEE: under *breast.*

**ductile** (dŭk′tĭl) [L. *ductilis,* fr. *ducere,* to lead] Capable of being elongated without breaking.

**duction** In ophthalmology, the rotation of an eye about an axis. This movement is controlled by the action of the extraocular muscles.

**ductless** [L. *ducere,* to lead, + AS. *loessa,* less] Having no duct; secreting only internally.

**ductless gland** A gland without ducts, secreting directly into capillaries one or more hormones that have specific effects on target organs or tissues. SEE: *endocrine gland; exocrine.*

**ductule** (dŭk′tūl) A very small duct.

***aberrant d.*** One of a group of small tubules associated with the epididymis. They end blindly, representing the vestigial remains of the caudal group of mesonephric tubules.

**ductulus** (dŭk′tū-lŭs) Ductule.

**ductus** (dŭk′tŭs) *pl.* **ductus** Duct.

***d. arteriosus*** A channel of communication between the main pulmonary artery and the aorta of the fetus.

***d. choledochus*** The common bile duct.

***d. cochlearis*** The cochlear duct. SYN: *scala media.*

***d. deferens*** The secretory duct of the testicle. It conveys sperm from the epididymis to the ejaculatory duct. SYN: *vas deferens.*

***d. epoophori longitudinalis*** Gartner's duct.

***d. hemithoracicus*** The ascending branch of the thoracic duct, opening into either the left lymphatic duct or close to the angle of union of the right subclavian and right internal jugular veins.

***d. hepaticus*** A duct about 3 in. (7.6 cm) long, formed by the union of the cystic and hepatic ducts. It carries bile to the intestine.

***d. hepaticus dexter*** The duct that originates in the right lobe of the liver and unites with the ductus hepaticus sinister to form the hepatic duct. It drains the right and caudate lobes.

***d. hepaticus sinister*** The duct that originates in the left lobe of the liver and unites with the ductus hepaticus dexter to form the hepatic duct. It drains the left and caudate lobes.

***patent d. arteriosus*** SEE: *patent ductus arteriosus.*

***d. prostaticus*** One of the ducts that carry secretions from the prostate into the urethra.

***d. reuniens*** The endolymph-containing canal of the inner ear that connects the saccule with the cochlear duct. SYN: *Hensen's canal.*

***d. utriculosaccularis*** Utriculosaccular duct.

***d. venosus*** The smaller, shorter, and posterior of two branches into which the umbilical vein divides after entering the abdomen. It empties into the inferior vena cava.

**Duffy system** A blood group consisting of two antigens determined by allelic genes. SEE: *blood group.*

**Duke Longitudinal Study** Three studies that focused on the normal aging process in middle-aged and older persons. The subjects were given periodic physical, mental, and social examinations at the Duke University Medical Center.

**Duke method** SEE: *bleeding time.*

**dull** [ME. *dul*] **1.** Not resonant on percussion. **2.** Not mentally alert. **3.** Having a boring personality.

**dullness 1.** Lack of normal resonance on percussion. **2.** The state of being dull.

***shifting d.*** An area of dullness, found on percussion of the abdominal cavity to shift as body position is changed. This indicates a collection of peritoneal fluid in the cavity.

**dumb** [AS.] Lacking the power or faculty to speak. SYN: *mute.*

**dumbness** Muteness.

**dumping 1.** In medical care, the practice of transferring a patient who is unable to pay for care to a hospital that accepts such patients. **2.** The abandoning of elderly individuals in hospital emergency departments.

**dumping syndrome** A syndrome marked by sweating and weakness after eating, occuring in patients who have had gastric resections. The exact cause is unknown but rapid emptying (dumping) of the stomach contents into the small intestine is associated with the symptoms. It is often ameliorated by a regimen of frequent small meals without fluids. Lying down after eating may help to slow the movement of food through the alimentary canal.

**Duncan's mechanism** The progress of placental separation inward from the edges, presenting the maternal surface of the placenta on expulsion. SEE: *Schulze mechanism.*

**duodenal** (dū-ō-dē'năl, dū-ŏd'ĕ-năl) [L. *duodeni,* twelve] Pert. to the duodenum.

**duodenal bulb** The area of the duodenum just beyond the pylorus.

**duodenal delay** Delay in the movement of food through the duodenum due to conditions such as inflammation of the lower portion of the intestine, which reflexly inhibits duodenal movements.

**duodenal ulcer** Damaged mucous membrane of the duodenum, usually accompanied by suppuration. Sometimes a bleeding sore is present, creating a danger of perforation. A duodenal ulcer heals slowly due to constant passage of irritating fluids, enzymes, and food over it. SEE: *peptic ulcer.*

**duodenectasis** (dū"ō-dĕn-ĕk'tă-sĭs) [" + Gr. *ektasis,* expansion] Chronic dilatation of the duodenum.

**duodenectomy** (dū"ō-dĕn-ĕk'tō-mē) [" + Gr. *ektome,* excision] Excision of part or all of the duodenum.

**duodenitis** (dū"ŏd-ĕ-nī'tĭs) [" + Gr. *itis,* inflammation] Inflammation of the duodenum.

**duodenocholecystostomy** (dū"ō-dē"nō-kō-lĭ-sĭs-tŏs'tō-mē) [" + Gr. *chole,* bile, + *kystis,* bladder, + *stoma,* mouth] Surgical formation of a passage between the duodenum and the gallbladder. SYN: *duodenocystostomy.*

**duodenocholedochotomy** (dū"ō-dē"nō-kō-lĕd-ō-kŏt'ō-mē) [" + Gr. *choledochos,* bile duct, + *tome,* incision] Surgical incision of the duodenum to reach the gallbladder.

**duodenocystostomy** Duodenocholecystostomy.

**duodenoenterostomy** (dū"ō-dē"nō-ĕn"tĕr-ŏs'tō-mē) [" + Gr. *enteron,* intestine, + *stoma,* mouth] The formation of a passage between the duodenum and the intestine.

**duodenogram** (dū-ŏd'ĕ-nō-grăm) [" + Gr. *gramma,* something written] A radiograph of the duodenum after it has been filled with a contrast medium.

**duodenography** (dū"ō-dē-nŏg'-ră-fē) [" + Gr. *graphein,* to write] Radiographic examination of the duodenum.

***hypotonic d.*** Radiographic examination of the duodenum after medication has been administered to halt the peristaltic action of the gastrointestinal tract.

**duodenohepatic** (dū-ŏd"ĕ-nō"hĕ-păt'ĭk) [" + Gr. *hepatos,* liver] Pert. to the duodenum and liver.

**duodenoileostomy** (dū"ō-dē"nō-ĭl"ē-ŏs'tō-mē) Surgical formation of a passage between the duodenum and the ileum.

**duodenojejunostomy** (dū"ō-dē"nō-jĕ-joo-nŏs'tō-mē) [" + *jejunum,* empty, + Gr. *stoma,* mouth] Surgical creation of a passage between the duodenum and the jejunum.

**duodenorrhaphy** (dū"ō-dĕ-nor'ă-fē) [" + Gr. *rhaphe,* seam, ridge] Suturing of the duodenum.

**duodenoscopy** (dū"ŏd-ĕ-nŏs'kō-pē) [" + Gr. *skopein,* to examine] Inspection of the duodenum with an endoscope.

**duodenostomy** (dū"ŏd-ĕ-nŏs'tō-mē) [" + Gr. *stoma,* mouth] Surgical creation of a permanent opening into the duodenum through the wall of the abdomen.

**duodenotomy** (dū"ŏd-ĕ-nŏt'ō-mē) [" + Gr. *tome,* incision] An incision into the duodenum.

**duodenum** (dū"ō-dē'nŭm, dū-ŏd'ĕ-nŭm) [L. *duodeni,* twelve] The first part of the small intestine, between the pylorus and the jejunum; it is 8 to 11 in. (20 to 28 cm) long. The duodenum receives hepatic and pancreatic secretions through the common bile duct. SEE: *duodenum; liver; pancreas; digestive system* for illus.

ANATOMY: The wall of the duodenum contains circular folds (plicae circulares) and villi, both of which increase the surface area. The microvilli of the epithelial cells are called the *brush border,* which also increases surface area for absorption. Intestinal glands (of Lieberkuhn) between the bases of the villi secrete digestive enzymes, and Brunner's glands in the submucosa secrete mucus. The common bile duct opens at the ampulla of Vater. The nerve supply is both sympathetic (the celiac plexus) and parasympathetic (the vagus nerves). Blood is supplied by branches of the hepatic and superior mesenteric arteries. SEE: *digestive system* for illus.

FUNCTION: Acid chyme enters the duodenum from the stomach, as do bile from the liver via the gallbladder and pancreatic juice from the pancreas. Bile salts emulsify fats; bile and pancreatic bicarbonate juice neutralize the acidity of the chyme. Pancreatic enzymes are lipase, which digests emulsified fats to fatty acids and glycerol; amylase, which digests starch to maltose; and trypsin, chymostrypsin, and carboxypeptidase, which continue the protein digestion begun in the stomach by pepsin. Intestinal enzymes are peptidases, which complete protein digestion to amino acids, and sucrase, maltase, and lactase, which digest dissacharides to monosaccharides. Some of these enzymes are in the brush border of the intestinal epithelium and are not secreted into the lumen. Three hormones are secreted by the duodenum when chyme enters. Gastric inhibitory peptide decreases gastric motility and secretions. Secretin stimulates the pancreas to secrete sodium bicarbonate and the liver to produce bile. Cholecystokinin stimulates secretion of enzymes from the pancreas and contraction of the gallbladder to propel bile into the common bile duct. Distension of the duodenum brings about reflex protein digestion, and secretion of sucrase, maltase, and lactase, which digest dissacharides to monosaccharides. Some of these enzymes function in the brush border rather than in the lumen of the intestine. Hormones secreted by the duodenum are gastric inhibitory peptide, secretin, and cholecystokinin; these influence the secretions or motility of other parts of the digestive tract.

The end products of digestion (amino acids, monosaccharides, fatty acids, glycerol, vitamins, minerals, and water) are absorbed into the capillaries or lacteals within the villi. Blood from the small intestine passes through the liver by way of the portal vein before returning to the heart.

**duplication, duplicature** [L. *duplicare,* to double] Doubling or folding of a part or an organ; the state of being folded.

**duplicitas** (dū-plĭs′ĭ-tăs) A fetal abnormality in which an organ or a part is doubled or apparently doubled.

**dupp** (dŭp) In cardiac auscultation, the expression for the second heart sound heard over the apex. This sound is shorter and of higher pitch than *lubb,* the first heart sound. SEE: *auscultation; heart.*

**Dupuytren, Baron Guillaume** (dū-pwē-trăn′) French surgeon, 1777–1835.

***D.'s contracture*** Contracture of palmar fascia usually causing the ring and little fingers to bend into the palm so that they cannot be extended. This condition tends to occur in families, after middle age, and more frequently in men. There is no correlation between occupation and development of this condition. It is associated with liver disease and long-term use of phenytoin. SEE: illus.

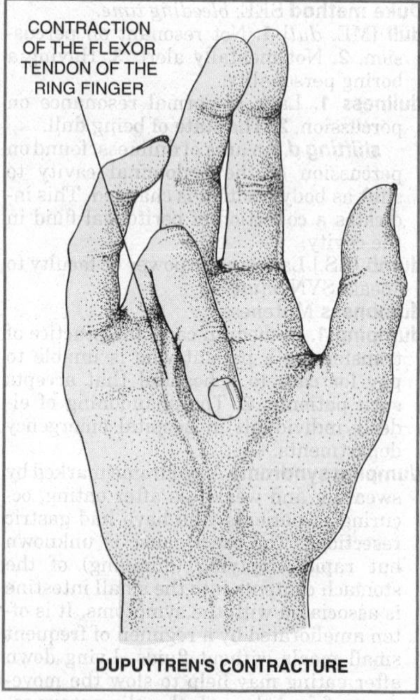

DUPUYTREN'S CONTRACTURE

ETIOLOGY: The cause is unknown.

TREATMENT: The tissue causing the contracture is removed surgically.

***D.'s fracture*** A fracture dislocation of the ankle. The talus is displaced upward.

**dura** (dū′ră) [L. *durus,* hard] The dura mater.

**dural** (dū′răl) [L. *durus,* hard] Pert. to the dura.

**dura mater** [L., hard mother] A fibrous connective tissue membrane, the outermost of the meninges covering the spinal cord (dura mater spinalis) and brain (dura mater cerebri or dura mater encephali). SEE: *pia mater; tentorium cerebelli.*

**duramatral** Dural.

**Durand-Nicolas-Favre disease** Lymphogranuloma venereum.

**duraplasty** [″ + Gr. *plassein,* to form] Plastic repair of the dura mater.

**duration 1.** The average length of time a disorder is present in a patient. **2.** In obstetrics, the time between the beginning and the end of one uterine contraction.

**durematoma** (dū″rĕm-ă-tō′mă) [″ + Gr. *haima,* blood, + *oma,* tumor] Accumulation of blood between the arachnoid and the dura.

**duritis** (dū-rī′tĭs) [″ + Gr. *itis,* inflammation] Inflammation of the dura. SYN: *pachymeningitis.*

**duroarachnitis** (dū″rō-ăr″ăk-nī′tĭs) [″ + Gr.

*arachne,* spider, + *itis,* inflammation] Inflammation of the dura and the arachnoid membrane.

**Duroziez' murmur** (dū-rō″zē-āz′) [Paul Louis Duroziez, Fr. physician, 1826–1897] The systolic and diastolic murmur heard over peripheral arteries in patients with aortic insufficiency. The murmur is audible when pressure is applied to the area just distal to the stethoscope.

**dust** Minute, fine particles of earth; any powder, esp. something that has settled from the air.

***blood d.*** Hemoconia.

***ear d.*** Fine calcareous bodies found in the gelatinous substance of the otolithic membrane of the ear; otoconium or otoliths.

***house d.*** The total of particles present in the air in a house. Materials included are mites, hairs, fibers, pollens, and smoke particles.

**dust cell** A macrophage in the walls of the alveoli of the lungs that ingests pathogens and particles of air pollution.

**dusting powder** Any fine powder for dusting on skin.

***absorbable d.p.*** Powder prepared from cornstarch. It is used as a lubricant for surgical gloves.

**Duverney's fracture** (dū-vĕr-nāz′) [Joseph G. Duverney, Fr. anatomist, 1648–1730] A fracture of the ilium.

**Duverney's gland** The vulvovaginal gland.

**D.V.M.** *Doctor of Veterinary Medicine.*

**dwarf** [AS. *dweorg,* dwarf] An abnormally short or undersized person.

***achondroplastic d.*** A type of dwarf characterized by a normal trunk but shortened extremities, a large head, and prominent buttocks.

***asexual d.*** A dwarf with deficient sexual development.

***hypophyseal d.*** A dwarf whose condition resulted from hypofunction of the anterior lobe of the hypophysis. SYN: *pituitary d.*

***infantile d.*** A dwarf with marked physical, mental, and sexual underdevelopment.

***micromelic d.*** A dwarf with very small limbs.

***ovarian d.*** A woman who is undersized due to absence or underdevelopment of the ovaries.

***phocomelic d.*** A dwarf with abnormally short diaphyses of either pair of extremities or of all four.

***physiological d.*** A person normally developed except for unusually short stature.

***pituitary d.*** Hypophyseal d.

***primordial d.*** A dwarf who has a selective deficiency of growth hormone but otherwise normal endocrine function.

***rachitic d.*** A dwarf whose condition is due to rickets.

***renal d.*** A dwarf whose condition is due to renal osteodystrophy.

***thanatophoric d.*** A dwarf whose condition is caused by generalized failure of endochondral bone formation. This condition is characterized by a large head, a prominent forehead, hypertelorism, a saddle nose, and short limbs extending straight out from the trunk. Most of these infants die soon after birth.

**dwarfism** The condition of being abnormally small. It may be hereditary or a result of endocrine dysfunction, deficiency diseases, renal insufficiency, diseases of the skeleton, or other causes.

**Dwyer instrumentation** A surgical procedure for stabilization of scoliosis. The spine is approached from the front and bolts are inserted transversely through each vertebra. A cable attached to the bolts is applied to the convexity of the curve and the vertebrae are pulled together.

**Dy** Symbol for the element dysprosium.

**dyad** [Gr. *duas,* pair] **1.** A pair. **2.** A pair of chromosomes formed by the division of a tetrad in meiosis. A dyad is a single chromosome that has already replicated for a subsequent division. **3.** In chemistry, a bivalent element or radical. **4.** In psychiatry, two people in an interactional situation.

**dyadic** Pert. to the social interaction between two people.

**Dycem** Registered trademark name for a nonslip material often used by persons with the use of only one arm to stabilize objects (such as plates) on tables and work surfaces.

**dyclonine hydrochloride** (dī′klō-nēn) A topical anesthetic used in otolaryngology.

**dye** Any substance that is of itself colored or that is used to impart color to another material, such as a thin slice of tissue prepared for microscopic examination. Dyes may also be employed in manufacturing test reagents used in medical laboratories.

**dying** The condition in which death seems imminent. SEE: *acceptance; advance directive; assisted suicide; death; death with dignity.*

Even though death is inevitable, persons in the medical care field receive almost no guidance or instruction in how to deal with the patient who asks, "Am I dying?", or with those related to the patient. The dying person may find it less difficult to discuss death with the physician than with family members or close associates. Another aspect of death, esp. in patients with incurable disease, is how society and the physician should deal with persons who ask for assistance in committing suicide. This problem has not been resolved in the U.S. In some countries, assisted suicide is legal.

Considering these difficult circumstances, the physician and all concerned health care workers must be prepared to provide emotional, physical, and spiritual support to the dying patient. This is done in a compassionate, open, and dignified way. Dying patients should not be isolated from their families. The family must be reassured that everything possible is being done for the dying person.

**dynamic** (dī-năm′ĭk) [Gr. *dynamis,* power] Pert. to vital force or inherent power; opposed to static.

**dynamics** The science of bodies in motion and their forces.

***group d.*** SEE: *group dynamics.*

***population d.*** SEE: *population dynamics.*

**dynamic splint** **1.** A protective appliance fabricated with moving parts to allow mobility by providing forces that substitute for weak or absent muscle strength. **2.** A spring-loaded appliance designed to exert a constant low-intensity stretch force on a stiff joint or an adaptively shortened musculotendinous unit.

**dynamogenic** [″ + *gennan,* to produce] Pert. to or caused by an increase of energy.

**dynamograph** (dī-năm′ō-grăf) [″ + *graphein,* to write] A device for recording muscular strength.

**dynamometer** (dī″nă-mŏm′ĕ-tĕr) [″ + *metron,* measure] **1.** A device for measuring muscular strength. **2.** A device for determining the magnifying power of a lens.

**dynamoneure** (dī-năm′ō-nūr) [″+ *neuron,* nerve] A motor spinal nerve cell.

**dynamoscope** (dī-năm′ō-skōp) [″ + *skopein,* to examine] An instrument for auscultation of muscles.

**dynamoscopy** (dī-năm-ŏs′kō-pē) **1.** Auscultation of muscles. **2.** Visual evaluation of the function of an organ or system.

**dyne** (dīn) [Gr. *dynamis,* power] The force needed for imparting an acceleration of 1 cm per second to a 1-g mass.

**dynein** A very large protein that has a molecular configuration resembling arms. Contraction of these arms facilitates the movement of cilia and flagella of bacteria. SEE: *immotile cilia syndrome; Kartagener's syndrome.*

**-dynia** Suffix meaning *pain.* SEE: *-algia.*

**dys-** [Gr.] Prefix meaning *bad, difficult, painful.*

**dysacousia, dysacusis, dysacousma** (dĭs″ă-koo′zē-ă, -koo′sĭs, -kooz′mă) [Gr. *dys,* bad, + *akousis,* hearing] **1.** Discomfort caused by loud noises. **2.** Difficulty in hearing.

**dysadrenalism** (dĭs″ăd-rē′năl-ĭzm) Disordered function or disease of the adrenal gland.

**dysantigraphia** (dĭs″ăn-tĭ-grăf′ē-ă) [″+ *anti,* against, + *graphein,* to write] Inability to copy writing or printed letters.

**dysaphia** (dĭs-ă′fē-ă) [″ + *haphe,* touch] Dullness of the sense of touch.

**dysaptation, dysadaptation** Impaired ability of the iris of the eye to accommodate to varying intensities of light.

**dysarthria** (dĭs-ăr′thrē-ă) [″ + *arthroun,* to utter distinctly] **1.** Difficult and defective speech due to impairment of the tongue or other muscles essential to speech. Mental function is intact. **2.** Inability to speak in which there is no defect in the ability to understand and, if literate, to read or write. The cause may be due to lower motor neuron disease, certain nervous system diseases, or cerebellar lesions.

**dysarthrosis** [″ + *arthrosis,* joint] Joint malformation or deformity.

**dysautonomia** (dĭs″aw-tō-nō′mē-ă) [″ + *autonomia,* freedom to use one's own laws] A rare hereditary disease involving the autonomic nervous system and characterized by mental retardation, motor incoordination, vomiting, frequent infections, and convulsions. It is seen almost exclusively in Ashkenazi Jews. SEE: *Mecholyl test.*

**dysbarism** (dĭs′băr-ĭzm) [″ + *barys,* heavy, + *-ismos,* condition] A symptom complex following exposure of the body to less than atmospheric pressure in air flight or an altitude chamber. When it occurs in severe form, it is sometimes called decompression sickness or bends.

**dysbasia** (dĭs-bā′zē-ă) [″ + *basis,* a step] Difficulty in walking, esp. when due to disease of the brain or spinal cord.

**dysboulia** (dĭs-bū′lē-ă) [″ + *boulē,* will] **1.** Inability to fix the attention; difficulty experienced in thinking; mind weariness. **2.** Weak and uncertain willpower.

**dyscalculia** (dĭs″kăl-kū′lē-ă) [″ + L. *calculare,* to compute] Disability with respect to using mathematics. Although this disorder is common, it is poorly understood.

**dyscephaly** (dĭs-sĕf′ă-lē) Malformation of the head and facial bones.

**dyschezia** (dĭs-kē′zē-ă) [″ + *chezein,* to defecate] Painful or difficult bowel movements.

**dyschiria** (dĭs-kī′rē-ă) [″ + *cheir,* hand] Inability to tell which side of the body has been touched. If referred to the wrong side it is called allochiria, or allesthesia. If referred to both sides it is called synchiria. SYN: *acheiria.*

**dyschondroplasia** (dĭs″kŏn-drō-plā′zē-ă) Chondrodysplasia.

**dyschroa, dyschroia** (dĭs-krō′ă, dis-kroy′ă) [″ + *chroia,* complexion] Discolored skin, esp. of the face; poor or bad complexion.

**dyschromatopsia** (dĭs″krō-mă-tŏp′sē-ă) [″ + *chroma,* color, + *opsis,* vision] Imperfect color vision.

**dyschromia** Discoloration, as of the skin.

***nail d.*** Discoloration of fingernails and toenails. Pigmented bands in the nails may be related to Addison's disease, Peutz-Jeghers syndrome, pregnancy, use of minocycline, radiotherapy, cytotoxic drugs, antimalarials, and zidovudine therapy in AIDS patients.

**dyschronism** (dĭs-krō′nĭzm) [″ + *chronos,* time] Disturbed time relation, esp. that occurring after transportation from one time zone to another that is 5 to 10 hr ahead or behind. This leads to disturbances of biological rhythms. SYN: *jet lag.*

**dyscoria** (dĭs-kō′rē-ă) [″ + *kore,* pupil] Abnormal form or shape of the pupil.

**dyscrasia** (dĭs-krā′zē-ă) [Gr. *dyskrasia,* bad temperament] An old term meaning abnormal mixture of the four humors. The word is now used as a synonym for disease.

**dysdiadochokinesia** (dĭs″dī-ăd″ō-kō-kĭ-nē′sē-ă) [″ + *diadochos,* succeeding, + *kinesis,* movement] Inability to quickly substitute antagonistic motor impulses to produce antagonistic muscular movements.

**dysembryoplasia** (dĭs-ĕm″brē-ō-plā′sē-ă) [″ + *embryon,* embryo, + *plassein,* to form] Fetal malformation occurring during growth of the embryo.

**dysenteric** (dĭs″ĕn-tĕr′ĭk) Pert. to dysentery.

**dysentery** (dĭs′ĕn-tĕr″ē) [″ + *enteron,* intestine] A term applied to various intestinal disorders, esp. of the colon, marked by inflammation of the mucous membrane.

SYMPTOMS: Dysentery is characterized by abdominal pain, tenesmus, and diarrhea with passage of mucus or blood.

ETIOLOGY: The cause is bacterial or viral infection, infestation by protozoa or parasitic worms, or chemical irritants.

***amebic d.*** Dysentery due to amebas.

***bacillary d.*** An acute infectious disease caused by bacteria of the genus *Shigella,* esp. *S. dysenteriae, S. boydii, S. flexneri,* and *S. sonnei.* It may occur sporadically or in epidemics. In addition to intestinal symptoms, a severe toxemia may occur due to exo- and endotoxins produced by the organisms.

***balantidial d.*** Dysentery caused by the ciliate protozoan *Balantidium coli.*

***malignant d.*** A form of dysentery in which symptoms are very pronounced and progress rapidly, usually terminating fatally.

***viral d.*** Dysentery caused by a virus.

**dysesthesia** (dĭs″ĕs-thē′zē-ă) [″ + *esthesia,* sensation] Abnormal sensations on the skin, such as a feeling of numbness, tingling, prickling, or a burning or cutting pain. SEE: *paresthesia.*

***auditory d.*** Abnormal discomfort from loud noises. SYN: *dysacousia.*

***d. pedis*** Severe itching and burning of the plantar surface of the feet and toes. This may occur as a reaction to heparin therapy.

**dysfunction** (dĭs-fŭnk′shŭn) [″ + L. *functio,* a performance] Abnormal, inadequate, or impaired action of an organ or part.

**dysgammaglobulinemia** Disproportion in the concentration of immunoglobulins in the blood. It may be congenital or acquired.

**dysgenesis** (dĭs-jĕn′ĕ-sĭs) [″ + *genesis,* generation, birth] Defective or abnormal development, particularly in the embryo.

***gonadal d.*** A congenital endocrine disorder caused by failure of the ovaries to respond to pituitary hormone (gonadotropin) stimulation. Clinically there is amenorrhea, failure of sexual maturation, and usually short stature. About one third of these patients have webbing of the neck and may have cubitus valgus. Intelligence may be impaired. SYN: *Turner's syndrome.*

ETIOLOGY: The cause is a defect in or absence of the second sex chromosome.

**dysgenic** [″ + *gennan,* to produce] Pert. to dysgenesis.

**dysgenitalism** [″ + L. *genitalia,* organs of reproduction, + Gr. *-ismos,* condition] A condition caused by abnormal genital development.

**dysgerminoma** (dĭs″jĕr-mĭn-ō′mă) [″ + L. *germen,* a sprout, + Gr. *oma,* tumor] A malignant neoplasm of the ovary.

**dysgeusia** (dĭs-gū′zē-ă) [″ + *geusis,* taste] Impairment or perversion of the gustatory sense so that normal tastes are interpreted as being unpleasant or completely different from the characteristic taste of a particular food or chemical compound. SEE: *cacogeusia; heterogeusia; hypogeusia, idiopathic; phantogeusia.*

**dysglobulinemia** (dĭs-glŏb″ū-lĭn-ē′mē-ă) [″ + L. *globulus,* globule, + Gr. *haima,* blood] Abnormality of the amount or quality of blood globulins.

**dysgnathia** (dĭs-nā′thē-ă) [″ + *gnathos,* jaw] Abnormality of the mandible and maxilla.

**dysgonesis** (dĭs″gō-nē′sĭs) [Gr. *dys,* bad, + *gone,* seed] **1.** A functional disorder of the genital organs. **2.** Poor growth of bacterial culture.

**dysgonic** Pert. to a bacterial culture of sparse growth.

**dysgraphia** (dĭs-grăf′ē-ă) [″ + *graphein,* to write] **1.** Inability to write properly, usually the result of a brain lesion. **2.** Writer's cramp.

**dyshidria** (dĭs-hĭd′rē-ă) [″ + *hidros,* sweat] Dyshidrosis.

**dyshidrosis** (dĭs-hī-drō′sĭs) [″ + ″ + *osis,* condition] **1.** A disorder of the sweating apparatus. **2.** A recurrent vesicular eruption on the skin of the hands and feet marked by intense itching. SEE: *pompholyx.*

TREATMENT: The control of sweating or proper absorption of perspiration is beneficial. For the feet, wearing absorbent socks and well-ventilated shoes and applying substances that reduce sweating helps to control symptoms. Individuals who do not wear shoes are rarely found to have this disorder. Acute attacks respond to treatment with a corticosteroid in an ointment combined with iodoquinol. This is applied at night with an occlusive dressing.

**dysidrosis** (dĭs-ī-drō′sĭs) Dyshidrosis.

**dyskaryosis** (dĭs-kăr″ē-ō′sĭs) Abnormality of the nucleus of a cell.

**dyskeratosis** (dĭs″kĕr-ă-tō′sĭs) [″ + *keras,* horn, + *osis,* condition] **1.** Epithelial alterations in which certain isolated malpighian cells become differentiated. **2.** Any alteration in the keratinization of the epithelial cells of the epidermis. This is characteristic of many skin disorders.

**dyskinesia** (dĭs″kĭ-nē′sē-ă) [″ + *kinesis,* movement] A defect in the ability to perform voluntary movement.

***biliary d.*** Failure of the sphincter of Oddi to relax normally. This prevents the flow of bile from the gallbladder to the intestinal tract.

***d. intermittens*** Limb disability occurring intermittently.

***tardive d.*** A condition of slow, rhythmical, automatic stereotyped movements, either generalized or in single muscle groups. These occur as an undesired effect of therapy with certain psychotropic drugs, esp. the phenothiazines.

***uterine d.*** Pain in the uterus on movement.

**dyskinetic** Concerning dyskinesia.

**dyslalia** (dĭs-lā′lē-ă) [″ + *lalein,* to talk] Impairment of speech due to a defect of the speech organs.

**dyslexia** (dĭs-lĕk′sē-ă) [″ + *lexis,* diction] An imprecise term concerning a condition in which an individual with normal vision is unable to interpret written language. The condition is more common in males and is usually noticed in children with reading difficulty in the first grade. These individuals can see and recognize letters but are unable to spell and write words. They have no difficulty recognizing the meaning of objects and pictures. Dyslexia is unrelated to intelligence. Some great intellects, including Thomas Edison, Albert Einstein, Woodrow Wilson, and Winston Churchill, are thought to have been dyslexic. SEE: *alexia.*

The exact cause is unknown. Recent evidence indicates that function of the left hemisphere of the brain of dyslexics is different from that of normal individuals. The results of other studies propose that, in dyslexics, there is a timing error in the reception of visual stimuli so that one of two major visual stimulus pathways is not received in the right line sequence.

**dyslogia** (dĭs-lō′jē-ă) [″ + *logos,* word, reason] Difficulty in expressing ideas.

**dysmasesis** (dĭs″mă-sē′sĭs) [″ + *masesis,* mastication] Difficulty in masticating.

**dysmaturity** A condition in which infants weigh less than would be expected for the known length of the gestational period. These infants are sometimes referred to as being small for date. SYN: *intrauterine growth retardation.*

**dysmegalopsia** [″ + *megas,* big, + *opsis,* vision] Inability to visualize correctly the size of objects; they appear larger than they really are.

**dysmelia** (dĭs-mē′lē-ă) [″ + *melos,* limb] Congenital deformity or absence of a portion of one or more limbs.

**dysmenorrhea** (dĭs″mĕn-ō-rē′ă) [″ + *men,* month, + *rhein,* to flow] Pain in association with menstruation. One of the most frequent gynecological disorders, it is classified as primary or secondary. An estimated 50% of menstruating women experience this disorder, and about 10% of these are incapacitated for several days each period. This disorder is the greatest single cause of absence from school and work among menstrual-age women. In the U.S., this illness causes the loss of an estimated 140,000,000 work hours each year. SEE: *premenstrual tension syndrome; Nursing Diagnoses Appendix.*

NURSING IMPLICATIONS: Young women experiencing discomfort or pain during menstruation are encouraged to seek medical evaluation to attempt to determine the cause. Support and assistance are offered to help the patient to deal with the problem. Application of mild heat to the abdomen may be helpful. A well-balanced diet and moderate exercise is encouraged. Noninvasive pain relief measures such as relaxation, distraction, guided imagery are employed, and the patient is referred for biofeedback training to control pain, and to support and self-help groups.

***congestive d.*** A condition caused by excessive fluid in the pelvis.

***inflammatory d.*** A condition caused by pelvic inflammation.

***membranous d.*** A severe spasmodic dysmenorrhea that is accompanied by the passage of a cast or partial cast of the uterine cavity.

***primary d.*** Dysmenorrhea not caused by a known pathological condition.

SYMPTOMS: The pain usually begins just before or at menarche. The pain is spasmodic and located in the lower abdomen, but it may also radiate to the back and thighs. Some individuals also experience nausea, vomiting, diarrhea, low back pain, headache, dizziness, and in severe cases, syncope and collapse. These symptoms may last from a few hours to several days but seldom persist for more than 3 days. They tend to decrease or disappear after the individual has experienced childbirth the first time, and to decrease with age. Primary dysmenorrhea is much more common than secondary dysmenorrhea.

ETIOLOGY: The exact cause is unknown, but uterine ischemia due to increased production of prostaglandins with increased contractility of the muscles of the uterus (i.e., the myometrium) is thought to be the principal mechanism. As in any disease or symptom, the individual's reaction to and tolerance of pain influences the extent of the disability experienced. Primary dysmenorrhea is not a behavioral or psychological disorder.

One study revealed that prevalence and severity of dysmenorrhea might have been reduced in those who used oral contraceptives, and that severity was increased in those who had long duration of menstrual flow, those who smoked, and those who had had early menarche. Exercise did not influence the prevalence or severity of dysmenorrhea.

DIAGNOSIS: A cramping, labor-like pain that starts just before or at the onset of menstruation is diagnostic of dysmenorrhea. The first attack occurs with or shortly after menarche and occurs subsequently only if preceded by ovulation; pelvic examination is normal. It is essential that secondary dysmenorrhea be ruled out.

TREATMENT: Effective drugs are oral contraceptives and nonsteroidal anti-inflammatory drugs including aspirin. These medicines should be taken in the appropriate dose 3 to 4 times a day and with milk to lessen the chance of gastric irritation.

***secondary d.*** A condition that frequently causes pain similar to that of primary dysmenorrhea, but usually begins some years after menarche. A history of the occurrence of pain in association with pelvic inflammatory disease, use of an intrauterine device, endometriosis, or fertility problems suggests the diagnosis of secondary dysmenorrhea.

TREATMENT: The underlying disease must be treated. Nonsteroidal anti-inflammatory drugs should be used in the meantime.

**dysmetria** (dĭs-mē′trē-ă) [Gr. *dys*, bad, + *metron*, measure] Inability to fix the range of a movement in muscular activity. Rapid and brusque movements are made with more force than necessary. Dysmetria is seen in cerebellar disorders.

**dysmetropsia** [″ + ″ + *opsis*, vision] Inability to visualize correctly the size and shape of things.

**dysmimia** (dĭs-mĭm′ē-ă) [″ + *mimos*, imitation] **1.** Inability to express oneself by gestures or signs. **2.** Inability to imitate.

**dysmnesia** (dĭs-nē′zē-ă) [″ + *mneme*, memory] Any impairment of memory.

**dysmorphophobia** (dĭs″mor-fō-fō′bē-ă) [″ + *morphe*, formed, + *phobos*, fear] Irrational fear of being deformed or the illusion that one is deformed.

**dysmyotonia** (dĭs″mī-ō-tō′nē-ă) [″ + *mys*, muscle, + *tonos*, tone] Muscle atony; abnormal muscle tonicity.

**dysnomia** A condition in which the patient forgets words or has difficulty finding words for written or oral expression.

**dysodontiasis** (dĭs″ō-dŏn-tī′ă-sĭs) [″ + *odous*, tooth, + *-iasis*, process] Painful or difficult dentition.

**dysomnia** (dĭs-ŏm′nē-ă) [″ + L. *somnus*, sleep] Any disturbance involving the amount, quality, or timing of sleep. SEE: *sleep*.

**dysontogenesis** (dĭs″ŏn-tō-jĕn′ĕ-sĭs) [″ + *ontos*, being, + *gennan*, to produce] Defective development of an organism, esp. of an embryo. **dysontogenetic,** *adj.*

**dysopia, dysopsia** (dĭs-ō′pē-ă, -ŏp′sē-ă) [″ + *opsis*, vision] Defective vision.

**dysosmia** (dĭs-ŏz′mē-ă) [″ + *osme*, smell] Distortion of normal smell perception.

**dysostosis** (dĭs″ŏs-tō′sĭs) [″ + *osteon*, bone, + *osis*, condition] Defective ossification.

***cleidocranial d.*** A congenital ossification of the skull with partial atrophy of the clavicles.

***craniocerebral d.*** A hereditary disease marked by ocular hypertelorism, exophthalmos, strabismus, widening of the skull, high forehead, beaked nose, and hypoplasia of the maxilla.

***mandibulofacial d.*** A condition marked by hypoplasia of the facial bones, downward sloping of the palpebral tissues, defects of the ear, macrostomia, and a fish-faced appearance. It occurs in two forms that are thought to be autosomal dominants.

***maxillofacial d.*** Hypoplasia of the maxillae and nasal bones resulting in a flattened face, elongated nose, and small maxillary arch with crowding or malocclusion of teeth. SYN: *Binder's syndrome; maxillofacial syndrome.*

**dysoxia** (dĭs-ŏk′sē-ă) [″ + L. *oxidum*] An abnormal metabolic condition in which tissues cannot make full use of the available oxygen.

**dysoxidizable** [″ + L. *oxidum*, oxide] Difficult to oxidize.

**dyspancreatism** [″ + *pankreas*, pancreas, + *-ismos*, condition] Impaired pancreatic function.

**dyspareunia** (dĭs″pă-rū′nē-ă) [″ + *pareunos*, lying beside] Occurrence of pain in the labia, vagina, or pelvis during or after sexual intercourse. This common condition has been difficult to investigate because most women do not discuss it with health care providers.

ETIOLOGY: Causes are infections in the reproductive tract, inadequate vaginal lubrication, uterine myomata, endometriosis, atrophy of the vaginal mucosa, psychosomatic disorders, and vaginal foreign bodies.

TREATMENT: Specific therapy is for primary disease; counseling is given with respect to appropriate vaginal and vulval lubrication. Vaseline is of no benefit.

**dyspepsia** (dĭs-pĕp′sē-ă) [″ + *peptein*, to digest] Imperfect or painful digestion; not a disease in itself but symptomatic of other diseases or disorders. It is marked by vague abdominal discomfort, a sense of fullness after eating, eructation, heartburn, nausea and vomiting, and loss of appetite. These symptoms may occur irregularly and in different patterns from time to time. The symptoms are increased in times of stress. SYN: *indigestion.*

***acid d.*** Dyspepsia due to excessive acidity of the stomach.

***alcoholic d.*** Dyspepsia caused by excessive use of alcoholic beverages.

***biliary d.*** A form of dyspepsia in which there is insufficient quantity or quality of bile secretion.

***cardiac d.*** A form of dyspepsia occurring during heart disease.

***gastric d.*** Dyspepsia caused by faulty stomach function.

***gastrointestinal d.*** Dyspepsia caused by faulty function of the stomach and intestines.

***hepatic d.*** Dyspepsia caused by liver disease.

***hysterical d.*** Dyspepsia present during hysterical attacks.

**dyspeptic** (dĭs-pĕp′tĭk) **1.** Affected with or pert. to dyspepsia. **2.** One afflicted with dyspepsia.

**dyspermasia** [″ + *sperma,* seed] Dyspermia.

**dyspermia** Difficult or painful emission of sperm during coitus.

**dysphagia** (dĭs-fā′jē-ă) [″ + *phagein,* to eat] Inability to swallow or difficulty in swallowing. SEE: *achalasia; cardiospasm.*

***d. constricta*** Dysphagia due to narrowing of the pharynx or esophagus.

***d. lusoria*** Dysphagia caused by pressure exerted on the esophagus by an anomaly of the right subclavian artery.

***oropharyngeal d.*** Difficulty in propelling food or liquid from the oral cavity into the esophagus.

***d. paralytica*** Dysphagia due to paralysis of the muscles of deglutition and of the esophagus.

***d. spastica*** Dysphagia resulting from a spasm of pharyngeal or esophageal muscles.

**dysphasia** (dĭs-fā′zē-ă) [″ + *phasis,* speech] Impairment of speech resulting from a brain lesion.

**dysphonia** (dĭs-fō′nē-ă) [″ + *phone,* voice] Difficulty in speaking; hoarseness.

***d. clericorum*** Hoarseness due to public speaking.

***d. puberum*** Change or breaking in the voice in boys during puberty.

***spasmodic d.*** Dysphonia due to spasmodic contraction of all of the muscles involved with speech production. Actions involving many of the same muscles (i.e., swallowing and singing) are usually unaffected. The condition is usually nonprogressive and is not thought to be due to psychological factors.

TREATMENT: In general, therapy has been ineffective. Injection of botulinum toxin into one or both thyroarytenoid muscles of the larynx has been used experimentally. The injections must be repeated several times a year.

**dysphoria** (dĭs-fō′rē-ă) [″ + *pherein,* to bear] An exaggerated feeling of depression and unrest without apparent cause; a mood of general dissatisfaction, unpleasantness, restlessness, anxiety, discomfort, and unhappiness.

**dysphrasia** (dĭs-frā′zē-ă) [Gr. *dys,* bad, + *phrasis,* speech] Impairment of speech due to a brain lesion. SYN: *dysphasia.*

**dysphylaxia** (dĭs-fĭ-lăk′sē-ă) [″ + *phylaxis,* protection] Waking too early from sleep.

**dyspigmentation** (dĭs″pĭg-mĕn-tā′shŭn) Abnormality of the skin or hair pigment.

**dyspituitarism** (dĭs″pĭ-tū′ĭ-tăr-ĭzm) [″ + L. *pituita,* mucus, + Gr. *-ismos,* condition] Any condition due to a disorder of the pituitary body.

**dysplasia** [″ + *plassein,* to form] Abnormal development of tissue. SYN: *alloplasia; heteroplasia.*

***anhidrotic d.*** A congenital condition marked by absent or deficient sweat glands, intolerance of heat, and abnormal development of teeth and nails.

***bronchopulmonary d.*** An iatrogenic chronic lung disease that develops in premature infants after a period of intensive respiratory therapy.

***cervical d.*** Abnormal changes in the tissues covering the cervix uteri.

***chondroectodermal d.*** A condition marked by defective development of bones, nails, teeth, and hair and by congenital heart disease. SYN: *Ellis–van Creveld syndrome.*

***hereditary ectodermal d.*** A form of anhidrotic dysplasia marked by few or absent sweat glands and hair follicles, smooth shiny skin, abnormal or absent teeth, nail deformities, cataracts or corneal alterations, absence of mammary glands, a concave face, prominent eyebrows, conjunctivitis, deficient hair growth, and mental retardation.

***monostotic fibrous d.*** Replacement of bone by fibrous tissue, marked by pain usually in the tibia or femur. The cause is unknown.

***polyostotic fibrous d.*** Replacement of bone by a vascular fibrous tissue, marked by difficulty in walking and multiple bone deformities and fractures. It usually commences in childhood. The cause is unknown.

**dyspnea** (dĭsp-nē′ă, dĭsp′nē-ă) [″ + *pnoē,* breathing] Air hunger resulting in labored or difficult breathing, sometimes accompanied by pain. It is normal when due to vigorous work or athletic activity. **dyspneic** (-nē-ĭc), *adj.*

SYMPTOMS: The symptoms are audible labored breathing, a distressed anxious expression, dilated nostrils, protrusion of the abdomen and expanded chest, gasping, and marked cyanosis.

ETIOLOGY: Dyspnea is caused by insufficient oxygenation of the blood resulting from disturbances in the lungs, low oxygen pressure of air, circulatory disturbances, and hemoglobin deficiency. Other causes may be acidosis, excessive carbon dioxide content of blood, lesions of the respiratory center, emotional excitation, hyperexcitability of the Hering-Breuer reflex, cardiac asthma, and orthopnea. It may be a subjective feeling.

NURSING IMPLICATIONS: The patient is assessed for airway patency, and a complete respiratory assessment is performed to identify additional signs and symptoms of respiratory distress and alleviating and aggravating factors. Arterial blood gas values are obtained if indicated, and oxygen saturation is monitored. The patient is placed in a high Fowler, orthopneic, or other comfortable position. Oxygen and medications are administered as prescribed, and the patient's response is evaluated and documented. The nurse remains with the patient until breathing becomes less labored and anxiety has decreased. When the patient is more comfortable, a more thorough interview and examination are conducted to obtain data about the patient's cardiopulmonary status and previous dyspneic episodes.

***cardiac d.*** Dyspnea due to cardiac insufficiency, as in acute myocardial infarction.

***expiratory d.*** Dyspnea as in asthma and bronchitis; wheezing and painful expiration. Secretions in the respiratory tract cause the sound.

***inspiratory d.*** Dyspnea due to interference with the passage of air to the lungs.

***paroxysmal nocturnal d.*** Attacks of shortness of breath that usually occur at night and awaken the patient. This is due to advanced forms of heart failure associated with elevations of pulmonary venous and capillary pressures. Previously, this condition was incorrectly termed cardiac asthma.

**dyspraxia** (dĭs-prăk′sē-ă) [″ + *prassein,* achieve] A disturbance in the programming, control, and execution of volitional movements. It cannot be explained by absence of comprehension, inadequate attention, or lack of cooperation; it is usually associated with a stroke, head injury, or any condition affecting the cerebral hemispheres.

**dysprosium** (dĭs-prō′sē-ŭm) SYMB: Dy. A metallic element of the yttrium group of rare earths with atomic number 66 and an atomic weight of 162.50.

**dysprosody** Lack of the normal rhythm, melody, and articulation of speech. This condition may be present in patients with parkinsonism.

**dysraphia, dysraphism** (dĭs-rā′fē-ă, -fĭzm) [″ + *rhaphe,* seam, ridge] In the embryo, failure of raphe formation or failure of fusion of parts that normally fuse.

***spinal d.*** A general term applied to failure of fusion of parts along the dorsal midline that may involve any of the following structures: skin, vertebrae, skull, meninges, brain, and spinal cord.

**dysreflexia** The state in which an individual with a spinal cord injury at T-7 or above experiences a life-threatening uninhibited sympathetic response of the nervous system to a noxious stimulus. SEE: *Nursing Diagnoses Appendix.*

**dysrhythmia** (dĭs-rĭth′mē-ă) [″ + *rhythmos,* rhythm] Abnormal, disordered, or disturbed rhythm.

***cardiac d.*** SEE: *Nursing Diagnoses Appendix.*

**dyssomnia** Sleep disorders characterized by a disturbance in the amount, quality, or timing of sleep. They include primary insomnia, primary hypersomnia, narcolepsy, breathing-related sleep disorders, altitude insomnia, food allergy insomnia, environmental sleep disorder, and circadian rhythm sleep disorders. SEE: *sleep; sleep disorder.*

**dysstasia** [″ + *stasis,* standing] Difficulty in standing.

**dystaxia** (dĭs-tăk′sē-ă) [″ + *taxis,* arrangement] Partial ataxia.

**dystectia** (dĭs-tĕk′shē-ă) [″ + L. *tectum,* roof] In the embryo, failure of closure of the neural tube. Deformities such as spina bifida cystica and meningocele are produced in this way.

**dysthanasia** An undignified and painful death due to the postponement of a merciful death.

**dysthymia** (dĭs-thī′mē-ă) [″ + *thymos,* mind] Dysthymic disorder. SEE: *Nursing Diagnoses Appendix.*

**dysthymic disorder** A chronically depressed mood that is present more than 50% of the time for at least 2 years in adults or 1 year for children or adolescents. These individuals describe themselves as being sad and "down in the dumps." SYN: *dysthymia.*

SYMPTOMS: The symptoms include poor appetite or overeating, insomnia or hypersomnia, low energy or fatigue, low self-esteem, poor concentration or difficulty making decisions, and feelings of hopelessness. The diagnosis of this disorder is not made if the patient has ever had a manic, hypomanic, or mixed manic and hypomanic episode.

TREATMENT: Treatment includes antidepressants including tricyclic medications and monoamine oxidase inhibitors. Newer second-generation antidepressants such as fluoxetine, bupropion, paroxetine, and sertraline have the advantage of having no anticholinergic side effects, do not cause weight gain, and do not have cardiac conduction effects.

**dysthyreosis** (dĭs″thī-rē-ō′sĭs) [″ + *thyreos,* shield, + *osis,* condition] Dysthyroidism.

**dysthyroidism** (dĭs-thī′roy-dĭzm) [″ + ″ + *eidos,* form, shape, + *-ismos,* condition] Imperfect development and function of the thyroid gland. SYN: *dysthyreosis.*

**dystocia** (dĭs-tō′sē-ă) [″ + *tokos,* birth] Difficult labor. It may be produced by either the size of the passenger (the fetus) or the small size of the pelvic outlet.

FETAL CAUSES: Large size of the fetus usually causes this condition. Other factors are malpositions of the fetus (transverse, face, brow, breech, or compound presentation), abnormalities of the fetus (hydrocephalus, tumors of the neck or abdomen, hydrops), and multiple pregnancy (interlocked twins).

MATERNAL CAUSES: *Uterus:* Causes include primary and secondary uterine inertia, congenital anomalies (bicornuate uterus), tumors (fibroids, carcinoma of the cervix), and abnormal fixation of the uterus by previous operation. *Bony pelvis:* Causes include flat or generally contracted pelvis, funnel pelvis, exostoses of the pelvic bones, and tumors of the pelvic bones. *Cervix uteri:* Causes include Bandl's contraction ring, a rigid cervix that will not dilate, and stenosis and stricture preventing dilatation. *Ovary:* Ovarian cysts may block the pelvis. *Vagina and vulva:* Causes include cysts, tumors, atresias, and stenoses. *Pelvic soft tissues:* A distended bladder or colon may interfere.

DIAGNOSIS: Dystocia generally can be detected by vaginal examination, ultrasound, and external pelvimetry before the patient goes into labor.

TREATMENT: Treatment varies according to the condition that causes the dystocia. The goal is correction of the abnormality in order to allow the fetus to pass. If this is not possible, operative delivery is necessary. SEE: *cesarean section.*

**dystonia** (dĭs-tō′nē-ă) [″ + *tonos,* tone] Prolonged muscle contractions that may cause twisting and repetitive movements or abnormal posture. These movements may be in the form of rhythmic jerks. The condition may progress in childhood, but progression is rare in adults. In children the legs are usually affected first.

ETIOLOGY: In most cases no cause can be discovered. The syndrome may be associated with a great variety of metabolic or neurological diseases and other conditions such as head trauma, viral encephalitis, stroke, brain tumor, toxic levels of manganese or carbon disulfide, wasp stings, and undesired side effects of drugs used in treating parkinsonism and antipsychotic medicines.

TREATMENT: Medicines are discontinued if they are implicated; specific diseases associated with the condition are treated. Forms of treatment include anticholinergic drugs; levodopa; injection of botulinum toxin in focal dystonias such as blepharospasm or torticollis; physiotherapy; and psychotherapy.

***d. musculum deformans*** A rare progressive syndrome that usually begins in childhood and in most patients is invariably progressive. It is marked by distorted twisting or movement of a part or all of the body. The posture may be bizarre and the position is sustained. The inherited pattern is seen in families from northern Europe. The patient remains mentally normal. The bizarre posture is abolished in sleep, but eventually it may persist even then. SYN: *torsion dystonia of childhood.*

ETIOLOGY: The cause is unknown.

TREATMENT: It is important that the patient not be treated as if the disease were due to hysteria or mental illness. There is no specific therapy but anticholinergics and reserpine may be of benefit. The most effective therapy has involved use of cryothalamectomy to destroy a portion of the ventrolateral nucleus of the thalamus.

**dystonic** Pert. to dystonia or hypertonicity or hypotonicity of tissues.

**dystopia** (dĭs-tō′pē-ă) [″ + *topos,* place] Malposition (1); displacement of any organ. **dystopic** (-tŏp′ik), *adj.*

***d. canthorum*** Lateral displacement of the inner canthi of the eyes.

**dystrophia** (dĭs-trō′fē-ă) Dystrophy.

**dystrophin** A protein of skeletal and cardiac muscle. Its precise function is unknown, but its production is impaired by the gene for Duchenne's muscular dystrophy.

**dystrophoneurosis** (dĭs-trŏf″ō-nū-rō′sĭs) [″ + *trephein,* to nourish, + *neuron,* nerve, + *osis,* condition] Defective nutrition caused by disease of the nervous system.

**dystrophy** (dĭs′trō-fē) [Gr. *dys,* bad, + *trephein,* to nourish] A disorder caused by defective nutrition or metabolism. **dystrophic** (-fĭk), *adj.*

***adiposogenital d.*** A condition marked by a peculiar type of obesity and hypogenitalism due to a disturbance in the hypothalamus, which controls food intake, and of the pituitary, which controls gonadal development. SYN: *Fröhlich's syndrome.*

***facioscapulohumeral muscular d.*** Landouzy-Déjérine d.

***Landouzy-Déjérine d.*** A hereditary form of progressive muscular dystrophy with onset in childhood or adolescence. It is marked by atrophic changes in the muscles of the shoulder girdle and face, inability to raise the arms above the head, myopathic facies, eyelids that remain partly open in sleep, and inability to whistle or purse the lips. SYN: *facioscapulohumeral muscular d.; Landouzy-Déjérine atrophy.*

***progressive muscular d.*** Spinal muscular atrophy.

***pseudohypertrophic muscular d.*** A hereditary disease usually beginning in childhood in which muscular ability is lost. At first there is muscular pseudohypertrophy, followed by atrophy.

**dysuria** (dĭs-ū′rē-ă) [″ + *ouron,* urine] Painful or difficult urination, symptomatic of numerous conditions. Dysuria may indicate cystitis; urethritis; infection anywhere in the urinary tract; urethral stricture; hypertrophied, cancerous, or ulcerated prostate in men; prolapse of the uterus in women; pelvic peritonitis and abscess; metritis; cancer of the cervix; dysmenorrhea; or psychological abnormalities. The condition may also be caused by certain medications, esp. opiates and medicines used to prevent motion sickness. Pain and burning may be caused by concentrated acid urine. SEE: *urinary tract infection.*

**dyszoospermia** (dĭs″zō-ō-spĕrm′ē-ă) [″ + ″ + *sperma,* seed] Imperfect formation of spermatozoa.

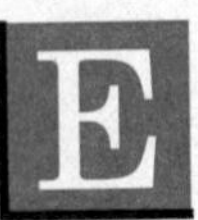

**E** *emmetropia; energy; Escherichia; eye.*

**$E_1$** *estrone.*

**$E_2$** *estradiol.*

**$E_3$** *estriol.*

**e** *electric charge; electron;* L. *ex,* from.

**ea** *each.*

**EACA** *epsilon-aminocaproic acid.*

**ead** L. *eadem,* the same.

**Eales' disease** (ēlz) [Henry Eales, Brit. physician, 1852–1913] Recurrent hemorrhages into the retina and vitreous, most commonly seen in men in the second and third decades of life. The cause is unknown.

**ear** [AS. *ear*] The organ of hearing, consisting of the external, the middle, and the internal ear. SEE: illus.; *Bárány's caloric test; hearing, functional test for; labyrinth* for illus.

EXAMINATION: Hearing ability may be estimated by asking the patient to repeat phrases or answer questions while the examiner faces away from the patient. For accuracy, however, hearing should be tested by using a properly calibrated audiometer. This is true esp. if the test of hearing acuity is done on an individual who works in a noisy environment. Comparing subsequent tests of hearing with the original or baseline record will determine the effect, if any, of the noisy work environment on the individual's ability to hear.

The examiner should also be alert to the color, size, and shape of the ear; any discharge from the middle or inner ear; tenderness on pressure in the front or back of the ear; inflammation or bulging of the drum; and perforation or scarring of the drum. Deafness may indicate wax in the external ear canals, blocked eustachian tubes, disorders of the vestibulocochlear nerve, disease of the middle ear, or the toxic effect of drugs. Pallor of ears, tongue, and gums indicates shock or anemia. Ringing in the ears may be noted in Ménière's disease and after use of certain drugs such as quinine or those containing salicylic acid (e.g., aspirin); it also occurs without any discernible cause. SYN: *auris.* SEE: *hearing, sensorineural.*

NURSING IMPLICATIONS: Patients are taught to keep their ears clean and protect them from trauma and infection by never inserting any object into the ear canal. Forceful nose blowing that can push secretions into the middle ear via the eustachian tube should be avoided. Overamplified music, noisy power tools, and hobbies involving exposure to the noise of firearms or other loud noises can cause hearing loss. Patients should wear sound-muffling ear plugs or muffs to protect against prolonged exposure to industrial or environmental noise. Hearing ability in patients receiving potentially ototoxic drugs is evaluated. Correct methods are taught for instillation of ear medications.

***Blainville's e.*** [Henri Marie Ducrotay de Blainville, Fr. scientist, 1777–1850] Congenital asymmetry of the ears.

***Cagot e.*** An ear without a lower lobe.

***cauliflower e.*** A colloquial term for a thickening of the external ear resulting from trauma that caused a hematoma. It is commonly seen in boxers. Plastic surgery may restore the ear to a normal shape.

***external e.*** The portion of the ear consisting of the auricle and external auditory canal, and separated from the middle ear by the tympanic membrane or eardrum. SYN: *auris externa.*

***foreign bodies in e.*** Objects that enter the ear accidentally or are inserted deliberately. These are usually insects, pebbles, beans, or peas.

SYMPTOMS: Foreign objects cause pain, ringing, or buzzing in the ear. A live insect usually causes a noise.

TREATMENT: A bright light should not be used to lure an insect from the ear canal; it may be stimulated to crawl deeper. Bland oil should be dropped in to float the insect out. In the case of a solid foreign body, oil or water should not be used, because it might either push the object farther into the ear or cause it to swell and become firmly embedded. Such foreign bodies in the ear do not constitute an emergency and should be left untreated until seen by a physician.

Water sometimes enters the ears of swimmers and does not flow out spontaneously. Usually, it can be dislodged by a sudden tap on the side of the head above the ear, or by introducing a long wisp of cotton, which draws it out by capillary action. Also, a few drops of 70% alcohol instilled in the canal will hasten evaporation of the so-called trapped water. Occasionally, this sensation of water in the ear is due not to water but to swelling of the cerumen. In such instances, a physician should be consulted.

***glue e.*** A condition caused by the chronic accumulation of a high-viscosity fluid in the middle ear, occurring principally in children who are 5 to 8 years old. It causes deafness, which can be treated by removal of the exudate.

***internal e.*** The portion of the ear consisting of the cochlea, containing the sensory receptors for hearing, and the vesti-

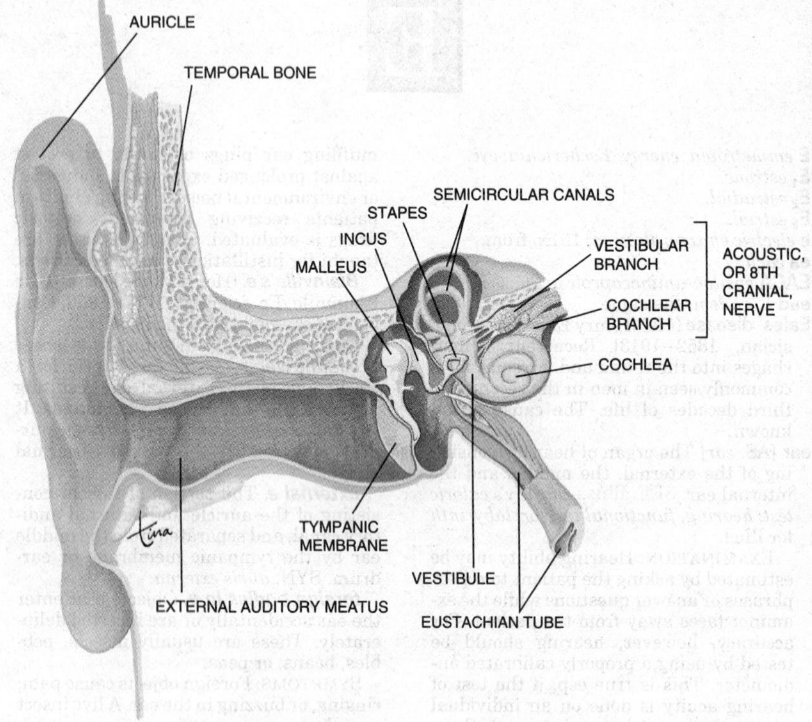


OUTER, MIDDLE, AND INNER **EAR**

bule and semicircular canals, which include the receptors for equilibrium and the sense of position. The internal ear is innervated by the vestibulocochlear nerve. SYN: *auris interna*.

***middle e.*** The tympanic cavity, an irregular air-filled space in the temporal bone. Anteriorly, it communicates with the eustachian tube, which forms an open channel between the middle ear and the cavity of the nasopharynx. Posteriorly, the middle ear opens into the mastoid antrum, which in turn communicates with the mastoid cells. Of the three potential openings into the middle ear, two—the tympanic membrane and the round window—are covered. The third one is the eustachian tube. Three ossicles (small bones) joined together, the malleus, incus, and stapes, extend from the tympanic membrane to the oval window. SYN: *auris media*. SEE: *eardrum; tympanum*.

***Mozart e.*** SEE: *Mozart ear*.

***nerve supply of e.*** *External:* The branches of the facial, vagus, and mandibular nerves and the nerves from the cervical plexus. *Middle:* The tympanic plexus and the branches of the mandibular, vagus, and facial nerves. *Internal:* The vestibulocochlear nerve.

***pierced e.*** An ear lobe that has been pierced with a needle so that a permanent channel will remain, permitting the wearing of an earring attached to the ear by a connector that passes through the channel.

***surfer's e.*** SEE: *surfer's ear*.

**earache** Pain in the ear. SYN: *otalgia; otodynia*.

**ear bone** One of the ossicles of the tympanic cavity: the malleus, incus, and stapes. SEE: *ear* for illus.

**eardrops** A medication in liquid form for instillation into the external ear canal.

Caution: Eardrops should not be used if the tympanic membrane is damaged or broken.

**eardrum** (ēr′drŭm) The membrane at the junction of the external auditory canal and the middle ear cavity. SYN: *tympanum*.

**ear oximeter** A device that determines the oxygen content of the blood flowing through the ear.

**ear plug** A device for preventing sound from entering the ear by occluding the external auditory canal.

Caution: Ear plugs should not be used during swimming because they may interfere with pressure equalization.

**earth 1.** The planet on which we live. The diameter of the earth at the equator is 7926 miles (12,755 km). It is 92.9 million miles (149.6 million km) from the sun, and it makes one revolution around the sun every 365.26 days. Its only natural satellite is the moon. **2.** The soil on the surface of the planet earth.

***alkaline e.*** A general term for the oxides of calcium, strontium, magnesium, and barium.

***diatomaceous e.*** Silica containing fossilized shells of microscopic algae with a siliceous or calcium-containing cell wall. It is used in insulating material and filters and as an absorbent.

***fuller's e.*** Clay that is similar to kaolin. It is used as an absorbent, as a filler in textiles, and in cosmetics.

**earth eating** Eating of clay or dirt, sometimes by children as a form of pica.

**ear thermometry** Determination of the temperature of the tympanic membrane by use of a device for rapidly sensing infrared radiation from the membrane. Commercially available devices do this in 3 sec. The convenience of assessing body temperature using this method is obvious, but if the probe is left in the ear canal for more than a few seconds, the reading may be abnormally low, owing to the condensation of moisture on the tip of the probe. SEE: *temperature.*

**ear tube** Grommet.

**earwax** (ēr′wăks) Cerumen.

**Easy Street Environments** Trade name for a type of simulated physical environment constructed in rehabilitation facilities. They provide realistic settings for learning and practicing functional daily living skills necessary for returning to the community, such as shopping for groceries.

**eat** [AS. *etan*] **1.** To devour, as food. **2.** To take solid food. **3.** To corrode.

**eating disorder** One of a subclass of disorders that includes any one of the multiple disturbances of eating behavior. Anorexia nervosa, bulimia, pica, and rumination disorder of infancy are included.

**Eaton agent** *Mycoplasma pneumoniae.*

**Eaton-Lambert syndrome** SEE: *Lambert-Eaton myasthenia syndrome.*

**Eberthella** (ā″bĕr-tĕl′ă) [Karl Joseph Eberth, Ger. pathologist, 1835–1926] Formerly a genus of bacteria; now classified under *Salmonella.*

**Ebner's glands** [A. G. Victor von Ebner, Austrian histologist, 1842–1925] Serous glands of the tongue usually found in the vicinity of the circumvallate papillae.

**Ebola virus hemorrhagic fever** [Ebola, Zaire, Africa] A viral disease marked by fever, systemic hemorrhage, and high mortality; it affects humans and monkeys and has appeared in epidemic form in Africa and Germany. The cause is one of three subtypes of viruses in the *Filoviridae* family that is distinguished by long threadlike strands of RNA. The animal or insect host (reservoir) has not been identified, limiting study of the disease. The three filoviruses known to cause disease in humans are the Marburg virus, identified in Germany in 1967; the Zaire virus, recognized in 1976; and the Sudan virus, identified in 1976. A fourth subtype, the Reston virus, identified in the U.S. in 1989, is fatal to monkeys, but did not produce disease in infected humans.

SYMPTOMS: Following an incubation period of 5 to 10 days, fever, myalgia, and headache begin abruptly, followed by some combination of nausea, vomiting, diarrhea, abdominal pain, cough, pharyngitis, conjunctivitis, lymphadenopathy, and jaundice. Petechiae and bleeding from mucous membranes and injection sites then appear. Central nervous system involvement is indicated by delirium and a decreased level of consciousness. A maculopapular rash on the trunk usually develops around day 5.

By day 10, the fever disappears, and patients either improve or die from irreversible hemorrhage and necrosis of the liver and other major organs. Severe organ necrosis marks the terminal stage. Mortality has ranged from 25% during the Marburg epidemic to approx. 60% for the Sudan virus and 90% during the Zaire epidemics.

TRANSMISSION: The Marburg virus is transmitted to humans from infected monkeys or their tissues. The source of infection for the first case of the epidemics in Zaire and Sudan is unknown. The virus spreads rapidly through contact with contaminated blood or body fluids. This occurs due to lack of isolation procedures and blood and body fluid precautions, and inadequate sterilization of syringes and needles. Transmission via airborne droplets has not been established.

TREATMENT: Currently no vaccines or drugs are effective against Ebola hemorrhagic fever viruses, and treatment is focused on supportive measures. Strict isolation and blood and body fluid precautions are essential to prevent the spread of the disease.

**ebonation** (ē″bō-nā′shŭn) [L. *e,* out, + AS. *ban,* bone] Removal of bony fragments from a wound.

**Ebstein's anomaly** (ĕb′stīnz) [Wilhelm Ebstein, Ger. physician, 1836–1912] A congenital heart condition resulting from downward displacement of the tricuspid valve from the annulus fibrosus. It causes fatigue, palpitations, and dyspnea.

**ebullism** (ĕb′ū-lĭzm) [L. *ebullire,* to boil over] Formation of water vapor in body tissue, which occurs when the body is exposed to extreme reduction in barometric pressure. SEE: *bends; decompression illness.*

**eburnation** (ĕb″ŭr-nā′shŭn) [L. *eburnus,* made of ivory] Changes in bone causing it to become dense and hard like ivory.

**eburneous** (ĕ-bŭr′nē-ŭs) Resembling ivory; ivory-colored.

**EBV** *Epstein-Barr virus.* SEE: *mononucleosis, infectious.*

**EC** *Enzyme Commission.*

**ecaudate** (ē-kaw′dāt) [L. *e,* without, + *cauda,* tail] Without a tail.

**ecbolic** (ĕk-bŏl′ĭk) [Gr. *ekbolikos,* throwing out] **1.** Hastening uterine evacuation by causing contractions of the uterine muscles. **2.** Any agent producing or hastening labor or abortion. SYN: *oxytocic.*

**ECC** *emergency cardiac care; external cardiac compression.*

**eccentric** (ĕk-sĕn′trĭk) [Gr. *ek,* out, + *kentron,* center] **1.** Proceeding away from a center. **2.** Peripheral. **3.** Departing from the usual, as in dress or conduct.

**eccentric muscle contraction** SEE: *muscle contraction, eccentric.*

**eccentro-osteochondrodysplasia** (ĕk-sĕn″trō-ŏs″tē-ō-kŏn″drō-dĭs-plā′zhē-ă) [Gr. *ekkentros,* from the center, + *osteon,* bone, + *chondros,* cartilage, + *dys,* bad, + *plassein,* to form] A pathological condition of bones caused by imperfect bone formation. Ossification occurs in several different centers instead of in one common center.

**ecchondroma** (ĕk-ŏn-drō′mă) [Gr. *ek,* out, + *chondros,* cartilage, + *oma,* tumor] A chondroma or cartilaginous tumor.

**ecchondrotome** (ĕk-ŏn′drō-tōm) [″ + ″ + *tome,* incision] A knife for excision of cartilage.

**ecchymosis** (ĕk-ĭ-mō′sĭs) *pl.* **ecchymoses** [″ + ″ + *osis,* condition] A skin discoloration consisting of large, irregularly formed hemorrhagic areas. The color is blue-black, changing in time to greenish brown or yellow. SEE: illus.

ETIOLOGY: The cause is extravasation of blood into skin or mucous membrane.

**ecchymotic** (-mŏt′ĭk), *adj.*

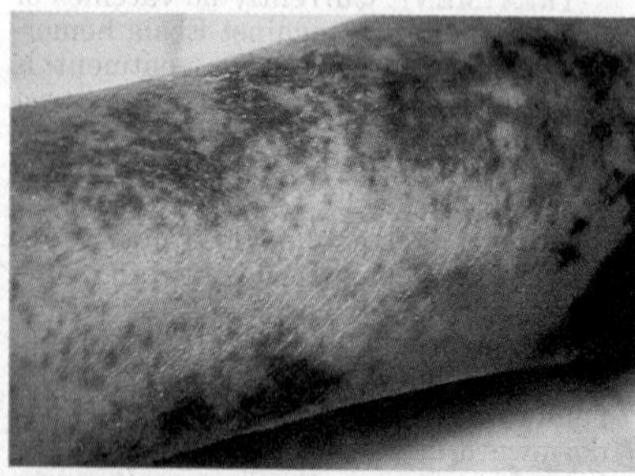

**ECCHYMOSIS** IN SKIN OF LEG

**eccrine** (ĕk′rĭn) [Gr. *ekkrinein,* to secrete] Pert. to secretion, esp. of sweat. SEE: *apocrine; endocrine; exocrine.*

**eccrine sweat gland** One of many glands distributed over the entire skin surface that, because they secrete sweat, are important in regulating body heat. The total number of glands ranges from 2 million to 5 million. There are over 400 per square centimeter on the palms and about 80 per square centimeter on the thighs. SEE: *sweat gland* for illus.; *apocrine sweat glands; sweat gland.*

**eccritic** (ĕk-krĭt′ĭk) [Gr. *ekkritikos*] **1.** Promoting excretion. **2.** An agent that promotes excretion.

**ecdysis** (ĕk′dĭ-sĭs) *pl.* **ecdyses** [Gr. *ekdysis,* getting out] **1.** The shedding or sloughing off of the epidermis of the skin. SYN: *desquamation.* **2.** The shedding (molting) of the outer covering of the body as occurs in certain animals such as insects, crustaceans, and snakes.

**ECF** *extracellular fluid.*

**ECG, ecg** *electrocardiogram.*

**echidnase** (ĕ-kĭd′nās) [Gr. *echidna,* viper] An enzyme, present in the venom of vipers, that produces inflammation.

**echidnin** (ĕ-kĭd′nĭn) **1.** The venom of poisonous snakes. **2.** The active principle present in snake venom.

**Echidnophaga** (ĕk″ĭd-nŏf′ă-gă) A genus of fleas belonging to the family Pulicidae.

***E. gallinacea*** The sticktight flea, an important flea pest of poultry. It collects in clusters on the heads of poultry and in the ears of mammals. It may infest humans, esp. children.

**Echinacea purpurea** (ĕk-ĭ-nā-sē′ah) A genus of native American plants of the family Compositae used as herbal remedies. Traditionally, these plants (also called coneflowers) have been used topically to promote wound healing and internally to improve the immune system. Studies indicate that there is some pharmacologic basis for the traditional uses of *Echinacea* species (e.g., extract of *E. purpurea* has been found to enhance immunologic activity), and no harmful side effects have been reported. However, no conclusions have been reached yet about its use as a therapeutic agent or about a safe dosage of over-the-counter supplements.

**echinate** (ĕk′ĭ-nāt) [Gr. *echinos,* hedgehog] **1.** Spiny. **2.** In agar streak, a growth with pitted or toothed margins along the inoculation line; in stab cultures, coiled growth with pointed outgrowths. SYN: *echinulate.*

**echinococcosis** (ĕ-kī″nō-kŏk-ō′sĭs, ĕk″ĭ-nō-kŏk-ō′sĭs) [″ + *kokkos,* berry, + *osis,* condition] Infestation with *Echinococcus.*

**echinococcotomy** (ĕ-kī″nō-kŏk-ŏt′ō-mē) [″ + ″ + *tome,* incision] An operation for evacuation of an echinococcal cyst.

**Echinococcus** (ĕ-kī″nō-kŏk′ŭs) *pl.* **Echinococci** A genus of tapeworms. They are minute forms consisting of a scolex and three or four proglottids.

***E. granulosus*** A species of tapeworms that infests dogs and other carnivores. Its

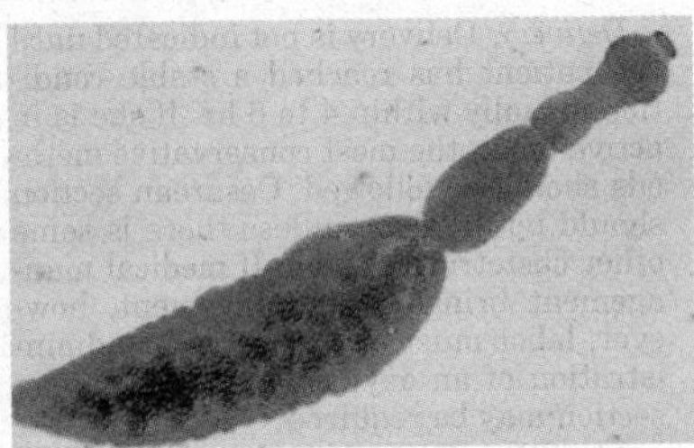

ECHINOCOCCUS GRANULOSUS
(ORIG. MAG. ×5)

larva, called a hydatid, develops in other mammals, including humans, and causes the formation of hydatid cysts in the liver or lungs. SEE: illus.; *hydatid.*

***E. hydatidosus*** A variety of *Echinococcus* characterized by development of daughter cysts from the mother cyst. SEE: *hydatid.*

**echinocyte** An abnormal erythrocyte with multiple, regular, spiny projections from the surface.

**Echinostoma** (ĕk″ĭ-nŏs′tō-mă) [″ + *stoma,* mouth] A genus of flukes characterized by a spiny body and the presence of a collar of spines near the anterior end. They are found in the intestines of many vertebrates, esp. aquatic birds. They occasionally occur as accidental parasites in humans.

**echinulate** (ĕ-kĭn′ū-lāt) A bacterial growth having pointed processes or spines. SYN: *echinate.*

**echo** (ĕk′ō) [Gr. *ekho*] A reverberating sound produced when sound waves are reflected back to their source.

***amphoric e.*** A sound, sometimes heard in auscultation of the chest, resembling the sound of air blown over the mouth of a bottle. SEE: *chest.*

**echocardiogram** (ĕk″ō-kăr′dē-ō-grăm″) The graphic record produced by echocardiography.

**echocardiography** (ĕk″ō-kăr″dē-ŏg′ră-fē) A noninvasive diagnostic method that uses ultrasound to visualize internal cardiac structures. All cardiac valves can be visualized, and the dimensions of each ventricle and the left atrium can be measured.

***dobutamine stress e.*** ABBR: DSE. A pharmacological imaging technique in which the heart is studied by use of echocardiography following intravenous infusion of dobutamine in an increasing dose. It is used to detect coronary artery disease and viable myocardium in patients with acute or chronic myocardial ischemia.

***Doppler e.*** SEE: *Doppler echocardiography.*

***multidimensional visualization e.*** An experimental echocardiographic technique using computer technology for three-dimensional visualization of cardiac structures. This becomes four-dimensional when time is used to impart the cinematic perception of motion.

***transesophageal e.*** ABBR: TEE. An invasive technique for obtaining echocardiographic images whereby probes are introduced into the esophagus where they provide information from several planes. TEE is useful in detecting cardiac sources of emboli, prosthetic heart valve malfunction, endocarditis, aortic dissection, cardiac tumors, and valvular and congenital heart disease.

**echoëncephalogram** (ĕk″ō-ĕn-sĕf′ă-lō-grăm″) Recording of the ultrasonic echoes of the brain, esp. useful in diagnosing conditions that cause a shift in the midline structures of the brain.

**echogenic bowel** A hyperechoic mass may be seen in the fetal abdomen. If ascites is not present, this is probably due to an enlargement of the fetal bowel. Finding this mass in the second trimester of pregnancy is thought to be associated with an increased and significant risk of an abnormal number of chromosomes (i.e., aneuploidy).

**echogram** (ĕk′ō-grăm) The record made by echography.

**echography** (ĕk-ŏg′ră-fē) [″ + *graphein,* to write] The use of ultrasound to photograph the echo produced when sound waves are reflected from tissues of different density. SEE: *ultrasonography.*

**echolalia** (ĕk-ō-lā′lē-ă) [″ + *lalia,* talk, babble] Involuntary parrot-like repetition of words spoken by others, often accompanied by twitching of muscles. It is frequently seen in catatonic schizophrenia.

**echolocation** The location of an object by the use of hearing to detect an echo and identify the position of obstructions.

**echomimia** (ĕk″ō-mĭm′ē-ă) [″ + *mimesis,* imitation] Imitation of the actions of others as seen in schizophrenia. SYN: *echopraxia.*

**echopathy** (ĕ-kŏp′ă-thē) [″ + *pathos,* disease, suffering] A neurosis marked by pathological repetition of another's actions and words.

**echophotony** (ĕk″ō-fŏt′ō-nē) [″ + *phos,* light, + *tonos,* tone] Mental association of certain sounds with particular colors.

**echopraxia** (ĕk″ō-prăk′sē-ă) [″ + *prassein,* to perform] Meaningless imitation of motions made by others. SYN: *echomimia.*

**echo sign** Repetition of the closing word of a sentence, a sign of epilepsy or other brain conditions.

**echothiophate iodide** (ĕk″ō-thī′ō-fāt) A cholinergic drug used topically in the eye for treatment of glaucoma. Trade name is Phospholine Iodide.

**ECHO virus** A virus belonging to the group originally known as *E*nteric *C*ytopatho-genic *H*uman *O*rphan group. They are associated with nonbacterial viral meningitis, enteritis, pleurodynia, acute respiratory infection, and myocarditis. More than 34 viruses were assigned to this group initially. Later some were reclassified. Types 10 and 28 were removed from the ECHO group and classed as reovirus 1 and rhinovirus 1, respectively.

**Eck's fistula** (ěks) [N. V. Eck, Russian physiologist, 1847–1908] An artificial communication between the portal vein and the inferior vena cava, used in experimental surgery in animals.

**eclampsia** (ĕ-klămp'sē-ă) [" + *lampein,* to shine] Coma and convulsive seizures between the 20th week of pregnancy and the end of the first week postpartum. It develops in 1 out of 200 patients with pregnancy-induced hypertension and is usually fatal if untreated. SEE: *hypertension, pregnancy-induced.*

SYMPTOMS: Convulsions are always present. There may be one or many, beginning with fixed eyeballs, rolling eyes, and twitching of the face, arms, and hands; the paroxysms then involve the entire body. Coma eventually follows. The pulse is rapid and bounding, the temperature usually rises to 103° or 104° F (39.4 or 40° C), and the blood pressure may be quite elevated. The patient may remain in coma until death. SEE: *hypertension, pregnancy-induced.*

ETIOLOGY: The cause is unknown. Eclampsia occurs more often in primigravidae. Pre-existing hypertension and glomerulonephritis are risk factors.

PATHOLOGY: Pathology is seen most frequently in the kidney, liver, brain, and placenta. The kidney shows degenerated tubal nephritis; the tubal epithelium shows cloudy swelling, fatty degeneration, and coagulation necrosis. The liver is enlarged and mottled, showing portal vein thrombosis and degeneration of the periphery of the lobules with subcapsular hemorrhages. Edema, hyperemia, thrombosis, and hemorrhages are present in the brain. The placenta shows infarcts, thromboses, and hemorrhages. There is also retinal edema.

TREATMENT: Prophylaxis is of primary importance. Good prenatal care is necessary, with careful, frequent observation and recording of the patient's blood pressure, urine output, and weight. Appropriate therapy should be instituted as soon as there are any abnormal findings, and the pregnancy should be terminated if therapy has been unsuccessful in reducing the signs of danger.

---

Caution: The routine use of diuretics in pregnancy is contraindicated because diuretics are of no benefit and may do considerable harm by masking signs and symptoms that would alert the patient and the physician to the onset of eclampsia.

---

*Delivery:* Delivery is not indicated until the patient has reached a stable condition, usually within 4 to 6 hr. If she is in active labor, the most conservative methods should be followed. Cesarean section should not be done unless there is some other obstetrical reason. If medical management brings no improvement, however, labor must be instituted by administration of an oxytocic agent. Cesarean section may be required.

NURSING IMPLICATIONS: Emergency care is provided during convulsions; prescribed medications are administered as directed, and patient and fetal responses are evaluated. Magnesium sulfate administration must be monitored because of the risk for toxicity; signs include absence of patellar reflexes, flushing, and muscle flaccidity. Calcium gluconate should be available at the bedside to counteract such effects. The patient and family are offered support and prepared for possible premature delivery. Although infants of mothers with eclampsia are usually small for gestational age, they sometimes fare better than other premature infants of similar weight because they have developed adaptive ventilatory and other responses to intrauterine stress. Assessments are continued every 4 hr for 48 hr after delivery. SEE: *Nursing Implications* under *hypertension, pregnancy-induced.*

**eclamptic** Rel. to, or of the nature of, eclampsia.

**eclamptogenic** (ěk-lămp"tō-jěn'ĭk) [Gr. *ek,* out, + *lampein,* to shine, + *gennan,* to produce] Causing eclampsia.

**eclectic** (ěk-lěk'tĭk) [Gr. *eklektikos,* selecting] Selecting what elements seem best from various sources.

**eclecticism** (ěk-lěk'tĭ-sĭzm) [" + *-ismos,* state of] A former system of medicine that treated disease through specific remedies for individual signs or symptoms rather than for distinct diseases. The remedies were principally botanical.

**ecmnesia** (ěk-nē'zē-ă) [Gr. *ek,* out, + *mnesis,* memory] Inability to remember recent events, as seen in senility. The long-term memory is not affected.

**ECMO** *extracorporeal membrane oxygenator.*

**ecocide** (ěk"ō-sīd') [Gr. *oikos,* house, + L. *caedere,* to kill] Willful destruction of some portion of the environment.

**E. coli.** *Escherichia coli.*

**ecological fallacy** In epidemiology, the erroneous attempt to determine from population studies the risk of a particular individual's developing a disease.

**ecological terrorism** The threat to use violent acts that would harm the quality of the environment in order to blackmail a group or society.

**ecology** (ē-kŏl'ō-jē) [Gr. *oikos,* house, + *logos,* word, reason] The science of the relations and interactions of the totality of organisms to their environment, including the relations and interactions of organisms to each other in that environment.

**ecomap** A family interview and assessment tool that delineates the needs, patterns, and relationships among family members and the environment.

**Economo's disease** Encephalitis lethargica.

**economy of movement** [Gr. *oikos,* house, + *nomos,* law] The efficient, energy-sparing motion or activity of the system or body.

**écorché** (ā″kor-shā′) [Fr.] A representation of an animal or human form without skin so that the muscles are clearly seen.

**ecosphere** (ĕk′ō-sfēr″) [Gr. *oikos,* house, + L. *sphera,* ball] The portions of the universe habitable by living organisms and plant life.

**ecostate** (ē-kŏs′tāt) [L. *e,* without, + *costa,* rib] Without ribs.

**ecosystem** (ĕk′ō-sĭs″tĕm) The smallest ecological unit; the living organisms and plants and their environment in a defined area.

**Ecotrin** Trade name for aspirin.

**écouvillonage** (ā-koo″vē-yŏ-năzh′) [Fr. *ecouvillon,* a stiff brush or swab] The cleansing and application of remedies to a cavity by means of a brush or swab.

**écrasement** (ā-krăz-mŏn′) [Fr.] Excision by means of an écraseur.

**écraseur** (ā-kră-zĕr′) [Fr., crusher] A wire loop used for excisions.

**EC space** *extracellular space.*

**ecstasy** (ĕk′stă-sē) [Gr. *ekstasis,* a standing out] **1.** An exhilarated, trancelike condition or state of exalted delight. **2.** A so-called designer drug, 3,4-methylenedioxymethamphetamine (MDMA). Research into the pharmacology and toxicology has been difficult because MDMA is an illicit drug. In addition, the product available on the street has been adulterated, and the dosage of pure drug that precipitates clinical conditions that result in hospitalization is unknown. Use of the drug has been associated with hyperthermia, disseminated intravascular coagulation, liver damage, hallucinations, convulsions, coma, and death.

TREATMENT: The immediate priorities are to control the convulsions, to measure the core temperature, and to reverse the hyperthermia by rapid rehydration and active cooling measures.

**ECT** *electroconvulsive therapy.*

**ectad** [Gr. *ektos,* outside, + L. *ad,* toward] Toward the surface; outward; externally.

**ectasia, ectasis** (ĕk-tā′sē-ă, ĕk′tă-sĭs) [Gr. *ek,* out, + *teinein,* to stretch] Dilatation of any tubular vessel.

***hypostatic e.*** Dilatation of a blood vessel from the pooling of blood in dependent parts, esp. the legs.

***e. iridis*** Small size of the pupil of the eye caused by displacement of the iris.

**ectatic** Distensible or capable of being stretched.

**ectental** [Gr. *ektos,* without, + *entos,* within] Pert. to the entoderm and ectoderm.

**ectental line** The point of the entodermal and ectodermal junction in the gastrula.

**ectethmoid** (ĕk-tĕth′moyd) [″ + *ethmos,* sieve, + *eidos,* form, shape] The lateral mass of the ethmoid bone.

**ecthyma** (ĕk-thī′mă) [Gr. *ek,* out, + *thyein,* to rush] A skin infection, usually a result of neglected treatment of impetigo. It is marked by shallow lesions with adherent crusts or scabs and may be followed by pigmentation and scarring. Treatment is the same as that for impetigo.

**ectiris** (ĕk-tī-rĭs) [Gr. *ektos,* outside, + *iris,* iris] The external portion of the iris.

**ecto-** [Gr. *ektos,* outside] Combining form meaning *outside.*

**ectoantigen** (ĕk″tō-ăn′tĭ-gĕn) [″ + *anti,* against, + *gennan,* to produce] **1.** An antigen assumed to have its origin in ectoplasm of bacterial cells. **2.** An antigen loosely attached to the surface of bacteria and capable of being separated from the bacterial cell.

**ectoblast** (ĕk′tō-blăst) [″ + *blastos,* germ] **1.** The ectoderm. **2.** Any outer membrane, such as the ectoderm.

**ectocardia** (ĕk′tō-kăr′dē-ă) [″+ *kardia,* heart] Displacement of the heart.

**ectocervix** (ĕk″tō-sĕr′vĭks) The portion of the canal of the uterine cervix that is lined with squamous epithelium. **ectocervical** (-sĕr′vĭ-kăl), *adj.*

**ectochoroidea** (ĕk″tō-kō-roy′dē-ă) [″ + *khorioeides,* choroid] The outer layer of the choroid coat of the eye.

**ectocolostomy** (ĕk″tō-kŏ-lŏs′tō-mē) [″ *kolon,* colon, + *stoma,* mouth] Surgical formation of an opening into the colon through the abdominal wall.

**ectocondyle** (ĕk″tō-kŏn′dĭl) [″ + *kondylos,* knuckle] The outer condyle of a bone.

**ectocornea** (ĕk-tō-kor′nē-ă) [″ + L. *corneus,* horny] The external layer of the cornea.

**ectocuneiform** (ĕk-tō-kū′nē-ĭ-form) [″+ L. *cuneus,* wedge, + *forma,* form] The external cuneiform bone.

**ectodactylism** (ĕk″tō-dăk′tĭl-ĭzm) [Gr. *ektrosis,* miscarriage, + *daktylos,* finger, + *ismos,* state of] Lack of a digit or digits.

**ectoderm** (ĕk′tō-dĕrm) [Gr. *ektos,* outside, + *derma,* skin] The outer layer of cells in the developing embryo. It produces skin structures, the teeth and glands of the mouth, the nervous system, organs of special sense, part of the pituitary gland, and the pineal and suprarenal glands. SYN: *epiblast.* SEE: *entoderm; mesoderm.* **ectodermal, ectodermic** (-ăl, -ĭk), *adj.*

**ectoentad** (ĕk″tō-ĕn′tăd) [″ + *entos,* within] From the outside inward.

**ectogenous** (ĕk-tŏj′ĕ-nŭs) [″ + *gennan,* to produce] **1.** Originating outside of a body or structure, as infection. **2.** Able to grow outside of the body, as a parasite.

**ectoglia** (ĕk-tŏg′lē-ă) [″ + *glia,* glue] The superficial embryonic layer in the beginning of the stratification of the medullary tube of the embryo.

**ectogony** (ĕk-tŏg′ō-nē) [″ + *gone,* seed] Influence of the embryo on the mother.

**ectolecithal** (ĕk″tō-lĕs′ĭ-thăl) [″ + *lekithos,* yolk] Pert. to an ovum having food yolk placed near the surface.

**ectomere** (ĕk′tō-mēr) [″ + *meros,* part] One of the blastomeres forming the ectoderm.

**ectomesoblast** (ĕk″tō-mĕs′ō-blăst) [″ + *mesos,* middle, + *blastos,* germ] A cell from which the ectoblast and mesoblast develop.

**ectomorph** (ĕk′tō-morf) [″ + *morphe,* form] A person with a body build marked by predominance of tissues derived from the ectoderm. The body is linear with sparse muscular development. SEE: *endomorph; mesomorph; somatotype.*

**-ectomy** (ĕk′tō-mē) [Gr. *ektome*] Combining form meaning *excision* of any anatomical structure.

**ectopagus** (ĕk-tŏp′ă-gŭs) [″ + *pagos,* something fixed] An abnormal fetus consisting of twins fused at the thorax.

**ectoparasite** (ĕk″tō-păr′ă-sīt″) [″ + Gr. *parasitos,* parasite] A parasite that lives on the outer surface of the body, such as fleas, lice, or ticks.

**ectoperitonitis** (ĕk″tō-pĕr″ĭ-tō-nī′tĭs) [″ + *peritonaion,* peritoneum, + *itis,* inflammation] Inflammation of the parietal layer of the peritoneum (the layer lining the abdominal wall).

**ectophyte** (ĕk′tō-fīt) [″ + *phyton,* plant] A parasite of vegetable origin growing on the skin.

**ectopia** (ĕk-tō′pē-ă) [Gr. *ektopos,* displaced] Malposition or displacement, esp. congenital, of an organ or structure.

***e. cordis*** A malposition of the heart in which it lies outside the thoracic cavity.

***e. lentis*** Displacement of the crystalline lens of the eye.

***e. pupillae congenita*** Congenital displacement of the pupil.

***e. renis*** Displacement of the kidney.

***e. testis*** Displacement of the testis.

***e. vesicae*** Displacement, esp. exstrophy, of the bladder.

***visceral e.*** An umbilical hernia.

**ectopic** (ĕk-tŏp′ik) In an abnormal position. Opposite of entopic.

**ectopic beat, complex** Electric stimulation of cardiac contractions beginning at a point other than the sinoatrial node.

**ectopic hormone production** The secretion of hormones by nonendocrine tissue. The term is not precise in that specific hormones may be produced by endocrine tissue at sites other than the usual endocrine gland. For example, gonadal hormones may be produced in the normal intestine, and thyrotropic hormone may be produced by the normal pancreas. Ectopically produced hormones may arise from both benign and malignant tumors. Ectopic sites may produce multiple hormones, such as adrenocorticotropic hormone, endorphins, and melanocyte-stimulating hormone.

**ectopic pregnancy** Implantation of the fertilized ovum outside of the uterine cavity. There is usually a poorly developed decidual reaction in the uterus. SEE: illus.; *pregnancy.*

SYMPTOMS: Symptoms include amenorrhea; tenderness, soreness, and pain on the affected side; and pallor, weak pulse, and signs of shock or hemorrhage. Pain may be reflected to the shoulder. Bluish discoloration of the umbilicus may be present.

*Unruptured:* Amenorrhea may or may not be present; there are vague pains in the abdomen, usually on one side, and irregular hemorrhage. The diagnosis at this stage can be made by the usual biological tests for pregnancy.

*Ruptured:* Without severe hemorrhage, there is intense pain in the lower abdomen with repeated fainting spells. Diagnosis is made by transvaginal needle puncture into the peritoneal cavity; this reveals free blood. If bleeding is severe and surgical therapy is not begun immediately, death may result.

LOCATIONS: *Abdominal:* The pregnancy is in the free abdominal cavity and attached to one of the abdominal viscera. *Interstitial:* The pregnancy is in the interstitial portion of the fallopian tube. *Ovarian:* The pregnancy is in the ovary. The ovarian and primary abdominal types are very rare. *Tubal:* The pregnancy is in the fallopian tube. This is the type most frequently encountered. The pregnancy may be situated in the interstitial, ampullar, or isthmic portion of the tube, the isthmic type being the most common. SEE: illus.

ETIOLOGY: Most ectopic pregnancies are associated with inflammatory conditions of the tube and other conditions that interfere mechanically with the downward passage of the ovum, such as diverticula, polypi in the tubal lumen, and peritoneal adhesions. Any variety of pregnancy or any combination of varieties may occur (e.g., uterine plus ectopic, bilateral ectopic).

DIAGNOSIS: Ectopic pregnancy must be differentiated from appendicitis, uterine pregnancy, acute salpingitis, twisting of the pedicle of an ovarian cyst, pedunculated fibroid tumor, and hemorrhage from a ruptured graafian follicle or corpus luteum cyst.

In some cases, the usual signs of pregnancy are present; however, in other cases, the patient may not even suspect that she is pregnant. If a woman with a history of normal ovulation is thought to be pregnant, the usual test for human chorionic gonadotropin (hCG) is done to help confirm the diagnosis. If the patient is thought to have an ectopic pregnancy, a transvaginal ultrasound study is done.

Conception stimulates production of hCG which, in turn, maintains the pro-

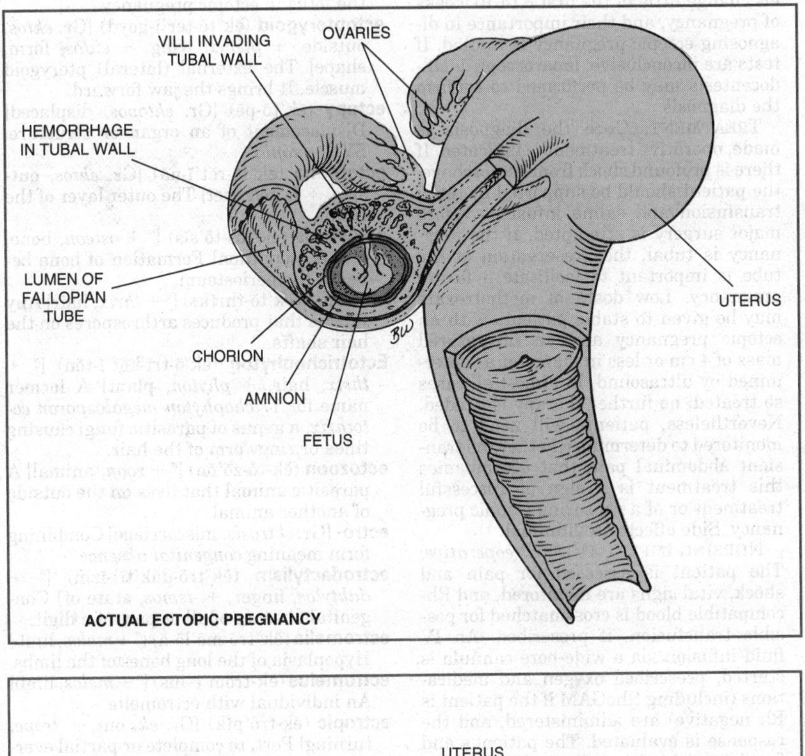

VILLI INVADING TUBAL WALL

OVARIES

HEMORRHAGE IN TUBAL WALL

LUMEN OF FALLOPIAN TUBE

UTERUS

CHORION

AMNION

FETUS

ACTUAL ECTOPIC PREGNANCY

UTERUS

ISTHMIC

AMPULLAR

INTRALIGAMENTOUS

INFUNDIBULAR

OVARIAN

FIMBRIAL

INTRAMURAL

CERVICAL

ABDOMINAL

VARIOUS SITES OF ECTOPIC PREGNANCY

ECTOPIC PREGNANCY

duction of progesterone by the corpus luteum; however, serum progesterone levels change little in the first 8 to 10 weeks of pregnancy, and their importance in diagnosing ectopic pregnancy is limited. If tests are inconclusive, laparoscopy or culdocentesis may be performed to confirm the diagnosis.

TREATMENT: Once the diagnosis is made, operative treatment is indicated. If there is profound shock from hemorrhage, the patient should be supported by blood transfusion and saline infusions before major surgery is attempted. If the pregnancy is tubal, the preservation of the tube is important to facilitate a future pregnancy. Low doses of methotrexate may be given to stable patients with an ectopic pregnancy and an unruptured mass of 4 cm or less in diameter as determined by ultrasound. In almost all cases so treated, no further therapy is needed. Nevertheless, patients will need to be monitored to determine whether the transient abdominal pain that accompanies this treatment is a sign of successful treatment or of a rupturing ectopic pregnancy. Side effects are minimal.

NURSING IMPLICATIONS: *Preoperative:* The patient is assessed for pain and shock, vital signs are monitored, and Rh-compatible blood is crossmatched for possible transfusion, if prescribed. An IV fluid infusion via a wide-bore cannula is started, prescribed oxygen and medications (including RhoGAM if the patient is Rh negative) are administered, and the response is evaluated. The patient's and family's wishes regarding religious rites for the products of conception are determined. Both patient and family are encouraged to express their feelings of fear, loss, and grief. Information regarding the condition and the need for surgical intervention is clarified.

*Postoperative:* Vital signs are monitored until stable, incisional dressings are inspected, vaginal bleeding is assessed, and the patient's physical and emotional reactions to the surgery are evaluated. Prescribed medications are administered. The griedving process is anticipated, and both the patient and family are referred for further counseling as needed. SEE: *Nursing Diagnoses Appendix.*

**ectopic rhythm** Any abnormal or irregular cardiac rhythm.

NURSING IMPLICATIONS: Cardiac rhythm is monitored, and appropriate action is taken for life-threatening dysrhythmias.

**ectopic secretion** (ĕk-tŏp′ĭk) The secretion of a hormone by a tumor arising from tissues that do not normally secrete the hormone.

**ectoplasm** [Gr. *ektos,* outside, + LL. *plasma,* form, mold] The outermost layer of cell protoplasm. **ectoplasmic, ectoplastic,** *adj.*

**ectopotomy** (ĕk-tō-pŏt′ō-mē) [Gr. *ektopos,* displaced, + *tome,* incision] Removal of the fetus in ectopic pregnancy.

**ectopterygoid** (ĕk″tō-tĕr′ĭ-goyd) [Gr. *ektos,* outside, + *pteryx,* wing, + *eidos,* form, shape] The external (lateral) pterygoid muscle. It brings the jaw forward.

**ectopy** (ĕk′tō-pē) [Gr. *ektopos,* displaced] Displacement of an organ or structure. SYN: *ectopia.*

**ectoretina** (ĕk″tō-rĕt′ĭ-nă) [Gr. *ektos,* outside, + L. *rete,* net] The outer layer of the retina.

**ectostosis** (ĕk-tŏs-tō′sĭs) [″ + *osteon,* bone, + *osis,* condition] Formation of bone beneath the periosteum.

**ectothrix** (ĕk′tō-thrĭks) [″ + *thrix,* hair] Any fungus that produces arthrospores on the hair shafts.

**Ectotrichophyton** (ĕk″ō-trī-kŏf′ĭ-tŏn) [″ + *thrix,* hair, + *phyton,* plant] A former name for *Trichophyton megalosporon ectothrix,* a genus of parasitic fungi causing tinea or ringworm of the hair.

**ectozoon** (ĕk-tō-zō′ŏn) [″ + *zoon,* animal] A parasitic animal that lives on the outside of another animal.

**ectro-** [Gr. *ektrosis,* miscarriage] Combining form meaning *congenital absence.*

**ectrodactylism** (ĕk″trō-dăk′tĭl-ĭzm) [″ + *daktylos,* finger, + *-ismos,* state of] Congenital absence of all or part of a digit.

**ectromelia** (ĕk″trō-mē′lē-ă) [″ + *melos,* limb] Hypoplasia of the long bones of the limbs.

**ectromelus** (ĕk-trŏm′ĕ-lŭs) [″ + *melos,* limb] An individual with ectromelia.

**ectropic** (ĕk-trō′pĭk) [Gr. *ek,* out, + *trope,* turning] Pert. to complete or partial eversion of a part, generally the eyelid.

**ectropion** (ĕk-trō′pē-ŏn) Eversion of an edge or margin, as the edge of an eyelid.

ETIOLOGY: Causes include old age, relaxation of skin, a cicatrix following trauma, infection, and palsy of the facial nerve.

**ectrosyndactyly** (ĕk″trō-sĭn-dăk′tĭ-lē) [″ + *syn,* together, + *dactylos,* finger] Congenital absence of one or more fingers; the remaining fingers are fused together.

**eczema** (ĕk′zĕ-mă) [Gr. *ekzein,* to boil out] An acute or chronic cutaneous inflammation with erythema, papules, vesicles, pustules, scales, crusts, or scabs alone or in combination. They may be dry or produce a watery discharge, with thickening, infiltration, and a variable amount of itching or burning. Eczema is more the description of a symptom than of a disease. SYN: *dermatitis.* SEE: *allergy.*

SYMPTOMS: Primary eczema is characterized by erythematous, papular, vesicular, or pustular lesions. In secondary eczema, the lesions evolve from the primary variety. Invasion by pathogenic organisms may cause suppuration.

ETIOLOGY: No class, age, or sex is exempt, but persons with thin, dry skin are more susceptible. The lesions are not infectious. Two classes of causes are external, or exciting (irritation; allergenic contact; reaction to exposure to certain microorganisms; occupational, nonoccupational, or chemical factors); and constitutional, or predisposing. The latter includes eczema caused by genetic and psychological factors.

TREATMENT: Treatment depends on the cause and therefore is highly individualized according to the causative agent, organism, or condition.

PROGNOSIS: Chronic eczema is amenable to treatment but prone to relapse and recurrence.

NURSING IMPLICATIONS: The patient should eliminate allergens from the diet and environment and avoid precipitating or exacerbating factors such as local irritants (wool, detergents, perfumes), extreme temperature changes, and emotional stress. The patient is taught about use and adverse effects of prescribed topical and systemic measures to relieve pruritus and inflammation. Measures such as wearing mittens and keeping nails short and smooth are instituted to decrease excoriation from scratching. The patient is instructed to bathe using tepid water and nonfat, nonperfumed soap, and to avoid soap altogether during exacerbations. The nurse avoids showing anxiety or revulsion when touching the patient's lesions during assessment or application of topical treatments. Universal precautions are followed during assessment and treatment. The patient is encouraged to verbalize and examine feelings about altered body image and may be referred for further counseling. SEE: *Nursing Diagnoses Appendix; Universal Precautions Appendix.*

***asteatotic e.*** SEE: *winter itch.*

***dyshidrotic e.*** Pompholyx.

***erythematous e.*** Dry, pinkish, ill-defined patches with itching and burning; slight swelling with tendency to spread and coalesce; branny scaling; roughness and dryness of skin. This type may become generalized.

***e. herpeticum*** Massive crops of vesicles that become pustular, occurring when herpes simplex virus infection occurs in a person, usually an infant, with pre-existing eczema. SYN: *Kaposi's varicelliform eruption.* SEE: *AIDS.*

***lichenoid e.*** Eczema with thickening of the skin.

***nummular e.*** Eczema with coin- or oval-shaped lesions. It is often associated with dry skin and worsens in dry weather. SEE: illus.

***pustular e.*** Follicular, impetiginous, or consecutive eczema including eczema rubrum (red, glazed surface with little oozing), eczema madidans (raw, red, and covered with moisture), eczema fissum (thick, dry, inelastic skin with cracks and fissures), squamous eczema (chronic on soles, legs, scalp; multiple circumscribed, infiltrated patches with thin, dry scales).

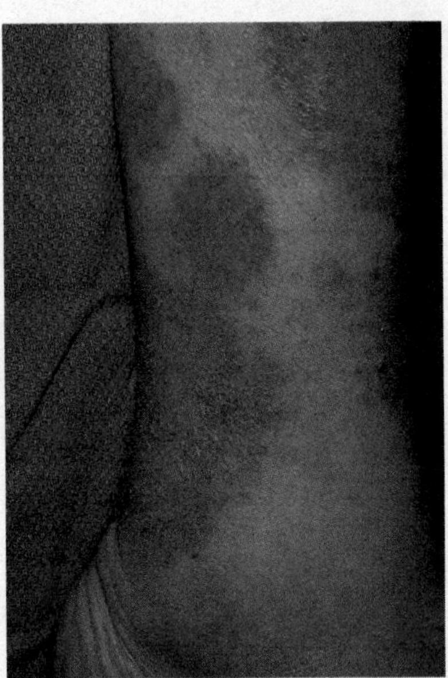

**NUMMULAR ECZEMA** ON LEG

***seborrheic e.*** Eczema marked by excessive secretion from the sebaceous glands. SYN: *seborrhea.*

**eczematous** (ĕk-zĕm′ă-tŭs) Marked by or resembling eczema.

**ED** *effective dose; erythema dose.*

**E.D.** *Emergency Department.*

**$ED_{50}$** The median effective dose, producing the desired effect in 50% of subjects tested.

**EDC** *expected date of confinement.*

**EDD** *expected date of delivery.*

**edema, oedema** (ĕ-dē′mă) *pl.* **edemas or edemata** [Gr. *oidema,* swelling] A local or generalized condition in which the body tissues contain an excessive amount of tissue fluid. Ascites and hydrothorax indicate accumulation of excess fluid in the peritoneal and pleural cavities, respectively. A generalized edema was previously termed dropsy.

ETIOLOGY: Edema may result from increased permeability of the capillary walls; increased capillary pressure due to venous obstruction or heart failure; lymphatic obstruction; disturbances in renal function; reduction of plasma proteins; inflammatory conditions; fluid and electrolyte disturbances, particularly those causing sodium retention; malnutrition; starvation; or chemical substances such as bacterial toxins, venoms, caustic substances, and histamine.

TREATMENT: Bedrest is desirable. Salt restriction is moderate or severe, depending on the degree of edema. Fluid intake may be restricted to as little as 600 ml in

24 hr. This prescription may be relaxed when free diuresis has been attained. Diuretics are effective when renal function is good and edema mild, and when any underlying abnormality of cardiac function, capillary pressure, or salt retention is being corrected simultaneously. One of various effective diuretics may be used. Diuretics are contraindicated in preeclampsia and in the true nephritic edema of acute diffuse glomerulonephritis. They are often useless in cardiac edema associated with advanced renal insufficiency. The diet in edema should be adequate in protein, high in calories, rich in vitamins, and low in salt. When diuresis appears, the patient may resume a normal diet. SEE: *decubitus ulcer*.

NURSING IMPLICATIONS: Edema is documented according to type (pitting, nonpitting, or brawny), extent, location, symmetry, and degree of pitting. Areas over bony prominences are palpated for edema by pressing with the fingertip for 5 sec, then releasing. The tissue should normally immediately rebound to its original contour, so the depth of indentation is measured and recorded. The patient is questioned about increased tightness of rings, shoes, waistlines of garments, belts, and so forth. Periorbital edema is assessed; abdominal girth and ankle circumference are measured; and the patient's weight and fluid intake and output are monitored. Fragile edematous tissues are protected from damage by careful handling and positioning and by providing and teaching about special skin care. Edematous extremities are mobilized and elevated to promote venous return, and lung sounds auscultated for evidence of increasing pulmonary congestion. Prescribed therapies, including sodium restriction, diuretics, protein replacement, and elastic stockings or other elastic support garments, are provided, and the patient is instructed in their use. **edematous** (-ăt-ŭs), *adj.*

***angioneurotic e.*** Old term for angioedema.

***brain e.*** Swelling of brain tissue due to accumulation of fluid. It may be caused by a tumor, toxic chemicals, or infections.

***e. bullosum vesicae*** A form of edema affecting the bladder.

***cardiac e.*** Accumulation of fluid due to congestive heart failure. It is most apparent in the dependent portion of the body.

***cerebral e.*** Brain e.

***dependent e.*** Edema or swelling of the part of the body below the heart. Thus, the legs are more edematous than are the upper arms.

***e. of the glottis*** Infiltration of the submucosa of the larynx with coughing, loss of voice, and a feeling of suffocation.

***high-altitude pulmonary e.*** ABBR: HAPE. Pulmonary edema that may occur in aviators, mountain climbers, or anyone exposed to decreased atmospheric pressure. SEE: *hypoxia*.

***inflammatory e.*** Edema associated with inflammation. The cause is assumed to be damage to the capillary endothelium. It is usually nonpitting and localized, and other signs of inflammation are present.

***laryngeal e.*** Edema of the larynx, usually resulting from allergic reaction and causing airway obstruction unless treated. Therapy consists of intravenous or intratracheal epinephrine, emergency tracheostomy, or both.

***malignant e.*** Edema marked by a rapid course and speedy destruction of tissue.

***e. neonatorum*** Edema in newborn, esp. premature, infants. This condition is usually transitory, involving the hands, face, feet, and genitalia, and rarely becomes generalized.

***pitting e.*** Edema, usually of the skin of the extremities. When pressed firmly with a finger, the skin maintains the depression produced by the finger.

***pulmonary e.*** Effusion of serous fluid into the alveoli and interstitial tissue of the lungs. The cause is weakening or failure of the left ventricle, which allows blood to back up and increase filtration pressure in the pulmonary capillaries. This is life-threatening. Acute pulmonary edema may be a sign of severe pulmonary or heart disease. The outcome will depend upon the success of treating the primary illness. SYN: *edema of lung*. SEE: *Nursing Diagnoses Appendix*.

SYMPTOMS: Symptoms include extreme dyspnea, rapid labored breathing, cough with frothy blood-stained expectoration, cyanosis, and cold extremities.

ETIOLOGY: Pulmonary edema is caused by weakening or failure of the left side of the heart; blood backs up in the pulmonary capillaries and increases filtration pressure. This may be caused by several conditions including hypoproteinemia, pulmonary infections, inhaled toxins, disseminated intravascular coagulation, narcotic overdose, pulmonary embolism, and high altitude.

TREATMENT: Therapy is directed toward altering the condition causing the difficulty. Usually this includes vigorous treatment of any heart condition, and administration of oxygen and morphine; in extreme cases phlebotomy may be required. Prior to this, tourniquets are applied to the limbs in an attempt to have the excess tissue fluid collect in the extremities rather than in the lungs.

NOTE: Tourniquets should be applied to only one limb at a time for 15 min, using sufficient pressure to block venous return but not enough to interfere with arterial blood flow to the limb.

PROGNOSIS: The outlook for these patients is grave. Often edema of the lungs is a final symptom of a fatal pulmonary disease.

***purulent e.*** Edema caused by suppurative infiltration.

***salt e.*** A form of edema caused by an increase of salt in the diet.

**edematogenic** (ĕ-dĕm″ă-tō-jĕn′ĭk) Causing edema.

**edentia** (ē-dĕn′shē-ă) [L. *e,* without, + *dens,* tooth] Absence of teeth.

**edentulous** (ē-dĕnt′ū-lŭs) Without teeth.

**edetate calcium disodium** (ĕd′ĕ-tāt) The disodium salt of ethylenediaminetetra-acetic acid. A chelating agent, it is used in diagnosing and treating lead poisoning. Trade names are Calcium Disodium Versenate and Versene CA.

**edetate disodium** (ĕd′ĕ-tāt dī-sō′dē-ŭm) A chelating agent, disodium dihydrogen ethylenediaminetetra-acetate dihydrate. It is used in treating hypercalcemia.

**edge** A margin or border.

***bevel e.*** A tooth edge produced by beveling.

***cutting e.*** An angled or sharpened edge for cutting, as an incisor tooth or the blade of a knife.

***denture e.*** The margin or border of a denture.

***incisal e.*** The sharpened edge of a tooth produced by occlusal wear; the labiolingual margin.

**edible** (ĕd′ĭ-bl) [L. *edere,* to eat] Suitable for food; fit to eat; nonpoisonous.

**edrophonium chloride** (ĕd″rō-fō′nē-ŭm) A cholinergic drug. Trade name is Tensilon. SEE: *edrophonium test.*

**edrophonium test** The use of edrophonium chloride to test for the presence of myasthenia gravis. The appropriate dose is injected intravenously; if there is no effect, a larger dose is given within 45 sec. A positive test demonstrates brief improvement in strength unaccompanied by lingual fasciculation. The test may also be used to determine an overdose of a cholinergic drug. An excessive dose of cholinergic drug produces weakness that closely resembles myasthenia. A very small dose of edrophonium chloride given intravenously worsens the weakness if it is due to cholinergic drug overdose and improves it if it is due to myasthenia gravis.

---

Caution: The test should not be performed unless facilities and staff for respiratory resuscitation are immediately available.

---

**EDTA** *ethylenediaminetetra-acetic acid.*

**education, fieldwork** The educational link between the classroom and service delivery settings that takes place in approved facilities under the supervision of a qualified professional.

**eduction** (ē-dŭk′shŭn) [L. *e,* out, + *ducere,* to lead] Emergence from a particular state or condition (e.g., coming out of the effects of general anesthesia). SEE: *induction* (4).

**EE** *coefficient of elastic expansion.*

**EEE** *eastern equine encephalitis.*

**EEG** *electroencephalogram.*

**EENT** *eyes, ears, nose, and throat.*

**EEOC** *Equal Employment Opportunity Commission.* A committee that enforces Title VII of federal regulations, which has guidelines that provide protection from sexual harassment and discrimination in the workplace.

**EFA** *essential fatty acid.*

**effacement** (ĕ-fās′mĕnt) In obstetrics, during the normal progress of delivery, the dilation of the cervix, enlarging the cross-sectional area of the canal to permit passage of the fetus.

**effect** (ĕ-fĕkt′) [L. *effectus,* to accomplish] The result of an action or force.

***additive e.*** The therapeutic effect of a combination of two or more drugs that is equal to the sum of the individual drug effects.

***Bainbridge e.*** SEE: *reflex, Bainbridge.*

***ceiling e.*** The optimal potential effect of a medication. This dose may not relieve the patient's symptoms. The frequent occurrence of side effects signals the provider to begin a different regimen.

***cumulative e.*** A drug effect that is apparent only after several doses have been given. It is caused by excretion or metabolic degradation of only a fraction of each dose given. Sometimes it is therapeutically desirable although this type of effect is usually avoided.

***fetal alcohol e.'s*** Mild to moderate physical or mental retardation or both, resulting from maternal alcohol abuse during the last trimester of pregnancy. Behavioral problems related to poor motor coordination and inadequate decision-making skills reflect interference with the refinement of brain functions that occurs as the fetus nears term. SEE: *defect, alcohol-related birth; fetal alcohol syndrome.*

***nonstochastic e.*** A radiation effect whose severity increases in direct proportion to the dose and for which there usually is a threshold. An example is radiation-induced cataracts.

***photoelectric e.*** An interaction between x-rays and matter in which the x-ray photon ejects an inner-shell electron, causing a cascade of outer-shell electrons to fill the hole. The changing of energy shells releases secondary radiation equal to the difference in the binding energies. This absorption reaction increases the patient dose and creates contrast on the radiographic film. It usually occurs at low photon energies.

***piezoelectric e.*** In ultrasound, a change of the mechanical action of the ceramic crystals into an electrical impulse. SEE: *triboluminescence.*

**effectiveness** (ĕ-fĕk′tĭv-nĕs) The ability to cause the expected or intended effect or result.

**effector** Any organ stimulated by motor nerve impulses; a muscle that contracts or a gland that secretes. SYN: *effector organ.*

**effector cell** An active cell of the immune system responsible for destroying or controlling foreign antigens. SEE: *leukocyte.*

**effector organ** Effector.

**effeminate** Pert. to a male who has the physical characteristics or mannerisms of a female.

**effemination** (ĕ-fĕm″ĭ-nā′shŭn) [L. *effeminare,* to make feminine] The production of female physical characteristics in a male. SYN: *feminization.*

**efferent** [L. *efferens,* to bring out] Carrying away from a central organ or section, as efferent nerves, which conduct impulses from the brain or spinal cord to the periphery; efferent lymph vessels, which convey lymph from lymph nodes; and efferent arterioles, which carry blood from glomeruli of the kidney. Opposite of afferent.

**efferent nerve** A nerve that carries impulses having one of the following effects: motor, causing contraction of muscles; secretory, causing glands to secrete; and inhibitory, causing some organs to become quiescent. SYN: *motor nerve.*

**effervesce** (ĕf″ĕr-vĕs′) [L. *effervescere,* to boil up] To boil or form bubbles on the surface of a liquid.

**effervescence** (ĕf-ĕr-vĕs′ĕns) Formation of gas bubbles that rise to the surface of a fluid.

**effervescent** Bubbling; rising in little bubbles of gas.

**efficacy** The ability to produce a desired effect.

**effleurage** (ĕf-loor-ăzh′) [Fr. *effleurer,* to touch lightly] Deep or gentle stroking in massage.

***abdominal e.*** Light stroking with the fingertips in a circular pattern from the symphysis pubis to the iliac crests, a Lamaze technique for coping with uterine contractions during the first stage of labor.

**efflorescence** (ĕf-flor-ĕs′ĕns) [L. *efflorescere,* to bloom] A rash; a redness of the skin. SYN: *exanthem.*

**efflorescent** Becoming powdery or dry from loss of water in crystallization.

**effluent** (ĕf′loo-ĕnt) [L. *effluere,* to flow out] **1.** A flowing out. **2.** Fluid material discharged from a sewage treatment or industrial plant.

**effluvium** (ĕf-loo′vē-ŭm) *pl.* **effluvia** A malodorous outflow of vapor or gas, particularly one that is toxic.

**effort** Expenditure of physical or mental energy.

**effort syndrome** A form of anxiety neurosis in which fatigue is the presenting symptom. The fatigue is increased by mild exertion and may be more pronounced in the morning. SEE: *neurosis.*

**effuse** (ĕ-fūs′) [L. *effusio,* pour out] Thin, widely spreading; applied to a bacterial growth that forms a very delicate film over a surface.

**effusion** (ĕ-fū′zhŭn) Escape of fluid into a part, as the pleural cavity, such as pyothorax (pus), hydrothorax (serum), hemothorax (blood), chylothorax (lymph), pneumothorax (air), hydropneumothorax (serum and air), and pyopneumothorax (pus and air).

***joint e.*** Increased fluid within a joint cavity. There may be increased production of synovial fluid following trauma or with some arthritic disease processes, or blood accumulating in the joint following trauma or surgery or due to hemophilia.

***pericardial e.*** Fluid in the pericardial cavity, between the visceral and the parietal pericardium. This condition may produce symptoms of cardiac tamponade.

***pleural e.*** Fluid in the thoracic cavity between the visceral and parietal pleura. It may be seen on a chest radiograph if it exceeds 300 ml.

**eflornithine** An antineoplastic and antiprotozoal drug. It has been used to treat African sleeping sickness (African trypanosomiasis). Trade name is Ornidyl.

**egesta** (ē-jĕs′tă) [L. *egere,* to cast forth] Waste matter eliminated from the body, esp. excrement.

**egg** [AS. *aeg*] **1.** The female sex cell or ovum, applied esp. to a fertilized ovum that is passed from the body and develops outside, as in fowls. **2.** The mammalian ovum.

***raw e.*** An egg in its fresh, uncooked state, esp. one intended for food. Human consumption of raw or inadequately cooked eggs has caused *Salmonella* infections. To kill *Salmonella* organisms, if present, eggs should be boiled for 7 min, fried for 3 min per side, or poached for 5 min. It is unsafe to use sauces or dressings made with raw eggs. Fresh eggs should be stored in the cold; cracked eggs should be discarded. SEE: *salmonellosis.*

**eglandulous** (ē-glănd′ū-lŭs) [L. *e,* out, + *glandula,* glandule] Without glands.

**ego** (ē′gō, ĕg′ō) [L. *ego,* I] In psychoanalysis, one of the three major divisions in the model of the psychic apparatus. The others are the id and superego. The ego is involved with consciousness and memory and mediates among primitive instinctual or animal drives (the id), internal social prohibitions (the superego), and reality. The psychiatric use of the term should not be confused with its common usage in the sense of self-love or selfishness. SEE: *id; superego.*

**egocentric** (ē″gō-sĕn′trĭk) [L. *ego,* I, + Gr. *kentron,* center] Pert. to a withdrawal from the external world with concentration on the inner self.

**egocentricity** The stage of cognitive development in which perception is almost exclusively from the child's own viewpoint and in the child's own way. This stage is characteristic of toddlers and early preschool children.

**ego-dystonic** (ē″gō-dĭs-tŏn′ĭk) [″ + Gr. *dys,* bad, + *tonos,* tension] Pert. to something repulsive to the individual's self-image.

**ego-integrity** The eighth stage in Erikson's developmental theory; the opposite of despair. It is the major psychic task of the mature elderly and is marked by a healthy unifying philosophy and the wisdom learned from experience. The individual feels vital, balanced, and whole in relation to the self and the world.

**egoism** (ē′gō-ĭzm) An inflated estimate of one's value or effectiveness.

**egomania** (ē″gō-mā′nē-ă) [″+ Gr. *mania,* madness] Abnormal self-esteem and self-interest.

**egophony** (ē-gŏf′ō-nē) [Gr. *aix,* goat, + *phone,* voice] An abnormal change in tone, somewhat like the bleat of a goat, heard in auscultation of the chest when the subject speaks normally. It is associated with bronchophony and may be heard over the lungs of persons with pleural effusion.

**ego strength** The ability of the ego to maintain its various functions, the prime one of which is to perceive reality and adapt to it.

**ego-syntonic** (ē″gō-sĭn-tŏn′ĭk) [″ + Gr. *syn,* together, + *tonos,* tension] Pert. to something that is consistent with the individual's self-image.

**egotism** (ē′gō-tĭzm) **1.** The tendency to regard oneself more highly than is warranted by the facts, and to boast of one's abilities or achievements. **2.** An inflated sense of self-importance; conceit. SEE: *egoism.*

**egotropic** (ē″gō-trŏp′ĭk) [L. *ego,* I, + Gr. *tropos,* a turning] Interested chiefly in one's self; self-centered.

**EGTA** *esophageal gastric tube airway.*

**Ehlers-Danlos syndrome** (ā′lĕrz-dăn′lŏs) [Edvard Ehlers, Danish dermatologist, 1863–1937; H. A. Danlos, Fr. dermatologist, 1844–1912] An inherited disorder of the elastic connective tissue. The characteristic soft velvety skin is fragile, hyperelastic, and bruises easily. Hyperextensibility of joints, visceral malformations, atrophic scars, pseudotumors, and calcified subcutaneous cysts are present.

ETIOLOGY: The cause is unknown.

TREATMENT: There is no specific therapy.

PROGNOSIS: Patients may be uncomfortable and inconvenienced by their disease, but the prognosis is good.

**Ehrenritter's ganglion** (ăr′ĕn-rĭt″ĕrs) [Johann Ehrenritter, Austrian anatomist, d. 1790] The superior ganglion of the glossopharyngeal nerve.

**ehrlichiosis, human granulocytic** [Paul Ehrlich, Ger. physician, 1854–1915. Awarded Nobel Prize in medicine in 1908] An infectious disease caused by members of the genus *Ehrlichia,* usually *E. chaffeensis* or *E. canis.* It was first reported in a human in the U.S. in 1947. Most patients give a history of tick bite; 80% of patients are male. Treatment is with tetracycline or doxycycline.

SYMPTOMS: Clinically, after a median incubation period of 7 days, the initial symptoms of fever, chills, headache, myalgia, and malaise appear. Later, nausea, anorexia, weight loss, diarrhea, altered mental state, lymphadenopathy, leukopenia, and altered liver function may be present. Less than half of the patients have a rash, which is seen more often in children than in adults. The fatality rate may be as high as 2%.

DIAGNOSIS: Serological tests are used; a polymerase chain reaction (PCR) applied to whole blood samples can confirm the diagnosis in 24 to 48 hr.

PREVENTION: Ticks should be avoided. If exposed to ticks, the body should be carefully searched for their presence and immediately removed.

**Ehrlich's side-chain theory** (ār′lĭks) [Paul Ehrlich] A theory, proposed to explain immune reactions, that compares the antigen-antibody reaction with a chemical structure having side chains or chemical receptors. Through these chemical receptors, the body cells combine with antigens that eventually are released as circulating antibodies.

**eicosanoid** One of the products of the metabolism of arachidonic acid. Prostaglandins, thromboxanes, and leukotrienes are some of the compounds formed.

**EID** *electroimmunodiffusion; electronic infusion device.*

**eidetic** (ī-dĕt′ĭk) [Gr. *eidos,* form, shape] Rel. to or having the ability of total visual recall of anything previously seen.

**eighth cranial nerve** The acoustic nerve. SYN: *vestibulocochlear nerve.*

**Eikenella corrodens** (ī″kĕn-ĕl′ă) A gram-negative rod normally present in the mouth.

**eikonometer** (ī″kō-nŏm′ĕ-tĕr) [Gr. *eikon,* image, + *metron,* measure] An optical instrument used in detecting aniseikonia.

**eikonometry** Determination of the distance of an object by measuring the image produced by a lens of known focus.

**eiloid** (ī′loyd) [Gr. *eilein,* to coil, + *eidos,* form, shape] Having a coil-like structure.

**Eimeria** (ī-mē′rē-ă) A genus of sporozoan parasites belonging to the class Telosporidia, subclass Coccidia. They are intracellular parasites living in the epithelial cells of vertebrates and invertebrates. They rarely are parasitic to humans.

***E. hominis*** A species that has been found in empyema in humans.

**einsteinium** (īn-stīn′ē-ŭm) [Albert Einstein, German-born U.S. physicist, 1879–1955] A radioactive element with atomic number 99 and an atomic weight of 254.0881. Its symbol is Es.

**EIP** *end-inspiratory pause.*

**Eisenmenger's complex** [Victor Eisenmenger, Ger. physician, 1864–1932] A congenital cyanotic heart defect consisting of ventricular septal defect, dextroposition of the aorta, pulmonary hypertension with pulmonary artery enlargement, and hypertrophy of the right ventricle.

**eisodic** (ī-sŏd′ĭk) [Gr. *eis,* into, + *hodos,* way] Centripetal or afferent, as nerve fibers of a reflex arc.

**ejaculate** The semen released during ejaculation.

**ejaculatio** (ē-jăk″ū-lā′shē-ō) [L.] Sudden expelling; ejaculation.

***e. praecox*** Premature ejaculation.

**ejaculation** (ē-jăk″ū-lā′shŭn) [L. *ejaculare,* to throw out] Ejection of the seminal fluid from the male urethra.

PHYSIOLOGY: Ejaculation consists of two phases: (1) the passage of semen and the secretions of the accessory organs (bulbourethral and prostate glands and seminal vesicles) into the urethra and (2) the expulsion of the seminal fluid from the urethra. The former is brought about by contraction of the smooth muscle of the ductus deferens and the increased secretory activity of the glands; the latter by the rhythmical contractions of the bulbocavernosus and ischiocavernosus muscles and the levator ani. The prostate discharges its secretions before those of the seminal vesicle. The sensations associated with ejaculation constitute the male orgasm. Ejaculation occurs without ejection of the seminal fluid from the male urethra in patients who have had a prostatectomy. In that case, the ejaculate is in the bladder.

Ejaculation is a reflex phenomenon. Afferent impulses arising principally from stimulation of the glans penis pass to the spinal cord by way of the internal pudendal nerves. Efferent impulses arising from a reflex center located in the upper lumbar region of the cord pass through sympathetic fibers in the hypogastric nerves and plexus to the ductus deferens and seminal vesicles. Other impulses arising from the third and fourth sacral segments pass through the internal pudendal nerves to the ischiocavernosus and bulbocavernosus muscles. Erection of the penis usually precedes ejaculation. Ejaculation occurs normally during copulation, masturbation, or as a nocturnal emission. The seminal fluid normally contains 60 million to 150 million sperm/ml. The volume of the ejaculation is from 2 to 5 ml. SEE: *orgasm; semen.*

***premature e.*** An imprecise term that usually indicates ejaculation occurring very shortly after the onset of sexual excitement, or ejaculation occurring before copulation or before the partner's orgasm.

***retrograde e.*** Ejaculation in which the seminal fluid is discharged into the bladder rather than outside through the urethra. Most occurrences of this condition follow prostatectomy. It is possible to retrieve the spermatozoa and then use them for artificial insemination.

**ejaculatory** Pert. to ejaculation.

**ejaculatory duct** The terminal portion of the seminal duct formed by the union of the ductus deferens and the secretory duct of the seminal vesicle.

**ejecta** (ē-jĕk′tă) [L. *ejectus,* thrown out, ejected] Material, espcially waste material, excreted by the body. SYN: *dejecta; egesta.*

**ejection** (ē-jĕk′shŭn) Removal, esp. sudden, of something.

***ventricular e.*** Forceful expulsion of blood from the ventricles of the heart.

**ejection fraction** In cardiac physiology, the percentage of the blood emptied from the ventricle during systole; it averages 60% to 70%.

**Ekbom's syndrome** [Karl A. Ekbom, Swedish neurologist, b. 1907] SEE: *restless legs syndrome.*

**EKG** Abbreviation for the German *elektrokardiogramm.* SEE: *electrocardiogram.*

**ekphorize** (ĕk′fō-rīz) [Gr. *ek,* out, + *phorein,* to bear] In psychiatry, to bring back the effect of a psychological experience in an attempt to repeat the experience in memory. SEE: *engram.*

**elaboration** (ē-lăb″ō-rā′shŭn) In body metabolism, the formation of complex compounds from simpler substances (e.g., formation of proteins from amino acids).

**elastance** The tendency of a material to return to its original form after having been deformed; the character or quality of such a material. SEE: *compliance* (1).

**elastase** (ē-lăs′tās) A pancreatic enzyme that cleaves amino acids from proteins in the presence of trypsin.

**elastic** (ē-lăs′tĭk) [Gr. *elastikos,* driven on, set in motion] Capable of being stretched and then returning to its original state.

***intermaxillary e.*** An elastic band used between the maxillary and mandibular teeth in orthodontic therapy; also called a maxillomandibular elastic.

***intramaxillary e.*** An elastic band used in a horizontal space closure by attachments within the same arch.

***vertical e.*** An elastic applied to arch brackets perpendicularly to the occlusal plane for approximating teeth.

**elastic bandage** A bandage that can be stretched on application to exert continuous local pressure.

**elastic cartilage** Yellow cartilage such as is found in the epiglottis, pharynx, external ears, and auditory tube.

**elasticity** (ē″lăs-tĭs′ĭ-tē) The quality of returning to original size and shape after compression or stretching.

**elastic skin** A rare condition in which there is unusual elasticity of the skin.

**elastic stocking** A stocking worn to apply pressure to the extremity, aiding the return of blood from the extremity to the heart through the deep veins. SEE:

*thrombosis, deep vein.*

**elastic tissue** Connective tissue supplied with elastic fibers, as found in the middle layer of arteries.

**elastin** (ē-lăs′tĭn) An extracellular connective tissue protein that is the principal component of elastic fibers in the middle layer of arteries.

**elastinase** (ē-lăs′tĭn-ās) An enzyme that dissolves elastin.

**elastofibroma** (ē-lăs″tō-fī-brō′mă) [″ + L. *fibra,* fiber, + Gr. *oma,* tumor] A benign soft tissue tumor that contains elastic and fibrous elements.

**elastoid** (ē-lăs′toyd) [″ + *eidos,* form, shape] Pert. to a substance formed by hyaline degeneration.

**elastoma** (ē″lăs-tō′mă) [″ + *oma,* tumor] A chronic disease of the skin; pseudoxanthoma.

**elastometer** (ē″lăs-tŏm′ĕ-tĕr) [″ + Gr. *metron,* measure] A device for measuring elasticity.

**elastometry** The measurement of tissue elasticity.

**elastorrhexis** (ē-lăs″tō-rĕk′sĭs) [″ + *rhexis,* rupture] Rupture of elastic tissue.

**elastose** (ē-lăs′tōs) A peptone resulting from gastric digestion of elastin.

**elation** (ē-lā′shŭn) [L. *elatus,* exalted] Joyful emotion. It is pathological when out of accord with the patient's actual circumstances.

**Elavil** Trade name for amitriptyline hydrochloride.

**elbow** (ĕl′bō) [AS. *eln,* forearm, + *boga,* bend] The joint between the arm and forearm. SEE: illus.

***golfer's e.*** A strain of the medial forearm muscles near their origin on the medial epicondyle of the humerus. SYN: *medial humeral epicondylitis.* SEE: *tennis elbow.*

***little league e.*** A form of overuse syndrome marked by inflammation of the medial condyle of the elbow. It is seen in adolescent baseball players, esp. in pitchers. In order to help prevent this condition, Little League Baseball regulations limit the time pitchers may play in any one game.

***tennis e.*** A strain of the lateral forearm muscles near their origin on the lateral epicondyle of the humerus. SYN: *lateral humeral epicondylitis.* SEE: *tennis elbow.*

**elbow conformer** A splint applied to prevent flexion contractures following burns to the upper extremity. The device is fabricated to conform to the anterior arm. Pressure is applied to the olecranon process by a soft, cupped pad.

**elbow jerk** Involuntary bending of the elbow caused by striking the tendon of the biceps or triceps muscle.

**elbow joint** The joint between the arm and the forearm. It includes the humeroulnar, humeroradial, and proximal radioulnar articulations. SEE: illus.

**elbow reflex** An involuntary response in the elbow region to stimulation of the biceps and triceps muscles. SEE: *biceps reflex; triceps reflex.*

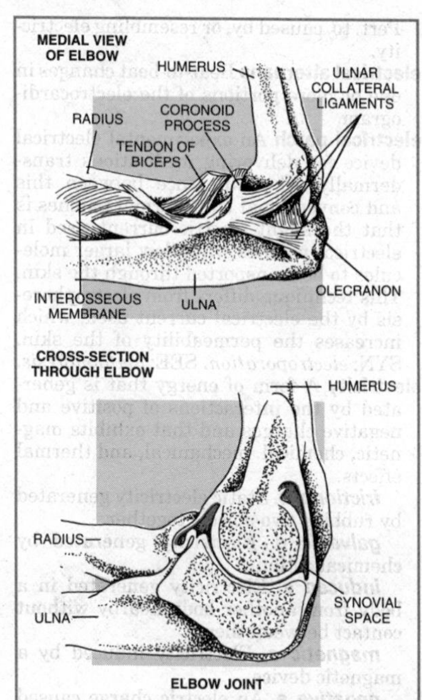


ELBOW JOINT

**elbow unit** A component of the upper-extremity prosthesis that permits the arm to bend at the elbow.

**eldercare** A service that an employer makes available to employees and retirees who may have caregiver responsibilities for an older relative or friend. Corporate eldercare helps caregivers to acquire needed products and services and to balance their caregiving responsibilities with their other commitments.

**elderly, frail** Older persons who cannot live independently and who are at high risk for even more severe disability. Underlying conditions may be osteoporosis, osteoarthritis, Parkinson's disease, and other muscular, endocrine, or neurological conditions. Side effects of medication and lifestyle factors may also contribute to disability.

**elective therapy** A treatment or surgical procedure not requiring immediate attention and therefore planned for the patient's convenience.

**Electra complex** [Gr. Elektra, Agamemnon's daughter, who helped assassinate her mother because of love for her father, whom the former had slain] In psychoanalysis, a group of symptoms due to suppressed sexual love of a daughter for her father. SEE: *Jocasta complex; Oedipus complex.*

**electric, electrical** [Gr. *elektron,* amber]

Pert. to, caused by, or resembling electricity.

**electrical alternans** Beat-to-beat changes in one or more portions of the electrocardiogram.

**electrical patch** An experimental electrical device for delivering medications transdermally. The difference between this and conventional transdermal patches is that the slight electric current used in electrical patches will allow larger molecules to be transported through the skin. This technique differs from electrophoresis by the electrical current used, which increases the permeability of the skin. SYN: *electroporation*. SEE: *iontophoresis*.

**electricity** A form of energy that is generated by the interactions of positive and negative charges and that exhibits magnetic, chemical, mechanical, and thermal effects.

***frictional e.*** Static electricity generated by rubbing two objects together.

***galvanic e.*** Electricity generated by chemical action.

***induced e.*** Electricity generated in a body from another body nearby without contact between them.

***magnetic e.*** Electricity induced by a magnetic device.

***negative e.*** An electric charge caused by an excess of negatively charged electrons.

***positive e.*** An electric charge caused by loss of negatively charged electrons.

***static e.*** Electricity generated by friction of certain materials.

**electric light baker** A device for warming a part, as in arthritis. SEE: *baker*.

**electric shock** Injury from electricity that varies according to type and strength of current and length and location of contact. Electric shocks range from trivial burns to complete charring and destruction of skin. They also may cause unconsciousness from paralysis of the respiratory center, fibrillation of the heart, or both. Approximately 1000 persons are electrocuted accidentally each year in the U.S., and 4000 persons are injured. Five percent of admissions to burn centers are related to electrical injury.

Whether or not an electric shock will cause death is influenced by the pathway the current takes through the body, the amount of current, and the skin resistance. Thus, a very small amount of electrical energy applied directly to the heart may be enough to stop its activity. As little as 100 micoramperes applied to the myocardium can cause ventricular fibrillation. Conversely, a very large amount of electrical energy may be unable to penetrate the dry calloused skin of the fingers and hands and thus will be harmless.

An effective current greater than 15 mA for alternating current and 75 mA for direct current causes muscle tissue to contract. A hand exposed to a sufficient electric current is unable to release its grip. Chest muscles are paralyzed and respiration ceases if sufficient current passes across the thorax.

*Emergency insulation:* Protection against such currents may be made with dry nonconductors such as folded newspapers, magazines, cardboard, wood, rubber, or clothing. These may be used to move the patient from the contact or to remove the wire from the patient. It is always preferable to turn off the current if possible. If patient is in water, the water is electrically charged and special precautions must be taken. On a humid or rainy day, ordinary insulators may contain sufficient moisture to conduct electricity. It is important to make sure that insulators are dry.

High-tension currents, such as those used with radiographic equipment, for long-distance conduction, or in special industrial locations, cannot be insulated by ordinary means. Such currents may penetrate or pass through rubber, paper, or strips of wood. A safe procedure is to ascertain the source of current and have it shut off; otherwise, multiple tragedies could result.

SYMPTOMS: Burns and loss of consciousness are symptoms of electrical injury.

FIRST AID: The victim should be freed carefully from the current source by means of nonconductors, or the current should be shut off. Prolonged artificial respiration may be necessary. SEE: *cardiopulmonary resuscitation; lightning safety rules; shock*.

**electro-, electr-** [Gr. *elektron*, amber] Prefix indicating a *relationship to electricity*.

**electroanalgesia** (ē-lĕk″trō-ăn″ăl-jē′zē-ă) [″ + *analgesia*, want of feeling] Relief from pain by application of low-intensity electric currents locally or through implanted electrodes.

**electroanesthesia** (ē-lĕk″trō-ăn″ĕs-thē′zē-ă) [″ + *an-*, not, + *aisthesis*, sensation] General anesthesia produced by a device that passes electricity of a certain frequency, amplitude, and wave form through the brain.

**electrobiology** (ē-lĕk″trō-bī-ŏl′ō-jē) [″ + *bios*, life, + *logos*, word, reason] The science of electrical phenomena in the living body.

**electrocardiogram** (ē-lĕk″trō-kăr′dē-ō-grăm″) [″ + *kardia*, heart, + *gramma*, something written] ABBR: ECG. A record of the electrical activity of the heart. It shows certain waves called P, Q, R, S, and T waves, and sometimes a U wave. The first, or P, wave is caused by the depolarization of the atrial muscle tissues, whose electrical changes in turn cause atrial contraction. The Q, R, and S waves (QRS complex) correspond to depolarization of ventricular muscle. The T wave corresponds to ventricular repolarization. The electrocardiogram gives important information concerning the spread of excitation to the different parts of the heart, and is of value in diagnosing cases of abnormal cardiac rhythm and myocardial damage. SEE: illus.

**electrocardiograph** (ē-lĕk″trō-kăr′dē-ō-grăf) [″ + ″ + *graphein,* to write] A device for recording changes in the electrical energy produced by the action of heart muscles.

**electrocardiography** The creation and study of graphic records (electrocardiograms) produced by electric currents originating in the heart.

**electrocardiophonograph** (ē-lĕk″trō-kăr″dē-ō-fō′nō-grăf) [Gr. *elektron,* amber, + *kardia,* heart, + *phone,* sound, + *graphein,* to write] A device for recording heart sounds.

**electrocautery** (ē-lĕk″trō-kaw′tĕr-ē) [″ + *kauterion,* branding iron] Cauterization using platinum wires heated to red or white heat by an electric current, either direct or alternating.

**electrochemistry** [″ + *chemeia,* chemistry] The science of chemical changes produced by electricity.

**electrocision** (ē-lĕk′trō-sĭ′zhŭn) [″ + L. *caedare,* to cut] Excision by electric current.

**electrocoagulation** (ē-lĕk″trō-kō-ăg″ū-lā′shŭn) [″ + L. *coagulare,* to thicken] Coagulation of tissue by means of a high-frequency electric current. The heat producing the coagulation is generated within the tissue to be destroyed.

**electrocochleography** (ē-lĕk″trō-kŏk-lē-ŏg′ră-fē) Measurement of electrical activity produced when the cochlea is stimulated. A needle electrode is passed through the eardrum and placed on the cochlea. The electrical activity is then recorded.

**electrocontractility** (ē-lĕk″trō-kŏn-trăk-tĭl′ĭ-tē) [″ + L. *contrahere,* to contract] Contraction of muscular tissue by electrical stimulation.

**electroconvulsive therapy** (ē-lĕk″trō-kŏn-vŭl′sĭv) ABBR: ECT. The use of an electric shock to produce convulsions. At one time, this form of therapy was used so indiscriminately that it fell into disfavor. There is, nevertheless, a place for this type of treatment in specific types of mental illness, esp. if acute depression and suicidal intentions are present.

**electrocorticography** (ē-lĕk″trō-kor″tĭ-kŏg′ră-fē) Recording of the electrical impulses from the brain by electrodes placed directly on the cerebral cortex.

**electrocution** (ē-lĕk″trō-kū′shŭn) [″ + L. *acutus,* sharpened] Destruction of life by means of electric current. SEE: *electric shock; lightning safety rules.*

**electrode** (ē-lĕk′trōd) [″ + *hodos,* a way] **1.** A medium intervening between an electric conductor and the object to which the current is to be applied. **2.** In electrotherapy, an instrument with a point or surface from which to discharge current to the body of a patient.

***active e.*** An electrode that is smaller than a dispersive electrode and produces stimulation in a concentrated area.

***calomel e.*** An electrode that develops a standard electric potential. It is used as a standard in determining the pH of fluids.

***carbon dioxide e.*** A blood gas electrode used to measure the carbon dioxide level of arterial blood. SYN: *Severinghaus electrode.*

***coated wire e.*** ABBR: CWE. A chemical sensor in some clinical laboratory analyzers that functions similarly to a pH electrode. SEE: *hydrogen e.; saturated calomel e.*

***depolarizing e.*** An electrode with greater resistance than the part of the body in the circuit.

***dispersive e.*** An electrode larger than an active electrode. It produces electrical stimulation over a large area.

***gas-sensing e.*** An electrode in which a gas-permeable membrane separates the test solution from an aqueous electrode solution in contact with an ion-selective electrode. Gas permeation of the membrane changes the chemical equilibrium within the electrolyte, and the ion-sensitive electrode detects this change.

***glass e.*** In chemistry, a chemical sensor that uses a glass membrane, as opposed to one that uses an organic or solid state membrane as the sensing surface.

***hydrogen e.*** An electrode that absorbs hydrogen gas; used in pH measurement.

***immobilized enzyme e.*** A chemical sensor that is highly selective due to a specific enzyme incorporated into its structure.

***indifferent e.*** Dispersive e.

***internal reference e.*** In chemistry, the metal electrode inside all chemical-sensing potentiometric electrodes.

***ion-selective e.*** A chemical transducer that yields a response to variations in the concentration of a given ion in solution.

***liquid membrane e.*** An electrode in which the sensing membrane is made up of a hydrophobic ion-exchange neutral carrier (ionophore) dissolved in a viscous, water-insoluble solvent. The liquid membrane is physically supported by an inert porous matrix such as cellulose acetate.

***multiple point e.*** Several sets of terminals providing for the use of several electrodes. SEE: *multiterminal.*

***negative e.*** A cathode; the pole by which electric current leaves the generating source.

***oxygen e.*** A blood gas electrode used to measure the partial pressure of oxygen ($PO_2$) in arterial blood. SYN: *Clark electrode.*

***$PO_2$ e.*** Oxygen e.

***point e.*** An electrode with an insulating handle at one end and a small metallic

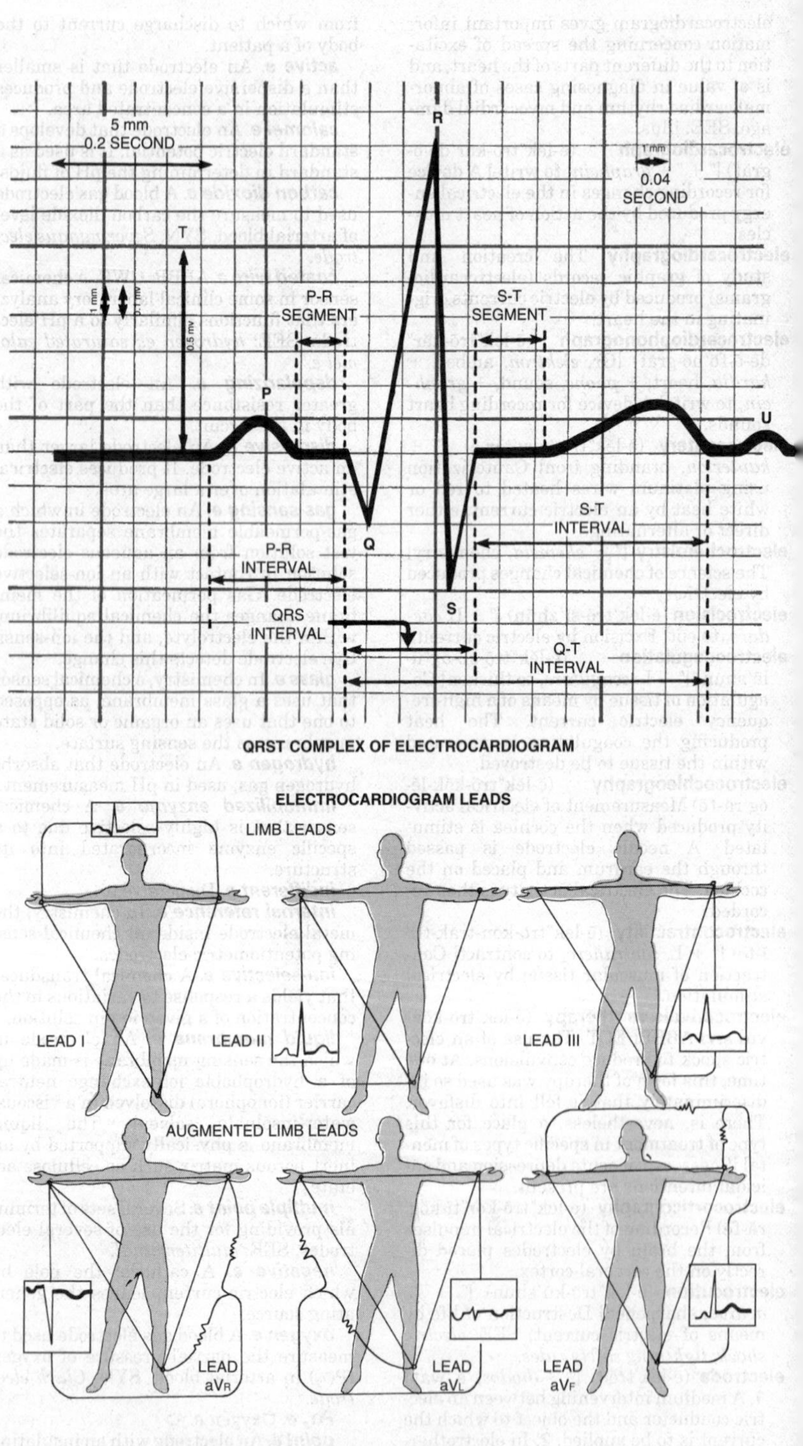

5 mm
0.2 SECOND
T
1 mm
0.1 mv
0.5 mv
P-R
SEGMENT
R
1 mm
0.04
SECOND
S-T
SEGMENT
P
U
Q
S-T
INTERVAL
P-R
INTERVAL
S
QRS
INTERVAL
Q-T
INTERVAL

QRST COMPLEX OF ELECTROCARDIOGRAM

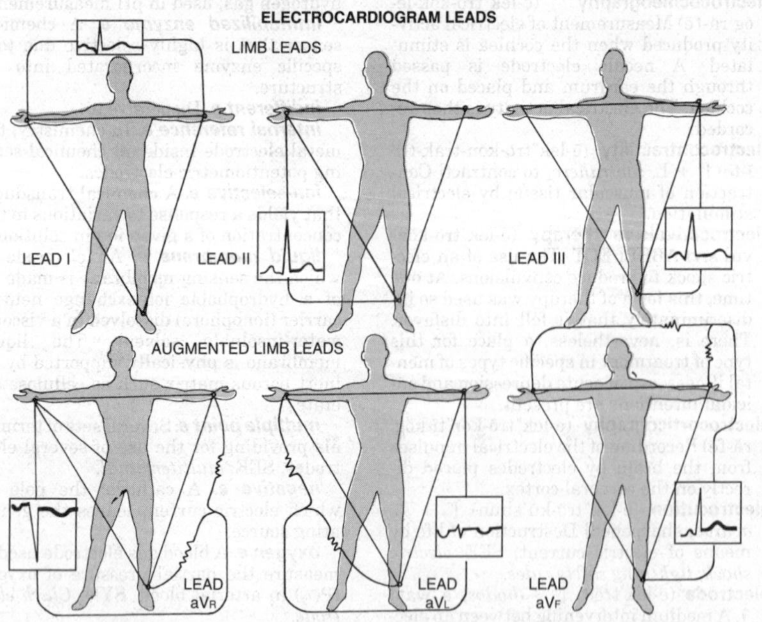

terminal at the other for use in applying static sparks.

***polymer membrane e.*** An electrode in which the sensing membrane is an organic polymer containing a hydrophobic ion-exchange neutral carrier (ionophore).

***positive e.*** An anode; the pole opposite a cathode.

***reference e.*** A chemical electrode whose cell potential remains fixed and against which an indicator electrode is compared. The most common reference electrode is the silver/silver chloride (Ag/AgCl) electrode.

***saturated calomel e.*** ABBR: SCE. One of two practical reference electrodes, used with a mercurous chloride (calomel) paste in pH and other potentiometric instruments. The other is the silver/silver chloride electrode. The calomel electrode has been the standard secondary reference electrode used in the laboratory since the introduction of the pH electrode.

***solid-state membrane e.*** An electrode in which the sensing membrane is made of a single crystal or pressed pellet containing the salt of the ion to be sensed.

***standard hydrogen e.*** ABBR: SHE. The standard reference electrode against which all others are measured. Its assigned electrode potential is 0.000 V.

***subcutaneous e.*** An electrode placed beneath the skin.

***surface e.*** An electrode placed on the surface of the skin or exposed organ.

***therapeutic e.*** An electrode used for introduction of medicines through the skin by ionization. SEE: *iontophoresis.*

**electrodesiccation** (ē-lĕk″trō-dĕs″ĭ-kā′shŭn) [Gr. *elektron,* amber, + L. *desiccare,* to dry up] The destructive drying of cells and tissue by means of short high-frequency electric sparks, as opposed to fulguration, the destruction of tissue by means of long high-frequency electric sparks. Electrodesiccation is used for hemostasis of very small capillaries or veins that have been severed during surgery.

**electrodiagnosis** The use of electrical and electronic devices for diagnostic purposes. This technique is helpful in almost all branches of medicine, but particularly in investigating the function of the heart, nerves, and muscles.

**electrodialysis** (ē-lĕk″trō-dī-ăl′ĭ-sĭs) *pl.* **electrodialyses** [″ + *dia-,* apart, + *lysis,* dissolution] A method of separating electrolytes from colloids by passing a current through a solution containing both.

**electrodynamometer** (ē-lĕk″trō-dī″nă-mŏm′ĕ-tĕr) [″ + *dynamis,* power, + *metron,* measure] An instrument that measures the strength of an electric current.

**electroencephalogram** (ē-lĕk″trō-ĕn-sĕf′ă-lō-grăm) [″ + *enkephalos,* brain, + *gramma,* something written] ABBR: EEG. A tracing on an electroencephalograph. SEE: illus.; *electroencephalography.*

**electroencephalograph** (ē-lĕk-trō-ĕn-sĕf′ă-lō-grăf) [″ + ″ + *graphein,* to write] An instrument for recording the electrical activity of the brain. SEE: *electroencephalography.*

**electroencephalography** Amplification, recording, and analysis of the electrical activity of the brain. The record obtained is called an electroencephalogram (EEG).

Electrodes are placed on the scalp in various locations. The difference between the electric potential of two sites is recorded. The difference between one pair or among many pairs at a time can be obtained. The most frequently seen pattern in the normal adult under resting conditions is the alpha rhythm of 8½ to 12 waves per sec. A characteristic change in the wave occurs during sleep, on opening the eyes, and during periods of concentration. Some persons who have intracranial disease will have a normal EEG and others with no otherwise demonstrable disease will have an abnormal EEG. Nevertheless, the use of this diagnostic technique has proved to be very helpful in studying epilepsy and convulsive disorders and in localizing lesions in the cerebrum. SEE: *rhythm, alpha; rhythm, beta; wave, theta.*

**electrogoniometer** (ē-lĕk″trō-gō″nē-ŏm′ĕ-tĕr) An electrical device for measuring angles of joints and their range of motion.

**electroimmunodiffusion** A laboratory method of identifying antigens in the blood by creating an artificial antigen-antibody reaction.

**electrolysis** (ē″lĕk-trŏl′ĭ-sĭs) [″ + *lysis,* dissolution] The decomposition of a substance by passage of an electric current through it. Hair follicles may be destroyed by this method. SEE: *depilatory technique.*

**electrolyte** (ē-lĕk′trō-līt) [″ + *lytos,* soluble] **1.** A solution that conducts electricity. **2.** A substance that, in solution, conducts an electric current and is decomposed by its passage. Acids, bases, and salts are common electrolytes. **3.** An ionized salt in blood, tissue fluids, and cells. These salts include sodium, potassium, and chlorine. SEE: illus.; table.

***amphoteric e.*** A solution that produces both hydrogen ($H^+$) and hydroxyl ($OH^-$) ions.

**electrolytes, direct measurement of** Measurement of serum ions, such as sodium, chloride, and potassium, without prior dilution of the sample. Direct measurement of electrolytes is considered to be more nearly accurate than measurement by indirect methods because it is not prone to error in cases of hyperlipidemia.

**electrolytes, indirect measurement of** Measurement of serum ions, such as sodium, chloride, and potassium, that employs a sample diluted prior to analysis. The method is prone to error in cases of hyperlipidemia.

## NORMAL AND ABNORMAL ELECTROENCEPHALOGRAM WAVE PATTERNS

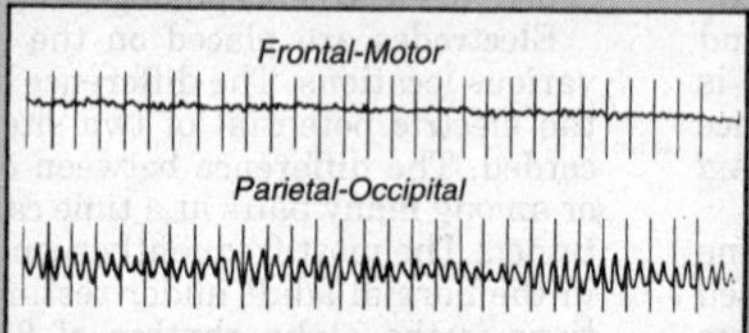


NORMAL ADULT
10/sec. activity in occipital area

PETIT MAL SEIZURE
Synchronous 3/sec. spikes and waves

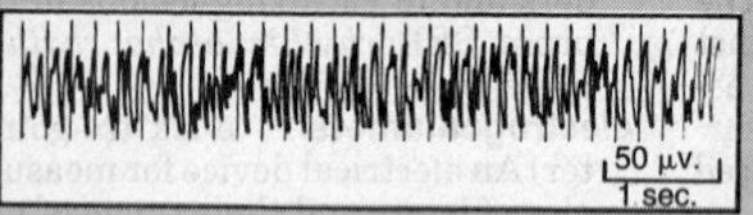


GRAND MAL SEIZURE
High-voltage spikes, generalized

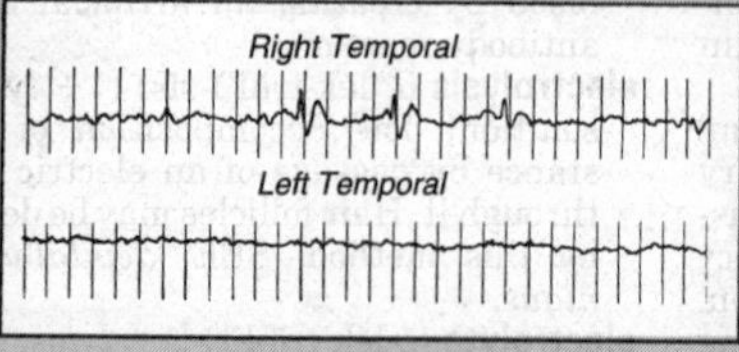


TEMPORAL LOBE EPILEPSY
Right temporal spike focus

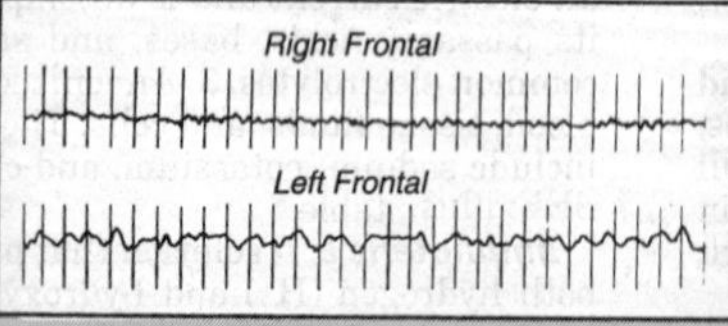


BRAIN TUMOR
Left frontal slow wave focus

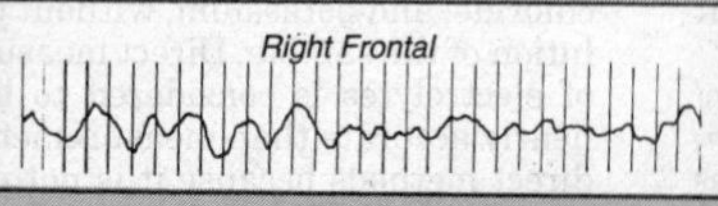


ENCEPHALITIS
Diffuse slowing

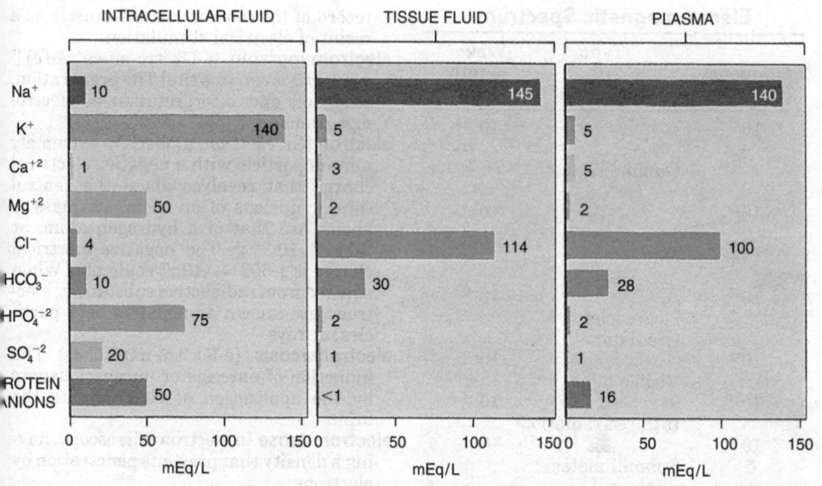


ELECTROLYTE CONCENTRATIONS IN BODY FLUIDS

**electrolytic** (ē-lĕk″trō-lĭt′ĭk) Caused by or rel. to electrolysis.

**electrolytic conduction** The passage of a direct current between metallic electrodes immersed in an ionized solution. In metals, the electric charges are carried by the electrons of inappreciable mass. In solutions, the electric charges are carried by electrolytic ions, each having a mass several thousand times as great as the electron. The positive ions move to the cathode and the negative ions to the anode.

**electromagnet** [″ + *magnes,* magnet] A magnet consisting of a length of insulated wire wound around a soft iron core. When an electrical current flows through the wire, a magnet is produced. **electromagnetic,** *adj.*

**electromagnetic induction** Generation of an electromotive force, in an insulated conductor moving in an electromagnetic field, or in a fixed conductor in a moving magnetic field.

**electromagnetic field** ABBR: EMF. All

### Electrolytes (Cations and Anions) in Plasma, Tissue Fluid, and Intracellular Fluid (ICF)

| | Plasma mEq/L Average | Tissue Fluid mEq/kg $H_2O$* Average | ICF mEq/kg $H_2O$ Average |
|---|---|---|---|
| **Cations** | | | |
| $Na^+$ | 140 | 144 | 5–10 |
| $K^+$ | 4 | 4 | 155 |
| $Ca^{2+}$ | 5 | 3 | 3 |
| $Mg^{2+}$ | 2 | 2 | 30 |
| Total | 151 | 153 | 193–198 |
| **Anions** | | | |
| $Cl^-$ | 103 | 114 | 5–10 |
| $HCO_3^-$ | 26 | 28 | 10 |
| Protein | 16 | 2 | 180† (Protein through Organic acids) |
| $HPO_4^{2-}$; $H_2PO_4^-$ | 2 | 1 | |
| $SO_4^{2-}$ | 1 | 4 | |
| Organic acids | 4 | 4 | |
| Total | 152 | 153 | 195–200 |

SOURCE: Adapted from Krupp, MA and Chatton, MJ (eds): Current Medical Diagnosis and Treatment 1982. Appleton and Lange, East Norwalk, CT, 1982.

* Concentrations derived by converting plasma concentrations to mEq/L of plasma fluid, accounting for nonfluid volume of plasma and applying Donnan factors of 0.96 for monovalent ions and 0.92 for divalent ions.

† Protein, organic phosphates, other organic compounds.

**Electromagnetic Spectrum**

| Frequency (Hz) | Type of Radiation | Wave-length (cm) |
|---|---|---|
| $10^{22}$ | | $10^{-12}$ |
| | Gamma rays | |
| $10^{19}$ | | $10^{-9}$ |
| | X-rays | |
| $10^{16}$ | | $10^{-6}$ |
| | Ultraviolet radiation | |
| $10^{15}$ | | $10^{-5}$ |
| | Visible light | |
| $10^{14}$ | | $10^{-4}$ |
| | Infrared radiation | |
| $10^{13}$ | | $10^{-2}$ |
| | Submillimeter waves | |
| $10^{12}$ | | $10^{-1}$ |
| | Microwaves | |
| $10^{9}$ | | 10 |
| | Television and radio waves | |
| $10^{4}$ | | $10^{6}$ |

forms of energy emanating from an electrical source and transmitted through the air. Included are the fields produced by light, radio, x-rays, and gamma rays. The higher the frequency of the fields produced, the more energy is contained. Thus, the radiated energy from the 60-cycle frequency of an ordinary household electric line is quite small. The long-range effects of prolonged exposure to EMF have been studied extensively. At present, the possible link between cause and effect concerning EMF and disease is poorly understood.

**electromagnetic spectrum** SEE: table; *spectrum, electromagnetic.*

**electromagnetism** Magnetism produced by an electric current.

**electromassage** [″ + Fr. *masser,* to massage] Massage combined with electrical treatment.

**electromotive** [″ + L. *motor,* mover] Pert. to the passage of electricity in a current or motion produced by it.

**electromotive force** ABBR: EMF. The energy (measured in volts) that causes a flow of electricity from one place to another, producing an electric current.

**electromyogram** (ē-lĕk″trō-mī′ō-grăm) [Gr. *elektron,* amber, + *mys,* muscle, + *gramma,* something written] A graphic record of the contraction of a muscle as a result of electrical stimulation.

**electromyography** (ē-lĕk″trō-mī-ŏg′ră-fē) [″ + ″ + *graphein,* to write] The preparation, study of, and interpretation of electromyograms.

**electron** [Gr. *elektron,* amber] An extremely minute particle with a negative electrical charge that revolves about the central core or nucleus of an atom. Its mass is about 1/1840 that of a hydrogen atom, or $9.11 \times 10^{-28}$ g. The negative electrical charge is $1.602 \times 10^{-19}$ coulombs. When emitted from radioactive substances, electrons are known as negative beta particles, or rays.

**electronarcosis** (ē-lĕk″trō-năr-kō′sĭs) The induction of narcosis or unconsciousness by the application of electricity to the brain.

**electron-dense** In electron microscopy, having a density that prevents penetration by electrons.

**electronegative** [″ + L. *negare,* to deny] Charged with negative electricity, which results in the attraction of positively charged bodies and the repulsion of negatively charged bodies.

**electroneurolysis** (ē-lĕk″trō-nū-rŏl′ĭ-sĭs) Destruction of a nerve by use of an electric needle.

**electronic** Pert. to electrons.

**electronic dental anesthesia** ABBR: EDA. In dentistry, the use of low levels of electric current to block pain signals en route to the brain. The patient controls the current through a hand-held box. The current creates no discomfort and, unlike local anesthesia, leaves no numbness to wear off once the dental work is completed. SEE: *patient-controlled analgesia.*

**electronic fetal monitoring** ABBR: EFM. The use of an electronic device to monitor vital signs of the fetus.

**electronic infusion device** ABBR: EID. A device for monitoring intravenous infusions. The device may have an alarm in case the flow is restricted because of an occlusion of the line. In that case, the alarm will sound when a preset pressure limit is sensed. The device can also signal that an infusion is close to completion. The pressure is regulated by the height at which the container is positioned above the level of the heart when the patient is lying flat. A height of 36 in. (91 cm) provides a pressure of 1.3 lb/sq in. (70 mm Hg). Most EIDs are equipped to stop the flow of the infused liquid if accidental free-flow occurs. SEE: *infusion pump.*

**electronics** The science of all systems involving the use of electrical devices used for communication, information processing, and control.

**electronic voice** SEE: *speech synthesizer.*

**electron microscope** SEE: *microscope, electron; microscope, scanning electron.*

**electron volt** SYMB: eV. The energy acquired by an electron as it passes through a potential of 1 V.

**electronystagmography** (ē-lĕk″trō-nĭs″tăg-mŏg′ră-fē) [″ + *nystagmos,* drowsiness, + *graphein,* to write] A method of recording nystagmus activity by detecting the electrical activity of the extraocular muscles. SEE: *nystagmus.*

**electro-oculogram** (ē-lĕk″trō-ŏk′ū-lō-grăm″) Recording of the electric currents produced by eye movements. SEE: *electroretinogram.*

**electropathology** (ē-lĕk″trō-pă-thŏl′ō-jē) [″ + *pathos,* disease, suffering, + *logos,* word, reason] Determination of the electrical reaction of muscles and nerves as a means of diagnosis.

**electrophobia** Irrational fear of electricity.

**electrophoresis** (ē-lĕk″trō-for-ē′sĭs) [″ + *phoresis,* bearing] The movement of charged colloidal particles through the medium in which they are dispersed as a result of changes in electrical potential. Electrophoretic methods are useful in the analysis of protein mixtures because protein particles move with different velocities depending principally on the number of charges carried by the particle. SEE: *diathermy; iontophoresis; -phoresis.*

**electrophrenic** (ē-lĕk″trō-frĕn′ĭk) Pert. to stimulation of the phrenic nerve by electricity.

**electrophrenic respiration** Application of intermittent electrical stimuli to cutaneous electrodes over the phrenic nerves in the neck to rhythmically stimulate respiration. This technique is used in patients whose respiratory center has been damaged.

**electrophysiology** (ē-lĕk″trō-fĭz″ē-ŏl′ō-jē) [″ + *physis,* nature, + *logos,* word, reason] A field of study that deals with the relationships of body functions to electrical phenomena (e.g., the effects of electrical stimulation on tissues, the production of electric currents by organs and tissues, and the therapeutic use of electric currents).

**electroporation** SEE: *electrical patch.*

**electropositive** [″+ L. *positivus,* to put, place] Charged with positive electricity, which results in the repulsion of bodies electrified positively and the attraction of bodies electrified negatively.

**electroresection** (ē-lĕk″trō-rē-sĕk′shŭn) Removal of tissue by use of an electric device such as a cautery.

**electroretinogram** (ē-lĕk″trō-rĕt′ĭ-nō-grăm) ABBR: ERG. A record of the action currents of the retina produced by visual or light stimuli.

**electroscission** (ē-lĕk″trō-sĭ′zhŭn) [″ + L. *scindere,* to cut] Division of tissues by electrocautery.

**electroscope** (ē-lĕk′trō-skōp) [″ + *skopein,* to examine] An instrument that detects intensity of radiation.

**electroshock** Shock produced by an electric current.

**electroshock therapy** The induction of convulsive seizures by the passing of an electric current through the brain. It is sometimes used in the treatment of acute depression. SEE: *electroconvulsive therapy.*

**electrosleep** Sleep produced by the passage of mild electrical impulses through parts of the brain. This technique has been used experimentally in treating insomnia and mental illness.

**electrostatic** [Gr. *elektron,* amber, + *statikos,* causing to stand] Pert. to static electricity.

**electrostatic unit** Any electrical unit of measure based on the attraction or repulsion of a static charge, as distinguished from an electromagnetic unit, which is defined in terms of the attraction or repulsion of magnetic poles.

**electrostimulation** (ē-lĕk″trō-stĭm″ū-lā′shŭn) Use of electric current to stimulate a tissue, such as muscle or bone. In the latter case, the stimulation is used experimentally to facilitate and hasten healing of fractures.

**electrosynthesis** (ē-lĕk″trō-sĭn′thĕ-sĭs) The use of electricity to synthesize chemical compounds.

**electrotherapy** The use of electricity in treating musculoskeletal dysfunction, pain, or disease. Also called *electrotherapeutics.*

**electrotonus** (ē-lĕk-trŏt′ō-nŭs) The change in the irritability of a nerve or muscle during the passage of an electric current.

**electrovalence** (ē-lĕk″trō-vā′lĕns) The ionic linkage between atoms in which each accepts or donates electrons so that each atom ends up with a completed electron shell.

**electuary** (ē-lĕk′tū-ă-rē) [Gr. *ekleikhein,* to lick up] A medicinal substance mixed with honey or sugar to form a paste suitable for oral consumption.

**eleidin** (ĕ-lē′ĭ-dĭn) [Gr. *elaion,* oil] An acidophilic substance present in the stratum lucidum of the epidermis of the palms and soles.

**element** [L. *elementum,* a rudiment] In chemistry, a substance that cannot be separated into substances different from itself by ordinary chemical processes. Elements exist in free and combined states. More than 100 have been identified.

Elements found in the human body include oxygen, aluminum, carbon, cobalt, hydrogen, nitrogen, calcium, phosphorus, potassium, sulfur, sodium, chlorine, magnesium, iron, fluorine, iodine, copper, manganese, and zinc.

***trace e.*** A chemical element present in the body or in the diet in extremely small amounts. Some are absolutely necessary for metabolism.

**eleosaccharum** (ĕl″ē-ō-săk′ă-rŭm) [″ + *sakcharon,* sugar] A mixture of powdered sugar with a volatile oil.

**elephantiasis** (ĕl″ĕ-făn-tī′ă-sĭs) [Gr. *elephas,* elephant, + *-iasis,* condition] A chronic condition marked by pronounced hypertrophy of the skin and subcutaneous tissues resulting from obstruction of the lymphatic vessels. The lower extremities and scrotum are the parts most frequently involved. SYN: *pachydermatosis.*

ETIOLOGY: Elephantiasis may be congenital (Milroy's disease) or the result of metastatic invasion of the lymph nodes by tumor cells. Inflammatory elephantiasis results from filariasis or local infection of the lymph nodes. Elephantiasis is caused by infection of the lymphatics by one of the three filiarial parasites of humans, *Wuchereria bancrofti, Brugia malayi,* or *Brugia timori.* It is common in tropical countries.

TREATMENT: There is no completely effective therapy, but diethylcarbamazine reduces the number of organisms in the peripheral blood. Surgery to treat hydrocele is indicated. Surgery is not effective in treating lymphedema of the legs.

***scrotal e.*** Elephantiasis that is mainly located in the scrotum. SYN: *chyloderma.*

**elephant man disease** Colloquial name for Recklinghausen's disease.

**elevation** (ĕl″ĕ-vā′shŭn) A raised area that protrudes above the surrounding area.

***tactile e.*** A small raised area of the palm and sole that contains a cluster of nerve endings.

**elevator** [L. *elevare,* to lift up] **1.** A curved retractor for holding the lid away from the globe of the eye. **2.** A retractor for raising depressed bones by levers or screws. **3.** An instrument of varying design for extracting teeth or removing root or bone fragments.

***periosteal e.*** A surgical instrument for separating the periosteum from the bone.

**eleventh cranial nerve** The motor nerve, made up of a cranial and a spinal part, that supplies the trapezius and sternomastoid muscles and the pharynx. The accessory portion joins the vagus to supply motor fibers to the pharynx, larynx, and heart. SYN: *accessory nerve; spinal accessory nerve.*

**eliminant** (ē-lĭm′ĭ-nănt) [L. *e,* out, + *limen,* threshold] **1.** Effecting evacuation. **2.** An agent aiding in elimination.

**eliminate** (ē-lĭm′ĭ-nāt) To expel; to rid the body of waste material.

**elimination 1.** Excretion of waste products by the skin, kidneys, lungs, and intestines. **2.** Leaving out, omitting, removing.

**elimination diet** A prescribed food plan used to determine which foods cause an allergic response. The patient starts with very few foods. If none of these causes sensitivity, one food is added to the diet. If that causes no reaction, another food is added, and so on. Offending foods discovered by this technique are then eliminated from the diet.

**ELISA** *enzyme-linked immunosorbent assay.*

**elixir** (ē-lĭk′sĕr) [L. from Arabic *al-iksir*] A sweetened, aromatic, hydroalcoholic liquid used in the compounding of oral medicines. Elixirs constitute one of the most common types of medicinal preparation taken orally in liquid form.

**Elixophyllin** Trade name for theophylline.

**ellipsis** (ē-lĭp′sĭs) [L. *ellīpsis* fr. Gr., a falling short, defective] In psychiatric therapy, omission by the patient of important words or ideas during treatment.

**ellipsoid** (ē-lĭp′soyd) Spindle-shaped.

**elliptocyte** (ē-lĭp′tō-sīt) An oval-shaped red blood cell. About 11% to 15% of red blood cells are normally oval, but in anemia and hereditary elliptocytosis, the percentage is increased to 25% to 100%. In birds, reptiles, and some other animals, the red cells are normally elliptocytes.

**elliptocytosis** (ē-lĭp″tō-sī-tō′sĭs) A condition in which the number of elliptocytes is increased. It occurs in some forms of anemia.

***hereditary e.*** A benign inherited condition in which the red blood cells are oval or elliptical. This anomaly occurs in about 1 in every 2000 births.

**Ellis–van Creveld syndrome** [Richard W.B. Ellis, Scot. physician, 1902–1966; Simon Creveld, Dutch physician, 1894–1977] A congenital syndrome consisting of polydactyly, chondrodysplasia with acromelic dwarfism, hydrotic ectodermal dysplasia, and congenital heart defects. It is thought to be transmitted as an autosomal trait. SYN: *chondroectodermal dysplasia.*

**elongation** (ē″lŏng-gā′shŭn) The condition of being extended or lengthened, or the process of extending.

**elope** To leave a hospital, esp. a psychiatric hospital, without permission.

**eluate** (ĕl′ū-āt) The material washed out by elution.

**eluent** (ē-lū′ĕnt) The solvent or dissolving substance used in elution.

**elution** (ē-lū′shŭn) [L. *e,* out, + *luere,* to wash] In chemistry, separation of one material from another by washing. If a material contains water-soluble and water-insoluble materials, the passage of water (the eluent) through the mixture will remove the portion that is water soluble (the eluate) and leave the water-insoluble residue.

**elutriation** (ē-lū-trē-ā′shŭn) [L. *elutriare,* to cleanse] The separation of insoluble particles from finer ones by decanting of the fluid.

**emaciate** (ē-mā′sē-āt) [L. *emaciare,* to make thin] To cause to become excessively lean.

**emaciated** Excessively thin or lacking in the normal amount of tissue.

**emaciation** The state of being extremely lean. SYN: *wasting.*

ETIOLOGY: Emaciation is caused by a number of conditions or diseases including Addison's disease, tuberculosis, anorexia nervosa, cancer, diabetes, suppuration, hyperthyroidism, chronic diarrhea, stricture of the esophagus, pyloric obstruction, parasites, loss of sleep, exophthalmic goiter, and starvation. SEE: *anorexia; marasmus; tabes; wasting.*

**emailloid** (ā-mī′loyd) [Fr. *email,* enamel, + Gr. *eidos,* form, shape] A tumor having its origin in tooth enamel.

**emanation** [L. *e,* out, + *manare,* to flow] **1.** Something given off; radiation; emission. **2.** A gaseous product of radioactive disintegration.

***actinium e.*** The radioactive gas given off by actinium; a radioactive isotope of actinium. SYN: *actinon.*

***radium e.*** The radioactive gas given off by radium. SYN: *radon.*

***thorium e.*** The radioactive gas given off by thorium. SYN: *thoron.*

**emancipated minor** A person legally under age but recognized by the state as having the legal capacity to consent for himself or herself. Criteria for being so categorized vary among the states.

**emasculation** (ē-măs″kū-lā′shŭn) [L. *emasculare,* to castrate] **1.** Castration. **2.** Excision of the entire male genitalia. **3.** Figuratively, the act of making powerless or ineffective.

**embalming** (ĕm-băm′ĭng) [L. *im-,* on, + *balsamum,* balsam] Preparing a body or part of a body for burial by injecting it with a preservative such as a 4% formaldehyde solution. This is usually done within 48 hr of death. Embalming the body of a person who had HIV infection or other infections transmissible by body fluids requires the use of universal precautions; the embalming fluid will destroy pathogenic organisms. Formaldehyde used in embalming does not represent an environmental hazard. SEE: *Universal Precautions Appendix.*

**embarrass** (ĕm-băr′ăs) To interfere with or compromise function.

**Embden-Meyerhof pathway** [Gustav G. Embden, Ger. biochemist, 1874–1933; Otto Fritz Meyerhof, Ger. biochemist, 1884–1951] A series of metabolic and enzymatic changes that occur in many plants and animals when glucose, glycogen, or starch is metabolized anaerobically to produce lactic acid. The process produces energy in the form of adenosine triphosphate (ATP).

**embedding** [″ + AS. *bedd,* to bed] In histology, the process by which a piece of tissue is placed in a firm medium such as paraffin to support it and keep it intact during the subsequent cutting into thin sections for microscopic examination.

**embolalia, embololalia** (ĕm″bō-lā′lē-ă, ĕm″bō-lō-lā′lē-ă) [Gr. *embolos,* thrown in, + *lalia,* babble] The meaningless language of the insane. SYN: *embolophrasia.*

**embole** (ĕm′bō-lē) [Gr. *emballein,* to throw in] **1.** Reduction of a dislocation. **2.** Formation of the gastrula by invagination.

**embolectomy** (ĕm″bō-lĕk′tō-mē) [″ + *ektome,* excision] Removal of an embolus from a vessel. It may be done surgically or by the use of enzymes that dissolve the clot. The latter method is used in treating acute myocardial infarction and in other areas where blood flow is obstructed by a blood clot. SEE: *tissue plasminogen activator.*

**embolic** Pert. to or caused by embolism.

**emboliform** [″ + L. *forma,* form] **1.** Resembling a nucleus. **2.** Wedge-shaped, as the nucleus emboliformis.

**embolism** (ĕm′bō-lĭzm) [″ + *-ismos,* condition] Obstruction of a blood vessel by foreign substances or a blood clot. Diagnosis depends on predisposing factors. Arteriosclerosis indicates thrombosis, whereas atrial fibrillation, bacterial endocarditis, or thrombophlebitis points to embolism. Embolism is usually due to blood clots. SEE: *tissue plasminogen inactivator.*

***air e.*** An embolism caused by an air bubble. SEE: *air embolism.*

SYMPTOMS: Symptoms include sudden onset of dyspnea, unequal breath sounds, hypotension, weak pulse, elevated central venous pressure, cyanosis, sharp chest pains, hemoptysis, a churning murmur over the precordium, and decreasing level of consciousness.

NURSING IMPLICATIONS: When an air embolism is suspected in the venous circulation, the patient should immediately be turned to the left with head down to trap air in the right side of the heart and maintained in this position for 20 to 30 min. The IV flow should be stopped if air is still in the line, and the air evacuated through the port nearest to the patient; otherwise, the rate of fluid flow should be slowed to keep the vein open, oxygen administered, and the physician notified.

*Prevention: All IV lines:* All air should be purged from the tubing before hookup and when changing solution bags or bottles. Air elimination filters should be used close to the patient. Infusion devices with air detection capability should be used, as well as locking tubing, locking devices for all connections, or taped connections. *Central lines:* To increase peripheral resistance and to help prevent air from entering the superior vena cava, the patient should be instructed to perform the Valsalva maneuver as the stylet is removed from the catheter, when the IV tubing is being attached, and when adapters or caps on the various ports are changed.

***amniotic e.*** The entry of a small amount of amniotic fluid through a tear in the placental membranes into the maternal circulation. The event can occur during labor, delivery, or placental separation. The contents of the fluid (e.g., shed fetal cells, meconium, lanugo, vernix) become nonthrombotic pulmonary emboli that induce thrombus formation. A major complication of amniotic fluid embolus is disseminated intravascular coagulation (DIC).

SYMPTOMS: The patient suddenly exhibits signs of a pulmonary embolus (e.g., severe chest pain, dyspnea, cyanosis, tachycardia, hypotension, and shock).

***drug e.*** A form of nonthrombotic obstruction to the pulmonary circulation. It is caused by intravenous use of drugs of abuse. The drug itself or a contaminant such as talc may induce thrombosis and obstruct the pulmonary vasculature.

***fat e.*** An embolism caused by globules of fat obstructing blood vessels. It frequently occurs after fracture of long and pelvic bones and may cause disseminated intravascular coagulation.

SYMPTOMS: Symptoms include agitation, restlessness, delirium, convulsions, coma, tachycardia, tachypnea, dyspnea, wheezing, blood-tinged sputum, copious production of white sputum, and fever, esp. during the first 12 to 24 hr after injury, when fat emboli are most likely to occur. Petechiae may appear on the buccal membranes, conjunctival sacs, and the chest and axillae. Laboratory values may show hypoxemia, decreased hemoglobin level, leukocytosis, thrombocytopenia, increased serum lipase, and fat globules in urine and sputum.

NURSING IMPLICATIONS: Long bone fractures are immobilized immediately. Patients at risk (i.e., those with fractures of long bones, severe soft tissue bruising, fatty liver injury, or multiple injuries) are assessed for symptoms of fat embolism. Chest radiograph reports are reviewed for evidence of mottled lung fields and right ventricular dilation, and the patient's electrocardiogram is checked for large S waves in lead I, large Q waves in lead III, and right axis deviation.

The patient is placed in the high Fowler's, orthopneic, or other comfortable position to improve ventilation; oxygen is supplied in high concentrations (unless otherwise contraindicated); and endotracheal intubation and mechanical ventilation are initiated as necessary. Prescribed pharmacological agents are administered; these may include steroids, heparin, and diazepam.

***paradoxical e.*** An embolism arising from the venous circulation that enters the arterial circulation by crossing from the right side of the heart to the left side through a patent foramen ovale or septal defect.

***pulmonary e.*** An obstruction of the pulmonary artery or one of its branches, usually caused by an embolus from thrombosis in a lower extremity. The risk of developing pulmonary embolism due to venous thrombosis in a lower extremity can be reduced by use of subcutaneously administered low doses of heparin before and following surgery. Also, various methods of preventing stasis in the leg veins are helpful in preventing embolism. They include active leg exercises, leg elevation, early ambulation following surgery, avoidance of prolonged bedrest and

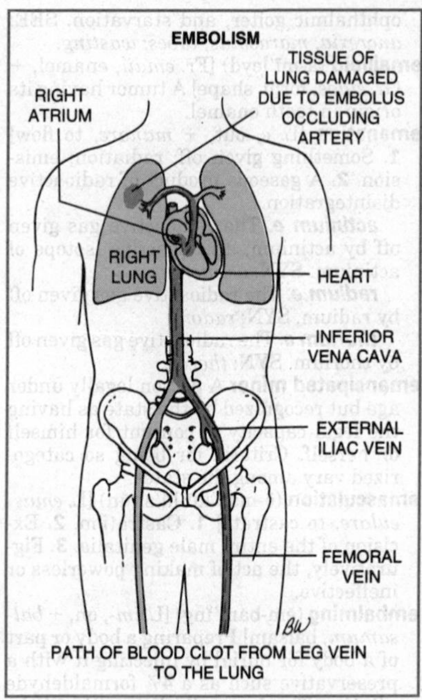

PATH OF BLOOD CLOT FROM LEG VEIN TO THE LUNG

sitting, adequate postoperative hydration, and intermittent leg compression with a pneumatic boot.

Infarction, with death of pulmonary tissue, is rare because the lung has three sources of oxygen: pulmonary circulation, bronchial arterial circulation, and air from the bronchi. SEE: illus.; *thrombosis, deep vein.*

SYMPTOMS: Symptoms include pleuritic or anginal chest pain, acute dyspnea, restlessness and apprehension, cough (possibly producing blood-tinged sputum), and low-grade fever. Adventitious lung sounds, pleural friction rub, tachypnea, tachycardia, and cardiac gallop rhythm or murmur may be present.

NURSING IMPLICATIONS: Venous stasis, thrombus formation, and thrombophlebitis are prevented in patients at risk by using elastic stockings or pneumatic dressings, venous return exercises, and early ambulation. Arterial blood gas values are monitored every 2 to 4 hr, and vital signs, cardiac rhythm, urine output, and level of consciousness are monitored every 1 to 2 hr, or as necessary. Signs of deterioration are reported.

The nurse assists with diagnostic studies and medical treatment, which consists of IV heparin by bolus and infusion and analgesics for pain, and ventilatory support with head-of-bed elevation, prescribed supplemental oxygen, and endotracheal intubation and mechanical ventilation as needed. As necessary, the patient is prepared physically and emotionally for surgery. All procedures and treatments, signs and symptoms of thrombophlebitis and pulmonary embolism, and safety measures for anticoagulant therapy are explained to the patient and family.

Women with a history of emboli should avoid use of oral contraceptive drugs. All patients with a history of emboli or related disorders are encouraged to walk, to exercise their legs, and to wear support or antiembolism hose if prescribed; crossing or massaging the legs should be avoided, however. SEE: *Nursing Diagnoses Appendix.*

***pyemic e.*** An embolism caused by purulent matter.

**embolophrasia** (ĕm″bŏ-lō-frā′zē-ă) [″ + *phrasis,* utterance] Meaningless speech. SYN: *embolalia.*

**embolotherapy** The use of any type of embolic material for therapeutic occlusion of a blood vessel. This technique is used to control bleeding, close fistulas or arteriovenous malformations, remove organs, and reduce tumors or varicoceles. Generally a catheter is threaded through the vascular system to the origin of the vessel to be occluded, and an agent is injected under fluoroscopic control.

**embolus** (ĕm′bō-lŭs) *pl.* **emboli** [Gr. *embolos,* stopper] A mass of undissolved matter present in a blood or lymphatic vessel and brought there by the blood or lymph current. Emboli may be solid, liquid, or gaseous. Other emboli may consist of bits of tissue, tumor cells, fat globules, air bubbles, clumps of bacteria, and foreign bodies. Emboli may arise within the body or gain entrance from outside. Occlusion of vessels from emboli usually results in the development of infarcts. SEE: *thrombosis; thrombus.*

***air e.*** An air bubble in a vein, the right atrium or ventricle, or a capillary.

***amniotic fluid e.*** An embolus that can occur naturally after a difficult labor or from oxytocin-induced hypertonic uterine contractions. A small tear in the amnion or chorion high in the uterus may allow fluid to leak into the chorionic plate and enter the maternal circulation through the venous system. Fluid can also enter at areas of placental separation or cervical tears; this condition occurs more often in multiparas. Although it has been thought that the signs and symptoms are caused by the leak of amniotic fluid into the maternal circulation, the validity of this explanation is in doubt.

SYMPTOMS: The symptoms are respiratory distress, circulatory collapse, acute hemorrhage, and cor pulmonale.

***coronary e.*** An embolus in one of the coronary arteries. It may be a complication of arteriosclerosis and may cause angina pectoris.

***pulmonary e.*** An embolus in the pulmonary artery or one of its branches.

**embolysis** (ĕm-bŏl′ĭ-sĭs) The dissolution of an embolus, esp. one due to a blood clot.

**embrace reflex** SEE: *Moro reflex.*

**embrasure** (ĕm-brā′zhŭr) [Fr., window opening from within] The space formed by the contour and position of adjacent teeth.

***buccal e.*** The embrasure spreading toward the cheek between the molar and premolar teeth.

***labial e.*** The embrasure opening toward the lips between the canine and incisor teeth.

***lingual e.*** The embrasure opening to the lingual sides of the teeth.

***occlusal e.*** The embrasure marked by the marginal ridge on the distal side of one tooth and that on the mesial side of the adjacent tooth, and the contact points.

**embryectomy** (ĕm″brē-ĕk′tō-mē) [Gr. *embryon,* something that swells in the body, + *ektome,* excision] Removal of an extrauterine embryo.

**embryo** (ĕm′brē-ō) [Gr. *embryon,* something that swells in the body] **1.** The young of any organism in an early stage of development. **2.** The stage in prenatal development of a mammal between the ovum and the fetus; in humans, the stage of development between the second and eighth weeks inclusive. SEE: illus.

DEVELOPMENT: *Zygote* (First week): Following fertilization, cells multiply (cleavage), resulting in the formation of a morula, which in turn develops into a blastocyst consisting of a trophoblast and inner cell mass. The trophoblast gives rise to the fetal membranes and placenta after the blastocyst enters the uterus and begins implantation. *Zygote* (Second week): Two cavities (amniotic cavity and yolk sac) arise within the inner cell mass. These are separated by the embryonic disk, which in the second week consists of an ectoderm and an endoderm layer. *Zygote* (Third week): A mesoderm layer forms between the ectoderm and endoderm layers, and these three germ layers develop into the embryo proper.

*Embryo* (Fourth through eighth weeks): The embryo increases in length from about 1.5 mm to 23 mm. The germ layers of the embryonic disk give rise to the principal organ systems, and the embryo begins to show human form. During this period of organogenesis, the embryo is particularly sensitive to the effects of viral infections of the mother (e.g., rubella) and toxic chemicals, including alcohol and tobacco smoke, and is sensitive to hypoxemia.

The epithelium of the alimentary canal, liver, pancreas, and lungs develops from endoderm. Muscle, all connective tissues, blood, lymphatic tissue and the epithelium of blood vessels, body cavities, kidneys, gonads, and suprarenal cortex develop from mesoderm. The epidermis, nervous tissue, hypophysis, and the epithelium of the nasal cavity, mouth, sali-

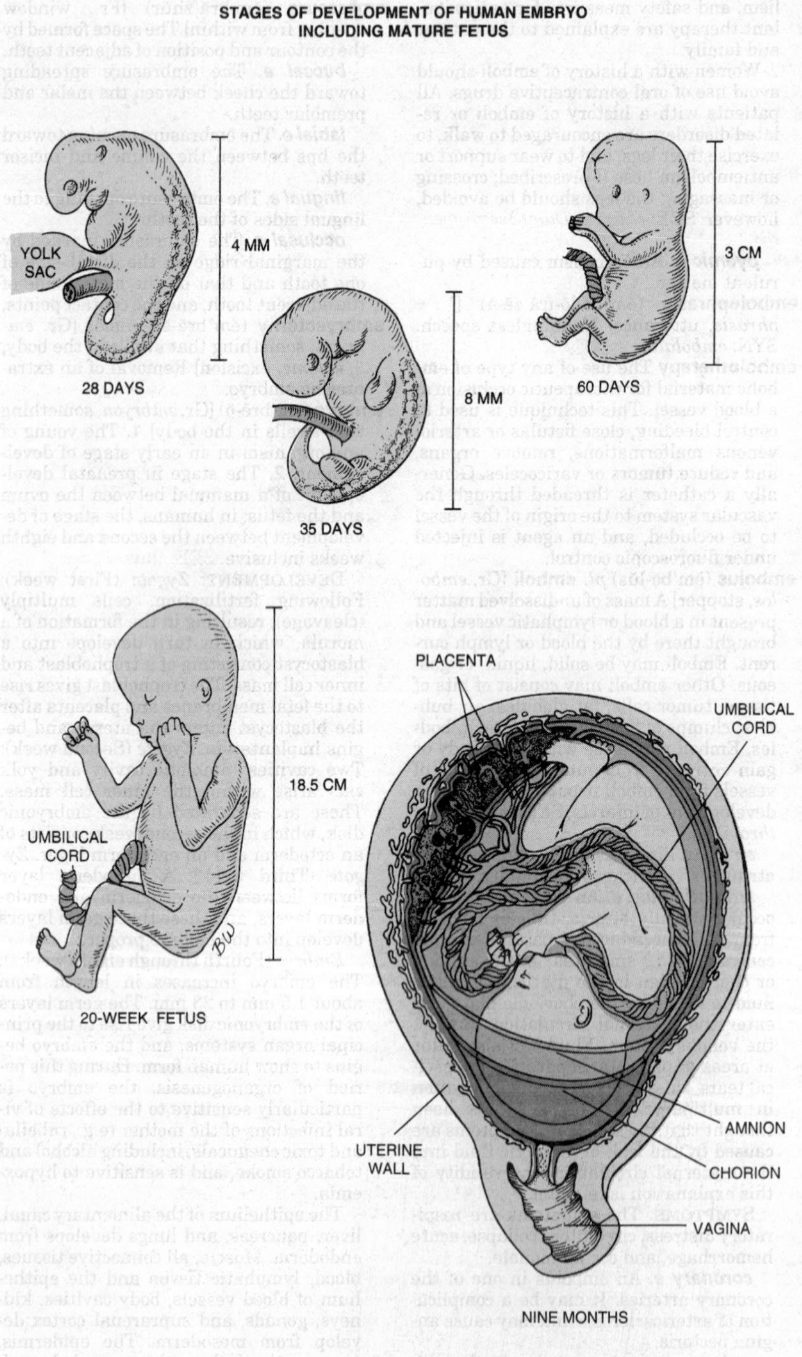

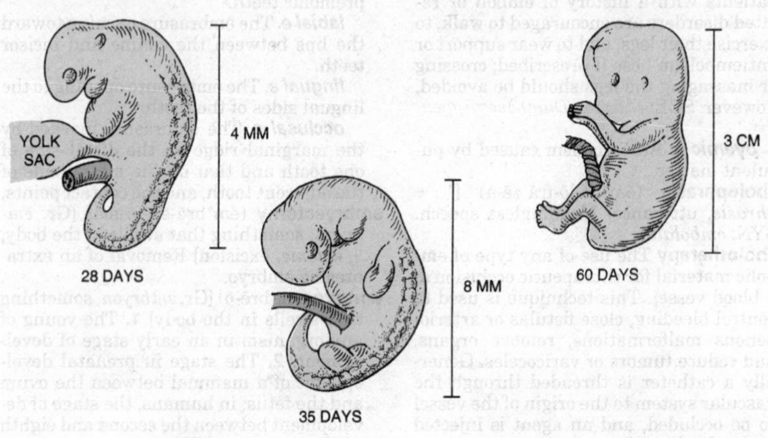
STAGES OF DEVELOPMENT OF HUMAN EMBRYO
INCLUDING MATURE FETUS
YOLK SAC
4 MM
28 DAYS
8 MM
35 DAYS
3 CM
60 DAYS
18.5 CM
UMBILICAL CORD
20-WEEK FETUS
PLACENTA
UMBILICAL CORD
AMNION
UTERINE WALL
CHORION
VAGINA
NINE MONTHS

vary glands, bladder, and urethra develop from ectoderm.

**embryocardia** (ĕm″brē-ō-kăr′dē-ă) [″ + *kardia,* heart] Heart action in which the first and second sounds are equal and resemble the fetal heart sounds; a sign of cardiac distress.

**embryocidal** (ĕm″brē-ō-sī′dăl) [Gr. *embryon,* something that swells in the body, + L. *cida,* killer] Pert. to anything that kills an embryo.

**embryoctony** (ĕm″brē-ŏk′tŏ-nē) [″ + *kteinein,* to kill] Destruction of the fetus in utero, as when delivery is impossible or during abortion. SEE: *craniotomy.*

**embryogenetic, embryogenic** [″ + *gennan,* to produce] Giving rise to an embryo.

**embryogeny** (ĕm″brē-ŏj′ĕ-nē) The growth and development of an embryo.

**embryography** [″ + *graphein,* to write] A treatise on the embryo.

**embryology** [″ + *logos,* word, reason] The science that deals with the origin and development of an individual organism.

**embryoma** (ĕm-brē-ō′mă) [″ + *oma,* tumor] A tumor consisting of derivatives of the embryonic germ layers but lacking in organization.

**embryonal** (ĕm′brē-ō-năl) Pert. to or resembling an embryo.

**embryonic** (ĕm″brē-ŏn′ĭk) [Gr. *embryon,* something that swells in the body] Pert. to or in the condition of an embryo.

**embryonic disk** The group of cells from which the embryo will develop. In humans, it is usually present as the inner cell mass of the blastocyst at the end of the first week of development after fertil-

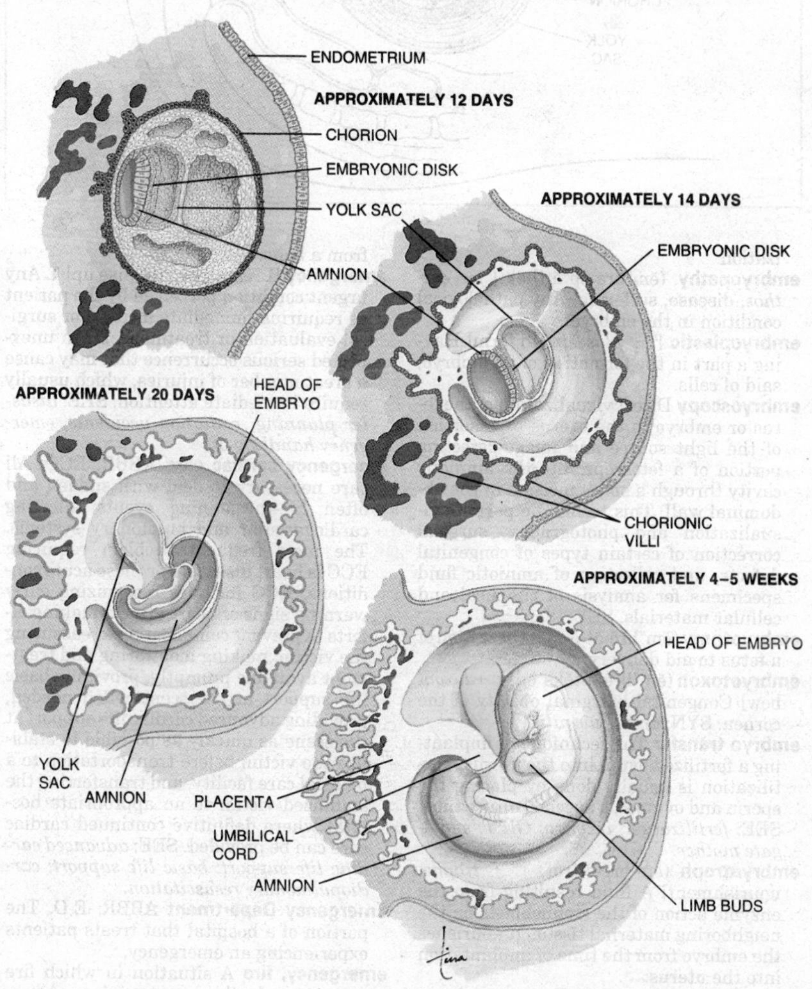


EMBRYONIC DEVELOPMENT

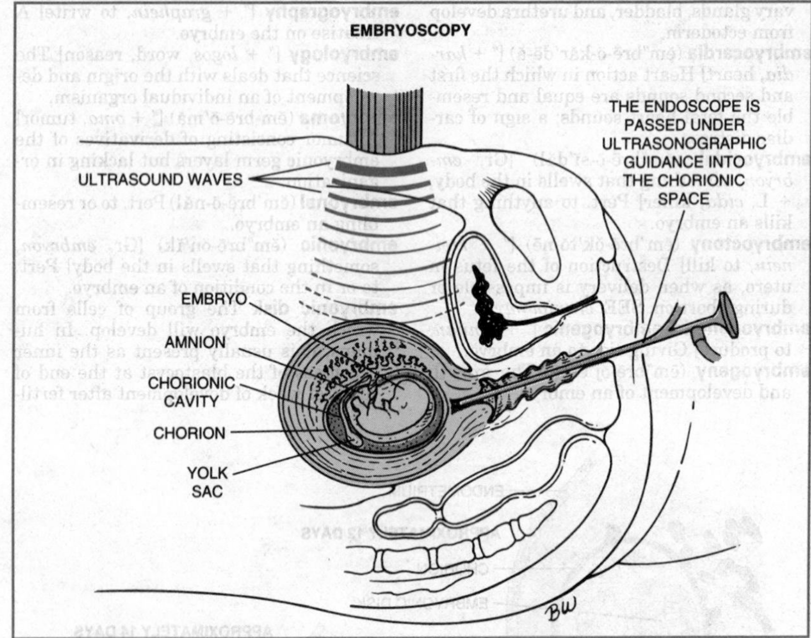


ization.

**embryopathy** (ĕm″brē-ŏp′ă-thē) [″ + *pathos,* disease, suffering] Any pathological condition in the embryo.

**embryoplastic** [″ + *plassein,* to form] Having a part in the formation of an embryo; said of cells.

**embryoscopy** Direct visualization of the fetus or embryo in the uterus by insertion of the light source and image-detecting portion of a fetoscope into the amniotic cavity through a small incision in the abdominal wall. This technique permits visualization and photography, surgical correction of certain types of congenital defects, and collection of amniotic fluid specimens for analysis of chemical and cellular materials. SEE: illus.

**embryotomy** (ĕm″brē-ŏt′ō-mē) Dissection of a fetus to aid delivery.

**embryotoxon** (ĕm″brē-ō-tŏks′ŏn) [″ + *toxon,* bow] Congenital marginal opacity of the cornea. SYN: *arcus juvenilis.*

**embryo transfer** The technique of implanting a fertilized ovum into the uterus. Fertilization is usually done by placing the sperm and ovum in a special culture tube. SEE: *fertilization, in vitro; GIFT; surrogate mother.*

**embryotroph** (ĕm′brē-ō-trōf) [″ + *trophe,* nourishment] A fluid resulting from the enzyme action of the trophoblasts on the neighboring maternal tissue. It nourishes the embryo from the time of implantation into the uterus.

**emedullate** (ē-mĕd′ū-lāt) [L. *e,* out, + *medulla,* marrow] To remove the marrow from a bone.

**emergency** [L. *emergere,* to raise up] **1.** Any urgent condition perceived by the patient as requiring immediate medical or surgical evaluation or treatment. **2.** An unexpected serious occurrence that may cause a great number of injuries, which usually require immediate attention. SEE: *disaster planning; radiation accidents, emergency handling of.*

**emergency cardiac care** ABBR: ECC. All care necessary to deal with sudden and often life-threatening events affecting cardiovascular and pulmonary systems. The most frequent problem requiring ECC is heart disease. For those acute conditions, ECC includes recognizing early warning signs of heart attack, making efforts to prevent complications, reassuring the victim, making monitoring and treatment available promptly, providing basic life support at the scene when needed, providing advanced cardiac life support at the scene as quickly as possible to stabilize the victim before transportation to a medical care facility, and transferring the stabilized victim to an appropriate hospital where definitive continued cardiac care can be provided. SEE: *advanced cardiac life support; basic life support; cardiopulmonary resuscitation.*

**Emergency Department** ABBR: E.D. The portion of a hospital that treats patients experiencing an emergency.

**emergency, fire** A situation in which fire may cause death or severe injury. A person whose clothing catches fire should be rolled in a rug or blanket to smother the flames. It may be necessary to trip a burning person to prevent running, which only fans the flames. If an individual is outdoors, rolling in the dirt will smother flames. SEE: *burn; gas; smoke inhalation; transportation of the injured.*

If the victim is trapped in a burning building, the occupied room should have the doors and windows closed to prevent cross-breezes from increasing the fire. The window should be opened only if the victim is to be rescued through it. Doors should be opened only a few inches to ascertain the possibility of escape. A burst of flame or hot air can push the door in and asphyxiate anyone in the room. Wet cloths or towels should be held over the mouth and nostrils to keep out smoke and gases.

Caution: In attempting to escape from an area filled with smoke or fire, it is important to crawl rather than run. The heat several feet above floor level may be lethal, but at floor level, it may be cool enough to tolerate. Even when crawling, it is important to proceed as quickly as possible. The toxic gas carbon monoxide is present in higher concentration at floor level because it is heavier than air.

**emergency kit** A kit containing the basic equipment and drugs needed to provide initial emergency care to individuals experiencing life-threatening conditions. Included are a stethoscope; a bag-valve-mask; oral airways, adult and pediatric; an infusion needle; a large-bore intravenous needle, 12-gauge for tracheal obstruction; appropriate sterile syringes and needles; tape; epinephrine 1:1000, 1-ml ampule; diazepam, 10-mg ampule; diphenhydramine hydrochloride, 50-mg ampule; 50% dextrose and water, 50-ml ampule; and a blood pressure cuff. Optional items are suction equipment; a small oxygen tank; laryngoscopes, adult and pediatric; endotracheal tubes of several sizes; 18- and 20-gauge intravenous catheters; normal saline, 250-ml bag; albuterol; atropine, 0.6 mg/ml ampule; nitroglycerin tablets; and morphine sulfate, 10-mg ampule.

**emergency medical identification** SEE: *Medic Alert.*

**Emergency Medical Service System** ABBR: EMS system. Services, including rescue operations, ambulance transportation, emergency department services, and public education, that are required as a result of an acute illness or injury. Other components of an effective EMS system include rescue and emergency care training, communications (including ambulance dispatch, hospital-to-EMS crew communication, and a centralized emergency telephone number, 911, for public access), continuing medical education, effective medical control and evaluation, disaster linkage with mutual aid agreements between neighboring communities. SEE: *disaster planning.*

**emergency medical technician** ABBR: EMT. An individual trained in techniques of administering emergency care in a variety of conditions, but esp. to heart attack, cardiac arrest, and trauma patients. EMTs function in an emergency medical service (EMS) system, are certified by the state after completing instruction, and work under the authority of a supervising physician (medical control), using treatment protocols approved by a medical advisory committee. In metropolitan areas, the EMT's equipment may include a system that allows communication with a hospital; some can transmit electrocardiograms for analysis by a physician. SEE: *Emergency Medical Service System; EMS medical control; EMS treatment protocol; paramedic.*

***emergency medical t.—basic*** ABBR: EMT—B. A basic-level technician who has successfully completed the U.S. Department of Transportation Medical Technician course.

***emergency medical t.—defibrillation*** ABBR: EMT—D. An emergency medical technician who is trained in defibrillation.

***emergency medical t.—intermediate*** ABBR: EMT—I. A technician trained to an intermediate level and able to perform some advanced life support skills, such as intravenous fluid administration or endotracheal intubation.

***emergency medical t.—paramedic*** ABBR: EMT—P. A technician trained to the highest level for delivery of prehospital care.

**emergency medicine** SEE: *medicine, emergency.*

**Emergency Nurses Association** A professional organization representing and certifying nurses who are proficient in emergency care.

**emergency readiness** Planning in advance for an unexpected crisis, esp. a natural disaster such as a flood or hurricane. The home should be inspected for potential hazards and those discovered should be corrected. Flammable materials such as paints, oils, and fuels should be isolated. Utility shut-off valves should be located and pointed out to all members of the household. It is important to know the location of the nearest public shelter and the time required to go there on foot and by car. Family members should be trained in basic life support techniques. Emergency telephone numbers, including names and telephone numbers of neighbors, should be posted and easily accessible. A first-aid kit should be available and restocked when supplies have been used. Fire extinguishers and flashlights should be in working condition. Supplies of food and water for least 3 days, and protective clothing and blankets, should be available. It is important to provide for the special needs of infants, the elderly, and the ill. Emergency drills should be practiced, including evacuation from the home by various routes in case the usual exits are blocked or surrounded by flames. SEE: *emergency, fire*.

**Emergency Room** ABBR: E.R. A seldom used term for Emergency Department.

**emergent** [L. *emergere,* to raise up] **1.** Growing from a cavity or other part. **2.** Sudden, unforeseen.

**emerging infectious disease** Any disease, such as tuberculosis or cholera, for which the steadily declining case rates of recent years have reversed and are now increasing. Also included in this class of illnesses are infectious diseases that were previously unrecognized because of their rarity or were caused by mutant strains of a pathogen. Examples are infections with human immunodeficiency virus, new strains of influenza virus, and multiple drug-resistant bacteria. Emerging pathogens in food or water include *Cryptosporidium*-associated diarrhea, and gastroenteritis due to *Escherichia coli* O157:H7. Hantavirus pulmonary syndrome is caused by a strain of virus that was not known to infect humans until the spring of 1993.

**emery** A granular mineral substance used as an abrasive.

**emesis** (ĕm′ĕ-sĭs) [Gr. *emein,* to vomit] Vomiting. It may be of gastric, systemic, nervous, or reflex origin or due to stimulation of the vomiting center. SEE: *antiemetic; aspiration; emetic; vomit; vomitus*.

NURSING IMPLICATIONS: The time of vomiting is obtained and documented in relation to when the patient ate. The presence of any aggravating factors such as pain, anxiety, the type of foods eaten, and noxious environmental stimuli, and the type of vomiting, amount, color, and characteristics of the emesis, are documented. Assistance is provided with oral hygiene, and antiemetics are administered, if prescribed, to control vomiting. If vomiting leaves the patient weak, dysphagic, or comatose, safety measures are instituted to prevent aspiration of vomitus into the lungs; these include placing the patient in a side-lying position with the head lowered and having suction and emergency tracheostomy equipment readily available.

***chemotherapy-induced e.*** Vomiting associated with chemotherapy regimens for cancer. Even though this side effect is usually self-limiting and seldom life-threatening, the prospect of it produces great anxiety. A number of agents are available for treating this condition.

***gastric e.*** Vomiting present in gastric ulcer, gastric carcinoma, acute gastritis, chronic gastritis, hyperacidity and hypersecretion, and pressure on the stomach.

***e. gravidarum*** Vomiting of pregnancy.

***irritation e.*** Vomiting caused by drugs, uremia, nephritis, some brain tumors, chloroform, or ether.

***nervous e.*** Vomiting resulting from tumor or abscess of the brain, seasickness, acute myelitis, meningitis, anemia or hyperemia of the brain, concussion or contusion of the brain, skull fracture, Ménière's disease, or migraine.

***reflex e.*** Vomiting caused by irritation of the fauces and pharynx, coughing, removal of viscous secretion from the nasopharynx, unpleasant odors and sights, shock, nervousness, anticipation, anxiety, hysteria, morning sickness, gastric crisis of tabes, or hiccoughs.

**emesis basin** SEE: under *basin*.

**emetic** (ĕ-mĕt′ĭk) [Gr. *emein,* to vomit] An agent that produces vomiting. An emetic may induce vomiting by its local effect, as do copper sulfate, zinc sulfate, mustard, and ipecac in small doses diluted in water; or by its effect on the central nervous system, as does apomorphine hydrochloride given parenterally. SEE: *vomiting; vomitus*.

ADMINISTRATION: The stomach contents should be diluted before an emetic is given. Emesis is much more likely to take place when the stomach is distended. Vomiting may be induced by drinking generous amounts of warm water, preferably warm soapy water, and by stimulating the uvula or posterior pharynx. Gastric lavage is preferable to emetics in treating patients who have swallowed poison because the poison may reinjure the esophagus and mouth as it is expelled from the stomach by vomiting. Emetics may be dangerous because of their own toxic effect, as in severe cardiovascular diseases, tuberculosis, advanced pregnancy, hernia, stomach ulcers, or corrosive poisoning. For these reasons, the indiscriminate use of chemical emetics is contraindicated.

---

Caution: Salt solutions should not be administered orally to induce vomiting. The absorbed salt can be lethal.

---

***direct e.*** An emetic that acts by its presence in the stomach (e.g., mustard).

***indirect e.*** An emetic that acts on the vomiting center of the brain (e.g., apomorphine).

**emetine** (ĕm′ĕ-tēn) [Gr. *emein,* to vomit] A powdered white alkaloid emetic obtained from ipecac.

***bismuth iodide e.*** A combination of emetine and bismuth containing about 20% emetine and 20% bismuth. The action and uses are the same as those of emetine.

***e. hydrochloride*** The hydrated hydrochloride of an alkaloid obtained from ipecac. It is used for the treatment of both intestinal and extraintestinal amebiasis. It should be used cautiously in elderly or debilitated patients. Children, pregnant women, and patients with serious organic disease should not receive emetine.

**emetism** [" + *-ismos,* condition of] Poisoning from an overdose of ipecac.

SYMPTOMS: Symptoms are acute inflammation of the pylorus, hyperemesis, diarrhea, and sometimes coughing and suffocation.

**emetocathartic** (ĕm"ĕ-tō-kă-thăr'tĭk) [" + *katharsis,* a purging] Producing both emesis and catharsis.

**emetology** (ĕm"ĕ-tŏl'ō-jē) [" + *logos,* word, reason] The study of the anatomy and physiology of vomiting.

**E.M.F.** *electromotive force; erythrocyte maturation factor.*

**EMG** *electromyogram.*

**-emia** Suffix meaning *blood.* SEE: *hema-; hemato-.*

**EMIC** *emergency maternal and infant care.*

**emic** (ē'mĭk) In anthropology and transcultural nursing, rel. to a type of disease analysis that focuses on the culture of the patient. The emic perspective emphasizes the subjective experience and cultural beliefs pertinent to the illness experience. For example, in psychiatric settings in the southeastern U.S., many patients believe that their illness is caused by a spell or curse from evil spirits. In these cases, a health care worker using an emic perspective would ask an indigenous health care provider to consult with the patient in addition to providing care within the traditional health care system. SEE: *etic.*

**emigration** [L. *e,* out, + *migrare,* to move] Passage of white blood corpuscles through the walls of capillaries and veins during inflammation.

**eminence** [" + *minere,* to hang on] A prominence or projection, esp. of a bone.

***arcuate e.*** A rounded eminence on the upper surface of the petrous portion of the temporal bone. SYN: *jugum petrosum.*

***articular e. of the temporal bone*** A rounded eminence forming the anterior boundary of the glenoid fossa.

***auditory e.*** A collection of gray matter on the floor of the fourth ventricle of the brain at its lower part, forming the deep origin of the auditory nerve.

***bicipital e.*** A tuberosity for insertion of the biceps muscle on the radius.

***blastodermic e.*** An elevated mass of cells of a developing ovum forming the blastoderm.

***canine e.*** A vertical ridge on the external surface of the maxilla.

***collateral e.*** An eminence between the middle and posterior horns in the lateral ventricle of the brain.

***e. of Doyère*** A slight elevation of muscular fiber corresponding to the entrance of a nerve fiber into the muscle.

***frontal e.*** A rounded prominence on either side of the median line and a little below the center of the frontal bone.

***germinal e.*** The mass of follicle cells that surrounds the ovum. SYN: *cumulus oophorus.*

***hypothenar e.*** An eminence on the ulnar side of the palm, formed by the muscles of the little finger.

***iliopectineal e.*** An eminence on the upper aspect of the pubic bone above the acetabulum, marking the junction of the bone with the ilium.

***intercondyloid e.*** A process on the head of the tibia lying between the two condyles.

***mamillary e.*** A projection of the inner pillars of the fornix. SYN: *corpus mamillare.*

***median e.*** The anterior bodies of the medulla oblongata separated by the anterior median fissure.

***nasal e.*** A prominence on the vertical portion of the frontal bone above the nasal notch and between the two superciliary ridges.

***occipital e.*** A protuberance on the occipital bone.

***olivary e.*** An oval projection at the upper part of the medulla oblongata above the extremity of the lateral column. SYN: *oliva; olivary body.*

***parietal e.*** A marked convexity on the outer surface of the parietal bone.

***portal e.*** One of the small median lobes on the lower surface of the liver.

***pyramidal e.*** An elevation on the mastoid wall of the tympanic cavity. It contains a cavity through which the stapedius muscle passes. SYN: *pyramid of the tympanum.*

***thenar e.*** An eminence formed by muscles on the palm below the thumb.

**eminentia** (ĕm"ĭn-ĕn'shē-ă) *pl.* **eminentiae** [L.] An eminence.

**emiocytosis** (ē"mē-ō-sī-tō'sĭs) [L. *emitto,* to send forth, + Gr. *kytos,* cell, + *osis,* condition] The process of movement of intracellular material to the outside. Granules join the cell membrane, which ruptures to allow the substance to be free in the intercellular fluid. SYN: *exocytosis.* SEE: *endocytosis; pinocytosis.*

**emissary** (ĕm'ĭ-să-rē) [L. *e,* out, + *mittere,* to send] **1.** Providing an outlet. **2.** An outlet.

**emissary vein** A small vein that pierces the skull and carries blood from the sinuses within the skull to the veins outside it.

**emission** (ē-mĭsh'ŭn) [L. *e,* out, + *mittere,* to send] An issuance or discharge; the sending forth or discharge of, for example, an atomic particle, an exhalation, or a light or heat wave.

***nocturnal e.*** The involuntary discharge of semen during sleep. SYN: *wet dream.*

***thermionic e.*** The process by which electrons are released from an x-ray filament after a current has been passed through it.

**emissivity** The ability of a substance or surface to emit radiant energy.

**EMIT** *Enzyme-multiplied immunoassay technique.*

**emit** To produce or release something (e.g., light, heat, or sound waves).

**EMLA** *eutectic mixture of local anesthetics.*

**EMLA Cream** A topical anesthetic composed of lidocaine and prilocaine. The cream is applied to the skin, covered with an occlusive bandage, and left in place for 1 to 2 hr. This anesthetizes the skin to a depth of about 5 mm so that superficial skin lesions can be removed without using any other form of anesthetic. Patients will not be aware of a needle piercing the skin; however, they will feel any tissue irritation caused by the fluid injected.

**emmenagogue** (ĕm-ĕn′ă-gŏg) [Gr. *emmena,* menses, + *agogos,* leading] A substance that promotes or assists the flow of menstrual fluid. SEE: *ecbolic.*

***direct e.*** An agent, such as a hormone, that affects the reproductive tract.

***indirect e.*** An agent that alters menstrual function by treatment of a primary illness.

**emmeniopathy** (ĕ-mē″nē-ŏp′ă-thē) [Gr. *emmena,* menses, + *pathos,* disease, suffering] Any disorder of menstruation.

**Emmet's operation** [Thomas A. Emmet, U.S. gynecologist, 1828–1919] **1.** Uterine trachelorrhaphy (i.e., suturing of a torn uterine cervix). **2.** Suturing of a lacerated perineum. **3.** Conversion of a sessile submucous tumor of the uterus into a pedunculated one. **4.** Surgical repair of a prolapsed uterus.

**emmetrope** (ĕm′ĕ-trōp) [Gr. *emmetros,* in measure, + *opsis,* sight] One endowed with normal vision. **emmetropic** (-trŏp′ĭk), *adj.*

**emmetropia** (ĕm″ĕ-trō′pē-ă) The normal condition of the eye in refraction in which, when the eye is at rest, parallel rays focus exactly on the retina. SEE: illus.; *astigmatism; myopia.*

**emollient** (ē-mŏl′yĕnt) [L. *e,* out, + *mollire,* to soften] An agent that softens and soothes the surface to which it is applied, usually the skin. SEE: *demulcent.*

**emotion** (ē-mō′shŭn) [L. *emovere,* to stir up] **1.** A passion or sensibility marked by physical changes in the body such as alteration in heart rate and respiratory activity, vasomotor reactions, and changes in muscle tone. **2.** A mental state or feeling such as fear, hate, love, anger, grief, or joy arising as a subjective experience rather than as a conscious mental effort. These feelings constitute the drive that brings about the affective or mental adjustment necessary to satisfy instinctive needs. Physiological changes invariably accompany alteration in emotion, but such change may not be apparent to either the person experiencing the emotion or an observer. **emotional** (-ăl), *adj.*

Frustration is normally associated with

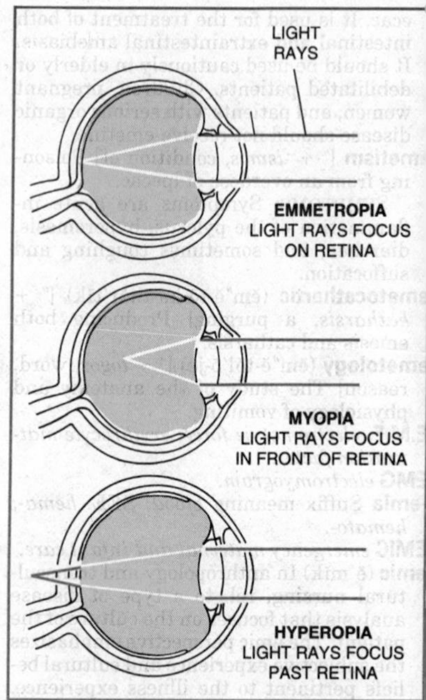


displeasure and intensified perception of personal need; the process of gratification is accompanied by pleasurable feelings that persist for a variable period in less intense form.

Anxiety or fear arises when one doubts one's ability to meet a situation adequately. Neutralization consists of flight from danger or a struggle (fight) to remove the threat. Civilized people may find a goal unattainable because their conditioned (moral) reactions cause them to regard the goal as socially objectionable; they may even deny the goal entirely. Thus, conflicts arise and the stage is set for the onset of psychogenic disease.

DISORDERS: Emotions are not felt in the same way by healthy persons as by those suffering from mental illness. In schizophrenia, there is a decrease of pleasure, hate, love, and other emotions. There is loss of ability to feel and express emotions such as love or hate. The patients are said to be blunted. The emotions they do show are not in harmony with their ideas. For example, they may smile while describing tortures and terrors.

Unhappiness is marked in manic depressive psychosis. It varies in degree and may lead to suicide. In the excited stage, undue happiness is marked. SEE: *anhedonia.*

**emotional need** An inner need regarding any of the emotions of love, fear, anxiety, sadness, loneliness, or anger. These needs may be understood and handled by the healthy individual, but are esp. difficult to cope with during illness or mental stress. The medical care team should be alert to the possibility that a patient's needs in these areas must be managed and treated. This is best done by demonstrating empathy for the patient and being close by when needed. In times of stress and anxiety, the therapy of holding an aged patient's hand has remarkable therapeutic effects. SEE: *TLC*.

**emotivity** (ē″mō-tĭv′ĭ-tē) One's capability for emotional response.

**empathy** (ĕm′pă-thē) Objective awareness of and insight into the feelings, emotions, and behavior of another person and their meaning and significance. It is not the same as sympathy, which is usually nonobjective and noncritical. **empathic** (-pă′thĭk), *adj.*

**emperor of pruritus** The itching that accompanies poison ivy dermatitis involving the anal area. It is so intense that it is called "the emperor of pruritus."

**emphysema** (ĕm″fĭ-sē′mă) [Gr. *emphysan,* to inflate] **1.** Pathological distention of interstitial tissues by gas or air. **2.** A chronic pulmonary disease marked by an abnormal increase in the size of air spaces distal to the terminal bronchiole with destructive changes in their walls. SYN: *chronic obstructive lung disease.* **emphysematous** (-ă-tŭs), *adj.*

SYMPTOMS: Symptoms may include a barrel chest and use of accessory muscles of ventilation; decreased tactile fremitus and inspiratory excursion; hyperresonance and decreased breath sounds; and adventitious sounds such as crackles and wheezing during inspiration, a prolonged expiratory phase with grunting, and distant heart sounds.

DIAGNOSIS: A precise diagnosis of emphysema is difficult to establish. Clinically the patient may have breathlessness only during exertion. A cough with production of sputum usually indicates chronic bronchitis.

TREATMENT: The patient should avoid contact with atmospheric pollution, esp. that caused by cigarette smoke. Treatment includes bronchodilators, mucolytic agents, weight reduction if the patient is obese, antibiotics for infections, and oxygen therapy only if this is clearly needed to prevent hypoxia.

Damaged lung tissue may be removed surgically and the area covered with a membrane to prevent air from leaking to the pleural space. This technique, called volume reduction, is being done experimentally in some medical centers.

NURSING IMPLICATIONS: A patent airway is maintained, and the patient is protected from environmental bronchial irritants such as smoke, automobile exhaust, aerosol sprays, and industrial pollutants. The nurse monitors the patient's weight and the results of arterial blood gas analysis, pulmonary function studies, and complete blood count. The patient is evaluated for infection and other complications, fatiguability, and the effects of the disease on functional capabilities. Oral fluid intake is increased to 3 L daily (or as permitted) to help loosen and liquify inspissated secretions. Prescribed medications are administered by parenteral or oral route or by inhalation.

Oral hygiene is provided after inhaled bronchodilator therapy, and the patient is taught how to use the inhaler. Prescribed inhalation therapy and chest physiotherapy, including postural drainage, clapping, and vibration, are scheduled at least 1 hr before or after meals; and the patient and family are instructed in their administration. After therapy, pulmonary toilet is provided.

The patient is encouraged to intersperse normal activities with rest periods. Respiratory infections can be prevented by avoiding contact with infectious persons; by using correct pulmonary hygiene procedures, including thorough hand washing; and by obtaining influenza and pneumococcus immunizations. Frequent small meals of easy-to-chew, easy-to-digest, high-calorie, high-protein foods and food supplements are encouraged. Small meals also reduce intra-abdominal pressure on the diaphragm and conserve energy.

The patient is taught diaphragmatic breathing to increase ventilatory efficiency, floppy-lipped breathing to keep small airways open, and expiratory exercises to improve functional capacity. Exposure to cold air may precipitate bronchospasm; the patient should cover the nose and mouth in cold, windy weather. A patient dependent on the hypoxic drive to initiate breathing is cautioned about the dangers of increased oxygen intake.

The patient and family are encouraged to voice their fears and concerns. Referral to support groups and services may be necessary. SEE: *Nursing Diagnoses Appendix.*

***interlobular e.*** The presence of air between the lobes of the lung.

***subcutaneous e.*** The presence of air in subcutaneous tissue.

**empiric** (ĕm-pĭr′ĭk) [Gr. *empeirikos,* skilled, experienced] **1.** Empirical. **2.** A practitioner whose skill or art is based on what has been learned through experience.

**empirical** (ĕm-pĭr′ĭk-ăl) Based on experience rather than on scientific principles.

**empiricism** (ĕm-pĭr′ĭs-ĭzm) [Gr. *empeirikos,* skilled, experienced, + *-ismos,* condition of] **1.** Experience, not theory, as the basis of medical science. **2.** Quackery.

**employment, supported** A program of paid work in integrated settings by persons with physical and mental disabilities. Ongoing training is provided by an interdisciplinary team of rehabilitation professionals, employers, and family members.

**emprosthotonos** (ĕm″prŏs-thŏt′ō-nŏs) [Gr. *emprosthen,* forward, + *tonos,* tension] A form of spasm in which the body is flexed forward, sometimes seen in tetanus and strychnine poisoning. Opposite of opisthotonos.

**empty follicle syndrome** In in vitro fertilization investigations, the absence of oocytes in the stimulated follicle of the ovary. This may be a cause of infertility in some individuals.

**empty-sella syndrome** A conditon, shown by lateral radiograph of the skull, in which the sella turcica, which normally contains the pituitary gland, is found to be empty. Clinically, patients may show no endocrine abnormality or may have signs of decreased pituitary function. The only treatment needed is hormonal replacement in those who demonstrate hypopituitarism. In autopsy studies, empty-sella syndrome has been found in about 5% of presumably normal persons. SEE: *pituitary gland.*

**empyema** (ĕm″pī-ē′mă) [Gr.] Pus in a body cavity, esp. in the pleural cavity (pyothorax). It is usually the result of a primary infection in the lungs.

SYMPTOMS: In the acute state, symptoms include chills, high fever, and sweating. The skin is gray and malar flushed, appetite is poor with marked malaise, and chest pain, cough, and emaciation are present. Dyspnea may ensue. Depending on the amount of fluid present (pleural effusion), pulmonary assessment may demonstrate unequal chest expansion, dullness to percussion, and decreased or absent breath sounds over the involved area. In the chronic state, weight loss, general malaise, and low-grade fever are present.

TREATMENT: Antibiotic therapy is administered into the cavity after pleural fluid is aspirated. The primary condition is treated. Surgical drainage may be necessary.

NURSING IMPLICATIONS: The nurse assists in providing drainage by thoracentesis or underwater-seal chest drainage with suction and provides prescribed preprocedure analgesia.

Vital signs are monitored, and the patient is observed for syncope throughout the procedure and for indications of pneumothorax (sudden-onset dyspnea and cyanosis) after the procedure. Prescribed local and systemic antibiotics and oxygen are also administered. Aseptic care of the chest tube insertion site and dressings is provided. Patency of the drainage system is maintained, drainage volume, color, and characteristics are documented, and the patient is protected from accidental dislodgement of the drainage tube. Increased fluid and protein are provided, and breathing exercises and use of incentive spirometry are encouraged. Home health care is arranged as necessary.

***interlobular e.*** A form of empyema with pus between the lobes of the lung.

**empyesis** (ĕm″pī-ē′sĭs) [Gr., suppuration] **1.** Any skin eruption marked by pustules. **2.** Any accumulation of pus. **3.** Hypopyon, or accumulation of pus in the anterior chamber of the eye.

**EMS** *emergency medical service.*

**EMS communication** A communication system that coordinates emergency medical care among ambulances, 911 (telephone) dispatch centers, and hospital emergency departments. Contact includes citizen to EMS, dispatcher to EMS crew, paramedic to doctor, and EMS crew to emergency department, as well as EMS to other public safety organizations (i.e., police, fire, and rescue). SEE: *disaster planning; EMS medical control.*

**EMS medical advisory committee** Representatives of medical groups that provide medical direction to the EMS system.

**EMS medical control** Physician direction of life support procedures performed by emergency medical technicians (EMT) and paramedics in prehospital care, including on-line and off-line supervision. *On-line:* The physician provides instruction via radio or telephone to an EMS crew. *Off-line:* The EMS crews receive direction and supervision via treatment protocols, case review, in-service training, and standing orders for treatment.

Medical control is also divided into prospective, immediate, and retrospective forms. *Prospective form:* Treatment protocols for EMTs are developed under a license from the medical director or medical advisory committee. *Immediate form:* Direct medical orders or consultation is given by radio or telephone (defined above as on-line control). *Retrospective form:* Call reports are reviewed to determine whether protocols have been followed.

**EMS medical director** The physician responsible for ensuring and evaluating the appropriate level of quality of care throughout an EMS system.

**EMS standing orders** Instructions preapproved by the medical advisory committee directing EMS crews to perform specific advanced life support measures *before* contacting a medical control physician. These orders are implemented in cases in which a delay in treatment could harm the patient (e.g., cardiac arrest).

**EMS treatment protocol** Written procedures for assessment, treatment, patient transportation, or patient transfer between hospitals. These procedures are part of the official policy of the EMS system and are approved by representatives of the medical advisory committee. The EMS treatment protocols may either be implemented as standing orders or require prior approval of a medical control physician.

**EMT** *emergency medical technician.*

**EMT–B** *emergency medical technician – basic.*

**EMT–D** *emergency medical technician – defibrillation.*

**EMT–I** *emergency medical technician – intermediate.*

**EMT–P** *emergency medical technician – paramedic.*

**emulsification** (ē-mŭl″sĭ-fĭ-kā′shŭn) [L. *emulsio,* emulsion, + *facere,* to make] **1.** The process of making an emulsion. **2.** The breaking down of large fat globules in the intestine into smaller, uniformly distributed particles, largely accomplished through the action of bile acids, which lower surface tension.

**emulsifier** Anything used to make an emulsion.

**emulsify** (ē-mŭl′sĭ-fī) To form into an emulsion.

**emulsion** [L. *emulsio*] **1.** A mixture of two liquids not mutually soluble. If they are thoroughly shaken, one divides into globules in what is called the discontinuous or dispersed phase; the other is then the continuous phase. Milk is an emulsion in which butterfat is the discontinuous phase. **2.** In radiology, the part of the radiographic film sensitive to radiation and containing the image after development.

***fat e.*** A combination of liquid, lipid, and an emulsifying system suitable for intravenous use. This isotonic solution should not be mixed with other materials given intravenously.

**emulsoid** (ē-mŭl′soyd) [″ + Gr. *eidos,* form, shape] A colloid in an aqueous solution in which the colloid has a marked attraction for water to the extent that the dispersoid contains large quantities of water. Examples are protoplasm, starch, soap, gelatin, and egg white.

**E.N.A.** *Emergency Nurses Association*; *extractable nuclear antigen.*

**enamel** (ĕn-ăm′ĕl) [O. Fr. *esmail,* enamel] The hard, white, dense substance forming a covering for the crown of the teeth. It is the hardest substance in the body. SYN: *enamelum.*

***aprismatic e.*** A thin surface layer of the tooth, thought to be solid without individual enamel rods or prisms.

***cervical e.*** Enamel at the neck of the tooth characterized by shorter enamel rods with more prominent incremental lines and perikymata.

***gnarled e.*** Enamel under the cusp of a tooth characterized by twisting, intertwining groups of enamel rods, thought to resist shearing forces.

***e. hypoplasia*** Incomplete development of tooth enamel, usually due to faulty calcium and phosphate metabolism.

***mottled e.*** A condition in which the enamel of the teeth acquires a mottled appearance, often as a result of excessive amounts of fluorides in water or foods. Mottling may also be caused by prolonged administration of tetracyclines to women during the first half of pregnancy, or to children while the teeth are developing. SEE: *fluorosis.*

**enamel organ** A cup-shaped structure that forms on the dental lamina of an embryo. It produces the enamel and serves as a mold for the remainder of the tooth. SEE: *morphogenesis.*

**enamel pearls** SEE: *pearls, enamel.*

**enamelum** Enamel.

**enanthem, enanthema** (ĕn-ăn′thĕm, -ăn-thē′mă) [Gr. *en,* in, + *anthema,* blossoming] An eruption on a mucous membrane. SEE: *exanthem; Koplik's spots; rash.* **enanthematous** (-thĕm′ă-tŭs), *adj.*

**enantio-** Combining form meaning *opposite.*

**enantiobiosis** (ĕn-ăn″tē-ō-bī-ō′sĭs) [Gr. *enantios,* opposite, + *bios,* life] The condition in which associated organisms are antagonistic to each other. SEE: *symbiosis.*

**enantiomorph** (ĕn-ăn′tē-ō-morf″) One of a pair of isomers, each of which is a mirror image of the other. They may be identical in chemical characteristics, but in solution one rotates a beam of polarized light in one direction and the other in the opposite direction. Isomers are called dextro if they rotate light to the right, and levo if they rotate light to the left.

**enarthrosis** (ĕn″ăr-thrō′sĭs) *pl.* **enarthroses** [Gr. *en,* in, + *arthron,* joint, + *osis,* condition] Ball-and-socket joint.

**en bloc** (ĕn blŏk) [Fr., as a whole] As a whole or as a lump; used to refer to surgical excision.

**encanthis** (ĕn-kăn′thĭs) [Gr. *en,* in, + *kanthos,* angle of the eye] An excrescence or new growth at the inner angle of the eye.

**encapsulation** [″ + *capsula,* a little box] **1.** Enclosure in a sheath not normal to the part. **2.** Formation of a capsule or a sheath about a structure.

**encatarrhaphy** (ĕn″kăt-ăr′ă-fē) [Gr. *enkatarrhaptein,* to sew in] Insertion of an organ or tissue into a part where it is not normally found.

**encephalalgia** (ĕn-sĕf″ăl-ăl′jē-ă) [Gr. *enkephalos,* brain, + *algos,* pain] Deep-seated head pain. SYN: *cephalalgia.*

**encephalatrophy** (ĕn-sĕf″ă-lăt′rō-fē) [″ + *a-,* not, + *trophe,* nourishment] Cerebral atrophy.

**encephalic** (ĕn″sĕf-ăl′ĭk) [Gr. *enkephalos,* brain] Pert. to the brain or its cavity.

**encephalitis** (ĕn-sĕf″ă-lī′tĭs) [″ + *itis,* inflammation] Inflammation of the brain.

ETIOLOGY: Encephalitis may be due to a specific disease entity such as rabies or an arthropod-borne virus (arbovirus), or it may occur as a sequela of influenza, measles, German measles, chickenpox, herpesvirus infection, smallpox, vaccinia, or other diseases.

SYMPTOMS: Symptoms include headache, muscle stiffness, malaise, sore throat, and upper respiratory tract problems. Neurological effects are nuchal rigidity and opisthotonos; changes in level of consciousness; increasing restlessness, projectile vomiting, convulsions, pupil irregularities, motor dysfunction, involuntary movements, and vital sign changes; and ptosis, diplopia, strabismus, tremor, exaggerated deep tendon reflexes, absent superficial reflexes, and extremity paresis or paralysis. Fever, nausea and vomiting, behavioral changes, and abnormal sleep patterns may also be present.

TREATMENT: Treatment includes support and therapy for the specific cause. SEE: *rabies*.

NURSING IMPLICATIONS: Fluid balance is monitored by measuring fluid intake and output and body weight to prevent dehydration and to avoid fluid overload and attendant cerebral edema. Prescribed drugs, including antiviral agents (in herpetic encephalitis), IV mannitol and corticosteroids, phenytoin or other anticonvulsants, sedatives, analgesics, and antipyretics are administered and evaluated for desired effects and adverse reactions (esp. those encountered when antiviral agents are administered intravenously).

Lights are dimmed to decrease headache, but without creating shadows, which increase the potential for hallucinations; and the delirious or confused patient is reoriented often. The patient at risk for seizures is protected from injury. Small, frequent meals, nutritional supplements, and nasogastric tube feedings or parenteral nutrition are provided. Oral hygiene is performed frequently. Stool softeners or a mild laxative is given as prescribed.

The patient is repositioned frequently to prevent neck discomfort and joint pain and to aid ventilatory excursions and secretion removal. Assistance is provided with range-of-motion exercises to maintain joint mobility and prevent contractures, as well as to enhance circulation and improve muscle tone. Assurance is offered to the patient's family that behavioral changes are usually transitory, although permanent problems may sometimes occur. Once the acute phase has subsided, the patient is referred for rehabilitative treatment of any residual effects. SEE: *Nursing Diagnoses Appendix*.

***acute disseminated e.*** Postinfection e.

***cortical e.*** Encephalitis of the brain cortex only.

***eastern equine e.*** Encephalitis, primarily viral, of birds and wild animals, transmitted to horses and humans by mosquitoes. It is more severe than other types of encephalitis. Outbreaks have occurred in the eastern and Gulf Coast states.

***epidemic e.*** Any form of encephalitis that occurs as an epidemic.

***equine e.*** A mosquito-borne type of viral encephalitis originally isolated as an encephalitis affecting horses.

***hemorrhagic e.*** Herpes encephalitis in which there is hemorrhage along with brain inflammation.

***herpes e.*** Encephalitis due to infection with herpes simplex virus. It is rare and frequently fatal. Some cases have been successfully treated with acyclovir.

***e. hyperplastica*** Acute encephalitis without suppuration.

***infantile e.*** A brain inflammation in the young that may cause cerebral palsy.

***Japanese (B type) e.*** A strain of encephalitis similar to St. Louis encephalitis but caused by a different strain of mosquito-borne virus. It occurs in summer and fall.

***lead e.*** Encephalitis due to lead poisoning.

***e. lethargica*** A disease of the nervous system thought to be caused by a virus. It is marked by lethargy, oculomotor paralysis, clonic and choreiform movements, rigidity, delirium, stupor, coma, and reversal of sleep rhythm. The disease first appeared pandemically in 1916 to 1917 and is now considered extinct. SYN: *Economo's disease*.

***e. neonatorum*** A form of encephalitis occurring within the first several weeks of life.

***e. periaxialis*** Inflammation of the white matter of the cerebrum, occurring mainly in the young.

***postinfection e.*** Encephalitis following a smallpox vaccination or one of the common communicable diseases, such as chickenpox. SYN: *acute disseminated e.*

***postvaccinal e.*** Acute encephalitis following vaccination.

***purulent e.*** Encephalitis characterized by abscesses in the brain.

***Russian spring-summer e.*** Encephalitis due to a tick-borne virus. Humans may also contract it by drinking goat milk.

***St. Louis e.*** A mosquito-borne viral encephalitis that first occurred epidemically in the summer of 1933 in and around St. Louis, Missouri. Now endemic in the U.S., Trinidad, Jamaica, Panama, and Brazil, it occurs most frequently during summer and early fall.

***toxic e.*** Encephalitis resulting from metal poisonings, such as lead poisoning.

***western equine e.*** A mild type of viral encephalitis that has occurred in the western U.S. and Canada.

**Encephalitozoon** A genus of the order Microsporidia. SEE: *microsporidiosis*.

**encephalocele** (ĕn-sĕf′ă-lō-sēl) [Gr. *enkephalos*, brain, + *kele*, hernia] A protrusion of the brain through a cranial fissure. SYN: *hydrencephalocele*.

**encephalocystocele** (ĕn-sĕf″ă-lō-sĭs′tō-sēl) [″ + *kystis*, sac, + *kele*, tumor, swelling] A hernia of the brain. The hernia sac is filled with cerebrospinal fluid.

**encephalogram** (ĕn-sĕf′ă-lō-grăm) [″ + *gramma*, something written] A radiograph of the brain, usually performed with air in the ventricles as a contrast medium. This procedure has been replaced by computed tomography and magnetic resonance imaging.

**encephalography** (ĕn-sĕf″ă-lŏg′ră-fē) [″ + *graphein,* to write] Radiography of the head, esp. examination following the introduction of air into the ventricles through a lumbar or cisternal puncture. This procedure is no longer performed. SEE: *encephalogram.*

**encephaloid** (ĕn-sĕf′ă-loyd) [″ + *eidos,* form, shape] **1.** Resembling the cerebral substance. **2.** A malignant neoplasm of brain-like texture.

**encephalolith** (ĕn-sĕf′ă-lō-lĭth) [″ + *lithos,* stone] A calculus of the brain.

**encephaloma** (ĕn-sĕf″ă-lō-mă) [″ + *oma,* tumor] A tumor of the brain.

**encephalomalacia** (ĕn-sĕf″ă-lō-mă-lā′sē-ă) [″ + *malakia,* softening] Cerebral softening.

**encephalomeningitis** (ĕn-sĕf″ă-lō-mĕn″ĭn-jī′tĭs) [″ + *meninx,* membrane, + *itis,* inflammation] Inflammation of the brain and its membranes.

**encephalomeningocele** (ĕn-sĕf″ă-lō-mĕ-nĭng′gŏ-sēl) [″ + ″ + *kele,* tumor, swelling] A protrusion of membranes and brain substance through the cranium.

**encephalomere** (ĕn-sĕf′ă-lō-mēr″) [″ + *meros,* part] A primitive segment of the embryonic brain. SYN: *neuromere.*

**encephalometer** (ĕn-sĕf″ă-lŏm′ĕ-tĕr) [″ + *metron,* measure] An instrument for measuring the cranium and locating brain regions.

**encephalomyelitis** (ĕn-sĕf″ă-lō-mī-ĕl-ī-′tĭs) [″ + *myelos,* marrow, + *itis,* inflammation] Acute inflammation of the brain and spinal cord.

***acute disseminated e.*** An acute disorder of the brain and spinal cord due to causes such as vaccination or acute exanthema. SYN: *postinfectious e.*

***benign myalgic e.*** An epidemic disease of unknown etiology marked by influenza-like symptoms, severe pain, and muscular weakness. SYN: *epidemic neuromyasthenia; Iceland disease.*

***equine e.*** A viral disease of horses that may be communicated to humans. It includes eastern and western equine encephalitis.

***postinfectious e.*** Acute disseminated e.

***postvaccinal e.*** Encephalomyelitis following smallpox vaccination.

**encephalomyeloneuropathy** (ĕn-sĕf″ă-lō-mī″ĕ-lō-nū-rŏp′ă-thē) Any disease involving the brain, spinal cord, and nerves.

**encephalomyelopathy** (ĕn-sĕf″ă-lō-mī″ĕl-ŏp′ă-thē) [″ + ″ + *pathos,* disease, suffering] Any disease of the brain and spinal cord.

**encephalomyeloradiculitis** (ĕn-sĕf″ă-lō-mī″ĕ-lō-ră-dĭk″ū-lī′tĭs) Inflammation of the brain, spinal cord, and nerve roots.

**encephalomyocarditis** (ĕn-sĕf″ă-lō-mī″ō-kăr-dī′tĭs) Any disease involving the brain and cardiac muscle.

**encephalon** (ĕn-sĕf′ă-lŏn) [Gr. *enkephalos,* brain] The brain, including the cerebrum, cerebellum, medulla oblongata, pons, diencephalon, and midbrain.

**encephalopathy** (ĕn-sĕf″ă-lŏp′ă-thē) [″ + *pathos,* disease, suffering] Any dysfunction of the brain.

***hepatic e.*** SEE: *hepatic coma.*

***HIV e.*** AIDS-dementia complex.

***portal-systemic e.*** ABBR: PSE. A brain dysfunction related to the shunting of blood around the liver and hepatic insufficiency. In this condition, substances that are toxic to the brain are not metabolized by the liver. Symptoms include dementia as well as neuromuscular abnormalities, metabolic slowing of the electroencephalogram, and elevated ammonia levels. SEE: *asterixis; hepatic coma.*

**encephalopyosis** (ĕn-sĕf″ă-lō-pī-ō′sĭs) [″ + *pyosis,* suppuration] An abscess of the brain.

**encephalospinal** [″ + L. *spina,* thorn, spine] Pert. to the brain and spinal cord.

**encephalotomy** (ĕn-sĕf″ă-lŏt′ō-mē) **1.** Brain dissection. **2.** Surgical destruction of the brain of a fetus to facilitate delivery.

**enchondroma** (ĕn″kŏn-drō′mă) [Gr. *en,* in, + *chondros,* cartilage, + *oma,* tumor] A benign cartilaginous tumor occurring generally where cartilage is absent, or within a bone, where it expands the diaphysis. SYN: *enchondrosis.*

**enchondrosarcoma** (ĕn-kŏn″drō-săr-kō′mă) [″ + ″ + *sarx,* flesh, + *oma,* tumor] A sarcoma made up of cartilaginous tissue.

**enchondrosis** (ĕn-kŏn-drō′sĭs) [″ + ″ + *osis,* condition] A benign cartilaginous outgrowth from bone or cartilaginous tissue. SYN: *enchondroma.*

**enclave** (ĕn′klāv) [Fr. *enclaver,* to enclose] A mass of tissue that becomes enclosed by tissue of another kind.

**enclitic** (ĕn-klĭt′ĭk) [Gr. *enklinein,* to lean on] Having the planes of the fetal head inclined to those of the maternal pelvis.

**encopresis** (ĕn-kō-prē′sĭs) [″ + *kopros,* excrement] A condition associated with constipation and fecal retention in which watery colonic contents bypass the hard fecal masses and pass through the rectum. This condition is often confused with diarrhea.

**encranial** [″ + *kranion,* cranium] Intracranial or within the cranium.

**enculturation** The process of transmitting to the members of the community the values, beliefs, and customs of the family, the cultural group, and the larger society.

**encysted** (ĕn-sĭst′ĕd) [″ + *kystis,* bladder, pouch] Surrounded by membrane; encapsulated. SYN: *saccate.*

**end** [AS. *ende*] A termination; an extremity.

**end-** SEE: *endo-.*

**endadelphos** (ĕnd″ă-dĕl′fŏs) [Gr. *endon,* within, + *adelphos,* brother] A congenitally deformed fetus whose twin is enclosed in the body or in a cyst on the fetus.

**Endamoeba** (ĕn″dă-mē′bă) *Entamoeba.*

**endangiitis, endangeitis** (ĕnd″ăn-jē-ī′tĭs) [Gr. *endon,* within, + *angeion,* vessel, + *itis,* inflammation] Inflammation of the endangium, or inner coat of a blood vessel. SYN: *endoangiitis; endoarteritis; endophlebitis.*

**endangium** (ĕn-dăn′jē-ŭm) [″ + *angeion,* vessel] The innermost layer, or intima, of a blood vessel.

**endaortitis** (ĕnd″ā-or-tī′tĭs) [″ + *aorte,* aorta, + *itis,* inflammation] Inflammation of the inner layer of the aorta.

**endarterectomy** (ĕnd″ăr-tĕr-ĕk′tō-mē) Surgical removal of the lining of an artery. It is performed on almost any major artery that is diseased or blocked, such as the carotid, femoral, or popliteal artery.

***carotid e.*** SEE: *carotid endarterectomy.*

**endarterial** (ĕnd″ăr-tē′rē-ăl) [″ + *arteria,* artery] **1.** Pert. to the inner portion of an artery. **2.** Within an artery.

**endarteritis, endoarteritis** (ĕnd-ăr-tĕr-ī′tĭs) [″ + ″ + *itis,* inflammation] Inflammation of the innermost layer (intima) of an artery, resulting from syphilis, trauma, pyogenic bacteria, or infective thrombi.

***e. deformans*** A condition in which the intima is thickened or replaced with atheromatous or calcareous deposits.

***e. obliterans*** Chronic progressive thickening of the intima leading to stenosis or obstruction of a lumen.

***syphilitic e.*** Endarteritis caused by syphilis.

**end artery** An artery that does not communicate with other arteries.

**endbrain** The telencephalon.

**end-bud** End-bulb.

**end-bulb** The terminal portion of a sensory nerve. SYN: *end-bud.*

***e. of Krause*** An encapsulated nerve ending found in the skin and mucous membranes.

**endemic** [Gr. *en,* in, + *demos,* people] Pert. to a disease that occurs continuously or in expected cycles in a population, with a certain number of cases expected for a given period. Examples include influenza and the common cold. The term is used in contrast to *epidemic.*

**endemoepidemic** (ĕn-dĕm″ō-ĕp-ĭ-dĕm′ĭk) [″ + ″ + *epi,* on, among, + *demos,* people] Endemic, but becoming epidemic periodically.

**endergonic** (ĕnd″ĕr-gŏn′ĭk) [Gr. *endon,* within, + *ergon,* work] Pert. to chemical reactions that require energy in order to occur.

**end feel** In physical therapy and rehabilitation, the feeling experienced by an evaluator when overpressure is applied to tissue at the end of the available range of motion. It is interpreted as abnormal when the quality of the feel is different from normal response at that joint. The feeling may be soft as when two muscle groups are compressed or soft tissues are stretched, firm as when a normal joint or ligament is stretched, or hard as when two bones block motion. Abnormal end feels may include a springy sensation when cartilage is torn within a joint, muscle guarding when a muscle involuntarily responds to acute pain, or muscle spasticity when there is increased tone due to an upper motor neuron lesion or when the feeling is different from that normally experienced for the joint being tested.

**end-foot** A terminal button; the enlarged end of a nerve fiber that terminates adjacent to the dendrite of another nerve cell.

**ending** The finish or final portion of a tissue or cell.

**endo-, end-** Prefix meaning *within.*

**endoaneurysmorrhaphy** (ĕn″dō-ăn″ū-rĭs-mor′ăf-ē) [Gr. *endon,* within, + *aneurysma,* aneurysm, + *rhaphe,* seam, ridge] Surgical opening of an aneurysmal sac and suturing of its orifice.

**endoangiitis** (ĕn″dō-ăn-jē-ī′tĭs) [″ + *angeion,* vessel, + *itis,* inflammation] Endangiitis.

**endoauscultation** (ĕn″dō-ăws″kŭl-tā′shŭn) [″ + L. *auscultare,* to listen to] Auscultation by an esophageal tube passed into the stomach or by a tube passed into the heart.

**endobiotic** (ĕn″dō-bī-ŏt′ĭk) [″ + *bios,* life] Pert. to an organism living parasitically in the host.

**endoblast** (ĕn′dō-blăst) [″ + *blastos,* germ] The immature cell that is the precursor of an endodermal cell.

**endocardiac, endocardial** [″ + *kardia,* heart] Within the heart or arising from the endocardium.

**endocarditis** (ĕn″dō-kăr-dī′tĭs) [″ + ″ + *itis,* inflammation] Inflammation of the lining membrane of the heart. It is usually confined to the covering of a valve and sometimes to the lining membrane of the chambers. It may be due to invasion of microorganisms or an abnormal immunological reaction.

SYMPTOMS: In acute infection, a great variety of symptoms may be present, including emobilization from the bacteria on the valves to any organ, bacteremia, and metastatic foci of infection. Fever, anorexia, weight loss, malaise, fatigue, vomiting, chills, and night sweats may be present.

TREATMENT: If the cause is bacterial invasion, appropriate antibiotic therapy should be used for as long as a month or, in the case of some organisms, several months.

NURSING IMPLICATIONS: During the acute phase, the patient rests in bed in a calm, quiet, environment. Assistance is provided with activities of daily living as necessary, and a commode is used to reduce cardiac work. Vital signs, including apical pulse, are monitored every 2 to 4 hr or more frequently. Cardiovascular status is assessed frequently.

If dyspneic, the patient is placed in the high Fowler's or orthopneic position. Prescribed antibiotic therapy is administered. Renal status, including blood urea nitrogen, creatinine clearance, and urine output, is monitored for evidence of renal emboli and drug toxicity. The patient is assessed for signs of embolization (hematuria, pleuritic chest pain, left upper quadrant abdominal pain, paresis), a common occurrence during the first 3 months of treatment, and taught to recognize and report such signs.

When the patient begins activity or ambulation, the pulse is checked before and after the activity. The patient is instructed to watch for and report fever, anorexia, and other signs of relapse occurring about 2 weeks after treatment stops. The importance of taking prescribed prophylactic antibiotics is emphasized. The patient is encouraged to express concerns about the effects of activity restrictions on responsibilities, routines, and lifestyle and is reassured that these restrictions are temporary. SEE: *Nursing Diagnoses Appendix.*

***acute bacterial e.*** Endocarditis that begins abruptly and progresses rapidly. It is usually caused by virulent organisms such as staphylococci or streptococci. SEE: *ulcerative e.*

***atypical verrucous e.*** Nonbacterial e.

***infective e.*** Endocarditis due to microorganisms.

***Libman-Sacks e.*** Nonbacterial e.

***malignant e.*** A fatal type of endocarditis that is usually secondary to suppurative inflammation elsewhere. SEE: *ulcerative e.*

***mural e.*** Endocarditis of the lining of the heart chambers but not including the heart valve.

***nonbacterial e.*** Endocarditis in which the accumulation of debris on the endocardium is associated with various wasting diseases.

***rheumatic e.*** Endocarditis that occurs following rheumatic fever.

***subacute bacterial e.*** A condition usually caused by colonization of the *Streptococcus viridans* group (mainly *S. salivarius, S. mitis, S. bovis, S. faecalis, S. sanguis*) in an abnormal heart or in valves damaged previously by rheumatic fever.

***syphilitic e.*** Endocarditis due to syphilis having extended from aortic involvement to the aortic valves.

***tuberculous e.*** Endocarditis involving the heart valves and caused by the tubercle bacillus.

***ulcerative e.*** A rapidly destructive form of acute bacterial endocarditis characterized by necrosis or ulceration of the valves and the growth of bacterial colonies on the valves.

***valvular e.*** Endocarditis affecting only the covering of the valves and not the lining of the heart chambers.

***vegetative e.*** Endocarditis associated with fibrinous clots on ulcerated valvular surfaces.

***verrucous e.*** Nonbacterial e.

***e. viridans*** Subacute bacterial e.

**endocardium** [Gr. *endon,* within, + *kardia,* heart] The endothelial membrane that lines the chambers of the heart and is continuous with the intima (the lining of arteries and veins).

**endocervical** (ĕn″dō-sĕr′vĭ-kăl) [″ + L. *cervix,* neck] Pert. to the endocervix.

**endocervicitis** (ĕn″dō-sĕr″vĭ-sī′tĭs) [″ + ″ + Gr. *itis,* inflammation] Inflammation of the mucous lining of the cervix uteri. It is usually chronic, due to infection, and accompanied by cervical erosion.

SYMPTOMS: A white or yellow mucoid discharge is symptomatic.

TREATMENT: Electrocauterization of the cervical lesion is performed. An antibiotic for local application may be prescribed. SEE: *carcinoma in situ.*

**endocervix** (ĕn″dō-sĕr′vĭks) [″ + L. *cervix,* neck] The lining of the canal of the cervix uteri.

**endochondral** (ĕn″dō-kŏn′drăl) [″ + *chondros,* cartilage] Within a cartilage.

**endochondral bone formation** One of the two types of bone formation in skeletal development. Each long bone is formed as a cartilage model before bone is laid down, replacing the cartilage.

**endochorion** (ĕn″dō-kō′rē-ŏn) [″ + *chorion,* chorion] The inner chorion; the vascular layer of the allantois.

**endocolitis** (ĕn″dō-kō-lī′tĭs) [″ + *kolon,* colon, + *itis,* inflammation] Inflammation of the mucosa of the colon. SEE: *colitis.*

**endocorpuscular** (ĕn″dō-kor-pŭs′kū-lăr) [″ + L. *corpusculum,* small body (corpuscle)] Within a corpuscle.

**endocranial** (ĕn″dō-krā′nē-ăl) [″ + *kranion,* cranium] **1.** Intracranial or within the cranium. **2.** Pert. to the endocranium.

**endocranium** (ĕn″dō-krā′nē-ŭm) The dura mater of the brain, which forms the lining membrane of the cranium.

**endocrine** (ĕn′dō-krīn, -krĭn, -krēn) [″ + *krinein,* to secrete] **1.** An internal secretion. **2.** Pert. to a gland that secretes directly into the bloodstream.

**endocrine gland** A ductless gland that produces an internal secretion discharged into the blood or lymph and circulated to all parts of the body. Hormones, the active principles of the glands, affect tissues more or less remote from their place of origin. In addition to their endocrine function, some glands produce an external secretion.

The endocrine glands include the hypophysis (pituitary gland), thyroid gland, parathyroid glands, adrenal (suprarenal) glands, islets of Langerhans of the pancreas, and gonads (ovaries and testes). In addition, the hypothalamus produces releasing hormones that affect the production of some other hormones. Other structures such as the gastrointestinal mucosa and the placenta have an endocrine func-

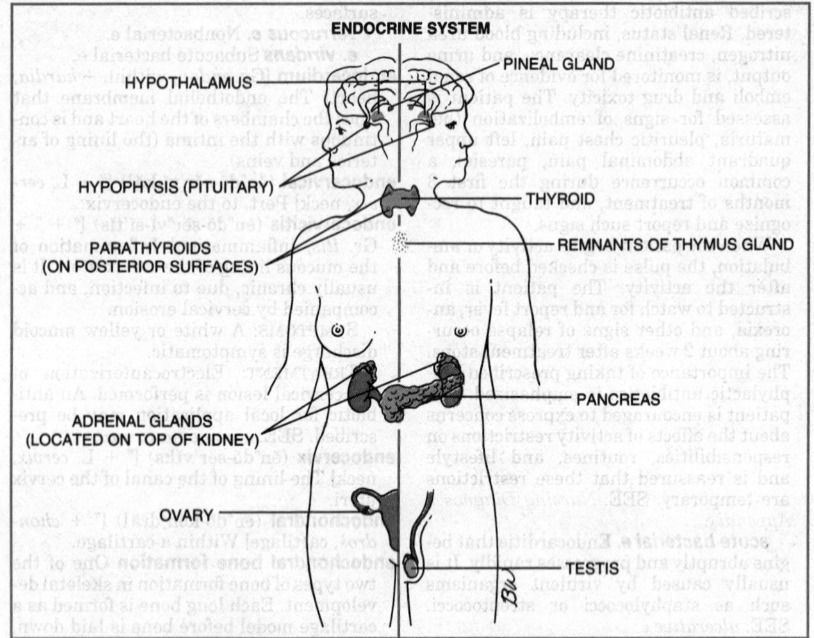


tion. SEE: illus.; table.

The hormones secreted by the ductless glands may have a specific effect on an organ or tissue or a general effect on the entire body, as in the case of the thyroid hormone, which affects metabolic rate. Among the physiological processes affected by hormones are metabolic rate and the metabolism of specific substances, growth and developmental processes, secretory activity of other endocrine glands, development and functioning of the reproductive organs, sexual characteristics and libido, development of personality and higher nervous functions, the ability of the body to meet conditions of stress, and resistance to disease.

Endocrine dysfunction may result from hyposecretion, in which an inadequate amount of hormone is secreted, or from hypersecretion, in which an excessive amounts of hormone is produced. Secretion of endocrine glands may be controlled by the nervous system, by chemical substances in the blood, or, in some cases, by other hormones. Many pathological conditions are caused by or associated with malfunction of the endocrine glands.

**endocrine neoplasm, multiple** SEE: *multiple endocrine neoplasm.*

**endocrino-** [Gr. *endon,* within, + *krinein,* to secrete] Combining form, *endocrine*.

**endocrinologist** A medical scientist skilled in endocrinology.

**endocrinology** (ĕn″dō-krĭn-ŏl′ō-jē) [″ + ″ + *logos,* word, reason] The science of the endocrine, or ductless, glands and their functions.

**endocrinopathy** (ĕn″dō-krĭn-ŏp′ă-thē) [″ + ″ + *pathos,* disease, suffering] Any disease resulting from disorder of an endocrine gland or glands. **endocrinopathic** (-krĭn″ō-pă′thĭk), *adj.*

**endocrinotherapy** (ĕn″dō-krĭn″ō-thĕr′ă-pē) [″ + ″ + *therapeia,* treatment] Treatment with endocrine preparations.

**endocyst** (ĕn′dō-sĭst) [″ + *kystis,* bladder, pouch] The innermost layer of any hydatid cyst.

**endocystitis** (ĕn′dō-sĭs-tī′tĭs) [″ + ″ + *itis,* inflammation] Inflammation of the mucous membrane of the bladder. SEE: *cystitis.*

**endocytosis** A method of ingestion of a foreign substance by a cell. The cell membrane invaginates to form a space for the material and then the opening closes to trap the material inside the cell. SEE: *emiocytosis; exocytosis; phagocytosis; pinocytosis.*

**endoderm** (ĕn′dō-dĕrm) [″ + *derma,* skin] The innermost of the three primary germ layers of a developing embryo. It gives rise to the epithelium of the digestive tract and its associated glands, the respiratory organs, bladder, vagina, and urethra. SYN: *hypoblast.* **endodermal** (-dĕrm′ăl), *adj.*

**Endodermophyton** (ĕn″dō-dĕr-mŏf′ĭ-tŏn) [″ + *derma,* skin, + *phyton,* a growth] The former name of a genus of parasitic fungi growing in the epidermis. It is now included in the genus *Trichophyton.*

**endodontia** (ĕn″dō-dŏn′shē-ă) [″ + *odous,*

**Principal Endocrine Glands**

| Name | Position | Function | Endocrine Disorders |
|---|---|---|---|
| Adrenal cortex | Outer portion of gland on top of each kidney | Steroid hormones regulate carbohydrate and fat metabolism and salt and water balance | Hypofunction: Addison's disease<br>Hyperfunction: Adrenogenital syndrome; Cushing's syndrome |
| Adrenal medulla | Inner portion of adrenal gland; surrounded by adrenal cortex | Effects mimic those of sympathetic nervous system; increases carbohydrate use of energy | Hypofunction: Almost unknown<br>Hyperfunction: Pheochromocytoma |
| Pancreas (endocrine portion) | Abdominal cavity; head adjacent to duodenum; tail close to spleen and kidney | Secretes insulin and glucagon, which regulate carbohydrate metabolism | Hypofunction: Diabetes mellitus<br>Hyperfunction: If a tumor produces excess insulin, hypoglycemia |
| Parathyroid | Four or more small glands on back of thyroid | Calcium and phosphorus metabolism; indirectly affects muscular irritability | Hypofunction: Tetany<br>Hyperfunction: Resorption of bone; renal calculi |
| Pituitary, anterior | Front portion of small gland below hypothalamus | Influences growth, sexual development, skin pigmentation, thyroid function, adrenocortical function through effects on other endocrine glands (except for growth hormone, which acts directly on cells) | Hypofunction: Dwarfism in child; decrease in all other endocrine gland functions except parathyroids<br>Hyperfunction: Acromegaly in adult; gigantism in child |
| Pituitary, posterior | Back portion of small gland below hypothalamus | Oxytocin increases uterine contraction<br>Antidiuretic hormone increases absorption of water by kidney tubule | Unknown<br>Hypofunction: Diabetes insipidus |
| Testes and ovaries | Testes—in the scrotum<br>Ovaries—in the pelvic cavity | Development of secondary sex characteristics; some effects on growth | Hypofunction: Lack of sex development or regression in adult<br>Hyperfunction: Abnormal sex development |
| Thyroid | Two lobes in anterior portion of neck | Increases metabolic rate; indirectly influences growth and nutrition | Hypofunction: Cretinism in young; myxedema in adult; goiter<br>Hyperfunction: Goiter; thyrotoxicosis |

tooth] Endodontics.

**endodontics** (ĕn″dō-dŏn′tĭks) The branch of dentistry concerned with diagnosis, treatment, and prevention of diseases of the dental pulp and its surrounding tissues.

**endodontist** A specialist in endodontics.

**endodontitis** (ĕn″dō-dŏn-tī′tĭs) [″ + *odous,* tooth, + *itis,* inflammation] Inflammation of the dental pulp. SYN: *pulpitis.*

**endodontologist** An endodontist.

**endoectothrix** (ĕn″dō-ĕk′tō-thrĭks) [″ + *ektos,* outside, + *thrix,* hair] Any fungus growth on and in the hair.

**endogamy** (ĕn-dŏg′ă-mē) [″ + *gamos,* marriage] **1.** The custom or tribal restriction of marriage within a tribe or group. **2.** In biology, reproduction by joining together gametes descended from the same ancestral cell.

**endogastritis** (ĕn″dō-găs-trī′tĭs) [″ + ″ + *itis,* inflammation] Inflammation of the lining membrane of the stomach.

**endogenic** (ĕn″dō-jĕn′ĭk) [″ + *gennan,* to produce] Endogenous.

**endogenous** (ĕn-dŏj′ĕ-nŭs) **1.** Produced or originating from within a cell or organism. **2.** Concerning spore formation within the bacterial cell. SYN: *endogenic.*

**endogenous opiate-like substance** SEE: *endorphin; enkephalin; opiate receptor.*

**endoglobar, endoglobular** (ĕn″dō-glōb′ăr, ĕn″dō-glŏb′ū-lăr) [Gr. *endon,* within, + L. *globulus,* a globule] Within the blood corpuscles.

**endognathion** (ĕn″dō-năth′ē-ŏn) [Gr. *endon,* within, + *gnathos,* jaw] A point in the inner segment of the intermaxillary bone, or premaxilla.

**endointoxication** (ĕn″dō-ĭn-tŏk″sĭ-kā′shŭn) [″ + L. *in,* into, + Gr. *toxikon,* poison] Poisoning due to an endogenous toxin.

**endolabyrinthitis** (ĕn″dō-lăb″ĭ-rĭn-thī′tĭs) [″ + *labyrinthos,* labyrinth, + *itis,* inflammation] Inflammation of the membranous labyrinth.

**Endolimax nana** (ĕn″dō-lī′măks nă′nă) [″ + *leimax,* meadow] A species of ameba inhabiting the intestines of humans, monkeys, and other mammals. It is usually nonpathogenic in humans and is found in the intestines of healthy persons.

**endolumbar** [″ + L. *lumbus,* loin] In the lumbar portion of the spinal cord.

**endolymph** (ĕn′dō-lĭmf) [″ + L. *lympha,* clear fluid] A pale transparent fluid within the membranous labyrinth of the inner ear. **endolymphatic** (-lĭm-făt′ĭk), *adj.*

**endolymphatic duct** A slender duct extending from the posterior surface of the saccule of the inner ear. It ends blindly in the petrous portion of the temporal bone as a dilated pouch, the endolymphatic sac.

**endolysin** (ĕn-dŏl′ĭ-sĭn) [″ + *lysis,* dissolution] A bacterial substance within a leukocyte that destroys bacteria.

**endomastoiditis** (ĕn″dō-măs″toy-dī′tĭs) [″ + *mastos,* breast, + *eidos,* form, shape, + *itis,* inflammation] Inflammation of the mucosa lining the mastoid cavity and cells.

**endometrial** (ĕn″dō-mē′trē-ăl) [″ + *metra,* uterus] Pert. to the lining of the uterus.

**endometrial cyst** An ovarian cyst or tumor lined with endometrial tissue, usually seen in ovarian endometriosis.

**endometrial dating** Microscopic examination of a suitable, stained specimen from the endometrium to establish the number of days to the next menstrual period. The dating is based on an ideal 28-day cycle. Thus, day 8 indicates menstruation is 20 days away, and day 23 that it is 5 days away. This system was devised by the late Dr. John Rock, a physician at Harvard Medical School, to enable gynecologists to visualize endometria being discussed without having to provide detailed descriptions of the material studied.

**endometrial jet washing** Collection of fluid that has been used to irrigate the uterine cavity. Cells present in the fluid are examined for evidence of malignancy. This method is used as a screening test for endometrial carcinoma.

**endometrioma** (ĕn″dō-mē″trē-ō′mă) [Gr. *endon,* within, + *metra,* uterus, + *oma,* tumor] A tumor containing shreds of ectopic endometrium. It is found most frequently in the ovary, the cul-de-sac, the rectovaginal septum, and the peritoneal surface of the posterior portion of the uterus.

**endometriosis** (ĕn″dō-mē″trē-ō′sĭs) [″ + ″ + *osis,* condition] The presence of functioning ectopic endometrial glands and stroma outside the uterine cavity. Characteristically, the endometrial tissue invades other tissues and spreads by local extension, intraperitoneal seeding, and vascular routes. The endometrial implants may be present in almost any area of the body. This condition is estimated to occur in 1% to 7% of women in the U.S. The fallopian tubes are common sites of ectopic implantation. Ectopic endometrial cells respond to the same hormonal stimuli as does the uterine endometrium. The cyclic bleeding and local inflammation surrounding the implants may cause fibrosis, adhesions, and tubal occlusion. Infertility may result. SEE: illus.

SYMPTOMS: No single symptom is diagnostic. Patients often complain of dysmenorrhea with pelvic pain, premenstrual dyspareunia, sacral backache during menses, and infertility. Dysuria may indicate involvement of the urinary bladder. Cyclic pelvic pain, usually in the lower abdomen, vagina, posterior pelvis, and back, begins 5 to 7 days before menses, reaches a peak, and lasts 2 to 3 days. Premenstrual tenesmus and diarrhea may indicate lower bowel involvement. There is no correlation between the degree of pain and the extent of involvement; many patients are asymptomatic.

ETIOLOGY: Although the cause is unknown, hypotheses are that either

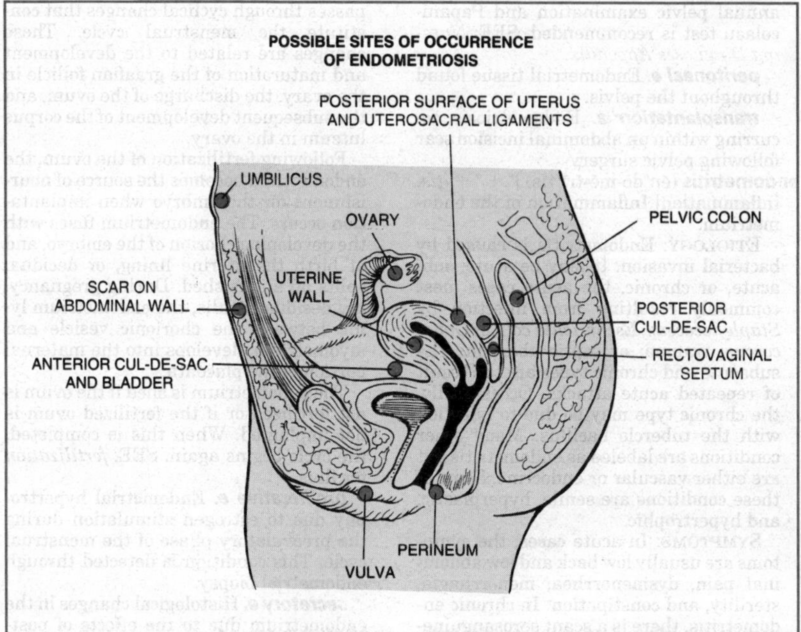


endometrial cell migration occurs during fetal development, or the cells shed during menstruation are expelled upward through the fallopian tubes.

DIAGNOSIS: Although history and findings of physical examination may suggest endometriosis, definitive diagnosis of endometriosis can be established only by direct visualization of ectopic lesions or by biopsy.

TREATMENT: Medical and surgical approaches may be used to preserve fertility and increase the woman's potential for achieving pregnancy. Pharmacological management includes the use of hormonal agents to induce endometrial atrophy by maintaining a chronic state of anovulation. Medroxyprogesterone inhibits ovulation and menstruation by inducing pseudopregnancy. Danazol inhibits pituitary release of gonadotropins. Gonadotropin-releasing hormone (GnRH) analogues inhibit release of follicle-stimulating hormone (FSH) and luteinizing hormone (LH). Methyltestosterone also has been used to cause endometrial atrophy and provide pain relief; however, ovulation and menstruation are not affected, and pregnancy may occur during therapy.

Conservative surgical management includes laparotomy, lysis of adhesions, and removal of aberrant endometrial cysts and implants to encourage fertility. The definitive treatment for endometriosis ends a woman's potential for pregnancy by removal of the uterus, tubes, and ovaries.

NURSING IMPLICATIONS: The laparoscopic procedure, used to confirm the diagnosis and to identify the disease stage, is explained to the patient. If excessive bleeding occurs with menses, the patient is monitored for signs and symptoms of anemia, and hemoglobin levels are checked.

Treatment options are explained and misconceptions corrected. Prescribed pharmacological treatment and analgesics are administered, and the patient is instructed about desired effects and adverse reactions. The patient is prepared physically and emotionally for surgery (laparoscopy with laser vaporization, laparotomy with excision of ovarian masses, or total hysterectomy with bilateral salpingo-oophorectomy.

The patient and her partner are encouraged to verbalize feelings and concerns about the disorder and its effect on their relationship. The need for open communication before and during intercourse to minimize discomfort and frustration is stressed. Assistance is provided to help the patient to develop effective coping strategies, and she and her partner are referred for additional counseling or to a support group, as necessary.

Adolescent girls with a narrow vagina or small vaginal meatus are advised to use sanitary napkins rather than tampons to help prevent retrograde flow. Because infertility is a possible complication, a patient who wants children is advised not to postpone childbearing. An annual pelvic examination and Papanicolaou test is recommended. SEE: *Nursing Diagnoses Appendix.*

***peritoneal e.*** Endometrial tissue found throughout the pelvis.

***transplantation e.*** Endometriosis occurring within an abdominal incision scar following pelvic surgery.

**endometritis** (ĕn″dō-mē-trī′tĭs) [″ + ″ + *itis,* inflammation] Inflammation of the endometrium.

ETIOLOGY: Endometritis is caused by bacterial invasion. It may be acute, subacute, or chronic, the acute cases most commonly resulting from infection by *Staphylococcus, Escherichia coli,* or *Gonococcus;* trauma; or septic abortion. The subacute and chronic types are the result of repeated acute attacks. Occasionally, the chronic type may be due to infection with the tubercle bacillus. Many other conditions are labeled as endometritis but are either vascular or endocrine. Some of these conditions are senile, hyperplastic, and hypertrophic.

SYMPTOMS: In acute cases, the symptoms are usually low back and low abdominal pain, dysmenorrhea, menorrhagia, sterility, and constipation. In chronic endometritis, there is a scant serosanguineous vaginal discharge. A positive diagnosis cannot be made without a curettage and a histological study of the recovered material. SEE: *cervix uteri; endometrium; uterus.*

***cervical e.*** Inflammation of the inner portion of the cervix uteri.

***decidual e.*** Inflammation of the mucous membrane of a gravid uterus.

***e. dissecans*** Endometritis accompanied by development of ulcers and shedding of the mucous membrane.

***puerperal e.*** Acute endometritis following childbirth.

**endometrium** (ĕn-dō-mē′trē-ŭm) [Gr. *endon,* within, + *metra,* uterus] The mucous membrane that lines the uterus. Histologically, it consists of a surface epithelium made up of a single layer of columnar cells, a few of which bear cilia. Invaginations of the epithelium form simple branched tubular glands that extend to the myometrium. The glands are separated by connective tissue resembling mesenchyme, which forms the stroma. There is no submucosa, the mucosa lying closely attached to the myometrium.

The endometrium is supplied by two types of arteries: straight, supplying the deeper third or basal layer of the endometrium, and spiral, supplying the spongy and compact layers. They penetrate between the glands and form a subepithelial capillary plexus. These arteries show marked changes in response to hormonal stimulation during the menstrual cycle.

Beginning with menarche and ending at menopause, the uterine endometrium passes through cyclical changes that constitute the menstrual cycle. These changes are related to the development and maturation of the graafian follicle in the ovary, the discharge of the ovum, and the subsequent development of the corpus luteum in the ovary.

Following fertilization of the ovum, the endometrium becomes the source of nourishment for the embryo when implantation occurs. The endometrium fuses with the developing chorion of the embryo, and at birth the uterine lining, or decidua, splits off and is shed. During pregnancy, the decidua basalis, the endometrium lying between the chorionic vesicle and myometrium, develops into the maternal portion of the placenta.

The endometrium is shed if the ovum is not fertilized or if the fertilized ovum is not implanted. When this is completed, the cycle begins again. SEE: *fertilization* for illus.

***proliferative e.*** Endometrial hypertrophy due to estrogen stimulation during the preovulatory phase of the menstrual cycle. This condition is detected through endometrial biopsy.

***secretory e.*** Histological changes in the endometrium due to the effects of postovulatory progesterone secretion by the corpus luteum. SEE: *defect, luteal phase; menstrual cycle.*

**endomorph** (ĕn″dō-morf′) [″ + *morphe,* form] A person with a body build marked by predominance of tissues derived from the endoderm. SEE: *ectomorph; mesomorph; somatotype.*

**endomyocarditis** (ĕn″dō-mī-ō-kăr-dī′tĭs) [″ + *mys,* muscle, + *kardia,* heart, + *itis,* inflammation] Inflammation of the endocardium and myocardium.

**endomysium** (ĕn″dō-mĭs′ē-ŭm) [″ + *mys,* muscle] A thin sheath of connective tissue, consisting principally of reticular fibers, that invests each striated muscle fiber and binds the fibers together within a fasciculus.

**endoneuritis** [″ + *neuron,* nerve, + *itis,* inflammation] Inflammation of the endoneurium.

**endoneurium** (ĕn″dō-nū′rē-ŭm) A delicate connective tissue sheath that surrounds nerve fibers with a fasciculus. SYN: *Henle's sheath.*

**endonuclease** (ĕn″dō-nū′klē-ās) An enzyme that cleaves the ends of polynucleotides.

***restriction e.*** One of many bacterial enzymes that inactivates foreign DNA but does not interfere with the cell's DNA. This type of enzyme is used to cleave strands of DNA at specific sites.

**endoparasite** (ĕn″dō-păr′ă-sīt) [″ + *para,* beside, + *sitos,* food] Any parasite living within its host.

**endopelvic** (ĕn″dō-pĕl′vĭk) [″ + L. *pelvis,* basin] Within the pelvis.

**endopelvic fasciae** The downward continuation of the parietal peritoneum of the abdomen to form the pelvic fasciae, which contribute to the support of the pelvic viscera.

**endopeptidase** (ĕn″dō-pĕp′tĭ-dās) A proteolytic enzyme that cleaves peptides in their centers rather than from their ends.

**endopericarditis** (ĕn″dō-pĕr″ĭ-kăr-dī′tĭs) [″ + *peri,* around, + *kardia,* heart, + *itis,* inflammation] Endocarditis complicated by pericarditis.

**endoperimyocarditis** (ĕn″dō-pĕr″ĭ-mī″ō-kăr-dī′tĭs) [″ + ″ + *mys,* muscle, + *kardia,* heart, + *itis,* inflammation] Inflammation of the pericardium, myocardium, and endocardium.

**endoperitonitis** (ĕn″dō-pĕr″ĭ-tō-nī′tĭs) [″ + *peritonaion,* peritoneum, + *itis,* inflammation] Inflammation of the peritoneum.

**endophasia** (ĕn″dō-fā′zē-ă) [″ + *phasis,* utterance] Formation of words by the lips without producing sound.

**endophasy** The silent process of thought and production of unuttered words. This function, called inner speech, is essential to thinking that is done with words. SEE: *exophasy*.

**endophlebitis** (ĕn″dō-flĕ-bī′tĭs) [″ + *phleps,* vein, + *itis,* inflammation] Inflammation of the inner layer or membrane of a vein. SYN: *endangiitis*.

***e. obliterans*** Endophlebitis causing obliteration of a vein.

***e. portalis*** Inflammation of the portal vein.

**endophthalmitis** (ĕn″dŏf-thăl-mī′tĭs) [″ + *ophthalmos,* eye, + *itis,* inflammation] Inflammation of the inside of the eye that may or may not be limited to a particular chamber (i.e., anterior or posterior).

**endoplasm** [″ + LL. *plasma,* form, mold] The central, more fluid portion of the cytoplasm of a cell. Opposed to ectoplasm.

**endoplasmic reticulum** A complex network of membranous tubules between the nuclear and cell membranes of the cell and cytoplasm, and sometimes to the cell exterior. They have been visualized with the electron microscope. One form with ribosome particles attached is called *granular* or *rough-surfaced endoplasmic reticulum*; another form that is free of ribosomes is called *agranular* or *smooth-surfaced endoplasmic reticulum*. Rough-surfaced endoplasmic reticulum transports proteins produced on the ribosomes; smooth endoplasmic reticulum synthesizes lipids. SYN: *ergastoplasm*. SEE: *cell* for illus.

**end organ** The expanded end of a nerve fiber in a peripheral structure.

***neuromuscular e.o.*** A spindle-shaped bundle of specialized fibers in which sensory nerve fibers terminate in muscles.

***neurotendinous e.o.*** A specialized tendon fasciculus in which sensory nerve fibers terminate in the tendon. SYN: *tendon spindle*.

***sensory e.o.*** An encapsulated termination of a nerve fiber that serves as a receptor. SEE: *receptor, sensory*.

**endorphin** (ĕn-dor′fĭn, ĕn′dor-fĭn) A polypeptide produced in the brain that acts as an opiate and produces analgesia by binding to opiate receptor sites involved in pain perception. The threshold for pain is therefore increased by this action. The most active of these compounds is beta-endorphin. SYN: *endogenous opiate-like substance*. SEE: *enkephalin; opiate receptor; substance P*.

**endorrhachis** (ĕn″dō-rā′kĭs) [Gr. *endon,* within, + *rhachis,* spine] The membrane lining the spinal canal. SYN: *dura mater*.

**endosalpingitis** (ĕn″dō-săl″pĭn-jī′tĭs) [″ + *salpinx,* tube, + *itis,* inflammation] Inflammation of the lining of the fallopian tubes.

**endosalpingoma** (ĕn″dō-săl″pĭn-gō′mă) An adenomyoma of the uterine tube.

**endosalpinx** (ĕn″dō-săl′pĭnks) [″ + *salpinx,* tube] The mucous membrane lining the uterine tube.

**endoscope** (ĕn′dō-skōp) [″ + *skopein,* to examine] A device consisting of a tube and optical system for observing the inside of a hollow organ or cavity. This observation may be done through a natural body opening or a small incision.

**endoscopic laser cholecystectomy** SEE: *laparoscopic laser cholecystectomy*.

**endoscopic retrograde cholangiopancreatography** ABBR: ERCP. Radiography following injection of a radiopaque material into the papilla of Vater. This is done through a fiberoptic endoscope guided by use of fluoroscopy. The procedure is helpful in determining the cause of jaundice. SEE: *jaundice; percutaneous transhepatic cholangiography*.

**endoscopy** (ĕn-dŏs′kō-pē) Inspection of body organs or cavities by use of an endoscope.

**endoskeleton** [″ + *skeleton,* skeleton] The internal bony framework of the body. Opposite of exoskeleton.

**endosome** (ĕn′dō-sōm) [″ + L. *soma,* body] The vacuole formed when material is absorbed in the cell by endocytosis. The vacuole fuses with lysosomes. SYN: *receptosome*.

**endospore** [″ + *sporos,* a seed] A thick-walled spore produced by a bacterium to enable it to survive unfavorable environmental conditions.

**endosteitis** (ĕn″dŏs-tē-ī′tĭs) [″ + *osteon,* bone, + *itis,* inflammation] Inflammation of the endosteum or the medullary cavity of a bone. SYN: *endostitis*.

**endosteoma** (ĕn-dŏs″tē-ō′mă) [″ + ″ + *oma,* tumor] A tumor in the medullary cavity of a bone.

**endosteum** (ĕn-dŏs′tē-ŭm) [″ + *osteon,* bone] The membrane lining the medullary cavity of a bone.

**endostitis** (ĕn″dŏs-tī′tĭs) [″ + ″ + *itis,* inflammation] Endosteitis.

**endostoma** (ĕn-dŏs-tō′mă) [″ + ″ + *oma,* tumor] An osseous tumor within a bone.

**endostosis** (ĕn″dŏs-tō′sĭs) [″ + ″ + *osis,* condition] The development of an endostoma.

**endotendineum** (ĕn″dō-tĕn-dĭn′ē-ŭm) [″ + L. *tendo,* tendon] The connective tissue in tendons between the bundles of fibers.

**endothelial** (ĕn″dŏ-thē′lē-ăl) [Gr. *endon,* within, + *thele,* nipple] Pert. to or consisting of endothelium.

**endothelin** One of several peptides derived from the vascular endothelium. These peptides have very potent and sustained vasoconstrictor and vasopressor actions as well as neuroendocrine and mitogenic effects. Under normal conditions, vascular tone is maintained by a variety of substances, but in pathological conditions, the endothelium can be activated to produce extreme vasoconstriction. The most potent of these vasoconstrictors is endothelin-1. The importance of endothelins in a variety of diseases is being investigated.

**endotheliocyte** (ĕn″dŏ-thē′lē-ō-sīt″) [″ + ″ + *kytos,* cell] An endothelial cell.

**endotheliocytosis** (ĕn″dŏ-thē″lē-ō-sī-tō′sĭs) [″ + ″ + ″ + *osis,* condition] An abnormal increase in endothelial cells.

**endotheliolysin** (ĕn″dŏ-thē-lē-ŏl′ĭ-sĭn) [″ + *thele,* nipple, + *lysis,* dissolution] An antibody found in snake venom that dissolves endothelial cells.

**endotheliolytic** (ĕn″dŏ-thē-lē-ō-lĭt′ĭk) Capable of destroying endothelial tissue.

**endothelioma** (ĕn″dŏ-thē-lē-ō′mă) [″ + *thele,* nipple, + *oma,* tumor] A malignant growth of lining cells of the blood vessels.

**endotheliomyoma** (ĕn″dŏ-thē″lē-ō-mī-ō′mă) [″ + ″ + *mys,* muscle, + *oma,* tumor] A muscular tumor with elements of endothelium.

**endotheliomyxoma** (ĕn″dŏ-thē″lē-ō-mĭks-ō′mă) [″ + ″ + *myxa,* mucus, + *oma,* tumor] A myxoma with elements of endothelium.

**endotheliosis** (ĕn″dō-thē″lē-ō′sĭs) Increased growth of endothelium.

**endotheliotoxin** (ĕn″dō-thē-lē-ŏ-tŏks′ĭn) [″ + ″ + *toxikon,* poison] A specific toxin that acts on endothelial capillary cells and causes hemorrhages.

**endothelium** (ĕn″dŏ-thē′lē-ŭm) [″ + *thele,* nipple] A form of squamous epithelium consisting of flat cells that line the blood and lymphatic vessels, the heart, and various other body cavities. It is derived from mesoderm. Endothelial cells are metabolically active and produce a number of compounds that affect the vascular lumen and platelets. Included are endothelium-derived relaxing factor (EDRF), prostacyclin, endothelium-derived contracting factors 1 and 2 (EDCF1, EDCF2), endothelium-derived hyperpolarizing factor (EDHF), and thrombomodulin. SEE: *intima.*

**endothelium-derived hyperpolarizing factor** ABBR: EDHF. A vasodilating substance released by the vascular endothelium. SEE: *endothelium.*

**endothelium-derived relaxing factor** ABBR: EDRF. An active vasodilator released by the vascular endothelium. It facilitates relaxation of vascular smooth muscle and inhibition of adhesion and aggregation of platelets. When the normal function of the endothelium is disrupted by mechanical trauma, hypertension, hypercholesterolemia, or atherosclerosis, less EDRF is released and the inhibition of platelet aggregation is decreased. In addition, the damaged vessels constrict. This favors the formation of thrombi. SEE: *endothelium.*

**endothermal, endothermic** [Gr. *endon,* within, + *therme,* heat] **1.** Storing up potential energy or heat. **2.** Absorbing heat. **3.** Pert. to absorption of heat during chemical reactions.

**endothermy** (ĕn′dō-thĕr″mē) An elevation of the temperature of deep body tissue in response to high-frequency current.

**endothrix** (ĕn′dō-thrĭks) [″ + *thrix,* hair] Any fungus growing inside the hair shaft.

**endotoscope** (ĕn-dō′tō-skōp) [″ + *ous,* ear, + *skopein,* to examine] An ear speculum. SYN: *otoscope.*

**endotoxemia** (ĕn″dō-tŏks-ē′mē-ă) Toxemia due to the presence of endotoxins in the blood.

**endotoxicosis** (ĕn″dŏ-tŏk″sĭ-kō′sĭs) [Gr. *endon,* within, + *toxikon,* poison, + *osis,* condition] Poisoning due to an endotoxin.

**endotoxin** A lipopolysaccharide that is part of the cell wall of gram-negative bacteria. It binds with CD4 receptors on leukocytes and endothelial cells. The linkage stimulates the release of interleukin-1 and tumor necrosis factors, initiating a systemic cascade of reactions that govern inflammation, cell-mediated immune responses, vascular tone, hematopoiesis, and wound healing. When large amounts of lipopolysaccharides are present, the clinical state of sepsis syndrome (septic shock) occurs. SEE: *inflammation; sepsis.*

**endotoxin shock** Shock due to release of endotoxins from bacteria. Endotoxins are present in the lipopolysaccharide (LPS) component of the cell wall of gram-negative bacteria. The LPS stimulates host responses that are beneficial but at the same time initiate toxic reactions that may lead to disseminated intravascular coagulation, widespread capillary damage, hypotension, acute respiratory distress syndrome, and fever. Unless these toxic reactions are treated vigorously, death may be the outcome.

TREATMENT: Supportive therapy is given for the shock; the source of gram-negative bacteria must be eradicated or removed. To be effective, these therapeutic measures must be instituted immediately, literally within minutes of when the patient is seen. Therapy with corticosteroids or nonsteroidal anti-inflammatory agents may be of help. The use of tissue necrosis antibodies is experimental. SEE: *shock; toxic shock syndrome.*

**endotracheal tube, cuffed** A tube, surrounded by an inflatable cuff, used inside the trachea to provide an airway through the trachea while preventing aspiration of foreign material into the bronchus. The tube is inflated after being placed in the trachea.

**endotracheitis** (ĕn″dō-trā-kē-ī′tĭs) [″ + *tracheia,* trachea, + *itis,* inflammation] Inflammation of the tracheal mucosa.

**endotrachelitis** (ĕn″dō-trā-kĕl-ī′tĭs) [″ + *trachelos,* neck, + *itis,* inflammation] Endocervicitis.

**endovasculitis** (ĕn″dō-văs″kū-lī′tĭs) [″ + L. *vasculum,* vessel, + Gr. *itis,* inflammation] Endangiitis.

**endplate** The terminal mass of a nerve fiber ending on a muscle cell.

***motor e.*** An ending in a striated muscle fiber. SYN: *myoneural junction.*

**end product** The final material or substance left at the completion of a series of reactions, either chemical or physical.

**end-stage** The final phase of a disease process.

**end-stage renal disease** The late stages of chronic renal failure. SEE: *hemodialysis; peritoneal dialysis; renal failure, acute; renal transplantation.*

**endurance** The ability to withstand extraordinary mental or physical stress for a prolonged period.

**endurance training** Physical training for athletic events requiring prolonged effort, such as running a marathon, swimming a long distance, or climbing mountains.

**endyma** (ĕn′dĭm-ă) [Gr., a garment] The membrane lining the cerebral ventricles and the central canal of the spinal cord. SYN: *ependyma.*

**enema** (ĕn′ĕ-mă) [Gr.] **1.** The introduction of a solution into the rectum and colon to stimulate bowel activity and cause emptying of the lower intestine, for feeding or therapeutic purposes, to give anesthesia, or to aid in radiographic studies. **2.** A solution introduced into the rectum.

***air contrast e.*** An enema in which two contrast agents, thick barium sulfate and air, are introduced simultaneously under fluoroscopic control followed by multiple radiographs of the colon. This technique produces better visualization of mucosal lining lesions, such as polyps or diverticula.

***barium e.*** The administration of a barium sulfate contrast medium under fluoroscopic control for visualization of the colon.

***cleansing e.*** An enema to empty the lower intestine or the colon. Fifteen to 60 ml should be used for an infant, 240 to 360 ml for a child, and 500 to 1000 ml (about 0.5 to 1 L) for an adult.

NURSING IMPLICATIONS: The procedure is explained to the patient and privacy ensured. All necessary equipment is assembled; the patient is placed in a left side-lying position with the right leg flexed and forward and draped to permit exposure of the rectum while protecting the patient's modesty.

The solution is checked for correct temperature, the tubing cleared of air, and the tip of the rectal tube lubricated and inserted 3 to 4 in. into the rectum. The container is positioned 12 to 18 in. above the rectum, and the solution is allowed to flow into the rectum slowly. The patient is coached to breathe slowly and deeply during the procedure to help relax abdominal muscles, and the flow is stopped for 30 sec if the patient complains of fullness or discomfort to prevent premature evacuation.

When the procedure is completed or the patient's urge to defecate is undeniable, the rectal tube is removed, and the patient is encouraged to lie still for a few moments to retain the enema for better results. The patient then is seated upright on a bedpan or assisted to the commode or toilet for defecation. After evacuation of the bowel contents, the patient's response is assessed, and the patient is assisted into a comfortable position. The amount and type of fluid administered and the amount, type, and consistency of the returned fluid and stool are documented.

***emollient e.*** An enema given to soothe and protect the intestinal mucosa by making a coating over the membranes. This allays local pain and irritation and acts as a vehicle for the rectal administration of drugs. It should be given at a temperature of about 105°F (40.6°C). The record must show whether the patient felt relieved and if and to what extent the solution was retained.

***high e.*** An enema designed to reach most of the colon. A rubber tube is inserted into the rectum to carry water as far as possible.

***lubricating e.*** An enema administered after an operation for hemorrhoids to soften the feces and lubricate the anal canal. When there is an impaction of feces, a lubricating enema may be given, followed in 2 hr by a cleansing enema. Warmed olive or mineral oil, 4 to 6 oz (120 to 180 ml), may be given. The patient should remain prone with hips elevated for 30 min following the enema to help retain the oil, thus aiding it in passing higher into the colon.

***medicinal e.*** An enema to which some drug or medication has been added on order of the attending physician. It may be given to medicate diseases of the rectum, sigmoid flexure, or colon or to aid in absorption of a medicine for its systemic effects, esp. if medication cannot be administered by mouth. It is necessary that this enema be retained and absorbed.

***nutrient e.*** An enema containing predigested foods for the purpose of giving sustenance to a patient unable to be fed otherwise. SYN: *nutritive e.*

***nutritive e.*** Nutrient e.

***one-two-three e.*** An enema consisting of 1 oz (30 ml) of magnesium sulfate, 2 oz (60 ml) of glycerine, and 3 oz (90 ml) of hot water. This mixture must be given with a small tube because of the small amount. The results following the injection are better if the solution is given very carefully, with assistance to help the patient retain it.

***physiological salt solution e.*** An enema consisting of a normal salt solution—5 g or 1 tsp of salt to 1 pint (473 ml) of water. The distention made by this enema excites peristalsis and evacuation. There is no harm in retaining this enema. Physicians often order its retention in treating dehydration.

***retention e.*** An enema that may be used to provide nourishment, medication, or anesthetic. It must be formulated from constituents that will not stimulate the nerve endings and reflexively promote peristalsis. It must necessarily consist of a small amount of solution, usually 100 to 240 ml.

NURSING IMPLICATIONS: The procedure is explained to the patient. Necessary equipment is assembled, and the patient is draped for privacy and assisted into a left side-lying position with the right knee flexed. The tubing is cleared of air, and the small tube is inserted 6 in. into the rectum and not removed (unless absolutely necessary) until the procedure is completed. The fluid is allowed to flow very slowly and stopped at intervals to aid retention. If the patient experiences an urge to defecate, the fluid flow is stopped until the urge passes. When the entire volume has been instilled, the tube is quickly withdrawn, the buttocks are compressed together for a few minutes to prevent evacuation, and the patient is encouraged to retain the enema for at least 30 min. The type and amount of fluid instilled, the patient's ability to retain it, and the amount, type, and consistency of the returned fluid and stool are documented.

***saline e.*** An enema consisting of normal saline solution or magnesium sulfate in warm water.

***soapsuds e.*** An enema consisting of prepared soapsuds or, if liquid soap is used, 30 to 1000 ml of water. Strong soapsuds should not be used because of the danger of injuring intestinal mucosa. Mild white soaps, such as castile, are best.

**energetics** (ĕn″ĕr-jĕt′ĭks) The study of energy, esp. in relation to human use of energy in the form of food and the expenditure of energy in work or athletic exercise.

**energy** (ĕn′ĕr-jē) [Gr. *energeia*] The capacity of a system for doing work or its equivalent in the strict physical sense. Energy is manifested in various forms: motion (kinetic energy), position (potential energy), light, heat, ionizing radiation, and sound.

Changes in energy may be physical, chemical, or both. Movement of a part of the body shortens and thickens the muscles involved and changes the position and size of cells temporarily, but intake of oxygen in the blood combined with glucose and fat creates a chemical change and produces heat (energy) and waste products within the cells; fatigue is produced in turn. SEE: *calorie; energy expenditure, basal.*

***conservation of e.*** The principle according to which energy cannot be created or destroyed, but is transformed into other forms.

***kinetic e.*** The energy of motion.

***latent e.*** Energy that exists but is not being used.

***potential e.*** Stored energy.

***radiant e.*** A form of energy transmitted through space without the support of a sensible medium. Radio waves, infrared waves, visible rays, ultraviolet waves, x-rays, gamma rays, and cosmic rays are energy in this form. SEE: *electromagnetic spectrum* for table.

**energy expenditure, basal** ABBR: BEE. The energy used by an individual doing no work. The BEE (expressed as Calories) may be calculated by using the Harris-Benedict equations. These account for sex, age, height, and weight. If the individual is sedentary, moderately active, or engaged in strenuous activity, 30%, 50%, or 100%, respectively, are added to the BEE. SEE: *diet; dietetics; food.*

The Harris-Benedict equation involves W (weight in kg), H (height in cm), and A (age in years). The formulae are:

For women: BEE $6.55 + (9.6 \times W) + (1.8 \times H) - (4.7 \times A)$

For men: BEE $6.6 + (13.7 \times W) + (5 \times H) - (6.8 \times A)$

Hospitalized patients who are non-stressed require 20% more calories than for basal needs.

Energy expended is increased by about 13% over basal needs for each degree centigrade of fever; burn and trauma patients require 40% to 100% more calories than for basal requirements.

**enervation** [L. *enervatio*] **1.** Deficiency in nervous strength; weakness. **2.** Resection or removal of a nerve.

**ENG** *electronystagmography.*

**engagement 1.** In obstetrics, the entrance of the fetal head or the part being presented into the superior pelvic strait. SYN: *lightening.* SEE: *labor.* **2.** In the behavioral sciences, a term often used to denote active involvement in everyday activities that have personal meaning.

**Engelmann's disk** [Theodor W. Engelmann, Ger. physiologist, 1843–1909] H band.

**energy field disturbance** A disruption of the flow of energy surrounding a person's being that results in a disharmony of the body, mind, and/or spirit. SEE: *Nursing Diagnoses Appendix.*

**engine** A device for converting energy into mechanical motion.

***dental e.*** A machine that rotates dental instruments.

***high-speed e.*** A machine that rotates a dental instrument in excess of 12,000 rpm.

***ultraspeed e.*** A machine that rotates a dental instrument at speeds from 100,000 to 300,000 rpm.

**engineering** In medical science, the practical application of principles of pure sciences such as physics or chemistry to medical problems. Branches of this science include human, dental, genetic, and biomechanical factors.

**engorged** (ĕn-gorjd′) [O. Fr. *engorgier,* to obstruct, to devour] Distended, as with blood or fluids.

**engorgement** Vascular congestion; distention.

**engram** (ĕn′grăm) [Gr. *engramm*] A durable protoplasmic mark or trace left by a stimulus in neural tissue.

**engrossment** An attitude of total focus on something or someone. In obstetrics, the term denotes attachment behavior exhibited by new fathers during initial contacts with their newborns.

**enhanced organized infant behavior, potential for** A pattern of modulation of the physiological and behavioral systems of functioning of an infant (i.e., autonomic, motor, state, organizational, self-regulatory, and attentional-interactional systems) that is satisfactory but that can be improved resulting in higher levels of integration in response to environmental stimuli. SEE: *Nursing Diagnoses Appendix.*

**enhancement** (ĕn-hăns′mĕnt) An increase in the effect of ionizing radiation on tissues, produced by the use of oxygen or other chemicals.

**enissophobia** (ĕn-ĭs″ō-fō′bē-ă) [Gr. *enissein,* to reproach, + *phobos,* fear] Fear of criticism, esp. for having committed a sin.

**enkephalin** (ĕn-kĕf′ă-lĭn) A pentapeptide produced in the brain. It acts as an opiate and produces analgesia by binding to opiate receptor sites involved in pain perception. The threshold for pain is therefore increased by this action. Enkephalins may have a role in explaining the withdrawal signs of narcotic addiction. SYN: *endogenous opiate-like substance.* SEE: *endorphin; opiate receptor.*

**enlargement** (ĕn-lărj′mĕnt) An increase in size of anything, esp. of an organ or tissue.

**enol** (ē′nŏl) A form that a ketone may take by tautomerism. A substance changes from an enol to a ketone by the oscillation of a hydrogen atom from the enol form to the ketone form.

**enolase** (ē′nō-lās) An enzyme present in muscle tissue that converts phosphoglyceric acid to phosphopyruvic acid.

**enology** (ē-nŏl′ō-jē) [Gr. *oinos,* wine, + *logos,* word, reason] The science of producing and evaluating wine. Also spelled *oenology*.

**enophthalmos** (ĕn″ŏf-thăl′mŭs) [Gr. *en,* in, + *ophthalmos,* eye] Recession of the eyeball into the orbit. Opposite of exophthalmos.

**enosimania** (ĕn″ŏs-ĭ-mā′nē-ă) [Gr. *enosis,* a quaking, + *mania,* madness] A mental state marked by excessive and irrational terror.

**enostosis** (ĕn″ŏs-tō′sĭs) [Gr. *en,* in, + *osteon,* bone, + *osis,* condition] An osseous tumor within the cavity of a bone.

**enriched** Having something extra added. For example, vitamins or minerals may be added to a food in order to *enrich* it.

**ensiform** (ĕn′sĭ-form) [L. *ensis,* sword, + *forma,* form] Xiphoid.

**ensisternum** (ĕn″sĭs-tĕr′nŭm) [″ + Gr. *sternon,* sternum] The lowest portion of the sternum. SYN: *xiphoid process.*

**enstrophe** (ĕn′strō-fē) [Gr. *en,* in, + *strephein,* to turn] Inversion; a turning inward, esp. of the eyelids.

**ENT** *ear, nose, and throat.*

**ent-** SEE: *ento-*.

**entad** (ĕn′tăd) [″ + L. *ad,* toward] Toward the inside; inwardly.

**ental** (ĕn′tăl) [Gr. *entos,* within] Pert. to the interior; inside; central.

**entamebiasis** (ĕn″tă-mē-bī′ă-sĭs) [″ + *amoibe,* change] Infestation with *Entamoeba.*

**Entamoeba** (ĕn″tă-mē′bă) A genus of parasitic amebae, several of which are found in the human digestive tract.

***E. buccalis*** E. gingivalis.

***E. coli*** A species of ameba normally found in the human intestinal tract. This species is nonpathogenic to humans.

***E. gingivalis*** A nonpathogenic species of ameba that inhabits the mouth.

***E. histolytica*** A pathogenic species of ameba, the cause of amebic dysentery and tropical liver abscess. SEE: illus.; *amebiasis.*

**enter-** SEE: *entero-*.

**enteral** (ĕn′tĕr-ăl) [Gr. *enteron,* intestine] Within or by way of the intestine.

**enteralgia** (ĕn″tĕr-ăl′jē-ă) [″ + *algos,* pain] Neuralgia or pain in the intestines; intestinal cramps or colic. SYN: *enterodynia.*

**enteral tube feeding** Feeding of the appropriate formula to a patient through a tube passed into the stomach or duodenum from the nasal passage (nasogastric or nasoduodenal tube), or by a gastrostomy or jejunostomy tube.

TYPES OF FORMULAS: *Intact nutrient:* These formulas are called “standard.” Because the nutrients are “whole,” they are appropriate for use whenever normal digestion takes place. They usally provide 1 kcal/ml and can be used orally. *Hydrolyzed nutrient:* In these formulas, the nutrients are “predigested” and are suitable for use whenever malabsorption is present or when the jejunum is the feeding site. These formulas are not appropriate

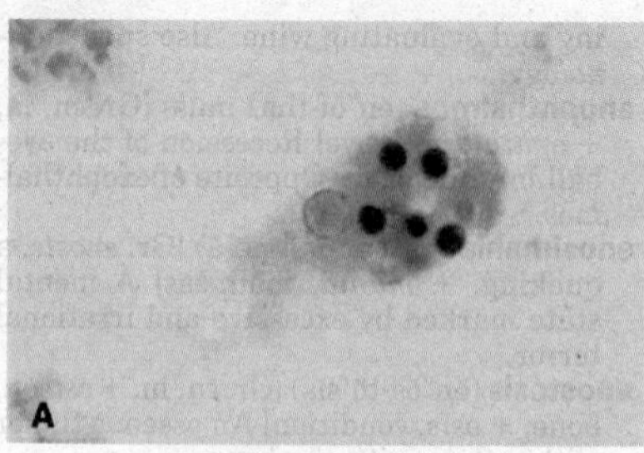


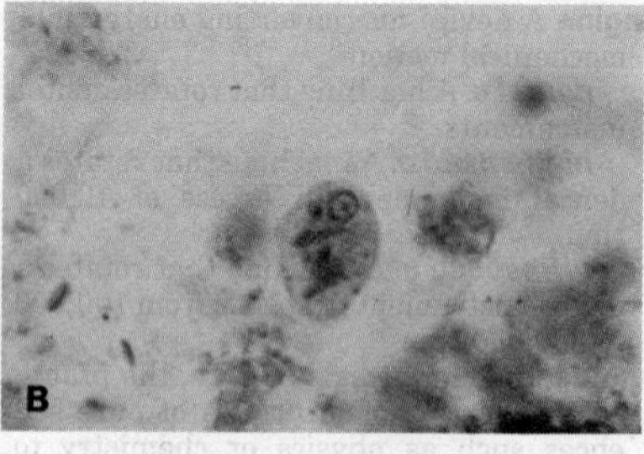


**ENTAMOEBA HISTOLYTICA (A)** TROPHOZOITE WITH FIVE INGESTED RED BLOOD CELLS (ORIG. MAG. ×1000), **(B)** CYST IN FECAL DEBRIS (ORIG. MAG. ×1000)

for oral use because of their taste. They are more expensive than intact nutrient formulas. *Elemental (defined):* Because nutrients in these formulas are in the simplest, most basic form, they are rapidly absorbed from the gut. These formulas are not appropriate for oral use. This type of formula is the most expensive. Formulas designed for specific diseases are available. *Modular:* Commercially produced nutritional products may be used as supplements to standard formulas. For example, the addition of a protein module would convert a standard formula to a high-protein formula.

METHODS OF DELIVERY: *Bolus administration:* Formula is delivered in four to six daily feedings by a large syringe attached to the feeding tube in the stomach. This type of delivery is the least well tolerated. *Intermittent infusion:* Formula is delivered four to six times daily over 30 to 60 min per feeding using a pump or gravity. This type of delivery is better tolerated. *Continuous drip:* An infusion pump delivers slow drips 16 to 24 hr/day. This is the best tolerated type of delivery.

**enterectomy** (ĕn″tĕr-ĕk′tō-mē) [″ + *ektome,* excision] Excision of a portion of the intestines.

**enteric** (ĕn-tĕr′ĭk) [Gr. *enteron,* intestine] Pert. to the small intestine.

**enteric bacilli** A broad term for bacilli present in the intestinal tract. Included are gram-negative non–spore-forming facultatively anaerobic bacilli such as *Escherichia, Shigella, Salmonella, Klebsiella,* and *Yersinia.* They may be present in the intestines of vertebrates as normal flora or pathogens.

**enteric-coated** Concerning a drug formulation in which tablets or capsules are coated with a special compound that does not dissolve until the tablet or capsule is exposed to the fluids in the small intestine.

**enteric fever** Typhoid fever.

**enteritis** (ĕn″tĕr-ī′tĭs) [″ + *itis,* inflammation] Inflammation of the intestines, particularly of the mucosa and submucosa of the small intestine. SEE: *Nursing Diagnoses Appendix.*

***regional e.*** SEE: *ileitis, regional.*

**entero-, enter-** [Gr. *enteron,* intestine] Combining form meaning *intestines.*

**enteroanastomosis** (ĕn″tĕr-ō-ăn-ăs″tō-mō′sĭs) [″ + *anastomosis,* opening] An intestinal anastomosis.

**enteroantigen** (ĕn″tĕr-ō-ăn′tĭ-jĕn) [″ + *anti,* against, + *gennan,* to produce] An antigen derived from the intestines.

**Enterobacter** A group of enteric gram-negative rods of the family Enterobacteriaceae that occur in soil, dairy products, water, sewage, and the intestinal tracts of humans and animals. Often they are secondary pathogens or produce opportunistic infections. In humans, many of these infections are hospital acquired (nosocomial).

***E. aerogenes*** A species of *Enterobacter* that occurs normally in the intestine of humans and other animals and is found in decayed matter, on grains, and in plants. The organism is important in causing urinary tract infections and intestinal disease when antibiotic therapy causes elimination of other organisms. It was formerly called *Aerobacter aerogenes.*

***E. agglomerans*** A species of *Enterobacter* formerly called *Erwinia.* It has been associated with serious systemic infections, particularly septicemia from contaminated intravenous fluids.

***E. cloacae*** A species of *Enterobacter* that, along with *E. agglomerans*, accounts for most nosocomial infections, esp. those due to intravenous line contamination.

**Enterobacteriaceae** (ĕn″tĕr-ō-băk-tē″rē-ā′sē-ē) A genus of gram-negative, non–spore-forming aerobes. Some are intestinal pathogens, others are usually normal colonizers of the human intestinal tract. Included in the family are *Shigella, Salmonella, Escherichia, Klebsiella, Proteus, Enterobacter,* and *Yersinia.*

**enterobiasis** (ĕn″tĕr-ō-bī′ă-sĭs) [Gr. *enteron,* intestine, + *bios,* life] Infestation with pinworms (*Enterobius vermicularis*). SYN: *oxyuriasis.*

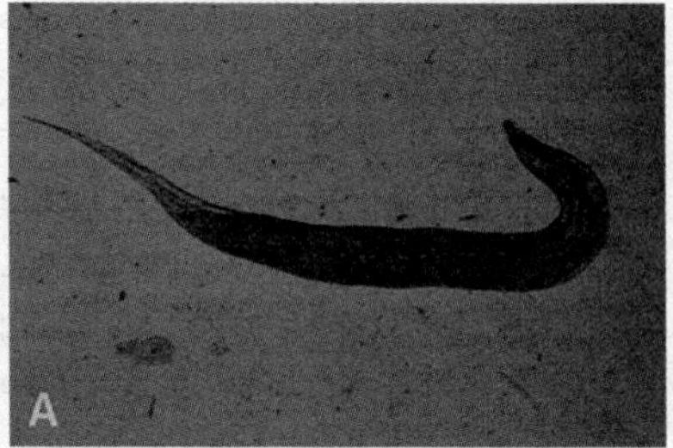


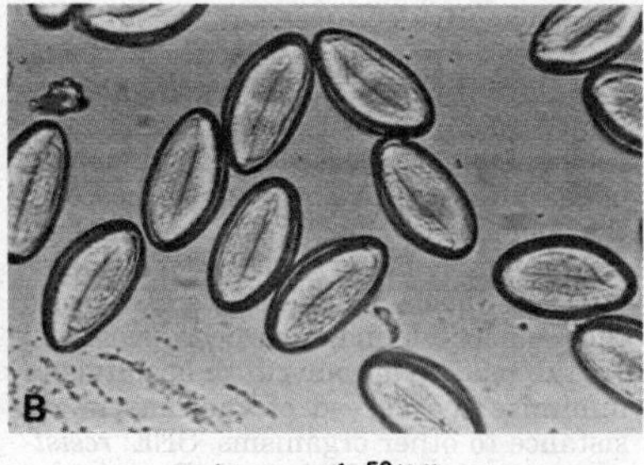


ENTEROBIUS VERMICULARIS (A) FEMALE (ORIG. MAG. ×10), (B) EGGS (ORIG. MAG. ×400)

**enterobiliary** (ĕn″tĕr-ō-bĭl′ē-ăr-ē) [″ + L. *bilis,* bile] Pert. to the intestines and the bile passages.

**Enterobius** (ĕn″tĕr-ō′bē-ŭs) [″ + *bios,* life] A genus of parasitic nematode worms, formerly *Oxyuris vermicularis.*

***E. vermicularis*** A species of nematode worms, the adult form of which inhabits the large intestine in humans. The genital organs and bladder may become infected in women, causing cystitis due to the bacteria that the female worm carries. Infestations cause irritation of the anal region and allergic reaction of the neighboring skin, accompanied by intense itching, which may result in loss of sleep, excessive irritability, and a secondary infection of the area around the anus as a result of the scratching. Distribution is worldwide. It is estimated that in temperate climates 20% of children have this condition. Female worms average 8 to 13 mm in length and males 2 to 5 mm. SYN: *pinworm.* SEE: illus.

DIAGNOSIS: The presence of adult worms in feces or on the anus confirms the diagnosis. Transparent, pressure-sensitive tape may be applied to the perianal area and then examined microscopically for eggs. This latter test is more likely to be positive in the morning before bathing.

TREATMENT: Pyrantel pamoate, albendazole, or mebendazole is effective. During treatment tight-fitting sleep wear should be used to prevent the eggs from contaminating the bedding. The house, bedding, and night clothes must be thoroughly cleaned daily for several days during treatment. Family recurrences may be prevented if the entire family is treated.

**enterocele** (ĕn′tĕr-ō-sēl) [″ + *keke,* hernia] **1.** A hernia of the intestine through the vagina. **2.** A posterior vaginal hernia.

**enterocentesis** (ĕn″tĕr-ō-sĕn-tē′sĭs) [″ + *kentesis,* puncture] Puncture of the intestine to withdraw gas or fluids.

**enterocholecystostomy** (ĕn″tĕr-ō-kō″lē-sĭs-tŏs′tō-mē) [″ + *chole,* bile, + *kystis,* bladder, + *stoma,* mouth] A surgically created opening between the gallbladder and small intestine. SYN: *cholecystenterostomy.*

**enterocholecystotomy** (ĕn″tĕr-ō-kō″lē-sĭs-tŏt′ō-mē) [″ + ″ + ″ + *tome,* incision] Incision of both the gallbladder and the intestine.

**enteroclysis** (ĕn″tĕr-ŏk′lĭ-sĭs) [″ + *klysis,* a washing out] **1.** Injection of a nutrient or medicinal liquid into the bowel. **2.** Irrigation of the colon with a large amount of fluid intended to fill the colon completely and flush it. SEE: *enema.* **3.** Radiography of the small bowel. A tube is advanced into the duodenum under fluoroscopic guidance and barium is given, followed by insufflation of the bowel with air.

**Enterococcus** (ĕn″tĕr-ō-kŏk′ŭs) A genus of gram-positive bacteria belonging to the family Streptococcaceae, formerly classified as part of the genus *Streptococcus,* but now classified as a separate genus. Of the 12 or more species, *E. faecalis* and *E. faecium* are found in the human gastrointestinal tract.

***vancomycin-resistant enterococci*** ABBR: VRE. A strain of *Enterococcus faecium* resistant to anti-infective agents, including penicillins, aminoglycosides, and vancomycin. These organisms have caused a major increase in nosocomial infections in patients who are critically ill, have received immunosuppressive therapy or multiple anti-infective drugs, have urinary or central venous catheters, have undergone abdominal or cardiothoracic surgery, or have had an extended hospital stay. The organism is transmitted by direct patient-to-patient contact or via contaminated hands or equipment used by health care workers.

Infection with VRE presents a major threat to susceptible patients because no consistently effective antimicrobial drug treatment has been identified, and because the resistant genes could be transferred to other gram-positive organisms, such as *Staphylococcus aureus,* making them more difficult to treat.

Preventing the spread of VRE involves early identification of the organism, isolation of patients in private rooms until three negative cultures have been taken at 1-week intervals, use of clean gowns and gloves by all persons entering the patient's room, careful handwashing after removal of gown and gloves, and storage of essential equipment (e.g., stethoscope, thermometer, tourniquets, commode, sphygmomanometer) in the room. Charts and flow sheets should not be taken into the room. Guidelines have been developed for the use of vancomycin in hospitals to minimize the spread of vancomycin resistance to other organisms. SEE: *resistance, antibiotic; Universal Precautions Appendix.*

**enterocolectomy** (ĕn″tĕr-ō-kō-lĕk′tō-mē) [″ + *kolon,* colon, + *ektome,* excision] Surgical removal of the terminal ileum, cecum, and ascending colon.

**enterocolitis** (ĕn″tĕr-ō-kō-lī′tĭs) [″ + ″ + *itis,* inflammation] Inflammation of the small intestine and colon. This serious condition may be acute enough to require immediate treatment of shock, regulation of electrolyte balance, and use of antibiotics.

***necrotizing e.*** ABBR: NEC. Severe damage to the intestinal mucosa of the preterm infant due to ischemia resulting from asphyxia or prolonged hypoxemia.

**enterocolostomy** (ĕn″tĕr-ō-kō-lŏs′tō-mē) [″ + ″ + *stoma,* mouth] A surgical joining of the small intestine to the colon.

**enterocutaneous** (ĕn″tĕr-ō-kū-tā′nē-ŭs) Pert. to communication between the skin and intestine.

**enterocyst** (ĕn′tĕr-ō-sĭst) [Gr. *enteron,* intestine, + *kystis,* bladder] A benign cyst of the intestinal wall.

**enterocystocele** (ĕn″tĕr-ō-sĭs′tō-sēl) [″ + *kele,* tumor, swelling] A hernia of the bladder wall and intestine.

**enterocystoma** (ĕn″tĕr-ō-sĭs-tō′mă) [″ + ″ + *oma,* tumor] A cystic tumor of the intestinal wall.

**enterocystoplasty** (ĕn″tĕr-ō-sĭs′tō-plăs″tē) [″ + ″ + *plastos,* formed] A plastic surgical procedure involving the use of a portion of intestine to enlarge the bladder.

**Enterocytozoon** A genus of the order Microsporidia. SEE: *microsporidiosis.*

**enterodynia** (ĕn″tĕr-ō-dĭn′ē-ă) [″ + *odyne,* pain] Enteralgia.

**enteroenterostomy** (ĕn″tĕr-ō-ĕn″tĕr-ŏs′tō-mē) [″ + *enteron,* intestine, + *stoma,* mouth] Surgical creation of a communication between two intestinal segments.

**enteroepiplocele** (ĕn″tĕr-ō-ē-pĭp′lō-sēl) [″ + *epiploon,* omentum, + *kele,* tumor, swelling] A hernia of the small intestine and omentum.

**enterogastritis** (ĕn″tĕr-ō-găs-trī′tĭs) [″ + *gaster,* belly, + *itis,* inflammation] Inflammation of the stomach (gastritis) and the intestines (enteritis).

**enterogastrone** (ĕn″tĕr-ō-găs′trōn) A hormone secreted by the intestinal mucosa that controls the release of food from the stomach into the duodenum by depressing gastric motility and secretion. A meal high in fat causes greater secretion of this hormone than a normal feeding does.

**enterogenous** (ĕn″tĕr-ŏj′ĕ-nŭs) [″ + *gennan,* to produce] Originating in the small intestines.

**enterohemorrhagic Escherichia coli** SEE: *Escherichia coli.*

**enterohepatic** (ĕn″tĕr-ō-hĕ-păt′ĭk) [″ + *hepar,* liver] Pert. to the intestines and liver.

**enterohepatitis** (ĕn″tĕr-ō-hĕp-ă-tī′tĭs) [″ + ″ + *itis,* inflammation] Inflammation of the intestine and liver.

**enterohydrocele** (ĕn″tĕr-ō-hī′drō-sēl) [″ + *hydor,* water, + *kele,* tumor, swelling] A hydrocele with a loop of intestine in the sac.

**enteroinvasive Escherichia coli** SEE: *Escherichia coli.*

**enterokinase** (ĕn″tĕr-ō-kī′nās) [″ + *kinesis,* movement] Previous term for enteropeptidase.

**enterology** [″ + *logos,* word, reason] The study of the intestinal tract.

**enterolysis** (ĕn″tĕr-ŏl′ĭ-sĭs) [″ + *lysis,* dissolution] Surgical therapy of intestinal adhesions.

**enteromegalia, enteromegaly** (ĕn″tĕr-ō-mĕ-gā′lē-ă, ĕn″tĕr-ō-mĕg′ă-lē) [″ + *megas,* large] Abnormal enlargement of the intestines. SYN: *megacolon.*

**Enteromonas hominis** (ĕn″tĕr-ŏm′ō-năs hŏm′ĭn-ĭs) A minute, flagellated protozoan parasite that lives in the intestine of humans. It is rare and considered nonpathogenic.

**enteromycosis** (ĕn″tĕr-ō-mī-kō′sĭs) [″ + *mykes,* fungus, + *osis,* diseased condition] A disease of the intestine resulting from bacteria or fungi.

**enteromyiasis** (ĕn″tĕr-ō-mī-ī′ă-sĭs) [″ + *myia,* fly] A disease caused by the presence of maggots (the larvae of flies) in the intestines.

**enteron** (ĕn′tĕr-ŏn) [Gr.] The alimentary canal.

**enteroneuritis** (ĕn″tĕr-ō-nū-rī′tĭs) [″ + *neuron,* nerve, + *itis,* inflammation] Inflammation of the intestinal nerves.

**entero-oxyntin** A hormone believed to be released by the small intestine in response to the presence of chyme. It is thought to cause the parietal (oxyntic) cells of the gastric mucosa to release hydrochloric acid.

**enteroparesis** (ĕn″tĕr-ō-păr′ē-sĭs) [″ + *paresis,* relaxation] Reduced peristalsis of the intestines followed by dilation of the walls.

**enteropathogen** (ĕn″tĕr-ō-păth′ō-jĕn) [″ + *pathos,* disease, suffering, + *gennan,* to produce] Any microorganism that causes intestinal disease.

**enteropathy** (ĕn″tĕr-ŏp′ă-thē) [″ + *pathos,* disease, suffering] Any intestinal disease.

***radiation e.*** Damage to the intestines due to radiation.

**enteropeptidase** (ĕn″tĕr-ō-pĕp′tĭ-dās) An enzyme of the duodenal mucosa that converts pancreatic trypsinogen to active trypsin. Formerly called *enterokinase*.

**enteropexy** (ĕn′tĕr-ō-pĕks″ē) [″ + *pexis*, fixation] Fixation of the intestine to the abdominal wall or to another portion of the intestine.

**enteroplegia** (ĕn″tĕr-ō-plē′jē-ă) [″ + *plege*, stroke] Paralysis of the intestines. SEE: *paralytic ileus*.

**enteroplex** (ĕn′tĕr-ō-plĕks) [″ + *plexis*, a weaving] An instrument for joining cut edges of intestines.

**enteroplexy** Surgical union of divided parts of the intestine. SYN: *enteroanastomosis*.

**enteroptosis** (ĕn″tĕr-ŏp-tō′sĭs) [″ + *ptosis*, a falling or dropping] Prolapse of the intestines or abdominal organs.

**enterorrhaphy** (ĕn″tĕr-or′ă-fē) [″ + *rhaphe*, seam, ridge] Stitching of an intestinal wound, or of the intestines to some other structure.

**enterorrhexis** (ĕn″tĕr-ō-rĕks′ĭs) [″ + *rhexis*, rupture] Rupture of the intestine.

**enteroscope** (ĕn′tĕr-ō-skōp″) [″ + *skopein*, to examine] A device for visually examining the inside of the intestines.

**enterosepsis** (ĕn″tĕr-ō-sĕp′sĭs) [″ + *sepsis*, decay] A condition in which bacteria in the intestines putrefy and produce intestinal sepsis. SEE: *enterotoxemia*.

**enterospasm** (ĕn′tĕr-ō-spăzm) [Gr. *enteron*, intestine, + *spasmos*, spasm] Intermittent painful contractions of the intestines.

**enterostasis** (ĕn″tĕr-ō-stā′sĭs) [″ + *stasis*, a standing] Cessation of or delay in the passage of food through the intestine.

**enterostenosis** (ĕn″tĕr-ō-stĕ-nō′sĭs) [″ + *stenosis*, a narrowing] Narrowing or stricture of the intestine.

**enterostomal therapist** ABBR: ET. An individual trained to teach patients proper methods of caring for an ostomy. The certification title is *certified enterostomal therapy nurse* (CETN).

**enterostomy** (ĕn″tĕr-ŏs′tō-mē) [″ + *stoma*, mouth] A surgically created opening into the stomach, duodenum, or jejunum for the insertion of a feeding tube.

**enterotoxemia** (ĕn″tĕr-ō-tŏk-sē′mē-ă) A condition in which bacterial toxins are absorbed from the intestine and circulate in the blood.

**enterotoxigenic** (ĕn″tĕr-ō-tŏk″sĭ-jĕn′ĭk) Producing enterotoxins, as in some strains of bacteria.

**enterotoxin** (ĕn″tĕr-ō-tŏk′sĭn) [″ + *toxikon*, poison] **1.** A toxin produced in or originating in the intestinal contents. **2.** An exotoxin specific for the cells of the intestinal mucosa. **3.** An exotoxin produced by certain species of bacteria that causes various diseases, including food poisoning and toxic shock syndrome.

**Enterovirus** A group of viruses that originally included poliovirus, coxsackievirus, and ECHO virus, which infected the human gastrointestinal tract. Enteroviruses are now classed as a genus of picornaviruses. SEE: *picornavirus*.

**enterozoic** (ĕn″tĕr-ō-zō′ĭk) [″ + *zoon*, animal] Pert. to parasites inhabiting the intestines.

**enthesitis** (ĕn-thĕ-sī′tĭs) Tenderness to palpation at the site of attachment of bone to a tendon, ligament, or joint capsule. It is usually caused by trauma to the area.

**enthlasis** (ĕn′thlă-sĭs) [Gr., dent caused by pressure] A depressed fracture of the skull.

**entire** (ĕn-tīr′) In bacteriology, the smooth, regular border of a bacterial colony.

**entity** (ĕn′tĭ-tē) [L. *ens*, being] **1.** A thing existing independently, containing in itself all the conditions necessary to individuality. **2.** Something that forms a complete whole, denoting a distinct condition or disease.

**ento-, ent-** [Gr. *entos*, within] Combining form meaning *within, inside*.

**entoblast** (ĕn′tō-blăst) [″ + *blastos*, germ] Endoblast.

**entocele** (ĕn′tō-sēl) [″ + *kele*, tumor, swelling] **1.** Internal hernia. **2.** Displacement of a part inwardly.

**entochondrostosis** (ĕn″tō-kŏn″drŏs-tō′sĭs) [″ + *chondros*, cartilage, + *osis*, condition] The development of bone within cartilage.

**entochoroidea** (ĕn″tō-kō-roy′dē-ă) [″ + *chorioeides*, choroid] The inner layer of the choroid of the eye. SYN: *lamina choriocapillaris*.

**entocone** (ĕn′tō-kōn) [″ + *konos*, cone] The inner posterior cusp of an upper molar tooth.

**entocornea** (ĕn″tō-kor′nē-ă) [″ + L. *corneus*, horny] The posterior limiting membrane of the cornea. SYN: *Descemet's membrane*.

**entoectad** (ĕn″tō-ĕk′tăd) [″ + *ektos*, without, + L. *ad*, toward] Proceeding outward from within.

**entome** (ĕn′tōm) [Gr. *en*, in, + *tome*, incision] A knife for division of urethral strictures.

**entomion** (ĕn-tō′mē-ŏn) [Gr. *entome*, notch] The tip of the mastoid angle of the parietal bone.

**entomology** (ĕn″tō-mŏl′ō-jē) [Gr. *entomon*, insect, + *logos*, word, reason] The study of insects.

***medical e.*** The branch of entomology that deals with insects and their relationship to disease, esp. of humans.

**entomophthoramycosis** (ĕn-tō-mŏf′thō-ră-mī-kō′sĭs) A disease caused by fungi of the class Zygomycetes, which includes two genera (*Conidiobolus* and *Basidiobolus*) responsible for human disease. *Conidiobolus* causes infections of the heart and face; *Basidiobolus* produces infections in other parts of the body.

SYMPTOMS: Clinically, there is swelling of the nose, perinasal tissues, and mouth. Nodular subcutaneous masses are palpable in the skin.

TREATMENT: A variety of antibiotics and oral antifungals have been used with variable success. Surgical therapy is used for the removal of nodules and reconstruction of grossly swollen and deformed tissues.

**entopic** [Gr. *en,* in, + *topos,* place] Normally situated; in a normal place. Opposite of ectopic.

**entoptic** (ĕn-tŏp′tĭk) [Gr. *entos,* within, + *optikos,* seeing] Pert. to the interior of the eye.

**entoptic phenomenon** A visual phenomenon arising from within the eye, marked by the perception of floating bodies, circles of light, black spots, and transient flashes of light. It may be due to the individual's own blood cells moving through the retinal vessels, or to floaters, which are small specks of tissue floating in the vitreous fluid. SEE: *Moore's lightning streaks; muscae volitantes; photopsia.*

Individuals may see imperfections of their own cornea, lens, and vitreous by looking at a white background through a pinhole held about 17 mm (4.3 in.) from the eye. The person sees a patch of light the size of which varies with the diameter of the pupil. The abnormalities are seen as shadows or bright areas. This method can be used also to see early discrete lens opacities.

**entoretina** (ĕn″tō-rĕt′ĭ-nă) [″ + L. *rete,* a net] The internal layer of the retina.

**entotic** (ĕn-tō′tĭk, ĕn-tŏt′ĭk) [″ + *ous,* ear] Pert. to the interior of the ear or to the perception of sound as affected by the condition of the auditory apparatus.

**entozoon** (ĕn″tō-zō′ŏn) *pl.* **entozoa** [″ + *zoon,* animal] Any animal parasite living within the body of another animal.

**entrails** The intestines of an animal.

**entrain** To alter the biological rhythm of an organism so that it assumes a cycle different from a 24-hour one.

**entrainment 1.** Control of heart rhythm by an external stimulus or with a cardiac pacemaker. **2.** The drawing of a second fluid into a stream of gas or fluid by the Bernoulli effect.

**entropion** (ĕn-trō′pē-ŏn) [Gr. *en,* in, + *trepein,* to turn] An inversion or turning inward of an edge, esp. the margin of the lower eyelid.

***cicatricial e.*** An inversion resulting from scar tissue on the inner surface of the lid.

***spastic e.*** An inversion resulting from a spasm of the orbicularis oculi muscles.

**entropionize** (ĕn-trō′pē-ō-nīz) To invert or correct by turning in.

**entropy** (ĕn′trŏ-pē) [Gr. *en,* in, + *trope,* a turning] **1.** The portion of energy within a system that cannot be used for mechanical work but is available for internal use. **2.** The quantity or degree of randomness, disorder, or chaos in a system.

**enucleate** (ē-nū′klē-āt) [L. *enucleare,* to remove the kernel of] **1.** To remove a part or a mass in its entirety. **2.** To destroy or take out the nucleus of a cell. **3.** To remove the eyeball surgically. **4.** To remove a cataract surgically.

**enucleation** (ē-nū″klē-ā′shŭn) Removal of an entire mass or part, esp. a tumor or the eyeball, without rupture.

**enucleator** (ĕ-nū′klē-ā-tor) An instrument for separating a tumor mass, such as a myoma.

**enuresis** (ĕn″ū-rē′sĭs) [Gr. *enourein,* to void urine] Involuntary discharge of urine after the age at which bladder control should have been established. In children, voluntary control of urination is usually present by 5 years of age. Nevertheless, nocturnal enuresis is present in about 10% of otherwise healthy 5-year-old children and 1% of normal 15-year-old children. Enuresis is slightly more common in boys than in girls and occurs more frequently in first-born children. This condition has a distinct family tendency. SEE: *nocturnal e.; bladder drill.*

ETIOLOGY: In most instances, there is no organic basis for persistent enuresis. These cases are probably due to inadequate or misguided attempts at toilet training. Also, emotional stress, such as the birth of a sibling, a death in the family, or separation from the family, may be associated with the onset of enuresis in a previously continent child. Conditions that may cause enuresis include urinary tract infection, increased fluid intake due to diabetes mellitus, any disease that interferes with the formation of concentrated urine, trauma to or disease of the spinal cord, and epilepsy.

TREATMENT: When no organic disease is present, the use of imipramine as a temporary adjunct may be helpful. This is usually given in a dose of 10 to 50 mg orally at bedtime, but the effectiveness may decrease with continued administration. The bladder may be trained to hold larger amounts of urine. This procedure has decreased the occurrence rate of enuresis. No matter what the cause, the child should not be made to feel guilty or ashamed, and the family and the child should regard enuresis as they would any other condition that lends itself to appropriate therapy. If the child tries too hard to control the condition, it may worsen. Conditioning devices that sound an alarm when bedwetting occurs should not be used unless prescribed by a health care professional familiar with the treatment of enuresis.

---

Caution: Imipramine is not recommended for children under 6 years of age. Blood counts should be taken at least monthly during therapy to detect the possible onset of granulocytosis.

---

***diurnal e.*** Urinary incontinence during the day. Its cause is usually pathological. It may be caused by muscular contractions brought about by laughing, coughing, or crying. It often persists for long periods, esp. after protracted illness. It occurs more commonly in women and girls.

***nocturnal e.*** Urinary incontinence during the night. It is irregular and unaccompanied by urgency or frequency. Adults who experience nocturnal enuresis should be evaluated for signs of neurological disorders. Incontinence may cease for several weeks only to return. This type is more common in boys than in girls.

Fluid should be restricted late in the day and diurnal voidings should be spaced at more than ordinary intervals. The child may be awakened once or twice in the night and, when fully awake, robed and walked to the bathroom. As improvement is noticed, the number of awakenings may be lessened. The foot of the bed may also be elevated. Electronic devices that awaken the child the moment the bed is wet are available. The use of desmopressin acetate nasal spray at bedtime has been successful in preventing formation of urine during the night. SEE: *enuresis.*

***primary e.*** Enuresis in which a child has never been dependably continent.

***secondary e.*** Enuresis in a child with no history of incontinence for a year or more.

**envelope** (ĕn′vĕ-lōp) A covering or container.

***nuclear e.*** Two parallel membranes containing a narrow perinuclear space and enveloping the nucleus of a cell. Before the advent of electron microscopy, the nucleus was thought to be surrounded by a single, thin membrane. SEE: *nuclear membrane.*

**envenomation** (ĕn-vĕn″ō-mā′shŭn) The introduction of poisonous venoms into the body by means of a bite or sting.

**environment** [O. Fr. *en-*, in, + *viron,* circle] The surroundings, conditions, or influences that affect an organism or the cells within it.

***neutrothermal e.*** Thermoneutral e.

***thermoneutral e.*** An environment with an ambient temperature that minimizes the risk of heat loss via conduction, convection, radiation, and evaporation; often used to protect newborns. SYN: *neutrothermal e.*

**environmental control unit** ABBR: ECU. An electronic device operated by persons with severe disabilities that permits remote control of various home functions, such as heating, lighting, telephone, television, doorlocks, drapes, and air conditioning.

**environmental interpretation syndrome, impaired** Consistent lack of orientation to person, place, time, or circumstances over more than 3 to 6 months, necessitating a protective environment. SEE: *Nursing Diagnoses Appendix.*

**envy** Unhappiness about or the wish to possess qualities, physical attributes, or belongings of someone else.

***penis e.*** SEE: *penis envy.*

**enzootic** (ĕn″zō-ŏt′ĭk) [Gr. *en,* in, + *zoon,* animal] An endemic disease limited to a small number of animals.

**enzygotic** (ĕn″zī-gŏt′ĭk) [Gr. *en,* in, + *zygon,* yoke] Developed from the same ovum.

**enzygotic twins** Twins developed from the same ovum. SYN: *monozygotic twins.* SEE: *twins, dizygotic.*

**enzyme** (ĕn′zīm) [″ + *zyme,* leaven] An organic catalyst produced by living cells but capable of acting outside cells or even in vitro. Enzymes are proteins that change the rate of chemical reactions without needing an external energy source or being changed themselves; an enzyme may catalyze a reaction numerous times. Enzymes are reaction specific in that they act only on certain substances (called substrates). The enzyme and its substrate or substrates form a temporary configuration, called an enzyme-substrate complex, that involves both physical shape and chemical bonding. The enzyme promotes the formation of bonds between separate substrates, or induces the breaking of bonds in a single substrate to form the product or products of the reaction. The human body contains thousands of enzymes, each catalyzing one of the many reactions that take place as part of metabolism.

Each enzyme has an optimum temperature and pH, at which it functions most efficiently. For most human enzymes, these would be body temperature and the pH of cells, tissue fluid, or blood. Enzyme activity can be impaired by extremes of temperature or pH, the presence of heavy metals (lead or mercury), dehydration, or ultraviolet radiation. Some enzymes require coenzymes (nonprotein molecules such as vitamins) to function properly; still others require certain minerals (iron, copper, zinc). Certain enzymes are produced in an inactive form (a proenzyme) and must be activated (e.g., inactive pepsinogen is converted to active pepsin by the hydrochloric acid in gastric juice).

ACTION: Of the many human enzymes, the digestive enzymes are probably the most familiar. These are hydrolytic enzymes that catalyze the addition of water molecules to large food molecules to split them into simpler chemicals. Often the name of the enzyme indicates the substrate with the addition of the suffix *-ase.* A lipase splits fats to fatty acids and glycerol; a peptidase splits peptides to amino acids. Some enzymes such as pepsin and trypsin do not end in *-ase*; they were named before this method of nomenclature was instituted.

Enzymes are also needed for synthesis reactions. The synthesis of proteins, nucleic acids, phospholipids for cell membranes, hormones, and glycogen all require one if not many enzymes. DNA polymerase, for example, is needed for

DNA replication, which precedes mitosis. Energy production also requires many enzymes. Each step in cell respiration (glycolysis, Krebs cycle, cytochrome transport system) reuqires a specific enzyme. Deaminases remove the amino groups from excess amino acids so that they may be used for energy. Long-chain fatty acids are split by enzymes into smaller compounds to be used in cell respiration. Blood clotting, the formation of angiotensin II to raise blood pressure, and the transport of carbon dioxide in the blood all require specific enzymes.

***activating e.*** An enzyme that catalyzes the attaching of an amino acid to the appropriate transfer ribonucleic acid.

***allosteric e.*** An enzyme whose activity can change when certain types of effectors, called allosteric effectors, bind to a nonactive site on the enzyme.

***amylolytic e.*** An enzyme that catalyzes the conversion of starch to sugar.

***angiotensin-converting e.*** ABBR: ACE. An enzyme normally found in the capillary endothelium throughout the vascular system. It converts angiotensin I (a part of the renin-angiotensin-aldosterone mechanism of the kidney) to angiotensin II, the final step in the renin-angiotensin mechanism. The latter stimulates aldosterone secretion and therefore sodium retention.

***autolytic e.*** An enzyme that produces autolysis, or cell digestion.

***bacterial e.*** An enzyme developed by bacteria.

***branching e.*** An enzyme, called a glycosyltransferase, that transfers a carbohydrate unit from one molecule to another.

***brush border e.*** An enzyme produced by the cells of the villi and microvilli (brush border) lining the small intestine.

***coagulating e.*** An enzyme that catalyzes the conversion of soluble proteins into insoluble ones. SYN: *coagulase*.

***deamidizing e.*** An enzyme that splits amine off amino acid compounds.

***debranching e.*** An enzyme, dextrin-1-6-glucosidase, that removes a carbohydrate unit from molecules that contain short carbohydrate units attached as side chains.

***decarboxylating e.*** An enzyme, such as carboxylase, that separates carbon dioxide from organic acids.

***digestive e.*** Any enzyme involved in digestive processes in the alimentary canal.

***extracellular e.*** An enzyme that acts outside the cell that produces it.

***fermenting e.*** An enzyme produced by bacteria or yeasts that brings about fermentation, esp. of carbohydrates.

***glycolytic e.*** An enzyme that catalyzes the oxidation of glucose.

***hydrolytic e.*** An enzyme that catalyzes hydrolysis.

***inhibitory e.*** An enzyme that blocks a chemical reaction.

***intracellular e.*** An enzyme that acts within the cell that produces it.

***inverting e.*** An enzyme that catalyzes the hydrolysis of sucrose.

***lipolytic e.*** An enzyme that catalyzes the hydrolysis of fats. SYN: *lipase*.

***mucolytic e.*** An enzyme that depolymerizes mucus by splitting mucoproteins. Examples are lysozyme and hyaluronidase. SYN: *mucinase*.

***oxidizing e.*** An enzyme that catalyzes oxidative reactions. SYN: *oxidase*.

***proteolytic e.*** An enzyme that catalyzes the conversion of proteins into peptides.

***redox e.*** An enzyme that catalyzes oxidation-reduction reactions.

***reducing e.*** An enzyme that removes oxygen. SYN: *reductase*.

***respiratory e.*** An enzyme, such as a cytochrome or a flavoprotein, that acts within tissue cells to catalyze oxidative reactions by releasing energy.

***splitting e.*** An enzyme that facilitates removal of part of a molecule.

***transferring e.*** An enzyme that facilitates the moving of one molecule to another compound. SYN: *transferase*.

***uricolytic e.*** An enzyme that catalyzes the conversion of uric acid into urea.

***yellow e.*** One of a group of flavoproteins involved in cellular oxidations.

**Enzyme Commission** ABBR: EC. An organization created in 1956 by the International Union of Biochemistry to standardize enzyme nomenclature.

**enzyme induction** The adaptive increase in the number of molecules of a specific enzyme secondary to either an increase in its synthesis rate or a decrease in its degradation rate.

**enzyme-linked immunosorbent assay** ABBR: ELISA. A rapid enzyme immunochemical assay method in which either an antibody or an antigen can be coupled to an enzyme. The resulting complex retains both immunological and enzymatic activity. The ELISA method can detect certain bacterial antigens and antibodies as well as hormones. The sensitivity is enhanced by the addition of an antibody to an enzyme such as alkaline phosphatase. An intense color reaction is produced. These assays are quite sensitive and specific as compared with the radioimmune assay (RIA) tests, and have the advantage of not requiring radioisotopes or the expensive counting apparatus.

**enzymology** (ĕn″zī-mŏl′ō-jē) The study of enzymes and their actions.

**enzymolysis** (ĕn-zī-mŏl′ĭ-sĭs) [Gr. *en*, in, + *zyme*, leaven, + *lysis*, dissolution] Chemical change or disintegration due to an enzyme.

**enzymopathy** (ĕn″zī-mŏp′ă-thē) Any disease involving an enzyme deficiency.

**enzymopenia** (ĕn-zī″mō-pē′nē-ă) Deficiency of an enzyme.

**enzymuria** (ĕn″zī-mū′rē-ă) [″ + ″ + *ouron*,

urine] The presence of enzymes in the urine.

**EOA** *esophageal obturator airway.*

**EOM** *extraocular muscles.*

**EOP** *external occipital protuberance.*

**eosin** (ē′ō-sĭn) [Gr. *eos,* dawn (rose-colored)] Any of several synthetic dyes, including bluish and yellow ones. They are used to stain tissues for microscopic examination.

**eosinoblast** (ē″ō-sĭn′ō-blăst) [″ + *blastos,* germ] A bone marrow cell that develops into a myelocyte. SYN: *myeloblast.*

**eosinopenia** (ē″ō-sĭn-ō-pē′nē-ă) [″ + *penia,* poverty] An abnormally small number of eosinophilic cells in the peripheral blood.

**eosinophil** (ē″ō-sĭn′ō-fĭl) [″ + *philein,* to love] A type of granulocytic white blood cell characterized by a polymorphic nucleus and cytoplasmic granules that stain with eosin or other acid stains. Although their activity is not entirely clear, eosinophils are known to destroy parasitic organisms and to play a major role in allergic reactions. They release some of the major chemical mediators that cause bronchoconstriction in asthma. Eosinophils make up 1% to 3% of the white cell count. SEE: *blood* for illus.; *leukocyte.*

**eosinophilia** (ē″ō-sĭn-ō-fĭl′ē-ă) [Gr. *eos,* dawn, + *philein,* to love] **1.** An unusual number of eosinophils in the blood. **2.** The characteristic of staining readily with eosin.

***urinary e.*** An increased amount of eosinophils in the urine.

**eosinophilia-myalgia syndrome, tryptophan-induced** Eosinophilia and severe myalgia seen in patients with a history of taking oral preparations of the amino acid L-tryptophan.

SYMPTOMS: There is abrupt onset, within a week or so, of pain, edema, and induration of the extremities, esp. the legs. Skin involvement includes alopecia, transient rash, and subjective weakness. The disease is disabling and chronic. Eosinophilia is greater than 1500 $\mu$l. To establish the diagnosis, it is necessary to exclude other diseases (e.g., infections or neoplasia) that could cause these findings. An outbreak that occurred in 1989 was most likely due to a chemical constituent associated with specific manufacturing conditions at one company.

TREATMENT: Treatment is supportive; tryptophan should be discontinued.

**eosinophilic** (ē″ō-sĭn-ō-fĭl′ĭk) Readily stainable with eosin.

**eosinophilous** (ē″ō-sĭn-ŏf′ĭ-lŭs) [″ + *philein,* to love] **1.** Easily stainable with eosin. **2.** Having eosinophilia.

**eosinotactic** (ē″ō-sĭn-ō-tăk′tĭk) [″ + *taktikos,* arranged] Attracting or repulsing eosinophilic cells.

**ep-** SEE: *epi-.*

**EPAP** *expiratory positive airway pressure.*

**epaxial** (ĕp-ăk′sē-ăl) [″ + L. *axis,* axis] Situated above or behind an axis.

**epencephalon** (ĕp″ĕn-sĕf′ă-lŏn) [″ + *enkephalos,* brain] The anterior portion of the embryonic hindbrain (rhombencephalon) from which the pons and cerebellum arise. SYN: *metencephalon.*

**ependyma** (ĕp-ĕn′dĭ-mă) [Gr. *ependyma,* an upper garment, wrap] The membrane lining the cerebral ventricles and central canal of the spinal cord. **ependymal,** *adj.*

**ependymitis** (ĕp″ĕn-dĭ-mī′tĭs) [″ + *itis,* inflammation] Inflammation of the ependyma.

**ependymoblast** (ĕp-ĕn′dĭ-mō-blăst) [″ + *blastos,* germ] An embryonic ependymal cell, or ependymocyte.

**ependymocyte** (ĕp-ĕn′dĭ-mō-sīt) [″ + *kytos,* cell] An ependymal cell.

**ependymoma** (ĕp-ĕn″dĭ-mō′mă) [″ + *oma,* tumor] A tumor arising from fetal inclusion of ependymal elements.

**ephebiatrics** (ĕ-fē-bē-ăt′rĭks) [Gr. *epi,* at, + *hebe,* youth, + *iatrikos,* healing] A branch of medicine dealing with adolescents.

**ephedrine** (ĕ-fĕd′rĭn, ĕf′ĕ-drēn) An alkaloid originally obtained from species of *Ephedra;* first isolated in 1887. In ancient Chinese medicine it was used as a diaphoretic and antipyretic. It was not until much later, however, that its action was studied and its valuable therapeutic properties were made known. It is a sympathomimetic drug usually produced synthetically. Its action is similar to that of epinephrine. Its effects, although less powerful, are more prolonged, and it exerts action when given orally, whereas epinephrine is effective only by injection. Ephedrine orally (or by injection) dilates the bronchial muscles, contracts the nasal mucosa, and raises the blood pressure. It is used chiefly for its bronchodilating effect in asthma, and for its constricting effect on the nasal mucosa in hay fever.

INCOMPATIBILITY: Calcium chloride, iodine, and tannic acid are incompatible with ephedrine.

***e. hydrochloride*** A more soluble salt of ephedrine, having the same action and uses.

***e. sulfate*** The salt of ephedrine and sulfuric acid. It occurs as fine white crystals or as a powder. Its action and uses are the same as those of ephedrine.

**ephelis** (ĕf-ē′lĭs) *pl.* **ephelides** [Gr. *ephelis,* freckle] A freckle.

**ephemeral** (ĕ-fĕm′ĕr-ăl) [Gr. *epi,* on, + *hemera,* day] Of brief duration.

**epi-, ep-** [Gr.] Prefix meaning *upon, over, at, in addition to, after.*

**epiandrosterone** (ĕp″ē-ăn-drŏs′tĕr-ōn) An androgenic hormone normally present in the urine.

**epiblast** (ĕp′ĭ-blăst) [Gr. *epi,* upon, + *blastos,* germ] The outer layer of cells of the blastoderm. SYN: *ectoderm.* **epiblastic** (-blăst′ik), *adj.*

**epiblepharon** (ĕp″ĭ-blĕf′ă-rŏn) [″ + Gr. *blepharon,* eyelid] A fold of skin that passes across the margin of either the upper or lower eyelid so that the eyelashes are pressed against the eye.

**epibole, epiboly** (ĕ-pĭb′ŏ-lē) [Gr. *epibole,* cover] Inclusion of the hypoblast within the epiblast due to swifter growth of the latter. SEE: *embole.*

**epibulbar** (ĕp″ĭ-bŭl′băr) Lying on the bulb of any structure; more specifically, located on the eyeball.

**epicanthus** [Gr. *epi,* upon, + *kanthos,* canthus] A vertical fold of skin extending from the root of the nose to the median end of the eyebrow, covering the inner canthus and caruncle. It is a characteristic of certain races and may occur as a congenital anomaly in others.

**epicardia** (ĕp″ĭ-kărd′ē-ă) [″ + *kardia,* heart] The abdominal portion of the esophagus extending from the diaphragm to the stomach, about 2 cm in length.

**epicardium** The serous membrane on the surface of the myocardium; the visceral layer of the pair of serous pericardial membranes.

**epichordal** (ĕp″ĭ-kord′ăl) [″ + *khorde,* cord] Located dorsad to the notochord.

**epichorion** (ĕp″ĭ-kō′rē-ŏn) [″ + *chorion*] The portion of the decidua of the placenta that covers the ovum.

**epicomus** (ē-pĭk′ō-mŭs) [″ + *kome,* hair] A congenital malformation consisting of a parasitic twin or head attached to the summit or vertex of the skull.

**epicondylalgia** (ĕp″ĭ-kŏn-dĭ-lăl′jē-ă) [″ + *kondylos,* condyle, + *algos,* pain] Pain in the elbow joint in the region of the epicondyles.

**epicondyle** (ĕp-ĭ-kŏn′dīl) [″ + *kondylos,* condyle] The eminence at the articular end of a bone above a condyle.

**epicondylitis** (ĕp″ĭ-kŏn″dĭ-lī′tĭs) [″ + ″ + *itis,* inflammation] Inflammation of the epicondyle of the humerus and surrounding tissues.

***lateral humeral e.*** Tennis elbow.

***medial humeral e.*** Golfer's elbow.

**epicranium** [″ + *kranion,* cranium] The soft tissue covering the cranium.

**epicranius** (ĕp″ĭ-krā′nē-ŭs) The occipitofrontal muscle and scalp.

**epicrisis** (ĕp′ĭ-krī″sĭs) [″ + *krisis,* crisis] A secondary turning point following the initial critical stage of a disease.

**epicritic** (ĕp-ĭ-krĭt′ĭk) [Gr. *epikritikos,* judging] **1.** Pert. to acute sensibility, such as that of the skin when it discriminates among degrees of sensation caused by touch or temperature. **2.** Pert. to an epicrisis. **3.** Something such as pain or itching that is well localized.

**epicystotomy** (ĕp″ĭ-sĭs-tŏt′ō-mē) [″ + ″ + *tome,* incision] A surgically created opening above the symphysis pubis into the bladder.

**epicyte** (ĕp′ĭ-sīt) [″ + *kytos,* cell] **1.** An epithelial cell. **2.** A cell membrane.

**epidemic** (ĕp″ĭ-dĕm′ĭk) [″ + *demos,* people] An infectious disease or condition that attacks many people at the same time in the same geographical area. SEE: *endemic; epizootic; pandemic.*

**epidemic viral gastroenteropathy** A disease that occurs in outbreaks affecting groups of people. The disease usually is self-limiting, but may cause severe dehydration and death. Symptoms include nausea, vomiting, diarrhea, mild fever, and abdominal pain.

ETIOLOGY: Norwalk-like agents are the causative organisms. Other viruses including rotavirus may cause this disease.

TREATMENT: Vigorous fluid replacement therapy is necessary, esp. in infections due to *Rotavirus.* This treatment may be lifesaving in infected children. Oral rehydration solutions are of distinct benefit and may be the only effective therapy available for infants and children in developing countries. SEE: *oral rehydration solution; oral rehydration therapy.*

**epidemiologist** (ĕp″ĭ-dē-mē-ŏl′ō-jĭst) A specialist in the field of epidemiology.

**epidemiology** (ĕp″ĭ-dē-mē-ŏl′ō-jē) [″ + *demos,* people, + *logos,* study] The study of the distribution and determinants of health-related states and events in populations, and the application of this study to the control of health problems. Epidemiology is concerned with the traditional study of epidemic diseases caused by infectious agents, and with health-related phenomena including accidents, suicide, climate, toxic agents such as lead, air pollution, and catastrophes due to ionizing radiation. SEE: *pharmacoepidemiology.* **epidemiological** (-ŏl-ŏ′jĭ-kăl), *adj.*

**epidermal growth factor** ABBR: EGF. An amino acid polypeptide that stimulates growth of several different cells, including keratinocytes. It has been used experimentally to promote wound healing.

**epidermatoplasty** (ĕp″ĭ-dĕr-măt′ō-plăs-tē) [″ + ″ + *plassein,* to mold] A surgical procedure grafting pieces of epidermis with the underlying layer of the corium.

**epidermis** (ĕp″ĭ-dĕr′mĭs) [″ + *derma,* skin] The outermost layer of the skin. SYN: *skin.* **epidermal, epidermic** *adj.*

**epidermitis** (ĕp″ĭ-dĕr-mī′tĭs) [″ + ″ + *itis,* inflammation] Inflammation of the superficial layers of the skin.

**epidermization** (ĕp″ĭ-dĕr″mĭ-zā′shŭn) **1.** Skin grafting. **2.** Conversion of the deeper germinative layer of cells into the outer layer of the epidermis.

**epidermodysplasia verruciformis** (ĕp″ĭ-dĕr″mō-dĭs-plā′sē-ă) Generalized warts of the skin.

**epidermoid** (ĕp″ĭ-dĕr′moyd) [Gr. *epi,* upon, + *derma,* skin, + *eidos,* form, shape] **1.** Resembling or pert. to the epidermis. **2.** A tumor arising from aberrant epidermal cells. SYN: *cholesteatoma.*

**epidermolysis** (ĕp″ĭ-dĕr-mŏl′ĭ-sĭs) [″ + ″ + *lysis,* dissolution] Loosening of the epidermis.

***e. bullosa*** A genetically transmitted form of epidermolysis marked by the for-

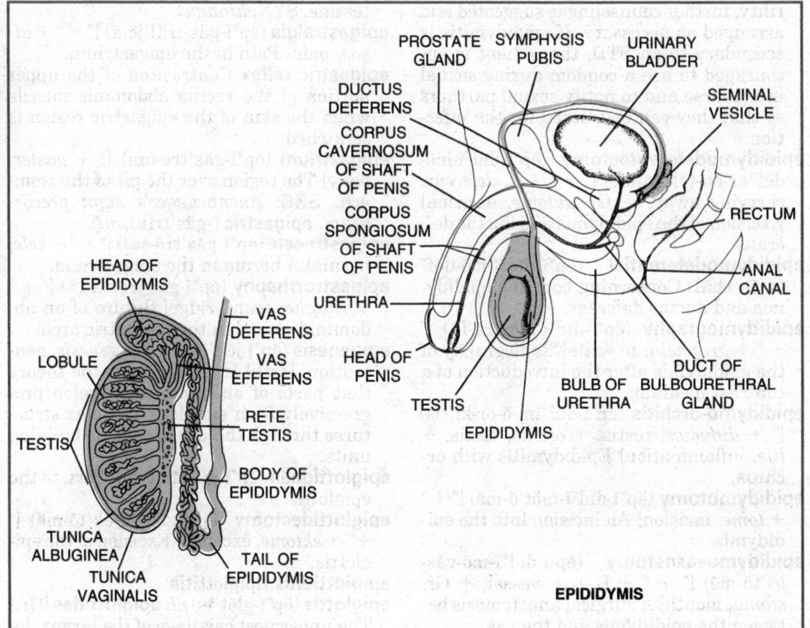

EPIDIDYMIS

mation of deep-seated bullae appearing after irritation or rubbing.

**epidermomycosis** (ĕp-ĭ-dĕr″mō-mī-kō′sĭs) [″ + ″ + *mykes,* fungus, + *osis,* condition] A skin disease caused by a fungus.

**Epidermophyton** (ĕp″ĭ-dĕr-mŏf′ĭ-tŏn) [″ + ″ + *phyton,* plant] A genus of fungi, similar to *Trichophyton* but affecting the skin and nails instead of the hair.

***E. floccosum*** The causative agent of certain types of tinea, esp. tinea pedis (athlete's foot), tinea cruris, tinea unguium, and tinea corporis.

**epidermophytosis** (ĕp″ĭ-dĕr-mō-fī-tō′sĭs) [″ + ″ + ″ + *osis,* condition] Infection by a species of *Epidermophyton.*

**epididymectomy** (ĕp″ĭ-dĭd″ĭ-mĕk′tō-mē) [″ + *didymos,* testis, + *ektome,* excision] Removal of the epididymis.

**epididymis** (ĕp″ĭ-dĭd′ĭ-mĭs) *pl.* **epididymides** A small oblong body resting on and beside the posterior surface of the testes, consisting of a convoluted tube 13 to 20 ft (3.97 to 6.1 m) long, enveloped in the tunica vaginalis, ending in the ductus deferens. It consists of the head (caput or globus major), which contains 12 to 14 efferent ducts of the testis, the body, and the tail (cauda or globus minor). It constitutes the first part of the secretory duct of each testis. The epididymis is supplied by the internal spermatic, deferential, and external spermatic arteries; it is drained by corresponding veins. SEE: illus.

**epididymitis** (ĕp″ĭ-dĭd″ĭ-mī′tĭs) [″ + *didymos,* testis, + *itis,* inflammation] Inflammation of the epididymis. SEE: *Nursing Diagnoses Appendix.*

SYMPTOMS: The symptoms are fever and chills, pain in the inguinal region, and a swollen epididymis.

ETIOLOGY: The cause may be a complication of infections and conditions associated with chlamydia, gonorrhea, syphilis, tuberculosis, mumps, prostatitis, urethritis, prostatectomy, or prolonged use of an indwelling catheter.

TREATMENT: Bedrest, support of the scrotum, and appropriate antibiotic therapy constitute the treatment of choice.

NURSING IMPLICATIONS: The patient is observed for signs of abscess formation (a localized hot, red tender area) or extension of the infection into the testes. Temperature is monitored, and adequate fluid intake maintained.

The nurse monitors the quality and pattern of pain; provides analgesics, noninvasive pain relief measures, and prescribed antibiotics and antipyretics; documents the patient's response; and instructs the patient in the use of these measures. If epididymitis is secondary to a sexually transmitted disease (STD), the disease is treated with the prescribed antibiotics.

The patient is encouraged to rest in bed with his legs slightly apart and with the testes elevated on a towel roll. Nonconstrictive, lightweight clothing should be worn until the swelling subsides. A scrotal support should be worn when the patient sits, stands, or walks.

If the patient faces the possibility of sterility, further counseling is suggested and arranged as necessary. If epididymitis is secondary to an STD, the patient is encouraged to use a condom during sexual intercourse and to notify sexual partners so that they can be treated for the infection.

**epididymodeferentectomy** (ĕp″ĭ-dĭd″ĭ-mō-dĕf″ĕr-ĕn-tĕk′tō-mē) [″ + ″ + L. *deferens,* carrying away, + Gr. *ektome,* excision] Excision of the epididymis and ductus deferens.

**epididymodeferential** (ĕp″ĭ-dĭd″ĭ-mō-dĕf″ĕr-ĕn′shăl) Concerning both the epididymis and ductus deferens.

**epididymography** (ĕp″ĭ-dĭd″ĭ-mŏg′ră-fē) [″ + ″ + *graphein,* to write] Radiography of the epididymis after the introduction of a contrast medium.

**epididymo-orchitis** (ĕp″ĭ-dĭd″ĭm-ō-or-kī′tĭs) [″ + *didymos,* testis, + *orchis,* testis, + *itis,* inflammation] Epididymitis with orchitis.

**epididymotomy** (ĕp″ĭ-dĭd″ĭ-mŏt′ō-mē) [″ + ″ + *tome,* incision] An incision into the epididymis.

**epididymovasostomy** (ĕp-ĭ-dĭd″ĭ-mō-văs-ŏs′tō-mē) [″ + ″ + L. *vas,* vessel, + Gr. *stoma,* mouth] A surgical anastomosis between the epididymis and the vas.

**epididymovesiculography** (ĕp″ĭ-dĭd″ĭ-mō-vĕ-sĭk″ū-lŏg′ră-fē) Radiography of the epididymis and seminal vesicle after introduction of a contrast medium.

**epidural** [Gr. *epi,* upon, + L. *durus,* hard] Located over or on the dura.

**epidural space** The space outside the dura mater of the brain and spinal cord.

**epifascial** (ĕp″ĭ-făsh′ē-ăl) On or above a fascia.

**epifolliculitis** (ĕp″ĭ-fŏl-lĭk″ū-lī′tĭs) [″ + L. *folliculus,* follicle, + Gr. *itis,* inflammation] Inflammation of the hair follicles of the scalp.

**epigaster** [″ + *gaster,* belly] An embryonic structure that develops into the large intestine. SYN: *hindgut.*

**epigastralgia** (ĕp″ĭ-găs-trăl′jē-ă) [″ + ″ + *algos,* pain] Pain in the epigastrium.

**epigastric reflex** Contraction of the upper portion of the rectus abdominis muscle when the skin of the epigastric region is scratched.

**epigastrium** (ĕp″ĭ-găs′trē-ŭm) [″ + *gaster,* belly] The region over the pit of the stomach. SEE: *Auenbrugger's sign; precordium.* **epigastric** (-găs′trĭk), *adj.*

**epigastrocele** (ĕp″ĭ-găs′trō-sēl) [″ + ″ + *kele,* hernia] A hernia in the epigastrium.

**epigastrorrhaphy** (ĕp″ĭ-găs-tror′ă-fē) [″ + ″ + *rhaphe,* seam, ridge] Suture of an abdominal wound in the epigastric area.

**epigenesis** (ĕp″ĭ-jĕn′ĕ-sĭs) [″ + *genesis,* generation, birth] In embryology, the theory that parts of an organism develop progressively from simple to complex structures through the use of cells as building units.

**epiglottidean** (ĕp″ĭ-glŏ-tĭd′ē-ăn) Pert. to the epiglottis.

**epiglottidectomy** (ĕp″ĭ-glŏt″ĭd-ĕk′tō-mē) [″ + ″ + *ektome,* excision] Excision of the epiglottis.

**epiglottiditis** Epiglottitis.

**epiglottis** (ĕp″ĭ-glŏt′ĭs) *pl.* **epiglottides** [Gr.] The uppermost cartilage of the larynx, located immediately posterior to the root of the tongue. It covers the entrance of the larynx when the individual swallows, thus preventing food or liquids from entering the airway. SEE: illus.

**epiglottitis** (ĕp″ĭ-glŏt-ī′tĭs) [″ + *itis,* inflammation] Inflammation of the epiglottis. This condition is most common in young children. If untreated, it may be so severe as to cause death. A more appropriate term for this condition is supraglottitis. SYN: *epiglottiditis.*

SYMPTOMS: Symptoms include sore throat, fever, croupy cough, drooling, cyanosis, and even coma.

TREATMENT: An airway is established

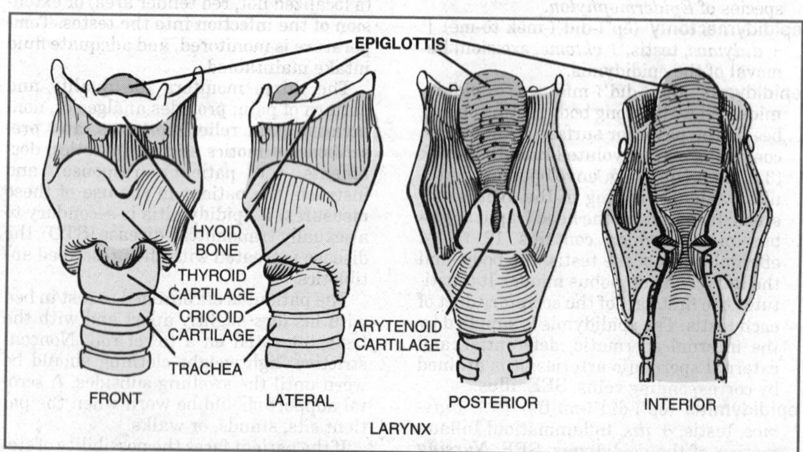

LARYNX

by tracheostomy if necessary. Appropriate antibiotics must be administered.

**epihyal** (ĕp-ĭ-hī'ăl) Pert. to the arch of the hyoid.

**epilate** (ĕp'ĭ-lāt) [L. *e*, out, + *pilus*, hair] To extract the hair by the roots.

**epilating** Depilating; extracting a hair.

**epilation** (ĕp-ĭ-lā'shŭn) **1.** Extraction of hair. SYN: *depilation; electrolysis*. **2.** Loss of hair due to exposure to ionizing radiation.

**epilemma** (ĕp-ĭ-lĕm'ă) [Gr. *epi*, upon, + *lemma*, husk] A neurilemma of small branches of nerve filaments.

**epilepsy** (ĕp'ĭ-lĕp"sē) [Gr. *epilepsia*, to seize] A recurrent paroxysmal disorder of cerebral function marked by sudden, brief attacks of altered consciousness, motor activity, or sensory phenomena. Convulsive seizures are the most common form of attack. Some but not all recurrent seizure patterns are due to epilepsy.

OCCURRENCE: Over 1 million persons in the U.S. are estimated to experience recurrent seizures. The estimated annual prevalence is 6.42 cases per 100,000 population.

ETIOLOGY: Attempts to find a cause for the sudden abnormal discharge of cerebral neurons is not possible in all types of epilepsy. In some cases, a brain tumor, scar tissue remaining from trauma to the brain, or a progressive neurological disease may be responsible. In the great majority of cases, however, no pathological basis for the seizures is evident, either during life or at autopsy. The latter type of seizure has been classed as "idiopathic." In certain circumstances (e.g., fever, convulsant drugs, hypoxia, or hypoglycemia in normal persons) the response may include one or more seizures. If these events are isolated and do not recur, these patients are not classed as having epilepsy.

SYMPTOMS: Symptoms may vary from the almost imperceptible alteration in consciousness, as in absence seizures (petit mal), to dramatic loss of consciousness, a cry, falling, tonic-clonic convulsions of all extremities, urinary and fecal incontinence, and amnesia for the event. Some attacks are preceded by an aura; others provide no warning. Other forms are limited to muscular contractions of a localized area or only one side of the body. SEE: *postictal confusion*.

TREATMENT: A thorough investigation is made to identify any remediable cause of the seizures. These would include metabolic diseases, endocrine system disturbances, cerebral tumors, abscess of the brain, and meningioma.

The patient must understand the illness and realize that he or she does not have to live as an invalid. Persons whose convulsions are controlled by medications can participate in sports. Most countries permit a person to drive an automobile if he or she has experienced no seizures for 6 months to 1 year. The family, physician, and associates should encourage the patient to work and live a normal life. If seizures are uncontrolled, however, automobile driving, swimming, operating unguarded machinery, and ladder climbing should not be allowed. Epileptics should not drink alcoholic beverages.

*Medical therapy* is available for prevention and control of seizures. Each type of epilepsy may require a specific therapeutic regimen. Antiepileptic drugs available include phenytoin, carbamazepine, phenobarbital, primidone, ethosuximide, methsuximide, clonazepam, valproate sodium, and trimethadione. In addition, if the seizures are related to a lesion in the brain, neurosurgical treatment is indicated. In treating epilepsy, it is important to know that no antiepileptic drug exists that is free of teratogenic potential or confusing drug interactions.

*Surgical therapy* is estimated to be indicated in 40% of partial epilepsy cases. About one third of patients treated at a center dedicated to this type of surgery were seizure free; another one third had marked reduction of seizures.

PROGNOSIS: Grand mal seizures can be controlled completely in about 50% of cases, and greatly reduced in frequency in another 35%. Petit mal can be controlled in 40% of cases, and frequency reduced in 35%. Psychomotor attacks can be controlled in 35% of cases, and frequency reduced in 50%. Virtually all epilepsy patients are normal between attacks.

The seizure disorders (epilepsy) were classified in 1970 and revised in 1981 according to the clinical form of the seizure and the EEG changes. The term *epilepsy* has a negative aspect, and for that reason it is advisable to use the term *seizure* when talking with the patient.

*Simple partial seizure:* The seizure is limited to a portion of the body with no loss of consciousness. The area involved may spread until the entire side is involved. This type of seizure, with motor, sensory, or autonomic signs, was originally called jacksonian epilepsy. *Complex partial seizure:* Episodic changes in behavior are accompanied by loss of consciousness. The seizure is preceded by an aura with complex hallucinations or sensory illusions. While unconscious, the patient may drive a car or continue to read a book, but will not respond to questions or commands. There is amnesia for the seizure, and recovery may take as long as 1 hour. *Secondary generalized partial seizure:* The seizure progresses from a simple or complex to a generalized form.

*Primary generalized seizure: Tonic-clonic (grand mal)*. This common seizure pattern is marked by sudden onset of unconsciousness, tonic contraction of muscles, loss of postural control, and a cry caused by contraction of the respiratory muscles forcing exhalation. This is followed by generalized contraction of the muscles of the four extremities. After 2 to 5 min of unconsciousness and subsidence of clonic contractions, the patient gradually regains consciousness. Fecal and urinary incontinence and biting of the tongue may occur. The patient is amnestic for the event and may not be completely functional for several days.

*Tonic seizure:* This type is quite similar to a generalized seizure, but with tonic rather than clonic muscular activity and possibly shorter duration. *Absence seizure (petit mal):* Activity ceases suddenly for a few seconds to several minutes. No fall or convulsive muscular contractions occur. The seizures begin in childhood, and patients often outgrow the condition. The patient is normal except for the seizures, which may occur as frequently as 100 times a day. *Atypical absence seizure:* This type is similar to an absence seizure in a patient who has other forms of generalized seizures. *Myoclonic seizure:* This type is marked by sudden and brief contractions of a single group of muscles or of the entire body. The patient falls but does not lose consciousness. *Atonic seizure:* Brief loss of consciousness and a fall occur without muscular contractions. *Infantile spasm:* This type of generalized seizure occurs in the first year of life. There are synchronous contractions of the muscles of the neck, trunk, and arms. About 90% of these children are mentally deficient. *Status epilepticus:* A series of grand mal seizures may occur when the patient is awake and active or during sleep, but consciousness is not completely regained between attacks. This serious condition requires therapy without delay. *Epilepsia partialis continua:* In this special type of focal motor status epilepticus, there is clonic twitching of one group of muscles. This is repeated at regular intervals of a few seconds and may persist for hours or indefinitely.

NURSING IMPLICATIONS: During a seizure, the patient is protected from injury and aspiration prevented. The area is cleared of hard objects, and the head cradled or something soft placed under it if the patient is on a hard surface, without restraining movement. Tight clothing is loosened and the patient turned to the side to allow the tongue to fall away from the airway and permit drainage of saliva.

If the nurse is present before the tonic phase begins, an oral airway, padded tongue blade, or other soft object may be inserted between the teeth; but no object should be forced between clenched teeth, because the teeth or the object may shatter and fragments be aspirated.

The nurse remains with the patient throughout the seizure, noting time of onset and duration; patient activity at the time of onset; sequence of events; sensory phenomena; motor activity; postural tone; laterality of movements; incontinence; tongue biting; pupillary, skin, or respiratory changes; and response after the seizure.

Comfort and reassurance are offered after the seizure; the patient is oriented to time and place, evaluated for understanding of what occurred, and informed of the seizure; and rest is provided as desired during the postictal period. The seizure's timing and events and the response are documented.

The condition and treatment are explained to the patient. Prescribed anticonvulsant therapy is administered and the patient assessed for toxicity. The importance of full cooperation with the treatment plan and of follow-up care is stressed.

The patient is encouraged to eat regular, well-balanced meals, because low blood glucose levels and inadequate vitamin intake can lead to seizures. The patient should get enough rest, because excessive fatigue can precipitate a seizure. The patient should also be alert for and eliminate triggering factors, such as hyperventilation, strong odors, flashing lights, loud noises, heavy musical beats, video games, and television. Alcohol intake should be limited, the first sign of fever treated, and stress controlled.

Further counseling and referral to local support groups may be necessary. The patient should wear or carry a medical identification tag. SEE: *Nursing Diagnoses Appendix.*

***Lennox-Gastaut syndrome e.*** Epilepsy with onset in early childhood. This type of epilepsy is characterized by a variety of seizure patterns and an abnormal electroencephalogram, and is frequently associated with developmental and mental retardation. Seizures are not controlled by the usual antiepileptic drugs; however, adjunctive therapy with felbamate may be beneficial.

***photogenic e.*** Convulsive attacks that occur as a result of intermittent light stimulus.

***reflex e.*** Recurrent epileptic seizures that occur in reaction to a specific stimulus, such as photic stimulation while looking at flashing lights or television, auditory stimulation while listening to specific musical compositions, tactile stimulation, or reading.

***sleep e.*** A spasmodic uncontrollable desire to sleep. SYN: *narcolepsy.*

***traumatic e.*** Epilepsy caused by trauma to the brain.

**epileptic** (ĕp″ĭ-lĕp′tĭk) [Gr. *epileptikos*] **1.** Concerning epilepsy. **2.** An individual suffering from attacks of epilepsy.

**epileptiform** (ĕp″ĭ-lĕp′tĭ-form) [Gr. *epilepsia,* to seize, + L. *forma,* form] Having the form or appearance of epilepsy.

**epileptogenic, epileptogenous** (ĕp″ĭ-lĕp-tō-jĕn′ĭk, -tŏj′ĕ-nŭs) [″ + *gennan,* to produce] Giving rise to epileptoid convulsions.

**epileptoid** [″ + *eidos,* form, shape] Resembling epilepsy. SYN: *epileptiform.*

**epileptology** [″ + *logos,* word, reason] The study of epilepsy.

**epiloia** (ĕp″ĭ-lŏy′ă) Tuberous sclerosis.

**epimandibular** (ĕp″ĭ-măn-dĭb′ū-lăr) [Gr. *epi,* upon, above, + L. *mandibulum,* jaw] Located on the lower jaw.

**epimer** (ĕp′ĭ-mĕr) One of a pair of isomers that differ only in the position of the hydrogen atom and the hydroxyl group attached to one asymmetrical carbon atom.

**epimere** (ĕp′ĭ-mēr) [Gr. *epi,* upon, + *meros,* apart] In embryology, the dorsal muscle-forming portion of the somite.

**epimerite** (ĕp″ĭ-mĕr′īt) [″ + *meros,* part] An organelle of certain protozoa by which they attach themselves to epithelial cells.

**epimorphosis** (ĕp″ĭ-mor′fō-sĭs) [″ + *morphoun,* to give shape, + *osis,* condition] Regeneration of a part of an organism by growth at the cut surface.

**epimysium** (ĕp″ĭ-mĭz′ē-ŭm) [″ + *mys,* muscle] The outermost sheath of connective tissue that surrounds a skeletal muscle. It consists of irregularly distributed collagenous, reticular, and elastic fibers, connective tissue cells, and fat cells. SYN: *perimysium externum.*

**epinephrine** (ĕp″ĭ-nĕf′rĭn) [″ + *nephros,* kidney] $C_9H_{13}NO_3$. A hormone secreted by the adrenal medulla in response to stimulation of the sympathetic nervous system. This substance and norepinephrine are the two active hormones produced by the adrenal medulla. Epinephrine causes some of the physiological expressions of fear and anxiety and has been found in excess in some anxiety disorders. Epinephrine is also produced by tissues other than the adrenal. Its effects are similar to those produced by stimulation of the sympathetic division of the autonomic nervous system. It is used therapeutically as a vasoconstrictor, to treat cardiac dysrhythmias, and to relax bronchioles; to check local hemorrhage and to relieve asthmatic attacks; and to prolong the action of local anesthetics by constricting blood vessels to prevent rapid absorption. Trade names are Adrenalin, Bronkaid Mist, Primatene Mist, and Sus-Phrine.

INCOMPATIBILITY: Epinephrine is incompatible with light, heat, air, iron salts, and alkalies. SYN: *adrenaline.*

**epinephritis** (ĕp″ĭ-nĕf-rī′tĭs) [″ + *nephros,* kidney, + *itis,* inflammation] Inflammation of an adrenal gland.

**epinephroma** (ĕp-ĭ-nĕ-frō′mă) [″ + ″ + *oma,* tumor] A lipomatoid tumor of the kidney. SYN: *hypernephroma.*

**epineural** (ĕp″ĭ-nū′răl) [″ + *neuron,* nerve] Located on a neural arch.

**epineurium** (ĕp″ĭ-nū′rē-ŭm) The general connective tissue sheath of a nerve. SEE: *nerve.*

**epiotic** (ĕp″ē-ŏt′ĭk) [″ + *ous,* ear] Located above the ear.

**epiotic center** The ossification center of the temporal bone, forming the upper and posterior part of the auditory capsule.

**epipastic** (ĕp″ĭ-păs′tĭk) [″ + *passein,* to sprinkle] Resembling a dusting powder.

**EpiPen** Trade name for an autoinjector of epinephrine, available by prescription for those allergic to insect stings. The EpiPen Jr. autoinjector is available for children.

**epipharynx** (ĕp″ĭ-făr′ĭnks) [″ + *pharynx,* throat] Nasopharynx.

**epiphenomenon** (ĕp″ĭ-fĕ-nŏm′ĕ-nŏn) [″ + *phainomenon,* phenomenon] An exceptional symptom or occurrence in a disease that is not related to the usual course of the disease.

**epiphora** (ĕ-pĭf′ō-ră) [Gr., downpour] An abnormal overflow of tears down the cheek due to excess secretion of tears or obstruction of the lacrimal duct.

**epiphyseolysis** (ĕp″ĭ-fĭz″ē-ŏl′ĭ-sĭs) [″ + ″ + *lysis,* dissolution] Separation of an epiphysis. Also spelled *epiphysiolysis.*

**epiphyseopathy** (ĕp″ĭ-fĭz-ē-ŏp′ă-thē) [″ + ″ + *pathos,* disease, suffering] **1.** Any disease of the pineal gland. **2.** Any disease of the epiphysis of a bone. Also spelled *epiphysiopathy.*

**epiphysis** (ĕ-pĭf′ĭ-sĭs) *pl.* **epiphyses** [Gr., a growing upon] **1.** In the developing infant and child, a secondary bone-forming (ossification) center separated from a parent bone in early life by cartilage. As growth proceeds (at a different time for each epiphysis), it becomes a part of the larger, or parent, bone. It is possible to judge the biological age of a child from the development of these ossification centers as shown radiographically. **2.** A center for ossification at each extremity of long bones. SEE: *diaphysis.* **3.** The end of a long bone. **epiphyseal, epiphysial** (ĕp″ĭ-fĭz′ē-ăl), *adj.*

**epiphysitis** (ĕ-pĭf″ĭ-sī′tĭs) [″ + *itis,* inflammation] Inflammation of an epiphysis, esp. that at the hip, knee, or shoulder in an infant.

**epipial** (ĕp″ĭ-pī′ăl) [″ + L. *pia,* tender] Situated on or above the pia mater.

**epiplocele** (ĕ-pĭp′lō-sēl) [Gr. *epiploon,* omentum, + *kele,* tumor, swelling] A hernia containing omentum.

**epiploenterocele** (ĕ-pĭp″lō-ĕn′tĕr-ō-sēl) [″ + *enteron,* intestine, + *kele,* tumor, swelling] A hernia consisting of omentum and intestine.

**epiploic** (ĕp″ĭ-plō′ĭk) [Gr. *epiploon,* omentum] Pert. to the omentum.

**epiploic foramen** The opening between the greater and lesser peritoneal cavities.

**epiploitis** (ĕ-pĭp″lō-ī′tĭs) [″ + *itis,* inflammation] Inflammation of the omentum.

**epiplomerocele** (ĕ-pĭp″lō-mē′rō-sēl) [″ + *meros,* thigh, + *kele,* tumor, swelling] A femoral hernia containing omentum.

**epiplomphalocele** (ĕ-pĭp″lŏm-făl′ō-sēl) [″ + *omphalos,* navel, + *kele,* hernia] An umbilical hernia with omentum protruding.

**epiploon** (ĕ-pĭp′lō-ŏn) [Gr., omentum] The omentum, esp. the greater omentum. SYN: *omentum.*

**epiplopexy** (ĕ-pĭp′lō-pĕks″ē) [″ + *pexis,* fixation] Suturing of omentum to the anterior abdominal wall.

**epiplosarcomphalocele** (ĕ-pĭp″lō-săr″kŏm-făl′ō-sēl) [″ + *sarx,* flesh, + *omphalos,* navel, + *kele,* tumor, swelling] An umbilical hernia with omentum protruding. SYN: *epiplomphalocele.*

**epiploscheocele** (ĕ-pĭp″lŏs-kē′ō-sēl) [″ + *oscheon,* scrotum, + *kele,* tumor, swelling] An omental hernia into the scrotum.

**epipygus** (ĕp″ĭ-pī′gŭs) [Gr. *epi,* upon, + *pyge,* buttocks] A developmental anomaly in which an accessory limb is attached to the buttocks. SEE: *pygomelus.*

**episclera** (ĕp″ĭ-sklē′ră) [″ + *skleros,* hard] The outermost superficial layer of the sclera of the eye.

**episcleral** (ĕp″ĭ-sklē′răl) **1.** Pert. to the episclera. **2.** Overlying the sclera of the eye.

**episcleritis** (ĕp″ĭ-sklē-rī′tĭs) [″ + *skleros,* hard, + *itis,* inflammation] Inflammation of the subconjunctival layers of the sclera.

**episioperineoplasty** (ĕ-pĭs″ē-ō-pĕr″ĭ-nē′ō-plăs″tē) [″ + *perinaion,* perineum, + Gr. *plassein,* to form] Plastic surgery of the perineum and vulva.

**episioperineorrhaphy** (ĕ-pĭs″ē-ō-pĕr″ĭ-nē-or′ă-fē) [″ + ″ + *rhaphe,* seam, ridge] Suturing of the vulva and perineum to support a prolapsed uterus.

NURSING IMPLICATIONS: The perineum is inspected at intervals to assess healing and to observe for indications of hematoma formation or infection. Perineal care is provided as needed, and the patient is taught correct perineal hygiene (i.e., wiping from front to back). To relieve pain, anesthetic sprays or creams are applied as prescribed, and local heat applied using a heat lamp, warm soaks, or sitz baths as prescribed, and the patient is taught to apply these therapies.

**episioplasty** (ĕ-pĭs″ē-ō-plăs′tē) [″ + *plassein,* to form] Plastic surgery of the vulva.

**episiostenosis** (ĕ-pĭs″ē-ō-stĕ-nō′sĭs) [″ + *stenosis,* narrowing] Narrowing of the vulvar opening.

**episiotomy** (ĕ-pĭs″ē-ŏt′ō-mē) [″ + *tome,* incision] Incision of the perineum at the end of the second stage of labor to avoid spontaneous laceration of the perineum and to facilitate delivery.

**episode** An occurrence that is one in a sequence of events.

**episome** (ĕp′ĭ-sōm) A bacterial element that can replicate either autonomously or in association with a chromosome. SEE: *plasmid.*

**epispadias** (ĕp″ĭ-spā′dē-ăs) [Gr. *epi,* upon, + *spadon,* a rent] A congenital opening of the urethra on the dorsum of the penis.

**episplenitis** (ĕp″ĭ-splē-nī′tĭs) [″ + *splen,* spleen, + *itis,* inflammation] Inflammation of the splenic capsule.

**epistasis** (ĕ-pĭs′tă-sĭs) [Gr., stoppage] **1.** A film that forms on urine that has been allowed to stand. **2.** The suppression of any discharge. SEE: *hypostasis.*

**epistaxis** (ĕp″ĭ-stăk′sĭs) [Gr.] Hemorrhage from the nose; nosebleed. SEE: *Kiesselbach's area.*

ETIOLOGY: Epistaxis may occur secondarily to local infections (vestibulitis, rhinitis, sinusitis), systemic infections (scarlet fever, typhoid), drying of nasal mucous membrane, trauma (including picking the nose), arteriosclerosis, hypertension, and bleeding tendencies associated with anemias.

TREATMENT: The patient should lie quietly, propped up in bed. Treatment includes cold compresses, epinephrine locally, and if necessary, cautery of the bleeding vessel. Posterior packing of the nasal cavity or balloon tamponade may be needed. The latter is done by inserting a Foley-like catheter into the nose and inflating the balloon after it is placed posteriorly. Traction is then applied to the catheter so that the vessels in the area are compressed. SEE: *nosebleed* for illus.

NURSING IMPLICATIONS: Airway clearance, level of discomfort and anxiety, and any prior history of nosebleeds are determined. The patient should be seated upright and leaning forward to prevent aspiration, and blood is expectorated to limit nausea and vomiting due to swallowed blood. Bleeding is controlled by pinching the nostrils against the nasal septum for 5 to 10 min while the patient breathes through the mouth. Pressure is applied across or under the upper lip, and cold over the nose or the nape of the neck to help stop bleeding. If a posterior packing or balloon tamponade is ordered, the nurse explains the procedure, administers prescribed presedation, assists with the procedure, assesses for hypoxemia, and administers supplemental oxygen by face mask as needed. The nares are inspected for pressure necrosis. The patient should avoid blowing or picking at the nose, and increased humidity may help to prevent bleeding if dryness is a factor. Simple measures are taught to help the patient stop a nosebleed at home.

**episternum** Upper portion of the sternum. SYN: *manubrium sterni.* **episternal,** *adj.*

**epitendineum** (ĕp″ĭ-tĕn-dĭn′ē-ŭm) [″ + L. *tendere,* to stretch] The fibrous sheath enveloping a tendon.

**epitenon** SEE: *epitendineum.*

**epithalamus** (ĕp″ĭ-thăl′ă-mŭs) [″ + *thalamos,* chamber] The uppermost portion of the diencephalon of the brain. It includes the pineal body, trigonum habenulae, habenula, and habenular commissure.

**epithelia** Pl. of *epithelium.*

**epithelial cancer** Epithelioma.

**epithelial diaphragm** The epithelial extension of Hertwig's root sheath that determines the number and size of tooth roots. It induces dentin formation locally as the root elongates. SEE: *Hertwig's root sheath.*

**epithelialization** (ĕp″ĭ-thē″lē-ăl-ī-zā′shŭn) The growth of skin over a wound.

**epithelial tissue** The cells that form the outer surface of the body and line the body cavities and the principal tubes and passageways leading to the exterior. These cells form the secreting portions of glands and their ducts and are important parts of certain sense organs. The cells of epithelial tissues lie in close approximation and contain very little intercellular substance. They are arranged in one or a few layers and are devoid of blood vessels. SEE: illus.; *tissue.*

**epitheliitis** (ĕp″ĭ-thē″lē-ī′tĭs) Overgrowth and inflammation of the mucosal epithe-

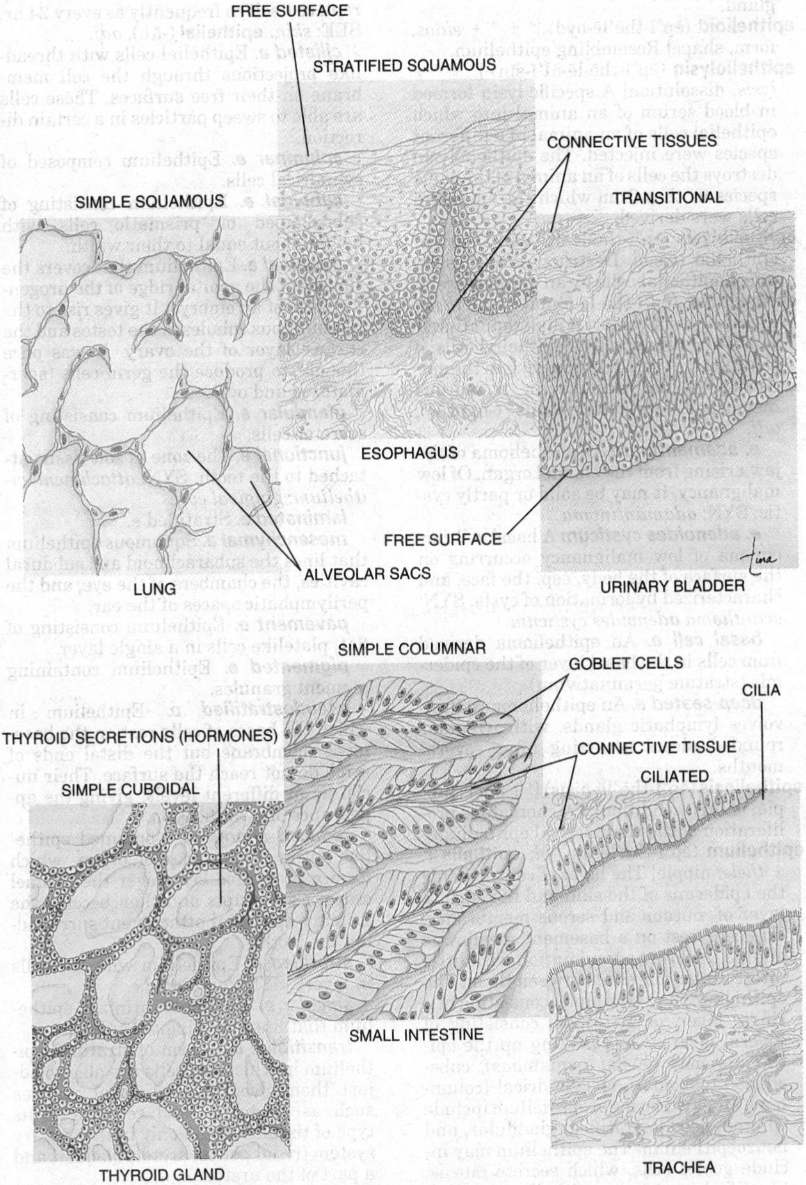

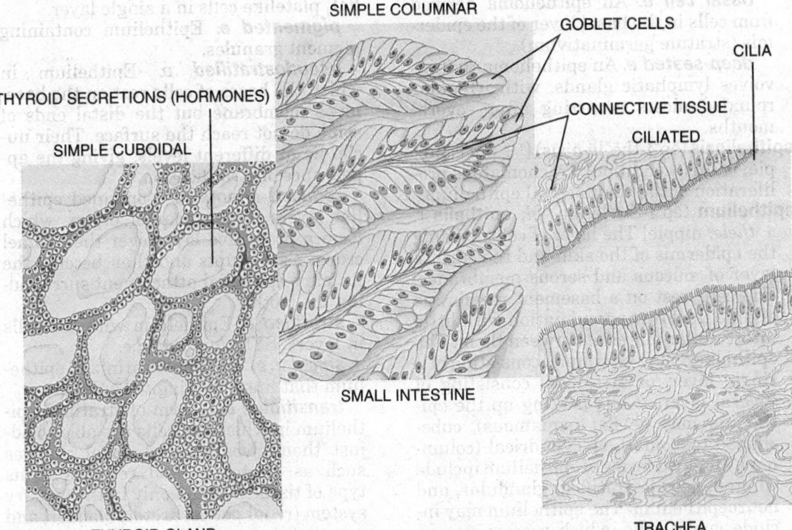


**EPITHELIAL TISSUES** (ORIG. MAG. ×430)

lium following injury such as is caused by ionizing radiation.

**epithelioblastoma** (ĕp″ĭ-thē″lē-ō-blăs-tō′mă) [″ + *thele,* nipple, + *blastos,* germ, + *oma,* tumor] An epithelial cell tumor.

**epitheliogenic, epitheliogenetic** (ĕp″ĭ-thē″lē-ō-jĕn′ĭk, -jĕ-nĕt′ĭk) [″ + ″ + *gennan,* to produce] Caused by epithelial proliferation.

**epithelioglandular** (ĕp″ĭ-thē″lē-ō-glăn′dū-lăr) Concerning the epithelial cells of a gland.

**epithelioid** (ĕp″ĭ-thē′lē-oyd) [″ + ″ + *eidos,* form, shape] Resembling epithelium.

**epitheliolysin** (ĕp″ĭ-thē-lē-ŏl′ĭ-sĭn) [″ + ″ + *lysis,* dissolution] A specific lysin formed in blood serum of an animal into which epithelial cells of an animal of a different species were injected. The epitheliolysin destroys the cells of an animal of the same species as that from which the epithelial cells were derived.

**epitheliolysis** (ĕp″ĭ-thē-lē-ŏl′ĭ-sĭs) Death of epithelial tissue. Destruction or dissolving of epithelial cells by an epitheliolysin.

**epithelioma** (ĕp″ĭ-thē-lē-ō′mă) [″ + *thele,* nipple, + *oma,* tumor] A malignant tumor consisting principally of epithelial cells; a carcinoma. A tumor originating in the epidermis of the skin or in a mucous membrane. **epitheliomatous** (-mă-tŭs), *adj.*

***e. adamantinum*** An epithelioma of the jaw arising from the enamel organ. Of low malignancy, it may be solid or partly cystic. SYN: *adamantinoma.*

***e. adenoides cysticum*** A basal cell carcinoma of low malignancy occurring on the surface of the body, esp. the face, and characterized by formation of cysts. SYN: *acanthoma adenoides cysticum.*

***basal cell e.*** An epithelioma derived from cells in the basal layer of the epidermis (stratum germinativum).

***deep-seated e.*** An epithelioma that involves lymphatic glands, with irregular rounded ulcers occurring after several months.

**epitheliosis** (ĕp″ĭ-thē″lē-ō′sĭs) [″ + *thele,* nipple, + *osis,* condition] Trachomatous proliferation of the conjunctival epithelium.

**epithelium** (ĕp″ĭ-thē′lē-ŭm) *pl.* **epithelia** [″ + *thele,* nipple] The layer of cells forming the epidermis of the skin and the surface layer of mucous and serous membranes. The cells rest on a basement membrane and lie in close approximation with little intercellular material between them. The epithelium may be simple, consisting of a single layer, or stratified, consisting of several layers. Cells making up the epithelium may be flat (squamous), cube-shaped (cuboidal), or cylindrical (columnar). Modified forms of epithelium include ciliated, pseudostratified, glandular, and neuroepithelium. The epithelium may include goblet cells, which secrete mucus. Stratified squamous epithelium may be keratinized for a protective function or abnormally keratinized in pathological response. Squamous epithelium is classified as endothelium, which lines the blood vessels and the heart, and mesothelium, which lines the serous cavities. Epithelium serves the general functions of protection, absorption, and secretion, and specialized functions such as movement of substances through ducts, production of germ cells, and reception of stimuli. Its ability to regenerate is excellent; it may replace itself as frequently as every 24 hr. SEE: *skin.* **epithelial** (-ăl.), *adj.*

***ciliated e.*** Epithelial cells with thread-like projections through the cell membrane on their free surfaces. These cells are able to sweep particles in a certain direction.

***columnar e.*** Epithelium composed of cylindrical cells.

***cuboidal e.*** Epithelium consisting of cube-shaped or prismatic cells with height about equal to their width.

***germinal e.*** Epithelium that covers the surface of the genital ridge of the urogenital folds of an embryo. It gives rise to the seminiferous tubules of the testes and the surface layer of the ovary. It was once thought to produce the germ cells (spermatozoa and ova).

***glandular e.*** Epithelium consisting of secretor cells.

***junctional e.*** The zone of soft tissue attached to the tooth. SYN: *attachment epithelium; gingival cuff.*

***laminated e.*** Stratified e.

***mesenchymal e.*** Squamous epithelium that lines the subarachnoid and subdural cavities, the chambers of the eye, and the perilymphatic spaces of the ear.

***pavement e.*** Epithelium consisting of flat, platelike cells in a single layer.

***pigmented e.*** Epithelium containing pigment granules.

***pseudostratified e.*** Epithelium in which the bases of cells rest on the basement membrane but the distal ends of some do not reach the surface. Their nuclei lie at different levels, giving the appearance of stratification.

***reduced enamel e.*** Combined epithelial layers of the enamel organ, which form a protective layer over the enamel crown as it erupts and then become the primary epithelial attachment surrounding the tooth.

***stratified e.*** Epithelium with the cells in layers. SYN: *laminated e.*

***sulcular e.*** The nonkeratinized epithelium that lines the gingival sulcus.

***transitional e.*** A form of stratified epithelium in which the cells are able to adjust themselves to mechanical changes such as stretching and recoiling. This type of tissue is found only in the urinary system (renal pelvis, ureter, bladder, and a part of the urethra).

**epitope** (ĕp′ĭ-tōp) Any component of an antigen molecule that functions as an antigenic determinant by permitting the attachment of certain antibodies. SYN: *antigenic determinant*. SEE: *paratope*.

**epitrichial layer** Epitrichium.

**epitrichium** (ĕp″ĭ-trĭk′ē-ŭm) [Gr. *epi*, upon, + *trichion*, hair] The superficial layers of the epidermis of the fetus. SYN: *epitrichial layer; periderm*.

**epitrochlea** (ĕp″ĭ-trŏk′lē-ă) [″ + *trochalia*, pulley] The inner condyle of the humerus. **epitrochlear**, *adj*.

**epiturbinate** (ĕp″ĭ-tĕr′bĭn-āt) [″ + L. *turbo*, top] The tissue on or covering the turbinate bone.

**epitympanum** (ĕp″ĭ-tĭm′pă-nŭm) [″ + *tympanon*, drum] The attic of the middle ear; the area above the drum membrane.

**epizoon** (ĕp″ĭ-zō′ŏn) *pl*. **epizoa** [″ + *zoon*, animal] An animal organism living as a parasite on the exterior of the host animal. **epizoic** (-zō′ĭk), *adj*.

**epizootic** Any disease of animals that attacks many animals in the same area.

**epoetin alfa** Synthetic human erythropoietin. Trade name is Epogen. SEE: *erythropoietin*.

**eponychium** (ĕp″ō-nĭk′ē-ŭm) [″ + *onyx*, nail] **1.** The horny embryonic structure from which the nail develops. **2.** The perionychium.

**eponym** (ĕp′ō-nĭm) [Gr. *eponymos*, named after] A name for anything (disease, organ, function, place) adapted from the name of a particular person or sometimes a geographical location (e.g., Haverhill fever, Lyme disease).

**epoophorectomy** (ĕp″ō-ō-fō-rĕk′tō-mē) [Gr. *epi*, upon, + *oophoron*, ovary, + *ektome*, excision] Removal of the parovarium.

**epoophoron** (ĕp″ō-ŏf′ō-rŏn) A rudimentary structure located in the mesosalpinx. Consisting of a longitudinal duct (duct of Gartner) and 10 to 15 transverse ducts, it is the remains of the upper portion of the mesonephros and is the homologue of the head of the epididymis in males. SYN: *parovarium; Rosenmüller body*.

**epoxide** (ĕ-pŏk′sīd) Any chemical compound that contains two carbon atoms joined to a single oxygen atom.

**epoxy** (ĕ-pŏk′sē) A general term for a polymer that contain molecules in which oxygen is attached to two different carbon atoms. These compounds are widely used as adhesives.

**epsilon-aminocaproic acid** A synthetic substance used to correct an overdose of certain fibrinolytic agents. It is also useful in treating excessive bleeding due to increased fibrinolytic activity in the blood.

**epsom salt** (ĕp′sŭm) Magnesium sulfate.

**EPSP** *excitatory postsynaptic potential*.

**Epstein-Barr virus** [M. A. Epstein, Brit. physician, b. 1921; Y. M. Barr, contemporary Canadian physician] ABBR: EBV. A member of the herpes virus family, discovered in 1964. It is one of the causes of infectious mononucleosis. In South African children, it is associated with Burkitt's lymphoma; in Asian populations, with nasopharyngeal carcinoma. Why the virus has these different and varied associations in different geographical areas is unknown.

**Epstein's pearls** [Alois Epstein, Czech. pediatrician, 1849–1918] In newborn infants, whitish-yellow accumulation of epithelial cells, or retention cysts, on the hard palate. They are harmless and disappear within a few weeks.

**epulis** (ĕp-ū′lĭs) *pl*. **epulides** [Gr. *epoulis*, a gumboil] **1.** A fibrous sarcomatous tumor having its origin in the periosteum of the lower jaw. **2.** A nonpathological softening and swelling of the gums due to hyperemia that begins during midtrimester pregnancy and subsides after delivery. In susceptible women, this condition tends to recur during subsequent pregnancies.

**epuloid** (ĕp′ū-loyd) [″ + *eidos*, form, shape] **1.** Like an epulis. **2.** A tumor of the jaw or gum resembling an epulis.

**epulosis** (ĕp″ū-lō′sĭs) [Gr. *epoulosis*] Cicatrization; a cicatrix.

**epulotic** (ĕp″ū-lŏt′ĭk) [Gr. *epoulotikos*] Promoting cicatrization.

**equation** [L. *aequare*, to make equal] **1.** The state of being equal. **2.** In chemistry, a symbolic representation of a chemical reaction.

***e. of motion*** A statement of the variables of pressure, volume, compliance, resistance, and flow for respiratory system mechanics.

***personal e.*** SEE: *personal equation*.

**equator** [L. *aequator*] A line encircling a round body and equidistant from both poles. **equatorial**, *adj*.

***e. of cell*** The boundary of a plane through which the division of a cell occurs.

***e. of crystalline lens, e. lentis*** The line that marks the junction of the anterior and posterior surfaces of the crystalline lens. The fibers of the suspensory ligament are attached to it.

***e. oculi*** An imaginary line encircling the bulb of the eye midway between the anterior and posterior poles.

**equatorial plate** The mass of chromosomes at the equator of the the nuclear spindle during karyokinesis.

**equi-** [L. *aequus*, equal] Prefix meaning *equal*.

**equianalgesic** A dose of one form of analgesic drug equivalent to another analgesic in pain-relieving potential. Knowing this equivalence permits the substitution of analgesics without undesired side effects.

**equilibrating** (ē-kwĭl′ĭ-brāt-ĭng) [L. *aequilibris*, in perfect balance] Maintaining equilibrium.

**equilibration** The modification of masticatory forces or occlusal surfaces of teeth to produce simultaneous occlusal contacts between upper and lower teeth, and to equalize the stress of occlusal forces of the supporting tissues of the teeth.

**equilibrium** [L. *aequus,* equal, + *libra,* balance] A state of balance; a condition in which contending forces are equal.

***nitrogenous e.*** A condition in which the nitrogen excreted equals the nitrogen intake.

***physiological e.*** A condition in which the egesta are equal to the ingesta.

***thermal e.*** A condition in which two substances exist at the same temperature and in which heat transfer is therefore in a steady state.

**equilin** (ĕk′wĭl-ĭn) [L. *equus,* horse] Crystalline estrogenic hormone derived from the urine of pregnant mares.

**equimolar** In the quantitative comparison of chemical substances, having the same molar concentration.

**equine** (ē′kwīn) [L. *equus,* horse] Concerning or originating from a horse.

**equinovarus** (ē-kwī″nō-vā′rŭs) [L. *equinus,* equine, + *varus,* bent inward] A form of clubfoot with a combinination of pes equinus and pes varus (i.e., walking without touching the heel to the ground and with the sole turned inward).

**equipotential** (ē″kwĭ-pō-tĕn′shăl) [L. *aequus,* equal, + *potentia,* ability] Having the same electric charge or physical strength.

**equivalence** (ē-kwĭv′ă-lĕns) [″ + *valere,* to be worth] The quality of being equal in power, force, or value.

**equivalent** (ē-kwĭv′a-lĕnt) **1.** Equal in power, force, or value. **2.** The amount of weight of any element needed to replace a fixed weight of another body.

***dose e.*** In radiology, the product of the absorbed dose and the quality factor. Expressed in rems or sieverts, it measures the effects of absorbing different types of radiation. SEE: *factor, quality.*

***metabolic e.*** ABBR: MET. A unit used to estimate the metabolic cost of physical activity. One MET equals the uptake of 3.5 ml of oxygen per kilogram of body weight per minute.

**equivalent weight** The weight of a chemical element that is equivalent to and can replace a hydrogen atom (1.008 g) in a chemical reaction.

**E.R.** *external resistance; Emergency Room.*

**Er** Symbol for the element erbium.

**eradication** Complete elimination of a disease, esp. one that is epidemic or endemic.

**Erben's reflex** (ĕrb′ĕnz) [Siegmund Erben, Austrian physician, b. 1863] Retardation of the pulse when the head and trunk are forcibly bent forward.

**erbium** (ĕr′bē-ŭm) A rare metallic element with atomic number 68, an atomic weight of 167.26, and a specific gravity of 9.051. Its symbol is Er.

**Erb's paralysis** [Wilhelm Heinrich Erb, Ger. neurologist, 1840–1921] Paralysis of the group of shoulder and upper arm muscles involving the cervical roots of the fifth and sixth spinal nerves. The arm hangs limp, the hand rotates inward, and normal movements are lost. SYN: *Erb's palsy.*

**Erb's point** The point on the side of the neck 2 to 3 cm above the clavicle and in front of the transverse process of the sixth cervical vertebra. Electrical stimulation over this area causes various arm muscles to contract.

**ERCP** *endoscopic retrograde cholangiopancreatography.*

**erectile** (ĕ-rĕk′tĭl) [L. *erigere,* to erect] Able to become erect.

**erectile tissue** Vascular tissue that becomes erect or rigid when filled with blood, as the clitoris, penis, or nipples.

**erection** The state of swelling, hardness, and stiffness observed in the penis and to a lesser extent in the clitoris, generally due to sexual excitement. It is caused by engorgement with blood of the corpora cavernosa and the corpus spongiosum of the penis in men and the corpus cavernosa clitoridis in women.

Erection is necessary in men for the natural intromission of the penis into the vagina but not for the emission of semen. The blood withdraws from the penis after ejaculation and the erection is reduced. Erection of the penis may occur as the result of sexual excitement, during sleep, or due to physical stimulation of the penis. Abnormal persistent erection of the penis due not to sexual excitement but to certain disease states is called priapism. SEE: *nocturnal emission; penile prosthesis.*

**erector** [L. *erigere,* to erect] A muscle that raises a body part.

**erector spinae reflex** Irritation of the skin over the erector spinae muscles causing contraction of the muscles of the back. SYN: *dorsal reflex; lumbar reflex.*

**eremophobia** (ĕr″ĕm-ō-fō′bē-ă) [Gr. *eremos,* solitary, + *phobos,* fear] Dread of being alone.

**erethism** (ĕr′ĕ-thĭzm) [Gr. *erethismos,* irritation] A group of psychological signs and symptoms associated with acute mercury poisoning. Included are restlessness, irritability, insomnia, difficulty in concentrating, and impaired memory. In severe cases, delirium and toxic psychosis may develop. SEE: *mercury poisoning.*

***e. mercurialis*** Mental illness occurring as a result of chronic mercury poisoning.

**erethismic** (ĕr″ĕ-thĭz′mĭk) Pert. to or causing erethism.

**erethisophrenia** (ĕr″ĕ-thĭ-zō-frē′nē-ă) [″ + *phren,* mind] Unusual mental excitability.

**ereuthrophobia** (ĕr″ū-thrō-fō′bē-ă) [Gr. *erythros,* red, + *phobos,* fear] Pathological fear of blushing. SYN: *erythrophobia.*

**ERG** *electroretinogram.*

**erg** [Gr. *ergon,* work] In physics, the amount of work done when a force of 1 dyne acts through a distance of 1 cm. One erg is roughly 1/980 gram-centimeter. That is, raising a load of 1 g against gravity the distance of 1 cm requires that a force of 980 dynes operate through a distance of 1 cm, and hence that 980 ergs of work be done.

**ergasiomania** (ĕr-gā″sē-ō-mā′nē-ă) [Gr. *ergasia,* work, + *mania,* madness] An abnormal desire to be busy at work.

**ergasiophobia** (ĕr-gā″sē-ō-fō′bē-ă) [″ + *phobos,* fear] Abnormal dislike for work of any kind or for assuming responsibility.

**ergastic** (ĕr-găs′tĭk) [Gr. *ergastikos*] Possessing potential energy.

**ergastoplasm** SEE: *endoplasmic reticulum.*

**ergocalciferol** (ĕr-gō-kăl-sĭf′ĕr-ŏl) Vitamin $D_2$, an activated product of ergosterol. It is used primarily in prophylaxis and treatment of vitamin D deficiency.

**ergogenic** (ĕr″gō-jĕn′ĭk) [Gr. *ergon,* work, + *gennan,* to produce] Having the ability to increase work, esp. to increase the potential for work output.

**Ergomar** Trade name for ergotamine tartrate.

**ergometer** (ĕr-gŏm′ĕ-tĕr) [″ + *metron,* measure] An apparatus for measuring the amount of work done by a human or animal subject.

***bicycle e.*** A stationary bicycle used in determining the amount of work performed by the rider.

**ergonomic aid** In athletic medicine, the questionable and often harmful use of various substances in an attempt to enhance performance. Some of these materials—such as blood transfusions, anabolic steroids, amphetamines, amino acids, and human growth hormone—are standard medicines approved for uses other than those intended by the athlete. Others are not only not indicated for any illness but may be harmful, esp. when the amount of the active ingredient in the product is unknown. Included in this latter group are cyproheptadine, taken to increase appetite, strength, and, allegedly, testosterone production; ginseng; pangamic acid; octacosanol, a 28-carbon straight-chain alcohol obtained from wheat germ oil, the biological effects of which are unknown; guarana, prepared from the seeds of the *Paulliania cupana* tree, used for its alleged ability to increase energy; gamma-oryzanol, an isomer of oryzanol extracted from rice bran oil, allegedly useful in decreasing recovery time after exercise; proteolytic enzymes (e.g., chymotrypsin, trypsin-chymotrypsin, and papain), the safety and efficacy of which have not been established, esp. when used with oral anticoagulants or by pregnant or lactating women; and bee pollen, which has shown no evidence of improving athletic performance. SEE: *anabolic agent; blood doping.*

**ergonomics** (ĕr″gō-nŏm′ĭks) [″ + *nomikos,* law] The science concerned with fitting a job to a person's anatomical, physiological, and psychological characteristics in a way that enhances human efficiency and well-being.

**ergonovine maleate** (ĕr″gō-nō′vĭn) An ergot derivative used in treating migraine, and in obstetrics to stimulate contractions of the uterus. Trade name is Ergotrate Maleate.

**ergophobia** (ĕr″gō-fō′bē-ă) [″ + *phobos,* fear] Morbid dread of working.

**Ergostat** Trade name for ergotamine tartrate.

**ergosterol** (ĕr-gŏs′tĕr-ŏl) The primary sterol, or fat, found in the cell membranes of fungi. It plays a role similar to that of cholesterol in human cell walls. Most antifungal drugs act on ergosterol to increase permeability of the cell wall of the fungus, promoting its destruction.

**ergot** (ĕr′gŏt) A drug obtained from *Claviceps purpurea,* a fungus that grows parasitically on rye. Several valuable alkaloids, such as ergotamine, are obtained from ergot.

**ergotamine** (ĕr-gŏt′ă-mēn) $C_{33}H_{35}O_5N_5$. A crystalline alkaloid derived from ergot.

***e. tartrate*** A white crystalline substance that stimulates smooth muscle of blood vessels and the uterus, inducing vasoconstriction and uterine contractions. It is used in the treatment of migraine. Trade names are Ergomar, Ergostat, and Gynergen.

**ergotherapy** (ĕr″gō-thĕr′ă-pē) [″ + *therapeia,* treatment] Work used as a treatment of disease.

**ergothioneine** (ĕr-gō-thī′ō-nēn) Thiolhistidine-betaine, a compound containing crystalline sulfur. It is found in ergot and red blood cells. SYN: *thioneine.*

**ergotism** (ĕr′gŏ-tĭzm) Poisoning resulting from excessive use of ergot or from eating food made from rye or wheat infected with the fungus *Claviceps purpurea.* It may be acute or chronic. SEE: *ergot poisoning.*

**ergot poisoning** A toxic reaction that may result from eating bread made with grain contaminated with the *Claviceps purpurea* fungus, or from an overdose of ergot.

SYMPTOMS: Symptoms appear several hours after ingestion. They include vomiting, burning, and cramping in the abdomen; great thirst; profound weakness; diarrhea; a slow, weak pulse; anesthesia, tingling, and twitching in the extremities; dilated pupils; occasionally convulsions; and anuria. If the patient survives, generalized gangrene, particularly of the extremities, may develop.

FIRST AID: Slurry of activated charcoal by mouth is followed by emesis or gastric lavage, instillation of a saline cathartic, and external heat. Amyl nitrite by inhalation counteracts arterial spasms; anticonvulsants are given if needed. SEE: *Poisons and Poisoning Appendix.*

**ergotrate** (ĕr′gō-trāt) An active principle isolated from ergot.

**Ergotrate Maleate** Trade name for ergonovine maleate.

**Erikson, Erik H.** [Ger.-born U.S. psychoanalyst, 1902–1993] A psychological theorist who proposed eight developmental stages from birth to late adulthood. In each stage, there is conflict between a specific psychosocial task and an opposing ego threat that must be resolved:

Birth to 1 year: Trust/mistrust
2 to 3 year: Autonomy/shame and doubt
4 to 5 year: Initiative/guilt
6 to 12 year: Industry/inferiority
13 to 18 year: Identity/role confusion
Young adult: Intimacy/isolation
Middle-aged adult: Generativity/self-absorption
Old adult: Ego integrity/despair

**Eristalis** (ĕr-ĭs'tă-lĭs) A genus of flies belonging to the family Syrphidae. The larva, called rat-tailed maggot (*E. tenax*), may cause intestinal myiasis in humans.

**erode** (ē-rōd') [L. *erodere*] **1.** To wear away. **2.** To eat away by ulceration.

**erogenous** (ĕr-ŏj'ĕ-nŭs) [Gr. *eros,* love, + *gennan,* to produce] Causing sexual excitement. SYN: *erotogenic.*

**erogenous zone** Any part of the body, touching or stroking of which can cause sexual excitement. SEE: *zone, erogenous.*

**eros 1.** In psychoanalysis, the collective instincts for self-preservation. **2.** Eros, the Greek god of love.

**E rosette test** A laboratory test performed to identify human T lymphocytes. When T lymphocytes combine with sheep red blood cells in a culture, a cluster of cells called a rosette forms. This test is often replaced by the use of monoclonal antibodies that identify the CD4 receptor specific for T cells.

**erosion** (ē-rō'shŭn) [L. *erodere,* to gnaw away] **1.** An eating away of tissue. **2.** External or internal destruction of a surface layer by physical or inflammatory processes.

***e. of cervix uteri*** The alteration of the epithelium on a portion of the cervix as a result of irritation by infection.

SYMPTOMS: In the early stages, the epithelium shows necrosis; in healing, there is a downgrowth of epithelium from the endocervical canal. If the growth is a single layer of tissue with a grossly granular appearance, it is called a simple granular erosion. If the growth is excessive and shows papillary tufts, it is called a papillary erosion. Histologically, the papillary erosion shows many branching racemose glands; their epithelium is the mucus-bearing cell with the nucleus at the base. In the healing process, squamous epithelium grows over the eroded area with one of the following results: the squamous cells replace the tissue beneath them completely, giving complete healing; the glands fill with squamous plugs and remain in that state; or the mouths of the glands are occluded by the squamous cells and nabothian cysts form. In the congenital type of erosion, the portio is covered by high columnar epithelium. SEE: *carcinoma in situ; Papanicolaou test.*

TREATMENT: Treatment consists of proper care of the cervix following delivery. Electrocauterization of the early erosion is usually curative. Cryotherapy may be used.

***dental e.*** The wearing away of the surface layer (enamel) of a tooth. SEE: *abrasion; attrition; bruxism.*

**erosive** (ē-rō'sĭv) **1.** Able to produce erosion. **2.** An agent that erodes tissues or structures.

**erotic** (ĕ-rŏt'ĭk) [Gr. *erotikos*] **1.** Stimulating sexual desire. **2.** Concerning sexual love. **3.** A person who stimulates sexual desire.

**eroticism** (ĕ-rŏt'ĭ-sĭzm) [" + *-ismos,* condition] Sexual desire.

***anal e.*** **1.** Sensations of pleasure experienced through defecation during a stage in the development of children. **2.** In psychiatry, fixation of the libido at the anal-erotic developmental stage. Personality traits associated with anal eroticism include cleanliness, frugality, and neatness, and an unusual interest in regularity of bowel movements.

***oral e.*** **1.** Sexual pleasure derived from use of the mouth. **2.** In psychiatry, fixation of the libido to the oral phase of development.

**erotogenic** (ĕ-rō"tō-jĕn'ĭk) [Gr. *eros,* love, + *gennan,* to produce] Producing sexual excitement. SEE: *zone, erogenous.*

**erotology** (ĕr"ŏ-tŏl'ō-jē) [" + *logos,* word, reason] The study of love and its manifestations.

**erotomania** (ĕ-rō"tō-, ĕ-rŏt"ŏ-mā'nē-ă) [" + *mania,* madness] The delusion in a man or woman that he or she is loved by a particular person. SYN: *erotomonomania.*

**erotomonomania** Erotomania.

**erotophobia** (ĕ-rō"tō-, ĕ-rŏt"ō-fō'bē-ă) [" + *phobos,* fear] An aversion to sexual love or its manifestations.

**erratic** [L. *errare,* to wander] Wandering, having an unpredictable or fluctuating course or pattern. SYN: *eccentric.*

**error** A mistake or miscalculation.

***inborn e. of metabolism*** Any inherited metabolic disease caused by the absence or deficiency of specific enzymes necessary to the metabolism of basic substances such as amino acids, carbohydrates, vitamins, or essential trace elements. Examples include phenylketonuria and hereditary fructose intolerance. SEE: *metabolism.*

***type I e.*** In statistics, experimental medicine, and epidemiology, erroneous rejection of a hypothesis.

***type II e.*** In statistics, experimental medicine and epidemiology, erroneous acceptance of a hypothesis.

**ERT** *estrogen replacement therapy.*

**eructation** (ĕ-rŭk-tā'shŭn) [L. *eructare*] Producing gas from the stomach, usually with a characteristic sound; belching.

**eruption** (ē-rŭp'shŭn) [L. *eruptio,* a breaking out] **1.** A visible breaking out, esp. of a skin lesion or rash accompanying a disease such as measles or scarlet fever. **2.** The appearance of a lesion such as redness or spotting on the skin or mucous membrane. **3.** The breaking of a tooth through the gum; the cutting of a tooth. **eruptive** (-tĭv), *adj.*

***active e.*** Movement of the tooth toward the occlusal plane.

***creeping e.*** A skin lesion marked by a tortuous elevated red line that progresses at one end while fading out at the other. It is caused by the migration into the skin of the larvae of certain nematodes, esp. *Ancylostoma braziliense* and *A. caninum,* which are present in ground exposed to dog or cat feces. SYN: *cutaneous larva migrans.*

***delayed e.*** The most common variation in the tooth eruption pattern. It may be due to crowding or to various genetic, endocrine, or physiological factors.

***drug e.*** A skin reaction resulting from ingestion of certain drugs such as iodides. SYN: *dermatitis medicamentosa.*

***fixed drug e.*** Erythematous skin lesions with hyperpigmentation of the area after the acute inflammation subsides. These result from exposure to certain drugs, including captopril, foscarnet, sulfonamides, tetracycline, and barbiturates. The lesions appear in the same location (i.e., fixed site) when the offending drug is administered again.

***passive e.*** Increased size of the clinical crown of a tooth by apical migration of the attachment epithelium and periodontium.

***serum e.*** An eruption that occurs following the injection of a serous fluid. It may be accompanied by chills and fever.

**eruptive stage** The stage of tooth eruption when the tooth is moving towards the occlusal plane prior to function. Root formation is coincident with eruption but is only one of several factors related to the mechanism of tooth eruption.

**erysipelas** (ĕr″ĭ-sĭp′ĕ-lăs) [Gr. *erythros,* red, + *pella,* skin] An acute febrile disease with localized inflammation and redness of the skin and subcutaneous tissue accompanied by systemic signs and symptoms. SEE: illus.

SYMPTOMS: The symptoms include fever, chills, nausea, vomiting, painful and warm skin, and hot, red lesions on the face and head that are usually seen within 24 to 48 hr. Bullae may develop.

ETIOLOGY: Group A streptococci are almost always the cause.

TREATMENT: Therapy is with penicillin or erythromycin, with cool magnesium sulfate solution compresses for the skin. Erysipelas may be fatal if untreated.

PROGNOSIS: The prognosis is excellent with treatment. Without treatment, nephritis, abscesses, and septicemia may develop.

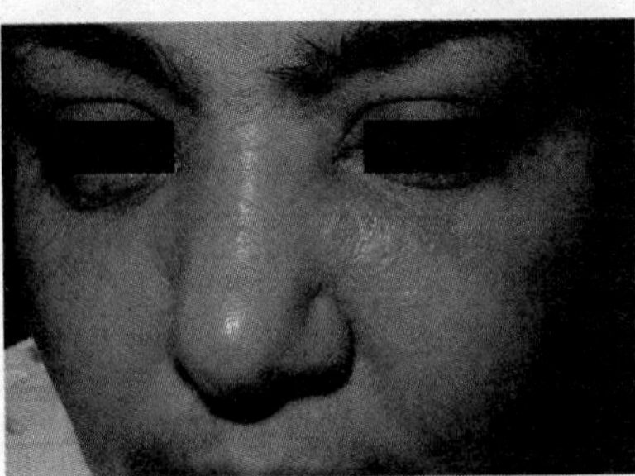

ERYSIPELAS

NURSING IMPLICATIONS: The patient is taught how and when to take prescribed antibiotics; the importance of adhering to the schedule and completing the course of treatment are stressed. During the acute phase, rest is prescribed, and affected body parts are elevated. The application of cool compresses to the affected parts is demonstrated, and its effect evaluated. Assistance is provided to help the patient and family to deal with fever, chills, nausea, and vomiting. If symptoms do not subside, medical follow-up is urged to detect complications early and to institute prescribed therapy. Hygienic measures such as thorough handwashing is encouraged to prevent the spread of infection to other members of the household.

**erysipelatous** (ĕr″ĭ-sĭ-pĕl′ă-tŭs) Of the nature of or pert. to erysipelas.

**erysipeloid** (ĕr-ĭ-sĭp′ĕ-loyd) [″ + ″ + *eidos,* form, shape] An infective dermatitis resembling erysipelas. Usually limited to the hands, it is marked by hyperemia, edema, and occasionally systemic complications.

ETIOLOGY: The cause is *Erysipelothrix rhusiopathiae,* usually acquired by handling shellfish, poultry, or meat.

TREATMENT: Penicillin or erythromycin is effective.

**Erysipelothrix rhusiopathiae** (ĕr″ĭ-sĭ-pĕl′ō-thrĭks) [″ + ″ + *thrix,* hair] A species of gram-positive, branching, filamentous, rod-shaped nonmotile bacteria. They cause erysipeloid.

**erysipelotoxin** (ĕr″ĭ-sĭp″ĕ-lō-tŏk′sĭn) The poisonous substance produced by *Streptococcus pyogenes,* the causative agent of erysipelas.

**erysiphake** (ĕr-ĭs′ĭ-făk) A small spoon-shaped device used in cataract surgery to remove the lens by suction.

**erythema** (ĕr″ĭ-thē′mă) [Gr., redness] A form of macula showing diffused redness of the skin. **erythematic, erythematous** (-thĕ-măt′ĭk, -thĕm′ă-tŭs), *adj.*

ETIOLOGY: The cause is capillary congestion, usually due to dilatation of the superficial arterioles as a result of some nervous mechanism within the body; inflammation; or some external influence such as heat, ionizing radiation, sunlight, or cold.

***e. ab igne*** Localized erythema due to exposure to heat.

***e. annulare*** Erythema that is annular, or ring shaped.

***e. chronicum migrans*** ABBR: ECM. An annular erythema following an insect bite, esp. that of the tick infected with the spirochete that causes Lyme disease. The erythema develops following the bite, and the annular inflamed border moves away from the site and becomes a large bluish-red area with a firm border. In time, multiple rings without a central bite may develop and produce intersecting patterns. This form of erythema is a marker for Lyme disease.

***e. induratum*** Chronic vasculitis of the skin occurring in young women. Hard cutaneous nodules break down to form necrotic ulcers and leave atrophic scars. SYN: *Bazin's disease.*

***e. infectiosum*** A mild, moderately contagious disease seen most commonly in school-age children. SYN: *Fifth disease.*

ETIOLOGY: The causative agent is human parvovirus B-19. Transmission is thought to be via respiratory secretions from infected patients; however, maternal-fetal transmission can occur and hydrops fetalis may result.

SYMPTOMS: Patients experience a mild, brief illness; complaints include fever, malaise, headache and pruritus. The characteristic erythema appears about 10 days later. Facial redness is similar to that which occurs when a child is slapped; however, circumoral redness is absent. Several days following initial erythema, a less distinct rash may appear on the extremities and trunk. The rash usually resolves within 1 week but may occur for several weeks when the patient is exposed to heat, cold, exercise, or stress. Adults may also experience arthralgia and arthritis, although these symptoms are less common in children. In addition, mild transient anemia, thrombocytopenia, and leukopenia may develop.

TREATMENT: Most patients require no specific therapy. Patients with coexisting chronic hemolytic anemia may experience transient aplastic crisis (TAC). These patients should be warned of the danger of exposure to parvovirus B-19 infection, informed of the early signs and symptoms, and instructed to seek medical consultation promptly if exposure is suspected. Patients with TAC may develop a life-threatening anemia that requires immediate blood transfusion or partial exchange transfusion.

***e. intertrigo*** Chafing.

***e. marginatum*** A form of erythema multiforme in which the center of the area fades, leaving elevated edges.

***e. multiforme*** ABBR: EM. A macular eruption with dark red papules, wheals,

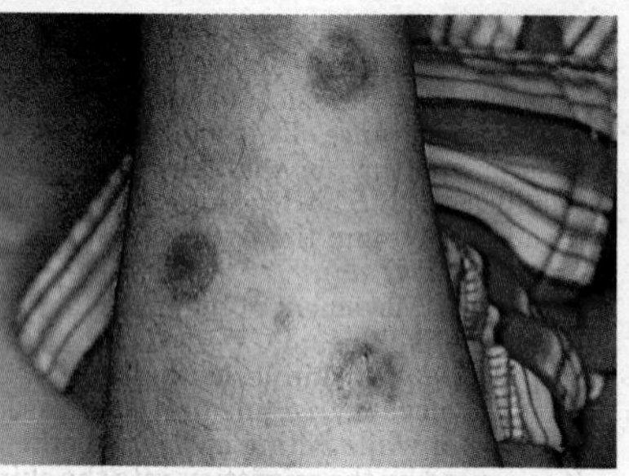

**ERYTHEMA MULTIFORME**

TYPICAL TARGET LESIONS ON ARM

vesicles, bullae, or tubercles. Usually on the extremities, including the palms and soles, it appears in successive eruptions of short duration. The eruption may appear in separate rings, concentric rings (called iris or target lesions), disk-shaped patches, distributed elevations, or figured arrangements. SEE: illus.

ETIOLOGY: The cause is presumed to be an immune reaction to antigens such as viruses or mycobacteria or to certain drugs. Stevens-Johnson syndrome is a severe form of EM in which there are bullae on the oral mucosa, pharynx, conjunctiva, and anal area.

TREATMENT: If the cause is known, the patient is treated accordingly.

***e. nodosum*** Red, painful nodules on the legs.

ETIOLOGY: In children, this condition is commonly caused by upper respiratory infection, esp. from streptococcus. In adults, streptococcal infections and sarcoidosis are the most common causes. This condition is also caused by certain drugs and food poisoning.

TREATMENT: Treatment consists of appropriate antibiotic therapy for infection, bedrest, and systemic corticosteroids to control lesions.

***punctate e.*** Erythema occurring in minute points, such as scarlet fever rash.

***e. toxicum neonatorum*** A benign, self-limited occurrence of firm, yellow-white papules or pustules from 1 to 2 mm in size present in about 50% of full-term infants. The cause is unknown, and the lesions disappear without need for treatment.

***e. venenatum*** A form of erythema caused by contact with a toxic substance.

**erythemogenic** (ĕr″ĭ-thē″mō-jĕn′ĭk) [″ + *gennan,* to produce] Producing erythema.

**erythr-** SEE: *erythro-.*

**erythralgia** (ĕr″ĭ-thrăl′jē-ă) [″ + *algos,* pain] Erythromelalgia.

**erythrasma** (ĕr″ĭ-thrăz′mă) A red-brown eruption in patches in the axillae and groin caused by *Corynebacterium minutissimum.*

**erythremia** (ĕr″ĭ-thrē′mē-ă) [″ + *haima,*

blood] Polycythemia vera.

**erythrism** (ĕr′ĭ-thrĭzm) [″ + *-ismos,* condition of] Red hair and beard with a ruddy complexion. **erythristic** (-thrĭs′tĭk), *adj.*

**erythrityl tetranitrate** (ĕ-rĭth′rĭ-tĭl) A drug used to dilate the coronary arteries, used in treating angina pectoris. Trade name is Cardilate.

**erythro-, erythr-** [Gr. *erythros*] Combining form meaning *red.*

**erythroblast** (ĕ-rĭth′rō-blăst) [″ + *blastos,* germ] Any form of nucleated red corpuscle. The earliest stages in the development are pronormoblast, basophilic normoblast, polychromatic normoblast, and orthochromatic normoblast. Nucleated red cells are not normally seen in the circulating blood. Erythroblasts contain hemoglobin. In the embryo they are found in blood islands of the yolk sac, body mesenchyma, liver, spleen, and lymph nodes; after the third month they are restricted to the bone marrow. **erythroblastic** (-blăs′tĭk), *adj.*

**erythroblastemia** (ĕ-rĭth″rō-blăs-tē′mē-ă) [″ + ″ + *haima,* blood] An excessive number of erythroblasts in the blood.

**erythroblastoma** (ĕ-rĭth″rō-blăs-tō′mă) [″ + *blastos,* germ, + *oma,* tumor] A tumor (myeloma) with cells resembling megaloblasts.

**erythroblastosis** (ĕ-rĭth″rō-blăs-tō′sĭs) [″ + ″ + *osis,* condition] A condition marked by erythroblasts in the blood.

***e. fetalis*** A hemolytic disease of the newborn marked by anemia, jaundice, enlargement of the liver and spleen, and generalized edema (hydrops fetalis). SEE: *hemolytic disease of the newborn.*

**erythrochloropia** (ĕ-rĭth″rō-klor-ō′pē-ă) [Gr. *erythros,* red, + *chloros,* green, + *ops,* eye] Partial color blindness with ability to see red and green, but not blue and yellow.

**erythrochromia** (ĕ-rĭth″rō-krō′mē-ă) [″ + *chroma,* color] Hemorrhagic red pigmentation of the spinal fluid.

**erythroclasis** (ĕr″ĕ-thrŏk′lă-sĭs) The splitting up of red blood cells.

**erythroclastic** (ĕ-rĭth-rō-klăs′tĭk) [″ + *klasis,* a breaking] Destructive to red blood cells.

**erythrocyanosis** (ĕ-rĭth-rō-sī″ă-nō′sĭs) [″ + *kyanos,* blue, + *osis,* condition] Red or bluish discoloration on the skin with swelling, itching, and burning.

**erythrocyte** (ĕ-rĭth′rō-sīt) [″ + *kytos,* cell] A mature red blood cell (RBC), or corpuscle. Each is a nonnucleated, biconcave disk averaging 7.7 μm in diameter. An RBC has a typical cell membrane and an internal stroma, or framework, made of lipids and proteins to which more than 200 million molecules of hemoglobin are attached. Hemoglobin is a conjugated protein consisting of a colored iron-containing portion (hematin) and a simple protein (globin). It combines readily with oxygen to form an unstable compound (oxyhemoglobin). The total surface

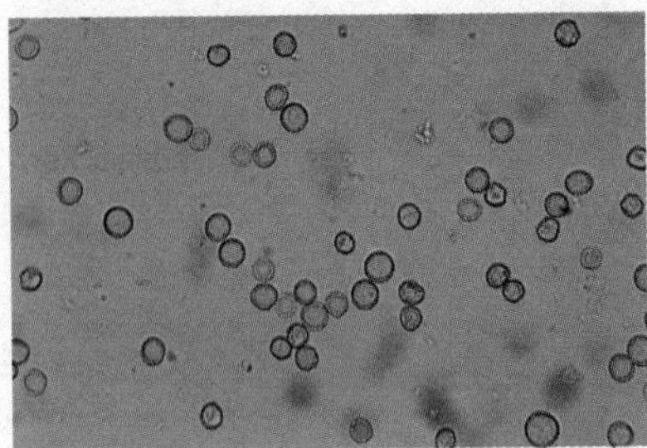

NORMAL **ERYTHROCYTES,** UNSTAINED (ORIG. MAG. ×400)

area of the RBCs of an average adult is 3820 sq m, or about 2000 times more than the total body surface area. SEE: illus. (Normal Erythrocytes); *blood cell* for illus.

NUMBER: In a normal person, the number of RBCs averages about 5,000,000 per microliter (5,500,000 for men and 4,500,000 for women). The total number in an average-sized person is about 35 trillion. The number per microliter varies with age (higher in infants), time of day (lower during sleep), activity and environmental temperature (increasing with both), and altitude. Persons living at altitudes of 10,000 ft (3048 m) or more may have an RBC count of 8,000,000 per microliter or more.

If an individual has a normal blood volume of 5 L (70 ml per kilogram of body weight) and 5,000,000 RBCs per $mm^3$ of blood, and the RBCs have an average life span of about 120 days, the red bone marrow must produce 2,400,000 RBCs per second to maintain this concentration of blood.

PHYSIOLOGY: The primary function of RBCs is to carry oxygen. The hemoglobin also contributes to the acid-base balance of the blood by acting as a buffer for the transport of carbon dioxide in the plasma as bicarbonate ions.

DEVELOPMENT: RBC formation (erythropoiesis) in adults takes place in the red bone marrow, principally in the vertebrae, ribs, sternum, diploë of cranial bones, and proximal ends of the humerus and femur. They arise from large nucleated stem cells (promegaloblasts), which give rise to pronormoblasts, in which hemoglobin appears. These produce normoblasts, which extrude their nuclei. RBCs at this stage possess a fine reticular network and are known as reticulocytes. This reticular structure is usually lost before the cells enter circulation as mature RBCs. The proper formation of RBCs depends on several factors, including healthy condition of the bone marrow; dietary substances such as iron, cobalt, and copper, all essential for the formation of hemoglobin; essential amino acids; and

RUBRIBLAST

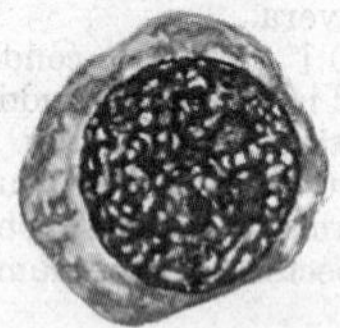

PRORUBRICYTE

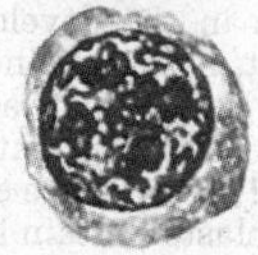

RUBRICYTE

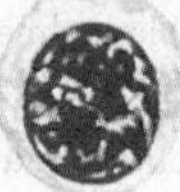

METARUBRICYTE

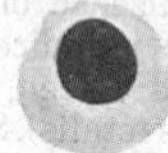

DIFFUSELY BASOPHILIC ERYTHROCYTE

ERYTHROCYTE

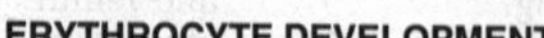

**ERYTHROCYTE DEVELOPMENT**

certain vitamins, esp. $B_{12}$ and folic acid (pteroylglutamic acid). SEE: illus. (Erythrocyte Development).

The average life span of an RBC is about 120 days. As RBCs age and become fragile, they are removed from circulation by macrophages in the liver, spleen, and red bone marrow. The protein and iron of hemoglobin are reused; iron may be stored in the liver until needed for the production of new RBCs in the bone marrow. The heme portion of the hemoglobin is converted to bilirubin, which is excreted in bile as one of the bile pigments.

VARIETIES: On microscopic examination, RBCs may reveal variations in the following respects: size (anisocytosis), shape (poikilocytosis), staining reaction (achromia, hypochromia, hyperchromia, polychromatophilia), structure (possession of bodies such as Cabot's rings, Howell-Jolly bodies, Heinz bodies; parasites such as malaria; a reticular network; or nuclei), and number (anemia, polycythemia). SEE: *blood, synthetic*.

***achromatic e.*** An RBC from which the hemoglobin has been dissolved; a colorless corpuscle.

***basophilic e.*** An RBC in which cytoplasm stains blue, indicating the presence of basophilic material. The staining may be diffuse (material uniformly distributed) or punctate (material appearing as pinpoint dots).

***crenated e.*** An RBC with a serrated or indented edge, usually the result of withdrawal of water from the cell, as occurs when cells are placed in hypertonic solutions.

***immature e.*** Any incompletely developed RBC.

***orthochromatic e.*** An RBC that stains with acid stains only, the cytoplasm appearing pink.

***polychromatic e.*** An RBC that does not stain uniformly.

**erythrocyte reinfusion** **1.** Infusion of blood into the person who donated it. This is usually done by obtaining one or two units of blood, separating the red blood cells and infusing them at a later date. **2.** Infusion with his or her own blood by a healthy person in an attempt to enhance athletic performance. SYN: *blood doping*.

**erythrocyte sedimentation rate** SEE: *sedimentation rate*.

**erythrocythemia** (ĕ-rĭth″rō-sī-thē′mē-ă) [Gr. *erythros,* red, + *kytos,* cell, + *haima,* blood] An enormous increase in circulating red blood cells. SEE: *erythremia; polycythemia vera*.

**erythrocytolysin** (ĕ-rĭth″rō-sī-tŏl′ĭ-sĭn) Anything that hemolyzes red blood cells.

**erythrocytolysis** (ĕ-rĭth″rō-sī-tŏl′ĭ-sĭs) [″ + ″ + *lysis,* dissolution] Dissolution of red blood cells with the escape of hemoglobin.

**erythrocytometer** (ĕ-rĭth″rō-sī-tŏm′ĕ-tĕr) [″ + ″ + *metron,* measure] An instrument for counting red blood cells.

**erythrocyto-opsonin** (ĕ-rĭth″rō-sī″tō-ŏp-sō′nĭn) [″ + ″ + *opsonein,* to buy food] A substance opsonic for red blood cells.

**erythrocytopenia** (ĕ-rĭth″rō-sī″tō-pē′nē-ă) [″ + ″+ *penia,* poverty] A deficiency in the number of red blood cells in the body. SYN: *erythropenia*.

**erythrocytopoiesis** Erythropoiesis.

**erythrocytorrhexis** (ĕ-rĭth″rō-sī″tō-rĕk′sĭs) [″ + ″ + *rhexis,* rupture] The breaking up of red blood cells with particles or fragments of the cells escaping into the plasma.

**erythrocytosis** (ĕ-rĭth″rō-sī-tō′sĭs) [″ + ″ + *osis,* increasing condition] An abnormal increase in the number of red blood cells in circulation, secondary to many disorders.

***spurious e., stress e.*** Gaisböck's syndrome.

**erythroderma** (ĕ-rĭth″rō-dĕr′mă) [″ + *derma,* skin] Abnormal redness of the skin, usually pert. to widespread areas of erythema. SYN: *erythrodermia*.

***e. desquamativum*** A disease of breast-fed infants. Resembling seborrhea, it is characterized by redness of the skin and development of scales.

***e. ichthyosiforme congenitum*** A congenital condition characterized by thickening and redness of the skin; it may resemble ichthyosis or lichen.

**erythrodermia** (ĕ-rĭth″rō-dĕr′mē-ă) Erythroderma.

**erythrodontia** (ĕ-rĭth″rō-dŏn′shē-ă) [″ + *odous,* tooth] Reddish-brown or yellow discoloration of the dentin of the teeth. This may be present in patients with congenital erythropoietic porphyria.

**erythrogenesis** (ĕ-rĭth″rō-jĕn′ĕ-sĭs) [″ + *genesis,* generation, birth] The development of red blood cells.

**erythroid** (ĕr′ĭ-throyd) [″ + *eidos,* form, shape] **1.** Reddish. **2.** Concerning the red blood cells.

**erythrokeratodermia** (ĕ-rĭth″rō-kĕr″ă-tō-dĕr′mē-ă) [″ + *keras,* horn, + *derma,* skin] Reddening and hardening of the skin.

**erythrokinetics** (ĕ-rĭth″rō-kĭ-nĕt′ĭks) [″ + *kinesis,* movement] The quantitative description of the production rate of red blood cells and their life span.

**erythroleukemia** (ĕ-rĭth″rō-loo-kē′mē-ă) [Gr. *erythros,* red, + *leukos,* white, + *haima,* blood] A variant of acute myelogenous leukemia with anemia, bizarre red blood cell morphology, erythroid hyperplasia in the bone marrow, and occasionally hepatosplenomegaly. The leukocyte count may be extremely high or quite low.

**erythromelalgia** (ĕ-rĭth″rō-mĕl-ăl′jē-ă) [″ + *melos,* limb, + *algos,* pain] A condition affecting the extremities, esp. the feet, marked by burning and throbbing sensations that come and go. SYN: *acromelalgia; erythralgia*.

**erythromelia** (ĕ-rĭth″rō-mē′lē-ă) [″ + *melos,* limb] Painless erythema of the extensor surfaces of the extremities.

**erythromycin** (ĕ-rĭth″rō-mī′sĭn) [″ + *mykes,* fungus] An antibiotic from *Streptomyces erythreus*. It is effective orally against many gram-positive and some gram-negative organisms.

**erythron** (ĕr′ĭ-thrŏn) [Gr. *erythros,* red] The blood as a body system including the circulating red cells and the tissue from which they originate.

**erythroneocytosis** (ĕ-rĭth″rō-nē″ō-sī-tō′sĭs) [″ + *neos,* new, + kytos, cell, + *osis,* condition] The presence of immature red blood cells in the peripheral blood.

**erythroparasite** (ĕ-rĭth″rō-păr′ă-sīt) [″ + *parasitos,* parasite] A red blood cell parasite.

**erythropenia** (ĕ-rĭth″rō-pē′nē-ă) [″ + *penia,* poverty] Erythrocytopenia.

**erythrophage** (ĕ-rĭth′rō-fāj) [″ + *phagein,* to eat] A phagocyte that destroys red blood cells.

**erythrophagia** Destruction of red blood cells

by phagocytes.

**erythrophile** (ĕ-rĭth'rō-fīl ["+ *philein,* to love]. An agent that readily stains red. **erythrophilous** (ĕr"ĭ-thrŏf'ĭ-lŭs), *adj.*

**erythrophobia** (ĕ-rĭth"rō-fō'bē-ă) [" + *phobos,* fear] **1.** Abnormal dread of blushing or fear of being diffident or embarrassed. **2.** Morbid fear of, or aversion to, anything red.

**erythrophose** (ĕ-rĭth'rō-fōz) [" + *phos,* light] Any red subjective perception of a bright spot. SEE: *phose.*

**erythropia, erythropsia** (ĕr"ĭ-thrō'pē-ă, -thrŏp'sē-ă) [" + *opsis,* vision] A condition in which objects appear to be red.

**erythroplasia** (ĕ-rĭth"rō-plā'zē-ă) [" + *plasis,* molding, forming] A condition characterized by erythematous lesions of the mucous membranes.

***e. of Queyrat*** [Louis A. Queyrat, Fr. physician, 1856–1953] A rare precancerous dermatosis of the genital mucosa that occurs predominantly in uncircumcised men. Treatment with topical application of 5% fluorouracil cream is usually effective.

**erythropoiesis** (ĕ-rĭth"rō-poy-ē'sĭs) [" + *poiesis,* making] The formation of red blood cells. **erythropoietic** (-ĕt'ĭk), *adj.*

**erythropoietin** (ĕ-rĭth"rō-poy'ĕ-tĭn) One of a specialized group of cytokines that is produced by the kidneys and stimulates the proliferation of red blood cells in the bone marrow. Other cytokines in the group stimulate production of other blood cells. Pharmacological erythropoietin (Epogen) is used in patients with depressed bone marrow function following cancer chemotherapy, bone marrow transplantation, and administration of zidovudine in HIV infection. SEE: *blood doping; cytokine; epoetin alfa.*

---

Caution: Athletes have used erythropoietin in an attempt to enhance performance. When the hormone is used without medical supervision and in large doses, it can cause an abnormal increase in red blood cell mass and may lead to death.

---

**erythroprosopalgia** (e-rĭth"rō-prō-sō-păl'jē-ă) [" + *prosopon,* face, + *algos,* pain] Neuropathy marked by redness and pain in the face.

**erythropsia** (ĕr-ĭ-thrŏp'sē-ă) [" + *opsis,* vision] A disorder of color vision in which all objects look red.

**erythropsin** (ĕ-rĭth-rŏp'sĭn) [" + *opsis,* vision] Pigment in the external portion of the rods of the retina. SYN: *rhodopsin.*

**erythrosine sodium** A dye used as a dental disclosing agent. It is applied to the teeth in a 2% solution or in soluble tablets, which are chewed. SEE: *disclosing agent.*

**erythrosis** (ĕr-ĭ-thrō'sĭs) [" + *osis,* condition] A reddish-purple discoloration of the skin and mucous membranes in polycythemia.

**erythrostasis** (ē-rĭth"rō-stā'sĭs) [" + *stasis,* standing still] Accumulation of red blood cells in vessels due to cessation of the blood flow. SEE: *sludged blood.*

**erythrotoxin** (ĕ-rĭth"rō-tŏk'sĭn) [" + *toxikon,* poison] An exotoxin that lyses red blood cells.

**erythruria** (ĕr-ĭ-thrū'rē-ă) [" + *ouron,* urine] Red color of the urine.

**Es** Symbol for the element einsteinium.

**escape** [O. Fr. *escaper*] **1.** To break out of confinement; to leak or seep out. **2.** The act of attaining freedom.

***vagal e.*** The occurrence of a ventricular contraction when the normal rhythmical beat of the heart has been stopped or inhibited by stimulation of the vagus nerve.

***ventricular e.*** The occurrence of single or repeated ventricular contractions from impulses arising in the atrioventricular node rather than the sinoauricular node. SYN: *nodal extrasystole.*

**escape phenomenon** The development of resistance to the effects of a continuously present stimulus.

**eschar** (ĕs'kăr) [Gr. *eschara,* scab] A slough, esp. one following a cauterization or burn. SEE: *escharotic.*

**escharotic** (ĕs-kăr-ŏt'ĭk) [Gr. *escharotikos*] An agent used to destroy tissue and to cause sloughing, which produces an eschar. Escharotics may be acids, alkalies, metallic salts, phenol or carbolic acid, carbon dioxide, or electric cautery.

**escharotomy** (ĕs-kăr-ŏt'ō-mē) [Gr. *eschara,* scab, + *tome,* incision] Removal of the eschar formed on the skin and underlying tissue of severely burned areas. This procedure can be life-saving when used to allow expansion of the chest and is also used to restore circulation to the extremities of patients in which the eschar forms a tight swollen band around the circumference of the limb.

**Escherichia** (ĕsh-ĕr-ĭk'ē-ă) A genus of bacteria belonging to the family Enterobacteriaceae, tribe Eschericheae. They are common inhabitants of the alimentary canal of humans and other animals.

**Escherichia coli** ABBR: *E. coli.* The colon bacillus. These short, plump, gram-negative, non–spore-forming motile bacilli are almost constantly present in the alimentary canal of humans and other animals. They are normally nonpathogenic in the intestinal tract. Outside the intestine and under certain conditions, particularly in the urinary tract, *E. coli* is responsible for infections in other systems and for enteritis in infants and adults. Certain enterotoxigenic strains are a principal cause of travelers' diarrhea. The presence of the bacilli in milk or water is an indicator of fecal contamination.

***enteroaggregative E.c.*** ABBR: EAggEC. A type of *E. coli* that causes persistent diarrhea.

***enterohemorrhagic E.c.*** ABBR: EHEC. The strain of *E. coli* that causes colitis with copious bloody discharges.

TREATMENT: Fluid and electrolyte balance should be maintained and an appropriate antibiotic given.

***enteroinvasive E.c.*** ABBR: EIEC. A type of *E. coli* that invades and multiplies in the epithelial cells of the distal ileum and colon. The clinical syndrome is the same as for *Shigella* infections.

TREATMENT: Fluid and electrolyte balance should be maintained and an appropriate antibiotic, usually trimethoprim-sulfamethoxazole, should be given.

***enteropathogenic E.c.*** ABBR: EPEC. A type of *E. coli* that produces infantile diarrhea.

TREATMENT: Fluid and electrolyte balance should be maintained and oral nonabsorbable antibiotics given. SEE: *oral rehydration therapy.*

***enterotoxigenic E.c.*** ABBR: ETEC. A type of *E. coli* that can cause diarrhea in infants and travelers. Fluid loss may be as severe as in cholera.

TREATMENT: Fluid and electrolyte balance should be maintained, and antidiarrheal medicines should be given in addition to trimethoprim-sulfamethoxazole or doxycycline. SEE: *diarrhea, travelers'; oral rehydration therapy.*

***E.c. O157:H7*** An enterohemorrhagic *E. coli* serotype that produces verotoxin, also called *Shiga-like toxin.* It was first recognized as a cause of an outbreak of hemorrhagic colitis in 1982. Since that time, a number of outbreaks have occurred in schools, nursing homes, day care centers, families, and communities. The organism may be present in undercooked meat, esp. hamburger; unpreserved apple cider; vegetables grown in cow manure; or contaminated water supplies. The infection may be spread from one person to another through food-to-food cross-contamination.

SYMPTOMS: Asymptomatic infection is common. In other cases, after the 3- to 8-day incubation period, an afebrile and self-limiting diarrhea occurs; however, the infection may progress to hemorrhagic colitis with bloody diarrhea, severe abdominal pain, and low-grade fever. Resolution usually occurs in 1 week. In 2% to 7% of cases, patients will develop hemolytic uremic syndrome (HUS); the mortality among patients who develop HUS ranges from 3% to 5%. The highest incidence of HUS is found among children and the elderly.

DIAGNOSIS: Without a high index of suspicion, diagnosis in either a lone case or an outbreak may be delayed. To prevent unnecessary diagnostic or therapeutic intervention, such as colonoscopy or colectomy, diagnosis be made as quickly as possible.

TREATMENT: The primary emphasis is on supportive therapy; antibiotic therapy is not beneficial. Dialysis is important if kidney failure occurs.

PREVENTION: Ground meat should be cooked until it reaches a temperature of 160°F (71.1°C) and the meat should not be pink in the center. Leftovers should be reheated to 165°F (73.3°C). Individuals who change a baby's diapers should thoroughly wash their hands immediately afterward. Food handlers must wash their hands after using the toilet.

**Escherich's reflex** (ĕsh'ĕr-ĭks) [Theodor Escherich, Ger. physician, 1857–1911] A pursing or muscular contraction of the lips resulting from irritation of the mucosa of the lips.

**eschrolalia** (ĕs-krō-lā'lē-ă) [Gr. *aischros,* indecent, + *lalia,* babble] Coprolalia.

**escorcin** (ĕs-kor'sĭn) A stain derived from escalin. It is used to stain and identify defects or injury of the cornea.

**esculent** (ĕs'kū-lĕnt) Suitable for use as food.

**escutcheon** (ĕs-kŭch'ăn) [L. *scutum,* a shield] The pattern of pubic hair growth. It is different in males and females.

**eserine** (ĕs'ĕr-ĭn) [*esere,* African name for the Calabar bean] Physostigmine.

**ESF** *erythropoietic stimulating factor.* SEE: *erythropoietin.*

**-esis** Suffix meaning *condition* or *state.* SEE: *-sis; -asis; -osis.*

**Esmarch's bandage** (ĕs'mărks) [Johannes F. A. von Esmarch, Ger. surgeon, 1823–1908] **1.** A triangular bandage. **2.** A rubber bandage used to control bleeding. Before surgery is begun, the bandage is applied tightly to the limb, commencing at the distal end and reaching above the site of operation, where a rubber tourniquet is firmly applied. The bandage is then removed, rendering the surgical area virtually bloodless. SEE: *bandage.*

Caution: The tourniquet must not be applied so tightly as to cause nerve damage and it must be removed in time to prevent injury caused by lack of blood flow to the distal tissues.

**esodic** (ē-sŏd'ĭk) [Gr. *es,* toward, + *hodos,* way] Pert. to sensory nerves conducting impulses toward the brain and spinal cord. SYN: *afferent; centripetal.*

**esoethmoiditis** (ĕs"ō-ĕth"moy-dī'tĭs) [Gr. *eso,* inward, + *ethmos,* sieve, + *eidos,* form, shape, + *itis,* inflammation] Inflammation of the membrane of ethmoid cells.

**esogastritis** (ĕs"ō-găs-trī'tĭs) [" + *gaster,* belly, + *itis,* inflammation] Inflammation of the gastric mucous membrane.

**esophagalgia** (ē-sŏf-ă-găl'jē-ă) [Gr. *oisophagos,* esophagus, + *algos,* pain] Pain in the esophagus.

**esophageal** (ē-sŏf"ă-jē'ăl) Pert. to the esophagus.

**esophageal apoplexy** SEE: *apoplexy, esophageal.*

**esophageal cancer** The presence of a malignancy in the esophagus. Esophageal cancer arises in the squamous epithelium in

98% of cases, with a few adenocarcinomas and fewer melanomas and sarcomas. About 50% of the squamous cell cancers occur in the lower portion of the esophagus, 40% in the midportion, and the remaining 10% in the upper or cervical esophagus. The disease is most common in men over age 60 and occurs worldwide, with more than 8,000 cases reported annually in the U.S. Esophageal cancer is also common in Japan, Russia, China, and the Middle East and has reached almost epidemic proportions in the Transkei region of South Africa.

Esophageal tumors usually are fungating and infiltrating, and in most cases, the tumor partially constricts the esophageal lumen. Regional metastasis occurs early by way of submucosal lymphatics, often fatally invading adjacent vital intrathoracic organs. The liver and lungs are the usual sites of distant metastases.

PREDISPOSING FACTORS: The cause of esophageal cancer is unknown; however, several predisposing factors have been identified. These include chronic irritation from heavy smoking or excessive use of alcohol; stasis-induced inflammation, as in achalasia or stricture; previous head and neck tumors; and nutritional deficiency, as in untreated sprue and Plummer-Vinson syndrome.

COMPLICATIONS: Direct invasion of adjoining structures may lead to severe complications, such as mediastinitis, tracheoesophageal or bronchoesophageal fistula (causing an overwhelming cough when swallowing liquids), and aortic perforation with sudden exsanguination. Other complications include an inability to control secretions, obstruction of the esophagus, and loss of lower esophageal sphincter control, which can result in aspiration pneumonia.

SIGNS AND SYMPTOMS: Early in the disease, the patient may report a feeling of fullness, pressure, indigestion, or substernal burning and may report using antacids to relieve gastrointestinal upset. Later, the patient may complain of dysphagia and weight loss. The degree of dysphagia varies, depending on the extent of the disease, ranging from mild dysphagia occurring only after eating solid foods (esp. meat) to difficulty in swallowing coarse foods and even liquids. The patient may complain of hoarseness (from laryngeal nerve involvement), a chronic cough (possibly from aspiration), anorexia, vomiting, and regurgitation of food. These latter symptoms result from the tumor size exceeding the limits of the esophagus. The patient may also complain of pain on swallowing or pain that radiates to the back. In the later stages of the disease, the patient will appear very thin, cachectic, and dehydrated.

DIAGNOSTIC TESTS: Radiography of the esophagus, with barium swallow and motility studies; chest radiography or esophagography; esophagoscopy; punch and brush biopsies; and exfoliative cytological tests; bronchoscopy; endoscopic ultrasonography of the esophagus; computed tomography scan; magnetic resonance imaging; liver function studies; a liver scan; and mediastinal tomography may be performed to delineate the tumor, confirm its type, reveal growth into adjacent structures, and reveal distant metastatic lesions.

TREATMENT: Because esophageal cancer usually is advanced when diagnosed, treatment is palliative to relieve disease effects. Treatment to keep the esophagus patent includes dilation, laser therapy, radiation therapy, and insertion of prosthetic tubes to bridge the tumor. Radical surgery can excise the tumor and resect either the esophagus alone or the stomach and esophagus. Chemotherapy and radiation therapy can slow the growth of the tumor. Gastrostomy or jejunostomy can help provide adequate nutrition. A prosthesis can be used to seal fistulae. Endoscopic laser treatment and bipolar electrocoagulation can help restore swallowing by vaporizing cancerous tissue; however, if the tumor is in the upper esophagus, the laser cannot be positioned properly. Analgesics provide pain control.

PROGNOSIS: Regardless of cell type, the prognosis for esophageal cancer is grim: 5-year survival rates are less than 5%, and most patients die within 6 months of diagnosis.

NURSING IMPLICATIONS: The patient is assessed for signs and symptoms as above. Food and fluid intake and body weight are monitored. All procedures are explained; the patient is prepared physically and emotionally for surgery and postsurgical care as indicated.

A high-calorie, high-protein diet is provided. Pureed or liquefied foods and commercially available nutritional supplements are offered as necessary. Enteral feedings and supplemental parenteral nutrition are administered as prescribed. The patient is placed in Fowler's position for meals and plenty of time is allowed to eat to prevent aspiration. Any regurgitation is documented, and oral hygiene is provided. Prescribed analgesics and noninvasive pain relief measures are provided.

When a gastrostomy tube is used, feedings are administered slowly by gravity in prescribed amounts (usually 200 to 500 ml), and the patient is given something to chew before and during each feeding to stimulate gastric secretions and promote some semblance of normal eating. The patient and family are taught about nutritional concerns (e.g., care of the feeding tube, including checking patency, administering the feeding, providing skin care at the insertion site, and keeping the patient upright during and immediately after feedings).

After surgery, vital signs and fluid and electrolyte balance (including intake and output) are monitored. The patient is observed for complications, such as infection, fistula formation, pneumonia, empyema, and malnutrition. If surgical resection with an esophageal anastomosis was performed, the patient is positioned flat on the back to prevent tension on the suture line and observed for signs of an anastomotic leak. If a prosthetic tube was inserted, the patient is monitored for signs of blockage or dislodgement, which can perforate the mediastinum or precipitate tumor erosion.

If chemotherapy is prescribed, the patient is monitored for complications such as bone marrow suppression and gastrointestinal reactions, adverse reactions are minimized by use of saline mouthwashes, extra periods of rest are encouraged, and prescribed medications are administered. If radiation therapy is used, the patient is monitored for complications such as esophageal perforation, pneumonitis, lung fibrosis, and spinal cord myelitis.

Expected outcomes of the prescribed therapies are explained to the patient and family, assurance is provided that pain will be managed, and the nurse stays with the patient during periods of anxiety or distress. The patient is encouraged to participate in care decisions.

The patient should resume as normal a routine as possible during recovery to maintain a sense of control and to reduce complications associated with immobility. Both patient and family are referred to appropriate organizations for information and support.

**esophageal obturator airway** ABBR: EOA. An airway device (primarily used in emergency medical service systems) in which the tube is blindly inserted into the esophagus, thereby blocking vomitus and permitting lung ventilation.

**esophageal varix** *pl.* **esophageal varices** A tortuous dilatation of an espohageal vein, esp. in the distal portion. It may be associated with any condition that causes chronic obstruction of venous drainage from the esophageal veins into the portal vein of the liver. Cirrhosis of the liver is frequently associated with this condition. SEE: *Mallory-Weiss syndrome; Müller maneuver.*

TREATMENT: The injection of sclerosing agents into or adjacent to the varices, or both, combined with the infusion of octreotide, a synthetic somatostatin analogue, for 5 days is more effective than sclerosing therapy alone.

**esophageal web** A group of thin membranous structures that include mucosal and submucosal coats across the esophagus. They may be congenital or may follow trauma, inflammation, or ulceration of the esophagus. SEE: *Plummer-Vinson syndrome.*

**esophagectasia, esophagectasis** (ē-sŏf″ă-jĕk-tā′sē-ă, -jĕk′tă-sĭs) [″ + *ektasis,* distention] Dilatation of the esophagus.

**esophagectomy** (ē-sŏf″ă-jĕk′tō-mē) [″ + *ektome,* excision] Excision of a part of the esophagus.

**esophagismus** (ē-sŏf-ă-jĭs′mŭs) [″ + *-ismos,* condition] Esophageal spasm.

**esophagitis** (ē-sŏf-ă-jī′tĭs) [″ + *itis,* inflammation] Inflammation of the esophagus. SEE: *acid reflux test.*

***reflux e.*** SEE: *gastroesophageal reflux; reflux disease.*

**esophagobronchial** (ĕ-sŏf″ă-gō-brŏng′kē-ăl) [″ + *bronchos,* windpipe] Concerning the esophagus and bronchus.

**esophagocele** (ē-sŏf′ă-gō-sēl) [″ + *kele,* tumor, swelling] A hernia of the esophagus.

**esophagodynia** (ē-sŏf″ă-gō-dĭn′ē-ă) [Gr. *oisophagos,* esophagus, + *odyne,* pain] Pain in the esophagus.

**esophagoenterostomy** (ē-sŏf″ă-gō-ĕn-tĕr-ŏs′tō-mē) [″ + *enteron,* intestine, + *stoma,* mouth] A surgical opening between the esophagus and intestine following excision of the stomach.

**esophagogastrectomy** (ĕ-sŏf″ă-gō-găs-trĕk′tō-mē) [″ + *gaster,* belly, + *ektome,* excision] Surgical removal of all or part of the stomach and esophagus.

**esophagogastroanastomosis** (ĕ-sŏf″ă-gō-găs″trō-ă-năs″tō-mō′sĭs) [″ + ″ + *anastomosis,* opening] A joining of the esophagus to the stomach.

**esophagogastroplasty** (ĕ-sŏf′ă-gō-găs′trō-plăs″tē) [″ + ″ + *plassein,* to form] Plastic repair of the esophagus and stomach.

**esophagogastroscopy** (ē-sŏf″ă-gō-găs-trŏs′kō-pē) [″ + ″ + *skopein,* to examine] Inspection of the esophagus and stomach by using an endoscope.

**esophagogastrostomy** (ē-sŏf″ă-gō-găs-trŏs′tō-mē) [″ + ″ + *stoma,* mouth] Formation of an opening between the esophagus and stomach.

**esophagojejunostomy** (ĕ-sŏf″ă-gō-jĕ-jū-nŏs′tō-mē) [″ + L. *jejunum,* empty, + Gr. *stoma,* mouth] The surgical anastomosis of a free end of the jejunum to the esophagus. It provides a bypass for food in cases of esophageal stricture.

**esophagomalacia** (ē-sŏf″ă-gō-mă-lā′sē-ă) [Gr. *oisophagos,* esophagus, + *malakia,* softness] Softening of the esophageal walls.

**esophagomycosis** (ē-sŏf″ă-gō-mī-kō′sĭs) [″ + *mykes,* fungus, + *osis,* condition] A bacterial or fungal disease of the esophagus.

**esophagomyotomy** (ĕ-sŏf″ă-gō-mī-ŏt′ō-mē) [″ + *mys,* muscle, + *tome,* incision] Cutting of the muscular coat of the esophagus, used in treating stenosis of the lower esophagus. SEE: *Schatzki ring.*

**esophagoplasty** (ē-sŏf′ă-gō-plăs″tē) [″ + *plassein,* to form] Repair of the esophagus by plastic surgery.

**esophagoplication** (ē-sŏf″ă-gō-plĭ-kā′shŭn)

[″ + L. *abplicare,* to fold] Surgical reduction of dilation of the esophagus by taking tucks in its walls.

**esophagoptosia, esophagoptosis** (ē-sŏf″ă-gŏp-tō′sē-ă, -sĭs) [″ + *ptosis,* a dropping] Relaxation and prolapse of the esophagus.

**esophagoscope** (ē-sŏf′ă-gō-skōp) [″ + *skopein,* to examine] An endoscope for examination of the esophagus.

**esophagospasm** (ē-sŏf′ă-gō-spăzm″) [″ + *spasmos,* a convulsion] A spasm of the esophagus.

**esophagostenosis** (ē-sŏf″ă-gō-stĕn-ō′sĭs) [″ + *stenosis,* act of narrowing] Stricture or narrowing of the esophagus.

**esophagostomy** (ē-sŏf-ă-gŏs′tō-mē) [″ + *stoma,* mouth] Surgical formation of an opening into the esophagus.

**esophagotome** (ē-sŏf′ă-gō-tōm) [″ + *tome,* incision] An instrument for forming an esophageal fistula.

**esophagotomy** (ē-sŏf-ă-gŏt′ō-mē) A surgical incision into the esophagus. SEE: *achalasia; cardiospasm; dysphagia.*

**esophagotracheal** (ĕ-sŏf″ă-gō-trā′kē-ăl) Concerning the esophagus and the trachea, or a communication between them.

**esophagus** (ē-sŏf′ă-gŭs) *pl.* **esophagi** [Gr. *oisophagos*] The muscular tube, about 9 to 9.75 in. (23 to 25 cm) long, that carries swallowed foods and liquids from the pharynx to the stomach. At the junction with the stomach is the lower esophageal or cardiac sphincter, which relaxes to permit passage of food, then contracts to prevent backup of stomach contents.

Foreign Body in Esophagus: A patient with a foreign body in the esophagus may complain of pain or an uncomfortable feeling deep in the chest. Foreign bodies are ordinarily not dangerous and usually pass safely through the alimentary tract in a few days. However, it may be dangerous to give cathartics or enemas. These patients should always be under the care of a physician. SEE: *Heimlich maneuver.*

First Aid: The article often can be dislodged if the patient is made to vomit by stimulation of the oral pharynx or back part of the throat with a finger.

**esophoria** (ĕs-ō-fō′rē-ă) [Gr. *eso,* inward, + *phorein,* to bear] **1.** The tendency of visual lines to converge. **2.** An inward turning, or the amount of inward turning, of the eye. Opposite of exophoria. SYN: *esotropia.* SEE: *heterotropia.*

**esosphenoiditis** (ĕs″ō-sfē-noyd-ī′tĭs) [″ + *sphen,* wedge, + *eidos,* form, shape, + *itis,* inflammation] Osteomyelitis of the sphenoid bone.

**esotropia** (ĕs-ō-trō′pē-ă) [″ + *tropos,* turning] Marked turning inward of the eye; crossed eyes.

**ESP** *extrasensory perception.*

**ESR** *electron spin resonance; erythrocyte sedimentation rate.*

**ESRD** *end-stage renal disease.*

**essence** [L. *essentia,* being or quality] **1.** The spirit or principle of anything. **2.** An alcoholic solution of volatile oil.

**essential** [L. *essentialis*] **1.** Pert. to an essence. **2.** Indispensable. **3.** Independent of a local abnormal condition; having no obvious external cause. SEE: *idiopathic.*

**EST** *electroshock therapy.* SEE: *electroconvulsive therapy.*

**ester** [L. *aether,* ether] In organic chemistry, a fragrant compound formed by the combination of an organic acid with an alcohol. This reaction removes water from the compound.

**esterase** (ĕs′tĕr-ās) Generic term for an enzyme that catalyzes the hydrolysis of esters.

**esterification** (ĕs-tĕr″ĭ-fĭ-kā′shŭn) The combination of an organic acid with an alcohol to form an ester.

**esthematology** (ĕs″thĕm-ă-tŏl′ō-jē) [Gr. *aisthema,* sensation, + *logos,* word, reason] The science of the sense organs and their function.

**esthesia** (ĕs-thē′zē-ă) [Gr. *aisthesis,* sensation] **1.** Perception; feeling; sensation. **2.** Any disease that affects sensation or perception.

**esthesiology** (ĕs-thē″zē-ŏl′ō-jē) [″ + *logos,* word, reason] The science of sensory phenomena.

**esthesiometer, aesthesiometer** (ĕs-thē-zē-ŏm′ĕ-tĕr) [″ + *metron,* measure] A device for measuring tactile sensibility.

**esthesioneurosis** (ĕs-thē″zē-ō-nū-rō′sĭs) [″ + *neuron,* nerve, + *osis,* condition] Any sensory impairment.

**esthesiophysiology** (ĕs-thē″sē-ō-fĭs-ē-ŏl′ō-jē) [″ + *physis,* nature, + *logos,* study] The physiology of the sense organs.

**esthesioscopy** (ĕs-thē″zē-ŏs′kō-pē) [″ + *skopein,* to examine] The testing of tactile and other forms of sensibility.

**estheticokinetic** (ĕs-thĕt″ĭ-kō-kĭn-ĕt′ĭk) [″ + *kinesis,* movement] Being both sensory and motor.

**esthetics** (ĕs-thĕt′ĭks) Aesthetics.

**estival** (ĕs′tĭ-văl) [L. *aestivus*] Pert. to or occurring in summer.

**estivoautumnal** [″ + *autumnalis,* pert. to autumn] Pert. to summer and autumn, formerly applied to a type of malaria.

**estradiol** (ĕs-tră-dī′ŏl) $C_{18}H_{24}O_2$, a steroid produced by the ovary and possessing estrogenic properties. Large quantities are found in the urine of pregnant women and of mares and stallions, the latter two serving as sources of the commercial product. Estradiol is effective when given subcutaneously or intramuscularly but not when given orally. It is converted to estrone in the body. SEE: *diethylstilbestrol; estrogen.*

***e. dipropionate*** An ester of estradiol.

**estrin** (ĕs′trĭn) Estrogen.

**estrinization** (ĕs″trĭn-ĭ-zā′shŭn) The production of vaginal epithelial changes characteristic of estrogen stimulation.

**estriol** (ĕs′trē-ŏl) $C_{18}H_{24}O_3$, an estrogenic

hormone considered to be the metabolic product of estrone and estradiol. It is found in the urine of women.

**estrogen** (ĕs′trō-jĕn) [Gr. *oistros,* mad desire, + *gennan,* to produce] Any natural or artificial substance that induces estrus and the development of female sex characteristics; more specifically, the estrogenic hormones produced by the ovary; the female sex hormones. Estrogens are responsible for cyclic changes in the vaginal epithelium and endometrium of the uterus. Natural estrogens include estradiol, estrone, and their metabolic product, estriol. When used therapeutically, estrogens are usually given in the form of a conjugate such as ethinyl estradiol, conjugated estrogens, or the synthetic estrogenic substance diethylstilbestrol. These preparations are effective when given by mouth.

Estrogens provide a satisfactory replacement hormone for treating menopausal symptoms and for reducing the risk of osteoporosis and cardiovascular disease in postmenopausal women. It is important to observe patients closely for any malignant changes in the breast or endometrium. Estrogen should be administered intermittently and in the lowest effective dose.

***conjugated e.*** Estrogenic substance, principally estrone and equilin, excreted in the urine of pregnant mares. Trade name is Premarin.

**estrogenic** (ĕs-trō-jĕn′ĭk) Causing estrus; acting to produce the effects of an estrogen.

**estrogen replacement therapy** ABBR: ERT. Administration of estrogen to women who have a deficiency of this hormone (e.g., menopausal and postmenopausal women) and women with hypothalamic amenorrhea. Estrogen is also used as adjunctive therapy for inoperable breast cancer and prostatic cancers.

Reported health benefits include a lowered risk of cardiovascular disorders (i.e., atherosclerosis, heart disease, and stroke), owing to improved cholesterol levels and blood lipid ratios; the level of high-density lipoproteins rises and that of low-density lipoproteins diminishes. Also, ERT is credited with retarding bone loss and lowering the risk of osteoporotic fractures. In addition, ERT relieves symptoms associated with menopause (e.g., hot flashes, diaphoresis, vaginal dryness, dyspareunia, moodiness, depression, and insomnia).

---

CAUTION: Women who have a history of thromboembolic disorders, impaired liver function, undiagnosed vaginal bleeding, or estrogen-stimulated tumors should not receive ERT. Estrogen replacement should be used with caution in women who have a family history of breast cancer or abnormal mammograms, who develop benign cystic breast disease while on ERT, or who have diseases of the liver, kidney, or gallbladder.

---

RISKS: An increased risk of uterine endometrial cancer has been linked with long-term use of estrogen. Controversy has surrounded a possible association with increased risk of breast cancer. Combined estrogen-progestin therapy provides the added benefit of lowered risk for development of estrogen-related malignancies. SEE: *estrogen, conjugated; hormone replacement therapy.*

**estrone** (ĕs′trōn) $C_{18}H_{22}O_2$. An estrogenic hormone found in the urine of pregnant women and mares. Also prepared synthetically, it is used in the treatment of estrogen deficiencies. It is less active than estradiol but more active than estriol. Trade name is Theelin.

**estropipate** Estrogen. The previously used name was *piperazine estrone citrate.* Trade name is Ogen.

**estrual** (ĕs′troo-ăl) [Gr. *oistros,* mad desire] Pert. to the estrus of animals.

**estruation** The sexually fertile period in animals; the so-called period of heat.

**estrus, oestrus** [Gr. *oistros,* mad desire] The cyclic period of sexual activity in nonhuman female mammals, marked by congestion of and secretion by the uterine mucosa, proliferation of vaginal epithelium, swelling of the vulva, ovulation, and acceptance of the male by the female. During estrus, the animal is said to be "in heat."

**estrus cycle** The sequence from the beginning of one estrus period to the beginning of the next. It includes proestrus, estrus, and metestrus followed by a short period of quiescence called diestrus.

**e.s.u.** *electrostatic unit.*

**état criblé** (ā-tă′ krēb-lā′) [Fr., sievelike state] Multiple irregular perforations of Peyer's patches of the intestines. These patches are characteristic of typhoid fever.

**etching** (ĕch′ĭng) [Ger. *ätzen,* to feed] Application of a corrosive or abrasive material to a glass or metal surface to create a pattern or design.

***acid e.*** A dental procedure used to roughen the surface of tooth enamel for better mechanical retention in bonding resin to the tooth structure.

**ethacrynic acid** A diuretic drug. Trade name is Edecrin.

**ethambutol hydrochloride** (ĕ-thăm′bū-tōl) A drug used in treating tuberculosis. It is used in combination with isoniazid.

**ethanol** (ĕth′ă-nŏl) Ethyl alcohol. SEE: *alcohol.*

**ethaverine hydrochloride** (ĕth″ă-vĕr′ēn) A drug used to relax the coronary artery. Its use is controversial.

**ethchlorvynol** (ĕth-klor′vĭ-nŏl) A sedative hypnotic drug that may produce addiction. Trade name is Placidyl.

**ethene** (ĕth-ēn′) $CH_2{=}CH_2$. Ethylene.

**ether** (ēth′ĕr) [Gr. *aither,* air] Any organic compound in which an oxygen atom links with carbon chains. The ether used for anesthesia is diethyl ether, $C_4H_{10}O$. As an anesthetic it causes postoperative nausea and profuse salivation. **ethereal** (ĕ-thē′rē-ăl), *adj.*

**ether anesthesia** $C_4H_{10}O$. Diethyl ether, the common ether previously used in anesthesia. It is rarely used now.

Caution: Ether is highly flammable and should be handled with great care. Also, it should not be stored once its container has been opened because toxic products form when ether is exposed to light.

**ether asphyxia** Suffocation during ether anesthetization. SEE: *resuscitation.*

**etherization** (ē″thĕr-ĭ-zā′shŭn) Administration of ether to induce anesthesia.

**etherize** (ē′thĕr-īz) To anesthetize by use of ether.

**ethics** [Gr. *ethos,* moral custom] A system of moral principles or standards governing conduct. SEE: *Declaration of Geneva; Declaration of Hawaii; Hippocratic oath; Nightingale Pledge; Prayer of Maimonides.*

***dental e.*** A system of principles governing dental practice; a moral obligation to render the best possible quality of dental service to the patient and to maintain an honest relationship with other members of the profession and people in general.

***medical e.*** A system of principles governing medical conduct. It deals with the relationship of a physician to the patient, the patient's family, fellow physicians, and society at large. SEE: *advance directive; do not attempt resuscitation; euthanasia; Hippocratic oath; living will.*

***nursing e.*** A system of principles governing the conduct of a nurse. It deals with the relationship of a nurse to the patient, the patient's family, associates and fellow nurses, and society at large. SEE: *Nightingale Pledge.*

**ethinamate** (ĕ-thĭn′ă-māt) A mild sedative and hypnotic drug.

**ethinyl estradiol** (ĕth′ĭ-nĭl) SEE: *estradiol.*

**ethionamide** (ĕ-thī″ŏn-ăm′īd) A drug used in treating tuberculosis. It is used in combination with other drugs. Trade name is Trecator-SC.

**ethionine** (ĕ-thī′ō-nĭn) A progestational agent used in some oral contraceptives.

**ethmoid** (ĕth′moyd) [Gr. *ēthmos,* sieve, + *eidos,* form, shape] Cribriform.

**ethmoidal** Pert. to the ethmoid bone or sinuses.

**ethmoid bone** A sievelike, spongy bone that forms a roof for the nasal fossae and part of the floor of the anterior fossa of the skull. It permits passage of the olfactory nerves to the brain and also contains three groups of air cavities, the ethmoid sinuses, which open into the nasal cavity.

**ethmoidectomy** (ĕth-moy-dĕk′tō-mē) [″ + *eidos,* form, shape, + *ektome,* excision] Excision of the ethmoid sinuses that open into the nasal cavity.

**ethmoiditis** (ĕth″moy-dī′tĭs) [″ + ″ + *itis,* inflammation] Inflammation of the ethmoidal sinuses. This may be acute or chronic.

SYMPTOMS: Symptoms include headache, acute pain between the eyes, and a nasal discharge.

**ethmoid sinus** An air cavity or space within the ethmoid bone, opening into the nasal cavity.

**ethnic** (ĕth′nĭk) [Gr. *ethnikos,* of a nation] Concerning groups of people within a cultural system who desire or are given a distinct classification based on traits such as religion, culture, language, or appearance.

**ethnobiology** (ĕth″nō-bī-ŏl′ō-jē) [Gr. *ethnos,* race, + *bios,* life, + *logos,* word, reason] The study of the biological characteristics of various races.

**ethnocentrism** **1.** A belief that one's own way of viewing and experiencing the world is superior to other perspectives; a mindset that judges the actions and beliefs of others according to one's own cultural background rules. **2.** In health care, a perspective that supports the worldview of the caretaker, rather than considering the patient's perspective of health and illness. **ethnocentric,** *adj.*

**ethnogerontology** The study of aging and population groups in reference to race, national origin, and cultural practices. Ethnogerontology addresses the causes, processes, heritage, and consequences specific to these groups.

**ethnography** (ĕth-nŏg′ră-fē) [″ + *graphein,* to write] The study of the culture of a single society. Data are gathered by direct observation during a period of residence with the group. SEE: *anthropology.*

**ethnology** (ĕth-nŏl′ō-jē) [″ + *logos,* word, reason] The comparative study of cultures using ethnographic data. SEE: *anthropology.*

**ethology** (ē-, ē-thŏl′ō-jē) [Gr. *ethos,* manners, habits, + *logos,* word, reason] The scientific study of the customs and behavior of animals in their natural habitat and in captivity.

**ethopropazine hydrochloride** (ĕth″ō-prō′pă-zēn) An autonomic nervous system blocking agent used in treating parkinsonism. Trade name is Parsidol.

**ethosuximide** (ĕth″ō-sŭk′sĭ-mīd) An anticonvulsant drug. Trade name is Zarontin.

**ethotoin** (ĕ-thō′tō-ĭn) An anticonvulsant that is little used because of its moderate effectiveness. Trade name is Peganone.

**ethyl** (ĕth′ĭl) [Gr. *aither,* air, + *hyle,* matter] In organic chemistry, the radical $C_2H_5$, which is contained in many compounds, including ethyl ether, ethyl alcohol, and ethyl acetate.

***e. acetate*** $C_4H_8O_2$. A colorless flammable liquid used as a solvent.

***e. alcohol*** $C_2H_6O$. Grain alcohol. SEE: *alcohol; Poisons and Poisoning Appendix.*

***e. aminobenzoate*** Benzocaine, a topical anesthetic.

***e. biscoumacetate*** An anticoagulant drug.

***e. chloride*** $C_2H_5Cl$. A very volatile liquid with a pleasant odor. When sprayed on the skin, it evaporates so quickly that the tissue is cooled immediately. Because of this property, the skin is anesthetized.

USES: Ethyl chloride is used as a topical local anesthetic in minor surgery. It is used only for very short periods.

**ethylamine** (ĕth″ĭl-ăm′ĭn) $CH_3CH_2NH_2$. An amine formed in the decomposition of certain proteins.

**ethylcellulose** (ĕth″ĭl-sĕl′ū-lōs) An ether of cellulose, used in preparing drugs.

**ethylene** (ĕth′ĭl-ēn) ABBR: ETO. $CH_2CH_2$. A flammable, explosive, colorless gas prepared from alcohol by dehydration. It is present in illuminating gas. It is colorless and has a sweetish taste but a pungent, foul odor. It is lighter than air and diffuses when liberated.

***e. glycol*** $C_2H_6O_2$. The simplest glycol; a colorless alcohol used as an antifreeze. SEE: *Poisons and Poisoning Appendix.*

***e. oxide*** ABBR: EtO. A chemical, $C_2H_4O$, that in its gaseous state is used to sterilize materials that cannot withstand heat or steam. It is also used as a fumigant.

**ethylene anesthesia** Ethylene given as a combination of oxygen 20%, cyclopropane 10%, and ethylene 70%. Because it is a rather weak anesthetic, it is not given alone.

PHYSICAL EFFECTS: Ethylene causes less alteration in the blood gases than nitrous oxide. Ethylene alone causes very little muscular relaxation; the blood pressure may rise and respiration is not depressed. Analgesia results before loss of hearing or complete unconsciousness. Nausea and vomiting seldom persist as long as 24 hr, but generally disappear before consciousness has returned.

ADVANTAGES: Ethylene is slightly stimulating to the cardiac and respiratory systems. It does not irritate mucous glands and kidneys. It has a short period of induction and allows a very rapid recovery. Cyanosis is absent and emesis is minimal.

DISADVANTAGES: Ethylene has an objectionable smell. It is highly flammable and explosive; lives have been lost because someone was careless and a spark was produced from some immediate source.

PRECAUTIONS: Ethylene should be stored where there is adequate ventilation. It should be administered away from fire, electrical appliances, or x-ray apparatus. To prevent sparks, all lights should be turned on before the tanks are brought into the room. Furniture should never be dragged or rolled into the room while the anesthetic is being given. The humidity of the room should be controlled during administration. Nylon clothing or undergarments should not be worn by anyone in the room; friction from the material may generate static electricity.

Ethylene does not combine as readily with air as do other volatile anesthetics, but floats around as clouds. The vapor rises in a cloudlike form and any gust of air may carry it out of the room; a devastating explosion will result if someone on the outside is smoking or if the fumes contact an electrical spark.

Ethylene always is stored in red tanks, oxygen in green tanks, nitrous oxide in blue tanks, and carbon dioxide in gray tanks.

**ethylenediamine** (ĕth″ĭ-lēn-dī′ă-mēn) Drug used as a solvent for theophylline; it is therefore present in aminophylline injection.

**ethylenediaminetetra-acetic acid** ABBR: EDTA. A chelating agent used in treating exposure to toxic chemicals.

**ethylnorepinephrine hydrochloride** (ĕth″ĭl-nor-ĕp″ĭ-nĕf″rĭn) An adrenergic drug used in treating asthma. Trade name is Bronkephrine.

**ethynodiol diacetate** (ĕ-thī″nō-dī′ōl) A progesterone used as an oral contraceptive in combination with an estrogen.

**ethynyl** (ĕth′ĭ-nĭl) An organic radical, HC≡C—.

**etic** (ē′tĭk) In anthropology and transcultural nursing, rel. to a kind of analysis that emphasizes the universal or culture-free aspects of disease. The categories of Western medicine may be viewed as etic classifications because objective measures are used to formulate a diagnosis irrespective of the patient's cultural and subjective perspectives. For example, hallucinations are classified as an "illness" from an etic perspective when, in fact, hallucinations may be a component of normal grieving in some cultures. SEE: *emic.*

**etio-** Combining form meaning *causation.*

**etiocholanolone** (ē″tē-ō-kō-lăn′ō-lōn) A steroid produced by testosterone catabolism. It is excreted in the urine.

**etiology** (ē″tē-ŏl′ō-jē) [Gr. *aitia,* cause, + *logos,* word, reason] **1.** The study of the causes of disease. **2.** The cause of a disease. **etiologic, etiological** (-ō-lŏj′ĭk, -ĭ-kăl), *adj.*

**etiotropic** (ē″tē-ō-trŏp′ĭk) [Gr. *aita,* cause, + *tropos,* turning] Directed against the cause of a disease; used of a drug or treatment that destroys or inactivates the causal agent of a disease. Opposite of nosotropic.

**ETO** *ethylene oxide.*

**etodolac** A nonsteroidal anti-inflammatory

agent. Trade name is Lodine.

**etretinate** A tretinoin drug used in the treatment of severe recalcitrant psoriasis. Trade name is Tegison.

Caution: Etretinate must not be used by women who are pregnant or who intend to become pregnant. It should be prescribed only by physicians knowledgeable in the systemic use of retinoids.

**etymology** (ĕt″ĭ-mŏl′ō-jē) [L. *etymon*, origin of a word, + *logos*, word, reason] The science of the origin and development of words. Most medical words are derived from Latin and Greek, but many of those from Greek have come through Latin and have been modified by it. Generally, when two Greek words are used to form one word, they are connected by the letter "o." Many medical words have been formed from one or more roots—forms used or adapted from Latin or Greek—and many are modified by a prefix, a suffix, or both. A knowledge of important Latin and Greek roots and prefixes will reveal the meanings of many other words. SEE: *Abbreviations Appendix; Prefixes and Suffixes Appendix.*

**Eu** Symbol for the element europium.

**eu-** [Gr. *eus*, good] Combining form meaning *healthy; normal; good; well.* SEE: also *normo-*.

**Eubacteriales** (ū″băk-tē-rē-ā′lēz) [Gr. *eus*, good, + *bakterion*, little rod] An order of bacteria that includes many of the microorganisms pathogenic to humans.

**Eubacterium** (ū″băk-tē′rē-ŭm) A genus of bacteria of the order Eubacteriales.

**eubiotics** (ū″bī-ŏt′ĭks) [″ + *bios*, life] The science of healthy and hygienic living.

**eucalyptol** (ū″kă-lĭp′tōl) [″ + *kalyptein*, to cover] A substance obtained from oil of eucalyptus. It has an aromatic odor and has been used in expectorants.

**eucalyptus oil** (ū-kă-lĭp′tŭs) Oil distilled from fresh eucalyptus leaves, used as an expectorant.

**eucapnia** (ū-kăp′nē-ă) [″+ *kapnos*, smoke] The presence of normal amounts of carbon dioxide in the blood.

**eucatropine hydrochloride** (ū-kăt′rō-pēn) An anticholinergic used as a mydriatic. It is applied topically to the eye.

**euchlorhydria** (ū″klor-hī′drē-ă) The presence of the normal amount of free hydrochloric acid in gastric juice.

**eucholia** (ū-kō′lē-ă) [″+ *chole*, bile] The normal condition of bile regarding its constituents and the amount secreted.

**euchromatin** (ū-krō′mă-tĭn) [″ + *chroma*, color] Unfolded or uncondensed portions of chromosomes during interphase. Transcription of DNA by messenger RNA occurs, and proteins are synthesized. SEE: *heterochromatin.*

**eucrasia** (ū-krā′sē-ă) [″ + *krasis*, mixture] Normal health; the state of the body in which all activities are in normal balance.

**eudiaphoresis** (ū″dī-ă-fō-rē′sĭs) [″ + *dia*, through, + *pherein*, to carry] Normal secretion of perspiration.

**eudiometer** (ū″dē-ŏm′ĕ-tĕr) [Gr. *eudia*, good weather, + *metron*, measure] An instrument for testing air purity and analyzing gases.

**eugenics** (ū-jĕn′ĭks) [″ + *gennan*, to produce] The study of improving a population by selective breeding in the belief that desirable traits will become more common and undesirable traits will be eliminated. Ths practice may have some validity in controlled animal populations, but it is considered unethical in humans.

**eugenol** (ū′jĕn-ŏl) A material obtained from clove oil and other sources. It is used as a topical analgesic in dentistry. It is also mixed with zinc oxide to form a material that hardens sufficiently to be used as a temporary dental filling.

**euglobulin** (ū-glŏb′ū-lĭn) A true globulin, or one that is insoluble in distilled water and soluble in dilute salt solution. SEE: *pseudoglobulin.*

**euglycemia** A normal concentration of glucose in the blood.

**euhydration** A normal amount of water in the body.

**eukaryon** (ū-kăr′ē-ŏn) [″ + *karyon*, nucleus] The nucleus of a eukaryote cell.

**eukaryote** (ū-kăr′ē-ōt) An organism in which the cell nucleus is surrounded by a membrane. SEE: *prokaryote.*

**Eulenburg's disease** (oyl′ĕn-bŭrgz) [Albert Eulenburg, Ger. neurologist, 1840–1917] Myotonia congenita.

**Eumycetes** (ū″mī-sē′tēz) [″+ *mykes*, fungus] A class of Thallophyta that includes all the true fungi.

**eunuch** (ū′nŭk) [Gr. *eune*, bed, + *echein*, to guard] A castrated man; one who has had his testicles removed, esp. before puberty so that secondary sexual characteristics do not develop. Absence of the male hormone produces certain symptoms, such as a high-pitched voice and loss of hair on the face. In Middle Eastern and some Asian countries, eunuchs were employed to guard the women of a harem.

**eunuchism** (ū′nŭk-ĭzm) [″ + ″ + *-ismos*, condition] A condition resulting from complete lack of male hormone. It may be due to atrophy or removal of the testicles.

***pituitary e.*** A condition produced by failure of the anterior lobe of the pituitary to secrete gonadotrophic hormones; secondary hypogonadism.

**eunuchoid** (ū′nŭ-koyd) [″ + ″ + *eidos*, form, shape] Having the characteristics of a eunuch, such as retarded development of sex organs, absence of beard and bodily hair, high-pitched voice, and striking lack of muscular development.

**eunuchoidism** (ū-′nŭk-oyd-ĭzm) [″ + ″ + ″ + *-ismos*, condition] Deficient production of the male hormone androgen by the testes.

**eupancreatism** (ū-păn′krē-ă-tĭzm) [Gr. *eus*,

good, + *pankreas,* pancreas, + *-ismos,* condition] The normal condition of the pancreas.

**eupepsia** [″ + *pepsis,* digestion] Normal digestion as distinguished from dyspepsia. **eupeptic,** *adj.*

**euphonia** (ū-fōn′ē-ă) [″ + *phone,* voice] The condition of having a normal clear voice.

**euphoria** (ū-for′ē-ă) [″ + *phoros,* bearing] **1.** A condition of good health. **2.** In psychiatry, an exaggerated feeling of well-being; mild elation.

**euphoriant** Something that induces euphoria.

**euplastic** (ū-plăs′tĭk) [″ + *plastikos,* formed] Healing quickly and well.

**euploidy** (ū-ploy′dē) [″ + *ploos,* fold, + *eidos,* form, shape] In genetics, the state of having complete sets of chromosomes.

**europium** (ŭ-rō′pē-ŭm) SYMB: EU. A rare element of the lanthanide series with atomic number 63 and an atomic weight of 151.96.

**Eurotium** (ū-rō′shē-ŭm) [Gr. *euros,* mold] A genus of molds.

**eury-** (ū′rē) [Gr. *eurys,* wide] Combining form meaning *broad.*

**eurycephalic** (ū″rē-sĕ-făl′ĭk) [″ + *kephale,* head] Having a broad or wide head.

**eustachian** (ū-stā′kē-ăn, -shĕn) [Bartolomeo Eustachio (Eustachi), It. anatomist, 1520–1574] Pert. to the auditory tube. SEE: *ear; eustachian tube.*

**eustachian catheter** An instrument for insertion into the eustachian tube.

**eustachianography** Radiography of the eustachian tube and middle ear after the introduction of a contrast medium.

**eustachian tube** The auditory tube, extending from the middle ear to the nasopharynx, 3 to 4 cm long and lined with mucous membrane. Occlusion of the tube leads to the development of otitis media. SYN: *otopharyngeal tube.* SEE: *politzerization.*

**eustachian valve** The valve at the entrance of the inferior vena cava.

**eustachitis** (ū″stā-kī′tĭs) Inflammation of the eustachian tube.

**eusystole** (ū-sĭs′tō-lē) [Gr. *eus,* good, + *systellein,* to draw together] A condition in which the systole of the heart is normal in time and force.

**eutectic** (ū-tĕk′tĭk) [Gr. *eutektos*] Easily melted.

**eutectic mixture** A mixture of two or more substances that has a melting point lower than that of any of its constituents.

**euthanasia** (ū-thă-nā′zē-ă) [Gr. *eus,* good, + *thanatos,* death] **1.** An easy, quiet, and painless death. **2.** The deliberate ending of life in individuals with an incurable disease. Ethical considerations are still being actively debated. One difficulty is determining the criteria by which the physician or society determines that the time has come to end the patient's life. SEE: *advance directive; assisted death; assisted suicide; death; death with dignity; do not attempt resuscitation; dying; hopelessly ill patients; living will.*

***involuntary e.*** Euthanasia performed without a competent person's consent.

***nonvoluntary e.*** Euthanasia provided to an incompetent person according to a surrogate's decision.

**euthenics** (ū-thĕn′ĭks) [Gr. *euthenia,* well-being] The science of improvement of a population through modification of the environment.

**Eutheria** A subclass of mammals with a true placenta.

**euthyroid** (ū-thī′royd) Having a normally functioning thyroid gland.

**Eutrombicula** (ū″trŏm-bĭk′ū-lă) A genus of mites.

**eutrophication** (ū-trŏf″ĭ-kā′shŭn) [Gr. *eutrophein,* to thrive] Alteration of the environment by increasing the nutrients required by one species to the disadvantage of other species in the ecosystem, esp. in an aquatic environment.

**ev, eV, EV** *electron volt.*

**evacuant** (ē-văk′ū-ănt) [L. *evacuans,* making empty] A drug that stimulates the bowels to move.

**evacuate** [L. *evacuatio,* emptying] **1.** To discharge, esp. from the bowels; to empty the uterus. **2.** To move patients from the site of an accident or catastrophe to a hospital or shelter.

**evacuation** (ē-văk″ū-ā′shŭn) **1.** The act of emptying, esp. the bowels. **2.** The material discharged from the bowels; stool. **3.** Removal of air from a closed container; production of a vacuum. **4.** The act of moving people to a safe place, esp. from a disaster or a war-torn area.

**evacuator** (ē-văk′ū-ā-tor) A device for emptying, as the bowels, or for irrigating the bladder and removing calculi.

**evagination** (ē-văj-ĭ-nā′shŭn) **1.** Emergence from a sheath. **2.** Protrusion of an organ or part. SEE: *invagination.* **evaginate** (-nāt), *adj.*

**evaluation** **1.** The judgment of anything. **2.** In medicine, consideration of the health and physical and mental capability and potential of a patient or a person considered to be healthy. **3.** The final step of the nursing process, essential in ensuring its quality and effectiveness. This step includes providing answers concerning the accuracy of the nursing diagnoses, the effectiveness of the nursing plan in meeting the needs of the patient, the usefulness of the nursing interventions in carrying out the plan, and the need for changing any aspects of the nursing process to improve the quality of care. SEE: *nursing assessment; nursing intervention; nursing process; planning; problem-oriented medical record.* **4.** In physical therapy, the procedures used to determine the condition of the patient before initiation of therapy, and change in status to determine the continued appropriateness or need for adaptation of the therapeutic program.

**evanescent** (ĕv″ă-nĕs′ĕnt) [L. *evanescere,* to

vanish] Not permanent; of brief duration.

**Evans blue** [Herbert M. Evans, U.S. anatomist, 1882–1971] A diazo dye occurring as a blue-green powder, very soluble in water. It is used intravenously as a diagnostic agent.

**Evans syndrome** [Robert S. Evans, U.S. physician, b. 1912] An autoimmune disease characterized by thrombocytopenia and hemolytic anemia.

**evaporation** [L. *e*, out, + *vaporare*, to steam] **1.** Change from liquid to vapor. **2.** Loss in volume due to conversion of a liquid into a vapor.

**evenomation** (ē-vĕn″ō-mā′shŭn) [L. *ex*, from, + *venenum*, poison] Removal of venom from a biting insect or reptile; removal of venom from the victim of a bite.

**eventration** (ē″vĕn-trā′shŭn) [L. *e*, out, + *venter*, belly] **1.** Partial protrusion of the abdominal contents through an opening in the abdominal wall. **2.** Removal of the contents of the abdominal cavity.

**eversion** (ē-vĕr′zhŭn) [″ + *vertere*, to turn] Turning outward. SEE: *chilectropion*.

**evidement** (ā-vēd-mŏn′) [Fr., a scooping out] Scraping away of diseased tissue.

**evidence** In forensic medicine, all the tangible items and record materials pertinent to the legal considerations.

***chain of custody of e.*** In legal and forensic medicine, the procedures for ensuring that specimens, data, or information important to legal proceedings are properly handled, labeled, and stored in a locked and secure place. If a biological specimen is stored, it may need to be frozen or refrigerated. Only authorized persons are allowed access to the stored material. When a specimen to be tested for drugs (e.g., urine, sputum, blood, or breath) is obtained from an individual, the person must be observed while passing or providing the specimen. In drug testing, samples are stored in duplicate so one will be available for retesting at a later date.

**evil** [AS. *yfel*] Disease or illness.

**eviration** (ē″vī-rā′shŭn) [L. *e*, out, + *vir*, man] **1.** Castration. **2.** In psychiatry, delusion in a man who thinks he has become a woman.

**evisceration** (ē-vĭs″ĕr-ā′shŭn) [″ + *viscera*, viscera] **1.** Removal of the viscera or of the contents of a cavity. **2.** Spilling out of abdominal contents resulting from wound dehiscence.

NURSING IMPLICATIONS: The patient's surgeon should be contacted immediately. The wound is covered with a sterile towel moistened with warm sterile physiological saline solution. Tension on the abdomen is decreased by placing the patient in the low Fowler's position and raising the knees or by instructing the patient to flex the knees and supporting them with a pillow. Vital signs are monitored, and fluid therapy is initiated via IV line. The patient is reassured and prepared for surgery.

**evisceroneurotomy** (ē-vĭs″ĕr-ō-nū-rŏt′ō-mē) [″ + ″ + Gr. *neuron*, nerve, + *tome*, incision] Scleral evisceration of the eye with division of the optic nerve.

**evocation** (ĕv″ō-kā′shŭn) [″ + *vocare*, to call] **1.** Re-creation by memory recall or by imagination. **2.** In the embryo, the induction or formation of a tissue in response to an evocator.

**evocator** In the embryo, a factor that controls morphogenesis.

**evoked response** The electroencephalographic record of electrical activity produced at one of several levels in the central nervous system by stimulation of an area of the sensory nerve system. Analysis of the response can provide important information concerning the function of the peripheral and central nervous systems. SEE: *brainstem auditory evoked potential; somatosensory evoked response; visual evoked response*.

**evolution** (ĕv″ō-lū′shŭn) [L. *e*, out, + *volvere*, to roll] A process of orderly and gradual change or development. More generally, any orderly and gradual process of modification whereby a system, whether physical, chemical, social, or intellectual, becomes more highly organized.

***theory of e.*** The theory that all species of plants and animals, including humans, have come into existence by gradual continuous change from earlier forms. SEE: *natural selection*.

**evulsion** SEE: *avulsion*.

**Ewing's tumor, Ewing's sarcoma** (ū′ĭngz [James Ewing, U.S. pathologist, 1866–1943]. A diffuse endothelioma or endothelial myeloma forming a fusiform swelling on a long bone.

**ex-** [L., Gr. *ex*, out] Combining form meaning *out; away from; completely*.

**exa-** In the International System, a combining form indicating $10^{18}$.

**exacerbation** (ĕks-ăs″ĕr-bā′shŭn) [″ + *acerbus*, harsh] Aggravation of symptoms or increase in the severity of a disease.

**exaltation** [L. *exaltare*, to lift up] A mental state characterized by feelings of grandeur, excessive joy, elation, and optimism; an abnormal feeling of personal well-being or self-importance.

**examination** [L. *examinare*, to examine] The act or process of inspecting the body and its systems to determine the presence or absence of disease. Terms employed indicate type of examination: physical, bimanual, digital, oral, rectal, obstetrical, roentgenological, cystoscopic.

Local physical examination includes specific parts and organs. Four procedures used are inspection, palpation, percussion, and auscultation. Laboratory examination includes urinalysis, blood tests, bacteriological cultures, and various special means of visualizing body spaces and organs and their functions. SEE: *abdominal examination*.

***bimanual e.*** SEE: *pelvic e.*

***dental e.*** Examination of the surfaces of teeth and dental fillings, usually with a sharp-pointed explorer to detect areas of demineralization or caries or failing margins of restorations. The depth of the gingival sulcus is also probed and measured around each tooth to assess the state of health of the periodontium.

***double-contrast e.*** A radiographic examination in which a radiopaque and a radiolucent contrast medium are used simultaneously to visualize internal anatomy.

***oral double-contrast e.*** A careful and thorough inspection and palpation of the mouth, tongue, cheek, and tissues of the neck to assess their condition. The floor of the mouth may be palpated bimanually to search for nodules or other irregularities. SEE: *oral diagnosis.*

***pelvic e.*** Physical examination of the vagina and adjacent organs by palpation by placing the fingers of one hand intravaginally and the other hand on the abdominal wall. In this way, tissues between the fingers of the two hands may be palpated. This is called a bimanual examination. Visual examination of the vagina and cervix is made by use of a speculum inserted intravaginally.

**examinations, National Board** Examinations administered to test the qualifications of medical, dental, and other professional students. Successful completion of the basic science and clinical parts of the examinations is required for licensure in most states.

**exanthem** (ĕks-ăn′thĕm) *pl.* **exanthems** [Gr. *exanthema,* eruption] Any eruption of the skin accompanied by inflammation, such as measles, scarlatina, or erysipelas. **exanthematous** (-ăn-thĕm′ă-tŭs), *adj.*

***e. subitum*** An acute disease of infants, probably due to a virus. It is marked by high fever for 3 or 4 days and sometimes by convulsions at the onset. A diffuse maculopapular rash usually appears just at the time the fever suddenly subsides. Treatment is symptomatic. SYN: *roseola infantum.* SEE: *convulsion.*

**exanthema** (ĕks-ăn-thē′mă) *pl.* **exanthemas, -mata** [Gr.] Exanthem.

**exanthrope** (ĕks′ăn-thrōp) [Gr. *ex,* out, + *anthropos,* man] A cause or source of a disease originating outside the body.

**exarticulation** (ĕks″ăr-tĭk-ū-lā′shŭn) [L. *ex,* out, + *articulus,* joint] **1.** Amputation of a limb through a joint. **2.** Excision of a part of a joint.

**excavation** (ĕks″kă-vā′shŭn) [″ + *cavus,* hollow] **1.** A hollow or depression. **2.** Formation of a cavity.

***atrophic e.*** A hollow or cupped appearance of the optic nerve head as seen by use of an ophthalmoscope.

***dental e.*** The preparation of a cavity in a tooth before filling.

***e. of optic nerve*** A slight depression in the center of the optic papilla, or disk, from which retinal vessels emerge. Depression is total in glaucoma as a result of high intraocular pressure.

***rectouterine e.*** The rectouterine pouch or pouch of Douglas.

**excavator** (ĕks′kă-vā″tor) An instrument for removing tissue or bone. It may be spoon-shaped if used on soft tissue and spoon-shaped with sharp edges if used in dentistry.

**excerebration** (ĕk″sĕr-ĕ-brā′shŭn) [″ + *cerebrum,* brain] Removal of the brain, esp. that of the dead fetus to facilitate delivery.

**excess, base** The difference between the normal and the actual buffer base in a blood sample.

**exchange 1.** To give up or substitute something for something else. **2.** In dietetics, the substitution of an equivalent amount of one food substance for another so that the caloric intake remains the same.

***cation e.*** The transfer of cations between those in a liquid medium and those in a solid polymer. The polymer is termed the cation exchanger. This technique is used in ion-exchange chromatography.

***sister chromatid e.*** The exchange of corresponding parts of homologous maternal and paternal chromosomes during the first meiotic division. This contributes to genetic diversity in the offspring. SYN: *crossing over.*

**exchange list** A grouping of foods to assist people on special diets. In each group, foods are listed in serving sizes that are interchangeable with respect to carbohydrates, fats, protein, and calories. The groups are starches and bread; meat; vegetables and fruit; milk; and fats. This approach is esp. useful in managing diets for diabetics.

**exchange transfusion** Transfusion and withdrawal of small amounts of blood repeated until the blood volume is almost entirely exchanged. It is used in infants born with hemolytic disease and dangerously high levels of serum bilirubin, in patients with uremia, and in some types of poisoning. SEE: *hemolytic disease of the newborn; kernicterus.*

**excipient** (ĕk-sĭp′ē-ĕnt) [L. *excipiens,* excepting] Any substance added to a medicine so that it can be formed into the proper shape and consistency; the vehicle for the drug.

**excise** (ĕk-sīz′) [L. *ex,* out, + *caedere,* to cut] To cut out or remove surgically.

**excision** (ĕk-sĭ′zhŭn) [L. *excisio*] The act of cutting away or taking out.

**excitability** [L. *excitare,* to arouse] Sensitivity to stimulation.

***muscle e.*** In a muscle fiber, the inducibility to contract. This is a function of the chemical state of the nerve membrane and the time since a previous stimulus was applied.

***nerve e.*** The property of a nerve to produce an action potential. This is a function of the permeability of the nerve membrane. The membrane is influenced by physical, chemical, and electrical forces. Also, the intensity of electrical stimuli influences the excitability of the nerve.

***reflex e.*** Sensitivity to reflex irritation.

**excitant** (ĕk-sīt'ănt) An agent that excites a special function of the body. According to their action, excitants are classified as motor, cerebral, and so forth. Amphetamine, cocaine, and strychnine are examples of medical excitants.

**excitation** [L. *excitatio*] **1.** The act of exciting. **2.** The condition of being stimulated or excited.

***direct e.*** Stimulation of a muscle physically or by placement of an electrode in it.

***indirect e.*** Stimulation of a muscle via its nerve.

**excitation wave** The wave of irritability originating in the sinoatrial node that sweeps over the conducting tissue of the heart and induces contraction of the atria and ventricles.

**exciting** Causing excitement.

**excitoglandular** (ĕk-sīt″ō-glăn'dū-lăr) [L. *excitare,* to arouse, + *glans,* kernel] Increasing glandular function.

**excitometabolic** (ĕk-sīt″ō-mĕt″ă-bŏl'ĭk) [″ + Gr. *metabole,* change] Inducing metabolic changes.

**excitomotor** (ĕk-sīt″ō-mō'tor) [″ + *motor,* moving] Pert. to increasingly rapid muscular activity.

**excitomuscular** (ĕk-sīt″ō-mŭs'kū-lăr) [″ + Gr. *mys,* muscle] Causing muscular activity.

**excitor** (ĕk-sī'tor) [L. *excitare,* to arouse] Something that incites to greater activity. SYN: *stimulant.*

**excitosecretory** (ĕk-sīt″ō-sē'krĕ-tor-ē) [″ + *secretio,* a hiding] Tending to produce secretion.

**excitotoxin** A neurotransmitter (e.g., glutamate or aspartate) that can cause cell death if its action is prolonged. These chemicals are thought to be important in damaging brain cells during ischemia.

**excitovascular** (ĕk-sī″tō-văs'kū-lăr) [″ + *vascularis,* pert. to a vessel] Increasing circulation activity.

**exclusion** (ĕks-kloo'zhŭn) [L. *exclusio,* fr. *ex,* out, + *claudere,* to shut] Shutting off or removing from the main part.

**excoriation** (ĕks-kō-rē-ā'shŭn) [″ + *corium,* skin] Abrasion of the epidermis or of the coating of any organ by trauma, chemicals, burns, or other causes.

**excrement** (ĕks'krĕ-mĕnt) [L. *excrementum*] Waste material passed out of the body, esp. feces. SEE: *excretion.* **excrementitious** (ĕks″krĕ-mĕn-tĭsh'ŭs), *adj.*

**excrescence** (ĕks-krĕs'ĕns) [L. *ex,* out, + *crescere,* to grow] Any abnormal growth from the surface of a part.

**excreta** (ĕks-krē'tă) [L.] Waste matter excreted from the body, including feces, urine, and perspiration. In some diseases, the excreta of the patient contains infectious material. This must be disinfected and handled carefully by hospital personnel. SEE: *AIDS; Universal Precautions Appendix.*

Pads made of absorbent materials should be placed under the patient who has involuntary discharges. When disposed of, the pads should be placed in sturdy plastic bags. In handling all infected discharges, the health care worker should wear rubber gloves and a face mask.

---

Caution: The following disinfecting materials should not come in contact with skin or eyes.

---

*Phenol:* A 5% solution should be used in quantity at least equal to the amount of the material to be disinfected.

*Chlorinated lime:* This substance should be dissolved in the proportion of 4 oz (120 ml) to 1 gal (3.8 L) of water. One qt (946 ml) of this solution should be used to disinfect each liquid discharge. For solid fecal matter, a stronger solution or a larger quantity is required.

**excrete** (ĕks-krēt') [L. *excretus,* sifted out] To expel or eliminate waste material from the body, blood, or organs.

**excretion** (ĕks-krē'shŭn) [L. *excretio*] **1.** Excreta. **2.** The elimination of waste products from the body.

ORGANS: *Intestines:* These produce indigestible residue, water, and bacteria. *Kidneys:* Water, nitrogenous substances (urea, uric acid, creatine, creatinine), mineral salts are excreted. *Respiratory system:* This produces carbon dioxide, water vapor, and other gases. *Skin:* A small amount of material is excreted through perspiration of water, salts, and minute quantities of urea. The excretory function of the skin is stimulated by kidney inactivity. In renal failure, diaphoretics, hot packs, and warm blankets stimulate skin, thus helping to avoid uremic coma.

**excretory** (ĕks'krē-tō-rē) [L. *excretus,* sifted out] Pert. to or bringing about excretion.

**excursion** (ĕks-kŭr'zhŭn) [L. *excursio*] **1.** Wandering from the usual course. **2.** The extent of movement of a part such as the extremities or eyes.

***diaphragmatic e.*** In respiration, the movement of the diaphragm from its level during full exhalation to its level during full inhalation. Normal diaphragmatic excursion is 3 to 5 cm bilaterally in adults and is determined by percussion over the thoracic area at the midscapular line.

**excurvation** (ĕks″kŭr-vā'shŭn) [Gr. *ex,* out, + L. *curvus,* bend] A curvature outward.

**excystation** (ĕk″sĭs-tā'shŭn) [″ + *kystis,* cyst] The escape of certain organisms (parasitic worms or protozoa) from an en-

**Exercise: Energy Required***

| Calories Required per Hour of Exercise | Activity† |
|---|---|
| 80 | Sitting quietly, reading |
| 200 | Golf with use of powered cart |
| 250 | Walking 3 miles/hr (4.83 km/hr); housework; light industry; cycling 6 miles/hr (9.7 km/hr) |
| 330 | Heavy housework; walking 3.5 miles/hr (5.6 km/hr); golf, carrying own bag; tennis, doubles; ballet exercises |
| 400 | Walking 5 miles/hr (8 km/hr); cycling 10 miles/hr (16.1 km/hr); tennis, singles; water skiing |
| 500 | Manual labor; gardening; shoveling |
| 660 | Running 5.5 miles/hr (8.9 km/hr); cycling 13 miles/hr (20.9 km/hr); climbing stairs; heavy manual labor |
| 1020 | Running 8 miles/hr (12.9 km/hr); climbing stairs with 30-lb (13.61-kg) load |

* These estimates are approximate and can serve only as a general guide. They are based on an average person who weighs 160 lb (72.58 kg).

† Energy requirements for swimming are not provided because of variables such as water temperature, whether the water is fresh or salt, buoyancy of the individual, and whether the water is calm or not.

closing cyst wall or envelope. This process occurs in the life cycle of an intestinal parasite after the encysted form is ingested.

**exencephalia** (ĕks″ĕn-sĕf-ā′lē-ă) [″ + *enkephalos,* brain] A congenital anomaly in which the brain is located outside the skull; a term for encephalocele, hydrencephalocele, and meningocele.

**exenteration** (ĕks-ĕn″tĕr-ā′shŭn) [″ + *enteron,* intestine] Evisceration.

**exercise** [L. *exercitus,* having drilled] A physical or mental activity performed to maintain, restore, or increase normal capacity. Physical exercise involves activities that maintain or increase muscle tone and strength, esp. to improve physical fitness or to manage a handicap or disability. SEE: table; *physical fitness; risk factor; sedentary lifestyle.*

Regular aerobic physical activity will increase exercise capacity, influence primary and secondary prevention of cardiovascular disease, increase the ability to use oxygen to derive energy for work, decrease myocardial oxygen demands for the same level of external work, favorably alter lipid and carbohydrate metabolism, and help to control weight gain and promote weight loss by using energy that might otherwise be stored as fat. An exercise program should include developing joint flexibility and muscle strength, esp. in the arms. This is of particular importance as people age. Exercise can have a beneficial effect in patients with depression or anxiety. It is thought to have a positive effect on mental health.

An exercise program should be neither begun or continued if the individual or the person prescribing the exercise program has evidence that the activity is painful or harmful. Persons have died while exercising, and heavy physical exertion may precede acute myocardial infarction, particularly in people who are habitually sedentary.

Mental exercise involves activities that maintain or increase cognitive faculties. Regular intellectual stimulation will improve concentration as well as integration and application of concepts and principles to problem solving; promote self-esteem and a positive self-concept; facilitate self-actualization; counteract depression associated with social isolation and boredom; and enhance the quality of life. This is particularly important during aging. SEE: *reminiscence therapy.*

Most of the negative aspects of aging can be either altered or diminished by a lifelong healthy lifestyle. For example, the loss of physical fitness and strength, an inevitable consequence of aging, can be altered by an individualized fitness and strength program. Progressive loss of bone mass due to osteoporosis either may be prevented or slowed by a program of regular exercise. Loss of cardiac fitness can be forestalled by an ongoing aerobic fitness program. Many cases of adult-onset diabetes can be controlled by exercise and an appropriate diet. Arthritic stiffness and loss of flexibility can be influenced favorably by exercise, for example, walking and jogging; for patients who experience joint pain with impact exercise, swimming is an alternative. Obesity and loss of muscle mass can be prevented or minimized.

Exercise stimulates release of endorphins, and people who participate in regular exercise programs express positive feelings toward living. Exercise programs can be adapted for patients who are confined to wheelchairs. An important consideration for any exercise program is that it be enjoyable. No matter how beneficial the program may be, if it is not enjoyable or rewarding, it will not be continued.

***active e.*** A type of bodily movement performed by voluntary contraction and relaxation of muscles.

***aquatic e.*** The use of a pool or tank of water for early exercise in the treatment of musculoskeletal injuries and for non- or partial weight-bearing activities in early rehabilitation training. SEE: *hydrotherapy.*

***assistive e.*** A type of bodily movement performed by voluntary contraction and relaxation of muscles with the aid of a therapist.

***blowing e.*** An exercise in which the patient blows into a tube connected to a bottle containing water. That bottle is attached to another bottle so that the air pressure produced forces water from the one into the other. This increases intrabronchial pressure, which tends to aid expansion of the lung. Research has indicated that emphysema cavities are irreversible. Thus, blowing exercise is used only to lessen the new formation of cavities. SEE: *atelectasis; empyema; pneumonia.*

***breathing e.*** Exercise that enhances the respiratory system by improving ventilation, strengthening respiratory muscles, and increasing endurance.

***Buerger's postural e.*** [Leo Buerger, U.S. physician, 1879–1943] An exercise used for circulatory disturbances of the extremities.

***Codman's e.*** A gentle, active exercise of the upper extremity following immobilization to reestablish range of motion and function following fracture. SYN: *pendulum e.; Codman's movements.*

***concentric e.*** An exercise in which the muscle action overcomes resistance or the muscle contracts. SEE: *muscle contraction, concentric; muscle contraction, eccentric.*

***corrective e.*** Use of specific exercises to correct deficiencies caused by trauma or inactivity.

***dynamic stabilization e.*** Stabilization e.

***eccentric e.*** An exercise in which there is overall lengthening of the muscle in response to an external resistance. SEE: *muscle contraction, concentric; muscle contraction, eccentric.*

***flexibility e.*** An exercise designed to increase range of motion and extensibility of muscle.

***free e.*** An exercise carried through with no external assistance.

***isokinetic e.*** An exercise, usually using a specially designed machine, that controls the velocity of muscle shortening or lengthening, so that the force generated by the muscle is maximal through the full range of motion.

***isometric e.*** Contraction and relaxation of a skeletal muscle or group of muscles in which the force generated by the muscle is equal to the resistance. There is no change in muscle length, and no movement results. SYN: *muscle-setting e.; static e.*

***isotonic e.*** An active muscle contraction in which the force exerted remains constant and muscle length changes.

***Kegel e.*** SEE: *Kegel exercise.*

***kinetic chain e.*** An exercise that requires the foot to apply pressure against a plate, pedal, or ground. This rehabilitation concept was determined by the anatomical functional relationship in the lower extremities. Kinetic chain exercises are more functional than open-chain exercises, in which the foot is off the ground and the force in generated by the muscles against a shin plate.

***muscle-setting e.*** Isometric e.

***passive e.*** A therapeutic exercise technique used to move a patient's joints through a range of motion without any effort on the part of the patient. It is accomplished by a therapist, an assistant, or the use of a machine. SYN: *passive motion; passive movement.*

***pelvic floor e.*** SEE: *Kegel exercise.*

***pendulum e.*** Codman's e.

***range-of-motion e.*** Movement of a joint through its available range of motion. It can be used to prevent loss of motion. SEE: illus.

***resistive e.*** A form of supervised exercise, with or without apparatus, that offers resistance to muscle action.

***stabilization e.*** The application of fluctuating resistance loads while the patient stabilizes the part being trained in a symptom-free position. Exercises begin easily so that control is maintained, and progress in duration, intensity, speed, and variety. SYN: *dynamic stabilization e.*

***static e.*** Isometric e.

***stretching e.*** A therapeutic exercise maneuver, using physiological principles, designed to increase joint range of motion or extensibility of pathologically shortened connective tissue structures.

***therapeutic e.*** A form of scientifically supervised exercise, with or without apparatus, for restoring normal function to diseased or injured tissues.

**exercise electrocardiogram** A record of the electrical activity of the heart taken during graded increases in the rate of exercise. SEE: *stress test.*

**exercise-induced asthma** SEE: *asthma, exercise-induced.*

**exercise prescription** An exercise schedule usually intended to increase the physical fitness of a previously sedentary individual who has recently had a serious illness such as myocardial infarction, or who is physically fit and wants to know the amount, frequency, and kind of exercise necessary to maintain fitness. The pre-

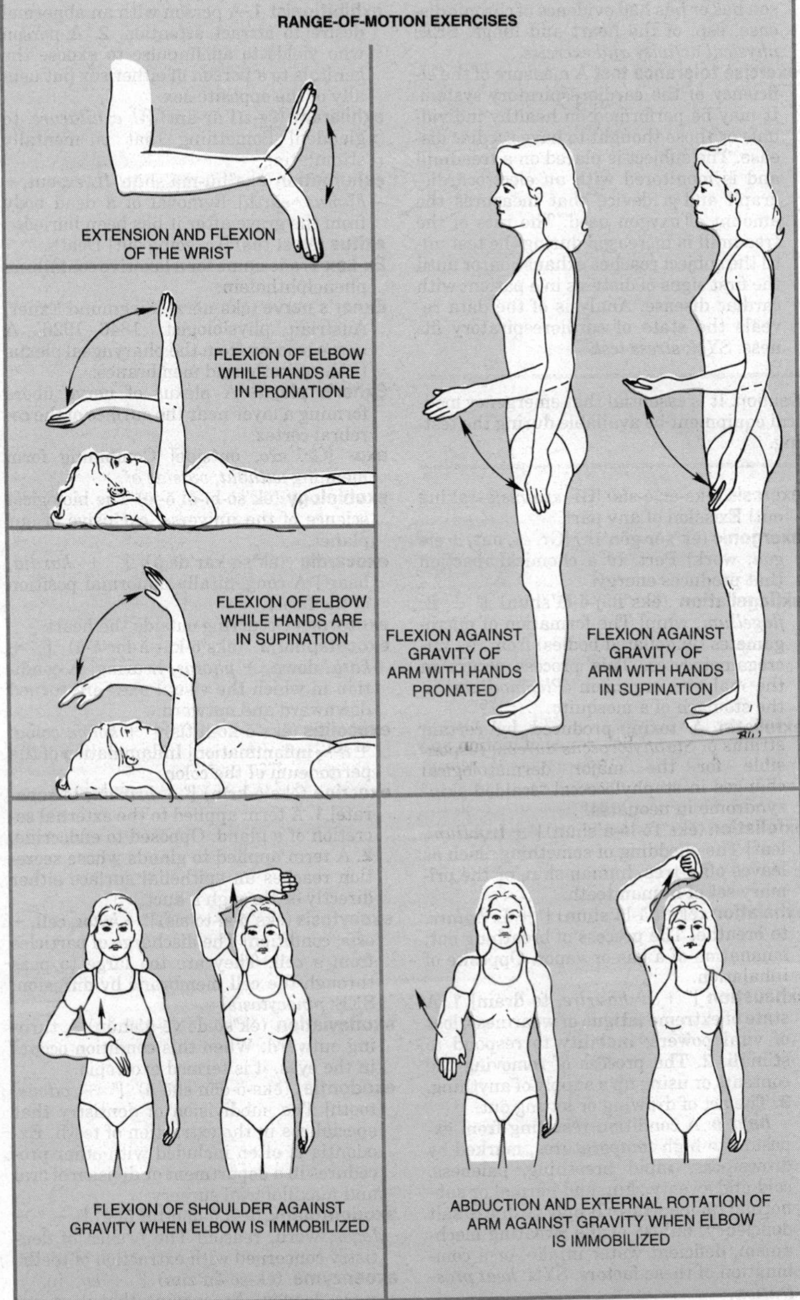
RANGE-OF-MOTION EXERCISES
EXTENSION AND FLEXION OF THE WRIST
FLEXION OF ELBOW WHILE HANDS ARE IN PRONATION
FLEXION OF ELBOW WHILE HANDS ARE IN SUPINATION
FLEXION AGAINST GRAVITY OF ARM WITH HANDS PRONATED
FLEXION AGAINST GRAVITY OF ARM WITH HANDS IN SUPINATION
FLEXION OF SHOULDER AGAINST GRAVITY WHEN ELBOW IS IMMOBILIZED
ABDUCTION AND EXTERNAL ROTATION OF ARM AGAINST GRAVITY WHEN ELBOW IS IMMOBILIZED

scription is individualized, taking into account the person's age and health status and the availability of facilities and adequate supervision, particularly if the person has or has had evidence of chronic disease, esp. of the heart and lungs. SEE: *physical activity and exercise.*

**exercise tolerance test** A measure of the efficiency of the cardiorespiratory system. It may be performed on healthy individuals or those thought to have cardiac disease. The subject is placed on a treadmill and is monitored with an electrocardiograph and a device that measures the amount of oxygen used. The rate of the treadmill is increased during the test until the subject reaches exhaustion, or until the first signs of distress in a patient with cardiac disease. Analysis of the data reveals the state of cardiorespiratory fitness. SYN: *stress test.*

---

Caution: It is essential that emergency medical equipment be available during the testing.

---

**exeresis** (ĕks-ĕr'ĕ-sĭs) [Gr. *exairesis,* taking out] Excision of any part.

**exergonic** (ĕk"sĕr-gŏn'ĭk) [Gr. *ex,* out, + *ergon,* work] Pert. to a chemical reaction that produces energy.

**exflagellation** (ĕks"flăj-ĕ-lā'shŭn) [" + L. *flagellum,* whip] The formation of microgametes (flagellated bodies) from the microgametocytes. This process occurs in the malarial organism *(Plasmodium)* in the stomach of a mosquito.

**exfoliatin** A toxin, produced by certain strains of *Staphylococcus aureus,* responsible for the major dermatological changes in staphylococcal "scalded skin" syndrome in neonates.

**exfoliation** (ĕks"fō-lē-ā'shŭn) [" + L. *folium,* leaf] The shedding of something, such as leaves off a tree, human skin, or the primary set of human teeth.

**exhalation** (ĕks"hă-lā'shŭn) [" + L. *halare,* to breathe] The process of breathing out; emanation of a gas or vapor. Opposite of inhalation.

**exhaustion** [" + L. *haurire,* to drain] **1.** A state of extreme fatigue or weariness; loss of vital powers; inability to respond to stimuli. **2.** The process of removing the contents or using up a supply of anything. **3.** The act of drawing or letting out.

***heat e.*** A condition resulting from exposure to high temperatures, marked by drowsiness, rapid breathing, paleness, cold and sweaty skin, and normal or subnormal temperature. It may be due to salt deficiency, failure of the sweating mechanism, deficient water intake, or a combination of these factors. SYN: *heat prostration.*

**exhibitionism** [" + Gr. *-ismos,* condition] **1.** A tendency to attract attention to oneself by any means. **2.** A psychoneurosis manifesting itself in an abnormal impulse that causes one to expose the genitals to a person of either sex but usually of the opposite sex.

**exhibitionist 1.** A person with an abnormal desire to attract attention. **2.** A person who yields to an impulse to expose the genitals to a person of either sex but usually of the opposite sex.

**exhilarant** (ĕg-zĭl'ăr-ănt) [L. *exhilarare,* to gladden] Something that is mentally stimulating.

**exhumation** (ĕks"hū-mā'shŭn) [L. *ex,* out, + *humus,* earth] Removal of a dead body from the grave after it has been buried.

**exitus** (ĕk'sĭ-tŭs) [L., going out] Death.

**Ex-Lax** Trade name for a laxative containing phenolphthalein.

**Exner's nerve** (ĕks'nĕrz) [Siegmund Exner, Austrian physiologist, 1846–1926] A nerve leading from the pharyngeal plexus to the cricothyroid membranes.

**Exner's plexus** A plexus of nerve fibers forming a layer near the surface of the cerebral cortex.

**exo-** [Gr. *exo,* outside] Combining form meaning *without; outside of.*

**exobiology** (ĕk"sō-bī-ŏl'ō-jē) The biological science of the universe, exclusive of our planet.

**exocardia** (ĕk"sō-kăr'dē-ă) [" + *kardia,* heart] A congenitally abnormal position of the heart.

**exocardial** Occurring outside the heart.

**exocataphoria** (ĕks"ō-kăt-ă-for'ē-ă) [" + *kata,* down, + *phoros,* bearing] A condition in which the visual axes are turned downward and outward.

**exocolitis** (ĕks"ō-kō-lī'tĭs) [" + *kolon,* colon, + *itis,* inflammation] Inflammation of the peritoneum of the colon.

**exocrine** (ĕks'ō-krĭn) [" + *krinein,* to separate] **1.** A term applied to the external secretion of a gland. Opposed to endocrine. **2.** A term applied to glands whose secretion reaches an epithelial surface either directly or through a duct.

**exocytosis** (ĕks"ō-sī-tō'sĭs) [" + *kytos,* cell, + *osis,* condition] The discharge of particles from a cell. They are too large to pass through the cell membrane by diffusion. SEE: *pinocytosis.*

**exodeviation** (ĕk"sō-dē"vē-ā'shŭn) A turning outward. When this condition occurs in the eyes, it is termed exotropia.

**exodontia** (ĕks-ō-dŏn'shē-ă) [" + *odous,* tooth] The subdivision of dentistry that specializes in the extraction of teeth. Exodontia is often included with other procedures in a department or division of oral and maxillofacial surgery.

**exodontology** (ĕks"ō-dŏn-tŏl'ō-jē) [" + " + *logos,* word, reason] The branch of dentistry concerned with extraction of teeth.

**exoenzyme** (ĕk-sō-ĕn'zīm) [" + *en,* in, + *zyme,* leaven] An enzyme that does not function within the cells that secrete it.

**exoerythrocytic** (ĕk"sō-ĕ-rĭth"rō-sī'tĭk) [" + *erythros,* red, + *kytos,* cell] Occurring outside the red blood cells. Part of the life cycle of the malaria parasite in a human host is inside the red cell; the rest is outside.

**exogamy** (ĕks-ŏg′ă-mē) [″ + *gamos,* marriage] **1.** Marriage outside a particular group. **2.** In biology, conjugation between protozoan gametes of different ancestry.

**exogastritis** (ĕks″ō-găs-trī′tĭs) [″ + *gaster,* belly, + *itis,* inflammation] Inflammation of the peritoneal coat of the stomach.

**exogenous** (ĕks-ŏj′ĕ-nŭs) [″ + *gennan,* to produce] Originating outside an organ or part.

**exohysteropexy** (ĕks″ō-hĭs′tĕr-ō-pĕks″ē) [″ + *hystera,* womb, + *pexis,* fixation] Fixation of the uterus by implanting the fundus into the abdominal wall.

**exomphalos** (ĕks-ŏm′fă-lŭs) [Gr. *ex,* out, + *omphalos,* navel] **1.** An umbilical protrusion. **2.** An umbilical hernia.

**exon** One of the coding regions of the DNA of genes. SEE: *intron.*

**exophasy** The expression of thought by spoken or written words and the understanding of spoken or written words of others. It is also called external speech. SEE: *endophasy.*

**exophoria** (ĕks″ō-fō′rē-ă) [″ + *phoros,* bearing] A tendency of the visual axes to diverge outward. Opposite of esophoria.

**exophthalmia** (ĕks″ŏf-thăl′mē-ă) [″ + *ophthalmos,* eye] Abnormal protrusion of the eyeball. SYN: *exophthalmos.*

**exophthalmic goiter** A condition marked by protrusion of the eyeballs, increased heart action, enlargement of the thyroid gland, weight loss, and nervousness. SYN: *thyrotoxicosis.* SEE: *hyperthyroidism.*

**exophthalmometer** (ĕk″sŏf-thăl-mŏm′ĕ-tĕr) A device for measuring the degree of protrusion of the eyeballs.

**exophthalmos, exophthalmus** (ĕks″ŏf-thăl′mŏs, -mŭs) Abnormal protrusion of eyeball. This may be due to thyrotoxicosis, tumor of the orbit, orbital cellulitis, leukemia, or aneurysm. **exophthalmic** (-mĭk), *adj.*

***pulsating e.*** Exophthalmos accompanied by pulsation and bruit due to an aneurysm behind the eye.

**exoplasm** (ĕk′sō-plăzm) [″ + LL. *plasma,* form, mold] Ectoplasm.

**exoserosis** (ĕks″ō-sĕr-ō′sĭs) [″ + *serum,* whey, + Gr. *osis,* condition] An oozing of serum or discharging of an exudate.

**exoskeleton** (ĕk″sō-skĕl′ĕ-tŏn) [″ + *skeleton,* a dried-up body] **1.** The hard outer covering of certain invertebrates such as the mollusks and arthropods. It is composed of chitin, calcareous material, or both. **2.** In vertebrates, the hard outer covering such as the shell of a turtle; more specifically, the hard parts of the body surface derived principally from the ectoderm. These include such structures as hair, hooves, horns, nails, feathers, and scales.

**exosmosis** (ĕks″ŏs-mō′sĭs) [″ + *osmos,* a thrusting, + *osis,* condition] Diffusion of a fluid outward, as from a blood vessel.

**exosplenopexy** (ĕks″ō-splēn′ō-pĕks-ē) [″ + *splen,* spleen, + *pexis,* fixation] Suturing of the spleen to an opening in the abdominal wall.

**exostosis** (ĕks″ŏs-tō′sĭs) *pl.* **exostoses** [″ + *osteon,* bone] A bony growth that arises from the surface of a bone, often involving the ossification of muscular attachments. SYN: *hyperostosis; osteoma; osteoncus.*

***e. bursata*** An exostosis arising from the epiphysis of a bone and covered with cartilage and a synovial sac.

***e. cartilaginea*** An exostosis consisting of cartilage underlying the periosteum.

***dental e.*** An exostosis on the root of a tooth.

***multiple osteocartilaginous e.*** A hereditary growth disorder marked by the development of multiple exostoses, usually on the diaphyses of long bones near the epiphyseal lines. It causes irregular growth of the epiphyses and often secondary deformities.

**exothermal, exothermic** [Gr. *exo,* outside, + *therme,* heat] Pert. to a chemical reaction that produces heat.

**exothymopexy** (ĕks″ō-thī′mō-pĕks″ē) [″ + *thymos,* thymus, + *pexis,* fixation] Suturing of an enlarged thymus gland to the sternum.

**exothyropexy** (ĕks″ō-thī′rō-pĕks″ē) Suturing of the thyroid gland and external fixation to induce atrophy.

**exotic** (ĕg-zŏt′ĭk) [Gr. *exotikos*] Not native; originating in another part of the world.

**exotoxin** (ĕks″ō-tŏks′ĭn) [Gr. *exo,* outside, + *toxikon,* poison] A poisonous substance produced by a microorganism and secreted into its surrounding medium. It can usually be recovered from the liquid medium in which the toxin-producing organisms have developed. Exotoxins generally are unstable, being sensitive to the effects of chemicals, light, and heat. They are produced by certain bacteria, including staphylococci, streptococci, and the tetanus bacteria. Different exotoxins affect different tissues of the host.

**exotropia** (ĕks″ō-trō′pē-ă) [″ + *tropos,* turning] Divergent strabismus; abnormal turning outward of one or both eyes.

**expander** (ĕk-spăn′dĕr) [L. *expandere,* to spread out] Something that increases the size, volume, or amount of something.

**expansive delusion** SEE: *delusion, expansive.*

**expected date of confinement** ABBR: EDC. The predicted date of childbirth. SEE: *pregnancy* for table.

**expectorant** (ĕk-spĕk′tō-rănt) [Gr. *ex,* out, + L. *pectus,* breast] An agent that facilitates removal of bronchopulmonary mucous membrane secretions. Expectorants are classed as sedative or stimulating. They include ammonium carbonate, ammonium chloride, and ipecac.

**expectoration** (ĕk-spĕk″tō-rā′shŭn) **1.** The

act or process of spitting out saliva or coughing up materials from the air passageways leading to the lungs. **2.** The expulsion of mucus or phlegm from the throat or lungs. It may be mucous, mucopurulent, serous, or frothy. In pneumonia, it is viscid and tenacious, sticks to anything, appears rusty, and contains blood. In bronchitis, it is frothy, often streaked with blood, and greenish-yellow from pus. In advanced tuberculosis, it varies from small amount of frothy fluid to abundant, offensive greenish-yellow sputum often streaked with blood. SEE: *sputum.*

**expel** (ěks-pěl′) [L. *expellere*] To drive or push out.

**experience 1.** To encounter something personally or undergo an event. **2.** The knowledge or wisdom obtained from one's own observations.

**experiment** [L. *experimentum,* to test] The scientific procedure used to test the validity of a hypothesis, gain further evidence or knowledge, or test the usefulness of a drug or type of therapy that has not been tried previously.

**expiration** (ěks″pĭ-rā′shŭn) [Gr. *ex,* out, + L. *spirare,* to breathe] **1.** Expulsion of air from the lungs in breathing. Normally the duration of expiration is shorter than that of inspiration. In general, if expiration lasts longer than inspiration, a pathological condition such as emphysema or asthma is present. SEE: *diaphragm* for illus.; *inspiration; respiration.* **2.** Death.

***active e.*** Expiration accomplished as a result of muscular activity, as in forced respiration. The muscles used in forced expiration are those of the abdominal wall (external and internal oblique, rectus, and transversus abdominis), the internal intercostalis, serratus posterior inferior, platysma, and quadratus lumborum.

***passive e.*** Expiration, performed during quiet respiration, that requires no muscular effort. It is brought about by the elasticity of the lungs, and by the ascent of the diaphragm and the weight of the descending chest wall, which compress the lungs.

**expiratory** (ěks-pī′ră-tor″ē) Pert. to expiration of air from the lungs.

**expiratory center** The part of the respiratory center in the medulla that controls expiratory movements.

**expire 1.** To breathe out or exhale. **2.** To die.

**explant** (ěks-plănt′) [″ + L. *planta,* sprout] To remove a piece of living tissue from the body and transfer it to an artificial culture medium for growth, as in tissue culture. Opposite of implant.

**explode** (ěks-plōd′) [L. *explodere,* fr. *ex,* out, + *plaudere,* to clap the hands] **1.** To burst or to have rapid onset, as an epidemic. **2.** To decompress suddenly, as a cavity. Explosive decompression occurs when the pressure in the cabin of an airplane flying at high altitude is suddenly decreased.

**exploration** [L. *explorare,* to search out] Examination of an organ or part by various means. **exploratory,** ***adj.***

**explorer** An instrument used in exploration, esp. a device used to locate foreign bodies or to define passageways in body sinuses or cavities.

***dental e.*** A sharp-pointed instrument used to detect unsound enamel, carious lesions, or imperfect margins of restorations in teeth.

**explosive decompression** SEE: *decompression, explosive.*

**explosive speech** Sudden loud utterance. SEE: *speech.*

**exponent** (ěks′pō-něnt) In mathematics, the number that indicates the power to which another number is to be raised. It is written as a superscript (e.g., $10^2$ or $x^2$ indicates that 10 and x are to be squared, or multiplied by themselves). The exponent can have any numerical value and may be positive or negative; it does not have to be a whole number. SEE: *Scientific Notation in Units of Measurement Appendix.*

**expose 1.** To open, as in surgically opening the abdominal cavity. **2.** To cause someone or something to lack heat or shelter. **3.** To place in contact with an infected person or agent. **4.** To display one's genitals publicly, esp. when members of the opposite sex are present. **5.** To deliver an amount of radiation.

**exposure** The amount of radiation delivered or received over a given area or to the entire body or object.

***acute e.*** Exposure to radiation that is of short duration and usually of high intensity.

***double e.*** Two exposures on one photographic or radiographic film.

***pulp e.*** An opening in the dentin that exposes the pulp of a tooth.

**express** [L. *expressare*] To squeeze out.

**expression 1.** Expulsion by pressure. **2.** Facial disclosure of feeling or a physical state. SYN: *facies.* SEE: *face.*

**expressivity** The extent to which a heritable trait is manifest in the individual carrying the gene.

**expulsion rate** In gynecology, the rate of spontaneous rejection of intrauterine contraceptive devices in the group of women who use them. It is usually expressed with respect to the time elapsed following implantation.

**expulsive** [L. *expellere,* to drive out] Having a tendency to expel.

**exsanguinate** (ěks-săn′gwĭn-āt) [Gr. *ex,* out, + *sanguis,* blood] To lose blood to the point at which life can no longer be sustained.

**exsanguination** (ěk-săn″gwĭn-ā′shŭn) The process of expressing blood from a part.

**exsanguine** (ěks-săn′gwĭn) Anemic; bloodless.

**exsiccant** (ěk-sĭk′ănt) [L. *exsiccare,* to dry out] **1.** Absorbing or drying up a discharge. **2.** An agent that absorbs moisture. **3.** A dusting or drying powder.

**exsiccation** (ĕk″sĭ-kā′shŭn) **1.** The process of drying up. **2.** In chemistry, removing the water from compounds or solutions. SYN: *desiccation.*

**exsorption** (ĕk-sorp′shŭn) Movement of material including cells and electrolytes from the blood to the lumen of the intestines. In pathological conditions such as intestinal obstruction, this process may greatly increase pressure inside the affected area of the intestinal tract.

**exstrophy** (ĕks′trō-fē) [″ + *strephein,* to turn] Congenital turning inside out of an organ. SYN: *eversion.*

***e. of bladder*** A congenital malformation in which the lower portion of the abdominal wall and the anterior wall of the bladder are missing and the bladder is everted through the opening. SYN: *ectopia vesicae.*

**exsufflation** (ĕk″sŭ-flā′shŭn) [″ + *sufflatio,* blown up] Forceful expulsion of air from a cavity by artificial means, such as use of a mechanical exsufflator.

**ext** L. *extractum,* extract.

**extemporaneous** [LL. *extemporaneus*] Not prepared according to formula but devised for the occasion.

**extend** (ĕk-stĕnd′) [Gr. *ex,* out, + L. *tendere,* to stretch] **1.** To straighten a leg or arm. **2.** To move forward. **3.** To increase the angle between the bones forming a joint.

**extended care facility** A medical care institution for patients who require long-term custodial or medical care, esp. for a chronic disease or one requiring prolonged rehabilitation therapy.

**extended family** Members of the immediate family plus grandparents and other relatives.

**extender** (ĕk-stĕn′dĕr) Something that increases duration or effect. The time required for absorption of some medicines given intramuscularly may be increased by injecting them with a substance such as an oil, which slows absorption.

***leg e.*** A device added to lengthen the legs of furniture (e.g., beds, tables) to accommodate the needs of persons in wheelchairs.

**extension** (ĕks-tĕn′shŭn) [L. *extensio*] **1.** The movement that pulls apart both ends of any part. **2.** A movement that brings the members of a limb into or toward a straight position. Opposite of flexion. **3.** The application of a pull (traction) to a fractured or dislocated limb.

***Buck's e.*** A method of producing traction by applying regular or flannel-backed adhesive tape to the skin and keeping it in smooth close contact by circular bandaging of the part to which it is applied. The adhesive strips are aligned with the long axis of the arm or leg, the superior ends being about 1 in. (2.5 cm) from the fracture site. Weights sufficient to produce the required extension are fastened to the inferior end of the adhesive strips by a rope that is run over a pulley to permit free motion.

**extensor** [L.] A muscle that extends a part.

**exterior** [L.] Outside of; external.

**exteriorize 1.** To expose a part temporarily in surgery. SEE: *marsupialization.* **2.** In psychiatry, to turn one's interests outward.

**extern** (ĕks′tĕrn) [L. *externus,* outside] A medical student, living outside a hospital, who assists in the medical and surgical care of patients. SEE: *intern.*

**external** Exterior; the opposite of medial or internal.

**external fixator** SEE: *fixator, external.*

**externalia** (ĕks″tĕr-nā′lē-ă) [L. *exter,* outside, + *genitalis,* genital] The external genitals.

**externalize** (ĕks-tĕr′nă-līz) **1.** In surgery, to provide exposure to the outside. **2.** In psychiatry, to direct one's inner conflicts to the outside rather than keeping them hidden inside.

**exteroceptive** (ĕks″tĕr-ō-sĕp′tĭv) [L. *externus,* outside, + *receptus,* having received] Pert. to the reception by end organs receiving stimuli from outside.

**exteroceptor** (ĕks″tĕr-ō-sĕp′tor) A sense organ (e.g., in the eye, ear, or skin) adapted for the reception of stimuli from outside the body.

**extima** (ĕks′tĭ-mă) [L., outermost] The outer layer of a structure. SEE: *intima.*

**extinction** [L. *exstinctus,* having extinguished] **1.** The process of extinguishing or putting out. **2.** The complete inhibition of a conditioned reflex through failure to reinforce it.

**extinguish** (ĕks-tĭng′gwĭsh) [L. *extinguere,* to render extinct] To abolish, esp. to remove a reflex, by surgical, psychological, or pharmacological means, depending on the type of reflex involved.

**extirpation** (ĕks-tĭr-pā′shŭn) [L. *extirpare,* to root out] Excision of a part; taking out by the roots.

**extorsion** (ĕks-tor′shŭn) [Gr. *ex,* out, + L. *torsio,* twisting] Rotation of an organ or limb outward.

**extra-** [L. *extra,* outside] Prefix meaning *outside of; in addition to; beyond.*

**extra-articular** [″ + *articulus,* joint] Outside a joint.

**extra beat** Extrasystole.

**extracapsular** (ĕks″tră-kăp′sū-lăr) Outside a capsule (e.g., a joint capsule or the capsule of the lens of the eye).

**extracellular** (ĕks″tră-sĕl′ū-lăr) Outside the cell.

**extracellular space** SEE: *space, extracellular.*

**extrachromosomal** Not connected to the chromosomes; exerting an effect other than through chromosomal action.

**extracorporeal** (ĕks″tră-kor-por′ē-ăl) [″ + *corpus,* body] Outside the body.

**extracorporeal membrane oxygenator** ABBR: ECMO. An external device that oxygenates blood delivered to it from the body and then returns it to the patient. It has been used experimentally in patients with acute respiratory failure.

**extracorporeal shock-wave lithotriptor** A device that breaks up kidney stones. The shock waves are focused on the stones, disintegrating them and permitting their passage in the urine. This technique is also used to treat gallstones. SEE: *calculus, renal; percutaneous ultrasonic lithotriptor.*

**extracorticospinal** (ĕks″tră-kor″tĭ-kō-spī′năl) Outside the corticospinal tract of the central nervous system.

**extracranial** (ĕks″tră-krā′nē-ăl) Outside the skull.

**extract** (ĕks-trăkt′, ĕks′trăkt) [L. *extractum*] **1.** To pull out or remove forcibly, as to extract a tooth. **2.** A solid or semisolid preparation made by removing the soluble portion of a compound by using water or alcohol as the solvent and evaporating the solution. **3.** The active principle of a drug obtained by distillation or chemical processes.

***alcoholic e.*** An extract in which alcohol is the solvent.

***aqueous e.*** An extract in which water is the solvent.

***aromatic fluid e.*** An extract made from an aromatic powder.

***compound e.*** An extract prepared from more than one drug or substance.

***ethereal e.*** An extract using ether as the vehicle.

***fluid e.*** An extract of a vegetable drug made into a solution. It contains medicinal components.

***liver e.*** A dry brown powder obtained from mammalian livers that contains the hematinic factor (antianemic factor) that stimulates erythropoiesis. This extract was important in the treatment of pernicious anemia until vitamin $B_{12}$ was discovered.

***powdered e.*** A dried, crushed extract.

***soft e.*** An extract with the consistency of honey.

***solid e.*** An extract made by evaporating the fluid part of a solution.

**extraction** [L. *extractum,* drawing out] **1.** Pulling out, as a tooth. **2.** The removal of the active portion of a drug from its vehicle.

***breech e.*** SEE: *delivery, breech.*

***extracapsular e.*** A basic surgical technique for cataract removal. The nucleus, cortex, and anterior capsule are removed; the posterior capsule is left intact. This is often done by phacoemulsification under local anesthesia using a microscope.

**extractive** (ĕks-trăk′tĭv) Something that has been extracted or removed.

**extractor** An instrument for removing foreign bodies. Varieties include esophageal, throat, bronchial, and tissue extractors.

***vacuum e.*** SEE: *vacuum extractor.*

**extractum** (ĕks-trăk′tŭm) *pl.* **extracta** [L., a drawing out] An extract. SEE: *fluidextract.*

**extracystic** (ĕks″tră-sĭs′tĭk) [L. *extra,* outside, + Gr. *kystis,* bladder] Outside or unrelated to a bladder or cystic tumor.

**extradural** (ĕks-tră-dū′răl) [″ + *durus,* hard] **1.** On the outer side of the dura mater. **2.** Unconnected with the dura mater.

**extraembryonic** (ĕks″tră-ĕm″brē-ŏn′ĭk) [″ + Gr. *embryon,* something that swells in the body] Apart from and outside the embryo (e.g., concerning the amnion).

**extragenital** (ĕks″tră-jĕn′ĭ-tăl) [″ + *genitalis,* genital] Outside or unrelated to the genital organs.

**extrahepatic** (ĕks″tră-hĕ-păt′ĭk) [L. *extra,* outside, + Gr. *hepatos,* liver] Outside or unrelated to the liver.

**extraligamentous** [″ + *ligare,* to bind] Outside or unrelated to a ligament.

**extramalleolus** (ĕks″tră-măl-lē′ō-lŭs) [″ + *malleolus,* little hammer] The external or lateral malleolus of the ankle.

**extramarginal** (ĕks″tră-măr′jĭ-năl) [″ + *margo,* margin] Pert. to subliminal consciousness.

**extramastoiditis** (ĕks″tră-măs″toyd-ī′tĭs) [″ + Gr. *mastos,* breast, + *eidos,* form, shape, + *itis,* inflammation] Inflammation of outside tissues contiguous to the mastoid process.

**extramedullary** (ĕks″tră-mĕd′ū-lă-rē) [″ + *medulla,* marrow] Outside or unrelated to any medulla, esp. the medulla oblongata.

**extramural** (ĕks″tră-mū′răl) [″ + *murus,* wall] Outside the wall of an organ or vessel.

**extraneous** (ĕks-trā′nē-ŭs) [L. *extraneus,* external] Outside and unrelated to an organism.

**extranuclear** [L. *extra,* outside, + *nucleus,* kernel] Outside a nucleus.

**extraocular** (ĕks″tră-ŏk′ū-lăr) [″ + *oculus,* eye] Outside the eye, as in extraocular eye muscles.

**extraocular eye muscle** ABBR: EOM. A muscle attached to the eyeball that controls eye movement and coordination. SEE: illus.

**extrapolar** [″ + *polus,* pole] Outside instead of between poles, as the electrodes of a battery.

**extrapolate** To infer a point between two given, or known, points on a graph or progression. Thus, if an infant weighed 20 lb at a certain age and 4 months later weighed 23 lb, it could be inferred that at a point halfway between the two time periods, the infant would have weighed 21.5 lb.

**extrapyramidal** (ĕks″tră-pĭ-răm′ĭ-dăl) Outside the pyramidal tracts of the central nervous system.

**extrapyramidal motor system** SEE: *system, extrapyramidal motor.*

**extrapyramidal syndrome** Any of several degenerative nervous system diseases that involve the extrapyramidal system and the basal ganglion of the brain. The

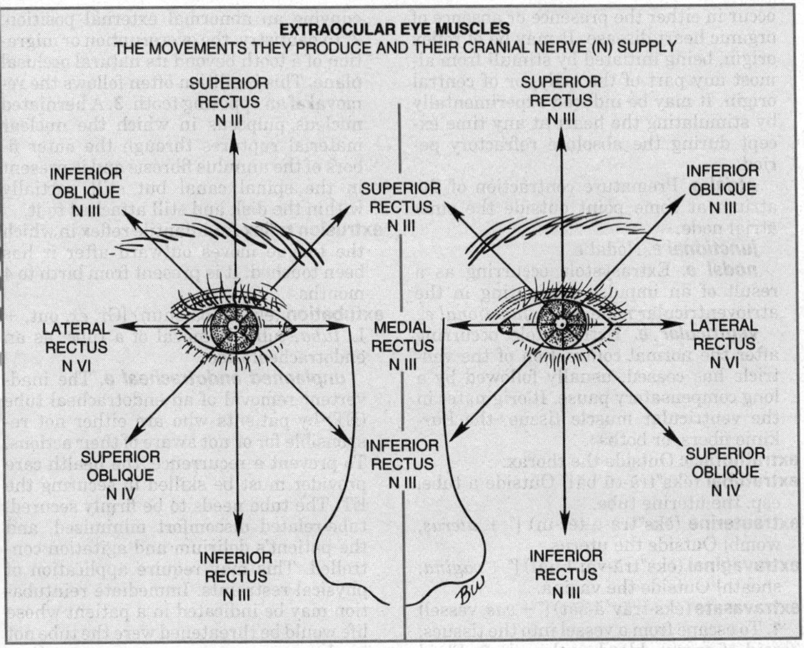

EXTRAOCULAR EYE MUSCLES
THE MOVEMENTS THEY PRODUCE AND THEIR CRANIAL NERVE (N) SUPPLY

SUPERIOR RECTUS N III
INFERIOR OBLIQUE N III
LATERAL RECTUS N VI
SUPERIOR OBLIQUE N IV
INFERIOR RECTUS N III
SUPERIOR RECTUS N III
MEDIAL RECTUS N III
INFERIOR RECTUS N III
SUPERIOR RECTUS N III
INFERIOR OBLIQUE N III
LATERAL RECTUS N VI
SUPERIOR OBLIQUE N IV
INFERIOR RECTUS N III

symptoms include tremors, chorea, athetosis, and dystonia. Parkinsonism is an extrapyramidal syndrome.

**extrasensory** Pert. to forms of perception, such as thought transference, that are not dependent on the five primary senses.

**extrasensory perception** ABBR: ESP. Perception of external events by other than the five senses.

**extrasystole** (ĕks″tră-sĭs′tō-lē) [″ + Gr. *systole,* contraction] Premature contraction of the heart. In humans, it is the result of some factor that initiates a stimulus in the impulse-conducting system. It may

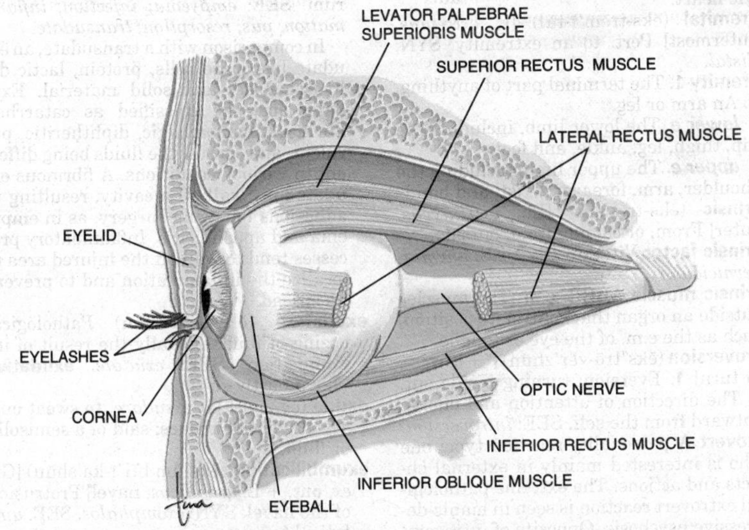


EXTRAOCULAR EYE MUSCLES

LATERAL VIEW, LEFT EYE (SUPERIOR OBLIQUE AND MEDIAL RECTUS NOT SHOWN)

occur in either the presence or absence of organic heart disease. It may be of reflex origin, being initiated by stimuli from almost any part of the body, or of central origin. It may be induced experimentally by stimulating the heart at any time except during the absolute refractory period.

***atrial e.*** Premature contraction of the atrium at some point outside the sinoatrial node.

***junctional e.*** Nodal e.

***nodal e.*** Extrasystole occurring as a result of an impulse originating in the atrioventricular node. SYN: *junctional e.*

***ventricular e.*** Extrasystole occurring after the normal contraction of the ventricle has ceased, usually followed by a long compensatory pause. It originates in the ventricular muscle tissue, the Purkinje fibers, or both.

**extrathoracic** Outside the thorax.

**extratubal** (ĕks″tră-tū′băl) Outside a tube, esp. the uterine tube.

**extrauterine** (ĕks″tră-ū′tĕr-ĭn) [″ + *uterus,* womb] Outside the uterus.

**extravaginal** (ĕks″tră-văj′ĭ-năl) [″ + *vagina,* sheath] Outside the vagina.

**extravasate** (ĕks-trăv′ă-sāt) [″ + *vas,* vessel] **1.** To escape from a vessel into the tissues, said of serum, blood, or lymph. **2.** Fluid escaping from vessels into surrounding tissue.

**extravasation** (ĕks-trăv″ă-sā′shŭn) The escape of fluids into the surrounding tissue. SYN: *suffusion.*

**extravascular** (ĕks″tră-văs′kū-lăr) [″ + *vasculum,* vessel] Outside a vessel.

**extraventricular** [″ + *ventriculus,* little belly] Outside any ventricle, esp. one of the heart.

**extremital** (ĕks-trĕm′ĭ-tăl) [L. *extremus,* outermost] Pert. to an extremity. SYN: *distal.*

**extremity 1.** The terminal part of anything. **2.** An arm or leg.

***lower e.*** The lower limb, including the hip, thigh, leg, ankle, and foot.

***upper e.*** The upper limb, including the shoulder, arm, forearm, wrist, and hand.

**extrinsic** (ĕks-trĭn′sĭk) [LL. *extrinsecus,* outer] From, or coming from, outside.

**extrinsic factor** Vitamin $B_{12}$. SEE: *anemia, pernicious.*

**extrinsic muscle** ABBR: e.m. The muscles outside an organ that control its position, such as the e.m. of the eye or tongue.

**extroversion** (ĕks″trō-vĕr′zhŭn) [″ + *vertere,* to turn] **1.** Eversion; turning inside out. **2.** The direction of attention and energy outward from the self. SEE: *introversion.*

**extrovert** A personality-reaction type; one who is interested mainly in external objects and actions. The extreme pathological extrovert reaction is seen in manic-depressive psychosis. Opposite of introvert.

**extrude** (ĕks-trūd′) [L. *extrudere,* to squeeze out] To push or force out.

**extrusion** (ĕks-troo′zhŭn) **1.** Something occupying an abnormal external position. **2.** In dentistry, the overeruption or migration of a tooth beyond its natural occlusal plane. This condition often follows the removal of an opposing tooth. **3.** A herniated nucleus pulposus in which the nuclear material ruptures through the outer fibers of the annulus fibrosis and is present in the spinal canal but still partially within the disk and still attached to it.

**extrusion reflex** An infantile reflex in which the tongue moves outward after it has been touched. It is present from birth to 4 months.

**extubation** (ĕks″tū-bā′shŭn) [Gr. *ex,* out, + L. *tuba,* tube] Removal of a tube, as an endotracheal tube.

***unplanned endotracheal e.*** The inadvertent removal of an endotracheal tube (ET) by patients who are either not responsible for or not aware of their actions. To prevent a recurrence, the health care provider must be skilled in securing the ET. The tube needs to be firmly secured, tube-related discomfort minimized, and the patient's delirium and agitation controlled. This may require application of physical restraints. Immediate reintubation may be indicated in a patient whose life would be threatened were the tube not in place.

**exuberant** (ĕg-zū′bĕr-ănt) [L. *exuberare,* to be very fruitful] **1.** Excessive, as in the increased and excessive growth of granulation tissue or bacterial culture. **2.** Joyful, happy.

**exudate** (ĕks′ū-dāt) [L. *exsudare,* to sweat out] Accumulated fluid in a cavity, matter that penetrates through vessel walls into adjoining tissue, or an oozing of pus or serum. SEE: *empyema; infection; inflammation; pus; resorption; transudate.*

In comparison with a transudate, an exudate has more cells, protein, lactic dehydrogenase, and solid material. Exudates may be classified as catarrhal, fibrinous, hemorrhagic, diphtheritic, purulent, and serous, the fluids being different in various conditions. A fibrinous exudate may wall off a cavity, resulting in adhesions following surgery, as in empyema and appendicitis. Inflammatory processes tend to wall off the injured area to localize the inflammation and to prevent its spread.

**exudation** (ĕks″ū-dā′shŭn) Pathological oozing of fluids, usually the result of inflammation. SEE: *exudate.* **exudative** (ĕks′ū-dā″tĭv), *adj.*

**exude** (ĕg-zūd′) [L. *exsudare,* to sweat out] To ooze out of tissues; said of a semisolid or fluid.

**exumbilication** (ĕks″ŭm-bĭl″ĭ-kā′shŭn) [Gr. *ex,* out, + L. *umbilicus,* navel] Protrusion of the navel. SYN: *exomphalos.* SEE: *umbilical hernia.*

**eye** [AS. *eage*] The organ of vision. SEE: illus.

ANATOMY: The eyeball has three lay-

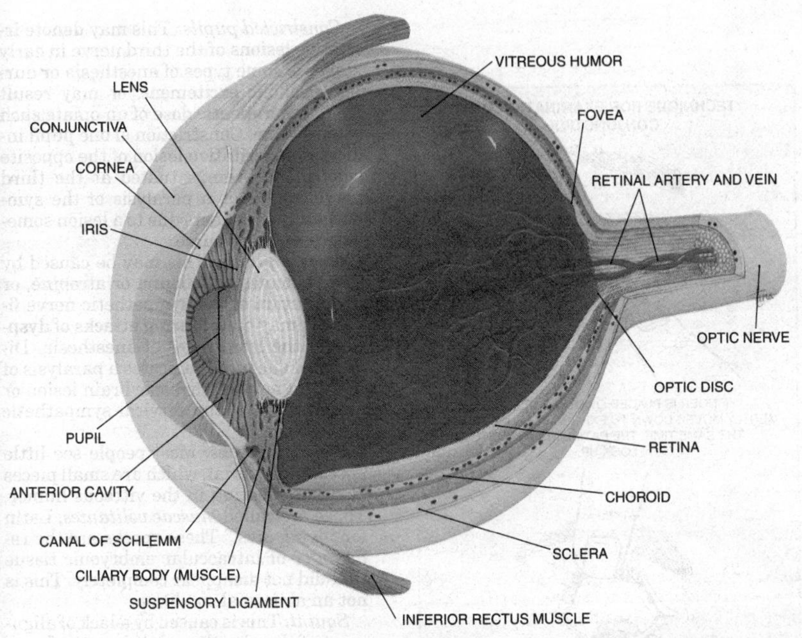


**ANATOMY OF THE EYE**

ers: the inner retina, which contains the photoreceptors; the middle uvea (choroid, ciliary body, and iris); and the outer sclera, which includes the transparent cornea. The eyeball contains two cavities. The smaller anterior cavity is in front of the lens and is further divided by the iris into an anterior chamber and a posterior chamber, both filled with watery (aqueous) humor. Behind the lens is the larger posterior cavity, which contains the jellylike vitreous body (humor). The lens is behind the iris, held in place by the ciliary body and suspensory ligaments. The visible portion of the sclera is covered by the conjunctiva, a membrane that continues as the lining of the eyelids. Six extrinsic muscles move the eyeball: the superior, inferior, medial, and lateral rectus muscles, and the superior and inferior oblique muscles.

*Nerve supply:* The eyeball is innervated by second cranial (optic) nerve. The eye muscles are supplied by third cranial (oculomotor), the fourth cranial (trochlear), and the sixth cranial (abducens) nerves. The lid muscles are supplied by the facial nerve to the orbicularis oculi and the oculomotor nerve to the levator palpebrae. Sensory fibers to the orbit are furnished by ophthalmic and maxillary fibers of the fifth cranial (trigeminal) nerve. Sympathetic postganglionic fibers originate in the carotid plexus, their cell bodies lying in the superior cervical ganglion. They supply the dilator muscle of the iris, lacrimal gland, and smooth muscle fibers in the eyelid. Parasympathetic fibers from the ciliary ganglion pass to the ciliary muscle and constrictor muscles of the iris.

PHYSIOLOGY: Light entering the eye passes through the cornea, then through the pupil, an opening in the iris, and on through the crystalline lens and the vitreous body to the retina. The cornea, aqueous humor, lens, and vitreous body are the refracting media of the eye. Changes in the curvature of the lens, brought about by its elasticity and contraction of the ciliary muscles, focus light rays on the retina, where they stimulate the rods and cones, the sensory receptors. The cones are concerned with color vision and the rods with vision in dim light. Sensory impulses pass through the optic nerve to the brain. The visual area of the cerebral cortex, located in the occipital lobe, registers them as visual sensations. The amount of light entering the eye is regulated by the iris; its constrictor and dilator muscles change the size of the pupil in response to varying amounts of light. The eye can distinguish nearly 8 million differences in color. As the eye ages, objects appear greener. The principal functions of the eye are color sense, light sense, movement, and form sense.

DIAGNOSIS: Following trauma to the head and in certain disease states, the size, shape, motion, and reactions of the pupils provide extremely important diagnostic information.

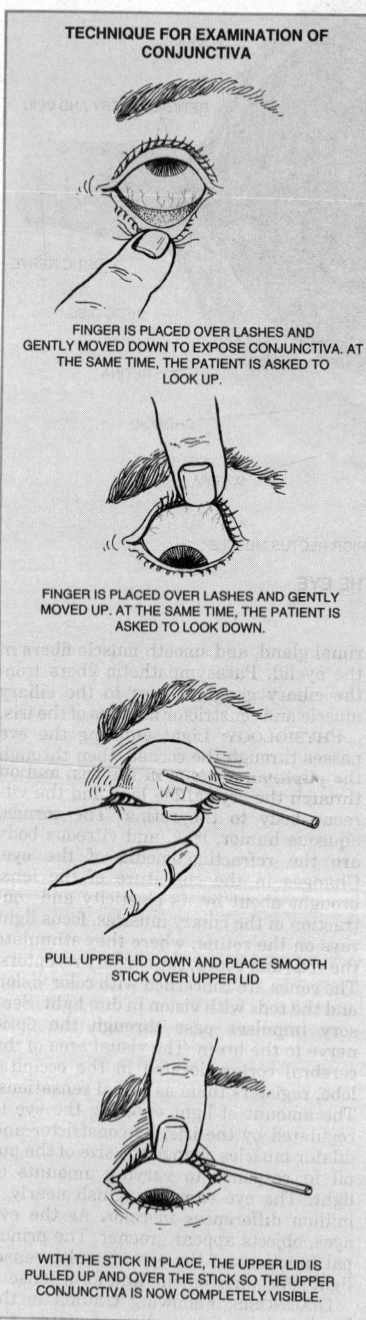


*Constricted pupils:* This may denote irritative lesions of the third nerve in early stages of some types of anesthesia or during alcoholic excitement, or may result from a therapeutic dose of an opiate such as morphine. Constriction of one pupil indicates an irritative lesion of the opposite side of the brain, situated at the third nerve nuclei, or a paralysis of the sympathetic nerve fibers due to a lesion somewhere in their course.

*Dilated pupils:* This may be caused by the medicines belladonna or atropine, or by irritation of the sympathetic nerve fibers. It may occur during attacks of dyspnea in the last stages of anesthesia. Dilation of one pupil indicates a paralysis of the third nerve from some brain lesion or an irritation of the cervical sympathetic nerve fibers.

*Floating specks:* Most people see little specks of material, which are small pieces of tissue, floating in the vitreous humor. These are called *muscae volitantes,* Latin for "flying flies." These specks are the remainder of intraocular embryonic tissue that did not disappear completely. This is not an abnormal condition.

*Squint:* This is caused by a lack of alignment of the visual axes. It is an unfavorable symptom in the course of a brain disease.

EYE COMPRESSES: *Cold compresses:* Cold compresses relieve congestion of eyelids, control intraocular hemorrhage, and are used occasionally for conjunctivitis and early lid injuries to prevent hemorrhage into tissues. The hands are scrubbed, and the compresses moistened with isotonic saline solution, wrung out with forceps, and placed on ice to chill. The compresses are placed over the lids and extended over the cheek and are changed every 2 or 3 min. Each compress may be used repeatedly if there is no pus. When pus is present, each compress may be used only once.

*Hot compresses:* Comfortably warm compresses are used to increase the blood supply to the eyelids and eyeballs and to relieve pain. The hands are scrubbed, and petroleum jelly is applied with a clean swab to the area where the compresses will be applied. The compresses are wrung dry with forceps, tested on the wrist, and applied with as much heat as the patient can tolerate. To increase blood supply to the eyelids, compresses are placed over the lids and extended over the cheeks; to increase blood supply to the eyeballs, they are placed over the lids and extended over the brow. New compresses are used for each application if pus is present. The eyelid is dried when the last compress is removed. SEE: *lacrimal apparatus*; *Universal Precautions Appendix.*

NURSING IMPLICATIONS: Visual acuity is assessed immediately. If the globe has been penetrated, a suitable eye shield, not an eye patch, is applied. A penetrating foreign body should not be removed. All medications, esp. corticosteroids, are withheld until the patient has been seen by an ophthalmologist.

The patient is assessed for pain and tenderness, redness and discharge, itching, photophobia, increased tearing, blinking, and visual blurring. When any prescribed topical eye medications (drops, ointments, or solutions) are administered, the hands are washed thoroughly, the head is turned slightly toward the affected eye, and the patient's cooperation is sought in keeping the eye wide open. Drops are instilled in the conjunctival sac (not on the orb), and pressure is applied to the lacrimal apparatus in the inner canthus as necessary to prevent systemic absorption. Ointments are applied along the palpebral border from the inner to the outer canthus, and solutions instilled from the inner to the outer canthus. Touching the dropper or tip of the medication container to the eye should be avoided, and hands should be washed immediately after the procedure.

Both patient and family are taught correct methods for instilling prescribed medications. Patients with visual defects are protected from injury, and family members taught safety measures. Patients with insufficient tearing or the inability to blink or close their eyes are protected from corneal injury by applying artificial tears and by gently patching the eyes closed. The importance of periodic eye examinations is emphasized. Persons at risk should protect their eyes from trauma by wearing safety goggles when working with or near dangerous tools or substances. Tinted lenses should be worn to protect the eyes from excessive exposure to bright light. Patients should avoid rubbing their eyes to prevent irritation or possibly infection. SEE: *eyedrops; tears, artificial.*

Caution: Corticosteroids should not be administered topically or systemically until the patient has been seen by a physician, preferably an ophthalmologist. *A red eye due to herpes simplex plus use of corticosteroids indicates risk for blindness in that eye.*

***aphakic e.*** An eye from which the crystalline lens has been removed.

***artificial e.*** A prosthesis for placement in the orbit of an individual whose eye has been removed. SEE: *ocularist.*

***black e.*** Ecchymosis of the tissues surrounding the eye.

***crossed e.*** Strabismus with deviation of the visual axis of one eye toward that of the other eye.

***dark-adapted e.*** An eye that has become adjusted for viewing objects in dim light; one adapted for scotopic, or rod, vision. Dark adaptation depends on the regeneration of a light-sensitive substance, rhodopsin, in the rods of the retina.

***e. deviation*** In eye muscle imbalance and "crossed eyes," the abnormal visual axis of the eye that is not aligned.

***dominant e.*** The eye to which a person unconsciously gives preference as a source of stimuli for visual sensations. The dominant eye is usually used in sighting down a gun or looking through a monocular microscope.

***dry e.*** SEE: *eye, dry.*

***exciting e.*** In sympathetic ophthalmia, the damaged eye, which is the source of sympathogenic influences.

***fixating e.*** In strabismus, the eye that is directed toward the object of vision.

***foreign body in e.*** This condition is manifested by pain, lacrimation, and spasm of the eye; later, redness, swelling, and occasionally headache occur. Infection may be carried into the eye, resulting in an ulcer of the cornea. Metal produces a chemical effect as it disintegrates, which affects the eyeball. A radiograph is sometimes used to detect tiny particles of metal, and an electromagnet to assist in removing them. Sympathetic ophthalmia, the transference of inflammation from the injured eye to the normal eye, may be produced by wounds that pierce the eyeball. Loss of vision in both eyes may result if the affected eye is not removed.

FIRST AID: Tearing often washes dust from the eye. Bringing the upper lid over the lower and directing the patient to roll the eye often deposits the dust on the margin of the lower lid.

Great care is necessary in removing larger particles. This should be done in a quiet, well-lighted place with clean, preferably sterile materials. One or two drops of a bland oil are then instilled into the eye. If the eye is inflamed, repeated comfortably warm compresses should be used.

If the patient cannot be taken care of at once, the eye should be bandaged to keep it closed and thus avoid scratching the conjunctiva. There should be no delay in having the speck removed, as serious injury to the eyeball or the vision may result. In general, the longer the foreign body remains in the eye, the deeper it becomes embedded.

***light-adapted e.*** An eye that has become adjusted to viewing objects in bright light; one adapted for photopic, or cone, vision. In this type of eye, most rhodopsin has been broken down.

***squinting e.*** An eye that deviates from the object of fixation in strabismus.

***sympathizing e.*** In sympathetic ophthalmia, the uninjured eye, which reacts to the pathological process in the injured eye.

***trophic ulceration of e.*** A noninfectious ulceration of the corneal epithelium of the eye due to repeated trauma.

**eyeball** The globe of the eye. Tension and position of the globe in relation to the orbit should be noted.

PATHOLOGY: Pathological conditions include enophthalmos (recession of the eyeball) and exophthalmos (protrusion of the eyeball).

**eyeball, voluntary propulsion of** The ability to voluntarily cause the globe of the eye to protrude by as much as 10 mm (0.4 in.). This is not harmful to the eye or visual acuity.

**eye bank** An organization that collects and stores corneas for transplantation.

**eyebrow** The arch over the eye; also its covering, esp. the hairs.

**eye contact** The meeting of the gaze of two persons; a direct look into the eyes of another.

**eyecup** **1.** The optic vesicle, an evagination of the embryonic brain from which the retina develops. **2.** A small cup that fits over the eye, used for bathing its surface.

**eyedrops** Any medicinal substance dropped in liquid form onto the conjunctiva.

In applying eyedrops, the head should be held back; the drops will not pass from under the upper lid to under the lower lid or vice versa. The smaller the eyedrops, the better. Too much liquid in the eye causes the patient to blink, and the medication is then washed away by the increased lacrimal secretion.

Caution: Many medicines are not absorbed from the conjunctiva; they may be readily absorbed from the nasolacrimal duct. For this reason, esp. in children, it is advisable to close off the duct by applying pressure to the inner canthus of the eye for a few minutes after each instillation. This is of particular importance with drugs such as belladonna to which young children are esp. sensitive.

**eye-gaze communicator** An electronic device that allows a person to control a computer by looking at words or commands on a video screen. A very low intensity light shines into one of the user's eyes. Reflections from the cornea and retina are picked up by a television camera. As the direction of the person's gaze moves, the relative position of the two reflections changes, and the computer uses this information to determine the area at which the person is looking. The computer then executes the command.

**eyeglass** A glass lens used to correct a defect in visual acuity or to prevent exposure to bright light if the lens is tinted. SEE: *glasses*.

**eyeground** The fundus of the eye, seen with an ophthalmoscope.

**eyelash** A stiff hair on the margin of the eyelid. SYN: *cilium*.

**eyelid** One of two movable protective folds that cover the anterior surface of the eyeball when closed. They are separated by the palpebral fissure. The upper (palpebra superior) is the larger and more movable. It is raised by contraction of the levator palpebrae superioris muscle. Angles formed at the inner and outer ends of the lids are known as the canthi. The cilia, or eyelashes, arise from the edges of the eyelids. The posterior surface is lined by the conjunctiva, a mucous membrane.

***drooping e.*** Ptosis of the eyelid.

***fused e.*** A congenital anomaly resulting from failure of the fetal eyelids to separate.

**eyelid closure reflex** Contraction of the orbicularis palpebrarum muscle with closure of lids resulting from percussion above the supraorbital nerve. SYN: *McCarthy's reflex; supraorbital reflex*.

**eye muscle imbalance** A pathological condition of the extraocular muscles of one or both eyes. It causes the eyes to be misaligned in one or more axes. SEE: *eye, crossed; esophoria; exophoria; squint; strabismus*.

**eyepiece** (ī'pēs) The portion of an optical device closest to the viewer's eye.

**eye protection** Use of goggles, plastic or glass face masks, or protective glasses to prevent injury to the eye during work or play in situations that could cause severe damage to the eye (e.g., work with a grinding machine, sports involving a small ball, fishing, or hiking in an area where tree branches must be dodged).

**eye stones** Very small stones placed in the conjunctival sac to remove a mobile foreign body from the eye.

**eyestrain** Tiredness of the eye due to overuse or use of an improper corrective lens.

**eyewash** Any suitable liquid material used to wash the eye (e.g., sterile physiological saline or sterile water).

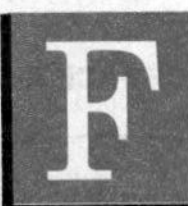

**F** 1. *Fahrenheit; femto-; field of vision; folic acid; formula; function.* 2. Symbol for the element fluorine.

**$F_1$** In genetics, the first filial generation, the offspring of a cross between two unrelated individuals.

**$F_2$** In genetics, the second filial generation, the offspring of a cross between two individuals of the $F_1$ generation.

**FA., F.A.** *fatty acid; filterable agent; first aid; fluorescent antibody.*

**F.A.A.N.** *Fellow of the American Academy of Nursing.*

**Fab** *fragment antigen binding.*

**fabella** (fă-bĕl′lă) *pl.* **fabellae** [L., little bean] Fibrocartilage or bone that sometimes develops in the head of the gastrocnemius muscle.

**fabism** (fā′bĭzm) [L. *faba,* bean, + Gr. *-ismos,* condition] Favism.

**fabrication** (făb″rĭ-kā′shŭn) [L. *fabricatus,* having built] A deliberately false statement told as if it were true. It is present in Korsakoff's syndrome.

**Fabry's disease** (fă′brēz) [J. Fabry, Ger. physician, 1860–1930] An inherited metabolic disease in which there is a galactosidase deficiency, which leads to accumulation of glycosphingolipids throughout the body. Clinically, by age 10, there is discomfort of the hands and feet with paresthesia or burning pain. There may be painful abdominal crises resembling other causes of acute abdominal pain. As these patients age, renal impairment may require dialysis or kidney transplant.

**F.A.C.C.P.** *Fellow of the American College of Chest Physicians.*

**F.A.C.D.** *Fellow of the American College of Dentists.*

**face** [L. *facies*] The anterior part of the head from the forehead to the chin, extending laterally to but not including the ears; the visage or countenance. SEE: illus.; *facial expression.*

ANATOMY: There are 14 bones in the face. The blood supply is bilateral from the facial, maxillary, and superficial temporal branches of the external carotid artery and the ophthalmic branch of the internal carotid artery. The veins include the exterior and interior jugular veins.

DIAGNOSIS: The following conditions affect the features: mouth breathing, chronic alcoholism, narcotic drug use, abdominal diseases, pain, fear, mental depression, fatigue, facial hemiplegia, cretinism, myxedema, congenital syphilis, exophthalmic goiter, paralysis agitans, encephalitis lethargica, locomotor ataxia, acromegaly, Down syndrome, acute diffuse peritonitis, dyspnea, hysteria, late stages of pulmonary tuberculosis, lobar pneumonia, renal diseases, typhoid fever, hippocratic facies.

*Brownish-yellow spots:* These are commonly called liver spots. They are seen in pregnancy, malignancies of the liver or uterus, and exophthalmic goiter. Cosmetics and facial irritants, sunburn, and exposure to weather are also factors. Liver spots occur in many diseases including Addison's disease, diabetes, hemochromatosis, pellagra, and acanthosis nigricans. They also occur in arsenic poisoning.

*Depigmentation:* This may be caused by vitiligo or scars.

*Yellowish discoloration:* Jaundice is due to an excess of bile pigments in the blood. Carotenemia may cause a similar discoloration.

*Cyanosis:* This may indicate deficient oxygenation of the blood, which may be due to acquired or congenital heart malformation, asthma, whooping cough, pulmonary tuberculosis, croup, tracheal obstruction, aneurysm, tumor, asphyxia, drug poisoning, emphysema, or dilation of the right side of the heart.

*Flushing:* Hyperemia may be either permanent or evanescent. If due to emotions or sunburn, it is temporary. Chronic flushing may be due to febrile diseases, pulmonary tuberculosis, convulsions, alcoholism, ovarian tumors, goiter, plethora, or hypertension.

*Pallor:* Absence of color may be due to use of cosmetics, excessive confinement indoors, malnourishment, anemia, hemorrhage, shock, or fright.

*Quivering chin:* Shaking of the chin is seen most often in children who are emotionally stressed and close to tears.

*Redness alternating with pallor:* This may be due to emotion such as anger, cerebrospinal meningitis, typhoid, menopause, or general vasomotor disturbance.

*Sallowness:* This symptom occurs in cachexia, cancer, lead poisoning, some anemias, Addison's disease, and diseases of the liver.

*Edema:* This is noted in cardiac, renal, and blood diseases; pneumothorax; mediastinal tumors; and aneurysm. Edema may be localized and evanescent due to urticaria, angioneurotic edema, or anaphylaxis. It is seen in thrombosis of the superior longitudinal sinus.

*Absence of expression from half the face with face drawn and distorted:* This indicates facial paralysis of the opposite side.

*Anxious or pinched look:* This expres-

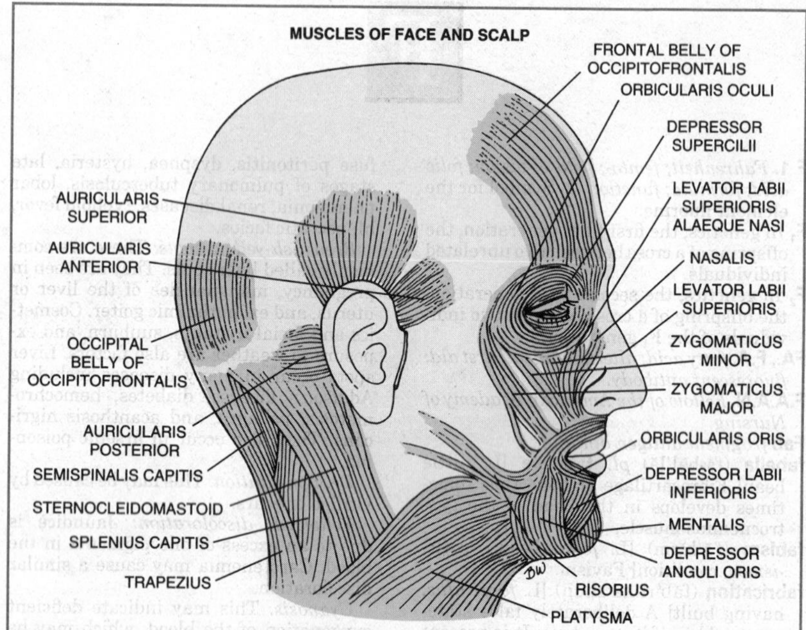


sion indicates anxiety, fear, or apprehension.

*Risus sardonicus:* A sardonic smile is caused by contraction or spasm of mouth muscles.

*Spasms:* These may be intermittent, continuous, bilateral, or unilateral. They may be due to dental disorders or diseases of the skin, nose, or eyes. They may be mimic or habit spasms; choreic, winking spasms; convulsive tic; or blepharospasm. Closure of the eyelids is caused by spasm of the orbicular muscles due to a disorder of the nerve supply or the eye muscles, or to eye disease. Spasm of the eyelids, chin, upper lips, or muscles of the face is seen in the early stages of meningitis. Tonic spasms are due to tetanus, paralysis, hysteria, or tic douloureux.

**moon f.** This full, round face is seen in Cushing's syndrome. It may also be a side effect of corticosteroid therapy.

**face-lift** A nonscientific term for plastic surgery of the face. SEE: *rhitidectomy.*

**FACEP** *Fellow of the American College of Emergency Physicians.*

**facet** (făs′ĕt) [Fr. *facette,* small face] A small, smooth area on a bone or other hard surface.

**wear f.** A line or plane worn on a tooth surface by attrition.

**facetectomy** (făs″ĕ-tĕk′tō-mē) [″ + Gr. *ektome,* excision] Surgical removal of the auricular facet of a vertebra.

**facet joint** One of the zygapophyseal joints of the vertebral column between the articulating facets of each pair of vertebrae.

**facial** [L. *facialis*] Pert. to the face.

**facial bones** The 14 bones that make up the face: maxillae (2); nasal (2); palatine (2); inferior nasal conchae (2); mandible (1); zygoma (2); lacrimal (2); vomer (1).

**facial center** The brain center that causes facial movements.

**facial expression** An appearance of the face conveying emotion or reaction. The human face has a great store and variety of expressions. Expressions may convey different meanings in different cultures. Also, certain disease states (e.g., schizophrenia) may limit the ability to interpret facial expression, and parkinsonism is associated with facial rigidity. In certain cultures a smile is to be expected, but in others it may be an infrequent facial expression.

**facial nerve** The seventh cranial nerve. A mixed nerve, it consists of efferent fibers supplying the facial muscles, the platysma muscle, the submandibular and sublingual glands; and afferent fibers from taste buds of the anterior two thirds of the tongue and from the muscles. The afferent fibers originate from the geniculate ganglion, and the motor and secretory fibers from nuclei in the pons. They are distributed throughout the ear, face, palate, and tongue. Branches are the tympanic, chorda tympani, posterior auricular, digastric, stylohyoid, temporal, zygomatic, malar, buccal, mandibular, and cervical. SEE: illus.; *cranial nerves.*

**facial paralysis** Loss of motion affecting the muscles of the face. The seventh cranial

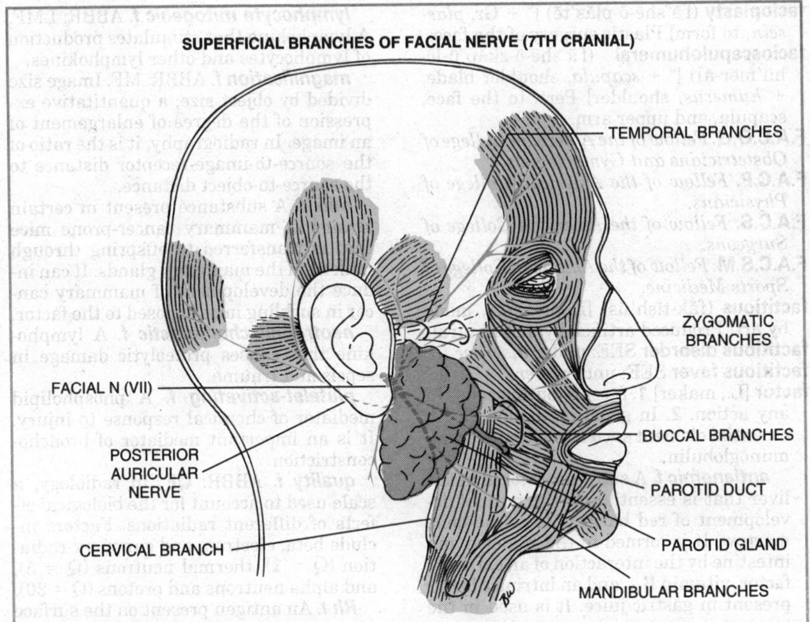


nerve is involved.

**facial reflex** In coma, contraction of facial muscles following pressure on the eyeball. SYN: *bulbomimic reflex; Mondonesi's reflex.*

**facial spasm** An involuntary contraction of muscles supplied by the facial nerve, involving one side of the face or the region around the eye. SEE: *cranial nerve; tic.*

**-facient** Suffix meaning *to make happen; to cause.*

**facies** (fā′shē-ēz) *pl.* **facies** [L] **1.** The face or the surface of any structure. **2.** The expression or appearance of the face.

***f. abdominalis*** A pinched, anxious, shrunken, and drawn expression seen with abdominal problems.

***adenoid f.*** A dull, lethargic appearance with open mouth, which may be due to hypertrophy of adenoids or to chronic mouth breathing.

***f. aortica*** The appearance seen in aortic valve insufficiency, with bluish sclerae, sunken cheeks, and sallow skin.

***f. hepatica*** The facies seen in liver disease. The skin is sallow, the conjunctivae yellow, and the eyeballs sunken.

***f. hippocratica*** The facies seen in those dying from long-continued illness or from cholera. The cheeks and temples are hollow, the eyes sunken, the complexion leaden, and the lips relaxed.

***f. leontina*** The lion-like facies seen in certain forms of leprosy.

***masklike f.*** An expressionless face with little or no animation, seen in parkinsonism.

***f. mitralis*** The facies seen in mitral insufficiency. Capillaries are more or less visible, and the cheeks are pink, although the patient is somewhat cyanotic.

***myopathic f.*** The facies due to muscular relaxation. The lids drop and the lips protrude.

***parkinsonian f.*** A masklike facies with infrequent eye blinking, characteristic of parkinsonism. The individual can move the face, but in repose it is expressionless.

**facilitation** (fă-sĭl″ĭ-tā′shŭn) [L. *facilis,* easy] **1.** The hastening of an action or process; esp., addition of the energy of a nerve impulse to that of other impulses activated at the same time. **2.** In neuromuscular rehabilitation, a generic term referring to various techniques that elicit muscular contraction through reflex activation.

***autogenic f.*** The process of inhibiting the muscle that generated a stimulus while providing an excitatory impulse to the antagonist muscle.

**facing** [L. *facies,* face] A veneer of restorative material used on a tooth or on a prosthesis to simulate a natural tooth.

**faciobrachial** (fā″shē-ō-brā′kē-ăl) [″ + Gr. *brachion,* arm] Pert. to the face and arm, esp. to juvenile muscular dystrophy.

**faciocervical** (fā″shē-ō-sĕr′vĭ-kăl) [″ + *cervix,* neck] Pert. to the face and neck, esp. to progressive dystrophy of facial muscles.

**faciolingual** (fā″shē-ō-lĭn′gwăl) [″ + *lingua,* tongue] Pert. to the face and tongue, esp. to paralysis of these.

**facioplasty** (fā″shē-ō-plăs′tē) [″ + Gr. *plassein,* to form] Plastic surgery of the face.

**facioscapulohumeral** (fā″shē-ō-skăp″ū-lō-hū′mĕr-ăl) [″ + *scapula,* shoulder blade, + *humerus,* shoulder] Pert. to the face, scapula, and upper arm.

**F.A.C.O.G.** *Fellow of the American College of Obstetricians and Gynecologists.*

**F.A.C.P.** *Fellow of the American College of Physicians.*

**F.A.C.S.** *Fellow of the American College of Surgeons.*

**F.A.C.S.M.** *Fellow of the American College of Sports Medicine.*

**factitious** (făk-tĭsh′ŭs) [L. *facticius,* made by art] Produced artificially; not natural.

**factitious disorder** SEE: under *disorder.*

**factitious fever** SEE: under *fever.*

**factor** [L., maker] **1.** A contributing cause in any action. **2.** In genetics, a gene. **3.** An essential element such as a vitamin or immunoglobulin.

***antianemic f.*** A substance stored in the liver that is essential for the normal development of red blood cells in the bone marrow. It is formed in the stomach and intestine by the interaction of an extrinsic factor, vitamin $B_{12}$, and an intrinsic factor present in gastric juice. It is used in the treatment of pernicious anemia.

***antihemophilic f.*** SEE: *antihemophilic factor.*

***autocrine motility f.*** A chemical released by neoplastic cells that induces motility, enabling the cells to metastasize.

***coagulation f.*** SEE: *coagulation factor.*

***eosinophil chemotactic f.*** A mediator released when mast cells are injured. This is in response to inflammation.

***heparin-binding epidermal growth f.*** ABBR: HB-EGF. A cytokine, classed as a monokine, that is involved in immune and inflammatory responses. It is produced by macrophages and stimulates production of smooth muscle cells and fibroblasts.

***hepatocyte growth f.*** ABBR: HGF. A cytokine, classed as a monokine, that is involved in immune and inflammatory responses. It is formed from platelets, fibroblasts, macrophages, endothelial cells, and smooth muscle cells. It stimulates growth of hepatocytes and increases migration and motility of various epithelial and endothelial cells.

***intrinsic f.*** A glycoprotein secreted by the parietal cells of the gastric mucosa. It is necessary for the absorption of ingested vitamin $B_{12}$. The absence of this factor leads to vitamin $B_{12}$ deficiency and pernicious anemia.

***lethal f.*** A gene or an abnormality in genetic composition that causes death of a zygote or of an individual before the reproductive age.

***leukocyte migration inhibition f.*** ABBR: LMIF. A lymphokine that inhibits movement of neutrophils.

***lymphocyte mitogenic f.*** ABBR: LMF. A lymphokine that stimulates production of lymphocytes and other lymphokines.

***magnification f.*** ABBR: MF. Image size divided by object size; a quantitative expression of the degree of enlargement of an image. In radiography, it is the ratio of the source-to-image-receptor distance to the source-to-object distance.

***milk f.*** A substance present in certain strains of mammary cancer-prone mice that is transferred to offspring through milk from the mammary glands. It can induce the development of mammary cancer in suckling mice exposed to the factor.

***neotrophil chemotactic f.*** A lymphokine that causes proteolytic damage in sepsis and trauma.

***platelet-activating f.*** A phospholipid mediator of chemical response to injury. It is an important mediator of bronchoconstriction.

***quality f.*** ABBR: QF. In radiology, a scale used to account for the biological effects of different radiations. Factors include beta, electron, and gamma x-radiation ($Q = 1$), thermal neutrons ($Q = 5$), and alpha neutrons and protons ($Q = 20$).

***Rh f.*** An antigen present on the surface of erythrocytes. SEE: *Rh blood group.*

**facultative** (făk′ŭl-tā″tĭv) [L. *facultas,* capability] **1.** Having the ability to do something that is not compulsory. **2.** In biology and particularly bacteriology, having the ability to live under certain conditions. Thus a microorganism may be facultative with respect to oxygen and be able to live with or without oxygen.

**facultative anaerobe** SEE: *anaerobe, facultative.*

**faculty 1.** A normal mental attribute or sense; ability to function. **2.** Persons employed as teachers at a college or university.

**FAD** *flavin adenine dinucleotide.*

**Faget's sign** [Jean C. Faget, Fr. physician, 1818–1884] A pulse slower than would be expected with the elevated temperature present. It may be seen in some viral infections.

**Fahrenheit scale** (făr′ĕn-hīt″) [Daniel Gabriel Fahrenheit, Ger.-Dutch physicist, 1686–1736] A temperature scale with the freezing point of water at 32° and the boiling point at 212°, indicated by F. SEE: table; *Celsius scale; Kelvin scale; thermometer; Units of Measurement Appendix.*

**fail safe** Pert. to the idea that a device, system, or program can be manufactured, planned, or conceived to prevent failure or malfunction, and to be problem free or infallible.

**failure** (fāl′yĕr) Inability to function, esp. loss of what was once present, as in failing eyesight or hearing.

***heart f.*** SEE: *heart failure.*

***kidney f.*** *Renal f.*

***liver f.*** The inability of the liver to function because of a disease process within

## Fahrenheit and Celsius Scales*

| F | C | F | C | F | C |
|---|---|---|---|---|---|
| 500° | 260° | 203° | 95° | 98° | 36.67° |
| 401 | 205 | 194 | 90 | 97 | 36.11 |
| 392 | 200 | 176 | 80 | 96 | 35.56 |
| 383 | 195 | 167 | 75 | 95 | 35 |
| 374 | 190 | 140 | 60 | 86 | 30 |
| 356 | 180 | 122 | 50 | 77 | 25 |
| 347 | 175 | 113 | 45 | 68 | 20 |
| 338 | 170 | 110 | 43.33 | 50 | 10 |
| 329 | 165 | 109 | 42.78 | 41 | 5 |
| 320 | 160 | 108 | 42.22 | 32 | 0 |
| 311 | 155 | 107 | 41.67 | 23 | −5 |
| 302 | 150 | 106 | 41.11 | 14 | −10 |
| 284 | 140 | 105 | 40.56 | 5 | −15 |
| 275 | 135 | 104 | 40.00 | −4 | −20 |
| 266 | 130 | 103 | 39.44 | −13 | −25 |
| 248 | 120 | 102 | 38.89 | −22 | −30 |
| 239 | 115 | 101 | 38.33 | −40 | −40 |
| 230 | 110 | 100 | 37.78 | −76 | −60 |
| 212 | 100 | 99 | 37.22 | | |

* To convert a Fahrenheit temperature to degrees Celsius, subtract 32 and multiply by 5/9. To convert a Celsius temperature to degrees Fahrenheit, multiply by 9/5 and add 32.

the liver or because of demands beyond its capability.

***metabolic f.*** Rapid failure of physical and mental functions ending in death.

***multisystem organ f.*** SEE: *multiple system organ failure.*

***renal f.*** Inability of the kidneys to function adequately. It may be partial, temporary, chronic, acute, or complete. SYN: *kidney f.*

***respiratory f.*** SEE: *respiratory failure, acute; respiratory failure, chronic.*

**failure to thrive** ABBR: FTT. A condition in which infants and children not only fail to gain weight but also may lose it. It is seen more often in institutionalized and retarded children. The organic causes include almost any severe chronic condition. The causes of nonorganic failure to thrive include starvation, emotional deprivation, and social disruption. SEE: *Nursing Diagnoses Appendix.*

**faint** [O. Fr. *faindre,* to feign] **1.** To feel weak as though about to lose consciousness. **2.** Weak. **3.** Syncope; loss of consciousness due to cerebral anemia or insufficient blood to the brain.

SYMPTOMS: Before the onset, the patient may be pale, weak, and dizzy, with cold perspiration and an uncomfortable abdominal sensation. The patient may fall to the ground unconscious. The pulse is usually weak and rapid and is often irregular.

FIRST AID: The individual must be placed in a horizontal position, preferably with the head low to facilitate blood flow to the brain. At the same time, it is essential to ensure that the airway is clear and that clothing is loose, esp. if a tight collar was being worn. It is important to ascertain that respiratory and cardiac functions are within normal limits. Fainting usually is of short duration and is counteracted by the supine position. Nevertheless the cause of the faint must be established before the episode is dismissed as being of no consequence. If recovery from fainting is not prompt, the patient should be moved to a hospital.

**faintness 1.** A sensation of impending loss of consciousness. SYN: *presyncope.* **2.** A sensation of weakness due to lack of food.

**faith healing** A cure accomplished by supplication to a divine being or power to the exclusion of medical or surgical therapy. Although this area is open to dangerous and fraudulent practice, the medical community cannot completely ignore the psychosomatic aspects of illness that this practice may affect positively.

**falcate** (făl′kāt) [L. *falx,* sickle] Sickle-shaped.

**falces** (făl′sēz) [L.] Plural of falx.

**falcial** (făl′shăl) Pert. to a falx.

**falciform** (făl′sĭ-form) [L. *falx,* sickle, + *forma,* form] Sickle-shaped.

**falciform ligament** The triangular ligament attached to the sides of the sacrum and coccyx by its base.

**falciform ligament of the liver** A wide, sickle-shaped reflection of the peritoneum that serves as a principal attachment of the liver to the diaphragm and separates the right and left lobes of the liver. Its broad attachment extends from the posterior superior portion of the liver to the anterior convex portion connected to the internal surface of the right rectus abdominis muscle. SYN: *falx ligamentosa.*

**falciform process** The portion of the falciform ligament along the inner margin of the ramus of the ischium.

**falcular** 1. Sickle-shaped. 2. Pert. to the falx cerebelli.

**fallectomy** (făl-ĕk'tō-mē) The surgical removal of part of a fallopian tube.

**falling drop** 1. In physical diagnosis, a metallic tinkle heard over the normal stomach and bowel when they are inflated. 2. A metallic tinkle heard over large cavities containing fluid and air, as in hydropneumothorax.

**fallophobia** An unofficial term for the shock of falling and the subsequent fear of falling again. It is often associated with post-fall syndrome in the elderly and can manifest itself as loss of independence and control, depression, and feelings of vulnerability and fragility. There are often concerns regarding death and dying and about becoming a burden to family and friends or requiring institutionalization.

**fallopian canal** (fă-lō'pē-ăn) [Gabriele Fallopio, It. anatomist, 1523–1562] A canal in the petrous portion of the temporal bone. The facial nerve passes through it.

**fallopian ligament** The round ligament of the uterus.

**fallopian tube** The tube or duct that extends laterally from the lateral angle of the fundal end of the uterus and terminates near the ovary. It conveys the ovum from the ovary to the uterus and spermatozoa from the uterus toward the ovary. Medially each tube opens into the uterus; distally, into the peritoneal cavity. Each lies in the superior border of the broad ligament of the uterus.

ANATOMY: The narrow region near the uterus, the isthmus, continues laterally as a wider ampulla. The latter expands to form the terminal funnel-shaped infundibulum, at the bottom of which lies a small opening, the ostium, through which the ovum enters the oviduct. Surrounding each ostium are several finger-like processes called fimbria extending toward the ovary. Each tube averages about 4½ in. (11.4 cm) in length and ¼ in. (6 mm) in diameter. Its wall consists of three layers: mucosa, muscular layer, and serosa. The epithelium of the mucosa consists of ciliated and nonciliated cells. Ciliary action aids in the movement of the ovum toward the uterus. The muscular layer comprises an inner circular and an outer longitudinal layer of smooth muscle. The serosa consists of connective tissue underlying the outermost layer of peritoneum. The blood supply is derived from branches of the uterine and ovarian arteries. The nerve supply is from the pelvic, ovarian, and uterine nerve plexuses, sending fibers to the tubes. SYN: *oviduct; uterine tube*. SEE: *genitalia, female* for illus; *uterus*.

**Fallot, tetralogy of** (făl-ō') [Etienne L. A. Fallot, Fr. physician, 1850–1911] A congenital condition characterized by a defect in the interventricular septum, pulmonary artery stenosis, dextroposition of the aorta, and right ventricular hypertrophy. Modern surgical therapy has made it possible to treat this condition effectively.

**fallotomy** (făl-ŏt'ō-mē) Division of the fallopian tubes. SYN: *salpingotomy*.

**fallout** Settling of radioactive fission products from the atmosphere after their release into the air following the explosion of an atomic bomb or device, or from a radiation accident such as could occur at any installation using radioactive materials.

**fall** 1. To drop accidentally to the floor or ground. 2. An accidental drop, usually caused by slipping or losing one's balance. In the elderly, falls are the leading cause of death. Approximately 30% of people 65 years of age or older fall each year. The yearly costs for acute care associated with fall-related injuries are estimated to be $10 billion. It is important for medical care providers to search for the cause or causes of the fall. Risk factors for falling include reduced visual acuity and hearing, vestibular dysfunction, peripheral neuropathy, musculoskeletal disorders including physical weakness, postural hypotension, and use of medicines such as antidepressants, sedatives, or vasodilators. Other specific risk factors include daily use of four or more prescription drugs, inability to transfer from bed or chair to bathtub or toilet, and being female. By careful clinical investigation, the cause of falls can be determined and appropriate steps taken to prevent them in the future.

Hazards in the home that increase the chances of falling are scatter rugs that are not secure or slip resistant, out-of-the-way light switches, cluttered access to paths through a room or entrance, poorly lighted steps and stairways, lack of handrails on the entire length of a stairway, and tubs and showers that are not fitted with sturdy grab bars and have slippery floors.

**false-negative** (făwls'nĕg'ă-tĭv) Concerning a test or procedure that indicates that an abnormality or disease is not present when in fact it is. SEE: *false-positive*.

**false-positive** (făwls'pŏs'ĭ-tĭv) Concerning a test or procedure that indicates that an abnormality or disease is present when in fact it is not. SEE: *false-negative*.

**false rib** One of the lower ribs (8, 9, and 10) that do not join the sternum directly. Their cartilage end connects to the cartilage of the seventh rib. The variation in the anatomy of the lower ribs may be considerable (i.e., there may be only two false ribs). SEE: under *rib; vertebra*.

**falsification** (făwl"sĭ-fĭ-kā'shŭn) The act of writing or stating what is not true.

***retrospective f.*** Deliberate or unconscious alteration of memory for past events or situations, a mental mechanism for ego preservation.

**falx** [L.] Any sickle-shaped structure.

***f. cerebelli*** A fold of the dura mater that forms a vertical partition between the hemispheres of the cerebellum.

***f. cerebri*** A fold of the dura mater that lies in the longitudinal fissure and separates the two cerebral hemispheres.

***f. inguinalis*** The conjoined, or conjoint, tendon that forms the origin of the transversus abdominis and internal oblique muscles.

***f. ligamentosa*** Falciform ligament of the liver.

**fames** (fā′mēz) [L.] Hunger.

**familial** [L. *familia,* family] Pert. to or common to the same family (e.g., a disease occurring more frequently in a family than would be expected by chance).

**familial Mediterranean fever** An inherited autosomal recessive disorder seen most commonly in Middle Eastern ethnic groups. It has also appeared in family clusters in persons of Irish or Italian descent. The attacks, which almost always include fever, first appear between the ages of 5 and 15. The syndrome includes some of the following: abdominal pain resembling peritonitis, chest pain of pleural or pericardial origin, erysipelas-like redness near the ankle, and joint involvement. Duration and frequency of attacks are unpredictable. Some of the patients develop amyloidosis. Otherwise, the prognosis is favorable although there is no specific therapy. SYN: *periodic fever.*

**familial periodic paralysis** A rare familial disease marked by attacks of flaccid paralysis, often at awakening. This condition is usually associated with hypokalemia, but is sometimes present when the blood potassium level is normal or elevated. In affected individuals the condition may be precipitated by administration of glucose in patients with hypokalemia, and by administation of potassium chloride in those with hyperkalemia.

Caution: These tests may cause cardiac or respiratory changes and should not be done by inexperienced physicians.

TREATMENT: Acetazolamide is used to prevent either hypokalemia or hyperkalemia. Oral potassium chloride is given in attacks accompanied by hypokalemia.

**family 1.** A group of individuals who have descended from a common ancestor. **2.** In biological classification, the division between an order and a genus. **3.** A group of people living in a household who share common attachments, such as mutual caring, emotional bonds, regular interactions, and common goals, which include the health of the individuals in the family.

***blended f.*** A common contemporary family group including children from previous and current relationships; often referred to as “yours, mine, and ours.”

***extended f.*** The basic or nuclear family plus close relatives.

***single-parent f.*** A family in which only one of the parents is living with the child or children.

**family care leave** Permission to be absent from work to care for a family member who is pregnant, ill, disabled, or incapacitated.

**family coping, ineffective: compromised** A state in which a usually supportive primary person (family member or close friend [significant other]) provides insufficient, ineffective, or compromised support, comfort, assistance, or encouragement that may be needed by the patient to manage or master adaptive tasks related to the patient’s health challenge. SEE: *Nursing Diagnoses Appendix.*

**family coping, ineffective: disabling** A state in which the behavior of a significant person (family member or other primary person) disables his or her own capacities and the patient’s capacities to effectively address tasks essential to either person’s adaptation to the health challenge. SEE: *Nursing Diagnoses Appendix.*

**family coping, potential for growth** A state in which the family member has effectively managed adaptive tasks involved with the patient’s health challenge and is exhibiting desire and readiness for enhanced health and growth in regard to self and in relation to the patient. SEE: *Nursing Diagnoses Appendix.*

**family planning** The spacing of conception of children according to the wishes of the parents rather than to chance. It is accomplished by practicing some form of birth control.

***symptothermal f.p.*** A fertility awareness method by which a woman plots her daily basal body temperature, cervical mucus characteristics, and common subjective complaints associated with ovulation (e.g., mittelschmerz) on a graph to identify the days of the menstrual cycle during which there is the highest potential for conception. The validity of this method is controversial.

**family practice** Comprehensive medical care with particular emphasis on the family unit, in which the physician’s continuing responsibility for health care is not limited by the patient’s age or sex nor by a particular organ system or disease entity.

Family practice is the specialty that builds on a core of knowledge derived from other disciplines, drawing most heavily on Internal Medicine, Pediatrics, Obstetrics and Gynecology, Surgery, and Psychiatry, and establishes a cohesive unit, combining the behavioral sciences with the traditional biological and clinical sciences. The core of knowledge encompassed by the discipline of Family Practice prepares the family physician for a unique role in patient management, problem solving, counseling, and as a personal physician who coordinates total health care delivery. (Definition supplied by The American Academy of Family Physicians.)

**family process, altered: alcoholism** The state in which the psychosocial, spiritual, and physiological functions of the family unit are chronically disorganized, leading to conflict, denial of problems, resistance to change, ineffective problem solving, and a series of self-perpetuating crises. SEE: *Nursing Diagnoses Appendix.*

**family processes, altered** The state in which a family that normally functions effectively experiences a dysfunction. SEE: *Nursing Diagnoses Appendix.*

**family therapy** Treatment of the members of a family together, rather than an individual "patient"; the family unit is viewed as a social system important to all of its members.

**famine** Pronounced scarcity of food, causing hunger and starvation. The worst famine of the 20th century occurred in China between 1959 and 1961 when between 15 million and 30 million people died. So far in the 1990s, Angola, Ethiopia, Liberia, Mozambique, Somalia, and Sudan have reported famines. Armed conflicts have been the major cause.

**Fanconi's syndrome** [Guido Fanconi, Swiss pediatrician, 1892–1979] **1.** Congenital hypoplastic anemia. **2.** Aminoaciduria associated with rickets due to failure of the proximal renal tubules or to dysfunction of the deamination process. Symptoms include rickets, polyuria, and growth failure. Dietary therapy is of some help but patients usually die before puberty.

**fang** [AS., to plunder] **1.** A sharp-pointed tooth. **2.** The root of a tooth.

**fango** (făn′gō) [Italian, mud] Mud obtained from thermal springs in Battaglia, Italy, used in treating rheumatism and gout.

**Fannia** (făn′ē-ă) A genus of small houseflies.

**fantast** (făn′tăst) [Gr. *phantasia,* imagination] A daydreamer.

**fantasy** (făn′tă-sē) [Gr. *phantasia,* imagination] The mechanism of creating in one's mind something that is unreal and may be disordered and weird. A fantasy may also be creative.

**FAOTA** *Fellow of the American Occupational Therapy Association.*

**FAPTA** *Fellow of the American Physical Therapy Association.*

**farad** (făr′ăd) [Michael Faraday, Brit. physicist, 1791–1867] A unit of electrical capacity. The capacity of a condenser that, charged with 1 coulomb, gives a difference of potential of 1 V. This unit is so large that 1 millionth of it has been adopted as a practical unit called a microfarad.

**faraday** (făr′ă-dā) The amount of electric charge associated with 1 g equivalent of an electrochemical reaction. It is equal to approx. 96,000 coulombs. SEE: *coulomb; farad.*

**faradic** Pert. to induced electricity.

**faradism** Therapeutic use of an interrupted current to stimulate muscles and nerves. Such a current is derived from the secondary, or induction, coil.

**faradization** **1.** The treatment of nerves or muscles with faradic current. **2.** The condition of nerves or muscles so treated.

**faradotherapy** Treatment of disease by faradic current.

**farcy** (făr′sē) [L. *farcire,* to stuff] A chronic form of glanders.

***button f.*** Farcy marked by dermal tubercular nodules.

**farina** (fă-rē′nă) [L.] Finely ground meal commonly made from wheat or other grain, used as cereal and flour.

**farinaceous** (făr″ĭ-nā′shŭs) **1.** Starchy. **2.** Pert. to flour.

**farmer's lung** A form of hypersensitivity alveolitis caused by exposure to moldy hay that has fermented. *Actinomyces micropolyspora faeni* and *Thermoactinomyces vulgaris* are the causative microorganisms. SEE: *alveolitis; bagassosis; hypersensitivity.*

**farpoint** The farthest point of vision at which objects can be seen distinctly with the eyes in complete relaxation.

**Farre's tubercles** (fărz) [John R. Farre, Brit. physician, 1775–1862] Carcinomatous masses on the surface of the liver.

**farsightedness** An error of refraction in which, with accommodation completely relaxed, parallel rays come to a focus behind the retina. Affected individuals can see distant objects clearly, but cannot see near objects in proper focus. SYN: *hyperopia.* **farsighted,** *adj.*

**fascia** (făsh′ē-ă) *pl.* **fasciae** [L., a band] A fibrous membrane covering, supporting, and separating muscles. It also unites the skin with underlying tissue. Fascia may be superficial, a nearly subcutaneous covering permitting free movement of the skin, or it may be deep, enveloping and binding muscles. **fascial,** *adj.*

***Abernethy's f.*** A layer of areolar tissue separating the external iliac artery from the iliac fascia over the psoas muscle.

***anal f.*** A fascia of connective tissue covering the levator ani muscle from the perineal aspect.

***aponeurotic f.*** A thick fascia that provides attachment for a muscle.

***Buck's f.*** The fascial covering of the penis, derived from Colles' fascia.

***Cloquet's f.*** The femoral fascia.

***Colles' f.*** The inner layer of the perineal fascia.

***cremasteric f.*** The fascia covering the cremaster muscle of the spermatic cord.

***cribriform f.*** The fascia of the thigh covering the saphenous opening.

***crural f.*** The deep fascia of the leg.

***deep f.*** Fascia that covers an individual muscle.

***deep cervical f.*** The fascia of the neck

covering the muscles, vessels, and nerves.

***dentate f.*** The gray matter in the cerebral dentate convolution of the brain. SYN: *gyrus, dentate.*

***endothoracic f.*** The fascia that separates the pleura of the lung from the inside of the thoracic cavity and the diaphragm. SYN: *extrapleural f.*

***extrapleural f.*** Endothoracic f.

***intercolumnar f.*** The fascia derived from the external abdominal ring sheathing the spermatic cord and testis.

***f. lata femoris*** The wide fascia encasing the hips and the thigh muscles.

***lumbodorsal f.*** Thoracolumbar f.

***pectineal f.*** The pubic section of the fascia lata.

***pelvic f.*** The fascia within the pelvic cavity. It is extremely important in maintaining normal strength in the pelvic floor. SEE: *diaphragm, pelvic.*

***perineal f.*** Three layers of tissue between the muscles of the perineum.

***pharyngobasilar f.*** The fascia lying between the mucosal and muscular layers of the pharyngeal wall. SYN: *pharyngeal aponeurosis.*

***plantar f.*** The fascia investing the muscles of the sole of the foot. SYN: *plantar aponeurosis.*

***Scarpa's f.*** The deep layer of the superficial fascia of the abdomen.

***superficial f.*** The areolar connective tissue and adipose tissue below the dermis of the skin. SYN: *subcutaneous tissue.*

***superficial cervical f.*** The fascia of the neck just inside the skin.

***thoracolumbar f.*** The fascia and aponeuroses of the latissimus dorsi, serratus posterior inferior, internal oblique, and transverse abdominis muscles, which provide support and stability for the lumbar spine in postural and lifting activities. The fascia attaches medially to the spinous processes of the vertebral column and inferiorly to the iliac crest and sacrum. SYN: *lumbodorsal f.*

***thyrolaryngeal f.*** The fascia covering the thyroid gland.

***f. transversalis*** The fascia located between the perineum and the transversalis muscle. It lines the abdominal cavity.

**fascial reflex** Muscular contraction resulting from percussing facial fascia.

**fasciaplasty** (făsh′ē-ă-plăs″tē) [″ + Gr. *plassein,* to form] Plastic surgery of a fascia.

**fascicle** (făs′ĭ-kl) [L. *fasciculus,* little bundle] A fasciculus.

**fascicular** (fă-sĭk′ū-lăr) **1.** Arranged like a bundle of rods. **2.** Pert. to a fasciculus.

**fasciculation** (fă-sĭk″ū-lā′shŭn) **1.** Formation of fascicles. **2.** Involuntary contraction or twitching of muscle fibers, visible under the skin. **3.** Spontaneous contractions of muscle fibers that do not cause movement at a joint.

**fasciculus** (fă-sĭk′ū-lŭs) *pl.* **fasciculi** A small bundle, esp. of nerve or muscle fibers; more specifically, a division of a funiculus of the spinal cord comprising fibers of one or more tracts. Sometimes the term is used as a synonym for *tract.* SYN: *fasciola.*

***f. cuneatus*** A triangular bundle of nerve fibers lying in the dorsal funiculus of the spinal cord. Its fibers enter the cord through the dorsal roots of spinal nerves and terminate in the medulla. SYN: *Burdach's tract; column of Burdach; root zone.*

***dorsolateral f.*** SEE: *tract, dorsolateral.*

***dorsal longitudinal f.*** A bundle of association fibers connecting the frontal lobe with the occipital and temporal lobes of the brain.

***fundamental f.*** The portion of the anterior column of the spinal cord continuing into the medulla oblongata.

***f. gracilis*** A bundle of nerve fibers, lying in the dorsal funiculus of the spinal cord medial to the fasciculus cuneatus, that conducts sensory impulses from the periphery to the medulla. SYN: *column of Goll; Goll's tract.*

***inferior longitudinal f.*** A bundle of association fibers connecting the occipital and temporal lobes of the brain.

***medial longitudinal f.*** A nerve fiber bundle running from the spinal cord to the upper portion of the midbrain.

***posterior longitudinal f.*** A nerve fiber bundle running between the corpora quadrigemina and the nuclei of the fourth and sixth spinal nerves.

***unciform f.*** Fibers within the sylvian fissure connecting the frontal and temporosphenoid lobes of the brain. SYN: *uncinate fasciculus.*

**fasciectomy** (făsh″ē-ĕk′tō-mē) [L. *fascia,* band, + Gr. *ektome,* excision] Excision of strips of fascia.

**fasciitis** (făs″ē-ī′tĭs) Inflammation of any fascia. SYN: *fascitis.*

***necrotizing f.*** Severe infection of the superficial or deep fascia surrounding muscles of an extremity or the trunk.

SYMPTOMS: The onset of illness is usually acute and progression is rapid. Initially there is severe pain, fever, chills, and malaise. These symptoms worsen as the infection spreads. If extensive surgical debridement, drainage, and antibiotics are not instituted early, the patient may die.

ETIOLOGY: Type I is caused by anaerobes of the genera *Bacteroides* or *Peptostreptococcus* combined with facultative anaerobes such as streptococci (other than group A) and bacteria such as *Escherichia coli* or other gram-negative organisms such as *Klebsiella, Enterobacter,* or *Proteus.* Type II, also called hemolytic streptococcal gangrene, is caused by group A streptococci alone or in combination with other species, usually *Staphylococcus aureus.*

**fasciodesis** (făsh″ē-ŏd′ĕ-sĭs) [″ + Gr. *desis,* binding] Surgical attachment of a fascia to a tendon or another fascia.

**Fasciola** (fă-sī′ō-lă) [L. *fasciola,* a band] A genus of flukes belonging to the class Trematoda.

***F. hepatica*** A species of flukes infesting the liver and bile ducts of cattle, sheep, and other herbivores; the common liver fluke. Infestation of watercress is a rare source of infection in humans. Intermediate hosts are snails belonging to the genus *Lymnaea*. SEE: illus.

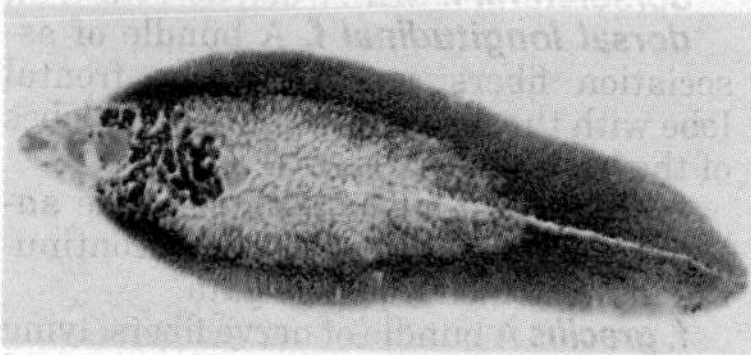

FASCIOLA HEPATICA (ORIG. MAG. ×2)

**fasciola** (fă-sī′ō-lă, fă-sē′ō-lă) *pl.* **fasciolae** [L., a band] A bundle of nerve or muscle fibers.

***f. cinerea*** The upper portion of the dentate fascia.

**fasciolar** (fă-sē′ō-lăr) Pert. to the fasciola cinerea.

**fasciolopsiasis** (făs″ē-ō-lŏp-sī′ă-sĭs) Infection of the body with a genus of trematode worms, *Fasciolopsis buski*. It is contracted by ingestion of plants grown in water infested by the intermediate host, snails.

SYMPTOMS: The symptoms are diarrhea, abdominal pain, anasarca, and eosinophilia.

TREATMENT: Treatment is with Praziquantel.

**Fasciolopsis buski** (făs″ē-ō-lŏp′sĭs) A fluke that infests the intestinal tract of certain mammals including humans. Symptoms include vomiting, anorexia, and diarrhea alternating with constipation. The number of flukes present may be sufficient to cause intestinal obstruction. The disease occurs in Asia, including central and southern China. SEE: illus.; *fasciolopsiasis.*

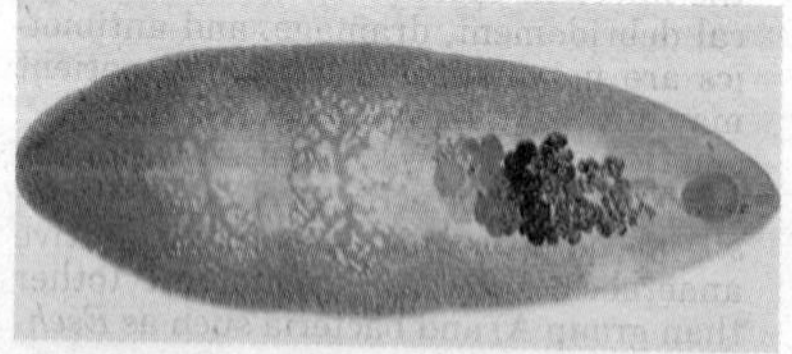

FASCIOLOPSIS BUSKI (ORIG. MAG. ×2)

**fascioplasty** (făsh′ē-ō-plăs″tē) [L. *fasciola,* a band, + Gr. *plassein,* to form] Plastic operation on a fascia.

**fasciorrhaphy** (făsh-ē-or′ă-fē) [″ + Gr. *rhaphe,* seam, ridge] Suturing of a fascia.

**fasciotomy** (făsh-ē-ŏt′ō-mē) [″ + Gr. *tome,* incision] Surgical incision and division of a fascia.

**fascitis** (fă-sī′tĭs) [″ + Gr. *itis,* inflammation] Fasciitis.

**FASRT** *Fellow of the American Society of Radiologic Technologists.*

**fast 1.** [AS. *faest,* fixed] Resistant to the effects or action of a chemical substance. **2.** [AS. *faestan,* to hold fast] Abstention from food, usually voluntary.

**fastidious** In microbiology, concerning an organism that has precise nutritional and environmental requirements for growth and survival.

**fastidium** (făs-tĭd′ē-ŭm) [L., aversion] Aversion to food or eating. Sometimes it is seen in hysteria.

**fastigium** (făs-tĭj′ē-ŭm) [L., ridge] **1.** The highest point. **2.** The fullest point of development of acute, infectious diseases when the temperature reaches the maximum. **3.** The most posterior portion of the fourth ventricle, formed by the junction of the anterior and posterior medullary vela projecting into the medullary substance of the cerebellum of the brain.

**fasting** [AS. *faestan,* to hold fast] Going without food. During fasting, the energy requirements of body metabolism are supplied by the oxidization of fats. If glucose is not supplied, the products of incomplete fat metabolism (fatty acids, diacetic acid, and acetone) produce ketosis and a mild acidosis. This condition occurs quickly in children because they have little glycogen reserve.

Caution: Unsupervised fasting to lose weight can cause death.

**fastness** [AS. *faest,* fixed] The ability of bacteria to resist stains or destructive agents.

**fat** [AS. *faett*] **1.** Adipose tissue of the body, which serves as an energy reserve. SEE: *heart; obesity.* **2.** Grease, oil. **3.** In chemistry, triglyceride ester of fatty acids; one of a group of organic compounds closely associated in nature with the phosphatides, cerebrosides, and sterols. The term *lipid* is applied in general to a fat or fatlike substance. Fats are insoluble in water but soluble in ether, chloroform, benzene, and other fat solvents. During hydrolysis, fats break down into fatty acids and glycerol (an alcohol). Fats are hydrolyzed by the action of acids, alkalies, lipases (fat-splitting enzymes), and superheated steam. **fatty** (făt′ē), *adj.*

CHEMICAL STRUCTURE: In the fat molecule, one molecule of glycerol is combined with three of fatty acids. Three fatty acids, oleic acid ($C_{18}H_{34}O_2$), stearic acid ($C_{18}H_{36}O_2$), and palmitic acid ($C_{16}H_{32}O_2$), constitute the bulk of fatty acids in neutral fats found in body tissues. According to the fatty acid with which the glycerol is combined, corresponding fats are triolein, tristearin, and tripalmitin. These three fats are the principal fats present in foods.

PHYSIOLOGY: The most important function of fats is as a form of stored or potential energy. In conjunction with carbohydrates, fats are protein sparers—dietary or body protein need not be used for energy production. Glycogen storage is sufficient to supply energy needs for about 12 hr, but in a 70-kg man of average build, 12 kg of stored fat (in the form of triglycerides) can supply energy needs for as long as 8 weeks. Subcutaneous fat provides a small amount of insulation against heat loss, and some organs such as the eyes and kidneys are cushioned by fat. The diglyceride phospholipids are part of all cell membranes. Dietary fat provides the essential fatty acids needed for normal growth.

Because certain fatty acids (linoleic, D-linolenic, and arachidonic) are necessary for formation of other products in the body and because the body does not synthesize them, they are classed as *essential fatty acids*. Linolenic acid can, however, be converted into other fatty acids including arachidonic acid. Arachidonic acid is of particular importance because it is essential to the formation of prostaglandins, thromboxanes, prostacyclins, and leukotrienes. These three essential fatty acids are obtainable in the diet from plant sources.

Animals fed a fat-free diet develop dermatitis and fail to grow; the liver becomes fatty, and there are neurological disturbances. These changes can be prevented or reversed by the addition of linoleic and linolenic acids to the diet. The human diet should consist of about 4% of the calories from linoleic and 1% from linolenic acids.

DIGESTION AND ABSORPTION: In the stomach, emulsified fats such as cream or egg yolk are acted on by gastric lipase; however, most fats undergo digestion in the intestine, where a pancreatic lipase, steapsin, hydrolyzes them to fatty acids and glycerol. The bile salts in bile are not enzymes; they emulsify fats and permit pancreatic lipase to digest them. Bile salts then make fatty acids soluble in water so that they may be readily absorbed. In the intestinal mucosa, fatty acids and glycerol combine to form neutral fats, then join to proteins to form chylomicrons, which enter the lacteals. In this form, they are carried in the lymph through the lymph vessels to the thoracic duct, which empties lymph into the blood.

METABOLISM: Absorbed fats are used in the following ways: oxidized to carbon dioxide and water to produce energy; stored in adipose tissue for energy production later; changed to phospholipids for cell membranes; converted to acetyl groups for the synthesis of cholesterol, from which other steroids are made; and used to make secretions such as sebum.

*Intermediary metabolism:* In the oxidation of fat to carbon dioxide and water, several intermediary substances (ketones) are formed. The principal ones are acetoacetic acid, betahydroxybutyric acid, and acetone. Excessive production of ketone bodies, which occurs when fats are incompletely oxidized, is called ketosis. This occurs esp. when there is an interference in carbohydrate metabolism, as in diabetes. Ketosis also occurs in starvation, certain fevers, pregnancy toxemias, and hyperthyroidism. Ketosis results in acidosis.

SOURCES: In addition to fat being absorbed from the intestine, body fat may arise from the conversion of carbohydrates (glucose) or proteins into fat. Fatty acids cannot be converted directly to glucose, but they are split into two-carbon acetyl groups that enter the Krebs cycle and thereby have the same energy-producing function as carbohydrates.

NUTRITION: Fats have a high caloric value, yielding about 9 kcal per gram as compared with about 4 kcal per gram for carbohydrates and proteins. The average diet of 3000 kcal may derive 40% of the caloric value from fats. Nutritionists and epidemiologists believe that decreasing dietary fat to 30% would decrease the risk of developing cancer, esp. of the colon, breast, and prostate.

In addition to their nutritive values, fats improve the taste and odor of foods, provide a feeling of satiety, and because of their high caloric content are of special importance in high-calorie diets. Fat-free fat substitutes that have been termed "designer fats" have been investigated for several decades. Whether they will play a major role in providing foods with fewer calories from fat has not been determined. SEE: table.

CONTRAINDICATIONS: Fat intake should be reduced in certain diseases such as hepatitis and in low-calorie diets.

**body f.** The portion of the human body that consists of fat. This is estimated in several ways: by determining body density by underwater weighing (hydrodensitometry), by calculating the ratio of weight in kilograms to height in meters squared (Quatelet index), and more recently, by estimating bioelectrical impedance of the body. None of these methods provides a precise indicator of body composition; however, bioelectrical impedance is the simplest, least expensive, and most nearly accurate.

**brown f.** Adipose tissue occurring primarily in the full-term newborn. It is located near major vessels. The fat produces heat metabolically and is therefore an important factor in temperature regulation. As the infant matures, shivering is established as a means of controlling body temperature. The brown fat either

**Food Sources of Saturated Fats**

| | |
|---|---|
| Meat products | Visible fat and marbling in beef, pork, and lamb, especially in prime-grade and ground meats, lard |
| Processed meats | Frankfurters |
| | Luncheon meats such as bologna, corned beef, liverwurst, pastrami, and salami |
| | Bacon, sausage, lard, suet, salt pork |
| Poultry and fowl | Chicken and turkey (mostly beneath the skin), cornish hens, duck, and goose |
| Whole milk and whole-milk products | Cheeses made with whole milk or cream, condensed milk, ice cream, whole-milk yogurt, all creams (sour, half-and-half, whipped) |
| Plant products | Coconut oil, palm-kernel oil, cocoa butter |
| Miscellaneous | Fully hydrogenated shortening and margarine, many cakes, pies, cookies, and mixes |

SOURCE: Lutz, CA and Przytulski, KR: Nutrition and Diet Therapy. FA Davis, Philadelphia, 1994.

involutes or becomes white fat. SEE: *tissue, brown adipose.*

***neutral f.*** Compounds of the higher fatty acids (palmitic, stearic, and oleic) with glycerol. They are the common fats of animal and plant tissues.

**fatal** (fāt'l) [L. *fatalis*] **1.** Inevitable. **2.** Causing death.

**fatality** A death, esp. from an accident or a disaster.

**fatigability** (făt″ĭ-gă-bĭl'ĭ-tē) The condition of becoming easily tired or exhausted.

**fatigue** (fă-tēg') [L. *fatigare,* to tire] **1.** A feeling of tiredness or weariness resulting from continued activity or as a side effect of some psychotropic drug. This overwhelming sustained sense of exhaustion results in a decreased capacity for physical and mental work. SEE: *Nursing Diagnoses Appendix.* **2.** The condition of an organ or tissue in which its response to stimulation is reduced or lost as a result of overactivity. **3.** To bring about fatigue.

Fatigue may be the result of excessive activity, which causes the accumulation of metabolic waste products such as lactic acid; malnutrition (deficiency of carbohydrates, proteins, minerals, or vitamins); circulatory disturbances such as heart disease or anemia, which interfere with the supply of oxygen and energy materials to tissues; respiratory disturbances, which interfere with the supply of oxygen to tissues; infectious diseases, which produce toxic products or alter body metabolism; endocrine disturbances such as occur in diabetes, hyperinsulinism, and menopause; psychogenic factors such as emotional conflicts, frustration, anxiety, neurosis, and boredom; or physical factors such as disability. Environmental noise and vibration contribute to the development of fatigue. SEE: *chronic fatigue syndrome.*

***acute f.*** Fatigue with sudden onset such as occurs following excessive exertion. It is relieved by rest.

***chronic f.*** Long-continued fatigue not relieved by rest, indicative of disease such as tuberculosis, diabetes, or other conditions of altered body metabolism. SEE: *chronic fatigue syndrome.*

***muscle f.*** The reduced capacity of a muscle to perform work as a result of repeated contractions and accumulation of lactic acid in anaerobic cell respiration. Fatigue may be partial or complete.

**fat overload syndrome** A rare complication of intravenous administration of fat emulsion. Symptoms include sudden elevation of the serum triglyceride level, fever, hepatosplenomegaly, coagulopathy, and dysfunction of other organs. Specific therapy is not available, but plasma exchange has been used experimentally.

**fat replacement** A substance developed to provide all the characteristics of fats but having either relatively few calories or none at all. Simplesse is the trade name for a fat replacement made of milk and egg white. It provides 1 to 2 kcal per gram. A calorie-free fat replacement has become available as the product Olestra. It has the same physical characteristics as fat but it is not digested by the body and is not absorbed from the gastrointestinal tract.

**fatty acid** A hydrocarbon in which one of the hydrogen atoms has been replaced by a carboxyl (COOH) group; a monobasic aliphatic acid made up of an alkyl radical attached to a carboxyl group.

Saturated fatty acids have single bonds in their carbon chain with the general formula $C_nH_{2n}O_2$. They include acetic, butyric, capric, caproic, caprylic, formic, lauric, myristic, palmitic, and stearic acids. Unsaturated fatty acids have one or more double or triple bonds in the carbon chain. They include those of the oleic series (oleic, tiglic, hypogeic, and palmitoleic) and the linoleic or linolic series (linoleic, linolenic, clupanodonic, arachidonic, hydrocarpic, and chaulmoogric). Fatty acids are insoluble in water. This would prevent their absorption from the intestines if the action of bile salts on the fatty acids did not enable them to be absorbed. SEE: *fat.*

***essential f.a.*** An unsaturated fatty acid (linoleic, linolenic, or arachidonic) that cannot be synthesized in the body and is considered essential to maintaining health. SEE: *digestion.*

***free f.a.*** ABBR: FFA. The form in which a fatty acid leaves the cell to be transported for use in another part of the body. These acids are not esterified. In the plasma they immediately combine with albumin.

***omega-3 (ω3) f.a.*** SEE: *acid, omega-3 fatty.*

***trans f.a.*** The solid fat produced by heating liquid vegetable oils in the presence of hydrogen and certain metal catalysts. This process of partial hydrogenation changes some of the unsaturated bonds to saturated ones. A positive association between intake of trans fatty acids and coronary artery disease and myocardial infarction has been observed, as has an association between blood levels of trans fatty acids and coronary artery narrowing. Regulations do not require food labels to provide information about food trans fatty acid content. Thus, the public has little basis for making informed decisions prior to purchasing and consuming products that contain trans fatty acids.

**fatty cast** Material seen in urine sediments. It is usually abnormal and consists of a mass of fat globules.

**fatty streak** SEE: *atherosclerosis.*

**fauces** (fŏ′sēz) [L.] The constricted opening leading from the mouth and the oral pharynx. It is bounded by the soft palate, the base of the tongue, and the palatine arches. The anterior pillars of the fauces are known as the glossopalatine arch, and the posterior pillars as the pharyngopalatine arch. SEE: *fossa.* **faucial** (-shăl), *adj.*

**fauna** (faw′nă) [L. *Faunus,* mythical deity of herdsmen] **1.** Animal life as distinguished from plant life. **2.** All the animals, including microscopic forms, in a specified area. SEE: *flora.*

**faveolate** (fā-vē′ō-lāt) [L. *faveolus,* little honeycomb] Honeycombed. SYN: *alveolate.*

**faveolus** (fā-vē′ō-lŭs) [L., little honeycomb] A depression or small pit, esp. on the skin. SYN: *foveola.*

**favism** (fā′vĭzm) [It. *fava,* bean, + Gr. *-ismos,* condition] A hereditary condition common in Sicily and Sardinia resulting from sensitivity to a species of bean, *Vicia faba.* It is marked by fever, acute hemolytic anemia, vomiting, and diarrhea, and may lead to prostration and coma. It is caused by ingestion of the beans or inhalation of the pollen of the plant by persons who have an inherited deficiency of the enzyme glucose-6-phosphate dehydrogenase.

**favus** (fā′vŭs) [L., honeycomb] A skin disease caused by the fungus *Trichophyton schoenleinii.* It is marked by pinhead- to pea-sized, cup-shaped, yellowish crusts (scutulum) over the hair follicles of the scalp and is accompanied by musty odor and itching. It may spread all over the body. SEE: *scutulum.*

**F.C.A.P.** *Fellow of the College of American Pathologists.*

**Fc fragment** A small piece of an immunoglobulin (an antibody) used by macrophages in processing and presenting foreign antigens to T lymphocytes. SEE: *immune response; macrophage processing.*

**Fc receptor** A receptor on phagocytes (neutrophils, monocytes, and macrophages) that binds Fc fragments of immunoglobulins G and E. SEE: *immunoglobulin; macrophage processing; phagocytosis.*

**F.D.** *fatal dose; focal distance.*

**F.D.A.** *Food and Drug Administration.*

**FDP** *fibrin degradation products.*

**Fe** [L. *ferrum*] Symbol for the element iron.

**fear** [AS. *faer*] A feeling of fright or dread related to an identifiable source which the individual validates. Primitively, fear is the emotional reaction to an environmental threat; it now also occurs frequently as an indicator of inner problems. Fear is present in anxiety disorders and depression. At the somatic level, hyperthyroidism and hyperadrenalism may strongly simulate fear. SEE: *emotion; Nursing Diagnoses Appendix; Phobias Appendix.*

**features** Any part of the face.

**febrifacient** (fĕb-rĭ-fā′sē-ĕnt) [L. *febris,* fever, + *facere,* to make] Producing fever.

**febrifugal** (fĕb-rĭf′ū-găl) [″ + *fugare,* to put to flight] Reducing fever.

**febrifuge** (fĕb′rĭ-fūj) Something that reduces fever. SYN: *antipyretic.*

**febrile** (fē′brĭl, fē′brīl, fĕb′rĭl) [L. *febris,* fever] Feverish; pert. to a fever. SEE: *fever.*

**febrile convulsion** A paroxysm of involuntary muscular contraction and relaxation associated with fever. About 3% to 5% of children experience a convulsion. Most do so in the period between 6 months and 2 to 3 years of age. Febrile convulsions are rare after ages 6 to 8. Boys are more susceptible than girls to this type of convulsion. A complete history and physical examination should include neurological appraisal for the possibility of another cause, such as tetany; epilepsy; acute lead encephalopathy; cerebral concussion, hemorrhage, or tumor; hypoglycemia; or poisoning with a convulsant drug. SEE: *epilepsy.*

TREATMENT: Appropriate therapy should be instituted to reduce the elevated body temperature. Oral diazepam may be administered while fever is present to prevent seizure recurrence. The measures to reduce the temperature must not be so vigorous as to cause hypothermia. Ice water baths and vigorous fanning with application of alcohol should not be used. The application of cool compresses with a gentle flow of air over the body is sufficient. A hypothermia blanket is also suitable. In the past, it was recommended that a child who had experienced a single febrile convulsion should have daily anticonvulsant therapy for 2 to 4 years. The efficacy and advisability of this have not been proved.

Caution: 1. If the fever is due to influenza or varicella, salicylates should not be administered; their use could increase the risk for developing Reye's syndrome. 2. Prolonged treatment with phenobarbital depresses cognitive function in children.

**febrile state** A term used to describe constitutional symptoms that accompany a rise in temperature. The pulse and respiration rate usually increase, with headache, pains, malaise, loss of appetite, concentrated and diminished urine, constipation, restlessness, insomnia, and irritability.

**febriphobia** (fĕb″rĭ-fō′bē-ă) [″ + Gr. *phobos,* fear] Anxiety or fear induced by a rise in body temperature.

**fecal impaction** The formation of a firm mass of feces in the distal colon or rectum. The size and firmness of the mass prevents its passage.

ETIOLOGY: Fecal impaction may be caused by congenital megacolon in children, psychiatric disorders, painful anal conditions that inhibit the patient's desire to defecate, intestinal obstruction, dehydration, immobility in elderly debilitated patients, spinal cord injury, rectal neoplasms, and use of narcotics.

TREATMENT: Manual extraction is the indicated and usual initial treatment. This may require local anesthesia. The impaction is fragmented by using a scissoring action of the fingers. After the impaction is fragmented, use of mild laxatives, such as mineral oil instilled into the rectum, provides lubrication and assists in passage of the fragments. Surgery is rarely required.

**fecalith** (fē′kă-lĭth) [″ + Gr. *lithos,* stone] A fecal concretion. SYN: *coprolith.*

**fecaloid** (fē′kă-loyd) [″ + Gr. *eidos,* form, shape] Resembling feces.

**fecaloma** (fē″kăl-ō′mă) [″ + Gr. *oma,* tumor] A large mass of accumulated feces in the rectum resembling a tumor. SYN: *scatoma.*

**fecaluria** (fē″kăl-ū′rē-ă) [″ + Gr. *ouron,* urine] Fecal matter in the urine.

**fecal vomit** Feces in vomitus. This occurs in strangulated hernia or intestinal obstruction preventing normal bowel movements.

**feces** (fē′sēz) [L. *faeces*] Body waste such as food residue, bacteria, epithelium, and mucus, discharged from the bowels by way of the anus. Also called *dejecta; excrement; excreta; stool.* **fecal** (fē′kăl), *adj.*

COMPOSITION: The total weight of the feces in a healthy man on a normal diet is 100 to 200 g daily. Of this, 65% is water and the remainder dry matter. Excreted nitrogen is less than 1.7 g daily. The feces are composed of food residue including undigested cellulose; water; secretions from the intestinal glands, stomach, and liver; indole; skatole; cholesterol; mucus and epithelial cells; purine bases; pigment; microorganisms; inorganic salts; and sometimes foreign substances. The normal reaction is neutral or slightly alkaline. The feces of infants usually are acid.

DIAGNOSIS: Inspection should include color, form, consistency, odor, and the presence of any observable foreign substances.

*Color:* Color may indicate various disorders. *Black* or *tarry* feces can indicate bleeding or hemorrhage into the gastrointestinal tract. *Tarry* describes feces containing digested blood or affected by drugs such as bismuth, iron, tannin, manganese, or charcoal. *Bloody:* Blood may indicate hemorrhoids, cancer of the rectum or colon, ulcers, fissures, abraded rectal membrane from dry feces, eroded rectal polypus, acute proctitis, foreign bodies, colitis, intussusception or strangulated hernia in children, typhoid fever, or phosphorus poisoning. *Clay-colored:* Clay color may denote impaired bile formation or obstruction, phosphorus poisoning, or yellow atrophy of the liver. *Green:* In general, green feces in children and infants indicate that the bowel contents have passed quickly through the intestinal tract.

*Form and consistency:* Feces are normally soft and formed. They are hard, nodular, or scybalous in constipation and fluid or mushy in diarrhea. Consistently flattened or ribbonlike feces indicate rectal obstruction or spastic colitis. They are greasy in jaundice.

*Mucus:* The amount should be noted. Mucus is present in both abnormal and normal circumstances. It may occur as superficial gelatinous streaks or blobs; mixed with the feces and only apparent after a thin paste is made with water; or mixed with blood as in dysentery. Mucus may be the principal component.

*Odor:* This varies with disease and dietary differences. Variations such as sour, pungent, or putrid odors occur in different diseases. SEE: *flatus. Offensive odor:* This occurs in jaundice, acute indigestion, enteritis, typhoid fever, and occasionally constipation. *Putrid odor:* This may be the result of syphilitic or carcinomatous ulceration of the rectum or gangrenous dysentery. *Sour odor:* The feces of infants normally smell sour.

*Parasites:* The presence of various intestinal parasites can be determined by examination of the feces. Gross examination may reveal nematodes (roundworms) or tapeworms; however, microscopic examination is necessary to determine the presence of protozoa, helminth ova, or larvae. Feces to be examined are collected in clean, dry containers. For microscopic examination, representative bits of feces or mucus are emulsified in saline solution on a clean slide, then spread evenly and covered with a coverglass. Diagnosis of pinworms is by examination of scrapings or contact slides from the anal and perianal regions.

**Fechner's law** (fĕk′nĕrz) [Gustav Theodor Fechner, Ger. psychologist, 1801–1887] A theory stating that the magnitudes of sensation produced by given stimuli form an arithmetical progression, the stimuli forming a geometrical progression.

**$Fe(C_3H_5O_3)_2$** Ferrous lactate; lactate of iron.

**$FeCl_2$** Ferrous chloride.

**$FeCl_3$** Ferric chloride.

**$FeCO_3$** Ferrous carbonate.

**fecula** (fĕk′ū-lă) [L. *faecula,* dregs] **1.** Sediment. **2.** Starch.

**feculent** (fĕk′ū-lĕnt) [L. *faeculentus*] Having sediment.

**fecund** Fertile.

**fecundate** (fē′kŭn-dāt) [L. *fecundare,* to bear fruit] To fertilize, impregnate, or render fertile.

**fecundation** (fē″kŭn-dā′shŭn) Impregnation; fertilization.

***artificial f.*** Impregnation by mechanical injection of the seminal fluid into the uterus. SYN: *artificial insemination.*

**fecundity** (fē-kŭn′dĭ-tē) Ability to produce offspring; fertility.

**feedback 1.** The influence of the output or result of a system on the input or stimulus. Feedback may be positive or negative. In positive feedback, the result of the process intensifies the stimulus (e.g., uterine contraction stimulates oxytocin secretion, which brings about increased contractions and increased oxytocin). In negative feedback, the result of the process reverses or shuts off the stimulus (e.g., a high blood glucose level stimulates insulin secretion, which lowers blood glucose, which in turn decreases insulin secretion). **2.** In psychiatry, the expressed verbal reaction or physical reaction (i.e., body language) of one person to another person's actions or behaviors.

**feeder** A device permitting independent eating by persons with severe motor control problems.

**feeding** [AS. *fedan,* to give food to] Taking or giving nourishment.

***artificial f.*** **1.** Providing a liquid food preparation through a tube passed into the stomach or the rectum. This is also done through gastrostomy or duodenostomy. SEE: *hyperalimentation.* **2.** Feeding of an infant with food other than mother's milk.

***enteral tube f.*** Feeding through a tube that extends through the mouth or nostril into the stomach, indicated for patients who cannot swallow or masticate food but who have functioning gastrointestinal tracts. The nasal method is used most often. It requires a much smaller tube and a little more dexterity but is less likely to be resisted successfully. A tube lubricated with glycerin is gently passed into pharynx and, avoiding the larynx, is passed into the stomach. Entry into the larynx may produce struggling and cyanosis.

---

Caution: Before feedings it is important to ascertain that the tube is in the stomach and not in the bronchus. This can be determined by aspirating the tube and observing for gastric contents or by listening to the end of the tube. If air comes out of the tube with each expiration, the tube is not in the stomach. If the position of the tube is in doubt, a small amount of air should be injected into it while the stomach area is being auscultated. If the tube is in the stomach, a gurgling should be heard as the air is injected. Foods or nutritional substances as ordered by the physician are fed slowly.

---

***forced f.*** Tube feeding to an individual who does not want to eat or to be fed by this means.

***intravenous f.*** The provision of total nutritional requirements intravenously; essential in treating some diseases. It is accomplished by carefully controlling the composition of fluid given with respect to total calories derived from protein hydrolysates, dextrose, and fat emulsions, and the electrolytes, minerals, and vitamins. Patients have been maintained for months on nothing but the nutrients and fluids given intravenously, usually through a major vein, such as the subclavian or the jugular. SEE: *total parenteral nutrition.*

***nasal f.*** SEE: *enteral tube f.*

***rectal f.*** The introduction of fluid nutrients into the colon through the rectum. This type of feeding is rarely used because little nourishment can be absorbed through the colon. Normal saline is often used with glucose; a 5% to 10% solution can be made by adding 15 to 30 g of sugar to 10 oz (300 ml) of normal saline. SYN: *nutritive enema.*

**feeding center** SEE: under *center.*

**feeling** [AS. *felan,* to feel] The conscious phase of nervous activity. The emotions are centrally stimulated and certain sensations are produced by excitation of peripheral nerves, including those of the special senses.

**Feen-A-Mint** Trade name of phenolphthalein.

**Feer's disease** (fārz) [Emil Feer, Swiss pediatrician, 1864–1955] Acrodynia.

**feet** [AS. *fet*] The pedal extremities of the legs. SEE: *foot.*

**Fehling's solution** (fā′lĭngz) [Hermann von Fehling, Ger. chemist, 1812–1885] A solution used to detect the presence of glucose in urine. It consists of equal parts of solutions A and B prepared as follows: Solution A (copper solution): 34.66 g of copper sulfate crystals dissolved in enough water to make 500 ml. Solution B (alkaline tartrate solution): 173 g of crystallized potassium sodium tartrate and 50 g of sodium hydroxide dissolved in enough water to make 500 ml. Equal portions of solutions A and B are mixed just before use. This mixture is then added to the urine sample and the liquid is boiled. If glucose is present, a cuprous oxide red precipitate is formed.

**Feingold diet** (fīn′gōld) [Benjamin Feingold, U.S. pediatrician, 1900–1982] A nutritional plan in which all foods containing artificial coloring, flavoring, and preserving materials are excluded. It is used in treating hyperactive children.

**fel** (fĕl) [L.] Bile.

**feline** (fē′līn) [L. *feles,* cat] Concerning cats.

**fellatio** (fĕl-ā′shē-ō) [L. *fellare,* to suck] Oral stimulation of the penis. SEE: *cunnilingus.*

**fellatrix, fellatrice** A woman who performs fellatio.

**felon** (fĕl′ŏn) [ME. *feloun,* malignant] An infection or abscess of the soft tissue of the terminal joint of a finger. SYN: *whitlow.*

**feltwork 1.** A fibrous network. **2.** A plexus of nerve fibrils.

**Felty's syndrome** (fĕl′tēz) [Augustus Roi Felty, U.S. physician, b. 1895] A group of pathological changes—splenomegaly, neutropenia, and in some cases anemia and thrombocytopenia—that can occur in patient with long-standing rheumatoid arthritis.

**female** [L. *femella,* little woman] **1.** An individual of the sex that produces ova or bears young. **2.** Characteristic of this sex. SEE: *genitalia, female.*

**female genital mutilation** A traditional practice in some African, Middle Eastern, and Southeast Asian cultures. The mutilation usually is performed between the ages of 1 week and 14 years. The procedure is performed by nonmedical personnel without benefit of anesthesia or sterile conditions. The most common procedures are removal of the clitoral prepuce, excision of the clitoris, removal of the labia minora and sometimes most of the labia majora; the two sides may be sutured together to occlude the vagina. Possible immediate complications include infection, tetanus, shock, hemorrhage, and death. The possible long-term physical and mental disabilities include chronic pelvic infection, keloids, vulvar abscesses, sterility, incontinence, depression, anxiety, sexual dysfunction, and obstetric complications. SEE: *circumcision, female.*

**female sexual arousal disorder** According to the DSM-IV, the essential feature of this condition is a persistent or recurrent inability to attain, or to maintain until completion of the sexual activity, an adequate vaginal lubrication-swelling response of sexual excitement. In order to establish this diagnosis, the disturbance must cause marked distress or interpersonal difficulty, and the difficulty cannot be attributed to a medical condition, substance abuse, or medications. SEE: *male erectile disorder.*

**feminine** (fĕm′ĭ-nĭn) Concerning or being of the female sex.

**feminism** [L. *femininus*] The development of female secondary sexual characteristics in a man. SEE: *gynecomastia.*

**feminization** The normal development of female secondary sexual characteristics, or the pathological development of these in a man.

***testicular f.*** An apparent female in whom the genetic sex is male. This condition is caused by the inability of the tissues to respond to the male hormone produced by the testicles. The external genitalia are rudimentary, and the testicles may be in the abdomen.

**femoral** (fĕm′or-ăl) [L. *femoralis*] Pert. to the femur.

**femoral artery** The artery that begins at the external iliac artery and terminates behind the knee as the popliteal artery on the inner side of the femur.

**femoral reflex** Extension of the knee and flexion of the foot resulting from irritation of the skin over the upper anterior third of the thigh.

**femoral vein** A continuation of the popliteal vein upward toward the external iliac vein.

**femorotibial** (fĕm″ō-rō-tĭb′ē-ăl) [″ + *tibia,* pipe] Pert. to the femur and tibia.

**femto-** [Danish *femten,* fifteen] In the metric system, a prefix indicating that the number following is to be multiplied by $10^{-15}$. Thus a femtogram is $10^{-15}$ g. SEE: *Metric System* in *Units of Measurement Appendix.*

**femur** (fē′mŭr) *pl.* **femora** [L.] The thigh bone. It extends from the hip to the knee and is the longest and strongest bone in the skeleton. SEE: illus.

**fenestra** (fĕ-nĕs′tră) *pl.* **fenestrae** [L., window] **1.** An aperture frequently closed by a membrane. **2.** An open area, as in the blade of a forceps. **fenestral** (-trăl), *adj.*

***f. cochleae*** The opening leading into the cochlea. It is closed by the secondary tympanic membrane. SYN: *f. rotunda; cochlear window; round window.*

***f. rotunda*** F. cochleae.

***f. vestibuli*** An oval opening on the inner wall of the middle ear, or tympanum, leading to the vestibule, into which the base of the stapes fits. SYN: *oval window.*

**fenestrated** (fĕn′ĕ-strāt-ĕd) Having openings.

**fenestration 1.** The condition of having a fenestra. **2.** An operation in which an artificial opening is made into the labyrinth of the ear. This procedure is performed to

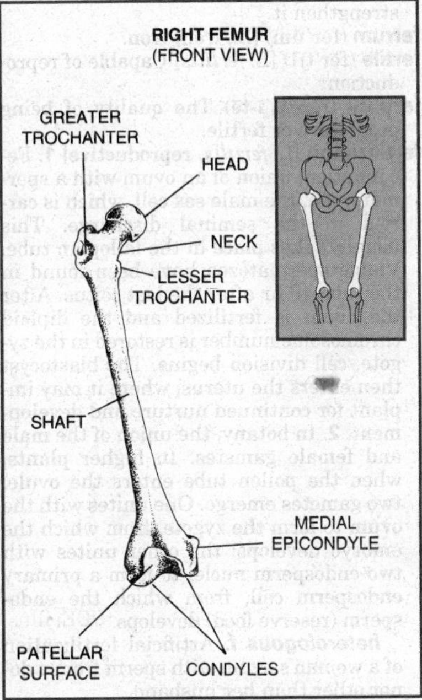


treat deafness associated with otosclerosis. **3.** An operation to open the mucoperiosteum and alveolar plate of bone over the root of an infected tooth to remove the inflammatory exudate and relieve pain.

**fenfluramine hydrochloride** (fĕn-floor′ă-mēn) An adrenergic agent. Trade name is Pondimin.

**fenoprofen calcium** (fĕn-ō-prō′fĕn) A nonsteroidal anti-inflammatory agent. Trade name is Nalfon.

**fentanyl citrate** (fĕn′tă-nĭl) A potent synthetic analgesic. Trade name is Sublimaze. SEE: *drug, designer*.

**feral** (fĕr′ŭl) [L. *fera,* wild animal] Existing in a wild, untamed, and undomesticated state.

**ferment** (fĕr-mĕnt′, fĕr′mĕnt) [L. *fermentum*] **1.** To decompose. **2.** A substance capable of inducing oxidative decomposition in other substances. **3.** A catalytic agent capable of inducing oxidative decomposition in substances with which it comes in contact.

**fermentation** The oxidative decomposition of complex substances through the action of enzymes or ferments, produced by microorganisms. Bacteria, molds, and yeasts are the principal groups of organisms involved. Fermentations of economic importance are those involved in the production of alcohol, alcoholic beverages, lactic and butyric acids, and bread.

***acetic f.*** Production of acetic acid by the bacterial oxidation of ethyl alcohol under aerobic conditions.

***alcoholic f.*** Production of ethyl alcohol from carbohydrates, usually through the action of yeasts.

***amylolytic f.*** Hydrolysis of starch with the formation of sugar.

***autolytic f.*** Disintegration of tissues after death due to enzymes present in the tissues.

***butyric f.*** Formation of butyric acid from bacterial action on carbohydrates under anaerobic conditions.

***citric acid f.*** Formation of citric acid from the action of molds on carbohydrates.

***invertin f.*** Conversion of cane sugar into glucose and fructose.

***lactic f.*** Formation of lactic acid from carbohydrates by bacterial action. The genera *Streptococcus* and *Lactobacillus* are the forms usually involved. Bacterial action is responsible for the souring of milk.

***oxalic acid f.*** Formation of oxalic acid from carbohydrates by the action of certain molds, esp. *Aspergillus*.

***propionic acid f.*** Formation of propionic acid from carbohydrates by the action of certain bacteria.

***viscous f.*** Production of gelatinous material by different forms of bacilli.

**fermium** (fĕr′mē-ŭm) [Enrico Fermi, It.-U.S. physicist and Nobel Prize winner, 1901–1954] SYMB: Fm. A radioactive element with atomic number 100 and an atomic weight of 257.

**ferning, fern pattern** The palm leaf (arborization) pattern that cervical mucus assumes when placed in a thin layer on a glass slide and allowed to dry. This is seen on microscopic examination of the slide. It occurs during only certain stages of the menstrual cycle. The pattern, caused by crystallization of the mucus as it dries, depends on the concentration of electrolytes, esp. sodium chloride. The salt concentration is determined by the amount of estrogen in the mucus. Ferning is usually seen at midcycle in normal menstruating women; therefore it may be helpful in determining the time of ovulation in women who have difficulty becoming pregnant. The mucus has a beaded (i.e., nonferning) pattern at other times in the cycle and during pregnancy. SYN: *cervical mucus*.

**-ferous** [L. *ferre,* to bear] Suffix meaning *producing*.

**ferri-, ferro-** [L. *ferrum,* iron] Prefix meaning *iron*.

**ferric 1.** Pert. to iron. SYN: *ferruginous*. **2.** Denoting a compound containing iron in its trivalent form.

***f. chloride*** $FeCl_3$, used principally in tincture form as an astringent.

**ferritin** (fĕr′ĭ-tĭn) An iron-phosphorus-protein complex containing about 23% iron. It is formed in the intestinal mucosa by the union of ferric iron with a protein, apoferritin. Tissues store iron in this form, principally in the reticuloendothelial cells of the liver, spleen, and bone marrow.

**ferrokinetics** (fĕr″rō-kĭ-nĕt′ĭks) [″ + Gr. *kinesis,* movement] The study of the absorption, use, storage, and excretion of iron.

**ferropexia** (fĕr-ō-pĕks′ē-ă) Iron fixation.

**ferroprotein** (fĕr″ō-prō′tē-ĭn) A protein combined with an iron-containing radical. Ferroproteins are important oxygen-transferring enzymes (e.g., Warburg's enzyme, cytochrome, oxidase).

**ferrotherapy** (fĕr″ō-thĕr′ă-pē) [″ + Gr. *therapeia,* treatment] The use of iron in treating anemia.

**ferrous** (fĕr′ŭs) [L. *ferrum,* iron] **1.** Pert. to iron. SYN: *ferruginous.* **2.** Denoting a compound containing bivalent iron.

***f. fumarate*** $C_4H_2FeO_4$, an iron preparation used to treat anemias.

***f. gluconate*** $C_{12}H_{22}FeO_{14}$, an iron preparation occurring as a yellowish powder or granules. It is used as a hematinic.

***f. sulfate*** $FeSO_4$; iron sulfate. It occurs as pale, bluish-green crystals and is taken orally as a hematinic. It is incompatible with alkalies, chlorides, tannic acid, and oxidizing agents.

**ferruginous** (fĕr-ū′jĭ-nŭs) [L. *ferrugo,* iron rust] **1.** Pert. to or containing iron. **2.** Having the color of iron rust.

**ferrule** (fĕr′ūl) [L. *viriola,* little bracelet] A band or ring of metal applied to the end of the root or crown of a tooth to strengthen it.

**ferrum** (fĕr′ŭm) [L., iron] Iron.

**fertile** (fĕr′tĭl) [L. *fertilis*] Capable of reproduction.

**fertility** (fĕr-tĭl′ĭ-tē) The quality of being productive or fertile.

**fertilization** [L. *fertilis,* reproductive] **1.** Fecundation; union of an ovum with a spermatozoon, the male sex cell, which is carried in the seminal discharge. This usually takes place in the fallopian tube. Viable spermatozoa have been found in the tube 48 hr after the last coitus. After the ovum is fertilized and the diploid chromosome number is restored in the zygote, cell division begins. The blastocyst then enters the uterus, where it may implant for continued nurture and development. **2.** In botany, the union of the male and female gametes. In higher plants, when the pollen tube enters the ovule, two gametes emerge. One unites with the ovum to form the zygote, from which the embryo develops; the other unites with two endosperm nuclei to form a primary endosperm cell, from which the endosperm (reserve food) develops. SEE: illus.

***heterologous f.*** Artificial fertilization of a woman's ovum with sperm from a donor other than her husband.

***homologous f.*** Artificial fertilization of a woman's ovum by her husband's sperm. The ovum and sperm are united while both are outside the body and then are

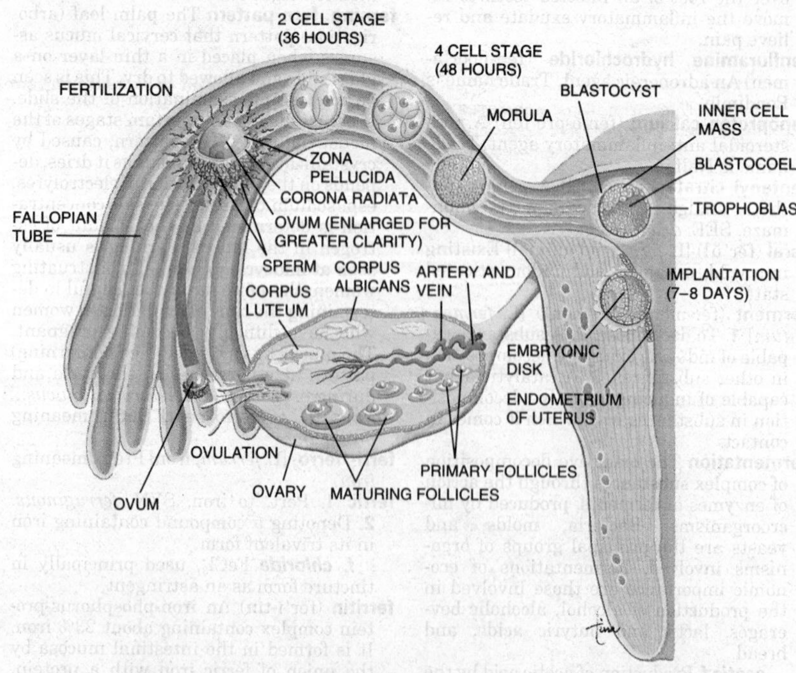


OVULATION, **FERTILIZATION**, AND EARLY EMBRYONIC DEVELOPMENT

placed intravaginally during the optimum time for fertilization.

***in vitro f.*** ABBR: IVF. Laboratory-produced conception; used to enable pregnancy in infertile women when sperm access to ova is prevented by structural defects in the fallopian tubes or by other factors. After drug-induced follicle maturation, a sample of ova and follicular fluid is removed surgically and mixed with a specimen of the partner's sperm for incubation. The resulting zygote is introduced into the woman's uterus for implantation. SEE: *embryo transfer; GIFT; ZIFT*.

**fester** (fĕs′tĕr) [L. *fistula*, ulcer] To become inflamed and suppurate.

**festinant** (fĕs′tĭ-nănt) Increasing in speed; accelerating.

**festinating gait** SEE: under *gait*.

**festination** (fĕs″tĭ-nā′shŭn) [L. *festinatio*] Abnormal and involuntary increase in speed of walking in an attempt to catch up with the center of gravity, which is displaced by the patient's leaning forward. It is seen in certain neurological diseases.

**festoon** (fĕs-toon′) [L. *festus*, festal] A carving in the base material of a denture that simulates the natural indentations of the gums.

**FET** *forced expiratory time.*

**fetal** (fē′tăl) Pert. to a fetus.

**fetal alcohol syndrome** ABBR: FAS. Birth defects in an infant born to a mother whose chronic alcoholism persisted during gestation. Shortly after birth such infants may exhibit signs of alcohol withdrawal. In addition, some have physical abnormalities (e.g., deficient growth and mental capacity). Other characteristic findings include a small head with multiple facial abnormalities: small eyes with short slits, a wide, flat nose bridge, a midface that lacks a groove between the lip and the nose, and a small jaw related to maxillary hypoplasia. Children often exhibit persistent growth retardation, hyperactivity, and learning deficits. SEE: *Nursing Diagnoses Appendix*.

**fetal assessment** SEE: *biophysical profile*.

**fetal circulation** The course of the flow of blood in a fetus. Oxygenated in the placenta, blood passes through the umbilical vein and ductus venosus to the inferior vena cava and from there to the right atrium. It then follows one of two courses: 1) through the foramen ovale to the left atrium and thence through the aorta to the tissues, or 2) through the right ventricle, pulmonary artery, and ductus arteriosus to the aorta and thence to the tissues. In either case the blood bypasses the lungs, which do not function before birth. Blood returns to the placenta through the umbilical arteries, which are continuations of the hypogastric arteries. At birth or shortly after, the ductus arteriosus and the foramen ovale close, establishing normal circulation. If either fails to close, the baby may be blue. SEE: illus.; *ductus arteriosus, patent*.

**fetal death** The demise of the fetus. This is suspected when the patient reports an absence of fetal movement. If fetal heart tones cannot be detected and there is no palpable fetal movement, real-time ultrasound is used to confirm the absence of cardiac activity. SYN: *fetal demise*.

**fetal demise** Fetal death. SEE: *Nursing Diagnoses Appendix*.

**fetal development** The growth and maturation of the fetus in utero. Fetal development of the fetus is divided into three periods: the preembryonic period begins with conception and ends on gestational day 14; the embryonic period encompasses gestational weeks 3 through 8; and the remainder of the pregnancy is known as the fetal period.

**fetal distress** A nonspecific clinical diagnosis indicating pathology in the fetus. The distress, which may be due to anoxia, is judged by fetal heart rate or biochemical changes in the amniotic fluid or fetal blood.

**fetal heart rate monitoring** The techniques used to determine the heart rate of the fetus. They include auscultation, use of an electronic device, or Doppler ultrasound. SEE: *Doppler echocardiography; fetal monitoring in utero*.

**fetal maturation** The natural processes of fetal growth and development that culminate in the birth of a full-term fetus. Body organs and systems arise from three primary germ layers (ectoderm, mesoderm, and entoderm) and rudimentary formation of all organ systems is completed by gestational week 16. Systems maturation essential to extrauterine survival begins during week 24 with beginning formation of pulmonary surfactant. Two critical events occur between weeks 26 and 29: the pulmonary vasculature becomes capable of gas exchange and the central nervous system becomes capable of controlling respiration. SEE: *preterm birth*.

**fetal membrane** SEE: *membrane, fetal*.

**fetal monitoring in utero** The techniques used to obtain information on the physical condition of the fetus. They include recording the fetal electrocardiogram, respiratory rate, and, by invasive techniques, blood gas and pH data. SEE: *amniocentesis; chorionic villus sampling; Doppler echocardiography; fetal heart rate monitoring*.

**fetal scalp blood sampling** The process of obtaining a small amount of blood from the fetal scalp for pH testing. When the monitor recording suggests fetal compromise during labor, the physician or nurse-midwife may elect to perform this procedure. The normal finding for fetal pH is at or above 7.25. Findings between 7.20 and 7.24 indicate a preacidotic state; if the pH is below 7.20, acidosis is present.

**fetal tissue transplant** A controversial ex-

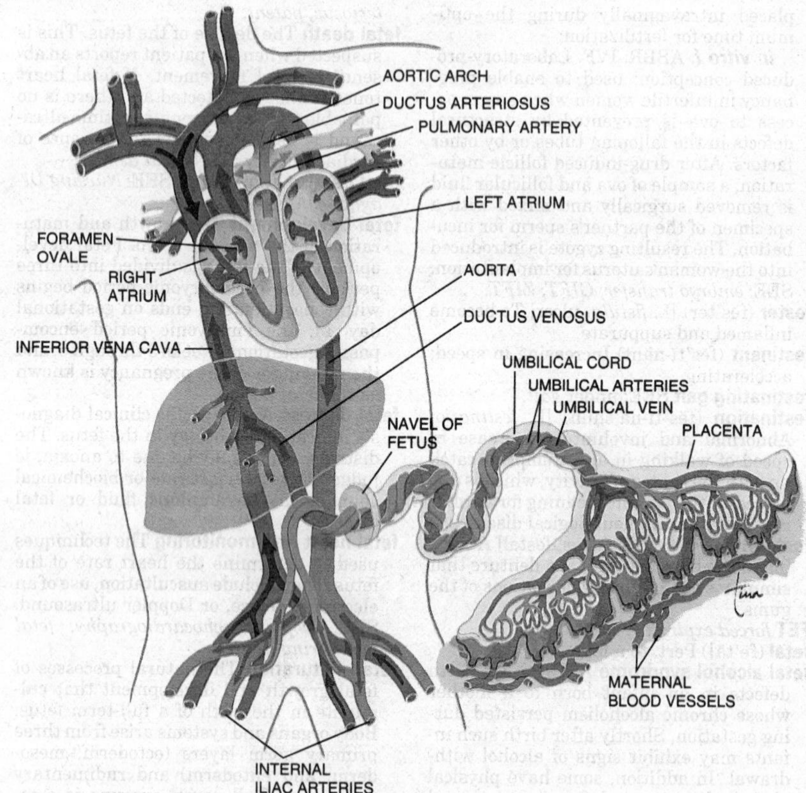


**FETAL CIRCULATION**

VESSELS THAT CARRY OXYGENATED BLOOD ARE RED

perimental technique in which tissue from a dead fetus is grafted into a patient in an attempt to treat or cure disease.

**fetal viability** The ability of a fetus to survive outside of the womb. Historically, a fetus was considered to be capable of living at the end of gestational week 20 when the mother had felt fetal movement (quickening) and the fetal heart tones could be auscultated with a fetoscope. In actuality, even with prompt and intensive neonatal support, a preterm fetus of less than 25 weeks' gestation has little chance of surviving outside of the womb. SEE: *viable.*

**feticide** (fē′tĭ-sīd) [″ + *cidus,* kill] Killing of a fetus. SEE: *infanticide.*

**fetid** (fē′tĭd) [L. *fetidus,* stink] Rank or foul in odor.

**fetish** (fē′tĭsh) [Portug. *feitico,* charm, sorcery] **1.** An object, such as an idol or charm, that is thought to have mysterious, magical, and supernatural power. **2.** In psychiatry, the love object of a person who suffers from fetishism.

**fetishism** (fē′tĭsh-, fĕt′ĭsh-ĭzm) [″ + Gr. *-ismos,* condition] **1.** Belief in some object as possessing power or capable of being a stimulus. **2.** Erotic stimulation or sexually arousing fantasies involving contact with nonliving objects, such as an article of dress or a braid of hair.

**fetochorionic** (fē″tō-kor-ē-ŏn′ĭk) [L. *fetus* + Gr. *chorion,* membrane] Pert. to the fetus and the chorion, or chorionic membrane, of the placenta.

**fetoglobulin** (fē″tō-glŏb′ū-lĭn) Fetoprotein.

**fetography** (fē-tŏg′ră-fē) Radiography of the fetus in utero. This procedure has been virtually replaced by ultrasound.

**fetology** (fē-tŏl′ō-jē) [″ + Gr. *logos,* word, reason] Study of the fetus.

**fetometry** (fē-tŏm′ĕ-trē) [L. *fetus* + Gr. *metron,* measure] Estimation of the size of a fetus or its head before delivery.

**fetoplacental** (fē″tō-plă-sĕn′tăl) [″ + *placenta,* a flat cake] Pert. to the fetus and its placenta.

**fetoprotein** (fē″tō-prō′tēn) An antigen present in the human fetus and in certain pathological conditions in adults. The amniotic fluid level can be used to evaluate

**Development of Fetal Tissue**

| Ectoderm | Mesoderm | Endoderm |
|---|---|---|
| Nervous tissue | Bone, cartilage, and other connective tissues | Epithelium of respiratory tract except nose |
| Sense organs | Male and female reproductive tracts | digestive tract except mouth and anal canal |
| Epidermis, nails, and hair follicles | Heart, blood vessels, and lymphatics | bladder except trigone |
| Epithelium of external and internal ear nasal cavity and sinuses mouth anal canal | Kidneys, ureters, trigone of bladder | Proximal portion of male urethra |
| Distal portion of male urethra | Pleura, peritoneum, and pericardium | Female urethra |
| | Skeletal muscle | Liver |
| | | Pancreas |

fetal development. Elevated serum levels are found in adults with certain kinds of liver diseases. SEE: *alpha-fetoprotein*.

**fetor** (fē′tor) [L.] Stench; an offensive odor.

***f. hepaticus*** A mousy odor in the breath of persons with severe liver impairment. SEE: *coma, hepatic*.

***f. oris*** Halitosis.

**fetoscope** An optical device, usually flexible and made of fiberoptic materials, used for direct visualization of the fetus in the uterus. SEE: *embryoscopy; fetoscopy*.

**fetoscopy** Direct visualization of the fetus in the uterus through a fetoscope. SEE: *embryoscopy*.

**fetotoxic** (fē″tō-tŏk′sĭk) [L. *fetus*, fetus, + Gr. *toxikon*, poison] Poisonous to the fetus. Materials considered potentially fetotoxic include alcohol, morphine, cocaine, salicylates, coumarin anticoagulants, sedatives, tetracyclines, thiazides, tobacco smoke, and large doses of vitamin K. SEE: *teratogenic; thalidomide*.

**fetus** (fē′tŭs) [L.] **1.** The latter stages of the developing young of an animal within the uterus or within an egg. **2.** In humans, the child in utero after completion of the eighth gestational week. Before that time it is called an embryo. SEE: table.

***f. amorphus*** A shapeless fetal anomaly, scarcely recognizable as a fetus.

***calcified f.*** A fetus that has died in utero and become hardened by calcium salts. SYN: *lithopedion*.

***harlequin f.*** A newborn with abnormal skin that resembles a thick horny armor, divided into areas by deep red fissures. These infants die within a few days. The condition is also known as ichthyosis fetalis and ichthyosiform erythroderma, which were once regarded as separate diseases but are now known to represent different degrees of severity of the same entity. SYN: *icthyosis congenita; icthyosis fetalis*.

***f. in fetu*** Parasitic f.

***mummified f.*** A dead fetus that has become dried and shriveled after resorption has failed to occur.

***f. papyraceus*** In a twin pregnancy, a dead fetus pressed flat by the development of the living twin.

***parasitic f.*** A small imperfect fetus, called a parasite, contained within the body of another fetus, the autosite. SYN: *f. in fetu*. SEE: *dermoid cyst*.

**FEV** *forced expiratory volume*.

**$FEV_1$** Forced expiratory volume in 1 sec. This is a form of timed vital capacity test. After full inspiration the person exhales as hard and fast as possible into a lightweight spirometer. The amount of air exhaled during the first second is recorded. The test results provide an excellent index of pulmonary function.

**fever** [L. *febris*] **1.** Abnormal elevation of temperature. The normal temperature taken orally is 98.6°F (37°C). Normal range may vary up to 1° above or 2° below this value. However, if a person whose normal temperature is 97.8°F (36.5°C) becomes ill, 98.6°F (37°C) could represent fever. Therefore it is not practical to attempt to designate a precise level of normal body temperature. Rectal temperature is 0.5° to 1.0°F higher than oral temperature. The basal energy expenditure is estimated to be increased about 12% for each degree centigrade of fever. SYN: *pyrexia*. SEE: *energy expenditure, basal; temperature*. **2.** A disease characterized by an elevation of body temperature, such as typhoid fever, yellow fever.

SYMPTOMS: Symptoms include a flushed face; hot, dry skin; anorexia; headache; nausea and sometimes vomiting; constipation and sometimes diarrhea; aching all over; and scant, highly colored urine. Delirium is possible if the temperature is over 105°F (40.5°C) or lower in some cases. Convulsions may follow, esp. in children, and may progress to coma. SEE: *convulsion*.

ETIOLOGY: Moderate increase in body temperature in children may result from minor causes and is of less significance than in adults. After childhood, fevers may be caused by a hot environment; generation of body heat by physical means such as exercise; neurogenic factors such as injury to the hypothalamus; dehydration such as occurs after excessive diuresis; many therapeutic drugs, which may cause fever as an undesired side effect; chemical substances such as caffeine or cocaine injected into the bloodstream; injection of proteins or their products; or breakdown of necrotic tissue (these are the aseptic fevers that follow surgery or coronary occlusion); infectious disease or inflammation (fever is caused by the breakdown of bacterial proteins or toxins liberated by the disease organisms that affect the heat-regulating centers); or severe hemorrhage.

TREATMENT: The traditional response to fever has been to take steps to lower the temperature. This was done by using antipyretic drugs such as aspirin or acetaminophen, cool baths, cooling blankets, or combinations of these. The rationale for such therapy is not clear, and the benefit to the patient's comfort is questionable. Except when due to causes such as dehydration, heatstroke, or heat exhaustion, fever may benefit the patient. It may be invalid to automatically assume that antipyretic therapy is indicated. In the presence of fever higher than 107°F, peripheral cooling alone may cause reflex vasoconstriction, which reduces heat loss. SEE: *Reye's syndrome.*

---

Caution: Aspirin and other salicylates are contraindicated for use as antipyretics or analgesics for children because of the increased risk of Reye's syndrome.

---

CLASSIFICATION: *Intermittent:* The temperature curve returns to normal during the day and reaches its peak in the evening. *Remittent:* The temperature fluctuates but does not return to normal. *Sustained:* The temperature remains elevated with little fluctuation. *Relapsing:* Periods of fever are interspersed with periods of normal temperature.

PERIODS: *Invasion or onset of fever:* The temperature rises until the maximum is reached. This period may be gradual as in typhoid or sudden as in scarlet fever. *Fastigium, or stadium:* The fever is more or less stationary, with variations often reaching the maximum observed in that illness. This is the highest point in the fever. *Defervescence:* The fever declines until the temperature is normal. When sudden, it is known as crisis, as in lobar pneumonia; when gradual, lysis, as in measles.

---

Caution: When evaluating a patient's temperature, it is necessary to remember that the thermometer may be inaccurate or that the patient may heat the thermometer to feign fever.

---

**childbed f.** An infection of the birth canal following trauma from childbirth. SYN: *sepsis, puerperal.*

**continuous f.** A sustained fever, as in scarlet fever, typhus, or pneumonia, with a slight diurnal variation.

**dengue f.** SEE: *dengue.*

**drug f.** Fever caused by the administration of a drug. Almost any drug can produce this undesired side effect in some individuals.

**factitious f.** Fever produced artificially by a patient. This is done by artificially heating the thermometer or by self-administered pyrogenic substances. An artificial fever may be suspected if the pulse rate is much less than expected for the degree of fever noted. This diagnosis should be considered in all patients in whom there is no other plausible explanation for the fever. Patients with this condition may have serious psychiatric problems. SYN: *psychogenic fever.* SEE: *disorder, factitious; malinger; Munchausen syndrome.*

**induced f.** Fever produced artificially to treat certain diseases such as central nervous system syphilis. Sustained fever of 105°F (40.5°C), or even higher, maintained for 6 to 8 or 10 hr may be induced by medical diathermy or injection of malarial parasites.

**intermittent f.** Fever in which symptoms disappear completely between paroxysms. SEE: *malaria; undulant fever.*

**neutropenic f.** In cancer therapy, fever associated with an abnormally low neutrophil level. Neutropenia may be caused by chemotherapy, aplastic anemia, bone marrow infiltration from malignancy, or bone marrow transplantation. The more severe the neutropenia, the greater the chance of infection and fever.

**periodic f.** Familial Mediterranean fever.

**phlebotomus f.** Sandfly fever.

**relapsing f.** Any of a group of acute infectious diseases caused by a variety of *Borrelia* and transmitted by head lice, body lice, and ticks of the genus *Ornithodorus.* Alternating periods of fever and normal temperature are typical of the disease. Treatment consists of a single dose of tetracycline, erythromycin, or procaine penicillin G and symptomatic treatment.

**remittent f.** Fever that never falls to a normal temperature but shows some diurnal variation. SEE: *malaria.*

**f. therapy** The use of artificially induced fever to treat disease. The induction of fever by injection of live malarial organisms has been beneficial in treating central nervous system syphilis. Contemporary management involves the use of specific drugs to induce a state of hyperthermia; however, hyperthermia treatment using microwave energy is not the same as fever therapy. SEE: *hyperthermia treatment*.

***f. of unknown origin*** ABBR: FUO. An illness of at least 3 weeks' duration with fever exceeding 38.3°C on several occasions and diagnosis not established after 1 week of hospital investigation. The main causes are systemic and localized infections, neoplasms, or collagen-vascular diseases such as rheumatoid arthritis, disseminated lupus erythematosus, and polyarteritis nodosa. Less common causes are granulomatous disease, inflammatory disease of the bowel, pulmonary embolization, drug fever, cirrhosis of the liver, and rare conditions such as Whipple's disease. Diseases such as AIDS, chronic fatigue syndrome, or Lyme disease may be added to the list of possible causes of FUO; however, better diagnostic methods may eliminate other diseases from the list. Some cases remain undiagnosed. SEE: *fever, factitious*.

**fever blister** An area of inflammation of the lips or mucous membrane of the mouth. The cause is herpes simplex virus, usually type I. SYN: *cold sore*.

**FFB** *fiberoptic bronchoscope*.

**F.F.D.** *focal-film distance*.

**$FH_4$** *5,6,7,8-tetrahydrofolic acid* (folacin).

**fiat** (fī'ăt) [L.] Let there be made, a term used in writing prescriptions.

**fiber** [L. *fibra*] **1.** A threadlike or filmlike element, as a nerve fiber. **2.** A neuron or its axonal portion. **3.** An elongated threadlike structure. It may be cellular as nerve fiber or muscle fiber, or may be a cellular product, as collagen, elastic, oxytalan, or reticular fiber. **4.** A slender cellulosic structure derived from plants such as cotton. SEE: *rayon, purified*.

***accelerator f.*** A fiber nerve pathway causing increased heart rate on stimulation.

***afferent f.*** A nerve fiber that carries sensory impulses to the central nervous system from receptors in the periphery.

***cholinergic f.*** Any preganglionic fiber, postganglionic parasympathetic fiber, postganglionic sympathetic fiber to a sweat gland, or efferent fiber to skeletal muscle.

***circular f.'s*** Collagen bundles in the gingiva that surround a tooth.

***dietary f.*** The components of food that resist chemical digestion. This category includes foods made up of cellulose, hemicellulose, lignin, gums, mucilages, and pectin. These substances add bulk to the diet to produce a large, bulky bowel movement.

Dietary fibers are classified according to their solubility in water. Water-insoluble fibers include cellulose, lignin, and some hemicelluloses. Natural gel-forming fibers such as gums, mucilages, and some hemicelluloses are water soluble. Most foods of plant origin contain both soluble and insoluble dietary fiber. Many disease processes such as hypertension, diabetes, hypercholesterolemia, polyps of the colon, colon cancer, gallstones, and irritable bowel syndrome have been investigated in regard to dietary fiber intake. These studies have not provided clear-cut evidence of benefit. It is clear, however, that dietary fiber, particularly if derived from wheat, oats, and other insoluble fiber sources, is useful in the prevention and treatment of constipation.

Foods rich in fiber include whole-grain foods, bran flakes, beans, fruits, leafy vegetables, nuts, root vegetables and their skins, and prunes, which also contain the laxative substance diphenolisatin.

***efferent f.*** A nerve fiber that carries motor impulses from the central nervous system to effector organs.

***gingival f.'s*** Collagen fibers that support the marginal or interdental gingiva and are adapted to the tooth surface.

***inhibitory f.*** A fiber whose nerve pathway slows heart action when stimulated.

***intercolumnar f.*** An intercrural fiber.

***interradicular f.'s*** The collagen fibers of the periodontal ligament in the interradicular area, attaching the tooth to alveolar bone.

***intrafusal muscle f.*** The structural component of the muscle spindle, made up of small skeletal muscle fibers at either end and a central noncontracile region where the sensory receptors are located.

***man-made f.*** A synthetic fiber made from chemicals (e.g., rayon or polyester). SYN: *synthetic f.*

***medullated f.*** Myelinated f.

***mossy f.*** Any of the afferent fibers to the cerebellar cortex. The fibers give off many collaterals, each ending in a glomerulus.

***motor f.*** Any of the axons of motor neurons that innervate skeletal muscles.

***muscle f.*** A muscle cell in striated, smooth, or cardiac muscle.

***myelinated f.*** A nerve fiber whose axon (dendrite) is wrapped in a myelin sheath. SYN: *medullated f.*

***nerve f.*** A neuron, although often used to mean *axon*. SEE: *nerve*.

***nonmedullated f.*** Unmyelinated f.

***oxytalan f.'s*** Bundles of thin, acid-resistant fibrils found in the periodontium.

***postganglionic f.*** The axon of a postganglionic neuron that passes from an autonomic ganglion to a visceral effector.

***principal f.'s*** The major fiber groups of the functioning periodontium. They attach the tooth to the bone and adjacent teeth.

***Purkinje f.*** Any of the atypical muscle fibers lying beneath the endocardium that form the impulse-conducting system of the heart.

***synthetic f.*** Man-made f.

***transseptal f.*** Any of the collagenous fibers that extend between the teeth and are embedded in the cementum of adjacent teeth.

***unmyelinated f.*** A nerve fiber that lacks a myelin sheath, although a neurilemma may be present in the peripheral nervous system. SYN: *nonmedullated f.*

**fibercolonoscope** (fī″bĕr-kō-lŏn′ō-skōp) A fiberoptic endoscope for examining the colon.

**fibergastroscope** (fī″bĕr-găs′trō-skōp) A fiberoptic endoscope for examining the stomach.

**fiberglass** Glass spun into fine fibers. It is used in the building industry for insulation. The fibers are irritating to the skin.

**fiber-illumination** (fī′bĕr-ĭl-loo″mĭn-ā″shŭn) The transmission of light to an object by use of fiberoptic bundles.

**fiberoptics** Flexible material of glass or plastic that transmits light along its course by reflecting it from the side or wall of the fiber. Use of this principle permits transmission of light, and therefore visual images, around sharp curves and corners. Devices that use fiberoptic materials are useful in endoscopic examinations.

**fiberscope** (fī′bĕr-skōp) A flexible endoscope that uses fiberoptics for visualization.

**fibra** (fī′bră) *pl.* **fibrae** [L.] A fiber.

**fibremia** (fī-brē′mē-ă) [″ + Gr. *haima,* blood] Fibrin formed in the blood, causing embolism or thrombosis. SYN: *inosemia.*

**fibril** (fī′brĭl) [L. *fibrilla*] **1.** A small fiber. **2.** A very small filamentous structure, often the component of a cell or a fiber.

***muscle f.*** Myofibril.

***nerve f.*** A delicate fibril found in the cell body and processes of a neuron. SYN: *neurofibril.*

**fibrilla** (fī-brĭl′ă) *pl.* **fibrillae** [L.] A fibril or small fiber.

**fibrillar, fibrillary** Pert. to or consisting of fibrils.

**fibrillated** (fī′brĭ-lāt′d) [L. *fibrilla,* little fiber] Composed of minute fibers. SYN: *fibrillar.*

**fibrillation** (fī″brĭl-ā′shŭn) **1.** Formation of fibrils. **2.** Quivering or spontaneous contraction of individual muscle fibers. **3.** An abnormal bioelectric potential occurring in neuropathies and myopathies.

***atrial f.*** Extremely rapid, incomplete contractions of the atria resulting in fine, rapid, irregular, and uncoordinated movements.

***ventricular f.*** The primary mechanism and arrhythmia seen in sudden cardiac arrest. Organized electrical activity and synchronized mechanical pumping activity are absent. The electrocardiogram shows a chaotic, wavy baseline. If ventricular fibrillation is not terminated rapidly with defibrillation, blood flow to the brain is cut off, causing brain damage. Untreated ventricular fibrillation leads to death. SEE: *defibrillation; pacemaker, artificial cardiac.*

**fibrillin** A protein constituent of connective tissue. It is present in skin, ligaments, tendons, and in the aorta. In Marfan's syndrome, there is reduced content of microfibrils that contain fibrillin. SEE: *elastin.*

**fibrillogenesis** (fī-brĭl″ō-jĕn′ĕ-sĭs) Formation of fibrils.

**fibrin** (fī′brĭn) [L. *fibra,* fiber] A whitish, filamentous protein formed by the action of thrombin on fibrinogen. The conversion of fibrinogen, a hydrosol, into fibrin, a hydrogel, is the basis for blood clotting. The fibrin is deposited as fine interlacing filaments containing entangled red and white blood cells and platelets, the whole forming a coagulum, or clot. SEE: *coagulation, blood.* **fibrinous,** *adj.*

**fibrin-fibrinogen degradation products** A group of soluble protein fragments produced by the proteolytic action of plasmin on fibrin or fibrinogen. These products impair the hemostatic process and are a major cause of hemorrhage in intravascular coagulation and fibrinogenolysis.

**fibrin glue** Fibrinogen concentrate combined with bovine fibrin. It may be applied topically where it acts as a hemostatic "glue." Commercial fibrin glue prepared from pooled human fibrinogen is unavailable in the U.S.

**fibrinocellular** (fī″brĭ-nō-sĕl′ū-lăr) Composed of fibrin and cells, as in certain exudates.

**fibrinogen** (fī-brĭn′ō-jĕn) [″ + Gr. *gennan,* to produce] A protein synthesized by the liver and present in blood plasma that is converted into fibrin through the action of thrombin and in the presence of calcium ions. This process is essential to blood clotting. Fibrinogen is also called factor I. SEE: *coagulation, blood; coagulation factor.*

**fibrinogenic, fibrinogenous** Producing fibrin.

**fibrinogenolysis** (fī″brĭ-nō-jĕ-nŏl′ĭ-sĭs) [″ + ″ + *lysis,* dissolution] Decomposition or dissolution of fibrin.

**fibrinogenopenia** (fī-brĭn″ō-jĕn″ō-pē′nē-ă) [″ + Gr. *gennan,* to produce, + *penia,* poverty] Reduction in the amount of fibrinogen in the blood, usually the result of a liver disorder.

**fibrinoid** (fī′brĭ-noyd) [″ + Gr. *eidos,* form, shape] Resembling fibrin.

**fibrinoid change** Alteration in connective tissues in response to immune reactions. The tissue becomes swollen, homogenous, and bandlike.

**fibrinoid material** A fibrinous substance that develops in the placenta, increasing in quantity as the placenta develops. Its origin is attributed to the degenerating decidua and trophoblast. It forms an incomplete layer in the chorion and decidua basalis and also occurs as small irregular patches on the surface of the chorionic villi. In late pregnancy it may have a striated, or canalized, appearance and is then termed *canalized fibrinoid*.

**fibrinolysis** (fī″brĭn-ŏl′ĭ-sĭs) A complicated system of biochemical reactions for lysis of clots in the vascular system. The principal physiological activator of the fibrinolytic system is tissue plasminogen activator. It converts plasminogen in a fibrin-containing clot to plasmin. The fibrin polymer is degraded by plasmin into fragments that are then scavenged by monocytes and macrophages. This process begins immediately after a clot forms. **fibrinolytic** (-ō-lĭt′ĭk), *adj.*

**fibrinopenia** (fī″brĭn-ō-pē′nē-ă) [″ + Gr. *penia,* poverty] Fibrin and fibrinogen deficiency in the blood.

**fibrinopeptide** (fī″brĭ-nō-pĕp′tīd) The substance removed by thrombin from fibrinogen during blood coagulation.

**fibrinosis** (fī-brĭ-nō′sĭs) [″ + Gr. *osis,* condition] Excess of fibrin in the blood.

**fibrin split products** The materials produced when the crosslinked fibrin in a blood clot is digested by plasmin.

**fibrinuria** (fī-brĭn-ū′rē-ă) [″ + Gr. *ouron,* urine] Passage of fibrin in the urine.

**fibro-** [L. *fibra*] Combining form meaning *fiber; fibrous tissues*.

**fibroadenia** (fī″brō-ă-dē′nē-ă) [L. *fibra,* fiber, + Gr. *aden,* gland] Fibrous degeneration of glandular tissue.

**fibroadenoma** (fī″brō-ăd″ĕ-nō′mă) [″ + ″ + *oma,* tumor] An adenoma with fibrous tissue forming a dense stroma.

**fibroadipose** [″ + *adeps,* fat] Containing fibrous and fatty tissue.

**fibroangioma** [″ + Gr. *angeion,* vessel, + *oma,* tumor] A fibrous tissue angioma.

**fibroareolar** Fibrocellular.

**fibroblast** (fī′brō-blăst) [″ + Gr. *blastos,* germ] Any cell or corpuscle from which connective tissue is developed; it produces collagen, elastin, and reticular protein fibers. SYN: *desmocyte; fibrocyte.*

**fibroblast growth factor** Any one of a group of proteins, usually intracellular, that have important angiogenic function and enhance wound healing and tissue repair. Overactivity of these factors has been associated with neoplasia.

**fibroblastoma** (fī″brō-blăs-tō′mă) [″ + ″ + *oma,* tumor] A tumor of connective tissue, or fibroblastic, cells.

**fibrocalcific** (fī″brō-kăl-sĭf′ĭk) Fibrous and partially calcified.

**fibrocarcinoma** (fī″brō-kăr″sĭ-nō′mă) [″ + Gr. *karkinos,* cancer, + *oma,* tumor] A carcinoma in which the trabeculae are resistant and thickened with granular degeneration of the cells.

**fibrocartilage** (fī″brō-kăr′tĭ-lĭj) [″ + *cartilago,* gristle] A type of cartilage in which the matrix contains thick bundles of white or collagenous fibers. It is found in the intervertebral disks.

**fibrocellular** (fī″brō-sĕl′ū-lăr) [″ + *cellula,* little cell] Containing fibrous and cellular tissue. SYN: *fibroareolar.*

**fibrochondritis** (fī″brō-kŏn-drī′tĭs) [″ + Gr. *chondros,* cartilage, + *itis,* inflammation] Inflammation of fibrocartilage.

**fibrochondroma** (fī″brō-kŏn-drō′mă) [″ + ″ + *oma,* tumor] A tumor of fibrous tissue and cartilage.

**fibrocyst** (fī′brō-sĭst) [″ + Gr. *kystis,* cyst] A fibrous tumor that has undergone cystic degeneration or has accumulated fluid in the interspaces.

**fibrocystic** (fī″brō-sĭs′tĭk) **1.** Consisting of fibrocysts. **2.** Fibrous with cystic degeneration.

**fibrocystoma** (fī″brō-sĭs-tō′mă) [″ + Gr. *kystis,* cyst, + *oma,* tumor] A fibroma combined with a cystoma.

**fibrocyte** (fī′brō-sīt) [″ + Gr. *kytos,* cell] A mature, older fiber-forming cell or fibroblast.

**fibrodysplasia** (fī″brō-dĭs-plā′sē-ă) [″ + Gr. *dys,* bad, + *plassein,* to form] Abnormal development of fibrous tissue.

**fibroelastic** (fī″brō-ē-lăs′tĭk) [″ + Gr. *elastikos,* elastic] Pert. to connective tissue containing both white nonelastic collagenous fibers and yellow elastic fibers.

**fibroelastosis** (fī″brō-ē″lăs-tō′sĭs) Overgrowth of fibroelastic tissue.

***endocardial f.*** Fibroelastosis of the endocardium, leading to cardiac failure.

**fibroenchondroma** (fī″brō-ĕn″kŏn-drō′mă) [″ + Gr. *en,* in, + *chondros,* cartilage, + *oma,* tumor] A benign cartilaginous tumor containing fibrous elements.

**fibroepithelioma** (fī″brō-ĕp″ĭ-thē″lē-ō′mă) [″ + Gr. *epi,* upon, + *thele,* nipple, + *oma,* tumor] A new growth containing fibrous and epithelial elements.

**fibroid** (fī′broyd) [″ + Gr. *eidos,* form, shape] **1.** Containing or resembling fibers. SEE: *degeneration.* **2.** A colloquial term for a fibroma, esp. of the uterus.

**fibroidectomy** (fī-broyd-ĕk′tō-mē) [″ + ″ + *ektome,* excision] Surgical removal of a fibroid tumor.

**fibrolipoma** (fī″brō-lĭ-pō′mă) [″ + Gr. *lipos,* fat, + *oma,* tumor] Lipofibroma.

**fibroma** (fī-brō′mă) *pl.* **fibromata** [″ + Gr. *oma,* tumor] A fibrous, encapsulated connective tissue tumor. It is irregular in shape, slow in growth, and has a firm consistency. Pressure or cystic degeneration may cause pain. Sometimes it occurs in the periosteum. It may affect the jaws, occiput, pelvis, vertebrae, ribs, long bones, or sternum. SYN: *fibroid.* **fibromatous** (-mă-tŭs), *adj.*

***f. of breast*** A benign, nonulcerative, painless breast tumor.

***interstitial f.*** A tumor in the muscular wall of the uterus that may grow inward and form a polypoid fibroid, or outward and become a subperitoneal fibroid. SEE: *uterine f.*

***intramural f.*** A tumor located in muscle tissue of the uterus between the peritoneal coat and endometrium.

***submucous f.*** A fibroma encroaching on

the endometrial cavity. It may be either sessile or pedunculated.

***subserous f.*** A fibroma, often pedunculated, lying beneath the peritoneal coat of the uterus.

***uterine f.*** A fibroid tumor of the uterus. It is the most common tumor found in women.

SYMPTOMS: Fibromata rarely cause symptoms before the age of 30. Although their cardinal symptoms are supposed to be dysmenorrhea, menorrhagia, and leukorrhea, these are found infrequently, and the symptomatology is directly related to the location of the tumor in the uterus. Thus, tumors that encroach on the bladder region cause frequency and dysuria, those pressing on the rectum cause rectal tenesmus, those that encroach on the endometrium may cause menorrhagia and dysmenorrhea, and very large subserous growths may be symptomless.

Use of oral contraceptives reduces the risk for uterine fibroma, as does cigarette smoking; obesity increases the risk. Fibromata may cause infertility because of their size or location. Whether or not fibromata enlarge during pregnancy is unclear. SEE: *dysmenorrhea; dysuria; menorrhagia; tenesmus.*

PATHOLOGY: The tumor may vary in diameter from a few millimeters to a size large enough to fill the entire abdominal cavity. Fibromata may be single or multiple. They usually increase in size during the reproductive years and may regress after menopause. They are completely enclosed by a fibrous connective tissue capsule containing the blood vessels that supply the tumor. They are subjected to numerous benign degenerations such as necrobiotic changes (red and gray degeneration), hyaline changes, telangiectatic and lymphangiectatic changes, calcareous degeneration, fatty degeneration, and infection. Occasionally a fibroma shows sarcomatous degeneration.

TREATMENT: Fibromata producing no symptoms should be left in place and the patient kept under observation. Medical treatment using luteinizing hormone–releasing hormone (LHRH) analogues will cause fibromata to shrink, but the growth returns when LHRH is discontinued. If there is evidence of unusually rapid growth, they should be removed. Small submucous tumors may be removed by electrocautery during hysteroscopy. Laser technique has been used to remove these tumors. If pregnancy is a possibility, tumors large enough to interfere with childbearing should be removed.

**fibromatosis** ( fī″brō-mă-tō′sĭs) [L. *fibra,* fiber, + Gr. *oma,* tumor, + *osis,* condition] The simultaneous development of many fibromata.

***f. gingivae*** An inherited condition marked by hypertrophy of the gums before the eruption of the teeth. Hypertrichosis is usually present.

***palmar f.*** Dupuytren's contracture.

**fibromectomy** (fī″brō-mĕk′tō-mē) [″ + Gr. *oma,* tumor, + *ektome,* excision] Removal of a fibroma.

**fibromembranous** (fī″brō-mĕm′bră-nŭs) [″ + *membrana,* web] Having both fibrous and membranous tissue.

**fibromuscular** (fī″brō-mŭs′kū-lăr) [″ + *musculus,* muscle] Consisting of muscle and connective tissue.

**fibromyalgia** [″ + Gr. *mys,* muscle, + *algos,* pain] Chronic pain in muscles and soft tissues surrounding joints. Efforts to classify this condition have resulted in the American College of Rheumatology criteria for classification of fibromyalgia, published in 1990. SYN: *fibromyitis; fibromyositis; fibrositis; tension myalgia.* SEE: table.

TREATMENT: Various approaches have been tried. Essential to the management of this condition are reassurance, elimination of contributing factors, physical therapy with the objective of restoring normal neuromuscular function, institution of a cardiovascular fitness program, and appropriate medications for sleep disturbances. Anti-inflammatory agents, including corticosteroids, have not been useful in the experience of some investigators. SEE: *trigger point; trigger zone.*

**fibromyitis** Fibromyalgia.

**fibromyoma** (fī″brō-mī-ō′mă) [″ + ″ + *oma,* tumor] **1.** A fibrous tissue myoma. **2.** A fibroid tumor of the uterus that contains more fibrous than muscle tissue.

**fibromyomectomy** (fī″brō-mī″ō-mĕk′tō-mē) [″ + ″ + *ektome,* excision] Removal of a fibromyoma from the uterus, leaving that organ in place.

**fibromyositis** Fibromyalgia.

**fibromyotomy** (fī″brō-mī-ŏt′ō-mē) [″ + ″ + *tome,* incision] Surgical incision of a fibroid tumor.

**fibromyxoma** (fī″brō-mĭk-sō′mă) [″ + Gr. *myxa,* mucus, + *oma,* tumor] A fibroma that has undergone partial myxomatous degeneration.

**fibromyxosarcoma** (fī″brō-mĭk″sō-săr-kō′mă) [″ + ″ + *sarkos,* flesh, + *oma,* tumor] **1.** A sarcoma containing fibrous and myxoid tissue. **2.** A sarcoma that has undergone mucoid degeneration.

**fibronectin** Any of a group of proteins present in blood plasma and extracellular matrix. The presence of fetal fibronectin in the cervical and vaginal secretions may be a marker for subsequent development of preterm labor.

**fibroneuroma** (fī″brō-nū-rō′mă) [″ + Gr. *neuron,* nerve, + *oma,* tumor] Neurofibroma.

**fibro-osteoma** (fī″brō-ŏs-tē-ō′mă) [″ + Gr. *osteon,* bone, + *oma,* tumor] A tumor containing bony and fibrous elements. SYN: *osteofibroma.*

**fibropapilloma** (fī″brō-păp-ĭ-lō′mă) [″ + *papilla,* nipple, + Gr. *oma,* tumor] A mixed fibroma and papilloma sometimes occur-

**The American College of Rheumatology 1990 Criteria for Classification of Fibromyalgia***

1. History of widespread pain

   *Definition:* Pain is considered widespread when all the following are present: pain in the left side of the body, pain in the right side of the body, pain above the waist, and pain below the waist. In addition, axial skeletal pain (cervical spine, anterior chest, thoracic spine, or low back) must be present. In this definition, shoulder and buttock pain is considered as pain for each involved side. "Low back" pain is considered lower segment pain.

2. Pain is 11 of 18 tender point sites on digital palpation

   *Definition:* On digital palpation, pain must be present in at least 11 of the following 18 tender point sites:

   *Occiput*—bilateral, at the suboccipital muscle insertions
   *Low cervical*—bilateral, at the anterior aspects of the intertransverse spaces at C5–7
   *Trapezius*—bilateral, at the midpoint of the upper border
   *Supraspinatus*—bilateral, at origins, above the scapular spine near the medial border
   *Second rib*—bilateral, at the second costochondral junctions, just lateral to the junctions on upper surfaces
   *Lateral epicondyle*—bilateral, 2 cm distal to the epicondyles
   *Gluteal*—bilateral, in upper outer quandrants of buttocks in anterior fold of muscle
   *Greater trochanter*—bilateral, posterior to the trochanteric prominence
   *Knee*—bilateral, at the medial fat pad proximal to the joint line

   Digital palpation should be performed with an approximate force of 4 kg.
   For a tender point to be considered "positive," the subject must state that the palpation was painful. "Tender" is not to be considered "painful."

SOURCE: American College of Rheumatology, Multicenter Criteria Committee, with permission.
* For classification purposes, patients will be said to have fibromyalgia if both criteria are satisfied. Widespread pain must have been present for at least 3 months. The presence of a second clinical disorder does not exclude the diagnosis of fibromyalgia.

ring in the bladder.

**fibroplasia** (fī″brō-plā′sē-ă) [″ + Gr. *plasis,* a molding] The development of fibrous tissue, as in wound healing.

***retrolental f.*** ABBR: RLF. Retinopathy of prematurity.

**fibroplastic** (fī″brō-plăs′tĭk) [″ + Gr. *plassein,* to form] Giving formation to fibrous tissue.

**fibropurulent** (fī″brō-pūr′ū-lĕnt) [″ + *purulentus,* festering] Pert. to pus that contains flakes of fibrous tissue.

**fibrosarcoma** (fī″brō-săr-kō′mă) [L. *fibra,* fiber, + Gr. *sarkos,* flesh, + *oma,* tumor] A spindle-celled sarcoma containing a large amount of connective tissue.

**fibrose** (fī′brōs) To form or produce fibrous tissue (e.g., a scar).

**fibroserous** (fī″brō-sē′rŭs) [″ + *serosus,* serous] Containing fibrous and serosal elements. The pericardium is such a tissue.

**fibrosis** (fī-brō′sĭs) [″ + Gr. *osis,* condition] Abnormal formation of fibrous tissue.

***arteriocapillary f.*** Arteriolar and capillary fibroid degeneration.

***diffuse interstitial pulmonary f.*** Idiopathic pulmonary f.

***idiopathic pulmonary f.*** A form of interstitial lung disease with a rapid deterioration in clinical course owing to diffuse interstitial pneumonitis or fibrosis. The etiology is unknown. Symptoms vary with the degree of the disease but include dyspnea, rapid respirations, anoxia, and weight loss with subsequent weakness and fatigue. At first pulmonary symptoms are not prominent unless there is bronchial involvement with exudate. As the disease progresses, finger clubbing, cyanosis, and heart failure develop. The disease is usually fatal 4 or 5 years after onset. SYN: *Hamman-Rich syndrome.*

DIAGNOSIS: The diagnosis is based on the characteristic clinical signs and symptoms. Definitive diagnosis, however, can be established only by open lung biopsy.

TREATMENT: Corticosteroids are usually beneficial but not curative. Supportive therapy consists of supplementary oxygen, antibiotics, and treatment for heart failure. Cyclophosphamide is also used to suppress the neutrophil component of inflammation.

***postfibrinosis f.*** Development of fibrosis in a tissue in which fibrin has been deposited.

***proliferative f.*** Formation of new fibrous tissue from connective tissue cells.

***pulmonary f.*** Formation of scar tissue in the connective tissue framework of the lungs following inflammation or pulmonary disease.

*f. uteri* Diffuse growth of fibrous tissue throughout the uterus.

**fibrositis** (fī-brō-sī′tĭs) [″ + Gr. *itis,* inflammation] Fibromyalgia.

**fibrotic** (fī-brŏt′ĭk) Marked by or pert. to fibrosis.

**fibrous plaques** SEE: *arteriosclerosis.*

**fibula** (fĭb′ū-lă) [L., pin] The outer and smaller bone of the leg from the ankle to the knee, articulating above with the tibia and below with the tibia and talus. It is one of the longest and thinnest bones of the body. **fibular,** *adj.*

**fibulocalcaneal** (fĭb″ū-lō-kăl-kā′nē-ăl) [L. *fibula,* pin, + *calcaneus,* pert. to the heel] Pert. to the fibula and calcaneus.

**ficin** (fī′sĭn) [L. *ficus,* fig] Sap from the fig tree. It contains an enzyme capable of hydrolyzing proteins.

**Fick, Adolf Eugen** German physician, 1829–1901.

*F. equation* F. principle.

*F.'s law* The rule stating that diffusion through a tissue membrane is directly proportional to the cross-sectional area, driving pressure, and gas coefficient and inversely proportional to tissue thickness.

*F. method* A method of determining cardiac output by calculating the difference in oxygen content of mixed venous and arterial blood. This figure is then divided into the total oxygen consumption.

*F. principle* In respiratory physiology, the rule stating that blood flow equals the amount of a substance absorbed in an organ divided by the difference in the amount of the substance entering and leaving the organ. Usually the substance is oxygen or a dye.

**F.I.C.S.** *Fellow of the International College of Surgeons.*

**FID** *flame ionization detector.*

**field** [AS. *feld*] A specific area in relation to an object.

*auditory f.* The space or distance within the limit of hearing.

*high-power f.* The portion of an object seen when the high-magnification lenses of a microscope are used.

*low-power f.* The portion of an object seen when the low-magnification lenses of a microscope are used.

*useful f. of view* ABBR: UFOV. A test of visual attention that measures the space in which an individual can receive information rapidly from two separate sources. It is a strong predictor of accidents in older drivers. This test has shown that training can expand the useful field of view and increase the visual processing speed of an elderly person.

*f. of vision* The portion of space that the fixed eye can see. SEE: *perimetry.*

**fifth cranial nerve** SEE: *trigeminal nerve.*

**fifth ventricle** The space separating the two layers of the septum pellucidum of the brain.

**fight-or-flight reaction of Cannon** [Walter B. Cannon, U.S. physiologist, 1871–1954] The generalized response to an emergency situation. This includes intense stimulation of the sympathetic nervous system and the adrenal gland. The heart and respiratory rates, blood pressure, and blood flow to muscles are increased. This response prepares the body to either flee or fight.

**FIGLU, FIGlu** *formiminoglutamic acid.*

**FIGLU excretion test** The test for folic acid deficiency. When histidine is administered to a patient with folic acid deficiency, formiminoglutamic (FIGLU) acid in the urine increases.

**FIGO staging system** The staging system for cancer of the cervix uteri developed by the International Federation of Gynecology and Obstetrics.

**figurate** (fĭg′ū-rāt) [L. *figuratum,* figured] Having a certain form, such as geographic, annular, or circular. This term applies to skin lesions associated with cutaneous diseases such as tinea or urticaria.

**figure** [L. *figura*] **1.** A body, form, shape, or outline. **2.** A number.

**filaceous** (fĭ-lā′shŭs) Composed of filaments.

**filament** [L. *filamentum*] **1.** A fine thread. **2.** A threadlike coil of tungsten found in the x-ray tube that is the source of electrons.

*axial f.* A fine filament forming the central axis of the tail of a spermatozoon.

**filamentous** Made up of long, interwoven or irregularly placed threadlike structures.

**filar** (fī′lăr) [L. *filum,* thread] Filamentous.

**Filaria** (fĭl-ā′rē-ă) [L. *filum,* thread] Term formerly applied to a genus of nematodes belonging to the superfamily Filarioidea.

*F. bancrofti* *Wuchereria bancrofti.*

*F. loa* *Loa loa.*

*F. medinensis* *Dracunculus medinensis.*

*F. sanguinis hominis* *Wuchereria bancrofti.*

**filaria** (fĭl-ā′rē-ă) *pl.* **filariae** [L. *filum,* thread] A long filiform nematode belonging to the superfamily Filarioidea. The adults live in vertebrates. In humans, they may be found in the lymphatic vessels and lymphatic organs, circulatory system, connective tissues, subcutaneous tissues, and serous cavities. Typically, the female produces larvae called microfilariae, which may be sheathed or sheathless. They reach the peripheral blood or lymphatic vessels, where they may be ingested by a blood-sucking arthropod (a mosquito, gnat, or fly). In the intermediate host, they transform into rhabditoid larvae that metamorphose into infective filariform larvae. These migrate to the proboscis and are deposited in or on the skin of the vertebrate host. SEE: *elephantiasis.* **filarial,** *adj.*

**filariasis** (fĭl-ă-rī′ă-sĭs) [″ + Gr. *-iasis,* condition] A chronic disease due to one of the filaria species. SEE: *elephantiasis*.

**filaricide** (fī-lăr′ĭ-sīd) [″ + *caedere*, to kill] Something that destroys *Filaria*. **filaricidal** (-sīd′ăl), *adj*.

**Filarioidea** (fĭ-lăr″ē-oy′dē-ă) A superfamily of filarial nematodes that parasitize many animal species, including humans. SEE: *filariasis*.

**file** (fīl) **1.** A metal device with a roughened surface. It is used for shaping bones and teeth. **2.** In computing, data stored in a specifically designated area of the computer's memory.

**filial generation** In genetics, the first offspring of a specific mating or crossmating. This is abbreviated $F_1$. Descendants resulting from $F_1$ matings are known as the $F_2$, or second, filial generation.

**filiform** (fĭl′ĭ-form) [″ + *forma*, form] **1.** In biology, pert. to a growth that is uniform along the inoculation line in stab or streak cultures. **2.** Hairlike; filamentous.

**fillet** (fĭl′ĕt) [Fr. *filet*, a band] **1.** A loop of thread, cord, or tape used to provide traction or suspension of tissue during surgery. **2.** Lemniscus.

**filling** (fĭl′ĭng) [AS. *fyllan*, to fill] **1.** The material used for insertion in a prepared tooth cavity, usually amalgam. **2.** The operation of filling tooth cavities.

**film** **1.** A thin skin, membrane, or covering. **2.** A thin sheet of material, usually cellulose and coated with a light-sensitive emulsion, used in taking photographs. **3.** In microscopy, a thin layer of blood or other material spread on a slide or coverslip.

***bite-wing f.*** A radiograph taken with a part of the film holder held between the teeth and the film parallel to the teeth. This technique permits films to be taken of several upper and lower teeth at the same time.

***spot f.*** A radiograph of a small anatomical area.

***x-ray f.*** A special photographic film with a sensitive emulsion layer that blackens in response to the light from intensifying screens. The emulsion has silver halide crystals immersed in gelatin. *Single-emulsion film* has the emulsion on one side of the cellulose base. It is used for digital, mammographic, and extremity imaging, in which high detail is necessary. *Duplitized film* has the emulsion on both sides of the cellulose base. It is used for general-purpose radiological studies.

**film badge** A badge containing film that is sensitive to x-rays. It is used to determine the cumulative exposure to x-rays of persons who work in radiology.

**filovaricosis** (fī″lō-văr-ĭ-kō′sĭs) [″ + *varix*, a dilated vein, + Gr. *osis*, condition] Dilatation or thickening of the axis cylinder of a nerve fiber.

**filter** [L. *filtrare*, to strain through] **1.** To pass a liquid through any porous substance that prevents particles larger than a certain size to pass through. **2.** A device for filtering liquids, light rays, or radiations. SEE: *absorption; osmosis*. **3.** Material, such as aluminum or molybdenum, inserted between the radiation source and the patient to absorb low-level radiation that would increase the dose.

***Berkefeld f.*** A diatomaceous earth filter that removes bacteria from solutions passed through it, but allows virus-sized particles to pass through into the filtrate.

***compensating f.*** In dentistry, a filter that shields less dense areas to produce a more nearly uniform radiographic image.

***high efficiency particulate air f.*** ABBR: HEPA filter. An air filter capable of removing 99.7% of particles greater than 0.3 μm in diameter.

***infrared f.*** A filter that permits passage of only infrared waves of a certain wavelength.

***membrane f.*** A filter made from biologically inert cellulose esters, polyethylene, or other porous materials.

***Millipore f.*** Trademark name of a filter with controlled pore size that separates particles above specific sizes from the solutions that flow through.

***optical f.*** A device that passes only a portion of the visible light spectrum. Absorption filters absorb the unwanted wavelengths. Interference filters employ the wave effects of constructive and destructive superposition to pass or inhibit appropriate wavelengths.

***Pasteur-Chamberland f.*** An unglazed porcelain filter capable of retaining bacteria and some viruses. Either pressure or suction is required to force or draw the liquid through the filter.

***umbrella f.*** A filter placed in a blood vessel to prevent emboli from passing that point. Once inserted, the device opens up like an umbrella. This technique has been used in the vena cava to prevent emboli in the veins from reaching the lungs.

***vena cava f.*** A wire apparatus inserted through a catheter into the inferior vena cava to prevent pulmonary emboli.

***wedge f.*** A filter used in radiography and radiation therapy to vary the intensity of the x-ray beam. This compensates for differences in the thicknesses of the parts being exposed to radiation.

***Wood's f.*** A glass screen allowing the passage of ultraviolet radiation and absorbing rays of visual light. It is used to diagnose certain dermatological conditions, esp. tinea capitis.

**filterable** [L. *filtrare*, to strain through] Capable of passing through the pores of a porcelain filter, through which bacteria cannot pass.

**filtrate** (fĭl′trāt) The fluid that has been passed through a filter. The residue is the precipitate.

***glomerular f.*** The fluid that passes from the blood through the capillary walls of the glomeruli of the kidney. It is a protein-free plasma from which urine is formed.

**filtration** (fĭl-trā′shŭn) The process of removing particles from a solution by allowing the liquid portion to pass through a membrane or other partial barrier. This contains holes or spaces that allow the liquid to pass but are too small to permit passage of the solid particles. SEE: *filter*.

***f. of x-ray photons*** The absorption of some longer-wavelength, low-energy x-ray photons by an absorbing medium placed in the path of the beam. Materials include aluminum, copper, molybdenum, and zinc.

**filum** (fī′lŭm) *pl.* **fila** [L.] A threadlike structure.

***f. coronaria*** A fibrous band extending from the base of the medial cusp of the tricuspid valve to the aortic annulus.

***f. terminale*** A long, slender filament at the end of the spinal cord.

**fimbria** (fĭm′brē-ă) *pl.* **fimbriae** [L., fringe] Any structure resembling a fringe or border.

***f. ovarica*** The longest fringelike extremity of a fallopian tube, extending from the infundibulum close to the ovary.

***f. tubae*** The fringelike portion at the abdominal end of a fallopian tube.

**fimbriate, fimbriated** (fĭm′brē-āt″, fĭm′brē-āt″ĕd) **1.** Having finger-like projections. **2.** Fringed.

**fimbriocele** (fĭm′brē-ō-sēl″) [″ + Gr. *kele*, tumor, swelling] A hernia including the fimbriated portion of the oviduct.

**fine motor skill** Any of the skills pert. to the synergy of small muscles, primarily in the hand, and related to manual dexterity and coordination.

**fineness** The proportion of pure gold in a gold alloy.

**finger** [AS.] One of the five digits of the hand.

***baseball f.*** Permanent flexion resulting from violent backward dislocation of the terminal phalanx onto the dorsum of the middle phalanx, as when an extended finger is struck on its tip. It is due to damage of the extensor tendon. SYN: *hammer f; mallet f.*

***clubbed f.*** An enlarged terminal phalanx of the finger. This may be present in chronic obstructive pulmonary disease, cyanotic congenital heart disease, carcinoma of the lung, bacterial endocarditis, and carcinoma of the thyroid. SYN: *hippocratic f.*

***dislocation of f.*** Displacement of a finger bone. This occurs only at a joint. If there has been a crushing injury, it should be treated as a fracture until radiography has been performed. Dislocations of a finger usually are easily diagnosed and quite easily reduced. They may be caused by blows, falls, and similar accidents.

First, it is important to ascertain that there is no fracture. Then the patient should be asked to steady and support the wrist (or have somebody else do so) for countertraction. The finger is grasped beyond the dislocated muscles and tendons and, with the free hand, the dislocated bone is slipped into place. A splint is applied from the tip of the finger well into the palm of the hand. The splint may be made of plastic, of tongue depressors, or temporarily of heavy cardboard.

---

Caution: No attempt should be made to reduce a dislocation of the thumb joint nearest the palm of the hand until radiography has ruled out the possibility of fracture.

---

***hammer f.*** Baseball f.

***hippocratic f.*** Clubbed f.

***jersey f.*** A traumatic avulsion of the insertion of the flexor digitorum profundus, caused by a forceful extension motion during an active muscular contraction. It is commonly seen in football players. As a tackler grabs a defender's jersey, the defender pulls the jersey out of the tackler's hand.

***mallet f.*** Baseball f.

***seal f.*** An infection of the finger caused by the bite of a seal. The infectious agent, which has not been identified, is carried in the blood of the seal. It is sensitive to tetracycline.

***webbed f.*** A congenital condition in which some or all of the fingers are fused; syndactylism.

**finger cot** A protective covering for a finger. It is usually made of plastic, rubber, metal, or leather. The injured finger is protected from trauma during the healing process. SYN: *finger-stall.*

**finger ladder** A device attached to a wall and in which notches are cut along an inclined line. The patient "walks" up this notched ladder by placing the fingertips in the notches. This self-stretching technique assists with shoulder flexion or abduction to maintain range of motion, and may be used to increase shoulder flexibility by stretching the extensors or adductors of the shoulder.

**fingernail** SEE: *nail.*

**fingerprint** An imprint made by the cutaneous ridges of the fleshy portion of the distal end of a finger. Fingerprints are used for identification because they are individually unique. SEE: illus.

**finger separator** Finger spreader.

**finger spelling** A method of communication used by persons with hearing or visual impairment in which words are spelled out letter by letter rather than depicted with single signs as in American Sign Language. Finger spelling can be done visually as well as tactually.

**finger splint** A padded strip of malleable metal used to immobilize a fractured finger. As an alternative, the injured finger is often "buddy taped" to an adjoining finger for support.

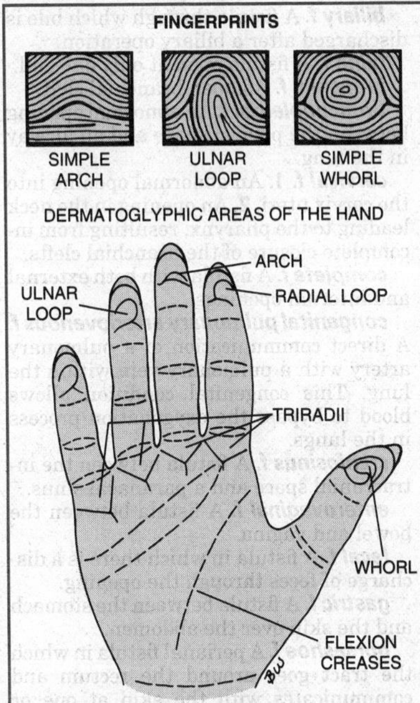


**finger spreader** An orthotic device, usually made of foam rubber, used to hold the thumb and fingers in extension while maintaining the normal arches of the hand. SYN: *finger separator.*

**finger spring** A device for assisting extension or flexion of finger joints.

**finger-stall** Finger cot.

**finger-to-nose test** A clinical test of cerebellar function. The patient stands with eyes closed and arms at the side and is asked to touch the nose with the tip of the finger.

**finite** Having limits or boundaries.

**Finklestein's test** A test involving lateral wrist flexion of the clenched fist, used to assist in the diagnosis of de Quervain's disease. The patient tucks the thumb in a closed fist, and the examiner deviates the fist ulnarly. Pain determines a positive result.

**$FIO_2$** *fractional concentration of oxygen.*

**fire** [AS. *fyr*] **1.** Flame that produces heat. **2.** Fever.

***St. Anthony's f.*** Former term for erysipelas.

**fire ant bite** SEE: under *bite.*

**fire-damp** Methane, $CH_4$, found in coal mines.

**first aid** The administration of emergency assistance to individuals who have been injured or otherwise disabled, prior to the arrival of a physician or transportation to a hospital or physician's office. First aid should never be a substitute for definitive medical care. SEE: *basic life support; burn; cardiopulmonary resuscitation; Universal Precautions Appendix.*

**first cranial nerves** The nerves supplying the nasal olfactory mucosa. They consist of delicate bundles of unmyelinated fibers, the fila olfactoria, which pass through the cribriform plate and terminate in the olfactory glomeruli of the olfactory bulb. The fila are the central processes of bipolar receptor neurons of olfactory mucous membrane. SYN: *olfactory nerves.*

**first-degree atrioventricular block** Cardiac dysrhythmia caused by delayed conduction through or from the atrioventricular node and marked by a prolonged PR interval. Usually no treatment is necessary.

**first intention healing** Healing that takes place when wound edges are held or sutured together without the formation of granulation tissue. SEE: *healing.*

**first responder** The first individual to arrive at the scene of an emergency.

**Fishberg concentration test** (fĭsh′bĕrg) [A. M. Fishberg, U.S. physician, b. 1898] A test of the ability of the kidneys to produce urine of high specific gravity.

**fishskin disease** A skin disease characterized by increase of the horny layer and deficient secretions. SYN: *ichthyosis.*

**fission** (fĭsh′ŭn) [L. *fissio*] **1.** Splitting into two or more parts. **2.** A method of asexual reproduction in bacteria, protozoa, and other lower forms of life. The cell or the body divides into two or more parts, each of which develops into a complete individual. **3.** Bombardment or splitting of the nucleus of a heavy atom to release energy and neutrons.

**fissiparous** (fĭ-sĭp′ă-rŭs) [L. *fissus,* cleft, + *parere,* to bring forth] Reproducing by fission.

**fissura** (fĭs-ū′ră) *pl.* **fissurae** [L.] A fissure.

**fissure** (fĭsh′ūr) [L. *fissura*] **1.** A groove, natural division, cleft, slit, or deep furrow in the brain, liver, spinal cord, and other organs. SYN: *fissura; sulcus.* **2.** An ulcer or cracklike sore. **3.** A break in the enamel of a tooth. **fissural,** *adj.*

***anal f.*** A linear ulcer on the margin of the anus.

***auricular f.*** A fissure of the petrous portion of the temporal bone.

***f. of Bichat*** The fissure below the corpus callosum in the cerebellum of the brain.

***branchial f.*** SEE: *cleft, branchial.*

***Broca's f.*** The fissure encircling the third left frontal convolution of the brain.

***Burdach's f.*** The fissure connecting the lateral surface of the insula and the inner surface of the operculum of the brain.

***calcarine f.*** The fissure extending from the occipital end of the cerebrum to the occipital fissure of the brain.

***callosomarginal f.*** A conspicuous fissure in the mesial surface of the cerebral hemisphere running above and concentric with the curved upper surface of the corpus callosum.

***central f.*** Rolando's f.

***Clevenger's f.*** The inferior temporal fissure of the brain.

***collateral f.*** The fissure on the inferior surface of the cerebral hemisphere separating the subcalcarine and subcollateral gyri.

***Henle's f.*** Any of the connective tissue areas between the muscular fibers of the heart.

***hippocampal f.*** The fissure extending from the posterior part of the corpus callosum to the tip of the temporal lobe of the brain.

***horizontal f.*** Transverse f. (3).

***inferior orbital f.*** The fissure at the apex of the orbit through which the infraorbital blood vessels and maxillary branch of the trigeminal nerve pass.

***interparietal f.*** The intraparietal sulcus.

***longitudinal f.*** **1.** The fissure on the lower surface of the liver. **2.** A fissure that separates the cerebral hemispheres; at its base is the corpus callosum, which connects the hemispheres.

***occipitoparietal f.*** The fissure between the occipital and parietal lobes of the brain.

***palpebral f.*** The opening separating the upper and lower eyelids.

***portal f.*** The opening into the undersurface of the liver. It continues into the liver as the portal canal.

***Rolando's f.*** The fissure separating the frontal and parietal lobes of the brain.

***sphenoidal f.*** The fissure separating the wings and body of the sphenoid bone.

***f. of Sylvius*** The fissure separating the frontal and parietal lobes from the temporal lobe of the brain.

***transverse f.*** **1.** The fissure between the cerebellum and cerebrum. **2.** The fissure on the lower surface of the liver that serves as the hilum transmitting vessels and ducts to the liver. **3.** The fissure that divides the upper right lobe of the lung from the middle right lobe. SYN: *transverse f.*

***umbilical f.*** The anterior portion of the longitudinal fissure of the liver. It contains the round ligament, the obliterated umbilical vein.

***Wernicke's f.*** The fissure dividing the temporal and parietal lobes from the occipital lobe of the brain.

***zygal f.*** A transverse cerebral sulcus that connects two parallel sulci. The three sulci are in the form of an H.

**fistula** (fĭs'tū-lă) [L., *fistula*, pipe] An abnormal tubelike passage from a normal cavity or tube to a free surface or to another cavity. It may result from congenital incomplete closure of parts or from abscesses, injuries, or inflammatory processes. **fistulous** (-lŭs), *adj.*

***anal f.*** A fistula near the anus.

***arteriovenous f.*** A fistula between an artery and a vein.

***biliary f.*** A fistula through which bile is discharged after a biliary operation.

***blind f.*** A fistula open at only one end.

***branchial f.*** An open branchial cleft.

***bronchopleural f.*** An abnormal opening between the pleural space and an airway in the lung.

***cervical f.*** **1.** An abnormal opening into the cervix uteri. **2.** An opening in the neck leading to the pharynx, resulting from incomplete closure of the branchial clefts.

***complete f.*** A fistula with both external and internal openings.

***congenital pulmonary arteriovenous f.*** A direct communication of a pulmonary artery with a pulmonary vein within the lung. This congenital condition allows blood to bypass the oxygenation process in the lungs.

***craniosinus f.*** A fistula between the intracranial space and a paranasal sinus.

***enterovaginal f.*** A fistula between the bowel and vagina.

***fecal f.*** A fistula in which there is a discharge of feces through the opening.

***gastric f.*** A fistula between the stomach and the skin over the abdomen.

***horseshoe f.*** A perianal fistula in which the tract goes around the rectum and communicates with the skin at one or more points.

***incomplete f.*** A fistula with only one opening, which leads to the skin (i.e., it does not communicate with an internal cavity or organ).

***metroperitoneal f.*** A fistula between the uterine and peritoneal cavities.

***parotid f.*** A fistula from the parotid gland to the skin surface.

***perineovaginal f.*** An opening from the vagina through the perineum.

***pilonidal f.*** A fistula beneath the skin at the lower end of the spinal column resulting from a pilonidal cyst.

***rectovaginal f.*** An opening between the rectum and the vagina.

***thyroglossal f.*** A midline fistula just above the thyroid that connects the openings in the skin to a persistent embryonic thyroglossal duct.

***umbilical f.*** A fistula between the umbilicus and the gut. It is usually due to nonclosure of the urachal duct.

***ureterovaginal f.*** A fistula between the ureter and the vagina.

***vesicouterine f.*** A fistula between the uterus and the bladder.

***vesicovaginal f.*** A fistula between the bladder and the vagina.

**fistulatome** (fĭs'tū-lă-tōm") [" + Gr. *tome*, incision] An instrument for incising a fistula.

**fistulectomy** (fĭs"tū-lĕk'tō-mē) [" + Gr. *ektome*, excision] Excision of a fistula.

**fistulization** (fĭs"tŭ-lī-zā'shŭn) [L. *fistula*, pipe] The process of becoming fistulous.

**fistuloenterostomy** (fĭs"tū-lō-ĕn-tĕr-ŏs'tō-mē) [" + Gr. *enteron*, intestine, + *stoma*, mouth] Surgical closure of a biliary fistula and formation of a new biliary passage into the intestine.

**fit** (fĭt) [AS. *fitt*] **1.** A sudden attack, convulsion, or paroxysm. SEE: *convulsion.* **2.** Modification of one structure to that of another, as in dental restoration.

**fitness, biological** The ability of an individual with a disease to produce or father children who survive to adult life and are themselves able to reproduce.

**fitness, physical** SEE: *physical fitness.*

**fix 1.** To treat tissues chemically so that the components and products of the cells are preserved for staining and microscopic examination. **2.** Slang for a dose of a drug of abuse. **3.** In film processing, the step that stops the development action, removes the undeveloped silver halide crystals, and makes the image permanent.

**fixation** [L. *fixatio*] **1.** The act of holding or fastening in a rigid position. The act of immobilizing or making rigid. **2.** Rigidity or immobility. **3.** A phase of Freudian psychosexual development in which the libido is arrested at an early or presexual level. **4.** Staining of microscopic specimens for examination. **5.** The process of making a film-recorded image permanent.

***binocular f.*** Focusing of both eyes on an object.

***complement f.*** The action of complement (a series of plasma proteins) on an antigen-antibody complex. In the body, it brings about lysis of cellular foreign antigens. Complement is the basis for complement fixation tests, which determine the presence of particular antibodies (or antigens) in a patient's serum. SEE: *complement.*

***external f.*** The use of external devices, such as pins, in fractured bone segments to keep them in place.

***f. of eyes*** Movement of the eyes so that the visual axes meet and the image of an object falls on corresponding points of each retina. This provides the most acute visualization of the object.

***field of f.*** The widest limits of vision in all directions within which the eyes can fixate.

***internal f.*** The use of internal wires, screws, or pins applied directly to fractured bone segments to keep them in place.

**fixation point** The fovea or point on the retina where the visual axes (lines) meet the point of clearest vision.

**fixative** (fĭk′să-tĭv) [L. *fixus,* fastened] **1.** A substance that firms or makes rigid. **2.** A substance used to preserve normal and pathological specimens for gross examination or for the sectioning and preparation of microscope slides.

**fixed-dose combination** Combining two or more drugs in one capsule or tablet. This is done to attempt to prevent the patient from taking only one of the drugs when two or more are prescribed. SEE: *directly observed therapy.*

**fixing** In histology, rapid killing of tissue elements so that their normal living form is preserved. It permits accurate and undistorted microscopic visualization of the tissues.

**Fl** *fluid.*

**flaccid** (flăk′sĭd) [L. *flaccidus,* flabby] Relaxed; flabby; having defective or absent muscular tone.

**flaccid paralysis** Paralysis marked by loss of muscle tone, loss or reduction of tendon reflexes, atrophy and degeneration of muscles, and reaction of degeneration. It is due to lesions of the lower motor neurons of the spinal cord.

**flagella** (flă-jĕl′ă) [L.] Pl. of flagellum.

**flagellant** (flăj′ĕ-lănt) [L. *flagellum,* whip] **1.** Pert. to a flagellum. **2.** Pert. to stroking in massage. **3.** One who practices flagellation.

**flagellate** (flăj′ĕ-lāt) **1.** Having one or more flagella. **2.** A protozoon with one or more flagella.

**flagellation** (flăj″ĕ-lā′shŭn) **1.** Whipping. **2.** Massage by strokes. **3.** A form of sexual aberration in which the libido is stimulated by whipping oneself, being whipped, or whipping someone else.

**flagelliform** (flă-jĕl′ĭ-form) [″ + *forma,* shape] Shaped like a flagellum.

**flagellum** (flă-jĕl′ŭm) *pl.* **flagella** [L., whip] A threadlike structure that provides motility for certain bacteria and protozoa (one, few, or many per cell) and for spermatozoa (one per cell).

**flag sign** A peculiar change in hair color in which the hair becomes discolored in a band perpendicular to its long axis. This is seen in kwashiorkor and indicates a period of severe malnutrition.

**Flagyl** Trade name for metronidazole.

**flail arm splint** ABBR: FAS. An upper-extremity orthotic device used to provide support and limited function, consisting of a shoulder-operated harness, a volar supporting structure made of low-temperature thermoplastic material, and a terminal device that allows the arm to grasp or stabilize objects.

**flail chest** A condition of the chest wall due to two or more fractures on each affected rib resulting in a segment of rib that is not attached on either end; the flail segment moves paradoxically in with inspiration and out during expiration.

**flail joint** A joint with excessive mobility usually due to paralysis of the muscles that control it.

**flammable** Burning easily.

**flange** (flănj) **1.** A border that projects above the main structure. **2.** In dentistry, the part of an artificial denture that extends from the imbedded teeth to the border of the denture.

**flank** [O. Fr. *flanc*] The part of the body between the ribs and the upper border of the ilium. The term also refers loosely to the outer side of the thigh, hip, and buttock.

SEE: *latus*.

**flannelmouth** A person whose speech is thick.

**flap** [Dutch *flappen,* to strike] **1.** A mass of partially detached tissue used in plastic surgery of an adjacent area or in covering the end of a bone after resection. **2.** An uncontrolled movement seen in some diseases. SEE: *asterixis*.

***amputation f.*** A flap of skin used to cover the end of a part left after an amputation.

***island f.*** A skin flap in which the edges are free but the center is attached and contains the vascular supply.

***jump f.*** A skin flap moved from place to place by successively cutting one end and attaching it to a new site.

***mucoperiosteal f.*** A flap of mucosal tissue, including the underlying periosteum, reflected from the bone during oral surgery.

***pedicle f.*** A flap made by suturing the edges to form a tube. Then one end of the tube is cut and sutured to another site. By use of the jump flap technique, such a flap may be moved a great distance in several stages.

***periodontal f.*** A section of soft tissue surgically separated from underlying bone and removed or repositioned to eliminate periodontal pockets or to correct mucogingival defects.

***skin f.*** A flap containing only skin.

***sliding f.*** Horizontal movement of a flap to cover a nearby raw area.

***tube f.*** A long pedicle flap. SEE: *pedicle f.*

**flare** A flush or spreading area of redness that surrounds a line made by drawing a pointed instrument across the skin. It is the second reaction in the triple response of skin to injury and is due to dilatation of the arterioles. SEE: *triple response.*

**flaring, nasal** Dilation of the nostrils during inspiration; a sign of respiratory distress.

**flash 1.** A hot flash. SEE: *menopause*. **2.** Excess material from a mold.

**flashback** The return of imagery and hallucinations after the immediate effects of hallucinogens have worn off. Hallucinations may occur for an extended period. They may be frightening or threatening or may consist only of perceptual distortion.

**flash method** A means of pasteurizing milk by rapidly raising its temperature to 178°F (80.1°C), maintaining it there for a few minutes, and rapidly chilling it until the temperature is 40°F (4.4°C).

**flash point** The temperature at which a substance bursts into flame spontaneously.

**flask** [LL. *flasco*] A small bottle with a narrow neck.

**flatfoot** Abnormal flatness of the sole and the arch of the foot. This condition may exist without causing symptoms or interfering with normal function of the foot. The inner longitudinal and anterior transverse metatarsal arches may be depressed. This condition may be acute, subacute, or chronic. SYN: *pes planus; splayfoot.*

***spasmodic f.*** Flatfoot in which the foot is held everted by spasmodic contraction of the peroneal muscle.

**flatness** Resonance heard on percussion over solid organs or when there is fluid in the thoracic cavity.

**flatplate** A radiograph requiring a frontal projection of the abdomen or other body part with the patient supine.

**flatulence** (flăt′ū-lĕns) [L. *flatulentus*] Excessive gas in the stomach and intestines. SEE: *distention; gastrointestinal decompression; paralytic ileus; Wangensteen tube.* **flatulent,** *adj.*

NURSING IMPLICATIONS: Bowel sounds are auscultated; abdominal girth is inspected, percussed, and measured for evidence of abdominal distention. The patient is questioned about the presence and location of any pain or cramping and the passage of flatus. Ambulation is encouraged to increase peristalsis. If the patient cannot ambulate or if ambulation is ineffective, the patient is turned from side to side (or as permitted by activity restrictions), and a lubricated tube is inserted 15 cm (6 in.) into the rectum and secured in place for 20 to 30 min. Unless contraindicated, local heat is applied to the lower abdomen. An enema is administered as prescribed to help the patient expel flatus and to relieve gaseous distention. If bowel sounds decrease or abdominal distention increases (as demonstrated by percussion, abdominal girth measurement, and increasing patient discomfort) and flatus is not passed, the physician is notified because the patient may be developing a paralytic ileus.

**flatus** (flā′tŭs) [L., a blowing] **1.** Gas in the digestive tract. **2.** Expelling of gas from a body orifice, esp. the anus. The average person excretes 400 to 1200 cc of gas each day. The gas passages may average a dozen a day in some persons and up to a hundred in others. Flatus from the lower intestinal tract contains hydrogen, methane, skatoles, indoles, carbon dioxide, and small amounts of oxygen and nitrogen. SEE: *borborygmus; eructation.*

Foods known for their ability to cause excess intestinal gas include beans, peas, lentils, cabbage, onions, Brussels sprouts, bananas, apples, raisins, apricots, high-fiber cereals, whole wheat products, milk and milk products, and sorbitol present in some dietetic foods.

TREATMENT: Some persons can control excess intestinal gas by avoiding foods they have found to be flatulogenic. Others in whom there is no distinct relationship to foods should be reassured that flatulence, although sometimes socially awkward or embarrassing, is not detrimental to health.

Administration of the enzyme alpha-D-galactosidase derived from *Aspergillus niger* may be effective in treating intestinal gas or bloating due to eating a variety of grains, cereals, nuts, and seeds of vegetables containing sugars such as raffinose or verbacose. This includes oats, wheat, beans, peas, lentils, foods containing soy, pistachios, broccoli, Brussels sprouts, cabbage, carrots, corn, onions, squash, and cauliflower. The enzyme is available as the tradenamed Beano in either liquid or tablet form.

***vaginal f.*** Expulsion of air from the vagina.

**flatus tube** A rectal tube to facilitate expulsion of flatus. It is used in cases of severe distention and before a saline enema.

NURSING IMPLICATIONS: The lubricated tube is inserted 15 cm (6 in.) into the patient's rectum and secured in place for 20 to 30 min. The patient is positioned on the right side (allowing gas to rise into the left descending colon and rectum) and turned from side to side as permitted. The tube may be reinserted every 2 to 4 hr as necessary until relief is obtained. Heat may also be applied to the lower abdomen (hot water bottle or heating pad) unless contraindicated. The degree of distention and passage of flatus are monitored to evaluate the effectiveness of the treatment.

**flatworm** A worm belonging to the phylum Platyhelminthes.

**flavescent** (flă-vĕs′ĕnt) Yellowish.

**flavin** (flā′vĭn) One of a group of natural water-soluble pigments occurring in milk, yeasts, bacteria, and some plants. All contain the flavin or isoalloxazine nucleus and are yellow. Flavin is present in riboflavin and Warburg's yellow enzyme.

**flavism** (flā′vĭzm) [L. *flavus,* yellow, + Gr. *-ismos,* condition] The condition of having a yellow tinge.

**flavivirus** (flă″vē-vī′rŭs) A genus of Togaviridae. They were previously called group B arboviruses. Viruses that cause yellow fever, certain types of encephalitis, and dengue are species in this genus.

**Flavobacterium** A genus of rod-shaped bacteria belonging to the Achromobacteraceae. They are found in soil and water and produce an orange-yellow pigment in cultures. *Flavobacterium meningosepticum* is esp. virulent for premature infants, in whom it causes meningitis. The fatality rate is high.

**flavone** (flā′vōn) The chemical from which the natural colors of many vegetables are derived.

**flavoprotein** One of a group of conjugated proteins that constitute the yellow enzymes essential in cellular respiration.

**flavor** (flā′vor) **1.** The quality of a substance that affects the sense of taste. It may also stimulate the sense of smell. **2.** A material added to a food or medicine to improve its taste.

**flaxseed** The seed of *Linum usitatissimum.* SYN: *linseed.*

**fl. dr.** *fluidram.*

**flea** (flē) [AS. *flea*] Any insect of the order Siphonaptera. Fleas are wingless, suck blood, and have legs adapted for jumping. Usually they are parasitic on warm-blooded animals including humans. Fleas of the genus *Xenopsylla* transmit the bacillus of plague *(Yersinia pestis)* from rats to humans. Fleas may transmit other diseases such as tularemia, endemic typhus, and brucellosis. They are intermediate hosts for the cat and dog tapeworms. SEE: illus.

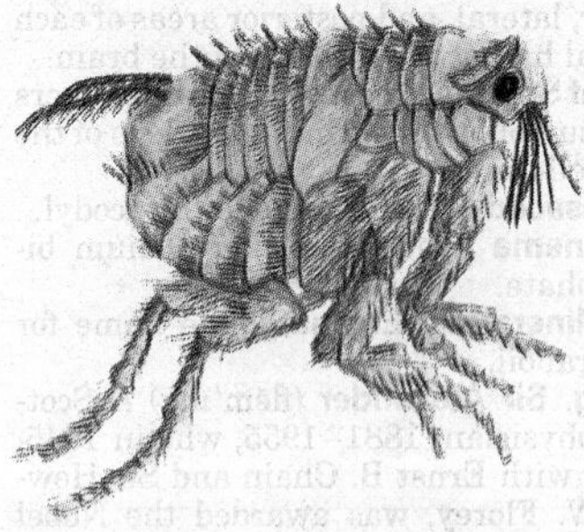

FLEA (XENOPSYLLA) (ORIG. MAG. ×15)

***f. bite*** A hemorrhagic punctum surrounded by erythematous and urticarial patches and caused by the injection of flea saliva.

TREATMENT: Ice applied to the site decreases the pain. Application of a corticosteroid cream may decrease the inflammatory response.

PREVENTION: The skin should be treated with an insect repellent available as a powder, spray, or oil for topical use.

***cat f.*** *Ctenocephalides felis.*

***chigger f.*** *Tunga penetrans.* SYN: *chigger; jigger; sand flea.*

***dog f.*** *Ctenocephalides canis.*

***human f.*** *Pulex irritans.*

***rat f.*** *Xenopsylla cheopis.*

**flea infestation** The harboring of fleas, esp. in a home with dogs or cats. It is possible to kill the flea population by treating the house for 24 hr by using naphthalene. This substance is available in flake form for use as a moth repellent. The flakes are spread on newspapers in the middle of each room, and the house is closed for 24 hr.

Caution: It is essential to disconnect all electrical equipment in the house prior to this procedure because an electrical spark could cause the fumes to explode. Any plants, pets, or humans could suffer adverse effects if they remain in the house during the treatment period. The house should be thoroughly ventilated afterwards to remove the fumes.

---

Another possibility is to drown the fleas by allowing them to jump into a shallow pan containing water and a detergent. The pan is left in the flea-infested area at night in a dark room except for a light over the pan. The fleas are attracted to the light and, when they jump, land in the water, where the detergent causes them to sink and drown.

**flecainide acetate** An antiarrhythmic drug. Trade name is Tambocor.

**Flechsig's areas** (flĕk'zĭgz) [Paul E. Flechsig, Ger. neurologist, 1847–1929] The anterior, lateral, and posterior areas of each lateral half of the medulla of the brain.

**fleece of Stilling** A meshwork of white fibers that surrounds the dentate nucleus of the cerebellum.

**Fleet Bisacodyl** Trade name for bisacodyl.

**Fleet Enema** Trade name for sodium biphosphate.

**Fleet Mineral Oil Enema** Trade name for mineral oil.

**Fleming, Sir Alexander** (flĕm'ĭng) A Scottish physician, 1881–1955, who in 1945, along with Ernst B. Chain and Sir Howard W. Florey, was awarded the Nobel Prize in medicine and physiology for the discovery of penicillin.

**flesh** [AS. *flaesc*] The soft tissues of the animal body, esp. the muscles. SEE: *carnivorous; meat.*

***examination of animal f.*** The inspection of animal meat intended for human consumption to determine its fitness to be sold and eaten. Animal flesh should be examined for color, consistency, proportion of fat, odor, and, after cooking, its taste. In general, it should be neither very pale nor dark purple; it may be marbled, firm, and elastic; it should be free from odor; and touching it should not moisten the finger.

NOTE: *Yellow:* This color may be produced by food eaten by the animal. In disease, it is due to animals having been jaundiced. *Brown:* This is rare except in old meat undergoing decomposition. *Dark purple:* This color may indicate that the animal died a natural death or suffered from acute fever, tuberculosis, or rinderpest. It should be avoided. *Dark reddish-brown:* This color may indicate the animal was hunted or overdriven; poisoned, drowned, or suffocated. Such meat is to be avoided. *Scarlet:* This rare color indicates arsenic or carbon monoxide poisoning. *Red:* The animal may have been poisoned or the meat frozen. *Green or violet:* This indicates the beginning of dangerous putrefaction. *Saffron:* This color is artificial. *Brilliant red:* This is due to poisonous bacteria. *Gray:* Usually found in sausages, gray is due to bacteria. *Phosphorescent:* Phosphorescence, not due to putrefaction, usually is found in fish and shellfish and is increased by heat. In meat, esp. veal, it may be caused by bacteria, and is generally transmitted from fish kept in the same place with meat. *White:* This color is rare except in veal. It is found in certain diseases and should be avoided.

***goose f.*** Cutis anserina.

***proud f.*** Excessive granular tissue in a wound or ulcer.

**Fletcher factor** A blood clotting factor, prekallikrein.

**fletcherism** [Horace Fletcher, U.S. dietitian, 1849–1919] Taking small amounts of food at a time. These small bites are chewed for a prolonged period prior to swallowing. SEE: *psomophagia.*

**Fletcher-Suit system** The most commonly used applicator for brachytherapy of gynecological malignancies.

**flex** [L. *flexus,* bent] To bend on itself, as a muscle.

**flexibilitas cerea** (flĕks″ĭ-bĭl'ĭ-tăs sē'rē-ă) [L.] A cataleptic state in which limbs retain any position in which they are placed. It is characteristic of catatonic patients. SEE: *catalepsy.*

**flexibility** [L. *flexus,* bent] The quality of bending without breaking; adaptability. SYN: *pliability.* **flexible,** ***adj.***

**flexile** (flĕks'ĭl) [L. *flexus,* bent] Pliant, flexible.

**flexion** (flĕk'shŭn) [L. *flexio*] **1.** The act of bending or condition of being bent in contrast to extension. SEE: *antecurvature.* **2.** Decrease in the angle between the bones forming a joint.

**flexor** (flĕks'or) [L.] A muscle that brings two bones closer together, causing flexion of the part or a decreased angle of the joint. Opposed to extensor.

**flexura** (flĕk-shoo'ră) [L.] A flexure.

**flexure** (flĕk'shĕr) [L. *flexura*] A bend.

***dorsal f.*** A convex curve in the thoracic area of the spine.

***duodenojejunal f.*** A curve at the meeting point of the jejunum and duodenum.

***hepatic f.*** Right colic f.

***left colic f.*** A bend at the transition point where the transverse colon becomes the descending colon. SYN: *splenic f.*

***right colic f.*** A bend at the transition point where the ascending colon becomes the transverse colon. SYN: *hepatic f.*

***sigmoid f.*** An S-like loop (in the left iliac fossa) of the descending colon as it joins the rectum. Former name for sigmoid colon. SEE: *colon* for illus.

***splenic f.*** Left colic f.

**flicker** The visual sensation of alternating intervals of brightness caused by rhythmic interruption of light stimuli.

**flicker phenomenon** A sensation of continuous light caused by an intermittent light stimulus produced at a certain rate.

**flight into disease** Ready adoption of a sick status to escape reality.

**flight into health** Voluntary and temporary suppression of mental or physical symptoms to prevent further psychoanalytic probing into the patient's psyche.

**flight of ideas** Continuous but fragmentary stream of talk. The general train of thought can be followed but direction is frequently changed, often by chance stimuli from the environment. This condition may be seen in acute manic states.

**flip-flop** A condition in which the reduction in fraction of inspired oxygen to reduce hypoxemia in infants causes a persistent and greater-than-expected decrease in oxygen tension ($PaO_2$).

**floater** (flō'tĕrs) [AS. *flotian,* float] A translucent speck that passes across the visual field. Floaters vary in size and shape. They are due to small bits of protein or cells floating in the vitreous. Most people have these benign materials in their eyes. SEE: *muscae volitantes.*

**floating** [AS *flota,* a raft] Moving about; out of normal location.

**floating kidney** A kidney movable from its normal bed of fat.

**floating ribs** The 11th and 12th ribs, which do not articulate with the sternum.

**floccillation, floccitation** (flŏk″sĭ-lā'shŭn, -tā'shŭn) [L. *floccilatio*] Semiconscious picking at bedclothes in association with fever, stupor, and delirium. SYN: *carphologia.*

**floccose** (flŏk'ōs) [L. *floccosus,* full of wool tufts] In biology, pert. to a growth consisting of short and densely but irregularly interwoven filaments.

**flocculation** (flŏk″ū-lā'shŭn) Gathering of the fine dispersed particles in a solution into larger, usually visible particles.

**flocculation reaction** Flocculation of a serum reaction.

**flocculence** (flŏk'ū-lĕns″) Resemblance to shreds or tufts of cotton.

**flocculent** (flŏk'ū-lĕnt) **1.** Resembling tufts or shreds of cotton. **2.** Pert. to a fluid or culture containing whitish shreds of mucus.

**flocculus** (flŏk'ū-lŭs) *pl.* **flocculi** [L., little tuft] **1.** A small tuft of woollike fibers. **2.** A lobe below and behind the middle peduncle of the cerebrum on each side of the median fissure. **floccular,** *adj.*

**flood 1.** A pathological uterine hemorrhage. **2.** Excessive menstrual bleeding.

**flooding** (flŭd'ĭng) **1.** A colloquial term for excessive menstrual flow. **2.** In treating phobias, repeated exposure to the disturbing ideas, situations, or conditions until these no longer produce anxiety.

**Flood's ligament** [Valentine Flood, Ir. surgeon, 1800–1847] A band of ligaments attached to the lower part of the lesser tuberosity of the humerus.

**floor** [AS. *flor*] The surface that forms the lower limit of a cavity or space, as the floor of the cranial cavity, fourth ventricle, mouth, nasal fossa, pelvis, or a cavity preparation in a tooth.

**floppy-valve syndrome** Mitral valve prolapse.

**flora** [L. *flos,* flower] **1.** Plant life as distinguished from animal life. **2.** Microbial life occurring or adapted for living in a specific environment, such as the intestinal, vaginal, oral, urinary tract, or skin flora. SEE: *fauna.*

***intestinal f.*** Bacteria present in the intestines. The chemical nature of the contents of the intestines varies according to the portion of the tract being considered. Bacteria do not exist in the intestines at birth but appear very shortly thereafter. These bacteria produce vitamins, esp. vitamin K, and inhibit the growth of pathogens. Certain antibiotics may cause drastic alterations in the number and kinds of bacteria present. SEE: *Clostridium difficile.*

***normal f.*** Potentially pathogenic organisms that are harmless in the body, including bacteria, fungi, and protozoa found on the skin and mucosa of the gastrointestinal and genitourinary tracts, that protect the body from pathogens. When one type of normal flora is destroyed, an overgrowth of others can occur. For example, when the bacteria are killed by antibiotics, fungal growth, usually from *Candida,* appears in the mouth, vagina, and moist skin folds, requiring treatment with an antifungal agent. Destruction of normal flora can also permit infection by more serious agents. SEE: *colitis, pseudomembranous; infection.*

The ability of the body to provide an environment that prevents overgrowth of certain species of bacteria is remarkable. The largest concentration of bacteria in humans is in the colon, where more than 400 genera may coexist. In the colon, anaerobic bacteria outnumber aerobic bacteria 1000:1, and there may be $10^{11}$ g of fecal material. The anaerobic gram-positive *Lactobacilli* may be concentrated in the vagina at the $10^5$ to $10^8$/ml level, but 20% of women have no detectable anaerobes in the vagina. In dental plague and gingival sulci, the bacteria may reach a concentration of $10^{12}$/ml.

**florid** [L. *floridus,* blossoming] Bright deep-red. The term describes skin coloration.

**floss 1.** A waxed or unwaxed tape or thread used to clean and remove plaque between teeth and below the gumline. SYN: *dental f.* **2.** To use dental floss or tape to remove plaque and calculus from the otherwise inaccessible dental surfaces between teeth.

***dental f.*** Floss (1).

**flour** [L. *flos,* flower] Finely ground meal obtained from wheat or other grain; any soft fine powder. SEE: *Nutritive Value of Foods Appendix.*

**flow** [AS. *flowan,* to flow] **1.** Movement with respect to time. **2.** The act of moving or running freely.

***laminar f.*** SEE: *laminar air flow.*

***peak f.*** The maximum amount of gas that can be exhaled with force after a maximum inspiration, measured in liters

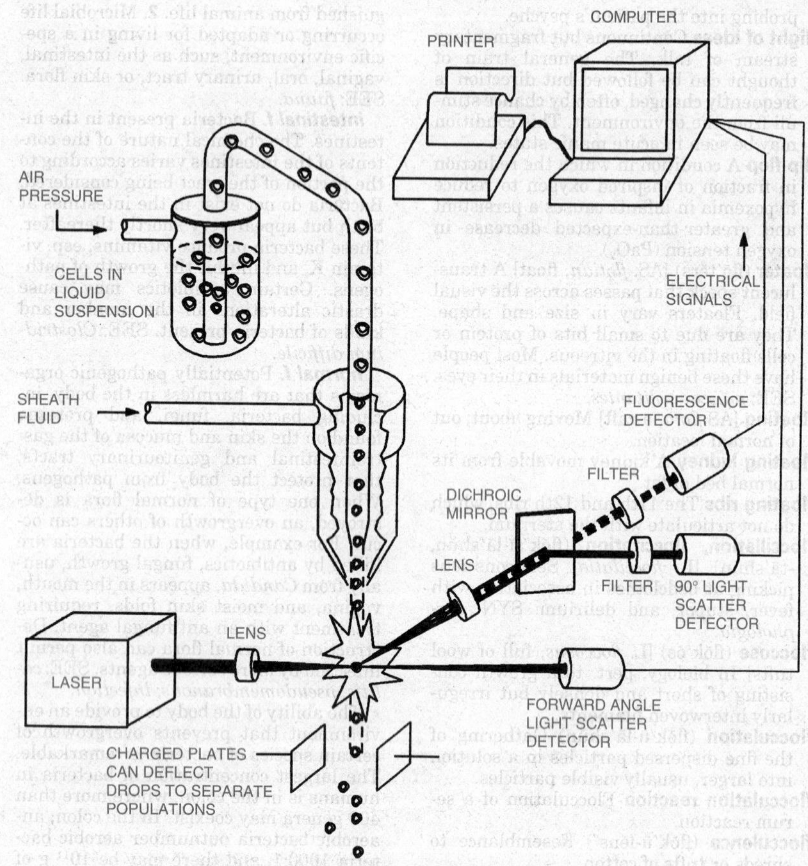


**FLOW CYTOMETRY**

**COMPONENTS OF A LASER-BASED FLOW CYTOMETER**

per minute.

***turbulent f.*** A movement of gas in disorderly currents, associated with high velocity and high density with increased tubing diameter.

**flow cell** A type of optical cell employed in photometers and cell counters through which the sample and any standards are passed for detection. SEE: *cytometry*.

**flow cytometry** SEE: illus.; *cytometry*.

**flowmeter** A device for measuring the movement of a gas or liquid. It is used esp. in monitoring the use of anesthetic gases.

**flow state** An altered state of consciousness in which the mind functions at its peak, time may seem distorted, and a sense of happiness seems to pervade that period. In such a state the individual feels alive and fully attentive to what is being done. This state is distinguished from strained attention, in which the person forces himself or herself to perform a task in which he or she has little interest.

**floxuridine** (flŏks-ŭr′ĭ-dēn) An antimetabolite used in treating certain forms of cancer.

**fl. oz.** *fluidounce*.

**flu** (floo) Influenza.

**fluctuant** (flŭk′chū-ănt) Varying or unstable. SEE: *fluctuation*.

**fluctuation** [L. *fluctuatio*] **1.** A variation from one course to another. **2.** A wavy impulse felt in palpation and produced by vibration of body fluid.

DIAGNOSIS: If fluctuation is felt over the lower abdomen, ascites usually is present. Fluctuation may be caused by peritoneal hemorrhage. If it is confined to a limited portion of the abdomen, tuberculous peritonitis may be implicated; over the central portion, bladder distention; in the lower abdomen in women, an ovarian cyst or pregnancy; in the right hypochondrium, a hydatid cyst, liver abscess, or distended gallbladder; over the left hypochondrium, cysts or abscess; above the

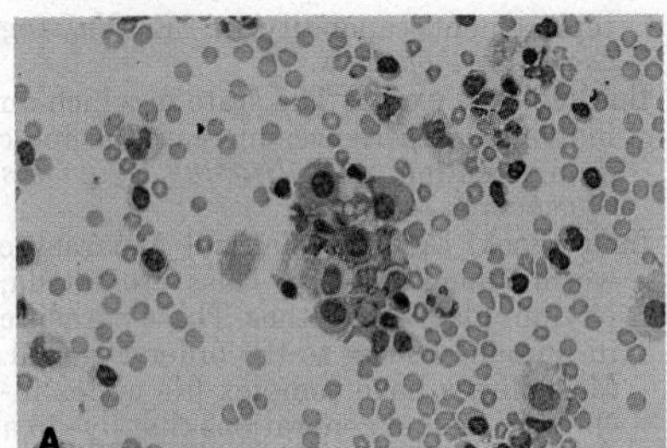

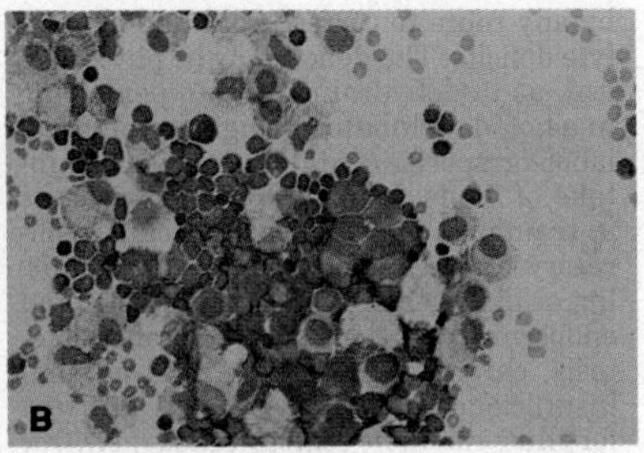


PLEURAL FLUID

(A) NORMAL FLUID WITH LYMPHOCYTES AND MONOCYTES (ORIG. MAG. ×500), (B) SMALL CELL CARCINOMA IN FLUID (ORIG. MAG. ×500)

umbilicus, a dilated colon or stomach partly filled with fluid and gas.

**flucytosine** (flū-sī′tō-sēn″) An antifungal drug. It is usually used with amphotericin B to decrease the emergence of resistant strains of yeasts and fungi. Trade name is Ancobon.

**fludrocortisone** (floo″drō-kor′tĭ-sōn) A synthetic corticosteroid.

***f. acetate*** A corticosteroid drug. Trade name is Florinef Acetate.

**fluid** [L. *fluidus*] A nonsolid, liquid, or gaseous substance. SEE: *secretion.*

***allantoic f.*** Fluid found in the fetal membrane that develops from the yolk sac.

***amniotic f.*** A clear yellowish fluid that fills the fetal membranes in pregnancy. Specific gravity is approx. 1.006. It is composed of albumin, salts (chiefly urea), and water, and suspended in it are lanugo, epidermal cells, vernix caseosa, and meconium. It is derived from the amnion. Its chief function is to protect the fetus. SEE: *amnion; meconium.*

***cerebrospinal f.*** Fluid found in the central canal of the spinal cord, the ventricles of the brain, and the subarachnoid space around the brain and spinal cord.

***crevicular f.*** In dentistry, the fluid that seeps through the gingival epithelium. It increases with gingival inflammation. SYN: *gingival f.*

***extracellular f.*** Tissue fluid or fluid occupying spaces between tissue cells. SYN: *interstitial f.*

***extravascular f.*** All the body fluids outside the blood vessels. They include tissue fluid, fluids within the serous and synovial cavities, cerebrospinal fluid, and lymph.

***gingival f.*** Crevicular f.

***interstitial f.*** Extracellular f.

***intracellular f.*** Fluid contained within cells and constituting about 50% of body weight.

***intraocular f.*** Fluid within the anterior and posterior chambers of the eye. SYN: *aqueous humor.*

***pleural f.*** Fluid secreted by serous membranes in the pleurae that reduces friction during respiratory movements of the lungs. SEE: illus.

***seminal f.*** Semen.

***serous f.*** Fluid secreted by serous membranes that reduces friction in the serous cavities (pleural, pericardial, and peritoneal).

***spinal f.*** Cerebrospinal fluid found in the spinal canal of the spinal cord.

***synovial f.*** Fluid contained within synovial cavities, bursae, and tendon sheaths. SYN: *synovia.*

**fluid balance** Regulation of the amount of water in the body. The balance is upset when fluids are lost by vomiting, diarrhea, bleeding, or dehydration. Treatment of fluid imbalance depends on the cause, the kind and quantity of fluids lost, and the state of renal function. SEE: *fluid replacement.*

**fluid diet** A nutritional plan for persons unable to chew and swallow solid food or for patients whose gastrointestinal tract must be free of solid matter.

**fluidextract, fluidextractum** [L. *fluidus,* fluid, + *extractum,* extract] A solution of the soluble constituents of vegetable drugs in which each cubic centimeter or milliliter represents 1 g of the drug. Fluidextracts contain alcohol as a solvent or preservative. Many of them form precipitates when water is added.

***aromatic cascara f.*** A liquid preparation of cascara sagrada, magnesium oxide, glycyrrhiza extract, saccharin, anise oil, coriander oil, methyl salicylate, alcohol, and water. It is used as a laxative.

***glycyrrhiza f.*** A liquid preparation of glycyrrhiza.

***ipecac f.*** A fluid preparation of the powdered rhizome and roots of *Cephaelis ipecacuanha* or *C. acuminata.* It is used as an emetic and expectorant.

**fluidounce** SYMB: f℥. An apothecaries' measure of fluid volume, equal to 8 fluidrams or 29.57 ml.

**fluidram** SYMB: fʒ. An apothecaries' measure of fluid volume, equal to 3.697 ml.

**fluid replacement** Administration of fluids

by any route to correct fluid and electrolyte deficits. The deficit may be physiological, as in dehydration due to perspiring in a hot, dry climate during hard physical labor or sports, or due to inadequate intake of fluids. It may be pathological, as in traumatic or septic shock, acute respiratory distress syndrome, severe vomiting or diarrhea or both, or metabolic and endocrine conditions such as diabetic ketosis, chronic renal failure, and adrenal insufficiency. SEE: *intravenous infusion* for illus; *catheter, central venous; central line; intravenous infusion; oral rehydration therapy; solution.*

The goal of fluid replacement is to correct both the fluid and the electrolyte (acid-base) imbalances. The oral route of replacement is used if possible. The intravenous, intraperitoneal, or subcutaneous routes are also used, with the intravenous route being used most frequently. Fluids may be isotonic, hypotonic, or hypertonic; may contain certain crystalloids (e.g., sodium, potassium, chloride or calcium); or may contain osmotically active substances (e.g., glucose, protein, starch, or a synthetic plasma volume expander such as dextran or hetastarch). The composition, rate of administration, and route depends on the clinical condition being treated.

---

Caution: A critically ill patient receiving fluid replacement should be monitored frequently to be certain that fluid overload is prevented and that the solution is flowing and not extravasating. This is esp. important in treating infants and small children.

---

**fluid retention** Failure to eliminate fluid from the body because of renal, cardiac, or metabolic disease, or combinations of these disorders. Excess salt is another cause of fluid retention, which maintains the proper chemical and physical properties of body fluids. A low-sodium diet is indicated in fluid retention. The advisability of using diuretics depends on the functional state of the kidneys.

**fluid volume deficit [active loss]** The state in which an individual experiences vascular, cellular, or intracellular dehydration (in excess of needs or replacement capabilities owing to active loss). SEE: *Nursing Diagnoses Appendix.*

**fluid volume deficit [regulatory failure]** The state in which an individual experiences vascular, cellular, or intracellular dehydration [in excess of needs or replacement capabilities owing to failure of regulatory mechanisms]. SEE: *Nursing Diagnoses Appendix.*

**fluid volume deficit, risk for** The state in which an individual is at risk of experiencing vascular, cellular, or intracellular dehydration [due to active or regulatory losses of body water in excess of needs or replacement capability]. SEE: *Nursing Diagnoses Appendix.*

**fluid volume excess** The state in which an individual experiences increased isotonic fluid retention. SEE: *Nursing Diagnoses Appendix.*

**fluke** (flook) [AS. *floc,* flatfish] A parasitic worm belonging to the class Trematoda, phylum Platyhelminthes. Those parasitic in humans belong to the order Digenea. Most flukes have complex life cycles including asexual generations that live in a mollusc (snail or bivalve). Stages of a typical fluke include adult, egg, miracidium, sporocyst, redia, cercaria, and metacercaria.

***blood f.*** A fluke of the genus *Schistosoma,* including *S. haematobium, S. mansoni,* and *S. japonicum.* Adults live principally in the mesenteric and pelvic veins. They cause schistosomiasis and schistosome dermatitis (swimmer's itch). SYN: *schistosome.*

***intestinal f.*** One of several species of flukes infesting the intestine in humans. They include *Gastrodiscoides hominis, Fasciolopsis buski, Heterophyes heterophyes,* and *Metagonimus yokogawai.*

***liver f.*** One of several species of fluke infesting the liver and bile ducts. Those infesting humans include *Clonorchis sinensis, Fasciola hepatica, Dicrocoelium dendriticum,* and *Opisthorchis felineus.* Adult liver flukes infest biliary and pancreatic ducts. The eggs pass from the body with the feces and continue their development in snails of the subfamily Buliminae (family Hydrobiidae). Cercariae emerge and infest numerous species of freshwater fishes in which they encyst. Infestation results from eating raw fish containing encysted metacercariae.

***lung f.*** A fluke that infests lung tissue. Only one species, *Paragonimus westermani,* is common in humans.

**flumina pilorum** (floo′mĭ-nă pī-lō′rŭm) [L., rivers of hair] **1.** The curved lines along which the hairs of the body are arranged, esp. in the fetus. **2.** Hairs lying in same direction.

**fluo-** Combining form meaning *flow.*

**fluocinolone acetonide** (floo-ō-sĭn′ō-lōn) A synthetic corticosteroid. Trade names are Fluonid and Synalar.

**Fluogen** Trade name for the influenza virus vaccine, trivalent.

**fluor albus** (floo′or ăl′bŭs) [L., white flow] A white discharge from the uterus or vagina. SYN: *leukorrhea.*

**fluorescein sodium** (floo″ō-rĕs′ē-ĭn) A red crystalline powder used chiefly for diagnostic purposes and for detecting foreign bodies or lesions in the cornea of the eye.

**fluorescence** (floo″ō-rĕs′ĕnts) The light-emitting property of certain substances when they are exposed to certain types of light radiation, usually ultraviolet. This phenomenon was first noted in fluorspar. The mechanism is absorption of shorter wavelengths and simultaneous emission of a longer wavelength that terminates with the cessation of the stimulus exciting radiation.

**fluorescent** (floo-ō-rĕs′ĕnt) **1.** In biology, having one color by transmitted light and another by reflected light. **2.** Luminous when exposed to other light rays.

**fluorescent antibody** ABBR: FA. An antibody that has been stained or marked by a fluorescent material. The fluorescent antibody technique permits rapid diagnosis of various infections.

**fluorescent polarization immunoassay** ABBR: FPIA. An antigen-antibody analysis using fluorescent-tagged molecules to measure both fluorescence and polarization of light. The technique is based on the principle that small molecules rotate rapidly and therefore emit randomly polarized fluorescence, whereas large molecules rotate slowly and produce highly polarized fluorescence.

**fluorescent screen 1.** A sheet of cardboard, paper, or glass coated with a material that fluoresces visibly, such as calcium tungstate. It is used in fluoroscopy, in which x-rays, radium rays, or electrons cause the object being examined to cast a shadow. **2.** A sheet of cardboard, paper, or glass, coated with anthracene or other fluorescing materials to reveal ultraviolet radiations. SYN: *intensifying screen.*

**fluorescent treponemal antibody-absorption test** ABBR: FTA-ABS. A test for syphilis using the fluorescent antibody technique.

**fluoridation** (floo″or-ĭ-dā′shŭn) The addition of fluorides to a water supply to prevent dental caries.

The development of dental caries in the deciduous and permanent teeth can be decreased by providing fluoride as a supplement in the drinking water, by topical application to the teeth, or by daily medication. There are several important considerations. Fluoride in excess daily dose discolors the teeth if the fluoride is ingested while the teeth are developing (i.e., from birth to 8 or 10 years). If fluoridated water is consumed during pregnancy, the deciduous teeth, which begin to mineralize during the fourth or fifth month in utero, incorporate that compound and become more resistant to caries. In the adult tooth, when enamel has lost mineral (white spot lesion), the remineralization is greatly enhanced by fluoride, which leads to the precipitation of calcium phosphate.

The rate of tooth loss in individuals receiving fluoride from infancy is only one fourth that of persons who receive no fluoride. The most certain and effective method of administering fluoride is by providing drinking water that contains 1 part per million, 1 mg/1000 ml, of fluoride. This will ensure a daily dose of fluoride of 0.25 to 0.50 mg per day.

Caution: Children drinking fluoridated water should not be given supplemental fluoride medication.

**fluoride** (floo′ō-rīd) A compound of fluorine, usually with a radical; a salt of hydrofluoric acid. Three preparations of fluoride-containing compounds are available for topical application to teeth for the prevention of decay. They are stannous fluoride, sodium fluoride, and acidulated phosphaste fluoride. Fluoride compounds are highly effective in preventing decay on the smooth surfaces of teeth.

***acidulated phosphate f.*** ABBR: APF. A fluoride compound available in solution and gel. It is recommended for use at a 1.23% concentration.

***sodium f.*** A stable, tasteless fluoride compound, NaF. It is recommended for use at a 2% concentration. The prepared solution has a basic pH.

***stannous f.*** An unstable acidic fluoride solution, $SnF_2$. It is recommended for use at an 8% concentration and has a bitter, metallic taste.

**fluoride dental treatment** The application of a fluoride solution or gel to the teeth as a means of controlling or preventing caries. SEE: *dental sealant.*

**fluoride poisoning** SEE: *Poisons and Poisoning Appendix.*

**fluorine** (floo′ō-rēn, floor′ēn) SYMB: F. A gaseous chemical element, atomic weight 18.9984, atomic number 9. It is found in the soil in combination with calcium. SEE: *fluoridation.*

**fluoroacetate** (floo″or-ō-ăs′ĕ-tāt) A salt of fluoroacetic acid. SEE: *Poisons and Poisoning Appendix.*

**fluoroapatite** A compound formed when tooth enamel is treated with appropriate concentrations of the fluoride ion. The modified hydroxyapatite is less acid soluble and therefore resistant to caries. Fluoroapatite is formed in bone, as well as in enamel and dentin of teeth, when fluoride is taken systemically.

**fluorocarbon** A general term for a hydrocarbon in which some of the hydrogen atoms have been replaced with fluorine. The use of such compounds in aerosol sprays was discontinued because of an adverse effect on the atmosphere.

**fluorometer** (floo-or-ŏm′ĕ-tĕr) **1.** A device for determining the amount of radiation produced by x-rays. **2.** A device for adjusting a fluoroscope to establish the location of the target more accurately and to produce an undistorted image or shadow. **3.** A clinical laboratory instrument used in many types of immunochemistry assays (e.g., fluorescent polarization immunoassay).

**fluorometholone** (floor″ō-mĕth′ō-lōn) A synthetic corticosteroid.

**fluorophor** A substance that tends to fluoresce, such as fluorescein.

**fluoroscope** (floo'or-ō-skōp) A device consisting of a fluorescent screen, mounted either separately or in conjunction with an x-ray tube, that shows the images of objects interposed between the tube and the screen. It has been replaced by the image intensifier for performing fluoroscopic studies.

**fluoroscopy** Examination of the body using a fluoroscope.

**fluorosis** (floo-or-ō'sĭs) Chronic fluorine poisoning, sometimes marked by mottling of tooth enamel. It often results from too much fluoride in drinking water.

**fluorouracil** (floor"ō-ŭr'ă-sĭl) An antimetabolite used in treating certain forms of cancer.

**fluoxetine hydrochloride** A tricyclic antidepressant drug. Trade name is Prozac.

**fluoxymesterone** (floo-ŏk"sē-mĕs'tĕr-ōn) An anabolic and androgenic hormone. Trade names are Ora-Testryl and Halotestin.

**fluphenazine enanthate** (floo-fĕn'ă-zēn) A phenothiazine-type tranquilizer. Trade name is Prolixin Enanthate.

**fluprednisolone** (floo"prĕd-nĭs'ō-lōn) A corticosteroid drug.

**flurandrenolide** (floor"ăn-drĕn'ō-līd) A corticosteroid drug.

**flurazepam hydrochloride** (floor-ăz'ĕ-păm) A sedative-hypnotic drug.

**flurothyl** (floor'ō-thĭl) A central nervous system stimulant.

**fluroxene** (floor-ŏks'ēn) An anesthetic agent administered by inhalation.

---

Caution: Fluroxene may be flammable and explosive.

---

**flush** [ME. *flusshen,* to fly up] **1.** Sudden redness of the skin. **2.** Irrigation of a cavity with water.

***hot f.*** A flush accompanied with a sensation of heat. It is common in neuroses and psychoneuroses and during menopause.

***malar f.*** A bright-colored flush over the malar area and cheekbones. It may be associated with any febrile disease.

**flutter** [AS. *floterian,* to fly about] A tremulous movement, esp. of the heart, as in atrial and ventricular flutter.

***atrial f.*** Atrial contractions of the heart at 200 to 400 per minute. In pure flutter a regular rhythm is maintained; in impure flutter the rhythm is irregular.

***diaphragmatic f.*** Rapid contractions of the diaphragm. They may occur intermittently or be present for an extended period. The cause is unknown.

***mediastinal f.*** Abnormal side-to-side motion of the mediastinum during respiration.

***ventricular f.*** Ventricular contractions of the heart at 250 per minute or more.

**Flutter device** A handheld device designed to facilitate clearance of mucus in hypersecretory lung disorders. Exhalation through the Flutter results in oscillations of expiratory pressure and airflow, which vibrate the airway walls, loosening mucus, decrease the collapsibility of the airways, and accelerate airflow. This facilitates movement of mucus up the airways. SEE: *cystic fibrosis.*

**flutter-fibrillation** Cardiac dysrhythmia alternating between atrial fibrillation and atrial flutter, or showing a pattern that could be either when seen on a cardiac monitor.

**flux** [L. *fluxus,* a flow] **1.** An excessive flow or discharge from an organ or cavity of the body. **2.** In physics, the flow rate of a liquid, particles, or energy. **3.** In dentistry, an agent that lowers the fusion temperature of porcelain. **4.** In metallurgy, a substance used to increase the fluidity of a molten metal and to prevent or reduce its oxidation. **5.** A substance that deoxidizes, cleans, and promotes the union of surfaces to be brazed, soldered, or welded together.

**fly** [AS. *fleoge*] An insect belonging to the order Diptera, characterized by possessing sucking mouth parts, one pair of wings, and incomplete metamorphosis, such as the mayfly, housefly, or dragonfly. The term is sometimes applied to insects belonging to other orders. SEE: *Diptera.*

***black f.*** A fly of the genus *Simulium.*

***flesh f.*** The Sarcophagidae.

***screwworm f.*** A fly belonging to the families Calliphoridae and Sarcophagidae.

***Spanish f.*** Cantharides.

***tsetse f.*** *Glossina palpalis;* the fly that transmits African sleeping sickness or trypanosomiasis.

***warble f.*** *Dermatobia.*

**Fm** Symbol for the element fermium.

**f.m.** L. *fiat mistura,* let a mixture be made. This abbreviation is used in prescription writing.

**foam** (fōm) [AS. *fam*] A mixture of finely divided gas bubbles interspersed in a liquid.

**focal** (fō'kăl) Pert. to a focus.

**focal infection** Infection occurring near a focus, such as the cavity of a tooth.

**focal lesion** A limited central lesion.

**focal spot** The area on the x-ray tube target that is bombarded with electrons to produce x-radiation.

**foci** (fō'sī) [L.] Pl. of focus.

**focus** [L. *focus,* hearth] *pl.* **foci 1.** The point of convergence of light rays or sound waves. **2.** The starting point of a disease process.

***real f.*** The point at which convergent rays intersect.

***virtual f.*** The point at which divergent rays would intersect if extended backward.

**FOD** *focus-object distance.* The distance from the target of an x-ray tube to the surface being radiographed.

**fog** Droplets suspended in a gas, as minute water droplets in air.

**fogging 1.** A method of testing vision, used particularly in testing astigmatism and in postcycloplegic examination, in which accommodation is relaxed by overcorrection. **2.** A method of intense application of an insecticide. The solution is nebulized and appears in the air as a fog. **3.** Unwanted density on radiographic film resulting from exposure to secondary radiation, light, chemicals, or heat.

**foil** A thin, pliable sheet of metal. In dentistry, various types of gold foil are used for restoring or preparing appliances.

**folacin** Folic acid.

**fold** [AS. *fealdan,* to fold] A ridge; a doubling back. SYN: *plica.*

***amniotic f.*** The folded edge of the inner fetal membrane where it rises over and finally encloses the embryo of birds, reptiles, and some mammals.

***aryepiglottic f.*** The ridgelike lateral walls of the entrance to the larynx.

***circular f.*** A macroscopic fold of the mucosa and submucosa of the small intestine that is arranged like accordian pleats.

***costocolic f.*** A ligament, arising from the peritoneum, that attaches the splenic flexure of the colon to the diaphragm.

***Douglas' f.*** A fold of peritoneum extending on each side to the base of the broad ligament. This forms the rectouterine space, called Douglas' pouch.

***gastric f.*** Any of the folds of mucosa, mostly longitudinal, in the empty stomach.

***genital f.*** A fold of skin in the embryo on each side of the genital tubercle that develops into the labia minora in females.

***glossoepiglottidean f.*** One of three mucous membrane folds between the base of the tongue and the epiglottis. SYN: *epiglottic plica.*

***gluteal f.*** The linear crease in the skin that separates the buttocks from the thighs.

***lacrimal f.*** A valvelike fold in the lower part of the nasolacrimal duct.

***mesouterine f.*** A fold of peritoneum supporting the uterus.

***mucobuccal f.*** The line of flexure where the oral mucosa passes from the maxilla or mandible to the cheek; the vestibule.

***mucolabial f.*** The line of flexure where the oral mucosa passes from the maxilla or mandible to the lip.

***mucosal f.*** A fold of mucosal tissue.

***nail f.*** A groove in the cutaneous tissue surrounding the margins and proximal edges of the nail.

***palmate f.*** Any of the ridges on the cervical canal of the uterus.

***semilunar f. of conjunctiva*** The fold of conjunctiva at the inner angle of the eye.

***transverse f. of rectum*** Any of the transverse mucosal folds of the rectum. SYN: *Houston's valve.*

***urogenital f.*** SEE: *ridge, urogenital.*

***ventricular f.*** The false vocal cord. SYN: *vestibular f.; vocal f.*

***vestibular f.*** Ventricular f.

***vestigial f.*** The ligament of the left superior vena cava. SYN: *Marshall's fold.*

***vocal f.*** Ventricular f.

**Foley catheter** [Frederic W.B. Foley, U.S. urologist, 1891–1966] A urinary tract catheter with a balloon attachment at one end. After the catheter is inserted, the balloon is filled with sterile water. Thus the catheter is prevented from leaving the bladder until the balloon is emptied.

**folia** (fō′lē-ă) [L.] Pl. of folium.

**foliaceous** (fō-lē-ā′shē-ŭs) [L. *folia,* leaves] Resembling or pert. to a leaf.

**folic acid** (fō′lĭk) A member of the vitamin B complex occurring naturally in green plant tissue, liver, and yeast. It is used in the treatment of megaloblastic and macrocytic anemias, malabsorption syndromes, sprue, and other disorders. Folic acid plays an important role in preventing neural tube defects (NTD); the U.S. Public Health Service recommends that all women of childbearing age in the U.S. who are capable of becoming pregnant should consume 0.4 mg of folic acid per day to reduce their risk of having a child affected with spina bifida or other NTDs. SEE: *neural tube defect.*

Caution: Folic acid should not be used to treat pernicious anemia because it does not protect patients against the development of changes in the central nervous system that accompany this type of anemia.

**folie** (fō-lē′) [Fr.] Mania; psychosis.

***f. à deux*** Occurrence of psychosis, usually of the paranoid type, at the same time in two closely associated persons. Rarely, more than two persons are involved.

***f. du doute*** Abnormal doubts about ordinary acts and beliefs; inability to decide on a definite course of action or conduct.

***f. du pourquoi*** Unreasonable and unrelenting questioning.

***f. gémellaire*** Psychosis occurring in both twins.

**folinic acid** The active form of folic acid. It is used in counteracting the effects of folic acid antagonists, and in treating anemia due to folic acid deficiency. Trade name is Calcium Folinate.

**folium** (fō′lē-ŭm) *pl.* **folia** [L., leaf] A thin, broad, leaflike structure.

***f. vermis*** A fold on the posterior part of the upper surface of the vermis of the cerebellum.

**folk medicine** SEE: under *medicine.*

**follicle** [L. *folliculus,* little bag] A small secretory sac or cavity. **follicular,** *adj.*

***aggregated f.'s*** A cluster of solitary lymph nodules or groups of nodules found chiefly in the ileum near its junction with the colon. They are circular or oval, about 1 cm wide and 2 to 3 cm long. They lie in the mucosa and submucosa and always occur on the side of the intestine opposite to the attachment of mesentery. In typhoid fever, they undergo hyperplasia and often become ulcerated. SYN: *Peyer's patch*.

***atretic f.*** An ovarian follicle that has undergone degeneration or involution.

***dental f.*** **1.** The connective tissue structure that encloses the developing tooth within the substance of the jaw prior to tooth eruption. **2.** The dental sac and its contents.

***gastric f.*** The glands in the gastric mucosa of the stomach.

***graafian f.*** The development of the primary oocyte in the cortex of the ovary to the stage at which the ovum is complete. SEE: *graafian follicle; ovary; ovum* for illus.

***hair f.*** An invagination of the epidermis that forms a cylindrical depression, penetrating the corium into the connective tissue that holds the hair root. Sebaceous glands, which secrete sebum, and tiny muscles (arrectores pili) that cause the hair to stand are attached to these follicles.

***lymph f.*** The densely packed collection of lymphocytes and lymphoblasts that make up the cortex of lymph glands.

***maturing f.*** A developing follicle of the ovary.

***nabothian f.*** A dilated cyst of the glands of the cervix uteri.

***ovarian f.*** A spherical structure in the cortex of the ovary consisting of an oogonium or an oocyte and its surrounding epithelial (follicular) cells. The follicles are of three types. The first type, or primary follicle, consists of an oogonium and a single layer of follicular cells. In the second type, or growing follicle, cells proliferate, forming several layers, and the first maturation division occurs. The third type, the vesicular (graafian) follicle, possesses a cavity (antrum) containing the follicular fluid (liquor folliculi). The oocyte lies in the cumulus oophorus, a mass of cells on the inner surface. The cells lining the follicle constitute the stratum granulosum. The follicle is a secretory structure producing estrogen and progesterone. SEE: *corpus luteum*.

***primordial f.*** An ovarian follicle consisting of the ovum enclosed in a single layer of cells.

***sebaceous f.*** An oil gland of the skin.

***solitary f.*** A single lymph nodule of the intestine.

***thyroid f.*** A spherical or ovoid structure, found in the thyroid gland, lined with a single layer of cuboidal epithelial cells, which secrete the thyroid hormone. The follicles are filled with colloid, a viscid substance rich in iodine.

***vesicular f.*** A follicle containing a cavity; a mature ovarian (graafian) follicle.

**follicle-stimulating hormone** ABBR: FSH. A hormone produced by the anterior pituitary. It stimulates ovarian follicle growth, estrogen secretion, and spermatogenesis in the testis.

**follicle-stimulating hormone and luteinizing hormone–releasing hormone** ABBR: FSH/LHRH. A hypothalamic hormone that stimulates the release of follicle-stimulating hormone and luteinizing hormone from the anterior pituitary.

**follicle-stimulating hormone–releasing hormone** ABBR: FSH-RH. A hypothalamic hormone that stimulates the release of follicle-stimulating hormone from the anterior pituitary. Also called *follicle-stimulating hormone–releasing factor*.

**follicular** Pert. to a follicle or follicles.

**follicular tonsillitis** Inflammation of the follicles on the surface of the tonsil, which become filled with pus.

**follicular tumor** A sebaceous cyst.

**folliculitis** (fō-lĭk″ū-lī′tĭs) [L. *folliculus,* little bag, + Gr. *itis,* inflammation] Inflammation of a follicle or follicles.

***f. barbae*** Ringworm of the beard.

***f. decalvans*** Purulent follicular inflammation of the scalp resulting in irregular alopecia and scarring.

SYMPTOMS: An initial inflammatory papule or pustule pierced by a hair appears at the mouth of the follicle. It is followed by crusting and desiccation, when it drops off with the loosened hair. Bald patches with a slightly depressed whitish center are surrounded by an inflamed margin. The inflammation extends peripherally.

ETIOLOGY: The disorder is thought to be caused by staphylococci. It affects mostly men between the second and fourth decades.

PATHOLOGY: Sebaceous gland atrophy and flattened papillae are seen.

TREATMENT: Treatment is external and consists of topical antibiotics or corticosteroids and frequent shampoos.

PROGNOSIS: Loss of hair in affected areas is permanent, although extension may be arrested.

***keloidal f.*** Chronic dermatitis with production of hard papules that join together to form keloid tissue.

**folliculogenesis, induction of** Stimulation of follicle development in the ovary by the use of drugs or hormones (e.g., clomiphene) or human menopausal gonadotropin. SEE: *fertilization, in vitro; gamete intrafallopian transfer*.

**folliculoma** (fō-lĭk″ū-lō′mă) [″ + Gr. *oma,* tumor] A tumor of the ovary originating in a graafian follicle in which the cells resemble those of the stratum granulosum.

**folliculose** (fō-lĭk′ū-lōs) Composed of follicles.

**folliculosis** (fō-lĭk″ū-lō′sĭs) [″ + Gr. *osis,* condition] The presence of an abnormal number of lymph follicles.

**folliculus** (fō-lĭk′ū-lŭs) *pl.* **folliculi** [L.] A follicle.

**follow-up** The continued care or monitoring of a patient after the initial visit or examination.

**Folvite** Trade name for folic acid.

**fomentation** (fō″mĕn-tā′shŭn) [L. *fomentatio*] A hot, wet application for the relief of pain or inflammation. SEE: *dressing, hot moist; stupe.*

**fomes** (fō′mēz) *pl.* **fomites** [L., tinder] Any substance that adheres to and transmits infectious material.

**fomites** (fō′mĭ-tēz) Pl. of fomes.

**Fontana's spaces** (fŏn-tă′năz) [Felice Fontana, It. scientist, 1730–1805] The spaces between the processes of the ligamentum pectinatum of the iris. These convey the aqueous humor.

**fontanel, fontanelle** (fŏn″tă-nĕl′) [Fr. *fontanelle,* little fountain] An unossified space or soft spot lying between the cranial bones of the skull of a fetus. SEE: illus.

***anterior f.*** The fontanel at the junction of the coronal, frontal, and sagittal sutures; closed by the end of the second year.

***posterior f.*** The triangular fontanel at the junction of the sagittal and lambdoid sutures; closed by the end of the first year.

**Fontan procedure** [Francois Maurice Fontan, Fr. surgeon, b. 1929] A procedure in which the right atrium is connected directly to the pulmonary artery, or alternatively, the superior venacava is joined directly to the inferior venacava or to the pulmonary arteries. In patients with complex congenital heart disease, this allows arterial oxygen saturation to return to normal.

**fonticulus** (fŏn-tĭk′ū-lŭs) [L., little fountain] A fontanel.

**food** [AS. *foda*] Any material that provides the nutritive requirements of an organism to maintain growth and physical well-being. SEE: *Nutritive Value of Foods Appendix; Recommended Daily Dietary Allowances Appendix.*

COURSE: *Alimentary canal:* Foods enter the mouth and in the buccal area are reduced to a pulp or semifluid mass through mastication and insalivation (the mixing of food with saliva). Swallowing, or deglutition, then occurs. In swallowing, the food mass, or bolus, passes into the pharynx and then through the esophagus to the stomach, the entrance to which is controlled by the cardiac sphincter of the esophagus.

*Stomach:* In the stomach the food is stored and mixed with gastric juice. This action combined with gastric acidity kills many of the microorganisms present in food. After the food attains a certain fluid consistency, it passes through the pyloric sphincter of the stomach into the small intestine.

*Small intestine:* In the first portion, or duodenum, the intestinal contents (now called chyme) are mixed with bile secreted by the liver and with pancreatic juice, both of which enter through the opening of the common bile duct. In the next two portions, the jejunum and ileum, the chyme is mixed with the intestinal juice secreted by the intestinal glands, or crypts of Lieberkühn. In the small intestine, digestion is completed and its end products (simple sugars, amino acids, fatty acids, and glycerol) are absorbed into the capillaries and lacteals of the intestinal mucosa.

*Large intestine:* Remaining material

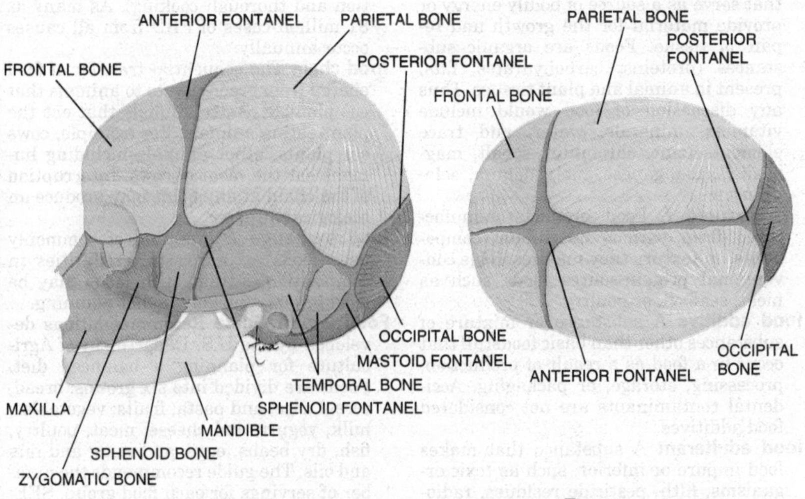


**FONTANELS** OF INFANT SKULL, **(A)** LATERAL VIEW, **(B)** SUPERIOR VIEW

passes from the small intestine into the large intestine (colon) through the ileocecal valve located at the junction of the ascending colon and the cecum, a blind pouch that terminates in the vermiform appendix. The material continues through the colon (ascending, transverse, descending, and sigmoid) to the rectum, from which it is discharged as feces through the anal canal at the anus, or anal orifice. Most of the water of the intestinal contents is absorbed in the large intestine. Digestive changes are limited to the action of bacteria, which brings about putrefaction and fermentation of incompletely digested foods.

***contamination of f.*** The presence of disease germs or infectious material in food, or the introduction of such substances into food. Food may cause illness by carrying pathogenic organisms such as those that cause enteritis *(Salmonella)* or tuberculosis, parasites such as those that cause trichinosis, or certain types of worms (e.g., roundworms, tapeworms).

***convenience f.*** Food in which one or more steps in preparation have been completed before the product is offered for retail sale. Examples include frozen vegetables, bake mixes, and heat-and-serve types of food.

***dietetic f.*** Food in which the nutrient content has been modified for use in special diets, esp. for diabetics.

***enriched f.*** Food in which the vitamin and mineral content has been increased by either addition or irradiation.

***medical f.*** A food formulated by the selective use of nutrients and manufactured for the dietary treatment of a specific condition.

***nutrient substances of f.*** Substances that serve as a source of bodily energy or provide material for the growth and repair of tissue. Foods are organic substances (proteins, carbohydrates, fats) present in animal and plant tissues. Thus any discussion of food would include vitamins, minerals, water, and trace elements (zinc, chromium, cobalt, magnesium, manganese, molybdenum, selenium).

***textured f.*** Food products manufactured from various nutritional components. In texture they may resemble conventional protein-source foods such as meat, seafood, or poultry.

**food additive** A substance or mixture of substances other than basic foodstuff that occur in a food as a result of production, processing, storage, or packaging. Accidental contaminants are not considered food additives.

**food adulterant** A substance that makes food impure or inferior, such as toxic organisms, filth, pesticide residues, radioactive fallout, any poisonous or deleterious substance, or any substance added to increase bulk or weight.

**food allergy** An allergic (i.e., immunological) reaction resulting from ingestion of a food to which a person has become sensitized. It is possible to become sensitive to almost any food; however, certain foods such as milk, eggs, wheat, shellfish, chocolate, and oranges are frequent offenders.

SYMPTOMS: Symptoms include urticaria (hives), certain eczemas, nausea, vomiting, diarrhea, and intestinal cramps. A syndrome (angioneurotic edema) characterized by a transient swelling of various body parts and intestinal spasm may result.

**Food and Drug Administration** ABBR: FDA. In the U.S., an official regulatory body for foods, drugs, cosmetics, and medical devices. It is a part of the U.S. Department of Health and Human Services.

**food and drug interactions** Drugs may interfere with absorption or use of food, particularly certain vitamins. Excess intake of food high in vitamin K may interfere with the action of anticoagulants. Prolonged use of antacids may cause phosphate depletion. SEE: *monoamine oxidase inhibitor*.

**food ball** Phytobezoar.

**food-borne disease** ABBR: FBD. A disease acquired by the ingestion of food contaminated with pathogens, usually bacteria and their toxins. These include *Staphylococcus, Clostridium botulinum, Salmonella, Shigella, Campylobacter, Listeria, Vibrio,* and *Escherichia*. Symptoms, treatment, and outcome depend on the causative agent and general health of the patient. The risks of FBD depend on the type of food; where it was produced; how it was handled, shipped, and stored prior to consumption; and the precautions taken by the consumer (proper refrigeration and thorough cooking). As many as 81 million cases of FBD from all causes occur annually.

**food chain** The sequential transfer of food energy from green plants to animals that eat plants, then to animals that eat the plant-eating animals. For example, cows eat plants; other animals including humans eat the meat of cows. Interruption of the chain at any point may produce an ecological disaster.

**food exchange** A grouping of commonly used foods according to similarities in composition so that such foods may be used interchangeably in diet planning.

**Food Group Guide** Recommendations developed by the U.S. Department of Agriculture for planning a balanced diet. Foods are divided into six groups: bread, cereal, rice, and pasta; fruits; vegetables; milk, yogurt, and cheese; meat, poultry, fish, dry beans, eggs, and nuts; and fats and oils. The guide recommends the number of servings for each food group. SEE: *Food Guide Pyramid*.

**Food Guide Pyramid** An annotated illustration of a pyramid published in 1993 by the

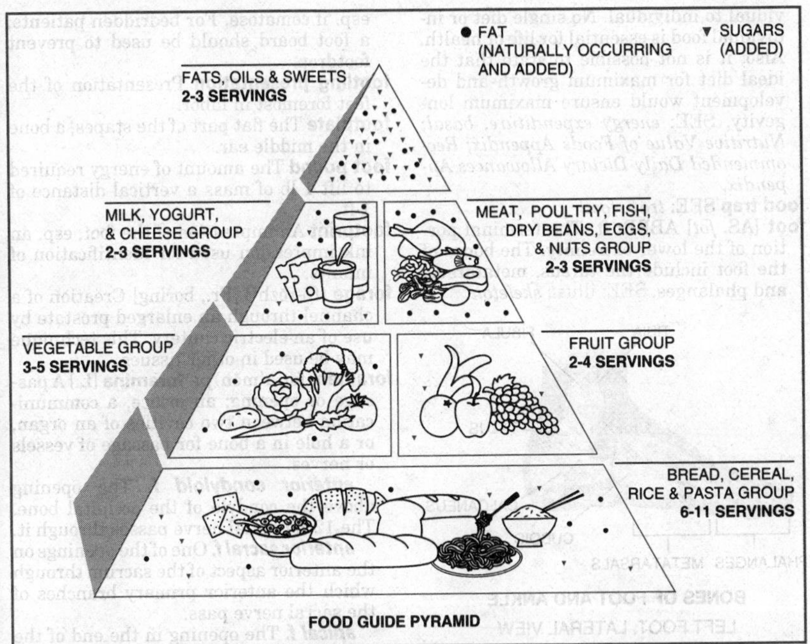

FOOD GUIDE PYRAMID

Source: U.S. Department of Agriculture, Human Nutrition Information Service.

U.S. Department of Agriculture. Classes of food are allotted space on the face of the pyramid and the number of daily servings advised for each class is given. SEE: illus.

**food hypersensitivity reaction** SEE: *food allergy*.

**food intolerance** An abnormal, nonimmunological response to ingested food. The basis for the intolerance may be pharmacological, metabolic, or toxic. Pharmacological intolerance is the body's reaction to a component of the food that produces druglike effects; metabolic intolerance is due to the effect of the food on the person's metabolism; and food toxicity is due to toxins in the food or released by microorganisms contaminating the food.

**food label** The information provided on a food package indicating the various nutrients, calories, and additives present in the food. U.S. Food and Drug Administration regulations have corrected some past inadequacies. For example, labels now list not only fat content, but the percentages of saturated and unsaturated fat.

**food poisoning** An imprecise term indicating an illness resulting from the ingestion of foods containing poisonous substances. True food poisoning includes poisoning resulting from mushrooms, shellfish, foods contaminated with poisonous insecticides or toxic substances such as lead or mercury, and milk sickness (due to milk from cows that have fed on certain poisonous plants). Also, poisoning may result from eating foods that have undergone putrefaction, decomposition, or poisoning from bacteria. SEE: *anisakiasis; fish poisoning*.

**food requirements** The need for various amounts and types of food according to a person's use of energy. It is assumed that an average healthy man (154 lb or 70 kg) performing light to moderate muscular work requires 2700 kcal/day, and that an average healthy woman (128 lb or 58 kg) requires 2000 kcal/day. These needs would be supplied in part by protein, but mostly by fat and carbohydrates. Persons in sedentary occupations require fewer calories. In general, adults require 1 g of protein per day for each kilogram of their ideal weight.

A diet made up of ordinary foods and supplying the necessary amounts of protein and energy undoubtedly supplies an abundance of mineral matter. The usual assumption is that a woman engaged in some moderately active occupation requires fewer calories each day because of her comparatively smaller build. On the basis of food energy required per kilogram of body weight, children and pregnant women are thought to require more food than adults. In patients with fever, basal energy expenditure is increased about 12% for each degree centigrade of fever.

The criteria for an adequate diet are difficult to define because food habits vary from one area to another and from individual to individual. No single diet or individual food is essential for life or health. Also, it is not possible to state that the ideal diet for maximum growth and development would ensure maximum longevity. SEE: *energy expenditure, basal; Nutritive Value of Foods Appendix; Recommended Daily Dietary Allowances Appendix.*

**food trap** SEE: *trap, food.*

**foot** [AS. *fot*] ABBR: ft. The terminal portion of the lower extremity. The bones of the foot include the tarsus, metatarsus, and phalanges. SEE: illus.; *skeleton.*

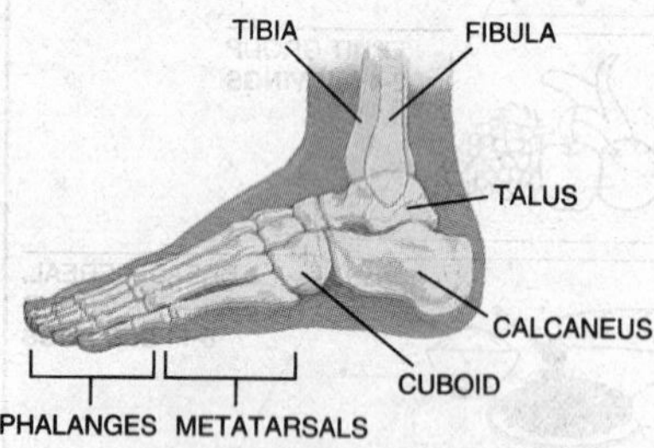


**BONES OF FOOT AND ANKLE**

LEFT FOOT, LATERAL VIEW

***arches of f.*** The four vaulted structures in the foot: the internal (medial) longitudinal, the outer (lateral) longitudinal, and two transverse.

***athlete's f.*** A fungal infection of the foot.

***cleft f.*** A condition in which a cleft extends between the digits to the metatarsal region, usually due to a missing digit and metatarsal.

***immersion f.*** A condition of the feet, resulting from prolonged immersion in cold water, in which pain and inflammation are followed by swelling, discoloration, and numbness.

***Madura f.*** SEE: *Madura foot.*

***march f.*** A spontaneous fracture of one of the metatarsal bones of the foot.

***trench f.*** Degeneration of the skin of the feet due to prolonged exposure to moisture. The condition may be prevented by ensuring that clean, dry socks are worn at all times. The feet do not have to be exposed to cold to develop this condition.

**foot board** A board or similar material placed at the foot end of a patient's bed. It is angled slightly away from the patient and extends up above the mattress. When used properly it helps to prevent footdrop. The patient should be positioned in bed so that when the legs are fully extended the soles of the feet just touch the board.

**foot-candle** An amount of light equivalent to 1 lumen per square foot.

**footdrop** Plantar flexion of the foot due to weakness or paralysis of the anterior muscles of the lower leg. It may occur in any patient who is in bed continuously, esp. if comatose. For bedridden patients, a foot board should be used to prevent footdrop.

**footling presentation** Presentation of the feet foremost in labor.

**footplate** The flat part of the stapes, a bone in the middle ear.

**foot pound** The amount of energy required to lift 1 lb of mass a vertical distance of 1 ft.

**footprint** An impression of the foot, esp. an ink impression used for identification of infants.

**forage** (fō-rŏzh′) [Fr., boring] Creation of a channel through an enlarged prostate by use of an electric cautery. This technique may be used in other tissues.

**foramen** (for-ā′mĕn) *pl.* **foramina** [L.] A passage or opening; an orifice, a communication between two cavities of an organ, or a hole in a bone for passage of vessels or nerves.

***anterior condyloid f.*** The opening above the condyle of the occipital bone. The 12th cranial nerve passes through it.

***anterior sacral f.*** One of the openings on the anterior aspect of the sacrum through which the anterior primary branches of the sacral nerve pass.

***apical f.*** The opening in the end of the root of a tooth through which the blood, lymphatic, and nerve supplies pass to the dental pulp.

***f. of Bochdalek*** The opening through the left side of the diaphragm between the abdomen and thorax. It is the most common site for a diaphragmatic hernia.

***epiploic f.*** The opening connecting the peritoneal cavity to its lesser sac. SYN: *f. of Winslow.*

***ethmoidal f.*** One of the openings in the medial wall of the orbit. The ethmoidal nerve and artery pass through these openings.

***external auditory f.*** The outer auditory meatus, through which sound waves travel to reach the tympanic membrane and the inner ear.

***greater sciatic f.*** The opening bounded by the hip bone, sacrum, and sacrotuberous ligament.

***incisive f.*** One of the small openings sometimes present in the incisive fossa of the hard palate. SYN: *palatine f.*

***infraorbital f.*** The opening in the maxilla through which the infraorbital branch of the maxillary nerve passes.

***internal auditory f.*** The opening in the petrous portion of the temporal bone through which the seventh and eighth cranial nerves pass.

***interventricular f.*** SEE: *Monro's foramen.*

***intervertebral f.*** The opening between adjacent articulated vertebrae for passage of nerves to and from the spinal cord.

***jugular f.*** The opening in the base of the skull through which pass the sigmoid and inferior petrosal sinus and the 9th, 10th, and 11th cranial nerves.

***lesser sciatic f.*** The opening bounded by the hip bone, sacrum, and sacrospinous ligament.

***lingual f.*** A small opening on the lingual surface of the mandible at the midline. It is surrounded by small bony protuberances called genial tubercles. The terminal branches of the mandibular nerve exit the bone through the lingual foramen and innervate the gingiva in the anterior portion of the mandible.

***Magendie's f.*** SEE: *Magendie's foramen.*

***f. magnum*** The opening in the occipital bone through which the spinal cord passes from the brain.

***mandibular f.*** The opening on the medial surface of the mandibular ramus through which the inferior alveolar vessels and nerve enter the mandibular canal.

***mastoid f.*** The opening in the mastoid part of the temporal bone. A small vein passes through it.

***mental f.*** The opening on the ventral surface of the body of the mandible. The mental nerve and artery exit through it for superficial distribution.

***Monro's f.*** SEE: *Monro's foramen.*

***obturator f.*** A large oval foramen below the acetabulum bounded by the pubis and ischium. SEE: *Magendie's foramen.*

***olfactory f.*** An opening in the ethmoid bone for passage of the olfactory nerves.

***optic f.*** An opening in the lesser wing of the sphenoid bone. The optic nerve and ophthalmic artery pass through it.

***f. ovale*** **1.** The opening between the two atria of the fetal heart. It usually closes shortly after birth as a result of hemodynamic changes related to respiration. If it remains open, the defect can be repaired surgically. **2.** The oval opening in the posterior margin of the great sphenoidal wing for the mandibular branch of the trigeminal nerve and the small meningeal artery.

***palatine f.*** Incisive f.

***palatine (greater and lesser) f.*** The openings of the palatine canals through which nerves pass to the mucosa of the hard and soft palate.

***posterior condyloid f.*** The opening behind the condyle of the occipital bone. A small vein passes through it.

***posterior sacral f.*** One of the openings on the posterior aspect of the sacrum through which the posterior primary branches of the sacral nerve pass.

***f. rotundum*** The opening in the great sphenoidal wing through which the maxillary branch of the trigeminal nerve passes.

***Scarpa's f.*** The opening behind the upper medial incisor tooth through which the nasopalatine nerve passes. This opening is not always present.

***sphenopalatine f.*** The opening between the palatine and sphenoid bones. It provides a passage from the pterygopalatine fossa to the nasal cavity for the sphenopalatine artery and nasal nerves.

***spinous f.*** The opening in the spine of the sphenoid bone through which the middle meningeal artery passes.

***supraorbital f.*** An opening sometimes present above the superior border of the orbit of the eye. The supraorbital nerve and vessels pass through it.

***thebesian f.*** One of the openings leading directly into the atria and ventricles of the heart. Very small thebesian veins empty into these openings.

***transverse f.*** An opening in the transverse process of a cervical vertebra.

***vena caval f.*** The opening in the diaphragm through which the vena cava and branches of the right vagus nerve pass.

***vertebral f.*** The large opening between the neural arch and the body of the vertebra that contains the spinal cord.

***f. of Vesalius*** An opening sometimes present in the sphenoid bone medial to the foramen ovale. A vein from the cavernous sinus passes through it.

***Weitbrecht's f.*** The opening in the articular capsule of the shoulder joint.

***f. of Winslow*** Epiploic f.

***zygomatico-orbital f.*** A small opening on the outer surface of the zygomatic bone through which the zygomatic nerve passes. There may be one or several openings.

**Forbes' disease** [Gilbert B. Forbes, U.S. pediatrician, b. 1915] Glycogen storage disease, type III.

**force** An external influence; a push or pull exerted on an object. The metric unit for force is the newton. One newton equals 0.225 lb of force.

***catabolic f.*** Energy produced by metabolism of food.

***centrifugal f.*** The force that impels a thing, or parts of it, outward from the center of rotation. SEE: *centrifuge.*

***electromotive f.*** ABBR: EMF. Energy that causes flow of electricity in a conductor. The energy is measured in volts.

***G f.*** The gravitational constant. In aerospace medicine, the term indicates the forces acting on the human body during acceleration in certain flight maneuvers. Thus a force of 2 positive G means that the aviator is being subjected to a force twice that of gravity with a doubling of weight in that condition (i.e., the force against the seat is 2 G). G force may be in any axis and may be negative or positive.

***maximum inspiratory f.*** ABBR: MIF. The output of the inspiratory muscles against a maximum stimulus, measured in centimeters of negative water pressure. It is measured by having the subject suck on a tube connected to a manometer. Also called *maximum inspiratory pressure; negative inspiratory force.*

***reserve f.*** The energy available above

that required for normal functioning of the heart.

***unit of f.*** An arbitrary measure of a certain amount of force. For example, a dyne is the amount of force acting continuously on a mass of 1 g that will accelerate the mass 1 cm per second per second.

**forced expiratory time** ABBR: FET. The time required to forcibly exhale a specified volume of air from the lung.

**forced expiratory volume** ABBR: FEV. The volume of air that can be expired after a full inspiration. The expiration is done as quickly as possible and the volume measured at precise times; at 1/2, 1, 2, and 3 sec. This provides valuable information concerning the ability to expel air from the lungs.

**forceps** (for′sěps) [L.] Pincers for holding, seizing, or extracting. There are many distinct types of forceps, varying according to the operation for which they are intended. In obstetrics, forceps application is classified according to the position of the fetal head when the forceps are applied (i.e., outlet forceps, low forceps, and midforceps). SEE: *station.*

***alligator f.*** Sturdy toothed forceps with a double clamp.

***Allis f.*** Forceps with curved, serrated edges. They are used to grasp tissue firmly.

***artery f.*** Forceps for holding ends of an artery to perform ligation.

***axis-traction f.*** Obstetrical forceps fitted with a handle that makes it possible to provide traction in line with the direction in which the head must be moved.

***bone f.*** Forceps for cutting bone and removing bone fragments.

***capsule f.*** Forceps for removing the capsule of the lens of the eye during cataract surgery.

***Chamberlen f.*** The original obstetrical forceps, named after the inventor Peter Chamberlen (1560–1631) or his son Peter (1601–1683). They kept their development secret until Hugh Chamberlen (1664–1726) disclosed it.

***clamp f.*** Any forceps with an automatic lock.

***dental f.*** Forceps of varying shapes for grasping teeth during extraction procedures.

***dressing f.*** Forceps for general use in dressing wounds and removing dead tissue and drainage tubes.

***Halsted's f.*** Mosquito f.

***Magill f.*** SEE: *Magill forceps.*

***mosquito f.*** A very small, delicately pointed hemostat. SYN: *Halsted's f.*

***needle f.*** Forceps for grasping and holding a needle.

***obstetrical f.*** Forceps used to extract the fetal head from the pelvis during delivery. They serve the dual purpose of allowing withdrawal force to be applied to the fetal head and protecting the head during the passage.

***rongeur f.*** Forceps used for cutting bone.

***tissue f.*** Forceps with tiny teeth for grasping delicate tissues.

***towel f.*** Forceps for clipping towels to the skin surrounding the site of the operative wound.

**forcipate** (for′sĭ-pāt) [L. *forceps,* tongs] Shaped like forceps.

**Fordyce-Fox disease** (for′dīs-fŏks′) [John Fordyce, U.S. dermatologist, 1858–1925; George Henry Fox, U.S. dermatologist, 1846–1937] A chronic pruritic papular eruption of areas of the skin that contain apocrine sweat glands. The intraepidermal ducts of the apocrine glands become obstructed and eventually rupture. The disease occurs mostly in persons 13 to 35 years of age and about 10 times more frequently in women than men. It does not occur before puberty. SYN: *Fox-Fordyce disease; miliaria, apocrine.*

TREATMENT: Several agents, including estrogens, corticosteroids, and topical tretinoin cream, have been used, but with little benefit.

**Fordyce's disease** (for′dī-sěs) [John Fordyce] Enlarged ectopic sebaceous glands in the mucosa of the mouth and genitals. They appear as small yellow spots, called Fordyce's spots. They are asymptomatic and are present in most people.

**Fordyce's spots** SEE: *Fordyce's disease.*

**forearm** [AS. *fore,* in front, + *arm,* arm] The portion of the arm between the elbow and wrist.

**forebrain** [″ + *bregen,* brain] The anterior portion of the brain of the embryo. SYN: *prosencephalon.*

**forefinger** The first (index) finger.

**forefoot** The part of the foot in front of the tarsometatarsal joint.

**foregut** [″ + *gut,* a pouring] The first part of the embryonic digestive tube from which the pharynx, esophagus, stomach, and duodenum are formed. SYN: *protogaster.*

**forehead** [AS. *forheafod*] The anterior part of the head below the hairline and above the eyes. SYN: *frons.*

**foreign body** Anything present at a site where it would not normally be found. Slivers, cinders, dirt, or small objects may lodge in the skin, ears, eyes, or nose or may be taken internally. If not removed, they may cause unsightly marks or tattooing of the skin and inflammation and infection of the tissue involved.

FIRST AID: *In skin:* The areas involved are cleaned carefully. Foreign material can be removed carefully piece by piece or by vigorous swabbing with gauze or a brush and a soapy solution. A sterile dressing should be used.

For removal of a small foreign body, the area is cleaned first with mild soap and warm water. A clean needle can be sterilized by heating it to a dull or bright red in a flame; this can be done with a single match. Because both ends of the needle get hot, it is wise to hold the far end in a nonconductor such as a fold of paper or a cork. The needle is allowed to cool. A black deposit on its surface should be disregarded; it is sterile carbon and does not interfere with the procedure. The needle is introduced at right angles to the direction of the sliver, and the sliver is lifted out. Most people attempt to stick the needle in the direction of the foreign body and consequently thrust many times before they manage to lift the sliver out. When the sliver is removed, an antiseptic is applied and the wound covered with a sterile dressing. Tetanus antitoxin or a tetanus booster may be required, depending on the history of immunization.

*In the ear:* Water is not introduced if any vegetable matter is in the ear because it may push the foreign body further into the ear or cause it to swell and become firmly embedded. A globule of ordinary glue can be placed on the end of a match stick or an applicator, gently introduced until it touches the foreign body, and removed gently.

If an insect is in the ear, loud buzzing, pain, and dizziness may result. The ear should be flooded with warm oil or water to let the insect float out.

*In the vagina:* A great variety of foreign bodies may be present in the vagina, esp. in children and in the insane. Also, it is possible to forget to remove a vaginal tampon, pessary, or contraceptive diaphragm. The treatment is to remove the foreign body. Antibiotic therapy is not usually necessary.

*In wounds:* Foreign bodies are often present in wounds. Generally they should be left undisturbed if a surgeon is available within a short time. If the foreign body is large, it might be embedded in large blood vessels or muscles. Removing it might result in much loss of blood or might break off splinters, rust particles, or dirt. Within a few moments, blood and the natural reaction of swelling would tend to fill in the wound and cover this foreign material, making it exceedingly difficult for the physician to care for the patient. Therefore it is much wiser to leave a large foreign body in position and obtain the services of a physician promptly.

**foreign body reaction** A localized inflammatory response to the presence of a foreign object in the skin or a body cavity.

**forelock** A lock of hair that grows on the forehead.

***white f.*** A white tuft of hair that grows on the forehead. It is associated with Waardenburg syndrome.

**forensic** (for-ĕn′sĭk) [L. *forensis,* public] Pert. to the law; legal.

**foreplay** Fondling of the sex partner to produce mutual sexual arousal and pleasure prior to intercourse.

**foreskin** [As. *fore,* in front, + O. Norse *skinn,* skin] The prepuce, the loose skin at and covering the end of the penis or clitoris like a hood. Excision of the prepuce constitutes circumcision. Smegma praeputii is secreted by Tyson's glands and collects under the foreskin. SEE: *circumcision.*

**forewaters** (for′wăt-ĕrz) The thin mucus secretion discharged from the vagina during pregnancy. It is produced by the uterine glands and is considered normal.

**forgetting** Inability to remember something previously known or learned. SEE: *memory.*

**fork** An elongated instrument that splits at the end to form two or more prongs.

***tuning f.*** **1.** A device that vibrates when struck at the forked end and thus can be heard and felt. It is used in testing the sensations of hearing, including bone conduction and vibration. **2.** A fork that vibrates at 256 cycles per second is suitable for use in hearing tests.

**form** The distinctive size, shape, and external appearance of anything.

***arch f.*** The shape of the dental arch when viewed in the horizontal plane.

**formaldehyde** (for-măl′dĕ-hīd) HCOH. A colorless, pungent, irritant gas commonly made by oxidation of methyl alcohol, the simplest member of the aldehyde group. An aqueous solution of 37% formaldehyde (formalin) is used as a preservative. This chemical has been shown to be carcinogenic in certain animals and may be carcinogenic in humans.

ACTION/USES: Formaldehyde is used as a disinfectant, preservative, or fumigant. A 10% solution is useful as an astringent. A 1% or 2% solution is used for cleansing dishes, instruments, or fabrics. Formaldehyde is a powerful disinfectant, esp. in gas form, because of its penetrating power, but it is active only in the presence of abundant moisture. A 1% to 2% solution is germicidal, but the action may require 20 to 30 min. Formaldehyde hardens tissues and is often used in histology for tissue preservation. It has a similar hardening effect on living skin; it is very irritating to mucous membranes and produces reddening, inflammation, and necrosis if applied repeatedly or continuously. It is sometimes used in soap for disinfection of the hands. A 10% solution is used for sterilizing feces, urine, and sputum; 5% to 10% is used for clothing and towels. SEE: *aldehyde; fumigation.*

**formaldehyde poisoning** Poisoning caused by ingestion of formaldehyde.

SYMPTOMS: Symptoms include local irritation of the eyes, nose, mouth, throat, respiratory and gastrointestinal tracts, and central nervous system, causing vertigo, stupor, abdominal pain, convulsions, unconsciousness, and renal damage. SEE: *Poisons and Poisoning Appendix.*

FIRST AID: Administration of 0.2% ammonia water changes formaldehyde into methenamine. This solution is given with large amounts of milk, water, and egg white. Then gastric lavage is used or vomiting induced. After that, milk is left in the stomach. Morphine may be needed for pain. Acidosis is treated with sodium bicarbonate. Shock and respiratory distress are treated as needed.

**formalin** (for'mă-lĭn) An aqueous solution of 37% formaldehyde. SEE: *aldehyde.*

**formate** (for'māt) A salt of formic acid.

**formatio** (for-mā'shē-ō) *pl.* **formationes** [L.] A structure with definite arrangement and shape.

***f. reticularis*** The dorsal part of the medulla oblongata.

**formation 1.** A structure, shape, or figure. **2.** The giving of form or shape to, or the development of, a structure.

***reticular f.*** A meshed structure formed of gray matter and interlacing fibers of white matter found in the medulla oblongata between the pyramids and the floor of the fourth ventricle of the brain. It is also present in the spinal cord, midbrain, and pons. Fibers from this structure are important in controlling or influencing alertness, waking, sleeping, and various reflexes. They are thought to activate the cerebral cortex independently of specific sensory or other neural systems. Thus reticular formation is part of the reticular activating (alerting) system.

**forme fruste** (form froost) *pl.* **formes frustes** [Fr., defaced] An aborted or incomplete form of disease arrested before running its course. Thus the disease appears in an atypical and indefinite form.

**formic** [L. *formica,* ant] Pert. to ants or to formic acid.

**formic acid** HCOOH. A clear, pungent liquid obtained from the oxidation of formaldehyde or wood alcohol. Originally it was obtained by distilling the bodies of red ants. It is the cause of the pain and swelling resulting from the bites or stings of certain insects.

**formic aldehyde** Formaldehyde.

**formication** A sensation as of insects creeping on the body; a form of paresthesia. This is one of the more common side effects of cocaine withdrawal.

**formiciasis** (for"mĭs-ī'ă-sĭs) [L. *formica,* ant, + Gr. *-iasis,* condition] Irritation caused by ant bites.

**formilase** (for'mĭ-lās) An enzyme that catalyzes conversion of acetic acid to formic acid.

**formiminoglutamic acid** ABBR: FIGLU. A chemical intermediate in the metabolism of histidine to glutamic acid. Folacin, $FH_4$, is an essential coenzyme for this reaction. If there is a deficiency of folic acid, excess amounts of formiminoglutamic acid appear in the urine.

**formol** (for'mŏl) Formaldehyde solution. SEE: *formalin.*

**formula** [L., a little form] **1.** A rule prescribing ingredients and proportions for the preparation of a compound. **2.** In chemistry, a symbolic expression of the constitution of a molecule. It consists of letters, each denoting one atom of one element, with subscripted numbers denoting the number of atoms present. Water, or $H_2O$, consists of two molecules of the element hydrogen and one of oxygen. It may also be written HOH or H—O—H.

Collections of atoms that constitute a group by themselves (radical) are often separated by periods or parentheses. In this case, figures prefixed or appended to the parentheses, or prefixed to an expression contained within periods, apply to all the symbols embraced by the parentheses or periods. In all other cases, a figure prefixed to a symbolic expression for a molecule, such as a coefficient in an algebraic formula, is a multiplier of all the symbols following.

***Arneth's f.*** A method of estimating the number of immature leukocytes by means of an elaborate differential blood count, on the basis of their shape and the number of lobes in the nucleus. It is seldom used.

***chemical f.*** SEE: *formula* (2).

***dental f.*** SEE: *dental formula.*

***empirical f.*** The formula of a compound that shows the atoms and their numbers in a molecule, as $H_2O$.

***molecular f.*** The chemical formula indicating the elements and the number of each present, but providing no information concerning their two- or three-dimensional arrangements in the formula. SEE: *stereochemical f.*

***official f.*** A formula in a pharmacopeia.

***spatial f.*** Stereochemical f.

***stereochemical f.*** A method of depicting chemical formulas so that the elements and their number are known as well as their position in space in relation to each other. SYN: *spatial f.*

***structural f.*** A formula of a compound that shows the relationship of the atoms in a molecule. The atoms are shown joined by valence bonds (e.g., H—O—H).

**formulary** [L. *formula,* a little form] A book of formulas.

***National F.*** ABBR: NF. A book that provides standards and specifications for drugs. Previously issued by the American Pharmaceutical Association, it is now published by the U.S. Pharmacopeial Convention, Inc.

**formyl** The radical of formic acid, HCO.

**fornicate 1.** [L. *fornicatus*] Arched or vaultlike. **2.** [L. *fornicari*] To have sexual intercourse with a partner to whom one is not married.

**fornication** Sexual intercourse between unmarried partners.

**fornices** (for'nĭ-sēz) [L.] Pl. of fornix.

**fornicolumn** [L. *fornix,* arch, + *columna,* column] The anterior pillar of the fornix uteri.

**fornicommissure** (for-nĭ-kŏm'ĭ-sūr) [" + *commissura,* a joining together] The commissure or body of the fornix uteri.

**fornix** [L., arch] **1.** A fibrous vaulted band connecting the cerebral lobes. **2.** Any vaultlike or arched body.

***f. conjunctivae*** The loose folds connecting the palpebral and bulbar conjunctivae.

***f. uteri*** The anterior and posterior spaces into which the upper vagina is divided. These recesses are formed by protrusion of the cervix uteri into the vagina. SYN: *f. vaginae.*

***f. vaginae*** F. uteri.

**Fort Bragg fever** [Fort Bragg, North Carolina, a U.S. military base] Pretibial fever.

**fortification spectrum** The appearance of a dark patch with a zigzag outline in the visual field, causing a temporary blindness in that portion of the eye. SYN: *teichopsia.*

**fortify** In food science technology, to add a substance to food to enhance its value as a food.

**Foscarnet** A drug used for treatment of cytomegalovirus (CMV) retinitis. CMV retinitis is present in about 20% of people with AIDS.

**Foshay's test** [Lee Foshay, U.S. physician, 1896–1961] Intradermal injection of a suspension of killed *Francisella tularensis,* the causative agent of tularemia. The appearance of an area of erythema at the injection site is considered a positive reaction.

**fossa** (fŏs′ă) *pl.* **fossae** [L.] A furrow or shallow depression.

***amygdaloid f.*** The depression containing the tonsil.

***articular f. of mandible*** The depression on the inferior surface of the temporal bone that accepts the condyle of the mandible. SYN: *articular f. of temporal bone; glenoid f.* (2); *mandibular f.*

***articular f. of temporal bone*** Articular f. of mandible.

***axillary f.*** The armpit (axilla).

***canine f.*** The wide, shallow depression on the external surface of the maxilla superolateral to the canine tooth. It serves as the origin of the levator anguli oris muscle.

***cerebral f.*** Any of several depressions on the inside floor of the cranium. SYN: *cranial f.*

***Claudius' f.*** The triangular area harboring the ovary.

***condylar f.*** The depression behind the occipital epicondyle.

***coronoid f.*** The depression on the anterior surface of the lower end of the humerus. During full flexion of the forearm, the coronoid process of the ulna fits into the depression.

***cranial f.*** Cerebral f.

***digastric f.*** The depression behind the lower margin of the mandible at the side of the symphysis menti. The anterior belly of the digastric muscle attaches here.

***epigastric f.*** The pit of the inside of the stomach.

***ethmoid f.*** SYN: *olfactory groove.*

***glenoid f.*** **1.** The depression on the scapula that provides space for articulation with the head of the humerus. **2.** The fossa of the temporal bone that articulates with the condyle of the mandible.

***hyaloid f.*** The depression on the anterior surface of the vitreous body of the eye. The lens is located there.

***hypophyseal f.*** The deep depression in the sphenoid bone in which the pituitary gland rests. SYN: *pituitary f.; sella turcica.*

***iliac f.*** One of the concavities of the iliac bones of the pelvis.

***incisive f.*** The depression on the anterior surface of the body of the maxilla medial to the root of the canine incisor tooth.

***infratemporal f.*** The shallow depression under and medial to the zygomatic arch. It contains the muscles of mastication, the first two parts of the maxillary artery, the pterygoid venous plexus, and branches of the mandibular nerve, the third division of the trigeminal nerve.

***intercondyloid f.*** The depression on the inferior surface of the femur between the femoral condyles. The cruciate ligaments pass through it.

***interpeduncular f.*** The deep groove in the anterior surface of the midbrain, between the cerebral peduncles. The third cranial nerve emerges here.

***ischiorectal f.*** The space on either side of the lower end of the rectum and anal canal. It is bounded laterally by the obturator internus muscle and the tuberosity of the ischium, medially by the levator ani and coccygeus muscles, and posteriorly by the gluteus maximus muscle.

***jugular f.*** The depression in the petrosal portion of the temporal bone for the jugular vein.

***lacrimal f.*** The hollow of the frontal bone that holds the lacrimal gland.

***lenticular f.*** The depression in the anterior surface of the vitreous for reception of the crystalline lens.

***mandibular f.*** The depression in the temporal bone into which the condyle of the mandible fits.

***mastoid f.*** The small triangular area between the posterior wall of the acoustic meatus and the posterior root of the zygomatic process of the temporal bone.

***nasal f.*** The cavity between the anterior opening to the nose and the nasopharynx.

***navicular f.*** The depression between the vulva and fourchette.

***olecranon f.*** The depression on the posterior surface of the lower end of the humerus. During full extension of the forearm, the olecranon process of the ulna fits into this depression.

***f. ovalis*** The opening in the fascia of the thigh through which the large saphenous vein passes.

***f. ovalis cordis*** The remnant of the embryonic foramen ovale in the right cardiac atrium.

***ovarian f.*** The depression in the parietal peritoneum of the pelvis that contains the ovary.

***piriform fossae*** The anatomical pockets of flesh on the lateral aspects of the pharynx.

***pituitary f.*** Hypophyseal f.

***popliteal f.*** The soft tissue depression posterior to the knee.

***Rosenmüller's f.*** The depression in the pharynx posterior to the opening of the eustachian tube.

***sphenomaxillary f.*** SEE: *pterygopalatine fossa.*

***sublingual f.*** A shallow depression on the inner surface of the body of the mandible above the anterior part of the mylohyoid ridge. It is occupied by the major salivary gland in the area, the sublingual gland.

***submandibular f.*** An oblong depression between the mylohyoid ridge and the inferior border of the medial surface of the body of the mandible. It is occupied by the submandibular gland. These were previously referred to as the submaxillary fossa and submaxillary gland.

***subpyramidal f.*** A depression in the inferior wall of the middle ear. It is inferior to the round window and posterior to the pyramid.

***supraspinous f.*** The concave triangular area above the spinous process of the posterior surface of the clavicle.

***f. supratonsillaris*** The space between the anterior and posterior pillars of the fauces above the tonsil.

***temporal f.*** The depression on the side of the skull below the temporal lines. It is deep to the zygomatic arch and continuous with the infratemporal fossa.

**fossae** (fŏs′ē) [L.] Pl. of fossa.

**fossette** (fŏ-sĕt′) [Fr.] **1.** A small depression or fossa. **2.** A small but deep corneal ulcer.

**fossula** (fŏs′ū-lă) A small fossa.

**foster care** The care of individuals in a group or private home. They are usually abandoned, orphaned, or delinquent children who are the responsibility of a governmental agency that provides the funds for their care.

***adult f.c.*** SEE: *adult foster care.*

**Fothergill's disease** (fŏth′ĕr-gĭlz) [John Fothergill, Brit. physician, 1712–1780] **1.** Scarlatina anginosa, an ulcerative sore throat present in severe scarlet fever. **2.** Trigeminal neuralgia.

**foulage** (foo-lŏzh′) [Fr.] Massage by kneading with pressure on the muscles.

**foundation, denture** The area on which a denture rests.

**fourchet, fourchette** (foor-shĕt′) [Fr. *fourchette,* a fork] A tense band or transverse fold of mucous membrane at the posterior commissure of the vagina, connecting the posterior ends of the labia minora. The fossa navicularis, a cul-de-sac anterior to the fourchette, separates it from the hymen. It disappears after defloration or parturition, leaving a more open vulva below and behind. SYN: *frenulum labiorum pudendi.* SEE: *vestibule of vagina.*

**fourth cranial nerve** A small mixed nerve exiting from the dorsal surface of the midbrain. It contains efferent motor fibers to the superior oblique muscle of the eye and afferent sensory fibers conveying proprioceptive impulses from the same muscle. SYN: *trochlear nerve.*

**fovea** (fō′vē-ă) *pl.* **foveae** [L.] A pit or cuplike depression. SEE: *fossa.*

***f. capitis*** The depression on the head of the femur for attachment of the ligamentum teres.

***f. centralis retinae*** In the eye, the pit in the middle of the macula lutea that contains only cones.

**foveate** (fō′vē-āt) [L. *foveatus*] Pitted; having depressions.

**foveation** (fō″vē-ā′shŭn) Pitting, as in smallpox.

**foveola** (fō-vē′ō-lă) *pl.* **foveolae** [L., little pit] A minute pit or depression.

**Fowler's position** [George R. Fowler, U.S. surgeon, 1848–1906] A semi-sitting position. The head of an adjustable bed can be elevated to the desired height to produce angulation of the body, usually 45° to 60°. The knees may or may not be bent. A wedge support can be used to elevate the patient's head and back if an adjustable bed is not available. The position is used to facilitate breathing and drainage and for the comfort of the bedridden patient while eating or talking.

NOTE: The hips (knees) may or may not be flexed in this position, which has three variations: high (sitting upright in bed), regular (head or torso elevated 45° or more), and low or semi-low (head and torso elevated to 30°).

**Fox-Fordyce disease** SEE: *Fordyce-Fox disease.*

**foxglove** (fŏks′glŏv) A common name for the plant *Digitalis purpurea,* from which the drug digitalis is obtained. Foxglove was mentioned in the writings of Welsh physicians in 1250 and by William Withering in a book published in 1785.

**Fr** Symbol for the element francium.

**fraction** [L. *fractio,* act of breaking] In biological chemistry, the separable part of a substance such as blood or plasma.

***f. of inspired oxygen*** ABBR: $FIO_2$. The concentration of oxygen in the inspired air, esp. that supplied as supplemental oxygen by mask or catheter. Concentrations of oxygen greater than 50% are toxic if administered for other than brief periods.

**fractional test meal** Extended examination of the stomach contents. First the residual contents are removed and then the test meal is given. After the meal, samples are removed every 15 min for 2 hr, examined, and submitted for chemical tests. Free hydrochloric acid, bile, blood, starch, mucus, and the total of acids are analyzed. Free hydrochloric and total acids are normally present in small amounts. In peptic ulcers there is a high acid curve. There is a low curve in carcinoma, and an absence of acid in pernicious anemia.

**fractionation** In radiation therapy, the process of spreading the total required treatment dose over an extended period.

**fracture** [L. *fractura,* break] **1.** Sudden breaking of a bone. **2.** A break in a bone. SEE: illus.

CAUSES: *Pathological:* In certain diseases and conditions such as osteomalacia, syphilis, and osteomyelitis, bones break spontaneously without trauma. *Direct violence:* The bone is broken directly at the spot where the force was applied, as in fracture of the tibia by being run over. *Indirect violence:* The bone is fractured by a force applied at a distance from the site of fracture and transmitted to the fractured bone, as fracture of the clavicle by falling on the outstretched hand. *Muscular contraction:* The bone is broken by a sudden violent contraction of the muscles.

SIGNS: Signs include loss of the power of movement, pain with acute tenderness over the site of fracture, swelling and bruising, deformity and possible shortening, unnatural mobility, and crepitus or grating that is heard when the ends of the bone rub together. It is important not to try to obtain these last two signs. Radiography should be used to find the type of fracture and the exact position of the bone fragments.

FIRST AID: In simple fractures, the limb or part must be kept immovable by means of splints. If proper wooden, plastic, or metal splints are unavailable, they may be improvised with magazines or folded newspapers. Clothing should not be removed unless there is dangerous hemorrhage. If it is necessary to remove clothing, the cloth should be cut away so as to disturb the area as little as possible.

If an upper extremity is fractured, it should be supported in a sling, and the patient may then walk. If a lower limb is injured, the patient should remain supine and make no attempt to walk.

TREATMENT: The physician reduces the fracture (places the fragments in proper position). The bone is kept in position by means of a cast until union has taken place. Then the limb is restored to complete function by physical therapy and exercise.

In compound fractures, any bleeding must be arrested before the fracture is treated. Open reduction may be required. The wound is then washed and cleaned with sterile saline. If the area is grossly contaminated, mild soap solution may be used provided it is thoroughly washed away with generous amounts of sterile saline. When the wound is clean, a sterile dressing is secured by a bandage. The bone may then be immobilized by external fixation until the wound heals.

Skeletal traction may be used instead of a cast or external fixator for certain fractures, such as femoral shaft fractures. Pins are placed in the bone and the bone ends are held in place by a system of pulleys and weights until bony union occurs.

If the bone does not heal, a weak electric current applied to the bone ends (bone stimulation) may promote healing.

---

Caution: First aid for fractures of the spine requires extreme care with respect to moving the patient. Unnecessary or improper movement may injure or even transect the spinal cord.

---

NURSING IMPLICATIONS: The fracture is immobilized by splinting the area, including the joints above and below the site. An open fracture is covered with a sterile or clean dressing. The extremity is elevated to minimize edema, and the patient's overall condition is monitored for shock and other complications. Prescribed analgesics are administered, and realistic reassurance is offered.

The patient is prepared physically and psychologically for closed or open reduction and fixation of the fracture. Vascular and neurological status of the limb distal to the fracture are monitored after immobilization with traction, casting, or fixation devices.

The patient is evaluated for fat embolism after long bone fractures, for infection in open fractures, for excessive blood loss and hypovolemic shock, and for delayed union or nonunion. The patient should report signs of impaired circulation (skin coldness, numbness, tingling, discoloration, and changes in mobility) and is taught the correct use of assistive devices (slings, crutches, walker). SEE: *Nursing Diagnoses Appendix.*

***avulsion f.*** Tearing of a piece of bone away from the main bone by the force of muscular contraction.

***Bennett's f.*** An intra-articular fracture at the base of the first metacarpal with subluxation of the carpometacarpal joint due to traction of the abductor pollicis longus muscle on the first metacarpal. This fracture usually requires percutaneous pinning to maintain reduction.

***bimalleolar f.*** A fracture of the medial and lateral malleoli of the ankle joint.

***blow-out f.*** A fracture of the floor of the orbit in which fragments are displaced downward by a blow to the eye.

***boxer's f.*** A fracture of the distal end of the fifth metacarpal with posterior dis-

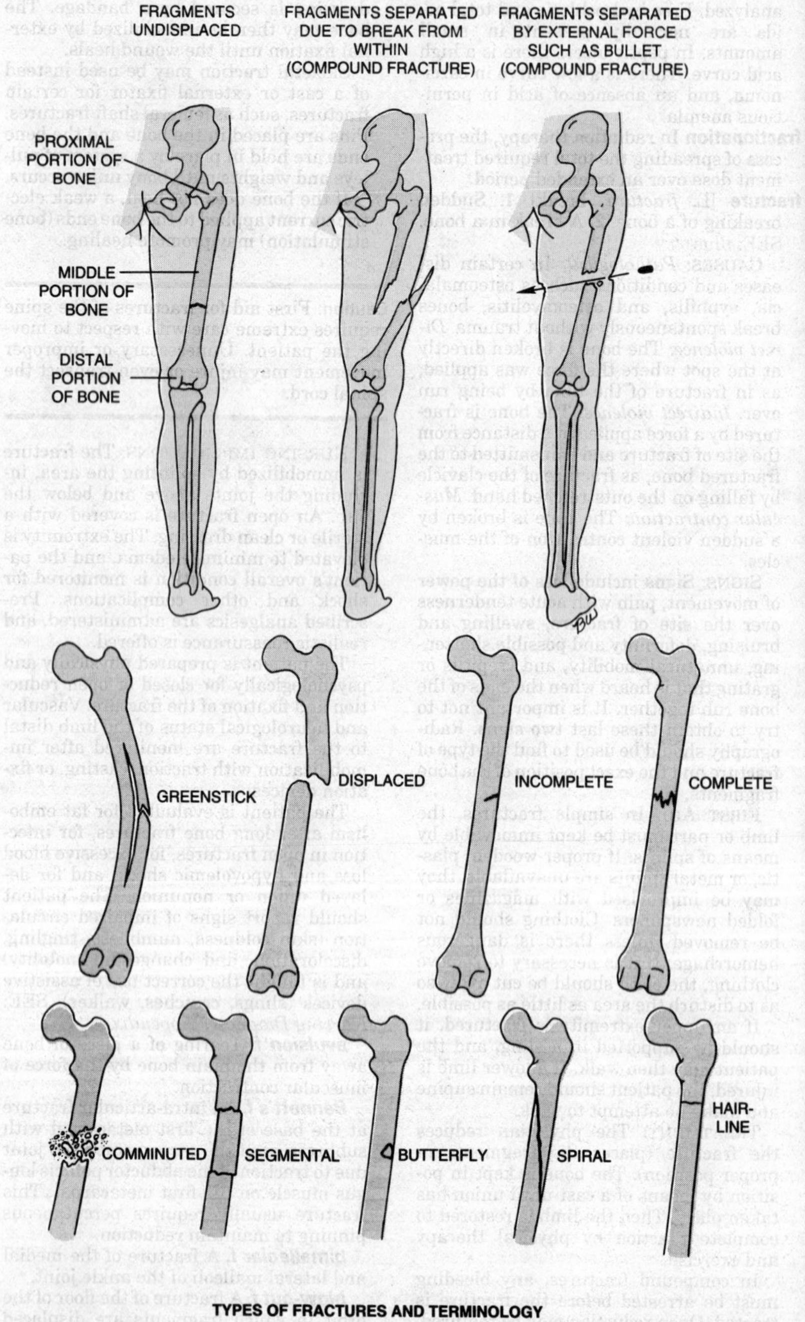

FRAGMENTS UNDISPLACED

FRAGMENTS SEPARATED DUE TO BREAK FROM WITHIN (COMPOUND FRACTURE)

FRAGMENTS SEPARATED BY EXTERNAL FORCE SUCH AS BULLET (COMPOUND FRACTURE)

PROXIMAL PORTION OF BONE

MIDDLE PORTION OF BONE

DISTAL PORTION OF BONE

GREENSTICK

DISPLACED

INCOMPLETE

COMPLETE

COMMINUTED

SEGMENTAL

BUTTERFLY

SPIRAL

HAIR-LINE

TYPES OF FRACTURES AND TERMINOLOGY

placement of the proximal structures.

***clay shoveler's f.*** A fracture of the base of the spinous process of the lower cervical spine associated with sudden flexion of the neck. It may also be caused by direct trauma.

***closed f.*** A fracture of the bone with no skin wound.

***comminuted f.*** A fracture in which the bone is broken or splintered into pieces.

***complete f.*** A fracture in which the bone is completely broken (i.e., neither fragment is connected to the other).

***complicated f.*** A fracture in which the bone is broken and has injured some internal organ, such as a broken rib piercing a lung.

***compound f.*** A fracture in which an external wound leads down to the site of fracture, or fragments of bone protrude through the skin. SYN: *open f.*

***compression f.*** A fracture of a vertebra by pressure along the long axis of the vertebral column.

***depressed f.*** A fracture in which a piece of the skull is broken and driven inward.

***diastatic f.*** A fracture that follows a cranial suture and causes it to separate.

***direct f.*** A fracture at a site where force was applied.

***dislocation f.*** A fracture near a dislocated joint.

***double f.*** Two fractures of the same bone.

***Duverney's f.*** A fracture of the ilium just below the anterior superior spine.

***epiphyseal f.*** A separation of the epiphysis from the bone between the shaft of the bone and its growing end. It occurs only in young patients.

***fatigue f.*** SEE: *stress fracture.*

***fissured f.*** A narrow split in the bone that does not go through to the other side of the bone.

***greenstick f.*** A fracture in which the bone is partially bent and partially broken, as when a green stick breaks. It occurs in children, esp. those with rickets.

***hairline f.*** A minor fracture in which all the portions of the bone are in perfect alignment. The fracture is seen on a radiograph as a very thin line between the two segments that does not extend entirely through the bone. SEE: *stress fracture.*

***hangman's f.*** The fracture produced when judicial hanging is done correctly. At the moment when the dropped victim fully extends the rope, the hangman knot causes fracture dislocation of the upper cervical spine and transection of the spinal cord or medulla. If the knot is not made or applied properly, death is usually due to asphyxia.

***impacted f.*** A fracture in which the bone is broken and one end is wedged into the interior of the other.

***incomplete f.*** A fracture in which the line of fracture does not include the whole bone. SEE: *stress fracture.*

***indirect f.*** A fracture distant from the place where the force was applied.

***intracapsular f.*** A fracture occurring within the capsule of a joint.

***intrauterine f.*** A fracture of a bone in the fetus in utero.

***Jones f.*** A transverse fracture of the proximal diaphysis, approx. three quarters of an inch from the base of the fifth metatarsal. This fracture is commonly confused with an avulsion fracture of the styloid process of the fifth metatarsal. The distinction is important because the true Jones fracture often results in a nonunion.

***lead pipe f.*** A fracture in which the bone is compressed and bent so that one side of the fracture bulges and the other side shows a slight crack.

***LeFort f.*** A fracture of one or more of the facial bones: maxillary, nasal, orbital, or zygomatic.

***march f.*** SEE: *stress fracture.*

***nightstick f.*** A nondisplaced transverse fracture of the ulna resulting from a direct blow.

***nonunion of f.*** SEE: *nonunion.*

***open f.*** Compound f.

***overriding f.*** A fracture in which the ends of the fractured bone slide past each other.

***pathological f.*** A fracture of a diseased or weakened bone produced by a force that would not have fractured a healthy bone. The underlying disease may be metastasis from the primary cancer, cancer of the bone, or osteoporosis.

NURSING IMPLICATIONS: The limbs and joints of at-risk patients are gently and carefully supported when repositioning, exercising, or mobilizing. If such patients fall or are otherwise injured, fracture is considered a potential cause or result.

***ping-pong f.*** A depressed fracture of the skull that resembles the indentation made by pressing firmly on a ping-pong ball.

***Pott's f.*** A fracture of the lower end of the fibula with outward displacement of the ankle and foot. The medial malleolus of the fibula may be fractured.

***pretrochanteric f.*** A fracture that passes through the greater trochanter of the femur.

***Rolando f.*** A comminuted intra-articular fracture of the base of the first metacarpal with distal fragment subluxation. This fracture is similar to a Bennett's fracture but with more comminution.

***simple f.*** A fracture without rupture of ligaments and skin.

***Smith's f.*** SEE: *Colles' fracture.*

***spiral f.*** A fracture that follows a helical line.

***spontaneous f.*** Pathological f.

***stellate f.*** A fracture in which cracks emerge from the central point.

***stress f.*** SEE: *stress fracture.*

***torus f.*** A fracture in which the bony cortex is not broken but is buckled.

***transcervical f.*** A fracture through the neck of the femur.

***transverse f.*** A fracture in which the fracture line is at right angles to the long axis of the bone.

***trimalleolar f.*** A fracture of the lateral and medial malleoli of the ankle joint with an additional fracture of the posterior edge of the distal tibia.

***tripod f.*** A fracture in which the zygoma is separated from its attachment to the maxilla and the temporal and frontal bones.

**fracture dislocation** SEE: *dislocation, fracture.*

**fragile X syndrome** A condition caused by an X-linked mutation associated with a fragile site near the tip of the long arm of the X chromosome. Most males and 30% of females with this syndrome are mentally deficient. This syndrome is the most common inherited cause of mental retardation. Males also develop greatly enlarged testicles (macro-orchidism), usually after puberty, but this change has been reported as early as 5 months of age.

**fragilitas** (fră-jĭl'ĭ-tăs) [L.] Fragility.

**fragility** A state of brittleness.

***capillary f.*** A breakdown of capillaries with hemorrhage into almost any site but most noticeably in the skin.

***erythrocyte f.*** An increased tendency of red blood cells to rupture when the salt content of the blood is decreased.

***f. of red blood cells*** The tendency of red blood cells to rupture. This is determined by subjecting the cells to different concentrations of saline in laboratory tests.

If red blood cells are placed in distilled water, they swell rapidly and burst because they normally are suspended in a solution of much greater osmotic pressure. This phenomenon is called hemolysis. If they are suspended in a solution of normal saline, the cells retain their normal shape and do not burst. If they are placed in successively weaker solutions of saline, a point is reached at which some of the cells burst and liberate their hemoglobin within a given length of time. Finally, at a given dilution, all the cells have burst within the allotted time, which is usually 2 hr. Normal blood cells begin to hemolyze in about 0.44% saline solution, and complete hemolysis occurs in about 0.35% solution.

**fragment** (frăg'mĕnt) A part broken off a larger entity.

***Fab f.*** A piece or fragment from an antibody that is digested and used by T cells to create antigen-specific receptors.

**fragment antigen binding** ABBR: Fab. A part of the antibody molecule that contains the antigen-binding site. It is obtained by enzymatic hydrolysis of the antibody.

**fragmentation** [L. *fragmentum*, detached part] Breaking up into pieces.

**frail elderly** Older individuals experiencing physical, mental, and emotional disability, any one of which could limit their independence and promote dependency on and require assistance from others. Such disabilities are seen more commonly in those 75 years of age or older.

**frambesia** (frăm-bē'zē-ă) [Fr. *framboise*, raspberry] Yaws.

**frambesioma** (frăm-bē-zē-ō'mă) [" + Gr. *oma*, tumor] The primary lesion of yaws in the form of a protruding nodule. This mother yaw appears at the site of inoculation of the causative agent, *Treponema pertenue.*

**frame** A supporting structure.

***Balkan f.*** A framework that fits over a bed. Weights suspended from the frame and connected through ropes and pulleys are used to produce continuous traction while permitting freedom of motion, thus maintaining desired immobilization of the part being treated.

***Bradford f.*** An oblong frame, about 7 × 3 ft (2.13 × 0.91 m), made of 1-in. (2.5-cm) pipe covered with movable canvas strips that run from one side of the frame to the other. It is used for patients with fractures or disease of the hip or spine, permitting them to urinate and defecate without moving the spine or changing position.

***quadriplegic standing f.*** A device for supporting a patient with all four extremities paralyzed.

***Stryker f.*** SEE: *Stryker frame.*

***trial f.*** An eyeglass frame for holding trial lenses while a person is being fitted for glasses.

**Franceschetti's syndrome** (frăn"chĕs-kĕt'ēz) [Adolphe Franceschetti, Swiss ophthalmologist, 1896–1968] Mandibulofacial dysostosis with hypoplasia of the facial bones, downward angulation of the palpebral fissures, macrostomia, ear defects, and defectively formed extremities. SYN: *Treacher Collins syndrome.*

**Franciscella tularensis** (frăn"sĭ-sĕl'ă too"lă-rĕn'sĭs) [Edward Francis, Tulare County, California] A short, nonmotile, encapsulated, non–spore-forming, gram-negative bacillus that causes tularemia in humans. Formerly classed as *Pasteurella tularensis.*

**francium** (frăn'sē-ŭm) [Named for France, the country in which it was discovered] SYMB: Fr. A radioactive metallic element occurring as a natural isotope. Its atomic number is 87; the atomic weight of the most stable isotope is 233.

**frank** Obvious, esp. in reference to a clinical sign or condition such as blood in the urine, sputum, or feces.

**Frankenhäuser's ganglion** (frăng'kĕn-hoy"zĕrs) [Ferdinand Frankenhäuser, Ger. gynecologist, 1832–1894] A nerve ganglion sometimes found in the lateral walls of the cervix uteri.

**Frankfort horizontal plane** A cephalometric plane joining the anthropometric landmarks of porion and orbitale; the reproducible position of the head when the upper margin of the ear openings and lower margin of the orbit of the eye are horizontal.

**Franklin glasses** [Benjamin Franklin, U.S. statesman and inventor, 1706–1790] Bifocal spectacles.

**Frank-Starling law** In respiratory physiology, the rule stating that cardiac output increases in proportion to the diastolic stretch of heart muscle fibers.

**fraternal twin** One of two offspring that have developed in the uterus at the same time, but are the result of independent fertilization of two ova. SYN: *dizygotic twin*. SEE: *monozygotic twin*.

**fratricide** (frăt′rĭ-sīd″) [L. *fratricidium*] Murder of one's brother or sister.

**Fraunhofer's lines** (frown′hōf-ĕrz) [Joseph von Fraunhofer, Ger. optician, 1787–1826] Absorption bands or lines seen in a spectrum, caused by the absorption of groups of light rays in their passage through solids, liquids, or gases.

**FRC** *functional residual capacity*.

**F.R.C.P.** *Fellow of the Royal College of Physicians*.

**F.R.C.P.(C.)** *Fellow of the Royal College of Physicians of Canada*.

**F.R.C.S.** *Fellow of the Royal College of Surgeons*.

**F.R.C.S.(C.)** *Fellow of the Royal College of Surgeons of Canada*.

**freckle** (frĕk′l) [O. Norse *freknur*] A small local brownish or yellowish pigmentation of the skin due to an accumulation of melanin. The likely cause is exposure to sun, which usually stimulates melanin production. SYN: *ephelis; lentigo*.

***Hutchinson's f.*** A noninvasive malignant melanoma.

**free association** **1.** The trend of thoughts when one is not under mental restraint or direction. **2.** The procedure in psychoanalysis that requires the patient to speak his or her thought flow aloud, word for word, without censorship.

**free base** A form of cocaine used by addicts. It is prepared by alkalinizing the hydrochloride salt, extracting it with an organic solvent such as ether, and then heating the extract to 90°C. The inhaled material is rapidly absorbed from the lung. SEE: *cocaine hydrochloride; crack; freebasing*.

**freebasing** The inhalation of a form of cocaine called free base. SEE: *cocaine hydrochloride; crack*.

**free medical clinic** A clinic that is established by the community rather than by a hospital and that provides free medical care. Such clinics are unusual in that their purpose is to deal with illnesses and conditions that are both medical and social.

**free radical** A molecule containing an odd number of electrons. These molecules contain an open bond or a half bond and are highly reactive. The odd electron is represented in the chemical formula by a dot. If two radicals react, both are eliminated; if a radical reacts with a nonradical, another free radical is produced. This type of event may become a chain reaction. In ischemic injury to tissues (e.g., myocardial infarction), free radical production may play an important role at certain stages in the progression of the injury.

The body has developed methods of defending against the harmful effects of free radicals. Superoxide dismutases, enzymes in mitochondria, and antioxidants are effective in counteracting the harmful effects of free radicals. SEE: *antioxidant; oxidative stress; superoxide; superoxide dismutase*.

**freeze-drying** Preservation of tissue by rapidly freezing the specimen and then dehydrating it in a high vacuum. SYN: *lyophilization*.

**freezing** [AS. *freosan*] **1.** Passing from a liquid to a solid state due to heat loss. **2.** Becoming stiff, rigid, and inflexible from cold. Frigidity of a limb can result from exposure to cold. Freezing is most common in the debilitated, the exhausted, and alcoholics who fall asleep in a location exposed to extreme cold. SEE: *frostbite; windchill factor*.

SYMPTOMS: Symptoms include pallor, cyanosis, and coldness. Unconsciousness usually develops.

FIRST AID: The frozen part is protected with a cradle and dry heat is applied at room temperature. Alternatively, the patient may be placed in tepid bath water. Sudden applications of intense heat are contraindicated; however, rapid rewarming in warm water at a temperature of 40° to 42°C (104° to 108°F) is mandatory. This is done until thawing is complete. After rewarming is accomplished, the patient receives analgesics for pain, tetanus prophylaxis, nonsteroidal anti-inflammatory agents, and intravenous penicillin for 48 to 72 hr.

**freezing mixture** A combination of 5 oz (150 ml) each of ammonium chloride and potassium nitrate and one part water, used for ice bags.

**freezing point** The temperature at which liquids freeze.

**Freiberg's infraction** (frī′bĕrgz) [Albert Henry Freiberg, U.S. surgeon, 1868–1940] Osteochondritis of the head of the second metatarsal bone of the foot.

**fremitus** (frĕm′ĭ-tŭs) [L.] Vibratory tremors, esp. those felt through the chest wall by palpation. Varieties include vocal or tactile, friction, hydatid, rhonchal or bronchial, cavernous on succussion, pleural, pericardial, tussive, and thrills. SEE: *palpation; thrill*.

***hydatid f.*** A tremulous sensation felt on palpating a hydatid tumor.

***tactile f.*** The vibration or thrill felt while the patient is speaking and the hand is held against the chest.

***tussive f.*** Vibrations felt when the hand is held against the chest when the patient coughs.

***vocal f.*** Vibrations of the voice transmitted to the ear during auscultation of the chest of a person speaking. In determining vocal fremitus, the following precautions should be observed: Symmetric parts of the chest are palpated with firm pressure. For comparison, the same pressure is used on both sides. The hands are applied as nearly parallel to the ribs as possible; the fremitus normally increases over the right apex. It is decreased in pleural effusions (air, pus, blood, serum, or lymph), emphysema, pulmonary collapse from an obstructed bronchus, pulmonary edema, and morbid growths of the lung.

**French scale** A system used to indicate the outer diameter of catheters and sounds. Each unit on the scale is approximatey equivalent to one third mm; thus a 21 French sound is 7 mm in diameter.

**frenectomy** (frē-nĕk′tō-mē) [L. *fraenum,* bridle, + Gr. *ektome,* excision] Surgical cutting of any frenum, usually the frenum of the tongue.

**frenotomy** (frē-nŏt′ō-mē) [″ + Gr. *tome,* incision] Division of any frenum, esp. for tongue-tie.

**frenuloplasty** (frĕn′ū-lō-plăs″tē) [″ + Gr. *plassein,* to form] Surgical correction of an abnormally attached frenulum.

**frenulum** (frĕn′ū-lŭm) *pl.* **frenula** [L., a little bridle] **1.** A small frenum. SYN: *vinculum.* **2.** A small fold of white matter on the upper surface of the anterior medullary velum extending to the corpora quadrigemina of the brain.

***f. clitoridis*** The union of the inner parts of the labia minora on the undersurface of the clitoris.

***f. of ileocecal valve*** The prolongation of the two lips of the ileocolic valve around the inner wall of the colon.

***f. labiorum pudendi*** The fold of membrane connecting the posterior ends of the labia minora.

***f. linguae*** F. of the tongue.

***f. of the lips, f. labialis oris*** The fold of mucous membrane extending from the middle of the inner surface of the lip to the alveolar mucosa. It is seen in both the upper and lower jaws.

***f. preputii*** The frenulum that unites the foreskin (prepuce) to the glans penis.

***f. of the tongue*** The frenulum that attaches the lower side of the tongue to the floor of the buccal cavity. At birth this may be tight, a condition called tongue-tie. SYN: *f. linguae.*

**frenum** (frē′nŭm) *pl.* **frena** [L. *fraenum,* bridle] A fold of mucous membrane that connects two parts, one more or less movable, and checks the movement of this part. SEE: *frenulum.* **frenal,** *adj.*

**frenzy** (frĕn′zē) [ME. *frenesie*] A state of violent mental agitation; maniacal excitement. SEE: *panic.*

**Freon** Trade name of a group of hydrocarbon gases previously used as a refrigerant and propellant in metered dose inhalers.

**frequency** [L. *frequens,* often] **1.** The number of repetitions of a phenomenon in a certain period or within a distinct population, such as the frequency of heartbeat, sound vibrations, or a disease entity. SEE: *incidence.* **2.** The rate of oscillation or alternation in an alternating current circuit, in contradistinction to periodicity in the interruptions or regular variations of current in a direct current circuit. Frequency is computed on the basis of a complete cycle, in which the current rises from zero to a positive maximum, returns to zero, descends to an opposite negative minimum, and returns to zero. **3.** The rate at which uterine contractions occur, measured by the time elapsed between the beginning of one contraction and the beginning of the next.

**F response** In electrodiagnostic study of spinal reflexes, the time required for a stimulus applied to a motor nerve to travel in the opposite direction up the nerve to the spinal cord and return.

**fretum** (frē′tŭm) [L.] A constriction.

**Freud, Sigmund** (froyd) A famous Austrian neurologist and psychoanalyst (1856–1939) whose teachings involved analysis of resistance and transference, and a procedure for investigating mental function by use of free-association dream interpretation. Freud did not consider psychoanalysis to be scientific. He believed that its real purpose was to elucidate the darkest recesses of the mind and soul and to enable individuals to integrate the emotional and intellectual sides of their nature (i.e., the forces of love and death) and to develop better knowledge of self and a level of maturity and peace of mind that would help the individual and others have better lives.

**freudian** (froy′dē-ăn) Pert. to Sigmund Freud's theories of unconscious or repressed libido, or past sex experiences or desires, as the cause of various neuroses, the cure for which is the restoration of such conditions to consciousness through psychoanalysis. SEE: *Freud, Sigmund.*

**freudian slip** [From Freudian psychology] A mistake in speaking or writing that is thought to provide insight into the individual's unconscious thoughts, motives, or wishes.

**Freund's adjuvant** (froynds) [Jules Thomas Freund, Hungarian-born U.S. immunologist, 1890–1960] A mixture of killed microorganisms, usually mycobacteria, in an oil and water emulsion. The material is administered to induce antibody formation. Because the oil retards absorption of the mixture, the antibody response is much greater than if the killed microorganisms were administered alone.

**friable** (frī'ă-b'l) [L. *friabilis*] Easily broken or pulverized.

**friction** [L. *frictio*] Rubbing. In massage, strong circular manipulations are always followed by centripetal stroking. In hydrotherapy, friction is used in drying patients after tonic baths, and in shampoos and drip sheet rubs.

***cross-fiber f.*** Deep transverse f.

***deep transverse f.*** A massage technique in which stroking is applied across the longitudinal direction of the tissues of muscles, tendons, ligaments or fascia to prevent adhesions, increase mobility of the tissue, and align new fibers along the lines of stress. SYN: *cross-fiber f.*

***dry f.*** Friction using no liquid.

***moist f.*** Friction using a liquid or oil.

**friction rub** The distinct sound heard when two dry surfaces are rubbed together. If the sound is loud enough, the condition producing the sound can also be felt.

***pericardial f.r.*** A friction rub that may be present in pericarditis, particularly when the disease process first starts.

***pleural f.r.*** The creaking, grating sounds made when inflamed pleural surfaces move during respiration. It is often heard only during the first day or two of a pleurisy. SEE: *pericardial friction rub.*

**Friedländer's bacillus** (frēd'lĕn-dĕrz) [Carl F. Friedländer, Ger. physician, 1847–1887] *Klebsiella pneumoniae,* a species of bacteria that causes pneumonia and is a secondary invader in bronchitis or sinusitis.

**Friedländer's disease** Endarteritis obliterans.

**Friedman's test** (frēd'mănz) [Maurice H. Friedman, U.S. physiologist, b. 1903] A pregnancy test in which the urine of the woman is injected into an unmated female rabbit. If the woman is pregnant, corpora lutea and corpora hemorrhagica form in the rabbit after 2 days. Tests that are less difficult to perform are available.

**Friedreich's ataxia** (frēd'rĭks) [Nikolaus Friedreich, Ger. neurologist, 1825–1882] An inherited degenerative disease with sclerosis of the dorsal and lateral columns of the spinal cord. It is accompanied by muscular uncoordination, speech impairment, lateral curvature of the spinal column, and peculiar swaying and irregular movements, with muscle paralysis esp. of the lower extremities. The onset is in childhood or early adolescence.

**Friedreich's sign 1.** Sudden collapse of the cervical veins that were previously distended at each diastole. The cause is an adherent pericardium. **2.** Lowering of the pitch of the percussion note that occurs over an area of cavitation during inspiration.

**fright** [AS. *fryhto*] Extreme sudden fear.

**frigid** (frĭj'ĭd) [L. *frigidus*] **1.** Cold. **2.** Irresponsive to emotion, applied esp. to the inability of a person to feel sexual desire. SEE: *impotence.*

**frigidity** (frĭ-jĭd'ĭ-tē) Inhibited sexual excitement during sexual activity. In men it manifests as partial or complete failure to attain or maintain erection until completion of the sex act.

In women there is partial or complete failure to attain or maintain the vaginal lubrication-swelling response of sexual excitement until completion of the sex act.

**frigolabile** (frĭg"ō-lā'bĭl) [L. *frigor,* cold, + *labilis,* unstable] Capable of being destroyed by low temperature.

**frigorific** (frĭg"ō-rĭf'ĭk) [L. *frigorificus*] Generating cold.

**frigorism** [L. *frigor,* cold, + Gr. *-ismos,* condition] Very poor blood circulation caused by long exposure to cold.

**frigostabile** (frĭg"ō-stā'b'l) [" + *stabilis,* firm] Incapable of being destroyed by low temperature.

**frigotherapy** (frĭg"ō-thĕr'ă-pē) [" + Gr. *therapeia,* treatment] The use of cold in treatment of disease. SYN: *cryotherapy.*

**frit** (frĭt) [It. *fritta,* fry] **1.** The material from which glass or the glazed portion of pottery is made. **2.** A similar material for making the glaze of artificial teeth.

**frog belly** A flaccid abdomen in children afflicted with rickets and atony of abdominal cells resulting from dyspepsia, accompanied by flatulence.

**frog face** Flatness of the face resulting from intranasal disease.

**Fröhlich's syndrome** (frā'lĭks) [Alfred Fröhlich, Austrian neurologist, 1871–1953] A condition characterized by obesity and sexual infantilism, atrophy or hypoplasia of the gonads, and altered secondary sex characteristics. It is caused by disturbance of the hypothalamus and hypophysis, usually secondary to a neoplasm. SYN: *adiposogenital dystrophy.*

**Froin's syndrome** (frō-ănz') [Georges Froin, Fr. physician, 1874–1932] The presence of yellow cerebrospinal fluid that coagulates rapidly. This is associated with any condition in which the fluid in the spinal canal is prevented from mixing with the cerebrospinal fluid in the ventricles.

**frolement** (frōl-mŏn') [Fr.] **1.** Very light friction with the hand in massage. SEE: *massage.* **2.** A sound resembling rustling heard in auscultation.

**Froment's sign** (frō-măz') [Jules Froment, Fr. physician, 1878–1946] Flexion of the distal phalanx of the thumb when a sheet of paper is held between the thumb and index finger. It indicates ulnar nerve palsy.

**Frommann's lines** (frŏm'ănz) [Carl Frommann, Ger. anatomist, 1831–1892] Transverse lines in the axis cylinder of medullated nerve fibers. They are demonstrated by staining with silver nitrate.

**frons** (frŏnz) [L.] The forehead.

**frontad** [L. *frons, front-,* brow, + *ad,* toward] Toward the frontal aspect.

**frontal** [L. *frontalis*] **1.** Anterior. **2.** Pert. to the forehead bone.

**frontal bone** The forehead bone.

**frontal lobe** Four main convolutions in front of the central sulcus of the cerebrum.

**frontal plane** A plane parallel to the long axis of the body and at right angles to the median sagittal plane.

**frontal sinuses** Two hollow spaces in the frontal bone lying above the orbits. They are lined with mucous membrane, contain air, and communicate with the middle nasal meatus by means of the nasofrontal duct.

**fronto-** [L. *frons,* brow] Combining form meaning *anterior; forehead.*

**frontomalar** (frŏn″tō-mā′lăr) [″ + *mala,* cheek] Pert. to the frontal and malar bones.

**frontomaxillary** (frŏn″tō-măx′ĭ-lār″ē) [″ + *maxilla,* jawbone] Pert. to the frontal and maxillary bones.

**frontoparietal** (frŏn″tō-pă-rī′ĕ-tăl) [″ + *parietalis,* pert. to a wall] Pert. to the frontal and parietal bones.

**frontotemporal** [″ + *tempora,* the temples] Pert. to the frontal and temporal bones.

**front-tap reflex** Contraction of the gastrocnemius muscle when stretched muscles of the extended leg are percussed.

**frost** [AS.] A frozen vapor deposit.

***uremic f.*** A deposit of urea crystals on the skin from evaporation of sweat in a patient whose kidneys are severely impaired, as in uremia.

**frostbite** Freezing or the effect of freezing of a body part. Exposed areas such as the ears, cheeks, nose, fingers, and toes are usually affected. SEE: *freezing; frostnip; Nursing Diagnoses Appendix.*

SYMPTOMS: Symptoms include tingling and redness followed by pallor and numbness of the affected area. There are three degrees: transitory hyperemia following numbness, formation of vesicles, and gangrene.

FIRST AID: The affected part should not be rubbed with snow, but should be rewarmed in water at 40° to 42°C (104° to 108°F). Tetanus prophylaxis, analgesics, nonsteroidal anti-inflammatory agents, and antibiotics are given if the area is blistered. The patient should be stimulated with orally administered hot fluids such as tea, coffee, or beef bouillon. The patient should not be allowed to smoke. Artificial respiration should be administered if the patient is unconscious. If sloughing of tissue occurs, treatment is the same as for a burn. Patients have been known to recover without loss of fingers or toes even when amputation seemed inevitable. SEE: *freezing* for treatment of frozen parts.

**frost-itch** Itching of the skin provoked by cold temperatures. SYN: *pruritus hiemalis.*

**frostnip** A mild form of cold injury. The reversible changes in areas farthest removed from the core of the body, such as the earlobes, cheeks, nose, fingers, and toes, consist of skin pallor and numbness. SEE: *frostbite.*

**frottage** (frō-tŏzh′) [Fr., rubbing] A massage technique using rubbing.

**frotteurism** Recurrent intense sexual urges and fantasies involving touching and rubbing against a nonconsenting person. These acts are usually performed in crowded places where arrest is unlikely. The perpetrators are usually young men. Persons who have acted on these urges are usually distressed about them.

**frozen section** The cutting of a thin piece of tissue from a frozen specimen to permit rapid examination under the microscope. This technique is usually used while the patient is still anesthetized. The surgeon's further action is influenced by the results of this rapid test.

**"frozen watchfulness"** The hopeless reproachful stare of battered children.

**F.R.S.** *Fellow of the Royal Society.*

**F.R.S.C.** *Fellow of the Royal Society (Canada).*

**fructofuranose** (frŭk″tō-fū′ră-nōs) The furanose form of fructose.

**fructokinase** (frŭk″tō-kī′nās) An enzyme that catalyzes transfer of high-energy phosphate from a donor to fructose.

**fructose** (frŭk′tōs) [L. *fructus,* fruit] Levulose; fruit sugar. A monosaccharide and a hexose, it has the same empirical formula as glucose, $C_6H_{12}O_6$, and is found in corn syrup, honey, fruit juices, and the syrup resulting from the inversion of sucrose, an invert sugar. It is metabolized to provide a source of energy or may be stored in the body after being converted to glycogen. SEE: *disaccharide.*

**fructose intolerance** Inability to metabolize the carbohydrate fructose due to a hereditary absence or deficiency of the enzyme 1-phosphofructaldolase. Clinical signs develop early in life. They include hypoglycemia, jaundice, hepatomegaly, vomiting, lethargy, irritability, and convulsions. Fructose can be identified in the urine. The fructose tolerance test should not be used because it can induce irreversible coma.

TREATMENT: Acute attacks are treated by glucose administration. For long-term therapy, all foods containing fructose (present in sweet fruits and sugar cane) and sucrose and sorbitol (the latter used as a sweetening agent in foods and drugs) must be eliminated from the diet.

**fructosemia** (frŭk″tō-sē′mē-ă) [″ + Gr. *haima,* blood] Fructose in the blood.

**fructoside** (frŭk′tō-sīd) A carbohydrate that yields fructose on hydrolysis.

**fructosuria** (frŭk″tō-sū′rē-ă) [″ + Gr. *ouron,* urine] Fructose in the urine.

**fruit** [L. *fructus,* fruit] **1.** The ripened ovary of a seed-bearing plant and the surrounding tissue, such as the pod of a bean, nut, grain, or berry. **2.** The edible product of a plant consisting of ripened seeds and the enveloping tissue. Fruits in general add bulk to the diet. This quality, and the presence of specific laxative substances in some cases, makes fruits helpful in treating constipation.

COMPOSITION: Carbohydrates in the form of fruit sugars are the chief nutritive value of fruits. Seventy-five percent of most fruits is a mixture of dextrose and levulose. Fruits are a good source of vitamins and minerals.

*Pectose bodies:* Pectose, the principle in fruits that causes them to jell, is found in unripe fruit; pectin is found in ripe fruit or fruit that has been cooked in a weak acid solution.

*Principal acids:* Acetic acid is found in wine and vinegar. Citric acid is found in lemons, oranges, limes, and citrons. Malic acid is found in apples, pears, apricots, peaches, and currants. Oxalic acid is found in rhubarb, sorrel, and cranberries. Tartaric acid is found in grapes, pineapples, and tamarinds. Salicylic acid is found in currants, cranberries, cherries, plums, grapes, and crabapples.

*Combined acids:* Citric and malic acid are found in raspberries, strawberries, gooseberries, and cherries. Citric, malic, and oxalic acid are found in cranberries.

**fruitarian** Someone who eliminates all foods from the diet except fruits, vegetable oils, nuts, and honey.

**frumentaceous** (froo-mĕn-tā′shŭs) [L. *frumentum,* grain] Resembling or pert. to grain.

**frustration** [L. *frustratus,* disappointed] **1.** Lack of an adequate outlet for the libido. **2.** The condition that results from the thwarting or prevention of acts that would satisfy or gratify physical or personality needs.

**FSH** *follicle-stimulating hormone.*

**FSH/LHRH** *follicle-stimulating hormone and luteinizing hormone–releasing hormone.*

**FSH-RF** *follicle-stimulating hormone–releasing factor.*

**FSH-RH** *follicle-stimulating hormone–releasing hormone.*

**ft** L. *fiat* or *fiant,* let there be made; *florentium,* former name for promethium; *foot.*

**FTA-ABS** *fluorescent treponemal antibody-absorption test for syphilis.*

**FTT** *failure to thrive.*

**5-FU** Trade name for fluorouracil.

**fuchsin** (fook′sĭn) A red dye that can be prepared in an acid or basic form.

**fucose** (fū′kōs) A mucopolysaccharide present in blood group substances and in human milk.

**fucosidosis** (fū″kō-sī-dō′sĭs) A hereditary disease resulting from absence of the enzyme required to metabolize fucosidase. Clinically, neurological deterioration begins shortly after a period of normal early development. Heart disease, thick skin, and hyperhidrosis develop and are followed by death at an early age.

**-fuge** [L. *fugare,* to put to flight] Suffix meaning *something that expels or drives away.*

**fugitive** (fū′jĭ-tĭv) [L. *fugitivus*] **1.** Temporary, transient. **2.** Wandering; pert. to inconstant symptoms.

**fugue** (fūg) [L. *fuga,* flight] A dissociative disorder in which the person acts normally but has almost complete amnesia for what happened when recovery occurs.

***psychogenic* f.** Sudden, unexpected travel away from one's home or place of work with inability to recall one's past. The individual may assume a partial or complete new identity. The condition is not due to organic brain disease. It may follow severe mental stress such as marital quarrels or a natural disaster. It is usually of short duration but can last for months. Recovery is the usual outcome without recurrences.

**fulcrum** The object or point on which a lever moves.

**fulgurant** (fŭl′gū-rănt) [L. *fulgurare,* to lighten] Coming and going intensely like a flash of light, as a shooting pain. SYN: *fulminant.*

**fulgurate** (fŭl′gū-rāt) To destroy or remove tissue by means of fulguration.

**fulguration** Destruction of tissue by means of long high-frequency electric sparks. SEE: *electrodesiccation.*

**fulling** [O. Fr. *fauler,* to fill] A movement in massage: kneading with the limb held between the hands, rolling it backward and forward.

**full term** In obstetrics, an infant born between the beginning of the 38th and the end of the 41st week of gestation. SYN: *term infant.*

**full width half maximum** ABBR: FWHM. A term used to describe the width of a peak or the bandpass of an emission or absorption spectrum in a laboratory photometer.

**fulminant, fulminating** (fool′-, fŭl′mĭ-nănt) [L. *fulminans*] Having a rapid and severe onset; coming in lightning-like flashes of pain, as in tabes dorsalis. SYN: *fulgurant.*

**fumarase** (fū′mă-rās) An enzyme present in many plants and animals. It catalyzes the production of L-malic acid from fumaric acid.

**fumaric acid** One of the organic acids in the citric acid cycle for the metabolism of the acetate produced from fats, carbohydrates, and proteins.

**fumes** [L. *fumus,* smoke] Vapors, esp. those with irritating qualities.

***nitric acid* f.** The vapors of nitric acid ($HNO_3$). They are used in various chemical processes. Poisoning is produced by the action of the corrosive fumes on the respiratory tract.

SYMPTOMS: Symptoms include choking, gasping, swelling of mucous membranes, tightness in the chest, pulmonary edema, cough, and shock. Symptoms may last for 1 week or more.

TREATMENT: The patient must be removed immediately from the fumes and good ventilation of the lungs maintained. Therapy is given for shock and pulmonary edema. Administration of oxygen under pressure using a mask may be required along with analgesics and anxiolytics as needed. Clothes must be removed if they are contaminated. Cortisone may be helpful in diminishing the inflammatory response of the lungs.

**fumigant** (fū′mĭ-gănt) [L. *fumigare,* to make smoke] An agent used in disinfecting a room. The substance produces fumes that are lethal to insects and rodents. Chemicals used include hydrogen cyanide gas, acrylonitrile, carbon tetrachloride, ethylene oxide, and methyl bromide.

---

Caution: All of these chemicals are highly toxic, potentially lethal, and in some cases explosive. They should be used only by persons skilled in their application.

---

**fumigation** (fū″mĭ-gā′shŭn) **1.** The use of poisonous fumes or gases to destroy living organisms, esp. rats, mice, insects, and other vermin. Fumigants are relatively ineffective against bacteria and viruses; consequently, terminal disinfection of the sickroom, formerly a common practice, has been discontinued. **2.** The disinfection of rooms by gases.

**fuming** [L. *fumus,* smoke] Having a visible vapor.

**function** (fŭng′shŭn) [L. *functio,* performance] **1.** The action performed by any structure. In a living organism this may pertain to a cell or a part of a cell, tissue, organ, or system of organs. **2.** The act of carrying on or performing a special activity. Normal function is the normal action of an organ. Abnormal activity or the failure of an organ to perform its activity is the basis of disease or disease processes. Structural changes in an organ are pathological and are common causes of malfunction, although an organ may function abnormally without observable structural changes. In humans, function can pertain to the manner in which the individual can perform successfully the tasks and roles required for everyday living.

**functional 1.** Pert. to function. **2.** A term describing various disturbances of function, such as a disturbance with no organic disease to account for the altered function.

**functional bleeding** SEE: under *bleeding.*

**functional disease** A general term for inorganic disease or a disease in which organic changes are not evident; a disturbance of the function of any organ.

**Functional Independence Measure** ABBR: FIM. An objectively scored measure of the ability of persons needing rehabilitation services to perform daily living tasks. These include self-care, sphincter control, mobility, locomotion, communication, and social cognition. Data from this scale have been collected from facilities across North America and correlated with several outcome variables. A version for use with children, WeeFIM, has been developed. SYN: *WeeFIM.*

**functional overlay** The emotional response to physical illness. It may take the form of a conversion or hysterical response, affective overreaction, prolonged symptoms of physical illness after signs of the illness have subsided, or combinations of these reactions. Functional overlay may appear to be the primary disease and require skillful diagnosis to determine the actual cause of illness.

**functional psychosis** A disorder exhibited in psychosis in which there is no apparent pathology of the central nervous system.

**functional residual capacity** ABBR: FRC. The amount of air remaining in the lungs after a normal resting expiration.

**functioning tumor** A tumor that is able to synthesize the same product as the normal tissues from which it arises, esp. an endocrine or nonendocrine tumor that produces hormones.

**funda** (fŭn′dă) [L., sling] A four-tailed bandage. **fundal,** *adj.*

**fundament** (fŭn′dă-mĕnt) [L. *fundamentum*] **1.** A foundation. **2.** The anus.

**fundectomy** (fŭn-dĕk′tō-mē) [L. *fundus,* base, + Gr. *ektome,* excision] Removal of the fundus of any organ.

**fundic** (fŭn′dĭk) Pert. to a fundus.

**fundiform** (fŭn′dĭ-form) [L. *funda,* sling, + *forma,* shape] Sling-shaped or looped.

**fundoplication** (fŭn″dō-plī-kā′shŭn) Surgical reduction of the opening into the fundus of the stomach, and suturing of the previously removed end of the esophagus to the opening. This technique is used in treating reflux of gastric contents into the esophagus.

**fundoscopy** (fŭn-dŏs′kō-pē) [L. *fundus,* base, + Gr. *skopein,* to examine] Examination, esp. visual, of the fundus of any organ. In ophthalmology, visual examination of the fundus of the eye. SYN: *ophthalmoscopy.*

**fundus** [L., base] **1.** The larger part, base or body of a hollow organ. **2.** The portion of an organ most remote from its opening. **fundic** (fŭn′dĭk), *adj.*

***f. of bladder*** The base of the urinary bladder, the portion closest to the rectum.

***f. of gallbladder*** The lower dilated portion of the gallbladder.

***f. oculi*** The posterior inner part of the eye as seen with an ophthalmoscope.

***f. of stomach*** The uppermost portion of the stomach, posterior and lateral to the entrance of the esophagus.

***f. tympani*** The floor of the tympanic cavity close to the jugular fossa. It contains the bulb of the internal jugular vein.

***f. uteri*** The body of the uterus above the openings of the fallopian tubes.

**funduscope** (fŭn′dŭs-skōp) [L. *fundus,* base, + Gr. *skopein,* to examine] A device for examining the fundus of the eye.

**fundusectomy** (fŭn″dŭs-ĕk′tō-mē) [″ + Gr. *ektome,* excision] Excision of the fundus of the stomach. SYN: *cardiectomy.*

**fungal septicemia** SEE: *fungemia.*

**fungate** (fŭn′gāt) [L. *fungus,* mushroom] To grow like a fungus.

**fungating** (fŭn′gāt-ĭng) Growing rapidly like a fungus; said of certain tumors.

**fungemia** (fŭn-jē′mē-ă) [″ + Gr. *haima,* blood] Pathogenic fungi in the blood. This condition may occur as a complication of parenteral hyperalimentation. SYN: *fungal septicemia.* SEE: *sepsis.*

**Fungi** (fŭn′jī) [L. *fungus,* mushroom] The kingdom of organisms that includes yeasts, molds, and mushrooms. Fungi grow as single cells, as in yeast, or as multicellular filamentous colonies, as in molds and mushrooms. They do not contain chlorophyll, so they are saprophytic (obtain food from dead organic matter) or parasitic (obtain nourishment from living organisms). Most fungi are not pathogenic, and the body's normal flora contains many fungi. SEE: illus.

Fungi that cause disease come from a group called fungi imperfecti. In immunocompetent humans they cause minor infections of the hair, nails, mucous membranes, or skin. In a person with a compromised immune system due to AIDS or immunosuppressive drug therapy, fungi are a source of opportunistic infections that can cause death.

**fungicide** (fŭn′jĭ-sīd) [L. *fungi,* mushrooms, + *cidus,* killing] An agent that kills fungi and their spores.

**fungiform** (fŭn′jĭ-form) [″ + *forma,* shape] Mushroom-shaped.

**fungiform papilla** Any of the small rounded eminences on the middle and anterior parts of the dorsum and esp. along the sides of the tongue.

**fungistasis** (fŭn-jĭ-stā′sĭs) [″ + Gr. *stasis,* a halting] A condition in which the growth of fungi is inhibited.

**fungistat** (fŭn′jĭ-stăt) [″ + Gr. *statikos,* standing] An agent that inhibits the growth of fungi. **fungistatic** (-stăt′ĭk), *adj.*

**fungitoxic** (fŭn″jĭ-tŏk′sĭk) Poisonous to fungi.

**fungoid** (fŭn′goyd) [″ + Gr. *eidos,* form, shape] Having the appearance of a fungus.

**fungosity** (fŭn-gŏs′ĭ-tē) A soft, spongy fungus-like growth.

**fungus** (fŭn′gŭs) *pl.* **fungi** [L., mushroom] **1.** An organism belonging to the kingdom Fungi; a yeast, mold, or mushroom. SEE: *Fungi.* **2.** A spongelike morbid growth on the body that resembles fungi. SEE: *actinomycosis.* **fungal, fungous,** *adj.*

**funic** (fū′nĭk) [L. *funis,* cord] Pert. to the umbilical cord.

**funicle** (fū′nĭ-k′l) [L. *funiculus,* little cord] Funiculus (1).

**funic souffle** A purring sound heard over the pregnant uterus and having the same rate as the fetal heartbeat. The sound is caused by blood flowing through vessels in the umbilical cord.

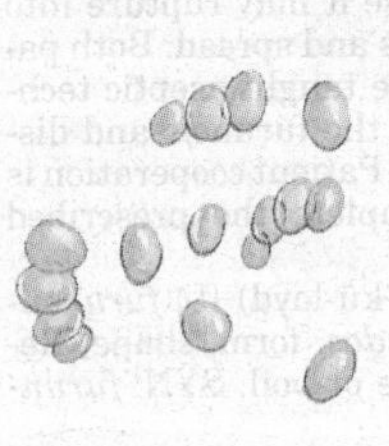
YEAST (×750)

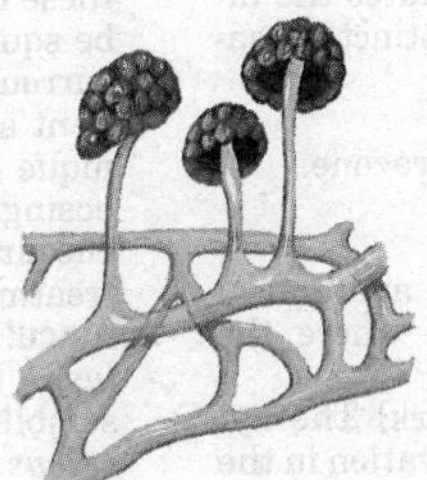
RHIZOPUS (×40)

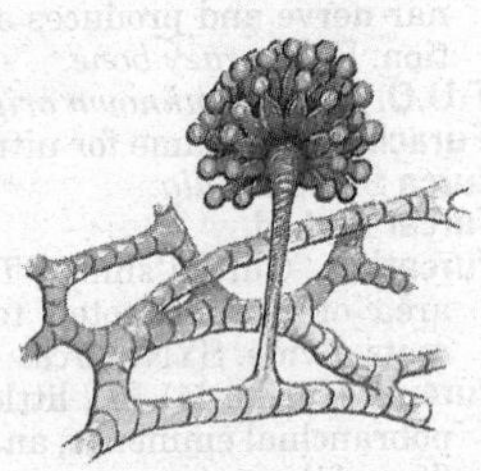
ASPERGILLUS (×40)

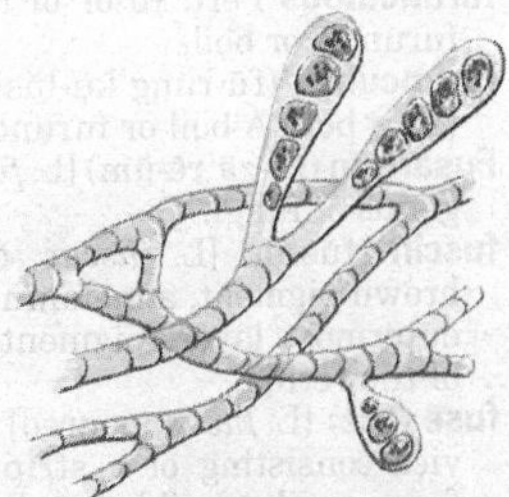
RINGWORM (×750)

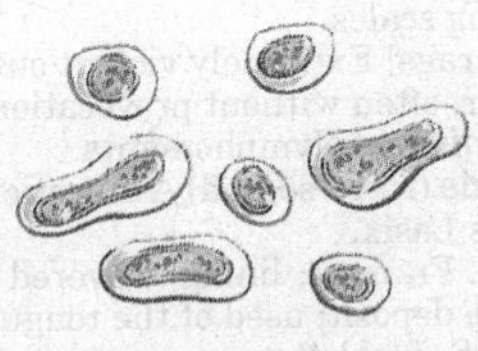
CRYPTOCOCCUS (×500)

FUNGI

**funicular** (fū-nĭk′ū-lăr) Pert. to the spermatic or umbilical cord.

**funicular process** The part of the tunica vaginalis that covers the spermatic cord.

**funiculitis** (fū-nĭk″ū-lī′tĭs) [″ + Gr. *itis,* inflammation] Inflammation of the spermatic cord.

**funiculopexy** (fū-nĭk′ū-lō-pĕks″ē) [″ + Gr. *pexis,* fixation] Suturing of the spermatic cord to the tissues in cases of undescended testicle.

**funiculus** (fū-nĭk′ū-lŭs) *pl.* **funiculi** [L., little cord] **1.** Any small structure resembling a cord. SYN: *funicle.* **2.** A division of the white matter of the spinal cord consisting of fasciculi, or fiber tracts, lying peripheral to the gray matter. The types of funiculi are dorsal, lateral, and ventral.

**funiform** (fū′nĭ-form) [L. *funis,* cord, + *forma,* shape] Cordlike.

**funipuncture** [L. *funis,* a cord, + *punctura,* to prick] Puncture of the vein of the umbilical cord to obtain a fetal blood sample. This is done in utero by using ultrasound technique to direct the needle.

**funis** (fū′nĭs) [L., cord] A cordlike structure, such as the spermatic cord or the umbilical cord.

**funisitis** Infection of the umbilical cord.

**funnel** [L. *fundere,* to pour] A conical device open at both ends for pouring liquid from one vessel into another.

**funnel breast, funnel chest** A congenital anomaly consisting of sternal depression of the chest walls so that the chest is funnel shaped.

**funny bone** The medial epicondyle of the humerus. It is so termed because pressure applied over this area stimulates the ulnar nerve and produces a distinct sensation. SYN: *crazy bone.*

**F.U.O.** *fever of unknown origin.*

**Furacin** Trade name for nitrofurazone.

**furca** SEE: *furcula.*

**furcal** Forked.

**furcation** (fŭr-kā′shŭn) The anatomical area of a multirooted tooth where the roots divide. SYN: *furca.*

**furcula** (fŭr′kū-lă) [L., little fork] The hypobranchial eminence, an elevation in the floor of the embryonic pharynx at the level of the third and fourth branchial arches. It gives rise to the epiglottis and the aryepiglottic folds. SYN: *furca.*

**furfur** [L., bran] Dandruff scales.

**furfuraceous** (fŭr-fū-rā′shŭs) Scaly or resembling scales.

**furor** [L., rage] Extremely violent outbursts of anger, often without provocation.

*f. femininus* Nymphomania.

**furosemide** (fū-rō′sĕ-mīd) A diuretic. Trade name is Lasix.

**furred** [O. Fr. *forre,* lining] Covered with a dustlike deposit; used of the tongue.

**furrow** [AS. *furh*] A groove.

*atrioventricular f.* The groove demarcating the atria of the heart from the ventricles.

*digital f.* Any of several transverse lines on the palmar surface of the fingers across the joints.

*gluteal f.* The vertical groove on the skin between the buttocks.

**furuncle** (fū′rŭng-k′l) [L. *furunculus*] An acute, deep-seated phlegmonous inflammation formed in the skin, usually ending in suppuration and necrosis. SYN: *boil; furunculus.* **furuncular** (fū-rŭng′kū-lăr), *adj.*

SYMPTOMS: The neck, axillae, face, buttocks, and breasts are common sites of predilection. The furuncle begins in a hair follicle or sudoriparous gland as a subcutaneous swelling or acuminate pustule around a hair shaft. The skin is smooth and shining, with pain and tenderness. The lesion may come to a head or become boggy and fluctuant, or regression may take place before suppuration, resulting in disappearance by absorption. The lesion ruptures spontaneously or following incision, discharging necrotic tissue and pus. Healing follows.

ETIOLOGY: The cause is usually a staphylococcal infection of follicular or sebaceous glands.

TREATMENT: Treatment consists of moist heat, incision after the lesion points (comes to a head), and an appropriate systemic antibiotic.

NURSING IMPLICATIONS: The patient is taught the importance of scrupulous personal and family hygiene to avoid spreading the infection to other locations or to other family members. The patient should not share towels or washcloths and should boil or otherwise disinfect these before reuse. A furuncle should not be squeezed because it may rupture into surrounding tissues and spread. Both patient and family are taught aseptic technique in caring for the furuncle and disposing of dressings. Patient cooperation is encouraged to complete the prescribed treatment regimen.

**furunculoid** (fū-rŭng′kū-loyd) [L. *furunculus,* a boil, + Gr. *eidos,* form, shape] Resembling a furuncle or boil. SYN: *furunculous.*

**furunculosis** (fū-rŭng″kū-lō′sĭs) [″ + Gr. *osis,* condition] A condition resulting from furuncles or boils.

**furunculous** Pert. to or of the nature of a furuncle or boil.

**furunculus** (fū-rŭng′kū-lŭs) *pl.* **furunculi** [L., a boil] A boil or furuncle.

**Fusarium** (fū-zā′rē-ŭm) [L. *fusus,* spindle] A genus of fungi.

**fuscin** (fŭs′ĭn) [L. *fuscus,* dark brown] A brown pigment, a melanin, present in the outermost layer (pigmented epithelium) of the retina.

**fuse** (fūz) [L. *fusus,* poured] **1.** A safety device consisting of a strip of wire made from easily fusible (meltable) metal of predetermined conductance. The metal fuses and breaks circuit when excess current passes through. **2.** To unite or blend together, as the coherence of adjacent body structures.

**fusible** (fū′zĭ-b'l) Capable of being melted.

**fusiform** (fū′zĭ-form) [L. *fusus,* spindle, + *forma,* shape] Tapering at both ends; spindle-shaped.

**fusimotor** (fū″sĭ-mō′tor) Pert. to the motor innervation of the intrafusal muscle fibers originating in the gamma efferent neurons of the anterior gray matter of the spinal cord.

**fusion** (fū′shŭn) [L. *fusio*] **1.** Meeting and joining together through liquefaction by heat. **2.** The process of fusing or uniting. **3.** The union of adjacent tooth germs to form an oversize tooth of abnormal configuration or two teeth partially fused at the crown or root.

***diaphyseal-epiphyseal f.*** Surgical obliteration of the epiphyseal line of a bone so that the epiphysis and diaphysis are joined.

***nuclear f.*** Joining of the nucleus of two atoms to form a larger nucleus. It occurs when temperatures reach millions of degrees.

***spinal f.*** Surgical fusion of two or more vertebrae. SYN: *spondylosyndesis.*

**Fusobacterium** A genus of non–spore-forming, nonencapsulated, nonmotile, gram-negative bacteria usually found in necrotic lesions of the mouth and bowel. *F. nucleatum* has been cultured from lesions of gangrenous stomatitis.

**fusocellular** [L. *fusus,* spindle, + *cellulus,* little cell] Spindle-celled.

**fusospirochetal** (fū″sō-spī-rō-kē′tăl) [″ + Gr. *speira,* coil, + *chaite,* hair] Pert. to fusiform bacilli and spirochetes.

**fusospirochetosis** (fū″sō-spī″rō-kē-tō′sĭs) [″ + ″ + ″ + *osis,* condition] Infection with fusiform bacilli and spirochetes.

**fustigation** (fŭs″tĭ-gā′shŭn) [L. *fustigatio*] In massage, beating with light rods.

**futility** In medical practice, the inappropriateness of a potential action to the best interest of the patient. The term is used esp. in cases in which the patient has previously directed that resuscitation efforts should not be used if a terminal illness develops. SEE: *advance directive.*

**FVC** *forced vital capacity.*

**F wave** Flutter waves in atrial fibrillation, detectable on the electrocardiogram at 250 to 350 per minute.

**FWB** *full weight bearing.*

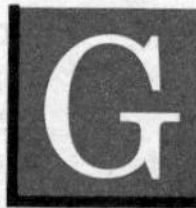

**γ 1.** The third letter of the Greek alphabet; gamma is the anglicized equivalent. **2.** Symbol for *microgram; immunoglobulin.*

**G 1.** The newtonian constant of gravitation. **2.** Symbol for giga, $10^9$, in SI units.

**g 1.** Symbol for the standard force of attraction of gravity, 980.665 m/sec², or about 32.17 ft/sec². **2.** *gingival; gram; gender.*

**Ga** Symbol for the element gallium.

**GABA** *gamma-aminobutyric acid.*

**gadfly** A fly belonging to the family Tabanidae that lays eggs under the skin of its victim, causing swelling simulating a boil. Multiple furuncles appear with hatching of larvae. SEE: *botfly.*

**gadolinium** (găd″ō-lĭn′ē-ŭm) SYMB: Gd. A chemical element of the lanthanide group, atomic weight 157.25, atomic number 64.

**GAF** *Global Assessment of Functioning.*

**gag 1.** A device for keeping the jaws open during surgery. **2.** To retch or cause to retch.

**gage** (gāj) Gauge.

**gain 1.** To increase in weight, strength, or health. **2.** In electronics, the term used to describe the amplification factor for a given circuit or device. **3.** The real or imagined positive effect of some action or situation. For example, an illness might allow a person to put off going to school or meeting some other obligation such as a court appearance.

***flux g.*** In radiographic image intensification, the ratio of the number of light photons at the output phosphor to the number of photons at the input phosphor.

***minification g.*** In radiographic image intensification, the ratio of the square of the input phosphor diameter to the square of the output phosphor diameter.

***primary g.*** In psychiatry, the relief of symptoms when the patient converts emotional anxiety to what he or she perceives as an organic illness (e.g., hysterical paralysis or blindness).

***secondary g.*** The advantage gained by the patient indirectly from illness, such as attention, care, and release from responsibility.

**Gaisböck's syndrome** (gīs′bĕks) [Felix Gaisböck, Ger. physician, 1869–1955] Benign erythrocytosis with no clinical findings associated with polycythemia. There is little evidence to support the view that this condition is a true clinical illness. Also called *stress erythrocytosis, spurious erythrocytosis, benign erythrocytosis,* and *pseudopolycythemia vera.*

**gait** (gāt) [ME. *gait,* passage] A manner of walking.

***antalgic g.*** A gait in which the patient experiences pain during the stance phase and thus remains on the painful leg for as short a time as possible.

***ataxic g.*** A gait marked by staggering and unsteadiness.

***cerebellar g.*** A staggering movement seen in cerebellar disease.

***double step g.*** A gait in which alternate steps are of a different length or at a different rate.

***drag-to g.*** A gait in which the crutches are advanced and the feet are dragged, rather than lifted, to the crutches.

***equine g.*** A gait marked by high steps, characteristic of tibialis anterior paralysis. In a rigid equinus posture of the ankle, the person walks on the toes. This is also seen in spastic gait patterns.

***festinating g.*** A gait characteristic of parkinsonism in which the patient walks on the toes as though pushed, starting slowly, increasing in speed, and possibly continuing until he or she grasps some object in order to stop.

***four-point g.*** A gait in which first the right crutch and the left foot are advanced consecutively, and then the left crutch and the right foot are moved forward.

***glue-footed g.*** A gait in which the individual has difficulty initiating the first step as if the feet were glued to the floor; once the gait is initiated, small, shuffling steps are taken. SYN: *magnetic g.*

***gluteus maximus g.*** Leaning of the trunk backward to keep the hip extended during the stance phase. It is caused by weakness of the gluteus maximus.

***gluteus medius g.*** Leaning of the trunk to the affected side during the stance phase. It is caused by paralysis of the gluteus medius muscle.

***helicopod g.*** A gait in which one or both feet describe a half circle with each step, sometimes seen in hysteria.

***hemiplegic g.*** A gait in which the patient abducts the paralyzed limb, swings it around, and brings it forward so that the foot comes to the ground in front. During the stance phase the patient bears very little weight on the involved leg.

***magnetic g.*** Glue-footed g.

***Parkinson's g.*** In patients with Parkinson's disease, a gait marked by short steps with the feet barely clearing the floor in a shuffling and scraping manner. As the steps continue, they may become successively more rapid. The posture is marked by flexion of the upper body with the spine bent forward, head down, and arms, elbows, hips, and knees bent. SEE: *festinating g.*

***quadriceps g.*** A gait in which the trunk leans forward at the beginning of the stance phase to lock the knee when the quadriceps femoris muscle is weak or paralyzed.

***scissor g.*** A gait in which the legs cross in walking, as seen in patients with an upper motor neuron lesion accompanied by spasticity.

***senile g.*** A gait marked by associated stooped posture, knee and hip flexion, diminished arm swinging, stiffness in turning, and broad-based, small steps. It is usually seen in the elderly.

***spastic g.*** A stiff movement in which the toes seem to catch and drag, the legs are held together, and the hips and knee joints are slightly flexed. It is seen in spastic paraplegia, sclerosis of the lateral pyramidal columns of the cord, tumor of the spinal cord, and arachnoiditis.

***spondylitic cervical myelopathic g.*** A spastic, shuffling gait due to increased muscle tone resulting from deep tendon reflexes below the level of compression.

***steppage g.*** A gait in which the foot is lifted high to clear the toes, there is no heel strike, and the toes hit the ground first. It is seen in anterior tibialis paralysis, peripheral neuritis, late stages of diabetic neuropathy, alcoholism, and chronic arsenic poisoning.

***swing-through g.*** A gait in which the crutches are advanced and the legs are swung between and ahead of the crutches.

***swing-to g.*** A gait in which the crutches are advanced and the legs are advanced to the crutches.

***tabetic g.*** A high-stepping ataxic walk in which the feet slap the ground. It is caused by tabes dorsalis.

***three-point g.*** A gait in which the crutches and the affected leg are advanced first, then the other leg.

***two-point g.*** A gait in which the right foot and left crutch are advanced simultaneously, then the left foot and right crutch are moved forward.

***waddling g.*** A gait in which the feet are wide apart and the walk resembles that of a duck. It occurs in coxa vara and double congenital hip displacement when lordosis is present. In late pregnancy, hormone-induced softening allows some pelvic movement at the sacroiliac and pubic symphysis articulations on ambulation. Compensatory widening of the stance results in the characteristic waddle.

**galact-** [Gr. *gala,* milk] SEE: *galacto-*.

**galactacrasia** [″ + *akrasia,* bad mixture] An abnormality of breast milk.

**galactagogue** (gă-lăk′tă-gŏg) [″ + *agogos,* leading] An agent that promotes the flow of milk.

**galactase** An enzyme or proteolytic ferment of milk.

**galactic** (gă-lăk′tĭk) Pert. to the flow of milk.

**galacto-, galact-** Combining form meaning *milk.*

**galactoblast** (gă-lăk′tō-blăst) [″ + *blastos,* germ] A body found in mammary acini that contains fat globules.

**galactocele** (gă-lăk′tō-sēl) [″ + *kele,* tumor, swelling] **1.** A cystic tumor of the female breast caused by occlusion of a milk duct. SYN: *galactoma; lactocele.* **2.** A hydrocele containing a milk-like liquid.

**galactokinase** (gă-lăk″tō-kī′nās) An enzyme that catalyzes the transfer of high-energy phosphate groups from a donor to D-galactose. D-galactose-1-phosphate is produced by this reaction.

**galactolipin** [″ + *lipos,* fat] A phosphorus-free lipid combined with galactose; a cerebroside.

**galactoma** (găl-ăk-tō′mă) [″ + *oma,* tumor] SEE: *galactocele* (1).

**galactopexy** (gă-lăk′tō-pĕk″sē) The fixation of galactose by the liver.

**galactophagous** (găl″ăk-tŏf′ă-gŭs) [″ + *phagein,* to eat] Feeding on milk.

**galactophore** (găl-ăk′tō-for) [″ + *pherein,* to bear] A milk duct.

**galactophoritis** (găl-ăk″tō-for-ī′tĭs) [″ + ″ + *itis,* inflammation] Inflammation of a milk duct.

**galactopoiesis** (gă-lăk″tō-poy-ē′sĭs) [″ + *poiesis,* forming] Milk production.

**galactopoietic** (gă-lăk″tō-poy-ĕt′ĭk) [″ + *poiein,* to make] **1.** Pert. to milk production. **2.** A substance that promotes galactopoiesis.

**galactorrhea** (gă-lăk″tō-rē′ă) [″ + *rhoia,* flow] **1.** The continuation of milk secretion at intervals after nursing has ceased. **2.** Excessive secretion of milk.

**galactosamine** (gă-lăk″tō-săm′ĭn) A derivative of galactose containing an amine group on the second carbon of the compound.

**galactose** (gă-lăk′tōs) A dextrorotatory monosaccharide or simple hexose sugar, $C_6H_{12}O_6$. Galactose is an isomer of glucose and is formed, along with glucose, in the hydrolysis of lactose. It is a component of cerebrosides. Galactose is readily absorbed in the digestive tract; in the liver it is converted to glucose and may be stored as glycogen.

**galactosemia** (gă-lăk″tō-sē′mē-ă) An inherited disorder marked by an inability to metabolize galactose because of a congenital absence of the enzyme galactose-1-phosphate uridyl transferase, which is needed to convert galactose to glucose. The diagnosis is confirmed by testing the newborn's urine for noncarbohydrate reducing substances. The infant with galactosemia will fail to thrive within a week after birth due to anorexia, vomiting, and diarrhea unless galactose and lactose are removed from the diet. If untreated, the disease may progress to starvation and death. Untreated children who do survive usually fail to grow, are mentally retarded, and have cataracts. If galactose is excluded from the diet early in life, the prognosis is good. Galactosemia can be diagnosed in utero by amniocentesis. If a pregnant woman is a known carrier, it is advisable that she exclude lactose and galactose from her diet.

**galactosidase** (gă-lăk″tō-sī′dās) An enzyme that catalyzes the metabolism of galactosides.

**galactoside** (gă-lăk′tō-sīd) A carbohydrate that contains galactose.

**galactostasis** (găl″ăk-tŏs′tă-sĭs) [″ + *stasis,* a stopping] The cessation or checking of milk secretion.

**galactosuria** (găl-ăk″tō-sū′rē-ă) [″ + *ouron,* urine] Galactose in the urine.

**galactotherapy** (gă-lăk″tō-thĕr′ă-pē) [″ + *therapeia,* treatment] **1.** Treatment of a nursing infant by drugs administered to the mother and excreted in her milk. **2.** Therapeutic use of milk, as a milk diet. SYN: *lactotherapy.*

**galactotoxin** (gă-lăk″tō-tŏks′ĭn) [″ + *toxikon,* poison] A toxic substance in milk produced by bacteria.

**galactozymase** (gă-lăk″tō-zī′mās) [″ + *zyme,* leaven] A starch-hydrolyzing enzyme in milk.

**galacturia** (găl-ăk-tū′rē-ă) [″ + *ouron,* urine] Chyluria.

**galea** (gā′lē-ă) [L. *galea,* helmet] **1.** A helmet-like structure. **2.** A type of head bandage.

***g. aponeurotica*** Epicranial aponeurosis.

**galeanthropy** (gā″lē-ăn′thrō-pē) [Gr. *gale,* cat, + *anthropos,* man] A delusion that one has become transformed into a cat.

**Galeazzi's sign** [Riccardo Galeazzi, It. orthopedic surgeon, 1866–1952] A clinical indication of congenital hip dislocation in infants and toddlers. With the child lying supine with the knees flexed and hips flexed at 90°, dislocation is present if one knee is higher than the other.

**Galen, Claudius** A noted Greek physician and medical writer, circa A.D. 130–200, residing in Rome, where he was physician to Emperor Marcus Aurelius. He is called the father of experimental physiology.

***G.'s veins*** The veins running through the tela choroidea formed by the joining of the terminal and choroid veins and forming the vena cerebri magna, which empties into the straight sinus of the brain.

**galenic** (gă-lĕn′ĭk) Pert. to Galen or his teachings.

**galenicals, galenics** (gă-lĕn′ĭ-kăls, -ĭks) **1.** Herb and vegetable medicines. **2.** Crude drugs and medicinals as distinguished from the pure active principles contained in them. **3.** Medicines prepared according to an official formula.

**galeophilia** (găl″ē-ō-fĭl′ē-ă) [Gr. *gale,* cat, + *philein,* to love] A fondness for cats.

**galeophobia** (găl″ē-ō-fō′bē-ă) [″ + *phobos,* fear] An abnormal aversion to cats.

**gall** [AS. *gealla,* sore place] **1.** An excoriation. **2.** The bitter liver secretion stored in the gallbladder; bile. It has no enzymes, but helps emulsify fats, stimulates the intestines, and multiplies the action of the pancreatic juice threefold. Gall is discharged through the cystic duct into the duodenum.

**gallamine triethiodide** (găl′ă-mīn trī″ē-thī′ō-dīd) A drug that inhibits transmission of nerve impulses across the myoneural junction of voluntary muscles. Trade name is Flaxedil.

**Gallant reflex** An infantile reflex in which the trunk curves toward the side of stimulation in a prone infant. It is present from birth to age 2 months.

**gallate** (găl′lāt) A salt of gallic acid.

**gallbladder** [AS. *gealla,* sore place, + *blaedre,* bladder] A pear-shaped sac on the underside of the right lobe of the liver that stores bile received from the liver. While in the gallbladder, bile is concentrated by removing water. About 500 to 600 ml of bile, approx. 82% water, is secreted each day. The bile is then discharged through the cystic duct, which is 3 to 4 in. (7.6 to 10.2 cm) long. The cystic duct, which is about 0.25 in. (6 mm) in diameter, joins the hepatic duct to form the common bile duct, which empties into the duodenum at the ampulla of Vater.

**gallium** (găl′ē-ŭm) [L. *Gallia,* Gaul] SYMB: Ga. A rare metal, small amounts of which are found in bauxite and zinc blends; atomic weight 69.72, atomic number 31. Gallium-68 ($^{68}$Ga) is used in studies involving use of radioactive materials. It has a half-life of 68 min.

**gallon** [Med. L. *galleta,* jug] Four liquid measure quarts; 231 cu in. or 3.79 L. In England the Imperial liquid gallon is 277.4 cu in. or 4.55 L.

**gallop rhythm** SEE: under *rhythm.*

**gallstone** [AS. *gealla,* sore place, + *stan,* stone] A concretion formed in the gallbladder or bile ducts. The most common type is the cholesterol-containing stone. Gallstones form when the bile contains more cholesterol than can be kept in solution. The cholesterol precipitates out to form gallstones. The incidence of gallstones in women is approx. twice that in men. Obesity increases the risk of developing gallstones. SEE: *Nursing Diagnoses Appendix.*

SYMPTOMS: A gallstone may remain dormant and produce little distress unless the gallbladder becomes inflamed and distended or unless the stone enters and is unable to pass through the biliary ducts, thus producing colic. The pain, which may radiate to the back and right shoulder, usually occurs several hours after eating, when the stomach is empty. Flatulence is a common symptom. Jaundice is usually absent.

TREATMENT: Analgesics are prescribed, with meperidine as the drug of choice. Morphine is thought to increase spasm of the sphincter of Oddi and thus is not used for pain relief. Persistent pain or enlargement of the gallbladder due to its distention with gallstones may require surgery. Chenodiol (chenodeoxycholic acid), taken orally, has been used to dissolve low-density, nonpigmented stones. The therapy may have to be continued for 18 months. Lithotripsy (i.e., extracorporeal shock-wave therapy) has been used to disintegrate gallstones.

---

Caution: Chenodiol is contraindicated in patients with liver disease. Liver function should be monitored in patients given chenodiol. Ursodiol (ursodeoxycholic acid), taken orally, is effective in treating cholesterol gallstones. Treatment may need to be continued for 1 year.

---

**GALT** *gut-associated lymphoid tissue.*

**Galton's whistle** [Sir Francis Galton, Brit. scientist, 1822–1911] A whistle used to test hearing.

**galvanic** [Luigi Galvani, It. physiologist, 1737–1798] Pert. to galvanism.

***g. battery*** A series of cells giving a combined effect of all the units and generating electricity by chemical reaction.

***g. current*** Direct electric current, usually from a battery.

***g. skin response*** SEE: under *response*.

**galvanism** (găl′vă-nĭzm) In dentistry, an electrochemical reaction occurring in the mouth when dissimilar metals used to restore teeth come into contact, producing a direct electric current that may cause pain.

**galvanization** (găl″văn-ī-zā′shŭn) Use of a galvanic current as a therapeutic measure.

**galvanometer** (găl″vă-nŏm′ĕ-tĕr) [″ + Gr. *metron,* measure] An instrument that measures electric current by electromagnetic action. SYN: *rheometer* (1).

**galvanopuncture** (găl″vă-nō-pŭng′chūr) [″ + L. *punctura,* puncture] Introduction of needles to complete a galvanic current.

**gam-** SEE: *gamo-*.

**gamete** (găm′ēt) [Gr. *gamein,* to marry] A mature male or female reproductive cell; the spermatozoon or ovum. **gametic** (-ĕt′ĭk), *adj.*

**gamete intrafallopian transfer** ABBR: GIFT. A procedure developed by Ricardo Asch, a contemporary U.S. physician, to assist couples who have an infertility problem. Through use of a laparoscope, ova are obtained from a mature follicle and then analyzed in a Petri dish. Sperm are placed in a separate Petri dish. If the two specimens are judged suitable for use, first an ovum, then a sperm, then another ovum are aspirated into a special catheter. The ova and sperm are then placed in the fallopian tube, where fertilization can occur naturally. SEE: *embryo transfer; fertilization, in vitro; zygote intrafallopian transfer.*

**gametocide** (găm′ĕ-tō-sīd″) [″ + L. *caedere,* to kill] An agent destructive to gametes or gametocytes, particularly those of malaria.

**gametocyte** (gă-mĕ′tō-sīt) [″ + *kytos,* cell] A stage of the malarial protozoon (*Plasmodium*) that reproduces in the blood of the Anopheles mosquito.

**gametogenesis** (găm″ĕt-ō-jĕn′ĕ-sĭs) [″ + *genesis,* generation, birth] Development of gametes; oogenesis or spermatogenesis.

**gametogony** (găm″ĕ-tŏg′ō-nē) The phase in the life cycle of the malarial parasite (*Plasmodium*) in which male and female gametocytes, which infect the mosquito, are formed.

**gametophyte** (găm′ĕ-tō-fīt) [″ + *phyton,* plant] In plants, the sexual (gamete-producing) generation that alternates with the asexual (spore-producing) generation.

**gamic** (găm′ĭk) [Gr. *gamein,* to marry] Sexual, esp. as applied to eggs that develop only after fertilization in contrast to those that develop without fertilization. SEE: *parthenogenesis.*

**gamma 1.** The third letter of the Greek alphabet, $\gamma$. **2.** In chemistry, the third of a series (e.g., the third carbon atom in an aliphatic chain).

**gamma-aminobutyric acid** ABBR: GABA. An amino acid inhibitory transmitter in the central nervous system.

**gamma benzene hexachloride** (găm′ă bĕn′zēn hĕk″să-klor′īd) A miticide used to treat scabies. Trade names are Kwell and Scabene. SYN: *lindane.*

**gammacism** An inability to pronounce "g" and "k" sounds correctly.

**Gammagee** Trade name for immune globulin.

**gamma globulin** A protein antibody formed by plasma cells in response to a foreign antibody. The ability to resist infection is related to the concentration of such proteins. SEE: *immunoglobulin.*

**gamma knife surgery** Radiosurgery in which an intracranial target can be destroyed by ionizing beams of radiation that are directed with stereotaxic precision. A surgical incision is not needed. The therapy is used to treat brain tumors and vascular lesions.

**gamma motor neuron** A small nerve originating in the anterior horns of the spinal cord that transmits impulses through type A gamma fibers to intrafusal fibers of the muscle spindle for muscle control.

**Gammar** Trade name for immune globulin.

**gammopathy** (găm-ŏp′ă-thē) A disease in which serum immunoglobulin is increased, as in myeloma, but Bence Jones protein is not present in the urine.

**gamo-, gam-** [Gr. *gamos,* marriage] Combining form meaning *marriage* or *sexual union.*

**gamogenesis** (găm″ō-jĕn′ĕ-sĭs) [″ + *genesis,* generation, birth] Sexual reproduction.

**gamont** (găm′ŏnt) [″ + *on,* being] A sexual

form of certain protozoa. SEE: *gametocyte.*

**gamophobia** (găm″ō-fō′bē-ă) [″ + *phobos,* fear] A neurotic fear of marriage.

**gampsodactylia** (gămp″sō-dăk-tĭl′ē-ă) [Gr. *gampsos,* curved, + *daktylos,* digit] Deformity of the toes causing them to resemble claws. SYN: *clawfoot.*

**ganciclovir** A synthetic antiviral drug used intravenously in treating cytomegalovirus retinitis in immunocompromised patients. Trade name is Cytovene. SEE: *cytomegalic inclusion disease.*

---

Caution: Ganciclovir is a potential carcinogen. Because of its mutagenic potential, women of childbearing age must use effective contraception during treatment. Male patients must practice barrier contraception during treatment and for at least 90 days afterward. Persons who care for patients receiving this drug must take appropriate precautions to prevent coming into contact with the drug, the patient's excreta, or the patient's used bed linens.

---

**ganglia** (găng′glē-ă) Pl. of ganglion.

**ganglial** (găng′lē-ăl) [Gr. *ganglion,* knot] Ganglionic.

**gangliated** (găng′lē-ā-tĕd) **1.** Having ganglia. **2.** Intermixed.

**gangliectomy** (găng″glē-ĕk′tō-mē) [″ + *ektome,* excision] Excision of a ganglion.

**gangliform** (găng′lĭ-form) [″ + L. *forma,* shape] Formed like a ganglion.

**gangliitis** (găng″glē-ī′tĭs) [″ + *itis,* inflammation] Inflammation of a ganglion.

**ganglioblast** (găng′glē-ō-blăst″) [″ + *blastos,* germ] An embryonic ganglion cell.

**gangliocyte** (găng′glē-ō-sīt″) [″ + *kytos,* cell] A ganglion cell.

**gangliocytoma** (găng″glē-ō-sī-tō′mă) [″ + ″ + *oma,* tumor] SYN: *ganglioneuroma.*

**ganglioglioma** (găng″glē-ō-glī-ō′mă) [″ + *glia,* glue, + *oma,* tumor] A ganglion-cell glioma.

**ganglioglioneuroma** (găng″glē-ō-glī″ō-nū-rō′mă) [″ + ″ + *neuron,* nerve, + *oma,* tumor] Ganglion cells, glia cells, and nerve fibers in a nerve tumor.

**ganglioma** (găng-lē-ō′mă) [″ + *oma,* tumor] **1.** A tumor of a lymphatic gland. **2.** A swelling of lymphoid tissue.

**ganglion** (găng′lē-ŏn) *pl.* **ganglia, ganglions** [Gr.] **1.** A mass of nervous tissue composed principally of neuron cell bodies and lying outside the brain or spinal cord (e.g., the chains of ganglia that form the main sympathetic trunks; the dorsal root ganglion of a spinal nerve). **2.** A cystic tumor developing on a tendon or aponeurosis. It sometimes occurs on the back of the wrist.

***abdominal g.*** Any ganglion located in the abdomen.

***aorticorenal g.*** A ganglion lying near the lower border of the celiac ganglion. It is located near the origin of the renal artery.

***Arnold's auricular g.*** Otic g.

***auricular g.*** Otic g.

***autonomic g.*** A ganglion of the autonomic nervous system.

***basal g.*** A mass of gray matter beneath the third ventricle consisting of the caudate, lentiform, and amygdaloid nuclei and the claustrum.

***basal optic g.*** A mass of gray matter beneath the third ventricle.

***cardiac ganglia*** Superficial and deep cardiac plexuses that contain autonomic nerves and branches of the left vagus nerve. They are located on the right side of the ligamentum arteriosus. SYN: *Wrisberg's ganglia.*

***carotid g.*** A ganglion formed by filamentous threads from the carotid plexus beneath the carotid artery.

***celiac g.*** One of a pair of prevertebral or collateral ganglia located near the origin of the celiac artery. Together they form a part of the celiac plexus.

***cephalic g.*** One of the parasympathetic ganglia (otic, pterygopalantine, and submandibular) in the head.

***cervical g.*** One of the three pairs of ganglia (superior, middle, inferior) in the cervical portion of the sympathetic trunk.

***cervicothoracic g.*** Stellate g.

***cervicouterine g.*** A ganglion near the uterine cervix. SYN: *Frankenhäuser's g.*

***ciliary g.*** A tiny ganglion in the rear portion of the orbit. It receives preganglionic fibers through the oculomotor nerve from the Edinger-Westphal nucleus of the midbrain. Six short ciliary nerves pass from it to the eyeball. Postganglionic fibers innervate the ciliary muscle, the sphincter of the iris, the smooth muscles of blood vessels of these structures, and the cornea. SYN: *lenticular g.; ophthalmic g.*

***coccygeal g.*** A ganglion located in the coccygeal plexus and forming the lower termination of the two sympathetic trunks; sometimes absent.

***collateral g.*** One of several ganglia of the sympathetic nervous system. They are in the mesenteric nervous plexuses near the abdominal aorta and include the celiac and mesenteric ganglia.

***Corti's g.*** A ganglion on the cochlear nerve.

***dorsal root g.*** Spinal g.

***false g.*** An enlargement on a nerve that does not contain a ganglion.

***Frankenhäuser's g.*** Cervicouterine g.

***gasserian g.*** Trigeminal g.

***geniculate g.*** A ganglion on the pars intermedia, the sensory root of the facial nerve. It lies in the anterior border of the anterior geniculum of the facial nerve.

***inferior mesenteric g.*** A prevertebral sympathetic ganglion located in the inferior mesenteric plexus near the origin of the inferior mesenteric artery.

***intervertebral g.*** Spinal g.

***jugular g.*** A ganglion located on the root of the vagus nerve and lying in the upper portion of the jugular foramen.

***lateral g.*** One of a chain of ganglia forming the main sympathetic trunk.

***lenticular g.*** Ciliary g.

***lumbar g.*** One of the ganglia usually occurring in fours in the lumbar portion of the sympathetic trunk.

***lymphatic g.*** A lymph node.

***nodose g.*** A ganglion of the trunk of the vagus nerve located immediately below the jugular ganglion. It connects with the spinal accessory nerve, the hypoglossal nerve, and the superior cervical ganglion of the sympathetic trunk.

***ophthalmic g.*** Ciliary g.

***otic g.*** A small ganglion located deep in the zygomatic fossa immediately below the foramen ovale. It lies medial to the mandibular nerve and supplies postganglionic parasympathetic fibers to the parotid gland. SYN: *Arnold's auricular g.; auricular g.*

***parasympathetic g.*** One of the ganglia on the cholinergic nerves of the parasympathetic nervous system, near or in the visceral effector.

***petrous g.*** A ganglion located on the lower margin of the temporal bone's petrous portion.

***pharyngeal g.*** A ganglion in contact with the glossopharyngeal nerve.

***phrenic g.*** One of a group of ganglia joining the phrenic plexus.

***renal g.*** One of a group of ganglia joining the renal plexus.

***sacral g.*** One of the four small ganglia located in the sacral portion of the sympathetic trunk that lie on the anterior surface of the sacrum and are connected to the spinal nerves by gray rami.

***Scarpa's g.*** Vestibular g.

***semilunar g.*** Trigeminal g.

***sensory g.*** One of the ganglia of the peripheral nervous system that transmit sensory stimuli.

***simple g.*** A cystic tumor in a tendon sheath. SYN: *wrist g.*

***spinal g.*** A ganglion located on the dorsal root of a spinal nerve. It contains the cell bodies of sensory neurons. SYN: *dorsal root g.; intervertebral g.*

***spiral g.*** A long, coiled ganglion in the cochlea of the ear. It contains bipolar cells, the peripheral processes of which terminate in the organ of Corti. The central processes form the cochlear portion of the acoustic nerve and terminate in the cochlear nuclei of the medulla.

***stellate g.*** A ganglion formed by joining of the inferior cervical ganglion with the first thoracic sympathetic ganglion. SYN: *cervicothoracic g.*

***submandibular g.*** A ganglion lying between the mylohyoideus and hyoglossus muscles and suspended from the lingual nerve by two small branches. Peripheral fibers pass to the submandibular, sublingual, lingual, and adjacent salivary glands.

***superior mesenteric g.*** A prevertebral ganglion of the sympathetic nervous system located near the base of the superior mesenteric artery. It lies close to the celiac ganglion and with it forms a part of the celiac plexus.

***suprarenal g.*** A ganglion situated in the suprarenal plexus.

***sympathetic g.*** One of the ganglia of the thoracolumbar (sympathetic) division of the autonomic nervous system. It includes vertebral or lateral ganglia (those forming the sympathetic trunk) and prevertebral or collateral ganglia, more peripherally located.

***temporal g.*** A tiny ganglion joining the anterior branches of the superior cervical ganglion.

***terminal g.*** A ganglion of the autonomic division of the nervous system that lies close to or within the organ innervated.

***thoracic g.*** One of 11 or 12 ganglia of the thoracic area of the sympathetic trunk.

***trigeminal g.*** A ganglion on the sensory portion of the fifth cranial nerve. SYN: *gasserian g.; semilunar g.*

***tympanic g.*** An enlargement on the tympanic portion of the glossopharyngeal nerve.

***vestibular g.*** A bilobed ganglion on the vestibular branch of the acoustic nerve at the base of the internal acoustic meatus. Its peripheral fibers begin in the maculae of the sacculus and utriculus and the cristae of the ampullae of the semicircular ducts. SYN: *Scarpa's g.*

***Wrisberg's ganglia*** Cardiac ganglia.

***wrist g.*** Simple g.

**ganglionated** Having or consisting of ganglia.

**ganglionectomy** (găng″lē-ō-nĕk′tō-mē) [Gr. *ganglion,* knot, + *ektome,* excision] Excision of a ganglion.

**ganglioneuroma** (găng″lē-ō-nū-rō′mă) [″ + *neuron,* nerve, + *oma,* tumor] A neuroma containing ganglion cells. SYN: *gangliocytoma.*

**ganglionic** (găng-lē-ŏn′ĭk) Pert. to or of the nature of a ganglion. SYN: *ganglial.*

**ganglionic blockade** Blocking of the transmission of stimuli in autonomic ganglia. Pharmacologically, this is done by using drugs that occupy receptor sites for acetylcholine and by stabilizing the postsynaptic membranes against the actions of acetylcholine liberated from presynaptic nerve endings. The usual effects of drugs that cause ganglionic blockade are vasodilatation of arterioles with increased peripheral blood flow; hypotension; dilation of veins with pooling of blood in tissues, decreased venous return, and decreased cardiac output; tachycardia; mydriasis; cycloplegia; reduced tone and motility of the gastrointestinal tract with consequent constipation; urinary retention; dry mouth; and decreased sweating. Ganglionic blocking drugs are not often used to treat hypertension but are used to treat autonomic hyperreflexia and to produce controlled hypotension during certain types of surgery. Several drugs are available for ganglionic blocking.

**ganglionitis** (găng″lē-ŏn-ī′tĭs) [″ + *itis,* inflammation] Inflammation of a ganglion.

**ganglionostomy** (găng″glē-ō-nŏs′tō-mē) [″ + *stoma,* mouth] Surgical incision of a simple ganglion.

**ganglioplegia** (găng″glē-ō-plē′jē-ă) [″ + *plege,* stroke] The failure of nervous stimuli to be transmitted by a ganglion. SEE: *blockade, ganglionic.*

**ganglioplegic** Any drug that prevents transmission of nervous impulses through sympathetic or parasympathetic ganglia. Such drugs have limited therapeutic applicability because of undesired side effects. They are useful in treating hypertensive crises. Because they decrease blood pressure, they are used to limit bleeding during certain surgical procedures.

**ganglioside** (găng′glē-ō-sīd) A particular class of glycosphingolipid present in nerve tissue and in the spleen.

**gangliosidosis** (găng″glē-ō-sī-dō′sĭs) *pl.* **gangliosidoses** An accumulation of abnormal amounts of specific gangliosides in the nervous system. SEE: *sphingolipidosis.*

**gangosa** (găng-gō′să) [Sp. *gangosa,* muffled voice] Ulceration of the nose and hard palate, seen in the late stage of yaws, leishmaniasis, or leprosy.

**gangrene** (găng′grēn) [Gr. *gangraina,* an eating sore] A necrosis, or death, of tissue or bone, usually resulting from deficient or absent blood supply. SEE: *necrosis.*

ETIOLOGY: Gangrene is usually caused by obstruction of the blood supply to an organ or tissue, possibly resulting from inflammatory processes, injury, or degenerative changes such as arteriosclerosis. It is commonly a sequela of boils, frostbite, crushing injuries, or diseases such as diabetes mellitus and Raynaud's disease. Emboli in large arteries in almost any part of the body can cause gangrene of the area distal to that point. The part that dies is known as a slough (for soft tissues) or a sequestrum (for bone). The dead matter must be removed before healing can take place.

***diabetic g.*** Gangrene, esp. of the lower extremities, occurring in some diabetics as a result of vascular pathology.

***dry g.*** Gangrene that results when the necrotic part has little blood and remains aseptic. This occurs when the arteries but not the veins are obstructed. The tissues dry and drop off, the process continuing for weeks or months. SEE: *Nursing Diagnoses Appendix.*

SYMPTOMS: Dry gangrene causes pain in the early stages. The affected part is cold and black and begins to atrophy. The most distal parts are generally affected first, the necrosis then spreading proximally. Dry gangrene is usually seen in arteriosclerosis associated with diabetes.

***embolic g.*** Gangrene arising subsequent to an embolic obstruction.

***gas g.*** Gangrene in a wound infected by a gas bacillus, the most common causative agent being *Clostridium perfringens.*

TREATMENT: Gas gangrene is treated with debridement of the wound site, antibiotics, and clostridial antitoxin. In some cases, surgical intervention may be necessary.

***idiopathic g.*** Gangrene of unknown etiology.

***inflammatory g.*** Gangrene associated with acute infections and inflammation.

***moist g.*** Gangrene that is wet as a result of tissue necrosis and bacterial infection. The condition is marked by serous exudation and rapid decomposition.

SYMPTOMS: At first the affected part is hot and red; later it is cold and bluish, starting to slough. Moist gangrene spreads rapidly and carries an offensive odor. Death may result in a few days.

***primary g.*** Gangrene developing in a part without previous inflammation.

***secondary g.*** Gangrene developing subsequent to local inflammation.

***symmetrical g.*** Gangrene on opposite sides of the body in corresponding parts, usually the result of vasomotor disturbances. It is characteristic of Raynaud's and Buerger's diseases.

***traumatic g.*** Gangrene resulting from extensive injuries.

**gangrenous** Pert. to gangrene.

**Ganser syndrome** (găn′zĕrz) [Sigbert J. M. Ganser, Ger. psychiatrist, 1853–1931] A factitious disorder in which the individual mimics behavior he or she thinks is typical of a psychosis (e.g., giving nonsense answers and doing things incorrectly). Although there may be amnesia, disturbance of consciousness, and hallucinations, the individual is not psychotic.

**gantry** (găn′trē) [Gr. *kanthēlios,* pack ass] **1.** The housing for the imaging source and detectors into which the patient is placed for computed tomography and magnetic resonance imaging. **2.** The portion of the radiation therapy machine (linear accelerator, cobalt unit) that houses the source of therapeutic particles.

**gap** [Old Norse *gap,* chasm] An opening or a break; an interruption in continuity.

***auscultatory g.*** A period of silence that sometimes occurs in the determination of blood pressure by auscultation. The exact cause is unknown. It may occur in patients with hypertension or aortic stenosis. SEE: *blood pressure.*

**gap junction** Minute pores between cells that provide pathways for intercellular communication. Originally described in muscle tissue, they are known to be present in most animal cells.

**Gardnerella vaginalis** [Herman Gardner, U.S. physician, d. 1947] A bacterium that may cause vaginitis in otherwise healthy women. Formerly called *Haemophilus vaginalis* or *Corynebacterium vaginale.*

**Gardnerella vaginalis vaginitis** Vaginitis caused by the bacterium *Gardnerella vaginalis* (formerly *Haemophilus vaginalis*). The bacilli are usually gram negative but may be gram variable in old cultures. The disease is probably transmitted sexually. Diagnosis is best made clinically rather than microbiologically because *Gardnerella* bacteria are often found in healthy, asymptomatic individuals. Clinically, there is a characteristic malodorous discharge, elevated vaginal pH, and wet preparation of vaginal epithelial cells that are heavily stippled with bacteria. These are called "clue cells." Mixing a 10% solution of potassium hydroxide with the vaginal secretion produces a fishy odor. Treatment is with oral metronidazole. Also, oral clindomycin, intravaginal metronidazole gel, and intravaginal clindamycin cream are effective. SYN: *bacterial vaginosis.* SEE: *clue cell.*

**Gardner's syndrome** [Eldon J. Gardner, U.S. geneticist, b. 1909] Familial polyposis of the colon associated with a high risk of developing carcinoma of the colon. Also present are multiple osteomas and soft-tissue tumors of the skin. The condition is inherited as an autosomal dominant trait.

**gargle** [Fr. *gargouille,* throat; but may be onomatopoeia for gargle] **1.** A throat wash. **2.** To wash out the mouth and throat by tipping the head back and allowing the fluid to accumulate in the back of the throat, while agitating it by the forceful expiration of air.

**gargoylism** (găr′goyl-ĭsm) Hurler's syndrome.

**garlic** [AS. *gar,* spear, + *leac,* the leek] An edible, strongly flavored bulb of *Allium sativum* used mainly for seasoning. The chemical allicin, responsible for the smell of garlic, is not evident until the clove is cut or crushed. The possibility that garlic has therapeutic properties has been investigated. The active ingredient in natural garlic may vary. Extracts of garlic contain very little allicin.

**garment, front-opening** Any female garment that opens from the front rather than the rear to increase dressing convenience for persons with limited function.

**Garré's disease** (găr-āz′) [Carl Garré, Swiss surgeon, 1858–1928] Chronic sclerosing osteitis or osteomyelitis due to pyogenic cocci.

**Garren gastric bubble** [Lloyd and Mary Garren, contemporary U.S. gastroenterologists] A deflated bladder that is placed in the stomach and then inflated; used to treat morbid obesity by reducing the effective volume of the stomach and thereby decreasing hunger.

**Gartner's duct** [Hermann T. Gartner, Danish surgeon and anatomist, 1785–1827] A small duct lying parallel to the uterine tube. It is a vestigial structure representing the persistent mesonephric duct. SYN: *duct of the epoophoron; ductus epoophori longitudinalis.*

**G.A.S.** *general adaptation syndrome.*

**gas** One of the basic forms of matter. Gas molecules are free and move swiftly in all directions. Therefore, a gas not only takes the shape of the containing vessel but expands and fills the vessel no matter what its volume. Among the common important gases are oxygen; nitrogen; hydrogen; helium; sewer gas, which contains carbon monoxide; carbon dioxide; the anesthetic gases; ammonia; and the poisonous war gases. Liquids and solids may release toxic fumes when heated. SEE: *war g.'s; anesthesia.*

***binary g.*** A toxic nerve gas formed by mixing two relatively harmless components. It was devised for use in chemical warfare. SEE: *war g.'s.*

***blood g.'s*** The principal gases found in the blood: oxygen, nitrogen, and carbon dioxide. They may be dissolved in the plasma or may exist in loose chemical combination with other compounds (e.g., oxygen combined with hemoglobin).

***Clayton g.*** SEE: *Clayton gas.*

***coal g.*** A flammable, explosive, toxic gas produced from the distillation of coal; used for heating and lighting. The principal constituents are methane, carbon monoxide, and hydrogen.

***digestive tract g.'s*** The gases found in the digestive tract, including oxygen, nitrogen, hydrogen, carbon dioxide, methane, and those produced by bacterial decomposition of proteins, such as hydrogen sulfide, indole, and skatole.

***illuminating g.*** A mixture of various combustible gases including hydrogen and carbon monoxide. Its poisonous effects are largely due to carbon monoxide.

***inert g.*** A gas that reacts little or not at all with other substances. Examples include helium, argon, neon, and krypton.

***intestinal g.*** One of several gaseous compounds, such as carbon dioxide, hydrogen, methane, methylmercaptan, and hydrogen sulfide, present in the intestinal tract. They are produced by digestive processes. SEE: *digestion; flatus.*

***laughing g.*** SEE: *nitrous oxide.*

***lewisite g.*** A poisonous gas that contains arsenic and smells like geraniums. Symptoms of poisoning are similar to those caused by vesicant gas, but begin abruptly and are usually less severe. Arsenic can be recovered from the serum of the blisters, and symptoms of arsenic poisoning may occur. The treatment is similar to that used for vesicant gas poisoning. SEE: *vesicant g.; war g.'s.*

***lung irritant g.*** A gas causing irritation of the lungs, such as chlorine or phosgene.

SEE: *Nursing Diagnoses Appendix.*

SYMPTOMS: Symptoms of poisoning include a burning sensation of the eyes, nose, and throat, bronchitis, and pneumonia. Pulmonary edema sometimes occurs, usually followed by death.

TREATMENT: The patient must be removed from exposure and a respirator applied. If the patient was exposed to phosgene (which smells like musty hay), symptoms may be delayed and the patient may collapse later. It is therefore important to provide complete rest and warmth and to remove the patient on a stretcher. Supplemental oxygen may be required over a fairly long period. SEE: *war g.'s.*

**marsh g.** Methane.

**mustard g.** Dichlorethyl sulfide, a poisonous gas used in warfare. SEE: *vesicant g.; war g.'s.*

**nerve g.** A gas that interferes with or prevents transmission of nerve impulses. SEE: *war g.'s.*

**nitric oxide g.** A toxic gas administered in very small concentrations during mechanical ventilation to treat persistent pulmonary hypertension.

**nose irritant g.** Diphenylchloroarsine, an irritant smoke. It causes intense pain in the nose, throat, and air passages, sneezing followed by headache and aching in the teeth and jaws, acute mental depression, and sometimes vomiting. The patient must be reassured that no permanent harm is done and should be warned against removing the respirator even though its use may worsen the symptoms. Nasal douching with warm sodium bicarbonate solution is helpful. SEE: *war g.'s.*

**sewer g.** A gas produced by decaying matter in sewage. It is toxic, usually flammable, and explosive.

**suffocating g.** Any of several war gases, such as phosgene or diphosgene, made from chlorine compounds. It irritates the bronchi and lungs, resulting in pulmonary edema. SEE: *lung irritant g.; war g.'s.*

**tear g.** A gas such as bromoacetone that irritates the conjunctiva and produces a flow of tears. Treatment is rarely necessary. When the victim is removed from the contaminated area, the symptoms tend to subside gradually. Irrigating the eyes with large amounts of clear water or physiological saline hastens recovery.

**toxic g.** Any harmful gas.

**vesicant g.** A type of gas that attacks the skin in every part of the body, causing blisters. Clothing and boots become contaminated and a source of danger. Mustard and lewisite gases are examples.

SYMPTOMS: Symptoms do not appear at once; their onset may be delayed 6 hr or longer. Eye pain, lacrimation, and discharge may be the first evidence. The eyelids swell and the patient becomes unable to see. A diffuse redness of the skin is followed by blistering and ulceration.

TREATMENT: Decontamination is essential and must be thorough. The eyes should be bathed freely with normal saline or plain water; a drop or two of castor oil prevents the lids from sticking together. No bandage should be worn. The patient should be scrubbed, if possible, under a hot or warm shower for 10 min. If blisters arise despite these precautionary measures, they should be treated with a mild antiseptic and a protective dressing.

PROGNOSIS: Healing is very slow, but generally complete if the correct treatment is begun promptly.

**vomiting g.** A gas, particularly chloropicrin, that induces emesis.

**war g.'s** Any chemical substances, whether solid, liquid, or vapor, used to produce poisonous gases with irritant effects. They can be classified as lacrimators, sternutators (sneeze causing), lung irritants, vesicants, and systemic poisons, such as nerve gas. Some gases have multiple effects.

War gases are known as nonpersistent (diffusing and dispersing fairly rapidly) or persistent (lingering and evaporating slowly).

FIRST AID: When giving first aid, the rescuer avoids becoming a casualty by taking appropriate precautions. All gas masks are checked to ensure that they are in working order. The rescuer first puts on his or her own mask, then fits masks to patients. The rescuer's skin is covered and exposed skin of persons at risk is flooded with water to flush off chemical contaminants if suspected.

NURSING IMPLICATIONS: Decontamination centers are essential to the rescue effort, and nurses are actively involved in the decontamination process. Thorough decontamination of patients, clothing, foot coverings, equipment, and even ambulances precedes admitting patients to emergency care areas to prevent unaffected persons in the area from becoming casualties.

**gas bacillus** SEE: *Clostridium perfringens.*

**gas chromotography** An analytical technique in which a sample is separated into its component parts between a gaseous mobile phase and a chemically active stationary phase.

**gas distention** Distention resulting from abnormal gaseous accumulation in the abdominal cavity. It may be acute, chronic, local, or general, and may involve the abdominal wall or intra-abdominal viscera in addition to the cavity. A preoperative enema may prevent postsurgical gas formation, a complication of surgery. It is usually limited to the lower part of the small intestine and all of the large intestine.

Cold fluids should be avoided. The patient's position should be changed often and a rectal tube inserted. An enema may be of benefit.

**gaseous** Having the nature or form of gas.

**gas exchange, impaired** The state in which the individual experiences an excess or deficit in oxygenation and/or carbon dioxide elimination at the alveolar-capillary membrane. [This may be an entity of its own, but it also may be an end result of other pathology with an interrelatedness between airway clearance and/or breathing pattern problems.] SEE: *Nursing Diagnoses Appendix.*

**gas gangrene** SEE: *gangrene, gas.*

**gasoline** A product of the destructive distillation of petroleum. Commercial gasolines may contain toxic additives such as tetraethyl lead or tricresyl phosphate.

---

Caution: Using the mouth to produce suction on a tube for siphoning gasoline from a tank is dangerous because the gasoline may be inhaled or swallowed.

---

**gasoline poisoning** The reaction of the body to ingested or inhaled gasoline.

SYMPTOMS: The symptoms of gasoline poisoning are giddiness, headache, intoxication, nervous disturbance, muscular tremors, difficulty in respiration, paralyses, convulsions, cyanosis, unconsciousness, and pulmonary hemorrhage. Usually no local stomach disturbance occurs unless the gasoline has been swallowed.

FIRST AID: The patient must breathe fresh air and should inhale oxygen and carbon dioxide. Artificial respiration is administered when necessary. After that, the symptoms are treated. If the clothing and skin have been grossly contaminated, all precautions to prevent sparks and open flames must be taken. Gasoline is highly flammable and is explosive when mixed with air.

**gasometric** (găs″ō-mĕt′rĭk) Pert. to the measurement of gases.

**gasometry** (găs-ŏm′ĕ-trē) Estimation of the amount of gas in a mixture.

**gasp** [Old Norse *geispa*] To catch the breath; to inhale and exhale with quick, difficult breaths; the act of gasping.

**gas pain** Abdominal pain caused by gas distention of all or part of the intestinal tract. It may be a sign of postsurgical paralytic ileus. SEE: *flatulence.*

**gasserectomy** (găs″ĕr-ĕk′tō-mē) The excision of a gasserian (trigeminal) ganglion. SEE: *ganglion, trigeminal.*

**gaster-** [Gr. *gaster,* belly] SEE: *gastro-.*

**gastero-** SEE: *gastro-.*

**Gasterophilus** (găs″tĕr-ŏf′ĭ-lŭs) A genus of botflies belonging to the family Oestridae, order Diptera. The larvae infest horses.

***G. hemorrhoidalis*** A species of botflies that infests the noses of horses.

***G. intestinalis*** A species of botflies that infests the stomachs of horses.

***G. nasalis*** The chin fly, which lays eggs on hair shafts on the lower lip and jaw of horses.

**gastorrhagia** (găs-tor-ā′jē-ă) [″ + *rhegnynai,* to burst forth] Gastrorrhagia.

**gastr-** SEE: *gastro-.*

**gastralgia** (găs-trăl′jē-ă) [″ + *algos,* pain] Pain in the stomach from any cause.

**gastratrophia** (găs″tră-trō′fē-ă) [″ + *atrophia,* atrophy] Atrophy of the stomach.

**gastrectasia, gastrectasis** [″ + *ektasis,* dilatation] Dilatation of the stomach, either acute or chronic.

SYMPTOMS: *Acute:* Severe, sudden pain is accompanied by collapse; a small, rapid pulse; subnormal temperature; upper abdominal pain resembling angina pectoris, and a distended, tympanic abdomen. Vomiting of fluids and eructation of gas occur. *Chronic:* The patient vomits food eaten several days before. The vomitus is sour and contains fatty acids, mucus, and bacteria.

ETIOLOGY: Gastrectasia is caused by pyloric obstruction, atony, overeating, omental hernia, or periduodenal adhesions.

**gastrectomy** (găs-trĕk′tō-mē) [″ + *ektome,* excision] The surgical removal of part or all of the stomach.

**gastric** (găs′trĭk) [Gr. *gaster,* stomach] Pert. to the stomach. SEE: *digestion; stomach.*

**gastric analysis** Analysis of the contents of the stomach to determine secretion quality, the amount of free and combined hydrochloric acid, and the absence or presence of blood, bile, bacteria, and fatty acids. The test is particularly helpful in suspected cases of gastric bleeding, gastric carcinoma, or pernicious anemia.

**gastric cancer** Adenocarcinoma of the stomach. Location by frequency of involvement is as follows: cardia, 10%; body and fundus, 10%; lesser curvature, 25%; greater curvature, 2% to 3%; and pyloric area, 50%, with rapid infiltration of the regional lymph nodes, omentum, liver, and lungs via the walls of the stomach, duodenum, and esophagus, the lymphatic system, adjacent organs, the bloodstream, and the peritoneal cavity. Although this form of cancer is common throughout the world in people of all races, the incidence of gastric cancer exhibits unexplained geographic, cultural, and gender differences, with the highest incidence in men over age 40 and high mortality in Japan, Iceland, Chile, and Austria.

Over the past 25 years, the incidence of gastric cancer in the U.S. has fallen 50%, with the resulting death rate now one third what it was 30 years ago. This decrease has been attributed (without proof) to the improved, well-balanced diets available to most people in the U.S. The prognosis for a particular patient depends on the stage of the disease at the time of diagnosis, but overall, the 5-year survival rate is about 15%.

PREDISPOSING CAUSES: Although the cause of gastric cancer is unknown, predisposing factors, such as gastritis with gastric atrophy, increase the risk. Genetic factors have been implicated. People with type A blood have a 10% increased risk, and the disease occurs more commonly in people with a family history of such cancer.

COMPLICATIONS: Malnutrition occurs when the stomach cannot digest protein, and gastrointestinal (GI) obstruction develops as the tumor enlarges. Iron deficiency anemia results as the tumor causes ulceration and bleeding. The tumor can interfere with the production of the intrinsic factor needed for vitamin $B_{12}$ absorption, resulting in pernicious anemia. As the cancer metastasizes to other structures, related complications occur.

SIGNS AND SYMPTOMS: In the early stages, the patient may experience pain in the back or in the epigastric or retrosternal areas that is relieved with nonprescription analgesics; however, this symptom may not be reported because of failure to recognize its significance. The patient typically reports a vague feeling of fullness, heaviness, and moderate abdominal distention after meals. Depending on the cancer's progression, the patient may report weight loss, resulting from appetite disturbance; nausea; and vomiting. Coffee-ground vomitus may be reported if the tumor is located in the cardia. Weakness and fatigue are common complaints.

If the tumor is located in the proximal area of the stomach, the patient may experience dysphagia. Palpation of the abdomen may disclose a mass. Also, the examiner may be able to palpate enlarged lymph nodes, esp. in the supraclavicular and axillary regions. Other assessment findings depend on the extent of the disease and the location of metastasis.

DIAGNOSTIC STUDIES: Gastric cancer is diagnosed by barium radiography of the GI tract with fluoroscopy, fiberoptic endoscope gastroscopy and biopsy, and gastric acid stimulation testing. Studies to rule out specific organ metastases include computed tomography scans, chest radiographs, liver and bone scans, and liver biopsy.

TREATMENT: Surgery to remove the tumor often is the treatment of choice. Excision of the lesion with appropriate margins is possible in more than one third of patients. Even in the patient whose disease is not considered surgically curable, resection eases symptoms and improves the potential benefits of the chemotherapy and radiation therapy that usually follow surgery. The nature and extent of the lesion determine the type of surgery. Surgical procedures include gastroduodenostomy, gastrojejunostomy, partial gastric resection, and total gastrectomy. If metastasis has occurred, the omentum and spleen may have to be removed.

Chemotherapy for GI tumors may help to control signs and symptoms and to prolong survival. Gastric adenocarcinomas respond to several agents, including fluorouracil, carmustine, doxorubicin, and mitomycin. Antispasmodics and antacids may help relieve GI distress. Antiemetics can control nausea, which intensifies as the tumor grows. In the more advanced stages, the patient may need sedatives and tranquilizers to control overwhelming anxiety. Opioid analgesics can relieve severe and unremitting pain.

If the patient has a nonresectable or partially resectable tumor, radiation therapy is effective if combined with chemotherapy. The patient should receive this therapy on an empty stomach. It should not be given preoperatively, because it may damage viscera and impede healing.

NURSING IMPLICATIONS: Nutritional intake is monitored and the patient weighed periodically. The patient is observed for malnutrition, anemia, and vitamin $B_{12}$ malabsorption, with complete blood count results and vitamin $B_{12}$ levels monitored. The patient is prepared physically and emotionally for surgery as necessary.

Throughout the course of the illness, a high-protein, high-calorie diet is provided to help the patient to avoid or recover from weight loss, malnutrition, and anemia. This diet also helps the patient to tolerate surgery, chemotherapy, and radiotherapy; promotes wound healing; and provides enough protein, fluid, and potassium to aid glycogen and body protein synthesis. Frequent small meals are offered, and iron-rich foods are included if the patient has an iron deficiency. Dietary supplements are provided as prescribed.

To stimulate a poor appetite, prescribed steroids, antidepressant drugs, or wine or brandy may be administered. Parenteral nutrition is given as prescribed. A prescribed antacid is administered to relieve heartburn and acid stomach, and a prescribed histamine$_2$-receptor antagonist, such as cimetidine or famotidine, to decrease gastric secretions. Prescribed opioid analgesics are also administered. The patient is instructed in use of all drugs.

Complications of radiation therapy include nausea, vomiting, alopecia, malaise, and diarrhea. Complications of chemotherapy include infection, nausea, vomiting, mouth ulcers, and alopecia. During radiation or chemotherapy, oral intake is encouraged to help relieve some of the adverse effects; orange or grapefruit juice, ginger ale, or other fluids and prescribed antiemetics are provided to minimize nausea and vomiting; and comfort measures and reassurance are offered as needed. The patient is advised to report persistent adverse reactions.

The patient is encouraged to follow normal routine as much as possible after recovery from surgery and during radiation therapy and chemotherapy. Activities that cause excessive fatigue should be stopped (at least temporarily) and rest periods incorporated. The patient should avoid crowds and people with known infections.

**gastric digestion** The phase of digestion that occurs in the stomach while food is being temporarily stored and mixed in it. The semisolid mass of food known as chyme is mixed with the salivary juices, and certain other substances are added from the stomach, including hydrochloric acid, mucus, pepsin, and some lipase. The general result of gastric digestion is the reduction of the ingested mass to a mushy gray mixture called acid chyme.

CHEMICAL ASPECTS: During a meal, stimuli from the brain are carried to the stomach by way of the vagal nerves. These stimuli are produced by the sensations of sight, smell, and taste. In addition, the stretching of the stomach wall stimulates the gastric glands, causing the hormone gastrin to be discharged from the pyloric region into the blood. The circulating gastrin reaches the gastric glands and causes them to secrete.

The food undergoes certain changes while in the stomach. Pepsin acts on high molecular weight proteins, hydrolyzing them to peptones, and also coagulates milk. Hydrochloric acid is essential for the activity of pepsin and is responsible for the antiseptic action of the gastric juice. SEE: *digestion*.

MOTOR ASPECTS: When food first enters the stomach, the stomach is relaxed; then it increases its pressure on the contents. The cardiac sphincter closes firmly to prevent regurgitation into the esophagus. Contractions of the pyloric region of the stomach become more forceful. At first the pyloric sphincter is closed; the result is physical mixing of the food and the beginning of chemical digestion. Then, at intervals, the pyloric sphincter relaxes to permit acid chyme to gradually enter the duodenum. How quickly the chyme leaves the stomach is influenced by the amount of the feeding, its osmotic character, and the amount of fat present. In general, a high-fat meal leaves the stomach more slowly than a low-fat meal. SEE: *digestion, duodenal*.

**gastric gland** One of the cardiac, fundic or oxyntic, and pyloric secretory glands of the stomach. These are tubular glands in the mucosa of the wall. The general result of gastric digestion is the reduction of the ingested mass to a mushy, gray mixture called acid chyme. Gastric glands contain zymogenic or peptic cells, which secrete pepsinogen, the inactive form of pepsin; parietal border or oxyntic cells, which secrete hydrochloric acid; and mucous cells found in the neck of the gland, which secrete mucin.

**gastric-inhibitory polypeptide** ABBR: GIP. A polypeptide hormone secreted by the duodenum and jejunum that inhibits motility and the secretion of gastric hydrochloric acid and pepsin and that stimulates insulin secretion. SEE: *enterogastrone*.

**gastric intramucosal pH** An experimental procedure to measure the pH of gastric mucosa to determine the adequacy of its oxygenation. The goal is to obtain an index of tissue oxygenation in general.

**gastric juice** The digestive secretion of the gastric glands of the stomach. It is a thin, colorless fluid containing pepsin, hydrochloric acid, mucin, small quantities of inorganic salts, the intrinsic factor of the antianemic principle, and lipase. It is strongly acid, having a pH of 0.9 to 1.5, its total acidity being equivalent to 10 to 50 ml of tenth-normal (10%) hydrochloric acid (free hydrochloric acid is from 0 to 30 ml of tenth-normal hydrochloric acid). The amount secreted in 24 hr varies greatly. The mixture of acid and pepsin has effects that neither substance has alone, acting on some proteins with remarkable speed.

DIAGNOSIS: *Achlorhydria:* Pernicious anemia is the most common cause of this finding in persons who do not have gastric cancer. *Carcinoma:* Bacteria, blood, and sometimes tumor cells are present; frequently no hydrochloric acid is found. *Hyperacidity:* This may indicate gastric ulcer. *Pus cells:* Severe stomach inflammation is present. *Red cells:* These have the same significance as pus cells, with the added evidence of hemorrhage.

**gastric lavage** Washing out of the stomach; used to empty the stomach when the contents are irritating, as in prolonged postanesthetic vomiting and some cases of regurgitant vomiting in acute intestinal obstruction. Lavage is also used to clean the cavity before gastric surgery, to remove poison when this treatment is indicated, and to remove a test meal.

NURSING IMPLICATIONS: The following equipment is assembled: plastic or rubber large-lumen nasogastric tube; ice in a bowl if a rubber tube is to be used; water-soluble lubricant; disposable irrigation set with bulb syringe; adhesive tape or other device; clamp, safety pins, and rubber band; gloves, and stethoscope; tissues; glass of water with straw; emesis basin; container for aspirant; at least 500 to 1000 ml of prescribed irrigating solution; and any specified antidote.

Physical restraints are applied as prescribed and required. The patient's clothing is removed and a hospital gown put on. If conscious and cooperative, the patient is placed in the high Fowler's position (head elevated 80 to 90 degrees), and the chest is covered with a water-impermeable bib or drape. If unconscious, the patient is positioned to prevent aspiration of stomach contents, and suction equipment is readily available.

The distance for tube insertion is measured by placing the tip of the tube at the tip of the patient's nose and extending the tube to the ear lobe and then to the xiphoid process. This location or the length of tubing that will remain outside the patient after insertion is marked on the tube. Nostril patency is checked and the nostril with the least obstruction used for the procedure. While the patient holds the emesis basin, the nurse lubricates the tip of the tube and inserts it. A downward and backward motion aids passage through the back of the nose and down into the nasopharynx, thus avoiding producing a gag reflex. The patient is instructed to dry-swallow during this phase of passage. The tube should not be forced. If obstruction is met, the tube is removed, the patient permitted to rest briefly, the tube relubricated, and the procedure attempted again. If the tube cannot be passed without traumatizing the mucosa, the physician is notified.

When the tube is in the nasopharynx, the patient is instructed to flex the neck slightly to bring the head forward. The glass of water (if permitted) is given to the patient, and the patient is encouraged to swallow the tube with small sips of water (or to dry swallow if water is not permitted). Rotating the tube toward the opposite nostril often helps direct toward the esophagus and away from the trachea. Placing the nondominant hand on the nose to secure the tube, the nurse advances it with the dominant hand as the patient swallows.

The back of the throat is periodically inspected for any evidence of coiled tubing, esp. if the patient is gagging or uncomfortable, or unconscious. When the tube has been passed, placement is verified by aspirating gastric contents with the bulb syringe or by injecting a small volume of air and auscultating over the epigastrium for a whooshing sound. The tube is then secured to the nostrils with adhesive tape or another securing device according to protocol.

---

Caution: Before any liquids are instilled into the stomach via the tube, the patient should be checked to ensure that the end of the tube is in the stomach and not in the bronchus. If proper placement is in doubt, a radiograph should be taken. In emergency situations, instilling 5 to 10 ml of sterile water will help to demonstrate tube placement; if the tube is in the bronchus, the cough reflex will be intact, and water will be returned in the air during expiration.

---

The irrigation fluid is instilled, and care is taken to prevent the entrance of air. A Y connector can be attached to the nasogastric tube, with one tubing exiting to the bulb syringe or irrigant container and the other to a drainage set. The return line is clamped, and the solution, usually 500 ml or more, instilled to distend the stomach and expose all areas to the solution. The large volume also dilutes harmful liquids and thins or dissolves other materials.

The patient is monitored throughout for retching. If retching occurs, the flow is stopped, suction is applied to the bulb syringe, or the drainage line is opened to remove some of the instilled fluid. The stomach is then drained, and the procedure repeated as necessary to cleanse and empty the stomach of harmful materials and irrigant. An antidote or activated charcoal slurry is then instilled as appropriate and prescribed.

A specimen of the aspirant is sent to the laboratory for analysis as directed. The tube may remain in place, attached to intermittent low suction as required, or be removed immediately after the procedure.

For removal, the tube is clamped securely. Any securing devices are removed, and the tube is rotated gently to ensure that it is freely moveable and then gently but steadily pulled outward and folded. The nurse's glove is then pulled off over the tube, and the second glove over the closed fist to effectively "double-bag" the tube. The patient is handed tissues to wipe the eyes and blow the nose and is assisted with oral hygiene. A fresh gown or linens are provided as necessary. The patient continues to be monitored for adverse effects of the toxic material.

The tube and prescribed suction are maintained as necessary, drainage is documented, comfort measures (oral misting, anesthetic throat sprays) are provided, and the patient is assessed for any complications.

**gastric ulcer** SEE: *ulcer, gastric.*

**gastrin** A hormone secreted by the mucosa of the pyloric area of the stomach and duodenum in various species of animals, including humans. The hormone is released into gastric venous blood, from which it flows into the liver and into the general circulation. When the hormone reaches the stomach glands, it stimulates gastric acid secretion. Gastrin causes the lower esophageal sphincter to contract and the ileocecal sphincter to relax. Also, it has a mild effect on small-intestine and gallbladder motility. Gastrin is released in response to partially digested protein, ethyl alcohol in about 10% concentration, and distention of the antrum of the stomach.

SEE: *Zollinger-Ellison syndrome.*

**gastrinoma** (găs″trĭn-ō′mă) The tumor associated with Zollinger-Ellison syndrome. SEE: *Zollinger-Ellison syndrome.*

**gastritis** (găs-trī′tĭs) [Gr. *gaster,* stomach, + *itis,* inflammation] Inflammation of the stomach; marked by epigastric pain or tenderness, nausea, vomiting, hematemesis, and systemic electrolyte changes if vomiting persists. The mucosa may be atrophic or hypertrophic.

ETIOLOGY: The cause is generally unknown. Gastritis may result from infection, excessive intake of alcoholic beverages, dietary indiscretions, or an excess or deficiency of hydrochloric acid. Pain in the stomach region may be due to causes other than gastritis, such as cancer.

NURSING IMPLICATIONS: Fluid intake and output and electrolyte and acid-base balance are monitored. If the patient is vomiting, prescribed antiemetics and replacement intravenous fluids are administered.

When the patient can tolerate oral feeding, a bland diet based on the patient's food preferences is begun. If nothing has been given by mouth, the patient is observed for returning symptoms when food is reintroduced. Small, frequent servings are offered. The patient is assisted to identify and eliminate foods that cause gastric upset. Antacids and other prescribed medications are administered and the patient is instructed in their use. If pain or nausea interferes with appetite, a prescribed analgesic or antiemetic is administered about 1 hr before meals.

If surgery is necessary, the patient is prepared physically and emotionally for the procedure.

The patient is educated about the disorder. A list of irritating foods and beverages is provided. The patient's questions are answered honestly, and emotional support is provided. Patients who smoke are encouraged to stop. Referral to a smoking cessation program or for nicotine patch therapy may be warranted.

The need for stress reduction is emphasized, and instruction is given in stress reduction techniques. Prophylactic medications should be taken as prescribed. Immediate medical attention should be sought for recurring symptoms such as nausea, vomiting, or hematemesis.

***acute g.*** Acute and sudden irritation of the gastric mucosa. This may be due to ingestion of toxic substances such as alcohol or poisons. The symptoms include moderate fever, anorexia, coated tongue, intense epigastic pain, persistent vomiting, thirst, and prostration. Therapy includes antisecretory drugs. For severe prolonged bleeding, surgery may be required. SEE: *Nursing Diagnoses Appendix.*

***atrophic g.*** Chronic gastritis with atrophied mucosa and glands. Patients with this type often are asymptomatic.

***chronic g.*** Prolonged continual or intermittent inflammation of the gastric mucosa. This may be due to systemic disease such as pernicious anemia, or use of tobacco products. Symptoms are usually absent, but one or more of the following may be present: mild nausea and anorexia; a sense of distention or fullness after eating a small meal; a bad taste in the mouth; mild or acute epigastric pain. The patient requires antispasmodics, antacids, reassurance, and sedatives. SEE: *Nursing Diagnoses Appendix.*

***giant hypertrophic g.*** Gastritis of unknown cause, marked by excessive proliferation of the stomach mucosal folds. SYN: *Ménétrier's disease.*

***toxic g.*** Gastritis due to any toxic agent, including poisons or corrosive chemicals.

**gastro-, gaster-, gastero-, gastr-** [Gr. *gaster,* stomach] Combining form meaning *stomach.*

**gastroanastomosis** (găs″trō-ăn-ăs″tō-mō′sĭs) [″ + *anastomosis,* outlet] The formation of a passage between the pyloric and cardiac ends of the stomach for relief of persistent hourglass contraction. SYN: *gastrogastrostomy.*

**gastrocamera** (găs″trō-kăm′ĕ-ră) A camera, small enough to be swallowed, used to photograph the inside of the stomach.

**gastrocardiac** (găs″trō-kăr′dē-ăk) [″ + *kardia,* heart] Concerning the stomach and heart.

**gastrocele** (găs′trō-sēl) [″ + *kele,* hernia] A hernia of the stomach.

**gastrocnemius** (găs″trŏk-nē′mē-ŭs) [″ + *kneme,* leg] The large muscle of the posterior portion of the lower leg. It is the most superficial of the calf muscles. It plantar flexes the foot and flexes the knee.

**gastrocoele** (găs′trō-sēl) Archenteron.

**gastrocolic** (găs″trō-kŏl′ĭk) [″ + *kolon,* colon] Pert. to the stomach and colon.

**gastrocolic omentum** SEE: *omentum, greater.*

**gastrocolitis** (găs″trō-kō-lī′tĭs) [″ + ″ + *itis,* inflammation] Inflammation of the stomach and colon.

**gastrocoloptosis** (găs″trō-kŏl″ŏp-tō′sĭs) [″ + ″ + *ptosis,* dropping] Downward prolapse of the stomach and colon.

**gastrocolostomy** (găs″trō-kŏl-ŏs′tō-mē) [″ + ″ + *stoma,* mouth] Establishment of a permanent passage between the stomach and colon.

**gastrocolotomy** (găs″trō-kō-lŏt′ō-mē) [″ + ″ + *tome,* incision] Incision into the stomach and colon.

**gastrocolpotomy** (găs″trō-kŏl-pŏt′ō-mē) [″ + *kolpos,* vagina, + *tome,* incision] An incision through the abdominal wall into the upper part of the vagina.

**gastrocutaneous** (găs″trō-kū-tā′nē-ŭs) [″ + L. *cutis,* skin] Concerning the stomach and skin, or a communication between the two.

**gastrodialysis** (găs″trō-dī-ăl′ĭ-sĭs) [″ + *dia,*

through, + *lysis,* dissolution] Dialysis (i.e., washing out) of the stomach to clear both the stomach and the blood of toxic materials secreted into the stomach.

**gastrodidymus** (găs″trō-dĭd′ĭ-mŭs) [″ + *didymos,* twin] Congenitally deformed twins united by a common abdominal cavity.

**gastrodisciasis** (găs″trō-dĭs-kī′ă-sĭs) Infestation by a fluke, *Gastrodiscoides hominis.*

**Gastrodiscoides** (găs″trō-dĭs-koy′dēz) A genus of flukes belonging to the family Gastrodiscidae, suborder Amphistomata.

***G. hominis*** A species of flukes commonly infesting hogs but occasionally found in humans.

**gastroduodenal** (găs″trō-dū″ō-dēn′ăl) [Gr. *gaster,* stomach, + L. *duodeni,* twelve] Rel. to the stomach and duodenum.

**gastroduodenitis** (găs″trō-dū-ŏd″ĕn-ī′tĭs) [″ + ″ + Gr. *itis,* inflammation] Inflammation of the stomach and duodenum.

**gastroduodenoscopy** (găs″trō-dū″ō-dĕ-nŏs′kō-pē) [″ + ″ + *skopein,* to examine] The use of an endoscope to visually examine the stomach and duodenum.

**gastroduodenostomy** (găs″trō-dū″ō-dĕn-ŏs′tō-mē) [″ + ″ + Gr. *stoma,* mouth] Excision of the pylorus of the stomach with anastomosis of the upper portion of the stomach to the duodenum. SYN: *Billroth I operation.*

**gastroenteralgia** (găs″trō-ĕn″tĕr-ăl′jē-ă) [″ + *enteron,* intestine, + *algos,* pain] Pain in the stomach and intestines.

**gastroenteric** (găs″trō-ĕn-tĕr′ĭk) Pert. to the stomach and intestines or to a condition involving both.

**gastroenteritis** (găs″trō-ĕn-tĕr-ī′tĭs) [″ + *enteron,* intestine, + *itis,* inflammation] Inflammation of the stomach and intestinal tract. SEE: *Nursing Diagnoses Appendix.*

***viral g.*** Gastroenteritis caused by waterborne or foodborne viruses including Norwalk virus, Norwalk-like viruses, astroviruses, caliciviruses, and rotaviruses. It is difficult to confirm these viral infections, and public health interventions needed to control outbreaks caused by these agents usually must be made before results of viral testing are available. The median incubation period is 24 to 48 hr and the median duration of the symptoms is 12 to 60 hr. Most patients will experience diarrhea, nausea, abdominal cramps, and vomiting. There is no specific treatment other than supportive therapy and fluid replacement.

**gastroenteroanastomosis** (găs″trō-ĕn″tĕr-ō-ă-năs″tō-mō′sĭs) The formation of a passage between the stomach and small intestine.

**gastroenterocolitis** (găs″trō-ĕn″tĕr-ō-kŏl-ī′tĭs) [″ + ″ + *kolon,* colon, + *itis,* inflammation] Inflammation of the stomach, small intestine, and colon.

**gastroenterocolostomy** (găs″trō-ĕn″tĕr-ō-kō-lŏs′tō-mē) [″ + ″ + ″ + *stoma,* mouth] The creation of a passage joining the stomach, small intestine, and colon.

**gastroenterology** (găs″trō-ĕn″tĕr-ŏl′ō-jē) [″ + ″ + *logos,* word, reason] The branch of medical science concerned with the study of the physiology and pathology of the stomach, intestines, and related structures, such as the esophagus, liver, gallbladder, and pancreas.

**gastroenteroptosis** (găs″trō-ĕn″tĕr-ŏp-tō′sĭs) [″ + ″ + *ptosis,* a dropping] Prolapse of the stomach and intestines.

**gastroenterostomy** (găs″trō-ĕn-tĕr-ŏs′tō-mē) [″ + *enteron,* intestine, + *stoma,* mouth] Surgical anastomosis between the stomach and small bowel. This operation is required for patients suffering from carcinoma or cicatricial stricture of the pyloric orifice of the stomach.

**gastroepiploic** (găs″trō-ĕp″ĭ-plō′ĭk) [″ + *epiploon,* omentum] Pert. to the stomach and greater omentum.

**gastroesophageal** (găs″trō-ē-sŏf″ă-jē′ăl) [″ + *oisophagos,* esophagus] Concerning the stomach and esophagus.

**gastroesophageal reflux** SEE: *acid-reflux disorder.*

**gastroesophageal reflux disease** ABBR: GERD. The reflux of acidic gastric contents into the lower esophagus. This may occur whenever the pressure in the stomach is greater than that in the esophagus and may be associated with obesity or pregnancy. This condition may cause esophagitis. SEE: *acid-reflux disorder.*

SYMPTOMS: Characteristic complaints include a persistent burning sensation after meals (heartburn) that is relieved by antacids, and postprandial regurgitation that is precipitated by bending over or by recumbency, esp. after eating fatty foods.

ETIOLOGY: Transient relaxation of the lower esophageal sphincter allows an upward escape of gastric acid.

TREATMENT: Pharmacological management includes histamine $H_2$ agonists to reduce secretion of gastric acid. Episodes are further reduced by decreasing fat intake and tobacco use, avoiding recumbency for 3 hr after eating, and elevating the head of the bed. Weight reduction by obese patients is helpful.

***chronic g.r.d.*** Persistent reflux of the acid gastric contents into the lower esophagus, causing heartburn.

TREATMENT: SEE: *gastroesophageal reflux disease.*

**gastroesophagitis** (găs″trō-ē-sŏf″ă-jī′tĭs) [″ + ″ + *itis,* inflammation] Inflammation of the stomach and esophagus.

**gastroesophagostomy** (găs″trō-ē-sŏf″ă-gŏs′tō-mē) [″ + ″ + *stoma,* mouth] The formation of a passage from the esophagus to the stomach.

**gastrofiberscope** (găs″trō-fī′bĕr-skōp) A flexible endoscope using fiberoptics for visual examination of the stomach.

**gastrogastrostomy** (găs″trō-găs-trŏs′tō-mē) [″ + *gaster,* stomach, + *stoma,* mouth] Gastroanastomosis.

**gastrogavage** (găs″trō-gă-văzh′) [″ + Fr. *gavage,* cramming] Artificial feeding through an opening into the stomach or a tube passed into the stomach.

**gastrogenic** (găs″trō-jĕn′ĭk) [″ + *gennan,* to produce] Originating in the stomach.

**gastrohepatic** [″ + *hepar,* liver] Pert. to the stomach and liver.

**gastrohepatitis** (găs″trō-hĕp-ă-tī′tĭs) [″ + ″ + *itis,* inflammation] The combination of gastritis and hepatitis.

**gastroileac** (găs-trō-ĭl′ē-ăk) [″ + L. *ileum,* groin] Pert. to the stomach and ileum.

**gastroileitis** (găs″trō-ĭl-ē-ī′tĭs) Inflammation of the stomach and ileum.

**gastroileostomy** (găs″trō-ĭl-ē-ŏs′tō-mē) A surgical anastomosis between the stomach and ileum.

**gastrointestinal** [″ + L. *intestinalis,* intestine] Pert. to the stomach and intestine.

**gastrointestinal bleeding** Bleeding from the gastrointestinal tract. This important sign requires prompt therapy and determination of its cause.

**gastrointestinal decompression** The removal of gases from the intestinal tract by use of suction through a tube inserted through the nostrils and into the digestive tract. SEE: *Wangensteen tube.*

**gastrojejunostomy** (găs-trō-jĕ-jū-nŏs′tō-mē) [″ + L. *jejunum,* empty, + Gr. *stoma,* mouth] Subtotal excision of the stomach with closure of the proximal end of the duodenum and side-to-side anastomosis of the jejunum to the remaining portion of the stomach. SYN: *Billroth II operation.*

**gastrolienal** (găs″trō-lī′ĕn-ăl) [″ + L. *lien,* spleen] Concerning the stomach and spleen.

**gastrolith** (găs′trō-lĭth) [″+ *lithos,* stone] A calculus in the stomach.

**gastrolithiasis** (găs″trō-lĭth-ī′ă-sĭs) The formation of calculi in the stomach.

**gastrology** (găs-trŏl′ō-jē) [″ + *logos,* word, reason] The study of function and diseases of the stomach.

**gastrolysis** (găs-trŏl′ĭ-sĭs) [″ + *lysis,* dissolution] Surgical breaking of adhesions between the stomach and adjoining structures.

**gastromalacia** (găs-trō-mă-lā′shē-ă) [″ + *malakia,* softening] A softening of the stomach walls.

**gastromegaly** (găs″trō-mĕg′ă-lē) [″ + *megas,* large] An enlargement of the stomach.

**gastromycosis** (găs″trō-mī-kō′sĭs) [″ + *mykes,* fungus, + *osis,* condition] A disease of the stomach caused by fungi.

**gastromyotomy** (găs″trō-mī-ŏt′ō-mē) [″ + *mys,* muscle, + *tome,* incision] An incision of the circular muscle fibers of the stomach.

**gastropancreatitis** (găs″trō-păn″krē-ă-tī′tĭs) [″ + *pan,* all, + *kreas,* flesh, + *itis,* inflammation] A simultaneous inflammation of the stomach and pancreas.

**gastroparalysis** (găs″trō-păr-ăl′ĭ-sĭs) [″ + *para,* beyond, + *lyein,* to loosen] Paralysis of the stomach. SYN: *gastroplegia.*

**gastropathy** (găs-trŏp′ă-thē) [″+ *pathos,* disease, suffering] Any disorder of the stomach.

**gastropexy, gastropexis** (găs′trō-pĕk″sē, -sĭs) [″+ *pexis,* fixation] Suturing of the stomach to the abdominal walls for correction of displacement.

**gastrophrenic** (găs″trō-frĕn′ĭk) [″+ *phren,* diaphragm] Rel. to the stomach and diaphragm.

**gastroplasty** (găs′trō-plăs″tē) [″ + *plassein,* to form] Plastic surgery of the stomach. This procedure has been used in several ways to decrease the size of the stomach to treat morbid obesity; its success is controversial.

**gastroplegia** (găs″trō-plē′jē-ă) [″+ *plege,* stroke] Gastroparalysis.

**gastroplication** (găs″trō-plī-kā′shŭn) [″+ L. *plicare,* to fold] Stitching of the walls of the stomach to reduce dilatation.

**gastroptosis** (găs″trō-tō′sĭs) [″+ *ptosis,* falling] Downward displacement of the stomach, which rarely causes symptoms or illness.

**gastropulmonary** (găs″trō-pŭl′mō-năr-ē) [″ + L. *pulmo,* lung] Concerning the stomach and lungs.

**gastropylorectomy** (găs″trō-pī″lor-ĕk′tō-mē) [″ + *pyloros,* pylorus, + *ektome,* excision] Excision of the stomach at the pyloric end.

**gastropyloric** Rel. to the stomach and pylorus.

**gastroradiculitis** (găs″trō-ră-dĭk″ū-lī′tĭs) [″ + L. *radix,* root, + Gr. *itis,* inflammation] Inflammation of the posterior spinal nerve roots, the sensory fibers of which supply the stomach.

**gastrorrhagia** (găs″trō-rā′jē-ă) [″ + *rhegnynai,* to burst forth] Hemorrhage from the stomach.

**gastrorrhaphy** (găs-tror′ă-fē) [″ + *rhaphe,* seam, ridge] **1.** Suture of an injured stomach wall. **2.** Gastroplication.

**gastrorrhexis** A rupture or tearing of the stomach.

**gastroschisis** (găs-trŏs′kĭ-sĭs) [″ + *schisis,* a splitting] A congenital fissure that remains open in the wall of the abdomen.

**gastroscope** (găs′trō-skōp) [″ + *skopein,* to examine] An endoscope for inspecting the stomach's interior.

**gastroscopy** (găs-trŏs′kō-pē) Examination of the stomach and abdominal cavity using a gastroscope.

**gastrospasm** (găs′trō-spăzm) [″ + *spasmos,* spasm] A spasm of the stomach.

**gastrosplenic** (găs″trō-splĕn′ĭk) [″ + *splen,* spleen] Of or pert. to the stomach and spleen.

**gastrostenosis** (găs″trō-stĕn-ō′sĭs) [″+ *stenosis,* narrowing] Contraction (stenosis) of the stomach.

*g. cardiaca* Stenosis of the cardiac orifice of the stomach.

*g. pylorica* Stenosis of the pylorus of the stomach.

**gastrostogavage** (găs-trŏs″tō-gă-văzh′) [″ + *stoma,* mouth, + Fr. *gaver,* to stuff] Feeding by means of a tube leading from outside the body into the stomach through a gastric fistula. SEE: *gavage.*

**gastrostolavage** (găs-trŏs″tō-lă-văzh′) [″ + Fr. *lavage,* fr. L. *lavare,* to wash] Irrigation of the stomach through a gastric fistula, or surgically constructed gastrostomy.

**gastrostoma** (găs-trŏs′tō-mă) [″ + *stoma,* mouth] A fistula of the stomach.

**gastrostomy** (găs-trŏs′tō-mē) Surgical creation of a gastric fistula through the abdominal wall, necessary in some cases of cicatricial stricture of the esophagus for the purpose of introducing food into the stomach.

NURSING IMPLICATIONS: The skin around the tube is inspected for signs of irritation or excoriation and kept clean, dry, and protected from excoriating gastric secretions. Tension on the tube that may cause the incision to widen and allow spillage of gastric secretions on the skin or into surrounding tissues is prevented.

Before the patient is fed, tube patency and position are assessed, and the volume of the remaining stomach contents is measured by aspirating the stomach. If the volume is greater than the amount permitted by protocol or physician's direction, feeding is withheld. After feedings, the tube is flushed with water to prevent clogging and promote hydration.

Assistance is provided with oral hygiene at intervals throughout the day to prevent dryness and parotitis. Both patient and family are taught correct techniques for tube and skin care and for feeding through the gastrostomy tube. SEE: *gastrostomy tube.*

***percutaneous endoscopic g.*** ABBR: PEG. A feeding ostomy. PEG tubes are inserted through the esophagus into the stomach with the aid of an endoscope and then pulled through a stab wound made in the abdominal wall.

**gastrostomy tube** A tube placed in the gastrostomy to provide a means of feeding the patient. The opening to the device is at skin level and does not protrude. It does not interfere with recreational and sexual activities. The device contains an antireflux valve to prevent expelled material from flowing back into the intestinal tract.

**gastrotherapy** (găs″trō-thĕr′ă-pē) [″ + *therapeia,* treatment] The treatment of gastric diseases.

**gastrothoracopagus** (găs″trō-thō″ră-kŏp′ă-gŭs) [″ + *thorax,* chest, + *pagos,* thing fixed] Congenitally deformed twins joined at the stomach and thorax.

**gastrotome** (găs′trō-tōm) [″ + *tome,* incision] An instrument for incising the stomach or abdomen.

**gastrotomy** (găs-trŏt′ō-mē) [″ + *tome,* incision] A gastric or abdominal incision.

**gastrotonometer** (găs″trō-tō-nŏm′ĕ-tĕr) [″ + *tonos,* tension, + *metron,* measure] An instrument for measuring intragastric pressure.

**gastrotympanites** (găs″trō-tĭm″pă-nī′tēz) [″ + *tympanites,* distention] Distention of the stomach by gas or air.

**gastrula** (găs′troo-lă) [L., little belly] The stage in embryonic development following the blastula in which the embryo assumes a two-layered condition. The outer layer is the ectoderm or epiblast; the inner layer, the endoderm or hypoblast. The latter lines a cavity, the gastrocoele or archenteron, that opens to the outside through an opening, the blastopore.

**gastrulation** (găs″troo-lā′shŭn) The development of the gastrula in the embryo.

**Gatch bed** [Willis Dew Gatch, U.S. surgeon, 1878–1962] A bed in which the patient can be raised and held in a half-sitting position.

**gatekeeper** A person who has been legally empowered by a patient to decide whether further medical assistance or care should be sought or allowed. Conflicts and problems may arise owing to the gatekeeper's financial interest in controlling costs and thus not referring the patient for further care. Ideally, the gatekeeper would be financially neutral and decions concerning medical care would be based solely on the needs of the patient.

**gatekeeping** In medical care, deciding the allocation, limitation, or rationing of services. Decisions are based on a variety of factors including need; cost; the potential for success of the proposed therapy; and the availability of facilities, staff, and equipment. SEE: *triage.*

**gate theory** The hypothesis that painful stimuli may be prevented from reaching higher levels of the central nervous system by stimulation of larger sensory nerves. This is one of the proposed explanations of the action of acupuncture.

**gating** In radiology, a procedure used to reduce image artifacts caused by involuntary motion.

***cardiac g.*** Medical image information consistently collected during a specific phase of the cardiac cycle.

***respiratory g.*** Medical image information consistently collected during a specific phase of respiration.

**gatism** (gā′tĭzm) [Fr. *gâter,* to spoil] Urinary or rectal incontinence.

**Gaucher, Philippe C. E.** (gō-shā′) French physician, 1854–1918.

***G.'s cell*** A large reticuloendothelial cell seen in Gaucher's disease, which contains a small, eccentrically placed nucleus and kerasin. SEE: illus.

***G.'s disease*** A chronic congenital disorder of lipid metabolism caused by a deficiency of the enzyme beta-glucocerebrosidase. The severe form is rare, but milder forms frequently occur, esp. in people of Jewish extraction. Fatty substances

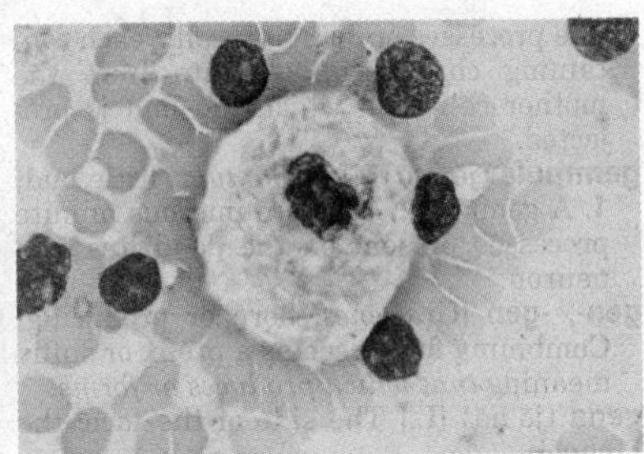

GAUCHER'S CELL (CENTER) IN BONE MARROW (ORIG. MAG. ×640)

called *glycosphingolipids* accumulate in the reticuloendothelial cells. SYN: *cerebroside lipoidosis.*

Three clinical subtypes of the disease exist. Type 1, comprising 99% of cases, is associated with an enlarged liver and spleen, increased skin pigmentation, and painful bone lesions. Enzyme replacement therapy is effective in this type. Type 2 is characterized by neurological symptoms including oculomotor apraxia, strabismus, and hypertonicity. These symptoms usually occur in the first year of life, with death following by age 18 months. Therapy is symptomatic. Type 3 is similar to type 2, but the onset of symptoms is much later and the course is longer. Therapy is symptomatic.

**gauge** (gāj) **1.** A device for measuring the size, capacity, amount, or power of an object or substance. **2.** A standard of measurement.

**Gault's reflex** (gawlts) Contraction of the orbicularis palpebrarum muscle to produce a blinking of the eye following a loud noise close to the ear. This reflex is tested in patients suspected of malingering to feign deafness. SEE: *malingerer.*

**gauntlet** (gawnt'lĕt) [Fr. *gant,* glove] A glovelike bandage that fits the hand and fingers.

**gauss** (gows) [Johann Carl F. Gauss, Ger. physicist, 1777–1855] The unit of intensity of a magnetic flux.

**Gauss' sign** (gows) [Carl J. Gauss, Ger. gynecologist, 1875–1957] An unusual mobility of the uterus in the early weeks of pregnancy.

**gauze** (gawz) [O. Fr. *gaze,* gauze] Thin, loosely woven muslin or similar material used for bandages and surgical sponges.

***absorbent g.*** Gauze made of absorbent material.

***antiseptic g.*** Gauze containing an antiseptic substance.

***aseptic g.*** Sterilized gauze, often packaged in an aseptic container, usually paper, and ready for use.

***petrolatum g.*** Sterilized absorbent gauze saturated with petrolatum.

**gavage** (gă-văzh') [Fr. *gaver,* to stuff] Feeding with a stomach tube or with a tube passed through the nares, pharynx, and esophagus into the stomach. The food is in liquid or semiliquid form at room temperature. SEE: *gastrostogavage.*

**Gavard's muscle** (gă-vărz') [Hyacinthe Gavard, Fr. anatomist, 1753–1802] The oblique muscular fibers of the stomach's coat.

**gay** Homosexual.

**gay bowel syndrome** Infectious diarrhea in homosexuals whose sexual activity includes penile penetration of the anus and rectum. *Shigella* as well as other pathogens have been associated with this syndrome.

**Gay's gland** [Alexander H. Gay, Russian anatomist, 1842–1907] A large sebaceous circumanal gland.

**Gay-Lussac's law** (gā"lū-săks') Charles' law.

**gaze** (gāz) **1.** To look or stare intently in one direction. **2.** The act of looking or staring intently in one direction.

**GB** *gallbladder.*

**Gd** Symbol for the element gadolinium.

**Ge** Symbol for the element germanium.

**Gee, Samuel J** (gē) British physician, 1839–1911.

***G.'s disease*** Infantile nontropical sprue. Also called *Gee-Herter disease; Gee-Herter-Heubner disease.*

**Gee-Thaysen disease** [Gee; Thorwald E.H. Thaysen, Danish physician, 1883–1936] Adult form of nontropical sprue.

**gegenhalten** (gā"gĕn-hălt'ĕn) [Ger.] In cerebrocortical disease, involuntary resistance to passive movement.

**Geigel's reflex** (gī'gĕlz) [Richard Geigel, Ger. physician, 1859–1930] The female reflex involving contraction of muscular fibers, adjacent to the superior portion of Poupart's ligaments, when the inner anterior aspect of the upper thigh is stroked. This reflex corresponds to the male cremasteric reflex.

**Geiger counter** (gī'gĕr) [Hans Geiger, Ger. physicist in England, 1882–1945] An instrument for detecting ionizing radiation.

**gel** (jĕl) [L. *gelare,* to congeal] A semisolid condition of a precipitated or coagulated colloid; jelly; a jelly-like colloid. It contains a large amount of water.

***aluminum hydroxide g.*** A white, viscous suspension of aluminum hydroxide used as an antacid.

**gelasmus** (jĕ-lăs'mŭs) [Gr. *gelasma,* a laugh] **1.** Spasmodic laughter of the insane. **2.** Hysterical laughter.

**gelate** (jĕl'āt) To cause formation of a gel.

**gelatin** (jĕl'ă-tĭn) [L. *gelatina,* gelatin] **1.** A derived protein obtained by the hydrolysis of collagen present in the connective tissues of the skin, bones, and joints of animals. It is used as a food, in the preparation of pharmaceuticals, and as a medium for culture of bacteria. **2.** The substance on an x-ray film in which the silver halide crystals are suspended in the radiographic emulsion.

***nutrient g.*** A bacterial culture medium composed of broth and gelatin.

**gelatiniferous** (jĕl″ăt-ĭn-ĭf′ĕr-ŭs) [″ + *ferre,* to bear] Producing gelatin.

**gelatinize** (jĕl-ăt′ĭn-īz) [L. *gelatina,* gelatin] To convert into gelatin.

**gelatinoid** (jĕl-ăt′ĭn-oyd) [″ + Gr. *eidos,* form, shape] Resembling gelatin.

**gelatinolytic** (jĕl-ăt″ĭn-ō-lĭt′ĭk) [″ + Gr. *lysis,* dissolution] Dissolving or splitting gelatin.

**gelatinous** (jĕl-ăt′ĭn-ŭs) Containing or of the consistency of gelatin.

**gelation** (jĕl-ā′shŭn) The transformation of a colloid from a sol into a gel.

**Gelfoam** Trade name for an absorbable gelatin sponge that acts as a hemostat. SEE: *sponge, gelatin.*

**Gellé's test** (zhĕl-āz′) [Marie Ernst Gellé, Fr. physician, 1834–1923] A test in which a tuning fork is connected with a rubber tube inserted in the ear. Pressure or suction in the tube is produced by an attached bulb. If the ear is normal, vibrations are felt.

**gelose** (jĕ′lōs) [L. *gelare,* to congeal] **1.** The gelatinous element of agar $(C_6H_{10}O_5)_n$. **2.** A bacterial culture medium.

**gelosis** (jĕl-ō′sĭs) A hard lump that is so firm as to appear frozen. It occurs esp. in muscle tissue.

**gelotherapy** (jĕl″ō-thĕr′ă-pē) [Gr. *gelos,* laughter, + *therapeia,* treatment] A method used to treat certain forms of mental illness by inducing laughter.

**gelotripsy** (jĕl′ō-trĭp″sē) [L. *gelare,* to congeal, + Gr. *tripsis,* a rubbing] The massaging away of indurated swellings.

**gemellipara** (jĕm″ĕl-lĭp′ă-ră) [L. *gemelli,* twins, + *parere,* to produce] One who has borne twins.

**gemellology** (gĕm″ĕl-ŏl′ō-jē) [L. *gemellus,* twin, + Gr. *logos,* study] The study of twins.

**gemellus** (jĕm-ĕl′ŭs) *pl.* **gemelli** [L., twin] Either of two muscles inserted in the obturator internus tendon.

**gemfibrozil** (jĕm-fī′brō-zĭl) A drug used to alter the blood lipids in order to delay the progress or development of atherosclerosis. Trade name is Lopid.

**geminate** (jĕm′ĭ-nāt) [L. *geminatus,* paired] In pairs.

**gemination** (jĕm-ĭ-nā′shŭn) **1.** The development of two teeth or two crowns within a single root. **2.** A doubling.

**gemistocyte** (jĕm-ĭs′tō-sīt) [Gr. *gemistos,* laden, full, + *kytos,* cell] In the central nervous system, a swollen astrocyte with an eccentric nucleus, seen adjacent to areas of edema or infarct.

**gemma** (jĕm′mă) [L., bud] **1.** A small budlike reproductive structure produced by lower forms of life. **2.** Any small budlike structure such as a taste bud or endbulb. SYN: *gemmule.*

**gemmation** (jĕm-mā′shŭn) [L. *gemmare,* to bud] Cell reproduction by budding. Budlike processes or daughter cells, each containing chromatin, separate from the mother cell from which the bud is projected.

**gemmule** (jĕm′ūl) [L. *gemmula,* little bud] **1.** A gemma. **2.** One of numerous minute processes present on the dendrites of a neuron.

**gen-, -gen** [Gr. *genes,* born or producing] Combining form used as a prefix or suffix meaning *that which produces or forms.*

**gena** (jē′nă) [L.] The side of the face; the cheek.

**genal** (jē′năl) Buccal.

**gender** [L. *genus,* kind] The sex of an individual (i.e., male or female).

**gender identification** Assignment of gender to a newborn. Genetic or chromosomal anomalies may create ambiguous genitalia, as may exposure of a female fetus to an androgenic hormone, or inhibition of androgen production or metabolism in a male fetus. In such cases, it is important to delay the final disposition until the chromosomal studies and endocrinological evaluation have been completed. These studies should be done as soon as possible.

***mistaken g.i.*** Assignment of incorrect gender to a newborn. This may lead to the individual's having a gender role opposite of the chromosomal sex.

**gender identity** The sex classification of an individual; an inner sense of maleness or femaleness influenced by culture, as opposed to sexual identity, which is biological.

***g.i. disorder*** SEE: under *disorder.*

**gender role** The characteristic lifestyle and behavior pattern of a person with respect to sexual and social conditions associated with being of a particular sex. Usually this behavior represents how the individual feels about his or her own sexual preference; it may not coincide with the true chromosomal and anatomical sexual differentiation of the person.

**gene** (jēn) *pl.* **genes** [Gr. *gennan,* to produce] The basic unit of heredity, made of DNA. Each gene occupies a certain location on a chromosome. Genes are self-replicating, ultramicroscopic structures capable under certain circumstances of producing a new trait; such a change is called a mutation. Hereditary traits are controlled by pairs of genes in the same position on a pair of chromosomes. These gene pairs, or alleles, may both be dominant or both be recessive in their expression of that trait. In either of those cases, the individual is homozygous for the trait controlled by that gene pair. If the gene pair consists of one dominant and one recessive gene, the individual is heterozygous for the trait controlled by that gene pair. SEE: illus. (Inheritance of Eye Color); *chromosome; DNA; RNA.*

***allelic g.'s*** Pairs of genes located at the same site on chromosome pairs.

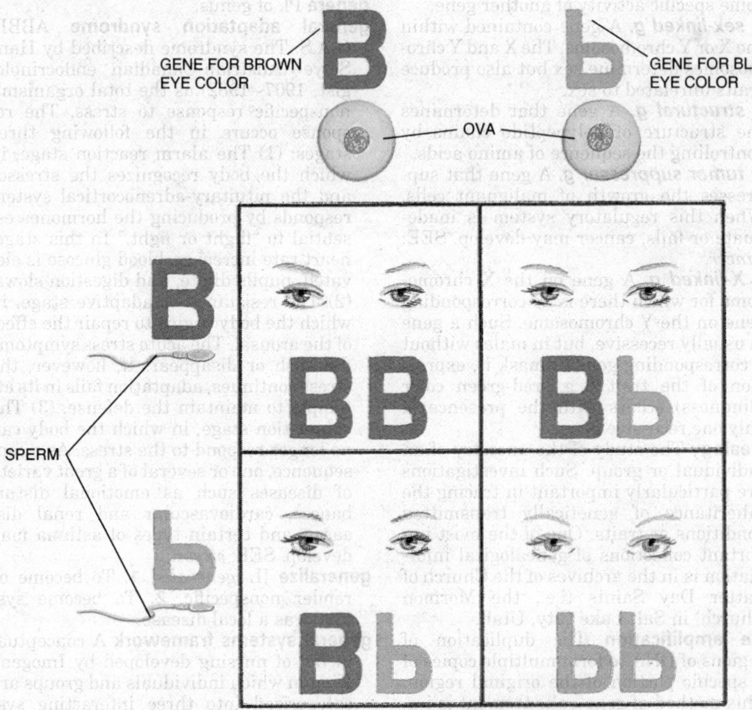


INHERITANCE OF EYE COLOR

***complementary g.'s*** Nonallelic, independent genes, neither of which will express its effect without the presence of the other.

***dominant g.*** A gene that expresses a trait without assistance from its allele.

***histocompatibility g.*** A gene that controls the specificity of the antigenic response of tissues.

***holandric g.*** A gene located in the nonhomologous portion of the Y chromosome of males.

***immune response g.*** A gene that controls the ability of lymphocytes to respond to specific antigens. SEE: *antigen; B cell; HLA complex; T cell.*

***inhibiting g.*** A gene that prevents the expression of another gene.

***lethal g.*** A gene that, when homozygous, brings about an effect that results in death, usually in utero.

***modifying g.*** A gene that influences or alters the effect of another gene.

***mutant g.*** An altered gene that permanently functions differently than it did before its alteration.

***operator g.*** One of certain genes believed to have a role in controlling the actions of other genes. SEE: *operon.*

***g. p53*** A gene thought to be important in controlling the cell cycle, DNA repair and synthesis, and programmed cell death (apoptosis). Mutations of p53 have occurred in almost half of all types of cancer arising from a variety of tissues. Mutant types may promote cancer and other forms may be important in tumor suppression.

***pleiotropic g.*** A gene that has multiple effects.

***recessive g.*** A gene that, in the presence of its dominant allele, does not express itself. A recessive trait may be apparent in the phenotype only if both alleles are recessive.

***regulator g.*** A gene that can control

some specific activity of another gene.

***sex-linked g.*** A gene contained within the X or Y chromosome. The X and Y chromosomes determine sex but also produce traits unrelated to sex.

***structural g.*** A gene that determines the structure of polypeptide chains by controlling the sequence of amino acids.

***tumor suppressor g.*** A gene that suppresses the growth of malignant cells. When this regulatory system is inadequate or fails, cancer may develop. SEE: *cancer*.

***X-linked g.*** A gene on the X chromosome for which there is no corresponding gene on the Y chromosome. Such a gene is usually recessive, but in males without a corresponding gene to mask it, expression of the trait (e.g., red-green color blindness) occurs with the presence of only one recessive gene.

**genealogy** The study of the ancestry of an individual or group. Such investigations are particularly important in tracing the inheritance of genetically transmitted conditions or traits. One of the most important collections of genealogical information is in the archives of the Church of Latter Day Saints (i.e., the Mormon Church) in Salt Lake City, Utah.

**gene amplification** The duplication of regions of DNA to form multiple copies of a specific portion of the original region. This method of gene enhancement is important in increasing a tumor cell's resistance to cytotoxic drugs, and in allowing multiple drug resistance to a wide range of unrelated drugs after resistance to a single agent has developed.

**gene mapping** Determining the hereditary information carried on the 23 pairs of human chromosomes, called the Human Genome Project. This requires determining the base pairs, or chemical code, of each of the estimated 60,000 to 100,000 human genes. The magnitude of this task can be appreciated by the fact that there are 3.5 billion base pairs in the human genome. Once a gene is mapped, that information may be used to compare abnormal genes with normal ones; molecular biological techniques then may be used to search for methods of treating and preventing conditions resulting from genetic abnormality. The book *Mendelian Inheritance in Man* contains a catalogue of human genes and genetic disorders. It is published by the Johns Hopkins University Press and is maintained and updated as part of the Human Genome Project. SYN: *genome mapping*. SEE: *gene splicing*.

**gene probe** In molecular biology, the technique of matching a short segment of DNA or RNA with the matching sequence of bases on a chromosome. Use of this method permits identification of the precise area on a chromosome responsible for the genetic abnormality being investigated. SEE: *gene splicing*.

**genera** Pl. of genus.

**general adaptation syndrome** ABBR: G.A.S. The syndrome described by Hans Selye (Austrian-Canadian endocrinologist, 1907–1982) as the total organism's nonspecific response to stress. The response occurs in the following three stages: (1) The alarm reaction stage, in which the body recognizes the stressor and the pituitary-adrenocortical system responds by producing the hormones essential to "flight or fight." In this stage, heart rate increases, blood glucose is elevated, pupils dilate, and digestion slows. (2) The resistance or adaptive stage, in which the body begins to repair the effect of the arousal. The acute stress symptoms diminish or disappear. If, however, the stress continues, adaptation fails in its attempts to maintain the defense. (3) The exhaustion stage, in which the body can no longer respond to the stress. As a consequence, one or several of a great variety of diseases such as emotional disturbances, cardiovascular and renal diseases, and certain types of asthma may develop. SEE: *stress*.

**generalize** [L. *generalis*] **1.** To become or render nonspecific. **2.** To become systemic, as a local disease.

**general systems framework** A conceptual model of nursing developed by Imogene King in which individuals and groups are categorized into three interacting systems—personal, interpersonal, and social—and in which the goal of nursing is to help people remain healthy so that they can function in their social roles. SEE: *Nursing Theory Appendix*.

**generation** (jĕn″ĕr-ā′shŭn) [L. *generare*, to beget] **1.** The act of reproducing offspring. **2.** A group of animals or plants the same distance removed from an ancestor, as the first filial ($F_1$) generation. SEE: *filial g.* **3.** The average period of time between the birth of parents and the birth of their children, which could be 16 to 20 years in some cultures and 20 to 25 years in others. Also the time would be different if only mothers were considered in computing this average, unless all marriages occurred between persons of the same age. **4.** The production of an electric current.

***alternate g.*** A mode of reproduction in which sexual generation alternates with an asexual generation, characteristic of all plants above the division Thallophyta. It also occurs in some of the lower animals.

***asexual g.*** Reproduction that occurs without the union of sexual elements or gametes, such as reproduction by fission or spore production.

***filial g.*** The offspring of a given mating or cross; $F_1$.

***parental g.*** In genetics, the generation in which a specific study is begun.

***sexual g.*** Reproduction by the union of male and female cells.

**generative** (jĕn′ĕr-ă-tĭv) Concerned in reproduction of, or affecting, the species.

**generator** (gĕn′ĕr-ā″tor) That which produces something, esp. a device that produces heat, electricity, or impulses.

***aerosol g.*** A device that produces minute particles from liquid materials such as medicines in solution. These particles may be used in inhalation therapy.

***electric g.*** A device that changes mechanical energy into electrical energy.

***flow g.*** A pneumatic engine that powers life-support equipment and uses a gauge of 5 to 50 lb/sq in. to supply gas to a ventilator circuit, allowing for a constant flow pattern.

***pressure g.*** A pneumatic engine that powers a life-support ventilator and incorporates a proportional meter, a motor-driven piston, or a blower. Pressure generators can adjust flow according to the patient's condition.

***pulse g.*** A device that produces stimuli intermittently; thus, a cardiac pacemaker requires this type of generator.

**generic** (jĕn-ĕr′ĭk) [L. *genus,* kind] **1.** General. **2.** Pert. to a genus. **3.** Distinctive.

**generic drugs** Nonproprietary drugs (i.e., not protected by a trademark). In the U.S., generic drugs are required to meet the same bioequivalency test as the original brand name drugs. Manufacturers of brand name drugs produce the majority of generic drugs and allow them to be sold without the original brand name. Generic and brand name drugs may experience manufacturing defects. More than 8000 generic drugs are available in the U.S. SYN: *nonproprietary name.*

**genesis** (jĕn′ĕ-sĭs) **1.** The act of reproducing; generation. **2.** The origin of anything.

**gene splicing** The use of micromanipulation techniques to insert a portion of a gene from one species into a gene from another species. This allows the altered gene to function in a different manner. From the practical standpoint, a gene that causes pathological changes could, by use of gene splicing, be changed to eliminate the portion of the gene responsible for the undesired effects. SEE: *recombinant DNA.*

**gene testing** The study of genetic material, as by amniocentesis, to attempt to diagnose and predict conditions caused by abnormalities of genes or chromosomes. This can be done on both plants and animals. These studies have allowed inherited diseases to be predicted prior to their clinical manifestations and, in some cases, prenatally.

**gene therapy** The replacement in a human of a defective or malfunctioning gene by introducing a gene that functions adequately and properly. This was first done in September 1990 by use of molecular biology techniques by Drs. R. Michael Blaese, W. French Anderson, and Kenneth W. Culver at the U.S. National Institutes of Health. The patient was a 4-year-old girl who lacked the ability to produce the specific enzyme adenosine deaminase (ADA) essential to keeping immune cells alive.

This type of therapy will permit use of vectors to introduce a repairing, or disease-correcting, gene into the tissue, a technique that may allow treatment of genetic diseases and cancer.

***somatic g.t.*** An experimental method of cloning genes and reintroducing them into cells for the purpose of correcting inherited disease. As this form of therapy develops so do ethical questions concerning its use: what diseases should be treated, and whether an individual could be treated to enhance his or her normal condition (e.g., to become a stronger or faster athlete).

**genetic** (jĕn-ĕt′ĭk) Pert. to reproduction.

**genetic burden** The impact of pathological changes (i.e., diseases and deaths) owing to inherited traits or diseases.

**genetic code** The code contained in the DNA of living cells (exception: the RNA-viruses) that determines the amino acid sequence of the cell's proteins and is passed on to offspring by way of egg and sperm. The code applies to all living things. SEE: *code, triplet.*

**genetic counseling** The application of knowledge about human genetics in providing advice to those concerned about the possibility of hereditary abnormality.

**genetic engineering** The synthesis, alteration, replacement, or repair of genetic material by synthetic means.

**geneticist** (jĕn-ĕt′ĭ-sĭst) [Gr. *gennan,* to produce] One who specializes in genetics.

**genetics** The study of heredity and its variation.

***biochemical g.*** The science of the biochemistry of genes and chemical influences on genes.

***clinical g.*** A clinical investigation of the importance of genetics in health and disease.

***molecular g.*** The study of genetics at the molecular level, in contrast to the study of entire genes or chromosomes. SEE: *gene splicing.*

**genetotrophic** (jĕ-nĕt″ō-trŏf′ĭk) Concerning genetics and nutrition.

**gene transfer** The transfer of a gene from one animal to another to repair an inherited defect in the recipient. This has not been done in human beings.

**Geneva Convention** Regulations concerning the status of those wounded in military action on land, established in 1864 by military powers meeting in Geneva, Switzerland. The sick and wounded and all those involved in their care, including physicians, nurses, corpsmen, ambulance drivers, and chaplains, were declared to be neutral and, therefore, would not be the target of military action. These provisions were expanded in 1868 to include naval military action. Much evidence in-

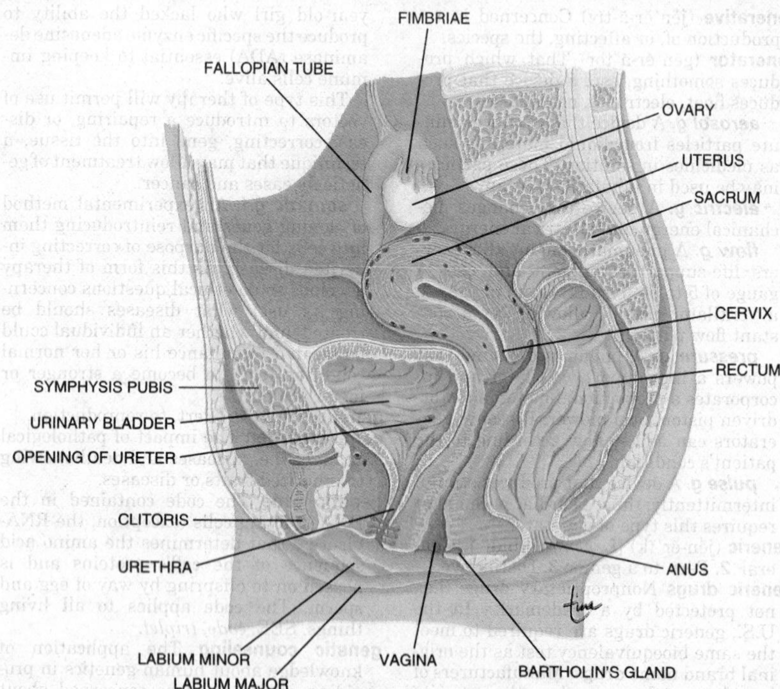


FEMALE GENITAL ORGANS
(MIDSAGITTAL SECTION)

dicates that warring nations have not always abided by the provisions of the Convention.

**genial** (jē′nē-ăl) [Gr. *geneion,* chin] Pert. to the chin.

**genic** (jĕn′ĭk) [Gr. *gennan,* to produce] Relating to or caused by genes.

**-genic** Suffix meaning *generation* or *production.*

**genicular** (jĕ-nĭk′ū-lăr) Concerning the knee.

**geniculate** (jĕ-nĭk′ū-lāt) [L. *geniculare,* to bend the knee] **1.** Bent, like a knee. **2.** Pert. to the ganglion or geniculum of the facial nerve.

**geniculate otalgia** Pain transmitted from the facial nerve to the ear.

**geniculocalcarine tract** Optic radiation.

**geniculum** (jĕn-ĭk′ū-lŭm) [L. *geniculum,* little knee] A structure resembling a knot or a knee, indicating an abrupt bend or angle in a small structure.

**genion** (jē′nē-ŏn) [Gr. *geneion,* chin] The apex of the mental spine of the mandible.

**genioplasty** (jē′nē-ō-plăs″tē) [″ + *plassein,* to form] Plastic surgery of the chin or cheek.

**genital** (jĕn′ĭ-tăl) [L. *genitalis,* belonging to birth] Pert. to the genitals.

**genital herpes** SEE: *herpes, genital.*

**genitalia, genitals** (jĕn-ĭ-tāl′ē-ă, jĕn′ĭ-tăls) Organs of generation; reproductive organs.

***ambiguous g.*** External genitalia that are not clearly distinguishable as being of either sexual form.

***female g.*** Reproductive organs of the female sex. The external genitalia collectively are termed the vulva or pudendum and include the mons veneris, labia majora, labia minora, clitoris, fourchet, fossa navicularis, vestibule, vestibular bulb, Skene's glands, glands of Bartholin, hymen and vaginal introitus, and perineum. The internal genitalia are the two ovaries, two fallopian tubes, uterus, and vagina. SEE: illus.

***male g.*** Reproductive organs of the male sex, including two bulbourethral (Cowper's) glands, two ejaculatory ducts, two glands producing spermatozoa (the testes or gonads), the penis with urethra, two seminal ducts (vasa deferentes or ducti deferentes), two seminal vesicles, two spermatic cords, the scrotum, and the prostate gland. SEE: illus.; *penis; prostate.*

**genital self-examination** SEE: *breast self-examination; testicle, self-examination of.*

**genito-** [L. *genitivus,* of birth, of generation] Combining form meaning reproduction.

**genitocrural** (jĕn″ĭ-tō-kroo′răl) Concerning

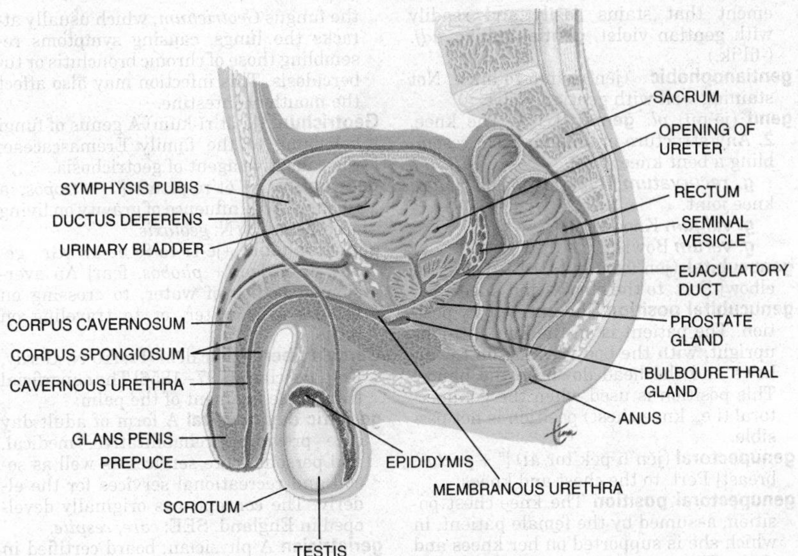


**MALE GENITAL ORGANS**
(MIDSAGITTAL SECTION)

the genitalia and leg. SYN: *genitofemoral*.

**genitofemoral** (jĕn″ĭ-tō-fĕm′or-ăl) Genitocrural.

**genitoplasty** (jĕn′ĭ-tō-plăs″tē) [L. *genitalis*, genital, + Gr. *plassein*, to form] Reparative surgery on the genital organs.

**genitourinary** (jĕn″ĭ-tō-ūr′ĭ-nār-ē) [″ + Gr. *ouron*, urine] Pert. to the genitals and urinary organs.

**genitourinary system** A system that includes the urinary organs (e.g, the kidneys, urinary bladder) and the organs of reproduction and their accessories. In males, the urethra is part of both the reproductive and urinary systems; in females, the systems are entirely separate.

**genius** (jēn′yŭs) **1.** The distinctive or inherent character of a disease. **2.** An individual with exceptional physical, mental, or creative power. SEE: *idiot-savant*.

**genocide** (jĕn′ō-sīd″) [Gr. *genos*, race, + L. *caedere*, to kill] The willful and planned murder of a particular social or ethnic group.

**genodermatosis** (jĕn″ō-dĕr-mă-tō′sĭs) [Gr. *gennan*, to produce, + *derma*, skin, + *osis*, condition] Any of a group of serious hereditary skin diseases such as hereditary angioedema, hereditary coporporphyria, hereditary telangectasia, tuberous sclerosis, Recklinghausen's disease, and Peutz-Jeghers syndrome.

**genogram** A family map of three or more generations that records relationships, deaths, occupations, and health and illness history.

**genome** (jē′nōm) The complete set of chromosomes, and thus the entire genetic information present in a cell.

**genome mapping** Gene mapping.

**genomic** Concerning the genome.

**Genoptic** A trade name for gentamicin sulfate.

**genotoxic** (jĕn″ō-tŏks′ĭk) [″ + *toxikon*, poison] Toxic to the genetic material in cells.

**genotoxic damage** Injury to the chromosomes of the cells. This may be determined by noting the number of micronuclei in the target tissues. When a cell with damaged genetic material divides, fragments of chromosomes and micronuclei remain in the cytoplasm.

**genotype** (jĕn′ō-tīp) [″ + *typos*, type] **1.** The total of the hereditary information present in an organism. **2.** The pair of genes present for a particular characteristic or protein. **3.** A type species of a genus. SEE: *phenotype*.

**gentamicin** (jĕn″tă-mī′sĭn) An antibiotic derived from the fungi of the genus *Micromonospora*.

***g. sulfate*** An antibiotic obtained from the actinomycete *Micromonospora purpurea*. Trade names include Garamycin and Genoptic Liquifilm.

**gentian** (jĕn′shŭn) Dried rhizome and roots of the plant *Gentiana lutea*.

***g. violet*** $C_{25}H_{30}ClN_3$. A dye derived from coal tar that is widely used as a stain in histology, cytology, and bacteriology. It is also used therapeutically as a topical anti-infective. Its chemical name is hexamethylpararosaniline chloride.

**gentianophil(e)** (jĕn′shăn-ō-fĭl, -fīl) An element that stains easily and readily with gentian violet. **gentianophilic,** *adj.* (-fil'ik.)

**gentianophobic** (jĕn"shăn-ō-fō'bĭk) Not staining well with gentian violet.

**genu** (jē'nū) *pl.* **genua** [L.] **1.** The knee. **2.** Any structure of angular form resembling a bent knee.

*g. recurvatum* Hyperextension at the knee joint.

*g. valgum* Knock-knee.

*g. varum* Bowleg.

**genucubital** (jĕn"ū-kū'bĭ-tăl) [" + *cubitus,* elbow] Pert. to the elbows and knees.

**genucubital position** The knee-elbow position. The patient is on the knees, thighs upright, with the body resting on the elbows and the head down on the hands. This position is used when the genupectoral (i.e., knee-chest) position is not possible.

**genupectoral** (jĕn"ū-pĕk'tor-ăl) [" + *pectus,* breast] Pert. to the chest and knees.

**genupectoral position** The knee-chest position, assumed by the female patient, in which she is supported on her knees and chest. This position is used for examination and treatment. SEE: *position* for illus.

**genus** (jē'nŭs) *pl.* **genera** [L. *genus,* kind] In taxonomy, the classification between the family and the species.

**genyplasty** (jĕn'ĭ-plăs"tē) [Gr. *genys,* jaw, + *plassein,* to form] Genioplasty.

**geobiology** (jē"ō-bī-ŏl'ō-jē) [Gr. *geo,* earth, + *bios,* life, + *logos,* word, reason] The study of terrestrial life.

**geode** (jē'ōd) [Gr. *geodes,* earthlike] A dilated lymph space.

**geographic distribution of disease** The relationship between the prevalence of a disease and specific geographical-environmental conditions. For example, goiter occurs in inland iodine-deficient areas, and pulmonary hypertension occurs in those who reside at high altitude. Certain infectious diseases, such as leprosy, leishmaniasis, and Chagas' disease, are endemic in specific tropical or subtropical areas.

**geographic tongue** Glossitis areata exfoliativa.

**geographic ulceration of the cornea** An ulcer of the cornea with an irregular and lobulated border.

**geomedicine** (jē"ō-mĕd'ĭ-sĭn) [Gr. *geo,* earth, + L. *medicina,* medicine] The study of the influence of geography and climate on health. SYN: *nosochthonography.*

**geophagia, geophagism, geophagy** (jē-ō-fā'jē-ă, -ŏf'ă-jĭzm, -ŏf'ă-jē) [" + *phagein,* to eat] A condition in which the patient eats inedible substances such as chalk, clay, or earth. SYN: *geotragia.* SEE: *pica.*

**geotaxis** (jē"ō-tăk'sĭs) [" + *taxis,* arrangement] Geotropism.

**geotragia** (jē"ō-trā'jē-ă) [" + *trogein,* to chew] Geophagia.

**geotrichosis** (jē"ō-trĭ-kō'sĭs) Infection by the fungus *Geotrichum,* which usually attacks the lungs, causing symptoms resembling those of chronic bronchitis or tuberculosis. This infection may also affect the mouth or intestine.

**Geotrichum** (jē-ŏt'rĭ-kŭm) A genus of fungi belonging to the family Eremascaceae; the causative agent of geotrichosis.

**geotropism** (jē"ŏt'rō-pĭzm) [" + *tropos,* a turning] The influence of gravity on living organisms. SYN: *geotaxis.*

**gephyrophobia** (jē-fī"rō-fō'bē-ă) [Gr. *gephyra,* bridge, + *phobos,* fear] An aversion to bodies of water, to crossing on bridges over water, or to traveling on boats.

**Gerdy's fibers** (zhĕr'dēz) [Pierre N. Gerdy, Fr. physician, 1797–1856] The superficial transverse ligament of the palm.

**geriatric day hospital** A form of adult day care providing rehabilitative, medical, and personal care services as well as social and recreational services for the elderly. The concept was originally developed in England. SEE: *care, respite.*

**geriatrician** A physician, board certified in geriatrics, who specializes in the care of elderly people.

**geriatrics** (jĕr"ē-ăt'rĭks) [Gr. *geras,* old age, + *iatrike,* medical treatment] The branch of medicine concerned with the problems of aging. Included are all aspects of aging, including physiological, pathological, psychological, economic, and sociological problems. The importance of geriatrics is emphasized by the fact that the expected lifespan is increasing. An estimated 25,000 persons in the U.S. are 100 years old or older, and by the year 2080 this number will increase to more than 1,000,000. Also called *geriatric medicine.* SEE: *gerontology.*

*dental g.* The special area of dentistry dealing with the problems of aging as it relates to dental illness and treatment.

**Gerlach's valve** (gĕr'lăks) [Joseph von Gerlach, Ger. anatomist, 1820–1896] An inconstant valve present at the opening of the vermiform process (appendix) into the cecum.

**germ** [L. *germen,* sprout, fetus] **1.** A microorganism, esp. one that causes disease. **2.** The first rudiment of a developing organ or part.

*dental g.* The embryonic structure that gives rise to the tooth. It consists of the enamel organ, dental papilla, and dental sac. SYN: *tooth bud.* SEE: *enamel organ.*

*hair g.* The rudimentary structure from which a hair develops. It consists of an ingrowth of epidermal cells called *hair peg,* which pushes into the corium.

*wheat g.* The vitamin-rich embryo of the wheat seed or kernel. It contains vitamin E, thiamine, riboflavin, and other vitamins.

**germanium** (jĕr-mā'nē-ŭm) [L. *Germania,* Germany] SYMB: Ge. A grayish-white metallic element of the silicon group.

Atomic weight is 72.59, atomic number is 32, and specific gravity is 5.323 (25°C).

**German measles** SEE: *rubella.*

**germ cell** SEE: *cell, germ.*

**germ epithelium** The ridge of epithelium in the embryo from which the sexual portions of the body are derived.

**germicidal** (jĕrm″ĭ-sī′dăl) [L. *germen,* sprout, + *caedere,* to kill] **1.** Destructive to germs. **2.** Pert. to an agent destructive to germs.

**germicide** (jĕr′mĭ-sīd) A substance that destroys microorganisms. Bacteria may be killed by boiling for 30 min, by dry heat at 160° to 170°C for 1 hr, and by steam at 121°C for 20 min. SEE: *antiseptic; disinfectant.*

**germinal** [L. *germen,* sprout] Pert. to a germ or reproductive cells (egg or sperm) or to germination.

**germinal center** A light area of lymphocytopoietic cells that occupies the center of lymphatic nodules of the spleen, tonsils, and lymph nodes.

**germinal disk** Blastoderm.

**germinal epithelium 1.** The epithelium that covers the surface of the genital ridge of an embryo. **2.** The epithelium that covers the surface of a mature mammalian ovary.

**germinal vesicle** Purkinje vesicle.

**germination** [L. *germinare,* to sprout] **1.** The development of an impregnated ovum into an embryo. **2.** The sprouting of the spore or seed of a plant.

**germinoma** (jĕr″mĭ-nō′mă) A neoplasm arising from germ cells in the testis or ovary.

**germ layers** Three primary cell layers in the embryo from which the organs and tissues develop. They are the ectoderm, mesoderm, and endoderm.

**germ plasm** The reproductive tissues.

**germ theory** The theory that certain diseases are the result of the presence of pathological microorganisms in the body.

**gero-** [Gr. *geras,* old age] Combining form meaning *old age.*

**gerontic** A combination of the scientific principles of aging with basic nursing methods to provide a comprehensive understanding. This broad concept relies on a logical scientific approach using specialized knowledge about aged persons.

**Gerontological Society of America** ABBR: GSA. An organization established in 1945 for the main purpose of promoting scientific study of aging. Researchers, practitioners, and educators are members. The society publishes *The Journal of Gerontology* and *The Gerontologist.*

**gerontology** (jĕ-rŏn-tŏl′ō-jē) [″ + *logos,* word, reason] The scientific study of the effects of aging and of age-related diseases on humans. SEE: *geriatrics.*

**gerontophilia** (jĕr″ŏn-tō-fĭl′ē-ă) [″ + *philein,* to love] A fondness or love for old people.

**gerontophobia** A fear of aging.

**gerontotherapeutics** (jĕr-ŏn″tō-thĕr″ă-pū′tĭks) [″ + *therapeia,* treatment] The therapy of the aged, the goal of which is to prevent, treat, or slow the onset of senescence.

**gerontoxon** (jĕ-rŏn-tŏks′ŏn) [″ + *toxon,* bow] Arcus senilis.

**geropsychiatry** A subspecialty of psychiatry dealing with mental illness in the elderly.

**Gerota's capsule** (gā-rō′tăz) [Dimitru Gerota, Rumanian anatomist, 1867–1939] The perirenal fascia.

**Gerstmann syndrome** [Josef Gerstmann, Austrian neurologist, 1887–1969] A neurological disorder resulting from a lesion in the left (or dominant) parietal area. Patients are unable to point or name different fingers, have confusion of the right and left sides of the body, and are unable to calculate or write. In addition, they may have word blindness and homonymous hemianopia.

**gestagen** (jĕs′tă-jĕn) Something that produces progestational effects. This general term is usually applied to natural or synthetic steroid hormones used to alter reproductive physiology.

**gestalt** (gĕs-tawlt′) [Ger. *Gestalt,* form] The concept that the configuration of objects and experience is present as a whole formation that cannot be analyzed by breaking it into its component parts.

***g. therapy*** A form of therapy that emphasizes the treatment of the person as a whole, with a focus on the reality of the present time and place and with an emphasis on personal growth and enhanced self-awareness.

**gestation** (jĕs-tā′shŭn) [L. *gestare,* to bear] In mammals, the length of time from conception to birth. The average gestation time is a species-specific trait. In humans, the average length, as calculated from the first day of the last normal menstrual period, is 280 days, with a normal range of 259 days (37 weeks) to 287 days (41 weeks). Infants born prior to the 37th week are considered premature and those born after the 41st week, postmature. SEE: *gestational assessment; pregnancy.*

***abdominal g.*** Ectopic gestation in which the embryo develops in the peritoneal cavity.

***cornual g.*** Gestation in an ill-developed cornu of a bicornuate uterus.

***ectopic g.*** Gestation in which the fetus develops outside the uterus.

***interstitial g.*** Tubal gestation in which the embryo is developed in a portion of the fallopian tube that traverses the wall of the uterus.

***multiple g.*** The presence of two or more embryos in the uterus. The incidence of this in the U.S. is about 1.5% of all births. Up to 40% of twin gestations are undiagnosed before labor and delivery. When twins are diagnosed by ultrasound early in the first trimester, in about half of these cases one twin will silently abort, and this may or may not be accompanied by bleeding. This has been termed the vanishing twin. The incidence of birth defects in each fetus of a twin pregnancy is twice that in singular pregnancies.

***plural g.*** Gestation in which there is more than one embryo.

***prolonged g.*** Gestation prolonged beyond the usual period.

***secondary g.*** Gestation in which the embryo becomes dislodged from the original seat of implantation and continues to develop in a new situation.

***secondary abdominal g.*** Extrauterine gestation in which the embryo, originally situated in the oviduct or elsewhere, has developed in the abdominal cavity.

***tubal g.*** Ectopic gestation in which the embryo grows in the fallopian tube.

***tuboabdominal g.*** Extrauterine gestation in which the embryonic sac is formed partly in the abdominal extremity of the oviduct and partly in the abdominal cavity.

***tubo-ovarian g.*** Extrauterine gestation in which the embryonic sac is partly in the ovary and partly in the abdominal end of the fallopian tube.

***uterotubal g.*** Gestation in which the ovum develops partially in the uterine end of the fallopian tube and partially within the cavity of the uterus.

**gestational assessment** Determination of the prenatal age of the fetus. This information is essential for obstetrical care because it influences the decision to intervene and at what time. The age has been estimated by evaluating the menstrual history, time of initial detection of fetal heart tones, and date the level of the fundus reaches the umbilicus. These methods are not precise, esp. if the date of the last menstrual period is either vaguely remembered or unknown.

Use of ultrasound to measure the crown-rump length in the first trimester, the biparietal diameter in the second trimester, and other measurements permits a more nearly precise estimate of gestational age. Even so, these techniques, because of biological variation of fetal size and early intrauterine growth failure, may not be consistently accurate. SEE: *Dubowitz tool.*

**gestation sac** The amnion and its contents.

**gestation time** The duration of a normal pregnancy for a particular species. SEE: *pregnancy* for table.

**gestosis** (jĕs-tō′sĭs) [L. *gestare,* to bear, + Gr. *osis,* condition] Any disorder of pregnancy.

**gesture 1.** A body movement that helps to express or conceal thoughts or emphasize speech. SEE: *body language.* **2.** An act, written or spoken, to indicate a feeling.

**geumaphobia** (gū″mă-fō′bē-ă) [Gr. *geuma,* taste, + *phobos,* fear] An abnormal dislike or fear of tastes.

**GFR** *glomerular filtration rate.*

**GH** *growth hormone.*

**Ghon's tubercle** (gănz) [Anton Ghon, Czech. pathologist, 1866–1936] A small, sharply defined shadow in radiographs of the lung seen in certain cases of pulmonary tuberculosis in children. It is usually the primary lesion of tuberculosis in children. The tubercle bacilli in the lesion may become encased in calcium and the only remaining sign of infection is a positive tuberculin skin test. Nevertheless, the mycobacterium tuberculosis organisms may remain viable and be the source of endogenous and generalized reinfection with the tubercle bacillus. Also called *Ghon's primary lesion.*

**GH-RH** *growth hormone–releasing hormone.*

**GI** *gastrointestinal.*

**Giannuzzi's cells** (jăn-noot′sēz) [Guiseppe Giannuzzi, It. anatomist, 1839–1876] Crescent-shaped groups of serous cells found in the mixed salivary glands. They appear as darkly staining cells forming a caplike structure on the alveoli.

**giant** [Gr. *gigas,* giant] An individual or structure much larger than normal.

**giant cell** A large cell with several nuclei, appearing to be made up of many cells, but not clearly outlined. It is found in both kinds of marrow, esp. in red marrow, and in the spleen. It is also found in tissues that are healing, around foreign bodies, and in the inflammatory reaction to tuberculosis. SYN: *megakaryocyte.*

**giant cell tumor 1.** A malignant or benign bone tumor that probably arises from connective tissue of the bone marrow. Histologically, it contains a vascular reticulum of stromal cells and multinucleated giant cells. **2.** A yellow giant cell tumor of a tendon sheath. **3.** Epulis. **4.** Chondroblastoma.

**giantism** (jī′ăn-tĭzm) Gigantism.

**Giardia** (jē-ăr′dē-ă) [Alfred Giard, Fr. biologist, 1846–1908] A genus of protozoa possessing flagella. They inhabit the small intestine of humans and other animals, are pear shaped, and have two nuclei and four pairs of flagella. They attach themselves to the cells of the intestinal mucosa, from which they absorb nourishment. Cysts can survive in water for up to 3 months. The concentration of chlorine routinely used in treating domestic water supplies does not kill *Giardia* cysts, but boiling water inactivates them.

***G. lamblia*** A species of *Giardia* found in humans, transmitted by ingestion of cysts in fecally contaminated water or food. *G. lamblia* organisms are found worldwide. They were formerly considered nonpathogenic, but evidence indicates that they interfere with fat absorption and cause giardiasis. The most common symptoms of *G. lamblia* infection are diarrhea, fever, cramps, anorexia, nausea, weakness, weight loss, abdominal distention, flatulence, greasy stools, belching, and vomiting. Onset of symptoms begins about 2 weeks after exposure;

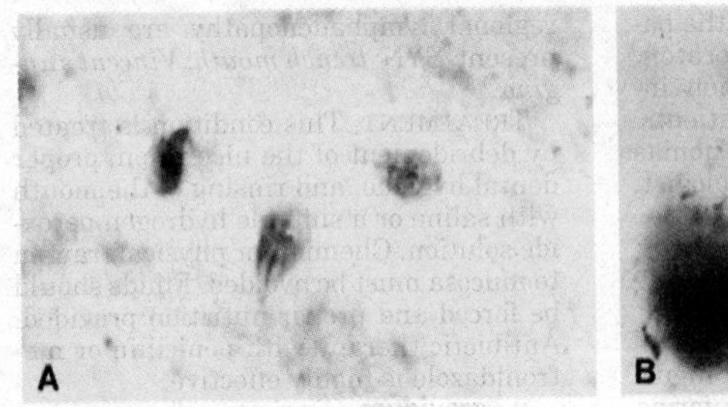


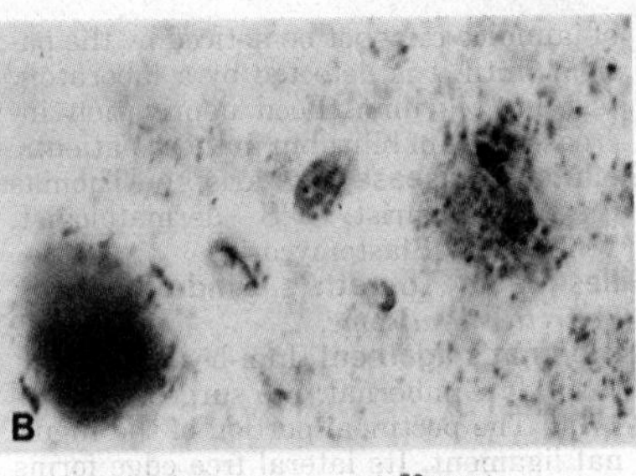


**GIARDIA LAMBLIA (A)** TROPHOZOITES (ORIG. MAG. ×1000), **(B)** CYSTS (ORIG. MAG. ×1000)

the disease may persist for up to 2 to 3 months.

There is no effective chemoprophylaxis for this disease. Metronidazole, tinidazole, and furazolidone are all effective in treating the illness. Furazolidone is often used to treat children because it is available in liquid form. Quinacrine is the drug of choice, but it is no longer produced in the U.S. SEE: *water, emergency preparation of safe drinking.*

DIAGNOSIS: Cysts or trophozoites are identified in feces. Three consecutive negative tests are required before the feces are considered to be negative. Duodenal contents can be examined by aspiration or string test, in which an ordinary string is swallowed and allowed to remain in the duodenum long enough for the protozoa to attach. On removal, it is examined for the presence of cysts or trophozoites. An antigen assay test is available for detecting *Giardia*. This involves either immunofluorescence or enzyme-linked immunoabsorbent assay. SEE: illus.

**giardiasis** (jī″ăr-dī′ă-sĭs) Infection with the flagellate protozoan *Giardia lamblia*.

**Gibbon's hydrocele** (gĭb′ŏns) [Quinton V. Gibbon, U.S. surgeon, 1813–1894] A hydrocele and large hernia combined.

**gibbosity** (gĭ-bŏs′ĭ-tē) [LL. *gebbosus*, humped] **1.** The condition of having a humpback. **2.** A hump or gibbus, as the deformity of Pott's disease.

**gibbous** (gĭb′bŭs) Humped; protuberant or hunchbacked.

**gibbus** (gĭb′ŭs) [L. *gibbosus*] Hump; protuberance.

**Gibney's boot, Gibney's bandage** (gĭb′nēz) [Virgil P. Gibney, U.S. surgeon, 1847–1927] A basket-weave bandage made of adhesive tape, used to treat ankle sprain or to support the ankle.

**Gibson's murmur** (gĭb′sŭnz) [George A. Gibson, Scot. physician, 1854–1913] A continuous cardiac murmur that increases in systole, occurring in patients with patent ductus arteriosus. It is heard best at the left of the sternum in the first and second intercostal spaces.

**giddiness** [AS. *gydig*, insane] Dizziness.

**Giemsa's stain** (gēm′zăs) [Gustav Giemsa, Ger. chemist, 1867–1948] A stain for blood smears, used for differential leukocyte counts and to detect parasitic microorganisms.

**Gifford's reflex** (gĭf′fords) [Harold Gifford, U.S. ophthalmologist, 1858–1929] Pupillary contraction resulting from endeavoring forcibly to close eyelids that are held apart.

**GIFT** *gamete intrafallopian transfer*.

**giga-** (jĭg′ă, jī′gă) In SI units, a prefix indicating that the entity following is to be multiplied by $10^9$. SEE: *Metric System in Units of Measurement Appendix*.

**gigantism** (jī′găn-tĭzm) [Gr. *gigas*, giant, + *-ismos*, state of] The excessive development of the body or a body part. SYN: *giantism*.

***acromegalic g.*** Gigantism characterized by overgrowth of the bones of the hands, feet, and face, owing to excessive production of the pituitary growth hormone after full skeletal growth has been attained.

***eunuchoid g.*** Gigantism accompanied by eunuchoid features and sexual insufficiency.

***normal g.*** Gigantism in which the bodily proportions and sexual development are normal, usually the result of hypersecretion of the growth hormone.

**gigantoblast** (jī-găn′tō-blăst) [″ + *blastos*, germ] A very large nucleated red corpuscle.

**gigantocyte** (jī-găn′tō-sīt) [″ + *kytos*, cell] **1.** A giant cell. **2.** A very large erythrocyte.

**Gigli's saw** (jēl′yēz) [Leonardo Gigli, It. gynecologist, 1863–1908] A wire saw originally used to cut the symphysis pubis to facilitate delivery of a fetus. This tool is now used to remove part of the skull in craniotomy and to transect bone in osteotomy.

**Gilbert's syndrome** (zhē1-bārz′) [Nicolas A. Gilbert, Fr. physician, 1858–1927] A benign, hereditary form of jaundice secondary to glucuronyl-transferase deficiency, resulting in elevated unconjugated bilirubin. There are no hemolytic changes. No treatment is necessary. The presence of jaundice may not be noticed by the patient until it is detected by a laboratory test for bilirubin. Food deprivation increases serum bilirubin in these patients.

**Gilchrist's disease** (gĭl'krĭsts) [Thomas Caspar Gilchrist, U.S. dermatologist, 1862–1927] Blastomycosis.

**Gilles de la Tourette's syndrome** SEE: *Tourette's syndrome.*

**Gimbernat's ligament** (hĭm-bĕr-năts') [Antonio de Gimbernat, Sp. surgeon, 1734–1790] The pectineal portion of the inguinal ligament. Its lateral free edge forms the medial portion of the femoral ring. SYN: *lacunar ligament.*

**ginger** A pungent, spicy material obtained from the root (rhizome) of the plant *Zingiber officinale* and used to flavor medicines and foods.

**gingiva** (jĭn-jī'vă, jĭn'jĭ-vă) [L.] The gum; the tissue that surrounds the necks of the teeth and covers the alveolar processes of the maxilla and mandible.

***alveolar g.*** The part of the gums that covers the alveolar process of the teeth.

***attached g.*** Gingiva lying between the free gingival groove and the mucogingival line. It is firmly attached by lamina propria to underlying periosteum, bone, and tooth.

***free g.*** The unattached portion of the gingiva. It forms part of the wall of the fissure surrounding the anatomical crown of a tooth.

***labial g.*** Gingiva covering the labial surfaces of the teeth.

***lingual g.*** Gingiva covering the lingual surfaces of the teeth.

***marginal g.*** The crest of the free gingiva surrounding the tooth like a collar. It is about 1 mm wide and forms the soft tissue portion of the gingival sulcus.

**gingival** (jĭn'jĭ-văl) [L. *gingiva,* gum] Rel. to the gums.

**gingivalgia** (jĭn"jĭ-văl'jē-ă) [" + Gr. *algos,* pain] Pain in the gums.

**gingival hypertrophy** SEE: under *hypertrophy.*

**gingivally** (jĭn'jĭ-văl"lē) Toward the gums.

**gingivectomy** (jĭn"jĭ-vĕk'tō-mē) [" + Gr. *ektome,* excision] Excision of diseased gingival tissue in surgical treatment of periodontal disease.

**gingivitis** (jĭn-jĭ-vī'tĭs) [" + Gr. *itis,* inflammation] Inflammation of the gums characterized by redness, swelling, and tendency to bleed. SYN: *ulitis.*

ETIOLOGY: Gingivitis may be local due to improper dental hygiene, poorly fitting dentures or appliances, or poor occlusion. It may accompany generalized stomatitis associated with mouth and upper respiratory infections. It may also occur in deficiency diseases such as scurvy, blood dyscrasias, or metallic poisoning.

***acute necrotizing ulcerative g.*** ABBR: ANUG. A painful pseudomembranous ulceration of the mucous membranes of the mouth and pharynx. Fever, malaise, and regional lymphadenopathy are usually present. SYN: *trench mouth; Vincent's angina.*

TREATMENT: This condition is treated by debridement of the ulceration, proper dental hygiene, and rinsing of the mouth with saline or a suitable hydrogen peroxide solution. Chemical or physical trauma to mucosa must be avoided. Fluids should be forced and proper nutrition provided. Antibiotic therapy with penicillin or metronidazole is highly effective.

***g. gravidum*** Gingivitis of pregnancy. The generalized hypertrophy of the gums characteristic of this disease may progress to tumor formation.

***hyperplastic g.*** Gingivitis associated with overgrowth of the gingiva. It may be caused by dental plaque or prolonged use of phenytoin.

***interstitial g.*** Inflammation of the gums and alveolar processes that precedes pyorrhea.

***phagedenic g.*** A rapidly spreading ulceration of the gums accompanied by extensive ulceration and sloughing of tissue.

**gingivoglossitis** (jĭn"jĭ-vō-glŏs-sī'tĭs) [" + Gr. *glossa,* tongue, + *itis,* inflammation] Inflammation of the gums and tongue. SYN: *stomatitis.*

**gingivolabial** (jĭn"jĭ-vō-lā'bē-ăl) Concerning the gums and lips.

**gingivoplasty** (jĭn'jĭ-vō-plăs"tē) [" + Gr. *plassein,* to form] Surgical correction of the gingival margin.

**gingivostomatitis** (jĭn"jĭ-vō-stō"mă-tī'tĭs) [" + Gr. *stoma,* mouth, + *itis,* inflammation] Inflammation of the gingival tissue and the mucosa of the mouth due to herpesvirus types I or II.

**ginglymoarthrodial** (jĭng"lĭ-mō-ăr-thrō'dē-ăl) [" + *arthrodia,* gliding joint] Pert. to a joint that is both hinged and arthrodial. SEE: *arthrodia.*

**ginglymoid** (jĭng'lĭ-moyd) [" + *eidos,* form, shape] Pert. to or shaped like a hinged joint.

**ginglymus** (jĭng'lĭ-mŭs) [Gr. *ginglymos,* hinge] A hinge joint; diarthrosis. SEE: *joint.*

**ginseng** (jĭn'sĕng) [Chinese *jen-shen,* man, man image] The root of the Chinese or American ginseng plant. Species of Asiatic ginseng are different from those in North America. Ginseng is used therapeutically by some cultures as an aphrodisiac or stimulant; however, the medical evidence to support such use is controversial.

Ginseng contains a large number of substances, the most important group of which is thought to be ginsenosides. Commercial ginseng products sold in several countries including the U.S. do not contain ginsenosides.

**Giraldés' organ** (hĭr-ăl-dās') [Joachim A. C. C. Giraldés, Portuguese surgeon in Paris, 1808–1875] Paradidymis.

**girdle** [AS. *gyrdel,* girdle] **1.** A zone or belt;

the waist. **2.** A structure that resembles a circular belt or band.

***pelvic g.*** The portion of the lower extremities to which the lower limbs are attached. It is composed of the two innominate or hip bones.

***shoulder g.*** The portion of the upper extremities to which the upper limbs are attached. It is composed of the two clavicles and two scapulae.

**girdle pain** Zonesthesia.

**girdle symptom** A symptom in tabes as of a tight girdle, such as a feeling of constriction about the chest; also found in compression of the cord owing to collapse of the vertebrae, as in Pott's disease.

**gitter cell** A macrophage present at sites of brain injury. The cells are packed with lipoid granules from phagositosis of damaged brain cells. SEE: *microglia.*

**gizzard** (gĭz′ărd) The very strong muscular stomach of certain birds. Food is mixed with gastric juice and macerated with the aid of small stones, called *grit,* that are ingested and remain in the gizzard.

**glabella** [L. *glaber,* smooth] The smooth surface of the frontal bone lying between the superciliary arches; the portion directly above the root of the nose. SYN: *intercilium; mesophryon.*

**glabrate, glabrous** [L. *glaber,* smooth] **1.** Bald. **2.** Smooth.

**glacial** (glā′shăl) [L. *glacialis,* icy] Glassy; resembling ice.

**gladiate** (glā′dē-āt) [L. *gladius,* sword] Xiphoid.

**glairy** Viscous; albuminous; mucoid.

**gland** [L. *glans,* acorn] **1.** A secretory organ or structure. **2.** A cell or a group of cells that can manufacture a secretion discharged and used in some other part of the body.

Glands may be structurally simple (consisting of one or a few secreting units) or compound (consisting of many secreting units whose secretions leave the gland by a common duct). Simple tubular glands may be straight, coiled, or branched. Glands consisting of one cell are called unicellular; those of more than one cell, multicellular.

On the basis of their secretion, glands may be mucous (those producing a viscous slimy secretion); serous (those producing a clear watery secretion); or mixed (those producing both).

Regarding the presence or absence of ducts, glands are exocrine (those having ducts that carry the secretions to an epithelial surface) and endocrine (those without ducts and whose secretions enter the blood or lymph). The latter are gonads or sex glands and pineal, pituitary, thyroid, parathyroid, thymus, and adrenal glands. The pancreas is both exocrine (digestive) and endocrine. The islets of Langerhans of the pancreas produce the endocrine insulin.

The secreting units may be tubular (elongated with a narrow lumen) or saccular (in the form of a sac or flask). If the lumen of the secreting portion is wide, it is termed an *alveolus;* if narrow, an *acinus*. Glands composed of these types of units are termed alveolar and acinar, respectively.

According to the manner of secretion, glands are merocrine (secretion forms within cells and is passed through cell membranes into excretory ducts); apocrine (secretion forms in apical ends of cells, which break off in and form a part of the secretion) such as the mammary gland; and holocrine (the entire cell with its contents is extruded as the secretion) such as sebaceous glands. SEE: *cell* for illus.

***accessory g.*** A small gland similar in function to another gland of similar structure some distance removed.

***acinotubular g.*** A gland structurally midway between an acinous and a tubular gland.

***acinous g.*** A gland whose secreting units are composed of saclike structures, each possessing a narrow lumen. SYN: *racemose g.*

***adrenal g.*** An endocrine gland lying above each kidney. SYN: *suprarenal g.*

***aggregate g.'s*** Peyer's patch.

***albuminous g.'s*** Digestive tract glands secreting a fluid containing albumin. SYN: *serous g.'s.*

***anal g.'s*** Glands in the region of the anus. SYN: *circumanal g.'s.*

***apocrine g.*** A gland whose cells lose some of their cytoplasmic contents in the formation of secretion. Examples include the mammary glands and some sweat glands. SEE: *eccrine sweat gland.*

***areolar g.'s*** SEE: *Montgomery's glands.*

***auricular g.'s*** External otic lymph nodes.

***axillary g.'s*** Axillary lymph nodes.

***Bartholin's g.*** SEE: *Bartholin's gland.*

***Blandin's g.'s*** SEE: *Blandin's glands.*

***Bowman's g.'s*** SEE: *Bowman's glands.*

***brachial g.'s*** Lymph nodes in the arm and forearm.

***bronchial g.'s*** Mixed glands lying in the submucosa of the bronchi and bronchial tubes.

***Bruch's g.'s*** Conjunctival lymph nodes in the lower lids.

***Brunner's g.'s*** SEE: *Brunner's glands.*

***buccal g.'s*** Acinous glands in the mucosa of the cheek.

***bulbourethral g.*** One of two small glands above the bulb of the corpus spongiosum whose secretion forms part of the seminal fluid. SYN: *Cowper's g.*

***cardiac g.'s*** Glands of the stomach near the cardiac orifice of the esophagus.

***carotid g.*** The carotid body.

***celiac g.'s*** Several lymph nodes anterior to the abdominal aorta.

***ceruminous g.'s*** Glands in the external auditory canal that secrete cerumen.

***cervical g.'s*** Lymph nodes in the neck. SYN: *jugular g.'s.*

***ciliary g.'s*** SEE: *Moll's glands.*

***circumanal g.'s*** Anal g.'s.

***Cobelli's g.'s*** Glands in the esophageal mucosa.

***coccygeal g.*** Luschka's g.

***compound g.*** A gland consisting of a number of branching duct systems that open into the main secretory duct.

***compound tubular g.*** A gland composed of numerous minute tubules leading to a lone duct.

***conglobate g.*** Lymph g.

***Cowper's g.*** Bulbourethral g.

***cutaneous g.'s*** Glands of the skin, esp. the sebaceous and sudoriferous glands. These include modified forms such as the ciliary, ceruminous, anal, preputial, areolar, and meibomian glands.

***cytogenic g.*** A gland that produces living cells, such as the testis or ovary.

***ductless g.*** A gland that lacks a secretory duct. SEE: *endocrine gland.*

***duodenal g.'s*** SEE: *Brunner's glands.*

***Ebner's g.'s*** Serous glands of the tongue located in the region of the vallate papillae, their ducts opening into the furrows surrounding the papillae.

***eccrine g.*** A simple sweat gland of the skin. SEE: *apocrine g.; eccrine sweat gland.*

***endocrine g.*** SEE: *endocrine gland.*

***Fraenkel's g.'s*** Tiny glands located below the margin of the vocal cords.

***fundic g.'s*** Glands of the body and fundus of the stomach; gastric glands, which secrete gastric juice.

***gastric g.*** Any of three different types of tubular excretory glands in the mucosa of the stomach wall: cardiac in the superior area, fundic or oxyntic in the fundus, and pyloric in the distal portion. Gastric glands contain zymogenic or peptic cells, which secrete pepsinogen, the inactive form of pepsin; parietal border or oxyntic cells, which secrete hydrochloric acid and intrinsic factor; and mucous cells, which secrete mucin. SYN: *peptic g.*

***Gay's g.'s*** Circumanal sebaceous glands.

***genal g.*** A gland in the buccal submucosa.

***genital g.'s*** The female ovaries and male testes.

***hair g.'s*** Sebaceous glands opening into each hair follicle.

***haversian g.'s*** Synovial g.'s.

***hepatic g.'s*** Lymph nodes located in front of the portal vein.

***holocrine g.*** SEE: *holocrine.*

***inguinal g.'s*** Lymph nodes in the inguinal region.

***interscapular g.*** Embryonic lymphatic tissue.

***interstitial g.*** Leydig cells.

***intestinal g.'s*** Simple or branched tubular glands of the intestine that secrete the succus entericus. These include Brunner's glands and crypts of Lieberkühn.

***jugular g.'s*** Cervical g.'s.

***Krause's g.'s*** Small glands in the conjunctiva of the eyelids.

***labial g.'s*** Multiple acinous glands between the mucosa of the lips and the opening on the inner lip.

***lacrimal g.*** The gland that secretes tears. It is a tubuloaveolar gland located in the orbit, superior and lateral to the eyeball, and consists of a large superior portion (pars orbitalis) and a smaller inferior portion (pars palpebralis).

***lactiferous g.*** Mammary g.

***lenticular g.*** One of the small masses of lymphatic tissue in the lamina propria of the pyloric region of the stomach.

***Lieberkühn's g.'s*** Lieberkühn crypt.

***lingual g.'s*** Glands of the tongue, including the anterior lingual glands (glands of Nuhn), posterior lingual glands (glands of von Ebner), and mucous glands at the root of the tongue.

***Littré's g.*** SEE: *Littré's gland.*

***lumbar g.'s*** Lymphatics located behind the peritoneal region and the lower section of the diaphragmatic posterior part.

***Luschka's g.*** A gland located near the coccygeal tip. SYN: *coccygeal g.*

***lymph g., lymphatic g.*** A node of lymphatic tissue, found along the path of a lymphatic vessel. SYN: *conglobate g.*

***mammary g.*** A compound alveolar gland that secretes milk. In women, these glands are made up of lobes and lobules bound together by areolar tissue. Each of the 15 to 20 main ducts, known as lactiferous ducts, discharges through a separate orifice on the surface of the nipple. The dilatations of the ducts form reservoirs for the milk during lactation. SYN: *lactiferous g.*

***meibomian g.'s*** Tarsal g.'s.

***merocrine g.*** A gland in which the cells remain intact during the elaboration and discharge of their secretion. SEE: *eccrine sweat gland.*

***mixed g.*** **1.** A gland that has both endocrine and exocrine function (e.g., the pancreas). **2.** A salivary gland that has both mucous and serous secretions, often with both cell types in the same acinus. SEE: *submandibular gland.*

***Moll's g.'s*** SEE: *Moll's glands.*

***Montgomery's g.'s*** SEE: *Montgomery's glands.*

***Morgagni's g.'s*** SEE: *Littré's g.'s.*

***muciparous g.'s*** Glands that secrete mucus.

***nabothian g.'s*** Dilated mucous glands in the uterine cervix.

***odoriferous g.'s*** Glands exuding odoriferous materials, as those around the prepuce or anus.

***olfactory g.'s*** Glands in the olfactory mucous membranes.

***oxyntic g.'s*** Gastric glands found in the fundus and body of the gastric mucosa.

***palatine g.'s*** Mucous glands in the tissue of the palate.

***palpebral g.'s*** Tarsal g.'s.

***parathyroid g.'s*** Several small endocrine glands about 6 mm long by 3 to 4 mm wide, on the back and lower edge of the thyroid gland or embedded within its substance. These glands secrete parathyroid hormone, which regulates calcium and phosphorus metabolism.

***paraurethral g.'s*** SEE: *Skene's glands.*

***parotid g.*** The largest of the salivary glands, located below and in front of the ear. It is a compound tubuloacinous serous gland. Its secreting tubules and acini are long and branched, and it is enclosed in a sheath, the parotid fascia. Saliva lubricates food and makes it easier to taste, chew, and swallow. SEE: *mumps.*

***peptic g.*** Gastric g.

***Peyer's g.'s*** Peyer's patch.

***pineal g.*** An endocrine gland in the brain, shaped like a pine cone and located in a pocket near the splenium of the corpus callosum. It is the site of melatonin synthesis, which is inhibited by light striking the retina. SEE: *melatonin.*

***pituitary g.*** SEE: *pituitary gland.*

***preputial g.*** SEE: *Tyson's gland.*

***prostate g.*** The male gland that surrounds the neck of the bladder and the urethra. It is partly glandular, with ducts opening into the prostatic portion of the urethra, and partly muscular. It secretes a thin, opalescent, slightly alkaline fluid that forms part of semen. The prostate consists of a median lobe and two lateral lobes measuring about $2 \times 4 \times 3$ cm and weighing about 20 g; it is enclosed in a fibrous capsule containing smooth muscle fiber in its inner layer. The nerve supply is from the inferior hypogastric plexus.

***pyloric g.'s*** Gastric glands near the pylorus that secrete gastric juice.

***racemose g.*** Acinous g.

***Rivinus' g.*** Sublingual g.

***salivary g.*** The parotid, sublingual, or submandibular salivary gland of the mouth.

***sebaceous g.*** A simple or branched alveolar gland that secretes sebum. It is found in the skin and its ducts usually open into hair follicles.

***sentinel g.*** An enlarged lymph gland caused by a pathological process in the area drained by the lymph channels leading to that gland.

***seromucous g.*** A mixed serous and muciparous gland.

***serous g.'s*** Albuminous g.'s.

***sex g.*** The ovary or testis.

***Skene's g.'s*** SEE: *Skene's glands.*

***sublingual g.*** The smallest salivary gland of the mouth. SYN: *Rivinus' gland.*

***submandibular g.*** The mixed seromucous salivary gland that lies below the mandible.

***sudoriferous g.'s*** Glands in the skin that secrete perspiration. SYN: *sweat g.'s.* SEE: *sweat glands* for illus.

***suprarenal g.*** Adrenal g.

***sweat g.'s*** Sudoriferous g.'s.

***synovial g.'s*** Glands that secrete synovial fluid. SYN: *haversian g.'s.*

***target g.*** Any gland affected by the action or secretion of another gland (e.g., the thyroid is a target gland of the pituitary).

***tarsal g.'s*** Glands in the eyelid that secrete a sebaceous substance that keeps the lids from adhering to each other. SYN: *meibomian g.'s; palpebral g.'s.*

***thymus g.*** The thymus body or thymus.

***thyroid g.*** A ductless gland located in the base of the neck on both sides of the lower part of the larynx and upper part of the trachea, consisting of two lateral lobes connected by an isthmus. Sometimes a third medial or pyramidal lobe extends upward from the isthmus. Histologically, a large number of closed vesicles, called *follicles*, contain the thyroglobulin, which in turn contains various active substances such as thyroxine. The thyroid gland is enlarged in goiter, and it may appear to pulsate owing to the increased blood supply.

***tracheal g.'s*** Acinous glands of the tracheal mucosa.

***tubular g.*** A gland whose terminal secreting portions are narrow tubes.

***Tyson's g.'s*** SEE: *Tyson's glands.*

***unicellular g.'s*** Mucus-secreting cells present in columnar or pseudostratified columnar epithelial tissue layers. They are called *goblet cells.*

***urethral g.'s*** SEE: *Littré's gland.*

***vaginal g.'s*** Acinous glands found in uppermost portion of the vaginal mucosa near the cervix, most of the vaginal mucosa being devoid of glands.

***vestibular g.'s*** Glands of the vaginal vestibule. They include the minor vestibular glands and the major vestibular glands (Bartholin's glands).

***vulvovaginal g.'s*** SEE: *Bartholin's gland.*

***Waldeyer's g.'s*** SEE: *Waldeyer's glands.*

***Weber's g.'s*** SEE: *Weber's glands.*

***g.'s of Zeis*** SEE: *Zeis glands.*

***Zuckerkandl's g.*** A tiny yellowish lobe occasionally seen between the geniohyoid muscles. It is an accessory thyroid gland.

**glanders** (glăn′dĕrz) A contagious infection caused by *Pseudomonas mallei* in horses, donkeys, and mules. It is communicable to humans, but no cases have occurred in the Western Hemisphere since 1938. Experience with the disease is limited, but sulfadiazine is the recommended therapy.

SYMPTOMS: Patients develop fever, inflammation of the skin and mucous membranes (esp. those of the nasal cavity), with formation of ulcers and abscesses. Small subcutaneous nodules develop, break down, and give rise to ulcers. Beginning as small areas, these tend to spread and coalesce and finally involve large areas that exude a viscid, mucopurulent discharge with a foul odor. The infection may occur in an acute or chronic form. In the acute septicemic form, prognosis is grave and the disease is almost invariably fatal.

**glandilemma** (glăn″dĭ-lĕm′ă) [L. *glans,* acorn, + Gr. *lemma,* sheath] The outer covering or capsule of a gland.

**glandula** (glăn′dū-lă) *pl.* **glandulae** Glandule.

**glandular** [L. *glandula,* little acorn] Pert. to or of the nature of a gland.

**glandular therapy** Treatment of disease with endocrine glands or their extracts. SYN: *organotherapy.*

**glandule** (glăn′dūl) A small gland. SYN: *glandula.*

**glans** [L. *glans,* acorn] A gland.

***g. clitoridis*** The head of the clitoris. SEE: *clitoris.*

***g. penis*** The bulbous end of the penis. SEE: *penis.*

**Glanzmann's thrombasthenia** (glănz′mănz) [Edward Glanzmann, Swiss pediatrician, 1887–1959] A rare congenital abnormality of blood platelets, characterized by easy bruising and epistaxis that sometimes requires blood transfusions. Bleeding is prolonged, clot retraction is diminished, and platelets do not aggregate during blood coagulation or after addition of adenosine diphosphate. The only therapy is platelet transfusions, which should be used only for treating severe bleeding.

**glare** [ME. *glaren,* to gleam] A condition causing temporary blurring of vision with possible permanent injury to the retina. The condition is caused by intense light (visible radiation) emanating from highly reflective objects (such as sunlight reflected on water or snow), or projected by an automobile headlight or by a therapeutic lamp. SEE: *dazzle.*

**glaserian artery** (glā-sē′rē-ăn) [Johann Heinrich Glaser, Swiss anatomist, 1629–1679] A branch of the internal maxillary artery that supplies the tympanum.

**glaserian fissure** A narrow slit posterior to the mandibular fossa of the temporal bone. The chorda tympani nerve passes through it.

**Glasgow Coma Scale** A scale for evaluating and quantitating the degree of coma by determining the best motor, verbal, and eye-opening response to standardized stimuli. Coma is diagnosed by the absence of motor, eye-opening, and verbal responses. A score of 7 or less indicates coma; 9 or greater excludes the diagnosis of coma. SEE: *coma; Trauma Score.*

**Glasgow Outcome Scale** A scale that predicts recovery and disability rather than survival in all types of brain injury. The scale is to be used at prescribed time intervals, such as 3 months, 6 months, and 1 year after injury. The Glasgow group reports the greatest recovery in the 6-month period after injury. The nurse (or other health-care practitioner) notes the patient's abilities at a particular time using this practical scale:

*Good outcome:* may have minimal disabling sequelae but returns to independent functioning comparable to preinjury level and a full-time job

*Moderate disability:* is capable of independent functioning but not of returning to full-time employment

*Severe disability:* depends on others for some aspect of daily living

*Persistive vegetative state:* has no obvious cortical functioning

*Dead*

**glass** [AS. *glaes*] A hard, brittle, amorphous, transparent material composed of silica and various bases.

***leaded g.*** Safety glass that contains lead, used in radiology to help protect technicians from x-rays.

***photochromic g.*** Glass that is manufactured to appear clear until light strikes it. When used in sunglasses, the lens becomes dark and reduces the amount of light transmitted, becoming clear again when no longer exposed to bright light.

***polarized g.*** Glass treated with a medium that permits the exiting light waves to vibrate in only one direction.

***safety g.*** A type of laminated glass that meets specific requirements concerning the force necessary to break it and is designed to break without shattering. Its use in automobiles reduces the risk of injury from broken glass.

***tempered g.*** Glass that has been heat-treated to increase the force required to break it.

***ultraviolet transmitting g.*** Glass designed to admit ultraviolet radiation through it. It transmits about half of the solar radiation, between the wavelengths of 290 and 320 nm.

***watch g.*** A shallow, saucer-like glass dish, resembling the glass cover widely used to cover the face of a large pocket watch.

**glasses** [AS. *glaes,* glass] **1.** A transparent refractive device worn to correct refraction errors in the patient's eyes. **2.** A device worn to protect eyes from glare or particles in the air. SYN: *eyeglass; spectacles.*

***bifocal g.*** Glasses in which the refracting power of the lower portion differs from that in the upper portion, the lower portion being used for viewing near objects or reading, the upper portion for distant objects. SYN: *Franklin glasses.*

***prism g.*** An optical device, used by persons who must lie supine for extended periods, to allow them to view objects in their environment without eye or neck strain. Prisms mounted on spectacle frames bend the image to make the feet visible while the person is looking straight ahead.

***safety g.*** Glasses using heat-treated

glass or impact-resistant plastic lenses. Their use serves to protect the eyes from dangerous slivers of glass that are produced when ordinary lenses are broken in an accident. Use of safety glass in manufacturing eyeglass lenses is mandatory in the U.S.

***trifocal g.*** Glasses with three different corrections in each lens: one each for near, intermediate, and far vision.

**glassy** Hyaline; vitreous; glasslike, smooth, and shiny.

**Glauber's salt** (glō'běrz) [Johann Rudolf Glauber, Dutch physician, 1604–1668] Sodium sulfate.

**glaucoma** (glaw-kō'mă) [L., cataract] A group of eye diseases characterized by increased intraocular pressure, resulting in atrophy of the optic nerve and possibly leading to blindness. Glaucoma is the third most prevalent cause of visual impairment and blindness in the U.S. Cataract and macular degeneration of aging are the two principal causes. An estimated 15 million residents of the U.S. have glaucoma; of these, 150,000 have bilateral blindness. The three major categories of glaucoma are closed-angle (acute) glaucoma, which occurs in persons whose eyes are anatomically predisposed to develop the condition; open-angle (chronic) glaucoma, in which the angle that permits the drainage of aqueous humor from the eye seems normal but functions inadequately; and congenital glaucoma, in which the intraocular pressure is increased for an unknown reason. The increased pressure causes the globe of the eye to be enlarged; a condition known as *buphthalmia*. The acute type of glaucoma often is attended by acute pain. The chronic type has an insidious onset. A normal tonometer reading ranges from 13 to 22. An initial visual dysfunction is loss of the mid-peripheral field of vision. The loss of central visual acuity occurs later in the disease.

ETIOLOGY: Glaucoma occurs when the aqueous humor drains from the eye too slowly to keep up with its production in the anterior chamber. Thus, narrowing or closure of the filtration angle that interferes with drainage through the canal of Schlemm causes intraocular fluid to accumulate, after which intraocular pressure increases. Glaucoma may develop, however, even if the filtration angle is normal and the canal of Schlemm appears to be functioning; the cause of this form of glaucoma is not known.

DIAGNOSIS: Glaucoma may not cause symptoms. It is detected usually by an abnormal intraocular pressure (IOP) measurement. The frequent need to change eyeglass prescriptions, vague visual disturbances, mild headache, and impaired dark adaptation may also be present. The standard for determining visual loss in glaucoma is the visual-field test.

Open-angle glaucoma causes mild aching in the eyes, loss of peripheral vision, haloes around lights, and reduced visual acuity (esp. at night) that is uncorrected by prescription lenses. Acute angle-closure glaucoma (an ophthalmic emergency) causes excruciating unilateral pain and pressure, blurred vision, decreased visual acuity, haloes around lights, diplopia, lacrimation, and nausea and vomiting due to increased IOP. The eyes may show unilateral circumcorneal injection, conjunctival edema, a cloudy cornea, and a moderately dilated pupil that is nonreactive to light.

TREATMENT: Nonoperative treatment includes the use of miotics (eserine, pilocarpine), timolol maleate, intravenous mannitol, and parenteral acetazolamide. Experimental studies indicate that marijuana alleviates the symptoms of severe glaucoma. Control of associated disorders such as diabetes should be maintained. Operative treatment includes paracentesis of the cornea, iridectomy (broad peripheral), cyclodialysis, anterior sclerotomy, sclerotomy with inclusion of the iris, as iridotasis or iridencleisis; sclerectomy. SEE: illus.; *ciliarotomy; trabeculoplasty.*

Caution: Acute glaucoma may be precipitated in patients with closed-angle glaucoma by dilating the pupils.

NURSING IMPLICATIONS: The nurse's hands should be washed thoroughly before touching the eye. Prescribed topical and systemic medications are administered and evaluated.

The patient is prepared physically and psychologically for diagnostic studies and surgery as indicated. If the patient has a trabeculectomy, prescribed cycloplegic drugs are administered to relax the ciliary muscle and decrease iris action.

Caution: In glaucoma patients, cycloplegic drops are given only after trabeculectomy and only in the eye that had the procedure. Administering drops in an eye affected with glaucoma can precipitate an acute attack in an eye already compromised by elevated IOP.

After any surgery, an eye patch and shield are applied to protect the eye, the patient is positioned with the head slightly elevated, and general safety measures geared to the patient's level of sensory alteration are instituted.

Patients with glaucoma need to know that the disease can be controlled, but not cured. Fatigue, emotional upsets, excessive fluid intake, and use of antihistamines may increase IOP. Signs and symptoms such as vision changes or eye pain should be reported immediately. Both pa-

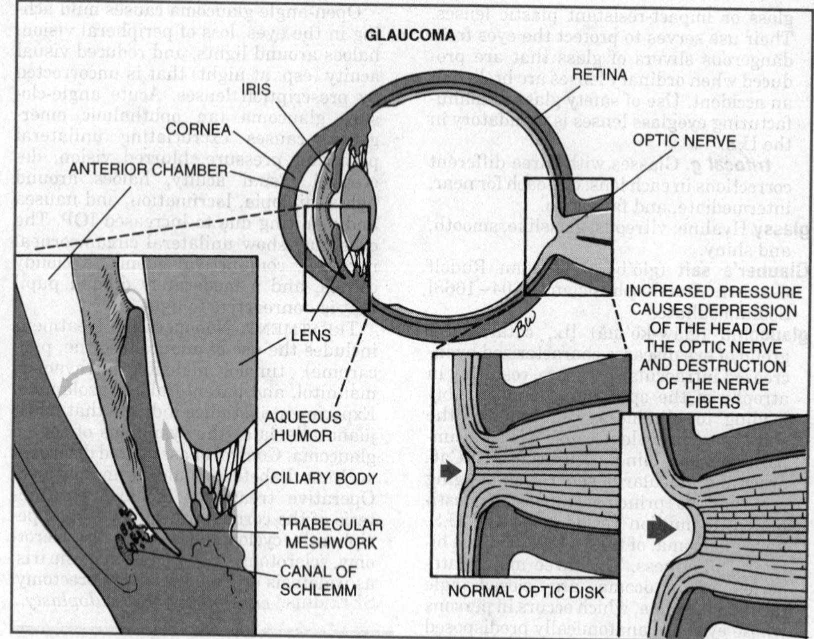


tient and family are instructed in correct techniques for eyedrop administration, the importance of strict adherence to the prescribed regimen, and adverse reactions to report.

Information is provided to the patient and family as needed. Referral is made to local organizations and support groups.

Public education is carried out to encourage glaucoma screening for early detection of the disease. Written information should be made available about detection and control of glaucoma. SEE: *Nursing Diagnoses Appendix.*

***absolute g.*** An extremely painful form of glaucoma in which the eye is completely blind and hard as stone, with an insensitive cornea, a shallow anterior chamber, and an excavated optic disk.

***chronic g.*** Glaucoma in which the tonometer indicates an intraocular pressure reading of up to 45 or 50, the anterior ciliary veins are enlarged, the cornea is clear, the pupil is dilated, and pain is present. During attacks vision is poor. The visual field may be normal. Cupping of the optic disk is not present in the early stages.

***closed-angle g.*** Glaucoma caused by a shallow anterior chamber and thus a narrow filtration angle through which the aqueous humor normally passes. Because the rate of movement of the aqueous is impaired, intraocular pressure increases. In general, headache, haloes around single sources of light, blurred vision, and eye pain are symptomatic. SYN: *narrow-angle glaucoma.*

***narrow-angle g.*** Closed-angle g.

***primary open-angle g.*** The most common type of glaucoma. It usually affects both eyes, and there is a characteristic change in the appearance of the optic disk. The cup (the depression in the center of the disk) is enlarged. Visual loss is determined by the visual-field test. Many patients with glaucoma have increased intraocular pressure but this is not considered essential to the diagnosis because some patients have normal intraocular pressure.

**glaucomatous** (glaw-kō′mă-tŭs) Pert. to glaucoma.

**GLC** *gas-liquid chromatography.*

**gleet** (glēt) A mucous discharge from the urethra in chronic gonorrhea.

**Glénard's disease** (glā-nărz′) [Frantz Glénard, Fr. physician, 1848–1920] The prolapse of one or more internal organs. SYN: *enteroptosis; splanchnoptosia.*

**glenohumeral** (glē″nō-hū′mĕr-ăl) [Gr. *glene,* socket, + L. *humerus,* humerus] Pert. to the humerus and the glenoid cavity.

**glenohumeral ligaments** Three ligaments in the shoulder.

**glenoid** (glē′noyd) [″ + *eidos,* form, shape] Having the appearance of a socket.

**glenoid cavity** The socket of the scapula that receives the head of the humerus below the acromion at the junction of the superior and axillary borders.

**glenoid fossa 1.** The fossa of the temporal bone that receives the condyle or capitulum of the mandible. **2.** A depression on the lateral portion of the scapula that forms part of the ball and socket articulation with the head of the humerus. SYN: *fossa, articular, of temporal bone; mandibular fossa.*

**glenoid labrum** The ring of fibrocartilaginous tissue around the glenoid cavity on the scapula. It deepens and increases the congruency of the articulating surface. SEE: *glenoid lip.*

**glenoid lip** A rim of fibrous tissue around the margin of the glenoid cavity.

**glia** (glī'ă) [Gr. *glia,* glue] The neuroglia; the nonnervous or supporting tissue of the brain and spinal cord.

**glia cells** Neuroglia cells, including astrocytes, oligodendroglia (oligoglia), and microglia. SEE: *cell; neuroglia.*

**gliacyte** (glī'ă-sīt) [" + *kytos,* cell] A neuroglia cell.

**gliadin** (glī'ă-dĭn) A water-insoluble protein present in the gluten of wheat. It is deficient in the essential amino acid lysine. The sticky mass that results when wheat flour and water are mixed is due to gliadin. In some individuals the intestinal mucosa lacks the ability to digest this substance, which therefore damages the intestinal lining and causes gluten-induced enteropathy.

**glial** (glī'ăl) Concerning glia or neuroglia.

**gliarase** (glī'ă-rās) [Gr. *glia,* glue] An astrocytic mass with incomplete fission of cytoplasm.

**glide 1.** To move in a smooth, virtually frictionless manner. **2.** Movement in a smooth, virtually frictionless manner. **3.** A joint mobilization technique in which the therapist applies a translatoric force against one of the bones of a joint causing it to move parallel to a defined treatment plane in the joint. This technique is used to maintain or increase joint play.

***mandibular g.*** The movement of the mandible in any direction as the teeth come into contact.

**glioblastoma** (glī"ō-blăs-tō'mă) [" + *blastos,* germ, + *oma,* tumor] A neuroglia cell tumor. SYN: *glioma.*

***g. multiforme*** A neoplasm of the central nervous system, esp. the cerebrum, consisting of a variety of cellular types.

**gliocyte** (glī'ō-sīt) [" + *kytos,* cell] A neuroglia cell.

**gliocytoma** (glī-ō-sī-tō'mă) [" + " + *oma,* tumor] A neuroglia cell tumor.

**gliogenous** (glī-ŏj'ĕ-nŭs) [" + *gennan,* to produce] Of the nature of neuroglia.

**glioma** (glī-ō'mă) *pl.* **gliomata** [" + *oma,* tumor] **1.** A sarcoma of neuroglial origin. **2.** A neoplasm or tumor composed of neuroglia cells. SYN: *glioblastoma; neurogli-oma.*

***g. retinae*** A malignant tumor of the retina that occurs in children and metastasizes late. SEE: *pseudoglioma.*

**gliomatosis** (glī"ō-mă-tō'sĭs) [" + " + *osis,* condition] The formation of a glioma, esp. a large one.

**gliomatous** (glī-ō'mă-tŭs) Affected with or of the nature of a glioma.

**gliomyoma** (glī"ō-mī-ō'mă) [" + *mys,* muscle, + *oma,* tumor] A mixed glioma and myoma.

**glioneuroma** (glī"ō-nū-rō'mă) [" + *neuron,* nerve, + *oma,* tumor] A tumor having the characteristics of glioma and neuroma.

**gliosarcoma** [" + *sarx,* flesh, + *oma,* tumor] A glioma combined with fusiform sarcoma cells.

**gliosis** (glī-ō'sĭs) [" + *osis,* condition] The proliferation of neuroglial tissue in the central nervous system.

**gliosome** (glī'ō-sōm) [" + *soma,* body] One of the rounded bodies seen in neuroglia cells.

**Glisson, Francis** (glĭs'ŭn) A British physician and anatomist, 1597–1677.

***G.'s capsule*** The outer capsule of fibrous tissue investing the liver.

***G.'s disease*** Rickets.

**glissonian cirrhosis** An inflammation of the peritoneal coat of the liver. SYN: *perihepatitis.*

**glissonitis** An inflammation of Glisson's capsule.

**Global Assessment of Relational Functioning Scale** ABBR: GARF scale. A measure of the degree to which a family meets the emotional and functional needs of its members.

**globi** (glō'bī) [L.] Pl. of globus.

**globin** (glō'bĭn) [L. *globus,* globe] **1.** A protein constituent of hemoglobin. **2.** One of a particular group of proteins.

**globoid** (glō'boyd) [" + Gr. *eidos,* form, shape] Resembling a globe. SYN: *spheroid.*

**globular** (glŏb'ū-lăr) [L. *globus,* a globe] Resembling a globe or globule; spherical.

**globule** (glŏb'ūl) [L. *globulus,* globule] Any small, rounded body.

**globulin** (glŏb'ū-lĭn) [L. *globulus,* globule] One of a group of simple proteins insoluble in pure water but soluble in neutral solutions of salts of strong acids. Examples include serum globulin, fibrinogen, myosinogen, and lactoglobulin.

***Ac g.*** Accelerator globulin; a globulin present in blood serum that speeds up the conversion of prothrombin to thrombin in the presence of thromboplastin and calcium ions.

***antihemophilic g.*** A clotting component present in the plasma that is essential for the normal agglutination and disintegration of blood platelets. It is deficient in the blood of hemophiliacs. SEE: *hemophilia.*

***antilymphocyte g.*** A globulin from a person who has become immunized to lymphocytes. It is used as an immunosuppressant.

***gamma g.*** The fraction of serum globulin with which most of the immune antibodies are associated. Most of the antibodies to viruses, bacterial agglutinogens, exotoxins, and injected foreign proteins are contained in the gamma globulin fraction. SEE: *immunoglobulin.*

***immune g.*** A sterile, nonpyrogenic solution of globulins normally present in human blood. It is used in passive immunization of nonimmune persons exposed to infectious hepatitis, poliomyelitis, mumps, rubella, rubeola, and varicella. The previously used name was human immune serum globulin. Trade names are Gamastan, Gamimune, Gammagee, Gammar, Immu-G, and Immuglobulin.

***Rh immune g.*** A solution of gamma globulin containing anti-Rh. Given to an Rh-negative mother within 72 hr after delivery of an Rh-positive infant, it destroys any Rh-positive red blood cells that may have entered maternal circulation before her immune system can produce anti-Rh antibodies. Also indicated in abortion done on an Rh-negative mother.

***$Rh_o$(D) immune g.*** Previously used name for Rh immune globulin.

***serum g.*** Any of the globulins present in blood plasma or serum; the fraction of the blood serum with which antibodies are associated. By electrophoresis, they can be separated into alpha, beta, and gamma globulins, which differ in their isoelectric points.

***varicella-zoster immune g.*** ABBR: VZIg. An immune globulin obtained from the blood of normal persons found to have high antibody titers to varicella-zoster. SEE: Prevention under *varicella.*

**globulinuria** (glŏb″ū-lĭn-ū′rē-ă) [L. *globulus,* globule, + Gr. *ouron,* urine] Globulin in the urine.

**globulose** (glŏb′ū-lōs) [L. *globulus,* globule] Albumose or protein produced by the digestion of globulins.

**globus** [L.] A globe or sphere.

***g. hystericus*** A lump in the throat in hysteria and other neuroses.

***g. major*** The head of the epididymis.

***g. minor*** The lower end of the epididymis.

***g. pallidus*** A pale section within the lenticular nucleus of the brain. SEE: *paleostriatum.*

**glomangioma** (glō-măn″jē-ō′mă) [L. *glomus,* a ball, + Gr. *angeion,* vessel, + *oma,* tumor] A benign tumor that develops from an arteriovenous glomus (cluster of blood cells) of the skin.

**glomectomy** (glō-mĕk′tō-mē) The surgical removal of a glomus.

**glomerate** (glŏm′ĕr-āt) [L. *glomerare,* to wind into a ball] Conglomerate, clustered, grouped.

**glomerular** (glō-mĕr′ū-lăr) [L. *glomerulus,* little ball] Pert. to a glomerulus; clustered.

**glomerular disease** Any of a large group of diseases that have basic pathological involvement of the glomerulus. They may be classified by clinical severity, by histological changes in the kidney, or by etiology. Etiological factors include *primary glomerular disease;* disease secondary to *systemic disease,* such as lupus erythematosus or polyarteritis; *infectious disease* such as streptococcal infection, malaria, syphilis, or schistosomiasis; *metabolic disease* such as diabetes or amyloidosis; *toxins* such as mercury, gold, or snake venom; *serum sickness;* and drug *hypersensitivity.*

Glomerular disease may also be associated with hereditary disorders (e.g., Alport's syndrome, Fabry's disease). SEE: *glomerulonephritis; kidney; nephritis; nephrotic syndrome.*

Clinical findings are those associated with the primary dysfunction and pathological changes in the glomerulus, which include proteinuria and hypertension. If protein loss exceeds 5 g/day, the nephrotic syndrome will develop.

**glomerulitis** (glō-mĕr″ū-lī′tĭs) [″ + Gr. *itis,* inflammation] An inflammation of glomeruli, esp. of the renal glomeruli.

**glomerulonephritis** (glō-mĕr″ū-lō-nĕ-frī′tĭs) [″ + Gr. *nephros,* kidney, + *itis,* inflammation] A form of nephritis in which the lesions involve primarily the glomeruli. This condition may be acute, subacute, or chronic. Acute glomerulonephritis, also known as acute nephritic syndrome, frequently follows infections, esp. those of the upper respiratory tract caused by particular strains of streptococci. It may also be caused by systemic lupus erythematosus, subacute bacterial endocarditis, cryoglobulinemia, various forms of vasculitis including polyarteritis nodosa, Henoch-Schönlein purpura, and visceral abscess. The condition is characterized by hematuria, proteinuria, red cell casts, oliguria, edema, pruritus, nausea, constipation, and hypertension. Investigation of serum complement and renal biopsy facilitates diagnosis and helps to establish the prognosis. SEE: *glomerular disease; glomerulonephritis, rapidly progressive; Nursing Diagnoses Appendix.*

NURSING IMPLICATIONS: Serum creatinine, blood urea nitrogen, and urine creatinine clearance levels are monitored, and the patient is assessed for electrolyte and acid-base imbalance. Fluid balance is monitored, and changes in the amount of edema, daily weight, and fluid intake and output are documented. Vital signs are monitored every 4 hr or as necessary, and skin is inspected for signs of breakdown. Skin care and frequent repositioning are provided.

The patient is instructed to limit activities during acute periods of hematuria, azotemia, gross edema, and hypertension; but self-care is encouraged as acute symptoms subside, depending on fatigue levels and changes in blood pressure. Appropriate diversional activities are encouraged. Instruction is provided in dietary and fluid restrictions; the importance of low-sodium, high-calorie meals with adequate (though at times restricted) protein content is stressed. Prescribed medications should be taken as scheduled.

The patient should avoid individuals with communicable illnesses and should report signs of infection, particularly urinary tract infections, immediately. The importance of keeping follow-up appointments is stressed. The patient's response is monitored, and the patient with severe renal dysfunction is prepared for dialysis.

***rapidly progressive g.*** ABBR: RPGN. Any glomerular disease in which there is rapid loss of renal function, usually damaging more than 50% of the glomeruli.

**glomerulopathy** (glō-mĕr″ū-lŏp′ă-thē) Any disease of the renal glomeruli.

**glomerulosclerosis** (glō-mĕr″ū-lō-sklē-rō′sĭs) Fibrosis of the renal glomeruli.

***diabetic g.*** A type of glomerulosclerosis seen in some cases of diabetes mellitus. Eosinophilic material is present in various parts of the glomerulus. SYN: *intercapillary g.*

***intercapillary g.*** Diabetic g.

**glomerulus** (glō-mĕr′ū-lŭs) *pl.* **glomeruli** [L.] **1.** One of the capillary networks that are part of the renal corpuscles in the nephrons of the kidney. Each is surrounded by a Bowman's capsule, the site of renal (glomerular) filtration, which is the first step in the formation of urine. SEE: *kidney* for illus. **2.** A group of twisted capillaries or nerve fibers.

***olfactory g.*** A rounded body found in the olfactory bulb, formed by the numerous terminal branches of the dendrites of a mitral cell intertwining with the terminal fibers of several olfactory receptor cells.

**glomoid** (glō′moyd) Appearing similar to a glomus.

**glomus** (glō′mŭs) [L., a ball] A small, round swelling made up of tiny blood vessels and found in stromata containing many nerve fibers.

***g. caroticum*** Carotid body.

***g. choroideum*** An enlargement of the choroid plexus at its entrance into the lateral ventricle.

***g. coccygeum*** The coccygeal body.

***periodontal g.*** The sensory endings of the periodontal ligament that provide acute sensitivity and reflex movements.

**glossa** [Gr. *glossa,* tongue] The tongue.

**glossal** Rel. to the tongue.

**glossalgia** (glŏs-săl′jē-ă) [″ + *algos,* pain] Glossodynia.

**glossectomy** (glŏs-ĕk′tō-mē) [″ + *ektome,* excision] Partial or complete excision of the tongue.

**Glossina** (glŏs-sī′nă) A genus of flies called tsetse flies, which includes about 20 species of bloodsucking flies that are confined principally to central and southern Africa. They transmit the trypanosomes *(Trypanosoma gambiense, T. rhodesiense),* the causative agents of sleeping sickness in humans, and other trypanosomes that infect wild and domestic animals. Important species are *Glossina palpalis, G. morsitans, G. tachinoides,* and *G. swynnertoni.* SEE: *sleeping sickness; Trypanosoma.*

**glossitis** (glŏs-sī′tĭs) [″ + *itis,* inflammation] An inflammation of the tongue.

***acute g.*** A form of glossitis associated with stomatitis. The tongue is covered with ulcers and is tender and painful. Another form affects the parenchyma of the tongue and is characterized by edema, which may spread to surrounding structures, producing asphyxia and necessitating tracheostomy.

SYMPTOMS: The tongue is painful and the saliva thick and viscid, making swallowing difficult. There is marked malaise and often fever.

TREATMENT: Acute glossitis is treated by maintaining oral cleanliness with frequent antiseptic mouthwashes, applying an anesthetic oral solution for pain, and following a bland or liquid diet.

***g. areata exfoliativa*** A condition of the tongue marked by numerous denuded patches on the dorsal surface coalescing into freeform shapes similar to the geographic areas on a map. SYN: *geographic tongue.*

***g. desiccans*** A painful, raw, and fissured tongue.

***herpetic geometric g.*** Herpes simplex virus type 1 infection of the tongue. This may be seen in immunocompromised patients. If it is associated with human immunodeficiency virus infection, acyclovir is an effective treatment.

***median rhomboid g.*** An inflammatory area, somewhat diamond-shaped, found on the dorsum of the tongue anterior to the vallate papillae.

***Moeller's g.*** A chronic superficial glossitis characterized by burning or pain and an increased sensitivity to hot and spicy foods. SYN: *glossodynia exfoliativa.*

***g. parasitica*** SEE: *tongue, black hairy.*

**glosso-** [Gr. *glossa,* tongue] Combining form meaning *tongue.*

**glossocele** (glŏs′sō-sēl) [″ + *kele,* swelling] A swelling and protrusion of the tongue resulting from disease or malformation.

**glossodynamometer** (glŏs″sō-dī″nă-mŏm′ĕ-tĕr) [″ + *dynamis,* power, + *metron,* measure] A device for measuring the strength of the tongue muscles.

**glossodynia** (glŏs″ō-dĭn′ē-ă) [″ + *odyne,* pain] Pain in the tongue. SYN: *glossalgia.* SEE: *burning mouth syndrome.*

***g. exfoliativa*** Moeller's glossitis.

**glossoepiglottic** (glŏs″ō-ĕp-ĭ-glŏt′ĭk) [″ + *epi,* upon, + *glottis,* back of tongue] Pert. to the ligament between the base of the tongue and the epiglottis.

**glossoepiglottidean** (glŏs″ō-ĕp-ĭ-glŏ-tĭd′ē-ăn) Rel. to the tongue and epiglottis.

**glossograph** (glŏs′ō-grăf) [″ + *graphein,* to write] An instrument for recording the tongue's movements during speech.

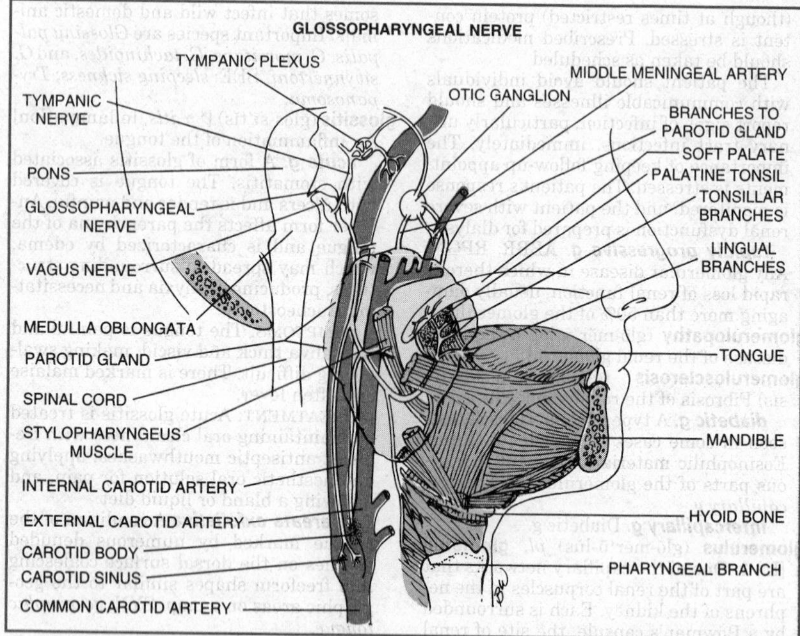


**glossohyal** (glŏs″ō-hī′ăl) [″ + *hyoeides,* U-shaped] Rel. to the tongue and hyoid bone. SYN: *hyoglossal.*

**glossokinesthetic** (glŏs″ō-kĭn″ĕs-thĕt′ĭk) [″ + *kinesis,* movement, + *aisthetikos,* perceptive] Pert. to movements of the tongue, esp. those in speech.

**glossolabial** (glŏs″ō-lā′bē-ăl) [″ + L. *labium,* lip] Pert. to the tongue and lips.

**glossolalia** (glŏs″ō-lā′lē-ă) [″ + *lalia,* babble] The repetition of senseless remarks not related to the subject or situation involved.

**glossology** (glŏ-sŏl′ō-jē) [″ + *logos,* word, reason] The study of the tongue and its diseases. SYN: *glottology.*

**glossopalatine** (glŏs″ō-păl′ă-tīn) Pert. to the tongue and palate.

**glossopathy** (glŏs-sŏp′ă-thē) [″ + *pathos,* disease, suffering] Any disease of the tongue.

**glossopharyngeal** (glŏs″ō-fă-rĭn′jē-ăl) [″ + *pharynx,* throat] Rel. to the tongue and pharynx.

**glossopharyngeal breathing** A technique of breathing in which the patient with inspiratory muscle weakness increases the volume of air breathed in by taking several "gulps" of air, closing the mouth, and forcing air into the lungs.

**glossopharyngeal nerve** The ninth cranial nerve, featuring special sensory (taste), visceral sensory, and motor functions. It originates by several roots from the medulla oblongata. Its distribution covers the pharynx, ear, meninges, posterior third of the tongue, and parotid gland. Branches include the carotid, tympanic, pharyngeal, lingual, tonsillar nerves, and the sinus nerve of Hering. SEE: illus.

**glossoplasty** (glŏs′ō-plăs″tē) [″ + *plassein,* to form] Reparative surgery of the tongue.

**glossoplegia** (glŏs″ō-plē′jē-ă) [″ + *plege,* stroke] Paralysis of the tongue, usually unilateral, which may result from cerebral hemorrhage, disease, or injury that involves the hypoglossal nerve.

**glossoptosis** (glŏs″ŏp-tō′sĭs) [″ + *ptosis,* a dropping] A dropping of the tongue downward out of normal position.

**glossopyrosis** (glŏs″ō-pī-rō′sĭs) [″ + *pyrosis,* a burning] A burning sensation of the tongue. SEE: *burning mouth syndrome.*

**glossorrhaphy** (glŏ-sor′ă-fē) [″ + *rhaphe,* seam, ridge] Suture of a wound of the tongue.

**glossospasm** (glŏs′ō-spăzm) [″ + *spasmos,* spasm] The spasmodic contraction of the muscles of the tongue.

**glossotomy** (glŏ-sŏt′ō-mē) [″ + *tome,* incision] An incision of the tongue.

**glossotrichia** (glŏs″ō-trĭk′ē-ă) [″ + *thrix,* hair] SEE: *tongue, hairy.*

**glossy** Smooth and shining.

**glottic** [Gr. *glottis,* back of tongue] Of or pert. to the tongue or glottis.

**glottis** (glŏt′ĭs) *pl.* **glottises or glottides** [Gr. *glottis,* back of tongue] The sound-producing apparatus of the larynx consisting of the two vocal cords and the intervening space, the rima glottidis. A leaf-shaped lid of fibrocartilage (the epiglottis) protects this opening. SEE: illus.

***edema of the g.*** An accumulation of

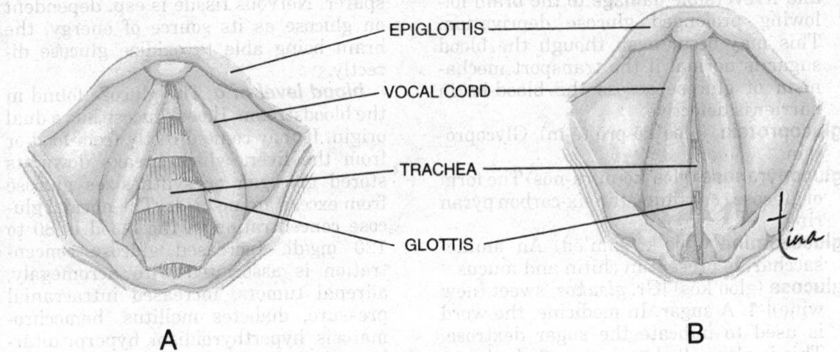


GLOTTIS AND VOCAL CORDS
**(A)** DURING BREATHING, **(B)** DURING SPEAKING

fluid in the tissues lining the larynx. It may result from irritation of the larynx from improper use of the voice, excessive use of tobacco or alcohol, chemical fumes, acute infections, or more serious conditions such as tuberculous or syphilitic laryngitis.

SYMPTOMS: Initially hoarseness, and later complete aphonia, characterize this condition. Other symptoms are extreme dyspnea, at first on inspiration only, but later on expiration also; stridulous respiration; and a barking cough when the epiglottis is involved.

**glottology** (glŏ-tŏl′ō-jē) [″ + *logos,* word, reason] Glossology.

**glove** A protective covering for the hand. In medical care the glove is made of a flexible impervious material that permits full movement of the hand and fingers. Gloves are used to protect both the operative site from contamination with organisms from the health care worker and the health care worker from contamination with pathogens from the patient. These factors are particularly important when the patient has a disease such as hepatitis B or AIDS. SEE: *Universal Precautions Appendix.*

---

Caution: It is not advisable to wash gloves and wear them again while treating another patient.

---

***edema control g.*** An elastic pressure-gradient glove designed to facilitate tissue healing following hand injury.

**gluc-** SEE: *gluco-.*

**glucagon** (gloo′kă-gŏn) A polypeptide hormone secreted by the alpha cells of the pancreas that increases the blood glucose level by stimulating the liver to change stored glycogen to glucose. It also increases the use of fats and excess amino acids for energy production. It is obtained from pork and beef pancreas glands. Parenteral administration of glucagon relaxes the smooth muscle of the stomach, duodenum, small bowel, and colon.

**glucagonoma** (glū″kă-gŏn-ō′mă) A malignant tumor of the alpha cells of the pancreatic islets of Langerhans. The principal signs and symptoms include weight loss, diabetes mellitus, skin rash, glossitis, elevated serum glucagon levels, and anemia. The treatment is surgical.

**gluco-, gluc-** Combining form denoting relationship to sweetness. SEE: *glyco-.*

**glucocerebroside** (gloo″kō-sĕr′ĕ-brō-sīd″) A cerebroside with the carbohydrate glucose contained in the molecule; present in tissues in those with Gaucher's disease.

**glucocorticoid** (gloo″kō-kort′ĭ-koyd) [Gr. *gleukos,* sweet (new wine), + L. *cortex,* + Gr. *eidos,* form, shape] A general classification of adrenal cortical hormones that are primarily active in protecting against stress and in affecting protein and carbohydrate metabolism. The most important glucocorticoid is cortisol (hydrocortisone). SEE: *mineralocorticoid.*

**glucofuranose** (gloo″kō-fū′ră-nōs) The form of glucose containing the furanose ring.

**glucogenesis** (gloo″kō-jĕn′ĕ-sĭs) The formation of glucose from glycogen.

**glucokinase** (gloo″kō-kī′nās) An enzyme in liver cells that in the presence of ATP catalyzes the conversion of glucose to glucose-6-phosphate. This is the first step in glycolysis, or the synthesis of glycogen from excess glucose.

**glucokinetic** (gloo″kō-kī-nĕt′ĭk) Acting to maintain the blood glucose level.

**Glucometer** A battery-operated device used to measure blood glucose from a few drops of blood obtained from the finger.

**gluconeogenesis** (gloo″kō-nē″ō-jĕn′ĕ-sĭs) [″ + *neos,* new, + *genesis,* generation, birth] Glyconeogenesis.

**glucopenia** (gloo″kō-pē′nē-ă) [″ + Gr. *penia,* lack] An abnormally low concentration of blood glucose.

**glucopenic brain injury** Disordered function

and irreversible damage to the brain following prolonged glucose deprivation. This may occur even though the blood sugar is normal if the transport mechanism of glucose across the blood-brain barrier is defective.

**glucoprotein** (gloo″kō-prō′tē-ĭn) Glycoprotein.

**glucopyranose** (gloo″kō-pī′ră-nōs) The form of glucose containing the six-carbon pyran ring.

**glucosamine** (gloo″kō-săm′ēn) An aminosaccharide present in chitin and mucus.

**glucose** (gloo′kōs) [Gr. *gleukos,* sweet (new wine)] **1.** A sugar. In medicine, the word is used to indicate the sugar dextrose. This is also called D-glucose. **2.** An intermediate in carbohydrate metabolism. SEE: *carbohydrate.*

Glucose is the most important carbohydrate in body metabolism. It is formed during digestion from the hydrolysis of disaccharides and polysaccharides, esp. starch. It is absorbed by the small intestine and circulates to the liver by way of the portal vein. In the liver, excess glucose is converted to glycogen (glycogenesis). The concentration of glucose in the blood is approx. 0.1% (100 mg/dl), the amount being maintained at a fairly constant level (80 to 120 mg/dl) through the action of insulin produced by the islets of Langerhans in the pancreas. Failure of the pancreas to produce adequate insulin results in hyperglycemia, in which the blood sugar (glucose) level may rise to 200 mg/dl or higher. When above the renal threshold (about 160 to 180 mg/dl), glucose appears in the urine (glycosuria). This is a symptom of diabetes. Overproduction of insulin or injection of insulin as in insulin shock treatment reduces the glucose level below normal, a condition known as hypoglycemia.

Within most cells, glucose is the primary energy source and is oxidized in cell respiration to carbon dioxide and water to produce energy in the form of adenosine triphosphate (ATP). The stages of cell respiration are glycolysis, which uses enzymes in the cell cytoplasm, and the Krebs cycle and the cytochrome transport system, which take place in the mitochondria. Insulin enables cells to take in glucose for use in energy production. Excess glucose may be converted to glycogen and stored in the liver and muscles; insulin and cortisol facilitate this process. The hormone glycogen (and epinephrine in stress situations) stimulates the liver to change glycogen back to glucose when the blood glucose level decreases. Any further excess glucose is converted to fat and stored in adipose tissue.

When the glucose level is below normal, fat stores are metabolized. Incomplete metabolism of fats leads to the formation of ketone bodies, also a symptom of diabetes. Blood glucose acts as a protein sparer. Nervous tissue is esp. dependent on glucose as its source of energy, the brain being able to oxidize glucose directly.

***blood level of g.*** The glucose found in the bloodstream. Blood glucose has a dual origin. It may come directly from food or from the liver, which breaks down its stored glycogen or synthesizes glucose from excess amino acids. The normal glucose concentration in the blood is 80 to 120 mg/dl. Increased glucose concentration is associated with acromegaly, adrenal tumors, increased intracranial pressure, diabetes mellitus, hemochromatosis, hyperthyroidism, hyperpituitarism, and hyperadrenalism. Decreased concentration is associated with Addison's disease, adenoma or carcinoma of the islets of Langerhans, cretinism, hyperinsulinism, hypopituitarism, hypothyroidism, insulin shock, muscular dystrophy, and myxedema.

***capillary blood g.*** ABBR: CBG. The level of circulating blood glucose as measured by glucometer analysis of a fingerstick sample. A common method of self-monitoring allows diabetic patients to participate actively in their own health management.

***liquid g.*** A thick, syrupy, sweet-tasting liquid obtained from the incomplete hydrolysis of starch, containing D-glucose (dextrose), dextrins, and other carbohydrates. It is used for nutritive purposes and in various pharmaceutical and food preparations.

**glucose-6-phosphate dehydrogenase** ABBR: G6PD. An enzyme that dehydrogenates glucose-6-phosphate to form 6-phospho-D-glucono-δ-lactone. This is the initial step in the pentose phosphate pathway of glucose catabolism.

**glucose-6-phosphate dehydrogenase deficiency** An inherited disorder that is transmitted as an autosomal recessive trait. It is present in the U.S in about 13% of black males and 2% of black females. The enzyme deficiency also occurs in Arabic, Mediterranean, and Asian ethnic groups. The enzyme is essential to maintaining the integrity of red blood cells, thus a deficiency of it causes nonimmune hemolytic anemia. There are many variants of the enzyme and great variation in severity of the disease. Some individuals do not have clinical symptoms until they are exposed to certain drugs such as antimalarials, antipyretics, sulfonamides, or to fava beans, or when they contract an infectious disease. In others the condition is present at birth. When present at birth, anemia, hepatomegaly, hypoglycemia, and interference with growth are present. In those who have the deficiency but are not affected until exposed to certain drugs or infections, hemolytic anemia and jaundice occur.

DIAGNOSIS: The clinical condition may

not be diagnostic, but laboratory tests for evidence of the enzyme deficiency are available.

TREATMENT: The only treatment is avoidance of drugs known to cause hemolysis and avoidance of fava beans if the individual is known to be sensitive to them.

**glucose polymer** A glucose saccharide mixture of 3% glucose, 7% maltose, 5% maltotriose, and 85% polysaccharides of 4 to 15 glucose units. Because it is virtually tasteless, its use as the source of glucose in the glucose tolerance test has improved patient acceptance. Trade name is Polycose. SEE: *glucose tolerance test.*

**glucose tolerance test** A test performed by giving a certain amount of glucose to a patient orally or intravenously. Blood samples are drawn at specified intervals, and the blood glucose level is measured in each sample. This determines the patient's ability to metabolize glucose. In suspected cases of hyperinsulinism, the test is prolonged to 6 hr, with blood samples drawn hourly and analyzed for sugar content. If the blood glucose level continues to drop after 3 hr, falling below 80 mg/dl, hyperinsulinism is indicated, although other conditions (e.g., hypoglycemia) may also produce a blood glucose deficiency.

Sometimes oral cortisone is administered 8½ hr and 2½ hr before giving the glucose. This is called the oral cortisone glucose tolerance test. The cortisone increases the demand for insulin and thus reveals any deficiency in insulin response. SEE: *glucose polymer.*

**glucosidase** (gloo-kō′sĭ-dās) An enzyme that catalyzes the hydrolysis of a glucoside.

**glucoside** (gloo′kō-sīd) A glycoside that on hydrolysis yields a sugar, glucose, and one or two additional products. Glucosides are numerous and widely distributed in plants. Many glucosides have medicinal properties (e.g., digitalin and strophanthin, present in digitalis and strophanthus, respectively, which have a specific effect on the heart). SEE: *glycoside.*

**glucosulfone sodium** (gloo″kō-sŭl′fōn) A derivative of dapsone used to treat leprosy.

**glucosuria** (gloo″kō-sū′rē-ă) [″ + *ouron,* urine] Glycosuria.

**glucuronic acid** SEE: under *acid.*

**β-glucuronidase** (gloo″kū-rŏn′ĭ-dās) An enzyme that splits glycosidic linkages in glucuronides. It is involved in cell division.

**glucuronide** (gloo-kū′rŏn-īd) The combination of glucuronic acid with phenol, alcohol, or any acid containing the carboxyl, COOH, group.

**glucuronyl transferase** An enzyme that converts unconjugated or indirect bilirubin to conjugated or direct bilirubin.

**glue-sniffing** The inhalation of vapor from types of glue or solvents that contain toxic chemicals such as benzene, toluene, or xylene. This produces an altered state of consciousness and occasionally death.

**Gluge's corpuscles** (gloo′gēz) [Gottlieb Gluge, Ger. pathologist, 1812–1898] Granular cells containing fat droplets, usually found in degenerating nervous tissue.

**glutamate** (gloo′tă-māt) A salt of glutamic acid.

**glutamic acid** (gloo-tăm′ĭk) [L. *gluten,* glue, + *am*monium] $COOH \cdot (CH_2)_2 \cdot CH(NH_2) \cdot COOH$. An amino acid formed in protein hydrolysis and an excitatory neurotransmitter in the central nervous system.

**glutamic-oxaloacetic transaminase** ABBR: GOT. The enzyme involved in the transfer of the amino group of glutamic acid to oxaloacetic acid to form α-ketoglutaric acid and aspartic acid. When cells of either the liver or the heart are injured, this enzyme's blood level is increased, thus providing a chemical indicator of hepatitis or myocardial tissue damage. SYN: *aspartate aminotransferase.*

**glutamic-pyruvic transaminase** ABBR: GPT. The enzyme involved in the transfer of the amino group of glutamic acid to pyruvic acid to form α-ketoglutaric acid and L-alanine. When cells of the liver are injured, this enzyme's blood level is increased, thus providing a chemical indicator of hepatitis. SYN: *alanine aminotransferase.*

**glutaminase** (gloo-tăm′ĭ-nās) An enzyme that catalyzes the breakdown of glutamine into glutamic acid and ammonia.

**glutamine** (gloo′tă-mĭn, -mēn″) A nonessential amino acid thought to play a major role in maintaining the integrity of the gastrointestinal mucosa, esp. during the hypermetabolic phase of the stress response. By enhancing cellular proliferation, it may reduce the incidence of bacterial translocation from the gut and improve absorption from the mucosa.

**γ-glutamyl transpeptidase** A tissue enzyme that is elevated in patients with many conditions involving hepatic damage, including that induced by alcohol; in patients with renal disease, pancreatitis, diabetes mellitus, coronary artery disease, or carcinoma of the prostate; and in individuals taking phenytoin and barbiturates.

**glutaral** (gloo′tă-răl) A solution of glutaraldehyde in sterile water.

**glutaraldehyde** (gloo″tă-răl′dĕ-hīd) **1.** A sterilizing agent effective against all microorganisms including viruses and spores. **2.** An excellent primary fixative agent for electron microscopy, usually followed by osmium in the preparation of material for transmission electron microscopy.

**glutathione** (gloo-tă-thī′ōn) [″ + Gr. *theion,* sulfur] A tripeptide of glutamic acid, cysteine, and glycine. Found in small quantities in active animal tissues, it takes up and gives off hydrogen and is fundamentally important in cellular respiration.

***reduced g.*** The form of glutaraldehyde present in red blood cells. It detoxifies hydrogen peroxide that forms either spontaneously or after drug administration, thus protecting red cells from injury due to this substance.

**gluteal** (gloo'tē-ăl) [Gr. *gloutos,* buttock] Pert. to the buttocks.

**gluten** [L., glue] Vegetable albumin, a protein that can be prepared from wheat and other grain.

**gluten-free diet** Elimination of gluten from the diet by avoiding all products containing wheat, rye, oats, or barley. Because gluten is present in many foods containing thickened sauces, the diet must be discussed with a dietitian.

**gluten-induced enteropathy** Nontropical sprue.

**glutethimide** (gloo-tĕth'ĭ-mīd) A hypnotic drug. Trade name is Doriden.

**glutinous** (gloo'tĭn-ŭs) [L. *glutinosus,* glue] Adhesive; sticky.

**glutitis** [Gr. *gloutos,* buttock, + *itis,* inflammation] An inflammation of the muscles of the buttocks.

**glyc-** SEE: *glyco-.*

**glycan** Polysaccharide.

**glycase** (glī'kās) [Gr. *glykys,* sweet] The enzyme that converts maltose into dextrose. SEE: *enzyme.*

**glycemia** (glī-sē'mē-ă) [" + *haima,* blood] Sugar or glucose in the blood.

**DL-glyceraldehyde** (glĭs"ĕr-ăl'dĕ-hīd) An aldose, $CHOCH(OH)CH_2OH$, produced by the metabolism of fructose in the liver.

**glyceride** (glĭs'ĕr-īd) [Gr. *glykys,* sweet] An ester of glycerin compounded with an acid.

**glycerin** (glĭs'ĕr-ĭn) $C_3H_8O_3$. A trihydric alcohol, trihydroxy-propane, present in chemical combination in all fats. It is a syrupy colorless liquid, soluble in all proportions in water and alcohol. It is made commercially by the hydrolysis of fats, esp. during the manufacture of soap, and is used extensively as a solvent, a preservative, and an emollient in various skin diseases. Given orally, it reduces intracranial pressure and, preoperatively, reduces intraocular pressure in glaucoma. SYN: *glycerol.*

**glycerol** (glĭs'ĕr-ŏl) [Gr. *glykys,* sweet] Glycerin.

**glyceryl** (glĭs'ĕr-ĭl) The trivalent radical $C_3H_5$ of glycerol.

***g. monostearate*** An emulsifying agent used in preparing creams and ointments.

***g. triacetate*** The previously used name for triacetin.

***g. trinitrate*** Nitroglycerin; a valuable medicine used to treat an angina pectoris attack or to prevent one if given before exercise.

NOTE: Tablets should be stored in tightly sealed, dark containers to prevent loss of potency.

**glycine** (glī'sēn, -sĭn) [Gr. *glykys,* sweet] $C_2H_5NO_2$. A nonessential amino acid. SYN: *aminoacetic acid.*

**glyco-, glyc-** (glī-kō) [Gr. *glykys,* sweet] Combining form indicating a relationship to sugars or the presence of glycerol or a similar substance. SEE: *gluco-.*

**glycocalyx** (glī"kō-kăl'ĭks) A thin layer of glycoprotein and oligosaccharides on the outer surface of cell membranes that contributes to cell adhesion and forms antigens involved in the recognition of "self."

**glycocholate** (glī"kō-kŏl'āt) A salt of glycocholic acid.

**glycocholic acid** SEE: *acid, glycocholic.*

**glycoclastic** (glī"kō-klăs'tĭk) [" + *klan,* to break] Pert. to the hydrolysis and digestion of sugars.

**glycogen** (glī'kŏ-jĕn) [" + *gennan,* to produce] $(C_6H_{10}O_5)\,x$. A polysaccharide commonly called animal starch, a whitish powder that can be prepared from mammalian liver and muscle and other animal tissues. Formation of glycogen from carbohydrate sources is called glycogenesis; from noncarbohydrate sources, glyconeogenesis. The conversion of glycogen to glucose is called glycogenolysis. SEE: *glycogen storage disease; glyconeogenesis.*

Glycogen is the form in which excess carbohydrate is stored in the liver and muscles; the hormones insulin and cortisol facilitate this process. When blood glucose decreases, the liver converts glucagon, or in stress situations, epinephrine. In cells, glucose is oxidized to carbon dioxide and water with the release of energy in the forms of ATP and heat. In muscle cells under anaerobic conditions, glucose is metabolized only to lactic acid, and oxygen is needed to convert lactic acid back to glucose, primarily in the liver.

**glycogenase** (glī-kō'jĕn-ās) A liver enzyme that hydrolyzes glycogen and whose end product is dextrose.

**glycogenesis** (glī"kō-jĕn'ĕ-sĭs) [" + *genesis,* generation, birth] The formation of glycogen from glucose. SEE: *glyconeogenesis.*

**glycogenetic** Pert. to the formation of glycogen.

**glycogenic** Rel. to glycogen.

**glycogenolysis** (glī"kō-jĕn-ŏl'ĭ-sĭs) [" + *gennan,* to produce, + *lysis,* dissolution] Conversion of glycogen into glucose in the liver and muscles.

**glycogenolytic** (glī"kō-jĕn"ō-lĭt'ĭk) [" + " + *lysis,* dissolution] Pert. to the hydrolysis of glycogen.

**glycogenosis** (glī"kō-jĕn-ō'sĭs) [" + " + *osis,* condition] A disorder associated with an abnormal accumulation of normal or abnormal forms of glycogen in tissue.

**glycogen storage disease** Any one of several heritable diseases characterized by the abnormal storage and accumulation of glycogen in the tissues, esp. in the liver. These diseases are grouped into various types according to the enzyme deficiency responsible.

***phosphorylase b kinase deficiency g.s.d.*** A form of glycogen storage disease caused by an x-linked deficiency of the kinase that activates phosphorylase. Previously called type VIa, VIII, or IX.

***g.s.d. type Ia*** A form of glycogen storage disease with onset usually in the first year of life. This autosomal recessive genetic disorder is due to a glucose-6-phosphatase deficiency. SYN: *von Gierke's disease.*

***g.s.d. type Ib*** A form of glycogen storage disease similar to type Ia but occurring at only one tenth its frequency. The disorder is due to a deficiency of glucose-6-phosphatase microsomal translocase.

***g.s.d. type II*** A form of glycogen storage disease caused by a deficiency of lysosomal $\alpha$-glucosidase.

***g.s.d. type III*** A form of glycogen storage disease caused by a deficiency of two debranching enzymes in liver and muscle tissues.

***g.s.d. type IV*** A form of glycogen storage disease caused by a branching enzyme deficiency. Liver and spleen enlargement and hepatic failure occur, followed by death. SYN: *Andersen's disease.*

***g.s.d. type V*** A form of glycogen storage disease caused by a muscle phosphorylase deficiency. SYN: *McArdle's disease.*

***g.s.d. type VI*** A form of glycogen storage disease caused by a deficiency of liver phosphorylase and characterized by growth retardation, hepatomegaly, hypoglycemia, and acidosis.

***g.s.d. type VII*** A form of glycogen storage disease caused by a deficiency of muscle phosphofructokinase and characterized by muscular weakness and cramping following exercise.

**glycogeusia** (glī″kō-jū′sē-ă) [Gr. *glykys,* sweet, + *geusis,* taste] A sweet taste.

**glycol** (glī′kōl, -kŏl) [″ + *alcohol*] Any one of the dihydric alcohols related to ethylene glycol, $C_2H_6O_2$.

**glycolipid(e)** (glī″kō-lĭp′ĭd) [″ + *lipos,* fat] A compound of fatty acids with a carbohydrate, containing nitrogen but not phosphoric acid. It is found in the myelin sheath of nerves.

**glycolysis** (glī-kŏl′ĭ-sĭs) [″ + *lysis,* dissolution] **1.** The series of reactions that convert a molecule of glucose into two molecules of pyruvic acid. **2.** The first stage of the cell respiration of a molecule of glucose, releasing a small amount of energy in the form of ATP.

**glycolytic** Pert. to glucose hydrolysis.

**glycometabolic** (glī″kō-mĕt-ă-bŏl′ĭk) [″ + *metabole,* change] Pert. to glucose metabolism.

**glycometabolism** (glī″kō-mĕ-tăb′ŏ-lĭzm) Use of glucose by the body. SEE: *metabolism.*

**glyconeogenesis** (glī″kō-nē″ŏ-jĕn′ĕ-sĭs) [″ + *neos,* new, + *genesis,* generation, birth] The formation of glycogen from noncarbohydrates such as fat or amino acids from protein. It occurs in the liver under such conditions as low carbohydrate intake or starvation. SYN: *gluconeogenesis.*

**glyconucleoprotein** (glī″kō-nū″klē-ō-prō′tē-ĭn) [″ + L. *nucleus,* kernel, + Gr. *protos,* first] A nucleoprotein so named to emphasize the presence of glucose units in the substance.

**glycopexic** (glī″kō-pĕks′ĭk) [″ + *pexis,* fixation] Pert. to the fixing or storing of glucose.

**glycopexis** (glī″kō-pĕk′sĭs) The storage of glycogen in the liver.

**glycophorin** (glī″kō-fō′rĭn) A glycoprotein that spans the bilipid layer of the red blood cell membrane. The outside end of this complex substance contains blood group antigens and sites to which some viruses attach. This protein provides the conduit through which anions pass in and out of the red blood cell.

**glycopolyuria** (glī″kō-pŏl″ē-ū′rē-ă) [″ + *polys,* much, + *ouron,* urine] Diabetes mellitus with moderately increased glucose but greatly increased uric acid in the urine.

**glycoprival, glycoprivous** (glī″kō-prī′văl, -vŭs) [″ + L. *privus,* deprived of] Lacking in or without carbohydrates.

**glycoprotein** (glī″kō-prō′tē-ĭn) [″ + *protos,* first] A compound consisting of a carbohydrate and protein. SYN: *glucoprotein.*

**glycoptyalism** (glī″kō-tī′ăl-ĭzm) [″ + *ptyalon,* saliva, + *-ismos,* condition] The excretion of glucose in the saliva. SYN: *melitoptyalism.*

**glycopyrrolate** (glī″kō-pĭr′rō-lāt) An anticholinergic drug. Trade name is Robinul.

**glycorrhachia** (glī-kō-rā′kē-ă) [″ + *rhachis,* spine] Glucose in the cerebrospinal fluid.

**glycosecretory** (glī″kō-sē-krē′tō-rē) [″ + L. *secretus,* separate] Pert. to or determining the formation of glycogen.

**glycosialia** (glī″kō-sī-ăl′ē-ă) [″ + *sialon,* saliva] Glucose in the saliva.

**glycosialorrhea** (glī″kō-sī″ăl-ō-rē′ă) [″ + ″ + *rhoia,* flow] Excessive secretion of saliva containing glucose.

**glycoside** A substance derived from plants that, on hydrolysis, yields a sugar and one or more additional products. Depending on the sugar formed, glycosides are designated glucosides or galactosides. SEE: *glucoside.*

**glycosphingolipids** (glī″kō-sfĭng″ō-lĭp′ĭds) A group of carbohydrate-containing fatty acid derivatives of ceramide. Three classes of these lipids are cerebrosides, gangliosides, and ceramide oligosaccharides. When the enzymes essential to the metabolism of these compounds are absent, the glycosphingolipids accumulate, particularly in the nervous system. Death is the usual outcome.

**glycostatic** (glī″kō-stăt′ĭk) [Gr. *glykys,* sweet, + *statikos,* standing] Acting to maintain the level of glucose in the body.

**glycosuria** (glī″kō-sū′rē-ă) [″ + *ouron,* urine] An abnormal amount of glucose in the urine. Traces of sugar, particularly glucose, may occur in normal urine but are not detected by ordinary qualitative methods. The presence of a reducing sugar found during routine urinalysis is suggestive of diabetes mellitus. It is found when the blood glucose level exceeds the renal threshold (about 170 mg/dl of blood). The fasting level of blood glucose is usually between 80 and 120 mg/dl of blood. SYN: *glucosuria.*

Glycosuria may result from pancreatic (insulin) insufficiency; disorders of the endocrine glands, esp. the hypophysis, adrenals, thyroid, or ovaries; excessive carbohydrate intake; excessive glycogenolysis; or reduction of the renal threshold.

***alimentary g.*** Glycosuria following ingestion of large amounts of starches or sugars.

***diabetic g.*** Glycosuria resulting from hyposecretion of insulin.

***emotional g.*** Glycosuria resulting from emotional states such as worry or anxiety.

***phloridzin g.*** Glycosuria resulting from the injection of phloridzin, which reduces the renal threshold for glucose.

***pituitary g.*** Glycosuria caused by dysfunction of the anterior pituitary.

***renal g.*** Glycosuria occurring when glucose is persistent and not accompanied by hyperglycemia and when the renal threshold for glucose is decreased.

**glycosylated hemoglobin** Hemoglobin $A_{1c}$.

**glycuronuria** (glĭ-kū″rō-nū′rē-ă) Glucuronic acid in the urine.

**glycyltryptophan** (glĭs″ĭl-trĭp′tō-făn) A dipeptide of glycine and tryptophan.

**glycyrrhiza** (glĭs-ĭ-rī′ză) [″ + *rhiza,* root] The dried root of *Glycyrrhiza glabra,* known commercially as Spanish licorice, used as an ingredient of glycyrrhiza fluidextract and glycyrrhiza syrup, both of which are used as flavoring agents in compounding medicine. This substance has a weak aldosterone-like effect. SEE: *licorice.*

**glyoxalase** (glē-ōk′să-lās) An enzyme that catalyzes the conversion of methylglyoxal to lactic acid by the addition of water.

**glyoxylic acid** An acid produced by the action of glycine oxidase on glycine or sarcosine.

**Glysennid** Trade name for sennosides A and B.

**GML** *glabellomeatal line.*

**gnashing** (năsh′ing) Grinding, as of the teeth. SEE: *bruxism.*

**gnat** (năt) Any of a number of small insects belonging to the order Diptera, suborder Orthorrhapha, including black flies, midges, and sandflies. It applies generally to insects smaller than mosquitoes.

***buffalo g.*** A small dipterous insect belonging to the genus *Simulium.*

**gnath-** SEE: *gnatho-.*

**gnathalgia** (năth-ăl′jē-ă) [Gr. *gnathos,* jaw, + *algos,* pain] Pain in the jaw. SYN: *gnathodynia.*

**gnathic** (năth′ĭk) [Gr. *gnathos,* jaw] Pert. to an alveolar process or to the jaw.

**gnathion** (năth′ē-ŏn) The lowest point of the middle line of the lower jaw; a craniometric point.

**gnathitis** (năth-ī′tĭs) [″ + *itis,* inflammation] Inflammation of the jaw or adjacent soft parts.

**gnatho-, gnath-** (năth′ō) [Gr. *gnathos,* jaw] Combining form meaning *jaw* or *cheek.*

**gnathocephalus** (năth″ō-sĕf′ă-lŭs) [″ + *kephale,* head] A malformed fetus in which the head consists principally of the jaws.

**gnathodynamometer** (năth″ō-dī″nă-mŏm′ĕ-tĕr) [″ + *dynamis,* power, + *metron,* measure] A device for measuring biting force. SYN: *occlusometer.*

**gnathodynia** (năth″ō-dĭn′ē-ă) [″ + *odyne,* pain] Gnathalgia.

**gnathoplasty** (năth′ō-plăs″tē) [″ + *plassein,* to form] Reparative surgery of the jaws or cheek.

**gnathoschisis** (năth-ŏs′kĭ-sĭs) [″ + *schizein,* to split] A congenital jaw cleft.

**Gnathostoma** (năth-ŏs′tō-mă) [″ + *stoma,* mouth] A genus of nematode worms that infest the stomach walls of domestic and wild animals. They occasionally infest humans.

**gnathostomiasis** (năth″ō-stō-mī′ă-sĭs) A form of visceral larva migrans infection of human tissues caused by the nematode parasite of dogs and cats, *Gnathostomiasis spinigerum.* Acquisition is by ingestion of undercooked fish and poultry containing the larvae. The parasite migrates through various body tissues and causes a transient inflammatory response and possibly abscess formation. If the brain is invaded, eosinophilic meningoencephalitis may develop and can be fatal. Travelers to areas such as the Orient where the condition is endemic are advised to avoid eating raw fish or undercooked fish or poultry.

TREATMENT: Therapy consists of surgical removal of lesions and administration of albendazole.

**gnosia** (nō′sē-ă) [Gr. *gnosis,* knowledge] The perceptive faculty of recognizing persons, things, and forms.

**gnotobiotics** (nō″tō-bī-ŏt′ĭks) [Gr. *gnotos,* known, + *bios,* life] The study of animals that have been raised in germ-controlled or germ-free surroundings.

**Gn-RH** *gonadotropin-releasing hormone.*

**goal** The desired outcome of actions to alter status or behavior. SEE: *nursing goal.*

**goblet cell** A type of secretory cell or unicellular gland found in the epithelium of the intestinal and respiratory tracts, which secretes mucus. Mucin droplets accumulate in the distal end of the cell, forming a large ovoid mass that swells the cell and distorts its shape. The free surface of the cell finally ruptures and liberates the mucus. SYN: *chalice cell; mucous cell.* SEE: *cell; gland; mucus; secretion.*

**goggle-eyed** Exophthalmic.

**goiter** (goy′tĕr) [L. *guttur,* throat] An enlargement of the thyroid gland, possibly due to a lack of iodine in the diet, thyroiditis, inflammation from infection, tumors, or hyperfunction or hypofunction of the thyroid gland. SYN: *struma.*

***aberrant g.*** A supernumerary goiter.

***acute g.*** A goiter that grows rapidly.

***adenomatous g.*** A goiter caused by the growth of an encapsulated adenoma.

***colloid g.*** A goiter in which there is a great increase of the follicular contents.

***congenital g.*** A goiter present at birth.

***cystic g.*** A goiter in which a cyst or cysts are formed, possibly resulting from the degeneration of tissue or liquefaction within an adenoma.

***diffuse g.*** A goiter in which the thyroid tissue is diffuse, in contrast to its nodular form as in adenomatous goiter.

***diving g.*** A movable goiter, located either below or above the sternal notch.

***endemic g.*** Goiter development in certain geographic localities, esp. where the iodine content in food and water is deficient. Goiters are more prevalent in fresh water and lake areas and less so on the sea coast, owing to the lack of iodine in fresh water. The treatment consists of iodine taken orally or in iodized salt.

***exophthalmic g.*** Goiter with exophthalmos. SEE: *Graves' disease.*

***fibrous g.*** A goiter with a hyperplastic capsule.

***intrathoracic g.*** A goiter in which a portion of the thyroid tissue lies within the thoracic cavity.

***lingual g.*** A hypertrophied mass forming a tumor at the posterior portion of the dorsum of the tongue.

***nodular g.*** A goiter that contains nodules.

***parenchymatous g.*** A usually diffuse goiter characterized by multiplication of cells lining the follicles or alveoli. Colloid is usually reduced and the follicular cavities assume various sizes and are often obliterated by the infoldings of their walls. Fibrous tissue may increase markedly. The iodine content of the gland is low.

***perivascular g.*** A goiter surrounding a large blood vessel.

***retrovascular g.*** A goiter that develops behind a large blood vessel.

***simple g.*** A goiter unaccompanied by constitutional symptoms.

***substernal g.*** An enlargement of the lower part of the thyroid isthmus.

***suffocative g.*** A goiter that causes shortness of breath owing to pressure.

***toxic g.*** An exophthalmic goiter or a goiter in which there is an excessive production of the thyroid hormone. SEE: *exophthalmic g.*

***vascular g.*** A goiter due to distention of the blood vessels of the thyroid gland.

**goitrogen** (goy′trō-jĕn) [L. *guttur,* throat, + *gennan,* to produce] A substance that causes goiters, occurring naturally in certain foods, including turnips, rutabagas, and cabbages.

**gold** SYMB: Au (from L. *aurum,* gold). A yellow metallic element; atomic weight 196.967; atomic number 79; specific gravity 19.32. Its salts have been used to treat early rheumatoid arthritis not adequately controlled by other anti-inflammatory agents or conservative therapy. Injection of radioactive gold, $^{198}$Au, is used to treat certain types of cancer and to help outline certain organs, as in liver scanning. SEE: *scanning.*

***g. alloy*** An alloy of gold with copper, silver, platinum, or other metals added for strength or hardness. Pure gold is rated 24 carats. A gold alloy that contains other metals is less than 24 carats. Thus, 18 parts of gold mixed with 6 parts of another metal would be rated as 18-carat gold.

***g. Au 198 injection*** A sterile colloidal solution of radioactive gold ($^{198}$Au) used as an antineoplastic.

***dental casting g. alloy*** A hard or extra-hard alloy used principally for dental crowns, inlays, clasps, splints, and orthodontic and prosthetic appliances.

***g. sodium thiomalate*** A water-soluble gold preparation used intramuscularly to treat rheumatoid arthritis with active joint inflammation. Trade name is Myochrysine.

**goldbeater's skin** A strong, thin membrane prepared from the cecum of the ox and previously used as a surgical dressing.

**Goldblatt kidney** [Harry Goldblatt, U.S. physician, 1891–1977] The kidney of a dog that has been deprived of part of its blood supply to induce hypertension experimentally. This condition may occur in humans as a result of vascular disease.

**gold standard** In medical care and experimental medicine, a therapeutic action, drug, or procedure that is the best available and with which other therapeutic actions, drugs, or procedures are compared to determine their efficacy.

**Golgi apparatus** (gŏl′jē) [Camillo Golgi, It. pathologist, 1843–1926] A lamellar membranous structure near the nucleus of almost all cells, best viewed by electron microscopy. It contains curved parallel series of flattened saccules that are often expanded at their ends. In secretory cells, the apparatus concentrates and packages the secretory product. Its function in other cells, although apparently important, is poorly understood.

**Golgi cell, Golgi neuron** A multipolar nerve cell in the cerebral cortex and posterior horns of the spinal cord. Type I possesses long axons; type II, short axons.

**Golgi tendon organ** ABBR: GTO. A spindle-shaped structure at junction of a muscle and a tendon. This structure is thought to function as a feedback system that senses muscle tension through tendon stretch, inhibits muscle contraction of the agonist, and facilitates contraction of the antagonistic muscle. The purpose of this mechanism, known as autogenic facilitation, is to prevent overuse and damage to the muscle and corresponding joint.

**Goll's tract** (gŏlz) [Friedrich Goll, Swiss anatomist, 1829–1903] The tract in the posterior white column of the spinal cord. SYN: *fasciculus gracilis.*

**Golytely** Trade name for polyethylene glycol electrolyte for gastrointestinal lavage solution.

**gomphosis** (gŏm-fō'sĭs) [Gr., bolting together] A conical process fitting into a socket in an immovable joint (e.g., a tooth in its bony socket in the alveolus).

**gon-** SEE: *gono-*.

**gonad** (gō'năd, gŏn'ăd) [Gr. *gone,* seed] **1.** The embryonic sex gland before differentiation into definitive testis or ovary. **2.** A generic term referring to the female sex glands, or ovaries, and the male sex glands, or testes. Each forms the cells necessary for human reproduction: spermatozoa from the testes, ova from the ovaries. SEE: *estrogen; ovary; testicle; testosterone.*

INTERNAL SECRETIONS: *Female:* The vesicular follicles of the ovaries secrete estrogen, which is important in regulating and controlling female reproductive function including the development of secondary sex characteristics. The corpus luteum produces progesterone, which helps to prepare the lining of the uterus (endometrium) to receive and assist in the implantation of the fertilized ovum. *Male:* The interstitial cells of the testes secrete the androgen testosterone, which stimulates metabolism, increases muscular strength, and influences the development of secondary sex characteristics.

Hormones from both sexes have been isolated and standardized and are used to treat conditions arising from an insufficiency of these hormones.

**gonadal** (gō'năd-ăl) Pert. to a gonad.

**gonadal dysgenesis** Turner's syndrome.

**gonadectomy** (gŏn-ă-dĕk'tō-mē) [Gr. *gonos,* genitals, + *ektome,* excision] The excision of a testis or ovary.

**gonadopathy** (gŏn"ă-dŏp'ă-thē) [" + *pathos,* disease, suffering] Any disease of the sexual glands.

**gonadotrophic, gonadotropic** (gŏn"ă-dō-trŏf'ĭk) [" + *trophe,* nourishment] Rel. to stimulation of the gonads.

**gonadotrophic hormone** Gonadotropin.

**gonadotropin** (gŏn"ă-dō-trō'pĭn) A gonad-stimulating hormone.

***anterior pituitary g.*** One of several hormones produced by the anterior lobe of the hypophysis, such as the follicle-stimulating hormone and luteinizing hormone in women and the interstitial cell–stimulating hormone in men.

***g.-releasing hormone*** ABBR: GnRH. The hormone produced in the hypothalamus that causes the pituitary to release the gonadotrophic substances luteinizing hormone and follicle-stimulating hormone. This hormone is used in treating endometriosis.

***human chorionic g.*** ABBR: hCG. A hormone, secreted in early pregnancy by the trophoblasts of the fertilized ovum, that maintains the corpus luteum during early pregnancy, stimulating it to secrete both estrogen and progesterone. Laboratory tests for hCG in maternal blood or urine are used as pregnancy tests and in follow-up assessments after treatment for hydatid mole and choriocarcinoma. SYN: *anterior pituitary hormone.*

**gonaduct** (gŏn'ă-dŭkt) [" + L. *ductus,* canal] The seminal duct or the oviduct.

**gonangiectomy** (gŏn"ăn-jē-ĕk'tō-mē) [Gr. *gone,* seed, + *angeion,* vessel, + *ektome,* excision] Vasectomy.

**gonarthritis** (gŏn"ăr-thrī'tĭs) [Gr. *gony,* knee, + *arthron,* joint, + *itis,* inflammation] Inflammation of the knee joint.

**gonarthromeningitis** (gŏn-ăr"thrō-mĕn-ĭn-jī'tĭs) [" + " + *meninx,* membrane, + *itis,* inflammation] Synovitis of the knee joint.

**gonarthrotomy** (gŏn"ăr-thrŏt'ō-mē) [" + " + *tome,* incision] Incision of the knee joint.

**gonatocele** (gŏn-ăt'ō-sēl) [" + *kele,* tumor, swelling] A tumor of the knee.

**gonecyst, gonecystis** (gŏn'ē-sĭst, gŏn-ē-sĭs'tĭs) [Gr. *gone,* seed, + *kystis,* a bladder] A seminal vesicle.

**gonecystitis** (gŏn"ĕ-sĭs-tī'tĭs) [" + " + *itis,* inflammation] Inflammation of the seminal vesicles.

**gonecystolith** (gŏn"ĕ-sĭs'tō-lĭth) [" + " + *lithos,* stone] A concretion or calculus in a seminal vesicle.

**Gongylonema** (gŏn"jĭ-lō-nē'mă) [Gr. *gongylos,* round, + *nema,* thread] A genus of nematode worms belonging to the suborder Spirurata, usually parasitic in the wall of the esophagus and stomach of domestic animals. Occasionally, they are parasitic in humans. *G. pulchrum* is the species most frequently involved.

**goniometer** (gō"nē-ŏm'ĕ-ter) [Gr. *gonia,* angle, + *metron,* measure] An apparatus to measure joint movements and angles. Various sizes and types of goniometers are available, including finger goniometers, bubble goniometers, gravity goniometers, and recording electrogoniometers.

**gonion** (gō'nē-ŏn) [Gr. *gonia,* angle] The point of the angle of the mandible or lower jaw.

**goniopuncture** (gō"nē-ō-pŭnk'tūr) A surgical procedure for allowing aqueous humor to drain from the eye, used in treating glaucoma.

**gonioscope** (gō'nē-ō-skōp) [" + *skopein,* to examine] An instrument for inspecting the angle of the anterior chamber of the eye and for determining ocular motility and rotation.

**goniosynechia** (gō′nē-ō-sĭ-nĕk′ē-ă) Adhesion of the iris to the cornea of the eye.

**goniotomy** (gō″nē-ŏt′ō-mē) [″ + *tome,* incision] A surgical procedure for removing obstructions to the free flow of aqueous humor into the canal of Schlemm of the eye.

**gono-, gon-** (gŏn′ō) [Gr. *gonos,* genitals] Combining form meaning *generation, genitals, offspring, semen.*

**gonococcal** (gŏn″ō-kŏk′ăl) [″ + *kokkos,* berry] Rel. to or caused by gonococci.

**gonococcal conjunctivitis** SEE: *conjunctivitis, gonorrheal.*

**gonococcemia** (gŏn″ō-kŏk-sē′mē-ă) [″ + ″ + *haima,* blood] Gonococci in the blood; gonococcal septicemia.

**gonococci** (gŏn″ō-kŏk′ sī) Pl. of gonococcus.

**gonococcic** (gŏn″ō-kŏk′sĭk) [″ + *kokkos,* berry] Pert. to the gonococcus.

**gonococcic smear** A smear using Gram's method and methylene blue. Gonococci, which appear in pairs and tetrads, are gram-negative and intracellular.

**gonococcus** (gŏn″ō-kŏk′ŭs) *pl.* **gonococci** [Gr. *gonos,* genitals, + *kokkos,* berry] The organism causing gonorrhea, a member of the species *Neisseria gonorrhoeae.* It is a gram-negative intracellular diplococcus that tends to occur in pairs. This bacterium may be found in or on the genitals and in blood, joints, heart, eyes, urine, feces, and boils. SEE: *gonorrhea.*

**gonocyte** (gŏn′ō-sīt) [″ + *kytos,* cell] The primitive reproductive cell.

**gonorrhea** (gŏn″ō-rē′ă) [″ + *rhoia,* flow] A specific, contagious, catarrhal inflammation of the genital mucous membrane of either sex, caused by infection by the gonococcus, *Neisseria gonorrhoeae.* The disease also may affect other structures of the body such as the heart, conjunctiva, oral mucosa, rectum, or joints. In women, it may involve the urethra, vulva, vulvovaginal glands, vagina, endocervix, Skene's glands, Bartholin's glands, or fallopian tubes. SEE: *safe sex; Nursing Diagnoses Appendix; Universal Precautions Appendix.*

SYMPTOMS: In men, symptoms include a yellow mucopurulent discharge from the penis resulting from inflammation of the urethra, which may become deep-seated and affect the prostate; slow, difficult, painful urination; and sometimes painful induration of the penis.

---

Caution: It was previously thought that gonorrhea in men was always symptomatic. Because this is not true, in suspected cases cultures for gonococci should always be taken. To be certain the patient is cured, the infected sites should be cultured 1 and 2 weeks after completion of treatment.

---

In women, gonorrhea may be asymptomatic, and, even when symptoms are present, they may not cause enough discomfort for the patient to seek medical care. Symptoms include one or more of the following: urethral or vaginal discharge; painful or frequent urination; lower abdominal pain; tenderness in the area of Bartholin's and Skene's glands; and acute pelvic inflammatory disease.

NOTE: In either sex, it is important to obtain results of a serological test for syphilis before starting antibiotic therapy, as penicillin therapy may mask an infection with syphilis. Also, it is important to test all sexual contacts of the patient for presence of gonorrhea and syphilis.

DIAGNOSIS: Gram's stain of the urethral discharge is almost 100% accurate in diagnosing gonorrhea in men. This is not true, however, for women. The material for diagnosis in women should be obtained from multiple sites including the cervix, vaginal vault, and urethra, and by milking Bartholin's and Skene's glands. The material should be inoculated without delay on Thayer-Martin medium. It is important to evaluate the patient for the presence of other sexually transmitted diseases, including syphilis and chlamydia.

PROPHYLAXIS: Prevention of gonorrhea is through use of condoms during sexual activity or avoidance of contact with infected persons. Following contact, penicillin should be administered immediately. All newborn infants should receive one drop of 1% silver nitrate in the conjunctival sac of each eye. If the mother has gonorrhea, both she and the infant should be treated with parenteral penicillin. SEE: *ophthalmia neonatorum.*

TREATMENT: Amoxicillin plus probenicid is the usual treatment, except in cases due to penicillinase-producing strains of *Neisseria gonorrhoeae.* In those individuals, the drug of choice is intramuscular spectinomycin or intramuscular cefoxitin with oral probenecid. Doxycycline or tetracycline must accompany the other drug to cure a concurrent chlamydial infection. Neither of these drugs alone is adequate therapy for gonorrhea; also, spectinomycin is not effective against pharyngeal gonococcal infection. In women, local therapy may be required for eradication of the foci of infection involving such structures as Skene's duct, Bartholin's glands, and the cervix. During pregnancy, combined ceftriaxone and erythromycin therapy is indicated to minimize the risk of teratogenesis. Spectinomycin may be prescribed for women who are allergic to ceftriaxone.

PROGNOSIS: The inflammation may clear up without serious results or may become chronic (involving deeper tissues and producing urethral stricture) or produce complications (prostatitis, epididymitis, orchitis, cystitis, arthritis, and endocarditis). In women, no case of acute gonorrhea should be considered cured until three successive negative smears from the cervix and Bartholin's and Skene's glands are obtained, at least two of which should be examined immediately after a menstrual period.

NURSING IMPLICATIONS: A history of allergies, esp. antibiotic sensitivity, is obtained. Universal precautions are observed.

Antibiotics should be taken as prescribed, and the full course of therapy completed. Moist heat or sitz baths should be taken as directed. The patient should avoid contact with his or her bodily discharges so that the eyes do not become contaminated. The patient should also refrain from sexual intercourse until the disease has been treated, because the infection will continue and can be transmitted until cultures become negative.

The patient's response to therapy is evaluated, and the patient is taught to recognize and report adverse drug reactions. The need for testing for other sexually transmitted diseases is discussed, as well as prevention of future infections and the importance of follow-up testing. All persons with whom the patient has had sexual contact should be tested and receive treatment, even if a culture is negative; and the case and known sexual contacts are reported to the local public health department for appropriate follow-up.

**gonorrheal** Of the nature of or pert. to gonorrhea.

**Gonyaulax** (gŏn″ē-aw′lăks) A genus of dinoflagellate that causes certain shellfish that eat them to become toxic. It is also one of the causes of "red tide" when present in massive numbers in the ocean. This condition has occurred on certain beaches of North America. Shellfish present in such water contain the toxin present in the dinoflagellate.

**gonycampsis** (gŏn″ĭ-kămp′sĭs) [Gr. *gony,* knee, + *kampsis,* bending] An abnormal curvature of the knee.

**gonycrotesis** (gŏn″ĭ-krō-tē′sĭs) [″ + *krotesis,* knocking] Knock-knee.

**gonyectyposis** (gŏn″ē-ĕk-tĭ-pō′sĭs) [″ + *ektyposis,* modeling in relief] Bowleg.

**gonyocele** (gŏn′ē-ō-sēl) [″ + *kele,* swelling] Tuberculous synovitis of the knee.

**gonyoncus** (gŏn″ē-ŏn′kŭs) [″ + *onkos,* tumor] A tumor of the knee.

**Goodell's sign** [William Goodell, U.S. gynecologist, 1829–1894] The softening of the cervix that occurs in pregnancy.

**Goodpasture's syndrome** [Ernest William Goodpasture, U.S. pathologist, 1886–1960] The rare syndrome of progressive glomerulonephritis, hemoptysis, and hemosiderosis. Death is usually due to renal failure.

**Good Samaritan Law** The legal stipulation for protection of those who give first aid in an emergency situation. The necessity for such legislation arose when physicians who assisted in giving emergency care were later accused of malpractice by the victim.

**gooseflesh** Piloerection.

**Gordon's reflex** [Alfred Gordon, U.S. neurologist, 1874–1953] The extension of the great toe on sudden pressure on the deep flexor muscles of the calf of the leg. It is present in pyramidal tract disease. SEE: *Babinski's reflex.*

**gorget** (gor′jĕt) [Fr. *gorge,* throat, because of shape of instrument] An instrument grooved to protect soft tissues from injury as a pointed instrument is inserted in a body cavity.

**goserelin acetate** A synthetic form of luteinizing hormone–releasing hormone. It is used to assist in treating prostate cancer by inhibiting pituitary gonadotropin secretions.

**Gossypium** (gŏ-sĭp′ē-ŭm) [L.] A genus of perennial shrub of the Malvaceae family, widely grown because of the cotton fiber derived from its seed covering. The bark of some species is diuretic, emmenagogic, and oxytocic. SEE: *cotton; gossypol.*

**gossypol** A toxic chemical present in cottonseed, which has been used experimentally as an infertility agent in men.

**gouge** (gowj) An instrument used for cutting away the hard tissue of bone.

**goundou** (goon′doo) [African] Periostitis of the nasal processes of the maxillae caused by prior infection with yaws or syphilis. The nasal bones become quite enlarged, and the orbit may be involved. The appearance of the nose has been characterized colloquially as "big nose" or "dog nose." SEE: *anakré.*

**gout** (gowt) [L. *gutta,* drop] A hereditary metabolic disease caused by hyperuricemia that is a form of acute arthritis and is marked by joint inflammation. Any joint may be affected, but gout usually begins in the knee or foot. SEE: *Nursing Diagnoses Appendix.*

SYMPTOMS: Most hyperuricemic persons are asymptomatic between acute attacks. When an attack of acute gouty arthritis does develop, it usually begins at night with moderate pain that increases in intensity to the point where no body position provides relief. Hypertension, back pain, low-grade fever, and joint inflammation may be present. Tophi may occur on the outer ears, hands, and feet.

ETIOLOGY: Gout is caused by excessive amounts of uric acid in the blood and deposits of urates of sodium in and around the joints. Several different metabolic abnormalities may cause the hyperuricemia. SEE: illus. (Uric Acid Crystals and White Blood Cells in Synovial Fluid).

TREATMENT: Colchicine or nonsteroidal anti-inflammatory agents are used to treat acute gout attacks. Long-term therapy aims at preventing hyperuricemia by

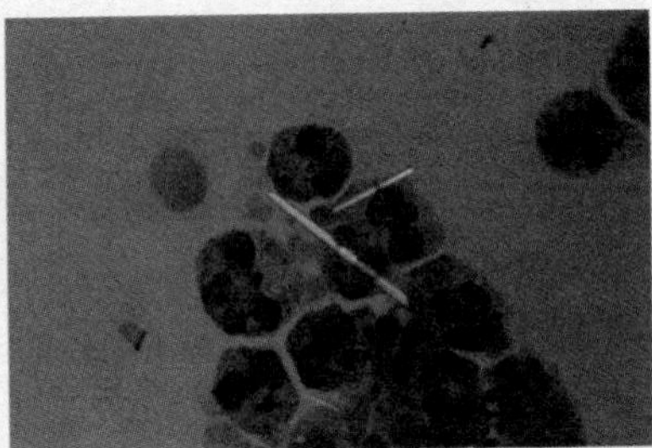

GOUT
URIC ACID CRYSTALS AND WHITE BLOOD CELLS IN SYNOVIAL FLUID (ORIG. MAG. ×500)

giving uricosuric drugs such as probenecid or allopurinol. Patients with gout have a tendency to form uric acid kidney stones. To help prevent this, fluids should be forced at the rate of 3 L/day. Because salicylates interact to interfere with the uricosuric action of either probenecid or allopurinol, they should be avoided. The diet should be well balanced and devoid of purine-rich foods.

NURSING IMPLICATIONS: During the acute phase, bedrest is prescribed for at least the first 24 hr, and affected joints are elevated and immobilized and protected by a bed cradle. Analgesics are administered and compresses (cold or warm) applied for pain relief, and the patient is taught about these measures. Colchicine, probenecid, or other prescribed drugs are administered. A low-purine diet is recommended, and the importance of gradual weight reduction if obesity is a factor is explained. If soft-tissue tophi are present, the patient should wear soft clothing to cover these areas and should use meticulous skin care and sterile dressings to prevent infection of open lesions.

Surgery may be required to excise or drain infected or ulcerated tophi, to correct joint deformities, or improve joint function. Even minor surgery may precipitate gout attacks (usually within 24 to 96 hr after surgery); therefore, the patient should be taught about this risk.

***abarticular g.*** Gout that involves structures other than the joints.

***chronic g.*** A persistent form of gout.

***lead g.*** Goutlike symptoms associated with lead poisoning. SYN: *saturnine g.*

***saturnine g.*** Lead g.

***tophaceous g.*** Gout marked by the development of tophi (deposits of sodium urate) in the joints, in the external ear, and about the fingernails.

**gouty** Of the nature of or rel. to gout.

**Gowers' sign, Gowers' maneuver** [Sir William R. Gowers, Brit. neurologist, 1845–1915] A clinical sign of muscular dystrophy in childhood, evidenced through children's use of their arms to push themselves erect by moving their hands up their legs and then their thighs. This action enables the child to stand from the kneeling position. It is indicative of weakness of the hip and knee extensors.

**Gowers' tract** (gow'ĕrz) A bundle of fibers from the posterior roots of the lateral tract of the spinal cord, reaching the cerebellum by way of the superior peduncle.

**G.P.** *general practitioner.*

**G6PD** *glucose-6-phosphate dehydrogenase.*

**gr** *grain.*

**graafian follicle** (grăf'ē-ăn) [Regnier de Graaf, Dutch physician and anatomist, 1641–1673] A mature vesicular follicle of the ovary. Beginning with puberty and continuing until the menopause, except during pregnancy, a graafian follicle develops at approx. monthly intervals. Each follicle contains a nearly mature ovum (an oocyte) that, on rupture of the follicle, is discharged from the ovary, a process called ovulation. Ovulation occurs usually about the 13th day of the menstrual cycle, dated from the first day of the menstrual period. Within the ruptured graafian follicle, the corpus luteum develops. Both the follicle and the corpus luteum are glands of internal secretion, the former secreting estrogens, and the latter, estrogen and progesterone. SEE: *ovum* for illus.

**grab bar** A bar attached to the wall to assist in climbing stairs or in using the bath, shower, or toilet.

**gracile** (grăs'ĭl) [L. *gracilis,* slender] Slender; slight.

**gracile nucleus** A mass of medullary gray matter terminating the funiculus gracilis.

**gracilis** (grăs'ĭ-lĭs) [L., slender] A long slender muscle on the medial aspect of the thigh.

**Gradenigo's syndrome** (gră-dĕn-ē'gōz) [Giuseppe Gradenigo, It. physician, 1859–1926] A syndrome involving the fifth and sixth cranial nerves. Ear pain, draining middle ear, and paralysis of the sixth cranial nerve are present. The lesion may be caused by inflammation or tumor of the petrous portion of the temporal bone. Appropriate antibiotics should be administered if the condition is due to an infection.

**gradient** (grā'dē-ĕnt) **1.** A slope or grade. **2.** An increase or decrease of varying degrees or the curve that represents such.

***alveolar/arterial g.*** ABBR: A/a gradient. The difference between the calculated oxygen pressure available and the arterial oxygen tension. It measures the efficiency of gas exchange, often expressed as the ratio a : A.

***average g.*** In sensitometry, a measure of the contrast of the film or film-screen system by determination of the slope of the sensitometric curve.

***axial g.*** A gradient of physiological or

metabolic activity exhibited by embryos and many adult animals, the principal one of which follows the main axis of the body, being highest at the anterior end and lowest at the posterior end.

**graduate** (grăd′ū-āt, -ăt) [L. *gradus,* a step] **1.** A vessel marked by lines for measuring liquids. **2.** One who has been awarded an academic or professional degree from a college or university.

**graduated** Marked by a series of lines indicating degrees of measurement, weight, or volume.

**graduated tenotomy** Partial surgical division of a tendon of an eye muscle.

**Graefe's sign** (grā′fēz) [Albrecht von Graefe, Ger. ophthalmologist, 1828–1870] Failure of the upper lid to follow a downward movement of the eyeball when the patient changes his or her vision from looking up to looking down. This is seen in Graves' disease (hyperthyroidism) with exophthalmos.

**graft** (grăft) [L. *graphium,* grafting knife] **1.** Tissue transplanted or implanted in a part of the body to repair a defect. A homograft is a graft of material from another individual of the same species. A heterograft is a graft of material from an individual of another species. **2.** The process of placing tissue from one site to another to repair a defect.

***allogeneic g.*** A graft from a genetically nonidentical donor of the same species as the recipient. SYN: *allograft.*

***autologous g.*** A graft taken from another part of the patient's body.

***avascular g.*** A graft in which vascular infiltration does not occur.

***bone g.*** A piece of bone usually taken from the tibia and inserted elsewhere in the body to replace another osseous structure. Bone storage banks have been established.

***cable g.*** A nerve graft made up of bundles of segments from an unimportant nerve. SYN: *rope g.*

***cadaver g.*** Grafting tissue, including skin, cornea, or bone, obtained from a body immediately after death.

***delayed g.*** A skin graft that is partially elevated and then replaced so that it may be moved later to another site.

***dermal g.*** A split-skin or full-thickness skin graft. The graft will grow hair and have active sweat and sebum glands.

***endovascular g.*** A graft implanted within an existing blood vessel.

***fascia g.*** A graft using fascia, usually removed from the fascia lata, for repairing defects in other tissues.

***fascicular g.*** A nerve graft in which each bundle of nerves is separately sutured.

***free g.*** A graft that is completely separated from its original site and then transferred.

***full-thickness g.*** A graft of the entire layer of skin without the subcutaneous fat.

***gingival g.*** A sliding graft employing the gingival papilla as the graft material.

***heterodermic g.*** A graft taken from a donor of another species.

***heteroplastic g.*** A graft taken from another person.

***heterotopic g.*** SEE: *transplant, heterotopic.*

***homologous g.*** A graft taken from a donor of the same species as the recipient.

***isologous g.*** A graft in which the donor and recipient are genetically identical (i.e., identical twins). SYN: *isograft.*

***lamellar g.*** A very thin corneal graft used to replace the surface layer of opaque corneal tissue.

***mesh g.*** A split-skin graft that contains multiple perforations or slits, which allow the graft to be expanded so that a much larger area is covered. The holes in the graft are covered by new tissue as the graft spreads.

***nerve g.*** The transplantation of a healthy nerve to replace a segment of a damaged nerve.

***Ollier-Thiersch g.*** SEE: *Ollier-Thiersch graft.*

***omental g.*** The use of a portion of the omentum to cover or repair a defect in a hollow viscus or to cover a suture line in an abdominal organ.

***ovarian g.*** The implantation of a section of an ovary into the muscles of the abdominal wall.

***pedicle g.*** A skin graft that is left attached at one end until the free end has begun to receive nourishment from the new site.

***periosteum g.*** The application of a piece of bone and its periosteum to another site.

***pinch g.*** A graft consisting of small bits of skin.

***postmortem g.*** Tissue taken from a body after death and stored under proper conditions to be used later on a patient requiring a graft of such tissue.

***punch g.*** A full-thickness graft, usually circular, for transplanting skin containing hair follicles to a bald area.

***rope g.*** Cable g.

***sieve g.*** A graft similar to a mesh graft in which a section of skin is removed except for small, regularly spaced areas that remain. The removed portion is used at the new site. The small remaining areas will grow to cover the entire area at the donor site.

***skin g.*** The use of small sections of skin from another body part or a donor to repair a defect or trauma of the skin, such as a large superficial burn. The skin surface at the receiving site should be clean and raw. The possibility that keratinocytes cultured from skin could be used to provide skin graft material is being investigated.

NURSING IMPLICATIONS: Before surgery, the nurse ensures that the patient's nutritional status is satisfactory and that hemoglobin and clotting time are within normal ranges, because these can affect healing. The donor and recipient sites are prepared according to protocol, and the postsurgical appearance of the wound and dressing and, if applicable, the need to immobilize the part after surgery are explained. Both patient and family receive support and encouragement. The graft is observed at regular intervals postoperatively for swelling or for development of hematoma and signs of purulent drainage. Appropriate aseptic technique is followed in applying dressings and compresses to prevent infection. Prophylactic antibiotics are administered as prescribed, and the graft site is immobilized to allow healing. Analgesics are administered as necessary to relieve pain. Before discharge, the nurse teaches the patient wound care and the need to keep the graft site clean, well lubricated, and away from sunlight for at least 6 months.

***split-skin g.*** A graft of a part of the skin thickness.

***sponge g.*** A small piece of sponge placed over an ulcerating part to stimulate epidermal growth.

***thick-split g.*** A graft of about half or more of the skin's thickness.

***Thiersch's g.*** SEE: *Thiersch's graft.*

***Wolfe's g.*** A graft using the whole skin thickness.

**grafting** The act of applying a graft of skin or tissue from a healthy site to an injured site.

**graft-versus-host reaction** ABBR: GVH. A pathological reaction to a bone marrow transplant in which the lymphocytes of the donated bone marrow destroy the "foreign" cells of the recipient. Recipients are immunodeficient after destruction of their own bone marrow in preparation for the transplant.

**Graham's law** (grā'ămz) [Thomas Graham, Brit. chemist, 1805–1869] A law stating that the rate of diffusion of a gas is inversely proportional to the square root of its density.

**grain** [L. *granum*] ABBR: gr. **1.** A weight; 0.065 of a gram. **2.** The seed or seedlike fruit of many members of the grass family, esp. corn, wheat, oats, and other cereals. **3.** Direction of fibers or layers. SYN: *granum.*

**gram** ABBR: g. A unit of weight (mass) of the metric system. It equals approx. the weight of a cubic centimeter or a milliliter of water. One gram is equal to 15.432 gr or 0.03527 oz (avoirdupois), 1000 g are equal to 1 kg. SEE: table.

***fat g.*** A standard measure of fat and the

**Gram Conversion into Ounces (Avoirdupois)***

| G | Oz | G | Oz | G | Oz | G | Oz |
|---|---|---|---|---|---|---|---|
| 1 | 0.03 | 30 | 1.06 | 59 | 2.08 | 88 | 3.10 |
| 2 | 0.07 | 31 | 1.09 | 60 | 2.12 | 89 | 3.14 |
| 3 | 0.11 | 32 | 1.13 | 61 | 2.15 | 90 | 3.17 |
| 4 | 0.14 | 33 | 1.16 | 62 | 2.18 | 91 | 3.21 |
| 5 | 0.18 | 34 | 1.20 | 63 | 2.22 | 92 | 3.24 |
| 6 | 0.21 | 35 | 1.23 | 64 | 2.26 | 93 | 3.28 |
| 7 | 0.25 | 36 | 1.27 | 65 | 2.29 | 94 | 3.31 |
| 8 | 0.28 | 37 | 1.30 | 66 | 2.33 | 95 | 3.35 |
| 9 | 0.32 | 38 | 1.34 | 67 | 2.36 | 96 | 3.38 |
| 10 | 0.35 | 39 | 1.37 | 68 | 2.40 | 97 | 3.42 |
| 11 | 0.39 | 40 | 1.41 | 69 | 2.43 | 98 | 3.46 |
| 12 | 0.42 | 41 | 1.44 | 70 | 2.47 | 99 | 3.49 |
| 13 | 0.45 | 42 | 1.48 | 71 | 2.50 | 100 | 3.53 |
| 14 | 0.49 | 43 | 1.51 | 72 | 2.54 | 125 | 4.41 |
| 15 | 0.53 | 44 | 1.55 | 73 | 2.57 | 150 | 5.30 |
| 16 | 0.56 | 45 | 1.59 | 74 | 2.61 | 175 | 6.18 |
| 17 | 0.60 | 46 | 1.62 | 75 | 2.64 | 200 | 7.05 |
| 18 | 0.63 | 47 | 1.65 | 76 | 2.68 | 250 | 8.82 |
| 19 | 0.67 | 48 | 1.69 | 77 | 2.71 | 300 | 10.58 |
| 20 | 0.70 | 49 | 1.73 | 78 | 2.75 | 350 | 12.34 |
| 21 | 0.74 | 50 | 1.76 | 79 | 2.79 | 400 | 14.11 |
| 22 | 0.77 | 51 | 1.80 | 80 | 2.82 | 450 | 15.87 |
| 23 | 0.81 | 52 | 1.83 | 81 | 2.85 | 454 | 16.00 |
| 24 | 0.84 | 53 | 1.87 | 82 | 2.89 | 500 | 17.64 |
| 25 | 0.88 | 54 | 1.90 | 83 | 2.93 | 600 | 21.16 |
| 26 | 0.91 | 55 | 1.94 | 84 | 2.96 | 700 | 24.69 |
| 27 | 0.95 | 56 | 1.97 | 85 | 3.00 | 800 | 28.22 |
| 28 | 0.99 | 57 | 2.01 | 86 | 3.03 | 900 | 30.75 |
| 29 | 1.02 | 58 | 2.04 | 87 | 3.07 | 1000 | 35.27 |

* 1 g is equal to 0.03527 oz (avoirdupois).

calories (9 kcal/g) contained. Counting and limiting fat grams is a method used in weight-reduction diets.

**gram-equivalent** In chemistry, the weight in grams of a substance that will react with 1 g of hydrogen.

**gramicidin** (grăm″ĭ-sī′dĭn) One of the antibiotics produced by *Bacillus brevis.*

**Gram's method** Gram stain.

**gram molecule** The weight in grams of a substance equal to its molecular weight.

**gram-negative** Losing the crystal violet stain and taking the color of the red counterstain in Gram's method of staining, a primary characteristic of certain microorganisms. SEE: *Gram stain.*

**gram-positive** Retaining the color of the crystal violet stain in Gram's method of staining. SEE: *Gram stain.*

**Gram stain** [Hans C. J. Gram, Danish physician, 1853–1938] A method of staining bacteria, important in their identification. SYN: *Gram's method.*

PROCEDURE: A film on a slide is prepared, dried, and fixed with heat. The film is stained with crystal violet for 1 min; rinsed in water, then immersed in Gram's iodine solution for 1 min. The iodine solution is rinsed off and the slide decolorized in 95% ethyl alcohol. The slide is then counterstained with dilute carbolfuchsin or safranine for 30 sec, after which it is rinsed with water, blotted dry, and examined. Gram-positive bacteria retain the violet stain and gram-negative bacteria adopt the red counterstain. SEE: illus.

NOTE: As a simple means of checking on the accuracy of the staining materials, a small amount of material from between one's teeth can be placed on the slide at the opposite end from that of the specimen being examined. As gram-negative and gram-positive organisms are always present in the mouth, that end of the slide should be examined first. If both types of organisms are seen, the specimen may then be examined.

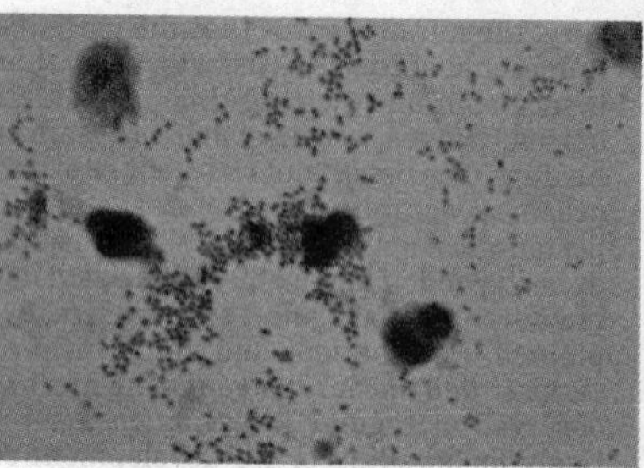

**GRAM STAIN**

GRAM-POSITIVE *STAPHYLOCOCCUS AUREUS* IN A PUS SMEAR (ORIG. MAG. ×500)

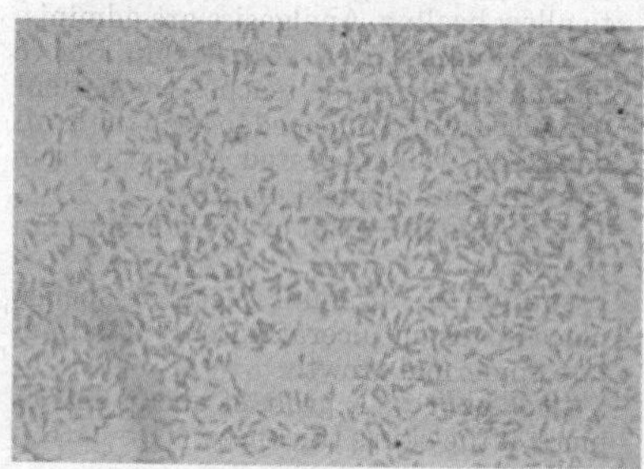

**GRAM STAIN**

GRAM-NEGATIVE *CAMPYLOBACTER JEJUNI* BACILLI (ORIG. MAG. ×500)

**Grancher's sign** (grăn-shăz′) [Jacques J. Grancher, Fr. physician, 1843–1907] The raised pitch of expiratory murmur in pulmonary consolidation.

**grandiose** (grăn′dē-ōs) In psychiatry, concerning one's unrealistic and exaggerated concept of self-worth, importance, wealth, and ability.

**grandiosity** An exaggerated sense of self-importance, power, or status.

**grand mal** SEE: *epilepsy.*

**granular** [L. *granulum,* little grain] **1.** Of the nature of granules. **2.** Roughened by prominences like those of seeds.

**granular cast** A coarse or fine granule, short and plump, sometimes yellowish, similar to a hyaline cast, and soluble in acetic acid. It is seen in inflammatory and degenerative nephropathies. SEE: *cast.*

**granulatio** (grăn″ū-lā′shē-ō) [L.] Granule.

**granulation 1.** The formation of granules or the condition of being granular. **2.** Fleshy projections formed on the surface of a gaping wound that is not healing by first intention or indirect union. Each granulation represents the outgrowth of new capillaries by budding from the existing capillaries and then joining up into capillary loops supported by cells that will later become fibrous scar tissue. Granulations bring a rich blood supply to the healing surface.

***arachnoidal g.*** Folds of the arachnoid layer of the cranial meninges that project through the inner layer of dura mater into the superior sagittal sinus and other venous sinuses of the brain. Through them, cerebrospinal fluid re-enters the bloodstream. SYN: *arachnoid villus; pacchionian body.*

***exuberant g.*** An excessive mass of granulation tissue formed in the healing of a wound or ulcer; proud flesh.

**granule** (grăn′ūl) [L. *granulum,* little grain] **1.** A small, grainlike body. **2.** In histology, a minute mass in a cell that has an outline but no apparent structure. SYN: *granulatio.*

***acidophil g.*** A granule that stains readily with acid dyes.

***albuminous g.*** A cytoplasmic granule

in many normal cells. It is not affected by ether or chloroform but disappears from view when acetic acid is added.

***amphophil g.*** Beta g.

***azurophil g.*** A small red or reddish-purple granule that easily takes a stain with azure dyes. Found in lymphocytes and monocytes, it is inconstant in number, being present in about 30% of the cells.

***basal g.*** Basal body.

***basophil g.*** A cellular granule that stains with a basic dye.

***beta g.*** An azurophil granule found in beta cells of the hypophysis or islets of Langerhans of the pancreas that stains with both acid and basic dyes. SYN: *amphophil g.*

***chromophil g.'s*** Nissl bodies.

***cone g.'s*** The nuclei of the cones, sensory cells of the retina. They form the outer zone of the outer nuclear layer of the retina.

***delta g.*** A small granule in the delta cells of the pancreas.

***eosinophil g.*** One of various granules that react with acid dyes. It is present in the eosinophils of the leukocytes.

***glycogen g.*** One of the minute particles of glycogen seen in liver cells following fixation.

***juxtaglomerular g.*** One of the secretory granules in the juxtaglomerular cells of the glomerulus of the kidney.

***Kölliker's interstitial g.*** A granule in the sarcoplasm of a striated muscle fiber.

***metachromatic g.*** An irregularly sized granule found in the protoplasm of numerous bacteria. It stains a different color from that of the dye used.

***Much's g.'s*** [Hans Christian Much, Ger. physician, 1880–1932] The granules sometimes seen in sputum from patients with tuberculosis. They do not stain with acid-fast stain but do take Gram stain. These particles are probably degenerated tubercle bacilli.

***neutrophil g.*** A granule such as those found in neutrophil leukocytes that stains with both basic and acid dyes, assuming a neutral tint.

***Nissl g.'s*** Nissl bodies.

***pigment g.*** A granule of coloring matter seen in pigment cells.

***Plehn's g.*** A basophilic granule seen in the conjugating form of *Plasmodium vivax.*

***protein g.*** A minute protein particle found in cells.

***rod g.*** A nucleus of the rod visual cell found in the external nuclear layer of the retina connected with the rods.

***Schüffner's g.*** [Wilhelm A.P. Schüffner, Ger. pathologist, 1867–1949] A coarse, red, polychrome methylene blue–staining granule found in parasitized erythrocytes of tertian malaria.

***secretory g.*** Zymogen g.

***seminal g.*** One of the minute particles in semen, supposed to derive from disintegrated nuclei in nutritive cells from seminiferous tubules.

***zymogen g.*** A granule present in gland cells, esp. the secretory cells of the pancreas, the chief cells of the gastric glands, and the serous cells of the salivary glands. It is the precursor of the enzyme secreted. SYN: *secretory g.*

**granuloblast** (grăn′ū-lō-blăst) [″ + Gr. *blastos,* germ] The mother cell of a granulocyte; a myeloblast found in bone marrow.

**granulocyte** (grăn′ū-lō-sīt″) [″ + Gr. *kytos,* cell] A granular leukocyte; a polymorphonuclear leukocyte (neutrophil, eosinophil, or basophil).

**granulocyte colony-stimulating factor** ABBR: G-CSF. A naturally occurring cytokine glycoprotein that stimulates the proliferation and functional activity of neutrophils. It is effective in treating bone marrow deficiency following cancer chemotherapy or bone marrow transplantation. The generic name is filgrastim; trade name is Neupogen. SEE: *colony-stimulating factor–1.*

**granulocyte-macrophage colony-stimulating factor** ABBR: GM-CSF. A naturally occurring cytokine glycoprotein that stimulates the production of neutrophils, monocytes, and macrophages. It is effective in treating bone marrow deficiency following cancer chemotherapy or bone marrow transplantation. The generic name is sargramostim; trade names are Leukine and Prokine. SEE: *colony-stimulating factor–1.*

**granulocytopenia** (grăn″ū-lō-sī″tō-pē′nē-ă) [″ + ″ + *penia,* poverty] An abnormal reduction of granulocytes in the blood. SYN: *granulopenia.*

**granulocytopoiesis** (grăn″ū-lō-sī″tō-poy-ē′sĭs) [″ + ″ + *poiein,* to form] The formation of granulocytes. SEE: illus.

**granulocytosis** (grăn″ū-lō-sī-tō′sĭs) [″ + ″ + *osis,* condition] An abnormal increase in the number of granulocytes in the blood.

**granuloma** [″ + Gr. *oma,* tumor] A tumor or growth that results when macrophages are unable to destroy foreign bodies and some mycobacteria. Large numbers of macrophages are drawn to the area over 7 to 10 days, surround the target, and enclose it. Other immune cells and fibroblasts become part of the inflammatory process and resulting growth. Granulomas are common in leprosy and tuberculosis, both of which are caused by mycobacteria.

***g. annulare*** A condition of the skin characterized by the development of reddish nodules arranged in a circle.

***apical g.*** Dental g.

***benign g. of the thyroid*** A lymphadenoma of the thyroid.

***coccidioidal g.*** A chronic, generalized granulomatous disease caused by the fungus *Coccidioides immitis.* SEE: *coccidioidomycosis.*

***dental g.*** A granuloma developing at

MYELOBLAST

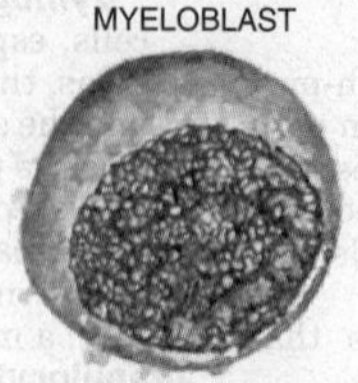

PROMYELOCYTE (PROGRANULOCYTE)

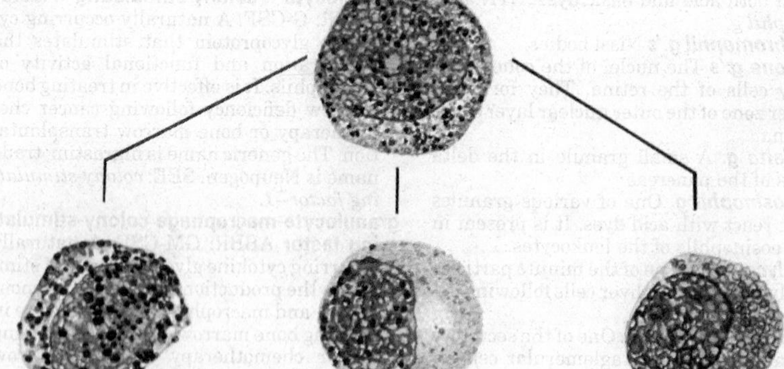

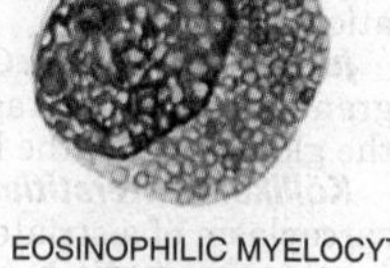

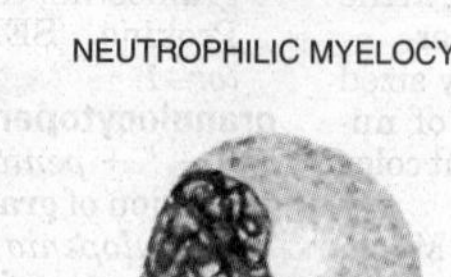

BASOPHILIC MYELOCYTE

NEUTROPHILIC MYELOCYTE

EOSINOPHILIC MYELOCYTE

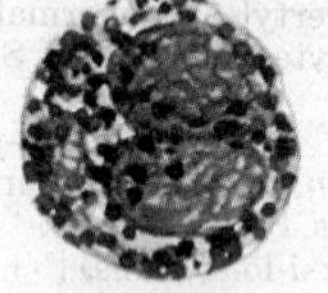

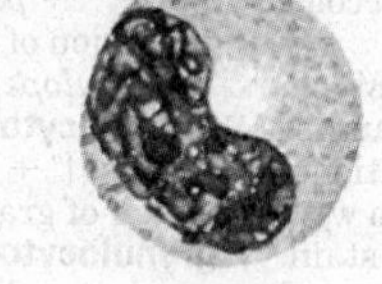

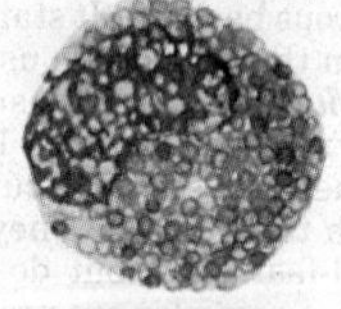

BASOPHILIC METAMYELOCYTE

NEUTROPHILIC METAMYELOCYTE

EOSINOPHILIC METAMYELOCYTE

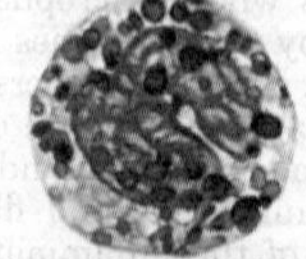

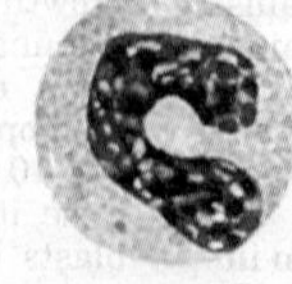

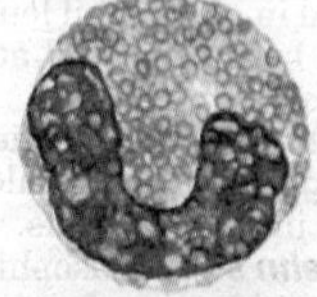

BASOPHILIC BAND

NEUTROPHILIC BAND

EOSINOPHILIC BAND

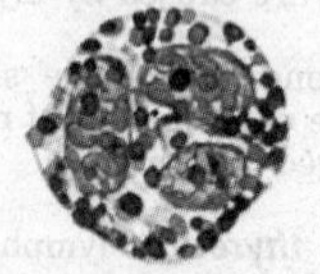

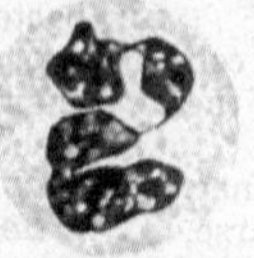

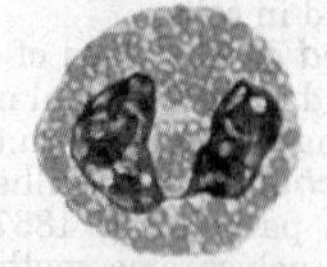

BASOPHILIC SEGMENTED

NEUTROPHILIC SEGMENTED

EOSINOPHILIC SEGMENTED

**GRANULOCYTOPOIESIS**

the tip of a tooth root, usually the result of pulpitis. It consists of a proliferating mass of chronic inflammatory tissue and possibly epithelial nests or colonies of bacteria. It may be encapsulated by fibrous tissue of the periodontal ligament. SYN: *apical g.; chronic apical periodontitis.*

**eosinophilic g.** A form of xanthomatosis accompanied by eosinophilia and the formation of cysts on bone.

**g. fissuratum** A circumscribed, firm, fissured, fibrotic tumor caused by chronic irritation. It may occur where hard objects such as dentures or the earpieces of glasses rub against the labioalveolar fold or the retroauricular fold, respectively. The tumor is not malignant and disappears when the irritating object is removed.

**foreign body g.** Chronic inflammation around foreign bodies such as sutures, talc, splinters, or gravel.

**g. fungoides** Mycosis fungoides.

**infectious g.** Any infectious disease in which granulomas are formed, such as tuberculosis or syphilis. Granulomas are also formed in mycoses and protozoan infections.

**g. inguinale** A granulomatous ulcerative disease in which the initial lesion commonly appears in the genital area as a painless nodule.

ETIOLOGY: This type of granuloma is caused by a short, gram-negative bacillus, *Calymmatobacterium granulomatis,* commonly called a Donovan body.

TREATMENT: Erythromycin, trimethoprim-sulfamethoxazole, or tetracyclines are used in treating this disease. Single-dose therapy with intramuscular ceftriaxone or oral ciprofloxacin may be effective.

**g. iridis** A granuloma that develops on the iris.

**lipoid g.** A granuloma that contains fatty tissue or cholesterol.

**lipophagic g.** A granuloma in which the macrophages have phagocytosed the surrounding fat cells.

**Majocchi's g.** Trichophytic g.

**malignant g.** Hodgkin's disease; lymphogranulomatosis.

**g. pyogenicum** A granuloma containing pyogenic organisms that develops at the site of a wound. It may also occur at the tips of the fingers along the sides of the nails or beneath the free edge of the nail. It bleeds easily and is usually painful to touch.

**swimming pool g.** Chronic skin infection with *Mycobacterium balnei,* an organism that may be present in unchlorinated swimming pools.

**g. telangiectaticum** A very vascular granuloma at any site, but esp. in the nasal mucosa or pharynx.

**trichophytic g.** A granuloma of the skin follicles and follicular areas of the legs. It is caused by fungi, usually *Trichophyton rubrum.* SYN: *Majocchi's g.*

**granulomatosis** (grăn″ū-lō″mă-tō′sĭs) [L. *granulum,* little grain, + Gr. *oma,* tumor, + *osis,* condition] The development of multiple granulomas.

**Wegener's g.** A rare disease of unknown etiology characterized by widespread granulomatous lesions of the bronchi, necrotizing arteriolitis, and glomerulonephritis.

**granulomatous** (grăn″ū-lŏm′ă-tŭs) Containing granulomas.

**granulopenia** (grăn″ū-lō-pē′nē-ă) [″ + Gr. *penia,* poverty] Granulocytopenia.

**granuloplasm** (grăn′ū-lō-plăzm) A granular cytoplasm.

**granuloplastic** (grăn″ū-lō-plăs′tĭk) [″ + Gr. *plassein,* to form] Developing granules.

**granulopoiesis** (grăn″ū-lō-poy-ē′sĭs) [″ + Gr. *poiein,* to make] The formation of granulocytes.

**granulopotent** (grăn″ū-lō-pō′tĕnt) [″ + *potentia,* power] Potentially capable of forming granules.

**granulosa** (grăn″ū-lō′să) A layer of cells in the theca of the graafian follicle.

**granulosis** (grăn″ū-lō′sĭs) [″ + Gr. *osis,* condition] A mass of minute granules.

**g. rubra nasi** A disease of the skin of the nose, characterized by a moist erythematous patch on numerous macules. The disease is caused by an inflammatory infiltration about the nose, with slightly elevated papules and dilated sweat glands.

**granum** (grā′nŭm) [L.] Grain.

**granzyme** Any of a family of proteases stored in the granules of cytotoxic T lymphocytes. They are involved in cytolytic functions.

**grape sugar** Dextrose.

**graph** (grăf) **1.** A visual presentation of statistical, clinical, or experimental data represented by a relationship between two sets of numbers or variables on the ordinate (y) (vertical) axis and the abscissa (x) (horizontal) axis. **2.** Any visual representation of a numerical relationship.

**-graph** [Gr. *graphos,* drawn or written; one who draws] Combining form used as a suffix meaning an instrument used to make a drawing or written record.

**graphesthesia** (grăf″ĕs-thē′zē-ă) [″ + *aisthesis,* sensation] The ability to recognize outlines, numbers, words, or symbols traced or written on the skin.

**graphite** (grăf′īt) [Gr. *graphein,* to write] A soft form of carbon.

**grapho-** [Gr. *graphein,* to write] Combining form meaning *writing.*

**graphology** (grăf-ŏl′ō-jē) [″ + *logos,* word, reason] The examination of handwriting of patients with diseases of the nerves, as a means of diagnosis or of analyzing a patient's personality.

**graphomotor** (grăf″ō-mō′tor) [″ + L. *motor,* mover] Pert. to movements involved in writing.

**graphophobia** (grăf″ō-fō′bē-ă) [″ + *phobos,*

fear] An abnormal fear of writing.

**graphorrhea** (grăf"ō-rē'ă) [" + *rhoia,* flow] The writing of many meaningless words and phrases.

**graphospasm** (grăf'ō-spăzm) [" + *spasmos,* spasm] Writer's cramp.

**GRAS List** A list of food additives *generally recognized as safe* by the U.S. Food and Drug Administration. SEE: *food additive.*

**grasp** A specific type of prehension involving the fingers, the palmar surface, or both. Types of grasp include cylindrical, as in holding a cylinder, where the fingers and palmar surface are in opposition; and ball grasp, as in holding a spherical object, where the fingers, thumb, and palmar surface surround an object.

***pincher g.*** The apposition of the thumb and index finger to pick up small objects. This fine motor skill is a developmental milestone usually attained by 10 months of age.

**grass** An artifact seen on oscilloscope tracings, esp. in hemodynamic monitoring, resembling the random addition of vertical lines to the pattern. In hemodynamic monitoring, this is caused by rapid movement of the end of the catheter, usually because of malplacement.

**grating** In spectrophotometry, the element used in a monochromator that disperses white light into the visible spectrum.

**grattage** (gră-tăzh') [Fr., a scraping] The removal of morbid growths by rubbing with a brush or harsh sponge.

**grave** [L. *gravis,* heavy] Serious; dangerous; severe.

**gravel** [Fr. *gravelle,* coarse sand] Crystalline dust or concretions of crystals from the kidneys; generally made up of phosphates, calcium, oxalate, and uric acid.

**Graves' disease** [Robert James Graves, Irish physician, 1796–1853] A disease complex of unknown etiology, although an autoimmune basis is suspected. The three major manifestations of this disease are hyperthyroidism with diffuse goiter (i.e., diffuse thyroid gland enlargement), ophthalmopathy, and dermopathy. All three manifestations may not be present at the same time; in some cases only one manifestation will be present. In other cases, each condition runs a course independent of the others. The disease is relatively common, esp. in middle age, and is more common in women than in men. SYN: *thyrotoxicosis.* SEE: *Grave's ophthalmopathy; hyperthyroidism; thyroidectomy; thyroid storm.*

SYMPTOMS: Symptoms include a hyperthyroidism manifesting as nervousness, emotional changes, a fine tremor of the fingers and tongue, insomnia, frequent bowel movements, profuse perspiration, and heat intolerance. The skin is warm and moist and has a velvety feel. Also present are weight loss and proximal muscle weakness. Women of menstrual age may have decreased menstrual blood loss or amenorrhea. The heart is affected and there may be a wide pulse pressure, tachycardia, atrial fibrillation, cardiac enlargement, and in some cases heart failure. The ophthalmopathy is manifest by an inflammatory filtrate of the orbit of the eye but not of the globe. Edema and fat infiltration accounts for the increased volume of the orbit and exophthalmos. The clinical signs include lid lag, visual stare, lid retraction, and an expression that resembles fright. In addition, conjunctivitis and periorbital swelling are present. All of this may lead to the complications of corneal ulcerations, optic neuritis, and optic atrophy. The dermopathy is characterized by areas of raised and thickened skin, usually over the dorsum of the hands and feet. The skin has a pebbly appearance (peau d'orange) and it may itch and be hyperpigmented.

DIAGNOSIS: The clinical signs and symptoms are diagnostic; however, if the diagnosis is in question, assay of various thyroid hormones will be of use in confirming the diagnosis.

TREATMENT: Drugs that limit the thyroid gland's output of thyroid hormone are effective as therapy. The thyroid gland may be removed surgically or it may be inactivated by use of radioactive iodine therapy.

NURSING IMPLICATIONS: A history documenting classic symptoms such as nervousness, heat intolerance, weight loss despite increased appetite, excessive sweating, diarrhea, tremor, and palpitations is obtained. Difficulty in concentrating, trouble climbing stairs, dyspnea on exertion and possibly at rest, anorexia, nausea and vomiting, and menstrual abnormalities may also be evident. The patient is observed for anxiousness and restlessness; for fine tremors of the fingers and tongue, shaky handwriting, clumsiness, emotional instability, and mood swings; for flushed skin and fine hair with premature graying and hair loss; and for fragile nails with distal separation from the nailbed. The patient is also observed for pretibial myxedema over the dorsum of the legs and feet, which produces raised, thickened skin that may be itchy, hyperpigmented, and unusually well demarcated from normal skin, with plaque-like or nodular lesions; and for generalized or localized muscle atrophy and acropachy.

Eyes are checked for infrequent blinking, a characteristic stare, and lid-lag, resulting from sympathetic overstimulation; as well as for exophthalmos, resulting from accumulated mucopolysaccharides and fluids in the retro-orbital tissues that force the eye outward. The conjunctiva may appear reddened, and the patient may have an impaired upward gaze, convergence, and strabismus due to ocular muscle weakness.

The thyroid gland is palpated for enlargement; the enlarged gland may feel asymmetrical, lobular, and three to four times normal size. The liver also may feel enlarged. The skin feels warm and moist, with a velvety texture; and tachycardia, characterized by a full, bounding pulse, is palpable. Hyperreflexia also is present. The patient is auscultated for blood pressure elevation, widened pulse pressure, cardiac dysrhythmias (paroxysmal supraventricular tachycardia or atrial fibrillation), and increased bowel sounds.

Assistance is provided to help the patient to cope with related anxiety, and the patient is encouraged to minimize emotional and physical stress and to balance rest and activity periods. A high-calorie, high-protein diet is recommended to treat increased protein catabolism. The patient is taught comfort measures to deal with elevated body temperature and G.I. complaints (abdominal cramping, frequent bowel movements); safety measures to protect the eyes from injury, including moistening the conjunctiva frequently with isotonic eye drops and wearing sunglasses to protect the eyes from light; and appropriate administration and safety procedures for iodide therapy, beta-blocker therapy, and propylthiouracil and methimazole therapy, as prescribed. Special instructions are provided for therapeutic use of radioactive iodide.

The patient is prepared physically and psychologically for surgery if planned, and postoperative care specific to thyroidectomy is provided. Regular medical follow-up is needed to detect and treat hypothyroidism, which may develop 2 to 4 weeks after surgery and after radioactive iodine therapy. The patient is advised of the possible need for lifelong replacement therapy, and should wear or carry a medical identification tag and keep a supply of medication with him or her at all times.

**Graves' ophthalmopathy** Ophthalmopathy associated with hyperthyroidism with the clinical characteristics of exophthalmos, periorbital edema, periorbital and conjunctival inflammation, decreased extraocular muscle mobility, and corneal injury. Accompanying these may be lacrimation, eye pain, blurring of vision, photophobia, diplopia, and loss of vision.

TREATMENT: The underlying hyperthyroidism must be treated. The patient should sleep with the head of the bed elevated. Methylcellulose eyedrops and diuretics will help to relieve eye discomfort. If the condition is severe and progressive, surgical decompression of the orbit will be required to treat impaired retinal function and exposure keratopathy. SEE: *goiter, exophthalmic.*

**gravid** (grăv'ĭd) [L. *gravida,* pregnant] Pregnant; heavy with child.

**gravida** (grăv'ĭ-dă) [L.] A pregnant woman.

**gravida macromastia** Rapid enlargement of the breasts during pregnancy. This may progress to cause severe distention with sloughing of breast tissue, bleeding, and infection. Surgical therapy may be required.

**gravidism** [L. *gravida,* pregnant, + Gr. *-ismos,* state of] The state of being pregnant.

**gravidity** (gră-vĭd'ĭ-tē) [L. *gravida,* pregnant] The total number of a woman's pregnancies.

**gravidocardiac** (grăv"ĭd-ō-kăr'dē-ăk) [" + Gr. *kardia,* heart] Pert. to cardiac disorders resulting from pregnancy.

**gravimetric** (grăv"ĭ-mĕt'rĭk) [L. *gravis,* heavy, + Gr. *metron,* measure] Determined by weight.

**gravistatic** (grăv"ĭ-stăt'ĭk) [" + Gr. *statikos,* causing to stand] Resulting from gravitation, as in a form of gravistatic pulmonary congestion.

**gravitation** [L. *gravitas,* weight] The force and movement tending to draw every particle of matter together, esp. the attraction of the earth for bodies at a distance from its center.

**gravity** **1.** The property of possessing weight. **2.** The force of the earth's gravitational attraction.

***specific g.*** ABBR: sp. gr. The weight of a substance compared with an equal volume of water. Water is used as a standard and is considered to have a specific gravity of 1 (1.000).

**gravity-induced loss of consciousness** ABBR: GLOC. The loss of consciousness due to positive gravity (G) forces. Certain aviation maneuvers produce increased downward force (i.e., positive G) that is measured as a multiple of the gravitational constant. When these forces are of sufficient intensity, blood flow to the brain is diminished, which, if continued, leads to unconsciousness.

**Gravlee jet washer** [Leland Clark Gravlee, Jr., U.S. obstetrician and gynecologist, 1928–1984] A proprietary device for irrigating the endometrial cavity with sterile isotonic saline and then removing the solution and dislodged cells. The cells are then stained and examined for evidence of malignancy.

**gray** ABBR: Gy. A measure of the quantity of ionizing radiation absorbed by any material per unit mass of matter. 1 Gy equals 100 rad. SEE: *radiation absorbed dose.*

**gray matter** SEE: *matter, gray.*

**gray syndrome of the newborn** The appearance of vomiting, lack of sucking response, irregular and rapid respiration, abdominal distention, and cyanosis in newborn infants treated at birth with chloramphenicol. Flaccidity and an ashen-gray color are present within 24 hr. About 40% of the patients die, most frequently on the fifth day of life.

---

Caution: Children less than 1 month of age

being treated with chloramphenicol should receive no more than 25 mg/kg of body weight each day.

---

**green** A color intermediate between blue and yellow, afforded by rays of wavelength between 492 and 575 nm. SEE: words beginning with *chloro-*.

***g. blindness*** Aglaucopsia.

***brilliant g.*** A derivative of malachite green, used in staining bacteria.

***indocyanine g.*** A dye used intravenously to determine blood volume.

***malachite g.*** A dye used as a stain and antiseptic.

***g. soap*** A potassium soap made by the saponification of suitable vegetable oils without the removal of glycerin.

***g. soap tincture*** Green soap to which lavender oil and alcohol have been added.

**Greenfield's disease** [J. Godwin Greenfield, Brit. neuropathologist, 1884–1958] Metachromatic leukodystrophy.

**grenz ray** [Ger. *Grenze,* boundary] X-radiation with an average wavelength of 2 angstroms. SEE: *ray.*

**grid 1.** A chart with an abscissa (x) (horizontal) axis and an ordinate (y) (vertical) axis on which to plot graphs. **2.** A device made of parallel lead strips, used to absorb scattered radiation during radiography of larger body parts.

***Fixott-Everett g.*** A plastic-embedded screen placed over dental radiographic film before x-ray exposure. It facilitates measurement of bone loss and other tissue changes.

**grief, chronic** Unresolved denial of the reality of a personal loss. Also called *dysfunctional grieving.* SEE: *grief reaction.*

**grief reaction** The emotional reaction that follows the loss of a love object. Somatic symptoms include easy fatigability, hollow or empty feelings in the chest and abdomen, sighing, hyperventilation, anorexia, insomnia, and the feeling of having a lump in the throat. Psychological symptoms begin with an initial stage of shock and disbelief accompanied by an inner awareness of mental discomfort, sorrow, and regret. These may be followed by tears, sobbing, and cries of pain. The duration of the reaction is variable.

**grieving, anticipatory** Intellectual and emotional responses and behaviors by which individuals (families, communities) work through the process of modifying self-concept based on the perception of potential loss. SEE: *Nursing Diagnoses Appendix.*

**grieving, dysfunctional** Extended, unsuccessful use of intellectual and emotional responses by which individuals (families, communities) attempt to work through the process of modifying self-concept based upon the perception of potential loss. SEE: *Nursing Diagnoses Appendix.*

**grinder** (grīn′dĕr) [AS. *grindan,* to gnash] A molar tooth. SYN: *dens molaris.*

**grinders' disease** Pneumoconiosis.

**grinding** A forceful rubbing together, as in chewing. SEE: *bruxism.*

***selective g.*** Altering and correcting the dental occlusion by grinding in accordance with what is required.

**grip, grippe** (grĭp) [Fr. *gripper,* to seize] Influenza.

**gripes** (grīps) [AS. *gripan,* to grasp] Intermittent severe pains in the bowels. SYN: *intestinal colic.*

**griping** An acute intermittent cramplike pain, esp. in the abdomen.

**griseofulvin** An oral antifungal antibiotic, esp. effective against ringworm.

**groin** [AS. *grynde,* abyss] The depression between the thigh and trunk; the inguinal region.

**grommet** (grŏm′ĭt) A device, also known as a ventilation tube, placed in an artificial opening in the tympanic membrane to permit air to flow freely between the inner ear and the external auditory canal. The prosthesis is used as a treatment adjunct in managing chronic otitis media with effusion. The routine use of grommets as part of the initial therapy for otitis media is not advised. Their use should be reserved for persistent or recurrent infections that have failed to respond to appropriate antibiotic therapy.

**groove** [MD. *groeve,* ditch] A long narrow channel, depression, or furrow. SYN: *sulcus.*

***bicipital g.*** The groove for the long tendon of the biceps brachii located on the anterior surface of the humerus.

***branchial g.*** A groove in the embryo that is lined with ectoderm and lies between two branchial arches.

***carotid g.*** A broad groove on the inner surface of the sphenoid bone lateral to the body. It lodges the carotid artery and the cavernous sinus.

***costal g.*** The groove on the lower internal border of a rib. It lodges the intercostal vessels and nerve. SYN: *subcostal g.*

***costovertebral g.*** A broad groove that extends along each side of a vertebra. It lodges the sacrospinalis muscle and its subdivisions.

***Harrison's g.*** The groove or line extending laterally from the xiphoid process of the sternum. It marks the attachment of the diaphragm to the costal margins and is seen in children with severe rickets.

***infraorbital g.*** The groove on the orbital surface of the maxilla that transmits the infraorbital vessels and nerve.

***labial g.*** The groove that develops in each of the primitive jaws. It gives rise to the vestibule separating the lips from the gums.

***lacrimal g.'s*** Two grooves, one on the posterior surface of the frontal process of the maxilla, and the other on the anterior surface of the posterior lacrimal crest of the lacrimal bone. These grooves lodge the lacrimal sac.

***laryngotracheal* g.** The groove along the ventral surface of the anterior portion of the embryonic gut that gives rise to the respiratory organs.

***malleolar* g.** The groove on the anterior surface of the distal end of the tibia that lodges tendons of the tibialis posterior and flexor digitorum longus musculi.

***meningeal* g.** One of several depressions on the internal surface of the cranial bones where blood vessels follow the meningeal and osseous structures of the skull.

***musculospiral* g.** Radial g.

***mylohyoid* g.** The groove on the inner surface of the mandible that runs obliquely forward and downward and contains the mylohyoid nerve and artery. In the embryo it lodges Meckel's cartilage.

***nasolacrimal* g.** The groove extending from the inner angle of the eye to the primitive olfactory sac in the embryo. It separates the maxillary and lateral nasal processes; its epithelial lining gives rise to the nasolacrimal duct.

***nasopalatine* g.** The groove on the vomer that lodges the nasopalatine nerve and vessels.

***neural* g.** A longitudinal groove on the dorsal surface of the embryo lying between the neural folds. On closure of the folds to form the neural tube, the groove becomes the cavity of the neural tube, eventually giving rise to the ventricles of the brain and the central canal of the spinal cord.

***obturator* g.** The groove at the superior and posterior angle of the obturator foramen through which pass the obturator vessels and nerve.

***olfactory* g.** A shallow groove on the superior surface of the cribriform plate of the ethmoid on each side of the crista galli. It contains the olfactory bulb.

***palatine* g.** One of several grooves on the inferior surface on the palatine process of the maxilla. They contain the palatine vessels and nerves.

***peroneal* g.'s** A shallow groove on the lateral aspect of the calcaneus and a deep groove on the inferior surface of the cuboid bone. Each transmits the tendon of the peroneus longus muscle.

***primitive* g.** In the embryo, a shallow groove in the primitive streak of the blastoderm, bordered by the primitive folds.

***pterygopalatine* g.** The groove on the maxillary surface of the perpendicular portion of the palatine bone that, with corresponding grooves on the maxilla and pterygoid process of the sphenoid, transmits the palatine nerve and descending palatine artery.

***radial* g.** A broad, shallow, spiraling groove on the posterior surface of the humerus. It transmits the radial nerve and the profunda branchi artery. SYN: *musculospiral g.*

***rhombic* g.** One of seven transverse grooves in the floor of the developing rhombencephalon of the brain. They separate the neuromeres.

***sagittal* g.** A shallow groove on the inner surface of the parietal bones that lodges the superior sagittal sinus. SYN: *sagittal sulcus.*

***sigmoid* g.** The groove on the inner surface of the mastoid portion of the temporal bone. It transmits the transverse sinus.

***subcostal* g.** Costal g.

***tympanic* g.** The groove at the bottom of the exterior auditory meatus that receives the inferior portion of the tympanic membrane.

***urethral* g.** The groove on the caudal surface of the genital tubercle or phallus bordered by the urethral folds. The latter close, transforming the groove into the cavernous urethra.

**gross** (grōs) [L. *grossus,* thick] **1.** Visible to the naked eye. **2.** Consisting of large particles or components; coarse or large.

**gross motor skills** Skills pert. to the synergy of large muscle groups, as in balancing, running, and throwing.

**ground 1.** Basic substance or foundation. **2.** Reduced to a powder; pulverized. **3.** In electronics, the negative or earth pole that has zero electrical potential.

**ground bundle** A bundle of nerve fibers that immediately surrounds the gray matter of the spinal cord. It is divided into three regions, the anterior, lateral, and posterior bundles, which lie in the corresponding funiculi. These consist principally of short descending fibers.

**group** [It. *gruppo,* knot] A number of similar objects or structures considered together (e.g., bacteria with similar metabolic characteristics). Atomic molecules and compounds with similar structures or properties are classified with certain groups.

***alcohol* g.** The hydroxyl, —OH, which imparts alcoholic characteristics to organic compounds. These may be in three forms: primary, $—CH_2OH$; secondary, ═CHOH; and tertiary, ≡COH.

***azo* g.** In chemistry, the group —N═N—.

***coli-aerogenes* g.** Coliform bacteria.

***colon-typhoid-dysentery* g.** The collective term for *Escherichia, Salmonella,* and *Shigella* bacteria.

**g. *dynamics*** In politics, sociology, and psychology, a study of the forces and conditions that influence the actions of the entire group as well as the relations of the individuals to each other in the group.

***peptide* g.** The —CONH— radical.

***prosthetic* g. 1.** In a conjugated protein, the nonprotein portion of the molecule. **2.** The nonprotein component of a coenzyme.

***resource utilization* g.** A grouping of nursing home patients according to diagnosis, treatment, and age for the purpose of providing adequate staff and ascertaining cost data. The primary use is for insurance reimbursement calculations.

***saccharide g.*** The monosaccharide unit, $C_6H_{10}O_5$, which is a component of higher polysaccharides.

***support g.*** Patients or families of patients with similar problems such as breast cancer, multiple sclerosis, alcoholism, or other life experiences, who meet to assist each other in coping with the problems and seeking solutions and ways of coping. The composition and focus of support groups varies. Some groups may be comprised of patients who are experiencing or have experienced the same disorder. Discussions often center on current treatments, resources available for assistance, and what individuals can do to improve or maintain their health. Other groups involve those who have experienced the same psychological and emotional trauma such as rape victims or persons who have lost a loved one. Benefits expressed by members include the knowledge that they are not alone but that others have experienced the same or similar problems and that they have learned to cope effectively.

**grouping** The classification of individual traits according to a shared characteristic.

***blood g.*** Classification of blood of different individuals according to agglutinating and hemolyzing qualities before making a blood transfusion. SEE: *blood groups; blood transfusion.*

**group therapy** A form of psychiatric treatment in which six to eight patients meet a specific number of times with a therapist. The value of this type of therapy is the opportunity for gaining insight into one's life experience.

**group transfer** An oxidation-reduction chemical reaction involving the exchange of chemical groups. A transferase enzyme is required.

**Grover's disease** [R. W. Grover, contemporary U.S. dermatologist] A common itchy (pruritic) condition of sudden onset, characterized by a few or numerous smooth or warty papules, vesicles, eczematous plaques, or shiny translucent nodules. The pruritus may be mild or severe and is aggravated by heat. Even though the condition is self-limiting, it may last months or years.

TREATMENT: The patient should be treated symptomatically. Heat and sweat-inducing activities should be avoided. Retinoic acid may be helpful.

**growing pains** An imprecise term indicating ill-defined pain, usually after bedtime, in the musculoskeletal system of young persons. There is no evidence that the pain is related to rapid growth.

TREATMENT: The child should be reassured and given aspirin, with application of local heat and massage. Quinine sulfate given before bedtime may help.

**growth** [AS. *growan,* to grow] The progressive development or increase in size of a living thing. This may be normal, as in growth of an embryo or child, or pathological, as in a cyst or benign or malignant tumor. Growth occurs by the synthesis of new protoplasm and multiplication of cells.

TYPES:

1. General body growth is seen in the increase in the physical size of the body and increase in the total weight of the muscles and various internal organs. Growth is usually slow and steady but has a marked acceleration just after birth and at the time of puberty (the "growth spurt").
2. Organs of the lymphoid type, such as the thymus and the lymph nodes, grow fastest early in life, reach their peak of development at about the age of 12 years, and then stop growing or regress.
3. The neural type of organ, such as the brain, cord, eye, and meninges, grows in childhood but is close to its adult size by the age of 8 years. This size is maintained without regression.
4. The genital type of growth is seen in the testes, ovaries, and other genitourinary structures. Their growth is the slowest of these four types in infancy, but at puberty they grow faster and cause the striking changes in appearance that make up the secondary sex characteristics. Not all of the organs of the body are included in these four types. Some structures, such as the mammary glands, have several cycles of growth and regression in a lifetime.

**growth curve** A graph of heights and weights of infants and children of various ages. Using a line to join the data points produces the curve. Usually the changes in height and weight are shown on the same chart.

**growth and development, altered** The state in which an individual demonstrates deviations in norms from his/her age group. SEE: *Nursing Diagnoses Appendix.*

**growth hormone, human synthetic** SEE: under *hormone.*

**gruel** [L. *grutum,* meal] Any cereal boiled in water.

**grumose, grumous** (groo'mōs, -mŭs) [L. *grumus,* heap] **1.** Made up of coarse granular bodies in the center. **2.** Lumpy, clotted.

**Grünfelder's reflex** (groon'fĕld-ĕrs) A fanlike spreading of the toes with upward flexion of the great toe, resulting from pressure over the posterior fontanel.

**gryposis** (grĭ-pō'sĭs) [G. *gryposis,* a crooking] Abnormal curvature of any part of the body, esp. the nails.

**GSA** *Gerontological Society of America.*

**GSR** *galvanic skin response.*

**G-suit** A coverall-type garment designed for use by aviators. It contains compartments that inflate and bring pressure on the legs and abdomen to prevent blood from pooling there. In aviators this helps to prevent unconsciousness caused by positive acceleration with resulting pooling of blood in the lower extremities. The suit has been used in medicine to treat postural hypotension. SEE: *MAST*.

**gt** L. *gutta,* a drop.

**gtt** L. *guttae,* drops.

**GU** *genitourinary*.

**guaiac** (gwī′ăk) [NL. *Guaiacum*] A resin obtained from trees of the genus *Guaiacum,* either *G. officinale* or *G. sanctum*. An alcoholic solution of guaiac is used to test for occult blood in feces.

**guaiacol** (gwī′ă-kōl) O-Methoxyphenol; a substance similar to phenol obtained by fractional distillation of creosote or by synthetic means. It is used as an antiseptic and germicide, intestinal antiseptic, and expectorant.

**guaifenesin** (gwī-fĕn′ĕ-sĭn) An expectorant. Trade name is Robitussin.

**guanethidine** (gwăn-ĕth′ĭ-dēn) A drug that depresses the function of postganglionic adrenergic nerves, thus inhibiting sympathetic nerve activity. It is used in treating hypertension.

***g. sulfate*** An adrenergic blocking agent used in treating hypertension.

**guanidine** (gwăn′ĭ-dēn) A crystalline organic compound, $(NH_2)_2C{=}NH$, found among the decomposition products of proteins.

**guanidinemia** (gwăn″ĭd-ĕn-ē′mē-ă) [*guanidine* + Gr. *haima,* blood] Guanidine in the blood.

**guanidoacetic acid** A chemical formed in the liver, kidney, and other tissues. It is then metabolized to form creatine.

**guanine** (gwă′nēn) $C_5H_5N_5O$. One of the purine bases in DNA and RNA. Purine bases are degraded to urate and excreted in the urine.

**guanosine** (gwăn′ō-sĭn) The nucleoside formed from guanine and ribosome. It is a major constituent of RNA and DNA.

**guard** A device for protecting something (e.g., a mouth guard or a face guard).

**guarded prognosis** A prognosis given by a physician when the outcome of a patient's illness is in doubt.

**guardian ad litem** [L.] In cases of child abuse, a guardian for the child appointed by the court to protect the best interests of the child.

**guardianship** A legal arrangement by which a person or institution assumes responsibility for an adult individual. When guardians are appointed, the individuals receiving the care are presumed to be incompetent and unable to care for themselves.

**guarding** A body defense method to prevent movement of an injured part, esp. spasm of abdominal muscles when an examiner attempts to palpate inflamed areas or organs in the abdominal cavity.

**gubernaculum** (gū″bĕr-năk′ū-lŭm) [L., helm] **1.** A structure that guides. **2.** A cordlike structure uniting two structures.

***g. dentis*** A connective tissue band that connects the tooth sac of an unerupted tooth with the overlying gum.

***g. testis*** A fibrous cord in the fetus that extends from the caudal end of the testis through the inguinal canal to the scrotal swelling. It plays a role in the descent of the testis into the scrotum.

**Gubler's line** (goob′lĕrz) [Adolphe Gubler, Fr. physician, 1821–1879] The level of superficial origin of the trigeminus or fifth nerve.

**Gubler's paralysis** A form of alternate hemiplegia in which a brainstem lesion causes paralysis of the cranial nerves on one side and of the body on the opposite side.

**Gubler's tumor** A fusiform swelling on the wrist in lead palsy.

**Gudden's inferior commissure** (gūd′ĕnz) [Bernard A. von Gudden, Ger. neurologist, 1824–1886] Fibers of the optic tract.

**Gudden's law** A law stating that, in the division of a nerve, degeneration in the proximal portion is toward the nerve cell.

**guidance** The act of guiding or counseling (e.g., of a patient).

**guide** A mechanical aid or device that assists in setting a course or directing the motion either of one's hand or of an instrument one holds.

**guide dog** A dog specifically trained to assist blind or partially sighted persons with mobility.

**guideline** An instructional guide or reference to indicate a course of action in a specified situation (e.g., critical care guideline).

**guidewire** A device used to assist in inserting, positioning, and moving a catheter. These wires vary in size, length, stiffness, composition, and shape of the end.

**guile** The use of deception or cunning in order to accomplish something.

**Guillain-Barré syndrome** (gē-yă′băr-rā′) [Georges Guillain, Fr. neurologist, 1876–1961; J. A. Barré, Fr. neurologist, b. 1880] ABBR: GBS. Acute, autoimmune inflammatory destruction of the myelin sheath covering peripheral nerves, causing rapid progressive symmetrical loss of motor function; the sensory nerves remain intact. Generally, an acute viral infection occurs 1 to 3 weeks before the onset of the syndrome. The virus triggers the production of autoantibodies that damage the myelin sheath, interfering with impulse conduction to muscle fibers. The damage is not uniform, but occurs in segments along the nerve between the nodes of Ranvier; a high degree of inflammation can destroy the nerve itself. SYN: *acute inflammatory demyelinating polyneuropathy; acute inflammatory polyradiculopathy*.

Paresthesia usually occurs first, followed by muscle weakness and flaccid paralysis that most commonly ascends from the extremities to the head; it becomes life threatening if respiratory muscles are affected. In descending GBS, paralysis occurs from the head down and causes respiratory distress more often.

The loss of motor function can occur over a few days or 2 to 3 weeks. A stable period of 10 to 14 days follows. Recovery requires 3 to 12 months. The syndrome may be mild, with only limited muscle weakness, or severe, producing full body paralysis; more severe cases may cause permanent residual weakness in the extremities.

TREATMENT: High-dose intravenous immunoglobulin (2 g/kg) given over 5 days is effective. Although other immunosuppressive drugs may be used during the early phase, corticosteroid use is controversial. Intravenous immune globulin is also effective. Other treatments are aimed at minimizing complications and supporting respiratory function.

NURSING IMPLICATIONS: The patient is assessed for cranial nerve involvement by observing and documenting difficulty in talking, chewing, and swallowing, and any signs of respiratory distress. Emergency measures are taken if either or both occur; emergency endotracheal intubation and tracheostomy equipment are kept available. The nurse monitors muscle function frequently as necessary, documenting the pattern and degree of loss and later the return. Vital signs and level of consciousness are also monitored.

Respiratory function is assessed. Arterial blood gas measurements are obtained as directed or as necessary. The nurse repositions the patient and encourages deep breathing and coughing. Respiratory support is initiated at the first sign of dyspnea, an emergency airway established, and mechanical ventilation initiated if respiratory failure is imminent.

Pain must be monitored closely to ensure that adequate analgesia is prescribed and administered. The patient may require increasing doses. Increases should be gradual to avoid respiratory depression.

Gentle passive range-of-motion exercises (in water if possible) are provided three to four times daily within the patient's pain limits. As the patient's condition stabilizes, gentle stretching and active-assisted exercises are provided.

Skin is inspected for signs of breakdown. To prevent decubiti, a strict 2-hr turning schedule is established, and alternating pressure pads are applied at points of contact. Care should be taken at each repositioning to ensure that the patient is covered sufficiently for warmth, since his or her temperature control center may be defective.

Fluid and electrolyte balance is maintained. To prevent aspiration, the head of the bed is elevated and the gag reflex tested before oral intake. If the gag reflex is impaired, nasogastric enteral feedings are provided until the reflex returns. The nurse encourages adequate fluid intake (2000 ml/day) orally, enterally, or if necessary, parenterally unless contraindicated. The bladder should be palpated and percussed to assess for urine retention. Either urinal or bedpan is offered every 3 to 4 hr, and manual pressure applied over the bladder. Intermittent urinary catheterization is instituted if necessary. To prevent or relieve constipation, prune juice and a high-bulk diet, stool softeners and laxatives, glycerin or bisacodyl suppositories, or enemas (as prescribed) are provided daily or on alternate days.

If the patient has facial paralysis, the nurse provides oral hygiene and eye care every 4 hr, protecting the corneas with shields and isotonic eye drops. If the patient cannot vocalize, the nurse establishes alternative methods of communication, such as eye blink or letter boards. The patient's legs are inspected regularly for signs of thrombophlebitis, and antiembolism devices are applied and anticoagulants given if prescribed.

The nurse explains the syndrome and provides emotional support to the patient and family. Diversional activities are provided and encouraged.

As the patient regains strength and can tolerate a vertical position (usually using a tilt table), blood pressure and pulse are monitored. Devices such as thigh-high elastic stockings and abdominal binder are applied as necessary to prevent postural hypotension.

Before discharge, the nurse assists the patient and family to develop an appropriate home care plan and makes appropriate referrals for home care as necessary. The patient and family are also taught the skills required for home care or are referred for instruction. SEE: *Nursing Diagnoses Appendix*.

**guillotine** (gĭl'ō-tēn) [Fr., instrument for beheading] An instrument for excising tonsils and laryngeal growths.

**guilt** (gĭlt) An emotion resulting from doing what is thought to be wrong, associated with self-reproach and the need for punishment. An excess or absence of guilt characterizes various psychiatric disorders.

**guinea pig** (gĭn'ē pĭg) **1.** A small rodent used in laboratory research. **2.** A colloquial term for persons being used in medical experiments.

**guinea worm** *Dracunculus medinensis.*

**Gull's disease** [Sir William W. Gull, Brit. physician, 1816–1890] Atrophy of the thyroid gland, which causes myxedema.

**gullet** [L. *gula,* throat] The esophagus.

**Gullstrand's slit lamp** (gŭl′străndz) [Allvar Gullstrand, Swedish ophthalmologist, 1862–1930] A device for illuminating the eye so that its anterior portion can be examined by microscope.

**gum 1.** A substance given out by or extracted from certain plants. It is sticky when moist but hardens on drying. Roughly, gum is any resin-like substance produced by plants. **2.** The fleshy substance or tissue covering the alveolar processes of the jaws. SYN: *gingiva.*

DIAGNOSIS: *Bleeding:* If the gums bleed easily, scurvy or inflammation, as in trench mouth or pyorrhea, is indicated. Silver poisoning causes the gums to turn *blue;* mercurial stomatitis or lead poisoning turns the gums *bluish red,* with a bluish line at the edge of the teeth. A *greenish line* at the edge of the teeth may indicate copper poisoning. A *purplish line or color* indicates scurvy. In youth, gingivitis, pyorrhea, or scurvy may cause a *red line. Spongy gums and ulceration* may indicate gingivitis, scurvy, stomatitis, leukemia, tuberculosis, or diabetes.

**gumboil** A gum abscess. SYN: *parulis.*

SYMPTOMS: The gum is red, swollen, tender, and very painful. A fluctuating swelling containing pus may appear, which may point and break or require incision.

ETIOLOGY: The abscess may be caused by a subperiosteal infection associated with a carious tooth. It may also be caused by irritation or injury by a denture.

TREATMENT: The patient should receive hot mouthwashes and applications over the gum or externally. The patient should be warned not to swallow pus. Frequent mouthwashes should continue after the lesion is evacuated.

**gumma** (gŭm′mă) [L. *gummi,* gum] A soft granulomatous tumor of the tissues characteristic of the tertiary stage of syphilis. Varying from a millimeter to a centimeter or more in diameter, it may be single or multiple and tends to be encapsulated. It consists of a central necrotic mass surrounded by an inflammatory zone and fibrosis. The necrotic portion may be firm or elastic, gelatinous or hyalinized. Infectious organisms may be present. The tumor occurs most frequently in the liver but may occur in other areas, such as the brain, testis, heart, skin, and bone. SEE: *syphilis.*

SYMPTOMS: Symptoms vary depending on the gumma location. Bursting of a gumma leads to a gummatous ulcer that is painless but slow to heal. The base is formed by a "wash-leather" slough, but surrounding tissues are healthy.

**gummatous** (gŭm′ă-tŭs) Having the character of a gumma.

**gummose** (gŭm′ōs) $C_6H_{12}O_6$. A sugar from animal gum.

**gummy** [L. *gummi,* gum] Sticky, swollen, puffy.

**Gunn's dots** (gŭnz) [Robert Marcus Gunn, Brit. ophthalmologist, 1850–1909] White spots on the retina of the eye, close to the macula.

**Gunn's syndrome** SEE: *Marcus Gunn syndrome.*

**gunshot wound** SEE: *wound, bullet.*

**gunstock deformity** SEE: under *deformity.*

**Günther's disease** [Hans Günther, Ger. physician, 1884–1956] Congenital erythropoietic porphyria.

**gurney** (gĕr′nē) A litter, equipped with wheels, used in hospitals for transporting patients.

**gustation** (gŭs-tā′shŭn) [L. *gustare,* to taste] The sense of taste.

**gustatory** (gŭs′tă-tō-rē) Pert. to the sense of taste.

**gustometry** (gŭs-tŏm′ĕ-trē) [" + Gr. *metron,* measure] The measurement of the acuteness of the sense of taste.

**gut** [AS.] **1.** The bowel or intestine. **2.** The primitive gut or embryonic digestive tube, which includes the foregut, midgut, and hindgut. **3.** Short term for catgut.

**gut-associated lymphoid tissue** ABBR: GALT. A term used for all lymphoid tissue associated with the gastrointestinal tract, including the tonsils, appendix, and Peyer's patches. GALT contains lymphocytes, primarily B cells, and is responsible for controlling microorganisms entering the body via the digestive system.

**Guthrie test** [Robert Guthrie, U.S. microbiologist, 1916–1995] A diagnostic test to detect phenylketonuria (PKU). It is required by law in most states. SEE: *phenylketonuria.*

**gutta** [L., a drop] ABBR: gt. (pl. *gtt.*) A drop. The amount in a drop varies with the nature of the liquid and its temperature. It is therefore not advisable to use the number of drops per minute of a solution as anything more than a general guide to the amount of material being administered intravenously.

**gutta-percha** (gŭt″ă-pĕr′chă) The purified dried latex of certain trees, used in dentistry as a temporary filling.

**guttate** [L. *gutta,* drop] Resembling a drop, said of certain cutaneous lesions.

**guttatim** (gŭt-tā′tĭm) [L.] Drop by drop.

**guttering** (gŭt′ĕr-ĭng) Cutting a channel or groove in a bone.

**guttur** (gŭt′ŭr) [L. *gutter,* throat] The throat.

**guttural** (gŭt′ŭ-răl) Pert. to the throat.

**gutturotetany** (gŭt″ŭr-ō-tĕt′ă-nē) [″ + Gr. *tetanos,* tension] A laryngeal spasm of the throat with temporary stutter.

**Guyon's canal** A tunnel on the ulnar side of the wrist formed by the hook of the hamate and pisiform bones. The ulnar nerve may be compressed at this site in long-distance bicyclists, by falling on the wrist, or by repetitive wrist actions.

**Guyon's sign** (gē-yŏnz′) [Felix J. C. Guyon, Fr. surgeon, 1831–1920] Ballottement of the kidney.

**GVHR** *graft-versus-host reaction*.
**Gwathmey's method** (gwăth′mēz) [James T. Gwathmey, U.S. surgeon, 1863–1944] The use of an anesthetic, consisting of ether and olive oil solution, placed in the rectum and colon, where it is absorbed.
**Gy** *gray* (unit of measure).
**gymnastics** [Gr. *gymnastikos,* pert. to nakedness] Systematic body exercise with or without special apparatus.

***ocular g.*** Systematic exercise of the eye muscles to improve muscular coordination and efficiency.

***Swedish g.*** A system of movements made by the patient against a resistance provided by the attendant, which was once used worldwide. It influenced the development of modern gymnastics.

**gymnophobia** (jĭm-nō-fō′bē-ă) [Gr. *gymnos,* naked, + *phobos,* fear] An abnormal aversion to viewing a naked body.
**gyn-** SEE: *gyneco-*.
**gynander** (jĭ-năn′dĕr, jī-, gī-) [Gr. *gyne,* woman, + *aner, andros,* man] Pseudohermaphrodite.
**gynandrism** (jĭ-năn′drĭzm) **1.** Male hermaphroditism. **2.** Partial female pseudohermaphroditism.
**gynandroid** (jĭ-năn′droyd, jī-, gī-) [″ + ″ + *eidos,* form, shape] An individual having sufficient hermaphroditic sexual characteristics to be mistaken for a person of the opposite sex.
**gynatresia** (jĭ-nă-trē′zē-ă, jī-, gī-) [″ + *a-,* not, + *tresis,* perforation] Congenital absence or closure of the vagina.
**gyne-** SEE: *gyneco-*.
**gynecic** (jĭ-nē′sĭk, jī, gī-) [Gr. *gyne,* woman] Pert. to women.
**gyneco-, gyno-, gyn-, gyne-** [Gr.] Combining form meaning *woman, female*.
**gynecogenic** (jĭn″ĕ-kō-jĕn′ĭk) [Gr. *gyne,* woman, + *gennan,* to produce] Producing female characteristics.
**gynecoid** (jĭn′ĕ-koyd) [″ + *eidos,* form, shape] Resembling the female of the species.
**gynecologic, gynecological** (gī″nĕ-kŏ-lŏj′ĭk, jī″-, jĭn″ĕ-; -ĭ-kăl) [″ + *logos,* word, reason] Pert. to gynecology, the study of diseases specific to women.
**gynecological operative procedures** Examination and surgery involving the femal reproductive tract. Included are pelvic examination, dilation and curettage, hysterectomy, tubal ligation, cautery of the cervix, and cesarean section.

NURSING IMPLICATIONS: *Preoperative:* The patient is prepared physically and emotionally for the procedure.

*Postoperative:* Vital signs are monitored frequently in the immediate postoperative period. If they deteriorate, the patient is assessed for shock or internal hemorrhage. Abdominal dressings are inspected for drainage, the presence of surgical drains is noted, the incision is assessed and redressed, and any vaginal drainage or perineal sutures are managed. A calm, quiet environment and light blankets are provided.

Ventilatory function is monitored; the patient is encouraged to breathe deeply and cough, and to use an inspirometer if prescribed, esp. if general anesthesia was used. Fluid and electrolyte balance is monitored, and intravenous fluid intake is maintained as prescribed until oral intake (clear liquids) is permitted and tolerated.

The nurse gently palpates and percusses the urinary bladder for evidence of urinary retention, offers the bedpan frequently to encourage urination, and documents the time and amount of each voiding. Intermittent catheterization is instituted for urinary retention (allowing no more than 12 hr to pass without urine output immediately postoperatively, then no more than 8 hr until the patient is able to void). Closed, continuous drainage is maintained via an indwelling catheter if the surgeon prefers or if the patient continues to be unable to void. The nurse assesses bowel activity and provides stool softeners as prescribed.

The nurse regularly assesses for signs of thrombophlebitis, encourages active leg exercises, and applies antiembolism stockings or pneumatic boots as prescribed. Early ambulation is encouraged.

**gynecologist** (gī″nĕ-kŏl′ō-jĭst, jī″-, jĭn″ĕ-) A physician who specializes in gynecology.
**gynecology** (gī″nĕ-kŏl′ō-jē, jī″-, jĭn″ĕ-) [″ + *logos,* word, reason] The study of the diseases of the female reproductive organs and the breasts.
**gynecomastia** (jī″nĕ-kō-măs′tē-ă, gī″-, jĭn″ĕ-) [″ + *mastos,* breast] Enlargement of breast tissue in the male. This may occur during three distinct age periods: transiently at birth, again beginning with puberty and declining during the late teenage years, and finally in adults between 50 and 80 years of age. The condition may be benign or may be associated with any one of a variety of clinical conditions or drugs.

TREATMENT: Therapy will depend on the cause, but it is important to keep in mind that gynecomastia has a high rate of spontaneous regression, and medical therapies are most effective during the active proliferative phase.

**gynecopathy** (jī-nĕ-kŏp′ă-thē, gī″-, jĭn″ĕ-) [″ *pathos,* disease, suffering] Diseases specific to women.
**gynecophonus** (jī″nĕ-kŏf′ŏn-ŭs, gī″-, jĭn″ĕ-) [″ + *phone,* voice] Having an effeminate voice.
**gynephobia** (jī″nĕ-fō′bē-ă, gī″-, jĭn″ĕ-) [″ + *phobos,* fear] An abnormal aversion to the company of women, or fear of them. **gynephobic,** *adj*.
**gynesic** (gī-nē′sĭk, jī-, jĭn-ē′-) [Gr. *gyne,* woman] Pert. to diseases of the female reproductive organs and breasts.
**gyno-** SEE: *gyneco-*.

**gynopathic** [" + *pathos,* disease, suffering] Pert. to diseases of the female reproductive organs and breasts.

**gynoplastics** [" + *plassein,* to form] Reparative surgery of the female genitalia.

**gypsies** A tightly knit cultural group whose origins were in India more than 500 years ago. They have migrated to Europe and the U.S. Many gypsies are nomadic. Medically they are prone to develop hypertension, diabetes, and occlusive vascular disease, some part of which may be related to their practice of inbreeding.

**gypsum** (jĭp'sŭm) [L.; G. *gypsos,* chalk] **1.** A natural form of hydrated calcium sulfate. When heated to 130°C, it loses its water and becomes plaster of paris. **2.** A hemihydrate of gypsum resulting from heating gypsum and allowing it to dehydrate in the presence of sodium succinate or calcium hydrochloride. This form is used as a dental stone in preparing investments for dental casting.

**gyrate** (jī'rāt) [Gr. *gyros,* circle] **1.** Ring-shaped, convoluted. **2.** To revolve.

**gyration** (jī-rā'shŭn) A rotary movement.

**gyre** (jīr) [Gr. *gyros,* circle] Gyrus.

**gyrectomy** (jī-rĕk'tō-mē) [" + *ektome,* excision] Surgical removal of a cerebral gyrus.

**gyrencephalic** (jī-rĕn-sĕ-făl'ĭk) [" + *enkephale,* head] Having a brain marked by numerous convolutions.

**gyri** (jī'rī) Pl. of gyrus.

**gyro-** [Gr.] Combining form meaning *circle, spiral, ring.*

**gyroma** (jī-rō'mă) [Gr. *gyros,* circle, + *oma,* tumor] An ovarian tumor consisting of a convoluted mass.

**gyrometer** (jī-rŏm'ĕ-ter) [" + *metron,* measure] A device for measuring the cerebral gyri of the brain.

**gyrose** (jī'rōs) In bacteriology, marked by circular or wavy lines. This term is applied to bacterial colonies.

**gyrospasm** (jī'rō-spăzm) [" + *spasmos,* a convulsion] A spasmodic rotary head movement.

**gyrus** (jī'rŭs) *pl.* **gyri** One of the convolutions of the cerebral hemispheres of the brain. The gyri are separated by shallow grooves (sulci) or deeper grooves (fissures). SYN: *gyre.* SEE: *convolution.*

***angular g.*** A gyrus of the parietal lobe that embraces the posterior end of the superior temporal sulcus.

***annectent g.*** Any of many short folds of gray matter formed as a result of short branches or twigs of sulci extending into adjacent gyri. They are not always present.

***anterior central g.*** A gyrus of the frontal lobe extending vertically between the precentral and central sulci.

***g.'s breves insulae*** Preinsular gyri of the brain.

***Broca's g.*** Inferior frontal g.

***callosal g.*** A large gyrus on the medial surface of the cerebral hemisphere that lies directly above the corpus callosum and arches over its anterior end.

***g. cerebelli*** A layer of the cerebellum.

***cingulate g.*** An arch-shaped convolution of the cingulum, curved over the surface of the corpus callosum, from which it is separated by the callosal sulcus.

***dentate g.*** A gyrus marked by indentations that lie on the upper surface of the hippocampal gyrus.

***g. fornicatus*** A gyrus on the medial surface of the cerebrum, which includes the gyrus cinguli, isthmus, hippocampus, hippocampal gyrus, and uncus.

***fusiform g.*** A gyrus beneath the collateral fissure joining the occipital and temporal lobes. SYN: *occipitotemporal g.*

***Heschl's g.*** A transverse temporal gyrus.

***hippocampal g.*** A gyrus between the hippocampal and collateral fissures.

***inferior frontal g.*** A convolution on the external surface of the frontal lobe of the cerebrum located between the sylvian fissure and the inferior frontal sulcus. SYN: *Broca's g.*

***lingual g.*** A gyrus between the calcarine and collateral fissures.

***g. longus insulae*** A lengthy gyrus composing the postinsula.

***middle frontal g.*** A gyrus between the superior and inferior frontal sulci.

***middle temporal g.*** A gyrus between the middle temporal sulcus and superior temporal sulcus.

***occipital g.*** Any of the gyri on the lateral surface of the occipital lobe. They are classified roughly into two groups, the inferior or lateral occipital gyri and the superior occipital gyri. They are not always present.

***occipitotemporal g.*** Fusiform g.

***orbital g.*** One of four gyri (anterior, posterior, lateral, and medial) forming the inferior surface of the frontal lobe.

***paracentral g.*** The area on the mesial aspect of the cerebrum; the paracentral lobule. It lies above the cingulate sulcus.

***parahippocampal g.*** A gyrus on the lower surface of each cerebral hemisphere between the hippocampal and collateral sulci.

***paraterminal g.*** A small area of the cerebral cortex anterior to the lamina terminalis and below the rostrum of the corpus callosum.

***parietal g.*** A gyrus on the lateral aspect of the parietal lobe. It includes the posterior central gyrus and the superior and inferior parietal gyri.

***postcentral g.*** A gyrus immediately posterior to the central sulcus of the cerebrum. It contains most of the general sensory area of the brain. SYN: *posterior central g.*

***posterior central g.*** Postcentral g.

***precentral g.*** A gyrus immediately anterior to the central sulcus of the cerebrum. It contains the motor area for initiation of voluntary movement.

***g. profundus cerebri*** One of the very deep gyri of the cerebrum.

***g. rectus*** A gyrus on the orbital aspect of the frontal lobe, located between the mesial margin and the olfactory sulcus.

***Retzius g.*** The supracallosal and subcallosal gyri.

***subcallosal g.*** A narrow band of gray matter on the medial surface of the hemisphere below the rostrum of the corpus callosum.

***superior frontal g.*** A convolution of the cerebral frontal lobe situated above the superfrontal fissure.

***supracallosal g.*** A rudimentary gyrus on the upper surface of the corpus callosum.

***supracallosus g.*** The gray matter layer covering the corpus callosum.

***supramarginal g.*** A gyrus in the inferior parietal lobule twisting about the upper terminus of the sylvian fissure.

***temporal g.*** One of the three gyri (superior, middle, inferior) on the lateral surface of the temporal lobe.

***uncinate g.*** The anterior hooked portion of the hippocampal gyrus.

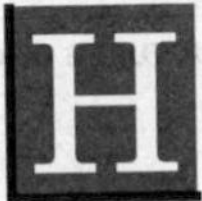

**H** Symbol for the element hydrogen.

**H, h** *haustus,* a draft of medicine; *height; henry; hora* or *hour; horizontal; hypermetropia.*

**h** Symbol for hecto, a term used in SI units.

***h.*** Symbol for Planck's constant.

**H+** Symbol for hydrogen ion.

**[H+** Symbol for hydrogen ion concentration.

**¹H** Symbol for protium.

**²H** Symbol for deuterium, an isotope of hydrogen.

**Ha** Symbol for hahnium.

**HAA** *hepatitis-associated antigen.*

**Haab's reflex** (hŏbz) [Otto Haab, Swiss ophthalmologist, 1850–1931] Contraction of pupils without alteration of accommodation or convergence when gazing at a bright object. It may indicate a cortical lesion.

**HaAg** *hepatitis A antigen.*

**habena** (hă-bē'nă) *pl.* **habenae** [L., rein] **1.** A frenum. **2.** Habenula. **habenal, habenar,** *adj.*

**habenula** (hă-bĕn'ū-lă) *pl.* **habenulae** [L., little rein, strap] **1.** A frenum or any reinlike or whiplike structure. **2.** A peduncle or stalk attached to the pineal body of the brain. Fibers that travel posteriorly along the dorsomedial border of the thalamus to the habenular ganglia (epithalamus) resemble reins. **3.** A narrow bandlike stricture. **habenular,** *adj.*

***h. urethralis*** One of two whitish bands between the clitoris and meatus urethra in young females.

**habenular** Pert. to the habenula, esp. the stalk of the pineal body.

***h. commissure*** A band of transverse fibers connecting the two habenular areas.

***h. trigone*** A depressed triangular area located on the lateral aspect of the posterior portion of the third ventricle. It contains a medial and lateral habenular nucleus.

**habilitation** (hă-bĭl″ĭ-tā'shŭn) The process of educating or training persons with disadvantage or disability to improve their ability to function in society.

**habit** [L. *habere, habitus,* to have, hold] **1.** A motor pattern executed with facility following constant or frequent repetition; an act performed at first in a voluntary manner but after sufficient repetition as a reflex action. Habits result from the passing of impulses through a particular set of neurons and synapses many times. **2.** A particular type of dress or garb. **3.** Mental or moral constitution or disposition. **4.** Bodily appearance or constitution, esp. as related to a disease or predisposition to a disease. SYN: *habitus* (1). **5.** Addiction to the use of drugs or alcohol (e.g., the drug habit or alcohol habit).

***chorea h.*** Habit spasm.

***h. disorder*** SEE: under *disorder.*

***masticatory h.*** An individual's sequence and pattern of jaw movement in chewing. It is influenced by the type of food, occlusal problems or missing teeth, personal habits, or state of mind and may be unilateral or bilateral. Under some conditions it would be recognized as clenching or bruxing habit. SEE: *bruxism.*

***h. spasm*** SEE: under *spasm.*

***h. training*** SEE: under *training.*

**habituation** The act of becoming accustomed to anything from frequent use or exposure. In drug addiction, the mental equivalent of physical tolerance and dependence on drugs.

**habitus** [L., habit] **1.** A physical appearance, body build, or attitude. **2.** A physical appearance that indicates a tendency for a person to develop a specific disease. SYN: *habit* (4).

**hachement** (hăsh-mŏn') [Fr., chopping] In massage, a chopping stroke with the edge of the hand.

**haem-** SEE: *hem-.*

**Haemadipsa** (hē″mă-dĭp'să) [Gr. *haima,* blood + *dipsa,* thirst] A genus of terrestrial leeches found in Asia that attach to humans and animals.

***H. ceylonica*** A species of leech found in certain humid, tropical areas.

**Haemagogus** (hē″mă-gŏg'ŭs) [″ + *agogos,* leading] A genus of mosquitoes that includes species that serve as vectors of yellow fever endemic in the Amazon region of South America. It is similar to *Aedes* species.

**Haemaphysalis** (hĕm″ă-fĭs'ă-lĭs) [″ + *physallis,* bubble] A genus of ticks including species that serve as vectors for tick-borne viral diseases including hemorrhagic fever.

**Haemophilus** (hē-mŏf'ĭl-ŭs) [″ + *philein,* to love] A genus of bacteria that require the growth factor X or V, or both, provided by blood. The small, nonmotile, gram-negative bacteria do not form spores. Because the V factor is destroyed by enzymes present in unheated red blood cells, chocolate agar is the preferred culture medium.

***H. aegyptius*** Koch-Weeks bacillus; the cause of one form of contagious conjunctivitis.

***H. ducreyi*** The causative organism of chancroid or soft chancre. SEE: *chancroid.*

***H. influenzae*** An organism found in respiratory infections and formerly thought to be the cause of influenza. It is a caus-

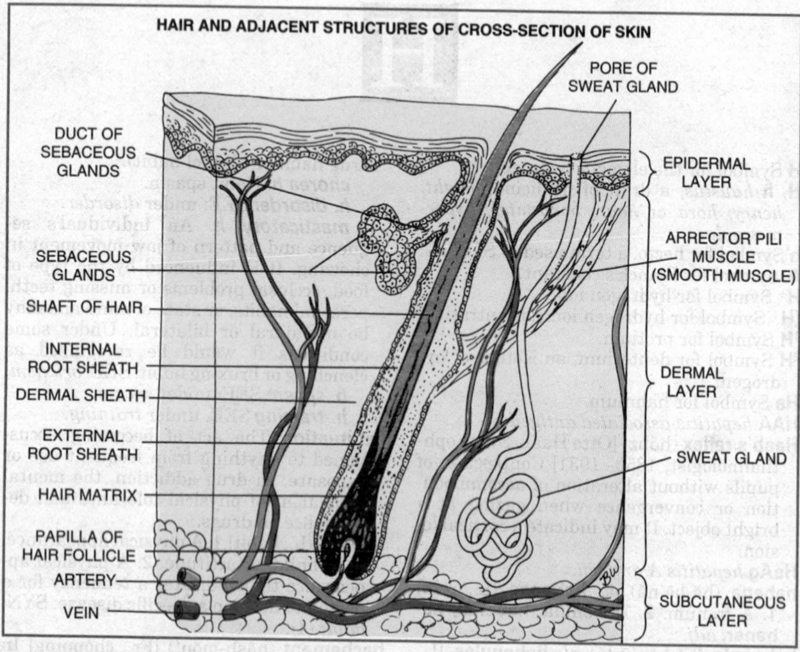


ative organism of respiratory infections, septicemia, and meningitis.

***H. influenzae type b infection*** ABBR: HIB. An important cause of meningitis, unusually in infants. In children, this organism also causes acute epiglottitis, pneumonia, septic arthritis, and cellulitis.

TREATMENT: A cephalosporin that penetrates into the cerebrospinal fluid, such as cefotaxime or ceftriaxone, should be used.

PREVENTION: Administer the form of HIB vaccine conjugated to an immunogenic protein carrier in three or four doses beginning at 2 months of age. Because the various forms of HIB vaccine are administered on different schedules, it is important to check the package insert for the appropriate scheduling information. Booster doses may be required. SEE: *vaccine* for table.

***H. vaginalis*** The former name for *Gardnerella vaginalis,* a bacterium that causes vaginitis.

**Haemosporidia** (hē″mō-spō-rĭd′ē-ă) An order of sporozoa that live in the blood cells of vertebrates and reproduce sexually in invertebrates; includes the genus *Plasmodium,* which causes malaria in humans.

**hafnium** (hăf′nē-ŭm) [L. *Hafnia,* Copenhagen] SYMB: Hf. A rare chemical element; atomic weight 178.49, atomic number 72, specific gravity 13.31.

**Hagedorn needle** (hă′gĕ-dorn) [Werner Hagedorn, Ger. surgeon, 1831–1894] A curved surgical needle with flattened sides.

**hahnium** (hăhn′ē-ŭm) [Named after Otto Hahn, Ger. scientist, 1879–1968] SYMB: Ha. Name proposed for the artificially made element 105.

**Hailey-Hailey disease** [W. H. Hailey, 1898–1967; H. E. Hailey, b. 1909, U.S. dermatologists] Benign familial pemphigus.

**hair** [AS. *haer*] **1.** A keratinized, threadlike outgrowth from the skin of mammals. **2.** Collectively, the threadlike outgrowths that form the fur of animals or that grow on the human body.

A hair is a thin, flexible shaft of cornified cells that develops from a cylindrical invagination of the epidermis, the hair follicle. Each consists of a free portion or shaft (scapus pili) and a root (radix pili) embedded within the follicle. The shaft consists of three layers of cells: the cuticle or outermost layer; the cortex, forming the main horny portion of the hair; and the medulla, the central axis. Hair color is due to pigment in the cortex. SEE: illus.

Hair in each part of the body has a definite period of growth, after which it is shed. In the adult human there is a constant gradual loss and replacement of hair. Hair of the eyebrows lasts only 3 to 5 months; that of the scalp 2 to 5 years. Baldness or alopecia results when replacement fails to keep up with hair loss. It may be hereditary or due to pathologic conditions such as infections or injury from irradiation. Also cytotoxic agents used in cancer chemotherapy may cause temporary loss of hair. SEE: *alopecia.*

***auditory h.*** An epithelial cell to which are attached delicate hairlike processes. These are present in the ear in the spiral organ of Corti, concerned with hearing; and in the crista ampullaris, macula utriculi, and macula sacculi, concerned with equilibrium.

***bamboo h.*** Trichorrhexis nodosa.

***beaded h.*** Swellings and constrictions in the hair shaft caused by a developmental defect known as monilethrix.

***burrowing h.*** A hair that grows horizontally under the skin, causing a foreign body reaction.

***gustatory h.*** One of several fine hairlike processes extending from the ends of gustatory cells in a taste bud. They project through the inner pore of a taste bud. SYN: *taste h.*

***ingrown h.*** A hair that reenters the skin, causing a foreign body reaction.

***kinky h.*** Short, sparse, kinky hair that may be poorly pigmented. The condition is associated with kinky hair disease.

***lanugo h.*** SEE: *lanugo.*

***moniliform h.*** Monilethrix.

***h. papilla*** A projection of the corium that extends into the hair bulb at the bottom of a hair follicle. It contains capillaries through which a hair receives nourishment.

***pubic h.*** Hair that appears over the pubes at the onset of sexual maturity.

***sensory h.*** Specialized epithelial cells with hairlike processes.

***tactile h.*** Hair that is capable of receiving tactile or touching stimuli.

***taste h.*** Gustatory h.

***terminal h.*** The long, coarse, pigmented hair of the adult.

***twisted h.*** Congenitally deformed hair that is short, brittle, and twisted.

**hair analysis** SEE: under *analysis.*

**hairball** Trichobezoar.

**hair bulb** SEE: under *bulb.*

**hair cell** SEE: under *cell.*

**hair follicle** SEE: under *follicle.*

**hair transplantation** SEE: under *transplantation.*

**hairy tongue** SEE: under *tongue.*

**halation** (hăl-ā′shŭn) [Gr. *alos,* a halo] A blurring of vision caused by light being scattered to the side of the source.

**halazone** (hăl′ă-zōn) A chloramine disinfectant. SEE: *water, emergency preparation of safe drinking.*

**Haldane effect** The oxygenation of hemoglobin, which lowers its affinity for carbon dioxide. SEE: *Bohr effect.*

**half-life 1.** Time required for half the nuclei of a radioactive substance to lose their activity by undergoing radioactive decay. **2.** Time it takes for a radioactive substance to reduce to one-half its energy due to metabolism and excretion. **3.** In biology and pharmacology, the time required by the body, tissue, or organ to metabolize or inactivate half the amount of a substance taken in. This is an important consideration in determining the proper amount and frequency of dose of drug to be administered. **4.** Time required for radioactivity of material taken in by a living organism to be reduced to half its initial value by a combination of radioactive decay and biological elimination.

**half-value layer** ABBR: HVL. The amount of lead, copper, cement, or material that would dissipate the beam of radiation by 50%. The number of half-value layers required for safety in blocking the area on a patient is five, because that represents 50% of 50% and 50% of that, and so forth. For example, 50% + 25% + 12.5% + 6.23% + 3.12% = 96.9%. Thus the patient would be shielded from all but about 3% of the radiation. (Examples of the thickness of material required to protect from radiation are 2 in. [5 cm] of lead or 2 ft [61 cm] of cement.)

**half-value thickness** The thickness of a substance that, when placed in the path of a given beam of rays, will lower its intensity to one half of the initial value.

**halfway house** A facility to house psychiatric patients who no longer need hospitalization but are not yet ready for independent living.

**halide** (hăl′īd) A compound containing a halogen (i.e., bromine, chlorine, fluorine, or iodine) combined with a metal or some other radical.

**halitosis** (hăl-ĭ-tō′sĭs) [L. *halitus,* breath, + Gr. *osis,* condition] Bad breath.

**halitus** (hăl′ĭ-tŭs) **1.** The breath. **2.** Warm vapor.

**Haller's anastomotic circle** (hăl′ĕrz) [Albrecht von Haller, Swiss physiologist, 1708–1777] The circle of arteries around the intraocular portion of the optic nerve. It is composed of branches of the posterior ciliary arteries.

**Hallervorden-Spatz disease, H.-S. syndrome** [Julius Hallervorden, 1882–1965; H. Spatz, 1888–1969, Ger. neurologists] An inherited, progressive, degenerative disease, beginning in childhood, of the globus pallidus, red nucleus, and reticular part of the substantia nigra of the brain. Clinically, characteristics include progressive rigidity, retinal degeneration, athetotic movements, and mental and, late in the disease, emotional retardation. There is no effective therapy.

**hallex** (hăl′ĕks) *pl.* **hallices** [L.] Hallux.

**Hallpike maneuver** [C. Hallpike, 20th century neurologist] A test performed to diagnose benign positional vertigo. The patient is moved from a sitting position to recumbency with the head tilted down 30° over the end of the bed and then 30° to one side. If a paroxysm of vertigo occurs, the test is positive. SEE: *vertigo, benign positional.*

**hallucination** (hă-loo-sĭ-nā′shŭn) [L. *hallucinari,* to wander in mind] In psychology, a false perception having no relation to reality and not accounted for by any exterior stimuli. It may be visual, tactile, auditory, gustatory, or olfactory. The patient's judgment may be impaired and he or she will not be able to distinguish between the real and the imagined.

Structural disease of the sensory organ and conducting mechanism may contribute to the formation of hallucinations (e.g., deafness following otitis media often is associated with tinnitus). An irritative lesion of the visual cortex may also produce hallucinations.

***auditory h.*** An imaginary perception of sounds, usually voices.

***extracampine h.*** A hallucination that arises from outside the normal sensory field or range, as people having the sensation of seeing something behind them.

***gustatory h.*** The sense of tasting something that is not present.

***haptic h.*** A hallucination pert. to touching the skin or to sensations of temperature or pain.

***hypnagogic h.*** A presleep phenomenon having the same practical significance as a dream but experienced during consciousness. It may include a sense of falling, of sinking, or of the ceiling moving.

***kinetic h.*** A sensation of flying or of moving the body or a part of it.

***microptic h.*** A hallucination in which things seem smaller.

***motor h.*** An imagined perception of movement.

***olfactory h.*** A hallucination involving the sense of smell.

***somatic h.*** A sensation of pain attributed to visceral injury.

***stump h.*** SEE: *phantom limb.*

***tactile h.*** A false sense of touching something.

***visual h.*** The sensation of seeing objects that are not really there.

**hallucinogen** (hă-loo′sĭ-nō-jĕn) [″ + Gr. *gennan,* to produce] A drug that produces hallucinations (e.g., LSD, peyote, mescaline, PCP, and sometimes ethyl alcohol).

**hallucinosis** (hă-loo″sĭn-ō′sĭs) [″ + Gr. *osis,* condition] The state of having hallucinations more or less persistently. SEE: *hallucination.*

***acute alcoholic h.*** Alcoholic psychosis marked by fear or anxiety and auditory hallucinations.

**hallus** Hallux.

**hallux** (hăl′ŭks) *pl.* **halluces** [L.] The great toe.

***h. dolorosus*** Pain in the metatarsophalangeal joint of the great toe resulting from flatfoot.

***h. flexus*** H. malleus.

***h. malleus*** Hammertoe of the great toe.

***h. rigidus*** A restriction or loss of motion of the joint connecting the great toe to the metatarsal. Pain occurs upon walking.

***h. valgus*** Displacement of the great toe toward the other toes.

***h. varus*** Displacement of the great toe away from the other toes.

**halo** [Gr. *halos,* a halo] **1.** The areola, esp. of the nipple. **2.** A ring surrounding the macula lutea in ophthalmoscopic images. **3.** A circle of light surrounding a shining body.

***Fick's h.*** A colored halo around light observed by some persons as a result of wearing contact lenses.

***glaucomatous h.*** The visual perception of rainbow-like colors around lights, caused by glaucoma-induced corneal edema.

***senile peripapillary h.*** A ring of choroidoretinal atrophy around the head of the optic nerve, a condition that may occur in the aged.

***h. symptom*** The perception of one or more colored circles around lights, seen by patients with glaucoma or with punctate lens opacities.

**halodermia** (hăl″ō-dĕr′mē-ă) A skin eruption caused by exposure to a halogen.

**halogen** (hăl′ō-jĕn) [Gr. *hals,* salt, + *gennan,* to produce] Any one of the elements (chlorine, bromine, iodine, fluorine, and astatine) forming Group VII of the periodic table. These elements have very similar chemical properties, combining with hydrogen to form acids and with metals to form salts.

**haloid** (hăl′oyd) [″ + *eidos,* form, shape] Resembling salt or a halogen.

**haloid salt** SEE: under *salt.*

**haloperidol** (hă″lō-pĕr′ĭ-dŏl) An antipsychotic drug used to treat psychotic disorders (e.g., schizophrenia) and Tourette's syndrome. Trade name is Haldol.

**halophilic** (hăl″ō-fĭl′ĭk) [″ + *philein,* to love] Concerning or having an affinity for salt or any halogen.

**halothane** (hăl′ō-thān) A fluorinated hydrocarbon used as a general anesthetic.

**Halsted's operation** (hăl′stĕdz) [William Stewart Halsted, U.S. surgeon, 1852–1922] **1.** An operation for inguinal hernia. **2.** A radical mastectomy for cancer of the breast.

**Halsted's suture** An interrupted suture for intestinal wounds.

**ham** [AS. *haum,* haunch] **1.** The popliteal space or region behind the knee. **2.** A common name for the thigh, hip, and buttock.

**hamartoma** (hăm-ăr-tō′mă) [Gr. *hamartia,* defect, + *oma,* tumor] A tumor resulting from new growth of normal tissues. The cells grow spontaneously, reach maturity, and then do not reproduce. Thus, the growth is self-limiting and benign.

***multiple h.*** A congenital malformation that presents a slowly growing mass of abnormal tissue in multiple sites. The tissues are appropriate to the organ in which the hamartomas are located but are not normally organized. They may appear in blood vessels as hemangiomata, and in the lung and kidney. They are not malignant but cause symptoms because of the space they occupy.

**hamartomatosis** (hăm″ăr-tō-mă-tō′sĭs) [″ +

" + *osis,* condition] Existence of multiple hamartomas.

**hamate** (hăm′ăt) Hooked; unciform. SYN: *hamular.*

***h. bone*** The medial bone in the distal row of carpal bones of the wrist. SYN: *hamatum; os hamatum; unciform bone.*

**hamatum** (hă-mā′tŭm) [L. *hamatus,* hooked] Hamate bone.

**hamaxophobia** [Gr. *amaxa,* a carriage, + *phobos,* fear] A fear of riding in a vehicle.

**Hamman, Louis** (hăm′ăn) U.S. physician, 1877–1946.

***H.'s disease*** Spontaneous mediastinal emphysema.

***H.'s syndrome*** Previously used term for idiopathic pulmonary fibrosis.

**hammer 1.** An instrument with a head attached crosswise to the handle for striking blows. **2.** The common name for the malleus, the hammer-shaped bone of the middle ear.

***dental h.*** A mallet or motor-driven hammer used for condensing direct-filling gold or silver amalgam during the placement of fillings in teeth.

***percussion h.*** A hammer with a rubber head used for tapping surfaces of the body in order to produce sounds for diagnostic purposes. SEE: *plexor.*

***reflex h.*** A hammer used for tapping body parts such as a muscle, tendon, or nerve in order to initiate certain reflex responses.

**hammer finger** A flexion deformity of the distal joint of a finger, caused by avulsion of the extensor tendon. SYN: *mallet finger.*

**hammertoe** A toe with dorsal flexion of the first phalanx and plantar flexion of the second and third phalanges. SYN: *hallux malleus.*

**hamster** A rodent, *Cricetus cricetus,* belonging to the family Cricetidae, common in Europe and western Asia. It is extensively used in medical research.

**hamstring** [AS. *haum,* haunch] **1.** One of the tendons that form the medial and lateral boundaries of the popliteal space. **2.** Any one of three muscles on the posterior aspect of the thigh, the semitendinosus, semimembranosus, and biceps femoris. They flex the leg and adduct and extend the thigh.

***inner h.*** One of the tendons of the semimembranosus, semitendinosus, and gracilis muscles.

***outer h.*** A tendon of the biceps femoris.

**Ham test** A test for diagnosing paroxysmal nocturnal hemoglobinuria, in which the red cells are assessed for resistance to lysis during incubation with acidified serum.

**hamular** (hăm′ū-lăr) [L. *hamulus,* a small hook] Hamate.

**hamulus** (hăm′ū-lŭs) *pl.* **hamuli** [L., a small hook] **1.** Any hook-shaped structure. **2.** The hooklike process on the hamate bone.

***h. cochleae*** The hooklike process at the tip of the osseous spiral lamina of the cochlea.

***h. lacrimalis*** The hooklike process on the lacrimal bone.

***h. pterygoideus*** The hooklike process at the tip of the medial pterygoid process of the sphenoid bone.

**hand** [AS.] The body part attached to the forearm at the wrist. It includes the wrist (carpus) with its eight bones, the metacarpus or body of the hand (ossa metacarpalia) having five bones, and the fingers (phalanges) with their 14 bones. In some occupations and recreational endeavors, workers use their hands as hammers, which may damage the ulnar nerve and artery, with consequent signs of ischemia and neuropathy. SYN: *manus.* SEE: illus.

***ape h.*** A deformity of the hand in which the thumb is permanently extended, usually caused by a median nerve injury. Paralysis and atrophy of the thenar muscles result.

***claw h.*** Clawhand.

***cleft h.*** A deformity of the hand in which the division between the fingers, particularly between the third and fourth, extends into the carpus.

***drop h.*** Wrist drop.

***functional position of h.*** The principle used in splint fabrication whereby the wrist is dorsiflexed 20 to 35 degrees, a normal transverse arch is maintained, and the thumb is in abduction and opposition and aligned with the pads of the four fingers. Proximal interphalangeal joints are flexed 45 to 60 degrees.

***lobster-claw h.*** Cleft h.

***obstetrician's h.*** The position of the hand in tetany with extension at the metacarpophalangeal and the interphalangeal joints, and adduction of the thumb. It is named for the position of the obstetrician's hand during vaginal examination.

***opera-glass h.*** A deformity of the hand caused by chronic arthritis in which the phalanges appear to be telescoped into one another like an opera glass.

***resting position of h.*** The principle used in splint fabrication whereby the forearm is midway between pronation and supination, the wrist is at 12 to 20 degrees dorsiflexion, and the phalanges are slightly flexed. The thumb is in partial opposition and forward.

***writing h.*** A deformity of the hand in which the tips of the thumb and first finger are touching and the other fingers are flexed as if holding a writing instrument. This is seen in paralysis agitans.

**H. and E.** *hematoxylin* and *eosin,* a stain used in histology.

**handedness** The tendency to use one hand in preference to the other. Preferential use of the left hand is called sinistrality and of the right hand dextrality.

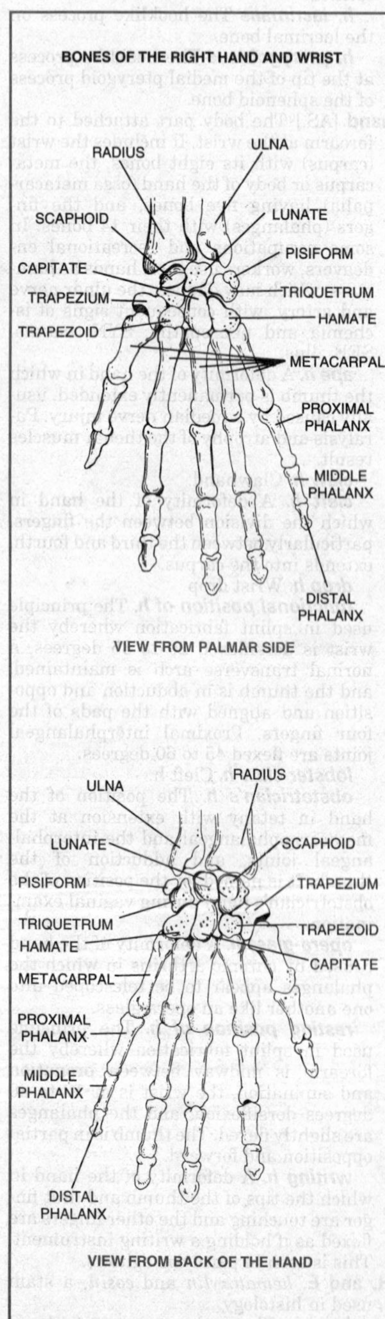


More than 90% of people are right-handed. Being left-handed may be hereditary or due to disease of the left cerebral hemisphere in early life. Left hemisphere dominance for language occurs in 95% of right-handed people and in 50% of those who are left-handed. A disturbance in language is produced in almost all right-handed persons by unilateral brain damage that affects the left hemisphere.

**hand-foot-and-mouth disease** A highly infectious disease characterized by painful ulcerative and vesicular lesions of the oral mucosa and tongue with vesicular lesions of the hands and feet. Various types of coxsackievirus group A, esp. type 16, and enterovirus 71 are the usual etiological agents. The disease is self limiting; however, infant death has occurred in rare cases.

**handicap** A disadvantage for a given individual, resulting from an impairment or disability, that limits or prevents the fulfillment of a role that is normal, depending on age, sex, and social and cultural factors, for that individual. SEE: *disability*.

**handle, built-up** The portion of an implement that has been increased in diameter to accommodate its use by persons with limited or weak grasp.

**handpiece** (hănd′pēs) A hand instrument used in dentistry. It contains a chuck for holding tools used in preparing teeth for restoration, polishing, and condensing. The tool may rotate or vibrate.

***air-bearing turbine h.*** A handpiece driven by compressed air, having a turbine and air bearings and capable of rotary speeds up to 400,000 rpm.

***contra-angle h.*** A handpiece with one or more bends so that the shaft of the rotary instrument is at an angle to the handpiece to reach less accessible areas of the mouth for dental work.

***high-speed h.*** A handpiece that operates at speeds about 12,000 rpm.

**Hand-Schüller-Christian disease** (hănd-shĭl′ĕr-krĭs′chăn) [Alfred Hand, Jr., U.S. pediatrician, 1868–1949; Artur Schüller, Austrian neurologist, b. 1874; Henry A. Christian, U.S. physician, 1876–1951] A rare disease of unknown cause in which lipids accumulate in the body and manifest as histiocytic granulomas in bone (particularly the skull), the skin, and viscera. Exophthalmos and diabetes insipidus may be present. The disease is seen in children and young adults. Adrenal cortical hormones have been of some help in treating the illness. SEE: *histiocytosis, Langerhans cell*.

**handsock** A type of glove that covers the hand but, because it has no individual spaces for the fingers, makes grasping objects difficult. Use of handsocks during infancy may inhibit the rate of development of hand skills.

**hanging drop culture** SEE: under *culture*.

**hangman's fracture** SEE: under *fracture.*

**hangnail** [AS. *ang-*, tight, painful, + *naegel,* nail] Partly detached piece of skin at root or lateral edge of finger or toenail.

**hangover** A nontechnical term for describing the malaise that may be present after ingestion of a considerable amount of an alcoholic beverage or other central nervous system depressant. Symptoms usually present upon awakening from a stuporous sleep include some if not all of the following: mental depression, headache, thirst, nausea, irritability, fatigue. Symptoms and their severity will vary with the individual. The presence of congeners in alcoholic beverages is thought to be related to the development of a hangover. There is no specific therapy. SEE: *alcoholism, acute; delirium tremens.*

**Hanot's disease** (ă-nōz') [Victor C. Hanot, Fr. physician, 1844–1896] Hypertrophic cirrhosis of the liver with jaundice.

**Hansen's bacillus** [Gerhard H. A. Hansen, Norwegian physician, 1841–1912] *Mycobacterium leprae,* the cause of leprosy, which Hansen discovered in 1871.

**Hansen's disease** Leprosy.

**Hantavirus** A genus of viruses of the family Bunyaviridae; the cause of epidemic hemorrhagic fever and hantavirus pulmonary syndrome. The natural reservoir is rodents.

**hantavirus pulmonary syndrome** ABBR: HPS. An acute pulmonary illness resembling acute respiratory distress syndrome mainly occurring in the southwestern U.S. The hantavirus is carried primarily by the deer mouse and spread by contact with the rodent's urine or feces, rodent bites, ingestion of water or food contaminated with the rodent's excreta or saliva, or inhaled as an airborne virus from rodent's living quarters and excreta. The case-fatality rate for people infected with this virus is between 40% and 50%, nearly 10 times higher than that for any previously known hantavirus. Patients have ranged from ages 12 through 69, with 60% between ages 20 and 39. All patients lived in or visited a rural area 6 weeks before becoming ill and were involved in activities associated with rodent contact, such as farming, hiking, or camping in rodent-infested areas, or living in rodent-infested dwellings. Transmission from person to person or by mosquitoes, fleas, or other arthropods has not been reported. Some question exists whether this syndrome is an autoimmune virus, because no cases have been identified in children under age 12, before autoimmune activity begins.

SYMPTOMS: Noncardiac pulmonary edema distinguishes the syndrome. Chief complaints include myalgia, fever, headache, nausea, vomiting, and cough. Respiratory distress typically follows the onset of a cough accompanied by a rising respiratory rate and increased heart rate. Fever, hypoxia, and in some patients, serious hypotension, typify the hospital course.

DIAGNOSIS: Diagnosis is based on clinical suspicion and by elimination of other infections with similar features; however, the Centers for Disease Control and Prevention and state health departments are able to perform definitive testing for hantavirus exposure and antibody formation. Laboratory tests usually reveal an elevated white blood cell count, with neutrophils predominating, myeloid precursors, and atypical lymphocytes; decreased platelet count; elevated partial thromboplastin time; and a normal fibrinogen level. Usually only minimal abnormalities in renal function occur, with serum creatinine levels no higher than 2.5 mg/dl (renal involvement and hemorrhagic features are associated with other hantavirus syndromes). Chest x-rays eventually show bilateral pulmonary interstitial infiltrates in almost all patients.

TREATMENT: Administration of ribavirin has been effective; otherwise, treatment is mainly supportive, consisting of maintaining adequate oxygenation; monitoring cardiopulmonary status; and using vasopressors, such as dopamine, to stabilize the patient's heart rate and blood pressure.

NURSING IMPLICATIONS: Vital signs, respiratory status, and arterial blood gas values are monitored. Fluid and electrolyte balance are also monitored and imbalances corrected by providing intravenous fluid therapy based on the results of hemodynamic evaluation; care is taken not to overhydrate the patient. A patent airway is maintained, by suctioning if necessary, and mechanical ventilation provided. Neurological status is assessed relative to hypoxemia. Emotional support is provided for the patient and family. All cases of hantavirus pulmonary syndrome must be reported to the state health department. Prevention guidelines focusing on ways to minimize the risk of contact with the rodent reservoir and rodent excreta and on rodent control are provided to persons at risk.

**hapalonychia** (hăp″ăl-ō-nĭk′ē-ă) [Gr. *hapalos,* soft, + *onyx,* nail] Onychomalacia.

**haphalgesia** (hăf″ăl-jē′zē-ă) [Gr. *haphe,* touch, + *algesis,* sense of pain] A sensation of pain upon touching the skin lightly or with a nonirritating object.

**haphephobia** (hăf″ē-fō′bē-ă) [″ + *phobos,* fear] An aversion to being touched by another person.

**haplodont** (hăp′lō-dŏnt) [″ + *odous,* tooth] Having teeth without ridges or tubercles on the crown.

**haploid** [Gr. *haploos,* simple, + *eidos,* form, shape] Possessing half the diploid or normal number of chromosomes found in somatic or body cells. Such is the case of the germ cells—ova or sperm—following the reduction divisions in gametogenesis, the haploid number being 23 in humans. SEE: *chromosome; diploid.*

**haploidy** (hăp′loy-dē) The state of being haploid.

**haplopia** (hăp-lō′pē-ă) [″ + *ops,* vision] Single vision; a condition in which an object viewed by two eyes appears as a single object, in contrast to diplopia, in which it appears as two objects.

**haplotype** The combination of several alleles in a gene cluster.

**hapten(e)** (hăp′tĕn, -tēn) [Gr. *haptein,* to seize] A substance that normally does not act as an antigen or stimulate an immune response but that can be combined with an antigen and, at a later time, initiate a specific antibody response on its own. SYN: *haptin.*

**haptic** (hăp′tĭk) [Gr. *haptein,* to touch] Tactile.

**haptics** The science of the sense of touch.

**haptin** (hăp′tĭn) Hapten.

**haptoglobin** (hăp″tō-glō′bĭn) A mucoprotein to which hemoglobin released from lysed red cells into plasma is bound. It is increased in certain inflammatory conditions and decreased in hemolytic disorders.

**hardening** [AS. *heardian,* to harden] **1.** Rendering a pathological or histological specimen firm or compact, for making thin sections for microscopic study. **2.** The development of increased resistance to extremes of environmental temperature. SEE: *acclimation.*

***h. of the arteries*** Colloquial expression used for arteriosclerosis.

**hardness 1.** A quality of water containing certain substances, esp. soluble salts of calcium and magnesium. These react with soaps, forming insoluble compounds that are precipitated out of solution, thus interfering with their cleansing action. **2.** The quality of x-rays determining their penetrating power. Hardness lessens as wavelengths become longer. **3.** The quality of firmness or density of a material imparted by the cohesion of the particles that compose it.

***h. of a gas tube*** A term used to qualify the condition of a tube according to the degree of rarefaction of the residual gas. The higher the vacuum, the harder the tube and the rays emitted, the higher the voltage required to cause a discharge with a cold cathode, and hence the shorter the wavelength of the resulting x-rays.

***h. number*** SEE: under *number.*

**harelip** [AS. *hara,* hare, + *lippa,* lip] Cleft lip.

***h. suture*** A twisted figure-of-eight suture used in the surgical correction of harelip.

**harlequin fetus** SEE: under *fetus.*

**harlequin sign** A benign transient color change seen in neonates in which one half of the body blanches while the other half becomes redder, with a clear line of demarcation.

**harmonic** In physics, concerning wave forms, an oscillation or frequency that is a whole number multiple of the basic frequency.

**harmony** (hăr′mō-nē) The condition of working or living together smoothly.

***functional occlusal h.*** The ideal occlusion of the teeth so that in all mandibular positions during chewing, the teeth will be functioning efficiently and without trauma to supporting tissues.

**harness** In postamputation rehabilitation, the part of an upper extremity prosthesis that fits around the shoulder and back to permit mechanical control of the terminal device and hold the socket firmly around the stump.

**harpoon** (hăr-poon′) [Gr. *harpazein,* to seize] A device with a hook on one end for obtaining small pieces of tissue such as muscle for examination.

**Harrison's groove** [Edwin Harrison, Brit. physician, 1779–1847] A depression on the lower edge of the thorax caused by the tug of the diaphragm, seen in rickets and any infant disease that tends to obstruct inspiration.

**Hartmann's solution** [Alexis F. Hartmann, U.S. pediatrician, 1849–1931] Lactated Ringer's injection used for fluid and electrolyte replacement. A sterile solution of 0.6 g of sodium chloride, 0.03 g of potassium chloride, 0.02 g of calcium chloride, and 0.31 g of sodium lactate diluted with water for injection to make 100 ml.

**Hartnup disease** [*Hartnup,* the family name of the first reported case] A rare hereditary metabolic disease in which absorption, excretion, and kidney resorption of amino acids, esp. tryptophan, is abnormal. Clinical signs resemble pellagra, with a rash that is worsened by exposure to sunlight.

**harvest** To obtain samples or remove bacteria or other microorganisms from a culture.

**Harvey, William** (hăr′vē) British physician, 1578–1657, who described the circulation of the blood.

**Hashimoto's thyroiditis** [Hakaru Hashimoto, Japanese surgeon, 1881–1934] A form of autoimmune thyroiditis that affects women eight times more often than men. Clinically there is an enlarged thyroid and hypothyroidism. The treatment is life-long replacement therapy with thyroid hormone.

**hashish** (hăsh′ĭsh) [Arabic, hemp, dried grass] A more or less purified extract prepared from the flowers, stalks, and leaves of the hemp plant *Cannabis sativa.* The gummy substance is smoked or chewed for its euphoric effects. SEE: *cannabis; marijuana.*

**Hasner's valve, H.'s fold** [Joseph R. Hasner, Prague ophthalmologist, 1819–1892] A fold of the mucous membrane at the opening of the nasolacrimal duct in the inferior meatus of the nasal cavity. SYN: *lacrimal* *plica.*

**Hassall's corpuscle** [Arthur H. Hassall, Brit. chemist and physician, 1817–1894] A spherical or oval body present in the medulla of the thymus. It consists of a central area of degenerated cells surrounded by concentrically arranged flattened or polygonal cells.

**Hatchcock's sign** Tenderness just beyond the angle of the jaws when the finger follows on the undersurface of the mandible toward the angle. This may be found in mumps before any swelling can be detected.

**hatchet, enamel** A hand-cutting instrument in which the blade is set continuously with the handle. The blade end has a bevel on one side and is used in dentistry to prepare cavities for restoration.

**haunch** (hawnsh) [Fr. *hanche*] The hips and buttocks.

**haustra** (haws'tră) [L. *haurire,* to draw, drink] Plural of haustrum.

***h. coli*** Haustrum.

**haustration** (haws-trā'shŭn) The process of formation of a haustrum.

**haustrum** (haw'strŭm) *pl.* **haustra** [L. *haurire,* to draw, drink] One of the sacculations of the colon caused by longitudinal bands that are shorter than the gut. SYN: *haustra coli.* **haustral** (haw'străl), *adj.*

**HAV** *hepatitis A virus.*

**Haverhill fever** (hā'vĕr-ĭl) [Haverhill, MA, U.S., where the initial epidemic occurred] A febrile disease transmitted to humans by rats, usually by rat bite. *Streptobacillus moniliformis* is the etiological agent. SYN: *rat-bite fever.*

**Havers, Clopton** British physician and anatomist (1650–1702) whose work is particularly remembered for its detailed description of the microscopic structure of bone. SEE: *haversian system.*

**haversian canal** SEE: under *canal.*

**haversian canaliculus** One of several delicate canals extending from the lacunae into the matrix of bone. It anastomoses with canaliculi of adjacent lacunae, forming a network of fine channels that communicate with haversian and Volkmann's canals and transmits nutrient materials.

**haversian gland** A minute gland projecting from the surface of the synovial tissue into the joint space, that secretes synovial fluid.

**haversian system** An architectural unit of bone consisting of a central tube (haversian canal) with alternate layers of intercellular material (matrix) surrounding it in concentric cylinders. Alternating layers of matrix and cells are called haversian lamellae. SEE: *bone.*

**hay fever** A type I hypersensitivity reaction or allergic disease of the mucous membranes of the nose and upper air passages induced by external irritation and causing inflammation, catarrh, watery discharges from the eyes, coryza, headache, and asthmatic symptoms. SYN: *allergic rhinitis; periodic rhinitis; pollinosis.* SEE: *Nursing Diagnoses Appendix.*

ETIOLOGY: Airborne pollens or occasionally fungus spores cause hay fever. The spring type of hay fever is due to pollens of trees such as oak, elm, hickory, and ash. The summer type is due to pollens of plants such as grasses, plantain, and sorrel. In the fall the allergy is caused principally by the pollen of ragweeds. Nonseasonal hay fever may result from inhalation of irritating substances including animal dander, dust from hay or straw, or house dust, or from ingestion of drugs or foods to which the individual is allergic.

TREATMENT: The patient should be removed from contact with the allergen or the allergen removed from the patient's environment. Filtration of air by masks and nasal filters may be helpful. Epinephrine, antihistamines, or other drugs are given orally or used as nose drops or nasal sprays. Antihistamines that are free of anticholinergic side effects (e.g., astemizole and terfenadine) are available. If nasal obstruction persists, inhaled corticosteroids should be tried. When it is not possible to avoid contact with the allergen, the patient may benefit from prophylactic treatment consisting of desensitization by injection of pollen extracts of allergens (other than food) to which he or she is sensitive.

---

Caution: Overuse of corticosteroids may damage the nasal mucosa, and absorption of the drug can cause adverse side effects.

---

**Hayflick's limit** [Leonard Hayflick, U.S. microbiologist, b. 1928] The number of cell divisions that will take place in human cell cultures prior to dying out. This is estimated to be about 50 cell divisions. Using data obtained from investigations of cell cultures, Dr. Hayflick estimated that the limit of life of human beings could be more than 100 years.

**Haygarth's deformities** [John Haygarth, Brit. physician, 1740–1827] Exostoses or bony tumors on joints in rheumatoid arthritis.

**hazardous material** ABBR: hazmat. A material handled in such a way that people coming into contact with it can suffer personal injury or property damage. The hazard of any material is determined by its chemical, physical, and biological properties and by the possibility of exposure to that material. SEE: *health hazard; permissible exposure limits; right-to-know law; toxic substance.*

**hazmat** Contraction for hazardous material.

**Hb** *hemoglobin.*

**HB Ag** *hepatitis B antigen.*

**HbCo** Carboxyhemoglobin.

**Hbg** *hemoglobin.*

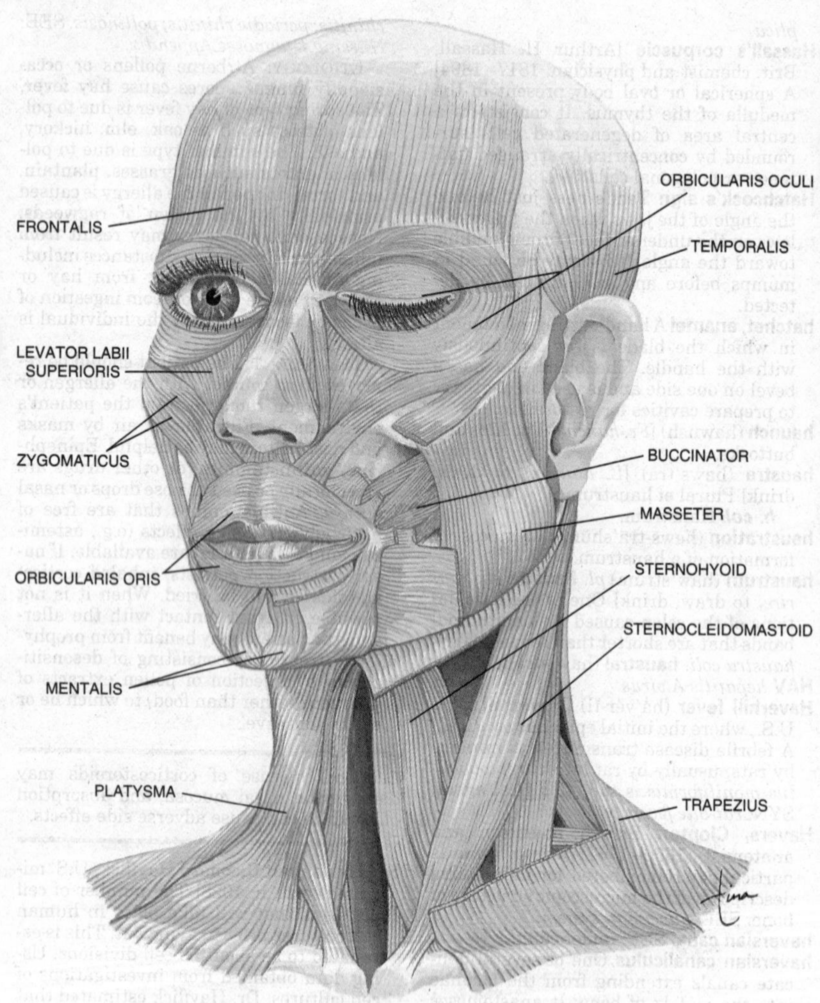


MUSCLES OF THE **HEAD** AND NECK (ANTERIOR VIEW)

**H2 blockers** SEE: *H2-receptor antagonists.*

**HBV** *hepatitis B virus.*

**HC Cream** Trade name for hydrocortisone cream.

**HCFA** *Health Care Financing Administration.*

**HCG** *human chorionic gonadotrophin.*

**HCl** *hydrochloric acid.*

**$HCO_3^-$** Chemical formula for bicarbonate ion.

**$H_2CO_3$** Chemical formula for carbonic acid.

**H.D.** *hearing distance.*

**HCV** *hepatitis C virus.*

**h.d.** L. *hora decubitus,* the hour of going to bed.

**HDCV** *human diploid cell vaccine* (for rabies).

**H. disease.** *Hartnup disease.*

**HDL** *high-density lipoprotein.*

**He** Symbol for helium.

**head** [AS. *heafod*] **1.** Caput; the part of the animal body containing the brain and organs of sight, hearing, smell, and taste and including the facial bones. SEE: illus. **2.** The proximal end of a bone. **3.** The larger extremity of any structure or body.

ABNORMALITIES: *An abnormal fixation* of the head may be caused by postpharyngeal abscess, arthritis deformans, swollen cervical glands, rheumatism, traumatism of the neck, sprains of cervical muscles, congenital spasmodic torticollis, caries of a molar tooth, burn scars, or eye muscle imbalance (hyperphoria). An inability to move the head may be due to caries of the cervical vertebrae and dis-

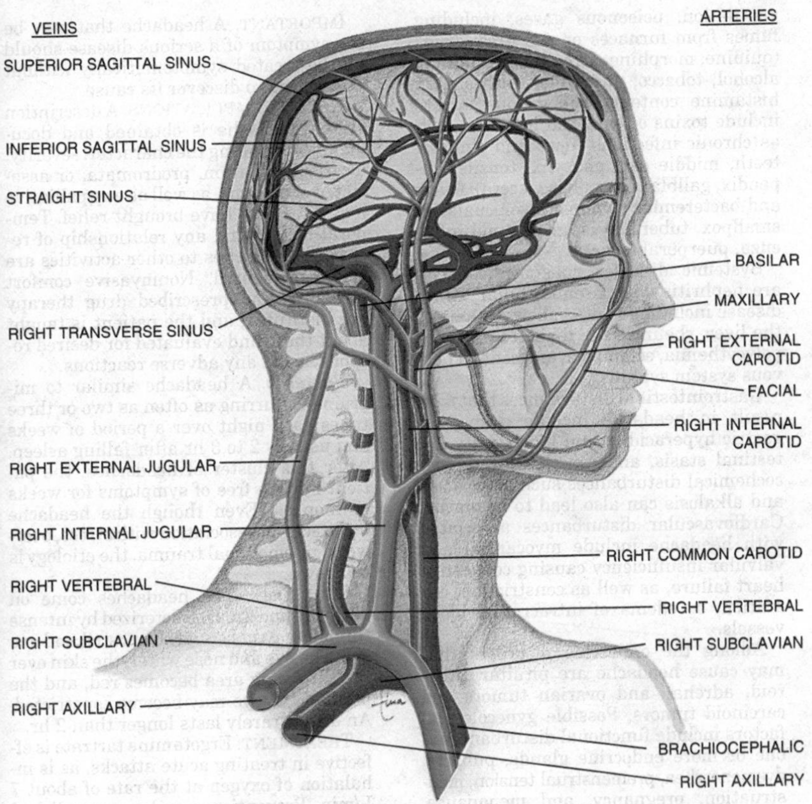


ARTERIES AND VEINS OF THE **HEAD** (RIGHT LATERAL VIEW)

eases of articulation between the occiput and atlas or paralysis of neck muscles.

*Abnormal movements* of the head include habit spasms such as nodding. Rhythmical nodding is seen in aortic regurgitation, chorea, and torticollis. A retracted head is seen in acute meningitis, cerebral abscess, tumor, thrombosis of the superior longitudinal sinus, acute encephalitis, laryngeal obstruction, tetanus, hydrophobia, epilepsy, spasmodic torticollis, strychnine poisoning, hysteria, rachitic conditions, and painful neck lesions at the back.

***after-coming h.*** Childbirth with the head delivered last.

***articular h.*** A projection on bone that articulates with another bone.

***nerve h.*** The optic disk.

**headache** [AS. *heafod,* head, + *acan,* to ache] An acute or chronic, diffuse pain in different portions of the head, not confined to any nerve distribution area. It may be frontal, temporal, or occipital, and may be confined either to one side of the head or to the region immediately over one eye. The character of pain may vary from dull and aching to acute and almost unbearable. It may be an intermittent intense pain, a throbbing pain, a pressure pain that feels as if the head will burst, or a penetrating pain driving through the head. Treatment depends entirely on the cause of the headache. SYN: *cephalalgia.* SEE: *migraine.*

ETIOLOGY: Transient acute headaches may be due to a variety of causes including diseases of the paranasal sinuses, teeth, eye, ear, nose, or throat; acute infections; or trauma to the head. Chronic headaches may be caused by a variety of conditions including physical, emotional, psychosomatic, or psychogenic factors; fevers; metabolic conditions; or exposure to toxic chemicals. The exact cause can be determined by thorough analysis of the data obtained from history, physical examination, tests, and laboratory studies, which may include roentgenography of the skull, electroencephalography, and metabolic studies.

Toxic factors leading to headache may be of exogenous or endogenous origin. Exogenous factors include foul air from poor ventilation; poisonous gases, including fumes from furnaces or gas fires; drugs (quinine, morphine, atropine, histamine); alcohol; tobacco; and wines with a high histamine content. Endogenous factors include toxins of bacterial infection such as chronic infections (nose and sinuses, teeth, middle ear, pharynx, tonsils, appendix, gallbladder, pelvic viscera); fever; and bacteremias (typhoid fever, malaria, smallpox, tuberculosis, grippe and influenza, puerperal fever).

Systemic diseases causing headache are nephritis with uremia, biliary tract disease including acute yellow atrophy of the liver, rheumatism, diabetes, anemia, polycythemia, eclampsia, and central nervous system syphilis.

Gastrointestinal disturbances that may result in headache include dyspepsia, gastric hyperacidity and hypoacidity, intestinal stasis, and constipation. Physicochemical disturbances such as acidosis and alkalosis can also lead to headache. Cardiovascular disturbances associated with headache include myocardial and valvular insufficiency causing congestive heart failure, as well as constriction, dilatation, or edema of intracranial blood vessels.

Among the endocrine disorders that may cause headache are pituitary, thyroid, adrenal, and ovarian tumors and carcinoid tumors. Possible gynecological factors include functional disturbances of one or more endocrine glands, puberty, dysmenorrhea, premenstrual tension, menstruation, pregnancy, and menopause. Psychoneurological factors causing headache are nervous exhaustion; worry, excitement, anger, or nervous tension; migraine; hysteria; epilepsy; and psychoneuroses.

Diseases of special sense organs (e.g., iritis, glaucoma, conjunctivitis; adenoids, deviated septum; middle ear infections can cause headache, as can organic brain disease causing pressure such as tumor, abscess, gumma, cyst, hydrocephaly, intracranial hemorrhage; subdural hematoma; intracranial vascular disease; arteriosclerosis; embolism, thrombosis, or aneurysm; encephalitis; various forms of meningitis and meningismus.

Almost any disturbance of body function may cause headache. Other causes are external pressure and constriction of the head; trauma to the head; sunstroke; motion sickness; irritation of mucous membrane of nose and sinuses by dust or pollen; fatigue (physical or mental); insomnia; and travel or ascent to an altitude sufficient to produce hypoxia. Spinal puncture or diagnostic examination involving injecting dyes or radioactive substances into cranial arteries or air into the ventricles of the brain may be followed by headache. Orgasm is a rare cause of headache.

IMPORTANT: A headache that may be the symptom of a serious disease should not be treated symptomatically without attempting to discover its cause.

NURSING IMPLICATIONS: A description of the headache is obtained and documented, including the character, severity, location, radiation, prodromata, or associated symptoms, as well as any palliative measures that have brought relief. Temporal factors and any relationship of recurring headaches to other activities are also documented. Noninvasive comfort measures and prescribed drug therapy are instituted, and the patient is taught about these and evaluated for desired responses and any adverse reactions.

***cluster h.*** A headache similar to migraine, occurring as often as two or three times each night over a period of weeks and usually 2 to 3 hr after falling asleep. After this cluster of headaches, the patient may be free of symptoms for weeks or months. Even though the headache may recur in association with stress, overwork, or emotional trauma, the etiology is unknown.

SYMPTOMS: The headaches come on abruptly and are characterized by intense throbbing pain behind the nostril and one eye. The eye and nose water, the skin over the throbbing area becomes red, and the pupil of the eye may become constricted. An attack rarely lasts longer than 2 hr.

TREATMENT: Ergotamine tartrate is effective in treating acute attacks, as is inhalation of oxygen at the rate of about 7 L/min. Prevention may be accomplished by use of methysergide, prednisone, or lithium.

***coital h.*** A headache that begins suddenly during coitus or immediately after orgasm. These are uncommon, occur more frequently in men than in women, and may last for minutes or hours. No significant underlying pathology exists.

***exertional h.*** An acute headache of short duration that appears after strenuous physical activity. Usually benign, it is relieved by aspirin and prevented by changing to a less strenuous exercise.

***histamine h.*** A headache resulting from ingestion of histamine (found in some wines), injection of histamine, or excessive histamine in circulating blood. This type of headache is due to dilatation of branches of the carotid artery. SEE: *cluster h.*

***postlumbar puncture h.*** A severe headache occurring in 10% to 40% of patients after lumbar puncture. It is thought to be related to the leakage of spinal fluid through the hole that fails to close when the needle is removed from the dura. The use of a small-gauge spinal puncture needle helps to prevent this headache.

TREATMENT: Bedrest in a completely flat and prone position (without a pillow), forced oral and intravenous fluids, and administration of cortical steroids are useful in treating the headache. If the headache persists in spite of therapy, it may be possible to stop the leakage of spinal fluid by injection of 10 ml of the patient's blood in the epidural space at the site of the lumbar puncture. The blood may "patch" the hole in the dura.

***tension h.*** **1.** A headache associated with chronic contraction of the muscles of the neck and scalp. **2.** A headache associated with emotional or physical strain.

***thundering h.*** A sudden acute headache that may accompany intracranial hemorrhage. Its absence, however, does not rule out intracranial hemorrhage.

**head banging** In children, a tension-discharging action in which the head is repeatedly banged against the crib; may be part of a temper tantrum.

**headgear 1.** A covering for the head, esp. a protective one, such as a helmet used by soldiers and a helmet used by those who participate in contact sports, auto racing, or aviation. **2.** Extraoral traction and anchorage used to apply force to the teeth and jaws.

**head-tilt chin-lift maneuver** A replacement for the head-tilt neck-lift maneuver for opening the airway in cardiopulmonary resuscitation. The head is tilted by gentle pressure to the forehead. The chin is lifted and brought forward with the fingers of the other hand.

**head trauma** Injury to the head, esp. to the scalp and cranium, that may be limited to soft tissue damage or may include the cranial bones and the brain.

**heal** (hēl) [AS. *hael,* whole] To cure; to make whole or healthy.

**healer 1.** One who heals. **2.** One who heals by use of an alternative method such as spiritual healing. SEE: *holistic medicine.*

**healing** The restoration to a normal mental or physical condition, esp. of an inflammation or a wound. SEE: illus.

*Healing by first intention:* This process closes the edge of a wound with little or no inflammatory reaction and in such a manner that little or no scar is left to reveal the site of the injury. New cells are formed to take the place of dead ones, and the capillary walls stretch across the wound to join themselves to each other in a smooth surface. New connective tissue may form an almost imperceptible but temporary scar. In repairing lacerations and surgical wounds, the goal is to produce a repaired area that will heal by first intention.

*Healing by second intention:* This is healing by granulation or indirect union. Granulation tissue is formed to fill the gap between the edges of the wound with a thin layer of fibrinous exudate. It excludes bacteria and aids in checking bleeding by the coagulation of the blood. Connective tissue cells support the new capillaries. This form of healing is slower than that by first intention, and its gray-red surface may become pale and flabby if the healing is too long delayed. If the granulations show above the surface, they may have to be removed with caustics. If the granulations first form at the top instead of the bottom of the wound, it may have to be kept open by drainage.

*Healing by third intention:* This type of healing, such as that of an ulcer or cavity, by filling with granulation tissue, usually leads to the formation of a scar.

COMPLICATIONS: These may result from the formation of a scar that interferes with the functioning of a part and possible deformity; the formation of a keloid, the result of overgrowth of connective tissue forming a tumor in the surface of a scar; necrosis of the skin and mucous membrane that produces a raw surface, which results in an ulcer; a sinus or fistula, which may be due to bacteria or some foreign substance remaining in the wound; proud flesh, which represents excessive growth of granulation tissue.

***holistic h.*** The total forces the body can muster to assist in repairing or attenuating pathological processes. Thus the responses of the immune system to inflammation, neoplasms, and trauma are examples of the body's self-healing process. A great number of factors are important in the holistic reaction of the body to disease. Both empirical and scientific evidence indicate that a patient's mental state plays an important part in influencing the outcomes of some illnesses and disabilities. Health care professionals can assist patients to sustain hope, have a positive outlook, and maintain motivation. SEE: Treatment under *cancer; grief reaction; hopelessness.*

**health** (hĕlth) [AS. *haelth,* wholeness] A condition in which all functions of the body and mind are normally active. The World Health Organization defines health as a state of complete physical, mental, or social well-being and not merely the absence of disease or infirmity. This definition is of limited usefulness when evaluating an individual and when asking who determines well-being, the health professional or the individual. Many persons enjoy a state of well-being even though they might be classed as unhealthy by others.

***bill of h.*** A public health certificate stating that passengers on a public conveyance or ship are free of infectious disease.

***board of h.*** A public body, appointed or elected, concerned with administering the laws pert. to the health of the public.

***h. care proxy*** A legal document that allows individuals to name someone they know and trust to make health care decisions for them if, for any reason and at any time, the individual becomes unable to make or communicate those decisions. Some states limit the age at which such a

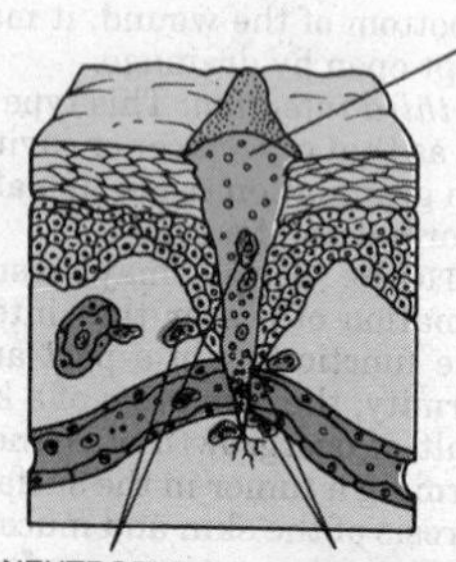


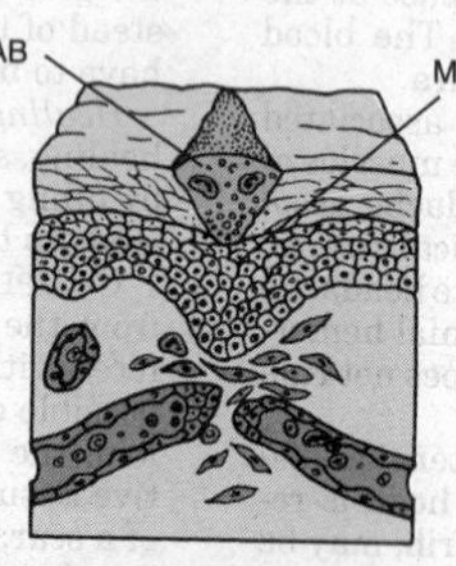


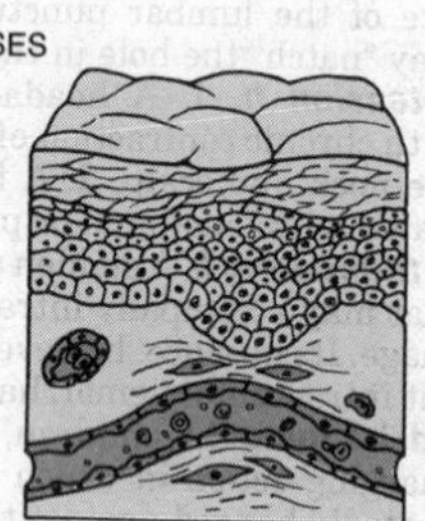


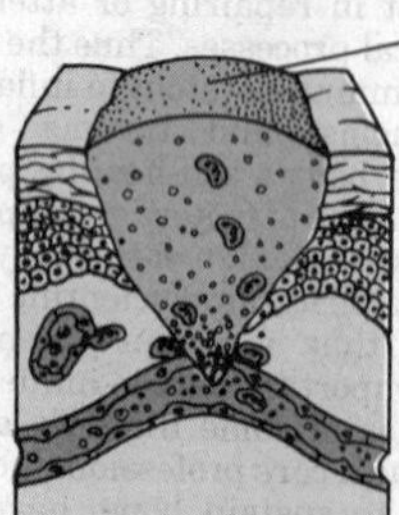


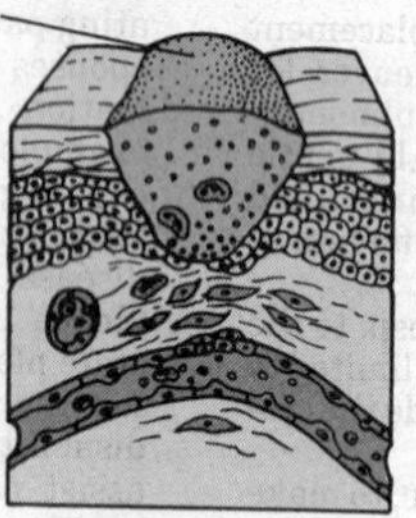


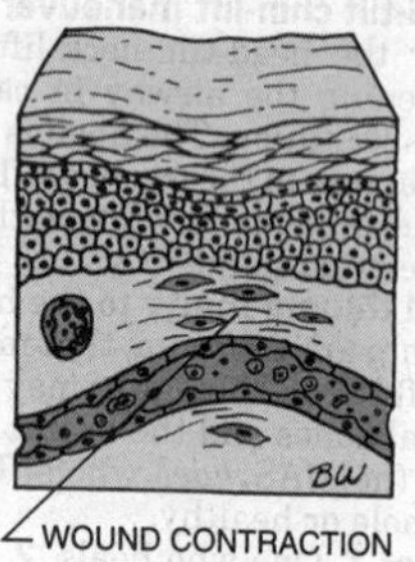


proxy may be established and prohibit certain persons, such as an estate administrator or an employee of a health care facility in which the person making the proxy is a resident, from being appointed to make health care decisions unless he or she is related to the person by blood, marriage, or adoption. SEE: *advance directive; do not attempt resuscitation; living will; donor card* for illus.

***h. certificate*** An official statement signed by a physician attesting to the state of health of a particular individual.

***department of h.*** The branch of a government (city, county, or nation) involved in the regulation and protection of the people's health.

***h. education*** An educational process or program designed for the improvement and maintenance of health. It is directed to the general public, in contrast to a health education program organized for instructing persons who will become health educators.

***h. hazard*** Literally, any thing, condition, or circumstance that may be or is harmful to health. With respect to chemicals, a substance is considered a health hazard if at least one study, conducted in accordance with established scientific principles, documents that acute or chronic effects may occur in connection with use of or exposure to that chemical. SEE: *hazardous material; permissible exposure limits; right to know law; toxic substance.*

***industrial h.*** The health of employees of industrial firms.

***mental h.*** In general, mental health is the absence of mental illness. This definition, of course, is vague because of the difficulty of providing a comprehensive definition of mental illness. Individuals are considered mentally healthy if they have adjusted to life in such a way that they are comfortable with their life situation and, at the same time, are able to live so that their behavior does not conflict with their associates or the rest of society. Inherent in this, for most individuals, are feelings of self-worth and accomplishment and the ability to be gainfully employed with sufficient reward for that employment to satisfy the economic needs required for their life situations. It is difficult but not impossible to be mentally healthy without being physically healthy.

***public h.*** The state of health of an entire community population, as opposed to that of an individual.

***h. risk appraisal*** An analysis of all that is known about a person's entire life situation including personal and family medical history, occupation, and social environment in order to estimate his or her risk of disability or death as compared with the national averages. The data used for comparison will vary with the patient's age, sex, ethnic background, and income, and the skill of the evaluator and the sensitivity and specificity of the tests used in the evaluation.

Assessments should include special diagnostic procedures such as mammography, prostate examination, Pap smear, electrocardiogram, tests for total serum lipids including cholesterol, tests for occult blood in feces, hearing tests, and stress tests as indicated and appropriate for the individual patient (i.e., health screening). SEE: *risk factors*.

***h. screening*** SEE: *h. risk appraisal*.

**Health Care Financing Administration** ABBR: HCFA. The division of the U.S. Department of Health and Human Services responsible for Medicare funding.

**healthful** Conducive to good health.

**health maintenance, altered** Inability to identify, manage, and/or seek out help to maintain health. SEE: *Nursing Diagnoses Appendix*.

**Health Maintenance Organization** ABBR: HMO. A prepaid health care program of group practice with comprehensive medical care being provided and with an emphasis on preventive medicine.

**health-seeking behaviors** A state in which an individual in stable health is actively seeking ways to alter personal health habits or the environment in order to move toward a higher level of health. Stable health status is defined as age-appropriate illness prevention measures achieved, client reports good or excellent health, and signs and symptoms of disease, if present, are controlled. SEE: *Nursing Diagnoses Appendix*.

**healthy** Being in a state of good health.

**healthy persons, medical evaluation of** The examination of healthy individuals in an attempt to determine their current state of health and to discover asymptomatic and latent indicators of disease that may develop later. In most economies, the benefits obtained weighed against the cost of such an evaluation make such medical evaluation inadvisable.

**hearing** [AS. *hieran*] The act or power of perceiving sound.

FUNCTION TESTS: Hearing acuity can be determined by measuring the distance at which a person can hear a certain sound such as a watch tick, by using audiometers, and by bone conduction. In audiometers, electrically produced sounds are conveyed by wires to a receiver applied to the subject's ear. Intensity and pitch of sound can be altered and are indicated on the dials. Results are plotted on a graph known as an audiogram. In bone conduction tests, a device such as a tuning fork or an apparatus that converts an electric current into mechanical vibrations is applied to the skull. This is of value in distinguishing between perceptive and conduction deafness. Conductive hearing loss may be diagnosed by use of the Weber test. Having the patient hum produces no difference in the sound heard if hearing is normal. The sound is perceived as louder in the ear with conductive hearing loss. SEE: *acoustic reflex threshold; audiogram; auditory evoked response; cochlear implant; ear; hearing impaired; Rinne test; Weber test*.

***h. aid*** A sound-amplifying apparatus used by those with impaired hearing. The modern electronic hearing aid may simply amplify sound or may be designed to attenuate certain portions of the sound signal and amplify others. The cost may vary from several hundred dollars to more than a thousand dollars. As a variety of hearing aids are available, it is important that patients buy the type most suitable for their needs and comfort. Patients should have a trial period prior to making the final decision to purchase the device.

***h. distance*** The distance at which a given sound can be heard. On the prairies and in Arctic air, a voice may be heard for 2 miles or more.

***h. hallucinations*** The subjective sensation of sound such as hearing voices when none actually exist.

***h. impaired*** A term used to describe individuals whose ability to hear has decreased to a degree that is noticeable by others as well as themselves.

***h. loss*** A decreased ability to perceive sounds as compared with what the individual or examiner would regard as normal. SEE: *audiogram; audiometry*.

**heart** (hărt) [AS. *heorte*] A hollow, muscular organ, the pump of the circulatory system. Its wall has three layers: the outer epicardium, a serous membrane; the mid-

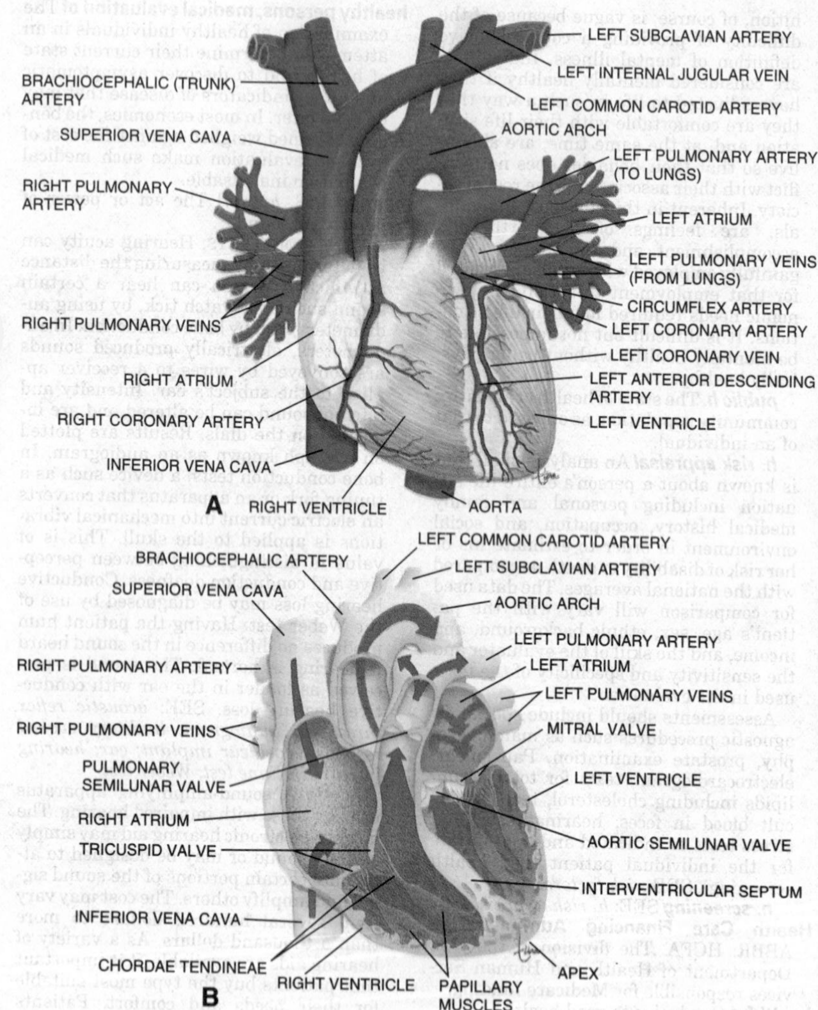


**THE HEART (A)** ANTERIOR VIEW, **(B)** FRONTAL SECTION

dle myocardium, made of cardiac muscle; and the inner endocardium, endothelium that lines the chambers and covers the valves. The heart is enclosed in a fibroserous sac, the pericardium; the potential space between the parietal pericardium and the epicardium is the pericardial cavity, which contains serous fluid to prevent friction as the heart beats. SEE: illus. (The Heart); *circulation, coronary* for illus.; *cardiomyopathy, hypertrophic*.

CHAMBERS: The upper right and left atria (singular: atrium) are thin-walled receiving chambers separated by the interatrial septum. The lower right and left ventricles are thick-walled pumping chambers separated by the interventricular septum; normally the right side has no communication with the left. The right side receives deoxygenated blood via the vena cavae from the body and pumps it to the lungs; the left side receives oxygenated blood from the lungs and pumps it via the aorta and arteries to the body. Contraction of the heart chambers is called systole; relaxation with accompanying filling with blood is called diastole. The sequence of events that occurs in a single heartbeat is called the cardiac cycle, with atrial systole followed by ventricular systole. For a heart rate of 70 beats per minute, each cycle lasts about 0.85 sec.

VALVES: In the healthy state, all four

cardiac valves prevent backflow of blood. The atrioventricular valves are at the openings between each atrium and ventricle; the tricuspid valve, between the right atrium and ventricle; and the bicuspid or mitral valve, between the left atrium and ventricle. The pulmonary semilunar valve is at the opening of the right ventricle into the pulmonary artery; the aortic semilunar valve is at the opening of the left ventricle into the aorta.

FUNCTION: In adults, the cardiac output varies from 5 L/min at rest to as much as 20 L/min during vigorous exercise. At the rate of 72 times each minute, the adult human heart beats 104,000 times a day, 38,000,000 times a year. Every stroke forces approx. 5 cu in. (82 ml) of blood out into the body, amounting to 500,000 cu in. (8193 L) a day. In terms of work, this is the equivalent of raising 1 ton (907 kg) to a height of 41 ft (12.5 m) every 24 hr.

BLOOD SUPPLY: The myocardium receives its blood supply from the coronary arteries that arise from the ascending aorta. Blood from the myocardium drains into several cardiac veins.

NERVE SUPPLY: The heart initiates its own beat, usually from 60 to 80 beats per minute, but the rate may change due to the cardiac centers in the medulla oblongata. Accelerator impulses are carried by sympathetic nerves. Preganglionic neurons in the thoracic spinal cord synapse with postganglionic neurons in the cervical ganglia of the sympathetic trunk; their axons continue to the heart. Sympathetic impulses are transmitted to the sinoatrial (SA) node, atrioventricular (AV) node, bundle of His, and myocardium of the ventricles, and increase heart rate and force of contraction. Inhibitory impulses are carried by the vagus nerves (parasympathetic). Preganglionic neurons (vagus) originating in the medulla synapse with postganglionic neurons in terminal ganglia in the wall of the heart. Parasympathetic impulses are transmitted to the SA and AV nodes and decrease the heart rate. Sensory nerves from the heart are for the sensation of pain, caused by an insufficient supply of oxygen to the myocardium. The sensory nerves for reflex changes in heart rate are the vagus and glossopharyngeal, which arise from pressoreceptors or chemoreceptors in the aortic arch and carotid sinus, respectively.

AUSCULTATION: This action reveals the intensity, quality, and rhythm of the heart sounds and detects any adventitious sounds, such as murmurs or pericardial friction. The two separate sounds heard by the use of a stethoscope over the heart have been represented by the syllables "lubb," "dupp." The first sound (systolic), which is prolonged and dull, results from the contraction of the ventricle, tension of the atrioventricular valves, and the impact of the heart against the chest wall, and is synchronous with the apex beat and carotid pulse. The first sound is followed by a short pause, and then the second sound (diastolic) is heard, resulting from the closure of the aortic and pulmonary valves. This sound is short and high pitched. After the second sound there is a longer pause before the first is heard again. A very useful technique for listening to the variation in sounds between one area and another is to move the stethoscope in small steps from site to site.

PROCEDURE: The patient should be recumbent when the examination begins. After all possible signs have been elicited, the examination should be repeated with the patient sitting, standing, or leaning forward, noting any variations from this change of position. Auscultation is performed first while the patient is breathing naturally, next while he or she holds the breath in both deep inspiration and expiration, and finally while the patient takes three or four forced inspirations. By listening over the entire thoracic cavity, the examiner should try to localize the points at which heart sounds, both normal and abnormal, are heard with the greatest intensity. The examination should proceed from below upward and from left to right.

The normal location of valves should be noted for auscultation. The aortic valve is in the third intercostal space, close to the left side of the sternum; the pulmonary valve is in front of the aorta, behind the junction of the third costal cartilage with the sternum, on the left side. The tricuspid valve is located behind the middle of the sternum about the level of the fourth costal cartilage. Finally, the mitral valve is behind the third intercostal space about 1 in. (2.5 cm) to the left of the sternum. SEE: illus.

Both heart sounds either are heard better or are actually accentuated in increased heart action from any cause, normal or abnormal, such as anemia, vigorous exercise, cardiac hypertrophy, thin chest walls, and lung consolidation as found in pneumonia. Accentuation of the aortic second sound results from hypertrophy of the left ventricle, increased arterial resistance as in arteriosclerosis with hypertension, or aortic aneurysm. Accentuation of the pulmonary second sound results from pulmonary obstruction as in emphysema, pneumonia, or hypertrophy of the right ventricle. Both heart sounds are poorly heard or are actually decreased in intensity in general obesity, general debility, degeneration or dilatation of the heart, pericardial or pleural effusion, and emphysema.

The reduplication of heart sounds is probably due to a lack of synchronous ac-

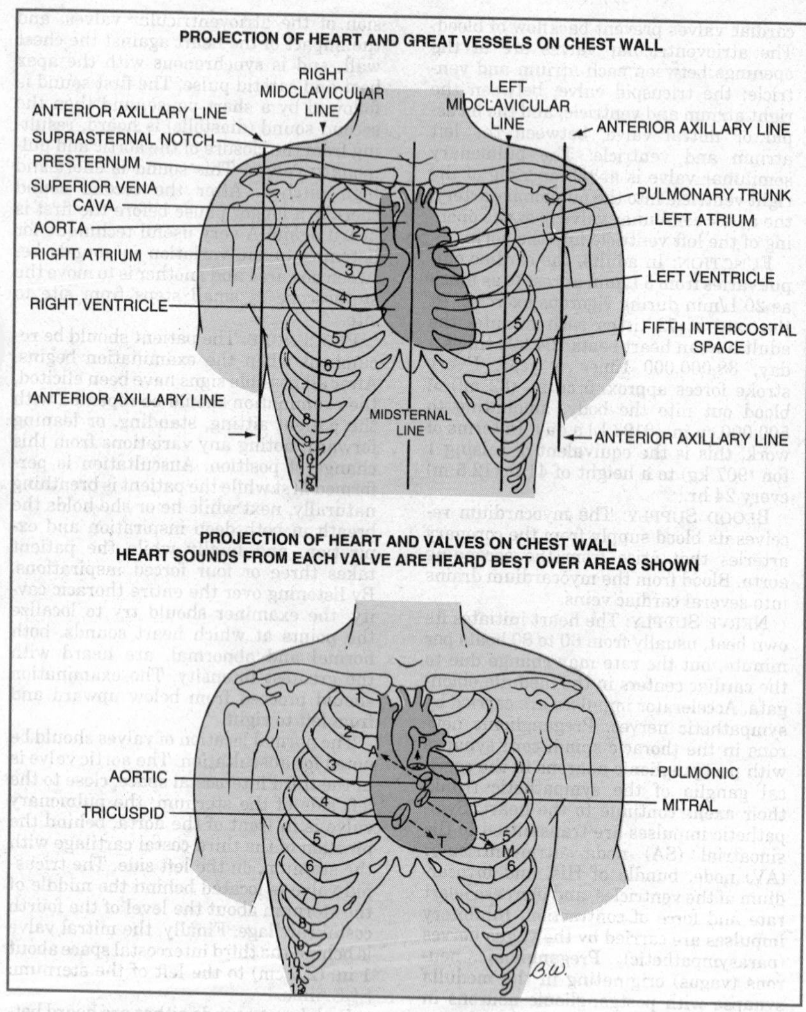


tion in the valves of both sides of the heart. It results from many conditions but notably from increased resistance in the systemic or the pulmonary circulation, as in arteriosclerosis and emphysema. It is also frequently noted in mitral stenosis and pericarditis.

A murmur, an abnormal sound heard over the heart or blood vessels, may result from obstruction or regurgitation at the valves following endocarditis; dilatation of the ventricle or relaxation of its walls rendering the valves relatively insufficient; aneurysm; a change in the blood constituents, as in anemia; roughening of the pericardial surfaces, as in pericarditis; and irregular action of the heart. Murmurs produced within the heart are termed endocardial; those outside, exocardial; those produced in aneurysms, bruits; those produced by anemia, hemic murmurs.

Hemic murmurs, which are soft and blowing and usually systolic, are heard best over the pulmonary valves. They are associated with symptoms of anemia.

An aneurysmal murmur, or bruit, is usually loud and booming, systolic, and heard best over the aorta or base of heart. It is often associated with an abnormal area of dullness and pulsation and with symptoms resulting from pressure on neighboring structures.

Pericardial friction sounds are superficial, rough, and creaking, to and fro in time, and not transmitted beyond the precordium. These sounds may be modified by the pressure of the stethoscope.

*Murmur intensity and configuration:* The intensity (loudness) of murmurs may be graded from I to VI as follows:

- Grade I–faint, can be heard only with intense listening in a quiet environment.
- Grade II–quiet but can be heard immediately.
- Grade III–moderately loud.
- Grade IV–quite loud; a thrill (like the purring of a cat) is usually felt over the heart.
- Grade V–loud enough to be heard with the stethoscope not completely in contact with the chest wall.
- Grade VI–loud enough to be heard with the stethoscope close to but not actually touching the chest.

The configuration of sound intensity of a murmur may begin low and rise in intensity (crescendo) or be relatively loud and then decrease in intensity (decrescendo) or some combination of those features; or may exhibit the same intensity from beginning to end.

PALPATION: This process not only determines position, force, extent, and rhythm of the apex beat, but also detects any fremitus or thrill. A thrill is a vibratory sensation likened to that received when the hand is placed on the back of a purring cat. Thrills at the base of the heart may result from valvular lesions, atheroma of the aorta, aneurysm, and roughened pericardial surfaces as in pericarditis. A presystolic thrill at the apex is almost pathognomonic of mitral stenosis. In children esp., a precordial bulge, substernal thrust, or apical heave suggests cardiac enlargement.

PERCUSSION: This procedure determines the shape and extent of cardiac dullness. The normal area of superficial or absolute percussion dullness (the part uncovered by the lung) is detected by light percussion and extends from the fourth left costosternal junction to the apex beat; from the apex beat to the juncture of the xiphoid cartilage with the sternum; and thence up the left border of the sternum. The normal area of deep percussion dullness (the heart projected on the chest wall) is detected by firm percussion and extends from the third left costosternal articulation to the apex beat; from the apex beat to the junction of the xiphoid cartilage with the sternum; and thence up the right border of sternum to the third rib. The lower level of cardiac dullness fuses with the liver dullness and can rarely be determined. The area of cardiac dullness is increased in hypertrophy and dilation of the heart and in pericardial effusion; it is diminished in emphysema, pneumothorax, and pneumocardium.

***abdominal h.*** A heart that is displaced into the abdominal cavity.

***armored h.*** A condition characterized by calcareous deposits in the pericardium.

***artificial h.*** A device that pumps the blood the heart would normally pump. It may be located inside or outside the body. SEE: *heart-lung machine.*

***athlete's h.*** Enlargement of the heart as a result of prolonged physical training (e.g., the aerobic exercise of running.) This is not known to be a predisposing factor for any form of heart disease.

***beriberi h.*** Heart failure due to deficiency of the vitamin thiamine.

***boatshaped h.*** A heart in which one ventricle is dilated and hypertrophied as a result of aortic regurgitation.

***bony h.*** A heart with calcareous patches in its walls and pericardium.

***cervical h.*** A heart that is displaced into the neck region.

***conduction system of the h.*** Specialized nervous tissue in the heart that conducts the electrical impulses throughout the heart. It consists of (in order of normal conduction) the sinoatrial node, the intra-atrial tracts, the atrioventricular node, the bundle of His, the right and left bundle branches, and the Purkinje fibers. SEE: illus.

***dilatation of the h.*** Enlargement of the heart caused by the stretching of its walls. Two types are dilatation with thickening of the walls and dilatation with thinning the walls. This condition is asymptomatic as long as the associated hypertrophy keeps pace with the dilatation. Otherwise, dyspnea, edema, and cough (signs of heart failure) occur.

***fatty degeneration of the h.*** A condition in which the myocardium has undergone fatty degeneration. All signs of heart failure are present (dyspnea; cough; weak, irregular pulse; edema; dyspepsia; and attacks of syncope). This condition carries an unfavorable prognosis: death may occur on slight exertion.

***fatty infiltration of the h.*** An abnormal amount of fat deposited in and upon the heart. Signs and symptoms include shortness of breath increased by exertion; weak but regular pulse; precordial distress; and a tendency to develop pulmonary congestion with resulting bronchitis. The prognosis depends on the cause of the condition. If the cause is correctable, the prognosis is favorable.

***fibroid h.*** Chronic myocarditis in which fibrous tissue develops within the muscular tissue of the heart. Signs and symptoms are the same as for fatty degeneration of heart. The condition depends on whether atheroma or sclerosis of coronary arteries exists.

***hypertrophy of the h.*** An enlargement of the heart caused by an increased size of the myocardium. It may be caused by exercise or a complication of hypertension (left ventricular hypertrophy). The myocardium increases in size by enlargement of each cell, not by an increase in number of cells.

***irritable h.*** Neurocirculatory asthenia or effort syndrome, characterized by

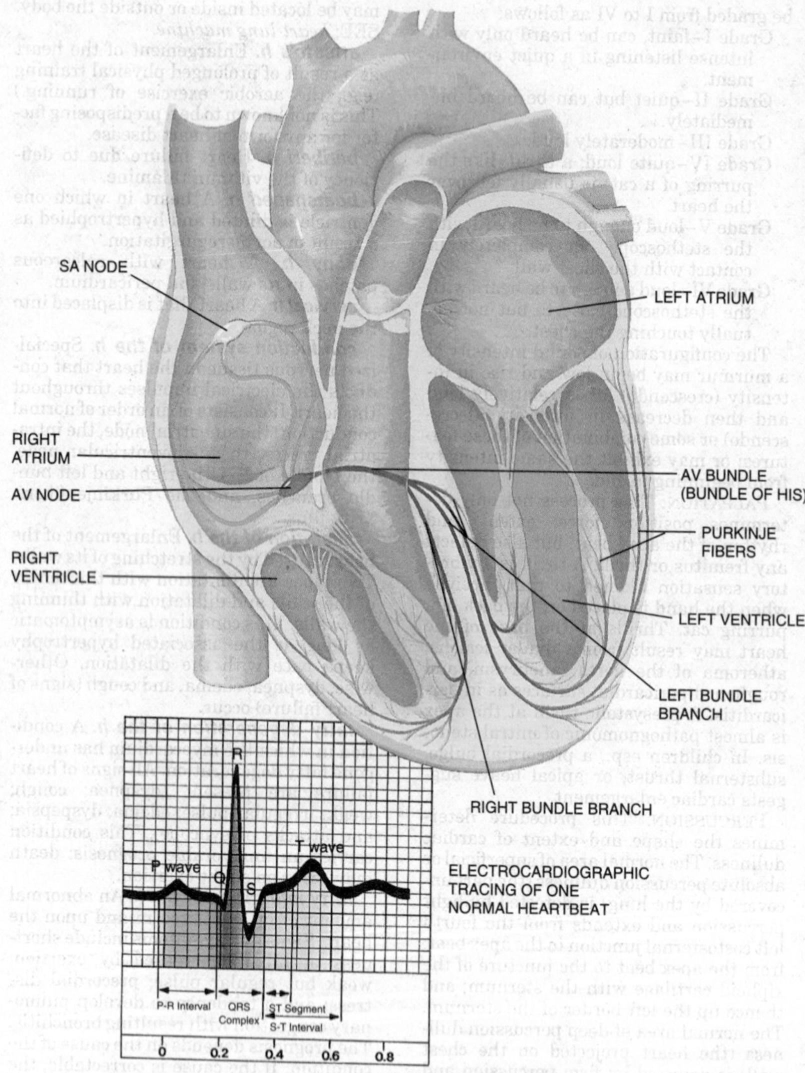


CONDUCTION SYSTEM OF THE HEART

breathlessness, palpitation, weakness, and exhaustion.

***left h.*** The left atrium and ventricle. The left atrium receives oxygenated blood from the lungs; the left ventricle pumps this blood into systemic circulation.

***palpitation of the h.*** A heartbeat that is easily noticed by the person; it is frequently rapid, irregular, or both. Causes include dyspepsia; mental or physical excitement; organic heart disease; hyperthyroidism; anemia; hysteria; independent neurosis; endocarditis, myocarditis, and pericarditis due to infection and trauma; circulatory disturbances; and disorders of metabolism, nutrition, and growth.

***right h.*** The right atrium and ventricle. The right atrium receives deoxygenated blood from the body; the right ventricle pumps this blood to the lungs.

**heart attack** Myocardial infarction.

**heartbeat** The rhythmic contraction of the heart.

**heart block** A condition in which the conductile tissue of the heart—the sinoatrial (SA) and atrioventricular (AV) nodes, bundle of His, and Purkinje fibers—fails to conduct impulses normally from the atrium to the ventricles. This alters the rhythm of the heartbeat, a condition known as arrhythmia. The condition may be present in several forms.

ETIOLOGY: Heart block is caused by structural changes, as from tumor or myocardial damage due to coronary artery occlusion. Toxic drug effects or the toxins of infections also contribute to this condition. Nutritional or endocrine factors may also play a role.

***atrioventricular h.b.*** SEE: *block, atrioventricular.*

***bilateral bundle branch h.b.*** SEE: *block, atrioventricular.*

***bundle branch h.b.*** A condition in which impulses are blocked in one of the branches of the bundle of His, resulting in ventricles beating out of rhythm with each other, which stimulates one ventricle to beat slightly before the other. SYN: *interventricular h.b.*

***complete h.b., third-degree h.b.*** A condition in which there is a complete dissociation between atrial and ventricular systoles. Ventricles may beat at a rate of 30 to 40 beats per minute while atria are beating the normal 70 beats per minute.

***congenital h.b.*** A type of heart block present at birth owing to improper development of the impulse-conducting system.

***fascicular h.b.*** A conduction defect in either or both of the subdivisions of the left bundle branch.

***first-degree h.b.*** A heart block in which the conduction time of impulses is prolonged but all atrial beats are followed by ventricular beats. It is usually recognized only by electrocardiograph by a prolonged P-R interval.

***interventricular h.b.*** Bundle branch h.b.

***partial h.b., second-degree h.b.*** A heart block in which one of two or three impulses passes from the atrium to the ventricle. Two variants exist, Wenckebach or Mobitz I and Mobitz II. In Wenckebach, the P-R intervals become progressively longer until a QRS complex is dropped, and the cycle repeats. In Mobitz II, a regular absence of QRS complexes occurs, with a constant length of P-R intervals.

***sinoatrial h.b.*** A partial or complete heart block characterized by interference in the passage of impulses from the sinoatrial node. SEE: *sick sinus syndrome.*

**heartburn** A burning sensation in the substernal area caused by reflux of acid contents of the stomach into the lower esophagus. This condition may occur in any person and it is known to occur in persons whose exercise program includes running, even if no food is present in the stomach. SYN: *brash; pyrosis.* SEE: *gastroesophageal reflux disease, chronic.*

NURSING IMPLICATIONS: Assess what the term means to the patient, exact location, time of occurrence in relation to food intake, duration, if position changes exaggerate discomfort, precipitating factors (such as type and amount of food), method of relief, and factors that aggravate the discomfort.

**heart disease** Any pathological condition of the heart.

***ischemic h.d.*** A lack of oxygen supply to the heart, with consequent altered cardiac function. The most common cause of myocardial ischemia is atherosclerosis of the coronary arteries. Depending upon several factors, including oxygen demand of the myocardium, degree of narrowing of the lumen of the arteries, and duration of the ischemia, the end result is temporary or permanent damage to the heart. SEE: *risk factors for h.d.; coronary arteries; coronary artery disease; coronary heart disease.*

***risk factors for h.d.*** Certain conditions and lifestyle variations that are more likely to be present in persons with ischemic heart disease than in the general population. These may be divided into those that are not reversible (aging, male sex, genetic factors); those that are reversible (tobacco use, hypertension, obesity, sedentary lifestyle, stress); and others that may or may not be reversible (hyperlipidemia, hyperglycemia, diabetes mellitus, decreased levels of high-density lipoproteins, and behavior patterns). SEE: *behavior patterns, types A and B.*

**heart failure 1.** A cessation of the heartbeat. **2.** A temporary or chronic syndrome or clinical condition resulting from failure of the heart to maintain adequate circulation of blood. This condition may result from failure of the right or left ventricle or both.

SYMPTOMS: Signs and symptoms of dyspnea, cardiac asthma, stasis in systemic or portal circulation, edema, cyanosis, and hypertrophy of the heart may occur, varying with the side of the heart affected.

ETIOLOGY: Causes include hypertension, infections, pericardial effusion, valvular insufficiency, coronary disease, congenital malformations, arteriosclerosis, constrictive pericarditis, atherosclerosis, and hyperthyroidism.

TREATMENT: The aim of therapy is to improve pump function by reversing the compensatory mechanisms producing the clinical effects. Heart failure usually can be controlled quickly by treatment consisting of diuresis with diuretics, such as furosemide, hydrochlorothiazide, spirinolactone, ethacrynic acid, bumetanide, or triamterene, to reduce total blood volume and circulatory congestion; bedrest in high Fowler's or orthopneic position; oxygen administration to increase oxygen delivery to the myocardium and other vital organ tissues; administration of inotropic drugs (e.g., digoxin) to strengthen myocardial contractility, sympathomimetics (e.g., dopamine and dobutamine) to treat acute situations or amrinone to increase contractility and cause arterial vasodilation, and vasodilators to increase cardiac output or angiotensin-converting enzyme inhibitors to decrease afterload; and antiembolism stockings to prevent venostasis and possible thromboembolism formation. After recovery, the patient usually must continue taking digoxin, diuretics, and potassium supplements and must remain under medical supervision. If the patient with valve dysfunction has recurrent acute heart failure, surgical replacement may be necessary.

NURSING IMPLICATIONS: The patient is assessed for signs and symptoms. Vital signs are monitored for increased heart and respiratory rates and for narrowing pulse pressure, and mental status is evaluated. The chest is auscultated for abnormal heart sounds and for lung crackles or gurgles. Daily weights are obtained to detect fluid retention, and the extremities are inspected for evidence of peripheral edema. Fluid intake and output are monitored (especially if the patient is receiving diuretics). Blood urea nitrogen and serum creatinine, potassium, sodium, chloride, and magnesium levels are monitored frequently. Continuous cardiac monitoring is provided during acute and advanced disease stages to identify and manage arrhythmias promptly. Calf pain and tenderness on foot dorsiflexion is noted. The patient is placed in high Fowler's position and on prescribed bedrest, and supplemental oxygen is administered as prescribed to ease the patient's breathing. Prescribed medications are administered and evaluated for desired responses and any adverse reactions, and the patient is instructed in their use. All patient activities are organized to maximize rest periods. To prevent deep venous thrombosis due to vascular congestion, the nurse assists with range-of-motion exercises and applies antiembolism stockings. Any deterioration in the patient's condition is documented and reported immediately. A diet high in potassium (to replace that lost through diuresis) is provided, including such potassium-rich foods as bananas, apricots, and orange juice, and the patient is instructed in this type of diet. To help curb fluid overload, the patient should avoid foods high in sodium content, such as canned and commercially prepared foods and dairy products. The importance of regular medical checkups is emphasized, and the patient is advised to notify the health-care practitioner if the pulse rate is unusually irregular, falls below 60, or increases above 120, or if the patient experiences palpitations, dizziness, blurred vision, shortness of breath, persistent dry cough, increased fatigue, paroxysmal nocturnal dyspnea, swollen ankles, decreased urine output, or a weight gain of 3 to 5 lb (1.4 to 2.3 kg) in 1 week.

***backward h.f.*** Heart failure in which venous return to the heart is reduced, resulting in venous stasis and congestion. This condition is due principally to right ventricular failure.

***congestive h.f.*** Condition characterized by weakness, breathlessness, abdominal discomfort, and edema in the lower portions of the body resulting from venous stasis and reduced outflow of blood from the left side of the heart. SEE: *dyspnea, paroxysmal nocturnal; Nursing Diagnoses Appendix.*

***forward h.f.*** Heart failure in which forward flow of blood to the tissues is inadequate owing either to inability of the left ventricle to pump sufficient blood or to insufficient blood arriving at the ventricle.

***high output h.f.*** Heart failure that occurs in spite of high cardiac output.

***left-sided h.f.*** Failure of the heart to maintain left ventricular output. SYN: *left ventricular h.f.*

***left ventricular h.f.*** Left-sided heart failure.

***low output h.f.*** Failure of the heart to maintain blood output.

***right-sided h.f.*** Failure of the heart to maintain right ventricular output. SYN: *right ventricular h.f.*

***right ventricular h.f.*** Right-sided heart failure.

**heart-lung machine** A device that maintains the functions of the heart and lungs while either or both are unable to continue to function adequately. The device pumps, oxygenates, and removes carbon dioxide from the blood. In animal studies and in open heart surgery, these machines take over the function of the heart and lungs while these organs are being treated or possibly replaced. The function of the heart-lung machine is also called heart-lung bypass.

**heart murmur** SEE: *murmur.*

**heart pump, nuclear-powered** An artificial heart powered by nuclear energy.

**heart rate** SEE: under *rate.*

**heart rate, target zone** A heart rate that is 50% to 75% of an individual's maximum heart rate. Persons who exercise for the purpose of attaining or maintaining physical fitness should attempt to exercise vigorously enough to produce a heart rate that is both safe and effective. When an exercise program is begun, the heart rate should be at the lower part of the 50% to 75% rate for the first few months. Then it should be gradually built up to 75%.

**heart reflex** SEE: under *reflex.*

**heart sounds** SEE: under *sound.*

**heart transplantation** SEE: under *transplantation.*

**heart valve, prosthetic** SEE: under *valve.*

**heat** [AS. *haetu*] **1.** The condition of being hot; warmth; opposite of cold. **2.** High

**Elimination of Body Heat**

The mode of elimination and the percentage of heat lost through each of the following is:

| | |
|---|---|
| Radiation | 55%* |
| Convection and conduction | 15% |
| Evaporation through skin | 24% |
| Warming inspired air | 2% |
| Warming ingested food and water, and loss through feces and urine | 1% |

* Figures are approximate and vary with physiological activity of the body, type of clothing worn, relative humidity, and degree of acclimitization to a particular environment.

temperature; generalized fever or localized warmth caused by an infection. Calor (fever), dolor (pain), rubor (redness), and tumor (swelling) are the four classic signs of inflammation. SEE: *febrile convulsions; fever* **3.** Sexual excitement in lower animals; period of such excitement. SYN: *estrus*. **4.** A form of energy that increases the temperature of surrounding tissues or objects by conduction, convection, or radiation. **5.** The sensation of warmth or an increase in temperature.

Heat is constantly being produced within the body as a result of exothermic chemical processes occurring in metabolic processes. Ultimately all heat produced in the body results from oxidative processes. Body temperature (normally 98.6°F or 37°C) is the result of a balance between heat production (thermogenesis) and heat loss (thermolysis). SEE: table.

The temperature of the body is not uniform. Oral temperatures range from 96.6° to 100°F (37° to 37.8°C). Axillary temperature is somewhat lower and rectal temperature is somewhat higher than oral temperature. SEE: *core temperature*.

Reducing the skin temperature reflexly constricts the blood vessels, thus reducing heat loss and conserving heat within the body. The application of heat reflexly dilates the blood vessels, thus increasing blood flow to the skin with consequent increase in heat loss.

Applying heat to the skin reflexly produces effects in the deeper portions of the body as well. It induces muscle relaxation, increases blood supply, and stimulates metabolic activity. Resultant physiological effects are hyperemia and sedation of sensory or motor activity. Application of moderate cold tends to produce the opposite effects.

Relaxation of muscular tissue results in relief of pain, which may be caused by rigidity and spasm in tissues. Local hot applications may have some reflex effect on deep organs. This is the basis of treating certain conditions by means of counterirritation such as that produced by liniments or mustard plaster.

***acclimatization to h.*** The adjustment of an organism to heat in the environment. Exposure to high environmental temperature requires a period of adjustment in order for the body to function efficiently. The amount of time required depends on the temperature, humidity, and duration of daily exposure. Significant physiological adjustments occur in 5 days and are completed within 2 weeks to a month.

***application of h.*** General application may use dry or moist heat. At first, the vessels in the skin contract slightly, which increases blood pressure. This makes patients feel that their head is full and bursting. However, this effect lasts only a short time, and discomfort can be avoided by applying a cold compress or ice bag to the head. The true effect follows immediately when the blood vessels in the skin are dilated owing to the relaxation of involuntary muscles contained in their walls. The skin is reddened, increased blood supply to the sweat glands causes them to act freely, and heat loss is accelerated. During a general application of heat the patient must be watched carefully, noting any apparent discomfort, state of pulse and respiration, and color, to be certain the patient does not become dehydrated or suffer heat exhaustion.

Caution: Heat should not be applied to extremities with reduced blood supply, as could be the case in most forms of arteriosclerosis or advanced diabetes.

Local application also may use dry or moist heat. Dry applications include hot water bottles, radiant heat, electric pads, and diathermy. Moist heat is considered more penetrating than dry heat, but this is due more to the fact that water-soaked materials lose heat slower than dry ones. The application should be approx. 120°F (48.9°C). Compresses may be kept warm by keeping hot water bottles at the proper temperature next to them. Do not use electric heating devices next to moist dressings. Devices that force hot water at a selected temperature through soft flexible tubing surrounding a part are available. These may be used to heat wet or dry compresses.

***conductive h.*** Heat transferred by conduction from a heat source to an object that is cold when the two materials are in contact with each other.

***convective h.*** The flow of heat to an object or part of the body by passage of heated particles, gas, or liquid from the heat source to the colder body.

***diathermy h.*** The source that, along with short-wave energy, converts electrical energy into heat.

***dry h.*** Heat that has no moisture. It may take the form of a hot dry pack, hot water bottle, electric light bath, heliotherapy, hot bricks, resistance coil, electric pad or blanket, hot air bath, or therapeutic lamp.

***h. of evaporation*** The heat absorbed per unit of mass when a substance is converted from a liquid to a gas, such as the change of water to steam when it is heated sufficiently. For water, the amount of heat required to transform water into steam is 540 kcal/g of water.

***initial h.*** Muscular heat produced during contraction when tension is increasing, during maintenance of tension, and during relaxation when tension is diminishing.

***latent h.*** SEE: *latent heat*.

***luminous h.*** Heat derived from light. This form may be tolerated better than other forms of radiation. Light may be converted into heat. Short infrared rays penetrate subcutaneous tissues to a greater extent than long invisible rays.

***mechanical equivalent of h.*** The value of heat units in terms of work units. One Calorie (kilocalorie) is equal to $4.1855 \times 10^4$ joules.

***moist h.*** Heat that has moisture content. It may be applied as hot bath pack, hot wet pack, hot foot bath, fomentations, poultices, or vapor bath. The patient should be observed for chill, fainting, dizziness, headache, collapse, increased pulse, and weakness. Cold applications to the head should be given during and after moist heat treatment. Opinions differ regarding the therapeutic use of heat versus cold.

***molecular h.*** The result of multiplying a substance's molecular weight by its specific heat.

***prickly h.*** Miliaria.

***radiant h.*** The heat given off from a heated body passing through the air in form of waves.

***specific h.*** The heat needed to raise the temperature of 1 g of a substance 1°C.

**heat cramp** An acute painful spasm of the voluntary muscles following hard physical work in a hot environment with inadequate fluid and salt intake. SEE: *heat exhaustion*.

FIRST AID: The patient should be moved to a cool place and given a salt solution (¼ tsp or 1 g of table salt in a glass of water) by mouth. The salt solution should be repeated at 5-min to 30-min intervals until the cramping stops.

PROPHYLAXIS: Heat cramps may be prevented by ingestion of 1 to 2 g (65 to 130 mg) of salt taken three or four times a day with at least two glasses (16 oz or ½ L) of water with each dose.

**heat exhaustion** An acute reaction to heat exposure, which differs from heatstroke. SEE: table.

SYMPTOMS: The patient experiences weakness, dizziness, nausea, and headache, and finally collapses. The skin is cold and clammy and the pupils are dilated. The body temperature is usually normal, but blood pressure may be decreased.

FIRST AID: The patient should be moved to a cool place and put in a head-low position. Clothing should be loosened. Intravenous infusion of isotonic saline is rarely needed. Prognosis is favorable if the patient is properly treated.

**heat gun** A device used in splint fabrication that produces heated air to render thermoplastic splinting materials malleable for fitting.

**heat labile** Thermolabile.

**heatstroke** An acute and dangerous reaction to heat exposure, characterized by high body temperature, usually above 105°F (40.6°C); cessation of sweating; headache; numbness; tingling and confusion prior to sudden delirium or coma; fast pulse; rapid respiratory rate; and usually elevated blood pressure. The basic defect is failure of the heat-regulating mechanisms of the body. SYN: *sunstroke*. SEE: *peritoneal dialysis; Nursing Diagnoses Appendix*.

TREATMENT: Effective therapy may save the patient's life. Without delay, the nude patient should be placed in a bathtub filled with ice-cold water. This will not cause pain, shock, or cutaneous vasoconstriction. The patient's temperature must be monitored carefully. The patient may be removed from the bath when the body temperature falls to 103°F (39.4°C). If cold water and a bathtub are not available, wet sheets should be placed on the nude body, while fanning the patient vigorously and massaging the skin. Because of its rapid cooling effect, alcohol should not be applied to the skin. The patient's temperature should be checked every 10 min and should not be allowed to fall below 101°F (38.5°C), to prevent changing hyperthermia to hypothermia. Careful observation of the patient for signs of fluid and electrolyte imbalance and renal failure will be required for several days. Peritoneal lavage using ice cold, sterile saline has also been used to treat heatstroke. SEE: *peritoneal dialysis*.

NURSING IMPLICATIONS: The nurse participates in efforts to educate the public about heat-related illnesses. Athletes and coaches are taught to recognize the signs and symptoms of heat problems and the importance of prevention and prompt treatment should they occur. Patients at particular risk (elderly, obese, diabetic, and cardiac patients; alcoholics, patients with chronic debilitating illnesses, and patients taking phenothiazine or anticholinergic drugs) are advised about hot weather precautions to avoid heat illnesses: wearing loose-fitting, lightweight clothing; taking frequent rest breaks, especially during strenuous activities; ingesting adequate amounts of fluids, in-

**Comparison of Heatstroke and Heat Exhaustion**

| Heatstroke | Heat Exhaustion |
|---|---|
| **Definition**<br>A condition or derangement of the thermoregulatory center due to exposure to the rays of the sun or very high temperatures. Loss of body heat is inadequate or absent. | **Definition**<br>A state of definite weakness produced by the excess loss of normal fluids and sodium chloride in the form of sweat. |
| **History**<br>Exposure to high environmental temperature; use of medications that increase heat production or inhibit perspiration. | **History**<br>Exposure to heat, usually indoors |
| **Differential Symptoms**<br>*Face:* Red, dry, and hot<br>*Skin:* Hot, dry, and no sweating<br>*Temperature:* High, 106° to 110°F (41.1° to 43.3°C)<br>*Pulse:* Full, rapid, strong, bounding<br>*Respirations:* Dyspneic, fast, sonorous<br>*Muscles:* Tense and possible convulsions<br>*Eyes:* Pupils are dilated but equal | **Differential Symptoms**<br>*Face:* Pale, cool, and moist<br>*Skin:* Cool, clammy, with profuse diaphoresis<br>*Temperature:* Usually not above 100°F (37.8°C)<br>*Pulse:* Weak, thready, and rapid<br>*Respirations:* Shallow and quiet<br>*Muscles:* Tense and contracted<br>*Eyes:* Pupils are normal; eyeballs may be soft |
| **Treatment**<br>Absolute rest with head elevated; keep body cool by any means available until hospitalized, but do not use alcohol applied to skin. Take temperature every 10 minutes, and do not allow it to fall below 101°F (38.5°C) to prevent hypothermia.<br>*Drugs:* Allow no stimulants; give infusions of normal saline (to force fluids). | **Treatment**<br>Keep patient quiet; head should be lowered to prevent orthostatic hypotension; keep body warm to prevent onset of shock.<br>*Drugs:* Salty fluids and fruit juices should be given frequently in small amounts. Intravenous isotonic saline will be required if patient is unconscious. |

cluding electrolyte solutions; avoiding hot environments as much as possible; using fans (and opening windows and doors) or air conditioner and seeking air-conditioned areas (shopping malls, public buildings such as libraries) for relief.

The patient admitted to the emergency department with heatstroke is assessed for weakness, dizziness, nausea, vomiting, blurred vision, and a history of specific cause. Using a rectal probe, the nurse monitors the patient's temperature; initially it may be 106°F (41.1°C) or higher. Skin is inspected and palpated for redness, diaphoresis, and heat (early stages), or gray coloration, dryness and heat (later stages). Respirations are monitored for evidence of hyperpnea, the pulse is palpated for rapidity, and blood pressure is auscultated for early elevations and later hypotension. Neurological status is assessed; the conscious patient may demonstrate dilated pupils, emotional lability, and confusion, with delirium, seizure, collapse, and unconsciousness occurring as the condition progresses. In late stages, the patient may manifest slow, deep respirations, progressing to Cheyne-Stokes respirations. Serum electrolyte levels are monitored for hyponatremia and hypokalemia, and arterial blood gas values for acid-base imbalances (respiratory alkalosis with compensatory metabolic acidosis). Laboratory studies are also monitored for leukocytosis, elevated blood urea nitrogen, hemoconcentration, hypocalcemia, hypophosphoremia, thrombocytopenia, increased bleeding and clotting times, fibrinolysis, and consumption coagulopathy; and urine studies for concentration (high specific gravity), with elevated protein levels, tubular casts, and myoglobinuria. Cooling procedures are instituted as necessary, including use of a hypothermia mattress and blanket and electronic temperature-regulating equipment if prescribed. The nurse places the unclothed patient in a lateral recumbent or knee-chest position to expose as much skin area as possible to the air and cooling equipment. Supportive measures are provided as necessary, including a patent airway, prescribed supplemental oxygen, and endotracheal intubation and mechanical ventilation. Adequate fluid intake is maintained, and intravenous fluid intake initiated as prescribed. Urinary output is monitored, and an indwelling urinary catheter inserted as necessary. Prescribed medications are administered to inhibit shivering. Cardiac and hemodynamic complications are monitored electronically and by central line measurements. The recovering patient is advised to avoid re-exposure to high temperatures because of the possibility of continued hypersensitivity. Preventive measures (as above) are taught. As necessary, the patient is referred to a social service agency for assistance with home cooling.

**heat unit** ABBR: HU. The amount of heat created at the anode during the production of x-ray photons. It is the product of the milliamperage times the seconds of exposure times the kilovoltage peak.

**heaves** (hēvs) Vomiting.

**heavy chain disease** ABBR: HCD. Any one of several abnormalities of immunoglobulins in which excessive quantities of alpha, gamma, delta, epsilon, or mu chains are produced. The immunoglobulins formed are incomplete, causing, in some cases, distinct clinical signs and symptoms including weakness, recurrent fever, susceptibility to bacterial infections, lymphadenopathy, hepatosplenomegaly, erythema, and edema of the soft palate; anemia, leukopenia, thrombocytopenia, eosinophilia, and abnormal protein electrophoretic patterns are also produced.

***alpha h.c.d.*** A form of heavy chain disease that is related to a malignancy known as Mediterranean lymphoma. The principal areas of involvement are the intestinal tract and rarely the respiratory tract. The symptoms and signs, which may come and go, include malabsorption, diarrhea, abdominal pains, and eventually weight loss. In some patients there is peripheral adenopathy and splenomegaly with no signs of intestinal or respiratory tract changes. The intestinal tract forms have been termed immunoproliferative small intestinal diseases (IPSID). Diagnosis is made through tests for the abnormal immunoglobulins. Chemotherapy may produce long-term remissions. SYN: *Seligmann's disease.*

***gamma h.c.d.*** A heavy chain disease that may affect persons of all ages from early childhood on. Clinically there is lymphadenopathy, hepatosplenomegaly, edema of the uvula, and infiltration of the skin and thyroid gland. Treatment includes therapy for the underlying disorders, including the particular type of lymphoma present. SEE: *heavy chain disease.*

***mu h.c.d.*** A heavy chain disease with presenting symptoms of a lymphoproliferative malignancy, especially chronic lymphocytic leukemia. Treatment focuses on the underlying disorders.

**Heberden's disease** (hē'bĕr-dĕnz) [William Heberden, Brit. physician, 1710–1801] Arthritis with deformity that begins in the fingers and progresses. The concomitant deformity is caused by ankylosis, exostosis, and atrophy of soft parts. SYN: *rheumatoid arthritis.*

**Heberden's nodes** Hard nodules or enlargements of the tubercles of the last phalanges of the fingers; seen in osteoarthritis.

**hebetude** [L. *hebet,* dull] Dullness or lethargy.

**hebotomy** (hē-bŏt'ō-mē) Pubiotomy.

**hecateromeric, hecatomeric** (hĕk"ă-tĕr"ō-mĕr'ĭk, hĕk"ă-tō-mĕr'ĭk) [Gr. *hekateros,* each of two, + *meros,* part] Having two processes on a spinal neuron, one supplying each side of the spinal cord.

**hecto-** [Gr. *hekaton,* hundred] In the metric system, a prefix indicating 100 times ($10^2$) the unit named. Thus, hectoliter ($10^2$ liters) is 100 L.

**hectogram** [" + *gramma,* small weight] One hundred grams, or 3.527 avoirdupois ounces.

**hectoliter** (hĕk'tō-lē"tĕr) [" + *litra,* a pound] One hundred liters.

**hectometer** (hĕk-tŏm'ĕ-tĕr) [" + *metron,* measure] One hundred meters.

**hedonism** (hēd'ŏn-ĭzm) [Gr. *hedone,* pleasure, + *-ismos,* condition] A theory or standard of conduct in which the principal object of life is pleasure. SYN: *pleasure principle.*

**heel** [AS. *huela,* heel] Rounded posterior portion of the foot under and behind the ankle. SYN: *calx.*

***h. bone*** Calcaneus.

***h. puncture*** A method for obtaining a blood sample from a newborn or premature infant.

---

Caution: The puncture should be made in the lateral or medial area of the plantar surface of the heel, while avoiding the posterior curvature of the heel. The puncture should go no deeper than 2.4 mm. Previous puncture sites should not be used.

---

***Thomas h.*** A corrective shoe in which the heel is approx. 12 mm longer and 4 to 6 mm higher on the medial edge. This produces varus of the foot and prevents depression of the head of the talus.

**HEENT** *head, eyes, ears, nose, throat.*

**Heerfordt's disease** (hār'forts) [C. F. Heerfordt, Danish ophthalmologist, 1871–1973] Uveoparotid fever, a form of sarcoidosis, marked by enlargement of the parotid gland, inflammation of the uveal tract, and prolonged low-grade fever.

**Hegar's sign** (hā'gărz) [Alfred Hegar, Ger. gynecologist, 1830–1914] A sign that may be present during the second and third months of pregnancy. On bimanual examination, the lower part of the uterus is easily compressed between the fingers placed in the vagina and those of the other hand over the pelvic area. This is due to the softening of lower segments of the uterus and to the fact that the fetus does not fill the uterine cavity at this stage, leaving an empty space in the lower part. The sign is not a positive one for pregnancy.

**Heidenhain's demilunes** (hī'dĕn-hīnz) [Rudolph Peter Heinrich Heidenhain, Ger. physiologist, 1834–1897] Crescent-shaped groups of serous cells at the base, or along the sides, of the mucous alveoli of the salivary glands, esp. sublingual and submandibular. SYN: *Giannuzzi's cells*.

**height** (hīt) [AS. *hiehthu*] The vertical distance from the bottom to the top of an organ or structure.

***h. of contour*** A line encircling a structure designating its greatest diameter in a specified plane. In dentistry, the term refers to the path of insertion or removal of a partial denture.

***fundal h.*** A measure of the uterine fundus, used in obstetrics. *Antepartum:* The distance between the symphysis pubis and the crown of the pregnant uterus, measured in centimeters, is used in assessing and confirming the estimated weeks of gestation. The fundus is first palpable at the level of the symphysis pubis during gestational week 12. SEE: *McDonald's rule. Postpartum:* The distance between the uterine fundus and the umbilicus, measured in fingerbreadths, is used in assessing the progress of uterine involution. After rising to the level of the umbilicus immediately after delivery, fundal height diminishes by approx. 1 fingerbreadth per postpartum day.

**Heimlich maneuver** (hīm'lĭk) [H. J. Heimlich, U.S. physician, b. 1920] A technique for removing a foreign body from the trachea or pharynx, where it is preventing air flow to the lungs. The obstruction usually is caused by a bolus of food. Also called *abdominal thrust maneuver*.

The maneuver consists of the rescuer applying subdiaphragmatic pressure by: (1) wrapping his or her arms around the victim's waist from behind; (2) making a fist with one hand and placing it against the victim's abdomen between the navel and the rib cage; and (3) clasping the fist with the free hand and pressing in with a quick forceful upward thrust. This procedure should be repeated several times if necessary. If one is alone and experiences airway obstruction caused by a foreign body, this technique could be self-applied.

If the person is supine, place the heel of one of your hands on the abdomen in the same position as described and then, with the other hand on top of that hand, exert a sudden upward pressure in the midline.

When the victim is a child and he or she can speak, breathe, or cough, the maneuver is unnecessary. If the maneuver is done it should be applied as gently as possible but still forcibly enough to dislodge the obstruction. The abdominal viscera of children are more easily damaged than those of adults.

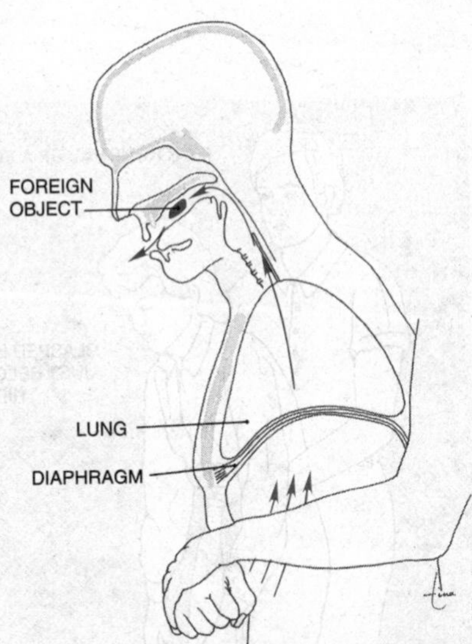


PHYSIOLOGY OF HEIMLICH MANEUVER

This treatment is quite effective in dislodging the obstruction by forcing air against the mass much as pressure from a carbonated beverage forcibly removes a cork or cap from a bottle. The average air flow produced is 225 L/min. SEE: illus.; *choking*.

**Heimlich sign** Grasping one's throat with the thumb and index finger to signal choking.

**Heineke-Mikulicz pyloroplasty** (hī'nĕ-kĕ-mĭk'ū-lĭch) [Walter Hermann Heineke, Ger. surgeon, 1834–1901; Johann von Mikulicz-Radecki, Polish surgeon, 1850–1905] Pyloroplasty of the stomach, done to enlarge the outlet of the stomach.

**Heinz bodies** [Robert Heinz, Ger. pathologist, 1865–1924] Granules in red blood cells caused by damage of the hemoglobin molecules, seen in premature infants, in certain forms of drug sensitivity, and in a certain type of hereditary hemolytic anemia. The bodies are best seen when the blood is stained with a special stain. SEE: illus.

**Heinz body anemia** Hemolytic anemia of infancy associated with the finding of Heinz bodies in the red blood cells.

**Heister, spiral valve of** (hī'stĕr) [Lorenz Heister, Ger. anatomist, 1683–1758] A spiral fold of the mucous membrane lining the cystic duct of the gallbladder. It serves to keep the lumen open.

**HeLa cells** SEE: under *cell*.

**helcoid** (hĕl'koyd) [Gr. *helkos*, ulcer, + *eidos*, form, shape] Resembling an ulcer.

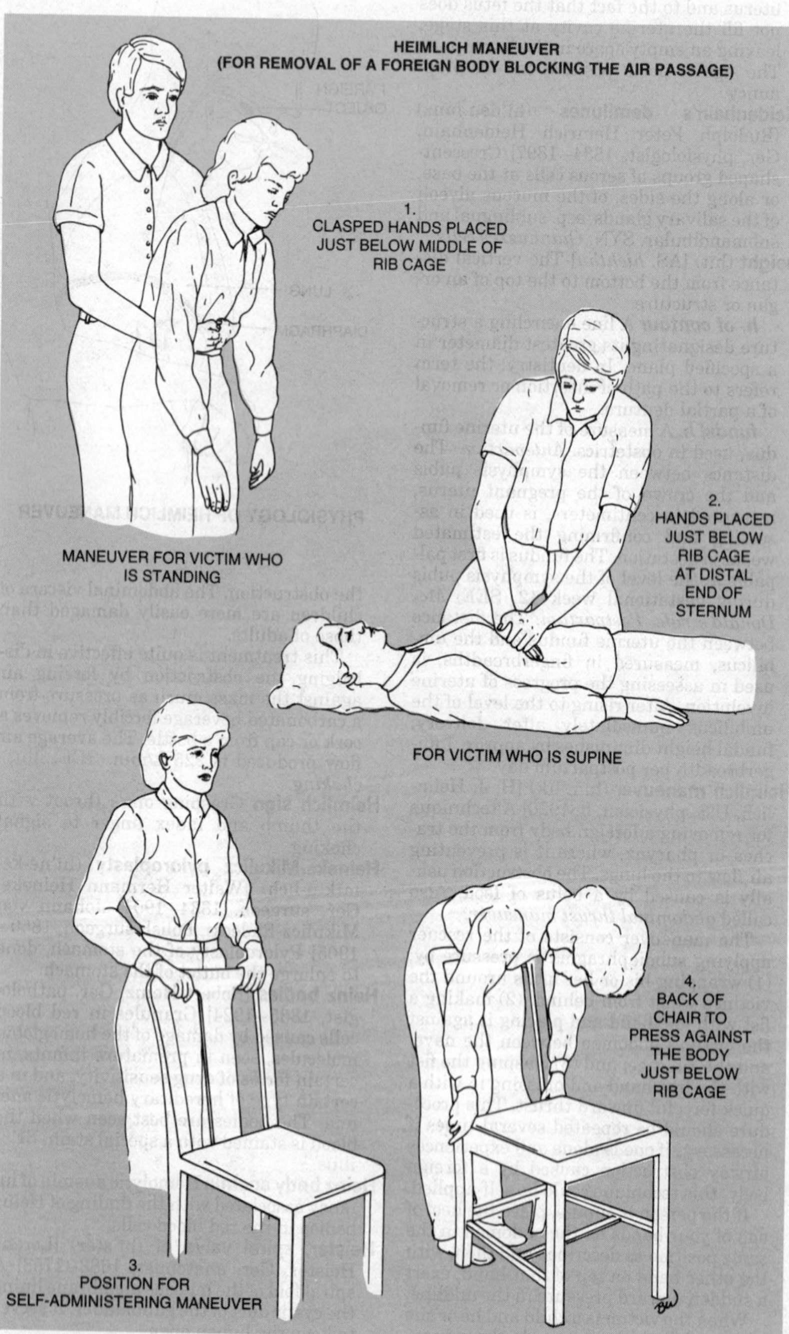
HEIMLICH MANEUVER
(FOR REMOVAL OF A FOREIGN BODY BLOCKING THE AIR PASSAGE)
1.
CLASPED HANDS PLACED
JUST BELOW MIDDLE OF
RIB CAGE
MANEUVER FOR VICTIM WHO
IS STANDING
2.
HANDS PLACED
JUST BELOW
RIB CAGE
AT DISTAL
END OF
STERNUM
FOR VICTIM WHO IS SUPINE
3.
POSITION FOR
SELF-ADMINISTERING MANEUVER
4.
BACK OF
CHAIR TO
PRESS AGAINST
THE BODY
JUST BELOW
RIB CAGE

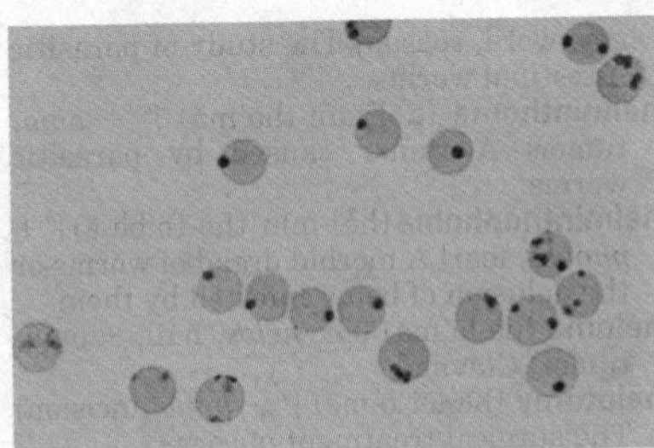

HEINZ BODIES (ORIG. MAG. ×500)

**helcology** (hĕl-kŏl′ō-jē) [″ + *logos*, word, reason] The study of ulcers.

**helcoma** (hĕl-kō′mă) [″ + *oma*, tumor] Ulcer of the cornea.

**helcosis** (hĕl-kō′sĭs) [″ + *osis*, condition] Ulceration.

**helianthine** (hē-lē-ăn′thĭn) Methyl orange used as an indicator in determining pH.

**helical** (hĕl′ĭ-kăl) In the shape of a helix.

**helicine** (hĕl′ĭ-sĭn) [Gr. *helix*, coil] **1.** Spiral. **2.** Pert. to a helix or coil.

***h. arteries*** Tortuous arteries in the cavernous tissue of the penis, clitoris, and uterus.

**Helicobacter pylori** A motile, gram-negative bacterium that causes some peptic ulcers, which are treated with combined antibiotics and agents to block gastric acid secretion.

DIAGNOSIS: Noninvasive diagnostic procedures include immunological tests of antibodies to *H. pylori* and urea breath tests. Invasive tests include endoscopy, gastric biopsy, and biopsy with bacterial culture for *H. pylori*.

**helicoid** (hĕl′ĭ-koyd) [″ + *eidos*, form, shape] Resembling a helix or spiral.

**helicopodia** (hĕl″ĭ-kō-pō′dē-ă) [″ + *pous*, foot] A peculiar movement in which the foot, when brought forward, drags and describes a partial arc, resulting in a gait such as that seen in spastic hemiplegia.

**helicotrema** (hĕl″ĭ-kō-trē′mă) [″ + *trema*, a hole] The opening at the tip of the cochlear canal where the scala tympani and scala vestibuli unite.

**heliophobia** (hē″lē-ō-fō′bē-ă) [Gr. *helios*, sun, + *phobos*, fear] An abnormal fear of the sun's rays, esp. by one who has suffered a sunstroke.

**heliotaxis** (hē-lē-ō-tăk′sĭs) [″ + *taxis*, arrangement] A reaction in plants that causes them to respond negatively or positively to the sunlight.

***negative h.*** A turning away from the sun.

***positive h.*** A turning toward the sun.

**heliotherapy** (hē″lē-ō-thĕr′ă-pē) [″ + *therapeia*, treatment] Exposure to sunlight for therapeutic purposes.

**heliotropism** (hē″lē-ŏt′rō-pĭzm) [″ + *trepein*, to turn, + *-ismos*, condition] The tendency of living organisms to turn or grow toward the sun.

**heliox** A therapeutic gas mixture of helium and oxygen.

**helium** (hē′lē-ŭm) [Gr. *helios*, sun] SYMB: He. A gaseous element; atomic weight 4.0026; atomic number 2. A liter of the gas at sea level pressure and 0°C weighs 0.1785 g. The second lightest element known, it is given off by radium and other radioactive elements in the form of charged helium ions known as alpha rays. Because of its low density, it is mixed with air or oxygen and used in the treatment of various respiratory disorders. Because of its low solubility, it is mixed with air supplied to workers laboring under high atmospheric pressure, as in caissons. When so used, it reduces the time required to adjust to increasing or decreasing air pressure and reduces the danger of bends.

**helix** (hē′lĭks) [Gr., coil] **1.** A coil or spiral. **2.** The margin of the external ear.

***Watson-Crick h.*** SEE: *Watson-Crick helix*.

**Heller's test** [Johann F. Heller, Austrian pathologist, 1813–1871] A test for the presence of albumin in urine. Pure nitric acid is poured into a clean test tube to a depth of ½ in. (13 mm) and carefully overlaid with an equal quantity of urine. The presence of albumin is indicated by the appearance of an opaque white ring at the junction of the fluids. Certain drugs in the urine and urates in highly concentrated specimens may give false-positive test results. SEE: *urine*.

**Hellin's law** [Dyonizy Hellin, Polish pathologist, 1867–1935] A law stating that twins occur once in 80 pregnancies, triplets once in 6400 ($80^2$) pregnancies, quadruplets once in 512,000 ($80^3$) pregnancies.

**HELLP** An acronym derived from the first letters of the terms that describe the following laboratory findings: Hemolysis, Elevated Liver enzymes, and Low Platelet count.

**HELLP syndrome** Severe pre-eclampsia characterized by hemolysis, elevated liver function, and low platelets. The syndrome occurs most commonly in the last trimester of pregnancy, often in association with severe pregnancy-induced hypertension. SEE: *pre-eclampsia*.

**helmet cell** An erythrocyte that has partially fragmented as if bitten off. It may be seen in peripheral blood in pulmonary embolism, certain carcinomas, glucose-6-phosphate dehydrogenase deficiency, and disseminated intravascular coagulation. Also called *bite cell*. SEE: illus.

**helminth** [Gr. *helmins*, worm] **1.** A wormlike animal. **2.** Any animal, either free-living or parasitic, belonging to the phyla Platy-

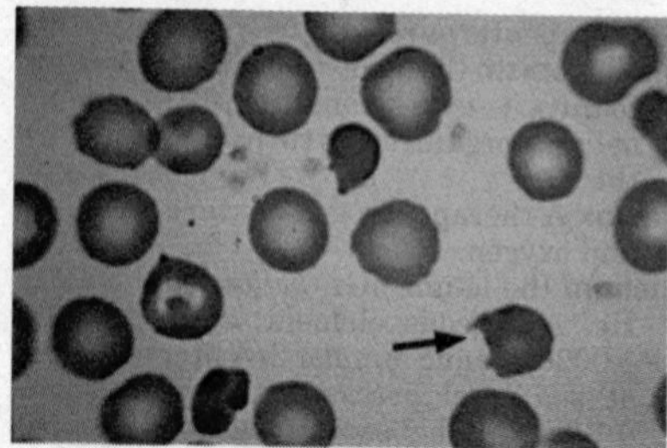

HELMET CELL (ARROW) (ORIG. MAG. ×640)

helminthes (flatworms), Acanthocephala (spinyheaded worms), Nemathelminthes (threadworms or roundworms), or Annelida (segmented worms). SEE: illus.

**helminthagogue** (hĕl-mĭnth′ă-gŏg) [″ + *agogos,* leading] Anthelmintic.

**helminthemesis** (hĕl-mĭn-thĕm′ĕ-sĭs) [″ + *emesis,* vomiting] The vomiting of intestinal worms.

**helminthiasis** (hĕl-mĭn-thī′ă-sĭs) [″ + *iasis,* condition] Having intestinal parasites or worms.

**helminthic** (hĕl-mĭn′thĭk) **1.** Pert. to worms. **2.** Pert. to that which expels worms. SYN: *anthelmintic; vermifugal.*

**helminthicide** (hĕl-mĭn′thĭ-sīd) [″ + L. *cidus,* kill] Anthelmintic.

**helminthoid** (hĕl-mĭn′thoyd) [″ + *eidos,* form, shape] Wormlike or resembling a worm.

**helminthology** (hĕl″mĭn-thŏl′ō-jē) [″ + *logos,* word, reason] The study of parasitic intestinal worms.

**helminthoma** (hĕl″mĭn-thō′mă) [″ + *oma,* tumor] A tumor caused by parasitic worms.

**helminthophobia** (hĕl-mĭn″thō-fō′bē-ă) [″ + *phobos,* fear] A morbid dread of worms or the delusion of being infested by them.

**heloma** (hē-lō′mă) [Gr. *helos,* nail, + *oma,* tumor] Clavus.

**helotomy** (hē-lŏt′ō-mē) [″ + *tome,* incision] The surgical treatment of corns.

**helper T cells** SEE: *cell, helper T.*

**helplessness** A state that may arise when a patient has a condition in which he or she is dependent on an outside source for life support. Such patients feel unable to alter their situation and experience anxiety owing to their inability to relieve their own discomfort. A fear of the necessary dependency on other people or even on mechanical supports may also be present. SEE: *giving-up; hopelessness; powerlessness.*

***learned h.*** A passive, rather fatalistic behavior based on the feeling that one is helpless. Lack of control in the elderly experiencing chronic illness and environmental and familial losses leads to a sense of passivity and acceptance.

**Helweg's bundle** (hĕl′vĕgz) [Hans K. S. Helweg, Danish physician, 1847–1901] A small tract passing from the olivary body to the anterior horn cells in the cervical region. Part of the extrapyramidal motor system.

**hem-, hema-, hemo-** [Gr. *haima,* blood] Combining form meaning *blood.* SEE: *he-*

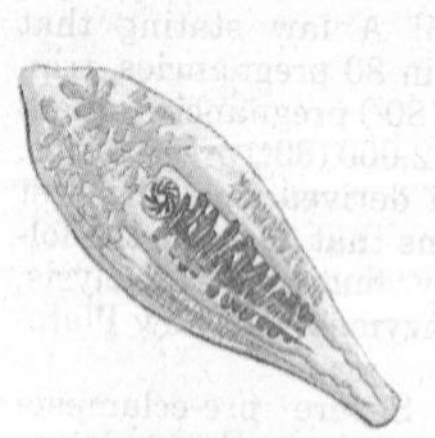

FLUKE (×4)

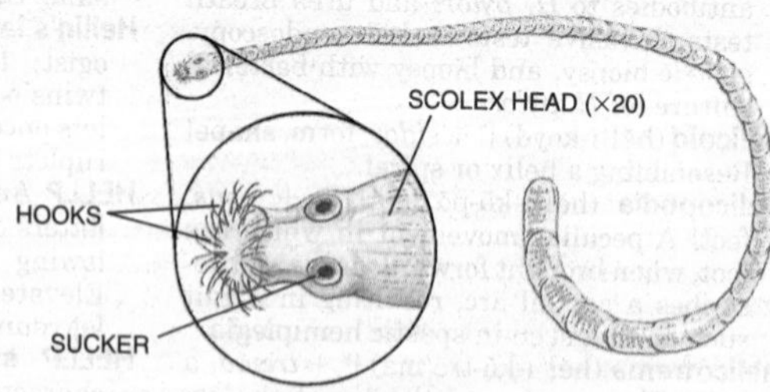


TAPEWORM (ACTUAL SIZE)

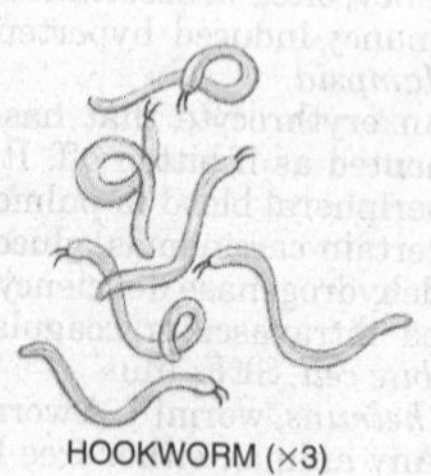

HOOKWORM (×3)

PINWORM (×2)

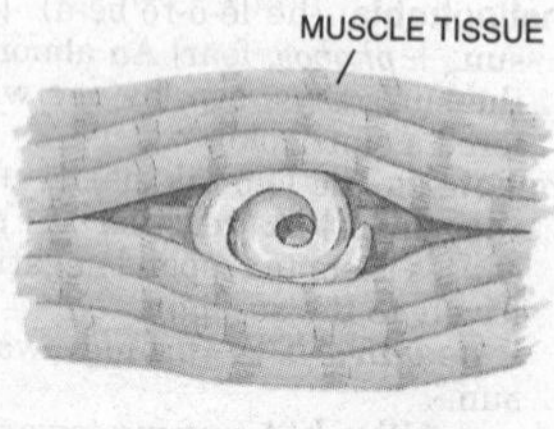


TRICHINELLA (×100)

REPRESENTATIVE HELMINTHS

*mat-*.

**hemachrosis** (hē″mă-, hĕm″ă-krō′sĭs) [″ + *chrosis,* coloring] Abnormal redness of blood. It is present in carbon monoxide poisoning.

**hemacytometer** (hē″mă-, hĕm″ă-sī-tŏm′ĭ-tĕr) [″ + *kytos,* cell, + *metron,* measure] Apparatus used in counting blood cells.

**hemacytozoon** (hē″mă-, hĕm″ă-sī-tō-zō′ŏn) [″ + ″ + *zoon,* animal] A protozoan parasite infesting red blood corpuscles.

**hemad** (hē′măd) [Gr. *haima,* blood, + L. *ad,* toward] Hemal (2).

**hemadsorption** (hĕm″ăd-sorp′shŭn) The adherence of red blood cells to other cells or surfaces.

**hemagglutination** (hĕm″ă-gloo-tĭ-nā′shŭn) [″+ L. *agglutinare,* to paste to] The clumping of red blood corpuscles.

***h. inhibition*** Prevention of hemagglutination by interaction or blocking of the antibody or virus that would otherwise cause it.

**hemagglutinin** (hĕm″ă-gloo′tĭ-nĭn) An antibody that induces clumping of red blood corpuscles.

***cold h.*** The agglutination of erythrocytes (usually from sheep) at low temperatures by the serum of patients with certain diseases.

***warm h.*** An agglutinin effective only at body temperature, 98.6°F (37°C).

**hemagogue** (hē″mă-, hĕm′ă-gŏg) [″ + *agogos,* leading] An agent that promotes the flow of blood, esp. menstrual flow. SEE: *emmenagogue*.

**hemal** (hē′măl) **1.** Pert. to the blood or blood vessels. **2.** Pert. to the ventral side of the body, in which the heart is located, as opposed to the neural or dorsal side. SYN: *hemad; hemic*.

***h. arch*** The ribs, breastbone, and portion of the vertebrae that, together, enclose the heart and viscera.

***h. gland*** H. node.

***h. node*** A body resembling a lymph node in structure but associated with blood vessels instead of lymph vessels; present in certain ungulates. SYN: *h. gland*.

**hemangiectasis** (hē″măn-, hĕm″ăn-jē-ĕk′tă-sĭs) [″ + *angeion,* vessel, + *ektasis,* dilatation] Dilatation of the blood vessels.

**hemangioblast** (hĕ-măn′jē-ō-blăst) [″ + ″ + *blastos,* germ] A mesodermal cell that can form either vascular endothelial cells or hemocytoblasts.

**hemangioblastoma** (hĕ-măn″jē-ō-blăs-tō′mă) [″ + ″ + *oma,* tumor] A hemangioma of the brain, usually in the cerebellum.

**hemangioendothelioblastoma** (hĕ-măn″jē-ō-ĕn″dō-thē″lē-ō-blăs-tō′mă) [″ + ″+ *endon,* within, + *thele,* nipple, + *blastos,* germ, + *oma,* tumor] A neoplasm of the epithelial cells that line the blood vessels.

**hemangioendothelioma** (hē″măn-jē-ō-ĕn″dō-thē-lē-ō′mă) [″ + ″ + ″ + ″ + *oma,* tumor] An overgrowth of the endothelium of the minute capillary vessels. It varies in size and is commonly seen in the capillary net of the cerebral meninges.

**hemangiofibroma** (hĕ-măn″jē-ō-fī-brō′mă) [″ + ″+ L. *fibra,* fiber, + Gr. *oma,* tumor] A fibrous hemangioma.

**hemangioma** (hē-măn″jē-ō′mă) *pl.* **hemangiomata** [″+ *angeion,* vessel, + *oma,* tumor] A benign tumor of dilated blood vessels.

**hemangiomatosis** (hē-măn″jē-ō-mă-tō′sĭs) [″ + ″ + *osis,* condition] Multiple angiomata of the blood vessels.

**hemangiopericytoma** (hĕ-măn″jē-ō-pĕr″ĕ-sī-tō′mă) A tumor arising in the capillaries, composed of pericytes.

**hemangiosarcoma** (hē-măn″jē-ō-săr-kō′mă) [″ + ″ + *sarkos,* flesh, + *oma,* tumor] A malignant neoplasm originating from the blood vessels. SYN: *angiosarcoma*.

**hemapheresis** SEE: *plasmapheresis*.

**hemapophysis** (hĕm-ă-pŏf′ĭ-sĭs) [″ + *apo,* from, + *physis,* growth] The portion of a developing vertebra that forms a rib and costal cartilage.

**hemarthros, hemarthrosis** (hĕm-ăr′thrōs, hĕm-ăr-thrō′sĭs) [″ + *arthron,* joint] A bloody effusion into the cavity of a joint.

**hemat-, hemato-** [Gr. *haimatos,* blood] Combining form meaning *blood*. SEE: *hem-*.

**hematapostema** (hĕm″ăt-ă-pŏs-tē′mă) [Gr. *haimatos,* blood, + *apostema,* abscess] An abscess that contains blood.

**hematemesis** (hĕm-ăt-ĕm′ĕ-sĭs) [″ + *emesis,* vomiting] The vomiting of blood. SEE: *hemoptysis* for table; *hemorrhage*.

SYMPTOMS: The blood is often clotted and mixed with food. Subsequent stools may be tarry. If of gastric origin, the blood is generally dark and acidic. If of pharyngeal origin, it is bright red and alkaline. If the blood loss is severe enough, shock and collapse may occur.

TREATMENT: The patient should lie down and be kept at absolute rest; should have nothing by mouth, but may be fed intravenously if necessary; and should be given no stimulants. Surgery may be necessary.

NURSING IMPLICATIONS: Vital signs are monitored. Vomitus is inspected and its character and quantity are documented, along with associated symptoms and state of alertness. The patient is supported in an upright position (or turned to one side) to prevent aspiration. Oral hygiene is provided after episodes of vomiting and as needed while the patient is not taking anything by mouth.

**hematencephalon** (hĕm″ăt-ĕn-sĕf′ă-lŏn) [″ + *enkephalos,* brain] A cerebral hemorrhage.

**hemathermal** (hĕm″ă-, hē″mă-thĕr′măl) [″ + *therme,* heat] Warm blooded; applied to animals whose blood remains at a fairly constant temperature.

**hemathidrosis, hematidrosis** (hē-măt″hĭ-drō′sĭs) [Gr. *haimatos,* blood, + *hidros,* sweat, + *osis,* condition] A condition in which sweat contains blood. SYN: *hematohidrosis; hemidrosis* (2).

**hematic** (hē-măt′ĭk) Hematinic.

**hematin** (hĕm′ă-tĭn) The nonprotein portion of the hemoglobin molecule wherein the iron is in the ferric ($Fe^{3+}$) rather than the ferrous ($Fe^{2+}$) state. SEE: *ferritin; heme.*

**hematinemia** (hē-mă-, hĕm-ă-tĭn-ē′mē-ă) Hematin in the circulating blood.

**hematinic** (hē-mă-, hĕm-ă-tĭn′ĭk) [Gr. *haima,* blood] **1.** Pert. to blood. **2.** An agent that facilitates blood formation, used in treating anemia. SYN: *hematic.*

**hemato-** SEE: *hemat-.*

**hematobilia** (hĕm″ă-tō-bĭl′ē-ă) [″ + L. *bilis,* bile] Blood in the bile or bile ducts.

**hematobium** (hē″mă-, hĕm″ă-tō′bē-ŭm) [″ + *bios,* life] Hemocytozoon.

**hematoblast** (hē′mă-, hĕm′ă-tō-blăst) [″ + *blastos,* germ] Hemocytoblast.

**hematocele** (hē′mă-, hĕm′ă-tō-sēl) [″ + *kele,* tumor, swelling] **1.** A blood cyst. **2.** The effusion of blood into a cavity. **3.** A swelling due to effusion of blood into the tunica vaginalis testis.

***parametric h.*** A tumor formed by blood effusion in the cul-de-sac of Douglas walled off by adhesions.

***pudendal h.*** A blood-filled swollen area of the labium.

**hematocelia** (hĕm″ă-tō-sē′ lē-ă) [″ + *koilia,* cavity] A hemorrhage into the peritoneal cavity.

**hematochezia** (hĕm″ă-tō-kē′zē-ă) [″+ *chezein,* to go to stool] The passage of stools containing red blood rather than tarry stools.

**hematochromatosis** (hĕm″ă-tō-krō″mă-tō′sĭs) [″ + *chroma,* color, + *osis,* condition] Hemochromatosis.

**hematochyluria** (hē″mă-, hĕm″ă-tō-kī-lū′rē-ă) [″ + *chylos,* juice, + *ouron,* urine] Blood and chyle in the urine.

**hematocolpos** (hē″mă-, hĕm″ă-tō-kŏl′pŏs) Retention of menstrual blood in the vagina, caused by an imperforate hymen.

**hematocrit** (hē-măt′ō-krĭt) [″ + *krinein,* to separate] **1.** A centrifuge for separating solids from plasma in the blood. **2.** The volume of erythrocytes packed by centrifugation in a given volume of blood. The hematocrit is expressed as the percentage of total blood volume that consists of erythrocytes or as the volume in cubic centimeters of erythrocytes packed by centrifugation of blood. Normal values at sea level: men, average 47%, range 40% to 54%; women, average 42%, range 37% to 47%; children, varies with age from 35% to 49%; newborn, 49% to 54%. SEE: *blood; buffy coat.*

**hematocyst** (hē′mă-, hĕm′ă-tō-sĭst) [Gr. *haimatos,* blood, + *kystis,* a bladder] **1.** Hemorrhage into a cyst or into the urinary bladder. **2.** A blood-filled cyst.

**hematocytoblast** (hĕm″ă-tō-sī′tō-blăst) [″ + ″ + *blastos,* germ] Hemocytoblast.

**hematocytometer** (hē″mă-, hĕm″ă-tō-sī-tŏm′ĕ-ter) [″ + ″+ *metron,* measure] A device for counting the number of blood cells in a given quantity of blood. SYN: *hemocytometer.*

**hematocytozoon** (hē″mă-, hĕm″ă-tō-sī-tō-zō′ŏn) [″ + ″ + *zoon,* animal] A parasite that lives in red blood cells.

**hematocyturia** (hē″mă-, hĕm″ă-tō-sī-tū′rē-ă) [″ + ″ + *ouron,* urine] Red blood cells in the urine; hematuria, as differentiated from hemoglobinuria.

**hematogenesis** (hē″mă-, hĕm″ă-tō-jĕn′ĕ-sĭs) [″ + *genesis,* generation, birth] Hematopoiesis.

**hematogenic, hematogenous** (hē″mă-, hĕm″ă-tō-jĕn′ĭk, -tŏj′ĕ-nŭs) [″ + *gennan,* to produce] **1.** Hematopoietic. **2.** Pert. to or originating in the blood.

**hematohidrosis** (hē″mă-, hĕm″ă-tō-hī-drō′sĭs) [″ + *hidros,* sweat, + *osis,* condition] Hemathidrosis.

**hematoidin** (hē″mă-, hĕm-ă-toy′din) The yellow crystalline substance, biliverdin, that remains when red blood cells are destroyed in bruised tissue.

**hematologist** (hē″mă-, hĕm″ă-tŏl′ō-jĭst) [″ + *logos,* word, reason] One who specializes in the study of the blood and in the diagnosis and treatment of disorders of blood and blood-forming tissues.

**hematology** (hē″mă-, hĕm″ă-tŏl′ō-jē) The science concerned with blood and the blood-forming tissues.

**hematolymphangioma** (hē″mă-, hĕm″ă-tō-lĭmf-ăn″jē-ō′mă) [″ + L. *lympha,* lymph, + Gr. *angeion,* vessel, + *oma,* tumor] A tumor consisting of dilated blood vessels and lymphatics. SYN: *hemolymphangioma.*

**hematolytic** (hĕm-ă-tō-lĭt′ĭk) Hemolytic.

**hematoma** (hē″mă-, hĕm-ă-tō′mă) [Gr. *haimatos,* blood, + *oma,* tumor] A swelling or mass of blood (usually clotted) confined to an organ, tissue, or space and caused by a break in a blood vessel.

***h. auris*** An effusion of blood, causing a hard swelling between perichondrium and the cartilage of the pinna of the ear. Common in fighters and wrestlers. SYN: *othematoma.* SEE: *cauliflower ear.*

***epidural h.*** A hematoma above the dura mater, usually arterial, except in posterior fossa.

***intracerebral h.*** A hemorrhage localized in one area of the brain.

***pelvic h.*** A hematoma present in the cellular tissue of the pelvis.

***subarachnoid h.*** A hemorrhage between the arachnoid membrane and the pia mater; usually caused by the rupture of a congenital intracranial aneurysm or berry aneurysm, hypertension, or trauma. It usually results from an arterial bleed.

***subdural h.*** A hematoma located beneath the dura, usually the result of a head injury.

***vulvar h.*** A hematoma occurring on the

vulva.

**hematomediastinum** (hē″mă-, hĕm″ă-tō-mē″dē-ă-stī′nŭm) [″ + L. *mediastinus*, in the middle] Hemomediastinum.

**hematometra** (hē″mă-, hĕm″ă-tō-mē′tră) [″ + *metra*, uterus] **1.** Hemorrhage in the uterus. **2.** An accumulation of menstrual blood in the uterus. SEE: *hematocolpos; hydrometra; pyometra*.

**hematomphalocele** (hē″mă-, hĕm″ăt-ŏm-făl′ō-sēl) [″ + *omphalos*, navel, + *kele*, tumor, swelling] The effusion of blood into an umbilical hernia.

**hematomyelia** (hē″mă-, hĕm″ă-tō-mī-ē′lē-ă) [″ + *myelos*, marrow] Hemorrhage of blood into the spinal cord.

**hematomyelitis** (hē″mă-, hĕm″ă-tō-mī″ĕl-ī′tĭs) [″ + ″+ *itis*, inflammation] An inflammation of the spinal cord accompanied by bloody effusion.

**hematonephrosis** (hē″mă-, hĕm″ă-tō-nĕ-frō′sĭs) [″ + *nephros*, kidney, + *osis*, condition] Hemonephrosis.

**hematopathology** [″ + *pathos*, disease, suffering, + *logos*, word, reason] The study of pathologic conditions of the blood.

**hematopericardium** (hē″mă-, hĕm″ă-tō-pĕr″ĭ-kăr′dē-ŭm) [″ + *peri*, around, + *kardia*, heart] A bloody effusion into the pericardial sac.

**hematoperitoneum** (hē″mă-, hĕm″ă-tō-pĕr″ĭ-tō-nē′ŭm) [″ + *peritonaion*, peritoneum] Hemoperitoneum.

**hematophagia** (hĕm″ă-tō-fā′jē-ă) **1.** The ingestion of blood. **2.** The destruction of blood cells by phagocytes.

**hematophagous** (hĕm-ă-tŏf′ă-gŭs) Living on blood.

**hematophilia** (hĕm″ă-tō-fĭ′ē-ă) [″ + *philein*, to love] Hemophilia.

**hematophobia** (hē″mă-, hĕm″ă-tō-fō′bē-ă) [″ + *phobos*, fear] Hemophobia.

**hematophyte** (hē′mă-, hĕm′ă-tō-fīt) [″ + *phyton*, plant] A plant organism or bacterium in the blood.

**hematoplastic** [″ + *plassein*, to form] Hematopoietic.

**hematopoiesis** (hē″mă-, hĕm″ă-tō-poy-ē′sĭs) [Gr. *haimatos*, blood, + *poiesis*, formation] The production and development of blood cells, normally in the bone marrow.

***extramedullary h.*** The production of blood cells in tissues other than bone marrow, which occurs in severe anemia and other diseases affecting the blood.

**hematopoietic** (hē″mă-, hĕm″ă-tō-poy-ĕt′ĭk) **1.** Pert. to the production and development of blood cells. **2.** A substance that assists in or stimulates the production of blood cells. SYN: *hematogenic; hematoplastic*.

***h. growth factors*** A group of at least seven substances involved in the production of blood cells, including several interleukins and erythropoietin.

***h. malignancies*** Cancers that arise from unregulated clonal proliferation of hematopoietic stem cells, such as leukemia and lymphoma. The individual cells, most of which are incompetent and useless, mature slowly and survive longer than normal. These conditions (leukemia and lymphoma) are lethal not because of the rapid production of new cells but due to the constant generation of defective new cells. SEE: *leukemia; lymphoma*.

***h. system*** The blood-forming organs, esp. bone marrow and the lymph nodes.

**hematoporphyrin** (hē″mă-, hĕm″ă-tō-por′fĭ-rĭn) [″ + *porphyra*, purple] Iron-free heme, a decomposition product of hemoglobin present in the urine in certain conditions.

**hematoporphyrinuria** (hē″mă-, hĕm″ă-tō-por″fĭ-rĭn-ū′rē-ă) [″ + ″ + *ouron*, urine] Hematoporphyrin in the urine.

**hematorrhachis** (hĕm-ă-tor′ă-kĭs) [″ + *rhachis*, spine] Hemorrhage into the spinal cord.

**hematosalpinx** (hē″mă-, hĕm″ă-tō-săl′pinks) [″ + *salpinx*, tube] Retained menstrual fluid in a fallopian tube. SYN: *hemosalpinx*.

**hematoscheocele** (hĕm-ă-tŏs′kē-ō-sēl) [″ + *oscheon*, scrotum, + *kele*, tumor, swelling] Blood accumulated in the scrotum.

**hematospermatocele** (hĕm″ă-tō-spĕr-măt′ō-sēl) [″ + *sperma*, seed, + *kele*, tumor, swelling] A blood-filled spermatocele.

**hematospermia** (hĕm″ă-tō-spĕr′mē-ă) Semen that contains blood. SYN: *hemospermia*.

***h. spuria*** Hematospermia coming from the prostatic urethra.

***h. vera*** Hematospermia coming from the seminal vesicles.

**hematostatic** (hĕm″ă-tō-stăt′ĭk) [Gr. *haimatos*, blood, + *stasis*, standing] **1.** Retaining blood in a part. **2.** Hemostatic.

**hematosteon** (hĕm-ă-tŏs′tē-ŏn) [″ + *osteon*, bone] Bleeding into the medullary cavity of a bone.

**hematothorax** (hĕm″ă-tō-thō′răks) [″ + *thorax*, chest] Hemothorax.

**hematotoxic** (hĕm″ă-tō-tŏk′sĭk) [″ + *toxikon*, poison] **1.** Pert. to septicemia. **2.** Toxic to blood cells.

**hematotropic** (hĕm″ă-tō-trŏp′ĭk) [″ + *tropos*, a turning] Having a special affinity for red blood cells.

**hematotympanum** (hĕm″ă-tō-tĭm′păn-ŭm) [″ + *tympanon*, drum] Blood in the middle ear.

**hematoxylin** (hĕm″ă-tŏk′sĭ-lĭn) $C_{16}H_{14}O_6$. A colorless crystalline compound obtained by ether extraction of the wood portion of the tree *Haematoxylon campechianum*. Upon oxidation it is converted into hematein, an oxidation product of hematoxylin, which stains certain structures a deep blue. An excellent nuclear stain, it is widely used in histological work.

**hematozoon** (hē″mă-, hĕm″ă-tō-zō′ŏn) [″ + *zoon*, animal] Any living organism in the blood. SYN: *hemozoon*.

**hematozymosis** (hē″mă-, hĕm″ă-tō-zī-mō′sĭs) [″ + *zymosis*, fermentation] Blood fermentation.

**hematuria** (hē″mă-, hĕm″ă-tū′rē-ă) [″ +

*ouron,* urine] Blood in the urine.

SYMPTOMS: Urine may be slightly smoky, reddish, or very red.

ETIOLOGY: Lesion of urinary tract; blood dyscrasia; contamination during menstruation or puerperium; prostatic disease; trauma; tumors; poisoning, esp. carbolic acid and cantharides; malaria, toxemias; or calculus in urinary tract.

DIAGNOSIS: If blood is well mixed with urine, it probably came from the kidneys. If clotted in tubular casts of ureters, it came from the kidneys and ureters. If passed at beginning of urination, from the urethra; if at the end, from the bladder.

NOTE: The occurrence of bright red blood in the urine and its appearance in the toilet bowl are quite frightening to the patient. The patient, physician, and nurse should realize that a very small amount of blood may cause the entire toilet bowl to appear to be full of blood.

***renal h.*** Hematuria in which the urine is smoky or sometimes bright red.

***urethral h.*** Hematuria in which bright red urine is present at the beginning of urination.

***vesical h.*** Hematuria in which the urine is not uniformly bright red.

**heme** (hēm) An iron-containing nonprotein portion of the hemoglobin molecule wherein the iron is in the ferrous ($Fe^{2+}$) state. SEE: *ferritin; hematin.*

**hemeralopia** (hĕm″ĕr-ăl-ō′pē-ă) [Gr. *hemera,* day, + *alaos,* blind, + *ops,* eye] Diminished vision in bright light. Term formerly erroneously applied to night blindness or nyctalopia. Nyctalopia indicates inability to see in dim light, though otherwise vision is normal.

In hemeralopia, the sight is poor in sunlight and in good illumination; it is good at dusk, at twilight, and in poor illumination. This is noted in albinism, retinitis with central scotoma, toxic amblyopia, coloboma of the iris and choroid, opacity of the crystalline lens or cornea, and in conjunctivitis with photophobia.

**hemi-** (hĕm′ē) [Gr.] Prefix meaning *half.*

**hemiacephalus** (hĕm″ē-ă-sĕf′ă-lŭs) [″ + *a-,* not, + *kephale,* head] A malformed fetus with a markedly defective head. SEE: *anencephalus.*

**hemiachromatopsia** (hĕm″ē-ă-krō-mă-tŏp′sē-ă) [″ + ″ + *chroma,* color, + *opsis,* vision] Color blindness in one-half, or in corresponding halves, of the vision field. SYN: *hemichromatopsia.*

**hemiageusia** (hĕm″ē-ă-gū′zē-ă) [″ + ″ + *geusis,* taste] Loss of sense of taste on one side of the tongue.

**hemialbumin** (hĕm″ē-ăl-bū′mĭn) [″ + L. *albumen,* white of egg] A product resulting from the digestion of albumin.

**hemialbumose** (hĕm″-ē-ăl′bū-mōs) An albumoid product from the digestion of certain proteins. It is found in bone marrow.

**hemialbumosuria** (hĕm″ē-ăl-bū″mō-sū′rē-ă) [″ + ″ + Gr. *ouron,* urine] Hemialbumose in the urine.

**hemialgia** (hĕm-ē-ăl′jē-ă) [″ + *algos,* pain] Pain in half of the body.

**hemiamaurosis** (hĕm″ē-ăm″ō-rō′sĭs) [″ + *amaurosis,* darkness] Hemianopia.

**hemiamblyopia** (hĕm″ē-ăm″blē-ō′pē-ă) [″ + *amblys,* dim, + *ops,* sight] Hemianopia.

**hemiamyosthenia** (hĕm″ē-ă″mī-ŏs-thē′nē-ă) [Gr. *hemi-,* half, + *a-,* not, + *mys,* muscle, + *sthenos,* strength] Absence of normal muscular power on one side of the body. SYN: *hemiparesis.*

**hemianacusia** (hĕm″ē-ăn″ă-kū′zē-ă) [″ + *an-,* not, + *akousis,* hearing] Deafness in one ear.

**hemianalgesia** (hĕm″ē-ăn-ăl-jē′zē-ă) [″ + ″ + *algos,* pain] Lack of sensibility to pain (analgesia) on one side of the body.

**hemianencephaly** (hĕm″ē-ăn″ĕn-sĕf′ă-lē) [″ + *an-,* not, + *enkephalos,* brain] Congenital absence of half of the brain.

**hemianesthesia** (hĕm″ē-ăn-ĕs-thē′zē-ă) [″ + ″ + *aisthesis,* sensation] Anesthesia of half of the body.

**hemianopia, hemianopsia** (hĕm″ē-ă-nŏ′pē-ă, -nŏp′sē-ă) [″ + *an-,* not, + *ops,* eye] Blindness in one-half of the visual field. SYN: *hemiamaurosis; hemiamblyopia.* **hemianopic,** *adj.*

***altitudinal h.*** Blindness in upper or lower half of the visual field of one or both eyes.

***binasal h.*** Blindness in the nasal half of the visual field in each eye.

***bitemporal h.*** Blindness in the temporal half of visual field in each eye.

***complete h.*** Blindness in half the visual field.

***crossed h.*** Either bitemporal or binasal hemianopsia. SYN: *heteronymous h.*

***heteronymous h.*** Crossed h.

***homonymous h.*** Blindness of nasal half of the visual field of one eye and temporal half of the other, or right-sided or left-sided hemianopsia of corresponding sides in both eyes.

***incomplete h.*** Blindness in less than half of the visual field of each eye.

***quadrant h.*** Blindness of symmetrical quadrant of the field of vision in each eye.

***unilateral h.*** Hemianopsia affecting only one eye.

**hemianosmia** (hĕm″ē-ăn-ŏs′mē-ă) [Gr. *hemi-,* half, + *an-,* not, + *osme,* smell] Loss of sense of smell in one nostril.

**hemiapraxia** (hĕm″ē-ă-prăks′ē-ă) [″ + *a-,* not, + *prassein,* to do] Incapacity to exercise purposeful movements on one side of the body.

**hemiarthrosis** (hĕm″ē-ăr-thrō′sĭs) [″ + *arthron,* joint, + *osis,* condition] A false articulation between two bones. SYN: *synchondrosis.*

**hemiasynergia** (hĕm″ē-ă″sĭn-ĕr′jē-ă) [″ + *a-,* not, + *syn,* with, + *ergon,* work] A lack of coordination of parts affecting one side of the body.

**hemiataxia** (hĕm″ē-ă-tăks′ē-ă) [″ + *ataxia,* lack of order] Impaired muscular coordination causing awkward movements of the affected side of the body.

**hemiathetosis** (hĕm″ē-ăth″ĕ-tō′sĭs) [″ + *athetos,* without fixed position, + *osis,* condition] Athetosis of one side of the body.

**hemiatrophy** (hĕm-ē-ăt′rō-fē) [″ + *atrophia,* atrophy] Impaired nutrition resulting in atrophy of one side of the body or of an organ or part.

**hemiballism** (hĕm-ē-băl′ĭzm) [″ + *balismos,* jumping] Jerking and twitching movements of one side of the body.

**hemiblock** (hĕm′ĭ-blŏk) In heart block, a failure of conduction in one of the two main divisions of the left branches of the conducting bundle.

**hemic** (hē′mĭk, hĕm′ĭk) [Gr. *haima,* blood] Pert. to blood; hemal (1).

**hemicanities** (hĕm″ē-kăn-ĭsh′ĭ-ēz) [Gr. *hemi-,* half, + L. *canities,* gray hair] Grayness of hair on one side only.

**hemicardia** (hĕm-ē-kăr′dē-ă) [″ + *kardia,* heart] Half of a four-chambered heart.

**hemicastration** (hĕm″ē-kăs-trā′shŭn) [″ + L. *castrare,* to prune] The removal of one ovary or testicle. At one time, removal of the left testicle was done on the erroneous assumption that sperm from the right testicle produced only sons.

**hemicellulose** (hĕm-ē-sĕl′ū-lōs) One of a group of polysaccharides that differ from cellulose in that they may be hydrolyzed by dilute mineral acids, and from other polysaccharides in that they are not readily digested by amylases. The group includes pentosans, galactosans (agar-agar), and pectins.

**hemicentrum** (hĕm-ē-sĕn′trŭm) [″ + *kentron,* center] Either lateral half of the centrum of a vertebra.

**hemicephalia** (hĕm″ē-sĕ-fā′lē-ă) [″ + *kephale,* head] The congenital absence of one half of the skull and brain.

**hemicephalus** (hĕm″ē-sĕf′ă-lus) A congenital deformity in which the child has only one cerebral hemisphere.

**hemicerebrum** (hĕm″ē-sĕr′ĕ-brŭm) [″ + L. *cerebrum,* brain] Half of the cerebral hemisphere.

**hemichorea** (hĕm-ē-kō-rē′ă) [″ + *choreia,* dance] Chorea affecting only one side of the body.

**hemichromatopsia** (hĕm″ē-krō-mă-tŏp′sē-ă) [″ + *chroma,* color, + *opsis,* vision] Hemiachromatopsia.

**hemicolectomy** (hĕm″ē-kō-lĕk′tō-mē) [″ + *kolon,* colon, + *ektome,* excision] Surgical removal of half or less of the colon.

**hemicorporectomy** (hĕm″ē-kor″pō-rĕk′tō-mē) [″ + L. *corpus,* body, + Gr. *ektome,* excision] Surgical removal of the lower half of the body.

**hemicrania** (hĕm-ē-krā′nē-ă) [″ + *kranion,* skull] **1.** Unilateral head pain, usually migraine. **2.** A malformation in which only one half of the skull is developed.

**hemicraniectomy** (hĕm″ē-krā-nē-ĕk′tō-mē) [″ + ″ + *ektome,* excision] The surgical division of the cranial vault from front backward, exposing half of the brain.

**hemicraniosis** (hĕm″ē-krā-nē-ō′sĭs) [″ + ″ + *osis,* condition] An enlargement of half of the cranium or face.

**hemidesmosome** The half of a desmosome produced by epithelial cells for attachment of basal surface of the cell to the underlying basement membrane or the enamel or cementum tooth surface in the case of junctional epithelium.

**hemidiaphoresis** (hĕm″ē-dī″ă-for-ē′sĭs) [″ + *dia,* through, + *pherein,* to carry] Sweating on one side of the body. SYN: *hemidrosis* (1); *hemihidrosis.*

**hemidiaphragm** (hēm″ĕ-dī′ă-frăm) [″ + ″ + *phragma,* wall] Half of the diaphragm.

**hemidrosis** (hĕm″ĭ-drō′sĭs) **1.** [″ + *hidrosis,* sweating] Hemidiaphoresis. **2.** [Gr. *haima,* blood, + *hidrosis,* sweating] Secretion of sweat containing blood. SYN: *hemathidrosis.*

**hemidysergia** (hĕm″ē-dĭs-ĕr′jē-ă) [Gr. *hemi-,* half, + *dys,* bad, + *ergon,* work] A lack of muscular coordination on one side of the body.

**hemidysesthesia** (hĕm″ē-dĭs-ĕs-thē′zē-ă) [″ + ″ + *aisthesis,* sensation] Impaired sensation of half of the body.

**hemidystrophy** (hĕm″ē-dis′trō-fē) [″ + ″ + *trophe,* nourishment] An inequality in development of the two sides of the body.

**hemiectromelia** (hĕm″ē-ĕk-trō-mē′lē-ă) [″ + *ektro,* abortion, + *melos,* limb] Deformed extremities on one side of the body.

**hemiepilepsy** (hĕm″ē-ĕp′ĭ-lĕp-sē) [″ + *epilepsia,* seizure] Epilepsy with convulsions confined to one side of the body.

**hemifacial** (hĕm″ē-fā′shăl) [″ + L. *facies,* face] Pert. to one side of the face.

**hemigastrectomy** (hĕm″ē-găs-trĕk′tō-mē) [″ + *gaster,* belly, + *ektome,* excision] Excision of half of the stomach.

**hemigeusia** (hĕm-ē-gū′sē-ă) [″ + *geusis,* taste] A loss of the sense of taste on one side of the tongue.

**hemiglossal** (hĕm″ē-glŏs′săl) [″ + *glossa,* tongue] Concerning one side of the tongue.

**hemiglossectomy** (hĕm″ē-glŏs-sĕk′tō-mē) [″ + ″ + *ektome,* excision] The surgical removal of one side of the tongue.

**hemiglossitis** [″ + ″ + *itis,* inflammation] Herpetic vesicular eruption on half of the tongue and the inner surface of the cheek.

**hemignathia** (hĕm″ē-năth′ē-ă) [″ + *gnathos,* jaw] Congenital absence of one half of the lower jaw.

**hemihepatectomy** (hĕm″ē-hĕp″ă-tĕk′tō-mē) [″ + *hepatos,* liver, + *ektome,* excision] The surgical removal of half of the liver.

**hemihidrosis** (hĕm″ē-hī-drō′sĭs) [″ + *hidros,* sweat, + *osis,* condition] Hemidiaphoresis.

**hemihydrate** A chemical compound with one molecule of water for every two molecules of the other substance. In dentistry, gypsum alpha hemihydrate is used for investing castings.

**hemihypalgesia** (hĕm″ē-hī″păl-jē′zē-ă) [″ +

*hypo,* under, + *algesis,* sense of pain] Partial anesthesia on one side of the body.

**hemihyperesthesia** (hĕm″ē-hī-pĕr-ĕs-thē′zē-ă) [″ + *hyper,* over, + *aisthesis,* sensation] Abnormal tactile and painful sensitiveness of one side of the body.

**hemihyperidrosis, hemihyperhidrosis** (hĕm″ē-hī-pĕr-ĭ-drō′sĭs, -hĭ-drō′sĭs) [″ + ″ + *hydrosis,* sweating] Excessive perspiration confined to one side of the body.

**hemihyperplasia** (hĕm″ē-hī″pĕr-plā′zē-ă) [″ + ″ + *plassein,* to form] The excessive development of one side or one half of the body or of an organ.

**hemihypesthesia, hemihypoesthesia** (hĕm″ē-hī″pĕs-thē′zē-ă, -pō-ĕs-thē′zē-a) [Gr. *hemi-,* half, + *hypo,* under, + *aisthesis,* sensation] Diminished sensibility on one side of the body.

**hemi-inattention** Unilateral visual inattention.

**hemikaryon** (hĕm″ē-kăr′ē-ŏn) [″ + *karyon,* nucleus] A cell nucleus with half the diploid number of chromosomes.

**hemilaminectomy** (hĕm″ē-lăm″ĭ-nĕk′tō-mē) [″ + L. *lamina,* thin plate, + Gr. *ektome,* excision] The surgical removal of the lamina of the vertebral arch on one side.

**hemilaryngectomy** (hĕm″ē-lăr″in-jĕk′tō-mē) [″ + *larynx,* larynx, + *ektome,* excision] The surgical removal of the lateral half of the larynx.

**hemilateral** [″ + L. *latus,* side] Relating to one side only.

**hemilesion** (hĕm″ē-lē′zhŭn) [″ + L. *laesio,* a wound] A lesion on one side of the body.

**hemilingual** (hĕm″ē-lĭng′gwăl) [″ + L. *lingua,* tongue] Affecting or concerning one lateral half of the tongue.

**hemimacroglossia** (hĕm″ē-măk″rō-glŏs′ē-ă) [″ + *makros,* large, + *glossa,* tongue] Enlargement of one lateral half of the tongue.

**hemimandibulectomy** (hĕm″ē-măn-dĭb-ū-lĕk′tō-mē) [″ + L. *mandibula,* lower jawbone, + Gr. *ektome,* excision] The surgical removal of half of the mandible.

**hemimelus** (hĕm″ĭ-mē′lŭs) [″ + *melos,* limb] A fetal malformation with defective development of the extremities, esp. the distal portion.

**hemin** (hē′mĭn) [Gr. *haima,* blood] A brownish-red crystalline salt of heme formed when hemoglobin is heated with glacial acetic acid and sodium chloride. The iron is present in the ferric ($Fe^{3+}$) state. Hemin is used in testing for presence of blood. SEE: *heme.*

**heminephrectomy** (hĕm″ē-nĕ-frĕk′tō-mē) [Gr. *hemi-,* half, + *nephros,* kidney, + *ektome,* excision] The excision or removal of a portion of a kidney.

**hemineurasthenia** (hĕm″ē-nū-răs-thē′nē-ă) [″ + *neuron,* nerve, + *astheneia,* weakness] Neurasthenia affecting one side of the body only.

**hemiopalgia** (hĕm″ē-ŏp-ăl′jē-ă) [″ + *ops,* eye, + *algos,* pain] Pain in one side of the head and the eye on that side.

**hemiopia** (hĕm-ē-ō′pē-ă) [″ + *ops,* eye] Hemianopia.

**hemiopic** (hĕm-ē-ŏp′ĭk) [″ + *ops,* eye] Pert. to hemiopia.

**hemipagus** (hĕm-ĭp′ă-gŭs) [″ + *pagos,* a thing fixed] Twins fused at the navel and thorax.

**hemiparalysis** [″ + *paralyein,* to disable] Hemiplegia.

**hemiparaplegia** (hĕm″ē-păr-ă-plē′jē-ă) [″ + ″ + *plege,* stroke] Paralysis of the lower half of one side or of one leg. This term is confusing because paraplegia indicates paralysis of both lower extremities.

**hemiparesis** (hĕm″ē-păr′ĕ-sĭs, hĕm-ē-păr-ē′sĭs) [″ + *paresis,* paralysis] Hemiplegia.

**hemiparesthesia** (hĕm″ē-păr-ĕs-thē′zē-ă) [″ + *para,* beyond, + *aisthesis,* sensation] Numbness of one side of the body.

**hemipelvectomy** (hĕm″ē-pĕl″vĕk′tō-mē) [″ + L. *pelvis,* basin, + Gr. *ektome,* excision] The surgical removal of half of the pelvis, and the leg.

**hemiplegia** (hĕm-ē-plē′jē-ă) [″ + *plege,* a stroke] Paralysis of only one side of the body. SYN: *hemiparalysis; hemiparesis.* SEE: *Benedikt's syndrome; paralysis; thalamic syndrome.*

SYMPTOMS: In individuals with hemiplegia, neglect is a symptom of parietal involvement. It is characterized by disturbed visual perception and neglect of one half of the body. The patient may fail to shave one side of the body, apply lipstick, or comb the hair on only one side. The patient may be able to recognize only one half of bilaterally and simultaneously presented stimuli. SEE: *anosognosia, visual.*

ETIOLOGY: Hemiplegia is caused by a brain lesion involving the upper motor neurons and resulting in paralysis of the opposite side of the body, which may result from disturbed blood flow to a portion of the brain. This may be due to cerebral hemorrhage, thrombosis, embolism, or tumor.

FIRST AID: The patient's head and shoulders should be elevated and he or she should be watched to ensure the tongue does not obstruct breathing. Stimulants should not be given. Patient should not be moved until someone competent in emergency medical care arrives.

NURSING IMPLICATIONS: The patient's neurological status is monitored, and evidence of deterioration or improvement documented. Respiratory status is assessed for evidence of decreased or adventitious breath sounds, and the patient is encouraged to breathe deeply and cough and to change position every 2 hr to prevent atelectasis and hypostatic pneumonia. Skin is inspected for evidence of incipient breakdown; the patient is turned frequently with care to avoid shearing forces, and special mattresses or beds may be used to prevent breakdown. Assistance is provided with active range-of-motion exercises to unaffected limbs and passive exercises to affected limbs. The patient is taught to use the unaffected limbs to move and exercise the affected limbs to maintain joint mobility and prevent contractures and to maintain muscle tone and strength. The nurse protects the patient from injury, using supportive devices to prevent subluxation or dislocation of affected joints. Fluid balance and nutritional status are monitored, and the patient is encouraged to maintain adequate nourishment and fluids; thickened liquids are offered if swallowing difficulties are present. Bowel and bladder functions are monitored, and nursing care measures and prescribed medical interventions instituted to prevent and manage urine retention or incontinence and constipation and straining at stool. Participation in activities of daily living is encouraged to the extent that the patient is able; additional time is allowed for such activities, with intermittent rest periods to prevent fatigue and frustration. Both patient and family are taught about assistive devices (e.g., sling, splint, walker), referral is made for physical and occupational therapy as appropriate, and rehabilitative care is explained. Both patient and family are encouraged to verbalize their fears and concerns, and accurate information, realistic reassurance, and emotional support are provided to assist with coping. A positive attitude and realistic goal setting are encouraged. Appropriate referrals to rehabilitation and home health care agencies are arranged.

***capsular h.*** Hemiplegia resulting from a lesion of the internal capsule of the brain.

***cerebral h.*** Hemiplegia caused by a brain lesion.

***facial h.*** Paralysis of the muscles on one side of the face.

***pontile h.*** Hemiplegia due to a lesion of the pons. The arm and leg on one side and the face on the opposite side are affected.

***spastic h.*** Hypertonus occurring in the muscles on half of the body. It is caused by cerebrovascular accident, cerebral hemorrhage, or head trauma.

***spinal h.*** Hemiplegia resulting from a lesion of the spinal cord. SEE: *Brown-Séquard's paralysis*.

**hemiplegic** (hĕm-ē-plē′jĭk) **1.** Pert. to hemiplegia. **2.** A colloquial reference to a patient having hemiplegia.

**Hemiptera** (hĕm-ĭp′tĕr-ă) [Gr. *hemi-*, half, + *pteron*, wing] The true bugs; an order of insects characterized by piercing and sucking mouth parts. The first pair of wings is leathery at the base and membranous at the tip; the second pair is membranous. Metamorphosis is incomplete. The order includes bedbugs, kissing bugs, and several other species that are pests or vectors of pathogenic organisms.

**hemipyocyanin** (hĕm″ē-pī″ō-sī′ă-nĭn) Antibacterial pigment produced by *Pseudomonas pyocyanea*.

**hemirachischisis** (hĕm″ē-ră-kĭs′kĭ-sĭs) [″ + *rhachis*, spine, + *schisis*, a splitting] Spina bifida occulta.

**hemisacralization** (hĕm″ē-sā″krăl-ī-zā′shŭn) The abnormal development of one half of the fifth lumbar vertebra so that it is fused with the sacrum.

**hemisection** (hĕm″ē-sĕk′shŭn) [″ + L. *sectio*, a cutting] Bisection.

**hemisomus** (hĕm″ē-sō′mŭs) [″ + *soma*, body] A fetus with the lateral half of the body either missing or malformed.

**hemispasm** (hĕm′ē-spăzm) [″ + *spasmos*, a convulsion] A spasm of only one side of the body or face.

**hemisphere** (hĕm′ĭ-sfēr) [″ + *sphaira*, sphere] Either half of the cerebrum or cerebellum.

***dominant h.*** The cerebral hemisphere with which the higher cortical functions, esp. those relating to speech and certain motor activities, are associated (i.e., the left hemisphere in right-handed individuals), a phenomenon known as cerebral dominance.

**hemispheric specialization** The differences in function affected by damage to either the right or left cerebral hemisphere. For example, right hemisphere damage may produce difficulties with visuoperceptual abilities whereas damage to the left hemisphere frequently results in difficulties with language, analytical thought, and abstract concepts. SEE: *stroke*.

**hemisyndrome** (hĕm″ē-sĭn′drōm) [″ + *syndrome*, a running with] A syndrome indicating a unilateral lesion of the spinal cord.

**hemithermoanesthesia** (hĕm″ē-thĕr″mō-ăn″ĕs-thē′zē-ă) [Gr. *hemi-*, half, + *therme*, heat, + *an-*, not, + *aisthesis*, sensation] The unilateral loss of sensitivity to heat and cold.

**hemithorax** (hĕm″ē-thō′răks) [″ + *thorax*, chest] One half of the chest.

**hemithyroidectomy** (hĕm″ē-thī″royd-ĕk′tō-mē) [″ + *thyreos*, shield, + *eidos*, form, shape, + *ektome*, excision] The surgical removal of one half of the thyroid gland tissue.

**hemitremor** (hĕm″ē-trĕm′or) A tremor present in one lateral half of the body.

**hemivertebra** (hĕm″ē-vĕr′tĕ-bră) The congenital absence of or the failure to develop half of a vertebra.

**hemizygosity** (hĕm″ē-zī-gŏs′ĭ-tē) [″ + *zygotos*, yoked] Possessing only one of the gene pair that determines a particular genetic trait.

**hemlock** [AS. *hemleac*] **1.** A species of evergreen plant. **2.** The volatile oil from either *Conium maculatum* or *Cicuta maculata* containing cicutoxin. Ingestion of these hemlock plants, esp. their roots, may cause fatal poisoning.

***h. poisoning*** Poisoning by hemlock ingestion, causing weakness, drowsiness, nausea, vomiting, difficult breathing, paralysis, and death.

TREATMENT: The stomach should be emptied by means of a stomach pump or an emetic. A cathartic should be given. Respiratory failure should be treated with artificial respiration and oxygen.

**Hemlock Society** An organization that has published information about suicide for terminally ill patients.

**hemo-** SEE: *hem-*.

**hemoagglutination** (hē″mō-ă-gloo″tĭ-nā′shŭn) [Gr. *haima,* blood, + L. *agglutinans,* gluing] The clumping of red blood corpuscles.

**hemoagglutinin** (hē″mō-ă-gloo′tĭ-nĭn) An agglutinin that clumps the red blood corpuscles.

**hemobilia** (hē″mō-bĭl′ē-ă) Blood in the bile or bile ducts.

**hemobilinuria** (hē″mō-bĭl-ĭn-ū′rē-ă) [″+ L. *bilis,* bile, + Gr. *ouron,* urine] Urobilin in the blood and urine.

**hemochromatosis** (hē″mō-krō″mă-tō′sĭs) [″ + *chroma,* color, + *osis,* condition] A genetic disease marked by excessive absorption and accumulation of iron in the body. The mechanism of this is unknown. It is not necessary to have a history of iron overload owing to excess iron intake or multiple blood transfusions for the disease to be present. Also, existence of the disease does not require the presence of symptoms or signs of illness. SYN: *bronze diabetes.*

SYMPTOMS: Persons who are symptomatic may experience weakness, weight loss, arthralgias, abdominal pain, palpitations, and impotence in males.

DIAGNOSIS: Physical findings include gray or bronzed skin, enlarged liver, arthritis, signs of congestive heart failure, and testicular atrophy in males. Laboratory studies indicate excess iron in liver cells, increased serum iron level, liver cirrhosis, and radiographic signs of joint disease, esp. in the fingers. SEE: illus.

TREATMENT: Treatment includes phlebotomy (i.e., removal of blood from the patient), done at regular intervals until the hematocrit returns to normal. This may require removal of as much as 500 ml of blood two times a week for several weeks. Maintenance therapy consists of removal of blood at 1- to 12-month intervals. Parenterally administered iron chelators such as deferoxamine are used if phlebotomy is not possible.

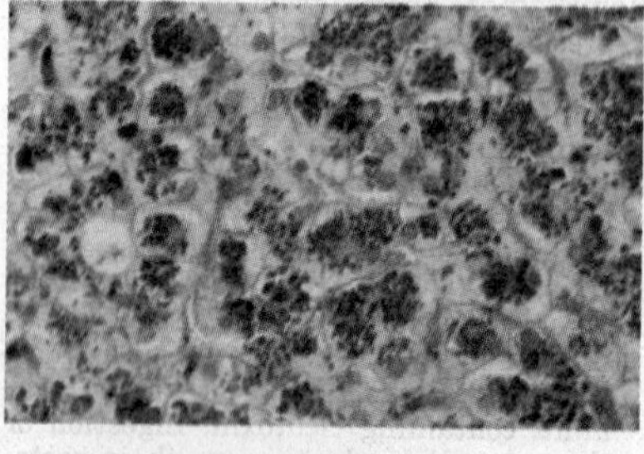

HEMOCHROMATOSIS

LIVER BIOPSY, EXCESS IRON STAINED GREEN

**hemochromogen** (hē″mō-krō′mō-jĕn) [″ + *chroma,* color, + *gennan,* to produce] A compound of heme with nitrogen-containing substances such as a protein.

**hemochromoprotein** (hē″mō-krō″mō-prō′tē-ĭn) Any protein combined with the blood pigment hemoglobin.

**hemoclip** A metal clip used to ligate blood vessels.

**hemoconcentration** A relative increase in the number of red blood cells resulting from a decrease in the volume of plasma.

**hemoconia** (hē″mō-kō′nē-ă) [Gr. *haima,* blood, + *konis,* dust] Minute colorless bodies in the blood thought to be the products of disintegration of red blood cells. SYN: *blood dust.*

**hemoconiosis** (hē″mō-kō″nē-ō′sĭs) [″+ ″ + *osis,* condition] Having an abnormal amount of hemoconia in the blood.

**hemocuprein** (hē″mō-kū′prē-ĭn) A blue copper-containing compound present in red blood cells.

**hemocyte** (hē′mō-sīt) [″ + *kytos,* cell] **1.** Any blood cell. **2.** A red blood cell.

**hemocytoblast** (hē″mō-sī′tō-blăst) [″ + ″ + *blastos,* germ] An undifferentiated stem cell found in the bone marrow and lymphatic tissue that may give rise to any type of blood cell. SEE: illus.

**hemocytology** (hē″mō-sī-tŏl′ō-jē) [″ + ″+ *logos,* word, reason] The study of the structure and function of blood cells.

**hemocytometer** (hē″mō-sī-tŏm′ĕ-tĕr) [″ + ″ + *metron,* measure] A device for determining the number of cells in a stated volume of blood.

**hemocytophagia** The phagocytic ingestion of red blood cells.

**hemocytotripsis** (hē″mō-sī″tō-trĭp′sĭs) [″ + ″ + *tribein,* to rub] The destruction of red blood cells caused by extreme pressure.

**hemocytozoon** (hē″mō-sī″tō-zō′ŏn) [″+ ″ + *zoon,* animal] A protozoan parasite of the blood cells. SYN: *hematobium.*

**hemodiagnosis** (hē″mō-dī″ăg-nō′sĭs) [″ + *dia,* through, + *gnosis,* knowledge] Examination of the blood for diagnostic purposes.

**hemodialysis** (hē″mō-, hĕm″ō-dī-ăl′ĭ-sĭs) [″ + ″+ *lysis,* dissolution] A method for providing the function of the kidneys by circulating blood through tubes made of semipermeable membranes. These dialyzing tubes are continually bathed by solutions that selectively remove unwanted material. This technique is lifesaving in patients in whom one or both kidneys are defective or absent. SEE: *hemoperfusion; Nursing Diagnoses Appendix.*

NURSING IMPLICATIONS: When caring

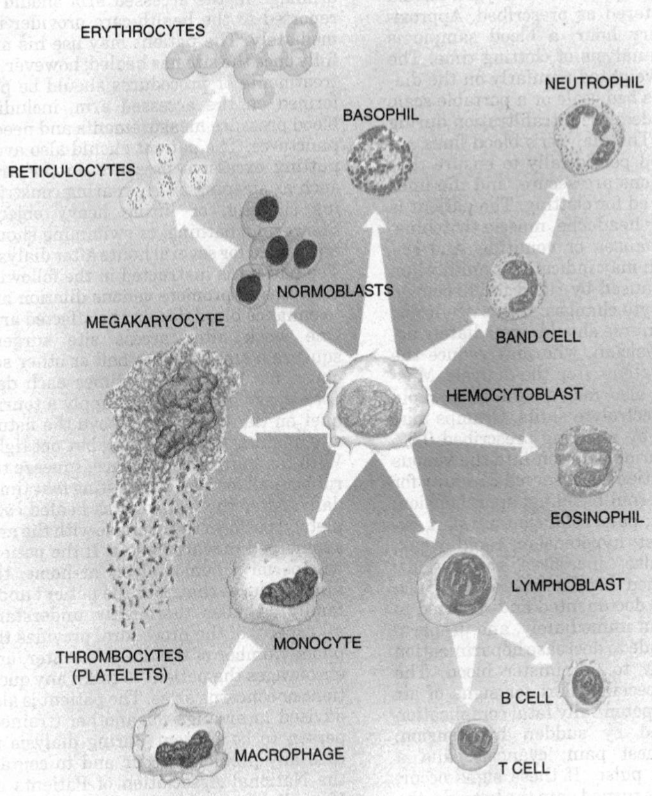


HEMOCYTOBLAST AND BLOOD CELLS

for a patient who is receiving hemodialysis, the nurse's primary responsibilities include patient teaching and monitoring for patient complications.

*Preprocedure:* If this is the patient's first hemodialysis session, the purpose of the treatment and expected results are explained. First, the patient undergoes a surgical procedure to create a vascular access. After the access site has been created and the patient is ready for dialysis, the patient's weight is obtained and vital signs checked; blood pressure should be measured in the nonaccessed arm while the patient is in both supine and standing positions. As prescribed, the hemodialysis equipment is prepared according to the manufacturer's guidelines and the institution's protocol. Strict aseptic technique is maintained to avoid introducing pathogens into the patient's bloodstream during treatment. The patient is placed in a supine or low Fowler position and made as comfortable as possible, with the venous access site well supported and resting on a sterile drape or sterile barrier shield.

*During the procedure:* The nurse follows Occupational Safety and Health Administration guidelines by wearing appropriate gloves and protective eye shields throughout the procedure. The patient is monitored continually throughout dialysis. Vital signs are checked and documented every 30 min to detect possible complications. Fever may indicate infection from pathogens in the dialysate or equipment and should be reported to the physician, who may prescribe an antipyretic, antibiotic, or both. Hypotension may indicate hypovolemia or a decreased hematocrit level; I.V. fluid supplements or blood should be administered as prescribed. Rapid respirations may signal hypoxemia; supplemental oxygen should be administered as prescribed. Approximately every hour, a blood sample is drawn for analysis of clotting time. The patient is weighted regularly on the dialyzing unit's bed scale or a portable scale to ensure adequate ultrafiltration during treatment. The dialyzer's blood lines are also checked periodically to ensure that all connections are secure, and the lines are monitored for clotting. The patient is assessed for headache, muscle twitching, backache, nausea or vomiting, and seizures, which may indicate disequilibrium syndrome caused by rapid fluid removal and electrolyte changes. If this syndrome occurs, the nurse should immediately notify the physician, who may reduce the blood flow rate or stop the dialysis. Muscle cramps also may result from rapid fluid and electrolyte shifts. Cramps may be relieved by injecting prescribed 0.9% sodium chloride solution into the venous line. The patient is observed carefully for signs of internal bleeding; apprehension; restlessness; pale, cold, clammy skin; excessive thirst; hypotension; rapid, weak, thready pulse; increased respirations; and decreased body temperature. Such findings are documented and reported to the physician immediately, and preparations are made to decrease heparinization and possibly to administer blood. The nurse is especially alert for signs of air embolism a potentially fatal complication characterized by sudden hypotension; dyspnea; chest pain; cyanosis; and a weak, rapid pulse. If these signs occur, the patient is turned onto the left side, the head of the bed lowered (to help keep air bubbles on the right side of the body, where they can be absorbed from the pulmonary vasculature), and the physician notified immediately.

*Postprocedure:* The venous access site is monitored for bleeding. If bleeding is excessive, pressure is maintained on the site and the physician notified. To prevent clotting and other blood flow problems, the arm used for venous access is not used for any other procedures, including I.V. line insertion, blood pressure monitoring, and venipuncture. At least four times daily, circulation at the access site is assessed by auscultating for a bruit and by palpating for a thrill; the patient is also instructed in these assessment techniques. An accurate record of the patient's food and fluid intake is maintained, and the patient is encouraged to cooperate with prescribed restrictions, such as limited protein, potassium, and sodium intake; increased caloric intake; and decreased fluid intake. The patient is instructed in care of the venous access site: cleaning the incision with hydrogen peroxide solution daily and keeping it dry until healing is complete (usually 10 to 14 days). Any pain, swelling, redness, or drainage in the accessed arm should be reported to the health-care provider immediately. The patient may use his arm fully once the site has healed; however, no treatments or procedures should be performed on the accessed arm, including blood pressure measurements and needle punctures. The patient should also avoid putting excessive pressure on the arm, such as sleeping on it, wearing constricting clothing, or lifting heavy objects. Showering, bathing, or swimming should be avoided for several hours after dialysis. The patient is instructed in the following exercises to promote venous dilation and to enhance blood flow in the affected arm: One week after access site surgery, squeeze a small rubber ball or other soft object for 15 min, four times each day. Two weeks after surgery, apply a tourniquet on the upper arm above the fistula site, making sure it is snug but not tight. With the tourniquet in place, squeeze the rubber ball for 5 min, repeating four times daily. After the incision has healed completely, perform the exercise with the arm submerged in warm water. If the patient will perform hemodialysis at home, the nurse ensures that both the patient and a family member thoroughly understand all aspects of the procedure, provides the phone number of the dialysis center, and encourages the patient to call if any questions or concerns arise. The patient is also advised to arrange for another (trained) person to be present during dialysis in case any problems occur and to contact the National Association of Patients on Hemodialysis and Transplantation or the National Kidney Foundation for information and support.

**hemodialyzer** (hē″mō-dī′ă-līz″ĕr) A device used in performing hemodialysis.

**hemodilution** (hē″mō-dī-lū′shŭn) An increase in blood plasma volume resulting in reduced relative concentration of red blood cells.

**hemodynamic monitoring** A general term for determining the functional status of the cardiovascular system as it responds to acute stress such as myocardial infarction and cardiogenic or septic shock. This is usually done by using a pulmonary artery catheter to directly measure intracardiac pressure changes, cardiac output, blood pressure, and heart rate. The data obtained permit the critical care team to follow the patient's course carefully and without delay.

**hemodynamics** (hē″mō-dī-năm′iks) [Gr. *haima,* blood, + *dynamis,* power] A study of the forces involved in circulating blood through the body.

**hemoendothelial** (hē″mō-ĕn-dō-thē′lē-ăl) Pert. to the relationship between blood of the mother and the endothelium of the chorionic vessels. SEE: *placenta.*

**Hemofil** Trade name for antihemophilic factor (AHF).

**hemofiltration** (hē″mō-fĭl-trā′shŭn) An ultrafiltration technique to remove excess accumulation of normal metabolic products from the blood. The technical aspects are similar to those of renal dialysis in that the blood flows from the body to the hemofilter and is then returned to the body.

Caution: Depending on the type of filter membrane used, essential materials may be removed from the blood. It is important to replace the excess crystalloids removed.

***continuous arteriovenous h.*** ABBR: CAVH. A technique using a hemofilter to facilitate removal of water, electrolytes, and small to medium molecular weight molecules from the vascular space. It is used in patients with renal failure or fluid overload.

**hemoflagellate** (hē″mō-flăj′ĕ-lāt″) [″ + L. *flagellum,* whip] Any flagellate protozoan of the blood. The most important genera are *Trypanosoma* and *Leishmania.*

**hemofuscin** (hē″mō-fū′sĭn) [″ + L. *fuscus,* brown] A brown pigment, derived from hemoglobin, which produces a reddish color in urine.

**hemoglobin** (hē″mō-, hĕm″ō-glō′bĭn) [″ + L. *globus,* globe] ABBR: Hb, Hbg, Hgb. The iron-containing pigment of the red blood cells which carries oxygen from the lungs to the tissues. The amount of hemoglobin in the blood averages 12 to 16 g/100 ml of blood in women, 14 to 18 g/100 ml in men, and somewhat less in children. When 1 g of hemoglobin can combine with 1.36 cc of oxygen, the resulting compound is oxyhemoglobin. Hemoglobin is a crystallizable, conjugated protein consisting of an iron-containing pigment called heme and a simple protein, globin. In the lungs it combines readily, by a process called oxygenation, with oxygen to form a loose, unstable compound called oxyhemoglobin. In the tissues where oxygen concentration is low and carbon dioxide concentration is high (low pH), hemoglobin releases its oxygen. An important chemical for oxygen release is 2,3-diphosphoglycerate. Hemoglobin also acts as a buffer for the hydrogen ions produced in red blood cells (RBCs) when carbon dioxide is converted to bicarbonate ions for transport in the plasma.

When old RBCs are phagocytized by macrophages in the liver, spleen, and red bone marrow, the iron of hemoglobin is reused immediately to produce new RBCs or is stored in the liver until needed. The globin is converted to amino acids for the synthesis of other proteins. The heme portion is of no further use and is converted to bilirubin, a bile pigment excreted by the liver in bile.

Hemoglobin combines with carbon monoxide to form the stable compound carboxyhemoglobin, which renders hemoglobin unable to bond with oxygen and results in hypoxia of tissues. Oxidation of the ferrous iron of hemoglobin to the ferric state produces methemoglobin.

Many different types of hemoglobin have been discovered. Study of these has facilitated the investigation of human genetics. Hemoglobin is named according to the way the amino acid components of the globin move when studied by electrophoresis. There are more than 100 different types of abnormal hemoglobin. SEE: *blood.*

ABNORMALITIES: Abnormal forms of hemoglobin are due to mutations. Because of the size of the hemoglobin molecule, the number of possible mutant forms is enormous, so only a few of the diseases caused by these forms can be described here.

***h. $A_{1c}$*** ABBR: Hb $A_{1c}$. Hemoglobin A that contains a glucose group linked to the terminal amino acid of the beta chains of the molecule. In diabetes mellitus, when the blood glucose level is optimally and carefully regulated over a long period, 5 to 6 weeks, the Hb $A_{1c}$ level is normal. If the blood glucose level has not been controlled (and has been abnormally elevated) in the preceding 5 to 6 weeks, the Hb $A_{1c}$ blood level is increased. SYN: *glycosylated h.*

***h. C disease*** A chronic hemolytic anemia with splenomegaly, arthralgias, and abdominal pain. SEE: illus.

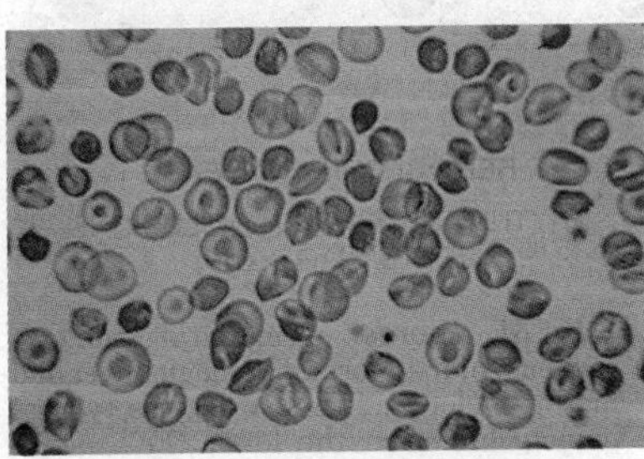

HEMOGLOBIN C DISEASE

TARGET CELLS (ORIG. MAG. ×400)

***h. E disease*** A mild form of hemolytic anemia observed in Southeast Asia natives.

***fetal h.*** The type of hemoglobin found in the erythrocytes of the normal fetus. It is capable of taking up and giving off oxygen at lower oxygen tensions than can the hemoglobin in adult erythrocytes. SEE: illus.

***glycosylated h.*** H. $A_{1c}$.

***h. H disease*** A chronic hemolytic anemia marked by hypochromic erythrocytes

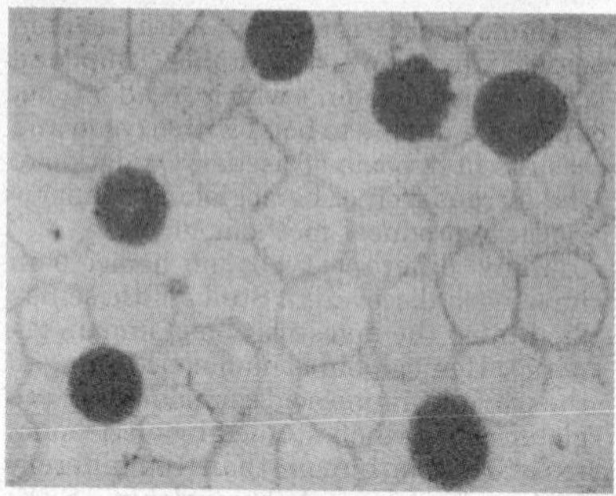

FETAL HEMOGLOBIN

HEMOGLOBIN F (RED) IN ERYTHROCYTES OF A NEWBORN; CLEAR CELLS INDICATE HEMOGLOBIN A

with inclusions that cause them to resemble golfballs. Sometimes called *thalassemia intermedia*. SEE: illus.

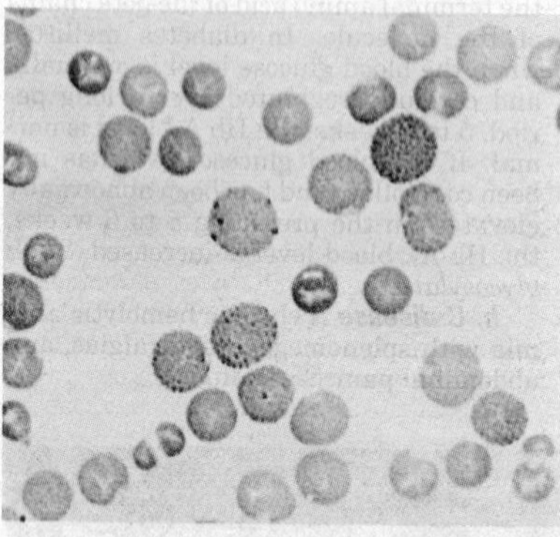

HEMOGLOBIN H DISEASE

ERYTHROCYTES WITH INCLUSIONS (ORIG. MAG. ×640)

***h. M disorder*** Congenital cyanosis caused by an abnormal hemoglobin called methemoglobin. The iron in this type of hemoglobin is in the ferric ($Fe^{3+}$) state and cannot combine with oxygen. Because patients with this condition also have an adequate amount of normal hemoglobin, the course of the disease is benign and no therapy is necessary.

***mean corpuscular h.*** ABBR: MCH. The hemoglobin content of the average red blood cell, usually expressed in picograms per red cell and calculated by multiplying the number of grams of hemoglobin/100 ml by 10 and dividing by the red cell count.

***h. S disease*** The first disease discovered to be due to a molecular abnormality of hemoglobin was sickle cell anemia. It is caused by the presence of an abnormal hemoglobin that, under certain conditions, alters its physical structure to cause red blood cells to assume a sickle shape. Patients with sickle cell trait are asymptomatic because they are genetically heterozygous for hemoglobin S. Those with sickle cell disease, however, are homozygous for hemoglobin S and are therefore symptomatic. SEE: *sickle cell anemia.*

***h. SC disease*** A disease of persons who have inherited two abnormal forms of hemoglobin, S and C. The symptoms include hematuria and pain in the bones, joints, abdomen, and chest.

**hemoglobinemia** (hē″mō-glō-bĭn-ē′mē-ă) [Gr. *haima,* blood, + L. *globus,* globe, + Gr. *haima,* blood] The presence of hemoglobin in the blood plasma.

**hemoglobinocholia** (hē″mō-glō″bĭn-ō-kō′lē-ă) [″ + ″ + Gr. *chole,* bile] Hemoglobin in the bile.

**hemoglobinolysis** (hē″mō-glō-bĭn-ŏl′ĭ-sĭs) [″ + ″ + Gr. *lysis,* dissolution] The dissolution of hemoglobin.

**hemoglobinometer** (hē″mō-glō-bĭn-ŏm′ĕ-ter) [″ + ″+ Gr. *metron,* measure] A device for determining the amount of hemoglobin in the blood.

**hemoglobinopathy** (hē″mō-glō″bĭ-nŏp′ă-thē) Any one of a group of diseases caused by or associated with the presence of one of several forms of abnormal hemoglobin in the blood. SEE: *hemoglobin.*

**hemoglobinophilic** (hē″mō-glō-bĭn-ō-fĭl′ĭk) [″ + ″ + Gr. *philein,* to love] Pert. to organisms that grow better in the presence of hemoglobin.

**hemoglobinous** (hē″mō-glō′bĭ-nŭs) Pert. to or containing hemoglobin.

**hemoglobinuria** (hē″mō-glō-bĭn-ū′rē-ă) [″ + L. *globus,* globe, + Gr. *ouron,* urine] The presence in urine of hemoglobin free from red blood cells. This condition occurs when the amount of hemoglobin from disintegrating red blood cells or from rapid hemolysis of red cells exceeds the ability of the blood proteins to combine with the hemoglobin.

ETIOLOGY: Causes of this condition include hemolytic anemia, scurvy, purpura, exposure to or ingestion of certain chemicals such as arsenic and phosphorus, typhus fever, and septicemia.

***cold h.*** Hemoglobinuria following local or general exposure to cold. SYN: *paroxysmal h.*

***epidemic h.*** Hemoglobinuria of the newborn characterized by jaundice, cyanosis, and fatty degeneration of heart and liver. SYN: *Winckel's disease.*

***intermittent h.*** Paroxysmal nocturnal hemoglobinuria.

***malarial h.*** Blackwater fever.

***march h.*** Hemoglobinuria that occurs following strenuous exercise (e.g., running a marathon).

***paroxysmal h.*** Intermittent, recurring attacks of hemoglobinuria following exposure to cold (cold hemoglobinuria) or strenuous exercise (march hemoglobinuria). Results from increased fragility of red blood cells or presence of a thermolabile autohemolysin.

***toxic h.*** Hemoglobinuria resulting from toxic substances such as muscarine or snake venom; toxic products of infectious diseases such as yellow fever, typhoid fever, syphilis, and certain forms of hemolytic jaundice; organisms such as *Plasmodium malariae,* which destroy red blood cells; foreign protein in blood as may follow blood transfusion.

**hemoglobinuric** (hē″mō-glō″bĭ-nū′rĭk) Relating to or marked by hemoglobinuria.

**hemolith** (hē′mō-lĭth) [″ + *lithos,* stone] A calculus in the wall of a blood vessel.

**hemolymph** (hē′mō-lĭmf″) [″ + L. *lympha,* lymph] Blood and lymph.

**hemolymphangioma** (hē″mō-lĭm-făn″jē-ō′mă) Hematolymphangioma.

**hemolysate** (hē-mŏl′ĭ-sāt) The product of hemolysis.

**hemolysin** (hē-mŏl′ĭ-sĭn) [″ + *lysis,* dissolution] A toxic agent or condition that destroys red blood cells. SYN: *hemotoxin.*

**hemolysis** (hē-mŏl′ĭ-sĭs) [″ + *lysis,* dissolution] The destruction of the membrane of red blood cells with the liberation of hemoglobin, which diffuses into the surrounding fluid. This may result from the effects of bacterial toxins, snake venoms, immune bodies (hemolysins), and hypotonic saline solutions. Their stroma is ruptured or dissolved and the hemoglobin is liberated into the plasma. As a result, the blood, examined grossly, appears to be more transparent and a richer red. Under the microscope, the dissolution of the red corpuscles can be observed. When hemolysis occurs within the blood vessels, the body cannot retain the hemoglobin, which is lost through the kidneys and turns the urine red, a condition called hemoglobinuria. Injection of a hypotonic saline solution or distilled water into the bloodstream induces hemolysis and may result in death. The red blood cells swell and become globular; their membranes rupture, freeing hemoglobin. All solutions injected intravenously must be isotonic with the blood. Hemolysis may result from infection by certain disease organisms (e.g., certain streptococci, staphylococci, and the tetanus bacillus). It also occurs in smallpox and diphtheria and following severe burns. SEE: *fragility of red blood cells.*

**hemolytic** (hē″mō-lĭt′ĭk) Pert. to the breaking down of red blood cells.

***h. anemia*** SEE: under *anemia.*

***h. disease of the newborn*** Neonatal disease characterized by anemia, jaundice, liver and spleen enlargement, and generalized edema (hydrops fetalis). SYN: *erythroblastosis fetalis.* SEE: *Rh blood group.*

ETIOLOGY: This disease is due to transplacental transmission of maternal antibody, usually evoked by maternal and fetal blood group incompatibility. Incompatibilities of the ABO system are common but are not severe because maternal antibodies are too large to cross the placenta readily. Rh incompatibility, however, can result in profound fetal anemia, causing death in utero.

Rh incompatibility may develop when an Rh-negative woman carries an Rh-positive fetus. At the time of delivery, fetal red blood cells may enter maternal circulation, stimulating antibody production against the Rh factor. In a subsequent pregnancy, these antibodies cross the placenta to the fetal circulation and destroy fetal red blood cells.

TREATMENT: In cases of Rh incompatibility, the condition can be controlled during pregnancy by following the anti-Rh titer of the mother's blood and the bilirubin level of the fetus by amniocentesis. These indices show whether the pregnancy should be allowed to go to full term and if intrauterine transfusion is indicated; or if labor should be induced earlier. Delivery should be as free of trauma as possible and the placenta should not be manually removed. The infant with hemolytic disease should be immediately seen by a physician who is capable of and has the facilities and blood supplies available for exchange transfusion. The use of $Rh_o$(D) immune globulin has been beneficial in preventing sensitization of an Rh-negative mother by an Rh-positive fetus, thus preventing hemolytic disease of the newborn in the next pregnancy.

***h. jaundice*** SEE: under *jaundice.*

***h. uremic syndrome*** An acute condition consisting of microangiopathic hemolytic anemia, thrombocytopenia, and acute nephropathy. Escherichia coli 0157:H7 is a causative agent that may be acquired from eating contaminated raw or rare hamburger or other meats. Children are most often affected. Onset may initially involve gastroenteritis and diarrhea or an upper respiratory tract infection. An acute phase of purpura, irritability, lethargy, and oliguria follows, continuing with splenomegaly, mild jaundice, seizures (in some patients), hepatomegaly, pulmonary edema, oliguria-anuria, cardiomegaly, and tachycardia. Urine may be dark yellow or brownish-red. The acute phase may last from 1 to 2 weeks in mild cases and much longer in severe cases.

TREATMENT: The treatment of this syndrome is for the renal failure and anemia. Transfusions may be needed, but the circulatory system should not be overloaded; thus, hemoglobin should not be increased beyond 7 to 8 g/dl.

PROGNOSIS: The usual outcome is complete recovery, but about 10% of patients develop end-stage renal disease.

**hemolyze** (hē′mō-līz) To produce hemolysis.

**hemomediastinum** (hē″mō-mē″dē-ă-stī′nŭm) [Gr. *haima,* blood, + L. *medias-*

*tinus,* in the middle] Effusion of blood into mediastinal spaces. SYN: *hematomediastinum.*

**hemometra** (hē″mō-mē′tră) [″ + *metra,* uterus] Hematometra.

**hemonephrosis** (hē″mō-nĕ-frō′sĭs) [″+ *nephros,* kidney, + *osis,* condition] Accumulation of blood in the renal pelvis. SYN: *hematonephrosis.*

**hemopathic** (hē″mō-păth′ĭk) [″ + *pathos,* disease, suffering] Relating or due to disease of the blood.

**hemopathology** (hē″mō-pă-thŏl′ō-jē) [″ + ″ + *logos,* word, reason] The science of blood disorders.

**hemoperfusion** The perfusion of blood through substances, such as activated charcoal or ion-exchange resins, to remove toxic materials. The blood is then returned to the patient. This technique differs from hemodialysis in that the blood is not separated from the chemicals or solutions by a semipermeable dialysis membrane. SEE: *hemodialysis.*

**hemopericardium** (hē″mō-pĕr″ĭ-kăr′dē-ŭm) [″ + *peri,* around, + *kardia,* heart] Accumulation of blood in the pericardial sac.

**hemoperitoneum** (hē″mō-pĕr″ĭ-tō-nē′ŭm) [″ + *peritonaion,* peritoneum] The effusion of blood into the peritoneal cavity.

**hemophage** (hē′mō-fāj) [″ + *phagein,* to eat] A cell that destroys red blood cells by phagocytosis.

**hemophagocyte** (hē″mō-făg′ō-sīt) [″ + ″ + *kytos,* cell] A phagocyte that ingests red blood cells.

**hemophagocytosis** (hē″mō-făg″ō-sī-tō′sĭs) [″ + ″ + ″ + *osis,* condition] The ingestion of red blood cells by phagocytes.

**hemophil** (hē′mŏ-fĭl) [″ + *philein,* to love] A type of bacteria that grows very well on agar that contains blood.

**hemophilia** (hē″mō-, hĕm″ō-fĭl′ē-ă) [″ + *philein,* to love] A hereditary blood disease marked by greatly prolonged coagulation time, with consequent failure of the blood to clot and abnormal bleeding, sometimes accompanied by swelling of the joints. It is a sex-linked trait transmitted by normal heterozygous females who carry the recessive gene and occurring almost exclusively in males. There are two main types of hemophilia, A and B; a third type, hemophilia C, is rare. The cause of hemophilia is a deficiency of a factor in plasma necessary for blood coagulation. The term *hemophilia* has been used to designate a variety of blood coagulation disorders. It should be used to refer to conditions in which a specific coagulation factor is lacking. SEE: *blood; Nursing Diagnoses Appendix.*

TREATMENT: There is no cure for hemophilia; however, the development of concentrated clotting factors VIII and IX has improved the prognosis for these patients. When hemorrhage occurs in patients with hemophilia A, coagulation factor VIII is given; factor IX is given when hemorrhage occurs in patients with hemophilia B. These factors are available from various sources and special care has been taken to be as sure as possible that they are free of the AIDS virus (HIV) and hepatitis viruses. Many persons with hemophilia learn to self-administer these factors to control bleeding episodes. Desmopressin (DDVAP) may be used to treat mild cases of hemophilia A. Hemophilia patients should avoid trauma and wear a bracelet indicating their condition. Information concerning hemophilia is available to the lay and medical public from the National Hemophilia Foundation, 110 Greene St., Suite 303, New York, NY 10012; (212) 219-8180.

---

Caution: Hemophilia patients should not be given aspirin, as its use can further complicate the bleeding tendency.

---

NURSING IMPLICATIONS: Vital signs are monitored, and the patient is assessed for signs and symptoms of decreased tissue perfusion (restlessness, anxiety, confusion, pallor, cool and clammy skin, chest pain, decreased urine output, hypotension, tachycardia). The skin, mucous membranes, and wounds are inspected for bleeding. Emergency care is provided for external bleeding, wounds cleaned, and gentle, consistent pressure applied to stop the bleeding. Safety measures are instituted to prevent injury, and the patient and family are instructed in these measures. The patient is assessed for development of hemarthrosis, and appropriate care is provided, which includes elevating the affected part, immobilizing the joint in a slightly flexed position, and applying ice intermittently. As necessary, deficient clotting factor or plasma is administered as prescribed until bleeding is controlled. The patient is monitored for adverse reactions to blood products, such as flushing, headache, tingling, fever, chills, urticaria, and anaphylaxis. Movement of the injured part is restricted, and exercise and weight bearing are prohibited for 48 hours until bleeding has stopped and swelling has subsided. Gentle passive range-of-motion exercises are then provided, gradually progressing to active-assisted and then active exercise. Prescribed analgesics are administered to control pain; however, I.M. injections are avoided as they may result in hematoma formation. The patient is cautioned against the use of aspirin, aspirin-containing medications, or other drugs that interfere with blood coagulation. Intracranial, muscle, subcutaneous, renal, and cardiac bleeding are monitored and managed according to protocols or as prescribed by the hematologist. Fluid balance is monitored throughout emergency situations, and adequate fluid replacement instituted as needed. Both patient and family are encouraged to verbalize their fears and concerns, and accurate information, realistic reassurance, and emotional support are provided. The nurse remains with the anxious or fearful patient or family. The patient may have been exposed to the human immunodeficiency virus (HIV) through contaminated blood; therefore, special support and information on infection control are provided to the patient and family. Gentle, careful, but thorough oral care is provided with a soft toothbrush or sponge-stick (toothette) to prevent inflamed gums and resultant bleeding, and the patient is instructed in this method of care. Regular dental examinations are recommended. Regular isometric exercise is encouraged to strengthen muscles, which in turn protects joints by reducing the incidence of hemarthrosis. Use of safety measures to protect the patient from injury (such as avoiding heavy lifting, contact sports, and falls and using power tools) is encouraged, while unnecessary restrictions that impair normal development are discouraged. The patient is encouraged to remain independent and self-sufficient, and assistance is provided to both patient and family to identify safe activities. Techniques are taught for managing bleeding episodes at home. The use of transfusion therapy is explained, and information is provided on all available methods of obtaining such therapy (including how to administer cryoprecipitate at home if appropriate). The seriousness of head injuries and the need for their immediate treatment are explained. Diversional activities and private time with family and friends are provided to help the patient overcome feelings of social isolation. The patient's and family's knowledge of the disease and its treatment, as well as the impact on the patient, siblings, and parent's marital relationship are continually assessed. Arrangements are made for the patient and family to talk with others in similar circumstances through local support groups and services, and they are referred to the National Hemophilia Foundation for further information. The patient should wear or carry a medical identification device identifying the illness and treatment.

***h. A*** Hemophilia due to a deficiency of blood coagulation factor VIII. SEE: *hemophilia.*

***h. B*** Hemophilia due to a deficiency of blood coagulation factor IX (plasma thromboplastin component). This condition can be treated with a lyophilized product that contains concentrated factor IX. SYN: *Christmas disease.* SEE: *hemophilia.*

***h. C*** Hemophilia due to a deficiency of blood coagulation factor XI.

**hemophiliac** (hē″mō-fĭl′ē-ăk) One afflicted with hemophilia.

**hemophilic** (hē″mō-fĭl′ĭk) **1.** Fond of blood, said of bacteria that grow well in culture media containing hemoglobin. **2.** Pert. to hemophilia or hemophiliacs.

**Hemophilus** Haemophilus.

**hemophobia** (hē″mō-fō′bē-ă) [Gr. *haima,* blood, + *phobos,* fear] An aversion to seeing blood or to bleeding.

**hemophthalmia, hemophthalmus** (hē″mŏf-thăl′mē-ă, -mŭs) [″ + *ophthalmos,* eye] An effusion of blood into the eye.

**hemopleura** (hē″mō-ploo′ră) Blood in the pleural space. SEE: *hemothorax.*

**hemopneumopericardium** (hē″mō-nū″mō-pĕr″ĭ-kăr′dē-ŭm) [″ + *pneuma,* air, + *peri,* around, + *kardia,* heart] Blood and air in the pericardial cavity.

**hemopneumothorax** (hē″mō-nū-mō-thō′răks) [″ + ″ + *thorax,* chest] Blood and air in the pleural cavity.

**hemopoiesis** (hē″mō-poy-ē′sĭs) [″ + *poiesis,* formation] Hematopoiesis.

**hemoprecipitin** (hē″mō-prē-sĭp′ĭ-tĭn) A precipitin in the blood.

**hemoprotein** (hē″mō-prō′tē-ĭn) Any protein combined with the heme blood pigment.

**hemopsonin** (hē″mŏp-sō′nĭn) [″ + *opsonein,* to buy food] An antibody that makes red blood cells more susceptible to phagocytosis.

**hemoptysis** (hē-mŏp′tĭ-sĭs) [″ + *ptyein,* to spit] The expectoration of blood arising from the oral cavity, larynx, trachea, bronchi, or lungs characterized by a sudden attack of coughing with production of salty sputum containing frothy bright red blood. Treatment consists of cold applications over the chest. SEE: table; *bleeding; hematemesis; hemorrhage; Nursing Diagnoses Appendix.*

Nursing Implications: Vital signs are monitored to determine the frequency of monitoring by the stability or instability of findings and by the patient's general condition. Universal precautions are used when expectorated blood and secretions are handled and when the patient is cleansed. Expectorated blood is inspected for amount, consistency, and color to assist in determining the site of bleeding. (Blood from the lungs is red and frothy; blood from the GI tract is dark red to black in color, depending on the location, size and speed of the bleed, and the amount of digestion occurring.) Expectorated blood and secretions are saved for the physician's inspection and possible laboratory analysis. A quiet, calm, and reassuring environment is maintained, and external warmth, but not excessive heat, is provided as necessary. The patient is placed on bedrest with the head slightly elevated, and turned toward the bleeding side if this is known. Oral care is provided as needed, and tepid fluids are administered as desired and tolerated. Coughing is discouraged; however, if the patient must cough, it should be done with an

**Comparison of Hemoptysis and Hematemesis**

| Hemoptysis | Hematemesis |
|---|---|
| Probable previous history of tuberculosis; possible embolism or infarction. | Probable previous history of gastric or duodenal trouble. |
| Blood is coughed up. | Blood is vomited. |
| Blood is frothy, bright red, and alkaline in reaction. | Blood is usually (not always) dark, usually not frothy, and acid in reaction. Often clotted. |
| Blood may be mixed with sputum. | Blood may be mixed with food. |
| There is some dyspnea, pain, and a tickling sensation in the chest, or pleuritic pain if pulmonary infarction occurs. | There is often nausea and pain referred to stomach. |

open glottis to avoid straining. Ice packs are applied locally as directed, and sedatives administered as prescribed.

***parasitic h.*** Spitting of blood resulting from infection of the lungs by *Paragonimus westermani,* a parasitic fluke.

**hemorrhage** (hĕm′ĕ-rĭj) [″ + *rhegnynai,* to burst forth] An abnormal, severe internal or external discharge of blood. It may be venous, arterial, or capillary from blood vessels into tissues, into or from the body. Venous blood is dark red and its flow is continuous. Arterial blood is bright red and flows in spurts. Capillary blood is reddish and exudes from the tissue.

SYMPTOMS: The diagnosis is obvious when the hemorrhage is visible. When it is internal, diagnosis is made from the patient's general condition: shock; weak, rapid, and irregular pulse; pallor; cold, moist skin.

NURSING IMPLICATIONS: The bleeding part is elevated as far above the head as possible, and pressure or a pressure dressing applied directly to the wound. Universal precautions are used for all procedures involving wound contact. If this is not effective, strong pressure is applied to the pressure point of the main artery supplying the wound. If a tourniquet is necessary to stop otherwise uncontrolled arterial bleeding, it should be tightened only enough to stop the bleeding and left in place until more definitive measures can be taken. The area distal to the wound (or tourniquet) is assessed for ischemic changes, and documents any deterioration of the distal limb. Vital signs are monitored, and fluid replacement is instituted as necessary according to protocol or as prescribed by the physician.

The nurse or emergency care provider may apply pneumatic splints or antigravity suits (G suit, MAST suit, antishock airpants) to delay the effects of internal hemorrhage during transportation. Such devices should not be deflated or removed until fluid replacement is initiated. The device should then be deflated proximally to distally, while appropriate measures are taken to prevent or control shock.

---

Caution: Universal precautions should be used. SEE: *Universal Precautions Appendix.*

---

***antepartum h.*** A hemorrhage appearing before the onset of labor.

***arterial h.*** A hemorrhage from an artery. In arterial bleeding, which is bright red, the blood ordinarily flows in waves or spurts; however, the flow may be steady if the torn artery is deep or buried.

FIRST AID: Almost all arterial bleeding can be controlled with direct pressure to the wound with gauze pads and elevation. Pressure should be applied for 20 min. If the blood soaks through, add more gauze to the wad, but do not remove the pads and replace with new ones as this will dislodge clots. A tourniquet is almost never needed and should be reserved for the rare conditions when the foregoing measures fail to stop the bleeding and the patient's life is in jeopardy. A tourniquet should be used only when the limb is considered sacrificable in order to save the patient's life. SEE: *bleeding, arterial* for table; *pressure points; tourniquet.*

***capillary h.*** Bleeding from minute blood vessels, present in all bleeding. When large vessels are not injured, capillary bleeding may be controlled by simple elevation and pressure with a sterile dry compress.

***carotid artery h.*** Hemorrhage from the carotid artery, usually accompanied by bleeding from the jugular veins. This type of hemorrhage can be fatal in a short time.

FIRST AID: The wound should be compressed with the thumbs placed transversely across the neck, both above and below the wound, and the fingers directed around the back of the neck to aid in compression. It may be more desirable to pack the wound with sterile gauze and compress it with the closed fist. Jugular vein wounds sometimes cause air embolism.

***cerebral h.*** The escape of blood into the tissues of the brain, which can be caused by hypertension, arteriosclerosis or atherosclerosis, rupture of an aneurysm, or trauma. SEE: *stroke.*

SYMPTOMS: This type of hemorrhage may cause unconsciousness, slow pulse, stertorous breathing, hemiplegia, and death. There may be speech disturbance, incontinence of the bladder and rectum, or constipation, depending on the area of brain damage.

TREATMENT: Supportive therapy is needed to maintain airway and oxygenation. The patient should be positioned properly to prevent nerve compression of the arms. Hydration and fluid and electrolyte balance should be maintained. Long-range therapy includes physical therapy, speech therapy, and counseling.

***fibrinolytic h.*** A hemorrhage due to a defect in the fibrin component in blood coagulation.

***gastrointestinal h.*** Bleeding into the intestinal tract.

***internal h.*** Hemorrhage into an area where it is not visible.

***intracranial h.*** Bleeding into the cranium.

***h. of the knee*** Bleeding from the knee.

TREATMENT: If the bleeding is at the knee or below, a pad should be applied with pressure. If the bleeding is behind the knee, a pad should be applied at the site and the leg bandaged firmly. The same precautions used with tourniquet (i.e., loosening at 12- to 15-min intervals) should be followed.

***lung h.*** Hemorrhage from the lung, with bright red and frothy blood, frequently coughed up.

***petechial h.*** Hemorrhage in the form of small rounded spots or petechiae occurring in the skin or mucous membranes.

***postmenopausal h.*** Bleeding from the uterus after menopause. It may be a sign of malignancy of the reproductive tract and should be carefully and thoroughly investigated without delay.

***postpartum h.*** Hemorrhage that occurs after childbirth. *Early postpartum hemorrhage* is defined as a blood loss of more than 500 ml of blood during the first 24 hr after delivery. The most common cause is loss of uterine tone caused by overdistention, prolonged or precipitate labor, uterine overstimulation, trauma, rupture, or inversion, lacerations of the lower genital tract, or blood coagulation disorder. *Late postpartum hemorrhage* occurs after the first 24 hr have passed. It usually is caused by retained placental fragments.

---

Caution: Universal precautions are essential. SEE: *Universal Precautions Appendix.*

---

NURSING IMPLICATIONS: During the first postpartum hour, the chance of hemorrhage is the greatest. To prevent hemorrhage, the mother's fundus is checked at least every 5 min and massaged. The mother's vital signs and vaginal discharge are checked every 15 min.

If hemorrhage begins, the uterus is elevated and held out of the pelvis by pushing the lower hand onto the abdomen above the symphysis pubis and by massaging the fundus with the upper hand to initiate and maintain a firmly contracted organ. If softness develops, massage is reinstituted immediately. A hand is kept on the uterus during treatment of hemorrhage to assess its condition and to massage it as indicated. Overmassage is contraindicated. The patient should keep her bladder empty. The physician may prescribe I.V. oxytocic drugs, plasma, or blood.

When ordered, well-diluted oxytocic drug therapy is administered by I.V. push followed by continuous I.V. oxytocic therapy in solution over 3 to 4 hr as prescribed. Methylergonovine or prostaglandin F2 may be ordered. Blood transfusions may be required to treat shock. The nurse prepares the patient for and assists the obstetrician with examination of the interior of the uterus for removal of retained products of conception or repair of lacerations. If lost blood fails to clot, coagulopathy may have developed, requiring prompt, life-saving treatment.

It is important to provide support and comfort for such a patient, who is understandably quite apprehensive. The nurse assures the patient that the newborn is well taken care of.

***primary h.*** A hemorrhage immediately following any trauma.

***retroperitoneal h.*** Bleeding into the retroperitoneal space.

***secondary h.*** **1.** A hemorrhage occurring some time after primary hemorrhage, usually caused by sepsis and septic ulceration into a blood vessel. It may occur after 24 hr or when a ligature separates, usually between the 7th and 10th days. **2.** Bleeding from the mother's uterus or the infant's umbilicus, resulting from a septic infection.

***stomach h.*** A hemorrhage into the stomach marked by dark blood, perhaps clotted or mixed with stomach contents, that is usually vomited. It may result from ruptured esophageal varices.

TREATMENT: Histamine-receptor type 2 ($H_2$) blockers and carafate should be given. Surgery may be required if the bleeding continues. If the hemorrhage is from the esophagus, compression of the bleeding site with a special intraesophageal tube balloon may be helpful.

***thigh h.*** Bleeding at the upper part of the thigh, near the groin.

TREATMENT: A pad or gauze should be inserted into the wound and pressure applied with the thumb in the center of the fold of the groin against the bone until the bleeding stops below the groin. Pad or tourniquet with pad under.

***typhoid h.*** A gross hemorrhage that occurs in approx. 10% of cases of typhoid that progress to the stage of gastrointestinal ulceration. Blood loss may reach 1000 ml. Single large hemorrhages or smaller successive ones may occur; the latter type are the most serious. Hemorrhages take place at the end of the second week and during the third week of the disease.

***unavoidable h.*** Ceaseless, painless bleeding from placenta previa.

***uterine h.*** Hemorrhage into the cavity of the uterus. The three types of pathologic uterine hemorrhage are essential uterine hemorrhage (metropathia haemorrhagica), which occurs with pelvic, uterine, or cervical diseases; intrapartum hemorrhage, which occurs during labor; and postpartum hemorrhage, which occurs after the third stage of labor. The latter may be caused by rupture, lacerations, relaxation of the uterus, hematoma, or retained products of conception including the placenta or membrane fragments.

ETIOLOGY: Common causes are trauma; congenital abnormalities; pathologic processes such as tumors; infections, esp. of the alimentary, respiratory, and genitourinary tracts; generalized vascular disorders such as various purpuras; coagulation defects; and retained products of conception following criminal or therapeutic abortion.

TREATMENT: Application of an umbrella pack will apply pressure to the uterine arterial supply. When a retained placenta is present and causing hemorrhage, it should be removed with uterine forceps. If the uterus is flaccid, it can usually be stimulated to contract by administering intravenous oxytocin. The patient may need transfusion and, in some cases, surgery to prevent fatal hemorrhage. SEE: *umbrella pack*.

***venous h.*** Hemorrhage of a vein, characterized by steady, profuse bleeding of rather dark blood.

FIRST AID: The patient should be kept quiet and relieved of anxiety. The bleeding part should be elevated if possible. A sterile pressure dressing should be applied directly over the wound. Elevation and pressure will control most venous bleeding. The patient should be watched closely for signs of shock. SEE: *tourniquet*.

***vicarious h.*** Hemorrhage from one part as a result of suppression of bleeding in another part. SEE: *vicarious menstruation*.

**hemorrhagenic** (hĕm″ō-ră-jĕn′ĭk) [″ + *rhegnynai*, to burst forth, + *gennan*, to form] Producing hemorrhage.

**hemorrhagic** (hĕm-ō-răj′ĭk) Pert. to or marked by hemorrhage.

***h. disease of the newborn*** Hemorrhaging due to an inadequate supply of prothrombin received from the mother or a delay in the establishment of the bacterial intestinal flora that produces vitamin K. Parenteral vitamin K given to the infant within 6 hr of birth prevents this condition.

***h. fever with renal syndrome*** An arthropod-borne viral disease caused by Hanta virus and marked by fever, thrombocytopenia, shock, and acute renal insufficiency. Treatment includes avoidance of excessive fluid administration, possible dialysis during the oliguric stage, and administration of plasma proteins or whole blood transfusion during the hemorrhagic phase.

***h. nephrosonephritis*** An acute infectious disease caused by the Hanta virus, with abrupt onset of fever that lasts 3 to 8 days, conjunctival injection, prostration, anorexia, and vomiting. Renal involvement may be mild or progress to acute renal failure, which may last several weeks. The mode of transmission is unknown but is apparently not from person to person. The incubation period varies from 9 to 35 days. Shock and renal failure should be treated symptomatically. There is no specific therapy. SYN: *epidemic hemorrhagic fever; Korean hemorrhagic fever*.

***viral h. fever*** ABBR: VHF. One of a group of diseases caused by arthropod-borne viruses, esp. the Bunyaviridae group, including Lassa, Marburg, Ebola, Rift Valley, and Congo-Crimean hemorrhagic fever viruses.

**hemorrhoid** (hĕm′ō-royd) [Gr. *haimorrhois*] A mass of dilated, tortuous veins in the anorectum involving the venous plexuses of that area. There are two kinds: external, those involving veins distal to the anorectal line; and internal, those involving veins proximal to the anorectal line. SYN: *piles*. SEE: illus.; *Nursing Diagnoses Appendix*.

TREATMENT: Therapy depends on the severity of the symptoms, not the extent of the hemorrhoids. In many instances, the only therapy required is improvement in anal hygiene and administration of stool softeners to prevent straining to have a bowel movement. The decision concerning the necessity of surgery or ligature with rubber bands should not be made until acute symptoms and inflammation have subsided, thus allowing tissues to regain their usual shape. SEE: *hemorrhoidectomy*.

***external h.*** One or more dilated veins at the junction of the anal mucosa with the anal skin. SEE: *hemorrhoid* for illus.

***internal h.*** One or more dilated veins of the lower rectum at the anorectal junction. SEE: *hemorrhoid* for illus.

***prolapsed h.*** The protrusion of an internal hemorrhoid through the anus.

***strangulated h.*** A prolapsed hemorrhoid that is trapped by the anal sphincter, thus cutting off blood flow to the vein in the hemorrhoid.

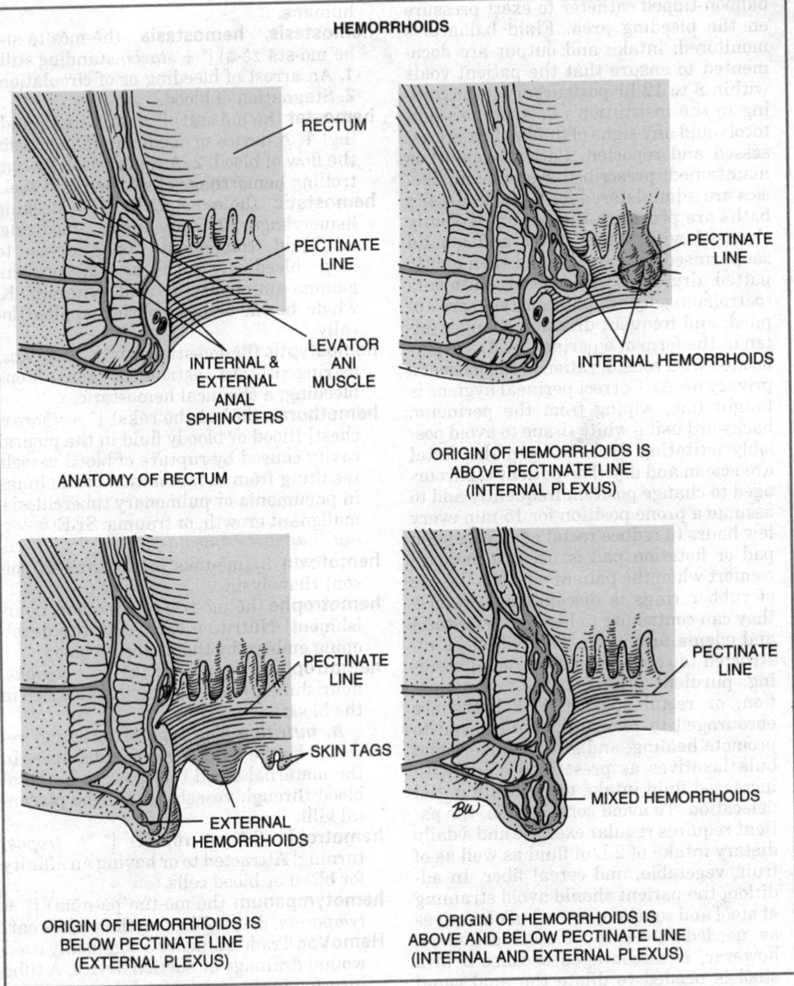


**hemorrhoidal** (hĕm-ō-roy′dăl) **1.** Relating to hemorrhoids. **2.** Pert. to certain anal arteries; arteria hemorrhoidalis.

**hemorrhoidectomy** (hĕm″ō-royd-ĕk′tō-mē) [Gr. *haimorrhois,* vein liable to bleed, + *ektome,* excision] The removal of hemorrhoids by one of several techniques including surgery, cryotherapy, infrared photocoagulation, laser surgery, or ligation by use of rubber bands, called surgical banding, applied to the base of the hemorrhoid. The latter method is used mostly for external hemorrhoids. SEE: *Nursing Diagnoses Appendix.*

NURSING IMPLICATIONS: *Preoperative:* The patient is prepared physically and emotionally for the surgery. The prescribed bowel preparation, which may include stool softeners, enema, and a low-residue diet, is provided. External hemorrhoids are assessed for size, evidence of bleeding, or the presence of drainage. Sitz baths are provided if prescribed, and the rectal area is cleansed and shaved (if shaving is part of the institution's or surgeon's protocol). The patient's knowledge of the procedure is determined, misconceptions are corrected, postoperative care and expected sensations are explained, a signed informed consent form is obtained, and prescribed preoperative sedation is administered.

*Postoperative:* Initially, vital signs are monitored hourly, then every 2 to 4 hr or as necessary. The rectal area is monitored hourly for bleeding during the early postoperative period, and excessive bleeding is reported and prescribed measures to reduce blood loss are instituted, such as inserting into the rectum and inflating a balloon-tipped catheter to exert pressure on the bleeding area. Fluid balance is monitored; intake and output are documented to ensure that the patient voids within 8 to 12 hr postsurgery (or according to the institution's or surgeon's protocol), and any signs of fluid deficit are assessed and reported. Patient comfort is maintained: prescribed systemic analgesics are administered for 24 to 48 hr; sitz baths are provided; the rectum is gently cleansed with warm water and a mild soap, rinsed thoroughly, and then gently patted dry; prescribed local ointments (petroleum jelly or analgesic type) are applied; and frequent dressing changes (often in the form of a perineal pad) are performed with consideration of the patient's privacy needs. Correct perineal hygiene is taught (i.e., wiping from the perineum backward using white tissue to avoid possibly irritating dyes) to keep the rectal area clean and dry. The patient is encouraged to change position frequently and to assume a prone position for 15 min every few hours to reduce rectal edema. A foam pad or flotation pad is used to increase comfort when the patient sits, but the use of rubber rings is discouraged, because they can contribute to local venous stasis and edema formation. The patient is instructed to report increased rectal bleeding, purulent drainage, fever, constipation, or rectal spasms. Sitz baths are encouraged to relieve discomfort and to promote healing, and stool softeners and bulk laxatives as prescribed along with increased fluid intake to facilitate initial defecation. To avoid constipation, the patient requires regular exercise and a daily dietary intake of 2 L of fluid as well as of fruit, vegetable, and cereal fiber. In addition, the patient should avoid straining at stool and continue to use bulk laxatives as needed. Overuse of stool softeners, however, is discouraged because a firm stool is needed to dilate the anal canal and to prevent formation of strictures.

**hemosalpinx** (hē″mō-săl′pĭnks) [Gr. *haima,* blood, + *salpinx,* tube] Hematosalpinx.

**hemosiderin** (hē″mō-sĭd′ĕr-ĭn) [″ + *sideros,* iron] An iron-containing pigment derived from hemoglobin from disintegration of red blood cells. It is one form in which iron is stored until it is needed for making hemoglobin.

**hemosiderosis** (hē″mō-sĭd-ĕr-ō′sĭs) [″+″ + *osis,* condition] A condition characterized by the deposition, esp. in the liver and spleen, of hemosiderin. It occurs in diseases in which there is marked red cell destruction such as hemolytic anemias, pernicious anemia, and chronic infection. SEE: *hemochromatosis.*

**hemospermia** (hē″mō-spĕr′mē-ă) [″ + *sperma,* seed] Hematospermia.

**Hemosporida** (hē-mō-spor-ĭ′dē-ă) [″ + *sporos,* seed] An order of parasites found in the blood of various animals, including humans.

**hemostasis, hemostasia** (hē-mŏs′tă-sĭs, hē″mō-stā′zē-ă) [″ + *stasis,* standing still] **1.** An arrest of bleeding or of circulation. **2.** Stagnation of blood.

**hemostat** (hē′mō-stăt) [″ + *statikos,* standing] **1.** A device or medicine that arrests the flow of blood. **2.** A compressor for controlling hemorrhage of a bleeding vessel.

**hemostatic** (hē″mō-stăt′ĭk) **1.** Checking hemorrhage. **2.** Any drug, medicine, or blood component that serves to stop bleeding, such as vasopressin, gamma-aminobutyric acid, vitamin K, whole blood, or epinephrine applied locally.

**hemostyptic** (hē-mō-stĭp′tĭk) [″ + *styptikos,* astringent] An astringent that stops bleeding; a chemical hemostatic.

**hemothorax** (hē″mō-thō′răks) [″ + *thorax,* chest] Blood or bloody fluid in the pleural cavity caused by rupture of blood vessels resulting from inflammation of the lungs in pneumonia or pulmonary tuberculosis, malignant growth, or trauma. SEE: *Nursing Diagnoses Appendix.*

**hemotoxin** (hē″mō-tŏks′ĭn) [″ + *toxikon,* poison] Hemolysin.

**hemotrophe** (hē′mō-trŏf) [″ + *trophe,* nourishment] Nutrition carried to the developing embryo by the maternal blood.

**hemotrophic** (hē-mō-trŏf′ĭk) [″ + *trophe,* nourishment] Pert. to nutrients carried in the blood.

***h. nutrition*** The type of nutrition received by the fetus through substances in the maternal blood that pass to the fetal blood through vessels within the placental villi.

**hemotropic** (hē-mō-trŏp′ĭk) [″ + *tropos,* turning] Attracted to or having an affinity for blood or blood cells.

**hemotympanum** (hē″mō-tĭm′pă-nŭm) [″ + *tympanon,* drum] Blood in the middle ear.

**HemoVac** Trade name for a commonly used wound drainage or suction device. A tube inserted in the wound leads to a reservoir for the fluid. Drainage is facilitated by gravity, suction, or vacuum.

**hemozoon** (hē″mō-zō′ŏn) Hematozoon.

**Henderson, Virginia** A nursing educator, born 1897, who developed a definition of nursing that was adopted by the International Council of Nurses. SEE: *Nursing Theory Appendix.*

**Henderson's Definition of Nursing** [Virginia Henderson, U.S. nursing educator, b. 1897] A definition, adopted by the International Council of Nurses, stating that the unique function of the nurse is to help sick or well individuals to perform activities that contribute to health, recovery, or a peaceful death. SEE: *Nursing Theory Appendix.*

**Henderson-Hasselbalch equation** [Lawrence Joseph Henderson, U.S. biochemist, 1878–1942; K. A. Hasselbalch, Danish physician, 1874–1962] An equation for stating the expression for the dissociation constant of an acid. In fluid and electrolyte balance, this important equation may be expressed in terms of the bicarbonate ($HCO_3^-$) system as: pH equals 6.1 + log $HCO_3^-/\alpha$ ($PaCO_2$) where $\alpha$ equals 0.03 mM/L/mm Hg at 38°C. At the normal pH of the blood, 7.4, the ratio of $HCO_3^-$ to $\alpha$ ($PaCO_2$) is 20 to 1.

**Henle, Friedrich G. J.** (hĕn′lē) German anatomist, 1809–1885.

***H.'s ampulla*** Ductus deferens dilatation just above the ejaculatory duct.

***H.'s fissure*** The fibrous tissue between the cardiac muscle fibers.

***H.'s layer*** The outer layer of cells of the inner root sheath of the hair follicle.

***H.'s ligament*** The conjoint tendon of the transversus abdominis muscle.

***H.'s loop*** The U-shaped portion of a renal tubule lying between the proximal and distal convoluted portions. It consists of a thin descending limb and a thicker ascending limb.

***H.'s membrane*** Bruch's layer forming inner boundary of the choroid of the eye.

***H.'s sheath*** Endoneurium.

***H.'s tubules*** The portion of the nephron following the proximal tubule. SEE: *nephron.*

**Henoch-Schönlein purpura** (hĕn′ōk-shān′lĭn) [Eduard H. Henoch, Ger. pediatrician, 1820–1910; Johann Lukas Schönlein, Ger. physician, 1793–1864] A form of allergic purpura with erythema, urticaria, and effusions of serum into subcutaneous or submucous tissue or viscera, accompanied by gastrointestinal and joint symptoms. The condition occurs mostly in children. Treatment is limited to supportive measures.

**henry** (hĕn′rē) [Joseph Henry, U.S. physicist, 1797–1878] A unit designating electrical inductance.

**Henry's law** (hĕn′rēz) [William Henry, Brit. chemist, 1774–1836] The law stating that the weight of a gas dissolved by a given volume of liquid at a constant temperature is directly proportional to the pressure.

**Hensen's cells** (hĕn′sĕns) [Victor Hensen, Ger. anatomist and physiologist, 1835–1924] Tall columnar cells that form the outer border cells of the organ of Corti of the cochlea.

**Hensen's disk** The band in the center of the A disk of a sarcomere of striated muscle. During contraction it appears lighter than the remaining portion and in its center, a dark stripe, the M line, is seen. SYN: *H band.*

**Hensen's stripe** A dark band on the undersurface of the tectorial membrane of the inner ear.

**HEPA filter** *high efficiency particulate air filter.*

**hepar** (hē′păr) [Gr. *hepatos,* liver] The liver.

**heparin** (hĕp′ă-rĭn) A polysaccharide that has been isolated from the liver, lung, and other tissues of domestic animals used for food. It is produced by mast cells and basophil leukocytes. It inhibits coagulation by forming an antithrombin that prevents conversion of prothrombin to thrombin and by preventing liberation of thromboplastin from blood platelets. Heparin is poorly absorbed from the gastrointestinal tract and is usually administered intravenously or subcutaneously as a sodium salt. Its action requires the presence of a cofactor found in plasma serum albumin.

USES: Heparin is used as an anticoagulant in the prevention and treatment of thrombosis and embolism. It is an important adjunct in the management of acute myocardial infarction and in the treatment of frostbite. The antagonist for an overdose is protamine sulfate 1%. Each milligram of protamine neutralizes approx. 100 USP heparin units.

***h. lock*** An intermittent infusion device that is used episodically for fluid or medication infusion. Heparin solution flushes are used to maintain its patency. SEE: *heparin lock flush solution.*

***h. lock flush solution*** A standard solution of heparin sodium labeled to indicate that it is intended for maintenance of patency of intravenous (IV) injection devices only and not for anticoagulant therapy. The standard concentration is 100 U/ml. The standard doses for a peripheral IV injection is 100 U or 1 ml and for a central IV injection, 3 ml every 8 to 12 hr.

***low molecular weight h.*** A particularly fast-acting, soluble form of heparin used in preventing deep vein thrombosis.

***h. sulfate*** A sulfurated mucopolysaccharide that accumulates in the connective tissue in abnormal amounts in some mucopolysaccharidoses. SEE: *mucopolysaccharidosis.*

**heparinize** (hĕp′ĕr-ĭ-nīz) To inhibit blood coagulation with heparin.

**hepat-** SEE: *hepato-.*

**hepatalgia** (hĕp″ă-tăl′jē-ă) [Gr. *hepatos,* liver, + *algos,* pain] Pain in the liver. SYN: *hepatodynia.* **hepatalgic** (hĕp″ă-tăl′jĭk), *adj.*

**hepatatrophia** (hĕp″ăt-ă-trō′fē-ă) [″ + *atrophia,* atrophy] Atrophy of the liver.

**hepatectomy** (hĕp″ă-tĕk′tō-mē) [″ + *ektome,* excision] Excision of part or all of the liver.

**hepatic** (hĕ-păt′ĭk) [Gr. *hepatikos*] Pert. to the liver.

***h. amebiasis*** SEE: under *amebiasis.*

***h. coma*** Impaired central nervous system function caused by liver disease. The disease permits venous blood to bypass portal circulation, thus allowing an accumulation of products in the blood that are usually metabolized by the liver (e.g., ammonia). Any situation associated with increased ammonia production promotes hepatic coma in patients with severely impaired liver function. These may include following a high-protein diet, gastrointestinal bleeding, fluid and electrolyte imbalance, infections, and drugs such as sedatives, tranquilizers, anesthetics, analgesics, diuretics, and alcohol.

SYMPTOMS: Symptoms of hepatic coma are impaired consciousness, sluggish or impaired speech, drowsiness, confusion, stupor, and coma. The patient will be unable to explain the meaning of simple sayings and may have difficulty telling the day of the week or month. Attempts at drawing simple figures will be unsuccessful. A "mousy" odor of the breath (fetor hepaticus) is usually present. A distinctive type of flapping tremor of the hand called asterixis occurs in severe cases. Ataxia may be present, along with altered deep tendon reflexes. An electroencephalogram will be abnormal, and the blood ammonia level will be elevated.

TREATMENT: A protein-restricted, high-carbohydrate diet should be given. The intestinal tract should be flushed free of blood, if present, by enemas or mild cathartics. Oral neomycin should be given to control the bacteria that favor ammonia production, and oral lactulose helps to decrease ammonia production in the intestinal tract. Exchange transfusions to remove ammonia from the blood are used, but have not been effective.

NURSING IMPLICATIONS: The patient's level of consciousness is assessed and documented frequently. Fluid and electrolyte balance is monitored by recording intake and output and by checking the patient's weight and measuring abdominal girth daily. Laboratory indicators or clinical signs of anemia (decreased hemoglobin levels), alkalosis (increased serum bicarbonate), G.I. bleeding (melena, hematemesis), and infection are monitored and reported immediately. The patient's serum ammonia level is also monitored for signs of deterioration or improvement. The nurse continually orients the patient to place and time and keeps a daily record of the patient's handwriting to evaluate the progression of neurological involvement. Prescribed medications are administered and evaluated for desired effects and any adverse reactions. A quiet atmosphere is provided and stressful activities discouraged to promote rest and comfort. Arrangements are made with the dietitian to provide a low-protein diet, with carbohydrates supplying most of the calories. Oral hygiene is provided as needed. If the patient is semicomatose or comatose, prescribed enteral feedings or parenteral nutrition are provided. Appropriate safety measures are used to protect the patient from injury; physical restraints should be avoided if at all possible. Sedatives should not be administered if the patient is semicomatose or comatose because they deepen the coma. Artificial tears or eye patches are used to protect the comatose patient's eyes from corneal injury due to drying. The family (and the patient if he or she can understand) is educated about the disease and its treatment; explanations of each treatment are repeated as the treatment is performed, even if the patient is comatose. If the patient has chronic encephalopathy, the mental and physical effects of the illness and signs and symptoms of worsening status or complications are explained to both patient and family, and they are advised to notify the physician should any of these occur. As the patient begins to recover, the low-protein diet and the prescribed drug regimen, including dosing schedule, desired effects, and adverse reactions to be reported, are explained to both patient and family. To reduce anxiety and frustration, both patient and family should be apprised that recovery from so severe an illness takes time. If the patient is in the terminal stages of encephalopathy, emotional support is offered to the family.

***h. duct*** The duct that carries bile out of the liver. It unites with the cystic duct from the gallbladder to form the common bile duct.

***h. encephalopathy*** SEE: *hepatic coma.*

***h. flexure*** The bend of the colon under the liver; the junction of the ascending and transverse colon.

***h. lobe*** A division of the liver.

***h. vein*** One of three vessels returning blood from the liver and discharging into the inferior vena cava.

**hepaticoduodenostomy** (hĕ-păt″ĭ-kō-dū″ō-dĕ-nŏs′tō-mē) [″ + L. *duodeni,* duodenum, + Gr. *stoma,* mouth] Hepatoduodenostomy.

**hepaticoenterostomy** (hĕ-păt″ĭ-kō-ĕn-tĕr-ŏs′tō-mē) [″ + *enteron,* intestine, + *stoma,* mouth] An operation to create an artificial opening between the hepatic duct and intestine.

**hepaticogastrostomy** (hĕ-păt″ĭ-kō-găs-trŏs′tō-mē) [″ + *gaster,* stomach, + *stoma,* mouth] An operation to create a passage between the hepatic duct and the stomach.

**hepaticojejunostomy** (hĕ-păt′ĭ-kō-jē″jū-nŏs′tō-mē) [″ + L. *jejunum,* empty, + Gr. *stoma,* mouth] The surgical joining of the hepatic duct and the jejunum.

**hepaticolithotomy** (hĕ-păt″ĭ-kō-lĭ-thŏt′ō-mē) The surgical removal of gallstones from the hepatic duct.

**hepaticolithotripsy** (hĕ-păt″ĭ-kō-lĭth′ō-trĭp-sē) [″ + *lithos,* stone, + *tripsis,* a crushing] Crushing of a biliary calculus in the hepatic duct.

**hepaticostomy** (hĕ-păt″ĭ-kŏs′tō-mē) [″ + *stoma,* mouth] The establishment of a permanent fistula into the hepatic duct.

**hepaticotomy** (hĕ-păt″ĭ-kŏt′ō-mē) [″ + *tome,* incision] An incision into the hepatic duct.

**hepatitis** (hĕp″ă-tī′tĭs) [″ + *itis,* inflammation] An inflammation of the liver. Although the most common cause is one of the five hepatitis viruses, it is also caused by other viruses, bacteria, parasites, and toxic reactions to drugs, alcohol, and chemicals. The primary clinical signs are jaundice and an enlarged liver (hepatomegaly).

PATHOLOGY: Damage to liver cells (hepatocytes) is caused by direct injury from the physical agent (e.g., carbon tetrachloride), the inflammatory process, cytotoxic T lymphocytes, or the formation of immune complexes between antigens and protective antibodies. During acute inflammation, the swollen hepatocytes are less able to detoxify drugs; produce clotting factors, cholesterol, plasma proteins, bile, and glycogen; store fat-soluble vitamins; and perform other functions. Hepatitis A and C may progress to fulminant hepatitis, which has a high mortality rate. Hepatitis B and C are more likely to cause significant fibrotic changes and have been associated with liver cancer.

SYMPTOMS: The clinical signs and symptoms of hepatitis are similar for all five viruses and are based on the stage of infection. The *prodromal stage* is marked by abrupt or gradual onset of general malaise, low-grade fever, anorexia, nausea and vomiting, muscle and joint pain, fatigue, headache, dark urine, clay-colored stools, and frequently, signs of an upper respiratory infection (pharyngitis, nasal discharge, and cough). This stage lasts a few days to 2 weeks. The *icteric stage* occurs 5 to 10 days after the prodromal stage begins. Patients develop jaundice, and the other symptoms worsen. Pruritis may also be present, and the liver is large and tender. Laboratory tests show elevations in serum bilirubin and two hepatic enzymes, aspartate transaminase and alanine aminotransferase. The *convalescent stage* begins as the jaundice begins to disappear, and the other signs and symptoms decrease.

NURSING IMPLICATIONS: Patients are generally not hospitalized unless there is significant liver damage; these patients require supportive physical and psychosocial care. Patients at home should be instructed about the nature and course of the illness, care and treatment, and signs and symptoms of complications. The patient should eat a well-balanced diet, drink adequate fluids, but avoid alcohol, and observe the color of urine and feces. Emphasis should be placed on the need for scrupulous attention to linens, dishes, handling of food, and so forth, to prevent the spread of hepatitis A to other household members. Intimate contact should be avoided until antigen and antibody serum levels are reduced. The patient should be encouraged to continue medical follow-up because recovery may require a considerable length of time. Emotional support and reassurance should be offered to the patient, as interference with the patient's habits and lifestyle may be considerable.

SEE: *cirrhosis; Nursing Diagnoses Appendix; Universal Precautions Appendix.*

***h. A*** Hepatitis caused by hepatitis A virus (HAV), an RNA virus without an envelope. Because it can be contracted through contaminated water or food, young adults and children in institutional settings and travelers in countries with minimal sanitation are at greatest risk for infection; small epidemics have been seen among persons eating at restaurants that served contaminated shellfish. The course of the illness is usually mild, although it can be severe; the acute stage resolves in about 2 weeks and complete recovery occurs in about 8 weeks. The two antibodies produced in response to hepatitis A antigen serve as markers for infection and provide immunity against reinfection. Previously called *infectious hepatitis.*

No drugs specifically treat hepatitis A; gamma globulin (immunoglobulin G) may be prescribed for family members and as prophylaxis for travelers. Preventive education focuses on good personal hygiene, especially handwashing, and use of judgment in choice of food and eating places. In some areas of the world, basic sanitation and the proper disposal of feces must be taught.

***acute anicteric h.*** Hepatitis marked by slight fever, gastrointestinal upset, and anorexia, but no jaundice.

***amebic h.*** The syndrome of a tender, enlarged liver; pain over the liver; fever; and leukocytosis in a patient with amebic colitis. This name is a misnomer in that the liver changes are not due to an infestation of that organ with amebae but are a part of the nonspecific reaction to the infection in the intestinal tract. Nevertheless, occasionally a liver abscess will develop and the walls of the abscess will contain amebae.

TREATMENT: Metronidazole plus iodoquinol, or chloroquine phosphate plus either emetine or dehydroemetine, are used to treat amebic hepatitis. These latter two drugs are toxic and should be given only if their course can be carefully observed by a cardiac monitor. The drugs should not be given to a patient who has cardiac disease or is pregnant. Needle aspiration of the abscess may be needed.

***h. antigen*** The original term for the Australian antigen, which is now called hepatitis B surface antigen (HBsAg). Its discovery made possible the differentiation of hepatitis B from other forms of viral hepatitis.

***h. B*** Hepatitis that tends to cause a severe acute infection and may progress to chronic infection and permanent liver damage. It is caused by hepatitis B virus (HBV), an enveloped, double-stranded DNA virus. Individuals at greatest risk for infection include intravenous drug abusers, homosexual men, infants born of

HBV-infected mothers, and health care workers. Blood banks now routinely screen for HBV antigens; this practice has greatly reduced the risk for infection in persons requiring multiple transfusions. Previously called *serum hepatitis*.

Three antigenic markers for HBV infection have been identified: HBsAg, a surface antigen on the viral envelope, is the earliest marker, appearing in the blood during incubation. The antigen HBeAg, from the protein capsid surrounding the DNA, also is a marker for active infection. Another core antigen, HBc, which does not circulate in the blood, stimulates the production of the primary antibodies against HBV. These antibodies are not protective and provide no immunity. Acute infection generally resolves in 4 to 6 months, and HBsAg markers disappear; anti-HBs and anti-HBe antibodies appear at this time and last for years. Approximately 5% to 10% of patients develop chronic infection, which lasts for more than 6 months. Serum titers of HBsAg and IgG anti-HBc are elevated in these patients; other markers increase with reactivation of the infection. The presence of HBsAg in the blood after the acute phase indicates that the individual is a carrier who can transmit the disease to others.

Hepatitis B infection can be prevented through a vaccine created using recombinant DNA technology. Complete protection requires two vaccinations 1 month apart and a third dose 4 months later; an elevated anti-HBs antibody titer indicates successful vaccination. All health care workers should be vaccinated, as should patients with renal disease requiring hemodialysis, police officers and other public safety workers, family members and sexual partners of those infected with HBV, and persons who travel extensively abroad. The Centers for Disease Control and Prevention recommends that pregnant women be tested for HBsAg so that newborns can be vaccinated. SEE: *h. B virus vaccine*.

---

Caution: Individuals who have not been vaccinated against HBV and receive a needlestick or mucous membrane contact with blood or other body secretions should contact their occupational health department. Hepatitis B virus immune globulin (HBIg) can be given to provide temporary protection.

---

***h. B core antigen*** ABBR: HBcAg. An antigen of the hepatitis B virus found only in liver cells. Tests for it (liver biopsy) or its antibody are helpful in the diagnosis of hepatitis B.

***h. Be antigen*** ABBR: HBeAg. An antigen of the hepatitis B virus; high levels indicate that a person is highly infectious.

***h. B immune globulin*** The standard solution consisting of globulins derived from blood plasma of human donors who have high titers of antibodies against hepatitis B surface antigen.

***h. B surface antigen*** ABBR: HBsAg. An antigen of hepatitis B virus; originally called hepatitis-associated antigen.

***h. B virus vaccine*** A recombinant vaccine used to vaccinate persons at high risk of coming in contact with hepatitis B carriers, or with blood or fluids from such individuals. Included in the high-risk group are health care workers, hemodialysis patients, police officers and other public safety workers, family members and sexual partners of those infected with HBV, and persons who travel extensively abroad.

***h. C*** An acute and chronic form of hepatitis caused by an RNA virus in the same family as yellow fever. Formerly called non-A, non-B hepatitis, it was discovered in 1989. It is similar in many ways to hepatitis B. The virus is spread through blood; sexual contact and mother-infant transmission are rare, perhaps because the level of virus in the blood is lower. However, the risk for infection from blood transfusions may be greater because antigens do not appear in the blood immediately after exposure. Presentation of the infection varies widely. Most acute infections are similar to those caused by HBV and resolve in about 4 months; some are asymptomatic; and others produce fulminant hepatitis. Almost 50% of patients develop chronic infections, and about 10% incur progressive hepatic fibrosis and cirrhosis. Alpha interferon has been effective in treating hepatitis C.

***chronic h.*** Hepatic inflammatory changes that continue for more than 6 months. The most common causes are hepatitis B and C viruses, but inflammation also occurs from alcohol, other drugs, toxic chemicals, or autoimmune processes. Chronic hepatitis may be asymptomatic and cause minimal liver damage, or actively progressive, eventually leading to cirrhosis and death. Alpha interferon is an effective treatment.

***h. D*** A form of hepatitis caused by a so-called "defective" virus that can produce infection only when HBV is present and therefore can be prevented by hepatitis B vaccination. Inflammatory changes in the liver are minimal; the virus is believed to kill cells by invasion. Hepatitis D antigens do not circulate and are found only in the nucleus of hepatocytes; antidelta antibodies in the blood are a marker for infection. Although hepatitis D usually appears simultaneously with acute hepatitis B, it also can cause a more severe infection in patients with chronic HBV infection. Also called *delta agent hepatitis*.

***h. E*** A form of hepatitis similar in presentation to hepatitis A that occurs primarily in Asia, Africa, and South America. Infection is most dangerous in pregnant women, for whom the mortality is approximately 20%. It is spread via contaminated food and water and, like hepatitis A, causes only acute infections; however, it is unclear if infection produces immunity.

***fulminant h.*** Hepatitis marked by the sudden onset of nausea and vomiting, chills, high fever, and severe and early jaundice. Significant liver damage produces the central nervous system changes of hepatic encephalopathy, coagulopathies, abnormalities in fluid and electrolyte imbalance, and cerebral edema. The mortality is high; death occurs usually within 10 days of onset. Causes include hepatitis A, B, C, and D; hypersensitivity to drugs and anesthetics (e.g., tetracycline and halothane); and toxic chemicals.

***infectious h.*** Term previously used for hepatitis A virus infection.

***serum h.*** Term previously used for hepatitis B virus infection.

***toxic h., drug-induced h.*** An inflammation of the liver caused by the entry of toxins or drugs into the body. Included in the great number of agents known to be able to cause this type of hepatitis are common drugs and chemicals (e.g., halothane, anabolic steroids, carbon tetrachloride, trichlorethylene) used in either the treatment of disease or in the workplace.

**hepatization** (hĕp″ă-tĭ-zā′shŭn) The second and third stages in consolidation in lobar pneumonia, in which the lung's surface looks like liver tissue.

**hepato-, hepat-** [Gr. *hepatikos*] Combining form meaning *liver*.

**hepatoblastoma** (hĕp″ă-tō-blăs-tō′mă) [″ + *blastos,* germ, + *oma,* tumor] A malignant teratoma of the liver.

**hepatocarcinogen** Anything that causes cancer of the liver.

**hepatocarcinoma** (hĕp″ă-tō-kăr″sĭn-ō′mă) [″ + *karkinos,* crab, + *oma,* tumor] Carcinoma of the liver.

**hepatocele** (hĕp′ă-tō-sĕl) [ + *kele,* tumor, swelling] Hernia of the liver.

**hepatocellular** (hĕp″ă-tō-sĕl′ū-lăr) Concerning the cells of the liver.

**hepatocholangiocystoduodenostomy** (hĕp″ă-tō-kō-lăn″jē-ō-sĭs″tō-dū″ō-dĕ-nŏs′tō-mē) [″ + *chole,* bile, + *angeion,* vessel, + *kystis,* bladder, + L. *duodenum,* duodenum, + Gr. *stoma,* mouth] The establishment of drainage of bile ducts into the duodenum through the gallbladder.

**hepatocholangioduodenostomy** (hĕp″ă-tō-kō-lăn″jē-ō-dū-ō-dĕ-nŏs′tō-mē) [″ + ″ + ″ + L. *duodenum,* duodenum, + Gr. *stoma,* mouth] The establishment of drainage of bile ducts into the duodenum.

**hepatocholangioenterostomy** (hĕp″ă-tō-kō-lăn″jē-ō-ĕn″tĕr-ŏs′tō-mē) [″ + ″ + ″ + *enteron,* intestine, + *stoma,* mouth] The establishment of a passage between the liver and intestine.

**hepatocholangiogastrostomy** (hĕp″ă-tō-kō-lăn″jē-ō-găs-trŏs′tō-mē) [″ + ″ + ″ + *gaster,* belly, + *stoma,* mouth] The establishment of drainage of bile ducts into the stomach.

**hepatocholangiostomy** (hĕp″ă-tō-kō-lăn-jē-ŏs′tō-mē) [″ + ″ + ″ + *stoma,* mouth] The establishment of free drainage by opening into the gall duct.

**hepatocholangitis** (hĕp″ă-tō-kō-lăn-jī′tis) [″ + ″ + ″ + *itis,* inflammation] An inflammation of the cells of the liver and bile ducts.

**hepatocolic** (hĕp″ă-tō-kŏl′ĭk) [″ + *kolon,* colon] Relating to the liver and colon.

**hepatocystic** (hĕp″ă-tō-sĭs′tĭk) [″ + *kystis,* bladder] Relating to the gallbladder or to both liver and gallbladder.

**hepatocyte** (hĕp′ă-tō-sīt) A parenchymal liver cell.

**hepatoduodenostomy** (hĕp″ă-tō-dū″ō-dĕ-nŏs′tō-mē) [″ + L. *duodenum,* duodenum, + Gr. *stoma,* mouth] The establishment of an opening from the liver (hepatic duct) into the duodenum. SYN: *hepaticoduodenostomy.*

**hepatoenteric** (hĕp″ă-tō-ĕn-tĕr′ĭk) [″ + *enteron,* intestine] Relating to the liver and intestines.

**hepatogastric** (hĕp″ă-tō-găs′trĭk) [Gr. *hepatikos,* liver, + *gaster,* belly] Relating to the liver and stomach.

**hepatogenous** (hĕp″ă-tŏj′ĕ-nŭs) Originating in the liver.

**hepatography** (hĕp″ă-tŏg′ră-fē) [″ + *graphein,* to write] Radiography of the liver, usually after injection of a radiographic contrast medium.

**hepatojugular** (hĕp″ă-tō-jŭg′ū-lăr) Concerning the liver and jugular vein.

**hepatolenticular** (hĕp″ă-tō-lĕn-tĭk′ū-lăr) [″ + L. *lenticula,* lentil, lens] Relating to the liver and lenticular nucleus of the eye.

***h. degeneration*** Wilson's disease.

**hepatolienography** (hĕp″ă-tō-lī″ĕ-nŏg′ră-fē) [″ + L. *lien,* spleen, + Gr. *graphein,* to write] Radiography of the liver and spleen, usually after intravenous injection of a contrast medium.

**hepatolienomegaly** (hĕp″ă-tō-lī″ĕ-nō-mĕg′ă-lē) [″ + ″ + *megas,* large] An enlargement of the liver and spleen.

**hepatolithectomy** (hĕp″ă-tō-lĭ-thĕk′tō-mē) [″ + *lithos,* stone, + *ektome,* excision] The surgical removal of a calculus from the liver.

**hepatolithiasis** (hĕp″ă-tō-lĭ-thī′ă-sĭs) [″ + ″ + *-iasis,* disease condition] A condition characterized by calculi or concretions in the liver.

**hepatologist** (hĕp″ă-tŏl′ō-jĭst) [″ + *logos,* word, reason] A specialist in diseases of the liver.

**hepatology** (hĕp″ă-tŏl′ō-jē) [″ + *logos,* word, reason] The study of the liver.

**hepatolytic** (hĕp″ă-tō-lĭt′ĭk) Destructive to tissues of the liver.

**hepatoma** (hĕp″ă-tō′mă) [″ + *oma,* tumor] A

term previously used to describe hepatocellular carcinoma.

**hepatomalacia** (hĕp″ă-tō-mă-lā′sē-ă) [″ + *malakia,* softening] A softening of the liver.

**hepatomegaly** (hĕp″ă-tō-mĕg′ă-lē) [″ + *megas,* large] An enlargement of the liver.

**hepatomelanosis** (hĕp″ă-tō-mĕl″ă-nō′sĭs) [″ + *melas,* black, + *osis,* condition] Pigmented deposits or melanosis in the liver.

**hepatomphalocele** (hĕp″ă-tŏm′fă-lō-sēl″) [Gr. *hepatikos,* liver, + *omphalos,* navel, + *kele,* tumor, swelling] The protrusion of a part of the liver, which is covered by a membrane, through the umbilicus.

**hepatonecrosis** (hĕp″ă-tō-nĕ-krō′sĭs) [″ + *nekrosis,* state of death] Gangrene of the liver.

**hepatonephric** (hĕp″ă-tō-nĕf′rĭk) [″ + *nephros,* kidney] Concerning the liver and kidney.

**hepatonephritis** (hĕp″ă-tō-nĕ-frī′tĭs) [″ + ″ + *itis,* inflammation] An inflammation of the liver and kidneys.

**hepatonephromegaly** (hĕp″ă-tō-nĕf″rō-mĕg′ă-lē) [″ + ″ + *megas,* large] Hypertrophy of the liver and kidneys.

**hepatoperitonitis** (hĕp″ă-tō-pĕr″ĭ-tō-nī′tĭs) [″ + *peritonaion,* peritoneum, + *itis,* inflammation] Perihepatitis.

**hepatopexy** (hĕp′ă-tō-pĕks″ē) [″ + *pexis,* fixation] Fixation of a movable liver to the abdominal wall.

**hepatopleural** (hĕp″ă-tō-ploo′răl) [″ + *pleura,* side] Concerning the liver and pleura.

**hepatopneumonic** (hĕp″ă-tō-nū-mŏn′ĭk) [″ + *pneumonikos,* of the lungs] Concerning the liver and lungs.

**hepatoportogram** (hĕp″ă-tō-por′tō-grăm) A radiograph of the portal vein and its hepatic branches after injection of a contrast medium.

**hepatoptosia, hepatoptosis** (hĕp″ă-tŏp-tō′sē-ă, -tō′sĭs) [″ + *ptosis,* a dropping] A downward displacement of the liver.

**hepatopulmonary** (hĕp″ă-tō-pŭl′mō-năr″ē) [″ + L. *pulmo,* lung] Relating to the liver and lungs.

**hepatorenal** (hĕp″ă-tō-rē′năl) [″ + L. *renalis,* kidney] Pert. to the liver and kidneys.

**hepatorrhaphy** (hĕp-ă-tor′ă-fē) [″ + *rhaphe,* seam, ridge] The suturing of a wound of the liver.

**hepatorrhexis** (hĕp″ă-tō-rĕks′ĭs) [″ + *rhexis,* rupture] A rupture of the liver.

**hepatoscan** (hĕp′ă-tō-skăn) A radioautograph of the liver.

**hepatoscopy** [″ + *skopein,* to examine] Inspection of the liver.

**hepatosplenitis** (hĕp″ă-tō-splĕ-nī′tĭs) [″ + *splen,* spleen, + *itis,* inflammation] An inflammation of the liver and spleen.

**hepatosplenography** (hĕp″ă-tō-splĕ-nŏg′ră-fē) [″ + ″ + *graphein,* to write] Radiographic examination of the liver and spleen.

**hepatosplenomegaly** (hĕp″ă-tō-splē″nō-mĕg′ă-lē) [″ + ″ + *megas,* large] An enlargement of the liver and spleen.

**hepatosplenopathy** (hĕp″ă-tō-splĕ-nŏp′ă-thē) [″ + ″ + *pathos,* disease, suffering] A disease that affects the liver and spleen.

**hepatotherapy** (hĕp″ă-tō-thĕr′ă-pē) [″ + *therapeia,* treatment] **1.** The treatment of liver disease. **2.** The use of liver or liver extract.

**hepatotomy** (hĕp″ă-tŏt′ō-mē) [″ + *tome,* incision] An incision into the liver.

**hepatotoxemia** (hĕp″ă-tō-tŏks-ē′mē-ă) [″ + *toxikon,* poison, + *haima,* blood] Autointoxication due to malfunctioning of the liver.

**hepatotoxic** Toxic to the liver.

**hepatotoxin** (hĕp″ă-tō-tŏk′sĭn) A cytotoxin specific for liver cells.

**heptachromic** (hĕp″tă-krō′mĭk) [Gr. *hepta,* seven, + *chroma,* color] Possessing normal color vision.

**heptapeptide** (hĕp″tă-pĕp′tīd) [″ + *peptein,* to digest] A polypeptide containing seven amino acids.

**heptaploidy** (hĕp′tă-ploy″dē) [″ + *ploos,* fold] Having seven sets of chromosomes.

**heptose** (hĕp′tōs) Any sugar containing seven carbon atoms in its molecule.

**heptosuria** (hĕp″tō-sū′rē-ă) [″ + *ouron,* urine] Heptose in the urine.

**herb** (ĕrb) [L. *herba,* grass] A plant with a soft stem containing little wood, esp. an aromatic plant used in medicine or seasoning. The plant usually produces seeds and then dies down at the end of the growing season.

**herbalist** One who attempts to promote healing or health through the use of herbs.

**herbicide** A substance (such as a chemical) that kills plants or inhibits plant growth.

***h. poisoning*** Poisoning due to the use of a toxic herbicide such as 2,4-D.

**herbivorous** (hĕr-bĭv′ō-rŭs) [″ + *vorare,* to eat] Vegetarian.

**herd** [AS. *heord*] Any large aggregation of people or animals.

***h. immunity*** SEE: under *immunity.*

**hereditary** (hĕ-rĕd′ĭ-tĕr-ē) [L. *hereditarius,* an heir] Pert. to a genetic characteristic transmitted from parent to offspring. SEE: *chromosome; gene.*

**heredity** (hĕ-rĕd′ĭ-tē) [L. *hereditas,* heir] The transmission of genetic characteristics from parent to offspring.

**heredo-** [L. *hereditas,* heir] Prefix meaning *heredity.*

**heredoataxia** (hĕr″ĕ-dō-ă-tăks′ē-ă) [″ + Gr. *ataxia,* lack of order] Friedreich's ataxia.

**heredodegeneration** (hĕr″ĕ-dō-dē-jĕn″ĕr-ā′shŭn) An inherited degeneration caused by defective or diseased hyaloplasm. It is seen in Marie's ataxia.

**heredofamilial** (hĕr″ĕ-dō-fă-mĭl′ē-ăl) Referring to any disease that occurs in families owing to the inherited defect or process to develop the condition.

**heredoimmunity** (hĕr″ĕ-dō-ĭ-mū′nĭ-tē) Inherited immunity.

**Hering, Heinrich Ewald** German physiologist, 1866–1948.

***H.'s nerves*** Afferent nerve fibers leading from the carotid sinus by way of the glossopharyngeal nerve to the brain. They are pressoreceptor nerves responding to changes in blood pressure that reflexly control heart rate. An increase in pressure diminishes heart rate.

***H.'s reflex*** A reflex inhibition of inspiration resulting from stimulation of pressoreceptors by inflation of the lungs.

**Hering, Karl Ewald K** (hĕr′ĭng) German physiologist, 1834–1918.

***H.'s theory*** A theory of color vision in which it is assumed that the retina possesses three photochemical substances that, depending on their decomposition or resynthesis, produce different color sensations by their stimulation of different nerve endings.

**heritable** Able to be inherited.

**heritage** The genetic and other characteristics transmitted to offspring.

**hermaphrodism** (hĕr-măf′rō-dĭzm) Hermaphroditism.

**hermaphrodite** (hĕr-măf′rō-dīt) [Gr. *Hermaphroditos,* mythical son of Hermes and Aphrodite, who was man and woman combined] An individual possessing genital and sexual characteristics of both sexes. The clitoris is usually enlarged, resembling the male penis. SYN: *androgyne.*

**hermaphroditism** (hĕr-măf′rō-dīt-ĭzm) A condition in which both ovarian and testicular tissue exist in the same individual, occurring rarely in humans. SYN: *hermaphrodism.* SEE: *intersex.*

***bilateral h.*** A condition in which an ovary and testicle are present on both sides.

***complex h.*** A form of hermophroditism in which the person has internal and external organs of both sexes.

***dimidiate h.*** Lateral h.

***false h.*** Pseudohermaphroditism.

***lateral h.*** A condition in which a testis is present on one side and an ovary on the other. SYN: *dimidiate h.*

***transverse h.*** Hermaphroditism characterized by having the outward organs of one sex and the internal organs of the other.

***true h.*** Hermaphroditism in which the individual possesses both ovarian and testicular glands.

***unilateral h.*** Hermaphroditism in which an ovary and a testis or an ovotestis are present on one side and either an ovary or a testis is present on the other side.

**hermetic** (hĕr-mĕt′ĭk) [L. *hermeticus*] Airtight.

**hernia** (hĕr′nē-ă) [L.] The protrusion or projection of an organ or a part of an organ through the wall of the cavity that normally contains it. SYN: *rupture* (2). SEE: *herniotomy.*

ETIOLOGY: Hernias may be caused by failure of certain normal openings to close during development; weakness resulting from debilitating illness, old age, or injury; prolonged distention as from tumors, pregnancy, or corpulence; and increased intra-abdominal pressure resulting from lifting heavy loads or coughing.

TREATMENT: Surgical or mechanical reduction is the treatment of choice. In very large hernias, mechanical devices or trusses may be used temporarily.

***abdominal h.*** A hernia through the abdominal wall.

***acquired h.*** A hernia that develops any time after birth in contrast to one that is present at birth (congenital hernia). This type of hernia is usually the result of excessive strain on the muscular wall, frequently occurring following injuries or operations.

***bladder h.*** The protrusion of the bladder or part of the bladder through a normal or abnormal orifice. SYN: *cystic h.*

***cerebral h.*** A hernia of the brain through the cranial wall.

***Cloquet's h.*** A type of femoral hernia. SEE: *femoral h.*

***complete h.*** A hernia in which the sac and its contents have passed through the aperture.

***concealed h.*** A hernia that is imperceptible when palpated.

***congenital h.*** A hernia existing from birth.

***crural h.*** A hernia that protrudes behind the femoral sheath.

***cystic h.*** Bladder h.

***diaphragmatic h.*** Herniation of abdominal contents into the thoracic cavity through an opening in the diaphragm. This may cause respiratory distress or strangulation and gangrene of the fundus of the stomach. The condition may be congenital, acquired (traumatic), or esophageal. In the latter, a portion of the stomach is pushed through the esophageal hiatus into the pleural cavity.

***direct h.*** Inguinal h.

***diverticular h.*** The protrusion of an intestinal congenital diverticulum.

***encysted h.*** A scrotal protrusion that, enveloped in its own sac, passes into the tunica vaginalis.

***epigastric h.*** A hernia of the intestine through an opening in the midline above the umbilicus.

***fascial h.*** Protrusion of muscular tissue through its fascial covering.

***fatty h.*** The protrusion of fatty tissue through the abdominal wall.

***femoral h.*** A descending of intestines through the femoral ring.

***hiatal h.*** The protrusion of the stomach upward into the mediastinal cavity through the esophageal hiatus of the diaphragm. SEE: illus.; *Nursing Diagnoses Appendix.*

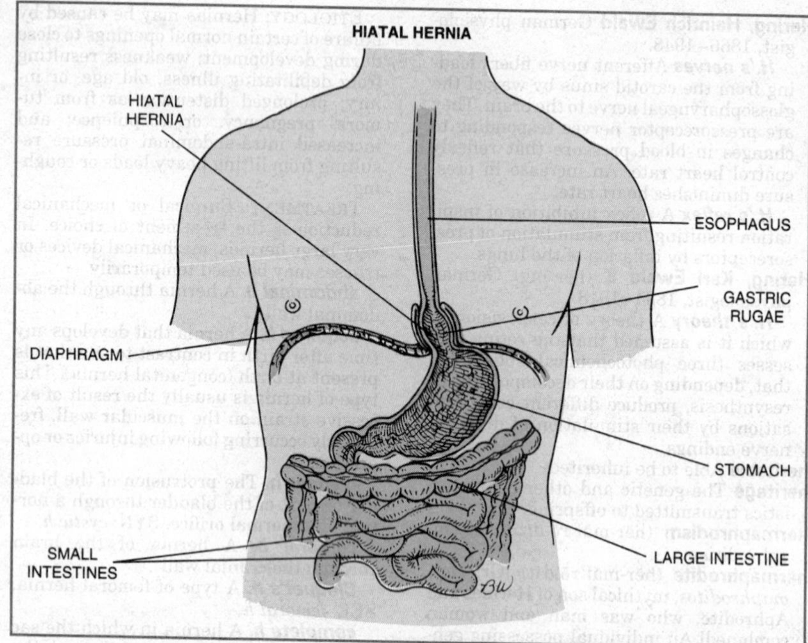


***incarcerated h.*** A hernia in which the bowel cannot be returned to the abdominal cavity, causing complete bowel obstruction.

***incisional h.*** A hernia through a surgical scar.

***incomplete h.*** A hernia that has not gone completely through the aperture.

***indirect h.*** Inguinal h.

***inguinal h.*** The protrusion of the hernial sac containing the intestine at the inguinal opening. In an indirect inguinal hernia, the sac protrudes through the internal inguinal ring into the inguinal canal, often descending into the scrotum. In a direct inguinal hernia, the hernial sac protrudes through the abdominal wall in the region of Hesselbach's triangle, a region bounded by the rectus abdominal muscle, inguinal ligament, and inferior epigastric vessels. Inguinal hernias account for about 80% of all hernias. SYN: *direct h.; indirect h.; lateral h.; medial h.; oblique h.*

NURSING IMPLICATIONS: *Preoperative:* The surgical procedure and expected sensations are explained to the patient; this discussion should be geared to the patient's age, level of comprehension, and type of hernia and planned repair. The nurse also explains that the surgery will relieve the discomfort from the hernia (once incisional pain is resolved). If the patient is undergoing elective surgery, recovery usually is rapid; if no complications occur, the patient probably will return home the same day as surgery and usually can resume normal activity within 4 to 6 weeks. If the patient is undergoing emergency surgery for a strangulated or incarcerated hernia, the patient may remain hospitalized for about a week and may have a nasogastric tube in place for a few days until G.I. function returns. Postoperative care treatments, procedures, and expected sensations are explained, and a signed informed consent form is obtained. The patient is prepared physically for surgery according to institutional protocol or surgeon's preference; this includes preparing the operative site, possibly administering a cleansing enema, restricting oral intake, and providing prescribed preoperative sedation.

*Postoperative:* Vital signs are monitored according to protocol until stable. Steps are taken to reduce pressure on the incision site: teaching the patient to get up from a lying or sitting position without straining the abdomen, instructing the patient to splint the incision when deep breathing, coughing, or sneezing, and reassuring the patient that coughing or sneezing will not cause the hernia to recur. Stool softeners are administered to prevent straining during defecation, and the patient is instructed in their use. Early ambulation is encouraged, but bending, lifting, pushing or pulling movements, driving a motor vehicle, or other strenuous activities should be avoided. The nurse ascertains that the patient voids within 12 hr after surgery. If swelling interferes with normal urination, an indwelling urinary catheter is inserted, or intermittent catheterization is performed as prescribed. Prescribed analgesics and noninvasive pain relief and comfort measures are provided; the latter include applying ice to the incision intermittently, or a scrotal bridge or truss before the patient ambulates. The dressing is checked regularly for drainage and the incisional site for local pain and inflammation, both of which may indicate infection, and the site is redressed according to protocol. The patient is assessed for other signs of infection, such as fever, chills, diaphoresis, malaise, lethargy, and pain and instructed to report any of these clinical signs to the surgeon, who may prescribe antibiotic therapy. The importance of keeping the incision site clean and dry and regular follow-up examinations to evaluate wound healing and the success of the repair is emphasized.

***inguinocrural h.*** A hernia that is both femoral and inguinal.

***internal h.*** A hernia that occurs within the abdominal cavity. It may be intraperitoneal or retroperitoneal.

***interstitial h.*** A form of inguinal hernia in which the hernial sac lies between the layers of the abdominal muscles.

***irreducible h.*** A hernia that cannot be returned to its original position out of its sac by manual methods. SEE: *incarcerated h.*

***labial h.*** The protrusion of a loop of bowel into the labium majus.

***lateral h.*** Inguinal h.

***lumbar h.*** A hernia in lumbar region or the loins.

***medial h.*** Inguinal h.

***mesocolic h.*** A hernia between the layers of the mesocolon.

***nuckian h.*** A hernia into the canal of Nuck.

***oblique h.*** Inguinal h.

***obturator h.*** A hernia through the obturator foramen.

***omental h.*** A hernia containing a portion of the omentum.

***ovarian h.*** The presence of an ovary in a hernial sac.

***perineal h.*** Perineocele.

***phrenic h.*** A hernia projecting through the diaphragm into one of the pleural cavities.

***posterior vaginal h.*** A hernia of Douglas' sac downward between the rectum and posterior vaginal wall. SYN: *enterocele* (2).

***properitoneal h.*** A hernia that protrudes through the peritoneum and into the abdominal wall.

***reducible h.*** A hernia that can be replaced by manipulation.

***retroperitoneal h.*** A hernia into the peritoneal sac extending behind the peritoneum into the iliac fossa.

***Richter's h.*** A hernia in which only a portion of intestinal wall protrudes, the main portion of the intestine being excluded from the hernial sac and the lumen remaining open.

***scrotal h.*** A hernia that descends into the scrotum.

***sliding h.*** A form of hernia that may develop and then return to normal as the viscus slides in and out of the sac of the hernia. This condition may occur with hiatal hernia or other types of abdominal hernias.

***strangulated h.*** A hernia so tightly constricted that gangrene results if surgery does not relieve it. It is not reducible by ordinary means.

***umbilical h.*** A hernia occurring at the navel, seen mostly in children. Usually it requires no therapy.

***uterine h.*** The presence of the uterus in the hernial sac.

***vaginal h.*** The hernial protrusion of the vaginal wall into the surrounding area, usually the pouch of Douglas.

***vaginolabial h.*** A hernia of a viscus into the posterior end of the labium majus.

***ventral h.*** A hernia through the abdominal wall. If stretching and thinning of an abdominal scar occur, pressure from the abdomen may cause protrusion of part of the gut. It is then protected only by a layer of thin scar tissue.

**hernial** (hĕr′nē-ăl) [L. *hernia,* rupture] Pert. to a hernia.

**herniated** Enclosed in or protruding like a hernia.

**herniation** (hĕr-nē-ā′shŭn) The development of a hernia.

***h. of nucleus pulposus*** Prolapse of the nucleus pulposus of a ruptured intervertebral disk into the spinal canal. This often results in pressure on a spinal nerve, which causes lower back pain that may radiate down the leg. SEE: illus.; *Nursing Diagnoses Appendix.*

NURSING IMPLICATIONS: A history is obtained of any unilateral low back pain that radiates to the buttocks, legs, and feet. When herniation follows trauma, the patient may report sudden pain, subsiding in a few days; then a dull, aching sciatic pain in the buttocks that increases with Valsalva's maneuver, coughing, sneezing, or bending. The patient may also complain of muscle spasms accompanied by pain that subsides with rest. The nurse inspects for a limited ability to bend forward, a posture favoring the affected side, and decreased deep tendon reflexes in the lower extremity. In later stages, muscle atrophy may be observed. Palpation may disclose tenderness over the region. Tissue tension assessment may reveal radicular pain from straight leg raising (with lumbar herniation) and increased pain from neck movement (with cervical herniation). Thorough assessment of the patient's peripheral vascular status, including posterior tibial and dorsalis pedis pulses and skin temperature of

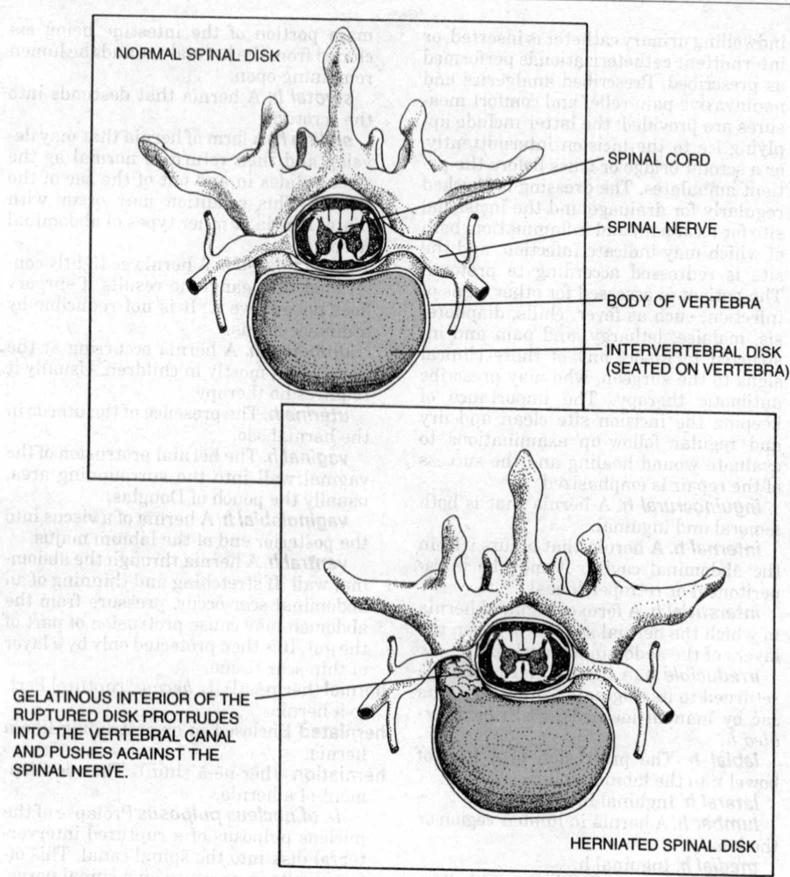


**NORMAL AND HERNIATED SPINAL DISKS**

the arms and legs, may help to rule out ischemic disease as the cause of leg numbness or pain.

The patient is prepared for diagnostic testing by explaining all procedures and expected sensations. Tests may include radiographic studies of the spine (to show degenerative changes and rule out other abnormalities), myelography (to pinpoint the level of herniation), computed tomography scanning (to detect bone and soft tissue abnormalities and possibly show spinal compression resulting from the herniation), magnetic resonance imaging (to define tissues in areas otherwise obscured by bone), electromyography (to confirm nerve involvement by measuring the electrical activity of muscles innervated by the affected nerves), and neuromuscular testing (to detect sensory and motor loss as well as leg muscle weakness). If the patient will undergo myelography, a history of allergies to iodides, iodine-containing substances, or seafood is obtained, because such allergies may indicate sensitivity to the radiopaque contrast agent used in the test. Prescribed sedation is administered before the test, fluid intake is encouraged before and after the test, intake and output are monitored, the patient is positioned with the head elevated, and the patient is observed for allergic reactions and seizure activity.

Pain status is monitored, prescribed analgesics are administered, the patient is taught about noninvasive pain relief measures (such as relaxation, transcutaneous nerve stimulation, distraction, heat or ice application, traction, bracing, or positioning), and patient's response to the treatment regimen is evaluated. During conservative treatment, neurological status is monitored (esp. in the first 24 hr after beginning treatment) for signs of deterioration, which may indicate a need for emergency surgery. Neurovascular assessments of the patient's affected and unaffected extremities (both legs or both arms) are performed to check color, motion, temperature, sensation, and pulses.

Vital signs are monitored, bowel sounds are auscultated, and the abdomen is inspected for distention. The disorder and the various treatment options are explained to the patient, including bedrest and pelvic (or cervical) traction, local heat application, an exercise program, antispasmodic and anti-inflammatory drug therapy, and surgery.

Both patient and family are encouraged to express their concerns about the disorder, questions are answered honestly, and support and encouragement are offered to assist the patient and family to cope with the frustration of impaired mobility and the discomfort of chronic back pain. The patient is encouraged to perform self-care to the extent that immobility and pain allow, to take analgesics before activities, and to allow adequate time to perform activities at a comfortable pace. Assistance is provided to help the patient to identify and perform care activities that promote rest and relaxation.

Antiembolism stockings are applied as prescribed, leg movement and exercises are encouraged as permitted, and a foot board or right-angle foam and Velcro foot support are provided as necessary to prevent footdrop. The nurse works closely with the physical therapist to ensure a consistent regimen of leg- and back-strengthening exercises. While the patient is restricted to bedrest (or in traction), the patient should increase fluid intake to prevent urinary stasis and breathe deeply, cough, and use incentive spirometry to avoid pulmonary complications. Skin care and a fracture bedpan are provided if the patient is not permitted bathroom or commode privileges.

As necessary, the patient is prepared physically and emotionally for surgery (such as laminectomy, spinal fusion, or microdiskectomy) according to institutional or surgeon's protocol, and a signed informed consent form is obtained. After microdiskectomy, bedrest is enforced for the prescribed period, the blood drainage system in use is managed, and the amount and color of drainage is documented. Any colorless moisture or excessive drainage should be reported; the former may indicate cerebrospinal fluid leakage. A log-rolling technique is used to turn the patient from side to side. Analgesics are administered as prescribed, especially 30 min before early attempts at sitting or walking. The nurse assists the patient with prescribed mobilization, provides a straight-backed chair, and explains any restrictions.

Before discharge, the nurse reviews proper body mechanics with the patient: bending at the knees and hips (never the waist), standing straight, and carrying objects close to the body. The patient is advised to lie down when tired and to sleep on the side (never on his abdomen) on an extra-firm mattress or a bed board. All prescribed medications are reviewed, including dosage schedules, desired actions, and adverse reactions to be reported. Referral for home health care or occupational therapy may be necessary to help the patient manage activities of daily living.

***tonsillar h.*** The protrusion of the cerebellar tonsils through the foramen magnum. It causes pressure on the medulla oblongata and may be fatal.

***transtentorial h.*** A herniation of the uncus and adjacent structures into the incisure of the tentorium of the brain. It is caused by increased pressure in the cranium. SYN: *uncal h.*

***uncal h.*** Transtentorial h.

**hernioenterotomy** (hĕr″nē-ō-ĕn″tĕr-ŏt′ō-mē) [″ + Gr. *enteron,* intestine, + *tome,* incision] Herniotomy and enterotomy done during the same surgical procedure.

**herniography** (hĕr″nē-ŏg′ră-fē) [″ + Gr. *graphein,* to write] The radiographical examination of a hernia after the introduction of a contrast medium.

**hernioid** (hĕr′nē-oyd) [″ + Gr. *eidos,* form, shape] Resembling a hernia.

**herniolaparotomy** (hĕr″nē-ō-lăp″ă-rŏt′ō-mē) [″ + Gr. *lapara,* loin, + *tome,* incision] Abdominal surgery for the treatment of hernia.

**hernioplasty** (hĕr′nē-ō-plăs″tē) [″ + Gr. *plassein,* to form] Surgical repair of a hernia.

**herniopuncture** (hĕr″nē-ō-pŭnk′chŭr) [″ + *punctura,* prick] The puncture of a hernia with a hollow needle to withdraw fluid or gas.

**herniorrhaphy** (hĕr-nē-or′ă-fē) [″ + Gr. *rhaphe,* seam, ridge] A surgical procedure for repair of a hernia.

**herniotomy** (hĕr-nē-ŏt′ō-mē) [″ + Gr. *tome,* incision] Surgery for the relief of hernia; an operation for the correction of irreducible hernia, esp. strangulated hernia.

**heroic measures** In medical practice, the undertaking of a procedure or therapy that is associated with an element of daring or boldness. Usually, such action is taken in an attempt to save a patient's life.

**heroin** (hĕr′ō-ĭn) A narcotic derived from morphine, whose importation, sale, and use are illegal in the U.S. SYN: *diacetylmorphine.* SEE: *drug addiction; endorphins.*

***h. toxicity*** Poisoning by heroin.

SYMPTOMS: Acute heroin poisoning causes euphoria, flushing, itching of the skin, miosis, drowsiness, decreased respiratory rate and depth, bradycardia, hypotension, and a decrease in body temperature. If the emergency condition is not treated without delay, cyanosis and death may result.

TREATMENT: To treat acute heroin toxicity, an airway must be established and maintained. Any false teeth should be removed and the mouth and pharynx cleaned of mucus or blood. Mouth-to-mouth or mouth-to-nose artificial respiration should be given if necessary. Any abnormality of cardiac function should be assessed and treated, using cardiac massage, defibrillator, or cardiac pacer as needed. Pulmonary edema should be treated with continuous positive-pressure respiration and oxygen therapy.

The opiate antagonist nalorphine hydrochloride should be given intravenously (use of the femoral or jugular vein may be necessary) according to package directions. A respiratory stimulant such as 3 to 5 ml of doxapram hydrochloride should also be given intravenously.

The caregiver should stay with the patient until he or she is fully responsive. A long-acting narcotic may continue its effect even after those of a short-acting antagonist have worn off. If the patient fails to respond to treatment, another cause for the coma should be sought. SEE: *Universal Precautions Appendix.*

**heroinism** (hĕr′ō-ĭn-ĭzm) [*heroin* + Gr. *-ismos,* condition] An addiction to heroin use. SEE: *drug addiction.*

**herpangina** (hĕrp-ăn-jī′nă, -ăn′jĭ-nă) [Gr. *herpes,* creeping skin disease, + L. *angina,* a choking] A benign infectious disease of children and, less commonly, of young adults. It occurs in epidemic form throughout the world, most often in summer and early fall. It is caused by one of several strains of group A coxsackievirus and rarely other enteroviruses.

SYMPTOMS: Sudden onset of fever, severe sore throat, nausea, vomiting, excess salivation, and malaise characterize the disease. The throat and posterior area of the mouth are covered with vesicles 1 to 2 mm in diameter that rupture and form ulcers.

TREATMENT: The treatment is symptomatic and supportive. There is no specific therapy, but recovery is prompt.

**herpes** (hĕr′pēz) [Gr. *herpes,* creeping skin disease] A word that was used to indicate vesicular eruption caused by a virus, esp. herpes simplex or herpes zoster, and the condition commonly called cold sore or fever blister. When used as a single word, "herpes" usually refers to herpes simplex. SEE: *Nursing Diagnoses Appendix.*

***h. corneae*** An inflammation of the cornea caused by herpesvirus.

***h. facialis*** A form of herpes simplex that occurs on the face.

***h. febrilis*** Herpes simplex of the lips and nasal mucosa.

***genital h.*** An infection of the genital and anorectal skin and mucosa with herpes simplex virus type 2. It is usually spread by sexual contact and is classed as a sexually transmitted disease. This viral infection may be transmitted to the fetus during delivery and may be fatal to the fetus. SEE: illus.

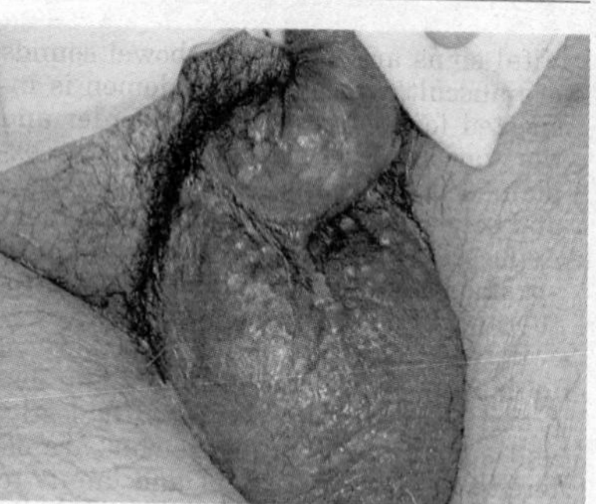

GENITAL HERPES
WIDESPREAD PRIMARY INFECTION

SYMPTOMS: Itching and soreness are usually present before a small patch of erythema develops. Then a vesicle appears, which erodes. Such vesicles are usually painful and heal in about 10 days. They may occur in any part of the genitalia.

TREATMENT: Topical acyclovir is beneficial in treating the initial infection. Oral acyclovir may reduce the frequency of subsequent lesions. Foscarnet is useful in treating acyclovir-resistant infections.

Caution: The lesions are highly contagious, and persons caring for the patient must avoid contact with the exudates. SEE: *Universal Precautions Appendix.*

***h. labialis*** A form of herpes simplex that occurs on the lips. SYN: *cold sore; fever blister.* SEE: illus.

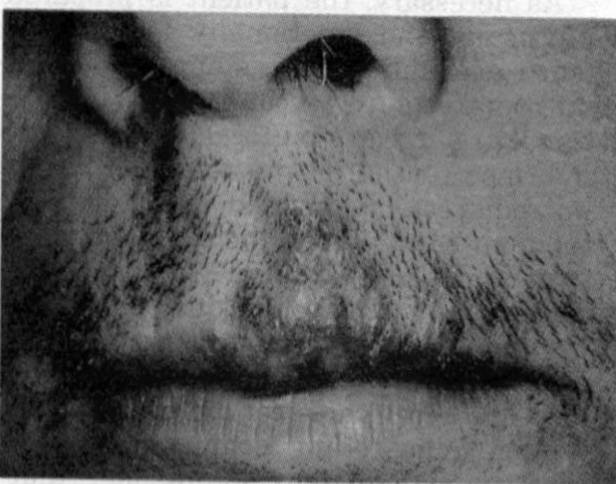

HERPES LABIALIS

***h. menstrualis*** Herpetic lesions appearing at the time of the menstrual period.

***ocular h.*** Herpes of the eye.

***h. simplex*** An infectious disease caused by herpes simplex virus type 1 or type 2. The disease is characterized by thin-walled vesicles that tend to recur in the same area, usually at a site where the mucous membrane joins the skin; however, they may be limited to the gingiva, oro-

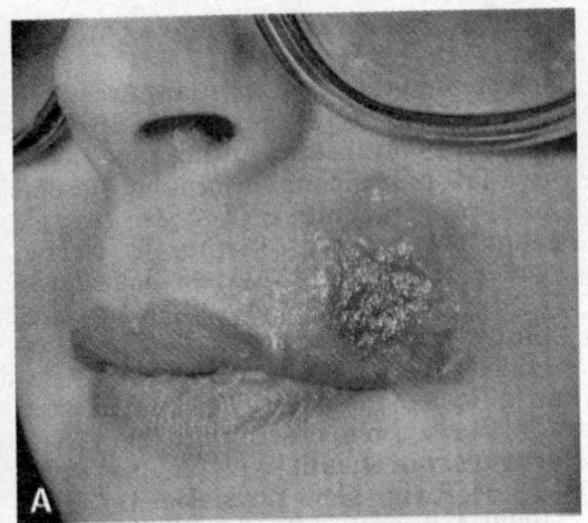

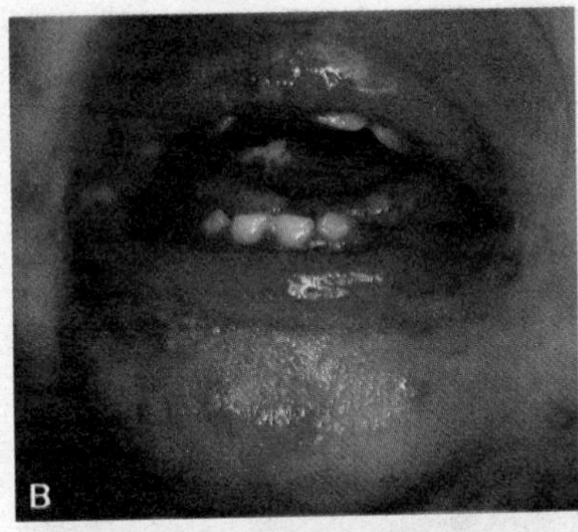

**HERPES SIMPLEX (A)** LOCALIZED AND **(B)** WIDESPREAD PRIMARY INFECTION

pharynx, or conjunctiva. In newborn infants, herpes simplex virus may cause meningoencephalitis or a panvisceral infection. In adults 5% to 7% of cases of aseptic meningitis are due to herpes simplex virus. SEE: illus.; *Nursing Diagnoses Appendix*.

TREATMENT: Acyclovir applied locally has been effective; oral acyclovir may prevent recurrences. Foscarnet is useful in treating acyclovir-resistant infections. Antibiotics may be helpful in treating secondary infections. Eye lesions should be treated by an ophthalmologist. Corticosteroids should never be used for ocular involvement.

***traumatic h.*** Herpes at a wound site.

***h. zoster*** An acute infectious viral disease. It is limited to humans and is marked by inflammation of the posterior root ganglia of only a few segments of the spinal or cranial peripheral nerves. A painful vesicular eruption occurs along the course of the nerve and is almost always unilateral. The trunk is the region most often affected, but the face may also be involved. The virus may cause meningitis, affect the optic nerve, or affect hearing. The herpes zoster virus is the chickenpox (varicella) virus that has remained dormant in nerves after recovery from chickenpox. It may be reactivated by the diminishing immune competency that comes with age or the physiological stress of disease. The incubation period is from 7 to 21 days. The total duration of the disease from onset to complete recovery varies from 10 days to 5 weeks. If all the vesicles appear within 24 hr, the total duration is usually short. In general, the disease lasts longer in adults than in children. It is estimated that about 50% of people who live to age 80 will have an attack of herpes zoster. This infection is more common in persons with a compromised immune system: the elderly, those with AIDS or illnesses such as Hodgkin's disease and diabetes, those taking corticosteroids or undergoing cancer chemotherapy.

The characteristic neuritis may develop into postherpetic neuralgia, esp. in patients older than 50 years of age. The pain may last for more than a month and may be stabbing; it is present along the affected nerves and it may intensify at night or when the individual is exposed to temperature changes. SYN: *shingles*. SEE: illus.; *h. zoster ophthalmicus; Nursing Diagnoses Appendix*.

TREATMENT: In most cases, the pain and itching can be treated symptomatically. The pain may be relieved by application of capsaicin cream (an extract of hot chili peppers). The antiviral drugs acyclovir or famciclovir are used. Each is most effective if administered within 3

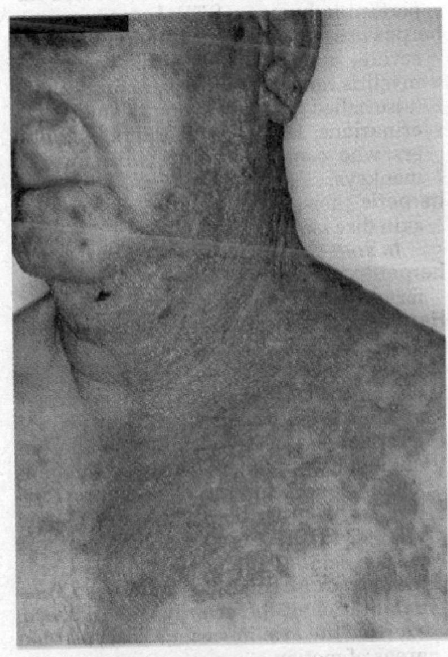

**HERPES ZOSTER (SHINGLES)**

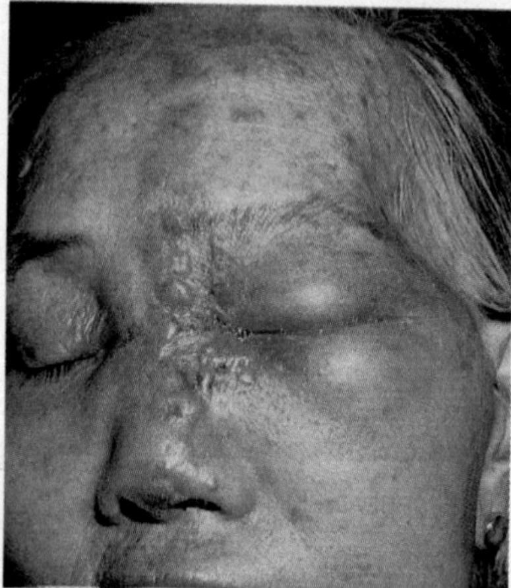

HERPES ZOSTER OPHTHALMICUS

days of onset. Antidepressants are also helpful.

***h. zoster ophthalmicus*** Herpes zoster affecting the first division of the fifth cranial nerve. The area of the face, eye, and nose supplied by this nerve is affected. Ocular complications can be quite serious. It is important that the eye be treated early with idoxuridine and that therapy be supervised by an ophthalmologist. Corticosteroids should never be used for ocular involvement. SEE: illus.

**herpesviruses** A family, *Herpesviridae,* of structurally similar viruses. Included in this family are a number of viruses important to humans. SEE: *herpes.*

**herpesvirus simian encephalomyelitis** A severe, almost always fatal, encephalomyelitis caused by the herpesvirus simiae (also called B virus). It occurs among veterinarians, laboratory workers, and others who come in contact with infected monkeys.

**herpetic** (hĕr-pĕt′ĭk) [Gr. *herpes,* creeping skin disease] Pert. to herpes.

***h. sore throat*** Herpetic tonsillitis.

**herpetiform** (hĕr-pĕt′ĭ-form) [″ + L. *forma,* form] Resembling herpes.

**Herplex Liquifilm** Trade name for idoxuridine.

**Herring bodies** [Percy T. Herring, Brit. physiologist, 1872–1967] Accumulation of neurosecretory material seen in the pars nervosa of the pituitary in the terminal nerve endings of the hypothalamus and hypophyseal tract. The neurosecretory material is thought to be a protein related to the hormones oxytocin and vasopressin.

**Herring track** An equipment item used in rehabilitation of the arm. It is designed to exercise the arm in various positions and areas of motion.

**hersage** (ār-săzh′) [Fr., a harrowing] The splitting of a nerve trunk into separate fibers.

**Herter's infantilism** [Christian Archibald Herter, U.S. physician, 1865–1910] A form of infantilism resulting from defective fat and calcium absorption. Resembles sprue in adults. SYN: *celiac disease.*

**Hertig-Rock embryos** [Arthur T. Hertig, U.S. pathologist, 1904–1990; John Rock, U.S. gynecologist, 1890–1984] Very beautifully preserved and dated embryos obtained experimentally in 1952.

**Hertig-Rock ovum** A fertilized human ovum 7 to 7½ days old, described in 1945.

**Hertwig's root sheath** [Wilhelm August Oscar Hertwig, Ger. physiologist, 1849–1922] A downgrowth of epithelium from the cervical loop of the enamel organ that induces dentin formation of the forming tooth root and determines its shape. The epithelial diaphragm, a horizontal extension of the Hertwig's root sheath, will determine the number and size of the tooth roots.

**hertz** [Heinrich R. Hertz, Ger. physicist, 1857–1894] ABBR: Hz. A unit of frequency equal to 1 cycle/sec.

**hesitancy** Involuntary delay in initiating urination. This symptom should not be ignored, because it may accompany serious disease of the urinary tract or prostate.

**hesperidin** (hĕs-pĕr′-ĭ-dĭn) A bioflavonoid present in orange and lemon peel.

**Hesselbach's hernia** (hĕs′ĕl-bŏks) [Franz K. Hesselbach, Ger. surgeon, 1759–1816] A lobated hernia that passes through the cribriform fascia.

**Hesselbach's triangle** SEE: under *triangle.*

**hetastarch** A synthetic polymer plasma volume expander composed of more than 90% amylopectin molecules. It has an average molecular weight of 450,000. Trade name is Hespan. SEE: *fluid replacement.*

**heter-** SEE: *hetero-.*

**heteradelphia** (hĕt″ĕr-ă-dĕl′fē-ă) [Gr. *heteros,* other, + *adelphos,* brother] Congenitally joined fetuses in which one twin is more nearly developed than the other.

**heteradenoma** (hĕt″ĕr-ăd-ĕ-nō′mă) *pl.* **heteradenomata** [″ + *aden,* gland, + *oma,* tumor] A glandular tumor arising from an area that does not usually contain glands.

**heterecious** (hĕt″ĕr-ē′shŭs) [″ + *oikos,* house] Denoting a parasite living on different hosts at different stages of development. SYN: *metoxenous.*

**heterecism** (hĕt″ĕr-ē′sĭzm) The state of being heterecious; the development of different cycles of existence on different hosts, said of certain parasites.

**heteresthesia** (hĕt″ĕr-ĕs-thē′zē-ă) [″ + *aisthesis,* sensation] The variation in degree (plus or minus) of sensory response to cutaneous stimuli.

**hetero-, heter-** [Gr. *heteros,* other] Prefix indicating *different; relationship to another.*

**heteroagglutination** (hĕt″ĕr-ō-ă-gloo″tĭ-nă′shŭn) The agglutination by one animal's serum of the red blood cells of an animal of another species.

**heteroagglutinin** (hět″ĕr-ō-ă-glū′tĭ-nĭn) **1.** Agglutinin formed as the result of an injection of an antigen from an animal of a different species. **2.** Agglutinin capable of agglutinating blood cells of other species of animals.

**heteroalbumose** (hět″ĕr-ō-ăl′bū-mōs) [″ + L. *albumen,* white of egg] Albumose insoluble in water but soluble in saline solutions or in acid or alkaline solutions. SYN: *hemialbumose.*

**heteroantibody** (hět″ĕr-ō-ăn″tĭ-bŏd′ē) An antibody corresponding to an antigen from another species.

**heteroantigen** (hět″ĕr-ō-ăn′tĭ-jĕn) An antigen in one species that produces a corresponding antibody in another species.

**heteroautoplasty** (hět″ĕr-ō-aw′tō-plăs-tē) [″ + *autos,* self, + *plassein,* to form] The grafting of skin from one person to that of another.

**heteroblastic** (hět″ĕr-ō-blăs′tĭk) [″ + *blastos,* germ] Originating in tissue of another kind; the opposite of homoblastic.

**heterocellular** (hět″ĕr-ō-sĕl′ū-lăr) Composed of different kinds of cells.

**heterocephalus** (hět″ĕr-ō-sĕf′ă-lŭs) [″ + *kephale,* head] Congenitally deformed fetus with two heads of unequal size.

**heterochiral** (hět″ĕr-ō-kī′răl) [″ + *cheir,* hand] Reversed as to right and left, but otherwise of the same form and size; said of images in a plane mirror and of the hands.

**heterochromatin** (hět″ĕr-ō-krō′mă-tĭn) [″ + *chroma,* color] Highly condensed or folded portions of chromosomes during interphase. They stain less distinctly than euchromatin. There is apparently no transcription of the DNA by messenger RNA (mRNA); these portions may be inactive genes. SEE: *euchromatin.*

**heterochromatosis** (hět″ĕr-ō-krō-mă-tō′sĭs) [″ + ″ + *osis,* condition] **1.** A pigmentation of the skin from foreign substances. **2.** Heterochromia.

**heterochromia** (hět″ĕr-ō-krō′mē-ă) A difference in color. SYN: *heterochromatosis* (2).

***h. iridis*** Different colors of the iris or sector of the iris in the two eyes. It may occur naturally or as a result of previous disease in the lighter-colored eye. Rarely it is associated with Waardenberg syndrome.

**heterochromosome** (hět″ĕr-ō-krō′mō-sōm) **1.** The X and Y or sex chromosomes. **2.** A chromosome containing material, heterochromatin, that stains differently from the remainder of the chromatin material.

**heterochromous** (hět″ĕr-ō-krō′mŭs) [″ + *chroma,* color] Having an abnormal difference in coloration.

**heterochronia** (hět″ĕr-ō-krō′nē-ă) [″ + *chronos,* time] Denoting an abnormal time for the occurrence of a phenomenon or production of a structure.

**heterochronic** (hět″ĕr-ō-krŏn′ĭk) Occurring at different or at abnormal times.

**heterochthonous** (hět″ĕr-ŏk′thō-nŭs) [Gr. *heteros,* other, + *chthon,* a particular land or country] Originating in a different place from where it was found.

**heterocinesia** (hět″ĕr-ō-sĭ-nē′zē-ă) [″ + *kinesis,* movement] Movements different from those the patient is instructed to make.

**heterocyclic** (hět″ĕr-ō-sīk′lĭk) [″ + *kyklos,* circle] Pert. to ring compounds that contain one or more elements other than carbon in the ring.

**heterodermic** (hět″ĕr-ō-dĕr′mĭk) [″ + *derma,* skin] Pert. to a method of skin grafting in which grafts are taken from another person.

**heterodont** (hět″ĕr-ō-dŏnt) [″ + *odous,* tooth] Having teeth of various shapes.

**heterodromus** (hět″ĕr-ŏd′rō-mŭs) [″ + *dromos,* running] Acting, arranged, or moving in the opposite direction.

**heterogametic** (hět″ĕr-ō-gă-mĕt′ĭk) [″ + *gamos,* marriage] Pert. to the production of unlike gametes, applied esp. to a male that produces two types of sperm, one containing the X chromosome, the other the Y chromosome. SEE: *homogametic.*

**heterogamy** (hět″ĕr-ŏg′ă-mē) The union of gametes that are dissimilar in size and structure. This union occurs in higher plants and animals. SEE: *isogamy.*

**heterogeneity** (hět″ĕr-ō-jĕ-nē′ĭ-tē) The quality of being heterogeneous.

**heterogeneous** (hět″ĕr-ō-jē′nē-ŭs) [″ + *genos,* type] Of unlike natures; composed of unlike substances; the opposite of homogeneous.

**heterogeneous vaccine** A vaccine made from some source other than the patient's own tissues or cells; the opposite of autogenous vaccine.

**heterogenesis** (hět″ĕ-rō-jĕn′ĕ-sĭs) [″ + *genesis,* generation, birth] The production of offspring that have different characteristics in alternate generations, as in the regular alternation of asexual with sexual reproduction. This characteristic is found in some fungi. SYN: *metagenesis.* SEE: *homogenesis.*

**heterogenetic** (hět″ĕ-rō-jĕ-nĕt′ĭk) Relative to heterogenesis.

**heterogeusia** (hět″ĕr-ō-gū′sē-ă) [″ + *geusis,* taste] The perception of an inappropriate quality of taste when food is present in the mouth or being chewed. The taste sensation is unexpected and unusual but not necessarily unpleasant.

**heterograft** (hĕt′ĕ-rō-grăft) [″ + L. *grapheim,* stylus] A graft taken from another individual or an animal of a different species from the one for whom it is intended. SEE: *autograft; graft; isograft.*

**heterography** (hět″ĕr-ŏg′ră-fē) [″ + *graphein,* to write] Writing different words from those the writer intended.

**heterohemagglutination** (hět″ĕr-ō-hĕm″ă-gloo″tĭ-nā′shŭn) The agglutination of red blood cells by hemagglutinins from another species.

**heterohemagglutinin** (hĕt″ĕr-ō-hĕm″ă-gloo′tĭ-nĭn) Hemagglutinin from one species that will agglutinate red blood cells from another species.

**heteroimmunity** (hĕt″ĕr-ō-ĭm-mū′nĭ-tē) Having immunity to an antigen from another species.

**heterokeratoplasty** (hĕt″ĕr-ō-kĕr′ă-tō-plăs″tē) [″ + *keras,* horn, + *plassein,* to form] Plastic surgery of the cornea using tissue from the cornea from another species.

**heterolalia** (hĕt″ĕr-ō-lā′lē-ă) [″ + *lalia,* babbling] Heterophasia.

**heteroliteral** (hĕt″ĕr-ō-lĭt′ĕr-ăl) In speaking, pert. to an incorrect letter being substituted for the correct one.

**heterologous** (hĕt″ĕr-ŏl′ō-gŭs) [″ + *logos,* word, reason] **1.** Made up of cell tissue not normal to the part. **2.** Obtained from a different individual or species, with respect to tissue, cells, or blood. SEE: *autologous; homologous.*

**heterolysin** (hĕt″ĕr-ŏl′ĭ-sĭn) [″ + *lysis,* solution] A lysin formed from an antigen from an animal of a different species. SEE: *autolysis; hemolysis.*

**heteromeric** (hĕt″ĕr-ō-mĕr′ĭk) [″ + *meros,* a part] **1.** Pert. to spinal neurons with processes extending to the opposite side of the spinal cord. **2.** Possessing a different chemical composition.

**heterometaplasia** (hĕt″ĕr-ō-mĕt″ă-plā′zē-ă) [″ + *meta,* beyond, + *plassein,* to form] The transformation of tissue into a type foreign to the part where it was produced.

**heterometropia** (hĕt″ĕr-ō-mē-trō′pē-ă) The ability of one eye to refract differently than the other, which produces perceived images of different sizes. The condition is probably prevalent in many individuals who are completely unaware of it.

**heteromorphosis** (hĕt″ĕr-ō-mor-fō′sĭs) [″ + *morphe,* form, + *osis,* condition] The regeneration of an organ different from the one that it replaced.

**heteromorphous** (hĕt″ĕr-ō-mor′fŭs) [″ + *morphe,* form] Deviating from the normal type.

**heteronomous** (hĕt″ĕr-ŏn′ō-mŭs) [″ + *nomos,* law] Abnormal; differing from type.

**heterophasia** (hĕt″ĕr-ō-fā′zē-ă) [″ + *phasis,* speech] Expression of meaningless words instead of those intended. SYN: *heterolalia; heterophemia.*

**heterophemia, heterophemy** (hĕt″ĕr-ō-fē′mē-ă, hĕt-ĕr-ŏf′ĕ-mē) [″ + *pheme,* speech] Heterophasia.

**heterophil(e)** (hĕt′ĕr-ō-fĭl, -fīl) [″ + *philein,* to love] **1.** In humans, the neutrophil leukocyte. **2.** Pert. to an antibody reacting with other than the specific antigen. **3.** Pert. to a tissue or microorganism that takes a stain other than the ordinary one.

**heterophilic** (hĕt″ĕr-ō-fĭl′ĭk) [Gr. *heteros,* other, + *philein,* to love] **1.** Having an affinity for something abnormal. **2.** Having an antibody response to an antigen other than the specific one.

**heterophonia** (hĕt″ĕr-ō-fō′nē-ă) [″ + *phone,* voice] A change of voice, esp. that which occurs at puberty.

**heterophoria** (hĕt″ĕ-rō-for′ē-ă) [″ + *phoros,* bearing] A tendency of the eyes to deviate from their normal position for visual alignment, esp. when one eye is covered; latent deviation or squint. This tendency is caused by an imbalance or weakness of the ocular muscles. SEE: *-phoria.*

**Heterophyes** (hĕt″ĕr-ŏf′ĭ-ēz) [″ + *phye,* stature] A genus of flukes belonging to the family Heterophyidae.

***H. heterophyes*** A species of intestinal fluke commonly infesting humans. In heavy infestations, it may cause diarrhea, nausea, and abdominal discomfort.

**heterophyiasis** (hĕt″ĕr-ō-fī-ī′ă-sĭs) [″ + ″ + *-iasis,* diseased condition] Infestation by any fluke belonging to the family Heterophyidae.

**Heterophyidae** A family of Trematoda (flukes) that infests the intestines of dogs, cats, and other mammals including humans. It includes the genera *Heterophyes, Haplorchis, Diorchitrema,* and *Metagonimus.* Infestations are common in Egypt and in the Far East. Intermediate hosts are snails; the cercaria encysting in fish, esp. mullets or frogs.

**heteroplasia** (hĕt″ĕr-ō-plā′zē-ă) [″ + *plassein,* to mold] The development of tissue at a location where that type of tissue would not normally occur. SYN: *alloplasia.*

**heteroplastic** (hĕt″ĕr-ō-plăs′tĭk) Relating to heteroplasia.

**heteroploid** (hĕt′ĕr-ō-ployd) [″ + *ploos,* fold] Possessing a chromosome number that is not a multiple of the haploid number common for the species.

**heteroprosopus** (hĕt″ĕr-ō-prō′sō-pŭs) [″ + *prosopon,* face] A congenitally deformed fetus having one head and two faces.

**heteropsia** (hĕt″ĕr-ŏp′sē-ă) [″ + *opsis,* vision] An inequality of vision in the two eyes.

**heteroptics** (hĕt″ĕr-ŏp′tĭks) A perversion of vision, such as seeing objects that do not exist or misinterpreting what is seen.

**heteropyknosis** (hĕt″ĕr-ō-pĭk-nō′sĭs) [″ + *pyknos,* dense, + *osis,* condition] The property whereby various parts of a chromosome stain with varying degrees of intensity. This is thought to be due to variations in the concentration of nucleic acid.

**heteroserotherapy** (hĕt″ĕr-ō-sē″rō-thĕr′ă-pē) [″ + L. *serum,* whey, + Gr. *therapeia,* treatment] Treatment by serum from another person.

**heterosexual** (hĕt″ĕr-ō-sĕk′shū-ăl) [″ + L. *sexus,* sex] **1.** Pert. to the opposite sex. **2.** A person whose sexual orientation is toward those of the opposite sex.

**heterosexuality** (hĕt″ĕr-ō-sĕk″shū-ăl′ĭ-tē) Sexual attraction for one of the opposite sex.

**heterosis** (hĕt-ĕr-ō′sĭs) [Gr., alteration] Greater strength, size, vigor, and growth rate seen in the first hybrid generation.

**heterosmia** (hĕt″ĕr-ŏs′mē-ă) [Gr. *heteros,* other, + *osme,* odor] The consistent perception of an inappropriate smell when an odorant is inhaled. The smell perceived is unusual and unexpected but not unpleasant. SYN: *allotriosmia.*

**heterotaxia** (hĕt″ĕr-ō-tăk′sē-ă) [″ + *taxis,* arrangement] An abnormal position of organs or parts. SEE: *dextrocardia; situs inversus viscerum.*

**heterotherm** (hĕt″ĕr-ō-thĕrm″) An animal whose temperature varies considerably in different situations. SEE: *heterothermy.*

**heterothermy** (hĕt′ĕr-ō-thĕr″mē) [″ + *therme,* heat] Condition in which an animal's temperature varies considerably in different situations, but is not poikilothermic.

**heterotopia** (hĕt″ĕr-ō-tō′pē-ă) [″ + *topos,* place] **1.** The development of a normal tissue in an abnormal location. **2.** The displacement of an organ or body part from its normal location.

**heterotopic** (hĕt″ĕr-ō-tŏp′ĭk) Misplaced; pert. to heterotopia.

**heterotopy** (hĕt″ĕr-ŏt′ō-pē) [″ + *topos,* place] Heterotopia (2).

**heterotoxin** (hĕt″ĕr-ō-tŏk′sĭn) [″+ *toxikon,* poison] A toxin introduced from outside the patient's body.

**heterotransplant** (hēt″ĕr-ō-trăns′plănt) [″ + L. *trans,* across, + *plantare,* to plant] An organ, tissue, or structure taken from an animal and grafted into, or on, another animal of a different species. Such transplants usually atrophy.

**heterotrichosis** (hĕt″ĕr-ō-trĭ-kō′sĭs) [″ + *trichosis,* growth of hair] The growth of different kinds or color of hairs on the scalp or body.

**heterotroph** (hĕt′ĕr-ō-trōf) [″ + *trophe,* food] An organism such as a human, requiring complex organic food in order to grow and develop; in contrast to plants, which can synthesize food from inorganic materials.

**heterotropia** (hĕt″ĕr-ō-trō′pē-ă) [″ + *tropos,* a turning] A manifest deviation of the eyes resulting from the absence of binocular equilibrium. SEE: *strabismus.*

**heterotypic** (hĕt″ĕr-ō-tĭp′ĭk) Concerning something of a different type than that which is being discussed or examined, esp. a tissue.

**heterovaccine** (hĕt″ĕr-ō-văk′sēn) [″ + L. *vaccinus,* pert. to a cow] A vaccine from a microbial source other than that causing the disease for which it is intended.

**heteroxenous** (hĕt″ĕr-ŏk′sē-nŭs) [″ + *xenos,* stranger] The property of a parasite that requires two different hosts in order to complete its life cycle.

**heterozygosis** (hĕt″ĕr-ō-zī-gō′sĭs) [″ + *zygone,* yoke, pair, + *osis,* condition] The state of having different alleles at a specific locus. SEE: *homozygosis.*

**heterozygote** (hĕt″ĕr-ō-zī′gōt) An individual with different alleles for a given characteristic. SEE: *allele.*

**heterozygous** (hĕt″ĕr-ō-zī′gŭs) Possessing different alleles at a given locus. SEE: *homozygous.*

**Heubner, Johann Otto L** (hoyb′nĕr) German pediatrician, 1843–1926.

***H.'s disease*** Syphilitic endarteritis of the brain.

***H.-Herter disease*** Nontropical sprue in infants.

**heuristic** (hū-rĭs′tĭk) [Gr. *heuriskein,* to find out, discover] Helping to discover or experiment, esp. the encouragement of students to learn through their own investigation.

**H.E.W.** U.S. Department of *H*ealth, *E*ducation, and *W*elfare. This agency is now the U.S. Department of Health and Human Services.

**hex-, hexa-** [Gr. *hex,* six] Prefix indicating *six.*

**hexabasic** [Gr. *hex,* six, + *basis,* base] An acid that contains six hydrogen (H) atoms that can be replaced by six hydroxyl (OH) radicals.

**hexachlorophene** (hĕks″ă-klō′rō-fēn) A bactericidal and bacteriostatic compound, used in emulsions and soaps for preoperative cleansing of the skin and for scrubbing the nurse's and surgeon's hands before surgery.

**hexachromic** [″ + *chroma,* color] Able to distinguish only six of the seven colors of the spectrum, or unable to distinguish violet from indigo.

**hexad** (hĕk′săd) **1.** Six similar things. **2.** An element with a valence of six.

**hexadactylism** (hĕks″ă-dăk′tĭl-ĭzm) [″ + *daktylos,* finger, + *-ismos,* condition] The presence of six fingers or six toes on one hand or foot.

**hexadecimal** (hĕks″ă-dĕs′ĭ-mŭl) [″ + L. *decimus,* tenth] In computers, a number system using base 16 rather than base 2 (binary) or 10 (decimal).

**hexafluorenium bromide** (hĕk″să-flūr-ĕn′ē-ŭm) A neuromuscular blocking agent.

**hexamethonium** (hĕks″ă-mĕ-thō′nē-ŭm) A compound that acts as a ganglionic blocking agent, used to treat hypertension.

**hexaploidy** (hĕk′să-ploy″dē) [″ + *ploos,* fold] A condition of having six sets of chromosomes.

**Hexapoda** (hĕks-ăp′ō-dă) [″ + *pous,* foot] Insecta.

**hexatomic** (hĕks″ă-tŏm′ĭk) [″ + *atomos,* indivisible] Pert. to a compound consisting of six atoms or one with six replaceable hydrogen or univalent atoms.

**hexavaccine** (hĕks″ă-văk′sēn) [″ + L. *vaccinus,* pert. to a cow] A vaccine made from six different microorganisms.

**hexavalent** (hĕks″ă-vā′lĕnt) [″ + L. *valere,* to have power] Having a chemical valence of six. SYN: *sexivalent.*

**hexavitamin** A standardized vitamin preparation containing vitamins A, D, C, and B, riboflavin, and niacinamide.

**hexokinase** (hĕks″ō-kī′nās) [″ + *kinein,* to move, + *-ase,* enzyme] An enzyme in cells that in the presence of ATP catalyzes the conversion of glucose to glucose-6-phosphate, the first step in glycolysis.

**hexosamine** (hĕk′sōs-ăm″ĭn) A sugar containing an amino group in place of a hydroxyl group (e.g., glucosamine).

**hexose** (hĕk′sōs) Any monosaccharide of the general formula $C_6H_{12}O_6$; the group includes glucose, fructose, and galactose.

**hexosephosphate** (hĕks″ōs-fŏs′fāt) [Gr. *hex,* six, + *phosphoros,* phosphorus] A phosphoric acid ester of glucose; one of several esters formed in the muscles and other tissues in the metabolism of carbohydrates.

**hexylresorcinol** (hĕks″ĭl-rĕ-sor′sĭ-nŏl) $C_{12}H_{18}O_2$. White needle-shaped crystals used as an anthelmintic.

**Hey's ligament** (hāz) [William Hey, Brit. surgeon, 1736–1819] The semilunar lateral margin (falciform margin) of the fossa ovalis, which lies between the iliac and pubic portions of the fascia lata.

**HF 1.** *Hageman factor;* blood coagulation factor XII. **2.** *high frequency.*

**Hf** Symbol for the element hafnium.

**HFJV** *high-frequency jet ventilation.*

**Hg** [L. *hydrargyrum*] Symbol for the element mercury.

**Hgb** *hemoglobin.*

**$HgCl_2$** Symbol for mercuric chloride; corrosive sublimate.

**$Hg_2Cl_2$** Symbol for mercurous chloride; calomel.

**HGE** *human granulocytic ehrlichiosis.*

**HGF 1.** *human growth factor.* **2.** *hyperglycemic-glycogenolytic factor* (glucagon).

**$HgI_2$** Symbol for mercuric iodide.

**HgO** Symbol for mercuric oxide.

**HgS** Symbol for mercuric sulfide.

**$HgSO_4$** Symbol for mercuric sulfate.

**HHb** *reduced hemoglobin (deoxyhemoglobin).*

**HHS** *U.S. Department of Health and Human Services.*

**5-HIAA** *5-hydroxyindoleacetic acid.*

**hiatal hernia** SEE: under *hernia.*

**hiatus** (hī-ā′tŭs) [L., an opening] **1.** An opening, a foramen. **2.** An aperture.

***h. aorticus*** An opening in the diaphragm through which pass the aorta and the thoracic duct.

***h. canalis facialis*** A hiatus of the canal for the greater petrosal nerve. SYN: *h. fallopii.*

***h. esophageus*** The opening in the diaphragm through which the esophagus passes.

***h. fallopii*** H. canalis facialis.

***h. maxillaris*** The opening of the maxillary sinus into the nasal cavity, located on the nasal surface of the maxillary bone.

***sacral h.*** The opening on the inferior-posterior surface of the sacrum into the sacral canal.

***h. semilunaris*** The groove in the external wall of the middle meatus of the nasal fossa into which the frontal sinus, maxillary sinus, and anterior ethmoid cells drain.

**hibernation** (hī″bĕr-nā′shŭn) [L. *hiberna,* winter] The condition of spending the winter asleep and in an almost comatose state. Some animals adapt to winter by this method.

***artificial h.*** A state of hibernation produced therapeutically by use of drugs alone or drugs and hypothermia. This greatly reduces the metabolic rate during procedures such as open heart surgery.

**hibernoma** (hī″bĕr-nō′mă) A rare multilobular encapsulated tumor that contains fetal fat tissue closely resembling the fat stored in the foot pads of hibernating animals.

**Hibiclens** Trade name for chlorhexidine gluconate.

**hiccup, hiccough** (hĭk′ŭp) [probably of imitative origin] A spasmodic periodic closure of the glottis following spasmodic lowering of the diaphragm, causing a short, sharp, inspiratory cough. SYN: *singultus.*

ETIOLOGY: It may be caused by indigestion, irritation of the diaphragm, alcoholism, new growths of the pleura, certain cerebral lesions, hysteria, or a disturbance of the phrenic nerve. If prolonged, it has serious significance.

TREATMENT: Hiccups may be treated by antiemetic drugs, rebreathing in a paper bag, briefly applying ice cubes to both sides of the neck at the level of the larynx, or inhalation of carbon dioxide. Stimulation of the nasopharynx with a soft rubber tube or placement of a thin coating of dry granulated sugar in the hypopharynx may also be tried. If these are not effective, anesthetization of the phrenic nerve may be helpful.

**Hickman catheter** A tunneled central venous catheter commonly used to administer solutions by central intravenous therapy for a prolonged period. Applications include total parenteral nutrition, antibiotic therapy, or blood transfusion.

**Hicks sign** Braxton Hicks sign.

**hidebound disease** [AS. *hyd,* a skin, + *bindan,* to tie up] Scleroderma.

**hidradenitis** (hī-drăd-ĕ-nī′tĭs) [Gr. *hidros,* sweat, + *aden,* gland, + *itis,* inflammation] An inflammation of the sweat glands.

**hidradenoma** (hī″drăd-ĕ-nō′mă) [″ + ″ + *oma,* tumor] Adenoma of the sweat glands.

**hidrocystoma** (hī″drō-sĭs-tō′mă) [″ + *kystis,* cyst, + *oma,* tumor] Hydrocystoma.

**hidropoiesis** (hī″drō-poy-ē′sĭs) [″ + *poiesis,* formation] The formation of sweat. **hidropoietic** (-poy-ĕt′ĭk), *adj.*

**hidrosadenitis** (hī″drōs-ăd″ĕ-nī′tĭs) [″ + *aden,* gland, + *itis,* inflammation] Hidradenitis.

**hidrosis** (hī-drō′sĭs) [″ + *osis,* condition] **1.** The formation and secretion of sweat. **2.** Excessive sweating.

**hidrotic** (hī-drŏt′ĭk) **1.** Causing the secretion of sweat. SYN: *diaphoretic; sudorific.* **2.** Any drug or medicine that induces sweating.

**hierarchy** (hī'răr-kē) The ordering or classification of anything in ascending or descending order of importance, or value in the case of numerical data. For example, the needs of a human being may be listed in order of importance, as air, water, food, health, protection from the elements and predators, security, esteem, and love.

**hierolisthesis** (hī"ĕr-ō-lĭs-thē'sĭs) [" + *olisthanein,* to slip] Displacement of the sacrum.

**hierophobia** (hī"ĕr-ō-fō'bē-ă) [Gr. *hieros,* sacred, + *phobos,* fear] An abnormal fear of sacred things or persons connected with religion.

**high-frequency jet ventilation** SEE: under *ventilation.*

**Highmore, antrum of** (hī'mor) [Nathaniel Highmore, Brit. surgeon, 1613–1685] The maxillary sinus. SEE: *antrocele.*

**Highmore's body** Mediastinum testis.

**hila** (hī'lă) [L.] Pl. of hilum.

**hilar** (hī'lăr) Concerning or belonging to the hilus.

**hilitis** (hī'lī'tĭs) [L. *hilus,* a trifle, + Gr. *itis,* inflammation] An inflammation of any hilum, esp. the hilum of the lung.

**hillock** (hĭl'ŏk) [ME. *hilloc*] A small eminence or projection.

***anal h.*** One of two small eminences that lie lateral and posterior to the cloacal membrane and, later, the anal fissure in the embryo.

***axon h.*** A small conical elevation on the cell body of a neuron from which the axon arises.

***seminal h.*** The colliculus seminalis.

**Hill sign** [Sir Leonard Erskine Hill, Brit. physiologist, 1866–1952] A sign used to determine aortic regurgitation. When the blood pressure in the leg is 20 to 40 mm Hg higher than in the arm, this sign is considered positive and indicative of aortic regurgitation.

**Hilton's law** [John Hilton, Brit. surgeon, 1804–1878] A law stating that the trunk of a nerve sends branches not only to a particular muscle but also to the joint moved by that muscle and to the skin overlying the insertion of the muscle.

**Hilton's line** A white line at the junction of the skin of the perineum and anal mucosa.

**Hilton's muscle** The aryepiglottic muscle.

**Hilton's sac** Laryngeal saccule.

**hilum** (hī'lŭm) *pl.* **hila** [L., a trifle] **1.** A depression or recess at the exit or entrance of a duct into a gland or of nerves and vessels into an organ. **2.** The root of the lungs at the level of the fourth and fifth dorsal vertebrae.

**hilus** (hī'lŭs) *pl.* **hili** [L.] Hilum.

**himantosis** (hī"măn-tō'sĭs) [Gr. *himantosis,* a long strap] An abnormal lengthening of the uvula.

**hindbrain** (hīnd'brān) [AS. *hindan,* behind, + *bragen,* brain] The most caudal of the three divisions of the embryonic brain. It differentiates into the metencephalon, which gives rise to the cerebellum and pons; and the myelencephalon, which develops into the medulla oblongata. SYN: *rhombencephalon.*

**hindfoot** (hīnd'foot) The posterior part of the foot consisting of the talus and calcaneus.

**hindgut** (hīnd'gŭt) The caudal portion of the entodermal tube, which develops into the alimentary canal. It gives rise to the ileum, colon, and rectum.

**hind-kidney** (hīnd-kĭd'nē) Metanephros.

**hinge joint** SEE: under *joint.*

**hip** [AS. *hype*] The region lateral to the ilium of the pelvic bone.

***congenital dislocation of the h.*** A congenital defect of the hip joint, probably caused by multifactorial effects of several abnormal genes.

***dislocation of the h.*** Physical displacement of the head of the femur from its normal location in the acetabulum. It is very often accompanied by a fracture, and it is extremely difficult even for a well-trained surgeon to distinguish a pure dislocation from a fracture dislocation without roentgenography.

SYMPTOMS: Pain, rigidity, and loss of function characterize this condition. The dislocation may be obvious by the abnormal position in which the leg is held or by seeing or feeling the head of the femur in an abnormal position.

DIAGNOSIS: The person has great difficulty in straightening the hip and leg after an accident. The knee on the injured side resistantly points inward toward the other knee. The dislocation is always accompanied by pain.

FIRST AID: The patient should be placed on a large frame or support, such as that used for a fractured back. In addition, a large pad such as a pillow should be placed under the knee of the affected side. The patient should be treated for shock if required.

***dislocation of the h. backward*** A dislocation of the hip onto the dorsum ilii or sciatic notch.

SYMPTOMS: The condition is characterized by an inward rotation of the thigh, with flexion, inversion, adduction, and shortening; pain and tenderness; and a loss of function and immobility.

TREATMENT: The patient should first be anesthetized and then laid in the dorsal position with the leg flexed on the thigh, and the latter upon the abdomen. The thigh is adducted and rotated outward. Circumduction is performed outwardly across the abdomen, and back to the straight position. Traction may be required.

***dislocation of the h. downward*** A rare type of hip dislocation that is treated with traction in the flexed position, followed by outward rotation and extension.

***dislocation of the h. forward*** A dislocation of the hip through the obturator foramen, on the pubis, in the perineum, or through a fractured acetabulum.

SYMPTOMS: Pain, tenderness, and immobility accompany this condition. Shortening is present in the pubic and suprapubic forms; lengthening in the obturator and perineal forms.

TREATMENT: Hyperextension and direct traction are used to treat this condition, followed by flexion, abduction with inward rotations, and adduction.

***fracture of the h.*** A very common occurrence in older persons, it is actually a fracture of the neck of the femur. It is estimated to occur in one of every three white women older than 85. Osteoporosis principally predisposes an elderly person to hip fracture.

***snapping h.*** A slipping around of the hip joint, sometimes producing an audible snapping sound.

***total replacement of h.*** SEE: *total hip replacement.*

**hip joint** SEE: under *joint.*

**hip-joint disease** Any disease of the hip joint, esp. tuberculosis.

**Hippel's disease; von Hippel-Lindau disease** (hĭp′ĕlz, vŏn hĭp′ĕl-lĭn′dow) [Eugen von Hippel, Ger. ophthalmologist, 1867–1939; Arvid Lindau, Swedish pathologist, 1892–1958] Angiomatosis of the retina and various areas of the body including the central nervous system, spinal cord, and visceral organs.

**hippocampal** (hĭp″ō-kăm′păl) [Gr. *hippokampos,* seahorse] Pert. to the hippocampus.

***h. formation*** Olfactory structures lying along the medial margin of the pallium. It includes the hippocampus, dentate gyrus, supracallosal gyrus, longitudinal striae, subcallosal gyrus, diagonal band of Broca, and hippocampal commissure.

**hippocampus** An elevation of the floor of the inferior horn of the lateral ventricle of the brain, occupying nearly all of it.

***digitations of h.*** Three or four shallow grooves on the anterior portion of the hippocampus.

***h. minor*** Calcar avis.

**Hippocrates** (hĭ-pŏk′ră-tēz) [ca. 460–375 B.C.] A Greek physician referred to as the Father of Medicine because he was the first healer to attempt to record medical experiences for future reference. By so doing he established the foundation for the scientific basis of medical practice. SEE: *Hippocratic oath.*

**hippocratic facies** The appearance of the face at the time of impending death, charactized by dark brown, livid, or lead-colored skin; hollow appearance of the eyes; collapse of the temples and sharpness of the nose.

**Hippocratic oath** The oath exacted of his students by Hippocrates: "I swear by Apollo the physician, and Aesculapius, and Hygeia, and Panacea, and all the gods and goddesses, that according to my ability and judgment, I will keep this oath and its stipulation—to reckon him who taught me this art equally dear to me as my parents, to share my substance with him, and to relieve his necessities if required; to look upon his offspring in the same footing as my own brothers, and to teach them this art if they shall wish to learn it, without fee or stipulation, and that by precept, lecture, and every other mode of instruction, I will impart a knowledge of the art to my own sons, and those of my teachers, and to disciples bound by a stipulation and oath according to the law of medicine, but to none other.

"I will follow that system of regimen which, according to my ability and judgment, I consider for the benefit of my patients, and abstain from whatever is deleterious and mischievous. I will give no deadly medicine to anyone if asked, nor suggest any such counsel; and in like manner I will not give to a woman a pessary to produce abortion. With purity and with holiness I will pass my life and practice my art. I will not cut persons laboring under the stone, but will leave this to be done by men who are practitioners of this work. Into whatever houses I enter, I will go into them for the benefit of the sick, and I will abstain from every voluntary act of mischief and corruption; and, further, from the seduction of females or males, of freemen and slaves. Whatever, in connection with my professional practice, or not in connection with it, I see or hear, in the life of men, which ought not to be spoken of abroad, I will not divulge, as reckoning that all such should be kept secret.

"While I continue to keep this Oath unviolated, may it be granted to me to enjoy life and the practice of this art, respected by all men, in all times. But should I trespass and violate this Oath, may the reverse be my lot." SEE: *Declaration of Geneva; Declaration of Hawaii; Nightingale Pledge; Prayer of Maimonides.*

**hippurase** (hĭp′ū-rās) Hippuricase.

**hippuria** (hĭ-pū′rē-ă) [Gr. *hippos,* horse, + *ouron,* urine] Large quantities of hippuric acid in the urine.

**hippuric acid** An acid formed and excreted by the kidneys. It is formed in the human body from the combination of benzoic acid and glycine, the synthesis taking place in the liver and to a limited extent in the kidney.

**hippuricase** (hĭ-pūr′ĭ-kās) An enzyme found in the liver, kidney, and other tissues that catalyzes the synthesis of hippuric acid from benzoic acid and glycine. SYN: *hippurase.*

**hippus** (hĭp′ŭs) [Gr. *hippos,* horse] The rhythmical and rapid dilatation and contraction of the pupils and spasmodic tremor of the iris seen in an aphakic eye or one with a subluxated lens. SYN: *iridodonesis.*

***respiratory h.*** A dilatation of the pupil during inspiration, and contraction on expiration.

**hircismus** (hĭr-sĭs′mŭs) A malodorous condition of the axillae caused by bacterial action on the sweat.

**hircus** (hĭr′kŭs) *pl.* **hirci** [L., goat] An axillary hair.

**Hirschberg's reflex** (hĭrsh′bĕrgz) [Leonard Keene Hirschberg, U.S. neurologist, b. 1877] Adduction of the foot when the sole at the base of the great toe is irritated.

**Hirschsprung's disease** (hĭrsh′sprŭngz) [Harald Hirschsprung, Dan. physician, 1830–1916] An extremely dilated colon, which is usually congenital but may occur in infancy or childhood. It is caused by a failure of development of the myenteric plexus of the rectosigmoid area of the large intestine. The colon above the inactive area of the sigmoid dilates, with accompanying chronic constipation, abdominal distention, and fecal impaction. SYN: *megacolon.* SEE: *megacolon, toxic.*

TREATMENT: Surgical excision of the affected bowel is the treatment of choice. The remaining normal colon is anastomosed to the anus.

**hirsute** (hŭr′sūt) [L. *hirsutus,* shaggy] Hairy.

**hirsuties** (hŭr-sū′shē-ēz) Hirsutism.

**hirsutism** (hŭr′sūt-ĭzm) Condition characterized by the excessive growth of hair or the presence of hair in unusual places, esp. in women. Hirsutism in women is usually caused by abnormalities of androgen production or metabolism. In patients who do not have an adrenal tumor, this condition may be treated symptomatically by shaving, depilatories, or electrolysis. The goal of medical therapy is to decrease androgen production. This may involve the use of various agents including hormones or an antiandrogen (cyproterone acetate).

**hirudicide** (hĭ-rū′dĭ-sīd) [L. *hirudo,* a leech, + *caedere,* to kill] Any substance that destroys leeches.

**hirudin** (hĭ-rū′dĭn) A substance present in the secretion of the buccal glands of the leech that prevents coagulation of the blood by inactivating thrombin.

**Hirudinea** (hĭr″ū-dĭn′ē-ă) A class of Annelida. This group is hermaphroditic, lack setae or appendages, usually have two suckers, and includes the bloodsucking leeches. A number of species, including *H. medicinalis,* were formerly used extensively for bloodletting. SEE: *leech.*

**hirudiniasis** (hĭr″ū-dĭn-ī′ă-sĭs) Infestation by leeches. SEE: *leech.*

***external h.*** A condition caused by leeches attaching themselves to the skin and sucking the blood. After the leeches drop off, bleeding may continue as a result of the action of hirudin. Bites may become infected or ulcerate.

***internal h.*** A condition resulting from accidental ingestion of leeches in drinking water. They may attach themselves to the wall of the pharynx, nasal cavity, or larynx.

**Hirudo** (hĭ-roo′dō) [L., leech] A genus of leeches belonging to the family Gnathobdellidae.

**His, Jr., Wilhelm** (hĭs) German physician, 1863–1934.

***bundle of H.*** The atrioventricular (AV) bundle, a group of modified muscle fibers, the Purkinje fibers, forming a part of the impulse-conducting system of the heart. It arises in the AV node and continues in the interventricular septum as a single bundle, the crus commune, which divides into two trunks that pass respectively to the right and left ventricles, fine branches passing to all parts of the ventricles. It conducts impulses from the atria to the ventricles, which initiates ventricular contraction.

***H. disease*** Trench fever.

**histaffine** (hĭs′tă-fēn) [Gr. *histos,* tissue, + L. *affinis,* having affinity for] Having an affinity for the tissues.

**histaminase** (hĭs-tăm′ĭ-nās) An enzyme widely distributed in the body that inactivates histamine.

**histamine** (hĭs′tă-mĭn, -mēn) A substance, produced from the amino acid histidine, which is normally present in the body. It exerts a pharmacological action when released from injured cells. The red flush of a burn is due to the local production of histamine. If histamine is injected intradermally and if circulation is normal, a triple response occurs. The first reaction is a small red spot that appears within a few seconds, reaches a maximum in about one minute, and then becomes bluish. This is followed by a wheal surrounded by a flare, suggesting a mosquito bite. The final reaction is the development of localized edema at the site of the small red spot, which lasts about 90 sec. Given intravenously, histamine stimulates gastric secretion and causes flushing of skin, lowered blood pressure, and headache. Blood pressure returns to normal in a short time because the circulatory system adjusts to the vascular changes and the histamine is inactivated.

The functions of histamine include increasing gastric secretion, increasing capillary permeability, and contracting the bronchial smooth muscle.

***h. blocking agent*** A drug that blocks the stimulation of cells by histamine. This type of agent acts by interfering with the action of histamine rather than by preventing its secretion. The two known classes, the $H_1$ receptor blocking agents and the $H_2$ receptor blocking agents, act at different receptor sites. Cimetidine is an example of an $H_2$ receptor blocking agent.

***h. phosphate*** Water-soluble colorless

crystals, sometimes called histamine acid phosphate or histamine diphosphate. It is used most frequently as a diagnostic agent in determining the acid-secreting power of the stomach.

***h. headache*** SEE: under *headache*.

**histaminemia** (hĭs-tăm″ĭ-nē′mē-ă) [*histamine* + Gr. *haima*, blood] Histamine in the blood.

**histenzyme** (hĭst-ĕn′zīm) [Gr. *histos*, tissue, + *en*, in, + *zyme*, leaven] A renal enzyme that splits up hippuric acid into benzoic acid and glycocol. SYN: *histozyme*.

**histidase** Histidine ammonia-lyase.

**histidine** (hĭs′tĭ-dĭn, -dēn) $C_6H_9N_3O_2$. An amino acid obtained by hydrolysis from tissue proteins and necessary for tissue repair and growth.

***h. ammonia-lyase*** A liver enzyme that catalyzes L-histidine with the resultant formation of urocanic acid and ammonia. Deficiency of this enzyme causes histidinemia.

**histidinemia** (hĭs″tĭ-dĭ-nē′mē-ă) A hereditary metabolic disease caused by lack of the enzyme histidine ammonia-lyase, which is normally present in the urine.

**histidinuria** (hĭs″tĭ-dĭ-nū′rē-ă) The presence of histidine in the urine.

**histioblast** (hĭs′tē-ō-blăst″) A tissue histiocyte.

**histiocyte** (hĭs′tē-ō-sīt″) [Gr. *histion*, little web, + *kytos*, cell] A monocyte that has become a resident in tissue. SYN: *histocyte; macrophage*.

**histiocytoma** (hĭs″tē-ō-sī-tō′mă) [″ + ″ + *oma*, tumor] A tumor containing histiocytes.

**histiocytosis** (hĭs″tē-ō-sī-tō′sĭs) [″ + ″ + *osis*, condition] An abnormal amount of histiocytes in the blood.

***Langerhans cell h.*** A number of clinical conditions, most commonly seen in infants and children, caused by disease of Langerhans cell histiocytes. These cells, which are characteristic of all of the variants of the disease, cause granulomas. The great variation in the signs and symptoms produced depends upon their location and how widely spread they are. Almost any organ system including the skeleton may be involved. These diseases were previously given names such as histiocytosis X, Hand-Schüller-Christian disease, Letterer-Siwe disease, and eosinophilic granuloma. Treatment may consist of surgical removal of bone lesions and radiation therapy for lesions threatening vital functions such as sight and hearing. Corticosteroids or cytotoxic agents are useful in controlling soft tissue disease and multiple skeletal lesions. Bone marrow transplantation has been used in recurrent and progressive Langerhans cell histiocytosis.

***lipid h.*** Niemann-Pick disease.

**histiogenic** (hĭs-tē-ō-jĕn′ĭk) [″ + *gennan*, to form] Histogenous.

**histo-** [Gr. *histos*, web, tissue] Combining form meaning *tissue*.

**histoblast** (hĭs′tō-blăst) [″ + *blastos*, germ] A tissue cell.

**histochemistry** (hĭs″tō-kĕm′ĭs-trē) The study of chemistry of the cells and tissues. It involves use of both light and electron microscopy and special chemical tests and stains.

**histoclastic** (hĭs″tō-klăs′tĭk) [″ + *klastos*, breaking] The ability to break down tissues, said of certain cells.

**histocompatibility** (hĭs″tō-kŏm-păt″ĭ-bĭl′ĭ-tē) The quality of certain tissues that have antigens of the same HLA complex, and, therefore, will not cause an immunological response if transplanted from one individual to another.

***h. locus antigen*** ABBR: HLA. One of the multiple antigens present on all nucleated cells in the body that identify the cells as "self." These markers determine the compatibility of tissue for transplantation. They are derived from genes at seven sites (loci) on chromosome 6, in an area called the major histocompatibility complex (MHC) and each histocompatibility antigen is divided into one of two MHC classes.

In humans, the proteins created in the MHC are called human leukocyte antigens (HLA) because these markers were originally found on lymphocytes. Each gene in the MHC has several forms or alleles. Therefore, the number of different histocompatibility antigens is huge, making it necessary to identify and match HLAs in donors and recipients involved in tissue and organ transplantation. The identification of HLAs is called tissue typing.

The identification of HLA sites on chromosome 6 has enabled researchers to correlate the presence of specific histocompatibility and certain autoimmune diseases including insulin-dependent diabetes mellitus, multiple sclerosis, some forms of myasthenia gravis, rheumatoid arthritis, and ankylosing spondylitis. SYN: *human leukocyte antigen*. SEE: *major histocompatibility complex*.

***h. gene*** One of the genes composing the HLA complex that determine the histocompatibility antigenic markers on all nucleated cells. These genes create the antigens by which the immune system recognizes "self" and, therefore, are important in determining the success of transplanted organs and tissues. Many different forms of one particular histocompatibility gene are found at the seven sites on chromosome 6. Each of these different forms is an allele. SEE: *h. locus antigen*.

**histocyte** (hĭs′tō-sīt) [″ + *kytos*, cell] Histiocyte.

**histodiagnosis** (hĭs″tō-dī″ăg-nō′sĭs) [″ + *dia*, through, + *gnosis*, knowledge] A diagnosis made from examination of the tissues, esp. by use of microscopy.

**histodifferentiation** (hĭs″tō-dĭf″ĕr-ĕn″shē-ă′shŭn) The process of cellular maturation in which a primitive cell develops into specific cellular tissue types.

**histogenesis** (hĭs-tō-jĕn′ĕ-sĭs) [″ + *genesis,* generation, birth] The development into differentiated tissues of the germ layer; the origin and development of tissue. **histogenetic** (hĭs″tō-jĕ-nĕt′ĭk), *adj.*

**histogenous** (hĭs-tŏj′ĕ-nŭs) Made by the tissues. SYN: *histiogenic.*

**histogram** (hĭs′tō-gram) [L. *historia,* observation, + Gr. *gramma,* something written] A graph showing frequency distributions.

**histohematin** (hĭs″tō-hĕm′ă-tĭn) [″ + *haima,* blood] A hemoglobin pigment in various tissues.

**histohematogenous** (hĭs″tō-hĕm″ă-tŏj′ĕ-nŭs) [″ + ″ + *gennan,* to form] Arising from the tissues and the blood.

**histoincompatible** Referring to tissues that are immunologically different enough to prevent their use for transplantation.

**histokinesis** (hĭs-tō-kĭ-nē′sĭs) [″ + *kinesis,* movement] Movement in the tissues of the body.

**histologist** (hĭs-tŏl′ō-jĭst) [″ + *logos,* word, reason] A specialist in the study of cells and microscopic tissues.

**histology** (hĭs-tŏl′ō-jē) The study of the microscopic structure of tissue. **histological** (hĭs″tō-lŏj′ĭ-kăl), *adj.*

***normal h.*** The microscopic study of healthy tissue.

***pathologic h.*** Histopathology.

**histolysis** (hĭs-tŏl′ĭ-sĭs) [″ + *lysis,* dissolution] Disintegration of the tissues. **histolytic** (hĭs″tō-lĭt′ĭk), *adj.*

**histoma** (hĭs-tō′mă) [″ + *oma,* tumor] A tumor composed of tissue.

**histone** (hĭs′tŏn, -tōn) [Gr. *histos,* web, tissue] One of the five kinds of proteins that are part of chromatin in eukaryotic cells. Their positive charge attracts the negatively charged DNA that is folded around them into units called nucleosomes. Histones also regulate some of the further folding of DNA in chromosomes about to undergo mitosis.

**histonuria** (hĭs-tōn-ū′rē-ă) [″ + *ouros,* urine] Excretion of histones in the urine.

**histopathology** (hĭs″tō-pă-thŏl′ō-jē) [″ + *pathos,* disease, suffering, + *logos,* word, reason] The microscopic study of diseased tissues. SYN: *pathologic histology.*

**histophysiology** (hĭs″tō-fĭz″ē-ŏl′ō-jē) [″ + *physis,* nature, + *logos,* word, reason] The study of the functions of cells and tissues.

**Histoplasma** (hĭs″tō-plăz′mă) [″ + LL. *plasma,* form, mold] A genus of parasitic fungi.

***H. capsulatum*** The causative agent of histoplasmosis. SEE: illus.

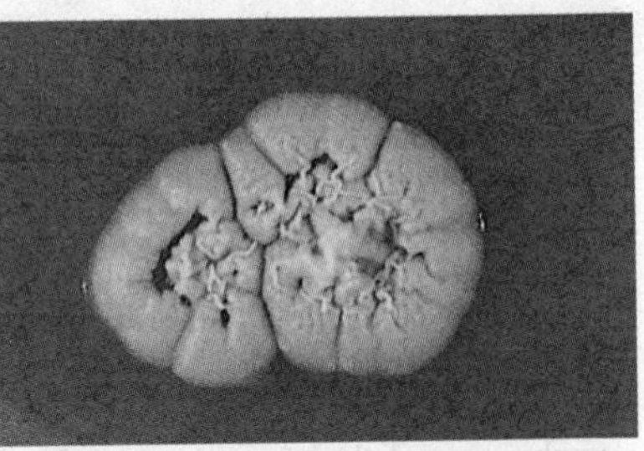

HISTOPLASMA CAPSULATUM IN CULTURE

**histoplasmin** (hĭs″tō-plăz′mĭn) An antigen prepared from cultures of *Histoplasma capsulatum* and used as a skin test for the diagnosis of histoplasmosis.

**histoplasmosis** (hĭs″tō-plăz-mō′sĭs) [″ + ″ + Gr. *osis,* condition] A systemic, fungal, respiratory disease caused by *Histoplasma capsulatum.* The reservoir for this fungus is in soil with a high organic content and undisturbed bird droppings, esp. that around old chicken houses; caves harboring bats; and starling, blackbird, and pigeon roosts.

SYMPTOMS: The signs and symptoms vary from those of a mild self-limited infection to a severe fatal disease. Immunocompromised persons are esp. susceptible. In the severe form there are fever, anemia, enlarged spleen and liver, leukopenia, pulmonary involvement, adrenal necrosis, and gastrointestinal tract ulcers. The treatment is intravenous amphotericin B.

NURSING IMPLICATIONS: Respiratory status is monitored every 8 hr (or more frequently as necessary) to assess for diminished breath sounds, pleural friction rub, or effusion; cardiovascular status every 8 hr (or more frequently as necessary) to document and immediately report any muffling of heart sounds, jugular vein distention, pulsus paradoxus, or other signs of cardiac tamponade; and neurological status every 8 hr (or more frequently as necessary) to document and report any changes in level of consciousness or any nuchal rigidity. The patient is assessed for signs and symptoms of hypoglycemia and hyperglycemia, indicating adrenal dysfunction. All stools are tested for occult blood, and its presence is documented and reported. Prescribed antifungal therapy (amphotericin B or ketaconazole) is administered and evaluated for desired effects and any adverse reactions. Because amphotericin B may cause pain, chills, fever, nausea, and vomiting, appropriate analgesics, antihistamines, antipyretics, and antiemetics are administered as prescribed. Small doses of meperidine or morphine sulfate may help reduce shaking chills. Such drug therapy should be administered in the early morning or late evening to avoid sedating the patient for the entire day. If needed, oxygen therapy is administered as prescribed, and rest periods are planned to assist the patient to conserve energy. The dietitian is consulted to construct an appetizing and nutritious diet incorporating the patient's food preferences; this diet is best offered in small, frequent meals rather than in three large ones. If the patient has oropharyngeal ulceration, soothing oral hygiene and soft, bland foods are provided. (Parenteral nutrition may be required if ulcerations are severe.) Emotional support is offered to the patient with chronic or disseminated histoplasmosis, and referral to a social worker, psychologist, or occupational therapist for further counseling and support may be necessary to help the patient cope with long-term therapy. The nurse assists parents of a child with this disease to arrange for home-bound instruction. The patient is advised that follow-up care on a regular basis will be required for at least a year. Cardiac and pulmonary signs and symptoms that may indicate effusions should be reported to the health care provider immediately. To help prevent histoplasmosis, persons in endemic areas are taught to watch for early signs of this infection and to seek treatment promptly. Persons who risk occupational exposure to contaminated soil are instructed to wear face masks.

**history** (hĭs'tō-rē) [Gr. *historia,* inquiry] A systematic record of past events as they relate to a person, a period, a country, or a particular group of people. A carefully taken medical, surgical, and occupational history will enable diagnosis in about 80% of patients. It is, therefore, essential that those involved in caring for and treating the sick be skilled in interviewing patients and that they cultivate listening to allow patients to answer without interruption.

***dental h.*** A record of all aspects of a person's oral health, previous evaluations and treatments, and the state of general physical and mental health. SEE: *oral diagnosis.*

***family h.*** A record of the state of health and medical history of members of the patient's immediate family, which may be of interest to the physician because of genetic or familial tendencies noted.

***medical h.*** The portion of a patient's life history, including ancestry and social, occupational, and medical information, that is important in diagnosing and caring for the medical or surgical condition or conditions present. This information, which is recorded in the patient's permanent record, may be obtained from all available sources if for some reason the patient is neither willing nor able to provide full details. The importance of an accurate and complete medical history for proper care of the patient cannot be overestimated. SEE: *nursing assessment* for illus.

***occupational h.*** A semistructured interview process used by occupational therapists to determine a person's roles, approach to tasks, and sense of identity.

**histothrombin** (hĭs"tō-thrŏm'bĭn) [" + *thrombos,* a clot] A thrombin derived from the connective tissue.

**histotoxic** (hĭs"tō-tŏk'sĭk) [" + *toxikon,* poison] Toxic to tissue.

**histotropic** (hĭs"tō-trŏp'ĭk) [" + *trope,* a turning] Having attraction for tissue cells, as certain parasites, stains, or chemicals.

**histozoic** (hĭs"tō-zō'ĭk) [" + *zoe,* life] Living within or on tissues, said of certain protozoan parasites.

**histozyme** (hĭs'tŏ-zīm) [" + *zyme,* leaven] A renal enzyme that converts hippuric acid into benzoic acid and glycine, causing fermentation.

**histrionic personality disorder** SEE: *personality, histrionic.*

**HIV** *human immunodeficiency virus.* SEE: *AIDS.*

**hives** (hīvz) [origin uncertain] Urticaria.

**HIV positive** SEE: *Nursing Diagnoses Appendix.*

**HL, Hl** *latent hyperopia.*

**hl** *hectoliter.*

**HLA** *histocompatibility locus antigen; human lymphocyte antigen.*

**HLA complex** SEE: *major histocompatibility complex.*

**Hm** *manifest hyperopia.*

**HMD** *hyaline membrane disease.*

**HMG** *human menopausal gonadotropin.*

**HMO** *Health Maintenance Organization.*

**$HNO_2$** Symbol for nitrous acid.

**$HNO_3$** Symbol for nitric acid.

**Ho** Symbol for the element holmium.

**$H_2O$** Symbol for water.

**$H_2O_2$** Symbol for hydrogen peroxide.

**hoarseness** [AS. *has,* harsh] A rough quality of the voice.

ETIOLOGY: Hoarseness may be caused by simple chronic inflammations secondary to chronic nasopharyngitis, chemical irritants, tobacco, or alcohol. Specific causes of chronic laryngitis include syphilis, tuberculosis, leprosy, neoplasms, papilloma, angioma, fibroma, singer's nodes, carcinoma, paralyses, overuse of the vocal cords, and prolapse of ventricle of larynx. Female virilization also usually causes hoarseness.

**Hochsinger's sign** (hōk'zĭng-ĕrz) [Karl Hochsinger, Austrian pediatrician, b. 1860] Closure of the fist in tetany when the inner side of the biceps muscle is pressed.

**Hodgkin's disease** (hŏj'kĭns) [Thomas Hodgkin, Brit. physician, 1798–1866] ABBR: HD. Solid tumor of the lymphoreticular system that may originate in any lymphoid tissue, but usually begins in lymph nodes of the supraclavicular, high cervical, or mediastinal area. Left untreated, the malignancy will invade adjacent areas and kill the patient by invading or obstructing vital organs. SEE: *lymphoma, non-Hodgkin's; Nursing Diagnoses Appendix.*

SYMPTOMS: The disease is characterized by painless enlargement of the lymph nodes beginning in the cervical region, then the axillary, inguinal, mediastinal, and mesenteric regions. There are signs of swelling due to pressure from lymphoid infiltration of blood vessels and organs such as the liver, heart, and spleen. Other symptoms include fever, night sweats, loss of appetite, and weight loss. Some patients experience severe pruritus.

DIAGNOSIS: The presence of the giant polypoid Reed-Sternberg (RS) cell in tissue obtained for biopsy is diagnostic.

INCIDENCE: The annual crude incidence of HD in the U.S. is 35 per million for white men and 26 per million for white women. The average age at diagnosis is 32 years, and the mortality rate is about 20%.

TREATMENT: The goal of therapy is cure, not palliation. More than 70% of patients are cured by the use of radiation and combination chemotherapy. One commonly used chemotherapy drug regimen is identified by the acronym MOPP and includes the drugs mechlorethamine, Oncovin (vincristine), procarbazine, and prednisone.

NURSING IMPLICATIONS: All procedures and treatments associated with the plan of care are explained. The patient is assessed for nutritional deficiencies and malnutrition by obtaining regular weights, by checking anthropomorphic measurements, and by monitoring appropriate laboratory studies (serum protein levels, transferrin levels) and, as necessary, anergy panels. The importance of maintaining good nutrition (aided by eating small, frequent meals of the patient's favorite food) and of drinking plenty of liquids is stressed. A well-balanced, high-calorie, high-protein diet is provided. The patient is observed for complications during chemotherapy, including anorexia, nausea, vomiting, mouth ulcers, alopecia, fatigue, and bone marrow depression; as well as for adverse reactions to radiation therapy, such as hair loss, anorexia, nausea, vomiting, and fatigue. Supportive care is provided as indicated for adverse reactions to chemotherapy or radiation therapy. Comfort measures are provided to promote relaxation, and periods of rest are planned because the patient will tire easily. Antiemetic drugs are administered as prescribed. The importance of gentle but thorough oral hygiene to prevent stomatitis is stressed. To control pain and bleeding, a soft toothbrush or sponge-stick, cotton swabs, and a soothing or anesthetic mouthwash such as a sodium bicarbonate mixture or viscous lidocaine are used as prescribed, petroleum jelly is applied to the lips; and astringent mouthwashes are avoided. The patient is advised to pace activities to counteract therapy-induced fatigue and taught relaxation techniques to promote comfort and rest and reduce anxiety. The patient should avoid crowds and any person with a known infection and should notify the health care provider if any signs or symptoms of infection develop. The nurse stays with the patient during periods of stress and anxiety. Emotional support is provided to the patient and family, and referral to local support groups may be necessary. Women of childbearing age should delay pregnancy until long-term remission occurs, because chemotherapy and radiation therapy can cause genetic mutations and spontaneous abortions. Because sudden withdrawal of prednisone is life-threatening, the health care provider should not change the dosage or discontinue the drug without consulting with the oncologist. As necessary, both patient and family are referred for respite or hospice care.

**Hodgson's disease** (hŏj'sŏnz) [Joseph Hodgson, Brit. physician, 1788–1869] Aneurysmal dilatation of the aorta.

**Hofbauer cell** (hŏf'bow-ĕr) [J. Isfred Isidore Hofbauer, U.S. gynecologist, 1878–1961] A histiocyte, believed to be phagocytic, found in the connective tissue of the chorionic villi.

**Hoffmann's reflex, Hoffmann's sign** [Johann Hoffmann, Ger. neurologist, 1857–1919] A sign of hyperactive tendon reflexes. Flicking the nail of the second, third, or fourth finger will cause flexion of these fingers and maybe the thumb if the reflex is present.

**hol-, holo-** [Gr. *holos,* entire] Combining form meaning *complete, entire,* or *homogenous.*

**holandric** (hŏl-ăn'drĭk) [" + *aner,* man] Transmitted only by a gene in the nonhomologous portion of the Y chromosome. SEE: *hologynic.*

**Holden's line** (hōl'dĕnz) [Luther Holden, Brit. anatomist, 1815–1905] A wrinkle or indistinct furrow in the groin at the junction of the thigh and the abdomen.

**holding area** An Emergency Department area in which patients are kept temporarily before being transferred to an intensive care unit.

**holism** (hōl'ĭzm) The philosophy based on the belief that, in nature, entities such as individuals and other complete organisms function as complete units that cannot be reduced to the sum of their parts. The philosophy was originally discussed by Jan C. Smuts. **holistic** (hō-lĭs'tĭk), *adj.*

**holistic medicine** SEE: under *medicine.*

**Hollenhorst plaques, Hollenhorst bodies** [R. W. Hollenhorst, U.S. ophthalmologist, b. 1913] Atheromatous plaques that have lodged in the retinal vessels after having been broken off from the lining of other vessels. They appear as shiny irregular patches in the vessels of the retina.

**hollow** (hŏl'ō) A depressed area, lower than the surrounding tissue.

***Sebileau's h.*** A depression in the floor

of the mouth between the tongue and the sublingual glands.

**hollow-back** Lordosis.

**Holmgren's test** (hōlm′grĕnz) [Alarik F. Holmgren, Swedish physiologist, 1831–1897] A test in which the patient matches colored skeins of yarn to test for color blindness.

**holmium** (hŏl′mē-ŭm) SYMB: Ho. A rare earth metal, whose atomic weight is 164.930 and atomic number is 67.

**holoacardius** (hŏl″ō-ă-kăr′dē-ŭs) [Gr. *holos,* entire, + *a-,* not, + *kardia,* heart] A congenitally deformed monozygotic twin fetus with no heart. The in utero circulation is obtained from the heart of the twin to which the deformed fetus is attached.

**holocrine** (hŏl′ō-krĭn) [″ + *krinein,* to secrete] Pert. to a secretory gland or its secretions consisting of altered cells of the same gland, the opposite of merocrine. SEE: *apocrine.*

**holodiastolic** (hŏl″ō-dī″ă-stŏl′ĭk) [″ + *diastellein,* to expand] Relating to the entire diastole, esp. a murmur that occurs during all of diastole.

**holoenzyme** (hŏl″ō-ĕn′zīm) [″ + *en,* in, + *zyme,* leaven] A type of enzyme consisting of a protein portion (apoenzyme) and a non-amino acid portion or prosthetic group. SEE: *apoenzyme; prosthetic group.*

**holography** (hŏl-ŏg′ră-fē) [″ + *graphein,* to write] A method of producing pictures in which the image appears as a three-dimensional representation of the original object. The picture obtained is called a hologram (i.e., whole message).

**hologynic** (hŏl″ō-jĭn′ĭk) [″ + *gyne,* woman] Transmitted only by a gene in the nonhomologous portion of the X chromosome. SEE: *holandric.*

**holophrase** A single word, usually a verb, used to convey a variety of meanings. It is common in the development of speech in toddlers.

**holophytic** (hŏl″ō-fĭt′ĭk) [″ + *phyton,* plant] Having plantlike characteristics, esp. in reference to protozoa that resemble plants in their metabolic processes.

**holoprosencephaly** (hŏl″ō-prŏs″ĕn-sĕf′ă-lē) [″ + *proso,* before, + *enkephalos,* brain] A congenital defect caused by an extra chromosome, either trisomy 13–15 or trisomy 18, which causes deficiency in the forebrain.

**holorachischisis** (hŏl″ō-ră-kĭs′kĭ-sĭs) [″ + *rhachis,* spine, + *schisis,* a splitting] Complete spina bifida.

**holosystolic** (hŏl″ō-sĭs-tŏl′ĭk) [″ + *systellein,* to draw together] Relating to the entire duration of systole.

**holotetanus, holotonia** (hŏl-ō-tĕt′ă-nŭs, hŏl″ō-tō′nē-ah) [″ + *tetanos,* tetanus, ″ + *tonos,* tension] A muscular spasm of the entire body.

**holotrichous** (hō-lŏt′rĭ-kŭs) [″ + *thrix,* hair] Covered entirely with cilia, said of certain protozoa and bacteria.

**holozoic** (hŏl″ō-zō′ĭk) [″ + *zoion,* animal] Resembling an animal as to its method of nutrition in which organic materials serve as a source of energy.

**Holter monitor** [Norman Jefferis Holter, U.S. biophysicist, 1914–1983] A portable device small enough to be worn by a patient during normal activity. It consists of an electrocardiograph and a recording system capable of storing up to 24 hr of recording of the individual's ECG record. It is particularly useful in obtaining a record of cardiac arrhythmia that would not be discovered by means of an ECG of only a few minutes' duration. This technique is limited in establishing or ruling out coronary artery disease; however, it is helpful in identifying intermittent arrhythmia or tachycardia, and in providing prognostic information in patients with various coronary disease syndromes.

**Holthouse's hernia** (hŏlt′howz-ĕs) [Carsten Holthouse, Brit. surgeon, 1810–1901] An inguinal hernia protruding along the folds of the groin.

**Holt-Oram syndrome** [Mary Clayton Holt, contemporary Brit. physician; Samuel Oram, contemporary Brit. physician] An inherited disorder, transmitted as an autosomal trait, that is marked by anomalies of the upper limbs and heart. Clinical manifestations vary from minimal radiographic changes to overt structural changes in the hands and arms and single or multiple atrial and ventricular defects that may be life-threatening.

**homalocephalus** (hŏm″ă-lō-sĕf′ă-lŭs) [Gr. *homalos,* level, + *kephale,* head] A person with a flat skull.

**Homans' sign** (hō′mănz) [John Homans, U.S. surgeon, 1877–1954] Pain in the calf when the foot is passively dorsiflexed. This is an early sign indicating venous thrombosis of the deep veins of the calf; however, diagnostic reliability is limited, that is, elicited calf pain may be associated with conditions other than thrombosis, and an absence of calf pain does not rule out thrombosis.

**homatropine hydrobromide** (hō-măt′rō-pēn) An antimuscarinic drug that acts like belladonna.

**homatropine methylbromide** An antimuscarinic drug that acts like belladonna.

**homaxial** (hō-măk′sē-ăl) [Gr. *homos,* same, + L. *axis,* axis] Having all axes alike, as a sphere.

**home assessment** An evaluation of the home environment of persons with disability, usually by an occupational therapist or home care specialist, for purposes of identifying architectural barriers and safety hazards and recommending modifications or devices for improving mobility, safety, and independent function.

**home maintenance management, impaired** Inability to independently maintain a safe, growth-promoting immediate environment. SEE: *Nursing Diagnoses Appendix.*

**homeo-** [Gr. *homoios,* like, similar] Prefix indicating *likeness; resemblance; constant unchanging state.*

**homeodynamics** A principle within the nursing theory of Martha Rogers, which suggests that human nature is dynamic, everchanging, and holistic. In contrast to homeostasis, in which we adapt to our environment, homeodynamics suggests that we interact with our environment. Nursing assessment then focuses on the patient's pattern, rhythm, and source of energy, rather than on his or her coping mechanisms and modes of adaptation.

**homeomorphous** (hō″mē-ō-mor′fŭs) [″ + *morphe,* form] Of like shape but different compositions.

**homeo-osteoplasty** (hō″mē-ō-ŏs′tē-ō-plăs″tē) [″ + *osteon,* bone, + *plassein,* to form] Grafting of a piece of bone that is like the one onto which it is grafted.

**homeopathist** (hō-mē-ŏp′ă-thĭst) One who practices homeopathy.

**homeopathy** (hō-mē-ŏp′ă-thē) [Gr. *homoios,* like, + *pathos,* disease] A school of medicine, founded by Dr. Samuel Christian Friedrich Hahnemann (1755–1843) in the late 18th century, based on the theory that large doses of drugs that produce symptoms of a disease in healthy people will cure the same symptoms when administered in small amounts. This is loosely based on the theory that "like cures like." SEE: *allopathy.* **homeopathic** (hō″mē-ō-păth′ĭk), *adj.*

**homeoplasia** (hō″mē-ō-plā′zē-ă) [″ + *plassein,* to form] The formation of new tissue similar to that already existing in a part.

**homeoplastic** (hō″mē-ō-plăs′tĭk) Relating to or resembling the structure of adjacent parts.

**homeostasis** (hō″mē-ō-stā′sĭs) [″ + *stasis,* a standing] The state of dynamic equilibrium of the internal environment of the body that is maintained by the ever-changing processes of feedback and regulation in response to external or internal changes. **homeostatic** (-stăt′ĭk), *adj.*

**homeotherapy** (hō″mē-ō-thĕr′ă-pē) [″ + *therapeia,* treatment] The treatment or prevention of disease using a substance similar but not identical to the active causative agent, such as jennerian vaccination.

**homeothermal** (hō″mē-ō-thĕr′măl) [″ + *therme,* heat] Pert. to a homoiotherm.

**homeotransplantation** (hō″mē-ō-trăns″plăn-tā′shŭn) [″ + L. *trans,* across, + *plantare,* to plant] Allotransplantation.

**homeotypical** (hō″mē-ō-tĭp′ĭ-kăl) [″ + *typos,* type] Resembling the typical or normal.

**homesickness** [AS. *ham,* home, + *seoc,* ill] Sadness, depression, and anxiety related to being away from home or loved ones.

**homicide** (hŏm′ĭ-sīd) [L. *homo,* man, + *caedere,* to kill] **1.** Murder. **2.** A murderer. **homicidal,** *adj.*

**hominid** (hŏm′ĭ-nĭd) [″ + *eidos,* form, shape] A primate of the Hominidae family. Humans are the only surviving species.

**Homo** (hō′mō) [L., man] A genus of primates of the family Hominidae. The sole existing species is humankind, *Homo sapiens.* Evidence from fossils indicates extinct species (e.g., *H. habilis, H. erectus, H. australopithecus*).

**homo-** [Gr. *homos,* same] Prefix meaning *the same* or *a likeness.*

**homoblastic** (hō″mō-blăs′tĭk) [″ + *blastos,* germ] Developing from a single type of tissue; the opposite of heteroblastic.

**homocentric** (hō″mō-sĕn′trĭk) [″ + *kentron,* center] Having the same center.

**homochronous** (hō-mŏk-rō′nŭs) [″ + *chronos,* time] Occurring at the same time or at the same age in each generation.

**homocysteine** (hō″mō-sĭs-tē′ĭn) An amino acid produced by the catabolism of methionine. With serine, it forms a complex that eventually produces cysteine and homoserine. There is evidence that a high level of homocysteine in the blood is associated with an increased risk of developing coronary artery disease. Blood homocysteine levels may be lowered by eating foods rich in folic acid, such as green leafy vegetables and fruits.

**homocystine** (hō″mō-sĭs′tĭn) A homologue of cystine formed by condensation of two molecules of homocystine.

**homocystinuria** (hō″mō-sĭs-tĭn-ū′rē-ă) An inherited disease caused by the absence of the enzyme essential to the metabolism of homocystine. Clinically the disease is similar to Marfan's syndrome. Patients are mentally retarded and have subluxated lenses, a tendency toward seizures, liver disease, and failure to grow at a normal rate.

**homocytotropic** (hō″mō-sī″tō-trŏp′ĭk) [″ + *kytos,* cell, + *tropos,* a turning] Having an affinity for cells of the same species.

**homodromous** (hō-mŏd′rō-mŭs) [″ + *dromos,* running] Moving in the same direction or toward the same goal.

**homoerotic** (hō″mō-ĕ-rŏt′ĭk) Homosexual (2).

**homogametic** (hō″mō-gă-mĕt′ĭk) [″ + *gamos,* marriage] Pert. to the production of one kind of gamete with regard to the sex chromosome. In humans, the XX female is the homogametic sex, as all ova produced contain the X chromosome. SEE: *heterogametic.*

**homogenate** (hō-mŏj′ĕ-nāt) The material obtained when something is homogenized.

**homogeneous** (hō″mŏ-jē′nē-ŭs) [″ + *genos,* kind] Uniform in structure, composition, or nature; the opposite of heterogeneous.

**homogenesis** (hō-mō-jĕn′ĕ-sĭs) [″ + *genesis,* generation, birth] Reproduction by the same process in succeeding generations; the opposite of heterogenesis.

**homogenize** (hō-mŏj′ĕ-nīz) To make homogeneous; to produce a uniform emulsion or suspension of two substances normally immiscible.

**homogentisuria** (hō″mō-jĕn″tĭ-sū′rē-ă) Alkaptonuria.

**homograft** (hō′mō-grăft) Allograft.

**homoiopodal** (hō″moy-ŏp′ō-dăl) [Gr. *homoios,* like, + *pous, pod-,* foot] Having only one kind of protruding process, as a dendrite in a nerve cell.

**homoiotherm** (hō-moy′ō-thĕrm) [″ + *therme,* heat] A warm-blooded organism that maintains a constant body temperature despite fluctuating environmental temperatures; the opposite of poikilotherm.

**homokeratoplasty** (hō″mō-ker′ă-tō-plăs″tē) A homograft of corneal tissue.

**homolateral** [Gr. *homos,* same, + L. *latus,* side] Ipsilateral.

**homologous** (hō-mŏl′ō-gŭs) [″ + *logos,* word, reason] Similar in fundamental structure and in origin but not necessarily in function (e.g., the arm of a man, forelimb of a dog, and wing of a bird). SEE: *heterologous.*

**homologous fertilization** SEE: under *fertilization.*

**homologous organs** Structures that are morphological equivalents, as the arm of a human and the forelimb of a quadruped; the penis of a man and the clitoris of a woman.

**homologue** (hŏm′ŏ-lŏg) **1.** An organ or part common to a number of species. **2.** One that corresponds to a part or organ in another structure. **3.** In chemistry, any member of a series that resembles the other members in action and general structure but has a constant compositional difference such as a methyl, $CH_3$, group.

**homology** (hō-mŏl′ō-jē) [″ + *logos,* word, reason] Similarity in structure but not necessarily in function; the opposite of analogy.

**homolysin** (hō-mŏl′ĭ-sĭn) [″+ *lysis,* dissolution] An agent in serum destructive to erythrocytes.

**Homonidae** [L. *homo,* man, + Gr. *ideos,* pert. to] A family of primates that includes ancient and modern humans.

**homonomous** (hō-mŏn′ō-mŭs) [″ + *nomos,* law] Pert. to parts arranged in a series that are similar in form and structure, as metameres of a segmented animal or the fingers and toes of a mammal.

**homonymous** (hō-mŏn′ĭ-mŭs) [″ + *onyma,* name] Having the same name.

**homophil** (hō-mō-fĭl) [″ + *philein,* to love] Pert. to an antibody reacting only with a specific antigen.

**homophile** (hō-mō-fīl′) Homosexual (1).

**homophobe** One who fears or dislikes homosexuals.

**homophobia** An abnormal fear of homosexuals.

**homoplastic** (hō″mō-plăs′tĭk) [″ + *plassein,* to form] Having a similar form and structure.

**Homo sapiens** (hō′mō sā′pē-ĕnz) [L. *homo,* man, + *sapiens,* wise, sapient] The species to which modern humans belong. SEE: *Homo.*

**homosexual** (hō″mō-sĕks′ū-ăl) [Gr. *homos,* same, + L. *sexus,* sex] **1.** One sexually attracted to another of the same sex. SYN: *homophile.* **2.** Pert. to attraction to another of the same sex. SYN: *homoerotic.* SEE: *AIDS; asexual; bisexual; heterosexual; lesbian.*

**homosexuality** (hō″mō-sĕks″ū-ăl′ĭ-tē) A condition in which the libido is directed toward one of the same sex.

**homostimulant** (hōm″ō-stĭm′ū-lănt) [″+ L. *stimulare,* to arouse] Stimulating the organ from which an extract is derived.

**homotherm** (hō′mō-thĕrm) [″ + *therme,* heat] An animal whose body temperature remains constant regardless of the temperature of the environment. SYN: *warm-blooded animal.* SEE: *poikilotherm.* **homothermal** (hōm″ō-thĕr′măl), *adj.*

**homotopic** (hōm″ō-tŏp′ĭk) [″ + *topos,* place] Occurring at the same site on the body.

**homotype** (hō′mō-tīp) [″ + *typos,* type] One organ or part similar in form and function to another, as one of two paired parts or organs.

**homotypic** (hō′mō-tĭp′ĭk) Of the same form and type.

**homovanillic acid** ABBR: HVA. A metabolite of catecholamine found in the urine of patients with neuroblastoma. The higher the amount before treatment, the better the prognosis for response to treatment.

**homozygosis** (hōm″ō-zī-gō′sĭs) [″ + *zygon,* yoke, pair, + *osis,* condition] The formation of a zygote by the union of gametes that have one or more identical alleles. SEE: *heterozygosis.*

**homozygote** (hōm″ō-zī′gōt) A homozygous individual; an individual developing from gametes with similar alleles and thus possessing like pairs of genes for a given hereditary characteristic.

**homozygous** (hōm″ō-zī′gŭs) **1.** Produced by similar alleles. **2.** Said of an organism when germ cells transmit nearly identical alleles as a result of inbreeding.

**homunculus** (hō-mŭn′kū-lŭs) [L. diminutive of *homo,* man] A dwarf in whom the body parts develop in their normal proportions.

**honey** [AS. *hunig*] A sweet thick liquid substance produced by bees from the nectar gathered from flowers and stored by them for food. The honey's color and flavor are determined by the flowers from which the nectar was obtained. Honey has been used by humans as a food since ancient times, when it was the principal source of sugar. One of the first fermented sources of alcohol was allegedly made from honey, to produce the alcoholic beverage called mead. About 80% of honey is levulose and dextrose, the remainder mostly water.

Honey was used as long as 4000 years ago for direct application to wounds. The ingredients in honey, including possible antibacterial substances derived from flowers that the bee has contacted, may account for the superiority of honey over granulated sugar in treating wounds.

Honey is not sterile. Its use in preparing infant's formula has caused botulism. SEE: *decubitus ulcer; propolis*.

**honorific** [L. *honorificus*, honor-making] To convey honor upon a person, esp. while writing or speaking about an individual. SEE: *pejorative*.

**hook** [AS. *hok*, an angle] **1.** A curved instrument. **2.** The terminal device in an upper extremity orthosis.

**hookworm** A parasitic nematode belonging to the superfamily Strongyloidea, esp. *Ancylostoma duodenale* and *Necator americanus*. SEE: illus.; *ancylostomiasis; uncinariasis*.

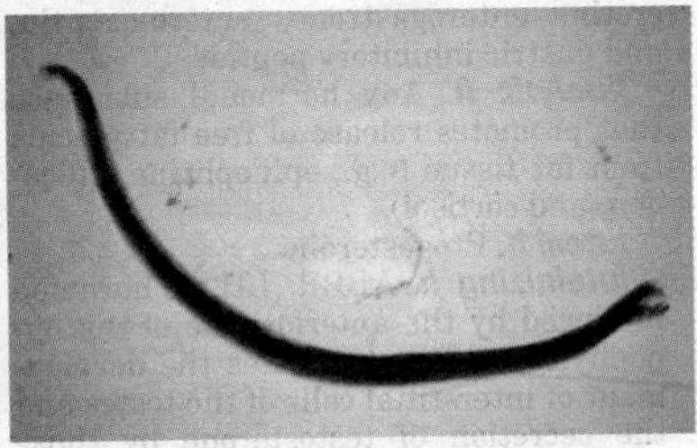

ADULT HOOKWORM (ORIG. MAG. ×10)

**Hoover sign** [Charles F. Hoover, U.S. physician, 1865-1927] A test used in suspected unilateral hysterical paralysis. The examiner places a hand under the heel of the paralyzed leg and asks the patient to raise the normal leg against resistance. In hysterical paralysis, the examiner will feel pressure against the hand under the allegedly paralyzed leg. In true paralysis, no pressure will be felt.

**hope** The expectation that something desired will occur. One of the mandates of medical care is not to destroy hope.

**hopelessness** A subjective state in which an individual sees limited or no alternatives or personal choices available and is unable to mobilize energy on own behalf. This reaction may occur in the patient or the health care personnel or both. In certain situations such as the grief reaction or mourning, a normal phase of feelings of despair, helplessness, and apathy occurs. If this continues for an inordinately long period, hopelessness develops. The alert medical and nursing team will be aware of the development of this reaction and take the appropriate action to prevent its continuation. When those responsible for providing medical care feel that a patient's condition is hopeless, they may give up trying to treat the patient effectively. SEE: *grief reaction; helplessness; Nursing Diagnoses Appendix*.

**hordeolum** (hor-dē'ō-lŭm) [L., barleycorn] Sty(e).

**horizontal** [L. *horizontalis*] **1.** Parallel to or in the plane of the horizon. **2.** A transverse plane of the body that is at right angles to the vertical axis of the body.

**hormesis** (hor-mē'sĭs) [Gr. *hormesis*, rapid motion] **1.** The stimulating effect of a small dose of a substance that is toxic in larger doses. **2.** The controversial hypothesis that very low doses of ionizing radiation may not be harmful and may even have beneficial effects.

**hormion** (hor'mē-ŏn) [Gr., little chain] The junction of the posterior border of the vomer with the sphenoid bone.

**hormonagogue** (hor-mōn'ă-gŏg) [Gr. *hormon*, urging on, + *agogos*, leading] Stimulating or increasing the production of a hormone.

**hormone** (hor'mōn) [Gr. *hormon*, urging on] **1.** A substance originating in an organ, gland, or body part that is conveyed through the blood to another body part, chemically stimulating that part to increase or decrease functional activity or to increase or decrease secretion of another hormone. **2.** The secretion of the ductless glands (e.g., insulin from the pancreas). SEE: *endocrine gland*. **hormonal** (hor-mō'năl), *adj.*

***adaptive h.*** A hormone produced in response to adapting to stress or some other powerful stimulus.

***adrenocortical h.*** A hormone secreted by the cortex of the adrenal gland. SEE: *adrenal gland*.

***adrenocorticotropic h.*** Corticotropin.

***adrenomedullary h.*** One of two hormones, epinephrine and norepinephrine, that are produced by the adrenal medulla.

***androgenic h.*** A hormone that regulates the development and maintenance of the male secondary sexual characteristics; an androgen. Androgens are secreted by the interstitial tissue of the testis and by the adrenal cortex of both sexes. Androgens include testosterone, androsterone, and dehydroandrosterone.

***anterior pituitary h.*** One of several hormones secreted by the anterior lobe of the hypophysis, including growth hormone; thyrotropic (TSH), gonadotropic, follicle-stimulating (FSH), interstitial cell-stimulating or luteotropic (ICSH or LH), prolactin; melanocyte-stimulating hormones; and corticotropin.

***antidiuretic h.*** A peptide hormone produced by the hypothalamus and stored in the posterior pituitary gland. It increases reabsorption of water by the kidneys, which contributes to normal blood volume and blood pressure and causes constriction of arterioles (pressor effect). SYN: *vasopressin*.

***calcitonin h.*** A hormone produced in the thyroid gland; it maintains a dense, hard bone matrix and lowers blood calcium level.

***corpus luteum h.*** Progesterone.

***cortical h.*** Adrenocortical h.

***corticotropin-releasing h.*** ABBR: CRH. A hormone released from the hypothalamus that acts on the anterior pituitary to increase secretion of adrenal corticotropin hormone (ACTH). Also, in response to stress, CRH causes hyperglycemia, increased oxygen consumption, increased cardiac output, and decreased sexual activity; suppresses release of growth hormone; diminishes gastrointestinal function; stimulates respiration; and causes behavioral changes.

***digestive h.*** Any of a group of hormones produced by the stomach or small intestine mucosa that stimulates various tissues via the bloodstream to release enzymes, produce fluids, or affect gastrointestinal motility. The digestive hormones are gastrin, motilin, secretin, cholecystokinin, enterogastrone, entero-oxyntin, and gastric inhibitory peptide.

***estrogenic h.*** A hormone that stimulates the development and maintenance of female sexual characteristics. Estrogens are secreted by the ovaries and the placenta in women and by the adrenal cortex in both sexes. Estrogenic hormones include estradiol, estrone, and estriol.

***follicle-stimulating h.*** ABBR: FSH. A hormone secreted by the anterior lobe of the hypophysis that stimulates maturation of the ovarian follicles in women. In the man, the hormone is important in maintaining spermatogenesis.

***follicle-stimulating h. releasing hormone*** ABBR: FSHRH. A hormone from the hypothalamus that regulates release of follicle-stimulating hormone.

***gastric h.*** Gastrin.

***gonadotropic h.*** An anterior pituitary hormone (follicle-stimulating hormone or luteinizing hormone) affecting the gonads.

***gonadotropin-releasing h.*** ABBR: GnRH. Luteinizing hormone releasing h.

***growth h.*** ABBR: GH. A hormone secreted by the anterior pituitary that regulates the cell division and protein synthesis necessary for normal growth. SYN: *somatotropin.*

The aging process usually includes loss of lean body mass, thinning of the skin, and increase in adipose tissue. These changes are probably related to the decline in secretion of growth hormone by the pituitary. This begins after age 30 and continues. The possibility that these age-related changes may be altered by administration of human growth hormone is being investigated.

***growth hormone-releasing h.*** ABBR: GH-RH. A hormone from the hypothalamus that stimulates the release of growth hormone from the anterior pituitary.

***human placental lactogen h.*** SEE: *lactogen, human placental.*

***immunoregulatory h.*** A hormone that influences components of the immune system, including the number and activity of the white blood cells. Hormones secreted by almost all of the glands in the body, particularly the hypothalamus and adrenal glands, are immunoregulatory. They include growth hormone, prolactin, thyroxine, and parathormone, as well as those secreted by and controlling the gonads.

***inhibitory h.*** One of a group of substances that inhibit the release of certain hormones from the pituitary. Somatostatin, which inhibits the release of growth hormone, is included in this group.

***interstitial cell-stimulating h.*** ABBR: ICSH. Luteinizing h.

***intestinal h.*** One of several hormones produced by the mucosa of the intestine; these include cholecystokinin, motilin, secretin, enterogastrone, entero-oxyntin, and gastric inhibitory peptide.

***lipolytic h.*** Any hormonal substance that promotes release of free fatty acids from fat tissue (e.g., epinephrine, glucagon, and cortisol).

***luteal h.*** Progesterone.

***luteinizing h.*** ABBR: LH. A hormone produced by the anterior lobe of the hypophysis, which stimulates the development of interstitial cells of the testes and the secretion of testosterone by those cells. In women, it stimulates ovulation (i.e., rupture of the mature ovarian follicle, transformation of the follicle into the corpus luteum, and secretion of progesterone and estrogen by the corpus luteum). SYN: *interstitial cell-stimulating h; luteotropin.*

***luteinizing hormone-releasing h.*** ABBR: LH-RH. A hormone from the hypothalamus that stimulates the release of luteinizing hormone from the anterior pituitary. SYN: *gonadotropin-releasing h.*

***luteotropic h.*** A hormone produced by the anterior lobe of the hypophysis that stimulates the secretion of progesterone by the corpus luteum.

***melanocyte-stimulating h.*** ABBR: MSH. A hormone of the anterior pituitary gland that causes pigmentation of the skin in humans.

***ovarian h.*** A hormone produced by the ovary. SEE: *estradiol; estriol; estrogen; estrone; progesterone.*

***pancreatic h.*** A hormone produced by the islets of Langerhans of the pancreas. SEE: *glucagon; insulin.*

***parathyroid h.*** A hormone secreted by the parathyroid glands that regulates blood levels of calcium and phosphorus. Its deficiency results in tetany. SEE: *parathormone.*

***placental h.*** One of the hormones secreted by the placenta; they include estrogen and progesterone, chorionic gonadotropin, a hormone similar to thyroid-stimulating hormone (TSH), melanocyte-stimulating hormone (MSH), and a variety of corticotropin.

***posterior pituitary h.*** One of the hormones secreted by the posterior lobe of the hypophysis, including vasopressin, which produces vasopressor and antidiuretic effects, and oxytocin, which stimulates contraction of smooth muscle of the uterus.

***progestational h.*** Progesterone.

***progesterone h.*** Progesterone.

***prolactin h.*** Prolactin.

***releasing h.*** One of a group of substances secreted by the hypothalamus that control or inhibit the release of various hormones. Thyrotropin-releasing hormone, gonadotropin-releasing hormone, dopamine, growth hormone–releasing hormone, corticotropin-releasing hormone, and somatostatin are included in this group. Dopamine and somatostatin act to inhibit release of the hormones they act upon.

***sex h.*** An androgenic or estrogenic hormone.

***somatotropic h.*** Somatotropin.

***somatotropin-releasing h.*** Growth hormone-releasing h.

***synthetic human growth h.*** A synthetic growth hormone made by using recombinant DNA techniques.

***testicular h.*** A hormone produced by the interstitial tissue of the testis (e.g., testosterone and inhibin, which is produced by the sustentacular cells).

***thyroid h.*** A hormone secreted by the follicles of the thyroid gland.

***thyrotropic h.*** Thyrotropin.

***thyrotropin-releasing h.*** ABBR: TRH. A hormone secreted by the hypothalamus that stimulates the anterior pituitary to release thyrotropin.

**hormonogenesis** (hor″mō-nō-jĕn′ĕ-sĭs) [″ + *genesis,* generation, birth] Hormonopoiesis. **hormonogenic** (-jĕn′ĭk), *adj.*

**hormonology** (hor″mō-nŏl′ō-jē) [″ + *logos,* word, reason] Clinical endocrinology.

**hormonopoiesis** (hor″mō-nō-poy-ē′sĭs) [″ + *poiesis,* formation] The production of hormones. SYN: *hormonogenesis.* **hormonopoietic** (-ĕt′ĭk), *adj.*

**hormonotherapy** (hor″mō-nō-thĕr′ă-pē) The therapeutic use of hormones.

**horn** A cutaneous outgrowth composed chiefly of keratin; a hornlike projection. SYN: *cornu.*

***h. of Ammon*** Hippocampus major.

***anterior h. of the spinal cord*** The horn-shaped portion of the gray matter of anterior part of the spinal cord. SEE: *spinal cord.*

***cicatricial h.*** A cutaneous horn originating in scar tissue.

***cutaneous h.*** A hard, horny outgrowth from the skin. It is slow-growing, benign, and may be small or large, 10 to 12 cm, in diameter.

***dorsal h.*** A posterior projection of the gray matter of the spinal cord.

***posterior h. of the spinal cord*** The horn-shaped portion of the gray matter of the posterior part of the spinal cord. SEE: *spinal cord.*

***sebaceous h.*** A hard protrusion from a sebaceous gland.

***ventral h.*** An anterior projection of the gray matter of the spinal cord.

***warty h.*** A hard outgrowth from a wart.

**Horner's syndrome** (hor′nĕrz) [Johann F. Horner, Swiss ophthalmologist, 1831–1886] A syndrome characterized by contraction of the pupil, partial ptosis of the eyelid, enophthalmos, and sometimes loss of sweating over one side of the face. The syndrome is caused by paralysis of the cervical sympathetic nerve trunk.

**horopter** (hō-rŏp′tĕr) [Gr. *horos,* limit, + *opter,* observer] The sum of all points in space that have a corresponding point on the retina of the eye.

**horripilation** (hor″ĭ-pĭ-lā′shŭn) [L. *horrere,* to bristle, + *pilus,* hair] Piloerection.

**horror** Intense fear, revulsion, or dread caused by seeing or hearing something that is terrifying, shocking, or perceived to be life-threatening to the individual or to others.

**horsepower** A unit of power equal to 745.7 watts, or 550 foot pounds per second.

**hospice** (hŏs′pĭs) An interdisciplinary program of palliative care and supportive services that addresses the physical, spiritual, social, and economic needs of terminally ill patients and their families. This care may be provided in the home or a hospice center. To obtain information about locating a hospice program call the National Hospice Organization at (800) 658-8898.

**hospital** [L. *hospitalis,* pert. to a guest] An institution for treatment of the sick and injured.

***base h.*** A hospital unit within the lines of an army that receives wounded and sick patients from the front and the line.

***camp h.*** An immobile military unit for the care of the sick and wounded in camp.

***evacuation h.*** A mobile advance hospital unit to replace field hospitals and supplement base hospitals.

***field h.*** A portable military hospital beyond the zone of conflict and the dressing stations.

***teaching h.*** A hospital concerned with instructing medical students, house officers (residents), and allied health personnel in conjunction with provision of medical care. The teaching programs may or may not be part of degree-granting programs, but most are part of a required curriculum for becoming licensed or eligible for certification in a medical or surgical specialty.

**hospitalism** [L. *hospitalis,* pert. to a guest, + Gr. *-ismos,* condition] **1.** The air of depression and apathy that often surrounds a group of seriously ill patients, esp. if they are in an overcrowded ward. **2.** A neurotic tendency to seek hospitalization and, once hospitalized, to resist being discharged.

**hospitalization** The removal of a patient to, and confinement in, a hospital.

**host** [L. *hospes,* a stranger] **1.** The organism from which a parasite obtains its nourishment. **2.** In embryology, the larger and more relatively normal of conjoined twins. **3.** In transplantation of tissue, the individual who receives the graft.

***accidental h.*** A host other than the usual or normal one.

***alternate h.*** Intermediate h. (1).

***h. defense mechanisms*** A complex interacting system that protects the host from endogenous and exogenous microorganisms. It includes physical and chemical barriers, inflammatory response, reticuloendothelial system, and immune responses. SEE: *cytokines; interleukin-1; interferon.*

***definitive h.*** **1.** The final host or the host in which the parasite reaches sexual maturity. SYN: *final h.* **2.** The vertebrate, when the intermediate host is an invertebrate.

***final h.*** Definitive h. (1).

***immunocompromised h.*** SEE: *immunocompromised.*

***intermediate h.*** **1.** The host in which a parasite passes through its larval or asexual stages of development. SYN: *alternate h.* **2.** The invertebrate host, when the final host is a vertebrate.

***h. of predilection*** The host preferred by a parasite.

***reservoir h.*** A host other than the usual or normal one, in which a parasite is capable of living and serving as a source of infestation.

***transfer h.*** An interim host that is not essential for the completion of the life cycle of the parasite.

**hostility** (hŏ-stĭl′ĭ-tē) In psychiatry, the manifestation of anger, animosity, or antagonism in a situation in which such a reaction is unwarranted. Hostility may be directed toward oneself, others, or inanimate objects. It is almost always a symptom of depression.

**hot** [AS. *hat,* hot] **1.** Possessing a high temperature. **2.** Actively conducting an electric current. **3.** Contaminated with dangerous radioactive material.

**hot flash** A symptom usually associated with menopause. SEE: *menopause.*

**hotline** A continuously managed telephone line for communicating with persons knowing about or experiencing a crisis, such as suicide contemplation, rape, child abuse, or illicit drug distribution.

**Hottentot apron** [Hottentot, southern African population] An excessive elongation of the labia minora seen in Hottentot women. SYN: *velamen vulvae.*

**hottentotism** (hŏt′ĕn-tŏt-ĭsm) [*Hottentot* + Gr. *-ismos,* condition] An abnormal form of stuttering.

**hot water bag** Rubber or plastic bag of various shapes and sizes for applying dry heat to circumscribed areas and for keeping moist applications warm.

**Hounsfield unit** In computerized tomography, a number or value that represents the attenuation of x-rays through a voxel (volume element) in the body and is assigned to the corresponding pixel (picture element) on the image. This number is relative to the standard, which is the absorption of x-rays in water.

**housefly** *Musca domestica,* a fly belonging to the order Diptera. It serves as a transmitter of organisms of many infectious diseases.

**housemaid's knee** SEE: under *knee.*

**house officer** An intern or resident appointed by a hospital to assist in providing medical care. This supervised individual receives medical training in order to meet the requirements for licensure or certification in a medical specialty. SEE: *hospital, teaching.*

**house physician** A physician, esp. an intern or resident, who is responsible for caring for patients under the direction of the medical and surgical staff.

**house staff** A nonspecific term for interns, residents, and other allied health professionals employed as part of the medical care team for a hospital. Their activities are supervised by the permanent hospital staff.

**house surgeon** ABBR: H.S. The senior surgical member of the hospital staff who acts in the absence of the attending surgeon.

**Houston's muscle** (hūs′tŏns) [John Houston, Irish surgeon, 1802–1845] The anterior part of the musculus bulbocavernosus of the penis.

**Houston's valve** One of the normal crescent-shaped folds of mucous membrane, or valves formed by them in the rectum.

**Howell-Jolly bodies** [William H. Howell, U.S. physiologist, 1860–1945; Justin Jolly, Fr. histologist, 1870–1953] Spherical granules seen in erythrocytes in slides of stained blood. They are thought to be nuclear particles. The bodies are seen in cases of congenital absence of the spleen; following splenectomy; in hemolytic anemia; in pernicious anemia; in thalassemia; and in leukemia. SEE: illus.

**Howship's lacuna** [John Howship, Brit. surgeon, 1781–1841] One of several small pits, grooves, or depressions found where bone is resorbed. It is usually occupied by osteoclasts. SEE: *osteoclast.*

**Howship's symptom** Paresthesia or pain in the obturator hernia on the inner side of the thigh.

**Hp** *haptoglobin.*

**HPG** *human pituitary gonadotropin.*

**HPL** *human placental lactogen.*

**HPLC** *high-pressure* or *high-performance liquid chromatography.*

**$HPO_3$** Metaphosphoric acid.

**$H_3PO_2$** Hypophosphorous acid.

**$H_3PO_3$** Phosphorous acid.

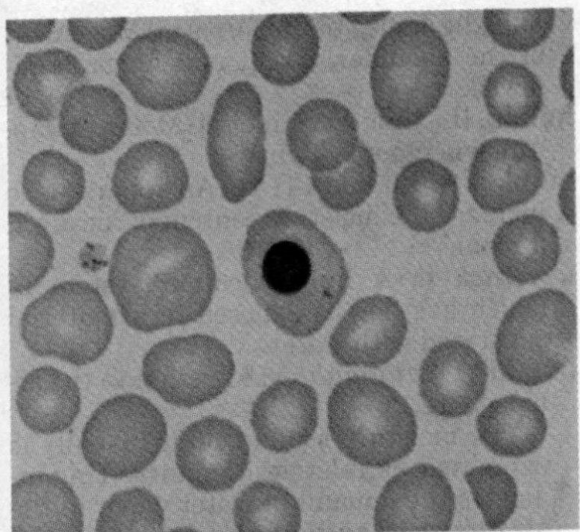

**HOWELL-JOLLY BODY** IN PERNICIOUS ANEMIA (ORIG. MAG. ×640)

**$H_3PO_4$** Orthophosphoric acid.

**$H_4P_2O_6$** Hypophosphoric acid.

**hr** *hour.*

**H2-receptor antagonists** Commonly termed H2 blocker; a chemical that blocks the interaction of histamine or acetylcholine with its receptors or parietal cells of the stomach. It acts as a potent inhibitor of gastric acid secretion. SEE: *hyperchlorhydria; peptic ulcer.*

**H reflex** [after Hoffmann who described it in 1918] In electrodiagnostic studies of spinal reflexes, the time required for a stimulus applied to a sensory nerve to travel to the spinal cord and return down the motor nerve. SEE: *F response.*

**H.S.** *house surgeon.*

**h.s.** *hora somni,* at bedtime.

**$H_2S$** Hydrogen sulfide.

**HSA** *human serum albumin.*

**$H_2SO_3$** Sulfurous acid.

**$H_2SO_4$** Sulfuric acid.

**H-substance** A substance similar to or identical with histamine.

**5-HT** *5-hydroxytryptamine,* serotonin.

**Ht** *total hypermetropia.*

**ht** *height.*

**HTLV-I** *human T-cell lymphotropic virus type I.*

**HTLV-II** *human T-cell lymphotropic virus type II.*

**HTLV-III** *human T-cell lymphotropic virus type III.*

**Hubbard tank** A tank of suitable size and shape for use in active or passive underwater exercises.

**hue** A property of each color that permits distinguishing it from another color.

**Huguier's canal** (ū-gē-āz′) [Pierre C. Huguier, Fr. surgeon, 1804–1873] The canal through which the chorda tympani nerve exits from the cranium.

**Huhner test** (hoon′ĕr) [Max Huhner, U.S. urologist, 1873–1947] Microscopic examination of a sample of cervical mucus taken shortly after sexual intercourse. Assessments include characteristics of the mucus as correlated with the phase of the woman's menstrual cycle, and the number and motility of the sperm in the endocervix.

**hum** A soft continuous sound.

***venous h.*** The sound from large veins in certain anemias.

**human** [L. *humanus,* human] Pert. to or characterizing men or women.

**human immunodeficiency virus** ABBR: HIV. A retrovirus of the subfamily lentivirus that causes acquired immunodeficiency syndrome (AIDS). The most common type of HIV is HIV-1, identified in 1984. HIV-2, first discovered in West Africa in 1986, causes a loss of immune function and the subsequent development of opportunistic infections identical to HIV-1 infections. The two types developed from separate strains of simian immunodeficiency virus. In the U.S., the number of individuals infected with HIV-2 is very small, but blood donations are screened for both types of HIV. SEE: *AIDS.*

**humanism** The concept that human interests, values, and dignity are of utmost importance. This is integral to the actions and thoughts of those who care for the sick.

**human papillomavirus** SEE: under *papillomavirus.*

**human T-cell lymphotropic virus type I** ABBR: HTLV-I. A virus associated with adult T-cell leukemia.

**human T-cell lymphotropic virus type II** ABBR: HTLV-II. A virus associated with hairy cell leukemia.

**human T-cell lymphotropic virus type III** ABBR: HTLV-III. The former name for human immunodeficiency virus.

**Humatin** Trade name for paromomycin sulfate.

**humectant** (hū-mĕk′tănt) [L. *humectus,* moist] A moistening agent.

**humeral** (hū′mĕr-ăl) [L. *humerus,* upper arm] Pert. to the humerus.

**humeroradial** (hū″mĕr-ō-rā′dē-ăl) [″ + *radius,* wheel spoke, ray] Pert. to the humerus and radius, esp. in comparison of their lengths.

**humeroscapular** (hū″mĕr-ō-skăp′ū-lăr) [″ + *scapula,* shoulder blade] Concerning the humerus and scapula.

**humeroulnar** (hū″mĕr-ō-ŭl′năr) [″ + *ulna,* elbow] Pert. to the humerus and ulna, esp. in comparison of their lengths.

**humerus** (hū′mĕr-ŭs) [L., upper arm] The upper bone of the arm from the elbow (articulating with the ulna and radius) to the shoulder joint, where it articulates with the scapula. SEE: illus.

***fracture of h.*** Physical injury of the humerus sufficient to fracture it. If the fracture is of the upper end of the humerus, the arm is abducted on a wire splint for about 4 weeks. Movements of the elbow and wrist are started early, and active movements of the shoulder are begun in about 3 weeks. SEE: *acromiohumeral;*

*capitellum; cubitus; glenoid cavity.*

In a fracture of the shaft and lower end of the humerus, the limb is put in a plaster cast in a position midway between pronation and supination with the humerus at right angles to the forearm. Movement of the shoulder, wrist, and finger is allowed.



**humid** [L. *humidus,* moist] Moist, damp, esp. when pert. to air.

**humidifier** (hū-mĭd′ĭ-fī″ĕr) An apparatus to increase the moisture content of the air in a room.

***wick h.*** A humidification system in which gas flow is exposed to a material saturated with water.

**humidity** [L. *humiditas*] Moisture in the atmosphere.

The moisture content of air usually is expressed as relative humidity. This indicates the amount of water vapor in the air compared with the maximum amount of moisture the air could contain at that temperature and atmospheric pressure. Air that is fully saturated with moisture has 100% relative humidity. When air that is fully saturated is cooled, the excess moisture condenses as in the case of dew or moisture on a cold glass in the summer.

If air was saturated at a temperature of 70°F (21.1°C), water would condense on all objects if the temperature fell to 68°F (20°C). At 90°F (32.2°C) air can contain almost twice as much water as it can at 70°F (21.1°C).

Moist air is less dense than completely dry air. This is another reason for humidifying oxygen or air used in inhalation therapy. Also humid air is much less irritating to the respiratory tract mucosa than dry air.

***absolute h.*** The actual mass of water vapor in a volume of gas, expressed as grams per cubic meter or milligrams per liter. It usually refers to ambient air.

***relative h.*** The ratio of the amount of water vapor present in an air sample to the amount that could be present if the sample were saturated with water vapor. This value is always influenced by the temperature of the air sample.

**humor** (hū′mor) [L. *humor,* fluid] Any fluid or semifluid in the body. **humoral** (-ăl), *adj.*

***aqueous h.*** The clear, watery fluid in the anterior and posterior chambers of the eye. It is produced by the ciliary processes and passes from the posterior to the anterior chamber, and then to the venous system by way of the canal of Schlemm.

***crystalline h.*** The fluidlike substance of the crystalline lens of the eye.

***vitreous h.*** The vitreous body; a semifluid, transparent substance occupying the space between the lens and retina.

**humpback** SEE: *kyphosis.*

**Humulin** Trade name for human insulin.

**hunchback** SEE: *kyphosis.*

**hunger** [AS. *hungur*] **1.** A sensation resulting from lack of food, characterized by a dull or acute pain referred to the epigastrium or lower part of chest. It is usually accompanied by weakness and an overwhelming desire to eat. Hunger pains coincide with powerful contractions of the stomach. Hunger is distinguished from appetite in that the latter is a pleasant sensation based on previous experience that causes one to seek food for the purpose of tasting and enjoying it. **2.** To have a strong desire.

***air h.*** Dyspnea; breathlessness.

***h. contractions*** Contractions occurring in the normal empty stomach, which may be painful. A series of such contractions is followed by a period of rest, after which the contractions may return with great intensity unless food is taken.

***h. pain*** Pain caused by a need for food, coinciding with powerful contractions of the stomach. It may be indicative of gastric disorder.

**Hunner's ulcer** (hŭn'ĕrz) [Guy LeRoy Hunner, U.S. surgeon, 1868–1957] Interstitial cystitis.

**Hunter's canal** [John Hunter, Scot. anatomist and surgeon, 1728–1793] Adductor canal.

**Hunter's disease** [Charles H. Hunter, Canadian physician, 1873–1955] Mucopolysaccharidosis II.

**hunterian chancre** Indurated, syphilitic chancre. SEE: *chancre.*

**Huntington's chorea, Huntington's disease** [George Huntington, U.S. physician, 1850–1916] An inherited disease of the central nervous system that usually has its onset between ages 25 and 55 (with the average age 35). Degeneration in the cerebral cortex and basal ganglia causes chronic progressive chorea (bizarre, involuntary dancelike movements) and mental deterioration, ending in dementia. The disease slowly progresses, and death usually results in 10 to 15 years from heart failure or an intercurrent infection such as pneumonia.

ETIOLOGY: In 1993, after decades of research, scientists discovered the gene that causes Huntington's disease. Because the disease is transmitted as an autosomal dominant trait, either sex can transmit or inherit it. Each child of a parent with the disease (usually born before the disease became evident) has a 50% chance of inheriting it; however, the child who does not inherit it cannot pass it on to his or her own children. Genetic counseling is important for any couple in which one individual has had a parent with this disease and thus may have inherited the defective gene.

SYMPTOMS: Assessment findings vary, depending on the disease progression. The patient's history usually shows a family history of the disorder, along with emotional and mental changes. The onset of Huntington's disease is insidious. The patient eventually becomes totally dependent through intellectual decline, emotional disturbances, and loss of musculoskeletal control. Potential complications include choking, aspiration, pneumonia, heart failure, and infections.

In the early stages, the patient is described as being clumsy, irritable, or impatient and subject to fits of anger and periods of suicidal depression, apathy, or elation. As the disease progresses, family members may report that the patient's judgment and memory have become impaired. Hallucinations, delusions, and paranoid thinking may occur. In later stages, emotional symptoms may subside, but eventually dementia does occur. The family describes a gradual loss of intellectual ability, although the patient seems to be aware that the symptoms result from the disease. The dementia does not always progress at the same rate as the chorea. The patient may be described as having a ravenous appetite, especially for sweets. In late stages, the patient may lose bladder and bowel control.

Inspection usually reveals choreic movements that are involuntary, purposeless, rapid, and often violent. In the early stages, the movements are unilateral and more prominent in the face and arms than in the legs. As the disease progresses, the choreic movements progress from mild fidgeting to grimacing, tongue smacking, dysarthria (indistinct speech), athetoid movements (especially of the hands) due to the emotional state, and torticollis. In later stages, the movements involve the entire body musculature. Writhing and twitching are constant, speech becomes intelligible, chewing and swallowing are difficult, and ambulation is impossible. In these late stages, the patient may appear emaciated and exhausted.

DIAGNOSIS: Positron emission tomography scanning and deoxyribonucleic acid analysis can detect Huntington's disease, but no reliable confirming test exists. However, the recent discovery of the causative gene opens the way for development of further tests to detect and predict the disease. Computed tomography scan, a secondary study, shows brain atrophy.

TREATMENT: Because no cure currently exists for this condition, treatment is supportive, protective, and based on the patient's symptoms. Tranquilizers, as well as chlorpromazine, haloperidol, or imipramine, help to control choreic movement, but cannot stop mental deterioration. They also alleviate discomfort and depression. However, tranquilizers increase rigidity. To control choreic movements without rigidity, choline may be prescribed. Psychotherapy to decrease anxiety and stress also may be helpful. The patient may require institutionalization because of mental deterioration.

NURSING IMPLICATIONS: Temperature and white blood cell count are monitored for early detection and correction of infection. Signs of neurological deterioration are assessed. The patient and family are educated about the disease and its genetic cause, and diagnostic tests and prescribed treatments are explained. Prescribed medication is administered and evaluated for desired responses and any adverse reactions, and the patient and family are instructed in its use. Self-care deficits are identified and physical support is provided for basic needs, such as hygiene, skin care, nutrition, and bowel and bladder care; support is increased as mental and physical deterioration make the patient increasingly immobile. The nurse encourages the patient to remain as independent as possible by providing short, explicit directions; demonstrations; and ample time to perform tasks that the patient can still manage. To help improve the patient's self-concept, the patient should participate in care as much as possible, and the nurse should assist the patient to adapt to any changes. The nurse provides psychological support to the patient and family by listening to their fears and concerns, by staying with them during stressful periods, and by answering questions honestly. If the patient has difficulty speaking, communications aids, such as an alphabet board, are provided, and sufficient time is allowed for the patient to communicate; the nurse should refrain from putting words into the patient's mouth. The nurse stays alert for possible suicide attempts and takes precautions to protect the patient from suicide or other self-inflicted injury. Physical restraints should be avoided, however, because they may cause the patient injury during violent, uncontrolled movements. If the patient has difficulty walking, the patient should use a walker to help maintain balance. If choreic movements are violent enough to cause injury, the nurse ensures that the patient is secure when sitting in a chair or wheelchair. If the patient is confined to bed, the nurse repositions him or her frequently (major changes every 2 hr, minor ones at least every 1/2 hr) and posts a turning schedule at the bedside. The nurse also assists the patient with range-of-motion exercises. The nurse helps to minimize the patient's risk for infection by thorough handwashing before providing care and by assisting the patient to wash the hands before and after meals and after urinating or defecating. The patient's head is elevated to 90 degrees when the patient is eating to reduce the risk of aspiration, and the nurse remains with the patient, reminding him or her to take only small amounts of food at one time. The urinary incontinent patient requires bladder elimination devices, such as an external condom catheter, incontinent pads and pants, and if absolutely necessary, an indwelling urinary catheter. The bowel incontinent patient requires pads or pants and bed protector pads. In either case, a record is kept of the patient's elimination habits, voiding or defecation needs anticipated, and the patient toileted on awakening, before and after meals, and before sleep. The nurse refers the patient for home healthcare follow-up and teaches the family to provide care at home. The family should obtain genetic counseling, because all offspring of an affected individual have a 50% chance of inheriting this disease. Both patient and family are also referred to appropriate community support agencies, such as social services and respite care services, and for outpatient psychiatric care and supportive psychiatric counseling and, as necessary, to long-term care facilities. In addition, they are referred to the Huntington's Disease Society of America for more information and support.

**Hunt's neuralgia, Hunt's syndrome** [Ramsey Hunt, U.S. neurologist, 1872–1937] Herpes zoster of the ganglion of the facial nerve. There is pain in the ear with a bloody serous discharge due to vesicles on the tympanic membrane. The face is paralyzed on the affected side, and the sense of taste is lost in the anterior two thirds of the tongue on the affected side.

**Hurler's syndrome** (hoor′lĕrz) [Gertrud Hurler, Ger. pediatrician, 1889–1965] Mucopolysaccharidosis I-H.

**Hürthle cells** (hĕr′tĕl) [Karl Hürthle, Ger. histologist, 1860–1945] Large eosinophil-staining cells occasionally present in the thyroid gland. SEE: *tumor, Hürthle cell.*

**Huschke, Emil** (hoosh′kēz) German anatomist, 1797–1858.

***H.'s auditory teeth*** Tiny, toothlike protuberances at the edge of the cochlear labium vestibulare.

***H.'s canal*** A canal formed by the juncture of the annulus tympanicus tubercules; usually present only during early childhood.

***H.'s foramen*** A perforation found in arrested development near the inner extremity of the tympanic plate.

***H.'s valve*** Plica lacrimalis.

**Hutchinson, Sir Jonathan** British surgeon, 1828–1913.

***H.-Gilford disease*** Progeria.

***H.'s patch*** Salmon patch.

***H.'s pupil*** A condition in which one pupil is dilated and the other is not. The pupil on the side of the lesion is dilated and the other is contracted. This condition is usually due to compression of the third cranial nerve in meningitis.

***H.'s teeth*** A congenital condition marked by pegged, lateral incisors and notched central incisors along the cutting edge. It is a sign of congenital syphilis.

***H.'s triad*** In congenital syphilis, the presence of interstitial keratosis, deafness, and Hutchinson's teeth.

**Huxley's layer** (hŭks′lēz) [Thomas H. Huxley, Brit. physiologist and naturalist,

1825–1895] The inner layer of nucleated cells forming the inner root sheath of a hair follicle.

**HVA** *homovanillic acid.*

**hyalin** (hī′ă-lĭn) [Gr. *hyalos,* glass] **1.** A clear substance present in tissues that have undergone amyloid degeneration. **2.** Material deposited in the glomerulus in certain forms of glomerulonephritis.

**hyaline** (hī′ă-lĭn) A histological term rather than a specific indicator of cell injury, referring to any alteration within cells or in the extracellular space that gives a homogeneous, glassy, pink appearance in reactive histological sections stained with hematoxylin and eosin. SYN: *hyaloid.*

**hyaline body** SEE: under *body.*

**hyaline cast** SEE: under *cast.*

**hyaline membrane disease** Respiratory distress syndrome of the newborn.

**hyalinization** (hī″ă-lĭn″ĭ-zā′shŭn) The development of an albuminoid mass in a cell or tissue.

**hyalinosis** (hī″ă-lĭn-ō′sĭs) [Gr. *hyalos,* glass, + *osis,* condition] Waxy or hyaline degeneration.

**hyalinuria** (hī″ă-lĭn-ū′rē-ă) [″ + *ouron,* urine] Hyalin present in the urine.

**hyalitis** (hī-ă-lī′tĭs) [″ + *itis,* inflammation] An inflammation of the hyaloid membrane of the vitreous humor. SYN: *hyaloiditis.*

***asteroid h.*** One of the spherical or star-shaped bodies in the vitreous of the eye, caused by inflammation.

***h. punctata*** A form of hyalitis marked by minute opacities in the vitreous humor.

***h. suppurativa*** A purulent inflammation of the vitreous humor.

**hyalo-** [Gr. *hyalos,* glass] Combining form indicating resemblance to glass.

**hyaloenchondroma** (hī″ă-lō-ĕn″kŏn-drō′mă) [″ + *en,* in, + *chondros,* cartilage, + *oma,* tumor] A chondroma composed of hyaline cartilage.

**hyalogen** (hī-ăl′ō-jĕn) [″ + *gennan,* to produce] A protein substance in cartilage and the vitreous humor.

**hyaloid** (hī′ă-loyd) [″ + *eidos,* form, shape] Hyaline, glassy.

**hyaloid artery** SEE: under *artery.*

**hyaloid canal** SEE: under *canal.*

**hyaloiditis** (hī″ă-loyd-ī′tĭs) [″ + *eidos,* form, shape, + *itis,* inflammation] Hyalitis.

**hyaloid membrane** SEE: under *membrane.*

**hyalomucoid** (hī″ă-lō-mū′koyd) [″ + L. *mucus,* mucus, + Gr. *eidos,* form, shape] Glycoprotein in the vitreous body.

**hyalonyxis** (hī″ă-lō-nĭk′sĭs) [″ + *nyxis,* puncture] The surgical procedure of puncturing the vitreous body.

**hyalophagia, hyalophagy** (hī″ă-lō-fā′jē-ă, -lŏf′ă-jē) [″ + *phagein,* to eat] The eating of glass.

**hyalophobia** (hī″ă-lō-fō′bē-ă) [″ + *phobos,* fear] A fear of touching glass.

**hyaloplasm** (hī′ă-lŏ-plăzm) [″ + LL. *plasma,* form, mold] The fluid portion of protoplasm; the basic ground substance, also called basic or fundamental protoplasm. SYN: *hyalotome.*

**hyalosis** (hī″ă-lō′sĭs) [″ + *osis,* condition] Pathologic changes in the vitreous humor of the eye.

***asteroid h.*** Suspended spherical white bodies, made of calcium salts, in the vitreous humor of the eye.

**hyalosome** (hī-ăl′ō-sōm) [″ + *soma,* body] An oval or round structure that resembles the nucleolus of a cell but stains only faintly.

**hyalotome** (hī-ăl′ō-tōm) [Gr. *hyalos,* glass] Hyaloplasm.

**hyaluronidase** (hī″ă-lūr-ŏn′ĭ-dās) An enzyme found in the testes and semen. It depolymerizes hyaluronic acid, thereby increasing the permeability of connective tissues by dissolving the substances that hold body cells together. It acts to disperse the cells of the corona radiata about the newly ovulated ovum, thus facilitating entry of the sperm.

**hybrid** (hī′brĭd) [L. *hybrida,* mongrel] The offspring of parents that are different, such as different species.

**hybridization** (hī′brĭd-ī-zā′shŭn) The production of hybrids by crossbreeding.

**hybridoma** (hī″brĭ-dō′mă) The cell produced by the fusion of an antibody-producing cell and a multiple myeloma cell. This hybrid cell is capable of producing a continuous supply of identical antibodies. SEE: *monoclonal antibody.*

**hydantoin** (hī-dăn′tō-ĭn) A colorless base, glycolyl urea, $C_3H_4N_2O_2$, derived from urea or allantoin.

**hydatid** (hī′dă-tĭd) [Gr. *hydatis,* watery vesicle] **1.** A cyst formed in the tissues, esp. the liver, resulting from the development of the larval stage of the dog tapeworm, *Echinococcus granulosus.* The cyst develops slowly, forming a hollow bladder from the inner surface of which hollow brood capsules are formed. These may be attached to the mother cyst by slender stalks or may fall free into the fluid-filled cavity of the mother cyst. Scolices form on the inner surface of the older brood capsules. Older cysts have a granular deposit of brood capsules and scolices called hydatid sand. Hydatids may grow for years, sometimes to an enormous size. Albendazole, a drug available only from its manufacturer, SmithKline Beecham, has been used to treat this disease. It is poorly absorbed, must be used for a prolonged period, and can be toxic to the liver. The cysts should be removed surgically. SEE: illus.; *echinococcosis.* **2.** A small cystic remnant of an embryonic structure.

***h. of Morgagni*** A cystlike remnant of the mullerian duct that is attached to the fallopian tube.

***sessile h.*** Morgagnian hydatid connected with a testicle.

***stalked h.*** Morgagnian hydatid connected with a fallopian tube.

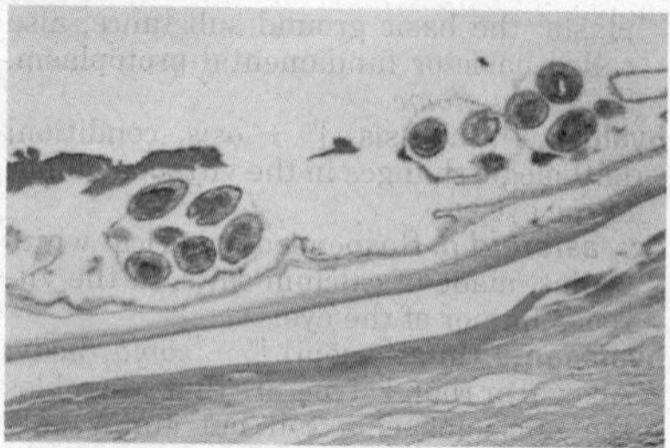


**HYDATID CYST** WITH THREE BROOD CAPSULES (ORIG. MAG. ×100)

**hydatidiform** (hī″dă-tĭd′ĭ-form) [″ + L. *forma,* shape] Having the form of a hydatid. SYN: *hydatiform.*

**hydatid mole** SEE: under *mole.*

**hydatidocele** (hī″dă-tĭd′ō-sēl) [″ + *kele,* tumor, swelling] A hydatid cyst of the scrotum or testicle.

**hydatidoma** (hī″dă-tĭd-ō′mă) [″ + *oma,* tumor] A tumor consisting of hydatids.

**hydatidosis** (hī″dă-tĭd-ō′sĭs) [Gr. *hydatis,* watery vesicle, + *osis,* condition] A condition caused by hydatid infestation.

**hydatidostomy** (hī″dă-tĭ-dŏs′tō-mē) [″ + *stoma,* mouth] The evacuation of a hydatid cyst by means of surgery.

**hydatiform** (hī-dăt′ĭ-form) [″ + L. *forma,* form] Hydatidiform.

**hydatism** (hī′dă-tĭzm) [″ + *-ismos,* condition] The sound produced by fluid in a cavity.

**hydr-** SEE: *hydro-.*

**hydradenitis** (hī″drăd-ĕn-ī′tĭs) [Gr. *hydros,* sweat, + *aden,* gland, + *itis,* inflammation] Inflammation of a sweat gland.

**hydradenoma** (hī″drăd-ĕ-nō′mă) [″ + ″ + *oma,* tumor] A tumor of a sweat gland.

**hydraeroperitoneum** (hī-dră″ĕr-ō-pĕr″ĭ-tō-nē′ŭm) [Gr. *hydor,* water, + *aer,* air, + *peritonaion,* peritoneum] A collection of fluid and gas in the peritoneal cavity.

**hydralazine hydrochloride** (hī-drăl′ă-zēn) An antihypertensive drug. Trade names are Apresoline Hydrochloride and Hydralyn.

**hydramnion, hydramnios** (hī-drăm′nē-ŏn, -ŏs) [″ + *amnion,* a caul on a lamb] An excess of amniotic fluid, which leads to an overdistention of the uterus and the possibility of malpresentation of the fetus. The normal amount is 500 to 1000 ml, but this may increase to 2500 ml and not be regarded as abnormal.

Amniotic fluid is secreted by the amnion. Fetal urine contributes to the volume after the fourth gestational month. Abnormal amounts of liquor amnii are probably caused by some abnormality of the fetus. Nearly half the cases are the result of a twin pregnancy. Hydramnion begins about the fifth month, with the uterus being large for the length of pregnancy. The pressure of the enlarged uterus gives rise to maternal breathlessness, edema, cyanosis, and varicose veins. The fetus may be felt bobbing about in the amniotic fluid, and the fetal heart is not easily heard.

TREATMENT: Amniocentesis is necessary to reduce the amount of amniotic fluid. Because the fluid is rapidly replenished, the procedure will have to be frequently repeated.

**hydranencephaly** (hī″drăn-ĕn-sĕf′ă-lē) [″ + *an-,* not, + *enkephalos,* brain] Internal hydrocephalus caused by congenital absence of the cerebral hemispheres.

**hydrarthrosis** (hī″drăr-thrō′sĭs) [″ + *arthron,* joint, + *osis,* condition] Serous effusion in a joint cavity; white swelling.

***intermittent h.*** Intermittent and usually painless swelling of the same joint, a condition that lasts for 3 to 5 days, affecting women more often than men. The period between attacks is commonly 2 to 4 weeks, during which time the joint is normal. The knee is the usual joint involved but the elbow, hip, and ankle also may be affected. No satisfactory treatment exists.

**hydrase** (hī′drās) An enzyme that catalyzes the addition or withdrawal of water from a compound without hydrolysis occurring.

**hydrate** (hī′drāt) A crystalline substance formed by water combining with various compounds.

**hydrated** (hī′drā-tĕd) [L. *hydratus*] Combined chemically with water, forming a hydrate.

**hydration** (hī-drā′shŭn) **1.** The chemical combination of a substance with water. **2.** The addition of water to a substance or tissue.

**hydraulics** (hī-draw′lĭks) [Gr. *hydor,* water, + *aulos,* pipe] The science of fluids.

**hydrazine** (hī′dră-zēn) **1.** $H_4N_2$. A colorless gas with a peculiar odor; soluble in water. **2.** One of a class derived from hydrazine.

**hydremia** (hī-drē′mē-ă) [Gr. *hydor,* water, + *haima,* blood] An excess of watery fluid in the blood.

**hydrencephalocele** (hī″drĕn-sĕf′ă-lō-sēl) [″ + *enkephalos,* brain, + *kele,* tumor] Hydroencephalocele.

**hydrencephalomeningocele** (hī″drĕn-sĕf″ă-lō-mĕ-nĭng′gō-sēl) [″ + ″ + *meninx,* membrane, + *kele,* tumor, swelling] A herniation through a defect in the skull. It contains brain substance and cerebrospinal fluid covered by meningeal tissues.

**hydrencephalus** (hī″drĕn-sĕf′ă-lŭs) Hydrocephalus.

**hydrepigastrium** (hī″drĕp-ĭ-găs′trē-ŭm) [″ + *epi,* upon, + *gaster,* belly] An accumulation of fluid between the peritoneum and the abdominal muscles.

**hydride** (hī′drīd) A chemical compound containing hydrogen and an element or radical.

**hydrion** (hī-drī′ŏn) The hydrogen ion ($H^+$).

**hydro-, hydr-** [Gr. *hydor,* water] Combining

form pert. to water or to hydrogen.

**hydroa** (hĭd-rō′ă) Any bullous skin eruption.

**hydroappendix** (hī″drō-ă-pĕn′dĭks) [″ + L. *appendere,* to hang upon] Watery fluid distending the vermiform appendix.

**hydrobilirubin** (hī″drō-bĭl″ĭ-roo′bĭn) [″ + L. *bilis,* bile, + *ruber,* red] A brownish-red bile pigment, derived from bilirubin, and thought to be identical with stercobilin and urobilin.

**hydrobromate** (hī″drō-brō′māt) [″ + *bromos,* stench] A salt of hydrobromic acid.

**hydrocalycosis** (hī″drō-kăl″ĭ-kō′sĭs) [″ + *kalyx,* cup, + *osis,* condition] Cystic dilation of the renal calix owing to obstruction.

**hydrocarbon** (hī″drō-kăr′bŏn) [″ + L. *carbo,* coal] A compound made up only of hydrogen and carbon.

***alicyclic h.*** A hydrocarbon that contains cyclic and straight-chain components.

***aliphatic h.*** A straight-chain hydrocarbon that contains no cyclic component.

***aromatic h.*** A hydrocarbon in which the carbon atoms are in a ring, or cyclic, configuration.

***cyclic h.*** A hydrocarbon in which the carbon atoms are in a ring configuration.

***saturated h.*** A hydrocarbon in which the carbon atoms are linked by a single electron pair and in which all valences are satisfied.

***unsaturated h.*** A hydrocarbon in which carbon atoms share two or three pairs of electrons.

**hydrocele** (hī′drō-sēl) [″ + *kele,* tumor, swelling] The accumulation of serous fluid in a saclike cavity, esp. in the tunica vaginalis testis.

***acute h.*** The most common hydrocele. The majority of cases occur suddenly between the second and fifth years, usually the result of inflammation of the epididymis or testis.

***cervical h.*** A hydrocele in the neck resulting from the accumulation of serous fluid in the persistent cervical duct or cleft.

***chronic h.*** A hydrocele usually seen in middle-aged men. It may result from filariasis.

***congenital h.*** A hydrocele present at birth, resulting from failure of closure of the vaginal process.

***encysted h.*** A hydrocele in the vaginal process in which openings to the scrotal and peritoneal cavities are closed.

***h. feminae*** A hydrocele in the labium majus or canal of Nuck. SYN: *h. muliebris.*

***h. hernialis*** A condition in which a hernia accompanies infantile or congenital hydrocele and peritoneal fluid accumulates in a hernial sac.

***infantile h.*** Peritoneal fluid in the tunica vaginalis and vaginal process with the latter closed at the abdominal ring.

***h. muliebris*** H. feminae.

***spermatic h.*** Spermatic fluid in the tunica vaginalis of the testes.

***h. spinalis*** Spina bifida cystica.

**hydrocelectomy** (hī″drō-sē-lĕk′tō-mē) [″ + ″ + *ektome,* excision] Surgical removal of a hydrocele.

**hydrocephalocele** (hī″drō-sĕf′ă-lō-sēl) [″ + *kephale,* head, + *kele,* tumor] Hydroencephalocele.

**hydrocephaloid** (hī″drō-sĕf′ă-loyd) [″ + ″ + *eidos,* form, shape] Resembling or pert. to hydrocephalus.

**hydrocephaloid disease** A condition resembling hydrocephalus, except that the fontanels of the infant are depressed owing to dehydration.

**hydrocephalus** (hī-drō-sĕf′ă-lŭs) [″ + *kephale,* head] The increased accumulation of cerebrospinal fluid within the ventricles of the brain, resulting from interference with normal circulation and with absorption of the fluid and esp. from destruction or blockage of the foramina of Magendie and Luschka. This may be caused by developmental anomalies, infection, injury, or brain tumors. In severe cases in children, the head is usually globular or pyramidal in shape. The face is disproportionately small with eyes hidden in sockets and turned upward. Sutures are separated with bulging fontanels and thin cranial bones. After the skull has formed in older individuals, there are headache, vomiting, choked disks, atrophy of the optic nerve, and mental disturbances. SYN: *hydrencephalus.* SEE: *Nursing Diagnoses Appendix.* **hydrocephalic,** *adj.*

TREATMENT: If hydrocephalus progresses, the condition is treated by a surgical procedure that uses a shunt through which the cerebrospinal fluid flows, connecting the ventricular system with a suitable cavity such as the peritoneal cavity.

PROGNOSIS: In untreated cases of congenital hydrocephalus, the outcome is fatal in about half of the patients. The prognosis for an uncomplicated course is excellent when hydrocephalus is promptly treated by use of a surgically instituted shunt.

NURSING IMPLICATIONS: *Preoperative:* The infant (or older child with fused cranium) is assessed for signs of increased intracranial pressure (ICP), such as frontal headache, nausea and vomiting that may be projectile, decreased level of consciousness, ataxia, and impaired intellectual functioning, and possibly incontinence. On inspection of the infant's head, bulging of the anterior fontanel may be observed before any increases in head circumference. Head circumference is measured and a picture drawn to indicate the measurement location for other staff members. The patient is also inspected for other characteristic findings, including distended scalp veins; thin, fragile, and shiny scalp skin; and underdeveloped neck muscles. In severe hydrocephalus, the parents may report a high-pitched, shrill cry; irritability; anorexia; and episodes of projectile vomiting. Inspection may reveal depression of the eye orbit, displacement of the eyes downward, and prominent sclera. On neurologic examination, abnormal muscle tone may be observed in the legs. The infant is monitored for such signs of neurological complications as seizure activity, irregular respirations, and bradycardia, and such changes are documented and reported immediately. If the infant's head is enlarged, the head position is changed frequently and assessed for skin breakdown. Placing a lambskin or foam or flotation (low pressure) pads under the infant's head may help to prevent skin breakdown and to provide comfort. The head of the bed is elevated 30 degrees to help alleviate increasing ICP. To prevent strqin on the infant's neck during movement, the head, neck, and shoulders are moved with his body as one unit. Oxygen is administered if prescribed, and suction equipment maintained at the bedside for use as necessary. Small, frequent feedings are provided to ensure adequate nutrition and to lessen vomiting by decreasing movement during and immediately after meals. The infant is fed slowly, with the head, neck, and shoulders resting on a pillow to lessen the strain of holding this weight on the arm. To prevent aspiration after feeding and to reduce the potential for hypostatic pneumonia, the infant is placed on the side and repositioned every 2 hr or propped in an infant seat. The infant's growth and development are monitored periodically. Calm, realistic reassurance and emotional support are offered to the parents, and they are encouraged to verbalize their concerns about the disease process, the surgery, and long-term rehabilitation of the child. The nurse encourages maternal-infant bonding where possible and holds, cuddles, and strokes the infant and speaks soothingly while providing care. The signed informed consent form is obtained, the patient prepared for surgery, and prescribed preoperative medications are administered.

*Postoperative:* Vital signs and neurological status are monitored hourly or as necessary according to institutional protocol or the surgeon's directions. In infants, the anterior fontanel is inspected for bulging or depression. The patient is positioned as directed by the surgeon, usually on the nonoperative side with the head level with the body. Fluid intake and output are monitored, and I.V. fluids are administered as prescribed. The patient is assessed for vomiting (an early sign of increased ICP and shunt malfunction). The patient is monitored for signs of infection (especially meningitis) such as fever, stiff neck, irritability, or tense fontanels. The area over the shunt tract is also inspected for redness, swelling, and other signs of local infection. Dressings are checked for drainage and the wound redressed as necessary using aseptic technique. The patient is also observed for other signs and symptoms of postoperative complications, such as adhesions, paralytic ileus, peritonitis, migration, intestinal perforation (with peritoneal shunt), and dehydration and septicemia. Prescribed analgesics are administered; the dose is carefully titrated to provide pain relief while still permitting adequate neurological assessment. The family is taught postoperative care measures, including watching for signs of shunt malfunction, infection, and paralytic ileus. The nurse explains that shunt insertion requires periodic surgery to lengthen the shunt as the child grows and that surgery also may be necessary to correct malfunctions or treat infection. The nurse helps the parents set goals consistent with the patient's ability and potential, explaining that they should focus on the child's strengths rather than weaknesses. Special education programs are also discussed with the parents; the infant's need for sensory stimulation appropriate to age is emphasized.

***communicating h.*** Hydrocephalus that maintains normal communication between the fourth ventricle and subarachnoid space.

***congenital h.*** A chronic type of hydrocephalus occurring in infancy.

***external h.*** An accumulation of fluid in subdural spaces.

***internal h.*** An accumulation of fluid within ventricles of the brain.

***noncommunicating h.*** Hydrocephalus in which a blockage at any location in the ventricular system prevents flow of cerebrospinal fluid to the subarachnoid space.

***normal pressure h.*** A type of hydrocephalus with enlarged ventricles of the brain with no increase in the spinal fluid pressure or no demonstrable block to the outflow of spinal fluid. Shunting fluids from the dilated ventricles to the peritoneal cavity may be helpful. SEE: *hydrocephalus.*

***secondary h.*** Hydrocephalus following injury or infections such as meningitis or syphilis.

**hydrochlorate** (hī″drō-klō′rāt) [Gr. *hydor,* water, + *chloros,* green] Any salt of hydrochloric acid.

**hydrochloric acid** An aqueous solution of hydrogen chloride (HCl), containing 35% to 38% HCl by weight. Crude commercial hydrochloric acid is known as muriatic acid.

This normal constituent of gastric juice is produced by the parietal (or oxyntic) cells of gastric glands. The HCl concentration in the stomach varies, depending on several factors, including rate of secretion of gastric juice and the type of food eaten.

It converts pepsinogen into pepsin and produces an acid medium favorable for the activity of pepsin; dissolves and disintegrates nucleoproteins and collagen; hydrolyzes sucrose; precipitates caseinogen; inhibits multiplication of bacteria, esp. putrefactive organisms that ferment lactic acid and certain pathogenic forms; stimulates secretion by the duodenum; inhibits the action of ptyalin and thus stops salivary digestion in the stomach.

The average amount of hydrochloric acid found in the food content of the stomach is small because of dilution and neutralization by alkaline contents. In pernicious anemia, hydrochloric acid is absent from the stomach (achlorhydria).

**hydrochloride** (hī″drō-klō′rīd) An alkaloid or other base combined with hydrochloric acid.

**hydrochlorothiazide** (hī″drō-klō″rō-thī′ă-zīd) A diuretic.

**hydrocholeretic** (hī″drō-kō″lĕr-ĕt′ĭk) Any agent that increases the output of bile without increasing the solids secreted in it.

**hydrocirsocele** (hī″drō-sĭr′sō-sēl) [″ + *kirsos,* varix, + *kele,* tumor, swelling] A hydrocele combined with varicose veins of the spermatic cord.

**hydrocodone bitartrate** (hī″drō-kō′dōn) An analgesic drug. Trade name is Vicodin.

**hydrocolloid** (hī″drō-kŏl′loyd) [″ + *kollodes,* glutinous] A colloidal suspension in which water is the liquid.

***h. dressing*** SEE: under *dressing.*

***irreversible h.*** A hydrosol of alginic acid whose physical state is changed by an irreversible chemical reaction, forming insoluble calcium alginate. This substance is called alginate or dental alginate.

**hydrocolpos** (hī″drō-kŏl′pŏs) [″ + *kolpos,* vagina] Retention cyst of the vagina containing watery, nonsanguineous fluid or mucus.

**hydrocortisone** (hī″drō-kor′tĭ-sōn) Pharmaceutical name for cortisol, an adrenocortical hormone produced by the adrenal cortex. It is closely related to cortisone in physiological effects. SYN: *cortisol.*

***h. acetate*** A form of corticosteroid that acts slowly over a long period.

**hydrocyanic acid** A colorless liquid that is a deadly poison. SYN: *hydrogen cyanide.* SEE: *cyanide poisoning.*

**hydrocyst** (hī′drō-sĭst) [Gr. *hydor,* water, + *kystis,* bladder] A cyst containing watery fluid.

**hydrocystoma** [″ + ″ + *oma,* tumor] A disease marked by small cysts that originate in the sweat glands. These cysts may appear on the face, esp. in women after middle age. SYN: *hidrocystoma.*

**hydrodensitometry** The weighing of an object immersed in water and subsequent measurement of the water displaced. The specific gravity of the body can be estimated from that information, and the percentage of the body fat can be estimated.

**hydrodiascope** (hī″drō-dī′ă-skōp) [″ + *dia,* through, + *skopein,* to examine] A device used to treat astigmatism.

**hydrodictiotomy** (hī″drō-dĭk″tē-ŏt′ō-mē) [″ + *diktyon,* retina, + *tome,* incision] A surgical procedure to correct retinal displacement.

**hydrodynamics** The study of fluids in motion.

**hydroencephalocele** (hī″drō-ĕn-sĕf′ă-lō-sēl) [″ + *enkephalos,* brain, + *kele,* tumor, swelling] Brain substance expanded into a watery sac protruding through a cleft in the cranium. SYN: *hydrencephalocele.*

**hydroflumethiazide** (hī″drō-floo″mĕ-thī′ă-zīd) A diuretic and antihypertensive drug.

**hydrogel** (hī′drō-jĕl) [″ + L. *gelare,* to congeal] A colloid containing hydrophilic polymers. Hydrogels are used in soft contact lenses and the treatment of burns.

**hydrogen** [″ + *gennan,* to produce] SYMB: H. An element existing as a colorless, odorless, and tasteless gas, possessing one valence electron; atomic weight 1.0079, atomic number 1, specific gravity 0.069. A liter of the gas at sea level and at 0°C weighs 0.08988 g. Three isotopes of hydrogen (protium, deuterium, and tritium) exist, having atomic weights of approx. 1, 2, and 3, respectively.

OCCURRENCE: Hydrogen is present in the sun and stars. Even though it is the most abundant element in the known universe, its concentration in the earth's atmosphere is only 0.00005%. Hydrogen occurs in its free state (in natural gases and volcanic eruptions) only in minute quantities. It occurs principally on the earth as hydrogen oxide (water, $H_2O$) and is a constituent of all hydrocarbons. It is present in all acids and in ionic form is responsible for the properties characteristic of acids. It is present in nearly all organic compounds and is a component of all carbohydrates, proteins, and fats.

USES: It is highly flammable and used in the oxyhydrogen flame in welding; in hydrogenation of oils for solidifying purposes; as a reducing agent; and in many syntheses.

***h. acceptor*** In oxidation-reduction reactions, a substance that receives hydrogen atoms from another substance, the donor. SEE: *h. donor; coenzyme.*

***h. cyanide*** Hydrocyanic acid.

***h. dioxide*** Hydrogen peroxide.

***h. donor*** In oxidation-reduction reactions, a substance that gives up hydrogen atoms to another substance, the acceptor. SEE: *h. acceptor.*

***h. iodide*** Hydriodic acid.

***h. ion*** SEE: under *ion.*

***h. sulfide*** $H_2S$. A poisonous, flammable, colorless compound with a characteristic odor of rotten eggs. SYN: *hydrosulfuric acid.* SEE: *Poisons and Poisoning Appendix.*

**hydrogenase** (hī′drō-jĕn-ās) An enzyme that catalyzes reduction by molecular hydrogen.

**hydrogenate** (hī'drō-jĕn-āt") To bring about a combination with hydrogen.

**hydrogenation** (hī"drō-jĕn-ā'shŭn) A process of changing an unsaturated fat to a solid saturated fat by the addition of hydrogen in the presence of a catalyst.

**hydrogen peroxide** $H_2O_2$. A colorless syrupy liquid with an irritating odor and acrid taste. It decomposes readily, liberating oxygen. Because light is particularly effective in decomposing $H_2O_2$, it should be stored in tightly sealed glass jars in a dark place. SYN: *hydrogen dioxide.*

USES: It is used as a commercial bleaching agent; as an oxidizing and reducing agent; and, in a 3% aqueous solution, as a mild antiseptic, germicide, and cleansing agent.

***solution of h.p.*** A standardized aqueous solution of hydrogen peroxide whose most important use is to kill bacteria. However, its germicidal activity has been greatly overrated. Organic matter tends to decompose it, and, as long as the solution effervesces when it is applied to a wound, there is no great destruction of bacteria.

A hydrogen peroxide solution is a valuable cleansing agent for suppurating wounds and inflamed mucous membranes. It is esp. useful for this purpose because of its development of gas that tends to loosen adherent deposits and detritus, which might otherwise form a breeding place for microorganisms.

Hydrogen peroxide solution is sometimes injected into deep cavities to determine the presence of pus, which will be indicated by effervescence. Because of its lack of toxicity, it is a favored disinfectant for application to various mucous membranes, esp. those of the nose and throat. Diluted with equal parts of water, it is used as a gargle in pharyngitis or a mouthwash in stomatitis.

**hydroglossa** (hī"drō-glŏs'ă) [Gr. *hydor,* water, + *glossa,* tongue] Ranula.

**hydrogymnastics** (hī"drō-jĭm-năs'tĭks) Underwater exercises.

**hydrohematonephrosis** (hī"drō-hĕm"ă-tō-nĕf-rō'sĭs) [" + *haima,* blood, + *nephros,* kidney, + *osis,* condition] Bloody urine distending the pelvis of the kidney.

**hydrokinetics** (hī"drō-kī-nĕt'ĭks) [" + *kinesis,* movement] The science of fluids in motion.

**hydrolabile** (hī"drō-lā'bĭl) Having the tendency to lose weight because of fluid loss possibly owing to gastrointestinal disease, or because of decreased salt or carbohydrate intake.

**hydrolase** (hī'drō-lās) An enzyme that causes hydrolysis.

**hydrology** (hī-drŏl'ō-jē) [" + *logos,* word, reason] The science of water in all its aspects.

**hydrolysate** (hī-drŏl'ĭ-sāt) That which is produced as a result of hydrolysis.

***protein h.*** The amino acids obtained from splitting proteins by hydrolysis; used as a source of amino acids in certain diets.

**hydrolysis** (hī-drŏl'ĭ-sĭs) [" + *lysis,* dissolution] Any reaction in which water is one of the reactants, more specifically the combination of water with a salt to produce an acid and a base, one of which is more dissociated than the other. It involves a chemical decomposition in which a substance is split into simpler compounds by the addition or the taking up of the elements of water. This kind of reaction occurs extremely frequently in life processes. The conversion of starch to maltose, of fat to glycerol and fatty acid, and of protein to amino acids are examples of hydrolysis, as are other reactions involved in digestion. A simple example is the reaction in which the hydrolysis of ethyl acetate yields acetic acid and ethyl alcohol: $C_2H_5C_2H_3O_2 + H_2O\ CH_3COOH + C_2H_5OH$. Usually such reactions are reversible; the reversed reaction is called esterification, condensation, or dehydration synthesis. SEE: *assimilation; enzyme.* **hydrolytic** (-drō-lĭt'ĭk), *adj.*

**hydrolyze** (hī'drō-līz) To cause to undergo hydrolysis.

**hydroma** (hī-drō'mă) [Gr. *hydor,* water, + *oma,* tumor] **1.** Hygroma. **2.** Any cyst containing a watery substance.

**hydromassage** A massage produced by a stream of water.

**hydromeiosis** (hī"drō-mī-ō'sĭs) [" + *meiosis,* dimunition] The swelling of the epidermis after it is exposed to water, with consequent blockage of the sweat ducts. This phenomenon limits fluid loss from sweating when the body is immersed in water.

**hydromeningitis** (hī"drō-mĕn"ĭn-jī'tĭs) [" + *meninx,* membrane, + *itis,* inflammation] **1.** An inflammation of membranes of brain with serous effusion. **2.** An inflammation of Descemet's membrane.

**hydromeningocele** (hī"drō-mĕn-ĭn'gō-sēl) [" + " + *kele,* tumor, swelling] Protrusion of the meninges or spinal cord in a sac of fluid.

**hydrometer** (hī-drŏm'ĕ-tĕr) [" + *metron,* measure] An instrument that measures the density of a liquid by the depth to which a graduated scale sinks into the liquid. SEE: *urinometer.*

**hydrometra** (hī"drō-mē'tră) [" + *metra,* uterus] The collection of watery fluid or mucus in the uterus.

**hydrometrocolpos** (hī"drō-mē"trō-kŏl'pŏs) [" + *metra,* uterus, + *kolpos,* vagina] The distention of the uterus by a collection of watery fluid.

**hydromicrocephaly** (hī"drō-mī"krō-sĕf'ă-lē) [" + *mikros,* small, + *kephale,* head] A condition in which the head is abnormally small and contains an increased amount of cerebrospinal fluid.

**hydromorphone hydrochloride** (hī"drō-mor'fōn) An analgesic drug.

**hydromphalus** (hī-drŏm′fă-lŭs) [″ + *omphalos,* navel] A watery tumor at the umbilicus.

**hydromyelia** (hī″drō-mī-ē′lē-ă) [″ + *myelos,* marrow] Increased fluid in the central canal of the spinal cord. SYN: *hydrorrhachis.*

**hydromyelocele** (hī″drō-mī-ĕl′ō-sēl) [″ + ″ + *kele,* tumor, swelling] The protrusion of a sac with cerebrospinal fluid through a defect in a wall of the spinal canal.

**hydromyelomeningocele** (hī″drō-mī″ĕ-lō-mĕ-nĭng′gō-sēl) [″ + *myelos,* marrow, + *meninx,* membrane, + *kele,* tumor, swelling] Spinal deformity in which a fluid-filled sac containing the spinal cord tissue and membranes protrudes through the spine.

**hydromyoma** (hī″drō-mī-ō′mă) [″ + *mys,* muscle, + *oma,* tumor] A cystic fibroid, usually uterine, filled with fluid.

**hydronephrosis** (hī″drō-nĕf-rō′sĭs) [″ + *nephros,* kidney, + *osis,* condition] A collection of urine in the renal pelvis owing to obstructed outflow, forming a cyst by production of distention and atrophy of the organ. SYN: *nephrydrosis.*

DIAGNOSIS: A large, fluctuating, soft mass is found in the region of the kidney, appearing and disappearing as retained urine passes into the ureters and bladder.

TREATMENT: Aspiration, nephrectomy, or nephrotomy may be needed, depending on the severity of the disease. Medical or surgical removal of the cause of the retention is indicated.

NURSING IMPLICATIONS: Renal function studies such as blood urea nitrogen, serum creatinine, and serum potassium levels are monitored daily. As appropriate, urine specific gravity is tested at the bedside. The condition, planned diagnostic procedures, and expected sensations are explained to the patient and family, and if the patient is scheduled for a surgical procedure, the surgeon's explanations of the planned procedure are reinforced, questions answered, and misconceptions corrected. The patient is prepared physically for the procedure according to institutional protocol or the surgeon's wishes, emotional support provided, postoperative care and activities are explained, a signed informed consent form is obtained, and prescribed preoperative sedation is administered. Postoperatively, intake and output, vital signs, and fluid and electrolyte balance are monitored (a rising pulse rate and cool, clammy skin may signal impending hypovolemia or hemorrhage and shock). Prescribed analgesics and noninvasive measures are used to relieve pain as necessary. Postobstructive diuresis may cause the patient to lose great volumes of dilute urine over hours or days along with excessive electrolyte loss. If this occurs, I.V. fluids are administered at a prescribed constant rate plus an amount equal to a given percentage of the patient's hourly urine output to safely replacing intravascular volume. The nurse consults with a dietitian to provide a diet consistent with the treatment plan while providing foods that the patient enjoys and will eat. If a nephrostomy tube has been inserted, the tube is irrigated as specifically prescribed, checked for patency, and never clamped or kinked. Meticulous skin care is provided to the tube entry site; if urine leaks around the tube, a protective skin barrier is provided to prevent excoriation, and the wound area is bagged to preserve the patient's dignity and to help prevent infection. If the patient will be discharged with the nephrostomy tube in place, the nurse teaches proper care of the tube and skin at the insertion site. Prescribed drug therapies, such as antibiotics, are administered, and the patient is taught about expected outcomes, adverse effects to be reported, and the necessity to complete the prescribed course of therapy even if feeling better. To prevent the progression of hydronephrosis to irreversible renal disease, older male patients (esp. ones with a family history of benign prostatic hyperplasia or prostatitis) should have routine medical checkups. The nurse teaches the patient to recognize and report symptoms of hydronephrosis, such as colicky pain, hematuria, or urinary tract infection.

**hydroparasalpinx** (hī″drō-păr″ă-săl′pĭnks) [Gr. *hydor,* water, + *para,* beside, + *salpinx,* tube] An accumulation of serous fluid in the accessory tubes of the fallopian tube.

**hydroparotitis** (hī″drō-păr″ō-tī′tĭs) [″ + ″ + *ous,* ear, + *itis,* inflammation] An accumulation of fluid in the parotid gland.

**hydropenia** (hī″drō-pē′nē-ă) [″ + *penia,* poverty] A deficiency of water in the body.

**hydropericarditis** [″ + *peri,* around, + *kardia,* heart, + *itis,* inflammation] A serous effusion accompanying pericarditis.

**hydropericardium** (hī″drō-pĕr″ĭ-kăr′dē-ŭm) Pericardial edema; a noninflammatory accumulation of water in the pericardial sac.

SYMPTOMS: Synptoms include distress in the region of the heart; diminished cardiac function with signs of heart failure; and dysphagia and dyspnea.

TREATMENT: Paracentesis is the treatment. Definitive therapy depends on the cause of the disease.

**hydroperinephrosis** (hī″drō-pĕr″ĭ-nĕ-frō′sĭs) [″ + *peri,* around, + *nephros,* kidney, + *osis,* condition] An accumulation of the serum of the connective tissue surrounding the kidney.

**hydroperion** (hī″drō-pĕr′ē-ŏn) [″ + ″ + *oon,* egg] Fluid present between the decidua capsularis and the decidua parietalis, occurring early in pregnancy.

**hydroperitoneum** (hī″drō-pĕr″ĭ-tō-nē′ŭm) [″ + *peritonaion,* peritoneum] Ascites.

**hydrophilia, hydrophilism** (hī-drō-fĭl′ē-ă, -drŏf′ĭ-lĭzm) [″ + *philein,* to love] The tendency of tissues to attract and hold water.

**hydrophilous** (hī-drŏf′ĭ-lŭs) Taking up moisture. SYN: *bibulous; hygroscopic.*

**hydrophobia** (hī-drō-fō′bē-ă) [Gr. *hydor,* water, + *phobos,* fear] **1.** A morbid fear of water. **2.** The common name for rabies. SYN: *lyssa; rabies.*

**hydrophobophobia** (hī″drō-fō″bō-fō′bē-ă) [″ + ″ + *phobos,* fear] A morbid fear of contracting hydrophobia (rabies), sometimes resulting in a hysterical condition resembling hydrophobia.

**hydrophthalmos** (hī″drŏf-thăl′mŏs) [″ + *ophthalmos,* eye] Distention of the eyeball owing to an accumulation of fluid within it. SEE: *glaucoma.*

**hydrophysometra** (hī″drō-fī″sō-mē′tră) [″ + *physa,* air, + *metra,* uterus] The presence of water and gas in the uterus.

**hydropic** (hī-drŏp′ĭk) [Gr. *hydropikos*] Edematous, or pert. to edema.

**hydropneumatosis** (hī″drō-nū″mă-tō′sĭs) [″ + *pneumatosis,* inflation] Liquid and gas in the tissues producing combined edema and emphysema.

**hydropneumopericardium** (hī″drō-nū″mō-pĕr-ĭ-kăr′dē-ŭm) [″ + ″ + *peri,* around, + *kardia,* heart] Serous effusion with gas in the pericardium.

**hydropneumoperitoneum** (hī″drō-nū″mō-pĕr″ĭ-tō-nē′ŭm) [″ + ″ + *peritonaion,* peritoneum] Gas and serous fluid in the peritoneal cavity.

**hydropneumothorax** (hī″drō-nū″mō-thō′răks) [″ + ″ + *thorax,* chest] Gas and serous effusion in the pleural cavity. SYN: *pneumohydrothorax.*

**hydrops, hydropsy** (hī′drŏps, -drŏp′sē) [Gr.] Edema.

***h. abdominis*** Ascites.

***endolymphatic h.*** Labyrinthine h.

***h. fetalis*** The clinical condition in infants of cardiac decompensation with hepatosplenomegaly, respiratory distress, and circulatory distress. This may be caused by erythroblastosis fetalis; infections; tumors; pulmonary, hepatic, or renal disease; diabetes mellitus; Gaucher's disease; or multiple congenital anomalies. SEE: *erythema infectiosum; erythroblastosis fetalis.*

***h. folliculi*** An accumulation of fluid in the graafian follicle of the ovary.

***h. gravidarum*** Edema accompanying pregnancy.

***labyrinthine h.*** Dilatation due to an accumulation of fluid in the endolymphatic space of the ear; a characteristic of Ménière's disease. SYN: *endolymphatic h.*

***h. tubae*** Hydrosalpinx.

***h. tubae profluens*** Intermittent hydrosalpinx.

**hydropyonephrosis** (hī″drō-pī″ō-nĕf-rō′sĭs) [Gr. *hydor,* water, + *pyon,* pus, + *nephros,* kidney, + *osis,* condition] Dilatation of the kidney pelvis with pus and urine.

**hydroquinone** (hī″drō-kwĭn′ōn) *p*-Dihydroxy benzene, a weak but safe depigmenting agent, used topically.

**hydrorheostat** (hī″drō-rē′ō-stăt) [″ + *rheos,* current, + *histanai,* to place] A device used to control the flow of electric current by changes in water resistance.

**hydrorrhachis** (hī-dror′ă-kĭs) [″ + *rhachis,* spine] Hydromyelia.

**hydrorrhachitis** (hī-dror-ă-kī′tĭs) [″ + ″ + *itis,* inflammation] A serous effusion from the spinal cord or its membranes, with inflammation of the cord.

**hydrorrhea** (hī″drō-rē′ă) [″ + *rhoia,* flow] Copious watery discharge from any part, as from the nose.

***h. gravidarum*** The discharge of a watery fluid from the vagina during pregnancy.

**hydrosalpinx** (hī″drō-săl′pĭnks) [″ + *salpinx,* tube] Distention of the fallopian tube by clear fluid. SYN: *hydrops tubae.*

***intermittent h.*** Edema of the fallopian tube in which the distention is so great that the tube is forced by the pressure to empty itself via the uterus. SYN: *hydrops tubae profluens.*

**hydrosarcocele** (hī″drō-săr′kō-sēl) [″ + *sarx,* flesh, + *kele,* tumor, swelling] A hydrocele with chronic swelling of the testis.

**hydroscheocele** (hī-drŏs′kē-ō-sēl″) [″ + *oscheon,* scrotum, + *kele,* tumor, swelling] A scrotal hernia that contains serous fluid.

**hydrosol** (hī′drō-sŏl) The fluid state of a colloidal solution (sol) in which the colloid particles, separated by water in a continuous phase, are free to move about. SEE: *hydrogel.*

**hydrosphygmograph** (hī″drō-sfĭg′mō-grăf) [″ + *sphygmos,* pulse, + *graphein,* to write] A sphygmograph with an indicator consisting of a column of water.

**hydrostat** (hī′drō-stăt) [″ + *statikos,* standing] A device that maintains the water level in a container at a predetermined level.

**hydrostatic** (hī″drō-stăt′ĭk) [″ + *statikos,* standing] Pert. to the pressure of liquids in equilibrium and to the pressure exerted on liquids.

***h. densitometry*** An underwater weighing technique for the determination of an individual's specific gravity. The amount of water displaced by the body is corrected for the air contained in the lungs, affording an accurate determination of body components (e.g., the percentage of fat). SYN: *h. weighing.*

***h. test*** A test to determine if a dead infant has breathed prior to death. The infant's lungs are put in water; if they float, prior breathing is proven.

***h. weighing*** H. densitometry.

**hydrostatics** (hī″drō-stăt′ĭks) The science of the properties of fluids in equilibrium.

**hydrosulfuric acid** Hydrogen sulfide.

**hydrosyringomyelia** (hī″drō-sĭr-ĭng″ō-mī-ē′lē-ă) [″ + *syrinx,* tube, + *myelos,* marrow] Distention of the central canal of the spinal cord with effusion of fluid and formation of cavities.

**hydrotaxis** (hī″drō-tăk′sĭs) [″ + *taxis,* arrangement] The response of an organism or cell toward or away from moisture. SEE: *hydrotropism.*

**hydrotherapist** (hī″drō-thĕr′ă-pĭst) One who specializes in hydrotherapy.

**hydrotherapy** (hī-drō-thĕr′ă-pē) [″ + *therapeia,* treatment] The scientific application of water in the treatment of disease. The therapeutic effects of hydrotherapy are as follows:

*Buoyancy:* This is used to treat conditions such as arthritis or paralysis, in which the buoyancy effects relieve the stress of weight bearing and allows freer motion.

*Brief hot tub and shower baths:* These relieve fatigue and produce a general relaxation.

*Cold baths and applications:* These cool the body or body part and stimulate it, esp. if followed by friction and percussion. The local application of cold contracts the small blood vessels.

*Cold and hot applications:* One followed by the other stimulates the cardiovascular system both generally and locally.

*Gradually elevated temperature of hot tub and vapor baths:* This produces general muscular relaxation.

*Hot baths:* These relax tissues, including capillaries of the skin, drawing blood from deeper tissues. They also relieve pain.

*Resistance:* The viscosity of the water causes resistance to movement and can be used for therapeutic exercise. The faster the movement, the greater the resistance.

*Whirlpool:* This is a water bath in which the water is agitated by water jets. Besides the benefits afforded by water temperature, buoyancy, and viscosity, whirlpool helps debride wounds.

**hydrothermic** (hī″drō-thĕr′mĭk) Concerning the effect of heated water.

**hydrothionammonemia** (hī″drō-thī″ō-năm″ō-nē′mē-ă) [″ + *theion,* sulfur, + *ammoniakos,* of Amen, from near whose temple it came, + *haima,* blood] The presence of ammonium sulfide in the blood.

**hydrothionemia** (hī″drō-thī″ō-nē′mē-ă) [″ + ″ + *haima,* blood] A condition caused by hydrogen sulfide in the blood.

**hydrothionuria** (hī″drō-thī″ō-nū′rē-ă) [″ + ″ + *ouron,* urine] The presence of hydrogen sulfide in the urine.

**hydrothorax** (hī″drō-thō′răks) [″ + *thorax,* chest] A noninflammatory collection of fluid in the pleural cavity, causing dyspnea, an absence of vesicular breath sounds, murmur, and flatness over the location of the fluid.

**hydrotis** (hī-drō′tĭs) [″ + *ous,* ear] A serous effusion in the internal ear or tympanum.

**hydrotropism** (hī″drō-trō′pĭzm) [″ + *trope,* a turning] The response of plants toward moisture (positive hydrotropism) or away from it (negative hydrotropism).

**hydrotubation** Injection of saline solution or liquid medication into the uterus and fallopian tubes to dilate or treat them.

**hydrotympanum** (hī″drō-tĭm′pă-nŭm) [″ + *tympanon,* drum] Edematous fluid in the middle ear.

**hydroureter** (hī″drō-ū-rē′tĕr) [″ + *oureter,* ureter] The distention of the ureter with fluid owing to obstruction.

**hydrous** (hī′drŭs) Containing water. SEE: *anhydrous.*

**hydrovarium** (hī″drō-vā′rē-ŭm) [″ + LL. *ovarium,* ovary] Edema or cyst of the ovary.

**hydroxide** (hī-drŏk′sīd) [″ + *oxys,* sour] A compound that contains the $OH^-$ group, such as NaOH (sodium hydroxide, or caustic soda).

**hydroxocobalamin** (hī-drŏk″sō-kō-băl′ă-mĭn) A naturally occurring form of vitamin $B_{12}$ used to treat $B_{12}$ deficiency.

**hydroxy acid** SEE: under *acid.*

**hydroxyamphetamine hydrobromide** (hī-drŏk″sē-ăm-fĕt′ă-mēn hī″drō-brō′mīd) An amphetamine with little ability to stimulate the central nervous system. It is used as a solution placed in the eye, where it has an ephedrine-like action. Trade name is Paredrine.

**hydroxyapatite** (hī-drŏk″sē-ăp′ă-tīt) The apatite form of calcium phosphate present with calcium carbonate in the bones and skeleton. In teeth it is soluble in the acids of soft drinks or carbohydrate fermentation, but it becomes decay-resistant fluoroapatite after combining with fluoride ions present in fluoridated water or fluoride supplement.

**hydroxybenzene** (hī-drŏk″sē-bĕn′zēn) Phenol.

**hydroxybutyric dehydrogenase** A serum enzyme whose level is elevated in myocardial infarction.

**hydroxychloroquine sulfate** (hī-drŏk″sē-klō′rō-kwĭn) An antimalarial drug. Trade name is Plaquenil Sulfate.

**25-hydroxycholecalciferol** (hī-drŏk″sē-kō″lē-kăl-sĭf′ĕ-rŏl) A vitamin D derivative.

**17-hydroxycorticosterone** (hī-drŏk″sē-kor″tĭ-kō-stĕr′ōn) Hydrocortisone.

**hydroxydione sodium succinate** (hī-drŏk″sē-dī′ōn) A steroid drug used intravenously as an anesthetic. It has no hormonal action.

**hydroxyl** Hydroxide.

**hydroxylase** (hī-drŏk′sĭ-lās) Any enzyme that catalyzes the introduction of hydrogen into a substrate.

**hydroxylysine** (hī″drŏk-sĭl′ĭ-sĭn) An amino acid found in collagen.

**hydroxyprogesterone caproate** (hī-drŏk″sē-prō-jĕs′tĕr-ōn) A progestational drug.

**hydroxyproline** (hī-drŏk″sē-prō′lĭn) An amino acid found in collagen.

**hydroxypropyl methycellulose** Cellulose hydroxypropyl methyl ester; a substance used to increase the viscosity of solutions.

**hydroxystilbamidine isethionate** (hī-drŏk″sē-stĭl-băm′ĭ-dēn) An antiprotozoal drug used in treating North American blastomycosis.

**5-hydroxytryptamine** (hī-drŏk″sē-trĭp′tă-mēn) Serotonin.

**hydroxyurea** (hī-drŏk″sē-ū-rē′ă) A cytotoxic drug.

**hydroxyzine hydrochloride** (hī-drŏk′sĭ-zēn) An antianxiety agent.

**hygiene** (hī′jēn) [Gr. *hygieinos*, healthful] The study of health and observance of health rules and the methods and means of preserving health.

***community h.*** That branch of hygiene that deals with the health of a large group of individuals such as in a city, state, or nation, and esp. with the control of communicable diseases.

***dental h.*** Oral h.

***industrial h.*** That branch of hygiene that deals primarily with health of industrial workers, esp. study, treatment, and prevention of occupational diseases.

***mental h.*** The science of developing and maintaining mental health and preventing mental illness.

***oral h.*** Preventive measures to avoid pathological conditions of the teeth and oral cavity. These include discontinuing the use of tobacco products, including "smokeless tobacco" (i.e., snuff); brushing the teeth and using dental floss daily; and removal of impacted food debris. Edentulous persons with partial restorations or false teeth should be sure that their appliances fit properly and are kept clean. An additional oral care measure that is important in the prevention of periodontal disease is the removal of plaque by a dental hygienist at least twice each year. SYN: *dental h.* SEE: *care, mouth; hygienist, dental; toothbrushing.*

**hygienic** (hī″jē-ĕn′ĭk) **1.** Pert. to health or its preservation. **2.** In a healthy condition.

**hygienist** (hī-jē′nĭst, hī′jē-ĕn-ĭst) A specialist in hygiene.

***dental h.*** An individual trained in dental prophylaxis who usually works under the supervision of a dentist. The hygienist is essential in patient education as well as in cleaning and polishing teeth. In some states hygienists' expanded duties include dental radiography, application of fluoride solutions, and placing and carving amalgam fillings.

**hygro-** Prefix meaning *moisture.*

**hygroblepharic** (hī″grō-blĕ-făr′ĭk) [″ + *blepharon*, eyelid] Any structure (such as the lacrimal gland) or agent that moistens the eye.

**hygroma** (hī-grō′mă) *pl.* **hygromas or hygromata** [″ + *oma*, tumor] A sac or bursa containing fluid.

***cystic h.*** A rapidly growing hygroma of lymphatic origin. It is usually located in the neck but may be in the thorax.

**hygrometer** (hī-grŏm′ĕ-tĕr) [″ + *metron*, measure] An instrument for measuring the amount of moisture in the air.

**hygroscopic** (hī-grō-skŏp′ĭk) [″ + *skopein*, to examine] **1.** Pert. to hygroscopy. **2.** Absorbing moisture readily. SYN: *bibulous; hydrophilous.*

**hygroscopy** (hī-grŏs′kō-pē) The estimation of the quantity of moisture in the atmosphere.

**hygrostomia** (hī-grō-stō′mē-ă) [″ + *stoma*, mouth] Ptyalism.

**hyla** (hī′lă) A lateral extension of the aqueductus cerebri.

**hyloma** (hī-lō′mă) [Gr. *hyle*, matter, + *oma*, tumor] A tumor composed of or in the hylic tissues, such as hypohyloma and mesohyloma.

**hymen** (hī′mĕn) [Gr.] A fold of mucous membrane that partially covers the entrance to the vagina. Contrary to folklore, the presence or absence (or rupture) of the hymen cannot be used to prove or disprove virginity or history of sexual intercourse. Pregnancy has been known to occur even when the hymen has not been entered. **hymenal** (-ăl), *adj.*

***annular h.*** A hymen with a ring-shaped opening in the center.

***h. biforis*** A hymen with two openings with a thick septum between.

***cribriform h.*** A hymen with many small perforations. SYN: *fenestrated h.*

***h. denticulatus*** A hymen with an opening with serrated edges.

***fenestrated h.*** Cribriform h.

***imperforate h.*** A hymen without an opening. Menstruation occurs, but the blood cannot escape from the vagina because of the obstruction of the hymen. The treatment is surgical incision of the hymen. SYN: *unruptured h.*

***lunar h.*** A hymen shaped like a crescent moon.

***ruptured h.*** A hymen that has been torn by coitus, injury, or surgery.

***septate h.*** A hymen in which the opening is separated by a thin septum.

***unruptured h.*** Imperforate h.

**hymenectomy** (hī″mĕn-ĕk′tō-mē) [″ + *ektome*, excision] **1.** In surgery and gynecology, the incision or removal of the hymen. **2.** The excision of a membrane.

**hymenitis** (hī-mĕn-ī′tĭs) [″ + *itis*, inflammation] The inflammation of the hymen or of a membrane.

**Hymenolepis** (hī″mĕ-nŏl′ĕ-pĭs) [″ + *lepis*, rind] A genus of tapeworm that is parasitic in birds and mammals.

***H. nana*** The dwarf tapeworm, a parasite in the intestine of rats and mice; also commonly found in humans. It averages about 1 in. (2.5 cm) in length and differs from other tapeworms in that it is capable of completing its life cycle within a single host. It causes severe toxic symptoms, esp. in children. SEE: illus.

**hymenology** (hī′mĕn-ŏl′ō-jē) [″ + *logos*, word, reason] The science of the membranes and their diseases.

**Hymenoptera** (hī″mĕn-ŏp′tur-ă) [Gr. *hymenopteros*, membrane-winged] An order of insects that includes ants, bees, hor-

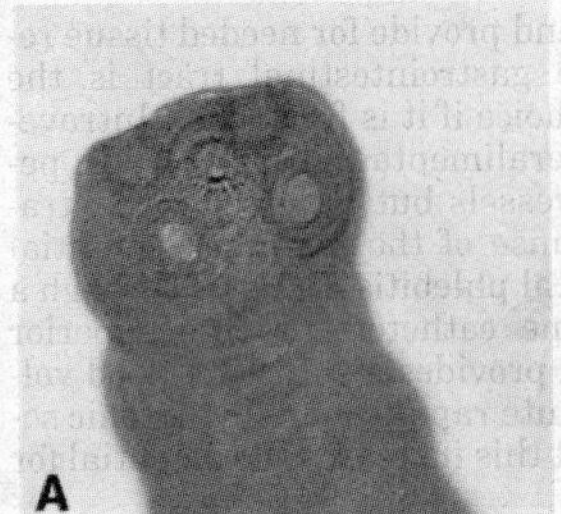


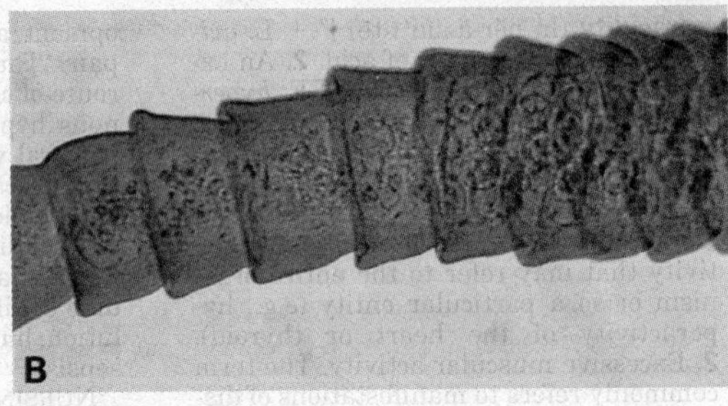


HYMENOLEPIS NANA (A) SCOLEX, (B) MATURE PROGLOTTIDS (ORIG. MAG. ×100)

nets, and wasps. SEE: *bite, insect; sting.*

**hymenorrhaphy** (hī″mĕn-or′ă-fē) [″ + *rhaphe*, seam, ridge] A plastic operation on the hymen to restore it to the preruptured state.

**hymenotome** (hī-mĕn′ō-tōm) [″ + *tome*, incision] A knife used to divide membranes.

**hymenotomy** (hī″mĕn-ŏt′ō-mē) **1.** An incision of the hymen. **2.** A dissection of a membrane.

**hyo-** [Gr. *hyoeides*, U-shaped] Prefix indicating connection with the hyoid bone.

**hyobasioglossus** (hī″ō-bā″sē-ō-glŏs′ŭs) [″ + *basis*, base, + *glossa*, tongue] The part of the hyoglossal muscle attached to the hyoid bone.

**hyoepiglottic, hyoepiglottidean** (hī″ō-ĕp″ĭ-glŏt′ĭk, hī″ō-ĕp″ĭ-glŏt-ĭd′ē-ăn) [″ + *epiglottis*, epiglottis] Relating to the hyoid bone and epiglottis.

**hyoglossal** (hī″ō-glŏs′ăl) [″ + *glossa*, tongue] **1.** Pert. to the hyoglossus. **2.** Extending to the tongue from the hyoid bone.

**hyoglossus** (hī″ō-glŏs′ŭs) A muscle arising from the body and greater cornu of the hyoid bone and inserted into the dorsum of the tongue. It draws the sides of the tongue down and retracts it.

**hyoid** (hī′oyd) [Gr. *hyoeides*, U-shaped] **1.** Shaped like the Gr. letter upsilon (*υ*). **2.** Pert. to the hyoid bone.

**hyoid bone** The horseshoe-shaped bone lying at the base of the tongue. SEE: illus.

**hyopharyngeus** (hī″ō-făr-ĭn′jē-ŭs) [″ + *pharynx*, throat] The middle pharyngeal constrictor.

**hyoscine hydrobromide** Previous name for scopolamine hydrobromide.

**hyoscyamus** (hī″ō-sī′ă-mŭs) [Gr. *hys*, a pig, + *kyamos*, bean] The dried leaves of the plant *Hyoscyamus niger;* a narcotic that also acts as an antispasmodic. A relative of atropine, hyoscyamus is also known as henbane.

**hyoscyamus poisoning** SEE: *atropine in Poisons and Poisoning Appendix.*

**hyp-** SEE: *hypo-.*

**hypacousia, hypacusia, hypacusis** (hī″pă-koo′sē-ă, -kū′sē-ă, -sĭs) [Gr. *hypo*, under, + *akousis*, hearing] Impaired hearing. SEE: *hearing; presbyacusia.*

**hypalgesia** (hī-păl-jē′zē-ă) [″ + *algesis*, sense of pain] A lessened sensitivity to pain; the opposite of hyperalgesia.

**hypamnios** (hī-păm′nē-ŏs) [″ + *amnion*, caul of a lamb] A deficiency in the amount of amniotic fluid. SEE: *oligohydramnios.*

**hypaxial** (hī-păks′ē-ăl) [″ + *axon*, axle] Situated beneath the body axis.

**hyper-** [Gr. *hyper*, over, above, excessive] Prefix meaning *above, excessive,* or *beyond.*

**hyperacid** (hī″pĕr-ăs′ĭd) [″ + L. *acidus*, sour] Containing too much acid.

**hyperacidaminuria** (hī″pĕr-ăs″ĭd-ăm-ĭn-ū′rē-ă) [″ + ″ + *amine* + Gr. *ouron*, urine] The presence of an excess of amino acids in the urine. SYN: *acidaminuria.*

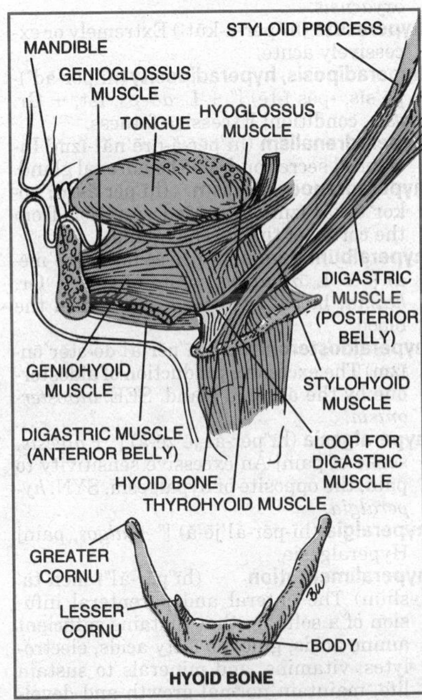


HYOID BONE

**hyperacidity** (hī″pĕr-ă-sĭd′ĭ-tē) [″ + L. *acidus,* sour] **1.** An excess of acid. **2.** An excess of acid in the stomach. SEE: *hyperchlorhydria.*

**hyperactive child syndrome** SEE: *attention-deficit hyperactivity disorder; hyperactivity.*

**hyperactivity 1.** Increased or excessive activity that may refer to the entire organism or to a particular entity (e.g., hyperactivity of the heart or thyroid). **2.** Excessive muscular activity. The term commonly refers to manifestations of disturbed behavior in children or adolescents characterized by constant overactivity, distractibility, impulsiveness, inability to concentrate, and aggressiveness. This condition is not easily defined because the claim that the child is hyperactive may be based on a low level of tolerance of the persons caring for the child. Hyperkinetic behavior usually lessens as a child grows older and usually disappears during adolescence. SEE: *attention-deficit hyperactivity disorder.*

Hyperactivity is caused by emotional disorders, central nervous system dysfunction, mental retardation, or an exaggeration of a normal personality trait.

**hyperacuity** (hī″pĕr-ă-kū′ĭ-tē) [Gr. *hyper,* over, above, excessive, + L. *acuitas,* sharpness] An abnormal acuteness of one of the special senses such as hearing or sight.

**hyperacusis** (hī″pĕr-ă-kū′sĭs) [″ + *akousis,* hearing] An abnormal sensitivity to sound, sometimes found in hysteria, in which hearing is abnormally acute. SYN: *oxyacusis.*

**hyperacute** (hī″pĕr-ă-kūt′) Extremely or excessively acute.

**hyperadiposis, hyperadiposity** (hī″pĕr-ăd″ĭ-pō′sĭs, -pŏs′ĭ-tē) [″ + L. *adeps,* fat, + Gr. *osis,* condition] Excessive fatness.

**hyperadrenalism** (hī″pĕr-ă-drē′năl-ĭzm) Increased secretion from the adrenal gland.

**hyperadrenocorticalism** (hī″pĕr-ă-drē″nō-kor′tĭ-kăl-ĭzm) Increased secretion from the cortex of the adrenal gland.

**hyperalbuminemia** (hī″pĕr-ăl-bū″mĭ-nē′mē-ă) [″ + L. *albumen,* white of egg, + Gr. *haima,* blood] Increased albumin in the blood.

**hyperaldosteronism** (hī″pĕr-ăl″dō-stĕr′ōn-ĭzm) The excessive production of aldosterone by the adrenal gland. SEE: *aldosteronism.*

**hyperalgesia** (hī″pĕr-ăl-jē′zē-ă) [″ + *algesis,* sense of pain] An excessive sensitivity to pain; the opposite of hypalgesia. SYN: *hyperalgia.*

**hyperalgia** (hī-pĕr-ăl′jē-ă) [″ + *algos,* pain] Hyperalgesia.

**hyperalimentation** (hī″pĕr-ăl″ĭ-mĕn-tā′shŭn) The enteral and parenteral infusion of a solution that contains sufficient amino acids, glucose, fatty acids, electrolytes, vitamins, and minerals to sustain life, maintain normal growth and development, and provide for needed tissue repair. The gastrointestinal tract is the route of choice if it is functional. Intravenous hyperalimentation may be via peripheral vessels but in lesser concentrations because of the increased potential for chemical phlebitis. Infusion through a central line catheter into the superior vena cava provides a sufficient blood volume to dilute rapidly more hypertonic solution, but this increases the potential for sepsis.

NURSING IMPLICATIONS: Vital signs, electrolyte values, and fluid balance (intake, output, and daily weight) are monitored for indications of fluid overload or dehydration. Urine specific gravity is measured, and the patient's urine is checked for the presence of glucose and acetone every 6 hours. If the hyperalimentation is enteral, the nurse is aware of where the distal end of the tube is placed (above or below the pyloric sphincter); auscultates for bowel sounds; inspects, percusses, and measures for abdominal distention; and assesses for, documents, reports, and treats nausea, vomiting, or diarrhea. As appropriate, stomach contents are monitored for residual volume. Tube patency as well as volume, rate, and type of feeding are maintained; comfort measures provided (oral misting, oral hygiene, and analgesic throat sprays); and any indications of infections due to long-term nasal tube placement, such as sinusitis, aspiration reflux chemical pneumonia, and other infections, are assessed. For example, sinusitis can occur because the tube impedes sinus drainage, allowing organisms to colonize the sinuses and resulting in fever and nasopurulent drainage. Chemical aspiration pneumonias often occur because of silent reflux regurgitation, resulting in acidic stomach contents and gram-negative organisms entering the respiratory tract. If hyperalimentation is via peripheral blood vessels, the nurse frequently assesses the insertion site for evidence of phlebitis; if via a central line, the nurse assesses the insertion site for signs of inflammation or infection, and the patient for signs and symptoms of sepsis. The insertion site is redressed and administration sets and connectors are changed according to institutional protocol; strict asepsis is maintained throughout these procedures. For all parenteral hyperalimentation, the flow-rate should never be sped up to "catch-up" an infusion that is behind unless this action is specifically prescribed by the physician. The physician is notified if the line becomes occluded or if fluids are stopped or slowed for any reason. The patient is assessed for hypoglycemia or fluid deficit. For all hyperalimentation: The patient is mobilized as possible. Nutritional status is monitored weekly; weight gain or loss, serum protein levels, transferrin levels, and anthropomorphic measurements are documented and reported as directed. The nurse maintains strict asepsis in handling fluids and equipment, being especially vigilant if the patient is immobile or paralyzed.

**hyperalkalinity** (hī″pĕr-ăl-kă-lĭn′ĭ-tē) A condition of excessive alkalinity.

**hyperaminoacidemia** (hī″pĕr-ăm″ĭ-nō-ăs″ĭ-dē′mē-ă) An abnormal amount of amino acids in the blood.

**hyperammonemia** (hī″pĕr-ăm″mō-nē′mē-ă) An excess amount of ammonia in the blood. SEE: *ammonia toxicity.*

***congenital h.*** An accumulation of an excess of ammonia in the body due to a congenital deficiency of enzymes, either carbamyl phosphate synthetase or ornithine transcarbamylase, essential to the metabolism of ammonia. Clinical signs of ammonia toxicity are present, including vomiting, lethargy, coma, and eventually death.

**hyperamylasemia** (hī″pĕr-ăm″ĭl-ās-ē′mē-ă) Increased blood amylase.

**hyperaphia** (hī″pĕr-ā′fē-ă) [″ + *haphe,* touch] An excessive sensitivity to touch. SYN: *hyperpselaphesia.* **hyperaphic** (hī-pĕr-ăf′ĭk), *adj.*

**hyperazotemia** (hī″pĕr-ăz″ō-tē′mē-ă) [″ + L. *azotum,* nitrogen, + Gr. *haima,* blood] An increased amount of nitrogenous substances such as urea in the blood.

**hyperazoturia** (hī″pĕr-ăz″ō-tū′rē-ă) [″ +″ + Gr. *ouron,* urine] An excessive amount of nitrogenous matter in the urine.

**hyperbaric chamber** SEE: under *chamber.*

**hyperbarism** (hī″pĕr-băr′ĭzm) The condition of being exposed to or having pressure greater than atmospheric pressure. Miners and deep sea divers are exposed to this condition. SEE: *bends; caisson disease.*

**hyperbetalipoproteinemia** (hī″pĕr-bā″tă-lĭp″ō-prō″tē-ĭn-ē′mē-ă) An excessive amount of $\beta$-lipoproteins in the blood. SEE: *hyperlipoproteinemia.*

**hyperbilirubinemia** (hī″pĕr-bĭl″ĭ-roo-bĭn-ē′mē-ă) [Gr. *hyper,* over, above, excessive, + L. *bilis,* bile, + *ruber,* red, + Gr. *haima,* blood] An excessive amount of bilirubin in the blood. In newborns, high bilirubin levels due to rapid destruction of red blood cells may be caused by maternal factors such as Rh or ABO incompatibility, prenatal use of certain therapeutic drugs, or intrauterine viral infection. Precipitating factors include neonatal sepsis, anoxia, polycythemia, postbirth cold stress and hypoglycemia, and congenital liver or gastrointestinal defects. SEE: *hemolytic disease of the newborn; incompatibility, ABO; isoimmunization; Nursing Diagnoses Appendix.*

**hyperbrachycephaly** (hī″pĕr-brăk″ē-sĕf′ă-lē) [″ + *brachys,* short, + *kephale,* head] An excessive degree of brachycephaly; having a cephalic index above 85.

**hypercalcemia** (hī″pĕr-kăl-sē′mē-ă) [″ + L. *calx,* lime, + Gr. *haima,* blood] An excessive amount of calcium in the blood. The causes of this condition include primary hyperthyroidism, lithium therapy, malignancies including solid tumors and hematological malignancies, vitamin D intoxication, hyperthyroidism, vitamin A intoxication, aluminum intoxication; and milk-alkali syndrome.

SYMPTOMS: Clinically, fatigue, depression, mental confusion, nausea, vomiting, constipation, increased urination, and possibly cardiac arrhythmia are present. A short Q-T interval is present on electrocardiographic study.

TREATMENT: Therapy is given for the causative condition.

***idiopathic h.*** A type of hypercalcemia seen in infants, caused by vitamin D intoxication. SEE: *bends.*

**hypercalciuria** (hī″pĕr-kăl″sē-ū′rē-ă) [″ +″ + Gr. *ouron,* urine] An excessive quantity of calcium in the urine.

**hypercapnia** (hī″pĕr-kăp′nē-ă) [″ + *kapnos,* smoke] An increased amount of carbon dioxide in the blood.

***permissive h.*** Intentional hypoventilation of a mechanically ventilated patient to minimize intrathoracic pressure.

**hypercarbia** Hypercapnia.

**hypercellularity** (hī″pĕr-sĕl″ū-lăr′ĭ-tē) An increased number of cells in any location, but esp. in the bone marrow.

**hypercementosis** (hī″pĕr-sē″mĕn-tō′sĭs) [″ + L. *cementum,* cement, + Gr. *osis,* condition] An overgrowth of tooth cement (cementum).

**hyperchloremia** (hī″pĕr-klō-rē′mē-ă) [″+ *chloros,* green, + *haima,* blood] An increase in the chloride content of the blood.

**hyperchlorhydria** (hī″pĕr-klor-hī′drē-ă) [″ + ″+ *hydor,* water] An excess of hydrochloric acid in the gastric secretion. It causes a burning sensation in the stomach in the absence of ingested foods. The amount secreted above what is needed to combine with albumoid and basic substances is known as free hydrogen chloride. SEE: *achlorhydria; gastrin; gastritis; $H_2$-receptor antagonists; hydrochloric acid; hypochlorhydria; peptic ulcer; Zollinger-Ellison syndrome.*

The ability of the stomach to produce hydrochloric acid can be evaluated clinically by administering pentagastrin or other chemicals that stimulate gastric production, such as histamine or betazole. The amount of acid produced is measured by aspirating the stomach four times at 15-minute intervals and analyzing each sample.

**hyperchloridation** (hī″pĕr-klō″rĭ-dā′shŭn) A dosing with large amounts of sodium chloride.

**hypercholesterolemia** (hī″pĕr-kō-lĕs″tĕr-ŏl-ē′mē-ă) [″ + *chole,* bile, + *stereos,* solid, + *haima,* blood] An excessive amount of cholesterol in the blood.

***familial h.*** A type of hyperlipoproteinemia, type IIA, in which the low-density lipoproteins are increased and the very low-density lipoproteins are normal. SEE: *hyperlipoproteinemia*.

**hypercholesterolia** (hī″pĕr-kō-lĕs″tĕr-ō′lē-ă) [″ + ″ + *stereos,* solid] Excessive cholesterol in the bile.

**hyperchromatic** (hī″pĕr-krō-măt′ĭk) [″ + *chroma,* color] Overpigmented.

**hyperchromatism** (hī″pĕr-krō′mă-tĭzm) [″ + ″ + *-ismos,* condition] **1.** Excessive pigmentation. **2.** The increased staining capacity of any structure.

**hyperchromia** (hī″pĕr-krō′mē-ă) Hyperchromatism.

**hyperchromic** (hī-pĕr-krō′mĭk) **1.** Pert. to excessive pigmentation. **2.** Intensely colored.

**hyperchylia** (hī″pĕr-kī′lē-ă) [Gr. *hyper,* over, above, excessive, + *chylos,* juice] An abnormal secretion of gastric juice.

**hyperchylomicronemia** (hī″pĕr-kī″lō-mī″krō-nē′mē-ă) The excessive accumulation of fat particles, chylomicrons, in the blood.

**hypercoagulability** (hīp″ĕr-kō-ăg″ū-lă-bĭl′ĭ-tē) An increased ability of anything to coagulate, but esp. the blood.

**hypercorticism** (hī″pĕr-kor′tĭ-sĭzm) An excessive production of adrenal cortical hormones in the body.

**hypercrinism** (hī″pĕr-krī′nĭsm) [″ + *krinein,* to separate, + *-ismos,* condition] A condition due to excessive activity of any endocrine gland.

**hypercryalgesia** (hī″pĕr-krī″ăl-jē′zē-ă) [″ + *kryos,* cold, + *algesis,* sense of pain] Hypercryesthesia.

**hypercryesthesia** (hī″pĕr-krī″ĕs-thē′zē-ă) [″ +″ + *aisthesis,* sensation] An excessive sensitivity to cold. SYN: *hypercryalgesia.*

**hypercupremia** (hī″pĕr-kū-prē′mē-ă) An increased level of copper in the blood. SEE: *Wilson's disease.*

**hypercyanotic** (hī″pĕr-sī″ă-nŏt′ĭk) Denoting extreme cyanosis.

**hyperdactylia** (hī″pĕr-dăk-tĭl′ē-ă) [Gr. *hyper,* over, above, excessive, + *daktylos,* finger] The state of having supernumerary fingers or toes.

**hyperdefecation** Increased stool frequency without an increase in stool weight above normal. This condition is not classed as diarrhea. It may be present in patients with irritable bowel syndrome, hyperthyroidism, or proctitis.

**hyperdicrotic** (hī″pĕr-dī-krŏt′ĭk) [″ + *dikrotos,* beating double] Abnormally dicrotic. SEE: *dicrotic.*

**hyperdynamia** (hī″pĕr-dī-nā′mē-ă) [″ + *dynamis,* force] Muscular restlessness or extreme violence.

***h. uteri*** Abnormal uterine contractions in labor.

**hypereccrisia, hypereccrisis** (hī″pĕr-ĕk-krĭs′ē-ă, -ĕk′krĭ-sĭs) [″+ *ekkrisis,* excretion] An abnormal amount of excretion. **hypereccritic** (-ĕk-krĭt′ĭk), *adj.*

**hyperemesis** (hī″pĕr-ĕm′ĕ-sĭs) [″ + *emesis,* vomiting] Excessive vomiting.

***h. gravidarum*** During pregnancy, nausea and vomiting severe enough to cause systemic effects such as acidosis, dehydration, and weight loss. About two of every 1000 pregnant women have this disease with such severity as to require hospitalization. If the severe form is untreated, it can be fatal. SEE: *morning sickness; Nursing Diagnoses Appendix.*

SYMPTOMS: This condition of unknown etiology may start as a simple vomiting of early pregnancy, but with combined vomiting, first of gastric contents and later of bile, chloride depletion and acidosis occur. Finally, with severe and continued vomiting, pathological changes in the liver take place.

TREATMENT: In early cases, effective therapy calls for rest in bed, with small amounts of carbohydrates taken frequently, a moderate restriction of fluids, and mild sedation and antiemetic drugs. In severe cases, the patient is hospitalized, with complete bedrest and no visitors until the vomiting ends and eating begins. The patient may initially have nothing by mouth for 24 hours, her nutritional and electrolyte balance maintained through parenteral fluids and proteins given as required. Rarely, nasogastric feeding or total parenteral nutrition is required.

The need to terminate the pregnancy should occur only rarely if the patient is properly treated early. When the patient improves, food taken by mouth should consist of a light solid diet given in frequent small feedings, with fruit juice or milk between feedings.

Caution: During therapy the patient's retinas should be monitored for evidence of hemorrhagic retinitis. If it occurs, the pregnancy should be terminated without delay. The death rate in patients with this complication is 50%.

**hyperemia** (hī″pĕr-ē′mē-ă) [″ + *haima,* blood] **1.** Congestion; an unusual amount of blood in a part. **2.** A form of macula; red areas on the skin that disappear on pressure. **3.** In physical therapy, an increase in the quantity of blood flowing through any part of the body, shown by redness of the skin caused by the application of heat.

***active h.*** Hyperemia caused by increased blood inflow. SYN: *arterial h.*

***arterial h.*** Active h.

***Bier's h.*** Passive hyperemia produced by application of an elastic bandage and by suction. SYN: *constriction h.*

***constriction h.*** Bier's h.

***leptomeningeal h.*** Pia-arachnoid congestion.

***passive h.*** Hyperemia caused by decreased drainage of blood. SYN: *venous h.*

***reactive h.*** The increased presence of blood in an area after restoration of blood flow following a decreased supply.

***venous h.*** Passive h.

**hyperemotivity** (hī″pĕr-ē″mō-tĭv′ĭ-tē) [Gr. *hyper,* over, above, excessive, + L. *emovere,* to disturb] Excessive emotivity or response to stimuli.

**hypereosinophilic syndrome, idiopathic** Persistent eosinophilia for which no cause can be found. This rare, worldwide disease is more common in men than in women. Almost any organ can be affected, but most patients have bone marrow, cardiac, and central nervous system involvement.

TREATMENT: Anticoagulants for patients with thromboembolic complication; corticosteroids. Patients unresponsive to corticosteroids have shown marked improvement when given cytotoxic agents such as hydroxyurea.

**hyperequilibrium** (hī″pĕr-ē″kwĭ-lĭb′rē-ŭm) [″ + L. *aequus,* equal, + *libra,* balance] A tendency to experience vertigo when making even slight turning movements.

**hypererethism** (hī″pĕr-ĕr′ĭ-thĭzm) [″ + *erethisma,* stimulation] Excessive irritability.

**hyperergasia** (hī″pĕr-ĕr-gā′sē-ă) [″ + *ergasia,* work] Unusual functional activity.

**hyperergia** (hī″pĕr-ĕr′jē-ă) An abnormal sensitivity to allergens.

**hyperergy** (hī′pĕr-ĕr″jē) [″ + *ergon,* energy] Hypersensitivity, or a condition in which there is an exaggerated response. SEE: *allergy; anaphylaxis.*

**hyperesophoria** (hī″pĕr-ĕs″ō-fō′rē-ă) [″ + *eso,* inward, + *phorein,* to bear] A tendency of the visual axis to deviate upward and inward owing to muscular imbalance; a form of heterophoria.

**hyperesthesia** (hī″pĕr-ĕs-thē′zē-ă) [″ + *aisthesis,* sensation] An increased sensitivity to sensory stimuli, such as pain or touch. SYN: *algesia; oxyesthesia.* **hyperesthetic** (-ĕs-thĕt′ĭk), *adj.*

***acoustic h.*** An abnormal sensitivity to sound.

***cerebral h.*** Hyperesthesia caused by a cerebral lesion.

***gustatory h.*** An oversensitivity of taste.

***muscular h.*** Muscular sensitivity to pain and fatigue.

***optic h.*** An abnormal sensitivity to light.

***h. sexualis*** An abnormal increase in libido.

***tactile h.*** An abnormal sensitivity of touch.

**hyperexophoria** (hī″pĕr-ĕks″ō-fō′rē-ă) [″ + *exo,* outward, + *phorein,* to bear] A tendency of the visual axis to deviate upward and outward owing to muscular imbalance; a form of heterophoria.

**hyperexplexia** An excessive reaction to being startled. SEE: *Tourette's syndrome; startle syndrome.*

**hyperextension** (hī″pĕr-ĕks-tĕn′shŭn) [″ + L. *extendere,* to stretch out] Extreme or abnormal extension.

**hyperfibrinogenemia** (hī″pĕr-fī-brĭn″ō-jĕ-nē′mē-ă) An increased amount of fibrinogen in the blood.

**hyperflexion** (hī″pĕr-flĕk′shŭn) Increased flexion of a joint, usually resulting from trauma.

**hyperfunction** [Gr. *hyper,* over, above, excessive, + L. *functio,* performance] Excessive activity.

**hypergalactia** (hī-pĕr-găl-ăk′shē-ă) [″ + *gala,* milk] Excessive milk secretion.

**hypergammaglobulinemia** (hī″pĕr-găm″ă-glŏb″ū-lĭ-nē′mē-ă) An excessive amount of gamma globulin in the blood.

**hypergamy** (hī-pĕr′gă-mē) [″ + *gamos,* marriage] The tendency of women to reproduce with men of equal or higher social standing.

**hypergenesis** (hī″pĕr-jĕn′ĕ-sĭs) [″ + *genesis,* generation, birth] *Hyperplasia.*

**hypergenitalism** (hī″pĕr-jĕn′ĭt-ăl-ĭzm) [″ + L. *genitalis,* genital] An excessive development of the genital organs, caused by disturbances in endocrine secretions of the adrenal gland or gonads or by hypothalamic disorders.

**hypergeusesthesia, hypergeusia** (hī″pĕr-gūs-ĕs-thē′sē-ă, -gū′sē-ă) [″ + *geusis,* taste + *aisthesis,* perception] An excessive acuteness of the sense of taste.

**hypergia** (hī-pĕr′jē-ă) A decreased sensitivity to allergens.

**hyperglandular** (hī″pĕr-glăn′dū-lăr) [″ + L. *glandula,* a little acorn] Having excessive glandular secretions.

**hyperglobulinemia** (hī″pĕr-glŏb″ū-lĭn-ē′mē-ă) [″ + L. *globulus,* a globule, + Gr. *haima,* blood] Excessive globulin in the blood.

**hyperglycemia** (hī″pĕr-glī-sē′mē-ă) [″ + *glykys,* sweet, + *haima,* blood] Increased blood sugar, as in diabetes. This condition increases susceptibility to infection and often precedes diabetic coma. SEE: *hypoglycemia.*

**hyperglyceridemia** (hī″pĕr-glĭs″ĕr-ĭ-dē′mē-ă) An accumulation of glycerides, esp. triglycerides, in the blood.

**hyperglycinemia** (hī″pĕr-glī″sĭ-nē′mē-ă) An accumulation of glycine in the blood. It is caused by a congenital defect in the ability to metabolize the amino acid glycine. There are at least six forms of this disease, all of which are associated with mental and growth retardation.

**hyperglycogenolysis** (hī″pĕr-glī″kō-jĕn-ŏl′ĭ-sĭs) [″ + ″ + *gennan,* to form, + *lysis,* dissolution] Excessive conversion of glycogen into glucose by hydrolysis.

**hyperglycorrhachia** (hī″pĕr-glī″kō-rā′kē-ă) [″ + *glykys,* sweet, + *rhachis,* spine] An excess of sugar in the cerebrospinal fluid.

**hypergnosia** (hī″pĕr-nō′sē-ă) [″ + *gnosis,* knowledge] A distorted or exaggerated perception, influenced by the unconscious projection of emotional subjective experiences.

**hypergonadism** (hī″pĕr-gō′năd-ĭzm) [″ + *gone,* seed, + *-ismos,* state of] Excessive hormonal secretion of the sex glands.

**hyperguanidinemia** (hī″pĕr-gwăn″ĭ-dĭn-ē′mē-ă) [″ + Sp. *guano,* dung, + *haima,* blood] An abnormal amount of guanidine in the blood.

**hyperhedonia, hyperhedonism** (hī″pĕr-hē-dō′nē-ă, -hē′dŏn-ĭzm) [Gr. *hyper,* over, above, excessive, + *hedone,* pleasure, + *-ismos,* state of] **1.** Abnormal pleasure in anything. **2.** Abnormal sexual excitement.

**hyperhidrosis** (hī″pĕr-hī-drō′sĭs) [″ + *hidros,* sweat, + *osis,* condition] Sweating greater than would be expected considering the temperature of the environment. SEE: *bromidrosis; sweat.*

ETIOLOGY: This symptom may be caused by functional overactivity of sweat glands due to debilitating disease or stimulants. Sweating is increased in rheumatic, malarial, relapsing, and septic fever. It occurs in neuralgia and migraine, and follows the ingestion of certain drugs and hot drinks. It affects the hands and feet locally in hysteria, fright, nervous irritability, and hyperthyroidism. Abnormal sweating may also be associated with hot flashes experienced during menopause.

TREATMENT: If the sweating is due to a systemic disease, appropriate therapy for that condition is indicated. If localized, application of a 20% solution of aluminum chloride hexahydrate in absolute alcohol at night using occlusive dressings is beneficial. The dressed sites must be dried before application and the salt washed away in the morning. Twice weekly treatment of the areas with tap water electrophoresis may be of benefit. In chronic cases that do not respond to therapy, thoracic sympathectomy may be required.

**hyperimmune** (hī″pĕr-ĭm-mūn′) A state of greater than normal immunity.

**hyperinflation** (hī″pĕr-ĭn-flā′shŭn) An excess of air in anything, esp. the lungs.

**hyperinosemia** (hī″pĕr-ī″nō-sē′mē-ă) [″ + *inos,* fiber, + *haima,* blood] An abnormal coagulability of the blood; an excess of fibrinogen in the blood.

**hyperinsulinism** (hī″pĕr-ĭn′sū-lĭn-ĭzm) [″ + L. *insula,* island, + Gr. *-ismos,* condition] An excessive amount of insulin in the blood.

SYMPTOMS: The symptoms associated with hyperinsulinism are consistent with those of hypoglycemia: hunger, weakness, sweating, staggering, diplopia, rarely convulsions, coma, and death.

ETIOLOGY: This condition may be caused by a tumor on islets of Langerhans or an excessive sensitivity of the islet tissue to an increase in blood sugar level. It may also be caused by an overdose of insulin. SEE: *insulin; insulin shock; shock.*

**hyperinvolution** (hī″pĕr-ĭn″vō-lū′shŭn) [″ + L. *involvere,* to enwrap] **1.** Reduction in the size of the uterus to below normal after childbirth. **2.** Reduction in size to below normal of any organ following hypertrophy. SYN: *superinvolution.*

***h. uteri*** Extreme atrophy of the uterus, seen following prolonged lactation or severe puerperal sepsis.

**hyperirritability** (hī″pĕr-ĭr″ĭ-tă-bĭl′ĭ-tē) An increased response to a stimulus.

**hyperisotonic** [″ + *isos,* equal, + *tonos,* tension] Said of one of two solutions that has the greater osmotic pressure. SYN: *hypertonic.*

**hyperkalemia** (hī″pĕr-kă-lē′mē-ă) [″ + L. *kalium,* potassium, + Gr. *haima,* blood] An excessive amount of potassium in the blood. SEE: *hypokalemia.*

ETIOLOGY: This condition is usually caused by inadequate excretion of potassium or the shift of potassium from tissues. Causes of inadequate secretion include acute renal failure, severe chronic renal failure, renal tubuar disorders, hypoaldosteronism, decreased renin secretion due to kidney disease or drugs (e.g., nonsteroidal anti-inflammatory agents, diuretics) that inhibit potassium excretion. The shift of potassium from tissues occurs in tissue damage due to trauma, hemolysis, digitalis poisoning, acidosis, and insulin deficiency.

SYMPTOMS: Clinically the most important changes are cardiac arrhythmias with high-peaked T waves; however, the Q-T interval in the electrocardiogram is not prolonged. Occasionally there may be muscle weakness.

TREATMENT: Mild hyperkalemia can be treated by eliminating the cause. Severe or progressive hyperkalemia is treated vigorously with rapid infusion of 10 to 30 ml of calcium gluconate over a period of 1 to 5 min under constant electrocardiographic monitoring. This infusion does not alter plasma potassium but counteracts the effect of potassium on the neuromuscular membranes. Administration of insulin and glucose or bicarbonate will reduce plasma potassium levels.

**hyperkeratinization** (hī″pĕr-kĕr″ă-tĭn″ĭ-zā′shŭn) [″ + *keras,* horn] A thickening of the horny layers of the skin, esp. of the palms and soles. It may be caused by vitamin A deficiency or chronic arsenic toxicity.

**hyperkeratomycosis** (hī″pĕr-kĕr″ă-tō-mī-kō′sĭs) [″ + ″ + *mykes,* fungus, + *osis,* condition] Hypertrophy of the horny layer of the epidermis resulting from a parasitic fungus.

**hyperkeratosis** [″ + ″ + *osis,* condition] **1.** An overgrowth of the cornea. **2.** An overgrowth of the horny layer of the epidermis.

***h. congenitalis*** Hyperkeratosis in the harlequin fetus.

***epidermolytic h.*** A congenital disorder characterized by hyperkeratosis, erythema, and blisters.

**hyperketonemia** (hī″pĕr-kē″tō-nē′mē-ă) Accumulation of an excess of ketone bodies in the blood.

**hyperketonuria** (hī″pĕr-kē-tō-nūr′ē-ă) An excessive quantity of ketones in the urine.

**hyperkinesia, hyperkinesis** (hī″pĕr-kĭ-nē′zē-ă, -nē′sĭs) [Gr. *hyper,* over, above, excessive, + *kinesis,* movement] Increased muscular movement and physical activity. In children it may be due to minimal brain dysfunction. SEE: *hyperactivity.*

**hyperlactation** (hī″pĕr-lăk-tā′shŭn) [″ + L. *lactare,* to suckle] Excessive milk secretion.

**hyperlipemia** (hī″pĕr-lĭp-ē′mē-ă) [″ + *lipos,* fat, + *haima,* blood] An excessive quantity of fat in the blood.

**hyperlipidemia** An increase of lipids in the blood.

**hyperlipoproteinemia** (hī″pĕr-lĭp″ō-prō″tē-ĭn-ē′mē-ă) Increased lipids in the blood resulting either from an increased rate of synthesis or from a decreased lipoprotein breakdown rate. The lipoproteins transport triglycerides and cholesterol in the plasma. Clinically, an increased lipoprotein level may cause atherosclerosis and pancreatitis. Hyperlipoproteinemias can develop as a result of a primary and heritable biochemical defect of either lipoprotein lipase activity or one of the cofactors essential to the function of that enzyme. They may also develop secondary to certain endocrine and metabolic disorders such as diabetes mellitus; glycogen storage disease, type I; Cushing's syndrome; acromegaly; hypothyroidism; anorexia; use of drugs such as alcohol, oral contraceptives, and glucocorticoids; renal disease; liver disease; immunological disorders; and stress. The hyperlipoproteinemias have been divided into five different lipoprotein patterns describing the changes found in the plasma. These patterns are not descriptive of specific diseases. SEE: *cholesterol; lipoprotein.*

NURSING IMPLICATIONS: The patient is assessed for signs and symptoms, and the patient's lipid profile is monitored regularly. The patient is also monitored for indications of coronary artery disease (CAD) and pancreatitis. Diagnostic procedures are explained. The nurse teaches the patient about the various components of the lipid profile and discusses the various means of lowering VLDL and LDL while increasing HDL levels. The patient should adhere to the prescribed diet, which is the fundamental part of the treatment regimen (usually 1000 to 1500 cal/day); avoid alcoholic beverages and excess sugar; minimize the intake of saturated fats (higher in meats, butter, coconut oil); and increase the intake of polyunsaturated fats (vegetable oils). Prescribed antilipemic drugs are administered and evaluated for desired effects and any adverse reactions, and the patient is taught about these drugs. Before administering a bile acid sequestrant, such as cholestyramine, to lower cholesterol levels, the nurse ascertains that the patient is not taking a drug whose absorption may be affected by bile acid sequestrance, such as beta-adrenergic blockers, digitoxin, diuretics, fat-soluble vitamins, folic acid, thiazides, thyroxine, or warfarin. If so, such drugs should be administered 1 hr before or 4 to 6 hr after the bile acid sequestrant. Dosage adjustment of such drugs may also be required, with readjustment when the bile acid sequestrant is discontinued. Taking cholesterol-reducing medication does not negate the need for dietary control. The nurse assists the patient with additional lifestyle changes, such as medically supervised exercise and smoking cessation, and refers the patient to safe, effective programs and support groups and for nicotine patch therapy, as needed. The patient is encouraged to verbalize fears concerning premature CAD, support is offered, a clear explanation of the treatment regimen is provided, and the patient and family are referred for further counseling as necessary. Women with elevated serum lipids should avoid oral contraceptives or other drugs that contain estrogens.

**hyperliposis** (hī″pĕr-lĭ-pō′sĭs) [″ + *lipos,* fat, + *osis,* condition] An abnormal amount of fat in the body.

**hyperlucency** In radiology, increased radiolucency.

**hypermastia** (hī″pĕr-măs′tē-ă) [″ + *mastos,* breast] **1.** Excessive enlargement of the breast in women or men. This condition may be unilateral. **2.** The presence of an abnormal number of mammary glands.

**hypermature** (hī″pĕr-mă-tūr′) [″ + L. *maturus,* ripe] **1.** Pert. to anything that has passed the stage of maturity. **2.** Overripe, as a cataract or abscess that has gone past the optimum time for incision.

**hypermelanosis** One of several disorders of melanin pigmentation resulting in increased melanin in either the epidermis (melanoderma), in which case the coloration is brown, or in the dermis, in which case it is blue or slate gray (ceruloderma). This disorder may be caused by a number of diseases and conditions, including pregnancy, ACTH-producing tumors, Wilson's disease, porphyria, biliary cirrhosis, chronic renal failure, certain drugs, suntanning, and chronic pruritus. SEE: *hypomelanosis.*

**hypermenorrhea** (hī″pĕr-mĕn″ō-rē′ă) [″ + *men,* month, + *rhoia,* flow] An abnormal increase in the duration or amount of menstrual flow.

**hypermetabolic state** (hī″pĕr-mĕt″ă-bŏl′ĭk) A condition of an abnormally increased rate of metabolism, seen in fever and in salicylate poisoning.

**hypermetabolism** (hī″pĕr-mĕ-tăb′ō-lĭzm) An increased rate of metabolism. SEE: *response, stress.*

***extrathyroidal h.*** An increased rate of metabolism not related to thyroid disease.

**hypermetaplasia** (hī″pĕr-mĕt″ă-plā′sē-ă) [″ + *meta-,* after, + *plassein,* to form]

Overactivity in tissue replacement or transformation from one type of tissue to another, as cartilage to bone.

**hypermetria** (hī″pĕr-mē′trē-ă) [Gr. *hyper,* over, above, excessive, + *metron,* measure] An unusual range of movement; motor incoordination in which muscular movement causes a person to overreach the objective.

**hypermetrope** (hī″pĕr-mĕt′rōp) [″ + ″ + *ops,* eye] Hyperope.

**hypermetropia** (hī″pĕr-mē-trō′pē-ă) Hyperopia. **hypermetropic** (-trŏp′ĭk), *adj.*

**hypermimia** (hī″pĕr-mĭm′ē-ă) [″ + *mimesis,* imitation] The use of a great number of gestures while speaking.

**hypermnesia** (hī″pĕrm-nē′zē-ă) [″ + *mneme,* memory] **1.** A great ability to remember names, dates, and details. **2.** An exaggeration of memory involving minute details of a past experience. It occurs in the manic phase of manic-depressive psychosis; in delirium and hypnoses; at the moment of shock and fright in life-threatening situations; with fever; during neurosurgical procedures involving temporal lobe stimulation; and following some brain injuries.

**hypermobility** (hī″pĕr-mō-bĭl′ĭ-tē) Excessive joint play (movement) that permits increased mobility. It is present in certain diseases of children such as Marfan's or Ehlers-Danlos syndromes.

**hypermorph** (hī′pĕr-morf) [″ + *morphe,* form] One whose length of limb and consequent standing height is high in proportion to the sitting height. SEE: *hypomorph; somatotype.*

**hypermotility** (hī″pĕr-mō-tĭl′ĭ-tē) [″ + L. *motio,* motion] Unusual or excessive movement. SYN: *hyperkinesia.*

**hypermyatrophy** (hī″pĕr-mī-ăt′rō-fē) [″ + *mys,* muscle, + *atrophia,* atrophy] An unusual wasting of muscle.

**hypermyesthesia** (hī″pĕr-mī″ĕs-thē′sē-ă) [″ + ″ + *aisthesis,* sensation] Muscular hyperesthesia.

**hypermyotonia** (hī″pĕr-mī″ō-tō′nē-ă) [″ + ″ + *tonos,* tone] Excessive muscular tonus.

**hypermyotrophy** (hī″pĕr-mī-ŏt′rō-fē) [″ + ″ + *trophe,* nourishment] Abnormal muscular development.

**hypernatremia** (hī″pĕr-nă-trē′mē-ă) [″ + L. *natron,* sodium, + Gr. *haima,* blood] An excess of sodium in the blood.

**hypernephroma** (hī″pĕr-nĕ-frō′mă) [″ + *nephros,* kidney, + *oma,* tumor] Renal cell carcinoma.

**hyperneurotization** (hī″pĕr-nū-rŏt″ĭ-zā′shŭn) [″ + *neuron,* nerve] Grafting of a motor nerve into a muscle that has an intact nerve supply.

**hypernitremia** (hī″pĕr-nī-trē′mē-ă) [″ + *nitron,* niter, + *haima,* blood] An excess of nitrogen in the blood.

**hypernutrition** (hī″pĕr-nū-trĭsh′ŭn) [″ + L. *nutrire,* to nourish] Overfeeding.

**hyperonychia** (hī″pĕr-ō-nĭk′ē-ă) [″ + *onyx,* nail] An overgrowth (hypertrophy) of the nails.

**hyperope** (hī′pĕr-ōp) [″ + *ops,* eye] One who is farsighted. SYN: *hypermetrope.*

**hyperopia** (hī″pĕr-ō′pē-ă) [″ + *ops,* eye] Farsightedness; a defect in vision in which parallel rays come to a focus behind the retina as a result of flattening of the globe of the eye or of an error in refraction. Symptoms include ocular fatigue and poor vision. SYN: *hypermetropia.* SEE: *emmetropia* for illus.

***absolute h.*** Hyperopia in which the eye cannot accommodate.

***axial h.*** Hyperopia caused by shortness of the eye's anteroposterior axis.

***facultative h.*** Hyperopia that can be corrected by accommodation.

***latent h.*** Hyperopia in which the error of refraction is overcome and disguised by ciliary muscle action.

***manifest h.*** Total amount of hyperopia that can be neutralized by a convex lens without interfering with clarity of vision.

***relative h.*** Hyperopia in which vision is clear only when excessive convergence is made.

***total h.*** Complete hyperopia combining both latent and manifest types; the amount of hyperopia present when accommodation is completely suspended by paralyzing the ciliary muscle, which is done by use of a cycloplegic drug.

**hyperorchidism** (hī″pĕr-or′kĭd-ĭzm) [Gr. *hyper,* over, above, excessive, + *orchis,* testicle, + *-ismos,* state of] An abnormal activity of testicular secretion.

**hyperorexia** (hī″pĕr-ō-rĕks′ē-ă) [″ + *orexis,* appetite] Abnormal hunger, usually satisfied by frequent small meals. It occurs in diabetes, hysteria, psychosis, helminthiasis, hyperthyroidism, brain tumors, convalescence from acute diseases, and diseases of the stomach in which hypermotility and hypersecretion are present. SYN: *bulimia.*

**hyperorthocytosis** (hī″pĕr-or″thō-sī-tō′sĭs) [″ + *orthos,* straight, + *kytos,* cell, + *osis,* condition] Increased white blood cells with normal proportion of various forms and without immature forms.

**hyperosmia** (hī″pĕr-ŏz′mē-ă) [″ + *osme,* smell] An abnormal sensitivity to odors.

***general h.*** Total h.

***partial h.*** Increased sensitivity to some odors.

***total h.*** Increased sensitivity to all odors. SYN: *general h.*

**hyperosmolarity** (hī″pĕr-ŏz″mō-lăr′ĭ-tē) Increased osmolarity of the blood.

**hyperostosis** (hī″pĕr-ŏs-tō′sĭs) [″ + *osteon,* bone, + *osis,* condition] An abnormal growth of osseous tissue. SYN: *exostosis; torus.*

***frontal internal h.*** An osteoma, usually multiple or arising from the internal area of the frontal bone.

***infantile cortical h.*** An increased growth of subperiosteal bone occurring most frequently in the mandible and clavicles, with fever and other systemic manifestations.

**hyperovaria** [Gr. *hyper,* over, above, excessive, + L. *ovarium,* ovary] Precocious sexual development in young girls owing to excessive ovarian secretion resulting from unusual and premature ovarian development.

**hyperovulation** The production of a large number of ova, usually in response to hormonal intervention. This is done in an attempt to improve the chance of pregnancy in a patient who has had difficulty conceiving.

**hyperoxaluria** (hī″pĕr-ŏk″să-lū′rē-ă) Increased oxalic acid in the urine.

***enteric h.*** Hyperoxaluria caused by disease of or surgical removal of the ileum.

***primary h.*** An inherited metabolic disease caused by a defect in glyoxalate metabolism. This causes an increased secretion of oxalate in the urine, renal calculi, renal failure, and generalized deficit of oxalate crystals in tissues.

**hyperoxemia** (hī″pĕr-ŏk-sē′mē-ă) [″ + *oxys,* sharp, + *haima,* blood] Increased acidity of the blood.

**hyperoxia** (hī″pĕr-ŏk′sē-ă) Increased oxygen in the blood.

**hyperoxygenation** (hī″pĕr-ŏk″sĭ-jĕn-ā′shŭn) The temporary administration of excess oxygen to a patient to prevent hypoxemia during subsequent therapeutic procedures.

**hyperpancreatism** (hī″pĕr-păn′krē-ă-tĭzm) [″ + *pankreas,* pancreas, + *-ismos,* condition] An abnormal amount of secretion from the pancreas.

**hyperparasitism** (hī″pĕr-păr′ă-sī″tĭzm) A condition in which a parasite lives in or upon another parasite.

**hyperparathyroidism** (hī″pĕr-păr″ă-thī′roy-dĭzm) [″ + *para,* beyond, + *thyreos,* shield, + *eidos,* form, shape, + *-ismos,* condition] A condition caused by increased activity of the parathyroid glands. SEE: *osteitis fibrosa cystica generalisata.*

**hyperpathia** [″ + *pathos,* disease, suffering] Hypersensitivity to sensory stimuli. Includes hyperesthesia, allodynia, and hyperalgesia.

**hyperphagia** [″ + Gr. *phagein,* to eat] Eating more food than required; gluttony. This symptom may be due to a lesion in the hypothalamus of the brain.

**hyperphalangism** (hī″pĕr-făl-ăn′jĭzm) [″ + *phalanx,* closely knit row, + *-ismos,* state of] Having an extra phalanx on a finger or toe. SYN: *polyphalangism.*

**hyperphasia** (hī″pĕr-fā′zē-ă) [″ + *phasis,* speech] An abnormal desire to talk.

**hyperphenylalaninemia** (hī″pĕr-fĕn″ĭl-ăl″ă-nĭ-nē′mē-ă) An increased amount of phenylalanine in the blood. SEE: *phenylketonuria.*

**hyperphonia** (hī″pĕr-fō′nē-ă) [″ + *phone,* voice] **1.** Stuttering or stammering due to irritability of the vocal cords. **2.** Explosive speech exhibited by those who stammer.

**hyperphoria** (hī″pĕr-fō′rē-ă) [″ + *phorein,* to bear] A tendency of one eye to turn upward.

**hyperphosphatasemia** (hī″pĕr-fŏs″fă-tă-sē′mē-ă) Increased alkaline phosphatase in the blood.

**hyperphosphatemia** (hī″pĕr-fŏs″fă-tē′mē-ă) [″ + L. *phosphas,* phosphate, + Gr. *haima,* blood] An abnormal amount of phosphorus in the blood. SYN: *hyperphospheremia.*

**hyperphosphaturia** (hī″pĕr-fŏs-fă-tū′rē-ă) [″ + ″ + Gr. *ouron,* urine] An increased amount of phosphates in the urine.

**hyperphospheremia** (hī″pĕr-fŏs-fĕr-ē′mē-ă) [″ + ″ + Gr. *haima,* blood] Hyperphosphatemia.

**hyperphrenia** (hī″pĕr-frē′nē-ă) [Gr. *hyper,* over, above, excessive, + *phren,* mind] **1.** Excessive mental activity, seen in the manic phase of manic-depressive psychosis. **2.** Mental ability and capacity much greater than normal.

**hyperpigmentation** (hī″pĕr-pĭg″mĕn-tā′shŭn) Increased pigmentation, esp. of the skin.

**hyperpituitarism** (hī″pĕr-pĭ-tū′ĭ-tăr-ĭsm) [″ + L. *pituita,* mucus, + Gr. *-ismos,* condition] A condition resulting from overactivity of the anterior lobe of the pituitary. SEE: *acromegaly; gigantism.*

**hyperplasia** (hī″pĕr-plā′zē-ă) [″ + *plassein,* to form] Excessive proliferation of normal cells in the normal tissue arrangement of an organ. SYN: *hypergenesis.* SEE: illus. **hyperplastic** (-plăs′tĭk), *adj.*

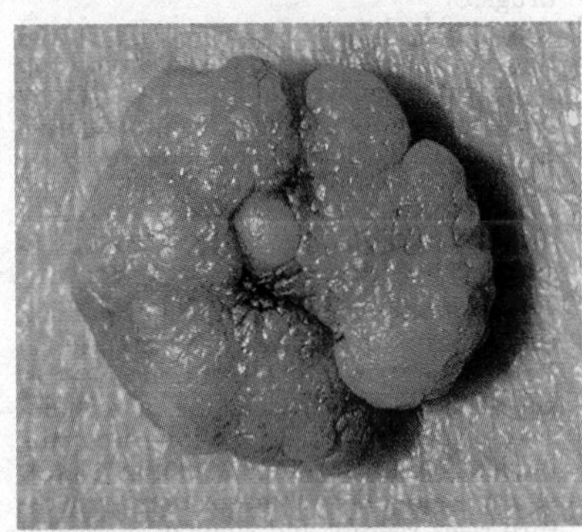

**HYPERPLASIA** OF DERMAL MOLE

***fibrous h.*** An increase in connective tissue cells after inflammation.

**hyperploidy** (hī″pĕr-ploy′dē) A condition of having one extra chromosome and thus not balanced sets of chromosomes. SEE: *Down syndrome; trisomy 21.*

**hyperpnea** (hī″pĕrp-nē′ă) [″ + *pnoia,* breath] An increased respiratory rate or breathing that is deeper than that usually experienced during normal activity. A certain degree of hyperpnea is normal after exercise; it may also be caused by pain, respiratory disease, febrile or cardiac disease, certain drugs, hysteria, or atmospheric conditions experienced at high altitude.

**hyperpraxia** (hī″pĕr-prăk′sē-ă) Excessive activity and restlessness seen in some mental disorders.

**hyperprolactinemia** (hī″pĕr-prō-lăk″tĭn-ē′mē-ă) An excess secretion of prolactin thought to be due to hypothalamic-pituitary dysfunction. This is usually associated with amenorrhea with or without galactorrhea.

**hyperprolinemia** (hī″pĕr-prō″lĭ-nē′mē-ă) An inherited metabolic disease of amino acid metabolism that results in an excess of proline in the body.

**hyperproteinemia** (hī″pĕr-prō″tē-ĭn-ē′mē-ă) [″ + *protos,* first, + *haima,* blood] An excess of protein in the blood plasma.

**hyperproteinuria** (hī″pĕr-prō″tē-ĭn-ū′rē-ă) [″ + ″ + *ouron,* urine] An excess of protein in the urine.

**hyperpselaphesia** (hī″pĕrp-sĕl″ă-fē′zē-ă) [Gr. *hyper,* over, above, excessive, + *pselaphesis,* touch] Hyperaphia.

**hyperptyalism** (hī″pĕr-tī′ăl-ĭzm) [″ + *ptyalon,* spittle] An excessive secretion of saliva. SYN: *hypersalivation.* SEE: *xerostomia.*

ETIOLOGY: Hyperptyalism may be due to pregnancy, stomatitis, rabies, exophthalmic goiter, menstruation, epilepsy, hysteria, nervous conditions, and gastrointestinal disorders. It may be induced by mercury, iodides, pilocarpine, and other drugs.

**hyperpyrexia** (hī″pĕr-pī-rĕks′ē-ă) [″ + *pyressein,* to be feverish] An elevation of body temperature above 106°F (41.1°C). It may be produced by physical agents such as hot baths, diathermy, or hot air or by reaction to infection caused by microorganisms. SYN: *hyperthermia* (1). **hyperpyretic, hyperpyrexial** (-rĕt′ĭk, -rĕk′sē-ăl), *adj.*

***malignant h.*** A severe form of pyrexia that occurs during the use of muscle relaxants and general inhalation anesthesia (usually succinylcholine and halothane) in those who have inherited this tendency as an autosomal dominant trait. During general anesthesia the temperature rises readily and signs of increased muscle metabolism appear. This condition progresses rapidly and, if left untreated, is fatal in 70% of patients. The condition may be diagnosed in susceptible persons by elevated creatine phosphokinase levels and histochemical studies on muscle biopsy, and by a history of exposure to halothane. If these individuals need anesthesia, they should have local anesthesia or neuroleptic anesthesia. SYN: *malignant hyperthermia.*

**hyperreactive** (hī″pĕr-rē-ăk′tĭv) Pert. to an increased response to stimuli.

**hyperreflexia** (hī″pĕr-rē-flĕk′sē-ă) [″ + L. *reflexus,* bent back] An increased action of the reflexes.

**hyperresonance** (hī″pĕr-rĕz′ō-năns) [″ + L. *resonare,* to resound] An increased resonance produced when an area is percussed.

**hypersalivation** (hī″pĕr-săl″ĭ-vā′shŭn) [″ + L. *salivatio,* salivation] Hyperptyalism.

**hypersecretion** (hī″pĕr-sē-krē′shŭn) [″ + L. *secretio,* separation] An abnormal amount of secretion.

**hypersensibility** (hī″pĕr-sĕn″sĭ-bĭl′ĭ-tē) [″ + L. *sensibilitas,* sensibility] Hypersensitivity.

**hypersensitive** (hī″pĕr-sĕn′sĭ-tĭv) [″ + L. *sensitivus,* sensitive] Excessively and abnormally susceptible to the action of a given agent, as pollen or foreign protein. SYN: *supersensitive.* SEE: *allergy; anaphylaxis; hay fever.*

**hypersensitivity** (hī″pĕr-sĕn″sĭ-tĭv′ĭ-tē) An abnormal sensitivity to a stimulus of any kind.

**hypersensitivity reaction** SEE: under *reaction.*

**hypersensitization** (hī″pĕr-sĕn″sĭ-tĭ-zā′shŭn) **1.** Producing or inducing increased sensitivity to an organism or drug. **2.** The condition of being highly sensitive to something.

**hypersomnia** (hī″pĕr-sŏm′nē-ă) [″ + L. *somnus,* sleep] Sleeping for excessive lengths of time. It may be associated with psychiatric illness, drug or alcohol use, or narcolepsy.

**hypersplenism** (hī″pĕr-splĕn′ĭzm) An increased activity of the spleen in which increased amounts of all types of blood cells are removed from the circulation.

**hypersthenia** (hī″pĕr-sthē′nē-ă) [Gr. *hyper,* over, above, excessive, + *sthenos,* strength] Abnormal strength or excessive tension of part or all of the body.

**hypersthenic** (hī″pĕr-sthĕn′ĭk) **1.** Denoting excessive strength or tension. **2.** Denoting a body habitus characterized by a broad, deep thorax, short thoracic cavity, and a large abdominal cavity; a massive build.

**hypersthenuria** (hī″pĕr-sthĕn-ū′rē-ă) [″ + *sthenos,* strength, + *ouron,* urine] The passage of abnormally concentrated urine, usually due to dehydration or excess loss of fluids in sweat.

**hypersusceptibility** (hī″pĕr-sŭ-sĕp″tĭ-bĭl′ĭ-tē) [″ + L. *suscipere,* to take up, + *-bilis,* able] An unusual susceptibility to a disease, pathologic conditions, chemicals, or parasites. SEE: *allergy; anaphylaxis.*

**hypersystole** (hī″pĕr-sĭs′tō-lē) [″ + *systole,* contraction] Unusual force or duration of systole. **hypersystolic** (-sĭs-tŏl′ĭk), *adj.*

**hypertelorism** (hī″pĕr-tĕl′or-ĭzm) [″ + *telouros,* distant] Abnormal distance between two paired organs, esp. the eyes.

**hypertensinogen** (hī″pĕr-tĕn-sĭn′ō-jĕn) A globulin present in blood plasma that, when acted upon by the enzyme renin, forms angiotensin. SYN: *renin substrate.*

**hypertension** (hī″pĕr-tĕn′shŭn) [″ + L. *tensio,* tension] **1.** Greater than normal tension or tonus. **2.** A condition in which the patient has a higher than normal blood pressure. SEE: *Nursing Diagnoses Appendix*. **hypertensive,** *adj.*

ETIOLOGY: The primary factor in hypertension is an increase in peripheral resistance resulting from vasoconstriction or narrowing of peripheral blood vessels. The specific etiology for this condition can be determined in only a small number of patients who have it; however, it is important to attempt to define the exact etiology because, if the disease is due to certain pathological states, definitive and curative therapy can be instituted. Causes in this category include coarctation of the aorta; hyperthyroidism with thyrotoxicosis; patent ductus arteriosus; arteriovenous fistula; pheochromocytoma; psychogenic causes; certain forms of renal disease, particularly when limited to one kidney; adrenal tumors; primary aldosteronism; and polycythemia. SEE: *blood pressure, indirect recording of; heart disease, risk factors; pseudohypertension.*

DIAGNOSIS: There are no precise rules concerning what blood pressure reading is considered to represent hypertension. In general, if on several separate occasions the systolic pressure is above 140 mm Hg or the diastolic above 90 mm Hg, the patient is considered to have elevated blood pressure. Normal systolic blood pressure is not 100 plus the individual's age. Coronary artery disease and cerebral vascular disease, the great causes of death and disability, are much more frequent in those who have elevated blood pressure than in those who are normotensive. On the other hand, a patient's blood pressure may register high merely because of being excited when the pressure is taken. For this reason it is advisable to take the pressure on several separate occasions to be certain that the true blood pressure is being obtained. SEE: *human growth hormone, synthetic; hypertensive crisis.*

TREATMENT: For patients with secondary hypertension, the cause is determined and treated appropriately. For example, patients who have hypertension associated with corticosteroid use may need to have their drug dosage decreased or discontinued.

NURSING IMPLICATIONS: To prevent or diagnose hypertension, periodic blood pressure checks are encouraged, patients are informed of their blood pressure reading and its meaning, and lifestyle changes that may prevent hypertension are encouraged, such as maintaining normal weight and regular exercise patterns, reducing or managing stress, limiting caffeine, and stopping smoking. Hypertensive patients are encouraged to have periodic examinations by their healthcare provider, to cooperate with prescribed medical and dietary therapies, to reduce other risk factors for cardiac disease, and to practice stress reduction and management techniques. The patient's knowledge of the condition is periodically assessed, and misconceptions corrected. The patient is taught about prescribed drug therapy, including safety measures pertaining to orthostatic hypotension and adverse reactions to report. Instruction is provided to the patient and family in the use of a sphygmomanometer to assess and document blood pressure at home on a continual basis following a consistent pattern (which provides more accurate baseline trends in the individual's readings).

***benign h.*** Hypertension that progresses slowly. The basic disease process may progress to the same endpoint as in malignant hypertension but at a slower rate.

***cuff-inflation h.*** A marked increase in blood pressure in association with inflation of the sphygmomanometer cuff. This does not represent true hypertension.

***essential h.*** Hypertension that develops without apparent cause. SYN: *primary h.*

***Goldblatt h.*** Hypertension that resembles renal hypertension produced in experimental animals by decreasing the blood flow to the kidney.

***intracranial h.*** ABBR: ICH. An increase in the pressure inside the skull from any cause such as a tumor, hydrocephalus, intracranial hemorrhage, trauma, infection, or interference with the venous flow from the brain. SEE: *hydrocephalus.*

---

Caution: Patients with intracranial hypertension should not undergo a lumbar puncture or any other procedure that decreases the cerebrospinal fluid pressure in the vertebral canal.

---

***malignant h.*** A form of hypertension that progresses rapidly, accompanied by severe vascular damage. It may progress to the point of death.

***portal h.*** Increased pressure in the portal vein caused by an obstruction of the flow of blood through the liver.

***pregnancy-induced h.*** ABBR: PIH. A complication of pregnancy marked by increasing hypertension, proteinuria, and edema. The diagnostic criteria are an increase of 30 mm Hg systolic or 15 mm Hg diastolic over the baseline pressure for the individual woman on two assessments with at least a 6-hr interval between measures. This condition occurs most commonly in the last trimester; however, it may manifest earlier in women with molar pregnancies. It may worsen rapidly and, if untreated, develop into eclampsia. SYN: *pre-eclampsia.* SEE: *eclampsia; HELLP syndrome.*

The cause is unknown; however, the incidence is higher among adolescent and older primigravidas, diabetics, and women with multiple pregnancy. Pathophysiology includes generalized vasospasm, damage to glomerular membranes, and hemoconcentration due to a fluid shift from intravascular to interstitial compartments. Characteristic complaints include sudden weight gain, severe headaches, and visual disturbances. Indications of increasing severity include complaints of epigastric or abdominal pain; generalized, presacral, and facial edema; oliguria; and hyperreflexia.

The treatment consists of bedrest, a high-protein diet, and medications including mild sedatives, antihypertensives, and intravenous anticoagulants if indicated. Complications are HELLP syndrome and eclampsia.

Nursing Implications: Pregnancy-induced hypertension (PIH) can be prevented by educating pregnant women about maternal and fetal nutritional needs and the importance of prenatal care in the early diagnosis and treatment of PIH, also called pre-eclampsia (the nonconvulsive form of the disorder) and eclampsia (the convulsive form of the disorder). The mother is taught to identify and report signs of PIH, such as headache, excessive weight gain, edema, and oliguria; the importance of keeping scheduled prenatal appointments is stressed.

The pregnant patient's blood pressure is monitored for levels greater than 140/90 mm Hg or for increases of 30 mm Hg systolic or 15 mm Hg diastolic (measured on two occasions more than 6 hours apart). Protein intake is monitored to ensure adequate maternal serum protein levels, normal oncotic pressure, limitation of edema formation, and normal fetal development. Foods high in sodium should be avoided, but excessive salt restriction, fluid restriction, and diuretic use may be harmful.

The patient is also assessed for albuminuria; weight gain greater than 3 lb (1.36 kg) per week in the second trimester or more than 1 lb (0.45 kg) per week in the third trimester; generalized edema, esp. of the face and hands, with pitting edema of the legs and ankles; hyporeflexia or hyperreflexia of the deep tendon reflexes, and clonus; and for oliguria as pre-eclampsia worsens. The patient may also complain of headaches, blurred vision or other visual disturbances, epigastric pain or heartburn, chest pressure, irritability, emotional tension, and decreased fetal activity.

Pre-eclampsia can suddenly progress to eclampsia, demonstrated by the onset of seizures, changes in breathing patterns, and onset of coma. Maternal vital signs, level of consciousness, fluid balance (assessing body weight daily in addition to intake and output), deep tendon reflex activity, headache unrelieved by analgesia, and fetal heart tones are monitored. Bedrest in a left side-lying position is prescribed to prevent venal caval and aortic compression and thereby to increase cardiac output and renal and uterine perfusion, and extremities are elevated to promote venous return. A quiet, calm, nonstimulating and nonstressful environment is created, a call bell is provided, full seizure precautions are in effect, and emergency medications and delivery equipment are available on standby.

The clinical state of the patient and fetus are continually evaluated; maternal vital signs are monitored. The patient is assessed for impending labor, and fetal and maternal responses to labor contractions are evaluated. The obstetrician is notified of any change in the patient's or the fetus' condition. Emergency care is provided during convulsions; prescribed medications are administered as directed, and patient and fetal response are evaluated. Magnesium sulfate administration needs to be carefully monitored because of the potential for toxicity; signs include absence of patellar reflexes, flushing, and muscle flaccidity. Calcium gluconate should be available at the bedside to counteract such effects.

Psychological support and assistance to develop effective coping strategies are provided to both patient and family, and they are prepared for possible premature delivery. Although infants of mothers with PIH are usually small for gestational age, but they sometimes fare better than other premature infants of similar weight because they have developed adaptive ventilatory and other responses to intrauterine stress. SEE: *Nursing Diagnoses Appendix.*

***primary h.*** Essential h.

***pulmonary h.*** Hypertension in the pulmonary arteries.

***renal h.*** **1.** Hypertension produced by kidney disease. The mechanism causing an increase in blood pressure is either alteration in the renal regulation of sodium and fluids or alteration in renal secretion of vasoconstrictors, which alter the tone of systemic or local arterioles. **2.** Hypertension produced experimentally by constriction of renal arteries. It is due to a humoral substance (renin) produced in an ischemic kidney.

***renal vascular h.*** Hypertension due to decreased blood flow to the kidney. The lack of blood supply is usually caused by stenosis of the renal artery, which can be corrected through surgery.

***white coat h.*** A colloquial term used to describe an episode of elevated blood pressure when the reading is taken by a physician. It is caused by anxiety regarding medical examination procedures or fear of possible findings.

**hypertensive** (hī″pĕr-tĕn′sĭv) Marked by a

rise in blood pressure.

***h. crisis*** Arbitrarily defined as severe elevation in diastolic blood pressure above 120 to 130 mm Hg. This is considered to be an emergency if there is evidence of rapid or progressive central nervous system, myocardial, hematological, or renal deterioration.

TREATMENT: Blood pressure must be reduced without delay by use of appropriate therapy, usually sodium nitroprusside (SNP), labetalol, and diazoxide. If the crisis is due to eclampsia, SNP may not be indicated because of risk to fetus. SEE: *cyanide poisoning*.

Caution: Infusion of SNP at the maximum dose rate of 8 μg/kg/min should never last more than 10 minutes.

**hyperthecosis** (hī″pĕr-thē-kō′sĭs) Hyperplasia of the theca interna of the ovary. Hirsutism, amenorrhea, and enlarged clitoris may be present.

**hyperthelia** (hī″pĕr-thē′lē-ă) [Gr. *hyper*, over, above, excessive, + *thele*, nipple] The presence of more than two nipples.

**hyperthermalgesia** (hī″pĕr-thĕrm″ăl-jē′zē-ă) [″ + *therme*, heat, + *algesis*, sense of pain] An unusual sensitivity to heat. SYN: *hyperthermoesthesia*.

**hyperthermia** (hī″pĕr-thĕr′mē-ă) [″ + *therme*, heat] Body temperature elevated above the normal range; an unusually high fever. SYN: *hyperpyrexia*. SEE: *Nursing Diagnoses Appendix*.

ETIOLOGY: Hyperthermia may be caused by heat stroke; central nervous system diseases; thyroid storm; infections including encephalitis, malaria, meningitis, or sepsis, esp. due to gram-negative organisms. To treat some diseases, hyperthermia can be artificially induced by the introduction of the malaria organism, injection of foreign proteins, or physical means.

NURSING IMPLICATIONS: Vital signs are monitored, symptoms assessed and documented, and prescribed therapies administered and the patient's responses documented. External covering is reduced to encourage heat loss through radiation without inducing chilling. The nurse bathes the patient with tepid water, which promotes reduction in surface temperature by convection and evaporation.

Caution: Rubbing alcohol should not be used to reduce fever.

Fluid intake is increased to 3 liters per day (unless otherwise restricted by cardiac or renal disorders) to replace fluids lost through diaphoresis, rapid ventilation, insensible loss, and metabolic increases. Frequent oral hygiene is provided because dehydration dries the oral mucosa. Bedrest is prescribed to reduce metabolic activities, and supplemental oxygen provided as prescribed to help meet these needs. Shivering and chilling are prevented because they further increase the patient's metabolic rate and body temperature. Prescribed antipyretics are administered and, the patient's response and any adverse reactions are monitored.

***malignant h.*** SEE: *hyperpyrexia, malignant*.

**hyperthermia treatment** The use of microwave energy to increase body temperature. This type of therapy, which is usually combined with chemotherapy or radiation, has been used in treating certain malignancies. SEE: *therapy, fever*.

**hyperthermoesthesia** (hī″pĕr-thĕrm″ō-ĕs-thē′zē-ă) [″ + ″ + *aisthesis*, sensation] Hyperthermalgesia.

**hyperthrombinemia** (hī″pĕr-thrŏm″bĭn-ē′mē-ă) [″ + *thrombos*, clot, + *haima*, blood] An excess of thrombin in the blood. This tends to promote intravascular clotting.

**hyperthymia** (hī″pĕr-thī′mē-ă) [″ + *thymos*, mind] Pathological sensitivity or excitability.

**hyperthyroidism** (hī″pĕr-thī′royd-ĭzm) [″ + *thyreos*, shield, + *eidos*, form, shape, + *-ismos*, state of] A disease of unknown etiology marked by sustained overproduction of thyroxine by the thyroid gland. When this continues, thyrotoxicosis results. SEE: *Graves' disease; Nursing Diagnoses Appendix*.

ETIOLOGY: The condition may result from various disorders such as nodular goiter, hyperemesis gravidarum, excess iodine ingestion, or pituitary adenoma; however, the most common cause is Graves' disease.

SYMPTOMS: In general, the signs and symptoms of Graves' disease are divided into two categories—those secondary to excessive stimulation of the sympathetic nervous system and those due to excessive levels of circulating thyroxine. The symptoms caused by sympathetic (adrenergic) stimulation include tachycardia, tremor, increased systolic blood pressure, hyperreflexia, eyelid lag (lagophthalmos), staring, palpitations, depression, nervousness, and anxiety. Symptoms caused by increased circulating thyroxine include increased metabolism, hyperphagia, weight loss, and some psychological disturbances.

TREATMENT: In Graves' disease, the adrenergic signs and symptoms respond to beta-adrenergic blocking agents. Definitive therapies include thyroidectomy, antithyroid drugs, and radioiodine, the latter being the preferred method.

NURSING IMPLICATIONS: Vital signs, fluid balance, and weight are monitored, and activity patterns documented. As necessary, neck circumference is measured to document progression of thyroid enlargement. Serum electrolyte levels are monitored, blood glucose levels checked for evidence of hyperglycemia and urine for glycosuria, and the ECG evaluated for arrhythmias and ST-segment changes. The nurse assesses for classic signs and symptoms (as above). The patient is assessed for indications of thyrotoxic crisis or heart failure. The patient's knowledge of the disorder is determined, misconceptions are corrected, and information on the condition, related problems, and symptom management is provided. Medical treatments, including radioactive iodine, are administered and evaluated for desired response and adverse reactions, and the patient is instructed about these treatments. If the patient has exophthalmos, isotonic eyedrops are instilled to moisten the conjunctivae, and sunglasses or eye patches are recommended to protect the eyes from light. A high-caloric, high-vitamin, high-mineral diet, including between-meal snacks and avoidance of caffeinated beverages, is encouraged. Frequency and characteristics of the patient's stools are checked, and related skin care is provided as needed. The patient should minimize physical and emotional stress and balance rest and activity periods, and wear loose-fitting cotton clothing. A cool, dim, quiet environment is also recommended. The patient is prepared physically and emotionally for surgery if needed. Both patient and family are reassured that mood swings and nervousness will subside with treatment. The patient is encouraged to verbalize feelings about changes in body image, assistance provided to help the patient to identify and develop positive coping strategies, emotional support offered, and referral for further counseling arranged as necessary. Life-long thyroid hormone replacement therapy will be necessary after surgical removal or radioactive iodine ablation treatment. The patient should wear or carry a medical identification device describing the condition and treatment and carry medication with him or her at all times.

**hyperthyrosis** (hī″pĕr-thī-rō′sĭs) Hyperthyroidism.

**hyperthyroxinemia** (hī″pĕr-thī-rŏk″sĭ-nē′mē-ă) An excess of thyroxine in the blood.

**hypertonia** (hī″pĕr-tō′nē-ă) [″ + *tonos*, tension] Hypertonicity.

**hypertonic** (hī″pĕr-tŏn′ĭk) **1.** Pert. to a solution of higher osmotic pressure than another. **2.** In a state of greater than normal tension or of incomplete relaxation, said of muscles; the opposite of hypotonic.

**hypertonicity** (hī″pĕr-tŏn-ĭ′sĭ-tē) An excess of muscular or arterial tonus or intraocular pressure. SYN: *hypertonia*.

**hypertonus** (hī″pĕr-tō′nŭs) Increased tension, as muscular tension in spasm.

**hypertrichophobia** (hī″pĕr-trĭk″ō-fō′bē-ă) [″ + ″ + *phobos*, fear] A fear of hair on the body.

**hypertrichophrydia** (hī″pĕr-trĭk″ŏ-frĭd′ē-ă) [″ + ″ + *ophrys*, eyebrow] Excessive thickness of the eyebrows.

**hypertrichosis** (hī″pĕr-trĭ-kō′sĭs) [″ + ″ + *osis*, condition] An excessive growth of hair, possibly caused by endocrine disease, esp. of the adrenal gland, and in women, disease of the ovary. SYN: *polytrichia; polytrichosis*.

**hypertriglyceridemia** (hī″pĕr-trī-glĭs″ĕr-ī-dē′mē-ă) An increased blood triglyceride level.

**hypertrophia** (hī″pĕr-trō′fē-ă) [Gr. *hyper*, over, above, excessive, + *trophe*, nourishment] Hypertrophy.

**hypertrophy** (hī-pĕr′trŏ-fē) [″ + *trophe*, nourishment] An increase in the size of an organ or structure, or of the body, owing to growth rather than tumor formation. This term is generally restricted to an increase in size or bulk not resulting from an increase in number of cells or tissue elements. It is sometimes used to apply to any increase in size as a result of functional activity. SYN: *hypertrophia*. SEE: *hyperplasia*. **hypertrophic** (hī″pĕr-trŏf′ĭk), *adj*.

***adaptive h.*** Hypertrophy in which an organ increases in size to meet increased functional demands, as the hypertrophy of the heart that accompanies valvular disorders.

***benign prostatic h.*** SEE: *benign prostatic hypertrophy*.

***cardiac h.*** An increase in size of the heart resulting from hypertrophy of muscle tissue, but without an increase in the size of the chambers.

***compensatory h.*** Hypertrophy resulting from increased function of an organ because of a defect or impaired function of the opposite of a paired organ.

***concentric h.*** Hypertrophy in which the walls of an organ become thickened without enlargement but with diminished capacity.

***eccentric h.*** Hypertrophy of an organ with dilatation.

***false h.*** Hypertrophy with degeneration of one constituent of an organ and its replacement by another.

***gingival h.*** Excess growth of the gingival tissue, possibly associated with prolonged phenytoin therapy.

***Marie's h.*** Chronic periostitis that causes the soft tissues surrounding the joints to enlarge.

***numerical h.*** Hypertrophy caused by an increase in structural elements.

***physiological h.*** Hypertrophy due to natural rather than pathological factors.

***pseudomuscular h.*** A disease, usually of childhood, characterized by paralysis, depending on degeneration of the muscles, which paradoxically become enlarged from a deposition of fat and connective tissue.

SYMPTOMS: This disease causes muscle weakness. The patient is awkward, stumbling and seeking support in walking. As paralysis increases, the muscles, particularly those of the calf, thigh, buttocks, and back, enlarge. The upper extremities are less frequently affected. When the patient stands erect, the feet are wide apart, the abdomen protrudes, and the spinal column shows a marked curvature with convexity forward. Rising from the recumbent position is accomplished by grasping the knees or by resting the hands on the floor in front, extending the legs and pushing the body backward. The gait is characterized by waddling. In a few years the paralysis becomes so marked that the patient is unable to leave the bed, which leads to further generalized muscular atrophy.

TREATMENT: Physical therapy helps to prevent contractures, but there is no effective therapy. The prognosis for this disease is unfavorable.

***simple h.*** Hypertrophy due to an increase in the size of structural parts.

***true h.*** Hypertrophy caused by an increase in the size of all the different tissues composing a part.

***ventricular h.*** Increased size and muscular content of the ventricular myocardium.

***vicarious h.*** Hypertrophy of an organ when another organ of allied function is disabled or destroyed.

**hypertropia** [Gr. *hyper,* over, above, excessive, + *tropos,* turning] Vertical strabismus upward. SYN: *strabismus sursum vergens.*

**hyperuricemia** (hī″pěr-ū″rĭs-ē′mē-ă) [″ + *ouron,* urine, + *haima,* blood] An abnormal amount of uric acid in the blood.

**hyperuricuria** (hī″pěr-ū″rĭk-ū′rē-ă) [″ + ″ + *ouron,* urine] An abnormal amount of uric acid in the urine.

**hypervalinemia** (hī″pěr-văl″ĭn-ē′mē-ă) An inherited condition caused by a deficiency of the enzymes essential to the metabolism of valine. The condition is marked by mental retardation, nystagmus, vomiting, and failure to thrive.

**hypervascular** (hī″pěr-văs′kū-lăr) [″ + L. *vasculus,* vessel] Excessively vascular.

**hyperventilation** (hī″pěr-věn″tĭ-lā′shŭn) [″ + L. *ventilatio,* ventilation] Increased minute volume ventilation which results in a lowered carbon dioxide ($CO_2$) level (hypocapnia). It is a frequent finding in many disease processes such as asthma, metabolic acidosis, pulmonary embolism, and pulmonary edema, and also in anxiety-induced states. SEE: *carpopedal spasm.*

TREATMENT: Treatment is directed at the underlying cause. Immediate therapy consists of decreasing the rate of loss of $CO_2$. This is best done by having the patient breathe through only one nostril, with the mouth closed. The patient can close one nostril by placing a finger against that side of the nose. This method is simpler than having the patient breathe into a paper bag over the head. After the acute phase of the hyperventilation episode has been treated it will be necessary to determine the underlying cause and provide appropriate therapy.

**hyperviscosity** (hī″pěr-vĭs-kŏs′ĭ-tē) [″ + L. *viscosus,* gummy] Excessive viscosity or exaggeration of adhesive properties. It is seen in anemias and inflammatory diseases.

**hypervitaminosis** (hī″pěr-vī″tă-mĭn-ō′sĭs) [″ + L. *vita,* life, + *amine* + Gr. *osis,* condition] A condition caused by an excessive intake of vitamins in the diet; most commonly due to excessive ingestion of vitamin pills.

**hypervolemia** (hī″per-vŏl-ē′mē-ă) [″ + L. *volumen,* volume, + Gr. *haima,* blood] A plethora of blood; an abnormal increase in the volume of circulating blood.

**hypesthesia** (hī″pĕs-thē′zē-ă) [Gr. *hypo,* under, beneath, below, + *aisthesis,* sensation] A lessened sensibility to touch; variant of hypoesthesia.

**hypha** (hī′fă) *pl.* **hyphae** [Gr. *hyphe,* web] A filament of mold, or part of a mold mycelium.

**hyphedonia** (hīp″hě-dō′nē-ă) [Gr. *hypo,* under, beneath, below, + *hedone,* pleasure] An abnormal diminution of pleasure in acts that should normally give pleasure.

**hyphema** (hī-fē′mă) [Gr. *hyphaimos,* suffused with blood] Blood in the anterior chamber of the eye, in front of the iris.

**Hyphomycetes** (hī″fō-mī-sē′tēz) [Gr. *hyphe,* web, + *mykes,* fungus] The Fungi Imperfecti; filamentous fungi with branched or unbranched threads. They do not have sexual spores.

**hypnagogic** (hĭp-nă-gŏj′ĭk) [Gr. *hypnos,* sleep, + *agogos,* leading] **1.** Inducing sleep or induced by sleep. SYN: *hypnotic.* SEE: *zones, hypnogenic* **2.** In psychology, pert. to hallucinations or dreams occurring just before loss of consciousness.

***h. state*** A transitional state between sleeping and waking, and the delusions that may result therefrom.

**hypnagogue** (hĭp′nă-gŏg) Concerning or causing sleep or drowsiness.

**hypno-** Combining form relating to sleep or hypnosis.

**hypnoanalysis** (hĭp″nō-ă-năl′ĭ-sĭs) [″ + *analysis,* a dissolving] Combined psychoanalytic therapy and hypnosis.

**hypnoanesthesia** (hĭp″nō-ăn″ĕs-thē′zē-ă) The use of hypnosis to produce anesthesia.

**hypnodontics** (hĭp″nō-dŏn′tĭks) The application of controlled suggestion and hypnosis to the practice of dentistry.

**hypnogenic** (hĭp″nŏ-jĕ-n′ĭk) [″ + *gennan,* to produce] Producing sleep.

**hypnoidal** (hĭp-noy′dăl) [″ + *eidos,* form, shape] Pert. to a condition between sleep and waking, resembling sleep.

**hypnoidization** (hĭp″noy-dī-zā′shŭn) [″ + *eidos,* form, shape] The induction of hypnosis.

**hypnolepsy** (hĭp′nŏ-lĕp″sē) [″ + *lepsis,* seizure] Narcolepsy.

**hypnonarcoanalysis** (hĭp″nō-năr″kō-ă-năl′ĭ-sĭs) A psychiatric interview combining hypnosis with drug-induced sedation or narcosis.

**hypnonarcosis** (hĭp″nō-năr-kō′sĭs) A combination of hypnosis and narcosis.

**hypnophobia** (hĭp″nō-fō′bē-ă) [″ + *phobos,* fear] A morbid fear of falling asleep.

**hypnopompic** (hĭp″nŏ-pŏm′pĭk) [″ + *pompe,* procession] Pert. to dreams or visual images persisting after sleep and before complete awakening.

**hypnosis** (hĭp-nō′sĭs) [″ + *osis,* condition] A subconscious condition in which the objective manifestations of the mind are more or less inactive, accompanied by an abnormal sensibility to suggestions. Hypnosis has been used to treat phobias and anxiety, and to manage pain. SEE: *autohypnosis; hypnotism; sleepwalking; somnambulism.*

**hypnotherapy** (hĭp″nō-thĕr′ă-pē) [″ + *therapeia,* treatment] Treatment by hypnotism or by inducing prolonged sleep.

**hypnotic** (hĭp-nŏt′ĭk) [Gr. *hypnos,* sleep] **1.** Pert. to sleep or hypnosis. **2.** An agent that causes an insensitivity to pain by inhibiting afferent impulses or by inhibiting the reception of sensory impressions in the cortical centers of the brain, thus causing partial or complete unconsciousness. Hypnotics include sedatives, analgesics, anesthetics, and intoxicants, and are sometimes called somnifacients and soporifics when used to induce sleep.

**hypnotism** (hĭp′nō-tĭzm) [″ + *-ismos,* condition] The act of inducing hypnosis.

**hypnotist** (hĭp′nō-tĭst) [Gr. *hypnos,* sleep] One who practices hypnotism.

**hypnotize** (hĭp′nō-tīz) To put under hypnosis.

**hypo** (hī′pō) [Gr. *hypo,* under, beneath, below] Popular name for hypodermic syringe or injection.

**hypo-, hyp-** [Gr. *hypo,* under, beneath, below] Prefix indicating *less than, below,* or *under.* SEE: *sub-.*

**hypoacidity** (hī″pō-ă-sĭd′ĭ-tē) [″ + L. *acidus,* sour] A condition of decreased acid in the stomach caused by lowered hydrochloric acid secretion. This condition may occur secondary to other disorders, such as stomach cancer or pernicious anemia. Hydrochloric acid should be given orally as treatment.

---

Caution: In order to protect the teeth, the patient should suck the acid solution through a straw.

---

**hypoacusis** (hī″pō-ă-kū′sĭs) [″ + *akousis,* hearing] Decreased sensitivity to sound stimuli.

**hypoadrenalism** (hī″pō-ăd-rē′năl-ĭzm) [″ + L. *ad,* to, + *renalis,* pert. to kidney, + Gr. *-ismos,* state of] Adrenal insufficiency.

**hypoadrenocorticism** (hī″pō-ă-drē″nō-kor′tĭ-sĭzm) Decreased secretion, or the effect of the adrenal cortical hormone.

**hypoaffectivity** (hī″pō-ăf′fĕk-tĭv′ĭ-tē) Decreased responsiveness to emotional stimuli. SEE: *obtund.*

**hypoalbuminemia** (hī″pō-ăl-bū″mĭn-ē′mē-ă) Decreased albumin in the blood.

**hypoaldosteronism** (hī″pō-ăl″dō-stēr′ōn-ĭzm) A condition characterized by decreased aldosterone in the blood associated with hypotension and increased salt excretion.

**hypoallergenic** [″ + *allos,* other, + *ergon,* work] Diminished potential for causing an allergic reaction.

**hypoazoturia** (hī″pō-ăz-ō-tū′rē-ă) [″ + L. *azotum,* nitrogen, + Gr. *ouron,* urine] Diminished urea in the urine.

**hypobaric** (hī″pō-băr′ĭk) [″ + *baros,* weight] Decreased atmospheric pressure. SEE: *bends; edema, high-altitude pulmonary.*

**hypoblast** (hī′pō-blăst) [″ + *blastos,* germ] The inner cell layer or endoderm, which develops during gastrulation. The external layer is called ectoderm. **hypoblastic** (hī-pō-blăs′tĭk), *adj.*

**hypocalcemia** (hī″pō-kăl-sē′mē-ă) [″ + L. *calx,* lime, + Gr. *haima,* blood] Abnormally low blood calcium. This condition is transient in severe sepsis; burns; acute renal failure; multiple transfusions with citrated blood; and medications such as protamine, heparin, and glucagon. Chronic hypocalcemia may be caused by chronic renal failure, hereditary or acquired hypoparathyroidism, vitamin D deficiency, pseudohypoparathyroidism, and hypomagnesemia. Clinical manifestations in chronic hypocalcemia include muscle spasm, carpopedal spasm, facial grimacing, possible convulsions, and mental changes such as irritability, depression, and psychosis. Treatment consists of appropriate therapy for the causative disease.

**hypocalciuria** (hī″pō-kăl″sē-ū′rē-ă) Decreased calcium in the urine.

**hypocapnia** (hī″pō-kăp′nē-ă) [Gr. *hypo,* under, beneath, below, + *kapnos,* smoke] A decreased amount of carbon dioxide in the blood. An excessively rapid rate of respiration will cause this.

**hypocarbia** (hī″pō-kăr′bē-ă) Hypocapnia.

**hypocellularity** (hī″pō-sĕl″ū-lăr′ĭ-tē) Decreased cell content of any tissue.

**hypochloremia** (hī″pō-klō-rē′mē-ă) [″ + *chloros,* green, + *haima,* blood] Deficiency of the chloride content of the blood. SYN: *chloropenia.*

**hypochlorhydria** (hī″pō-klor-hī′drē-ă) [″ + ″ + *hydor,* water] Hypoacidity. SEE: *achlorhydria; hyperchlorhydria.*

**hypochlorite** A salt of hypochlorous acid used in household bleach and as an oxidizer, deodorant, and disinfectant.

**hypochlorite salt poisoning** SEE: *Poisons and Poisoning Appendix.*

**hypochlorization** (hī″pō-klō″rĭ-zā′shŭn) Diminished sodium chloride in the diet; used in treating hypertension and certain kidney diseases.

**hypochloruria** (hī″pŏ-klor-ū′rē-ă) [″ + *chloros,* green, + *ouron,* urine] Diminution of chlorides in the urine.

**hypocholesteremia** (hī″pō-kō-lĕs-tĕr-ē′mē-ă) [″ + *chole,* bile, + *stereos,* solid, + *haima,* blood] Decreased blood cholesterol.

**hypochondria** (hī″pō-kŏn′drē-ă) [″ + *chondros,* cartilage] An abnormal concern about one's health, with the false belief of suffering from some disease, despite medical reassurance to the contrary. This is a common symptom among depressed patients. The certainty of this diagnosis in an elderly person is complicated by the presence of physical disabilities and diseases and the increase of social stress factors that accompany the aging process. SYN: *hypochondriasis.*

**hypochondriac** (hī″pō-kŏn′drē-ăk) **1.** Pert. to the region of the hypochondrium or the the upper lateral region on each side of the body and below the thorax; beneath the ribs. **2.** An individual with an abnormal and excessive interest in and fear of disease, esp. in persons who are otherwise healthy. **hypochondriacal** (-kŏn-drī′ă-kăl), *adj.*

***h. region*** Hypochondrium.

**hypochondriasis** (hī″pō-kŏn-drī′ă-sĭs) [″ + *chondros,* cartilage, + *-iasis,* diseased condition] Hypochondria.

**hypochondrium** (hī″pō-kŏn′drē-ŭm) The part of the abdomen beneath the lower ribs on each side of the epigastrium.

**hypochromasia** (hī″pō-krō-mā′sē-ă) [″ + *chroma,* color] Decreased hemoglobin in the red blood cells.

**hypochromatism** (hī″pō-krō′mă-tĭzm) [″ + *chroma,* color] **1.** Decreased or lack of color. **2.** Decreased pigment in a cell, esp. its nucleus. **3.** Decreased hemoglobin in the red cells.

**hypochromatosis** (hī″pō-krō-mă-tō′sĭs) [″ + ″ + *osis,* condition] The disappearance of the chromatin or nucleus in a cell. SYN: *chromatolysis.*

**hypochromia** (hī″pō-krō′mē-ă) A condition of the blood in which the red blood cells have a reduced hemoglobin content. **hypochromic** (-krōm′ĭk), *adj.*

**hypochylia** (hī″pō-kī′lē-ă) [Gr. *hypo,* under, beneath, below, + *chylos,* juice] Lack of normal secretion of gastric juice.

**hypocomplementemia** (hī″pō-kŏm″plĕ-mĕn-tē′mē-ă) Decreased complement in the blood.

**hypocondylar** (hī″pō-kŏn′dĭ-lăr) [″ + *kondylos,* condyle] Below a condyle.

**hypocone** (hī″pō-kōn) [″ + *konos,* cone] The distolingual cusp of an upper molar tooth.

**hypoconid** (hī″pō-kō′nĭd) The distobuccal cusp of a lower molar tooth.

**hypoconulid** The distal, or fifth, cusp of the mandibular first molar tooth. SEE: *hypoconid.*

**hypocorticism** (hī″pō-kor′tĭ-sĭzm) Decreased adrenal cortical hormone.

**hypocrinism** (hī″pō-krī′nĭzm) [″ + *krinein,* to separate, + *-ismos,* condition] Deficient secretion of any gland, esp. an endocrine gland.

**hypocupremia** (hī″pō-kū-prē′mē-ă) Decreased copper in the blood.

**hypocyclosis** (hī″pō-sī-klō′sĭs) [″ + *kyklos,* circle] Deficient accommodation of the eye.

***ciliary h.*** A weakness of the ciliary muscle.

***lenticular h.*** A lack of elasticity in the crystalline lens.

**hypocythemia** (hī″pō-sī-thē′mē-ă) [″ + *kytos,* cell, + *haima,* blood] A decrease in the number of blood cells, esp. red blood cells.

**hypodactylia** (hī″pō-dăk-tĭl′ē-ă) [″ + *daktylos,* finger] Having less than the normal number of fingers or toes.

**Hypoderma** (hī″pō-dĕr′mă) [″ + *derma,* skin] A genus of warble flies of the family Oestridae. The larvae of some species attack cattle and, rarely, humans. They cause a subcutaneous channel of inflammation as they burrow under the skin. SEE: *larva migrans, cutaneous.*

**hypodermatomy** (hī″pō-dĕr-măt′ō-mē) [″ + *derma,* skin, + *tome,* incision] Subcutaneous incision or section, as of a muscle or tendon.

**hypodermiasis** (hī″pō-dĕr-mī′ă-sĭs) [″ + ″ + *-iasis,* condition] Infection with *Hypoderma.*

**hypodermic** (hī″pō-dĕr′mĭk) [″+ *derma,* skin] Under or inserted under the skin, as a hypodermic injection. It may be given subcutaneously (under the skin), intracutaneously (into the skin), intramuscularly (into a muscle), intraspinally (into the spinal canal), or intravascularly (into a vein or artery). It is given to secure prompt action of a drug when the drug cannot be taken by mouth, when it may not be readily absorbed in the stomach or intestines, when it might be changed by the action of the gastric secretions, or to act as an anesthetic about the site of injection. SEE: *anesthesia, local.*

---

Caution: When the injected substance is not intended for intravascular injection, the syringe plunger should be pulled back after the needle is inserted to determine if the needle is in a vein or artery. If blood is obtained, the needle must be repositioned and the procedure repeated. It may be necessary to use a fresh needle and syringe. Because medicines not intended for intravenous injection produce serious undesired effects when given by this route, do not inject the medicine if the needle is in a vessel. If the medicine is to be injected into an artery or vein, it must not be administered unless pulling back on the plunger permits blood freely to enter the syringe.

---

***intracutaneous h.*** Injection into the skin.

***intramuscular h.*** Injection given in the gluteal or lumbar muscular region. This route is used when a drug is not easily absorbed, when it is irritating, or when a large quantity of liquid is to be used.

***intraspinal h.*** Injection into the spinal canal.

***intravenous h.*** Injection into a vein, the usual site being the median basilic or median cephalic vein of the arm.

***subcutaneous h.*** Injection given just under the skin, usually in the outer surface of the arm and forearm.

**hypodermoclysis** (hī″pō-dĕr-mŏk′lĭ-sĭs) [Gr. *hypo,* under, beneath, below, + *derma,* skin, + *klysis,* a washing out] Injection of fluids into the subcutaneous tissues to supply the body with liquids quickly, as after shock, hemorrhage, or diarrhea; it may be given in any condition in which it is impossible to give sufficient water by mouth, by rectum, or by vein.

When it is necessary to maintain a larger amount of water in the tissues in order to keep up proper metabolism, hypodermoclysis may be ordered. The purpose is about the same as that of intravenous infusions. Physiological salt solution (normal salt solution) is usually used because it is compatible with the constituents of the blood. Other solutions are given by this method as preferred by the attending physician. If the solution is not of the correct osmolarity, hemolysis may occur. The solution must be at the proper temperature, from 108° to 115°F (42.2° to 46.1°C), in the flask because it cools rapidly while passing through the tubing.

The site of the injection may be in the loose tissues at the base of the breasts; in the thighs or buttocks (being careful to avoid the large blood vessels); in the axillary line (esp. for men); beneath the skin of the abdomen (halfway between the navel and the anterior superior spine); and intraperitoneally in children. The inner aspect of the thighs should be used as an injection site only with great caution because of its proximity to the femoral vessels.

**hypodontia** (hī″pō-dŏn′shē-ă) Diminished development, or absence, of teeth.

**hypodynamia** (hī″pō-dī-nā′mē-ă) [″ + *dynamis,* power] Diminished muscular power or energy. SEE: *adynamia.*

**hypoeccrisia** (hī″pō-ĕk-krĭs′ē-ă) [″ + *ek,* out, + *krisis,* separation] Diminished excretion of waste material.

**hypoeccritic** (hī″pō-ĕk-krĭt′ĭk) **1.** Retarding normal excretion. **2.** Pert. to insufficient or defective excretion.

**hypoeosinophilia** (hī″pō-ē″ō-sĭn″ō-fĭl′ē-ă) [Gr. *hypo,* under, beneath, below, + *eos,* dawn, + *philein,* to love] A diminished quantity of eosinophil leukocytes in the blood.

**hypoergasia** (hī″pō-ĕr-gā′sē-ă) [″ + *ergon,* work] Decreased functional activity.

**hypoergia** (hī″pō-ĕr′jē-ă) **1.** A mild allergy owing to decreased allergic response. **2.** A diminished response to any stimulus. **hypoergic** (-ĕr′jĭk), *adj.*

**hypoergy** (hī″pō-ĕr′jē) [″ + *ergon,* work] Hyposensitivity to allergens.

**hypoesophoria** (hī″pō-ĕs″ō-fō′rē-ă) [″ + *eso,* inward, + *phorein,* to bear] A downward and inward deviation of the eye.

**hypoesthesia** (hī″pō-ĕs-thē′zē-ă) [″ + *aisthesis,* sensation] A dulled sensitivity to touch.

**hypoexophoria** (hī″pō-ĕks-ō-fō′rē-ă) [″ + *exo,* outward, + *phorein,* to bear] A downward and outward deviation of the eye.

**hypoferremia** (hī″pō-fĕ-rē′mē-ă) Iron deficiency as indicated by diminished iron in the blood.

**hypofibrinogenemia** (hī″pō-fī-brĭn″ō-jĕ-nē′mē-ă) Decreased fibrinogen in the blood.

**hypofunction** (hī″pō-fŭnk′shŭn) Decreased function.

**hypogalactia** (hī″pō-gă-lăk′shē-ă) [″ + *gala,* milk] Deficient milk production.

**hypogammaglobulinemia** (hī″pō-găm″ă-glŏb″ū-lĭ-nē′mē-ă) The lack of one or more of the five classes of antibodies or immunoglobulins caused by defective B lymphocyte function. Patients are highly susceptible to infections from pyogenic organisms (staphylococci, streptococci, and *Pseudomonas aeruginosa*). They are treated with intravenous gamma globulin (100 to 200 mg/kg monthly) and antibiotics specific to the causative organism when infections occur.

***acquired h.*** A form of hypogammaglobulinemia that usually appears after childhood. The cause of the defective B cells is unknown. It is often associated with autoimmune disorders. Patients generally live a relatively normal life span.

***congenital h.*** A hereditary, sex-linked form of hypogammaglobulinemia that appears in male infants at approximately 6 months of age, by which time the maternal immunoglobulins have disappeared from the infant's blood.

**hypogastric** (hī″pō-găs′trĭk) [″ + *gaster,* belly] Pert. to the lower middle of the abdomen or to the hypogastrium.

***h. artery*** Arteria iliaca interna.

***h. plexus*** Sympathetic nerve plexus in the pelvis.

***h. region*** The hypogastrium. SEE: *abdominal regions.*

**hypogastrium** (hī″pō-găs′trē-ŭm) The region below the umbilicus or navel, between the right and left inguinal regions.

**hypogenesis** (hī″pō-jĕn′ĕ-sĭs) [Gr. *hypo,* under, beneath, below, + *genesis,* generation, birth] Cessation of growth or development at an early stage, causing defective structure. SEE: *ateliosis*.

**hypogenitalism** (hī″pō-jĕn′ĭ-tăl-ĭzm) [″ + L. *genitalis*, a genital, + Gr. *-ismos*, condition] A condition in which the genital organs are underdeveloped. It is characterized by reduced size of genital organs, failure of testes to descend in some cases, and incomplete development of secondary sex characteristics. SEE: *hypogonadism*.

**hypogeusia** (hī″pō-gū′sē-ă) [″ + *geusis*, taste] A blunting of the sense of taste.

***idiopathic h.*** A syndrome of unknown cause, consisting of decreased taste and olfactory acuity, and with or without perverted taste (dysgeusia) and smell. In experimental studies, certain trace elements such as zinc added to the diet appear to correct some of the symptoms.

**hypoglossal** (hī″pō-glŏs′ăl) [″ + *glossa*, tongue] Situated under the tongue.

***h. alternating hemiplegia*** Medulla lesion paralyzing the tongue by involving the 12th nerve fibers as they course through the uncrossed pyramid. The pathology may extend across the midline or dorsally, involving the medial fillet, causing contralateral anesthesia.

***h. nerve*** A mixed cranial nerve, carrying afferent proprioceptive impulses as well as efferent motor impulses. It originates in the medulla oblongata and distributes impulses to the extrinsic and intrinsic muscles of the tongue. SYN: *twelfth cranial nerve*.

**hypoglottis** (hī″pō-glŏt′ĭs) The undersurface of the tongue.

**hypoglycemia** (hī″pō-glī-sē′mē-ă) [″ + *glykys*, sweet, + *haima*, blood] A deficiency of blood sugar. SEE: *Nursing Diagnoses Appendix*. **hypoglycemic** (-sē′mĭk), *adj*.

SYMPTOMS: Hypoglycemia is characterized by acute fatigue, restlessness, malaise, marked irritability, and weakness. Severe cases result in mental disturbances, delirium, coma, and possibly death. SEE: *diabetes mellitus* for table; *coma; hyperglycemia; hyperinsulinism; insulinoma; neuroglycopenia*.

ETIOLOGY: Hypoglycemia may be caused by hyperfunction of the islets of Langerhans; injection of an excessive quantity of insulin, or failure to eat after taking insulin; often precipitated by increased energy need, as in exercise. If the diabetic ingests alcohol, the insulin dose needs to be adjusted.

FIRST AID: If the patient is awake with an intact gag reflex and can swallow, give sugar in the form of juice or a candy bar. If the patient is unresponsive, do not put anything in his or her mouth, as it could be aspirated. Intravenous glucose is given if the patient is unconscious, even though the cause may be other than hypoglycemia.

NURSING IMPLICATIONS: Signs of hypoglycemia are monitored and reported in high-risk patients. If possible, blood glucose level (with a glucometer at the bedside) is measured to verify the severity of hypoglycemia before providing corrective treatment. The nurse corrects such episodes quickly and implements measures to protect the unconscious patient, such as maintaining a patent airway. Prescribed medications are administered. The purpose, preparation, procedure, and expected sensations for any diagnostic tests are explained. Hypoglycemic episodes need to be prevented or treated promptly if they do occur to avoid severe complications. The nurse ensures that the patient understands the signs and symptoms and key dangers of hypoglycemia and urges the patient to note signs and symptoms typically experienced. Once it occurs, the patient may quickly lose his ability to think clearly. If this should happen while the patient drives a car or operates machinery, a serious accident could result. The patient taking beta-blockers may experience only CNS-related symptoms. Family, friends, and co-workers also should be taught to recognize this patient's warning signs so that immediate treatment can be instituted. The nurse reviews with the patient and family treatment measures they should follow if the patient experiences a hypoglycemic episode. If conscious, the patient should consume a readily available source of glucose, such as five to six pieces of hard candy; 4 to 6 oz of apple juice, orange juice, cola, or other soft drink; or 1 tbsp of honey or grape jelly. If unconscious, the patient should receive a subcutaneous injection of glucagon; therefore, the patient's family should be taught how to administer the glucagon injection. If hypoglycemic episodes do not respond to treatment or if they occur frequently, either the patient or family should notify the physician. The patient should follow the prescribed diet to prevent a rapid drop in blood glucose levels. A dietitian can help the patient to understand the necessary diet and to develop a dietary plan that includes foods that the patient enjoys while avoiding simple carbohydrates. The patient should eat small meals throughout the day, and bedtime snacks also may be necessary to keep blood glucose at an even level. The patient should avoid delays in mealtimes, as well as alcohol and caffeine, because they may trigger severe hypoglycemic episodes. If the patient is obese and has impaired glucose tolerance, the nurse suggests ways that the patient can restrict caloric intake and lose weight and assists in finding a weight loss support group as necessary. The patient with fasting hypoglycemia should not postpone or skip scheduled meals or snacks and should call the physician for instructions if he or she does not feel well enough to eat. The nurse helps the patient to identify factors that can precipitate a hypoglycemic episode, such as poor diet, stress, or not cooperating with a diabetes mellitus treatment regimen and suggests ways of changing or avoiding each of these factors. As necessary, the nurse teaches the patient stress reduction techniques and encourages him or her to join a support group. Precautions need to be taken when the patient exercises; for example, he should consume extra calories and not exercise alone or at a time when the blood glucose level is likely to drop. The patient should carry a source of fast-acting carbohydrate, such as hard candy, at all times. The patient should wear or carry a medical identification device describing the condition and emergency treatment measures. For the patient with pharmacological hypoglycemia from insulin or antidiabetic agents, the nurse reviews the essentials of managing diabetes mellitus. As warranted, the patient is taught about prescribed drug therapy or surgery; when surgery becomes necessary, the patient is prepared physically and emotionally for the procedure and postoperative care provided (as for a patient undergoing other intra-abdominal surgery, with added blood glucose level concerns). Because hypoglycemia is a chronic disorder, the patient should have periodic medical checkups. Both patient and family are encouraged to discuss their concerns about the patient's condition and treatment, emotional support is offered, and questions are answered honestly.

**hypoglycemic agents, oral** Sulfonylurea compounds that cause a decrease in blood sugar (e.g., acetohexamide, tolbutamide, and chlorpropamide). There is no proof that their use in diabetes mellitus helps prevent the long-term complications of diabetes.

---

Caution: The sulfonylureas should be used only in patients with diabetes of the insulin-independent type who cannot be treated with diet alone and are unwilling or unable to take insulin if weight reduction and dietary control fail.

---

**hypoglycemic shock** SEE: under *shock.*

**hypoglycogenolysis** (hī″pō-glī″kō-jĕn-ŏl′ĭ-sĭs) [Gr. *hypo,* under, beneath, below, + *glykys,* sweet, + *gennan,* to produce, + *lysis,* dissolution] Defective hydrolysis of glycogen (glycogenolysis).

**hypoglycorrhachia** (hī″pō-glī″kō-rā′kē-ă) [″ + ″ + *rhachis,* spine] A decreased amount of glucose in the cerebrospinal fluid. It usually occurs in meningitis.

**hypognathous** (hī-pŏg′nă-thŭs) [″ + *gnathos,* jaw] Having a lower jaw smaller than the upper jaw.

**hypogonadism** (hī″pō-gō′năd-ĭzm) [″ + *gone,* semen, + *-ismos,* condition] Defective internal secretion of the gonads.

**hypogonadotropic** (hī″pō-gŏn″ă-dō-trŏp′ĭk) Concerning or caused by a deficiency of gonadotropin.

**hypohepatia** (hī″pō-hĕ-pă′tē-ă) [″ + *hepar,* liver] Deficient liver function.

**hypohidrosis** (hī″pō-hī-drō′sĭs) [″ + *hidros,* sweat, + *osis,* condition] Diminished perspiration.

**hypohyloma** (hī″pō-hī-lō′mă) [″ + *hyle,* matter, + *oma,* tumor] A tumor formed by embryonic tissue. It is derived from hypoblastic tissue.

**hypoinsulinism** [″ + L. *insula,* island, + Gr. *-ismos,* condition] Diabetes mellitus.

**hypoisotonic** (hī″pō-ī″sō-tŏn′ĭk) [″ + *isos,* equal, + *tonos,* tension] Hypotonic.

**hypokalemia** (hī″pō-kă-lē′mē-ă) [″ + Mod. L. *kalium,* potash, + Gr. *haima,* blood] Extreme potassium depletion in the circulating blood, commonly manifested by episodes of muscular weakness or paralysis, tetany, and postural hypotension. SYN: *hypopotassemia.* SEE: *hyperkalemia.* **hypokalemic** (-lē′mĭk), *adj.*

ETIOLOGY: Causes include deficient potassium intake or excess loss of potassium due to vomiting, diarrhea, or fistulas; metabolic acidosis; diuretic therapy; aldosteronism; excess adrenocortical secretion; renal tubule disease; and alkalosis.

SYMPTOMS: The clinical signs are mostly neuromuscular with generalized weakness. Sudden development of hypokalemia may lead to almost total paralysis. On physical examination the weakness is obvious and deep tendon reflexes are decreased or absent. Electrocardiographic changes include flattening and inversion of the T wave, prominent U wave, and depression of the ST segment. Cardiac arrhythmias may occur, esp. in patients taking digitalis.

TREATMENT: Therapy consists of increased dietary intake of potassium and supplemental potassium chloride in elixir or tablet form.

---

Caution: Enteric-coated potassium chloride can cause small bowel ulceration.

---

**hypokinesia** (hī″pō-kĭ-nē′zē-ă) [″ + *kinesis,* movement] Decreased motor reaction to stimulus. **hypokinetic** (-nĕt′ĭk), *adj.*

**hypolemmal** (hī″pō-lĕm′ăl) [″ + *lemma,* sheath] Situated below a sheath or membrane.

**hypoleydigism** (hī″pō-lī′dĭg-ĭzm) Decreased secretion of androgen by the interstitial (Leydig) cells of the testicles.

**hypolipidemic** (hī″pō-lĭp″ĭ-dē′mĭk) Decreasing the lipid concentration of the blood.

**hypoliposis** (hī″pō-lĭ-pō′sĭs) [″ + *lipos,* fat, + *osis,* condition] A deficiency of fat in the tissues.

**hypologia** (hī-pō-lō′jē-ă) [″ + *logos,* word, reason] A cerebral symptom marked by inadequate speech.

**hypolymphemia** (hī″pō-lĭm-fē′mē-ă) [″ + L. *lympha,* lymph, + Gr. *haima,* blood] Decreased amount of lymphocytes in the blood, with a normal number of leukocytes.

**hypomagnesemia** (hī″pō-măg″nĕ-sē′mē-ă) Decreased magnesium in the blood. Clinically, it is accompanied by increased neuromuscular irritability.

**hypomania** (hī″pō-mā′nē-ă) [″ + *mania,* madness] Mild mania and excitement, with a moderate change in behavior.

**hypomastia** (hī-pō-măs′tē-ă) [″ + *mastos,* breast] A condition of having abnormally small breasts. SYN: *hypomazia.*

**hypomazia** (hī″pō-mā′zē-ă) [″ + *mazos,* breast] Hypomastia.

**hypomelanosis** One of several disorders of melanin pigmentation in which melanin in the epidermis is decreased or absent. It may be caused by albinism, chronic protein deficiency, burns, trauma, or vitiligo. SEE: *hypermelanosis.*

**hypomenorrhea** (hī″pō-mĕn-ō-rē′ă) [″ + *men,* month, + *rhoia,* flow] A deficient amount of menstrual flow, but with regular periods. SEE: *oligomenorrhea.*

**hypomere** (hī′pō-mēr) [″ + *meros,* part] The portion of the mesoderm that later forms the pleuroperitoneal walls. SEE: *epimere; mesomere.*

**hypometabolism** (hī″pō-mĕ-tăb′ō-lĭzm) [″ + *metabole,* change, + *-ismos,* condition] A lowered metabolism.

**hypometria** (hī″pō-mē′trē-ă) [″ + *metron,* measure] A shortened range of movement.

**hypometropia** (hī″pō-mĕ-trōp′ē-ă) [″ + ″ + *ops,* eye] Myopia or nearsightedness.

**hypomnesia, hypomnesis** (hī″pŏm-nē′zē-ă, -nē′sĭs) [″ + *mnesis,* memory] Impaired memory.

**hypomobility** Restricted joint movement (play) that limits normal range of motion; the opposite of hypermobility.

**hypomorph** (hī′pō-morf) [″ + *morphe,* form] An individual with disproportionately short legs with respect to the length of the trunk; the opposite of hypermorph. SEE: *somatotype.*

**hypomotility** (hī″pō-mō-tĭl′ĭ-tē) [″ + L. *motus,* moved] Hypokinesia.

**hypomyotonia** (hī″pō-mī″ō-tō′nē-ă) [″ + *mys,* muscle, + *tonos,* tension] Lacking in muscular tonus.

**hypomyxia** (hī″pō-mĭks′ē-ă) [″ + *myxa,* mucus] A diminished secretion of mucus.

**hyponanosoma** (hī″pō-năn-ō-sō′mă) [″ + *nanos,* dwarf, + *soma,* body] Extreme dwarfism.

**hyponatremia** (hī″pō-nă-trē′mē-ă) [″ + L. *natron,* sodium, + Gr. *haima,* blood] A decreased concentration of sodium in the blood.

**hyponeocytosis** (hī″pō-nē″ō-sī-tō′sĭs) [″ + *neos,* new, + *kytos,* cell, + *osis,* condition] A decreased number of leukocytes (leukopenia) with immature cells in the blood.

**hyponoia** (hī″pō-noy′ă) [″ + *nous,* mind] Diminished or sluggish mental activity.

**hyponychium** (hī-pō-nĭk′ē-ŭm) [Gr. *hypo,* under, beneath, below, + *onyx,* nail] Nailbed. SYN: *matrix unguis.*

**hyponychon** (hī-pŏn′ĭ-kŏn) [″ + *onyx,* nail] An extravasation of blood beneath the nail.

**hypo-orthocytosis** (hī″pō-or″thō-sī-tō′sĭs) [″ + *orthos,* regular, + *kytos,* cell, + *osis,* condition] Leukopenia with normal proportions of white blood cells.

**hypopallesthesia** (hī″pō-păl″ĕs-thē′zē-ă) [″ + *pallein,* to shake, + *aisthesis,* sensation] Decreased ability to perceive vibratory sense.

**hypopancreatism** (hī″pō-păn′krē-ă-tĭzm) [″ + *pankreas,* pancreas, + *-ismos,* condition] Diminished activity of the pancreas.

**hypoparathyreosis** (hī″pō-păr-ă-thī-rē-ō′sĭs) [″ + *para,* beside, + *thyreos,* shield, + *osis,* condition] Hypoparathyroidism.

**hypoparathyroidism** (hī″pō-păr-ă-thī′royd-ĭzm) [″ + ″ + ″ + *eidos,* form, shape, + *-ismos,* condition] A condition caused by an insufficient or absent secretion of the parathyroid glands. SYN: *hypoparathyreosis.* SEE: *Nursing Diagnoses Appendix.*

**hypopepsia** (hī″pō-pĕp′sē-ă) [″ + *pepsis,* digestion] Impaired digestion owing to lack of pepsin.

**hypopepsinia** (hī″pō-pĕp-sĭn′ē-ă) Deficient pepsin in the gastric juice.

**hypoperistalsis** (hī″pō-pĕr″ĭ-stăl′sĭs) Diminished peristalsis. SEE: *paralytic ileus.*

**hypophalangism** (hī″pō-fă-lăn′jĭzm) The state of having fewer than the normal number of fingers or toes.

**hypopharynx** (hī″pō-făr′ĭnks) [″ + *pharynx,* throat] The lower portion of the pharynx that opens into the larynx anteriorly and the esophagus posteriorly. SYN: *laryngopharynx.*

**hypophonesis** (hī″pō-fō-nē′sĭs) [″ + *phone,* voice] A diminished or fainter sound in auscultation or percussion.

**hypophonia** (hī″pō-fō′nē-ă) An abnormally weak voice resulting from incoordination of speech muscles, including weakness of muscles of respiration.

**hypophoria** (hī″pō-fō′rē-ă) [″ + *phorein,* to bear] The tendency of one visual axis to fall below the other one.

**hypophosphatasia** (hī″pō-fŏs″fă-tā′zē-ă) Signs and symptoms of rickets due to a deficiency of alkaline phosphatase. There are four forms of this condition: lethal perinatal, infantile, childhood, and adult. The perinatal and infantile forms are inherited as autosomal recessive traits. The inheritance pattern of the childhood and adult forms is unknown. In the adult form, signs and symptoms may not become apparent until middle age, but there may be a history of early loss of either deciduous or permanent teeth and short stature. No treatment is available.

**hypophosphatemia** (hī″pō-fŏs″fă-tē′mē-ă) [″ + L. *phosphas,* phosphate, + Gr. *haima,* blood] Abnormally decreased amount of phosphates circulating in the blood.

**hypophosphaturia** (hī″pō-fŏs″fă-tū′rē-ă) [″ + ″ + Gr. *ouron,* urine] Decreased excretion of phosphate in the urine.

**hypophrenia** (hī″pō-frē′nē-ă) [″ + *phren,* mind] Mental deficiency. **hypophrenic,** *adj.*

**hypophrenic** (hī″pō-frĕn′ĭk) [″ + *phren,* diaphragm, mind] **1.** Mental deficiency. **2.** Below the diaphragm.

**hypophyseal** (hī″pō-fĭz′ē-ăl) [″ + *physis,* growth] Pert. to the hypophysis or pituitary.

**hypophysectomy** (hī-pŏf″ĭ-sĕk′tō-mē) [″ + ″ + *ektome,* excision] Excision of the hypophysis cerebri.

**hypophyseoportal** (hī″pō-fĭz″ē-ō-por′tăl) Concerning the portal system of the pituitary gland. SEE: *system, hypophyseoportal.*

**hypophyseoprivic** (hī″pō-fĭz″ē-ō-prĭv′ĭk) Deficiency of hormone secretion from the pituitary.

**hypophysis** (hī-pŏf′ĭ-sĭs) *pl.* **hypophyses** [Gr., an undergrowth] **1.** An undergrowth. **2.** The pituitary body or gland. An endocrine gland lying in the sella turcica of the sphenoid bone. It consists of two portions, the adenohypophysis (anterior lobe) and the neurohypophysis (posterior lobe), which are attached to the hypothalamus of the brain by the hypophyseal stalk. SEE: *pituitary gland.*

***h. cerebri*** Pituitary gland.

***pharyngeal h.*** A small structure anterior to the pharyngeal bursa. It is derived from the lower portion of Rathke's pouch and occasionally gives rise to a cyst or tumor.

**hypophysitis** (hī-pŏf″ĭ-sī′tĭs) [Gr. *hypo,* under, beneath, below, + *physis,* growth, + *itis,* inflammation] An inflammation of the pituitary body.

**hypopigmentation** (hī″pō-pĭg″mĕn-tā′shŭn) Diminished pigment in a tissue.

**hypopinealism** (hī″pō-pĭn′ē-ăl-ĭzm) [″ + L. *pineus,* pert. to pine cone, + Gr. *-ismos,* condition] Diminished secretion of the pineal gland.

**hypopituitarism** (hī″pō-pĭ-tū′ĭ-tă-rĭzm) [″ + L. *pituita,* mucus, + Gr. *-ismos,* condition] A condition resulting from diminished secretion of pituitary hormones, esp. those of the anterior lobe. SEE: *Sheehan's syndrome.*

**hypoplasia** (hī″pō-plā′zē-ă) [″ + *plasis,* formation] Underdevelopment of a tissue organ or body. SEE: *tissue.*

**hypopnea** (hī″pō-nē′ă) [″ + *pnoia,* breath] Decreased rate and depth of breathing.

**hypoporosis** (hī″pō-pō-rō′sĭs) [″ + *poros,* callus, + *osis,* condition] Deficient development of a callus at the site of a bone fracture.

**hypoposia** (hī″pō-pō′zē-ă) [″ + *posis,* drinking] A decreased intake of fluids.

**hypopotassemia** (hī″pō-pō″tăs-sē′mē-ă) [″ + *potassium* + Gr. *haima,* blood] Hypokalemia.

**hypoproteinemia** (hī″pō-prō″tē-ĭn-ē′mē-ă) [″ + *protos,* first, + *haima,* blood] A decrease in the amount of protein in the blood.

**hypoprothrombinemia** (hī″pō-prō-thrŏm″bĭn-ē′mē-ă) [″ + L. *pro,* for, + Gr. *thrombos,* clot, + *haima,* blood] A deficiency of blood clotting factor II (prothrombin) in the blood.

**hypopselaphesia** (hī″pŏp-sĕl-ă-fē′zē-ă) [″ + *pselaphesis,* touch] Blunted tactile sense.

**hypoptyalism** (hī″pō-tī′ăl-ĭzm) [″ + *ptyalon,* saliva, + *-ismos,* condition] Decreased salivary secretion.

**hypopyon** (hī-pō′pē-ŏn) [″ + *pyon,* pus] Pus in the anterior chamber of the eye in front of the iris but behind the cornea, seen in corneal ulcer.

**hyporeactive** (hī″pō-rē-ăk′tĭv) A decreased response to stimuli.

**hyporeflexia** (hī″pō-rē-flĕk′sē-ă) [″ + L. *reflexus,* bent back] A diminished function of the reflexes.

**hyposalivation** (hī″pō-săl″ĭ-vā′shŭn) An abnormal decrease in flow of saliva.

**hyposcleral** (hī″pō-sklē′răl) Beneath the sclera of the eye.

**hyposecretion** (hī″pō-sē-krē′shŭn) Lowered amount of secretion.

**hyposensitive** (hī″pō-sĕn′sĭ-tĭv) [″ + L. *sentire,* to feel] Having a reduced ability to respond to stimuli.

**hyposensitization** (hī″pō-sĕn″sĭ-tĭ-zā′shŭn) The production of hyposensitivity.

**hyposialadenitis** (hī″pō-sī″ăl-ăd-ĕ-nī′tĭs) [Gr. *hypo,* under, beneath, below, + *sialon,* saliva, + *aden,* gland, + *itis,* inflammation] Inflammation of the submandibular salivary gland.

**hyposmia** (hī-pŏz′mē-ă) [″ + *osme,* smell] A defect in sense of smell.

**hyposmolarity** (hī-pŏz″mō-lăr′ĭ-tē) Decreased osmolar concentration, esp. of the blood or urine.

**hyposomnia** (hī″pō-sŏm′nē-ă) A decreased ability to sleep. SEE: insomnia, under *sleep, disorders of.*

**hypospadia, hypospadias** (hī″pō-spā′dē-ă, -ăs) [″ + *span,* to draw] **1.** An abnormal congenital opening of the male urethra upon the undersurface of the penis. **2.** A urethral opening into the vagina.

**hypostasis** (hī″pŏs′tă-sĭs) [″ + *stasis,* a standing] **1.** A diminished blood flow or circulation. **2.** A deposit of sediment owing to decreased flow of a body fluid such as blood or urine. **hypostatic,** *adj.*

**hypostatic** (hī″pō-stăt′ĭk) [″ + *statikos,* standing] **1.** Of or pert. to hypostasis. **2.** In genetics, hidden or suppressed, said of a gene whose effect is suppressed by the presence of another gene.

**hyposteatolysis** (hī″pō-stē-ă-tŏl′ĭ-sĭs) [″ + *stear,* fat, + *lysis,* dissolution] Diminished emulsification of fats during digestion.

**hyposthenic** (hī-pŏs-thĕn′ik) **1.** Debilitant. **2.** A body habitus characterized by a long, shallow thorax, a long thoracic cavity, a long, narrow abdominal cavity, and a slender build.

**hyposthenuria** (hī″pŏs-thĕn-ū′rē-ă) [″ + *sthenos,* strength, + *ouron,* urine] The secretion of urine of low specific gravity, chiefly in chronic nephritis.

***tubular h.*** Hyposthenuria resulting from disease of the renal tubule epithelial cells.

**hypostomia** (hī″pō-stō′mē-ă) [″ + *stoma,* mouth] A congenital defect in which the mouth is abnormally small.

**hypostosis** (hĭp″ŏs-tō′sĭs) [″ + *osteon,* bone, + *osis,* condition] Deficient bone development.

**hypostypsis** (hī″pō-stĭp′sĭs) [″ + *stypsis,* a contracting] The state of being slightly astringent. **hypostyptic** (-stĭp′tĭk), *adj.*

**hyposynergia** (hī″pō-sĭn-ĕr′jē-ă) [″ + *syn,* together, + *ergon,* work] Poor coordination.

**hypotelorism** (hī″pō-tĕl′ō-rĭzm) [″ + *telouros,* distant] Abnormally decreased distance between paired organs, esp. the eyes.

**hypotension** [″ + L. *tensio,* tension] **1.** A deficiency in tonus or tension. **2.** A decrease of the systolic and diastolic blood pressure to below normal. This occurs in shock, in hemorrhages, infections, fevers, cancer, anemia, neurasthenia, and Addison's disease; in debilitating or wasting diseases; and in approaching death. SEE: *blood pressure, chronic low.*

***orthostatic h., postural h.*** Hypotension occurring when a person who experiences it assumes an upright position from a supine position.

***postprandial h.*** A decrease in systolic blood pressure of 20 mm Hg or more within 2 hr of the start of a meal. This may cause syncope, falls, dizziness, weakness, angina pectoris, or stroke. This condition occurs most often in the elderly and in persons with autonomic failure. Change in posture may increase the severity of the condition but postprandial hypotension is a different entity than postural hypotension.

**hypotensive** Characterized by or causing low blood pressure.

**hypothalamus** (hī″pō-thăl′ă-mŭs) [″ + *thalamos,* chamber] The portion of the diencephalon comprising the ventral wall of the third ventricle below the hypothalamic sulcus and including structures forming the ventricular floor, including the optic chiasma, tuber cinereum, infundibulum, and mamillary bodies. It lies beneath the thalamus and laterally is continuous with the subthalamic regions. It contains neurosecretions that are important to the control of certain metabolic activities, such as maintenance of water balance, sugar and fat metabolism, regulation of body temperature, and secretion of releasing and inhibiting hormones. It is the chief subcortical region for the integration of sympathetic and parasympathetic activities. SEE: *hormone, releasing.*

**hypothenar** (hī-pŏth′ĕ-năr) [″ + *thenar,* palm] The fleshy prominence on the inner side of the palm next to the little finger. SYN: *hypothenar eminence.*

**hypothermal** (hī″pō-thĕr′măl) [″ + *therme,* heat] **1.** Tepid. **2.** Subnormal temperature.

**hypothermia** (hī″pō-thĕr′mē-ă) **1.** The state in which an individual's body temperature is reduced below normal range.

In newborns, hypothermia elicits a sudden increase in metabolic rate, higher demands for oxygen and energy, and mobilization of brown fat deposits to produce heat. Physiological demands rapidly exceed the limited energy reserves and can result in hypoglycemia, hyperbilirubinemia, and metabolic acidosis. SEE: *Nursing Diagnoses Appendix.* **2.** A technique for lowering the body temperature, usually between 78° and 90°F (26° and 32.5°C), to reduce oxygen need during surgery (esp. cardiovascular and neurological procedures) and in hypoxia, to reduce blood pressure, and to alleviate hyperpyrexia. SEE: *hyperthermia.*

***accidental h.*** Hypothermia due to causes other than those resulting from a systemic disorder such as shock, trauma, or carcinoma. This form of hypothermia may be lethal in anyone, esp. the elderly. It may occur in those exposed for prolonged periods to the cold (i.e., skiers, hunters, sailors, swimmers, climbers, the indigent, homeless persons in winter, and alcoholics).

SYMPTOMS: This type of hypothermia is characterized in the elderly by impaired speech, disorientation, and a generalized lethargy. Hypothermia depresses the central nervous system. Initially tachycardia occurs, followed by bradycardia and atrial and ventricular dysrhythmias. Respirations are increased at first and then depressed, and renal function is depressed after initial diuresis.

TREATMENT: Many persons with hypothermia will not be near available comprehensive medical care. Nevertheless, immediate steps should be taken to prevent further heat loss, then rewarming can begin. The patient should be immobilized. Massage of the extremities is contraindicated, and warm stimulant fluids by mouth are of no help. However, the administration of warm heated air is of benefit, as is warmed 5% dextrose in normal saline given intravenously. Plans to transport the patient to a hospital should be made. SEE: *frostbite.*

---

Caution: Oral thermometers are likely to be inaccurate in the cold, outdoors. No one should be assumed dead until warming techniques have been used.

---

***h. blanket*** A specially designed blanket for cooling patients with hyperthermia. It has flexible tubing between the layers of cloth, and cold water is pumped through the tubing.

**hypothesis** (hī-pŏth′ĕ-sĭs) *pl.* **hypotheses** [″ + *thesis,* a placing] **1.** An assumption not proved by experiment or observation. It is assumed for the sake of testing its soundness or to facilitate investigation of a class of phenomena. **2.** A conclusion drawn before all the facts are established and tentatively accepted as a basis for further investigation.

***null h.*** The assumption or hypothesis that the observed difference between two groups of patients studied is accidental or due to chance and is not due to one of the groups having received a benefit from treatment.

**hypothrombinemia** (hī″pō-thrŏm-bĭn-ē′mē-ă) [″ + *thrombos,* clot, + *haima,* blood] A deficiency of thrombin in the blood.

**hypothymia** (hī″pō-thī′mē-ă) [″ + *thymos,* mind] A decreased emotional response to stimuli.

**hypothymism** (hī″pō-thī′mĭzm) [″ + ″ + *-ismos,* condition] Decreased activity of the thymus.

**hypothyroid** (hī″pō-thī′royd) [″ + *thyreos,* shield, + *eidos,* form, shape] Marked by insufficient thyroid secretion.

**hypothyroidism** (hī″pō-thī′royd-ĭzm) A condition due to deficient thyroid secretion, resulting in a lowered basal metabolism; a lesser degree of cretinism. SEE: *thyroid function tests; Nursing Diagnoses Appendix.*

SYMPTOMS: Symptoms may include obesity; dry skin and hair, both of which become lusterless; low blood pressure; slow pulse; sluggishness of all functions; depressed muscular activity; intolerance of cold; and goiter.

TREATMENT: Replacement therapy is necessary, with natural or synthetic thyroid hormone preparations. If dietary iodine is deficient, the amount of it in the diet should be increased.

NURSING IMPLICATIONS: The patient is assessed for indications of decreased metabolic rate; easy fatigability; cool, dry, and scaly skin; hypercarotenemia; hair and eyebrow loss; brittle nails, facial puffiness and periorbital edema; paresthesias; ataxias; cold intolerance; bradycardia; reduced cardiac output; aching muscles and joint stiffness; changes in bowel habits; irregular menses; and decreased libido. Vital signs, fluid intake, urine output, and weight are monitored. Cardiac and breath sounds are auscultated, chest pain or dyspnea is noted, and the extremities and back inspected for dependent and sacral edema. Mental and neurological status is monitored. Diagnostic tests are performed, and each test and expected sensations are explained. Prescribed long-term hormone replacement and other medical therapies aimed at restoring a normal metabolic state are administered, and the patient is instructed about these therapies. Assistance is provided to help the patient and family to deal with the psychosocial and psychomotor effects of decreased metabolism. The patient's activity level is increased gradually as treatment proceeds, while adequate rest continues to be provided to avoid fatigue and to decrease myocardial oxygen demand. Body system problems such as venous congestion, pulmonary complications, and constipation are assessed, prevented, and managed. Gastrointestinal and cardiac complications are monitored and reported. The nurse protects the patient from chilling, infections, traumas, and other physical and psychological stressors. Weight loss is encouraged, meticulous skin care provided, and layered dressing recommended to combat cold intolerance. The patient is encouraged to verbalize feelings and concerns about body image changes, and assistance is provided to help the patient to identify strengths, to develop positive coping strategies, and to develop interests that foster a positive self-image. The patient should wear or carry a medical identification device describing the condition and its treatment and carry medications at all times. Desired outcomes include: understanding of and cooperation with treatment regimen, restoration of normal activity level, absence of complications, evidence of positive body image and good self-esteem.

**hypotonia** (hī″pō-tō′nē-ă) [″ + *tonos,* tone] **1.** Reduced tension; relaxation of arteries. **2.** Loss of tonicity of the muscles or intraocular pressure.

**hypotonic** (hī-pō-tŏn′ĭk) **1.** Pert. to defective muscular tone or tension. **2.** Pert. to a solution of lower osmotic pressure than that of a reference solution or of an isotonic solution.

**hypotrichosis** (hī″pō-trĭ-kō′sĭs) [″ + *thrix,* hair, + *osis,* condition] An abnormal deficiency of hair.

**hypotrophy** (hī-pŏt′rŏ-fē) [″ + *trophe,* nourishment] Atrophy.

**hypotropia** (hī″pō-trō′pē-ă) [″ + *trope,* a turning] Vertical strabismus downward.

**hypotympanotomy** (hī″pō-tĭm″pă-nŏt′ō-mē) Surgical incision of the hypotympanum.

**hypotympanum** (hī″pō-tĭm′pă-nŭm) The part of the middle ear beneath the level of the tympanic membrane.

**hypouricuria** (hī″pō-ū-rĭ-kū′rē-ă) [″ + *ouron,* urine, + *ouron,* urine] Deficient uric acid in the urine.

**hypovenosity** (hī″pō-vĕn-ŏs′ĭ-tē) [″ + L. *venosus,* pert. to a vein] Incomplete development of the venous system in an area, resulting in atrophy or degeneration.

**hypoventilation** (hī″pō-vĕn″tĭ-lā′shŭn) [″ + L. *ventilatio,* ventilation] Reduced rate and depth of breathing that causes an increase in carbon dioxide.

**hypovitaminosis** (hī″pō-vī″tă-mĭn-ō′sĭs) [″ + L. *vita,* life, + *amine* + Gr. *osis,* condition] A condition caused by a lack of vitamins in the diet.

**hypovolemia** (hī″pō-vō-lē′mē-ă) [″ + L. *vol-*

*umen,* volume] Diminished blood volume.

**hypovolia** (hī″pō-vō′lē-ă) Decreased water content.

**hypoxanthine** (hī″pō-zăn′thĭn, -thēn) [″ + *xanthos,* yellow] A purine derivative, $C_5H_4N_4O$, in muscles and tissues in a stage of uric acid formation. It is formed during protein decomposition. Hypoxanthine is normal in urine in small amounts.

**hypoxemia** (hī-pŏks-ē′mē-ă) [″ + *oxygen* + *haima,* blood] Decreased oxygen tension (concentration) in the blood, measured by arterial oxygen partial pressure ($PaO_2$) values. It is sometimes associated with decreased oxygen content. SEE: *hypoxia; respiration.*

**hypoxia** (hī″pŏks′ē-ă) **1.** An oxygen deficiency. **2.** A decreased concentration of oxygen in the inspired air. SEE: *anoxia; hypoxemia; posthypoxia syndromes.*

***altitude h.*** Hypoxia due to insufficient oxygen content of inspired air at high altitudes.

***anemic h.*** Hypoxia due to a decrease in hemoglobin concentration or in the number of erythrocytes in the blood.

***anoxic h.*** Hypoxia due to disordered pulmonary mechanisms of oxygenation; may be due to reduced oxygen supply, respiratory obstruction, reduced pulmonary function or inadequate respiratory movements.

***cerebral h.*** Lack of oxygen supply to the brain, usually due to cardiopulmonary arrest. If nothing is done to treat this condition, irreversible anoxic damage to the brain begins after 4 to 6 minutes and sooner in some cases. If basic resuscitation measures are begun before the end of this period, the onset of cerebral death may be postponed. SEE: *cardiopulmonary resuscitation.*

***histotoxic h.*** Hypoxia due to inability of the tissues to use oxygen. SEE: *cyanide.*

***hypokinetic h.*** Stagnant h.

***stagnant h.*** Hypoxia due to insufficient peripheral circulation, as occurs in cardiac failure, shock, arterial spasm, and thrombosis. SYN: *hypokinetic h.*

**hypoxic lap swimming** A practice by competitive swimmers of holding their breath for a number of laps in order to increase the tolerance to oxygen debt during races. The practice is potentially dangerous and may lead to drowning.

**hypsarrhythmia** (hĭp″săr-ĭth′mē-ă) [Gr. *hypsi,* high, + *a-,* not, + *rhythmos,* rhythm] An abnormal electroencephalographic pattern of persistent generalized slow waves and very high voltage. Clinically it is often associated with infantile spasm and progressive mental deterioration. The etiology is unknown.

**hypsibrachycephalic** (hĭp″sē-brăk″ē-sĕ-făl′ĭk) [Gr. *hypsi,* high, + *brachys,* broad, + *kephale,* head] Having a broad and high skull.

**hypsicephalic** (hĭp″sē-sĕ-făl′ĭk) [″ + *kephale,* head] Having a skull with a cranial index greater than 75.1 degrees. SYN: *hypsistenocephalic; hypsocephalous.*

**hypsicephaly** (hĭp-sē-sĕf′ă-lē) The condition of having a skull with a cranial index greater than 75.1 degrees.

**hypsiconchous** (hĭp″sē-kŏng′kŭs) [″ + *konche,* shell] Having an orbital index of about 85 degrees.

**hypsiloid** (hĭp′sĭ-loyd) [Gr. *upsilon,* U or Y, + *eidos,* form] Hyoid.

***h. ligament*** Iliofemoral ligament.

**hypsistenocephalic** (hĭp″sē-stĕn″ō-sĕ-făl′ĭk) [″ + *stenos,* narrow, + *kephale,* head] Hypsicephalic.

**hypsocephalous** (hĭp″sō-sĕf′ă-lŭs) [Gr. *hypsos,* height, + *kephale,* head] Hypsicephalic.

**hypsokinesis** (hĭp″sō-kĭ-nē′sĭs) [″ + *kinesis,* movement] A tendency to fall backward when standing; seen in paralysis agitans.

**hypsophobia** (hĭp″sō-fō′bē-ă) [″ + *phobos,* fear] Acrophobia.

**hyster-** SEE: *hystero-.*

**hysteralgia** (hĭs-tĕr-ăl′jē-ă) [Gr. *hystera,* womb, + *algos,* pain] Uterine pain. SYN: *hysterodynia.*

**hysterectomy** (hĭs-tĕr-ĕk′tō-mē) [″ + *ektome,* excision] Surgical removal of the uterus through the abdominal wall or vagina. The presence of benign or malignant tumors is the most frequent reason for hysterectomy. SEE: illus.; *Nursing Diagnoses Appendix.*

In preparation for abdominal hysterectomy, the patient is placed in the dorsal position. The table is ready to be tipped into the Trendelenburg position. As soon as the incision is made through the peritoneum, the table should be put into Trendelenburg position. This procedure is the same for all abdominopelvic surgery, as the Trendelenburg position allows the intestines and abdominal organs to fall away from pelvis, so that they may be easily packed off and isolated from the surgical field with large pads or a large roll of packing.

NURSING IMPLICATIONS: *Preoperative:* The patient is prepared physically and emotionally for the surgery; the procedure, expected sensations, postoperative care, and the need for patient cooperation are explained. The surgeon's prescribed preparatory protocol is carried out, a signed informed consent form obtained, and prescribed presedation administered.

*Postoperative:* Vital signs are monitored, abdominal dressings and the vaginal introitus inspected for drainage, bleeding, or signs of hemorrhage, the perineal pad is changed frequently, and the incision wound redressed according to protocol. Breath sounds are auscultated, and respiratory complications prevented by encouraging the patient to breathe deeply and cough every 1 to 2 hours, by using prescribed incentive spirometry, by splinting the incision, and by turning the patient side to side every 2 hours until able to ambulate. Prescribed analgesia is administered to prevent postoperative discomfort, or the patient is taught how to administer patient-controlled analgesia, and the patient's response evaluated.

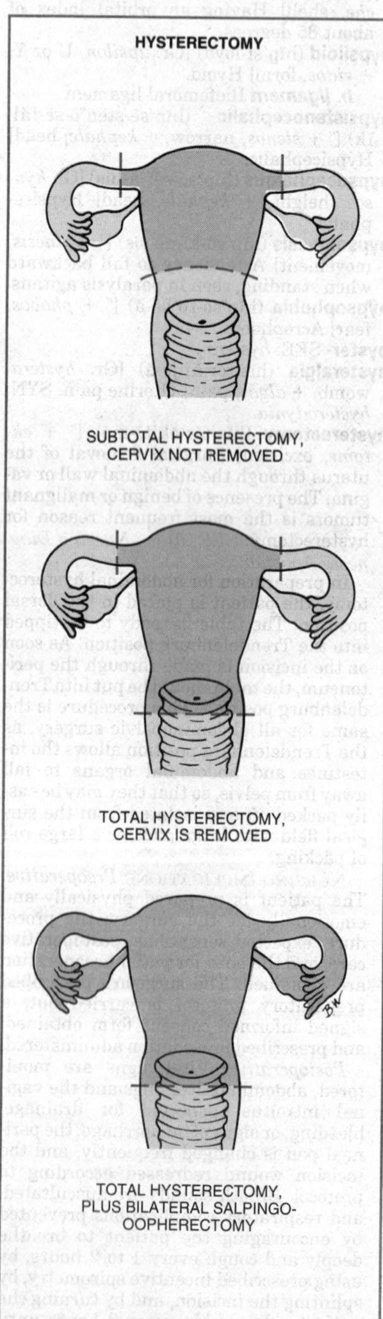


Prescribed I.V. fluid and electrolyte therapy are maintained, and the patient is assessed for nausea and vomiting and treated with prescribed antiemetics until oral intake is tolerated. Nasogastric drainage is maintained if present, and bowel sounds assessed because paralytic ileus can develop. The patient is assessed for bladder distention and catheterized according to institutional or surgeon's protocol; urinary output is monitored from an indwelling catheter, and bladder emptying and residual urine volume is assessed when the catheter is removed. A rectal tube, ambulation, and analgesics and cholinergics are used as prescribed to assist the patient to deal with gaseous distention. Prescribed perineal care is provided to increase comfort and to aid healing (sitz baths, ice packs, heat lamps). Thigh-high antithromboembolitic devices (pneumatic dressings or elastic stockings) are employed as prescribed, and leg exercises and early ambulation are encouraged to prevent venous stasis that may result in phlebitis or deep vein phlebothrombosis. Signs and symptoms of thrombophlebotic complications are assessed, including changes in calf or thigh size, redness, warmth, or local discomfort. A high-protein, high vitamin C diet is provided to encourage healing once the G.I. tract is functional. The nurse teaches the patient to maintain good nutrition and adequate fluid intake and to report vaginal bleeding, wound infections, and prolonged gastrointestinal or urinary tract complaints. Tub baths, douching, and coitus usually are restricted until after a postoperative evaluation by the surgeon. The patient is encouraged to increase walking time and distance gradually; to avoid prolonged sitting; and to avoid heavy lifting, rapid walking, or dancing, because these activities can lead to pelvic congestion. The rationale for hormonal replacement after ovary removal, if prescribed, is explained, and such therapy is initiated when the patient is able to tolerate oral intake. The patient may experience depression or irritability temporarily because of abrupt hormonal fluctuations, and the family is encouraged to respond calmly and with understanding. Both patient and spouse are encouraged to verbalize their fears and concerns about altered femininity and sexuality (which are myths); about loss or grief, to assist them in developing positive coping strategies; and about follow-up chemotherapy and radiation if these are required. Desired outcomes include: evidence of incisional healing, normal G.I. and bladder function, absence of complications, and understanding of and cooperation with prescribed follow-up treatment regimens.

***abdominal h.*** The removal of the uterus through an abdominal incision.

***cesarean h.*** The surgical removal of the uterus at the time of cesarean section.

***Porro h.*** SEE: *Porro's operation.*

***radical h.*** The surgical removal of the uterus, tubes, ovaries, adjacent lymph nodes, and part of the vagina.

***subtotal h.*** The surgical removal of the uterus, leaving the cervix in place. SYN: *supracervical h.; supravaginal h.*

***supracervical h.*** Subtotal h.

***supravaginal h.*** Subtotal h.

***total abdominal h.*** Removal of the uterus, including the cervix, through an abdominal incision.

***vaginal h.*** The surgical removal of the uterus through the vagina.

**hysteresis** (hĭs″tĕr-ē′sĭs) [Gr., a coming too late] **1.** The failure of related phenomena to keep pace with each other. **2.** The failure of the manifestation of an effect to keep up with its cause. **3.** The difference between inflation and deflation of the lung, shown as a pressure volume difference.

**hystereurynter** (hĭs″tĕr-ū-rĭn′tĕr) [Gr. *hystera,* uterus, + *eurynein,* to stretch] Metreurynter.

**hysteria** (hĭs-tĕ′rē-ă) [Gr. *hystera,* uterus] A mental disorder, usually temporary, presenting somatic symptoms, simulating almost any type of physical disease. The condition occurs in the absence of organic disease to account for the symptoms.

The mental attitude is calm. Easy laughing and crying episodes may be present, possibly without any apparent explanation, sometimes occurring during sleep. Episodic states known as fugues occur (sleepwalking is similar, occurring in sleep). In these disorders, certain dissociated (repressed) ideas, emotions, and goals develop a reality sufficient to constitute a secondary personality that functions apart from the primary one. When the primary consciousness reasserts itself, the patient forgets the secondary state.

NOTE: Currently accepted nomenclature for mental disorders does not include the term *hysteria;* nevertheless, it has been in use for centuries and is included here for historical reasons. SEE: *mass psychogenic illness; somatization disorder.*

SYMPTOMS: Symptoms include emotional instability, various sensory disturbances, and a marked craving for sympathy, which sometimes leads to fraud.

ETIOLOGY: As in most psychic disturbances the causes of this disorder are variable, but may be related to emotional and physical stress.

TREATMENT: The patient should be put in a quiet place devoid of spectators. Cold applications to the head, face, and neck are helpful. Quiet, firm suggestions are important. Sedatives are to be used only under the direction of a physician.

***anxiety h.*** Hysteria combined with an anxiety neurosis.

***conversion h.*** An apparent loss of physical function, but with no organic basis for signs and symptoms such as deafness, blindness, tunnel vision, paralysis, anesthesia, parathesias, or aphonia. SYN: *conversion disorder.* SEE: *gain, primary; gain, secondary.*

***epidemic h.*** Hysteria in a group of people, usually closely associated in a school or workplace. The inciting incident might be a rumor or an unaccustomed odor (e.g., paint fumes in a workplace). Vomiting by an individual who has just eaten in a public place (e.g., a school cafeteria) may lead to a hysterical reaction by others eating there who feel that the food they ate was toxic. SYN: *mass h.* SEE: *mass psychogenic illness.*

***major h.*** Very severe hysteria accompanied by epileptiform convulsions.

***mass h.*** Epidemic h.

***rabies h.*** SEE: *rabies.*

**hysteriac** (hĭs-tĕr′ē-ăk) [Gr. *hystera,* womb] A hysterical person.

**hysteric, hysterical** Pert. to hysteria.

**hystericoneuralgic** (hĭs-tĕr″ĭk-o-nū-răl′jĭk) [″ + *neuron,* nerve, + *algos,* pain] Pert. to pain of hysterical origin, but resembling neuralgia.

**hystero-, hyster-** [Gr. *hystera,* womb] Combining form meaning *uterus* or *hysteria.* SEE: *metro-; utero-.*

**hysterobubonocele** (hĭs″tĕr-ō-bū-bŏn′ō-sēl) [″ + *boubon,* groin, + *kele,* tumor, swelling] An inguinal hernia surrounding the uterus.

**hysterocele** (hĭs′tĕr-ō-sēl) [″ + *kele,* tumor, swelling] A hernia of the uterus, esp. when gravid.

**hysterocystocleisis** (hĭs″tĕr-ō-sĭs″tō-klī′sĭs) [″ + *kystis,* a bladder, + *kleisis,* closure] An operation fastening the cervix uteri to the wall of the bladder.

**hysterodynia** (hĭs″tĕr-ō-dĭn′ē-ă) [″ + *odyne,* pain] Hysteralgia.

**hysterogastrorrhaphy** (hĭs″tĕr-ō-găs-tror′ă-fē) [″ + *gaster,* belly, + *rhaphe,* seam, ridge] Fixation of the uterus to the gastric wall.

**hysterogenic** (hĭs″tĕr-ō-jĕn′ĭk) [″ + *gennan,* to produce] Causing hysteria.

**hysterogram** (hĭs′tĕr-ō-grăm) A radiograph of the uterus after injection of a contrast medium.

**hysterography** (hĭs″tĕ-rŏg′ră-fē) [″ + *graphein,* to write] A recording of the frequency and intensity of contractions of the uterus.

**hysteroid** (hĭs′tĕr-oyd) [″ + *eidos,* form, shape] Resembling or pert. to hysteria.

**hysterolaparotomy** (hĭs″tĕr-ō-lăp″ă-rŏt′ō-mē) [″ + *lapara,* flank, + *tome,* incision] A uterine incision through the abdominal wall; abdominal hysterectomy.

**hysterolith** (hĭs′tĕr-ō-lĭth) [″ + *lithos,* stone] A calculus in the uterus.

**hysterolysis** (hĭs″tĕr-ŏl′ĭ-sĭs) [″ + *lysis,* dissolution] An operation to loosen the uterus from its adhesions.

**hysterometer** (hĭs″tĕ-rŏm′ĕ-tĕr) [″ + *metron,* measure] A device for measuring the uterus.

**hysterometry** (hĭs″tĕ-rŏm′ĕ-trē) Measurement of the size of the uterus.

**hysteromyoma** (hĭs″tĕr-ō-mī-ō′mă) [Gr. *hystera,* womb, + *mys,* muscle, + *oma,* tumor] A myoma or fibromyoma of the uterus.

**hysteromyomectomy** (hĭs″tĕr-ō-mī″ō-mĕk′tō-mē) [″ + ″ + *ektome,* excision] Excision of a uterine fibroid.

**hysteromyotomy** (hĭs″tĕr-ō-mī-ŏt′ō-mē) [″ + ″ + *tome,* incision] Uterine incision for removal of a solid tumor.

**hystero-oophorectomy** (hĭs″tĕr-ō-ō″ō-for-ĕk′tō-mē) [″ + *oon,* egg, + *phoros,* bearing, + *ektome,* excision] Removal of the uterus and of one or both ovaries.

**hysteropathy** (hĭs″tĕr-ŏp′ă-thē) [″ + *pathos,* disease, suffering] Any uterine disorder.

**hysteroptosia, hysteroptosis** (hĭs″tĕr-ŏp-tō′sē-ă, -sĭs) [″ + *ptosis,* a dropping] Prolapse of the uterus. SYN: *procidentia.*

**hysterorrhaphy** (hĭs-tĕr-or′ă-fē) [″ + *rhaphe,* seam, ridge] Suture of the uterus.

**hysterorrhexis** (hĭs″tĕr-ō-rĕk′sĭs) [″ + *rhexis,* rupture] Rupture of the uterus, esp. when pregnant.

**hysterosalpingectomy** (hĭs″tĕr-ō-săl″pĭn-jĕk′tō-mē) [″ + *salpinx,* tube, + *ektome,* excision] Surgical removal of the uterus and fallopian tubes.

**hysterosalpingography** (hĭs″tĕr-ō-săl″pĭn-gŏg′ră-fē) [″ + ″ + *graphein,* to write] Radiography of the uterus and oviducts after injection of a contrast medium.

**hysterosalpingo-oophorectomy** (hĭs″tĕr-ō-săl-pĭng″gō-ō″ō-for-ĕk′tō-mē) [″ + ″ + *oon,* egg, + *phoros,* bearing, + *ektome,* excision] The surgical removal of the uterus, oviducts, and ovaries.

**hysterosalpingostomy** (hĭs″tĕr-ō-săl″pĭng-ŏs′tō-mē) [″ + ″ + *stoma,* mouth] Anastomosis of the uterus with the distal end of the fallopian tube after excision of a strictured portion of the tube.

**hysteroscope** (hĭs′tĕr-ō-skōp) [″ + *skopein,* to examine] An instrument for examining the uterine cavity.

**hysteroscopy** (hĭs″tĕr-ŏs′kō-pē) Inspection of the uterus by use of a special endoscope. SEE: *hysteroscope.*

**hysterospasm** (hĭs′tĕr-ō-spăzm″) [Gr. *hystera,* womb, + *spasmos,* a convulsion] A uterine spasm.

**hysterostomatocleisis** (hĭs″tĕr-ō-stō″mă-tō-klī′sĭs) [″ + *stoma,* mouth, + *kleisis,* closure] An operation for vesicovaginal fistula, consisting of closure of the cervix uteri and making the vesical and uterine cavities into a common cavity by means of the opening between them.

**hysterostomatomy** (hĭs″tĕr-ō-stō-măt′ō-mē) [″ + ″ + *tome,* incision] The surgical enlargement of the os uteri; incision of the os or cervix uteri.

**hysterotomy** (hĭs-tĕr-ŏt′ō-mē) **1.** Incision of the uterus. **2.** Cesarean section.

**hysterotracheloplasty** (hĭs″tĕr-ō-trā′kĕl-lō-plăs″tē) [″ + ″ + *plassein,* to form] Plastic surgery or repair of the cervix.

**hysterotrachelorrhaphy** (hĭs″tĕr-ō-trā″kĕl-or′ă-fē) [″ + ″ + *rhaphe,* seam, ridge] Plastic surgery of a lacerated cervix by paring the edges and suturing them together.

**hysterotrachelotomy** (hĭs″tĕr-ō-trā″kĕl-ŏt′ō-mē) [″ + ″ + *tome,* incision] A surgical incision of the neck of the uterus.

**hysterovagino-enterocele** (hĭs″tĕr-ō-văj″ĭn-ō-ĕn′tĕr-ō-sēl) [″ + L. *vagina,* sheath, + Gr. *enteron,* intestine, + *kele,* tumor, swelling] A hernia surrounding the uterus, vagina, and intestines.

**Hz** *hertz.*

**HZV** *herpes zoster virus.*

# I

**I 1.** Symbol for the element iodine. **2.** Symbol for the quantity of electricity expressed in amperes.

**$^{131}$I** Radioactive iodine; atomic weight 131.

**$^{132}$I** Radioactive iodine; atomic weight 132.

**i** *optically inactive.*

**-ia** Suffix indicating a condition, esp. an abnormal state.

**IABC** *intra-aortic balloon counterpulsation.*

**IABP** *intra-aortic balloon pump.*

**I.A.D.R.** *International Association for Dental Research.*

**IAET** *International Association for Enterostomal Therapy.*

**I and O** *intake and output.*

**ianthinopsia** (ī-ăn″thĭ-nŏp′sē-ă) [Gr. *ianthinos,* violet colored, + *opsis,* vision] An abnormality of vision in which all objects appear to be violet.

**-iasis** [Gr.] Suffix, the same as or interchangeable with *-osis,* meaning the state or condition of, particularly with respect to a pathological condition. SEE: *-asis; -sis.*

**-iatric** (ī-ăt′rĭk) [Gr. *iatrikos,* medical] Combining form used as a suffix referring to *medicine, the medical profession,* or *physicians.*

**iatro-** [Gr. *iatros,* physician] Combining form indicating relationship to medicine or a physician.

**iatrogenesis** (ī″ăt-rō-jĕn′ĕs-ĭs) [″ + *gennan,* to produce] Any adverse mental or physical condition induced in a patient through the effects of treatment by a physician or surgeon. For example, chemotherapy, often used to attenuate or cure a cancer, initiates a process that causes the individual to become severely ill. In an elderly person, a fall can lead to the use of restraints and bedrest, which can cause thrombophlebitis. The use of a Foley catheter for incontinence can create a urinary tract infection and septic shock. **iatrogenic** (ī″ăt-rō-jĕn′ĭk), *adj.*

**iatrology** (ī″ă-trŏl′ō-jē) [″ + *logos,* word, reason] Medical science.

**IBC** *iron-binding capacity.*

**IBD** *inflammatory bowel disease.*

**IBS** *irritable bowel syndrome.*

**ibuprofen** A nonsteroidal anti-inflammatory agent with antipyretic and analgesic properties. Although its exact mechanism of action is unknown, it does not stimulate the pituitary-adrenal system. It is used in treating chronic symptomatic rheumatoid arthritis and osteoarthritis. This drug has antiprostaglandin activity and is useful in treating primary dysmenorrhea. Trade names are Advil, Motrin, and Nuprin.

Caution: All nonsteroidal anti-inflammatory agents may cause bleeding from the intestinal tract.

**IBW** *ideal body weight.*

**IC** *inspiratory capacity.*

**-ic** A suffix indicating *characteristic of* or *relating to.*

**ICD** *intrauterine contraceptive device; International Classification of Diseases.*

**ice** (īs) [AS. *is*] A solid form of water. Water becomes ice at a temperature of 32°F (0°C) and may be chilled lower than the freezing point. An ice bag, cap, collar, and cravat are devices for holding ice to be applied to a patient to obtain the effect of continuous cold in a circumscribed area. The part so treated should always be covered with several thicknesses of cloth to prevent cold injury to the tissues.

***i. bag*** A flexible, watertight bag with a sealable opening large enough to permit ice cubes or chipped ice to be added. It is used in any condition requiring local application of cold. In an emergency any sturdy, flexible plastic bag can be used, sealing the open end with a knot. A simple ice pack can be made at home by mixing 3 cups of water and 1 cup of rubbing alcohol in a resealable plastic bag and placing the sealed mixture in the freezer for 8 to 12 hours. The solution will not freeze but will attain a gel-like consistency that molds to the body part on which it is used.

Caution: Dry ice should not be placed in an ice bag.

***dry i.*** Carbon dioxide cooled to the point at which it becomes solid, which occurs at −110°F (−78.9°C). It is used as a commercial refrigerant and for therapeutic refrigeration in the treatment of certain skin conditions, including warts. SEE: *carbon dioxide.*

***i. massage*** Application of ice to obtain a therapeutic numbing effect. Paper cups containing water previously frozen are preferable. The cups are rubbed over a localized area in small circles for 5 to 10 minutes in order to numb the part and prepare it for deep pressure or deep transverse friction massage. Ice massage is also used to treat traumatized tissues and joints.

Caution: Direct application of ice may damage the area; ice should be placed in cloth.

***i. treatment*** The use of ice applied either directly or in a suitable container to cool an injured area. Ice therapy, at least in the first 24 to 48 hours after injury, is believed to be much more beneficial than heat in treating superficial bruises, contusions, and sprains. The application of cold or of ice water in immediate treatment of a burn helps to reduce the extent of inflammation and pain.

**iceberg phenomenon** The term for recognition of the gross conditions and diseases and failure to recognize the great majority of conditions that are mild and do not become clinically apparent.

**Iceland disease** Benign myalgic encephalomyelitis.

**Iceland moss** An edible lichen of the genus *Cetraria,* which contains a form of starch; a slightly tonic demulcent.

**ICF** *intracellular fluid.*

**ichor** (ī'kor) [Gr. *ichor,* serum] Thin, fetid discharge from an ulcer or from a wound.

**ichorous** (ī'kor-ŭs) [Gr. *ichor,* serum] Resembling ichor or watery pus.

**ichthammol** (ĭk'thă-mŏl) A reddish-brown viscous fluid obtained by the destructive distillation of certain bituminous shale. The distillate is sulfonated and the final compound contains 10% organic sulfonates. It is used as a mild antiseptic and local stimulant in certain skin diseases. Trade name is Ichthyol.

**ichthyism, ichthyismus** (ĭk'thē-ĭzm, ĭk"thē-ĭz'mŭs) [Gr. *ichthys,* fish, + *-ismos,* condition] Poisoning from eating decomposed or toxic fish. SEE: *tetrodotoxin.*

**ichthyo-** [Gr. *ichthys,* fish] Combining form meaning *fish.*

**ichthyoacanthotoxism** (ĭk"thē-ō-ă-kăn"thō-tŏk'sĭzm) [" + *akantha,* thorn, + *toxikon,* poison, + *-ismos,* condition] A toxin or venom present in the sting, spines, or "teeth" of certain venomous fish.

**ichthyohemotoxin** (ĭk"thē-ō-hē"mō-tŏk'sĭn) [" + *haima,* blood, + *toxikon,* poison] A toxin present in the blood of certain poisonous fish.

**ichthyoid** (ĭk'thē-oyd) [" + *eidos,* form, shape] Fishlike.

**ichthyology** (ĭk"thē-ŏl'ō-jē) [" + *logos,* word, reason] The study of fish.

**ichthyootoxin** (ĭk"thē-ō"ō-tŏk'sĭn) [" + *oon,* egg, + *toxikon,* poison] A toxin present in the roe of certain fish.

**ichthyophagous** (ĭk"thē-ŏf'ă-gŭs) [" + *phagein,* to eat] Subsisting on fish.

**ichthyophobia** (ĭk-thē-ō-fō'bē-ă) [" + *phobos,* fear] An abnormal aversion to fish.

**ichthyosarcotoxin** (ĭk"thē-ō-săr"kō-tŏk'sĭn) [" + *sarx,* flesh, + *toxikon,* poison] A toxin present in the flesh of certain fish.

**ichthyosis** (ĭk"thē-ō'sĭs) [" + *osis,* condition] A condition in which the skin is dry and scaly, resembling fish skin. Because ichthyosis is so easily recognized, a variety of diseases have been called by this name.

A mild nonhereditary form is called xeroderma. This is often seen on the legs of older patients, esp. during dry weather during the winter months. It may be more prevalent in those who bathe frequently, thus causing excessive dryness of the skin.

TREATMENT: The application of lotions or ointments that soften and soothe the skin provide symptomatic relief for all forms of ichthyosis. Dry scales can be removed by applying a combination of 6% salicylic acid in a gel containing propylene glycol, ethyl alcohol, hydroxy propylene cellulose, and water. This is most effective when applied to moistened skin at night, and covered with an occlusive dressing. Soaps should be used sparingly.

***i. congenita*** Harlequin fetus. SEE: under *fetus.*

***i. fetalis*** I. congenita.

***i. hystrix*** Linear nevus. The skin contains bands or lines of rough, thick, warty, hypertrophic papillary growths.

***lamellar i. of newborn*** A rare form of inherited ichthyosis with lamellar desquamation.

***i. vulgaris*** A hereditary form of ichthyosis that includes two genetically distinct types. Dominant ichthyosis vulgaris is produced by an autosomal dominant gene. Characterized by dry, rough, scaly skin, it is not present at birth and is usually noticed between the ages of one and four. Many cases improve in later life.

The second type is sex-linked ichthyosis vulgaris. It is present only in males and is transmitted by the female as a recessive gene. Onset of scattered large brown scales is seen in early infancy. The scalp may be involved, but the face is spared except for the sides and in front of the ear. There is little tendency for this condition to improve with age.

**ichthyotic** (ĭk"thē-ŏt'ĭk) [Gr. *ichthys,* fish] Relating to ichthyosis.

**ichthyotoxicology** (ĭk"thē-ō-tŏk"sĭ-kŏl'ō-jē) [" + *toxikon,* poison, + *logos,* word, reason] The study of poisons and toxins produced by certain fish.

**ichthyotoxin** (ĭk"thē-ō-tŏk'sĭn) [" + *toxikon,* poison] Any toxin present in fish.

**ICIDH** *International Classification of Impairment, Disability and Handicap.*

**icing 1.** A technique of cutaneous stimulation using ice (12° to 17°C) to evoke or facilitate reflex muscular responses in patients with central nervous system dysfunction. **2.** Application of ice to a recently traumatized area in order to reduce pain and swelling.

**ICN** *International Council of Nurses.*

**ICP** *intracranial pressure.*

**ICS** *intercostal space.*

**I.C.S.** *International College of Surgeons.*

**ICSH** *interstitial cell-stimulating hormone.* Luteinizing hormone.

**ictal** (ĭk'tăl) [L. *ictus,* a blow or stroke] Pert.

to or caused by a sudden attack or stroke such as epilepsy. SEE: *postictal.*

**icteric** (ĭk-tĕr′ĭk) [Gr. *ikteros,* jaundice] Pert. to jaundice.

**icteroanemia** (ĭk″tĕr-ō-ă-nē′mē-ă) [″ + *an-,* not, + *haima,* blood] Icterus associated with anemia, hemolysis, and splenic enlargement.

**icterogenic, icterogenous** (ĭk″tĕr-ō-jĕn′ĭk, -ŏj′ĕn-ŭs) [″ + *gennan,* to produce] Causing jaundice.

**icterohemoglobinuria** (ĭk″tĕr-ō-hē″mō-glō″bĭ-nū′rē-ă) [″ + *haima,* blood, + L. *globus,* globe, + Gr. *ouron,* urine] Concerning icterus and hemoglobinuria.

**icterohepatitis** (ĭk″tĕr-ō-hĕp-ă-tī′tĭs) [″ + *hepar,* liver, + *itis,* inflammation] Liver inflammation with jaundice.

**icteroid** (ĭk′tĕr-oyd) [″ + *eidos,* form, shape] Resembling jaundice; yellow-hued.

**icterus** (ĭk′tĕr-ŭs) [Gr. *ikteros,* jaundice] Jaundice.

***i. gravis neonatorum*** Hemolytic disease of the newborn. SEE: *erythroblastosis fetalis; kernicterus; phototherapy; transfusion, exchange.*

***hemolytic i.*** A rare chronic form of icterus, frequently congenital, with periodic attacks of intense hemolysis. SYN: *nonobstructive i.*

SYMPTOMS: The symptoms resemble those of obstructive icterus. The condition is sometimes found in acute yellow atrophy, the anemias, and infectious fevers. The spleen is enlarged.

***i. neonatorum*** Physiologic jaundice of the newborn.

***nonobstructive i.*** Hemolytic i.

***obstructive i.*** Jaundice caused by obstruction to the flow of bile in the common or hepatic duct. This may result from cholangitis, carcinoma, gallstones, cirrhosis of liver, cysts, parasites in ducts, pressure by tumors, or hepatic abscess.

SYMPTOMS: The condition is characterized by skin, mucous membrane, sclera, and secretions stained yellow, first noticed in the conjunctivae. The stool is light or clay-colored, the urine dark, the pulse slow, and the temperature slightly subnormal. In extreme cases, delirium, convulsions, and coma result.

**ictus** [L., stroke] A blow or sudden attack.

***i. cordis*** The heartbeat.

***i. epilepticus*** Epileptic convulsion.

***i. sanguinis*** Apoplexy; cerebrovascular accident.

**ICU** *intensive care unit.*

**ID** *identification; infective dose; inside diameter; intradermal.*

**$ID_{50}$** The infective dose of microorganisms that will produce illness in 50% of the individuals who receive that dose.

**id** [L. *id,* it; later translators of Freud's writings believed that the word *es* should have been translated to *it* and not to id] In psychiatry, one of the three divisions of the psyche, the others being the ego and superego. The id is the obscure, inaccessible part of our personality that serves as a repository of instinctual drives continually striving for expression. Expression is manifested as an impulse to obtain satisfaction for the instinctive needs in accordance with the pleasure-pain principle.

**id** L. *idem,* the same.

**-id** [Gr. *eidos,* form, shape] Suffix indicating certain secondary skin eruptions that appear some distance from site of primary infection. If the etiological agent of primary infection is known, the secondary lesion is designated by adding -id, as in tuberculid and trichophytid.

**IDDM** *insulin-dependent diabetes mellitus.*

**idea** [Gr., form] A mental image; a concept.

***autochthonous i.*** A thought that comes into the mind independent of a train of thoughts, in an unaccountable way.

***compulsive i.*** A persistent, obsessional impulse or thought.

***dominant i.*** An idea that controls all one's actions and thoughts.

***fixed i.*** An idea that completely dominates the mind despite evidence to the contrary; a delusion. SYN: *idée fixe.*

***flight of i.'s*** Rapid speech, often disconnected and incoherent, occurring in certain mental diseases.

***i. of reference*** An impression that the conversation or actions of others have reference to oneself.

**ideal** [L. *idea,* model] A goal or endeavor regarded as a standard of perfection.

**ideation** (ī-dē-ā′shŭn) The process of thinking; formation of ideas. It slows down in dementias, depressions, and other organic brain diseases, and in narcotic intoxications; but speeds up in the early stage of some types of intoxications. It is unduly active in manic-depressive states.

**idée fixe** (ē-dā′ fēks′) [Fr.] Fixed idea. SEE: under *idea.*

**identical** [L. *identicus,* the same] Exactly alike.

**identification** [″ + *facere,* to make] **1.** A kind of daydream, as in identification of oneself with the hero of a book or play. **2.** The process of determining the sameness of a thing or person with that described or known to exist. **3.** A defense mechanism, operating unconsciously, by which a person patterns himself or herself after some other person. This plays a major role in personality development.

***dental i.*** The use of the unique characteristics of a person's teeth or dental work as recorded in dental charts, radiographs, and records to establish the person's identity.

***palm and sole system of i.*** A system based on prints of the palmar surface of the hand and the plantar surface of the foot. SEE: *dermatoglyphics.*

**identity** (ī-dĕn′tĭ-tē) **1.** The concept that each individual has of his or her body in space and his or her thought processes in relation to the social and intellectual environment. **2.** The physical and mental characteristics by which an individual is known and recognized.

***ego i.*** The sense of self that provides a unity of personality.

***gender i.*** One's self-concept with respect to being male or female, or being confused about one's true sexual identity.

***i. testing*** SEE: *paternity analysis.*

**ideo-** [Gr. *idea,* form] Prefix pert. to mental images.

**ideogenous, ideogenetic** (ĭd-ē-ŏj′ĕn-ŭs, -ō-jĕ-nĕt′ĭk) [″ + *gennan,* to produce] Stimulated by an idea.

**ideology** (ī″dē-ŏl′ō-jē) [″ + *logos,* word, reason] **1.** The science of ideas or thought. **2.** A system or schema of ideas; a philosophy.

**ideomuscular** (ī″dē-ō-mŭs′kū-lăr) [″ + L. *musculus,* muscle] **1.** Indicating muscular activity produced in connection with a thought. **2.** Concerning both ideation and muscular activity.

**idio-** [Gr. *idios,* own] Prefix indicating *individual, distinct,* or *unknown.*

**idiocy** [Gr. *idiotes,* ignorant person] A severe mental deficiency, usually due to an arrest in development, or defective development, as opposed to the loss of mental competence. The cause, which occurs either in utero or in the first years after birth, may be genetic or traumatic, or due to severe disease. SEE: *mental retardation.*

***cretinoid i.*** Endemic idiocy accompanied by goiter. SEE: *cretinism.*

***hydrocephalic i.*** Idiocy accompanied by chronic hydrocephalus.

***microcephalic i.*** Idiocy accompanied by microcephalia.

***traumatic i.*** Idiocy caused by an injury received in infancy or in early childhood.

**idioglossia** (ĭd″ē-ō-glŏs′ē-ă) [″ + *glossa,* tongue] An inability to articulate properly, so that the sounds emitted are like those of an unknown language.

**idiogram** (ĭd′ē-ō-grăm″) [″ + *gramma,* something written] The graphic representation of the karyotype, or chromosome complement of a cell.

**idioisolysin** (ĭd″ē-ō-ī-sŏl′ĭ-sĭn) [″ + *isos,* equal, + *lysis,* dissolution] A hemolysin active against the cells of an individual of the same species.

**idiolysin** (ĭd″ē-ŏl′ĭ-sĭn) [″ + *lysis,* dissolution] A lysin normally present in the blood.

**idiopathic** (ĭd″ē-ō-păth′ĭk) [″ + *pathos,* disease, suffering] Pert. to conditions without clear pathogenesis, or disease without recognizable cause, as of spontaneous origin.

**idiopsychological** (ĭd″ē-ō-sī″kō-lŏj′ĭk-ăl) [″ + *psyche,* mind, + *logos,* word, reason] Concerning ideas produced in one's own mind.

**idiosyncrasy** (ĭd″ē-ō-sĭn′kră-sē) [″ + *syn,* together, + *krasis,* mixture] **1.** Special characteristics by which persons differ from each other. **2.** That which makes one react differently from others; a peculiar or individual reaction to an idea, action, drug, food, or some other substance through unusual susceptibility. **idiosyncratic** (-sĭn-krăt′ĭk), *adj.*

***drug i.*** An unusual response to a drug. It can manifest as an accelerated, toxic, or inappropriate response to the usual therapeutic dose of a drug.

***i. of effect*** When doses of a drug that would have a known and predictable effect instead cause a toxic or opposite effect, an unusual effect, or no effect.

**idiot** [Gr. *idiotes,* ignorant person] Former term for a person with severe mental deficiency. SEE: *idiocy; mental retardation.*

**idiotic** Like an idiot; said of an idea or action.

**idiotope** A single antigenic determinant on a variable region of an antibody or T-cell receptor. A set of idiotopes make up the idiotype.

**idiotrophic** (ĭd″ē-ō-trŏf′ĭk) [Gr. *idios,* own, + *trophe,* nourishment] Capable of securing its own nourishment.

**idiotropic** (ĭd″ē-ō-trŏp′ĭk) [″ + *trope,* a turning] Egocentric.

**idiot-savant** (ēd-jō′să-vănt) [Fr., learned idiot] An individual who is generally mentally retarded but has the ability to do complicated tasks such as play instruments, recall dates, or accurately and rapidly perform mathematical calculations. SEE: *autism.*

**idiotype** (ĭd″ē-ō-tīp′) [Gr. *idios,* own, + *typos,* type] In immunology, the set of antigenic determinants (idiotopes) on an antibody that make that antibody unique. It is associated with the amino acids of immunoglobulin light and heavy chains. **idiotypic** (-tĭp′ĭk), *adj.*

**idiovariation** (ĭd″ē-ō-văr″ē-ā′shŭn) [″ + L. *variare,* to vary] A mutation that occurs without known cause.

**idioventricular** (ĭd″ē-ō-vĕn-trĭk′ū-lăr) [″ + L. *ventriculus,* little belly] Pert. to the cardiac ventricle alone when dissociated from the atrium. A heart rhythm that arises in the ventricle is an example.

**IDM** *infant of diabetic mother.*

**idoxuridine** (ī-dŏks-ūr′ĭ-dēn) ABBR: IDU. 5-iodo-2′deoxyuridine; used to treat herpesvirus infections of the eye.

**IDU** *5-iodo-2′deoxyuridine; idoxuridine.*

**Ifosfamide** A cytotoxic agent used in treating metastatic germ-cell testicular cancer. This drug is usually given with mesna to help reduce the toxicity of its metabolites. Trade name is Ifex. SEE: *mesna; testicular cancer, germ-cell.*

**IgA** *immunoglobulin A.*

**IgD** *immunoglobulin D.*

**IgE** *immunoglobulin E.*

**IgG** *immunoglobulin G.*

**IgM** *immunoglobulin M.*

**ignatia** (ĭg-nā′shē-ă) [L.] The seeds of a climbing plant native to the Philippine Islands, which contain about 3% strychnine and brucine.

**igniextirpation** (ĭg″nē-ĕks″tĭr-pā′shŭn) [L. *ignis,* fire, + *exstirpare,* to root out] Cautery excision.

**ignis** (ĭg′nĭs) [L., fire] Moxa.

***i. infernalis*** Ergotism.

**I.H.** *infectious hepatitis.*

**IHS** *Indian Health Service.*

**ILD** *interstitial lung disorder.*

**ilea** Plural of ileum.

**ileac** (ĭl′ē-ăk) **1.** Pert. to the ileum. **2.** Pert. to ileus.

**ileal** (ĭl′ē-ăl) Pert. to the ileum.

**ileal conduit** SEE: under *conduit.*

**ileectomy** (ĭl″ē-ĕk′tō-mē) [L. *ileum,* ileum, + Gr. *ektome,* excision] Excision of the ileum.

**ileitis** (ĭl″ē-ī′tĭs) [″ + Gr. *itis,* inflammation] An inflammation of the ileum. The mucosa becomes inflamed and ulcerates, the affected portion becoming thick, rigid, and edematous, and the lumen progressively narrowed. The lymph glands enlarge and the adjacent mesentery becomes thickened. The condition is found most often in the terminal ileum but may spread to other parts of the bowel and to the cecum. Adhesions may be formed. Pain is centered around the umbilicus and right lower abdominal quadrant. Abdominal distention is present. Diarrhea may alternate with constipation, and vomiting may occur.

***regional i.*** A nonspecific, chronic, inflammatory, granulomatous lesion involving the terminal ileum. It is nontuberculous. The disease may extend over many years with exacerbations and remissions of diarrhea, abdominal pain, anemia, loss of weight, fistula formation, and eventually obstructive intestinal symptoms. Stools are soft and gray or brown, with abundant fecal particles. Any part of the gastrointestinal tract may be involved, but the ileum is the principal site. The cause is unknown. SYN: *Crohn's disease; regional enteritis.* SEE: *disease, inflammatory bowel.*

TREATMENT: The treatment is dietary and symptomatic with respect to the anemia and dehydration. Corticosteroids are indicated in acute attacks. Very low daily doses may be of benefit when the acute attack is over. Antibiotics are needed for bacterial complications. If symptoms persist or intestinal obstruction recurs, resection of the inflamed bowel may be palliative but not curative.

NURSING IMPLICATIONS: The nurse obtains a history for fatigue, fever, abdominal pain, diarrhea, (usually without obvious bleeding), and checks for weight loss. Usually the patient reports a gradual onset of symptoms, with periods of exacerbation and remission. The diarrhea may worsen after emotional upset or after ingestion of poorly tolerated foods, such as milk, fatty foods, and spices. The patient also may report anorexia, nausea, and vomiting. The patient typically describes the pain as steady, colicky, or cramping, and occurring in the right lower quadrant. The nurse inspects the patient's stools, which may appear soft or semiliquid, without gross blood (distinguishing the disorder from the bloody diarrhea of ulcerative colitis). Palpation may reveal tenderness in the right lower quadrant, and may also reveal an abdominal mass indicative of adherent loops of bowel. The nurse documents fluid intake and output (including the amount of stools), and weighs the patient daily. The nurse monitors hydration and serum electrolyte levels, and maintains fluid and electrolyte balance. The nurse monitors hemoglobin and hematocrit levels, checks stools for occult blood, and is alert for signs of intestinal bleeding. The nurse monitors for complications, assessing for fever and pain on urination, signaling bladder fistula; and for abdominal pain, fever, and a hard distended abdomen, indicating intestinal obstruction or rupture. The nurse provides emotional support to the patient and family, listening to the patient's concerns, and helping him or her to cope with body image disturbances. The nurse plans care to include rest periods throughout the day, and stresses the importance of adequate rest to the patient, explaining that limiting physical activity helps to reduce intestinal motility and promote healing. The nurse provides, and teaches the patient and family about, a diet high in proteins, calories, and vitamins, offering frequent, small meals throughout the day rather than three large ones. The nurse encourages the patient to avoid irritating foods, including milk products, spicy, fried, or high-residue foods, raw vegetables and fruits, and whole-grain cereals. The nurse also advises avoiding carbonated, caffeinated, and alcoholic beverages (because they increase intestinal activity). If the patient is receiving parenteral nutrition, the nurse monitors his or her condition closely and provides meticulous entry site care. The nurse administers and teaches the patient about prescribed medications (such as steroids, immunosuppressant agents, sulfasalazine, metronidazole, antidiarrheals, and narcotic analgesics), vitamins, iron supplements, and blood transfusions as prescribed. The nurse evaluates for desired effects and assesses for adverse reactions, teaching the patient about reactions to be reported. The nurse provides hygienic care, including frequent oral care if oral intake is restricted, and careful care of the anal region after each bowel movement. The nurse keeps a clean, covered bedpan or commode within the patient's reach, and ventilates the room to eliminate odors. The nurse teaches the patient and family about the disease: its symptoms, treatment, and complications. The nurse encourages the patient to identify and reduce sources of stress within his or her life, teaching stress-management techniques or referring for counseling. If the patient smokes, the nurse encourages him or her to stop, and refers to a smoking-cessation program or for nicotine patch therapy, if warranted, pointing out the smoking can aggravate the disease by altering bowel motility. The nurse explains and prepares the patient for prescribed diagnostic studies. As indicated, the nurse prepares the patient for surgery, providing procedural and sensation information and explaining postoperative care concerns.

**ileo-** (ĭl″ē-ō) [L. *ileum*] Combining form indicating relationship to the ileum.

**ileocecal** (ĭl′ē-ō-sē′kăl) [″ + *caecus*, blind] Relating to the ileum and cecum.

**ileocecostomy** (ĭl″ē-ō-sē-kŏs′tō-mē) [″ + ″ + Gr. *stoma*, opening] The surgical formation of an opening between the ileum and cecum.

**ileocecum** (ĭl″ē-ō-sē′kŭm) The ileum and cecum combined.

**ileocolic** (ĭl″ē-ō-kŏl′ĭk) [″ + Gr. *kolon*, colon] Pert. to the ileum and colon.

**ileocolitis** (ĭl″ē-ō-kō-lī′tĭs) [″ + ″ + *itis*, inflammation] An inflammation of the mucous membrane of the ileum and colon. SEE: *Nursing Diagnoses Appendix*.

**ileocolostomy** (ĭl″ē-ō-kō-lŏs′tō-mē) [″ + ″ + *stoma*, mouth] An anastomosis between the ileum and the colon.

**ileocolotomy** (ĭl″ē-ō-kō-lŏt′ō-mē) [″ + ″ + *tome*, incision] An incision of the ileum and colon.

**ileocystoplasty** (ĭl″ē-ō-sĭst′ō-plăs″tē) [″ + Gr. *kystis*, bladder, + *plassein*, to form] The use of a portion of the ileum to increase the size of the bladder.

**ileocystostomy** (ĭl″ē-ō-sĭs-tŏs′tō-mē) [″ + ″ + *stoma*, mouth] The surgical formation of an opening between the ileum and bladder.

**ileoileostomy** (ĭl″ē-ō-ĭl″ē-ŏs′tō-mē) [″ + *ileum*, small intestine, + Gr. *stoma*, mouth] The surgical formation of an opening between two parts of the ileum.

**ileoproctostomy** (ĭl″ē-ō-prŏk-tŏs′tō-mē) [″ + Gr. *proktos*, rectum, + *stoma*, mouth] The establishment of an opening between the ileum and rectum. SYN: *ileorectostomy*.

**ileorectal** (ĭl″ē-ō-rĕk′tăl) [″ + *rectum*, rectum] Concerning the ileum and rectum.

**ileorectostomy** (ĭl″ē-ō-rĕk-tŏs′tō-mē) [″ + ″ + Gr. *stoma*, mouth] Ileoproctostomy.

**ileorrhaphy** (ĭl″ē-or′ă-fē) [″ + Gr. *rhaphe*, seam, ridge] Surgical repair of the ileum.

**ileosigmoidostomy** (ĭl″ē-ō-sĭg″moyd-ŏs′tō-mē) [″ + Gr. *sigma*, letter S, + *eidos*, form, shape, + *stoma*, mouth] A surgical opening between the ileum and sigmoid flexure.

**ileostomy** (ĭl′ē-ŏs′tō-mē) [″ + Gr. *stoma*, mouth] The creation of a surgical passage through the abdominal wall into the ileum. The fecal material drains into a bag worn on the abdomen. SEE: *Nursing Diagnoses Appendix*.

***urinary i.*** The surgical formation of an opening between the ileum and the urinary bladder.

**ileotomy** (ĭl″ē-ŏt′ō-mē) [″ + Gr. *tome*, incision] An incision into the ileum.

**ileotransversostomy** (ĭl″ē-ō-trăns″vĕr-sŏs′tō-mē) [″ + *transversus*, crosswise, + Gr. *stoma*, mouth] Connection of the ileum with the transverse colon.

**ileum** (ĭl′ē-ŭm) *pl.* **ilea** [L., ileum] The lower three fifths of the small intestine from the jejunum to the ileocecal valve. Its length varies in men from 31 ft 6 in. (9.6 m) to 15 ft 6 in. (4.72 m). SEE: *abdominal regions* and *digestive system* for illus.

***duplex i.*** A congenital doubling of the ileum.

**ileus** (ĭl′ē-ŭs) [Gr. *eileos*, a twisting] An intestinal obstruction. The term originally meant colic due to intestinal obstruction. It is characterized by an acute obstruction causing sudden pain that is paroxysmal at first, and then continuous; constipation; persistent fecal vomiting; abdominal distention; and collapse. SEE: *Nursing Diagnoses Appendix*.

***adynamic i.*** Ileus caused by intestinal muscle paralysis. SYN: *i. paralyticus*.

***dynamic i.*** Ileus caused by intestinal muscle contraction.

***mechanical i.*** Ileus produced by an obstruction.

***meconium i.*** Ileus of the newborn owing to obstruction of the bowel with meconium.

***i. paralyticus*** Adynamic i.

***postoperative i.*** Ileus resulting from handling the bowel during surgery, anesthesia, electrolyte imbalance, or wound infection.

***spastic i.*** Ileus due to spasm of a segment of the intestine.

**ilia** Pl. of ilium.

**iliac** [L. *iliacus*, pert. to ilium] Relating to the ilium.

***i. crest*** The hip; the upper free margin of the ilium.

***i. fascia*** Transversalis fascia over the anterior surface of the iliopsoas muscle.

***i. fossa*** One of the concavities of the iliac bones of the pelvis.

***i. region*** The inguinal region on either side of the hypogastrium.

***i. spine*** One of four spines of the ilium, namely the anterior and posterior inferior spines and the anterior and posterior superior spines.

**ilio-** [L. *ilium*, flank] Combining form indicating relationship to the ilium or flank.

**iliococcygeal** (ĭl″ē-ō-kŏk-sĭj′ē-ăl) [″ + Gr. *kokkyx*, coccyx] Concerning the ilium and coccyx.

**iliocolotomy** (ĭl″ē-ō-kō-lŏt′ō-mē) [″ + Gr. *kolon*, colon, + *tome*, incision] A opening into the colon in the iliac or inguinal region.

**iliocostal** (ĭl″ē-ō-kŏs′tăl) [″ + *costa*, rib] Joining or concerning the ilium and ribs.

**iliofemoral** (ĭl″ē-ō-fĕm′or-ăl) [″ + *femoralis,* pert. to femur] Pert. to the ilium and femur.

**iliohypogastric** (ĭl″ē-ō-hī″pō-găs′trĭk) [″ + Gr. *hypo,* under, + *gaster,* stomach] Concerning the ilium and hypogastrium.

**ilioinguinal** (ĭl″ē-ō-ĭn′gwĭ-năl) [″ + *inguinalis,* pert. to groin] Pert. to the groin and iliac regions.

**iliolumbar** (ĭl″ē-ō-lŭm′bar) [″ + *lumbus,* loin] Pert. to the iliac and lumbar regions.

**iliopagus** (ĭl″ē-ŏp′ă-gŭs) [″ + Gr. *pagos,* thing fixed] Twins joined in the iliac region.

**iliopectineal** (ĭl″ē-ō-pĕk-tĭn′ē-ăl) [L. *ilium,* flank, + *pecten,* a comb] Concerning the ilium and pubes.

**iliopelvic** (ĭl″ē-ō-pĕl′vĭk) [″ + *pelvis,* basin] Concerning the iliac area and pelvis.

**iliopsoas** (ĭl″ē-ō-sō′ăs) [″ + Gr. *psoa,* loin] The compound iliacus and psoas magnus muscles.

**iliosacral** (ĭl″ē-ō-sā′krăl) [″ + *sacralis,* pert. to the sacrum] Concerning the sacrum and ilium.

**iliosciatic** (ĭl″ē-ō-sī-ăt′ĭk) [″ + *sciaticus,* pert. to the ischium] Concerning the ilium and ischium.

**iliospinal** (ĭl″ē-ō-spī′năl) [″ + *spinalis,* pert. to the spine] Concerning the ilium and spinal column.

**iliothoracopagus** (ĭl″ē-ō-thō″ră-kŏp′ă-gŭs) [″ + Gr. *thorax,* chest, + *pagos,* thing fixed] Twins joined from pelvis to thorax.

**ilioxiphopagus** (ĭl″ē-ō-zī-fŏp′ă-gŭs) [″+ Gr. *xiphos,* sword, + *eidos,* form, shape, + *pagos,* thing fixed] Twins joined from the pelvis to the xiphoid process.

**ilium** (ĭl′ē-ŭm) *pl.* **ilia** [L., groin, flank] **1.** One of the bones of each half of the pelvis. It is the superior and widest part and serves to support the flank. In the child, before fusion with adjacent pelvic bones, it is a separate bone. SYN: *os ilium.* **2.** The flank. SEE: *sacroiliac.*

**Ilizarow method** [G. A. Ilizarow, Siberian surgeon, 1921-1992] Lengthening a bone by cutting through the outer layer but not into the marrow cavity. The two ends are held in place for a week and then slowly pulled apart with an external fixator device. This is known as distraction. The bone may be lengthened by about 1 mm/day. After lengthening is complete, the device is left in place for at least a month to allow complete healing of the bone. The bone is radiographically evaluated for completeness of healing before the device is removed.

**ill** (ĭl) [Old Norse *illr,* bad] Sick; not healthy; diseased.

**illaqueation** (ĭl″ăk-wē-ā′shŭn) [L. *illaqueare,* to ensnare] Turning an inverted eyelash by drawing a loop of thread behind it.

**illiterate** Being unable to read and write or to use written language as in understanding graphs, charts, tables, maps, symbols, and formulas.

**illness** (ĭl′nĭs) [Old Norse *illr,* bad, + AS. *-ness,* state of] **1.** The state of being sick. **2.** An ailment.

***catabolic i.*** Rapid weight loss with loss of body fat and muscle mass that frequently accompanies short-term, self-limiting conditions such as infection or injury. This condition may be associated with diabetic ketoacidosis, multiple organ system failure, and chemotherapy or radiation therapy for cancer.

TREATMENT: Inflammation should be reduced and appropriate nutrients provided.

***catastrophic i.*** An unusually prolonged or complex illness, esp. one that requires a large expenditure of money for the medical care involved.

***folk i.*** Any disorder known by a specific name among cultural groups outside the context of conventional medicine. Often the culture has causal explanations for these illnesses, as well as preventive and treatment measures. Several such disorders exist in the Hispanic American culture; these are diagnosed and treated by folk healers called *curandieros.*

***functional i.*** An illness for which no organic explanation is present. SYN: *functional disease.* SEE: *organic disease.*

***mental i.*** Any disorder that affects the mind or behavior.

***psychosomatic i.*** SEE: *somatoform disorder.*

***terminal i.*** An illness that, because of its nature or because of the specific circumstances of the patient, will result in the death of the patient, esp. cancers for which there is little hope that therapeutic interventions will be helpful.

**illumination** (ĭl-lū-mĭn-ā′shŭn) [L. *illuminare,* to light up] The lighting up of a part for examination or of an object under a microscope.

***axial i.*** Light transmitted along the axis of a microscope. SYN: *central i.*

***central i.*** Axial i.

***dark-field i.*** The illumination of an object under a microscope in which the central or axial light rays are stopped and the object is illuminated by light rays coming from the sides, which causes the object to appear light against a dark background. This technique is used to observe extremely small objects such as spirochetes or colloid particles.

***direct i.*** The illumination of an object under a microscope by directing light rays upon its upper surface.

***focal i.*** Concentration of light on an object by means of a mirror or a system of lenses.

***oblique i.*** Illumination of an object from one side.

***transmitted light i.*** Illumination in which the light is directed through the object. Light may come directly from a light source or be reflected by a mirror.

**illusion** [L. *illusio*] An inaccurate perception; a misinterpretation of sensory impressions, as opposed to a hallucination, which has no basis in reality. Vague stimuli are conducive to the production of illusions, but essentially it is a disorder of ideation. If an illusion becomes fixed, it is said to be a delusion.

***optical i.*** A visual impression that is inaccurate with respect to the reality of the viewed object.

**illusional** Pert. to, or of the nature of, an illusion.

**I.M.** *intramuscular(ly).*

**im-** Prefix that is used in place of *in-* before words beginning with *b, m,* or *p.*

**I.M.A.** *Industrial Medical Association.*

**ima** (ī'mă) [L.] Lowest.

**image** (ĭm'ĭj) [L. *imago,* likeness] **1.** A mental picture representing a real object. **2.** A more or less accurate likeness of a thing or person. **3.** A picture of an object such as that produced by a lens or mirror.

***body i.*** The concept an individual has of his or her physical self. Many individuals have inappropriate self-images. For example, some obese individuals have the body image of a much less obese person.

***direct i.*** A picture produced from rays that are not yet focused. SYN: *virtual i.*

***double i.*** A perceived image that occurs in strabismus when the visual axes of the eyes are not directed toward the same object. SYN: *false i.* SEE: *diplopia.*

***false i.*** Double i.

***i. intensifier*** A special x-ray tube used during fluoroscopic imaging that increases the brightness of an image. This increased brightness is controlled by image minification and electron acceleration. The minified image can be viewed directly, coupled with a television camera, or imaged by serial or digital radiography. The quality of the image is better than that of an unintensified fluoroscopic image.

***inverted i.*** An image that is turned upside down.

***latent i.*** In radiology, the image on an exposed radiograph that is invisible because it has not been developed.

***mirror i.*** An image of an object reflected in a mirror, in which right and left are reversed. The term is also used to indicate the similarity of chemical substances or persons with quite similar personalities and looks (e.g., identical twins).

***radiographic i.*** An x-ray image created on a fluorescent screen or photographic film by x-rays passed through a structure or tissue.

***real i.*** The image formed by convergence of rays of light from an object.

***virtual i.*** Direct i.

**imagery** (ĭm'ĭj-rē) [L. *imago,* likeness] **1.** Imagination; the calling up of events or mental pictures. Mental imagery may be of various types. **2.** A form of distraction in which the patient is stimulated to visualize or think about pleasant or desirable feelings, sensations, or events. This is done to divert the patient's attention away from pain.

***active i.*** The conscious formation of a mental picture. This may be used by a patient to counter tense feelings or to imagine that an unwanted symptom is disappearing.

***auditory i.*** A mental image of sounds that can be recalled, as thunder or wind.

***smell i.*** A mental concept of odor sensations previously experienced; often very weak.

***tactile i.*** A mental image of the way an object feels.

***taste i.*** A mental concept of taste sensations previously experienced; often very weak.

***visual i.*** A mental concept of an object seen previously. This is probably the commonest type of imagery. SEE: *afterimage.*

**imagination** [L. *imago,* likeness] The formation of mental images of things, persons, or situations that are wholly or partially different from those previously known or experienced.

**imaging** The production of a picture, image, or shadow that represents the object being investigated. In diagnostic medicine the classic technique for imaging is x-ray examination. Techniques using computer-generated images produced by x-ray, ultrasound, magnetic resonance, or infrared are also available.

***digital subtraction i.*** In radiology, use of electronic means to subtract portions of the radiograph image in order to better visualize the object.

**imago** (ĭ-mā'gō) [L., likeness] **1.** An image or shadow. **2.** A memory, esp. of a loved one, developed during childhood that has become clouded by idealism and imagination, and is therefore not always correct. **3.** The adult, sexually mature form of an insect.

**imbalance** [L. *in-,* not, + *bilanx,* two scales] Lack of balance; the state of inequality in power between opposing forces.

***autonomic i.*** An imbalance between sympathetic and parasympathetic divisions of the autonomic nervous system, esp. as pertains to vasomotor reactions.

***sympathetic i.*** Vagotonia.

***vasomotor i.*** Excessive vasoconstriction or vasodilation resulting from impulses to blood vessels.

**imbecile** (ĭm'bĕ-sĭl) [L. *imbecillus,* feeble] Former term for an individual with severe mental deficiency. SEE: *mental retardation.*

**imbecility** Former term for a state of severe mental deficiency.

**imbed** [L. *in,* in, (put) into, + AS. *bedd,* bed] In histology, to surround with a firm substance, such as paraffin, preparatory to cutting sections. SEE: *embedding.*

**imbibition** (ĭm"bĭ-bĭsh'ŭn) [" + *bibere,* to drink] The absorption of fluid by a solid body or gel.

**imbricated, imbrication** (ĭm′brĭ-kāt-ĕd, ĭm″brĭ-kā′shŭn) [L. *imbricare,* to tile] **1.** Overlapping, as tiles. **2.** The overlapping of aponeurotic layers in abdominal surgery.

**Imferon** Trade name for iron dextran.

**imidazole** (ĭm″ĭd-ăz′ōl″) An organic compound, $C_3H_4N_2$, characterized structurally by the presence of the heterocyclic ring that occurs in histidine and histamine.

**imide** (ĭm′ĭd) A compound with the bivalent atom group (NH).

**imipramine hydrochloride** (ĭ-mĭp′ră-mēn) A tricyclic antidepressant drug, also used to treat enuresis in children over 6 years of age.

**immature** (ĭm″mă-tūr′) [L. *in-,* not, + *maturus,* ripe] Not fully developed or ripened.

**immediate** [″ + *mediare,* to be in middle] Direct; without intervening steps.

**immedicable** (ĭ-mĕd′ĭ-kă-b′l) [L. *immedicabilis*] Incurable; pert. to that which cannot be healed.

**immersion** (ĭm-ĕr′shŭn) [L. *in,* into, + *mergere,* to dip] **1.** Placing a body under water or other fluid. **2.** In microscopy, the act of immersing the objective (then called an immersion lens) in water or oil, preventing total reflection of rays falling obliquely upon peripheral portions of the objective.

***i. foot*** Damage to the entire foot owing to continued exposure to water or to moisture. It can occur in a hot or cold climate in a situation in which it is not possible to maintain proper foot hygiene. Symptoms of numbness, tingling, and leg cramping are present. From military experience, it was found that the condition could be prevented by changing to dry socks as frequently as required. SEE: *trench foot.*

***homogeneous i.*** Immersion in which the stratum of air between objective and cover glass is replaced by a medium that deflects as little as possible the rays of light passing through the cover glass.

**immiscible** (ĭ-mĭs′ĭ-bl) [L. *in-,* not, + *miscere,* to mix] Pert. to that which cannot be mixed, as oil and water.

**immobilization** [″ + *mobilis,* movable] The making of a part or limb immovable.

NURSING IMPLICATIONS: The patient is assessed for development of any of the complications of immobilization, such as pneumonia, thrombophlebitis, renal calculi, urinary tract infections, constipation, decubitus ulcers, muscle atrophy, and contracture formation. Lung and heart sounds are auscultated, fluid balance and nutritional and dietary fiber intake monitored, bowel sounds auscultated, and bowel and bladder function are assessed.

Nursing interventions to prevent such complications include having the patient deep breathe and cough every 2 hours, using incentive spirometry if prescribed; completely change position every 2 hours, with lesser position changes in between; wear antithromboembolic devices; do quadriceps setting, gluteal muscle setting, and range-of-motion exercises at least daily; ensure good body hygiene; maintain nutrition, including adequate dietary fiber, protein, and vitamin C intake; and increase fluid intake to 3 liters daily, unless otherwise restricted by renal or cardiac disorders. Skin care is provided, the skin is inspected daily for redness and signs of breakdown, intact areas are gently massaged to increase circulation, and low-pressure foam or flotation pads or mattresses are applied as needed. The nurse ensures that blood supply to the extremities is not restricted by any appliance or by tight bedcovers, distal neurovascular and circulatory status is evaluated for the presence of pulses, changes in size of extremities, and pallor or other changes in color, as well as for paresthesias or paralysis, temperature changes, and pain.

**immortality** The ability of some cells, particularly cancer cells, to reproduce indefinitely. Normal human cells have a finite life expectancy. They may divide for a few dozen generations, but eventually stop reproducing and die.

**immotile cilia syndrome** An inherited condition marked by reduced fertility in women and sterility in men. This condition is due to the absence or deficiency of the dynein arms of the cilia, causing them to beat ineffectively. The normal motion of the cilia is 1000 cycles/min. SEE: *dynein; Kartagener's syndrome.*

**immune** (ĭm-ūn′) [L. *immunis,* safe] Protected from or resistant to a disease or infection by a pathogenic organism as a result of the development of antibodies or cell-mediated immunity.

***i. body*** Antibody.

***i. complex*** A substance formed when antibodies attach to antigens to destroy them. These complexes circulate in the blood and may eventually attach to the walls of blood vessels, producing a local inflammatory response. Immune complexes form in type III hypersensitivity reactions and are involved in the development of glomerulonephritis, serum sickness, arthritis, and vasculitis, which may be called immune-complex diseases.

***mucosal i. system*** The clusters of lymphoid cells beneath the mucosal endothelium of the gastrointestinal, respiratory, and genitourinary tracts. It has two parts: organized and diffuse. The organized part (the mucosal-associated lymphoid tissue of the gastrointestinal and respiratory tracts) is composed of nodules containing lymphocytes and macrophages that are activated by ingested or inhaled microorganisms. The diffuse part is composed of loose clusters of macrophages and mature B and T lymphocytes found within the folds of the intestinal walls. The B cells secrete antibodies, primarily immunoglobulin A; the T cells directly lyse microorganisms.

The mucosal immune system is augmented by the presence of normal microflora; peristalsis and cilia, which move mucus outward; and various chemicals, such as gastric acid and pancreatic enzymes, that destroy pathogens. Normally all of these components must be functioning to prevent infection. SEE: *gut-associated lymphoid tissue; immunoglobulin A.*

***primary i. response*** The initial reaction to an immunogen, during which T and B lymphocytes are activated and antibodies specific to the antigen are produced. This reaction is considered relatively weak but produces large numbers of antigen-specific memory cells.

***i. reaction*** **1.** A demonstrated antigenic response to a specific antibody. **2.** The specific reaction of host cells to antigenic stimulation. SEE: *i. response.*

***i. response*** The body's reaction to foreign antigens so that they are neutralized or eliminated, thus preventing damage. It requires that the body recognize the antigen as "nonself," or foreign. *Cell-mediated immune response* involves the production of lymphocytes by the thymus (T cells) in response to antigen exposure. This reaction is important in delayed hypersensitivity; rejection of tissue transplants; response to malignant growths; and in some infections. In *humoral immune response* plasma lymphocytes (B cells) are produced in response to antigen exposure with subsequent antibody formation. This response can produce immunity or hypersensitivity. *Nonspecific immune response,* or inflammation, is the response of the body's tissues and cells to injury from any source (e.g., trauma, organisms, chemicals, ischemia). The initial response of the immune system to any threat, it involves vascular, chemical, and white blood cell activities. *Specific immune response* is required when inflammation is inadequate to cope with injury or invasion by an organism. It is directed and controlled by T cells and B cells. Cellular immunity refers to the T cell response; humoral immunity is the term previously used to refer to B cell response. SEE: *B-cell–mediated immunity; T-cell–mediated immunity.*

***secondary i. response*** The rapid, strong response by T and B cells to a second or subsequent appearance of an immunogen. This occurs because of the availability of T and B lymphocyte memory cells.

***i. system*** The lymphatic tissues, organs, and physiological processes that identify an antigen as abnormal or foreign and prevent it from harming the body. The skin, mucosa, normal flora of the gastrointestinal tract and skin, and chemicals contained in tears, sebaceous glands, gastric acid, and pancreatic enzymes protect the body from pathogen invasion. The bone marrow produces white blood cells (WBCs), the primary internal defense. Lymphoid tissues, including the thymus gland, spleen, and lymph nodes, influence the growth, maturation, and activation of WBCs; lymphoid tissue in the gastrointestinal and respiratory tracts and mucous membranes contain WBCs for site-specific protection. Finally, physiologically active protein mediators, called cytokines, help regulate the growth and function of immunologically active cells.

*Effects of stress:* Investigations of the influence of stress on susceptibility to disease have shown that in some, but not all individuals, who experienced undesirable events, the possibility of onset of illness was increased. A decrease in the usual number of pleasant events was a stronger predictor of susceptibility to illness than was an increase in unpleasant ones. Negative experiences included criticism, frustration, irritating encounters with fellow workers, deadlines, heavy workload, and burdensome and unpleasant chores or errands. Even though the concept that stress lowers resistance to disease appears to apply only to some individuals, the explanation of this mechanism has not been established.

**immune globulin** A sterile solution of globulins containing many antibodies normally present in human blood, used in passive immunization of nonimmune persons exposed to diseases such as infectious hepatitis, poliomyelitis, mumps, rubella, rubeola, and varicella.

***cytomegalovirus i.g. intravenous*** An immune globulin preparation suitable for use intravenously to treat primary cytomegalovirus disease associated with kidney transplantation.

***intramuscular i.g.*** A preparation of immune globulin for intramuscular use. It is used prophylactically before or soon after exposure to hepatitis A. It is not indicated in patients with clinical manifestations of hepatits A or in those exposed more than 2 weeks previously. It is also used in prevention or modification of measles (rubeola) and in patients with immunoglobulin deficiency.

***intravenous i.g.*** ABBR: IVIG. An immune globulin preparation used intravenously in patients with immunodeficiency syndromes and in immunosuppressed recipients of bone marrow transplants. In conjunction with aspirin, it is the standard of care for children during the first 10 days of Kawasaki disease to prevent the development of coronary aneurysms. The risks of using IVIG are minimal.

IVIG is used to treat idiopathic thrombocytopenic purpura and Guillain-Barré syndrome, as well as to prevent bacterial infections in patients with hypogammaglobulinemia or recurrent infections associated with B-cell chronic lymphocytic leukemia.

***tetanus i.g.*** An immune globulin used for patients with unknown histories of active tetanus immunization who present with wounds that might be contaminated with tetanus spores, or ones who present with symptoms of tetanus.

***$Rh_o$(D) i.g.*** An immune globulin preparation that suppresses the immune response of nonsensitized $Rh_o$(D) negative individuals who receive $Rh_o$(D) positive blood as the result of fetomaternal transfusion (as a consequence of abdominal trauma, amniocentesis, abortion, or full-term delivery) or due to a transfusion error. SEE: *Rh blood group.*

---

Caution: $Rh_o$(D) immune globulin should not be injected intravenously.

---

***varicella-zoster i.g.*** ABBR: VZIG. An immune globulin, primarily immunoglobulin, used for passive immunization of susceptible immunodeficient individuals after significant exposure to varicella. VZIG does not modify established varicella-zoster infections.

---

Caution: VZIG should not be injected intravenously.

---

**immunifacient** (ĭ-mū″nĭ-fā′shĕnt) [″ + *facere,* to make] Making immune.

**immunity** [L. *immunitas*] The state of being immune to or protected from a disease, esp. an infectious disease. This state is usually induced by having been exposed to the antigenic marker on an organism that invades the body or by having been immunized with a vaccine capable of stimulating production of specific antibodies. SEE: *autoimmune disease; immune response; immunodeficiency disease, severe combined; immunoglobulin; vaccine.*

***acquired i.*** Immunity resulting from the development of active or passive immunity, as opposed to natural or innate immunity.

***active i.*** Immunity resulting from the development within the body of antibodies or sensitized T lymphocytes that neutralize or destroy the infective agent. This may result from the immune response to an invading organism or from inoculation with a vaccine containing a foreign antigen. SEE: *immune response; vaccination.*

***B-cell–mediated i.*** SEE: *humoral i.*

***cell-mediated i.*** The regulatory and cytotoxic activities of T cells during the specific immune response. This process requires about 36 hr to reach its full effect. SYN: *T-cell–mediated i.* SEE: illus.; *humoral i.*

*Physiological Actions:* Unlike B cells, T cells cannot recognize foreign antigens on their own. A foreign antigen is recognized by a macrophage that engulfs it and displays part of the antigen on its surface next to a histocompatibility or "self" antigen (macrophage processing). The presence of these two markers plus the secretion of a cytokine, interleukin-1 (IL-1), by macrophages and other antigen-presenting cells activates CD4+/CD8− T cells (helper T cells), which regulate the activities of other cells involved in the immune response.

CD4+ T cells secrete interleukin-2 (IL-2), which stimulates the activity of natural killer cells, cytotoxic T cells, and B cells, and promotes proliferation of CD4+ T cells so that the invading pathogen can be destroyed or neutralized. Gamma interferon, also secreted by CD4+ T cells, enhances macrophage cytotoxicity and antigen processing. T-cell–mediated immunity plays a significant role in the rejection of transplanted tissues and in tests for allergies (delayed hypersensitivity reaction).

***congenital i.*** Immunity present at birth. It may be natural or acquired, the latter depending on antibodies received from the mother's blood.

***herd i.*** Immune protection through vaccination of a portion of a population, which may reduce the spread of a disease by limiting the number of potential hosts for the pathogen.

***humoral i.*** Immunity mediated by antibodies in body fluids such as plasma or lymph. These antibodies are synthesized and secreted by B cells, which protect the body against infection or reinfection by common organisms (e.g., streptococci and staphylococci). B cells are stimulated by direct contact with a foreign antigen and differentiate into plasma cells (which produce antibodies against the antigen) and memory cells (which enable the body to quickly produce these antibodies if the same antigen appears at a later time). B cell differentiation is also stimulated by interleukin-2 (IL-2), secreted by T4 cells, and by foreign antigens processed by macrophages. SYN: *B-cell–mediated i.* SEE: illus.; *cell-mediated i.*

***local i.*** Immunity limited to a given area or tissue of the body.

***natural i.*** Immunity programmed in the DNA, also called genetic immunity. Some pathogens cannot infect certain species because the cells are not suitable environments (e.g., the measles virus cannot reproduce in canine cells; therefore dogs have natural immunity to measles).

***passive i.*** Immunity acquired by the introduction of preformed antibodies into an unprotected individual. This can occur through injection or in utero from antibodies that pass from the mother to the

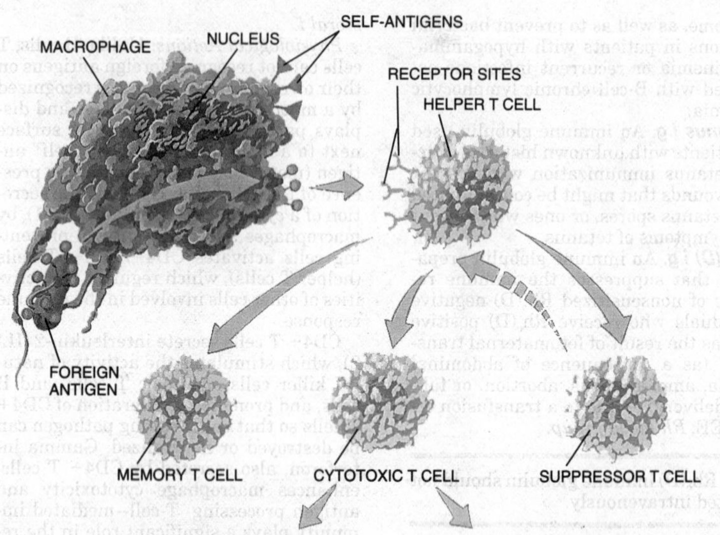


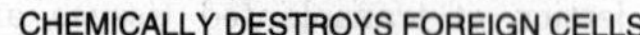


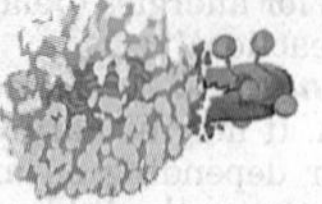


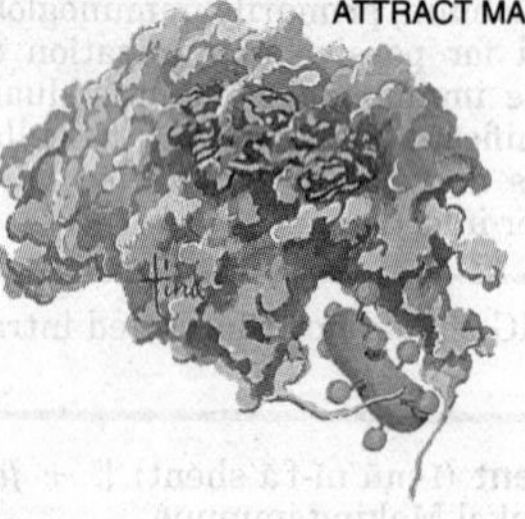

CELL-MEDIATED IMMUNITY

fetus through the placenta. It may also be acquired by the newborn by ingesting the mother's milk.

***T-cell–mediated i.*** SEE: *cell-mediated i.*

**immunization** [L. *immunitas,* immunity] The process of creating immunity to a specific disease in an individual. SEE: table; *vaccination; vaccine.*

**immunoassay** (ĭm″ū-nō-ăs′sā) [L. *immunis,* safe, + O. Fr. *assai,* trial] Measuring the protein and protein-bound molecules that are concerned with the reaction of an antigen with its specific antibody. SEE: *immunoelectrophoresis; immunofluorescence; radioimmunoassay.*

**immunobiology** (ĭm″ū-nō-bī-ŏl′ō-jē) [″ + Gr. *bios,* life, + *logos,* word, reason] The study of immune phenomena in biological systems, including the immune response to infectious diseases, transplantation of organs, allergy, autoimmunity, and cancer.

**immunochemistry** (ĭm″ū-nō-kĕm′ĭs-trē) [″ + Gr. *chemeia,* chemistry] The chemistry of immunization; the chemistry of antigens, antibodies, and their relation to each other.

**immunocompetence** (ĭm″ū-nō-kŏm′pĕ-tĕns) The ability of the body's immune system to respond to pathogenic organisms and tissue damage. This ability may be diminished by drugs specifically developed to inhibit immune cell function (e.g., chemotherapeutic agents used to treat leukemia and drugs used to prevent organ transplant rejections), by diseases that attack elements of the immune system, or overwhelming infections. SEE: *immunocompromised.*

**immunocompromised** Having an immune system incapable of reacting to pathogens or tissue damage. This may be due to a genetic disorder, disease process, or drugs such as corticosteroids or immunosuppressive agents given to treat a disorder that inhibits immune function. SYN: *immunodeficient*. SEE: *AIDS; compromised host; immunocompetence.*

**immunoconglutinin** (ĭm″ū-nō-kŏn-gloo′tĭ-nĭn) [″ + *conglutinare,* to glue together] A protein used in the laboratory. It binds with complement factor 3, a significant part of an antigen-antibody immune complex. It is used to assess the number of

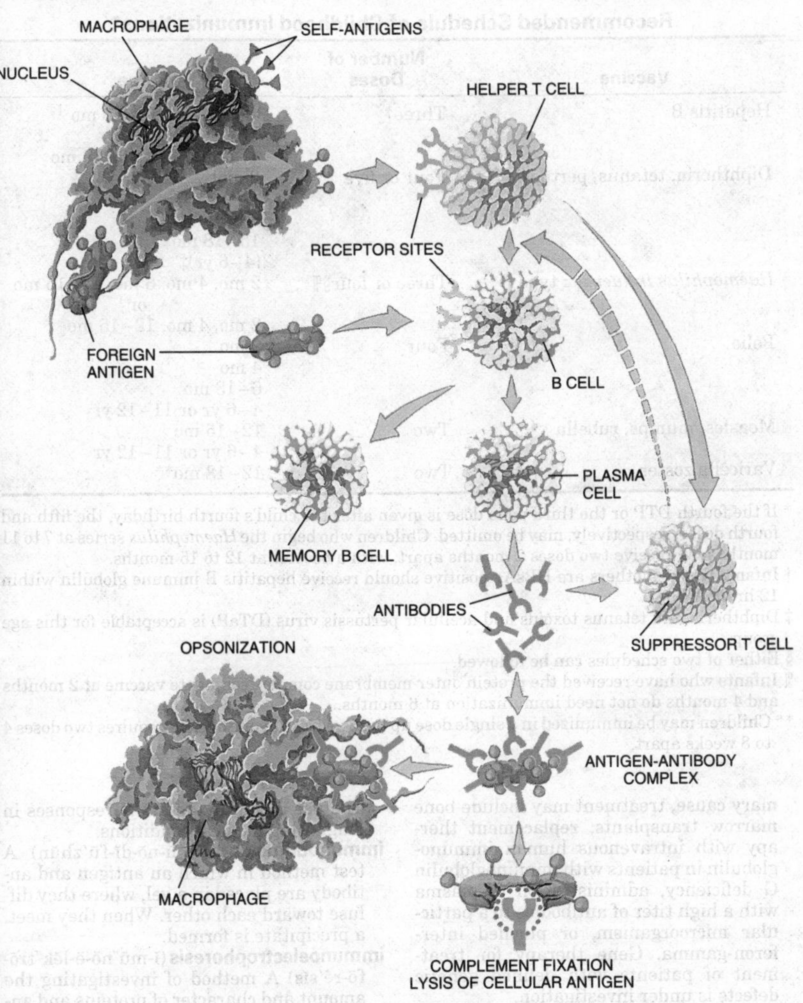


HUMORAL IMMUNITY

immune complexes in blood, which may be related to immunologic activity.

**immunocytoadherence** A laboratory test used to identify antibody-bearing cells by the formation of rosettes composed of red blood cells and those cells bearing antibodies.

**immunodeficiency** (ĭm″ū-nō-dĕ-fĭsh′ĕn-sē) Decreased or compromised ability to respond to antigenic stimuli by appropriate cellular immunity reaction. This state may be secondary to loss of immunoglobulins or an abnormality of B- or T-cell lymphocytes. SEE: *AIDS; immunocompetence.* **immunodeficient,** *adj.*

***primary i.*** A disorder due to abnormalities in the development and maturation of immune system cells, resulting in increased susceptibility to infection (e.g., recurrent pyogenic infections, which occur with defects of humoral immunity). Primary immunodeficiencies include X-linked agammaglobulinemia, severe combined immunodeficiency, and Wiskott-Aldrich syndrome.

**immunodeficiency disease, primary** A broad class of immunodeficiency syndromes that may be congenital, spontaneously acquired, or a result of therapeutic intervention that attempts to prevent rejection of transplanted tissues or organs. In most cases, the clinical manifestations are unusual susceptibility to infection, development of autoimmune disease, and lymphoreticular malignancies. SEE: *immunodeficiency disease, severe combined.*

TREATMENT: Depending on the pri-

## Recommended Schedule of Childhood Immunizations*

| Vaccine | Number of Doses | Age |
|---|---|---|
| Hepatitis B | Three† | Birth, 2 mo, 6–18 mo<br>or<br>1–2 mo, 4 mo, 6–18 mo |
| Diphtheria, tetanus, pertussis | Four or five | 2 mo<br>4 mo<br>6 mo<br>15–18 mo‡<br>(4–6 yr)‡ |
| *Haemophilus influenzae* type B | Three or four§¶ | 2 mo, 4 mo, 6 mo, 12–15 mo<br>or<br>2 mo, 4 mo, 12–15 mo |
| Polio | Four | 2 mo<br>4 mo<br>6–18 mo<br>4–6 yr or 11–12 yr |
| Measles, mumps, rubella | Two | 12–15 mo<br>4–6 yr or 11–12 yr |
| Varicella zoster | Two | 12–18 mo** |

* If the fourth DTP or the third polio dose is given after the child's fourth birthday, the fifth and fourth doses, respectively, may be omitted. Children who begin the *Haemophilus* series at 7 to 11 months may receive two doses 2 months apart, with a booster at 12 to 15 months.

† Infants whose mothers are HBsAg positive should receive hepatitis B immune globulin within 12 hr after birth.

‡ Diphtheria and tetanus toxoids and acellular pertussis virus (DTaP) is acceptable for this age group.

§ Either of two schedules can be followed.

¶ Infants who have received the protein outer membrane complex conjugate vaccine at 2 months and 4 months do not need immunization at 6 months.

** Children may be immunized in a single dose up to 13 years. Anyone over 13 requires two doses 4 to 8 weeks apart.

mary cause, treatment may include bone marrow transplants, replacement therapy with intravenous human immunoglobulin in patients with immunoglobulin G deficiency, administration of plasma with a high titer of antibodies to a particular microorganism, or purified interferon-gamma. Gene therapy for treatment of patients with defined genetic defects is under investigation.

**immunodeficiency disease, severe combined** ABBR: SCID. Any of a group of inherited autosomal or x-linked recessive disorders in which there is partial or complete dysfunction of the immune system. To prevent lethal infectious diseases from developing in children afflicted with SCID, they are kept in a protected environment, and have therefore been called "bubble babies." No single pathogenic mechanism is common to all patients with SCID. In one form, the cause is a deficiency of the enzyme adenosine deaminase. Those patients may be treated parenterally with enzyme replacement therapy provided by the drug pegademase bovine. The treatment must be continued for life. SEE: *adenosine deaminase conjugated with polyethylene glycol; immunodeficiency disease, primary.*

**immunodeficient** Immunocompromised.

**immunodiagnosis** (ĭm″ū-nō-dī″ăg-nō′sĭs) The use of specific immune responses in diagnosing medical conditions.

**immunodiffusion** (ĭm″ū-nō-dĭ-fū′zhŭn) A test method in which an antigen and antibody are placed in a gel, where they diffuse toward each other. When they meet, a precipitate is formed.

**immunoelectrophoresis** (ĭ-mū″nō-ē-lĕk″trō-fō-rē′sĭs) A method of investigating the amount and character of proteins and antibodies in body fluids by using electrophoresis.

**immunofluorescence** (ĭm″ū-nō-floo″ō-rĕs′ĕns) The detection of antibodies by using special proteins labeled with fluorescein. If the specific organism or antibody that is being searched for is present, it is observed as a fluorescent material when examined microscopically while illuminated with a fluorescent light source.

**immunogen** (ĭ-mū-nō-jĕn) [″ + Gr. *gennan,* to produce] A substance capable of producing an immune response. Proteins and polysaccharides may be strong immunogens, but lipids and nucleic acids may also be immunogenic. SEE: *antigen.*

**immunogenetics** (ĭm″ū-nō-jĕ-nĕt′ĭks) [″ + Gr. *gennan,* to produce] The study of genetics by use of immune responses, including investigations of immunoglobulins and histocompatibility antigens.

**immunogenic** (ĭm″ū-nō-jĕn′ĭk) Capable of

inducing an immune response. This response depends on the properties of both the immunogen and the host. It is essential that the host recognize that the immunogen is foreign (i.e., nonself).

**immunogenicity** (ĭm″ū-nō-jĕ-nĭs′ĭ-tē) The capacity to induce a detectable immune response.

**immunoglobulin** (ĭm″ū-nō-glŏb′ū-lĭn) ABBR: Ig. One of a family of closely related though not identical proteins capable of acting as antibodies. All antibodies are immunoglobulins, but researchers have not yet determined if all immunoglobulins have antibody functions.

***i. A*** ABBR: IgA. The principal immunoglobulin in exocrine secretions such as milk, respiratory and intestinal mucin, saliva, and tears. This is probably important in protecting mucosal surfaces from invasion by pathogenic bacteria and viruses. Its presence in colostrum helps to protect the suckling newborn from infection.

***i. D*** ABBR: IgD. An immunoglobulin that is present on the surface of B lymphocytes and acts as an antigen receptor.

***i. E*** ABBR: IgE. An immunoglobulin that attaches to mast cells in the respiratory and intestinal tracts and plays a major role in allergic reactions. About 50% of patients with allergies have increased IgE levels. IgE is also important in the formation of reagin, a type of immunoglobulin gamma E (IgGE), found in the blood of individuals with an atopic hypersensitivity.

***i. G*** ABBR: IgG. The principal immunoglobulin in human serum. Because it moves across the placental barrier, IgG is important in producing immunity in the infant before birth. It is the major antibody for antitoxins, viruses, and bacteria. It also activates complement and serves as an opsonin. As gamma globulin, IgG may be given to provide temporary resistance to hepatitis or other diseases.

***intravenous i.*** ABBR: IVIG. An immunoglobulin product, administered intravenously, that contains concentrated human immunoglobulin, primarily IgG. IVIG is approved as replacement therapy in patients with primary immunodeficiencies, Kawasaki syndrome, chronic lymphocytic leukemia, and idiopathic thrombocytopenic purpura, and in those undergoing bone marrow transplantation.

***i. M*** ABBR: IgM. An immunoglobulin formed in almost every immune response during the early period of the reaction. IgM controls the A, B, O blood group antibody responses and is the most efficient antibody in stimulating complement activity. Its size prevents its moving across the placenta to the fetus.

**immunohematology** (ĭ-mū-nō-hēm″ă-tŏl′ō-jē) [L. *immunis,* safe, + Gr. *haima,* blood, + *logos,* word, reason] The study of blood diseases including certain autoimmune diseases by use of immunological techniques.

**immunoincompetency** An inability to produce an immune response. SEE: *immunodeficiency.*

**immunological therapy** The use of natural and synthetic substances to stimulate or suppress the cell-mediated immune response and inflammation, or to interfere with the growth of malignant neoplasms. The use of cytokines such as interferons and interleukin-2, and monoclonal antibodies obtained in a laboratory, may increase specificity of action so that only targeted cells are affected.

***stimulation i.t.*** The therapeutic use of agents that stimulate immune function (immunostimulators). Attenuated solutions of mycobacterium Bacille Calmette-Guérin, which stimulates macrophage, lymphocyte, and interleukin-1 activity, and *Streptococcus pyogenes,* which enhances macrophage and natural killer cell function, have been used with limited success as adjunct cancer therapy. New techniques have enabled researchers to isolate hormones from the thymus gland, where T lymphocytes mature, to treat viral infections and cancers. Their clinical effectiveness has not been established.

More definitive data have come from the use of laboratory-prepared cytokines, the protein mediators of immune responses. The interferons and interleukin-2 are used to treat some cancers; transforming growth factor beta seems to enhance wound healing, erythropoietin is used to treat several types of anemia, and granulocyte and macrophage colony-stimulating factors increase white blood cell production in the bone marrow following cancer chemotherapy or bone marrow transplantation.

Several biochemical immunostimulators have resulted from the intensive research that has accompanied the appearance of the AIDS pandemic.

***suppressive i.t.*** Any of the methods used to block abnormal or excessive immune responses. Research efforts have produced several means of blocking these responses, now recognized as the source of pathology in a broad range of diseases.

*Corticosteroids,* the most widely known anti-inflammatory agents, increase the number of neutrophils in the blood but decrease their aggregation at inflammatory sites, decrease the number and function of other white blood cells, and inhibit cytokine production. They are most effective during an acute flareup of a chronic autoimmune disease and in conjunction with other agents because they do not adequately block autoantibodies when used alone.

*Cytotoxic drugs* kill all white blood cells and their precursors and were originally developed as anticancer agents. However, low-dose methotrexate is now known to be effective in reducing the symptoms and the need for corticosteroids in chronic inflammatory diseases such as rheumatoid arthritis, Crohn's disease, psoriasis, and asthma.

*Cyclosporin* selectively inhibits CD4+ or helper T cells and is used extensively to block rejection of transplanted tissue. A new drug, tacrolimus (FK 506), acts in a similar manner.

*Intravenous gamma globulin* inhibits phagocytosis of platelets in idiopathic thrombocytopenic purpura and is the primary treatment in children. Because it seems to inhibit natural killer cells and augment CD8+ T cells, it has been used for other autoimmune diseases, such as myasthenia gravis, but its clinical effectiveness has not been determined.

*Monoclonal antibodies* are laboratory-created antibodies developed from a single cell line that block specific cytotoxic T cells, the mediators that activate these cells, and the adhesion molecules that bind and transfer signals from cytokines. They are being tested in the treatment of cancers and transplant rejection.

*Plasmapheresis,* the separation and removal of plasma containing autoantibodies (AAb), is most effective against disorders in which the AAbs are tissue specific, such as myasthenia gravis, and those in which more AAbs are found in the blood than in extravascular spaces.

**immunologist** (ĭm″ū-nŏl′ō-jĭst) An individual whose special training and experience is in immunology.

**immunology** (ĭm″ū-nŏl′ō-jē) [″ + Gr. *logos,* word, reason] The study of the components of the immune system and their function. SEE: *immune system.* **immunologic** (ĭm″ū-nō-lŏj′ĭk), *adj.*

**immunomagnetic technique** An experimental technique involving the use of magnetic microspheres in treating bone marrow in order to purge malignant cells.

**immunomodulation** The ability to change immune responses. SEE: *therapy, immunological.*

**immunopathology** (ĭm″ū-nō-pă-thŏl′ō-jē) The study of tissue alterations that result from immune or allergic reactions.

**immunoprecipitation** (ĭm″ū-nō-prē-sĭp″ĭ-tā′shŭn) The formation of a precipitate when an antigen and antibody interact.

**immunoproliferative** (ĭm″ū-nō-prō-lĭf′ĕr-ă-tĭv) The proliferation of cells and tissues involved in producing antigens.

**immunoprotein** (ĭm″ū-nō-prō′tē-ĭn) [″ + Gr. *protos,* first] Any protein or substance that confers immunity.

**immunoreactant** (ĭ-mū″nō-rē-ăk′tănt) Any of the substances involved in immunologic reactions, including immunoglobulins, complement components, and specific antigens.

**immunoreaction** (ĭ-mū″nō-rē-ăk′shŭn) The reaction of an antibody to an antigen.

**immunoselection** (ĭm″ū-nō-sĕ-lĕk′shŭn) The selective survival of cell lives owing to their having the least amount of cell surface antigenicity. This aspect allows those cells to escape the destructive activity of either antibodies or immune lymphoid cells.

**immunosenescence** The effect of age on the immune system and host defense mechanisms. The clinician caring for an elderly patient can assume that the individual has defective host defenses, is at greater risk for developing an infectious disease, and has greater risk of morbidity and mortality. Immunosenescence markedly affects the outcomes of many illnesses that have an age-related incidence, such as emphysema, postoperative infection, urinary tract infection, diabetes, bowel inflammation, and infections in areas with decreased blood perfusion.

**immunostimulator** (ĭm″ū-nō-stĭm′ū-lā-tōr) SEE: *therapy, immunological.*

**immunosuppression** (ĭm″ū-nō-sū-prĕsh′ŭn) Prevention of the activation of immune responses.

**immunosuppressive** (ĭm″ū-nō-sū-prĕs′ĭv) Acting to suppress the body's natural immune response to an antigen.

***i. agent*** SEE: *therapy, immunological.*

**immunosurgery** (ĭ-mū″nō-sĕr′jĕr-ē) The use of specific antigenic substances in surgical therapy.

**immunosurveillance** (ĭm″ū-nō-sĕr-vā′lĕns) The immune system's recognition and destruction of newly developed abnormal cells that arise from mutations of cell lines. This would occur in cancer cells that contained new antigens.

**immunotherapy** (ĭm″ū-nō-thĕr′ă-pē) [″ + Gr. *therapeia,* treatment] Use of the body's immune system to counteract the side effects of treatment, especially cancer chemotherapy. Monoclonal antibodies, interferon, interleukins, and colony-stimulating factors are used. Also called *biological therapy* or *immunological therapy.*

***adoptive i.*** Culturing of a patient's blood lymphocytes in vitro with interleukin-2 and subsequent reinfusion in the patient. This therapy stimulates endogenous responses or replaces suppressed components of the immune system. It is used in patients who have become immunodeficient from cancer.

**immunotoxin** (ĭm″ū-nō-tŏk′sĭn) [″ + Gr. *toxikon,* poison] Toxic agents that can be attached to antibody molecules and, because of this enhanced toxicity, used to combat tumor cells. This technique has been used to eliminate malignant tumors in the bone marrow.

**immunotransfusion** (ĭ-mū″nō-trăns-fū′zhŭn) [″ + *trans,* across, + *fusus,* poured] Transfusion of blood that contains known antibodies.

**Imodium** Trade name for loperamide hydrochloride. An antiperistaltic drug used in treating diarrhea. SEE: *diarrhea, travelers'*.

**impacted** [L. *impactus,* pressed on] Pressed firmly together so as to be immovable. This term may be applied to a fracture in which the ends of the bones are wedged together, a tooth so placed in the jaw bone that eruption is impossible, a fetus wedged in the birth canal, cerumen, calculi, or accumulation of feces in the rectum.

**impaction** (ĭm-păk′shŭn) [L. *impactio,* a pressing together] A condition of being tightly wedged into a part, as when the eruption of a tooth is blocked by other teeth; the overloading of an organ, as the feces in the bowels.

***food impaction i.*** The forcing of food into the interproximal spaces of teeth by chewing (vertical impaction) or by tongue and cheek pressure (horizontal impaction).

**impairment** Any loss or abnormality of psychological, physiological, or anatomical structure or function.

**impaled object** A foreign body that penetrates the skin and remains imbedded in the body tissue. Such objects should not be removed outside of the operating room because hemorrhage may occur if vessels were damaged in such a way that the foreign body, while in place, prevents hemorrhage. Instead, impaled objects should be stabilized to prevent movement, and allowed to remain in place while the patient is transported to the hospital.

**impalpable** (ĭm-păl′pă-b'l) [L. *in-,* not, + *palpare,* to touch] Felt with difficulty, if at all; hardly perceptible to the touch.

**impar** (ĭm′păr) [L., unequal] Azygous.

**imparidigitate** (ĭm-păr″ĭ-dĭj′ĭ-tāt) [″ + *digitus,* finger] Having an uneven number of fingers or toes.

**impatent** (ĭm-pā′tĕnt) [″ + *patere,* to be open] Closed; not patent.

**impedance** (ĭm-pē′dăns) [L. *impedire,* to hinder] Resistance met by alternating currents in passing through a conductor; consists of resistance, reactance, inductance, or capacitance. The resistance due to the inductive and condenser characteristics of a circuit is called reactance.

***acoustic i.*** Resistance to the transmission of sound waves.

**imperative** [L. *imperativus,* commanding] Obligatory; not controlled by the will; involuntary.

**imperception** [L. *in-,* not, + *percipere,* to perceive] The inability to form a mental picture; lack of perception.

**imperforate** (ĭm-pĕr′fō-rāt) [″ + *per,* through, + *forare,* to bore] Without an opening.

**imperforation** Atresia.

**impermeable** [L. *in-,* not, + *permeare,* to pass through] Not allowing passage, as of fluids; impenetrable.

**impervious** [L. *impervius*] Unable to be penetrated.

**impetiginous** (ĭm″pĕ-tĭj′ĭ-nŭs) [L. *impetiginosus*] Relating to or resembling impetigo.

**impetigo** (ĭm-pĕ-tī′gō, -tē′gō) [L.] An inflammatory skin disease marked by isolated pustules, which become crusted and rupture. It occurs principally around the mouth and nostrils and is usually caused by staphylococcal or streptococcal infection, or both. SEE: *Nursing Diagnoses Appendix.*

***bullous i.*** A rare infection, usually occurring in infants, caused by a strain of *Staphylococcus aureus* that produces a toxin that splits the epidermis. SEE: illus.

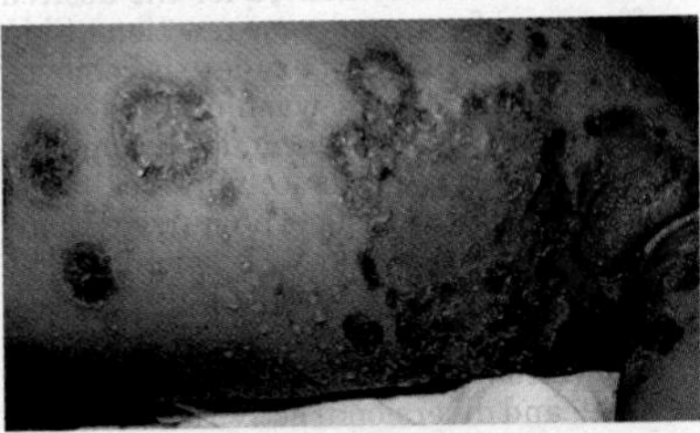

BULLOUS IMPETIGO

***i. contagiosa*** A contagious form of impetigo, to which children are esp. susceptible, caused by streptococci or staphylococci.

SYMPTOMS: Discrete, thin-walled vesicles and bullae, which become pustular and thin-crusted, appear in crops. They may be flat and umbilicated with no tendency to rupture, and they are filled with a straw-colored fluid. They dry up as thin yellow crusts. SEE: illus.

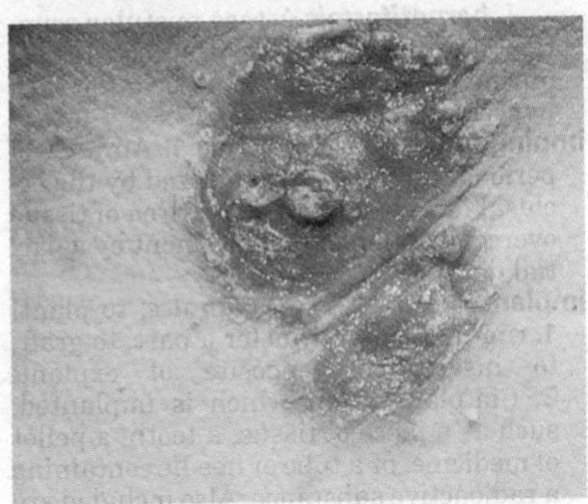

IMPETIGO CONTAGIOSA IN AXILLA

TREATMENT: An appropriate systemic antibiotic should be given. Either cephalexin or a $\beta$-lactamase–resistant penicillin is the drug of choice. Crusts can be removed by applying room-temperature aqueous soaks.

NURSING IMPLICATIONS: Care is provided in an isolation setting, or the patient or parent is taught to care for the condition at home. Appearance, location, and distribution of lesions are inspected and documented, along with any associated symptoms (pruritus, pain) and associated regional lymphadenopathy, as well as risk factors for developing the disease, such as anemia, malnutrition, and impaired skin integrity. Vesicle fluid is obtained for Gram's stain to confirm the infection and for culture and sensitivity to determine the most appropriate treatment, but prescribed treatment is begun without waiting for the culture results. Prescribed systemic antibiotics are administered and evaluated for the desired effects and for any adverse reactions. Skin is kept clean and dry; exudate is removed 2 to 3 times daily by washing the lesions with soap and water and by applying warm saline soaks or compresses to remove stubborn crusts. The nurse encourages the patient to avoid scratching. The fingernails should be cut and, if necessary, mittens applied to prevent further injury from scratching. Comfort is provided, and diversional activities appropriate to the patient's developmental stage are encouraged to distract the patient from local discomforts. The patient and parents are taught about care of the lesions; the importance of not sharing washcloths, towels, or bed linens; the need for thorough hand washing, and the importance of early diagnosis and treatment of any purulent eruption to limit spread to others. The school nurse or the employer are notified of the infection, and family members are checked for evidence of impetigo. The patient can return to school or work when all lesions have healed.

***i. herpetiformis*** A rare pustular eruption of unknown etiology that occurs esp. during pregnancy and in association with hypocalcemia.

**impingement** (ĭm-pĭnj′mĕnt) **1.** An area of periodontal tissue traumatized by the occlusal force of a tooth. **2.** An area of tissue overcompaction or displacement by a partial denture.

**implant** [L. *in-*, into, + *plantare,* to plant] **1.** (ĭm-plănt′) To transfer a part, to graft, to insert; the opposite of explant. **2.** (ĭm′plănt) That which is implanted, such as a piece of tissue, a tooth, a pellet of medicine, or a tube or needle containing a radioactive substance. Also included are liquid and solid plastic materials used to augment tissues or to fill in areas traumatically or surgically removed. Artificial joints are another example of an implant. SEE: *mammaplasty, augmentation.*

***bone i.*** The use of implanted materials to repair bone or to cover implanted objects such as artificial hips or tooth implants.

***brain i.*** Transplantation of tissue into the brain to treat a disease. Implantation of tissue from the adrenal gland into the caudate nucleus (of the nondominant side of the brain) has been done experimentally to treat Parkinson's disease.

***dental i.*** In dentistry, a prosthetic device in any of several shapes. It is implanted into oral tissues beneath the mucosa or the periosteal layer, or within the bone to support or hold a fixed or removable prosthesis. SEE: illus.

***interstitial i.*** The insertion of an applicator containing a radioactive source directly into a tumor to deliver a high radiation dose while sparing the surrounding tissues.

***intracavitary i.*** The insertion of an applicator containing a radioactive source directly into a hollow organ to deliver a high radiation dose to the organ while sparing the surrounding tissues.

***radioactive i.*** SEE: *brachytherapy; interstitial i.; intracavitary i.*

***tooth i.*** The placement of artificial teeth directly into the jawbone or into a frame attached to the jawbone. In some cases, an implant is used to stabilize a loose tooth. This is done by placing an implant through the natural tooth into the jaw. Subperiosteal implants rest on the jawbone, and the gingival tissue grows over the framework; and artificial teeth are attached to the framework. SEE: *implantation; reimplantation.*

**implantation** (ĭm″plăn-tā′shŭn) [″ + *plantare,* to plant] **1.** The grafting of tissue or the insertion of an organ such as tooth, skin, or tendon into a new location in the body. **2.** Embedding of the developing blastocyst in the uterine mucosa 6 or 7 days after fertilization.

***hypodermic i.*** The introduction of an implant under the skin; usually a solid substance placed by forcing a small amount out of a hypodermic needle.

***teratic i.*** The union of an abnormal fetus with a nearly normal fetus.

**implosion** A violent collapse inward.

***i. flooding*** A method of treating fear due to a phobia by exposing the person to the worst possible phobic situation. The fear is experienced at maximum intensity for up to an hour until the patient is no longer capable of experiencing further fear. The phobic situation is imagined in the first sessions and later produced in reality. SEE: *phobic desensitization.*

**imponderable** [L. *in-*, not, + *pondus,* weight] Incapable of being weighed or measured.

**impostors, medical** Persons who practice medicine without a license and who have not graduated from an accredited medical school.

**impotence, impotency** [″ + *potentia,* power] A weakness, esp. pert. to the inability of a man to achieve or maintain an erection. An adult's age has no specific etiological influence on sexual potency. The etiology of impotence with respect to attributing

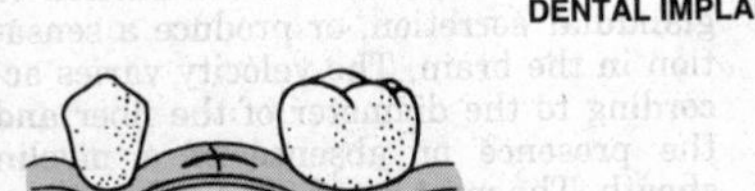


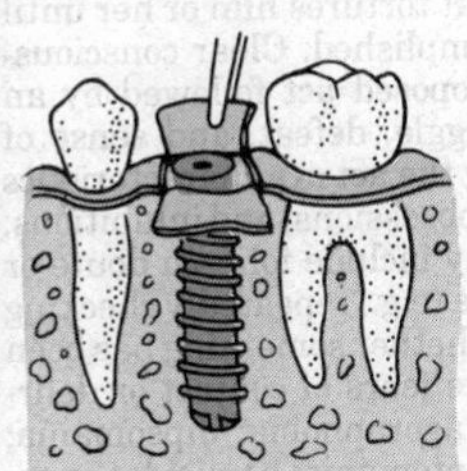


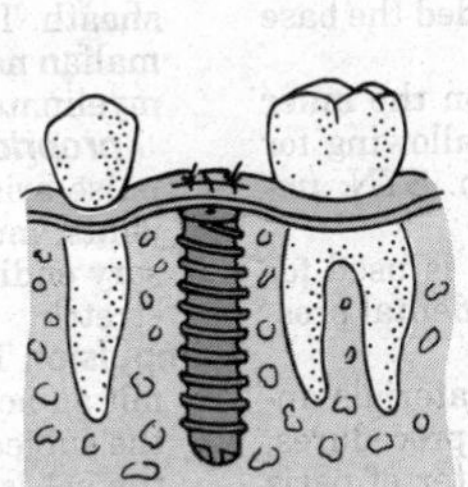


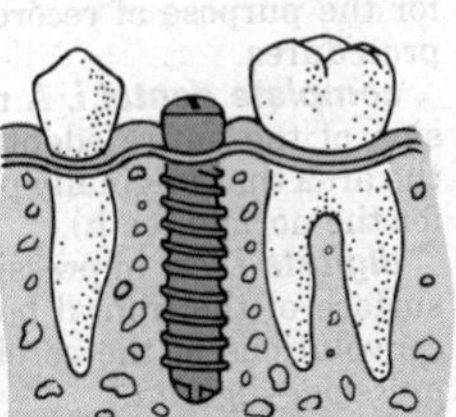


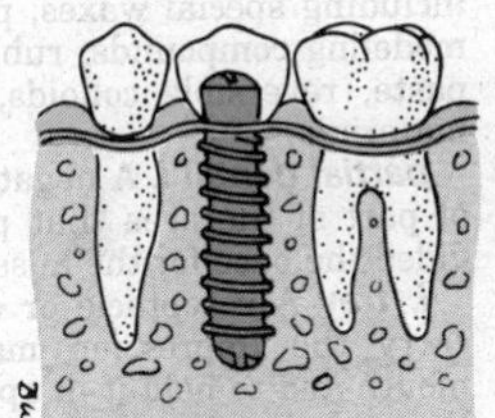


the cause to physical conditions or psychiatric disorders may be tested in men by measuring nocturnal penile tumescence (NPT). This involves monitoring frequency and intensity of erections that normally accompany rapid eye movement sleep. There is no appreciable decline in those with psychogenic impotence. SYN: *impotentia*. SEE: *penile prosthesis; sex therapy; sexual dysfunction; sexual stimulant.*

TREATMENT: For treatable conditions, specific therapy is needed. Particularly useful in patients with vascular insufficiency and neurological impairment, and possibly in those with psychogenic impotence, is intracavernosal injection of vasoactive drugs such as papaverine, phentolamine, or prostaglandin E. The patient may inject these drugs. Self-injection is not appropriate in patients with poor manual dexterity, poor visual acuity, or morbid obesity.

***anatomical i.*** Impotence caused by a genital defect.

***atonic i.*** Impotence resulting from paralysis of nerves supplying the penis.

***functional i.*** Impotence not due to an organic or anatomical defect; usually of psychogenic origin. The individual may experience impotence with one or more sexual partners, but not with others.

***neurogenic i.*** Impotence due to central nervous system lesions, paraplegia, or diabetic neuropathy.

***pharmacological i.*** Impotence due to the side effects of certain drugs and medications (e.g., alcohol, cytotoxic agents, barbiturates, beta blockers, marijuana, cimetidine, clonidine, guanethidine, immunosuppressives, lithium, opiates, phenothiazine, some antihypertensive agents, some diuretics, antidepressants, and anticholinergics).

***psychic i.*** Psychogenic i.

***psychogenic i.*** Impotence caused by emotional factors rather than organic disease. Before making this diagnosis, it is important to know what medicines the patient is taking that could cause impotence. SYN: *psychic i.* SEE: *male erectile disorder.*

***vasculogenic i.*** Impotence due to an inadequate supply of arterial blood to the corpora cavernosa of the penis.

**impotent** (ĭm′pō-tĕnt) **1.** Unable to copulate. **2.** Sterile; barren.

**impotentia** (ĭm″pō-tĕn′shē-ă) [L.] Impotence.

**impregnate** (ĭm-prĕg′nāt) [L. *impregnare,* to make pregnant] **1.** To render pregnant; to fertilize an ovum. **2.** To saturate.

**impregnated 1.** Rendered pregnant. **2.** Saturated.

**impregnation** (ĭm″prĕg-nā′shŭn) [L. *impregnare,* to make pregnant] **1.** Fertilization of an ovum. SYN: *fecundation.* **2.** Saturation.

***artificial i.*** Artificial insemination.

**impression** [L. *impressio*] **1.** A hollow or depression in a surface. **2.** An effect produced upon the mind by external stimuli. **3.** The imprint of all or part of the dental arch, individual teeth, or cavity preparations, using appropriate dental materials, for the purpose of records or restorative procedures.

***complete dental i.*** A negative impression of the entire edentulous area (e.g., the area that originally provided the base for the normal teeth).

***digitate i.*** An impression on the inner surface of the frontal bone, allowing for convolutions of the cerebrum. SYN: *impressione digitata.*

***final i.*** An impression that is used for making the master cast for a dental prosthesis.

***i. materials*** A variety of materials appropriate for different dental procedures, including special waxes, plaster of paris modeling compounds, rubber, zinc oxide paste, reversible colloids, and alginate materials.

***partial dental i.*** A negative impression of part of the area that previously provided the base for the missing teeth.

***i. tray*** A receptacle or device used to carry the impression material to the mouth and to hold it in apposition to the tissues being recorded.

**impressione digitata** Digitate impression.

**imprinting** A special type of learned response that occurs in some animals at a critical period in their development. For example, goslings mothered by a hen may adopt the hen as if she were their mother.

**impulse** (ĭm′pŭls) [L. *impulsus*] **1.** The act of driving onward with sudden force. SEE: *conation.* **2.** An incitement of the mind, prompting an unpremeditated act (e.g., impulse buying). **3.** In physiology, a change transmitted through certain tissues, esp. nerve fibers and muscles, resulting in physiological activity or inhibition.

***cardiac i.*** **1.** The heartbeat felt at the left side of the chest over the apex of the heart; this is a physical impulse. **2.** The electrical impulse transmitted over the conducting pathway of the heart that is responsible for the contraction of the muscular tissue of the heart. SEE: *heart.*

***ectopic i.*** A cardiac impulse arising in some part of the heart other than the sinoatrial node.

***enteroceptive i.*** An afferent nerve impulse arising from stimuli originating in receptors located in internal organs.

***excitatory i.*** An impulse that stimulates activity.

***exteroceptive i.*** An afferent nerve impulse arising from stimuli originating in sense organs located on the body surface.

***inhibitory i.*** An impulse that lessens activity.

***nerve i.*** A self-propagated electrical change transmitted along the membrane of a nerve fiber. At the end of the axon of the nerve fiber, the electrical impulse stimulates the release of a neurotransmitter, which may stimulate or inhibit another electrical impulse in another nerve fiber, cause muscle contraction or glandular secretion, or produce a sensation in the brain. The velocity varies according to the diameter of the fiber and the presence or absence of a myelin sheath. The most rapid conducting mammalian neurons (50 to 80 m/sec) are large, myelinated neurons.

***proprioceptive i.*** An afferent nerve impulse arising from stimuli originating in joints, muscles, or tendons, or other sensory endings that respond to pressure or stretch.

**impulsion** The idea to do something or commit an act or crime, suddenly imposed on the subject, that tortures him or her until the act is accomplished. Clear consciousness of the proposed act followed by an agonizing struggle, defeat, and sense of relief following the act are characteristics of impulsions, obsessions, and inhibitions. Impulsions may include folie du doute or doubting mania (e.g., repeatedly checking to determine whether something has been done); obsessive fears of contact or delirium of touch; agoraphobia; dipsomania; pyromania; kleptomania; homicidal or suicidal impulsion; onomatomania; arithmomania; exhibitionism.

**IMV** *intermittent mandatory ventilation; intermittent mechanical ventilation.*

**In** Symbol for the element indium.

**in- 1.** [L. *in,* into] Prefix indicating *in, inside, within;* and also *intensive action.* **2.** [L. *in-,* not] Prefix indicating *negative.*

**inaction** (ĭn-ăk′shŭn) [L. *in-,* not, + *actio,* act] Failure of or decreased response to a stimulus.

**inactivate** [″ + *activus,* acting] To render inactive, esp. the alteration or destruction of an enzyme system or a biologically active agent such as a microorganism or antigen.

**inactivation** Rendering anything inert by using heat or other means.

***i. of complement*** Loss of activity caused by heating serum to about 55°C (131°F) for ½ hour.

**inanimate** [″ + *animatus,* alive] **1.** Not alive; not animate. **2.** Dull, lifeless.

**inanition** (ĭn″ă-nĭsh′ŭn) [L. *inanis,* empty] A debilitated condition caused by a lack of sufficient food material essential to the body, such as in starvation or malabsorption syndrome. This condition may also be due to causes other than the food supply, such as malabsorption, or to other diseases of the gastrointestinal system that prevent absorption of food.

**inappetence** (ĭn-ăp′ĕ-tĕns) [″ + *appetere,* to long for] A lack of craving or desire, esp. for food.

**Inapsine** Trade name for droperidol.

**inarticulate** [″ + *articulus,* joined] **1.** Not jointed; without joints. **2.** Unable to pronounce distinct syllables or express oneself intelligibly. **3.** Not given to expressing oneself verbally.

**in articulo mortis** (ĭn ăr-tĭk′ū-lō mor′tĭs) [L.]

At the very moment of death.

**inassimilable** (ĭn″ă-sĭm′ĭ-lă-b′l) [″ + *assimilis,* to make similar] Not capable of being used by the body for nutrition.

**inattention, unilateral** Unilateral visual inattention.

**inattention, unilateral visual** Lack of attention or unresponsiveness to stimuli presented on the side opposite a damaged brain hemisphere. This condition occurs in patients with injury to one hemisphere. It is one in a larger category of visual-spatial deficits following brain injury. SYN: *altitudinal neglect; hemi-inattention; hemispatial neglect; visual inattention; unilateral inattention; unilateral spatial agnosia.*

**inattention, visual** Unilateral visual inattention.

**inborn** Innate or inherent, said of characteristics both structural and functional that are inherited or developed during intrauterine development.

**inbreeding** [″ + AS. *bredan,* to cherish] Mating of closely related individuals.

**incandescent** [L. *incandescere,* to glow] Glowing with light; white hot.

**incapacitate** Being made incapable of some function, act or strength. This may be purely physical or intellectual or both.

**incaparina** A mixture of cereal grains and oilseed meals of a given range of protein and quality fortified with vitamins and minerals. It was developed at the Institute of Nutrition of Central America and Panama (INCAP) and distributed in Latin American countries for feeding young children to prevent kwashiorkor and other forms of malnutrition.

**incarcerated** [L. *incarcerare*] Imprisoned, confined, constricted, as an irreducible hernia.

**incarceration** **1.** Legal confinement. **2.** The imprisonment of a part; constriction, as in a hernia.

**incasement** Becoming surrounded by a structure or wall.

**inception** [L. *inceptio,* taking in, beginning] **1.** The beginning of anything. **2.** Ingestion. **3.** Intussusception.

**incest** (ĭn′sĕst) [L. *incestus,* unchaste, incest] Coitus between close blood relatives.

**incidence** [L. *incidens,* falling upon] **1.** The frequency of occurrence of any event or condition over a period of time and in relation to the population in which it occurs, as incidence of a disease. SEE: *prevalence.* **2.** The falling or impinging upon, touching, or affecting in some way.

**incident** **1.** A happening, event, or occurrence. **2.** Falling or striking, as a ray of light.

**incineration** (ĭn-sĭn″ĕr-ā′shŭn) [L. *in,* into, + *cineres,* ashes] Destruction by fire; cremation.

**incipient** (ĭn-sĭp′ē-ĕnt) [L. *incipere,* to begin] Beginning; coming into existence.

**incisal** (ĭn-sī′zăl) Relating to or involving cutting.

**incise** (ĭn-sīz′) [L. *incisus*] To cut, as with a sharp instrument.

**incised** (ĭn-sīzd′) Cut cleanly, as with a knife.

**incision** (ĭn-sĭzh′ŭn) [L. *incisio*] A cut made with a knife, esp. for surgical purposes.

**incisive** (ĭn-sī′sĭv) [L. *incisivus*] **1.** Cutting; having the power of cutting. **2.** Relating to the incisor teeth.

**incisive bone** An obsolete term for the part of the maxilla that supports the incisor teeth and was derived from the median nasal process embryologically; commonly called the premaxilla.

**incisor** (ĭn-sī′zor) [L., a cutter] **1.** That which cuts. **2.** That which applies to the incisor teeth. **3.** One of the cutting teeth; the four front teeth in each jaw of the adult. SEE: *dentition.*

***central i.*** One of two upper and lower incisors adjacent to the midsagittal plane.

**incisura** (ĭn-sī-sū′ră) *pl.* **incisurae** [L.] **1.** An incision. **2.** Incisure; notch; emargination; indentation at the edge of any structure.

***i. angularis gastrica*** A fold or notch on the distal end of the lesser curvature of the stomach.

**incisure** (ĭn-sīz′ūr) [L. *incisura,* a cutting into] A notch or slit.

***i. of Rivinus*** Tympanic incisure.

***i. of Schmidt-Lanterman*** One of several oblique lines on medullated nerve fiber sheaths.

**incitant** (ĭn-sīt′ănt) [L. *incitarē,* to set in motion] The stimulus that sets off a reaction, disease, or incident.

**inclination** [L. *inclinere,* to slope] Leaning from the normal or from the vertical, as a tooth or the pelvis.

**inclinometer** (ĭn″klĭ-nŏm′ĕ-ter) [″ + Gr. *metron,* measure] A device for measuring ocular diameter from vertical and horizontal lines.

**inclusion** [L. *inclusus,* enclosed] Being enclosed or included.

***i. blennorrhea*** Inclusion conjunctivitis of the newborn.

***i. body*** One of several bodies present in the nucleus or cytoplasm of certain cells in cases of infection by certain viruses. SEE: *Negri body.*

***cell i.*** The lifeless, temporary constituent of the protoplasm of a cell. SEE: *cell.*

***i. conjunctivitis*** Inflammation of the conjunctiva of the eye due to the organism *Chlamydia trachomatis.* SEE: *ophthalmia neonatorum.*

***dental i.*** A tooth unable to erupt because of excessive surrounding tissue. SEE: *impacted tooth.*

***fetal i.*** Malformed twins in which one, the parasite, is completely enclosed within the other, its host or autosite. SEE: *teratoma.*

**incoagulability** (ĭn″kō-ăg″ū-lă-bĭl′ĭ-tē) [L. *in-,* not, + *coagulare,* to congeal] Not coagulable.

**incoherence** (ĭn″kō-hĕr′ĕns) [″ + *cohairens,* adhering] An inability to express oneself coherently or to present ideas in a related order.

**incoherent** (ĭn″kō-hē′rĕnt) Not coherent or understandable.

**incombustible** [″ + *combustus,* burned] Incapable of being burned.

**incompatibility** [L. *incompatibilis*] **1.** The quality of not being suitable for mixture. It can be applied to a state that renders admixture of medicines unsuitable through chemical action or interaction, insolubility, formation of poisonous or explosive compounds, difference in solubility, or antagonistic action. **2.** The quality of not being mixed without chemical changes, or without countering the action of other ingredients in a compound. **3.** The condition of not being in harmony with one's surroundings or associates, esp. a spouse or friend.

***ABO i.*** An antigen-antibody immune response to alien red blood cells. Transfusion reactions occur most commonly in people with type O blood. People with type A blood carry antigens on their red cells and form anti-B antibodies. Those with type B blood carry B antigens and form anti-A antibodies. The patient's immune system perceives the donor cells as being threatening foreign proteins and produces antibodies to destroy them by agglutination and hemolysis.

*Obstetrics:* Transplacental fetal-maternal transfusion occurs when fetal blood cells escape into the maternal circulation, eliciting antibody formation. Maternal antibodies then cross the placenta into the fetal circulation, attack, and destroy red blood cells, as evidenced by neonatal bilirubinemia and jaundice. The reaction usually is mild and requires no treatment.

***physiological i.*** A condition in which one or more substances in a mixture have a physiological action antagonistic to that of one of the other compounds.

**incompatible** **1.** Not capable of uniting. **2.** Antagonistic in action, said of some drugs. **3.** Not being in harmony with one's environment, situation, or associates, esp. a spouse or friend.

**incompetence, incompetency** [L. *in-*, not, + *competere,* to be suitable] An inadequate ability to perform the function or action normal to an organ or part.

***aortic i.*** Regurgitation of blood through the aortic valve.

***ileocecal i.*** An inability of the ileocecal valve to stop the return of the material from the colon to the ileum.

***mental i.*** The mental inability to retain charge of one's self or possessions.

***muscular i.*** An imperfect closure of one of the atrioventricular valves due to weak action of papillary muscles.

***pyloric i.*** A weakness of the pyloric sphincter, which permits undigested food to leave the stomach and enter the duodenum.

***relative i.*** Excessive dilatation of a cardiac cavity, rendering it impossible for the cardiac valves leading in and out of the chamber to close perfectly.

***valvular i.*** Leaky condition of one or more cardiac valves permitting regurgitation of blood at the time the valves should be completely closed.

**incompetent** **1.** One legally unable to execute a contract, such as a brain-damaged individual or one with marked mental retardation or insanity. **2.** The inability to perform necessary activities and tasks expected of one's life roles.

**incompressible** [″ + *compressus,* pressed together] Compact; not compressible.

**incontinence** [″ + *continere,* to stop] The inability to retain urine, semen, or feces because of loss of sphincter control or cerebral or spinal lesions. SEE: *bladder drill; continence.*

TREATMENT: The specific therapy needed for urinary incontinence depends on the cause. Symptomatic management of urinary incontinence is facilitated by use of one of several different types of leakproof underpants, absorbent panty liners, highly absorbent perineal pads, or collection devices.

***active i.*** A discharge of feces and urine in the normal way at regulated intervals but involuntarily.

***fecal i.*** Failure of the anal sphincter to prevent involuntary expulsion of gas, liquid, or solids from the lower bowel. This type of incontinence is a common and often debilitating condition in elderly patients. SEE: *encopresis.*

***functional i.*** The state in which an otherwise continent individual experiences an involuntary, unpredictable passage of urine. A number of medications, including various diuretics, narcotics, sedatives, and anticholenergics may cause this condition, as may stroke or severe arthritis. SEE: *Nursing Diagnoses Appendix.*

***giggle i.*** The occurrence of involuntary uncontrollable passage of urine induced by laughter. Laughter triggers full-scale micturition that cannot be stopped, often until the bladder is empty, even if the laughter stops. It starts at about age five to seven years and tends to improve or disappear with increasing age. This condition, which may be due to a central nervous system disease, is distinct from stress urinary incontinence. SEE: *stress urinary i.*

***intermittent i.*** Loss of control of the bladder upon sudden pressure or movement, because of interruption of the voluntary path above the lumbar center.

***i. of milk*** Galactorrhea.

***overflow i.*** Incontinence characterized by small frequent voidings due to overfilling of the bladder or to a bladder with pathologically decreased volume.

***paralytic i.*** The constant voiding of

small amounts of urine and feces owing to defective nervous control of sphincters.

***passive i.*** A form of urinary incontinence; instead of emptying normally, the full bladder allows urine to drip away upon pressure.

***reflex i.*** The state in which an individual experiences an involuntary loss of urine, occurring at somewhat predictable intervals when a specific bladder volume is reached. SEE: *Nursing Diagnoses Appendix.*

***stress urinary i.*** ABBR: SUI. An inability to prevent escape of small amounts of urine during stress such as laughing, coughing, sneezing, lifting, or sudden movement. SEE: *Nursing Diagnoses Appendix.*

DIAGNOSIS: Direct observation of urine loss while coughing is a reliable method of establishing this diagnosis. The urine should be cultured to rule out urinary tract infection. This phenomenon should be investigated to be certain that it is not caused by a structural abnormality.

TREATMENT: In addition to using devices to absorb urine that escapes, therapy consists of behavioral modification, pharmacological treatment, and surgical management. Behavioral therapy includes bladder training, timed voiding, prompted voiding, and pelvic muscle exercises. Pharmacotherapy includes oxybutyrin hydrochloride, propartheline bromide, and imipramine hydrochloride. Surgery may restore anatomic support of the urethra or compensate for a poorly functioning urethral sphincter. SEE: *bladder drill; Kegel exercise.*

NURSING IMPLICATIONS: The patient is taught Kegel exercises to strengthen pubococcygeal muscles and encouraged to practice the exercises at frequent intervals throughout the day, as well as during urination (by stopping and starting the urinary stream intermittently). The vulvae and introitus should be kept clean and dry and odor-free, and commercial barrier products should be used to protect clothing. To avoid isolation, the patient should continue or resume usual activities while using protective barriers. The nurse periodically evaluates the patient's response to the exercise regimen.

***total i.*** The state in which an individual experiences a continuous and unpredictable loss of urine. SEE: *Nursing Diagnoses Appendix.*

***urge i.*** The state in which an individual experiences involuntary passage of urine occurring soon after a strong sense of urgency to void. This does not refer to a similar sensation due to an excessively full bladder. SEE: *Nursing Diagnoses Appendix.*

***i. of urine*** Intermittent or complete absence of ability to control loss of urine from the bladder.

TREATMENT: Therapy will depend upon the cause. Information on this subject may be obtained from Health for Incontinent People at (800) 251-3337. SEE: *Kegel exercise; urinary stress i.*

**incoordinate** [L. *in-*, not, + *coordinare,* to arrange] **1.** Not able to make coordinated muscular movements. **2.** Unable to adjust one's work harmoniously with others.

**incoordination** (ĭn″kō-or″dĭ-nā′shŭn) An inability to produce harmonious, rhythmic, muscular action that is not due to weakness. The condition may be sensory, owing to failure of afferent impulses to be transmitted from muscles, bones, and joints to coordination centers; or it may be motor, owing to disturbance in tone or harmony between simultaneously acting muscle groups. SYN: *asynergy*. SEE: *disdiadochokinesia.*

**incorporation** [L. *in,* into, + *corporare,* to form into a body] Combining two ingredients to form a homogenous mass.

**increment** (ĭn′krĕ-mĕnt) [L. *incrementum*] **1.** An increase or addition in number, size, or extent; an enlargement. **2.** Something added or gained. **3.** The beginning portion of a uterine contraction between baseline and acme. Increasing strength of contraction is shown by the upslope record recorded by the fetal monitor.

**incrustation** [L. *in,* on, + *crusta,* crust] The formation of crusts or scabs.

**incubation** (ĭn″kū-bā′shŭn) [L. *incubare,* to lie on] **1.** The interval between exposure to infection and the appearance of the first symptom. SYN: *latent period* (2). SEE: table. **2.** In bacteriology, the period of culture development. **3.** The development of an impregnated ovum. **4.** The care of a premature infant in an incubator.

**incubator 1.** An enclosed crib, in which the temperature and humidity may be regulated, for care of premature babies. **2.** An apparatus for providing suitable atmospheric conditions for culturing bacteria or for maintaining eggs until they hatch.

**incubus** (ĭn′kū-bŭs) [L. *incubare,* to lie upon] A nightmare.

**incudal** (ĭng′kū-dăl)[L. *incus,* anvil] Relating to the incus.

**incudectomy** (ĭng″kū-dĕk′tō-mē) [″ + Gr. *ektome,* excision] The surgical removal of all or part of the incus of the middle ear.

**incudiform** (ĭn-kū′dĭ-form) [″ + *forma,* shape] Anvil-shaped.

**incudomalleal** (ĭng″kū-dō-măl′ē-ăl) [″ + *malleus,* a hammer] Pert. to the incus and malleus their articulation in the tympanum; in the middle ear.

**incudostapedial** (ĭn″kū-dō-stă-pē′dē-ăl) [″ + *stapes,* a stirrup] Pert. to the incus and stapes and their articulation in the tympanum; in the middle ear.

**incurable** [L. *in-*, not, + *curare,* to care for] Not capable of being cured.

**incurvation** (ĭn″kŭr-vā′shŭn) [L. *incurvare,* to bend in] State of being bent or curved in.

**incus** (ĭng′kŭs) *pl.* **incudes** [L., anvil] In the

**Incubation and Isolation Periods in Common Infections***

| Infection | Incubation Period | Isolation of Patient† |
|---|---|---|
| AIDS | Unclear; antibodies appear within 1–3 months of infection; T cell counts probably drop in 1–3 years. Symptoms appear in 5–12 years. Median incubation in infants is shorter than in adults. | Protective isolation if T cell count is very low; enteric precautions with severe diarrhea; private room only necessary with severe diarrhea, bleeding, copious blood tinged sputum if patient has poor personal hygiene habits |
| Bloodstream (bacteremia fungemia) | Variable; usually 2–5 days | Contact: private room; gloves and masks; gowns as needed for dealing with drainage or body fluids |
| Brucellosis | Highly variable, usually 5–21 days; may be months | None |
| Chickenpox | 2–3 weeks | 1 week after vesicles appear or until vesicles become dry |
| Cholera | A few hours to 5 days | Enteric precautions |
| Common cold | 12 hr–5 days | None |
| Diphtheria | Usually 2–5 days | Until two cultures from nose and throat, taken at least 24 hr apart, are negative; cultures to be taken after cessation of antibiotic therapy |
| Dysentery, amebic | From a few days to several months, commonly 2–4 weeks | None |
| Dysentery, bacillary (shigellosis) | 12–96 hr | As long as stools remain positive |
| Encephalitis, mosquito-borne | 5–15 days | None |
| Giardiasis | 3–25 days or longer; median 7–10 days | Enteric precautions |
| Gonorrhea | 2–7 days; may be longer | No sexual contact until cured |
| Hepatitis A | 15–50 days | Enteric (gloves with infected material; gowns as needed to protect clothing) |
| Hepatitis B | 45–180 days | Blood and body fluid precautions (gloves and plastic gowns for contact with infective materials; mask if risk of coughing or sneezing exists) |
| Hepatitis C | 14–180 days | As for hepatitis B |
| Hepatitis D | 2–8 weeks | As for hepatitis B |
| Hepatitis E | 15–64 days | Enteric precautions |
| Influenza | 1–3 days | As practical |
| Legionella | 2–10 days | None |
| Lyme disease | 3–32 days after tick bite | None |

*Table continued on following page*

**Incubation and Isolation Periods in Common Infections*** (Continued)

| Infection | Incubation Period | Isolation of Patient† |
|---|---|---|
| Malaria | 12 days for *Plasmodium falciparum;* 8–14 days for *P. vivax, P. ovale;* 7–30 days for *P. malariae* | Protection from mosquitoes |
| Measles (rubeola) | 8–13 days from exposure to onset of fever; 14 days until rash appears | From diagnosis to 7 days after appearance of rash; strict isolation from children under 3 years |
| Meningitis, meningococcal | 2–10 days | Until 24 hr after start of chemotherapy |
| Mononucleosis, infectious | 4–6 weeks | None; disinfection of articles soiled with nose and throat discharges |
| Mumps | 12–25 days | Until the glands recede |
| Paratyphoid fevers | 3 days–3 months; usually 1–3 weeks; 1–10 days for gastroenteritis | Until 3 stools are negative |
| Plague | 2–8 days | Strict; danger of airborne spread (pneumoniae plague) |
| Pneumonia, pneumococcal | Believed to be 1–3 days | Enteric precautions in hospital. Respiratory isolation may be required. |
| Poliomyelitis | 3–35 days | 1 week from onset |
| Puerperal fever, streptococcal | 1–3 days | Transfer from maternity ward |
| Rabies | Usually 2–8 weeks; rarely as short as 9 days or as long as 7 years | Strict for duration of illness; danger to attendants |
| Rubella (German measles) | 16–18 days with range of 14–23 days | None; no contact with nonimmune pregnant women |
| Salmonellosis | 6–72 hr, usually 12–36 hr | Until stool cultures are salmonella free on two consecutive specimens collected in 24-hr period |
| Scabies | 2–6 weeks before onset of itching in patients without previous infections; 1–4 days after re-exposed | Patient is excused from school or work until day after treatment |
| Scarlet fever | 1–3 days | 7 days; may be ended in 24 hr |
| Syphilis | 10 days–10 weeks; usually 3 weeks | None; but for hospitalized patients, universal precautions for body secretions |
| Tetanus | 4 days–3 weeks | None |
| Toxic shock syndrome | Unknown but may be as brief as several hours | None |
| Trachoma | 5–12 days | Until lesions disappear, but usually not practical |
| Tuberculosis | 4–12 weeks to demonstrable primary lesion or significant tuberculin reactions | Variable, depending on conversion of sputum to negative after specific therapy and on ability of patient to understand and carry out personal hygiene methods |

*Table continued on following page*

**Incubation and Isolation Periods in Common Infections*** (Continued)

| Infection | Incubation Period | Isolation of Patient† |
|---|---|---|
| Tularemia | 2–14 days | None |
| Typhoid fever | Usually 1–3 weeks | Until 3 cultures of feces and urine are negative. These should be taken not earlier than 1 month after onset. |
| Typhus fever | 7–14 days | None |
| Whooping cough | Usually 6–20 days | Respiratory isolation for known cases; for suspected cases, removal from contact with infants and young children |

* SEE: *Universal Precautions Appendix.*
† Universal precautions and handwashing are assumed.

middle ear, the middle of the three ossicles in the tympanum; the anvil. SEE: *ear* for illus.

***lenticular process of i.*** The long process of the incus, a middle ear ossicle. It articulates with the head of the stapes. SYN: *orbiculare.*

**incyclophoria** (ĭn-sī″klō-for′ē-ă) [L. *in-*, not, + Gr. *kyklos,* circle, + *phoros,* bearing] Median or negative cyclophoria in which the affected eye, when covered, turns inward about its anteroposterior axis.

**incyclotropia** (ĭn-sī″klō-trō′pē-ă) [″ + ″ + *tropos,* turning] Cyclotropia in which the eye turns inward toward the nose even when both eyes are open.

**in d** L. *in dies,* daily.

**indentation** [L. *in,* in, + *dens,* tooth] A depression or hollow.

**independent living** The term used by many disabled persons and professionals that emphasizes the rehabilitation goals of active community involvement and assuming responsibility for directing one's own life.

**independent living skills** Activities of daily living.

**independent practice associations** ABBR: IPA. A method of arranging for medical care wherein the individual has a contract with office-based practitioners who agree to see patients on a prenegotiated fee schedule.

**index** (ĭn′dĕks) *pl.* **indexes, indices** [L., an indicator] **1.** The forefinger. **2.** The ratio of the measurement of a given substance with that of a fixed standard.

***alveolar i.*** Gnathic i.

***cardiac i.*** The cardiac output of blood expressed (as liters per minute) divided by the body surface area (expressed in square meters).

***i. case*** The initial individual whose condition led to investigation of a hereditary disorder. SEE: *cohort.*

***cephalic i.*** Skull breadth multiplied by 100 and divided by the length of the skull.

***cerebral i.*** The ratio of greatest transverse to the greatest anteroposterior diameter of the cranium.

***chemotherapeutic i.*** The ratio of the toxicity of a drug, expressed as maximum tolerated dose per kilogram of body weight to the minimal curative dose per kilogram of body weight. This index is used in judging the safety and effectiveness of drugs used in treating parasitic diseases.

***DMF i.*** The index of dental health and caries experience based on the number of DMF teeth or tooth surfaces. D indicates the number of decayed teeth, M the missing teeth, and F the filled or restored teeth.

***glycemic i.*** An index used to quantitate the speed and degree of change in blood sugar that results from ingesting foods of the same weight and carbohydrate, fat, and protein content as compared with an equivalent amount of glucose. Tests to determine the index for individual foods may not be valid when that food is ingested as part of a normal mixed-content meal.

***gnathic i.*** A measure of the degree of projection of the upper jaw by finding the ratio of the distance from the nasion to the basion to that of the basion to the alveolar point multiplying by 100. SYN: *alveolar i.*

***leukopenic i.*** In allergic individuals, a test of sensitivity to foods. A precipitous decrease in the white blood cell count within 90 minutes after ingestion of the test food indicates that the food is incompatible with that individual.

***opsonic i.*** A ratio of the number of bacteria that are ingested by leukocytes contained in the serum of a normal individual, compared with the number ingested by leukocytes in the patient's own blood serum.

***oral hygiene i.*** ABBR: OHI. A popular indicator developed in 1960 to determine oral hygiene status in epidemiological studies. The index consists of an oral debris score and a calculus score. Six indicator teeth are examined for soft deposits and calculus. Numerical values are assigned to the six indicator teeth according to the extraneous deposits present. The scores are added and divided by the number of surfaces examined to calculate the average oral hygiene score.

***pelvic i.*** The ratio of pelvic conjugate and transverse diameters.

***periodontal (Ramfjord) i.*** An extensive consideration of the periodontal status of six teeth by evaluating gingival condition, depth of gingival sulcus or pocket, plaque or calculus, attrition, tooth mobility, and extent of tooth contact.

***phagocytic i.*** The average number of bacteria ingested by each leukocyte after incubation of the bacteria in a mixture of serum and bacterial culture.

***refractive i.*** SEE: under *refraction*.

***respiratory i.*** The ratio of the alveolar-arterial oxygen tension to the arterial partial pressure of oxygen.

***sulcus bleeding i.*** ABBR: SBI. A sensitive measure of gingival condition that involves probing of all sulci. The score is based on six defined criteria. It is calculated by counting the number of sulci with bleeding, dividing by the total number of sulci, and multiplying by 100.

***therapeutic i.*** The maximum tolerated dose of a drug divided by the minimum curative dose.

***thoracic i.*** The ratio of the thoracic anteroposterior diameter to the transverse diameter.

***vital i.*** The ratio of the number of births to the number of deaths in a population over a stated period of time.

***Index Medicus*** A publication of the National Library of Medicine that lists biomedical and health sciences journal articles by title, subject, field, and country of publication. More than 2000 journals and periodicals are indexed.

**indican** (ĭn′dĭ-kăn) **1.** Potassium salt of indoxylsulfate, found in sweat and urine, and formed when intestinal bacteria convert tryptophan to indole. **2.** In plants, a yellow glycoside, the precursor of the dye indigo.

**indicanemia** (ĭn″dĭ-kăn-ē′mē-ă) [*indican* + Gr. *haima,* blood] Indican in the blood.

**indicant** (ĭn′dĭ-kănt) **1.** Something such as a sign or symptom that points to the presence of a disease. **2.** Something such as loss of a symptom or sign that indicates that the treatment of the disease is proper and effective.

**indicanuria** (ĭn″dĭ-kăn-ū′rē-ă) [″ + Gr. *ouron,* urine] An excess of indoxylsulfate of potassium, a derivative of indole, in urine. It is found in small quantities in normal urine. SEE: *urocyanosis*.

**indication** [L. *indicare,* to show] A sign or circumstance that indicates the proper treatment of a disease.

***causal i.*** An indication provided by the knowledge of the cause of a disease.

***symptomatic i.*** An indication provided by the symptoms of a disease rather than because of precise knowledge of the actual disease process (e.g., a patient may be given aspirin or antibiotics without knowing the cause of the symptoms of headache or fever).

**indicator** [L. *indicare,* to show] In chemical analysis, a substance that can be used to determine pH. In a more general sense, any substance that can be used to determine the completeness of a chemical reaction, as in volumetric analysis. Its uses include (1) in the titration of ammonia and other weak bases; (2) in Topfer's reagent, for determining free acid in gastric juice; and (3) in the titration of weak acids and determination of combined acid in gastric juice. SEE: table.

**indifferent** [L. *in-,* not, + *differre,* to differ] **1.** Neutral; tending in no specific direction. **2.** Not responsive to normal stimuli; apathetic. **3.** Pert. to cells that have not differentiated.

**indigenous** (ĭn-dĭj′ĕn-ŭs) [L. *indigenus,* born in] Native to a country or region.

**indigestible** (ĭn″dĭ-jĕs′tĭ-bl) [L. *in-,* not, + *digerere,* to separate] Not digestible.

**indigestion** [″ + *digerere,* to separate] Incomplete or imperfect digestion, usually accompanied by one or more of the following symptoms: pain, nausea and vomiting, heartburn, acid regurgitation, accumulation of gas, and belching. SYN: *dyspepsia*.

**indigitation** (ĭn-dĭj″ĭ-tā′shŭn) [L. *in,* in, +

## Colors of Indicators of pH

| | Color | | |
|---|---|---|---|
| | **Toward Acid** | **Toward Alkali** | **Range of pH** |
| Methyl yellow | Red | Yellow | 2.9–4.0 |
| Congo red | Blue | Red | 3.0–5.2 |
| Methyl orange | Red | Yellow | 3.1–4.4 |
| Methyl red | Red | Yellow | 4.2–6.2 |
| Litmus | Red | Blue | 4.5–8.3 |
| Bromcresol purple | Yellow | Purple | 5.2–6.8 |
| Bromothymol blue | Yellow | Blue | 6.0–7.6 |
| Phenol red | Yellow | Red | 6.8–8.4 |
| Phenolphthalein | Colorless | Pink | 8.2–10.0 |

*digitus,* finger] Intussusception.

**indigo** A blue dye obtained from plants or made synthetically.

**Indigo Carmine** Trade name for indigotindisulfonate.

**indigotindisulfonate sodium** (ĭn″dĭ-gō″tĭn-dī-sŭl′fō-nāt) A dye used in testing renal function. Trade name is Indigo Carmine.

**indisposition** [L. *in-*, not, + *dispositus,* arranged] A mild disorder; any slight or temporary illness.

**indium** (ĭn′dē-ŭm) [L. *indicum,* indigo] SYMB: In. A rare metallic element; atomic weight 114.82; atomic number 49; specific gravity 7.31.

**indium-111 ($^{111}$In)** An isotope of indium with a half-life of 2.8 days; used in radioactive tracer studies.

**individuation** (ĭn″dĭ-vĭd″ū-ā′shŭn) **1.** During development, the emergence of specific and individual structures and functions. **2.** The process by which a healthy, integrated personality is developed.

**indocyanine green** A dye used in testing hepatic and renal function. Trade name is Cardio-Green.

**indolaceturia** (ĭn″dō-lăs″ē-tū′rē-ă) [*indole* + L. *acetum,* vinegar, + Gr. *ouron,* urine] The excretion of an increased amount of indoleacetic acid in the urine. This occurs in patients with phenylketonuria and may also be increased by eating serotonin-containing foods (e.g., bananas).

**indole** (ĭn′dōl) $C_8H_7N$. A substance found in feces. It is the product of bacterial decomposition of tryptophan and is partially responsible for the odor of feces. In intestinal obstruction it is absorbed and eliminated in the urine in the form of indican.

**indolent** (ĭn′dō-lĕnt) [LL. *indolens,* painless] **1.** Indisposed to action. **2.** Inactive; not developing; sluggish.

**indologenous** (ĭn″dō-lŏj′ĕn-ŭs) [*indole* + Gr. *gennan,* to produce] Causing the production of indole.

**indoluria** (ĭn″dōl-ū′rē-ă) [″ + Gr. *ouron,* urine] The presence of indole in the urine.

**indomethacin** (ĭn″dō-mĕth′ă-sĭn) An anti-inflammatory, analgesic, and antipyretic drug. Its primary use is in rheumatoid arthritis, ankylosing spondylitis, and degenerative joint disease when salicylates are ineffective or cannot be tolerated. Because of the high incidence and severity of side effects associated with prolonged administration, its use as a mild antipyretic or analgesic is not recommended. It has been used in treating attacks of arthritis due to gout. Indomethacin is also useful in stimulating the closure of patent ductus arteriosus in premature infants who are otherwise healthy. It inhibits uterine activity and has been used to prevent premature labor.

**indoxyl** (ĭn-dŏk′sĭl) [Gr. *indikon,* indigo, + *oxys,* sharp] $C_8H_7NO$. An oily substance sometimes found in the urine of apparently healthy individuals, formed from the decomposition of tryptophan by intestinal bacteria.

**indoxylemia** (ĭn-dŏk″sĭl-ē′mē-ă) [″ + ″ + *haima,* blood] Indoxyl in the blood.

**indoxyluria** (ĭn″dŏk-sĭl-ū′rē-ă) [″ + ″ + *ouron,* urine] The excretion of indoxyl in the urine.

**induced** (ĭn-dūsd′) [L. *inducere,* to lead in] Produced; caused.

**inducer** (ĭn-dūs′ĕr) In chemistry, a compound that increases the concentration of another molecule; in molecular biology, something that facilitates the development of a gene. SEE: *catalyst.*

**inductance** That property of an electric circuit by virtue of which a varying current induces an electromotive force in that circuit or a neighboring circuit. The unit of inductance, or self-induction, is the henry.

**induction** (ĭn-dŭk′shŭn) [L. *inductio,* leading in] **1.** The process of causing or producing, as induction of labor with oxytocic drugs in cases of uterine dysfunction. **2.** The generation of an electric current in a conductor by electricity in another conductor near it. **3.** In embryology, the production of a specific morphogenic effect by a chemical substance from one part of the embryo to another. SYN: *evocation.* **4.** In anesthesia, the period from the initial inhalation or injection of an anesthetic gas or drug until optimum level of anesthesia is reached.

**inductor** (ĭn-dŭk′tĕr) **1.** Any substance that causes cells exposed to it to differentiate into an organized tissue. **2.** In electronics, a component that employs the principles of electromagnetic induction. It is used in filter circuits and transformers.

**inductothermy** Treatment of disease by artificial production of fever by electromagnetic induction.

**indulin** (ĭn′dū-lĭn) Any one of a group of dyes used in histology.

**indulinophil(e)** (ĭn″dū-lĭn′ō-fĭl, -fīl) The state of being readily stained with indulin.

**indurate** (ĭn′dū-rāt) [L. *in,* in, + *durus,* hard] **1.** To harden. **2.** Hardened.

**indurated** Hardened.

**induration** (ĭn′dū-rā″shun) **1.** The act of hardening. **2.** An area of hardened tissue. SEE: *sclerosis; skin.* **indurative** (-dūr-ā″tĭv), *adj.*

***black i.*** Anthracosis of the lung.

***brown i.*** Pigmentation and fibrosis of the lung as a result of chronic venous congestion of the lung.

***cyanotic i.*** Induration from long continued venous hyperemia, pressure on vessels causing transudation of blood and serum, and formation of a dark, hard mass. In the liver or spleen it leads to absorption of the parenchyma with formation of scar tissue.

***granular i.*** Fibrosis of an organ such as the liver or kidney in which small fibrotic granules are present.

***gray i.*** Pneumonia with fibrosis of the lung and no pigmentation.

***red i.*** Chronic interstitial pneumonia with severe congestion.

**indusium** (ĭn-dū′zē-ŭm) [L., tunic] A membranous covering.

***i. griseum*** A rudimentary gyrus located on the upper surface of the corpus callosum. SYN: *supracallosal gyrus.*

**indwelling** Inside the body; said of invasive diagnostic or therapeutic devices; pert. to a catheter, drainage tube, or other device that remains inside the body for a prolonged time.

**inebriant** (ĭn-ē′brē-ănt) [L. *inebrius,* drunken] **1.** Any intoxicant. **2.** Making drunk.

**inebriate** To make drunk or to become intoxicated.

**inebriation** (ĭn-ē″brē-ā′shŭn) Intoxication.

**inelastic** [L. *in-,* not, + Gr. *elastikos,* elastic] Not elastic.

**inert** (ĭn-ĕrt′) [L. *iners,* unskilled, idle] **1.** Not active; sluggish. **2.** In chemistry, having little or no tendency or ability to react with other chemicals.

**inertia** (ĭn-ĕr′shē-ă) [L., inactivity] **1.** In physics, the tendency of a body to remain in its state (at rest or in motion) until acted upon by an outside force. **2.** Sluggishness; a lack of activity.

***uterine i.*** An absence or weakness of uterine contractions in labor.

**in extremis** (ĭn ĕks-trē′mĭs) [L.] At the point of death.

**infancy** The very early period of life in which the child is still unable to walk or to feed itself. SEE: *infant.*

**infant** [L. *infans*] A liveborn fetus from time of birth through the completion of one year of age. SEE: *neonate.*

*Development:* For three days after birth a baby loses weight; in the next four days, however, a baby should regain the loss and weigh as much as at birth.

The average weekly weight gain in the first three months is 210 g for boys and 195 g for girls; from three to six months it is 150 g for both girls and boys; from six to nine months, 90 g for boys and 105 g for girls; from 9 to 18 months 60 g for both sexes; and from 18 to 24 months 45 g, both sexes.

The newborn is aware of shadow, movement, and voice. By the fourth week the infant lifts the head momentarily; by the 16th week, holds the head erect, coos, or laughs; walks with hands held by the 52nd week; and by the 15th month, toddles alone and may have a vocabulary of a few words. SEE: *psychomotor and physical development of infant.*

*Respiration:* At birth, respirations are 40 to 50/min; during the first year, 20 to 40/min; during the fifth year, 20 to 25/min; during the 15th year, 15 to 20/min. SEE: *pulse; respiration; temperature.*

*Temperature:* Normal (rectal) temperature may have a daily variation of 1° to 1.5°C (1.8° to 2.7°F). It is usually highest between 5 and 8 P.M. and lowest between 3 and 6 A.M. There is therefore no specific normal temperature, but the values given should be regarded as ranging around the value of 37.6°C (99.7°F) when the temperature is taken rectally. Infants have poorly developed temperature-regulating mechanisms, and need to be protected from chilling and overheating.

***post-term i.*** An infant born after the beginning of the 42nd week of gestation (longer than 288 days).

***premature i.*** Preterm i. SEE: *Nursing Diagnoses Appendix.*

***preterm i.*** An infant born before the completion of 37 weeks (259 days) of gestation. SEE: *prematurity.*

***i. stimulation*** The use of various techniques to provide multisystems input to neonates and infants identified with or at risk for developmental delay. The purpose is to create an environment that provides the stimulation necessary for normal development.

***term i.*** An infant born between the beginning of the 38th week through the 41st week of gestation (260 to 287 days).

**infant feeding pattern, ineffective** A state in which an infant demonstrates an impaired ability to suck or to coordinate the suck-swallow response. SEE: *Nursing Diagnoses Appendix.*

**infanticide** (ĭn-făn′tĭ-sīd) [LL. *infanticidium*] The killing of an infant.

**infantile** (ĭn′făn-tīl) [Fr. *infantilis*] Pert. to infancy or an infant.

**infantilism** (in-făn′tĭl-ĭzm, ĭn′făn-tĭl-ĭzm″) [″ + Gr. *-ismos,* condition] **1.** A condition in which the mind and body make slow development and the individual fails to attain adult characteristics. It is characterized by mental retardation, stunted growth, and sexual immaturity. **2.** Childishness.

***angioplastic i.*** Infantilism due to defective development of the vascular system.

***Brissaud's i.*** Cretinism.

***cachectic i.*** Infantilism caused by chronic infection or poisoning.

***celiac i.*** Infantilism caused by intestinal malabsorption due to intolerance to gluten in the diet.

***dysthyroidal i.*** Infantilism caused by a defective thyroid.

***hepatic i.*** Infantilism combined with cirrhosis of the liver.

***hypophyseal i.*** Hypophyseal dwarfism. SYN: *pituitary i.*

***intestinal i.*** Infantilism associated with a chronic intestinal disorder, causing poor growth.

***myxedematous i.*** Cretinism.

***pituitary i.*** Hypophyseal dwarfism.

***renal i.*** Infantilism caused by a defect in renal function.

***sex i.*** The continuation of childish traits, esp. sex characteristics, beyond the age of puberty.

***symptomatic i.*** Infantilism caused by poor tissue development.

***universal i.*** Infantilism marked by dwarfed stature and an absence of secondary sexual characteristics.

**infarct** [L. *infarctus*] An area of tissue in an organ or part that undergoes necrosis following cessation of the blood supply. This may result from occlusion or stenosis of the supplying artery or, more rarely, from occlusion of the vein that drains the tissue.

***anemic i.*** An infarct in which blood pigment is lacking or decoloration has occurred. SYN: *pale i.; white i.*

***bland i.*** An infarct in which infection is absent.

***calcareous i.*** An infarct in connective tissue in which calcareous salts have been deposited.

***cicatrized i.*** An infarct that has been replaced or encapsulated by fibrous tissue.

***hemorrhagic i.*** Red i.

***infected i.*** Infarcted tissue that has been invaded by pathogenic organisms. SYN: *septic i.*

***pale i.*** Anemic i.

***red i.*** An infarct that is swollen and red as a result of hemorrhage. SYN: *hemorrhagic i.*

***septic i.*** Infected i.

***uric acid i.*** An infarct in the kidney caused by obstruction of the renal tubules by uric acid crystals.

***white i.*** Anemic i.

**infarction 1.** The formation of an infarct. **2.** An infarct.

***cardiac i.*** Myocardial i.

***cerebral i.*** An infarction in the brain due to failure of blood supply to the area.

***evolution of i.*** The normal healing process after myocardial infarction; seen on ECG as progressive changes in the S-T segment.

***extension of i.*** An increase in the size of a myocardial infarction, occurring after the initial infarction and usually accompanied by a return of acute symptoms, such as angina unrelieved by appropriate medicines.

***myocardial i.*** An infarction in the cardiac muscle, usually resulting from formation of a thrombus in the coronary arterial system.

The immediate therapeutic need involves assuring the patient that comprehensive care will be given and at the same time instituting whatever needs to be done to put the patient at rest and to arrange for immediate transport to a hospital, doctor's office, or any place where appropriate therapy may be provided. Sublingual nitroglycerin is indicated. Intramuscular morphine may be required for pain. Because the majority of deaths occur in the first several hours following infarction, it is essential that treatment not be delayed. SEE: *tissue plasminogen inactivator.*

***placental i.*** A localized necrotic area caused by abruption. SEE: *abruptio placentae.*

***pulmonary i.*** An infarction in the lung usually resulting from pulmonary embolism. Immediate therapy includes control of pain, oxygen administered continuously by mask, intravenous heparin (unless patient has a known blood clotting defect), and treatment of circulatory collapse (shock) if present.

***silent myocardial i.*** An actual infarction of the myocardium, but with none of the signs or symptoms of this condition.

**infect** [ME. *infecten*] To cause pathogenic organisms to be present in or upon, as to infect a wound.

**infection** (ĭn-fĕk′shŭn) The presence and growth of a microorganism that produces tissue damage. The extent of infection depends on the number and virulence of the organisms and the ability of the body to contain or destroy them. Infection is usually accompanied by inflammation, but inflammation may occur without infection. SEE: table.

Infectious diseases are the leading cause of death in the world. Important weapons in a country's defense against infections are its disease surveillance system and an effective laboratory system for validating the presence of a disease. In the U.S., the Centers for Disease Control and Prevention provide these services.

SYMPTOMS: The signs and symptoms of localized infection are those of inflammation. The five classic symptoms listed by early medical writers are dolor (pain), calor (heat), rubor (redness), tumor (swelling), and functio laesa (disordered function). Vasodilation produces redness and warmth in surface infections as blood is brought to the area from the body's interior. Edema is due to increased vascular permeability as plasma containing white blood cells (WBCs) moves into the tissues to neutralize or kill the organism. The pressure of the edema on nerve endings and the release of kinins from the WBCs causes pain; edema also causes dysfunction when it interferes with movement of an extremity, slows blood flow, or inhibits normal cell function. Pus forms in an infection if the organism is pyogenic. Fever, another common sign, is due to the effect of interleukin-1 and tumor necrosis factors on the hypothalamus.

ETIOLOGY: The most common pathogenic organisms are bacteria, mycobacteria, viruses, fungi, protozoa, chlamydiae, mycoplasmas, spirochetes, rickettsiae, and helminths. Persons without adequate WBCs, those who are malnourished, the very young or very old, those receiving immunosuppressive therapy, and those with severe trauma or burns are at increased risk for infection.

TRANSMISSION: To spread from one person to another, the organism must

## Fungal Infections

| Disease | Causative Organisms | Structures Infected | Microscopic Appearances |
|---|---|---|---|
| ***Superficial Fungal Infections*** | | | |
| Epidermophytosis (dhobie itch, etc.) | *Epidermophyton* (*floccosum*, etc.) | Inflamed patches in inguinal, axillary, and interdigital folds; hairs not affected | Long, wavy, branched and segmented hyphae and spindle-shaped cells in stratum corneum |
| Favus (tinea favosa) | *Trichophyton schönleini* | Yellow disks in epidermis around a hair; all parts of body; nails | Vertical hyphae and spores in epidermis; sinuous branching mycelium and chains in hairs |
| Ringworm (tinea, otomycosis) | *Microsporum* (*audouinii*, etc.) | Horny layer of epidermis and hairs, chiefly of scalp | Fine septate mycelium inside hairs and scales; spores in rows and mosaic plaques on hair surface |
| | *Tricophyton* (*tonsurans*, etc.) | Hairs of scalp, beard, and other parts; nails | Mycelium of chained cubical elements and threads in and on hairs; often pigmented |
| Thrush and other forms of candidiasis | *Candida albicans* | White patches on tongue, mouth, throat; lesions of vagina and skin | Yeastlike budding cells and oval thick-walled bodies in lesion |
| ***Systemic Fungal Infections*** | | | |
| Aspergillosis | *Aspergillus fumigatus* | Lungs | Y-shaped branching of septate hyphae |
| Blastomycosis | *Blastomyces brasiliensis, B. dermatitidis* | Skin and lungs | Yeastlike cells demonstrated in lesion |
| Candidiasis | *Candida albicans* | Esophagus, lungs, peritoneum, mucous membranes | Small thin-walled ovoid cells |
| Coccidiodomycosis | *Coccidioides immitis* | Respiratory tract | Nonbudding spores containing many endospores, in sputum |
| Cryptococcosis | *Cryptococcus neoformans* | Meninges, lungs, bone, skin | Yeastlike fungus having gelatinous capsule; demonstrated in spinal fluid |
| Histoplasmosis | *Histoplasma capsulatum* | Lungs | Oval, budding, uninucleated cells |
| Nocardiosis | *Nocardia asteroides* | Lungs, brain, subcutaneous tissues | Closely resemble bacteria; found in pus |

leave the body of one infected person and invade that of the other; respiratory secretions, mucosal secretions, and feces are the most common routes. The pathogen enters the body by (1) inhalation of airborne organisms; (2) ingestion into the gastrointestinal tract from contaminated food, water, or utensils; and (3) by direct contact with a normally protected part of the body (by contamination of instruments during invasive procedures, exposure of underlying tissues through burns or trauma, via contaminated blood, or through an insect bite). Within hospitals, organisms are readily carried among patients (cross infection) by health care providers if handwashing protocols are not followed.

The body's defenses against infection begin with mechanisms that block entry of the organism into the skin or the respiratory, gastrointestinal, or genitourinary tract. These defenses include (1) chemicals (e.g., lysozymes in tears, fatty acids in skin, gastric acid, and pancreatic enzymes in the bowel), (2) mucus that traps the organism, (3) clusters of antibody-producing B lymphocytes (e.g., tonsils, Peyer's patches), and (4) bacteria and fungi (normal flora) on skin and mucosal surfaces that destroy more dangerous organisms. In patients receiving immunosuppressive drug therapy, the normal flora can become the source of opportunistic infections. Also, one organism can impair external defenses and permit another to enter; for example, viruses can enhance bacterial invasion by damaging respiratory tract mucosa.

The body's second line of defense is the nonspecific immune response, inflammation. The third major defensive system, the specific immune response, depends on lymphocyte activation, during which B and T cells recognize specific antigenic markers on the organism. B cells produce immunoglobulins (antibodies) and T cells orchestrate a multifaceted attack by cytotoxic cells. SEE: *cell, B; cell, T; inflammation.*

SPREAD: Once organisms have gained entry into internal tissues, they have many different ways of spreading. Warm, moist areas such as mucosa promote growth, allowing organisms to spread quickly along the peritoneum, meninges, and pleura. Some organisms produce enzymes that damage cell walls, enabling them to move rapidly from cell to cell. Others enter the lymphatic channels; if they can overcome WBC defenses in the lymph nodes, they move into the bloodstream to multiply at other sites. This phenomenon is frequently seen with pyogenic organisms, which create abscesses far from the initial entry site. Viruses or rickettsiae, which live only inside cells, use red or white blood cells to travel through the blood; many viruses that damage a fetus during pregnancy (e.g., rubella and cytomegalovirus) travel via the blood.

TREATMENT: A sample of infected tissue, blood, urine, stool, or sputum is placed in a culture medium so that the organism can grow and be identified in the laboratory. Different anti-infective drugs are placed on the growth to determine which is most effective in killing the organism. This procedure is known as a culture and sensitivity test. Many organisms have shown the ability to develop mechanisms that block the action of anti-infective drugs, requiring continued development of new agents.

***acute i.*** An infection that appears suddenly and may be of brief or prolonged duration.

***air-borne i.*** An infection caused by inhalation of pathogenic organisms in the air.

***apical i.*** An infection located at the tip of the root of a tooth.

***blood-borne i.*** An infection transmitted through contact with the blood of an infected individual, such as hepatitis or AIDS. This contact may also be through a medical or dental procedure in which a blood-contaminated instrument is inadvertently used after inadequate sterilization. SEE: *needle-stick injuries; Universal Precautions Appendix.*

***chronic i.*** An infection having a protracted course.

***concurrent i.*** The existence of two or more infections at the same time. SEE: *superinfection.*

***contagious i.*** Infectious disease easily transmitted by casual cutaneous contact or respiratory droplets. Usually refers to those that are easily transmitted and commonly seen, such as influenza or chickenpox.

***cross i.*** The transfer of an infectious organism or disease from one patient in a hospital to another.

***cryptogenic i.*** The invasion of bacteria without outward evidence of entry into the body. SEE: *infection.*

***droplet i.*** An infection acquired by the inhalation of a microorganism in the air, esp. one added to the air by someone's breath or cough.

***local i.*** An infection that has not spread but remains contained near the entry site.

***low-grade i.*** A loosely used term for a subacute or chronic infection with only mild inflammation and without pus formation.

***nosocomial i.*** An infection that is acquired during hospitalization.

***opportunistic i.*** **1.** Any infection that results from a defective immune system that cannot defend against pathogens normally found in the environment. Common types include bacterial (*Clostridium difficile*), fungal (*Candida albicans*), and protozoan (*Pneumocystis carinii*). Opportunistic infections are seen in patients receiving large doses of steroids or other immunosuppressive drugs, or in patients with acquired immunodeficiency syndrome (AIDS). **2.** An infection that results when resident flora proliferate and infect a body site in which they are normally present or at some other location. In healthy humans, the millions of bacteria in and on the body do not cause infection or disease. Host defenses and interaction with other microorganisms prevent excess growth of potential pathogens. A great number of factors, many poorly understood, may alter this healthy state and allow a normal bacterial resident to proliferate and cause disease. SEE: *AIDS; immunocompromised.*

***protozoal i.*** An infection with a protozoon (e.g., malaria).

***pyogenic i.*** An infection resulting from pus-forming organisms.

***risk for i.*** The state in which an individual is at increased risk for being invaded by pathogenic organisms. SEE: *Nursing Diagnoses Appendix.*

***secondary i.*** An infection made possible by a primary infection that lowers the host's resistance (e.g., bacterial pneumonia following influenza).

***subacute i.*** An infection intermediate between acute and chronic.

***subclinical i.*** An infection that is immunologically confirmed but does not show clinical symptoms in the individual.

***systemic i.*** An infection in which the infecting agent or organisms are throughout the body rather than restricted to a local area as in an abscess.

**infectious** (ĭn-fĕk′shŭs) [ME. *infecten,* infect] **1.** Capable of being transmitted with or without contact. **2.** Pert. to a disease caused by a microorganism. **3.** Producing infection.

**infecundity** (ĭn-fē-kŭn′dĭ-tē) [L. *infecunditas,* sterility] Barrenness; an inability to conceive.

**inferior** (ĭn-fē′rē-or) [L. *inferus,* below] **1.** Beneath; lower. **2.** Used medically in reference to the undersurface of an organ or indicating a structure below another structure.

**inferiority complex** SEE: under *complex.*

**infertility** The inability or diminished ability to produce offspring. Reproductive assessment is warranted when a couple fails to achieve pregnancy during 1 yr of unprotected intercourse, or when a woman repeatedly fails to carry a pregnancy to fetal viability. The condition may be present in either or both partners and may be reversible. Diagnostic investigation includes special tests of both partners as well as a complete physical examination. Some factors responsible for infertility are immature or abnormal reproductive systems, anomalies of other organs in that vicinity, infections, endocrine dysfunction, and emotional problems. Fertility also may be affected by a great number of therapeutic drugs, substances of abuse, certain pesticides, and use of tobacco products. SEE: *embryo transfer; fertilization in vitro; gamete intrafallopian transfer; tuboplasty, transcervical balloon.*

***secondary i.*** Infertility in which one or more pregnancies have occurred before the present condition of infertility.

**infest** [L. *infestare,* to attack] To overrun to a harmful extent; said esp. of parasites.

**infestation** The harboring of animal parasites, esp. macroscopic forms such as worm endoparasites and arthropod ectoparasites.

**infibulation** (ĭn-fĭb-ū-lā′shŭn) [L. *in,* in, + *fibula,* clasp] The process of fastening, as in joining the lips of wounds by clasps. Also, suturing together of the labia of women to prevent sexual intercourse.

**infiltrate** (ĭn-fĭl′trāt, ĭn′fĭl-trāt) [″ + *filtrare,* to strain through] **1.** To pass into or through a substance or a space. **2.** The material that has infiltrated.

**infiltration** (ĭn″fĭl-trā′shŭn) The process of a substance passing into and being deposited within the substance of a cell, tissue, or organ. Examples of infiltration include that of a tissue or organ by blood corpuscles and that of a cell by fatty particles. Infiltration must not be confused with degeneration; in the latter condition the foreign substances are from changes within the cell.

***amyloid i.*** The infiltration of tissue or viscera with a glycoprotein.

***anesthesia i.*** The injection of an anesthetic solution directly into the tissue. SEE: *anesthesia.*

***calcareous i.*** Deposits of calcium or magnesium salts within a tissue.

***cellular i.*** An infiltration of cells, esp. blood cells, into tissues; invasion by cells of malignant tumors into adjacent tissue.

***fatty i.*** A deposit of fat in the tissues, or oil or fat globules in the cells.

***glycogenic i.*** Glycogen deposit in cells.

***lymphocytic i.*** An infiltration of tissue by lymphocytes.

***pigmentary i.*** An infiltration of pigments.

***purulent i.*** Pus cells in a tissue.

***serous i.*** An infiltration with lymph.

***urinous i.*** An infiltration with urine.

***waxy i.*** Amyloid degeneration.

**infinite distance** **1.** A distance without limits. **2.** In ophthalmology, the assumption that the light rays coming from a point of a distance beyond 20 ft (6.1 m) are practically parallel and accommodation is unnecessary.

**infirm** [L. *infirmis*] Weak or feeble, esp. from old age or disease.

**infirmary** [L. *infirmarium*] A small hospital; a place for the care of sick or infirm persons.

**infirmity** **1.** Weakness. **2.** A sickness or illness.

**inflammation** [L. *inflammare,* to flame

## Mediating Factors in Inflammation

| Factors | Source | Effect |
|---|---|---|
| Arachidonic acid metabolites (prostaglandins and leukotrienes) | Phospholipids of cell membranes, especially mast cells | Primary mediators of late-stage (> 6 hrs) inflammation; increase dilation and permeability of blood vessels; stimulate neutrophil adhesion to endothelial tissue; bronchoconstriction; anaphylaxis |
| Bradykinin | Kinin system of plasma proteins | Primary mediator of prolonged (> 1 hr) inflammation; vasodilation and increased permeability of blood vessels; pain; release of leukotrienes and prostaglandins |
| Complement proteins | Macrophages; liver endothelium | Increase vasodilation and vascular permeability; coat antigens to enhance phagocytosis; attract neutrophils; destroy pathogens |
| Histamine and serotonin | Mast cells Basophils | Primary mediators of early (≤ 30 min) inflammation; rapid dilation and increase in permeability of venules; bronchoconstriction; stimulation of prostaglandin production |
| Interleukin 1 (IL-1) | Macrophages; B cells, dendritic cells, neutrophils, other nucleated cells | Increases production and activity of other chemical mediators, phagocytes and lymphocytes; promotes release of acute phase proteins; causes fever |
| Interleukin 8 (IL-8) | T lymphocytes; monocytes | Attracts neutrophils and more T cells |
| Platelet-activating factor (PAF) | Platelets | Releases chemical mediators; activates neutrophils; dilates and increases permeability of vessels |
| Transforming growth factor $\beta$ (TFG$\beta$) | Activated macrophages and T lymphocytes | Attracts neutrophils and monocytes; stimulates growth of connective tissue; inhibits other mediators |
| Tumor necrosis factors (TFN$\alpha$) | Activated macrophages and some lymphocytes | Increase synthesis of other cytokines; induce formation of new blood vessels; increase adhesion of neutrophils to endothelium; cause fever and cachexia |

within] The nonspecific immune response that occurs in reaction to any type of bodily injury. It is a stereotyped response that is identical whether the injurious agent is a pathogenic organism, foreign body, ischemia, physical trauma, ionizing radiation, electrical energy, or extremes of temperature. Inflammation is a conservative process modified by whatever produces the reaction, but it should not be confused with infection; the two are relatively different conditions, although one may arise from the other. The reactions produced during inflammation and repair may be harmful (e.g., hypersensitivity reactions, the processes that lead to rheumatoid arthritis, and excess scar formation). SEE: table; *autoimmune disease; infection.* **inflammatory,** *adj.*

SYMPTOMS: The cardinal signs of inflammation include rubor (redness), calor (heat), tumor (swelling), and dolor (pain). In addition, fever commonly occurs with extensive inflammation.

*Process:* The first step in inflammation is local vasodilation that increases blood flow (causing redness and heat), followed by increased vascular permeability that enables plasma to move out of the capillaries and into the tissues, producing local edema and pain secondary to pressure on nerve endings. Neutrophils, and later monocytes, move out of the bloodstream and into the injured tissues. Chemical mediators are released by the leukocytes and tissues to continue the inflammatory response. The arrival of additional neutrophils and macrophages (chemotaxis) is also stimulated by the release of mediators. Following destruction of the organism or control of the damage, tissue repair can begin. If the inflammatory response is inadequate to deal with the invading organisms, the specific immune response is required.

Chemical mediators in inflammation include histamine, kinins, complement, and arachidonic acid metabolites. These promote continued vasodilation, capillary permeability, and the emigration of neutrophils. Interleukin-1 (IL-1) is released by macrophages during inflammation, which stimulates the activity of other white blood cells and produces fever. Interferons may be released by the leukocytes if the invading organism is a virus.

Inflammation is implied in the name of any disease ending with "itis" (e.g., appendicitis, bronchitis, cholecystitis), as well as other pathologic disorders (e.g., adult respiratory distress syndrome, which occurs as the result of massive neutrophil aggregation, and emphysema, which occurs following chronic inflammation of the alveoli). However, most inflammation occurs as a normal part of the immune response, not as a pathologic response. It is only when inflammation occurs inappropriately, as in autoimmune disorders, or when it is prolonged or overwhelming that it is considered pathologic.

***acute i.*** Inflammation of rapid onset and rapid resolution. The majority of the response is usually over within 12 hours.

***chronic i.*** Inflammation that is usually less intense and of prolonged duration. It may be characterized by chronically elevated white blood cell count, low-grade fever, and pain.

***exudative i.*** An inflammatory process in which the fluid leaving the capillaries is rich in plasma proteins.

***fibrinous i.*** Inflammation in which the exudate is rich in fibrin.

***granulomatous i.*** An inflammation characterized by granulomas; seen esp. in tuberculosis, syphilis, and some fungal infections.

***hyperplastic i.*** Inflammation characterized by excess production of young fibrous tissue. SYN: *proliferative i.*

***interstitial i.*** Inflammation involving principally the noncellular or supporting elements of an organ.

***proliferative i.*** Hyperplastic i.

***pseudomembranous i.*** Inflammation in which a pseudomembrane is formed. It is due to a toxin that necrotizes the tissues, and is seen in the oral, nasal, and respiratory tract tissues in diphtheria.

***purulent i.*** Inflammation in which pus is formed. SYN: *suppurative i.*

***serous i.*** Inflammation of a part with serous exudate, or inflammation of a serous membrane.

***subacute i.*** Mild inflammatory process with minimal signs and symptoms. It may progress to a chronic process and, over time, do serious damage.

***suppurative i.*** Purulent i.

***ulcerative i.*** The formation of an ulcer over an area of inflammation.

**inflammatory** [L. *inflammare,* to flame within] Pert. to or marked by inflammation.

**inflation** (ĭn-flā′shŭn) [L. *in,* into, + *flare,* to blow] The distention of a part by air, gas, or liquid.

**inflator** (ĭn-flā′tor) A device for forcing air into an organ. This may be done for diagnostic or therapeutic purposes.

**inflection** (ĭn″flĕk′shŭn) [″ + *flectere,* to bend] **1.** An inward bending. **2.** A change of tone or pitch of the voice; a nuance.

**influenza** (ĭn″floo-ĕn′ză) [It., influence] An acute, contagious respiratory infection characterized by the sudden onset of fever, chills, headache, myalgia, and sometimes prostration. Coryza, cough, and sore throat are common. The incubation period is 1 to 3 days. It is usually a self-limited disease that lasts from 2 to 7 days. Differential diagnosis includes typhoid fever, cerebrospinal meningitis, and, rarely, pulmonary tuberculosis. SYN: *flu.* SEE: *cold; Nursing Diagnoses Appendix.* **influenzal** (-zăl), *adj.*

SYMPTOMS: Signs and symptoms begin abruptly with lassitude, malaise, chilliness, severe pain in the head and back, and fever from 101° to 103°F (38.3° to 39.4°C). The prostration is usually out of proportion to the fever. The eyes are injected, and sneezing, hoarseness, and a hard paroxysmal cough develop. Coryza is moderate to severe. Less frequently, gastrointestinal symptoms including anorexia, nausea, vomiting, and diarrhea are present.

ETIOLOGY: The causative agent is a virus of which several types, A, B, and C, and subtypes, such as $H_0N_1$ ($A_0$ human); $H_1N_1$ ($A_1$); $H_2N_2$ ($A_2$); $H_3N_2$ ($A_{HK}$, $A_3$); $H_{SW}N_1$ (swine); $H_{eq}N$ (2 equine); and $N_{av}N$ (8 avian), have been identified. The influenza virus has shown great genetic variation. This ability provides the basis for development of epidemics in populations that have previously been exposed to influenza caused by other subtypes.

EPIDEMIOLOGY: Influenza is usually more prevalent in the winter and spring.

The disease is spread by discharges from the mouth and nose of infected persons. It may occur sporadically, epidemically, or pandemically. Young healthy adults appear to be particularly susceptible. The very young and the very old are most at risk of dying. Even during an epidemic, the number of infected people who remain asymptomatic is higher than those who are symptomatic. The influenza virus is the only organism that still causes acute nationwide epidemics.

COURSE: Influenza ordinarily lasts from 4 to 5 days and may terminate by crisis or speedy lysis. The pulse rate is usually not increased in proportion to the fever; it may be 90 to 100 beats per minute. The blood pressure is low; nosebleed is not uncommon. Examination of the blood demonstrates a leukopenia. Urinalysis generally demonstrates the presence of albumin and casts. Even though fairly rapid recovery is the rule, some patients experience lassitude for weeks or even months after the acute phase disappears.

The principal complications are secondary bacterial infections of the nasal sinuses, middle ear, and lungs.

PREVENTION: Available vaccines reduce the incidence rate if they contain the inactivated virus of the strain causing the disease. The vaccine should be given to the elderly and to persons who have chronic diseases, esp. of the heart or lungs. The vaccine does not produce permanent immunity. Amantadine and rimantadine are effective in preventing influenza A.

TREATMENT: The treatment is symptomatic, with forced fluids, bedrest, antipyretics, analgesics, and nasal decongestants. Antibiotics are not indicated unless a secondary bacterial infection develops. Amantadine or rimantadine, if given early in the course of the disease, is helpful in treating influenza A.

PROGNOSIS: As a rule, the outcome is favorable in the absence of pulmonary complications. In patients with cyanosis, severe nerve disturbances, or bloody expectoration, prognosis is extremely guarded.

Death may occur, but mostly in infants under one year old, in those over 60, or in those with a chronic disease. SEE: *Reye's syndrome*.

NURSING IMPLICATIONS: For the hospitalized patient, the nurse follows respiratory and blood and body fluid precautions. Vital signs and fluid balance are monitored. Respiratory function is assessed for signs and symptoms of developing pneumonia, such as crackles, increased fever, chest pain, dyspnea, and coughing accompanied by purulent or rusty-colored sputum. Prescribed analgesics, antipyretics, and decongestants are administered. Bedrest and increased oral fluid intake are encouraged, and I.V. fluids administered if prescribed. Cool, humidified air is provided, and the humidifier water is changed daily to prevent Pseudomonas superinfections; oxygen therapy is administered if necessary. The nurse assists the patient to return to normal activities gradually. Mouthwash or warm saline gargles are provided to ease throat soreness. The patient is taught proper disposal of tissues and correct and thorough hand-washing techniques to prevent spread of the virus. The patient treated at home is taught about all of the above supportive care measures as well as about signs and symptoms of serious complications to be reported. Influenza immunizations are discussed with patients; high-risk patients and health-care workers should get an annual inoculation in late fall. The composition of each year's vaccine is based on an estimate of the viruses expected to be present, which is based in part on the previous year's virus, and the vaccine is usually about 75% effective. Patients with allergies should be evaluated for chicken, feathers, or egg allergies, because the vaccine is made from chick embryos. An antiviral agent (amantadine) is an effective alternative for persons infected with influenza A virus. The vaccine also is not recommended for pregnant women, unless they have chronic diseases and are highly susceptible to influenza. Possible adverse reactions include discomfort at the inoculation site, fever, malaise, and rarely, Guillain-Barré syndrome.

***Asian i.*** Influenza caused by a variant strain of influenza virus type A.

**infolding** Process of enclosing within a fold; an operation employed in the treatment of stomach ulcer in which the walls on either side of the lesion are sutured together.

**infra-** [L. *infra,* below, underneath] Prefix meaning *below; under; beneath; inferior to; after.*

**infra-axillary** (ĭn″fră-ăks′ĭl-ă-rē) [″ + *axilla,* little axis] Below the axilla.

**infrabulge** (ĭn′fră-bŭlj) The surfaces of the tooth gingival to the height of contour.

**infraclavicular** (ĭn″fră-klă-vĭk′ū-lăr) [″ + *clavicula,* little key] Below the clavicle.

**infracortical** (ĭn″fră-kor′tĭ-kăl) [″ + *cortex,* rind] Beneath the cortex of any organ.

**infracostal** (ĭn″fră-kŏs′tăl) [″ + *costa,* rib] Below the rib.

**infracotyloid** (ĭn″fră-kŏt′ĭ-loyd) [″ + Gr. *kotyloeides,* cup shaped] Beneath the cotyloid cavity of the acetabulum of the hip.

**infraction** (ĭn-frăk′shŭn) [L. *infractus,* to destroy] An incomplete fracture of a bone in which parts do not become displaced.

**infradentale** A craniometric landmark; it is the bony point between the mandibular central incisors. SEE: *cephalometry.*

**infradiaphragmatic** (ĭn″fră-dī″ă-frăg-măt′ĭk) Subdiaphragmatic.

**infraglenoid** (ĭn″fră-glē′noyd) [L. *infra,* below, underneath, + Gr. *glene,* cavity, + *eidos,* form, shape] Subglenoid.

**infraglottic** (ĭn″fră-glŏt′ĭk) [″ + Gr. *glottis,* back of tongue] Below the glottis.

**infrahyoid** (ĭn″fră-hī′oyd) [″ + Gr. *hyoeides,* U-shaped] Below the hyoid bone.

**inframammary** [″ + *mamma,* breast] Below the mammary gland.

**inframandibular** (ĭn″fră-măn-dĭb′ū-lăr) [″ + *mandibula,* lower jawbone] Below the lower jaw (mandible).

**inframarginal** [″ + *margo,* a margin] Below any edge or margin.

**inframaxillary** [″ + *maxilla,* jawbone] Below the upper jaw (maxilla).

**infranuclear** (ĭn″fră-nū′klē-ăr) [″ + *nucleus,* kernel] In the nervous system, peripheral to a nucleus.

**infraocclusion** [″ + *occlusio,* a shutting up] Location of a tooth below the line of occlusion.

**infraorbital** (ĭn-fră-or′bĭ-tăl) [″ + *orbita,* track] Beneath the orbit.

**infrapatellar** (ĭn″fră-pă-tĕl′ăr) [″ + *patella,* a small plate] Below the patella.

**infrapsychic** (ĭn″fră-sī′kĭk) [″ + Gr. *psyche,* mind] Below the level of consciousness; automatic.

**infrapubic** [″ + *pubes,* hair covering pubic area] Below the pubis.

**infrared** Lying outside the red end of the visible spectrum.

**infrascapular** [″ + *scapula,* shoulder blade] Beneath the shoulder blade.

**infrasonic** (ĭn″fră-sŏn′ĭk) [L. *infra,* below, underneath, + *sonus,* sound] Sound wave frequency lower than those normally heard.

***i. recorder*** A device that can be used to determine blood pressure by detecting and recording the subaudible oscillations of the arterial wall under an occluding cuff. The resulting values are comparable to those determined by use of an intra-arterial catheter. SEE: *blood pressure, indirect measurement of; pseudohypertension.*

**infraspinous** [″ + *spina,* thorn] Beneath the scapular spine.

**infrasternal** [″ + Gr. *sternon,* chest] Beneath the sternum.

**infratemporal** (ĭn″fră-tĕm′pō-răl) [″ + *temporalis,* pert. to the temple] Below the temporal fossa of the skull.

**infratonsillar** (ĭn″fră-tŏn′sĭ-lăr) [″ + *tonsilla,* almond] In the pharynx below the tonsils.

**infratrochlear** (ĭn″fră-trŏk′lē-ăr) [″ + *trochlea,* pulley] Beneath the trochlea.

**infraumbilical** (ĭn″fră-ŭm-bĭl′ĭ-kăl) [″ + *umbilicus,* a pit] Below the umbilicus.

**infraversion** (ĭn″fră-vĕr′zhŭn) [″ + *versio,* a turning] A downward deviation of the eye.

**infundibulectomy** (ĭn″fŭn-dĭb″ū-lĕk′tō-mē) [L. *infundibulum,* funnel, + Gr. *ektome,* excision] Surgical excision of the infundibulum of any structure or organ, esp. the heart.

**infundibuliform** (ĭn″fŭn-dĭb′ū-lĭ-form) [″ + *forma,* form] Funnel-shaped.

***i. fascia*** The membranous layer investing the spermatic cord.

**infundibulopelvic** (ĭn″fŭn-dĭb″ū-lō-pĕl′vĭk) [″ + *pelvis,* basin] Concerning the infundibulum and pelvis of an organ, esp. the kidney.

**infundibulum** (ĭn″fŭn-dĭb′ū-lŭm) [L.] **1.** A funnel-shaped passage or structure. **2.** The tube connecting the frontal sinus with the middle nasal meatus. **3.** The stalk of the pituitary gland. **4.** Any renal pelvis division. **5.** The cavity formed by the fallopian fimbriae. **6.** The terminus of a bronchiole. **7.** The terminus at the upper end of the cochlear canal. **8.** The conelike upper anterior angle at the right cardiac ventricle from which the pulmonary artery arises. SYN: *conus arteriosus.*

***ethmoidal i.*** The area in the middle meatus of the nose. The anterior ethmoidal air cells and the frontal nasal duct from the frontal sinus open into this area.

***i. of hypothalamus*** Infundibulum of the hypothalamus. It extends from the stalk of the hypothalamus to the posterior lobe of the hypothalamus.

***i. of the uterine tube*** The funnel-shaped opening at the lateral end of the uterine tube.

**infusible 1.** [L. *in-,* not, + *fusio,* fusion] Not capable of being fused or melted. **2.** [L. *in,* into, + *fundere,* to pour] Capable of being made into an infusion.

**infusion** (ĭn-fū′zhŭn) [L. *infusio*] **1.** Steeping a substance in hot or cold water in order to obtain its active principle. **2.** The product obtained from the process of steeping. **3.** Any liquid substance (other than blood) introduced into the body via a vein for therapeutic purposes.

***bone marrow i.*** A method of obtaining immediate vascular access, esp. in children. Access is obtained by percutaneous insertion of a bone marrow aspiration needle into the marrow cavity of a long bone, usually into the proximal tibia. Once access is gained, substances may be injected into the bone marrow where they are absorbed almost immediately into the general circulation. This avenue of access does not collapse in the presence of shock or peripheral circulatory collapse.

***continuous hepatic artery i.*** ABBR: CHAI. The use of an infusion pump to provide a continuous supply of chemotherapeutic agents to the hepatic artery to control metastases from colorectal cancer. Chemotherapy with CHAI offers a limited benefit to patients. SEE: *infusion pump.*

***continuous i.*** A controlled method of prolonged drug administration that includes the ability to control the delivery rate. This system permits the drug to be available to the body at a prescribed level. It has proved to be more effective than other regimens in the treatment of certain neoplastic diseases, including acute leukemia.

***intravenous i.*** The injection into a vein

of a solution to secure a route for the administration of drugs or for the replacement of fluid lost from bleeding. SEE: illus.

SOLUTIONS: Many liquid preparations are given by intravenous infusion. Those commonly used include isotonic saline, Ringer's lactated, dextrose 5% in water, and potassium chloride 0.2% in 5% dextrose. The quantity depends on the needs of the patient. The solution is usually given continuously at the rate of 1 to 2 or more liters per day. In severe shock, however, rapid infusion of up to 4 L may be necessary.

SITE: Intravenous infusion is usually given in the arm, to the median basilic or median cephalic vein, but veins at various other sites may be used. Preparation is the same as for intravenous injection, except that a needle or cannula is used. The vein must be exposed if a cannula is used. Introduction of solution should be at the rate required to deliver the needed amount of fluid and contained electrolytes, medicines, or nutrients in a prescribed time.

***subcutaneous i.*** The infusion of solutions into the subcutaneous space.

**infusion pump** A pump used to infuse material into an artery or vein, which is beneficial in overcoming arterial resistance or administering thick solutions. Also, it allows the rate of administration to be controlled. SEE: *electronic infusion device.*

***electronic implantable i.p.*** ABBR: EIIP. A type of infusion pump implanted in the body rather than being located outside the body. The pump is implanted in a subcutaneous pocket and is connected to a dedicated catheter leading to the appropriate compartment or site. The pump may be programmable or nonprogrammable.

**Infusoria** (ĭn-fū-sō′rē-ă) The former name of a class of Protozoa, now called Ciliata.

**ingesta** (ĭn-jĕs′tă) [L. *in,* into, + *gerere,* to carry] Food and drink received into the body through the mouth.

**ingestant** (ĭn-jĕs′tănt) [" + *gerere,* to carry] Any substance such as food and drink taken orally.

**ingestion** The process of taking material (particularly food) into the gastrointestinal tract or the process by which a cell takes in foreign particles.

**Ingrassia's apophysis** (ĭn-gră′sē-ăs) [Giovanni Filippo Ingrassia, It. anatomist, 1510–1580] One of the lesser wings of the sphenoid.

**ingredient** (ĭn-grē′dē-ĕnt) [L. *ingredi,* to enter] Any part of a compound or a mixture; a unit of a more complex substance.

**ingrowing** [L. *in,* into, + AS. *growan,* to grow] Growing inward so that a portion that is normally free becomes covered.

**inguen** (ĭn′gwĕn) *pl.* **inguina** [L.] The groin.

**inguinal** (ĭng′gwĭ-năl) [L. *inguinalis,* pert. to the groin] Pert. to the region of the groin.

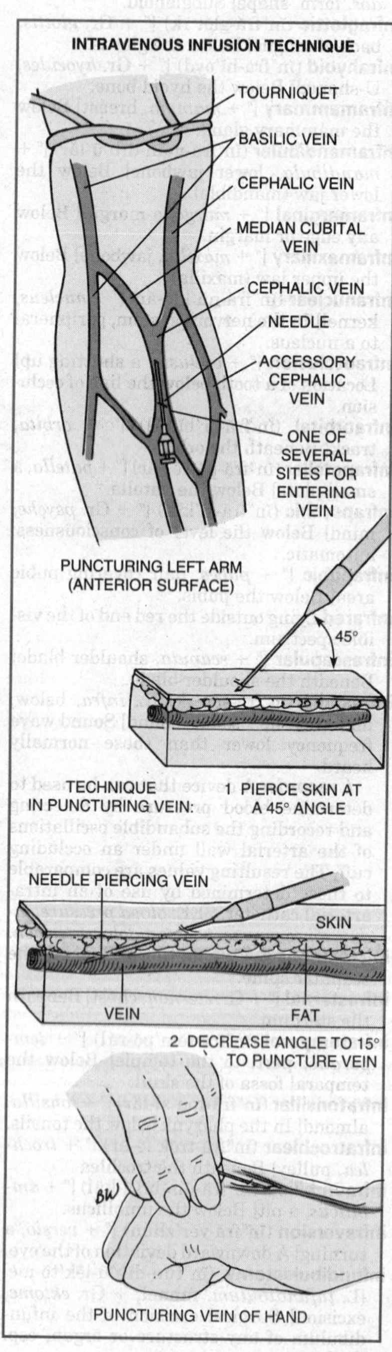

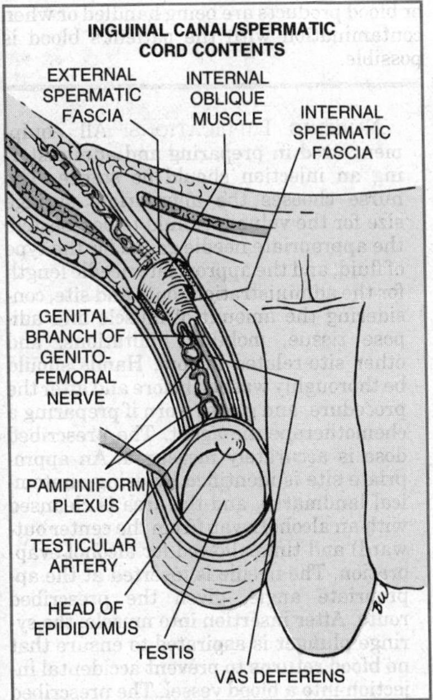


***i. canal*** Canalis inguinalis; a narrow, somewhat elongated opening in the lower lateral portion of the abdominal wall, extending from the abdominal (internal) inguinal ring to the subcutaneous (external) inguinal ring. It is an oblique passageway about 1½ in. (3.8 cm) long. In men it transmits the spermatic cord and the ilioinguinal nerve, and in women, the round ligament of the uterus and the ilioinguinal nerve. It forms a channel through which an indirect inguinal hernia descends. SEE: illus.

***i. reflex*** The reflex in women that resembles the cremasteric reflex in men.

***i. region*** The iliac region on either side of the pubes. SYN: *groin.*

**inguinal ring** The interior opening of the inguinal canal (abdominal inguinal ring) and the end of the inguinal canal (subcutaneous inguinal ring).

**inguinocrural** (ĭng″gwĭ-nō-kroo′răl) [L. *inguen,* groin, + *cruralis,* pert. to the leg] Concerning the inguinal and thigh areas.

**inguinolabial** (ĭng″gwĭ-nō-lā′bē-ăl) [″ + *labialis,* pert. to the lips] Concerning the inguinal and labial areas.

**inguinoscrotal** (ĭng″gwĭ-nō-skrō′tăl) [″ + *scrotum,* a bag] Concerning the inguinal and scrotal areas.

**INH** *isoniazid.*

**inhalant** [L. *inhalare,* to inhale] A medication or compound suitable for inhaling.

**inhalation** (ĭn″hă-lā′shŭn) [L. *inhalatio*] **1.** The act of drawing breath, vapor, or gas into the lungs; inspiration. **2.** The introduction of dry or moist air or vapor into the lungs for therapeutic purposes, such as aromatic spirits of ammonia used to overcome fainting.

SUBSTANCES: A mixture of oxygen and carbon dioxide is inhaled to relieve depressed breathing. Steam inhalations are given to reduce dryness of mucous membranes and to provide heat and moisture to the lung membranes.

**inhale** (in-hāl′) [L. *inhalare*] To draw in the breath; to inspire.

**inhaler 1.** A device for administering medicines by inhalation. **2.** One who inhales.

***metered-dose i.*** ABBR: MDI. A device used for self-administration of exact doses of aerosolized drugs.

**inherent** (ĭn-hĕr′ĕnt) [L. *inhaerens,* to inhere] Belonging to anything naturally, not as a result of circumstances, and existing as an essential character of something. SYN: *innate* (1); *intrinsic* (1).

**inheritance** (ĭn-hĕr′ĭ-tăns) [L. *inhereditare,* to inherit] The sum total of all that is inherited; that which is the result of genetic material (DNA) contained within the ovum and sperm.

***alternative i.*** The inheritance of a trait from one parent.

***extrachromosomal i.*** Inherited traits governed by mechanisms other than by chromosomes.

***holandric i.*** Inherited traits carried only by men; thus, the operative gene is on the Y chromosome.

***hologynic i.*** Transmission of traits from mothers only to daughters.

***multifactorial i.*** The inheritance of traits influenced by a number of genetic and nongenetic factors, none of which has a major effect.

***sex-influenced i.*** Inherited traits for which the genes are on autosomes, but their expression is influenced by the sex chromosomes (e.g., the reproductive organs).

***sex-limited i.*** A trait that can be expressed in only one sex.

***sex-linked i.*** The inheritance of traits regulated by either of the sex chromosomes, X or Y.

**inherited** Body traits and genetic make-up received as a result of genetic transmission rather than acquired.

**inhibin** (ĭn-hĭb′ĭn) A hormone that inhibits the secretion of follicle-stimulating hormone by the anterior pituitary gland. In women, inhibin is secreted throughout the menstrual cycle and in pregnancy but is normally not present in postmenopausal women. It is, however, elevated in most postmenopausal women with mucinous carcinomas of the ovary and in some women with other types of epithelial ovarian tumors. SEE: *cancer, ovarian.*

**inhibited sexual excitement** SEE: *frigidity.*

**inhibition** (ĭn″hĭ-bĭsh′ŭn) [L. *inhibere,* to restrain] **1.** The repression or restraint of a function. **2.** In physiology, a stopping of an action or function of an organ, as in the slowing or stopping of the heart produced by electrical stimulation of the vagus. **3.** In psychiatry, restraint of one mental process almost simultaneously by another opposed mental process; an inner impediment to free thought and activity.

***competitive i.*** Inhibiting the function of an active material by competing for the cell receptor site. SYN: *selective i.*

***contact i.*** The inhibition of cell division caused by the close contact of similar cells.

***noncompetitive i.*** The inhibition of enzyme activity resulting only from the concentration of the inhibitor.

***psychic i.*** The arrest of an impulse, thought, action, or speech. SYN: *suppression.*

***selective i.*** Competitive i.

**inhibitor** That which inhibits (e.g., a chemical substance that stops enzyme activity or a nerve that suppresses activity of an organ innervated by it).

***ACE i.*** A drug that blocks the effects of angiotensin-converting enzyme, preventing the formation of angiotensin II and therefore preventing a rise in blood pressure.

***monoamine oxidase i.*** SEE: *monoamine oxidase inhibitor.*

**inhibitory** (ĭn-hĭb′ĭ-tō-rē) Restraining, preventing.

**iniencephalus** (ĭn′ē-ĕn-sĕf′ă-lŭs) [Gr. *inion,* back of the head, + *enkephalos,* brain] A congenitally deformed fetus in which the brain substance protrudes through a fissure in the occiput, so that the brain and spinal cord occupy a single cavity.

**inion** (ĭn′ē-ŏn) [Gr.] External occipital protuberance. SEE: *antinion.* **iniac, inial** (ĭn″ē-ăk, -ăl), *adj.*

**iniopagus** (ĭn″ē-ŏp′ă-gŭs) [″ + *pagos,* thing fixed] Twins fused at the occiput.

**iniops** (ĭn′ē-ŏps) [″ + *ops,* eye] A double deformity in which two fetuses are joined from the posterior thorax up, so that one complete face is anterior, with the suggestion of a face posteriorly.

**initial** (ĭn-ĭsh′ăl) [L. *initium,* beginning] Relating to the beginning or commencement of a thing or process.

**initis** (ĭn-ī′tĭs) [Gr. *inos,* fiber, + *itis,* inflammation] **1.** An inflammation of fibrous tissue. SYN: *fibrositis.* **2.** An inflammation of a tendon. SYN: *tendinitis.* **3.** An inflammation of a muscle. SYN: *myositis.*

**inject** [L. *injicere,* to throw in] To introduce fluid into the body or its parts artificially.

**injectable** Capable of being injected.

**injected** [L. *injectus,* thrown in] **1.** Filled by injection of fluid. **2.** Congested.

**injection** (ĭn-jĕk′shŭn) **1.** The forcing of a fluid into a vessel, tissue, or cavity intramuscularly or under the skin. **2.** A solution introduced in this manner. **3.** The state of being injected; congestion. SEE: *AIDS; Universal Precautions Appendix.*

---

Caution: Gloves should be worn when blood or blood products are being handled or when contamination with the patient's blood is possible.

---

NURSING IMPLICATIONS: All equipment used in preparing and administering an injection should be sterile. The nurse chooses the appropriate syringe size for the volume of fluid to be injected, the appropriate needle gauge for the type of fluid, and the appropriate needle length for the administration route and site, considering the amount of muscle and adipose tissue, mobility limitations, and other site-related factors. Hands should be thoroughly washed before and after the procedure, and gloves worn if preparing a chemotherapeutic agent. The prescribed dose is accurately measured. An appropriate site is identified by using anatomical landmarks, and the area is cleansed with an alcohol swab (from the center outward) and time allowed for alcohol evaporation. The needle is inserted at the appropriate angle, given the prescribed route. After insertion into muscle, the syringe plunger is aspirated to ensure that no blood returns to prevent accidental injection into a blood vessel. The prescribed medication is injected slowly, then the needle is removed, and pressure is applied to the site with a dry sponge. When removing a needle after administering an intravenous injection, the nurse lessens the chance of bleeding into soft tissue by applying firm pressure while elevating the site above heart level for several minutes. The needle should not be recapped; both the needle and syringe should be destroyed and disposed of according to protocol. The injection time and site, any untoward responses to the injection, desired effects, and adverse reactions to the particular drug injected are recorded.

***epidural i.*** The injection of anesthetic solution or other medicine into the epidural space of the spinal cord.

***fractional i.*** The process of injecting small amounts at a time until the total injection is complete.

***hypodermic i.*** The term originally indicating injection of a substance beneath the skin. It is preferable, however, to specify the route of administration (e.g., intramuscular). SEE: *anesthesia, local.*

***intra-alveolar i.*** Infiltration method of anesthesia where the anesthetic is introduced into the soft tissues adjacent to the tooth.

***intracardial i.*** Injection into the heart.

***intracutaneous i.*** Injection into the skin, used in giving serums and vaccines when a local reaction is desired.

***intralingual i.*** The injection of medicines into the tongue, usually done as an emergency measure when a vein suitable for use is not available because of circulatory collapse.

***intramuscular i.*** Injection into intramuscular tissue, usually the anterior thigh, deltoid, or buttocks. No more than 4 ml should be injected at one time into an adult with normal musculature; in children and adults with underdeveloped musculature, no more than 2 ml should be injected at one time. SEE: illus.

***intraosseous i.*** The injection of anesthetic solution directly into the cancellous bone of the alveolar process adjacent to the tooth, to produce a localized effect.

***intraperitoneal i.*** Injection into the peritoneal cavity.

***intravenous i.*** Injection into a vein. The insertion of a needle requires a degree of skill that is easily obtained if proper instruction is obtained. The vein may be distended by applying a tourniquet with sufficient pressure to stop venous return but not arterial flow. The tourniquet is applied several inches above the injection site. If the patient does not have vascular collapse, the arterial pulse can be palpated; if not, the tourniquet is too tight. Heat applied to the area for 15 minutes before starting the injection will also help distend the vessels. The use of a needle attached to a 5- or 10-ml syringe will greatly facilitate controlling the course of the needle. It is best to insert the needle into the vein with the bevel side facing out and then, after the needle is in the vein, to rotate it so that the bevel is face in. There will be resistance as the needle goes through one side of the vein wall. The vein should be entered with the needle making only a narrow angle with the long axis of the vein. This will help to prevent pushing the needle completely through the vein. SEE: *cutdown*; *infusion, interosseous; Universal Precautions Appendix*.

NOTE: In patients with collapsed veins it may be possible to make the veins apparent by placing a tourniquet around the arm or leg and then inserting a 23- or 25-gauge catheter into a tiny superficial vein. Instillation of sterile intravenous fluid into the vein while the catheter is in place will distend the entire larger vein proximal to the small vein. A larger needle or catheter can then be inserted into the larger vein.

***jet i.*** The technique of injecting medicines and vaccines through the skin without puncturing it. A nozzle ejects a fine spray of liquid at such speed as to penetrate but not harm the skin. The procedure is harmless and is esp. useful in immunizing a great number of persons quickly and economically. Hypospray is the trade name for a device used in this procedure.

***rectal i.*** An instillation (i.e., not an injection) into the rectum; an enema.

***sclerosing i.*** The injection into a vessel or into a tissue of a substance that will bring about obliteration of the vessel or hardening of the tissues.

***spinal i.*** Injection into the spinal canal.

***subcutaneous i.*** Injection beneath the skin. The usual site is the skin over the deltoid, the upper outer arm.

***vaginal i.*** An instillation (i.e., not an in-

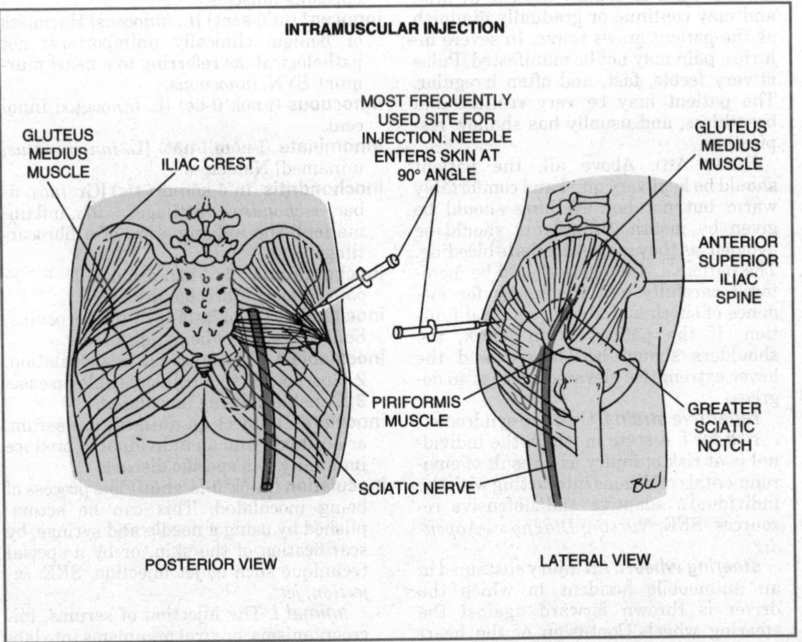

jection) into the vagina; a douche.

***Z-track i.*** An injection technique in which the surface (skin and subcutaneous) tissues are pulled and held to one side before the needle is inserted deep into the muscle in the identified site. The medication is injected slowly, followed by a 10-second delay, at which time the needle is removed and the tissues are quickly permitted to resume their normal position. This provides a Z-shaped track, which makes it difficult for the injected irritating drug to seep back into subcutaneous tissues.

**injector** A device for making injections.

***jet i.*** SEE: *injection, jet.*

***pressure i.*** A device that delivers a substance to be injected over a specified time or at a specified pressure.

**injury** [L. *injurius,* unjust] Trauma or damage to some part of the body. SEE: *transportation of the injured.*

SYMPTOMS: Various symptoms may occur, depending on the nature, extent, and severity of the damage. If the injury is severe, there may be signs of shock with progressive fall in blood pressure; subnormal temperature; shallow, rapid breathing; and cold, clammy, pale skin.

***internal i.*** Any injury not visible from the outside, as injury to the organs occupying the thoracic, abdominal, or cranial cavities.

SYMPTOMS: Symptoms vary depending on the structures involved. Ordinarily, profound shock is present. The patient is pale, cold, and perspiring freely; has an anxious expression; and may be semicomatose. Pain is usually intense at first, and may continue or gradually diminish as the patient grows worse. In severe injuries, pain may not be manifested. Pulse is very feeble, fast, and often irregular. The patient may be very restless and breathless, and usually has shallow respiration.

FIRST AID: Above all, the patient should be kept very quiet and comfortably warm but not hot. Nothing should be given by mouth. Stimulants should be avoided, as they may exacerbate bleeding. The patient's vital signs should be monitored carefully and frequently for evidence of shock and altered cerebral function. If the patient is in shock, the shoulders should be lowered and the lower extremities elevated at least 45 degrees.

***repetitive strain i.*** Overuse syndrome.

***risk for i.*** A state in which the individual is at risk of injury as a result of environmental conditions interacting with the individual's adaptive and defensive resources. SEE: *Nursing Diagnoses Appendix.*

***steering wheel i.*** An injury sustained in an automobile accident in which the driver is thrown forward against the steering wheel. Contusion of the heart and rib cage trauma may result.

***traumatic brain i.*** ABBR: TBI. Preferred term for injury to the head that involves neurological damage.

**inlay** (ĭn'lā) [L. *in,* in, + AS. *lecgan,* to lay] A solid filling made to the precise shape of a cavity of a tooth and cemented into it; usually the inlay is made of casting alloy, but it may be porcelain.

**inlet** A passage leading to a cavity.

***i. of pelvis*** The upper pelvic entrance between the sacral promontory and the superior aspect of the symphysis pubis.

**INN** *International Nonproprietary Names,* a list of pharmaceuticals published periodically by the World Health Organization.

**innate** (ĭn-nāt') [" + *natus,* born] **1.** Belonging to the essential nature of something. SYN: *inherent; intrinsic.* **2.** Existing at birth.

**innervate** (ĭn-nĕr'vāt, ĭn'ĕr-vāt) [" + *nervus,* nerve] To stimulate a part, as the nerve supply of an organ.

**innervation** (ĭn"ĕr-vā'shŭn) **1.** The stimulation of a part through the action of nerves. **2.** The distribution and function of the nervous system. **3.** The nerve supply of a part.

***collateral i.*** Development of the nerve supply in a nerve tract adjacent to the original nerve supply that has been injured or destroyed.

***double i.*** Innervation of an organ with both sympathetic and parasympathetic fibers.

***reciprocal i.*** Innervation of muscles, as around a joint, in which contraction of one set of muscles leads to the relaxation of opposing muscles.

**innocent** (ĭn'ō-sĕnt) [L. *innocens*] Harmless or benign; clinically unimportant; not pathological (as referring to a heart murmur). SYN: *innocuous.*

**innocuous** (ĭ-nŏk'ū-ŭs) [L. *innocuus*] Innocent.

**innominate** (ĭ-nŏm'ĭ-nāt) [L. *innominatus,* unnamed] Nameless.

**inochondritis** (ĭn"ō-kŏn-drī'tĭs) [Gr. *inos,* fiber, + *chondros,* cartilage, + *itis,* inflammation] The inflammation of a fibrocartilage.

**inochondroma** (ĭn"ō-kŏn-drō'mă) [" + " + *oma,* tumor] Fibrochondroma.

**inoculability** (ĭn-ŏk"ū-lă-bĭl'ĭ-tē) [" + *oculus,* bud] The state of being inoculable.

**inoculable 1.** Transmissible by inoculation. **2.** Susceptible to a transmissible disease. **3.** Capable of being inoculated.

**inoculate** To inject an antigen, antiserum, or antitoxin into an individual to produce immunity to a specific disease.

**inoculation** (ĭn-ŏk"ū-lā'shŭn) The process of being inoculated. This can be accomplished by using a needle and syringe, by scarification of the skin, or by a special technique such as jet injection. SEE: *injection, jet.*

***animal i.*** The injection of serums, microorganisms, or viral organisms into laboratory animals for the purpose of immunizing them or of investigating the effects of the inoculated material on them.

**inoculum** (ĭn-ŏk′ū-lŭm) [L.] A substance introduced by inoculation.

**inocyst** (ĭn′ō-sĭst) [Gr. *inos,* fiber, + *kystis,* a bladder] A fibrous capsule.

**inocyte** (ĭn′ō-sīt) [″ + *kytos,* cell] Fibroblast.

**inogenesis** (ĭn″ō-jĕn′ĕ-sĭs) [″ + *genesis,* generation, birth] The formation of fibrous tissue.

**inogenous** (ĭn-ŏj′ĭ-nŭs) [″ + *gennan,* to produce] Forming or produced from tissue.

**inoglia** (ĭn-ŏg′lē-ă) [″ + *glia,* glue] The supporting tissue of fibroblasts.

**inohymenitis** (ĭn″ō-hī″mĕn-ī′tĭs) [″ + *hymen,* membrane, + *itis,* inflammation] The inflammation of any fibrous membrane or of an aponeurosis.

**inomyositis** (ĭn″ō-mī″ō-sī′tĭs) [″ + *mys,* muscle, + *itis,* inflammation] Fibromyositis.

**inomyxoma** (ĭn″ō-mĭk-sō′mă) [″ + *myxa,* mucus, + *oma,* tumor] Fibromyxoma.

**inoneuroma** (ĭn″ō-nū-rō′mă) [″ + *neuron,* nerve, + *oma,* tumor] Fibroneuroma.

**inoperable** [L. *in-,* not, + *operari,* to work] Unsuitable for surgery. In the case of a tumor, the disease may have spread so extensively as to make surgery useless, or the patient's general condition may be so poor that surgery could result in the patient's death.

**inorganic** [L. *in-,* not, + Gr. *organon,* an organ] **1.** In chemistry, occurring in nature independently of living things; sometimes considered to indicate chemical compounds that do not contain carbon. **2.** Not pert. to living organisms.

**inosculate** [L. *in,* in, + *osculum,* little mouth] Anastomose.

**inosculation** (ĭn-ŏs″kū-lā′shŭn) Anastomosis.

**inose** (ĭn′ōs) Inositol.

**inosemia** (ĭn-ō-sē′mē-ă) [Gr. *inos,* fiber, + *haima,* blood] **1.** An excessive amount of fibrin in the blood. **2.** The presence of inositol in the blood.

**inosite** (ĭn′ō-sīt) Inositol.

**inositis** (ĭn″ō-sī′tĭs) [″ + *itis,* inflammation] Inflammation of fibrous tissue.

**inositol** (ĭn-ŏs′ĭ-tŏl) $C_6H_6(OH)_6$. Hexahydroxycyclohexane, a sugar-like crystalline substance found in the liver, kidney, skeletal muscle, and heart muscle, as well as in the leaves and seeds of most plants. It is part of the vitamin B complex. Deficiency of inositol in experimental animals results in hair loss, eye defects, and growth retardation. Its significance in human nutrition has not been established. SYN: *inose; inosite.*

**inosituria** (ĭn″ō-sĭ-tū′rē-ă) [*inositol* + Gr. *ouron,* urine] Inosuria (2).

**inosuria** (ĭn-ō-sū′rē-ă) **1.** [Gr. *inos,* fiber, + *ouron,* urine] Fibrinous excess in urine. **2.** [*inositol* + Gr. *ouron,* urine] Inositol in the urine. SYN: *inosituria.*

**inotropic** (ĭn″ō-trŏp′ĭk) [Gr. *inos,* fiber, + *trepein,* to influence] Influencing the force of muscular contractility.

**inpatient** A patient who is hospitalized. SEE: *outpatient.*

**inquest** [L. *in,* into, + *quaerere,* to seek] **1.** In legal medicine, an official examination and investigation into the cause, circumstance, and manner of sudden, unexpected, violent, or unexplained death. **2.** The act of inquiring.

**insalivation** [″ + *saliva,* spittle] The process of mixing saliva with food, as in chewing.

**insane** (ĭn-sān′) [″ + *sanus,* sound] Mentally deranged; pert. to insanity.

**insanitary** Not conducive to health; unhealthful, esp. pert. to filth.

**insanity** [L. *insanitas,* insanity] An imprecise term indicating a severe mental disorder such as a psychosis; now obsolete except as a legal term. In legal medicine, the state or mental condition characterized by the inability to distinguish between right and wrong, possession of delusions or hallucinations that prevent individuals from looking after their own affairs with ordinary prudence or that render them a menace to others, or actions resulting from impulses of such intensity that they cannot be resisted. SEE: *neurosis; psychosis.*

During lucid intervals, an insane person may enter into a legal contract, marriage, business, or buying and selling, providing at the time he or she is capable of entering into such matters with an understanding of all that is implied. The mental capacity at the time determines the validity of such acts and not the condition before or after.

***i. defense*** In legal and forensic medicine, the premise that an insane individual who commits a crime is not legally responsible for that act.

**insatiable** (ĭn-sā′shē-ă-b′l) [L. *insatiabilis*] Incapable of being satisfied or appeased.

**inscriptio** (ĭn-skrĭp′shē-ō) [L.] **1.** Inscription. **2.** A band or line. SYN: *intersection.*

***i. tendinea*** A tendinous band traversing a muscle.

**inscription** (ĭn-skrĭp′shŭn) [L. *in,* upon, + *scribere,* to write] The body of a prescription, which gives the names of the drug(s) prescribed and the dosage. SYN: *inscriptio* (1).

**insect** [L. *insectum*] The common name for any of the class Insecta of the phylum Arthropoda. Insects of medical importance are flies, mosquitoes, lice, fleas, ticks, spiders, scorpions, bees, hornets, and wasps. For more information see entries for individual insects.

**Insecta** A class of the phylum Arthropoda characterized by three distinct body divisions (head, thorax, abdomen), three pairs of jointed legs, trachea, and usually two pairs of wings. Insects are of medical significance in that some are parasitic; some serve as carriers or vectors of pathogenic organisms; and some are annoying pests causing injury by their bites or stings. SYN: *Hexapoda.*

**insecticide** (ĭn-sĕk′tĭ-sīd) [L. *insectum,* insect, + *caedere,* to kill] **1.** An agent used to exterminate insects. **2.** Destructive to insects.

**insectifuge** (ĭn-sĕk′tĭ-fūj) [″ + *fugare,* to put to flight] An insect repellant.

**Insectivora** (ĭn″sĕk-tĭv′ō-ră) [″ + *vorare,* to devour] An order of small mammals, including moles and shrews.

**insectivore** (ĭn-sĕk′tĭ-vor) A member of the order Insectivora.

**insecurity** Feelings of helplessness, apprehension, and vulnerability, and an inability to cope with situations or people.

**insemination** (ĭn-sĕm″ĭn-ā′shŭn) [L. *in,* into, + *semen,* seed] **1.** The discharge of semen from the penis into the vagina during coitus. **2.** The fertilization of an ovum.

***artificial i.*** ABBR: AI. The introduction of viable sperm into the vagina, cervical canal, or uterus by artificial means. SEE: *impregnation.*

***heterologous artificial i.*** ABBR: AID. Artificial insemination in which the semen is obtained from a donor other than the husband or partner.

***homologous artificial i.*** ABBR: AIH. Artificial insemination in which the semen is obtained from the husband or partner.

**insenescence** (ĭn″sē-nĕs′ĕns) [″ + *senescens,* growing old] The process of growing old or the approaching of old age.

**insensible** [L. *in-,* not, + *sensibilis,* appreciable] **1.** Unconscious; without feeling or consciousness. **2.** Not perceptible.

**insertion** [L. *in,* into, + *serere,* to join] **1.** The movable attachment of the distal end of a muscle, which produces shape changes or skeletal movement when the muscle contracts. **2.** The placement or implanting of something into something else (e.g., in dentistry, the process of placing a filling or inlay in a cavity preparation or placing dentures or other prostheses in the mouth).

***velamentous i.*** The attachment of the umbilical cord to the edge of the placenta.

**insheathed** (ĭn-shēthd′) [″ + AS. *sceath,* sheath] Enclosed, as by a sheath or capsule. SYN: *encysted.*

**insidious** (ĭn-sĭd′ē-ŭs) [L. *insidiosus,* cunning] Indicative of a disease that comes on in such a manner (lacking symptoms) as to make the patient unaware of its onset.

**insight** **1.** Self-understanding. **2.** In psychiatry, the patient's comprehension that he or she is mentally ill; and awareness of the character of the illness or of the unconscious factors responsible for the emotional conflict involved.

**in situ** (ĭn sī′tū, sĭt′ū) [L.] **1.** In position, localized. **2.** In the normal place without disturbing or invading the surrounding tissue.

**insolation** (ĭn″sō-lā′shŭn) [L. *insolare,* to expose to the sun] **1.** Any exposure to the rays of the sun. **2.** Heatstroke or sunstroke. SEE: *heat; heat exhaustion; hyperpyrexia.*

In the past it was felt that exposure to the sunlight was a powerful therapeutic measure. It is now known that exposure to excess sunlight on either an acute or a chronic basis may be unwise. Acute overexposure leads to severe sunburn of the skin. People with light skin who experience chronic exposure to the sun have an increased chance of developing malignant neoplasms of the skin.

**insoluble** (ĭn-sŏl′ū-b′l) [L. *insolubilis*] Incapable of solution or of being dissolved.

**insomnia** Prolonged or abnormal inability to sleep. SEE: *sleep, disorders of.*

***fatal familial i.*** ABBR: FFI. An inherited, rapidly progressive prion disease of middle or later life. Signs and symptoms include intractable insomnia, autonomic dysfunction, endocrine disturbances, dysarthria, myoclonus, coma, and death. There is no specific therapy. SEE: *prion disease.*

**insomniac** (ĭn-sŏm′nē-ăk) One who has insomnia.

**insorption** (ĭn-sorp′shŭn) [L. *in,* into, + *sorbere,* to suck in] The passage of material into the blood, as when substances move from the gastrointestinal tract into the bloodstream.

**inspect** [L. *inspectare,* to examine] To examine visually.

**inspection** Visual examination of the external surface of the body as well as of its movements and posture. SEE: *abdomen; chest; circulatory system.*

**inspiration** (ĭn″spĭr-ā′shŭn) [L. *in,* in, + *spirare,* to breathe] Inhalation; drawing air into the lungs; the opposite of expiration. The average rate is 12 to 18 respirations per minute in a normal adult at rest. SEE: *diaphragm* for illus.; *respiration.*

Inspiration may be costal or abdominal, the latter being deeper. The breaking point for breath holding is quite variable. Some professional divers and others are able to prolong it for more than two minutes. The muscles involved in inspiration are the external intercostals, diaphragm, levatores costarum, pectoralis minor, scaleni, serratus posterior, superior sternocleidomastoid, and sometimes the platysma.

***crowing i.*** The peculiar noise heard in laryngismus stridulus or spasmodic croup. SEE: *croup, spasmodic.*

***forcible i.*** Inspiration in which the muscles of inspiration are assisted by inspiration auxiliaries (i.e., muscles attached to the chest that by contraction increase the volume of the thoracic cavity directly or indirectly by furnishing fixed support whereby other muscles may act more advantageously). If movements become excessively labored, every muscle in the body that can either directly or indirectly increase the capacity of the thorax is brought into coordinate action.

***full i.*** Inspiration in which the lungs are filled as completely as possible (voluntarily, as in determining the amount of complemental air, or involuntarily, as in cardiac dyspnea).

***sustained maximal i.*** A deep-breathing maneuver that mimics the normal physiological sigh mechanism. The patient inspires from a resting expiratory level up to maximum inspiratory capacity, with a pause at end inspiration.

**inspirator** (ĭn′spĭ-rā″tor) A type of respirator or inhaler.

**inspiratory** (ĭn-spīr′ă-tor″e) Pert. to inspiration.

***i. capacity*** The maximum amount of air a person can breathe in after a resting expiration.

***i. hold*** A ventilating maneuver in which the delivered volume of gas is held in the lung for a while before expiration; called a plateau or ledge at end inspiration. Also called *grunt breathing*.

**inspirometer** (ĭn″spĭ-rŏm′ĕ-tĕr) [″ + ″ + Gr. *metron,* measure] A device for determining the amount of air inspired.

**inspissate** (ĭn-spĭs′āt) [L. *inspissatus,* thickened] To thicken by evaporation or absorption of fluid.

**inspissated** (ĭn-spĭs′ā-tĕd) Thickened by absorption, evaporation, or dehydration.

**inspissation** (ĭn-spĭ-sā′shŭn) **1.** Thickening by evaporation or absorption of fluid. **2.** Diminished fluidity or increased thickness.

**instability** The lack of ability to maintain alignment of bony segments, usually due to torn or lax ligaments and weak muscles.

**instar** Any one of the various stages of insect development during successive molts.

**instep** The arched medial portion of the foot.

**instillation** (ĭn″stĭl-ā′shŭn) [L. *in,* into, + *stillare,* to drop] Slowly pouring or dropping a liquid into a cavity or onto a surface.

**instillator** An apparatus for introducing, drop by drop, liquids into a cavity.

**instinct** (ĭn′stĭngkt) [L. *instinctus,* instigation] The inherited tendency for the members of specific species to react to certain environmental conditions and stimuli in a particular way. The nature of the reaction has enabled the individuals and species involved to adapt and survive through many generations. Instincts are best understood when considered against the evolutionary background of the individuals and species being observed. Freud spoke of instinct, but current psychoanalytic terminology would refer to the forces Freud described as drive instead of instinct.

***death i.*** In psychoanalytic theory, the unconscious will to destroy oneself; the counterinstinct for the instinct to live.

***herd i.*** The basic drive to be associated with a group.

**instinctive** Determined by instinct.

**Institute of Electrical and Electronic Engineers** ABBR: IEEE. An organization partially responsible for standards regulating electrical devices and equipment.

**institutionalization** A process in which individuals who live together gradually develop certain unhealthy patterns of behavior and thought (e.g., assumption of illness and depression apathy, behaviors frequently associated with nursing home institutionalization). The current movement in medicine and nursing is away from institutionalism in an attempt to create a more normalized home environment.

**institutional review board** ABBR: IRB. A board whose members are independent of the hospital or medical institution involved. It is established to oversee the plans for conducting medical investigations involving human subjects. The purpose of the board is to protect the rights of those subjects. SEE: *informed consent.*

**instruction 1.** A direction or command. **2.** The act of teaching or furnishing information.

***dental hygiene i.*** A program in which patients are taught the methods of oral hygiene and the importance of plaque control through proper toothbrushing, flossing, and appropriate nutrition.

**instrument** (ĭn′stroo-mĕnt) [L. *instrumentum,* tool] **1.** A mechanical device. **2.** A special tool for accomplishing specific tasks. Thus a reflex hammer, microscope, stethoscope, cystoscope, and surgeon's scalpel are all examples of instruments.

***care and sharpening of i.*** *Cleansing.* After surgery, the instruments should be collected, counted, and disassembled. First they should be rinsed with warm water to remove any blood, and next, washed with hot water and soap. They should then be placed under the hot water faucet while boiling water is run on and through them. They should be dried at once with gauze. To remove rust, cleanser should be used sparingly; otherwise, the surface of the instrument will be damaged in the course of time.

Reliable bacterial sterilization of instruments before an operation can always be ensured by boiling in a 1% solution of sodium bicarbonate for 15 minutes. This helps to prevent rusting of the instruments. The dipping of an instrument into alcohol or even pure carbolic acid cannot be relied upon to sterilize it.

---

Caution: Boiling water does not kill the hepatitis viruses. To be certain that these viruses are destroyed, either autoclaving or the use of some chemical method of sterilization such as ethylene oxide gas is required.

---

*Sharpening.* Washita stone is best for sharpening dull instruments because it cuts away the metal faster. Arkansas stone is better for finishing. Glycerin is a suitable lubricant. The entire edge of the knife should be covered in one sweep. The knife should be held so that the edge of the blade is at an angle of 30 degrees. Blunt instruments should be kept highly polished by rubbing with fine emery paper and polishing with rouge and chamois skin or gauze. Emery paper should not be used on saws. Silver instruments should not come in contact with rubber or be exposed to the atmosphere. They should be wrapped in dry gauze.

***dental i.*** Any instrument used in the practice of dentistry including a variety of hand or machine-driven cutting instruments for soft and calcified tissues, forceps, elevators, clamps, reamers, wire pliers, pluggers, carvers, explorers, and other instruments unique to the dental specialties: oral surgery, endodontics, orthodontics, periodontics, prosthodontics, restorative dentistry, and so on.

**instrumental** **1.** Pert. to instruments. **2.** Important in achieving a result or goal.

***i. activities of daily living*** ABBR: IADL. Those daily living skills, such as shopping, cooking, cleaning, and child care, that are necessary for maintaining the home environment.

**instrumentarium** (ĭn′stroo-mĕn-tā′rē-ŭm) Instruments required for a surgical or other procedure.

**instrumentation** **1.** The use of instruments and their care. **2.** The accomplishment of a task by use of instruments (e.g., removal of a foreign body from the bronchus by means of a bronchoscope).

***biomedical instrumentation*** The use of mechanical and electronic devices in medical diagnosis, therapy, or measurement.

**insufficiency** (ĭn″sŭ-fĭsh′ĕn-sē) [L. *in-*, not, + *sufficiens*, sufficient] The condition of being inadequate for a given purpose.

***adrenal i.*** Decreased or abnormally low production of adrenal cortical hormone by the adrenal gland, a condition resulting in Addison's disease.

***aortic i.*** An imperfect closure of the aortic valve.

***cardiac i.*** An inability of the heart to function adequately.

***coronary i.*** Diminished blood flow through the coronary arteries of the heart.

***gastric i.*** An inability of the stomach to empty itself.

***hepatic i.*** An inability of the liver to function properly.

***ileocecal i.*** Failure of the ileocecal valve to prevent the back flow of intestinal contents from the cecum to the ileum.

***mitral i.*** A condition in which the mitral valve fails to close completely with each heartbeat. SEE: *facies mitralis.*

***muscular i.*** A condition in which a muscle is unable to exert its normal force and bring about normal movement of the part to which it is attached.

***i. of ocular muscles*** An absence of dynamic equilibrium of ocular muscles.

***pulmonary valvular i.*** Failure of the pulmonary valve between the right atrium and right ventricle of the heart to close completely.

***renal i.*** An inability or reduced capacity of the kidney to remove waste products from the blood at the normal rate.

***respiratory i.*** Inadequate oxygen intake associated with abnormal breathing and signs and symptoms of distress due to hypoxia.

***thyroid i.*** Hypothyroidism.

***uteroplacental i.*** Inadequate blood flow through the placental intervillous spaces to enable sufficient transmission of nutrients, oxygen, and fetal wastes. It may be caused by diminished maternal cardiac output due to anemia, heart disease, regional anesthesia, or supine hypotension; vasoconstriction due to chronic or pregnancy-related hypertension or uterine overstimulation; vasospasm due to pregnancy-induced hypertension; vascular sclerosis due to maternal diabetes or collagen disease; or intrauterine infection.

***valvular i.*** Imperfect cardiac valve closure, permitting leakage of blood.

***venous i.*** A failure of the valves of the veins to function, which interferes with venous return to the heart.

**insufflate** [L. *insufflare*, to blow into] **1.** To blow into, as in the lungs of a newborn infant. **2.** To blow a medicated powder or medicinal vapor into a cavity.

**insufflation** The act of blowing a vapor or powder into a cavity, as the lungs.

***perirenal i.*** The instillation of air into the perirenal space in order to visualize the adrenal gland better on radiographic studies.

***tubal i.*** Rubin's test.

**insufflator** (ĭn′sŭ-flā″tor) A device for blowing powders into a cavity.

**insula** (ĭn′sū-lă) [L.] **1.** The central lobe of the cerebral hemisphere. It is a triangular area of the cerebral cortex lying in the floor of the lateral fissure. SYN: *island of Reil.* **2.** Any round cutaneous body or patch.

**insular** (ĭn′sū-lăr) [L. *insula*, island] Relating to any insula, as in pancreatic islets.

**insulation** [L. *insulare*, to make into an island] **1.** The protection of a body or substance with a nonconducting medium to prevent the transfer of electricity, heat, or sound. **2.** The material or substance that insulates.

**insulator** That which insulates. Specifically, a substance or body that prevents the transmission of electricity to surrounding objects by conduction; anything that exerts great resistance to the passage of an electric current by conduction. The electrical resistance of an insulator is expressed in ohms. SEE: *nonconductor.*

**insulin** [L. *insula*, island] **1.** A hormone secreted by the beta cells of the islets of Langerhans of the pancreas. It can be readily crystallized as a zinc salt, although nickel, calcium, and cobalt also are effective. It is a protein with a molecular weight of approx. 5700. Insulin secretion is stimulated by a high blood glucose level, such as occurs after meals. Insulin is essential for the use of glucose by cells to produce energy; it lowers the blood glucose level. Inadequate secretion results in the inability of cells to take in glucose. The cells in the liver are unable to produce and store glycogen. This condition is diabetes mellitus, characterized by hyperglycemia and glycosuria. Impaired use of glucose increases the use of fats for energy, which may lead to ketoacidosis. SEE: illus.; Etiology at *diabetes mellitus*. **2.** A protein, obtained from the pancreas of healthy bovine and porcine animals used for food by humans, that affects the metabolism of glucose. **3.** A preparation used in the medical treatment of diabetes, made either synthetically or from animal pancreas, usually pork or beef. Insulin was first discovered and used successfully in diabetes by Sir F.G. Banting. Insulin administration is not a cure for diabetes, nor is it necessary in every case of diabetes. Insulin, when injected (it is not active orally) into an individual with diabetes, produces the following effects: normal storage of glycogen in the liver and muscle tissue; reduction in blood sugar level by facilitating metabolism of glucose; disappearance of ketosis and hyperlipemia; prevention of excessive breakdown of protein; and increase in respiratory quotient.

DOSAGE: The insulin dosage should always be expressed in units. There is no average dose of insulin for diabetics; each patient must be assessed and treated individually.

ADMINISTRATION: Insulin preparations are divided into three categories according to how quickly they act and their potency and duration following subcutaneous administration. The types include fast-, intermediate-, and long-acting. Examples of these are given in the subentries. Syringes for use by blind diabetics are available. SEE: table.

---

**Caution: Persons taking insulin should wear an easily seen bracelet or necklace indicating that they have diabetes and take insulin. This will facilitate diagnosis and treatment in case of coma due to insulin. SEE:** ***Medic Alert.***

---

STORAGE: The FDA requires that all

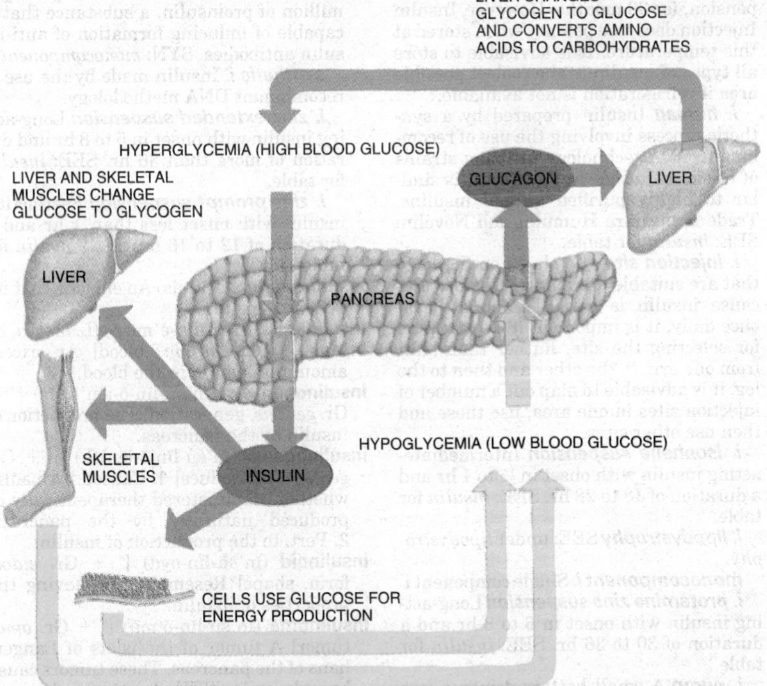


COMPLEMENTARY FUNCTIONS OF **INSULIN** AND GLUCAGON

**Duration of Effect of Various Insulins When Given by Subcutaneous Injection***

| Type of Insulin | Synonym or Trade Name | Onset | Maximum | Duration |
|---|---|---|---|---|
| | | (Given in Hours) | | |
| Insulin | Insulin. May be derived from one of several animals (e.g., pork, beef, ox). | 0.5–1.0 | 2–3 | 5–7 |
| Insulin human | Humulin; Novolin | 0.5–1.0 | 2–3 | 5–7 |
| Insulin isophane suspension | NPH Iletin | 1–2 | 6–12 | 18–24 |
| Insulin protamine zinc suspension | Insulin Protamine Zinc | 4–6 | 14–20 | 24–36 |
| Insulin zinc extended suspension | Ultralente Insulin | 4–6 | 16–18 | 20–36 |
| Insulin zinc prompt suspension | Semilente Iletin | 0.5–1 | 2–8 | 12–16 |
| Insulin zinc suspension | Lente Insulin | 1–2 | 6–12 | 18–24 |

* These times are "average" and may be quite different in an individual patient.

preparations of insulin contain instructions *to keep in a cold place and to avoid freezing.* Stored at room temperature, Insulin Zinc Prompt Suspension, Insulin Zinc Suspension, and Insulin Zinc Extended Suspension retain their potency for 24 months; Insulin Protamine Zinc Suspension and Insulin Isophane Suspension, for 36 months. However, Insulin Injection does lose potency when stored at this temperature. It is advisable to store all types of insulin in the coolest possible area if refrigeration is not available.

***i. human*** Insulin prepared by a synthetic process involving the use of recombinant DNA technology utilizing strains of *Escherichia coli.* In its effect it is similar to highly purified animal insulins. Trade names are Humulin and Novolin. SEE: *insulin* for table.

***i. injection site*** The places on the body that are suitable for injecting insulin. Because insulin is administered at least once daily, it is important to have a plan for selecting the site. Rather than shift from one arm to the other and then to the leg, it is advisable to map out a number of injection sites in one area, use those and then use other sites.

***i. isophane suspension*** Intermediate-acting insulin with onset in ½ to 1 hr and a duration of 18 to 28 hr. SEE: *insulin* for table.

***i. lipodystrophy*** SEE: under *lipodystrophy.*

***monocomponent i.*** Single component i.

***i. protamine zinc suspension*** Long-acting insulin with onset in 6 to 8 hr and a duration of 30 to 36 hr. SEE: *insulin* for table.

***i. pump*** A small battery-driven pump that delivers insulin subcutaneously into the abdominal wall. The pump can be programmed to deliver varying doses of insulin in accordance with changes in need for insulin during different conditions (e.g., prior to eating).

***i. resistance*** SEE: under *resistance.*

***i. shock*** SEE: under *shock.*

***single component i.*** Highly purified insulin that contains less than 10 parts per million of proinsulin, a substance that is capable of inducing formation of anti-insulin antibodies. SYN: *monocomponent i.*

***synthetic i.*** Insulin made by the use of recombinant DNA methodology.

***i. zinc extended suspension*** Long-acting insulin with onset in 5 to 8 hr and duration of more than 36 hr. SEE: *insulin* for table.

***i. zinc prompt suspension*** Fast-acting insulin with onset less than 1 hr and a duration of 12 to 16 hr. SEE: *insulin* for table.

**insulinase** (ĭn′sū-lĭn-ās) An enzyme that inactivates insulin.

**insulinemia** (ĭn-sū-lĭn-ē′mē-ă) [L. *insula,* island, + Gr. *haima,* blood] An excess amount of insulin in the blood.

**insulinogenesis** (ĭn″sū-lĭn-ō-jĕn′ĕ-sĭs) [″ + Gr. *genesis,* generation] The production of insulin by the pancreas.

**insulinogenic** (ĭn″sū-lĭn″ō-jĕn′ĭk) [″ + Gr. *gennan,* to produce] **1.** Caused by insulin whether administered therapeutically or produced naturally by the pancreas. **2.** Pert. to the production of insulin.

**insulinoid** (ĭn′sū-lĭn-oyd) [″ + Gr. *eidos,* form, shape] Resembling or having the properties of insulin.

**insulinoma** (ĭn″sū-lĭn-ō′mă) [″ + Gr. *oma,* tumor] A tumor of the islets of Langerhans of the pancreas. These tumors cause hypoglycemia. SEE: *hypoglycemia; neuroglycopenia.*

**insulitis** (ĭn″sū-lī′tĭs) [″ + Gr. *itis,* inflammation] Inflammation of the islets of Langerhans of the pancreas. In insulin dependent diabetes mellitus, the islets in the pancreas contain cells with enlarged nuclei, some degranulated beta cells, and a chronic inflammatory infiltrate.

**insulopathic** (ĭn″sū-lō-păth′ĭk) [″ + Gr. *pathos,* disease, suffering] Relating to or caused by abnormal insulin secretion.

**insult** In medicine, an injury or trauma.

**insusceptibility** (ĭn″sŭ-sĕp″tĭ-bĭl′ĭ-tē) [L. *in,* not, + *suscipere,* to take up] Immunity or lack of susceptibility to infection or disease.

**intake** (ĭn-tāk′) That which is taken in, esp. food and liquids.

***i. and output*** ABBR: I and O. A record of the oral and parenteral intake of foods and fluids; and of all output including urine, feces, vomitus, and, if required, an estimate of fluid loss as a result of perspiration.

**Intal** Trade name for cromolyn sodium.

**integration** (ĭn″tĕ-grā′shŭn) [L. *integrare,* to make whole] The bringing together of various parts or functions so that they function as a harmonious whole.

***primary i.*** The early recognition of the body and its psyche as apart from one's environment.

***secondary i.*** The process involved in developing the adult personality so that the individual coordinates the components into unified and socialized action.

**integrin** The receptor on cell surfaces that links with proteins and chemical mediators to enhance cell-to-cell communication. SEE: *cytokine; interleukin.*

**integrity** To be in an undiminished or unimpaired state.

**integument** (ĭn-tĕg″ū-mĕnt) [L. *integumentum,* a covering] A covering; the skin, consisting of the corium or dermis, and epidermis.

**integumentary** (ĭn-tĕg-ū-mĕn′tă-rē) Relating to the integument.

**intellect** [L. *intelligere,* to understand] The mind, or understanding; conscious brain function.

**intellectual 1.** Pert to the mind. **2.** Possessing intellect.

**intellectualization** (ĭn″tĕ-lĕk″chū-ăl-ĭ-zā′shŭn) The analysis of personal or social problems on an intellectual basis despite the individual's personal and emotional reactions to those problems.

**intelligence** [L. *intelligere,* to understand] The capacity to comprehend relationships; the ability to think, to solve problems and adjust to new situations. The use of a single test to estimate the intelligence of persons from different social, racial, cultural, or economic backgrounds, however, is unreliable.

***artificial i.*** SEE: *Computer Glossary.*

**intelligence quotient** SEE: under *quotient.*

**intensifying** [L. *intensus,* intense, + *facere,* to make] Making intense; magnifying.

***i. screen*** SEE: under *screen.*

**intensity 1.** A state of increased force or energy. **2.** The strength of uterine labor contractions at acme. Palpation identifies contractions as mild, moderate, or strong by indentability. Contraction strength can be measured in millimeters of mercury by insertion of a saline-filled intrauterine pressure catheter attached to a transducer.

**intensive** (ĭn-tĕn′sĭv) Relating to or marked by intensity.

**intensive care unit** ABBR: ICU. A special hospital unit for patients who, because of the nature of their illness, injury, or surgical procedure, require almost continuous monitoring by specially trained staff. In large hospitals, units may be devoted to a single group of patients such as surgical cases, compromised newborns, or patients with burns, trauma, emergency cardiac care needs, or infectious diseases.

**intention** (ĭn-tĕn′shŭn) [″ + *tendere,* to stretch] **1.** A natural process of healing. **2.** Goal or purpose.

***first i.*** Healing without granulation or suppuration.

***second i.*** Healing by adhesion of two granulated surfaces.

***third i.*** Healing of an ulcer, wound, or cavity by filling with granulation tissue and by cicatrization. SEE: *granulation; resolution.*

**inter-** [L.] Prefix meaning *in the midst, between.*

**interacinar** (ĭn″tĕr-ăs′ĭ-năr) [L. *inter,* between, + *acinus,* grape] Located between acini of a gland.

**interaction, dielectric** A term used to quantitate the electrical polarity or dipole moment of a molecule. SEE: *dipole.*

**interaction, drug** SEE: *drug interaction.*

**interalveolar** (ĭn″tĕr-ăl-vē′ō-lăr) [″ + *alveolus,* little tub] Between the alveoli, esp. the alveoli of the lungs.

**interarticular** [″ + *articulus,* joint] **1.** Between two joints. **2.** Situated between two articulating surfaces.

**interarytenoid** (ĭn″tĕr-ăr″ē-tē′noyd) [″ + Gr. *arytaina,* ladle, + *eidos,* form, shape] Between the arytenoid cartilages of the larynx.

**interatrial** (ĭn″tĕr-ā′trē-ăl) [″ + *atrium,* hall] Between the atria of the heart. SYN: *interauricular.*

**interauricular** (ĭn″tĕr-aw-rĭk′ū-lăr) [″ + *auricula,* little ear] Interatrial.

**interbrain** [″ + AS. *braegen,* brain] Diencephalon.

**intercadence** (ĭn″tĕr-kā′dĕns) [″ + *cadere,* to fall, die] A supernumerary pulse wave between two regular heartbeats.

**intercalary, intercalated** (ĭn-tĕr′kă-lĕr″ē, -kăl-āt-ĕd) [″ + *calare,* to call] **1.** Inserted or interposed between. SYN: *extraneous; interposed.* **2.** Pert. to an upstroke on a pulse tracing that comes between two heartbeats.

**intercanalicular** (ĭn″tĕr-kăn″ă-lĭk′ū-lăr) [″ + *canalicularis,* pert. to a canaliculus] Between the canaliculi of a tissue.

**intercapillary** (ĭn″tĕr-kăp′ĭ-lār-ē) [″ + *capillaris,* hairlike] Between the capillaries.

**intercarpal** (ĭn″tĕr-kăr′păl) [″ + Gr. *karpalis,* pert. to the carpus] Between the carpal bones.

**intercartilaginous** (ĭn″tĕr-kăr″tĭ-lăj′ĭ-nŭs) [″ + *cartilago,* cartilage] Connecting or between cartilages. SYN: *interchondral.*

**intercavernous** (ĭn″tĕr-kăv′ĕr-nŭs) [″ + L. *caverna,* a hollow] Between the cavernous sinuses.

**intercellular** (ĭn″tĕr-sĕl′ū-lăr) [″ + *cella,* compartment] Between the cells of a structure.

***i. junctions*** The microscopic space between cells. These spaces are important in assisting the transfer of small molecules across capillary walls. These junctions may be widened by chemical or physical factors and are acted on by chemical mediators of inflammation to increase vascular permeability.

**intercerebral** (ĭn″tĕr-sĕr′ē-brăl) [″ + *cerebrum,* brain] Between the two cerebral hemispheres. SYN: *interhemicerebral.*

**interchange** In dispensing drugs, the use of a generic form of the drug in place of the proprietary form. Some states mandate that prescriptions be filled using generic drugs unless the instructions specifically indicate “interchange not permitted.”

**interchondral** (ĭn″tĕr-kŏn′drăl) [″ + Gr. *chondros,* cartilage] Intercartilaginous.

**intercilium** (ĭn″tĕr-sĭl′ē-ŭm) [″ + *cilium,* eyelash] Glabella.

**interclavicular** (ĭn″tĕr-klă-vĭk′ū-lăr) [″ + *clavicula,* clavicle] Between the clavicles.

**intercoccygeal** (ĭn″tĕr-kŏk-sĭj′ē-ăl) [″ + Gr. *kokkyx,* coccyx] Between the segments of the coccyx.

**intercolumnar** (ĭn″tĕr-kō-lŭm′năr) [″ + *columna,* column] Between columns.

**intercondylar, intercondyloid, intercondylous** [″ + Gr. *kondylos,* knuckle] Between two condyles.

**intercostal** [″ + *costa,* rib] Between the ribs.

**intercostobrachial** (ĭn″tĕr-kŏs″tō-brā′kē-ăl) [″ + ″ + *brachium,* arm] Pert. to the intercostal space and the arm, as the posterior lateral branch of the second intercostal nerve supplying the skin of the arm, or a similar branch of the third intercostal nerve; formerly called intercostohumeralis.

**intercostohumeral** (ĭn″tĕr-kŏs-tō-hū′mĕr-ăl) [″ + ″ + *humerus,* upper arm] Concerning or connecting an intercostal space and the humerus.

**intercourse** [L. *intercursus,* running between] The social interaction between individuals or groups; communication.

***sexual i.*** Coitus.

**intercricothyrotomy** (ĭn″tĕr-krī″kō-thī-rŏt′ō-mē) [L. *inter,* between, + Gr. *krikos,* ring, + *thyreos,* shield, + *tome,* incision] The surgical separation of the cricothyroid membrane in order to incise the larynx.

**intercristal** (ĭn″tĕr-krĭs′tăl) [″ + *crista,* crest] Between two crests of a bone, organ, or process.

**intercrural** (ĭn″tĕr-krū′răl) [″ + *crus,* limb] Between two crura.

**intercurrent** [″ + *currere,* to run] **1.** Intervening. **2.** Pert. to a disease attacking a patient with another disease.

**intercuspation** [″ + *cuspis,* point] The cusp-to-fossa relation of the upper and lower posterior teeth in occlusion. SYN: *intercusping.* SEE: *occlusion.*

**intercusping** Intercuspation.

**interdent** A specially designed knife used for removing interdental tissue.

**interdental** [″ + *dens,* tooth] Between adjacent teeth in the same arch. SYN: *interproximal.* SEE: *interocclusal.*

**interdentium** (ĭn″tĕr-dĕn′shē-ŭm) The space between any two contiguous teeth.

**interdigitation** [″ + *digitus,* digit] **1.** Interlocking of toothed or finger-like processes. **2.** Processes so interlocked.

**interdisciplinary** Involving or overlapping of two or more health care professions in a collaborative manner or effort.

**interest checklist** An assessment approach used by occupational therapists to determine an individual’s unique play and leisure interests.

**interfascicular** (ĭn″tĕr-făs-ĭk′ū-lăr) [″ + *fasciculus,* bundle] Between fasciculi.

**interfemoral** [″ + *femoralis,* pert. to the thigh] Between the thighs.

**interference** [″ + *ferire,* to strike] **1.** Clashing or colliding. **2.** A dental occlusion that interferes with harmonious movement of the mandible.

***i. of impulses*** A condition in which two excitation waves, upon approaching each other and meeting in any part of the heart, are mutually extinguished.

**interferometer** (ĭn″tĕr-fĕr-ŏm′ĕ-tĕr) An optical device that acts on the interference of two beams of light, permitting examination of the structure of spectral lines. It is also used in examining prisms of lenses for faults.

**interferon** (ĭn-tĕr-fēr′ŏn) ABBR: IFN. Any of a group of glycoproteins with antiviral activity. The antiviral type I interferons (alpha and beta interferons) are produced by leukocytes and fibroblasts in response to invasion by a pathogen, particularly a virus. These interferons enable invaded cells to produce class I major histocompatibility complex (MHC) surface antigens, increasing their ability to be recognized and killed by T lymphocytes. They also inhibit virus production within infected cells. Type I alpha interferon is used to treat condyloma acuminata, chronic hepatitis B and C, and Kaposi’s sarcoma. Type I beta interferon is used to treat multiple sclerosis.

Type II gamma interferon is distinctly different from and less antiviral than the other interferons. It is a lymphokine, excreted primarily by CD8+ T cells and the helper T subset of CD4+ cells that stimulates several types of antigen-presenting cells, particularly macrophages, to release class II MHC antigens that enhance CD4+ activity. It is used to treat chronic granulomatous disease. SEE: *cell, antigen-presenting; macrophage.*

**interfibrillar, interfibrillary** (ĭn″tĕr-fĭb′rĭ-lăr, -rĭ-lăr″ē) [″ + *fibrilla,* a small fiber] Between fibrils.

**interfilamentous** (ĭn″tĕr-fĭl″ă-mĕn′tŭs) [″ + *filamentum,* filament] Between filaments.

**interfilar** (ĭn-tĕr-fī′lăr) [″ + *filum,* thread] Between the fibrils of a reticulum.

**interganglionic** [″ + *ganglion,* a swelling] Between ganglia.

**intergemmal** (ĭn″tĕr-jĕm′ăl) [″ + *gemma,* bud] Between taste buds.

**interglobular** [″ + *globulus,* globule] Between globules.

**intergluteal** (ĭn″tĕr-gloo′tē-ăl) [″ + Gr. *gloutos,* buttock] Between the buttocks.

**intergonial** An anthropometric line between the tips of the two angles of the mandible.

**intergyral** (ĭn″tĕr-jī′răl) [″ + Gr. *gyros,* circle] Between the cerebral gyri.

**interhemicerebral** (ĭn″tĕr-hĕm″ĭ-sĕr′ĕ-brăl) [″+ Gr. *hemi,* half, + L. *cerebrum,* brain] Intercerebral.

**interictal** (ĭn″tĕr-ĭk′tăl) [″ + *ictus,* a blow] Between seizures.

**interior** [L. *internus,* within] The internal portion or area of something; situated within.

**interischiadic** (ĭn″tĕr-ĭs″kē-ăd′ĭk) [L. *inter,* between, + Gr. *ischion,* hip] Between the ischia of the pelvis.

**interkinesis** (ĭn″tĕr-kĭ-nē′sĭs) [″ + Gr. *kinesis,* movement] The interval between the first and second meiotic divisions of cells.

**interlabial** Between the lips or any two labia.

**interlamellar** (ĭn″tĕr-lă-mĕl′ăr) [″ + *lamella,* layer] Between lamellae.

**interleukin** ABBR: IL. A type of cytokine that enables communication among leukocytes and other cells active in inflammation or the cell-mediated immune response. The result is a maximized response to a microorganism or other foreign antigen. SEE: *cell-mediated immunity; cytokine; inflammation.*

***i.-1*** ABBR: IL-1. A cytokine released by almost all nucleated cells that activates the growth and function of neutrophils, lymphocytes, and macrophages; promotes the release of additional mediators that influence immune responses; enhances production of cerebrospinal fluid; and modulates certain adrenal, hepatic, bone, and vascular smooth muscle cell activity. Interleukin-1 and tumor necrosis factors, whose actions are almost identical to those of IL-1, are involved in fever production and other systemic effects of inflammation. SEE: *tumor necrosis factors.*

***i.-2*** ABBR: IL-2. A cytokine released primarily by activated CD4+ helper T lymphocytes. It is a major mediator of T cell proliferation, promotes production of other cytokines, enhances natural killer cell function, and is a cofactor for immunoglobulin secretion. SYN: *T-cell growth factor.*

***i.-3*** ABBR: IL-3. A cytokine produced by activated T cells that promotes proliferation of bone marrow stem cells.

***i.-4*** ABBR: IL-4. A cytokine released by activated T cells and mast cells that stimulates lymphocyte production and inhibits macrophage activation.

***i.-5*** ABBR: IL-5. A cytokine produced by T cells, eosinophils and mast cells that acts as the primary stimulant for eosinophil production. SEE: *basophil; eosinophil.*

***i.-6*** ABBR: IL-6. A lymphokine produced by many cell types, including mononuclear phagocytes, T cells, and endothelial cells. It mediates the acute phase response, enhances B cell production and differentiation to immunoglobulin secreting plasma cells, and stimulates megakaryocyte production. SEE: *acute phase reactions; lymphokine.*

***i.-7*** ABBR: IL-7. A cytokine produced by bone marrow stromal cells. It stimulates growth of B cell precursors, thymocyte development, and macrophage activation.

***i.-8*** ABBR: IL-8. A cytokine produced by many cell types. It acts as a neutrophil chemoattractant.

***i.-9*** ABBR: IL-9. A cytokine produced by CD4+ cells and T cells. It is a cofactor for production of some CD4+ and T cell clones and promotes mast cell growth.

***i.-10*** ABBR: IL-10. A cytokine derived from mononuclear phagocytes, CD4+ cells, T cells, and keratinocytes. It inhibits cytokine synthesis by macrophages, T cells, and natural killer cells, and enhances B cell growth and secretion of immunoglobulin.

***i.-11*** ABBR: IL-11. A cytokine produced by bone marrow stromal cells. It mediates acute phase protein synthesis, enhances B cell growth and differentiation to plasma cells, and promotes megakaryocyte production.

***i.-12*** ABBR: IL-12. A cytokine produced by mononuclear phagocytes and B cells. It induces interferon gamma production from T cells and natural killer cells, and enhances T cell and natural killer cell cytotoxicity.

***i.-13*** ABBR: IL-13. A cytokine produced by T cells. It induces major histocompatibility class II expression on mononuclear phagocytes and B cells, B cell proliferation, and immunoglobulin production.

***i.-14*** ABBR: IL-14. A cytokine produced by T lymphocytes. It stimulates proliferation of activated B lymphocytes and inhibits immunoglobulin secretion from activated B lymphocytes.

**interlobar** (ĭn″tĕr-lō′băr) [″ + *lobus,* lobe] Between lobes.

**interlobitis** (ĭn″tĕr-lō-bī′tĭs) [″ + ″ + Gr. *itis,*

inflammation] Inflammation of the pleura separating the pulmonary lobes.

**interlobular** (ĭn″tĕr-lŏb′ū-lăr) [″ + *lobulus,* lobule] Between the lobules of an organ.

**intermalleolar** (ĭn″tĕr-mă-lē′ō-lăr) [″ + *malleolus,* little hammer] Between the malleoli.

**intermammary** (ĭn″tĕr-măm′ă-rē) [″ + *mamma,* breast] Between the breasts.

**intermamillary** (ĭn″tĕr-măm′ĭ-lăr″ē) [″ + *mammilla,* nipple] Between the nipples of the breasts.

**intermarriage** [″ + *maritare,* to marry] **1.** Marriage between persons from two distinct populations. **2.** Marriage between related individuals.

**intermaxillary** [″ + *maxilla,* jawbone] **1.** Between the two maxillae, as in an intermaxillary suture. **2.** Formerly meaning between the two jaws.

**intermediary** (ĭn″tĕr-mē′dē-ăr-ē) [″+ *medius,* middle] **1.** Situated between two bodies. **2.** Occurring between two periods of time.

**intermediate** (ĭn″tĕr-mē′dē-ĭt) [″ + *medius,* middle] Between two extremes; sequentially, after the beginning and before the end.

**intermedin** (ĭn″tĕr-mē′dĭn) A substance secreted by the pars intermedia of the pituitary. It is important in controlling pigment cells of the skin of some reptiles, fish, and amphibians.

**intermediolateral** [″ + ″ + *latus,* side] Intermediate but not central.

**intermedius** (ĭn″tĕr-mē′dē-ŭs) [″ + *medius,* middle] The middle of three structures.

**intermembranous** (ĭn″tĕr-mĕm′bră-nŭs) [″ + *membrana,* membrane] Between membranes.

**intermeningeal** (ĭn″tĕr-mĕn-ĭn′jē-ăl) [″ + *meninx,* membrane] Between the meninges.

**intermenstrual** (ĭn″tĕr-mĕn′stroo-ăl) [″ + Gr. *men,* month] Between the menses or menstrual periods.

**intermetacarpal** (ĭn″tĕr-mĕt″ă-kăr′păl) [″ + Gr. *meta,* beyond, + *karpos,* wrist] Between the carpal bones.

**intermission** [″ + *mittere,* to send] **1.** The interval between two paroxysms of a disease. **2.** A temporary cessation of symptoms.

**intermittence** [″ + *mittere,* to send] **1.** A condition marked by intermissions in the course of a disease or of a process. **2.** A loss of one or more pulse beats.

**intermittent** (ĭn″tĕr-mĭt′ĕnt) Suspending activity at intervals; coming and going.

**intermittent positive-pressure breathing** SEE: under *breathing.*

**intermural** (ĭn″tĕr-mū′răl) [L. *inter,* between, + *murus,* wall] Between the walls or sides of an organ.

**intermuscular** [″ + *musculus,* muscle] Between muscles.

**intern** (ĭn′tĕrn) [L. *internus,* within] A physician or surgeon on a hospital staff, usually a recent graduate receiving a year of postgraduate training before being eligible to be licensed to practice medicine. SEE: *extern.*

**internal** [L. *internus,* within] Within the body; within or on the inside; enclosed; inward; the opposite of external.

**internal injury** SEE: under *injury.*

**internalization** (ĭn-tĕr″năl-ĭ-zā′shŭn) The unconscious mental mechanism in which the values and standards of society and one's parents are taken as one's own.

**internal medicine** SEE: under *medicine.*

**internarial** (ĭn″tĕr-nā′rē-ăl) [L. *inter,* between, + *nares,* nostrils] Between the nares.

**internasal** (ĭn″tĕr-nā′zăl) [″ + *nasus,* nose] Between the nasal bones.

**internatal** (ĭn″tĕr-nā′tăl) [″ + *nates,* buttocks] Between the buttocks.

**International Association for Dental Research** ABBR: I.A.D.R. An association founded in 1920 to provide research in dental science and application of research to develop better treatment and oral health.

**International Classification of Diseases** ABBR: ICD. A codification of diseases, injuries, causes of death, and procedures including operations and diagnostic and nonsurgical procedures. The ICD's principal use is to standardize reporting of illness, death, and procedures. The publication is essential to the compilation of statistical information about diseases in a format that allows international comparison of those data.

**International Classification of Impairment, Disability and Handicap** ABBR: ICIDH. A standard originated by the World Health Organization for classifying and coding conditions requiring rehabilitation.

**international normalized ratio** ABBR: INR. A system of standardizing the prothrombin time (PT) in oral anticoagulant control, introduced by the World Health Organization in 1983, and increasingly used in the 1990s. The system is based upon the determination of an International Normalized Ratio (INR) which provides a common basis for communication of PT results and interpretations of therapeutic ranges. The INR is derived from calibrations of commercial thromboplastin reagents against a sensitive human brain thromboplastin, the IRP. For the three commercial rabbit brain thromboplastins currently used in North America, a PT ratio of 1.3 to 2.0 is equivalent to an INR of 2.0 to 4.0. For other thromboplastins, the INR can be calculated as INR = (observed PT ratio)$^{ISI}$, where the ISI is the calibration factor and is available from the manufacturers of the thromboplastin reagent.

NURSING IMPLICATIONS: The nurse uses the INR in managing oral anticoagulant (warfarin) therapy. Therapeutically, the INR should be maintained at 2.0 to 3.0 for prophylaxis and treatment of venous thromboembolism and for long-term therapy in atrial fibrillation.

**International Psychogeriatric Association** ABBR: IPA. An organization of health care professionals and scientists with an interest in the behavioral and biological aspects of mental health in the elderly.

**International Symbol of Access** A symbol used to identify buildings and facilities that are barrier-free and therefore accessible to disabled persons with restricted mobility, including wheelchair users. SEE: illus.

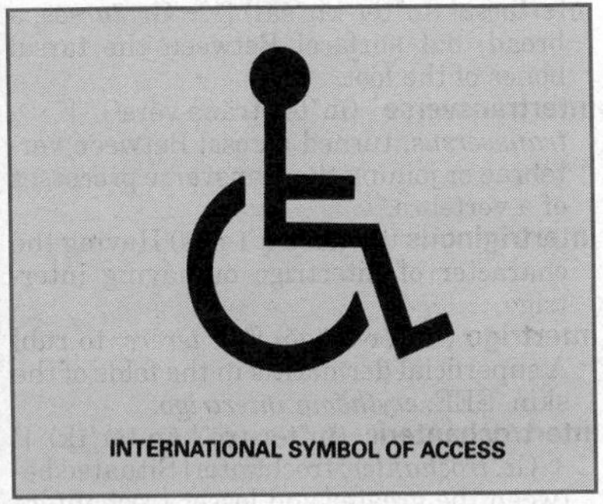
INTERNATIONAL SYMBOL OF ACCESS

**International System of Units** ABBR: SI. An internationally standardized system of units. The basic quantity measured and the names of the units are meter (length), kilogram (mass), second (time), ampere (electric current), kelvin (temperature), candela (luminous intensity), and mole (amount of a substance). All other units of measurement are derived from these seven basic units. SEE: *SI Units Appendix.*

**interneuron** (ĭn″tĕr-nū′rŏn) [L. *inter,* between, + Gr. *neuron,* nerve] A neuron of the central nervous system that transmits impulses from sensory to motor neurons or to other interneurons. SYN: *association neuron.*

**internist** A physician who specializes in internal medicine.

**internode** [″ + *nodus,* knot] The space between adjacent nodes.

**internship** (ĭn′tĕrn-shĭp) The period an intern spends in training, usually in a hospital.

**internuclear** (ĭn″tĕr-nū′klē-ăr) [″ + *nucleus,* a kernel] **1.** Between nuclei. **2.** Between outer and inner nuclear layers of the retina.

**internuncial** (ĭn″tĕr-nŭn′shē-ăl) [″ + *nuncius,* messenger] Acting as a connecting medium.

**interocclusal** (ĭn″tĕr-ŏ-kloo′zăl) [L. *inter,* between, + *occlusio,* a shutting up] Between the occlusal surfaces or cusps of opposing teeth of the maxillary and mandibular arches. SEE: *interdental; interproximal.*

**interoceptive** [L. *internus,* within, + *capere,* to take] In nerve physiology, concerned with sensations arising within the body itself, as distinguished from those arising outside the body.

**interofective** (ĭn″tĕr-ō-fĕk′tĭv) [″ + *afficere,* to influence] Pert. to that which concerns the interior of an organism.

**interoinferior** (ĭn″tĕr-ō-ĭn-fē′rē-or) [″ + *inferus,* below] Pert. to an inward and downward position.

**interolivary** [L. *inter,* between, + *oliva,* olive] Between the olivary bodies.

**interorbital** [″ + *orbita,* orbit] Between the orbits.

**interosseous** [″ + *os,* bone] Situated or occurring between bones, as muscles, ligaments, or vessels; specific muscles of the hands and feet.

**interpalpebral** (ĭn″tĕr-păl′pĕ-brăl) [″ + *palpebra,* eyelid] Between the eyelids.

**interparietal** (ĭn″tĕr-pă-rī′ĕ-tăl) [″ + *paries,* wall] **1.** Between walls. **2.** Between the parietal bones. **3.** Between the parietal lobes of the cerebrum.

**interparoxysmal** (ĭn″tĕr-păr″ŏk-sĭz′măl) [″ + Gr. *paroxysmos,* spasm] Between paroxysms.

**interpeduncular** (ĭn″tĕr-pĕ-dŭnk′ū-lăr) [L. *inter,* between, + *pedunculus,* peduncle] Between peduncles.

**interpersonal** Concerning the relations and interactions between persons.

**interphalangeal** (ĭn″tĕr-fă-lăn′jē-ăl) [″ + Gr. *phalanx,* closely knit row] In a joint between two phalanges.

**interphase 1.** The stage of a cell between mitotic divisions during which DNA replication takes place. **2.** The area or zone where two phases of a substance, such as a gas and a liquid, contact each other.

**interpolation** (ĭn-tĕr″pō-lā′shŭn) **1.** In surgery, the transfer of tissues from one site to another. **2.** In statistics, the calculation of an intermediate value from the observed values larger and smaller than the unknown intermediate.

**interposed** (ĭn′tĕr-pōzd) Inserted between parts.

**interpretation 1.** In psychotherapy, the deeper analysis of the meaning and significance of what the patient says or does. It is explained to the patient to help provide insight. **2.** In dentistry or radiology, the study and analysis of a diagnostic radiograph and the integration of the findings with the case history and the laboratory and clinical evidence.

**interproximal** [″ + *proximus,* next] Between two adjoining surfaces. SYN: *interdental.*

**interpubic** (ĭn-tĕr-pū′bĭk) [″ + *pubes,* pubes] Between the pubic bones.

**interpupillary** [″ + *pupilla,* pupil] Between the pupils.

**interradicular** Between the roots of teeth; the furcation area.

**interrenal** (ĭn″tĕr-rē′năl) [L. *inter,* between, + *ren,* kidney] Between the kidneys.

**interrogatory** In law, a written question sent by one party to another requesting information about issues and witnesses surrounding the allegations in a lawsuit.

**interscapilium** (ĭn″tĕr-skă-pĭl′ē-ŭm) [″ + *scapula,* shoulder blade] The area between the shoulders or scapulae. SYN: *interscapulum.*

**interscapular** Between the scapulae.

**interscapulum** (ĭn-tĕr-skăp′ū-lŭm) Interscapilium.

**intersection** The site where one structure crosses another or joins a similar structure.

**intersegmental** (ĭn″tĕr-sĕg-mĕn′tăl) [″ + *segmentum,* a portion] Between segments.

**interseptal** (ĭn″tĕr-sĕp′tăl) [″ + *saeptum,* a partition] Between two septa.

**intersex** (ĭn′tĕr-sĕks) An individual having both male and female secondary sexual characteristics. The term is descriptive but has little or no diagnostic value. Determination of sex in individuals who appear to have both male and female characteristics is complex. The diagnosis should be made after careful study of the chromosomes and of the gross and microscopic anatomical findings. SEE: *hermaphrodite; hermaphroditism.*

***female i.*** A genetic female with external sexual characteristics of both sexes.

***male i.*** A genetic male with external sexual characteristics of both sexes.

***true i.*** An individual whose genetic sex may be either male or female and whose sexual characteristics are of both sexes.

**intersexuality** (ĭn″tĕr-sĕks″ū-ăl′ĭ-tē) The varying expression of male and female physical and sexual characteristics in the same individual. SEE: *intersex.*

**interspace 1.** The space between two similar parts, as between two ribs. **2.** In radiology, the distance between the lead strips in a grid. It may contain organic material or aluminum.

**interspinal** (ĭn-tĕr-spī′năl) [″ + *spinalis,* pert. to the spine] Between two spinous processes of the spine.

**interstice** (ĭn-tĕr′stĭs) [L. *interstitium*] The space or gap in a tissue or structure of an organ. SYN: *interstitium.*

**interstitial** (ĭn″tĕr-stĭsh′ăl) **1.** Placed or lying between. **2.** Pert. to interstices or spaces within an organ or tissue.

***i. lung disorders*** ABBR: ILD. A large group of diseases with different causes but with the same or similar clinical and pathological changes. These are due to chronic, nonmalignant, noninfectious diseases of the lower respiratory tract characterized by inflammation and disruption of the walls of the alveoli. This manifests clinically as a limitation in the ability of the lungs to transfer oxygen from the alveoli to the pulmonary capillary bed. Patients with these disorders are dyspneic first in connection with exercise and, later, as the disease progresses, even at rest.

Approx. 180 different types of ILD exist, not all of which have a known cause. Known causes include inhalation of irritating or toxic environmental agents such as organic dusts, fumes, vapors, aerosols, and inorganic dusts; drugs; radiation; aspiration pneumonia; and residual acute respiratory distress syndrome. SEE: *idiopathic pulmonary fibrosis.*

**interstitium** (ĭn″tĕr-stĭsh′ē-ŭm) [L.] Interstice.

**intersystole** (ĭn″tĕr-sĭs′tō-lē) [L. *inter,* between, + Gr. *systole,* contraction] The period between the end of the atrial systole and the commencement of the ventricular systole.

**intertarsal** (ĭn″tĕr-tăr′săl) [″ + Gr. *tarsos,* a broad, flat surface] Between the tarsal bones of the foot.

**intertransverse** (ĭn″tĕr-trăns-vĕrs′) [″ + *transversus,* turned across] Between vertebrae or joining the transverse processes of a vertebra.

**intertriginous** (ĭn″tĕr-trĭj′ĭ-nŭs) Having the character of intertrigo or having intertrigo.

**intertrigo** (ĭn″tĕr-trī′gō) [″ + *terere,* to rub] A superficial dermatitis in the folds of the skin. SEE: *erythema intertrigo.*

**intertrochanteric** (ĭn″tĕr-trō″kăn-tĕr′ĭk) [″ + Gr. *trochanter,* trochanter] Situated between the greater and lesser trochanters of the femur.

**intertubular** (ĭn″tĕr-tū′bū-lăr) [″ + *tubulus,* tubule] Between or among tubules.

**interureteral, interureteric** (ĭn″tĕr-ū-rē′tĕr-ăl, ĭn″tĕr-ū″rē-tĕr′ĭk) [″ + Gr. *oureter,* ureter] Between the two ureters.

**intervaginal** (ĭn″tĕr-văj′ĭ-năl) [″ + *vagina,* sheath] Between sheaths.

**interval** [″+ *vallum,* a breastwork] **1.** A space or time between two objects or periods. **2.** A break in the course of disease or between paroxysms.

***atriocarotid i.*** In a venous pulse tracing, the interval between the onset of the presystolic wave (a) and that of the systolic wave (c). It indicates the time required for impulses to travel from the SA node to the ventricle, normally about 0.2 sec.

***atrioventricular (AV) i.*** An interval between the beginning of atrial systole and ventricular systole, measured in humans by an electrocardiogram.

***cardioarterial i.*** The time between the apex beat and radial pulsation.

***contraction i.*** The period between uterine contractions. Relaxation of the uterine muscle replenishes the blood flow to the muscle and to the intervillous spaces of the placenta.

***focal i.*** The distance between the anterior and posterior focal points of the eyes.

***isometric i.*** Presphygmic i.

***lucid i.*** A brief remission of symptoms in a psychosis.

***postsphygmic i.*** The interval between closure of the semilunar valves and opening of atrioventricular valves.

***P-R i.*** In the electrocardiogram, the period between the onset of the P wave and the beginning of the QRS complex.

***presphygmic i.*** The brief period between the beginning of ventricular systole and opening of the semilunar valves. SYN: *isometric i.*

***Q-R i.*** In the electrocardiogram, the period between the onset of the QRS complex and the peak of the R wave.

***QRS i.*** In the electrocardiogram, the interval between the beginning of the Q wave and the end of the S wave. The normal interval is less than 0.12 sec.

***QRST i.*** The ventricular complex of the electrocardiogram. SEE: *electrocardiogram* for illus.

***Q-T i.*** In the electrocardiogram, the interval between the beginning of the Q wave and the end of the T wave.

**intervalvular** (ĭn″tĕr-văl′vū-lăr) [L. *inter,* between, + *valva,* leaf of a folding door] Between valves, esp. the heart valves.

**intervascular** [″ + *vasculum,* a vessel] Between blood vessels.

**intervention** (ĭn″tĕr-vĕn′shŭn) One or more actions taken in order to modify an effect.

***crisis i.*** In psychiatry, the immediate institution of all appropriate forms of therapy for an individual experiencing a personal crisis.

***life-sustaining i.*** Any modern method, medicine, or device used to prolong life. Whether and when to use these interventions is a matter of great concern and controversy. Courts have ruled that making the decision not to intervene does not mean that the person making the decision is a murderer, nor is it considered suicide if the patient makes the decision. SEE: *advance directive; living will.*

***nursing i.*** SEE: *nursing intervention.*

**interventricular** [″ + *ventriculum,* a small cavity] Between the ventricles.

**intervertebral** [″ + *vertebra,* joint] Between two adjacent vertebrae.

**intervillous** (ĭn″tĕr-vĭl′ŭs) [″ + *villus,* tuft] Between villi.

**intestinal** [L. *intestinum,* intestine] Pert. to the intestines. SEE: *digestion; intestine.*

***i. obstruction*** SEE: *under obstruction.*

***i. perforation*** SEE: *perforation of stomach or intestine.*

**intestine** (ĭn-tĕs′tĭn) [L. *intestinum*] The alimentary canal extending from the pylorus to the anus. It is divided into the small intestine and large intestine or colon. SYN: *intestinum.*

PALPATION: A fecal accumulation feels similar to a tumor but is hard and resistant; however, if one finger is pressed steadily on a fecal mass for one or two minutes, the mass will indent. Fecal accumulations most frequently collect in the descending colon.

PERCUSSION: In normal conditions, the large intestine furnishes a more amphoric percussion sound than the stomach. When the large intestine is filled with liquid or solid accumulations, their location can be marked out on the surface by dullness on percussion. Because these accumulations most frequently occur in the descending colon, the percussion sound over this portion is usually less resonant than over the ascending or transverse colon.

***large i.*** The large intestine extends from the ileum to the anus and is about 1.5 m (5 ft) in length. It absorbs water, minerals, and vitamins from the intestinal contents and eliminates undigested material during defecation. The mucosa has no villi but contains glands that secrete mucus. Hyperactivity of the colon may cause diarrhea.

The first part of the large intestine is the cecum, a pouch on the right side into which the ileum empties. Attached to the cecum is the vermiform appendix, about 7.5 to 10.4 cm (3 to 4 in.) long. The colon is approx. 1.5 m (5 ft) long. The ascending colon extends from the cecum upward to the undersurface of the liver, where it turns left (hepatic flexure) and becomes the transverse colon, which continues toward the spleen and turns downward (splenic flexure) to become the descending colon. At the level of the pelvic brim, the descending colon turns inward in the shape of the letter S and is then called the sigmoid colon. The rectum, about 10.2 to 12.7 cm (4 to 5 in.) long, is the straight part that continues downward; the last 2.5 cm (1 in.) is called the anal canal, which surrounds the anus.

***small i.*** The first part of the small intestine is the duodenum, approx. 8 to 11 in. (20 to 28 cm) long, which receives chyme from the stomach through the pyloric orifice, and by way of the common bile duct, bile from the liver and gallbladder and pancreatic juice from the pancreas. The second part is the jejunum, about 9 ft (2.8 m) long. The third part is the ileum, about 13 ft (4 m) long. The ileum opens into the cecum of the large intestine, and the ileocecal valve prevents backup of intestinal contents.

The wall of the small intestine has circular folds (plicae circulares), which are folds of the mucosa and submucosa that look like accordian pleats. The mucosa is further folded into villi, which look like small (0.5 to 1.5 mm long) projections. The free surfaces of the epithelial cells have microscopic folds called microvilli that are collectively called the brush border. All of the folds increase the surface area for absorption of the end products of digestion. Intestinal glands (of Lieberkühn) between the bases of the villi secrete enzymes. The duodenum has submucosal Brunner's glands that secrete mucus. Enzymes secreted by the small intestine are peptidases, which complete protein digestion, and sucrase, maltase, and lactase, which digest disaccharides to monosaccharides. Some of these enzymes function in the brush border rather than in the lumen of the intestine. Hormones secreted by the duodenum are gastric inhibitory peptide, secretin, and cholecystokinin; these influence secretions or motility of other parts of the digestive tract.

The end products of digestion (amino acids, monosaccharides, fatty acids, glycerol, vitamins, minerals, and water) are absorbed into the capillaries or lacteals within the villi. Blood from the small intestine passes through the liver by way of the portal vein before returning to the heart. SEE: *digestive system* for illus.; *duodenum; liver; pancreas.*

**intestinum** (ĭn″tĕs-tī′nŭm) *pl.* **intestina** [L.] Intestine.

**intima** (ĭn′tĭ-mă) [L.] The innermost layer of the wall of an artery. It consists of a continuous layer of endothelial cells. Normally these cells serve as a barrier that controls the entry of substances from the lumen of the vessel into the wall of the artery. However, materials may pass this barrier by means of transport systems. The endothelial cells secrete substances that are important in blood coagulation and in controlling relaxation and contraction of the smooth muscle tissue in the middle layer of the vessel. As the normal artery ages, the intima thickens due to an increase in lipid material.

**intimal** (ĭn′tĭ-măl) Pert. to the inner layer of a blood vessel, the intima.

**intimitis** (ĭn″tĭ-mī′tĭs) [L. *intima,* innermost, + Gr. *itis,* inflammation] Inflammation of an intima.

**intolerance** [L. *in-,* not, + *tolerare,* to bear] An inability to endure, or an incapacity for bearing, pain or the effects of a drug or other substance.

**intorsion** (ĭn-tor′shŭn) [L. *in,* toward, + *torsio,* twisting] Rotation of the eye inward toward the nose on the anterioposterior axis of the eye. In this condition, twelve o'clock on the corneal margin would be closer to the nose than normal.

**intoxicant** (ĭn-tŏks′ĭ-kănt) An agent that produces intoxication.

**intoxication** [L. *in,* in, + Gr. *toxikon,* poison] **1.** The state of being intoxicated, esp. of being poisoned by a drug or toxic substance. **2.** Intoxicated from overindulgence in alcoholic beverages.

The determination of alcohol content of the blood (i.e., ethyl alcohol or the alcohol present in commercial beverages such as beer, wine, and whiskey) is frequently of value in the diagnosis of alcohol intoxication, esp. in differentiating it from other disorders. Normally the alcohol content of body tissues and fluids is negligible. Upon ingestion, alcoholic fluids are absorbed slowly or quickly, depending upon the amount swallowed, presence of food in the stomach, and rate of gastric emptying. The amount of alcohol found in each milliliter of blood also depends on body size. Thus, if 70-kg (154-lb) and 90-kg (198-lb) individuals drink the same amount of alcohol in the same time and under similar conditions, the alcohol concentration in each milliliter of blood will be least in the person who weighs the most.

The amount of alcohol present in expired air also provides an estimate of the alcohol content of the blood. The amount of alcohol present in the blood does not provide completely valid information about the degree of intoxication because of the ability of the central nervous system to adapt to alcohol. SEE: *alcoholism; Breathalyzer.*

***water i.*** Excess intake or undue retention of water. SEE: *brain edema.*

SYMPTOMS: Clinically, abdominal cramps, dizziness, lethargy, nausea, vomiting, convulsions, and coma may be present. In obstetrics, patient complaints of headache, drowsiness, and confusion may indicate water intoxication. Objective findings include signs of edema and decreased urinary output.

ETIOLOGY: Causes include excess ingestion of water, intravenous administration of hypotonic solutions or oxytocin, excess tap water enemas, hypothalamic tumors, cerebral concussion, or excess secretion of antidiuretic hormone. This condition has also been reported in endurance athletes who take in as much as 12 quarts of water during an event such as a marathon without replacing the salt lost in their perspiration.

**intra-** [L.] Prefix meaning *within.*

**intra-abdominal** [L. *intra,* within, + *abdomen,* belly] Within the abdomen.

**intra-acinous** (ĭn-tră-ăs′ĭ-nŭs) [″ + *acinus,* grape] Within an acinus.

**intra-alveolar** Inside the alveoli.

**intra-aortic balloon counterpulsation** ABBR: IABC. The use of a balloon attached to a catheter inserted through the femoral artery into the descending thoracic aorta to produce alternating inflation and deflation during diastole and systole, respectively. This permits lowering resistance to aortic blood flow during systole and increasing resistance during diastole. The result is to decrease the work of the heart and increase blood flow to the coronary arteries. The balloon is inflated with helium. This method is useful in treating shock. SEE: *Nursing Diagnoses Appendix.*

NURSING IMPLICATIONS: *Patient preparation:* If time permits, the nurse explains to the patient that the cardiologist will place a special catheter into the aorta to help the heart pump more easily, and provide specific procedural and sensation information. The nurse explains that the catheter will be connected to a large console beside the bed that has an alarm system, and that a nurse will promptly answer any alarms. The nurse explains that the console normally makes a pumping sound, and ensures that the patient understands that this does not mean that his heart is not beating. The nurse also explains that because of the catheter, the patient will not be able to sit up, bend the knee, or flex the hip more than 30 degrees. The nurse explains that the patient will continue on the cardiac monitor, and will have a central line (pulmonary artery catheter), arterial line and peripheral I.V. line in place. If the procedure is to be performed at the bedside, the nurse gathers the appropriate equipment, including a surgical tray for percutaneous catheter insertion, heparin solution, normal saline solution, the IABC catheter, and the pump console. The nurse prepares the femoral insertion site according to agency protocol, ascertains that a signed informed consent for the procedure has been obtained, and provides the patient with emotional support throughout the procedure.

*Monitoring and aftercare:* Following agency protocol or physician orders, the nurse sets the console to regulate the rate of inflation and deflation of the balloon based on the ECG or the arterial waveform. (If the patient has no intrinsic heart rate, the pump may be set to its own intrinsic rate.) The nurse uses strict aseptic technique in caring for the catheter insertion site and connections, and frequently inspects the site for bleeding or inflammation. If bleeding occurs at the insertion site, the nurse applies direct pressure over it and notifies the cardiologist. The nurse maintains the catheterized leg in correct body alignment and prevents hip flexion. The nurse maintains head elevation at no more than 30 degrees, to prevent upward migration of the catheter and occlusion of the left subclavian artery. If the balloon does occlude the artery, the nurse might expect to note a diminished left radial pulse and a patient report of dizziness. (Incorrect balloon placement also may occlude the renal artery, causing flank pain or a sudden drop in urine output.) The nurse also periodically assesses distal pulses, and documents the color, temperature, and capillary refill of the patient's extremities. The nurse assesses the affected leg's warmth, color, pulses, and the patient's ability to move the toes at 30-minute intervals for the first 4 hours after insertion, then hourly for the duration of IABC. (Often, arterial flow to the involved extremity diminishes during insertion, but the pulse should strengthen once pumping begins.)

If the patient is receiving heparin or low-molecular-weight dextran to inhibit thrombosis, the nurse keeps in mind that he is still at risk for thrombus formation, and observes for such indications as a sudden weakening of pedal pulses, pain and motor or sensory loss. The nurse also maintains adequate hydration to help prevent thrombus formation. As prescribed, the nurse applies antiembolism stockings for 8 hours, then removes them, inspects and palpates the legs, and reapplies the stockings. The nurse encourages active range-of-motion exercises every 2 hours for the arms, the unaffected leg, and the affected ankle.

An alarm on the console may detect gas leaks from a damaged or ruptured balloon. If the alarm sounds, or if the nurse observes blood in the catheter, the nurse should shut down the pump console and immediately place the patient in Trendelenburg's position to prevent an air (gas) embolus from reaching the brain, then notify the cardiologist.

Once the signs and symptoms of left ventricular failure have diminished, and the patient requires only minimal pharmacological support, the patient will be gradually weaned from IABC. Then to discontinue IABC, the cardiologist or a designate will deflate the balloon, clip the sutures, and remove the catheter, allowing the site to bleed for 5 seconds to expel clots. The nurse then applies direct pressure to the site for 30 minutes, followed by a pressure dressing. The nurse evaluates the site for bleeding and hematoma formation hourly for the next 4 hours.

**intra-arterial** [″ + Gr. *arteria,* artery] Within the artery(ies).

**intra-articular** (ĭn″tră-ăr-tĭk′ū-lăr) [″ + *articulus,* little joint] Within a joint.

**intra-atrial** (ĭn″tră-ā′trē-ăl) [″ + Gr. *atrion,* hall] Within one or more atria of the heart.

**intrabronchial** (ĭn″tră-brŏng′kē-ăl) [″ + Gr. *bronchos,* windpipe] Within a bronchus.

**intrabuccal** (ĭn″tră-bŭk′ăl) [″ + *bucca,* cheek] Within the tissue of the cheek or within the mouth.

**intracanalicular** (ĭn″tră-kăn″ă-lĭk′ū-lăr) [″ + *canalicularis,* pert. to a canaliculus] Within a canaliculus.

**intracapsular** [″ + *capsula,* little box] Within a capsule.

***i. extraction*** The basic surgical technique for cataract removal, in which the nucleus, cortex, and capsule are removed as one unit. SEE: *cataract.*

**intracardiac** Within the heart.

**intracarpal** (ĭn″tră-kăr′păl) [″ + Gr. *karpalis,* pert. to the carpus] Within the wrist.

**intracartilaginous** (ĭn″tră-kăr″tĭ-lăj′ĭn-ŭs) [″ + *cartilago,* gristle] Within a cartilage or cartilaginous tissue.

**intracath** A device for facilitating the introduction of an intravenous catheter. An inflexible needle is surrounded by a catheter. They are inserted into the vein as a unit; then the needle is removed. This allows the catheter to be inserted further in the vein. The traditional intracath has been replaced by the angiocath or central venous line.

**intracellular** (ĭn″tră-sĕl′ū-lăr) [″ + *cellula,* cell] Within the cell.

**intracerebellar** (ĭn″tră-sĕr″ĕ-bĕl′ăr) [″ +

*cerebellum,* little brain] Within the cerebellum of the brain.

**intracerebral** (ĭn″tră-sĕr′ĕ-brăl) [″ + *cerebrum,* brain] Within the main portion of the brain, the cerebrum.

**intracervical** (ĭn″tră-sĕr′vĭ-kăl) [″ + *cervicalis,* pert. to the neck] In the cervical canal of the uterus.

**intracisternal** (ĭn″tră-sĭs-tĕr′năl) [″ + *cisterna,* cavity] Within a cistern of the brain.

**intracostal** (ĭn″tră-kŏs′tăl) [″+ *costa,* rib] On the inner surface of a rib.

**intracranial** [″ + Gr. *kranion,* skull] Within the cranium or skull.

**intractable** (ĭn-trăk′tă-b′l) Incurable or resistant to therapy.

**intracutaneous** [″ + *cutis,* skin] Within the substance of the skin. SYN: *intradermal.*

**intracystic** [″ + Gr. *kystis,* bladder] Within a bladder or cyst.

**intrad** (ĭn′trăd) Inwardly; toward the inner part.

**intradermal** (ĭn″tră-dĕr″măl) [″ + Gr. *derma,* skin] ABBR: ID. Intracutaneous.

**intraduct** (ĭn′tră-dŭkt) [″ + *ductus,* a canal] Within a duct.

**intraduodenal** (ĭn″tră-dū″ō-dē′năl) [″ + *duodeni,* twelve] Within the duodenum.

**intradural** (ĭn-tră-dū′răl) [″ + *durus,* hard] Within or enclosed by the dura mater.

**intraepidermal** (ĭn″tră-ĕp″ĭ-dĕr′măl) [L. *intra,* within, + Gr. *epi,* upon, + *derma,* skin] Within the epidermis.

**intraepithelial** (ĭn″tră-ĕp″ĭ-thē′lē-ăl) [″ + ″ + *thele,* nipple] Within the epithelium or located between its cells.

**intrafebrile** [″ + *febris,* fever] During the febrile stage. SYN: *intrapyretic.*

**intrafilar** (ĭn-tră-fī′lăr) [″ + *filum,* thread] Within a network or reticulum.

**intragastric** [″ + Gr. *gaster,* belly] Within the stomach.

***i. balloon*** An inflatable device placed in the stomach in an uninflated state. Once in place, it is inflated. This method of treating obesity has not been effective on a long-term basis.

**intragemmal** (ĭn″tră-jĕm′ăl) [″ + *gemma,* bud] Within a bud or the expanded ending of a nerve, as a taste bud.

**intraglandular** [″ + *glans,* acorn] Within a gland.

**intragyral** (ĭn″tră-jī′răl) [″ + Gr. *gyros,* circle] Within a gyrus of the brain.

**intrahepatic** (ĭn″tră-hĕ-păt′ĭk) [″+ Gr. *hepatikos,* pert. to the liver] Within the liver.

**intraintestinal** [″ + *intestinum,* intestine] Within the intestine.

**intralaryngeal** (ĭn″tră-lă-rĭn′jē-ăl) [″ + Gr. *larynx,* larynx] Within the larynx.

**intralesional** (ĭn″tră-lē′zhŭn-ăl) [″ + *laesio,* a wound] Within a lesion.

**intraligamentary** [″ + *ligamentum,* a binding] Within the leaves of a ligament; usually used in referring to fibroid tumors or cysts of the ovary that have grown within the broad ligament.

**intraligamentous** Within a ligament.

**intralingual** Within the tongue.

**intralobar** (ĭn″tră-lō′băr) [″ + *lobus,* a lobe] Within a lobe.

**intralobular** (ĭn″tră-lŏb′ū-lăr) [″ + *lobulus,* a lobule] Within a lobule.

**intralocular** (ĭn″tră-lŏk′ū-lăr) [″+ *loculus,* a cavity] Within the cavity of any structure.

**intralumbar** [″ + *lumbus,* loin] Within the lumbar region or portion of the spinal cord.

**intraluminal** (ĭn″tră-lū′mĭ-năl) [″ + *lumen,* light] Intratubal.

**intramastoiditis** (ĭn″tră-măs″tŏyd-ī′tĭs) [″ + Gr. *mastos,* breast, + *eidos,* form, shape, + *itis,* inflammation] An inflammation of the antrum and mastoid process. SYN: *endomastoiditis.*

**intramedullary** (ĭn″tră-mĕd′ū-lār″ē) [″ + *medullaris,* marrow] **1.** Within the medulla oblongata of the brain. **2.** Within the spinal cord. **3.** Within the marrow cavity of a bone.

**intramural** [″ + *murus,* a wall] Within the walls of a hollow organ or cavity.

**intramuscular** [″ + *musculus,* a muscle] ABBR: IM. Within a muscle.

**intranasal** [″ + *nasus,* nose] Within the nasal cavity.

**intranatal** [″ + *natalis,* birth] Occurring during birth.

**intraocular** [″ + *oculus,* eye] Within the eyeball.

**intraoperative** (ĭn″tră-ŏp′ĕr-ă″tĭv) [L. *intra,* within, + *operativus,* working] Occurring during surgery.

**intraoral** [″ + *oralis,* pert. to the mouth] Within the mouth.

**intraorbital** [″ + *orbita,* mark of a wheel] Within the orbit.

**intraosseous** (ĭn″tră-ŏs′ē-ŭs) [″ + *os,* bone] Within the bone substance.

**intraosseous infusion** The emergency infusion of fluids, blood, or medications, when intravenous access is not available, into the tibia in young children. SEE: illus.

**intraovarian** (ĭn″tră-ō-vā′rē-ăn) [″ + *ovarium,* ovary] Within the ovary.

**intraparietal** (ĭn″tră-pă-rī′ĕ-tăl) [″ + *paries,* wall] **1.** Within the parietal lobe of the cerebrum. **2.** Intramural.

**intrapartal** The period from the onset of labor to its termination, marked by delivery of the placenta.

**intrapartum** (ĭn″tră-păr′tŭm) [″ + *partus,* birth] Happening during childbirth.

**intrapelvic** (ĭn″tră-pĕl′vĭk) [″ + *pelvis,* basin] Within the pelvis.

**intraperitoneal** [″ + Gr. *peritonaion,* peritoneum] Within the peritoneal cavity.

**intraplacental** (ĭn″tră-plă-sĕn′tăl) [″ + *placenta,* a flat cake] Within the placenta.

**intrapleural** [″ + Gr. *pleura,* rib] Within the pleural cavity.

**intrapontine** (ĭn″tră-pŏn′tĭn) [″ + *pons,* bridge] Within the pons varolii.

**intrapsychic, intrapsychical** (ĭn″tră-sī′kĭk, -kĭ-kăl) [″ + Gr. *psyche,* mind] Having a mental origin or basis, such as conflicts

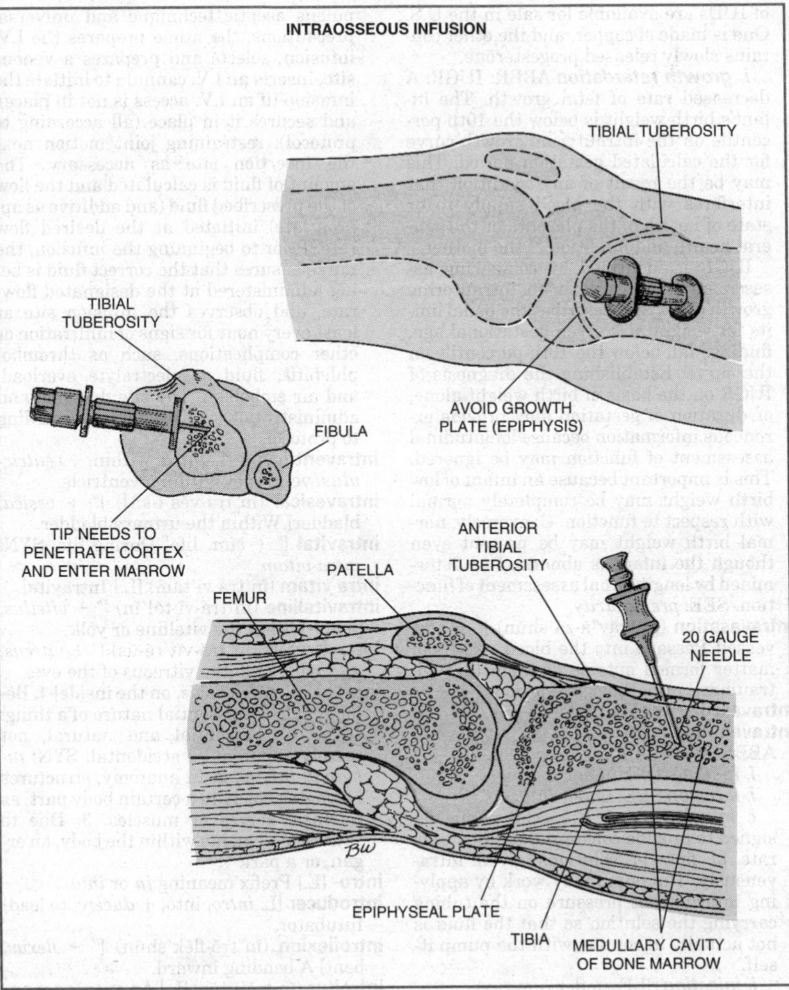


and complexes.

**intrapulmonary** [″ + *pulmo,* lung] Within the lung substance.

**intrapyretic** (ĭn″tră-pī-rĕt′ĭk) [″ + Gr. *pyretos,* fever] Intrafebrile.

**intrarectal** (ĭn″tră-rĕk′tăl) [″ + *rectum,* straight] Within the rectum.

**intrarenal** (ĭn″tră-rē′năl) [″ + *renalis,* pert. to the kidney] Within the kidney.

**intraretinal** (ĭn″tră-rĕt′ĭ-năl) [″ + *retina,* retina] Within the retina of the eye.

**intrascrotal** (ĭn″tră-skrō′tăl) [″ + *scrotum,* a bag] Within the scrotum.

**intraspinal** [L. *intra,* within, + *spina,* thorn] **1.** Ensheathed; within a sheath. **2.** Within the spinal canal.

**intrathecal** (ĭn″tră-thē′kăl) [″ + Gr. *theke,* sheath] **1.** Within the spinal canal. **2.** Within a sheath.

**intrathoracic** (ĭn″tră-thō-răs′ĭk) [″ + Gr. *thorax,* chest] Within the thorax.

**intratracheal** (ĭn″tră-trāk′ē-ăl) [″ + Gr. *tracheia,* trachea] Introduced into, or inside, the trachea.

**intratubal** [″ + *tubus,* hollow tube] Within a tube, esp. the fallopian tube. SYN: *intraluminal.*

**intratympanic** (ĭn″tră-tĭm-păn′ĭk) [″ + Gr. *tympanon,* drum] Within the tympanic cavity.

**intrauterine** (ĭn″tră-ū′tĕr-ĭn) [″ + *uterus,* womb] Within the uterus.

***i. contraceptive device*** ABBR: IUCD or IUD. A device made in a variety of shapes and from several different materials, including plastic and copper, and placed in the uterus for a prolonged period of time to prevent conception. Because of undesired side effects, the use of IUDs in the U.S. has declined. Two types of IUDs are available for sale in the U.S. One is made of copper, and the other contains slowly released progesterone.

***i. growth retardation*** ABBR: IUGR. A decreased rate of fetal growth. The infant's birth weight is below the 10th percentile on the intrauterine growth curve for the calculated gestation period. This may be the result of any condition that interferes with the blood supply to or state of health of the placenta or the general health and nutrition of the mother.

IUGR is identified by comparing assessment findings with an intrauterine growth chart that describes the usual limits for weight at a given gestational age; findings fall below the 10th percentile on the curve. Establishing the diagnosis of IUGR on the basis of birth weight alone, or duration of gestation may provide erroneous information because longitudinal assessment of function may be ignored. This is important because an infant of low birth weight may be completely normal with respect to function. Conversely, normal birth weight may be present even though the infant is abnormal as determined by longitudinal assessment of function. SEE: *prematurity*.

**intravasation** (ĭn-trăv″ă-zā′shŭn) [″ + *vas,* vessel] Passage into the blood vessels of matter formed outside of them through traumatic or pathological lesions.

**intravascular** Within blood vessels.

**intravenous** (ĭn-tră-vē′nŭs) [″ + *vena,* vein] ABBR: IV. Within or into a vein.

***i. feeding*** SEE: under *feeding*.

***i. infusion*** SEE: under *infusion*.

***i. infusion pump*** A special pump designed to provide constant but adjustable rate of flow of solutions given intravenously. The pump may work by applying intermittent pressure on the tubing carrying the solution so that the fluid is not actually in contact with the pump itself.

***i. injection*** SEE: under *injection*.

***i. treatment*** Intravenous injection or infusion. *Injection* is the use of a needle attached to a hypodermic syringe to instill a single dose of medicine. An *infusion* is the introduction of a solution in a larger quantity—250 to 500 ml by means of a bottle connected to the needle by a plastic or rubber tubing. The rate of infusion may be regulated by adjusting the number of drops per minute. Flow is usually by gravity but can be given under pressure.

---

Caution: Intravenous infusions should be discontinued or infusion fluid replenished when the bottle being administered is depleted. If this is not done, it is possible for air to be introduced into the bloodstream. Clotting of blood in the needle occurs when the infusion is not continuous.

---

NURSING IMPLICATIONS: Using scrupulous aseptic technique and universal precautions, the nurse prepares the I.V. infusion, selects and prepares a venous site, inserts an I.V. cannula to initiate the infusion (if an I.V. access is not in place), and secures it in place (all according to protocol), restraining joint motion near the insertion site as necessary. The amount of fluid is calculated and the flow of the prescribed fluid (and additive as appropriate) initiated at the desired flow rate. Prior to beginning the infusion, the nurse ensures that the correct fluid is being administered at the designated flowrate, and observes the infusion site at least every hour for signs of infiltration or other complications, such as thrombophlebitis, fluid or electrolyte overload, and air embolism. The site dressing and administration set are changed according to protocol.

**intraventricular** [L. *intra,* within, + *ventriculus,* ventricle] Within a ventricle.

**intravesical** (ĭn″tră-vĕs′ĭ-kăl) [″ + *vesica,* bladder] Within the urinary bladder.

**intravital** [″ + *vita,* life] During life. SYN: *intra vitam*.

**intra vitam** (ĭn′tră vī′tăm) [L.] Intravital.

**intravitelline** (ĭn″tră-vī-tĕl′ĭn) [″ + *vitellus,* yoke] Within the vitelline or yolk.

**intravitreous** (ĭn″tră-vĭt′rē-ŭs) [″ + *vitreus,* glassy] Within the vitreous of the eye.

**intrinsic** [L. *intrinsicus,* on the inside] **1.** Belonging to the essential nature of a thing. It is both essential and natural, not merely apparent or accidental. SYN: *inherent; innate*. **2.** In anatomy, structures belonging solely to a certain body part, as intrinsic nerves or muscles. **3.** Due to causes or elements within the body, an organ, or a part.

**intro-** [L.] Prefix meaning *in* or *into*.

**introducer** [L. *intro,* into, + *ducere,* to lead] Intubator.

**introflexion** (ĭn″trō-flĕk′shŭn) [″ + *flexus,* bent] A bending inward.

**introitus** (ĭn-trō′ĭ-tŭs) [L.] An opening or entrance into a canal or cavity, as the vagina.

***i. canalis sacralis*** The terminal opening of the spinal canal at the end of the sacrum.

***i. laryngis*** The upper opening of the larynx.

***i. vaginae*** The exterior orifice of the vagina.

**introjection** [″ + *jacere,* to throw] In psychoanalysis, identification of the self with another or with some object, the victim assuming the supposed feelings of the other personality.

**intromission** (ĭn″trō-mĭsh′ŭn) [″ + *mittere,* to send] An insertion or placing of one part into another, esp. insertion of the penis into the vagina.

**intromittent** (ĭn-trō-mĭt′ĕnt) Conveying or injecting into a cavity or body.

**intron** The noncoding space between the discrete coding regions (exons) of the

DNA of the gene.

**introspection** [″ + *spicere,* to look] Looking within, esp. examination of one's own mind.

**introsusception** (ĭn″trō-sŭ-sĕp′shŭn) [″ + *suscipere,* to receive] Intussusception.

**introversion** (ĭn″trō-vĕr′shŭn) [″ + *versio,* a turning] **1.** Turning inside out of a part or organ. **2.** The condition of an introvert; preoccupation with one's self.

**introvert 1.** A personality-reaction type characterized by withdrawal from reality, fantasy formation, and stress on the subjective side of life adjustments, seen pathologically in extreme form in schizophrenia. **2.** To turn one's psychic energy inward upon oneself.

**intubate** (ĭn′tū-bāt) [L. *in,* into, + *tuba,* a tube] To insert a tube in a part, esp. the larynx. SEE: *catheterization.*

**intubation** (ĭn″tū-bā′shŭn) The insertion of a tube into any hollow organ, as into the larynx or trachea through the glottis for entrance of air, or to dilate a stricture.

POSITION: The patient, who is usually anesthetized, should be placed so that body, neck, and head are kept aligned. Neck hyperextension may aid in endotracheal intubation.

***endotracheal i.*** The insertion of an endotracheal tube through the nose or mouth into the trachea to maintain the airway, to administer an anesthetic gas or oxygen, or to aspirate secretions.

***nasogastric i.*** SEE: *gastric lavage.*

***nasotracheal i.*** The insertion of an endotracheal tube through the nose and into the trachea. Unlike orotracheal intubation, the tube is passed "blindly" without using a laryngoscope to visualize the glottic opening. Because this technique may be used without hyperextension, it is useful when the patient has cervical spinal trauma and with patients who have clenched teeth. SEE: *endotracheal i.*

**intubator** A device for controlling, directing, and placing an intubation tube within the trachea, blood vessel, or heart (as in Swan-Ganz catheter placement). SYN: *introducer.*

**intuition** Knowing something without going through a rational process of thinking.

**intumesce** (ĭn-tū-mĕs′) [L. *intumescere*] To enlarge or swell.

**intumescence 1.** A swelling. **2.** The process of enlarging. SYN: *tumefaction.*

**intumescent** (ĭn-tū-mĕs′ĕnt) Swelling or becoming enlarged.

**intussusception** (ĭn″tŭ-sŭ-sĕp′shŭn) [L. *intus,* within, + *suscipere,* to receive] The slipping of one part of an intestine into another part just below it; becoming ensheathed. It is noted chiefly in children and usually occurs in the ileocecal region. Prognosis is good if surgery is performed immediately; but mortality is high if this condition is left untreated more than 24 hours. SYN: *introsusception; invagination.* SEE: *ileus.*

**intussusceptum** (ĭn″tŭ-sŭ-sĕp′tŭm) [L.] The inner segment of intestine that has been pushed into another segment.

**intussuscipiens** (ĭn″tŭ-sŭ-sĭp′ē-ĕns) [L.] The portion of intestine that receives the intussusceptum.

**Inuit** [Eskimo people] People native to Arctic America.

**inulase** (ĭn′ū-lās) An enzyme that converts inulin to levulose.

**inulin** A polysaccharide found in plants that yields levulose when hydrolyzed. It is used to study renal function.

**inunction** (ĭn-ŭngk′shŭn) [L. *in,* into, + *unguere,* to anoint] An ointment or medicated substance rubbed into the skin to secure a local or a more general systemic effect.

**in utero** (ĭn ū′tĕr-ō) [L.] Within the uterus.

**in vacuo** (ĭn văk′ū-ō) [L.] Within a cavity or a space from which air has been exhausted.

**invaginate** (ĭn-văj′ĭn-āt) [L. *invaginatio*] **1.** To ensheath. **2.** To insert one part of a structure within a part of the same structure. **3.** In embryology, to grow in or from an ingrowth or inpocketing, esp. the ingrowth of the wall of the blastula, which results in the formation of the gastrula.

**invaginated** Enclosed in a sheath; ensheathed.

**invagination** Intussusception.

**invalid** [L. *in-,* not, + *validus,* strong] **1.** Not well; weak. **2.** A sickly person, particularly one confined to a bed or wheelchair.

**invasion** [L. *in,* into, + *vadere,* to go] **1.** The period of a disease that follows the entrance of infective organisms and precedes the appearance of symptoms. **2.** The entrance of bacteria or other infectious organisms into the body and their distribution to the tissues.

**invasive** Tending to spread, esp. the tendency of a malignant process or growth to spread into healthy tissue.

***i. procedure*** A procedure in which the body cavity is entered (e.g., by use of a tube, needle, device, or even ionizing radiation) or any other invasion that could interfere with bodily function.

**inventory** Any list of items, esp. items to describe an individual's personality.

**invermination** [″ + *vermis,* worm] Infestation by intestinal worms.

**inversion** (ĭn-vĕr′zhŭn) [L. *inversio,* to turn inward] **1.** The reversal of a normal relationship. **2.** A turning inside out of an organ (e.g., the uterus). **3.** In chemistry, the process of converting sucrose (which rotates the plane of polarized light to the right) into a mixture of dextrose and levulose (which rotates the plane to the left). The resulting mixture is called invert sugar, and the enzyme that catalyzes this conversion is called invertase. SEE: *enzyme.*

***uterine i.*** A condition in which the uterus is turned inside out so that the internal surface protrudes into the vagina or beyond it.

**invert** (ĭn-vĕrt′) To turn inside out or upside down.

**invertase** (ĭn-vĕr′tās) An enzyme that changes a disaccharide into a monosaccharide, such as cane sugar into invert sugar. SYN: *invertin; sucrase; zymose.*

**invertebrate** [L. *in-*, not, + *vertebratus*, vertebrate] **1.** Without a backbone. **2.** Species of animals that do not have a backbone.

**invertin** (ĭn-vĕr′tĭn) Invertase.

**invertor** (ĭn-vĕr′tor) A muscle that rotates a part inward.

**investing** [L. *in*, into, + *vestire*, to clothe] **1.** Ensheathing, encircling with a sheath or coating, as tissue; surrounding. **2.** In dentistry, the complete or partial covering of an object (e.g., a tooth, denture, wax form, or crown) with a suitable material before processing, soldering, or casting.

**investment** A covering or sheath.

***dental casting i.*** A material combining principally a form of silica and a bonding agent. The bonding substance may be gypsum or silica phosphate according to the casting temperature.

**inveterate** [″ + *vetus*, old] Chronic; firmly seated, as a disease or a habit.

**inviscation** (ĭn″vĭs-kā′shŭn) [L. *in*, among, + *viscum*, slime] The mixing of saliva with food during chewing.

**in vitro** (ĭn vē′trō) [L., in glass] In glass, as in a test tube. An in vitro test is one done in the laboratory, usually involving isolated tissue, organ, or cell preparations. SEE: *in vivo.*

**in vivo** (ĭn vē′vō) [L., in the living body] In the living body or organism. An in vivo test is one performed on a living organism. SEE: *in vitro.*

**involucre, involucrum** (ĭn′vō-lū″kĕr, ĭn″vō-lū′krŭm) [″ + *volvere*, to wrap] **1.** A sheath or covering. **2.** The covering of newly formed bone enveloping the sequestrum in infection of the bone.

**involuntary** [L. *in-*, not, + *voluntas*, will] Independent of or even contrary to volition.

**involution** (ĭn″vō-lū′shŭn) [″ + *volvere*, to roll] **1.** A turning or rolling inward. **2.** The reduction in size of the uterus after childbirth. **3.** The retrogressive change in vital processes after their functions have been fulfilled, such as the change that follows the menopause. **4.** A backward change. **5.** The diminishing of an organ in vital power or in size. **6.** In bacteriology, digression from the usual morphological type such as occurs in certain bacteria, esp. when grown under unfavorable conditions; degeneration.

***i. of uterus*** The return of the uterus to normal size after childbirth.

***senile i.*** The atrophy of an organ or part from old age.

**involutional** (ĭn-vō-lū′shŭn-ăl) Concerning involution or a turning inward.

**Io** Symbol for the element ionium.

**iocetamic acid** A radiopaque agent used in certain radiographical studies. Trade name is Cholebrine.

**Iodamoeba** (ī″ō-dă-mē′bă) A genus of amebas found in the intestinal tract. Their cysts are peculiar in that they are shaped irregularly, the nucleus usually is single, and they possess a vacuole filled with glycogen that stains brown in iodine.

***I. bütschlii*** A small, sluggish ameba found in the large intestine of humans, as well as in monkeys and pigs. It is usually nonpathogenic.

**iodide** (ī′ō-dīd) A compound of iodine containing another radical or element, as potassium iodide.

***cesium i.*** A phosphor used in radiographical image intensifiers that emits light when struck by radiation.

***sodium i. I 125 solution*** A standardized solution of radioactive iodide, $^{125}$I.

**iodinate** (ī-ō′dĭ-nāt) To combine with iodine.

**iodinated I 131 albumin injection** A standardized preparation of albumin iodinated with the use of radioactive iodine, $^{131}$I.

**iodine** (ī′ō-dīn, ī′ō-dēn) [Gr. *ioeides*, violet colored] SYMB: I. A nonmetallic element belonging to the halogen group; atomic weight 126.904; atomic number 53; specific gravity (solid, 20°C) 4.93. It is a black crystalline substance with a melting point of 113.5°C; it boils at 184.4°C, giving off a characteristic violet vapor. Sources of iodine include vegetables, esp. those growing near the seacoast; iodized salt; and seafoods, esp. liver of halibut and cod, or fish liver oils.

FUNCTION: Iodine is part of the hormones triiodothyronine ($T_3$) and thyroxine ($T_4$), and prevents goiter by enabling the thyroid gland to function normally. The amount of iodine in the entire body averages 50 mg, of which 10 to 15 mg is found in the thyroid. The adult daily requirement for iodine is from 100 to 150 $\mu$g. Growing children, adolescents, pregnant women, and those under emotional strain need more than this amount of iodine.

DEFICIENCY SYMPTOMS: Iodine deficiency in the diet may lead to simple goiter characterized by thyroid enlargement and hypothyroidism. In young children, this deficiency may result in retardation of physical, sexual, and mental development, a condition called cretinism.

***i. poisoning*** SEE: *Poisons and Poisoning Appendix.*

***protein-bound i.*** Iodine that is attached to serum protein.

***radioactive i.*** SYMB: $^{131}$I. An isotope of iodine with an atomic weight of 131; used in diagnosis of thyroid disorders and in the treatment of toxic goiter and thyroid carcinoma.

***tincture of i.*** A solution of 2% iodine and 2.4% sodium iodide diluted in 50% ethyl alcohol. It is used as a disinfectant for the skin and as a germicide. It may be used to make contaminated water safe for drinking. Adding three drops of tincture of iodine to a quart of water will kill amebas and bacteria within 30 minutes, and the water will still be palatable. If water to be treated by this method is cloudy or turbid, it should be allowed to settle; then the clear portion should be decanted and treated with iodine.

**iodinophilous** (ī″ō-dĭn-ŏf′ĭ-lŭs) [Gr. *ioeides,* violet colored, + *philos,* love] Easily stained with iodine.

**iodipamide meglumine injection** A combination of iodipamide and meglumine used to aid in x-ray examination of the gallbladder. Trade name is Cholografin Meglumine.

**iodipamide sodium I 131** Radioactive chemical used in examining body organs and cavities. Trade name is RadioCholografin.

**iodism** (ī′ō-dĭzm) A condition induced by prolonged and excessive use of iodine or its compounds.

**iodize** To administer or impregnate with iodine.

**5-iodo-2′-deoxyuridine** ABBR: IDU. Idoxuridine.

**iododerma** (ī-ō″dō-dĕr′mă) [″ + *derma,* skin] Dermatitis due to iodine.

**iodoform** (ī-ō′dō-form) [Gr. *ioeides,* violet colored, + L. *forma,* form] $CHI_3$. A yellow crystalline substance with a disagreeable odor, produced by the action of iodine on acetone in the presence of an alkali. Used topically, it has mild antibacterial action.

**iodoformism** (ī′ō-dō-form″ĭzm) [″ + ″+ Gr. *-ismos,* state of] Poisoning caused by iodoform.

**iodoglobulin** (ī″ō-dō-glŏb′ū-lĭn) [″ + L. *globus,* globe] A globulin protein that contains iodine.

**iodohippurate sodium I 131 injection** (ī-ō″dō-hĭp′ū-rāt) A radioactive dye used in testing renal function. Trade name is Hippuran I 131.

**iodophilia** (ī″ō-dō-fĭl′ē-ă) [″ + *philein,* to love] A condition in which certain cells, esp. polymorphonuclear leukocytes, when stained, show a pronounced affinity for iodine. These cells turn a brownish-red color. It is seen in pathologic conditions such as acute infections and anemia.

***extracellular i.*** Iodophilia in which substances in the plasma outside the cells are colored.

***intracellular i.*** Iodophilia in which color changes occur within the cells.

**iodophor** (ī-ō′dō-for) A combination of iodine and a solubilizing agent or carrier that liberates free iodine in solution. Some forms are used as general antiseptics; they are less irritating than elemental forms of iodine. SEE: *povidone-iodine.*

**iodopsin** In cones of the retina, the photopsin molecule and retinal, the functional photopigment.

**iodopyracet** (ī-ō″dō-pī′ră-sĕt) A radiopaque medium used in intravenous pyelography and urography. Trade name is Diodrast.

**iodoquinol** (ī-ō″dō-kwĭn′ŏl) $C_9H_5I_2NO$. An antiamebic agent used in the treatment of amebiasis and *Trichomonas hominis* infection of the intestines. Its previously used name was diiodohydroxyquin. Trade name is Yodoxin. Outside the U.S. this drug is sold under several names.

---

Caution: The use of this drug has been associated with production of a severe disease of the central nervous system called subacute myelo-optic neuropathy.

---

**iodotherapy** [Gr. *ioeides,* violet colored, + *therapeia,* treatment] The use of iodine medication, as in treating goiter due to iodine deficiency.

**IOML** *infraorbitomeatal line;* a line through the infraorbital margin and the external auditory meatus.

**ion** [Gr. *ion,* going] An atom or group of atoms that has lost one or more electrons and has a positive charge, or has gained one or more electrons and has a negative charge. In aqueous solutions, ions are called electrolytes because they permit the solution to conduct electricity. Positive ions such as sodium, potassium, magnesium, and calcium are called cations; negative ions such as chloride, bicarbonate, and sulfate are called anions. In body fluids, ions are available for reactions (e.g., calcium ions from food may be combined with carbonate ions to form calcium carbonate, part of bone matrix). SEE: *electrolyte* for table.

Ions occur in gases, esp. at low pressures, under the influence of strong electrical discharges, x-rays, and radium; in solutions of acids, bases, and salts.

***dipolar i.*** An ion that contains both positive and negative charges.

***hydrogen i.*** A hydrogen atom that has lost an electron. It has a positive charge, and its symbol is $H^+$.

**ion-exchange resins** Synthetic organic substances of high molecular weight. They replace certain negative or positive ions that they encounter in solutions.

**ionic** [Gr. *ion,* going] Pert. to ions.

**ionium** (ī-ō′nē-ŭm) A natural radioactive isotope of thorium. It has a mass number of 230.

**ionization** The dissociation of compounds (acids, bases, salts) into their constituent ions.

**ionize** To separate into ions; ionization.

**ionogen** (ī-ŏn′ō-jĕn) [Gr. *ion,* going, + *gennan,* to produce] Anything that can be ionized.

**ionophore** A chemical material that has a high affinity for ions. Ionophores are used in ion-selective electrode (ISE) membranes.

**ionotherapy** (ī″ŏn-ō-thĕr′ă-pē) [″ + *therapeia,* treatment] Iontophoresis.

**iontophoresis** (ī-ŏn″tō-fō-rē′sĭs) [″ + *phorein,* to carry] **1.** The process of electric current traveling through a salt solution, causing migration of the metal (positive) ion to the negative pole and the radical (negative) ion to the positive pole. **2.** The introduction of various ions into tissues through the skin by means of electricity. SYN: *ionic medication; ionotherapy; iontotherapy*. SEE: *electrical patch.*

**iontoradiometer** (ī-ŏn″tō-rā″dē-ŏm′ĭ-tĕr) [″ + L. *radius,* ray, + Gr. *metron,* measure] An instrument for measuring the amount and intensity of roentgen rays.

**iontotherapy** (ī-ŏn″tō-thĕr′ă-pē) [″ + *therapeia,* treatment] Iontophoresis.

**IOP** *intraocular pressure.*

**iopanoic acid** A radiopaque dye used in radiographic studies of the gallbladder.

**iophendylate** (ī″ō-fĕn′dĭ-lāt) A radiopaque material used in myelography.

**iophobia** (ī″ō-fō′bē-ă) [Gr. *ios,* poison, + *phobos,* fear] **1.** Toxicophobia. **2.** Fear of touching any rusty object.

**iotacism** (ī-ō′tă-sĭzm) [Gr. *iota,* letter i] Defective utterance marked by the constant substitution of an ē sound (Greek iota) for other vowels.

**iothalamate meglumine injection** (ī-ō-thăl′ă-māt) A radiopaque material used in investigating arteries of the brain as well as in the rest of the body, and in studying kidney function.

**I.P.** *intraperitoneal; isoelectric point.*

**ipecac** (ĭp′ĕ-kăk) The dried root of the plant ipecacuanha, grown in Brazil. It is the source of emetine and is used as an emetic. SEE: *Poisons and Poisoning Appendix.*

**I.P.L.** *interpupillary line;* the line between the center of both pupils.

**ipodate calcium** (ī′pō-dāt) A radiopaque material used in radiographical studies of the gallbladder.

**ipodate sodium** A radiopaque material used in radiographical studies of the gallbladder.

**IPPB** *intermittent positive-pressure breathing.*

**IPPV** *intermittent positive-pressure ventilation.*

**ipratropium bromide** An anticholinergic administered by inhalation, used in treating asthma.

**iproniazid** (ī″prō-nī′ă-zĭd) An antitubercular drug.

**ipsi-** [L. *ipse,* same] Combining form meaning *the same.*

**IPSID** *immunoproliferative small intestinal disease.*

**ipsilateral** (ĭp″sĭ-lăt′ĕr-ăl) [″ + *latus,* side] On the same side; affecting the same side of the body; the opposite of crossed, contralateral. For example, when the right patellar tendon is tapped, an ipsilateral knee-jerk is observed on the same side. In paralysis, this term is used to describe findings appearing on same side of the body as the brain or spinal cord lesion producing them. SYN: *homolateral.*

**IPSP** *inhibitory postsynaptic potential.*

**IQ** *intelligence quotient.*

**IR** *infrared.*

**I.R.** *internal resistance.*

**Ir** Symbol for the element iridium.

**iralgia** (ĭr-ăl′jē-ă) [Gr. *iris,* colored circle, + *algos,* pain] Iridalgia.

**irascible** (ĭ-răs′ĭ-b′l) [LL. *irascibilis*] Marked by outbursts of temper or irritability; easily angered.

**IRB** *institutional review board.*

**irid-** [Gr. *iridos,* colored circle] Combining form indicating relationship to the iris of the eye.

**iridadenosis** (ĭr″ĭd-ăd-ĭn-ō′sĭs) [L. *iris,* colored circle, + Gr. *aden,* gland, + *osis,* condition] A glandular infection of the iris.

**iridal** (ī′rĭd-ăl) Iridic.

**iridalgia** (ī″rĭd-ăl′jē-ă) [″ + *algos,* pain] Pain felt in the iris. SYN: *iralgia.*

**iridectome** (ĭr″ĭ-dĕk′tōm) [″ + *tome,* incision] An instrument for cutting the iris in iridectomy.

**iridectomesodialysis** (ĭr″ĭ-dĕk″tō-mēs″ō-dī-ăl′ĭ-sĭs) [″ + *ektome,* excision, + *mesos,* middle, + *dialysis,* loosening] The formation of an artificial pupil, by separating adhesions on the inner margin of the iris.

**iridectomize** (ĭr″ĭd-ĕk′tō-mīz) [″ + *ektome,* excision] To excise a portion of the iris.

**iridectomy** The surgical removal of a portion of the iris.

***optical i.*** Iridectomy performed to make an artificial pupil.

**iridectropium** (ĭr-ĭ-dĕk-trō′pē-ŭm) [″ + *ektrope,* a turning aside] Partial eversion of the iris.

**iridemia** (ĭr-ĭ-dē′mē-ă) [″ + *haima,* blood] Bleeding from the iris.

**iridencleisis** (ĭr″ĭ-dĕn-klī′sĭs) [″ + *enklein,* to lock in] An operation for relieving increased intraocular pressure, as in glaucoma, in which the iris and a portion of the limbus are excised to allow increased volume of the aqueous humor under the conjunctiva.

**iridentropium** (ĭr″ĭ-dĕn-trō′pē-ŭm) [″ + *en,* in, + *tropein,* to turn] Partial inversion of the iris.

**irideremia** (ĭr″ĭd-ĕr-ē′mē-ă) [″ + *eremia,* lack] Aniridia.

**irides** (ĭr′ĭ-dēz) [Gr.] Plural of iris.

**iridescence** (ĭr″ĭ-dĕs′ĕns) [L. *iridescere,* to gleam like a rainbow] Having the capability to disperse light into the colors of the spectrum.

**iridesis** (ĭ-rĭd′ĕ-sĭs) [″ + *desis,* a binding] Repositioning the pupil by bringing a portion of the iris through an incision in the cornea. SYN: *iridodesis.*

**iridic** (ĭ-rĭd′ĭk) [Gr. *iris,* colored circle] Relating to the iris. SYN: *iridal; iritic.*

**iridium** (ī-rĭd′ē-ŭm) [Gr. *iris,* colored circle] SYMB: Ir. A white, hard metallic element; atomic weight, 192.2; atomic weight 77.

**irido-** [Gr. *iridos,* colored circle] Combining form pert. to the iris.

**iridoavulsion** (ĭr″ĭ-dō-ăv-ŭl′shŭn) [″ + L. *avulsio,* a pulling away from] A tearing away of the iris.

**iridocapsulitis** (ĭr″ĭd-ō-kăp-sū-lī′tĭs) [″ + L. *capsula,* little box, + Gr. *itis,* inflammation] Iritis with inflammation of the capsule of the lens.

**iridocele** (ī-rĭd′ō-sēl) [″ + *kele,* tumor, swelling] Protrusion of a portion of the iris through a defect in the cornea.

**iridochorioiditis, iridochoroiditis** (ĭr″ĭ-dō-kō″rē-oy-dī′tĭs, ĭr″ĭ-dō-kō-roy-dī′tĭs) [″ + *chorioeides,* skinlike, + *itis,* inflammation] An inflammation of both iris and choroid.

**iridocoloboma** (ĭr″ĭd-ō-kŏl″ō-bō′mă) [″ + *koloboma,* mutilation] Congenital defect or fissure of the iris.

**iridoconstrictor** (ĭr″ĭ-dō-kŏn-strĭk′tor) A muscle or drug that acts to constrict the pupil of the eye.

**iridocyclectomy** (ĭr″ĭ-dō-sī-klĕk′tō-mē) [″ + *kyklos,* circle, + *ektome,* excision] Surgical removal of the iris and ciliary body.

**iridocyclitis** (ĭr″ĭd-ō-sī-klī′tĭs) [″ + ″ + *itis,* inflammation] An inflammation of the iris and ciliary body.

***heterochromic i.*** An inflammation of the iris that leads to depigmentation.

**iridocyclochoroiditis** (ĭr″ĭ-dō-sī″klō-kō″roy-dī′tĭs) [″ + ″ + *chorioeides,* skinlike, + *itis,* inflammation] An inflammation of the iris, ciliary body, and choroid of the eye.

**iridocystectomy** (ĭr″ĭ-dō-sĭs-tĕk′tō-mē) [″ + *kystis,* bladder, + *ektome,* excision] Surgical removal of a cyst from the iris.

**iridodesis** (ĭr-ĭ-dŏd′ĕ-sĭs) [″ + *desis,* a binding] Iridesis.

**iridodiagnosis** [″ + *dia,* through, + *gnosis,* knowledge] Diagnosis of disease by examination of the iris.

**iridodialysis** (ĭr″ĭd-ō-dī-ăl′ĭ-sĭs) [″ + *dialysis,* loosening] Separation of the outer margin of the iris from its ciliary attachment.

**iridodilator** [″ + L. *dilatare,* to dilate] A substance causing dilatation of the pupil.

**iridodonesis** (ĭr″ĭd-ō-dō-nē′sĭs) [″ + *donesis,* tremor] Hippus.

**iridokeratitis** (ĭr″ĭ-dō-kĕr″ă-tī′tĭs) [″ + *keras,* horn, + *itis,* inflammation] An inflammation of the iris and cornea.

**iridokinesis** (ĭr″ĭd-ō-kĭn-ē′sĭs) [Gr. *iridos,* colored circle, + *kinesis,* movement] The contracting and expanding movements of the iris.

**iridoleptynsis** (ĭr″ĭ-dō-lĕp-tĭn′sĭs) [″ + *leptynsis,* attenuation] Thinning or atrophy of the iris.

**iridology** (ĭr″ĭ-dŏl′ō-jē) [″ + *logos,* word, reason] The study of changes in the iris during the course of a disease.

**iridomalacia** (ĭr″ĭd-ō-mă-lā′shē-ă) [″ + *malakia,* softness] A softening of the iris.

**iridomedialysis** (ĭr″ĭd-ō-mē-dē-ăl′ĭ-sĭs) [″ + L. *medius,* in middle, + Gr. *dialysis,* loosening] A separation of the inner marginal adhesions of the iris. SYN: *iridomesodialysis.*

**iridomesodialysis** (ĭr″ĭd-ō-mĕs″ō-dī-ăl′ĭ-sĭs) [″ + *mesos,* middle, + *dialysis,* loosening] Iridomedialysis.

**iridomotor** [″ + L. *motor,* that which moves] Relating to movements of the iris.

**iridoncus** (ĭr-ĭ-dong′kŭs) [″ + *onkos,* bulk] Swelling of the iris.

**iridoparalysis** [″ + *paralyein,* to disable] Iridoplegia.

**iridoparelkysis** (ĭr″ĭ-dō-păr-ĕl′kĭ-sĭs) [″ + *parelkysis,* protraction] Surgically induced prolapse of the iris in order to displace the pupil artificially.

**iridopathy** (ĭr″ĭ-dŏp′ă-thē) [″ + *pathos,* disease, suffering] Disease of the iris.

**iridoperiphacitis, iridoperiphakitis** (ĭr″ĭ-dō-pĕr″ĭ-fă-sī′tĭs, -pĕr″ĭ-fă-kī′tĭs) [″ + *peri,* around, + *phakos,* lens, + *itis,* inflammation] An inflammation of the iris and anterior portion of the capsule of the lens.

**iridoplegia** (ĭr″ĭd-ō-plē′jē-ă) [″ + *plege,* stroke] Paralysis of the sphincter of the iris. SYN: *iridoparalysis.*

***accommodative i.*** An inability of the iris to contract when stimulated by increased light intensity.

***complete i.*** Iridoplegia in which the iris fails to respond to any stimulation; seen in Adie's pupil.

***reflex i.*** The absence of light reflex, with retention of the accommodation reflex (Argyll Robertson pupil).

**iridoptosis** (ĭr″ĭ-dŏp-tō′sĭs) [″ + *ptosis,* a falling] Prolapse of the iris.

**iridopupillary** (ĭr″ĭ-dō-pū′pĭ-lĕr″ē) [″ + L. *pupilla,* pupil] Concerning the iris and the pupil of the eye.

**iridorrhexis** (ĭr″ĭd-ō-rĕk′sĭs) [″ + *rhexis,* rupture] Rupture of the iris, or a tearing of the iris away from its attachment.

**iridoschisis** (ĭr″ĭ-dŏs′kĭ-sĭs) [″ + *schisis,* a splitting] Separation of the stroma of the iris into two layers with disintegration of the anterior layer.

**iridosclerotomy** (ĭr″ĭd-ō-sklē-rŏt′ō-mē) [″ + *skleros,* hard, + *tome,* incision] Piercing of the sclera and the border of the iris.

**iridosteresis** (ĭr″ĭ-dō-stē-rē′sĭs) [″ + *steresis,* loss] Removal of the iris or a portion of it.

**iridotasis** (ĭr-ĭ-dŏt′ă-sĭs) [″ + *tasis,* a stretching] A stretching of the iris in the treatment of glaucoma.

**iridotomy** (ĭr-ĭ-dŏt′ō-mē) [″ + *tome,* incision] An incision of the iris without excising a portion, done for the purpose of making a new aperture in the iris when the pupil is closed. This is indicated in eyes that had been operated on for cataract but that have lost their sight through subsequent iridocyclitis. SYN: *iritomy; irotomy.*

**iris** [Gr.] The colored contractile membrane suspended between the lens and the cornea in the aqueous humor of the eye, separating the anterior and posterior chambers of the eyeball and perforated in the center by the pupil. By contraction and dilatation it regulates the amout of light that enters the eye. SEE: *aniridia; choroidoiritis; heterochromia iridis; irid-; iris, chromatic asymmetry of; rubeosis iridis.*

ANATOMY: The free inner edge rests on the lens when the pupil is constricted or partially dilated. The iris contains two sets of smooth muscle fibers, the sphincter pupillae (circular fibers), about 1 mm wide; and the dilator pupillae (meridionally arranged fibers), extending from the sphincter pupillae to the outer edge of the iris. The former, supplied through the oculomotor nerve with parasympathetic fibers derived from the ciliary ganglion, constricts the pupil; the latter, supplied by sympathetic fibers from the superior cervical ganglion, dilates the pupil. The color of the iris depends on the pigment in the stroma cells and in the cells of the retinal layers. However, the color may change due to some medications.

***i. bombé*** A condition seen in annular posterior synechia. The iris is bulged forward by the pressure of the aqueous humor, which cannot reach the anterior chamber.

***chromatic asymmetry of i.*** A difference in color between the two irides (heterochromia). For example, one may be blue or gray and the other brown. The asymmetry may occur in early iritis or cyclitis, or may be present without an associated pathological process.

***piebald i.*** A dark discoloration in an irregularly shaped area. It may be in one or both eyes.

**Irish moss** Carrageen.

**irisopsia** (ī″rĭs-ŏp′sē-ă) [Gr. *iris,* colored circle, + *opsis,* vision] A visual defect in which colored circles are seen around lights.

**iritic** (ĭ-rĭt′ĭk) [Gr. *iris,* colored circle] Iridic.

**iritis** [″ + *itis,* inflammation] An inflammation of the iris.

SYMPTOMS: In iritis, there are pain, photophobia, lacrimation, and diminution of vision. The iris appears swollen, dull, and muddy; the pupil contracted, irregular, and sluggish in reaction.

TREATMENT: One percent atropine is used, as an ointment or in drop form, frequently enough to keep the pupil dilated. Cortisone or hydrocortisone is used systemically as well as topically. If the primary disease causing the iritis is known, it should be treated; however, the etiological factor is usually not known.

Caution: Corticosteroids should be prescribed only by an ophthalmologist.

***plastic i.*** Iritis in which the fibrinous exudate forms new tissue.

***purulent i.*** Iritis with a purulent exudate.

***secondary i.*** Iritis in which the inflammation has spread from neighboring parts, as in diseases of the cornea and sclera.

***serous i.*** Iritis in which serum forms the exudate.

**iritoectomy** (ī″rĭ-tō-ĕk′tō-mē) [″ + *ektome,* excision] In cataract treatment, excision of the part of the iris that is inflamed and occluding the pupil.

**iritomy** (ĭ-rĭt′ō-mē) [″ + *tome,* incision] Iridotomy.

**iron** (ī′ĕrn) [AS. *iren;* L. *ferrum*] SYMB: Fe. A metallic element widely distributed in nature; atomic weight 55.847, atomic number 26. Compounds (oxides, hydroxides, salts) exist in two forms: ferrous, in which iron has a valence of two ($Fe^{++}$), and ferric, in which it has a valence of three ($Fe^{+++}$). It is widely used in the treatment of certain forms of anemia. Iron is essential for the formation of chlorophyll in plants, although it is not a constituent of chlorophyll. It is part of the hemoglobin and myoglobin molecules. SEE: *ferritin.*

FUNCTION: Iron, as part of hemoglobin, is essential for the transport of oxygen in the blood; it is also part of some of the enzymes needed for cell respiration. Men's bodies have approx. 3.45 g of iron and women approx. 2.45 g, distributed as follows: 60% to 70% in hemoglobin; 10% to 12% in myoglobin and enzymes; and, as ferritin, 29% in men and 10% in women, stored in the liver, spleen, and bone marrow. Iron is stored in the tissues principally as ferritin. It is absorbed from the food in the small intestine and passes, in the blood, to the bone marrow. There, it is used in making hemoglobin, which is incorporated into the red corpuscles. A corpuscle, after circulating in the blood for approx. 120 days, is destroyed, and its iron is used over again.

Men require from 0.5 to 1.0 mg of iron a day. A woman of menstrual age requires about twice this amount. During pregnancy and lactation from 2 to 4 mg of iron per day is required. Before puberty and after menopause, women require no more iron than men. Because only a fraction of the iron present in food is absorbed, it is necessary to provide from 15 to 30 mg of iron in the diet to be certain that 1 to 4 mg will be absorbed.

In the first few months of life, infants will use up most of their iron stores, and the typical diet or formula may not have sufficient iron to replenish those stores. It is therefore important to add iron-containing foods to an infant's diet by age 6 months.

Manganese, copper, and cobalt are necessary for the proper use of iron. Copper is stored in the body and reused repeatedly.

There are two broad types of dietary iron. About 90% of iron from food is in the form of iron salts and is called nonheme iron, which is poorly absorbed. The other 10% of dietary iron is in the form of heme iron, which is derived primarily from the hemoglobin and myoglobin of meat and is well absorbed. Iron absorption is influenced by other dietary factors. About 50% of iron from breast milk is absorbed but only about 10% of iron in whole cow's milk is absorbed. The reasons for the higher bioavailability of iron in breast milk are unknown. Ascorbic acid, meat, fish, and poultry enhance absorption of nonheme iron. Bran, oxalates, vegetable fiber, tannins in tea, and phosphates inhibit absorption of iron. Orange juice doubles the absorption of iron from the meal and tea decreases it by 75%.

DEFICIENCY SYMPTOMS: Iron deficiency is characterized by anemia, lowered vitality, pale complexion, conjunctival pallor, retarded development, and a decreased amount of hemoglobin in each red cell.

NOTE: Sometimes a disturbance in iron metabolism occurs, in which an iron-containing pigment, hemosiderin, and hemofuscin are deposited in the tissues, leading to hemochromatosis. Excessive deposition of hemosiderin in the tissues, such as may occur as a result of excessive breakdown of red cells, is called hemosiderosis. SEE: *hemochromatosis*.

SOURCES: The following foods provide iron in the diet: almonds, asparagus, bran, beans, Boston brown bread, cauliflower, celery, chard, dandelions, egg yolk, graham bread, kidney, lettuce, liver, oatmeal, oysters, soybeans, and whole wheat. Other good sources are apricots, beets, beef, cabbage, cornmeal, cucumbers, currants, dates, duck, goose, greens, lamb, molasses, mushrooms, oranges, parsnips, peanuts, peas, peppers, potatoes, prunes, radishes, raisins, rhubarb, pineapple, tomatoes, and turnips.

**iron dextran injection** A preparation of iron suitable for parenteral use.

Caution: At the time of intravenous use, one or two drops are administered over a 5-minute period to determine whether any signs of anaphylaxis appear.

**iron lung** Drinker respirator.

**iron poisoning** SEE: under *poisoning*.

**iron sorbitex injection** A preparation of iron suitable for parenteral use.

**iron storage disease** Hemochromatosis.

**irotomy** (ī-rŏt′ō-mē) [Gr. *iris,* colored circle, + *tome,* incision] Iridotomy.

**irradiate** (ĭ-rā′dē-āt) [L. *in,* into, + *radiare,* to emit rays] **1.** To expose to radiation. **2.** To treat with high-energy x-rays or other forms of radiation. SEE: *irradiation.*

**irradiating** Diverging or spreading out from a common center.

**irradiation 1.** The diagnostic or therapeutic application of x-ray photons, nuclear particles, high-speed electrons, ultraviolet rays, or other forms of radiation to a patient. **2.** The application of a form of radiation to an object or substance to give it therapeutic value or increase that which it already has. **3.** A phenomenon in which a bright object on a dark background appears larger than a dark object of the same size on a bright background. **4.** The spreading in all directions from a common center (e.g., nerve impulses, the sensation of pain).

***interstitial i.*** Therapeutic irradiation by insertion into the tissues of capillary tubes or beads containing radon. It may be temporary or permanent.

***i. of reflexes*** The spread of a reflex to an increasing number of motor units upon increasing the strength of the stimulus.

**irrational** Contrary to what is reasonable or logical; used to describe behavior that cannot be explained by normal reasoning.

**irreducible** (ĭr″rē-dū′sĭ-bl) [L. *in-,* not, + *re,* back, + *ducere,* to lead] Not capable of being reduced or made smaller, as a fracture or dislocation.

**irreversible** Not being possible to reverse.

**irrigate** [L. *in,* into, + *rigare,* to carry water] To wash out with a fluid.

**irrigation** The cleansing of a canal by flushing with water or other fluids; the washing of a wound. The solutions used for cleansing should be sterile and have an approximate temperature slightly warmer than body temperature (100° to 115°F or 37.8° to 46.1°C). SYN: *lavage.* SEE: *gastric lavage.*

***bladder i.*** Washing out of the bladder to treat inflammation or infection or to maintain patency of a urinary catheter. The irrigation may be intermittent or continuous. Normal saline is commonly used.

NURSING IMPLICATIONS: The necessary sterile equipment and the prescribed irrigant are assembled. The patient is prepared physically and emotionally for the procedure: the procedure and expected sensations are explained, and emotional and physical warmth and security are provided by draping the patient to preserve privacy. A catheter is inserted into the urinary bladder according to protocol; placement is determined by onset of urinary drainage. The prescribed volume of irrigant is instilled by bulb syringe; the catheter clamped to allow the solution to remain in the bladder for the prescribed period of time; then the catheter is unclamped to allow the irrigant to flow out of the bladder by gravity drainage into a collecting basin. The irrigation is repeated the prescribed number of times, and the character of the irrigation solution returned and the presence of any mucus, blood, or other material visible in the drainage is noted and then the catheter removed. The time of the procedure, the type and volume of irrigant instilled, the type and volume of return, and the patient's response to the procedure are documented. If intermittent or continuous bladder irrigation is required, the nurse inserts a three-lumen indwelling catheter, in which the first lumen leads to the inflation balloon, the second lumen is for instillation of irrigating fluid, and the third lumen provides a channel to a closed drainage system.

***colonic i.*** Flushing of the colon with water. This procedure is done to wash out material in the colon and to cleanse the bowel as high as possible.

***continuous bladder i.*** ABBR: CBI. A constant flow of normal saline or another bladder irrigant through a three-way urinary catheter to keep the catheter patent. It is typically used postoperatively following a transurethral resection of the prostate gland.

**irrigator** A device with a hose attachment used to flush or wash a part or cavity with fluids.

**irritability** [L. *irritabilis,* irritable] **1.** Excitability. **2.** An ability to respond in a specific way to a change in environment, a property of all living tissue. **3.** A condition in which a person, organ, or a part responds excessively to a stimulus. **4.** A quick response to annoyance; impatience.

***muscular i.*** The normal response of muscle to a stimulus.

***nervous i.*** The response of a nerve to a stimulus.

**irritable 1.** Capable of reacting to a stimulus. **2.** Sensitive to stimuli.

**irritable bowel syndrome** SEE: under *syndrome.*

**irritant** An agent that, when used locally, produces a more or less local inflammatory reaction. Anything that induces or gives rise to irritation, such as iodine.

***i. poison*** One of a large number of poisons of great variety, not including the corrosive acids or alkalies. They cause pain in the mouth, esophagus, and stomach; nausea; vomiting; great thirst; abdominal cramping; bloody diarrhea; and diminished urine output. SEE: *Poisons and Poisoning Appendix.*

**irritation** [L. *irritatio*] **1.** A reaction to that which is irritating. It is important to distinguish between irritation and sensitization. For example, a substance contacting the skin may cause no irritation when initially applied but can cause a sensitization reaction that will not become obvious until the material is applied the second time. SEE: *allergen; sensitization.* **2.** An extreme reaction to pain or pathological conditions. **3.** A normal response to stimulus of a nerve or muscle.

***spinal i.*** A neurasthenic condition characterized by tenderness along the spinal column, numbness and tingling in the limbs, and susceptibility to fatigue.

***sympathetic i.*** The response of an organ to irritation in another organ.

**irritative** Pert. to that which causes irritation.

**ischemia** (ĭs-kē′mē-ă) [Gr. *ischein,* to hold back, + *haima,* blood] A local and temporary deficiency of blood supply due to obstruction of the circulation to a part.

***intestinal i.*** SEE: *angina, intestinal.*

***myocardial i.*** Inadequate flow of blood to the heart leading to angina pectoris and, if untreated, to myocardial infarction. About half of the deaths that occur in the U.S. each year are caused by ischemic heart disease, and about half of these deaths occur suddenly. Myocardial ischemia may be treated by use of drugs (i.e., nitroglycerin, beta adrenergic blockers, calcium entry blockers), by the use of surgical procedures such as coronary artery bypass, or by dilating the coronary arteries by use of the procedure of percutaneous transluminal coronary angioplasty. SEE: *angina pectoris, stable; angina pectoris, unstable; Prinzmetal's angina.*

**ischesis** (ĭs-kē′sĭs) Suppression of a discharge, esp. a normal one.

**ischia** (ĭs′kē-ă) [L.] Pl. of ischium.

**ischiac, ischiadic** (ĭs′kē-ăk, ĭs-kē-ăd′ĭk) Sciatic.

**ischial** (ĭs′kē-ăl) [Gr. *ischion,* hip] Pert. to the ischium.

**ischialgia** (ĭs″kē-ăl′jē-ă) [″ + *algos,* pain] Sciatica.

**ischiatic** (ĭs″kē-ăt′ĭk) [Gr. *ischion,* hip] Sciatic.

**ischiatitis** (ĭs″kē-ă-tī′tĭs) [″ + *itis,* inflammation] Sciatic nerve inflammation.

**ischidrosis** (ĭs″kĭ-drō′sĭs) [Gr. *ischein,* to hold back, + *hidrosis,* sweat] The suppression of perspiration.

**ischio-** [Gr. *ischion,* hip] Combining form meaning *ischium.*

**ischioanal** (ĭs″kē-ō-ā′năl) [″ + L. *anus,* anus] Concerning the ischium and anus.

**ischiobulbar** (ĭs″kē-ō-bŭl′băr) [″ + L. *bulbus,* bulb] Relating to the ischium and urethral bulb.

**ischiocapsular** (ĭs″kē-ō-kăp′sū-lăr) [″ + L. *capsula,* capsule] Concerning the ischium and capsule of the hip.

**ischiocavernosus** (ĭs″kē-ō-kă″vĕr-nō′sŭs) [″ + L. *cavernosus,* cavernous] A muscle extending from the ischium to the penis or clitoris and assisting in their erection.

**ischiocele** (ĭs′kē-ō-sēl) [″ + *kele,* tumor, swelling] A hernia through the sciatic notch.

**ischiococcygeus** (ĭs″kē-ō-kŏk-sĭj′ē-ŭs) [″ + *kokkyx,* coccyx] **1.** The coccygeus muscle. **2.** The posterior portion of the levator ani.

**ischiodynia** (ĭs″kē-ō-dĭn′ē-ă) [″ + *odyne,* pain] Pain in the ischium.

**ischiofemoral** (ĭs″kē-ō-fĕm′or-ăl) [″ + L. *femur,* thigh] Relating to the ischium and femur.

**ischiofibular** (ĭs″kē-ō-fĭb′ū-lăr) [″ + L. *fibula,* pin] Relating to the ischium and fibula.

**ischiohebotomy** (ĭs″kē-ō-hē-bŏt′ō-mē) [″ + *hebe,* pubes, + *tome,* incision] Surgical division of the ascending ramus of the pubes and the ischiopubic ramus. SYN: *ischiopubiotomy.*

**ischioneuralgia** (ĭs″kē-ō-nū-răl′jē-ă) [″ + *neuron,* nerve, + *algos,* pain] Sciatica.

**ischionitis** (ĭs″kē-ō-nī′tĭs) [″ + *itis,* inflammation] Inflammation of the tuberosity of the ischium.

**ischiopubic** (ĭs″kē-ō-pū′bĭk) [″ + L. *pubes,* the pubes] Relating to the ischium and pubes.

**ischiopubiotomy** (ĭs″kē-ō-pū″bē-ŏt′ō-mē) Ischiohebotomy.

**ischiorectal** (ĭs″kē-ō-rĕk′tăl) [″ + L. *rectus,* straight] Pert. to the ischium and rectum.

**ischiosacral** (ĭs″kē-ō-sā′krăl) [″ + L. *sacralis,* pert. to the sacrum] Concerning the ischium and sacrum.

**ischiovaginal** (ĭs″kē-ō-văj′ĭ-năl) [″ + L. *vagina,* sheath] Concerning the ischium and vagina.

**ischium** (ĭs′kē-ŭm) *pl.* **ischia** [Gr. *ischion,* hip] The lower portion of the innominate or hip bone.

**ischogalactic** (ĭs″kō-gă-lăk′tĭk) [Gr. *ischein,* to hold back, + *gala,* milk] Antigalactic.

**I.S.C.L.T.** *International Society of Clinical Laboratory Technologists.*

**iseikonia** (īs″ī-kō′nē-ă) [Gr. *isos,* equal, + *eikon,* image] Isoiconia.

**island** [AS. *igland,* island] A structure detached from surrounding tissues or characterized by difference in structure; an islet.

***blood i.*** A small area of blood accumulation present in the yolk sac of the early embryo.

***i.'s of Calleja*** Groups of densely packed, small cells in the cortex of the gyrus hippocampi. SYN: *islets of Calleja.*

***i.'s of Langerhans*** Islets of Langerhans.

***pancreatic i.'s*** Islets of Langerhans.

***i. of Reil*** The insula, a lobe of the cerebral cortex comprising a triangular area lying in the floor of the lateral or sylvian fissure. It is overlapped and hidden by the gyri of the fissure, which constitute the operculum of the insula.

**islet** (ī′lĕt) A tiny isolated mass of one kind of tissue within another type.

***i.'s of Calleja*** Islands of Calleja.

***i.'s of Langerhans*** Clusters of cells in the pancreas. They are of three types: alpha, beta, and delta cells. The alpha cells secrete glucagon, which raises the blood glucose level; the beta cells secrete insulin, which lowers it; and the delta cells secrete somatostatin, an inhibitor of growth hormone secretion. Destruction or impairment of function of the islets of Langerhans may result in diabetes or hypoglycemia. SYN: *islands of Langerhans; pancreatic islands.*

***Walthard's i.'s*** Embryological nests of epithelial-like cells in the superficial part of the ovaries, tubes, and uterine ligaments. They may also appear as minute cysts. Brenner's tumor is thought to arise from these islets.

**-ism** [Gr. *-ismos*] Suffix meaning *condition* or *theory of*; *principle* or *method.*

**I.S.O.** *International Standards Organization.*

**iso-** [Gr. *isos,* equal] Combining form meaning *equal.*

**isoagglutination** (ī″sō-ă-gloo″tĭ-nā′shŭn) [″ + L. *agglutinare,* to glue to] Agglutination of red blood cells by agglutinins from the blood of another member of the same species. SYN: *isohemagglutination.*

**isoagglutinin** (ī″sō-ă-glū′tĭn-ĭn) [″ + L. *agglutinare,* to glue to] An antibody in a serum that agglutinates the blood cells of those of the same species from which it is derived. SEE: *agglutinin; blood group; isohemagglutinin.*

**isoagglutinogen** (ī″sō-ă-ğlū-tĭn′ō-jĕn) One of two substances designated A and B that may be present on the surface of red blood cells. Cells containing these substances become agglutinated when mixed with serum containing corresponding isoagglutinins (anti-A or anti-B). SEE: *blood groups.*

**isoanaphylaxis** (ī″sō-ăn″ă-fĭ-lăk′sĭs) [″ + *ana,* against, + *phylaxis,* protection] Anaphylaxis produced by serum from another member of the same species.

**isoantibody** (ī″sō-ăn′tĭ-bŏd″ē) An antibody produced in response to an isoantigen.

**isoantigen** (ī″sō-ăn′tĭ-jĕn) [″ + L. *anti,* against, + *gennan,* to produce] A substance present in certain individuals that stimulates antibody production in other members of the same species but not in the donor (e.g., blood group isoantigens that are harmless to the donor but may produce severe antibody response in a recipient of a different blood group or type). SYN: *alloantigen.*

**isobar** (ī′sō-băr) [″ + *baros,* weight] In chemistry, one of two or more chemical bodies having the same atomic weight but different atomic numbers.

**isobaric** (ī″sō-băr′ĭk) Specific gravity equal to that with which it is being compared. For example, an anesthetic solution used in spinal anesthesia, if isobaric, would be of the same specific gravity as the spinal fluid.

**isobucaine hydrochloride** (ī″sō-bū′kān) A local anesthetic agent.

**isocaloric** (ī″sō-kă-lō′rĭk) [″ + L. *calor,* heat] Containing the same number of calories as the food or diet with which it is being compared.

**isocarboxazid** (ī″sō-kăr-bŏk′să-zĭd) An antidepressant drug. Trade name is Marplan.

**isocellular** [″ + L. *cellula,* cell] Composed of equal and similar cells.

**isochromatic** (ī″sō-krō-măt′ĭk) [″ + *chroma,* color] **1.** Having the same color. **2.** Of uniform color.

**isochromatophil(e)** (ī″sō-krō-măt′ō-fĭl, -fīl) [″ + ″ + *philein,* to love] Having the same affinity for a dye.

**isochromosome** (ī″sō-krō′mō-sōm) [″ + ″ + *soma,* body] A chromosome with arms that are morphologically identical and contain the same genetic loci. This is the result of the transverse rather than the longitudinal splitting of a chromosome.

**isochronal** (ī-sŏk′rō-năl) [″ + *chronos*, time] Acting in uniform time, or taking place at regular intervals.

**isochronia** (ī″sō-krō′nē-ă) [Gr. *isos*, equal, + *chronos*, time] The correspondence of events with respect to time, rate, or frequency.

**isochroous** (ī-sŏk′rō-ŭs) [″ + *chroa*, color] Isochromatic (2).

**isocitrate dehydrogenase** (ī″sō-cĭt′rāt dē″hī-drŏj′ĕn-ās) An enzyme present in tissues. It catalyzes the conversion of isocitric acid to $\alpha$-ketoglutaric acid.

**isocolloid** (ī-sō-kŏl′oyd) [″ + *kollodes*, glutinous] A colloid having the same composition in every transformation.

**isocomplement** [″ + L. *complere*, to complete] Complement from an individual of the same species.

**isocoria** (ī″sō-kō′rē-ă) [″ + *kore*, pupil] Equality of size of both pupils. SEE: *anisocoria*.

**isocortex** (ī″sō-kor′tĕks) [″ + L. *cortex*, bark] The nonolfactory portion of the cerebral cortex. It is composed of six layers of fibrous and cellular tissue having a similar distribution pattern. Phylogenetically, it is the new part of the pallium. SYN: *neocortex; neopallium*.

**isocytosis** (ī″sō-sī-tō′sĭs) [″ + *kytos*, cell, + *osis*, condition] Cells of equal size.

**isocytotoxin** (ī″sō-sī″tō-tŏk′sĭn) [″ + ″ + *toxikon*, poison] Cytotoxin destructive to homologous cells of the same species.

**isodactylism** (ī-sō-dăk′tĭl-ĭzm) [″ + *daktylos*, finger] A condition of having fingers or toes of equal length.

**isodiametric** (ī″sō-dī-ă-mĕt′rĭk) [″ + *dia*, across, + *metron*, measure] Having equal diameters.

**isodontic** (ī″sō-dŏn′tĭk) [″ + *odous*, tooth] Having teeth of equal size.

**isodose** (ī′sō-dōs) In radiology, equal doses of radiation received by different areas of the body.

***i. curve*** In radiation therapy, a graph on which the points plot areas or levels of equal radiation dose.

**isodynamic** (ī″sō-dī-năm′ĭk) [″ + *dynamis*, power] Having equal power.

**isoelectric** (ī″sō-ē-lĕk′trĭk) [″ + *elektron*, amber] Having equal electric potentials.

**isoenergetic** [Gr. *isos*, equal, + *energeia*, energy] Showing equal force or activity.

**isoenzyme** (ī″sō-ĕn′zīm) [″ + *en*, in, + *zyme*, leaven] One of several forms in which an enzyme may exist in various tissues. Although the isoenzymes are similar in catalytic qualities, they may be separated from each other by special chemical tests. SYN: *isozyme*. SEE: *lactic dehydrogenase*.

**isoetharine hydrochloride** (ī-sō-ĕth′ă-rēn) A sympathomimetic drug used as a bronchodilator.

**isoflurophate** (ī-sō-floo′rō-fāt) An anticholinesterase drug used in treating glaucoma as well as atony of the smooth muscle of the intestinal tract and urinary bladder.

**isogamete** (ī″sō-găm′ēt) [″ + *gamete*, wife, *gametes*, husband] **1.** A cell that reproduces through conjugation or fusion with a similar cell. **2.** A gamete of the same size as the one with which it fuses or unites.

**isogamy** (ī-sŏg′ă-mē) [″ + *gamos*, marriage] Reproduction resulting from the conjugation of isogametes or identical cells.

**isogeneic** (ī″sō-jĕn-ē′ĭk) Syngeneic.

**isogeneric** (ī″sō-jĕ-nĕr′ĭk) [″ + L. *genus*, kind] Of the same kind; concerning or obtained from members of the same genus.

**isogenesis** (ī″sō-jĕn′ĕ-sĭs) [″ + *genesis*, generation, birth] A similarity in morphological development.

**isogenic** (ī″sō-jĕn′ĭk) Isologous.

**isograft** [″ + L. *graphium*, grafting shoot] A graft taken from another individual or animal of the same genotype as the recipient. SEE: *autograft*.

**isohemagglutination** (ī″sō-hĕm″ă-gloo″tĭ-nā′shŭn) [″ + *haima*, blood, + L. *agglutinare*, to glue to] Isoagglutination.

**isohemagglutinin** (ī″sō-hĕm″ă-glū′tĭn-ĭn) [″ + *haima*, blood, + L. *agglutinare*, to glue to] A substance normally present in most human blood serum; responsible for the clumping of corpuscles observed when incompatible bloods are mixed. The clumping is ascribed to the interaction of an agglutinogen in the corpuscles with a specific agglutinin in the foreign serum. In transfusions, the corpuscles of the donor are exposed to an overwhelming quantity of the recipient's plasma; therefore, the agglutinogen content of the donor's corpuscles and the agglutinin content of the recipient's serum are the factors that determine compatibility. Assuming that there are but two possible agglutinogens, red corpuscles from a given donor may contain both, either, or neither. If the agglutinin alpha can react only with agglutinogen A, a table can be constructed to illustrate which blood types will be compatible or incompatible with other types. SEE: *agglutinin; agglutinogen*.

**isohemolysin** (ī″sō-hē-mŏl′ĭ-sĭn) [″ + ″ + *lysis*, dissolution] A substance that destroys red blood corpuscles of animals of the same species from which it is obtained. SEE: *hemolysin*.

**isohemolysis** (ī″sō-hē-mŏl′ĭ-sĭs) The destruction of red blood corpuscles produced by an isolysin; the action of an isohemolysin. SYN: *isolysis*. SEE: *hemolysis*.

**isohypercytosis** (ī″sō-hī″pĕr-sī-tō′sĭs) [″ + *hyper*, over, above, excessive + *kytos*, cell, + *osis*, condition] A condition in which the total number of white blood cells is increased but the proportions of the polymorphonuclear leukocytes remain stable.

**isoiconia** (ī″sō-ī-kō′nē-ă) [Gr. *isos*, equal, + *eikon*, image] Equality of both retinal images. SYN: *iseikonia*.

**isoiconic** (ī″sō-ī-kŏn′ĭk) Having equal retinal images.

**isoimmunization** [″ + L. *immunis*, safe] Immunization of an individual against the blood of an individual of the same species, esp. the development of Rh-negative agglutinins in an Rh-negative mother in response to agglutinogens present in transfused Rh-positive blood or developed in an Rh-positive fetus.

**isolate** [It. *isolato,* isolated] **1.** To separate or detach from other persons, as during an infectious disease. **2.** In chemistry, to obtain a substance in pure form from the mixture or solution that contains it.

**isolation 1.** The fear of interrelating with another individual. **2.** The separation of infected persons or animals from others for the period of communicability to prevent or limit direct or indirect transmission of the infectious agent. In contrast, quarantine applies to restriction on healthy contacts of an infectious agent. SEE: *incubation* for table; *infectious i.; protective i.; quarantine; Universal Precautions Appendix.*

NURSING IMPLICATIONS: The rules to be followed for achieving isolation are based on the mode of transmission of the particular organism; for example, if the organism is spread by droplet, then all items that come in contact with the patient's upper respiratory tract are isolated and destroyed or disinfected. Those in contact with the patient are also protected from droplet transmission by wearing protective barriers such as special masks (and if necessary by goggles, gowns, caps, boots, and gloves) by careful and thorough hand washing, and by keeping the hands away from the nose and mouth, because the hands of those in contact with the patient are the most common means of transmitting infection. On leaving the patient area, the nurse, other care provider, or family member unties the lower gown tie (if worn); removes gloves (if worn); washes hands; unties the upper gown tie; removes the gown, stripping and folding it inside out as it is removed; removes mask, goggles, boots, and cap, and immediately places them in an appropriate container. The nurse then rewashes the hands. Most agencies use disposable equipment in the care of an isolated patient as far as is possible. Contaminated disposables are double-bagged for safe-disposal, usually by incineration. Contaminated linens and other non-disposable equipment are also double-bagged and marked "isolation," so that they will be properly decontaminated or disinfected on receipt by the laundry or supply service. Laboratory specimens also are double-bagged and marked with the particular type of isolation, so that personnel handle them appropriately. Center for Disease Control and Prevention recommendations and institutional procedure are followed for the specific type of isolation that is in effect. The purpose of the isolation precautions is explained to the patient and family to decrease their fears and to increase their cooperation, and the family and other visitors are taught how to use and discard the required barriers and especially how to thoroughly wash their hands. When the at-risk patient requires protection from others, equipment going to the patient is disposable or sterilized, and human contacts wear barriers that may be clean or sterile depending on the circumstances and protocol. After use, these items are handled in the agency's usual manner, with no special care necessary beyond that defined in universal precautions.

***infectious i.*** An isolation technique that protects health care personnel from a patient who has or is suspected of having an infectious disease.

***protective i.*** Isolation in which the patient is being protected from potentially harmful bacteria in the environment. This is particularly important in caring for immunodeficient patients such as those undergoing transplantation surgery. SYN: *reverse i.*

***reverse i.*** Protective i.

***i. ward*** A hospital ward in which patients suffering from communicable disease may be kept apart from the rest of the patients.

**isoleucine** (ī″sō-lū′sēn) An amino acid formed during hydrolysis of fibrin and other proteins. It is essential in the diet.

**isologous** (ī-sŏl′ō-gŭs) Genetically identical. In transplantations, being isologous (or isogenic) indicates the absence of any tissue incompatibility between the recipient of tissue and the tissue or organ itself. SYN: *isogenic; syngeneic.*

**isolophobia** (ī″sō-lō-fō′bē-ă) [It. *isolato,* isolated, + Gr. *phobos,* fear] The fear of being alone. SEE: *agoraphobia.*

**isolysis** (ī-sŏl′ĭ-sĭs) Isohemolysis. **isolytic** (ī-sō-lĭt′ĭk), *adj.*

**isomer** (ī′sō-mĕr) [Gr. *isos,* equal, + *meros,* part] One of two or more chemical substances that have the same molecular formula but different chemical and physical properties owing to a different arrangement of the atoms in the molecule. Dextrose is an isomer of levulose. SEE: *polymer.*

**isomerase** (ī-sŏm′ĕr-ās) Any enzyme that catalyzes the isomerization of its substrate. For example, phosphoglucose isomerase interconverts glucose and fructose-6-phosphate. SEE: *isomerism.*

**isomeric** (ī″sō-mĕr′ĭk) Pert. to isomerism.

**isomerism** (ī-sŏm′ĕr-ĭzm) The state of being composed of compounds of the same number of atoms but having different atomic arrangement in the molecule. SEE: *metamerism; polymerism.*

**isomerization** (ī-sŏm″ĕr-ī-zā′shŭn) The conversion of one chemical substance to an isomer. SEE: *isomer; isomerism.*

**isometric** [″ + *metron,* measure] Having

equal dimensions. SEE: *isotonic* (2).

***i. contraction phase*** The first phase in contraction of the ventricle of the heart in which ventricular pressure increases but there is no decrease in volume of contents because semilunar valves are closed.

**isometropia** (ī″sō-mĕ-trō′pē-ă) [″ + ″ + *ops,* eye] Same refraction of the two eyes.

**isomorphism** (ī-sō-mor′fĭzm) [″+ *morphe,* form, + *-ismos,* state of] A condition marked by possession of the same form.

**isomorphous** (ī″sō-mor′fŭs) Possessing the same shape.

**isoniazid** (ī″sō-nī′ă-zĭd) ABBR: INH. $C_6H_7N_3O$. An odorless compound occurring as colorless or white crystals or as a white crystalline powder. It is an antibacterial, used principally in treating tuberculosis. The antidote for isoniazid overdose is pyridoxine. SYN: *isonicotinoylhydrazine.*

**isonicotinoylhydrazine** (ī″sō-nĭk″ō-tĭn″ō-ĭl-hī′dră-zēn) Isoniazid.

**isonormocytosis** (ī″sō-nor″mō-sī-tō′sĭs) [″ + L. *norma,* rule, + Gr. *kytos,* cell, + *osis,* condition] The state of having the normal amount and proportion of varieties of leukocytes.

**isopathy** (ī-sŏp′ă-thē) [Gr. *isos,* equal, + *pathos,* disease, suffering] Isotherapy.

**isophoria** (ī″sō-fō′rē-ă) [″ + *phorein,* to carry] Equal tension of vertical muscles of each eye with visual lines in the same horizontal plane; absence of hyperphoria and hypophoria.

**isopia** (ī-sō′pē-ă) [″ + *ops,* vision] Equal vision in the eyes.

**isoplastic** (ī″sō-plăs′tĭk) [″ + *plastos,* formed] Removed from one individual and transplanted to another of the same species, as a graft. SEE: *isograft.*

**isoprecipitin** (ī″sō-prē-sĭp′ĭ-tĭn) [″ + L. *praecipitare,* to cast down] A precipitin that reacts with antigens from other members of the same species but which are genetically dissimilar.

**isopropamide iodide** (ī″sō-prō′pă-mīd) A synthetic antimuscarinic drug with actions similar to those of belladonna.

**isopropanol** (ī″sō-prō′pă-nŏl) Isopropyl alcohol.

**isoproterenol hydrochloride** (ī″sō-prō″tĕ-rē′nŏl) A sympathomimetic amine used to relieve bronchoconstriction in asthma and also as a cardiac stimulant in heart block.

Caution: Overdosage administered by inhalation can be fatal.

**isopters** (ī-sŏp′tĕrz) [″ + *opter,* observer] Lines on a chart of the field of vision that connect points of equal visual acuity.

**isopyknosis** (ī″sō-pĭk-nō′sĭs) [″ + *pyknosis,* condensation] Having uniform density, esp. being in a state of equal condensation as in comparing different chromosomes.

**isoserotherapy** (ī″sō-sē″rō-thĕr′ă-pē) [″ + L. *serum,* whey, + Gr. *therapeia,* treatment] Treatment with serum from an individual who has had the same disease as the patient.

**isoserum** (ī″sō-sē′rŭm) A serum from a person who has had the disease for which a patient is to receive treatment.

**isosexual** (ī″sō-sĕks′ū-ăl) Concerning or characteristic of the same sex.

**isosmotic** (ī″sŏs-mŏt′ĭk) [″ + *osmos,* impulsion] Having the same total concentration of osmotically active molecules or ions in solution as the solution or body fluid to which it is being compared. SEE: *isotonic* (1).

**isosorbide dinitrate tablets** (ī″sō-sor′bīd) An antianginal drug used sublingually.

**Isospora** (ī-sŏs′pō-ră) [″ + *sporos,* spore] A genus of Sporozoa belonging to the order Coccidia.

***I. hominis*** A parasitic, nonpathogenic protozoon inhabiting the small intestine in humans.

**isospore** (ī′sō-spor) [Gr. *isos,* equal, + *sporos,* spore] A nonsexual spore from plants with only one kind of spore. It grows to maturity without conjugating.

**isosthenuria** (ī″sŏs-thĕn-ū′rē-ă) [″ + *sthenos,* strength, + *ouron,* urine] A condition of the urine being of a uniform specific gravity and osmolarity despite variations in fluid intake; a sign of marked impairment of renal function.

**isostimulation** [″ + L. *stimulare,* to goad] Stimulation of an animal by the use of antigenic material derived from another animal of the same species.

**isotherapy** (ī″sō-thĕr′ă-pē) [″ + *therapeia,* treatment] The treatment of a disease by administering the active causative agent of the same disease. SYN: *isopathy.*

**isothermal** [″ + *therme,* heat] Having equal temperature.

**isothermognosis** (ī″sō-thĕrm″ŏg-nō′sĭs) [″ + ″ + *gnosis,* knowledge] Abnormal perception in which stimulations by pain, heat, and cold are all felt as heat.

**isotone** (ī′sō-tōnz) One of several nuclides with the same number of neutrons but a different number of protons in their nuclei.

**isotonia** (ī″sō-tō′nē-ă) [″ + *tonos,* tone] The state of equal osmotic pressure of two or more solutions or substances.

**isotonic** (ī″sō-tŏn′ĭk) **1.** Relating to the maintenance of a constant amount resistive force during muscular contraction. **2.** Having equal pressure. SEE: *isometric.*

**isotonicity** (ī″sō-tō-nĭs′ĭ-tē) The state or condition of being isotonic.

**isotope** (ī′sō-tōp) [″ + *topos,* place] One of a series of chemical elements that have nearly identical chemical properties but different atomic weights and electric charge. Many isotopes are radioactive.

***i. cisternography*** The use of a radioactive tracer to investigate the circulation of cerebrospinal fluid. A tracer such as $^{131}I$ serum albumin is injected in the lumbar subarachnoid space. Flow of the tracer toward the head and into areas of the brain can be recorded by means of serial scintillation scanning. This technique is useful in studying hydrocephalus.

***radioactive i.*** An isotope in which the nuclear composition is unstable.

***stable i.*** An isotope that does not undergo radioactive decay and become another element.

**isotretinoin** A keratolytic agent used in treating acne.

---

Caution: This medicine should not be used by pregnant women or those who are sexually active and at risk of becoming pregnant.

---

**isotropic** (ī″sō-trŏp′ĭk) [″ + *tropos,* a turning] **1.** Possessing similar qualities in every direction. **2.** Having equal refraction.

**isotropy** (ī-sŏt′rō-pē) The state of being isotropic.

**isotype** In immunology, one of the determinants on the immunoglobulin molecule that distinguish among the main classes of antibodies of a given species. They are the same for all normal individuals of that species. SEE: *idiotype.*

**isotypical** (ī-sō-tĭp′ĭ-kăl) [″ + *typos,* mark] Belonging to the same variety or classification.

**isovalericacidemia** (ī″sō-vă-lĕr″ĭk-ăs″ĭ-dē′mē-ă) An inherited metabolic disease affecting leucine metabolism. Isovaleric acid accumulates in the blood during periods of increased amino acid metabolism (i.e., during infections or following ingestion of proteins). Coma and death may occur.

**isoxsuprine hydrochloride** (ī-sŏk′sū-prēn) A vasodilator drug whose therapeutic usefulness has not been established. Trade name is Vasodilan.

**isozyme** (ī′sō-zīm) Isoenzyme.

**issue** (ĭsh′ū) [ME.] **1.** Offspring. **2.** A suppurating sore maintained by a foreign body in the tissue to act as a counterirritant. **3.** A discharge of pus or blood.

**isthmectomy** (ĭs-mĕk′tō-mē) [Gr. *isthmos,* isthmus, + *ektome,* excision] Excision of an enlarged isthmus, esp. of the thyroid gland.

**isthmian** (ĭs′mē-ăn) Relating to an isthmus.

**isthmitis** (ĭs-mī′tĭs) [″ + *itis,* inflammation] An inflammation of the throat or fauces.

**isthmoparalysis** (ĭs″mō-pă-răl′ĭ-sĭs) [″ + *para,* beyond, + *lyein,* to loosen] Paralysis of the muscles of the fauces. SYN: *isthmoplegia.*

**isthmoplegia** (ĭs″mō-plē′jē-ă) [″ + *plege,* a stroke] Isthmoparalysis.

**isthmospasm** (ĭs′mō-spăzm″) [″ + *spasmos,* a convulsion] Isthmian spasm of the fallopian tubes.

**isthmus** (ĭs′mŭs) *pl.* **isthmuses, isthmi** [Gr. *isthmos,* isthmus] **1.** A narrow passage connecting two cavities. **2.** A narrow structure connecting two larger parts. **3.** A constriction between two larger parts of an organ or anatomical structure.

***aortic i.*** A constriction in the fetal aorta between the ductus arteriosus and left subclavian artery. The condition sometimes persists to adulthood.

***i. of eustachian tube*** I. tubae auditivae.

***i. faucium*** A constriction connecting the posterior mouth cavity proper with the pharynx.

***i. glandulae thyroideae*** A narrow portion of the thyroid gland connecting the left and right lobes. SYN: *i. of thyroid.*

***pharyngeal i.*** I. pharyngonasalis.

***i. pharyngonasalis*** The opening between the nasopharynx and oral pharynx. SYN: *pharyngeal i.*

***i. of thyroid*** I. glandulae thyroideae.

***i. tubae auditivae*** The narrowest portion of the eustachian tube. SYN: *i. of eustachian tube.*

***i. tubae uterinae*** The constricted portion (the medial third) of the uterine (fallopian) tube nearest the uterus. SYN: *i. of uterine tube.*

***i. uteri*** A slight constriction on the surface of the uterus midway between the uterine body and the cervix. SYN: *i of uterus.*

***i. of uterine tube*** I. tubae uterinae.

***i. of uterus*** I. uteri.

**itch** [ME. *icchen*] **1.** Pruritus. **2.** Scabies.

***baker's i.*** A rash that occurs on the hands and forearms of bakers. It may be due to mechanical or chemical factors.

***barber's i.*** Tinea barbae.

***dhobie i.*** Tinea cruris.

***grain i.*** Dermatitis caused by mites in stored grain.

***grocer's i.*** Dermatitis caused either by mites in grain or cheese, or by sugar.

***ground i.*** A local irritation produced by penetration of the skin of the foot by hookworm larvae, esp. *Necator americanus.* SYN: *ancylostomiasis.*

***jock i.*** Tinea cruris.

***seven-year i.*** Scabies.

***swimmer's i.*** Dermatitis that develops after swimming in water containing the larval form of schistosomes. SYN: *water i.*

***water i.*** Swimmer's i.

***winter i.*** Pruritus hiemalis.

**itching** Pruritus; irritation of the skin, causing desire to rub or scratch the part. Itching is a frequent manifestation of systemic disease and may cause more distress than pain; no specific drugs relieve itching. Some systemic diseases associated with itching are drynesss and itching of the skin in hypothyroidism; warm, moist itching skin in thyrotoxicosis; mucocutaneous candidiasis in diabetes mellitus; Hodgkin's disease; water-induced itching associated with polycythemia vera; high concentration of bile salts due to decreased bile excretion; and uremia.

**-ite** [Gr.] **1.** Suffix meaning *of the nature of.*

2. In chemistry, a salt of an acid having the termination *-ous.*

**iter** (ī′tĕr) [L.] A passageway between two anatomical parts. **iteral** (-ăl), *adj.*

**iteroparity** (ĭt″ĕr-ō-păr′ĭ-tē) [L. *iterare,* to repeat, + *parere,* to bear] The state of reproducing more than once in a lifetime.

**ithycyphosis, ithyokyphosis** (ĭth″ĭ-sī-fō′sĭs, ĭth″ē-ō-kī-fō′sĭs) [Gr. *ithys,* straight, + *kyphos,* humped] Kyphosis with backward projection of the spine.

**ithylordosis** (ĭth″ĭ-lor-dō′sĭs) [″ + *lordosis,* a bending forward] Lordosis without lateral curvature of the spine.

**-itis** (ī′tĭs) [Gr.] Suffix meaning *inflammation of.*

**ITP** *immune thrombocytopenic purpura.*

**I.U.** *immunizing unit; international unit.*

**IUCD** *intrauterine contraceptive device.*

**IUD** *intrauterine device.*

**IUGR** *intrauterine growth retardation.*

**IV** *intravenous(ly).*

**IVC** *intravenous cholangiography.*

**IVCD** *intraventricular conduction defect.* In electrocardiography, this term is used to refer to abnormal conduction in ventricular muscle. SEE: *bundle branch block.*

**ivermectin** An antiparasitic drug used in veterinary medicine. It is used to treat human onchocerciasis (river blindness). The drug is also being used experimentally as part of the therapeutic protocol for colorectal carcinoma. Trade names are Eqvalan and Ivomec.

**IVF** *in vitro fertilization.*

**IVIG** *intravenous immunoglobulin.*

**IVP** *intravenous pyelogram.*

**IV push.** The administration of medicine intravenously by quick and forcible injection.

**IVT** *intravenous transfusion.*

**IVU** *intravenous urography.*

**Ivy method** SEE: *bleeding time.*

**ivy poisoning** SEE: *poison ivy dermatitis.*

**Ixodes** (ĭks-ō′dēz) [Gr. *ixodes,* like birdlime] A genus of ticks of the family Ixodidae, many of which are parasitic on humans and animals. SEE: illus.

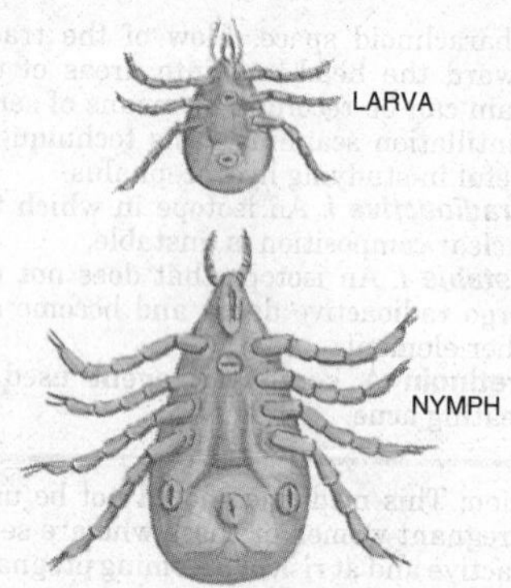


**IXODES TICK** (ORIG. MAG. ×12)

**ixodiasis** (ĭks″ō-dī′ă-sĭs) **1.** Lesions of the skin caused by tick bites. **2.** Any disease caused by ticks, as Rocky Mountain spotted fever.

**ixodic** (ĭks-ŏd′ĭk) Pert. to or caused by ticks.

**Ixodidae** (ĭks-ŏd′ĭ-dē) A family of ticks belonging to the order Acarina, class Arachnida, comprising the hard-bodied ticks including the genera *Amblyomma, Boophilus, Dermacentor, Haemaphysalis, Hyalomma, Ixodes,* and *Rhipicephalus.* All are parasitic and of significance as pests or as transmitters of disease in domestic animals and humans. Among the diseases transmitted by ticks are Rocky Mountain spotted fever, relapsing fever, tularemia, and Lyme disease.

**Ixodides** (ĭks-ŏd′ĭ-dēz) Ticks.

**Ixodoidea** (ĭks″ō-doy′dē-ă) A superfamily of Acarina, the ticks, in which the adults have a thick cuticle.

**ixomyelitis** (ĭks″ō-mī-ĕ-lī′tĭs) [Gr. *ixodes,* like birdlime, + *myelos,* marrow, + *itis,* inflammation] An inflammation of the spinal cord in the lumbar region.

# J

**J** Symbol for joule.

**Jaboulay's amputation** (zhă″boo-lāz′) [Mathieu Jaboulay, Fr. surgeon, 1860–1913] Amputation of the thigh and removal of the hip bone.

**Jaboulay's button** Two cylinders that may be screwed together for lateral intestinal anastomosis without the use of sutures.

**jacket** [O. Fr. *jacquet,* jacket] A bandage usually applied to the trunk to immobilize the spine or correct deformities.

***porcelain j.*** A jacket crown tooth restoration made of porcelain.

***Sayre's j.*** A plaster-of-paris jacket used as a support for a deformity of the spinal column.

**jackscrew** A threaded screw used for expanding the dental arch or for positioning bone fragments after a fracture.

**jacksonian epilepsy** [John Hughlings Jackson, Brit. neurologist, 1835–1911] A localized form of epilepsy with spasms confined to one part or one group of muscles. SEE: *epilepsy.*

**Jackson's syndrome** A dysfunction of cranial nerves X through XII caused by medullary lesions, resulting in unilateral muscle paralysis in the head, the mouth including the soft palate, and the vocal cords.

**Jacob, Arthur** Irish ophthalmologist, 1790–1874.

***J.'s membrane*** The retinal layer of rods and cones.

***J.'s ulcer*** Rodent ulcer.

**Jacobson, Ludwig** Danish anatomist, 1783–1843.

***J.'s cartilage*** One of two narrow longitudinal cartilages lying along the anterior inferior border of the nasal septum. They are rudimentary in humans.

***J.'s nerve*** Tympanic nerve.

***J.'s organ*** Organ of Jacobson.

***J.'s sulcus*** A portion of the middle ear containing branches of the tympanic plexus.

**Jacquemier's sign** (zhăk-mē-āz′) [Jean Jacquemier, Fr. obstetrician, 1806–1879] Blue or purple color of the vaginal mucosa; a presumptive sign of pregnancy.

**jactatio** (jăk-tā′shē-ō) [L., tossing] Restless tossing of the head and body; seen in acute illness. SYN: *jactitation.*

***j. capitis nocturna*** A form of sleep disturbance characterized by nocturnal head-banging.

**jactitation** (jăk″tĭ-tā′shŭn) [L. *jactitatio,* tossing] Jactatio.

**Jaeger's test types** (yā′gĕrz) [Eduard Jaeger, Ritter von Jaxtthal, Austrian ophthalmologist, 1818–1884] Lines of type of various sizes, printed on a card for testing near vision. The smallest type read at the closest distance is recorded.

**jamais vu** (zhăm′ā voo) [Fr., never seen] The subjective mental sensation of being in a completely strange environment when in familiar surroundings; may be associated with temporal lobe lesions. SEE: *déjà vu.*

**James fibers** [T. N. James, U.S. cardiologist and physiologist, b. 1925] A pathway for conduction of cardiac impulses so that they bypass the atrioventricular node. This alternate fiber pathway permits preexcitation of the ventricle with resultant tachycardia.

**Janeway lesion** [Edward Gamaliel Janeway, U.S. physician, 1841–1911] A small, painless, red-blue macular lesion a few millimeters in diameter; found on the palms and soles in acute bacterial endocarditis. SEE: *Roth's spots.*

**janiceps** (jăn′ĭ-sĕps) [L. *Janus,* a two-faced god, + *caput,* head] A deformed embryo having a face on both the anterior and the posterior aspects of the single head.

**Jansky-Bielschowsky syndrome** (jăn′skē-bē-ăl-show′skē) [Jan Jansky, Czech physician, 1873–1921; Max Bielschowsky, Ger. neuropathologist, 1869–1940] Early juvenile cerebral sphingolipidosis. SEE: *sphingolipidosis.*

**jar 1.** A container made of glass, plastic, or other sturdy material. It is usually taller than it is wide and may be cylindrical, square, or another shape. **2.** To move suddenly, as in a jolt or shock.

***bell j.*** A glass vessel with an opening at only one end.

***heel j.*** The production of pain by having the patient stand on tiptoes and suddenly bring the heels to the floor. This may be diagnostic of tuberculosis of the spine, pelvic inflammatory disease in women, or renal calculus.

**jargon** (jăr′gŭn) [O. Fr., a chattering] **1.** Paraphasia. **2.** The technical language or specialized terminology of those in a specific profession or group.

**Jarvis' snare** [William C. Jarvis, U.S. laryngologist, 1855–1895] A snare for removing growths in the nasal cavities.

**jaundice** (jawn′dĭs) [Fr. *jaune,* yellow] A condition characterized by yellowness of the skin, whites of eyes, mucous membranes, and body fluids owing to deposition of bile pigment resulting from excess bilirubin in the blood (hyperbilirubinemia). It may be caused by obstruction of bile passageways, excess destruction of red blood cells (hemolysis), or disturbances in the functioning of liver cells.

Jaundice may indicate a benign curable disease, such as a gallstone blocking the common duct, or carcinoma of the head of the pancreas involving the opening of the bile duct into the duodenum. It is therefore important to make the correct diagnosis.

The diagnostic studies to determine the cause of jaundice include noninvasive procedures such as ultrasonography and computed tomography, in addition to clinical laboratory studies and expert clinical evaluation. Invasive studies include cholangiography, endoscopic retrograde cholangiopancreatography (ERCP), or percutaneous transhepatic cholangiography (PTC).

In the newborn, severe jaundice may damage the cells of the basal ganglia and the brainstem, and may lead to deafness, cerebral palsy, or death. Depending on its cause, which may be red cell (Rh) incompatibility or septicemia, jaundice in the newborn may be treated with exchange transfusion, phototherapy, or both. SYN: *icterus*. SEE: *bilirubin* for illus.; *hemolytic disease of the newborn; kernicterus; phototherapy; transfusion, exchange.*

**acholuric j.** Jaundice without bile pigment in the urine.

**breastfeeding j.** An exaggerated physiological jaundice of the newborn. It may result initially from hemoconcentration due to inadequate fluid intake.

**breast milk j.** Hyperbilirubinemia resulting from pregnanediol or free fatty acids that inhibit bilirubin conjugation. Serum bilirubin level usually peaks above 20 ml/dl by 14 to 21 days of age. Some pediatricians recommend stopping breastfeeding for 24 to 36 hr if the level exceeds 20 ml/dl. If the infant's bilirubin level drops rapidly, the mother may resume nursing.

**cholestatic j.** Jaundice due to failure of bile to reach the duodenum, possibly caused by blockage of the flow of bile or by liver cell changes.

**congenital j.** Jaundice occurring at or shortly after birth owing to maldevelopment of the biliary apparatus.

**hematogenous j.** Hemolytic j.

**hemolytic j.** A rare chronic form of jaundice that results from increased destruction of red blood cells. The serum bilirubin may be only slightly elevated even though bile pigment production may be increased to as much as six times normal. The bilirubin, which is mostly unconjugated and therefore insoluble in water, does not appear in the urine. The spleen is usually enlarged. SYN: *hematogenous j.; hemolytic icterus.*

**hemorrhagic j.** Leptospiral j.

**hepatocanalicular j.** Jaundice resulting from changes in the bile canaliculi, with the liver cells remaining relatively normal.

**hepatocellular j.** Jaundice resulting from disease of the liver cells. SYN: *parenchymatous j.*

**hepatogenous j.** Jaundice due to disease of the liver.

**infectious j.** Infectious hepatitis.

**leptospiral j.** Jaundice present with leptospirosis. SYN: *hemorrhagic j.*

**j. of newborn** Nonpathological jaundice affecting newborns. It manifests 48 to 72 hr after birth, lasts only a few days, and does not require therapy. SYN: *icterus neonatorum.*

**nonhemolytic j.** Jaundice due to abnormal metabolism of bilirubin, and not to excessive destruction of red blood cells.

**obstructive j.** Jaundice due to a mechanical impediment in the flow of bile from the liver to the duodenum. SYN: *obstructive icterus.*

**pathological j. of newborn** Jaundice occurring during the first 24 hr after birth. It is caused by the destruction of red blood cells by maternal antibodies generated by previous fetal-maternal transfusion. SEE: *isoimmunization.*

**parenchymatous j.** Hepatocellular j.

**posthepatic j.** Jaundice resulting from obstruction of flow of bile ducts; may be incomplete or complete.

**regurgitation j.** Jaundice due to bile entering the lymph channels of the liver and thence being conveyed to the blood; may result from biliary obstruction or lesions involving bile capillaries.

**retention j.** Jaundice resulting from the inability of liver cells to remove bile pigment from circulation.

**spirochetal j.** An acute infectious disease caused by one of several spirochetes, including *Leptospira interrogans icterohaemorrhagiae*. SYN: *Weil's disease.*

**toxic j.** Jaundice resulting from bacterial toxins or poisons such as phosphorus, arsphenamine, or carbon tetrachloride.

**Javelle water** (zhŭ-vĕl′) [Javel, a city now part of Paris] An aqueous solution of potassium or sodium hypochlorite used as a bleach and disinfectant.

**jaw** [ME. *iawe*] Either or both of the maxillary and mandibular bones, bearing the teeth and forming the mouth framework. SEE: illus.

**cleft j.** An early embryonic malformation resulting in lack of fusion of the right and left mandible into a single bone.

**crackling j.** Noise in the normal or diseased temporomandibular joint during movement of the jaw. SYN: *crepitation.*

**dislocation of j.** Traumatic or spontaneous displacement of the mandible. Jaw dislocations are uncomfortable and may be extremely embarrassing to the patient. They may occur on either side, in which instance the tip of the jaw is pointed away from the dislocation. On the unaffected side, just in front of the ear, may be felt a little hollow or depression that is often tender. If both sides of the jaw are dislocated, the jaw is pushed downward and backward. In either event, there is pain and difficulty in speech and the condition

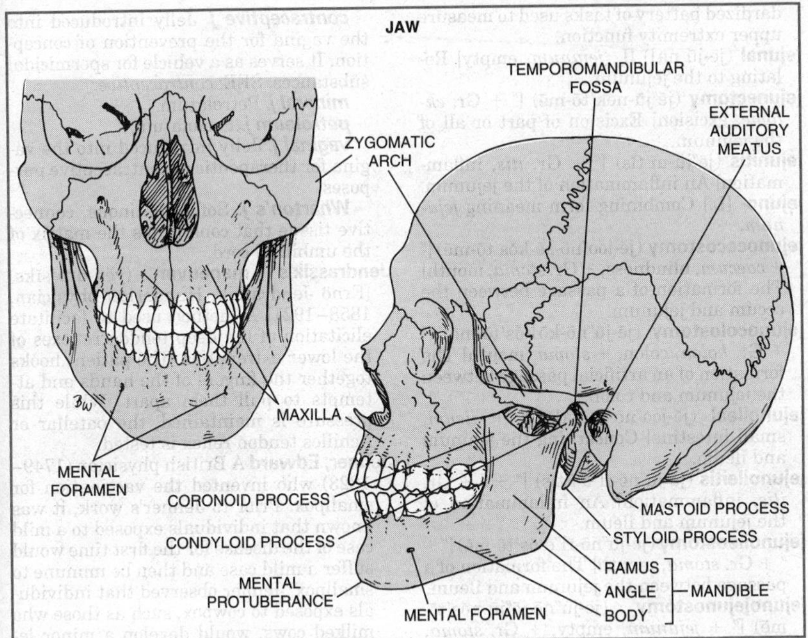


is often accompanied by shock. Backward dislocation of the jaw is rare.

CAUSES: Jaw dislocation is usually caused by a blow to the face or by keeping the mouth open for long periods as in dental treatment, but occasionally may be caused by chewing large chunks of food, yawning, or hearty laughing. A fall or blow on the chin could cause dislocation, but backward dislocation seldom occurs without fracture or extreme trauma.

REDUCTION: These dislocations are reduced by placing well-padded thumbs inside of the mouth on the lower molar (back) teeth with the fingers running along the outside of the jaw as a lever. The thumbs should press the jaw downward and backward. The jaw will glide posteriorly over the ridge of bone (articular eminence), which can be felt, and just as this occurs the jaw usually snaps into place. When this motion is noted, the thumbs should be moved laterally toward the cheeks to keep them from being crushed between the molars.

This snapping into place is due to an involuntary spasm of the muscles, which pulls the jaw as though an overstretched rubber band were attached to it. Following the reduction, an immobilizing bandage or double cravat should be applied.

---

Caution: It is important that the hands be protected by heavy gloves to prevent trauma by the teeth. SEE: *Universal Precautions Appendix*.

---

***lumpy j.*** Actinomycosis.

***swelling of j.*** In the lower jaw, a condition that may be due to alveolar abscess, a cyst, gumma, sarcoma, or actinomycosis. In the upper jaw, this sign may occur in alveolar abscess, parotid tumor, parotitis, carcinoma, sarcoma, necrosis of bone, or disease of antrum.

**jaw thrust** A maneuver that manually displaces the jaw to establish an airway during resuscitation. The person performing the maneuver stands at the patient's head and places his or her hands on the sides of the neck to hold the head in traction. The thumbs are then used to push up on the angles of the mandible.

***modified j.t.*** A maneuver used to open the airway of an unconscious patient that omits hyperextension in cases where possible cervical spine injury has occurred. The jaw is jutted forward, moving the tongue away from the hypopharynx.

**jaw winking** Voluntary movement of the lower face causing unilateral contraction of the orbicularis oculi muscle. This may be seen in patients who have recovered from Bell's palsy. SEE: *Marcus Gunn syndrome*.

**JCAH** *Joint Commission on the Accreditation of Hospitals.*

**J.C.A.H.O.** *Joint Commission on Accreditation of Healthcare Organizations.*

**Jebsen-Taylor Hand Function Test** A standardized battery of tasks used to measure upper extremity function.

**jejunal** (jē-jū'năl) [L. *jejunum,* empty] Relating to the jejunum.

**jejunectomy** (jē"jū-nĕk'tō-mē) [" + Gr. *ektome,* excision] Excision of part or all of the jejunum.

**jejunitis** (jē"jŭ-nī'tĭs) [" + Gr. *itis,* inflammation] An inflammation of the jejunum.

**jejuno-** [L.] Combining form meaning *jejunum.*

**jejunocecostomy** (jĕ-joo"nō-sē-kŏs'tō-mē) [" + *caecum,* blindness, + Gr. *stoma,* mouth] The formation of a passage between the cecum and jejunum.

**jejunocolostomy** (jē-jū"nō-kōl-ŏs'tō-mē) [" + Gr. *kolon,* colon, + *stoma,* mouth] The formation of an artificial passage between the jejunum and colon.

**jejunoileal** (jĕ-joo"nō-ĭl'ē-ăl) [" + *ileum,* small intestine] Concerning the jejunum and ileum.

**jejunoileitis** (jē-jū"nō-ĭl"ē-ī'tĭs) [" + " + Gr. *itis,* inflammation] An inflammation of the jejunum and ileum.

**jejunoileostomy** (jē-jū"nō-ĭl"ē-ŏs'tō-mē) [" + " + Gr. *stoma,* mouth] The formation of a passage between the jejunum and ileum.

**jejunojejunostomy** (jē-jū"nō-jē"jū-nŏs'tō-mē) [" + *jejunum,* empty, + Gr. *stoma,* mouth] The formation of a passage between two parts of the jejunum.

**jejunorrhaphy** (jĕ"joo-nor'ă-fē) [" + Gr. *rhaphe,* seam, ridge] Surgical repair of the jejunum.

**jejunostomy** (jē"jū-nŏs'tō-mē) [" + Gr. *stoma,* mouth] Surgical creation of a permanent opening into the jejunum.

***needle catheter j.*** ABBR: NCJ. A jejunostomy created by using a needle to insert a catheter into the jejunum. It is intended exclusively for feeding for a maximum of 6 weeks.

***percutaneous endoscopic j.*** ABBR: PEJ. A jejunostomy created for feeding purposes with the use of an endoscope and guide wire.

**jejunotomy** (jē"jū-nŏt'ō-mē) [" + Gr. *tome,* incision] Surgical incision into the jejunum.

**jejunum** (jē-jū'nŭm) [L., empty] The second portion of the small intestine extending from the duodenum to the ileum. It is about 8 ft (2.4 m) long, comprising about two fifths of the small intestine.

***inflammation of j.*** Pathological inflammatory changes that may occur in bacterial infections of the intestinal tract or in regional enteritis. It is characterized by absence of diarrhea, colic, distention of the abdomen, borborygmus, and flocculent or semisolid stools containing undigested food, unchanged bile, and some mucus.

**jelling** In arthritis, becoming stiff and "fixed" in any position in which movement does not occur for a prolonged period.

**jelly** [L. *gelare,* to freeze] A thick, semisolid, gelatinous mass.

***contraceptive j.*** Jelly introduced into the vagina for the prevention of conception. It serves as a vehicle for spermicidal substances. SEE: *contraceptive.*

***mineral j.*** Petrolatum.

***petroleum j.*** Petrolatum.

***vaginal j.*** Jelly introduced into the vagina for therapeutic or contraceptive purposes.

***Wharton's j.*** Soft, gelatinous, connective tissue that constitutes the matrix of the umbilical cord.

**Jendrassik's maneuver** (yĕn-dră'sĭks) [Ernö Jendrassik, Hungarian physician, 1858–1921] A method used to facilitate elicitation of the deep tendon reflexes of the lower extremities. The patient hooks together the fingers of the hands and attempts to pull them apart. While this pressure is maintained, the patellar or Achilles tendon reflex is tested.

**Jenner, Edward** A British physician (1749–1823) who invented the vaccination for smallpox. Prior to Jenner's work, it was known that individuals exposed to a mild case of the disease for the first time would suffer a mild case and then be immune to smallpox. Jenner observed that individuals exposed to cowpox, such as those who milked cows, would develop a minor lesion and then be immune to smallpox. From this observation he developed a vaccine from cowpox lesions, now known to be the vaccinia virus, which provides immunity to smallpox.

**Jenner's stain** [Louis Jenner, Brit. physician, 1866–1904] Eosin methylene blue stain.

**jerk** (jĕrk) **1.** A sudden muscular movement. **2.** Certain reflex actions resulting from striking or tapping a muscle or tendon. SEE: *reflex.*

***Achilles j.*** Ankle j.

***ankle j.*** Contraction of the calf muscles produced by tapping the stretched Achilles tendon. SYN: *Achilles j.*

***biceps j.*** A reflex contraction of the biceps brachii produced by tapping over the insertion of the tendon at the head of the radius. Usually, the evaluator places a thumb against the tendon and taps the nail of the thumb to elicit the reflex.

***elbow j.*** An involuntary extension of forearm produced by external stimulation of the stretched triceps tendon.

***jaw j.*** A movement resulting from tapping the mandible when the jaw is half open. It may be increased when there are bilateral supranuclear cerebral lesions.

***knee j.*** The extension of the lower leg upon striking the patellar tendon when the knee is flexed at a right angle. Knee jerk is absent in locomotor ataxia, infantile paralysis, meningitis, destructive lesions of the lower part of the spinal cord, and certain forms of paralysis. It is increased in lesions of pyramidal areas, brain tumors, spinal irritability, and cerebrospinal sclerosis. SYN: *patellar-ten-*

*don reflex*. SEE: *reflex, knee-jerk*.

***tendon j.*** The contraction of a muscle after tapping its tendon.

***triceps surae j.*** Ankle j.

**jet lag** SEE: *desynchronosis*.

**jig** A mechanical device used to maintain a stable, correct relationship between a piece of work and a tool, or between components during assembly.

**jigger** Common name for parasitic fleas called *Tunga penetrans*. SEE: *chiggers*.

**jimson weed** Stramonium.

**jitters** (jĭt′ĕrz) Shakes.

**Jobst pressure garment** An elastic garment fabricated to apply varying pressure gradients to an area. It may be worn over severely burned areas for the purpose of reducing hypertrophic scarring as wounds heal or may be used to prevent or control lymphedema in the arms or legs.

**Job's syndrome** [Job, Biblical character] Recurrent infections of the skin related to impaired defenses, the precise nature of which are unclear.

**Jocasta complex** (jō-kăs′tă) [Jocasta, mythical character who was the wife and mother of Oedipus] The psychological or emotional fixation of a mother toward her son. SEE: *Oedipus complex*.

**Joffroy's reflex** (zhŏf-rwhăz′) [Alexis Joffroy, Fr. physician, 1844–1908] A twitching of the gluteal muscles when pressure is made against the buttocks.

**Joffroy's sign 1.** The absence of facial muscle contraction when the eyes turn upward in exophthalmic goiter. **2.** An inability to do simple sums in arithmetic; an early sign of general paralysis in organic brain syndrome.

**jogger's heel** An irritation of the fibrous and fatty tissue covering the heel. The condition is due to the type of running characteristic of jogging, in which the heel strikes the surface first, rather than that of sprinting, in which the toes strike first. Persons prone to develop this may diminish the risk by wearing pads on their heels and by running on surfaces softer than wood, concrete, or asphalt.

**jogging** Running for enjoyment or to maintain physical fitness. In contrast to running, jogging is not a competitive exercise.

**Johnson, Dorothy** A nursing educator, born 1919, who developed the Behavioral System Model of Nursing. SEE: *Nursing Theory Appendix*.

**joint** [L. *junctio*, a joining] An articulation. The point of juncture between two bones. A joint is usually formed of fibrous connective tissue and cartilage. It is classified as being immovable (synarthrosis), slightly movable (amphiarthrosis), or freely movable (diarthrosis). *Synarthrosis* is a joint in which the two bones are separated only by an intervening membrane, such as the cranial sutures. *Amphiarthrosis* is a joint having a fibrocartilaginous disk between the bony surfaces (symphysis), such as the symphysis pubis; or one with a ligament uniting the two bones (syndesmosis), such as the tibiofibular articulation. *Diarthrosis* is a joint in which the adjoining bone ends are covered with a thin cartilaginous sheet and joined by ligament lined by a synovial membrane, which secretes a lubricant. SYN: *arthrosis* (1). SEE: illus.

Joints are also grouped according to motion: ball and socket (enarthrosis); hinge (ginglymus); condyloid; pivot (trochoid); gliding (arthrodia); and saddle joint.

Joints can move in four ways: *gliding*, in which one bony surface glides on an-

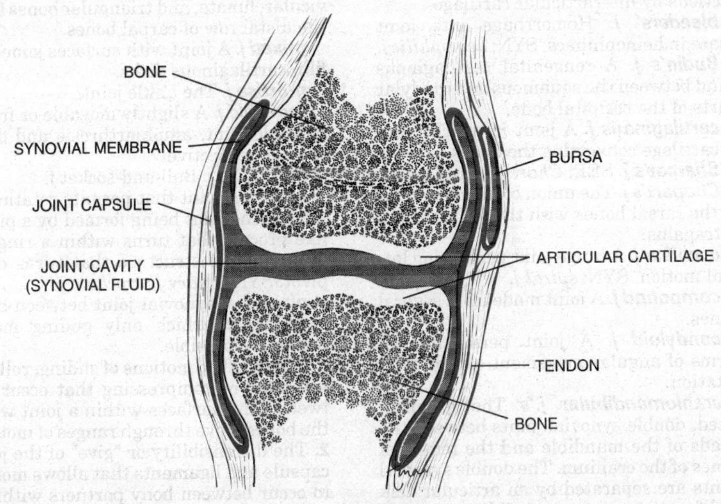


SYNOVIAL JOINT

other without angular or rotatory movement; *angular,* occurring only between long bones, increasing or decreasing the angle between the bones; *circumduction,* occurring in joints composed of the head of a bone and an articular cavity, the long bone describing a series of circles, the whole forming a cone; and *rotation,* in which a bone moves about a central axis without moving from this axis. Angular movement, if it occurs forward or backward, is called flexion or extension, respectively; away from the body, abduction; and toward the median plane of the body, adduction.

Because of their location and constant use, joints are prone to stress, injury, and inflammation. The main diseases affecting the joints are rheumatic fever, rheumatoid arthritis, osteoarthritis, and gout. Injuries are contusions, sprains, dislocations, and penetrating wounds.

The Appendix contains information about principal joints. For joints not listed here, SEE: *Joints Appendix.*

**amphidiarthrodial j.** A joint that is both ginglymoid and arthrodial.

**j. approximation** A rehabilitation technique whereby joint surfaces are compressed together while the patient is in a weight-bearing posture for the purpose of facilitating cocontraction of muscles around a joint.

**arthrodial j.** Diarthrosis permitting a gliding motion. SYN: *gliding j.*

**ball-and-socket j.** A joint in which the round end of one bone fits into the cavity of another bone. SYN: *enarthrodial j.; multiaxial j.; polyaxial j.*

**biaxial j.** A joint possessing two chief movement axes at right angles to each other.

**bilocular j.** A joint separated into two sections by interarticular cartilage.

**bleeders' j.** Hemorrhage into joint space in hemophiliacs. SYN: *hemophilic j.*

**Budin's j.** A congenital cartilaginous band between the squamous and condylar parts of the occipital bone.

**cartilaginous j.** A joint in which there is cartilage connecting the bones.

**Charcot's j.** SEE: *Charcot's joint.*

**Chopart's j.** The union of the remainder of the tarsal bones with the os calcis and astragalus.

**cochlear j.** A hinge joint permitting lateral motion. SYN: *spiral j.*

**compound j.** A joint made up of several bones.

**condyloid j.** A joint permitting all forms of angular movement except axial rotation.

**craniomandibular j.'s** The encapsulated, double synovial joints between the heads of the mandible and the temporal bones of the cranium. The double synovial joints are separated by an articular disk and function as an upper gliding joint and a lower modified hinge or ginglymoid joint. SYN: *temporomandibular j.'s.*

**diarthrodial j.** A joint characterized by the presence of a cavity within the capsule separating the bony elements, thus permitting considerable freedom of movement.

**dry j.** Arthritis of the chronic villous type.

**elbow j.** The hinge joint between the humerus and the ulna.

**ellipsoid j.** A joint having two axes of motion through the same bone.

**enarthrodial j.** Ball-and-socket j.

**false j.** False joint formation subsequent to a fracture.

**fibrous j.'s** Joints connected by fibrous tissue.

**flail j.** A joint that is extremely relaxed, the distal portion of the limb being almost beyond the control of the will.

**ginglymoid j.** A synovial joint having only forward and backward motion, as a hinge. SYN: *hinge j.; ginglymus.*

**gliding j.** Arthrodial j.

**hemophilic j.** Bleeders' j.

**hinge j.** Ginglymoid j.

**hip j.** A stable ball-and-socket type of joint in which the head of the femur fits into the acetabulum of the hip bone.

**immovable j.** Synarthrosis.

**intercarpal j.'s** Articulations formed by the carpal bones in relation to one another.

**irritable j.** A recurrent joint inflammation of unknown cause.

**knee j.** The joint formed by the femur, patella, and tibia.

**j. mice** Free bits of cartilage or bone present in the joint space, esp. the knee joint. These are usually the result of previous trauma, and may or may not be symptomatic.

**midcarpal j.** A joint separating the navicular, lunate, and triangular bones from the distal row of carpal bones.

**mixed j.** A joint with surfaces joined by fibrocartilaginous disks.

**mortise j.** The ankle joint.

**movable j.** A slightly movable or freely movable joint, amphiarthrosis and diarthrosis, respectively.

**multiaxial j.** Ball-and-socket j.

**pivot j.** A joint that permits rotation of a bone, the joint being formed by a pivotlike process that turns within a ring, or by a ringlike structure that turns on a pivot. SYN: *rotary j.; trochoid j.*

**plane j.** A synovial joint between bone surfaces, in which only gliding movements are possible.

**j. play 1.** The motions of sliding, rolling, spinning, or compressing that occur between bony surfaces within a joint when the bones move through ranges of motion. **2.** The distensibility or "give" of the joint capsule and ligaments that allows motion to occur between bony partners within a joint.

**polyaxial j.** Ball-and-socket j.

***j. protection*** A technique for minimizing stress on joints, including proper body mechanics and the avoidance of continuous weight-bearing or deforming postures.

***receptive j.*** Saddle j.

***rotary j.*** Pivot j.

***saddle j.*** A joint in which the opposing surfaces are reciprocally concavoconvex. SYN: *receptive j.*

***shoulder j.*** The ball-and-socket joint between the head of the humerus and the glenoid cavity of the scapula.

***simple j.*** A joint composed of two bones.

***spheroid j.*** A multiaxial joint with spheroid surfaces.

***spiral j.*** Cochlear j.

***sternoclavicular j.*** The joint space between the sternum and the medial extremity of the clavicle.

***subtalar j.'s*** The three articular surfaces on the inferior surface of the talus.

***synarthrodial j.*** Synarthrosis.

***synovial j.*** A joint in which the articulating surfaces are separated by synovial fluid. SEE: *joint* for illus.

***tarsometatarsal j.*** A joint composed of three arthrodial joints, the bones of which articulate with the bases of the metatarsal bones.

***temporomandibular j.'s*** Craniomandibular j.'s.

***trochoid j.*** Pivot j.

***ulnomeniscal-triquetral j.*** The functional articulation of the distal ulna, articular disc, and triquetrum. The disc may subluxate following injury or with arthritis and block supination of the forearm.

***uniaxial j.*** A joint moving on a single axis.

***unilocular j.*** A joint with a single cavity.

**Joint Review Committee for Respiratory Therapy Education** ABBR: JRCRTE. An organization that establishes standards and oversees educational programs in respiratory therapy.

**Jones criteria** [T.D. Jones, U.S. physician, 1899–1954] The criteria for diagnosis of acute rheumatic fever. SEE: *rheumatic fever.*

**joule** (jūl) [James Prescott Joule, Brit. physicist, 1818–1889] ABBR: J. The work done in one second by a current of one ampere against a resistance of one ohm. One kilogram calorie (kcal or Calorie) is equal to 4185.5 J. One calorie (small calorie) equals 4.1855 J.

**JRA** *juvenile rheumatoid arthritis.*

**JRCEDMS** *Joint Review Committee on Education in Diagnostic Medical Sonography.*

**JRCERT** *Joint Review Committee on Education in Radiologic Technology.*

**JRCRTE** *Joint Review Committee for Respiratory Therapy Education.*

**judgment** The use of available evidence or facts to formulate a rational opinion or to make a correct decision. Judgment may be impaired by mental illness, medications, fatigue, or bias.

**jugal** [L. *jugalis,* of a yoke] **1.** Connected or united as by a yoke. **2.** Pert. to the malar or zygomatic bone.

**jugale** (jū-gā′lē) The point at the margin of the zygomatic process.

**jugomaxillary** (joo″gō-măk′sĭ-lār″ē) Concerning the maxilla and the zygomatic bone.

**jugular** (jŭg′ū-lăr) [L. *jugularis*] Pert. to the throat.

***j. vein*** Any of several large veins that return blood to the heart from the head and neck. The external jugular vein receives the blood from the exterior of the cranium and the deep parts of the face. It lies superficial to the sternocleidomastoid muscle as it passes down the neck to join the subclavian vein. The internal jugular vein receives blood from the brain and superficial parts of the face and neck. It is directly continuous with the transverse sinus, accompanying the internal carotid artery as it passes down the neck, and joins with the subclavian vein to form the innominate vein. The jugular veins are more prominent during expiration than during inspiration and are also prominent during cardiac decompensation.

When the patient is sitting or in a semirecumbent position, the height of the jugular veins and their pulsations can provide an accurate estimation of central venous pressure and give important information about cardiac compensation.

**jugulate** (jŭg′ū-lāt) [L. *jugulare,* to cut the throat] To quickly arrest a process or disease by therapeutic measures.

**jugulation** (jŭg″ū-lā′shŭn) The sudden arrest of a disease by therapeutic means.

**jugulum** (jŭg′ū-lŭm) [L.] Neck or throat.

**jugum** (jū′gŭm) *pl.* **juga** [L., a yoke] **1.** A ridge or furrow connecting two points. **2.** A type of forceps.

***j. penis*** A forceps for temporarily compressing the penis.

***j. petrosum*** An eminence on the petrous section of the temporal bone showing the position of the superior semicircular canal. SYN: *arcuate eminence.*

**juice** [L. *jus,* broth] Liquid excreted, secreted, or expressed from any part of an organism.

***alimentary j.*** Digestive secretion.

***gastric j.*** A secretion of the stomach, consisting of water, salts, pepsin, and free hydrochloric acid.

***intestinal j.*** Alkaline secretion that contains peptidases and enzymes to complete the digestion of disaccharides. SEE: *digestion.*

***pancreatic j.*** A clear, viscid, alkaline digestive juice of the pancreas poured into the duodenum. It contains the enzymes trypsin, amylase, and lipase or steapsin.

**Jumping Frenchmen of Maine** A condition characterized by a sudden, single, sometimes violent movement or cry that occurs in response to a sharp unexpected sound

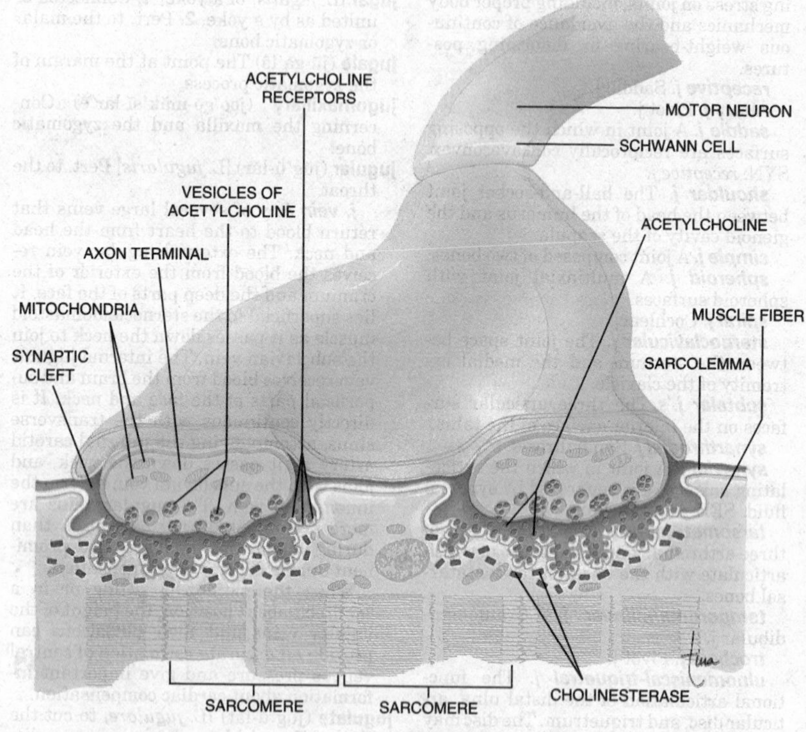


MYONEURAL JUNCTION

or touch. The individual may also blurt out whatever was being thought of at the time of the stimulus. The condition may begin in childhood and be lifelong. It has been most frequently described in persons of French descent living in Maine, but may occur in a person of almost any nationality or geographic location. The cause is unknown and there is no effective therapy. SEE: *Tourette's syndrome; miryachit; startle syndrome.*

**junction** (jŭnk′shŭn) [L. *junctio,* a joining] The place of union or coming together of two parts or tissue layers.

***amelodentinal j.*** Dentinoenamel j.

***atrioventricular j.*** The area of cardiac conduction pathway composed of the AV node and bundle of His.

***cementodentinal j.*** The interface of dentin and cementum of the tooth. SYN: *dentinocemental j.*

***cementoenamel j.*** The line around the tooth that marks the boundary between the crown and root of the tooth; the interface between enamel and cementum.

***dentinocemental j.*** Cementodentinal j.

***dentinoenamel j.*** The plane or interface between the dentin of the tooth and the enamel crown; histological sections show it to be a scalloped boundary at the site of the basement membrane which separated the cell layers that formed the calcified enamel and dentin. SYN: *amelodentinal j.*

***dentogingival j.*** The interface and zone of attachment between the gingiva and enamel or cementum of the tooth. It holds in place the junctional or attachment epithelium.

***interneuronal j.*** Synapse.

***liquid j.*** The point in a potentiometric reference electrode measurement system at which the reference solution makes contact with the test solution. An example is pH reference electrode.

***mucocutaneous j.*** The junction between the skin and a mucous membrane.

***mucogingival j.*** A scalloped, indistinct boundary between the gingiva and the oral mucosa on the alveolar process. The coral color of gingiva may be contrasted with the more vascular oral mucosa. Also called the mucogingival line.

***myoneural j.*** The axon terminal of a motor neuron, synaptic cleft, and sarcolemma of a muscle cell. SYN: *neuromuscular j.* SEE: illus.; *motor endplate.*

***neuromuscular j.*** Myoneural j.

***sclerocorneal j.*** The meeting point between the sclera and the cornea marked on the external surface of the eyeball by the outer scleral sulcus.

***squamocolumnar j.*** The point in the cervical canal at which the squamous and columnar epithelia meet. As most cervical cancers begin in this area, it is important to obtain cells from this location for the Pap test.

***tight j.*** A part of the junctional complex at the lateral interface between epithelial cells; also called zonula occludens.

**junctura** (jŭnk-tū′ră) *pl.* **juncturae** [L., a joining] Suture of bones; articulation.

**Jung, Carl Gustave** [Swiss psychiatrist, 1875–1961] The founder of the Jungian school of analytic psychology. In his early career, Jung was associated with Sigmund Freud. Later they disagreed about certain aspects of psychoanalytic theory.

**juniper tar** (joo′nĭ-pĕr) A volatile oil obtained from the wood of *Juniperus oxycedrus.* It is used in shampoos and bath emulsions.

**jurisprudence** (joor″ĭs-proo′dĕns) [L. *juris prudentia,* knowledge of law] The scientific study or application of the principles of law and justice.

***dental j.*** The application of the principles of law as they relate to the practice of dentistry, to the obligations of the practitioners to their patients, and to the relations of dentists to each other and to society in general. This term and forensic dentistry are sometimes used as synonyms, but some authorities consider the first as a branch of law and the second as a branch of dentistry.

***medical j.*** The application of the principles of law as they relate to the practice of medicine, to the obligations of the practitioners to their patients, and to the relations of physicians to each other and to society in general.

***nursing j.*** The application of the principles of law as they relate to the practice of nursing, to the obligations of nurses to their patients, and to the relations of nurses with each other and with other health care professionals.

**jury-mast** (jūr′ē-măst) [L. *jurare,* to be right, + AS. *masc,* a stick] An apparatus for support of the head in diseases of the spine.

**Juster's reflex** [Emile Juster, 20th century Fr. neurologist] Finger extension instead of flexion when palm of hand is irritated.

**justo major** (jŭs′tō mā′jor) [L.] Bigger than normal, as a pelvis.

**justo minor** (jŭs′tō mī′nor) [L.] Smaller than normal, as a pelvis.

**juvenile** (jū′vĕ-nīl″) [L. *juvenis,* young] **1.** Pert. to youth or childhood. **2.** Young; immature.

**juxta-** [L., near] Prefix indicating *proximity.*

**juxta-articular** (jŭks″tă-ăr-tĭk′ū-lăr) [″ + *articulus,* joint] Situated close to a joint.

**juxtaglomerular** (jŭks″tă-glō-mĕr′ū-lăr) [″ + *glomus,* ball] Near or adjacent to a glomerulus.

**juxtaposition** (jŭks″tă-pō-zĭ′shŭn) [″ + *positio,* place] Apposition.

**juxtapyloric** (jŭks″tă-pī-lor′ĭk) [″ + Gr. *pyloros,* pylorus] Near the pylorus or pyloric orifice.

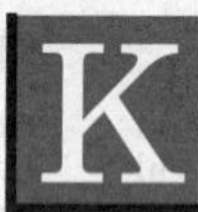

**K** [L. *kalium*] Symbol for the element potassium.

**K, k 1.** Symbol for the Greek letter *kappa*. **2.** Used in some formulas in chemistry and physics to indicate a constant or value that does not change. **3.** Kelvin temperature scale. **4.** Symbol for kilo.

**Kader's operation** (kă′dĕrs) [Bronislaw Kader, Polish surgeon, 1863–1937] The surgical formation of a gastric fistula with the feeding tube inserted through a valve-like flap.

**kaif** (kĭf) [Arabic, quiescence] A dreamy, tranquil state induced by drugs.

**kainophobia** (kī-nō-fō′bē-ă) [Gr. *kainos*, new, + *phobos*, fear] Neophobia.

**kaiserling** (kī′zĕr-lĭng) [Karl Kaiserling, Ger. pathologist, 1869–1942] A liquid used in preserving pathological specimens.

**kakidrosis** (kăk-ĭ-drō′sĭs) [Gr. *kakos*, bad, + *hidrosis*, sweat] Bromidrosis.

**kakke** (kŏk′kā) [Japanese] Beriberi.

**kakosmia** (kăk-ŏz′mē-ă) [Gr. *kakos*, bad, + *osme*, smell] Cacosmia.

**kala azar** (kă′lă ă-zăr′) [Hindi, black fever] An infectious disease, common in the rural parts of tropical and subtropical areas of the world. There are several types, which differ as to preference for children or adults, incidence in domestic animals, and transmitting agent. The disease is characterized by lesions of the reticuloendothelial system, esp. the liver and spleen, and it is often fatal. The incubation period is generally 2 to 6 months, however the range is from 10 days to more than a year. SYN: *visceral leishmaniasis.*

Etiology: Kala azar is caused by *Leishmania donovani*, an intracellular flagellated protozoon. The organism is transmitted by the bite of infected sandflies of the genus *Phlebotomus*.

Prophylaxis: The sandflies that transmit the organisms can be controlled by use of insecticides that have residual action. In addition, elimination of breeding grounds of the flies is helpful, as is avoidance of animals that are known reservoirs. If exposure to flies is inevitable, protective clothing should be worn.

Treatment: Various forms of pentavalent antimonial compounds are used, but treatment failures are common. The combination of allopurinol with pentavalent antimonials is more effective than antimonials alone. Amphotericin B given for up to 8 weeks has been successful in treating patients who do not respond to antimony compounds

**kaligenous** (kā-lĭj′ĕ-nŭs) [″ + Gr. *gennan*, to produce] Forming potash.

**kalimeter** (kă-lĭm′ĕ-ter) [″ + Gr. *metron*, measure] Alkalimeter.

**kaliopenia** (kă″lē-ō-pē′nē-ă) [L. *kalium*, potassium, + Gr. *penia*, poverty] Hypokalemia; decreased potassium in the blood.

**kaliuresis** (kă″lē-ū-rē′sĭs) [L. *kalium*, potassium, + Gr. *ouresis*, urination] The excretion of potassium in the urine.

**kallidin** (kăl′ĭ-dĭn) A plasma kinin. SEE: *kinin.*

**kallikrein** (kăl-ĭ-krē′ĭn) [Gr. *kallikreas*, pancreas] An enzyme normally present in blood plasma, urine, and body tissue in an inactive state. When activated, kallikrein is one of the most potent vasodilators. It forms kinin.

**kallikreinogen** (kăl″ĭ-krī′nō-jĕn) [″ + *gennan*, to produce] The precursor of kallikrein in blood plasma.

**kanamycin sulfate** (kăn″ă-mī′sĭn) An antibiotic.

**Kanner syndrome** [Leo Kanner, Austrian psychiatrist in the U.S., b. 1894] Infantile autism.

**kaolin** (kā′ō-lĭn) [Fr., from Mandarin Chinese *kao*, high, + *ling*, mountain] A yellow-white or gray clay powder occurring in a natural state as a form of hydrated aluminum silicate. It is used internally as an absorbent, externally as a protective by absorbing moisture. SYN: *China clay.*

**kaolinosis** (kā″ō-lĭn-ō′sĭs) Pneumonoconiosis caused by inhaling kaolin particles.

**Kaopectate** Trade name for a combination product containing kaolin.

**Kaposi, Moritz K.** (kăp′ō-sē″) Austrian physician, 1837–1902. Originally his name was Moritz Kohn.

***K.'s disease*** Xeroderma pigmentosum.

***K.'s sarcoma*** ABBR: KS. A vascular malignancy that is often first apparent in the skin or mucous membranes but may involve the viscera. Once a rare disease seen usually in elderly men, in recent years the incidence of Kaposi's sarcoma has risen dramatically along with the incidence of acquired immunodeficiency syndrome (AIDS). Currently, it is the most common AIDS-related tumor. Characterized by obvious, colorful lesions, Kaposi's sarcoma causes structural and functional damage. When associated with AIDS, it progresses aggressively, involving the lymph nodes, the viscera, and possibly the gastrointestinal tract. SEE: *AIDS.*

Etiology: The exact cause of Kaposi's sarcoma is unknown, but the disease may be due to immunosuppression. Genetic or hereditary predisposition also is suspected.

Symptoms: The health history frequently reveals that the patient has AIDS. If the sarcoma advances beyond the early stages or if a lesion breaks down, the patient may report pain. Usually, however, the lesions remain painless unless they impinge on nerves or organs. On inspection, the examiner may observe several lesions in various shapes, sizes, and colors (ranging from red-brown to dark purple). The lesions occur most commonly on the skin, buccal mucosa, hard and soft palates, lips, gums, tongue, tonsils, conjunctiva, and sclera. In advanced disease the lesions may join, becoming one large plaque. Untreated lesions may appear as large, ulcerative masses. The patient may exhibit dyspnea, especially if pulmonary involvement is present. Palpation and inspection may also disclose edema from lymphatic obstruction. Auscultation may reveal wheezing and hypoventilation. Respiratory distress usually results from bronchial obstruction. The most common extracutaneous sites are the lungs and G.I. tract (esophagus, oropharynx, and epiglottis).

DIAGNOSIS: Usually, the patient will undergo a tissue biopsy to determine the lesion's type and stage. Then a computed tomography scan may be performed to look for metastasis.

TREATMENT: Radiation therapy, chemotherapy, and drug therapy with biological response modifiers are local treatment options. Radiation therapy offers palliation of symptoms, including pain from obstructing lesions in the oral cavity or extremities and edema caused by lymphatic blockage. Intralesional therapy includes application of liquid nitrogen and injection of small amounts of dilute vinblastine directly into the KS lesion. Chemotherapy includes combinations of doxorubicin, vinblastine, and vincristine. The biological response modifier interferon Alfa-2b may be prescribed in AIDS-related KS. It reduces the number of lesions but is ineffective in advanced disease.

NURSING IMPLICATIONS: The nurse inspects the patient's skin every shift for new lesions and skin breakdown. The patient is monitored for signs and symptoms of respiratory distress or G.I. dysfunction. The nurse reinforces the physician's explanation of treatments, ensuring that the patient understands the adverse reactions and their management. Prescribed drug therapies are administered and evaluated for desired effects, and adverse reactions such as anorexia, nausea, vomiting, and diarrhea are assessed for and managed. Prescribed analgesics are administered for pain as necessary, and noninvasive pain relief measures such as distraction, relaxation techniques, positioning, and imagery are used to enhance the patient's comfort. Infection prevention techniques are explained and basic hygiene measures to prevent infection (especially important if the patient also has AIDS) are demonstrated. The nurse listens to the patient's fears and concerns, answers questions honestly, and stays with the patient during periods of stress or anxiety. The patient should participate in care planning, self-care management, and decision making as much as possible. High-calorie, high-protein meals are often better tolerated as small, frequent meals rather than as three large ones. The nurse consults with a dietitian to plan meals around the patient's treatment schedule. Prescribed antiemetics and sedatives are administered as needed, and I.V. fluids or parenteral nutrition is provided if the patient is unable to eat. Frequent rest periods are provided, because the patient tires easily. The patient shares feelings about appearance, and assistance is offered to help the patient to adjust to changes in body image. The nurse offers emotional support to the patient and family to help them cope with the diagnosis and prognosis and provides opportunities for them to discuss their concerns. The need for ongoing treatment and care is stressed. As appropriate, the nurse refers the patient (and family) to available social services and support groups, and for terminal (hospice) care.

***K.'s varicelliform eruption*** A skin disease resulting from infection with herpes simplex or vaccinia virus in the presence of another skin disease such as eczema.

**karaya gum** (kăr′ā-ă) The dried gum from *Sterculia* plants, which becomes gelatinous when moist. It is used as an adhesive and as a bulk laxative.

**Karman catheter** [Harvey Karman, U.S. psychologist, b. 1924] A catheter used for suction curettage of the uterus.

**Karnofsky Index, Karnofsky Scale** [D.A. Karnofsky, 20th century physician] A means to clinically estimate a patient's physical state, performance, and prognosis. The scale is from 100, perfectly well, to 0, dead. It has been used in studying cancer and chronic illness.

**Kartagener's syndrome** (kăr′tă-gā″nĕrz) [Manes Kartagener, Swiss physician, 1897–1975] A hereditary syndrome consisting of bronchiectasis, maldevelopment of the sinuses, and transposition of the viscera. SEE: *immotile cilia syndrome.*

**karyo-, kary-** [Gr. *karyon,* kernel] Prefix referring to a cell's nucleus. SEE: also *caryo-.*

**karyochromatophil** (kăr″ē-ō-krō-măt′ō-fĭl) [″ + *chroma,* color, + *philein,* to love] Having a nucleus that stains.

**karyochrome** (kăr′ē-ō-krōm″) The cell of a nerve with an easily staining nucleus.

**karyocyte** (kăr′ē-ō-sīt) [″ + *kytos,* cell] Normoblast, the nucleated red blood cell.

**karyogamy** (kăr-ē-ŏg′ă-mē) [″ + *gamos,* marriage] The union of nuclei in cell conjugation.

**karyogenesis** (kăr″ē-ō-jĕn′ĕ-sĭs) [″ + *genesis,* generation, birth] The formation and development of a cell nucleus.

**karyokinesis** (kăr″ē-ō-kĭn-ē′sĭs) [″ + *kinesis,* movement] The equal division of nuclear material that occurs in cell division. SEE: *cytokinesis; mitosis.*

**karyokinetic** (kăr″ē-ō-kĭ-nĕt′ĭk) **1.** Pert. to karyokinesis. **2.** Ameboid.

**karyoklasis** (kăr″ē-ŏk′lă-sĭs) [″ + *klasis,* a breaking] Disintegration of the cell nucleus.

**karyolobism** (kăr″ē-ō-lō′bĭzm) [″ + L. *lobus,* lobe, + Gr. *-ismos,* state of] A condition in which the nucleus of a cell is lobed, as in polymorphonuclear leukocytes.

**karyolymph** [″ + L. *lympha,* lymph] Fluid in meshes of the nucleus; now known to contain active submicroscopic components of the nucleoplasm. Thus the terms karyolymph and nuclear sap do not describe clearly definable entities and should not be used. SEE: *cell; organelle.*

**karyolysis** (kăr-ē-ŏl′ĭ-sĭs) [″ + *lysis,* dissolution] Chromatolysis. **karyolytic** (-ō-lĭt′ĭk), *adj.*

**karyomegaly** (kăr″ē-ō-mĕg′ă-lē) [″ + *megas,* large] An abnormal enlargement of the cell nucleus.

**karyomere** (kăr′ē-ō-mēr″) [″ + *meros,* part] **1.** Chromomere (1). **2.** A vesicle containing only a small portion of the nucleus.

**karyomicrosome** (kăr″ē-ō-mī′krō-sōm) [″ + *mikros,* small, + *soma,* body] **1.** Any one of the small particles in the karyoplasm. **2.** Any one of the small tangible bodies or segments of chromatin fiber.

**karyomitosis** (kăr″ē-ō-mī-tō′sĭs) [″ + *mitos,* thread, + *osis,* condition] Karyokinesis.

**karyomorphism** (kăr-ē-ō-mor′fĭzm) [″ + *morphe,* form, + *-ismos,* state of] The form of a cell nucleus.

**karyon** (kăr′ē-ŏn) [Gr.] The nucleus of a cell.

**karyophage** (kăr′ē-ō-fāj) [Gr. *karyon,* kernel, + *phagein,* to eat] An intracellular protozoan parasite that destroys the nucleus of a cell.

**karyopyknosis** (kăr″ē-ō-pĭk-nō′sĭs) [″ + *pyknos,* thick, + *osis,* condition] Shrinkage of the nucleus of the cell with condensation of the chromatin.

**karyorrhexis** (kăr″ē-ō-rĕk′sĭs) [″ + *rhexis,* rupture] Fragmentation of the chromatin in nuclear disintegration.

**karyosome** (kăr′ē-ō-sōm) [″ + *soma,* body] Irregular clumps of nondividing chromatin material seen in the nuclei of cells. SYN: *chromocenter.*

**karyostasis** (kăr″ē-ŏs′tă-sĭs) [″ + *stasis,* standing] The resting stage of a cell nucleus.

**karyotheca** (kăr″ē-ō-thē′kă) [″ + *theke,* sheath] The enveloping membrane of a cell nucleus.

**karyotype** (kăr′ē-ō-tīp) [″ + *typos,* mark] A photomicrograph of the chromosomes of a single cell, taken during metaphase, when each chromosome is still a pair of chromatids. The chromosomes are then arranged in numerical order, in descending order of size. SEE: *chromosome* for illus.

**karyozoic** (kăr″ē-ō-zō′ĭk) [″ + *zoon,* animal] Living in the cell nucleus, as would occur with an intracellular protozoal parasite.

**Kasabach-Merritt syndrome** [Haig H. Kasabach, U.S. pediatrician, 1898–1943; Katherine K. Merritt, U.S. physician, b. 1886] Capillary hemangioma associated with thrombocytopenic purpura.

**Kasai procedure** [named for a province in Zaire] Hepatic portoenterostomy. Also called *Kasai hepatoportoenterostomy.*

**Kashin-Beck disease** [N. I. Kashin, Russian physician, 1825–1872; E. V. Beck (Bek)] Endemic polyarthritis limited to certain areas of Asia. It is believed to be a form of mycotoxicosis caused by eating grain contaminated with the fungus *Fusarium sporotrichiella.*

**kata-** [Gr. *kata,* down] Prefix meaning *down, reversing process, wrongly, back, destruction, against.* SEE: *cata-.*

**kataplasia** (kăt-ă-plā′sē-ă) Cataplasia.

**katathermometer** (kăt″ă-thĕr-mŏm′ĕ-ter) [″ + *therme,* heat, + *metron,* measure] A device consisting of two thermometers, one a dry bulb and the other a wet bulb. Both are heated to 110°F (43.3°C) and the time required for each thermometer to fall from 100° to 90°F (37.8° to 32.2°C) is noted. The dry bulb gives the cooling power by radiation and convection, the wet bulb by radiation, convection, and evaporation. Attempts to use this type of thermometer to measure wind velocity have been unsuccessful.

**kathisophobia** (kăth″ĭ-sō-fō′bē-ă) [Gr. *kathizein,* to sit down, + *phobos,* fear] A fear of sitting down, and subsequent inability to sit still.

**katophoria** (kăt″ō-fō′rē-ă) Katotropia.

**katotropia** (kăt″ō-trō′pē-ă) [Gr. *kata,* down, + *tropos,* a turning] A tendency of the eyeball to deviate downward. SYN: *katophoria.*

**katzenjammer** (kăts′ĕn-yăm′ĕr) [Ger. *katzen,* cats, + *jammer,* distress, misery] German word meaning hangover.

**kava** [Tongan, bitter] **1.** Root of *Piper methysticum,* a tropical shrub. **2.** A Polynesian beverage made from the root of *Piper methysticum.* It has the effect of a tranquilizer and muscle relaxant with caffeinelike properties. Continued use may cause a scaly skin disease.

**Kawasaki disease** [Tomsaku Kawasaki, contemporary Japanese pediatrician] An acute febrile disease of children that resembles scarlet fever. The fever is present on the first day of the illness and may last from 1 to 3 wk. The child is irritable, lethargic, and has bilateral congestion of the conjunctivae. The oral mucosa is deep red, and strawberry tongue is prominent. Lips are dry, cracked, and red. On the third to fifth day, the palms and soles are distinctly red, the hands and feet are edematous. The skin on the tips of the fingers and toes peels in layers. A macular erythematous rash free of crusts and vesicles spreads from the extremities to the trunk. Cervical lymphadenopathy is present in the first 3 days and lasts more than 3 weeks. The disease is rarely fatal in the acute phase, but children may die suddenly from coronary artery disease some years later. This disease was previously called *mucocutaneous lymph node syndrome*. SEE: *toxic shock syndrome; Nursing Diagnoses Appendix*.

TREATMENT: Treatment is supportive. If given within 10 days of onset of fever, immune gamma globulin I.V. in high doses and aspirin will decrease the risk of coronary artery dilation and aneurysms. Antibiotics and corticosteroids are not beneficial. Frequent follow-up care in the first 2 months to detect heart disease is important, as is prolonged low-dose aspirin therapy to help prevent platelet aggregation.

**Kayser-Fleischer ring** SEE: *Wilson's disease*.

**KBr** Potassium bromide.

**kc** *kilocycle*.

**K cells** A type of T lymphocyte activated by an antigen-antibody reaction that directly lyses (kills) infected cells.

**$KC_2H_3O_2$** Potassium acetate.

**KCl** Potassium chloride.

**KClO** Potassium hypochlorite.

**$KClO_3$** Potassium chlorate.

**$K_2CO_3$** Potassium carbonate.

**kc.p.s., kc/s** *kilocycles per second*.

**keep vein open** ABBR: KVO. An order indicating that a vein be kept open so that subsequent intravenous (IV) solutions or medicines can be administered. The implication is that even though IV medication is not needed at the moment, the line carrying IV solutions should remain functional. This is done using the lowest possible infusion rate.

**kefir, kefyr** (kĕf'ĕr) [Caucasus region of Russia] A preparation of curdled milk made originally in the Caucasus by adding kefir grains to milk.

**Kegel exercise** [A. H. Kegel, contemporary U.S. physician] An exercise for strengthening the pubococcygeal and levator ani muscles. Basically, the patient tightens those muscles that could be used in attempting to prevent defecation or urination. Dr. Kegel placed a bulb in the vagina and attached it to a manometer. While doing the exercises, the patient could observe the pressure increase and decrease as the muscles were contracted and relaxed. For this technique to be effective, it is imperative that the patient receive detailed instruction. The muscles should be contracted for 10 to 20 sec at least 4 times a day. The exercises may be done at any time. Increase in the strength of the muscles helps to control urinary and fecal incontinence, aids in the childbirth process, and may enhance the pleasure derived from sexual intercourse. SEE: *incontinence, stress urinary*.

**Keith's bundle, Keith's node** (kēths) [Sir Arthur Keith, Brit. anatomist, 1866–1955] Sinoatrial node of the heart.

**Keith-Wagener-Barker classification** Classification of the funduscopic findings in hypertensive patients. Grades 1 to 4 indicate progressive pathological changes. Grade 1 is moderate narrowing of the retinal arterioles; grade 2 indicates retinal hemorrhages in addition to arteriolar narrowing; in grade 3 there are cotton-wool exudates; grade 4 shows papilledema.

**kelis** (kē'lĭs) [Gr., blemish] Keloid.

**Kell blood group** One of the human blood groups. It is composed of three forms of antigens present on the surface of the red blood cells. SEE: *blood groups*.

**Kelly's pad** [Howard A. Kelly, U.S. surgeon, 1858–1943] A drainage pad for the operating table or bed made by wrapping one end of a rubber sheet over a rolled small blanket, forming a bolster. The bolster is twisted round like a horseshoe to form the pad, the free part of the sheet forming the apron. A commercial inflatable rubber pad of horseshoe shape may be used in the same way.

**keloid** (kē'lŏyd) [Gr. *kele*, tumor, + *eidos*, form, shape] Scar formation in the skin following trauma or surgical incision. Tissue response is out of proportion to the amount of scar tissue required for normal repair and healing. The result is a raised, firm, thickened red scar that may grow for a prolonged period of time. The increase in scar size is due to deposition of an abnormal amount of collagen into the tissue. Blacks are esp. prone to developing keloids.

TREATMENT: The injection of a corticosteroid into the scar has been effective in some patients. Laser therapy has been tried, as have pharmacological agents that interfere with collagen synthesis.

***acne k.*** A keloid that develops at the site of an acne pustule.

**keloidosis** (kē"loy-dō'sĭs) [" + " + *osis*, condition] The formation of keloids.

**kelotomy** (kē-lŏt'ō-mē) [" + *tome*, incision] An operation for strangulated hernia through tissues of the constricting neck.

**kelp 1.** Any member of the brown seaweeds of the order Laminariales. **2.** The ash of seaweed from which potassium and iodine salts are prepared.

**Kelvin scale** [Lord (William Thompson) Kelvin, Brit. physicist, 1824–1907] ABBR: K. The temperature scale in which absolute zero is equal to minus 273° on the Celsius scale. On the Kelvin scale the freezing point of water is 273°K, and the boiling point 373°K.

**Kempner rice-fruit diet** (kĕmp'nĕr) [Walter Kempner, U.S. physician, b. 1903] A rigid salt-restriction diet used in treating hypertension. It consists of rice, fruit, and sugar for no more than 2000 kcal/day and 7 mEq of sodium per day.

**Kendrick Extrication Device** ABBR: KED. A flexible vest-type device used to immobilize the head and neck of a seated patient (i.e., in a car).

**Kenny treatment** [Sister Elizabeth Kenny, Australian nurse, 1886–1952] Physical therapy used in treating poliomyelitis. The regimen consists of application of hot, moist packs to affected muscles and early re-education of muscles, first through passive exercise and then by active movements as soon as possible. Rigid fixation of paralyzed limbs is discouraged.

**kenophobia** (kĕn″ō-fō′bē-ă) [Gr. *kenos,* empty, + *phobos,* fear] A fear of empty spaces.

**Kent's bundles** [Albert Frank Stanley Kent, Brit. physiologist, 1863–1958] Accessory conduction fiber bundles in the heart which rapidly convey atrial impulses across the atrioventricular tissue. They are usually present in the Wolff-Parkinson-White syndrome.

**kerasin** (kĕr′ă-sĭn) A cerebroside isolated from brain tissue.

**keratalgia** (kĕr″ă-tăl′jē-ă) [Gr. *keras,* horn, + *algos,* pain] Neuralgia of the cornea.

**keratectasia** (kĕr″ă-tĕk-tā′sē-ă) [″ + *ektasis,* extension] Conical protrusion of the cornea.

**keratectomy** (kĕr-ă-tĕk′tō-mē) [″ + *ektome,* excision] Excision of a portion of the cornea.

**keratiasis** (kĕr-ă-tī′ă-sĭs) [″ + *-iasis,* condition] Horny wart formations on the skin.

**keratic** (kĕr-ăt′ĭk) **1.** Horny. **2.** Relating to the cornea.

***k. precipitates*** Inflammatory cells of the anterior chamber of the eye that adhere to the endothelial surface of the cornea. These precipitates may be large, heavy, and fat or small and punctate.

**keratin** (kĕr′ă-tĭn) An extremely tough protein substance in hair, nails, and horny tissue; insoluble in water, weak acids, or alkalis; and unaffected by most proteolytic enzymes. The fibrous protein is produced by keratinocytes and may be hard or soft.

***hard k.*** Keratin found in the hair and nails.

***soft k.*** Keratin found in the epidermis of the skin as the flexible, tough stratum corneum in the form of flattened non-nucleated scales which slough continually.

**keratinase** (kĕr′ă-tĭ-nās) An enzyme that hydrolyzes the protein keratin.

**keratinization** The process of keratin formation that takes place within the keratinocytes as they progress upward through the layers of the epidermis of skin to the surface stratum corneum. This process may occur normally on moist oral mucosa during chewing. Pathological changes (keratoses) may occur due to an autosomal dominant gene, or environmental trauma (e.g., the heat or toxins of tobacco or other carcinogens).

**keratinize** (kĕr′ă-tĭn-īz) [Gr. *keras,* horn] To become hard or horny; usually said of tissue.

**keratinocyte** (kĕ-răt′ĭ-nō-sīt) [″ + *kytos,* cell] Any one of the cells in the skin that synthesize keratin.

***cultured k.'s*** Keratinocytes that are cultured so that a small biopsy sample from uninjured skin may grow as a sheet and expand to have a surface area 1000 to 10,000 times the area of the sample. The sheet can be used to cover wounds such as burns. The culture technique requires 2 to 3 wk and the regeneration of tissue below the sheet may not be complete for 5 to 6 months.

**keratinous** (kĕr-ăt′ĭ-nŭs) Pert. to or composed of keratin.

**keratitis** (kĕr-ă-tī′tĭs) [″ + *itis,* inflammation] Inflammation of the cornea, which is usually associated with decreased visual acuity. Pain is the most common symptom.

ETIOLOGY: The inflammation may be caused by microorganisms, trauma, or immune-mediated reactions.

TREATMENT: Therapy depends upon the causative organism or other causes (e.g., removal of a foreign body from the cornea).

NURSING IMPLICATIONS: Because of the seriousness of this condition, patients experiencing eye inflammation or pain should seek immediate medical attention. The nurse assesses for a history of recent upper respiratory infection accompanied by cold sores; questions the patient about pain, central vision loss, sensitivity, the sensation of a foreign body in his eye, photophobia, and blurred vision; and inspects for loss of normal corneal luster and inflammation. The patient should refrain from rubbing the eye because this can result in complications. Prescribed therapies are administered, and the patient is instructed in their use. When making contact with the eyes or ocular drainage in the case of the patient whose keratitis is from herpes simplex the nurse or other care provider should wear gloves. Warm compresses are applied as prescribed to relieve pain. If the patient complains of photophobia, the use of dim lighting or sunglasses is recommended. The patient should follow the prescribed medical regimen carefully for the entire course and return for follow-up examination. In patient-teaching, the correct instillation of prescribed eye medications and the importance of thorough handwashing are emphasized. A well-balanced diet is recommended because nutritional deficiencies can increase susceptibility to this condition. Stress, traumatic injury, fever, colds, and overexposure to the sun may trigger a flare-up of keratitis. Both patient and family are taught about safety precautions pertaining to visual sensory or perceptual alterations. The nurse encourages the patient and family to verbalize their fears and concerns, offers appropriate information, and provides emotional support and reassurance.

***band-shaped k.*** A white or gray band extending across the cornea.

***k. bullosa*** The formation of large, quite resistant blebs with increased tension in the cornea of blind trachomatous eyes.

***dendritic k.*** Superficial branching corneal ulcers.

***k. disciformis*** A gray, disk-shaped opacity in the middle of the cornea.

***fascicular k.*** A corneal ulcer resulting from phlyctenules that spread from limbus to center of cornea accompanied by fascicle of blood vessels.

***herpetic k.*** Vesicular keratitis in herpes zoster.

***hypopyon k.*** A serpent-like ulcer with pus in the anterior chamber of the eye.

***interstitial k.*** A deep form of nonsuppurative keratitis with vascularization, occurring usually in syphilis and rarely in tuberculosis. It commonly occurs between ages 5 and 15. Symptoms include pain, photophobia, lacrimation, and loss in vision. SYN: *parenchymatous k.*

***lagophthalmic k.*** Drying due to air exposure of the cornea resulting from a defective closure of the eyelids.

***mycotic k.*** Keratitis produced by fungi.

***neuroparalytic k.*** The dull and slightly cloudy insensitive cornea seen in lesions of the fifth nerve.

***parenchymatous k.*** Interstitial k.

***phlyctenular k.*** Circumscribed inflammation of the conjunctiva and cornea accompanied by the formation of small projections called phlyctenules, which consist of accumulations of lymphoid cells. The phlyctenules soften at the apices, forming ulcers.

***punctate k.*** Cellular deposits on the posterior surface of the cornea seen in diseases of the uveal tract.

***purulent k.*** Keratitis with the formation of pus.

***sclerosing k.*** A triangular opacity in the deeper layers of the cornea, associated with scleritis.

***superficial punctate k.*** Small gray spots in the superficial layers of the cornea beneath Bowman's membrane. This occurs in young persons.

***trachomatous k.*** Pannus.

***traumatic k.*** Keratitis caused by a wound of the cornea.

***xerotic k.*** Softening, desiccation, and ulceration of cornea resulting from dryness of the conjunctiva.

**kerato-, kerat-** [Gr. *keras,* horn] Combining form indicating *horny substance* or *cornea.*

**keratoacanthoma** (kĕr″ă-tō-ăk″ăn-thō′mă) [″ + *akantha,* thorn, + *oma,* tumor] A papular lesion filled with a keratin plug that can resemble squamous cell carcinoma. It is benign and usually subsides spontaneously within 6 months. SEE: illus.

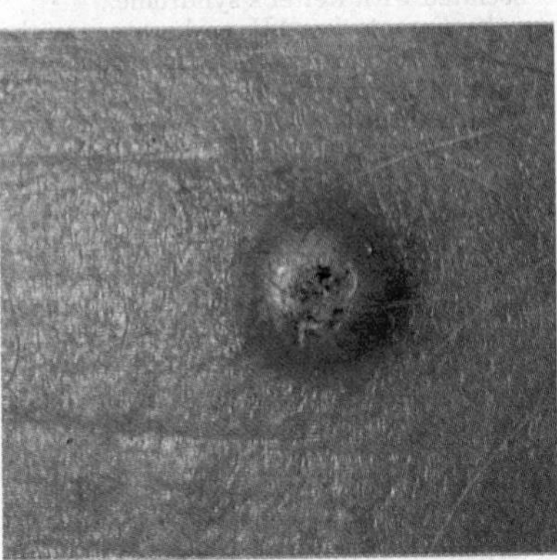

EARLY **KERATOACANTHOMA** ON FOREHEAD

**keratocele** (kĕr-ăt′ō-sēl) [″ + *kele,* tumor, swelling] The protrusion or herniation of Descemet's membrane through a weakened or absent corneal stroma as a result of injury or ulcer.

**keratoconjunctivitis** (kĕr″ă-tō-kŏn-jŭnk″tĭ-vī′tĭs) Inflammation of the cornea and the conjunctiva.

***epidemic k.*** An acute, self-limited keratoconjunctivitis caused by a highly infectious adenovirus.

***flash k.*** Painful keratoconjunctivitis resulting from exposure of the eyes to intense ultraviolet irradiation. Arc welders whose eyes are not properly protected will develop this acute condition.

***phlyctenular k.*** Acute inflammation of areas of the conjunctiva owing to an allergic response of a portion of the cornea or conjunctiva to an unknown allergen. The inflamed area is called a phlyctenule. Symptoms include photophobia, pain, lacrimation, conjunctival injection, and diminished visual acuity.

***k. sicca*** Dryness with hyperemia of the conjunctiva owing to decreased lacrimal function. The corneal epithelium may be thickened and visual acuity impaired. The condition is treated by use of artificial tears solution. SYN: *dry eyes; xerophthalmia.* SEE: *Schirmer's test; Sjögren's syndrome.*

**keratoconus** (kĕr-ă-tō-kō′nŭs) [″ + *konos,* cone] Conical protrusion of the center of the cornea, without inflammation. This occurs most often in pubescent females.

**keratocyte** (kĕr′ă-tō-sīt) A red blood cell of normal cell volume that is deformed with two or more horn-shaped points.

**keratoderma** (kĕr″ă-tō-dĕr′mă) [″ + *derma,* skin] A localized or disseminated disease of the horny layer of the skin.

***k. blennorrhagica*** Prominent hyperkeratotic scaling lesions of the palms, soles, and penis; around the nails; and occasionally in other areas. This condition is associated with Reiter's syndrome.

***k. climactericum*** Hyperkeratosis of the palms and soles of women, which may occur during menopause.

**keratodermatitis** (kĕr″ă-tō-dĕr″mă-tī′tĭs) [″ + ″ + *itis,* inflammation] Inflammation of the horny layer of the skin with proliferation.

**keratodermia** Hypertrophy of the stratum corneum or horny layer of the epidermis, esp. on the palms of hands and soles of feet, producing a horny condition of the skin. SYN: *hyperkeratosis.*

**keratogenous** (kĕr-ă-tŏj′ĕ-nŭs) [″ + *gennan,* to produce] Causing horny tissue development.

**keratoglobus** (kĕr″ă-tō-glō′bŭs) [″ + L. *globus,* circle] A globular protrusion and enlargement of the cornea, seen in congenital glaucoma.

**keratohelcosis** (kĕr″ă-tō-hĕl-kō′sĭs) [″ + *helkosis,* ulceration] Corneal ulceration.

**keratohemia** (kĕr″ă-tō-hē′mē-ă) [″ + *haima,* blood] Deposits of blood in the cornea of the eye.

**keratohyalin** A substance present in the form of granules in the cytoplasm of cells in the stratum granulosum of keratinized mucosa or epidermis of the skin.

**keratoid** (kĕr′ă-toyd) [″ + *eidos,* form, shape] Horny; resembling corneal tissue.

**keratoiditis** (kĕr″ă-toyd-ī′tĭs) [″ + ″ + *itis,* inflammation] Inflammation of the cornea.

**keratoiritis** (kĕr″ă-tō-ī-rī′tĭs) [″ + *iris,* iris, + *itis,* inflammation] Inflammation of the cornea and iris.

**keratoleptynsis** (kĕr″ă-tō-lĕp-tĭn′sĭs) [″ + *leptynein,* to make thin] A cosmetic operation performed on a sightless eye. The procedure involves removing the corneal surface and covering the area with bulbar conjunctiva.

**keratoleukoma** (kĕr″ă-tō-lū-kō′mă) [″ + *leukos,* white, + *oma,* tumor] White corneal opacity.

**keratolysis** (kĕr-ă-tŏl′ĭ-sĭs) [″ + *lysis,* dissolution] **1.** A loosening of the horny layer of the skin. **2.** Shedding of the skin at regular intervals.

***pitted k.*** Hyperkeratotic areas of the soles and palms with erosion and pitting. The etiology is unknown but may involve infection with *Corynebacterium* or *Actinomyces.* It occurs mostly in barefooted adults in the tropics.

**keratolytic** (kĕr″ă-tō-lĭt′ĭk) **1.** Relating to or causing keratolysis. SYN: *desquamative.* **2.** An agent that causes or promotes keratolysis.

**keratoma** (kĕr″ă-tō′mă) [″ + *oma,* tumor] Keratosis (2).

**keratomalacia** (kĕr″ă-tō-mă-lā′shē-ă) [″ + *malakia,* softness] Softening of the cornea seen in early childhood owing to deficiencies of vitamin A. SYN: *xerotic keratitis.*

**keratome** (kĕr′ă-tōm) [″ + *tome,* incision] A knife for incising the cornea. SYN: *keratotome.*

**keratometer** (kĕr-ă-tŏm′ĕ-ter) [″ + *metron,* measure] An instrument for measuring the curves of the cornea.

**keratometry** (kĕr″ă-tŏm′ĕ-trē) [″ + *metron,* measure] Measurement of the cornea.

**keratomileusis** (kĕr″ă-tō-mĭ-loo′sĭs) [″ + *smileusis,* carving] Plastic surgery of the cornea in which a portion is removed and frozen and its curvature reshaped; then it is reattached to the cornea.

**keratomycosis** (kĕr″ă-tō-mī-kō′sĭs) [″ + *mykes,* fungus, + *osis,* condition] Fungus growth on the cornea.

**keratonosis** (kĕr″ă-tō-nō′sĭs) [″ + *nosos,* disease] Any noninflammatory disease or deformity of the horny layer of the skin.

**keratonyxis** (kĕr″ă-tō-nĭks′ĭs) [″ + *nyssein,* to puncture] A corneal puncture, esp. surgical puncture.

**keratopathy** (kĕr″ă-tŏp′ă-thē) [″ + *pathos,* disease] Any disease of the cornea.

***band k.*** Band-shaped calcium deposits in the superficial layer of the cornea and Bowman's membrane. This occurs with chronic intraocular inflammation and with systemic diseases in which there is hypercalcemia.

**keratoplasty** (kĕr′ă-tō-plăs″tē) [″ + *plassein,* to form] Plastic operation on the cornea. SEE: *lens, corneal contact.*

***optic k.*** The removal of a corneal scar and replacement with corneal tissue.

***refractive k.*** Treatment of myopia or hyperopia by removing a portion of the cornea, freezing it in order to reshape it surgically to correct refractive error, and then replacing it after it has thawed. SEE: *keratomileusis.*

***tectonic k.*** Use of corneal tissue to replace that lost because of trauma or disease.

**keratoprotein** (kĕr″ă-tō-prō′tē-ĭn) [″ + *protos,* first] The protein of the hair, nails, and epidermis.

**keratorrhexis** (kĕr″ă-tō-rĕks′ĭs) [″ + *rhexis,* rupture] Corneal rupture.

**keratoscleritis** (kĕr″ă-tō-sklĕr-ī′tĭs) [″ + *skleros,* hard, + *itis,* inflammation] Inflammation of both cornea and sclera.

**keratoscope** (kĕr′ăt-ō-skōp) [″ + *skopein,* to examine] An instrument for examination of the cornea.

**keratoscopy** Examination of the cornea and its reflection of light.

**keratose** (kĕr′ă-tōs) [Gr. *keras,* horn] Horny.

**keratosis** (kĕr-ă-tō′sĭs) *pl.* **keratoses** [″ + *osis,* condition] **1.** Horny growth. **2.** Any condition of the skin characterized by the formation of horny growths or excessive development of the horny growth. SYN: *keratoma.*

***actinic k.*** A horny, premalignant lesion of the skin caused by excess exposure to sunlight. The regular use of sunscreens prevents the development of solar keratoses and will most probably reduce the risk of skin cancer. SYN: *solar k.* SEE: *sunscreen.*

***k. climactericum*** A skin disease occurring in women during menopause, characterized by a circumscribed hyperkeratosis of the palms and soles.

***k. follicularis*** Darier's disease.

***k. nigricans*** Acanthosis nigricans.

***oral k.*** Keratinization of the mucosa of the mouth to an unusual extent, or in locations normally not keratinized, as a result of an inherited autosomal dominant gene or the more common effect of tobacco and other carcinogens.

***k. palmaris et plantaris*** A congenital abnormality of the palms and soles, characterized by a dense thickening of the keratin layer in these regions.

***k. pharyngis*** Horny projections from the pharyngeal tonsils and adjacent lymphoid tissue.

***k. pilaris*** Chronic inflammatory disorder of area surrounding the hair follicles. The etiology is unknown.

SYMPTOMS: The disorder is characterized by an accumulation of horny material at follicular orifices of persons with rough, dry skin. It is most pronounced in winter on lateral aspects of thighs and upper arms with possible extension to legs, forearms, and scalp.

TREATMENT: There is no specific therapy, but keratolytic lotions may be of some value.

***k. punctata*** Discrete horny projections from the sweat pores of the palms and soles.

***seborrheic k.*** A benign skin tumor that may be pigmented. It is composed of immature epithelial cells and is quite common in the elderly. Its etiology is unknown.

SYMPTOMS: Keratoid, nevoid, acanthoid, or verrucose types occur in the elderly and in those with longstanding dry seborrhea, on the face, scalp, interscapular or sternal regions, and backs of the hands. The yellow, gray, or brown sharply circumscribed lesions are covered with a firmly adherent scale, greasy or velvety on the trunk or scalp but harsh, rough, and dry on the face or hands. The tendency as time passes is for the lesions to increase in number. It is doubtful that they ever become malignant.

TREATMENT: Thorough curettage is quite effective. This leaves a flat surface that becomes covered with normal skin within about one week. Pedunculated lesions can be removed surgically. Cautery may produce scarring; therefore, it should not be used. SYN: *wart, seborrheic.*

***k. senilis*** Dry, harsh skin of the aged.

***solar k.*** Actinic k.

**keratotome** (kĕr-ăt′ō-tōm) [″ + *tome,* incision] Keratome.

**keratotomy** (kĕr-ă-tŏt′ō-mē) Incision of the cornea.

***radial k.*** Surgical therapy for nearsightedness. Very shallow, bloodless, hairline, radial incisions are made in the outer portion of the cornea where they will not interfere with vision. This allows the cornea to flatten and to help correct the nearsightedness. About two thirds of patients undergoing this procedure will be able to eliminate the use of glasses or contact lenses.

**keraunoneurosis** (kĕ-raw″nō-nū-rō′sĭs) [Gr. *keraunos,* lightning, + *neuron,* nerve, + *osis,* condition] A neurosis caused by fear of a thunderstorm or stroke of lightning.

**keraunophobia** (kĕ-raw″nō-fō′bē-ă) [″ + *phobos,* fear] Fear of thunder and lightning.

**Kerckring's folds** (kĕrk′rĭngz) [Theodorus Kerckring, Dutch anatomist, 1640–1693] Valvulae conniventes of the small intestine.

**kerectomy** (kē-rĕk′tō-mē) [Gr. *keras,* horn, + *ektome,* excision] Excision of a portion of the cornea.

**kerion** (kē′rē-ŏn) [Gr., honeycomb] In tinea capitis, an inflammatory, boggy mass containing broken hairs and oozing purulent material from follicular orifices. This is a rare, delayed hypersensitivity to fungal antigens that may result in permanent hair loss. SEE: illus.

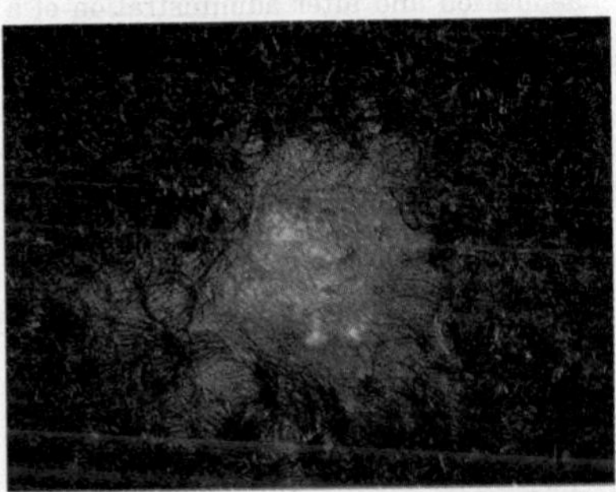

KERION

**Kerley lines** [P. J. Kerley, Brit. radiologist, b. 1900] Lines present on chest roentgenograms of patients with any disease that causes thickening or infiltration of the interlobular septa. Those in the costophrenic angle area are called Kerley B lines, and those extending peripherally from the hilum are termed Kerley A lines. Kerley C lines are fine lines in the middle of pulmonary tissue.

**kernicterus** (kĕr-nĭk′tĕr-ŭs) [Ger.] A form of icterus neonatorum occurring in infants during the second to eighth day of life. The basal ganglia and other areas of the brain and spinal cord are infiltrated with bilirubin, a yellow substance produced by the breakdown of hemoglobin. The prognosis is quite poor if the condition is left untreated. For prevention and treatment, SEE: *erythroblastosis fetalis; hemolytic disease of the newborn; phototherapy.*

**Kernig's sign** (kĕr′nĭgz) [Vladimir Kernig, Russ. physician, 1840–1917] A symptom of meningitis evidenced by reflex contraction and pain in the hamstring muscles when attempting to extend the leg after flexing the thigh upon the body.

**kerosene** (kĕr′ō-sēn) A flammable liquid fuel distilled from petroleum. It is used as a solvent as well as a fuel source. SEE: *Poisons and Poisoning Appendix*.

**Ketaject** Trade name for ketamine hydrochloride.

**Ketalar** Trade name for ketamine hydrochloride.

**ketamine hydrochloride** A nonbarbiturate substance, $C_{13}H_{16}ClNO \cdot HCl$, that is used intravenously or intramuscularly to produce anesthesia. The patient becomes cataleptic and may seem awake but is unaware of the environment and unresponsive to pain. Because the laryngeal reflexes are depressed, an endotracheal tube is used to prevent aspiration. Most frequently used for diagnostic procedures and minor operations in which muscle relaxation is not required. SEE: *anesthesia, dissociative.*

NURSING IMPLICATIONS: Ketamine should be administered on an empty stomach to prevent vomiting and possible aspiration and after administration of a prescribed anticholinergic to reduce saliva flow. The patient should reawaken in a quiet area with minimal stimulation to reduce the severity of hallucinations and delirium. Premedication with prescribed diazepam or a narcotic also may reduce the severity of symptoms during the recovery period. The nurse warns the patient about the possibility of flashback-type hallucinations within 24 hr of having received ketamine anesthesia. Blood pressure is monitored for hypertension, and respiratory status for airway patency, depressed laryngeal and pharyngeal reflexes, respiratory depression, and apnea. Resuscitative equipment is made (or kept) readily available. The patient should not be discharged after recovery from anesthesia unless accompanied by a responsible adult. The patient should not drive or operate other motorized equipment for 24 hr after anesthesia.

**ketoacidosis** (kē″tō-ă″sĭ-dō′sĭs) [Ger. *keton,* alter. of *azeton,* acetone, + L. *acidus,* sour, + Gr. *osis,* condition] Acidosis due to an excess of ketone bodies.

**ketoaciduria** (kē″tō-ăs″ĭ-dū′rē-ă) [″ + ″ + Gr. *ouron,* urine] The presence of keto acids in the urine.

**ketogenesis** (kē-tō-jĕn′ĕ-sĭs) [″ + Gr. *genesis,* generation, birth] The production of ketones or acetone substances.

**ketolysis** (kē-tŏl′ĭ-sĭs) [″ + Gr. *lysis,* dissolution] The dissolution of acetone or ketone bodies. **ketolytic,** *adj.*

**ketone** (kē′tōn) A substance containing the carbonyl group (C═O) attached to two carbon atoms. Acetone, $C_3H_6O$, is an example of a simple ketone.

***k. body*** SEE: under *body*.

***k. threshold*** The level of ketone in the blood above which ketone bodies appear in the urine.

**ketonemia** (kē″tō-nē′mē-ă) [″ + Gr. *haima,* blood] The presence of acetone bodies in the blood, which causes the characteristic fruity breath odor in ketoacidosis.

**ketonuria** (kē-tō-nū′rē-ă) [″ + Gr. *ouron,* urine] Acetone bodies in the urine.

**ketoplasia** (kē-tō-plā′sē-ă) [″ + Gr. *plassein,* to form] The formation or excretion of ketones.

**ketoplastic** [″ + Gr. *plastikos,* formed] Pert. to ketoplasia or to the formation of ketones.

**ketose** A carbohydrate containing the ketones.

**ketosis** (kē-tō′sĭs) [″ + Gr. *osis,* condition] The accumulation in the body of the ketone bodies: acetone, beta-hydroxybutyric acid, and acetoacetic acid. It is frequently associated with acidosis. Ketosis results from the incomplete metabolism of fatty acids, usually from carbohydrate deficiency or inadequate use, and is commonly observed in starvation, high-fat diet, and pregnancy; following ether anesthesia; and most significantly in inadequately controlled diabetes mellitus. Large quantities of these ketone bodies may be eliminated in the urine (ketonuria). Ketosis is easily determined by testing for the presence of acetone or diacetic acid in the urine. Ketonuria is an early sign of acidosis in patients with diabetes mellitus.

**17-ketosteroid** One of a group of neutral steroids having a ketone group in carbon position 17. They are produced by the adrenal cortex and gonads and appear normally in the urine. Among them are androsterone, dehydroisoandrosterone, corticosterone, and 11-hydroxyisoandrosterone. A greater than normal or less than normal excretion in the urine is indicative of certain endocrine disorders. SEE: *perhydrocyclopentanophenanthrene.*

**ketosuria** (kē″tō-sū′rē-ă) Presence of ketone bodies in the urine. SEE: *ketosis.*

**ketotic** Pert. to ketosis.

**keV** *kiloelectron volts.*

**Key-Retzius foramina** (kē′rĕt′zē-ŭs) [Ernst A. H. Key, Swedish physician, 1832–1901; Gustav Magnus Retzius, Swedish anatomist, 1842–1919] Passages in the pia mater carrying the choroid plexus to the fourth ventricle.

**kg** *kilogram.*

**kg-m** *kilogram-meter.*

**$KHCO_3$** Potassium bicarbonate.

**$KHSO_4$** Potassium bisulfate.

**kHz** *kilohertz.*

**KI** Potassium iodide.

**kidney** [ME. *kidenei*] One of a pair of purple-brown organs situated at the back (retroperitoneal area) of the abdominal cavity; each is lateral to the spinal column.

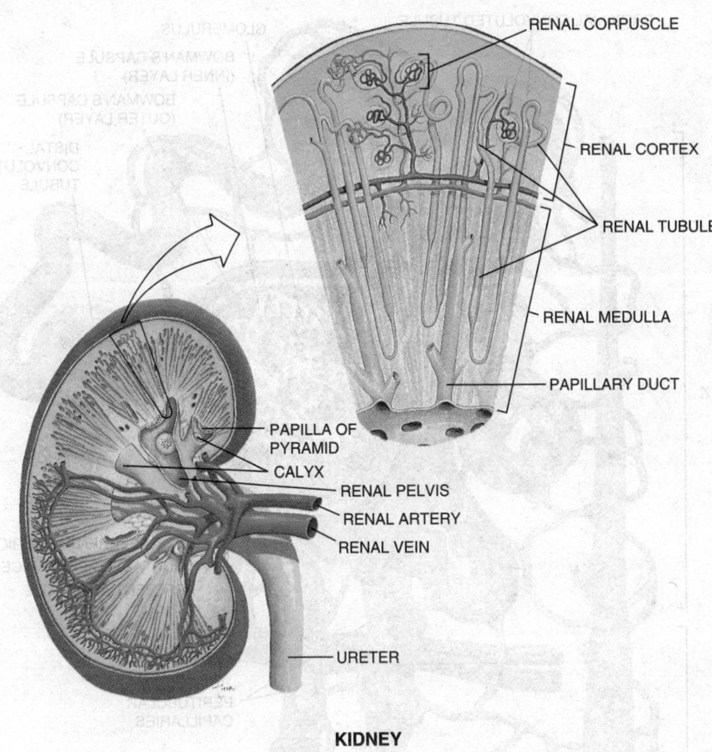


**KIDNEY**
(FRONTAL SECTION)

The kidneys form urine from blood plasma. They are the major regulators of the water, electrolyte, and acid-base content of the blood and, indirectly, all body fluids.

ANATOMY: The top of each kidney is opposite the 12th thoracic vertebra; the bottom is opposite the third lumbar vertebra. The right kidney is slightly lower than the left one. Each kidney weighs 113 to 170 g (4 to 6 oz), and each is about 11.4 cm (4½ in.) long, 5 to 7.5 cm (2 to 3 in.) broad, and 2.5 cm (1 in.) thick. The kidneys in the newborn are about three times as large in proportion to body weight as they are in the adult.

Each kidney is surrounded by adipose tissue and by the renal fascia, a fibrous membrane that helps hold the kidney in place. On the medial side of a kidney is an indentation called the hilus or hilum, at which the renal artery enters and the renal vein and ureter emerge. The microscopic nephrons are the structural and functional units of the kidney; each consists of a renal corpuscle and renal tubule with associated blood vessels. In frontal section, the kidney is composed of two areas of tissue and a medial cavity. The outer renal cortex is made of renal corpuscles and convoluted tubules. The renal medulla consists of 8 to 18 wedge-shaped areas called renal pyramids; they are made of loops of Henle and collecting tubules. Adjacent to the hilus is the renal pelvis, the expanded end of the ureter within the kidney. Urine formed in the nephrons is carried by a papillary duct to the tip (papilla) of a pyramid, which projects into a cuplike calyx, an extension of the renal pelvis. SEE: illus. (Kidney).

NEPHRON: The nephron consists of a renal corpuscle and renal tubule. The renal corpuscle is made of a capillary network called a glomerulus surrounded by Bowman's capsule. The renal tubule extends from Bowman's capsule. The parts, in order, are as follows: proximal convoluted tubule, loop of Henle, distal convoluted tubule, and collecting tubule, all of which are surrounded by peritubular capillaries. SEE: illus. (Nephron and Blood Vessels).

FORMATION OF URINE: Urine is formed by filtration, reabsorption, and secretion. As blood passes through the glomerulus, water and dissolved substances are filtered through the capillary walls and the inner or visceral layer of Bowman's capsule; this fluid is now called glomerular

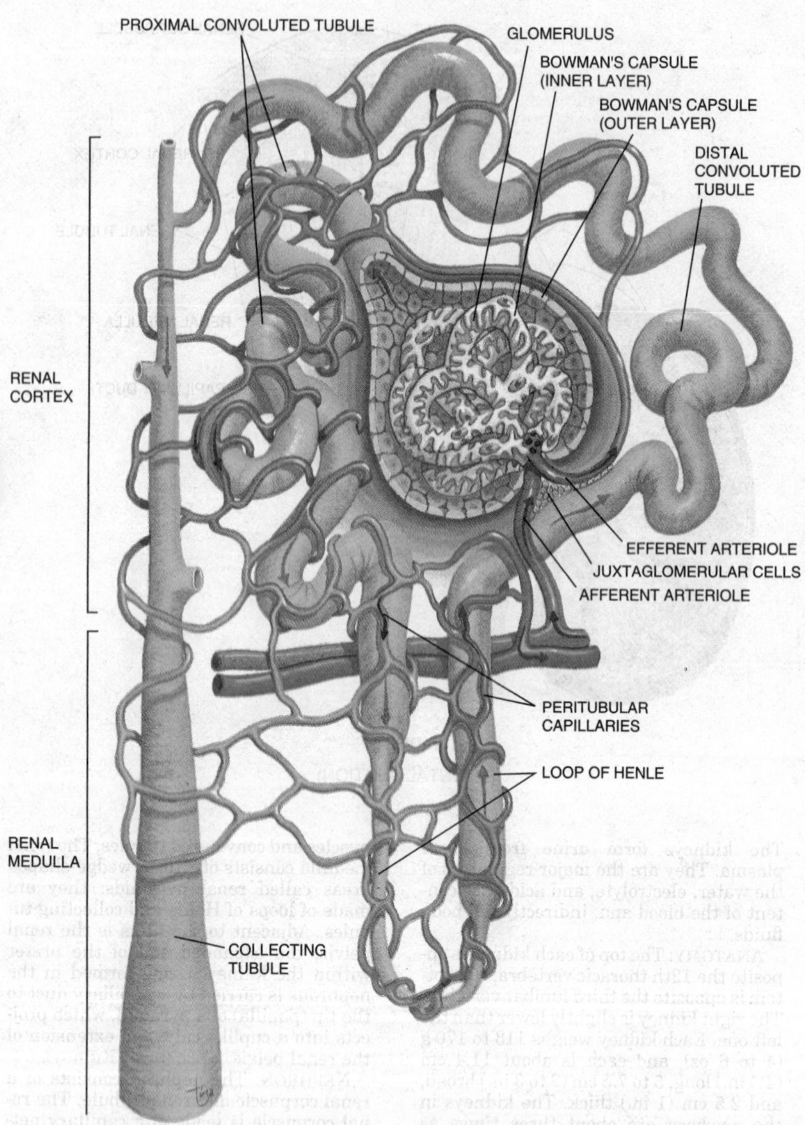


**NEPHRON AND BLOOD VESSELS**

filtrate. Blood cells and large proteins are retained within the capillaries. Filtration is a continuous process; the rate varies with blood flow through the kidneys and daily fluid intake and loss. As the glomerular filtrate passes through the renal tubules, useful materials such as water, glucose, amino acids, vitamins, and minerals are reabsorbed into the peritubular capillaries. Most of these have a renal threshold level, that is, a limit to how much can be reabsorbed, but this level is usually not exceeded unless the blood level of these materials is above normal. Reabsorption of water is regulated directly by antidiuretic hormone and indirectly by aldosterone. Most waste products remain in the filtrate and become part of the urine. Hydrogen ions, creatinine, and the metabolic products of medications may be actively secreted into the filtrate to become part of the urine. The collecting tubules unite to form papillary ducts that empty urine into the calyces of the renal pelvis,

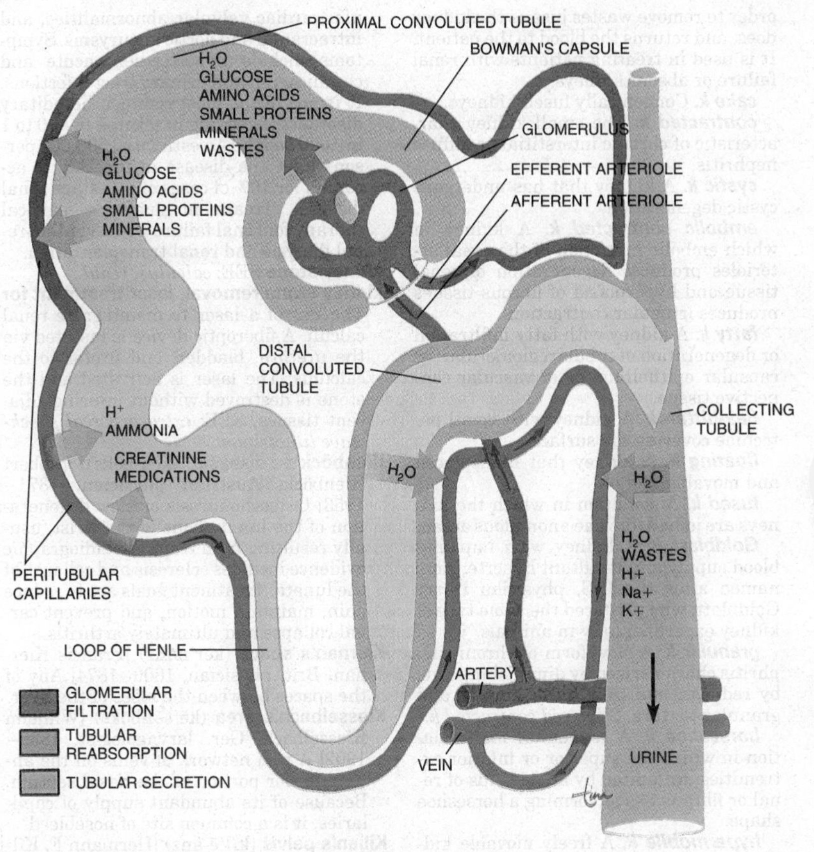


**FORMATION OF URINE**

from which it enters the ureter and is transported to the urinary bladder. Periodically the bladder is emptied (a reflex subject to voluntary control) by way of the urethra; this is called micturition, urination, or voiding. If a normally hydrated individual ingests a large volume of aqueous fluids, in about 45 minutes a sufficient quantity will have been excreted into the bladder to cause the urge to urinate. SEE: illus. (Formation of Urine).

URINE: Urine is about 95% water and about 5% dissolved substances. The dissolved materials include minerals, esp. sodium, the nitrogenous waste products urea, uric acid, and creatinine, and other metabolic end products. The volume of urine excreted daily varies from 1000 to 2000 ml (averaging 1500 ml). The amount varies with water intake, nature of diet, degree of body activity, environmental and body temperature, age, blood pressure, and many other factors. Pathological conditions may affect the volume and nature of the urine excreted. However, patients with only one kidney have been found to have normal renal function even after half of that kidney was removed because of cancer. There is no evidence that forcing fluids is detrimental to the kidneys.

NERVE SUPPLY: The nerve supply consists of sympathetic fibers to the renal blood vessels. These promote constriction or dilation, esp. of arteries and arterioles.

DISORDERS: Symptoms of a kidney disorder include lumbar pain, renal colic, fever, disturbances in micturition (anuria, oliguria, or pain on micturition), presence of blood or pus in the urine, tenderness or swelling in costovertebral region, enlargement or diminution in size of kidney, and edema. SEE: *dialysis*; *glomerulonephritis*; *nephropathy*; *nephritis*; *renal failure*.

EXAMINATION: The kidneys are examined by palpation, intravenous pyelography, CT scan, cystoscopy, retrograde cystoscopy, or panendoscopy.

***amyloid k.*** A kidney infiltrated with amyloid. SYN: *waxy k.*

***artificial k.*** A device that receives blood from the patient, treats it by dialysis in order to remove wastes just as the kidney does, and returns the blood to the patient. It is used in treating patients with renal failure or absent kidneys.

***cake k.*** Congenitally fused kidneys.

***contracted k.*** The small kidney characteristic of chronic interstitial or diffuse nephritis.

***cystic k.*** A kidney that has undergone cystic degeneration.

***embolic contracted k.*** A kidney in which embolic infarction of the renal arterioles produces degeneration of renal tissue and hyperplasia of fibrous tissues produces irregular contraction.

***fatty k.*** A kidney with fatty infiltration or degeneration of tubular, glomerular, or capsular epithelium, or of vascular connective tissue.

***flea-bitten k.*** A kidney with small petechiae covering the surface.

***floating k.*** A kidney that is displaced and movable.

***fused k.*** A condition in which the kidneys are joined into one anomalous organ.

***Goldblatt k.*** A kidney with impaired blood supply and resultant hypertension; named after the U.S. physician Harry Goldblatt, who produced the same type of kidney experimentally in animals.

***granular k.*** A slow form of chronic nephritis characterized by diminishing size; by redness; and by a hard, fibrous, and granular texture. SYN: *red contracted k.*

***horseshoe k.*** A congenital malformation in which the superior or inferior extremities are united by an isthmus of renal or fibrous tissue, forming a horseshoe shape.

***hypermobile k.*** A freely movable kidney. SYN: *wandering k.*

***movable k.*** A kidney that is not firmly attached owing to lack of support of fatty tissue and perinephric fascia. SYN: *nephroptosis.*

***polycystic k.*** A kidney bearing many cysts. SEE: *kidney disease, polycystic.*

***red contracted k.*** Granular k.

***sacculated k.*** A condition in which the kidney has been absorbed and only the distended capsule remains.

***sponge k.*** A condition characterized by the presence of multiple small cysts in the renal parenchyma.

***syphilitic k.*** Kidney with fibrous bands running across it, also caseating gummata, as a result of syphilis.

***wandering k.*** Hypermobile k.

***waxy k.*** Amyloid k.

**kidney disease, polycystic** ABBR: PKD. An inherited renal disorder transmitted as an autosomal recessive trait in infants and as an autosomal dominant trait in adults. PKD was previously termed *adult polycystic kidney disease.* It is characterized by cyst formation in ductal organs, particularly the kidney and liver, and by gastrointestinal and cardiovascular abnormalities. Included are colonic diverticula, cardiac valvular abnormalities, and intracranial and aortic aneurysms. Symptoms include hypertension, acute and chronic pain, and urinary tract infections. It is one of the most common hereditary disorders, occurring in about 1 in 400 to 1 in 1000 people. An estimated 500,000 persons have the disease in the U.S. It accounts for 10% of cases of end-stage renal disease. Treatment includes medical therapy for renal failure with eventual renal dialysis and renal transplantation.

**kidney stone** SEE: *calculus, renal.*

**kidney stone removal, laser treatment for** The use of a laser to disintegrate renal calculi. A fiberoptic device is inserted via the urethra, bladder, and ureter to the calculus. The laser is activated and the stone is destroyed without injuring adjacent tissues. SEE: *extracorporeal shock-wave lithotriptor.*

**Kienböck's disease** (kēn′bĕks) [Robert Kienböck, Austrian physician, 1871–1953] Osteochondrosis or slow degeneration of the lunate bone of the wrist; usually resulting from trauma. Radiographic evidence includes sclerosis and collapse of the lunate. Treatment goals are to reduce pain, maintain motion, and prevent carpal collapse and ultimately arthritis.

**Kiernan's space** (kēr′nănz) [Francis Kiernan, Brit. physician, 1800–1874] Any of the spaces between the lobes of the liver.

**Kiesselbach's area** (kē′sĕl-bŏks) [Wilhelm Kiesselbach, Ger. laryngologist, 1839–1902] A rich network of veins on the anteroinferior portion of the nasal septum. Because of its abundant supply of capillaries, it is a common site of nosebleed.

**Kilian's pelvis** (kĭl′ē-ănz) [Hermann F. Kilian, Ger. gynecologist, 1800–1863] Pelvis spinosa.

**kilo-** [Fr.] Combining form indicating *1000.*

**kilobase** ABBR: kb. Unit indicating the length of a nucleic acid sequence. One kb is 1000 nucleotide sequences long.

**kilocalorie** ABBR: C, kcal. A unit of measure for heat. In nutrition, a kilocalorie is known as a large Calorie and is always written with a capital C. SEE: *calorie.*

**kilocycle** (kĭl′ō-sī″k′l) ABBR: kc. One thousand cycles; previous name for kilohertz.

**kilogram** [Fr. *kilo,* a thousand, + *gramme,* a weight] ABBR: kg. One thousand grams or 2.2 lb avoirdupois. A unit of mass, not a unit of force. SEE: *newton; pascal; SI Units Appendix.*

**kilogram-meter** ABBR: kg-m. The work required to raise one kilogram one meter.

**kilohertz** ABBR: kHz. In electricity, a unit of 1000 cycles; formerly called kilocycle.

**kilojoule** ABBR: kJ. One thousand joules.

**kiloliter** (kĭl′ō-lē″tĕr) [Fr. *kilolitre*] ABBR: kl. One thousand liters.

**kilomegacycles** $10^9$ cycles/sec (i.e., 1000 megacycles/sec).

**kilometer** [Fr. *kilometre*] ABBR: km. One thousand meters, or 3281 feet (roughly 0.62 mile).

**kilopascal** (kĭl″ō-păs-kăl′) [Fr. *kilo,* a thousand, + *Pascal,* Fr. scientist] ABBR: kPa. In SI units, a unit of pressure equal to 1000 pascals. Attempts to have blood pressure expressed in kPa have not been accepted. SEE: *pascal.*

**kilounit** (kĭl″ō-ū′nĭt) One thousand units.

**kilovolt** [Fr. *kilo,* a thousand, + *volt*] ABBR: kV. One thousand volts.

**kilovoltage peak** The highest voltage occurring during an electrical cycle.

**kilowatt** ABBR: kW. A unit of electrical energy equal to 1000 watts.

**Kimmelstiel-Wilson syndrome** [Paul Kimmelstiel, Ger. physician, 1900–1970; Clifford Wilson, Brit. physician, b. 1906] A syndrome that may develop in patients in whom diabetes mellitus has been present for several years. Hypertension, glomerulonephrosis, edema, and retinal lesions are present and arteriosclerosis of the renal artery is a common complication. SEE: *diabetes.*

**kinanesthesia** (kĭn-ăn-ĕs-thē′zē-ă) [Gr. *kinesis,* movement, + *an-,* not, + *aisthesis,* sensation] The inability to perceive the extent of a movement or direction, resulting in ataxia.

**kinase** (kĭn′ās) An enzyme that catalyzes the transfer of phosphate from ATP to an acceptor.

***protein k.*** SEE: *protein kinase.*

**kinematics** [Gr. *kinematos,* movement] The branch of biomechanics concerned with description of the movements of segments of the body without regard to the forces that caused the movement to occur. SEE: *arthrokinematics; osteokinematics.*

**kinematograph** (kĭn″ĕ-măt′o-grăf) A device for viewing photographs of objects in motion; used in studying the motion of organs such as the heart and lungs, and the gastrointestinal tract.

**kineplastic** (kĭn″ĭ-plăs′tĭk) [Gr. *kinein,* to move, + *plastikos,* formed] Pert. to kineplasty.

**kineplasty** A form of amputation enabling the muscles of the stump to impart motion to an artificial limb. SEE: *Boston arm; cineplastics.*

**kinesalgia** (kĭn″ĕ-săl′jē-ă) [Gr. *kinesis,* movement, + *algos,* pain] Pain associated with muscular movement.

**kinescope** (kĭn′ĕ-skōp) [″ + *skopein,* to examine] A device for testing the refraction of the eye. A slit of variable width moves as the patient observes a fixed object.

**kinesia** (kī-nē′sē-ă) Sickness caused by motion, as seasickness, car sickness.

**kinesiatrics** (kĭ-nē″sē-ăt′rĭks) [″ + *iatrikos,* curative] Kinesitherapy.

**kinesics** (kī-nē′sĭks) Systematic study of the body and the use of its static and dynamic position as a means of communication. SEE: *body language.*

**kinesimeter** (kĭn″ĕ-sĭm′ĕ-tĕr) [″ + *metron,* measure] An apparatus for determining the extent of movement of a part.

**kinesiodic** (kĭ-nē″sē-ŏd′ĭk) [″ + *hodos,* path] Pert. to paths through which motor impulses pass.

**kinesiology** (kĭ-nē″sē-ŏl′ō-jē) [″ + *logos,* word, reason] The study of muscles and body movement. SEE: *biomechanics.*

**kinesioneurosis** (kĭ-nē″sē-ō-nū-rō′sĭs) [″ + *neuron,* nerve, + *osis,* condition] A functional disorder marked by tics and spasms. SEE: *Tourette's syndrome.*

***external k.*** Kinesioneurosis affecting external muscles.

***vascular k.*** Kinesioneurosis of the vasomotor system.

***visceral k.*** Kinesioneurosis affecting muscles of internal organs.

**kinesiotherapy** (kĭ-nē″sē-ō-thĕr′ă-pē) [″ + *therapeia,* treatment] Kinesitherapy.

**kinesis** (kĭn-ē′sĭs) [Gr.] Motion.

**kinesitherapy** [″ + *therapeia,* treatment] Treatment by movements or exercises. SYN: *kinesiatrics; kinesiotherapy; kinetotherapy.* SEE: *physical therapy.*

**kinesthesia** (kĭn″ĕs-thē′zē-ă) [″ + *aisthesis,* sensation] The ability to perceive extent, direction, or weight of movement. **kinesthetic,** *adj.*

**kinesthesiometer** (kĭn″ĕs-thē-zē-ŏm′ĕ-tĕr) [″ + ″ + *metron,* measure] An instrument for testing the ability to determine the position of the muscles.

**kinetic** (kĭ-nĕt′ĭk) [Gr. *kinesis,* motion] Pert. to or consisting of motion.

**kinetics** The forces acting on the body during movement and the interactions of sequence of motion with respect to time and forces present.

**kinetochore** A protein disk attached to the DNA of the centromere that connects a pair of chromatids during cell division. A spindle fiber is in turn attached to the kinetochore.

**kinetotherapy** (kĭ-nĕt″ō-thĕr′ă-pē) [″ + *therapeia,* treatment] Kinesitherapy.

**King, Imogene** A nursing educator who developed the General Systems Framework and Theory of Goal Attainment. SEE: *Nursing Theory Appendix.*

**kingdom** [AS. *cyningdom*] The largest of the five categories in the classification of living organisms. There are five kingdoms: Procaryotae (Monera), Protista, Fungi, Plantae, and Animalia. SEE: *taxonomy.*

**kinin** (kī′nĭn) [Gr. *kinesis,* movement] A general term for a group of polypeptides that have considerable biological activity. They are capable of influencing smooth muscle contraction; inducing hypotension; increasing the blood flow and permeability of small blood capillaries; and inciting pain.

**kininases, plasma** Plasma carboxypeptidases that inactivate plasma kinins.

**kininogen** A substance that produces a kinin when acted on by certain enzymes.

**kink** [Low Ger. *kinke,* a twist in rope] An unnatural angle or bend in a duct or tube such as the intestine, umbilical cord, or ureter.

**kino-** (kī′nō) [Gr. *kinein,* to move] Combining form meaning *movement.*

**kinocilium** (kī″nō-sĭl′ē-ŭm) [″ + L. *cilium,* eyelash] Protoplasmic filament on the cell surface.

**kinship** (kĭn′shĭp) The descendants from a common ancestor.

**Kirschner wire** (kērsh′nĕrz) [Martin Kirschner, Ger. surgeon, 1879–1942] Steel wire placed through a long bone in order to apply traction to the bone.

**Kisch's reflex** (kĭsh′ĕs) [Bruno Kisch, Ger. physiologist, 1890–1966] Auriculopalpebral reflex.

**kitasamycin** (kĭt″ă-să-mī′sĭn) An antibiotic substance produced by *Streptomyces kitasatoensis.* It is also called *leucomycin.*

**KJ** *knee jerk.*

**KK** *knee kick* (knee jerk).

**kl** *kiloliter.*

**Klebsiella** (klĕb″sē-ĕl′ă) [T. A. Edwin Klebs, Ger. bacteriologist, 1834–1913] A genus of bacteria of the family Enterobacteriaceae. These short, plump, gram-negative bacilli form capsules but not spores. They are frequently associated with respiratory infections and may cause urinary tract infections.

***K. ozaenae*** A species found in ozena.

***K. pneumoniae*** Friedländer's bacillus.

***K. rhinoscleromatis*** A species that can cause rhinoscleroma, a destructive granuloma of the nose and pharnyx.

**Klein-Bell ADL Scale** In rehabilitation, an objectively scored measure of functional independence, which includes items related to self-care, mobility and communication.

**klepto-** (klĕp′tō) [Gr. *kleptein,* to steal] Combining form meaning *stealing, theft.*

**kleptolagnia** (klĕp″tō-lăg′nē-ă) [″ + *lagneia,* lust] Sexual gratification derived from stealing.

**kleptomania** (klĕp-tō-mā′nē-ă) [″ + *mania,* madness] Impulsive stealing, the motive not being in the intrinsic value of the article to the individual. In almost all cases, the individual has enough money to pay for the stolen goods. The stealing is done without prior planning and without the assistance of others. There is increased tension before the theft and a sense of gratification while committing the act.

**kleptomaniac 1.** Pert. to kleptomania. **2.** A psychopathic personality suffering from impulsive stealing.

**kleptophobia** (klĕp-tō-fō′bē-ă) [″ + *phobos,* fear] Morbid fear of stealing.

**Klieg eye** (klēg) [after John H. Kliegl, Ger. manufacturer, 1869–1959] Conjunctivitis, lacrimation, and photophobia from exposure to the intense lights used in making motion pictures or television films.

**Klinefelter's syndrome** (klīn′fĕl-tĕrs) [Harry F. Klinefelter, Jr., U.S. physician, b. 1912] Congenital endocrine condition of primary testicular failure usually not evident before puberty. The classic form is associated with the presence of an extra X chromosome. The testes are small and firm, and gynecomastia, abnormally long legs, and subnormal intelligence usually are present. In variant forms the chromosomal abnormalities vary and the severity and number of abnormal findings are diversified. The syndrome is estimated to occur in one of 700 live male births. Diagnosis may be confirmed by chromosomal analysis of tissue culture.

**Klippel's disease** (klĭ-pĕlz′) [Maurice Klippel, Fr. neurologist, 1858–1942] Weakness or pseudoparalysis due to generalized arthritis.

**Klippel-Feil syndrome** [Maurice Klippel; André Feil, Fr. physician, b. 1884] A congenital anomaly characterized by a short wide neck; low hairline, esp. on the back of the neck; reduction in the number of cervical vertebrae; and fusion of the cervical spine. The central nervous system also may be affected.

**klismaphilia** The derivation of sexual pleasure by receiving enemas.

**Klumpke's paralysis** (kloomp′kĕz) [Madame Augusta Déjérine-Klumpke, Fr. neurologist, 1859–1927] Atrophic paralysis of the forearm.

**Klüver-Bucy syndrome** [Heinrich Klüver, Ger.-born U.S. neurologist, 1897–1979; Paul C. Bucy, U. S. neurologist, b. 1904] Behavioral syndrome usually following bilateral temporal lobe removal. It is characterized by loss of recognition of people, loss of fear, rage reactions, hypersexuality, memory deficit, and overreaction to certain stimuli.

**km** *kilometer.*

**kMc** *kilomegacycle.*

**$KMnO_4$** Potassium permanganate.

**Knapp's forceps** (năps) [Herman J. Knapp, U.S. ophthalmologist, 1832–1911] A forceps with roller-like blades for expressing trachomatous granulations on the palpebral conjunctiva.

**kneading** (nēd′ĭng) [AS. *cnedan*] Pétrissage.

**knee** [AS. *cneo*] **1.** The anterior aspect of the leg at the articulation of the femur and tibia and the articulation itself, covered anteriorly with the patella or kneecap. It is formed by the femur, tibia, and patella. SEE: illus. **2.** Any structure shaped like a semiflexed knee. SYN: *geniculum.*

***Brodie's k.*** A chronic fungoid synovitis of the knee joint in which the affected parts become soft and pulpy.

***dislocation of k.*** Displacement of the knee. Dislocations in themselves are unusual. The so-called dislocation of the knee is usually due to various injuries of the joint and of the complicating structures of the knee, such as the tearing of the crushed tendons or ligaments, or the slipping of cartilages. Dislocations should be treated either by a straight splint, as in a fracture of the kneecap, or by two splints, one on either side of the knee, as in a fracture involving the knee joint. The patient should be transported to a hospital as quickly as possible.

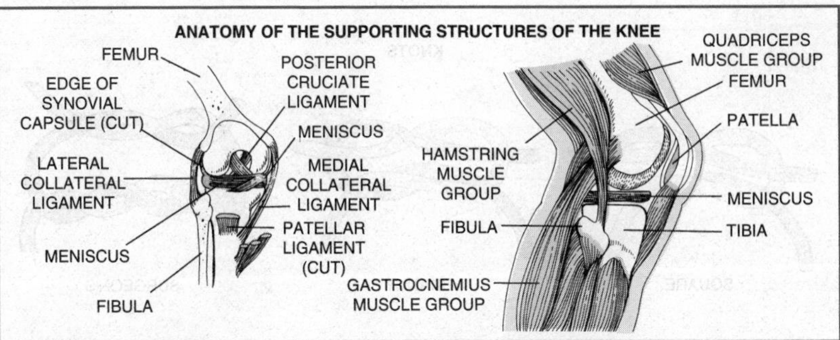


***game k.*** A lay term for internal derangement of the knee joint, characterized by pain or instability, locking, and weakness. It is usually the result of a torn internal cartilage, a fracture of the tibial spine, or an injury to the collateral or cruciate ligaments.

FIRST AID: The knee should be immobilized with a posterior splint. Surgical exploratory arthrotomy or arthroscopy may be necessary.

***housemaid's k.*** An inflammation of the bursa anterior to the patella, with accumulation of fluid therein. It may be seen in those who have to kneel frequently or continually while working.

***k. of internal capsule*** The curve at the meeting place of the anterior and posterior limbs of the internal capsule of the brain.

***jumper's k.*** An overuse syndrome, marked by chronic inflammation and infrapatellar tendinitis, resulting from repetitive jumping or leg extension exercises. It is commonly seen in basketball and volleyball players. The usual treatment is nonsteroidal anti-inflammatory drugs, rest, and phonophoresis.

***locked k.*** A condition in which the leg cannot be extended. It is usually due to displacement of semilunar cartilage.

***replacement of k.*** Replacement of the knee joint, particularly useful in treating patients with severe disabling arthritis of the knee. When done by those skilled in the technique, total knee replacement relieves pain in more than 95% of patients and improves function in more than 90%.

***runner's k.*** A general term describing several overuse conditions resulting from excessive running. These may involve the extensor mechanism and other musculotendinous insertions. Patellar tendinitis (jumper's knee), patellofemoral dysfunction, iliotibial band syndrome, and pes anserinus tendinitis or bursitis have all been called by this term.

**kneecap** The patella.

**Kneipp cure** (nīp) [Rev. Father Sebastian Kneipp, Ger. priest, 1821–1897] The application of water in various forms and degrees of temperature in the cure of disease, esp. wading in cold, dewy grass. SEE: *hydrotherapy*.

**kneippism** (nīp'ĭzm) Walking barefoot in dewy grass or bathing in cold water as a form of hydrotherapy.

**knemometry** (nē-mŏm'ĕt-rē) [Gr. *kneme*, shinbone, + *metron*, measure] A precise method of determining the length of a limb, esp. the lower leg. It has been used to record the effect of administering growth hormone to children with deficiency of the hormone.

**knife** (nīf) [AS. *cnif*] A cutting instrument.

***electric k.*** A knife that functions by use of a high-frequency cutting current.

***gold k.*** A special contra-angle knife used to trim a gold filling in a tooth.

***interdental k.*** A double-ended knife used in periodontal surgery for removing tissue between teeth.

***periodontal k.*** A surgical knife with a scaler-shaped blade whose entire perimeter is a cutting edge. It is used in gingivectomy and other periodontal surgery.

***plaster k.*** A stout knife used for cutting and trimming plaster study models in dental practice.

**knitting** [AS. *cnyttan*, to make knots] The process of healing by uniting pieces of a fractured bone.

**$KNO_3$** Potassium nitrate; niter; saltpeter.

**knob** (nŏb) [ME. *knobbe*] A protuberance on a surface or extremity; a mass or nodule.

**knock-knee** A condition in which knees are very close to each other and the ankles are apart. SYN: *genu valgum*.

**Knoop hardness test** A test of surface hardness using a stylus with a pyramidal diamond indenter. The long diagonal of the resulting indentation determines the hardness, expressed as the Knoop hardness number, of the substance. The test is used often in dentistry.

**knot** [AS. *cnotta*] **1.** An intertwining of a cord or cordlike structure to form a lump or knob. **2.** In surgery, the intertwining of the ends of a suture, ligature, bandage, or sling so that the ends will not slip or become separated. SEE: illus.; *square knot*. **3.** In anatomy, an enlargement forming a knoblike structure.

***false k.*** An external bulging of the um-

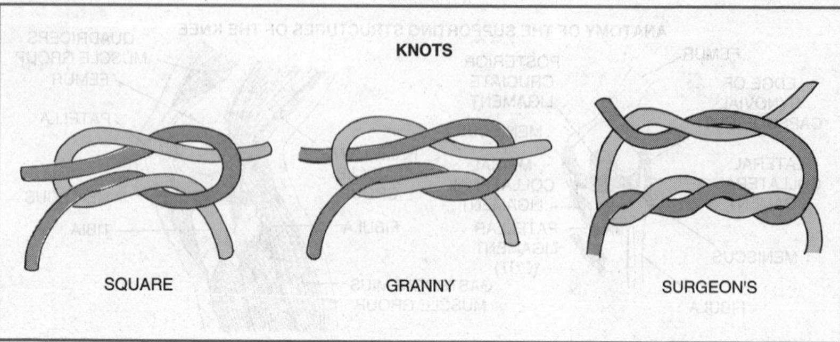


bilical cord, resulting from the coiling of the umbilical blood vessels.

***granny k.*** A double knot in which the ends of the cord do not lie parallel, but alternate being over and under each other. SEE: *knot* for illus.

***Hensen's k.*** A knoblike structure at the anterior end of the primitive streak. SEE: *primitive streak.*

***primitive k.*** Hensen's k.

***square k.*** A double knot in which the ends of the second knot are in the same place as the ends of the first knot. SEE: *knot* for illus.; *square knot.*

***surgeon's k.*** A double knot in which the cord is passed through the first loop twice. SEE: *knot* for illus.

***syncytial k.*** A protuberance formed by many nuclei of the syntrophoblast and found on the surface of a chorionic villus.

***true k.*** A knot formed by the fetus slipping through a loop of the umbilical cord.

**knowledge deficit** Lack of specific information necessary for the patient and significant other(s) to make informed choices regarding condition/therapies/treatment plan. SEE: *Nursing Diagnoses Appendix.*

**knuckle** (nŭk′ĕl) [Middle Low Ger. *knokel*] Prominence of the dorsal aspect of any of the phalangeal joints, esp. of the distal heads of the metacarpals when the fist is clenched.

***k. pad*** A discrete fibromatous pad appearing over a finger joint. It usually appears between the ages of 15 and 30. The etiology is unknown but trauma is not a significant factor.

**K.O.C.** *cathodal opening contraction.*

**Koch, Heinrich Herman Robert** (kōk) German bacteriologist, 1843–1910.

***K.'s bacillus*** Mycobacterium tuberculosis.

***K.'s law*** The criterion used in proving an organism is the cause of a disease or lesion: the microorganism in question is regularly found in the lesions of the disease; pure cultures can be obtained from it. When inoculated into susceptible animals, pure cultures can reproduce the disease or pathological condition; and the organism can be obtained again in pure culture from the inoculated animal. SYN: *K.'s postulate.*

***K.'s phenomenon*** A local inflammatory reaction resulting from injection of tuberculin into the skin of a person who has been previously exposed to the tubercle bacillus.

***K.'s postulate*** K.'s law.

**Koch, Walter** (kōk) German surgeon, b. 1880.

***K.'s node*** The atrioventricular node.

**kocherization** (kōk″ĕr-ī-zā′shŭn) An operative technique used in opening the duodenum to expose the ampulla of the common bile duct.

**Kocher's reflex** (kō′kĕrz) [Theodor Kocher, Swiss surgeon, 1841–1917] A contraction of abdominal muscles following moderate compression of the testicle.

**Koebner phenomenon** [Heinrich Koebner, Ger. dermatologist, 1838–1904] The appearance of a skin lesion as a result of nonspecific trauma (e.g., sunlight, burn, operative wound). It will appear at the trauma site and may be of a type found elsewhere on the skin. It may be seen in lichen planus or eczema but is particularly characteristic of psoriasis. The lesion must be sufficient to act on the papillary and epidermal layers of the skin and will appear in 3 to 18 days following the trauma.

**KOH** Potassium hydroxide.

**Köhler's disease** (kă′lĕrz) [Alban Köhler, Ger. physician, 1874–1947] **1.** Aseptic necrosis of the navicular bone of the wrist. **2.** Osteochondrosis of the head of the second metatarsal bone of the foot.

**Kohler's syndrome** Pain in the midfoot with accompanying point tenderness over the navicular bone, with increased density and narrowing of the tarsal navicular on radiographs. Most patients respond to 6 weeks' cast immobilization and there are no long-term sequela.

**Kohlman Evaluation of Living Skills** ABBR: KELS. A standard assessment for determining the ability of an individual to perform self-care and community living tasks. The assessment includes an interview and tasks that measure self-care, safety and health, money management, transportation and telephone use, and work and leisure behaviors.

**Kohlrausch's fold** (kōl'rowsh-ĕs) [Otto L. B. Kohlrausch, Ger. physician, 1811–1854] The rectal valve; one of the horizontal folds of the mucosa of the rectum. SYN: *Houston's valves; plica, transverse, of the rectum.*

**Kohnstamm's phenomenon** (kōn'stămz) [Oscar Kohnstamm, Ger. physician, 1871–1917] Aftermovement.

**koilocyte** (koy'lō-sīt) [Gr. *koilos,* hollow, + *kytos,* cell] An abnormal cell of the squamous epithelium of the cervix. It is associated with infection with human papillomavirus and the eventual development of cervical intraepithelial neoplasia.

**koilocytotic atypia** (koy"lō-sī-tŏt'ĭk ā-tĭp'ē-ă) [" + " + *osis,* condition, + *a-,* not, + *typicalis,* typical] Abnormality of the top layers of the epithelium of the uterine cervix wherein the cells undergo vacuolization and enlargement. SEE: *koilocyte.*

**koilonychia** (koy-lō-nĭk'ē-ă) [" + *onyx,* nail] Dystrophy of the fingernails in which they are thin and concave with raised edges. This condition is sometimes associated with iron-deficiency anemia. It is often called *spooning of nails.* SEE: illus.

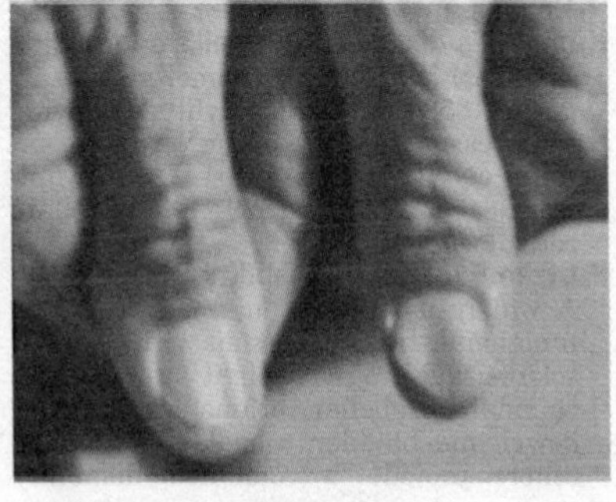

KOILONYCHIA

**koilosternia** (koy"lō-stĕr'nē-ă) [" + Gr. *sternon,* sternum] Condition in which the chest has a funnel-like depression in the middle of the thoracic wall.

**kolp-** [Gr. *kolpos,* vagina] Prefix meaning *vagina.*

**Kondoleon's operation** (kŏn-dō'lē-ŏnz) [Emmanuel Kondoleon, Gr. surgeon, 1879–1939] The surgical removal of layers of subcutaneous tissue to relieve elephantiasis.

**koniocortex** (kō"nē-ō-kor'tĕks) [Gr. *konis,* dust, + L. *cortex,* rind] The cortex of the sensory areas, so named because of its granular appearance.

**koniology** [" + *logos,* word, reason] Coniology.

**koniometer** (kō-nē-ŏm'ĕ-ter) [" + *metron,* measure] A device for estimating amount of dust in the air.

**koniosis** (kō-nē-ō'sĭs) [" + *osis,* condition] Coniosis.

**Koplik's spots** [Henry Koplik, U.S. pediatrician, 1858–1927] Small red spots with blue-white centers on the oral mucosa, particularly in the region opposite the molars; a diagnostic sign in measles before the rash appears. Not infrequently, the spots disappear as the rash develops.

**kopophobia** (kŏp"ō-fō'bē-ă) [Gr. *kopos,* fatigue, + *phobos,* fear] Abnormal fear of fatigue or exhaustion.

**Korányi's sign** (kō-răn'yēz) [Friedrich von Korányi, Hung. physician, 1828–1913] Increased resonance on percussion of the dorsal spine, a sign of pleural effusion.

**koro** (kō'rō) In China and Southeast Asia, a hysterical phobia that the penis will retract into the abdomen. The individual believes that once the penis disappears completely, he will die.

**koronion** (kō-rō'nē-ŏn) [Gr. *korone,* crest] Apex of coronoid process of the mandible.

**Korotkoff's sounds** (kō-rŏt'kŏfs) [Nikolai S. Korotkoff, Russ. physician, 1874–1920] Sounds heard in auscultation of blood pressure. SEE: *blood pressure.*

**Korsakoff's syndrome** (kor'să-kŏfs) [Sergei S. Korsakoff, Russ. neurologist, 1854–1900] A personality disorder characterized by a psychosis with polyneuritis, disorientation, muttering delirium, insomnia, illusions, and hallucinations; painful extremities, rarely a bilateral wrist drop, more frequently bilateral foot drop with pain or pressure over the long nerves. It may occur as a sequel to chronic alcoholism. SYN: *polyneuritic psychosis.*

**kosher** (kō'shĕr) [Hebrew *kasher,* proper] Pert. to food prepared and served according to Jewish dietary laws.

**koumiss** (koo'mĭs) [Tartar *kumyz*] Fermented cow's milk or substance used for fermenting cow's milk; also spelled kumiss and kumyss.

**Kr** Symbol for the element krypton.

**Krabbe's disease** (krăb'ēz) [Knud H. Krabbe, Danish neurologist, 1885–1961] Globoid cell leukodystrophy due to the accumulation of galactocerebroside in the tissues, resulting from a deficiency of galactocerebrosidase. Clinically, the infant develops seizures, deafness, blindness, cachexia, paralysis, and marked mental deficiency. Survival beyond 2 years is rare.

**Kraepelin's classification** (krā'pă-lĭnz) [Emil Kraepelin, Ger. psychiatrist, 1856–1926] A classification of mental illness into two groups: the manic-depressive and the schizophrenic.

**krait** (krāt) A small venomous snake of the genus *Bungarus,* indigenous to India.

**kraurosis** (krŏ-rō'sĭs) [Gr. *krauros,* dry] Atrophy and dryness of the skin and any mucous membrane, esp. of the vulva. The subcutaneous fat of the mons pubis and labia disappears, clitoris and prepuce atrophy, and stenosis of the vaginal orifice is common. Fissures may develop.

***k. penis*** Kraurosis in which the glans

penis atrophies and becomes shriveled.

***k. vulvae*** An atrophic disease affecting the female external genitalia, seen most often in older women. Characterized by severe itching and a white marble-like appearance of the skin, frequently with excoriations. If untreated, the skin may undergo malignant degeneration. SYN: *Breisky's disease; leukoplakia vulvae.*

**Krause, Karl** (krowz) German anatomist, 1797–1868.

***K.'s gland*** A small mucous acinous gland located beneath the fornix conjunctivae. This accessory lacrimal gland opens into the fornix.

***K.'s valve*** A fold of mucous membrane of the lacrimal sac at the junction of the lacrimal duct. SYN: *Beraud's valve.*

**Krause, Wilhelm** (krowz) German anatomist, 1833–1910.

***K.'s end bulb*** One of the widely distributed encapsulated nerve endings present superficially in the skin, cornea, and organs such as the testicles.

***K.'s membrane*** A thin, dark disk that transversely crosses through and bisects the clear zone of a striated muscle and bisects the clear zone (isotropic disk) of a striated muscle fiber. The portion between two disks constitutes a sarcomere. SYN: *Z disk.*

**Krebs cycle** [Sir Hans Krebs, Ger. biochemist, 1900–1981, co-winner of a Nobel prize in 1953. He lived and worked in Britain.] A complicated series of reactions in the body involving the oxidative metabolism of pyruvic acid and liberation of energy. It is the main pathway of terminal oxidation in the process of which not only carbohydrates but proteins and fats are utilized. SYN: *citric acid cycle; tricarboxylic acid cycle.* SEE: illus.

**kringle** A subunit of plasminogen consisting of 80 amino acids in a loop structure.

**Krönig's area** (krā'nĭgz) [Georg Krönig, Ger. physician, 1856–1911] Resonant region in the thorax over the apices of the lungs.

**Krukenberg's chopsticks** [Hermann Krukenberg, Ger. surgeon, 1863–1935] A condition occurring after surgical separation of the remaining ulna and radius of a forearm stump after traumatic removal of a lower arm. This allows the ulna and radius to act as crude pincers (i.e., chopsticks).

**Krukenberg's tumor** (kroo'kĕn-bĕrgz) [Frederick Krukenberg, Ger. pathologist, 1871–1946] A malignant tumor of the ovary, usually bilateral and frequently secondary to malignancy of the gastrointestinal tract. Histologically, these tumors consist of myxomatous connective tissue and cells having a signet ring arrangement of their nuclei. The epithelial tissue resembles malignancy of the original site.

**krypton** (krĭp'tŏn) [Gr. *kryptos,* hidden] SYMB: Kr. A gaseous element found in small amounts in the atmosphere; atomic weight 83.80; atomic number 36.

**$K_2SO_4$** Potassium sulfate.

**KT-1000** A testing device that measures the laxity of the anterior cruciate ligament and determines clinical instability by comparison with the normal opposite knee.

**KUB** *kidneys, ureters, bladder;* pert. to anteroposterior projection films of the abdomen.

**kubisagari** (koo-bĭs″ă-gă'rē) [Japanese, hang-head] Ptosis and bulbar weakness in nutritionally deficient children; endemic in Japan. A similar disorder was observed in prisoners of war in Japan. Parenteral administration of thiamine has been beneficial.

**Kufs' disease** [H. Kufs, Ger. psychiatrist, 1871–1955] The adult form of cerebral sphingolipidosis. The onset of symptoms is between 21 and 26 years of age. The disease is diagnosed by the development of dementia, myoclonic jerks, blindness, and retinitis pigmentosa.

**Kugelberg-Welander disease** [Eric Klaus Henrik Kugelberg, 1913–1983; L. Welander, b. 1909; Swedish neurologists] Juvenile spinal muscular atrophy.

**kumiss, kumyss** (koo'mĭs) [Tartar *kumyz*] Koumiss.

**Kümmell's disease, Kümmell's spondylitis** (kĭm'ĕlz) [Hermann Kümmell, Ger. surgeon, 1852–1937] Spondylitis following compression fracture of the vertebrae.

**Kupffer cell** (koop'fĕrz) [Karl W. von Kupffer, Ger. anatomist, 1829–1902] Stellate reticuloendothelial cell.

**Kurtzke Expanded Disability Status Scale** A widely used scale for measuring the functional status of persons with multiple sclerosis. Ratings on eight systems (pyramidal, cerebellar, brainstem, sensory, bowel and bladder, visual, mental, and other) provide a combined disability score.

**kuru** (koo'roo) A rapidly progressive neurological disease that is invariably fatal. The disease affects mostly adult women and children of both sexes belonging to the Fore tribe of New Guinea. This disease is probably due to a transmissible slow infection (rather than a slow virus). It is transmitted by the practice of ingesting tissue from an infected individual who has died (ritual cannibalism) and rubbing infected tissues over the bodies of the women and children kin to the victim. With the decline of this practice, the incidence of kuru has decreased.

**Kussmaul, Adolph** (koos'mowl) German physician, 1822–1902.

***K.'s breathing*** A very deep gasping type of respiration associated with severe diabetic acidosis and coma.

***K.'s disease*** Periarteritis nodosa.

**kv** *kilovolt.*

**KVO** *keep vein open.*

**kvp** *kilovoltage peak.*

**kwashiorkor** (kwăsh-ē-or'kor) [Ghana, Af-

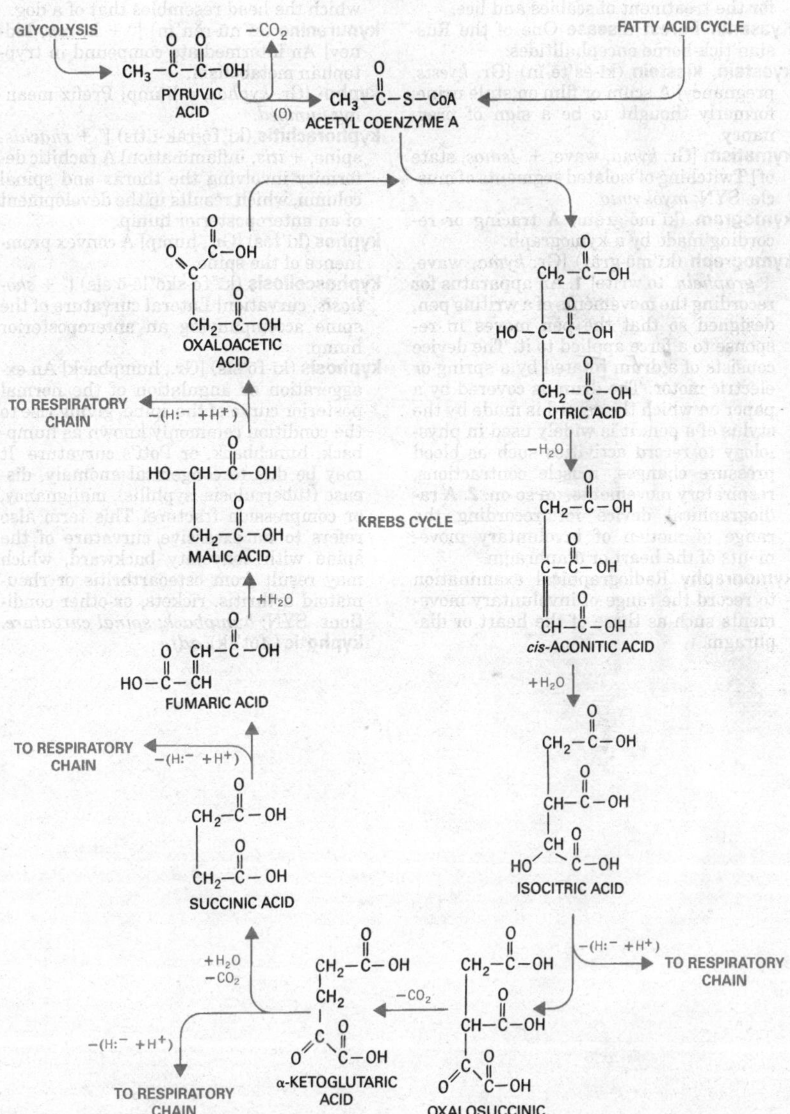


rica, deposed child, i.e., child that is no longer suckled] A severe protein-deficiency type of malnutrition of children. It occurs after the child is weaned. The clinical signs are, at first, a vague type of lethargy, apathy, or irritability and, later, failure to grow, mental deficiency, inanition, increased susceptibility to infections, edema, dermatitis, and liver enlargement. The hair may have a reddish color.

TREATMENT: In addition to dietary therapy, the acute problems of infections, diarrhea, poor renal function, and shock need immediate attention. At first the diet must be carefully supervised to prevent overloading the system with calories or protein. In the first weeks of therapy, the child may lose weight owing to the loss of edema. If the disease has been severe and longstanding, the child may never attain full growth and mental development.

**Kwell** Trade name of a shampoo and lotion for the treatment of scabies and lice.

**Kyasanur Forest disease** One of the Russian tick-borne encephalitides.

**kyestein, kiestein** (kī-ĕs′tē-ĭn) [Gr. *kyesis,* pregnancy] A scum or film on stale urine; formerly thought to be a sign of pregnancy.

**kymatism** [Gr. *kyma,* wave, + *-ismos,* state of] Twitching of isolated segments of muscle. SYN: *myokymia.*

**kymogram** (kī′mō-grăm) A tracing or recording made by a kymograph.

**kymograph** (kī′mō-grăf) [Gr. *kyma,* wave, + *graphein,* to write] **1.** An apparatus for recording the movements of a writing pen, designed so that the pen moves in response to a force applied to it. The device consists of a drum rotated by a spring or electric motor. The drum is covered by a paper on which the record is made by the stylus of a pen. It is widely used in physiology to record activities such as blood pressure changes, muscle contractions, respiratory movements, an so on. **2.** A radiographical device for recording the range of motion of involuntary movements of the heart or diaphragm.

**kymography** Radiographical examination to record the range of involuntary movements such as those of the heart or diaphragm.

**kynocephalus** (kī″nō-sĕf′ă-lŭs) [Gr. *kyon,* dog, + *kephale,* head] A deformed fetus in which the head resembles that of a dog.

**kynurenine** (kī″nū-rĕn′ĭn) [″ + L. *ren,* kidney] An intermediate compound in tryptophan metabolism.

**kypho-** [Gr. *kyphos,* a hump] Prefix meaning *humped.*

**kyphorachitis** (kī″fō-răk-ī′tĭs) [″ + *rhachis,* spine, + *itis,* inflammation] A rachitic deformity involving the thorax and spinal column, which results in the development of an anteroposterior hump.

**kyphos** (kī′fŏs) [Gr., hump] A convex prominence of the spine.

**kyphoscoliosis** (kī″fō-skō″lē-ō′sĭs) [″ + *skoliosis,* curvation] Lateral curvature of the spine accompanying an anteroposterior hump.

**kyphosis** (kī-fō′sĭs) [Gr., humpback] An exaggeration or angulation of the normal posterior curve of the spine, giving rise to the condition commonly known as humpback, hunchback, or Pott's curvature. It may be due to congenital anomaly, disease (tuberculosis, syphilis), malignancy, or compression fracture. This term also refers to an excessive curvature of the spine with convexity backward, which may result from osteoarthritis or rheumatoid arthritis, rickets, or other conditions. SYN: *humpback; spinal curvature.* **kyphotic** (-fŏt′ĭk), *adj.*

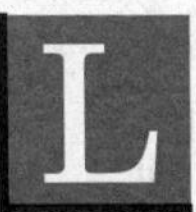

**Λ, λ** The Greek symbol for lambda.

**L, l** *Lactobacillus; Latin; left; left eye; length; lethal; light sense; liter.*

**$L_+$** Symbol for limes tod.

**L1, L2, etc.** *first lumbar nerve, second lumbar nerve,* and so forth.

**$L_0$** Symbol for limes nul.

**L-** In biochemistry, a symbol used as a prefix to indicate the carbon atom is symmetrical (or achiral) and that only three dissimilar groups attach to it. The names of such compounds would be preceded by L-. SEE: D-.

**LA** *left atrium.*

**La** Symbol for the element lanthanum.

**lab 1.** German for the enzyme rennin. **2.** Colloquial for laboratory.

**Labbé's vein** (lăb-āz′) [Léon Labbé, Fr. surgeon, 1832–1916] The vein that connects the superficial middle cerebral vein and the transverse sinus of the brain.

**label** The attachment of a radioactive marker or other chemical to a biologically active substance such as a drug or body chemical (such as glucose, protein, or fat). The metabolic fate of the labeled material may be investigated by detecting the presence of the label in various body sites or in excretions. The label material itself is chosen so that it does not alter the metabolism or action of the substance being investigated. SEE: *tracer.*

**labeling** SEE: *tag, radioactive; tagging.*

**la belle indifference** [Fr., beautiful indifference] An unrealistic degree of indifference to, or complacency about, gross symptoms of hysterical anesthesia or paralysis. It is seen in the conversion reaction.

**labetalol hydrochloride** An alpha- and beta-adrenergic blocking agent used in treating hypertension. SEE: *hypertensive crisis.*

**labia** (lā′bē-ă) [L.] Plural of labium.

***l. majora*** The two folds of skin and adipose tissue lying on either side of the vaginal opening and forming the lateral borders of the vulva. Their medial surfaces unite anteriorly above the clitoris to form the anterior commissure; posteriorly they are connected by a poorly defined posterior commissure. They are separated by a cleft, the rima pudendi, into which the urethra and vagina open. In young girls, their medial surfaces are in contact with each other, concealing the labia minora and vestibule. In older women, the labia minora may protrude between them.

***l. minora*** The two thin folds of integument that lie just inside the vestibule of the vagina and between the labia majora and the hymen. They enclose the vestibule. Anteriorly each divides into two smaller folds that unite with similar folds from the other side and enclose the clitoris, the more anterior one forming the prepuce (preputium clitoridis) of the clitoris and the posterior one the frenulum clitoridis. In young girls, they are hidden entirely by the labia majora.

**labial** (lā′bē-ăl) [L. *labialis*] Pert. to the lips.

**labialism** (lā′bē-ăl-ĭzm) [L. *labium,* lip, + Gr. *-ismos,* state of] Defective speech in which sounds influenced by the position of the lips are stressed.

**labile** (lā′bīl) [L. *labi,* to slip] Not fixed; unsteady; easily disarranged; rapidly shifting and changing emotions.

***heat l.*** Thermolabile.

**lability** (lă-bĭl′ĭ-tē) The state of being unstable or changeable.

***emotional l.*** Excessive emotional reactivity associated with frequent changes or swings in emotions and mood.

**labioalveolar** (lā″bē-ō-ăl-vē′ō-lăr) [L. *labium,* lip, + *alveolus,* little hollow] Pert. to the lips and tooth sockets.

**labiocervical** (lā″bē-ō-sĕr′vĭ-kl) [″ + *cervix,* neck] Pert. to the buccal surface of the lips and the neck of a tooth.

**labiochorea** (lā″bē-ō-kō-rē′ă) [″ + Gr. *choreia,* dance] A spasm of the lips in chorea, causing stammering.

**labioclination** (lā″bē-ō-klī-nā′shŭn) [″ + Gr. *klinein,* to slope] In dentistry, deviation of a tooth from the normal vertical toward the labial side.

**labiodental** (lā″bē-ō-dĕn′tăl) [″ + *dens,* tooth] **1.** Concerning the lips and teeth, esp. the labial surface of a tooth. **2.** Referring to the pronunciation of certain letters that require interaction of the teeth and lips.

**labiogingival** (lā″bē-ō-jĭn′jĭ-văl) [″ + *gingiva,* gum] Concerning the lips and gums or referring to the labial and gingival surfaces of a tooth.

**labioglossolaryngeal** (lā″bē-ō-glŏs″ō-lăr-ĭn′jē-ăl) [″ + Gr. *glossa,* tongue, + *larynx,* larynx] Pert. to the lips, tongue, and larynx.

**labioglossopharyngeal** (lā″bē-ō-glŏs″ō-făr-ĭn′jē-ăl) [″ + ″ + *pharynx,* throat] Pert. to the lips, tongue, and pharynx.

**labiomental** (lā″bē-ŏ-mĕn′tăl) [″ + *mentum,* chin] Pert. to the lower lip and chin.

**labiomycosis** (lā″bē-ō-mī-kō′sĭs) [″ + Gr. *mykes,* fungus, + *osis,* condition] Any disease of the lips caused by the presence of a fungus.

**labionasal** (lā″bē-ō-nā′zăl) [″ + *nasus,* nose] Concerning the nose and lips.

**labiopalatine** (lā″bē-ō-păl′ă-tīn) [″ + *palatum,* palate] Relating to the lips and palate.

**labioplasty** (lā′bē-ō-plăs″tē) [″ + Gr. *plassein,* to form] Cheiloplasty.

**labiotenaculum** (lā″bē-ō-tĕn-ăk′ū-lŭm) [″ + *tenaculum,* a hook] An instrument for holding the lips during an operation.

**labioversion** (lā″bē-ō-vĕr′zhŭn) [″ + *versio,* a turning] The state of being twisted in a labial direction, esp. a tooth.

**labium** (lā′bē-ŭm) *pl.* **labia** [L.] A lip or a structure like one; an edge or fleshy border.

***l. cerebri*** The margin of the cerebral hemispheres overlapping the corpus callosum.

***l. inferius oris*** The lower lip.

***l. majus*** SEE: *labia majora.*

***l. minus*** SEE: *labia minora.*

***l. minus pudendi*** SEE: *labia minora.*

***l. oris*** The skin and muscular tissue surrounding the mouth; the lips of the mouth.

***l. superius oris*** The upper lip.

***l. tympanicum*** The outer edge of the organ of Corti.

***l. urethrae*** The lateral margin of the meatus urinarius externus.

***l. uteri*** The thickened margin of the cervix uteri.

***l. vestibulare*** The vestibular or inner edge of the organ of Corti.

**labor** [L., work] The physiological process by which the fetus is expelled from the uterus into the vagina and then to the outside of the body. SYN: *childbirth; parturition.* SEE: illus.

Approx. 95% of normal full-term babies are born 265 to 300 days from the first day of the last menstrual period. The average duration of a normal pregnancy is 282 days.

Traditionally, labor is divided into three stages, but *lightening* most often occurs up to 4 weeks before the onset of labor in primigravid women. It may occur during labor in a woman who has borne a previous child or children. The shape of the abdomen changes, with the lower portion becoming more pendulous and the costal area looking flatter. This change is due to the presenting part having descended into the pelvis to the level of the ischial spines.

*First Stage (stage of dilatation):* This is the period from the onset of regular uterine contractions to full dilation and effacement of the cervix. This stage averages 12 hours in primigravidas and 8 hours in multiparas.

The identification of this stage is particularly important to women having their first baby. Its diagnosis is complicated by the fact that many women experience false labor pains, which may begin as early as 3 to 4 weeks before the onset of true labor. False labor pains are quite irregular, are usually confined to the lower part of the abdomen and groin, and do not extend from the back around the abdomen as in true labor. False labor pains do not increase in frequency with time and are not made more intense by walking. The conclusive distinction is made by determining the effect of the pains on the cervix. False labor pains do not cause effacement and dilatation of the cervix as do true labor pains. SEE: *Braxton Hicks sign.*

A reliable sign of impending labor is *show.* The appearance of a slight amount of vaginal blood-tinged mucus is a good indication that labor will begin within the next 24 hours. The loss of more than a few milliliters of blood at this time, however, must be regarded as being due to a pathological process. SEE: *placenta previa.*

*Second Stage (stage of expulsion):* This period lasts from complete dilatation of the cervix through the birth of the fetus, averaging 50 minutes in primigravidas and 20 minutes in multigravidas. Labor pains are severe, occur at 2- or 3-minute intervals, and last from a little less than 1 minute to a little more than 1½ minutes.

Rupture of the membranes (bag of waters) usually occurs during the early part of this stage, accompanied by a gush of amniotic fluid from the vagina. The muscles of the abdomen contract involuntarily during this portion of labor. The patient directs all her strength to bearing down during the contractions. She may be quite flushed and perspire. As labor continues the perineum bulges and, in a head presentation, the scalp of the fetus appears through the vulvar opening. With cessation of each contraction, the fetus recedes from its position and then advances a little more when another contraction occurs. This continues until more of the head is visible and the vulvar ring encircles the head. This is called *crowning.*

At this time the decision is made concerning an incision in the perineum (i.e., episiotomy) to facilitate delivery. If done, it is most commonly a midline posterior episiotomy. When the head is completely removed from the vagina it falls posteriorly; later the head rotates as the shoulders turn to come through the pelvis. There is usually a gush of amniotic fluid as the shoulders are delivered.

*Third Stage (placental stage):* This is the period following the birth of the fetus through expulsion of the placenta and membranes. As soon as the fetus is delivered, the remainder of the amniotic fluid escapes. It will contain a small amount of blood. Uterine contractions return, and usually within 8 to 10 minutes the placenta and membranes are delivered. After this, there is a certain amount of bleeding from the uterus. The amount may vary from 100 to 500 ml or more, but the average is 200 ml.

The amount of blood loss will vary directly with the size of the fetus. The probability that blood loss will exceed 500 ml is less than 5% if the fetus weighs 5 lb

## SEQUENCE OF LABOR AND CHILDBIRTH

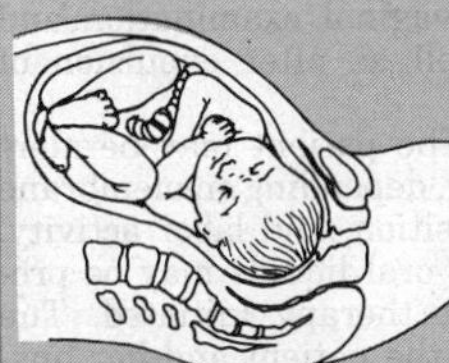

1. LABOR BEGINS, MEMBRANES INTACT.

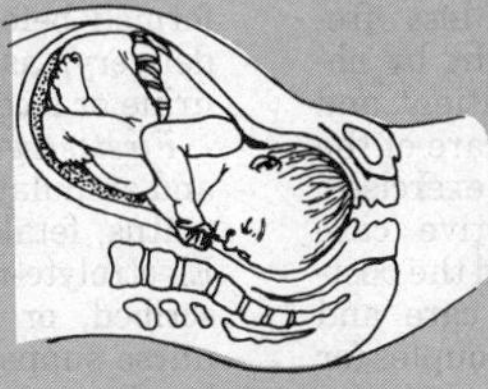

2. EFFACEMENT OF CERVIX, WHICH IS NOW PARTIALLY DILATED.

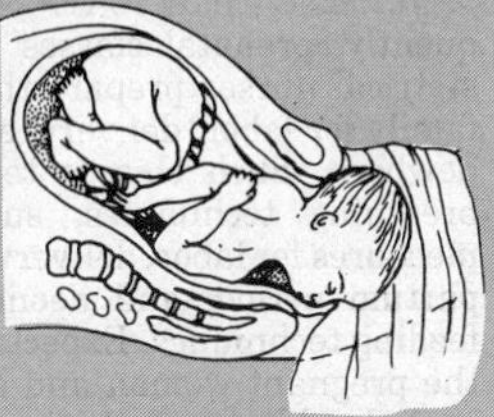

3. HEAD IS ROTATED, PARTIALLY EXTENDED, AND NOW PRESENTS. MEMBRANES ARE RUPTURED.

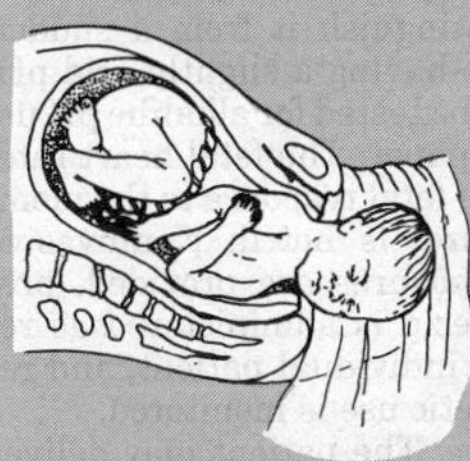

4. HEAD IS ALMOST DELIVERED.

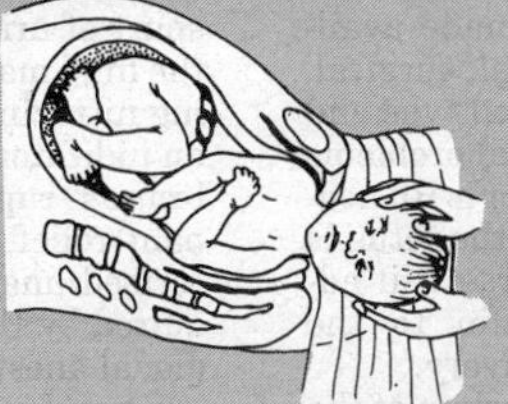

5. DELIVERY OF HEAD.

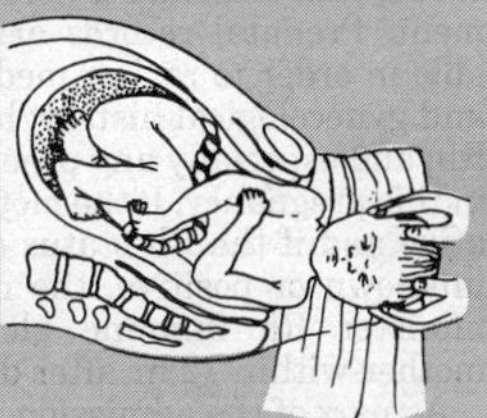

6. DELIVERY OF SHOULDERS.

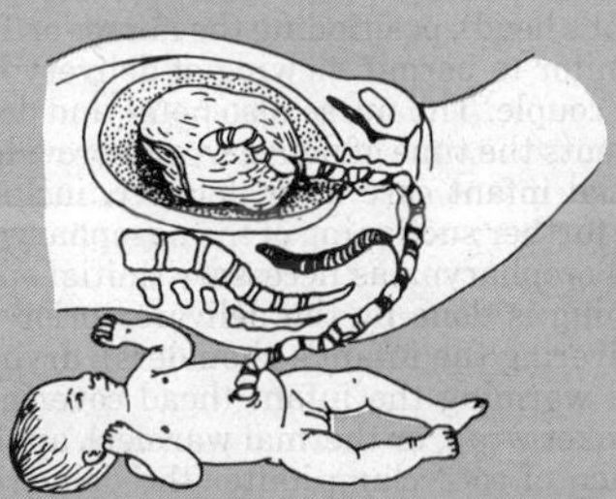

7. DELIVERY OF INFANT IS COMPLETE. UTERUS BEGINS TO CONTRACT.

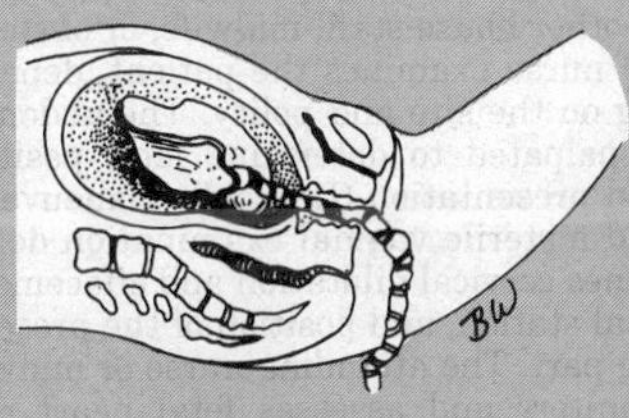


8. UMBILICAL CORD HAS BEEN TIED AND CUT. PLACENTA HAS BEGUN TO SEPARATE FROM UTERUS.

(2268 gm) or less. The chances that blood loss will exceed 500 ml is 25% if the fetus weighs more than 9 lb (4082 gm). Other factors such as episiotomy or perineal laceration will also affect the amount of blood loss. SEE: *birthing chair; Credé's method* for assisting the expulsion of the placenta.

NURSING IMPLICATIONS: Most frequently, prenatal classes taught by obstetrical nurses prepare the patient and family for labor, delivery, and care of the newborn. Such classes teach exercises; breathing techniques; supportive care measures for labor, delivery, and the postpartum period; and neonatal care and feeding techniques. Expectant couples (or the pregnant woman and a support person) should attend classes together. The goals of expectant parent education are the birth of a healthy infant and a positive experience for the couple. Labor and delivery may take place in a hospital, birthing center, or at home. Hospitals offer care in traditional labor and delivery rooms and, increasingly, in birthing rooms that simulate a homelike environment. Prenatal records are made available in order to review medical, surgical, and gynecological history; blood type and Rh; and especially any prenatal problems in this pregnancy. If the mother is Rh negative and if the Rh status of the fetus is unknown or positive, the nurse will administer Rh immune globulin to the mother within 72 hr after delivery.

As part of the admission workup of the laboring woman, the nurse assesses vital signs, height and weight, fetal heart tone and activity, and labor status (i.e., condition of membranes, show, onset time of regular contractions, contraction frequency and duration, and patient anxiety, pain, or discomfort). Initial laboratory studies are carried out according to protocol. The obstetrician, resident physician or other house staff, midwife, or obstetrical nurse examines the patient, depending on the site and policy. The abdomen is palpated to determine fetal position and presentation (Leopold's maneuvers), and a sterile vaginal examination determines cervical dilatation and effacement, fetal station, and position of the presenting part. The attending nurse or midwife monitors and assesses fetal heart rate and the frequency and duration of contractions, using palpation and a fetoscope. The frequency of assessment and repetition of vaginal examination are determined by the patient's labor stage and activity and by fetal response. In the past, admission to a labor suite usually included a perineal shave and enema in preparation for delivery, but these procedures have been largely discontinued and are currently done only if prescribed for a particular patient. The patient should urinate and have a bowel movement, if possible. Bladder distension is to be avoided, but catheterization is carried out only if all other efforts to encourage voiding in a patient with a distended bladder fail. The perineum is cleansed (protecting the vaginal introitus from entry of cleansing solutions) and kept as clean as possible during labor. Special cleansing is performed before vaginal examination and delivery, as well as after expulsion of urine or feces.

*First stage:* The patient may be alert and ambulating, depending on membrane status, fetal position, and labor activity. Electrolyte-rich oral liquids may be prescribed, or I.V. therapy initiated. The nurse supports the patient and her husband or other support person and monitors the progress of the labor and the response of the fetus, notifying the obstetrician or midwife of any abnormal findings. When membranes rupture spontaneously or are ruptured artificially by the midwife or obstetrician, the color and volume of the fluid and the presence of meconium staining or unusual odor are noted. To distinguish it from a sudden spurt of urine having a slightly acid pH, the fluid may be tested for alkaline pH using nitrazine paper. The fetal heart rate, an indicator of fetal response to the membrane's rupture, is noted. Noninvasive pain relief measures are provided, prescribed analgesia is administered as required by the individual patient, and regional anesthetic use is monitored.

*Second stage:* The patient may deliver in any previously agreed-on position, including lithotomy or modified lithotomy, sitting, or side lying, in a birthing chair, birthing bed, or on a delivery table. The nurse continues to monitor the patient and fetus, prepares the patient for delivery (cleansing and draping); sets up delivery equipment; and supports the father or support person (positioned near the patient's head), positioning the mirror or TV monitor to permit viewing of delivery by the couple. The nurse also notes and documents the time of delivery, and provides initial infant care after delivery, including further suctioning of the nasopharynx and oropharynx as necessary (initial suctioning is done by the deliverer prior to delivering the infant's shoulders), drying and warming the infant (head covering, blanket wrap, or thermal warmer), application of cord clamp (after the deliverer double-clamps the cord and cuts between the clamps), and positive identification (footprints of infant and thumb prints or fingerprints of mother, and application of numbered ankle and wrist band to the infant and wrist band to the mother). Eye prophylaxis for gonorrhea may be delayed up to 2 hr to facilitate eye contact and to enhance maternal-infant bonding, or may be refused by the parents, on signing of an informed consent. An Apgar score of the infant's overall condition is obtained at 1 min and 5 min after the birth. The infant in good condition is placed on the mother's chest or abdomen or put to breast, and the couple is encouraged to inspect and interact with the infant. An infant in distress is hurried to the nursery, usually with the father attending, so that specialized care can be provided by nursery and neonatal-nurse specialists, and pediatrician. In extreme cases (and at parental request), the infant may be baptized by the nurse or by a chaplain or other Christian minister, and photographs may be taken to assist the parents in dealing with the life, critical time, and possible death of the infant.

*Third stage:* The nurse continues to monitor the status of the patient and the fundus through delivery of the placenta and membranes (documenting the time), examination of the vagina and uterus for trauma or retained products, and repair of any laceration or surgical episiotomy. The placenta is examined to ascertain that no fragments remain in the uterus. The perineal area is cleansed, and the mother assisted to a comfortable position and covered with a warm blanket.

*Fourth stage:* The nurse continues to observe the patient closely and is alert for hemorrhage or other complications through frequent assessment, including monitoring vital signs, palpating the fundus for firmness and position in relation to the umbilicus at intervals (determined by agency policy or patient condition), and massaging the fundus gently or administering prescribed oxytocic drugs to maintain uterine contraction and to limit bleeding. The character (including presence, size, and number of clots) and volume of vaginal discharge or lochia are assessed periodically; the perineum is inspected and ice applied as prescribed, and the bladder is inspected, palpated, and percussed for distention. The patient is encouraged to void, and catheterization is performed only if absolutely necessary. The nurse notifies the obstetrician or midwife if any problems occur or persist. This period also is used for parent-infant bonding, because the infant is usually awake for the first hour or so after delivery. The mother can breast-feed if desired, and the couple can inspect the infant. The nurse supports the couple's responses to the newborn, as well as to the labor and delivery experience. The infant is then taken to the nursery for initial infant care.

*Early postpartum period:* Once the infant's temperature has stabilized, measurements have been taken (length, head and chest circumference, weight), and other prescribed care carried out, the infant may be returned to the mother's side (in its crib carrier). The nurse continues to assess the mother's physical and psychological status after delivery, checking the fundus, vulva, and perineum according to policy; inspects the mother's breasts and assists the mother with feeding or measures to prevent lactation as desired; helps the mother to deal with other responsibilities of motherhood; and carries out the mandated maternal teaching program, including providing written information for later review by the patient. In hospitals or birthing centers, the nurse prepares the mother for early discharge to the home setting and arranges for follow-up care as needed and available. In many settings, the nurse makes follow-up calls or visits to the mother during the early post-partum period or encourages the patient to call in with concerns, or the patient may receive follow-up visits by a nurse from her health maintenance organization. The mother may also be referred to support groups, such as the La Leche League, Nursing Mothers' Club, and others as available in the particular community.

***active l.*** Regular uterine contractions with increasing dilatation of the cervix and descent of the presenting part.

***arrested l.*** Failure of labor to proceed through the normal stages. This may be due to uterine inertia, obstruction of the pelvis, or systemic disease.

***artificial l.*** Induced l.

***augmented l.*** Induced l.

***back l.*** Labor involving malposition of the fetal head with the occiput opposing the mother's sacrum. The laboring woman experiences severe back pain. SEE: *occiput posterior, persistent.*

***complicated l.*** Labor occurring with an accompanying abnormal condition such as hemorrhage or inertia.

***dry l.*** Labor after most of the amniotic fluid has been drained away. It is usually associated with premature rupture of the membranes.

***dysfunctional l.*** Failure to progress in a normal pattern of labor.

***false l.*** Uterine contractions occurring before the onset of actual labor. These contractions eventually subside. SEE: under *labor; Braxton Hicks sign.*

***induced l.*** The use of oxytocics or other methods to stimulate uterine contractions before they would normally occur. Uterine contractions may be stimulated by gently squeezing the nipples. SYN: *artificial l.; augmented l.* SEE: *Nursing Diagnoses Appendix.*

Caution: Oxytocin should be used only intravenously, using a device that permits precise control of flow rate. While oxytocin is being administered, the fetal heart rate and uterine contractions should be monitored electronically.

***instrumental l.*** Labor completed by mechanical means, such as the use of forceps.

***missed l.*** **1.** False l. **2.** Labor in which true labor pains begin but subside. This may be a sign of a dead fetus or extrauterine pregnancy.

***normal l.*** Progressive dilatation and effacement of the cervix with descent of the presenting part.

***obstructed l.*** Interference with fetal passage through the birth canal. Causes include fetal malposition, malpresentation, and cephalopelvic disproportion.

***precipitate l.*** Labor of less than 3 hours' duration, marked by sudden onset and rapid cervical effacement and dilation.

***premature l.*** Preterm l.

***preterm l.*** Labor that begins between 20 and 38 weeks' gestation. Causes include uterine structural abnormalities, overdistension related to multiple pregnancy or hydramnios, infection, substance abuse, dehydration, pregnancy-induced hypertension, diabetes, and cardiovascular or renal disease. Actions to interrupt preterm labor are attempted if cervical dilation exceeds 4 cm. Bedrest is advised to reduce pressure against the cervix. Fluids are administered orally or intravenously to improve hydration. Pharmacological management includes administration of tocolytic drugs; if delivery can be delayed for 24 to 48 hr, corticosteroids may be given to stimulate fetal production of pulmonary surfactant. Home management of preterm labor requires extensive patient teaching to ensure accurate external fetal monitoring, self-administration of tocolytic drugs, and recognition of signs and symptoms that should be reported immediately. SYN: *premature l.* SEE: *premature rupture of membranes; prematurity; Nursing Diagnoses Appendix.*

***prodromal l.*** The initial changes that precede actual labor, usually occurring 24 to 48 hr before the onset of labor. Some women report a surge of energy. Findings include lightening, excessive mucoid vaginal discharge, softening and beginning effacement of the ripe cervix, scant bloody show associated with expulsion of the mucus plug, and diarrhea.

***prolonged l.*** Abnormally slow progress of labor, lasting more than 20 hr. SEE: *dystocia.*

***spontaneous l.*** Labor that is completed without mechanical or operative interference.

***stage I l.*** SEE: *labor; Nursing Diagnoses Appendix.*

***stage II l.*** SEE: *labor; Nursing Diagnoses Appendix.*

***trial of l.*** Permitting labor to continue long enough to determine if normal birth appears to be possible.

**laboratory** (lăb′ră-tor″ē) [L. *laboratorium*] A room or building equipped for scientific experimentation, research, testing, or clinical studies of materials, fluids, or tissues obtained from patients.

**Laborde's method** (lă-bordz′) [Jean B. V. Laborde, Fr. physician, 1830–1903] Stimulation of the respiratory center in asphyxiation by a series of rhythmical traction movements upon the tongue.

**labret** (lā′brĕt) [L. *labrum,* lip] Among some primitive peoples, a distinctive plug of ivory, bone, stone, or bottle top worn in a hole artificially produced in the lips of adolescent boys.

**labrocyte** (lăb′rō-sīt) [Gr. *labros,* greedy, + *kytos,* cell] A mast cell.

**labrum** (lā′brŭm) *pl.* **labra** [L., lip] **1.** Lip or liplike structure. **2.** The upper lip of an insect.

**labyrinth** (lăb′ĭ-rĭnth) [Gr. *labyrinthos,* maze] **1.** A series of intricate communicating passages. **2.** Within the inner ear, the bony and membranous labyrinths, which contain the receptors for hearing and equilibrium. SEE: illus.

***bony l.*** Osseous l.

***ethmoidal l.*** The lateral mass of the ethmoid bone, which includes the superior and middle conchae and encloses the ethmoidal air cells. SYN: *olfactory l.*

***membranous l.*** The structure in the osseous labyrinth consisting of the utricle and saccule of the vestibule, three semicircular ducts, and the cochlear duct, all filled with endolymph.

***olfactory l.*** Ethmoidal l.

***osseous l.*** The structure that consists of the vestibule, three semicircular canals, and cochlea. SYN: *bony l.*

**labyrinthectomy** (lăb-ĭ-rĭn-thĕk′tō-mē) [″ + *ektome,* excision] Excision of the labyrinth.

**labyrinthine** (lăb-ĭ-rĭn′thĭn) **1.** Pert. to a labyrinth. **2.** Intricate or involved, as a labyrinth. **3.** Pert. to speech that wanders aimlessly and unconnectedly from subject to subject, as seen in schizophrenia.

**labyrinthitis** (lăb″ĭ-rĭn-thī′tĭs) [″ + *itis,* inflammation] An inflammation (acute or chronic) of the labyrinth; otitis interna. Symptoms include vertigo, vomiting, and nystagmus. The condition may be caused by primary infection; trauma; complication of influenza, otitis media, or meningitis. SEE: *Ménière's disease.*

**labyrinthotomy** (lăb″ĭ-rĭn-thŏt′ō-mē) [″ + *tome,* incision] Surgical incision into the labyrinth.

**labyrinthus** (lăb″ĭ-rĭn′thŭs) [L., Gr. *labyrinthos,* maze] A labyrinth.

**lac** (lăk) [L.] **1.** Milk. **2.** Milky medicinal substance.

**lacerable** (lăs′ĕr-ă-b′l) [L. *lacerare,* to tear] Having the capability of being lacerated.

**lacerate** (lăs′ĕr-āt) [L. *lacerare,* to tear] To tear, as into irregular segments.

**lacerated** Torn; broken.

**laceration** A wound or irregular tear of the flesh.

***l. of cervix*** Bilateral, stellate, or unilateral tear of the cervix uteri caused by

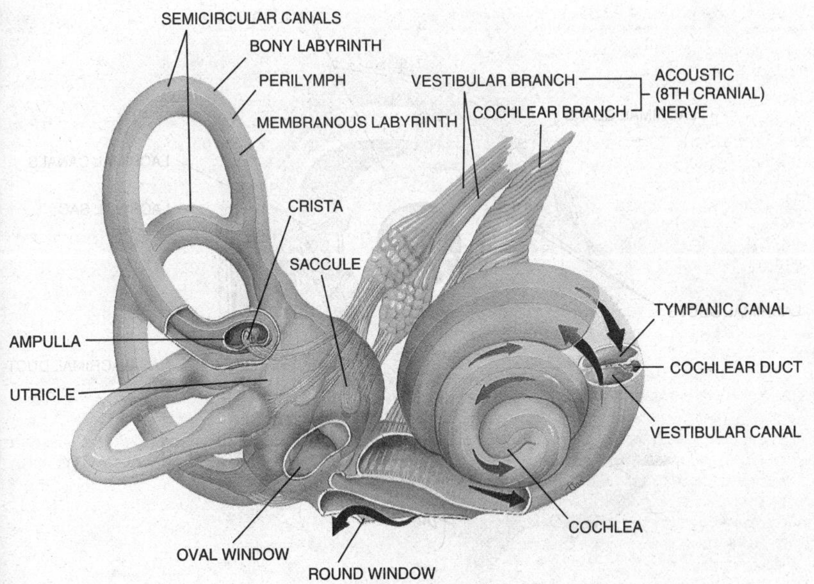


**LABYRINTHS OF INNER EAR**

ARROWS IN COCHLEA INDICATE PATH OF VIBRATIONS

childbirth.

***l. of perineum*** An injury of the perineum caused by childbirth. If it extends through the sphincter ani muscle, it is considered complete or fourth degree. SEE: *episiotomy*.

**lacertus** (lă-sĕr′tŭs) [L., lizard] **1.** The muscular part of the arm. **2.** A muscular or fibrous band.

***l. cordis*** A muscular tissue band on the inner cardiac surface. SYN: *trabeculae carneae cordis*.

***l. fibrosus*** An aponeurotic band from the biceps tendon to the bicipital or semilunar fascia of forearm.

**Lachman test** A sensitive test to evaluate the integrity of the anterior cruciate ligament of the knee. The examiner stands on the side being examined and grasps the tibia at the level of the tibial tubercle while stabilizing the femur with the other hand. The patient relaxes the leg while the examiner holds the knee flexed at 30° and pulls forward on the tibia. Excessive motion and no discernible end point determine a positive result.

**laciniate** (lă-sĭn′ē-āt) [L. *lacinia*, fringe] Being jagged or fringed.

**lacrima** (lăk′rĭ-mă) [L.] Tear fluid from eye.

**lacrimal** (lăk′rĭm-ăl) [L. *lacrima*, tear] Pert. to the tears.

***l. apparatus*** Structures concerned with the secretion and conduction of tears. It includes the lacrimal gland and its secretory ducts, lacrimal canaliculi, lacrimal sac, and nasolacrimal duct, which empties into the nasal cavity. SEE: illus.

Patency of the lacrimal duct may be tested by placing a dilute solution of sugar in the conjunctival sac; if the duct is patent, the individual will report the sensation of sweetness in the mouth; if not, the sugar will not be perceived.

**lacrimation** [L. *lacrima*, tear] The secretion and discharge of tears.

***test for l.*** Schirmer's test.

**lacrimator** A substance that increases the flow of tears.

**lacrimatory** (lăk′rĭ-mă-tō″rē) Causing the production of tears.

**lacrimonasal** (lăk″rĭ-mō-nā′zăl) [″ + *nasus*, nose] Concerning the nose and lacrimal apparatus.

**lacrimotome** (lăk′rĭ-mō-tōm) [″ + Gr. *tome*, incision] A cutting instrument used for incising the lacrimal sac or duct.

**lacrimotomy** (lăk″rĭm-ŏt′ō-mē) [″ + Gr. *tome*, incision] Incision of lacrimal duct.

**lactacid** Lactic acid.

**lactacidemia** (lăk-tăs″ĭ-dē′mē-ă) [″ + ″ + Gr. *haima*, blood] An accumulation of an excess of lactic acid in the blood. It occurs normally following strenuous and prolonged exercise. SYN: *lacticemia*.

**lactaciduria** (lăkt-ă-sĭd-ū′rē-ă) [″ + ″ + Gr. *ouron*, urine] Lactic acid excreted in the urine.

**lactagogue** (lăk′tă-gŏg) [″ + Gr. *agogos*, leading] Galactagogue.

**lactalbumin** [″ + *albumen*, coagulated white of egg] The albumin of milk and cheese; a soluble simple protein. Lactalbumin is

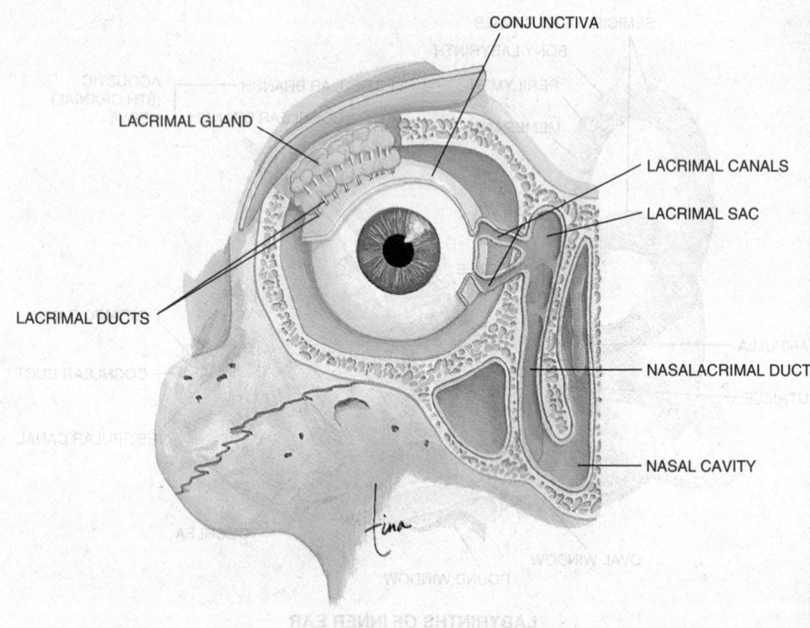


**LACRIMAL APPARATUS**

(ANTERIOR VIEW OF RIGHT EYE)

present in higher concentration in human milk than in cow's milk. When milk is heated, the lactalbumin coagulates and appears as a film on the surface of the milk.

**lactam** (lăk′tăm) An organic chemical that contains the —NH—CO group in a ring form. It is formed by the removal of a molecule of water from certain amino acids.

**β-lactamase-resistant antibiotics** Antibiotics that are resistant to the action of β-lactamase. This property makes them effective against microbial organisms that produce β-lactamase.

**β-lactamases** (bā″tă-lăk′tă-mās) A group of enzymes that act on certain antibodies to inactivate them.

**lactase** [″ + *-ase,* enzyme] An intestinal sugar-splitting enzyme converting lactose into dextrose and galactose; found in intestinal juice. SEE: *enzyme; maltase; sucrase; sugar.*

**lactate** (lăk′tāt) **1.** Any salt derived from lactic acid. **2.** To secrete milk.

**lactate dehydrogenase** Lactic dehydrogenase.

**lactation** (lăk-tā′shŭn) [L. *lactatio,* a suckinq] **1.** The period of suckling in mammals. **2.** The function of secreting milk.

DIET: During lactation the mother needs additional calcium to offset her loss of milk, as well as an adequate intake of calories, fluids, and protein. Fruits, vegetables, and whole-grain cereal should also be included in the diet.

***l. amenorrhea method*** ABBR: LAM. The method of causing decreased fertility in a woman by nursing a child for a lengthy period (several years or more). In general, the longer a woman breastfeeds, the longer ovulation is delayed. The questionable reliability of this method of contraception is compromised further by partial breastfeeding. In addition, most breastfeeding women ovulate before their first postpartum menses and within 4 to 18 months after delivery.

**lacteal** (lăk′tē-ăl) [L. *lacteus,* of milk] **1.** Pert. to milk. **2.** A lymphatic capillary in a villus of the small intestine that takes up chyle and passes it to the lymph circulation and, by way of the thoracic duct, to the blood vascular system. SEE: *lymph.*

**lactic** (lăk′tĭk) [L. *lac,* milk] Pert. to milk.

**lactic dehydrogenase** ABBR: LDH. An enzyme present in various tissues and serum that is important in catalyzing the oxidation of lactate. In humans, LDH is present in several molecular forms called isoenzymes. Some LDH isoenzymes are present in certain tissues to a greater extent than in others. When one of these particular tissues is damaged, an isoenzyme of LDH is released into the blood. In that case, determination of the pattern of LDH isoenzymes in serum may help to identify which tissue has been damaged. SYN: *lactate dehydrogenase.*

**lacticemia** (lăk-tĭ-sē′mē-ă) [″ + Gr. *haima,* blood] Lactacidemia.

**lactiferous** (lăk-tĭf′ĕr-ŭs) [″ + *ferre,* to bear] Secreting and conveying milk.

**lactification** (lăk″tĭ-fĭ-kā′shŭn) [″ + *facere,* to make] Lactic acid production.

**lactifuge** (lăk′tĭ-fūj) [″ + *fugare,* to expel] **1.** Stopping milk secretion. **2.** An agent stopping milk secretion.

**lactigenous** (lăk-tĭj′ĕn-ŭs) [″ + Gr. *gennan,* to produce] Producing milk.

**lactigerous** (lăk-tĭj′ĕr-ŭs) [″ + *gerere,* to carry] Secreting or conveying milk.

**lactinated** (lăk′tĭ-nāt″ĕd) Containing or prepared with lactose, or milk sugar.

**lactivorous** (lăk-tĭv′or-ŭs) [″ + *vorare,* to devour] Living on milk.

**Lactobacillus** (lăk-tō-bă-sĭl′ŭs) [″ + *bacillus,* little rod] A genus of bacteria belonging to the family Lactobacillaceae. These bacteria are gram-positive, nonmotile, rod-shaped organisms that do not produce spores and are acid resistant. They produce lactic acid from carbohydrates and are responsible for the souring of milk.

***L. acidophilus*** An organism that produces lactic acid by fermenting the sugars in milk. It is found in milk and in the feces of bottle-fed infants and adults whose diets include a high milk content. It is also present in carious teeth, saliva, and the vagina.

***L. bulgaricus*** A bacillus found in fermented milk. Milk fermented with this organism is known as Bulgarian milk.

***L. casei*** A bacillus found in milk and cheese.

***L. helveticus*** A bacillus found in Swiss cheese.

**lactocele** (lăk′tō-sēl) [″ + Gr. *kele,* tumor, swelling] Galactocele.

**lactoferrin** An enzyme released in phagocytosis by neutrophils and macrophages that combines with iron in the blood. As a result, the iron is unavailable to invading pathogens that require iron for their reproduction.

**lactogen** (lăk′tō-jĕn) [L. *lac,* milk, + Gr. *gennan,* to produce] Any substance that stimulates milk production. SEE: *prolactin.*

***human placental l.*** ABBR: HPL. A hormonal substance produced by the placenta and released to maternal blood. It acts in the last stage of gestation to prepare the breasts for milk production. It is no longer present in the maternal circulation 2 days after delivery.

**lactogenic** [″ + Gr. *gennan,* to produce] Inducing the secretion of milk.

**lactoglobulin** (lăk″tō-glŏb′ū-lĭn) [″ + *globulus,* globule] A protein found in milk. Casein and lactoglobulin are the most common proteins in cow's milk.

***immune l.'s*** Antibodies present in the colostrum.

**lactometer** (lăk-tŏm′ĕ-tĕr) [″ + Gr. *metron,* measure] A device for determining the specific gravity of milk.

**lacto-ovo-vegetarian** (lăk″tō-ō″vō-vĕj″ĕ-tā′rē-ăn) A person who is a vegetarian but also includes eggs and dairy products in the diet.

**lactophosphate** (lăk″tō-fŏs′fāt) [″ + *phosphas,* phosphate] A salt derived jointly from lactic and phosphoric acids.

**lactoprotein** (lăk″tō-prō′tē-ĭn) [″ + Gr. *protos,* first] Any protein present in milk.

**lactorrhea** (lăk-tō-rē′ă) [″ + Gr. *rhoia,* flow] The discharge of milk between nursings and after weaning of offspring. SYN: *galactorrhea.*

**lactose 1.** A disaccharide that on hydrolysis yields glucose and galactose. Bacteria can convert it into lactic and butyric acids, as in the souring of milk. The milk of mammals contains 4% to 7% lactose. Its presence in the urine may be indicative of obstruction to flow of milk after cessation of nursing. Commercial lactose is a fine white powder that will not dissolve in cold water. **2.** A sugar, $C_{11}H_{22}O_{11}$, obtained from evaporation of cow's milk. It is used in manufacturing tablets and as a diluent.

***l. intolerance*** An intolerance to milk and some dairy products. It is characterized by gastrointestinal symptoms associated with malabsorption of food. The intolerance may be congenital or have a later onset, beginning at several years of age.

Those who believe that they have a severe form of this condition may mistakenly attribute various abdominal symptoms to lactose intolerance. Although lactose intolerance may exist when lactose intake is limited to the equivalent of 240 ml of milk or less a day, symptoms are likely to be negligible and the use of lactose-digestive aids unnecessary.

ETIOLOGY: A deficiency of the enzyme lactase, which is essential to the absorption of lactose from the intestinal tract, causes this intolerance. The deficiency may be present in the newborn or acquired as an adult.

TREATMENT: The patient should limit milk consumption to one glass or less each day, determined by the patient's reaction. Yogurt may be consumed instead of milk. Enzyme tablets containing lactose to predigest milk are helpful.

**lactosuria** (lăk-tō-sū′rē-ă) [″ + Gr. *ouron,* urine] The presence of milk sugar (lactose) in the urine, a condition that occurs frequently during pregnancy and lactation.

**lactotherapy** (lăk-tō-thĕr′ă-pē) [″ + Gr. *therapeia,* treatment] SYN: *galactotherapy.*

**lactovegetarian 1.** Pert. to milk and vegetables. **2.** One who lives on a diet of milk, other dairy products, and vegetables.

**lactulose** A synthetic disaccharide, 4-*O*-β-D-galactopyranosyl-D-fructofuranose, that is not hydrolyzed or absorbed in humans. It is metabolized by bacteria in the colon with the production of organic acids and is used to treat the encephalopathy that develops in patients with advanced cirrhosis of the liver. The unabsorbed sugar produces diarrhea, and the acid pH helps to contain ammonia in the feces.

**lacuna** (lă-kū′nă) *pl.* **lacunae** [L., a pit] **1.** A small pit, space, or cavity. **2.** The space occupied by cells of calcified tissues (e.g., cementocytes, chondrocytes, and osteocytes). **lacunar** (-năr), *adj.*

***absorption l.*** Howship's l.

***Howship's l.*** A pit or groove in bone where resorption or dissolution of bone is occurring; usually contains osteoclasts. SYN: *absorption l.*

***intervillous l.*** A space in the placenta occupied by maternal blood and into which fetal placenta villi project.

***l. laterales*** Irregular diverticula on either side of the superior sagittal sinus of the brain into which the arachnoidal granulations project.

***l. magna*** The largest pitlike recess in the fossa navicularis of the distal end of the male urethra.

***l. pharyngis*** Pit at pharyngeal end of the eustachian tube.

***trophoblastic l.*** An irregular cavity in the syntrophoblast that develops into intervillous spaces or lacunae. SEE: *intervillous l.*

***l. of the urethra*** One of several recesses in the mucous membrane of the urethra, esp. along the floor and in the bulb. They compose the openings of the urethral glands.

***l. vasorum*** Space for passage of femoral vessels to the thigh.

**lacunae** (lă-kū′nē) [L.] Pl. of lacuna.

**lacunula, lacunule** (lă-kū′nū-lă, -nūl) [L., little pit] A small or minute lacuna.

**lacus** (lā′kŭs) [L., lake] A collection of fluid in a small hollow or cavity.

***l. lacrimalis*** The space at the medial canthus of the eye where tears collect.

**LAD** *left anterior descending* (branch of the left coronary artery).

**Laënnec's cirrhosis** (lā″ĕ-nĕks′) [René T. H. Laënnec, Fr. physician and the inventor of the stethoscope, 1781–1826] Cirrhosis of the liver associated with chronic excessive alcohol ingestion. SYN: *hobnail liver.* SEE: *liver, cirrhosis of.*

**Laënnec's pearls** Round gelatinous masses seen in asthmatic sputum.

**Laënnec's thrombus** Globular thrombus in the heart.

**Laetrile** Amygdalin; a glycoside derived from pits or other seed parts of plants, including apricots and almonds. Amygdalin contains sufficient cyanide to be fatal when taken in large doses. Laetrile, also known as vitamin $B_{17}$, has no known therapeutic or nutritional value. There is no evidence that it is effective in treating cancer. SYN: *amygdalin.*

---

Caution: Those who administer Laetrile should be prepared to treat acute cyanide poisoning. Signs of chronic cyanide poisoning (weakness of the arms and legs and disorders of the central nervous system) should also be kept in mind.

---

**Lafora, Gonzalo R** (lă-fō′ră) Spanish physician, 1887–1971.

***L.'s bodies*** Cytoplasmic inclusion bodies that are made of acid mucopolysaccharides and are present in neuronal tissue of the brain in familial myoclonus epilepsy.

***L.'s disease*** Familial progressive epilepsy.

**lag 1.** The period of time between the application of a stimulus and the resulting reaction. **2.** The early period following bacterial inoculation into a culture medium, characterized by slow growth. SYN: *lag phase; latent period.*

**lageniform** (lă-jĕn′ĭ-form) [L. *lagena,* flask, + *forma,* shape] Flask-shaped.

**lagophthalmos, lagophthalmus** (lăg″ŏf-thăl′mŏs, -mŭs) [Gr. *lagos,* hare, + *ophthalmos,* eye] An incomplete closure of the palpebral fissure when an attempt is made to shut the eyelids. This results in exposure and injury to the bulbar conjunctiva and cornea. This condition is caused by contraction of a scar of the eyelid, facial nerve injury, atony of the orbicularis palpebrarum, or exophthalmos. Incomplete closure of the lids during sleep is seen in hysteria, in exhausted adults, and often in healthy children.

***nocturnal l.*** Failure of the eyelids to remain closed during sleep, which may be an etiological factor in chronic keratitis.

**la grippe** (lă grĭp′) [Fr.] Influenza.

**laity** (lā′ĭ-tē) [Gr. *laos,* the people] Individuals who are not members of a particular profession such as law, dentistry, medicine, or the ministry.

**LAK cell** *lymphokine-activated killer cell.* SEE: under *cell.*

**lake** [L. *lacus*] A small cavity of fluid. SYN: *lacus.*

***lacrimal l.*** The small pouch formed by the junction of the conjunctiva at the medial canthus of the eye.

***venous l.*** A small subcutaneous bleb filled with blood. It may be present on the lips, mouth or ears.

**laked** A term used to describe the blood in hemolysis or disintegration of the red blood corpuscles, freeing the hemoglobin into the blood plasma.

**laking** The freeing of hemoglobin from red blood corpuscles.

**LAL** *limulus amebocyte lysate.*

**La Leche League** An organization whose purpose is to promote breastfeeding. The address is 9616 Minneapolis Avenue, Franklin Park, Illinois 60131.

**laliatry** (lăl-ī′ă-trē) [Gr. *lalia,* talk, + *iatria,* therapy] The study and treatment of speech disorders and defects.

**lallation** (lă-lā′shŭn) [L. *lallatio*] A babbling form of stammering; an infantile form of speech.

**lalopathology** (lăl″ō-pă-thŏl′ō-jē) [″ + *pathos,* disease, + *logos,* word, reason] The medical area concerned with speech pathology.

**lalopathy** (lă-lŏp′ă-thē) [″ + *pathos,* disease] Any disorder of the speech.

**lalophobia** (lăl″ō-fō′bē-ă) [″ + *phobos,* fear] A morbid reluctance to speak owing to fear of stammering or committing errors.

**laloplegia** (lăl-ō-plē′jē-ă) [″ + *plege,* a stroke] A paralysis of the speech muscles without affecting the action of the tongue.

**lalorrhea** (lăl″ō-rē′ă) [″ + *rhoia,* flow] An abnormal flow of speech.

**Lamarck's theory** (lă-mărks′) [Jean Baptiste P. A. Lamarck, Fr. naturalist, 1744–1829] The theory, popular in the 19th century but now rejected, that evolutionary changes are the result of environmental changes, and that acquired characteristics are inherited and passed on to descendants. SEE: *natural selection.*

**Lamaze technique, Lamaze method** (lă-măz′) [Fernand Lamaze, Fr. obstetrician, 1890–1957] A method of psychoprophylaxis for childbirth in which the mother is instructed in breathing techniques that permit her to facilitate delivery by relaxing at the proper time with respect to the involuntary contractions of abdominal and uterine musculature. Those who are able to use the method require little if any anesthesia during delivery. SEE: *labor.*

**lambda** (lăm′dă) [Gr.] **1.** A letter in the Greek alphabet (Λ, λ); also signified by the letter L or l. **2.** The point or angle of junction of the lambdoid and sagittal sutures.

**lambdacism** (lăm′dă-sĭzm) [Gr. *lambdakismos*] **1.** Stammering of the "l" sound. **2.** An inability to pronounce the "l" sound properly. **3.** Substitution of "l" for "r" in speaking.

**lambdoid, lambdoidal** (lăm′doyd, lăm-doyd′ăl) [Gr. *lambda,* + *eidos,* form, shape] Shaped like the Greek letter Λ.

**lambert** [Johann H. Lambert, Ger. physicist, 1728–1777] A unit of brightness equal to that seen when a perfectly diffusing surface radiates or reflects one lumen of light per square centimeter. SEE: *lumen* (2).

**Lambert-Eaton myasthenia syndrome** [Edward Howard Lambert, U.S. physiologist, b. 1915; Lee McKendree Eaton, U.S. physician, 1905–1958] A type of myasthenia associated with muscle weakness, hyporeflexia, and autonomic dysfunction. About half of the cases are associated with oat cell carcinoma of the lung.

**lame** [AS. *lama*] Disabled in one or more limbs, esp. in a leg or foot, impairing normal locomotion. It may also be applied to a weak or painful condition, such as a lame back.

**lamella** (lă-mĕl′ă) *pl.* **lamellae** [L., a little plate] **1.** A thin plate or scale. **2.** A medicated disk of gelatin inserted under the lower eyelid and against the eyeball; used as a local application to the eye.

***bone l.*** A thin layer of ground substance of osseous tissue.

***circumferential l.*** A layer of bone that underlies the periosteum.

***concentric l.*** The plate of bone surrounding a haversian canal. SYN: *haversian l.*

***enamel l.*** Microscopic cracks or calcification imperfections in the enamel surface of a tooth. They may be shallow or extend into the underlying dentin and occur as a developmental defect or a microfracture caused by temperature change or shearing forces.

***ground l.*** Interstitial l.

***haversian l.*** Concentric l.

***interstitial l.*** The bone lamella filling the irregular spaces within the haversian system. SYN: *ground l.*

***medullary l.*** An osseous lamella surrounding and forming the wall of the medullary cavity of tubular bones.

***periosteal l.*** The bone lamella next to and parallel with the periosteum, forming the external portion of bone.

***triangular l.*** The small fibrous lamina between the choroid plexuses of the third ventricle of the brain.

***vitreous l.*** Bruch's membrane.

**lamellar** (lă-mĕl′ăr) **1.** Arranged in thin plates or scales. **2.** Pert. to the lamella.

**lameness** Limping, abnormal gait, or hobbling resulting from partial loss of function in a leg. The symptom may be due to maldevelopment, injury, or disease.

**lamina** (lăm′ĭ-nă) *pl.* **laminae** [L.] **1.** A thin flat layer or membrane. **2.** The flattened part of either side of the arch of a vertebra.

***alar l.*** The alar plate of the spinal cord in the human embryo, which later becomes the sensory portion.

***anterior elastic l.*** Bowman's membrane.

***basal l.*** **1.** The basal plate of the spinal cord in the human embryo, which later becomes the motor portion. **2.** A mucopolysaccharide layer on the basal surface of epithelial cells which separates them functionally from the underlying connective tissue of the body.

***l. basalis choroideae*** Bruch's membrane.

***l. basilaris ductus cochlearis*** The membranous portion of the spiral lamina of the cochlea of the inner ear.

***Bowman's l.*** Bowman's membrane.

***l. cartilaginis cricoideae*** The posterior portion of the cricoid cartilage.

***l. choriocapillaris*** The middle layer of the choroid, containing close mesh of capillaries.

***l. cribrosa*** The cribriform plate of the ethmoid bone.

***l. cribrosa sclerae*** The portion of sclera forming a sievelike plate through which pass fibers of the optic nerve to the retina.

***dental l.*** A U-shaped downgrowth of the oral epithelium in both the maxillary and mandibular regions that forms into enamel organs which produce the teeth. SEE: *enamel organ.*

***l. dura*** A radiographical term describing the compact bone (alveolar bone proper) that surrounds the roots of teeth. In a state of health, it appears on a radiograph as a dense radiopaque line.

***epithelial l.*** The epithelial layer covering the choroid layer of the eye.

***l. fusca sclerae*** The layer of thin pigmented connective tissue on the inner surface of the sclera of the eye.

***internal medullary l.*** The layer of white substance that divides the gray substance of the thalamus into three parts: anterior, medial, and lateral.

***interpubic fibrocartilaginous l.*** Part of the articulation of the pubic bones, connecting the opposing surfaces of these bones.

***labial l.*** A thickened band of epithelium that grows from the ectodermal covering of the primitive jaw. The ectodermal plate splits and separates the lip from the gum. SYN: *vestibular l.*

***l. multiformis*** The polymorphic layer of the isocortex of the cerebral cortex.

***l. papyracea*** A thin, smooth plate of bone on the lateral surface of the ethmoid bone; it forms part of the orbital plate.

***perpendicular l.*** A thin sheet of bone forming the perpendicular plate of the ethmoid bone. It supports the upper portion of the nasal septum.

***l. propria mucosae*** The thin layer of areolar connective tissue, blood vessels, and nerves that lies immediately beneath the surface epithelium of mucous membranes.

***pterygoid l.*** One of the internal and external laminae that make up the pterygoid process of the sphenoid bone. They are areas of attachment for the muscles of mastication.

***rostral l.*** A continuation of the rostrum of the corpus callosum and the terminal lamina of the third ventricle of the brain.

***l. suprachoroidea*** The outermost layer of the choroid.

***terminal l.*** The thin sheet of tissue forming the anterior border of the third ventricle.

***l. of vertebral arch*** One of the laminae extending from the pedicles of the vertebral arches and fusing together to form the dorsal portion of the arch. The spinous process extends from the center of these laminae.

***vestibular l.*** Labial l.

***l. vitrea*** Bruch's membrane.

***l. zonalis*** The outer or plexiform layer of the isocortex of the brain.

**laminae** (lăm′ĭ-nē) Pl. of lamina.

**laminagram** (lăm′ĭ-nă-grăm) [L. *lamina,* thin plate, + Gr. *gramma,* something written] A roentgenogram taken of a section of the body, so that the area being investigated appears as if only a slice through the tissue is depicted. SEE: *tomogram.*

**laminagraph** (lăm′ĭ-nă-grăf) [″ + Gr. *graphein,* to write] An x-ray technique for producing a laminagram.

**laminagraphy** (lăm″ĭ-năg′ră-fē) [″ + Gr. *graphein,* to write] The study of body tissues by use of laminagrams. SEE: *tomography.*

**laminar** Made up of or pert. to laminae.

***l. air flow*** Filtered air moving along separate parallel flow planes to surgical theaters, nurseries, bacteriology work areas, or food preparation areas. This method of air flow helps to prevent bacterial contamination and collection of hazardous chemical fumes in areas where they would pollute the work environment.

**Laminaria digitata** (lăm-ĭ-năr′ē-ă dĭj-ĭ-tā′tă) A genus of kelp or seaweed that, when dried, has the ability to absorb water and expand with considerable force. It has been used to dilate the uterine cervical canal in induced abortion.

**laminarin** (lăm″ĭ-nā′rĭn) A polysaccharide obtained from *Laminaria* species of seaweed. It consists principally of glucose residues.

**laminated** (lăm′ĭn-āt″ĕd) [L. *lamina,* thin plate] Arranged in layers or laminae.

**lamination** (lăm″ĭn-ā′shŭn) Layer-like arrangement.

**laminectomy** (lăm″ĭ-nĕk′tō-mē) [″ + Gr. *ektome,* excision] The excision of a vertebral posterior arch, usually to remove a lesion or herniated disc. SEE: *Nursing Diagnoses Appendix.*

NURSING IMPLICATIONS: *Preoperative:* The patient's knowledge of the procedure is determined, misconceptions are corrected, additional information is provided as necessary, and a signed informed consent form is obtained. A baseline assessment of the patient's neurological function and of lower extremity circulation is documented. The nurse discusses postoperative care concerns, demonstrates maneuvers such as log-rolling, assures the patient of the availability of pain relief medications on request, and prepares the patient for surgery according to the surgeon's or institutional protocol.

*Postoperative:* Vital signs and neurovascular status (motor, sensory, and circulatory) are monitored, antiembolism stockings or pneumatic dressings are applied if prescribed. The dressing is inspected for bleeding or cerebrospinal fluid leakage, either problem is documented and reported immediately, and the incision is redressed as necessary and directed with the use of scrupulous aseptic technique. The patient is maintained in a supine position, with the head flat or no higher than 45 degrees according to the surgeon's preference, for the prescribed time period (usually 1 to 2 hr), then repositioned side to side every 2 hr by log-rolling the patient with a pillow between the legs to prevent twisting and hip adduction and to maintain spinal alignment. Deep breathing (with use of an inspirometer if prescribed) is encouraged, and assistance is provided with range-of motion, gluteal muscle setting, and quadriceps setting exercises. Adequate assistance should be available when the patient is permitted to dangle, stand, and ambulate in the early postoperative period. Prescribed anti-inflammatory, muscle-relaxant, and antibiotic agents are administered, and noninvasive measures in addition to prescribed analgesia are provided to prevent and relieve incisional discomfort. The nurse monitors fluid balance by administering prescribed I.V. fluids and by assessing urine output. The patient is encouraged to void within 8 to 12 hr postsurgery and is assessed for bladder distention, which may indicate urinary retention; however, catherization is instituted only after other nursing measures to promote voiding have been tried. The abdomen is auscultated for return of bowel sounds, and adequate oral nutrition is provided when G.I. function has returned.

*Rehabilitative and home care:* Incisional care techniques are taught to the patient and family, and the importance of checking for signs of infection (increased local pain and tenderness, redness, swelling, and changes in the amount or character of any drainage) and of reporting these to the surgeon is stressed. A gradual increase in the patient's activity level is encouraged, usually including a walking regimen and rest periods as prescribed by the surgeon and physical therapist. The nurse reviews any prescribed exercises (pelvic tilts, leg raising, toe pointing) and discusses and reinforces prescribed activity restrictions, usually including sitting for prolonged periods, lifting heavy or moderately heavy objects, bending over, and climbing long flights of stairs. Proper body mechanics are taught to lessen strain and pressure on the spine; these include maintaining proper body alignment and good posture and sleeping on a firm mattress. Involvement in an exercise program is encouraged after 6 wk, beginning with gradual strengthening of abdominal muscles. The patient should schedule and keep a follow-up appointment with the surgeon and communicate any concerns to the surgeon (if necessary) before that visit.

**laminitis** (lăm-ĭn-ī′tĭs) [″ + Gr. *itis,* inflammation] The inflammation of a lamina.

**laminotomy** (lăm″ĭ-nŏt′ō-mē) [″ + Gr. *tome,* incision] A division of one of the vertebral laminae.

**lamp** [Gr. *lampein,* to shine] A device for producing and applying light, heat, radiation, and various forms of radiant energy for the treatment of disease.

***infrared l.*** Heat lamp; a lamp that develops a high temperature, emitting infrared rays. The rays penetrate only a short distance (5 to 10 mm) into the skin. Its principal effect is to cause heating of the skin.

***slit l.*** A lamp constructed so that an intense light is emitted through a slit; used for examination of the eye.

***sun l.*** A lamp that produces ultraviolet light. SYN: *ultraviolet l.*

***ultraviolet l.*** Sun l.

**lamprophonia** (lăm″prō-fō′nē-ă) [Gr. *lampros,* clear, + *phone,* voice] A marked distinctness or clearness of voice.

**lamprophonic** (lăm″prō-fŏn′ĭk) Possessing a clear voice.

**lanatoside C** (lăn-ăt′ō-sīd) A glycoside of *Digitalis lanata;* an agent used for digitalization.

**lance** (lăns) [L. *lancea*] **1.** A two-edged surgical knife. **2.** To incise with a lancet.

**Lancefield classification** (lăns′fēld) [Rebecca Craighill Lancefield, U.S. bacteriologist, 1895–1981] A classification of hemolytic streptococci into various groups according to antigenic structure.

**lancet** (lăn′sĕt) [L. *lancea,* lance] A pointed surgical knife with two edges.

**lancinating** (lăn′sĭ-nāt″ĭng) [L. *lancinare,* to tear] Sharp or cutting, as pain.

**L and A** Abbreviation for the reaction of the pupils of the eye to *light* and *accommodation.*

**Landau reflex** An infantile reflex in which the body flexes when the head is passively flexed forward in a prone position. It appears normally at 3 months and is absent in children with cerebral palsy and gross motor retardation.

**landmark** A recognizable skeletal or soft tissue structure used as a reference point in measurements or in describing the location of other anatomical structures. SEE: *cephalometry; craniometry.*

***bony l.*** A structure or spot on a bone that serves as a reference for measurement.

***cephalometric l.*** A bony point that serves in living persons or radiographs for measurements of the head or face or orientation of the head in certain positions.

***craniometric l.*** A bony point or area on the skull used for measurements or orientation of the skull.

***orbital l.*** A cephalometric point located at the lowest point of the orbital margin.

***radiographic l.*** A cephalometric, craniometric, or soft tissue landmark used for orientation or measurements.

***soft tissue l.*** An area or point on a soft tissue that serves as a point of reference for measurements of the body or its parts.

**Landouzy-Déjérine dystrophy** (lăn-dū-zē′ dĕ″zhĕ-rēn′) [Louis T. J. Landouzy, Fr. physician, 1845–1917; Joseph Jules Déjérine, Fr. neurologist, 1849–1917] A slowly progressive dystrophy involving principally the musculature of the face and shoulders. SYN: *dystrophy, facioscapulohumeral muscular*.

TREATMENT: Therapy is supportive; no specific therapy is known. The patient should be encouraged to maintain as full and normal a life as possible and to avoid prolonged bed rest.

**Landry-Guillain-Barré syndrome** Guillain-Barré syndrome.

**Landsteiner's classification** (lănd'stī-nĕrz) [Karl L. Landsteiner, Austrian-born U.S. biologist, 1868–1943; Nobel prize winner in medicine in 1930] A classification of blood types designating O, A, B, and AB based on the presence of antigens on the erythrocytes.

**Lane's kinks** [Sir William Arbuthnot Lane, Brit. surgeon, 1856–1943] Bending or twisting of the last few centimeters of the ileum with external adhesions between the folded loops of intestines. This may cause intestinal obstruction.

**Langerhans' islands** SEE: *islets of Langerhans*.

**Langer's lines** (lăng'ĕrz) [Carl (Ritter von Edenberg) Langer, Austrian anatomist, 1819–1887] The structural orientation of the fibrous tissue of the skin. They form the natural cleavage lines that, though present in all body areas, are visible only in certain sites such as the creases of the palm. These lines are of particular importance in surgery. Incisions made parallel to them make a much smaller scar upon healing than those made at right angles to the lines. SEE: illus.

**Langer's muscle** Muscular fibers from insertion of the pectoralis major muscle, over the bicipital groove to the insertion of the latissimus dorsi.

**Lange's test** (lăng'ĕz) [Carl Lange, Ger. physician, 1883–1953] A test for diagnosis of cerebrospinal syphilis by the degree of gold precipitation in varying concentrations of colloidal gold solution and spinal fluid.

**Langhans' layer** (lăng'hăns) [Theodor Langhans, Ger. pathologist, 1839–1915] A cellular layer present in the chorionic villi of the placenta. SYN: *cytotrophoblast*.

**language** A group of words written or spoken used in accordance with a system common to people of the same community or country and of the same cultural background. The use of language, spoken or written, permits a person to attempt to influence the behavior of another and to express the result of thought processes.

**languor** (lăng'gĕr) [L. *languere*, to languish] A feeling of weariness or exhaustion as from illness; lack of vigor or animation; lassitude.

**laniary** (lăn'ē-ā"rē) [L. *laniare*, to tear to pieces] Adapted or designed for tearing, as the canine teeth.

**lanolin** (lăn'ō-lĭn) [L. *lana*, wool] The purified, fatlike substance obtained from the wool of sheep; used as an ointment base.

***anhydrous l.*** Wool fat containing not more than 0.25% water; used as an ointment base that has the ability to absorb water.

**Lanoxin** Trade name for digoxin.

**lanthanum** (lăn'thă-nŭm) SYMB: La. A metallic element; atomic weight 138.906; atomic number 57. It is one of a group of elements called lanthanides.

**lanuginous** (lă-nū'jĭn-ŭs) Covered with lanugo.

**lanugo** (lă-nū'gō) [L. *lana*, wool] **1.** Downy hair covering the body. **2.** Fine downy hairs that cover the body of the fetus, esp. when premature.

**LAO** *left anterior oblique* position.

**laparectomy** (lăp"ă-rĕk'tō-mē) [Gr. *lapara*, flank, + *ektome*, excision] Excision of strips or gores in the abdominal wall to relieve extreme weakness of the abdominal muscles.

**laparo-** [Gr. *lapara*, flank] Combining form pert. to the flank and to operations through the abdominal wall.

**laparocele** (lăp'ă-rō-sēl) [" + *kele*, tumor, swelling] An abdominal hernia.

**laparocholecystotomy** (lăp"ăr-ō-kōl"ē-sĭs-tŏt'ō-mē) [" + *chole*, bile, + *kystis*, bladder, + *tome*, incision] An incision into the gallbladder through the abdominal wall.

**laparocolectomy** (lăp"ă-rō-kō-lĕk'tō-mē) [" + *kolon*, colon, + *ektome*, excision] Colectomy.

**laparocolostomy, laparocolotomy** (lăp"ăr-ō-kō-lŏs'tō-mē, lăp"ăr-ō-kō-lŏt'ō-mē) [" + " + *stoma*, mouth] The formation of a permanent opening into the colon through the abdominal wall.

**laparocystectomy** (lă"pă-rō-sĭs-tĕk'tō-mē) [" + *kystis*, bladder, + *ektome*, excision] The removal of an extrauterine fetus or a cyst through an abdominal incision.

**laparocystidotomy** (lăp"ăr-ō-sĭst-ĭ-dŏt'ō-mē) [" + " + *tome*, incision] An incision of the bladder through the abdominal wall.

**laparocystotomy** (lăp"ăr-ō-sĭs-tŏt'ō-mē) An incision of the abdomen to remove the contents of a cyst or an extrauterine fetus.

**laparoenterostomy** (lăp"ă-rō-ĕn"tĕr-ŏs'tō-mē) [" + *enteron*, intestine, + *stoma*, mouth] The formation of an artificial opening into the intestine through the abdominal wall.

**laparoenterotomy** (lăp"ăr-ō-ĕn"tĕr-ŏt'ō-mē) [" + " + *tome*, incision] An opening into the intestinal cavity by incision through the loins.

**laparogastroscopy** (lăp"ă-rō-găs-trŏs'kō-pē) [" + *gaster*, belly, + *skopein*, to examine] Inspection of the inside of the stomach after gastrotomy.

**laparogastrostomy** (lăp"ăr-ō-găs-trŏs'tō-mē) [" + " + *stoma*, mouth] The surgical formation of a permanent gastric fistula through the abdominal wall. SYN: *celiogastrostomy*.

**laparogastrotomy** (lăp"ă-rō-găs-trŏt'ō-mē) [" + " + *tome*, incision] An incision into the stomach through the abdominal

LANGER'S LINES

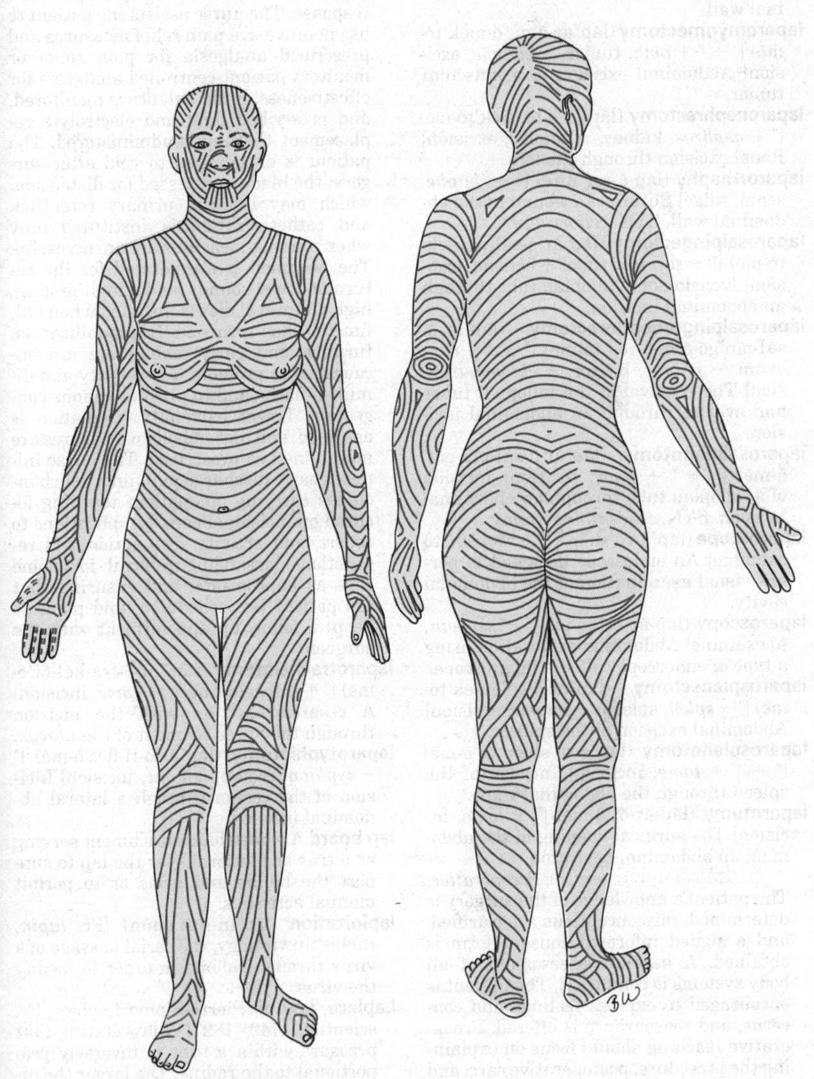

wall. SYN: *celiogastrotomy.*

**laparohepatotomy** (lăp″ăr-ō-hĕp″ă-tŏt′ō-mē) [″ + *hepar,* liver, + *tome,* incision] An incision of the liver through the abdominal wall.

**laparohystero-oophorectomy** (lăp″ăr-ō-hĭs″tĕr-ō-ō″ō-for-ĕk′tō-mē) [″ + ″ + *oon,* ovum, + *phoros,* bearer, + *ektome,* excision] The removal of the uterus and ovaries through an abdominal incision.

**laparohysteropexy** (lăp″ăr-ō-hĭs′tĕr-ō-pĕks-ē) [″ + ″ + *pexis,* fixation] Abdominal fixation of the uterus.

**laparohysterosalpingo-oophorectomy** (lăp″ăr-ō-hĭs″tĕr-ō-săl-pĭn″gō-ō″ō-fō-rĕk′tō-mē) [″ + *hystera,* womb, + *salpinx,* tube, + *oon,* ovum, + *phoros,* bearer, + *ektome,* excision] The removal of the uterus, fallopian tubes, and ovaries through an abdominal incision.

**laparohysterotomy** (lăp″ăr-ō-hĭs″tĕr-ŏt′ō-mē) [″ + ″ + *tome,* incision] Surgery of the uterus through an abdominal incision. SEE: *cesarean section.*

**laparoileotomy** (lăp″ăr-ō-ĭl-ē-ŏt′ō-mē) [″ + L. *ileum,* ileum, + Gr. *tome,* incision] An abdominal incision into the ileum.

**laparomyitis** (lăp″ăr-ō-mī-ī′tĭs) [″ + *mys,*

muscle, + *itis,* inflammation] Inflammation of the muscular portion of the abdominal wall.

**laparomyomectomy** (lăp″ăr-ō-mī″ō-mĕk′tō-mē) [″ + ″ + *oma,* tumor, + *ektome,* excision] Abdominal excision of a muscular tumor.

**laparonephrectomy** (lăp″ăr-ō-nĕ-frĕk′tō-mē) [″ + *nephros,* kidney, + *ektome,* excision] Renal excision through the loin.

**laparorrhaphy** (lăp-ă-ror′ă-fē) [″ + *rhaphe,* seam, ridge] Suture of a wound in the abdominal wall. SYN: *celiorrhaphy.*

**laparosalpingectomy** (lăp″ăr-ō-săl-pĭn-jek′tō-mē) [″ + *salpinx,* tube, + *ektome,* excision] Excision of a fallopian tube through an abdominal incision.

**laparosalpingo-oophorectomy** (lăp″ăr-ō-săl-pĭn″gō-ō″ŏf-ō-rĕk′tō-mē) [″ + ″ + *oon,* ovum, + *phoros,* bearer, + *ektome,* excision] The removal of the fallopian tubes and ovaries through an abdominal incision.

**laparosalpingotomy** (lăp″ăr-ō-săl-pĭn-gŏt′ō-mē) [″ + ″ + *tome,* incision] Incision of a fallopian tube through an abdominal incision. SYN: *celiosalpingectomy.*

**laparoscope** (lăp′ă-rō-skōp″) [″ + *skopein,* to examine] An endoscope designed to permit visual examination of the abdominal cavity.

**laparoscopy** (lăp-ăr-ŏs′kō-pē) [″ + *skopein,* to examine] Abdominal exploration using a type of endoscope called a laparoscope.

**laparosplenectomy** (lăp″ăr-ō-splēn-ĕk′tō-mē) [″ + *splen,* spleen, + *ektome,* excision] Abdominal excision of the spleen.

**laparosplenotomy** (lăp″ăr-ō-splēn-ŏt′ō-mē) [″ + ″ + *tome,* incision] Incision of the spleen through the abdominal wall.

**laparotomy** (lăp-ăr-ŏt′ō-mē) [″ + *tome,* incision] The surgical opening of the abdomen; an abdominal operation.

NURSING IMPLICATIONS: *Preoperative:* The patient's knowledge of the surgery is determined, misconceptions are clarified, and a signed informed consent form is obtained. A baseline assessment of all body systems is conducted. The patient is encouraged to express feelings and concerns, and reassurance is offered. Preoperative teaching should focus on explaining the procedure, postoperative care, and expected sensations. Physical preparation of the patient is carried out according to institutional or surgeon's protocol regarding diet, shaving of abdomen and pubic area, enemas, douches, and collecting of urine specimens, and thigh-high antiembolism or pneumatic dressings are applied as prescribed.

*Postoperative:* Vital signs and dressing status are monitored; the latter includes checking any drains in place and for the presence of vaginal bleeding if applicable. Ventilatory status is assessed by auscultating for adventitious or decreased breath sounds, and respiratory toilet (deep breathing, coughing, incentive spirometry, oral hygiene, and repositioning) is provided as determined by the patient's response. The nurse assists the patient to use noninvasive pain relief measures and prescribed analgesia for pain relief or monitors patient-controlled analgesia for effectiveness. Fluid balance is monitored, and prescribed fluid and electrolyte replacement therapy is administered. The patient is encouraged to void after surgery, the bladder assessed for distention, which may indicate urinary retention, and catheterization is instituted only when nursing measures are unsuccessful. The abdomen is auscultated for the return of bowel sounds, and a high-protein, high vitamin C diet is initiated when G.I. function has returned. Leg mobilization, turning, and early ambulation are encouraged to promote G.I. activity and diminish flatus and to prevent venous congestion. Lower extremity circulation is assessed, and antiembolism measures are maintained as prescribed. The nurse initiates early discharge planning, which includes carrying out patient teaching focused on incisional care, complications to report, and activity resumption and restrictions; arranging referral for home care as appropriate; and ensuring that the patient has scheduled (and plans to keep) a follow-up appointment with the surgeon.

**laparotrachelotomy** (lăp″ăr-ō-trā-kĕl-ŏt′ō-mē) [″ + *trachelos,* neck, + *tome,* incision] A cesarean section with the incision through the lower segment of the uterus.

**laparotyphlotomy** (lăp″ăr-ō-tĭ-flŏt′ō-mē) [″ + *typhlon,* cecum, + *tome,* incision] Incision of the cecum through a lateral abdominal incision.

**lap board** A wheelchair attachment serving as a tray or platform over the lap to support the hands and arms or to permit manual activities.

**lapinization** (lăp″ĭn-ī-zā′shŭn) [Fr. *lapin,* rabbit] In virology, the serial passage of a virus through rabbits in order to modify the virus.

**Laplace, law of** [Pierre-Simon Laplace, Fr. scientist, 1749–1827] A law stating that pressure within a tube is inversely proportional to the radius. The larger the diameter of a tubular structure, the less chance that it will rupture when subjected to an increase in pressure. So, for example, when pressure in the colon is increased due to obstruction, the right colon, which has a larger diameter than the left colon, would be at less risk of perforation than the left.

**lard** [L. *lardum,* fat] Purified fat from the hog. The sole nutrient is fat; a 100-g portion contains 902 kcal.

***benzoinated l.*** Lard containing 1% benzoin, used as a vehicle for certain types of topically applied medicines.

**lardaceous** (lăr-dā′shŭs) [L. *lardum,* fat] Resembling lard; waxy, fatty.

**large for gestational age** ABBR: LGA. Term used of a newborn whose birth weight is above the 90th percentile on the intrauterine growth curve. Such babies should be monitored for signs of hypoglycemia during the first 24 hr after birth.

**large loop excision of the transformation zone** ABBR: LLETZ. Obtaining a biopsy of the uterine cervix in patients in whom the colposcopic examination or Pap smear indicates the area is abnormal. The tissue is obtained by use of an electrically heated wire loop. Obtaining tissue in this manner has been used to treat noninvasive carcinoma of the cervix. SYN: *loop electrode excision procedure.*

**larva** [L., mask] **1.** General term applied to the developing form of an insect after it has emerged from the egg and before it transforms into a pupa, from which it emerges as an adult. **2.** The immature forms of other invertebrates such as worms. **larval** (lăr′văl), *adj.*

***l. currens*** A type of larva migrans. The organism, *Strongyloides stercoralis,* travels subcutaneously at the rate of about 10 cm an hour rather than at the slow rate of larva migrans.

***cutaneous l. migrans*** A skin lesion characterized by a tortuous elevated red line that progresses at one end while fading out at the other. It is caused by the subcutaneous migration of the larvae of certain nematodes, esp. *Ancylostoma braziliense* and *A. caninum,* that occur as accidental invaders of humans.

***visceral l. migrans*** Toxocariasis.

**larvate** [L. *larva,* mask] Hidden, concealed, as an atypical or hidden symptom.

**larvicide** [″ + *caedere,* to kill] An agent that destroys insect larvae.

**larviphagic** (lăr″vĭ-fā′jĭk) [″ + Gr. *phagein,* to eat] Consuming larva, as is done by certain fish.

**laryngalgia** (lăr-ĭn-găl′jē-ă) [Gr. *larynx,* larynx, + *algos,* pain] Neuralgia of the larynx.

**laryngeal** (lăr-ĭn′jē-ăl) [Gr. *larynx,* larynx] Pert. to the larynx.

**laryngectomee** (lăr″ĭn-jĕk′tō-mē) [″ + *ektome,* excision] An individual whose larynx has been removed.

**laryngectomy** (lăr″ĭn-jĕk′tō-mē) [″ + *ektome,* excision] Excision of the larynx. SEE: *Nursing Diagnoses Appendix.*

NURSING IMPLICATIONS: *Preoperative:* The nurse prepares the patient for vocal and airway changes and for other functional losses after surgery and supplements explanations with diagrams and samples of required equipment. Postsurgical communication methods most appropriate for and agreeable to the particular patient (e.g., simple sign language, flash cards, magic slate, alphabet board) are explained. The postoperative setting and care are described to the patient, including assessment measures, therapies, equipment, procedures, and expected sensations. Nutritional modalities (parenteral, enteral via tube feeding, then oral feeding) are also explained. Both patient and family are encouraged to verbalize their feelings and concerns, and realistic reassurance and information are provided. The nurse supports the patient through anticipatory grieving and refers the patient as necessary for further psychological or religious support. Once the signed informed consent form is obtained, the nurse prepares the patient for surgery according to the surgeon's or institutional protocol.

*Postoperative:* Vital signs are monitored, especially ventilatory rate and effort, as well as level of consciousness, arterial blood gas values, peripheral oxygen saturation levels, and the status of dressings and drains. The airway is assessed for patency, the laryngostomy tube gently (but not deeply) suctioned, as well as the oral cavity and nose as needed, crust formation is prevented by increasing humidity and fluid intake, and frequent oral hygiene and assistance in managing saliva are provided. The nurse positions the patient as prescribed (usually with the head elevated to 30 to 45 degrees and the patient turned on the side) and supports the patient's neck posteriorly during movement. Fluid balance is monitored, prescribed replacement therapy provided, and urination encouraged. Protein-rich, high vitamin C nutrition is provided via the prescribed route to aid healing. The nurse anticipates and attends to the patient's needs by providing noninvasive measures and prescribed analgesics to relieve pain; by allowing time for communication; and by reassuring the patient that verbal communication ability will be reestablished through surgically implanted prostheses, speech therapy for esophageal speech, or external mechanical and electronic artificial larynges. The nurse supports the patient and family through their grief over real losses (including usual voice, laughing and crying sounds, whistling, sucking ability, sense of smell, nose blowing, and activities such as swimming) and assists the patient to deal with problems due to body image changes and altered self-esteem. The patient is assessed for early complications such as respiratory distress due to edema, infection, dehydration, and hemorrhage (remembering to check the posterior aspect of the neck as well as dressings, drains, and vital signs); and for later ones such as fistula formation, tracheal stenosis, and carotid artery rupture. The patient is prepared for possible follow-up therapies, such as radiation and chemotherapy. The nurse prepares the patient for early discharge by teaching self-care activities and complications to be reported, by referring the patient for home health care or other professional services as appropriate (such as psychological counseling if he becomes severely depressed), and by ensuring that the patient has scheduled (and plans to keep) a follow-up appointment with the surgeon or oncologist. Participation of both patient and family in support groups and informational services (e.g., American Speech-Learning-Hearing Association, American Cancer Society, International Association of Laryngectomees, Lost Chord Club) is encouraged, as is a rapid return to employment, with the assistance of social service agencies if employment changes are required.

**laryngismal** (lăr″ĭn-jĭs′măl) [″ + *-ismos,* condition] Concerning or resembling affliction with laryngeal spasm.

**laryngismus** (lăr″ĭn-jĭs′mŭs) [″ + *-ismos,* condition] Spasm of the larynx.

**laryngitic** (lăr-ĭn-jĭt′ĭk) [Gr. *larynx,* larynx] **1.** Resulting from laryngitis. **2.** Relating to laryngitis.

**laryngitis** (lăr-ĭn-jī′tĭs) [″ + *itis,* inflammation] Inflammation of the larynx. SEE: *croup; Nursing Diagnoses Appendix.*

***acute catarrhal l.*** Acute congestive laryngitis; catarrhal inflammation of laryngeal mucosa and the vocal cords. It is characterized by hoarseness and aphonia and occasionally pain on phonation and deglutition. It may be caused by improper use or overuse of the voice, exposure to cold and wet, extension from infections in nose and throat, inhalation of irritating vapors and dust, or systemic diseases such as whooping cough or measles.

TREATMENT: Treatment includes complete rest of the voice, promotion of diaphoresis, liquid or soft diet, steam inhalations, and codeine or nonnarcotic cough suppressants for pain and cough. If the laryngitis is viral, no specific therapy exists; if bacterial, appropriate antibiotics should be given. If acute or chronic bronchitis is present, treatment of that condition will help control laryngitis.

***atrophic l.*** Laryngitis leading to diminished secretion and atrophy of the mucous membrane. Symptoms are a tickling sensation in the throat, hoarseness, cough, and dyspnea when the crusts are thick and accumulate on the vocal cords, narrowing the breathing aperture. Inhalants and medicated sprays should be used to loosen the crusts, along with strict attention to associated nose and throat pathology.

***chronic l.*** A type of laryngitis caused by a recurrent irritation, or following the acute form. It is often secondary to sinus or nasal pathology, improper use of the voice, excessive smoking or drinking, or neoplasms. The patient experiences a tickling in the throat, huskiness of the voice, and dysphonia. The treatment involves correcting the preexisting nose and throat pathology, discontining alcohol and tobacco use, and avoiding excessive use of the voice.

***croupous l.*** Laryngitis occurring mainly in infants and young children and characterized by a barky cough, hoarseness, and stridor.

***diphtheritic l.*** Invasion of the larynx by diphtheria bacilli, usually with formation of a membrane.

***membranous l.*** Laryngitis characterized by inflammation of the larynx, with the formation of a false, nondiphtheritic membrane.

***syphilitic l.*** A chronic form of laryngitis caused by syphilis. It is characterized by hoarseness, cough, simple catarrh, formation of broad condylomata, follicular hyperplasia, syphiloma, and syphilitic perichondritis. Secondary syphilis is a diffuse infection, with mucous patches spread over large areas of the larynx. In tertiary syphilis, the gummatous lesion can occur in any part of larynx. There is marked redness over the infiltrated area as well as in the surrounding mucous membrane. When breakdown occurs, the resultant ulceration is deep with sharp edges. Pain is usually absent and fixation of the cord is late. Cicatrization and deformity follow healing of gumma. The appropriate antibiotic therapy for syphilis should be given.

***tuberculous l.*** Laryngitis secondary to pulmonary tuberculosis. Patients have hoarseness, aphonia, pain in swallowing, and cough. Lesions may be located in the interarytenoid area, vocal cords, epiglottis, or false cords. Lesions are relatively pale; ulceration occurs early.

**laryngo-** [Gr. *larynx,* larynx] Combining form pert. to the larynx.

**laryngocele** (lăr-ĭn′gō-sēl) [″ + *kele,* tumor, swelling] A congenital air sac connected to the larynx. Its presence is normal in some animals but abnormal in humans.

**laryngocentesis** (lăr-ĭn″gō-sĕn-tē′sĭs) [″ + *kentesis,* puncture] Incision or puncture of the larynx.

**laryngoedema** A swelling of the larynx, caused by an allergic reaction. It requires immediate endotracheal intubation or tracheostomy.

**laryngofissure** (lăr-ĭng″gō-fĭsh′ūr) [″ + L. *fissura,* a cleft] The operation of opening the larynx by a median line incision through the thyroid cartilage.

**laryngogram** (lă-rĭng′gō-grăm) [″ + *gramma,* something written] A radiograph of the larynx.

**laryngograph** (lăr-ĭng′ō-grăf) [″ + *graphein,* to write] A device for making a record of laryngeal movements.

**laryngography** (lăr″ĭn-gŏg′ră-fē) **1.** A description of the larynx. **2.** Radiography of the larynx using a radiopaque contrast medium.

**laryngologist** (lăr″ĭn-gŏl′ō-jĭst) [″ + *logos,* word, reason] A specialist in laryngology.

**laryngology** The specialty of medicine concerned with the pharynx, throat, larynx, nasopharynx, and tracheobronchial tree.

**laryngomalacia** (lăr-ĭng″gō-mă-lā′shē-ă) [″ + *malakia,* softness] A softening of the tissues of the larynx.

**laryngometry** (lăr″ĭn-gŏm′ĕ-trē) [″ + *metron,* measure] The systematic measurement of the larynx.

**laryngoparalysis** (lăr-ĭn″gō-păr-ăl′ĭ-sĭs) [″ + *paralyein,* to disable at one side] Paralysis of the muscles of the larynx.

**laryngopathy** (lăr″ĭn-gŏp′ă-thē) [″ + *pathos,* disease] Any disease of the larynx.

**laryngopharyngeal** (lăr-ĭn″gō-făr-ĭn′jē-ăl) [″ + *pharynx,* throat] Relating jointly to the larynx and pharynx.

**laryngopharyngectomy** (lăr-ĭn″gō-făr-ĭn-jĕk′tō-mē) [″ + ″ + *ektome,* excision] Removal of the larynx and pharynx.

**laryngopharyngeus** (lă-rĭng″gō-fă-rĭn′jē-ŭs) The muscle that constricts the inferior pharynx.

**laryngopharyngitis** (lăr-ĭn″gō-făr-ĭn-jī′tĭs) [″ + ″ + *itis,* inflammation] Inflammation of the larynx and pharynx.

**laryngopharyngography** (lă-rĭng″gō-fă-rĭn-jŏg′ră-fē) [″ + ″ + *graphein,* to write] Radiographical examination of the larynx and pharynx when filled with air.

**laryngopharynx** (lăr-ĭn″gō-făr′ĭnks) [Gr. *larynx,* larynx, + *pharynx,* throat] Hypopharynx.

**laryngophony** (lăr″ĭn-gŏf′ō-nē) [″ + *phone,* voice] Voice sounds heard in auscultating the pharynx.

**laryngophthisis** (lăr″ĭng-gŏf′thĭ-sĭs) [″ + *phthisis,* a wasting] Tuberculosis of the larynx.

**laryngoplasty** (lăr-ĭn′gō-plăs″tē) [″ + *plassein,* to form] Plastic reparative surgery of the larynx.

**laryngoplegia** (lă-rĭng″gō-plē′jē-ă) [″ + *plege,* stroke] Paralysis of the laryngeal muscles.

**laryngorhinology** (lăr-ĭn″gō-rĭn-ŏl′ō-jē) [″ + *rhis,* nose, + *logos,* word, reason] The branch of medical science concerned with diseases of the larynx and nose.

**laryngorrhagia** (lăr″ĭn-gō-rā′jē-ă) [″ + *rhegnynai,* to flow forth] Laryngeal hemorrhage.

**laryngorrhea** (lăr″ĭn-gō-rē′ă) [″ + *rhoia,* flow] Excessive discharge of laryngeal mucus.

**laryngoscleroma** (lăr-ĭn″gō-sklĕ-rō′mă) [″ + *skleros,* hard, + *oma,* tumor] Scleroma affecting the larynx.

**laryngoscope** (lăr-ĭn′gō-skōp) [″ + *skopein,* to examine] An instrument used for examining the larynx.

**laryngoscopic** (lăr″ĭn-gō-skŏp′ik) [″ + *skopein,* to examine] Pert. to observation of the interior of the larynx with the aid of a small long-handled mirror. SEE: *laryngoscopy.*

**laryngoscopist** (lăr″ĭng-gŏs′kō-pĭst) [″ + *skopein,* to examine] An individual trained in laryngoscopy.

**laryngoscopy** (lăr″ĭn-gŏs′kō-pē) Visual examination of the interior of the larynx.

NURSING IMPLICATIONS: The patient's knowledge of the procedure is determined, misconceptions are corrected, and additional information about the procedure and expected sensations are provided as necessary. Once the signed informed consent form has been obtained, the nurse prepares the patient for the procedure according to the institutional or surgeon's protocol. The nurse assists the physician as necessary during the procedure and provides reassurance to the patient. After the procedure, the patient is placed in the semi-Fowler position, and vital signs are monitored until stable. Oral intake is withheld until the patient's swallowing reflex has returned, usually within 2 to 8 hr. An emesis basin is provided for spitting saliva, and sputum is inspected for blood and excessive bleeding reported. Application of an ice collar helps to minimize edema; subcutaneous crepitus around the face or neck should be reported immediately, because it may indicate tracheal perforation. The patient should not cough, clear the throat, or smoke for at least 24 hr to prevent irritation.

***direct l.*** Laryngoscopy using a laryngeal speculum or laryngoscope.

***indirect l.*** Laryngoscopy using a mirror.

**laryngospasm** (lăr-ĭn′gō-spăzm) [″ + *spasmos,* a convulsion] Spasm of the laryngeal muscles.

**laryngostenosis** (lăr-ĭng″gō-stĕ-nō′sĭs) [″ + *stenosis,* a narrowing] Stricture of the larynx.

***compression l.*** Stricture of the larynx owing to outside causes such as abscess, tumor, or goiter.

***occlusion l.*** Stricture of the larynx owing to congenital bands or membranes, foreign bodies, tumors, cicatricial contraction following ulceration as in diphtheria and tertiary syphilis, penetrating wounds, or corrosive fluid. Patients experience dyspnea, esp. on inspiration and exertion, with loud breathing that becomes a stridulous choking respiration; weak rapid pulse; and anxious, cyanotic face. Treatment depends on the cause. Tracheotomy is often necessary.

**laryngostomy** (lăr-ĭn-gŏs′tō-mē) [″ + *stoma,* mouth] Establishing a permanent opening through the neck into the larynx.

**laryngostroboscope** (lăr″ĭn-gō-strō′bō-skōp) [″ + *strobos,* whirl, + *skopein,* to view] An instrument for inspecting vibration of the vocal cords.

**laryngotomy** (lăr-ĭn-gŏt′ō-mē) [″ + *tome,* incision] Incision of the larynx.

***inferior l.*** Surgical incision of the larynx through the cricoid cartilage.

***median l.*** Surgical incision of the larynx through the thyroid cartilage.

***subhyoid l.*** Surgical incision of the larynx through the thyroid membrane. SYN: *superior l.*

***superior l.*** Subhyoid l.

**laryngotracheal** (lă-rĭng″gō-trā′kē-ăl) [″ + *tracheia,* trachea] Concerning the larynx and trachea.

**laryngotracheitis** (lăr-ĭn″gō-trā-kē-ī′tĭs) [″ + ″ + *itis,* inflammation] An inflammation of the larynx and trachea.

**laryngotracheobronchitis** (lă-rĭng″gō-trā″kē-ō-brŏng-kī′tĭs) [″ + ″ + *bronchos,* windpipe, + *itis,* inflammation] Inflammation of the larynx, trachea, and bronchi.

**laryngotracheotomy** (lăr-ĭn″gō-trā-kē-ŏt′ō-mē) [″ + ″ + *tome,* incision] Incision of the larynx with section of upper tracheal rings.

**laryngoxerosis** (lăr-ĭn″gō-zĕr-ō′sĭs) [″ + *xeros,* dry, + *osis,* condition] Abnormal dryness of the larynx.

**larynx** (lăr′ĭnks) *pl.* **larynges** [Gr.] A musculocartilaginous organ at the upper end of the trachea below the root of the tongue, lined with ciliated mucous membrane; part of the airway and the organ of voice. SEE: illus.

STRUCTURE: The larynx consists of nine cartilages bound together by an elastic membrane and moved by muscles. The cartilages include three single (cricoid, thyroid, and epiglottic) and three paired (arytenoid, corniculate, and cuneiform). The extrinsic muscles include the omohyoid, sternohyoid, sternothyroid, and several others; intrinsic muscles include the cricothyroid, external and internal thyroarytenoid, transverse and oblique arytenoid, and external and internal thyroarytenoid. The cavity of the larynx contains two pairs of folds, the ventricular folds (false vocal cords) and the vocal folds (true vocal cords), and is divided into three regions (vestibule, ventricle, and inferior entrance to the glottis). An opening between the true vocal folds forms a narrow slit, the rima glottidis or glottis.

NERVES: The larynx is innervated from the interior and external branches of superior laryngeal nerve.

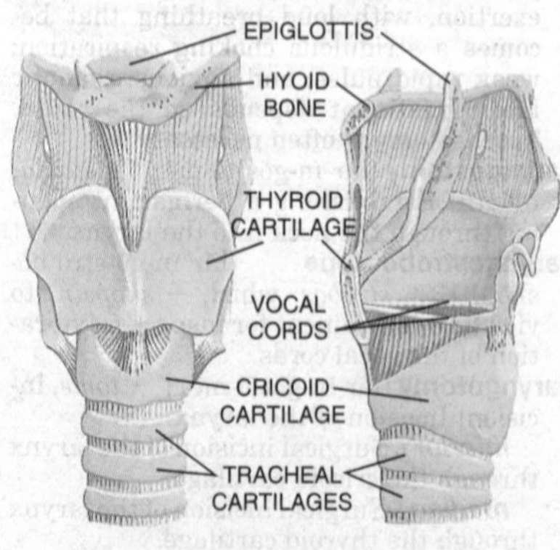


**LARYNX**
**(A)** ANTERIOR VIEW, **(B)** MIDSAGITTAL SECTION

BLOOD SUPPLY: Inferior thyroid, branch of thyroid axis and superior thyroid, branch of external carotid.

***foreign bodies in l.*** The presence of a foreign body in the upper airway. Common culprits include red meat, hard candy, and coins.

SYMPTOMS: Symptoms are violent spasmodic cough and dyspnea, fixed pain at a particular spot, and loss of voice.

NURSING IMPLICATIONS: The American Heart Association current recommendations for aspiration of a foreign body include recognition of foreign body obstruction. If the patient is able to speak or cough, the rescuer should not interfere with the patient's attempts to expel the object. If the patient is unable to speak, cough, or breathe, the rescuer should apply the Heimlich maneuver 6 to 10 times rapidly in succession. Using air already in the lungs, the thrusts create an artificial cough to propel the obstructing object out of the airway. If the patient loses consciousness, the rescuer lowers him or her carefully to the floor, while protecting the head and neck, and continues the effort by applying abdominal thrusts 6 to 10 times from a position kneeling astride the victim's thighs. The rescuer also initiates CPR for unconscious victims as required, based on assessment of airway, breathing, and circulation. After the abdominal thrusts, the rescuer opens the airway and attempts to remove visible obstructions by sweeping the airway and then attempts to ventilate the patient. For an obese or pregnant victim or a child, the rescuer administers chest thrusts applied to the middle of the sternum rather than abdominal thrusts. For an infant, the rescuer uses back blows before chest thrusts. Emergency tracheotomy or cricothyrotomy may be required.

**Lasègue's sign** (lă-sĕgz′) [Ernest C. Lasègue, Fr. physician, 1816–1883] In sciatica, pain and discomfort in the back when the fully extended leg of the supine patient is gently raised.

**laser** (lā′zĕr) Acronym for *l*ight *a*mplification by *s*timulated *e*mission of *r*adiation. A device that emits intense heat and power at close range. The instrument converts various frequencies of light into one small and extremely intense unified beam of one wavelength radiation. The laser can be focused on a very small target. Lasers that provide short pulses of light rather than a continuous beam have been found to cause less damage to normal tissue. Lasers have multiple treatment applications. In ophthalmology, they are used in treating retinal detachment and diabetic retinopathy; in cardiology, experimentally to vaporize arterial blockage; in dermatology, to obliterate blood vessels, for superficial removal of warts and skin cancers, to remove excess tissue in enlarged noses, for superficial removal of pigmented conditions (brown spots) and port-wine nevus, and for removal of tattoos; in gynecology, to remove vulval lesions, including genital warts; in gastroenterology, to control bleeding in the gastrointestinal tract; in surgery and dentistry, to remove tumors. A variety of lasers are used depending upon the wavelength and power required, including argon, carbon dioxide, copper vapor, dye, excimer, helium-neon, ion, krypton, neomydium:yttrium-aluminum garnet, and ruby lasers.

***l. cane*** An experimental cane that helps a blind person detect objects ahead of, above, and below his or her path.

**Lassa fever** [Lassa, city in Africa] A disease caused by arenavirus, first reported in Nigeria in 1969. A reservoir for the virus is a rat, *Mastomys natalensis,* indigenous to Africa.

SYMPTOMS: Patients have abrupt onset of high fever that is continuous or intermittent and spiking, with generalized myalgia, chest and abdominal pain, headache, sore throat, cough, dizziness with flushing of the face, conjunctival injection, nausea, diarrhea, and vomiting. Hemorrhagic areas of the skin and mucous membranes may appear on the fourth day. Mortality of those in Africa with this disease varies from 16% to 45%.

TREATMENT: Ribavirin given in the first week of illness and continued for 10 days has been very effective in reducing the death rate. This medicine should also be given orally for 10 days prophylactically to those who have been percutaneously exposed to the virus. Patients are isolated in special isolation units that filter the air leaving the room and maintain negative pressure. All sputum, blood, excreta, and objects that the patient has contacted are disinfected. SEE: *Universal Precautions Appendix.*

**lassitude** (lăs'ĭ-tūd) [L. *lassitudo,* weariness] Weariness; exhaustion.

**LAT** *licensed athletic trainer.*

**latah** (lă'tă) A type of mental disorder that occurs in people of Southeast Asia, esp. in women, marked by imitative behavior, coprolalia, echolalia, and automatic obedience. It may be provoked by startling, tickling, or frightening the patient.

**LATC** *licensed athletic trainer, certified.*

**latchkey children** Children who have a key to their home, needed for when they return home when no adult is present to supervise them. These children are at a higher risk of accidents, abusing drugs, and smoking cigarettes.

**latency** (lā'tĕn-sē) [L. *latens,* lying hidden] State of being concealed, hidden, inactive, or inapparent.

***sleep l.*** The amount of time between reclining in bed and the onset of sleep.

**latent 1.** Lying hidden. **2.** Quiet; not active.

***l. content*** In psychology, that part of a dream or unconscious mental content that cannot be brought into the objective consciousness through any effort of will to remember.

**latent heat** The caloric or heat energy absorbed by matter changing from solid to liquid or from liquid to vapor with no change in temperature.

***l.h. of fusion*** The heat required to convert 1 g of a solid to a liquid at the same temperature. For example, the process of converting 1 g of ice at 0°C to water at 0°C requires 80 kcal, and until it is completed there will be no rise in the temperature.

***l.h. of vaporization*** The heat required to change 1 g of a liquid at its boiling point to vapor at the same temperature. The latent heat of steam is 540 kcal; therefore, when steam cools to liquid, each gram gives out 540 kcal. This explains why a scald from steam is much more severe than one caused by boiling water.

**laterad** (lăt'ĕr-ăd) [L. *latus,* side, + *ad,* toward] Toward a side or lateral aspect.

**lateral** (lăt'ĕr-ăl) [L. *lateralis*] Pert. to the side.

**lateralis** (lăt"ĕr-ā'lĭs) [L.] Located away from the mid-plane of the body.

**laterality** (lăt"ĕr-ăl'ĭ-tē) The condition of being on one side or toward the side; used to specify which side of the body or brain is dominant.

***crossed l.*** Mixed dominance of certain body parts so that the left arm and right leg would be dominant.

***dominant l.*** Preferential dominance and use of the parts of one side of the body such as the eye, arm, leg, or hand.

**latericeous, lateritious** (lăt"ĕr-ĭsh'ŭs) [L. *later,* brick] Resembling brick dust.

**lateroabdominal** (lăt"ĕr-ō-ăb-dŏm'ĭ-năl) [L. *lateralis,* pert. to side, + *abdomen,* belly] Concerning the side of the body and the abdominal area.

**laterodeviation** (lăt"ĕr-ō-dē"vē-ā'shŭn) [" + *deviare,* to turn aside] Deviation or displacement to one side.

**lateroduction** (lăt"ĕr-ō-dŭk'shŭn) [" + *ducere,* to lead] Movement to one side, esp. of the eye.

**lateroflexion** (lăt"ĕr-ō-flĕk'shŭn) [" + *flexis,* bending] Bending or curvature toward one side.

**laterognathism** Asymmetry of the mandible owing to retarded growth, fractures, tumors, or soft tissue atrophy or hypertrophy.

**lateroposition** (lăt"ĕr-ō-pō-zĭsh'ŭn) [" + *positio,* position] Displacement to one side.

**lateropulsion** (lăt"ĕr-ō-pŭl'shŭn) [L. *lateralis,* pert. to side, + *pulsus,* driving] In cerebellar and labyrinthine disease, the involuntary tendency to fall to one side.

**laterotorsion** (lăt"ĕr-ō-tor'shŭn) [" + *torsio,* a twisting] Twisting to one side.

**lateroversion** (lăt"ĕr-ō-vĕr'shŭn) [" + *versio,* a turning] A tendency or a turning toward one side.

**lathyrism** (lăth'ĭ-rĭzm) [Gr. *lathyros,* vetch] A disease presumably caused by eating certain plants of the genus *Lathyrus*. It is characterized by irreversible muscular weakness and paraplegia.

**lathyrogen** (lăth′ĭ-rō-jĕn) [″ + *gennan*, to produce] Something that produces lathyrism.

**Latino** A person residing in the U.S. whose nationality group, or the country in which the person or person's parents or ancestors were born, is a Latin American country in the Western Hemisphere.

**latissimus** (lă-tĭs′ĭ-mŭs) [L., widest] Denoting a broad anatomical structure such as a muscle.

**latitude** In radiology, a range of exposure that would produce a technically correct radiograph.

**latrine** (lă-trēn′) [L. *latrina*] A toilet, particularly one in a military camp.

***pit l.*** A type of latrine installed outdoors and used where it is impractical to provide a standard, flushing-type toilet. The structure may be manufactured and installed so that odors and flies are not a problem.

**latrodectism** (lăt″rō-dĕk′tĭzm) [*Latrodectus* + Gr. *-ismos*, condition] The toxic reaction to the bite of spiders of the genus *Latrodectus*. SEE: *spider, black widow*.

**Latrodectus** (lăt″rō-dĕk′tŭs) [L. *latro*, robber, + Gr. *daknein*, biting] A genus of small black spiders belonging to the family Theridiidae.

***L. mactans*** Black widow spider.

**LATS** *long-acting thyroid stimulator*.

**lattice** (lăt′ĭs) **1.** A network or framework formed by structures intertwined usually at right angles with each other. **2.** In physics, the arrangement of atoms in a crystal.

**latus** (lā′tŭs) *pl.* **latera** [L., broad] The side; the flank.

**latus, lata, latum** (lā′tŭs, lā′tă, lāt′ŭm) [L., broad] Broad, as the uterine broad ligament.

**laudable** [L. *laudabilis*, praiseworthy] Commendable; healthy; normal; formerly said erroneously of pus.

**laudanum** (lăw′dăn-ŭm) Tincture of opium. SEE: *morphine*.

**laugh** (lăf) [ME. *laughen*, to laugh] **1.** The sound produced by laughing. SYN: *risus*. **2.** To express emotion, usually happiness or mirth, by a series of inarticulate sounds. Typically the mouth is open and a wide smile is present.

***sardonic l.*** Risus sardonicus.

**laughing gas** SEE: under *gas*.

**laughter** (lăf′tĕr) A series of inarticulate sounds produced as an expression of emotion, usually happiness or mirth. The role of humor and laughter in promoting a positive attitude and health and in preventing the progress of some diseases has been documented. This does not mean that laughter and a positive attitude can substitute for proven medical therapy.

***compulsive l.*** Laughter without cause, occurring in certain psychoses, esp. schizophrenia.

***l. reflex*** Uncontrollable laughter resulting from tickling or the pretense of tickling.

**Laurence-Moon-Biedl syndrome** (law′rĕns-moon′bē′dĕl) [John Zachariah Laurence, Brit. ophthalmologist, 1829–1870; Robert C. Moon, U.S. ophthalmologist, 1844–1914; Arthur Biedl, Prague endocrinologist, 1869–1933] The combination of girdle-type obesity, sexual underdevelopment, mental retardation, retinal degeneration, polydactyly, and deformity of the skull. The condition is inherited as an autosomal recessive trait.

**lavage** (lă-văzh′) [Fr., from L. *lavare*, to wash] Washing out of a cavity. SYN: *irrigation*.

***gastric l.*** Washing out of the stomach using a stomach tube or catheter. The purpose of the procedure is to remove and dilute irritants or poisons and to cleanse the stomach preoperatively or postoperatively. Solutions such as sterile water, normal saline, 1% to 5% sodium bicarbonate, or activated charcoal may be used. The latter is particularly helpful in certain types of poisoning in which intubation will not damage the esophagus or stomach. No more than 10 oz of the solution at a temperature of 105°F (40.6°C) should be used at a time, the procedure repeated until fluid runs clear. The procedure should be performed before breakfast. The patient should be semirecumbent or positioned low enough to prevent inhalation of returning fluid. In poisoning, the siphoned fluid should be saved for examination. If the patient is unconscious, a mouth gag should be used. SEE: *colonic irrigation; irrigation, bladder*.

> Caution: It is important to ascertain that the tube or catheter is in the stomach rather than the bronchus.

**law** [AS. *laga*, law] **1.** Scientifically, a statement that is found to hold true uniformly for a whole class of natural occurrences. **2.** A body of rules, regulations, and legal opinions of conduct and action that are made by controlling authority and are legally binding.

***all-or-none l.*** The weakest stimulus capable of producing a response produces the maximum response contraction in cardiac and skeletal muscles and nerves.

***Avogadro's l.*** SEE: *Avogadro's law*.

***Bell's l.*** SEE: *Bell's law*.

***biogenetic l.*** Ontogeny recapitulates phylogeny (i.e., an individual in its development recapitulates stages in its evolutionary development). SYN: *Haeckel's l.*

***Boyle's l.*** SEE: *Boyle's law*.

***Charles' l.*** SEE: *Charles' law*.

***Courvoisier's l.*** SEE: *Courvoisier's law*.

***l. of definite proportions*** Two or more elements when united to form a new substance do so in a constant and fixed proportion by weight.

***Fechner's l.*** SEE: *Fechner's law.*

***Gay-Lussac's l.*** SEE: *Charles' law.*

***Graham's l.*** SEE: *Graham's law.*

***Haeckel's l.*** Biogenetic l.

***l. of the heart*** Other things being equal, the stroke volume of the heart varies as the extent of diastolic filling or the energy of contraction is a function of the initial length of the muscle fibers.

***Hilton's l.*** SEE: *Hilton's law.*

***Hooke's l.*** The stress used to stretch or compress a body is proportional to the strain as long as the elastic limits of the body have not been exceeded.

***l. of the intestine*** Moderate distention of the intestine at a point causes relaxation below (aborally to the point) and contraction above.

***inverse-square l.*** A law stating that the intensity of radiation or light at any distance is inversely proportional to the square of the distance between the irradiated surface and a point source. Thus, a light with a certain intensity at a 4-ft distance will have only one-fourth that intensity at 8 ft and would be four times as intense at a 2-ft distance.

***Koch's l.*** SEE: *Koch's law.*

***l. of Magendie*** SEE: *Bell's law.*

***Marey's l.*** The heart rate varies inversely with arterial blood pressure (i.e., a rise or fall in arterial blood pressure brings about, respectively, a slowing or speeding up of heart rate).

***Mariotte's l.*** SEE: *Boyle's law.*

***l. of mass action*** In chemical reactions, the amount of change taking place is proportional to the action mass of the reacting substance.

***Mendel's l.'s*** SEE: *Mendel's laws.*

***l. of multiple proportions*** When two substances unite to form a series of chemical compounds, the proportions in which they unite are simple multiples of one another or of one common proportion.

***Nysten's l.*** SEE: *Nysten's law.*

***periodic l.*** The physical and chemical properties of chemical elements are periodic functions of atomic weight. A natural classification of elements is made according to their atomic weight. When arranged in order of their atomic weight or atomic number, elements show regular variations in most of their physical and chemical properties.

***l. of reciprocal proportions*** In chemistry, the proportions in which two elementary bodies unite with a third one are simple multiples or simple fractions of the proportions in which these two bodies unite with each other.

***reciprocity l.*** Any milliamperage multiplied by an exposure time setting that gives the same milliamperage-second outcome should give the same density to the film. For example, 100 mA at 1 sec should give a density equivalent to that produced by 200 mA at 0.5 sec. In radiographic film screen technology, the reciprocity law does not hold at long exposure times because of leser film density.

***Rubner's l.'s*** **1.** Law of constant energy consumption: rapidity of growth is proportional to intensity of the metabolic process. **2.** Law of constant growth quotient: the same proportional part, or growth quotient, of total energy is used for growth.

***l. of specificity of nervous energy*** Excitation of a receptor always gives rise to the same sensation, regardless of the nature of the stimulus.

***Sutton's l.*** SEE: *Sutton's law.*

***Waller's l. of degeneration*** If a spinal nerve is completely divided, the distal portion undergoes fatty degeneration.

***Weber's l.*** The increase in stimulus necessary to produce the smallest perceptible increase in sensation bears a constant ratio to the strength of the stimulus already acting.

***Wolff's l.*** Changes in form and function of bones result in definite changes in their internal structure.

**lawrencium** (lă-rĕn′sē-ŭm) [Ernest O. Lawrence, U.S. physicist, 1901–1958] SYMB: Lr. A synthetic transuranic chemical element; atomic weight of most stable isotopes is 260; atomic number is 103.

**lax** (lăks) [L. *laxus,* slack] **1.** Without tension. **2.** Loose and not easily controlled; said of bowel movements.

**laxative** (lăk′să-tĭv) [L. *laxare,* to loosen] A food or chemical substance that acts to loosen the bowels (i.e., facilitate passage of bowel contents at time of defecation), and, therefore, to prevent or treat constipation. Laxatives may act by increasing peristalsis by irritating the intestinal mucosa, lubricating the intestinal walls, softening the bowel contents by increasing the amount of water in the intestines, and increasing the bulk of the bowel contents. Many individuals feel that it is essential to have one or more bowel movements a day, and if they do not, they may develop the habit of taking some form of laxative daily. They should be instructed that missing a bowel movement is not harmful and bowel movements do not necessarily occur at regular intervals. SYN: *aperient; cathartic; purgative.* SEE: *constipation; enema.*

---

Caution: A sudden change in bowel habits may be the first sign of a malignancy of the intestinal tract. When this happens, the individual should consult a physician without delay.

---

***l. regimen*** The diet may be modified to avoid chronic constipation by maintaining an adequate volume of food; eating high-bulk foods that contain a high fiber content; eating foods that tend to stimulate bowel activity such as stewed fruits and vegetables; maintaining adequate fluid intake; and participating in regular exercise. In addition, foods that the individual has found to cause constipation should be avoided. Some persons are esp. liable to be constipated by certain cheeses.

**laxator** (lăk-sā′tor) [L. *laxare,* to loosen] That which has a relaxing effect.

***l. tympani*** One of two muscles or ligaments of the malleus of the inner ear.

**layer** (lā′ĕr) [ME. *leyer*] A stratum; a thin sheetlike structure of more or less uniform thickness.

***ameloblastic l.*** The enamel layer of the tooth. SYN: *enamel l.*

***bacillary l.*** The rod and cone layer of the retina of the eye.

***basal l.*** The outermost layer of the uterine endometrium lying next to the myometrium.

***blastodermic l.*** Germ l.

***choriocapillary l.*** Lamina choriocapillaris.

***claustral l.*** The layer of gray matter between the external capsule and insula.

***clear l.*** The stratum lucidum of the skin.

***columnar l.*** A layer of tall, narrow epithelial cells forming a covering or lining.

***compact l.*** The compact surface layer of the uterine endometrium.

***cuticular l. of epithelium*** A striated layer secreted by and covering the free surface of an epithelial sheet, esp. that on the surface of columnar epithelium of the intestine.

***enamel l.*** Ameloblastic l.

***ependymal l.*** The inner layer of cells of the embryonic neural tube.

***ganglionic l.*** **1.** The fifth layer of the cerebral cortex. **2.** The inner layer of ganglion cells in the retina whose axons form the fibers of the optic nerve.

***germ l.*** One of the three primary layers of the developing embryo from which the various organ systems develop. SYN: *blastodermic l.* SEE: *ectoderm; endoderm; mesoderm.*

***germinative l.*** The innermost layer of the epidermis, consisting of a basal layer of cells and a layer of prickle cells (stratum spinosum). SYN: *malpighian l.; stratum germinativum.*

***granular exterior l.*** The second layer of the cerebellar cortex, lying within the molecular layer and separated from it by a single row of Purkinje cells; consists principally of granule cells.

***granular interior l.*** The fourth layer of the cerebral cortex, consisting principally of closely packed stellate cells.

***half-value l.*** In radiology, the thickness of an absorber that will reduce by one-half the intensity of a beam of radiation.

***Henle's l.*** SEE: *Henle's layer.*

***horny l.*** Outermost layer of the skin, consisting of clear, dead, scalelike cells, those of the surface layer being constantly desquamated. SYN: *stratum corneum.*

***Huxley's l.*** SEE: *Huxley's layer.*

***Langhans' l.*** SEE: *Langhans' layer.*

***malpighian l.*** Germinative l.

***mantle l.*** The middle layer of the neural tube of the developing embryo.

***molecular l.*** **1.** The outermost layer of the cerebral or cerebellar cortex. **2.** The inner or outer plexiform layer of the retina.

***nervous l.*** The nerve-containing portion of the retina of the eye.

***odontoblastic l.*** The layer of connective tissue cells at the outer edge of the pulp where they produce the dentin of the tooth.

***osteogenetic l.*** SEE: *Ollier's layer.*

***outer nuclear l.*** The layer of the retina containing the nuclei of the visual cells (rods and cones).

***papillary l.*** The superficial layer of the corium lying immediately under the epidermis into which it extends, forming dermal papillae.

***pigment l.*** The outermost layer of the retina. Cells contain a pigment called fuscin.

***prickle cell l.*** Stratum spinosum epidermidis; the layer between the granular and basal layers of the skin. Prickle cells are present in this layer. SYN: *spinous l.*

***Purkinje l.*** SEE: *Purkinje layer.*

***l. of pyramidal cells*** The exterior pyramidal layer; the third layer of the cerebral cortex.

***reticular l.*** The inner layer of the corium lying beneath the papillary layer.

***l. of rods and cones*** The layer of the retina of the eye next to the pigment layer. It contains the rods and cones.

***somatic l.*** In the embryo, a layer of extraembryonic mesoderm that forms a part of the somatopleure, the outer wall of the coelom.

***spinous l.*** Prickle cell l.

***splanchnic l.*** In the embryo, a layer of extraembryonic mesoderm that with the endoderm forms the splanchnopleure.

***spongy l.*** Middle layer of the uterine endometrium; contains dilated portions of uterine glands. SYN: *stratum spongiosum.*

***subendocardial l.*** The layer of loose connective tissue immediately under the endocardium that binds it to the myocardium; contains fibers of the conducting system of the heart.

***subendothelial l.*** The layer of fine fibers and fibroblasts lying immediately under the endothelium of the tunica intima of larger arteries and veins.

***Tomes' granular l.*** The layer of interglobular dentin beneath the dentinocemental junction in the root of a tooth.

***Weil's basal l.*** A relatively cell-free zone just below the odontoblastic layer in the dental pulp. It is also called subodontoblastic layer; cell-free zone of Weil; cell-poor zone.

***zonal l. of hypothalamus*** The layer of myelinated fibers covering the thalamus of the brain.

**lb** *pound.*

**LBBB** *left bundle branch block.*

**LD** *lethal dose.*

**$LD_{50}$** The *median lethal dose* of a substance, which will kill 50% of the animals receiving that dose. Dose is usually calculated on amount of material given per gram or kilogram of body weight or amount per unit of body surface area.

**LDH** *lactic dehydrogenase.*

**LDL** *low-density lipoprotein.*

**L-dopa** L-3,4-dihydroxyphenylalanine. A drug used in the treatment of Parkinson's disease. SYN: *levodopa.*

**LDRP** An acronym for Labor, Delivery, Recovery, Postpartum that describes a maternity unit designed for family-centered care. Women in labor and their families complete normal childbearing experiences in one homelike room. The newborn may remain at the bedside thoughout the stay.

**L.E.** *lupus erythematosus.*

**leachate** Water that has passed through a material and in doing so becomes contaminated with substances dissolved in the water. These substances are the leachates, a term used esp. in describing water that has passed through waste disposal sites.

**leaching** (lēch′ĭng) [AS. *leccan,* to wet] Extraction of a substance from a mixture by washing the mixture with a solvent in which only the desired substance is soluble. SYN: *lixiviation.*

**lead** (lēd) [AS. *laedan,* to guide] **1.** Insulated wires connecting a monitoring device to a patient. **2.** A conductor attached to an electrocardiograph. The three common leads are lead I, right arm to left arm; lead II, right arm to left leg; lead III, left arm to left leg. These are known as standard leads, bipolar limb leads, or indirect leads. SEE: *electrocardiogram* for illus.

***bipolar l.*** In electrocardiography, any lead that consists of one electrode at one body site and another at a different site. A standard limb lead, I, II, or III, is a bipolar lead.

***esophageal l.*** A lead that is placed in the esophagus.

***limb l.*** Any lead, unipolar or bipolar, in which a limb is the location of one of the electrodes.

***precordial l.*** A lead having one electrode placed over the precordium, the other over an indifferent region.

***unipolar l.*** In electrocardiography, any lead that consists of one electrode placed on the chest wall overlying the heart, where potential changes are of considerable magnitude, and the other (distant or indifferent electrode) placed in a site where potential changes are of small magnitude.

**lead** (lĕd) [L. *plumbum*] SYMB: Pb. A metallic element whose compounds are poisonous; atomic weight 207.2, atomic number 82, specific gravity 11.35. Accumulation and toxicity occur if more than 0.5 mg/day is absorbed. Any level of lead in the blood is abnormal. Most cases of lead poisoning occur in children who live in homes in which the paint contains lead. Children who eat the paint develop signs of lead toxicity. SEE: *acute l. encephalopathy; lead poisoning, acute; lead poisoning, chronic; pica.*

***l. acetate*** A lead compound that is used in solution as an astringent.

***acute l. encephalopathy*** A syndrome seen mostly in children, following the rapid absorption of a large amount of lead. Initially there is clumsiness, vertigo, ataxia, falling, headache, insomnia, restlessness, and irritability. As the syndrome progresses, forceful vomiting, excitement, confusion, convulsions, and coma will occur. A sudden and marked increase in intracranial pressure accompanies these symptoms. Sequelae include permanent damage to the central nervous system, causing mental retardation, EEG abnormalities, cerebral palsy, and optic atrophy.

TREATMENT: Lead exposure should be discontinued. Corticosteroids and intravenous mannitol, 20% solution, will relieve increased intracranial pressure. Lead can be removed from the body by giving dimercaprol (BAL) and calcium disodium edetate in a carefully administered dose schedule. Convulsions may be controlled with phenobarbital, hydantoin, or diazepam. Hydration should be maintained with intravenous administration of fluids, while avoiding sodium-containing materials. Oral fluids or food should not be given for at least 3 days.

***l. line*** SEE: under *line.*

***l. monoxide*** A reddish-brown compound used to prepare lead subacetate.

***l. pipe contraction*** Cataleptic condition during which limbs remain in any position in which placed.

**lead poisoning, acute** The ingestion or inhalation of a large amount of lead, causing abdominal pain, metallic taste in mouth, anorexia, vomiting, diarrhea, headache, stupor, convulsions, and coma. SEE: *Nursing Diagnoses Appendix.*

TREATMENT: Adequate urine flow should be established; convulsions may be controlled with diazepam. Calcium disodium edetate and dimercaprol are administered to remove lead from the body. After acute therapy is completed, penicillamine is given orally for 3 to 6 months for children and up to 2 months for adults. The exposure to lead should be reduced or eliminated.

---

Caution: Patients receiving penicillamine

therapy must be monitored weekly for adverse reactions, including diffuse erythematous rashes, angioneurotic edema, proteinuria, and neutropenia. Penicillamine is contraindicated in patients with a history of penicillin sensitivity, renal disease, or both.

---

**lead poisoning, chronic** The chronic ingestion or inhalation of lead, damaging the central and peripheral nervous systems, the blood-forming organs, and the gastrointestinal tract. Early symptoms include loss of appetite, weight loss, anemia, vomiting, fatigue, weakness, headache, lead line on gums, apathy or irritability, and a metallic taste in the mouth. Later, symptoms of paralysis, sensory loss, incoordination and vague pains develop. Laboratory diagnosis is made through evidence of anemia; blood lead level above 5 $\mu$g/dl; elevated free erythrocyte protoporphyrin (FEP); increased excretion of lead in urine; characteristic x-ray changes in the ends of growing bones. SEE: *Nursing Diagnoses Appendix.*

TREATMENT: Lead exposure should be eliminated and an adequate diet with added vitamins provided. If hematological disorders are present, penicillamine should be given as if poisoning were acute.

NURSING IMPLICATIONS: A history is obtained to determine environmental, work-related, or folk remedy related sources of lead ingestion or inhalation, and preparations are made for their removal. (In many states, removal of household lead must be done by licensed specialists, not homeowners, following state regulations. The Centers for Disease Control and Prevention and local poison control centers provide relevant information. A 1-cm square chip of lead-based paint may contain a thousand times the usual safe daily ingestion of lead.) A history is obtained of pica; recent behavioral changes, particularly disinterest in play; and behavioral problems such as aggression and hyperirritability. The patient is assessed for developmental delays or loss of acquired skills, especially speech. Central nervous system signs indicative of lead toxicity may be irreversible. In the younger child, the nurse assesses for at-risk characteristics such as the high level of oral activity in late infancy and toddlerhood; small stature, which enhances inhalation of contaminated dust and dirt in areas heavily contaminated with lead; and nutritional deficiencies of calcium, zinc, and iron, the single most important predisposing factor for increased lead absorption. In older children, the nurse assesses for gasoline sniffing, which is especially prevalent among children in some cultures. The nurse assesses parent-child interaction for indications of inadequate child care, including poor hygienic practices, insufficient feeding to promote adequate nutrition, infrequent use of medical facilities, insufficient rest, less use of resources for child stimulation, less affection, and immature attitudes toward maintaining discipline. Prescribed chelating agent(s) are administered to mobilize lead from the blood and soft tissues by enhancing its deposition in bones and its excretion in urine. A combination of drugs may result in fewer side effects and better removal of lead from the brain. If encephalopathy is present, fluid volume is restricted to prevent additional cerebral edema. Injections are administered intramuscularly, and injection sites are rotated for painful injections (which may include simultaneous procaine injection for local anesthesia). The child is allowed to express pain and anger, and physical and emotional comfort measures are provided to relieve related distress. In the absence of encephalopathy, injections are administered intravenously, and hydration is maintained. The patient is evaluated for desired drug effects (measured by blood levels and urinary excretion of lead) and for signs of toxicity from the chelating agents. As necessary, prescribed anticonvulsants are administered to control seizures, which are often severe and protracted, an antiemetic for nausea and vomiting, a hemopoietic for anemia, an antispasmodic for muscle cramps, and analgesic and muscle relaxant agents for muscle and joint pain. Serum electrolytes are monitored daily, and renal function is evaluated by frequent urinalysis. Cleansing enemas are administered when lead is visible in the G.I. tract (or for episodes of acute lead ingestion). Adequate nutrition is provided, and coexisting nutritional deficiencies are corrected, by administering prescribed supplemental iron, for example. An active, active-assisted, or passive range-of-motion exercise program is established to maintain joint mobility and prevent muscle atrophy. The nurse educates and supports the parents to prevent recurrence and educates the public about the dangers of lead ingestion, the importance of screening young (especially preschool) children at risk, the signs and symptoms indicative of toxicity, and the need for treatment.

**lean** (lēn) [AS. *hlaene,* without flesh] Without flesh, emaciated.

***l. body mass*** The weight of the body minus the fat content.

**learning** A change in behavior or skill level that follows gaining experience and practice.

***educative l.*** The concept of learning as a process in which the learner makes judgments, gains foresights and insights, identifies patterns, and finds meanings. It is characteristic of the paradigm shift in nursing education and health teaching.

***latent l.*** Learning that is inapparent to

the individual at the time it occurs but later becomes evident when the learning is facilitated beyond what would be expected in the area of the original learning.

***motor l.*** The processes related to the aquisition and retention of skills associated with movement. They are influenced by practice, experience, and memory.

***programmed l.*** A system of education in which information is presented in small increments and one does not progress to the next step until a correct answer is provided. This may be done by use of a machine or may be self-administered by use of a workbook. SEE: *Skinner box.*

**Leber's disease** (lā'běrz) [Theodor Leber, Ger. ophthalmologist, 1840–1917] A hereditary form of atrophy of the optic nerve that affects males.

**Leber's plexus** A plexus of venules in the eye between Schlemm's canal and Fontana's spaces.

**Leboyer method** (lĕ-boy-yā') [Frederick Leboyer, Fr. obstetrician, b. 1918] A procedure for childbirth that emphasizes the provision of a gentle and peaceful environment for the birth process. Central to this method is the physical contact between the mother and the child immediately after delivery. The infant is given a warm bath at this time. Caressing and massaging the infant begins immediately and is continued daily for several months. The method is believed to facilitate the child's mental and physical development.

**Lecat's gulf** (lā-kăz') [Claude Nicholas Lecat, Fr. surgeon, 1700–1768] The hollow of the bulbous portion of the urethra.

**L.E. cell** Abbreviation for *lupus erythematosus* cell, a mature neutrophilic polymorphonuclear leukocyte that contains the phagocytosed nucleus of another cell. It is characteristic but not diagnostic of lupus erythematosus.

This distinctive cell may form when the blood of patients with systemic lupus erythematosus is incubated and further processed according to a specified method. The plasma of some patients contains an antibody to the nucleoprotein of leukocyte nuclei. These altered nuclei, which are swollen, pink, and homogenous, are ingested by phagocytes. These are the L.E. cells. The ingested material, when stained properly, is lavender and displaces the nucleus of the phagocyte to the edge of the cell wall. The L.E. cell phenomenon can be demonstrated in most patients with systemic lupus erythematosus but is not essential for diagnosis. SEE: illus.; *lupus erythematosus, systemic.*

**lecithal** (lěs'ĭ-thăl) [Gr. *lekithos,* egg yolk] Concerning the yolk of an egg.

**lecithin** (lěs'ĭth-ĭn) [Gr. *lekithos,* egg yolk] A phospholipid (phosphoglyceride) that is part of cell membranes; also found in blood and egg yolk. On hydrolysis, it yields stearic acid, glycerol, phosphoric acid, and choline on hydrolysis.

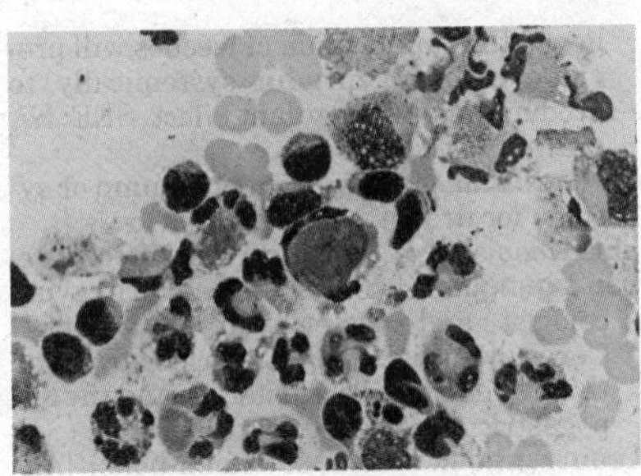

L.E. CELL (CENTER) (ORIG. MAG. ×1000)

**lecithinase** (lěs'ĭ-thĭn-ās) An enzyme that catalyzes the decomposition of lecithin.

***cobra l.*** An enzyme present in certain snake venoms.

**lecithin : sphingomyelin ratio** ABBR: L:S ratio. The ratio of lecithin to sphingomyelin in the amniotic fluid. It is used to assess maturity of the fetal lung. Until about the 34th week of gestation the lungs produce less lecithin than sphingomyelin. As the fetal lungs begin to mature, they produce more lecithin than sphingomyelin. Delivery before the reversal of the ratio is associated with an increased risk of hyaline membrane disease in the infant. The use of this test enables the obstetrician to determine the optimum time for elective termination of pregnancy.

**lecithoblast** (lěs'ĭ-thō-blăst") [" + *blastos,* germ] One of the cells that proliferates to form the yolk sac.

**lecithoprotein** (lěs"ĭ-thō-prō'tē-ĭn) [" + *protos,* first] A protein in which lecithin is part of the conjugate.

**lectin** (lěk'tĭn) [L. *legere,* to pick and choose] One of several plant proteins that stimulate lymphocytes to proliferate. Phytohemagglutinin and concanavalin A are lectins. SEE: *mitogen.*

**lectual** (lěkt'ū-ăl) [L. *lectus,* bed] Pert. to a bed or couch.

**LED** *light-emitting diode.*

**leech** (lētch) [AS. *laece*] A bloodsucking water worm, belonging to the phylum Annelida, class Hirudinea. It is parasitic on humans and other animals, producing a condition known as hirudiniasis. Leeches were used as a means of bloodletting, a practice common up to the middle of the 19th century but now almost completely abandoned. The worms are a source of hirudin, an anticoagulating principle secreted by their buccal glands. In modern times leeches have been used to evacuate periorbital hemorrhage (black eye) and to remove congested venous blood from the suture lines of reimplanted fingers. In addition to hirudin, leech saliva contains several active substances including inhibitors of platelet aggregation. It is not believed that application of leeches will provide sufficient hirudin systemically to produce an anticoagulant effect. SEE: *Hirudinea; hirudiniasis.*

***artificial l.*** Cup and suction pump or syringe for drawing blood.

**LEEP** *loop electrocautery excision procedure.*

**Lee's ganglion** (lēz) [Robert Lee, Brit. gynecologist and obstetrician, 1793–1877] Cervical uterine ganglion formed from the third and fourth sacral nerves and the hypogastric and ovarian plexuses.

**Leeuwenhoek's disease** (lū'ĕn-hōks) [Antoni van Leeuwenhoek, Dutch microscopist, 1632–1723] Repetitive involuntary contractions of the diaphragm and accessory muscles of respiration. The patient complains of shortness of breath and epigastric pulsations. The disease is caused by an abnormality of the respiratory control system of the brainstem.

TREATMENT: Diphenylhydantoin may be effective. If not, section of the phrenic nerve may be necessary. SYN: *respiratory myoclonus.*

**left** The opposite of right. SYN: *sinistral.*

**left-handedness** The condition of being more adept in use of left hand. SYN: *sinistrality.*

**leg** (lĕg) [ME.] One of the two lower extremities, including the femur, tibia, fibula, and patella; specifically, the part between the knee and ankle. SEE: illus.

***badger l.*** Inequality in the length of the legs.

***baker l.*** Genu valgum.

***bandy l.*** Genu varum.

***Barbados l.*** Elephantiasis of the legs.

***bayonet l.*** An uncorrected backward displacement of the knee bones, followed by ankylosis at the joint.

***bird l.*** A reduction in the size of the leg as a result of atrophy of the muscles.

***milk l.*** Phlegmasia alba dolens.

***restless l.*** A sense of uneasiness and uncomfortableness of the legs that comes on at bedtime. Moving the legs tends to relieve the condition. This syndrome is sometimes present at the onset of renal colic as a result of renal calculi.

***scissor l.*** Crossed-leg deformity, a result of double hip disease, in which the patient walks with the legs swinging across the midline with each step.

***white l.*** Phlegmasia alba dolens.

**legal** Pert. to or according to the law.

**Legg-Calvé-Perthes disease** (lĕg'kăl-vā' pĕr'tĕz) [Arthur T. Legg, U.S. surgeon, 1874–1939; Jacques Calvé, Fr. orthopedist, 1875–1954; Georg C. Perthes, Ger. surgeon, 1869–1927] Legg's disease.

**Legg's disease** (lĕgz) [Arthur T. Legg] Osteochondritis of the upper femoral epiphysis. SYN: *coxa plana; Legg-Calvé-Perthes disease.*

**leggings** (lĕg'gĭngs) [ME. *leg,* leg] Sterile leg coverings used on patients while in operating room.

**Legionella pneumophila** The gram-negative, rod-shaped bacterium that causes Legionnaires' disease. SEE: *Legionnaires' disease.*

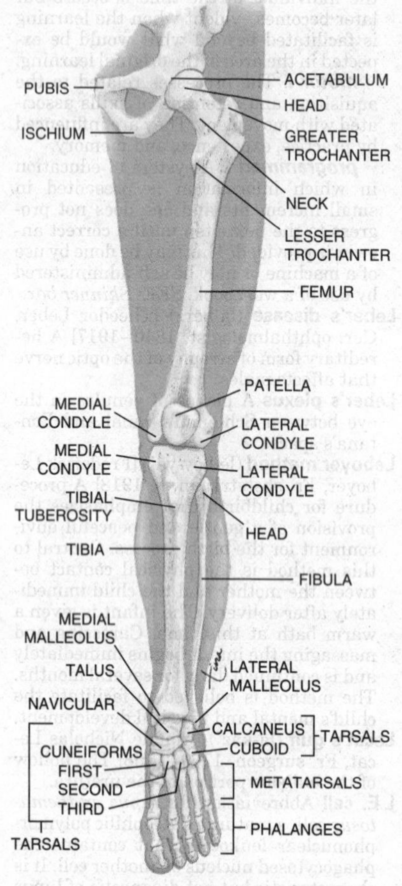


BONES OF THE **LEG** AND FOOT (ANTERIOR VIEW)

**legionellosis** Legionnaires' disease.

**Legionnaires' disease** [after individuals stricken while attending an American Legion convention in Philadelphia, PA, in 1976] A severe, often fatal disease characterized by pneumonia, dry cough, myalgia, and sometimes gastrointestinal symptoms. It may occur in epidemics or sporadically and has become an important cause of nosocomial pneumonia. As the disease progresses, dysfunction of other major organs and, in fatal cases, eventually cardiovascular collapse occurs. SYN: *legionellosis.*

ETIOLOGY: A gram-negative bacillus not previously recognized as an agent of human disease causes this disease. The organism, which has been termed *Legionella pneumophila,* causes the disease

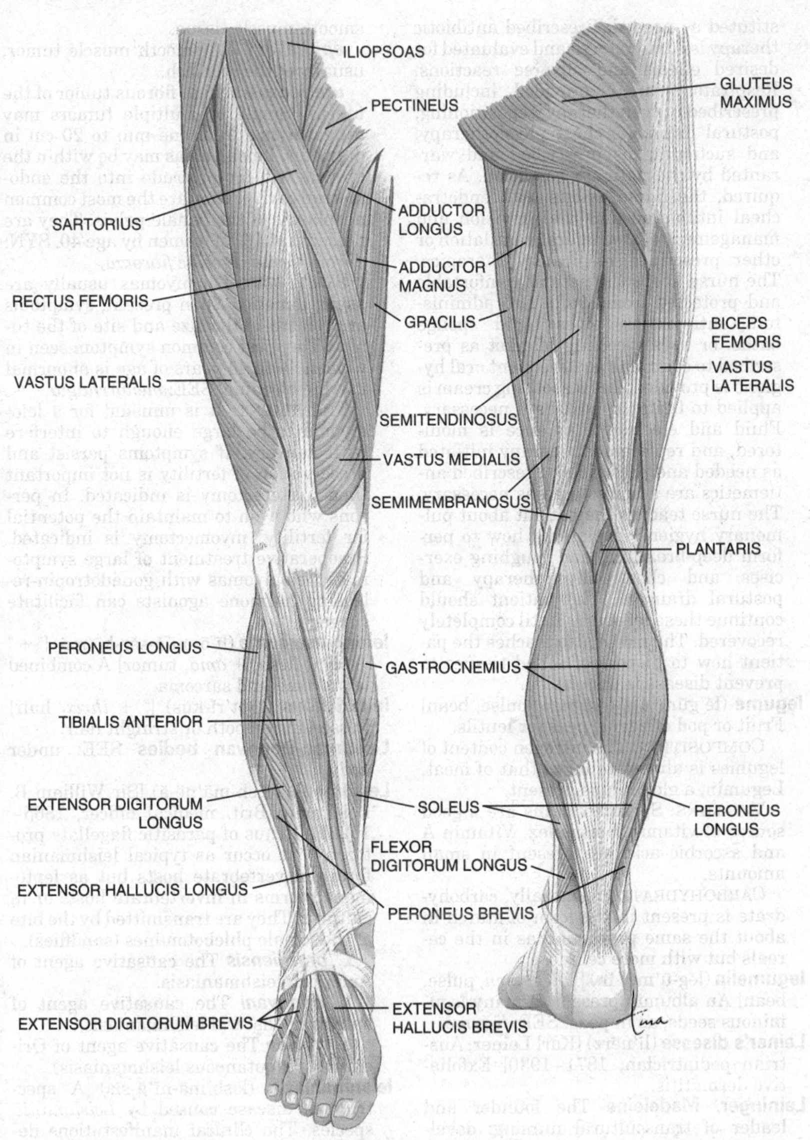


**MUSCLES OF THE LEG**

when it is inhaled from aerosols produced by water cooling towers, air conditioning units, water faucets, shower heads, humidifiers, and contaminated respiratory therapy equipment. Person-to-person transmission does not occur.

TREATMENT: Erythromycin given early in the course of the disease and for a prolonged period is the drug of choice. Rifampin is also of benefit.

NURSING IMPLICATIONS: Respiratory status is monitored, including chest wall expansion, depth and pattern of ventilations, cough and chest pain, and restlessness, which may indicate hypoxemia. Vital signs, arterial blood gas levels, hydration, and color of lips and mucous membranes are also monitored. The nurse is alert for signs of shock (decreased blood pressure; tachycardia with weak, thready pulse; diaphoresis; and cold, clammy skin). Level of consciousness is monitored for signs of neurological deterioration, and seizure precautions are instituted as needed. Prescribed antibiotic therapy is administered and evaluated for desired effects and adverse reactions. Respiratory care is provided, including prescribed oxygen therapy, repositioning, postural drainage, chest physiotherapy, and suctioning as prescribed and warranted by the patient's condition. As required, the nurse assists with endotracheal intubation and the provision and management of mechanical ventilation or other prescribed respiratory therapies. The nurse keeps the patient comfortable and protected from drafts and administers antipyretics, gives tepid sponge baths, or uses a cooling blanket as prescribed to control fever. Frequent oral hygiene is provided, and a soothing cream is applied to irritated nostrils if necessary. Fluid and electrolyte balance is monitored, and replacement therapy initiated as needed and prescribed. Prescribed antiemetics are administered as necessary. The nurse teaches the patient about pulmonary hygiene, explaining how to perform deep-breathing and coughing exercises and chest physiotherapy and postural drainage. The patient should continue these measures until completely recovered. The nurse also teaches the patient how to dispose of soiled tissues to prevent disease transmission.

**legume** (lĕ′gūm) [L. *legumen,* pulse, bean] Fruit or pod of beans, peas, or lentils.

COMPOSITION: The nitrogen content of legumes is almost equal to that of meat. Legumin, a globulin, is present.

VITAMINS: Sprouted beans are a good source of vitamin B complex. Vitamin A and ascorbic acid are present in small amounts.

CARBOHYDRATES: Generally, carbohydrate is present in the form of starch in about the same proportion as in the cereals but with more cellulose.

**legumelin** (lĕg-ū′mĕl-ĭn) [L. *legumen,* pulse, bean] An albumin present in many leguminous seeds, as in peas. SEE: *legume.*

**Leiner's disease** (lī′nĕrz) [Karl Leiner, Austrian pediatrician, 1871–1930] Exfoliative dermatitis.

**Leininger, Madeleine** The founder and leader of transcultural nursing; developed the Theory of Cultural Care Diversity and Universality. SEE: *Nursing Theory Appendix.*

**leio-** [L. *leios,* smooth] Combining form meaning *smooth.*

**leiodermia** (lī″ō-dĕr′mē-ă) [Gr. *leios,* smooth, + *derma,* skin] Dermatitis characterized by abnormal glossiness and smoothness of the skin.

**leiomyofibroma** (lī″ō-mī″ō-fī-brō′mă) [″ + *mys,* muscle, + L. *fibra,* fiber, + Gr. *oma,* tumor] A benign tumor composed principally of smooth muscle and fibrous connective tissue.

**leiomyoma** (lī″ō-mī-ō′mă) [″ + ″ + *oma,* tumor] A myoma consisting principally of smooth muscle tissue.

***epithelioid l.*** A smooth muscle tumor, usually of the stomach.

***uterine l.*** A benign fibrous tumor of the uterus. Single or multiple tumors may range in size from one mm to 20 cm in diameter. Leiomyomas may be within the uterine wall or protrude into the endometrial cavity. They are the most common neoplasms of the female pelvis. They are present in 40% of women by age 40. SYN: *fibroid tumor; uterine fibroma.*

SYMPTOMS: Leiomyomas usually are asymptomatic. When present, symptoms are related to the size and site of the tumor. The most common symptom seen in women 40 to 45 years of age is abnormal uterine bleeding. SEE: *menorrhagia.*

TREATMENT: It is unusual for a leiomyoma to be large enough to interfere with delivery. If symptoms persist and preservation of fertility is not important then hysterectomy is indicated. In persons who wish to maintain the potential for fertility, myomectomy is indicated. Preoperative treatment of large symptomatic leiomyomas with gonadotropin-releasing hormone agonists can facilitate surgery.

**leiomyosarcoma** (lī″ō-mī″ō-săr-kō′mă) [″ + ″ + *sarx,* flesh, + *oma,* tumor] A combined leiomyoma and sarcoma.

**leiotrichous** (lī-ŏt′rĭ-kŭs) [″ + *thrix,* hair] Possessing smooth or straight hair.

**Leishman-Donovan bodies** SEE: under *body.*

**Leishmania** (lēsh-mā′nē-ă) [Sir William B. Leishman, Brit. medical officer, 1865–1926] A genus of parasitic flagellate protozoa that occur as typical leishmanian forms in vertebrate hosts but as leptomonad forms in invertebrate hosts or in cultures. They are transmitted by the bite of the female phlebotomines (sandflies).

***L. braziliensis*** The causative agent of American leishmaniasis.

***L. donovani*** The causative agent of kala azar (visceral leishmaniasis).

***L. tropica*** The causative agent of Oriental sore (cutaneous leishmaniasis).

**leishmaniasis** (lēsh″mă-nī′ă-sĭs) A spectrum of disease caused by *Leishmania* species. The clinical manifestations depend upon a number of factors including the parasite's invasiveness and pathogenecity, as well as the host's genetically determined immune responses. The clinical syndromes are visceral (kala azar), cutaneous, and mucosal; a single *Leishmania* species can produce different clinical syndromes, and each of the syndromes can be caused by more than one species. Leismaniasis is transmitted by the bite of infected female sandflies. SEE: *kala azar.*

TREATMENT: Various forms of pentavalent antimonial compounds are used, but treatment failures are common. Pentamide is effective but is more toxic than pentavalent antimonials. Other drugs have been found to be effective but are not used because of their toxicity or undesired side effects.

***American l.*** Mucocutaneous l.

***cutaneous l.*** An ulcerating, chronic, nodular skin lesion prevalent in Asia and the tropics and due to infection with *Leishmania tropica.* SYN: *Aleppo boil; Oriental sore.*

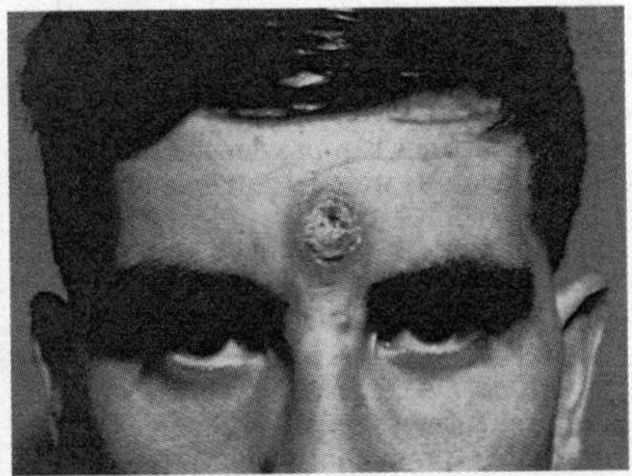

MUCOCUTANEOUS LEISHMANIASIS

CUTANEOUS LESION CAUSED BY *L. BRAZILIENSIS*

***mucocutaneous l.*** A form of cutaneous leishmaniasis, involving principally the nasopharynx and mucocutaneous membranes, found in parts of Central and South America. The causative organism is *Leishmania braziliensis* transmitted by sandflies, usually of the genus *Lutzomyia.* SYN: *American leishmaniasis.* SEE: illus.

***visceral l.*** Kala azar.

**lema** (lē′mă) [Gr. *leme*] The dried secretion of the tarsal glands that collects in the inner canthus of the eye. SYN: *sebum palpebrale.*

**lemmocyte** (lĕm′ō-sīt) [Gr. *lemma,* husk, + *kytos,* cell] A cell that becomes a neurilemma cell. SEE: *nerve fiber.*

**lemniscus** (lĕm-nĭs′kŭs) *pl.* **lemnisci** [Gr. *lemniskos,* a ribbon] A bundle of sensory fibers (lateral or exterior and median or interior) in the medulla and pons.

**lemon** [Persian *limun,* lemon] Fruit of the tree *Citrus limon,* containing citric acid. Lemons contain enough ascorbic acid to prevent or treat scurvy. Lemon may be used in place of vinegar, spices, and aromatic substances by those who cannot use such items.

---

Caution: Food faddists who drink large quantities of lemon juice by sucking directly from the raw fruit may develop erosion of the enamel of their teeth.

---

**lemostenosis** [″ + *stenosis,* act of narrowing] Stricture of the esophagus.

**length** The measurement of the distance between two points.

***basialveolar l.*** The distance from the basion of the foramen magnum of the skull to the intermaxillary suture of the jaw.

***basinasal l.*** The distance from the basion of the foramen magnum of the skull to the center of the suture between the frontal and nasal bones.

***crown-heel l.*** In the embryo, fetus, or newborn, the distance from the crown of the head to the heel.

***crown-rump l.*** In the embryo, fetus, or newborn, the distance from the crown of the head to the apex of the buttocks.

***focal l.*** In optics, the distance from the lens to the point of focus of light rays passing through the lens.

***l. of stay*** The number of days between admission and discharge from an inpatient care facility.

***wave l.*** In the line of progression of a wave, the distance from one point on the wave to the same point on the next wave. The length of a wave determines whether or not the wave is a visible light, x-ray, gamma, or radio wave.

**Lennox-Gastaut syndrome** A complex form of epilepsy marked by early childhood onset, poorly controlled multiple seizure types, slow-spike electroencephalographic waves, and a high incidence of mental retardation.

**lens** (lĕnz) [L. *lens,* lentil] **1.** A transparent refracting medium; usually made of glass. **2.** The crystalline lens of the eye.

***achromatic l.*** A lens that corrects chromatic aberration.

***aplanatic l.*** A lens that corrects spherical aberrations.

***apochromatic l.*** A lens that corrects both spherical and chromatic aberrations.

***biconcave l.*** A lens that has a concave surface on each side. SEE: *biconcave* for illus.

***biconvex l.*** A lens that has a convex surface on each side. SEE: *biconvex* for illus.

***bifocal l.*** A corrective lens containing upper and lower segments, each with a different power. The main lens is for distant vision; the secondary lens is for near vision.

***bifocal contact l.*** A contact lens that contains two corrections in the same lens.

***concave spherical l.*** A lens formed of prisms with their apices together, which is, therefore, thin at the center and thick at the edge. This type of lens is used in myopia.

***contact l.*** A device made of various materials, either rigid or flexible, that fits over the cornea or part of the cornea to supplement or alter the refractive ability of the cornea or the lens of the eye. Contact lenses of any type require special care with respect to storage when they are not being worn, directions for insertion and removal, and the length of time they can be worn. The manufacturer's or dispensing health care worker's instructions should be read and followed. Failure to do this could result in serious eye diseases. Wearing contact lenses while swimming is inadvisable.

***convexoconcave l.*** A lens with a convex surface on one side and a concave surface on the opposite side.

***convex spherical l.*** A lens formed of prisms with their bases together, which is, therefore, thick at the center and thin at the edge. This type of lens is used in hyperopia.

***corneal contact l.*** A type of contact lens that adheres to and covers only the cornea.

***crystalline l.*** A transparent colorless biconvex structure in the eye, enclosed in a capsule, and held in place just behind the pupil by the suspensory ligament. It consists principally of lens fibers that at the periphery are soft, forming the cortex lentis, and in the center of harder consistency, forming the nucleus lentis. Beneath the capsule on the anterior surface is a thin layer of cells, the lens epithelium. The shape is changed by the ciliary muscle to focus light rays on the retina.

***cylindrical l.*** A segment of a cylinder parallel to its axis, used in correcting astigmatism.

***disposable contact l.*** A soft contact lens worn for a week or two and then discarded.

***extended wear contact l.*** A contact lens made of materials that permit permeation of gas (i.e., oxygen) so that there is less chance for corneal irritation.

***hard contact l.*** A contact lens made of rigid translucent materials.

***implanted l.*** Intraocular l.

***intraocular l.*** ABBR: IOL. An artificial lens usually placed inside the capsule of the lens to replace the one that has been removed. A lens is removed because of some abnormality such as a cataract. If the original lens capsule is present and an IOL is placed inside it, the surgical procedure is called *posterior chamber IOL implantation.* If the capsule has been removed in a previous surgical procedure, the IOL may be placed in front of the iris, directly adjacent to the cornea. This is called *anterior chamber IOL implantation.* In another procedure, the IOL is implanted behind the iris. Which method of IOL implantation produces the best results is being investigated. SYN: *implanted l.* SEE: *cataract.*

***oil immersion l.*** A special lens with oil placed between the lens and the object being visualized. This produces a higher magnification than would be the case if the oil were not used.

***omnifocal l.*** An eyeglass lens whose power to alter light rays varies from the top to the bottom of the lens, permitting a smooth transition from one power lens to the other as one moves the eyes. This is in contrast to an eyeglass lens with the usual two-component bifocal lens.

***orthoscopic l.*** A lens that produces no distortion of the periphery of the image.

***soft contact l.*** A contact lens made of flexible, translucent materials. These lenses are more comfortable, can be worn longer, and are harder to displace than hard lenses, but there are disadvantages. They may not provide the same degree of visual acuity as hard lenses and they require more cleaning and disinfection. Tear production may be decreased, esp. in older patients. The soft lenses may need to be replaced every 6 to 18 months. Corneal infections can prevent further use of soft lenses, as well as causing permanent loss of vision.

***spherical l.*** A lens in which all surfaces are spherical.

***trial l.*** Any lens used in testing the vision.

***trifocal l.*** A corrective eyeglass lens containing three segments—for near, intermediate, and distant vision.

**lentectomy** (lĕn-tĕk′tō-mē) [L. *lens,* lentil, + Gr. *ektome,* excision] Surgical removal of the lens of the eye.

**lenticonus** (lĕn″tĭ-kō′nŭs) [″ + *conus,* cone] Conical protrusion of the anterior or posterior surface of the lens.

**lenticular** [L. *lenticularis,* lentil] **1.** Lens shaped. SYN: *lentiform.* **2.** Pert. to a lens.

**lenticulostriate** (lĕn-tĭk″ū-lō-strī′āt) [″ + *striatus,* streaked] Relating to the lenticular nucleus and corpus striatum.

**lenticulothalamic** Pert. to the lenticular nucleus and the thalamus.

**lentiform** (lĕnt′ĭ-form) [L. *lens,* lentil, + *forma,* shape] Lenticular (1).

**lentigines** (lĕn-tĭ′jĭn-ēz) Flat, brown spots appearing on aged exposed skin, frequently on the back of the hands due to the accumulation of lipofuscin in tissues as one ages. Although commonly called "liver spots," they are not related to liver disease. SEE: illus.

**lentiginosis** (lĕn-tĭj″ĭ-nō′sĭs) [L. *lentigo,* freckle, + Gr. *osis,* condition] The presence of multiple lentigines. SEE: *lentigo.*

**lentiginous** (lĕn-tĭj′ĭn-ŭs) [L. *lentigo,* freckle] **1.** Affected by lentigo. **2.** Covered with very small dots.

**lentiglobus** (lĕn″tĭ-glō′bŭs) [L. *lens,* lentil, + *globus,* sphere] A lens of the eye that has extreme anterior spherical bulging.

**lentigo** (lĕn-tī′gō) *pl.* **lentigines** [L., freckle] Freckle. SEE: illus.

***l. maligna*** A noninvasive malignant melanoma. SYN: *Hutchinson's freckle.*

***l. senilis*** Flat, brown spots appearing on the exposed skin of aged white people, frequently on the back of the hands, due to the accumulation of lipofuscin in tissues during the aging process. Although commonly called "liver spots," they are not related to liver disease. They are uniformly tan to dark brown and range from 1 mm to more than 1 cm in size.

**lentitis** (lĕn-tī′tĭs) [L. *lens,* lentil, + Gr. *itis,*

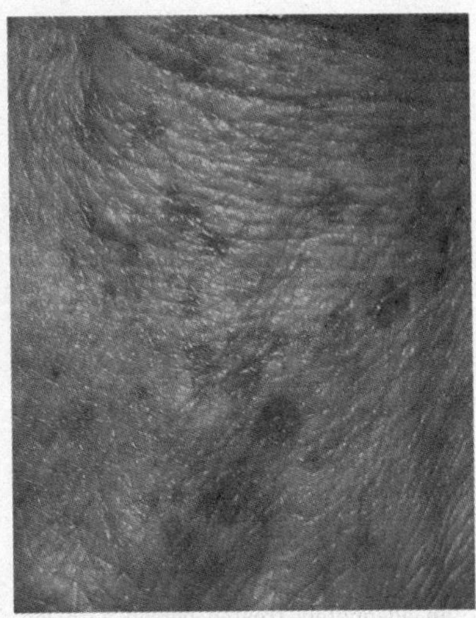

LENTIGINES
TYPICAL EARLY OCCURRENCE ON BACK OF HAND

inflammation] Phakitis.

**lentivirus** [L. *lentus,* slow] A group of retroviruses that cause slowly developing diseases. Human immunodeficiency virus (HIV), the virus that causes acquired immunodeficiency syndrome (AIDS), is included in this group of viruses.

**leontiasis** (lē″ŏn-tī′ă-sĭs) [Gr. *leon,* lion, + *-iasis,* condition] Lionlike appearance of the face seen in certain diseases, esp. lepromatous leprosy. SYN: *facies leontina; leonine facies.*

***l. ossea*** Enlargement and distortion of facial bones, giving one the appearance of a lion. The condition is rare and not fatal.

**Leopold's maneuver** [Christian Gerhard Leopold, Ger. physician, 1846–1911] In obstetrics, the use of four steps in palpating the uterus in order to determine the position and presentation of the fetus.

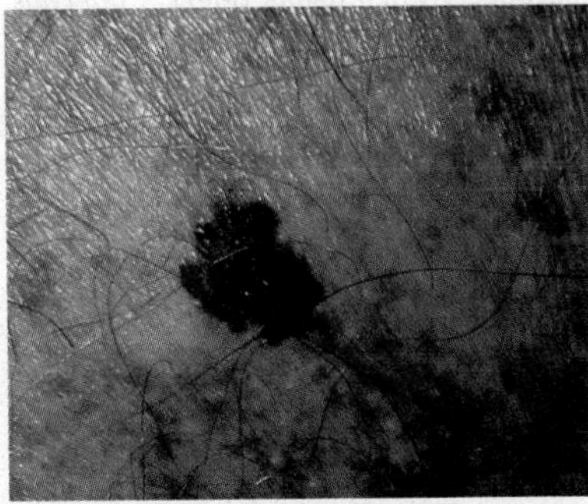

**LENTIGO** AND HYPERPIGMENTATION OF SUN-DAMAGED SKIN

**leper** (lĕp′ĕr) [Gr. *lepros,* scaly] A person afflicted with leprosy.

**lepidic** (lĕ-pĭd′ĭk) [Gr. *lepis,* scale] Concerning scales, or a scaly covering.

**lepido-** [Gr. *lepis,* scale] Combining form meaning *flakes* or *scales.*

**Lepidoptera** (lĕp″ĭ-dŏp′tĕr-ă) [″ + *pteron,* feather, wing] An order of the class Insecta that includes the butterflies, moths, and skippers; characterized by scaly wings, sucking mouth parts, and complete metamorphosis.

**lepidosis** (lĕp″ĭ-dō′sĭs) [″ + *osis,* condition] Any scaly or desquamating eruption such as pityriasis.

**lepothrix** (lĕp′ō-thrĭks) [″ + *thrix,* hair] A condition in which the shaft of the hair is encased in hardened, scaly, sebaceous matter.

**lepra** (lĕp′ră) [Gr. *lepra,* leprosy] A term formerly used for leprosy. It is now used to indicate a reaction that occurs in leprosy patients consisting of aggravation of lesions accompanied by fever and malaise. It can occur in any form of leprosy and may be prolonged.

***l. alba*** A form of lepra in which the skin is anesthetic and white, associated with different forms of paralysis.

***l. Arabum*** True or nodular leprosy.

***l. maculosa*** A form of lepra with pigmented cutaneous areas.

**leprechaunism** (lĕp′rĕ-kŏn″ĭzm) A hereditary disease in which the elfin features of the face are accompanied by retardation of physical and mental development, a variety of endocrine disorders, emaciation, and susceptibility to infections. SYN: *Donohue's syndrome.*

**leprid** (lĕp′rĭd) [Gr. *lepra,* leprosy, + *eidos,* form, shape] A leprous cutaneous lesion.

**leprology** (lĕp-rŏl′ō-jē) [″ + *logos,* word, reason] The study of leprosy and methods of treating it.

**leproma** (lĕp-rō′mă) [″ + *oma,* tumor] A cutaneous nodule or tubercle characteristic of leprosy.

**lepromatous** (lĕp-rō′mă-tŭs) Concerning lepromas. SEE: *leprosy.*

**leprosarium** An institution for the care of lepers.

**leprostatic** (lĕp″rō-stăt′ĭk) [″ + *statikos,* standing] **1.** Inhibiting the growth of *Mycobacterium leprae.* **2.** An agent that inhibits the growth of *M. leprae.*

**leprosy** (lĕp′rō-sē) [Gr. *lepros,* scaly] A chronic communicable disease caused by the acid-fast *Mycobacterium leprae.* It may occur at any age, and in various clinical forms. The two principal forms are lepromatous and tuberculoid. Incubation time ranges from 1 to 30 years but is usually 3 to 5 years. SYN: *Hansen's disease.*

The *lepromatous* (LL) form is characterized by skin lesions and symmetrical involvement of peripheral nerves with anesthesia, muscle weakness, and paralysis. In this form, the lesions are limited to the cooler portions of the body such as skin, upper respiratory tract, and testes. In *tuberculoid* (TT) leprosy, which is usually benign, the nerve lesions are asymmetrical and skin anesthesia is an early occurrence. Visceral involvement is not seen. Because of the anesthesia, rats have been able to remove digits while the patient sleeps. For some time this loss of digits was thought, erroneously, to be due to spontaneous amputation as a part of the disease process.

Lepromatous leprosy is much more contagious than the tuberculoid form. In the latter, *M. leprae* are found in lesions only rarely except during reactions.

Between the two major forms are *borderline* (BB) and *indeterminate* leprosy. In the borderline group, the clinical and bacteriological features represent a combination of the two principal types. In the indeterminate group, there are fewer skin lesions and bacteria are much less abundant in the lesions. In many respects, this infection resembles tuberculosis and for many years was regarded as incurable; this is no longer considered to be valid.

SYMPTOMS: Onset is very gradual. The first signs of infection are usually skin changes, but they may be so nonspecific and slow to progress as to go unrecognized for years.

DIAGNOSIS: Biopsy of a suspected skin lesion is used for diagnosis. The bacilli may not be present in tuberculoid lesions. In vitro tests of the immunological response can be accomplished by the lymphocyte transformation test and the leukocyte migration inhibition test.

COMPLICATIONS: Bacterial skin infections, ulcers, and traumatic amputation of fingers owing to anesthesia may occur. Tuberculosis is a much more common complication in untreated cases of lepromatous leprosy than in the tuberculoid form. Amyloidosis may be the cause of death in advanced cases.

TREATMENT: Dapsone (4,4′-diaminodiphenyl sulfone, DDS) is the form of sulfone used, but widespread development of sulfone resistance necessitates combined chemotherapy treatment with dapsone, rifampin, and clofazimine.

Treatment may be complicated by an acute reversal reaction in tuberculoid or indeterminate forms of leprosy in which the lesions become erythematous and edematous and may become necrotic and ulcerated. Also, the erythema nodosum leprosum (ENL) reaction may develop. This occurs most commonly during the end of the first year of therapy. In this reaction, multiple painful red nodules develop and then may become ulcerated and necrotic; they may last a short time, but new lesions appear. The ENL reaction may be of short or long duration. Thalidomide is the drug of choice for treatment of the ENL reaction. Severe reactions may also require corticosteroid therapy. Thalidomide does not alter the primary disease. This drug is available in the U.S. from Gillis W. Long Hansen's Disease Center, Carville, LA 70721, (800) 642–2477. Thalidomide is contraindicated in women of childbearing age.

The management of patients with leprosy is complex and may require expert consultation. Such assistance may be obtained by contacting physicians in Carville.

Segregation of patients in colonies or hospitals until bacterial test results have been negative for 6 months is not the preferred or effective method of isolating patients. Ambulatory treatment of patients at general clinics has been found to be much more effective. Patients are usually not infectious after 3 months of therapy with dapsone or clofazimine, and after 3 days of rifampin. Thus, children need not be removed from the household in which an adequately treated person with leprosy resides.

PROGNOSIS: With proper therapy, esp. if given at the earliest time possible, the outlook is favorable.

**leprotic** (lĕp-rŏt′ĭk) [Gr. *lepra,* leprosy] Leprous.

**leprous** (lĕp′rŭs) **1.** Pert. to leprosy. **2.** Affected by leprosy. SYN: *leprotic.*

**lepto-** [Gr. *leptos,* thin, fine, slim] A combining form meaning *thin, fine, slight, delicate.*

**leptocephalia** (lĕp″tō-sĕ-fā′lē-ă) [Gr. *leptos,* slender, + *kephale,* head] Having an abnormally vertically elongated, narrow skull.

**leptocephalus** An individual possessing an abnormally vertically elongated, narrow skull.

**leptochromatic** (lĕp″tō-krō-măt′ĭk) [″ + *chromatin*] Having a fine chromatin network.

**leptocyte** (lĕp′tō-sīt) [″ + *kytos,* cell] Target cell.

**leptocytosis** (lĕp″tō-sī-tō′sĭs) [″ + ″ + *osis,* condition] The presence of target cells in the blood.

**leptodactyly** (lĕp″tō-dăk′tĭ-lē) [″ + *daktylos,* finger] Abnormally slim fingers.

**leptomeninges** (lĕp″tō-mĕn-ĭn′jēs) *sing.,* **leptomeninx** [″ + *meninx,* membrane] The pia mater and arachnoid as distinct from the dura mater, because of their thinner and more delicate structure.

**leptomeningitis** (lĕp″tō-mĕn-ĭn-jī′tĭs) [″ + ″ + *itis,* inflammation] Inflammation of the pia and arachnoid membranes, caused by the tubercle bacillus, spirochete of syphilis, and other organisms. SEE: *meningitis.*

SYMPTOMS: Patients have an acute headache, pain in the back, spinal rigidity, irritability, and drowsiness ending in coma. Clinically, it cannot be distinguished from pachymeningitis. SYN: *piarachnitis.*

**leptomeningopathy** (lĕp″tō-mĕn″ĭn-gŏp′ă-thē) [″ + ″ + *pathos,* disease] A disease of the leptomeninges of the brain.

**leptomeninx** Sing. of leptomeninges.

**leptonema** (lĕp″tō-nē′mă) [″ + *nema,* thread] The early stage of prophase in meiosis. At this stage the chromatin contracts into long, thin filaments. SEE: *cell division.*

**leptophonia** (lĕp″tō-fō′nē-ă) [″ + *phone,* voice] Weakness or feebleness of the voice.

**leptoprosopia** (lĕp″tō-prō-sō′pē-ă) [″ + *prosopon,* face] Narrowness of the face.

**leptorhine, leptorrhine** (lĕp′tor-rīn) [″ + *rhis,* nose] Having a very thin or slender nose.

**leptoscope** (lĕp′tō-skōp) [″ + *skopein,* to examine] An optical device for measuring the thickness of cell membranes.

**Leptospira** (lĕp-tō-spī′ră) [″ + *speira,* coil] A genus of thin, spiral, and hook-ended spirochetes.

***L. interrogans icterohaemorrhagiae*** Serotype causing infectious, hemorrhagic, spirochetal jaundice (Weil's disease).

**leptospire** (lĕp′tō-spīr) Any organism belonging to the genus *Leptospira.*

**leptospirosis** (lĕp″tō-spī-rō′sĭs) [″ + ″ + *osis,* condition] Condition resulting from *Leptospira* infection.

**leptospiruria** (lĕp″tō-spĭr-ū′rē-ă) [″ + ″ + *ouron,* urine] The presence of *Leptospira* organisms in the urine.

**leptotene** (lĕp′tō-tēn) [″ + *tainia,* ribbon] The initial stage of the prophase of cell division. The chromosomes become visible as separate entities but are not yet paired.

**leptothricosis** (lĕp″tō-thrī-kō′sĭs) [″ + *thrix,* hair] Disease caused by the gram-negative bacillus *Leptothrix.*

**Leptus autumnalis** Parasitic mite larvae causing itch and sometimes wheals. SEE: *chiggers.*

**leresis** (lĕ-rē′sĭs) [Gr.] Loquacity in old age; garrulousness.

**Leriche's syndrome** (lĕ-rēsh′ĕz) [René Leriche, Fr. surgeon, 1879–1955] Occlusion of the abdominal aorta by a thrombus at its bifurcation. This causes intermittent ischemic pain (i.e., claudication), in the lower extremities and buttocks, impotence, and absent or diminished femoral pulses.

**Leri's pleonosteosis** (lā′rēz) [André Leri, Fr. physician, 1875–1930] A form of hereditary physical malformation characterized by upward slanting palpebral fissures, broad thumbs, short stature, and flexion contractures of the fingers.

**lesbian** (lĕs′bē-ăn) [Gr. *lesbios,* pert. to island of Lesbos] **1.** Pert. to lesbianism or sexual orientation in women toward those of their own sex. SEE: *bisexual; homosexual.* **2.** One who practices lesbianism.

**lesbianism** Sexual desire of women for one of their own sex. It was named for the Island of Lesbos, where the practice of lesbianism was reputed to have been widespread in ancient days. SYN: *sapphism.*

**Lesch-Nyhan disease** [M. Lesch, b. 1939, William Leo Nyhan, b. 1926, U.S. pediatricians] An inherited metabolic disease that affects only males, in whom mental retardation, aggressive behavior, self-mutilation, and renal failure are exhibited. Biochemically there is excess uric acid production owing to a virtual absence of an enzyme essential for purine metabolism.

**lesion** (lē′zhŭn) [L. *laesio,* a wound] **1.** A circumscribed area of pathologically altered tissue. **2.** An injury or wound. **3.** A single infected patch in a skin disease.

Primary or initial lesions include macules, vesicles, blebs or bullae, chancres, pustules, papules, tubercles, wheals, and tumors. Secondary lesions are the result of primary lesions. They may be crusts, excoriations, fissures, pigmentations, scales, scars, and ulcers.

***degenerative l.*** A lesion caused by or showing degeneration.

***diffuse l.*** A lesion spreading over a large area.

***discharging l.*** **1.** A brain lesion that discharges nervous impulses. **2.** A lesion that discharges an exudate.

***focal l.*** A lesion of a small definite area.

***gross l.*** A lesion visible to the eye without the aid of a microscope.

***indiscriminate l.*** A lesion affecting separate systems of the body.

***initial l. of syphilis*** A hard chancre. SEE: *chancre; syphilis.*

***irritative l.*** A lesion that stimulates or excites activity in the part of the body where it is situated.

***local l.*** A lesion of nervous system origin giving rise to local symptoms.

***lower motor neuron l.*** An injury occurring in the anterior horn cells, nerve roots, or peripheral nervous system that results in diminished reflexes, flaccid paralysis, and atrophy.

***peripheral l.*** A lesion of the nerve endings.

***primary l.*** The first lesion of a disease, esp. used in referring to chancre of syphilis.

***structural l.*** A lesion that causes a change in tissue.

***systemic l.*** A lesion confined to organs of common function.

***toxic l.*** A lesion resulting from poisons or toxins from microorganisms.

***vascular l.*** A lesion of a blood vessel.

**LET** *linear energy transfer.* A measure of the rate of energy transfer from ionizing radiation to soft tissue.

**lethal** [Gr. *lethe,* oblivion] Pert. to or that which causes death.

**lethargic** (lĕ-thăr′jĭk) [Gr. *lethargos,* drowsiness] **1.** Affected with lethargy. **2.** Relating to lethargy. **3.** Sluggish.

**lethargy** (lĕth′ăr-jē) [Gr. *lethargos,* drowsiness] A condition of functional torpor or sluggishness; stupor.

***African l.*** Sleeping sickness. SEE: *encephalitis lethargica*.

***hysteric l.*** The sleep of hypnotic lethargy, the state in which many cases of apparent death and resurrection are found.

***induced l.*** A hypnotic trance.

***lucid l.*** The retention of intellect but loss of willpower with a consequent total lack of muscular response. The subject knows what is going on, may resent it, but is unable to exercise sufficient will to bring about muscular defense.

**lethe** (lē′thē) [Gr., oblivion] Amnesia.

**lethologica** (lĕth-ō-lŏj′ĭ-kă) [Gr. *lethe,* forgetfulness, + *logos,* word, reason] The temporary inability to remember a word, name, or intended action.

**Letterer-Siwe disease** (lĕt′ĕr-ĕr-sī′wē) [Erich Letterer, Ger. physician, b. 1895; S. August Siwe, Ger. physician, 1897–1966] A histiocytosis syndrome characterized by proliferation of histiocytes in the viscera and bones. It begins before age 3 and is fatal if untreated. The spleen and liver are enlarged, and there is widespread pulmonary infiltration. There is bone marrow failure accompanied by fever and severe infections. The skin is involved and a variety of lesions are present, including papulovesicular eruption and inflamed pruritic lesions around the anal and vaginal areas. The cause is unknown and there is no specific treatment, but cortisone is used to control lung pathology. It is believed that this disease, eosinophilic granuloma of bone, Hand-Schüller-Christian syndrome, histiocytosis X, and reticuloendotheliosis share a common pattern of the development of granulomatous lesions with histiocytic proliferation. SEE: *histiocytosis, Langerhans cell.*

**Leu** *leucine.*

**leuc-** SEE: *leuk-.*

**leucine** (loo′sĭn) [Gr. *leukos,* white] An amino acid, $C_6H_{13}NO_2$, found among the products of digestion of proteins. It is present in body tissues and is essential for normal growth and metabolism.

**leucine aminopeptidase** ABBR: LAP. A proteolytic enzyme present in the pancreas, liver, and small intestine. Its serum level is elevated in disease of the pancreas, esp. acute pancreatitis, and in obstruction of the common bile duct.

**leucinosis** (loo″sĭn-ō′sĭs) [″ + *osis,* condition] An excess of leucine in the body, thus producing leucine in the urine.

**leucinuria** (loo″sĭn-ū′rē-ă) [″ + *ouron,* urine] The presence of leucine in urine.

**leucitis** (loo-sī′tĭs) [″ + *itis,* inflammation] Scleritis.

**leucovorin calcium** (loo″kō-vō′rĭn) The calcium salt of folinic acid. It is used in the treatment of megaloblastic anemias. It is also used to antagonize the effect of methotrexate on normal cells when methotrexate is being used to treat malignancies. When so used, large doses of leucovorin are required and the optimum timing and dosage are difficult to establish. This use is called leucovorin "rescue."

**leuk-** [Gr. *leukos,* white] Combining form signifying *white, colorless,* or relating to *leukocytes.*

**leukapheresis** (loo″kă-fĕ-rē′sĭs) [″ + *aphairesis,* removal] The separation of leukocytes from blood, which are then transfused back into the patient.

**leukemia** (loo-kē′mē-ă) [Gr. *leukos,* white, + *haima,* blood] A malignancy of the blood-forming cells in the bone marrow. These become widespread throughout the body but esp. in the liver, spleen, and lymph nodes. The leukemias are classified according to their cell type (i.e., lymphoid or myeloid). In most patients, the cause is unknown, but risk factors include certain environmental factors such as ionizing radiation as well as exposure to certain chemicals. Some chemotherapeutic agents combined with radiation also are associated with an increased risk of leukemia. The human T-cell virus type I causes adult T-cell leukemia. Other viruses have been suspected as causes of leukemia, but this has not been proven. It is estimated that in the U.S. the incidence of leukemia is 13 per 100,000 people per year. The pathological changes are a result of a deficit in the number of normal blood cells (red blood cells, white blood cells, platelets), invasion of vital organs by the leukemic cells, and systemic disturbances such as weight loss. SEE: *Nursing Diagnosis Appendix.*

SYMPTOMS: Clinical findings such as anemia, fatigue, lethargy, fever, and bone and joint pain may be present. Physical findings include combinations of pallor, petechiae, or purpura; mucous membrane bleeding; enlarged liver, spleen, and kidneys; and tenderness over the sternum and other bones.

DIAGNOSIS: In most types of leukemia, the abnormal blood cell present in the bone marrow provides valuable diagnostic information.

NOTE: Leukemias have been classified and reclassified as additional information became available; and that process will, no doubt, continue. The leukemias described are common but do not include the many subcategories of this malignant disease.

NURSING IMPLICATIONS: The nurse develops a plan of care that emphasizes comfort, minimizes the effects of chemotherapy, promotes preservation of veins, manages complications, and provides teaching and psychological support. Because so many of these patients are children, sensitivity to their emotional needs and to those of their families is especially important in development of the plan of care. Before treatment begins, an appropriate rehabilitation program is established for the patient during remission. To develop a trusting relationship that promotes communication, the nurse allows the patient and family to express their anger, anxiety, fear, and depression and explains the course of the disease to the patient and family. Drug therapy is tailored to the type of leukemia; most patients require a combination of drugs. Instruction is given in the drugs that the patient is to receive, including their adverse reactions and the measures that can be taken to prevent or alleviate these effects. Prescribed chemotherapy is administered. If the patient receives daunorubicin or doxorubicin, the nurse observes for early signs of cardiotoxicity, such as arrhythmias and signs of heart failure. Steps are taken to prevent hyperuricemia, a possible result of rapid, chemotherapy-induced leukemic cell lysis. The patient should receive about 1/2 gal (2 L) of fluid daily, and acetazolamide, sodium bicarbonate, and allopurinol are administered as prescribed. Urine pH level is checked frequently; it should be above 7.5. The patient is assessed for a rash or other hypersensitivity reaction to allopurinol. If the chemotherapy causes weight loss and anorexia, the patient will need to eat and drink high-caloric, high-protein foods and beverages; foods should be provided in small, frequent meals to help the patient to cope with loss of appetite. If the chemotherapy and adjunctive prednisone result in weight gain, the patient is referred to a dietitian for dietary counseling. The patient should use a soft toothbrush or sponge-stick and avoid hot, spicy foods and commercial mouthwashes, which can irritate mouth ulcers resulting from chemotherapy. The patient's oral cavity is checked daily for ulceration and the rectal area daily for induration, swelling, erythema, perianal skin discoloration, and drainage. Frequent mouth care with saline rinses and prescribed soothing, analgesic rinses helps to control mouth ulceration. The skin and perianal region are kept clean, and mild lotions or creams are applied to prevent drying and cracking. The nurse thoroughly cleans the skin before all invasive procedures, uses strict aseptic technique when starting an I.V. line, and changes sets according to protocol. If the patient requires total parenteral nutrition, scrupulous catheter care is provided. Complete blood count and platelet count are monitored for evidence of deterioration or improvement. The nurse observes for signs of meningeal infiltration (confusion, lethargy, and headache), signifying the need for intrathecal chemotherapy. If the patient is receiving intrathecal chemotherapy, the patient is placed in Trendelenburg's position for 30 minutes after drug instillation, and the lumbar puncture site is checked frequently for bleeding or oozing of clear fluid. The patient is kept supine for 4 to 6 hr and receives adequate fluids. Temperature is monitored every 4 hr; an elevation over 101°F (38.3°C) and a decreased white cell count signify a need for prompt antibiotic therapy. The nurse teaches the patient and family to recognize signs of infection (fever, chills, sore throat, cough) and urges them to report these to the oncologist immediately. To control infection, the nurse places the patient in a private room and imposes reverse isolation if necessary (although the benefits of reverse isolation are controversial). Care is coordinated so that the patient does not come into contact with staff members who are caring for patients with infections or infectious diseases. Use of an indwelling urinary catheter should be avoided, because it provides an avenue for infection. Staff members and visitors are routinely screened for contagious diseases, and any signs of infection in the patient are documented and reported. The patient is monitored for bleeding. If bleeding occurs, ice compresses and pressure are applied and the extremity is elevated. The nurse should avoid giving aspirin or aspirin-containing drugs or rectal suppositories, taking a rectal temperature, or performing a digital rectal examination. Because the patient may not have enough platelets in his blood for proper clotting, the patient and family are taught to recognize the signs of abnormal bleeding (bruising, petechiae). The patient learns the steps to prevent bleeding, and if it occurs, to control it by applying direct pressure and ice to the bleeding areas and is urged to report excessive or uncontrolled bleeding to the oncologist. Prescribed analgesics are administered as needed, and noninvasive pain relief techniques and comfort measures such as position changes, cutaneous stimulation, distraction, relaxation breathing, and imagery are used to alleviate any discomfort. The effects of analgesics and other pain relief measures are evaluated. To minimize stress, a calm, quiet atmosphere conducive to rest and relaxation is provided. Flexibility is maintained with regard to patient care routines and visiting hours (especially if the patient is a child), so that the patient has time to be with family and friends or to play or do schoolwork. The nurse should assist the patient to limit activities, however, and plan rest periods during the day. Both patient and family are encouraged to participate in care as much as possible. If the patient receives cranial irradiation, the nurse explains the treatment procedure and expected sensations, potential benefits, possible adverse reactions, and steps to relieve them. If the patient needs a bone marrow transplant, the nurse reinforces the oncologist's explanation of the treatment, its potential benefits, and any adverse reactions and prepares the patient for transplantation according to institutional or oncologist's

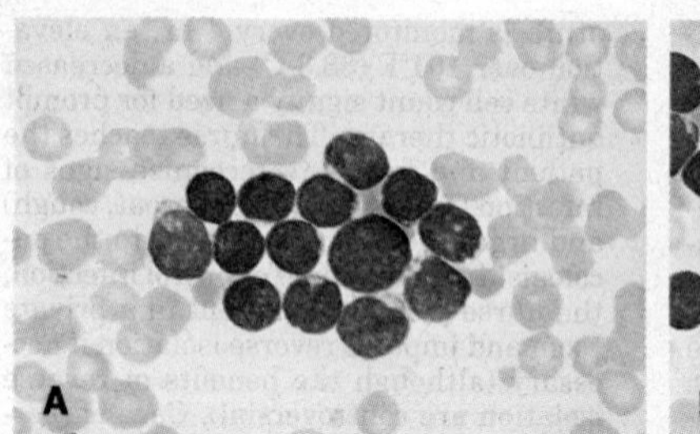

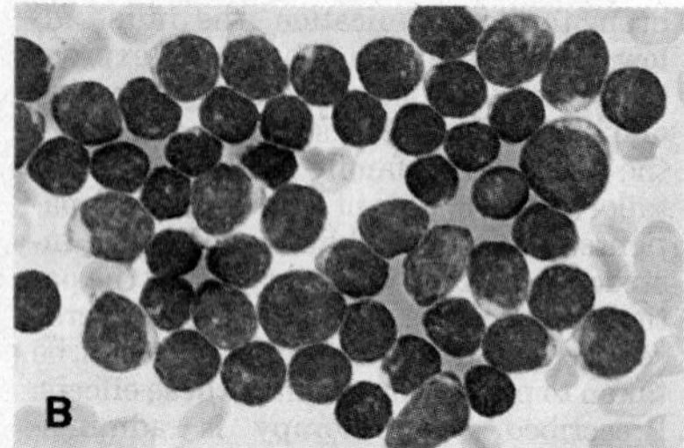

ACUTE LYMPHOCYTIC LEUKEMIA

**(A)** PERIPHERAL BLOOD (ORIG. MAG. ×640), **(B)** BONE MARROW (ORIG. MAG. ×640)

protocol. Total-body irradiation and the chemotherapy given before transplantation are explained, as well as the post-transplantation course. Referral is made to social service agencies, home health-care agencies, and support groups such as the American Cancer Society. If the patient does not respond to treatment and has reached the terminal phase of the disease, supportive nursing care will be needed, including steps taken to manage pain, fever, and bleeding. The nurse keeps the patient comfortable and provides emotional support to the patient and family. As the patient wishes, arrangements are made for religious counseling. Options such as home or hospice care are discussed with the patient and family.

***acute lymphoblastic l.*** Acute lymphocytic l.

***acute lymphocytic l.*** ABBR: ALL. A form of leukemia accounting for 30% of all childhood cancers. It is the most common malignancy affecting children. Its highest incidence is in children between 1 to 5 years of age. It is more common in whites and slightly more frequent in males. SYN: *acute lymphoblastic l.* SEE: illus.

SYMPTOMS: The onset of symptoms may be slowly progressive or acute and rapid. The most common presenting symptoms are those due to anemia, fatigue, lethargy, fever, and bone and joint pain. Physical findings include combinations of pallor, petechiae, or purpura; mucous membrane bleeding; enlarged liver, spleen, and kidneys; and tenderness over the sternum and other bones.

DIAGNOSIS: ALL is diagnosed by the presence of lymphoblasts in the bone marrow. The minimum number required is 25%.

TREATMENT: Therapy includes bone marrow transplantation and a combination of prednisone and cytotoxic agents.

PROGNOSIS: It is estimated that 70% of children will be cured.

***acute myelogenous l.*** ABBR: AML. Acute nonlymphocytic l.

***acute nonlymphocytic l.*** ABBR: ANLL. A group of malignancies of the bone marrow. The bone marrow contains nonlymphoid immature or blast cells. As is typical of virtually all leukemias, the morbidity and mortality are caused by deficits in normal blood cells and impairment of their function, invasion of vital organs, and systemic disturbances such as weight loss. ANLL occurs in both children and adults. Treatment includes cytotoxic chemotherapy alone and bone marrow transplantation after chemotherapy with or without total body irradiation. The very young and the elderly have the worst prognosis.

***chronic lymphocytic l.*** ABBR: CLL. A type of leukemia in which abnormal cells arise from within the lymphoid matura-

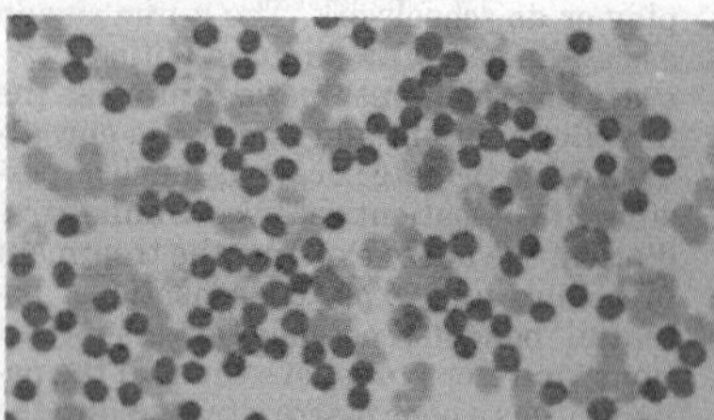

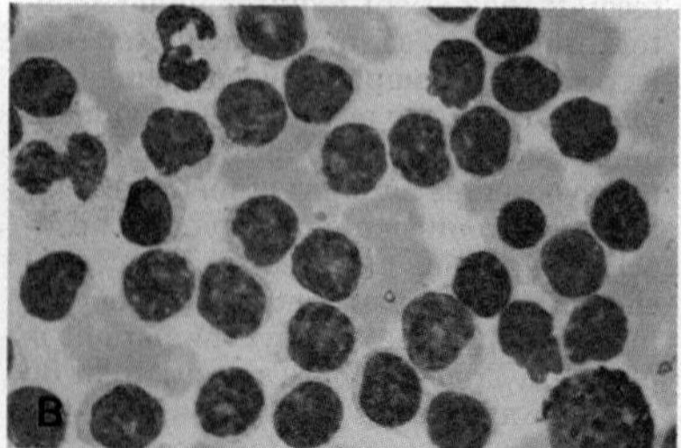

CHRONIC LYMPHOCYTIC LEUKEMIA

**(A)** PERIPHERAL BLOOD (ORIG. MAG. ×400), **(B)** BONE MARROW (ORIG. MAG. ×640)

tional pathways. It commonly occurs in white men older than 50. The prognosis is poor. SEE: illus.

***chronic myelogenous l.*** ABBR: CML. Chronic myeloid l.

***chronic myeloid l.*** ABBR: CML. A malignancy characterized by a considerable and sustained increase in the number of white blood cells. Almost all cases have a small group G chromosome called the Philadelphia or Ph[1] chromosone in the bone marrow cells. CML can occur at any age but the frequency increases steadily with age, and men are affected more commonly than women. Clinically the signs and symptoms are quite similar to those described for acute lymphocytic leukemia. Busulfan is the drug of choice for treatment. The average survival time is from 1 to 3 or more years.

***hairy cell l.*** ABBR: HCL. A malignant, lymphoproliferative disease characterized by pancytopenia, splenomegaly, and abnormal mononuclear cells with irregular cytoplasmic projections. These so-called hairy cells are esp. evident in the spleen. The median age of patients is 50 to 55 years with a range of 24 to 80; and the male to female ratio is about 4:1. Most of the clinical manifestations are owing to the decrease in blood cells and splenomegaly. SEE: illus.

SYMPTOMS: Patients exhibit weight loss, hypermetabolism with accompanying increased sweating, and abdominal discomfort due to the enlarged spleen.

TREATMENT: Treatment includes splenectomy and chemotherapy with alpha-interferon, pentostatin, or cladribine. These drugs have been impressive in improving the outlook of patients in whom the disease continued to progress after splenomegaly. Interferon has been used successfully to treat CML.

PROGNOSIS: Prior to the availability of the chemotherapeutic agents, the mean survival time was 4.6 years for nonsplenectomized patients and 6.4 for those who had splenectomy. The use of chemotherapy in HCL patients may permit longer survival times.

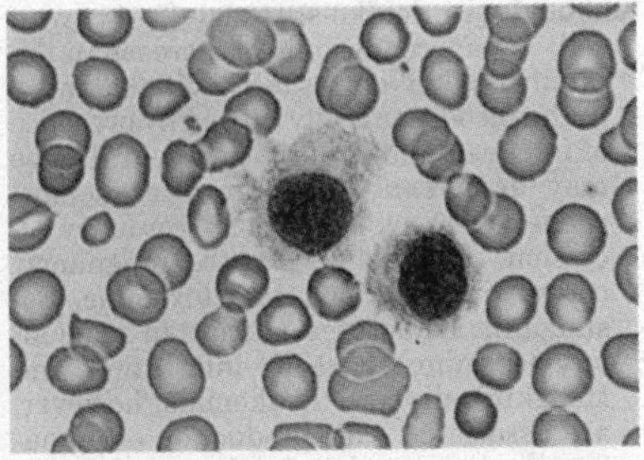

LYMPHOCYTES IN **HAIRY CELL LEUKEMIA** (ORIG. MAG. ×640)

**leukemic** (loo-kēm′ĭk) [″ + *haima,* blood] **1.** Relating to leukemia. **2.** Affected with leukemia.

**leukemid** (loo-kē′mĭd) Any nonspecific skin lesion associated with leukemia. The lesions may or may not contain leukemia cells.

**leukemogenesis** (loo-kē″mō-jĕn′ĕ-sĭs) [″ + ″ + *genesis,* generation, birth] The induction of leukemia.

**leukemoid** (loo-kē′moyd) [″ + ″ + *eidos,* form, shape] Having symptoms of leukemia that are actually caused by other conditions.

**leukin** (loo′kĭn) A thermostable bactericidal substance present in leukocytes.

**leuko-** SEE: *leuk-*.

**leukoagglutinin** (loo″kō-ă-gloo′tĭ-nĭn) [″ + L. *agglutinans,* gluing] An antibody that agglutinates white blood cells.

**leukocidin** (loo-kō-sī′dĭn) [″ + L. *caedere,* to kill] A bacterial toxin that destroys leukocytes.

**leukocoria, leukokoria** White or abnormal pupillary reflex. This reflex may be present in infants and children who have retinoblastoma, cataract, retinal detachment, and intraocular infections. Patients with this reflex should be referred to an ophthalmologist without delay.

**leukocyte** (loo′kō-sīt) [″ + *kytos,* cell] A white blood cell or corpuscle (WBC). There are two types: granulocytes (those possessing, in their cytoplasm, large granules that stain different colors under a microscope) and agranulocytes (those lacking granules). Granulocytes include basophils, eosinophils, and neutrophils. Agranulocytes include monocytes and lymphocytes. Clinically, granulocytes are often referred to as "polys" because they are all polymorphonuclear (multilobed nuclei); whereas agranulocytes are mononuclear (one nucleus). SEE: *blood* for illus.

Neutrophils, 55% to 70% of all WBCs, are the most numerous phagocytic cells and are a primary effector cell in inflammation. Eosinophils, 1% to 3% of total WBCs, destroy parasites and are involved in allergic reactions. Basophils, less than 1% of all WBCs, contain granules of histamine and heparin and are part of the inflammatory response to injury. Monocytes, 3% to 8% of all WBCs, become macrophages and phagocytize pathogens and damaged cells, esp. in the tissue fluid. Lymphocytes, 20% to 35% of all WBCs, have several functions: recognizing foreign antigens, producing antibodies, suppressing the immune response to prevent excess tissue damage, and becoming memory cells.

Leukocytes are formed from the undifferentiated stem cells, that give rise to all blood cells. Those in the red bone marrow may become any of the five kinds of WBCs. Those in the spleen and lymph nodes may become lymphocytes or monocytes. Those in the thymus become lymphocytes called T-lymphocytes.

FUNCTION: Leukocytes are the primary effector cells against infection and tissue damage. They not only neutralize or destroy organisms, but also act as scavengers, cleaning up damaged cells by phagocytosis to initiate the repair process. Leukocytes travel by ameboid movement and are able to penetrate tissue and then return to the bloodstream. Their movement is directed by chemicals released by injured cells, a process called chemotaxis. After coming in contact with and recognizing an antigen, neutrophils or macrophages phagocytize (engulf) it in a small vacuole that merges with a lysosome, to permit the lysosomal enzymes to digest the phagocytized material. When leukocytes are killed along with the pathogenic organisms they have destroyed, the resulting material is called pus, commonly found at the site of localized infections. Pus that collects because of inadequate blood or lymph drainage is called an abscess.

*Microscopic examination:* Leukocytes can be measured in any bodily secretion. They are normally present in blood and, in small amounts, in spinal fluid and mucus. The presence of WBCs in urine, sputum, or fluid drawn from the abdomen is an indication of infection or trauma. The type of WBC present is identified by the shape of the cell or by the use of stains (Wright's) to color the granules: granules in eosinophils stain red, those in basophils stain blue, and those in neutrophils stain purple.

Clinically, serum WBC counts are important in detecting infection or immune system dysfunction. The normal WBC level is 5000 to 10,000/$mm^3$. An elevated (greater than 10,000) leukocyte count (leukocytosis) indicates an acute infection or disease process (such as certain types of leukemia), whereas a decrease in the number of leukocytes (less than 5000) indicates either immunodeficiency or an overwhelming infection that has depleted WBC stores. In addition to the total WBC count, the differential count is also frequently important. A differential count measures the percent of each type of WBC (e.g., neutrophils, monocytes, lymphocytes). The differential also measures the number of immature cells of each cell type as an indication of production by the bone marrow. Immature cells are called "blasts" (e.g., lymphoblasts, myeloblasts). During an infection, the number of blasts is increased as large numbers of immature cells are released. SEE: *inflammation.*

***acidophilic l.*** Eosinophilic l.

***agranular l.*** Nongranular l.

***basophilic l.*** A leukocyte with cytoplasmic granules that stain with basic dyes, turning a deep purple with Wright's stain. This leukocyte constitutes 0% to 0.75% of the white cell count.

***eosinophilic l.*** A granular leukocyte with cytoplasmic granules that stain with acid dyes, appearing reddish when stained with Wright's stain. It constitutes 1% to 3% of the white cell count. SYN: *acidophilic l.*

***granular l.*** A leukocyte containing granules in cytoplasm.

***heterophilic l.*** A neutrophilic leukocyte of certain animals whose granules stain with an acid stain.

***lymphoid l.*** Nongranular l.

***neutrophilic l.*** A leukocyte with fine cytoplasmic granules that do not stain with acid or basic stains but have an affinity for neutral stains.

***nongranular l.*** An agranulocyte; a lymphocyte or monocyte. SYN: *agranular l.*

***polymorphonuclear l.*** ABBR: PMN. A white blood cell that possesses a nucleus composed of two or more lobes or parts; also called a *granulocyte* (neutrophil, eosinophil, basophil). Neutrophils, the most numerous polymorphonuclear leukocytes, are the most important phagocytic cells in the body. Clinically, polymorphonuclear leukocytes are often referred to as "polys."

**leukocytic** (loo″kō-sĭt′ĭk) [″ + *kytos,* cell] Pert. to leukocytes.

**leukocytoblast** (loo″kō-sī′tō-blast) [″ + ″ + *blastos,* germ] A cell from which a leukocyte arises.

**leukocytogenesis** (loo″kō-sī″tō-jĕn′ĕ-sĭs) [″ + *kytos,* cell, + *genesis,* generation, birth] Leukopoiesis.

**leukocytoid** (loo′kō-sī″toyd) [″ + ″ + *eidos,* form, shape] Resembling a leukocyte.

**leukocytolysin** A lysin that destroys leukocytes. SEE: *leukocidin.*

**leukocytolysis** (loo″kō-sī-tŏl′ĭ-sĭs) [″ + *kytos,* cell, + *lysis,* dissolution] Destruction of leukocytes.

**leukocytoma** (loo″kō-sī-tō′mă) [″ + ″ + *oma,* tumor] **1.** A tumor composed of cells resembling leukocytes. **2.** A tumor-like mass of leukocytes.

**leukocytopenia** (loo″kō-sī″tō-pē′nē-ă) [″ + ″ + *penia,* want] Leukopenia.

**leukocytopoiesis** (loo″kō-sī″tō-poy-ē′sĭs) [″ + ″ + *poiein,* to make] The formation of white blood cells.

**leukocytosis** (loo″kō-sī-tō′sĭs) [″ + *kytos,* cell, + *osis,* condition] An increase in the number of leukocytes (above 10,000/$mm^3$) in the blood, generally caused by presence of infection and usually transient. It also may accompany or occur after hemorrhage, extensive operations, coronary occlusion, malignant growth, pregnancy, certain intoxications, and toxemias. Eosinophilic leukocytosis occurs in some allergies, animal parasite infestation, and Hodgkin's disease. Leukemias, however, are associated with production of immature leukocytes due to abnormal blood-forming organs. Leukocytosis is present in most bacterial infections but not usually in those caused by a virus. In leukocytosis the numbers of white cells may vary from a 50% increase to many times more than normal. In leukemia there may be as many as 1 million white cells/mm$^3$. Leukocytosis is early and marked in severe infections when the patient's resistance is good; if infection and resistance are less marked it appears later to a lesser degree and disappears more quickly. Leukocytosis may occur in unusually virulent infections such as diphtheria, pneumonia, and sepsis. SEE: *leukopenia.*

***basophilic l.*** An increase in the basophils in the blood.

***mononuclear l.*** An increase in the monocytes in the blood.

***pathological l.*** Leukocytosis due to a disease such as an infection.

**leukocytotaxis** (loo″kō-sī″tō-tăk′sĭs) [Gr. *leukos,* white, + *kytos,* cell, + *taxis,* arrangement] The movement of leukocytes either toward or away from an area such as a traumatized or infected site.

**leukocytotoxin** (loo″kō-sī″tō-tŏk′sĭn) [″ + ″ + *toxikon,* poison] A toxin that destroys leukocytes.

**leukocyturia** (loo″kō-sī-tū′rē-ă) [″ + ″ + *ouron,* urine] Leukocytes in the urine.

**leukoderma** (loo-kō-dĕr′mă) [″ + *derma,* skin] Deficiency of skin pigmentation, esp. in patches. SEE: *vitiligo.*

***syphilitic l.*** Macular depigmentation, esp. of the skin of the neck and shoulders, seen in late syphilis.

**leukodystrophy** (loo″kō-dĭs′trō-fē) An incurable disease of the central nervous system in which the formation of the myelin is abnormal. This may be due to a specific biochemical defect.

***metachromatic l.*** A type of hereditary leukodystrophy caused by a deficiency of the enzyme cerebroside sulfatase, an enzyme that is essential for the degradation of sulfatide. Deficiency of the enzyme allows excess deposition of sulfatide in nerve tissues. Clinical signs of this disease usually appear at about 1 year of age. They include gait disturbance, inability to learn to walk, spasticity of the limbs, hyperreflexia, dementia, and eventually death. The disease, for which there is no specific therapy, is usually fatal by age 10.

**leukoedema** (loo″kō-ĕ-dē′mă) [″ + *oidema,* swelling] A benign leukophakia-like abnormality of the mucosa of the mouth or tongue. The affected areas are opalescent or white, and wrinkled.

**leukoencephalitis** (loo″kō-ĕn-sĕf-ă-lī′tĭs) [″ + *enkephalos,* brain + *itis,* inflammation] Inflammation of the white matter of the brain.

**leukoencephalopathy, progressive multifocal** ABBR: PML. Widespread demyelinating lesions of the brain, brainstem, and cerebellum caused by the JC virus (the initials of the first patient from whom the virus was isolated). It is usually associated with chronic neoplastic diseases including Hodgkin's disease, chronic lymphocytic leukemia, and lymphosarcoma. It also occurs as a complication of AIDS and in immunocompromised patients. Clinically there is paralysis, blindness, aphasia, ataxia, dysarthria, dementia, confusional states, and coma. There is no treatment. Death occurs 3 to 6 months after onset of neurological symptoms.

**leukoerythroblastosis** (loo″kō-ĕ-rĭth″rō-blăs-tō′sĭs) [″ + *erythros,* red, + *blastos,* germ, + *osis,* condition] Anemia due to any condition that causes the bone marrow to be infiltrated and thus inactivated.

**leukokeratosis** (loo″kō-kĕr-ă-tō′sĭs) [″ + *keras,* horn, + *osis,* condition] Leukoplakia.

**leukokoria** (loo″kō-kō′rē-ă) [″ + *kore,* pupil] Leukocoria.

**leukokraurosis** (loo″kō-kraw-rō′sĭs) [″ + *krauros,* dry, + *osis,* condition] Kraurosis vulvae.

**leukolymphosarcoma** (loo″kō-lĭm″fō-săr-kō′mă) [″ + L. *lympha,* lymph, + Gr. *sarx,* flesh, + *oma,* tumor] Lymphosarcoma cell leukemia.

**leukoma** (loo-kō′mă) [″ + *oma,* tumor] A white, opaque corneal opacity.

***l. adherens*** A corneal scar with incarcerated iris tissue.

**leukomatous** (loo-kō′mă-tŭs) [Gr. *leukos,* white, + *oma,* tumor] **1.** Pert. to leukoma. **2.** Suffering from leukoma.

**leukomyelitis** (loo″kō-mī-ĕ-lī′tĭs) [″ + *myelos,* marrow, + *itis,* inflammation] Inflammation of the white matter of the spinal cord.

**leukomyelopathy** (loo″kō-mī-ĕl-ŏp′ă-thē) [″ + ″ + *pathos,* disease] Disease involving the white matter of the spinal cord.

**leukonecrosis** (loo″kō-nĕ-krō′sĭs) [″ + *nekrosis,* state of death] Dry, light-colored, or white gangrene.

**leukonychia** (loo″kō-nĭk′ē-ă) [″ + *onyx,* nail] White spots or streaks on the nails. SYN: *canities unguium.*

**leukopathia** (loo″kō-păth′ē-ă) [″ + *pathos,* disease] **1.** The absence of pigment in the skin. SEE: *leukoderma.* **2.** A disease involving leukocytes.

***l. unguium*** Leukonychia.

**leukopedesis** (loo″kō-pĕ-dē′sĭs) [″ + *pedan,* to leap] The passage of leukocytes through the walls of the blood vessels.

**leukopenia** (loo″kō-pē′nē-ă) [″ + *penia,* lack] Abnormal decrease of white blood corpuscles usually below 5000/mm$^3$. A great number of drugs may cause leukopenia, as can failure of the bone marrow. SYN: *granulocytopenia; leukocytopenia.*

**leukoplakia** (loo″kō-plā′kē-ă) [″ + *plax,* plate] Formation of white spots or patches on the mucous membrane of the tongue or cheek. The spots are smooth, irregular in size and shape, hard, and occasionally fissured. The lesions may become malignant.

***l. buccalis*** Leukoplakia of the mucosa

of the cheek.

***l. lingualis*** Leukoplakia of the tongue.

***l. vulvae*** An atrophic disease affecting the female external genitalia seen most often in older women. It is characterized by severe itching and a white marble-like appearance of the skin, frequently with excoriations. Without medical intervention, the skin may undergo malignant degeneration. SYN: *kraurosis vulvae.*

**leukoplasia** (loo-kō-plā′zē-ă) Leukoplakia.

**leukopoiesis** (loo″kō-poy-ē′sĭs) [″ + *poiesis,* formation] Leukocyte production. SYN: *leukocytogenesis.*

**leukopoietic** (loo″kō-poy-ĕt′ĭk) [″ + *poiein,* to make] Forming leukocytes.

**leukopsin** A substance formed in the rods of the retina from rhodopsin under the influence of light.

**leukorrhagia** (loo″kō-rā′jē-ă) [″ + *rhegnynai,* to burst forth] Leukorrhea.

**leukorrhea** (loo″kō-rē′ă) [″ + *rhoia,* flow] Usually white or yellow mucous discharge from the cervical canal or the vagina. Frequently a so-called physiological leukorrhea may be constantly present but somewhat increased preceding and following menstruation, and during sexual excitement. It may be of considerable concern to the young girl at the time of menarche if she has not been told that this white fluid would tend to collect on the vulvae. Leukorrhea may be abnormal if it is increased in amount, has a change in color, is malodorous, or contains blood.

SYMPTOMS: There are usually indications of acute inflammation—pain, heat, and redness of parts involved. Pain exists in the groin, hypogastrium, sacral regions, and small of the back. The urethra is often implicated, causing painful micturition. Symptoms that may occur in connection with chronic leukorrhea are innumerable. Discharge may be of any consistency: thin and watery or viscid and tenacious; and it may or may not have a foul odor.

ETIOLOGY: Leukorrhea is caused by pathological states of the endocervix and vagina, including infection by *Trichomonas vaginalis, Candida albicans,* and other pathogens.

TREATMENT: If the condition is due to a specific microorganism, treatment with an appropriate antibiotic is needed. In general, douches are ineffective in curing the cause of this symptom. If caused by senile changes in the vagina, estrogen-containing cream or ointment applied locally is quite effective.

**leukosarcoma** (loo″kō-săr-kō′mă) [Gr. *leukos,* white, + *sarx,* flesh, + *oma,* tumor] A variation of malignant lymphoma in which the blood cells become leukemic.

**leukotactic** (loo″kō-tăk′tĭk) [″ + *taxis,* arrangement] Possessing the power of attracting leukocytes.

**leukotaxis** (loo″kō-tăks′ĭs) Possessing the power of attracting (positive leukotaxis) or repelling (negative leukotaxis) leukocytes.

**leukotomy** (loo-kŏt′ō-mē) [″ + *tome,* incision] Lobotomy.

**leukotoxic** (loo″kō-tŏks′ĭk) [″ + *toxikon,* poison] Destructive to leukocytes.

**leukotoxin** (loo″kō-tŏk′sĭn) [″ + *toxikon,* poison] Leukocytotoxin.

**leukotrichia** (loo″kō-trĭk′ē-ă) [″ + *thrix,* hair] Whiteness of the hair. SYN: *canities.*

**leukotriene** Any of a group of arachidonic acid metabolites that functions as a chemical mediator of inflammation. Leukotrienes C4, D4, and E4 are derived from the precursor molecule leukotriene A4. All are synthesized by cells in response to inflammation or tissue injury. LT have been implicated in the development of the inflammation responses in asthma, psoriasis, rheumatoid arthritis, and inflammatory bowel disease. They are extremely powerful bronchoconstrictors and vasodilators and mediate the adverse vascular and bronchial effects of systemic anaphylaxis.

**leukous** (loo′kŭs) [Gr. *leukos,* white] White, esp. relating to the skin.

**levallorphan tartrate** (lĕv″ăl-lor′făn) A narcotic antagonist used to counteract morphine or opioid-induced respiratory depression. Trade name is Lorfan.

**levamisole hydrochloride** An antihelminthic drug originally used in veterinary medicine and now as adjuvant therapy in treating metastatic colorectal cancer. Trade name is Tramisol.

**levarterenol bitartrate** (lĕv″ăr-tĕ-rē′nŏl bī-tăr′trāt) Previously used name for norepinephrine bitartrate. A sympathomimetic agent that, due to its vasopressor effect, may be useful in treating hypotension that accompanies shock. It is usually administered intravenously because it is rapidly inactivated. Trade name is Levophed.

**levator** (lē-vā′tor) *pl.* **levatores** [L., lifter] **1.** A muscle that raises or elevates a part; opposite of depressor. **2.** An instrument that lifts depressed portions.

***l. ani*** A broad muscle that helps to form the floor of the pelvis.

***l. palpebrae superioris*** A muscle that elevates the upper eyelid.

**LeVeen shunt** [Harry LeVeen, U.S. surgeon, b. 1917] A shunt from the peritoneal cavity to the venous circulation; used to help control ascites by allowing ascitic fluid to enter the venous circulation.

**level of activities** In the nervous system, the levels corresponding to different stages of development into which connector neurons are grouped: spinal cord level, medullary level, midbrain level, basal ganglial level, and cortical level. Each level is responsible for certain activities but is controlled by the one above it.

**level of health care** SEE: *system, health care.*

**lever** (lĕv′ĕr, lē′vĕr) [L. *levare,* to raise] A rigid bar used to modify direction, force, and motion. A type of simple machine that provides the user with a mechanical advantage. Levers are used to facilitate the moving and lifting of objects too heavy or awkward for one to move unassisted.

**Levine, Myra** A nursing educator who developed the Conservation Model of Nursing. SEE: *Nursing Theory Appendix*.

**Levin's tube** (lĕ-vĭnz′) [Abraham L. Levin, U.S. physician, 1880–1940] A catheter that is usually introduced through the nose and extends through the stomach into the duodenum. It is used to help prevent accumulation of intestinal liquids and gas during and after intestinal surgery.

**levitation** [L. *levitas*, lightness] The subjective sensation of rising in the air or moving through the air unsupported. It occurs in dreams, altered states of consciousness, and certain mental disorders.

**levocardia** (lē″vō-kăr′dē-ă) [L. *laevus*, left, + Gr. *kardia*, heart] A term describing the normal position of the heart when other viscera are inverted. SEE: *dextrocardia*.

**levocarnitine** An amino acid-derived drug used in treating primary carnitine deficiency. SEE: *carnitine*.

**levoclination** (lē″vō-klī-nā′shŭn) [″ + *clinatus*, leaning] Torsion or twisting of the upper meridians of the eyes to the left. SYN: *levotorsion* (2).

**levocycloduction** (lē″vō-sī″klō-dŭk′shŭn) [″ + Gr. *kyklos*, circle, + L. *ducere*, to lead] Levoduction.

**levodopa** L-3,4-dihydroxyphenylalanine. A drug used in the treatment of Parkinson's disease. Also called L-dopa.

**levoduction** (lē″vō-dŭk′shŭn) [L. *laevus*, left, + *ducere*, to lead] Movement or drawing toward the left, esp. of an eye. SYN: *levocycloduction*.

**Levopa** Trade name for levodopa.

**levophobia** (lĕv″ō-fō′bē-ă) [″ + Gr. *phobos*, fear] A morbid dread of objects on the left side of the body.

**levorotation** (lē″vō-rō-tā′shŭn) [″ + *rotare*, to turn] Levotorsion (1).

**levorotatory** (lē″vō-rō′tă-tor-ē) Causing to turn toward the left, applied esp. to substances that turn polarized light rays to the left.

**levorphanol tartrate** (lēv-or′fă-nŏl) A synthetic analgesic that acts similarly to morphine.

**levothyroxine sodium** (lē″vō-thī-rŏk′sēn) The sodium salt of the natural isomer of thyroxine used in treating thyroid deficiency.

**levotorsion, levoversion** (lē″vō-tor′shŭn, lē″vō-vĕr′shŭn) [″ + *torsio*, a twisting] **1.** A twisting to the left. SYN: *levorotation*. **2.** Levoclination.

**levulinic acid** An acid formed when certain simple sugars are acted on by dilute hydrochloric acid.

**levulose** SEE: *fructose*.

**levulosemia** (lĕv″ū-lō-sē′mē-ă) [″ + Gr. *haima*, blood] The presence of fructose in the blood.

**levulosuria** (lĕv″ū-lō-sū′rē-ă) [″ + Gr. *ouron*, urine] The presence of fructose in the urine.

**lewisite** (lū′ĭ-sīt) [Warren Lee Lewis, U.S. chemist, 1878–1943] A toxic gas similar in action to mustard gas, used in warfare to disable and kill. It acts as a vesicant in the lungs. Dimercaprol is the treatment drug of choice.

**Lewy bodies** [Frederic H. Lewy, Ger. neurologist, 1885–1950] Neuronal cells with pigmented inclusion bodies. They are found in the brain in the substantia nigra and locus ceruleus, esp. in Parkinson's disease.

**Leydig cell** (lī′dĭg) [Franz von Leydig, Ger. anatomist, 1821–1908] One of the interstitial tissue cells in the testicles that produce testosterone.

**L.F.A.** *left frontoanterior* fetal position.

**L-forms** [named for *Lister* Institute] Spontaneous variants of bacteria that replicate as spherically structured, filterable elements with defective or absent cell walls. They are filterable because of their flexibility rather than their size. Stable forms may grow for an indefinite time in a wall-less state. Organisms of the unstable form are capable of regenerating their cell walls and reverting to their antecedent bacterial form. The ability of L-forms to cause disease is unknown. SYN: *L-phase variants*.

**L.F.P.** *left frontoposterior* fetal position.

**L.F.T.** *left frontotransverse* fetal position.

**LGA** *large for gestational age*.

**LH** *luteinizing hormone*.

**Lhermitte's sign** (lār′mīts) [Jacques Jean Lhermitte, Fr. neurologist, 1877–1959] The symptom (rather than a sign) of a pain resembling a sudden electric shock throughout the body produced by flexing the neck. It is caused by trauma to the cervical portion of the spinal cord, multiple sclerosis, cervical cord tumor, or cervical spondylosis.

**LHRH** *luteinizing hormone–releasing hormone*.

**Li** Symbol for the element lithium.

**liability** Legal responsibility. A health care provider is legally responsible for actions that fail to meet the standard of care, thereby causing potential harm to the patient.

**Liberty Mutual elbow** Boston arm.

**libidinous** (lĭ-bĭd′ĭ-nŭs) [L. *libidinosus*, pert. to desire] Characterized by sexual desires.

**libido** (lĭ-bī′dō, -bē′dō) [L., desire] **1.** The sexual drive, conscious or unconscious. Some drugs used therapeutically, including beta blockers, clonidine, diuretics, lithium, major tranquilizers, methyldopa, oral contraceptives, and sedatives, may have libido-reducing side effects. **2.** In psychoanalysis, the energy or force that is the driving force of human behavior. It has been variously identified as the sex urge, desire to live, desire for pleasure or satisfaction.

**Libman-Sacks disease** (lĭb′măn-săks′) [Emanuel Libman, U.S. physician, 1872–1946; Benjamin Sacks, U.S. physician 1896–1939] Verrucous, nonbacterial endocarditis.

**lice** Pl. of louse.

**licensure** In the health care professions, the granting of permission—official, legal, or both—to perform professional actions in various fields such as medicine or nursing that may not be legally done by persons who do not have such permission. Qualification for a license in health care is usually determined by an official body representing the state or federal government.

***individual l.*** In the health care profession, licensure of an individual to perform certain medical actions.

***institutional l.*** In the health care business, the licensing of institutions such as hospitals, clinics, or corporations to perform certain medical care functions.

***mandatory l.*** Licensure that regulates the practice of a profession such as nursing or medicine by requiring compliance with the licensing statute if an individual engages in activities defined within the scope of that profession.

**licentiate** (lī-sĕn′shē-ăt) **1.** An individual who practices a profession by the authority granted by a license. **2.** In some countries, a medical practitioner who has no medical degree.

**lichen** (lī′kĕn) [Gr. *leichen,* lichen] **1.** Any form of papular skin disease; usually denoting lichen planus. **2.** In botany, any one of numerous plants consisting of a fungus growing symbiotically with certain algae. They form characteristic scaly or branching growths on rocks or barks of trees.

***myxedematous l.*** Generalized eruption of asymptomatic nodules caused by mucinous deposits in the upper layers of the skin and in vessels and organs.

***l. nitidus*** A rare skin condition characterized by small, chronic, asymptomatic papules that are usually pink and are usually located only on the penis, abdomen, and flexor surfaces of the elbows and palms.

***l. pilaris*** L. spinulosus.

***l. planopilaris*** A form of lichen planus in which white shiny follicular papules are present along with the usual plane papules.

***l. planus*** Inflammatory pruritic skin lesions. The cause of this disease is unknown, but exposure to some chemicals may cause similar lesions on the skin. Prognosis is prolonged but favorable.

SYMPTOMS: The condition begins with pinhead-sized papules, reddish or violaceous, glistening, then coalescing, forming rough, scaly patches; acute, subacute, or chronic itching; usually symmetrical

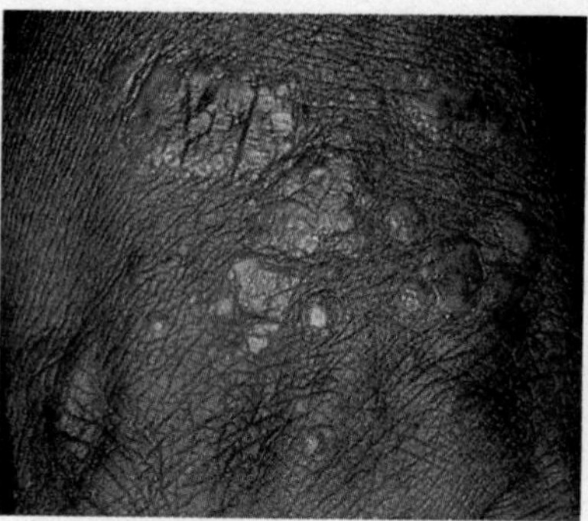

LICHEN PLANUS

lesions on the flexor surface of the arms, trunk, and genitalia, and on the oral and vaginal mucosa. According to type of lesion the disease may be lichen planus atrophicus, erythematosus, hypertrophicus, linearis, or ruber moniliformis. SEE: illus.

TREATMENT: The disease, for which there is no specific therapy, is self-limiting but may last years, or recur. If exposure to a chemical is related to the onset of the disease, discontinue exposure to it. Local symptomatic therapy for itching and occlusive dressing with corticosteroid cream will be helpful. If mucosal lesions are severe, systemic corticosteroids are indicated.

***l. ruber moniliformis*** Large verrucous lesions of lichen planus arranged as the beads in a necklace.

***l. ruber planus*** L. planus.

***l. sclerosus et atrophicus*** A chronic skin eruption consisting of discrete or confluent flat-topped ivory-white papules, each of which contains a black keratotic plug. The lesions may be associated with intractable itching, esp. when they are in the anal and genital areas. Kraurosis vulvae is frequently associated with this disease.

***l. scrofulosus*** An eruption of tiny punctate reddish-brown papules arranged in circles or groups in young persons with tuberculosis. The lesions are caused by the spread of the tubercle bacilli through the blood to the skin.

***l. simplex chronicus*** An itching papular eruption that is circumscribed and located on skin that has become thickened and pigmented owing to the rubbing of it. SEE: illus.; *neurodermatitis* for illus.

***l. spinulosus*** A form of lichen with a spine developing in each follicle. SYN: *l. pilaris; keratosis pilaris.*

***l. striatus*** A papular eruption usually seen on one extremity of a child. It is arranged in linear groups and consists of pink papules. The disease, though self-limiting, may last for a year or longer.

***l. tropicus*** A form of lichen with red-

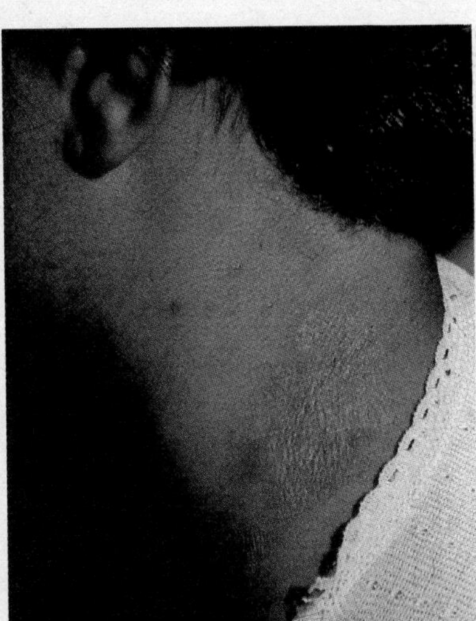

LICHEN SIMPLEX CHRONICUS

ness and inflammatory reaction of the skin. SYN: *miliaria rubra; prickly heat.*

**lichenification** (lī-kĕn″ĭ-fĭ-kā′shŭn) [Gr. *leichen,* lichen, + L. *facere,* to make] **1.** Cutaneous thickening and hardening from continued irritation. **2.** The changing of an eruption into one resembling a lichen.

**lichenoid** (lī′kĕn-oyd) [″ + *eidos,* form, shape] Resembling lichen.

**Lichtheim's syndrome** (lĭkt′hīmz) [Ludwig Lichtheim, Ger. physician, 1845–1928] Subacute combined degeneration of the spinal cord associated with pernicious anemia.

**licorice** (lĭk′ĕr-ĭs, -ĕr-ĭsh) [ME.] A dried root of *Glycyrrhiza glabra* used as a flavoring agent, demulcent, and mild expectorant. Glycyrrhiza is prepared from licorice. Ingestion of large amounts of licorice can cause salt retention, excess potassium loss in the urine, and elevated blood pressure. SYN: *glycyrrhiza.*

**lid** [ME.] An eyelid.

**lidocaine** (lī′dō-kān) A local anesthetic drug. Trade name is Xylocaine.

***l. hydrochloride*** A local anesthetic that is also used intravenously to treat certain cardiac arrhythmias, esp. ventricular dysrhythmias.

**lie, transverse** A position of the fetus in utero in which the long axis of the fetus is across the long axis of the mother. SEE: *presentation* for illus.

**Lieberkühn crypt** (lē′bĕr-kēn) [Johann N. Lieberkühn, Ger. anatomist, 1711–1756] One of the simple tubular glands present in the intestinal mucosa. In their epithelium are found goblet cells, cells of Paneth, and argentaffin cells. The glands form minute invaginations opening between the bases of the villi. They lie in the lamina propria, their blind ends extending to the muscularis mucosa. In the large intestine they are longer and contain few if any Paneth cells and more goblet cells. They are arranged vertically with much regularity. SYN: *intestinal glands; Lieberkühn's glands.*

**lie detector** SEE: *polygraph.*

**lien** (lī′ĕn) [L.] The spleen.

***l. accessorius*** Accessory spleen.

***l. mobilis*** Floating spleen.

**lienal** (lī-ē′năl) [L. *lien,* spleen] Splenic.

**lienitis** (lī″ĕ-nī′tĭs) [″ + Gr. *itis,* inflammation] Splenitis.

**lienocele** (lī-ē′nō-sēl) [″ + Gr. *kele,* tumor, swelling] Splenocele.

**lienography** (lī″ē-nŏg′ră-fē) [″ + Gr. *graphein,* to write] Radiographical examination of the spleen after introduction of a contrast medium.

**lienomalacia** (lī-ē″nō-mă-lā′shē-ă) [″ + Gr. *malakia,* softening] Splenomalacia.

**lienomedullary** (lī-ē″nō-mĕd′ū-lăr-ē) [″ + *medulla,* marrow] Relating to both spleen and bone marrow.

**lienomyelogenous** (lī-ē″nō-mī-ĕl-ŏj′ĕ-nŭs) [″ + Gr. *myelos,* marrow, + *gennan,* to produce] Derived from both spleen and bone marrow.

**lienomyelomalacia** (lī-ē″nō-mī″ĕl-ō-mă-lā′shē-ă) [″ + ″ + *malakia,* softening] Softening of the spleen and bone marrow.

**lienopancreatic** (lī-ē″nō-păn″krē-ăt′ĭk) [″ + Gr. *pankreas,* pancreas] Relating to the spleen and pancreas.

**lienorenal** (lī-ē″nō-rē′năl) [″ + *renalis,* pert. to kidney] Relating to the spleen and kidney.

**life** (līf) [AS.] **1.** The state of being alive; a quality manifested by metabolism, growth, reproduction, and adaptation to environment; a state in which the organs of an animal or plant are capable of performing all or any of their functions. **2.** The time between the birth or inception and the death of an organism. Biologically, the life of a system begins at the moment of conception and ends at death; however, for legal and other reasons the definition of when life begins and death occurs has been subject to a variety of interpretations. SEE: *death.* **3.** The sum total of those properties that distinguish living things (animals or plants) from nonliving inorganic chemical matter or dead organic matter.

***l. expectancy*** The number of years that an average person of a given age may be expected to live, according to mortality tables. The data from which such tables are constructed may be obtained as much as two decades or more before their publication. This is particularly true for data used for insurance purposes. SEE: tables.

***l. extension*** The concept that certain types of intervention may allow a person to live longer than would have been the case if those interventions had not been

### Expectation of Life in Years, by Race, Sex, and Age: 1992

| Age in 1990 (years) | White | | Black | |
|---|---|---|---|---|
| | Male | Female | Male | Female |
| Birth | 73.2 | 79.8 | 65.0 | 73.9 |
| 5 | 68.9 | 75.4 | 61.4 | 70.3 |
| 10 | 64.0 | 70.4 | 56.5 | 65.4 |
| 15 | 59.1 | 65.5 | 51.7 | 60.4 |
| 20 | 54.3 | 60.6 | 47.2 | 55.6 |
| 25 | 49.7 | 55.7 | 42.9 | 50.8 |
| 30 | 45.1 | 50.9 | 38.7 | 46.1 |
| 35 | 40.5 | 46.0 | 34.5 | 41.4 |
| 40 | 36.0 | 41.2 | 30.5 | 37.1 |
| 45 | 31.5 | 36.5 | 26.7 | 32.7 |
| 50 | 27.1 | 31.9 | 23.0 | 28.5 |
| 55 | 22.9 | 27.5 | 19.5 | 24.5 |
| 60 | 19.1 | 23.2 | 16.3 | 20.8 |
| 65 | 15.5 | 19.3 | 13.5 | 17.4 |
| 70 | 12.4 | 15.6 | 11.0 | 14.3 |
| 75 | 9.6 | 12.2 | 8.9 | 11.4 |
| 80 | 7.2 | 9.2 | 6.8 | 8.6 |
| 85 and over | 5.3 | 6.6 | 5.1 | 6.3 |

SOURCE: Adapted from U.S. Bureau of the Census: Statistical Abstract of the United States: 1995, 115th edition. Washington, DC, 1995.

used. Examples would be in the areas of nutrition, exercise, abstinence from cigarettes, and not driving while intoxicated.

***l. review therapy*** A type of insight-oriented therapy that was first described by Robert Butler in 1964. The therapy has a psychoanalytical theoretical base and is focused on conflict resolution. It is usually conducted with persons who are near the end of their life cycle. The therapeutic process allows the patients to review their lives, come to terms with conflict, gain meaning from their lives, and die peacefully.

***l. satisfaction*** One's attitudes concerning one's present life situation and the

### Expectation of Life at Birth, 1970 to 1993, and Projections, 1995 to 2010*

| Year | Total | | White | | Black and Other | |
|---|---|---|---|---|---|---|
| | Male | Female | Male | Female | Male | Female |
| 1970 | 67.1 | 74.7 | 68.0 | 75.6 | 61.3 | 69.4 |
| 1975 | 68.8 | 76.6 | 69.5 | 77.3 | 63.7 | 72.4 |
| 1980 | 70.0 | 77.4 | 70.7 | 78.1 | 65.3 | 73.6 |
| 1981 | 70.4 | 77.8 | 71.1 | 78.4 | 66.2 | 74.4 |
| 1982 | 70.8 | 78.1 | 71.5 | 78.7 | 66.8 | 74.9 |
| 1983 | 71.0 | 78.1 | 71.6 | 78.7 | 67.0 | 74.7 |
| 1984 | 71.1 | 78.2 | 71.8 | 78.7 | 67.2 | 74.9 |
| 1985 | 71.1 | 78.2 | 71.8 | 78.7 | 67.0 | 74.8 |
| 1986 | 71.2 | 78.2 | 71.9 | 78.8 | 66.8 | 74.9 |
| 1987 | 71.4 | 78.3 | 72.1 | 78.9 | 66.9 | 75.0 |
| 1988 | 71.4 | 78.3 | 72.2 | 78.9 | 66.7 | 74.8 |
| 1989 | 71.7 | 78.5 | 72.5 | 79.2 | 66.7 | 74.9 |
| 1990 | 71.8 | 78.8 | 72.7 | 79.4 | 67.0 | 75.2 |
| 1991 | 72.0 | 78.9 | 72.9 | 79.6 | 67.3 | 75.5 |
| 1992 | 72.3 | 79.1 | 73.2 | 79.8 | 67.7 | 75.7 |
| 1993 | 72.1 | 78.9 | 73.0 | 79.5 | 67.4 | 75.5 |
| Projection†: 1995 | 72.8 | 79.7 | 73.7 | 80.3 | 68.2 | 76.8 |
| 2000 | 73.2 | 80.2 | 74.3 | 80.9 | 68.3 | 77.5 |
| 2005 | 73.8 | 80.7 | 74.9 | 81.4 | 69.1 | 78.1 |
| 2010 | 74.5 | 81.3 | 75.6 | 82.0 | 69.9 | 78.7 |

* In years. Excludes deaths of nonresidents of the United States.

† Based on middle mortality assumptions.

SOURCE: Adapted from U.S. Bureau of the Census: Statistical Abstract of the United States: 1995, 115th edition. Washington, DC, 1995.

extent to which one is either content or discontent. It is sometimes used simultaneously with morale, successful aging, and well-being.

***l. satisfaction index*** ABBR: LSI. A self-reporting instrument measuring life satisfaction in the elderly. A total of five rating scales are used.

***l. span*** The maximal obtainable age by a member of a species.

***l. table*** A statistical table that estimates the life expectancy of individuals in a particular population. The data used to establish the table come from records of the age of death of the individuals in that same population.

**lifestyle** The pattern of living and behavior of an individual, society, or culture, esp. as it distinguishes individuals concerned or included in the groups from other individuals or groups.

**life support** The use of any technique, therapy, or device to assist in sustaining life. SEE: *basic l.s.*

***advanced cardiac l.s.*** ABBR: ACLS. A procedure that includes basic life support (BLS), plus the use of adjunctive equipment to support ventilation, establishment of an IV fluid lifeline, drug administration, cardiac monitoring, defibrillation, control of cardiac arrhythmias, and postresuscitation care. ACLS requires the supervision of a physician in person at the scene of the emergency, direct communication with one, or an alternative method of communication previously defined by the physician, such as standing orders. Patients in whom field resususcitation (i.e., prehospital ACLS) fails are usually rushed to a local emergency department where resuscitation attempts are continued, though few of these patients survive. SEE: *basic life support; cardiopulmonary resuscitation; emergency cardiac care.*

***advanced l.s.*** ABBR: ALS. The use of advanced airway procedures, drug administration, cardiac monitoring, defibrillation/cardioversion, or invasive procedures by emergency medical technicians to attempt to save the lives of the critically ill or injured in a prehospital setting.

***advanced trauma l.s.*** ABBR: ATLS. Treatment measures necessary to stabilize a seriously injured patient.

***basic l.s.*** ABBR: BLS. The phase of cardiopulmonary resuscitation (CPR) and emergency cardiac care that either (1) prevents circulatory or respiratory arrest or insufficiency by prompt recognition and early intervention or by early entry into the emergency care system or both; or (2) externally supports the circulation and respiration of a victim of cardiac arrest through CPR. When cardiac or respiratory arrest occurs, BLS should be initiated by anyone present who is familiar with CPR. SEE: *advanced cardiac life support; bag-valve-mask resuscitator; cardiopulmonary resuscitation; emergency cardiac care; Heimlich maneuver.*

***withholding l.s.*** Removal of or not giving medical interventions, with the expectation that the patient will die as a result.

**life-sustaining therapy** Therapy of a critically ill patient that, if discontinued, would cause the patient to die.

**ligament** (lĭg′ă-mĕnt) [L. *ligamentum,* a band] **1.** A band or sheet of strong fibrous connective tissue connecting the articular ends of bones, binding them together and facilitating or limiting motion. **2.** A thickened portion or fold of peritoneum or mesentery that supports a visceral organ or connects it to another viscus. **3.** A band of fibrous connective tissue connecting bones, cartilages, and other structures and serving to support or attach fascia or muscles. **4.** A cordlike structure representing the vestigial remains of a fetal blood vessel.

***accessory l.*** A ligament that supplements another, esp. one on the lateral surface of a joint. This type of ligament lies outside of and independent of the capsule of a joint.

***acromioclavicular l.*** The ligament supporting the acromioclavicular joint; it joins the acromial process of the scapula and the distal end of the clavicle and in combination with the coracoclavicular ligaments, holds the clavicle down.

***alar l.*** One of a pair of ligaments that stabilize the dens of the second vertebra to the occipital bone of the skull, limiting side flexion and rotation of the head.

***annular l.*** A circular ligament, esp. one enclosing a head or radius or one holding the footplate of the stapes in the fenestra vestibuli.

***anterior talofibular l.*** The ligament of the ankle that connects the lateral talus and fibular malleolus, preventing anterior displacement of the talus in the mortisse. This ligament is injured with an inversion movement and is the most commonly injured ligament of the ankle.

***apical l.*** A single median ligament extending from the odontoid process to the occipital bone.

***arcuate l.'s*** The lateral, medial, and exterior ligaments that extend from the 12th rib to the transverse process of the first lumbar vertebra, to which the diaphragm is attached.

***arterial l.*** A fibrous cord extending from the pulmonary artery to the arch of the aorta, the remains of the ductus arteriosus of the fetus.

***auricular l.'s*** The anterior, posterior, and superior auricular ligaments uniting the external ear to the temporal bone.

***broad l. of liver*** A wide, sickle-shaped fold of peritoneum, attached to the lower surface of the diaphragm, the internal surface of the right rectus abdominis muscle, and the convex surface of the liver.

***broad l. of uterus*** The folds of peritoneum attached to lateral borders of the uterus from insertion of the fallopian tube above to the pelvic wall. It consists of two leaves between which are found the remnants of the wolffian ducts, cellular tissues, and the major blood vessels of the pelvis.

***capsular l.'s*** Heavy fibrous structures, lined with synovial membrane and surrounding articulations.

***carpal l.'s*** The ligaments uniting the carpal bones.

***caudal l.*** The ligament formed by bundles of fibrous tissue uniting dorsal surfaces of the two lower coccygeal vertebrae and superjacent skin.

***check l.*** A ligament that restrains the motion of a joint, esp. the lateral odontoid ligaments.

***collateral l.*** One of the ligaments that provide medial and lateral stability to joints. They include the medial (ulnar) and lateral (radial) collateral ligaments at the elbow, the medial (tibial) and lateral (fibular) collateral ligaments at the knee, the medial (deltoid) and lateral collateral ligaments at the ankle, and the collateral ligaments of the fingers.

***conoid l.*** The posterior and inner portion of the coracoclavicular ligament.

***coracoacromial l.*** The broad triangular ligament attached to the outer edge of the coracoid process of the scapula and the tip of the acromion.

***coracoclavicular l.*** The ligament uniting the clavicle and coracoid process of the scapula.

***coracohumeral l.*** The broad ligament connecting the coracoid process of the scapula to the greater tubercle of the humerus.

***coronary l. of liver*** A fold of peritoneum extending from the posterior edge of the liver to diaphragm.

***costocolic l.*** The ligament attaching the splenic flexure of the colon to the diaphragm.

***costocoracoid l.*** The ligament joining the first rib and coracoid process of the scapula.

***costotransverse l.'s*** The ligaments uniting the ribs with the transverse processes of vertebrae.

***costovertebral l.'s*** Ligaments uniting the ribs and vertebrae.

***cricopharyngeal l.*** A ligamentous bundle between the upper and posterior border of the cricoid cartilage and the anterior wall of the pharynx.

***cricothyroid l.*** The ligament uniting cricoid and thyroid cartilages and the location for the horizontal incision (called coniotomy) to prevent choking.

***cricotracheal l.*** The ligamentous structure uniting the upper ring of the trachea and the cricoid cartilage.

***cruciate l.*** **1.** The ligament of the ankle passing transversely across the dorsum of the foot that holds tendons of the anterior muscle group in place. **2.** A cross-shaped ligament of the atlas consisting of the transverse ligament and superior and inferior bands, the former passing upward and attaching to the margin of the foramen magnum, the latter passing downward and attaching to the body of the atlas. **3.** The ligament of the knee that originates on the anterior portion of the femur in the intercondylar notch and inserts on the posterior aspect of the tibial plateau. It prevents posterior translation of the tibia on the femur and, in combination with the anterior cruciate ligament, provides rotary stability to the knee.

***cruciform l.*** A structure consisting of one ligament crossing another.

***crural l.*** Inguinal l.

***deltoid l.*** The interior lateral ligament of the ankle.

***dentate l.*** A fibrous band of pia mater extending the length of the spinal cord on each side between the spinal nerves. It has a scalloped appearance as it pierces the arachnoid to attach to the dura mater at regular intervals.

***dentoalveolar l.*** Periodontal l.

***falciform l. of liver*** A wide, sickle-shaped fold of peritoneum attached to the lower surface of the diaphragm, internal surface of the right rectus abdominis muscle, and convex surface of the liver.

***fundiform l. of penis*** The ligament extending from the lower portion of the linea alba and Scarpa's fascia to the dorsum of the penis.

***gastrophrenic l.*** A fold of peritoneum between the esophageal end of the stomach and the diaphragm.

***Gimbernat's l.*** SEE: *Gimbernat's ligament.*

***gingivodental l.*** The part of the periodontal ligament that extends into the gingiva and blends with the connective tissue lamina propria.

***glenohumeral l.'s*** Fibers of the coracohumeral ligament passing into the joint and inserted into the inner and upper part of the bicipital groove.

***glenoid l.*** The ligament that extends between the palmar surfaces of phalanges and the corresponding metacarpal bone.

***glossoepiglottidean l.*** The elastic band from the base of the tongue to the epiglottis in the middle glossoepiglottidean fold.

***Henle's l.*** The lateral extension of the tendinous insertion of the rectus abdominis muscle. It is posterior to the falx inguinalis.

***hepaticoduodenal l.*** A fold of peritoneum from the transverse fissure of the liver to the vicinity of the duodenum and right flexure of colon, forming the anterior boundary of the foramen of Winslow.

***iliofemoral l.*** The bundle of fibers forming the upper and anterior portion of the capsular ligament of the hip joint. This ligament extends from the ilium to the intertrochanteric line. SYN: *Y ligament.*

***iliolumbar l.*** The ligament extending from the fourth and fifth lumbar vertebrae to the iliac crest.

***iliopectineal l.*** A portion of the pelvic fascia attached to the iliopectineal line and to the capsular ligament of the hip joint.

***infundibulopelvic l.*** Suspensory l. of ovary.

***inguinal l.*** The ligament extending from the anterior superior iliac spine to the pubic tubercle. It forms the lower margin of aponeurosis of the exterior oblique muscle. SYN: *crural l.; Poupart's l.*

***interclavicular l.*** The bundle of fibers between the sternal ends of the clavicles, attached to the interclavicular notch of the sternum.

***interspinal l.*** The ligament extending from the superior margin of a spinous process of one vertebra to the lower margin of the one above.

***ischiocapsular l.*** In the hip, the ligament extending from the ischium to the ischial border of the acetabulum.

***lacunar l.*** SEE: *Gimbernat's ligament.*

***lateral occipitoatlantal l.*** The ligament on each side between the transverse processes of the atlas and the jugular process of the occipital bone.

***lateral odontoid l.*** One of the strong ligaments extending between the sides of the odontoid process of the axis of the spinal column and the inner sides of condyles of the occipital bone.

***lateral l.'s of liver*** Folds of peritoneum extending from the lower surface of the diaphragm to adjacent borders of the right and left lobes of the liver. SYN: *triangular l.'s of liver.*

***lateral umbilical l.*** The fibrous cord extending from the bladder to the umbilicus. It represents the obliterated interior iliac artery of the fetus.

***Lisfranc's l.'s*** SEE: *Lisfranc's ligament.*

***Lockwood's l.*** SEE: *Lockwood's ligament.*

***medial l.*** A broad ligament that connects the medial malleolus of the tibia to the tarsal bones.

***median umbilical l.*** The fibrous cord extending from the apex of the bladder to the umbilicus. It represents the remains of the urachus of the fetus.

***meniscofemoral l.'s*** Two small ligaments of the knee, one anterior and one posterior. The anterior one attaches to the posterior area of the lateral meniscus and the anterior cruciate ligament. The posterior one attaches to the posterior area of the lateral meniscus and the medial condyle of the femur.

***middle costotransverse l.*** A ligament consisting of parallel fibers extending between a vertebra and its adjacent rib.

***nephrocolic l.'s*** Fibrous strands that connect the kidneys with the ascending and descending colon.

***nuchal l.*** The upward continuation of the supraspinous ligament, extending from the seventh cervical vertebra to the occipital bone.

***palpebral l.'s*** Two ligaments, medial and lateral, extending from tarsal plates of the eyelids to the frontal process of the maxilla and the zygomatic bone respectively.

***patellar l.*** A strong, flat band securing the patella to the tibia. It is a continuation of the tendon of the quadriceps femoris muscle.

***pectineal l.*** A triangular-shaped ligament that extends from the medial end of the inguinal ligament and the pectineal line of the pubis.

***periodontal l.*** ABBR: PDL. The connective tissue attached to the cementum on the outer surface of a dental root and the osseous tissue of the alveolar process. The periodontal ligament holds the teeth in the sockets of the bone. SYN: *dentoalveolar l.; alveolar periosteum.*

***Petit's l.*** SEE: *Petit's ligament.*

***phrenocolic l.*** A fold of peritoneum joining the left colic flexure of the colon to the adjacent costal portion of the diaphragm.

***popliteal arcuate l.*** The ligament on the posterolateral side of the knee, extending from the head of the fibula to the joint capsule.

***Poupart's l.*** Inguinal l.

***pterygomandibular l.*** The band of fiber extending between the apex of the internal pterygoid plate of the sphenoid bone and the posterior extremity of the internal oblique line of the mandible.

***pubic arcuate l.'s*** The ligaments connecting the pubic bones at the symphysis pubis, including anterior and superior pubic ligaments and the arcuate (inferior) ligament.

***pulmonary l.*** A fold of pleura that extends from the hilus of the lung to the base of the medial surface of the lung.

***rhomboid l. of clavicle*** A strong structure extending from the tuberosity of the clavicle to the outer surface of the cartilage of the first rib.

***round l. of femur*** The ligament of the head of the femur that is attached to the anterior superior part of the fovea of the head of the femur and to the sides of the acetabular notch.

***round l. of liver*** A fibrous cord extending upward from the umbilicus and enclosed in lower margin of the falciform ligament; represents obliterated left umbilical vein of the fetus.

***round l. of uterus*** One of the ligaments attached to the uterus immediately below and in front of the entrance of the fallopian tube. Each extends laterally in the broad ligament to the pelvic wall, where it passes through inguinal ring, terminating in the labium majora.

***sacroiliac l.'s*** Two ligaments, the anterior and posterior, that connect sacrum and ilium.

***sacrospinous l.*** The ligament extending from the spine of the ischium to the sacrum and coccyx in front of the sacrotuberous ligament.

***sacrotuberous l.*** The ligament extending from the tuberosity of the ischium to the posterior superior and inferior iliac spines and to the lower part of the sacrum and coccyx.

***sphenomandibular l.*** The ligament attached superiorly to the spine of the sphenoid and inferiorly to the lingula of the mandible.

***spiral l. of cochlea*** The thickened periosteum of the peripheral wall of the osseous cochlear canal. The basilar membrane is attached to its inner surface.

***stylohyoid l.*** A thin fibroelastic cord between the lesser cornu of the hyoid bone and the apex of the styloid process of the temporal bone.

***stylomandibular l.*** A thin fibrous band of tissue extending between the styloid process of the temporal bone and the lower part of the posterior border of the ramus of the mandible. SYN: *stylomaxillary l.*

***stylomaxillary l.*** Stylomandibular l.

***suprascapular l.*** A thin fibrous band of tissue extending from the base of the coracoid process of the scapula to the inner margin of the suprascapular notch.

***supraspinal l.*** A ligament uniting the apices of the spinous processes of the vertebrae.

***suspensory l.*** A ligament suspending an organ.

***suspensory l. of axilla*** The continuation of the clavipectoral fascia down to attach to the axillary fascia.

***suspensory l. of lens*** The zonula ciliaris (ciliary zonule); the fibers holding the crystalline lens in position.

***suspensory l. of ovary*** A ligament extending from the tubal end of the ovary laterally to the pelvic wall. It lies in the layers of the broad ligament in which the ovarian artery is found. SYN: *infundibulopelvic l.*

***suspensory l. of penis*** A triangular bundle of fibrous tissue extending from the anterior surface of the symphysis pubis and adjacent structures to the dorsum of the base of the penis.

***suspensory l.'s of uterus*** The broad ligaments, the round ligaments, and the rectouterine folds of the uterus.

***sutural l.'s*** Thin, fibrous layers interposed between articulating surfaces of bones united by suture.

***temporomandibular l.*** The thickened portion of the joint capsule that passes from the articular tubercle at the root of the zygomatic arch to attach to the subcondylar neck of the mandible.

***tendinotrochanteric l.*** A ligament that forms a part of the capsule of the hip joint.

***transverse crural l.*** The ligament lying on the anterior surface of the leg just above the ankle.

***transverse humeral l.*** A fibrous band that bridges the bicipital groove of the humerus in connecting the lesser and greater tuberosities.

***transverse l. of atlas*** A strong ligament passing over the odontoid process of the axis.

***transverse l. of hip joint*** A ligamentous band extending across the cotyloid notch of the acetabulum.

***transverse l. of knee joint*** A fibrous band extending from the anterior margin of the external semilunar fibrocartilage of the knee to the extremity of the internal semilunar fibrocartilage.

***trapezoid l.*** The anterior exterior portion of the coracoclavicular ligament.

***triangular l.'s of liver*** Lateral l.'s of liver.

***uterorectosacral l.*** One of the ligaments that arise from the sides of the cervix and pass upward and backward, passing around the rectum, to the second sacral vertebra. They are enclosed within the rectouterine folds, which demarcate the borders of the rectouterine pouch.

***uterosacral l.*** SEE: *Petit's ligament.*

***venous l. of liver*** A solid fibrous cord representing the obliterated ductus venosus of the fetus. It lies between the caudate and left lobes of the liver and connects the left branch of the portal vein to the inferior vena cava.

***ventricular l. of larynx*** The lateral free margin of the quadrangular membrane. It is enclosed within and supports the ventricular fold.

***vesicouterine l.*** The ligament that attaches the anterior aspect of the uterus to the bladder.

***vestibular l.*** A thin fibrous band attached anteriorly to the lamina of the thyroid cartilage and posteriorly to the anterior portion of the arytenoid cartilage.

***vocal l.*** The thickened free edges of the elastic cone extending from the thyroid angle to the vocal processes of arytenoid cartilages. They support the vocal folds.

***Weitbrecht's l.*** SEE: *Weitbrecht's ligament.*

***yellow l.*** One of the ligaments connecting the laminae of adjacent vertebrae.

**ligamenta** Pl. of ligamentum.

**ligamentopexis** (lĭg″ă-mĕn″tō-pĕks′ĭs) [L. *ligamentum,* band, + Gr. *pexis,* fixation] Suspension of the uterus on the round ligament.

**ligamentous** (lĭg″ă-mĕn′tŭs) [L. *ligamentum,* band] **1.** Relating to a ligament. **2.** Like a ligament.

**ligamentum** (lĭg″ă-mĕn′tŭm) *pl.* **ligamenta** [L., a band] Ligament.

**ligand** (lī′gănd, lĭg′ănd) [L. *ligare,* to bind] **1.** In chemistry, an organic molecule attached to a central metal ion by multiple bonds. **2.** In immunology, a small molecule bound to another chemical group or molecule.

**ligase** (lī′gās, lĭg′ās) The general term for a class of enzymes that catalyze the joining of the ends of two chains of DNA.

**ligate** (lī′gāt) To apply a ligature.

**ligation** (lī-gā′shŭn) The application of a ligature.

***rubber-band l.*** Application of a rubber band around a superficial bit of tissue such as a hemorrhoid. Because the blood supply is cut off, the tissue dies and sloughs off.

**ligature** (lĭg′ă-chūr) [L. *ligatura,* a binding] **1.** Process of binding or tying. **2.** A band or bandage. **3.** A thread or wire for tying a blood vessel or other structure in order to constrict or fasten it. The cord or material used may be catgut, synthetic suture materials such as nylon or Dacron, polyglycolic acid, or natural fibers such as silk or cotton. Sometimes strips of fascia obtained from the patient are used as a ligature. SEE: *suture.*

**light** (līt) [AS. *lihtan,* to shine] The sensation produced by electromagnetic radiation that falls on the retina. Radiant energy producing a sensation of luminosity on the retina is limited to a wavelength of about 400 nm (extreme violet) to 770 nm (extreme red). SEE: *laser; ray; seasonal affective disorder.*

***l. adaptation*** Changes that occur in a dark-adapted eye in order for vision to occur in moderate or bright light. Principal changes are contraction of the pupil and bleaching of visual purple in the rods. Bright sunlight is 30,000 times the intensity of bright moonlight, but the eye adapts so that visual function is possible under both conditions. SEE: *night vision; vision.*

***axial l.*** Light with rays parallel to each other and to the optic axis.

***cold l.*** Any form of light that is not perceptibly warm. The heat of ordinary light rays is dissipated when they are passed through some medium such as quartz.

***l. difference*** The difference between the two eyes with respect to sensitivity to light intensity.

***diffused l.*** Rays broken by refraction.

***idioretinal l.*** The sensation of light when there are no retinal stimuli to produce that sensation. SYN: *intrinsic l.*

***intrinsic l.*** Idioretinal l.

***oblique l.*** Light that strikes a surface obliquely.

***polarized l.*** Light in which waves vibrate in one direction only.

***reflected l.*** Light rays that are thrown back by an illuminated object such as a mirror.

***refracted l.*** Rays bent from their original course.

***l. sense*** One of the three parts of visual function, the other parts being color sense and form sense. It is tested by visual field examination. SEE: *color sense; form sense.*

***l. therapy*** Phototherapy.

***transmitted l.*** Light that passes through an object.

***white l.*** Light that contains all of the visible wavelengths of light.

***Wood's l.*** SEE: *Wood's rays.*

**lightening** [AS. *leohte,* not heavy] The descent of the presenting part of the fetus into the pelvis. This often occurs 2 to 3 weeks before the first stage of labor begins. It may not occur in multiparas until active labor begins. SYN: *engagement.* SEE: *labor.*

**light-headedness** The feeling of dizziness or of being about to faint; a possible sign of postural hypotension. SEE: *vertigo, benign positional.*

**lightning** The discharge of atmospheric electricity from cloud to cloud or from cloud to earth. About 100 lightning strokes hit the earth every second. Thirty percent of persons struck by lightning die. SEE: *lightning safety rules.*

**lightning safety rules** Rules that, if followed, could reduce the estimated 100 deaths that occur annually in the U.S. from electrocution due to lightning. During a lightning storm one should remain indoors, but should not stay near open doors, fireplaces, radiators, or appliances. Plug-in electric equipment such as hair dryers, electric toothbrushes, or electric razors should not be used. One should not take laundry off clotheslines or work on fences, computers or word processors, telephones or telephone lines, power lines, pipelines, or structural steel construction, or metal objects such as fishing rods or golf clubs. When outdoors, one should avoid hilltops; in a forest, shelter should be sought in a low area under a thick growth of small trees. Open spaces, wire fences, metal clotheslines, exposed sheds, and all electrically conductive elevated objects should be avoided. Persons should get out of water and off small boats, but stay in an automobile if traveling. If an electrical charge is evidenced by hair standing on end or tingling of the skin, one should immediately squat down with feet touching each other and hands clasped around the knees. No part of the rest of the body should touch the ground. This may prevent being struck by lightning. It is important to be aware that when lightning occurs, the charge that may be as much as 100 million volts of current is trying to find a direct path to the ground and the one with the least resistance. Trees conduct electricity better than air, and metal and water conduct better than trees. Lightning will strike the tallest object. One should not be the tallest object during a storm and should not stand close to good conductors.

**lightning streaks, Moore's** SEE: *Moore's*

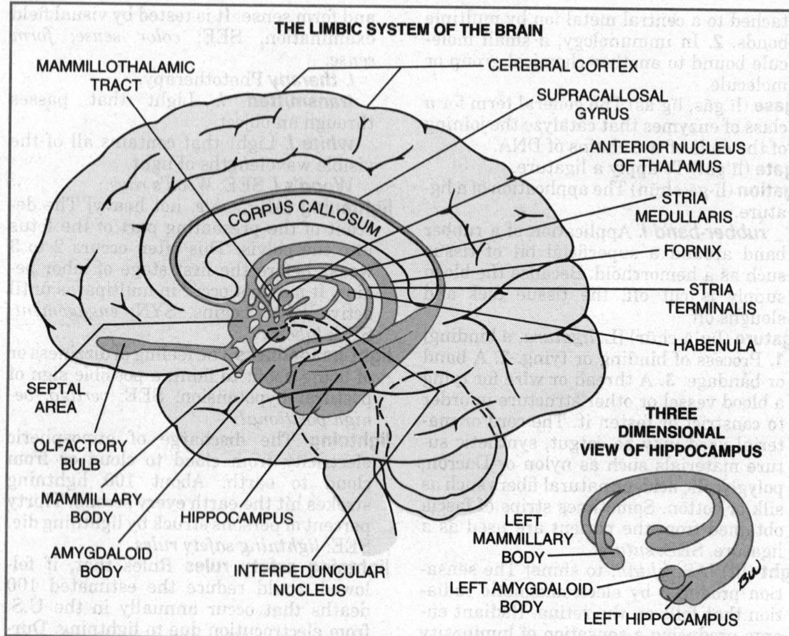


*lightning streaks.*

**lignin** (lĭg′nĭn) A polysaccharide present in plants that combines with cellulose to form the cell walls.

**lignocaine** (lĭg′nō-kān) A local anesthetic. SEE: *lidocaine hydrochloride*.

**lignoceric acid** A saturated, naturally occurring fatty acid, $C_{24}H_{48}O_2$, present in certain foods, including peanuts.

**limb** (lĭm) [AS. *lim*] **1.** An arm or leg. **2.** An extremity. **3.** A limblike extension of a structure.

***anacrotic l.*** The ascending portion of the pulse wave.

***anterior l. of internal capsule*** The lenticulocaudate portion that lies between the lenticular and caudate nuclei.

***ascending l. of renal tubule*** The portion of the tubule between the bend in Henle's loop and the distal convoluted section.

***catacrotic l.*** The descending portion of the pulse wave.

***descending l. of renal tubule*** The portion of the tubule between the proximal convoluted section and the bend in Henle's loop.

***pectoral l.*** The arm.

***pelvic l.*** The lower extremity.

***phantom l.*** SEE: *sensation, phantom.*

***l. replantation*** The surgical reattachment of a traumatically amputated limb or part.

***thoracic l.*** The upper extremity.

**limbic** (lĭm′bĭk) [L. *limbus,* border] Pert. to a limbus or border. SYN: *marginal.*

***l. system*** A group of brain structures, including the hippocampus, amygdala, dentate gyrus, cingulate gyrus, gyrus fornicatus, the archicortex, and their interconnections and connections with the hypothalamus, septal area, and a medial area of the mesencephalic tegmentum. The system is activated by motivated behavior and arousal, and it influences the endocrine and autonomic motor systems. SEE: illus.

**limbus** (lĭm′bŭs) *pl.* **limbi** [L., border] The edge or border of a part.

***l. alveolaris*** **1.** The upper free edge of the alveolar process of the mandible. **2.** The lower free edge of the alveolar process of the maxilla. SYN: *arcus alveolaris maxillae.*

***l. conjunctivae*** The edge of the conjunctiva overlapping the cornea.

***l. corneae*** The edge of the cornea where it unites with the sclera.

***corneoscleral l.*** In the eye, a transitional dome 1 or 2 mm wide where the cornea joins the sclera and conjunctiva.

***l. fossae ovalis*** The thickened margin of the fossae ovalis, esp. the rim of the septum secundum bounding the fossa.

***l. laminae spiralis osseae*** A thickening of the periosteum of the osseous spiral lamina of the cochlea to which the tectorial membrane is attached.

***l. palpebrales anteriores*** The anterior margin of the free edge of the eyelids from which the cilia or eyelashes grow.

***l. palpebrales posteriores*** The posterior margin of the free edge of the eyelids; the region of transition of skin to conjunctival mucous membrane.

***l. sphenoidalis*** Ridge on anterior portion of upper surface of sphenoid bone.

**lime** (līm) [AS. *lim*, glue] Calcium oxide, CaO. A substance obtained from limestone. Calcium oxide is prepared from limestone, $CaCO_3$, by heating it sufficiently to drive off the carbon dioxide. When lime is mixed with water, heat is produced. Lime is an ingredient of cement and mortar. SYN: *calcium oxide; quicklime*. SEE: *calcium*.

Caution: Lime should not come into contact with one's eyes or be inhaled.

***chlorinated l.*** A substance resulting from chlorination of slaked lime, consisting chiefly of calcium chloride and calcium hypochlorite. It is used principally as a disinfectant and in aqueous solution as a bleaching agent.

***slaked l.*** The substance produced when lime is allowed free access to water and carbon dioxide from the atmosphere. It is a mixture of calcium hydroxide, $Ca(OH)_2$, and calcium carbonate, $CaCO_3$.

***soda l.*** A combination of calcium oxide and sodium hydroxide.

***sulfurated l.*** A solution of lime, sublimated sulfur, and water, used as a topical solution in treating skin disease.

***l. water*** Alkaline solution of calcium hydroxide, $Ca(OH)_2$, in water; a weak base used as an antacid.

**lime** [Fr.] The fruit of *Citrus aurantifolia*, the juice of which is antiscorbutic.

**limen** (lī'mĕn) *pl.* **limina** [L.] Entrance; threshold.

***l. nasi*** The boundary line between the bony and cartilaginous portion of the nasal cavity. It is also at this point that the nasal cavity proper and the vestibule of the nose meet.

***l. of insula*** The portion of the cortex of the brain that provides a threshold to the insula. The middle cerebral artery passes over this threshold to extend to the insula.

**limes nul** SYMB: $L_0$. The greatest amount of toxin that, when mixed with 1 unit of antitoxin and injected into a guinea pig weighing 250 g, will cause no local reaction.

**limes tod** SYMB: $L_+$. The least amount of toxin that, when mixed with 1 unit of antitoxin and injected into a guinea pig weighing 250 g, will kill it within 96 hr.

**limestone** A rock formed of organic fossil remains of shells, composed mostly of calcium carbonate. SEE: *lime*.

**liminal** (lĭm'ĭ-năl) [L. *limen*, threshold] Hardly perceptible; relating to a threshold as of consciousness or vision. SEE: *subliminal*.

**limit** (lĭm'ĭt) **1.** A boundary. **2.** A point or line beyond which something cannot or may not progress.

***assimilation l.*** The amount of carbohydrate that can be absorbed or ingested without causing glycosuria.

***audibility l.*** The limits of sound frequencies at both the low and high ends of the sound scale beyond which sound cannot be heard. The lower limit is approx. 8 to 16 Hz (cycles per second) and the upper limit between 12,000 and 20,000 Hz, depending on various factors, including age. In general, the upper limit of audible sound decreases with age.

***elastic l.*** The extent to which something may be stretched or bent and still have the ability to return to its original shape.

***l. of flocculation*** The amount of a toxin or toxoid that causes the most rapid flocculation when combined with its antitoxin.

***Hayflick's l.*** SEE: *Hayflick's limit*.

***l. of perception*** The smallest object that can be detected by the eye. Such an object usually subtends a visual image of 1 minute. This produces a retinal image slightly larger than the diameter of a retinal cone (i.e., about 0.004 mm). SYN: *normal limit of visual acuity*.

***quantum l.*** The minimum wavelength present in the spectrum produced by x-rays.

***ventilator l.*** A secondary ventilator alarm or stop mechanism that prevents a specific variable from exceeding a preset parameter.

**limitans** (lĭm'ĭ-tăns) [L. *limitare*, to limit] **1.** A term used in conjunction with other words to denote limiting. **2.** Membrane limitans.

**limitation** (lĭm"ĭ-tā'shŭn) The condition of being limited.

***l. of motion*** The restriction of movement or range of motion of a part or joint, esp. that imposed by disease or trauma to joints and soft tissues.

**limnology** [Gr. *limne*, pool, + *logos*, study] The scientific study of all of the features of a body of fresh water such as a pond, lake, or river that are important ecologically (i.e., potability, pH, degree of pollution, mineral content, and variation with seasonal and climatic changes).

**limonene** (lĭm'ō-nēn) An essential oil derived from orange or lemon peel. It is used as a flavoring agent in cough syrups.

**limp** To walk with abnormal, jerky movements.

**lincomycin hydrochloride** (lĭn"kō-mī'sĭn) An antibiotic obtained from *Streptomyces lincolnensis*.

**lincture, linctus** (lĭnk'tūr, -tŭs) [L. *linctus*, a licking] A thick, sweet, syrupy medicinal preparation given for its effect on the throat, usually sipped but may be licked or sucked as with a throat lozenge.

**lindane** (lĭn'dān) SYN: *gamma benzene hexachloride*.

**Lindau's disease** (lĭn'dowz) [Arvid Lindau, Swedish pathologist, 1892–1958] Lindau-von Hippel disease.

**Lindau-von Hippel disease** (lĭn′dow-vŏn-hĭp′ĕl) [Arvid Lindau; Eugen von Hippel, Ger. ophthalmologist, 1867–1939] Angiomata of the retina and cysts and angiomata of the brain and certain visceral organs.

**line** (līn) [L. *linea*] **1.** Any long, relatively narrow mark. **2.** A boundary or outline. **3.** A wrinkle. **4.** In anthropometry or cephalometry, an imaginary line connecting two anatomical points. This is necessary to establish a plane or an axis. **5.** A catheter attached to a patient, as an intravenous line or arterial line.

***abdominal l.*** A line indicating abdominal muscle boundaries.

***absorption l.*** A black line in the continuous spectrum of light passing through an absorbing medium.

***alveolobasilar l.*** The line from basion to alveolar point.

***alveolonasal l.*** The line from alveolar point to nasion.

***auriculobregmatic l.*** The line from auricular point to bregma.

***axial l.*** A line running in the main axis of the body or part of it. The axial line of the hand runs through the middle digit; the axial line of the foot runs through the second digit.

***axillary l.'s*** Anterior, posterior, and midaxillary lines that extend downward from the axilla.

***base l.*** The line from the infraorbital ridge through the middle of the external auditory meatus to midline of occiput.

***basiobregmatic l.*** The line from basion to bregma.

***Baudelocque's l.*** SEE: *Baudelocque's diameter.*

***Beau's l.'s*** SEE: *Beau's lines.*

***biauricular l.*** A line over the vertex from one auditory meatus to the other.

***blue l.*** Lead l.

***canthomeatal l.*** An imaginary line extending from the canthus of the eye to the center of the external auditory meatus. SYN: *orbitomeatal line.*

***cement l.*** The refractile boundary of an osteon of the haversian system of a bone.

***cervical l.*** **1.** A line of junction of cementum and enamel of a tooth. **2.** A line on the neck of the tooth where the gum is attached.

***cleavage l.'s*** Langer's lines.

***costoarticular l.*** The line from sternoclavicular joint to a point on the 11th rib.

***costoclavicular l.*** The line midway between the nipple and the sternum border.

***l. of demarcation*** A line of division between healthy and diseased tissue.

***Douglas' l.*** A crescent-shaped line at the lower limit of the posterior sheath of the rectus abdominis muscle. It is sometimes indistinct.

***epiphyseal l.*** A line at the junction of the epiphysis and diaphysis of a long bone. It is at this junction that bone growth occurs. SYN: *epiphyseal disk.*

***l. of fixation*** An imaginary line drawn from the subject viewed to the fovea centralis.

***gingival l.*** A line determined by the extent of coverage of the tooth by gingiva. The shape of the gingival line is similar to the curvature of the cervical line but they rarely coincide. It is also called the free gingival margin.

***glabelloalveolar l.*** An imaginary line through the glabella on the frontal bone and the alveolar process of the maxilla.

***glabellomeatal l.*** An imaginary line that extends from the glabella to the center of the external auditory meatus and is used for radiographical positioning of the skull.

***gluteal l.'s*** Three lines—anterior, posterior, and inferior—on the exterior surface of the ilium.

***gum l.*** Gingival l.

***iliopectineal l.*** The bony ridge marking the brim of the pelvis.

***incremental l.*** One of the lines seen in a microscopic section of tooth enamel. They resemble growth lines in a tree.

***incremental l. of Retzius*** Periodic dark lines seen in the enamel of a tooth that represent occasional metabolic disturbances of mineralization.

***incremental l. of von Ebner*** Very light lines in the dentin of a tooth that represent the boundary between the layers of dentin produced daily.

***inferior nuchal l.*** One of two curved ridges on the occipital bone extending laterally from the exterior occipital crest. SEE: *superior nuchal l.*

***infraorbitomeatal l.*** An imaginary line from the inferior orbital margin to the external auditory meatus, used for radiographical positioning of the skull.

***interauricular l.*** A line joining the two auricular points.

***intercondylar l.*** The transverse ridge joining condyles of the femur above the intercondyloid fossa.

***intermediate l. of ilium*** The ridge on the crest of the ilium between the inner and outer lips.

***interpupillary l.*** An imaginary line between the centers of the eyes, used for radiographical positioning of the skull.

***intertrochanteric l.*** The ridge on the posterior surface of the femur exterior between the greater and lesser trochanters.

***intertuberal l.*** The line joining the inner borders of the ischial tuberosities below the small sciatic notch.

***Langer's l.'s*** SEE: *Langer's lines.*

***lateral supracondylar l.*** One of two ridges on the posterior surface of the distal end of the femur, formed by diverging lips of the linea aspera. SEE: *medial supracondylar l.*

***lead l.*** An irregular dark line in the gingival margin. The line is present in chronic lead poisoning and is caused by the deposition of lead in that portion of the gum. SYN: *blue l.*

***lip l.*** The highest or lowest point the lips reach on the teeth or gums during a broad smile.

***M l.*** In striated muscle, the thin, dark line in the center of an H band of a sarcomere. It contains the protein that connects the thick (myosin) filaments. SYN: *M disk.*

***mamillary l.*** An imaginary vertical line through the center of the nipple.

***mammary l.*** An imaginary horizontal line from one nipple to the other.

***medial supracondylar l.*** One of two ridges on the posterior surface of the distal end of the femur, formed by diverging lips of the linea aspera. SEE: *lateral supracondylar l.*

***median l.*** An imaginary line joining any two points in the periphery of the median plane of the body or one of its parts.

***mentomeatal l.*** An imaginary line from the mental point of the mandible to the external auditory meatus, used in radiography of the skull.

***milk l.*** SEE: *ridge, mammary.*

***mucogingival l.*** SEE: *junction, mucogingival.*

***mylohyoid l.*** A ridge on the inner surface of the mandible. It extends from a point beneath the mental spine upward and back to the ramus past the last molar. The mylohyoid muscle and the superior constrictor muscle of the pharynx attach to this ridge.

***nasobasilar l.*** A line through the basion and nasion.

***oblique l. of fibula*** The medial crest of posteromedial border; a line extending from the medial side of the head and terminating distally at the interosseous crest.

***oblique l. of mandible*** The ridge on the outer surface of the lower jaw.

***oblique l. of radius*** The faint ridge on the anterior surface passing downward and laterally from the radial tuberosity.

***orbitomeatal l.*** The imaginary line running through the mid-orbit and external auditory meatus.

***l.'s of Owen*** [Sir Richard Owen, Brit. anatomist, 1804–1892] Occasional prominent growth lines or bands in the dentin of a tooth. They provide a record of the growth of the coronal or radicular dentin.

***parasternal l.*** The line midway between the nipple and the border of the sternum.

***pectineal l.*** The line on the posterior surface of the femur extending downward from the lesser trochanter. It is the portion of the iliopectineal line formed by the os pubis.

***popliteal l. of femur*** An oblique line on the posterior surface of the tibia.

***popliteal l. of tibia*** A line on the posterior surface of the tibia, extending obliquely downward from the fibular facet on the lateral condyle to the medial border of the bone.

***resting l.*** A smooth cement line seen in microscopic sections that separates old bone from newly formed bone.

***reversal l.*** A cement line seen in microscopic sections of bone that shows scallops and irregularites representing earlier bone resorption. Resorption to that point occurred before the process reversed and new bone was formed by apposition. SEE: *Howship's lacunae.*

***scapular l.*** The line extending downward from the lower angle of the scapula.

***semilunar l.*** Spigelian line.

***Shenton's l.*** SEE: *Shenton's line.*

***sight l.*** The line from the center of the pupil to a viewed object.

***spigelian l.*** SEE: *spigelian line.*

***sternal l.*** The medial line of the sternum.

***sternomastoid l.*** The line from between the heads of the sternomastoid muscle to the mastoid process.

***superior nuchal l.*** One of two curved ridges on the occipital bone extending laterally from the exterior occipital crest. SEE: *inferior nuchal l.*

***supraorbital l.*** The line across the forehead above the root of the exterior angular process of the frontal bone.

***temporal l. of frontal bone*** Two curved lines on the lateral surface of the skull, passing upward and backward from the zygomatic process of the frontal bone and terminating posteriorly at the supramastoid crest.

***umbilicopubic l.*** The portion of median line extending from the umbilicus to the symphysis pubis.

***visual l.*** The line that extends from object to macula lutea passing through the nodal point. SYN: *visual axis.*

***Z l.*** In striated muscle, the end boundary of a sarcomere to which the thin filaments (actin) are directly attached. SYN: *Z disk.*

***Zöllner's l.'s*** Parallel lines, usually three long ones, with a series of short lines drawn at regular intervals across one of the lines at approx. 60 degrees. Similar lines are drawn across the second line at the angle of approx. 120 degrees. Short lines are drawn across the third at the same angle as on the first lines. These lines produce the optical illusion that the long lines are converging or diverging.

**linea** (lĭn′ē-ă) *pl.* **lineae** [L. *linea*, line] An anatomical line.

***l. alba*** The white line of connective tissue in the middle of the abdomen from sternum to pubis.

***l. albicantes*** Lines seen on the abdomen, buttocks, and breasts, frequently caused by pregnancy, obesity, or prolonged adrenal cortical hormone therapy but may occur as the result of abdominal distention from any cause. SYN: *striae atrophicae.*

***l. aspera*** A longitudinal ridge on the posterior surface of the middle third of the femur.

***l. costoarticularis*** A line between the sternoclavicular articulation and the point of the 11th rib.

***l. nigra*** A dark line or discoloration of the abdomen that may be seen in pregnant women during the latter part of term. It runs from above the umbilicus to the pubes.

***l. semilunaris*** Spigelian line.

***l. splendens*** A thickening of the pia mater extending along the anterior median surface of the spinal cord. It ensheaths the anterior spinal artery.

***l. sternalis*** The median line of the sternum.

***l. striae atrophicae*** Striae atrophicae.

***l. terminalis*** A bony ridge on the inner surface of the ilium continued on to the pubis that divides the true and false pelvis.

***l. transversae ossis sacri*** Ridges formed by lines of union of the fifth sacral vertebrae.

**linear** (lĭn′ē-ăr) [L. *linea,* line] Pert. to or resembling a line.

***l. energy transfer*** A measure of the rate of energy transfer from ionizing radiation to soft tissue.

**linearity** In radiography, the production of a constant amount of radiation for different combinations of milliamperage and exposure time.

**liner** (līn′ĕr) Anything applied to the inside of a hollow body or structure.

***cavity l.*** A layer of material applied to a cavity preparation to protect the pulp of the tooth. It is usually a suspension of zinc phosphate or calcium hydroxide and is used to neutralize the acidity of the base or cement material.

***soft l.*** The material applied to the underside of a denture to provide a soft surface contact with the oral tissues. Some acrylic or silicone resins have been made resilient and are used as liners. This material is also called cushion liner or resilient liner.

**lingua** (lĭng′gwă) *pl.* **linguae** [L.] The tongue or a tonguelike structure.

***l. frenata*** Ankyloglossia.

***l. geographica*** Geographic tongue.

***l. nigra*** Hairy tongue.

***l. plicata*** Fissured tongue.

**lingual** (lĭng′gwăl) [L. *lingua,* tongue] **1.** Pert. to the tongue. **2.** Tongue-shaped. SYN: *linguiform.* **3.** In dentistry, pert. to the tooth surface that is adjacent to the tongue.

**linguiform** (lĭng′gwĭ-form) [″ + *forma,* shape] Tongue-shaped. SYN: *lingual* (2).

**lingula** (lĭng′gū-lă) [L., little tongue] A tongue-shaped process, esp. lingula cerebelli.

***l. cerebelli*** A tonguelike process of the cerebellum prolonged forward on the upper surface of the superior medullary velum.

***l. of lung*** The projection of lung that separates the cardiac notch from the inferior margin of the left lung.

***l. of mandible*** The projection of bone that forms the medial boundary of the mandibular foramen and gives attachment to the sphenomandibular ligament.

***l. of sphenoid*** The ridge between the body and ala magna of the sphenoid.

**lingulectomy** (lĭng″gū-lĕk′tō-mē) [L. *lingula,* little tongue, + Gr. *ektome,* excision] Surgical removal of the lingula of the upper lobe of the left lung.

**linguo-** [L. *lingua,* tongue] Combining form meaning *tongue.*

**linguoclasia** (lĭng′gwō-klā′zē-ă) [L. *lingua,* tongue, + Gr. *klasis,* destruction] Displacement of a tooth toward the tongue.

**linguoclination** (lĭng′gwō-klī-nā′shŭn) [″ + *clinatus,* leaning] Angulation of a tooth in its vertical axis toward the tongue.

**linguodental** Relating to the tongue and teeth, such as the speech sound "th," which is produced with the aid of the tongue and teeth.

**linguodistal** (lĭng″gwō-dĭs′tăl) [″ + *distare,* to be distant] Concerning the distal part of a tooth and the tongue.

**linguogingival** (lĭng″gwō-jĭn′jĭ-văl) [″ + *gingiva,* gum] Concerning the tongue and the gingiva, or pert. to the lingual and gingival walls of a cavity preparation.

**linguomesial** Pert. to the lingual and mesial surfaces of a tooth or the lingual and mesial walls of a cavity preparation.

**linguo-occlusal** (lĭng″gwō-ŏ-kloo′zăl) [″ + *occludere,* to shut up] Concerning or bounded by the lingual and occlusal surfaces of a tooth.

**linguopapillitis** (lĭng″gwō-păp″ĭ-lī′tĭs) [″ + *papilla,* nipple, + Gr. *itis,* inflammation] Small ulcers of the papillae of the edge of the tongue.

**linguopulpal** Pert. to the lingual and pulpal surfaces of a cavity preparation.

**linguoversion** (lĭng″gwō-vĕr′zhŭn) [″ + *versio,* a turning] Displacement of a tooth toward the tongue.

**liniment** [L. *linimentum,* smearing substance] A liquid containing a medicament and oil, alcohol, or water for use externally. It may be applied by the friction method or on a bandage.

***camphor l.*** A preparation of camphor and a suitable vehicle, such as an oil, that is used topically as an irritant.

***medicinal soft soap l.*** A tincture of green soap.

**linimentum** (lĭn-ĭ-mĕn′tŭm) [L.] Liniment.

**linitis** (lĭn-ī′tĭs) [Gr. *linon,* flax, + *itis,* inflammation] Inflammation of the lining of the stomach.

***l. plastica*** Linitis with thickening of the wall of the stomach, usually due to neoplastic tissue. SYN: *leather-bottle stomach.*

**linkage** In genetics, the association between distinct genes that occupy closely situated loci on the same chromosome. This results in an association in the inheritance of these genes.

***sex l.*** A genetic characteristic that is located on the X or Y chromosome.

**linseed** [AS. *linsaed*] Seed of the common flax, *Linum usitatissimum;* the source of linseed oil. Linseed is used as a demulcent and emollient. SYN: *flaxseed.*

**lint** (lĭnt) [L. *linteum,* made of linen] **1.** Linen scraped until soft and wooly for dressing wounds. **2.** Cotton fiber. **3.** Household dust.

**lintin** (lĭn′tĭn) Prepared absorbent cotton; fabric used in dressings.

**liothyronine sodium** (lī″ō-thī′rō-nēn) Sodium salt of triiodothyronine; used in treating hypothyroidism. SEE: *thyroid function tests.*

**lip-** SEE: *lipo-.*

**lip** [AS. *lippa*] **1.** A soft external structure that forms the boundary of the mouth or opening to the oral cavity. SYN: *labium (or labia) oris.* **2.** One of the lips of the pudendum (labium majus or minus). **3.** A liplike structure forming the border of an opening or groove.

PATHOLOGY: *Chancre:* It is not unusual to have the initial lesion of syphilis appear on the lip of the mouth as an indurated base with a thin secretion and accompanied by enlargement of the submaxillary glands. *Condyloma latum:* This appears as a mucous patch, flattened, coated with gray exudate, with strictly delimited area, usually at the angle of the mouth. *Eczema:* This is characterized by dry fissures, often covered with a crust, bleeding easily, and occurring on both lips. *Epithelioma:* This may be confused with chancre. It seldom appears before the age of 40, but there are exceptions. It may appear as a common cold sore, a painless fissure, or other break of the lower lip. A crust or scab covers the lesion, leaving a raw surface if removed. Pain does not appear until the lesion is well advanced. It is much more common on the lower lip than on the upper. *Herpes:* These lesions may appear on the lips in pneumonia, typhoid, common cold, other febrile diseases, and idiopathically. *Tuberculous ulcer:* This type of ulcer is located at the inner portion of the lip, close to the angle of the mouth. Pathological examination is necessary for verification.

DIAGNOSIS: Examination is considered to be incomplete unless the lips are everted to expose buccal surfaces. *Bluish or purplish:* This sign may appear in the aged, in those exposed to great cold, and in carbon monoxide poisoning. *Dry:* Mouth dryness may be seen in fevers or be caused by drugs such as atropine, by thirst, or by mouth breathing. *Fissured:* This may occur after exposure to cold, in avitaminosis, and in children with congenital syphilis. The dribbling of saliva and a toothless condition may cause fissures in the corners of the mouth. *Pale:* Pallor may be seen in anemia and wasting diseases, in prolonged fever, and after a hemorrhage. *Rashes:* These may be manifestations of typhoid fever, meningitis, or pneumonia. Mucous patches may appear in secondary syphilis, chancre, cancer, and epithelioma.

***cleft l.*** SEE: *cleft lip.*

***double l.*** A redundant fold of mucous membrane in the mouth on either side of the midline of the lip.

***glenoid l.*** A thickened fibrocartilaginous structure surmounting the margin of the acetabulum.

***Hapsburg l.*** A thick, overdeveloped lower lip.

***oral l.'s*** Upper and lower lips that surround the mouth opening and form the anterior wall of the buccal cavity.

***tympanic l.*** The lower border of the sulcus spiralis internus of the cochlea.

***vestibular l.*** The upper border of the sulcus spiralis internus of the cochlea.

**lipacidemia** (lĭp″ăs-ĭ-dē′mē-ă) [Gr. *lipos,* fat, + L. *acidus,* acid, + Gr. *haima,* blood] Excess fatty acids in the blood.

**lipaciduria** (lĭp″ăs-ĭ-dū′rē-ă) [″ + ″ + Gr. *ouron,* urine] Fatty acids in the urine.

**liparocele** (lĭp′ă-rō-sēl) [″ + *kele,* tumor, swelling] **1.** A scrotal hernia containing fat. **2.** A fatty tumor.

**lipase** (lī′pās, lĭ′pās) [″ + *-ase,* enzyme] A lipolytic or fat-splitting enzyme found in the blood, pancreatic secretion, and tissues. Emulsified fats of cream and egg yolk are changed in the stomach to fatty acids and glycerol by gastric lipase. SEE: *digestion; enzyme.*

***pancreatic l.*** Steapsin.

**lipasuria** (lĭp″ăs-ū′rē-ă) [″ + ″ + Gr. *ouron,* urine] Lipase in the urine.

**lipectomy** (lĭ-pĕk′tō-mē) [″ + *ektome,* excision] Excision of fatty tissues.

***suction l.*** SEE: *liposuction.*

**lipedema** (lĭp″ĕ-dē′mă) [″ + *oidema,* swelling] Swelling of the skin, esp. of the lower extremity, owing to accumulation of fat and fluid subcutaneously.

**lipemia** (lĭ-pē′mē-ă) [″ + *haima,* blood] An abnormal amount of fat in the blood.

***alimentary l.*** An accumulation of fat in the blood after eating.

***l. retinalis*** A condition in which retinal vessels appear reddish white or white; found in cases of hyperlipidemia. SEE: *hyperlipoproteinemia.*

**lipid(e)** (lĭp′ĭd, -īd) [Gr. *lipos,* fat] Any one of a group of fats or fatlike substances, characterized by their insolubility in water and solubility in fat solvents such as alcohol, ether, and chloroform. The term is descriptive rather than a chemical name such as protein or carbohydrate. It includes true fats (esters of fatty acids and glycerol); lipoids (phospholipids, cerebrosides, waxes); and sterols (cholesterol, ergosterol). SEE: *fat; lipoprotein.*

**lipidemia** A syndrome of painful accumulation of fat in the legs. The ankles are spared, but the fatty tissue may hang over them. Treatment includes weight control to prevent further gain and weight reduction. Liposuction may be of benefit. SYN: *painful fat syndrome.* SEE: *liposuction.*

**lipid histiocytosis** Niemann-Pick disease.

**lipidosis** Any disorder of fat metabolism.

***arterial l.*** Arteriosclerosis.

***cerebroside l.*** Gaucher's disease.

**lipiduria** (lĭp″ĭ-dū′rē-ă) [″ + Gr. *ouron,* urine] Lipids in the urine.

**Lipiodol** (lĭp-ī′ō-dŏl) [″ + L. *oleum,* oil] Trade name for an iodized oil used as a contrast medium in radiographical studies.

**lipo-, lip-** [Gr. *lipos,* fat] Combining form meaning *fat.* SEE: *adipo-; steato-.*

**lipoarthritis** (lĭp″ō-ărth-rī′tĭs) [″ + *arthron,* joint, + *itis,* inflammation] An inflammation of the fatty tissues of the joints.

**lipoatrophia, lipoatrophy** (lī″pō-ă-trō′fē-ă, lī″pō-ăt′rō-fē) [″ + *a-,* not, + *trophe,* nourishment] Atrophy of fat tissue. This condition may occur at the site of insulin injection. SEE: *lipodystrophy.*

**lipoblast** (lĭp′ō-blăst) [″ + *blastos,* germ] An immature fat cell.

**lipoblastoma** (lĭp″ō-blăs-tō′mă) [″ + ″ + *oma,* tumor] A benign tumor of the fatty tissue. SYN: *lipoma.*

**lipocardiac** (lĭp″ō-kăr′dē-ăk) [″ + *kardia,* heart] **1.** Pert. to fatty heart degeneration. **2.** One who suffers from fatty degeneration of the heart.

**lipocele** (lĭp′ō-sēl) [″ + *kele,* tumor, swelling] The presence of fatty tissue in a hernia sac. SYN: *adipocele; liparocele.*

**lipochondrodystrophy** (lĭp″ō-kŏn″drō-dĭs′trō-fē) [″ + *chondros,* cartilage, + *dys,* bad, + *trephein,* to nourish] Mucopolysaccharidosis I.

**lipochondroma** (lĭp″ō-kŏn-drō′mă) [″ + ″ + *oma,* tumor] A tumor that is both fatty and cartilaginous.

**lipochrome** (lĭp′ō-krōm) [″ + *chroma,* color] Any one of a group of fat-soluble pigments (e.g., carotene, the fat-soluble yellow pigment found in carrots, sweet potatoes, egg yolk, butter, body fat and corpus luteum).

**lipocyte** SEE: *cell, fat.*

**lipodystrophy** (lĭp″ō-dĭs′trō-fē) [″ + *dys,* bad, + *trophe,* nourishment] Disturbance or defectiveness of fat metabolism.

***insulin l.*** A complication of insulin administration characterized by changes in the subcutaneous fat at the site of injection. The changes may take the form of atrophy or hypertrophy; rarely are both types present in the same patient. Atrophy develops in as many as one third of children and women who use insulin regularly, but rarely in men. The subcutaneous fat appears to have melted away and leaves a saucer-like depression. Hypertrophy at the injection site occurs in the form of a spongy localized area. This type of complication of insulin administration is slightly more common in males than in females. It is usually associated with a history of prolonged use of the same injection site.

***intestinal l.*** A disease characterized principally by fat deposits in intestinal and mesenteric lymphatic tissue, fatty diarrhea, loss of weight and strength, and arthritis.

***progressive l.*** A pathological condition in which there is progressive, symmetrical loss of subcutaneous fat from the upper part of the trunk, face, neck, and arms.

***trochanteric l.*** Excess accumulation of fatty tissue over the thighs, commonly known as saddlebag thighs.

**lipofibroma** (lĭp″ō-fī-brō′mă) [″ + L. *fibra,* fiber, + Gr. *oma,* tumor] A lipoma having much fibrous tissue. SYN: *fibrolipoma.*

**lipofuscin** (lĭp″ō-fŭs′sĭn) [″ + L. *fuscus,* brown] One of a class of insoluble lipid pigments present in cardiac and smooth muscle cells. It is known as aging pigment. It is the indigestible residue of portions of the cell that have been injured and phagocytosed. This is frequently seen in cells undergoing atrophy. Its presence is not injurious to the cell. SEE: *atrophy, brown; radical, free.*

**lipofuscinosis** (lĭp″ō-fū″sĭn-ō′sĭs) [″ + ″ + Gr. *osis,* condition] Abnormal deposition of lipofuscin in tissues.

**lipogenesis** (lĭp″ō-jĕn′ĕ-sĭs) [Gr. *lipos,* fat, + *genesis,* generation, birth] Fat formation.

**lipogenetic, lipogenic** (lĭp″ō-jĕ-nĕt′ĭk, lĭp″ō-jĕn′ĭk) Producing fat. SYN: *lipogenous.*

**lipogenous** (lĭp-ŏj′ĕ-nŭs) Lipogenetic.

**lipogranuloma** (lĭp″ō-grăn-ū-lō′mă) [″ + L. *granulum,* granule, + Gr. *oma,* tumor] Inflammation of fatty tissue with granulation and development of oily cysts.

**lipogranulomatosis** (lĭp″ō-grăn″ū-lō-mă-tō′sĭs) [″ + ″ + ″ + *osis,* condition] A disorder of fat metabolism in which a nodule of fat undergoes central necrosis and the surrounding tissue becomes granulomatous.

**lipoid** (lĭp′oyd) [″ + *eidos,* form, shape] **1.** Similar to fat. **2.** Lipid.

**lipoidosis** (lĭp-oy-dō′sĭs) [″ + ″ + *osis,* condition] Condition in which lipids accumulate in excessive quantities in body tissue. SYN: *lipidosis.* SEE: *xanthomatosis.*

***arterial l.*** Arteriosclerosis.

***cerebroside l.*** A familial disease characterized by deposition of glucocerebroside in cells of the reticuloendothelial system. SYN: *Gaucher's disease.*

**lipoiduria** (lĭp″oy-dū′rē-ă) [″ + ″ + *ouron,* urine] Lipoids in the urine.

**lipolipoidosis** (lĭp″ō-lĭp″oy-dō′sĭs) [″ + *lipos,* fat, + *eidos,* form, shape, + *osis,* condition] Infiltration of fats and lipoids into a tissue.

**lipolysis** (lĭp-ŏl′ĭ-sĭs) [″ + *lysis,* dissolution] The decomposition of fat.

**lipolytic** (lĭp-ō-lĭt′ĭk) Relating to lipolysis.

***l. digestion*** The conversion of neutral fats by hydrolysis into fatty acids and glycerol; fat splitting.

**lipoma** (lĭ-pō′mă) [Gr. *lipos,* fat, + *oma,* tumor] A fatty tumor. It is frequently found in multiple but is not metastatic. SYN: *adipoma*. SEE: *chondrolipoma*.

***l. arborescens*** An abnormal treelike accumulation of fatty tissue in a joint.

***cystic l.*** A lipoma containing cysts.

***diffuse l.*** A lipoma not definitely circumscribed.

***l. diffusum renis*** A condition in which fat displaces parenchyma of the kidney.

***l. durum*** A lipoma in which there is marked hypertrophy of the fibrous stroma and capsule.

***nasal l.*** A fibrous growth of the subcutaneous tissue of the nostrils.

***osseous l.*** A lipoma in which the connective tissue has undergone calcareous degeneration.

***l. telangiectodes*** A rare form of lipoma containing a large number of blood vessels.

**lipomatoid** (lĭ-pō′mă-toyd) [″ + ″ + *eidos*, form, shape] Similar to a lipoma.

**lipomatosis** (lĭp″ō-mă-tō′sĭs) [″ + *oma*, tumor + *osis*, condition] A condition marked by the excessive deposit of fat in a localized area. SYN: *liposis; obesity*.

***l. renis*** Lipoma diffusum renis.

**lipomatous** (lĭp-ō′mă-tŭs) **1.** Of the nature of lipoma. **2.** Affected with lipoma.

**lipomeningocele** (lĭp″ō-mĕ-nĭng′gō-sēl) [″ + *meninx*, membrane, + *kele*, tumor, swelling] A meningocele associated with lobules of fat tissue.

**lipomeria** (lī″pō-mē′rē-ă) [Gr. *leipein*, to leave, + *meros*, a part] In a deformed fetus, the congenital absence of a limb.

**lipometabolism** (lĭp-ō-mĕ-tăb′ŏl-ĭzm) [″ + ″ + *-ismos*, condition] Fat metabolism.

**lipomyoma** (lĭp″ō-mī-ō′mă) [″ + *mys*, muscle, + *oma*, tumor] A myoma containing fatty tissue.

**lipomyxoma** (lĭp″ō-mĭks-ō′mă) [″ + *myxa*, mucus, + *oma*, tumor] A mixed lipoma and myxoma. SYN: *myxolipoma*.

**lipopenia** (lĭp″ō-pē′nē-ă) [″ + *penia*, poverty] A deficiency of lipids. **lipopenic** (-nĭk), *adj*.

**lipopeptid, lipopeptide** (lĭp″ō-pĕp′tĭd, -tīd) A complex of lipids and amino acids.

**lipophagia, granulomatous** (lĭp″ō-fā′jē-ă) Intestinal lipodystrophy.

**lipophagy** (lĭ-pŏf′ă-jē) The ingestion of fat cells by phagocytes.

**lipophanerosis** (lĭp″ō-făn″ĕ-rō′sĭs) [″ + *phaneros*, visible, + *osis*, condition] The alteration of fat in a cell so that it becomes visible as droplets.

**lipophil** (lĭp′ō-fĭl) [″ + *philein*, to love] **1.** Having an affinity for fat. **2.** Absorbing fat.

**lipophilia** (lĭp″ō-fĭl′ē-ă) [″ + *philos*, love] Affinity for fat.

**lipopolysaccharide** (lĭp″ō-pŏl″ē-săk′ă-rīd) The linkage of molecules of lipids with polysaccharides.

**lipoprotein** Conjugated proteins consisting of simple proteins combined with lipid components: cholesterol, phospholipid, and triglyceride. Most plasma lipids do not circulate in an unbound state but are chemically linked with proteins. These large molecules are categorized with respect to their chemical properties and densities as determined by ultracentrifugation. Analysis of their concentrations and proportions in the blood can provide important clues as to their role in certain diseases, particularly cardiovascular abnormalities, hypertension, atherosclerosis, and coronary artery disease. Lipoproteins are classified as very low-density (VLDL), low-density (LDL), intermediate-density (IDL) and high-density (HDL). It is thought that individuals with high blood levels of HDL are less predisposed to coronary heart disease than those with high blood levels of VLDL or LDL. SEE: *hyperlipoproteinemia*.

***alpha l.*** High-density l.

***high-density l.*** ABBR: HDL. Plasma lipids bound to albumin, consisting of lipoproteins. They contain more protein than either very low-density lipoproteins or low-density lipoproteins. High-density lipoprotein cholesterol is the so-called good cholesterol; therefore a high level is desirable. SYN: *alpha l.*

***intermediate-density l.*** ABBR: IDL. Plasma lipids bound to albumin, consisting of lipoproteins with less protein than high-density, but more than low-density, lipoproteins.

***l. lipase*** ABBR: Lp(a). An enzyme produced by many tissues. It is present on capillary walls where it is activated to hydrolyze fat (chylomicrons) and very low-density lipoprotein (VLDL) to monoglycerides to free fatty acids and intermediate-density lipoprotein (IDL). This enzyme, similar to plasminogen, is an important regulator of lipid and lipoprotein metabolism. Even though the physiological functions of Lp(a) and apo(a) are not fully understood, there is a positive association of plasma Lp(a) with premature myocardial infarction. Deficiency of this enzyme leads to an increase in chylomicrons and VLDLs, and to low levels of high-density lipoproteins (HDL). Diseases associated with acquired causes of decreased lipoprotein lipase include acute ethanol ingestion, diabetes mellitus, hypothyroidism, chronic renal failure, and nephrotic syndrome.

***low-density l.*** ABBR: LDL. Plasma lipids bound to albumin, consisting of lipoproteins that contain more protein than the very low-density lipoproteins.

***very low-density l.*** ABBR: VLDL. Plasma lipids bound to albumin and consisting of chylomicrons and prelipoproteins. This class of plasma lipoproteins contains a greater ratio of lipid than the low-density lipoproteins and is the least dense.

**liposarcoma** (lĭp″ō-săr-kō′mă) [Gr. *lipos*, fat, + *sarx*, flesh, + *oma*, tumor] A malignant tumor derived from embryonal lipoblastic cells.

**liposis** (lĭ-pō′sĭs) [″ + *osis,* condition] Adiposis.

**liposoluble** (lĭp″ō-sŏl′ū-b′l) [″ + L. *solubilis,* soluble] Soluble in fats.

**liposome** (lĭp′ō-sōm) [″ + *soma,* body] The sealed concentric shells formed when certain lipid substances are in an aqueous solution. As it forms, the liposome entraps a portion of the solution in the shell. Liposomes may be manufactured and filled with a variety of medications. These have been used to deliver substances to particular organs. These drug forms may be more effective and less toxic than drugs given by other means.

**lipostomy** (lī-pŏs′tō-mē) [Gr. *leipein,* to fail, + *stoma,* mouth] Congenital absence or extreme smallness of the mouth.

**liposuction** The removal of subcutaneous fat tissue with a blunt-tipped cannula introduced into the fatty area through a small incision. Suction is then applied and fat tissue removed. Liposuction is a form of plastic surgery intended to remove adipose tissue from localized areas of fat accumulation as on the hips, knees, buttocks, thighs, face, arms, or neck. To be cosmetically successful, the skin should be elastic enough to contract after the underlying fat has been removed. Liposuction will not benefit dimpled or sagging skin or flabby muscles. There are no health benefits to liposuction, and as with any surgery there may be risks such as infection, severe postoperative pain, or a result that is unsatisfactory to the patient. SYN: *suction lipectomy.*

**lipotropic** (lĭp-ō-trŏp′ĭk) [″ + *trope,* a turning] Having an affinity for lipids, as with certain dyes (e.g., Sudan III, which stains fat readily).

***l. factors*** Compounds that promote the transportation and use of fats and help to prevent accumulation of fat in the liver.

**lipotropism, lipotropy** (lĭ-pŏt′rō-pĭzm, -pē) [″ + *trope,* a turn, + *-ismos,* condition] **1.** Having the action of removing fat deposits in the liver. **2.** An agent that acts to remove fat from the liver.

**lipovaccine** (lĭp″ō-văk′sēn) A vaccine suspended in vegetable oil.

**lipoxidase** (lĭ-pŏk′sĭ-dās) An enzyme that catalyzes the oxidation of the double bonds of an unsaturated fatty acid.

**lipoxygenase** (lĭ-pŏks′ĭ-jĕ-nās) Lipoxidase.

**Lippes loop** (lĭ′pēz) [Jacob Lippes, U.S. obstetrician, b. 1924] A type of intrauterine contraceptive device.

**lipping** (lĭp′ĭng) A growth of bony tissue beyond the joint margin in degenerative joint disease.

**lippitude** (lĭp′ĭ-tūd) [L. *lippitudo,* fr. *lippus,* blear-eyed] Blepharitis.

**lip reading** Interpreting what is being said by watching the speaker's lip and facial movements and expression. This method is used very effectively by deaf people.

**lipuria** (lĭ-pū′rē-ă) [Gr. *lipos,* fat, + *ouron,* urine] Fat in the urine.

**liquefacient** (lĭk″wĕ-fā′shĕnt) [L. *liquere,* to flow, + *facere,* to make] **1.** An agent that converts a solid substance into a liquid. **2.** Converting a solid into a liquid.

**liquefaction** (lĭk″wĕ-făk′shŭn) **1.** The conversion of a solid into a liquid. **2.** The conversion of solid tissues to a fluid or semifluid state.

**liquescent** (lĭk-wĕs′sĕnt) [L. *liquescere,* to become liquid] Becoming liquid. SYN: *deliquescent.*

**liquid** (lĭk′wĭd) [L. *liquere,* to flow] **1.** Flowing easily. **2.** The state of matter in which a substance flows without being melted. SEE: *emulsion; liquefacient; liquefaction.*

***l. measure*** A measure of liquid capacity.

**liquid crystal display** ABBR: LCD. A type of electronic display unit used on devices from watches to clinical laboratory instruments. It is very efficient and consumes little energy or power.

**liquor** (lĭk′ĕr) [L.] **1.** Any liquid or fluid. **2.** An alcoholic beverage. **3.** A solution of medicinal substance in water.

***l. amnii*** The amniotic fluid, a clear watery fluid that surrounds the fetus in the amniotic sac. SEE: *hydramnion.*

***l. folliculi*** The fluid contained in the graafian follicle.

***l. sanguinis*** Blood serum or plasma.

***l. solution*** An aqueous solution of nonvolatile substances presenting the greatest variety in strength, character, and method of preparation. These solutions are usually very active medicinal preparations.

**Lisch nodule** [K. Lisch, contemporary Ger. scientist] A melanocytic hamartoma projecting from the surface of the iris of the eye. It is a well-defined, dome-shaped elevation that is clear to yellow or brown. These growths, which do not cause ophthalmological complications, may be seen without magnification, but examination with use of a slit lamp is needed to differentiate them from nevi of the iris. Lisch nodules are found only in patients with neurofibromatosis, type 1.

**Lisfranc's dislocation** (lĭs-frănks′) [Jacques Lisfranc, Fr. surgeon, 1790–1847] A dislocation of the tarsometatarsal joints of the foot by direct or indirect mechanisms. Accompanying fracture is common.

**Lisfranc's ligament** The ligament joining the first cuneiform bone of the ankle to the second metatarsal.

**lisping** (lĭsp′ĭng) [AS. *wlisp,* lisping] A substitution of sounds owing to a defect in speech, as of the "th" sound for "s" and "z."

**lissencephalous** (lĭs″sĕn-sĕf′ă-lŭs) [Gr. *lissos,* smooth, + *enkephalos,* brain] Pert. to a condition in which the brain is smooth owing to failure of cerebral gyri to develop.

**lissotrichy** (lĭs-sŏt′rĭ-kē) [″ + *thrix,* hair] The condition of having straight hair.

**Lister, Baron Joseph** (lĭs′tĕr) British surgeon, 1827–1912, who developed the technique of antiseptic surgery. Without this technique, modern surgery would not be possible.

**Listeria** A genus of gram-positive, non-spore forming coccobacilli that may be found singly or in filaments. They are normal soil inhabitants.

**Listeria monocytogenes** The causative agent of listeriosis. This species lives in soil or the intestines of animals and may contaminate food, esp. milk or meat. Its growth is not inhibited by refrigeration.

**listeriosis, listerosis** (lĭs-tĕr″ē-ō′sĭs, lĭs″tĕr-ō′sĭs) A disease affecting many domestic animals, wild animals, and humans, caused by *Listeria monocytogenes,* a soil saprophyte that becomes pathogenic for animals or humans under favorable circumstances (e.g., pregnancy, immunosuppression, or extremes of age). The most common manifestation in the adult is meningitis. The disease may be transmitted transplacentally to the fetus, in which case it may cause spontaneous abortion. In newborns, the disease is much more serious than in the adult. The mortality may be 100% when it occurs in the first 4 days. Although humans have a high degree of resistance to the bacteria, hygienic precautions should be taken when handling infected animals.

TREATMENT: Initially, the patient should receive ampicillin and an aminoglycoside antibiotic. If the patient is allergic to penicillin, trimethoprim or sulfamethoxazole should be used.

**liter** (lē′tĕr) [Fr. *litre,* liter] Metric fluid measure; equivalent to 1000 ml, 270 fl drams, 61 cu in., 33.8 fl oz, or 1.0567 qt. The volume occupied by 1 kg of water at 4°C and 760 mm Hg pressure. SEE: *metric system.*

NOTE: It is common to define a liter as 1000 cc. This is almost but not quite correct because 1 ml is equal to 1.000028 cc. Thus, liquid volume should be expressed in milliliters rather than in cubic centimeters.

**literate** Being able to read and write, and to use written language as in understanding graphs, charts, tables, maps, symbols, and formulas.

**lith-** SEE: *litho-.*

**lithectasy** (lĭth-ĕk′tă-sē) [Gr. *lithos,* stone, + *ektasis,* dilatation] The removal of a calculus from the bladder through the dilated urethra.

**lithectomy** (lĭ-thĕk′tō-mē) [″ + *ektome,* excision] The surgical removal of a calculus.

**lithemia** (lĭth-ē′mē-ă) [″ + *haima,* blood] An excess of lithic or uric acid in the blood owing to imperfect metabolism of the nitrogenous substances.

**lithiasis** (lĭth-ī′ă-sĭs) **1.** The formation of calculi and concretions. **2.** Uric acid diathesis.

***l. biliaris*** Gallstone.

***l. nephritica*** Stone formation in the kidneys. SYN: *nephrolithiasis; renal calculus.* SEE: *calculus, renal.*

***l. renalis*** Kidney stone. SEE: *calculus, renal.*

**lithic acid** (lĭth′ĭk) Uric acid.

**lithicosis** (lĭth″ĭ-kō′sĭs) [Gr. *lithikos,* made of stone] Stone cutters' silicosis; pneumoconiosis.

**lithium** (lĭth′ē-ŭm) [Gr. *lithos,* stone] SYMB: Li. A metallic element; atomic weight 6.941; atomic number 3.

***l. carbonate*** A drug that is particularly useful in treating the manic phase of manic-depressive disorders and bipolar disorder. Given orally it is readily absorbed and eliminated at a fast rate for 5 to 6 hr and much more slowly over the next 24 hr. It is essential to monitor the blood level of the drug in patients taking this therapy; samples should be taken 8 to 10 hr after the last dose and at intervals after medication. SEE: *bipolar disorder.*

A dose of 1200 mg each day is initially given and adjusted as needed to produce a plasma level of 0.8 mEq/L. When the dose has been found to produce the optimal plasma concentration, blood analysis is done every 3 months. Plasma levels of 2 mEq/L or more cause serious toxic effects including stupor or coma, muscular rigidity, marked tremor, and, in some cases, epileptic seizure.

Side effects including fatigue, weakness, fine tremor of the hands, nausea and vomiting, thirst, dry mouth, and polyuria may be noticed in the first week of therapy. Most will disappear, but the thirst, polyuria, and tremor tend to persist. Dry mouth may be severe enough to promote dental decay.

---

Caution: Decreased dietary sodium intake lowers the excretion rate of lithium. It should not be administered to patients following a salt-free diet. The risk of toxicity is very high in patients with significant renal or cardiovascular disease, severe debilitation, dehydration, sodium depletion, or in patients receiving diuretics.

---

**litho-, lith-** [Gr. *lithos,* stone] Combining form meaning *stone* or *calculus.*

**lithocenosis** (lĭth″ō-sĕn-ō′sĭs) [″ + *kenosis,* evacuation] The removal of crushed fragments of calculi from the bladder.

**lithoclast** (lĭth′ō-klăst) [″ + *klastos,* broken] Forceps for breaking up large calculi.

**lithoclasty** (lĭth′ō-klăs″tē) The crushing of a stone into fragments that may pass through natural channels.

**lithocystotomy** (lĭth″ō-sĭs-tŏt′ō-mē) [″ + *kystis,* bladder, + *tome,* incision] Incision of the bladder to remove a calculus.

**lithogenesis** (lĭth″ō-jĕn′ĕ-sĭs) [″ + *gennan,* to produce] Formation of calculi.

**lithokelyphopedion** (lĭth″ō-kĕl″ĭ-fō-pē′dē-ŏn) [″ + *kelyphos,* sheath, + *paidion,* child] Calcification of both the fetus and the membranes of a lithopedion.

**lithokelyphos** (lĭth″ō-kĕl′ĭ-fŏs) [″ + *kelyphos,* sheath] A type of lithopedion in which only the membranes are calcified.

**lithokonion** (lĭth″ō-kō′nē-ŏn) [″ + *konios,* dusty] Lithomyl.

**litholabe** (lĭth′ō-lāb) [″ + *lambanein,* to hold] A device for holding a calculus during its removal.

**litholapaxy** (lĭth-ŏl′ă-păks″ē) [Gr. *lithos,* stone, + *lapaxis,* evacuation] The operation of crushing a stone in the bladder followed by immediate washing out of the crushed fragments through a catheter. SEE: *percutaneous ultrasonic lithotriptor.*

**lithology** (lĭth-ŏl′ō-jē) [″ + *logos,* word, reason] The science dealing with calculi.

**litholysis** (lĭth-ŏl′ĭ-sĭs) [″+ *lysis,* dissolution] Dissolving of calculi.

**lithometer** (lĭth-ŏm′ĕ-tĕr) [″ + *metron,* measure] An instrument for estimating the size of calculi.

**lithometra** (lĭth-ō-mē′tră) [″ + *metra,* uterus] Uterine tissue ossification.

**lithomyl** (lĭth′ō-mĭl) [″ + *myle,* mill] An instrument for crushing a vesical stone. SYN: *lithokonion.*

**lithonephritis** (lĭth″ō-nĕ-frī′tĭs) [″+ *nephros,* kidney, + *itis,* inflammation] An inflammation of the kidney because of a calculus.

**lithonephrotomy** (lĭth″ō-nē-frŏt′ō-mē) [″ + *nephros,* kidney, + *tome,* incision] An incision of the kidney for removal of a renal calculus.

**lithopedion** (lĭth″ō-pē′dē-ŏn) [″ + *paidion,* child] A uterine or extrauterine fetus that has died and become calcified. SYN: *ostembryon; osteopedion.*

**lithotome** (lĭth′ō-tōm) [″ + *tome,* incision] An instrument for performing lithotomy.

**lithotomy** (lĭth-ŏt′ō-mē) [″ + *tome,* incision] The incision of a duct or organ, esp. of the bladder, for removal of a calculus.

NURSING IMPLICATIONS: A dietary history is obtained to identify factors contributing to calculus formation. Noninvasive measures and prescribed analgesic agents are provided to relieve pain. Fluid balance is monitored, and unless otherwise contraindicated by cardiac or renal status, fluid intake of 4 L/day is recommended to maintain a urine output of 3 to 4 L/day, which aids in the passage of small calculi (up to 5 mm in diameter) and prevents ascending infections. Supplemental I.V. fluids are provided if the patient is unable to tolerate the required volume by mouth. Vital signs and laboratory studies are monitored for signs of infection, and prescribed antibiotics are administered. The nurse prepares the patient for lithotripsy or surgery, as indicated, by explaining postoperative equipment, care procedures, and expected sensations. Any incisions are assessed for drainage and healing, the character and amount of drainage are documented, and a ureteral catheter or nephrotomy tube, if prescribed, is irrigated. Using aseptic techniques, the nurse protects surrounding skin from excoriation by redressing frequently. All urine is strained for evidence of calculi and any solid material is sent for analysis. Based on laboratory analysis of the calculus, the nurse teaches the patient to check urinary pH and about dietary regimens to change the urinary pH or to control hyperuricemia, as indicated, and about other prescribed regimens to prevent recurrence.

***bilateral l.*** A lithotomy performed with the incision across the perineum.

***high l.*** A lithotomy performed through a suprapubic incision.

***lateral l.*** A lithotomy performed with the incision from the front of the rectum to one side of the raphe.

***median l.*** A lithotomy performed with the incision in the median line in front of the anus.

***rectal l.*** A lithotomy performed through the rectum.

***vaginal l.*** A lithotomy performed with the incision through the vaginal wall.

**lithotony** (lĭth-ŏt′ō-nē) [Gr. *lithos,* stone, + *teinein,* to stretch] The removal of a calculus through a small bladder incision that is instrumentally dilated.

**lithotresis** (lĭth″ō-trē′sĭs) [″ + *tresis,* boring] The drilling or boring of holes in a calculus to facilitate crushing.

**lithotripsy** (lĭth′ō-trĭp″sē) [″ + *tribein,* to rub] **1.** The application of physical force to crush a calculus in the bladder or urethra. **2.** The production of shock waves by use of an external energy source in order to crush renal calculi.

**lithotriptic** (lĭth-ō-trĭp′tĭk) **1.** Pert. to lithotripsy. **2.** An agent that dissolves calculi.

NOTE: There are no substances that have this capability and are harmless to the patient.

**lithotriptor** (lĭth′ō-trĭp″tor) [″ + *tripsis,* friction] A device for breaking up renal calculi.

***percutaneous ultrasonic l.*** A device that uses ultrasound to break up kidney stones and gallstones. The sound waves are applied to the outside of the body and penetrate to the calculi.

**lithotriptoscopy** (lĭth″ō-trĭp-tŏs′kō-pē) [″ + ″ + *skopein,* to examine] The crushing of a renal calculus under direct vision by using a lithotriptoscope.

**lithotrity** (lĭth-ŏt′rĭ-tē) The crushing of a calculus to small fragments in the bladder.

**lithous** (lĭth′ŭs) [Gr. *lithos,* stone] Relating to a calculus or stone. SYN: *calculous.*

**lithoxiduria** (lĭth″ŏks-ĭ-dū′rē-ă) [″ + L. *oxidum,* oxide, + Gr. *ouron,* urine] The presence of xanthic oxide in the urine.

**lithuria** (lĭth-ū′rē-ă) [″ + *ouron,* urine] An excess of uric acid or urates in the urine.

**litigation** A lawsuit or legal action that determines the legal rights and remedies of the person or party.

**litmus** (lĭt′mŭs) A blue dyestuff made by treating coarsely powdered lichens, such as those of the genus *Roccella,* with ammonia.

***l. paper*** Chemically prepared blue paper that is turned red by acids and remains blue in alkali solutions; pH range is 4.5 to 8.5. SEE: *indicator.*

**litter** (lĭt′tĕr) [O. Fr. *litiere,* offspring at birth, bed] **1.** A stretcher for carrying the wounded or the sick. **2.** The young produced at one birth by a multiparous mammal.

**Little's disease** [William John Little, Brit. physician, 1810–1894] Congenital spastic paralysis on both sides (diplegia), although it may be paraplegic or hemiplegic in form.

SYMPTOMS: The child may be delayed in developing sphincter control and is usually mentally normal. Symptoms include stiff, awkward movements; legs crossed and pressed together; arm(s) adducted; forearm(s) flexed; hand(s) pronated; scissors gait.

ETIOLOGY: The cause is unknown. Efforts to implicate hypoxemia in utero have not been successful.

**Littré's gland** (lē′trz) [Alexis Littre, Fr. surgeon, 1658–1725] Urethral gland.

**littritis** (lĭt-trī′tĭs) An inflammation of the urethral glands.

**Litzmann's obliquity** [Karl K. T. Litzmann, Ger. gynecologist, 1815–1890] Posterior parietal presentation of the fetal head during labor. SYN: *posterior asynclitism.*

**lived experience** The subjective perception of one's health or illness experience. The term is associated with Rosemary Parse's nursing theory of Man-Living-Health and emphasizes the nurse's need to understand the personal health experience of patients, rather than to collect data from patients as objects.

**livedo** (lĭv-ē′dō) [L. *livedo,* lividness] A patchy or general bluish discoloration of the skin, as a bruise. SYN: *lividity.*

***l. reticularis*** Semipermanent bluish mottling of the skin of the legs and hands. It is aggravated by exposure to cold.

**liver** ( lĭv′ĕr) [AS. *lifer*] The largest organ in the body, approx. 21 to 22.5 cm in its greatest transverse diameter, 15 to 17.5 cm in its greatest vertical height, and 10 to 12.5 cm in its anteroposterior depth, weighing 1200 to 1600 g. It is situated on the right side beneath the diaphragm; occupies the right hypochondrium, epigastrium, and part of the left hypochrondrium; and is level with the bottom of the sternum. Its undersurface is concave and covers the stomach, duodenum, hepatic flexure of colon, right kidney, and adrenal capsule. The liver secretes bile and is the site of a great many metabolic functions. SEE: illus.

ANATOMY: The liver has four lobes, five ligaments, and five fissures and is covered by a tough fibrous membrane, Glisson's capsule, which is thickest at the transverse fissure. At this point the capsule carries the blood vessels and hepatic duct, which enter the organ at the hilus. Strands of connective tissue originating from the capsule enter the liver parenchyma and form the supporting network of the organ and separate the functional units of the liver, the hepatic lobules.

The many intrahepatic bile ducts converge and anastomose, finally forming the secretory duct of the liver, the hepatic duct, which joins the cystic duct from the gallbladder to form the common bile duct or the ductus choledochus, which enters the duodenum at the papilla of Vater. A ring of smooth muscle at the terminal portion of the choledochus, the sphincter of Oddi, permits the passage of bile into the duodenum by relaxing. The bile leaving the liver enters the gallbladder, where it undergoes concentration principally through loss of water absorbed by the gallbladder mucosa. When bile is needed in the small intestine for digestive purposes, the gallbladder contracts and the sphincter relaxes, thus permitting escape of the viscid gallbladder bile. Ordinarily, the sphincter of Oddi is contracted, shutting off the duodenal entrance and forcing the bile to enter the gallbladder after leaving the liver.

The functional units of the liver are the liver lobules, six-sided aggregations of hepatocytes permeated by capillaries called sinusoids. Lining these sinusoids are Kupffer cells, the macrophages of the liver.

BLOOD SUPPLY: The blood supply consists of oxygenated blood from the hepatic artery, a branch of the celiac artery, and blood from all the digestive organs and spleen by way of the portal vein. The end products of digestion and other materials thus pass through the liver before entering general circulation.

NERVE SUPPLY: The nerve supply consists of parasympathetic fibers from the vagi and sympathetic fibers from the celiac plexus via the hepatic nerve.

FUNCTION: The only digestive function of the liver is the production of bile, which emulsifies fats in the small intestine; 800 to 1000 ml of bile is secreted in 24 hr, and the secretion rate is greatly increased during digestion of meals high in fats.

*Metabolic functions:* Synthesis of vitamin K-dependent plasma proteins: albumin, globulin carrier molecules, and the clotting factors including prothrombin, fibrinogen, and others. *Amino acid metabolism:* Synthesis of the nonessential amino acids, deaminates excess amino acids for use in energy production, and from the amino groups forms urea, which will be excreted by the kidneys. *Carbohydrate metabolism:* Monosaccharides other than glucose are changed to glucose; excess glucose is converted to glycogen and

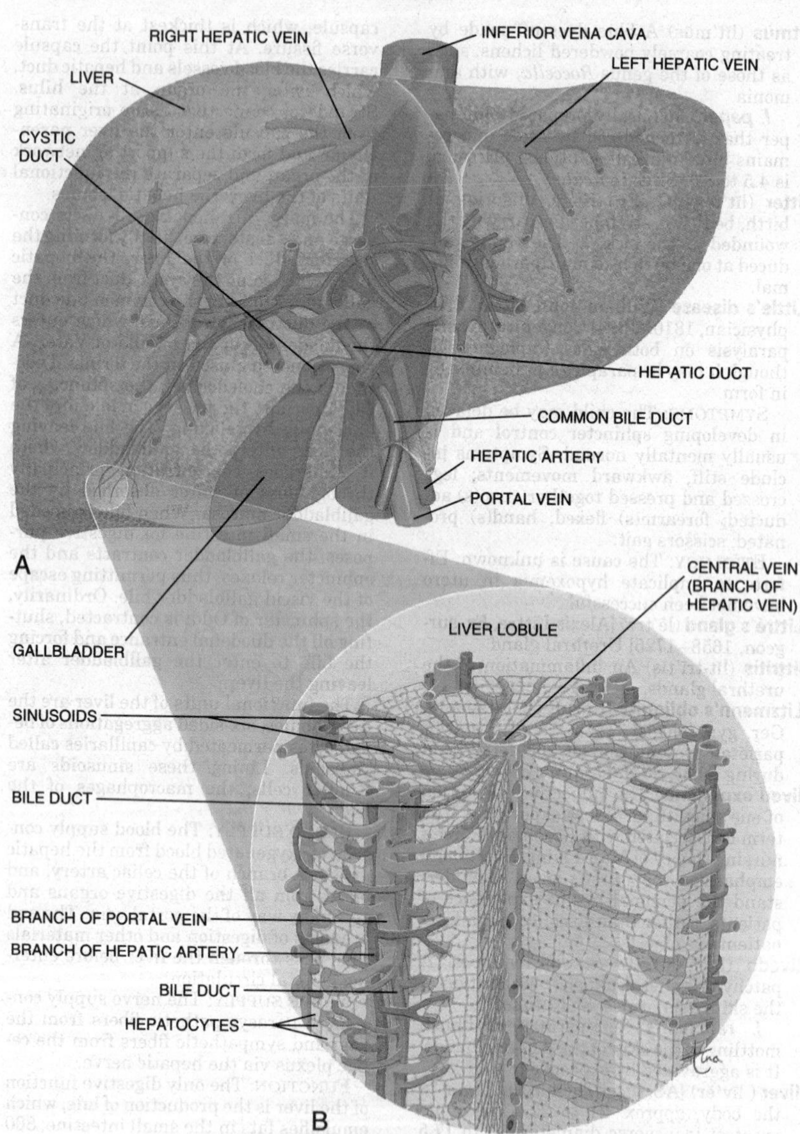


**(A) LIVER AND GALLBLADDER, (B) LOBULE**

stored until needed. *Fat metabolism:* Cholesterol is synthesized; lipoproteins for the transport of fat to other tissues are synthesized; fatty acids are converted to acetyl groups or ketones to be used for energy production. *Phagocytosis:* The Kupffer cells (macrophages) phagocytize bacteria or other pathogens, and old red blood cells. *Excretion:* The bile pigments bilirubin and biliverdin, formed from the hemoglobin of old red blood cells by the liver, spleen, and red bone marrow, are excreted into bile, as is excess cholesterol, to be eliminated in feces. *Detoxification:* The liver produces enzymes to convert potentially harmful substances into less toxic ones. The former include ammonia, indole, and skatole from the intestine; alcohol; and medications. *Storage:* The minerals iron and copper, the fat-soluble vitamins A, D, E, and K, and vitamin $B_{12}$ are stored in the liver. SEE: *hepatitis*; *test, liver function.*

***abscess of l.*** A localized collection of

pus in the liver caused by pathogenic bacteria, esp. pyogenic organisms such as those of *Streptococcus* and *Staphylococcus*; trauma; or infection by *Entamoeba histolytica*.

SYMPTOMS: The patient will have temperature elevated in the evening, low in the morning; sweats and chills; and an enlarged, painful, tender liver, which may be bulging and fluctuating. Pus may be obtained by aspiration.

PROGNOSIS: Embolic (multiple) abscesses are generally fatal. Traumatic abscesses, or those due to an amebic dysentery, may terminate favorably after spontaneous or induced evacuation.

***acute yellow atrophy of l.*** A rare and grave disease, characterized anatomically by a rapid destruction of the liver tissues, and manifested by jaundice and hemorrhages, a reduction in the size of the liver, and marked cerebral phenomena. It is usually due to viral hepatitis B infection or to a toxic reaction to a drug. SYN: *fulminant hepatitis*. SEE: *asterixis; hepatic coma*.

SYMPTOMS: The patient will have malaise, slight fever, nausea, vomiting, jaundice, severe headache, tremor, delirium, convulsions, and coma. Urine is scanty and contains albumin, blood, and casts. Renal failure may occur. Hemorrhages are common, the skin may be covered with ecchymoses, and bleeding from the mucous membranes may occur. Hepatic dullness is diminished; splenic dullness is increased. Treatment is symptomatic. The disease is generally fatal.

***amyloid l.*** An enlargement of liver caused by the deposition of an albuminoid substance. SYN: *lardaceous liver*.

SYMPTOMS: The patient will have a failure of general health, with anemia. The liver is enlarged, smooth, firm, and painless. The spleen and kidneys share in the degeneration, so the spleen is enlarged and the urine albuminous.

TREATMENT: Therapy must be directed to the causal disease, usually prolonged suppuration, syphilis, tuberculosis, or chronic malaria. The prognosis is unfavorable.

***biliary cirrhotic l.*** Cirrhosis of the liver caused by fibrous tissue formed, as a result of infection or obstruction of the bile ducts.

***cancer of l.*** Malignancy of the liver that results either from spread from a primary source or from primary tumor of the liver itself. The former is the more frequent cause. Male sex and heredity are predisposing factors. The liver is the most usual site of metastatic spread of tumors that disseminate through the bloodstream. Chronic hepatitis B is a risk factor for primary liver cancer. Treatment is symptomatic. The disease is fatal; the prognosis for survival is from a few months to 1 yr.

SYMPTOMS: The disease causes severe pain and tenderness; cachexia (i.e., loss of weight); and pressure symptoms. Jaundice is common. The liver is enlarged, its surface is nodular, and a central depression or umbilications can often be detected. Symptoms of the primary growth are present. Fever is generally absent, but secondary perihepatitis or suppuration of cancerous nodules may produce it.

***cirrhosis of l.*** Generalized pathology of the liver with disturbed normal architecture of the lobes as a result of infiltration of fibrous tissue and nodule formation. These changes are accompanied by impaired liver function. Spider nevi may be present on the skin. The disease can progress to the stage of complete liver failure. SEE: *asterixis; hepatic coma; spider nevus*.

SYMPTOMS: Symptoms include abdominal swelling due to ascites, jaundice, weakness, weight loss, anorexia, nausea, fetor hepaticus, and mild continuous fever. As cirrhosis progresses, portal blood finds new channels, and the superficial abdominal veins enlarge, notably about the umbilicus, forming the so-called caput medusae; hemorrhoids and esophageal varices result from the same cause. In the final stages, hepatic encephalopathy develops. This is due in part to substances including ammonia absorbed from the intestines that have not been metabolized by the liver. These reach the brain and produce encephalopathy. Clinically, the patient is mentally dulled, and may have hallucinations. A peculiar type of flapping tremor may be elicited when the patient maintains the hands in an extended position. SEE: *asterixis*.

ETIOLOGY: In the U.S., the most frequent cause is chronic alcoholism. About 20% of those who drink alcohol heavily for a 5- to 10-year period develop cirrhosis. The disease may occur also in individuals with no history of alcoholism. It can develop due to contact with toxic substances such as methotrexate, methanol, halothane, or oxyphenisatin. Other causes include chronic hepatitis B or C; metabolic disorders, including glycogen storage diseases, tyrosinosis, thalassemia, and hemochromatosis; heart disease with chronic passive congestion of the liver; biliary obstruction; and intestinal bypass surgery complications. Prognosis is unfavorable after the disease has progressed.

TREATMENT: Therapy depends on the etiology. Major complications that occur regardless of etiology include portal hypertension, upper gastrointestinal tract bleeding, ascites, and hepatic coma.

***cysts of l.*** Simple cysts, usually small and single; hydatid cysts; or cysts associated with cystic disease of the liver, a rare condition usually associated with congenital cystic kidneys. SEE: *Echinococcus granulosus; hydatid*.

***fatty l.*** Degenerative changes in liver

cells owing to fat deposits in the cells.

***l. flap*** Asterixis.

***floating l.*** An easily displaced liver. SYN: *wandering l.*

***foamy l.*** The presence of gas bubbles in the liver as a result of infection with anaerobic bacteria. This produces a honeycomb appearance in the liver tissue.

***hobnail l.*** Degeneration of the liver characterized by fatty changes, fibrous scarring, nodular degeneration, and atrophy of the liver with the surface covered with brown or yellow nodules. This condition is seen in chronic alcoholism and malnutrition.

***inflammation of l.*** Hepatitis.

***lardaceous l.*** Amyloid l.

***nutmeg l.*** Chronic passive congestion of the liver, which produces a reddened central portal area and a yellowish periportal zone.

***l. spots*** Lentigo senilis.

***wandering l.*** Floating l.

**liver transplantation** The grafting of liver tissue from one person to another. This can be done so that the transplanted organ is an auxiliary at an ectopic site to the host's liver or in the usual location after the removal of the host's liver. The procedure has been used to treat a number of benign diseases and to replace cirrhotic livers. Reproductive function including a normal outcome of pregnancy is possible after liver transplantation, but pregnancy should be avoided for at least 6 months following transplantation.

**livid** (lĭv′ĭd) [L. *lividus,* lead-colored] **1.** Ashen, cyanotic. **2.** Discolored, black and blue.

**lividity** (lĭ-vĭd′ĭ-tē) **1.** Skin discoloration, as from a bruise or venous congestion. SYN: *livor.* **2.** The state of being livid.

***postmortem l.*** Livedo that may be present beginning after death.

**living will** An advance directive, prepared when an individual is alive, competent, and able to make decisions, regarding acceptance and refusal of future health care. The ethical questions surrounding medical decisions to administer or withhold life-saving treatments without the patient's collaboration have generated widespread controversy. The Institute of Society, Ethics, and the Life Sciences (i.e., the Hastings Center) has developed guidelines for termination of treatment. Further, in many states, hospitals have developed admission forms that require the patient to specify a preference regarding such measures and also regarding organ donation. It is not unusual for the medical care team either to be unaware of the patient's living will or for them to choose to ignore it. This is likely to occur when the patient expires and the staff feel resuscitation is indicated. When this happens, the staff should be informed without delay that the patient had left instructions that such measures should not be used. SEE: *advance directive.*

**livor** (lī′vor) [L., a black-and-blue spot] Lividity (1).

***l. mortis*** A cutaneous dark spot on a dependent portion of a cadaver resulting from gravitational pooling of blood.

**lixiviation** (lĭks″ĭv-ē-ā′shŭn) [L. *lixivia,* lye] Leaching.

**L.L.E.** *left lower extremity.*

**LLETZ** *large loop excision of the transformation zone.*

**LLQ** *left lower quadrant* (of abdomen).

**L.M.A.** *left mentoanterior* fetal position.

**L.M.P.** *left mentoposterior* fetal position; *last menstrual period.*

**L.M.T.** *left mentotransverse* fetal position.

**L.O.A.** *left occipitoanterior* fetal position.

**load 1.** The weight supported or force imposed. **2.** A substance given to test body function, esp. metabolic function. SEE: *loading test.*

**loading, bicarbonate** The ingestion of sodium bicarbonate in an effort to neutralize excessive lactic acid produced in the muscles during exercise. The purpose is to decrease muscle soreness and fatigue.

**loading, carbohydrate** SEE: *carbohydrate loading.*

**loading, glycogen** A dietary regimen used to fill the body's glycogen storage areas (i.e., the liver and muscles). SEE: *carbohydrate loading.*

**loaiasis** Loiasis.

**Loa loa** (lō′ă) [W. African] The African eyeworm, a species of filarial worm that infests the subcutaneous tissues and conjunctiva of humans. Its migration causes itching and a creeping sensation. Sometimes it causes itchy edematous areas known as Calabar swellings. It is transmitted by flies of the genus *Chrysops.* SEE: illus.

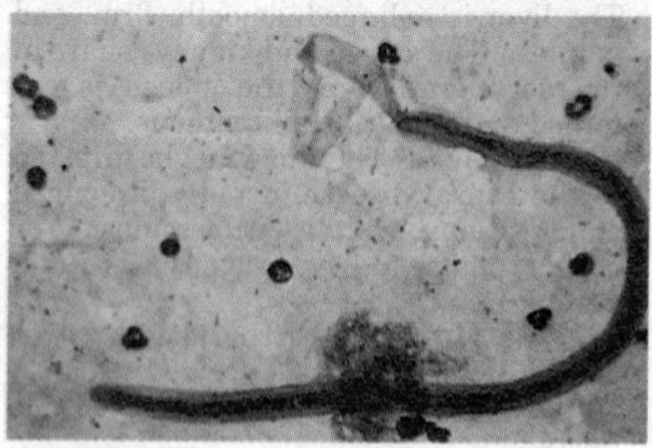

LOA LOA IN BLOOD (ORIG. MAG. ×400)

**lobar** (lō′băr) [Gr. *lobos,* lobe] Pert. to a lobe.

**lobate** (lō′bāt) [L. *lobatus,* lobed] **1.** Pert. to a lobe. **2.** Having a deeply undulated border. **3.** Producing lobes.

**lobe** (lōb) [Gr. *lobos,* lobe] **1.** A fairly well-defined part of an organ separated by boundaries, esp. glandular organs and the brain. **2.** A major part of a tooth formed by a separate calcification center.

***accessory l. of parotid*** A small lobe,

variable in size, on the anterior surface of the parotid gland superior to the exit of the parotid duct.

***anterior l. of hypophysis*** The anterior portion of the hypophysis or pituitary gland, consisting of the pars distalis and pars tuberalis.

***azygos l.*** An anomalous lobe at the apex of the right lobe of the lung.

***caudate l. of liver*** Spigelian l.

***central l.*** The island of Reil, which forms the floor of the lateral cerebral fossa. SYN: *insular l.*

***l.'s of cerebrum*** The frontal, parietal, occipital, and temporal lobes and the insula or island of Reil (central lobe).

***l. of ear*** The lower portion of the auricle having no cartilage.

***flocculonodular l.*** The lobe of the cerebellum consisting of the flocculi, nodulus, and their connecting peduncles.

***frontal l.*** The anterior part of a cerebral hemisphere in front of the central and sylvian fissures.

***hepatic l.*** A lobe of the liver.

***insular l.*** Central l.

***lateral l.'s of prostate*** The portions of the prostate located on each side of the urethra.

***lateral l.'s of thyroid gland*** The two main portions of the thyroid, one on each side of the trachea, united below by the thyroid isthmus.

***limbic l.*** The marginal section of a cerebral hemisphere on the medial aspect. SYN: *gyrus fornicatus.*

***l. of lungs*** One of the large divisions of the lungs: superior and inferior lobes of the left lung; superior, middle, and inferior lobes of the right lung.

***l. of mamma*** One of the 15 to 20 divisions of the glandular tissue of the breast separated by connective tissue and each possessing a duct (lobar duct) opening via the nipple.

***occipital l.*** The posterior region of a cerebral hemisphere that is shaped like a three-sided pyramid.

***olfactory l.*** The olfactory bulb and tract. SYN: *rhinencephalon.* SEE: *olfactory nerve* for illus.

***orbital l.'s*** The convolutions above the orbit.

***l. of pancreas*** A round aggregation of glandular tissue separated by connective tissue.

***parietal l.*** The division of each cerebral hemisphere lying beneath each parietal bone.

***posterior l. of hypophysis*** The posterior portion of the pituitary gland, consisting of the pars intermedia and the processus infundibuli (pars nervosa).

***prefrontal l.*** The frontal portion of the frontal lobe of the brain.

***l.'s of prostate*** The lateral lobes and the middle lobe of the prostate gland.

***pyramidal l. of thyroid*** A portion of the thyroid gland extending upward from the isthmus. It is extremely variable in size.

***quadrate l. of liver*** An oblong elevation on the lower surface of the liver.

***Riedel's l.*** An anomalous tonguelike extension from the right lobe of the liver to the gallbladder.

***spigelian l.*** The irregular quadrangular portion of liver behind the fissure for the portal vein and between the fissures for the vena cava and ductus venosus. SYN: *caudate l. of liver.*

***temporal l.*** The portion of the cerebral hemisphere lying below the lateral fissure of Sylvius. It is continuous posteriorly with the occipital lobe.

**lobectomy** (lō-bĕk′tō-mē) [Gr. *lobos,* lobe, + *ektome,* excision] The surgical removal of a lobe of any organ or gland.

**lobeline** (lŏb′ĕ-lēn) The chief constituent of lobelia.

**lobi** Pl. of lobus.

**lobitis** (lō-bī′tĭs) [″ + *itis,* inflammation] Inflammation of a lobe.

**Loboa loboi** Fungus that causes keloidal blastomycosis (Lobo's disease). It has been identified in tissues but has not been cultured.

**Lobo's disease** Keloidal blastomycosis. SEE: *blastomycosis.*

**lobotomy** (lō-bŏt′ō-mē) [Gr. *lobos,* lobe, + *tome,* incision] The incision of a lobe; this procedure was used at one time to treat some forms of mental disturbances that did not respond to other treatments. It is accomplished by a small bilateral trephination in the plane of the coronal suture through which the white matter of the brain is sectioned; the diencephalon, esp. the hypothalamic area, is disconnected from the prefrontal cortex by section of the white fiber connecting pathways subcortically in a plane passing adjacent to the anterior tip of the lateral ventricle and the posterior margin of the sphenoid wing.

**Lobstein's disease** (lōb′stīnz) [John Georg Friedrich Lobstein, Ger. surgeon, 1777–1835] Osteogenesis imperfecta.

**lobular** (lŏb′ū-lăr) [L. *lobulus,* small lobe] Lobulate.

**lobulate, lobulated** (lŏb′ū-lāt, -lāt-ĕd) **1.** Consisting of lobes or lobules. **2.** Pert. to lobes or lobules. **3.** Resembling lobes. SYN: *lobular.*

**lobule** (lŏb′ūl) [L. *lobulus,* small lobe] A small lobe or primary subdivision of a lobe. It is typical of the pancreas and major salivary glands and may be represented on the surface by bumps or bulges as seen on the thyroid gland.

***central l. of cerebellum*** A small lobe at anterior part of the superior vermiform process.

***l.'s of epididymis*** Conelike divisions of the head of the epididymis formed by the much-coiled distal ends of the efferent ducts of the testis.

***l. of kidney*** Subdivision of the renal cortex consisting of a medullary ray and surrounding glandular tissue.

***l. of liver*** A structural unit consisting of hepatic cells arranged in irregular, branching, and interconnected groups and anastomosing blood channels (sinusoids) surrounding a central vein. It is polyhedral and contains branches of portal vein, hepatic artery, and interlobular bile ducts at its periphery.

***l.'s of lung*** Physiological units of the lung consisting of a respiratory bronchiole and its branches (alveolar ducts, alveolar sacs, and alveoli).

***paracentral l.*** The superior convolution of the ascending frontal and parietal convolutions of the brain, forming a union of both.

***parietal l.*** One of two subdivisions of the parietal lobe of the brain. The superior parietal lobule comprises the posterior part of the upper portion, and the inferior parietal lobule comprises a lateral area continuous with temporal and occipital lobes.

***primary pulmonary l.*** The functional unit of the lung. It includes the respiratory bronchiole, alveolar ducts, sacs, and alveoli. SYN: *respiratory lobe.*

***l.'s of testis*** Pyramidal divisions separated from each other by incomplete partitions called septula. Each consists of one to three coiled seminiferous tubules.

***l.'s of thymus*** Subdivisions of a lobe, each consisting of a cortex and medulla.

**lobuli** Pl. of lobulus.

**lobulus** (lŏb'ū-lŭs) *pl.* **lobuli** [L.] A lobule or small division of a lobe.

**lobus** (lō'bŭs) *pl.* **lobi** [L.] Lobe.

**L.O.C.** *level of consciousness.*

**local** (lō'kăl) [L. *locus,* place] Limited to one place or part.

**localization** (lō-kăl-ĭ-zā'shŭn) **1.** Limitation to a definite area. **2.** Determination of the site of an infection. **3.** Relation of a sensation to its point of origin.

***cerebral l.*** Determination of centers of various faculties and functions in particular parts of the brain.

**localized** (lō'kăl-īzd) Restricted to a limited region.

**localizer** An apparatus, usually opaque or laser, used for finding foreign bodies or exact anatomical locations during radiography.

**locator** (lō'kā-tĕr) A device for locating or discovering an object such as a foreign body.

**lochia** (lō'kē-ă) [Gr. *lochia*] The discharge from the uterus of blood, mucus, and tissue during the puerperal period. For the first 6 days postpartum it is distinctly blood-tinged and is known as lochia rubra or lochia cruenta. Over the following 3 or 4 days the discharge becomes brown and is known as lochia serosa. After this it becomes yellow, then turning to white, and is known as lochia alba. It is diminished or suppressed in the presence of high fever. If the odor is offensive, it is the result of contamination with saprophytic organisms. The patient should be positioned so as to favor drainage. **lochial** (-ăl), *adj.*

***l. alba*** The white postpartum vaginal discharge that is no longer blood-tinged. SYN: *l. purulenta.*

***l. cruenta*** The bloody postpartum vaginal discharge. SYN: *l. rubra.*

***l. purulenta*** L. alba.

***l. rubra*** L. cruenta.

***l. serosa*** A thin, watery postpartum vaginal discharge.

**lochiocolpos** (lō"kē-ō-kŏl'pŏs) [Gr. *lochia,* discharge following childbirth, + *kolpos,* vagina] Distention of the vagina resulting from retention of lochia.

**lochiometra** (lō"kē-ō-mē'tră) [" + *metra,* uterus] Retention of lochia in the uterus.

**lochiometritis** (lō"kē-ō-mē-trī'tĭs) [" + " + *itis,* inflammation] Puerperal inflammation of the uterus.

**lochiorrhagia** (lō'kē-ō-rā'jē-ă) [" + *rhegnynai,* to break forth] Excessive flow of lochia.

**lochiorrhea** (lō"kē-ō-rē'ă) [" + *rhoia,* flow] Abnormal flow of lochia.

**lochioschesis** (lō"kē-ŏs'kĕ-sĭs) [" + *schesis,* retention] Retention or suppression of the lochia.

**lochometritis** (lō"kō-mē-trī'tĭs) [" + *metra,* uterus, + *itis,* inflammation] Lochiometritis.

**loci** [L.] Pl. of locus.

**Locke's solution, Locke-Ringer's solution** [Frank S. Locke, Brit. physician, 1871–1949; Sydney Ringer, Brit. physiologist, 1835–1910] A solution used in experiments in physiology. It contains sodium, potassium, calcium, and magnesium chlorides; sodium bicarbonate, dextrose, and water.

**lockjaw** Tonic spasm of muscles of jaw. SEE: *tetanus; trismus.*

**lock, saline** An intermittent infusion device used episodically to administer fluids and medications. Its patency is maintained by periodic saline flushes. SEE: *heparin lock flush solution.*

**Lockwood's ligament** [Charles B. Lockwood, Brit. surgeon, 1856–1914] The suspensory ligament of the eyeball.

**locomotion** (lō"kō-mō'shŭn) [L. *locus,* place, + *movere,* to move] Movement or the power of movement from one place to another.

**locomotor** (lō"kō-mō'tor) Pert. to locomotion.

**locomotorium** (lō"kō-mō-tō'rē-ŭm) The locomotor apparatus of the body.

**locular** (lŏk'ū-lăr) [L. *loculus,* a small space] Loculated.

**loculated** (lŏk'ū-lāt-ĕd) Containing or divided into loculi. SYN: *locular.*

**loculi** (lŏk'ū-lī) Pl. of loculus.

**loculus** (lŏk'ū-lŭs) *pl.* **loculi** [L.] A small space or cavity.

**locum tenens** (lō'kŭm tĕn'ĕns) [L. *locus,* place, + *tenere,* to hold] A substitute; a physician who temporarily substitutes for another.

**locus** (lō′kŭs) *pl.* **loci** [L. *locus,* a place] **1.** A spot or place. **2.** In genetics, the site of a gene on a chromosome.

***l. ceruleus*** A dark-colored depression in the floor of the fourth ventricle of the brain at its upper part.

***l. of control*** A term used in reference to an individual's sense of mastery or control over events. Persons with an internal locus of control are more apt to believe that they can influence events, whereas those with an external locus of control tend to believe that events are dictated by fate. These respective orientations can influence a person's practice of health-related behaviors.

***l. niger*** Substantia nigra.

**Loeffler's bacillus** (lĕf′lĕrz) [Friedrich August Johannes Loeffler (Loffler), Ger. bacteriologist, 1852–1915] Corynebacterium diphtheriae.

**Löffler's endocarditis** (lĕf′lĕrz) [Wilhelm Löffler, Swiss physician,1887–1972] Endocarditis of unknown etiology, associated with eosinophilia and fibroplastic thickening of the endocardium.

**logadectomy** (lŏg″ă-dĕk′tō-mē) [Gr. *logades,* the whites of the eyes, + *ektome,* excision] Excision of a portion of the conjunctiva.

**logaditis** (lŏg″ă-dī′tĭs) [″ + *itis,* inflammation] Scleritis.

**logagnosia** (lŏg″ăg-nō′sē-ă) [Gr. *logos,* word, reason, + *a-,* not, + *gnosis,* knowledge] A type of aphasia in which words are seen but not identified with respect to their meaning. SEE: *aphasia.*

**logagraphia** (lŏg-ă-grăf′ē-ă) [″ + ″ + *graphein,* to write] Agraphia.

**logamnesia** (lŏg-ăm-nē′zē-ă) [″ + *amnesia,* forgetfulness] Aphasia of a sensory character; the inability to recognize spoken or written words.

**logaphasia** (lŏg″ă-fā′zē-ă) [″ + *a-,* not, + *phasis,* speaking] Motor aphasia, usually the result of a cerebral lesion.

**logasthenia** (lŏg″ăs-thē′nē-ă) [″ + ″ + *sthenos,* strength] Mental impairment characterized by a defective ability to understand the spoken word.

**logoklony** (lŏg′ō-klŏn-ē) [″ + *klonein,* to agitate] Intermittent repetition of the last syllable of a word.

**logokophosis** (lŏg″ō-kō-fō′sĭs) [″ + *kophosis,* deafness] Wernicke's aphasia.

**logomania** (lŏg-ō-mā′nē-ă) [″ + *mania,* madness] Logorrhea.

**logoneurosis** (lŏg″ō-nū-rō′sĭs) [″ + *neuron,* nerve, + *osis,* condition] Any neurosis marked by speech disorders.

**logopathia** (lŏg-ō-păth′ē-ă) [″ + *pathos,* disease, suffering] Any disorder of speech arising from derangement of the central nervous system.

**logopedia** (lŏg″ō-pē′dē-ă) [″ + *pais,* child] The science dealing with speech defects and their correction.

**logoplegia** (lŏg-ō-plē′jē-ă) [″ + *plege,* stroke] Paralysis of the speech organs.

**logorrhea** (lŏg″ō-rē′ă) [″ + *rhoia,* flow] The repetitious, continuous, and excessive flow of speech seen in insanity. SYN: *logomania.*

**logospasm** (lŏg′ō-spăzm) [″ + *spasmos,* a convulsion] Spasmodic word enunciation.

**-logy** [Gr. *logos,* word, reason] Combining form used as a suffix meaning *science or study of.* SEE: *-ology.*

**loiasis** (lō-ī′ă-sĭs) Infestation with *Loa loa.*

**loin** (loyn) [O. Fr. *loigne,* long part] The lower part of the back and sides between the ribs and pelvis. SYN: *lumbus.*

**lomustine** (lō-mŭs′tēn) A chemotherapeutic agent used in treating certain neoplastic conditions; also called *CCNU.*

**loneliness** Literally, the condition of being alone. Medically, it is the important state of being frightened, anxious, depressed, or sad because of the lack of companionship, esp. of a particular person or group (i.e., one may experience loneliness even though in the presence of people).

***risk for l.*** A subjective state in which an individual is at risk of experiencing vague dysphoria. SEE: *Nursing Diagnoses Appendix.*

**Long, Crawford Williamson** U.S. physician, 1815–1878, who in 1842 first administered an anesthetic during surgery.

**long-acting thyroid stimulator** ABBR: LATS. A serum globulin that causes hyperfunction of the thyroid. There are probably other similar substances involved in affecting the thyroid gland in thyrotoxicosis.

**longevity** (lŏn-jĕv′ĭ-tē) [L. *longaevus,* aged] Long duration of life.

**longing** A persistent desire or craving for something, usually that which is remote or unattainable.

**longissimus** (lŏn-jĭs′ĭ-mŭs) [L.] An anatomical term indicating a long structure.

**longitudinal** (lŏn″jĭ-tū′dĭ-năl) [L. *longitudo,* length] Parallel to the long axis of the body or part.

**longsightedness** Hyperopia.

**longus** (lŏng′gŭs) [L.] An anatomical term indicating a long structure.

**loop** [ME. *loupe*] A curve or bend in a cord or cordlike structure, forming roughly an oval.

***l.'s of capillary*** Minute blood vessels in the papillae of the skin.

***cervical l.*** The part of an enamel organ in which the inner enamel epithelium is continuous with the outer enamel epithelium. This establishes the limit of enamel formation and therefore represents the site of the cementoenamel junction. The cells of the cervical loop become Hertwig's epithelial root sheath, induce dentinogenesis, and determine the number, size, and shape of the tooth roots.

***closed l.*** A biological system in which a substance produced affects the output of the substance by a feedback mechanism.

***Henle's l.*** The descending and ascending loops of the renal tubule.

***Lippes l.*** SEE: *Lippes loop.*

**loop electrode excision procedure** ABBR: LEEP. A technique for resecting abnormal cervical tissue. Following an abnormal Pap smear, thin wire loop electrodes are used to excise the affected or suspicious area. LEEP provides a specimen suitable for histologic evaluation.

**loosening of association** A sign of disordered thought processes in which the person speaks with frequent changes of subject, and the content is only obliquely related, if at all, to the subject matter. This may be seen in mania or schizophrenia.

**L.O.P.** *left occipitoposterior* fetal position.

**loperamide hydrochloride** Generic name for Imodium.

**lophotrichea** (lŏf-ō-trĭk′ē-ă) [Gr. *lophos,* tuft, + *thrix,* hair] Microorganisms possessing flagella in tufts.

**lophotrichous** (lŏf-ŏt′rĭ-kŭs) Having bunches of flagella at one end.

**lordoscoliosis** (lor″dō-skō″lē-ō′sĭs) [Gr. *lordosis,* bending, + *skoliosis,* curvation] Forward curvation of the spine complicated by lateral curvature.

**lordosis** (lor-dō′sĭs) [Gr.] Abnormal anterior convexity of the lumbar spine.

**L.O.T.** *left occipitotransverse* fetal position.

**lotion** (lō′shŭn) [L. *lotio*] A liquid medicinal preparation for local application to, or bathing of, a part.

***calamine l.*** SEE: *calamine.*

***white l.*** A combination of 4% zinc sulfate with 4% sulfurated potash.

**LOTR** *Licensed Occupational Therapist.*

**loudness** Sound intensity. SEE: *decibel.*

**Louis-Bar syndrome** (loo-wē′băr) [Denise Louis-Bar, 20th century European physician] Ataxia-telangiectasia.

**loupe** (loop) [Fr.] A magnifying lens used in the form of a monocular or binocular lens. Surgeons, dentists, jewelers, and watchmakers frequently use this device.

**louse** [AS. *lus*] Pediculus. SEE: illus.

***body l.*** Pediculus humanus corporis.

***crab l.*** Phthirus pubis.

***head l.*** Pediculus humanus capitis.

**lousiness** Pediculosis.

**lovastatin** A drug used to control the level of cholesterol in the blood by inhibiting the synthesis of cholesterol. Trade name is Mevacor.

**love** [ME.] **1.** Concern and affection for another person. This may be to such a degree as to cause individuals to risk losing their lives in their concern for the safety, care, and well-being of another. **2.** In psychiatry, love may be equated with pleasure, particularly as it applies to the gratifying sexual experiences between individuals.

**Loven's reflex** (lō-vānz′) [Otto Christian Loven, Swed. physician, 1835–1904] Vasodilation with a corresponding increase in the size of an organ, resulting from stimulation of an afferent nerve or organ.

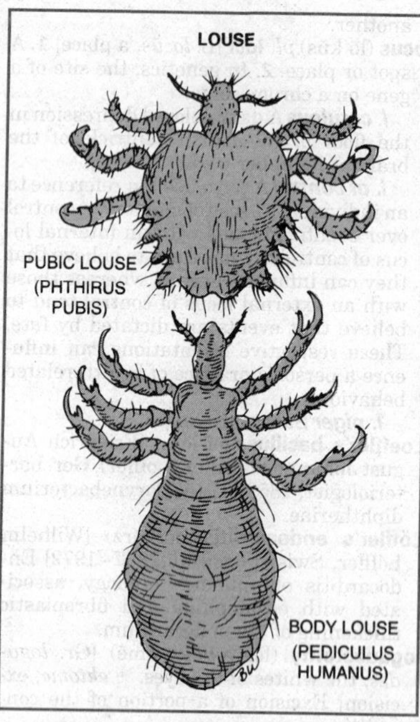


**low birth weight** ABBR: LBW. Abnormally low weight of a newborn, usually less than 2500 g. A 280-g infant has survived, but with physical and mental impairment.

Identifying mothers at risk for delivery of LBW infants involves careful assessment. Demographic factors include maternal age (adolescence) and non-white race; the highest risk occurs in primiparas under the age of 15. A review of the mother's history often finds low birth weight or prepregnancy weight, previous preterm delivery or spontaneous abortion, delivery of other LBW newborns, or fetal exposure to diethylstilbestrol. Cigarette smoking or abuse of other substances (i.e., alcohol or narcotics) may be involved. Other factors include height less than 60 in. and weight less than 80% of standard weight for height, diabetes with vascular changes, *Chlamydia trachomatis* genital tract infections, and urinary tract infections.

**Lowe's syndrome** (lōz) [Charles U. Lowe, U.S. pediatrician, b. 1921] Oculocerebrorenal dystrophy characterized by hypotonia, loss of reflexes, mental deterioration, glaucoma, cataracts, and renal tubular dysfunction. The syndrome is transmitted as a sex-linked recessive.

**low-level radiation** SEE: *radiation, low-level.*

**lox** *liquid oxygen.*

**loxarthron** (lŏks-ăr′thrŏn) [Gr. *loxos,* slanting, + *arthron,* joint] Oblique deformity of a joint without dislocation.

**loxia** (lŏks′ē-ă) [Gr., slanting] Torticollis.

**Loxosceles** (lŏks-ŏs′sĕ-lēz) A genus of spiders, family Loxoscelidae, which includes the brown recluse spider.

**loxoscelism** (lŏk-sŏs′sĕ-lĭzm) The disease produced by the bite of the brown recluse spider, *Loxosceles laeta* or *L. reclusa.* Symptoms include a painful red vesicle that eventually becomes gangrenous and sloughs off. Complications may include hemolytic anemia or renal failure and may be fatal.

**loxotomy** (lŏks-ŏt′ō-mē) [″ + *tome,* incision] Amputation by oblique section.

**lozenge** (lŏz′ĕnj) [Fr.] A small, dry, medicinal solid to be held in mouth until it dissolves. SYN: *troche.*

**Lp(a)** *lipoprotein (a).*

**L-phase variants** L-forms.

**L.P.N.** *licensed practical nurse.*

**LPO** *left posterior oblique* position.

**Lr** Symbol for the element lawrencium.

**L.R.C.P.** *licentiate of the Royal College of Physicians.*

**L.R.C.S.** *licentiate of the Royal College of Surgeons.*

**LRF** *luteinizing hormone releasing factor.*

**L.S.A.** *left sacroanterior* fetal position.

**L.Sc.A.** *left scapuloanterior* fetal position.

**L.Sc.P.** *left scapuloposterior* fetal position.

**LSD** *lysergic acid diethylamide.*

**LSI** *life satisfaction index.*

**L.S.P.** *left sacroposterior* fetal position.

**L/S ratio** *lecithin/sphingomyelin ratio.*

**L.S.T.** *left sacrotransverse* fetal position.

**LTC** *long-term care.*

**LTH** *luteotropic hormone.*

**Lu** Symbol for the element lutetium.

**lubb-dupp** (lŭb-dŭp′) The two sounds heard in auscultation marking a complete cycle of the heart. The pause following the cycle is slightly longer than that between the two sounds. SEE: *auscultation.*

**lubricant** (loo′brĭ-kănt) [L. *lubricans*] An agent, usually a liquid oil, that reduces friction between parts that brush against each other as they move. Joints are lubricated by synovial fluid.

**Lucas-Championnière's disease** (lū-kă′shaw″pē-ŏn-ē-ayrz′) [J. M. M. Lucas-Championnière, Fr. surgeon, 1843–1913] Pseudomembranous bronchitis.

**lucent** [L. *lucere,* to shine] Shining, translucent, clear.

**lucid** (lū′sĭd) [L. *lucidus,* clear] Clear, esp. applied to clarity of the mind.

***l. interval*** A period of normal mental functioning between attacks of mental illness or cerebral trauma. In head trauma, the period of being awake after the injury until coma develops. A lucid interval is common in epidural and subdural hematomas.

**lucidity** (lū-sĭd′ĭ-tē) The quality of clearness or brightness, esp. with regard to mental conditions.

**luciferase** (loo-sĭf′ĕr-ās) An enzyme that acts on luciferins to oxidize them and cause bioluminescence. It is present in certain organisms (e.g., fireflies, other insects) that emit light either continuously or intermittently.

**luciferin** (loo-sĭf′ĕr-ĭn) The general term for substances present in some organisms, which become luminescent when acted on by luciferase.

**lucifugal** (loo-sĭf′ū-găl) [L. *lux,* light, + *fugere,* to flee from] Repelled by bright light.

**lucipetal** (loo-sĭp′ĭ-tăl) [″ + *peter,* to seek] Attracted by bright light.

**lucotherapy** (lū″kō-thĕr′ă-pē) [″ + Gr. *therapeia,* treatment] Phototherapy.

**Ludwig's angina** (lūd′vĭgz) [Wilhelm F. von Ludwig, Ger. surgeon, 1790–1865] A suppurative inflammation of subcutaneous connective tissue adjacent to a submaxillary gland.

**L.U.E.** *left upper extremity.*

**Luer-Lok syringe** (lū′ĕr-lŏk′) A syringe made to permit rapid and firm attachment of the needle.

**lues** (lū′ēz) [L.] Syphilis.

**luetic** (lū-ĕt′ĭk) Syphilitic.

**Lugol's solution** (lū′gŏlz) [Jean G. A. Lugol, Fr. physician, 1786–1851] A strong iodine solution used in iodine therapy, consisting of iodine 5 g, potassium iodide 10 g, and water to make 100 ml.

**LUL** *left upper lobe* (of the lung).

**lumbago** (lŭm-bā′gō) [L. *lumbus,* loin] A general nonspecific term for dull, aching pain in the lumbar region of the back. SYN: *lumbodynia.*

**lumbar** (lŭm′băr) [L. *lumbus,* loin] Pert. to the loins; the part of the back between the thorax and pelvis.

***l. puncture*** A puncture made by placing an aspiration needle into the subarachnoid space of the spinal cord, usually in the lumbar area at the level of the fourth intervertebral space. This procedure is done to inject an anesthetic solution, to measure the pressure of the cerebrospinal fluid (CSF), or to obtain a sample of CSF for determining its constituents (e.g., pathogens, blood, proteins, excess white blood cells). The information obtained is esp. helpful in diagnosing bacterial meningitis and central nervous system syphilis. SYN: *spinal puncture.* SEE: illus.; *cerebrospinal fluid; cisternal puncture; headache; Queckenstedt's sign.*

NOTE: This procedure may be lethal if it is done in the presence of increased intracranial pressure. When the pressure in the spinal canal is decreased, the brainstem may herniate into the foramen magnum of the base of the skull.

PROCEDURE: Medication, dissolved in previously removed cerebrospinal fluid, or anesthetics for cord blocking may be cautiously introduced. The area is cleansed and painted with antiseptic. A sterile puncture needle of small gauge (22) is then readily passed directly in the midline, to and through the dura. When the stylet is removed, spinal fluid will es-

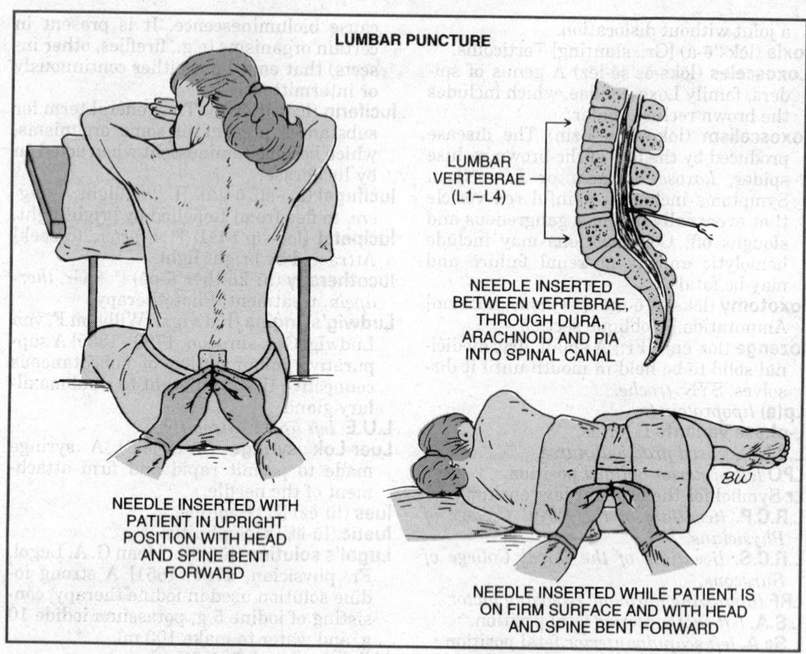


cape and can be collected in two or three tubes for examination. When the procedure is completed, the patient must be instructed to lie flat in a prone position for 6 to 12 hr. This will greatly reduce the possibility of developing a postlumbar puncture headache. This type of headache is related to continued leakage of fluid from the spinal canal. The use of a small-gauge needle will lessen the chance that spinal fluid will continue to seep from the spinal canal after the needle is removed, thus diminishing the possibility of development of postspinal tap headache. The injection of a small amount of the patient's blood epidurally at the site of the puncture forms a "patch" that will help to prevent loss of cerebrospinal fluid through the puncture hole.

NURSING IMPLICATIONS: The procedure, expected sensations, and the patient's role are explained to reassure the patient, and a signed informed consent form is obtained. Required equipment is assembled and prepared. The patient is positioned on his left side near the right edge of the bed or examining table, with the back to the operator. The nurse assists the patient to flex the thighs on the trunk and to lower the head to the chest, bowing the back as far as possible, and then holds the patient in this position. Alternately, the patient may be placed in a sitting position, with the head, neck, and thoracic spine flexed and the legs dangling over the far side of the bed or table. When this position is used, the nurse stands in front of the patient to provide support. The nurse assists the operator as necessary throughout the procedure by numbering and capping specimen tubes for laboratory examination and by applying jugular vein pressure as directed. An impervious adhesive dressing is applied to prevent leakage of spinal fluid, perhaps using a collodion or blood patch. Reassurance and direction is provided to the patient throughout the procedure.

After the procedure, the nurse assesses vital signs and neurological status, particularly observing for signs of paralysis, weakness, or loss of sensation in the lower extremities. To decrease the chance of headache, oral intake (for spinal fluid replacement and equalization of pressures) is encouraged, and the patient should remain in bed in a prone position for 4 to 24 hr (per operator or institutional protocol). While the patient should not lift his head, he or she can move it (and himself or herself) from side to side. Noninvasive pain relief measures and prescribed analgesia are provided if headache occurs.

ARTICLES NECESSARY: Sterilized lumbar puncture needles, gloves and mask for the physician and assistants, antiseptic for the skin, sterilized gauze and sponge, sterile towel, 5 ml of 0.5% solution of procaine hydrochloride, and two sterile test tubes will be needed. If spinal fluid pressure is to be determined, sterile manometer tubes and a 3-way stopcock adapter for connecting the manometer to the spinal puncture needle will be required.

***l. region*** Each side of umbilical region above the iliac region and below the hypochondriac region.

**lumbarization** (lŭm″băr-ĭ-zā′shŭn) Nonfusion of the first sacral vertebra with the sacrum, therefore functioning as an additional (sixth) lumbar vertebra.

**lumbo-** [L. *lumbus,* loin] Combining form pert. to the loins.

**lumboabdominal** (lŭm″bō-ăb-dŏm′ĭ-năl) [″ + *abdomen,* belly] Concerning the lateral and frontal areas of the abdomen.

**lumbocolostomy** (lŭm″bō-kō-lŏs′tō-mē) [″ + Gr. *kolon,* colon, + *stoma,* mouth] Colostomy by lumbar incision.

**lumbocolotomy** (lŭm″bō-kō-lŏt′ō-mē) [″ + ″ + *tome,* incision] Incision into the colon through the lumbar region.

**lumbocostal** (lŭm″bō-kŏs′tăl) [″ + *costa,* rib] Relating to the loins and ribs.

**lumbodynia** (lŭm″bō-dĭn′ē-ă) [″ + Gr. *odyne,* pain] Lumbago.

**lumboiliac** (lŭm″bō-ĭl′ē-ăk) [″ + *iliacus,* pert. to ilium] Concerning the lumbar and inguinal areas. SYN: *lumboinguinal.*

**lumboinguinal** (lŭm″bō-ĭng′gwĭ-năl) [″ + *inguinalis,* pert. to the groin] Lumboiliac.

**lumbosacral** Pert. to the lumbar vertebrae and the sacrum.

**lumbrical** (lŭm′brĭ-kăl) [L. *lumbricus,* earthworm] Vermiform.

**lumbricalis** One of the worm-shaped muscles of the hand or foot.

**lumbricide** (lŭm′brĭ-sīd) [″ + *caedere,* to kill] An agent that kills lumbricoid worms (i.e., ascarides or intestinal worms).

**lumbricoid** (lŭm′brĭ-koyd) [″ + Gr. *eidos,* form, shape] Resembling a roundworm.

**lumbricosis** (lŭm″brĭ-kō′sĭs) [″ + Gr. *osis,* condition] The state of being infested with lumbricoid worms.

**Lumbricus** (lŭm-brī′kŭs) A genus of worms that includes earthworms.

**lumbricus** (lŭm-brī′kŭs) Ascaris lumbricoides.

**lumbus** [L.] The loin; the part of the back between the thorax and pelvis.

**lumen** (lū′mĕn) *pl.* **lumina** [L., light] **1.** The space within an artery, vein, intestine, or tube. **2.** A unit of light, the amount of light emitted in a unit solid angle by a uniform point source of one international candle. SEE: *light unit; candela.*

**luminal** (lū′mĭ-năl) Relating to the lumen of a tubular structure, such as a blood vessel.

**luminescence** (loo″mĭ-nĕs′ĕns) **1.** Production of light without production of heat. SEE: *bioluminescence* **2.** In radiology, the light produced by a fluorescent phosphor when exposed to radiation.

**luminiferous** (loo″mĭ-nĭf′ĕr-ŭs) [L. *lumen,* light, + *ferre,* to bear] Producing or conveying light.

**luminometer** A luminescence photometer used to assay chemiluminescent and bioluminescent reactions. It is used clinically to assay for bacteria and living cells.

**luminophore** (loo′mĭ-nō-for″) [″ + Gr. *phoros,* bearing] A chemical present in organic compounds that permits luminescence of those compounds.

**luminous** (loo′mĭ-nŭs) Emitting light.

**lumirhodopsin** (loo″mĭ-rō-dŏp′sĭn) A chemical in the retina of the eye, intermediate between rhodopsin and all-*trans*-retinal plus opsin, formed during the bleaching of rhodopsin by exposure to light.

**lumpectomy** (lŭm-pĕk′tō-mē) [*lump* + Gr. *ektome,* excision] Surgical removal of a tumor from the breast, esp. to remove only the tumor and no other tissue or lymph nodes.

**lunacy** (lū′nă-sē) [L. *luna,* moon] An obsolete term for insanity. Insanity was formerly thought to be affected by the moon.

**lunar** Pert. to the moon, a month, or silver.

**lunate** **1.** Moon-shaped or crescent. **2.** A bone in the proximal row of the carpus. SYN: *semilunar bone.*

**lunatic** (lū′nă-tĭk) [L. *luna,* moon] An obsolete term for a person with an unsound mind. SEE: *lunacy.*

**lung** (lŭng) [AS. *lungen*] One of two cone-shaped spongy organs of respiration contained within the pleural cavity of the thorax. SEE: illus.; *alveolus* for illus.

ANATOMY: The lungs are connected with the pharynx through the trachea and larynx. The base of each lung rests on the diaphragm and each lung apex rises from 2.5 to 5 cm above the sternal end of the first rib, the collarbone, supported by its attachment to the hilum or root structures. The lungs include the lobes, lobules, bronchi, bronchioles, alveoli or air sacs, and pleural covering.

The right lung has three lobes and the left two. In men, the right lung weighs approx. 625 g, the left 570 g. The lungs contain 300,000,000 alveoli and their respiratory surface is about 70 sq m. Respirations per minute are 12 to 20 in an adult. The total capacity of the lung varies from 3.6 to 9.4 L in men and 2.5 to 6.9 L in women.

The left lung has an indentation, called the cardiac depression, for the normal placement of the heart. Behind this is the hilum, through which the blood vessels, lymphatics, and bronchi enter and leave the lung.

Air travels from the mouth and nasal passage to the pharynx and the trachea. Two main bronchi, one on each side, extend from the trachea. The main bronchi divide into smaller bronchi, one for each of five lobes. These further divide into a great number of smaller bronchioles. The pattern of distribution of these into the segments of each lobe is important in pulmonary and thoracic surgery. There are about 10 bronchopulmonary segments in the right lung and eight in the left, the actual number varying. There are 50 to 80 terminal bronchioles in each lobe. Each of these divides into two respiratory bronchioles, which in turn divide to form two

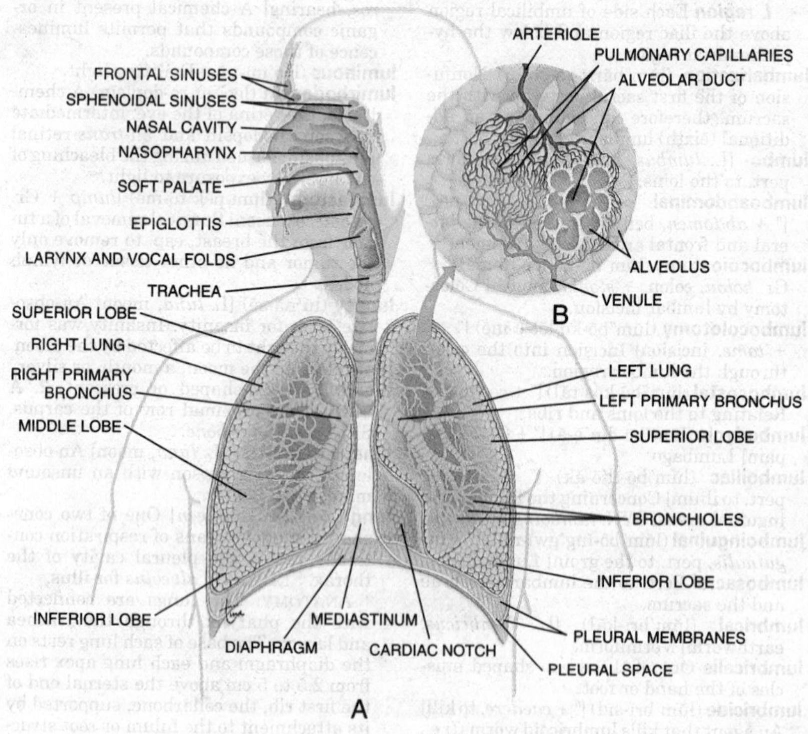


**LUNGS**

**(A) ANTERIOR VIEW OF UPPER AND LOWER RESPIRATORY TRACTS, (B) ALVEOLI AND PULMONARY CAPILLARIES**

to 11 alveolar ducts. The alveolar sacs and alveoli arise from these ducts. The spaces between the alveolar sacs and alveoli are called atria.

In the alveolus, blood and inspired air are separated only by the cell of the alveolus and that of the pulmonary capillary. This respiratory membrane is thin (0.07 to 2.0 $\mu$m) and permits oxygen to diffuse into the blood and carbon dioxide to diffuse from the blood to the air.

NERVE SUPPLY: The lungs are innervated by parasympathetic fibers via the vagus nerve and sympathetic fibers from the anterior and posterior pulmonary plexuses to the walls of the bronchial tree.

BLOOD VESSELS: The bronchial arteries and veins circulate blood to the bronchial tree. The pulmonary arteries and veins circulate the blood involved in gas exchange.

FUNCTION: The primary purpose of the lung is to bring air and blood into intimate contact so that oxygen can be added to the blood and carbon dioxide removed from it. This is achieved by two pumping systems, one moving a gas and the other a liquid. The blood and air are brought together so closely that only approx. 1 $\mu$m ($10^{-6}$ m) of tissue separates them. The volume of the pulmonary capillary circulation is 150 ml, but this is spread out over a surface area of approx. 750 sq ft (69.68 sq m). This capillary surface area surrounds 300 million air sacs called alveoli. The blood that is low in oxygen but high in carbon dioxide is in contact with the air that is high in oxygen and low in carbon dioxide for less than 1 second. SEE: *respiratory defense function.*

***l. abscess*** Circumscribed suppuration of the lung. The prognosis is fair, except in embolic abscesses. SEE: *empyema.*

SYMPTOMS: This condition is characterized by high and irregular fever, rigors, sweats, and pallor; dyspnea, cough, and purulent expectoration. There may be bubbling rales and later cavernous breathing and pectoriloquy.

TREATMENT: The basic cause of the abscess should be treated. Therapy includes a high protein, high vitamin diet and surgical drainage of the abscess.

***acute edema of l.*** Pulmonary edema.

***blast l.*** The shredding-type effect that takes place in the alveolar surfaces of the lung caused by the shock of an explosion or blast, which can cause alveolar contusion.

***brewer's l.*** A respiratory condition caused by the mold *Aspergillus* that produces allergies in otherwise healthy people and serious sinusitis, pneumonia, and fungemia in patients with neutropenia.

***compliance of l.'s*** A measure of the distensibility of the lungs. It is expressed as the change in volume of the lungs in liters when the transpulmonary pressure is changed by 1 cm of water pressure. Normally this measure is between 0.08 and 0.33 L/cm of water. It is reduced by anything that obstructs the normal flow of air in and out of the lungs, whether caused by changes in the airway or by the mechanical forces that move the ribs and diaphragm.

***l. inflammation*** Pneumonia.

***iron l.*** Drinker respirator.

***shock l.*** A diffuse lung injury, causing reduced perfusion, pulmonary edema, and alveolar collapse, associated with adult respiratory distress syndrome. SYN: *wet l.*

***l. surfactant*** Pulmonary surfactant.

***l. transplantation*** Grafting of a donor lung into patients with end-stage lung disease. Most patients who have a single- or double-lung transplant survive.

***wet l.*** Shock l.

**lung collapse** A condition resulting from a lowering of intrapulmonic pressure or an increase in intrathoracic pressure. It may be focal, involving only a few lobules, or massive, involving an entire lobe or the complete lung. It may result from obstruction of the bronchial tubes (obstructive atelectasis) or pressure upon the lung by air or fluid in the pleural cavity, an intrathoracic tumor, or a greatly enlarged heart (compressive atelectasis). Air may be introduced artificially into the pleural cavity (artificial pneumothorax) or derived from emphysematous lesions. Collapse may occur in the newborn as a result of blockage of bronchioles by mucus or from failure of the lung to distend because of weak inspiratory movements. The prognosis depends on the extent of collapse and the gravity of the preexisting disease. SYN: *atelectasis; pneumothorax*. SEE: *auscultation; chest; emphysema; tuberculosis.*

SYMPTOMS: In a sudden collapse, there is pronounced dyspnea and circulatory collapse. When collapse is gradual, symptoms may be less pronounced or even nonexistent.

TREATMENT: In the newborn, the excess mucus should be aspirated from the bronchus and the lung gently inflated with a catheter. In acquired varieties, the original disease should be directly treated.

***hypostatic l.c.*** Congestion of the dependent portions of the lungs, occurring in asthenic diseases that necessitate a protracted recumbent position.

SYMPTOMS: Dyspnea, cough, and scanty expectoration characterize this condition. Slight dullness to percussion, and feeble bronchial breathing are also present.

TREATMENT: Development of congestion should be prevented by frequent change in position, by deep breathing exercises, and by assisted ventilation if required.

***passive l.c.*** Lung congestion resulting from obstruction to the flow of blood from the lungs to the heart. Dyspnea, hard cough, mucous expectoration containing pigmented cells, slight dullness, and feeble breathing will be present.

**lungworm** (lŭng′wĕrm) Any of the nematodes that infest the lungs of humans and animals.

**lunula** (lū′nū-lă) *pl.* **lunulae** [L., little moon] **1.** A crescent-shaped area. **2.** An active area of nailbed growth at the base of the fingernails and toenails. The cells develop and keratinize to form nails.

***l. of valves of heart*** One of two narrow portions on the free edges of the semilunar valves on each side of the nodulus.

**lupiform** (lū′pĭ-form) [L. *lupus*, wolf, + *forma*, shape] Resembling lupus.

**lupoid** (loo′poyd) [″ + Gr. *eidos*, form, shape] **1.** Resembling lupus. **2.** Boeck's sarcoid.

**lupous** (lū′pŭs) **1.** Pert. to lupus. **2.** Affected with lupus.

**lupus** (lū′pŭs) [L., wolf] Originally any chronic, progressive, usually ulcerating, skin disease. In current usage when the word is used alone, it has no precise meaning.

***discoid l. erythematosus*** ABBR: DLE. A chronic disease of the skin characterized by remissions and exacerbations of a scaling, red, macular rash. These lesions contain plugged follicles and are atrophic. In one form, the lesions are above the chin, and in the second form, on the rest of the body. The disease is limited to the skin in 90% of patients, but may eventually develop into systemic lupus erythematosus. Thought to be an autoimmune disorder, it is approx. five times more common in females than in males. SEE: *systemic l. erythematosus.*

TREATMENT: The patient should avoid exposure to the sun. Skin lesions should be treated with topical corticosteroids, but overuse of these preparations should be avoided.

***l. pernio*** Skin lesions sometimes present in sarcoidosis. They are hard, blue-purple, swollen, shiny lesions of the nose, cheeks, lips, ears, fingers, and knees.

***systemic l. erythematosus*** ABBR: SLE. A chronic autoimmune inflammatory disease involving multiple organ systems and marked by periods of exacerbation and remission. Its name is derived from the characteristic butterfly (malar) rash over the nose and cheeks that resembles a wolf's face. The disease is most prevalent in nonwhite women of childbearing age. SYN: *septic shock.* SEE: *Nursing Diagnoses Appendix.*

SYMPTOMS: Patients present with a wide diversity of clinical signs but polyarthralgia, polyarthritis, glomerulonephritis, fever, malaise, normocytic anemia, and vasculitis of small vessels of the hands and feet causing peripheral neuropathy are the most common. Other signs include skin rashes after exposure to sunlight, pleuritic pain, interstitial lung disease, pericarditis, myocarditis, gastrointestinal ulcerations, and other problems caused by inflammatory changes of the blood vessels or connective tissue.

DIAGNOSIS: Formerly, the presence of lupus erythematosus cells was considered the most significant diagnostic laboratory test. Currently, testing focuses on antinuclear antibodies that attack the nuclei of cells, anti-DNA antibodies, various other autoantibiodies, and low blood levels of complement. Diagnosis can be made if four or more of the following are present either at one time or sequentially: butterfly rash; characteristic discoid skin lesion; Raynaud's phenomenon; development of a skin rash on exposure to sunlight; oral or nasopharyngeal ulceration; arthritis without deformity; positive test results for autoantibodies, lupus cells, and anti-DNA and anti-Sm antigens; a chronic false-positive serological test for syphilis; chronic pleuritis or pericarditis; proteinurea greater than 0.5 g/day or cellular casts in the urine; psychosis; convulsions; and hemolytic anemia; white blood cell count less than 4000 $mm^3$; lymphocyte count less than $1500/mm^3$; or thrombocytopenia of less than $100,000/mm^3$. Many drugs can cause the appearance of signs and symptoms of SLE; the most common of these are procainamide and hydralazine. The appearance of antinuclear antibodies in the serum, fever, and rash are considered diagnostic; these disappear when the drug is discontinued.

ETIOLOGY: Although the complete etiology is unknown, SLE is classified as an autoimmune disease in which B lymphocytes produce autoantibodies that attack cells, possibly due to a genetic defect in B cells or an abnormality in the T cell-mediated immune response. Other predisposing factors under study include environmental triggers and the role played by low serum complement levels.

PATHOLOGY: Autoantibodies react with self-antigens to form immune complexes in such large numbers that they cannot be excreted; the immune complexes precipitate within blood vessels, producing inflammation and disrupting the flow of blood and oxygen to tissues.

TREATMENT: There is no cure and complete remissions are rare. Nevertheless, about 25% of patients have mild disease and do not require glucocorticoids. Nonsteroidal anti-inflammatory drugs should be used to control symptoms. The dermatologic manifestations may respond to antimalarials, but patients must be closely observed for retinal damage. Other treatments for the skin rash include sunscreens, quinacrine, retinoids, and dapsone. Life-threatening and severely disabling conditions should be treated with high doses of glucosteroids and supplemental calcium to minimize osteoporosis, which may be an undesired side effect of long-term glucocorticoid use. The cytotoxic agents azathioprine, chlorambucil, and cyclophosphamide are used in treating active disease and reducing flares.

PROGNOSIS: The prognosis depends on which organ systems are involved, how severely they are damaged, and how rapidly the disease progresses. Five-year survival rates are high (80% to 90%), but the average long-term survival is less than 15 years.

NURSING IMPLICATIONS: Patient education related to the disease and treatment is essential in any chronic disease. The purpose, proper dosage, use, and side effects of drugs should be taught. Patients need emotional support to help cope with changes in appearance because of skin lesions or when high-dose corticosteroids are given. Patients should be taught to wear clothing and hats that block direct sunlight and to maintain a diet high in potassium and protein. The nurse should help establish a regimen for adequate relief of both the musculoskeletal pain and chronic fatigue experienced by most patients. Additional support and teaching depends on the organ system most affected by the disease. Over time, patients with severe progressive disease need assistance in coping with the probability of an early death.

***l. vulgaris*** Tuberculosis of the skin; characterized by patches that break down and ulcerate, leaving scars on healing.

**LUQ** *left upper quadrant* of abdomen.

**Luque wires** Wires used in the surgical procedure for the stabilization of scoliosis. Transverse traction on each vertebra is accomplished by wrapping flexible wires around the affected vertebrae and attaching the wires to flexible rods.

**Lust's reflex** (lŭsts) [Franz Alexander Lust, Ger. pediatrician, b. 1880] Dorsal flexion and abduction of the foot resulting from percussion of the external branch of the sciatic nerve.

**luteal** [L. *luteus,* yellow] Pert. to the corpus luteum, its cells, or its hormone.

**lutein** (lū'tē-ĭn) Yellow pigment derived from the corpus luteum, egg yolk, and fat cells or lipochromes.

**luteinic** (loo″tē-ĭn′ĭk) Concerning the corpus luteum of the ovary.

**luteinization** (lū″tē-ĭn-ī-zā′shŭn) The process of development of the corpus within a ruptured graafian follicle.

**Lutembacher's syndrome** (loo′tĕm-băk″ĕrz) [René Lutembacher, Fr. physician, 1884–1916] Atrial septal defect of the heart with mitral stenosis.

**luteolysin** (loo″tē-ō-lī′sĭn) [L. *luteus,* yellow, + Gr. *lysis,* dissolution] Something that promotes death of the corpus luteum.

**luteoma** (lū″tē-ō′mă) [L. *luteus,* yellow, + Gr. *oma,* tumor] An ovarian tumor containing lutein cells.

**luteotropin** (loo″tē-ō-trō′pĭn) Luteinizing hormone.

**lutetium** (lū-tē′shē-ŭm) SYMB: Lu. A rare element; atomic weight 174.97; atomic number 71.

**luteum** (lū′tē-ŭm) [L.] Yellow.

***corpus l.*** A yellow cellular mass in the ovary that forms after the graafian follicle has erupted. It enlarges if pregnancy occurs, and secretes estrogen and progesterone that maintain early pregnancy. If pregnancy does not occur the follicle atrophies. SEE: *fertilization* for illus.

**Lutz-Splendore-Almeida disease** [A. Lutz, Brazilian physician, 1855–1940; A. Splendore, contemp. Italian physician; Floriano P. de Almeida, Brazilian physician, b. 1898] South American blastomycosis.

**lux** (lŭks) [L., light] A unit of light intensity equivalent to 1 lumen/sq m.

**luxation** (lŭks-ā′shŭn) [L. *luxatio,* dislocation] **1.** Displacement of organs or articular surfaces; dislocation of a joint. SEE: *subluxation* **2.** In dentistry, injury to supporting tissues that results in the loosening of the teeth with rotation or partial displacement.

**Luys' body** (lū-ēz′) [Jules-Bernard Luys, Fr. physician, 1828–1898] A small mass of gray matter lying on the dorsal surface of the peduncle dorsolateral to the substantia nigra of the brain. Luys' nucleus is located in the posterior portion of the thalamus.

**LV** *left ventricle.*

**LVEDP** *left ventricular end-diastolic pressure.*

**L.V.N.** *licensed vocational nurse.*

**lyase** (lī′ās) The class name for enzymes (as decarboxylase, aldolase, and synthases) that remove chemical groups other than by hydrolysis.

**lycanthropy** (lī-kăn′thrō-pē) [Gr. *lykos,* wolf, + *anthropos,* man] A mania in which one believes oneself to be a wild beast, esp. a wolf.

**lycopene** (lī′kō-pēn) The red carotenoid pigment found in tomatoes and other red fruits and berries.

**lycopenemia** (lī″kō-pĕ-nē′mē-ă) [*lycopene* + Gr. *haima,* blood] A type of carotenemia caused by eating excessive amount of foods that contain lycopene.

**lycoperdonosis** (lī″kō-pĕr″dŏn-ō′sĭs) [Gr. *lykos,* wolf, + *perdesthai,* to break wind, + *osis,* condition] A respiratory disease caused by inhaling large quantities of spores from the mature mushroom commonly called puffball. *Lycoperdon* is the genus of fungi to which most puffballs belong.

**lycopodium** (lī-kō-pō′dē-ŭm) A yellow powder formed from spores of *Lycopodium clavatum,* a club moss. It is used as a dusting powder and as a desiccant, and absorbent.

**lye** (lī) [AS. *leag*] **1.** Liquid from leaching of wood ashes. **2.** Any strong alkaline solution, esp. sodium or potassium hydroxide. SEE: *alkali; potassium hydroxide; sodium hydroxide.*

**lye poisoning** SEE: *Poisons and Poisoning Appendix.*

**lying-in 1.** The puerperal state. **2.** Being hospitalized for the purpose of childbearing.

**Lyme disease, Lyme arthritis** [Lyme, CT, U.S.A., where the disease was originally described] ABBR: LD. A multisystem disorder caused by the tick-transmitted spirochete *Borrelia burgdorferi.* After an incubation period of 3 to 32 days, usually in summer when ticks are most active, stage 1 begins with a characteristic expanding skin lesion, called erythema migrans, at the site of the tick bite. The tick (*Ixodes dammini*) is so small and the initial bite so mild that the patient may not recall having been bitten. The patient may also have flulike symptoms and headache at this time. SEE: *Nursing Diagnoses Appendix.*

The disseminated infection, stage 2, begins within the next few days to weeks. During that time, the spirochete may spread to many other skin sites and to the heart, joints, and nervous system. Symptoms may include severe headache, mild neck stiffness, meningitis, Bell's palsy, joint and muscle pain, cardiac arrhythmias, lymphadenopathy, profound fatigue, and lethargy. Even without treatment, these symptoms either improve or disappear within several weeks.

Stage 3 begins months after the onset of the infection. In patients who have not received an antibiotic, 60% will develop arthritis. The symptoms of arthritic involvement of the large joints may be intermittent for a period of weeks to months. The arthritic changes in the joints may become chronic.

Lyme disease occurs throughout the U.S. and both sexes and patients of any age may be infected. Transplacental transmission of the spirochete has been reported in mothers who had Lyme disease during the first trimester of pregnancy. The infection has been transmitted by blood transfusion.

TREATMENT: Treatment includes doxycycline or amoxicillin, but doxycycline should not be given to children or pregnant women. Arthritis may respond to 30 days of oral antibiotic therapy, but parenteral therapy is more effective for neurologic abnormalities.

PROGNOSIS: When treated early, results are good. If the disease is treated late, convalesence is prolonged, but complete recovery is the usual outcome in the majority of patients.

**lymph** (lĭmf) [L. *lympha*] An alkaline fluid found in the lymphatic vessels and the cisterna chyli. It is usually a clear, transparent, colorless fluid; however, in vessels draining the intestines it may appear milky owing to the presence of absorbed fats. It differs from blood in that red blood corpuscles are absent and the protein content is lower. Osmotic pressure is slightly higher than in blood plasma; viscosity, slightly less. Specific gravity is 1.016 to 1.023.

Lymph may vary considerably in composition in different parts of the body. In peripheral vessels, it is similar to blood plasma except that the protein content is usually much lower. Lymph contains proteins (serum albumin, serum globulin, serum fibrinogen), salts, organic substances (urea, creatinine, neutral fats, glucose), and water. Cells present are principally lymphocytes, formed in the lymph nodes and other lymphatic organs. Lymph from the intestines (called chyle) contains fats and other substances absorbed from the intestines.

Lymph is formed in tissue spaces all over the body and is gathered into small vessels that carry it centrally. All lymph eventually enters into either the thoracic duct or right lymph duct, each terminating at the junction of the internal jugular and subclavian veins, where the lymph reenters the bloodstream. The thoracic duct commences in the abdomen as a dilated sac, the cisterna (receptaculum) chyli, which receives lymph vessels from the lower limbs and the pelvic viscera including the stomach and intestines. It continues upward through the thorax, receiving intercostal lymph vessels, and near its termination, it receives the left subclavian trunk, draining the left upper extremity, and the left jugular trunk, draining the left side of head and neck. The right lymph duct drains the right sides of the thorax, head, and neck. SEE: *lymphatic system* for illus.

As lymph flows through the lymph vessels toward the subclavian veins, it passes through lymph nodes, which contain macrophages to phagocytize bacteria or other pathogens that may be present.

***l. channel*** L. sinus.

***l. follicle*** An irregular and inconstant aggregation of lymphocytes, usually seen in the lamina propria of a mucosal layer; an old term for lymph node.

***inflammatory l.*** An exudate due to inflammation.

***intercellular l.*** Tissue fluid.

***l. node*** One of many small kidney-shaped organs of lymphoid tissue that lie at intervals along the lymphatic vessels. It contains large numbers of lymphocytes and macrophages connected by a loose fibrin net and serves as a filter for lymph, destroying microorganisms and abnormal cells through direct lysis or phagocytosis. An increase in the size of the node (lymphadenopathy) indicates a high level of activity during infection.

Lymph nodes occur singly or in closely connected chains. Prominent chains lie in the neck, axilla, groin, and mesentery, where they filter lymphatic flow from the head, arms, pelvis and legs, and gastrointestinal tract, respectively. The white blood cells within the node initiate both the nonspecific inflammatory response and the specific immune response to eliminate foreign antigens.

Lymph nodes consist of multiple compartments through which the lymph travels. Lymph enters the node through the afferent vessels along the larger outer rim. It passes through the subcapsular sinus, which is lined with macrophages, into the primary and secondary folllicles of the cortex. Follicles are collections of lymphocytes that shift and change as needed in response to the antigens presented. They contain both immature and mature B and T cells. The particular antibody-producing or activated lymphocyte needed to destroy the antigen matures and proliferates rapidly. Lymph then passes through the paracortex and the medulla, which contain mature T and B cells, B memory cells, and macrophages, before exiting through the efferent vessel. Antibodies produced in the node travel via the lymph to the blood for distribution throughout the body. SEE: illus; *immune response; inflammation; lymph; lymphocyte.*

**lymphadenectasis** (lĭm-făd″ĕ-nĕk′tă-sĭs) [L. *lympha,* lymph, + Gr. *aden,* gland, + *ektasis,* dilatation] Dilatation or distention of a lymph node.

**lymphadenectomy** (lĭm-făd″ĕ-nĕk′tō-mē) [″ + ″ + *ektome,* excision] Surgical removal of a lymph node.

**lymphadenia** (lĭm″fă-dē′nē-ă) Hyperplasia affecting lymph nodes.

***l. ossea*** Bone marrow hyperplasia accompanied by Bence Jones protein in the urine. This disease is characterized by neuralgic pains followed by painful swellings on the ribs and skull and the possible occurrence of spontaneous fractures.

**lymphadenitis** (lĭm-făd″ĕn-ī′tĭs) [″ + ″ + *itis,* inflammation] An inflammation of the lymph nodes. SYN: *adenolymphitis.*

SYMPTOMS: The disease is characterized by a marked increase of tissue, with possible suppuration. Swelling, pain, and tenderness are present. The disease usually accompanies lymphangitis.

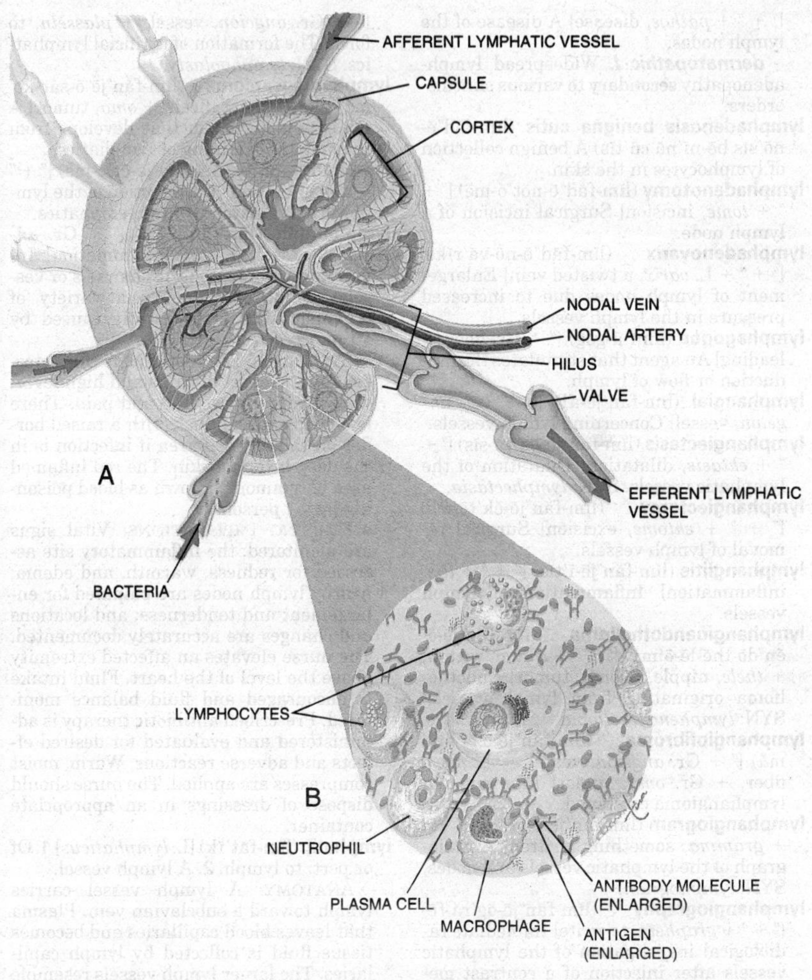


**LYMPH NODE**

**(A)** SECTION THROUGH A LYMPH NODE, **(B)** MICROSCOPIC DETAIL OF DESTRUCTION OF BACTERIA

ETIOLOGY: The condition is caused by drainage of bacteria or toxic substances into the lymph nodes. The etiology may be specific, as when caused by the organisms of typhoid, syphilis, or tuberculosis, or nonspecific, in which the causative organism is not identified.

TREATMENT: Hot, moist dressings should be applied. Incision and drainage are necessary if abscesses occur. Antibiotics should be given as indicated.

***tuberculous l.*** Tuberculosis of the lymph nodes, caused by *Mycobacterium tuberculosis*. Symptoms include a possible loss of weight and strength. There is a gradual onset of the disease and enlargement of lymph nodes. Nodes may become adherent and necrotic, and may discharge pus through the skin. The disease is treated with antituberculosis drugs.

**lymphadenocele** (lĭm-făd′ĕ-nō-sēl″) [″ + ″ + *kele,* tumor, swelling] A cyst of a lymph node.

**lymphadenogram** (lĭm-făd′ĕ-nō-grăm″) [″ + ″ + *gramma,* something written] A radiograph of a lymph gland.

**lymphadenography** (lĭm-făd″ĕ-nŏg′ră-fē) [″ + ″ + *graphein,* to write] Radiography of the lymph glands after injection of radiopaque material.

**lymphadenoid** (lĭm-făd′ĕ-noyd) [″ + ″ + *eidos,* form, shape] Resembling a lymph node or lymph tissue.

**lymphadenopathy** (lĭm-făd″ĕ-nŏp′ă-thē)

[" + " + *pathos,* disease] A disease of the lymph nodes.

***dermatopathic l.*** Widespread lymphadenopathy secondary to various skin disorders.

**lymphadenosis benigna cutis** (lĭm-făd"ĕ-nō'sĭs bē-nī'nă cū'tĭs) A benign collection of lymphocytes in the skin.

**lymphadenotomy** (lĭm-făd"ĕ-nŏt'ō-mē) [" + " + *tome,* incision] Surgical incision of a lymph node.

**lymphadenovarix** (lĭm-făd"ĕ-nō-vā'rĭks) [" + " + L. *varix,* a twisted vein] Enlargement of lymph nodes due to increased pressure in the lymph vessels.

**lymphagogue** (lĭmf'ă-gŏg) [" + Gr. *agogos,* leading] An agent that stimulates the production or flow of lymph.

**lymphangial** (lĭm-făn'jē-ăl) [" + Gr. *angeion,* vessel] Concerning lymph vessels.

**lymphangiectasis** (lĭm-făn"jē-ĕk'tă-sĭs) [" + " + *ektasis,* dilatation] Dilatation of the lymphatic vessels. SYN: *lymphectasia.*

**lymphangiectomy** (lĭm-făn"jē-ĕk'tō-mē) [" + " + *ektome,* excision] Surgical removal of lymph vessels.

**lymphangiitis** (lĭm-făn"jē-ī'tĭs) [" + " + *itis,* inflammation] Inflammation of lymph vessels.

**lymphangioendothelioma** (lĭm-făn"jē-ō-ĕn"dō-thē-lē-ō'mă) [" + " + *endon,* within, + *thele,* nipple, + *oma,* tumor] Endothelioma originating from lymph vessels. SYN: *lymphendothelioma.*

**lymphangiofibroma** (lĭm-făn"jē-ō-fī-brō'mă) [" + Gr. *angeion,* vessel, + L. *fiber,* fiber, + Gr. *oma,* tumor] Fibroma and lymphangioma combined.

**lymphangiogram** (lĭm-făn'jē-ō-grăm) [" + " + *gramma,* something written] A radiograph of the lymphatic vessels and nodes. SYN: *lymphogram.*

**lymphangiography** (lĭm-făn"jē-ŏg'ră-fē) [" + " + *graphein,* to write] Immediate radiological investigation of the lymphatic vessels after injection of a contrast medium via cutdown, usually on the dorsum of the hand or foot. Delayed films are taken to visualize the nodes. This technique has been replaced by computed tomography and magnetic resonance imaging. SYN: *lymphography.*

**lymphangiology** (lĭm-făn"jē-ŏl'ō-jē) [" + " + *logos,* word, reason] The branch of medical science concerned with the lymphatic system.

**lymphangioma** (lĭm-făn"jē-ō'mă) [" + " + *oma,* tumor] A tumor composed of lymphatic vessels.

***cavernous l.*** Dilated lymph vessels filled with lymph.

***cystic l.*** Multilocular cysts filled with lymph. The condition is usually congenital.

**lymphangiophlebitis** (lĭm-făn"jē-ō-flĕ-bī'tĭs) [" + " + *phleps,* vein, + *itis,* inflammation] Inflammation of the lymphatic vessels and veins.

**lymphangioplasty** (lĭm-făn'jē-ō-plăs"tē) [" + Gr. *angeion,* vessel, + *plassein,* to form] The formation of artificial lymphatics. SYN: *lymphoplasty.*

**lymphangiosarcoma** (lĭm-făn"jē-ō-săr-kō'mă) [" + " + *sarx,* flesh, + *oma,* tumor] A malignant neoplasm that develops from the endothelial lining of lymphatics.

**lymphangiotomy** (lĭm-făn"jē-ŏt'ō-mē) [" + " + *tome,* incision] **1.** Dissection of the lymphatics. **2.** Anatomy of the lymphatics.

**lymphangitis** (lĭm"făn-jī'tĭs) [" + Gr. *angeion,* vessel, + *itis,* inflammation] Inflammation of lymphatic channels or vessels. It may be due to a variety of organisms but is frequently caused by streptococci.

SYMPTOMS: The condition is characterized by the onset of chills and high fever, with moderate swelling and pain. There is a deep general flush with a raised border on the affected area if infection is in the deep layers of skin. The red inflamed area is commonly known as blood poisoning by lay persons.

NURSING IMPLICATIONS: Vital signs are monitored; the inflammatory site assessed for redness, warmth, and edema; nearby lymph nodes are palpated for enlargement and tenderness; and locations and changes are accurately documented. The nurse elevates an affected extremity above the level of the heart. Fluid intake is encouraged and fluid balance monitored. Prescribed antibiotic therapy is administered and evaluated for desired effects and adverse reactions. Warm, moist compresses are applied. The nurse should dispose of dressings in an appropriate container.

**lymphatic** (lĭm-făt'ĭk) [L. *lymphaticus*] **1.** Of or pert. to lymph. **2.** A lymph vessel.

ANATOMY: A lymph vessel carries lymph toward a subclavian vein. Plasma that leaves blood capillaries and becomes tissue fluid is collected by lymph capillaries. The larger lymph vessels resemble veins in that they have valves to prevent backflow of lymph. These larger vessels anastomose to form either the thoracic duct or the right lymphatic duct, which empty lymph into the blood in the left and right subclavian veins, respectively. The lymph capillaries within the villi of the small intestine (lacteals) absorb the fat-soluble end products of digestion (chyle), which are transported in the form of chylomicrons to the blood by the larger lymphatic vessels.

***afferent l.*** Any of the small vessels carrying lymph to a lymph node.

***l. capillary*** One of the smallest lymphatic vessels. These thin-walled tubes consist of a single layer of endothelium ending blindly in a swollen or rounded end, and form a dense network in most tissues of the body. They are generally slightly larger in diameter than blood capillaries. Because they collect interstitial fluid, the composition of the lymph

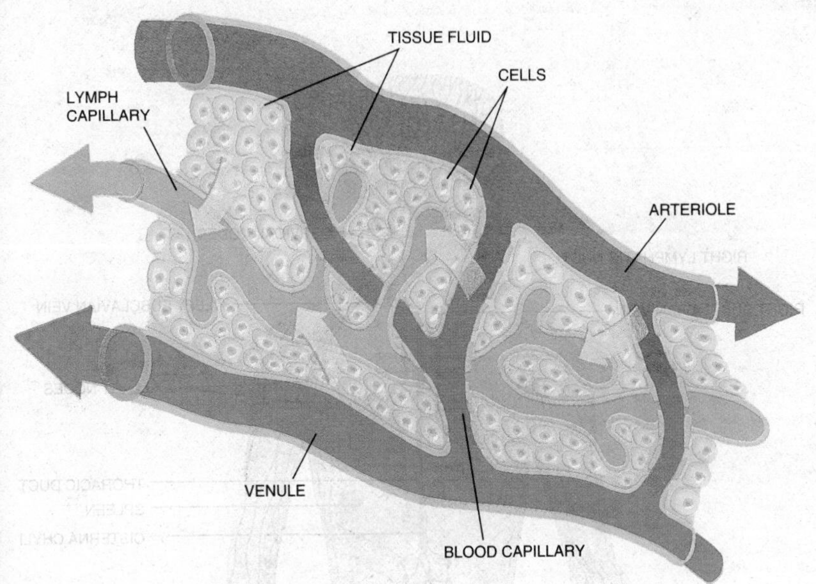


LYMPHATIC CAPILLARIES IN TISSUE SPACES

ARROWS INDICATE MOVEMENT OF PLASMA, LYMPH, AND TISSUE FLUID

varies according to the tissue being drained. Intestinal lymphatics contain fatty materials during digestion; those from the liver contain proteins. Lymphatic capillaries unite to form larger lymphatic vessels, which drain into lymph nodes drained by efferent lymph vessels, which carry lymph via the thoracic duct and right lymphatic duct into the venous blood in the left and right subclavian veins, respectively. SEE: illus.

***efferent l.*** Any of the small vessels carrying lymph from a lymph node.

***l. system*** The system that includes all the lymph vessels that collect tissue fluid and return it to the blood (lymph capillaries, lacteals, larger vessels, the thoracic duct, and the right lymphatic duct), and the organs made of lymphatic tissue (lymph nodes and nodules, the spleen, and the thymus) that produce lymphocytes and monocytes, defend against pathogens, and provide immunity. SEE: illus.; *lymph.*

**lymphaticostomy** (lĭm-făt″ĭ-kŏs′tō-mē) [L. *lymphaticus,* lymphatic, + Gr. *stoma,* mouth] The making of a permanent aperture into a lymphatic duct.

**lymphatitis** (lĭm″fă-tī′tĭs) [″ + Gr. *itis,* inflammation] An inflammation of the lymphatic system.

**lymphatolysis** (lĭm″fă-tŏl′ĭ-sĭs) [″ + Gr. *lysis,* dissolution] Destruction of lymphatic vessels or tissue.

**lymphatolytic** (lĭm″fă-tō-lĭt′ĭk) Destructive to lymphatics.

**lymphectasia** (lĭmf″ĕk-tā′zē-ă) [L. *lympha,* lymph, + Gr. *ektasis,* dilatation] Lymphangiectasis.

**lymphedema** (lĭmf-ĕ-dē′mă) [″ + Gr. *oidema,* swelling] An abnormal accumulation of tissue fluid (potential lymph) in the interstitial spaces. The mechanism for this is either impairment of normal uptake of lymph by the lymphatic vessels or excessive production of lymph caused by venous obstruction that increases capillary blood pressure. Stagnation of tissue fluid encourages infection and consequent inflammatory response. When allowed to continue, elephantiasis or sclerodermatous changes may develop. After surgery for cancer of the breast, lymphedema of the hand and arm on the operated side may occur. This may develop weeks or even many months after surgery. Radiation therapy for breast cancer and adjacent nodes may cause lymphedema by damaging the lymph vessels that pass through lymph nodes. Following breast surgery swelling of the arm and hand may take 6 weeks to subside. If it persists after that time, then lymphedema is most probably the cause. Isometric and range-of-motion exercises of the arm and hand should be started postoperatively when the surgeon feels this is safe. Those exercises will help lymph fluid to escape from the swollen area. Routine procedures such as obtaining blood pressure and venipunctures should be done on the unaffected arm. Leg surgery may also

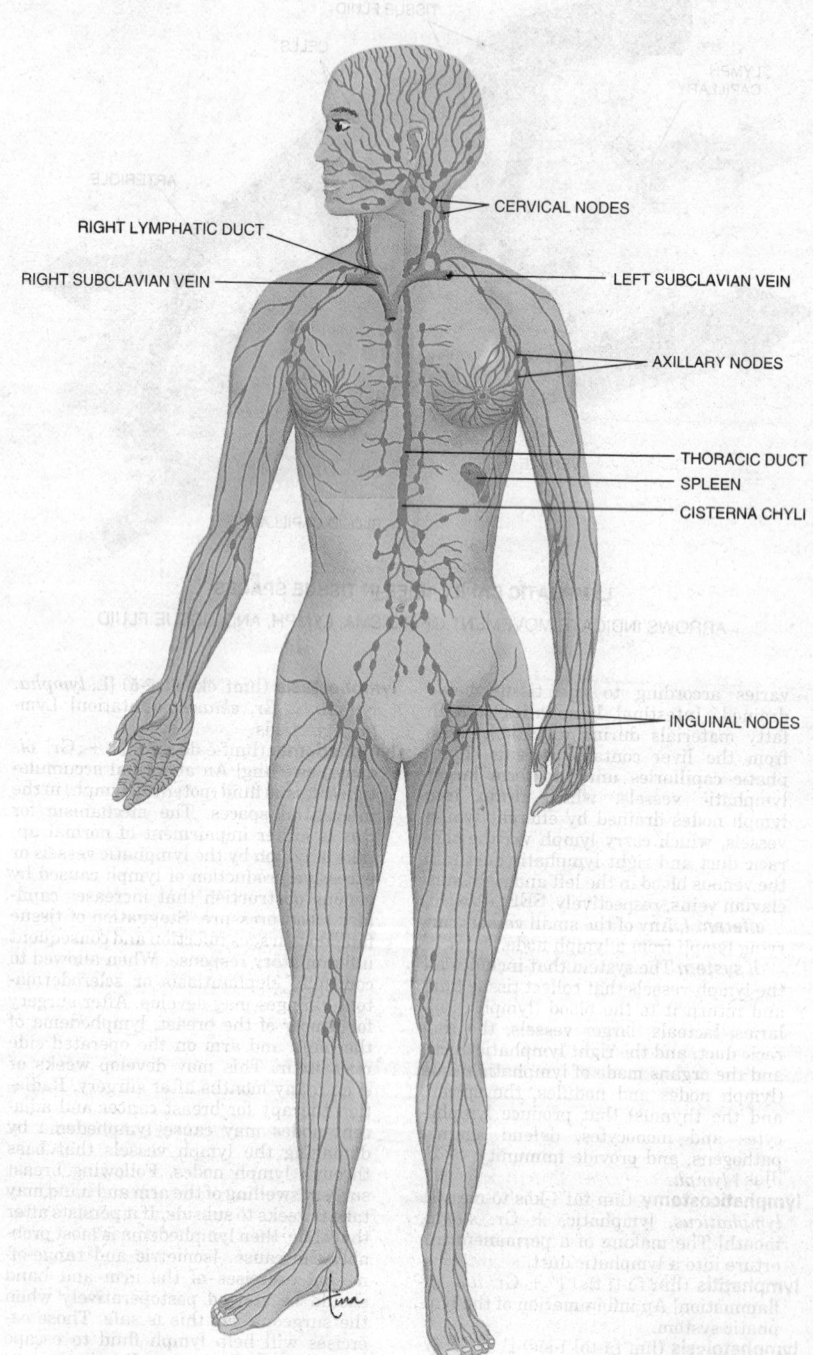


THE LYMPHATIC SYSTEM

cause lymphedema. SEE: *blockade, lymphatic; elephantiasis; pump, lymphedema.*

***congenital l.*** Chronic pitting edema of the lower extremities. SYN: *Meige-Milroy's disease.*

**lymphendothelioma** (lĭmf″ĕn-dō-thē-lē-ō′mă) [″ + Gr. *endon,* within, + *thele,* nipple, + *oma,* tumor] Tumor from proliferation and dilatation of lymphatics with overgrowth of myxomatous tissue.

**lymphization** (lĭm″fī-zā′shŭn) Production of lymph.

**lymphoblast** (lĭm′fō-blăst) [″ + Gr. *blastos,* germ] An immature cell that gives rise to a lymphocyte.

**lymphoblastic** (lĭm″fō-blăs′tĭk) [″ + Gr. *blastos,* germ] Concerning a lymphoblast. SYN: *lymphocytoblast.*

**lymphoblastoma** (lĭm″fō-blăst-ō′mă) [″ + ″ + *oma,* tumor] Lymphosarcoma.

**lymphoblastomatosis** (lĭm″fō-blăs″tō-mă-tō′sĭs) [″ + ″ + *oma,* tumor, + *osis,* condition] A condition produced by lymphoblastomas.

**lymphoblastosis** (lĭm″fō-blăs-tō′sĭs) [″ + ″ + *osis,* condition] An excessive number of lymphoblasts in the blood.

**lymphocele** (lĭm′fō-sēl) [L. *lympha,* lymph, + Gr. *kele,* tumor, swelling] A cyst that contains lymph.

**lymphocytapharesis** [″ + Gr. *aphairesis,* removal] Removal of lymphocytes from the blood after it has been withdrawn. The blood is then returned to the donor.

**lymphocyte** (lĭm′fō-sīt) [L. *lympha,* lymph, + Gr. *kytos,* cell] A cell present in the blood and lymphatic tissue. Less than 1% are present in the circulating blood. These cells travel from the blood to the lymph and lymph nodes and back into the circulation. Small lymphocytes are 6 to 9 μm and the largest ones 9 to 15 μm in diameter. There are a number of different types of lymphocytes with respect to function, but these cannot be differentiated by microscopic examination. Lymphocytes are derived from the stem cells from which all blood cells arise. They are the main means of providing the body with immune capability. This is done by means of humoral immunity produced by B cells and cell-mediated immunity produced by T cells. The total cell mass of lymphocytes is about equivalent to that of the liver. In the circulating blood, lymphocytes constitute 20% to 44% of the total white cells. SEE: illus.; *blood* for illus.; *cell, plasma; immunity, cell-mediated; immunity, humoral*

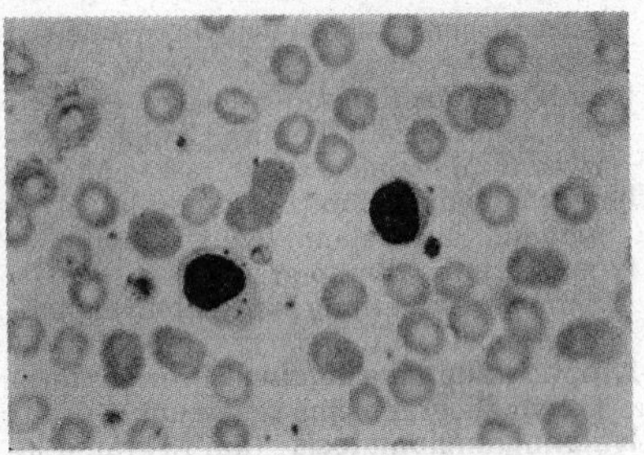

NORMAL LARGE AND SMALL LYMPHOCYTES (ORIG. MAG. ×500)

***activated l.*** A lymphocyte that has been stimulated by exposure to a specific antigen or by macrophage processing so that it is capable of responding to a foreign antigen by neutralizing or eliminating it.

***l. activation*** The use of an antigen (or mitogen in vitro) to stimulate lymphocyte metabolic activity.

***B l.*** A lymphocyte formed from pluripotent stem cells in the bone marrow that migrates to the spleen, lymph nodes, and other peripheral lymphoid tissue where it comes in contact with foreign antigens and becomes a mature functioning cell. Mature B cells are able to independently identify foreign antigens and differentiate into antibody-producing plasma cells or memory cells; their activity also may be stimulated by IL-2 (previously called B-cell growth factor). Plasma cells are the only source of immunoglobulins (antibodies). Memory cells enable the body to produce antibodies quickly when it is invaded by the same organism at a later date. SYN: *B cell.* SEE: *B-cell–mediated immunity; immune response.*

***T l.*** A lymphocyte that develops in the bone marrow and then migrates to the thymus, where it begins to mature. T cells circulate throughout the body and are essential for the specific immune response. Subpopulations of T cells include helper (T4) cells, suppressor (T8) cells, and two types of cytotoxic cells, natural killer cells and cytotoxic T cells. SYN: *T cell.* SEE: *immune response; T-cell–mediated immunity.*

**lymphocytoblast** (lĭm″fō-sī′tō-blăst″) [″ + ″ + *blastos,* germ] Lymphoblast.

**lymphocytopenia** (lĭm″fō-sīt″ō-pē′nē-ă) [″ + ″ + *penia,* lack] A deficiency of lymphocytes in the blood.

**lymphocytopoiesis** (lĭm″fō-sīt″ō-poy-ē′sĭs) [″ + ″ + *poiesis,* production] Lymphocyte production.

**lymphocytosis** (lĭm″fō-sī-tō′sĭs) [″ + ″ + *osis,* condition] An excess of lymph cells in the blood.

**lymphocytotoxin** (lĭm″fō-sīt″ō-tŏks′ĭn) [″ + ″ + *toxikon,* poison] A toxin destructive to lymphocytes.

**lymphoduct** (lĭm′fō-dŭkt) [″ + *ducere,* to lead] A lymph vessel.

**lymphoepithelioma** (lĭm″fō-ĕp″ĭ-thē-lē-ō′mă) [″ + Gr. *epi,* at, + *thele,* nipple, + *oma,* tumor] A poorly differentiated squamous cell carcinoma that involves the lymphoid tissue of the tonsils and nasopharynx.

**lymphogenesis** (lĭm″fō-jĕn′ĕ-sĭs) [″ + Gr.

*genesis,* generation, birth] Production of lymph.

**lymphogenous** (lĭm-fŏj′ĕn-ŭs) [″ + Gr. *gennan,* to produce] **1.** Forming lymph. **2.** Derived from lymph.

**lymphoglandula** (lĭm″fō-glăn′dū-lă) [″ + *glandula,* little gland] Lymph gland.

**lymphogram** (lĭm′fō-grăm) [″ + Gr. *gramma,* something written] Lymphangiogram.

**lymphogranuloma inguinale** Previous term for lymphogranuloma venereum.

**lymphogranulomatosis** (lĭm″fō-grăn-ū-lō″mă-tō′sĭs) [″ + *granulum,* granule, + Gr. *oma,* tumor, + *osis,* condition] **1.** Infectious granuloma of the lymphatics. **2.** Hodgkin's disease.

**lymphogranuloma venereum** (lĭm″fō-grăn″ū-lō′mă) [″ + ″ + Gr. *oma,* tumor] ABBR: LGV. An infectious venereal disease caused by group A *Chlamydiae* (*C. trachomatis*) and rarely group B (*C. psittaci*). Usually the diagnosis is based on clinical findings, but a skin reaction to injected killed organisms may help to confirm such evidence. Tetracyclines cure the acute clinical signs but do not affect the previous scarring. SYN: *lymphogranuloma inguinale; lymphopathia venereum.*

SYMPTOMS: From 7 to 12 days after exposure, a vesicle similar to that caused by herpes will appear, usually on the genitals. This ruptures and heals painlessly. Then from 1 to 8 weeks later, the regional lymph nodes enlarge, become tender, and may suppurate. These enlarged glands are called buboes. They heal and leave scars that may obstruct lymph channels. The perirectal lymph nodes in women may scar and cause rectal obstruction.

***l.v. antigen*** An antigen used in a skin test for lymphogranuloma venereum.

**lymphography** (lĭm-fŏg′ră-fē) [L. *lympha,* lymph, + Gr. *graphein,* to write] Lymphangiography.

**lymphoid** (lĭm′foyd) [″ + Gr. *eidos,* form, shape] Resembling lymph or lymph tissue.

***l. cell*** Lymphocyte.

**lymphoidectomy** (lĭm″foyd-ĕk′tō-mē) [″ + ″ + *ektome,* excision] Surgical removal of lymphoid tissue.

**lymphokine** (lĭm′fō-kīn) A cytokine released by lymphocytes, including many of the interleukins, gamma interferon, tumor necrosis factor beta, and chemokines. SEE: *cytokine.*

**lymphokinesis** (lĭm″fō-kī-nē′sĭs) [″ + Gr. *kinesis,* motion] **1.** Circulation of lymph in the lymphatic system. **2.** Movement of lymph in the semicircular canals of the inner ear.

**lymphology** (lĭm-fŏl′ō-jē) [″ + Gr. *logos,* word, reason] The science of the lymphatics.

**lymphoma** A usually malignant lymphoid neoplasm.

***Burkitt's l.*** A form of malignant, non-Hodgkin's lymphoma that causes bone-destroying lesions of the jaw. The Epstein-Barr virus is the causative agent. It was initially reported from central Africa.

***cutaneous T cell l.*** ABBR: CTCL. A group of non-Hodgkin's lymphomas that includes mycosis fungoides and Sézary syndrome. The former is the cutaneous form and the latter consists of both cutaneous and systemic involvement.

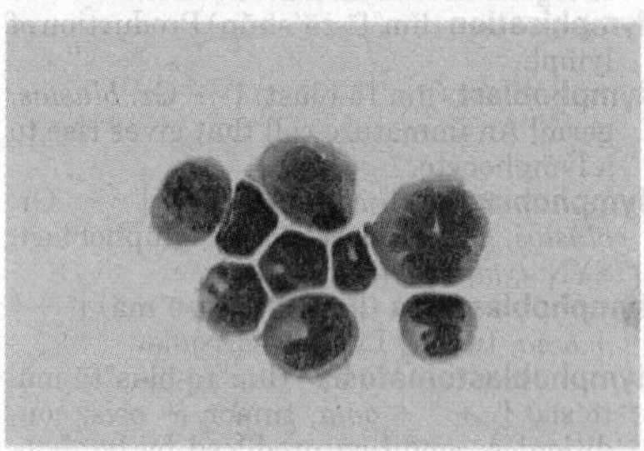

LYMPHOMA CELLS (ORIG. MAG. ×1000)

***non-Hodgkin's l.*** ABBR: NHL. A group of malignant solid tumors of lymphoid tissues. SEE: illus.; *Hodgkin's disease.*

SYMPTOMS: Painless lymphadenopathy in two thirds of patients is the most frequent presenting symptom. Others have fever, night sweats, loss of 10% or more of body weight in the 6 months before presenting with symptoms of infiltration into nonlymphoid tissue. Additional involvement is in peripheral areas such as epitrochlear nodes, the tonsillar area, and bone marrow. NHL is 50% more frequent in men than in women of similar age. In most cases the cause of NHL is unknown, but patients who have received immunosuppressive agents have a more than 100 times greater chance of developing NHL, probably owing to the immunosuppressive agents activating tumor viruses. Some patients taking a hydantoin anticonvulsant develop pseudolymphomas, which resolve when the drug is stopped.

Classification of NHL is unsettled but includes various types of malignant lymphomas, including low grade, intermediate grade, high grade, and miscellaneous. The last category includes, among others, mycosis fungoides.

TREATMENT: Specific therapy depends on the type, grade, and stage of the NHL. Radiation and combinations of chemotherapy are of benefit. Monoclonal antibodies to remove NHL tumor cells are used.

***non-Hodgkin's T cell l.*** Lymphoma that arises directly from the thymus.

**lymphomatoid** (lĭm-fō′mă-toyd) [L. *lympha,* lymph, + Gr. *oma,* tumor, + *eidos,* form, shape] Resembling lymphoma.

**lymphomatosis** (lĭm″fō-mă-tō′sĭs) [″ + ″ + *osis,* condition] General lymphatic engorgement; deposition of lymphomata throughout the body.

**lymphomatous** (lĭm-fō′mă-tŭs) **1.** Pert. to a lymphoma. **2.** Affected with lymphomata.

**lymphomyxoma** (lĭm″fō-mĭk-sō′mă) [″ + Gr. *mys,* muscle, + *oma,* tumor] A soft, nonmalignant tumor that contains lymphoid tissue.

**lymphopathia venereum** Lymphogranuloma venereum.

**lymphopathy** (lĭm-fŏp′ă-thē) [″ + Gr. *pathos,* disease] Any disease of the lymphatic system.

**lymphopenia** (lĭm-fō-pē′nē-ă) [″ + Gr. *penia,* a lack] A deficiency of lymphocytes in the blood.

**lymphoplasmapheresis** [″ + Gr. *aphairesis,* removal] The removal of lymphocytes and plasma from the blood after it has been withdrawn. The blood is then returned to the donor.

**lymphoplasty** (lĭm′fō-plăs″tē) [″ + Gr. *plassein,* to form] Lymphangioplasty.

**lymphopoiesis** (lĭm″fō-poy-ē′sĭs) [″ + Gr. *poiesis,* production] The formation of lymphocytes or of lymphoid tissue.

**lymphopoietic** (lĭm″fō-poy-ĕt′ĭk) [″ + Gr. *poiein,* to produce] Forming lymphocytes.

**lymphoproliferative** (lĭm″fō-prō-lĭf′ĕr-ă-tĭv) Concerning the proliferation of lymphoid tissue.

**lymphoreticular** (lĭm″fō-rĕ-tĭk′ū-lăr) [″ + *reticula,* net] Pert. to reticuloendothelial cells of the lymph node.

***l. disorder*** One of a great variety of poorly understood and inadequately classified diseases of the lymphoreticular system. Included are self-limited proliferation of lymph glands, lymphocytes, and monocytes; infectious mononucleosis; benign abnormalities of immunoglobulin synthesis; leukemias; lymphomas such as Hodgkin's disease, lymphosarcoma, reticulum cell sarcoma, and mycosis fungoides; malignant proliferative response or abnormal immunoglobulin synthesis such as plasma cell myeloma, macroglobulinemia, and amyloidosis; histiocytosis; and lipid storage disease.

**lymphoreticulosis, benign, of inoculation** (lĭm″fō-rē-tĭk″ū-lō′sĭs) [″ + ″ + Gr. *osis,* condition] Cat scratch disease.

**lymphorrhagia** (lĭm″fō-rā′jē-ă) [″ + Gr. *rhegnynai,* to burst forth] Flow of lymph from ruptured lymph vessels. SYN: *lymphorrhea.*

**lymphorrhea** (lĭm″fō-rē′ă) [″ + Gr. *rhoia,* flow] Lymphorrhagia.

**lymphorrhoid** (lĭm′fō-royd) Dilated lymph channels that resemble hemorrhoids.

**lymphosarcoma** (lĭm″fō-săr-kō′mă) [″ + Gr. *sarx,* flesh, + *oma,* tumor] A malignant disease of the lymphatic tissue. Clinically it may be quite similar to Hodgkin's disease. Diagnosis is made by biopsy rather than by clinical examination. SYN: *lymphoblastoma.*

**lymphosarcomatosis** (lĭm″fō-săr″kō-mă-tō′sĭs) [″ + ″ + ″ + *osis,* condition] A condition characterized by the development of lymphosarcoma.

**lymphostasis** (lĭm″fŏs′tă-sĭs) [″ + Gr. *stasis,* a stoppage] Stoppage of the flow of lymph.

**lymphotaxis** (lĭm″fō-tăk′sĭs) [″ + Gr. *taxis,* arrangement] The effect of attracting or repelling lymphocytes.

**lymphotome** (lĭm′fō-tōm) [″ + Gr. *tome,* incision] An instrument for removing glandular growths from tonsils and adenoids.

**lymphotoxin** (lĭm″fō-tŏk′sĭn) [″ + Gr. *toxikon,* poison] A lymphokine that is produced by activated lymphocytes. The toxin affects a variety of cells.

**lymphotrophy** (lĭm-fŏt′rō-fē) [″ + Gr. *trophe,* nourishment] Lymph nourishment of cells in regions devoid of blood vessels.

**lymphotropic** Attracted to lymph cells. For example, human immunodeficiency virus and human T-cell leukemia-lymphoma virus are lymphotropic for CD4+ lymphocytes and Epstein-Barr virus is lymphotropic for B lymphocytes.

**lymphuria** (lĭm-fū′rē-ă) [″ + Gr. *ouron,* urine] Lymph in the urine.

**lyo-** [Gr. *lyein,* to dissolve] Combining form meaning *dissolved* or *loose.*

**lyochrome** (lī′ō-krōm) [″ + *chroma,* color] Flavin.

**lyoenzyme** (lī″ō-ĕn′zīm) [″ + *en,* in, + *zyme,* leaven] An extracellular enzyme.

**lyogel** (lī′ō-jĕl) A gel containing much water.

**Lyon hypothesis** (lī′ŏn) [Mary Lyon, Brit. geneticist, b. 1925] The idea that one of the X chromosomes of the female is inactivated during embryogenesis and becomes hyperpyknotic. This chromosome forms, in the cell nucleus, the sex chromatin mass, or Barr body. This X chromosome remains in this state throughout the cell's progeny so that in the adult only one X chromosome is active in each cell.

**lyophilization** (lī-ŏf″ĭ-lī-zā′shŭn) The process of rapidly freezing a substance at an extremely low temperature and then dehydrating the substance in a high vacuum. SYN: *freeze-drying.*

**lyosorption** (lī″ō-sorp′shŭn) [″ + *sorbere,* to suck in] The absorption, in a colloid, of a substance on the surface of the particles in the dispersed phase.

**lypressin** (lī-prĕs′ĭn) A posterior pituitary hormone obtained from the pituitary glands of healthy pigs. It is used as an antidiuretic. Trade name is Diapid. SEE: *vasopressin*

**lyra** (lī′ră) [L., Gr., *lyre*] One of several anatomical structures so called because of their resemblance to the shape of a lyre.

**lysate** (lī′sāt) **1.** The products of hydrolysis. **2.** Material produced when cells are lysed by the actions of agents such as chemicals, enzymes, or physical agents.

**lyse** (līz) [Gr. *lysis,* dissolution] To kill.

**lysemia** (lī-sē′mē-ă) [″ + *haima,* blood] Lysis of red blood cells with release of hemoglobin into the plasma.

**lysergic acid diethylamide** ABBR: LSD. A derivative of an alkaloid in ergot. LSD is used legally only for experimental purposes. It is used illegally for its hallucinogenic effects.

**lysimeter** (lī-sĭm′ĕ-tĕr) [Gr. *lysis,* dissolution, + *metron,* measure] An apparatus for determining solubilities of various substances.

**lysin** (lī′sĭn) A specific antibody acting destructively on cells and tissues. SEE: *antibody.*

**lysine** (lī′sēn) An amino acid that is a hydrolytic cleavage product of digested protein. It is essential for growth and repair of tissues.

***l. acetate*** An amino acid.

***l. hydrochloride*** An amino acid.

**lysinogen** (lī-sĭn′ō-jĕn) [Gr. *lysis,* dissolution, + *gennan,* to produce] An antibody that forms lysins.

**lysis** (lī′sĭs) [Gr., dissolution] **1.** The gradual decline of a fever or disease; the opposite of crisis. **2.** The destruction of blood cells by a lysin, as when a rabbit's red corpuscles are dissolved by a dog's serum.

**-lysis 1.** Combining form meaning *dissolution* or *decomposition of.* **2.** In medicine, combining form indicating *reduction* or *relief of.*

**lysocephalin** (lī″sō-sĕf′ă-lĭn) Partial hydrolysis of a cephalin. It can be caused by the action of cobra venom.

**lysogen** (lī′sō-jĕn) [″ + *gennan,* to produce] Something capable of producing a lysin.

**lysogenesis** (lī″sō-jĕn′ĕ-sĭs) [″ + *genesis,* generation, birth] The production of cell-dissolving substances known as lysin.

**lysogenic** (lī-sō-jĕn′ĭk) [″ + Gr. *gennan,* to produce] Producing lysins.

**lysogeny** (lī-sŏj′ĕ-nē) A special type of virus-bacterial cell interaction maintained by a complex cellular regulatory mechanism. Bacterial strains freshly isolated from their natural environment may contain a low concentration of bacteriophage. This phage will lyse other related bacteria. Cultures that contain these substances are said to be lysogenic.

**Lysol** (lī′sŏl) A proprietary preparation of a mixture of cresols. Because of its potential for causing toxicity, its use should be confined to disinfecting inanimate objects, feces, and urine. SEE: *Lysol poisoning*

***L. poisoning*** When swallowed, Lysol causes corrosion, edema of the lungs, immobility of pupils, and collapse. Vomiting may occur. Death sometimes occurs after symptoms have abated.

TREATMENT: The stomach should be promptly emptied by emesis and lavage if the esophagus is not injured. Shock and convulsions are treated symptomatically. Acidosis is corrected and an airway maintained. Tracheotomy should be performed if indicated.

**lysolecithin** (lī″sō-lĕs′ĭ-thĭn) A substance obtained from lecithin through the action of an enzyme present in cobra venom. It exerts a powerful hemolytic action.

**lysosome** (lī′sō-sōm) A cell organelle that is part of the intracellular digestive system. Inside its limiting membrane, it contains a number of hydrolytic enzymes capable of breaking down proteins and certain carbohydrates. Lysomal enzymes contribute to the digestion of pathogens phagocytized by a cell, and also to the tissue damage that accompanies inflammation.

**lysozyme** (lī′sō-zīm) [Gr. *lysis,* dissolution, + *zyme,* leaven] An enzyme found in phagocytes, neutrophils, and macrophages, and in tears, saliva, sweat and other body secretions, that destroys bacteria by breaking down their walls.

**lyssa** (lĭs′să) [Gr., frenzy] Obsolete term for rabies.

**Lyssavirus** The genus of the family Rhabdoviridae, which includes the rabies virus.

**lyssoid** (lĭs′oyd) [Gr. *lyssa,* frenzy, + *eidos,* form, shape] Resembling lyssa or rabies.

**lyssophobia** (lĭs-ō-fō′bē-ă) [″ + *phobos,* fear] **1.** Hysteria resembling that of rabies. **2.** Fear of rabies.

**lytic** (lĭt′ĭk) Relating to lysis or a lysin.

**lyze** (līz) [Gr. *lysis,* dissolution] To bring about lysis.

# M

**μ** [*mu,* the twelfth letter of the Greek alphabet] Symbol for micro-, a prefix indicating one-millionth ($10^{-6}$) of the quantity (e.g., μg or 0.000001 g).

**μμ** Symbol for micromicro-; micromicron.

**μm** Symbol for micrometer.

**M** *master* or *medicine* in professional titles; *mille,* a thousand; *misce,* mix; *molar.*

**m** *meter* and *minim;* in chemistry, for *meta-,* and for *mol* or *mole.*

**mμ** Symbol for millimicron.

**MA** *mental age.*

**M.A.** *Master of Arts.*

**ma** *milliampere.*

**Maalox** Trade name for magnesia and alumina tablets.

**MAC** *maximum allowable concentration.*

**Mace** A proprietary substance for which the name is an acronym for *m*ethylchloroform chloro-*ace*tophenone, a chemical compound used at one time in riot control because of its ability to irritate the eyes. Now it is considered too toxic for that purpose. SEE: *IDU.*

TREATMENT: A 0.1% aqueous solution of idoxuridine (IDU) should be instilled into the eye. Contact lenses must be removed immediately.

**macerate** (măs′ĕr-āt) To soften by steeping or soaking in water; usually pertains to the skin.

**maceration** (măs-ĕr-ā′shŭn) [L. *macerare,* to make soft] **1.** The process of softening a solid by steeping in a fluid. **2.** The dissolution of the skin of a dead fetus retained in utero.

**Mache unit** (mă′kĕ) [Heinrich Mache, Austrian physicist, 1876–1954] ABBR: M.u., or German, M.E. A unit of measurement of the concentration of radium emanation.

**machine** Any mechanical device or apparatus.

**Machover test** SEE: *Draw-a-Person test.*

**macies** (mā′shē-ēz) [L., wasting] Atrophy, wasting, emaciation.

**macr-** SEE: *macro-.*

**macrencephalia, macrencephaly** (măk-rĕn″sĕ-fā′lē-ă, -sĕf′ă-lē) [Gr. *makros,* large, + *enkephalos,* brain] Abnormally large size of the brain.

**macro-, macr-** [Gr. *makros,* large] Combining form meaning *large* or *long.*

**macroamylase** (măk″rō-ăm′ĭ-lās) A form of amylase with a molecular weight much greater than ordinary amylase. The macroamylase molecule is too large to be excreted by the glomerulus of the kidney. It is clinically important because the routine blood amylase study of an individual with macroamylase in the blood would indicate amylase to be elevated, possibly leading the physician to believe that the patient required therapy for a disease of the pancreas or the gastrointestinal tract. In such a patient, the urinary amylase would be within normal limits, which would not be true if the elevation of blood amylase were due to an actual increase in amylase present.

**macroamylasemia** (măk″rō-ăm″ĭl-ă-sē′mē-ă) Macroamylase in the serum. The presence of increased amounts of macroamylase in the blood has not been correlated with a specific single disease state.

**macrobiosis** (măk″rō-bī-ō′sĭs) [Gr. *makros,* large, + *biosis,* life] Longevity.

**macrobiota** (măk″rō-bī-ō′tă) The macroscopic living organisms, flora and fauna, of an area.

**macroblepharia** (măk″rō-blĕ-fā′rē-ă) [Gr. *makros,* large, + *blepharon,* eyelid] Abnormal largeness of the eyelid.

**macrobrachia** (măk″rō-brā′kē-ă) [″ + *brachion,* arm] Abnormal size or length of the arm.

**macrocardius** (măk″rō-kăr′dē-ŭs) [″+ *kardia,* heart] An individual with an abnormally large heart; caused by congenital heart disease.

**macrocephalia, macrocephaly** (măk″rō-sĕ-fā′lē-ă, -sĕf′ă-lē) [″ + *kephale,* head] Abnormally large size of the head. It is found in acromegaly, hydrocephalus, rickets, osteitis deformans, leontiasis ossea, myxedema, leprosy, and pituitary disturbances. **macrocephalic, macrocephalous** (-sĕf′ă-lŭs), *adj.*

**macrocheilia** (măk″rō-kī′lē-ă) [″ + *cheilos,* lip] Abnormal size of a lip characterized by swelling of the glands of the lip. It is a congenital condition. SYN: *macrolabia.*

**macrocheiria** (măk-rō-kī′rē-ă) [″ + *cheir,* hand] Excessive size of the hands.

**macroconidium** (măk″rō-kō-nĭd′ē-ŭm) A large conidium or exospore.

**macrocornea** (măk-rō-kor′nē-ă) [″ + L. *cornu,* horn] Abnormal size of the cornea. SYN: *megalocornea.*

**macrocyst** (măk′rō-sĭst) [″ + *kystis,* bladder] A large cyst.

**macrocyte** [″ + *kytos,* cell] Abnormally large erythrocyte exceeding 10 microns in diameter.

**macrocythemia, macrocytosis** (măk″rō-sī-thē′mē-ă, măk″rō-sī-tō′sĭs) [″ + ″ + *haima,* blood] Condition in which erythrocytes are larger than normal.

**macrodactylia** (măk″rō-dăk-tĭl′ē-ă) [″ + *daktylos,* finger] Excessive size of one or more digits.

**macrodontia** (măk″rō-dŏn′shē-ă) [″ + *odous,* tooth] Abnormal increase in size of the teeth.

**macroesthesia** (măk″rō-ĕs-thē′zē-ă) [Gr.

*makros,* large, + *aisthesis,* sensation] State in which objects seen or felt appear to be greatly magnified.

**macrofauna** (măk″rō-faw′nă) The animal life visible to the naked eye in a particular location or area.

**macroflora** (măk″rō-flō′ră) The plant life visible to the naked eye in a particular location or area.

**macrogamete** (măk″rō-găm′ĕt) [″ + *gamete,* wife] A large immobile reproductive cell formed in certain protozoa and simple plants. It corresponds to the ovum in higher forms.

**macrogametocyte** (măk″rō-gă-mē′tō-sīt) A large nonmotile reproductive cell developing from the merozoite of certain protozoans. Macrogametocytes are found in red blood cells infected with the female form of the malarial parasite. SEE: *Plasmodium.*

**macrogenitosomia praecox** (măk″rō-jĕn″ĭ-tō-sō′mē-ă prē′kŏks) [″ + L. *genitalis,* genital, + Gr. *soma,* body, + L. *praecox,* early] Abnormal size of genitalia in the developing fetus due to excess androgens (male hormones) from the fetal adrenal. In the female, this causes pseudohermaphroditism, and in the male, enlarged external genitalia.

**macrogingivae** (măk″rō-jĭn-jī′vē) [″ + L. *gingiva,* gum] Hypertrophy of the gums.

**macroglia** (măk-rŏg′lē-ă) [″ + *glia,* glue] Astrocyte.

**macroglobulin** (măk″rō-glŏb′ū-lĭn) A globulin of high molecular weight over about 400 kilodaltons. Macroglobulin is normally present in the blood but is increased in disease states such as multiple myeloma, collagen disorders, cirrhosis of the liver, and amyloidosis.

**macroglobulinemia** (măk-rō-glŏb″ū-lĭn-ē′mē-ă) ABBR: WM. Presence of globulins of high molecular weight in serum.

***Waldenström's m.*** Macroglubulinemia marked by excess production of immunoglobulin M (IgM), predominating in the elderly. Peak incidence is in the sixth and seventh decades. The disease is more common in men. Symptoms include anemia due to infiltration of the bone marrow with lymphocytes and plasma cells, weight loss, neurological disturbances, blurred vision, bleeding disorders, cold sensitivity, generalized lymphadenopathy, chronic lymphocytic leukemia, and hyperviscosity of the blood.

TREATMENT: Plasmaphoresis to remove the excess IgM from the blood. This may require removing 4 to 6 units of plasma a day until blood viscosity returns to normal, and it needs to be continued until chemotherapy is effective. Reduction of tumor mass by use of cytotoxic agents; symptomatic therapy for complications.

**macroglossia** [Gr. *makros,* large, + *glossa,* tongue] Hypertrophied condition of the tongue; a congenital disorder.

**macrognathia** (măk-rō-nā′thē-ă) [″ + *gnathos,* jaw] Abnormal size of the jaw.

**macrography** (măk-rŏg′ră-fē) [″ + *graphein,* to write] Writing with large letters.

**macrogyria** [″ + *gyros,* circle] Excessively large size of convolutions (gyri) of the cerebral hemispheres.

**macrolabia** (măk-rō-lā′bē-ă) [″ + L. *labium,* lip] Abnormal size of a lip. SYN: *macrocheilia.*

**macroleukoblast** (măk″rō-lū′kō-blăst) [″ + *leukos,* white, + *blastos,* germ] A large leukoblast.

**macrolymphocyte** (măk″rō-lĭmf′ō-sīt) [″ + L. *lympha,* lymph, + Gr. *kytos,* cell] A large lymphocyte.

**macromastia** (măk-rō-măs′tē-ă) [″ + *mastos,* breast] Abnormally large breasts.

**macromelia** [″ + *melos,* limb] Abnormally large size of the limbs.

**macromelus** (măk-rŏm′ĕ-lŭs) [″ + *melos,* limb] An individual with abnormally large extremities.

**macromere** (măk′rō-mēr) [″ + *meros,* a part] A blastomere of large size.

**macromethod** (măk′rō-mĕth″ŏd) Chemical examinations or analyses wherein ordinary quantities of the material being studied are used.

**macromolecule** (măk″rō-mŏl′ĕ-kūl) A large molecule such as a protein, polymer, or polysaccharide.

**macromonocyte** (măk″rō-mŏn′ō-sīt) A large monocyte.

**macromyeloblast** (măk″rō-mī′ĕ-lō-blăst) [″ + *myelos,* marrow, + *blastos,* germ] A large myeloblast.

**macronormoblast** (măk″rō-nor′mō-blăst) [″ + L. *norma,* rule, + Gr. *blastos,* germ] A large nucleated red blood corpuscle.

**macronucleus** (măk″rō-nū′klē-ŭs) A nucleus that occupies most of the cell.

**macronutrient** Any essential nutrient required in large amounts in a balanced diet, such as carbohydrates, proteins, and fats. SEE: *micronutrient; trace element.*

**macronychia** (măk″rō-nĭk′ē-ă) [″ + *onyx,* nail] Abnormal length or thickness of the fingernails or toenails.

**macropathology** (măk″rō-pă-thŏl′ō-jē) Pathological changes in gross anatomical structures.

**macrophage, macrophagus** (măk′rō-fāj, măk-rŏf′ă-gŭs) [″ + *phagein,* to eat] A monocyte that has left the circulation and settled and matured in a tissue. Macrophages are found in large quantities in the spleen, lymph nodes, alveoli, and tonsils. About 50% of all macrophages are found in the liver as Kupffer cells. They are also present in the brain as microglia, in the skin as Langerhans cells, in bone as osteoclasts, as well as in serous cavities and breast and placental tissue. Along with neutrophils, macrophages are the major phagocytic cells of the immune system. They have the ability to recognize and ingest all foreign antigens through receptors on the surface of their cell membranes; these antigens are then destroyed by lysosomes. Their placement in the peripheral lymphoid tissues enables macrophages to serve as the major scavengers of the blood, clearing it of abnormal or old cells and cellular debris as well as pathogenic organisms.

Macrophages also serve a vital role by processing antigens and presenting them to T cells, activating the specific immune response. They also release many chemical mediators that are involved in the body's defenses, including interleukin-1 and complement. SEE: illus.; *macrophage processing; monocyte; phagocytosis; tumor necrosis factor.*

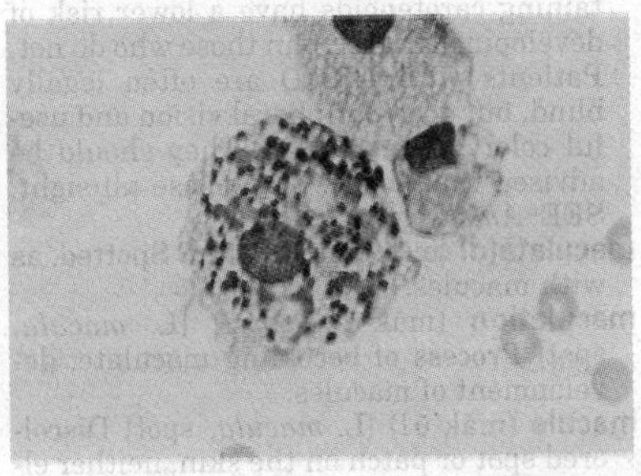

**MACROPHAGE** WITH HEMOSIDERIN GRANULES (ORIG. MAG. ×1000)

***m. activating factor*** ABBR: MAF. A lymphokine that stimulates macrophages to change in appearance and metabolic activities and to become more effective killers of certain microbial cells. Macrophages stimulated by MAF can kill tumor cells.

***m. chemotactic factor*** ABBR: MCF. A lymphokine released by T and B cell lymphocytes in response to an antigen. It attracts macrophages to the site of the invading antigen.

***m. colony stimulating factor*** ABBR: M-CSF. A hematopoietic growth factor that stimulates monocytes to form colonies.

***m. migration inhibiting factor*** ABBR: MIF. A lymphokine that blocks the migration of macrophages in culture.

***m. processing*** The mechanism by which foreign antigens are taken into the macrophage by phagocytosis and broken up. Part of the antigen is then displayed on the surface of the macrophage next to a histocompatibility or "self" antigen activating T lymphocytes and the specific immune response. T lymphocytes are unable to recognize or respond to most antigens without macrophage assistance.

**macrophagocyte** (măk″rō-făg′ō-sīt) A large phagocyte.

**macrophallus** (măk″rō-făl′ŭs) [Gr. *makros,* large, + *phallos,* penis] Abnormally large penis.

**macrophthalmia** (măk″rŏf-thăl′mē-ă) [″ + *ophthalmos,* eye] Abnormally large eyeball.

**macroplasia** (măk″rō-plā′zē-ă) [″ + *plasis,* forming] Abnormally large size of a part or specific tissue.

**macropodia** (măk-rō-pō′dē-ă) [″ + *pous,* foot] Abnormally large feet.

**macropolycyte** (măk″rō-pŏl′ē-sīt) [″ + *polys,* many, + *kytos,* cell] A large polymorphonuclear leukocyte with a multisegmented nucleus.

**macropromyelocyte** (măk″rō-prō-mī′ĕ-lō-sīt) A large promyelocyte.

**macroprosopia** (măk″rō-prō-sō′pē-ă) [″ + *prosopon,* face] Large facial features.

**macropsia** (măk-rŏp′sē-ă) [″ + *opsis,* vision] Macroesthesia.

**macrorhinia** (măk-rō-rīn′ē-ă) [″ + *rhis,* nose] Excessive size of the nose, either congenital or pathological.

**macroscelia** (măk-rō-sē′lē-ă) [″ + *skelos,* leg] Abnormally large legs.

**macroscopic** (măk-rō-skŏp′ĭk) [″ + *skopein,* to examine] Large enough to be seen by the naked eye. Opposite of microscopic.

**macroscopy** (măk-rŏs′kō-pē) Examination of an object with the naked eye.

**macrosigmoid** (măk″rō-sĭg′moyd) Abnormally large sigmoid colon.

**macrosmatic** (măk″rŏs-măt′ĭk) [″ + *osmasthai,* to smell] Having an abnormally keen sense of smell.

**macrosomatia, macrosomia** (măk″rō-sō-mā′shē-ă, măk-rō-sō′mē-ă) [Gr. *makros,* large, + *soma,* body] Abnormally large body.

***fetal m.*** In a newborn, birth weight above the 90th percentile on the intrauterine growth curve. SEE: *large for gestational age.*

**macrospore** (măk′rō-spor) The larger spore type in certain fungi and protozoa with two spores.

**macrostereognosis** (măk″rō-stē″rē-ō-nō′sĭs) [″ + *stereos,* solid, + *gnosis,* knowledge] A misperception that objects appear to be larger than they are.

**macrostomia** (măk-rō-stō′mē-ă) [″ + *stoma,* mouth] Excessively large mouth.

**macrostructure** (măk′rō-strŭk″tūr) The gross structure of an entity.

**macrothrombocyte** [″ + *thrombos,* clot, + *kytos,* cell] A large platelet seen in some rare disorders of platelets.

**macrothrombocytopenia** [″ + ″ + ″ + *penia,* lack] Deficiency of macrothrombocytes. SEE: *Alport's syndrome.*

**macrotia** (măk-rō′shē-ă) [″ + *ous,* ear] Abnormally large ears.

**macrotooth** An abnormally enlarged tooth.

**macula** (măk′ū-lă) *pl.* **maculae** [L., spot] **1.** A small spot or colored area. SEE: *roseola.* **2.** A macule. **macular** (-lăr), *adj.*

***maculae acusticae*** The site of the hair cells (receptors) in the wall of the saccule and utricle of the inner ear. These receptors respond to changes in the pull of gravity (position of the head) and generate impulses carried by the vestibular branch of the acoustic nerve. They include the macula sacculi and macula utriculi.

***m. acustica sacculi*** M. sacculi.

***m. acustica utriculi*** M. utriculi.

***m. albida*** A white mark found on the visceral layer of the peritoneum or epicardium in some contagious diseases.

***m. atrophica*** A glistening white spot on the skin due to atrophy.

***m. caerulea*** A steel-gray or blue stain of epidermis without elevation. It does not disappear on pressure and occurs esp. with pediculosis pubis or flea bites.

***cerebral m.*** A reddened line that becomes deeper and persists for some time when the fingernail is drawn across the skin, esp. in tuberculous meningitis. SYN: *tache cérébrale.*

***m. corneae*** An opaque spot in the cornea.

***m. cribrosa*** One of several tiny foramina in the wall of the vestibule of the bony labyrinth of the ear through which pass filaments of the acoustic nerve.

***m. densa*** A group of cells in the wall of the distal renal tubule, next to the juxtaglomerular cells, that are sensitive to changes in the salt concentration of the filtrate in the tubule.

***m. flava laryngis*** A small yellow spot at the ventral end of each vocal cord formed by a small mass of elastic tissue or, sometimes, cartilage.

***m. folliculi*** The point on the ovarian follicle where it ruptures.

***m. germinativa*** The germinal area in eggs with large yolks.

***m. gonorrhoeica*** A red spot at the orifice of the Bartholin's gland; seen in gonorrheal vulvitis.

***m. lutea retinae*** A yellow spot in the center of the retina approx. 2 mm lateral to the exit of optic nerve. It contains a pit, fovea centralis, where the retina is reduced to a layer of closely packed cones, which functions as the area of most acute vision (central vision).

***m. sacculi*** The site of the hair cells in the saccule; receptors stimulated by the pull of gravity. These cells generate impulses carried by the vestibular branch of the acoustic nerve. SYN: *m. acustica sacculi.*

***m. utriculi*** The site of the hair cells in the utricule; receptors stimulated by the pull of gravity. These cells generate impulses carried by the vestibular branch of the acoustic nerve. SYN: *m. acustica utriculi.*

**macular atrophy** SEE: under *atrophy.*

**macular degeneration** Degeneration of the macular area of the retina of the eye, an area important in the visualization of fine details. Although this may be related to the toxic effects of drugs such as chloroquine or phenothiazine, the cause of the most common type—age-related macular degeneration (ARMD)—is unknown. This condition, the leading cause of visual impairment in persons over age 50, can lead to loss of central vision, making it difficult to read or do fine work, such as threading a needle. If this condition is due to growth of blood vessels under the retina and it is diagnosed early, the loss of vision can be arrested by using laser therapy to destroy the vessels. Test for loss of central vision may be done by using the Amsler grid. The patient looks at the grid with each eye separately. If central vision is impaired, the lines will appear wavy instead of straight. This condition will not, in itself, result in total blindness. Some vision is retained, making self-care possible.

Reportedly, people who eat foods containing carotenoids have a lower risk of developing ARMD than those who do not. Patients with ARMD are often legally blind, but good peripheral vision and useful color vision remain. They should be advised that they will not lose all sight. SEE: *Amsler grid.*

**maculate(d)** (măk′ū-lāt, -lāt-ĕd) Spotted, as with macules.

**maculation** (măk-ū-lā′shŭn) [L. *macula,* spot] Process of becoming maculate; development of macules.

**macule** (măk′ūl) [L. *macula,* spot] Discolored spot or patch on the skin, neither elevated nor depressed, of various colors, sizes, and shapes. Macules include hyperemia, roseola, erythema, telangiectasis, nevi vasculosi, areola, achromia, chloasma, purpura, petechiae, ecchymoses, vibices, albinism, vitiligo, lentigines, nevi pigmentosi, nevi spili, and discolorations.

Macules occur in pellagra, pityriasis rosea, pediculosis corporis, rubella, scurvy, serum sickness, peliosis, anemia, leukemia, cancer, infectious diseases, erysipelas, acne rosacea, nevus pigmentosus, vitiligo, leprosy, morphea, and facial hemiatrophy. SYN: *macula.*

**maculopapular** (măk″ū-lō-păp′ū-lăr) **1.** Consisting of or pert. to macules and papules. **2.** An eruption consisting of both macules and papules.

**maculopathy** (măk″ū-lŏp′ă-thē) [″ + Gr. *pathos,* disease] Retinal pathology involving the macula of the eye.

**mad 1.** Not rational. SYN: *insane.* **2.** Angry. **3.** Rash, foolish, frantic. **4.** Suffering from infection with rabies. SYN: *rabid.*

**madarosis** (măd-ă-rō′sĭs) [Gr. *madaros,* bald] Loss of eyelashes or eyebrows.

**madder** (măd′ĕr) Root of the plant *Rubia tinctorum,* a source of the red dye alizarin.

**Madelung's deformity** [Otto W. Madelung, Strasbourg surgeon, 1846–1926] Displacement of the hand to the radial side due to relative overgrowth of the ulna.

**Madelung's disease** Generalized symmetrical deposits of fatty tissue (lipomas) on the upper back, shoulders, and neck. SYN: *Madelung's neck.*

**madescent** (măd-ĕs′ĕnt) [L. *madescere,* to become moist] Slightly moist or becoming so.

**Madura foot** [from Madur district in India where disease was first described in 1842] A local painless lesion—called a mycetoma—of an exposed area, such as bare feet. It consists of swollen tissue, sinuses filled with pus, and microbial colonies (called grains) embedded in the pustular tissues. Mycetomas may occur in any body part. It is usually found in adult males who work outside and have poor or no medical care for wounds. SYN: *maduromycosis.*

ETIOLOGY: Various fungi including eumycetoma and actinomycetes. In the U.S., the most frequent cause is *Pseudallescheria boydii.*

TREATMENT: The antibiotic given depends on the specific organism involved. Clindamycin is used for actinomycetoma. Ketoconazole or itraconazole have been used in eumycetomas. Surgery should not be necessary, but treatment will be needed for at least 10 months.

**maduromycosis** (măd-ū″rō-mī-kō′sĭs) A chronic fungal infection of the foot or hand characterized by marked swelling and development of nodules, vesicles, abscesses, and sinuses. A type of mycetoma.

**mafenide acetate** (măf′ĕn-īd) An antibacterial of the sulfonamide class, used topically in cream form for treating burns.

**magaldrate** (măg′ăl-drāt) Aluminum magnesium hydroxide sulfate; used as an antacid.

**magenblase syndrome** [Ger. *Magen,* stomach, + *Blase,* bubble] Accumulation of swallowed air in the stomach that leads to postprandial fullness and pressure. Radiograph of the stomach will reveal a large gastric bubble.

**Magendie's foramen** (mă-jĕn′dēz) [François Magendie, Fr. physiologist, 1783–1855] The median of three openings in the roof of the 4th ventricle. It is in front of the cerebellum and behind the pons varolii, connecting the ventricle with the subarachnoid space.

**magenstrasse** (măg″ĕn-străs′ĕ) [″ + *Strasse,* street] A groove along the lesser curvature of the stomach from cardia to pylorus.

**magenta** (mă-jĕn′tă) The dye basic fuchsin.

**maggot** Larva of an insect, esp. the softbodied footless larva of flies (order Diptera). Many are parasitic, giving rise to myiasis.

**maggot treatment** A method of treating septic wounds. In the 1930s, scientific studies indicated that neglected and infected compound fractures were aided in healing when blowfly maggots accidentally infested the wounds. The maggots removed necrotic tissue and left healthy granulating tissue. Modern therapy, including antibiotics, has made this method of treating wounds and osteomyelitis obsolete. Nevertheless, it is possible to culture sterile blowfly maggots for this use. In severe skin infections when all other forms of therapy have failed, this method has been used.

**magic thinking** The feeling that thoughts or actions have the ability to cause actions or effects that would defy the normal laws of cause and effect.

**Magill forceps** Angulated forceps used during direct laryngoscopy to remove a foreign body from an obstructed airway.

**magistery** (măj′ĭs-tĕr″ē) [L. *magister,* master] **1.** Specially compounded remedy. **2.** A precipitate.

**magma** (măg′mă) [Gr.] **1.** Mass left after extraction of principal. **2.** Salve or paste. **3.** A suspension of finely divided material in a small amount of water.

**magnesia** (măg-nē′zē-ă) [magnetic stone found in Magnesia, region of ancient Thessaly] Magnesium oxide. MgO.

***milk of m.*** Aperient composed of magnesium hydroxide and water.

**magnesia and alumina (tablets)** An antacid preparation composed of aluminum hydroxide and magnesium hydroxide. Trade name is Maalox.

**magnesium** [L.] SYMB: Mg. At. wt. 24.312; at. no. 12; sp. gr. 1.738. A white mineral element found in soft tissue, muscles, bones, and to some extent in the body fluids. It is a naturally occurring element on earth, being extracted from well and sea water. The human body contains approx. 25 g of magnesium, most of which is in the bones. Muscles contain less of it than they do of calcium. Concentration of magnesium in the blood serum is between 1.5 and 2.5 mEq/L.

Magnesium is widely distributed in foods; therefore, deficiency rarely occurs. It is obtained in sufficient quantities in whole grains, fruits, and vegetables. A typical diet contains 200 to 400 mg, but very little of this is absorbed. Deficiency may be present in patients with chronic diarrhea or diseases that interfere with absorption.

FUNCTION: Magnesium is a component of enzymes required for synthesis of adenosine triphosphate (ATP) and for the release of energy from ATP. It is also a component of enzymes involved in muscle contraction and protein synthesis.

DEFICIENCY: Tetany quite similar to that produced by hypocalcemia, weakness, and mental depression.

EXCESS: An excess is usually caused by intravenous magnesium replacement or decreased renal excretion due to renal disease. Bradycardia, hypotension, decreased level of consciousness, and muscle weakness are common symptoms. In severe hypermagnesemia, cardiac arrest may occur. Treatment includes diet therapy and diuretics if renal function is present.

***m. carbonate*** $MgCO_3 \cdot 3H_2O$. A bulky, white, odorless powder. Taken by mouth to neutralize acid in stomach.

***m. chloride*** $MgCl_2 \cdot 6H_2$. Used in treating electrolyte disturbances and in dialysis solutions.

*m. gluconate* A medicine used to replace magnesium in the body.

*m. hydroxide* $Mg(OH)_2$. A bulky white powder that, in aqueous suspension, is called milk of magnesia. Used as a laxative and an antacid.

*m. oxide* MgO. Calcined magnesia. Light magnesia. A white, very bulky powder. In Great Britain, it is called light magnesium oxide. It is used as an antacid and laxative.

*m. salicylate* An antipyretic and analgesic. Trade name is Magan.

*m. sulfate* $MgSO_4 \cdot 7H_2O$. Small colorless crystals with a bitter saline taste; used as a cathartic, anticonvulsant, and topically as an anti-inflammatory agent. The intravenous form is used to manage pregnancy-induced hypertension and to halt preterm labor. SYN: *epsom salt.*

INCOMPATIBILITY: Ammonium chloride, soapsuds enema, quinine, ferric chloride, sulfanilamide.

**magnet** [Gr. *magnes*, magnet] Any body that has the property of attracting iron. This may be a natural iron oxide or a mass of iron or steel that has this property given to it artificially. A piece of iron may be magnetized by passage of an electric current through an insulated wire wound around it. **magnetic,** *adj.*

**magnetic cortical stimulation** The induction of painless electrical current within the brain to detect abnormalities in cortical motor neuron function.

**magnetic field** The space permeated by the magnetic lines of force surrounding a permanent magnet or coil of wire carrying electric current.

**magnetic lines of force** The lines indicating the direction of the magnetic force in the space surrounding a magnet or constituting a magnetic field.

**magnetic microsphere** SEE: under *microsphere.*

**magnetic resonance imaging** ABBR: MRI. A type of diagnostic radiography using electromagnetic energy. Certain atomic nuclei with an odd number of neutrons, protons, or both are subjected to a radiofrequency pulse, causing them to absorb and release energy. The resulting current passes through a radiofrequency receiver and is then transformed into an image. This technique is valuable in providing soft-tissue images of the central nervous and musculoskeletal systems. New imaging techniques allow visualization of the vascular system without the use of contrast agents. However, agents are available for contrast enhancement. Magnetic resonance imaging is contraindicated in patients with cardiac pacemakers or ferromagnetic aneurysmal clips in place. SEE: illus.; *brain* for illus.; *positron emission tomography.*

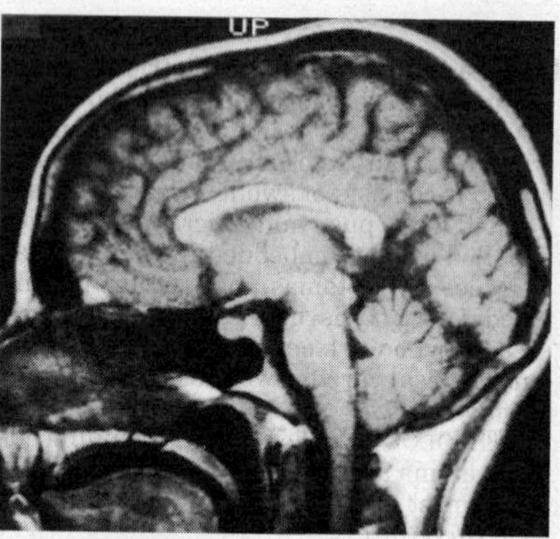


MAGNETIC RESONANCE IMAGING

MIDSAGITTAL SECTION OF BRAIN OF NORMAL YOUNG SUBJECT

NURSING IMPLICATIONS: Metal may become damaged during testing; therefore, the nurse establishes whether the patient has metal anywhere on or in the body. Patients should not wear metal objects such as jewelry, hair ornaments, or watches, for example. Patients who have had surgical procedures after which metal clips, pins, or other hardware remain in the body should not have the test. During testing, the patient lies on a flat surface that is moved inside a tube encompassing a magnet. The patient must lie as still as possible. No discomfort occurs as a result of the test. Sounds heard during the test come from the pulsing of the magnetic field as it scans the body. Confinement during the 30 to 90 min required for testing may frighten the patient, but the patient can talk to staff by microphone. Relaxation techniques are also taught for use during the test.

**magnetism** (măg′nĕ-tĭzm) [Gr. *magnes*, magnet, + *-ismos*, condition] The property of repulsion and attraction of certain substances that have magnetic properties. SEE: *magnet.*

**magnetoelectricity** (măg-nē″tō-ē″lĕk-trĭs′ĭ-tē) [″ + *elektron*, amber] Electricity generated by use of magnets.

**magnetometer** (măg″nĕ-tŏm′ĕ-tĕr) [″ + *metron*, measure] Device for measuring magnetic fields.

**magneton** (măg′nĕ-tŏn) The unit of nuclear magnetic force.

**magnetotherapy** (măg-nē″tō-thĕr′ă-pē) [″ + *therapeia*, treatment] Application of magnets or magnetism in treating diseases. There is no evidence that such therapy is effective.

**magnetropism** (măg-nĕt′rō-pĭzm) [″ + *trope*, a turn] The change in direction of growth of a plant or organism in response to the action of a magnetic field.

**magnification** (măg-nĭ-fĭ-kā′shŭn) [L. *mag-*

*nus,* great, + *facere,* to make] Process of increasing apparent size of an object, esp. under a microscope.

**magnitude** Size, extent, or dimensions.

**magnum** [L.] **1.** Large or great. **2.** Old term for capitate bone (os magnum), the largest of the carpals.

**Mahaim fibers** [I. Mahaim, contemporary Fr. physician] Fibers for conducting cardiac impulses. They connect the proximal main atrioventricular bundle to the septal myocardium and permit ventricular pre-excitation with resultant tachycardia.

**maim** (mām) [ME. *maymen,* to cripple] **1.** To injure seriously; to disable. **2.** To deprive of the use of a part, such as an arm or leg.

**main** (măn) [Fr.] Hand.

***m. en griffe*** Clawhand.

**mainstreaming** Term referring to the philosophy of educating children with disabling conditions in natural settings so as not to deprive them of normal social experiences and conditions.

**maintainer** Something that supports or keeps another thing in existence or continuity.

***space m.*** Device fashioned to keep teeth separated when placed across an edentulous segment of the dental arch. It may consist of bands, bars, springs, or other materials, and is cemented or soldered to orthodontic bands or crowns on the adjacent teeth.

**Majocchi's disease** (mă-yŏk'ēz) [Domenico Majocchi, It. physician, 1849–1929] Ring-shaped purple eruption of lower limbs. SYN: *purpura annularis telangiectodes.*

**Majocchi's granuloma** Allergic granulomata of the skin due to fungal infections.

**major histocompatibility complex** ABBR: MHC. A group of genes on chromosome 6 that code for the antigens that determine tissue and blood compatibility. In humans, histocompatibility antigens are called human leukocyte antigens (HLA) because they were originally discovered in large numbers on lymphocytes. There are thousands of combinations of HLA antigens. Class I MHC antigens (HLA-A, HLA-B, and HLA-C) are found on all nucleated cells and platelets. Class II antigens (HLA-DR, HLA-DQ, and HLA-DP) are found on lymphocytes and antigen processing cells and are important in the specific immune response. In tissue and organ transplantation, the extent to which the HLA or "tissue type" of the donor and recipient match is a major determinant of the success of the transplant.

**makro-** SEE: words beginning with *macro-.*

**mal** (măl) [Fr., from L. *malum,* an evil] A sickness or disorder.

***m. de mer*** Seasickness.

**mal-** Combining form meaning *ill, bad, poor.*

**mala** (mā'lă) [L. *mala,* cheek] **1.** The cheek. **2.** The cheekbone. **malar** (mā'lăr), *adj.*

**malabsorption syndrome** Disordered or inadequate absorption of nutrients from the intestinal tract, esp. the small intestine. The syndrome may be associated with or due to a number of diseases, including those affecting the intestinal mucosa, such as infections, tropical sprue, gluten enteropathy, pancreatic insufficiency, or lactase deficiency. It may also be due to surgery such as gastric resection and ileal bypass or to antibiotic therapy such as neomycin. SEE: *gluten-induced enteropathy; irritable bowel syndrome; lactose intolerance.*

**malacia** (mă-lā'shē-ă) [Gr. *malakia,* softening] Abnormal softening of tissues of an organ or of tissues themselves.

**malacoplakia** (măl″ă-kō-plā'kē-ă) [Gr. *malakos,* soft, + *plax,* plaque] Existence of soft patches in mucous membrane of a hollow organ.

***m. vesicae*** Soft, funguslike patches on mucosa of the bladder and ureters.

**malacosarcosis** (măl″ă-kō-săr-kō'sĭs) [″ + *sarx,* flesh, + *osis,* condition] Softness of tissue, esp. muscular.

**malacosteon** (măl-ă-kŏs'tē-ŏn) [″ + *osteon,* bone] Softening of the bones. SYN: *osteomalacia.*

**malacotomy** (măl-ă-kŏt'ō-mē) [Gr. *malakos,* soft, + *tome,* incision] Incision of soft areas of the body, esp. of the abdominal wall.

**maladie de Roger** (măl″ă-dē') [Henry L. Roger, Fr. physician, 1809–1891] Congenital interventricular septal defect.

**maladjusted** Poorly adjusted; unhappy or unsuccessful because of inability or failure to adjust to life's stresses. Marked by depression, anxiety, and irritability.

**malady** (măl'ă-dē) [Fr. *maladie,* illness, from L. *malum,* an evil] A disease or disorder. SYN: *disease.*

**malaise** (mă-lāz') [Fr.] Discomfort, uneasiness, or indisposition, often indicative of infection.

**malalignment** (măl″ă-līn'mĕnt) Improper alignment of structures such as teeth or the portions of a fractured bone. SEE: *malocclusion.*

**malar bone** A four-pointed bone on each side of the face, uniting the frontal and superior maxillary bones with the zygomatic process of the maxilla. SYN: *cheekbone; mala; zygoma; zygomatic bone.*

**malaria** (mă-lā'rē-ă) [It. *malaria,* bad air] An acute and sometimes chronic infectious disease due to protozoa of the genus *Plasmodium* in red blood cells. Malaria is transmitted to a human by the bite of an infected female Anopheles mosquito. The mosquito becomes infected by ingesting the blood of a human infected with malaria. SEE: *Anopheles.* **malarial, malarious** (-ăl, -ŭs) *adj.*

Of the 1.8 billion persons at risk of malaria worldwide, there are an estimated 500 million clinical cases and nearly 3.5 million deaths each year. It is therefore one of the most important infectious diseases in the world. Malaria has not been

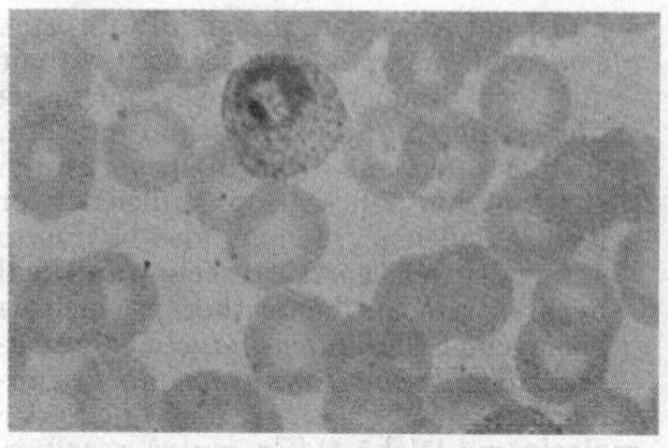


PLASMODIUM VIVAX SPOROZOITE

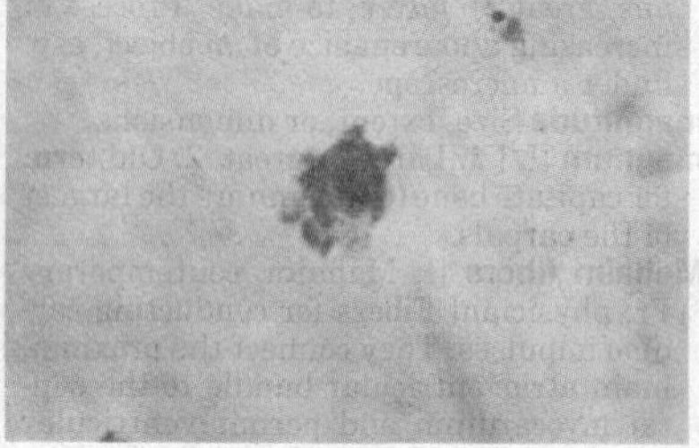


PLASMODIUM VIVAX SCHIZONT FORMING MEROZOITES

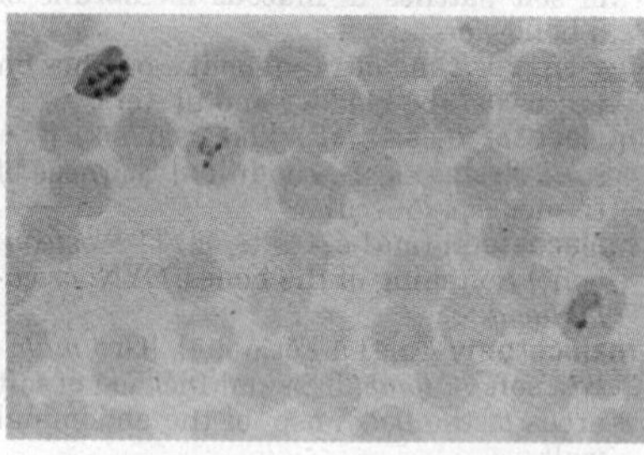


PLASMODIUM MALARIAE MEROZOITES

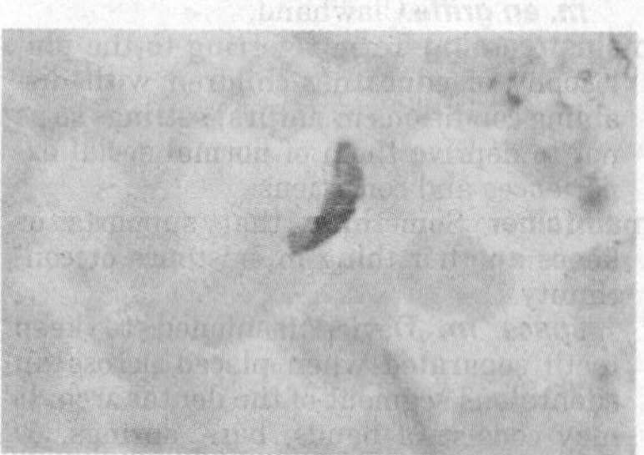


PLASMODIUM FALCIPARUM GAMETOCYTE

**MALARIA-CAUSING ORGANISMS** (ORIG. MAG. ×1000)

endemic in the U.S. since the 1940s; however, hundreds of cases are contracted in endemic zones and imported to this country each year.

The parasites undergo an asexual cycle in humans and a sexual cycle in mosquitoes. Sporozoites injected into a human by the bite of a mosquito or by blood transfusion go through an exoerythrocytic cycle in tissue cells, such as liver cells, where they undergo schizogony. After an incubation period (7 to 10 days for *P. falciparum*, 8 to 14 days for *P. vivax* and *P. ovale*, 7 to 30 days for *P. malariae*) they invade erythrocytes, where they undergo several divisions (schizogony), forming many merozoites. These break free and invade other corpuscles. The destruction of corpuscles with liberation of pigment and waste products brings on the characteristic paroxysms of chills and fever.

After several generations of schizonts, some merozoites develop into microgametocytes and macrogametocytes, which, when sucked up by a mosquito feeding on the human, undergo further development. The microgametocytes produce several flagellated bodies that unite with a macrogamete to form a zygote. This elongates, forming a vermicule or ookinete, which penetrates the stomach wall of the mosquito, forming an oocyst in which sporozoites develop. The oocyst bursts when mature, liberating sporozoites into the body cavity, through which the sporozoites then make their way to salivary glands. They are discharged through salivary ducts when the mosquito bites a human. SEE: illus.

SYMPTOMS: Initially, the symptoms are nonspecific and resemble those of a minor febrile illness with malaise, headache, fatigue, abdominal discomfort, and muscle aches, followed by fever and chills. The three stages of the malarial paroxysm are the defining characteristics of the illness. In the first (or chill) stage, patients complain of feeling cold and experience shaking chills that last from a few minutes to several hours. During the second (or hot) stage, minimal sweating occurs, although temperature rises to as high as 104°F (40°C); this stage lasts for several hours, and patients are at risk for febrile convulsions and hyperthermic brain damage. The patient may also exhibit tachycardia, hypotension, cough, headache, backache, nausea, abdominal pain, vomiting, diarrhea, and altered consciousness. The third (sweating) stage begins within 2 to 6 hr. In this period, the sweating is marked as the fever subsides, and is followed by profound fatigue and by sleep. If untreated, malarial paroxysms caused by *Plasmodium ovale* or *Plasmodium vivax* will occur cyclically every 48 hr (tertiary malaria). If due to *Plasmodium malariae,* paroxysms will occur every 72 hr (quartan malaria). Infections with *P. falciparum* may have a 48-hr cycle of paroxysms, but continuous fever is more characteristic. A severe form of falciparum malaria (cerebral malaria) is characterized by coma and, in spite of treatment, is associated with a 20% mortality rate in adults and 15% in children. About 10% of children who survive cerebral malaria have persistent neurologic deficits. Residual deficits in adults who survive this form of malaria are unusual. Progressive, possibly severe anemia and enlargement of the spleen are characteristic of all forms of malaria.

A rare but serious hematologic complication of malaria is acute intravascular hemolytic anemia, associated with infection with *P. falciparum*. This condition is called blackwater fever because of the accompanying hemoglobinuria.

ETIOLOGY: The causative organism, four species of a sporozoan, *Plasmodium (P. vivax, P. falciparum, P. malariae, P. ovale),* is transmitted through bites of infected female mosquitoes of the genus *Anopheles*. Inadvertent transfusion of blood from persons with malaria, or needle sharing among drug addicts, may infect the recipient. Malaria contracted by either of these means does not recur once it is effectively treated. Congenital malaria is acquired when the protozoa pass from maternal to fetal circulation.

DIAGNOSIS: Identification of the parasites in the blood is diagnostic.

PREVENTION: Pools of standing or stagnant water, in which mosquitoes breed, should be eliminated. Individuals can protect themselves from mosquito bites by wearing protective clothing, using a bed net, and applying a topical insecticide to exposed skin.

PROPHYLAXIS: Chemoprophylaxis is begun 1 week prior to arriving in an endemic area, is continued throughout the stay, and for 4 weeks after leaving the area. Chemoprophylaxis is never entirely effective; thus, malaria should always be considered when treating patients who have a febrile illness and who have traveled to an endemic area, even if they have taken prophylactic antimalaria drugs. The drug(s) advised for prophylaxis depend on the sensitivity of local parasites and whether infection is likely. Because of the changing sensitivity of the malaria parasites to drugs, it is not possible to be certain that a particular drug will be effective in all endemic areas. The prophylactic drugs used for *P. falciparum* are usually effective in preventing infections with *P. ovale* and *P. vivax*. For nonimmune individuals traveling in areas where malaria is due to chloroquine-resistant *P. falciparum,* mefloquine is effective for prophylaxis. Its safety for use in pregnancy has not been established. In areas where *P. falciparum* is chloroquine-sensitive, chloroquine is the drug of choice. Chloroquine may be used prophylactically during pregnancy.

TREATMENT: All forms of malaria including chloroqine-resistant *P. falciparum* may be treated with orally administered quinine sulfate plus pyrimethamine-sulfadoxine. Other drugs that may be used include quinine sulfate plus either tetracycline or clindamycin; mefloquine; or halofantrine. All forms of malaria except choroquine-resistant *P. falciparum* may be treated with chloroquine phosphate. Relapses of *P. ovale* or *P. vivax* may be prevented with primaquine phosphate.

Severe malaria due to chloroquine-resistant *P. falciparum* will require treatment with intravenous quinine. Exchange transfusion may be needed. There is no vaccine for malaria.

NURSING IMPLICATIONS: Nurses in primary health care settings in endemic areas need to work toward prompt detection and effective treatment of malaria. In such areas, suppressive and prophylactic drugs may be needed to control the disease. Other precautions include using mosquito nets, covering as much of the body as possible with clothing, and using mosquito repellent to reduce chances of being bitten. Travelers to endemic areas should take appropriate prophylactic medications before leaving, during the visit, and for a time afterwards to avoid infection. They also need to know that the time between dusk and dawn is the most dangerous for bites, because the insects feed during that time.

***cerebral m.*** Falciparum malaria in which the brain is affected due to tendency of parasites to agglutinate, resulting in clogging of capillaries, which leads to coma or sometimes sudden death.

***double quartan m.*** Malaria in which two concurrent cycles result in fever occurring on two successive days.

***falciparum m.*** Malaria caused by *Plasmodium falciparum*. More prevalent in the tropics. Symptoms more severe than in other types but runs a shorter course without relapses.

***quartan m.*** Malaria with short and less severe paroxysms. Sporulation occurs each 72 hr, causing seizures every 4 days. Caused by *Plasmodium malariae*.

***quotidian m.*** Malaria in which paroxysms occur with daily periodicity due to 24-hr sporulation of two groups of *P. vivax*. Abrupt rise and fall of temperature.

***tertian m.*** Malaria in which sporulation occurs each 48 hr. Symptoms more common during the day. Paroxysms divided into chill, fever, and sweating stages. Cold stage is usually 10 to 15 min but may last an hour or more. Febrile stage varies from 4 to 6 hr. Benign tertian malaria is caused by *Plasmodium vivax,* malignant tertian malaria by *Plasmodium falciparum.*

***triple quartan m.*** Malaria in which three concurrent cycles result in fever occurring every day.

***vivax m.*** Malaria caused by *Plasmodium vivax.* It is the most common form of malaria. Marked by frequent recurrence.

**malariacidal** (mă-lā″rē-ă-sī′dăl) [It. *malaria,* bad air, + L. *caedere,* to kill] Having the property of killing malaria parasites.

**malariology** (mă-lār-ē-ŏl′ō-jē) The scientific study of malaria.

**malariotherapy** (mă-lār-ē-ō-thĕr′ă-pē) A now obsolete method of treating syphilis of the central nervous system by injecting malarial organisms into the body. The organisms produce hyperthermia, which is then terminated by administration of an antimalarial.

**Malassezia** (măl″ă-sē′zē-ă) [Louis Charles Malassez, Fr. physiologist, 1842–1909] A genus of fungi.

**malassimilation** (măl″ă-sĭm-ĭ-lā′shŭn) [L. *malus,* ill, + *assimilatio,* making like] Defective, incomplete, or faulty assimilation, esp. of nutritive material. SEE: *malabsorption syndrome.*

**malate** (mā′lāt) A salt or ester of malic acid.

**malathion** (măl″ă-thī′ŏn) An effective pesticide.

**maldigestion** (măl″dī-jĕs′chŭn) Disordered digestion.

**male** [O. Fr.] **1.** Masculine. **2.** The sex that has organs for producing sperm for fertilization of ova.

**male erectile disorder** Essentially, the persistent or recurrent inability to attain, or to maintain until completion of the sexual activity, an adequate erection. The disturbance causes marked distress or interpersonal difficulty. The difficulty cannot be attributed to a medical condition, substance abuse, or medications. SEE: *impotence; female sexual arousal disorder.*

**malemission** (măl″ē-mĭsh′ŭn) [L. *malus,* evil, + *e,* out, + *mittere,* to send] Failure of semen to be ejaculated from the urinary meatus during coitus.

**maleruption** (măl-ē-rŭp′shŭn) Incorrect eruption of teeth.

**malformation** (măl-for-mā′shŭn) [″ + *formatio,* a shaping] Deformity; abnormal shape or structure, esp. congenital.

***tooth m.*** Abnormalities of size and shape that usually occur during the morphodifferentiation stage of tooth formation. Incomplete matrix formation or mineralization will also result in defective teeth that may or may not be abnormal in shape initially.

**malfunction** (măl-fŭnk′shŭn) Defective function.

**malic** (mā′lĭk, măl′ĭk) [L. *malum,* apple] Pert. to apples.

**malic acid** SEE: under *acid.*

**malice** (măl′ĭs) [L. *malus,* bad] Desire or intent to harm someone or to see others suffer.

**malign** (mă-līn′) [ME. *maligne*] Tending to injure or harm; malignant.

**malignancy** (mă-lĭg′năn-sē) [L. *malignus,* of bad kind] **1.** State of being malignant. **2.** A neoplasm or tumor that is cancerous as opposed to benign. SYN: *virulence.*

**malignant** (mă-lĭg′nănt) Growing worse; resisting treatment, said of cancerous growths. Tending or threatening to produce death; harmful. SYN: *virulent.*

**malinger** (mă-lĭng′ĕr) [Fr. *malingre,* weak, sickly] To feign illness, usually to arouse sympathy, to escape work, or to continue to receive compensation. SEE: *factitious disorder; Munchausen syndrome.*

**malingerer** (mă-lĭng′gĕr-ĕr) **1.** One who pretends to be ill or suffering from a nonexistent disorder to arouse sympathy. **2.** One who pretends slow recuperation from a disease once suffered in order to continue to receive benefits of medical insurance and work absence.

**malinterdigitation** (măl″ĭn-tĕr-dĭj″ĭ-tā′shŭn) Abnormal intercuspal relation of the upper and lower teeth. SEE: *overbite; underbite.*

**malleable** (măl′ē-ă-bl) [L. *mallere,* to hammer] Having the property of being shaped by pressure.

**malleation** (măl-lē-ā′shŭn) Spasmodic action of the hands in which they seem drawn to strike any near object, as spasmodic rapping against thighs or furniture. SEE: *tic.*

**malleoincudal** (măl″ē-ō-ĭng′kū-dăl) [L. *malleus,* hammer, + *incus,* anvil] Concerning or pert. to the malleus and incus.

**malleolus** (măl-ē′ō-lŭs) *pl.* **malleoli** [L. *malleolus,* little hammer] The protuberance on both sides of the ankle joint, the lower extremity of the fibula being known as the lateral malleolus and lower end of the tibia as the medial malleolus. **malleolar** (-ō-lăr), *adj.*

***external m.*** Process on outer edge of fibula at lower end.

***internal m.*** Round process on inner edge of tibia at lower end.

**malleotomy** (măl″ē-ŏt′ō-mē) [″ + Gr. *tome,* incision] **1.** Division of the malleus of the inner ear. **2.** Severing the ligaments attached to the malleoli of the ankle.

**mallet** A hammer-like tool to condense amalgam or direct filling gold.

**mallet finger** SEE: *finger, hammer.*

**mallet toe** SEE: *hammertoe.*

**malleus** (măl′ē-ŭs) *pl.* **mallei** [L., hammer] The largest of the three auditory ossicles in the middle ear. It is attached to the eardrum and articulates with the incus. SEE: *ear.*

**Mallophaga** (măl-ŏf′ă-gă) [Gr. *mallos,* wool, + *phagein,* to eat] An order of insects that

## Physical Signs of Malnutrition and Deficiency State

| Infants and Children | Adolescents and Adults |
|---|---|
| Lack of subcutaneous fat | Red swollen lingual papillae |
| Wrinkling of skin on light stroking | Glossitis |
| Poor muscle tone | Papillary atrophy of tongue |
| Pallor | Stomatitis |
| Rough skin (toad skin) | Spongy, bleeding gums |
| Hemorrhage of newborn, vitamin K deficiency | Muscle tenderness in extremities |
| Bad posture | Poor muscle tone |
| Nasal area is red and greasy | Loss of vibratory sensation |
| Sores at angles of mouth, cheilosis | Increase or decrease of tendon reflexes |
| Rapid heartbeat | Hyperesthesia of skin |
| Red tongue | Purpura |
| Square head, wrists enlarged, rib beading | Dermatitis: facial butterfly, perineal, scrotal, vulval |
| Vincent's angina, thrush | Thickening and pigmentation of skin over bony prominences |
| Serious dental abnormalities | Nonspecific vaginitis |
| Corneal and conjunctival changes | Follicular hyperkeratosis of extensor surfaces of extremities |
| **Adolescents and Adults** | Rachitic chest deformity |
| | Anemia not responding to iron |
| Nasolabial sebaceous plugs | Fatigue of visual accommodation |
| Sores at angles of mouth, cheilosis | Vascularization of cornea |
| Vincent's angina | Conjunctival changes |
| Minimal changes in tongue color or texture | |

SOURCE: Committee on Medical Nutrition, National Research Council.

includes biting lice.

**Mallory-Weiss syndrome** [G. Kenneth Mallory, U.S. pathologist, b. 1900; Soma Weiss, U.S. internist, 1898–1942] Hemorrhage from the upper gastrointestinal tract due to a tear in the mucosa of the esophagus or gastroesophageal junction. The syndrome is associated with chronic alcoholism and is usually preceded by severe vomiting. SEE: *cirrhosis; Nursing Diagnoses Appendix.*

**malnutrition** (măl″nū-trĭ′shŭn) Any disorder of nutrition causing a lack of necessary or proper food substances in the body or improper absorption and distribution of them. Malnutrition may be due to a deficient diet or deficient breakdown, assimilation, or utilization of food. SEE: table.

***protein-energy m.*** Malnutrition due to inadequate intake of calories or protein, or both. It is usually seen in children younger than 5 years of age. SYN: *protein-calorie malnutrition.* SEE: *kwashiorkor.*

**malocclusion** Malposition and imperfect contact of the mandibular and maxillary teeth.

***classification of m.*** The designation by Angle of the types of malocclusion based on the relative positions of the first molar in the two arches when in occlusion: *Class I*—normal anteroposterior relationship but with crowding and rotated teeth. *Class II*—the lower arch is distal to the upper arch on one or both sides; the lower first molar is distal to the upper first molar. *Class III*—the lower arch is anterior to the upper arch on one or both sides; the lower first molar is anterior to the upper first molar.

**malonylurea** (măl″ō-nĭl-ū′rē-ă) Barbituric acid. SEE: *acid, barbituric.*

**malpighian body** (măl-pĭg′ē-ăn) [Marcello Malpighi, It. anatomist, founder of histology, 1628–1694] **1.** Renal corpuscle consisting of a glomerulus enclosed in Bowman's capsule. **2.** Lymph nodule found in the spleen.

**malpighian capsule** A spherical body found in cortex of kidney consisting of a glomerulus and Bowman's capsule. SYN: *corpuscle, renal.* SEE: *nephron.*

**malpighian layer** Inner layer of the epidermis that includes both stratum germinativum and stratum spinosum.

**malposition** (măl-pō-zĭ′shŭn) [L. *malus,* evil, + *positio,* placement] **1.** Faulty or abnormal position or placement, esp. of the body or one of its parts. **2.** Abnormal position of the fetal presenting part in relation to the maternal pelvis. SEE: *occiput posterior, persistent.*

**malpractice** [″ + Gr. *praxis,* an action] Incorrect or negligent treatment of a patient by persons responsible for health care, such as physicians, dentists, and nurses.

**malpresentation** [″ + *praesentatio,* a presenting] Abnormal position of the fetus, making natural delivery difficult or impossible. SEE: *presentation* for illus.

**malrotation** (măl″rō-tā′shŭn) Failure during embryogenesis of normal rotation of all or a portion of an organ or system, esp. the viscera.

**malt** [AS. *mealt*] Germinated grain, usually

barley, used in manufacture of ale and beer. Contains carbohydrates (dextrin, maltose), a diastase, and proteins. Used as a food, esp. in wasting diseases.

**Malta fever** Brucellosis.

**maltase** (mawl'tās) [AS. *mealt,* grain] An enzyme of the small intestine that acts on maltose, converting it by hydrolysis to glucose. SEE: *digestion; enzyme.*

**malt extract** A viscous, light brown fluid obtained from malt steeped in water.

**maltose** (mawl'tōs) $C_{12}H_{22}O_{11}$. A disaccharide present in malt, malt products, and sprouting seeds. It is formed by the hydrolysis of starch and is converted into glucose by the enzyme maltase. SYN: *malt sugar*. SEE: *carbohydrate.*

**maltosuria** (mawl"tō-sūr'ē-ă) [" + Gr. *ouron,* urine] Presence of maltose in urine.

**malt sugar** Maltose.

**malturned** Abnormally turned, said of a tooth having turned on its long axis.

**malunion** [L. *malus,* evil, + *unio,* oneness] Growth of the fragments of a fractured bone in a faulty position, forming an imperfect union.

**mamanpian** (mă-măn"pē-ăn') [Fr. *maman,* mother, + *pian,* yaw] A mother yaw.

**mamelon** (măm'ĕ-lŏn) [Fr., nipple] One of three rounded protuberances present on the cutting edge of an incisor tooth when it erupts. These are worn away by use.

**mamill-** SEE: words beginning with *mammill-*.

**mamma** (măm'ă) *pl.* **mammae** [L., breast] A glandular structure beneath the skin in the female that secretes milk. In the human female, there are normally two, situated over the anterolateral area between the third and sixth ribs. The nipple of each breast extends from the glandular tissue through the surface of the skin. SYN: *breast; mammary gland.*

**mammal** (măm'ăl) An animal of the class Mammalia, characterized by having breasts, from which milk is available for the nourishment of the newborn.

**mammalgia** (măm-ăl'jē-ă) [L. *mamma,* breast, + Gr. *algos,* pain] Pain in the breast. SYN: *mastalgia; mastodynia.*

**mammaplasty** (măm'ă-plăs"tē) [" + Gr. *plassein,* to form] Plastic surgery of the breast. Also spelled *mammoplasty.*

***augmentation m.*** Plastic surgical procedure to increase the size of the breast(s) or to make an artificial breast to replace one surgically removed. This is usually done by implanting a soft plastic material in an impervious cover or by implanting a gel.

---

Caution: The long-term health risks of some of the implant materials are unknown.

---

***reduction m.*** Plastic surgery of the breast to decrease and reshape the breast(s).

**mammary** (măm'ă-rē) [L. *mamma,* breast] Pert. to the breast.

**mammary glands** Compound glands of the female breast that can secrete milk. They are made up of lobes and lobules bound together by areolar tissue. The main ducts number 15 to 20 and are known as lactiferous ducts, each one discharging through a separate orifice upon the surface of the nipple. The dilatations of the ducts form reservoirs for the milk during lactation. The pink, or dark-colored, skin around the nipple is called the areola. SYN: *mammae.*

**mammectomy** SEE: *mastectomy.*

**mammillated** (măm'mĭl-lā-tĕd) Having protuberances like a nipple.

**mammilliplasty** (măm-mĭl'ĭ-plăs"tē) [" + Gr. *plassein,* to form] Plastic operation on a nipple. SYN: *theleplasty.*

**mammillitis** (măm"mĭl-ī'tĭs) [" + Gr. *itis,* inflammation] Inflammation of a nipple. SYN: *acromastitis; thelitis.*

**mammitis** SEE: *mastitis.*

**mammogram** (măm'ō-grăm) [" + Gr. *gramma,* something written] X-ray of the breast.

**mammography** (măm-ŏg'ră-fē) [" + Gr. *graphein,* to write] Use of radiography of the breast to diagnose breast cancer. This technique has increased the rate of early detection. Mammography is capable of detecting 85% to 90% of existing breast cancers. Despite the increased exposure to radiation, mammography is recommended as a screening technique for breast cancer. Women in the high-risk group for breast cancer (ages 40 to 49) should have the examination every 1 to 2 years. Women over age 50 should have the examination every year. Use of mammography as a diagnostic tool does not mean that a careful periodic physical examination should be omitted. This is esp. true for women with dense, fibrous breast tissue, in which lesions are difficult to detect.

Because having two radiologists evaluate a mammogram (double reading) leads to discovery of more cancers than if only one reads it, it is advisable to have each mammogram read by two radiologists. Double reading increases the rate of cancer detection by 15%. Also, no clinician should rely on the mammogram to determine whether a palpable abnormality is benign or malignant. That should be determined clinically, with tests including biopsy of suspicious lesions.

**mammoplasty** SEE: *mammaplasty.*

**mammose** (măm'ōs) [L. *mammosus*] **1.** Having unusually large breasts. **2.** Shaped like a breast.

**mammotomy** SEE: *mastotomy.*

**mammotrophic** (măm"ō-trŏf'ĭk) [" + Gr. *trophe,* nourishment] To have the effect of stimulating size or function of the breast.

**man** [AS. *mann*] **1.** Member of the human species, *Homo sapiens.* **2.** Male member of the species as distinguished from female.

**3.** The human race, collectively; mankind. SEE: words beginning with *anthro-*.

**managed care** A variety of methods of financing and organizing the delivery of health care in which costs are contained by controlling the provision of services. Physicians, hospitals, and other health care agencies contract with the system to accept a predetermined monthly payment for providing services to patients enrolled in a managed care plan. Enrollee access to care is limited to the physicians and other health care providers who are affiliated with the plan. In general, managed care attempts to control costs by overseeing and, perhaps, altering the behavior of their providers. Clinical decision making is influenced by a variety of administrative incentives and constraints. Incentives affect the health care provider's financial return for professional services. Constraints include specific rules, regulations, practice guidelines, diagnostic and treatment protocols, or algorithms. Care is affected further by quality assurance procedures and utilization reviews. SEE: *cost awareness; cost-effectiveness; gatekeeper; Health Maintenance Organization; managed competition; resource-based relative value scale.*

**managed competition** In health care practice, the requirement that health care organizations compete with each other in terms of price and quality of delivered services. SEE: *managed care; resource-based relative value scale.*

**manchette** (măn-chĕt′) [Fr., a cuff] A circular band consisting of microtubules around the caudal pole of developing sperm.

**manchineel** (măn″kĭ-nēl′) [Sp. *manzanilla,* small apple] A tree, *Hippomane mancinella,* native to tropical America that contains a milky, poisonous sap. Contact with the sap causes blistering of the skin. The fruit is also poisonous.

**mancinism** (măn′sĭn-ĭzm) [L. *mancus,* crippled] State of being left-handed.

**Mandelamine** Trade name for methenamine mandelate.

**mandelic acid** SEE *acid, mandelic.*

**mandible** (măn′dĭ-bl) [L. *mandibula,* lower jawbone] The horseshoe-shaped bone forming the lower jaw. SYN: *mandibula.* SEE: illus. **mandibular** (măn-dĭb′ū-lăr), *adj.*

**mandibula** SEE: *mandible.*

**mandibular reflex** SEE: under *reflex.*

**mandibulopharyngeal** (măn-dĭb″ū-lō-fă-rin′jē-ăl) [″ + Gr. *pharynx,* throat] Concerning the mandible and pharynx.

**mandrel, mandril** (măn′drĕl) Handle that holds a dental tool so that it may be easily positioned by the operator. A spindle or shaft designed to fit a dental handpiece for the purpose of using a variety of tools for grinding, polishing or buffing.

**mandrin** (măn′drĭn) [Fr.] A guide or stylet for a flexible catheter.

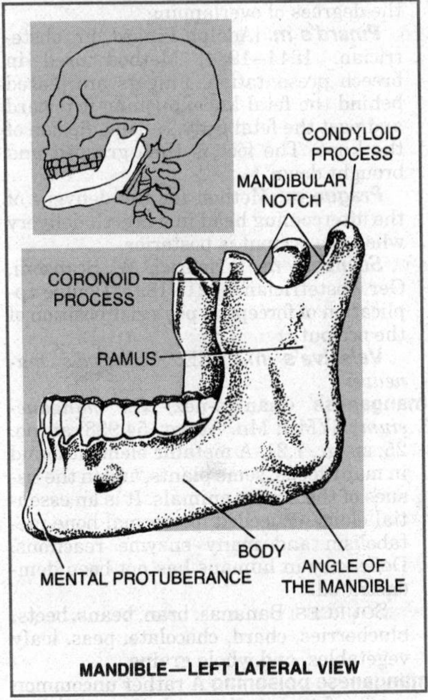

MANDIBLE—LEFT LATERAL VIEW

**maneuver** [Fr. *manoeuvre,* from L. *manu operari,* to work by hand] **1.** Any dexterous or skillful procedure. **2.** In obstetrics, manipulation of the fetus to aid in delivery. SEE: *labor.*

***Credé's m.*** SEE: *Credé's method.*

***Heimlich m.*** SEE: *Heimlich maneuver.*

***Leopold's m.*** SEE: *Leopold's maneuver.*

***Mauriceau-Smellie m.*** [François Mauriceau, Fr. obstetrician, 1637–1709; William Smellie, Brit. obstetrician, 1697–1763] Method employed to deliver the aftercoming head in breech presentation. The baby is held over the right arm, and the index finger of the right hand is introduced into the mouth of the child and applied over the maxilla; two fingers of the other hand are then hooked over the neck, grasping the shoulders. Downward traction is made until the occiput appears under the symphysis pubis. The body of the child is then raised up toward the mother's abdomen and the mouth, nose, brow, and occiput are successively brought over the perineum.

***Müller's m.*** SEE: *Müller's maneuver.*

***Munro Kerr m.*** [John Munro Kerr, Scot. obstetrician, 1868–1955] Method for determining the presence of disproportion between the fetal head and the maternal pelvis. The fetal head is pushed into the pelvis with the right hand on the abdomen while, with two fingers of the left hand in the vagina, the possibilities of engagement of the head are noted. At the same time the thumb of the left hand feels over the brim of the pelvis to determine the degrees of overlapping.

***Pinard's m.*** [Adolph Pinard, Fr. obstetrician, 1844–1934] Method used in breech presentation. Fingers are placed behind the fetal knee, pushing it toward and past the fetal body, causing flexion of the knee. The foot is then grasped and brought down.

***Prague m.*** Method for the delivery of the aftercoming head in a breech delivery when the occiput is posterior.

***Scanzoni m.*** [Friedrich W. Scanzoni, Ger. obstetrician, 1821–1891] Double application of forceps in posterior position of the occiput.

***Valsalva's m.*** SEE: *Valsalva's maneuver.*

**manganese** (măn′gă-nēz) [L. *manganesium*] SYMB: Mn. At. wt. 54.938; at. no. 25; sp. gr. 7.21. A metallic element found in many foods, some plants, and in the tissues of the higher animals. It is an essential element needed for normal bone metabolism and many enzyme reactions. Deficiency in humans has not been demonstrated.

SOURCES: Bananas, bran, beans, beets, blueberries, chard, chocolate, peas, leafy vegetables, and whole grains.

**manganese poisoning** A rather uncommon cause of toxicity in workers exposed to manganese on a regular basis.

SYMPTOMS: Muscular weakness, peculiar gait, tremors, central nervous system disturbances, salivation.

**mange** (mānj) A cutaneous communicable disease of domestic animals, including dogs and cats. A number of mites, such as *Chorioptes, Demodex, Psoroptes,* and *Sarcoptes* are causative agents. In humans, this condition is known as scabies.

**mania** (mā′nē-ă) [Gr., madness] **1.** Mental disorder characterized by excessive excitement. **2.** A form of psychosis characterized by exalted feelings, delusions of grandeur, elevation of mood, psychomotor overactivity, and overproduction of ideas. SEE: *psychosis, manic-depressive.*

***histrionic m.*** Dramatic gestures, expressions, and speech in certain psychiatric states.

***religious m.*** Mania resulting from excessive religious fervor.

***transitory m.*** Attacks of severe frenzy, of short duration.

***unproductive m.*** Behavior characteristic of mania with lack of spontaneity in speech or muteness, sometimes seen in manic-depressive psychosis. SEE: *alcoholism.*

**-mania** Suffix meaning *frenzy* or *madness.*

**maniac** (mā′nē-ăk) Person afflicted by mania.

**maniacal** (mă-nī′ă-kl) **1.** Relating to or characterized by mania. **2.** Afflicted with mania.

**manic** (măn′ĭk) Mood state characterized by excessive energy, poor impulse control, psychosis, agitation, flight of ideas, frenzied movement, and decreased sleep.

**manic-depressive psychosis** SEE: under *psychosis.*

**manifest** To reveal in an obvious manner.

**manifestation** The demonstration of the presence of a sign, symptom, or alteration, esp. one that is associated with a disease process.

**manifest squint** Tropia.

**manikin** [D. *manneken,* little man] A model of the human body or its parts, used esp. in teaching anatomy and nursing procedures.

**maniphalanx** (măn″ĭ-fā′lănks) [L. *manus,* hand, + Gr. *phalanx,* closely knit row] A phalanx, or finger, of the hand. SEE: *pedphalanx.*

**manipulation** [L. *manipulare,* to handle] **1.** Conscious or unconscious process by which one person attempts to influence another person in order to obtain his or her own needs or desires. **2.** A joint mobilization technique, usually involving a rapid thrust or stretching a joint with the patient under anesthesia. SEE: *joint manipulation.* **3.** A method of realigning a fractured long bone with manual pressure, traction or angulation.

***joint m.*** Passive therapeutic techniques used to stretch restricted joints or reposition a subluxation. The techniques are sometimes applied with rapid thrust movements and may be applied with the patient under anesthesia to ensure maximum relaxation. SEE: *mobilization, joint.*

**manna** (măn′ă) [L.] **1.** The sweet juice obtained from the flowering ash, *Fraxinus ornus.* **2.** General term applied to sweetish juices obtained from a variety of plants.

**mannans** (măn′ănz) Any of several polysaccharides of mannose.

**mannerism** A peculiar modification or exaggeration of style or habit of dress, speech, or action.

**mannitol** (măn′ĭ-tŏl) A carbohydrate that may be obtained from plant sources. It is used as an osmotic diuretic, to reduce cerebrospinal fluid pressure, and in prophylaxis of acute renal failure.

**Mannkopf's sign** [Emil W. Mannkopf, Ger. physician, 1836–1918] Pulse acceleration exhibited on pressing a painful point. The sign is not present in feigned pain.

**mannose** (măn′ōs) A polysaccharide present in certain plants. It is an aldohexose.

**mannoside** (măn′ō-sīd) A glycoside of mannose.

**mannosidosis** (măn″ōs-ĭ-dō′sĭs) An inborn error of metabolism in which the deficiency of α-mannosidase is associated with mental deficiency, kyphosis, enlarged tongue, abnormal lymphocytes, and accumulation of mannose in tissues.

**manometer** (măn-ŏm′ĕt-ĕr) [Gr. *manos,* thin, + *metron,* measure] Device for determining liquid or gaseous pressure. The measurement is expressed in millimeters of either mercury or water, or in torr.

***saline m.*** Manometer that uses a special hollow tube shaped like the letter U and open at both ends. The tube is partially filled with saline. Pressure is determined by connecting one end of the U tube to the system in which pressure is to be measured. The pressure, in millimeters of saline, is the measured distance between the fluid level in one side of the U tube and that in the other side.

**Mansonella** (măn″sō-nĕl′ă) A genus of filarial nematodes.

***M. ozzardi*** A species found in humans in Central and South America and the Caribbean. It is transmitted by blackflies and midges. The parasites are unsheathed and most patients are asymptomatic.

**mansonelliasis** (măn″sō-nĕl-ī′ă-sĭs) [*Mansonella* + Gr. *-iasis,* condition] Infection in humans with *Mansonella ozzardi.*

**Mansonia** (măn-sō′nē-ă) A genus of mosquitoes found in tropical countries that transmit microfilariae to humans.

**mantle** [AS. *mentel,* a garment] A covering structure or layer.

***dentin m.*** The narrow zone of dentin that is first formed in the crown and root of a tooth.

**Mantoux test** (măn-tū′) [Charles Mantoux, Fr. physician, 1877–1947] An intradermal (intracutaneous) injection of 0.1 ml of intermediate strength Purified Protein Derivative (PPD). The needle is removed after a brief delay in order to minimize leakage of the PPD at the puncture site. Within 24 to 72 hr, the injected area becomes hard (indurated) and 10 mm in diameter if either an active or inactive tuberculous infection is present. Induration of 5 to 10 mm is doubtful, and a reaction of less than 5 mm is considered to be negative. SEE: *tuberculosis.*

**manual** (măn′ū-ăl) [L. *manus,* hand] **1.** Pert. to the hands. **2.** Performed by or with the hands.

**manual muscle test** A technique for estimating the relative strength of specific muscles. Rating categories and values include normal (5), good (4), fair (3), poor (2), trace (1), and zero (0). A grade of fair is based on the ability of the muscle to move the part through its full range of motion against gravity; a grade of poor is based on the ability to move through the range with gravity eliminated. Higher grades are then based on the muscles' ability to maintain an isometric contraction against resistance.

**manubrium** (mă-nū′brē-ŭm) *pl.* **manubria** [L., handle] Any handle-shaped structure.

***m. sterni*** The upper segment of the sternum articulating with the clavicle and first pair of costal cartilages.

**manudynamometer** (măn″ū-dī″nă-mŏm′ĕ-tĕr) [L. *manus,* hand, + Gr. *dynamis,* force, + *metron,* measure] A device for measuring the force of a thrust.

**manus** (mā′nŭs) *pl.* **manus** [L.] The hand.

**MAO** *monoamine oxidase.*

**map** A graphic presentation in two dimensions of the location of all or part of an area.

***genetic m.*** SEE: *gene map.*

***linkage m.*** Map of chromosomes indicating the relationship of genes to each other on the chromosome.

**maple bark disease** A pneumonitis caused by inhalation of spores from the mold *Cryptostroma corticale,* which is present under the bark of logs cut from maple tree.

**maple syrup urine disease** An inherited metabolic disease involving defective amino acid metabolism; so named because of the characteristic odor of the urine and sweat. The amino acids involved are leucine, isoleucine, valine, and alloisoleucine. Clinically there is rapid deterioration of the nervous system in the first few months of life and then death at an early age.

TREATMENT: Controlling the intake of the involved amino acids; exchange transfusion; and peritoneal dialysis.

**mapping** Location of the genes on a chromosome.

**marantology** (mă″răn-tŏl′ō-jē) [Gr. *marasmos,* a dying away, + *logos,* word, reason] Study, care, and treatment of debilitated, elderly, and chronically ill patients whose outlook for recovery is poor.

**marasmus** (măr-ăz′mŭs) Emaciation and wasting in an infant due to malnutrition. Causes include caloric deficiency secondary to acute diseases, esp. diarrheal diseases of infancy, deficiency in nutritional composition, inadequate food intake, malabsorption, child abuse, failure-to-thrive syndrome, deficiency of vitamin D, or scurvy. SYN: *wasting.* SEE: *kwashiorkor; malnutrition, protein-energy.* **marantic, marasmic** (mă-răn′tĭk, mă-răz′mĭk), *adj.*

SYMPTOMS: Extreme wasting. Failure to gain weight is followed by a loss of weight. Brain and skeletal growth continues, resulting in a long body and a large head in proportion to weight. Subcutaneous fat is minimal, the eyes are sunken, and tissue turgor is lost. The skin appears loose and sags. The infant is not active, muscles are flabby and relaxed, and the cry is weak and shrill.

TREATMENT: Initial feedings should be small and low in calories, because digestive capacity is poor. Diluted formula or breast milk is best. The amount of calories and protein, carbohydrates, and fat should be increased gradually. The goal for protein intake is 5 g/kg of body weight per day. If diarrhea due to disaccharidase deficiency is present, a low-lactose diet will be of benefit. Parenteral fluid therapy is indicated if shock or fluid and electrolyte imbalance exists.

PROGNOSIS: Death occurs in 40% of affected children.

**marble bone disease** Osteopetrosis.

**Marburg virus disease** [Marburg, Germany] This frequently fatal disease is caused by a virus classed as a member of the family *Filoviridae*. Clinically this disease is identical to that caused by the Ebola virus. SEE: *Ebola virus hemorrhagic fever*.

**marc** (mărk) [Fr.] The residue remaining after a drug has been percolated. SEE: *percolation*.

**Marchiafava-Micheli syndrome** (măr″kē-ă-fă′vă-mē-kā′lē) [Ettore Marchiafava, It. pathologist, 1847–1935; F. Micheli, It. clinician, 1872–1937] A rare hemolytic anemia associated with paroxysmal nocturnal hemoglobinuria.

**Marcus Gunn pupil** [Robert Marcus Gunn, Brit. ophthalmologist, 1850–1909] A pupil of the eye that responds by constricting more to an indirect than a direct light.

**Marcus Gunn syndrome** [Robert Marcus Gunn] A congenital condition in which a ptotic eyelid retracts briefly when the mouth is opened or the jaw moved to one side. The person appears to wink each time the jaw is opened. SEE: *jaw winking*.

**Marfan's syndrome** [Bernard-Jean Antonin Marfan, Fr. physician, 1858–1942] A hereditary condition of connective tissue, bones, muscles, ligaments, and skeletal structures.

SYMPTOMS: Irregular and unsteady gait, tall lean body type with long extremities including fingers and toes, abnormal joint flexibility, flat feet, stooped shoulders, and dislocation of the optic lens. The aorta will usually be dilated and may become sufficiently weakened to allow an aneurysm to develop. SEE: *arachnodactyly*.

NURSING IMPLICATIONS: Patients with this condition are encouraged to seek medical attention promptly for complications. Because complications are serious, the patient's lifestyle must be continually monitored. Reassurance and support are given on a continual basis.

**margarine** Butter substitute made from refined vegetable oils or a combination of vegetable oils and fats. Coloring material and vitamins A and D are added. It contains 7.2 kcal/g.

**margin** [L. *marginalis*, border] **1.** A boundary, such as the edge of a structure of the anatomy. SYN: *margo*. **2.** In dentistry, the apical extent or boundary of enamel adjacent to the cementum of the tooth root; the junction of a restoration with the cavosurface angle of a prepared cavity in enamel.

***gingival m.*** The most coronal part of the gingiva surrounding a tooth.

**marginal** (măr′jĭn-ăl) Concerning a margin or border. SYN: *limbic*.

**margination** (măr″jĭ-nā′shŭn) Adhesion of leukocytes to the walls of blood vessels in the first stages of inflammation.

**marginoplasty** (mar-jĭn′ō-plăs″tē) [L. *marginalis*, border, + Gr. *plassein*, to mold] Plastic surgery of a border, as of an eyelid.

**margo** (măr′gō) *pl.* **margines** [L.] A border or edge.

***m. acutus*** Sharp margin of the heart extending from the apex to the right.

***m. obtusus*** Portion of a line extending from apex to root of the pulmonary artery that lies along the rounded left side of the left ventricle.

**Marie's ataxia** (mă-rēz′) [Pierre Marie, Fr. neurologist, 1853–1940] Hereditary cerebellar ataxia caused by bilateral cortical atrophy of the cerebellum.

**Marie's disease** Chronic condition with enlargement of bones and soft tissues of hands, feet, and face. SYN: *acromegaly*.

**Marie's sign** Hand tremor seen in exophthalmic goiter.

**marijuana, marihuana** (măr″ĭ-wă′nă) The dried flowering tops of *Cannabis sativa*, the hemp plant. SYN: *cannabis*. SEE: *hashish*. There is controversy over the effects of marijuana. This substance has dose-related effects on mood, perception, and psychomotor coordination. Driving and other machine-operating skills may therefore be seriously affected. Users of marijuana have impairment of short-term memory, and its use slows learning. Depending on the dose of the drug and the underlying psychological conditions of the user, marijuana may cause transient episodes of confusion, anxiety, or even frank toxic delirium. Its use may exacerbate pre-existing mental illness, esp. schizophrenia. Long-term, relatively heavy use may be associated with behavioral disorders and a kind of ennui called the amotivational syndrome, but it is not known whether use of the drug is a cause or a result of this condition. Transient symptoms occur on withdrawal, indicating that the drug can lead to physical dependence. There has been considerable interest in the effects of marijuana on pregnancy and fetal growth but because substance abusers often abuse more than a single substance, it is difficult to evaluate the effects of individual substances on the outcome of pregnancy or fetal development.

Because marijuana smoke contains many of the components of tobacco smoke, prolonged heavy smoking of marijuana leads to impaired pulmonary function. The possibility that chronic marijuana use is associated with an increased risk of developing lung cancer exists, but it has not been proved because most people who smoke marijuana also smoke cigarettes.

Marijuana, its constituents, or its derivatives may be useful in the acute treatment of glaucoma and in the control of the severe nausea and vomiting caused by cancer chemotherapy.

The most important psychoactive substance in cannabis is delta-9-tetrahydrocannabinol. This chemical, dronabinol, is approved for use in treating nausea and vomiting associated with cancer chemotherapy in patients who have failed to respond adequately to conventional antiemetic treatment, and treatment of anorexia associated with weight loss in patients with acquired immunodeficiency syndrome. Marijuana itself is not approved for medical use.

Caution: Dronabinol is highly abusable. Prescriptions are limited to the amount necessary for a single cycle of chemotherapy.

**Marinol** Trade name for dronabinol, the principal psychoactive substance present in *Cannabis sativa* (marijuana). SEE: *marijuana*.

**mark** [AS. *mearc*] Any nevus, bruise, cut, or spot on the surface of a body.

***birth- m.*** SEE: *birthmark; nevus*.

***port-wine m.*** Nevus flammeus.

***strawberry m.*** Nevus vascularis.

**marker 1.** A device or substance used to indicate or mark something. **2.** An identifying characteristic or trait that allows apparently similar materials or disease conditions to be differentiated.

***fecal m.*** A substance, such as carmine, ingested to mark the beginning and end of fecal collection periods.

***genetic m.*** An identifiable physical location on a chromosome (e.g., a gene or segment of DNA with no known coding function) whose inheritance can be monitored.

**Marlex mesh** A monofilament, biologically inert mesh used in surgical procedures to help cover or strengthen areas, as in hernia repair.

**marrow** [AS. *mearh*] The soft tissue occupying the medullary cavities of the sternum, long bones, some haversian canals, and spaces between trabeculae of cancellous or spongy bone. Marrow is of two types: red and yellow. The yellow marrow is found esp. in the medullary cavity of the long bones; the red marrow is found in spongy bones.

***gelatinous m.*** Yellow marrow of old or emaciated persons, almost devoid of fat and having a gelatinous consistency.

***red m.*** Marrow found in spongy bone that produces all the types of blood cells. SEE: illus.

***spinal m.*** The spinal cord.

***yellow m.*** Marrow found in the medullary canal of long bones. Consists principally of fat cells and connective tissue. It does not participate in hematopoiesis.

**marrow aspiration** Procedure using a special aspirating needle to obtain a specimen of bone marrow for examination. The material is usually obtained from the upper portion of the sternum or the iliac crest. Examination of the stained marrow is helpful in diagnosing a great number of blood disorders, infections, and malignant diseases.

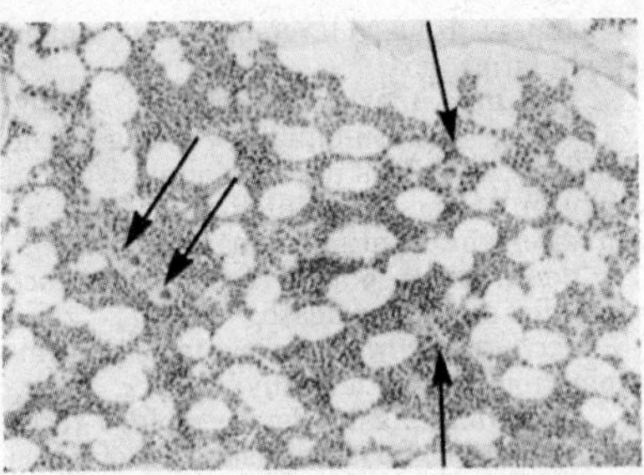

NORMAL RED BONE MARROW

ARROWS INDICATE MEGAKARYOCYTES (ORIG. MAG. ×200)

**marrow transplantation** SEE: *bone marrow transplantation*.

**Marsh's test** [James Marsh, Brit. chemist, 1789–1846] A test to detect the presence of arsenic.

**marsupialization** (măr-sū″pē-ăl-ĭ-zā′shŭn) [L. *marsupium*, pouch] Process of raising the borders of an evacuated tumor sac to the edges of the abdominal wound and stitching them there to form a pouch. The interior of the sac suppurates and gradually closes by granulation.

**marsupium** (măr-sū′pē-ŭm) [L., pouch] **1.** Scrotum. **2.** A sac or pouch that serves to hold the young of a marsupial.

**MAS, mAs** *milliampere-second*.

**masculation** (măs-kū-lā′shŭn) [L. *masculus*, a male] Development of male secondary sexual characteristics.

**masculine** (măs′kū-lĭn) **1.** Pert. to the male sex. **2.** Having male characteristics. SYN: *virile*.

**masculinization 1.** The normal development of secondary male sex characteristics that occur at puberty. **2.** The abnormal development of masculine characteristics in the female. This may be caused by certain testosterone-producing tumors, medication that contains testosterone, or anabolic steroids. SYN: *virilization*.

**masculinovoblastoma** (măs″kū-lĭn-ō″vō-blăs-tō′mă) A benign ovarian tumor that microscopically resembles adrenocortical tissue and usually results in masculinization.

**maser** Acronym for *m*icrowave *a*mplification by *s*timulation *e*mission of *r*adiation. A device that produces a small, nondiverging radiation beam. SEE: *laser*.

**mask** [Fr. *masque*] **1.** A covering for the face that serves as a protective barrier. SEE: *Universal Precautions Appendix*. **2.** The immobile appearance of the face occurring in certain pathological conditions. **3.** To conceal or prevent detection.

***aerosol m.*** A mask used for the therapeutic administration of a nebulizer, humidity, or high air flow with oxygen enrichment. It has a large-bore inlet and an exhalation port.

***BLB m.*** A mask invented by Boothby, Lovelace, and Bulbulian, working at the Mayo Clinic. It is used for administering oxygen to persons at high altitudes (e.g., aviators) or to patients during anesthesia.

***death m.*** A plaster cast of the face molded soon after death.

***ecchymotic m.*** Cyanotic facies accompanying traumatic asphyxia.

***face m.*** A plastic device molded to fit over the face for administration of gases or humidified air.

***HAFOE m.*** *high air flow with oxygen enrichment m.*

***high air flow with oxygen enrichment m.*** ABBR: HAFOE mask. Term applied to Venturi-type devices. SEE: *Venturi mask.*

***Hutchinson's m.*** A feeling of compression over the face as though one is wearing a mask.

***luetic m.*** Blotchy brown pigmentation of cheeks, forehead, and temples, seen in tertiary syphilis.

***nonrebreathing m.*** An oxygen administration device with one-way valves for inspiration and expiration and a reservoir bag; used to attain high concentrations of oxygen.

***oxygen m.*** Any device that provides low-flow administration of oxygen or other therapeutic gas. It includes a simple, partial rebreathing type and a nonrebreathing type.

***Parkinson's m.*** Immobile, expressionless facial appearance resulting from paralysis agitans (Parkinson's disease).

***pocket face m.*** A folding mask that can be carried in a pocket and used for artificial ventilation. Some pocket face masks have an inlet for oxygen.

***m. of pregnancy*** Pigmented areas seen on the face of some pregnant women. SYN: *chloasma gravidarum; melasma gravidarum.*

***ventilation m.*** A face mask device that applies mechanical ventilation.

**masked** Concealed, esp. as in masked infection. For example, women exposed to rubella during the first trimester of pregnancy may be given immune globulin. This may prevent clinical symptoms of rubella in the mother, yet the fetus may be adversely affected and born with congenital defects.

**Maslach Burnout Inventory** ABBR: MBI. A self-reporting questionnaire that measures the frequency and intensity of burnout in the allied health professions. It assesses three aspects of burnout: emotional exhaustion, dehumanization, and lack of a sense of personal accomplishment. It is used to assess professionals who work extensively with cognitively impaired people.

**Maslow, Abraham H.** [U.S. psychologist, 1908–1970] Articulator of a theory of human motivation based on a synthesis of holistic and dynamic principles. His major work, *Motivation and Personality* (1954), was completed while he was a professor at Brandeis University.

***M.'s theory of human motivation*** A theory stating that human existence is based on needs that arise in hierarchal order: physiological needs such as hunger; safety needs; love, affection, and belonging needs; self-respect and self-esteem needs; and self-actualization. Although the term self-actualization was coined by Kurt Goldstein in 1939, Maslow believed that the ultimate destiny of mankind was self-actualization or a tendency to become everything that one is capable of becoming. Humans' realization of themselves occurs not only by thinking but also by the realization of all instinctive and emotional capacities as they move toward optimal physical, emotional, and spiritual health, which he called transcendence. A contemporary of Carl Rogers, Maslow is considered one of the major theorists of humanistic psychology.

**masochism** (măs′ō-kĭzm) [Leopold von Sacher-Masoch, Austrian novelist, 1835–1895] A general orientation to life based on the belief that suffering relieves guilt and leads to a reward. Opposite of sadism. SEE: *algolagnia; flagellation.*

***sexual m.*** Sexual excitement produced in an individual by being humiliated or hurt by another.

**masochist** (măs′ō-kĭst) A person who derives pleasure from masochism.

**mass** [L. *massa*] **1.** A quantity of material, such as cells, that unite or adhere to each other. **2.** Soft solid preparation for internal use and of such consistency that it may be molded into pills. **3.** A fundamental scalar property of an object that describes the amount of acceleration an object will have when a given force is applied to it. The metric unit of mass is the kilogram. One kilogram equals 2.205 pounds. SEE: *weight.*

***cell m.*** An aggregation of cells that serves as the primordium (anlage) of a future organ or part.

***epithelial m.*** Inner portion of a developing gonad enclosed within the germinal epithelium.

***inner cell m.*** In embryology, the group of cells within the blastocyst from which the embryo, yolk sac, and amnion develop. SEE: *blastocyst.*

***interfilar m.*** The fluid portion of the protoplasm.

***intermediate cell m.*** A plate of nonsegmented mesoderm lying lateral to the segments (somites) and connecting them to the nonsegmented lateral mesoderm. SYN: *nephrotome.*

**massa** [L.] Mass.

***m. intermedia*** The middle commissure of the brain, an inconstant mass of gray matter extending across the third ventricle and connecting adjacent surfaces of the thalami.

**massage** [Gr. *massein*, to knead] Manipulation, methodical pressure, friction, and kneading of the body.

***auditory m.*** Massage of the eardrum.

***cardiac m.*** Manual compression of the heart to restore heartbeat after heart has stopped. This is accomplished by applying pressure over the sternum (closed chest massage) or through an incision in the chest wall (open chest massage), forcing blood out of the heart and, when pressure is removed, allowing the heart to fill as if it were beating. SEE: *cardiopulmonary resuscitation*.

***electrovibratory m.*** Massage by means of an electric vibrator.

***general m.*** Centripetal stroking in connection with some muscular kneading from the toes upward. Used in connection with baths lasting 30 to 40 min. As soon as a part is massaged, it should be given a few passive rotary movements and afterwards covered up.

***introductory m.*** Massage consisting of centripetal strokings around an affected part when it is impossible to apply treatment directly to the part.

***local m.*** Massage confined to particular parts.

***vapor m.*** Treatment of a cavity by a medicated and nebulized vapor under interrupted pressure.

***vibratory m.*** Massage by rapidly repeated tapping of the affected surface by means of a vibrating hammer or sound.

**masseter** (măs-sē′tĕr) [Gr. *maseter*, chewer] The muscle that closes the mouth and is the principal muscle in mastication. SEE: *Muscles Appendix*.

**masseur** (mă-soor′) [Fr.] **1.** A man who gives massages. **2.** An instrument for massaging.

**masseuse** (mă-sooz′) [Fr.] A woman who gives massages.

**massive** (măs′sĭv) [Fr. *massif*] Bulky; consisting of a large mass; huge.

**massive collapse of the lung** Collapse due to obstruction of a main bronchus by a mucous plug, foreign body, or a tension pneumothorax. SEE: *lung; pneumothorax*.

SYMPTOMS: Dyspnea, cyanosis, shock, and pain in chest, esp. in patients who have suffered severe shock and collapse after abdominal operation or thyroidectomy.

TREATMENT: If caused by mucus, therapy consists of carbon dioxide inhalation, breathing exercises, antibiotics, and oxygen. If due to foreign body, the treatment is removal of the foreign body.

**mass number** SEE: under *number*.

**mass psychogenic illness** The occurrence of psychogenic illnesses in a related group of people over a short period of time. Historical sources described tarantism, the dancing mania reported in Italy in the 15th to 17th centuries, and dancing mania in Germany and the Netherlands. The condition is poorly understood but somatic complaints (e.g., headache, dizziness, nausea, dry mucous membranes, sleepiness, weakness, numbness, and chest tightness) are frequently reported. SYN: *mass hysteria*. SEE: *hysteria, epidemic; mass sociogenic illness*.

**mass sociogenic illness** ABBR: MSI. An unexplained, self-limiting illness characterized by onset of a group of symptoms in persons in a social setting such as a school, work place, church, or military group. The onset is usually rapid and may include dizziness, weakness, headache, abdominal pain, rash, itching, blurred vision, nausea and vomiting, and fainting. There are no laboratory studies to confirm an etiologic agent. Resolution of the mass illness occurs when those affected are reassured that it is not due to a toxic substance or disease. SEE: *mass psychogenic illness*.

**MAST** *medical antishock trousers; military antishock trousers*. SEE: *anti-G suit*.

**mastadenitis** (măst-ăd-ĕ-nī′tĭs) [Gr. *mastos*, breast, + *aden*, gland, + *itis*, inflammation] A mammary gland inflammation.

**mastadenoma** (măst″ă-dĕ-nō′mă) [″ + ″ + *oma*, tumor] A tumor of the breast.

**mastalgia** (măst-ăl′jē-ă) [″ + *algos*, pain] Pain in the breast. SYN: *mammalgia; mastodynia*.

**mastatrophia, mastatrophy** (măst-ă-trō′fē-ă, măst-ăt′rō-fē) [″ + *atrophia*, want of nourishment] Atrophy of breasts.

**mast cell** [Gr. *masten*, to feed] A large tissue cell resembling basophil that does not circulate in the blood. It contains hydrolytic enzymes, 5-hydroxytryptamine, and serotonin, which basophils do not. Mast cells are present around blood vessels of the skin and in bone marrow. They can be stimulated by factors derived from microorganisms to produce histamine, arachidonic metabolites, and proteinase. They are also important in producing the signs and symptoms of immediate hypersensitivity reactions (e.g., drug anaphylaxis, urticaria, insect stings, allergic reactions, and certain forms of asthma). SEE: illus.

**mastectomy** (măs-tĕk′tō-mē) [Gr. *mastos*,

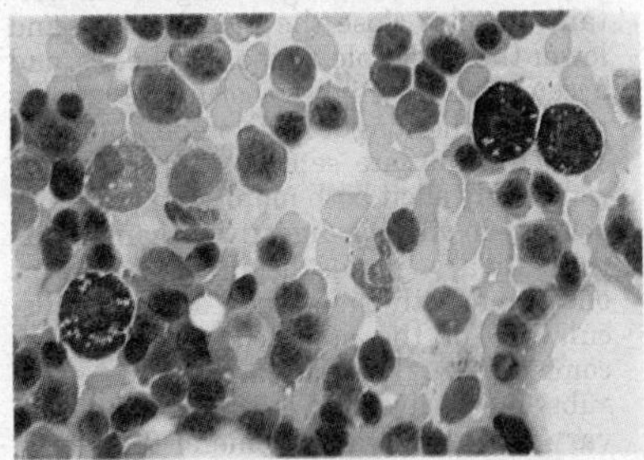

THREE **MAST CELLS** (DARK) IN BONE MARROW (ORIG. MAG. ×640)

breast, + *ektome,* excision] Excision of the breast. SEE: *Nursing Diagnoses Appendix.*

NURSING IMPLICATIONS: The nurse provides emotional support for the woman undergoing diagnostic studies and encourages discussion of treatment options. Vital signs and the quantity and character of wound drainage are monitored. The patient is positioned with affected arm elevated on a pillow until the drain is removed, and active and passive exercise of the arm is encouraged to prevent joint contracture and muscle shortening. Prescribed pain medication is provided as ordered. Support is provided to help the patient and family to cope with the diagnosis and subsequent grief response and to adjust to changes in body image and self-concept. The patient is taught protective measures for lymphedema and offered information about breast prostheses and reconstructive surgery.

***radical m.*** Treatment of breast cancer in which the breast, involved skin, pectoral muscles, axillary lymph nodes, and subcutaneous fat are removed. SEE: *lumpectomy.*

***simple m.*** Treatment of breast cancer in which the breast, nipple, areola, and the involved overlying skin is removed. SEE: *lumpectomy.*

**Master two-step test** [Arthur Matthew Master, U.S. physician, 1895–1973] A standardized exercise test used to assess cardiac function. The patient repeatedly walks up and down two steps 9 in. high. The electrocardiogram is monitored during the study, and the exercise is stopped if abnormal changes appear. Though useful, the test has been replaced with use of a treadmill. SEE: *exercise tolerance test.*

**masthelcosis** (măs″thĕl-kō′sĭs) [Gr. *mastos,* breast, + *helkosis,* ulceration] Ulceration of the breast.

**mastic** (măs′tĭk) A resin obtained from the tree *Pistacia lentiscus.* It has been used in industry and in coating tablets.

**mastication** (măs-tĭ-kā′shŭn) [L. *masticare,* to chew] Chewing. The physical breaking up of food and mixing with saliva in the mouth is the first stage of digestion. Certain muscles close the mouth, raise and lower the mandible, tense the cheeks, and accomplish the highly coordinated movements of the tongue. The smell and taste of food stimulate sensory nerves, which reflexively elicit both motor and secretory activity in various digestive organs. Thus the salivary glands begin to secrete at once, and both the glands and the musculature of the stomach gradually become active. The saliva dissolves some substances, hydrolyzes (due to the salivary enzyme ptyalin) some of the starch to maltose, and lubricates material to be swallowed. **masticatory** (măs′tĭk-ă-tō″rē), *adj.*

**Mastigophora** (măs″tĭ-gŏf′ō-ră) Formerly a division of protozoa characterized by one or more flagella. Now called Zoomastigophora, a phylum of the kingdom Protista.

**mastigote** (măs′tĭ-gōt) A member of the protozoon group formerly called Mastigophora.

**mastitis** (măs-tī′tĭs) [Gr. *mastos,* breast, + *itis,* inflammation] Inflammation of the breast. This condition is most common in women during breastfeeding in the second or third postpartum week; however, it may occur at any age. SEE: *Nursing Diagnoses Appendix.*

SYMPTOMS: The earliest sign is a triangular flush generally underneath the breast. There may be a high temperature and pulse rate.

ETIOLOGY: May be due to entry of disease-producing germs through the nipple. In most cases there is a crack or abrasion of the nipple. Infection begins in one lobule but may extend to other areas.

TREATMENT: Local therapy includes application of local heat and appropriate antibiotics. Beta-lactamase stable penicillin is used if the infection is due to *Staphylococcus aureus.* If an abscess forms, incision and drainage will be necessary.

NURSING IMPLICATIONS: The importance of personal hygiene and general care of the breast is emphasized for breast-feeding mothers. Mothers are encouraged to get adequate rest and take copious fluids.

***cystic m.*** Mastitis resulting in formation of cysts that give the breast a nodular feeling upon palpation.

***interstitial m.*** Inflammation of connective tissue of the breast.

***parenchymatous m.*** Inflammation of the secreting tissue of the breast.

***puerperal m.*** Mastitis, often accompanied by suppuration, occurring in the later portion of puerperium. Breast may become indurated due to retention of milk.

***stagnation m.*** Painful distention of breast occurring during early lactation. SYN: *caked breast.*

**mastocarcinoma** (măst″ō-kăr-sĭn-ō′mă) [″ + *karkinos,* crab, + *oma,* tumor] Carcinoma of the breast.

**mastochondroma** (măst″ō-kŏn-drō′mă) [″ + *chondros,* cartilage, + *oma,* tumor] Cartilaginous breast tumor.

**mastocyte** (măs′tō-sīt) [Gr. *masten,* to feed, + *kytos,* cell] Mast cell.

**mastocytoma** (măs″tō-sī-tō′mă) [″ + ″ + *oma,* tumor] An accumulation of mast cells that resembles a neoplasm.

**mastocytosis** (măs″tō-sī-tō′sĭs) [″ + ″ + *osis,* condition] A general term for a variety of rare disorders in which there is proliferation of mast cells systemically and in the skin. Lesions present on the skin are termed urticaria pigmentosa. Firm stroking of the skin lesion will cause the area to become raised and pruritic with surrounding erythema; this is Darier's sign.

In addition to the skin manifestations, systemic mastocytosis is marked by infiltration of mast cells into the bone marrow, abdominal organs, and lymph nodes. Many of the signs and symptoms of this illness are due to the mast cells releasing granules containing histamine, prostaglandins, and arachidonic metabolites.

**mastodynia** (măst-ō-dĭn'ē-ă) [Gr. *mastos,* breast, + *odyne,* pain] Pain in the breast. SYN: *mammalgia; mastalgia.*

**mastography** [" + *graphein,* to write] Roentgenography of the breasts.

**mastoid** (măs'toyd) [" + *eidos,* form, shape] **1.** Shaped like a breast. **2.** The mastoid process of temporal bone. **3.** Pert. to mastoid process. **mastoidal** (măs-toy'dăl), *adj.*

**mastoidale** (măs-toy-dā'lē) The lowest point of the mastoid process.

**mastoidalgia** (măs-toyd-ăl'jē-ă) [Gr. *mastos,* breast, + *eidos,* form, shape, + *algos,* pain] Pain in the mastoid.

**mastoid antrum** SEE: under *antrum.*

**mastoid cells** SEE: under *cell.*

**mastoidectomy** [" + " + *ektome,* excision] Excision of mastoid cells. Rarely indicated since advent of antibiotics. May be simple, involving exenteration of the air cells of the mastoid process alone, or radical, involving the middle ear. SEE: *Nursing Diagnoses Appendix.*

NURSING IMPLICATIONS: Wound dressing is inspected at frequent intervals and reinforced as necessary. Aseptic technique is used during dressing changes. The nurse observes for bright red blood, neck stiffness, vomiting, dizziness, disorientation, headache, and facial paralysis. If any of these symptoms occur, the physician is notified immediately. Deafness will occur in the affected ear if the ossicles were removed during surgery.

**mastoideocentesis** (măs-toyd"ē-ō-sĕn-tē'sĭs) [" + " + *kentesis,* puncture] Surgical puncture of the mastoid process and subsequent paracentesis of mastoid cells.

**mastoiditis** (măs-toyd-ī'tĭs) [" + " + *itis,* inflammation] Inflammation of the air cells of the mastoid process.

SYMPTOMS: Fever, chills, tenderness over emissary vein, leukocytosis, sepsis.

TREATMENT: Surgical. Myringotomy and antibiotics, mastoidectomy.

COMPLICATIONS: Complications include perisinuous abscess, periphlebitis, and lateral sinus thrombosis. Involvement is metastatic through blood vessels without erosion of the sinus plate or extension of suppuration directly through the sinus plate into the sinus. Injury to the facial nerve is also possible.

***Bezold's m.*** Abscess underneath insertion of sternocleidomastoid muscle due to pus breaking through the mastoid tip.

***m. externa*** Inflammation of the periosteum of the mastoid process.

***sclerosing m.*** Mastoiditis in which there is thickening and hardening of trabeculae between mastoid cells.

**mastoidotomy** (măs-toyd-ŏt'ō-mē) [" + " + *tome,* incision] Incision into the mastoid process.

**mastoid portion of temporal bone** Portion of the temporal bone lying behind the external opening of the ear and below the temporal line and containing mastoid cells and antrum. Its inner surface bears a deep, curved, sigmoid groove that contains a part of the transverse sinus in which the opening of the mastoid foramen is visible.

**mastoid process** Nipple-shaped process of mastoid portion of temporal bone extending downward and forward behind the external auditory meatus. It serves for attachment of sternocleidomastoid, splenius capitis, and longissimus capitis muscles.

**mastology** (măs-tŏl'ō-jē) [" + *logos,* word, reason] The branch of medicine concerned with study of the breast.

**mastomenia** (măs-tō-mē'nē-ă) [" + *menes,* menses] Vicarious menstruation from the breast.

**mastoncus** (măst-ŏng'kŭs) [" + *onkos,* bulk] Any tumor of the breast.

**masto-occipital** (măs"tō-ŏk-sĭp'ĭ-tăl) Relating to the mastoid process and occipital bone.

**mastoparietal** (măs"tō-pă-rī'ĕ-tăl) Concerning the mastoid process and the parietal bone.

**mastopathy** (măs-tŏp'ă-thē) [Gr. *mastos,* breast, + *pathos,* disease] Any disease of the mammary glands.

**mastopexy** (măs'tō-pĕks-ē) [" + *pexis,* fixation] Correction of a pendulous breast by surgical fixation and plastic surgery. SYN: *mazopexy.*

**mastoplasia** (măst-ō-plā'zē-ă) [" + *plassein,* to form] Degenerative hyperplasia of mammary gland tissue. SYN: *mazoplasia.*

**mastoplasty** (măs'tō-plăs"tē) [" + *plassein,* to form] Plastic surgery of the breast.

**mastoptosis** (măs"tō-tō'sĭs) [" + *ptosis,* a dropping] Pendulous breasts.

**mastorrhagia** (măs-tor-ā'jē-ă) [" + *rhegnynai,* to burst forth] Hemorrhage from the breast.

**mastoscirrhus** (măs-tō-skĭr'ŭs) [" + *skirros,* hardness] Hardening of the breast.

**mastosquamous** (măs-tō-skwā'mŭs) Relating to the mastoid process and the squamous portion of the temporal bone.

**mastostomy** (măs-tŏs'tō-mē) [" + *stoma,* mouth] Incision into the breast in order to drain a cyst or obtain tissue for microscopic study.

**mastotomy** (măs-tŏt'ō-mē) Surgical incision of a breast. SYN: *mammotomy.*

**masturbate** (măs'tĕr-bāt) [L. *masturbari,* fr. *manus,* hand, + *stuprare,* to defile] To practice masturbation.

**masturbation** (măs"tĕr-bā'shŭn) Stimulation of genitals or other erogenous areas, usually to orgasm, by some means other than sexual intercourse.

At one time practicing masturbation was believed to cause a great variety of mental and physical disorders. There is no scientific basis for such beliefs. Reports that masturbation is practiced by an increasing number of persons of all ages and of both sexes probably reflect a fear of contracting AIDS from casual sexual contact. SEE: *AIDS; safe sex.*

**match** [ME. *macche,* lamp wick] A narrow strip of wood tipped with a compound that ignites by friction. Lucifer matches usually are made of phosphorus and potassium chlorate. Safety matches contain antimony, sulfide, and potassium chlorate and must be lit by striking a rough surface.

**matching 1.** Comparison in order to select objects or persons with similar characteristics. **2.** Being identical, equal, or exactly alike.

***m. of blood*** Technique and procedure for determining the immunologic and genetic characteristics of the patient's blood so that appropriate blood may be used for transfusion. SEE: *blood groups.*

***cross-m.*** Technique of determining the compatibility of the patient's blood with that of blood being considered for use in transfusion. SEE: *blood groups.*

**match poisoning** Gastrointestinal irritation caused by ingesting or sucking on the heads of matches.

FIRST AID: The stomach should be washed out with water or very dilute potassium permanganate. Repeated catharsis should be done. SEE: *phosphorus poisoning.*

**maté** (mă-tā′) [Sp., vessel for preparing leaves] Tea made from the leaves of *Ilex paraguayensis.* Contains caffeine and tannin.

USES: Diaphoretic and diuretic when taken in large quantities.

**mater** (mā′tŭr) [L., mother] The tissue coverings of the brain and spinal cord. SYN: *meninges.*

***dura m.*** SEE: *dura mater.*

***pia m.*** SEE: *pia mater.*

**materia alba** (mă-tē′rē-ă ăl′bă) [L., white matter] White cheeselike deposit along gum line about the necks of teeth, consisting of mucus, epithelial cells, food particles, leukocytes, and microorganisms.

**material** The substance from which something may be made, constructed, or created.

***base m.*** The basic ingredient in a denture. It may be a polymer, shellac, or metal.

***impression m.*** Any material used to make an impression of teeth.

**material safety data sheet** ABBR: MSDS. Descriptive sheet that accompanies a chemical or a chemical mixture. The sheet provides identity of the material, physical hazard (e.g., flammability), and acute and chronic health hazards associated with contact with or exposure to the compound. It is estimated that there are almost 600,000 hazardous chemical products in American workplaces. SEE: *right to know law.*

**materia medica** (mă-tē′rē-ă mĕd′ĭ-kă) [L., medical matter] **1.** That branch of science dealing with the sources, preparation, dosage, and uses of all drugs used in the treatment of diseases. SYN: *pharmacology.* **2.** A substance used to prepare a medicine.

**maternal** [L. *maternus*] **1.** Relating to the mother. **2.** From a mother.

**maternal deprivation syndrome** Emotional, physical, and nutritional neglect of an infant or young child as a result of the premature loss or absence of the mother. Children suffering from this syndrome are emotionally disturbed, withdrawn, apathetic, and retarded in growth and development.

**maternal mortality rate** SEE: under *rate.*

**maternity** (mă-tĕr′nĭ-tē) **1.** Motherhood. **2.** The obstetrical department of a hospital.

**mating** [ME. *mate,* companion] Pairing of male and female, esp. for reproduction.

***assortative m.*** Pairing of male and female that is controlled in some manner.

***random m.*** Pairing of male to female when each individual has the same chance of mating with those of other genetic make-up.

**matricide** [L. *mater,* mother, + *caedere,* to kill] Killing one's mother.

**matrilineal** (mā″trĭ-lĭn′ē-ăl) [L. *mater,* mother, + *linea,* line] Concerning descent through the female line.

**matrix** (mā′trĭks) *pl.* **matrices** [L.] **1.** The basic substance from which a thing is made or develops. **2.** The intercellular material of a tissue. **3.** Mold for casting amalgams in dental restoration.

***m. unguis*** Nailbed.

**matrixitis** (mā-trĭks-ī′tĭs) Inflammation of the nailbed. SYN: *onychia.* SEE: *paronychia.*

**matter 1.** Anything that occupies space. May be gaseous, liquid, or solid. **2.** Pus.

***gray m.*** Nerve tissue composed mainly of the cell bodies of neurons rather than their myelinated processes. The term is generally applied to the gray portions of the central nervous system, which include the cerebral cortex, basal ganglia, and nuclei of the brain, and the gray columns of the spinal cord, which form an H-shaped region surrounded by white matter. Sympathetic ganglia and nerves may also be gray. SYN: *substantia grisea.*

***white m.*** The white substance of spinal cord and brain, consisting principally of nerve fibers (myelinated and unmyelinated). SYN: *substantia alba.*

**maturate** (măt′ū-rāt) [L. *maturus,* ripe] **1.** To ripen; to mature. **2.** To suppurate.

**maturation** (măt″ū-rā′shŭn) **1.** Maturing;

ripening, as a graafian follicle. **2.** Suppuration. **3.** The process in the development of germ cells (spermatozoa and ova) occurring in spermatogenesis or oogenesis in which the number of chromosomes is reduced from the diploid number to the haploid number (one half of diploid). Includes two cell divisions. SEE: *oogenesis; spermatogenesis.* **4.** The completion of the mineralization pattern or crystalline structure of calcified tissues.

***enamel m.*** The process of changing from about 30% inorganic mineral in enamel matrix of the teeth to the 96% inorganic content in mature enamel; maturation is accomplished by the ameloblast cells over a long period, with a decrease in water and organic content, and an increase in mineral content and size or density of hydroxyapatite crystals.

**mature** (mă-tūr′) **1.** Fully developed or ripened. **2.** To become fully developed.

**mature minor rule** Regulations in some states that allow the practitioner to treat minors without parental consent if the minor is deemed to be capable of understanding the nature and consequences of the treatment and if the treatment is of benefit to the minor.

**maturity** State of completed growth; fully developed; time when an individual becomes capable of reproducing.

**matutinal** (mă-tū′tĭ-năl) [L. *matutinalis,* morning] Pert. to morning or occurring early in the day, such as morning sickness.

**Maurer's dots** (mow′ĕrz) [Georg Maurer, Ger. physician in Sumatra, b. 1909] Coarse stippling of the red cells seen in malaria, caused by *Plasmodium falciparum.*

**maxilla** [L., jawbone] A paired bone with several processes that forms the skeletal base of most of the upper face, roof of the mouth, sides of the nasal cavity, and floor of the orbit. The alveolar process of the maxilla supports the teeth, which is the basis for calling the maxilla the upper jaw. SEE: *skull* for illus; *skeleton.*

**maxillary** (măk′sĭ-lĕr″ē) Pert. to the upper jaw.

**maxillary sinus** SEE: under *sinus.*

**maxillitis** (măks″ĭl-ī′tĭs) [L. *maxilla,* jawbone, + Gr. *itis,* inflammation] Inflammation of the maxilla.

**maxillodental** (măk-sĭl″ō-dĕn′tăl) [″ + *dens,* tooth] Concerning the maxilla and the teeth it supports.

**maxillofacial** (măks-ĭl″ō-fā′shăl) Pert. to the maxilla and face.

**maxillofacial syndrome** Facial defects resulting from improper ossification of the fetal cartilages in the facial area.

**maxillojugal** (măk-sĭl″ō-jū′găl) Concerning the maxilla and zygomatic bone.

**maxillomandibular** (măk-sĭl″ō-măn-dĭb′ū-lăr) [″ + *mandibula,* lower jawbone] Concerning the maxilla and mandible.

**maxillopalatine** (măk-sĭl″ō-păl′ă-tīn) Concerning the maxilla and palatine bone.

**maxillotomy** (măk″sĭ-lŏt′ō-mē) [″ + Gr. *tome,* incision] Surgical incision of the maxilla.

**maximum** (măks′ĭ-mŭm) *pl.* **maxima** [L. *maximus,* greatest] **1.** The greatest quantity or effect. **2.** Height of a disease. **maximal** (-măl), *adj.*

**maximum allowable concentration** ABBR: MAC. The upper limit of concentration of certain atmospheric contaminants allowed in the workplace.

**maximum breathing capacity** ABBR: MBC. The greatest amount of air that can be breathed in a specified period, usually 30 sec. It is expressed in liters of air per minute.

**maximum permissible dose** SEE: under *dose.*

**May Hegglin anomaly** An autosomal-dominant inherited blood disorder marked by the presence of Dohle bodies in granulocyte leukocytes. Platelets vary in size and may be decreased in number. Purpura and excessive bleeding may occur, although some affected persons are asymptomatic.

**Mayo-Robson's point** [Arthur Mayo-Robson, Brit. surgeon, 1853–1933] A point just above and to right of the umbilicus where pressure causes tenderness in pancreatic disease.

**maze** A labyrinth of communicating paths.

**mazopexy** SEE: *mastopexy.*

**mazoplasia** SEE: *mastoplasia.*

**M.B.** *Bachelor of Medicine.*

**m.b.** Prescription sign meaning L. *misce bene,* mix well.

**MBC** *maximum breathing capacity.*

**MBD** *minimal brain dysfunction; minimal brain damage.*

**M.C.** **1.** *Master of Surgery.* **2.** *Medical Corps.*

**mc** Former abbreviation for *millicurie.*

**McArdle's disease** [Brian McArdle, Brit. pediatrician, b. 1911] One of the glycogen storage diseases (type V) in which there is an abnormal accumulation of glycogen in muscle tissue due to deficiency of myophosphorylase B. Symptoms include pain, fatigability, and muscle stiffness after prolonged exertion.

**McBurney's incision** [Charles McBurney, U.S. surgeon, 1845–1913] Abdominal incision employed in appendectomy. The incision is made parallel to the path of the external oblique muscle, 1 to 2 in. (2.5 to 5.1 cm) away from the anterosuperior spine of the right ilium, through the external oblique to the internal oblique and transversalis, separating their fibers.

**McBurney's point** Point 1 to 2 in. (2.5 to 5.1 cm) above the anterosuperior spine of the ilium, on a line between the ilium and umbilicus, where pressure produces tenderness in acute appendicitis.

**McBurney's sign** Tenderness and rigidity at McBurney's point, probably indicative of appendicitis.

**McCarthy's reflex** [Daniel J. McCarthy,

U.S. neurologist, 1874–1958] Contraction of orbicularis palpebrarum with closure of lids resulting from percussion above the supraorbital nerve.

**McCormac's reflex** Adduction of one leg resulting from percussion of the patellar tendon of the opposite leg.

**McCune-Albright syndrome** Albright's syndrome.

**McDonald's rule** A formula for determining the expected height of the fundus of the pregnant uterus during the second and third trimesters by gestational week. Fundal height in centimeters multiplied by 8/7 equals the gestational age. Comparing assessment findings with the expected normal measurement for gestational week may indicate a need for ultrasound to rule out intrauterine growth retardation, multiple pregnancy, or hydramnios.

**mcg** *microgram.*

**MCH** *mean corpuscular hemoglobin.*

**mc.h.** *millicurie hour.*

**MCHC** *mean corpuscular hemoglobin concentration.*

**μCi** *microcurie.*

**MCi** *megacurie.*

**mCi** *millicurie.*

**McMurray's sign** [Thomas P. McMurray, Brit. orthopedic surgeon, 1887–1949] Production of a pronounced click during manipulation of the tibia with the leg flexed when the meniscus has been injured.

**MCP** *metacarpophalangeal joint.*

**MCS** *multiple chemical sensitivity.*

**MCV** *mean corpuscular volume.*

**M.D.** [L. *Medicinae,* Doctor] *Doctor of Medicine.*

**Md** Symbol for the element mendelevium.

**MDI** *metered-dose inhaler.*

**MDR** *multiple drug resistance.*

**meal** (mēl) [AS. *mael,* measure, meal] **1.** Portion of food eaten at a particular time to satisfy the appetite. **2.** The edible portion of any cereal grain that has been coarsely ground, as in corn meal.

**Meals on Wheels** A government-funded program that provides home-delivered meals to elderly Americans.

**mean** In statistics, the average of the values. SEE: *mean, arithmetic; median.*

***arithmetic m.*** The result obtained by adding all of the values given and dividing by the number of items that were added. SYN: *average; mean.* SEE: *median.*

**measles** (mē'zls) [Dutch *maselen*] A highly communicable disease characterized by fever, general malaise, sneezing, nasal congestion, brassy cough, conjunctivitis, spots on the buccal mucosa (Koplik's spots), and a maculopapular eruption over the entire body caused by the rubeola virus. The occurrence of measles before the age of 6 months is relatively uncommon, because of passively acquired maternal antibodies from the immune mother. SYN: *rubeola.*

An attack of measles almost invariably confers permanent immunity. Active immunization can be produced by administration of measles vaccine, preferably that containing the live attenuated virus, although measles vaccine containing the inactivated virus is available for individuals in whom the live attenuated type is contraindicated. Passive immunization is afforded by administration of gamma globulin. SEE: *Nursing Diagnoses Appendix.*

SYMPTOMS: The onset of symptoms is gradual; symptoms include coryza, rhinitis, drowsiness, loss of appetite, and gradual elevation of temperature for first 2 days, when fever may rise to 101° to 103°F (38.3° to 39.4°C). Koplik's spots appear on the buccal mucosa opposite the molars on the second or third day. Photophobia and cough soon develop, although some recession in the temperature may occur. About the fourth day, fever usually reaches a higher elevation than previously, at times as high as 104° to 106°F (40° to 41.1°C). With this recurrence, the rash appears.

Eruption first appears on the face, first as small maculopapular lesions that increase rapidly in size and coalesce in places, often causing a swollen, mottled appearance. The rash extends to the body and extremities and in some areas may resemble the rash of scarlet fever.

A cough, present at this time, is due to bronchitis produced by the inflammatory condition of the mucous membranes that undoubtedly corresponds to the rash seen on the skin. Ordinarily, the rash lasts 4 to 5 days; as it subsides, the temperature declines. Consequently, 5 days after the appearance of the rash, the temperature should be normal or about normal in uncomplicated cases. Early in the disease, leukopenia, esp. of polymorphonuclear cells, may be present.

COMPLICATIONS: Encephalitis is a grave complication. Of those who develop encephalitis, about one in eight will die, about half will have permanent central nervous system injury, and the remainder will recover completely. Bronchopneumonia is a serious complication of measles. Otitis media, followed by mastoiditis, brain abscess, or even meningitis, is not rare. Cervical adenitis with marked cellulitis sometimes leads to fatal consequences. Tracheitis and laryngeal stenosis, due to edema of glottis, are sometimes seen in the course of measles. Eye complications are not common in measles, although a marked conjunctivitis usually occurs.

DIFFERENTIAL DIAGNOSIS: The differential diagnosis includes scarlet fever and German measles. If the measles patient is observed prior to the appearance of a rash, or sometimes even after a rash has developed, a diagnosis may be based on the presence of Koplik's spots.

Hemorrhagic spots are also seen on the hard palate and mucous membrane many times before a rash is evident on the skin. These spots probably correspond to the typical maculopapular eruption of the disease.

INCUBATION: The incubation period ranges from 7 to 18 days, with the average being approx. 10 days.

PROGNOSIS: The prognosis is usually favorable in the well-nourished child, but the seriousness of the possible complications of measles should not be minimized.

PREVENTION: All children who have not had measles or who have not been vaccinated previously should be immunized with live attenuated measles vaccine at 9 months of age and again at or about 15 months. Measles vaccine is often given in conjunction with mumps and/or rubella virus vaccine. SEE: under *vaccine*.

Live attenuated vaccine is contraindicated in pregnancy, leukemia, lymphomas, and other generalized neoplasms; when agents that depress resistance such as steroids and antimetabolites are being given; during severe illness; in active tuberculosis that is not being treated; in individuals with neomycin, duck, or egg sensitivity; and after blood transfusion or injection of immune serum globulin. In these latter two cases, a 12-week waiting period is necessary before administering the vaccine.

Persons who were born after 1956 and are traveling to foreign countries should be vaccinated with live attenuated measles vaccine 1 to 2 weeks prior to departure.

Measles immune serum globulin given for passive protection later than the third day of the incubation period may extend the incubation period instead of preventing measles.

NURSING IMPLICATIONS: The nurse advises immunization of children to prevent measles. Patients who contract the disease remain isolated from diagnosis until 4 days after appearance of the rash. Bedrest, isolation, and a quiet, calm environment are provided. A dimly lit room can help to counteract the effects of photophobia, should it occur. Eye secretions are removed with warm saline or water. The child should avoid rubbing the eyes. Adequate hydration is maintained, and antipyretics and tepid sponge baths are administered as ordered. A cool mist vaporizer is used to relieve cough and coryza. Antipruritic medication is applied as ordered to prevent itching. The parents are taught about the importance of handwashing and care of contaminated articles. The nurse assesses for complications of otitis media, pneumonia, brochiolitis, laryngotracheitis with obstructive edema, and encephalitis.

***black m.*** A severe form of measles in which the eruption is dark due to an effusion of blood into the skin. SYN: *hemorrhagic m.*

***German m.*** Rubella.

**measly** (mē′zlē) Description of pork that is infected with the cysticerci of *Taenia solium* or *saginata*.

**measure** (mĕ′zhūr) [L. *mensura,* a measuring] **1.** The dimensions, capacity, or quantity of anything that can be so evaluated. Length, area, volume, and mass are basic properties of matter and materials that can be measured. **2.** To determine the extent of length, area, mass, or volume of a substance or object. SYN: *mensuration.* **3.** A device used in measuring, for example, a marked tape or a graduated beaker. SEE: *Weights and Measures Appendix.*

**meat** [AS. *mete,* food] The flesh of animals, including poultry, that is used for food.

Meat from animals is a source of vitamins, esp. those of the B complex (thiamine, riboflavin, niacin). Pork is esp. rich in thiamine. Liver has an unusually high vitamin content, esp. of vitamin A. The glandular organs such as liver and kidney contain a considerably higher percentage of certain mineral elements and vitamins than are found in other forms of meat.

Most meats have the same nutritive value but differ greatly in flavor and tenderness. Muscle contains about 20% protein, 20% fat, and 60% water. Lean meat is rich in phosphorus, potassium, and iron; it has a good percentage of other minerals but is deficient in calcium. In all meats, the acid-forming elements are decidedly in excess of those that are base-forming.

Many myths about meat have been repudiated. For instance, one kind of meat is as easily digested as another and tough meat is just as nutritious as tender meat.

**meatometer** (mē-ă-tŏm′ĕt-ĕr) [L. *meatus,* passage, + Gr. *metron,* measure] Device for measuring the size of a passage or opening.

**meatorrhaphy** (mē″ă-tor′ăf-ē) [″ + Gr. *rhaphe,* seam, ridge] Suture of the severed end of the urethra to the glans penis following surgical procedure to enlarge the meatus.

**meatoscope** (mē-ăt′ō-skōp) [″ + Gr. *skopein,* to examine] A speculum for examining a meatus.

**meatoscopy** (mē-ă-tŏs′kō-pē) [″ + Gr. *skopein,* to examine] Instrumental examination of a meatus, esp. the meatus of the urethra.

**meatotome** (mē-ăt′ŏ-tōm) [″ + Gr. *tome,* incision] Knife with probe or guarded point for enlarging a meatus by direct incision.

**meatotomy** (mē″ă-tŏt′ō-mē) Incision of urinary meatus to enlarge the opening.

**meatus** (mē-ā′tŭs) *pl.* **meatus** [L.] A passage or opening. **meatal** (mē-ā′tăl), *adj.*

***m. acusticus externus*** External auditory canal from the eardrum to the external ear.

***m. acusticus internus*** Canal in the petrous portion of temporal bone, through which pass the cochlear and vestibular nerves.

***external auditory m.*** The lateral, outer opening of the external auditory canal.

***internal auditory m.*** The most medial opening of the internal auditory canal, located on the posterior surface of the petrous portion of the temporal bone.

***m. nasi communis*** Common nasal cavity on either side of septum, into which three meatus open.

***m. nasi inferior*** Space beneath inferior turbinate or concha of the nose.

***m. nasi medius*** Space beneath middle turbinate or concha of the nose.

***m. nasi superior*** Space beneath superior turbinate or concha of the nose.

***m. nasopharyngeus*** Posterior portion of nasal cavity, which communicates with the nasopharynx.

***m. urinarius*** External opening of the urethra.

**mebendazole** (mě-běn′dă-zōl) A broad-spectrum antihelmintic. It is used in treating tapeworm infections and is the drug of choice in treating *Ascaris lumbricoides, Trichuris trichuria,* hookworm, and *Strongyloides stercoralis.*

Caution: This drug should not be used during pregnancy.

**mebutamate** (mě-bū′tă-māt) A sedative-hypnotic that also has antihypertensive action.

**mecamylamine hydrochloride** (měk″ă-mĭl′ă-mĭn) An antihypertensive of the ganglionic blocking agent type.

**mechanical rectifier** A device that, by changing contacts at the proper moment in a cycle, changes alternating current into pulsating direct current.

**mechanics** [Gr. *mechane,* machine] The science of force and matter.

***dynamic m.*** The continuous automated analysis of simultaneous measurements of lung variables affecting mechanical ventilation.

**mechanism** **1.** Involuntary and consistent response to a stimulus. **2.** A habit or response pattern formed to achieve a result. **3.** A machine or machinelike structure.

***countercurrent m.*** Mechanism used by the kidneys, making it possible to excrete excess solutes in the urine with little loss of water from the body.

***cycling m.*** The component of a ventilator that ends the inspiratory phase of mechanical ventilation of the lungs.

***defense m.*** SEE: *defense mechanism.*

***Duncan's m.*** Delivery of the placenta from the uterus with the rough side presenting first.

***m. of injury*** The manner by which an injury occurred. The most common type of injuries are due to movement or motion, as in abrasion rapid forward deceleration, rapid vertical deceleration, and projectile penetration.

**mechanoreceptor** (měk″ă-nō-rē-sěp′tor) A receptor that receives mechanical stimuli such as pressure from sound or touch.

**mechanotherapy** (měk″ăn-ō-thěr′ă-pē) [Gr. *mechane,* machine, + *therapeia,* treatment] Use of various types of mechanical apparatus to perform passive movements and to exercise various parts of the body.

**mechlorethamine** (měk″lor-ěth′ă-mēn) A cytotoxic of the nitrogen mustard type.

**Mecholyl test** A test of parasympathetic nervous system function. A 2% solution of methacholine (Mecholyl) is instilled in the conjunctival sac. The pupil constricts if the patient has a parasympathetic disorder, such as familial dysautonomia.

**Meckel, Johann Friedrich (the elder)** (měk′ěl) German anatomist, 1724–1774.

***M.'s ganglion*** Ganglion located in the sphenomaxillary fossa giving off nerves to eyes, nose, and palate. SYN: *sphenopalatine ganglion.*

***M.'s space*** Area in dura holding the gasserian (trigeminale) ganglion.

**Meckel, Johann Friedrich (the younger)** (měk′ěl) German anatomist, 1781–1833, grandson of J. F. Meckel, the elder.

***M.'s cartilage*** A cartilaginous bar about which the mandible develops.

***M.'s diverticulum*** A congenital sac or blind pouch sometimes found in lower portion of the ileum. It represents the persistent proximal end of the yolk stalk. Sometimes it is continued to the umbilicus as a cord or as a tube forming a fistulous opening at the umbilicus. Strangulation may cause intestinal obstruction. SEE: *diverticulitis.*

**meckelectomy** (měk-ěl-ěk′tō-mē) Excision of Meckel's ganglion.

**meclizine hydrochloride** (měk′lĭ-zēn) Antiemetic esp. effective for control of nausea and vomiting of motion sickness.

**meclocycline sulfosalicylate** An antibacterial used topically.

**meconium** (mě-kō′nē-ŭm) [Gr. *mekonion,* poppy juice] **1.** Opium; poppy juice. **2.** First feces of a newborn infant, made up of salts, liquor amnii, mucus, bile and epithelial cells. This substance is greenish black, almost odorless, and tarry. The first meconium stool should appear during the first 24 hr. Meconium should persist for about 3 days.

**meconium aspiration syndrome** ABBR: MAS. The aspiration of meconium by the newborn prior to delivery. The presence of meconium in the trachea or a chest x-ray consistent with the appearance of aspirated meconium with overdistention of the chest establishes the diagnosis. SEE: *meconium.*

TREATMENT: At time of birth, remove pharyngeal and tracheal meconium by use of gentle suction; assisted pulmonary ventilation as needed.

**meconium ileus** Ileus due to impacted meconium in the intestines. It is usually associated with newborn children with cystic fibrosis.

**meconium staining, meconium show** Fetal defecation while in utero at time of labor that occurs with fetal distress. It is composed of thick, mucous-pasty material that must be suctioned before newborn takes first breath or the material may be aspirated.

**M.E.D.** *minimal effective dose; minimal erythema dose.*

**medi-** [L.] Prefix indicating *middle.*

**media** (mē′dē-ă) [L.] **1.** Pl. of medium. **2.** The middle or muscular layer of an artery or vein. SYN: *tunica media.*

**mediad** (mē′dē-ăd) [L. *medium,* middle, + *ad,* toward] Toward the median line or plane of the body.

**medial** [L. *medialis*] **1.** Pert. to middle. **2.** Nearer the medial plane.

**medialis** (mē″dē-ā′lĭs) [L.] Term indicating something is close to the midline of the body.

**medial tibial syndrome** Shinsplints.

**median** (mē′dē-ăn) [L. *medianus*] **1.** Middle; central. **2.** In statistics, a number obtained by arranging the given series in order of magnitude and taking the middle number; one then has an equal number of values above and below that number. Thus, in the series 5, 7, 8, 9, 10, the median is 8. SYN: *mesial.* SEE: *mean.*

**median line** SEE: under *line.*

**median nerve** SEE: under *nerve.*

**median plane** SEE: under *plane.*

**mediastinal** (mē″dē-ăs-tī′năl) [L. *mediastinalis*] Relating to the mediastinum.

**mediastinitis** (mē″dē-ăs″tĭ-nī′tĭs)[″ + Gr. *itis,* inflammation] Inflammation of tissue of the mediastinum.

**mediastinography** (mē″dē-ăs″tĭ-nŏg′ră-fē) [″ + Gr. *graphein,* to write] X-raying of the mediastinum.

**mediastinopericarditis** (mē-dē-ăs″tĭ-nō-pĕr″ĭ-kăr-dī′tĭs) [″ + Gr. *peri,* around, + *kardia,* heart, + *itis,* inflammation] Inflammatory condition of the mediastinum and pericardium.

**mediastinoscopy** (mē″dē-ăs″tĭ-nŏs′kō-pē) [″ + *skopein,* to examine] Endoscopic examination of the mediastinum.

**mediastinotomy** (mē″dē-ăs″tĭ-nŏt′ō-mē) [″ + *tome,* incision] Surgical incision of the mediastinum.

**mediastinum** (mē″dē-ăs-tī′nŭm) *pl.* **mediastina** [L., in the middle] **1.** A septum or cavity between two principal portions of an organ. **2.** The mass of organs and tissues separating the lungs. It contains the heart and its large vessels, trachea, esophagus, thymus, lymph nodes, and connective tissue.

***m. testis*** The thickened portion of the tunica albuginea on posterior surface of the testis. SYN: *corpus highmorianum.*

**mediate** (mē′dē-āt) **1.** Accomplished by indirect means. **2.** Between two parts or sides.

**mediation** (mē″dē-ā′shŭn) The action of a mediating agent.

**mediator** (mē′dē-ā″tŏr) **1.** That which acts to mediate. The mediator may be a person, a nerve, a chemical substance, or a cellular substance. **2.** A neutral third party who facilitates agreements by helping both sides to identify their needs and work toward agreeable solutions.

**medic 1.** Medical corpsman. SEE: *corpsman.* **2.** Slang for paramedic.

**medicable** (mĕd′ĭ-kă-bl) [L. *medicari,* to heal] Possibly responsive to therapy; curable.

**Medicaid** In the U.S., a government program for providing medical care for those who are unable to afford it. The program is jointly funded by the federal and state governments.

**medical** (mĕd′ĭ-kăl) **1.** Pert. to medicine or the study of the art and science of caring for those who are ill. **2.** Requiring therapy with medicines as distinct from surgical treatment.

**medical access** The right or ability of an individual to obtain medical and health care services.

**medical assistant** An individual who assists a qualified physician in an office or other clinical setting, performing administrative tasks (such as those of secretary, receptionist, or bookkeeper) and technical duties (vital signs, height, weight, laboratory tests) as delegated and in accordance with state laws governing medical practice.

**medical audit** A systematic approach to reviewing, analyzing, and evaluating medical care in order to identify discrepancies in the quality of care and to provide a mechanism for improving that quality. SEE: *medical outcomes study.*

**medical corpsman** SEE: *corpsman.*

**medical device** Any article or health care product intended for use in the diagnosis of disease or other condition or for use in the care, treatment, or prevention of disease. The article does not achieve any primary intended purpose by chemical action or by being metabolized. Examples include crutches, wheelchairs, electrodes, pacemakers, catheters, intraocular lenses, and catamenial products.

**Medic Alert** A nonprofit organization that provides a bracelet or pendant with an emblem on which is contained information and a warning in case of emergency. The company also keeps a file of the medical information and provides an emergency phone number that medical personnel can call collect. The purpose is the prevention of a serious or fatal mistake in rendering aid or medical care to an injured or unconscious person who may have an additional condition or allergy (e.g., diabetes, penicillin allergy). Applications may be obtained from Medic Alert, P.O. Box 1009, Turlock, CA 95381. Persons wishing to donate organs may

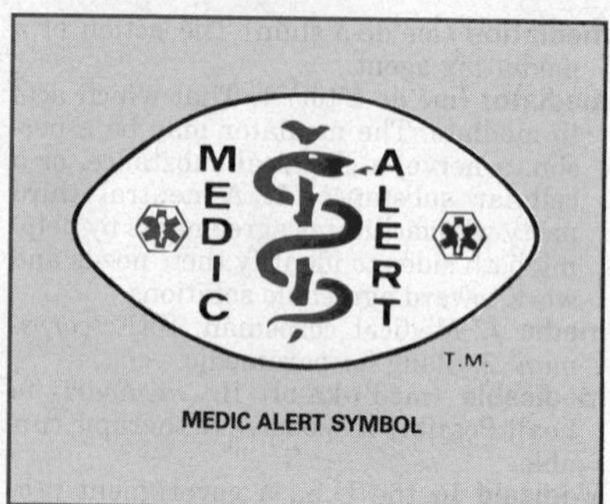

MEDIC ALERT SYMBOL

also acquire an emblem from the Medic Alert company stating that fact. SEE: illus.

**medical examiner** A physician who is trained and qualified for the task of investigating the cause of death and the circumstances surrounding it. Training usually includes study of pathology and forensic medicine. The examiner is empowered by governmental agencies to represent them, and is expected to make a comprehensive report of findings to judicial or police authorities. The skill of a medical examiner is esp. important in investigating deaths wherein malpractice, homicide, suicide, or other criminal actions are suspected of being a contributing factor. SEE: *coroner; death investigation; forensic medicine.*

**medical grand rounds** A medical education procedure, used esp. in teaching hospitals, in which all aspects of a patient's condition, management, and problems encountered are presented to faculty members, medical students, and health care workers. This provides an opportunity for all concerned to ask questions and provide comments on the patient's diagnosis, care, and clinical program. The patient is usually, but not always, present during the conference. This method of teaching was begun in America by Sir William Osler at Johns Hopkins Hospital, Baltimore, Maryland. SEE: *clinicopathological conference.*

**medical history** SEE: under *history.*

**medical informatics** The application of information technology and processing to all aspects of medical knowledge, practice, and management, including medical education and research. This process is facilitated by computer technology.

**medical jurisprudence** SEE: *jurisprudence, medical.*

**medical outcomes study** ABBR: MOS. Studies designed to provide valid comparisons between medical care processes and outcomes as they are affected by system of care and clinician's specialty, as well as by patients' diagnoses and the levels of severity of illness. Thus, MOS provides a model for monitoring the results of medical care. SEE: *medical audit.*

**medical preparations** Medicinal substance prepared or made ready for use.

SOLID SUBSTANCES: Capsule or capsula, confection, extract, lozenge, lamella, ointment, plaster, powder or pulvis, pill or pilula, paper, suppository or suppositorium, tablet or tabella.

FLUIDS: Fluidextract, tincture infusion, decoction, wine, oleoresin.

SUSPENSIONS: Mixture, emulsion.

SOLUTIONS: Water, mucilage, solution or liquor, elixir, syrup, spirit, glycerite, vinegar.

MISCELLANEOUS: Liniment or linimentum, oleate or oleatum.

**medical problems of musicians** SEE: *musicians, medical problems of.*

**medical record** A written transcript of information obtained from a patient, guardian, or medical professionals concerning a patient's health history, diagnostic tests, diagnoses, treatment, and prognosis.

**medical record, problem-oriented** SEE: *problem-oriented medical record.*

**medical transcriptionist** A person who makes a typed record from the data and information available from the physician's dictated material concerning the patient's medical records. An individual who has met the requirements of the American Association of Medical Transcription is certified by that body as a Certified Medical Transcriptionist.

**medical waste** Infectious or physically dangerous medical or biological waste. Included are discarded blood and blood products; waste from pathology department, including body parts, tissues, or fluids discarded during surgery or at autopsy; contaminated animal carcasses; animal body parts and bedding; sharps; discarded preparations made from genetically altered living organisms and their products. SEE: *sharps; Universal Precautions Appendix.*

**medicament** [L. *medicamentum*] A medicine or remedy.

**medicamentosus** (mĕd″ĭ-kă-mĕn-tō′sŭs) Concerning drugs.

**Medicare** In the U.S. a federal program of medical and hospital care for the elderly. In Canada, the system of national health insurance operates under the jurisdiction of the provinces and provides for coverage of 100% of qualified residents. Medical and hospital services covered by the provincial health insurance plans must guarantee reasonable access.

**medicate** (mĕd′ĭ-kāt) [L. *medicatus*] **1.** To treat a disease with drugs. **2.** To permeate with medicinal substances.

**medication** (mĕd-ĭ-kā′shŭn) **1.** Medicinal substance. **2.** Treatment with remedies. **3.** Impregnation with medicine.

***hypodermic m.*** Treatment by injection of medicine into the body through the skin, using a syringe and needle.

***intravenous m.*** The injection of a sterile solution of a drug or an infusion into a vein.

***ionic m.*** Introduction of ions of drugs into body tissues through the skin by means of electricity. SEE: *cataphoresis; iontophoresis* (2).

***sublingual m.*** Treatment with an agent, usually in tablet form, placed under the tongue.

***substitutive m.*** Medical therapy to cause a nonspecific inflammation to counteract a specific one.

**medication errors** Administering the wrong medicine, administering an incorrect dose of a medicine, failing to administer a prescribed medicine, or administering the medicine either at the incorrect time or via the incorrect route. Every effort should be made to prevent errors in medication. It is essential that the nurse, physician, and pharmacist cooperate and communicate concerning medication. In addition, the following will help to avoid errors: Administer no drug without an order; identify drug and amount in each dose unit; be certain that the name of the medicine ordered is spelled precisely as that on the label—if in doubt, do not administer until the question is resolved; do not use outdated medicines; if drug appears unusual due to discoloration or precipitation, do not use; administer medicine at the time specified or as close to that time as possible—if there is a delay, document it; identify patient; do not leave medication at bedside; permit patient to self-administer medicines only if permitted by physician's written order; unless authorized by physician, do not use drugs patient brought to hospital; if an alert patient questions the drug's identity or appropriateness for use, recheck the identity of the patient and the drug; if patient refuses medication, document this on chart and notify the physician responsible for the care of the patient at that time.

**medication route** The way that a drug is introduced into the body. The route of administration is chosen according to the speed of absorption desired and the site of action of the medication. Some medications are formulated for a specific route only and must be given in that manner. It is important that medicines be administered as directed by the manufacturer. Various routes of administration used are as follows:

*Oral* and *enteral* administration require that the medication not be destroyed by the environment of the stomach and digestive enzymes. It is too slow if rapid absorption is required, and cannot be used if the patient is vomiting. Rectal administration in the form of liquids or suppositories circumvents this problem in enteral administration.

*Mucosal* routes of administration other than the above include absorption through the nasal mucosa, the buccal mucosa, sublingually, or the bronchioles, the latter usually achieved through inhalation of an aerosol. Vaginal or rectal administration are also mucosal routes of medication.

*Percutaneous* administration is used for iontophoresis or by direct absorption through the skin.

*Parenteral* administration is used when a drug cannot be given by mouth. The speed of absorption varies greatly with the specific route used, which may be subcutaneous, intravenous, intramuscular, intra-arterial, intraperitoneal, intrathecal, intracardiac, or intrasternal.

**medicinal** (mĕ-dĭ′sĭn-ăl) [L. *medicina,* medicine] Pert. to medicine.

**medicinal enema** SEE: under *enema.*

**medicine 1.** A drug or remedy. **2.** The act of maintenance of health, and prevention and treatment of disease and illness. **3.** Treatment of disease by medical, as distinguished from surgical, treatment.

***aerospace m.*** Branch of medicine concerned with the selection of individuals for duty as pilots or crew members for flight and space missions. Includes study of the pathology and physiology of persons and animals who travel in airplanes and spacecraft in the earth's atmosphere and in outer space.

***alternative m.*** SEE: *alternative medicine.*

***clinical m.*** Observation and treatment at the bedside; the practice of medicine in the clinical setting as distinguished from laboratory science.

***community m.*** Medical care directed toward service of the entire population of the community, with emphasis on preventive medicine.

***cookbook m.*** SEE: *cookbook medicine.*

***dental m.*** Branch of medicine concerned with the preservation and treatment of the teeth and other orofacial tissues. It includes preventive measures such as oral hygiene, as well as restorative procedures or prostheses and surgery. The results are widespread, including better nutrition and digestion from restored and balanced occlusion, and improved mental health from the control of oral and dental infections that often are overlooked but jeopardize the success of other medical treatments.

***disaster m.*** Large-scale application of emergency medical services in a community following a natural or man-made catastrophe. The aim is to save lives and restore every survivor to maximum health as promptly as possible. Its success depends on prompt sorting of patients according to their immediate needs and prognosis. SEE: *triage.*

***emergency m.*** Branch of medicine specializing in emergency care of the acutely ill and injured. Board-certified physicians who successfully complete a residency and qualifying examination may use the abbreviation F.A.C.E.P. (Fellow of the American College of Emergency Physicians). SEE: *certified emergency nurse; Emergency Nurses Association; F.A.C.E.P.*

***environmental m.*** Branch of medicine concerned with the effects of the environment (temperature, rainfall, population size, pollution, radiation) on humans.

***experimental m.*** The scientific study of disease or pathological conditions through experimentation on laboratory animals or through clinical research.

***family m.*** Area of medical specialization concerned with providing or supervising the medical care of all members of the family.

***folk m.*** Use of home remedies for treatment of diseases.

***forensic m.*** Medicine in relation to the law; as in autopsy proceedings, or the determination of time or cause of death, or in the determination of sanity. Also, the legal aspects of medical ethics and standards. SYN: *legal m.*

***group m.*** **1.** Practice of medicine by a group of physicians, usually consisting of specialists in various fields who pool their services and share laboratory and roentgenography facilities. Such a group is commonly called a clinic. **2.** Securing of medical services by a group of individuals who, on paying definite sums of money, are entitled to certain medical services or hospitalization in accordance with prearranged rules and regulations.

***high-tech m.*** The recent advances in medical knowledge and technique that have resulted in improved diagnostic, therapeutic, and rehabilitative procedures.

***holistic m.*** The comprehensive and total care of a patient. In this system, the needs of the patient in all areas, such as physical, emotional, social, spiritual, and economic, are considered and cared for. SEE: *holism.*

***industrial m.*** Occupational m.

***internal m.*** Branch of medicine that treats diseases of the internal organs by other than surgical means. In effect, internal medicine is based on experimental work in physiology and physiochemistry and the implication that investigators and practitioners in the specialty have special training, knowledge, and skills.

***legal m.*** Forensic m.

***nuclear m.*** Branch of medicine involved with the use of radioactive substances for diagnosis, therapy, and research.

***occupational m.*** ABBR: OC. Branch of medical specialization in which the object is to investigate, prevent, and treat diseases peculiar to persons whose environment includes their work spaces. It is a form of environmental medicine.

***patent m.*** A drug or medical preparation that is protected by patent and sold without a physician's prescription. The law requires that it be labeled with names of active ingredients, the quantity or proportion of the contents, and directions for its use, and that it not have misleading statements as to curative effects on the label. SEE: *nonproprietary name; prescription; proprietary medicine.*

***physical m.*** Treatment of disease by physical agents such as heat, cold, light, electricity, manipulation, or the use of mechanical devices.

***preclinical m.*** **1.** Preventive medicine. **2.** Term used to indicate the first 2 years of medical school training, during which there is little or no exposure to patients for teaching purposes.

***preventive m.*** SEE: *preventive medicine.*

***proprietary m.*** SEE: *proprietary medicine.*

***psychosomatic m.*** Branch of medicine that recognizes the importance of mind-body interrelationship in all illnesses, on which therapy and management are based.

***socialized m.*** Practice of medicine under control and direction of a government agency. The cost of medical care under this plan is usually financed by levying taxes or through a national medical insurance program.

***sports m.*** Field of medicine concerned with all aspects of physiology, pathology, and psychology as they apply to persons who participate in sports, whether at the recreational, amateur, or professional level. An important facet of sports medicine is the application of medical knowledge to the prevention of injuries in those who participate in sports.

***tropical m.*** Branch of medical science that deals principally with diseases common in tropical or subtropical regions, esp. diseases of parasitic origin.

***veterinary m.*** Branch of medical science that deals with diagnosis and treatment of diseases of animals.

**medicine man** Shaman.

**medicinerea** (mĕd″ĭ-sĭn-ē′rē-a) [L. *medius,* middle, + *cinerea,* ashen] Internal gray matter of the claustrum and lenticula of the brain.

**medicochirurgical** (mĕd″ĭ-kō-kī-rŭr′jĭ-kăl) [L. *medicus,* medical, + Gr. *cheir,* hand, + *ergon,* work] Concerning both medicine and surgery.

**medicolegal** (mĕd″ĭ-kō-lē′găl) [″ + *legalis,* legal] Relating to medical jurisprudence or forensic medicine.

**medicomechanical** (mĕd″ĭ-kō-mĕ-kăn′ĭ-kăl) Concerning both medical and mechanical aspects of treating patients.

**medicopsychology** (mĕd″ĭ-kō-sī-kŏl′ō-jē) The relationship of medicine to the mind or to mental illness.

**medicornu** (mĕd″ĭ-kor′nū) [L. *medius,* middle, + *cornu,* horn] The inferior horn of the lateral ventricle of the brain.

**Medina worm** *Dracunculus medinensis.*

**medio-** [L. *medius,* middle] Prefix meaning *middle.*

**mediocarpal** (mē″dē-ō-kăr′păl) Concerning the middle part of the carpal bone.

**mediolateral** (mē″dē-ō-lăt′ĕr-ăl) Concerning the middle and side of a structure.

**medionecrosis** (mē″dē-ō-nē-krō′sĭs) [″ + *nekrosis,* state of death] Necrosis of the tunica media of a blood vessel.

**mediopontine** (mē″dē-ō-pŏn′tīn) [″ + *pons,* bridge] Relating to the center of the pons varolii.

**mediotarsal** (mē″dē-ō-tăr′săl) Relating to the middle of the tarsus.

**medisect** (mē′dĭ-sĕkt) [″ + *secare,* to cut] To cut on the median line of the body or structure.

**meditation** The art of contemplative thinking.

***transcendental m.*** ABBR: TM. A type of meditation based on ancient Hindu practices in which an individual tries to relax by sitting quietly for regular periods while repeating a mantra. The value of TM in treating various conditions is under investigation. SEE: *relaxation response.*

**Mediterranean fever, familial** A disease originally common in people of the Middle East, but now seen in various parts of the world. This familial disease is characterized by short attacks of fever, signs of peritonitis, pleuritis, and arthritis. In the past, the most frequent cause of death was amyloidosis, which occurred as the disease progressed. The use of prophylactic colchine has greatly reduced the number of attacks and prevents amyloidosis. SYN: *recurrent polyserositis.*

**medium** (mē′dē-ŭm) *pl.* **media 1.** An agent through which an effect is obtained. **2.** Substance used for the cultivation of microorganisms or cellular tissue. SYN: *culture m.* **3.** Substance through which impulses are transmitted.

***clearing m.*** A substance that renders histological specimens transparent.

***culture m.*** A substance on which microorganisms may grow. Those most commonly used are broths, gelatin, and agar, which contain the same basic ingredients.

***defined m.*** In bacteriology, a medium in which the composition is accurately defined and carefully controlled. One use of this culture medium is to investigate the influence of altering ingredients on bacterial cell growth characteristics.

***dispersion m.*** A liquid in which a colloid is dispersed.

***nutrient m.*** A fortified culture medium with added nutrient materials.

***radiolucent m.*** A substance injected into an anatomical structure to decrease the density, producing a dark area on the radiograph.

***radiopaque m.*** A substance injected into a cavity or region or passed through the gastrointestinal tract to increase the density, producing a light area on the radiograph.

***refracting m.*** The fluids and transparent tissues of the eye that refract light rays passing through them toward the retina.

***separating m.*** In dentistry, a substance applied to the surface of an impression or mold to prevent interaction of the materials and to facilitate their separation after casting. SYN: *separating agent.*

**medium-chain triglycerides** SEE: under *triglycerides.*

**medius** (mē′dē-ŭs) [L.] Middle. Indicating the middle one of three similar structures.

**MEDLARS** [*Med*ical *L*iterature *A*nalysis and *R*etrieval *S*ystem] A computerized system of databases and data banks available from the National Library of Medicine. A person may search the computer files to produce a list of publications (bibliographic citations) or retrieve factual information on a specific question. MEDLARS databases cover medicine, nursing, dentistry, veterinary medicine, and the preclinical sciences. They are used by universities, medical schools, hospitals, government agencies, commercial and nonprofit organizations, and private individuals. MEDLARS includes two computer subsystems, ELHILL and TOXNET, comprising more than 40 on-line databases with about 14 million references.

**MEDLINE** [*MED*LARS on *line*] The computer-accessible bibliographic database of the National Library of Medicine. It is the system that links telephone lines to the MEDLARS databases. It includes references that appear in *Index Medicus, Index to Dental Literature,* and the *International Nursing Index.* SEE: *MEDLARS.*

**medrogestone** SEE: *progestin* (2).

**medroxyprogesterone acetate** (mĕd-rŏk″sē-prō-jĕs′tĕr-ōn) A progestational agent. It is used intramuscularly in appropriate dose and is effective for as long as 90 days.

**medrysone** (mĕd′rĭ-sōn) A corticosteroid used in a 1% suspension in ophthalmology.

**medulla** (mĕ-dŭl′lă) *pl.* **medullae** [L.] **1.** The marrow. **2.** Inner or central portion of an organ in contrast to the outer portion or cortex. **medullary** (mĕd′ū-lār-ē), *adj.*

***adrenal m.*** Inner portion of the adrenal gland. It is composed of chromaffin tissue and secretes epinephrine and norepinephrine. SEE: *adrenal gland.*

***m. of hair*** Central axis of a hair.

***m. of kidneys*** SEE: *pyramid, renal.*

***m. nephrica*** SEE: *pyramid, renal.*

***m. oblongata*** The lowest part of the brainstem, continuous with the spinal cord above the level of the foramen magnum of the occipital bone. It regulates heart rate, breathing, blood pressure, and other reflexes, such as coughing, sneezing, swallowing, and vomiting.

***m. ossium*** Marrow in bone.

***m. of ovary*** Central portion of the ovary composed of loose connective tissue, blood vessels, lymphatics, and nerves.

***m. spinalis*** Spinal cord.

**medullated** (mĕd′ū-lāt″ĕd) Covered by or containing marrow; myelinated.

**medullated nerve fiber** SEE: under *nerve fiber*.

**medullation** Acquiring a myelin sheath.

**medullectomy** (mĕd″ū-lĕk′tō-mē) [L. *medulla*, marrow, + Gr. *ektome*, excision] Surgical excision of a part of the medulla of the brain.

**medullitis** (mĕd-ū-lī′tĭs) [″ + Gr. *itis*, inflammation] Inflammation of marrow. SYN: *myelitis*.

**medullization** (mĕd″ū-lī-zā′shŭn) Abnormal conversion to marrow.

**medulloadrenal** (mē-dŭl″ō-ă-drē′năl) [″ + *ad*, to, + *ren*, kidney] Concerning the medulla of the adrenal gland.

**medulloarthritis** (mĕ-dŭl″ō-ăr-thrī′tĭs) [L. *medulla*, marrow, + Gr. *arthron*, joint, + *itis*, inflammation] Inflammation of marrow elements of bone ends.

**medulloblast** (mĕ-dŭl′ō-blăst) [″ + Gr. *blastos*, germ] An immature cell of the neural tube that may develop into either a nerve or neuroglial cell.

**medulloblastoma** (mĕ-dŭl″ō-blās-tō′mă) [″ + Gr. *blastos*, germ, + *oma*, tumor] A soft infiltrating malignant tumor of the roof of the fourth ventricle and cerebellum. The tumor often invades the meninges.

**medulloepithelioma** (mĕ-dŭl″ō-ĕp″ĭ-thēl-ē-ō′mă) [″ + Gr. *epi*, upon, + *thele*, nipple, + *oma*, tumor] Tumor composed of retina epithelium and of neuroepithelium. SYN: *glioma; neuroepithelioma*.

**MedWatch** A voluntary and confidential program of the Food and Drug Administration (FDA) for monitoring the safety of drugs, biologicals, medical devices, and nutritional products such as dietary supplements, medical foods, and infant formulas. The FDA provides forms for reporting adverse events associated with any of these products. Health professionals may obtain the form by calling 1-800-332-1088. Information may be faxed to the FDA by calling 1-800-332-0178.

**Mees lines** [R. A. Mees, 20th century Dutch scientist] Transverse white lines that appear above the lunula of the fingernails about 5 weeks after exposure to arsenic.

**mefenamic acid** An analgesic and antipyretic that also has anti-inflammatory action.

**mega-** [Gr. *megas*, large] **1.** Combining form meaning *of great size* or *large*. SEE: words beginning with *mega-* and *megalo-*. **2.** Indicates 1 million ($10^6$) when used in combination with terms indicating units of measure; thus a megaton is 1 million tons.

**megabladder** (mĕg″ă-blăd′ĕr) [″ + AS. *blaedre*, bladder] Permanent abnormal enlargement of the urinary bladder. SYN: *megalocystis*.

**megacardia** SYN: *cardiomegaly*.

**megacephalic** SEE: *megalocephalic*.

**megacolon** (mĕg-ă-kō′lŏn) [″ + *kolon*, colon] Extremely dilated colon. The condition is usually congenital, but is also known to develop in infancy or childhood. SEE: *Hirschsprung's disease*.

***toxic m.*** A severe complication of ulcerative colitis marked by dilatation of the colon. Because of the possibility of rupture of the colon, which is associated with about a 50% mortality rate, this condition requires immediate therapy. Treatment can include nasogastric suction, intravenous corticosteroid therapy, nothing by mouth, and an appropriate broad-spectrum antibiotic. If no significant improvement is obtained with medical therapy within 48 hr, emergency colectomy should be performed.

**megacurie** (mĕg″ă-kū′rē) [″ + *curie*] ABBR: Mc. A unit of radioactivity equal to $10^6$ curies.

**megadontia** (mĕg″ă-dŏn′shē-ă) [″ + *odous, odont-*, tooth] Possessing very large teeth.

**megadose** A dose of a nutrient, such as a vitamin supplement, that is 10 times greater than the recommended daily allowance for that nutrient.

**megadyne** (mĕg′ă-dīn) A unit equal to 1 million dynes. SEE: *dyne*.

**megaesophagus** (mĕg″ă-ē-sŏf′ă-gŭs) [″ + *oisophagos*, esophagus] A grossly dilated esophagus usually associated with achalasia.

**megahertz** (mĕg′ă-hĕrtz) ABBR: MHz. One million cycles per second, or $10^6$ hertz.

**megakaryoblast** (mĕg″ă-kăr′ē-ō-blăst) An immature megakaryocyte.

**megakaryocyte** (mĕg″ă-kăr′ē-ō-sīt″) [″ + *karyon*, nucleus, + *kytos*, cell] Large bone marrow cell with large or multiple nuclei that gives rise to blood platelets essential for the clotting mechanism of blood. SYN: *giant cell*. SEE: illus.

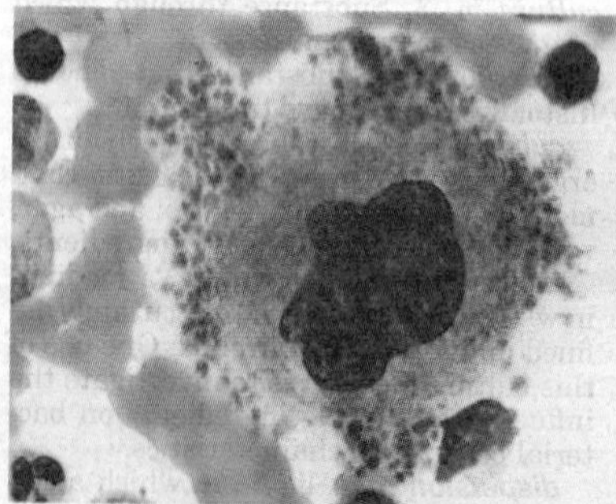

**MEGAKARYOCYTE** IN BONE MARROW FRAGMENTING INTO PLATELETS (ORIG. MAG. ×640)

**megakaryocytosis** (mĕg″ă-kăr″ē-ō-sī-tō′sĭs) [″ + ″ + ″ + *osis*, condition] An increased number of megakaryocytes in the bone marrow; presence of megakaryocytes in the blood.

**megalencephaly** (mĕg″ăl-ĕn-sĕf′ă-lē) [″ + *enkephalos,* brain] Abnormally large size of the brain, usually accompanied by mental deficiency.

**megalo-** [Gr. *megas,* large] Combining form meaning *great* or *large.*

**megaloblast** (mĕg′ă-lō-blăst) [″ + *blastos,* germ] A large, nucleated, abnormal red blood corpuscle, from 11 to 20 μm in diameter, oval and slightly irregular. It is found in the blood in cases of pernicious anemia.

**megalocephalic** (mĕg-ă-lō-sĕf-ăl′ĭk) [″ + *kephale,* head] Having an abnormally large head. SYN: *macrocephalic; megacephalic.*

**megalocephaly** (mĕg″ă-lō-sĕf′ă-lē) [″ + *kephale,* head] **1.** Abnormal size of the head. SYN: *macrocephaly.* **2.** A rare disease characterized by hyperostosis of bones of the skull. SYN: *leontiasis ossea.*

**megalocheiria** (mĕg″ă-lō-kī′rē-ă) [″ + *cheir,* hand] Abnormally large hands.

**megalocornea** (mĕg″ă-lō-kor′nē-ă) [″ + L. *cornu,* horn] Abnormally enlarged cornea due to a developmental anomaly. SYN: *macrocornea.*

**megalocystis** SEE: *megabladder.*

**megalocyte** (mĕg′ă-lō-sīt) [″ + *kytos,* cell] A larger than average red blood corpuscle.

**megalodactyly** (mĕg″ă-lō-dăk′tĭ-lē) [″ + *daktylos,* finger] Having very large fingers or toes.

**megalodontia** (mĕg″ă-lō-dŏn′shē-ă) [″ + *odous,* tooth] Having abnormally large teeth.

**megaloesophagus** SEE: *megaesophagus.*

**megalomania** (mĕg″ă-lō-mā′nē-ă) [″ + *mania,* madness] A psychosis characterized by ideas of personal exaltation and delusions of grandeur.

**megalonychosis** (mĕg′ă-lō″nĭ-kō′sĭs) [″ + *onyx,* nail] Hypertrophy of the nails.

**megalophthalmus** (mĕg″ă-lŏf-thăl′mŭs) [″ + *ophthalmos,* eye] Abnormally large eyes.

**megalopodia** (mĕg″ă-lō-pō′dē-ă) [″ + *pous,* foot] Abnormally large feet.

**megaloscope** (mĕg′ă-lō-skōp″) [″ + *skopein,* to examine] A large magnifying lens; a speculum fitted with a magnifying lens.

**megalosyndactyly** (mĕg′ă-lō-sĭn-dăk′tĭl-ē) [″ + *syn,* with, + *daktylos,* finger] A condition in which the fingers or toes are of large size and webbed.

**megaloureter** (mĕg″ă-lō-ū-rē′tĕr, -ūr′ē-tĕr) [″ + *oureter,* ureter] Increase in diameter of the ureter.

**-megaly** [Gr. *megas,* large] Combining form indicating an enlargement of a specified body part.

**megaprosopia** (mĕg″ă-prŏs′ō-pŭs) [″ + *prosopon,* face] Possessing a large face.

**megarectum** (mĕg-ă-rĕk′tŭm) [″ + L. *rectum,* straight] Excessive dilatation of the rectum.

**megaseme** (mĕg′ă-sēm) [″ + *sema,* sign] Having an orbital aperture with an index exceeding 89, said of a skull.

**megavitamin** (mĕg″ă-vī′tă-mĭn) A dose of one or more vitamins that is much in excess of the normal daily requirements.

**megavolt** (mĕg′ă-vōlt) One million, $10^6$, volts.

**megestrol acetate** (mĕ-jĕs′trōl) A synthetic progestin that is also used in treating certain neoplasms. Trade name is Megace.

**meglumine** (mĕg′lū-mēn) A radiopaque compound used in x-ray studies.

***m. antimonate*** A drug used in treating leishmaniasis.

**megohm** (mĕg′ōm) One million, $10^6$, ohms.

**megophthalmos** SEE: *megalophthalmus.*

**meibomian cyst** (mī-bō′mē-ăn) [Heinrich Meibom, Ger. anatomist, 1638–1700] Chalazion.

**meibomian gland** SEE: *gland, tarsal.*

**meibomitis** (mī-bō″mī′tĭs) Inflammation of the meibomian glands.

**Meigs' syndrome** [Joe V. Meigs, U.S. gynecologist, 1892–1963] Benign tumor of the ovary associated with ascites and pleural effusion.

**meio-** [Gr. *meioun,* diminution] Combining form indicating decrease in size or number. SEE: words beginning with *mio-.*

**meiogenic** (mī″ō-jĕn′ĭk) [Gr. *meiosis,* diminution, + *gennan,* to produce] Causing meiosis.

**meiosis** (mī-ō′sĭs) [Gr., diminution] A process of two successive cell divisions, producing cells, egg or sperm, that contain half the number of chromosomes in somatic cells. When fertilization occurs, the nuclei of the sperm and ovum fuse and produce a zygote with the full chromosome complement. SEE: illus.; *chromosome; mitosis; oogenesis* for illus.

**Meissner's corpuscle** (mīs′nĕrz) [Georg Meissner, Ger. histologist, 1829–1905] An encapsulated end-organ of touch found in dermal papillae close to the epidermis. Each is an ovoid body containing endings of myelinated and unmyelinated nerve fibers. They are most numerous in the hairless portions of the skin, esp. the volar surface of hands, fingers, feet, and toes; they are also present in the lips, eyelids, nipples, and the tip of the tongue.

**Meissner's plexus** An autonomic plexus in the submucosa of the alimentary tube that regulates secretions of the mucosa.

**melagra** (mĕl-ă′gră) [Gr. *melos,* limb, + *agra,* seizure] Pain of muscular origin in the limbs.

**melalgia** (mĕl-ăl′jē-ă) [″ + *algos,* pain] Pain of neural origin in the limbs.

**melancholia** (mĕl-ăn-kō′lē-ă) [Gr. *melankholia,* sadness] A severe depression with a dull, uninterested affect and lack of interest in activities that would normally be pleasurable. There may be agitation or retardation. Weight loss, anorexia, insomnia, and worsening of the symptoms may occur in the early morning.

***affective m.*** Melancholia observed in depressed phase of manic-depressive psychoses. SEE: *psychosis, manic-depressive.*

***climacteric m.*** Melancholia occurring at the time of menopause.

***involutional m.*** A depressive psychosis that occurs during the involutional period (40 to 55 years of age in women; 50 to 65 in men). There is usually no previous history of mental illness. Characteristic symptoms include depression; delusions of sin, guilt, or poverty; an obsession with death; imagined gastrointestinal tract disease; and sometimes delusions of being persecuted. The patient feels agitated and dejected. The condition may be successfully treated with antidepressant drugs or

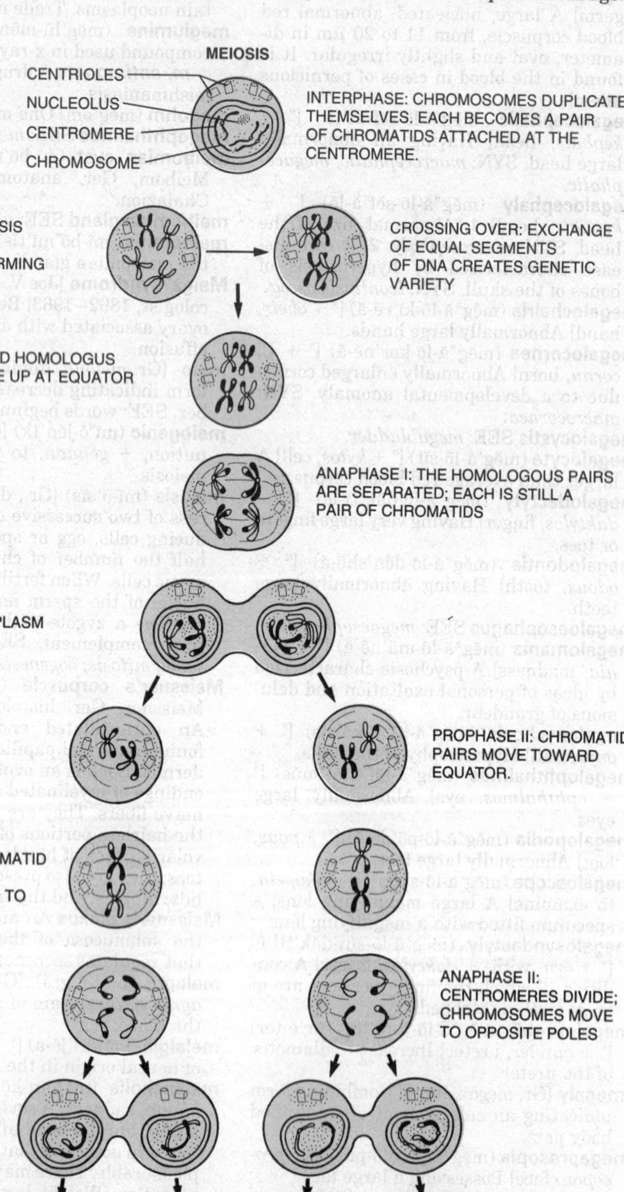

electroconvulsive therapy.

***panphobic m.*** Melancholia characterized by dread of everything.

***suicidal m.*** Impulse to commit suicide combined with melancholia.

**melanephidrosis, melanidrosis** (mĕl″ăn-ĕf″ĭ-drō′sĭs, mĕl″ăn-ĭd-rō′sĭs) [″ + *ephidrosis,* sweating] A form of chromidrosis in which the sweat is black.

**melaniferous** (mĕl″ăn-ĭf′ĕr-ŭs) [″ + L. *ferre,* to carry] Containing melanin or some other black pigment.

**melanin** [Gr. *melas,* black] The pigment produced by melanocytes that gives color to hair, skin, the substantia nigra of the brain, and the choroid of the eye. Exposure to sunlight stimulates melanin production. It can be prepared chemically. It is present in some cancers, such as melanoma. **melanoid** (mĕl′ă-noyd), *adj.*

**melano-** [Gr. *melas,* black] Prefix meaning *black, black color,* or *darkness.*

**melanoameloblastoma** (mĕl″ă-nō-ă-mĕl″ō-blăs-tō′mă) [″ + O. Fr. *amel,* enamel, + Gr. *blastos,* germ, + *oma,* tumor] Melanotic neuroectodermal tumor.

**melanoblast** (mĕl′ăn-ō-blăst″, mĕl-ăn′ō-blăst) [″ + *blastos,* germ] A cell originating from the neural crest that differentiates into a melanocyte.

**melanoblastoma** (mĕl″ă-nō-blăs-tō′mă) [″ + ″ + *oma,* tumor] A tumor containing melanin.

**melanocyte** (mĕl′ăn-ō-sīt, mĕl-ăn′ō-sīt) [″ + *kytos,* cell] A melanin-forming cell. Those of the skin are found in the lower epidermis.

**melanocytoma** (mĕl″ă-nō-sī-tō′mă) [″ + *kytos,* cell, + *oma,* tumor] A rare pigmented benign tumor of the optic disk.

**melanoderma** (mĕl″ăn-ō-dĕr′mă) A patchy or generalized skin discoloration caused by either an increase in the production of melanin by the normal number of melanocytes or an increase in the number of melanocytes. SYN: *melanopathy.*

**melanodermatitis** (mĕl″ă-nō-dĕr″mă-tī′tĭs) [″ + ″ + *itis,* inflammation] Dermatitis in which an excess of melanin is deposited in the involved area.

**melanoepithelioma** (mĕl″ăn-ō-ĕp″ĭ-thē-lē-ō′mă) [″ + *epi,* upon, + *thele,* nipple, + *oma,* tumor] A malignant epithelioma containing melanin.

**melanogen** (mĕ-lăn′ō-jĕn) [″ + *gennan,* to produce] A colorless substance that may be converted into melanin.

**melanogenesis** (mĕl″ăn-ō-jĕn′ĕ-sĭs) [″ + *genesis,* generation, birth] Formation of melanin.

**melanoglossia** (mĕl″ăn-ō-glŏs′ē-ă) [″ + *glossa,* tongue] Black tongue.

**melanoleukoderma** (mĕl″ăn-ō-lū″kō-dĕr′mă) [″ + *leukos,* white, + *derma,* skin] Mottled skin.

***m. colli*** Mottled skin of the neck sometimes seen in syphilis. SYN: *collar of Venus; syphilitic leukoderma; venereal collar.*

**melanoma** (mĕl″ă-nō′mă) [″ + *oma,* tumor] A malignant, darkly pigmented mole or tumor of the skin. The four types of cutaneous melanoma are superficial spreading melanoma, lentigo maligna melanoma, acral lentiginous melanoma, and nodular melanoma. The first three of these tend to grow superficially and expand radially, and do not penetrate deeply. Nodular melanoma is deeply invasive and quite likely to metastasize. Malignant melanoma was the cause of death of 7200 persons in the U.S. in 1995. SEE: illus.

ETIOLOGY: Excessive exposure to the sun, esp. in light-skinned people; however, having dark or black skin is no guarantee of protection against melanoma. Heredity may also be important. The lesion of melanoma is characterized by its asymmetry, irregular border, and lack of uniform color. The diameter is usually greater than 6 mm (about ¼ in.). Also, the

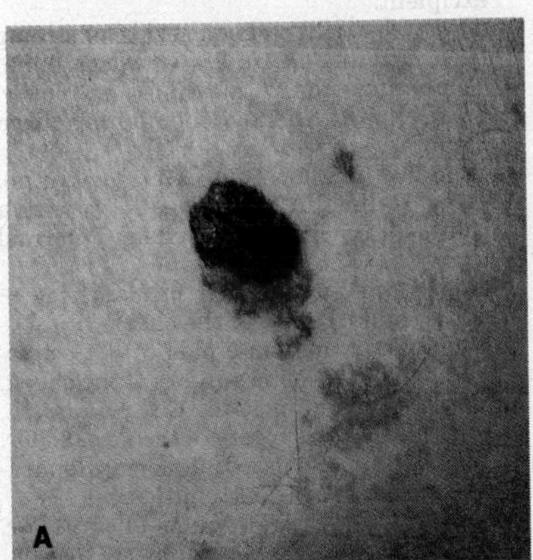


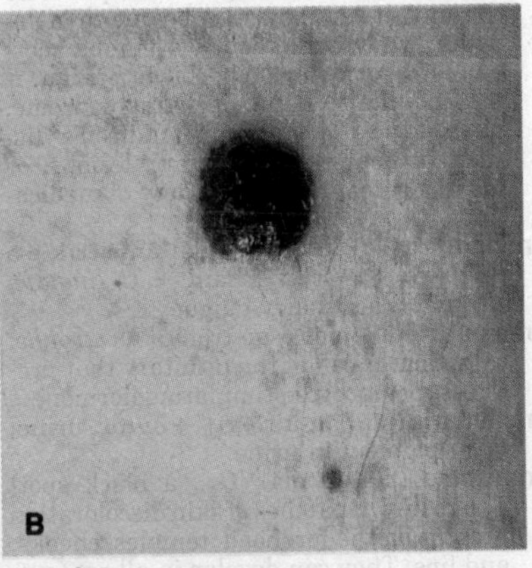


**MELANOMA, (A)** SUPERFICIAL SPREADING AND **(B)** NODULAR

following should be considered as a warning of melanoma: change in surface appearance or size of a mole; scaliness; oozing; bleeding; itchiness, tenderness, or pain.

PREVENTION: Avoid sun or, if exposure is necessary, use sunscreen on exposed areas of skin.

TREATMENT: Early detection is essential for successful treatment by surgical removal.

**melanomatosis** (mĕl″ă-nō″mă-tō′sĭs) [″ + ″ + *osis,* condition] Formation of numerous melanomas on or beneath the skin.

**melanonychia** (mĕl″ă-nō-nĭk′ē-ă) [″ + *onyx,* nail] Black pigmentation of the nails.

**melanopathy** SEE: *melanoderma.*

**melanophage** (mĕl′ă-nō-fāj″) [″ + *phagein,* to eat] A phagocytic cell that contains ingested melanin.

**melanophore** (mĕl′ăn-ō-for) [″ + *phoros,* bearing] Cell containing dark pigment.

**melanoplakia** (mĕl″ăn-ō-plā′kē-ă) [″ + *plax,* a flat plain] Condition marked by pigmented patches on the tongue and buccal mucosa.

**melanosarcoma** (mĕl″ă-nō-săr-kō′mă) [″ + *sarx,* flesh, + *oma,* tumor] Sarcoma containing melanin.

**melanoscirrhus** (mĕl″ă-nō-skĭr′ŭs) [Gr. *melas,* black, + *skirros,* hardness] Black-pigmented cancer; an unusual form of melanoma.

**melanosis** (mĕl-ăn-ō′sĭs) [″ + *osis,* condition] **1.** Unusual deposit of black pigment in different parts of body. **2.** Disorder of pigment metabolism.

***m. lenticularis*** SEE: *xeroderma pigmentosum.*

**melanosome** (mĕl′ă-nō-sōm″) [″ + *soma,* body] The pigment granule produced by melanocytes.

**melanotic 1.** Black. **2.** Pert. to melanosis.

**melanotic macule** A small, brown to black lesion of the oral mucosa that is usually less than 1 cm in diameter, solitary, and asymptomatic. In most instances, this type of macule is benign and requires no therapy. It can, however, be due to melanoma, which will require vigorous therapy without delay. When it is benign, it may be due to Peutz-Jeghers syndrome, physiologic pigmentation, Addison's disease, or healing of traumatic lesions, or may be secondary to a variety of medications.

**melanotrichia linguae** (mĕl″ăn-ō-trĭk′ē-ă lĭng′gwē) [″ + *thrix,* hair, + L. *linguae,* tongue] Black, hairy tongue.

**melanotroph** (mĕl′ă-nō-trōf″) [″ + *trophe,* nutrition] A cell of the pituitary that produces melanocyte-stimulating hormone.

**melanuria** (mĕl-ăn-ū′rē-ă) [″ + *ouron,* urine] Dark pigment in urine.

**melasma** (mĕl-ăz′mă) [Gr., a black spot] Tan to brown patches of skin discoloration present on the forehead, temples, cheeks, and lips. They can develop in all races on sun-exposed areas. While they are usually idiopathic, they may occur in association with pregnancy or use of oral contraceptives. Women are more frequently affected than men. Retinoic acid has been used for treatment. Exposure to the sun should be avoided.

**melatonin** (mel″ă-tō′nĭn) A hormone produced by the pineal gland in mammals. In humans, it may be involved in the onset of puberty and may influence sleep-waking cycles.

**melena** (mĕl′ĕ-nă, mĕl-ē′nă) [Gr. *melaina,* black] Black, tarry feces due to action of intestinal secretions on free blood. Common in the newborn. **melenic, melenotic** (mĕl-ĕ-nŏt′ĭk), *adj.*

***m. neonatorum*** Melena in the newborn.

**melicera, meliceris** (mĕl-ĭ-sēr′ă, -ĭs) [Gr. *meli,* honey, + *keros,* wax] **1.** Cyst containing matter of honey-like consistency. **2.** Viscid, syrupy.

**melioidosis** (mē″lē-oy-dō′sĭs) [Gr. *melis,* a distemper of asses, + *eidos,* form, shape, + *osis,* condition] An acute or chronic disease due to *Pseudomonas pseudomallei* (formerly called *Malleomyces pseudomallei).* Acute form causes pneumonia, multiple abscesses, septicemia, and possibly death.

**melissophobia** (mĕ-lĭs″ō-fō′bē-ă) [Gr. *melissa,* bee, + *phobia,* fear] Abnormal fear of bees.

**melitemia** (mĕl-ĭ-tē′mē-ă) [ + *haima,* blood] Abnormal amount of sugar in the blood.

**melitensis** (mĕl-ĭ-tĕn′sĭs) Undulant fever; brucellosis.

**melitis** (mĕl-ī′tĭs) [Gr. *melon,* cheek, + *itis,* inflammation] Inflammation of the cheek.

**melitoptyalism** (mĕl″ĭ-tō-tī′ăl-ĭzm) [Gr. *meli,* honey, + *ptyalon,* saliva] Excretion of saliva containing glucose. SYN: *glycoptyalism.*

**melituria** (mĕl-ĭ-tū′rē-ă) [″ + *ouron,* urine] Presence of sugar in the urine.

**mellitum** (mĕ-lī′tŭm) [L.] A pharmaceutical preparation with honey as the vehicle or excipient.

**melo-, mel- 1.** [Gr. *melon,* cheek] Combining form meaning *cheek.* **2.** [Gr. *melos,* limb] Combining form meaning *extremity.* **3.** [Gr. *meli,* honey] Combining form meaning *honey.*

**melomelus** (mē-lŏm′ē-lŭs) [Gr. *melos,* limb, + *melos,* limb] A malformed fetus with a rudimentary limb attached to a normal limb.

**meloncus** (mĕl-ŏn′kŭs) [Gr. *melon,* cheek, + *onkos,* bulk] Tumor of the cheek.

**melonoplasty** (mĕl′ŏn-ō-plăs″tē) [″ + *plassein,* to form] Plastic surgery of the cheek.

**meloplasty** (mĕl′ō-plăs-tē) **1.** [″ + *plassein,* to form] Plastic surgery of the face. **2.** [Gr. *melos,* limb, + *plassein,* to form] Reparative surgery of the extremities.

**melorheostosis** (mĕl″ō-rē″ŏs-tō′sĭs) [Gr. *melos,* limb, + *rhein,* to flow, + *osteon,* bone, + *osis,* condition] A rare disease of long bones in which new bone formation resembles a candle with wax dripping down the sides.

**meloschisis** (mĕ-lŏs′kĭ-sĭs) [Gr. *melon,* cheek, + *schistos,* divided] A congenitally cleft cheek.

**melotia** (mĕ-lō′shē-ă) [″ + *ous,* ear] Congenital displacement of the ear on the cheek.

**melphalan** (mĕl′fă-lăn) An antineoplastic drug of the nitrogen mustard class.

**melting point** Temperature at which conversion of a solid to a liquid begins.

**member** [L. *membrum*] An organ or part of the body, esp. a limb.

**membrane** (mĕm′brān) [L. *membrana*] A thin, soft, pliable layer of tissue that lines a tube or cavity, covers an organ or structure, or separates one part from another.

***alveolocapillary m.*** The structures and substances through which gases must pass as they diffuse from air to blood (oxygen) or blood to air (carbon dioxide), including the alveolar fluid and surfactant, cell of the alveolar wall, interstitial space (tissue fluid), and cell of the capillary wall. SEE: illus.

***alveolodental m.*** SEE: *periodontium*.

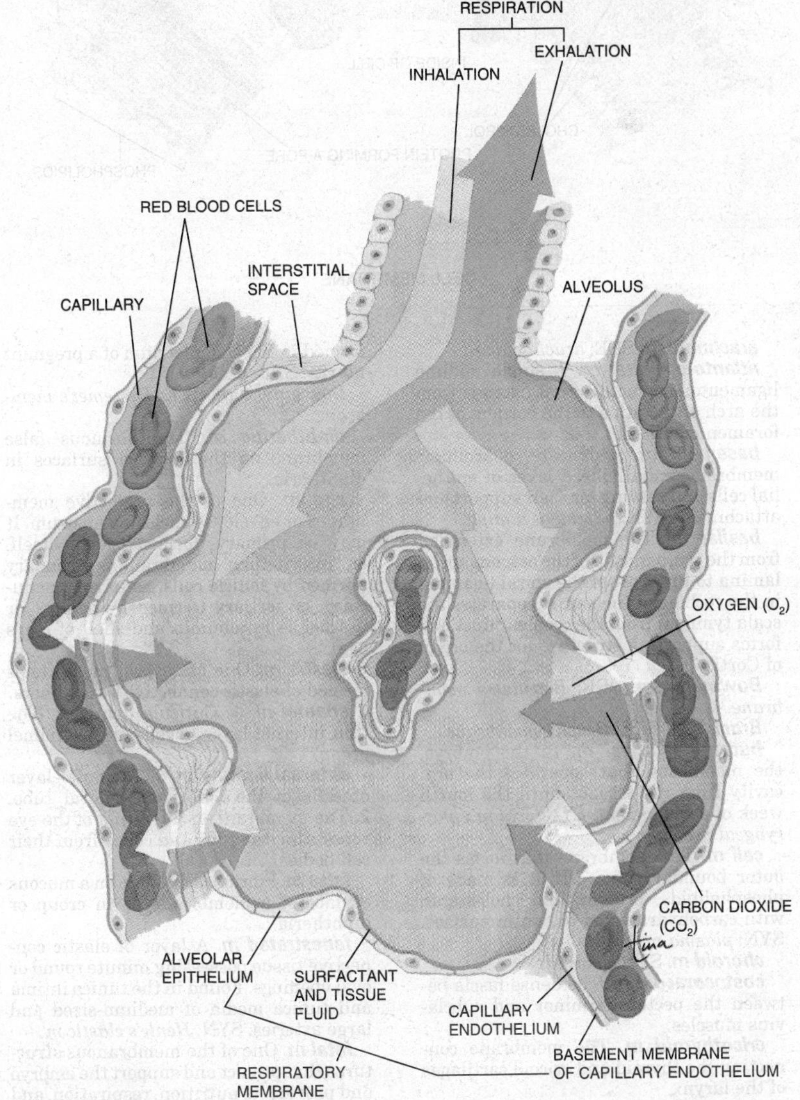


**ALVEOLOCAPILLARY MEMBRANE**

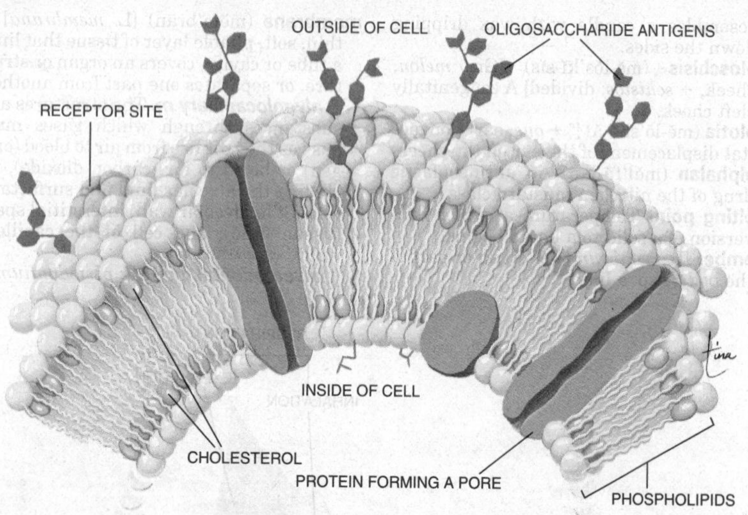


CELL MEMBRANE

***arachnoid m.*** SEE: *arachnoidea.*

***atlanto-occipital m.*** A single midline ligamentous structure that extends from the arch of the atlas to the borders of the foramen magnum.

***basement m.*** A delicate, noncellular membrane underlying a layer of epithelial cells and serving for their support and attachment. SYN: *basement lamina.*

***basilar m.*** The membrane extending from the tympanic lip of the osseous spiral lamina to the crest of the spiral ligament in the cochlea of the ear. It separates the scala tympani from the cochlear duct and forms supporting structure for the organ of Corti.

***Bowman's m.*** SEE: *Bowman's membrane.*

***Bruch's m.*** SEE: *Bruch's membrane.*

***buccopharyngeal m.*** In the embryo, the membrane that separates the oral cavity from the foregut until the fourth week of development. SYN: *oral m.; pharyngeal m.*

***cell m.*** The membrane that forms the outer boundary of a cell; it is made of phospholipids, protein, and cholesterol, with carbohydrates on the outer surface. SYN: *plasma m.* SEE: illus.

***choroid m.*** SEE: *choroid.*

***costocoracoid m.*** The dense fascia between the pectoralis minor and subclavius muscles.

***cricothyroid m.*** The membrane connecting the thyroid and cricoid cartilages of the larynx.

***croupous m.*** False m.

***decidual m.*** One of the membranes formed in the endometrium of a pregnant uterus. SEE: *decidua.*

***Descemet's m.*** SEE: *Descemet's membrane.*

***diphtheritic m.*** The fibrinous false membrane on the mucous surfaces in diphtheria.

***egg m.*** One of the protective membranes or envelopes enclosing an ovum. It may be primary (formed by egg itself, as in vitelline membrane), secondary (formed by follicle cells, as in zona pellucida), or tertiary (formed by oviduct or uterus, as in albumin and shell of hen's egg).

***elastic m.*** One of several membranes formed of elastic connective tissue fibers.

***enamel m.*** **1.** Cuticula dentis. **2.** The thin internal layer of cells of the enamel organ.

***external limiting m.*** **1.** The outer layer of cells of the embryonic neural tube. **2.** The membrane in the retina of the eye separating the rods and cones from their cell bodies.

***false m.*** Fibrinous exudate on a mucous surface of a membrane, as in croup or diphtheria.

***fenestrated m.*** A layer of elastic connective tissue possessing minute round or oval openings. Found in the tunica intima and tunica media of medium-sized and large arteries. SYN: *Henle's elastic m.*

***fetal m.*** One of the membranous structures that protect and support the embryo and provide its nutrition, respiration, and excretion. The structures are yolk sac, allantois, amnion, chorion, decidua, and placenta.

***fibrous m.*** A membrane composed entirely of connective tissue. Examples include the fasciae, aponeuroses, perichondrium, periosteum, dura mater, and the capsules of some organs.

***glassy m.*** **1.** The transparent capsule that separates membrana granulosa from the theca of the graafian follicle. **2.** The internal layer of a hair follicle separating the epithelial and connective tissues.

***glial cell m.*** An extremely delicate membrane, formed of foot plates of astrocytes, that surrounds all the blood vessels in the brain, spinal cord, and the lining of the pia mater, separating these vessels from the nervous tissue proper. This membrane is thought to be one of the components of the blood-brain barrier.

***Henle's elastic m.*** Fenestrated m.

***homogeneous m.*** A fine membrane covering villi of the placenta.

***Huxley's m.*** SEE: *Huxley's layer.*

***hyaline m.*** **1.** Basement lamina. **2.** The membrane between the outer root sheath of a hair follicle and the inner fibrous layer.

***hyaloid m.*** The membrane that envelops the vitreous humor.

***hyoglossal m.*** A transverse fibrous membrane uniting tongue to hyoid bone.

***interosseous m.*** **1.** A fibrous membrane in the arm connecting ulna to radius. **2.** A fibrous membrane in the leg connecting tibia to fibula.

***internal limiting m.*** **1.** The inner layer of ependymal cells lining the embryonic neural tube. **2.** The glial membrane forming the innermost layer of the retina and the iris.

***ion-selective m.*** The ion-selective component in an ion-selective electrode. It uses a modified and highly selective ion-exchange mechanism.

***Krause's m.*** SEE: *Krause's membrane.*

***laryngeal mucous m.*** The mucous membrane, glands, and cilia that characterize the surface covering within the larynx.

***lingual mucous m.*** The mucosa covering the tongue.

***masticatory mucous m.*** The mucosa of the mouth involved in the masticatory process. It is characterized by a keratinized surface epithelium, and includes the hard palate, gingiva, and dorsum of the tongue.

***medullary m.*** Endosteum.

***mucous m.*** SEE: *mucous membrane.*

***nasal mucous m.*** The mucosa lining the nasal cavity and characterized by pseudostratified ciliated columnar epithelium with goblet mucous gland cells.

***Nasmyth's m.*** SEE: *Nasmyth's membrane.*

***nictitating m.*** A third eyelid present in lower vertebrates and represented in humans by a fold of the conjunctiva, the plica semilunaris.

***nuclear m.*** Either of two layered membranes surrounding the nucleus of a cell. Prior to the advent of electron microscopy, the nucleus was thought to be surrounded by a single thin membrane. SEE: *nuclear envelope.*

***obturator m.*** A fibrous membrane closing the obturator foramen.

***olfactory m.*** The membrane in the upper part of the nasal cavity that contains olfactory receptors.

***oral m.*** Buccopharyngeal m.

***oronasal m.*** A double epithelial layer separating the nasal pits from the embryonic oral cavity.

***otolithic m.*** A layer of gelatinous substance containing otoconia or otoliths, found on the surface of maculae in the inner ear.

***palatal mucous m.*** The mucosa covering the hard and soft palatal surfaces within the mouth. The hard palate has heavily keratinized epithelium and copious mucous glands or fat in the submucosa. The mobile soft palate contains muscle in addition to mucous glands, and is much less keratinized on the surface.

***peridental m.*** An old term used to describe the periodontal ligament.

***periodontal m.*** Periodontium.

***permeable m.*** A membrane that permits the passage of water and certain substances in solution. SEE: *osmosis; selectively permeable m.; semipermeable m.*

***pharyngeal m.*** Buccopharyngeal m.

***pharyngeal mucous m.*** The mucosa that lines the funnel-shaped pharynx. The mucosa varies according to the adjacent area, with pseudostratified epithelium in the region of the nasal cavity, stratified squamous epithelium near the oral cavity, and ciliated stratified columnar or pseudostratified epithelium in the region of the laryngeal opening. The lower pharynx is lined by stratified squamous epithelium, as it is continuous with the esophagus.

***placental m.*** The membrane of the placenta that separates the maternal blood from fetal blood.

***plasma m.*** Cell m.

***pseudoserous m.*** A membrane resembling a serous membrane but differing in structure as the endothelium.

***pupillary m.*** The transparent membrane closing the fetal pupil. If it persists after birth, it is known as persistent pupillary membrane.

***pyogenic m.*** The granular lining of an abscess or fistula.

***pyophylactic m.*** The lining membrane of an abscess cavity separating it from healthy tissue.

***quadrangular m.*** The upper portion of the elastic membrane of the larynx extending from the aryepiglottic folds to the level of the ventricular folds below.

***Reissner's m.*** SEE: *Reissner's membrane.*

***respiratory m.*** Alveolocapillary m.

***Ruysch's m.*** SEE: *Ruysch's membrane.*

***Scarpa's m.*** SEE: *Scarpa's membrane.*

***schneiderian m.*** SEE: *schneiderian membrane.*

***Schwann's m.*** SEE: *Schwann's cell.*

***selectively permeable m.*** A membrane that allows one substance, such as water, to pass through more readily than another, such as salt or sugar.

***semipermeable m.*** A membrane that allows passage of water but not substances in solution. SEE: *osmosis.*

***serous m.*** A membrane consisting of mesothelium lying on a thin layer of connective tissue that lines the closed cavities (peritoneal, pleural, and pericardial) of the body and is reflected over the organs in the cavity. Serous fluid, similar to lymph, decreases friction between the two layers.

***Shrapnell's m.*** SEE: *Shrapnell's membrane.*

***submucous m.*** Submucosa.

***synovial m.*** The membrane lining the capsule of a joint and secreting synovial fluid. SYN: *synovium.*

***tectorial m.*** The thin, jelly-like membrane projecting from vestibular lip of osseous spiral lamina and overlying the spiral organ of Corti of the ear.

***thyrohyoid m.*** The membrane joining the hyoid bone and the thyroid cartilage.

***tympanic m.*** The membrane serving as the lateral wall of the tympanic cavity and separating it from the external acoustic meatus. SYN: *eardrum.* SEE: *ear thermometry; tympanum.*

***unit m.*** The three-layered structure of cell membranes and intracellular membranes.

***vestibular mucous m.*** The mucosa of the oral vestibule with its nonkeratinized stratified squamous epithelium, elastic lamina propria, and seromucous labial glands.

***virginal m.*** The tissue surrounding the entrance to the vagina. SYN: *hymen.*

***vitelline m.*** The membrane that forms the surface layer of an ovum. SYN: *yolk m.; zona pellucida.*

***vitreous m.*** **1.** The inner membrane of the choroid. **2.** The innermost layer of the connective tissue sheath surrounding a hair follicle. SYN: *Descemet's m.*

***yolk m.*** Vitelline m.

**membranectomy** (mĕm″brăn-nĕk′tō-mē) [L. *membrana,* membrane, + Gr. *ektome,* excision] Surgical removal of a membrane.

**membranelle** (mĕm″bră-nĕl′) A thin membrane composed of fused cilia and present in the buccal area of some ciliated protozoa.

**membrane potential** SEE: under *potential.*

**membraniform** (mĕm-brā′nĭ-form) Resembling or of the nature of a membrane. SYN: *membranoid; membranous.*

**membranocartilaginous** (mĕm″brăn-ō-kăr-tĭ-lăj′ĭ-nŭs) **1.** Pert. to both membrane and cartilage. **2.** Derived from both membrane and cartilage.

**membranoid** (mĕm′bră-noyd) [L. *membrana,* membrane, + Gr. *eidos,* form, shape] Resembling a membrane. SYN: *membraniform; membranous.*

**membranous** Membranoid.

**memory** [L. *memoria*] The mental registration, retention, and recall of past experience, knowledge, ideas, sensations, and thoughts. Registration of experience is favored by clear comprehension during intense consciousness. Memory for specific details differs greatly with individuals and with the content of the event. Thus, exciting, unusual, or novel events are easily remembered, but those that are dull or ordinary are quickly forgotten. Memory recall, esp. its intentional recall, means the reproduction of a memory in consciousness. Clear comprehension greatly favors retention. Recall may fail because the memory has been obliterated or because one does not wish to remember the stream of ideas. Various memory defects occur in many diseases.

In general, disease states in the aged are more important in having an adverse affect on memory than is merely having attained advanced age.

Memory is confused or obliterated in maniacal states, lively in paranoia, and abolished in senile psychosis and organic brain disease, but undisturbed in depressions. In dementia from senile causes, there is accurate memory for remote events but little or none for recent occurrences.

The precise neurophysiological, biochemical, molecular, and emotional factors important in memory are being investigated; but so far, how the individual stores and recalls material in and from the brain is poorly understood.

Maintenance of the quality of memory can be achieved by the use of various methods of exercising memory. It is helpful to establish habits such as writing things down and keeping all essential items, such as keys and eyeglasses, in the same place. Remaining mentally active and being willing to abandon old habit patterns are essential components for keeping the memory exercised. Forgetting is a natural event at any age. It is important to keep in mind that whatever information is sought will probably be remembered in time.

***anterograde m.*** Ability to remember events occurring in the remote past but not those occurring recently. SYN: *anterograde amnesia.*

***declarative m.*** The memory function and capability that permits an individual to express ideas stored in the brain's memory. SEE: *procedural m.*

***false m.*** An inaccurate or incomplete remembrance of a past event. Memory accuracy, validity, and reliability are affected by the following factors: age; serious illness, injury, or psychological trauma; prolonged medication therapy or use of a substance of abuse; mental retardation; mental illness; anxiety; preoccupation; fatigue; guilt and fear of penalty; and coercion and incentive to testify falsely. These factors must be considered when evaluating the reliability of patient-reported memories.

**_immediate m._** Memory for events or information in the immediate past. SEE: *digit span test.*

**_impaired m._** The state in which an individual experiences the inability to remember or recall bits of information or behavioral skills. Impaired memory may be attributed to pathophysiological or situational causes that are either temporary or permanent. SEE: *Nursing Diagnoses Appendix.*

**_long-term m._** Recall of experiences, or of information gained, in the distant past.

**_procedural m._** The memory capability that permits an individual to perform activities. This type of memory is usually preserved when other memory functions are lost. SEE: *declarative m.*

**_recovered m._** A memory recalled after having been forgotten. Recall may be the result of psychotherapy or suggestion. However, not all instances of recovered memory are accurate. SEE: *false m.*

**_retrograde m._** Ability to recall events of recent occurrence but lacking ability to recall knowledge with which patient had previously been familiar. SYN: *retrograde amnesia.*

**_selective m._** Choice an older individual makes to remember only the pleasant memories of the past or those that are ego-protective.

**_short-term m._** Recall of events in the immediate past.

**MEN** *multiple endocrine neoplasia.*

**menacme** (măn-ăk′mē) [Gr. *men*, month, + *akme*, top] **1.** The time between menarche and menopause. **2.** The height of the menstrual activity of a woman.

**menadiol sodium diphosphate** A synthetic water-soluble vitamin with the same activity as natural vitamin K. It is used as an antihemorrhagic agent in hypoprothrombinemia or hemorrhagic disorders due to hypoprothrombinemia.

**menadione** (měn″ă-dī′ōn) A synthetic drug that acts like vitamin K. It is used parenterally in oil or orally in tablet form.

---

Caution: Menadione powder is irritating to the respiratory tract and skin. In alcoholic solution, it is a vesicant.

---

**_m. sodium bisulfite_** Synthetic vitamin K.

**menarche** (měn-ăr′kē) [Gr. *men*, month, + *arche*, beginning] The initial menstrual period, normally occurring between the 9th and 17th year. The average age of menarche in the U.S. is 12.8 years. SEE: *adrenarche; puberty.* **menarchal, menarcheal, menarchial** *adj.*

**mendelevium** (měn-dě-lē′vē-ŭm) SYMB: Md. At. wt. 256; at. no. 101. A transuranium element.

**mendelism** (měn′děl-ĭzm) The principles of heredity expressed in Mendel's laws.

**Mendel's laws** [Gregor Johann Mendel, Austrian monk, 1822–1884] By carefully studying the heredity characteristics of garden peas, Mendel was able to explain the transmission of certain traits from one generation to the next.

Most inherited characteristics are controlled by the interaction of two genes, one from each parent. During meiosis, parent cells divide and contribute half their chromosome complement to the egg or sperm. After fertilization, the zygote contains a pair of each chromosome; each pair has genes for the same traits at corresponding locations. Alternate forms of the gene for a specific trait are called *alleles*, which may be dominant or recessive. SEE: *allele; chromosome; gamete; gene; meiosis.*

*Mendel's law of segregation* states that as the gametes are formed, the gene pairs separate and do not influence each other.

*Mendel's law of dominance* resulted from his observation that crossing a tall strain of peas with a short strain resulted in the expression of the dominant trait, in this case tallness. Thus, some alleles will dominate others in physical expression.

*Mendel's law of independent assortment* states that traits controlled by different gene pairs (such as height and color) pass to the offspring independently of each other.

**Mendel's reflex** [Kurt Mendel, Ger. neurologist, 1874–1946] Dorsal flexion of second to fifth toes upon percussion of the dorsum of the foot.

**Ménétrier's disease** (mān″ā-trē-ārz′) [Pierre Ménétrier, Fr. physician, 1859–1935] SEE: *gastritis, giant hypertrophic.*

**menhidrosis, menidrosis** (měn-hī-drō′sĭs, měn″ĭ-drō′sĭs) [Gr. *men*, month, + *hidros*, sweat] Vicarious menstruation through the sweat glands.

**Ménière's disease** (mān″ē-ārz′) [Prosper Ménière, Fr. physician, 1799–1862] A recurrent and usually progressive group of symptoms including progressive deafness, ringing in the ears, dizziness, and a sensation of fullness or pressure in the ears. The attacks occur suddenly and may last for as long as 24 hr. When one ear is affected, the other ear will become involved in approx. 50% of the cases.

ETIOLOGY: The etiology is unknown, but edema of the membranous labyrinth has been found in autopsy studies.

TREATMENT: In acute attacks, bedrest is the most effective treatment. Also ef-

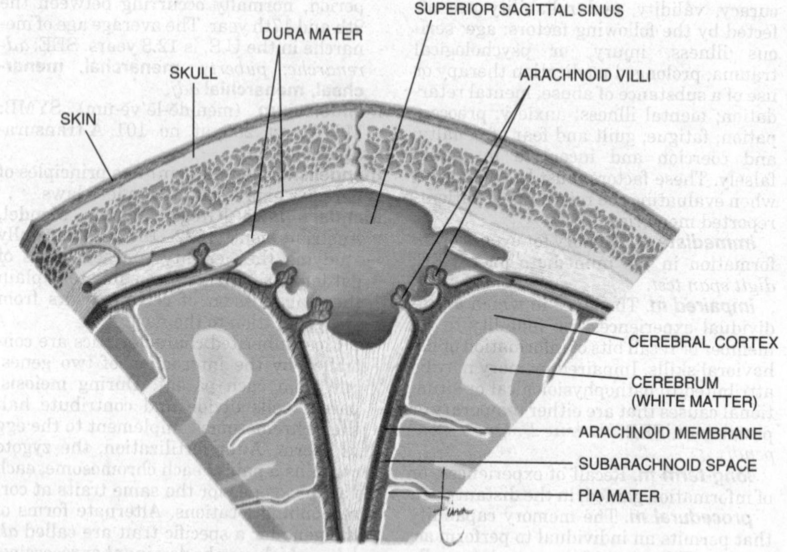


MENINGES

FRONTAL SECTION OF TOP OF SKULL

fective are antihistamines, sedatives, discontinuation of smoking, and, rarely, surgical treatment. A low-salt diet (less than 2 g/day) and diuretics may be of benefit.

**mening-** SEE: *meningo-*.

**meningeocortical** (mĕ-nĭn″jē-ō-kor′tĭ-kăl) [Gr. *meninx*, membrane, + L. *corticalis*, pert. to cortex] Concerning the meninges and cortex of the brain.

**meningeorrhaphy** (mĕ-nĭn″jē-or′ă-fē) [″ + *rhaphe*, seam, ridge] Suture of membranes, esp. those of the brain and spinal cord.

**meninges** (mĕn-ĭn′jēz) *sing.*, **meninx** [Gr.] **1.** Membranes. **2.** The three membranes covering the spinal cord and brain: dura mater (external), arachnoid (middle), and pia mater (internal). SEE: illus. **meningeal** (mĕn-ĭn′jē-ăl), *adj.*

**meningioma** (mĕn-ĭn″jē-ō′mă) [Gr. *meninx*, membrane, + *oma*, tumor] A slow-growing tumor that originates in the arachnoidal tissue.

**meningiomatosis** (mĕ-nĭn″jē-ō-mă-tō′sĭs) [″ + ″ + *osis*, condition] Multiple meningomas.

**meningism** (mĕn-ĭn′jĭzm) [″ + *-ismos*, condition] Irritation of the brain and spinal cord with symptoms simulating meningitis, but without actual inflammation.

**meningismus** Meningism.

**meningitis** (mĕn-ĭn-jī′tĭs) *pl.* **meningitides** [Gr. *meninx*, membrane, + *itis*, inflammation] Inflammation of the membranes of the spinal cord or brain. SEE: illus.; *choriomeningitis; Kernig's sign; leptomeningitis; pachymeningitis; Universal Precautions Appendix*. **meningitic** (mĕn-ĭn-jĭt′ĭk), *adj.*

***acute aseptic m.*** A nonpurulent form of meningitis often due to viral infection. It usually runs a short, benign course ending with recovery.

***acute meningococcal m.*** Meningitis caused by various serogroups of *Neisseria meningitidis*, a gram-negative coccus. SEE: *Nursing Diagnoses Appendix*.

SYMPTOMS: Symptoms include moderate and irregular fever, loss of appetite, constipation, intense headache, intolerance to light and sound, contracted pupils, delirium, retraction of head, convulsions, and coma.

TREATMENT: Strict isolation techniques must be followed when the causa-

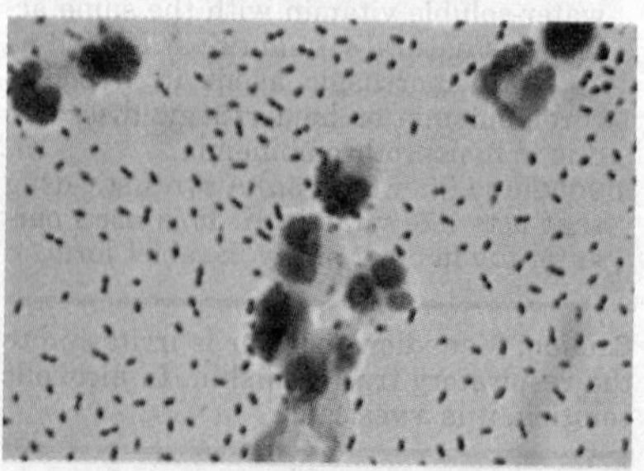

MENINGITIS

STREPTOCOCCUS PNEUMONIAE IN CEREBROSPINAL FLUID (ORIG. MAG. ×400)

tive organism is meningococcus. SEE: *Universal Precautions Appendix.*

Early administration of antibiotics is essential. Intravenous penicillin G should be used if possible. If the patient is allergic to penicillin, cephalosporins such as cefotaxime or ceftriaxone may be used.

Supportive measures for shock and other complications, such as disseminated intravascular coagulation (DIC), congestive heart failure, and metabolic acidosis, should be initiated. Patient will need cardiac vascular monitoring in an intensive care unit. A potentially lethal complication is acute adrenal insufficiency. SEE: *Waterhouse-Friderichsen syndrome.*

DIET: A fluid diet will be necessary during the acute stage, but a general diet should be given later. Tube feeding is necessary with stuporous patients, and children and some adults may have to be fed with a spoon or a medicine dropper.

PROGNOSIS: Prompt diagnosis and appropriate therapy lead to a favorable prognosis.

PREVENTION: Meningococcal polysaccharide vaccines A, C, Y, and W135 are highly effective in preventing the disease. For epidemic control, chemoprophylaxis may be initiated by using sulfadiazine or rifampin for close contacts of the patients.

---

Caution: The meningococci may be resistant to sulfonamides. The vaccines are of little benefit in children under 2 years of age.

---

NURSING IMPLICATIONS: The patient remains isolated for at least 24 hr after initiation of antibiotic therapy. If the causative organism is meningococcus, strict isolation techniques are observed. Fluids are forced and a high-protein diet is provided. Antipyretics and tepid sponge baths are administered as ordered. Contaminated articles are disposed of in a double bag. Neurological status is monitored for changes in level of consciousness and for increases in intracranial pressure. The nurse provides personal hygiene and intervenes to prevent complications due to immobility. Gentle position changes are performed to reduce excessive stimulation. Artificial airway, suction, and oxygen are readily available. A quiet, dark atmosphere is provided, and siderails are padded to reduce the risk of injury. Prescribed analgesics are administered and cool compresses are applied to the forehead to relieve headache. Intravenous fluids or tube feedings are administered as ordered, and intake and ouput are monitored. The nurse assesses for complications such as shock, respiratory distress, and disseminated intravascular coagulation.

***aseptic m.*** Inflammation of the meninges that may be due to injection of air or drugs into the subarachnoid space.

***basal m.*** Inflammation of the meninges at the base of the brain, usually due to tuberculosis.

***cerebral m.*** Acute or chronic inflammation of the meninges of the brain.

***cerebrospinal m.*** Inflammation of the meninges of the brain and spinal cord.

***pneumococcal m.*** A purulent form of meningitis caused by *Streptococcus pneumoniae;* the most common cause of meningitis in adults.

***m. serosa circumscripta*** Meningitis accompanied by the formation of cystic accumulations of fluid that simulate tumors.

***serous m.*** Meningitis with serous exudation into the cerebral ventricles.

***spinal m.*** Inflammation of the spinal cord membranes.

***traumatic m.*** Meningitis resulting from trauma to the meninges.

***tuberculous m.*** An acute inflammation of the cerebral meninges caused by the tubercle bacillus.

SYMPTOMS: Loss of weight, gradual wasting of strength, evening rise of temperature, restlessness, irritability, and sleeplessness may exist for some time before acute symptoms manifest. Acute symptoms are severe headache, occasional convulsions, delirium, vomiting, fever, and optic neuritis.

**meningitophobia** (mĕn″ĭn-jĭt″ō-fō′bē-ă) [Gr. *meninx,* membrane, + *phobos,* fear] A condition simulating meningitis, caused by the fear of contracting meningitis.

**meningo-, mening-** (mĕn-ĭn′gō) [Gr. *meninx,* membrane] Combining form denoting relationship to the meninges (membranes covering the spinal cord or brain).

**meningoarteritis** (mĕn-ĭn″gō-ăr″tĕr-ī′tĭs) [″ + *arteria,* artery, + *itis,* inflammation] Inflammation of the meningeal arteries.

**meningocele** (mĕn-ĭn′gō-sēl) [″ + *kele,* tumor, swelling] Congenital hernia in which the meninges protrude through a defect in the skull or spinal column.

**meningococcal vaccine** SEE: under *vaccine.*

**meningococcemia** (mĕn-ĭn″gō-kŏk-sē′mē-ă) [″ + *kokkos,* berry, + *haima,* blood] Meningococci in the circulating blood.

**meningococcidal** (mĕ-nĭng″gō-kŏk-sī′dăl) [″ + ″ + L. *caedere,* to kill] Lethal to meningococci.

**meningococcus** (mĕn-ĭn″gō-kŏk′ŭs) *pl.* **meningococci** A microorganism of the species *Neisseria meningitidis,* the causative agent of epidemic cerebral meningitis (cerebrospinal fever, spotted fever).

**meningocortical** (mĕn-ĭn″gō-kor′tĭ-kăl) Pert. to the meninges and the cortex of the brain.

**meningocyte** (mĕ-nĭng′gō-sīt) [″ + *kytos,* cell] A macrophage of the meninges of the brain.

**meningoencephalitis** (mĕn-ĭn″gō-ĕn-sĕf″ă-lī′tĭs) [″ + *enkephalos,* brain, + *itis,* inflammation] Inflammation of the brain and its meninges. The usual cause is a bacterial infection, but free-living amebae such as the species of *Naegleria* and *Acanthamoeba,* have also caused this condition.

***primary amebic m.*** Inflammation of brain and meninges caused by free-living amebae ordinarily found in water, soil, and decaying vegetation. Organisms that can cause primary amebic meningoencephalitis include *Naegleria fowleri, Acanthamoeba culbertsoni,* and other species of *Acanthamoeba.* The amebae are acquired by swimming in freshwater lakes and sniffing water into the nasal cavities.

SYMPTOMS: Similar to those of acute meningococcal meningitis.

TREATMENT: For *Naegleria* infections, amphotericin B, miconazole, and rifampin are effective if given early in the disease, but diagnosis of this rare disease is often delayed and few patients survive. *Acanthamoeba* species are sensitive to pentamidine, propamidine, ketoconazole, miconazole, neomycin, and flucytosine.

**meningoencephalocele** (měn-ĭn″gō-ĕn-sĕf′ăl-ō-sēl) [″ + ″ + *kele,* tumor, swelling] Hernial protrusion of brain and meninges through a defect in the skull.

**meningoencephalomyelitis** (měn-ĭn″gō-ĕn-sĕf″ăl-ō-mī-ĕl-ī′tĭs) [″ + ″ + *myelos,* marrow, + *itis,* inflammation] Inflammation of the brain and spinal cord, and their meninges.

**meningoencephalopathy** (mĕ-nĭng″gō-ĕn-sĕf″ă-lŏp′ă-thē) [″ + ″ + *pathos,* disease] Disease of the meninges and brain.

**meningomalacia** (mĕn-ĭn″gō-mă-lā′shē-ă) [″ + *malakia,* softening] Softening of any membrane.

**meningomyelitis** (měn-ĭn″gō-mī″ĕl-ī′tĭs) [″ + *myelos,* marrow, + *itis,* inflammation] Inflammation of spinal cord and its enveloping membranes.

**meningomyelocele** (mĕ-nĭng″gō-mī′ĕ-lō-sēl″) [″ + ″ + *kele,* tumor, swelling] Hernia of the spinal cord and membranes through a defect in the vertebral column.

**meningomyeloradiculitis** (mĕ-nĭng″gō-mī″ĕ-lō-ră-dĭk″ū-lī′tĭs) [″ + ″ + L. *radicula,* radicle, + Gr. *itis,* inflammation] Inflammation of the meninges and the roots of spinal or cranial nerves.

**meningo-osteophlebitis** (mĕ-nĭng″gō-ŏs″tē-ō-flĕ-bī′tĭs) [″ + *osteon,* bone, + *phleps,* vein, + *itis,* inflammation] Parosteitis and inflammation of the veins of the bone.

**meningopathy** (mĕn-ĭn-gŏp′ă-thē) [″ + *pathos,* disease, suffering] Any pathological condition of the meninges.

**meningoradicular** (mĕ-nĭng″gō-ră-dĭk′ū-lăr) [″ + L. *radicula,* radicle] Concerning the meninges and spinal and cerebral nerve roots.

**meningoradiculitis** (mĕ-nĭng″gō-ră-dĭk″ū-lī′tĭs) [″ + ″ + Gr. *itis,* inflammation] Inflammation of the meninges and roots of the spinal nerves.

**meningorhachidian** (mĕn-ĭn″gō-ră-kĭd′ē-ăn) [″ + *rhachis,* spine] Concerning the spinal cord and meninges.

**meningorrhagia** (mĕn-ĭn″gō-rā′jē-ă) [″ + *rhegnynai,* to burst forth] Hemorrhage of the cerebral or spinal membrane.

**meningorrhea** (mĕn-ĭn″gō-rē′ă) [″ + *rhoia,* flow] Effusion of blood on or between the meninges.

**meningotyphoid** (mĕn-ĭn″gō-tī′foyd) Typhoid fever with symptoms of meningitis.

**meningovascular** (mĕn-ĭn″gō-văs′kū-lăr) Pert. to blood vessels of the meninges.

**meninx** (mē′nĭnks) *pl.* **meninges** [Gr., membrane] **1.** Membrane. **2.** Any of the three membranes investing the spinal cord and brain: dura mater (external), arachnoid (middle), and pia mater (internal).

**meniscectomy** (mĕn″ĭ-sĕk′tō-mē) [″ + *ektome,* excision] Removal of meniscus cartilage of the knee. SEE: *Nursing Diagnoses Appendix.*

NURSING IMPLICATIONS: After surgery, the nurse checks the dressing, peripheral pulses, and sensory and motor status of the affected area every 2 hr. Knee immobility is maintained for a specified period. Although dependent on the procedure, use of crutches with partial weight bearing may begin in 1 to 2 days. The affected leg is kept elevated to prevent or reduce swelling, and ice is applied to control swelling. The patient may begin active and passive range-of-motion exercises as early as the third postoperative day. On discharge, the patient is advised to continue to perform appropriate exercises at home and begin a gradual return to normal activities. Physical therapy to help restore muscle strength and range of motion is also indicated. The nurse encourages follow-up visits to the physician.

**meniscitis** (mĕn″ĭ-sī′tĭs) [Gr. *meniskos,* crescent, + *itis,* inflammation] Inflammation of an interarticular cartilage, esp. the medial and lateral menisci of the knee joint.

**meniscocyte** (mĕn-ĭs′kō-sīt) [″ + *kytos,* cell] A crescent-shaped red blood cell. SYN: *sickle cell.*

**meniscus** (mĕn-ĭs′kŭs) *pl.* **menisci** [Gr. *meniskos,* crescent] **1.** Convexoconcave lens. **2.** Interarticular fibrocartilage of crescent shape, found in certain joints, esp. the lateral and medial menisci (semilunar cartilages) of the knee joint. **3.** The curved upper surface of a liquid in a container.

***m. articularis*** Crescent-shaped interarticular fibrocartilage found in certain synovial joints.

**Menkes disease** Metabolic defect blocking the absorption of copper in the gastrointestinal tract. SEE: *kinky hair disease.*

**meno-** Pert. to menses or menstruation.

**menometrorrhagia** (mĕn″ō-mĕt-rō-rā′jē-ă) [Gr. *men,* month, + *metra,* womb, + *rhegnynai,* to burst forth] Irregular or excessive menstrual bleeding. SEE: *menorrhagia.*

**menopause** (mĕn′ō-pawz) [″ + *pausis,* cessation] The period that marks the permanent cessation of menstrual activity, usually occurring between the ages of 35 and 58. The menses may stop suddenly, there may be a decreased flow each month until a final cessation, or the interval between periods may be lengthened until complete cessation is accomplished. Natural menopause will occur in 25% of women by age 47, in 50% by age 50, 75% by age 52, and in 95% by age 55. Menopause due to surgical removal of the ovaries has occurred in almost 30% of U.S. women who are 50 years of age or older. Women with short menstrual cycles may reach menopause as much as two years earlier than women with long cycles. Cigarette smoking has an effect on menopause, causing it to occur 1 to 2 years prematurely. SYN: *change of life; climacteric.* SEE: *osteoporosis; perimenopause.*

SYMPTOMS: The symptoms associated with menopause begin soon after the ovaries stop functioning. This is true whether menopause occurs naturally or is due to surgical removal of the ovaries or failure of the pituitary gland to function. Symptoms, which may last from a few months to years, vary from being hardly noticeable to being severe. Included are vasomotor instability, nervousness, hot flashes (flushes), chills, excitability, fatigue, apathy, mental depression, crying episodes, insomnia, palpitation, vertigo, headache, numbness, tingling, myalgia, urinary disturbances such as frequency and incontinence, and various disorders of the gastrointestinal system. The long-range effects of lower estrogen levels are osteoporosis and atherosclerosis.

Hot flashes (flushes) may start with an aura preceding abdominal discomfort and perhaps a chill, quickly followed by a feeling of heat moving toward the head. Next the face becomes red, then there is sweating followed by exhaustion. The cause of hot flashes is not completely understood. Although the popular myth is that sexual desire and activity inevitably decrease following menopause, there is little to support this. Sexual desire may remain at the premenopause level or be increased due to the lack of fear of pregnancy. If sexual activity decreases, it is most probably due to the lack of a socially acceptable, sexually capable partner.

TREATMENT: Hormone replacement therapy (HRT) may be required. This therapy should consist of estrogen combined with progestin. Therapy using estrogen alone has been found to promote endometrial hyperplasia. HRT is contraindicated in those with a history of an estrogen-dependent breast tumor, thromboembolic disease, or acute liver disease. Decisions regarding use of HRT require identifying the relative benefits and risks of treatment for the individual woman. Important considerations include the benefits of delaying the development of osteoporosis, reducing the risk of osteoporotic fractures, and lowering the risk of heart attacks and strokes, as well as the potential risk for development of estrogen-related malignancies. Another important consideration is the alteration in the quality of life associated with the use of HRT as perceived by the individual patient. If menopause is the result of surgical removal of the ovaries, it is possible that estrogen therapy will reduce the risk of coronary disease. Yearly pelvic examination should include Papanicolaou test for cancer of the uterus and cervix. SEE: *estrogen replacement therapy; hormone replacement therapy.*

NURSING IMPLICATIONS: Because women may experience a variety of symptoms during this period, their nature, severity, and personal impact need to be determined. Menopause is explained as a normal phase in the reproductive cycle. If the woman experiences severe symptoms, a physician may need to assess the patient. The woman is encouraged to maintain a diet high in calcium, vitamins, and minerals. The advantages and disadvantages of estrogen replacement therapy are discussed. The nurse offers emotional support and reassurance, as symptoms can be distressing and frightening, and provides written follow-up information and self-help resources.

***artificial m.*** Menopause occurring subsequent to surgical removal of ovaries, x-ray irradiation, or radium implantation into the uterus.

***male m.*** SEE: *climacteric.*

***premature m.*** Natural or artificial menopause occurring before age 35.

***surgical m.*** Artificial m.

**menoplania** (mĕn-ō″plā′nē-ă) [″ + *plane,* deviation] Menstruation through other than the normal outlet, as through the nose. SYN: *vicarious menstruation.*

**menorrhagia** (mĕn″ō-rā′jē-ă) [″ + *rhegnynai,* to burst forth] Excessive bleeding at the time of a menstrual period, either in number of days or amount of blood or both. SEE: *hemorrhage, uterine.*

ETIOLOGY: Menorrhagia may be caused by endocrine disturbances, hypertension, diabetes mellitus, blood dyscrasias, chronic nephritis, retroversion or retroflexion of the uterus, intramural or submucous fibroids of the uterus, uterine adenomyosis, fibrosis of the uterus with hyperplastic changes of the endometrium, erosions or polyps of the cervix uteri, acute salpingitis, acute or chronic metritis, or acute endometritis.

**menorrhalgia** (mĕn-ō-răl′jē-ă) [″ + *rhoia,* flow, + *algia,* pain] Painful menstruation or pelvic pain accompanying menstruation, sometimes a symptom of endometriosis. SYN: *dysmenorrhea.*

**menostasis** (mĕn-ŏs′tă-sĭs) [″ + *stasis,*

standing still] Suppression of the menses.

**menostaxis** (mĕn″ō-stăk′sĭs) [″ + *staxis*, dripping] Prolonged menstruation.

**menotropins** (mĕn″ō-trō′pĭns) A combination of follicle-stimulating hormone (FSH) and luteinizing hormone (LH) used to treat infertility by promoting growth and maturation of the follicle of the ovary. Menotropins is obtained from the urine of postmenopausal women. A standard extract is used with human chorionic gonadotropin (HCG) to induce ovulation. Trade name is Pergonal.

**menoxenia** (mĕn-ŏk-sē′nē-ă) [″ + *xenos*, strange] Abnormal menstruation.

**menses** (mĕn′sēz) [L., month] The monthly flow of bloody fluid from the endometrium.

**menstrual cramps** SEE: *cramps, menstrual; dysmenorrhea.*

**menstrual cycle** The periodically recurrent series of changes occurring in the uterus and associated sex organs (ovaries, cervix, and vagina) associated with menstruation and the intermenstrual period. The human cycle averages 28 days in length, measured from the beginning of menstruation. The menstrual cycle is, however, quite variable in length, even in the same person from month to month. Variations in the length of the cycle are due principally to variation in the length of the proliferative phase. SEE: illus.

The menstrual cycle is divided into four phases characterized by histological changes that take place in the uterine endometrium. They are:

*Proliferative Phase:* Following blood loss from the endometrium, the uterine epithelium is restored to normal; the endometrium becomes thicker and more vascular; the glands elongate. During this period, the ovarian follicle is maturing and secreting estrogens. The phase is terminated by the rupture of the follicle and the liberation of the ovum at about 14 days before next menstrual period begins.

*Luteal or Secretory Phase:* The endometrium increases in thickness; the glands become more tortuous and produce an abundant secretion containing glycogen. The coiled arteries make their appearance; the endometrium becomes edematous; the stroma becomes compact. During this period, the corpus luteum in an ovary is developing and secreting progesterone. This phase lasts 10 to 14 days.

*Premenstrual or Ischemic Phase:* If pregnancy has not occurred, the coiled arteries constrict and the endometrium becomes anemic and shrinks a day or two before menstruation. The corpus luteum of the ovary begins involution. This phase lasts about 2 days and is terminated by the opening up of constricted arteries, the breaking off of small patches of endometrium, and the beginning of menstruation with the flow of menstrual fluid.

*Menstruation:* A period of uterine bleeding accompanied by shedding of the endometrium. This phase averages 4 to 5 days in length.

The menstrual cycle in normal women may be altered by pregnancy, by taking

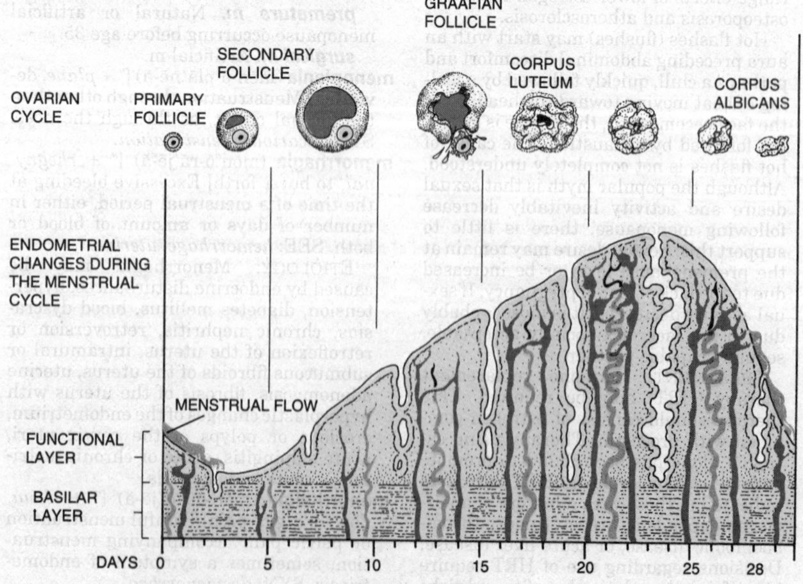

MENSTRUAL CYCLE

birth control pills, or by using an intrauterine device (IUD). In general, taking birth control pills decreases the amount of flow and use of an IUD increases it.

**menstrual epilepsy** Epileptic convulsions that tend to occur at certain times during the menstrual period. SEE: *epilepsy*.

**menstrual extraction** Vacuum or suction curettage of the uterus done just prior to the date of the next menstrual period. The procedure, performed using carefully controlled suction and a soft flexible catheter, is used to be certain the menstrual period is induced, even though the uterus may contain a fertilized ovum.

**menstrual regulation** Vacuum or suction curettage of the uterus done within the first two weeks following the expected date of the onset of menstruation. If the amenorrhea was due to pregnancy, the procedure is classed as a form of fertility control.

**menstrual synchrony** The valid observation that women living in close association, as in dormitories, may develop menstrual cycles in which the various phases are synchronized for that group.

**menstruant** (mĕn′stroo-ănt) [L. *menstruare,* to discharge the menses] **1.** In the condition of menstruating. **2.** One who menstruates.

**menstruate** (mĕn′stroo-āt) To discharge menses.

**menstruation** (mĕn-stroo-ā′shŭn) [L. *menstruare,* to discharge the menses] The periodic discharge of a bloody fluid from the uterus, occurring at more or less regular intervals during the life of a woman from the age of puberty to menopause. The discharge contains altered blood with normal, hemolyzed, and sometimes agglutinated, red blood cells, disintegrated endometrial and stroma cells, and glandular secretions. In general, menstrual blood does not coagulate, but the passage of occasional clots is not unusual. Menstruation is brought on by reduced production of ovarian hormones, esp. progesterone, that results from involution of the corpus luteum following failure of the ovum to become fertilized. SYN: *catamenia*. SEE: *ovary* for illus; *lactation amenorrhea method; menstrual cycle*.

Menstruation has its onset at puberty (9 to 17 years of age). The length of the menstrual flow varies from 3 to 7 days, averaging 4 to 5 days, and occurs on an average every 27 to 28 days, although the time may vary from 18 to 40 days. Menstruation ceases during pregnancy, may or may not cease during lactation, and ceases permanently with the completion of menopause. Its failure to occur may result from congenital abnormalities, physical disorders (disease, obesity, malnutrition), or emotional or hormonal disturbances, esp. diseases involving the ovaries, hypophysis, thyroid, or adrenal glands.

Blood loss during the menstrual period is the most common single cause of iron deficiency in women. In healthy women, the blood loss is about 44 ml each menstrual period, and the upper limit of normal is about 80 ml per menstrual period. Blood loss varies considerably among women; it is usually constant from one period to the next in the same individual. Menstrual blood flow is increased by the use of certain intrauterine contraceptive devices and is reduced by the use of oral contraceptives. Estimating menstrual blood loss from interviewing women is difficult because many women are poor judges of the volume of their flow. A rough estimate of blood loss may be made by querying the number, type, and amount of saturation of tampons or sanitary pads used each day of the period. When noting the number of pads or tampons used daily, the historian should determine the reason for changes; some women may change for reasons other than pad saturation.

Indications of excessive or abnormal menstrual flow include a need to change saturated tampons or pads hourly; passage of clots, esp. when larger than 2 cm in diameter or occurring on other than the first full day of menses; and duration of flow exceeding 7 days in one or more cycles. SEE: *sanitary napkin; tampon, menstrual*.

*Menstrual irregularities:* An absence of flow when normally expected is called *amenorrhea;* scanty flow is known as *oligomenorrhea;* painful menstruation is *dysmenorrhea*. Excessive loss of blood is termed *menorrhagia;* loss of blood during intermenstrual periods is known as spotting or *metrorrhagia*. **menstrual** (mĕn′stroo-ăl), *adj*.

***anovulatory m.*** Menstruation occurring without discharge of ovum from ovary, i.e., without ovulation.

***retrograde m.*** Backflow of menstrual fluid through the fallopian tubes into the peritoneal cavity.

***suppressed m.*** Failure of menstruation to occur when normally expected.

***vicarious m.*** Menstruation from a site other than the uterus when the menstrual flow is expected.

**menstruum** (mĕn′stroo-ŭm) [L. *menstruus,* menstrual fluid] A solvent; a medium. It was once believed that menstrual fluid had solvent qualities. SEE: *vehicle*.

**mensual** (mĕn′sū-ăl) [L. *mensis,* month] Monthly.

**mensuration** (mĕn-sū-rā′shŭn) [L. *mensuratio*] The process of measuring.

**mental 1.** [L. *mens,* mind] Relating to the mind. **2.** [L. *mentum,* chin] Relating to the chin.

**mental age** SEE: under *age*.

**mental deficiency** SEE: *mental retardation*.

**mental disorder** SEE: under *disorder*.

**mental fog** Clouding of consciousness, usu-

ally with some loss of memory.
**mental health** SEE: under *health.*
**mental hygiene** SEE: under *hygiene.*
**mental illness** SEE: under *illness.*
**mentality** Mental power or activity.
**Mental Measurements Yearbook** A widely used index of commercially published, standardized tests.
**mental retardation** Below-normal intellectual function that has its cause or onset during the developmental period and usually in the first years after birth. There are impaired learning, social adjustment, and maturation. The causes may be, but do not have to be, genetic. Rubella in the first trimester of pregnancy may be associated with mental retardation. Intrauterine trauma or infection may also cause this condition. Methods for judging mental competence and the degree of disability due to mental retardation are controversial, and there is disagreement concerning the validity of tests that purport to detect what is called intelligence quotient (IQ). Tests such as Wechsler Preschool and Primary Scale of Intelligence-Revised (WPPSI-R), the Stanford-Binet Intelligence Scale, edition 4; and McCarthy Scales of Children's Abilities have been more reliable in assessing IQ than were earlier tests. Tests for IQ provide no insight into why an individual makes a certain score. SEE: *intelligence quotient; Nursing Diagnoses Appendix.*

---

Caution: Because the measurement of IQ may be inaccurate, its value should not be the sole basis for classifying an individual's intellectual state or potential.

---

**mental status** SEE: under *status.*
**mentation** (mĕn-tā′shŭn) Mental activity. It is possible to determine the level of mental activity that occurs during sleep by studying eye movements observed through the closed eyelids and by monitoring the electrical activity of the brain by use of electroencephalography. SEE: *REM.*
**menthol** $C_{10}H_{20}O$. An alcohol obtained from oil of peppermint or other mint oils. Menthol may be prepared synthetically. It occurs in crystalline form. When applied to the skin in a 0.25% to 2% solution, it is an antipruritic.
**menton** (mĕn′tŏn) [L. *mentum,* chin] A craniometric landmark, being the lowest point of the mandibular symphysis seen in a lateral radiograph. Similar to, but not necessarily the same as, gnathion, which is the lowest point of the mandible in the midline as palpated in the living.
**mentulagra** (mĕn″tū-lăg′ră) [L. *mentula,* penis, + Gr. *agra,* seizure] Painful involuntary erection of the penis, sometimes curved. SYN: *priapism.* SEE: *chordee; Peyronie's disease.*
**mentulate** (mĕn′tū-lāt) [L. *mentula,* penis] Possessing a large penis.
**mentulomania** (mĕn″tū-lō-mā′nē-ă) [″ + Gr. *mania,* madness] Mental state characterized by addiction to masturbation.
**mentum** [L.] The chin. SYN: *genion.*
**MEOS** *microsomal ethanol oxidizing system.*
**mepacrine hydrochloride** (mĕp′ă-krĭn) Quinacrine hydrochloride. An antimalarial drug.
**mepazine** (mĕp′ă-zēn) An antipsychotic.
**mepenzolate bromide** (mĕ-pĕn′zō-lāt) An anticholinergic used as an antispasmodic in treating peptic ulcer. Its action mimics belladonna.
**meperidine hydrochloride** (mĕ-pĕr′ĭ-dēn) A narcotic analgesic sold under the trade name of Demerol.
**mephentermine sulfate** (mĕ-fĕn′tĕr-mēn) A drug used for its pressor effect in treating hypotension.
**mephenytoin** (mĕ-fĕn′ĭ-tō-ĭn) An anticonvulsive that is used in the lowest concentration possible in combination with other drugs. This is done because of its toxicity.
**mephitic** [L. *mephiticus, mephitis,* foul exhalation] Noxious, foul, as a poisonous odor.
**mephobarbital** (mĕf″ō-băr′bĭ-tăl) An anticonvulsant and sedative of the barbiturate class.
**mepivacaine hydrochloride** (mĕ-pĭv′ă-kān) A local anesthetic.
**meprednisone** (mĕ-prĕd′nĭ-sōn) An adrenocorticosteroid.
**meprobamate** (mĕ-prō′bă-māt) A tranquilizing agent, used for relief of anxiety and mental tension. SEE: *Poisons and Poisoning Appendix.*
**meprylcaine hydrochloride** (mĕp′rĭl-kān) A local anesthetic.
**mEq** *milliequivalent.*
**meralgia** (mĕr-ăl′jē-ă) [Gr. *meros,* thigh, + *algos,* pain] Pain in the thigh.
***m. paresthetica*** Pain and hyperesthesia on the outer femoral surface from lesion or disease of the external cutaneous nerve of the thigh.
**merbromin** (mĕr-brō′mĭn) An organic mercury compound used as a topical antiseptic.
**mercaptan** (mĕr-kăp′tăn) Any organic chemical that contains the —SH radical. It is formed when the oxygen of an alcohol is replaced by sulfur.
**mercaptomerin sodium injection** (mĕr-kăp″tō-mĕr′ĭn) A diuretic of the organomercurial type.
**mercaptopurine** (mĕr-kăp″tō-pū′rēn) An antineoplastic and immunosuppressive agent used in treating acute leukemia.
**Mercier's bar** (mĕr-sē-āz′) [Louis A. Mercier, Fr. urologist, 1811–1882] A curved fold at the neck of the bladder forming the posterior margin of the trigonum vesicae.
**mercurial** (mĕr-kū′rē-ăl) [L. *mercurialis*] **1.** Pert. to mercury. **2.** A substance containing mercury.
**mercurial diuretics** A class of organic mer-

curial compounds that produce diuresis.

**mercurialism** (mĕr-kū′rē-ăl-ĭzm) [L. *mercurius,* mercury, + Gr. *-ismos,* condition] Chronic poisoning by mercury. Seen as a result of continuous administration of mercury or occurs in persons who work with the metal or inhale its vapors.

SYMPTOMS: Soreness of gums and loosening of teeth; increased salivation; fetor of breath; griping, and diarrhea.

**mercurialized** (mĕr-kū′rē-ăl-īzd) **1.** Impregnated with mercury. **2.** Influenced by or treated with mercury.

**mercurial palsy** SEE: under *palsy.*

**mercurial rash** SEE: under *rash.*

**mercuric** (mĕr-kū′rĭk) Relating to bivalent mercury.

***m. chloride*** $HgCl_2$. A highly toxic inorganic salt of mercury. SYN: *mercury bichloride.*

***yellow m. oxide*** HgO. A yellow to orange powder used in ointments as an antibacterial agent.

**mercuric chloride poisoning** Acute toxic reaction to ingested or inhaled salt of mercury. This form of mercury may also be absorbed through the skin. SYM: *Acute:* Severe gastrointestinal irritation with pain, cramping, constriction of the throat, vomiting, and a metallic taste in the mouth. Stronger solution causes a white coating due to coagulation. Abdominal pain may be so severe as to cause fainting, bloody diarrhea, bloody vomitus, scanty or absent urine output, prostration, convulsions, and unconsciousness. Death from uremia is the usual outcome unless treatment is begun immediately.

*Chronic:* Halitosis, loosening of teeth, fever, urinary difficulties, nausea, diarrhea, sore tongue, paralysis, weakness, and death.

FIRST AID: Evacuate the stomach and wash out with milk or a baking soda solution made by dissolving a teaspoonful of sodium bicarbonate in 6 oz (177 ml) of water. Treatment with BAL (British antilewisite) should begin as soon as possible after poisoning has occurred. Maintain fluid and electrolyte balance. SEE: *Poisons and Poisoning Appendix.*

**mercurous** (mĕr-kū′rŭs, mĕr′kū-rŭs) Relating to monovalent mercury.

***m. chloride*** HgCl. A heavy white powder previously used in small doses in medicine as a laxative. SYN: *calomel.*

**mercurous chloride poisoning** Acute toxic reaction to ingestion or absorption through the skin of the mercury salt, mercurous chloride. Acute poisoning is rare because it is poorly absorbed. Symptoms include increased salivation, abdominal discomfort, and diarrhea. SEE: *mercuric chloride in Poisons and Poisoning Appendix.*

**mercury** (mĕr′kū-rē) [L. *mercurius*] SYMB: Hg. A metallic element with an atomic weight of 201 and an atomic number of 80. It is insoluble in ordinary solvents but soluble in hydrochloric acid on boiling. It is a silvery liquid at room temperature. Mercury forms two series of salts: mercurous, in which it has a valence of one (univalent), and mercuric, in which it has a valence of two (bivalent).

***ammoniated m.*** A topical antiseptic used in treating certain skin diseases.

---

Caution: Chronic use can cause mercury poisoning. Use should be avoided in infants.

---

***m. bichloride*** Mercuric chloride.

**mercury in amalgam (dental) fillings** SEE: *amalgam, dental.*

**mercury poisoning** Systemic toxicity produced by inhalation of mercury vapor. At one time, mass of mercury was used to treat constipation. The possibility of mercury poisoning through the swallowing of mercury in a broken thermometer is remote. Symptoms and treatment are the same as for mercuric chloride poisoning. SEE: *erethism mercurialis; mercuric chloride; mercuric chloride in Poisons and Poisoning Appendix.*

**mercy** (mĕr′sē) [L. *merces,* reward] In medicine, the compassionate provision of relief or mitigation of physical pain, mental suffering, or psychological distress. Mercy is not being used if patients in pain are given narcotics or analgesics "by the clock." That is, even though the patient is in obvious pain, the prescribed narcotic is not given until the dictated amount of time has elapsed since the last dose.

**meridian** (mĕ-rĭd′ē-ăn) An imaginary line encircling a globular body at right angles to its equator and passing through the poles, or half of such a line. **meridional,** *adj.*

***m. of eye*** A circle passing through anterior and posterior poles of the eyeball.

**merinthophobia** (mĕr-ĭn″thō-fō′bē-ă) [Gr. *merinthos,* a cord, + *phobia,* fear] Morbid fear of being tied.

**merispore** (mĕr′ĭ-spor) [Gr. *meros,* a part, + *sporos,* seed] A secondary spore resulting from the division of another spore.

**meristic** (mĕr-ĭs′tĭk) [Gr. *meristikos,* fit for dividing] Bilaterally symmetrical.

**meroacrania** (mĕr″ō-ă-krā′nē-ă) [Gr. *meros,* a part, + *a-,* not, + *kranion,* skull] Congenital absence of a part of the cranium.

**meroblastic** (mĕr-ō-blăst′ĭk) [″ + *blastos,* germ] Pert. to a type of ovum containing considerable yolk or a type of cleavage in which cleavage divisions are restricted to the protoplasmic region of the animal pole.

**merocele** (mĕr′ō-sēl) [″ + *kele,* tumor, swelling] Femoral hernia.

**merocoxalgia** (mĕr″ō-kŏk-săl′jē-ă) [″ + L. *coxa,* hip, + Gr. *algos,* pain] Painful condition of the thigh and hip.

**merocrine** (mĕr′ō-krĭn) [″ + *krinein,* to separate] Denoting a type of secretion in which the glandular cell remains intact during the process of elaborating and discharging its product. SEE: *apocrine; eccrine; holocrine*.

**merodiastolic** (mĕr″ō-dī-ă-stŏl′ĭk) Concerning a part of the diastole of the cardiac cycle.

**merogenesis** (mĕr″ō-jĕn′ĕ-sĭs) [Gr. *meros*, a part, + *genesis*, generation, birth] Multiplication or reproduction by segmentation.

**merogony** (mĕ-rŏg′ō-nē) [″ + *gonos*, procreation] Incomplete development of fragments of an ovum.

**meromelia** (mĕr″ō-mē′lē-ă) [″ + *melos*, limb] Partial absence of a limb.

**meromicrosomia** (mĕr″ō-mī″krō-sō′mē-ă) [″ + *mikros*, small, + *soma*, body] Abnormal smallness of some part or structure of the body.

**meromyosin** (mĕr″ō-mī′ō-sĭn) Either of the subunits produced by tryptic digestion of myosin.

**meropia** (mĕr-ō′pē-ă) [″ + *ops*, vision] Partial blindness.

**merorhachischisis** (mĕ″rō-ră-kĭs′kĭ-sĭs) [″ + *rhachis*, spine, + *schisis*, a splitting] Fissure of a portion of the spinal cord. SYN: *mesorhachischisis*.

**merosmia** (mĕr-ŏs′mē-ă) [″ + *osme*, odor] Inability to detect certain odors.

**merosystolic** (mĕr″ō-sĭs-tŏl′ĭk) [″ + *systole*, a contraction] Concerning a part of the systole of the cardiac cycle.

**merotomy** (mĕr-ŏt′ō-mē) [″ + *tome*, incision] Division into sections or segments.

**merozoite** (mĕr″ō-zō′īt) [″ + *zoon*, animal] A body formed by segmentation or breaking up of a schizont in asexual reproduction of certain sporozoans, such as *Plasmodium*. When formed, merozoites are liberated and invade other corpuscles, where they repeat the process of schizogony or develop into gametocytes.

**merozygote** (mĕr″ō-zī′gōt) [″ + *zygotos*, yoked together] A bacterial mechanism of gene transfer in which part of the genome, or chromosome complement, is transferred into an intact recipient cell.

**Merthiolate** Trade name for thimerosal.

**mesad** Mesiad.

**mesal** Mesial.

**mesangium** (mĕs-ăn′jē-ŭm) The suspensory structure of the renal glomerulus. **mesangial,** *adj.*

**mesaortitis** (mĕs″ā-or-tī′tĭs) [″ + *aorte*, aorta, + *itis*, inflammation] Inflammation of the middle aortic layer.

**mesarteritis** (mĕs-ăr-tĕr-ī′tĭs) Inflammation of the tunica media or middle layer of an artery.

**mesaticephalic** (mĕs-ăt″ĭ-sĕf-ăl′ĭk) [Gr. *mesatos*, medium, + *kephale*, brain] Having a skull with a cephalic index of 75 to 79.9.

**mesatipellic, mesatipelvic** (mĕs-ăt″ĭ-pĕl′lĭk, -pĕl′vĭk) [″ + *pella*, bowl] Having a pelvis of medium size with an index between 90 and 95.

**mescaline** (mĕs′kă-lēn) A poisonous alkaloid, the active ingredient of the mescal buttons of the cactus plant *Lophophora williamsii*, that causes hallucinations, esp. those involving color and sound.

**mescalism** (mĕs′kă-lĭzm) Intoxication produced by ingesting mescal.

**mesectoderm** (mĕs-ĕk′tō-derm) Migratory cells derived from ectoderm, esp. from the neural crest of the cephalic area in young embryos, that become pigment cells.

**mesencephalitis** (mĕs″ĕn-sĕf″ă-lī′tĭs) [″ + *enkephalos*, brain, + *itis*, inflammation] Inflammation of the mesencephalon.

**mesencephalon** (mĕs-ĕn-sĕf′ă-lŏn) [″ + *enkephalos*, brain] The midbrain. One of three primitive cerebral vesicles from which develop the corpora quadrigemina, the crura cerebri, and the aqueduct of Sylvius. **mesencephalic,** *adj.*

**mesencephalotomy** (mĕs″ĕn-sĕf″ă-lŏt′ō-mē) [″ + ″ + *tome*, incision] Surgical incision of the midbrain, usually done to relieve intractable pain.

**mesenchyme** (mĕs′ĕn-kīm) [″ + *enchyma*, infusion] A diffuse network of cells forming the embryonic mesoderm and giving rise to connective tissues, blood and blood vessels, the lymphatic system, and cells of the mononuclear phagocyte system. SYN: *mesenchyma*. **mesenchymal, mesenchymatous,** *adj.*

**mesenchymoma** (mĕs″ĕn-kī-mō′mă) A neoplasm containing a mixture of mesenchymal and fibrous tissue.

**mesenterectomy** (mĕs″ĕn-tĕ-rĕk′tō-mē) [″ + *enteron*, intestine, + *ektome*, excision] Surgical removal of the mesentery.

**mesenteriopexy** (mĕs″ĕn-tĕr′ē-ō-pĕk″sē) [″ + *enteron*, intestine, + *pexis*, fixation] Surgical attachment of a torn mesentery.

**mesenteriorrhaphy** (mĕs″ĕn-tĕr-ē-or′ă-fē) [″ + ″ + *rhaphe*, seam, ridge] Suturing of the mesentery. SYN: *mesorrhaphy*.

**mesenteriplication** (mĕs″ĕn-tĕr″ĭ-plĭ-kā′shŭn) [″ + ″ + L. *plicare*, to fold] Shortening the mesentery by taking tucks in it surgically.

**mesenteritis** (mĕs″ĕn-tĕr-ī′tĭs) [″ + ″ + *itis*, inflammation] Inflammation of the mesentery.

**mesenteron** (mĕs-ĕn′tĕr-ŏn) Middle portion of the embryonic digestive tract.

**mesentery** (mĕs′ĕn-tĕr″ē) [″ + *enteron*, intestine] Commonly, the peritoneal fold that encircles the small intestine and connects it to the posterior abdominal wall. Other abdominal organs, however, also have a mesentery. SYN: *mesenterium*. **mesenteric** (mĕs″ĕn-tĕr′ĭk), *adj.*

**MESH** *Me*dical *S*ubject *H*eadings. A list of the medical words used in storing and retrieving medical references by the U.S. National Library of Medicine. SEE: *MEDLARS*.

**mesiad, mesad** (mē′zē-ăd, mē′săd) [Gr. *mesos*, middle, + L. *ad*, toward] Toward the median plane of a body or part.

**mesial, mesal** (mē′zē-ăl, mē′săl) Toward the middle point or midline plane. In dentistry, ventral or nearer to the center of the dental arch.

**mesial drift** The natural tendency for teeth to move in a mesial direction within the dental arch to maintain tight interproximal contacts between adjacent teeth. Also called physiological tooth movement. SEE: *tooth migration, pathologic; tooth migration, physiologic; tooth movement.*

**mesio-** [Gr. *mesos,* middle] **1.** A combining form meaning *toward the middle.* **2.** In dentistry, a combining form pert. to the ventral surface of teeth or ventrally toward the center of the dental arch.

**mesiobuccal** (mē″zē-ō-bŭk′kăl) Concerning the mesial and buccal surfaces of a tooth or the surfaces involved in a cavity in the tooth.

**mesiobucco-occlusal** (mē″zē-ō-bŭk″kō-ŏ-kloo′zăl) Concerning the mesial, buccal, and occlusal surfaces of a tooth.

**mesiobuccopulpal** (mē″zē-ō-bŭk″kō-pŭl′păl) Concerning the mesial, buccal, and pulpal sides of a tooth cavity.

**mesiocervical** (mē″zē-ō-sĕr′vĭ-kăl) Concerning the mesial surface of the neck of a tooth.

**mesioclusion** (mē″zē-ō-kloo′zhŭn) Malocclusion of the lower teeth. They are located in front of their normal position with respect to the upper teeth.

**mesiodens** (mē′zē-ō-dĕnz) A supernumerary tooth, often paired, that has a small, cone-shaped crown and a short root. It appears between the maxillary central incisors.

**mesiodistal** (mē″zē-ō-dĭs′tăl) Concerning the mesial and distal surfaces of a tooth.

**mesiogingival** (mē′zē-ō-jĭn′jĭ-văl) Concerning the mesial and gingival walls of a tooth cavity.

**mesiolabial** (mē″zē-ō-lā′bē-ăl) Concerning the mesial and labial surfaces of a tooth or cavity.

**mesiolingual** (mē″zē-ō-lĭng′gwăl) Concerning the mesial and lingual surfaces of a tooth or cavity.

**mesiolinguo-occlusal** (mē″zē-ō-lĭng′gwō-ŏ-kloo′zăl) Concerning the mesial, lingual, and occlusal surfaces of a tooth.

**mesiolinguopulpal** (mē′zē-ō-lĭng″gwō-pŭl′păl) Concerning the mesial, lingual, and pulpal sides of a tooth cavity.

**mesion** (mē′sē-ŏn) [Gr. *mesos,* middle] The imaginary plane dividing the body into right and left symmetric halves. SYN: *meson* (2).

**mesiopulpal** (mē″zē-ō-pŭl′păl) Concerning the mesial and pulpal sides of a tooth cavity.

**mesioversion** (mē″zē-ō-vĕr′zhŭn) Displacement of a tooth posteriorly in the dental arch.

**mesiris** (mĕs-ī′rĭs) Middle portion of the iris.

**mesmerism** (mĕs′mĕr-ĭzm) [Franz Anton Mesmer, Austrian physician, 1734–1815] Originally Mesmer's theory of animal magnetism, mesmerism now means therapeutics employing hypnotism or hypnotic suggestion. **mesmeric** (mĕs-mĕr′ĭk), *adj.*

**mesna** A detoxifying agent used to inhibit the hemorrhagic cystitis induced by ifosamide. SEE: *ifosfamide.*

**meso-** [Gr. *mesos,* middle] **1.** Combining form meaning *middle.* **2.** In anatomy, combining form pert. to a mesentery. **3.** In medicine, combining form meaning *secondary* or *partial.*

**mesoappendicitis** Inflammation of the mesoappendix.

**mesoappendix** (mĕs″ō-ă-pĕn′dĭks) [Gr. *mesos,* middle, + L. *appendix,* an appendage] Mesentery of the vermiform appendix.

**mesoblast** (mĕs′ō-blăst) [″ + *blastos,* germ] Mesoderm.

**mesobronchitis** (mĕs″ō-brŏng-kī′tĭs) Inflammation of the middle layer of the bronchi.

**mesocardia** (mĕs″ō-kăr′dē-ă) [″ + *kardia,* heart] Location of the heart in the midline of the thorax. This position is normal in the fetal stage, but a malposition after birth.

**mesocardium** (mĕs-ō-kăr′dē-ŭm) An embryonic mesentery supporting the heart. The dorsal mesocardium connects the heart to the foregut, and the ventral mesocardium connects the heart to the central body wall.

**mesocarpal** (mĕs″ō-kăr′păl) Mediocarpal.

**mesocecum** (mĕs″ō-sē′kŭm) [″ + L. *caecum,* blindness] Part of the mesentery that connects the cecum to the right iliac fossa.

**mesocele** (mĕs′ō-sēl) [″ + *koilia,* hollow] Sylvian aqueduct in the brain.

**mesocephalic** (mĕs″ō-sĕ-făl′ĭk) [″ + *kephale,* head] **1.** Pert. to the midbrain. **2.** Having a medium-sized head, with a cranial index of 76.0 to 80.9.

**mesocephalon** (mĕs″ō-sĕf′ă-lŏn) Mesencephalon.

**mesocolon** (mĕs″ō-kō′lŏn) [″ + *kolon,* colon] Mesentery connecting the colon with the posterior abdominal wall. **mesocolic** (mĕs″ō-kŏl′ĭk), *adj.*

**mesocolopexy** (mĕs″ō-kō′lō-pĕk″sē) [″ + ″ + *pexis,* fixation] The suturing of tucks in the mesocolon to shorten it in order to correct unneeded mobility and ptosis.

**mesocoloplication** (mĕs″ō-kō″lō-plī-kā′shŭn) [″ + ″ + L. *plicare,* to fold] Plication of the mesocolon for stabilization.

**mesocord** A portion of umbilical cord attached to the placenta by means of an amniotic fold.

**mesocuneiform** (mĕs″ō-kū′nē-ĭ-form) The intermediate cuneiform bone of the ankle.

**mesoderm** (mĕs′ō-dĕrm) [″ + *derma,* skin] A primary germ layer of the embryo lying between ectoderm and endoderm. From it arise all connective tissues; muscular, skeletal, circulatory, lymphatic, and urogenital systems; and the linings of the body cavities. SEE: *ectoderm; entoderm.* **mesodermic, mesodermal,** *adj.*

***axial m.*** Portion of the mesoderm that gives rise to the notochord and prechordal plate.

***extraembryonic m.*** Mesoderm lying outside the embryo proper and involved in the formation of amnion, chorion, yolk sac, and body stalk.

***intermediate m.*** Mesoderm lying between somite and lateral mesoderm, and giving rise to embryonic and definitive kidneys and their ducts. SYN: *mesomere; nephrotome.*

***lateral m.*** Unsegmented mesoderm lying lateral to the intermediate mesoderm. In it develops a cavity (coelom), separating it into layers (somatic and splanchnic mesoderm). SYN: *hypomere.*

***paraxial m.*** Mesoderm lying immediately lateral to the neural tube and notochord.

***somatic m.*** The outer layer of the lateral mesoderm. It becomes intimately associated with the ectoderm, forming the somatopleure, from which the ventral and lateral walls of the embryo develop.

***splanchnic m.*** The inner layer of the lateral mesoderm. It becomes intimately associated with the entoderm, forming the splanchnopleure, from which the gut and the lungs and their coverings arise.

**mesodiastolic** (mĕs″ō-dī″ă-stŏl′ĭk) Mid-diastole of the heartbeat sequence.

**mesodont** (mĕs′ō-dŏnt) Having teeth of medium size; a dental index of 42 to 43.9.

**mesoduodenum** (mĕs″ō-dū″ō-dē′nŭm) Mesentery connecting the duodenum to the abdominal wall.

**mesoepididymis** (mĕs″ō-ĕp″ĭ-dĭd′ĭ-mĭs) A fold of the tunica vaginalis that is not always present. It binds the epididymis to the testicle.

**mesogastrium** (mĕs″ō-găs′trē-ŭm) [″ + *gaster,* belly] **1.** The umbilical region. **2.** The part of the mesentery of the embryo attached to the primitive stomach. **mesogastric** (-trĭk), *adj.*

**mesoglia** (mĕ-sŏg′lē-ă) Phagocytes present in the neuroglia, probably arising in the mesoderm.

**mesogluteus** (mĕs″ō-gloo′tē-ŭs) The gluteus medius muscle. **mesogluteal** (-ăl), *adj.*

**mesognathion** (mĕs-ŏg-nā′thē-ŏn) A point in the lateral portion of the intermaxillary bone or premaxilla.

**mesognathous** Having a facial profile that protrudes slightly from the vertical line between nasion and gnathion. SEE: *prognathous.*

**mesohyloma** (mĕs″ō-hī-lō′mă) [″ + *hyle,* matter, + *oma,* tumor] Tumor derived from the mesothelium.

**mesoileum** (mĕs″ō-ĭl′ē-ŭm) The mesentery of the ileum.

**mesojejunum** (mĕs″ō-jē-jū′nŭm) The mesentery of the jejunum.

**mesolymphocyte** (mĕs″ō-lĭm′fō-sīt) A medium-sized lymphocyte.

**mesomere** (mĕs′ō-mēr) [″ + *meros,* part] **1.** Portion of the mesoderm between epimere and hypomere. SYN: *mesoderm, intermediate; nephrotome.* **2.** A blastomere that is intermediate in size between a micromere and a macromere.

**mesometritis** (mĕs-ō-mē-trī′tĭs) [″ + *metra,* uterus, + *itis,* inflammation] Myometritis.

**mesometrium** (mĕs″ō-mē′trē-ŭm) **1.** The uterine musculature. **2.** The broad ligament below the mesovarium. **mesometric, mesometrial,** *adj.*

**mesomorph** (mĕs′ō-morf) A body build characterized by predominance of tissues derived from the mesoderm (i.e., muscle, bone, and connective tissues); a well-proportioned individual. SEE: *ectomorph; endomorph; somatotype.*

**meson** (mĕs′ŏn, mē′sŏn) [Gr. *mesos,* middle] **1.** Particle of mass intermediate between that of the electron and that of the proton. Mesons of more than one variety and of positive, neutral, and negative charges occur. SYN: *mesotron.* **2.** Mesion.

**mesonasal** (mĕs″ō-nā′zăl) In the middle of the nose.

**mesonephric duct** SEE: under *duct.*

**mesonephric tubules** SEE: under *tubule.*

**mesonephroma** (mĕs″ō-nē-frō′mă) [″ + *nephros,* kidney, + *oma,* tumor] A relatively rare tumor derived from mesonephric cells developing in reproductive organs, esp. the ovary, or the genital tract.

**mesonephros** (mĕs″ō-nĕf′rŏs) *pl.* **mesonephroi** A type of kidney that develops in all vertebrate embryos of classes above the Cyclostomes. It is the permanent kidney of fishes and amphibians but is replaced by the metanephros in reptiles and mammals. SYN: *wolffian body.* **mesonephric** (mĕs″ō-nĕf′rĭk), *adj.*

**mesoneuritis** (mĕs-ō-nū-rī′tĭs) [″ + *neuron,* nerve, + *itis,* inflammation] Inflammation of the substance of a nerve or of its lymphatics.

**meso-ontomorph** (mĕs″ō-ŏn′tō-morf) A broad, husky body type.

**mesopexy** (mĕs′ō-pĕks″ē) [″ + *pexis,* fixation] Surgery to attach a torn mesentery.

**mesophile** (mĕs′ō-fīl) [″ + *philein,* to love] Organisms preferring moderate temperatures, as some bacteria, which develop best at temperatures between 15° and 43°C. **mesophilic** (mĕs-ō-fĭl′ĭk), *adj.*

**mesophlebitis** (mĕs″ō-flĕ-bī′tĭs) Inflammation of the medial layer of the wall of a vein.

**mesophragma** (mĕs″ō-frăg′mă) [″ + *phragmos,* a fencing in] A band in the center of the A band in the myofibrils of a striated muscle.

**mesophryon** (mĕs-ŏf′rē-ŏn) [″ + *ophrys,* eyebrow] The smooth surface of the frontal bone lying between the superciliary arches; the portion directly above the root of the nose. SYN: *glabella; metopion.*

**mesopia** (mĕs-ŏp′ē-ă) Ability to see at low levels of light (e.g., at twilight). **mesopic** (mĕs-ŏp′ĭk), *adj.*

**mesopneumon** (mĕs″ō-nū′mŏn) [″ + *pneumon,* lung] Meeting point of two pleural layers at the hilus of the lung.

**mesoporphyrin** $C_{34}H_{38}O_4N_4$. An iron-free derivative of hemin.

**mesoprosopic** (mĕs″ō-prō-sŏp′ĭk) [″ + *prosopon,* face] Having a face of moderate width with a facial index of 90.

**mesopulmonum** (mĕs″ō-pŭl-mō′nŭm) The mesentery of the lung.

**mesorchium** (mĕs-or′kē-ŭm) [″ + *orchis,* testicle] Peritoneal fold that holds the fetal testes in place.

**mesorectum** (mĕs″ō-rĕk′tŭm) Mesentery of the rectum.

**mesorhachischisis** (mĕs″ō-ră-kĭs′kĭ-sĭs) [″ + *rhachis,* spine, + *schisis,* a splitting] Merorhachischisis.

**mesoridazine** (mĕs″ō-rĭd′ă-zēn) An antipsychotic.

**mesoropter** (mĕs-ō-rŏp′tĕr) [″ + *horos,* boundary, + *opter,* observer] Normal eye position with muscles at rest.

**mesorrhaphy** (mĕs-or′ă-fē) [″ + *rhaphe,* seam, ridge] Mesenteriorrhaphy.

**mesorrhine** (mĕs′ō-rīn) [″ + *rhis,* nose] Having a nasal index variously quoted to range between 48 and 53.

**mesosalpinx** (mĕs″ō-săl′pĭnks) [″ + *salpinx,* tube] The free margin of the upper division of the broad ligament within which lies the oviduct.

**mesoseme** (mĕs′ō-sēm) [″ + *sema,* sign] Possessing an orbital index between 83 and 89.

**mesosigmoid** (mĕs-ō-sĭg′moyd) Mesentery of the sigmoid flexure.

**mesosigmoiditis** (mĕs″ō-sĭg″moy-dī′tĭs) Inflammation of the sigmoid colon.

**mesosigmoidopexy** (mĕs″ō-sĭg-moy′dō-pĕk″sē) Surgical fixation of the sigmoid colon.

**mesoskelic** (mĕs-ō-skĕl′ĭk) [″ + *skelos,* leg] Having legs of medium length.

**mesosome** (mĕs′ō-sōm) [″+ *soma,* body] In some bacteria, one or more large irregular convoluted invaginations of the cytoplasmic membrane.

**mesosternum** (mĕs″ō-stĕr′nŭm) [″ + *sternon,* chest] The middle (second) section of the sternum.

**mesosystolic** (mĕs″ō-sĭs-tŏl′ĭk) Midsystolic portion of the cardiac cycle.

**mesotarsal** (mĕs″ō-tăr′săl) Mediotarsal.

**mesotendineum** (mĕs″ō-tĕn-dĭn′ē-ŭm) The part of the synovial sheath of a tendon that connects the lining of the tendon sheath to the fibrous sheath covering the tendon. SYN: *mesotendon.*

**mesotendon** Mesotendineum.

**mesothelioma** (mĕs″ō-thē-lē-ō′mă) A rare malignant tumor of the mesothelium of the pleura, pericardium, or peritoneum.

**mesothelium** (mĕs″ō-thē′lē-ŭm) [″ + *epi,* at, + *thele,* nipple] The layer of cells derived from the mesoderm lining the primitive body cavity. In the adult, it becomes the epithelium covering the serous membranes. **mesothelial** (mĕs″ō-thē′lē-ăl), *adj.*

**mesothenar** (mĕs″ō-thē′năr) [″ + *thenar,* palm] The adductor pollicis muscle.

**mesothorium** (mĕs″ō-thō′rē-ŭm) The first two disintegration products of thorium.

**mesotron** A subatomic particle of weight intermediate between light particles (electrons) and heavy particles (protons). SYN: *meson* (1).

**mesouranic** (mĕs″ō-ū-răn′ĭk) Having a palatal index between 110 and 114.9.

**mesovarium** (mĕs″ō-vā′rē-ŭm) The portion of the peritoneal fold that connects the anterior border of the ovary to the posterior layer of the broad ligament.

**mestranol** (mĕs′tră-nōl) An estrogen used in combination with progestational drugs in some birth control pill formulations.

**MET** *metabolic equivalent.*

**meta-** (mĕt′ă) [Gr. *meta,* after, beyond, over] **1.** Prefix denoting change or transformation, or following something in a series. **2.** In chemistry, a prefix indicating the 1,3 position of benzene derivatives.

**meta-analysis** A statistical procedure for combining data from a number of studies and investigations in order to analyze the therapeutic effectiveness of specific treatments and plan future studies. Data obtained from combined studies must be compatible in order to be evaluated by this method.

**metabiosis** (mĕt′ă-bī-ō′sĭs) [″+ *biosis,* way of life] Dependence of an organism for its existence on another. SYN: *commensalism.* SEE: *symbiosis.*

**metabolic balance** SEE: under *balance.*

**metabolic body size** Body weight in kilograms to the three-fourths power ($kg^{0.75}$), representative of the active tissue mass or metabolic mass of an individual.

**metabolic equivalent** ABBR: MET. SEE: under *equivalent.*

**metabolic failure** SEE: under *failure.*

**metabolic gradient** A gradient in metabolic activity that exists in certain structures, such as the small intestine from duodenum to ileum or in embryos from animal to vegetal poles, in which metabolic activity is highest in one region and becomes progressively lower away from this region.

**metabolic rate** The rate of utilization of energy. This is usually measured at a time when the subject is completely at rest and in a fasting state. Energy used is calculated from the amount of oxygen used during the test. SEE: *basal metabolic rate; metabolism, basal.*

**metabolism** [Gr. *metaballein,* to change, + *-ismos,* state of] The sum of all physical and chemical changes that take place within an organism; all energy and material transformations that occur within living cells. It includes material changes (i.e., changes undergone by substances during all periods of life, such as growth, maturity, and senescence) and energy changes (i.e., all transformations of chemical energy of foodstuffs to mechanical energy or heat). Metabolism involves two fundamental processes: anabolism (assimilation or building-up processes) and catabolism (disintegration or tearing-down processes). Anabolism is the conversion of ingested substances into the constituents of protoplasm; catabolism is the breakdown of substances into simpler substances, the end products usually being excreted. **metabolic** (mĕt″ă-bŏl′ĭk), *adj.*

***basal m.*** Lowest level of energy expenditure. It is determined when the body is at complete rest. For an average person, basal metabolism is measured in various ways. In terms of large calories (Cal), measurement is about 1500 to 1800 per day; in terms of body weight, measurement is 1 Cal/kg per hour; in terms of body surface, measurement is 40 Cal/sq m per hour.

***carbohydrate m.*** The sum of the physical and chemical changes involved in the breakdown and synthesis of carbohydrates in the body. All carbohydrates are digested to monosaccharides and absorbed as such principally in the form of hexoses, of which glucose is the principal one. In the liver and muscles, glucose may be converted to glycogen. In all cells, glucose is oxidized to carbon dioxide and water with energy released in the forms of ATP and heat. These reactions require the presence of insulin and other hormones. In the process, many intermediate compounds are formed, among them lactic acid.

***constructive m.*** The building-up processes by which complex substances are synthesized. SYN: *anabolism; assimilation.*

***destructive m.*** The breakdown or decomposition of substances into their simple constituents. SYN: *catabolism.*

***fat m.*** The digestion of fats to fatty acids and glycerol. Following absorption they may be reconverted to neutral fats and stored as adipose tissue or oxidized to carbon dioxide and water with the release of energy. Fats may be formed from excess carbohydrates or excess dietary amino acids. In the utilization of fats, the liver plays an important role in the desaturation of fatty acids. Fat metabolism also involves the formation and utilization of substances related to fats, such as sterols and phospholipids.

***general m.*** All processes involved in utilization of substances entering the body.

***intermediary m.*** The series of intermediate compounds formed during digestion before the final excretion or oxidation products are formed or eliminated from the body.

***muscle m.*** SEE: *muscle metabolism.*

***protein m.*** The digestion of proteins to amino acids and absorption as such. In the body, these are synthesized into body proteins, which form an integral part of protoplasm; thus, they are essential for normal growth, development, and repair of tissues. Those not utilized thus are deaminized (i.e., the amino, $NH_2$, group is removed). This results in the production of urea, which is excreted; the remainder, a fatty acid residue (COOH), may be converted to a simple carbohydrate and oxidized to produce energy.

***purine m.*** Metabolism involving nucleic acids, present in nuclei of cells, in which they are combined with proteins to form nucleoproteins. In the breakdown of nucleic acid, uric acid, one of the end products, is formed.

**metabolite** (mĕ-tăb′ō-līt) Any product of metabolism.

**metabolize** (mĕ-tăb′ō-līz) [Gr. *metaballein,* to change] To alter the character of a food substance by metabolic reactions.

**metacarpal** [Gr. *meta,* after, beyond, over, + *karpos,* wrist] **1.** Pert. to the bones of the metacarpus. **2.** Any of the bones of the metacarpus. SEE: *hand.*

**metacarpectomy** (mĕt″ă-kăr-pĕk′tō-mē) [″ + ″ + *ektome,* excision] Surgical excision or resection of one or more metacarpal bones.

**metacarpophalangeal** (mĕt″ă-kăr″pō-fă-lăn′jē-ăl) Concerning the metacarpus and the phalanges.

**metacarpus** (mĕt″ă-kăr′pŭs) [″ + *karpos,* wrist] The five metacarpal bones of the palm of the hand. SEE: *carpometacarpal.*

**metacentric** (mĕt″ă-sĕn′trĭk) Term indicating a chromosome with the centromere in the median position, making the arms of the chromosome equal in length.

**metacercaria** (mĕt″ă-sĕr-kā′rē-ă) The encysted stage in the life of a trematode. This stage occurs in an intermediate host prior to transfer to the definitive host.

**metachromasia, metachromatism** (mĕtă-krō-mā′zē-ă, -krōm′ă-tĭzm) [Gr. *meta,* change, + *chroma,* color] Condition in which different components of the same tissue stain different colors or shades of color. The colors are different from that of the dye used. **metachromatic** (mĕt″ă-krō-măt′ĭk), *adj.*

**metachromatic granules** SEE: *granule, metachromatic.*

**metachromatic leukodystrophy** SEE: under *leukodystrophy.*

**metachromophil** (mĕt-ă-krōm′ō-fĭl) [″ + *chroma,* color, + *philein,* to love] Not reacting normally to staining.

**metachrosis** (mĕt-ă-krō′sĭs) The ability to change color in some animals, as in the chameleon.

**metacone** [Gr. *meta,* after, beyond, over, + *konos,* cone] The distobuccal cusp of an upper molar tooth.

**metaconid** (mĕt-ă-kŏn′ĭd) The mesiolingual cusp of a lower molar tooth.

**metaconule** (mĕt-ă-kŏn′ūl) The distal intermediate cusp of an upper molar tooth.

**metagenesis** [″ + *genesis,* generation, birth] Alternation of generations, esp. involving regular alternation of sexual with asexual reproduction, as seen in some fungi.

**Metagonimus** (mĕt″ă-gŏn′ĭ-mŭs) [″ + *gonimos,* productive] A genus of flukes belonging to the family Heterophyidae.

***M. yokogawai*** A species of intestinal flukes common in the Middle and Far East that normally infests the intestines of dogs, cats, and other animals, but is also commonly found in humans. Intermediate hosts are snails and fish, esp. a species of trout, *Plecoglossus altivelis.*

**metainfective** (mĕt″ă-ĭn-fĕk′tĭv) Occurring subsequent to an infection.

**metakinesis** (mĕt″ă-kĭ-nē′sĭs) Moving apart, esp. the moving of the two chromatids of each chromosome away from each other as they move to opposite poles in the anaphase of mitosis.

**metalbumin** (mĕt-ăl-bū′mĭn) The mucin present in ovarian cysts. SYN: *pseudomucin.*

**metal fume fever** A syndrome resembling influenza produced by inhalation of excessive concentrations of metallic oxide fumes such as zinc oxide or antimony, arsenic, brass, cadmium, cobalt, copper, iron, lead, magnesium, manganese, mercury, nickel, or tin. It occurs in persons whose occupations lead to exposure to these metals. This disorder is also called brass founder's fever (brass chills) and spelter's fever (zinc chills). SEE: *polymer fume fever.*

SYMPTOMS: The onset of symptoms is usually delayed. There are chills, weakness, lassitude, and profound thirst, followed some hours later by sweating and anorexia. Occasionally, there is mild inflammation of the eyes and respiratory tract. The symptoms are more acute at the beginning of the work week than at the end. This is felt to be due to the individual's adapting to the fumes as exposure continues.

FIRST AID: Therapy includes fresh air and symptomatic treatment.

**metallesthesia** (mĕt″ăl-ĕs-thē′sē-ă) [Gr. *metallon,* metal, + *aisthesis,* sensation] Recognition of metals by touching them.

**metallic 1.** Pert. to metal. **2.** Composed of or resembling a metal.

**metallic tinkling** A peculiar ringing or bell-like auscultatory sound in pneumothorax over large pulmonary cavities.

**metalloenzyme** (mĕ-tăl″ō-ĕn′zīm) An enzyme that contains a metal ion in its structure.

**metallophilia** (mĕ-tăl″ō-fĭl′ē-ă) [″ + *philein,* to love] The property of some tissues of binding certain metal salts.

**metallophobia** (mĕ″tăl-ō-fō′bē-ă) [″ + *phobos,* fear] Abnormal fear of metals and metallic objects and of touching them.

**metalloporphyrin** (mĕ-tăl″ō-por′fĭ-rĭn) Porphyrin combined with a metal, such as iron with heme to form hemoglobin, or with magnesium to form chlorophyll.

**metalloprotein** (mĕ-tăl″ō-prō′tē-ĭn) A protein bound with metal ions.

**metallotherapy** (mĕt″ăl-ō-thĕr′ă-pē) [″ + *therapeuein,* to heal] Treatment of disease by applying metals to the affected part.

**metallurgy** (mĕt″ăl-ŭr′jē) [″ + *ergon,* work] Science of obtaining metals from their ores, refining them, and making them into various shapes and forms.

**metamer** (mĕt′ă-mĕr) Something similar to but different from something else (e.g., isomers of chemical compounds).

**metamere** (mĕt′ă-mēr) [Gr. *meta,* after, beyond, over, + *meros,* part] One of a series of similar segments arranged in a linear series and making up the body of an animal such as an earthworm.

**metamerism** (mĕ-tăm′ĕr-ĭzm) **1.** Isomerism. **2.** Isomerism consisting of segments or metameres. **metameric** (mĕt-ă-mĕr′ĭk), *adj.*

**metamorphopsia** (mĕt″ă-mor-fŏp′sē-ă) [Gr. *meta,* after, beyond, over, + *morphe,* form, + *opsis,* vision] In ophthalmology, visual distortion of objects, which may be due to refractive errors (esp. astigmatism), retinal disease, choroiditis, detachment of retina, or tumors of retina and choroid.

**metamorphosis** (mĕt″ă-mor′fō-sĭs) [″ + *morphosis,* bringing into shape] **1.** A change in form or structure, esp. the transition from one form to another as in complete metamorphosis of an insect (egg, larva, pupa, adult). **2.** In pathology, a degenerative change.

***fatty m.*** Transformation of fat by infiltration or degeneration.

***platelet m.*** Fusion of platelets during blood coagulation.

***retrograde m.*** Degeneration.

***structural m.*** Platelet m.

**Metamucil** Trade name for a laxative preparation made of a hydrophilic mucilloid from psyllium seed husk.

**metamyelocyte** (mĕt″ă-mī-ĕl′ō-sīt) A transitional cell intermediate in development between a myelocyte and a mature granular leukocyte. SYN: *juvenile cell.*

**metanephrine** (mĕt″ă-nĕf′rĭn) An inactive metabolite of epinephrine.

**metanephrogenic** (mĕt″ă-nĕf′rō-jĕn′ĭk) [″ + *nephros,* kidney, + *gennan,* to produce] Concerning the part of the caudal mesoderm of the embryo that forms metanephric tubules of the kidney.

**metanephros** (mĕt″ă-nĕf′rŏs) *pl.* **metanephroi** [″ + *nephros,* kidney] The permanent kidney of amniotes (reptiles, birds, and mammals). Part of the metanephros develops from the caudal portion of the intermediate cell mass or nephrotome; the remaining portion is derived from a bud of the mesonephric duct.

**metaneutrophil** (mĕt-ă-nū′trō-fĭl) [″ + L. *neuter,* neither, + Gr. *philein,* to love] Not staining normally with neutral dyes.

**metaphase** (mĕt′ă-fāz) [″ + *phasis,* an appearance] The second stage of mitosis in which the pairs of chromatids line up on the equator of the cell. Each pair is connected at the centromere, which is attached to a spindle fiber. Metaphase follows prophase and precedes anaphase, in which the chromatids become chromosomes and are pulled to opposite poles of the cell. SEE: *cell division* for illus; *mitosis.*

**metaphrenia** (mĕt″ă-frē′nē-ă) [″ + *phren,* mind] The mental state of turning away from family interests toward personal goals such as business.

**metaphysis** (mĕ-tăf′ĭ-sĭs) *pl.* **metaphyses** [Gr. *meta,* after, beyond, over, + *phyein,* to grow] The portion of a developing long bone between the diaphysis, or shaft, and the epiphysis; the growing portion of a bone. **metaphyseal,** *adj.*

**metaphysitis** (mĕt″ă-fĭs-ī′tĭs) [″ + ″ + *itis,* inflammation] Inflammation of the metaphysis of a bone.

**metaplasia** (mĕt″ă-plā′zē-ă) [″+ *plassein,* to form] Conversion of one kind of tissue into a form that is not normal for that tissue. **metaplastic** (mĕt-ă-plăs′tĭk), *adj.*

***myeloid m.*** Development of marrow tissue at sites in which it would not normally occur.

**metapophysis** (mĕt″ă-pŏf′ĭ-sĭs) [″+ *apophysis,* a process] Mammillary process on the superior articular processes of a vertebra.

**metaprotein** Derived protein resulting from the action of acids or alkalies, in which the molecule is changed to form protein insoluble in neutral solvents but soluble in alkalies and weak acids. SEE: *protein.*

**metaproterenol sulfate** (mĕt″ă-prō-tĕr′ĕ-nōl) An adrenergic stimulant used to treat bronchospasm and bronchial asthma. It is effective when given by inhalation.

**metaraminol bitartrate** (mĕt″ă-răm′ĭ-nōl) A drug used for its pressor effect in treating hypotension.

**metarteriole** (mĕt″ăr-tē′rē-ōl) A small vessel connecting an arteriole to a venule from which true capillaries are given off. SYN: *precapillary.*

**metarubricyte** A normoblast, the last nucleated stage in the development of an erythrocyte. SEE: *erythrocyte* for illus.

**metastasis** (mĕ-tăs′tă-sis) *pl.* **metastases** [″ + *stasis,* stand] **1.** Movement of bacteria or body cells (esp. cancer cells) from one part of the body to another. **2.** Change in location of a disease or of its manifestations or transfer from one organ or part to another not directly connected.

The usual application is to the manifestation of a malignancy as a secondary growth arising from the primary growth in a new location. The malignant cells may spread through the lymphatic circulation, the bloodstream, or avenues such as the cerebrospinal fluid. **metastatic** (mĕt″ă-stăt′ĭk), *adj.*

**metastasize** (mĕ-tăs′tă-sīz) To invade by metastasis.

**metastatic survey** Procedure in which various structures of the body are investigated, esp. by x-ray or imaging, to demonstrate any spread of cancer.

**metasternum** (mĕt″ă-stĕr′nŭm) Xiphoid process of the sternum.

**metatarsal** (mĕt″ă-tăr′săl) **1.** Concerning the metatarsal arch of the foot. **2.** Any of the bones of the metatarsus.

**metatarsalgia** (mĕt″ă-tăr-săl′jē-ă) [″ + *tarsos,* a broad flat surface, + *algos,* pain] Severe pain or cramp in anterior portion of metatarsus. SEE: *Morton's disease.*

**metatarsectomy** (mĕt″ă-tăr-sĕk′tō-mē) [″ + ″ + *ektome,* excision] Removal of the metatarsus or a metatarsal bone.

**metatarsophalangeal** (mĕt″ă-tăr″sō-fă-lăn′jē-ăl) [″ + ″ + *phalanx,* closely knit row] Concerning the metatarsus and phalanges of the toes.

**metatarsus** (mĕt″ă-tăr′sŭs) [″ + *tarsos,* a broad flat surface] The region of the foot between the tarsus and phalanges that includes the five metatarsal bones. SEE: *foot.*

**metatarsus primus varus** Inturning of the first metatarsal bone of the foot.

**metatarsus varus** A congenital deformity of the foot involving adduction of the forefoot. When the child walks, the foot toes in. SEE: illus.

**metathalamus** (mĕt″ă-thăl′ă-mŭs) [″ + *thalamos,* a chamber] The posterior part of the thalamus including the two geniculate bodies.

**metathesis** (mĕ-tăth′ĕ-sĭs) [″ + *thesis,* placement] **1.** A changing of places. **2.** Forcible transference of a disease process from one part to another where it will be more accessible for treatment or where it causes less inconvenience. **3.** Double decomposition of two chemical compounds.

**metatrophia** (mĕt-ă-trō′fē-ă) [″ + *trophe,* nourishment] **1.** A wasting due to malnutrition. **2.** A change in diet.

**metatypical** (mĕt″ă-tĭp′ĭ-kăl) Tissue elements similar to those of other tissues at the same site, but having components that are not in a normal pattern.

**metaxalone** (mĕ-tăks′ă-lōn) A centrally acting skeletal muscle relaxant. Trade name is Skelaxin.

**metazoa** [″ + *zoon,* animal] A term used for the multicellular animals, in contrast to unicellular forms called protozoa.

**Metchnikoff's theory** (mĕch′nĭ-kŏfs) [Elie Metchnikoff, Russian biologist and zoologist in France, 1845–1916] The theory that the body is protected against infection by cells, such as leukocytes and phagocytes, that attack and destroy invading microorganisms. SEE: *phagocytosis.*

**metencephalon** (mĕt″ĕn-sĕf′ă-lŏn) [Gr. *meta,* after, beyond, over, + *enkephalos,* brain] The anterior portion of the embryonic rhombencephalon, from which the cerebellum and pons arise. SEE: *hindbrain.*

**meteorism** (mē′tē-or-ĭzm) [Gr. *meteorizein,* to raise up] Distention of the abdomen or

METATARSUS VARUS

LEFT FOOT

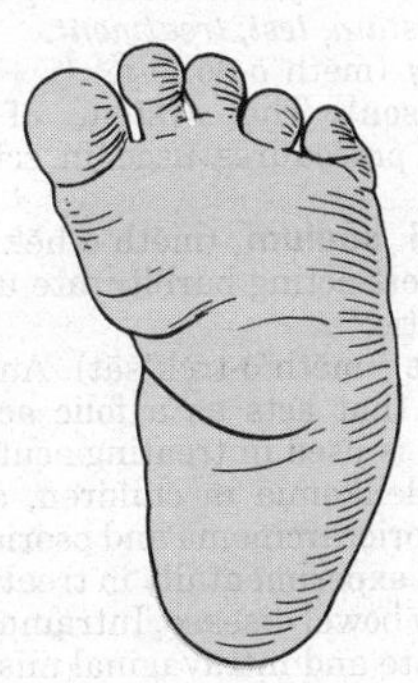
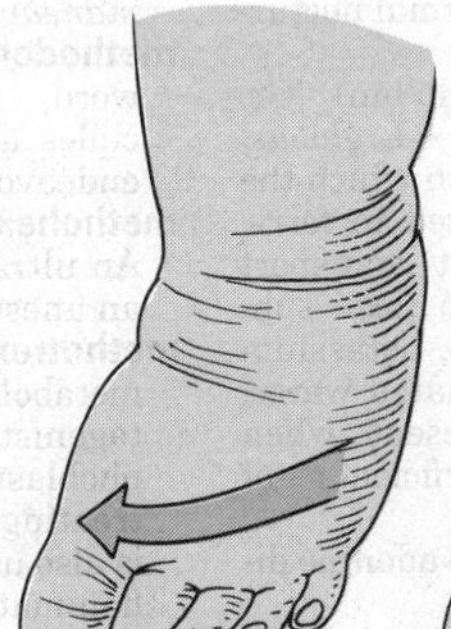
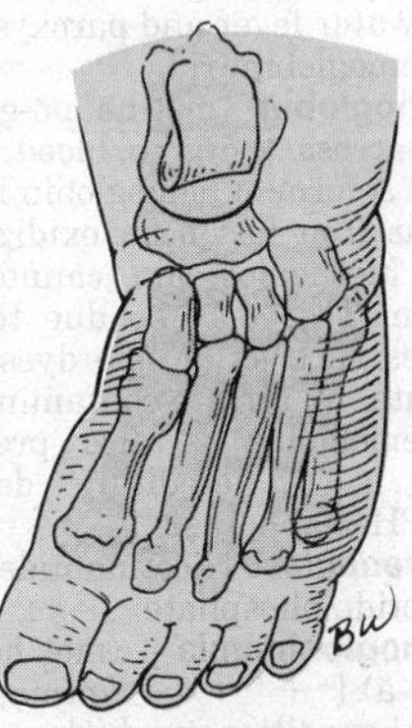


intestines due to the presence of gas. SYN: *tympanites*.

**meteoropathy** (mē″tē-ĕ-rŏp′ă-thē) [″ + *pathos*, disease, suffering] Illness due to climatic conditions.

**meteorotropism** (mē″tē-ĕ-rŏt′rō-pĭzm) The influence of meteorological events on biological conditions and events, such as death rate, disease incidence, and birth rate. **meteorotropic** (mē″tē-ĕ-rō-trŏp′ĭk), *adj*.

**meter** (mē′tĕr) [Gr. *metron*, measure] A linear standard of measurement in the Système International d' Unités (SI system) that is equal to about 39.37 inches. Also spelled *metre* in certain European countries.

**metergasis** (mĕt″ĕr-gā′sĭs) [Gr. *meta*, change, + *ergon*, work] Change or alteration in function.

**metestrus** (mĕ-tĕs′trŭs) [″ + L. *oistros*, mad desire] Period following estrus and preceding diestrus. SEE: *estrus; oestrus*.

**methacholine chloride** (mĕth″ă-kō′lēn) A parasympathomimetic bronchoconstrictor similar to acetylcholine, used as an aerosol in different strengths in airway challenge tests.

Caution: This substance should be used only for diagnostic purposes under the supervision of a physician trained in and thoroughly familiar with all aspects to the technique. Emergency resuscitation devices and medication should be available to treat respiratory distress.

**methadone hydrochloride** A synthetic analgesic with potency equal to that of morphine, but with a narcotic action that is weaker than that of morphine. Methadone is a habit-forming agent, and its use should be carefully supervised. It is used in the treatment of drug dependence due to use of opium derivatives.

**methamphetamine hydrochloride** (mĕth″ăm-fĕt′ă-mēn) A sympathicomimetic agent with central nervous system activity. It has a high potential for abuse. As with almost any drug of abuse, an overdose can be lethal.

**methane** $CH_4$. A colorless, odorless, inflammable gas. It is produced as a result of putrefaction and fermentation of organic matter. SYN: *marsh gas*.

**methanol** $CH_3OH$. A poisonous, volatile, inflammable alcohol that may be mistaken for ethyl alcohol. If ingested, it can cause blindness and death. SYN: *methyl alcohol; wood alcohol*. SEE: *methyl alcohol in Poisons and Poisoning Appendix*.

**methantheline bromide** (mĕ-thăn′thĕ-lēn) An anticholinergic that acts similarly to belladonna.

**methaqualone hydrochloride** (mĕ-thă′kwă-lōn) A hypnotic and sedative that has become a drug of abuse. Because of the potential for abuse of this drug, it is no longer distributed in the U.S.

**methazolamide** (mĕth″ă-zō′lă-mīd) A carbonic acid inhibitor used in treating glaucoma.

**methdilazine** (měth-dī′lă-zēn) An antihistamine and antipruritic.

**methemalbumin** (mět″hěm-ăl-bū′mĭn) The abnormal combination of heme with albumin instead of globulin. It is present in blackwater fever and paroxysmal nocturnal hemoglobinuria.

**methemoglobin** (mět-hē″mō-glō′bĭn) [Gr. *meta,* across, + *haima,* blood, + L. *globus,* globe] A form of hemoglobin in which the ferrous iron has been oxidized to ferric iron. Methemoglobin cannot transport oxygen. This may be due to toxic substances such as aniline dyes, potassium chlorate, or nitrate-contaminated water. Methemoglobin is also present when there is a hereditary deficiency of NADPH-diaphorase.

***m. reductase*** Nicotinamide adenine dinucleotide phosphate.

**methemoglobinemia** (mět″hē-mō-glōb″ĭ-nē′mē-ă) [″ + ″ + ″ + *haima,* blood] The clinical condition in which more than 1% of hemoglobin in blood has been oxidized to the ferric ($Fe^{3+}$) form. The principal sign is cyanosis because the oxidized hemoglobin is incapable of transporting oxygen.

***congenital m.*** Condition due to a hereditary deficiency of NADH-diaphorase.

**methemoglobinuria** (mět″hē-mō-glōb″ĭ-nū′rē-ă) [″ + ″ + ″ + *ouron,* urine] Presence of methemoglobin in the urine.

**methenamine** (měth-ěn′ă-mēn) A urinary antiseptic. Methenamine was previously called hexamethylenamine.

***m. mandelate*** A urinary antiseptic that derives its activity from the release of formaldehyde. Trade name is Mandelamine.

USES: In the treatment of urinary tract infection, esp. pyelitis and cystitis. It is necessary that the acidity of the urine be controlled. Thus, an acidifying agent such as ammonium chloride is usually required to maintain a urine pH of 5.5. This drug should not be used as the sole therapeutic agent in acute urinary tract infections.

**methene** Methylene.

**methicillin-resistant Staphylococcus aureus** ABBR: MRSA. *Staphylococcus aureus* organisms that are resistant to the antibacterial action of methicillin, a form of penicillin.

**methicillin sodium** (měth″ĭ-sĭl′ĭn) A semisynthetic penicillinase-resistant penicillin.

**methimazole** (měth-ĭm′ă-zōl) A drug that inhibits the synthesis of thyroid hormones. It is used in treating hyperthyroidism.

**methiodal sodium** (měth-ī′ō-dăl) A radiopaque compound used in x-ray examination of the urinary tract.

**methionine** (měth-ī′ō-nīn) $C_5H_{11}NO_2S$. A sulfur-bearing compound; an essential amino acid.

**methocarbamol** (měth″ō-kăr′bă-mōl) A centrally acting muscle relaxant. Trade name is Robaxin.

**method** [Gr. *methodos*] The systematic manner, procedure, or technique in performing details of an operation, tests, treatment, or any act. SEE: *algorithm; maneuver; stain; test; treatment.*

**methodology** (měth″ŏ-dŏl′ō-jē) [″ + *logos,* word, reason] The system of principles and procedures used in scientific endeavors.

**methohexital sodium** (měth″ō-hěk′sĭ-tăl) An ultrashort-acting barbiturate used as an anesthetic.

**methotrexate** (měth″ō-trěk′sāt) An antimetabolite that acts as a folic acid antagonist. It is used in treating acute lymphoblastic leukemia in children, and in treating choriocarcinoma and psoriasis. It is also used experimentally in treating inflammatory bowel disease. Intramuscular methotrexate and intravaginal misoprostol (RU 486) have been used experimentally to induce abortion and in treating ectopic pregnancy. It was previously called amethopterin. Trade names are Mexate and Folex.

**methotrimeprazine** (měth″ō-trī-měp′ră-zēn) A tranquilizer and analgesic.

**methoxamine hydrochloride** (mě-thŏk′să-mēn) An adrenergic used to maintain blood pressure in hypotensive states by causing vasoconstriction. It is also used to end attacks of paroxysmal atrial tachycardia.

**methoxsalen** (mě-thŏk′să-lěn) A psoralen used in treating vitiligo, eczema, mycosis fungoides, and psoriasis. Trade name is Oxsoralen. SEE: *psoralen; psoriasis; PUVA therapy; trioxsalen.*

**methoxyflurane** (mě-thŏk″sē-floo′rān) A general anesthetic administered by inhalation for procedures of short duration. Its renal toxicity prevents its being used for prolonged anesthesia.

**methoxyphenamine hydrochloride** (mě-thŏk″sē-fěn′ă-mēn) A beta-2–specific antiasthmatic bronchodilator. Trade name is Orthoxine.

**methscopolamine bromide** (měth″skō-pŏl′ă-mēn) An anticholinergic drug used in treating gastric hyperacidity and hypermotility. Trade name is Pamine.

**methsuximide** (měth-sŭk′sĭ-mīd) An anticonvulsant used in treating epilepsy. Trade name is Celontin.

**methyclothiazide** (měth″ĭ-klō-thī′ă-zīd) An antihypertensive and diuretic.

**methyl** (měth′ĭl) [Gr. *methy,* wine, + *hyle,* wood] In organic chemistry, the radical $CH_3$, seen, for instance, in the formula for methyl alcohol, $CH_3OH$.

***m. alcohol*** SEE: under *alcohol.*

***m. mercury*** An organic mercury compound produced by marine and soil bacteria. The level of methyl mercury increases in fish as it increases in polluted water. It is toxic to humans, esp. children.

*m. orange* A dye used as a pH indicator.

*m. purine* An oxidation product of purine. Includes caffeine, theophylline and theobromine. SEE: *aminopurine; oxypurine.*

*m. salicylate* Wintergreen oil. It is produced synthetically or from distillation of leaves of sweet birch, has a characteristic odor, and is commonly used in liniment or ointment form for use as a topical analgesic balm and counterirritant.

*m. violet* Stain employed in histology and bacteriology.

**methyl alcohol poisoning** Acute toxic reaction to ingested methyl alcohol. Symptoms include depression, weakness, nausea, headache, abdominal cramping, difficult breathing, cold sweats, coma, and convulsions. This type of poisoning may be confused with cerebrovascular accident. Blindness, which often follows, may appear in several hours to several days, and it may be permanent.

TREATMENT: Gastric lavage should be used or vomiting induced. This is effective only if given within 2 hr after ingestion of the alcohol. An intravenous alkali solution (5% sodium bicarbonate) is administered in large amounts; supportive therapy is given. To prevent formation of formic acid, ethanol is given in a 5% dextrose and water solution. This is continued in adults until a blood level of about 100 mg/dl of ethanol is obtained, and then it is maintained at that level. This ethyl alcohol will help to prevent metabolism of methyl alcohol to its toxic and acid metabolites. Hemodialysis may be necessary. SEE: *Poisons and Poisoning Appendix.*

**methylate** (měth'ĭ-lāt) **1.** A compound of methyl alcohol and a base. **2.** To introduce the methyl group, $CH_3$, into a chemical compound. **3.** To mix with methyl alcohol.

**methylation** (měth″ĭ-lā'shŭn) The addition of methyl groups to a compound.

**methylcellulose** A tasteless powder that becomes swollen and gummy when wet. Methylcellulose is used as a bulk substance in foods and laxatives and as an adhesive or emulsifier.

**methylcytosine** (měth″ĭl-sī'tō-sĭn) A derivative of pyrimidine present in some nucleic acids.

**methyldopa** (měth″ĭl-dō'pă) An antihypertensive used in treating essential hypertension.

**methyldopate hydrochloride** (měth″ĭl-dō'pāt) An antihypertensive used in treating essential hypertension. Trade name is Aldomet Ester Hydrochloride.

**methylene** (měth'ĭ-lēn) The chemical radical $=CH_2$.

**methylene blue** (měth'ĭ-lēn) A dark green dye available as a crystalline powder. It produces a distinct blue stain. It is used for treatment of severe methemoglobinemia.

**methylenophil** (měth″ĭ-lěn'ō-fĭl) Something that stains easily with methylene blue.

**methylergonovine maleate** (měth″ĭl-ĕr″gō-nō'vēn) A drug of the ergot alkaloid type. It is used to stimulate uterine contractions and to treat migraine. Trade name is Methergine.

**methylmalonic acidemia** An inherited metabolic disease caused by inability to convert methylmalonic acid to succinic acid. Clinically, signs are failure to grow, mental retardation, and severe metabolic acidosis. One form of the disease will respond to vitamin $B_{12}$ given either in utero or to the mother prior to delivery.

**methylparaben** (měth″ĭl-păr'ă-běn) An antifungal agent used as a preservative in pharmaceuticals.

**methylphenidate hydrochloride** (měth″ĭl-fěn'ĭ-dāt) A drug that is chemically related to amphetamine. It is used in treating narcolepsy and attention deficit disorder.

**methylprednisolone** (měth″ĭl-prěd'nĭ-sō-lōn) An adrenal corticosteroid.

**methylrosaniline chloride** (měth″ĭl-rō-zăn'ĭ-lĭn) Previously used name for gentian violet.

**methyltestosterone** (měth″ĭl-těs-tŏs'těr-ōn) An androgenic steroid hormone.

**methyltransferase** (měth″ĭl-trăns'fěr-ās) An enzyme that catalyzes the transfer of a methyl group from one compound to another.

**methylxanthine** A group of naturally occurring agents present in caffeine, theophylline, and theobromine. They act on the central nervous system by stimulating the myocardium, relaxing smooth muscle, and promoting diuresis.

**methysergide maleate** (měth″ĭ-sěr'jīd) A vasoconstrictor used in the prevention and treatment of vascular headaches. Its use is indicated for patients suffering from one or more severe vascular headaches per week or those suffering from vascular headaches so severe that preventive therapy is indicated regardless of their frequency. Trade name is Sansert. SEE: *carcinoid syndrome; serotonin.*

**metmyoglobin** (mět-mī″ō-glō'bĭn) Myoglobin with the ferrous ion in the heme oxidized to the ferric ion.

**metocurine iodide** (mět″ō-kū'rēn) A skeletal muscle relaxant used as an adjuvant in surgical anesthesia and electroshock therapy.

Caution: An overdose may be lethal due to prolonged apnea and cardiac collapse. This drug should be used only by those familiar with its pharmacology and where facilities and staff for respiratory and cardiovascular resuscitation are immediately available.

**metol** Monomethy-*p*-aminophelol sulfate, one of two developing agents used in dental radiographic developing solutions. Its primary function is to act quickly to bring out the shades of gray in a radiographic image.

**metonymy** (mĕ-tŏn′ĭ-mē) [Gr. *meta,* after, beyond, over, + *onyma,* name] Mental confusion exhibited by an individual's use of a word that is not the precise term intended but of similar meaning (e.g., rifle in place of war; apple in place of ball).

**metopagus** (mĕ-tŏp′ă-gŭs) [Gr. *metopon,* forehead, + *pagos,* thing fixed] Conjoined twins united at the forehead.

**metopic** (mē-tŏp′ĭk) [Gr. *metopon,* forehead] Relating to the forehead.

**metopion** (mē-tō′pē-ŏn) Craniometric point in forehead midway between frontal eminences. SYN: *glabella.*

**metopism** (mĕt′ō-pĭzm) Persistence of the metopic suture in an adult.

**metoprolol tartrate** A beta-blocking agent.

**metoxenous** (mĕt″ŏk-sē′nŭs) [Gr. *meta,* change, + *xenos,* host] Denoting a parasite living on different hosts at different stages of development. SYN: *heterecious.*

**metoxeny** (mĕt-ŏk′sĕ-nē) Condition of being metoxenous.

**metr-** (mē′tr) [Gr.] SEE: *metro-.*

**metralgia** (mē-trăl′jē-ă) [Gr. *metra,* uterus, + *algos,* pain] Uterine pain. SYN: *hysteralgia; hysterodynia; uteralgia.*

**metratonia** (mē″tră-tō′nē-ă) Uterine atony occurring after childbirth.

**metre** (mē′tĕr) [Gr. *metron,* measure] Meter.

**metrectasia** (mē″trĕk-tā′zē-ă) [Gr. *metra,* uterus, + *ektasis,* extension] Dilatation of a nonpregnant uterus.

**metrectopia** (mē″trĕk-tō′pē-ă) [″ + *ektopos,* displaced] Displacement of the uterus.

**metreurynter** (mē-troo-rĭn′tĕr) [″ + *eurynein,* to stretch] An inflatable bag that is inserted in the os uteri and distended to dilate the cervix. SYN: *hystereurynter.*

**metreurysis** (mē-troo′rĭ-sĭs) Dilatation of the cervix uteri with the metreurynter.

**metria** (mē′trē-ă) Inflammation of the uterus during pregnancy.

**metric system** A system of weights and measures based on the meter (about 39.37 in.) as the unit of measurement, the gram (about 15.432 g) as the unit of weight, and the liter (about 1.057 qt liquid or 0.908 qt dry measure) as the unit of volume.

CONVERSION RULES: (Approximate) To change grams (g) to grains (gr), multiply grams by 15. To change grains to grams, divide by 15. To change grams to avoirdupois ounces (oz), divide by 28.35. To change fluid ounces to milliliters, multiply by 30. SEE: *avoirdupois measure; troy weight; Weights and Measures Appendix.*

**metriocephalic** (mĕt″rē-ō-sĕ-făl′ĭk) [Gr. *metrios,* moderate, + *kephale,* head] A skull with a vertical index of 72 to 76.9.

**metritis** (mĕ-trī′tĭs) [Gr. *metra,* uterus, + *itis,* inflammation] Inflammation of the uterus. Metritis is designated endometritis if the endometrium is involved and myometritis if the musculature (myometrium) is involved.

***chronic m.*** Metritis with an increase in fibrous tissue and infiltration of lymphocytes.

**metro-, metr-** [Gr. *metra,* uterus] Combining form meaning *uterus.*

**metrocarcinoma** (mē″trō-kăr-sĭ-nō′mă) [″ + *karkinos,* cancer, + *oma,* tumor] Uterine carcinoma.

**metrocele** (mē′trō-sēl) [″ + *kele,* tumor, swelling] Uterine hernia.

**metrocolpocele** (mē″trō-kŏl′pō-sēl) [″ + *kolpos,* vagina, + *kele,* tumor, swelling] Protrusion of the uterus into the vagina, which pushes the vaginal wall downward. SEE: *procidentia.*

**metrocystosis** (mē″trō-sĭs-tō′sĭs) [″ + *kystis,* cyst, + *osis,* intensive] Formation of uterine cysts.

**metrofibroma** (mē-trō-fī-brō′mă) [″ + L. *fibra,* fiber, + *oma,* tumor] Uterine fibroma.

**metromalacia** (mē″trō-măl-ā′shē-ă) [″ + *malakia,* softness] Softening of the uterus.

**metromalacosis** (mē″trō-măl-ă-kō′sĭs) [″ + ″ + *osis,* condition] Softening of uterine tissues.

**metronidazole** Antiprotozoal used in treating infections due to *Trichomonas vaginalis* or *Giardia lamblia,* and in treating amebiasis. It may cause gastrointestinal upset, and unpleasant metallic taste, and darkening of the urine. Trade name is Flagyl.

Caution: This drug may depress the level of white blood cells. Drinking alcohol while taking it may cause abdominal pain, nausea, or vomiting, and central nervous system symptoms such as vertigo, dizziness, and ataxia.

**metronoscope** (mĕ-trŏn′ō-skōp) A device for exposing written material to the eye at timed intervals in order to facilitate development of reading skills and speed.

**metroparalysis** (mē″trō-pă-răl′ĭ-sĭs) [Gr. *metra,* uterus, + *paralyein,* to disable] Uterine paralysis during or immediately following childbirth.

**metropathia hemorrhagica** (mē″trō-păth′ē-ă hĕm″ō-răj′ĭk-ă) [″ + *pathos,* disease, + *haima,* blood, + *rhegnynai,* to burst forth] A condition of the uterus characterized by hemorrhage, usually accompanied by hypertrophy of the endometrium.

**metroperitoneal** (mē″trō-pĕr″ĭ-tō-nē′ăl) [″ + *peritonaion,* peritoneum] Concerning the uterus and the peritoneum.

**metroperitonitis** (mē″trō-pĕr″ĭ-tō-nī′tĭs) [″ + ″ + *itis,* inflammation] Inflammation of uterus and surrounding peritoneum.

**metrophlebitis** (mē″trō-flē-bī′tĭs) [″ + *phleps,* vein, + *itis,* inflammation] Inflammation of the uterine veins.

**metroplasty** (mē″trō-plăs′tē) [″ + *plastikos,*

formed] Plastic surgery on the uterus. SYN: *uteroplasty.*

**metroptosis** (mē-trō-tō′sĭs) [″ + *ptosis,* a dropping] Downward displacement or prolapse of the uterus.

**metrorrhea** (mē″trō-rē′ă) [″ + *rhoia,* flow] Abnormal uterine discharge.

**metrorrhexis** (mē″trō-rĕk′sĭs) [″ + *rhexis,* rupture] Rupture of the uterus.

**metrosalpingitis** (mē″trō-săl″pĭn-jī′tĭs) [″ + *salpinx,* tube, + *itis,* inflammation] Inflammation of the uterus and oviducts.

**metrosalpingography** (mē″trō-săl″pĭng-gŏg′ră-fē) [″ + ″ + *graphein,* to write] Radiography of the uterus and the fallopian tubes after the injection of air or an opaque medium into them.

**metrostenosis** (mē″trō-stĕn-ō′sĭs) [″ + *stenosis,* contraction] Contraction or narrowing of the uterine cavity.

**metrotomy** (mē-trŏt′ō-mē) Incision of the uterus. SYN: *hysterotomy.*

**metrourethrotome** (mĕt″rō-ū-rē′thrō-tōm) [Gr. *metron,* measure, + *ourethra,* urethra, + *tome,* incision] Device for incising the urethra and measuring depth to be incised.

**-metry** [Gr. *metrein,* to measure] Suffix meaning *to measure.*

**metyrapone** (mĕ-tēr′ă-pōn) A drug that inhibits adrenocortical secretion from the adrenal gland. It is used to treat excessive adrenocortical hormone secretion and to test the function of the adrenal gland.

**metyrapone test** Diagnostic test to assess ACTH and cortisol production.

**Mev, mev** *million electron volts.*

**Meynert's commissure** (mī′nĕrts) [Theodor H. Meynert, Austrian neurologist, 1833–1892] Fibrous tract extending from the subthalamic body to the base of the third ventricle.

**Meynet's nodes** (mā-nāz′) [Paul C. H. Meynet, Fr. physician, 1831–1892] In rheumatic disease, nodules attached to the tendon sheaths and joints.

**M.F.D.** *minimum fatal dose.*

**μg** *microgram.*

**Mg** Symbol for the element magnesium.

**mg** *milligram.*

**mgh** *milligram hour.* Dosage of radiation obtained by application of 1.0 mg radium for 1 hr.

**MHC** *major histocompatibility complex.*

**mho** (mō) [ohm spelled backward] Siemens.

**MHz** *megahertz.*

**MI** *myocardial infarction.*

**MIC** *minimal inhibitory concentration.*

**mica** (mī′kă) [L.] **1.** A crumb. **2.** A mineral composed of various silicates of metals. It occurs in thin, laminated scales.

**micella, micelle** (mī-sĕl′ă, mī-sĕl′) One of the ultramicroscopic units of protoplasm.

**miconazole nitrate** (mĭ-kŏn′ă-zōl) An antifungal agent used for vaginal infections. Trade name is Monistat.

**micr-** SEE: *micro-.*

**micra** Pl. of micron.

**micrencephalon** (mī″krĕn-sĕf′ă-lon) [Gr. *mikros,* small, + *enkephalos,* brain] **1.** Cerebellum. **2.** Smallness of the brain; cretinism.

**micrencephaly** (mī″krĕn-sĕf′ă-lē) Abnormal smallness of the brain. **micrencephalous** (mī″krĕn-sĕf′ă-lŭs), *adj.*

**micro-, micr-** [Gr. *mikros,* small] SYMB: μ. Combining form denoting small size or extent; 1 millionth of a unit (i.e., 1 microgram is 1 millionth of a gram).

**microabscess** (mī″krō-ăb′sĕs) [″ + L. *abscessus,* a going away] A very small abscess.

**microaerophilic** (mī″krō-ā′ĕr-ō-fĭl″ĭk) [″ + *aer,* air, + *philein,* to love] Growing at low amounts of oxygen; said of certain bacteria.

**microaerosol** A fine aerosol whose particles are of uniform size, usually less than 1 μm in diameter.

**microanalysis** An analytical examination of minute amounts of material.

**microanatomy** Histology.

**microaneurysm** (mī″krō-ăn′ū-rĭzm) [″ + *aneurysma,* a widening] A microscopic aneurysm.

**microangiitis** (mī″krō-ăn″jē-ī′tĭs) An inflammation of very small blood vessels.

**microangiopathy** (mī″krō-ăn″jē-ŏp′ă-thē) [″ + *angeion,* vessel, + *pathos,* disease, suffering] Pathology of small blood vessels.

***thrombotic m.*** The formation of thrombi in small blood vessels.

**microangioscopy** (mī″krō-ăn″jē-ŏs′kō-pē) [″ + ″ + *skopein,* to examine] The use of microscopy to diagnose pathological changes in capillaries.

**microatelectasis** Microscopic collapse of alveoli that does not involve the airways and may not appear on radiographic examination.

**microbalance** (mī′krō-băl″ăns) A scale or balance for measuring very small weight changes.

**microbe** (mī′krōb) [″ + *bios,* life] A unicellular or small multicellular organism including bacteria, protozoa, some algae and fungi, viruses, and some worms. SEE: *microorganism.* **microbial, microbic** (mī-krō′bē-ăl, mī-krōb′ĭk), *adj.*

**microbicide** (mī-krō′bĭ-sīd) [″ + *bios,* life, + L. *cidus,* kill] An agent that kills microbes. **microbicidal** (mī-krō″bĭ-sī′dăl), *adj.*

**microbiological antagonism** SEE: under *antagonism.*

**microbiology** (mī″krō-bī-ŏl′ō-jē) [″ + *bios,* life, + *logos,* word, reason] Scientific study of microorganisms.

**microbiophobia** (mī″krō-bī″ō-fō′bē-ă) [″ + ″ + *phobos,* fear] Abnormal fear of microbes.

**microbiota** (mī″krō-bī-ō′tă) Microscopic organisms of an area. SEE: *macrobiota.* **microbiotic** (mī″krō-bī-ŏt′ĭk), *adj.*

**microblepharism, microblephary** (mī″krō-blĕf′ăr-ĭzm, -ăr-ē) [″ + *blepharon,* eyelid] Condition of having abnormally small eyelids.

**microbrachia** (mī″krō-brā′kē-ă) [″ + *brachion,* arm] Abnormally small arms.

**microbrachius** (mī″krō-brā′kē-ŭs) [″ + *brachion,* arm] A fetus with abnormally small arms.

**microcardia** (mī″krō-kăr′dē-ă) [Gr. *mikros,* small, + *kardia,* heart] Unusual smallness of the heart.

**microcentrum** (mī″krō-sĕn′trŭm) [″ + *kentron,* center] **1.** Centrosome. **2.** Motor or dynamic center of a cell.

**microcephalia** (mī″krō-sĕf-ā′lē-ă) [″ + *kephale,* head] Microcephaly.

**microcephalus** (mī″krō-sĕf′ă-lŭs) Individual with an exceptionally small head.

**microcephaly** (mī″krō-sĕf′ă-lē) Abnormal smallness of head (below 1350 cc capacity) often seen in mental retardation. **microcephalic, microcephalous** (mī″krō-sĕf-ăl′ĭk, mī″krō-sĕf′ă-lŭs), *adj.*

**microcheilia** (mī″krō-kī′lē-ă) [Gr. *mikros,* small, + *cheilos,* lip] Abnormal smallness of the lips.

**microchemistry** (mī″krō-kĕm′ĭs-trē) [″ + *chemeia,* chemistry] Branch of chemistry analyzing specimens of minute quantity.

**microcheiria, microchiria** (mī″krō-kī′rē-ă) [″ + *cheir,* hand] Abnormal smallness of the hands.

**microcinematography** (mī″krō-sĭn″ĕ-mă-tŏg′ră-fē) [″ + *kinema,* motion, + *graphein,* to write] Motion pictures of microscopic objects.

**microcirculation** (mī″krō-sĭr″kū-lā′shŭn) Blood flow in the very small vessels (arterioles, capillaries, and venules). **microcirculatory,** *adj.*

**Micrococcaceae** (mī″krō-kŏk-ā′sē-ē) A family of bacteria belonging to the order Eubacteriales and containing the genera *Micrococcus, Sarcina,* and *Staphylococcus.*

**Micrococcus** (mī″krō-kŏk′ŭs) [Gr. *mikros,* small, + *kokkos,* berry] A genus of spherical gram-positive bacteria belonging to the family Micrococcaceae. Cells occur singly or in irregular groups.

**micrococcus** (mī″krō-kŏk′ŭs) *pl.* **micrococci** An organism of the genus *Micrococcus.*

**microcolon** Abnormally small colon.

**microcoria** (mī″krō-kō′rē-ă) [″ + *kore,* pupil] Smallness of the pupil of the eye.

**microcornea** Abnormally small cornea.

**microcoulomb** (mī″krō-koo′lŏm) A microunit of current electricity; one-millionth part ($10^{-6}$) of a coulomb.

**microcrystalline** (mī″krō-krĭs′tăl-īn, -ēn) Composed of microscopic crystals.

**microcurie-hour** The radiation produced by radioactive decay at the rate of $3.7 \times 10^4$ atoms per second.

**microcyst** (mī′krō-sĭst) A very small cyst.

**microcyte** A small erythrocyte or red blood corpuscle less than 5 $\mu$m in diameter.

**microdactylia, microdactyly** (mī″krō-dăk-tĭl′ē-ă, -dăk′tĭ-lē) [″ + *daktylos,* digit] Abnormal smallness of the fingers or toes.

**microdissection** (mī″krō-dī-sĕk′shŭn) [″ + L. *dissectio,* a cutting apart] Dissection with the aid of a microscope, esp. by utilization of a micromanipulator.

**microdont** (mī′krō-dŏnt) [″ + *odous,* tooth] Possessing very small teeth.

**microdontia** (mī″krō-dŏn′shē-ă) [″ + *odous,* tooth] Having abnormally small teeth or a single small tooth.

**microdontism** (mī″krō-dŏn′tĭzm) [″ + ″ + *-ismos,* condition] Microdontia.

**microelectrophoresis** Electrophoresis of minute quantities of a solution.

**microembolus** (mī″krō-ĕm′bō-lŭs) [″ + *embolos,* plug] A very small embolus.

**microencapsulation** Very small capsules that contain an active ingredient. The coating of the capsule is designed to disintegrate within the body in order to release the active ingredient.

**microencephaly** (mī″krō-ĕn-sĕf′ă-lē) [″ + *enkephalos,* brain] Micrencephaly.

**microenvironment** The environment at the microscopic or cellular level.

**microerythrocyte** (mī″krō-ĕ-rĭth′rō-sīt) [″ + *erythros,* red, + *kytos,* cell] Microcyte.

**microfarad** (mī-krō-făr′ăd) A microunit of electrical capacity; one millionth of a farad.

**microfauna** (mī″krō-faw′nă) In a specific location, the animal life that is microscopic in size.

**microfibril** (mī″krō-fī′brĭl) A very small fibril.

**microfiche** (mī′krō-fēsh″) [Gr. *mikros,* small, + Fr. *fiche,* index card] A sheet of microfilm that enables a large number of library data and medical records to be stored in a small space.

**microfilament** (mī″krō-fĭl′ă-mĕnt) Submicroscopic elements of the cell.

**microfilaremia** (mī″krō-fĭl″ă-rē′mē-ă) Presence of microfilariae in the blood.

**microfilaria** (mī″krō-fī-lā′rē-ă) The embryos of filarial worms. Microfilariae are present in the blood and tissues of one infected with filariasis and are of importance in the diagnosis of filarial infections.

**microfilm** A film containing a greatly reduced photoimage of printed or graphic matter.

**microflora** (mī″krō-flō′ră) In a specific area, the plant life that is visible by use of a microscope.

**microgamete** (mī-krō-găm′ēt) [″ + *gametes,* spouse] Male element in conjugation of protozoa.

**microgamy** (mī-krŏg′ă-mē) Union of male and female cells in certain lower forms.

**microgastria** (mī″krō-găs′trē-ă) [″ + *gaster,* stomach] Unusual smallness of the stomach.

**microgenia** (mī″krō-jĕn′ē-ă) [″ + *geneion,* chin] Abnormal smallness of the chin.

**microgenitalism** (mī″krō-jĕn′ĭ-tăl-ĭzm) [″ + L. *genitalia,* genitals, + Gr. *-ismos,* condition] Abnormal smallness of the external genitalia.

**microglia** (mī-krŏg′lē-ă) [″ + *glia,* glue] Cells of the central nervous system (CNS) present between neurons or next to capillaries. These cells may function as macrophages when they migrate to damaged CNS tissue. SEE: *gitter cell.*

**microgliacyte** (mī″krŏg′lē-ă-sīt) [″ + ″ + *kytos,* cell] An embryonic cell of the microglia.

**microglioma** (mī″krō-glī-ō′mă) [″ + ″ + *oma,* tumor] A tumor composed of microglial cells.

**microglossia** (mī-krō-glŏs′ē-ă) [″ + *glossa,* tongue] Abnormally small tongue.

**micrognathia** (mī-krō-nā′thē-ă) [″ + *gnathos,* jaw] Abnormal smallness of jaws, esp. the lower jaw.

**microgonioscope** (mī″krō-gō′nē-ō-skōp) [″ + *gonia,* angle, + *skopein,* to examine] Device for measuring the angles of the anterior chamber of the eye. It is used in studying glaucoma.

**microgram** ABBR: $\mu$g or mcg. One-millionth part of a gram; one-thousandth part of a milligram.

**micrograph** (mī′krō-grăf) [Gr. *mikros,* small, + *graphein,* to write] **1.** Apparatus for magnifying and recording minute movements. **2.** Photograph of an object seen through a microscope. SYN: *photomicrograph.*

**micrography** (mī-krŏg′ră-fē) **1.** Study of the physical appearance and characteristics of microscopic objects. **2.** Study of an object by use of a microscope.

**microgyria** (mī-krō-jĭr′ē-ă) [″ + *gyros,* circle] Abnormal smallness of cerebral convolutions.

**microgyrus** (mī″krō-jī′rŭs) [″ + *gyros,* circle] A small, malformed gyrus of the brain.

**microhematuria** The detection of red blood cells in the urine on microscopic examination of a urine specimen. Even though this finding in asymptomatic persons may, in 20% to 25% of cases, represent a pathologic process, the remaining cases may be unexplained. In the normal individual, about 1500 erythrocytes are excreted in the urine each minute.

**microhepatia** (mī″krō-hē-păt′ē-ă) [″ + *hepar,* liver] Abnormally small size of the liver.

**microhm** (mī′krōm) A microunit of electrical resistance; one-millionth of an ohm.

**microincineration** Determination of the presence and distribution of inorganic matter in tissues by subjecting a microscopic section of tissue to high temperatures, which destroys organic matter and leaves mineral matter as ash.

**microinjection** Injection of substances into cells or minute vessels by means of a micropipette.

**microinvasion** (mī″krō-ĭn-vā′zhŭn) Invasion of the cellular tissue adjacent to a carcinoma in situ. **microinvasive,** *adj.*

**microleakage** The seepage of oral fluids containing bacteria and debris between the walls of a tooth cavity and the restoration or cement layer.

**microlentia** (mī″krō-lĕn′shē-ă) Microphakia.

**microlesion** (mī″krō-lē′zhŭn) A very small lesion.

**microliter** (mī′krō-lē″tĕr) One-millionth part of a liter.

**microlith** (mī′krō-lĭth) [″ + *lithos,* stone] A very tiny calculus.

**microlithiasis** (mī″krō-lĭ-thī′ă-sĭs) [″ + ″ + *-iasis,* process] The development of minute calculi.

***pulmonary alveolar m.*** Deposition of microscopic concretions throughout the lungs.

**micromanipulation** The use of minute instruments and magnification aids to perform surgical or other procedures on tissues. SEE: *gene splicing; micromanipulator; microsurgery.*

**micromanipulator** An apparatus by which extremely minute pipettes or needles can be manipulated under a microscope for microdissection, microinjection, or microsurgery.

**micromazia** (mī-krō-mā′zē-ă) [Gr. *mikros,* small, + *mastos,* breast] Abnormally small size of the breasts.

**micromelia** (mī″krō-mē′lē-ă) [″ + *melos,* limb] Abnormally small or short limbs.

**micromelus** (mī-krŏm′ĕ-lŭs) [″ + *melos,* limb] One who has abnormally small or short limbs.

**micromere** (mī′krō-mēr) [″ + *meros,* part] A small blastomere.

**micrometer** ABBR: $\mu$m. **1.** (mī′krō-mē-ter) One millionth of a meter ($10^{-6}$); one thousandth of a millimeter (0.001 mm). SYN: *micron.* **2.** (mī-krŏm′ĕ-tĕr) Device used for measuring small distances.

**micromethod** (mī″krō-mĕth′ŏd) Any chemical or physical procedure involving small amounts of material or tissue.

**micrometry** (mī-krŏm′ĕ-trē) [″ + *metron,* measure] Use of device, esp. a micrometer, to measure small objects or thickness.

**micromicro- (**$\mu\mu$**)** Prefix formerly used to indicate one trillionth ($10^{-12}$). The term currently used is *pico.*

**micromicrogram** (mī″krō-mī′krō-grăm) ABBR: $\mu\mu$g. One millionth of a microgram. Now called a picogram, or $10^{-12}$ gram.

**micromicron** (mī″krō-mī′krŏn) ABBR: $\mu\mu$. Former name for picometer or $10^{-12}$ meter.

**micromillimeter** (mī-krō-mĭl′ĭ-mē-tĕr) ABBR: $\mu$mm. One millionth of a millimeter. SYN: *millimicron.*

**micromole** (mī′krō-mōl) One millionth, $10^{-6}$, of a mole. SEE: *mole* (1).

**micromolecular** (mī″krō-mō-lĕk′ū-lăr) Composed of small molecules.

**Micromonospora** (mī″krō-mō-nŏs′por-ă) A genus of actinomycetes belonging to the family Streptomycetaceae.

**micromyelia** (mī″krō-mī-ē′lē-ă) [″ + *myelos,* marrow] Abnormally small-sized or short spinal cord.

**micromyeloblast** (mī-krō-mī′ĕl-ō-blăst) [″ + *myelos,* marrow, + *blastos,* germ] A small, immature myelocyte, often the predomi-

nating cell in myeloblastic leukemia.
**micromyelolymphocyte** (mī″krō-mī″ĕ-lō-lĭm′fō-sīt) [″ + ″ + L. *lympha,* lymph, + Gr. *kytos,* cell] Micromyeloblast.
**micron** SEE: *micrometer* (1).
**microneedle** Extremely minute needle used in a micromanipulator for microdissection.
**micronize** To pulverize a substance into particles only a few micra in size.
**micronodular** (mī″krō-nŏd′ū-lăr) Having small nodules.
**micronucleus** (mī-krō-nū′klē-ŭs) *pl.* **micronuclei** [″ + L. *nucleus,* kernel] **1.** A small nucleus. **2.** The smaller of the two nuclei of Ciliata considered as containing the inheritable germ substance.
**micronutrient** (mī″krō-nū′trē-ĕnt) An essential nutrient required only in small amounts.
**micronychia** (mī″krō-nĭk′ē-ă) [″ + *onyx,* nail] Possessing abnormally small nails.
**microorganism** (mī-krō-or′găn-ĭzm) [″ + *organon,* organ, + *-ismos,* condition] Minute living body not perceptible to the naked eye, esp. a bacterium or protozoon.

Microorganisms may be carried from one host to another as follows:

*Animal sources:* Some organisms are pathogenic for animals as well as humans and may be communicated to humans through direct, indirect, or intermediary animal hosts.

*Airborne:* Pathogenic microorganisms in the respiratory tract may be discharged from the mouth or nose into the air and settle on food, dishes, or clothing. They may carry infection if they resist drying.

*Contact infections:* Direct transmission of bacteria from one host to another, as in sexually transmitted diseases.

*Foodborne:* Food and water may contain pathogenic organisms acquired from the handling the food by infected persons or through fecal or insect contamination.

*Fomites:* Inanimate objects such as linens, books, cooking utensils, or clothing that can harbor microorganisms and could serve to transport them from one location to another.

*Human carriers:* Persons who have recovered from an infectious disease remain carriers of the organism causing the infection and may transfer the organism to another host.

*Insects:* Insects may be physical carriers, such as the housefly, or act as intermediate hosts, such as the Anopheles mosquito.

*Soilborne:* Spore-forming organisms in the soil may enter the body through a cut or wound. Vegetables and fruits, esp. root crops, need thorough cleansing before being eaten raw.

***pathologic m.*** Any disease-causing microorganism. Includes rickettsias, bacteria, viruses, spirochetes, yeasts, molds, protozoons, and some helminths.

**micropannus** Pathological condition in which a vascular sheet of tissue covers the corner of the eye. SEE: *pannus.*
**microparasite** (mī″krō-păr′ă-sīt) A parasitic microorganism.
**micropathology** (mī″krō-păth-ŏl′ō-jē) [Gr. *mikros,* small, + *pathos,* disease, + *logos,* word, reason] The use of a microscope to study diseases caused by microorganisms.
**micropenis** (mī″krō-pē′nĭs) An abnormally small penis. SYN: *microphallus.*
**microphage, microphagus** (mī′krō-fāj, mī-krŏf′ă-gŭs) [″ + *phagein,* to eat] A small phagocyte.
**microphagocyte** (mī″krō-făg′ō-sīt) [″ + ″ + *kytos,* cell] Microphage.
**microphakia** (mī″krō-fā′kē-ă) [″ + *phakos,* lens] Abnormally small crystalline lens. SYN: *microlentia.*
**microphallus** (mī-krō-făl′ŭs) [″ + *phallos,* penis] Micropenis.
**microphobia** (mī-krō-fō′bē-ă) [″ + *phobos,* fear] Abnormal fear of small objects.
**microphone** (mī′krō-fōn) [″ + *phone,* voice] Device for detecting and converting sound energy into an electronic signal, which is then transmitted.
**microphonia** (mī-krō-fō′nē-ă) Weakness of the voice.
**microphonoscope** (mī″krō-fō′nō-skōp) [Gr. *mikros,* small, + *phone,* voice, + *skopein,* to examine] Form of binaural stethoscope for magnifying sound.
**microphotograph** (mī″krō-fō′tō-grăf) [″ + *phos,* light, + *graphein,* to write] **1.** A photograph of extremely small size. **2.** A photograph on microfilm. **3.** A photomicrograph.
**microphthalmia, microphthalmus** (mī-krŏf-thăl′mē-ă, -mŭs) [″ + *ophthalmos,* eye] Abnormally small size of one or both eyes.
**micropipette, micropipet** An extremely small pipette used for measuring small amounts of fluid substances.
**microplasia** (mī″krō-plā′zē-ă) [″ + *plassein,* to form] Failure to attain full size, as in dwarfism.
**microplethysmography** (mī″krō-plĕth″ĭs-mŏg′ră-fē) [″ + *plethysmos,* increase, + *graphein,* to write] Detection of small changes in the volume of a part due to alteration in blood flow.
**micropodia** (mī-krō-pō′dē-ă) [″ + *pous,* feet] Unusually small size of the feet.
**micropolariscope** (mī″krō-pōl-ăr′ĭ-skōp) A microscope with a polarizer.
**microprobe** (mī′krō-prōb) A very small probe, suitable for use in microsurgery.
**microprojection** Projection of images of microscopic objects upon a screen.
**microprosopia** (mī″krō-prō-sō′pē-ă) [″ + *prosopon,* face] Abnormal smallness of the face.
**micropsia** (mī-krŏp′sē-ă) [″ + *opsis,* vision] Visual disorder in which objects seem smaller than they actually are. Seen in paralysis of accommodation, retinitis, and choroiditis.
**micropuncture** (mī″krō-pŭnk′chŭr) A very

small incision or puncture of a structure such as a single cell.

**micropus** (mī-krō′pŭs) [″ + *pous,* feet] One with unusually small feet.

**micropyle** (mī′krō-pīl) [″ + *pyle,* gate] The opening in the ovum for entrance of the spermatozoon. Seen in the ova of some animals.

**microradiography** (mī″krō-rā″dē-ŏg′ră-fē) Technique of x-raying microscopic objects. The pictures are usually enlarged.

**microrefractometer** (mī″krō-rē″frăk-tŏm′ĕ-tĕr) Refractometer used to study cells, esp. red blood cells.

**microrespirometer** (mī″krō-rĕs″pĭ-rŏm′ĕ-tĕr) Device for measuring oxygen consumption of minute amounts of tissue.

**microrhinia** (mī″krō-rĭn′ē-ă) [″ + *rhis,* nose] Abnormal smallness of the nose.

**microscelous** (mī-krŏs′kĕ-lŭs) [″ + *skelos,* leg] Having abnormally short legs.

**microscope** (mī′krō-skōp) [″ + *skopein,* to examine] Optical instrument that greatly magnifies minute objects. **microscopic, microscopical** (mī-krō-skŏp′ĭk, -ĭ-kăl), *adj.*

***binocular m.*** A microscope possessing two eyepieces or oculars.

***compound m.*** A microscope with two or more lenses or lens systems for use in observing very small bodies.

***dark-field m.*** A microscope by which objects invisible through an ordinary microscope may be seen by means of powerful side illumination. SYN: *ultramicroscope.* SEE: *illumination, dark-field.*

***electron m.*** A microscope that uses streams of electrons deflected from their course by an electrostatic or electromagnetic field for the magnification of objects. The final image is viewed on a fluorescent screen or recorded on a photographic plate. Because of greater resolution, images may be magnified up to 400,000 diameters. SEE: *scanning electron m.*

***light m.*** A microscope that uses ordinary light to allow viewing of the object.

***operating m.*** A microscope designed for use during surgery involving small tissue such as nerves, vessels, the inner ear, or fallopian tubes. SEE: *microsurgery.*

***phase m.*** A compound microscope to which a diffraction or phase plate and a specialized condenser diaphragm have been added. These additional elements make it possible to view details of objects characterized by differences in refractive index and thus delineate a change of phase, such as brightness or color. This microscope is particularly useful for viewing living cells and observing cytoplasmic organelles. Buccal smears of desquamated epithelial cells, food debris, and spirochetes viewed through this microscope easily convince dental patients that better oral hygiene is essential.

***polarization m.*** A microscope for examining specimens that polarize light or have double refraction.

***scanning electron m.*** ABBR: SEM. An electron microscope that scans the image point by point and displays the image on a photographic film or television screen. The SEM, unlike other types of microscopes, allows a three-dimensional view of the tissue, and tissues do not need to be extensively handled and prepared in order to be visualized. The magnification ranges from 20 to 100,000 times.

***simple m.*** A microscope with a single magnifying lens.

***slit-lamp m.*** A microscope with slit illumination for examining the eye, esp. the cornea.

***stereoscopic m.*** A binocular microscope with an objective lens for each eyepiece, permitting objects to be viewed stereoscopically.

***ultraviolet m.*** A microscope using ultraviolet radiations as a light source and having an optical system for transmitting them. Used in observing specimens that fluoresce, such as tissues stained with a fluorescent dye.

***x-ray m.*** A microscope using x-rays to reveal the structure of objects through which light cannot pass. The image is usually reproduced on film.

**microscopy** (mī-krŏs′kŏp-ē) Inspection with a microscope.

**microsecond** (mī′krō-sĕk″ŭnd) One-millionth ($10^{-6}$) of a second.

**microseme** (mī′krō-sēm) [Gr. *mikros,* small, + *sema,* sign] Possessing an orbital index of less than 83.

**microsmatic** (mī″krŏs-măt′ĭk) [″ + *osmasthai,* to smell] Having a poorly developed sense of smell.

**microsome** (mī′krō-sōm) Ribosome.

**microspectrophotometry** (mī″krō-spĕk″trō-fō-tŏm′ĕ-trē) Method for the histochemical study of substances present in cells, such as nucleic acid, based on absorption in the ultraviolet spectrum. This method permits quantitative and qualitative studies of certain cellular components.

**microspectroscope** [″ + L. *spectrum,* image, + Gr. *skopein,* to examine] A combined spectroscope and microscope.

**microsphere** Minute container suitable for implantation or injection into the body or circulatory system. Microspheres may be used for delivering medicines to certain sites or, if radioactive, to study the blood flow to an area. If microspheres are used as a drug-delivery system, the container is designed to be dissolved in body fluids.

***magnetic m.'s*** Microscopic magnetic particles that are used experimentally in autologous bone marrow transplant. The particles are coated with or coupled to antibodies and exposed to certain types of malignant cells in order to bind to them. The microspheres so bound can be removed by passing the cells through a magnetic field.

**microspherocyte** (mī″krō-sfē′rō-sīt) [″ +

*sphaira,* globe, + *kytos,* cell] Small, sphere-shaped red blood cells seen in certain kinds of anemia.

**microspherocytosis** (mī″krō-sfē″rō-sī-tō′sĭs) [″ + ″ + *osis,* condition] Spherocytosis; marked by an excessive number of microspherocytes.

**microsplanchnic** (mī″krō-splănk′nĭk) Having a relatively small abdominal cavity in comparison with the rest of the body.

**microsplenia** (mī-krō-splē′nē-ă) [″ + *splen,* spleen] Abnormal smallness of the spleen.

**microsporid** (mī-krŏs′pō-rĭd) A skin eruption distant from the site of infection with *Microsporum* and due to hypersensitivity to the organism.

**microsporidiosis** Intracellular spore-forming protozoa that infect many animals and are known to cause human disease, esp. in those with AIDS. The genera of microsporidia implicated are *Encephalitozoon, Pleistophora, Septata, Nosema,* and *Enterocytozoon.* They may be related to a variety of pathological conditions, including diarrhea, wasting, keratoconjunctivitis, peritonitis, myositis, and hepatitis. Treatment is symptomatic. There is no known specific therapy.

**microsporosis** (mī″krō-spō-rō′sĭs) Ringworm infection due to fungi of the genus *Microsporum.*

**Microsporum** (mī″krŏs′por-ŭm) A genus of fungi that causes disease of the skin, hair, and nails.

***M. audouini*** The causative agent of tinea capitis (ringworm of scalp).

***M. canis*** The causative agent of ringworm in cats and dogs. It may be easily transmitted to children.

**microstomia** (mī-krō-stō′mē-ă) [″ + *stoma,* mouth] Abnormal smallness of the mouth.

**microstrabismus** (mī″krō-stră-bĭs′mŭs) [″ + *strabismos,* a squinting] Movement of the eyes in divergent directions or at different speeds. These movements are too small and too quick to be seen, but they have been detected through analysis of high-speed motion pictures.

**microsurgery** Surgery in which various types of magnification, specialized instrumentation, fine sutures, and meticulous techniques are used to repair, anastomose, or restore tissues.

**microthelia** (mī″krō-thē′lē-ă) [″ + *thele,* nipple] Abnormal smallness of nipples.

**microtia** (mī-krō′shē-ă) [″ + *ous,* ear] Unusually small size of the auricle or external ear.

**microtome** (mī′krō-tōm) [″ + *tome,* incision] Instrument for preparing thin sections of tissue for microscopic study. SYN: *histotome.*

***freezing m.*** Microtome equipped to cut frozen tissues.

***sliding m.*** Microtome in which the tissue being sectioned slides along a track.

**microtomy** (mī-krŏt′ō-mē) The process of incising thin sections of tissues.

**microtonometer** (mī″krō-tō-nŏm′ĕ-tĕr) Device for determining oxygen and carbon dioxide concentration in blood.

**microtrauma** (mī″krō-traw′mă) A very small lesion.

**microtropia** (mī″krō-trō′pē-ă) [″ + *trope,* a turning] Strabismus with very small deviation, usually less than 4°.

**microtubule** (mī″krō-tū′būl) An elongated (200 to 300 Å), hollow or tubular structure present in the cell. Microtubules are important in helping certain cells maintain their rigidity, in converting chemical energy into work, and in providing a means of transporting substances in different directions within a cell. They increase in number during mitosis.

**microtus** (mī-krō′tŭs) [″ + *ous,* ear] Individual with very small ears.

**microvasculature** (mī″krō-văs′kū-lă-chur) The very fine blood vessels of the body. **microvascular** (mī″krō-văs′kū-lăr), *adj.*

**microvillus** (mī″krō-vĭl′ŭs) *pl.* **microvilli** [L., tuft of hair] A microscopic fold from the free surface of a cell membrane. Microvilli greatly increase the exposed surface area of the cell. SEE: *border, brush.*

**microvolt** One millionth of a volt.

**microwave** (mī′krō-wāv) That portion of the radio wave spectrum between a wavelength of 1 mm and 30 cm.

***m. oven*** An oven that uses microwave energy for cooking food. This method of food preparation may not kill microorganisms, esp. when used to reheat.

**miction** (mĭk′shŭn) Urination.

**micturate** (mĭk′tū-rāt) [L. *micturire*] To pass urine from the bladder. SYN: *urinate.*

**micturition** (mĭk-tū-rĭ′shŭn) Urination.

**micturition syncope** SEE: under *syncope.*

**MICU** *medical intensive care unit.*

**MID** *minimum infective dose.*

**midazolam hydrochloride** A benzodiazepine used to produce sedation for brief diagnostic or endoscopic procedures and as sedation prior to general anesthesia. Use of this drug has been associated with respiratory depression and respiratory arrest. If given intravenously, it should be used in a setting in which continuous monitoring of respiratory and cardiac function is done. Resuscitative drugs and trained personnel should be immediately available.

**midbody** (mĭd′bŏd-ē) Microtubules that appear as a granule between daughter cells during telophase of mitosis.

**midbrain** [AS. *mid,* middle, + *braegen,* brain] The corpora quadrigemina, the crura cerebri, and aqueduct of Sylvius, which connect the pons and cerebellum with the hemispheres of the cerebrum. It contains reflex centers for eye and head movements in response to visual and auditory stimuli. SYN: *mesencephalon.*

**midcarpal** (mĭd-kăr′păl) **1.** Between the two rows of carpal bones. **2.** Mediocarpal.

**middle age** An imprecise term indicating

someone is about 40 to 60 years of age.

**middle lobe syndrome** Atelectasis, bronchiectasis, or chronic pneumonitis of the middle lobe of the right lung, possibly due to calcified lymph nodes compressing the right middle lobe bronchus.

**midge** (mĭj) [ME. *migge*] Small, gnat-like flies including those from the families Chironomidae and Ceratopogonidae. Some cause painful bites.

**midget** A nontechnical term for a very small person; an adult who is perfectly formed but has not attained and will not attain normal size.

**midgut** [AS. *mid,* middle, + *gut,* intestine] The midportion of the embryonic gut that opens ventrally into the yolk stalk.

**midline** (mĭd'līn) Any line that bisects a structure that is bilaterally symmetrical.

**midoccipital** (mĭd"ŏk-sĭp'ĭ-tăl) In the middle of the occiput.

**midpain** (mĭd'pān) Intermenstrual pain. SEE: *mittelschmerz.*

**midplane** (mĭd'plān) **1.** The plane bisecting a symmetrical structure. **2.** In obstetrics, the plane of least dimensions in the pelvic outlet.

**midriff** (mĭd'rĭf) [" + *hrif,* belly] The diaphragm; the middle region of the torso.

**midsection** (mĭd-sĕk'shŭn) [" + L. *secare,* to cut] A section through the middle of a structure.

**midsternum** (mĭd-stĕr'nŭm) The largest and middle portion of the sternum.

**midstream specimen** A urine specimen collected during the passage of the urine after the flow has begun and prior to the end. It is done to obtain a specimen with little contamination from bacteria in the urethra.

**midtarsal** (mĭd-tăr'săl) Between the two rows of bones that make up the tarsus of the foot.

**midwife** [" + *wif,* wife] SEE: *nurse midwife.*

**midwifery** (mĭd-wīf'ĕr-ē) The practice of assisting at childbirth. SYN: *obstetrics.*

**MIF** *maximum inspiratory force.*

**mifepristone** An antiprogesterone steroid used as an abortifacient. SYN: *RU 486.*

**migraine** (mī'grān) [Fr. from Gr. *hemikrania,* half skull] A familial disorder marked by periodic, usually unilateral, pulsatile headaches that begin in childhood or early adult life and tend to recur with diminishing frequency in later life. There are two closely related syndromes comprising what is known as migraine. They are classic migraine (migraine with aura) and common migraine (migraine without aura). The classic type may begin with aura, which consists of episodes of well-defined, transient focal neurologic dysfunction that develops over the course of minutes and may last an hour. Visual symptoms include seeing stripes, spots, or lines and scotomata. In most people, the aura precedes the headache; however, occasionally the aura will appear or recur at the height of the headache. Prior to the onset of symptoms, some persons experience mood changes, fatigue, difficulty thinking, depression, sleepiness, hunger, thirst, urinary frequency, or altered libido. Others report a feeling of well-being, increased energy, clarity of thought, and increased appetite, esp. for sweets. The headache follows. Pain usually is confined on one side but occasionally is bilateral. Nausea and vomiting may be present and may last a few hours or a day or two. Common migraine has a similar onset with or without nausea. Light and noise sensitivity are present in both types. In the general population, migraine is present in an estimated 3.5% of males and 7.4% of females. During their reproductive years, women experience a much higher rate of migraine, and their headaches tend to occur during periods of premenstrual tension and fluid retention. Many patients link their attacks to ingesting certain foods, exposure to glare, or to sudden changes in barometric pressure. SEE: *Nursing Diagnoses Appendix.*

ETIOLOGY: A family history of migraine will be found in over half of the patients. Migraine may be precipitated by allergic hypersensitivity or emotional disturbances. At one time, it was believed that red wine was less likely than white wine to be tolerated by persons with migraine because of a higher concentration of tyramine in red wine. It is now known that tyramine is present in about the same concentration in both red and white wine. However, phenolic flavonoids are much higher in red wine than in white wine. This may account for persons with migraine tolerating white wine better than red wine. In cases of migraine with aura, there is reduced regional cerebral blood flow in the posterior portion of the cerebral hemisphere, usually on the same side as the headache.

DIAGNOSIS: The International Headache Society (IHS) defines migraine without aura as at least five attacks unrelated to organic disease, with a duration of 4 to 72 hr, and pain characterized by at least two of the following: unilateral location, pulsating quality, moderate to severe intensity, or aggravation by routine physical activity; and at least one associated symptom: nausea and vomiting, or photophobia and phonophobia (sensitivity to noise). The IHS defines migraine with aura as at least two attacks unrelated to organic disease with at least one reversible aura symptom indicating focal cerebral cortical or brainstem dysfunction; at least one symptom developing over more than 4 min, or two or more symptoms in succession; and no single aura symptom lasting more than 60 min. The headache may precede, be concurrent with, or follow (within 60 min) the aura.

TREATMENT: The best therapy is prevention. Ideally, migraine is prevented by taking ergotamine tartrate and promethazine daily. These drugs will prevent migraines in more than 50% of patients treated. Acute attacks that are mild may be controlled with acetylsalicylic acid, an equivalent amount of another nonnarcotic analgesic, or small doses of codeine. For severe attacks, ergotamine tartrate is effective. If nausea and vomiting are a problem, the drug may be given subcutaneously or intramuscularly, or an uncoated tablet of ergotamine tartrate may be held under the tongue until it is dissolved. This may be repeated every half hour until the headache is gone or a total of 8 mg is taken. Ergotamine may also be administered by inhaler or rectal suppository. A single dose of promethazine (Phenergan) will help prevent side effects and relax the patient. If this regimen fails, codeine or Demerol will control the pain. Pregnant patients and those with vascular disease should not be given ergotamine because of the danger of arterial spasm. Sumatriptan is a suitable alternative to ergotamine therapy.

NURSING IMPLICATIONS: The nurse monitors the nature and character of the patient's pain, helps the patient to relax by creating a quiet environment, and teaches the patient techniques for coping with discomfort. Prescribed medications are administered and evaluated for desired effects and any adverse reactions. To enhance the effects of medications and pain relief, noninvasive pain relief measures should be instituted before pain becomes severe.

**migration** (mī-grā′shŭn) [L. *migrare,* to move from place to place] Movement from one location to another. **migratory,** *adj.*

***internal m. of ovum*** Passage of the ovum from the ovary through the fallopian tube to the uterus.

***m. of leukocytes*** Passage of white blood corpuscles through walls of capillaries. SYN: *diapedesis.*

***m. of teeth*** The movement of teeth during eruption or out of their normal position in the dental arch because of periodontal disease or missing adjacent teeth.

***m. of testicle*** Descent of testicle into the scrotum. SYN: *descensus testis.*

**mikro-** SEE: words beginning with *micro-*.

**Mikulicz's drain** (mĭk′ū-lĭch″ĕs) [Johann von Mikulicz-Radecki, Polish surgeon, 1850–1905] A large-scale capillary drain that also serves as a tampon to arrest bleeding. It consists of a tubular piece of iodoform gauze of requisite size, placed in a cavity and filled with narrow strips of plain gauze until the necessary degree of compression is secured. This is used if there is parenchymatous oozing. SYN: *Mikulicz's tampon.*

**Mikulicz's mask** Gauze-covered frame worn over nose and mouth during performance of operation.

**Mikulicz's pad** Folded gauze pad for packing off the viscera in abdominal operations and used as a sponge in general.

**Mikulicz's syndrome** Chronic infiltration with lymphocytes and painless enlargement of lacrimal and salivary glands.

**mildew** [AS. *mildeaw*] Lay term for a discoloration or superficial coating on various materials caused by the growth of fungi. Occurs in damp conditions.

**milia** (mĭl′ē-ă) Pl. of milium.

**miliaria** (mĭl-ē-ā′rē-ă) [L. *milium,* millet] The blockage of sweat glands due to bacterial damage of cells in the lumen. This blockage causes sweat to escape into the epidermis. The tiny blisters that form may go unnoticed; however, as the sweat penetrates deeper in the epidermis, the area becomes painful and itching is intense. Acute inflammation of the sweat glands will result if the obstruction persists. The three forms of miliaria (sudamina, rubra, and profunda) represent different levels of obstruction of the sweat glands. SYN: *heat rash; miliaria rubra; prickly heat.* SEE: illus.

SYMPTOMS: The sudden appearance of patches of small, red papules. The patches usually appear on the trunk and are accompanied by itching, burning, and fever of short duration. The papules may become eczematous if irritated.

ETIOLOGY: Exposure to excessive heat, skin irritants, immoderate clothing, and tendency to hyperhidrosis.

TREATMENT: Cool and dry the area, and avoid conditions that cause sweating. Calamine lotion helps to relieve symptoms. **miliary** (mĭl′ē-ă-rē), *adj.*

***apocrine m.*** Fordyce-Fox disease.

***m. crystallina*** Sudamen.

***m. profunda*** Form of miliaria seen almost exclusively in the tropics, frequently following attacks of miliaria rubra. The

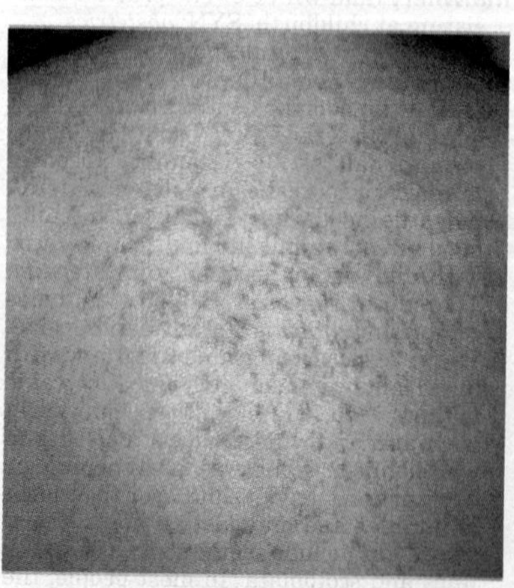

**MILIARIA**
SKIN OF BACK

affected area is covered with pale, firm, painless papules 1 to 3 mm across. These papules do not cause itching.

**miliary tubercle** SEE: under *tubercle.*

**miliary tuberculosis** SEE: under *tuberculosis.*

**milieu** (mē-lyŭ') [Fr.] Environment.

***m. interieur*** Internal environment of the extracellular fluids of the body.

**milieu therapy** SEE: under *therapy.*

**military antishock trousers** ABBR: MAST. SEE: *anti-G suit.*

**milium** (mĭl'ē-ŭm) *pl.* **milia** [L., millet seed] White pinhead-size, keratin-filled cyst. In the newborn, milia occur on the face and, less frequently, on the trunk, and usually disappear within several weeks. Treatment consists of the use of mechanical keratolytics (pumice stone, soap), salicylic acid and sulfur ointment, or incision and expression of contents.

***colloid m.*** Tiny papule formed beneath the epidermis due to colloid degeneration.

**milk** [AS. *meolc*] A secretion of the mammary glands for the nourishment of the young. The amount of food substances vary from animal to animal.

COMPOSITION: Milk from cows consists of water, organic substances, and mineral salts. *Organic substances:* Proteins: The principal proteins are caseinogen, lactoalbumin, and lactoglobulin; in the presence of calcium ions, soluble caseinogen is converted into insoluble casein by the action of acids, rennet, or pepsin. This brings about the curdling of milk. Lactoglobulin is identical with serum globulin of the blood and hence contains maternal antibodies. Carbohydrates: Lactose (milk sugar) is the principal sugar, although small quantities of other sugars are present. Fats: The principal fats are glycerides of oleic, palmitic, and myristic acids. Smaller quantities of stearic acid and short-chain fatty acids with carbon chains of $C_4$ to $C_{24}$ are present. Sterols and phosphatides (lecithin and cephalin) are also present. Churning causes the fat globules to unite into a solid mass and separate from the whey to form butter. *Mineral salts:* The principal cations are calcium, potassium, and sodium; the principal anions are phosphate and chloride. Citrates and lactates are present in small quantities. Milk is low in iron and magnesium.

*Vitamins:* Vitamin A and those of the B complex (thiamine, riboflavin, and pantothenic acid) are present in adequate quantities to meet the needs of a growing child. Milk is low in vitamins C and D.

On standing at room temperature for several hours, milk sours as a result of the action of lactic acid bacilli on lactose converting it into lactic acid. When the pH reaches 5.34, coagulation occurs, resulting in production of a curd. The remaining watery portion is called whey.

Milk contains antibodies that are present in the mother's blood and a number of enzymes (catalase, oxidase, reductase, phosphatase).

***acidophilus m.*** Milk inoculated with *Lactobacillus acidophilus,* a bacterium that grows best in an acid medium. Acidophilus milk is used to modify the bacterial flora of the digestive tract in persons with gastrointestinal disorders.

***breast m.*** Milk obtained from the mammary glands of the human breast. Human breast milk that is collected and refrigerated immediately may be used for up to 5 days. If it is collected, frozen, and stored at −17.7°C (0°F), it is safe for 6 months.

***butter m.*** That portion of milk left after removal of butter following churning.

***casein m.*** Milk prepared with a large quantity of casein and fat but little sugar and salts.

***condensed m.*** Partly evaporated and sweetened milk.

***cow's m.*** Milk obtained from cows.

***evaporated m.*** Cow's milk that has been concentrated by evaporating some of the water. It can be canned after pasteurization and stored for long periods of time. SEE: *lactic acid evaporated m.*

***goat's m.*** Milk obtained from goats and given to infants who cannot tolerate cow's milk. It should be pasteurized before use.

***homogenized m.*** Milk that has been processed in such as manner that fats are combined with the body of the milk and the cream does not separate.

***instant dry nonfat m.*** Dried skimmed milk that may be stored at room temperature until needed and then reconstituted by adding water to the granules.

***lactic acid evaporated m.*** Evaporated milk to which sugar and lactic acid have been added. To prepare this milk, add 17 oz (503 ml) of water to 13 oz (384 ml) of evaporated milk, 2 level tbsp (1 oz or 28 g) of granulated sugar, and 3 tbsp (45 ml) of vinegar. This mixture contains 77 Cal per 100 ml and may be used for normal infants from birth to 12 months. The sugar is omitted for older children, which reduces the calories to about 67 per 100 ml (20 per ounce).

***low fat m. 1%*** Cow's milk with 1% fat, which represents 22% of the calories.

***low fat m. 2%*** Cow's milk with 2% fat, which represents 35% of the calories.

***modified m.*** Milk altered so that its composition more closely approximates that of human milk.

***mother's m.*** Breast m.

***nonfat m.*** Skim m.

***pasteurized m.*** Milk heated to a specified temperature for a precise length of time and then cooled rapidly. This process kills pathogenic bacteria without appreciably altering the taste of the milk. SEE: *pasteurization.*

***protein m.*** Milk modified to be high in protein and low in carbohydrate and fat content.

***red m.*** Milk contaminated by blood,

chromogenic bacteria, or plant pigments.

***ropy m.*** Milk that has become viscid due to formation of vegetable gums from carbohydrates or mucin-like substances from proteins as a result of bacterial action.

***skim m.*** Cow's milk from which the fat has been removed.

***sour m.*** Milk with lactic acid caused by lactic acid-producing bacteria.

***sterilized m.*** Milk that has been boiled to kill bacteria.

***vegetable m.*** **1.** The latex of plants. **2.** A synthetic milk prepared from juices of various plants, such as soybean.

***vitamin D m.*** Milk in which vitamin D content has been increased by addition of concentrates, ultraviolet irradiation, or feeding of irradiated yeast to milk-producing animals.

***whole m.*** Milk that has not been altered except for pasteurization. The fat content is 3.3%, which represents 51% of the calories present.

***witch's m.*** Milk secreted by the newly born infant's breast, stimulated by the lactating hormone circulating in the mother.

**milk-alkali syndrome** Elevated blood calcium without an increase in calcium or phosphate in the urine, renal insufficiency, and alkalosis due to prolonged intake of excessive amounts of milk and soluble alkali. This condition is usually found as an undesired side effect of treating a peptic ulcer. SYN: *Burnett's syndrome.*

**milk of bismuth** A suspension of bismuth hydroxide and bismuth subcarbonate in water, used as an antacid. Previously used name was bismuth magma.

**milker's nodules** SEE: under *nodule.*

**milk fever** Fever due to infection suffered during the puerperium.

**milking** Removal of the contents of a tubular structure, such as the urethra, by compressing the tube with the fingers and moving them along the course of the tube and away from the origin of the urethra. This maneuver forces material out of the tube that might not otherwise be seen or available for study. SEE: *strip.*

**milk leg** Phlegmasia alba dolens.

**milk of magnesia** Magnesium hydroxide in suspension, used as an antacid and a cathartic. Previously used name was magnesia magma.

**Milkman's syndrome** (mĭlk′mănz) [Louis A. Milkman, U.S. roentgenologist, 1895–1951] Failure of reabsorption of phosphate by the renal tubules. This failure causes a special type of demineralization of bones that produces a transverse striped area of multiple pseudofractures in roentgenograms of the bones.

**milk teeth** SEE: under *teeth.*

**milk tumor** Retention of milk in the mammary gland.

**Miller-Abbott tube** [Thomas Grier Miller, U.S. physician, 1886–1981; William Osler Abbott, U.S. physician, 1902–1943] A double-channel intestinal tube used to relieve intestinal obstruction. Inserted through a nostril, the tube is passed through the stomach into the small intestine.

**Miller Assessment for Preschoolers** [Lucy Jane Miller, Ph.D., contemporary occupational therapist] ABBR: M.A.P. A widely used standardized developmental screening test for youngsters from 2 to 5 years of age. It contains sensory, motor, and cognitive performance items.

**milli-** [L. *milli,* thousand] Prefix used in metric system to denote one-thousandth ($10^{-3}$).

**milliammeter** Ammeter registering in milliamperes. SEE: *ammeter.*

**milliampere** (mĭl″ē-ăm′pēr) ABBR: ma. One-thousandth of an ampere.

**milliampere minute** An electrical unit of quantity, equivalent to that delivered by 1 milliampere in 1 min.

**milliampere seconds** ABBR: MAS. In radiography, the milliamperage of the exposure multiplied by the time of the exposure in seconds. This factor determines the exposure of the radiograph.

**millibar** (mĭl′ĭ-băr) One thousandth of a bar, which is 100 newtons/sq m. The normal atmospheric pressure of 14.7 lb/sq in. is equal to 1013 millibars.

**millicoulomb** (mĭl″ĭ-koo′lŏm) ABBR: mC. A unit of electric current, one thousandth ($10^{-3}$) of a coulomb.

**millicurie** (mĭl″ĭ-kū′rē) ABBR: mCi. One thousandth of a curie. A practical unit of dosage for a radioactive source: 1 mCi of a radioactive substance applied for 1 hr.

**millicurie-hour** ABBR: mCi-hr. A practical unit of dosage for radon: 1 mCi of radon applied for 1 hr. The biological effect depends on time, filtration, and distance.

**milliequivalent** ABBR: mEq. One thousandth of a chemical equivalent. The concentration of electrolytes in a certain volume of solution is usually expressed as milliequivalent per liter (mEq/L). It is calculated by multiplying the milligrams per liter by the valence of the chemical and dividing by the molecular weight of the substance.

**milligram** (mĭl′ĭ-grăm) ABBR: mg. One thousandth of a gram.

**millilambert** (mĭl″ĭ-lăm′bĕrt) One thousandth of a lambert, a unit of light intensity. About one foot-candle, but more accurately, it is 0.929 lumens per square foot.

**milliliter** ABBR: ml. One thousandth of a liter. For practical purposes, a milliliter is equivalent to 1 cu cm. The term milliliter (ml) is used when referring to *liquid* volume; cubic centimeter (cc) is used when referring to the volume of a gas.

**millimeter** ABBR: mm. One thousandth of a meter.

**millimicro- (m$\mu$)** Prefix formerly used to indicate one billionth ($10^{-9}$). The term currently used is *nano.*

**millimicrocurie** (mĭl″ĭ-mī″krō-kū′rē) A nanocurie, or $10^{-9}$ curie.

**millimicrogram** (mĭl″ĭ-mī′krō-grăm) A nanogram, or $10^{-9}$ g.

**millimicron** (mĭl-ĭ-mī′krŏn) ABBR: m$\mu$. One thousandth of a micron; one millionth of a millimeter. Nanometer is the preferred term.

**millimole** (mĭl′ĭ-mōl) ABBR: mM or mmol. One thousandth of a mole.

**milling-in** A method of adjusting the occlusion of teeth by moving them against each other while an abrasive substance is between them.

**millinormal** (mĭl″ĭ-nor′măl) The strength of a solution equal to one-thousandth normal.

**milliosmole** (mĭl″ē-ŏs′mōl) One thousandth of an osmole. The osmotic pressure equal to one thousandth of the molecular weight of a substance divided by the number of ions that the substance forms in a liter of solution.

**millipede** (mĭl′ĭ-pēd) A wormlike arthropod with two pairs of legs on each body segment. Some produce an irritating venom.

**millirem** ABBR: mrem. One thousandth of a rem.

**milliroentgen** ABBR: mR. One thousandth of a roentgen.

**millisecond** (mĭl″ĭ-sĕk′ŏnd) One thousandth of a second.

**millivolt** (mĭl′ĭ-vōlt) One thousandth of a volt.

**milphae** (mĭl′fē) [Gr. *milphai*] Loss of eyebrow hair.

**milphosis** (mĭl-fō′sĭs) [Gr.] Loss of eyelashes.

**Milroy's disease** (mĭl′roys) [William Forsyth Milroy, U.S. physician, 1855–1942] Chronic hereditary lymphedema of the legs.

**Milwaukee brace** A brace made of strong, lightweight materials. It extends from a chin cup with neck pad to the pelvis, and is used to correct minimal-curve scoliosis.

**mimesis** [Gr.] Imitation, mimicry. Term applied to a disease that exhibits symptoms of another disease or to conditions in hysteria that simulate organic disease. **mimetic, mimic** (mī-mĕt′ĭk, mĭm′ĭk), *adj.*

**mimmation** (mĭ-mā′shŭn) A form of stuttering in which the "m" sound is inappropriately used.

**min** *minim; minimum; minute.*

**Minamata disease** (mĭn″ă-maw′tă) [Minamata Bay, Japan] A neurological disease due to ingestion of alkyl mercury, an organic mercury compound used in industrial processes. SYN: *yushi.*

SYMPTOMS: Clinical findings are paresthesias, loss of peripheral vision, dysarthria, ataxia, tremors, excessive salivation, sweating, and mental disturbances.

ETIOLOGY: This condition is caused by the ingestion of contaminated seafood.

PROGNOSIS: The prognosis is poor; death may occur.

**mind** [AS. *gemynd*] Psyche. Integration and organization of functions of the brain resulting in the ability to perceive surroundings, to have emotions, imagination, memory, and will, and to process information in an intelligent manner. The quality and quantity of the functions of the mind vary with experience and development.

**mineral** [L. *minerale*] **1.** An inorganic element or compound occurring in nature, esp. one that is solid. **2.** Inorganic; not of animal or plant origin. **3.** Impregnated with minerals, as mineral water. **4.** Pert. to minerals.

**mineral acid** Inorganic acid.

**mineral compounds** Compounds of mineral elements. Many such chemicals are present in the body. SEE: *acid-base balance; buffer.*

FUNCTION: Minerals are essential constituents of all cells; they form the greater portion of the hard parts of the body (bone, teeth, nails); they are essential components of respiratory pigments, enzymes, and enzyme systems; they regulate the permeability of cell membranes and capillaries; they regulate the excitability of muscular and nervous tissue; they are essential for regulation of osmotic pressure equilibria; they are necessary for maintenance of proper acid-base balance; they are essential constituents of secretions of glands; they play an important role in water metabolism and regulation of blood volume.

Mineral salts and water are excreted daily from the body. These must be replaced through food intake. Daily requirements for principal minerals for a normal adult are as follows: calcium and phosphorus, 800 to 1200 mg; copper, 1.5 to 3 mg; iodine, 150 $\mu$g (micrograms); magnesium, 280 to 400 mg; potassium, 2000 mg; sodium, about 500 mg. Daily intake of sodium chloride should be limited to 6 g (2.4 g of sodium) or less each day. Requirements are greater for growing children and pregnant women and in certain pathological conditions. SEE: *Recommended Daily Dietary Allowances Appendix.*

**mineralization** (mĭn″ĕr-ăl-ī-zā′shŭn) Normal or abnormal deposition of minerals in tissues.

**mineralocorticoid** (mĭn″ĕr-ăl-ō-kor′tĭ-koyd) A steroid hormone (e.g., aldosterone) of the adrenal cortex predominantly involved in the regulation of fluid and electrolytes by its effects on ion transport and on the renal tubules.

**mineral oil** SEE: *petrolatum, liquid.*

**mineral spring** A spring in which water contains mineral salts that are thought to have a therapeutic value in certain diseases, but usually the principal action is as a cathartic. SYN: *spa.*

**mineral water** Water that contains sufficient inorganic salts to cause it to have therapeutic properties.
**minification** In radiography, the reduction in the size of a fluoroscopic image to intensify the brightness of that image.
**minim** (mĭn′ĭm) [L. *minimum,* least] ABBR: m; min. One sixtieth of a fluidram, or 0.06 ml.
**minimal** (mĭn′ĭ-măl) Least; the smallest possible.
**minimal brain damage** SEE: *attention-deficit hyperactivity disorder.*
**minimal brain dysfunction** ABBR: MBD. SEE: *attention-deficit hyperactivity disorder.*
**minimal cerebral dysfunction** SEE: *attention-deficit hyperactivity disorder.*
**minimal change disease** SEE: *nephrotic syndrome.*
**Mini–Mental State Examination** ABBR: MMSE. A commonly used assessment tool to quantify a person's cognitive ability. It assesses orientation, registration, attention and calculation, and language. Scoring is from 0 to 30, with 30 indicating intact cognition.
**minimum** (mĭn′ĭ-mŭm) *pl.* **minima** Least quantity or lowest limit. SEE: *threshold.*
**minimum daily requirements** ABBR: MDR. The daily requirements of vitamins and minerals needed to prevent symptoms of deficiency. SEE: *Recommended Daily Dietary Allowances Appendix.*
**Minimum Data Set** ABBR: MDS. A comprehensive computer-compatible form for assessment of nursing home residents covering 13 key clinical areas. It was developed as a result of the Omnibus Reconciliation Act of 1987 and mandated for use in nursing homes in the U.S. Resident assessment protocols are used to identify multiple "triggers" for the assessment of various conditions. The form must be completed within 14 days of admission to a nursing home. SEE: *Nursing Minimum Data Set.*.
**minimum dose** SEE: under *dose.*
**minimum lethal dose** SEE: under *dose.*
**Minin light** (mĭn′ĭn) [A.V. Minin, early 20th century Russian surgeon] A special lamp that produces violet or ultraviolet light.
**mini-stroke** Transient ischemic attack.
**Minnesota Multiphasic Personality Inventory** ABBR: MMPI. SEE: *personality testing.*
**minocycline hydrochloride** (mĭ-nō-sī′klēn) An antibiotic of the tetracycline class.
**minor** A person not of legal age and thus requiring consent for medical, surgical, or dental care. The legal age in the U.S. varies from state to state.

***emancipated m.*** A person not of legal age who is in the armed services, married, the mother of a child whether married or not, or has left home and is self-sufficient. Some state legislatures do not require such an individual to have parental consent to receive medical or surgical care, or advice on contraception or abortion.

**Minot-Murphy diet** (mī′nŏt) [George R. Minot, U.S. physician, 1885–1950; William P. Murphy, U.S. physician, b. 1892] Diet for pernicious anemia containing large quantities of liver.
**minoxidil** A drug used to promote hair growth. Trade name is Rogaine.
**minute volume** SEE: under *volume.*
**mio-** (mī′ō) [Gr. *meion,* less] Combining form meaning *less, smaller.*
**miocardia** (mī-ō-kăr′dē-ă) [″ + *kardia,* heart] Decreasing heart volume during systolic contraction. SYN: *systole.*
**miodidymus** (mī″ō-dĭd′ĭ-mŭs) [″ + *didymos,* twin] A fetus with two heads joined at the occiput.
**miolecithal** (mī″ō-lĕs′ĭ-thăl) [″ + *lekithos,* egg yolk] Pert. to an egg with a small amount of yolk.
**miopus** (mī′ō-pŭs) [″ + *ops,* face] Conjoined twins with one having a rudimentary face.
**miosis** (mī-ō′sĭs) [Gr. *meiosis,* a lessening] Abnormal contraction of the pupils, possibly due to irritation of the oculomotor system or paralysis of dilators. Miosis occurs in certain fevers, congestion of iris, typhus, early stages of meningitis, some forms of drug poisoning, brain lesions, and sunstroke.
**miotic 1.** An agent that causes the pupil to contract, such as eserine or pilocarpine. **2.** Pert. to or causing contraction of the pupil. **3.** Diminishing.
**MIP** *maximum inspiratory pressure.*
**miracidium** (mī″ră-sĭd′ē-ŭm) *pl.* **miracidia** [Gr. *meirakidion,* lad] The ciliated free-swimming larva of a digenetic fluke. On emerging from an ovum, it penetrates a snail of a particular species and metamorphoses into a sporocyst. SEE: *fluke.*
**miracle, medical** The unexplained spontaneous regression of a medical condition thought to be invariably fatal or incurable or both. Such miracles have been claimed after sick persons have visited the shrine in Lourdes, France. The Roman Catholic Church has carefully investigated alleged miracles at Lourdes and has found that since 1858, when the story of Lourdes began, some of the spontaneous regressions meet their criteria for classification as miracles.

Miracles may be negative in that healthy persons may become ill and die without any reasonable explanation.

**mire** (mēr) [L. *mirari,* to look at] A test object on the ophthalmometer, the images of which denote the amount of astigmatism.
**mirror** [Fr. *miroir*] A polished surface that reflects light and thus reproduces visible images of objects in front of it.

***dental m.*** An instrument commonly used for viewing occlusal and distal surfaces of teeth. SYN: *mouth mirror.*

**mirror writing** Writing in which letters and words are reversed and appear as in a mirror.

**miryachit** (mĭr-ē′ă-chĭt) [Russian] A type of "jumping disorder" seen in Siberia, the symptoms of which are similar to those of the Jumping Frenchmen of Maine. Also spelled myriachit. SYN: *saltatory spasm.*

**misandry** [Gr. *miso,* hatred, + *andros,* man] Aversion to or hatred of males. SEE: *misogyny.*

**misanthropy** (mĭs″ăn′thrō-pē) [″ + Gr. *anthropos,* man] Hatred of mankind.

**miscarriage** [″ + L. *carrus,* cart] Lay term for termination of pregnancy at any time before the fetus has attained the potential for extrauterine viability. It usually refers specifically to expulsion of the fetus in the period between fourth month and viability. SYN: *abortion, spontaneous.*

**misce** (mĭs′ē) [L., mix] ABBR: M. A direction on prescriptions that instructs the pharmacist to mix the ingredients.

**miscegenation** (mĭs″ĕ-jē-nā′shŭn) [L. *miscere,* to mix, + *genus,* race] Sexual relations or marriage between those of different races.

**miscible** (mĭs′ĭ-bl) Capable of being mixed.

**misery** Extreme mental or emotional unhappiness.

**misinformation** Data or information concerning a patient that may be assumed erroneously to be accurate (e.g., laboratory data that are inaccurate, historical data from the patient or the family that are unreliable, and transcription errors in recording data). In some instances, misinformation is knowingly presented to, or the truth withheld from, the physician by the patient in order to conceal something that would be personally embarrassing or incriminating.

**misogamy** (mĭ-sŏg′ă-mē) [″ + *gamos,* marriage] Aversion to marriage.

**misogynist** (mĭs-ŏj′ĭ-nĭst) [″ + *gyne,* woman] One who hates women.

**misogyny** (mĭs-ŏj′ĭn-ē) Aversion to or hatred of females. SEE: *misandry.*

**misologia** (mĭs-ō-lō′jē-ă) [Gr. *miseio,* to hate, + *logos,* word, reason] Aversion to mental activity.

**misoneism** (mĭ-sō-nē′ĭzm) [″ + *neos,* new] Aversion to new things or new ideas; conservatism.

**misopedia** (mĭ-sō-pē′dē-ă) [″ + Gr. *pais,* child] Abnormal dislike of children or the young.

**Misoprostol** Anti-ulcerative used as prophylaxis against drug-induced gastrointestinal bleeding. SEE: *nonsteroidal anti-inflammatory drug.*

**misrepresentation** The act of modifying a patient's reports to change the status of his or her condition to facilitate the patient's obtaining benefits such as insurance or disability, or of withholding certain portions of his or her medical history from a third party such as a potential employer. To comply with patient requests such as these is unethical and in some cases is a criminal act.

**mist** Mistura.

**mister** In England and other parts of the British Commonwealth, the title of address of a surgeon.

**mistura** (mĭs-tū′ră) Mixture.

**Mitchell's disease** (mĭch′ĕlz) [Silas Weir Mitchell, U.S. neurologist, 1829–1914] Erythromelalgia.

**mite** (mīt) [AS.] A minute arachnid, a member of the order Acarina. Some mites are parasitic and cause conditions such as asthma, mange, and scabies; some serve as vectors of disease organisms and as intermediate hosts for certain Cestodes.

***dust m.*** A type of mite, *Dermatophagoides pteronyssinum* or *D. farinae,* that ingests shed human skin cells. They are a common cause of allergic reactions, including asthma.

***follicle m.*** A mite that lives in hair follicles and sebaceous glands. SYN: *Demodex folliculorum.*

***harvest m.*** A mite, similar in appearance to scabies, that lives in grain stems, grasses, and bushes. It is common in the southern U.S. The larvae attach to the skin and inject a secretion that causes itching. SYN: *chigger.*

***itch m.*** *Sarcoptes scabiei.* SEE: *scabies.*

***mange m.*** A mite belonging to the families Sarcoptidae and Psoroptidae, and causing mange in many species of animals. SEE: *mange; scabies.*

***red m.*** Redbug or chigger; a member of the family Thrombiculidae. SEE: *chigger.*

**mithridatism** (mĭth′rĭ-dāt″ĭzm) [Mithridates, king of Pontus, 132–63 B.C., supposed to have acquired immunity in this fashion] Immunity to a poison acquired by taking it in doses of gradually increasing size.

**miticide** (mī′tĭ-sīd) [AS. *mite,* mite, + L. *caedere,* to kill] A substance that kills mites.

**mitigated** (mĭt′ĭ-gāt-ĕd) [L. *mitigare,* to soften.] Diminished in severity. SYN: *allayed; moderated.*

**mitis** (mī′tĭs) [L.] Mild.

**mitleiden** Psychosomatic pregnancy-related symptoms of nausea, fatigue, and backache experienced by the expectant father.

**mitochondrion** (mīt″ō-kŏn′drē-ŏn) *pl.* **mitochondria** [Gr. *mitos,* thread, + *chondros,* cartilage] Cell organelles of rod or oval shape 0.5$\mu$m in diameter. They can be seen by using phase-contrast or electron microscopy. They contain the enzymes for the aerobic stages of cell respiration and thus are the sites of most ATP synthesis. SEE: *cell; organelle* for illus.

**mitogen** (mī′tō-jĕn) A plant-derived protein substance that is used in the laboratory to stimulate cell division (mitosis). It is frequently used in vitro to study the proliferation of lymphocytes from blood drawn during a research study. The most commonly used mitogens are phytohemagglutinin and concanavalin A. SEE: *concanavalin A; lectin; phytohemagglutinin.*

***pokeweed m.*** ABBR: PWM. A mitogen

isolated from the pokeweed plant, *Phytolacca americana.* In the presence of T lymphocytes, it has the capacity to induce primed B lymphocytes to proliferate and differentiate into plasma cells. The B lymphocytes are also influenced by PWM.

**mitogenesis** (mī″tō-jĕn′ĕ-sĭs) [″ + *osis,* condition, + *genesis,* generation, birth] The production of cell mitosis.

**mitoma, mitome** [Gr. *mitos,* thread] A fine network support or framework of protoplasm in a cell.

**mitomycin** (mī″tō-mī′sĭn) An antibiotic with antineoplastic action.

**mitoplasm** (mī′tō-plăzm) [″ + *plassein,* to form] The chromatic substance in a cell nucleus.

**mitosis** (mī-tō′sĭs) *pl.* **mitoses** [″ + *osis,* condition] Type of cell division of somatic cells in which each daughter cell contains the same number of chromosomes as the parent cell. Mitosis is the process by which the body grows and dead somatic cells are replaced. Mitosis is a continuous process divided into four phases: prophase, metaphase, anaphase, and telophase. SEE: illus.; *meiosis.*

*Prophase:* the chromatin granules of the nucleus stain more densely and become organized into chromosomes. These first appear as long filaments, each consisting of two identical chromatids, the result of DNA replication. Each pair of chromatids is joined at a region called the centromere, which may be central or toward one end. As prophase progresses, the chromosomes become shorter and more compact and stain densely. The nuclear membrane and the nucleoli disappear. At the same time, the centriole divides and the two daughter centrioles, each surrounded by a centrosphere, move to opposite poles of the cell. They are connected by fine protoplasmic fibrils, which form an achromatic spindle.

*Metaphase:* the chromosomes (paired chromatids) arrange themselves in an equatorial plane midway between the two centrioles.

*Anaphase:* the chromatids (now called daughter chromosomes) diverge and move toward their respective centrosomes. The end of their migration marks the beginning of the next phase.

*Telophase:* the chromosomes at each pole of the spindle undergo changes that are the reverse of those in the prophase, each becoming a long, loosely spiraled thread. The nuclear membrane re-forms and nucleoli reappear. Outlines of chromosomes disappear, and chromatin appears as granules scattered throughout the nucleus and connected by a lightly staining net. The cytoplasm becomes separated into two parts, resulting in two complete cells. This is accomplished in animal cells by constriction in the equatorial region; in plant cells, a cell plate that gives rise to the cell membrane forms in a similar position. The period between two successive divisions is called interphase.

Mitosis is of particular significance in that genes are distributed equally to each daughter cell and a fixed number of chromosomes is maintained in all somatic cells of an organism. **mitotic** (mī-tŏt′ĭk), *adj.*

***heterotypic m.*** The first or reduction division in the maturation of germ cells.

***homeotypic m.*** The second or equational division in the maturation of germ cells.

**mitosome** (mī′tō-sōm) [Gr. *mitos,* thread, + *soma,* body] **1.** Chromatin mass in a cellular nucleus. **2.** A body giving rise to the middle portion of the spermatozoon.

**mitotane** (mī′tō-tān) An adrenal cytotoxic agent that can cause adrenal inhibition without destroying the cells of the adrenal cortex. It is used in treating inoperable adrenocortical carcinoma. Trade name is Lysodren.

**mitral** (mī′trăl) **1.** Pert. to the bicuspid or mitral valve. **2.** Shaped like a miter.

**mitral commissurotomy** Surgical procedure for treating stenosis of the mitral valve of the heart. Patients may undergo an open or a closed procedure. The open procedure involves the use of a cardiopulmonary bypass pump and is considered the treatment of choice.

NURSING IMPLICATIONS: The nurse provides general care for the patient undergoing open heart surgery. The types of access lines and endotrachial and drainage tubes in place after surgery, as well as the reasons for their use, are explained. The type of postoperative pain to be expected is also explained, and the patient is encouraged to report pain before it becomes severe to maintain a comfortable state necessary for healing. The nurse supports the patient and family throughout recovery. After discharge, the patient begins a gradual return to activity. Regular medical follow-up and participation in a cardiac rehabilitation program, if recommened by the physician, should be encouraged.

**mitral disease** Disease of the mitral valve. SEE: *heart.*

**mitralization** (mī″trăl-ī-zā′shŭn) Straightening of the left border of the heart due to mitral valve disease, as seen in the anteroposterior view of an x-ray of the heart.

**mitral murmur** SEE: under *murmur.*

**mitral orifice** SEE: under *orifice.*

**mitral regurgitation** SEE: under *regurgitation.*

**mitral stenosis** Narrowing of the mitral orifice, obstructing free flow from atrium to ventricle. SEE: *Nursing Diagnoses Appendix.*

**mitral valve** The cardiac valve between the left atrium and left ventricle; the bicuspid valve.

**mitral valve prolapse** A common and occasionally serious condition in which the cusp or cusps of the mitral valve prolapse into the left atrium during systole. In patients without evidence of mitral regurgitation, there are usually no symptoms, but in some patients, nonanginal chest pain, palpitations, dyspnea, and fatigue may be present. On auscultation, there is a murmur at the apex that is present during all of systole (holosystolic). Sometimes only a midsystolic click and late systolic murmur are heard.

TREATMENT: Simple prolapse requires no therapy, but if mitral regurgitation is present, antibiotic prophylaxis is indicated during surgical and dental procedures. If heart failure develops, surgery

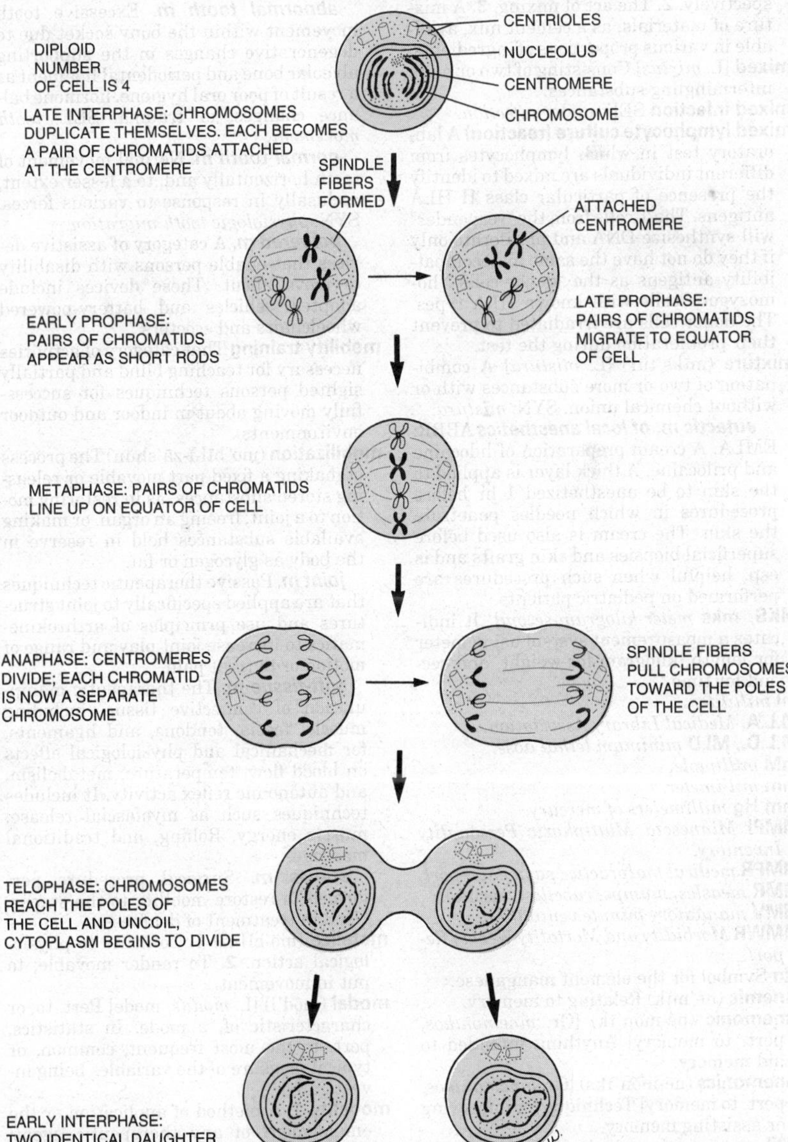

should be considered.

**mittelschmerz** (mĭt'ĕl-shmārts) [Ger.] Abdominal pain midway between menstrual periods, occurring at time of ovulation and from the ovulation site. SYN: *mid-pain.*

**Mittendorf's dot** [20th century U.S. physician] A gray dot on the posterior lens capsule. It is the remnant of the fetal hyaloid artery of the eye.

**mix** (mĭks) [L. *mixtus,* to mix] **1.** To put things, substances, or people together in solution, a collection, or an assembly, respectively. **2.** The act of mixing. **3.** A mixture of materials, as a cement mix, available in various proportions of ingredients.

**mixed** [L. *mixtus*] Consisting of two or more intermingling substances.

**mixed infection** SEE: under *infection.*

**mixed lymphocyte culture (reaction)** A laboratory test in which lymphocytes from different individuals are mixed to identify the presence of particular class II HLA antigens. The T cells from the "responder" will synthesize DNA and proliferate only if they do not have the same histocompatibility antigens as the "donor cells," homozygous cells with known HLA types. The donor cells are irradiated to prevent their proliferation during the test.

**mixture** (mĭks'tūr) [L. *mistura*] A combination of two or more substances with or without chemical union. SYN: *mistura.*

***eutectic m. of local anesthetics*** ABBR: EMLA. A cream preparation of lidocaine and prilocaine. A thick layer is applied to the skin to be anesthetized 1 hr before procedures in which needles penetrate the skin. The cream is also used before superficial biopsies and skin grafts and is esp. helpful when such procedures are performed on pediatric patients.

**MKS, mks** *meter-kilogram-second.* It indicates a measurement system using meter for length, kilogram for weight, and second for time.

**ml** *milliliter.*

**M.L.A.** *Medical Library Association.*

**M.L.D., MLD** *minimum lethal dose.*

**mM** *millimole.*

**mm** *millimeter.*

**mm Hg** *millimeters of mercury.*

**MMPI** *Minnesota Multiphasic Personality Inventory.*

**MMPR** *medical malpractice payment report.*

**MMR** *measles, mumps, rubella* (vaccine).

**MMV** *mandatory minute ventilation.*

**MMWR** *Morbidity and Mortality Weekly Report.*

**Mn** Symbol for the element manganese.

**mnemic** (nē'mĭk) Relating to memory.

**mnemonic** (nē-mŏn'ĭk) [Gr. *mnemonikos,* pert. to memory] Anything intended to aid memory.

**mnemonics** (nē-mŏn'ĭks) [Gr. *mnemonikos,* pert. to memory] Technique for improving or assisting memory.

**MNL** *mononuclear leukocyte* (e.g., monocytes and macrophages).

**M.O.** *Medical Officer.*

**Mo** Symbol for the element molybdenum.

**mo** *month.*

**mobile** [L. *mobilis*] Movable.

**mobile arm support** A device for support of the forearm, usually mounted on a wheelchair, that assists weak shoulder and elbow muscles in positioning the hand, as in feeding. SYN: *balanced forearm orthosis; ball bearing feeder.*

**mobile spasm** Athetosis.

**mobility** [L. *mobilitas*] State or quality of being mobile; facility of movement.

***abnormal tooth m.*** Excessive tooth movement within the bony socket due to degenerative changes in the supporting alveolar bone and periodontal ligament as a result of poor oral hygiene, hormone balance changes, or trauma. SEE: *tooth movement.*

***normal tooth m.*** Normal movement of teeth horizontally and, to a lesser extent, occlusally in response to various forces. SYN: *physiologic tooth migration.*

***powered m.*** A category of assistive devices that enable persons with disability to move about. These devices include adapted vehicles and battery-powered wheelchairs and scooters.

**mobility training** That category of activities necessary for teaching blind and partially sighted persons techniques for successfully moving about in indoor and outdoor environments.

**mobilization** (mō"bĭl-ĭ-zā'shŭn) The process of making a fixed part movable or releasing stored substances, as in restoring motion to a joint, freeing an organ, or making available substances held in reserve in the body as glycogen or fat.

***joint m.*** Passive therapeutic techniques that are applied specifically to joint structures and use principles of arthrokinematics to increase joint play and range of motion or to treat pain.

***soft-tissue m.*** The therapeutic manipulation of connective tissue, including muscle, fascia, tendons, and ligaments, for mechanical and physiological effects on blood flow, temperature, metabolism, and autonomic reflex activity. It includes techniques such as myofascial release, muscle energy, Rolfing, and traditional massage.

***stapes m.*** Surgical procedure performed to restore mobility to the stapes. Used in treatment of deafness.

**mobilize** (mō'bĭl-īz) **1.** To incite to physiological action. **2.** To render movable; to put in movement.

**modal** (mōd'l) [L. *modus,* mode] Pert. to, or characteristic of, a mode. In statistics, pert. to the most frequent, common, or typical measure of the variables being investigated.

**modality** **1.** A method of application or the employment of any therapeutic agent; limited usually to physical agents and devices. **2.** Any specific sensory stimulus such as taste, touch, vision, pressure, or hearing.

***physical agent m.*** A form of therapy used in rehabilitation that produces a change in soft tissue through light, water, temperature, sound, or electricity. These include transcutaneous electrical nerve stimulation units, ultrasound, whirlpool, hot and cold packs, and other modalities.

**mode** (mōd) [L. *modus,* measure, mode] **1.** In statistics, the value or item of the class occurring most frequently in a series of variables. **2.** In respiratory therapy, any of several approaches to continuous mechanical ventilation including volume- and pressure-targeted application with full or partial ventilatory support.

***assist-control m.*** A type of mechanical ventilation with a minimum frequency of respirations determined by ventilator settings. It also permits the patient to initiate ventilation.

***control m.*** Continuous mandatory ventilation using a preset pattern that does not require patient intervention.

**model 1.** A pattern or form used to make a replica, as a cast or impression of teeth in dentistry. **2.** A person or thing worthy of emulation or imitation. **3.** A framework or system for organizing and representing hypotheses or theories.

***animal m.*** The study of anatomy, physiology, or pathology in laboratory animals in order to apply the results to human function and disease.

***conceptual m.*** A set of abstract and general concepts and statements about those concepts. Also called *conceptual framework, conceptual system,* and *paradigm.*

***conceptual m. of nursing*** Nursing m.

***m. of human occupation*** A conceptual framework for viewing occupational therapy practice, aimed at improving the patient's organization of time, overall function, and adaptation as reflected in the performance of occupations. Within this framework, intervention includes strategies for fostering skill development and habit changes through role acquisition, improved self-image, and environmental changes.

***nursing m.*** A conceptual model that refers to global ideas about people, their environments and health, and nursing.

***study m.*** A diagnostic cast of an impression of the dental arches or a part thereof, trimmed with the arches articulated and the edges perpendicular to the occlusal plane. The study model serves as the basis for construction of dental appliances, dentures, or orthodontic treatment.

**modeling** A form of behavior therapy involving the patient's acquisition of social behavior and mental response by following the example of associates, esp. parents and siblings.

**model trimmer** SEE: under *trimmer.*

**moderated** Mitigated.

**modification** (mŏd″ĭ-fĭ-kā′shŭn) The act or result of changing something, such as the shape or character of an object or structure.

**modified jaw thrust** SEE: *jaw thrust, modified.*

**modifier** In medicine, esp. in therapeutics and clinical medicine, use of or addition of something that alters that to which it is added.

***biological response m.*** A substance, such as an interferon, produced in the body that may stimulate the immune system. Such substances may be useful in treating cancer.

**modiolus** (mō-dī′ō-lŭs) [L., hub] Central pillar or axial part of cochlea extending from the base to the apex.

**modulation** (mŏd″ū-lā′shŭn) **1.** The alteration in function or status of something in response to a stimulus or altered chemical or physical environment. **2.** In electronics, the manner in which a signal is used to vary either the amplitude, frequency, or phase of a normally constant carrier signal; a method of coding information onto a carrier.

**modulus** (mŏj′ŭ-lŭs) [L., a small measure] In physics, a constant or coefficient that indicates to what extent a substance possesses some property.

**modus operandi** Method of performing an act.

**Moebius' (Möbius') disease** (mē′bē-ŭs) [Paul J. Moebius, Ger. neurologist, 1853–1907] Migraine accompanied by paralysis of the oculomotor nerves.

**Moebius' sign** A symptom of Graves' disease in which one eye converges and the other diverges when one looks at the tip of one's nose.

**Moebius' syndrome** Maldevelopment of the cranial nerves resulting in unbalanced movements of the facial muscles.

**mogilalia** (mŏj-ĭ-lā′lē-ă) [Gr. *mogis,* with difficulty, + *lalia,* chatter] Any speech defect, as stuttering.

**mogiphonia** (mōj-ĭ-fō′nē-ă) [″ + *phone,* voice] Difficulty in emitting vocal sounds.

**Mohrenheim's space** (mor′ĕn-hīmz) [Baron J. J. Freiherr von Mohrenheim, Austrian surgeon, 1759–1799] Space between the pectoralis major and deltoid muscles just beneath the clavicle.

**Mohs' chemosurgery technique** [Frederic Edward Mohs, U.S. surgeon, 1910–1979] A method of excising tumors of the skin. The tumor tissue is fixed in place and a layer is removed. That portion is then examined microscopically. This procedure is repeated until the entire tumor is removed. Use of this technique ensures complete removal. It is esp. useful in treating basal cell epitheliomas.

**moiety** (moy′ĕ-tē) [Fr. *moitié,* fr. L. *medietas,* middle] **1.** One of two equal parts. **2.** A portion of something that has been divided.

**moist** (moyst) Damp, wet.

**mol** Mole (1).

**molal** (mō′lăl) One mole of solute per kilogram of solvent. SEE: *mole* (1).

**molality** (mō-lăl′ĭ-tē) The number of moles of a solute per kilogram of solvent.

**molar 1.** [L. *molaris,* grinding] A grinding or back tooth, one of three on each side of each jaw. The first permanent molar erupts between 6 and 7 years; the second between the 13th and 16th years. The third molars (wisdom teeth) are extremely variable, usually erupting between 18th and 25th years; however, they may erupt later or not at all. SEE: *dentition* for table; *teeth*. **2.** [L. *moles,* a mass] Pert. to a mass; not molecular. **3.** Pert. to a mole. **4.** Gram-molecule. SYN: *mole* (1).

***impacted m.*** A tooth that is unable to erupt into its place in normal occlusion, usually due to crowding by other teeth. This condition is commonly related to the third molar, or wisdom tooth.

***mulberry m.*** A malformed first molar with dwarfed cusps and aggregations of enamel globules around the surface so that the crown has the appearance of a berry. This condition is seen in congenital syphilis and other diseases.

**molariform** (mŏl-ăr′ĭ-form) Resembling a molar tooth.

**molarity** The number of gram molecular weights (moles) of a substance per liter of solution. Thus 1/M (also expressed as 1 M) means 1 mole of a substance per liter, and 0.1/M indicates 0.1 mole/L.

**molar solution** SEE: under *solution*.

**mold 1.** A fuzzy coating due to growth of a fungus on the surface of decaying vegetable matter or on nonorganic objects. **2.** Any one of a group of parasitic or saprophytic fungi that cause mold, such as black molds (Mucorales) and blue and green molds (Aspergillales), the latter including *Penicillium,* the source of the antibiotic penicillin. **3.** To shape a mass or the container in which the mass is shaped.

**molding 1.** Shaping of the fetal head to adapt itself to the pelvic inlet. **2.** A protective border used in plastic surgery. **3.** The casting of a reproduction.

***border m.*** In dentistry, the shaping of impression material at the edges by the oral tissues.

**mole** (mōl) **1.** [Ger. *Mol,* abbr. for *Molekulargewicht,* molecular weight] In the Système International d' Unités (SI system), 1 mole of a substance contains as many atoms as exist in 0.012 kg of carbon 12. **2.** [L. *moles,* a shapeless mass] A uterine mass arising from a poorly developed or degenerating ovum. **3.** [AS. *mael*] A congenital discolored spot elevated above the surface of the skin. Avoidance of irritation renders most moles harmless. SYN: *nevus*. SEE: illus.; *melanoma; racemose*.

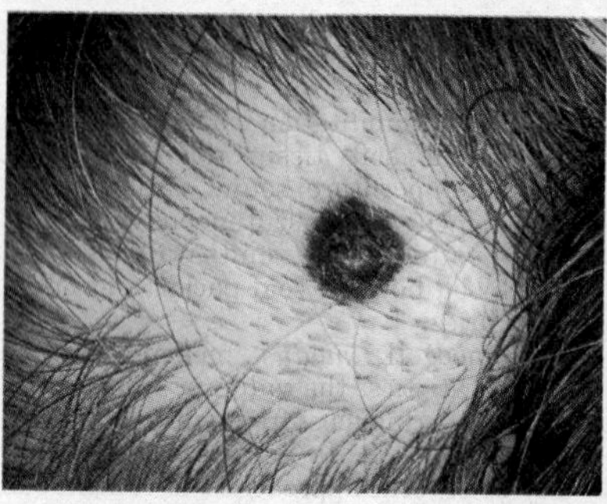

**MOLE ON SCALP**

Caution: Removal of a mole by tying a thread around it should not be attempted. Removal should be done by a physician.

NURSING IMPLICATIONS: The patient is encouraged to regularly inspect areas of the skin that have moles and consult a physician about any mole that changes color or shows signs of growth or changes in appearance, as such changes may indicate neoplasm.

***blood m.*** A mass made up of blood clots, membranes, and placenta, retained following abortion.

***Breus m.*** [Karl Breus, Austrian physician, 1852–1914] Malformation of the ovum; a decidual tuberous subchorional hematoma.

***carneous m.*** Blood mole that assumes a fleshlike appearance when retained in uterus for some time. SYN: *fleshy m.*

***false m.*** Mole formed from a uterine tumor or polypus.

***fleshy m.*** Carneous m.

***hydatid m.*** A polycystic mass in which the chorionic villi have undergone cystic degeneration, resulting in rapid growth of the uterus with hemorrhage. It is thought to be caused by abnormal postfertilization replication of spermatozoal chromosomes. Complete and partial moles differ in karyotype. Complete moles show an absence of ovum chromosomes and a duplication of spermatozoal chromosomes. Partial moles exhibit either karyotype 69 XXY or karyotype 69 XYY due to the presence of the ovum X chromosome.

Signs include a fundal height higher than that consistent with gestational age, absence of fetal heart tones, dark brown to bright red vaginal discharge, expulsion of cystic vesicles, elevated gonadotropin level, hyperemesis gravidarum, and pregnancy-induced hypertension before 24 weeks. Ultrasonography reveals uterine cystic vessels filling the uterus. The treatment is vacuum evacuation of the uterus followed by curettage.

***pigmented m.*** Nevus pigmentosus.

***stone m.*** A fleshy mole that has undergone calcareous degeneration in the uterus.

***true m.*** A mole representing the degenerated embryo or fetus.

***vascular m.*** Hemangioma.

***vesicular m.*** Hydatid m.

**molecular biology** SEE: under *biology*.

**molecular disease** Disease due to a defect in a single molecule. The abnormal hemoglobin molecule found in persons with sickle cell anemia causes the abnormally shaped red cells characteristic of this disease.

**molecular layer** SEE: under *layer*.

**molecular lesion** Defect or absence of a basic organic molecule that is of sufficient importance to cause disease. Sickle cell anemia is an example of this type of lesion.

**molecular weight** SEE: under *weight*.

**molecule** (mŏl′ĕ-kūl) [L. *molecula,* little mass] **1.** The smallest quantity into which a substance may be divided without loss of its characteristics. **2.** A chemical combination of two or more atoms that form a specific chemical compound.

Combinations of dissimilar atoms form chemical compounds. In normal molecules, the positive and negative electrical charges balance exactly. Excess or deficiency of either positive or negative charge by the loss or acquisition of electrons results in the formation of an ion.

A molecule is designated by the number of atoms it contains, as monatomic (one atom); diatomic (two); triatomic (three); tetratomic (four); pentatomic (five); or hexatomic (six). SEE: *cleavage.* **molecular** (mō-lĕk′ū-lăr), *adj.*

**molimen** (mō-lī′mĕn) *pl.* **molimina** [L., effort] Effort to establish any normal function, esp. that necessary to establish the menstrual flow.

**Moll's glands** [Jacob Anthoni Moll, Dutch ophthalmologist, 1832–1914] Modified sweat glands at border of eyelids. SYN: *ciliary glands.*

**Mollusca** A phylum of animals that includes the bivalves (mussels, oysters, clams), slugs, and snails. Snails serve as intermediate hosts for many parasitic flukes. Oysters, clams, and muscles, esp. if inadequately cooked, may transmit the hepatitis A virus or bacterial pathogens.

**molluscum** (mŏ-lŭs′kŭm) [L., soft] A mildly infective skin disease marked by tumor formations on the skin. **molluscous** (mŏ-lŭs′kŭs), *adj.*

***m. contagiosum*** A common, mildly contagious form of molluscum that is caused by a large virus of the pox group. It affects mainly children and young adults. The condition is marked by the presence of small, waxy, globular, umbilicated epithelial tumors commonly found on the face, eyelids, breasts, genitalia, or inner surface of the thighs. The tumors are a few mm to 3 cm in diameter and contain solid or semifluid caseous matter that can be expressed on pressure. They heal without scarring, though they may suppurate and break down. Treatment consists of incision and expression of contents, followed by application of tincture of iodine. SEE: illus.

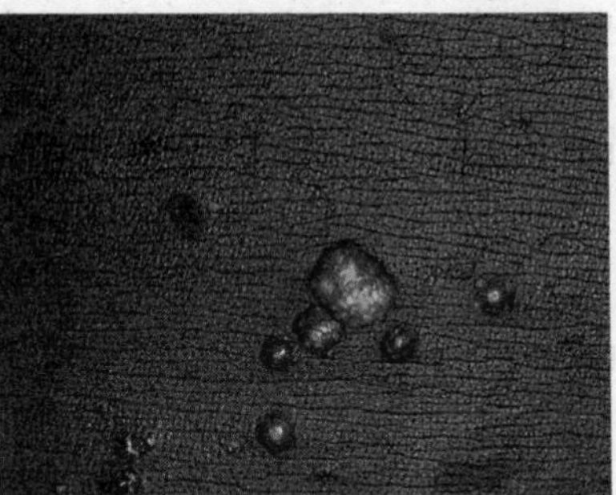

**MOLLUSCUM CONTAGIOSUM**

**mollusk, mollusc** Any member of the phylum Mollusca.

**molt** To shed a covering such as feathers or skin that is replaced by new growth.

**mol. wt.** *molecular weight.*

**molybdenum** (mō-lĭb′dĕ-nŭm) SYMB: Mo. At. wt. 95.94; at. no. 42. A hard, heavy, metallic element.

**molysmophobia** (mō-lĭz″mō-fō′bē-ă) [Gr. *molysma,* stain, + *phobia,* fear] Abnormal fear of contamination or infection. SYN: *mysophobia.*

**momentum** (mō-mĕn′tŭm) [L.] **1.** In physics, the description of a quantity obtained by multiplying the mass of a body by its linear velocity. **2.** Force of motion acquired by a moving object as a result of continuance of its motion; impetus.

**momism** [Coined by Phillip Wylie in his book *A Generation of Vipers*] In American culture, undue dependence on one's mother, esp. in very early life. This was alleged to cause the individual to be immature.

**monad** [Gr. *monas,* a unit] **1.** A univalent element. **2.** A unicellular organism. **3.** One of the four components of a tetrad.

**monamide** (mŏn-ăm′ĭd) Monoamide.

**monamine** (mŏn-ăm′ĭn) Monoamine.

**monarthric** (mŏn-ăr′thrĭk) [Gr. *monos,* single, + *arthron,* joint] Monarticular.

**monarthritis** (mŏn″ăr-thrī′tĭs) [″ + ″+ *itis,* inflammation] Arthritis affecting a single joint.

**monarticular** (mŏn-ăr-tĭk′ū-lăr) Concerning or affecting one joint. SYN: *monarthric.*

**monaster** (mŏn-ăs′tĕr) [″ + *aster,* star] Single starlike figure formed in mitosis.

**monathetosis** (mŏn″ăth-ē-tō′sĭs) [″ + *athetos,* not fixed, + *osis,* condition] Athetosis affecting a single limb.

**monatomic** (mŏn″ă-tŏm′ĭk) [″ + *atomos,* indivisible] **1.** Concerning a single atom. **2.** Univalent.

**monaural** (mŏn-aw′răl) Concerning or affecting one ear.

**monaxon** (mŏn″ăk′sŏn) [″ + Gr. *axon,* axis] A neuron with one axon.

**Monday chest tightness** In the early stage of byssinosis, chest tightness due to decreased respiratory function caused by exposure to cotton dust on the first day of the work week, which is usually Monday. SEE: *byssinosis; metal fume fever.*

**Mondonesi's reflex** (mŏn-dō-nā′zēz) [Filippo Mondonesi, It. physician] In coma, contraction of facial muscles following pressure on the eyeball. SYN: *bulbomimic reflex; facial reflex.*

**Mondor's disease** (mŏn′dorz) [Henri Mondor, Fr. physician, 1885–1962] Thrombosis and sclerosis of a subcutaneous vein or veins in the breast and chest wall. The long, firm, tender cordlike or stringlike structure extends from the breast up into the axilla or down toward the epigastrium. The condition may occur after trauma or appear without apparent cause. Although a benign, self-limiting disease, its appearance may be confused with breast cancer.

**Monera** Prokaryotae.

**monesthetic** (mŏn″ĕs-thĕt′ĭk) [Gr. *monos,* single, + *aisthesis,* sensation] Affecting only one of the senses.

**monestrous** (mŏn-ĕs′trŭs) Having a single estrous cycle in a single sexual season.

**Monge's disease** [Carlos Monge, Peruvian physician, 1884–1970] SEE: *mountain sickness, chronic.*

**mongolian spot** SEE: under *spot.*

**mongolism** (mŏn′gōl-ĭzm) An inaccurate and inappropriate term for Down syndrome.

**mongoloid** (mŏn′gō-loyd) **1.** Concerning Mongols. **2.** Characterized by mongolism (i.e., Down syndrome).

**monilethrix** (mŏn-ĭl′ĕ-thrĭks) [L. *monile,* necklace, + Gr. *thrix,* hair] A genetic defect of the hair shaft in which the hair becomes beaded and brittle. The defect usually appears by the second month of life. There is no effective treatment.

**Monilia** [L. *monile,* necklace] Former name for the genus of fungi now called *Candida.*

**monilial** (mō-nĭl′ē-ăl), *adj.*

**moniliasis** (mō″nĭ-lī′ă-sĭs) Candidiasis.

**moniliform** (mŏn-ĭl′ĭ-form) [″ + *forma,* shape] Resembling a necklace or string of beads.

**moniliid** (mō-nĭl′ē-ĭd) A skin eruption due to hypersensitivity to a *Candida* infection in another part of the body.

**monitor** (mŏn′ĭ-tor) [L., one who warns] **1.** One who observes a condition, procedure, or apparatus, esp. one responsible for detecting and preventing malfunction. **2.** A device that provides a warning if that which is being observed fails or malfunctions. **3.** To check by using an electronic device.

***apnea m.*** SEE: *apnea monitoring.*

***blood pressure m.*** SEE: *blood pressure monitor.*

***cardiac m.*** Monitor of heart function, providing visual and audible record of heartbeat.

***continuous ambulatory electrocardiographic m.*** SEE: *Holter monitor.*

***fetal m.*** **1.** Monitor that detects and displays fetal heartbeat. **2.** Assessment of fetus in utero with respect to its heart rate by use of electrocardiogram or by chemical analysis of the amniotic fluid or fetal blood. SEE: *fetal heart rate monitoring; fetal monitoring in utero.*

***Holter m.*** SEE: *Holter monitor.*

***personal radiation m.*** Small device carried by an individual to measure the accumulated radiation dosage over a period of time. SEE: *dosimeter.*

***pregnancy m.*** An electronic device connected to the abdomen to monitor uterine contractions. If the monitoring is done in the home, the information can be transmitted by phone to a health care professional who will provide analysis and advice. The use of these devices for home monitoring is controversial with respect to their efficacy.

***respiratory m.*** SEE: *respiratory function monitoring.*

***temperature m.*** Monitor for measuring and recording temperature of the body or some particular portion of the body.

***unit m.*** In radiation therapy, a calibrated unit of dose that determines the length of the treatment.

**mono-, mon-** [Gr. *monos,* single] Prefix meaning *one, single.*

**monoacidic** (mŏn″ō-ă-sĭd′ĭk) Having one replaceable hydroxyl (OH) group.

**monoamide** An amide with only one amide group.

**monoamine** An amine with only one amine group.

**monoamine oxidase inhibitor** ABBR: MAO inhibitors. One of a group of drugs that are effective in treating depression. The mode of action of MAO inhibitors, in addition to inhibiting monoamine oxidase, is not clearly understood. Because of the toxic potential, MAO inhibitors should be used with caution. Hypertensive crises have been observed in persons who eat certain kinds of cheese or chicken liver or drink chianti wine while taking MAO inhibitors. SEE: *tyramine.*

**monobacillary** (mŏn″ō-băs′ĭ-lă″rē) Concerning a single species of bacilli.

**monobacterial** (mŏn″ō-băk-tē′rē-ăl) Concerning a single species of bacteria.

**monobasic** (mŏn-ō-bā′sĭk) [″ + *basis,* a base] Having only one hydrogen atom replaceable by a metal or positive radical.

**monobenzone** (mŏn″ō-bĕn′zōn) A drug used topically in treating hyperpigmentation conditions. Trade name is Benoquin.

**monoblast** (mŏn′ō-blăst) [″ + *blastos,* germ] A cell that gives rise to a monocyte.

**monoblastoma** (mŏn″ō-blăs-tō′mă) [″ + ″ + *oma,* tumor] A neoplasm that contains both monoblasts and monocytes.

**monoblepsia** (mŏn-ō-blĕp′sē-ă) [″ + *blepsis,* sight] **1.** Condition in which vision is more distinct when only one eye is used, hence tendency to close one eye to see clearly. **2.** A type of color blindness in which only one color can be seen.

**monobrachius** (mŏn″ō-brā′kē-ŭs) [″ + *brachion,* arm] **1.** State of having only one arm. **2.** Fetus with only one arm.

**monobromated** (mŏn″ō-brō′māt-ĕd) Pert. to chemical compound with only one atom of bromine in each molecule.

**monocalcic** (mŏn-ō-kăl′sĭk) Pert. to a chemical compound containing only one atom of calcium in the molecule.

**monocardian** (mŏn-ō-kăr′dē-ăn) [″ + *kardia,* heart] An animal possessing a heart with only one atrium and one ventricle.

**monocelled** (mŏn′ō-sĕld) Composed of a single cell.

**monocephalus** (mŏn″ō-sĕf′ă-lŭs) [″ + *kephale,* head] A congenitally deformed fetus with duplicated parts except for the head.

**monochord** (mŏn′ō-kord) [″ + *chorde,* cord] A single-string instrument used for testing upper tone audition.

**monochorea** (mŏn″ō-kō-rē′ă) [″ + *choreia,* dance] Chorea affecting a single part.

**monochorionic** (mŏn-ō-kor″ē-ŏn′ĭk) Possessing a single chorion, as in the case of identical twins.

**monochromasy** (mŏn″ō-krō-mā′sē) Monochromatism.

**monochromatic** (mŏn″ō-krō-măt′ĭk) [″ + *chroma,* color] **1.** Having one color. **2.** A color-blind person to whom all colors appear to be of one hue.

**monochromatism** (mŏn″ō-krō′mă-tĭzm) [Gr. *monos,* single, + *chroma,* color, + *-ismos,* condition] Complete color blindness in which all colors are perceived as shades of gray. SYN: *monochromasy.*

**monochromatophil** (mŏn″ō-krō-măt′ō-fĭl) [″ + ″ + *philein,* to love] A cell or tissue that accepts only one stain.

**monochromator** (mŏn-ō-krō′mā-tor) A spectroscope modified for selective transmission of a narrow band of the spectrum.

**monoclinic** (mŏn″ō-klin′ĭk) [″ + *klinein,* to incline] Pert. to crystals in which the vertical axis is inclined to one lateral axis but at right angles to the other.

**monoclonal** (mŏn″ō-klōn′ăl) Arising from a single cell.

**monoclonal antibody** A type of antibody derived from hybridoma cells. Such antibodies are of exceptional purity and specificity. They are being used to identify many infectious organisms and hormones such as human chorionic gonadotropin. In addition, they are used in tissue and blood typing, to identify tumor antigens, and experimentally to treat autoimmune diseases, B-cell lymphomas, and pancreatic cancer. SEE: *hybridoma; monoclonal antibody therapy.*

**monoclonal antibody therapy** Treatment with artificially produced proteins that bind to tissue antigens. Because the antibodies are derived from one cell line (monoclonal), they are highly specific to one particular antigen. This means that they can be designed to target specific tumor or immune cells for destruction. In clinical trials, for example, monoclonal antibodies attached to radioactive isotopes can deliver radiation directly to tumors.

Most commercially produced monoclonal antibodies are derived from B-lymphocyte mouse cells. A mouse is injected with the antigen from the tissue targeted for destruction and develops an immune response to the antigen. Next, B lymphocytes (lymph cells that secrete antibodies) are removed from the mouse's spleen and are manipulated so that they will grow in a culture medium. As they grow, they secrete antibodies. Antibodies are isolated from the culture medium and injected into the patient, where they seek out and mark the target tissue for destruction, either by the patient's own immune system or by drugs or radioactive isotopes bonded to the monoclonal antibodies.

One product available now is muromonab-CD3 (Orthoclone OKT3), which treats transplant patients showing signs of organ rejection. It is believed to block T cells, the immune cells responsible for transplant rejection.

**monococcus** (mŏn-ō-kŏk′ŭs) [″ + *kokkos,* berry] A form of coccus existing singly instead of as part of the usual group or chain.

**monocontaminated** (mŏn″ō-kŏn-tăm′ĭ-nāt″ĕd) Infected with a single species of organism.

**monocrotic** (mŏn″ō-krŏt′ĭk) [″ + *krotos,* beat] Indicating a single pulse wave with no notches in it.

**monocular** (mŏn-ŏk′ū-lar) [″ + L. *oculus,* eye] **1.** Concerning or affecting one eye. **2.** Possessing a single eyepiece, as in a monocular microscope.

**monoculus** (mŏn-ŏk′ū-lŭs) **1.** A bandage for shielding one eye. **2.** A fetus with only one eye. SYN: *cyclops.*

**monocyclic** (mŏn″ō-sī′klĭk) Concerning one cycle.

**monocyesis** (mŏn″ō-sī-ē′sĭs) [″ + *kyesis,* pregnancy] Pregnancy with a single fetus.

**monocyte** (mŏn′ō-sīt) [″ + *kytos,* cell] A mononuclear phagocytic white blood cell derived from the myeloid stem cells. Monocytes circulate in the blood stream for about 24 hr and then move into tissues, at which point they mature into macrophages, which are long lived. Monocytes and macrophages are one of the first lines of defense in the inflammatory process. This network of fixed and mobile phagocytes that engulf foreign antigens and cell debris is commonly called the macrophage system. SEE: illus.; *blood* for illus.; *macrophage.* **monocytic** (mŏn-ō-sĭt′ĭk), *adj.*

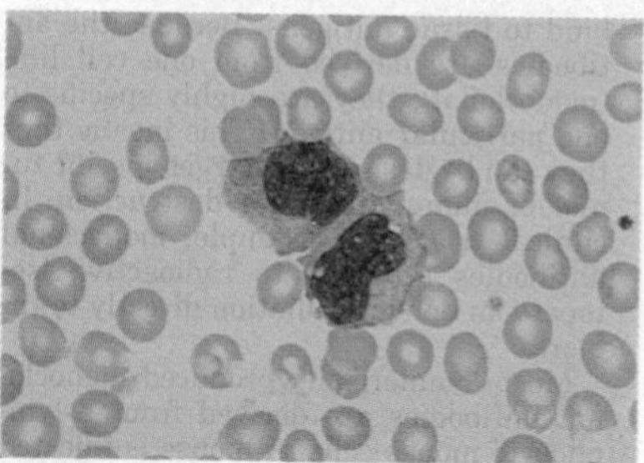

MONOCYTES (ORIG. MAG. ×640)

**monocytopenia** (mŏn″ō-sī″tō-pē′nē-ă) [″ + *kytos,* cell, + *penia,* lack] Diminished number of monocytes in the blood.

**monocytosis** (mŏn″ō-sī-tō′sĭs) [″ + ″ + *osis,* condition] Excessive number of monocytes in the blood.

**monodactylism** (mŏn-ō-dăk′tĭl-ĭzm) [″ + *daktylos,* digit] Condition, usually congenital, of having only one digit on a hand or foot. Also called monodactyly or monodactylia.

**monodal** (mŏn-ō′dăl) [″ + *hodos,* road] Connected with one terminal of a resonator so that the patient acts as a capacitor for entrance and exit of high-frequency currents.

**monodermoma** (mŏn″ō-dĕr-mō′mă) [″ + *derma,* skin, + *oma,* tumor] A neoplasm originating in one germinal layer.

**monodiplopia** (mŏn″ō-dĭ-plō′pē-ă) [″ + *diploos,* double, + *ops,* eye] Double vision in one eye only.

**monoecious** (mŏn-ē′shŭs) [″ + *oikos,* house] Pert. to the presence of functioning male and female sex organs in the same individual.

**monogamy** (mō-nŏg′ă-mē) [″ + *gamos,* marriage] The practice of being married to only one person at a time.

**monogenesis** (mŏn″ō-jĕn′ĕ-sĭs) [Gr. *monos,* single, + *genesis,* generation, birth] **1.** Production of offspring of only one sex. **2.** The theory that all organisms arise from a single cell. **3.** Asexual reproduction.

**monogerminal** (mŏn″ō-jĕr′mĭ-năl) Produced from a single ovum.

**monogony** (mō-nŏg′ō-nē) [″ + *gone,* seed] Asexual reproduction.

**monograph** (mŏn′ō-grăf) [″ + *graphein,* to write] A treatise dealing with a single subject.

**monogyny** (mō-nŏj′ă-nē) [″ + *gyne,* woman] Practice whereby a male has only one female mate.

**monohybrid** [″ + L. *hybrida,* mongrel] Offspring of a cross between parents differing in a single character.

**monohydrated** (mŏn-ō-hī′drāt-ĕd) [″ + *hydor,* water] United with only one molecule of water.

**monohydric** (mŏn″ō-hī′drĭk) Having a single replaceable hydrogen atom.

**monoideaism, monoideism** (mŏn″ō-ī-dē′ă-ĭzm, -dē′ĭzm) [″ + *idea,* idea] Preoccupation with only one idea; a slight degree of monomania.

**monoinfection** (mŏn″ō-ĭn-fĕk′shŭn) Infection with a single species of organism.

**monoiodotyrosine** (mŏn″ō-ī-ō″dō-tī′rō-sēn) An amino acid intermediate in the synthesis of thyroxine and triiodothyronine.

**monokine** A chemical mediator released by monocytes and macrophages during the immune response. Monokines affect the growth and activity of other white blood cells. Interleukin-1 is an important monokine. SEE: *cytokine; inflammation; interleukin-1; lymphokine; paracrine.*

**monolayer** (mŏn″ō-lā′ĕr) Having a single layer, esp. of cells growing in culture.

**monolocular** (mŏn″ō-lŏk′ū-lar) [″ + L. *loculus,* a small chamber] Having only one cell or cavity. SYN: *unilocular.*

**monomania** (mŏn-ō-mā′nē-ă) [″ + *mania,* madness] Mental illness characterized by distortion of thought processes concerning a single subject or idea.

**monomaniac** One afflicted with monomania.

**monomastigote** (mŏn-ō-măs′tĭ-gōt) [″ + *mastix,* whip] Mastigote possessing only one flagellum.

**monomelic** (mŏn-ō-mĕl′ĭk) [″ + *melos,* limb] Affecting a single limb.

**monomer** (mŏn′ō-mĕr) Any molecule that can be bound to similar molecules to form a polymer.

**monomeric** (mŏn-ō-mĕr′ĭk) [″ + *meros,* part] Consisting of, or affecting, a single piece or segment of a body.

**monometallic** (mŏn″ō-mĕ-tăl′ĭk) Containing a single atom of a metal per molecule.

**monomicrobic** (mŏn″ō-mī-krō′bĭk) Concerning organisms of a single species.

**monomolecular** (mŏn″ō-mō-lĕk′ū-lăr) Concerning one molecule.

**monomorphic** (mŏn-ō-mor′fĭk) [″ + *morphe,* form] Unchangeable in form; keeping the same form throughout every stage of development.

**monomyoplegia** (mŏn″ō-mī″ō-plē′jē-ă) [″ + *mys,* muscle, + *plege,* stroke] Paralysis of only one muscle.

**monomyositis** (mŏn″ō-mī-ō-sī′tĭs) [″ + ″ + *itis,* inflammation] Inflammation of only one muscle.

**mononeural** (mŏn-ō-nū′răl) [″ + *neuron,* nerve] Supplied by or concerning a single nerve.

**mononeuritis** (mŏn″ō-nū-rī′tĭs) [″ + ″ + *itis,* inflammation] Inflammation of a single nerve.

***m. multiplex*** Inflammation of nerves in separate body areas.

**mononeuropathy** (mŏn″ō-nū-rŏp′ă-thē) [″ + ″ + *pathos,* disease, suffering] Disease of a single nerve.

***hypertrophic m.*** Neuropathy associated with enlargement and tenderness of two or three nerves of the head and neck

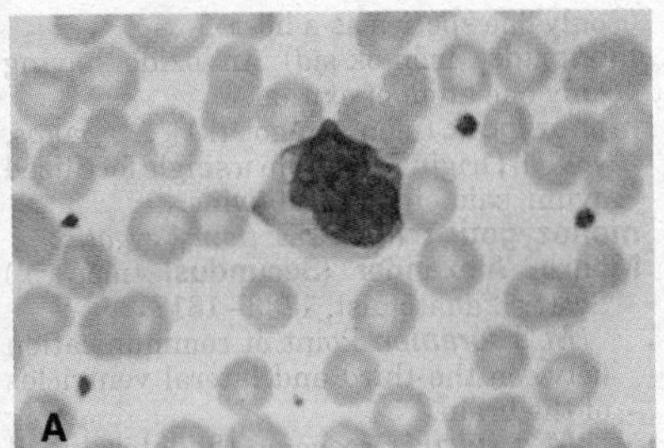
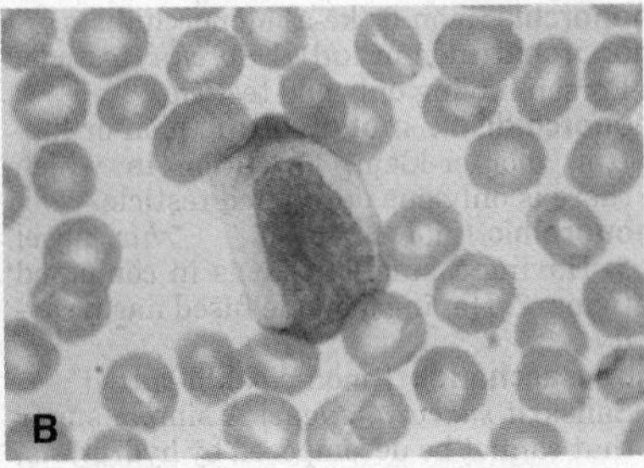

MONONUCLEOSIS

ATYPICAL LYMPHOCYTES

area. The nerves may appear to be a neurofibroma, but biopsy will provide the correct diagnosis.

**mononuclear** (mŏn-ō-nū′klē-ăr) [″ + L. *nucleus,* kernel] Having one nucleus, particularly a blood cell such as a monocyte or lymphocyte. SYN: *uninuclear.*

**mononuclear phagocyte system** ABBR: MPS. The modern name for reticuloendothelial system.

**mononucleosis** (mŏn-ō-nū″klē-ō′sĭs) [″ + *nucleus,* kernel, + *osis,* condition] Presence of an abnormally high number of mononuclear leukocytes in the blood. SEE: illus.

***infectious m.*** An acute infectious disease that affects primarily lymphoid tissue. The cause of most cases of infectious mononucleosis is the Epstein-Barr virus; however, 10% to 20% of cases are caused by other viruses, esp. cytomegalovirus. SYN: *glandular fever.* SEE: *Epstein-Barr virus; Nursing Diagnoses Appendix.*

SYMPTOMS: After the incubation period, which may be as long as 4 to 7 weeks, flu-like symptoms, fever, sore throat, fatigue, enlarged and often tender lymph nodes, and enlarged spleen with a great increase of atypical or abnormal mononuclear leukocytes in the blood develop. A skin rash may appear.

DIAGNOSIS: Serologic testing for heterophil antibodies will identify about 90% of cases of adults with the Epstein-Barr virus. However, this test is often negative in children less than 4 years of age. Abnormal liver function will be present in about 90% of cases.

TREATMENT: There is no specific therapy for infectious mononucleosis. For serious complications (e.g., hemolytic anemia, pharyngeal swelling interfering with swallowing), cortisone is indicated.

NURSING IMPLICATIONS: During the acute phase, the patient is encouraged to refrain from activity and maintain adequate rest to reduce fatigue and malaise. The patient may resume activity that does not involve heavy exertion after 1 to 2 weeks. Most patients can resume their normal activity level in 4 to 6 weeks. If spleen enlargement is present, extra caution is required, for example, avoiding heavy lifting and contact sports, to prevent traumatizing or rupture of the spleen.

**mononucleotide** (mŏn″ō-nū′klē-ō-tīd″) A product resulting from hydrolysis of nucleic acid, containing phosphoric acid combined with a glucoside or pentoside. SYN: *nucleotide.*

**monoparesis** (mŏn-ō-păr-ē′sĭs) [Gr. *monos,* single, + *paresis,* weakness] Paralysis of a single part of the body.

**monoparesthesia** (mŏn″ō-păr-ĕs-thē′sē-ă) [″ + *para,* beside, + *aisthesis,* sensation] Paresthesia of only one region or limb.

**monophagia** (mŏn-ō-fā′jē-ă) [″ + *phagein,* to eat] **1.** Appetite for only one kind of food. Said esp. of insects. **2.** The habit of eating only one meal a day.

**monophasia** (mŏn-ō-fā′zē-ă) [″ + *phasis,* speech] Inability to utter anything but one word or phrase repeatedly.

**monophobia** (mŏn-ō-fō′bē-ă) [″ + *phobos,* fear] Abnormal fear of being alone.

**monophyletic** (mŏn″ō-fī-lĕt′ĭk) [″ + *phyle,* tribe] Originating from a single source. Opposite of polyphyletic.

**monophyletism** (mŏn″ō-fī′lĕ-tĭzm) Concerning the concept that all blood cells are derived from a single stem cell.

**monophyodont** (mŏn″ō-fī′ō-dŏnt) [″ + *phyein,* to grow, + *odous,* tooth] Having a single, permanent set of teeth.

**monoplasmatic** (mŏn″ō-plăz-măt′ĭk) [″ + LL. *plasma,* form, mold] Made up of a single substance or tissue.

**monoplast** (mŏn″ō-plăst) [″ + *plastos,* formed] A single-cell type of organism that does not change during its life cycle.

**monoplegia** (mŏn-ō-plē′jē-ă) [″ + *plege,* stroke] Paralysis of a single limb or a single group of muscles. **monoplegic,** *adj.*

**monopodia** (mŏn″ō-pō′dē-ă) [″ + *pous,* foot] Condition of having only one foot; usually the two feet are fused.

**monopolar** (mŏn-ō-pōl′ăr) [″ + L. *polus,* pole] Having one pole. SYN: *unipolar.*

**monopsychosis** (mŏn″ō-sī-kō′sĭs) [Gr. *monos,* single, + *psyche,* mind, + *osis,* condition] Monomania.

**monorchia** (mŏn-or′kē-ă) Monorchidism.

**monorchid** (mŏn-or′kĭd) [″ + *orchis,* testicle] Person having only one testicle.

**monorchidism, monorchism** (mŏn-or′kĭd-ĭzm, mŏn′or-kĭzm) Condition in which there is only one descended testicle.

**monorhinic** (mŏn″ō-rĭn′ĭk) [″ + *rhis,* nose] **1.** Having a single nose, as in conjoined twins. **2.** Having a single fused nasal cavity.

**monosaccharide** (mŏn-ō-săk′ă-rīd) [″ + Sanskrit *sarkara,* sugar] A simple sugar that cannot be decomposed by hydrolysis, such as fructose, galactose, or glucose.

**monosodium glutamate** ABBR: MSG. $C_5H_8NNaO_4 \cdot H_2O$. Sodium salt of glutamic acid. A white crystalline substance used to flavor foods, esp. meats. When ingested in large amounts, it may cause chest pain, a sensation of facial pressure, headaches, burning sensation, and excessive sweating, commonly called Chinese restaurant syndrome. Allergy to monosodium glutamate is common, and those persons who are allergic should avoid eating foods containing this ingredient. The use of MSG to enhance the flavor of foods prepared for infants is controversial. MSG is sold under various names, such as Ajinomoto, Accent, Vetsin.

**monosome** (mŏn′ō-sōm) [″ + *soma,* body] An accessory chromosome that, without dividing, goes into only one of the daughter cells; the unpaired sex chromosome.

**monosomy** (mŏn′ō-sō″mē) Condition of having one member of a chromosome pair missing.

**monospasm** (mŏn′ō-spăzm) [″ + *spasmos,* convulsion] Spasm of a single limb or part.

**monospermy** (mŏn′ō-spĕr″mē) [″ + *sperma,* seed] Fertilization by a single spermatozoon entering an ovum.

**monostotic** (mŏn″ŏs-tŏt′ĭk) [″ + *osteon,* bone] Concerning a single bone.

**monosubstituted** (mŏn″ō-sŭb′stĭ-tūt″ĕd) Having only a single molecule replaced.

**monosymptomatic** (mŏn″ō-sĭmp-tō-măt′ĭk) [″ + *symptomatikos,* pert. to symptom] Having only one dominant symptom.

**monosynaptic** (mŏn″ō-sĭ-năp′tĭk) Transmitted through only a single synapse.

**monosyphilide** (mŏn-ō-sĭf′ĭl-ĭd) [″ + Fr. *syphilide,* syphilitic lesion] Characterized by a single syphilitic lesion.

**monotocous** (mō-nŏt′ō-kŭs) [Gr. *monos,* single, + *tokos,* birth] Producing a single offspring per birth.

**monotricha** (mō-nŏt′rĭ-kă) [″ + *thrix,* hair] Bacteria having a single flagellum at one pole.

**monotrichous** (mŏn-ŏt′rĭ-kŭs) Pert. to or having a single flagellum.

**monovalent** (mŏn-ō-vā′lĕnt) [″ + L. *valere,* to have power] Having the combining power of a single hydrogen atom. SYN: *univalent* (1).

**monoxenous** (mō-nŏks′ĕn-ŭs) [″ + *xenos,* stranger] Said of a parasite that requires only one species as a host.

**monoxide** (mŏn-ŏk′sīd) An oxide having only one atom of oxygen.

**monozygotic** (mŏn″ō-zī-gŏt′ĭk) [″ + *zygotos,* yoked] Originating from a single fertilized ovum, said of identical twins.

**monozygotic twins** SEE: *twins, zygotic.*

**Monro, Alexander (Secundus)** (mŏn-rō′) Scottish anatomist, 1733–1817.

***M.'s foramen*** Point of communication between the third and lateral ventricles of the brain.

***M.'s sulcus*** Groove on the lateral wall of the third ventricle from the opening to the lateral ventricle to the opening of the cerebral aqueduct of the brain.

**mons** (mŏns) *pl.* **montes** [L., mountain] An anatomical eminence above the surface of the body.

***m. pubis*** A pad of fatty tissue and coarse skin overlying the symphysis pubis. After puberty it is covered with hair.

***m. veneris*** M. pubis.

**Monteggia's fracture** (mŏn-tĕj′ăz) [Giovanni B. Monteggia, It. surgeon, 1762–1815] Fracture of the upper portion of the ulna with dislocation of the radial head.

**Montgomery, William F.** Irish obstetrician, 1797–1859.

***M.'s glands*** Large sebaceous and rudimentary milk glands present in the areola surrounding the nipple of the female breast. SYN: *M.'s tubercles; areolar glands.*

***M.'s tubercles*** M.'s glands.

**Montgomery straps** Adhesive straps affixed to the skin arranged opposite to each other, and with the middle ends turned back on each other, so that gauze straps can be placed between holes of each end of the middle of the paired tapes. This provides a method of securing a bandage and subsequently changing it without having to replace the tape each time. SEE: illus.

**month, lunar** Four calendar weeks (28 days), a measurement of time used in obstetrics. Pregnancy is calculated in terms of 10 lunar months.

**monticulus** (mŏn-tĭk′ū-lŭs) *pl.* **monticuli** [L., little mountain] A protuberance.

***m. cerebelli*** In the cerebellum, protuberance of the superior vermis, the anterior portion of which is called the culmen and the posterior portion, the declive.

**mood** [AS. *mod,* mind, feeling] A pervasive and sustained emotion that may have a major influence on a person's perception of the world. Examples of mood include depression, joy, elation, anger, and anxiety. SEE: *affect.*

**mood disorder** Any mental disorder that has a disturbance of mood as the predominant feature. In DSM-IV, these have been divided into mood episodes, mood disorders, and specifications describing either the most recent mood episode or the course of recurrent episodes. Mood disorders, including dysthymic disorder, are divided into the depressive disorders

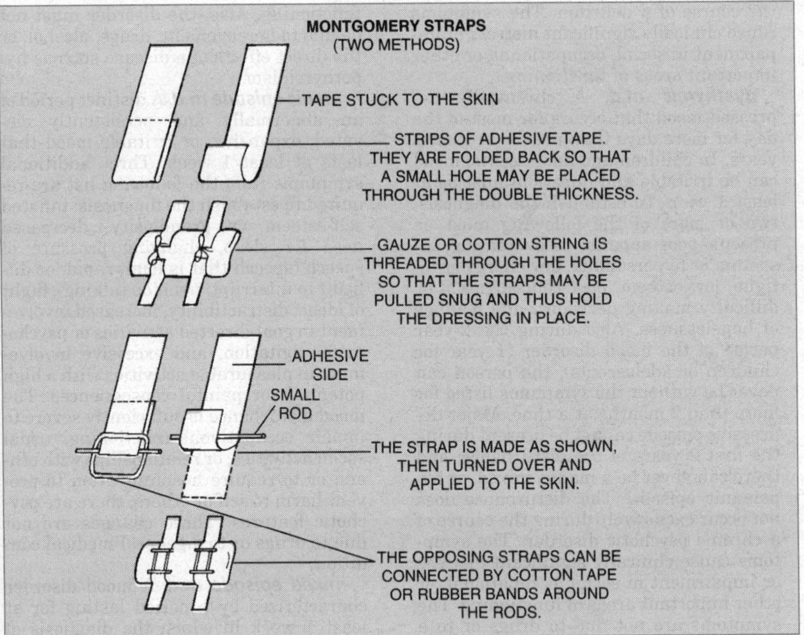


(unipolar depression), the bipolar disorders, and two disorders based on etiology (i.e., those due to a general medical condition or substance-induced mood disorder). Depressive disorders are distinguished from the bipolar disorders by the fact that there is no history of ever having had a manic, mixed, or hypomanic episode. Bipolar I disorder and bipolar II disorder involve the presence of or history of manic episodes, mixed episodes, or hypomanic episodes usually with presence of or history of major depressive episodes. SEE: *Nursing Diagnoses Appendix.*

***bipolar I m.d.*** A mood disorder characterized by the presence of only one manic episode and no past major depressive episodes that is not better accounted for by a psychotic disorder. The classes or specifiers of bipolar I disorder include mild, moderate, severe without psychotic features, severe with psychotic features, in partial remission, in full remission, with catatonic features, and with postpartum onset.

***bipolar II m.d.*** A mood disorder characterized by the occurrence of one or more major depressive episodes accompanied by at least one hypomanic episode. If manic or mixed episode mood disorders are present, the diagnosis of bipolar I cannot be supported. Episodes of substance-induced mood disorder or a mood disorder due to drugs or toxin exposure preclude the diagnosis of bipolar II mood disorder. In addition, the symptoms must cause clinically significant distress or impairment in social, occupational, or other important areas of functioning. The specifiers “hypomanic” or “depressed” are used to indicate the current or most recent episode.

***cyclothymic m.d.*** A diagnosis of exclusion in which for at least 2 years there has been the presence of numerous periods of hypomanic symptoms and numerous periods with depressive symptoms that do not meet the criteria for major depressive episode. During the 2-year period, the person cannot be without the symptoms mentioned for more than 2 months at a time. In addition, no major depressive episode, manic episode, or mixed episode can be present during the first 2 years of the disturbance. The symptoms cannot be accounted for by a psychosis and are not due to drugs or a general medical condition. The symptoms cause clinically significant distress or impairment in social, occupational, or other important areas of functioning.

***m.d. due to a general medical disorder*** A prominent and persistent disturbance in mood characterized by either or both of the following: markedly diminished interest or pleasure in all, or almost all, activities and elevated, expansive, or irritable mood. The clinical and laboratory findings are consistent with attributing the cause to a direct physiological consequence of the general medical condition. The condition is not better accounted for by another mental disorder. The disturbance does not occur exclusively during the course of a delirium. The symptoms cause clinically significant distress or impairment in social, occupational, or other important areas of functioning.

***dysthymic m.d.*** A chronically depressed mood that occurs for most of the day for more days than not for at least 2 years. In children and adolescents, mood can be irritable and duration must be at least 1 year. To establish the diagnosis, two or more of the following must be present: poor appetite or overeating, insomnia or hypersomnia, low energy or fatigue, low esteem, poor concentration or difficulty making decisions, and feelings of hopelessness. Also during the 2-year period of the mood disorder (1 year for children or adolescents), the person can never be without the symptoms listed for more than 2 months at a time. Major depressive episode cannot be present during the first 2 years of the disturbance, and there can never be a manic, mixed, or hypomanic episode. The disturbance does not occur exclusively during the course of a chronic psychotic disorder. The symptoms cause clinically significant distress or impairment in social, occupational, or other important areas of functioning. The symptoms are not due to drugs or to a general medical condition.

***hypomanic episode m.d.*** A mood disorder characterized by a period of persistently elevated, expansive, or irritable mood lasting for at least 4 days. Three or more of the following must be present: inflated self-esteem, decreased need for sleep, talking more than usual, flight of ideas or feeling that thoughts are racing, distractibility, increase in goal-directed activities, and excessive involvement in pleasurable activities with a high potential for painful consequences. The episode is not severe enough to cause marked impairment in social or occupational functioning or to necessitate hospitalization; there are no psychotic features. These changes are not due to drugs or to a general medical condition.

***major depressive episode m.d.*** A mood disorder characterized by a period of at least 2 weeks of depressed mood or the loss of interest or pleasure in nearly all activities. In children and adolescents, the mood may be irritable rather than sad. Establishing the diagnosis requires the presence of at least four of the following: changes in appetite, weight, sleep, and psychomotor activity; decreased energy; feelings of worthlessness or guilt; difficulty thinking, concentrating, or making decisions; or recurrent thoughts of death, or plans for or attempts to commit suicide. The symptoms must persist for most of the day, nearly every day, for at least 2 consecutive weeks. The episode must be accompanied by clinically significant distress or impairment in social, occupational, or other important areas of functioning. Also, the disorder must not be due to bereavement, drugs, alcohol, or the direct effects of a disease such as hypothyroidism.

***manic episode m.d.*** A distinct period of an abnormally and persistently elevated, expansive, or irritable mood that lasts at least 1 week. Three additional symptoms from the following list are required to establish the diagnosis: inflated self-esteem or grandiosity, decreased need for sleep, changing pressure of speech (speech that is loud, rapid, or difficult to interrupt; nonstop talking), flight of ideas, distractibility, increased involvement in goal-directed activities or psychomotor agitation, and excessive involvement in pleasurable activities with a high potential for painful consequences. The mood disturbance is sufficiently severe to impair occupational functioning, usual social activities, or relationships with others, or to require hospitalization to prevent harm to self or others; there are psychotic features. These changes are not due to drugs or to a general medical condition.

***mixed episode m.d.*** A mood disorder characterized by a period lasting for at least 1 week in which the diagnosis of manic episode and major depressive episode are met nearly each day. SEE: *major depressive m.d.; manic episode m.d.*

***substance-induced m.d.*** A prominent and persistent disturbance in mood characterized by either or both of the following: depressed mood or markedly diminished interest or pleasure in all, or almost all, activities and elevated, expansive, or irritable mood. The clinical and laboratory findings must support that either the symptoms developed during, or within a month of, substance intoxication or withdrawal, or that the medication (i.e., substance) is etiologically related to the disturbance. The condition cannot be better accounted for by a mood disorder that is not substance induced. The disturbance does not occur exclusively during the course of a delirium. The symptoms cause clinically significant distress or impairment in social, occupational, or other important areas of functioning.

**mood swings** Periods of variation in how one feels, changing from a sense of well-being to one of depression. This occurs normally, but may become abnormally intense in persons with manic-depressive states.

**moon face** SEE: under *face.*

**Moore's lightning streaks** [Robert F. Moore, Brit. ophthalmologist, 1878–1963] The perception of zigzag flashes of light in the peripheral field of vision that occurs in the dark, esp. in older persons. These flashes are due to vitreous tags on the retina. The condition is benign. SEE: *coruscation.*

**Moraxella lacunata** (mor-ăx-ĕl'ă) A gram-negative coccobacillus that is a cause of conjunctivitis in humans.

**morbid** (mor′bĭd) [L. *morbidus,* sick] **1.** Diseased. **2.** Pert. to disease. **3.** Preoccupied with unwholesome ideas and circumstances.

**morbidity** [L. *morbidus,* sick] **1.** State of being diseased. **2.** The number of sick persons or cases of disease in relationship to a specific population. SEE: *incidence.*

***compression of m.*** Shortening of the period or proportion of long-term disability by elimination of a chronic disease.

***expansion of m.*** Increase in the number of years and proportion of disability by the elimination of a fatal disorder, such as cancer or heart disease.

**Morbidity and Mortality Weekly Report** ABBR: MMWR. The weekly report published by the Centers for Disease Control, Atlanta, Georgia, of illness and death rates for a variety of diseases. Prominent in the material are statistics on communicable diseases in each state, territory, and 121 major cities in the U.S. Articles concerning outbreaks of disease or accidents appear in the MMWR, sometimes including reports of importance to public health due to international events.

**morbidity rate** SEE: under *rate.*

**morbific** (mor-bĭf′ĭk) [″ + *facere,* to make] Causing or producing disease.

**morbilli** (mor-bĭl′ī) [L. *morbillus,* little disease] Measles. **morbillous** (mor-bĭl′ŭs), *adj.*

**morbilliform** [″ + *forma,* shape] Resembling measles or its rash.

**morcellation, morcellement** (mor-sĕl-ā′shŭn, -ā-mŏn′) [Fr. *morceller,* to subdivide] Method of removing a fetus, tumor, or organ by pieces.

**mordant** (mor′dănt) [L. *mordere,* to bite] A substance that fixes a stain or dye, as alum and phenol.

**mores** (mō′rāz) [L.] Habits and customs of society. Usually those that come to be regarded as being essential to the survival and well-being of the society.

**Morgagni, Giovanni B.** (mor-găn′yē) Italian pathological anatomist, 1682–1771. **morgagnian** (mor-găn′yē-ăn), *adj.*

***M.'s caruncle*** The middle prostatic lobe.

***M.'s cataract*** Cataract that is hypermature with a softened cortex and a hard nucleus.

***M.'s hydatid*** Cystlike remains of müllerian duct attached to testicle or oviduct.

***M.'s hyperostosis*** Hyperostosis of the frontal bones of the head, possibly associated with obesity, headache, amenorrhea, diabetes, multiple endocrine abnormalities, and various neuropsychiatric disturbances. SYN: *frontal internal hyperostosis.*

***M.'s rectal columns*** Vertical ridges in the upper half of the anal canal produced by infolding mucosa over a venous plexus.

***M.'a ventricle*** Ventriculus laryngis. SEE: *ventricle of larynx.*

**morgagnian cyst** SEE: under *cyst.*

**Morganella morganii** [Harry de R. Morgan, Brit. physician, 1863–1931] A gram-negative intestinal bacillus that may cause urinary tract infections, wound infections, bacteremia, meningitis, keratitis, and acute enteritis.

**morgue** (morg) [Fr.] A place for holding dead bodies until they are identified or claimed for burial.

**moria** (mō′rē-ă) [Gr. *moria,* folly] **1.** Simple dementia. **2.** Foolishness. SEE: *witzelsucht.*

**moribund** (mor′ĭ-bŭnd) [L. *moribundus*] In a dying condition; dying.

**morning care** Care provided for a patient, which includes taking temperature, pulse, and respiration, assistance with oral hygiene and bathing, changing bed linen, and providing breakfast.

**morning sickness** The nausea and vomiting that affect some women during first few months of pregnancy, particularly in the morning. Typically it starts after 4 to 6 weeks of gestation, reaches a peak in incidence and severity by 8 to 12 weeks, and usually resolves spontaneously by the 16th week. It is the most common complaint of the first few months of pregnancy and is probably due to the hormonal changes incident to pregnancy. Mild or moderate nausea and vomiting is present in 70% of pregnancies. SYN: *nausea gravidarum.*

SYMPTOMS: Symptoms vary from simple morning sickness to pernicious vomiting of pregnancy. Headache, dizziness, and exhaustion also may be experienced. Simple morning sickness usually clears up without treatment in 1 to 3 weeks; in rare cases, a more serious condition develops. Severe morning sickness (hyperemesis gravidarum) results in dehydration, electrolyte disturbances, and weight loss. SEE: *hyperemesis gravidarum.*

TREATMENT: Treatment is symptomatic. Dietary management will help in most cases. Frequent small feedings of bland foods such as crackers, broths, and clear soups may be beneficial. If the sickness persists, an antinausea medicine suitable for use during pregnancy is usually effective. Antihistamines and other drugs have been tried, and they may be helpful, but carefully controlled studies have not been done.

---

Caution: The use of any drug during pregnancy should be carefully evaluated prior to its administration to avoid possible damage to the fetus.

---

NURSING IMPLICATIONS: The patient is advised that this condition is experienced by many women during the first trimester of pregnancy and that it usually subsides after this period. The nurse encourages the use of dietary remedies such as dry crackers, low-fat soups, and other foods to reduce nausea and vomiting. For severe symptoms or symptoms that do not subside, medications may be prescribed; however, management by other means is always considered first because of the possible adverse effects of prescription drugs on the fetus.

**morning stiffness** Generalized joint and muscle stiffness that is present on awakening. It tends to subside as activity is increased during the day. The stiffness is associated with various types of inflammatory arthritis.

**moron** [Gr. *moros,* stupid] A feebleminded person, not beyond the intellectual development level of age 12, or an IQ of 50 to 70. The term is outmoded, and affected persons are now referred to as mildly retarded. SEE: *mental retardation.*

**Moro reflex** [Ernst Moro, Ger. pediatrist, 1874–1951] A reflex seen in infants in response to stimuli, such as that produced by suddenly striking the surface on which the infant rests. The infant responds by rapid abduction and extension of the arms followed by an embracing motion (adduction) of the arms. SYN: *embrace reflex; startle reflex.*

**morphea** (mor-fē′ă) [Gr. *morphe,* form] A rare skin disease of unknown etiology, characterized by sclerosis of the skin that may be localized or widespread. There is no specific treatment, but physical therapy or infiltration with cortisone solution may help to prevent contractures.

***generalized m.*** A severe form of localized morphea. There are multiple indurated plaques, hyperpigmentation, and possible muscle atrophy. It is not associated with systemic disease. The disease may become inactive in 3 to 5 years.

***localized m.*** A localized form of scleroderma that does not progress to the systemic form of the disease.

**morpheme** (mor′fēm) The smallest meaningful unit in phonetics. SEE: *phoneme.*

**morphia** Morphine.

**morphine** (mor′fēn) [L. *morphina,* from *Morpheus,* god of dreams or sleep] The principal alkaloid found in opium, occurring as bitter colorless crystals.

***m. sulfate*** The sulfate of an alkaloid obtained from opium and occurring as feathery white crystals, incompatible with alkalies, tannic acid, and iodides. This form of morphine is the one usually used as an analgesic and sedative.

---

Caution: Morphine sulfate is used by drug addicts due to its action on the central nervous system. For this reason, its security in the hospital and pharmacy must be strictly maintained.

---

**morphine poisoning** Acute toxic reaction to injected or inhaled morphine sulfate. SEE: *Poisons and Poisoning Appendix.*

SYMPTOMS: Symptoms include brief mental exhilaration, then languor, followed by weariness, sleepiness, and pinpoint pupils. There is a rapid forcible pulse that becomes slow and feeble. Respirations are slow and shallow. Unconsciousness occurs, from which the patient may be aroused only with difficulty. Muscles become relaxed, reflexes are diminished, and temperature is low. The skin is pale, cold, and moist, and the pupils are dilated. If the dose was large enough, coma and death follow.

TREATMENT: Establish airway and provide ventilation. Give a narcotic antagonist such as naloxone, which is the treatment of choice, in small doses, and repeat if necessary at 30-min intervals. Pulmonary edema may occur; treat with positive-pressure respiration.

**morphinism** (mor′fĭn-ĭzm) [L. *morphina,* morphine, + *-ismos,* condition] Morbid condition due to habitual or excessive use of morphine. SEE: *morphine poisoning.*

**morphodifferentiation** The stage of tooth formation that determines the shape and size of the tooth crown. SEE: *enamel organ.*

**morphogenesis** (mor″fō-jĕn′ĕ-sĭs) [Gr. *morphe,* form, + *genesis,* generation, birth] Various processes occurring during development by which the form of the body and its organs is established. SYN: *morphosis.* **morphogenetic** (mor″fō-jĕn-ĕt′ĭk), *adj.*

**morphogenetic process** Any of the processes by which morphogenesis is accomplished, including cell migration, cell aggregation, localized growth, splitting (delamination and cavitation), and folding (invagination and evagination).

**morphogenetic substance** Chemical substance present in eggs or early embryos that induces morphologic differentiation. SEE: *induction.*

**morphography** (mor-fŏg′ră-fē) [″ + *graphein,* to write] The classification of organisms by form and structure.

**morphology** (mor-fŏl′ō-jē) [Gr. *morphe,* form, + *logos,* word, reason] The science of structure and form of organisms without regard to function.

**morphometry** (mor-fŏm′ĕ-trē) [″ + *metron,* measure] The measurement of forms.

**morphosis** (mor-fō′sĭs) Morphogenesis.

**morphovar** [*morpho*logical *var*iation] Variants within a species defined by variation in morphological characteristics. SEE: *biovar; serovar.*

**morpio, morpion** (mor′pē-ō, -pē-ŏn) [L.] The crab louse, *Phthirus pubis,* that infests the pubic area. SEE: *lice.*

**Morquio's syndrome** (mor-kē′ōz) [Louis Morquio, Uruguayan physician, 1867–1935] Mucopolysaccharidosis IV.

**morrhuate sodium injection** (mor′ū-āt) A sclerosing agent used intravenously to obliterate varicose veins.

**morsal** (mor′săl) [L. *morsus,* bite] Involved

in biting and chewing, as the occlusal surfaces of teeth.

**morsulus** (mor′sū-lŭs) [L. dim. of *morsus,* bite] Troche.

**mortal** [L. *mortalis*] **1.** Causing death. **2.** Subject to death.

**mortality 1.** The condition of being mortal. **2.** The death rate; the ratio of the number of deaths to a given population.

***fetal m.*** The number of fetal deaths per 1000 live births, usually per year.

***infant m.*** The number of death of children younger than 1 year per 1000 live births per year.

***maternal m.*** The number of deaths of women during childbearing per 100,000 births.

***neonatal m.*** The number of deaths of infants younger than 28 days per 1000 live births per year.

***perinatal m.*** The number of fetal deaths plus the number of deaths of infants younger than 7 days per 1000 live births per year.

**mortality table** A compilation in tabular form of the death rate at specific ages of the population being studied. Tables also may be constructed to include other demographic data (e.g., race or a causative agent or event such as childbearing or accident). This information allows comparison of the death rates of different populations.

**mortar** [L. *mortarium*] Vessel with a smooth interior in which crude drugs are crushed or ground with a pestle.

**mortician** [L. *mors,* death] Undertaker; person trained to prepare the dead for burial.

**mortification** SEE: *gangrene; necrosis.*

**mortinatality** (mor″tĭ-nā-tăl′ĭ-tē) [″ + *natus,* birth] Natimortality.

**mortise joint** Ankle.

**Morton's disease, Morton's syndrome** (mor′tŭnz) [Dudley J. Morton, U.S. orthopedist, 1884–1960] Congenital short, hypertrophied second metatarsal bone with tenderness over the head of that bone, callosities under the second and third metatarsals, and pain and tenderness of the metatarsal area.

**Morton's foot syndrome** Morton's disease.

**Morton's neuralgia** [Thomas G. Morton, U.S. surgeon, 1835–1903] Pain in the metatarsal area due to a fallen transverse arch with pressure on the lateral plantar nerve. SYN: *metatarsalgia.*

**Morton's neuroma** A neuroma-like mass of the neurovascular bundle of the intermetatarsal spaces.

**mortuary** (mor′chū-ā-rē) [L. *mortuarium,* a tomb] **1.** Temporary place for keeping dead bodies before burial. SYN: *morgue.* **2.** Relating to the dead or to death.

**morula** (mor′ū-lă) [L. *morus,* mulberry] Solid mass of cells, resembling a mulberry, resulting from cleavage of an ovum. SEE: *fertilization* for illus.

**morulation** (mor″ū-lā′shŭn) The formation of morula.

**moruloid** (mor′ū-loyd) [″ + Gr. *eidos,* form, shape] **1.** A bacterial colony made up of a mass resembling a mulberry. **2.** Resembling a mulberry.

**Morvan's disease** (mor′vănz) [Augustin M. Morvan, Fr. physician, 1819–1897] A form of syringomyelia, in which there are trophic changes in the extremities with formation of slowly healing lesions.

**MOS** *medical outcomes study.*

**mosaic 1.** A pattern made up of many small segments. **2.** Genetic mutation wherein the tissues of an organism are of different genetic kinds even though they were derived from the same cell. SEE: *chimera.*

**mosaic bone** SEE: under *bone.*

**mosaicism** (mō-zā′ĭ-sĭzm) Presence of cells of two different genetic materials in the same individual.

**mOsm** *milliosmole.*

**mosquito** [Sp., little fly] A blood-sucking insect belonging to the order Diptera, family Culicidae. Important genera are *Anopheles, Culex, Aedes, Haemagogus, Mansonia,* and *Psorophora.* They are vectors of many diseases, including malaria, filariasis, yellow fever, dengue, viral encephalitis, and dermatobiasis.

**mosquitocide** [″ + L. *caedere,* to kill] An agent that is lethal to mosquitoes or their larvae.

**mosquito forceps** SEE: under *forceps.*

**moss 1.** Any low-growing green plant of the class Musci. **2.** In general, any one of a number of lichens and seaweeds.

***sphagnum m.*** Peat moss. It has been used as a surgical bandage and by some primitive people as a form of external menstrual protection.

**mossy cell** SEE: under *cell.*

**mossy fibers** SEE: under *fiber.*

**mother** [AS. *modor*] **1.** Female parent. **2.** A structure that gives rise to others.

***biological m.*** SEE: *biological mother; surrogate parenting.*

***surrogate m.*** A woman who, through in vitro fertilization, gives birth to a child to which she may not have a genetic relationship.

**mother cell** SEE: under *cell.*

**mother cyst** SEE: under *cyst.*

**mother's mark** A birthmark. SEE: *mark.*

**motile** (mō′tĭl) [L. *motilis,* moving] Having spontaneous movement.

**motilin** A hormone secreted by the mucosa of the small intestine. It stimulates the gastrointestinal muscles to contract, promoting peristalsis and motility. SEE: *secretin.*

**motility** (mō-tĭl′ĭ-tē) The power to move spontaneously.

**motion** (mō′shŭn) [L. *motio,* movement] **1.** A change of place or position; movement. **2.** Evacuation of the bowels. **3.** Matter evacuated from bowels. SEE: words beginning with *cine-* and *kine-.*

***active m.*** Movement caused by the patient's own intention.

***continuous passive m.*** ABBR: CPM.

The postsurgical use of an electromechanical device to move the hand repeatedly through a prescribed range of motion. The purpose is to prevent joint stiffness and adhesions and promote circulation and healing. SYN: *continuous passive range of motion.*

Caution: Patients should be monitored closely during use of these devices.

***passive m.*** Movement as the result of the attendant's causing the part to be moved.

**motion sickness** A syndrome of physiological responses to real or apparent motion to which a person is not adapted. This may occur in many forms of transport, such as ships, aircraft, and automobiles. Motion sickness is also experienced in flight simulators and the microgravity of space travel. The condition can be produced in the absence of motion as in visualization of motion while viewing widescreen movies. It is estimated that more than 90% of inexperienced ship passengers become seasick in very rough weather conditions. Susceptibility to motion sickness is highest between the ages of 2 and 12; there is a significant decline between 12 and 21 years of age, and the incidence is very low in the elderly.

SYMPTOMS: The principal symptom of motion sickness is nausea, and the main signs are pallor, sweating, and vomiting. Other responses include apathy, general discomfort, headache, increased salivation and prostration.

ETIOLOGY: Changing the rate of motion that acts on the labyrinth of the inner ear causes motion sickness. There may be a psychological component to the causation of motion sickness, in that some individuals may develop anxiety when exposed to unfamiliar modes of travel.

TREATMENT: Prior to traveling, persons prone to motion sickness should avoid bulky, greasy meals, particularly if there is little time to digest them before beginning the trip. Susceptible persons should be seated in the most stable part of the aircraft, boat, or vehicle, and avoid head movement and reading. A number of different forms of desensitization have been used to prevent motion sickness. Antimotion sickness medications include diphenhydramine, meclizine, diazepam, and scopolamine. The last drug may be administered via a dermal patch applied 4 hr before departure.

Caution: Sedatives for treating motion sickness should be mild enough to not interfere with mental and physical function when the person arrives at the destination.

**motivation** (mō″tĭ-vā′shŭn) The internal drive or externally arising stimulus to action or thought.

**motive** (mō′tĭv) The mental condition or state that affects, alters, or stimulates behavior.

**motofacient** (mō″tō-fā′shĕnt) Producing motion.

**motoneuron** (mō″tō-nū′rŏn) A neuron that carries impulses to muscle tissue to stimulate contraction, or to glandular tissue to stimulate secretion. SYN: *motor neuron.*

***lower m.'s*** Peripheral motor neurons that originate in the ventral gray columns of the spinal cord and terminate in skeletal muscles.

***peripheral m.'s*** Motor neurons that transmit stimuli to skeletal muscles.

***upper m.'s*** Neurons of the cerebral cortex that conduct stimuli from the motor cortex of the brain to motor nuclei of cerebral nerves or the ventral gray columns of the spinal cord.

**motor** [L. *motus,* moving] **1.** Causing motion. **2.** A part or center that induces movements, as nerves or muscles. **motorial** (mō-tor′ē-ăl), *adj.*

**motor aphasia** SEE: under *aphasia.*

**motor area** SEE: under *area.*

**motor endplate** SEE: under *endplate.*

**motor fiber** SEE: under *fiber.*

**motor nerve** SEE: under *nerve.*

**motor neuron** Motoneuron.

**motor neuron disease** One of several types of disease of the motoneurons, including progressive muscular atrophy, primary lateral sclerosis, progressive bulbar paralysis, and amyotrophic lateral sclerosis. These diseases are characterized by degeneration of anterior horn cells of the spinal cord, the motor cranial nerve nuclei, and the corticospinal tracts. They occur principally in males. In the U.S., amyotrophic lateral sclerosis is better known as Lou Gehrig's disease.

**motorpathy** (mō-tor′păth-ē) [L. *motus,* moving, + Gr. *pathos,* disease, suffering] Kinesitherapy.

**motor point** SEE: under *point.*

**motor sense** SEE: *sense, muscular.*

**motor speech area** SEE: *Broca's area.*

**motor test meal** The use of various techniques to monitor the progress of food through the gastrointestinal tract.

**motor unit** SEE: under *unit.*

**mottled enamel** SEE: under *enamel.*

**mottling** (mŏt′lĭng) [ME. *motteley,* many colored] Condition that is marked by discolored areas.

**moulage** (moo-lăzh′) [Fr.] **1.** A wax model or reproduction of the configuration of some part of the anatomy such as the face or nose, or of a pathological skin lesion. **2.** Molding of a wax model.

**mounding** [origin uncertain] The rising of a lump, as the mounding of a wasting muscle when struck a quick, firm blow. SYN: *myoedema* (1).

**mount** (mownt) [ME. *mounten,* to mount] **1.** To place on a support or backing. **2.** To place specimens or sections in special containers or on slides for study.

***x-ray m.*** A stiff cardboard folder with windows in which radiographs of teeth in the dental arches are placed in sequence for examination and diagnosis.

**mountain fever** Condition occurring in individuals ascending to high altitudes (over 10,000 ft or 3,048 m) or to those subjected to rarefied atmospheres. It is due to anoxia resulting from reduced oxygen tension. SEE: *bends.*

SYMPTOMS: euphoria, tachycardia, headache, nausea, increased respiratory rate, fatigue, and cerebral disorders (loss of memory, errors of judgment).

**mountain sickness, chronic** The slow onset of symptoms in persons who reside at high altitude for several years. Included are florid color that turns to cyanosis during mild exertion, apathy, fatigue, and headache. Persons between ages 40 and 60 are most likely to be affected. The symptoms subside when the person returns to sea level. SYN: *Monge's disease.*

**mounting** (mownt′ĭng) **1.** The arrangement of specimens on slides, frames, chart boards, display boards, or any background for study. **2.** In dentistry, the attachment of a cast of the mandible or maxilla to an articulator.

**mourning** [AS. *murnan*] Normal grief usually produced by the death of a loved one. Mourning is not synonymous with depression or melancholia. SEE: *grief reaction.*

**mouse** (mows) **1.** A small rodent of the genus *Mus*. Mice are used extensively in research. **2.** A small piece of tissue that has become free or unattached, esp. in a body cavity or joint.

***joint m.*** Fragment of synovial membrane or cartilage becoming free in the joint space due to trauma or osteoarthritis.

***New Zealand black m.*** ABBR: NZB m. A mouse bred for the genetic trait of spontaneously developing autoimmune hemolytic anemia.

***nude m.*** A mutant mouse, completely devoid of hair and lacking T lymphocytes, bred for use in immunological investigations.

**mouse unit** SEE: *Allen-Doisy unit.*

**mouth** [AS. *muth*] **1.** The opening of any cavity. **2.** The cavity within the cheeks, containing the tongue and teeth, and communicating with the pharynx. SYN: *buccal cavity; oral cavity.* SEE: illus.

ABNORMALITIES: *Tongue:* dry, coated, smooth, strawberry, large, pigmented, geographic, deviated, tremulous, sore. *Gums and teeth:* gingivitis, sordes, lead line, pyorrhea, atrophy, hypertrophy, dental caries, alveolar abscesses. *Mucous membranes and other parts of mouth:* eruptions accompanying exanthematous diseases, stomatitis, canker sores, herpes simplex, thrush, trench mouth, cysts, tumors, carcinoma, lesions of syphilis such as chancre, mucous patches, gumma, lesions of tuberculosis, abscesses.

Disorders of the mouth cavity may be indications of purely local diseases or they

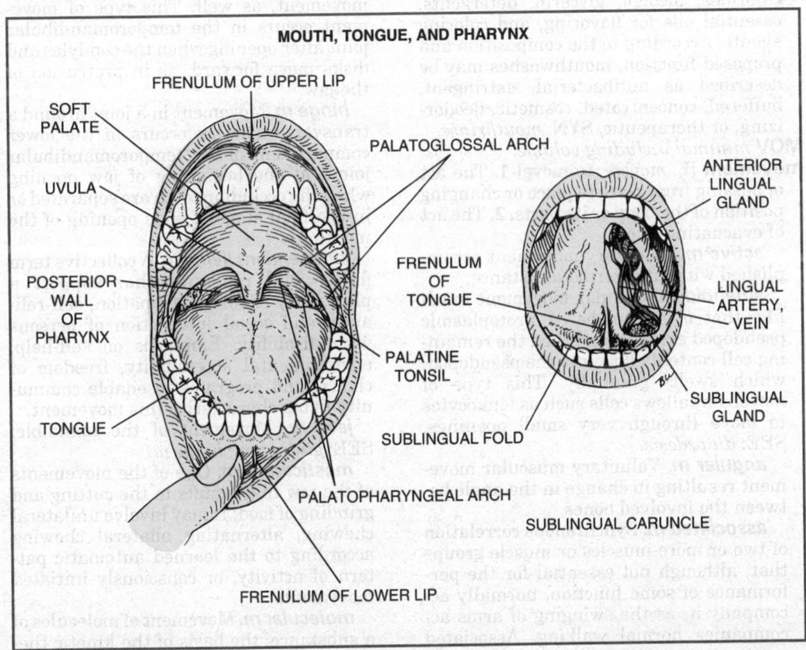

may be symptoms of systemic disturbances such as dehydration, pernicious anemia, nutritional deficiencies, esp. avitaminosis.

Rashes of the mouth may indicate stomatitis, measles, or scarlet fever. Rashes on lips may indicate typhoid fever, meningitis, or pneumonia. In secondary syphilis, chancre, cancer, and epithelioma, mucous patches appear.

EXAMINATION: In addition to visual examination, careful digital examination should be made because it reveals areas of tenderness and alterations of texture characteristic of leukoplakia, cancer, cystic swellings, and lymphadenopathy.

Excessive moisture of the mouth is seen in stomatitis, irritation of the vagus nerve, ingestion of irritating drugs or foods, nervous disorders, teething, seeing appetizing foods, and smelling pleasant odors. SEE: *burning mouth syndrome.*

***trench m.*** SEE: *trench mouth.*

**mouth guard** A removable dental appliance used to protect the teeth and investing tissues during contact sports. SEE: *occlusal guard.*

**mouthrinse** Mouthwash.

**mouthstick** Adapted device consisting of a stick attached to a molded dental mouthpiece that permits page turning and other tasks through head movement.

**mouthwash** A medicated solution used to cleanse or treat diseases of the oral mucosa, reduce halitosis, or add fluoride to the teeth for control or prevention of dental caries. It may contain various chemical compounds, such as fluoride or zinc chlorides, alcohol, glycerin, detergents, essential oils for flavoring, and coloring agents. According to the composition and proposed function, mouthwashes may be described as antibacterial, astringent, buffered, concentrated, cosmetic, deodorizing, or therapeutic. SYN: *mouthrinse.*

**MOV** *minimal occluding volume.*

**movement** [L. *movere,* to move] **1.** The act of passing from place to place or changing position of the body or its parts. **2.** The act of evacuating feces.

***active m.*** Voluntary movement accomplished without external assistance.

***ameboid m.*** Cellular movement much like that of an ameba. A protoplasmic pseudopod extends, and then the remaining cell contents flow into the pseudopod, which swells gradually. This type of movement allows cells such as leukocytes to move through very small openings. SEE: *diapedesis.*

***angular m.*** Voluntary muscular movement resulting in change in the angle between the involved bones.

***associated m.*** Synchronous correlation of two or more muscles or muscle groups that, although not essential for the performance of some function, normally accompany it, as the swinging of arms accompanies normal walking. Associated movements are characteristically lost in cerebellar disease.

***autonomic m.*** Spontaneous, involuntary movement independent of external stimulation.

***bodily m.*** Movement of a tooth by natural or orthodontic forces so that the crown and root maintain their same vertical axis. SEE: *rotational m.; tipping m.*

***brownian m.*** SEE: *brownian movement.*

***cardinal m.'s of labor*** Changes in the position of the fetal head as it descends through the birth canal and exits the mother's body. Flexion, internal rotation, and extension enable the descending head to accommodate to the dimensions of the maternal pelvis. External rotation occurs as the head exits the mother's body.

***ciliary m.*** Rhythmic movement of the cilia of a ciliated cell or epithelium. SYN: *vibratile m.*

***circus m.*** A phenomenon appearing after injury to a corpus striatum, optic thalamus, or crus cerebri, and causing an odd circular gait.

***disorders of m.*** Hemiplegia, ataxia, monoplegia, tremors, rigors, chorea, athetosis, convulsions, spasm (clonic or tonic), reflex (hysterical, habit spasm, tics), and spastic paralysis. These disorders may be due to injury or disease of muscle, nerve ending, motor nerve, spinal cord, or the brain.

***fetal m.*** Muscular movements performed by the fetus in utero.

***gliding m.*** Movement of one surface over another without angular or rotatory movement, as well. This type of movement occurs in the temporomandibular joint after opening when the condyles and disks move forward, as in protrusion of the jaw.

***hinge m.*** Movement in a joint around a transverse axis, as occurs in the lower compartment of the temporomandibular joints at the beginning of jaw opening when the occluding teeth are separated or in the final stage of wide opening of the mouth.

***independent living m.*** A collective term for societal programs that support a philosophy of full participation, self-reliance, and social integration of persons with disability. Emphasis on self-help, environmental accessibility, freedom of choice, and programs to enable community living characterize this movement.

***jaw m.*** Movement of the mandible. SEE: *gliding m.; hinge m.*

***masticatory m.*** One of the movements of the jaw that results in the cutting and grinding of food. It may involve unilateral chewing, alternating bilateral chewing according to the learned automatic pattern of activity, or consciously initiated movements.

***molecular m.*** Movement of molecules of a substance, the basis of the kinetic theory of matter. SEE: *brownian movement.*

**orthodontic m.** Movement of teeth by orthodontic appliances for aesthetics or to correct malocclusions. Such movement depends on remodeling of the bony socket, which usually occurs without resorption of the tooth root unless excessive force has been used.

**passive m.** Movement of the body or a part due to outside forces.

**pendular m.'s** Swaying movements of the intestines caused by rhythmic contractions of the longitudinal muscles of the walls of the intestines.

**peristaltic m.** Peristalsis.

**physiological m.** A movement that is normally executed by muscles that are under voluntary control such as flexion, extension, abduction, adduction, and rotation. It is also known as physiological motion.

**respiratory m.** Any movement resulting from the contraction of respiratory muscles or occurring passively as a result of elasticity of the thoracic wall or lungs. SEE: *compliance* (1); *expiration; inspiration; respiration.*

**m. of restitution** A partial rotation of the fetal head in cases of head presentation.

**rotational m.** Movement around an axis, as in hinge movement of the temporomandibular joint or rotation of a tooth around its longitudinal axis in tooth movement or extraction. SEE: *bodily m.; tipping m.*

**saccadic m.'s** Jerky movements of the eyes as they move from one point of fixation to another.

**segmenting m.** Movement of the intestine in which annular constrictions occur, dividing the intestine into ovoid segments.

**tipping m.** Movement of a tooth crown while the root apex remains essentially stationary, resulting in an inclination of the axis of the tooth in one direction. SEE: *bodily m.; rotational m.*

**triplanar m.** Movement occurring around an oblique axis in all three body planes.

**vermicular m.** The wormlike movements of peristalsis.

**vibratile m.** Ciliary m.

**moxa** (mŏk′sa) [Japanese] A soft, combustible substance to be burned on skin, popular in eastern Asia and Japan as a cautery and counterirritant. SEE: *moxibustion.*

**moxalactam disodium** An antibacterial drug.

**moxibustion** (mŏks-ĭ-bŭs′chŭn) [″ + L. *combustus,* burned] Cauterization and counterirritation by means of a cylinder or cone of cotton wool, called a moxa, placed on the skin and fired at the top.

**Mozart ear** [Wolfgang Amadeus Mozart, Austrian composer, 1756–1791. Alleged to have had this deformity] Deformity of the ear in which the antihelix is fused with the crura of the helix.

**M.P.D.** *maximum permissible dose.*

**M.P.H.** *Master of Public Health.*

**M.P.N.** *most probable number* (of bacteria present in a quantity of solution, esp. water).

**MPS** *mucopolysaccharidosis.*

**MR** *magnetic resonance.*

**mR** *milliroentgen.*

**MRCP** *Member of the Royal College of Physicians.*

**MRCP(C)** *Member of the Royal College of Physicians of Canada.*

**MRCS** *Member of the Royal College of Surgeons.*

**MRCS(C)** *Member of the Royal College of Surgeons of Canada.*

**mrem** *millirem.*

**MRI** *magnetic resonance imaging.*

**M.R.L.** *Medical Record Librarian.*

**mRNA** *messenger RNA.*

**MRSA** *methicillin-resistant Staphylococcus aureus.*

**$\mu$s** Symbol for microsecond.

**MS** *multiple sclerosis.*

**M.S.** *Master of Surgery; Master of Science.*

**ms** *millisecond.*

**msec** *millisecond.*

**MSH** *melanocyte-stimulating hormone.*

**M.S.N.** *Master of Science in Nursing.*

**MSVC** *maximum sustainable ventilatory capacity.* SEE: *ventilation, maximum sustainable.*

**M.T.** *medical technologist.*

**M.u.** *Mache unit.*

**mu** (mū) [Gr. $\mu$, letter m] SYMB: $\mu$; u. Symbol used for the prefix *micro-* which stands for multiplication by $10^{-6}$. Thus, $\mu$m would stand for $10^{-6}$ m.

**m.u.** *mouse unit.*

**muc-** SEE: *muco-.*

**mucedin** (mū′sĕ-dĭn) [L. *mucedo,* mucus] A substance obtained from gluten.

**muci-** SEE: *muco-.*

**muciform** (mū′sĭ-form) [″ + *forma,* shape] Appearing similar to mucus.

**mucigen** (mŭ′sĭ-jĕn) [″ + Gr. *gennan,* to produce] A substance present in mucous cells that, upon being extruded from the cell, is converted into mucin.

**mucigenous** (mū-sĭj′ĕn-ŭs) Muciparous.

**mucilage** (mū′sĭ-lĭj) [L. *mucilago,* moldy juice] Thick, viscid, adhesive liquid, containing gum or mucilaginous principles dissolved in water, usually employed to suspend insoluble substances in aqueous liquids or as a demulcent. **mucilaginous** (mū-sĭl-ăj′ĭn-ŭs), *adj.*

**mucilloid** (mū′sĭl-loyd) A mucilaginous preparation.

**psyllium hydrophilic m.** Mucilloid prepared from psyllium seeds. It is used as a bulk-type laxative.

**mucin** (mū′sĭn) [L. *mucus,* mucus] A glycoprotein found in mucus. It is present in saliva and bile, in salivary glands, and in the skin, connective tissues, tendon, and cartilage. Mucin is formed from mucigen and forms a slimy solution in water. **mucinoid** (mū'sĭn-oyd), *adj.*

**mucinase** (mū'sĭ-nās) Any enzyme that acts on mucin.

**mucinemia** (mū"sĭn-ē'mē-ă) [" + Gr. *haima,* blood] Accumulation of mucin in the blood.

**mucinogen** (mū-sĭn'ō-jĕn) [" + Gr. *gennan,* to produce] A glycoprotein that forms mucin.

**mucinolytic** (mū"sĭ-nō-lĭt'ĭk) [" + Gr. *lysis,* dissolution] Capable of hydrolyzing or dissolving mucin.

**mucinuria** (mū-sĭn-ū'rē-ă) [" + Gr. *ouron,* urine] Presence of mucin in the urine.

**muciparous** (mū-sĭp'ăr-ŭs) [" + *parere,* to bring forth, to bear] Producing or secreting mucus. SYN: *mucigenous.*

**muco-, muc-, muci** [L. *mucus,* mucus] Combining form meaning *mucus.*

**mucocele** (mū'kō-sēl) [" + Gr. *kele,* tumor, swelling] **1.** Enlargement of the lacrimal sac. **2.** A mucous cyst. **3.** A mucous polypus. **4.** Cystic disease of the air cavities of the cranial bones causing erosion of the bone.

**mucociliary** Pert. to ciliated mucosa.

**mucocutaneous** (mū"kō-kū-tā'nē-ŭs) [" + *cutis,* skin] Concerning mucous membrane and the skin. SYN: *mucodermal.*

**mucocutaneous lymph node syndrome** Kawasaki disease.

**mucodermal** (mū-kō-dĕr'măl) Mucocutaneous.

**mucoenteritis** (mū"kō-ĕn-tĕr-ī'tĭs) [" + Gr. *enteron,* intestine, + *itis,* inflammation] Inflammation of intestinal mucosa.

**mucoglobulin** (mū"kō-glŏb'ū-lĭn) [" + *globulus,* globule] A type of glycoprotein.

**mucoid** (mū'koyd) [" + Gr. *eidos,* form, shape] **1.** Glycoprotein similar to mucin. **2.** Muciform similar to mucus.

**mucokinesis** Any therapeutic technique that removes excessive or abnormal secretions from the respiratory tract.

**mucolytic** Pert. to a class of agents that liquefy sputum or reduce its viscosity. SEE: *cystic fibrosis.*

**mucomembranous** (mū"kō-mĕm'bră-nŭs) [" + *membrana,* membrane] Concerning mucous membrane.

**mucoperiosteum** (mū"kō-pĕr"ē-ŏs'tē-ŭm) Periosteum that has a mucous surface; or mucous and periosteal surfaces combined to form a membrane.

**mucopolysaccharidase** (mū"kō-pŏl"ē-săk'ă-rī-dās) An enzyme that catalyzes the hydrolysis of polysaccharides.

**mucopolysaccharide** (mū"kō-pŏl"ĭ-săk'ă-rīd) A group of polysaccharides, containing hexosamine and sometimes proteins, that forms chemical bonds with water. The thick gelatinous material is found in many places in the body, forming intercellular ground substance and basement membranes of cells and found in mucous secretions and synovial fluid.

**mucopolysaccharidosis** ABBR: MPS. A group of inherited disorders characterized by a deficiency of enzymes that are essential for the degradation of the mucopolysaccharides heparan sulfate, dermatan sulfate, and keratan sulfate. These chemicals are excreted in excess quantities in the urine, and they usually accumulate in reticuloendothelial cells, endothelial cells, intimal smooth muscle cells, and fibroblasts throughout the body. Clinical changes are not usually apparent at birth, but the inherited defect can be diagnosed prior to birth by culturing amniotic fluid cells and testing them for specific enzyme activity. The test may yield either false-positive or false-negative results. After birth, the conditions may be diagnosed by testing cultured skin fibroblasts for specific enzymes.

***m. IH*** Hurler's syndrome. MPS due to a deficiency of the enzyme α-L-iduronidase with accumulation of dermatan sulfate and heparan sulfate. Clinically, there are lens opacities, coarse facies, skeletal dysplasia, hepatosplenomegaly, and mental deficiency.

***m. IHS*** Hurler-Scheie syndrome. An intermediate form of MPS between MPS IH and MPS IS, due to the same enzyme deficiency. Mental development may be normal.

***m. IS*** Scheie's syndrome. MPS due to the same enzyme defect as MPS IH and with similar clinical characteristics, except mental deficiency is absent.

***m. II*** Hunter's disease. MPS due to a deficiency of the enzyme L-iduronosulfate sulfatase. Clinically, there are retinal degeneration without corneal clouding, mental retardation, joint stiffness, skeletal dysplasia, cardiac lesions, and deafness.

***m. III*** Sanfilippo's disease. This MPS has been further differentiated into Sanfilippo A, B, C, or D, on the basis of the specific enzyme deficiency present in each form. Clinically, it may not be possible to distinguish the types. Present are moderate coarse facies, severe mental deficiency, and mild hepatosplenomegaly. Corneal clouding is absent and growth is normal.

***m. IV*** Morquio's syndrome. MPS due to a deficiency of the enzyme *N*-acetylgalactosamine-6-sulfatase. Clinically, there are dwarfism, thoracolumbar gibbus (hunchback), kyphoscoliosis, coarse facies, cardiac lesions, moderate hepatosplenomegaly, and joint hypermobility.

***m. V*** Former designation for mucopolysaccharidosis IS.

***m. VI*** Maroteaux-Lamy syndrome. MPS due to a deficiency of the enzyme *N*-acetylgalactosamine-4-sulfatase. Clinically, MPS VI is similar to MPS IH, except intelligence is normal.

***m. VII*** Glucuronidase deficiency disease. MPS due to a deficiency of β-glucuronidase. Clinically, MPS VII is quite similar to MPS IH, except intelligence may be normal.

**mucopolysacchariduria** (mū″kō-pŏl″ē-săk′ă-rĭ-dū′rē-ă) Mucopolysaccharides in the urine.

**mucoprotein** (mū″kō-prō′tē-ĭn) A complex of protein and mucopolysaccharide. Usually, the polysaccharide contains hexosamine.

***Tamm-Horsfall m.*** SEE: *Tamm-Horsfall mucoprotein.*

**mucopurulent** (mū-kō-pūr′ū-lĕnt) [L. *mucus,* mucus, + *purulentus,* made up of pus] Consisting of mucus and pus.

**Mucor** (mū′kor) [L.] A genus of mold fungi seen on dead and decaying matter. Some species can cause infections of external ear, skin, and respiratory passageways. SEE: *mucormycosis.*

**mucoriferous** (mū″kor-ĭf′ĕr-ŭs) [L. *mucor,* mold, + *ferre,* to carry] Covered with mold or a moldlike substance.

**mucormycosis** (mū″kor-mī-kō′sĭs) [″ + Gr. *mykes,* fungus, + *osis,* condition] Mycosis usually caused by fungi of the family Mucoraceae of the class Zygomycetes. These fungi have an affinity for blood vessels, in which they cause thrombosis and infarction. The form of this disease that affects the head and face usually causes paranasal sinus infections, esp. during periods of ketoacidosis in persons with diabetes mellitus. This form may also disseminate to the brain. The pulmonary form of the disease causes infarcts of the lung; the gastrointestinal form causes mucosal ulcers and gangrene of the stomach. The disease is contracted by inhalation or ingestion of the fungus by susceptible individuals. Most persons have a natural resistance to the fungus, accounting for the rarity of the disease. SYN: *zygomycosis.*

TREATMENT: Control or prevention of diabetic acidosis, administration of amphotericin B, and resection of necrotic tissue.

**mucorrhea** [″ + *rhoia,* to flow] Increased cervical discharge at ovulation, usually covering a span of 3 to 4 days. The discharge has the character and appearance of raw egg white. SEE: *spinnbarkeit.*

**mucosa** (mū-kō′să) *pl.* **mucosae** [L., mucous] A mucous membrane or moist tissue layer that lines the hollow organs and cavities of the body. Specifically, it consists of an epithelial covering with its basement membrane and a connective tissue layer often called lamina propria. The tissue lining the alimentary canal also contains a smooth muscle layer called the muscularis mucosae. The type of epithelium, thickness, and presence or absence of glands varies with the function or location of the mucosa. **mucosal** (mū-kō′săl), *adj.*

***alveolar m.*** A thin, nonkeratinized mucosal layer covering the alveolar process and loosely attached to underlying bone. It is continuous with the mucosa of the cheek, lips, tongue, and palate.

***buccal m.*** The lining of the cheeks of the oral cavity. It is characterized by stratified squamous non-keratinized epithelium that may become keratinized in local areas due to cheek-biting. It may also contain ectopic sebaceous glands. SEE: *Fordyce's disease.*

***lingual m.*** The keratinized, papillated covering of the dorsum of the tongue that contains nerve endings for the sense of taste.

***masticatory m.*** Those areas of the mucosa of the mouth that have become keratinized due to the friction and abrasion of the masticatory process, esp. the gingivae and hard palate.

***nasal m.*** The mucosa lining the nasal cavity and paranasal sinuses, characterized by pseudostratified ciliated columnar epithelium with goblet cells. Nasal mucosa functions to warm and hydrate the air inspired and by ciliary action to exteriorize mucus-entrapped dust and debris.

***oral m.*** The mucous membrane lining the oral cavity and described by its location on the gingiva, hard palate, soft palate, cheek, vestibule, lip, tongue, and pharyngeal area.

**mucosanguineous** (mū″kō-săn-gwĭn′ē-ŭs) [″ + *sanguineus,* bloody] Containing mucus and blood.

**mucoserous** (mū″kō-sēr′ŭs) Composed of mucus and serum.

**mucositis** (mū″kō-sī′tĭs) [″ + Gr. *itis,* inflammation] Inflammation of a mucous membrane. SEE: *gingivitis, acute necrotizing ulcerative.*

**mucosocutaneous** (mū-kō″sō-kū-tā′nē-ŭs) Concerning a mucous membrane and the skin.

**mucostatic** (mū″kō-stăt′ĭk) [″ + *statikos,* standing] Stopping the secretion of mucus.

**mucous** (mū′kŭs) **1.** Having the nature of or resembling mucus. **2.** Secreting mucus. **3.** Depending on presence of mucus.

**mucous colitis** SEE: *irritable bowel disease.*

**mucous membrane** The membrane lining passages and cavities communicating with the air, consisting of a surface layer of epithelium, a basement membrane, and an underlying layer of connective tissue (lamina propria). Mucus-secreting cells or glands are usually present in the epithelium but may be absent. In humans, mucous membranes and the skin provide effective mechanisms for preventing the entry of pathogens. Mucous membranes are normally colonized with nonpathogenic organisms that discourage colonization by pathogens because the resident organisms compete for the nutrients essential to their survival. Some mucosal surfaces in the digestive tract have special characteristics that tend to repel or kill organisms, such as the extremely high acid level on the mucosa of the stomach. SEE: *bacterial adherence.*

Noninvasive examination of membranes should reveal the degree of moisture, cyanosis, pallor, hyperemia, pigmentation, lesions or their absence, and hemorrhage. Pallor is seen in all anemias. If temporary, it may indicate shock or vasomotor spasm, or it may occur in severe hemorrhages. Blanching and flushing alternately accompany aortic regurgitation.

Hyperemia or excessive redness of the mucous membranes is indicative of certain pathological changes in particular tissues. For example: *Buccal mucous membrane:* Due to decayed teeth, traumatism, stomatitis. SEE: *mouth. Nasal mucosa:* Ulceration of nose, rhinitis, inflammation. SEE: *nose. Eyes (local irritation):* Foreign body, ulcer, inflammation. SEE: *jaundice.* Dryness is seen in fevers, chronic gastritis, some liver disturbances, excitement, shock, prostration, fatigue, thirst, and certain drugs.

**mucous polyp** Small growth from mucous lining of the cervix or uterus.

**mucoviscidosis** (mū″kō-vĭs″ĭ-dō′sĭs) Cystic fibrosis.

**mucus** (mū′kŭs) [L.] A viscid fluid secreted by mucous membranes and glands, consisting of mucin, leukocytes, inorganic salts, water, and epithelial cells. A good example is the almost ropy secretion from the sublingual and submandibular glands.

***cervical m.*** The discharge secreted by the endocervical glands of the uterine cervix. Characteristic assessment findings correlate with normal hormonal changes of the menstrual cycle that influence the type and amount of mucus secreted. Immediately before ovulation, high estrogen levels stimulate secretion of a large amount of thin, watery mucus that is hospitable to sperm transit. After ovulation, high progesterone levels stimulate secretion of a thick, viscous mucus that is less hospitable to sperm. SEE: *fern pattern; spinnbarkeit.*

**mull** (mŭl) To grind or pulverize.

**Müller, Heinrich** (mül′ĕr) German anatomist, 1820–1864.

***M.'s fibers*** Fine fibers of neuroglia cells that form supporting elements of the retina.

***M.'s muscle*** **1.** Circular fibers of ciliary muscle. **2.** The superior tarsal muscle of the eyelid. **3.** Smooth muscle covering the sphenomaxillary fissure.

***M.'s trigone*** Portion of tuber cinereum folding over the optic chiasm.

**Müller, Johannes P.** (mül′ĕr) German physician, 1801–1858.

***M.'s ducts*** Embryonic tubes from which the oviducts, uterus, and vagina develop in the female; in the male, they atrophy. SYN: *müllerian ducts.*

***M.'s maneuver*** Inspiratory effort with a closed glottis at the end of expiration. This technique is used during radiographic studies to produce negative intrathoracic pressure and cause engorgement of blood vessels, thus allowing visualization of esophageal varices.

***M.'s ring*** Muscular ring at the junction of the cervical canal and the gravid uterus.

***M.'s tubercle*** Projection on the dorsal wall of the cloaca at which Müller's ducts terminate.

**mult-, multi-** [L. *multus*] Prefix meaning *many, much.*

**multangular** Having many angles.

**multangular bone, greater** The first or outermost of the distal row of carpal bones. SYN: *trapezium.*

**multangular bone, lesser** The second in distal row of carpal bones. SYN: *trapezoid bone.*

**multiallelic** (mŭl″tē-ă-lĕl′ĭk) Concerning a large number of genes affecting hereditary characteristics.

**multiarticular** (mŭl″tē-ăr-tĭk′ū-lăr) [L. *multus,* many, + *articulus,* joint] Concerning, having, or affecting many joints. SYN: *polyarticular.*

**multicapsular** (mŭl″tĭ-kăp′sū-lăr) [″ + *capsula,* a little box] Composed of many capsules.

**multicellular** (mŭl″tĭ-sĕl′ū-lăr) [″ + *cellula,* small chamber] Consisting of many cells.

**Multiceps** A genus of tapeworms.

**multicuspid, multicuspidate** (mŭl″tĭ-kŭs′pĭd, -pĭ-dāt) [″ + *cuspis,* point] Having several cusps.

**multidisciplinary** Relating to multiple fields of study involved in the care of patients. The term suggests that the various disciplines are working in collaboration, but in a parallel mode of interaction. Each distinctive discipline is accountable and responsible for its tasks and functions regarding patient care.

**multifactorial** The result of many factors, as in a disease resulting from the combined effects of several components.

**multifamilial** (mŭl″tĭ-fă-mĭl′ē-ăl) Concerning a familial disease that affects children in several generations.

**multifid** (mŭl′tĭ-fĭd) [″ + *fidus,* from *findere,* to split] Divided into many sections.

**multifocal** (mŭl″tĭ-fō′kăl) Concerning or arising from many locations.

**multiform** (mŭl′tĭ-form) [″ + *forma,* shape] Having many forms or shapes. SYN: *polymorphic; polymorphous.*

**multiglandular** (mŭl″tĭ-glănd′ū-lar) [″ + *glandula,* a little acorn] Concerning several glands.

**multigravida** (mŭl″tĭ-grăv′ĭ-dă) [″ + *gravida,* pregnant] A woman who is experiencing her second pregnancy or who has been pregnant more than once. The number of pregnancies may be recorded as gravida II, gravida III, and so on. SEE: *multipara.*

**multi-infarct dementia** SEE: under *dementia.*

**multi-infection** (mŭl″tĭ-ĭn-fĕk′shŭn) [L. *multus,* many, + *infectio,* an infection] A mixed infection with several organisms developing at the same time.

**multilobular** (mŭl″tĭ-lŏb′ū-lar) [″ + *lobulus,* a small lobe] Formed of or possessing many lobules.

**multilocular** (mŭl″tĭ-lŏk′ū-lar) [″ + *loculus,* a cell] Having many cells or compartments.

**multimammae** (mŭl″tĭ-măm′mē) [″ + *mamma,* breast] Polymastia.

**multinodal** (mŭl-tĭ-nō′dăl) Having many nodes or knots.

**multinodular** (mŭl-tĭ-nŏd′ū-lar) [″ + *nodulus,* little knot] Possessing many nodules or small knots.

**multinuclear, multinucleate** (mŭl-tĭ-nū′klē-ăr, -āt) Possessing several nuclei. SYN: *polynuclear; polynucleate.*

**multipara** (mŭl-tĭp′ă-ră) [″ + *parere,* to bring forth, to bear] A woman who has borne more than one viable fetus, whether or not the offspring were alive at birth. The number of deliveries may be recorded as para II, para III, and so on. SEE: *multigravida.*

***grand m.*** A woman who has given birth seven or more times.

**multiparity** (mŭl-tĭ-păr′ĭ-tē) The condition of having borne more than one child.

**multiparous** (mŭl-tĭp′ăr-ŭs) Having borne more than one child.

**multiphasic screening** SEE: *screening test, multiphasic.*

**multiple** (mŭl′tĭ-pl) [L. *multiplex,* many folded] **1.** Consisting of or containing more than one; manifold. **2.** Occurring simultaneously in various parts of the body.

**multiple drug resistance** A lack of expected therapeutic response to several disease-specific pharmaceutical agents, esp. antibiotics. In cancer therapy, resistance to a wide range of unrelated drugs may occur after resistance to a single agent has developed. SEE: *gene amplification.*

**multiple endocrine neoplasia** ABBR: MEN. An inherited genetic defect that produces hyperplasia or malignant tumors in several endocrine glands. This group of diseases has been classed according to the glands affected. In MEN type I (MEN I), there are tumors of the parathyroid, pituitary, and islet cells of the pancreas. SYN: *Wermer's syndrome.* MEN type II (MEN II) is characterized by medullary thyroid carcinoma, pheochromocytoma, and parathyroid hyperplasia. SYN: *Sipple syndrome.* MEN type III (MEN III) is quite similar to MEN II, but there are marked facial aberrations with neuromas of the conjunctiva, labial mucosa, tongue, larynx, and gastric intestinal tract.

**multiple malformation syndrome** Developmental anomalies of two or more systems in the fetus. These may be caused by chromosome and genetic abnormalities, or by teratogens including certain drugs and chemicals. In attempting to determine the etiology, it is important to obtain a complete family history and history of exposure to known teratogens and infectious diseases. SEE: *amniotic band disruption sequence syndrome.*

**multiple myeloma** SEE: under *myeloma.*

**multiple personality** SEE: under *personality.*

**multiple sclerosis** SEE: under *sclerosis.*

**Multiple Sleep Latency Test** SEE: *narcolepsy.*

**multiple systems organ failure** ABBR: MSOF. Progressive failure of two or more organ systems due to acute, usually generalized clinical conditions and mediated by the body's inability to sufficiently activate its defense mechanisms. Organs fail because of this generalized defense system malfunction, rather than as isolated incidents. The clinical signs will be consistent with failure of organ systems such as the lungs, kidneys, circulatory system, liver, central nervous system, gastrointestinal system, or hematologic system. SEE: *acute respiratory distress syndrome; disseminated intravascular coagulation.*

NURSING IMPLICATIONS: Closely monitor patients at risk and help to prevent MSOF by prompt recognition and correction of perfusion problems, infection, and organ dysfunction. Assess for indicators of hypermetabolic hyperdynamic state as the body tries to compensate for the initial insult. This will be followed by a hypodynamic, decompensated state with imbalances in oxygen supply and demand, maldistribution of circulating volume, and metabolic abnormalities, resulting in organ failure. Common problems are pulmonary, cardiovascular, renal, and hepatic, often followed or accompanied by gram-negative sepsis and disseminated intravascular coagulation (DIC). Appropriate medical interventions will be initiated for each failing system's problems. Nursing responsibilities include monitoring vital signs and assessing diagnostic study results, coordinating and carrying out prescribed therapies and evaluating patient responses while simultaneously assessing for adverse effects, protecting the patient from nosocomial infections and environmental stressors, and providing emotional support for patient and family through this type of devastating illness, which has a 90% mortality rate.

**multipolar** (mŭl-tĭ-pōl′ăr) [L. *multus,* many, + *polus,* a pole] **1.** Possessing more than two poles. **2.** Possessing more than two processes, said of neurons.

**multirooted** In dentistry, referring to a tooth having several roots.

**multisynaptic** (mŭl″tē-sĭ-năp′tĭk) Polysynaptic.

**multiterminal** [″ + Gr. *terma,* a limit] Providing several sets of terminals, making possible the use of several electrodes.

**multivalent** (mŭl-tĭ-vā′lĕnt) [″ + *valere,* to have power] **1.** Having ability to combine with more than two atoms of a univalent element or radical **2.** Active against several strains of an organism.

**mummification** (mŭm″mĭ-fĭ-kā′shŭn) [Arabian *mumiyaa,* mummy, + L. *facere,* to make] **1.** Mortification producing a hard, dry mass. SYN: *dry gangrene.* **2.** Drying and shriveling of a body, as a dead and retained fetus.

**mumps** (mŭmps) An acute, contagious, febrile disease marked by inflammation of the parotid glands and other salivary glands. The causative agent is the mumps virus. SYN: *parotitis.* SEE: *Nursing Diagnoses Appendix.* The incubation period is 12 to 25 days. The period of communicability ranges from 6 to 7 days before development of parotitis to 9 days following development. Exposed nonimmune people should be considered infectious from the 12th through the 25th day after exposure.

SYMPTOMS: The onset of symptoms is gradual. There may be chills, malaise, headache, pain below the ears, moderate fever of 101° to 102°F (38.3° to 38.9°C) or higher followed by swelling of one or both parotid glands. Usually, swelling in one gland is subsiding as the other swells. Swelling is below and in front of the ear. The lobe of the ear is sometimes pushed forward, surrounding tissues are edematous, and the features may be greatly distorted. Movements of the jaw are painful and restricted. Saliva may be increased or diminished. In a third of cases only one parotid gland is involved. Occasionally, the parotid glands seem to escape, and swelling is confined to the submaxillary gland. Swelling usually lasts from 5 to 7 days.

COMPLICATIONS: Complications usually develop about the time the swelling in the parotids subsides. The most common complication in the postpubertal male is orchitis, which occurs in about 20% to 30% of cases. In the female, common complications are oophoritis and mastitis. In rare cases, permanent impairment of hearing follows an attack of mumps. Meningoencephalitis has been estimated to occur in 10% of patients.

DIFFERENTIAL DIAGNOSIS: Cases of symptomatic parotitis may be excluded. Instances of trauma, infections about teeth and mouth, or a blocking of Stensen's duct may suggest mumps.

TREATMENT: Treatment consists of bedrest, a soft diet, and administration of analgesics for headache and general malaise. Cold local applications may control swelling of testicles in orchitis.

PROGNOSIS: The outcome is favorable, although the possibility of sexual sterility may occur in rare instances of bilateral orchitis.

NURSING IMPLICATIONS: The nurse encourages immunization in children older than 12 months to prevent the disease and, if mumps occur, isolation of the patient to promote recovery and prevent transmission of the disease to others. The patient's temperature is monitored, and nursing and other measures are used to reduce high fever. Good hydration and rest are encouraged. If the patient has pain from swollen glands, the nurse applies heat or cold as effective for pain relief, encourages a liquid or soft diet to reduce pain on swallowing, and administers analgesics as indicated. The patient is observed for signs and symptoms of complications, and is encouraged to begin gradual resumption of activity as symptoms subside.

**mumps skin test antigen** A standardized suspension of sterile formaldehyde-inactivated mumps virus. It is used in diagnosing mumps.

**mumps virus vaccine live** A sterile preparation of attenuated mumps virus used to immunize against mumps.

**Munchausen syndrome** (mĕn-chow′zĕn) [Baron Karl F. H. von Munchausen, fictional 18th century baron created by Rudolph Raspe] A type of malingering or factitious disorder in which the patient may practice self-multilation and deception in order to feign illness. When detected, such patients leave one hospital and appear in the emergency room of another. Patients of this type are seldom recognized in time to receive psychiatric diagnoses and therapy, which they need. SEE: *disorder, factitious.*

**Munchausen syndrome by proxy** The fabrication of symptoms or physical evidence of another's illness, or the deliberate causing of another's illness, to gain medical attention.

**mural** (mū′răl) [L. *murus,* a wall] Pert. to a wall of an organ or part.

**muramidase** An enzyme found in blood cells of the granulocytic and monocytic series. Its serum and urine level is increased in patients with acute or chronic leukemia. It is also normally present in saliva, sweat, and tears. Formerly called lysozyme.

**Murchison-Pel-Ebstein fever** (mŭr′chĭ-sŏn-pĕl-ĕb′stīn) [Charles Murchison, Brit. physician, 1830–1879; Pieter K. Pel; Wilhelm Ebstein] Pel-Ebstein fever.

**muriate** (mūr′ē-āt) [L. *muria,* brine] Former term for chloride.

**muriatic acid** (mū″rē-ăt′ĭk) Hydrochloric acid.

**murine** (mū′rĭn) [L. *mus,* mouse] Concerning rodents, esp. rats and mice.

**murmur** [L.] An abnormal sound heard on auscultation of the heart and adjacent large blood vessels. Murmurs range in sound from soft and blowing to loud and booming and may be heard during systole, diastole, or both. A murmur does not necessarily indicate organic pathology, and heart disease may not be associated with the production of a murmur. Air in the lungs may simulate sounds similar to heart murmurs. SEE: *heart.*

***anemic m.*** Hemic m.

***aneurysmal m.*** A whizzing systolic sound heard over an aneurysm.

***aortic obstructive m.*** A harsh systolic murmur heard with and after the first heart sound. It is loudest at the base.

***aortic regurgitant m.*** A blowing and hissing following the second heart sound.

***apex m.*** An inorganic murmur over the apex of the heart.

***arterial m.*** A soft flowing murmur that is synchronous with the pulse.

***Austin Flint m.*** SEE: *Austin Flint murmur.*

***bronchial m.*** A murmur heard over large bronchi, resembling respiratory laryngeal murmur.

***cardiac m.*** A sound arising due to blood flow through the heart.

***cardiopulmonary m.*** A murmur caused by movement of the heart against the lungs.

***continuous m.*** A continuous murmur that extends through systole and diastole.

***crescendo m.*** A murmur that progressively builds up in intensity and then suddenly subsides.

***Cruveilhier-Baumgarten m.*** A murmur heard on the abdominal wall over the collateral veins connecting the caval and portal veins.

***diastolic m.*** A murmur occurring during dilation of the heart.

***Duroziez' m.*** SEE: *Duroziez' murmur.*

***ejection m.*** A systolic murmur that is most intense at the time of maximum flow of blood from the heart. This murmur is associated with pulmonary and aortic stenosis.

***endocardial m.*** An abnormal sound produced by any cause and arising within the heart.

***exocardial m.*** A cardiac murmur produced outside the cavities of the heart.

***extracardiac m.*** Exocardial m.

***friction m.*** A murmur caused by an inflamed mucous surface rubbing against another, as in pericarditis.

***functional m.*** A murmur occurring in the absence of any pathological change in the structure of the heart valves or orifices. It does not indicate organic disease of the heart, and may disappear upon a return to health. It must not be mistaken for true pathological murmurs.

***Gibson's m.*** SEE: *Gibson's murmur.*

***Graham Steell's m.*** [Graham Steell, Brit. physician, 1867–1942] A high-pitched diastolic murmur heard best along the left sternal border. It is caused by backflow (regurgitation) of blood through the dilated pulmonary valve of the heart. This type of murmur is usually associated with severe pulmonary hypertension.

***heart m.*** Cardiac m.

***hemic m.*** A sound heard on auscultation of anemic persons without valvular lesions and resulting from an abnormal, usually anemic, blood condition.

***holosystolic m.*** Pansystolic m.

***machinery m.*** Gibson's murmur.

***mitral m.*** A murmur produced at the orifice of the mitral (bicuspid) valve.

***musical m.*** A cardiac murmur with sounds that have an intermittent harmonic pattern.

***organic m.*** A murmur due to structural changes.

***pansystolic m.*** A heart murmur heard throughout systole.

***pericardial m.*** A friction sound produced within the pericardium.

***physiologic m.*** Functional m.

***prediastolic m.*** Systolic m.

***presystolic m.*** A murmur occurring just before systole, due to mitral or tricuspid obstruction.

***pulmonary m.*** A murmur produced at the orifice of the pulmonary artery.

***regurgitant m.*** A murmur due to leakage or backward flow of blood through a dilated valvular orifice.

***seagull m.*** A murmur that resembles the cry of a seagull; sometimes associated with aortic insufficiency.

***Still's m.*** A benign, functional midsystolic murmur heard in children. The maximum sound is heard over the left lower sternal border.

***systolic m.*** A murmur heard during contraction of the heart due to obstruction of the flow of blood at one or several of the heart valves or in the aorta.

***to-and-fro m.*** A pericardial murmur heard during both systole and diastole.

***tricuspid m.*** A murmur produced at the orifice of the tricuspid valve and caused by stenosis or incompetency of the valve.

***vascular m.*** A murmur occurring over a blood vessel.

***vesicular m.*** Normal breath sounds.

**Murphy's button** [John B. Murphy, U.S. surgeon, 1857–1916] Mechanical device used for intestinal anastomosis consisting of two button-like hollow cylinders. Each cylinder is sutured to an open end of the intestine, then they are fitted together. After firm union of the ends of the intestine, the sutures separate and the cylinders are passed in stools.

**Murphy's sign** Pain on deep inspiration when an inflamed gallbladder is palpated by pressing the fingers under the rib cage.

**Mus** (mŭs) [L., mouse] A genus of rodents including mice and rats.

***M. musculus*** The common house mouse.

**Musca** (mŭs′kă) [L., fly] A genus of flies belonging to the order Diptera, family Muscidae.

***M. domestica*** The common house fly, a transmitting agent for the causative organisms of typhoid fever, bacillary and amebic dysentery, cholera, trachoma, and many other diseases.

**muscae volitantes** (mŭs′sē vōl-ĭ-tăn′tēz) [L., flitting flies] Black specks seen float-

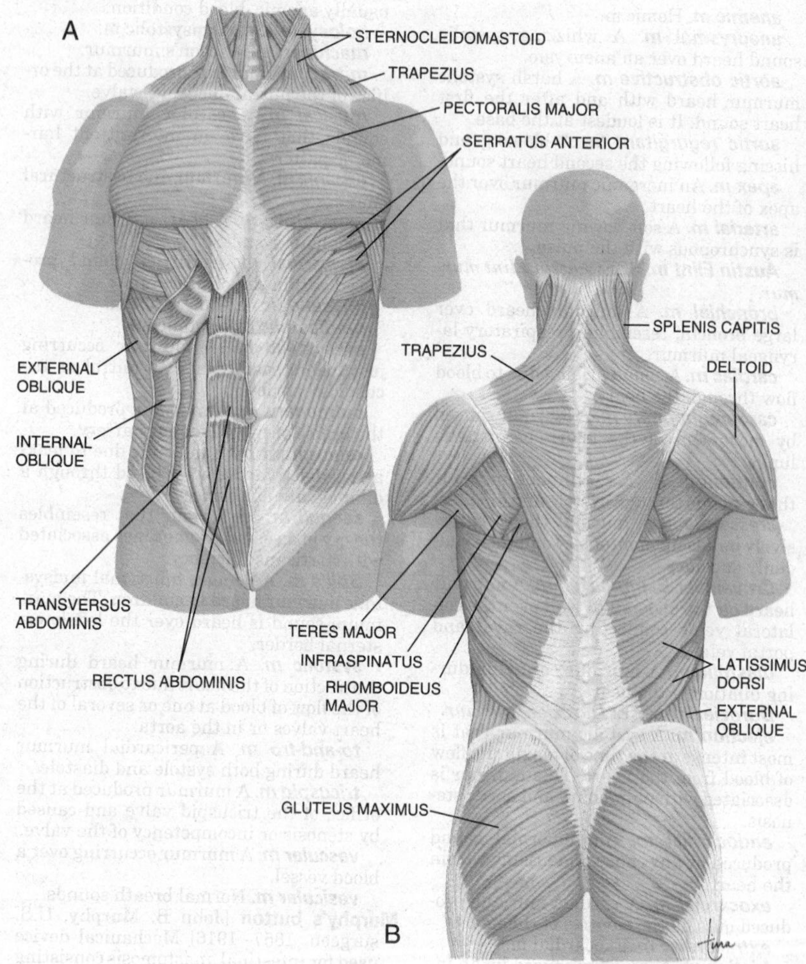


**MUSCLES OF THE TRUNK, (A)** ANTERIOR AND **(B)** POSTERIOR

ing in the vitreous humor of the eye. They are sometimes apparent to the individual. This benign phenomenon is present in most individuals. SYN: *floaters*.

**muscarine** (mŭs′kă-rĭn) [L. *muscarius*, pert. to flies] A highly toxic organic compound present in *Amanita muscaria* (fly agaric mushroom). SEE: *mushroom and toadstool poisoning; amanita in Poisons and Poisoning Appendix*.

**muscarinic** Pert. to the effect of acetylcholine on parasympathetic ganglionic affector sites.

**muscegenetic** (mŭs″ē-jĕ-nĕt′ĭk) [L. *musca*, fly, + Gr. *genesis*, generation, birth] Causing muscae volitantes.

**muscicide** (mŭs′ĭ-sīd) [″ + *cidus*, killing] Lethal to flies.

**muscle** (mŭs′ĕl) [L. *musculus*] A type of tissue composed of contractile cells or fibers that effects movement of an organ or part of the body. The outstanding characteristic of muscular tissue is its ability to shorten or contract. It also possesses the properties of irritability, conductivity, and elasticity. Muscle tissue possesses little intercellular material; hence, its cells or fibers lie close together. SYN: *musculus*. SEE: illus. (Muscles of the Trunk); *leg* for illus; *arm; cell; face*.

TYPES: Three types of muscle occur in the body, differentiated on the basis of histologic structure. These muscle types are smooth, skeletal (striated), and cardiac. SEE: illus. (Muscle Tissues); table; *Muscles Appendix*.

*Smooth (Involuntary):* Smooth muscle is found principally in the internal or-

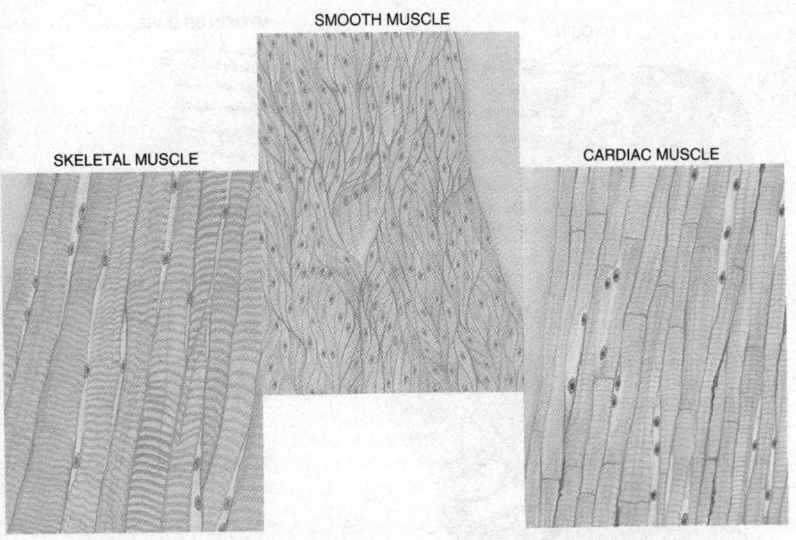


**MUSCLE TISSUES** (ORIG. MAG. ×430)

gans, esp. the digestive tract, respiratory passages, urinary and genital ducts, urinary bladder, gallbladder, and walls of blood vessels. It lacks the cross striations characteristic of other types of muscle. This type of muscle tissue is called involuntary because it is not under conscious control. Smooth muscle cells are fusiform or spindle-shaped, each containing a central nucleus. The cells are usually arranged in sheets or layers, but may occur as isolated units in connective tissue.

*Striated, Skeletal (Voluntary):* Striated muscle is found in all skeletal muscles. It also occurs in the tongue, pharynx, and upper portion of esophagus. Since movement is under conscious control, this type of muscle tissue is called voluntary. The cytoplasm (sarcoplasm) contains numerous myofibrillae. The cytoplasmic cell membrane is called the sarcolemma. Muscle fibers are grouped into bundles called fasciculi, each of which is surrounded by a sheath or connective tissue called perimysium. The fibers within a fasciculus are surrounded by and held together by delicate reticular fibrils forming the endomysium.

*Cardiac:* Cardiac muscle fibers branch and anastomose, forming a continuous network or syncytium. At intervals, prominent bands or intercalated disks cross the fibers. Certain nerve fibers, called Purkinje fibers, form the impulse-conducting system of the heart.

ANATOMY: Muscle is a contractile organ consisting of tissue that allows movement of parts of the body, especially a structure composed of striated (voluntary) muscle that is attached to a part of

**Comparison of Properties of Three Types of Muscle**

| | Smooth | Cardiac | Striated |
|---|---|---|---|
| Synonyms | Involuntary<br>Nonstriated<br>Visceral | Myocardium | Voluntary<br>Skeletal |
| Fibers | | | |
| Length (in micrometers) | 50–200 | | 25,000 |
| Thickness (in micrometers) | 4–8 | | 75 |
| Shape | Spindles | | Cylinders |
| Markings | No striation | Striation | Marked striation |
| Nuclei | Single | Single | Multiple |
| Effects of cutting related nerve | Slight | Nervous regulation of heart rate is lost | Complete paralysis |

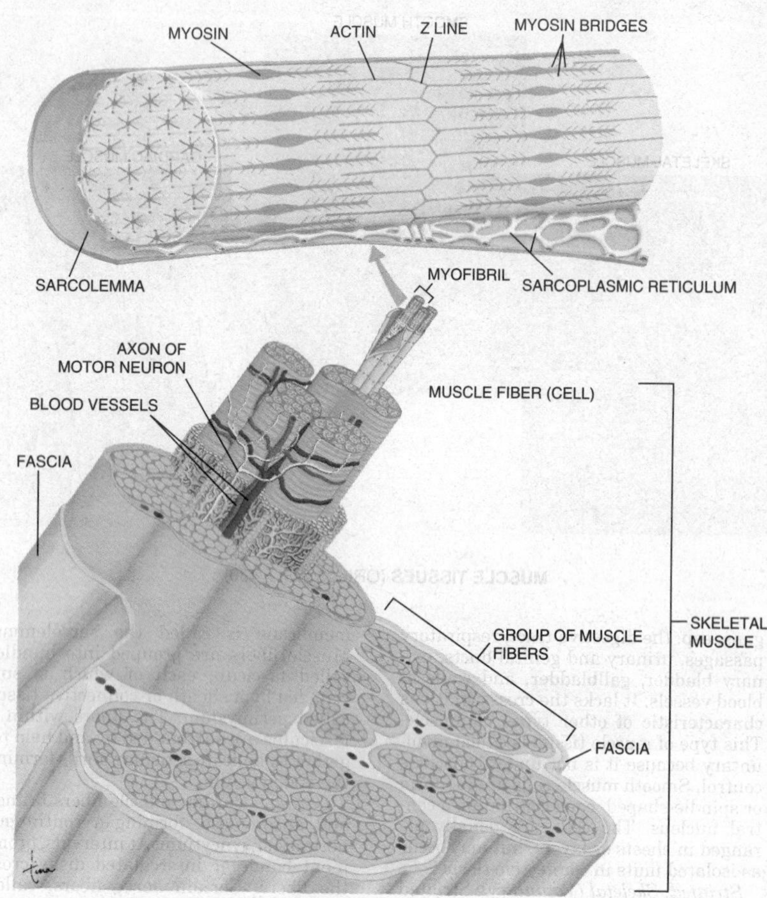


**SKELETAL MUSCLE**

the skeleton. A typical muscle consists of a central fleshy portion or belly and its attachments. One end called the head is attached to a fixed structure termed the origin; the other end is attached to a movable part called the insertion. Some muscles are spindle-shaped; others form flat sheets or bands. Muscles may be attached directly to the periosteum of the bones, or they may be attached by means of tough cords of connective tissue (tendons) or broad flat sheets (aponeuroses). The connective tissue enclosing a muscle is called epimysium; it is continuous with the deep fascia. SEE: illus. (Skeletal Muscle).

BLOOD SUPPLY: Obtained from small blood vessels that enter the muscular tissue and subdivide into capillaries that permeate throughout.

NERVE SUPPLY: *Voluntary:* These muscles are innervated by somatic branches of cranial or spinal nerves; it is because of this that the skeletal muscles are under conscious control. *Involuntary:* Smooth and cardiac muscles receive their nerve supply from autonomic nervous system and function involuntarily without conscious control.

***abductor m.*** A muscle that draws away from the midline.

***adductor m.*** A muscle that draws toward the midline.

***agonist m.*** A muscle that is the prime mover.

***antagonist(ic) m.*** A muscle that counteracts the action of another muscle.

***antigravity m.'s*** Muscles that pull against the constant force of gravity to maintain posture.

***appendicular m.*** One of the skeletal muscles of the limbs.

***arrector pili m.*** Arrectores pilorum.

***articular m.*** A muscle attached to the capsule of a joint.

***axial m.*** A skeletal muscle of the head

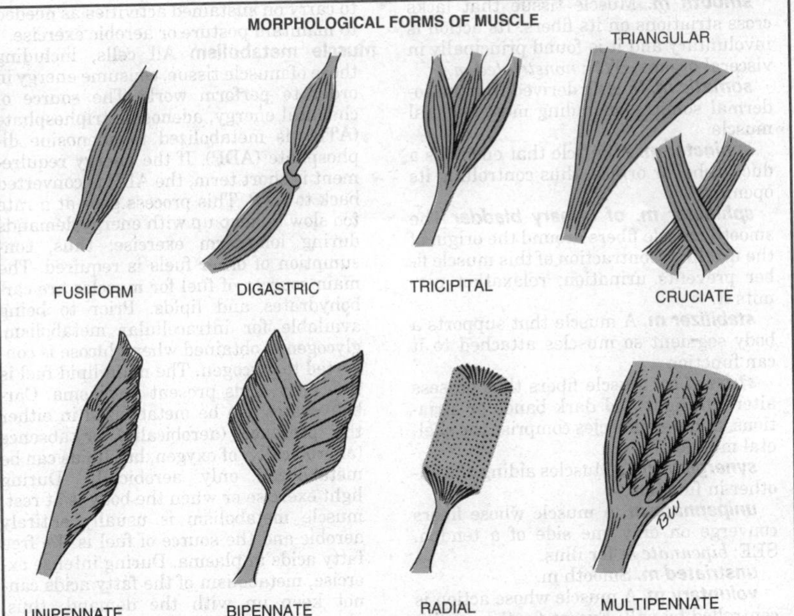


or trunk.

***bipennate m.*** A muscle in which the fibers converge toward a central tendon on both sides. SEE: illus.

***constrictor m. of pharynx*** A muscle that constricts the pharynx.

***digastric m.*** A muscle that lowers the jaw. SEE: *bipennate m.* for illus.

***extensor m.*** A muscle that extends a part.

***external intercostal m.'s*** The outer layer of muscles between the ribs, originating on the lower margin of each rib and inserted on the upper margin of the next rib. During inspiration, they draw adjacent ribs together, pulling them upward and outward, and increasing the volume of the chest cavity.

***extraocular eye m.'s*** SEE: *extraocular eye muscles*.

***extrinsic m.*** A muscle whose origin lies outside the part moved.

***fixation m.*** A muscle that steadies a part so that more precise movements in a related structure may be accomplished.

***flexor m.*** A muscle that bends a part.

***fusiform m.*** A muscle resembling a spindle. SEE: *bipennate m* for illus.

***internal intercostal m.'s*** The muscles between the ribs, lying beneath the external intercostals. During expiration, they pull the ribs downward and inward, decreasing the volume of the chest cavity and contributing to a forced exhalation.

***intrinsic m.*** A muscle that has both its origin and insertion within a structure, as intrinsic muscles of the tongue, eye, hand, or foot.

***involuntary m.*** A muscle not under conscious control; mainly smooth muscle.

***mastication m.'s*** The four pairs of muscles that move the mandible and provide the primary forces of mastication; the masseter, temporalis, medial pterygoid, and lateral pterygoid muscles.

***mimetic m.'s*** Superficial muscles of the facial region controlling skin movement that produce the facial expressions. SYN: *muscles of facial expression*.

***multipennate m.*** A muscle with several tendons of origin and several tendons of insertion, in which fibers pass obliquely from a tendon of origin to a tendon of insertion on each side. SEE: *bipennate m* for illus.

***nonstriated m.*** Smooth m.

***obturator m.*** Either of the two muscles on each side of the pelvic region that rotate the thighs outward.

***papillary m.*** A cylindrical muscle of the interior of the heart that arises from the floor of each ventricle. It is attached to the chordae tendinae, which anchor the flaps of the atrioventricular valves during ventricular systole.

***pectinate m.*** A muscle on the inner surface of the right atrium of the heart, giving it a ridged appearance.

***postaxial m.*** A muscle on the posterior or dorsal aspect of a limb.

***preaxial m.*** A muscle on the anterior or ventral aspect of a limb.

***skeletal m.*** A mainly striated muscle that is connected to a bone.

***smooth m.*** Muscle tissue that lacks cross striations on its fibers. Its action is involuntary and it is found principally in visceral organs. SYN: *nonstriated m.*

***somatic m.*** Muscle derived from mesodermal somites, including most skeletal muscle.

***sphincter m.*** A muscle that encircles a duct, tube, or orifice, thus controlling its opening.

***sphincter m. of urinary bladder*** The smooth muscle fibers around the origin of the urethra. Contraction of this muscle fiber prevents urination; relaxation permits it.

***stabilizer m.*** A muscle that supports a body segment so muscles attached to it can function.

***striated m.*** Muscle fibers that possess alternate light and dark bands or striations. Striated muscles comprise the skeletal muscles.

***synergistic m.'s*** Muscles aiding one another in function.

***unipennate m.*** A muscle whose fibers converge on only one side of a tendon. SEE: *bipennate m* for illus.

***unstriated m.*** Smooth m.

***voluntary m.*** A muscle whose action is controlled by will. Except for the cardiac muscle, all striated muscles are voluntary.

**muscle compartment syndrome** Compression of nerves, vessels, and tissue within a fascial compartment causing the production of nerve damage, ischemia, edema, and muscle contractures. SEE: *carpal tunnel syndrome.*

**muscle contraction, concentric** Contraction of a muscle in which the extended muscle is shortened. An example would be pulling the body up by grasping a bar over the head.

**muscle contraction, eccentric** Contraction of a muscle in which the tensed muscle lengthens. An example would be the lowering of the body from a position in which the body was supported by the flexed arms, i.e., holding on to a bar above the head.

**muscle cramps** Painful involuntary contractions of muscles. They may be due to ischemia of the muscle(s), dehydration, or electrolyte imbalance.

Cramps associated with exercise may be alleviated, if not abolished, by flexing (stretching) the involved muscle group. At the same time, gentle massage to the area will help.

Nocturnal cramps may be prevented by use of quinine. There is not enough quinine in tonic water to make it effective.

**muscle fiber** SEE: under *fiber.*

**muscle fiber types, fast twitch and slow twitch** Types of fibers found in skeletal muscle. Fast twitch fibers are more abundant in muscles requiring intensive activity for short periods of time. Slow twitch oxidative fibers resist fatigue and are able to carry on sustained activities as needed to maintain posture or aerobic exercise.

**muscle metabolism** All cells, including those of muscle tissue, consume energy in order to perform work. The source of chemical energy, adenosine triphosphate (ATP), is metabolized to adenosine diphosphate (ADP). If the energy requirement is short term, the ADP is converted back to ATP. This process goes at a rate too slow to keep up with energy demands during long-term exercise; thus, consumption of other fuels is required. The main sources of fuel for muscles are carbohydrates and lipids. Prior to being available for intracellular metabolism, glycogen is obtained when glucose is converted to glycogen. The main lipid fuel is free fatty acids present in plasma. Carbohydrates can be metabolized in either the presence (aerobically) or absence (anerobically) of oxygen, but lipids can be metabolized only aerobically. During light exercise or when the body is at rest, muscle metabolism is usually entirely aerobic and the source of fuel is the free fatty acids in plasma. During intense exercise, metabolism of the fatty acids cannot keep up with the demand; thus, glycogen is used. However, as intense exercise continues, glycogen stores are exhausted and free fatty acids become the principal source of energy. Trained athletes have an increased ability to metabolize fatty acids as compared with sedentary individuals. This permits athletes to exercise longer and at higher work rates than would be the case if they were not trained. Athletic trainers found that muscle glycogen stores could be increased by what is known as carbohydrate loading. This regimen will permit the athlete to exercise for a much longer period than would be possible if carbohydrate loading had not been done prior to exercising. SEE: *carbohydrate loading.*

**muscle soreness** The onset of muscular discomfort within 24 to 48 hours following unaccustomed exercise or of exercise of greater intensity than usual.

**muscular** [L. *muscularis*] **1.** Pert. to muscles. **2.** Possessing well-developed muscles.

**muscular contractions, graduated 1.** The mechanism by which all smooth, coordinated muscle activity occurs. Normally controlled involuntarily by the central nervous system, motor units are recruited and stimulated at an intensity needed to accomplish a desired activity. **2.** Contractions accomplished by use of electric current of varying strength and duration. This method is used in muscles with an intact nerve supply when muscles are atonic, wasted away, or when voluntary exercise is not feasible, and in denervated muscles, as in cases following nerve injury or poliomyelitis.

**muscular dystrophy** SEE: *dystrophy, pro-*

*gressive muscular.*
**muscularis** (mŭs-kū-lā′rĭs) [L.] The smooth muscle layer of an organ or tubule.
  ***m. mucosae*** Unstriated muscular tissue layer of mucous membrane.
**musculature** [L. *musculus,* muscle] The arrangement of muscles in the body or its parts.
**musculo-** [L. *musculus,* muscle] Combining form meaning *muscle.*
**musculoaponeurotic** (mŭs-kū-lō-ăp″ō-nū-rŏt′ĭk) Composed of muscle and an aponeurosis of fibrous connective tissue.
**musculocutaneous** (mŭs″kū-lō-kū-tān′ē-ŭs) [″ + *cutis,* skin] **1.** Pert. to the muscles and skin. **2.** Supplying or affecting the muscles and skin. **3.** The specific nerve from the brachial plexus that innervates the coracobrachialis, biceps branchii, and brachialis muscles and provides cutaneous sensory distribution to the forearm.
**musculofascial** (mŭs″kū-lō-făsh′ē-ăl) Composed of muscle and fascia.
**musculomembranous** (mŭs″kū-lō-mĕm′brān-ŭs) Pert. to or consisting of muscle and membrane.
**musculophrenic** (mŭs″kū-lō-frĕn′ĭk) Pert. to muscles of the diaphragm.
**musculoskeletal** (mŭs″kū-lō-skĕl′ĕ-tăl) Pert. to the muscles and skeleton.
**musculospiral** (mŭs″kū-lō-spī′răl) [″ + *spira,* coil] Concerning the musculospiral (radial) nerve.
**musculotendinous** Composed of both muscle and tendon.
**musculotropic** (mŭs″kū-lō-trŏp′ĭk) [″ + Gr. *tropikos,* turning] Affecting, acting on, or having an affinity for muscular tissue.
**musculus** [L.] Muscle.
**mushroom** [Fr. *mousseron*] Umbrella-shaped fungus belonging to the class Basidiomycetes. Mushrooms grow on decaying vegetable matter and are generally found in woods and dark, damp places. Some of the poisonous varieties are commonly called toadstools. SEE: *toadstool.*
  COMPOSITION: Mushrooms are low in carbohydrates and fats, and high in protein. Their relationship and similarity to poisonous fungi are so close that only those who are thoroughly capable of distinguishing the poisonous varieties from the edible ones should attempt to gather and eat them.
**mushroom and toadstool poisoning** Poisoning resulting from ingestion of mushrooms such as *Amanita muscaria,* which contains muscarine, or other species that contain phalloidine, a component of the amanita toxin. SEE: *amanita in Poisons and Poisoning Appendix.*
**musicians, medical problems of** Profession-related injuries, most commonly overuse injuries involving muscle-tendon units. The pain associated with this type of injury may be mild or severe enough to prevent use of the affected part. Those who play string instruments have more difficulty than those who use percussion instruments; women are more commonly affected than men. Focal dystonias may involve the hands or the muscles of the face and lips, and may be severe. Stress and anxiety may interfere with or prevent performing.
  TREATMENT: Treatment consists of rest for physical difficulties and beta-adrenergic blocking agents for stress and anxiety.
**musicogenic** (mū″zĭ-kō-jĕn′ĭk) [L. *musica,* music, + *gennan,* to produce] Caused by music, esp. epileptic convulsions.
**musicogenic epilepsy** Epilepsy in which the convulsive attacks are induced by music. SEE: *epilepsy.*
**musicomania** [″ + Gr. *mania,* madness] Insane love of music.
**musicotherapy** [″ + *therapeia,* treatment] Treatment of disease, esp. mental illness, with music.
**musk** (mŭsk) [Sanskrit *muska,* testicle] An oily secretion obtained from the musk bag, a gland beneath the abdominal skin of the male musk deer. It has a very strong odor and is used in manufacturing perfume.
**mussel** A freshwater bivalve mollusc belonging to the class Pelecypoda.
**mussel poisoning** Poisoning common on the Pacific coast of the United States resulting from eating mussels or clams that have ingested a poisonous dinoflagellate that is not destroyed by cooking. Mussel poisoning may occur from June to October.
**Musset's sign** (mū-sāz′) [Louis C. A. de Musset, Fr. poet, 1810–1857] Repetitive jerking movements of the head and neck, in synchrony with ventricular contractions of the heart, seen in advanced aortic incompetence or aortic aneurysm.
**mustard** [Fr. *moustarde*] Yellow powder of mustard seed used as a counterirritant, rubefacient, emetic, stimulant, and condiment. SEE: *plaster.*
  ***nitrogen m.*** SEE: *nitrogen mustards.*
**mustard gas** Dichlorodiethyl sulfide, a war gas that causes burns and destruction of tissue either topically or if inhaled.
**mutacism** (mū′tă-sĭzm) A form of speech impediment in which the "m" sound is often substituted for other sounds.
**mutagen** (mū′tă-jĕn) [L. *mutare,* to change, + Gr. *gennan,* to produce] Any agent that causes genetic mutations. Many medicines, chemicals, and physical agents such as ionizing radiations and ultraviolet light have this ability. SEE: *teratogen.*
**mutagenesis** (mū″tă-jĕn′ĕ-sĭs) The induction of genetic mutation. SEE: *mutation; teratogenesis.*
**mutant** (mū′tănt) [L. *mutare,* to change] A variation of genetic structure that breeds true.
**mutase** (mū′tās) [″ + *ase,* enzyme] **1.** Enzyme that accelerates oxidation-reduction reactions through activation of oxygen and hydrogen. **2.** A food preparation made

from leguminous plants high in protein content.

**mutation** (mū-tā′shŭn) **1.** Change; transformation; instance of such change. **2.** Permanent variation in genetic structure with offspring differing from parents in a characteristic; differentiated from gradual variation through many generations. **3.** A change in a gene potentially capable of being transmitted to offspring.

***induced m.*** Mutation resulting from exposure to x-rays, radioactive substances, and certain drugs and chemicals.

***natural m.*** Mutation occurring without artificial external intervention. Natural mutation is thought to be a primary factor in evolutionary change.

***somatic m.*** Mutation occurring in somatic cells.

**mute** (mūt) [L. *mutus*, dumb] **1.** One who is unable to speak. **2.** Without the ability to speak.

***deaf m.*** One who is unable to hear or speak.

**mutilate** [L. *mutilatus,* to maim] To deprive of a limb or a part; to maim or disfigure.

**mutilation** (mū″tĭ-lā′shŭn) Maiming; the act of removing or destroying a conspicuous or essential part or organ.

**mutism** (mū′tĭzm) [L. *mutus,* dumb] **1.** Condition of being unable to speak. **2.** Persistent inhibition of speech seen in some severe forms of mental disorder.

***akinetic m.*** The condition of being immobile and silent while partially or fully awake. This may be due to a tumor in certain areas of the brain or to hydrocephalus.

***hysterical m.*** Inability to speak due to hysteria.

**mutualism** (mū′tū-ăl-ĭzm) [L. *mutuus,* exchanged] A form of symbiosis in which organisms of two different species live in close association to the mutual benefit of each.

**mutualist** (mū′tū-ăl-ĭst) Organism associated with another organism to the mutual benefit of each.

**μV** Symbol for microvolt.

**M.V.** *Medicas Veterinarius.* Latin for veterinary physician.

**mv** *millivolt.*

**M.W.I.A.** *Medical Women's International Association.*

**my-, myo-** [Gr. *mys,* muscle] Prefix denoting *muscle.*

**myalgia** (mī-ăl′jē-ă) [″ + *algos,* pain] Tenderness or pain in the muscles; muscular rheumatism. SYN: *myodynia; myosalgia.*

***tension m.*** Fibromyalgia.

**myasis** (mī-ā′sĭs) [Gr. *myia,* a fly] Myiasis.

**myasthenia** (mī-ăs-thē′nē-ă) [Gr. *mys,* muscle, + *astheneia,* weakness] Muscular weakness and abnormal fatigue. **myasthenic,** *adj.*

***angiosclerotic m.*** Vascular changes producing excessive muscular fatigue.

***m. gravis*** ABBR: MG. An autoimmune disease marked by skeletal muscle fatigability due to an abnormality in the synaptic junction between nerve and muscle fiber. Autoantibodies combine with autoantigens on acetylcholine receptors that lie on muscle fiber end plates. These immune complexes and their associated inflammation destroy the receptors, decreasing the amount of acetylcholine the muscle can receive. Acetylcholine deficiency limits muscle fiber contraction, and muscular activity produces rapid fatigue and loss of strength; resting the muscle restores it to full power until it is used again. Patients with myasthenia gravis often have tumors or hyperplasia of the thymus gland, the site of T lymphocyte maturation and proliferation; however, the role of T cells in the production of autoantibodies against the acetylcholine receptors in unclear. SEE: *autoantibody; autoantigen; Nursing Diagnoses Appendix.*

SYMPTOMS: Clinical signs include drooping of the upper eyelid (ptosis) and double vision (diplopia) due to fatigue and weakness in the extraocular muscles, and difficulty chewing and swallowing from impaired facial and pharyngeal muscles.

TREATMENT: The primary treatment is plasmapheresis to remove many autoantibodies from the blood, followed by removal of the thymus gland (thymectomy). Symptomatic treatment includes use of neostigmine, corticosteroids, and immunosuppressants such as azathioprine and cyclosporine. Short-term immunotherapies, including plasma exchange and intravenous immune globulin, are indicated when weakness is not adequately controlled by anticholinesterase drugs.

NURSING IMPLICATIONS: The nurse explains the diagnosis, nature of the disease process, and treatment and provides emotional support and reassurance. Activity-planning commensurate with capabilities is encouraged to help the patient conserve energy. Positive coping behaviors are reinforced. Regular medical follow-up, early reporting of any untoward symptoms, and family assistance and support are encouraged.

**myatonia** (mī-ă-tō′nē-ă) Deficiency or loss of muscular tone.

***m. congenita*** Oppenheim's disease.

**myatrophy** (mī-ăt′rō-fē) Muscular wasting.

**myc-, myco-** [Gr. *mykes,* fungus] Combining form meaning *fungus.*

**mycelioid** (mī-sē′lē-oyd) [″ + *helos,* nail, + *eidos,* form, shape] Moldlike; resembling mold colonies in which filaments radiate from a center, said of bacterial colonies.

**mycelium** (mī-sē′lē-ŭm) [Gr. *mykes,* fungus, + *helos,* nail] The mass of filaments (hyphae) that constitutes the vegetative body of fungi such as molds.

**mycetes** (mī-sē′tēz) The fungi.

**mycethemia** (mī-sĕ-thē′mē-ă) [″ + *haima,* blood] Fungi in the blood.

**mycetism, mycetismus** (mī′sĕ-tĭzm, mī-sĕtĭz′mŭs) [″ + *-ismos*, condition] Poisoning from eating fungi, esp. poisonous mushrooms.

**mycetogenetic** (mī-sē″tō-jĕn-ĕt′ĭk) [″ + *gennan*, to produce] Induced by fungi.

**mycetoma** (mī-sĕ-tō′mă) [″ + *oma*, tumor] A syndrome caused by a variety of aerobic actinomycetes and fungi. It is characterized by swelling and suppuration of subcutaneous tissues and formation of sinus tracts, with granules present in the pus draining from the tracts. These tracts usually appear on the lower body.

TREATMENT: Sulfones, trimethoprim-sulfamethoxazole, or sulfonamides may benefit lesions caused by actinomycetes. If lesions are due to fungi, there is no specific therapy.

**mycobacteriosis** (mī″kō-băk-tē″rē-ō′sĭs) An infection caused by any mycobacterium.

**Mycobacterium** [″ + *bakterion*, little rod] A genus of acid-fast organisms, belonging to the Mycobacteriaceae family, which includes the causative organisms of tuberculosis and leprosy. The organisms are slender, nonmotile, gram-positive rods and do not produce spores or capsules.

Species include *M. africanum, M. avium intracellulare, M. bovis, M. chelonei, M. fortuitum, M. gastri, M. gordonae, M. kansasii, M. marinum, M. scrofulaceum, M. terrae, M. triviale, M. smegmatis*, and *M. xenopi*.

***M. bovis*** The organism that causes tuberculosis in cows.

***M. kansasii*** A cause of tuberculosis-like pulmonary disease in humans.

***M. leprae*** The causative agent of leprosy.

***M. marinum*** An atypical mycobacterium that produces skin infection resembling sporotrichosis. The organism has been cultured from tropical fish aquariums. SEE: *swimming pool granuloma*.

***M. tuberculosis*** The causative agent of tuberculosis in mammals. SEE: illus.

**mycocidin** (mī″kō-sī′dĭn) An antibiotic derived from molds of the family Aspergillaceae.

**mycoderma** [Gr. *mykos*, mucus, + *derma*, skin] Mucous membrane.

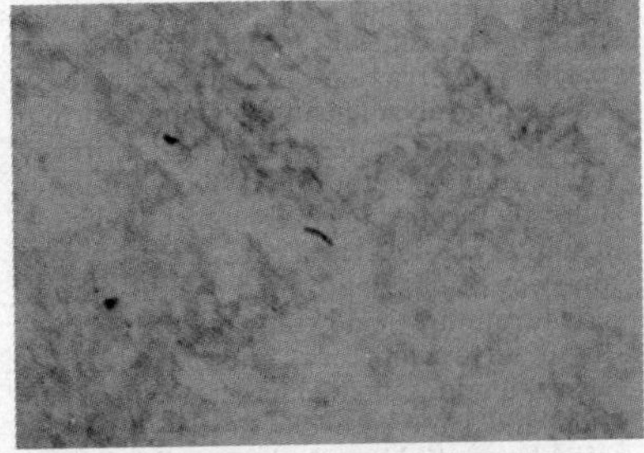

**MYCOBACTERIUM TUBERCULOSIS IN SPUTUM** (ORIG. MAG. ×500)

**mycoid** (mī′koyd) [″ + *eidos*, form, shape] Fungus-like.

**mycology** (mī-kŏl′ō-jē) [″ + *logos*, word, reason] The science and study of fungi.

**mycophthalmia** (mī-kŏf-thăl′mē-ă) Ophthalmia resulting from fungus infection.

**Mycoplasma** A group of bacteria that lack cell walls and are highly pleomorphic. There are more than 70 organisms in this group, including 12 species that infect humans. *M. hominis* can cause genital tract infections; *M. pneumoniae* can cause infections of the upper respiratory tract and the lungs (i.e., mycoplasma pneumonia).

TREATMENT: Tetracycline or erythromycin are effective for treatment of *M. pneumoniae* and *M. hominis* infections.

**mycosis** (mī-kō′sĭs) [″ + *osis*, condition] Any disease induced by a fungus.

***m. fungoides*** A non-Hodgkin's form of cutaneous T-cell lymphoma of unknown etiology. In a similar cutaneous T-cell lymphoma, Sézary syndrome, there is systemic and cutaneous involvement, whereas in mycosis fungoides, skin manifestations predominate.

SYMPTOMS: Appearance of urticarial, erythematous, or eczematous patches of irregular shape and size, with well-defined margins, usually on the scalp and the skin of the trunk, accompanied by intense itching. Frequently the patches become hypertrophic and firm, and hard, sessile, or pedunculated nodules of varying size develop on them. These nodules eventually break down and form ulcers that contain sensitive, fungating granulation tissue, and discharge thin pus and serum.

In addition to the cutaneous changes, lesions may be present throughout the body. Infection of the lesions may be fatal.

TREATMENT: A variety of therapeutic approaches including topical chemotherapy, phototherapy, photopheresis, systemic chemotherapy, monoclonal antibody therapy, and interferons may be used alone or in combination.

***superficial m.*** Any of a group of fungus infections of the skin. Included in this group are erythrasma, tinea barbae, tinea capitis, tinea corporis, tinea cruris, tinea favosa, tinea pedis, tinea unguium, and trichomycosis axillaris.

***systemic m.*** Any of a group of deep fungus infections involving various bodily systems or regions. Included in this group are aspergillosis, blastomycosis, chromoblastomycosis, coccidioidomycosis, cryptococcosis, geotrichosis, histoplasmosis, maduromycosis, moniliasis, mucormycosis, nocardiosis, penicilliosis, rhinosporidiosis, and sporotrichosis. SEE: illus.

**mycostasis** (mī-kŏs′tă-sĭs) [Gr. *mykes*, fungus, + *stasis*, standing] Stopping the growth of fungi.

**mycostat** (mī′kō-stăt) [″ + *statikos*, standing] Any agent that stops the growth of fungi.

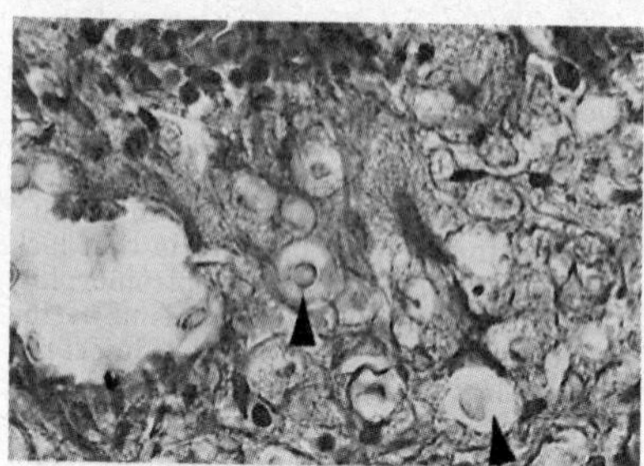

**SYSTEMIC MYCOSIS**

CRYPTOCOCCOSIS OF LUNG; ARROWS INDICATE FUNGUS (ORIG. MAG. ×450)

**mycotic** (mī-kŏt′ĭk) Caused by or infected with fungus; concerning mycosis.

**mycotoxicosis** (mī″kō-tŏk″sĭ-kō′sĭs) [″ + *toxikon,* poisoning, + *osis,* condition] Disease either caused by toxins on molds or produced by molds.

**mycotoxins** Substances produced by mold growing in food or animal feed and causing illness or death when ingested by humans or animals. SEE: *ergotism.*

**mycterophonia** (mĭk″tĕr-ō-fō′nē-ă) [Gr. *mykter,* nostril, + *phone,* voice] Phonation in which the voice possesses a nasal quality.

**mydaleine** (mĭd-ā′lē-ēn) [Gr. *mydaleos,* moldy] A poisonous ptomaine formed in putrefied visceral organs, acting mainly on the heart.

**mydriasis** (mĭd-rī′ă-sĭs) [Gr.] Pronounced or abnormal dilation of the pupil.

ETIOLOGY: Causes include fright, sudden emotion, first and third stages of anesthesia, drugs, coma, hysteria, botulism, and irritation of the cervical sympathetic nerve.

***alternating m.*** Mydriasis that affects one eye, then the other.

***paralytic m.*** Mydriasis resulting from paralysis of oculomotor nerve.

***spastic m.*** Mydriasis resulting from overactivity of the dilator muscle of the iris or of sympathetic nerves supplying that muscle.

***spinal m.*** Mydriasis resulting from irritation of, or a lesion in, the ciliospinal center of spinal cord.

**mydriatic** (mĭd-rē-ăt′ĭk) **1.** Causing pupillary dilatation. **2.** A drug that dilates the pupil, such as atropine, cocaine, ephedrine, euphthalmine, and homatropine. In certain eye diseases, it is essential that the pupil be dilated during the course of treatment to prevent adhesions of the pupils.

**myectomy** (mī-ĕk′tō-mē) [Gr. *mys,* muscle, + *ektome,* excision] Excision of a portion of a muscle.

**myel-** SEE: *myelo-.*

**myelalgia** (mī-ĕl-ăl′jē-ă) [Gr. *myelos,* marrow, + *algos,* pain] Pain in the spinal cord or its membranes.

**myelapoplexy** (mī″ĕl-ăp′ō-plĕks-ē) [″ + *apoplexia,* stroke] Hemorrhagic effusion into the spinal cord.

**myelatelia** (mī″ĕl-ă-tē′lē-ă) [″ + *ateleia,* imperfection] Myelodysplasia.

**myelauxe** (mī-ĕl-awks′ē) [″ + *auxe,* increase] Abnormal enlargement of spinal cord.

**myelencephalon** (mī″ĕl-ĕn-sĕf′ă-lŏn) [Gr. *myelos,* marrow, + *enkephalos,* brain] The most posterior portion of the embryonic hindbrain (rhombencephalon), which gives rise to the medulla oblongata.

**myelic** Pert. to the spinal cord.

**myelin** The phospholipid-protein of the cell membranes of Schwann cells (parasympathetic nervous system) and oligodendrocytes (central nervous system) that forms the myelin sheath of neurons. It acts as an electrical insulator and increases the velocity of impulse transmission. SEE: *neuron* for illus. **myelinic** (mī-ĕl-ĭn′ĭk), *adj.*

**myelination** (mī″ĕl-ĭn-ā′shŭn) [Gr. *myelos,* marrow] Myelinization.

**myelinization** (mī″ĕl-ĭn-ĭ-zā′shŭn) Process of acquiring a myelin sheath for nerve fibers. SYN: *myelination.*

**myelinoclasis** (mī″ĕ-lĭn-ŏk′lă-sĭs) [″ + *klasis,* breaking] Process of destruction of myelin.

**myelinogenetic** (mī″ĕl-ĭn-ō-jĕn-ĕt′ĭk) [″ + *gennan,* to produce] Producing myelin or a myelin sheath.

**myelinolysis** (mī″ĕ-lĭn-ŏl′ĭ-sĭs) [″ + *lysis,* dissolution] Destruction of the myelin sheaths of nerves.

**myelinopathy** Degeneration of the myelin sheaths of neurons, esp. in the central nervous system. SEE: *multiple sclerosis.*

**myelinosis** (mī″ĕl-ĭn-ō′sĭs) [″ + *osis,* condition] Fatty degeneration during which myelin is produced.

**myelitis** (mī-ĕ-lī′tĭs) [″ + *itis,* inflammation] **1.** Inflammation of bone marrow. SEE: *osteomyelitis.* **2.** Inflammation of the spinal cord. SEE: *poliomyelitis.*

SYMPTOMS: Symptoms include moderate fever (101° to 103°F or 38.3° to 39.4°C), loss of appetite, and constipation, followed by pain in the back radiating into the limbs. Various forms of paresthesia, such as numbness, tingling, or burning, may be present. Frequently a sense of painful constriction (girdle pain) also develops. Paralysis soon develops and may become more or less complete. Initially, there may be retention of feces, followed later by incontinence. Decubiti (bedsores) are likely to develop if care is not taken to prevent them. Death may result in a few days from upward extension and involvement of respiratory muscles. In rare cases, a spontaneous arrest of inflammation and slow recovery follow, accompanied by partial paralysis. **myelitic** (mī-ĕl-ĭt′ĭk), *adj.*

***acute m.*** A simple acute form of myelitis that develops following injury.

***acute ascending m.*** Myelitis that moves progressively upward in the spinal cord.

***acute transverse m.*** An acute form of myelitis involving the entire thickness of the spinal cord, developing subsequent to injury to the spinal cord.

***bulbar m.*** Myelitis involving the medulla oblongata.

***central m.*** Inflammation of the gray matter of the spinal cord.

***compression m.*** Myelitis caused by pressure on the spinal cord, as by a hemorrhage or tumor.

***descending m.*** Myelitis affecting successively lower areas of the spinal cord.

***disseminated m.*** Inflammation of several separate areas of the spinal cord.

***focal m.*** Myelopathy of small areas of the spinal cord.

***hemorrhagic m.*** Myelitis with hemorrhage.

***sclerosing m.*** Myelopathy wherein there is hardening of the spinal cord.

***transverse m.*** Myelitis involving the whole thickness of the spinal cord, but limited longitudinally.

***traumatic m.*** Myelitis due to spinal cord injury.

**myelo-, myel-** [Gr. *myelos,* marrow] Combining form meaning *spinal cord, bone marrow.*

**myeloblast** (mī′ĕl-ō-blăst) [″ + *blastos,* germ] Immature bone marrow cell that develops into a myelocyte. It matures to develop into a promyelocyte, and eventually into a granular leukocyte.

**myeloblastemia** (mī″ĕl-ō-blăst-ē′mē-ă) [″ + ″ + *haima,* blood] The occurrence of myeloblasts in the blood.

**myeloblastoma** (mī″ĕl-ō-blăst-ō′mă) [″ + ″ + *oma,* tumor] A tumor containing myeloblasts; seen in the myelogenic form of leukemia.

**myeloblastosis** (mī″ĕ-lō-blăs-tō′sĭs) [″ + ″ + *osis,* condition] Excess production of myeloblasts and their presence in circulating blood.

**myelocele** (mī′ĕ-lō-sēl) [″ + *kele,* tumor, swelling] A form of spina bifida with spinal cord protrusion.

**myelocyst** (mī′ĕl-ō-sĭst) [″ + *kystis,* bladder] Cyst arising from the rudimentary medullary canal of the spinal cord.

**myelocystocele** (mī″ĕl-ō-sĭst′ō-sēl) [″ + ″ + *kele,* tumor, swelling] Protrusion of spinal cord substance through a defect in the canal.

**myelocystomeningocele** (mī″ĕl-ō-sĭst″ō-mĕn-ĭn′gō-sēl) [″ + *kystis,* bladder, + *meninx,* membrane, + *kele,* tumor, swelling] Combined myelocystocele and meningocele.

**myelocyte** (mī′ĕl-ō-sīt) [″ + *kytos,* cell] A large cell in red bone marrow from which leukocytes are derived.

**myelocythemia** (mī″ĕl-ō-sī-thē′mē-ă) [″ + ″ + *haima,* blood] Myelocytosis.

**myelocytic** (mī″ĕl-ō-sĭt′ĭk) Characterized by presence of, or pert. to, myelocytes.

**myelocytosis** (mī″ĕl-ō-sī-tō′sĭs) [″ + ″ + *osis,* condition] Presence of an excess number of myelocytes in the blood. SYN: *myelocythemia.*

**myelodysplasia** (mī″ĕl-ō-dĭs-plā′zē-ă) [″ + *dys,* bad, + *plassein,* to form] Defective formation of the spinal cord. SYN: *myelatelia.*

**myeloencephalic** (mī″ĕl-ō-ĕn-sĕf-ăl′ĭk) [″ + *enkephalos,* brain] Concerning the spinal cord and the brain.

**myeloencephalitis** (mī″ĕl-ō-ĕn-sĕf″ă-lī′tĭs) [″ + ″ + *itis,* inflammation] Inflammation of the spinal cord and the brain.

**myelofibrosis** (mī″ĕ-lō-fī-brō′sĭs) Replacement of bone marrow by fibrous tissue.

**myelogenesis** (mī″ĕl-ō-jĕn′ĕ-sĭs) [″ + *genesis,* generation, birth] **1.** Development of the brain and the spinal cord. **2.** Development of the myelin sheath of nerve fiber.

**myelogenic, myelogenous** (mī-ĕ-lō-jĕn′ĭk, -lŏj′ĕn-ŭs) [″ + *gennan,* to produce] Producing or originating in marrow.

**myelogeny** (mī″ĕ-lŏj′ĕ-nē) Maturation of the myelin sheaths during the development of the central nervous system.

**myelogram** (mī′ĕ-lō-grăm) [″ + *gramma,* something written] **1.** A radiograph of the spinal cord and associated nerves. **2.** A differential count of bone marrow cells.

**myelography** (mī-ĕ-lŏg′ră-fē) [″ + *graphein,* to write] Radiography of the spinal cord and associated nerves after intrathecal injection of a radiopaque, water-soluble contrast medium. This technique has limited use, owing to computed tomography and magnetic resonance imaging.

***air m.*** Myelography using a radiolucent contrast medium, usually air or oxygen.

**myeloid** (mī′ĕ-loyd) [″ + *eidos,* form, shape] **1.** Medullary; marrowlike. **2.** Resembling a myelocyte, but not necessarily originating from bone marrow.

**myeloidosis** (mī″ĕ-loy-dō′sĭs) [″ + ″ + *osis,* condition] Development of myeloid tissue.

**myelolysis** (mī″ĕ-lŏl′ĭs-sĭs) [″ + *lysis,* dissolution] Dissolution of myelin.

**myeloma** (mī-ĕ-lō′mă) [″ + *oma,* tumor] A tumor originating in cells of the hematopoietic portion of bone marrow.

***multiple m.*** A neoplastic disease characterized by the infiltration of bone and bone marrow by myeloma cells forming multiple tumor masses that lead to pathological fractures. The condition is usually progressive and generally fatal. Symptoms include anemia, renal lesions, and high globulin levels in blood. Multiple myeloma is common in sixth decade of life and occurs more frequently in males than in females by a ratio of 3:1. SYN: *myelomatosis.* SEE: illus.

TREATMENT: Individual painful bone lesions are irradiated; hemibody irradiation is also used, first to the upper half of the body, then, 6 weeks later, to the lower

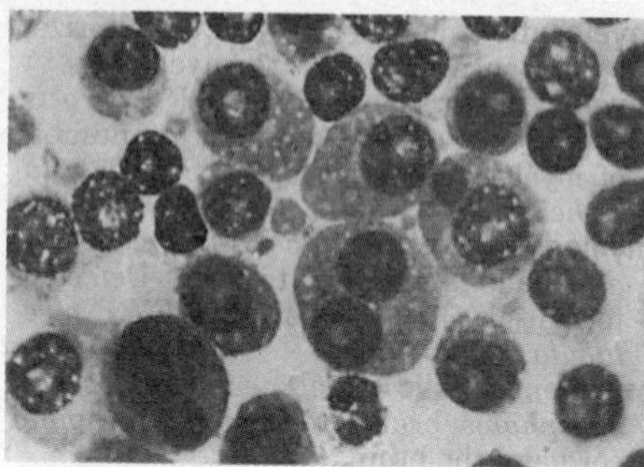
MULTIPLE MYELOMA (ORIG. MAG. ×600)

half. Standard chemotherapy includes the use of melphalan, cyclophosphamide, and carmustine. Melphalan is usually given with prednisone.

**myelomalacia** (mī″ĕ-lō-mă-lā′shē-ă) [Gr. *myelos,* marrow, + *malakia,* softening] Abnormal softening of the spinal cord.

**myelomatosis** (mī″ĕl-ō-mă-tō′sĭs) [″ + *oma,* tumor, + *osis,* intensive] Multiple myeloma.

**myelomeningocele** (mī″ĕ-lō-mĕn-ĭn′gō-sēl) [″ + ″ + *kele,* tumor, swelling] Spina bifida with a portion of the spinal cord and membranes protruding.

**myelomere** (mī′ĕ-lō-mēr) [″ + *meros,* part] A segment of the developing spinal cord.

**myeloneuritis** (mī″ĕ-lō-nū-rī′tĭs) [″ + *neuron,* nerve, + *itis,* inflammation] Neuromyelitis.

**myelopathy** (mī-ĕ-lŏp′ă-thē) [″ + *pathos,* disease, suffering] Any pathological condition of the spinal cord.

***ascending m.*** Myelopathy that ascends along the spinal cord toward the head.

***descending m.*** Myelopathy that descends along the spinal cord toward the feet.

***focal m.*** Myelopathy of small areas.

***sclerosing m.*** Myelopathy in which there is hardening of the spinal cord.

***transverse m.*** Myelopathy extending across the spinal cord.

***traumatic m.*** Myelopathy due to trauma to the spinal cord.

**myelopetal** (mī-ĕ-lŏp′ĕt-ăl) [″ + L. *petere,* to seek for] Proceeding toward the spinal cord, said of certain nerve impulses.

**myelophthisis** (mī-ĕ-lŏf′thĭ-sĭs) [″ + *phthisis,* a wasting] **1.** Atrophy of the spinal cord. **2.** Replacement of the bone marrow by a disease process such as a neoplasm.

**myeloplegia** (mī″ĕl-ō-plē′jē-ă) [Gr. *myelos,* marrow, + *plege,* stroke] Paralysis of spinal origin.

**myelopoiesis** (mī″ĕl-ō-poy-ē′sĭs) [″ + *poiein,* to form] Development of bone marrow or formation of cells derived from bone marrow.

***ectopic m.*** Extramedullary m.

***extramedullary m.*** Development of myeloid elements (erythrocytes and granular leukocytes) in regions other than bone marrow. SYN: *ectopic myelopoiesis.*

**myelopore** An opening in the spinal cord.

**myeloproliferative** (mī″ĕ-lō-prō-lĭf″ĕr-ā′tĭv) Concerning abnormal proliferation of bone marrow elements either in the bone marrow or extramedullary.

**myeloradiculitis** (mī″ĕ-lō-ră-dĭk″ū-lī′tĭs) [″ + L. *radiculus,* rootlet, + Gr. *itis,* inflammation] Inflammation of the spinal cord and the dorsal roots of spinal nerves.

**myeloradiculodysplasia** (mī″ĕ-lō-rā-dĭk″ū-lō-dĭs-plā′sē-ă) [″ + ″ + Gr. *dys,* bad, + *plassein,* to form] Congenital abnormality of the spinal cord and spinal nerve roots.

**myeloradiculopathy** (mī″ĕ-lō-ră-dĭk″ū-lŏp′ă-thē) [″ + ″ + Gr. *pathos,* disease, suffering] Disease of the spinal cord and spinal nerves.

**myelorrhagia** (mī-ĕ-lō-rā′jē-ă) [″ + *rhegnynai,* to burst forth] Hemorrhage into the spinal cord.

**myelorrhaphy** (mī-ĕl-or′ă-fē) [″ + *rhaphe,* seam, ridge] Suture of a cut or wound of the spinal cord.

**myelosarcoma** (mī″ĕl-ō-săr-kō′mă) [″ + *sarx,* flesh, + *oma,* tumor] Sarcoma composed of bone marrow cells and tissue. SYN: *osteosarcoma.*

**myelosarcomatosis** (mī″ĕ-lō-săr-kō″mă-tō′sĭs) [″ + ″ + ″ + *osis,* condition] Disseminated myelosarcomas.

**myeloschisis** (mī″ĕ-lŏs′kĭ-sĭs) [″ + *schisis,* a splitting] Cleft spinal cord resulting from failure of the neural tube to close. SEE: *rachischisis; spina bifida cystica.*

**myelosclerosis** (mī″ĕ-lō-sklĕr-ō′sĭs) [″+ *sklerosis,* hardening] Sclerosis of the spinal cord.

**myelosis** (mī-ĕ-lō′sĭs) [″ + *osis,* condition] Formation of a myeloma or medullary tumor.

***erythremic m.*** A malignancy involving the erythropoietic tissue. Symptoms and signs include anemia, fever, hepatosplenomegaly, bleeding tendency, and abnormal cells in the circulating blood.

**myelospongium** (mī″ĕ-lō-spŏn′jē-ūm) [Gr. *myelos,* marrow, + *spongos,* sponge] Embryonic network from which the neuroglia arises.

**myelosuppression** (mī″ĕ-lō-sŭ-prĕsh′ŭn) Inhibition of bone marrow function.

**myelotome** (mī-ĕl′ō-tōm) [″ + *tome,* incision] Instrument used to dissect the spinal cord.

**myelotomy** (mī-ĕl-ŏt′ō-mē) Surgical severance of nerve fibers of the spinal cord.

**myelotoxic** (mī-ĕl-ō-tŏk′sĭk) [″ + *toxikon,* poison] **1.** Destroying bone marrow. **2.** Pert. to or arising from diseased bone marrow.

**myelotoxin** (mī″ĕl-ō-tŏk′sĭn) Toxin that destroys marrow cells.

**myenteric reflex** SEE: under *reflex.*

**myenteron** (mī-ĕn′tĕr-ŏn) The smooth muscle layer of the intestine. **myenteric** (mī″ĕn-tĕr′ĭk), *adj.*

**Myerson's sign** [Abraham Myerson, U.S. neurologist, 1881–1948] In Parkinson's disease, repeated blinking of the eyes in response to tapping the forehead, nasal bridge, or maxilla.

**myesthesia** (mī″ĕs-thē′zē-ă) [Gr. *mys,* muscle, + *aisthesis,* sensation] Muscle sense; consciousness of muscle contraction.

**myiasis** (mī′ă-sĭs) [Gr. *myia,* fly, + *-sis,* condition] Condition resulting from infestation by the larvae (maggots) of flies. Infestation may be cutaneous, intestinal, atrial (within a cavity such as mouth, nose, eye, sinus, vagina, urethra), via a wound, or external.

**myiocephalon** (mī″yō-sĕf′ă-lŏn) [″ + *kephale,* head] Extrusion of a part of the iris through a tear in the cornea.

**myiodesopsia** (mī″ē-ō-dĕs-ŏp′sē-ă) [Gr. *myiodes,* flylike, + *opsis,* vision] Condition in which spots are seen before the eyes. SEE: *muscae volitantes.*

**myiosis** (mī-yō′sĭs) [″ + *osis,* condition] Myiasis.

**mylodus** A molar tooth.

**mylohyoid** (mī″lō-hī′oyd) [Gr. *myle,* mill, + *hyoid,* U-shaped] **1.** Pert. to the hyoid bone and the molar teeth. **2.** The paired muscles attached to the mandible that fuse in the midline and form the floor of the mouth.

**myo-** [Gr. *mys,* muscle] Combining form meaning *muscle.*

**myoalbumin** (mī″ō-ăl-bū′mĭn) [″ + L. *albus,* white] Albumin found in muscular tissue.

**myoalbumose** (mī″ō-ăl′bū-mōs) A protein derived from muscle.

**myoarchitectonic** (mī″ō-ăr″kĭ-tĕk-tŏn′ĭk) [Gr. *mys,* muscle, + *architekton,* master workman] Pert. to or resembling structural arrangement of muscle or of fibers.

**myoatrophy** (mī-ō-ăt′rō-fē) Muscular wasting.

**myoblast** (mī′ō-blăst) [″ + *blastos,* germ] An embryonic cell that develops into muscle fiber cell.

**myoblastoma** (mī″ō-blăs-tō′mă) [″ + ″ + *oma,* tumor] A tumor consisting of cells resembling myoblasts.

**myobradia** (mī″ō-brā′dē-ă) [″ + *bradys,* slow] Slow muscular reaction to stimulation.

**myocardial, myocardiac** (mī-ō-kăr′dē-ăl, -ăk) [″ + *kardia,* heart] Concerning the myocardium.

**myocardial infarction** ABBR: MI. A condition caused by partial or complete occlusion of one or more of the coronary arteries. SYN: *heart attack.* SEE: *Nursing Diagnoses Appendix.*

SYMPTOMS: The symptoms include prolonged heavy pressure or squeezing pain in the center of the chest behind the sternum. Typically, the patient will describe this by clenching a fist and holding it over the heart to demonstrate the character of the pain. The pain may spread or be localized to the shoulder, neck, arm, fourth and fifth fingers of the left hand, the back, the teeth, or the jaw. These symptoms may be accompanied by nausea and vomiting, sweating, and shortness of breath. At least one third of myocardial infarctions are clinically unrecognized. These are called silent, atypical, or unrecognized infarctions. Patients who have silent infarctions and have a history of angina pectoris have a greater risk of dying of coronary heart disease than do those who have history of angina and a recognized heart attack.

It is imperative that medical care be instituted without delay. Many MI patients not treated prior to reaching the hospital die. Delaying specific therapy may cause loss of life. Immediate administration of life support measures may be necessary. SEE: *echocardiography, dobutamine stress.*

DIAGNOSIS: Prompt diagnosis of acute MI in the first several hours after an attack is made by analyzing the concentration of the enzyme creatine kinase in the blood. An increase in the blood level of this enzyme can confirm the diagnosis of infarction as early as 2 hr after the onset of chest pain.

TREATMENT: After stabilization, therapy should be provided in a coronary care unit. Complete bed rest is initially indicated, with monitoring of electrocardiography (ECG) and oxygen therapy if indicated. Pain is treated with intravenous (IV) morphine, supplemented with continuous drip IV nitroglycerine if the pain continues. The addition of an angiotensin converting enzyme inhibitor to the therapeutic regimen in the early phase of an acute MI can be safe and effective and may reduce the risk of subsequent fatal and nonfatal cardiovascular events. Arrhythmias should be treated with appropriate drugs. Hypotension should be treated by elevating foot of bed or use of vasopressors or both.

Removal of the blockage of coronary artery(ies) should be attempted. This can be done by immediate use of thrombolytic agents such as streptokinase or tissue plasminogen activator (tPA). After the patient's condition is stabilized, percutaneous transluminal angioplasty may be done. SEE: *angina; artificial respiration; cardiopulmonary resuscitation; reperfusion.*

NURSING IMPLICATIONS: All diagnostic and treatment procedures are briefly explained to reduce stress and anxiety. Cardiac rhythm, rate, and conduction are monitored on a lead that provides easily identifiable P and R waves (a 12-lead ECG should be included). Location, radiation, quality and severity, and frequency of chest pain are documented. Prescribed oxygen and analgesic medications (mainly IV) are administered and evaluated for desired effects. Vital signs and hemodynamic status are monitored according to protocol or as required by the patient. An IV access is established and maintained for emergency therapy, such as administration of cardiac and diuretic drugs and implementation of other emergency measures according to protocol or as prescribed for the patient's problems. The nurse promotes rest and provides support throughout the acute phase of the illness. Both patient and family are taught about required lifestyle and diet modifications and the need for long-term drug therapy. A cardiac rehabilitation program based on graduated activity to increase cardiac work is prescribed and evaluated, and the patient is encouraged to continue participation in the program after discharge. Stress testing is explained. The nurse assists the patient with grief connected to changes in health status and self-concept.

**myocardial insufficiency** Inability of the heart to perform its usual function, eventually resulting in cardiac failure.

**myocardial ischemia** SEE: under *ischemia.*

**myocardiograph** (mī″ō-kăr′dē-ō-grăf) [″ + ″ + *graphein,* to write] Instrument for recording heart movements.

**myocardiopathy** (mī″ō-kăr″dē-ŏp′ă-thē) [″ + ″ + *pathos,* disease, suffering] Any disease of the myocardium.

**myocarditis** (mī″ō-kăr-dī′tĭs) [″ + *kardia,* heart, + *itis,* inflammation] Inflammation of the myocardium. SEE: *cardiomyopathy; Nursing Diagnoses Appendix.*

SYMPTOMS: Apex beat is extremely weak and rapid, pulse is irregular and weak, there is tenderness over precordium, and percussion is negative. Auscultation reveals that the first heart sound resembles the second heart sound, being high pitched and wanting in muscular quality. The electrocardiogram may be normal or show only non-specific ST-T wave abnormalities.

ETIOLOGY: Myocarditis may be associated with a number of conditions, including many types of bacterial, fungal, protozoal, and viral infections, heat stroke, and ionizing radiation. It commonly occurs after rheumatic fever and diphtheria. The specific cause may be unknown.

NURSING IMPLICATIONS: Complete bedrest is prescribed until symptoms resolve. A light diet including foods to prevent constipation and a stress-free environment are provided. Electocardiogram and cardiac status are assessed frequently for signs of increased cardiac workload and fatigue. If these occur, more frequent rest periods are provided. Prescribed antibiotics are administered, and immediate treatment is instituted for progressive or life-threatening dysrhythmias. Activity is increased gradually after the acute phase. During the recovery period, the patient should avoid travel to high altitudes, frequent stair climbing, and stress.

**myocardium** (mī-ō-kăr′dē-ŭm) [″ + *kardia,* heart] The middle layer of the walls of the heart, composed of cardiac muscle.

**myocele** (mī′ō-sēl) [″ + *kele,* tumor, swelling] Muscular protrusion through a muscle sheath.

**myocelitis** (mī″ō-sē-lī′tĭs) [″ + ″ + *itis,* inflammation] Inflammation of abdominal muscles.

**myocellulitis** (mī″ō-sĕl-ū-lī′tĭs) [″ + L. *cellula,* little chamber, + Gr. *itis,* inflammation] Myositis combined with cellulitis.

**myoceptor** (mī′ō-sĕp″tor) [″ + L. *capere,* to take] The endplates of a nerve supplying a muscle.

**myocerosis** (mī″ō-sē-rō′sĭs) [″ + *keros,* wax] Waxy degeneration of a muscle or muscular tissue. SYN: *myokerosis.*

**myochorditis** (mī″ō-kor-dī′tĭs) [″ + *chorde,* cord, + *itis,* inflammation] Inflammation of the muscles of the vocal cord.

**myochrome** (mī′ō-krōm) [″ + *chroma,* color] **1.** Any muscle pigment. **2.** Cytochrome C.

**myochronoscope** (mī″ō-krō′nō-skōp) [″ + *chronos,* time, + *skopein,* to examine] Device used for timing a muscular contraction.

**myoclonia** (mī-ō-klō′nē-ă) Myoclonus.

**myoclonus** (mī-ŏk′lō-nŭs) [″ + *klonos,* tumult] Twitching or clonic spasm of a muscle or group of muscles.

***m. multiplex*** Condition marked by persistent and continuous muscular spasms in unrelated muscles. SYN: *paramyoclonus multiplex.*

***nocturnal m.*** Involuntary limb movements (e.g., twitching) during the night. SEE: *leukemia; restless legs syndrome.*

***palatal m.*** Rapid clonus of one or both sides of the palate.

**myocoele** (mī′ō-sēl) [″ + *koila,* hollow] Cavity within a somite of an embryo.

**myocolpitis** (mī″ō-kŏl-pī′tĭs) [″ + *kolpos,* vagina, + *itis,* inflammation] Inflammation of vaginal muscular tissue.

**myocomma** (mī-ō-kŏm′mă) *pl.* **myocommata** [″ + *komma,* cut] Septum dividing the myotomes.

**myocyte** (mī′ō-sīt) [″ + *kytos,* cell] A muscular tissue cell.

**myocytoma** (mī″ō-sī-tō′mă) [″ + ″ + *oma,* tumor] Tumor containing muscle cells.

**myodemia** (mī-ō-dē′mē-ă) [″ + *demos,* fat] Fatty degeneration of muscular tissue. Muscular fiber cells become filled with fat granules and are ultimately destroyed.

**myodiastasis** (mī″ō-dī-ăs′tă-sĭs) [Gr. *mys,* muscle, + *diastasis,* separation] Division or rupture of a muscle.

**myodiopter** (mī″ō-dī-ŏp′tĕr) The force of ciliary muscle contraction needed to increase the refraction of the eye one diopter more than when the eye is at rest.

**myodynamia** (mī″ō-dī-năm′ē-ă) [″ + *dynamis,* force] Muscular force or strength.

**myodynamometer** (mī″ō-dī″nă-mŏm′ĕt-ĕr) [″ + ″ + *metron,* measure] Device for measurement of muscular strength.

**myodynia** (mī″ō-dĭn′ē-ă) [″ + *odyne,* pain] Muscle pain. SYN: *myalgia.*

**myodystrophy** (mī″ō-dĭs′trō-fē) [″ + ″ + *tro-*

*phe,* nutrition] Muscular dystrophy.

**myoedema** (mī″ō-ĕ-dē′mă) [″+ *oidema,* swelling] **1.** Mounding. **2.** Edema of a muscle.

**myoelastic** Pert. to muscle and elastic tissue.

**myoelectric** Pert. to the electrical properties of muscles.

**myoelectric prosthesis** SEE: under *prosthesis.*

**myoendocarditis** (mī″ō-ĕn″dō-kăr-dī′tĭs) [″ + *endon,* within, + *kardia,* heart, + *itis,* inflammation] Inflammation of the cardiac muscular wall and membranous lining.

**myoepithelial cell** SEE: under *cell.*

**myoepithelioma** (mī″ō-ĕp″ĭ-thē″lē-ō′mă) [″ + *epi,* upon, + *thele,* nipple, + *oma,* tumor] A slow-growing tumor of the sweat gland.

**myoepithelium** (mī″ō-ĕp″ĭ-thē′lē-ŭm) [″ + ″ + *thele,* nipple] Tissue containing contractile epithelial cells. **myoepithelial** (mī″ō-ĕp″ĭ-thē′lē-ăl), *adj.*

**myofasciitis** (mī″ō-făs″ē-ī′tĭs) [″ + L. *fascia,* band, + Gr. *itis,* inflammation] Inflammation of a muscle and its fascia.

**myofibril, myofibrilla** (mī-ō-fī′brĭl, -fī-brĭl′lă) [″ + L. *fibrilla,* a small fiber] A microscopic fibril found in muscle cells, grouped into bundles that run parallel to the long axis of the cell. It is made of myofilaments of myosin and actin, the contractile proteins.

**myofibroma** (mī″ō-fī-brō′mă) [″+ L. *fibra,* fiber, + Gr. *oma,* tumor] Tumor containing muscular and fibrous tissue.

**myofibrosis** (mī″ō-fī-brō′sĭs) [″+ ″+ Gr. *osis,* condition] Increase of connective or fibrous tissue with degeneration of muscular tissue.

**myofibrositis** (mī″ō-fī″brō-sī′tĭs) [Gr. *mys,* muscle, + L. *fibra,* fiber, + Gr. *itis,* inflammation] Inflammation of the perimysium, the fibrous tissue that encloses muscle tissue.

**myofilament** (mī″ō-fĭl′ă-mĕnt) A filament within the myofibrils of muscle cells. Thick ones are made of myosin; thin ones are made of actin, troponin, and tropomyosin.

**myofunctional** (mī″ō-fŭnk′shŭn-ăl) Concerning muscle function.

**myogelosis** (mī″ō-jē-lō′sĭs) [″ + L. *gelare,* to congeal] Abnormal hardening of a portion of muscle.

**myogenesis** (mī-ō-jĕn′ĕ-sĭs) [″ + *genesis,* generation, birth] Formation of muscular tissue, esp. in embryos.

**myogenetic, myogenic** (mī-ō-jĕn′ĕt′ĭk, mī-ō-jĕn′ĭk) [″ + *gennan,* to produce] Originating in muscle.

**myoglia** (mī-ŏg′lē-ă) [″ + *glia,* glue] A fibrous network in muscular tissue resembling neuroglia in appearance.

**myoglobin** The iron-containing protein found in muscle cells that stores oxygen for use in cell respiration.

**myoglobinuria** (mī″ō-glō″bĭn-ū′rē-ă) Myoglobin in the urine. It may occur following muscular activity, trauma, or as a result of a deficiency of muscle phosphorylase.

**myoglobulin** (mī″ō-glŏb′ū-lĭn) [″ + L. *globulus,* globule] A coagulable globulin present in muscular tissue.

**myognathus** (mī-ŏg′nă-thŭs) [″+ *gnathos,* jaw] Deformed individual with a rudimentary conjoined twin.

**myogram** [″ + *gramma,* something written] Tracing made by the myograph of muscular contractions.

**myograph** (mī′ō-grăf) [″+ *graphein,* to write] Instrument for tracing movements caused by muscular contractions. **myographic** (mī-ō-grăf′ĭk), *adj.*

**myographic tracing** A myogram or muscular tracing.

**myography** (mī-ŏg′ră-fē) **1.** Recording of muscular contractions by a myograph. **2.** Description of the muscles and their action.

**myohematin** (mī″ō-hĕm′ă-tĭn) Cytochrome C.

**myohemoglobin** (mī″ō-hē″mō-glō′bĭn) ABBR: MHb. Myoglobin.

**myoid** (mī′oyd) [Gr. *mys,* muscle, + *eidos,* form, shape] Resembling muscle.

**myoidema** (mī-oy-dē′mă) [″ + *oidema,* swelling] Myoedema.

**myoischemia** (mī″ō-ĭs-kē′mē-ă) [″+ *ischein,* to hold back, + *haima,* blood] Localized deficiency of blood supply in muscle tissue.

**myokerosis** (mī″ō-kē-rō′sĭs) [″ + *keros,* wax, + *osis,* condition] Myocerosis.

**myokinase** (mī″ō-kĭn′ās) An enzyme present in muscle that catalyzes the synthesis of adenosine triphosphate.

**myokinesimeter** (mī″ō-kĭn″ĕ-sĭm′ĕ-tĕr) [″ + *kinesis,* movement, + *metron,* measure] A device for measuring muscle activity.

**myokinesis** (mī″ō-kĭn-ē′sĭs) [″ + *kinesis,* movement] **1.** Muscular activity. **2.** Surgical displacement of muscular fibers.

**myokymia** (mī-ō-kĭm′ē-ă) [″ + *kyma,* wave] Twitching of isolated segments of muscle. The condition may be functional; however, it is also seen in organic diseases and general paresis. SYN: *kymatism.*

**myolemma** (mī″ō-lĕm′ă) [″ + *lemma,* sheath] Sarcolemma.

**myolipoma** (mī″ō-lī-pō′mă) [″+ *lipos,* fat, + *oma,* tumor] Muscle tissue tumor containing fatty elements.

**myology** (mī-ŏl′ō-jē) [″+ *logos,* word, reason] The science or study of the muscles and their parts.

**myolysis** (mī-ŏl′ĭ-sĭs) [″ + *lysis,* dissolution] Fatty degeneration and infiltration with destruction of muscular tissue accompanied by separation and disappearance of muscle cells.

**myoma** (mī-ō′mă) *pl.* **myomas** or **myomata** [″ + *oma,* tumor] A tumor containing muscle tissue. SEE: *chondromyoma.* **myomatous** (-tŭs), *adj.*

***m. striocellulare*** Rhabdomyoma.

***m. telangiectodes*** Angiomyoma.

***m. uteri*** Fibroid tumor of the uterus.

**myomalacia** (mī″ō-mă-lā′sē-ă) [Gr. *mys,* muscle, + *malakia,* softening] Softening of muscular tissue.

***m. cordis*** Softening of the heart muscle.

**myomatosis** (mī″ō-mă-tō′sĭs) [″ + *oma,* tumor, + *osis,* condition] The development of multiple myomas.

**myomectomy** (mī″ō-mĕk′tō-mē) [″ + *oma,* tumor, + *ektome,* excision] **1.** Removal of a portion of muscle or muscular tissue. **2.** Removal of a myomatous tumor, generally uterine, usually by abdominal section, leaving the uterus in place. SYN: *myomotomy.*

**myomelanosis** (mī″ō-mĕl-ă-nō′sĭs) [″ + *melanosis,* blackening] Abnormal darkening of muscle tissue.

**myomere** (mī′ō-mēr) [″ + *meros,* part] Myotome (2).

**myometer** (mī-ŏm′ĕt-ĕr) [″ + *metron,* measure] Device for measurement of muscular contractions.

**myometrial** Concerning the myometrium.

**myometritis** (mī″ō-mē-trī′tĭs) [″ + *metra,* uterus, + *itis,* inflammation] Inflammation of the muscular wall of the uterus. SYN: *mesometritis.*

**myometrium** (mī″ō-mē′trē-ŭm) The smooth muscle layer of the uterine wall, forming the main mass of the uterus.

**myomotomy** (mī″ō-mŏt′ō-mē) [″ + ″ + *tome,* excision] Myomectomy (2).

**myon** [Gr. *mys,* muscle] A single muscle unit.

**myonecrosis** (mī″ō-nĕ-krō′sĭs) [″ + *nekrosis,* state of death] Necrosis of muscle tissue.

**myonephropexy** (mī″ō-nĕf′rō-pĕk″sē) [″ + *nephros,* kidney, + *pexis,* fixation] Fixation of a movable kidney by attaching it to a portion of muscular tissue with sutures.

**myoneural** Pert. to muscle and nerve, esp. nerve terminations in muscles.

**myoneuralgia** (mī″ō-nū-răl′jē-ă) [″ + *neuron,* nerve, + *algos,* pain] Muscle pain.

**myoneural junction** SEE: under *junction.*

**myoneurasthenia** (mī″ō-nūr″ăs-thē′nē-ă) [″ + ″ + *astheneia,* weakness] Relaxed condition of muscular system associated with neurasthenia.

**myoneuroma** (mī″ō-nū-rō′mă) [″ + ″ + *oma,* tumor] Neuroma partially composed of muscular elements.

**myonymy** (mī-ŏn′ĭ-mē) [″ + *onoma,* name] Nomenclature of muscles.

**myoparalysis** (mī″ō-pă-răl′ĭ-sĭs) Paralysis of a muscle.

**myoparesis** (mī″ō-păr′ĕ-sĭs) Weakness or incomplete paralysis of a muscle.

**myopathic facies** SEE: under *facies.*

**myopathy** (mī-ŏp′ă-thē) [″ + *pathos,* disease, suffering] Any disease or abnormal condition of striated muscle. **myopathic** (mī-ō-păth′ĭk), *adj.*

***centronuclear m.*** Myopathy in which the muscle fibers resemble those seen in fetal development. The nuclei of the cells are surrounded by a clear zone. SYN: *myotubular myopathy.*

***distal m.*** Myopathy of the hands.

***myotubular m.*** Centronuclear m.

***nemaline m.*** Congenital nonprogressive weakness, esp. of the proximal muscles. The muscles are thin and resemble rods.

***ocular m.*** Hereditary dystrophy of the extraocular muscles. This may progress to complete paralysis of these muscles.

***thyrotoxic m.*** A chronic disease characterized by progressive muscular weakness and atrophy and hyperthyroidism.

**myope** (mī′ōp) [Gr. *myein,* to shut, + *ops,* eye] One afflicted with myopia (nearsightedness).

**myopericarditis** (mī″ō-pĕr-ĭ-kar-dī′tĭs) [Gr. *mys,* muscle, + *peri,* around, + *kardia,* heart, + *itis,* inflammation] Inflammation of the pericardium and cardiac muscular wall.

**myopia** [Gr. *myein,* to shut, + *ops,* eye] An error in refraction in which light rays are focused in front of the retina, enabling the person to see distinctly for only a short distance. A negative (concave) lens of proper strength will correct this condition. SYN: *nearsightedness.* SEE: *emmetropia* for illus. **myopic** (mī-ŏp′ĭk), *adj.*

***axial m.*** Myopia due to elongation of the axis of the eye.

***chromic m.*** Color blindness only when viewing distant objects.

***curvature m.*** Myopia due to the curvature of the eye's refracting surfaces.

***index m.*** Myopia resulting from abnormal refractivity of the media of the eye.

***malignant m.*** Progressive myopia leading to retinal detachment and blindness. SYN: *pernicious m.*

***pernicious m.*** Malignant m.

***prodromal m.*** Myopia, seen in incipient cataract, in which reading without glasses becomes possible.

***progressive m.*** Myopia that increases steadily during adult life.

***space m.*** Myopia occurring when the eye is attempting to focus on an object but all that is visible is a complete noncontrasting material, such as may occur when looking into dense fog (e.g., while piloting an airplane). No image is produced on the retina.

***stationary m.*** Myopia that ends after adult growth is attained.

***transient m.*** Myopia seen in spasm of accommodation, as in acute iritis or iridocyclitis.

**myopic crescent** SEE: under *crescent.*

**myoplasm** (mī′ō-plăzm) [Gr. *mys,* muscle, + LL. *plasma,* form, mold] The contractile part of the muscle cell, as differentiated from the sarcoplasm.

**myoplastic** (mī′ō-plăs′tĭk) [″ + *plassein,* to form] Pert. to the plastic use of muscle tissue or plastic surgery on muscles.

**myoplasty** (mī-ō-plăs″tē) Plastic surgery of muscle tissue.

**myoporthosis** (mī″ŏp-or-thō′sĭs) Correction of myopia (nearsightedness).

**myopsychopathy** (mī″ō-sī-kŏp′ă-thē) [″ + *psyche,* mind, + *pathos,* disease, suffering] Any muscle dysfunction associated with mental disorder.

**myoreceptor** (mī″ō-rē-sĕp′tor) A proprioceptor in the muscle.

**myorrhaphy** (mī-or′ă-fē) [Gr. *mys,* muscle, + *rhaphe,* a sewing] Suture of a muscle. SYN: *myosuture.*

**myorrhexis** (mī-or-ĕk′sĭs) [″ + *rhexis,* a rupture] Rupture of a muscle.

**myosalpingitis** (mī″ō-săl-pĭn-jī′tĭs) [″ + *salpinx,* tube, + *itis,* inflammation] Inflammation of the muscular tissue of a fallopian tube.

**myosarcoma** (mī″ō-sar-kō′mă) [″ + *sarx,* flesh, + *oma,* tumor] A malignant tumor derived from myogenic cells.

**myosclerosis** (mī″ō-sklĕr-ō′sĭs) [″ + *skleros,* hardening] Hardening of muscle.

**myosin** [Gr. *mys,* muscle] A protein present in muscle fibrils and constituting about 65% of total muscle protein. It consists of long chains of polypeptides joined to each other by side chains. The molecular structure of myosin is thought to be responsible for the properties of muscle tissue, namely, birefringence, double refraction, contractility, and elasticity. Myosin and actin are the contractile proteins in muscle fibers. SEE: *sarcomere.*

**myosinose** (mī-ŏs′ĭn-ōs) A proteose resulting from the hydrolysis of myosin.

**myosinuria** (mī″ō-sĭn-ū′rē-ă) The presence of myosin in the urine. SYN: *myosuria.*

**myositis** (mī-ō-sī′tĭs) [″ + *itis,* inflammation] Inflammation of muscle tissue, esp. voluntary muscles, possibly caused by infection, trauma, diathetic states, or infestation by parasites. SYN: *myitis.* SEE: *fibromyalgia.*

***epidemic m.*** Bornholm disease; epidemic pleurodynia.

***m. fibrosa*** Myositis accompanied by infiltration of fibrous tissue.

***interstitial m.*** Myositis with hyperplasia of connective tissue.

***multiple m.*** Polymyositis.

***m. ossificans*** Myositis marked by ossification of muscles.

***parenchymatous m.*** Myositis of the substance of a muscle.

***m. purulenta*** Suppurative myositis with abscesses; caused by bacterial infection.

***traumatic m.*** Myositis due to physical injury. The condition may be simple, with accompanying pain and swelling, or may be suppurative.

***m. trichinosa*** Myositis due to infestation with trichinae. SYN: *trichinous myositis.*

**myospasm** (mī′ō-spăzm) [″ + *spasmos,* a convulsion] Spasmodic contraction of a muscle.

**myosteoma** (mī-ŏs″tē-ō′mă) [″ + *osteon,* bone, + *oma,* tumor] A bony growth found in muscle tissue.

**myosthenometer** (mī″ō-sthĕn-ŏm′ĕ-tĕr) [″ + *sthenos,* strength, + *metron,* measure] Device for measuring muscle power.

**myostroma** (mī″ō-strō′mă) [″ + *stroma,* mattress] The framework of muscle tissue.

**myosuria** (mī-ō-sū′rē-ă) [″ + *ouron,* urine] Myosinuria.

**myosuture** (mī″ō-sū′chūr) [″ + L. *sutura,* sewing] Myorrhexis.

**myotactic** (mī″ō-tăk′tĭk) [″ + L. *tactus,* touch] Pert. to muscle or kinesthetic sense.

**myotasis** (mī-ŏt′ă-sĭs) [″ + *tasis,* stretching] Stretching of a muscle. **myotatic,** *adj.*

**myotatic reflex** Stretch reflex.

**myotenontoplasty** (mī″ō-tĕn-ŏn′tō-plăst″ē) [″ + *tenon,* tendon, + *plassein,* to form] Tenomyoplasty; tenontomyoplasty.

**myotenositis** (mī″ō-tĕn-ō-sī′tĭs) [″ + ″ + *itis,* inflammation] Inflammation of a muscle and its tendon.

**myotenotomy** (mī″ō-tĕn-ŏt′ō-mē) [″ + ″ + *tome,* incision] Division of the tendon of a muscle.

**myotherapy** A method for relaxing muscle spasm, improving circulation, and alleviating pain. Pressure is applied, using elbows, knuckles, or fingers, and held for several seconds to defuse "trigger points." The success of this method depends upon the use of specific corrective exercises of the freed muscles. The method was developed by Bonnie Pruden in 1976.

**myothermic** (mī″ō-thĕrm′ĭk) [Gr. *mys,* muscle, + *therme,* heat] Pert. to rise in muscle temperature due to its activity.

**myotome** (mī′ō-tōm) [″ + *tome,* incision] **1.** Instrument used for cutting muscles. **2.** That portion of an embryonic somite that gives rise to somatic (striated) muscles. SYN: *myomere.*

**myotomy** (mī-ŏt′ō-mē) Surgical division or anatomical dissection of muscles.

**myotonia** (mī″ō-tō′nē-ă) [″ + *tonos,* tension] Tonic spasm of a muscle or temporary rigidity after muscular contraction. **myotonic,** *adj.*

***m. atrophica*** M. dystrophica.

***m. congenita*** A benign disease characterized by tonic spasms of the muscles induced by voluntary movements. The condition is usually congenital and is transmitted from one generation to another. SYN: *Oppenheim's disease; paramyotonia disease; Thomsen's disease.*

SYMPTOMS: The disease appears in early childhood and is manifested by a tonic spasm of the muscles every time the muscles are used. In a few minutes, rigidity wears away and the movements become free from repeated contractions, the muscles becoming firm and extremely well developed.

TREATMENT: Quinine or procainamide are indicated for relief of myotonia. Neostigmine is contraindicated. Avoidance of obesity is important.

PROGNOSIS: The disease is incurable, but may improve with age.

***m. dystrophica*** A hereditary disease characterized by muscular wasting, myotonia, and cataract. SYN: *m. atrophica; Steinert's disease.*

**myotonic** Pert. to tonic muscular spasm, as differentiated from myokinetic spasm.

**myotonus** (mī-ŏt′ō-nŭs) A tonic muscle spasm with temporary rigidity.

**myotrophy** (mī-ŏt′rō-fē) [″ + *trophe,* nourishment] Nutrition of muscle tissues.

**myotropic** (mī″ō-trŏp′ĭk) [″ + *trope,* a turn] Attracted to muscle tissue.

**myotube** (mī′ō-tūb) The developing stage of skeletal muscle. The central nucleus occupies most of the cell.

**myovascular** (mī″ō-văs′kū-lăr) Concerning muscles and their blood supply.

**myriachit** (mĭr-ē′ă-chĭt) [Russian] Myryachit.

**Myriapoda** (mĭr-ē-ăp′ō-dă) [Gr. *myrios,* numberless, + *pous,* foot] Group of arthropods including millipedes and centipedes.

**myriapodiasis** (mĭr″ē-ăp-ō-dī′ă-sĭs) Infestation with one of the Myriapoda class of anthropods.

**myricin** (mĭr′ĭ-sĭn) A chemical obtained from beeswax.

**myringa** (mĭr-ĭn′gă) [L.] The tympanic membrane.

**myringectomy** (mĭr-ĭn-jĕk′tō-mē) [″ + Gr. *ektome,* excision] Myringodectomy.

**myringitis** (mĭr-ĭn-jī′tĭs) [L. *myringa,* drum membrane, + Gr. *itis,* inflammation] Inflammation of the tympanic membrane (eardrum).

***m. bullosa*** Myringitis with serous or hemorrhagic blebs or vesicular inflammation of the eardrum and adjacent wall.

**myringodectomy** (mĭr-ĭn″gō-dĕk′tō-mē) [″ + Gr. *ektome,* excision] Excision of a part of or the entire tympanic membrane. SYN: *myringectomy.*

**myringomycosis** (mĭr-ĭn″gō-mī-kō′sĭs) [″ + Gr. *mykes,* fungus, + *osis,* condition] Inflammation of the tympanic membrane resulting from infection by parasitic fungi. SYN: *otomycosis.*

**myringoplasty** (mĭr-ĭn′gō-plăst″ē) [″ + Gr. *plassein,* to form] Plastic surgery of the tympanic membrane.

**myringotome** (mĭ-rĭn′gō-tōm) [″ + Gr. *tome,* incision] Surgical knife used for incising the tympanic membrane.

**myringotomy** (mĭr-ĭn-gŏt′ō-mē) Incision of the tympanic membrane. This procedure is most often performed on children with acute otitis media. Tympanostomy tubes are often placed in the opening made by the incision. SEE: *Nursing Diagnoses Appendix.*

NURSING IMPLICATIONS: Because this procedure is most often performed on young children in response to a recurring condition, the nurse teaches parents to recognize the signs of otitis media and to seek medical assistance when their child complains of pain or they observe the child experiencing pain to prevent spontaneous rupture of the eardrum. The parents are advised that tubes inserted after myringotomy gradually come out of the eardrum, and that the child should not swim in the early period after surgery.

**myrmecia** (mŭr-mē′shē-ă) [Gr. *myrmex,* ant] A dome-shaped wart.

**myrmecology** Study of ants.

**myrrh** (mŭr) [Gr. *myrra*] A gum resin used by man for many centuries. In antiquity, myrrh was cherished as a constituent of incense and perfume. Its most important use today is as an aromatic astringent mouthwash. Tincture of myrrh provides symptomatic relief when applied to canker sores.

**mysophilia** (mī″sō-fĭl′ē-ă) Erotic interest in body excretions.

**mysophobia** (mī″sō-fō′bē-ă) [Gr. *mysos,* filth, + *phobos,* fear] Abnormal aversion to dirt or contamination. SYN: *molysmophobia.*

**mytacism** (mī′tă-sĭzm) [Gr. *mytakismos* from Gr. letter $\mu$] Excessive or incorrect use of the letter *m* in writing, or the *m* sound in speaking.

**mythomania** (mĭth″ō-mā′nē-ă) [Gr. *mythos,* myth, + *mania,* madness] Abnormal tendency to lie and exaggerate.

**mythophobia** (mĭth″ō-fō′bē-ă) [″ + *phobos,* fear] Abnormal dread of making a false or incorrect statement.

**mytilotoxin** (mĭt″ĭ-lō-tŏk′sĭn) A neurotoxin present in certain mussels.

**myxadenitis** (mĭks″ăd-ĕn-ī′tĭs) [Gr. *myxa,* mucus, + *aden,* gland, + *itis,* inflammation] Inflammation of a mucous gland.

***m. labialis*** Cheilitis glandularis.

**myxadenoma** (mĭks″ăd-ē-nō′mă) [″ + ″ + *oma,* tumor] **1.** A tumor with the structure of a mucous gland. SYN: *myxoadenoma.* **2.** A tumor of glandular structure containing mucous elements.

**myxangitis** (mĭks″ăn-jī′tĭs) [″ + *angeion,* vessel, + *itis,* inflammation] Inflammation of mucous gland ducts.

**myxedema** (mĭks-ĕ-dē′mă) [Gr. *myxa,* mucus, + *oidema,* swelling] A condition resulting from hypofunction of the thyroid gland. SEE: *Nursing Diagnoses Appendix.* **myxedematous** (mĭks-ĕ-dĕm′ă-tŭs), *adj.*

SYMPTOMS: Symptoms include decreased metabolic rate, low radioactive iodine uptake by the thyroid gland, decreased protein-bound iodine, anemia, myxedematous facies, large tongue, slow speech, puffiness of hands and face, coarse and thickened edematous skin, loss and dryness of hair, mental apathy, drowsiness, and sensitivity to cold.

ETIOLOGY: Possible causes are iodine deficiency in the diet, surgical excision or atrophy of the thyroid gland, or excessive use of antithyroid drugs. Myxedema may occur secondary to hypofunction of the anterior pituitary and is complicated by adrenal and gonadal deficiencies.

TREATMENT: Therapy consists of administration of thyroid hormone replacement.

***childhood m.*** Myxedema occurring before puberty.

***operative m.*** Myxedema following removal of the thyroid gland. SYN: *cachexia strumipriva.*

***pituitary m.*** Myxedema occurring secondary to anterior pituitary hypofunction.

***pretibial m.*** Edema of the anterior surface of the legs following hyperthyroidism and exophthalmos.

**myxedematoid** (mĭks-ĕ-dēm′ă-toyd) [Gr. *myxa,* mucus, + *oidema,* swelling, + *eidos,* form, shape.] Resembling myxedema.

**myxo-, myx-** [Gr. *myxa*] Combining form denoting *mucus.*

**myxoadenoma** (mĭks″ō-ăd-ē-nō′mă) [″ + *aden,* gland, + *oma,* tumor] Myxadenoma (1).

**Myxobacterales** (mĭks″ō-băk-tĕ-rā′lēz) An order of bacteria found in soil and dung. It is characterized by a slimy spreading colony.

**myxochondrofibrosarcoma** (mĭks″ō-kŏn″drō-fi″brō-săr-kō′mă) A malignant tumor composed of myxomatous, chondromatous, fibrous, and sarcomatous elements.

**myxochondroma** (mĭks″ō-kŏn-drō′mă) A benign tumor composed of myxomatous and chondromatous elements.

**myxocystoma** (mĭks″ō-sĭs-tō′mă) [Gr. *myxa,* mucus, + *kystis,* cyst, + *oma,* tumor] A benign cystic tumor containing mucus.

**myxocyte** (mĭk′sō-sīt) [″ + *kytos,* cell] A characteristic cell of mucous tissue.

**myxoedema** (mĭks″ĕ-dē′mă) [″ + *oidema,* swelling] Myxedema.

**myxoenchondroma** (mĭks″ō-ĕn-kŏn-drō′mă) [″ + *en,* in, + *chondros,* cartilage, + *oma,* tumor] A cartilaginous tissue tumor that has undergone partial mucous degeneration.

**myxofibroma** (mĭks″ō-fī-brō′mă) [″ + L. *fibra,* fiber, + Gr. *oma,* tumor] Tumor composed of mucous and fibrous elements.

**myxofibrosarcoma** (mĭk″sō-fī″brō-săr-kō′mă) [″ + ″ + Gr. *sarx,* flesh, + *oma,* tumor] Fibrosarcoma that contains primitive mesenchymal tissue.

**myxoglioma** (mĭk″sō-glī-ō′mă) [Gr. *myxa,* mucus, + *glia,* glue, + *oma,* tumor] Tumor composed of myxomatous and gliomatous elements.

**myxoid** (mĭk′soyd) [″ + *eidos,* form, shape] Similar to or resembling mucus.

**myxolipoma** (mĭk″sō-lĭ-pō′mă) [″ + *lipos,* fat, + *oma,* tumor] Mucous tumor with fatty tissue elements. SYN: *lipomyxoma.*

**myxoma** (mĭk-sō′mă) *pl.* **myxomas or myxomata** [″ + *oma,* tumor] Tumor composed of mucous connective tissue similar to that present in the embryo or umbilical cord. Cells are stellate or spindle-shaped and separated by mucoid tissue. The tumors are usually soft, gray, lobulated, and translucent and are not completely encapsulated. Myxomas may be pure or of mixed types involving other types of tissue.

***cartilaginous m.*** Chondromyxoma.

***cystic m.*** A tumor with parts fluid enough to resemble cysts.

***enchondromatous m.*** A tumor with nodules of hyaline cartilage.

***erectile m.*** Myxoma containing an excess of vessels, resembling an angioma.

***fibrous m.*** Fibromyxoma.

***intracanalicular m.*** Myxoma that develops in the interstitial connective tissue of the breasts.

***odontogenic m.*** A tumor of the jaw that appears to arise from mesenchymal tissue.

***telangiectatic m.*** Myxoma of highly vascular structure. SYN: *vascular m.*

***vascular m.*** Telangiectatic m.

**myxomatosis** (mĭk″sō-mă-tō′sĭs) [″ + ″ + *osis,* condition] **1.** Formation of multiple myxomas. **2.** Myxomatous degeneration.

**Myxomycetes** (mīk″sō-mī-sē′tēz) [Gr. *myxa,* mucus, + *mykes,* fungus] A class of organisms that includes slime molds. The organisms are of uncertain classification, but are thought to be fungus-like. SEE: *Myxobacterales.*

**myxoneuroma** (mĭks″ō-nū-rō′mă) [″ + *neuron,* nerve, + *oma,* tumor] Tumor composed of mucous and nerve tissue elements.

**myxopapilloma** (mĭk″sō-păp″ĭl-ō′mă) [″ + L. *papilla,* nipple, + Gr. *oma,* tumor] A tumor containing myxomatous and papillomatous elements.

**myxorrhea** (mĭk-sō-rē′ă) [″ + *rhoia,* flow] Free discharge from mucous surfaces. SYN: *blennorrhea.*

***m. gastrica*** Excessive mucous secretion in the stomach.

***m. intestinalis*** Excessive secretion of mucus from the bowels.

**myxosarcoma** (mĭk″sō-săr-kō′mă) [″ + *sarx,* flesh, + *oma,* tumor] Tumor containing myxomatous and sarcomatous elements, having undergone partial degeneration. **myxosarcomatous** (mĭk″sō-săr-kō′mă-tŭs), *adj.*

**myxospore** (mĭks′ō-spor) [″ + *sporos,* seed] A spore embedded in a gelatinous mass; seen in some fungi and protozoa.

**Myxosporidia** (mĭks-ō-spor-ĭd′ē-ă) Parasitic sporozoans most commonly found in the epithelial cells of lower vertebrates.

**myxovirus** Any of a family of viruses including those that cause influenza. SEE: *paramyxovirus.*

**Myzomyia** (mī″zō-mī′ă) [Gr. *myzan,* to suck, + *myia,* fly] Subgenus of anopheline mosquitoes. Some species transmit malarial parasites.

**Myzorhynchus** (mī″zō-rĭng′kŭs) [″ + *rhynchos,* snout] Subgenus of anopheline mosquitoes. Some species transmit malarial parasites.

# N

**N 1.** Symbol for the element nitrogen. **2.** *normal,* esp. with reference to solutions.

**n 1.** Symbol for *index of refraction.* **2.** *nasal; number.*

**$^{15}N$** Symbol for radioactive isotope of nitrogen.

**NA** *nicotinic acid; Nomina Anatomica; numerical aperture; nurse's aide.*

**Na** [L. *natrium*] Symbol for the element sodium.

**NAACOG** *Nurses Association of the American College of Obstetricians and Gynecologists.*

**nabothian cyst** (nă-bō′thē-ăn) [Martin Naboth, Ger. anatomist and physician, 1675–1721] A cystic formation caused by closure of the ducts of the nabothian glands in the cervix uteri as a result of healing of an erosion.

**NaBr** Sodium bromide.

**NaCl** Sodium chloride.

**NaClO** Sodium hypochlorite.

**$Na_2CO_3$** Sodium carbonate.

**nacreous** (nā′krē-ŭs) [L. *nacer,* mother of pearl] Having an iridescent pearl-like luster, as bacterial colonies.

**N.A.D.** *no appreciable disease.*

**NAD** *nicotinamide adenine dinucleotide.*

**$NAD^+$** *nicotinamide adenine dinucleotide,* oxidized form.

**NADH** *nicotinamide adenine dinucleotide,* reduced form.

**NADP** *nicotinamide adenine dinucleotide phosphate.*

**$NADP^+$** *nicotinamide adenine dinucleotide phosphate,* oxidized form.

**NADPH** *nicotinamide adenine dinucleotide phosphate,* reduced form.

**Naegele, Franz Carl** (nā′gĕ-lē) German obstetrician, 1777–1851.

***N.'s obliquity*** Anterior parietal presentation of the fetal head in labor. SYN: *anterior asynclitism.*

***N.'s pelvis*** An obliquely contracted pelvis in which the conjugate diameter assumes an oblique direction. The condition is caused by disease in infancy.

***N.'s rule*** A system used to estimate the date of onset of labor by counting back exactly 90 days from the day the last menstrual period began and adding seven days to that date.

**Naegleria** A genus of amebic protozoa present in soil, ground water, and sewage. One species, *N. fowleri,* is the causative agent of a lethal form of meningoencephalitis. SEE: *acanthamebiasis; meningoencephalitis.*

**N.A.E.M.S.P.** *National Association of EMS Physicians.*

**N.A.E.M.T.** *National Association of Emergency Medical Technicians.*

**NaF** Sodium fluoride.

**nafcillin sodium** (năf-sĭl′ĭn) A semisynthetic penicillin that is penicillinase-resistant. Trade names are Nafcil and Unipen.

**$NaHCO_3$** Sodium bicarbonate.

**$NaHSO_3$** Sodium bisulfite.

**nail** [AS. *naegel*] **1.** A rod made of metal, bone, or solid material used to attach the ends or pieces of broken bones. **2.** A horny cell structure of the epidermis forming flat plates upon the dorsal surface of the fingers and toes. SYN: *onyx; unguis.* SEE: illus.

A fingernail or toenail consists of a body composed of keratin (the exposed portion) and a root (the proximal portion hidden by the nail fold), both of which rest on the nailbed (matrix). The latter consists of epithelium and corium continuous with the epidermis and dermis of the skin of the nail fold. The crescent-shaped white area near the root is called the lunula. The epidermis extending from the margin of the nail fold over the root is called eponychium; that underlying the free border of the distal portion is called hyponychium.

A nail grows in length and thickness through cell activity in the stratum germinativum of the root. The average rate of growth in fingernails is about 1 mm per week. Growth is slower in toenails and slower in summer than in winter. Nail growth varies with age and is affected by disease and certain hormone deficiencies. The onset of a disease that briefly interferes with nail growth and development may be estimated by measuring the distance of the line (Beau's line) across the nail from the root of the nail.

DIFFERENTIAL DIAGNOSIS: Changes in the nails, such as ridges, may occur after a serious illness or indicate defective nu-

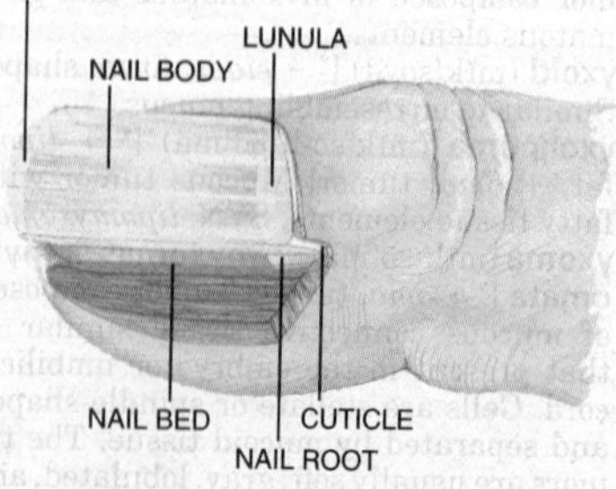


NAIL

(LONGITUDINAL SECTION)

trition. In achlorhydria and hypochromic anemia, excessively spoon-shaped nails that are depressed in the center may occur. In chronic pulmonary conditions and congenital heart disease, a spongy excess of soft tissue at the base of the nails may be associated with clubbed fingers. Atrophy may occur as a result of hereditary or congenital tendencies. Permanent atrophy may follow injuries, scars from disease, frostbite, nerve injuries, and hyperthyroidism. Nail shedding is due to the same causes. Fragile or split nails often occur as a congenital condition or may be due to prolonged contact with chemicals or too frequent buffing or filing of the flat surface of the nail during manicuring. In a healthy person brittle nails are usually caused by exposure to solvents, detergents, and soaps. The brittleness disappears when the external causes are avoided. Dry, malformed nails may be due to trophic changes resulting from injury to a nerve or a finger or from neuritis, Raynaud's disease, pulmonary osteoarthropathy, syphilis, onychia, scleroderma, acrodermatitis, or granuloma fungoides of the fingers. Transverse lines (Beau's lines) may result from previous interference of nail matrix growth. These lines may be caused by local or systemic conditions. The approximate date of the lesion may be determined, because it takes 4 to 6 months for the fingernail to be replaced. Chancre may be suspected if a small indolent ulcer appears near the nail, esp. if indurated and associated with enlarged lymph glands above the inner condyle. Quincke's capillary pulsation, indicated by a rhythmic flushing and blanching under the nails, is seen most frequently in aortic regurgitation and often in anemia.

Discoloration of nails is seen in various medical conditions. *Black* discoloration may be seen in diabetic gangrene, as well as some other forms of gangrene. *Blue-black* discoloration is a common condition due to hemorrhage caused by bleeding diseases, such as hemophilia, or trauma. This condition may be painful and can be relieved by drilling a small hole in the nail at the site of the hemorrhage. A dental drill, the heated tip of a paper clip, or a similar rigid wire of small diameter may be used. *Brown* discoloration may be due to arsenic poisoning. *Brownish-black* discoloration often indicates chronic mercury poisoning, due to the formation of sulfide of mercury in the tissues. *Cyanosis* of the nails usually indicates anemia, poor circulation, or venous stasis. *Green* staining of the nail fold or under the nail is associated with the growth of *Pseudomonas* in a wet area. *Slate* discoloration is an early manifestation of argyria, and intake of silver should be stopped at once. *White* spots or striate lesions may be due to trauma and are more frequently seen in women. Transverse white bands in all nails may be a sign of acute or chronic arsenic poisoning or, rarely, of thallium acetate poisoning. SEE: *Mees lines.*

***clubbing of n.*** SEE: *clubbing.*

***eggshell n.*** A condition in which the nail plate is soft and semitransparent, bends easily, and splits at the end. The condition is associated with arthritis, peripheral neuritis, leprosy, and hemiplegia. It may be the only visible sign of late syphilis.

***fungal infection of n.*** Infection of a nail by one of a number of fungi. Systemic therapy with griseofulvin or itraconazole is helpful, but they may need to be used 6 to 12 months for fingernails and 12 to 18 months for toenails.

***habit deformity n.*** Disruption of the nail surface by the habit of abrading or stroking that area. This produces a wavy or washboard-like nail surface.

***hang n.*** Broken epidermis at the edge of a nail.

***ingrown n.*** Growth of the nail edge into the soft tissue, thus causing inflammation and sometimes an abscess. Ingrown nails may be due to improper paring of the nails or pressure on a nail edge from improperly fitted shoes. In many cases, this condition may be prevented by cutting the nails straight across rather than curved.

***intermedullary n.*** A surgical rod inserted into the intermedullary canal to act as an immobilization device to hold the two ends of a fractured long bone in position.

***reedy n.*** A nail marked by longitudinal fissures.

***Smith-Petersen n.*** A three-flanged nail employed to fix fractures of the neck of the femur.

***splitting n.*** A troublesome condition in which the brittle nails split easily. Polishing, buffing, or abrading the nail surface will weaken the nail; thus, these practices should be discouraged. Brittle nails should be soaked, preferably in bath oil, prior to cutting them.

***spoon n.*** A nail with a depressed center and elevated lateral edges. This condition may follow trauma to the nail fold or iron deficiency anemia or may develop naturally. SYN: *koilonychia.* SEE: *koilonychia* for illus.

**nailbed** The portion of a finger or toe covered by the nail. SYN: *nail matrix.*

**nail biting** A nervous affliction or neurosis in which the free edges of the nails are bitten down. SYN: *onychophagy.*

**nail fold** SEE: under *fold.*

**nail groove** The space between the nail wall and the nailbed.

**nailing** Fixing fragments of bone by use of a nail.

**nail matrix** Nailbed.

**nail-patella syndrome** Onycho-osteodysplasia.

**nail root** Proximal portion of nail covered by

nail fold.

**nail wall** Epidermis covering edges of the nail. SYN: *vallum unguis.*

**naked** (nā′kĕd) [AS *naced,* nude] Uncovered, exposed to view, nude, bare, devoid of clothing.

**nalidixic acid** An antibiotic used in treating certain urinary tract infections.

**nalorphine hydrochloride** (năl-or′fēn) A narcotic antagonist used in the treatment of certain kinds of narcotic overdose, esp. with morphine.

**naloxone hydrochloride** (năl-ŏks′ōn) A drug that prevents or reverses the action of morphine and other opioid drugs. Its most important use is treatment of narcotic overdose.

**naltrexone** An opioid antagonist used to treat addiction to opium-derived drugs. It is also approved to treat alcohol dependence.

Caution: Naltrexone may cause liver damage when given in large doses.

**NANDA** *North American Nursing Diagnosis Association.*

**nandrolone decanoate** (năn′drō-lōn) An anabolic androgenic steroid.

**nandrolone phenpropionate** An anabolic androgenic steroid.

**nanism** (nā′nĭzm) [L. *nanus,* dwarf, + Gr. *-ismos,* condition] Dwarfism.

***symptomatic n.*** Nanism with deficient dentition, sexual development, and ossification.

**nano-** (nā′nō) [L. *nanus,* dwarf] **1.** Prefix indicating one billionth ($10^{-9}$) of the unit following; thus, a nanogram is one billionth ($10^{-9}$) of a gram. **2.** Combining form indicating dwarfism (nanism).

**nanocephaly** (nā-nō-sĕf′ă-lē) [″ + Gr. *kephale,* head, + *-ismos,* condition] Microcephaly. **nanocephalous** (nā-nō-sĕf′ă-lŭs), *adj.*

**nanocormia** (nā″nō-kor′mē-ă) [L. *nanus,* dwarf, + Gr. *kormos,* trunk] Abnormal smallness of thorax or body.

**nanocurie** (nā″nō-kū′rē) A unit of radioactivity equal to $10^{-9}$ curie.

**nanogram** One billionth ($10^{-9}$) of a gram.

**nanoid** (nā′noyd) [″ + Gr. *eidos,* form, shape] Dwarflike.

**nanomelus** (nā-nŏm′ĕ-lŭs) [″ + Gr. *melos,* limb] Micromelus.

**nanometer** (nā″nō-mē′tĕr) A unit of length equal to $10^{-9}$ meter.

**nanomole** One billionth ($10^{-9}$) mole.

**nanophthalmia** (năn″ŏf-thăl′mē-ă) [″ + Gr. *ophthalmos,* eye] Microphthalmia.

**nanosecond** (nā″nō-sĕk′ŏnd) A unit of time measurement equal to $10^{-9}$ second.

**nanosoma, nanosomia** (nā″nō-sō′mă, nā-nō-sō′mē-ă) [L. *nanus,* dwarf, + Gr. *soma,* body] Dwarfism.

**nanosomus** (nā-nō-sō′mŭs) A person of stunted size; a dwarf.

**nanous** (nā′nŭs) [L. *nanus,* dwarf] Dwarfed or stunted.

**nanukayami** (nă″nū-kă-yă′mē) A form of leptospirosis present in Japan.

**NaOH** Sodium hydroxide.

**nap** (năp) [AS. *hnappian,* nap] **1.** To slumber. **2.** A short sleep; a doze. SEE: *sleep.*

**napalm** (nā′pălm) [from *na*phthene + *palm*itate] Gasoline made thick or jelly-like for use in incendiary bombs and flame throwers.

**napalm burn** SEE: under *burn.*

**nape** (nāp, năp) The back of the neck. SYN: *nucha.*

**napex** (nā′pĕks) Scalp beneath the occipital protuberance.

**naphazoline hydrochloride** (năf-ăz′ō-lēn) A vasoconstrictor drug used topically as a nasal decongestant and as an ophthalmic mydriatic or vasoconstrictor.

**naphtha** (năf′thă) **1.** A volatile inflammable liquid distilled from carbonaceous substances. **2.** Petroleum, esp. more volatile varieties.

**naphthalene** (năf′thă-lēn) $C_{10}H_8$. A hydrocarbon, one of principal constituents of coal tar. It is used as a disinfectant, in moth balls, and in the manufacture of dyes and explosives. SEE: *Poisons and Poisoning Appendix.*

**naphthol** (năf′thōl) $C_{10}H_8O$. Petroleum substance used as an antiseptic and in certain dyes. It is prepared from naphthalene.

**N.A.P.N.A.P.** *National Association of Pediatric Nurse Associates and Practitioners.*

**N.A.P.N.E.S.** *National Association for Practical Nurse Education and Services.*

**N.A.P.T.** *National Association of Physical Therapists.*

**narcissism** (năr′sĭs-ĭzm) [Narcissus, a Gr. mythical character who fell in love with his own reflection] **1.** Self-love or self-admiration. **2.** Sexual pleasure derived from observing one's own naked body. **narcissistic** (năr-sĭs-sĭst′ĭk), *adj.*

**narcissistic object choice** Selection of another like one's own self as the object of love, friendship, or liking.

**narco-** [Gr. *narke,* numbness] Combining form meaning *numbness, stupor.*

**narcoanalysis** (năr″kō-ă-năl′ĭ-sĭs) [″ + *analysis,* a dissolving] A form of psychotherapy in which light anesthesia is produced by use of I.V. barbiturates. Patients are encouraged to talk about their experiences and may discuss events that would ordinarily be suppressed. SYN: *narcosynthesis.*

**narcoanesthesia** (nar″kō-ăn-ĕs-thē′zē-ă) Anesthesia produced by a narcotic, as scopolamine and morphine.

**narcohypnia** (năr″kō-hĭp′nē-ă) [Gr. *narke,* numbness, + *hypnos,* sleep] Numbness following sleep.

**narcohypnosis** (năr″kō-hĭp-nō′sĭs) Stupor or deep sleep produced by hypnosis.

**narcolepsy** (năr′kō-lĕp″sē) [Gr. *narke,* numbness, + *lepsis,* seizure] A chronic ailment consisting of recurrent attacks of drowsiness and sleep during daytime. More than 125,000 people in the U.S. have narcolepsy. The patient is unable to control these spells of sleep but is easily awakened. These attacks may be distinguished from ordinary drowsiness following a meal by the frequency of occurrence of attacks in narcolepsy, their irresistibility, and their happening in unusual circumstances, such as while eating, standing, or conversing. About 40% of the patients will have some form of cataplexy, (i.e., sudden loss of muscle tone brought on by some strong emotion such as laughter, surprise, or anger). The knees may buckle, the head will fall forward, and the person may fall to the ground but remain conscious. SEE: *sleep disorder*. **narcoleptic** (năr-kō-lĕp′tĭk), *adj.*

DIAGNOSIS: Findings from the daytime Multiple Sleep Latency Test include an average sleep of less than 5 min and the appearance of REM sleep during two or more of five naps. Sleep latencies of less than 10 min and sleep-onset REM periods during nocturnal polysomnographic studies are also found. Human leukocyte antigen (HLA) typing shows HLA-DR2 and DQw6 in approx. 90% of people with narcolepsy.

Narcolepsy occurs in families and is probably controlled by a specific gene. It is also present as a familial disorder in cats, certain breeds of dogs, ponies, quarterhorses, and Brahma bulls. Except for frequent sleep patterns, the electroencephalogram is normal.

TREATMENT: Symptomatic treatment with drugs such as ephedrine or dextroamphetamine sulfate or methylphenidate hydrochloride is indicated. In addition, 15-minute naps planned to coincide with the known time of occurrence of drowsiness will help.

---

Caution: Patients with this illness must be warned to avoid participation in activities that require constant alertness (e.g., driving, employment as a security guard). Drivers with narcolepsy should, at the first sign of drowsiness, park the vehicle and take a nap.

---

NURSING IMPLICATIONS: Patients with this condition are taught to enhance safety through care in driving and other activities in which falling asleep may endanger both the patient's and others' lives. Support is given for distressing symptoms. The nurse encourages the patient to seek medical attention to assist in coping with symptoms.

**narcosis** [Gr. *narkosis,* a benumbing] Unconsciousness or stupor produced by drugs.

***basal n.*** Initial narcosis produced by sedatives used prior to administration of a general anesthetic.

***carbon dioxide n.*** Personality changes, confusion, and coma due to an increase in carbon dioxide content of the blood. This may occur during oxygen therapy during which the concentration of administered oxygen becomes high enough to cause an actual decrease in respirations that allows enough carbon dioxide to cause narcosis. This may be treated by decreasing but not discontinuing the rate of administration of oxygen, or by assisted ventilation.

***medullary n.*** General anesthesia induced by a local anesthetic injected into the sheath of the spinal cord in lumbar region. SYN: *spinal anesthesia.*

**narcosynthesis** (năr″kō-sĭn′thĕ-sĭs) [″ + *synthesis,* synthesis] Narcoanalysis.

**narcotic** [Gr. *narkotikos,* benumbing] **1.** Producing stupor or sleep. **2.** An older term for a drug that depresses the central nervous system, thus relieving pain and producing sleep. Most narcotics are habit-forming. Excessive use produces unconsciousness, stupor, coma, and possibly death. Opium, morphine, codeine, papaverine, and heroin are examples of narcotics. The newer term is *opioid analgesic.* SEE: *pain.*

**narcotic addict** One who has become physiologically or psychologically dependent upon narcotics. SEE: *drug addiction.*

**narcotic poisoning** Poisoning caused by narcotic or sleep-producing drugs such as opium and its derivatives, chloral combinations, or barbital and its myriad subvarieties.

SYMPTOMS: Symptoms include depression, slowing of heart rate and respiration, and sleep, followed by coma.

FIRST AID: The drugs should be removed by gastric lavage. Administration of nalorphine is indicated if poisoning is due to a derivative of opium, such as morphine.

**narcotism** (năr′kō-tĭzm) [Gr. *narke,* stupor, + *-ismos,* condition] An addiction to the use of narcotics. Addiction may be said to exist when discontinuance causes abstinence symptoms that are speedily relieved by a dose of the drug.

TREATMENT: Treatment is ordinarily successful only during hospitalization. Relapses are frequent, and the adoption of an alternate philosophy of life is of prime importance.

**narcotize** [Gr. *narkotikos,* benumbing] To place under the influence of a narcotic.

**naris** (nā′rĭs) *pl.* **nares** [L.] The nostril. SEE: *nose.*

***anterior n.*** External nostril.

***posterior n.*** The opening between the nasal cavity and the nasopharynx.

**narrowing** Decreasing the width or diameter of some space or channel (e.g., narrowing of the size of the coronary arteries), usually due to some pathological process.

**NASA** *National Aeronautics and Space Administration.*

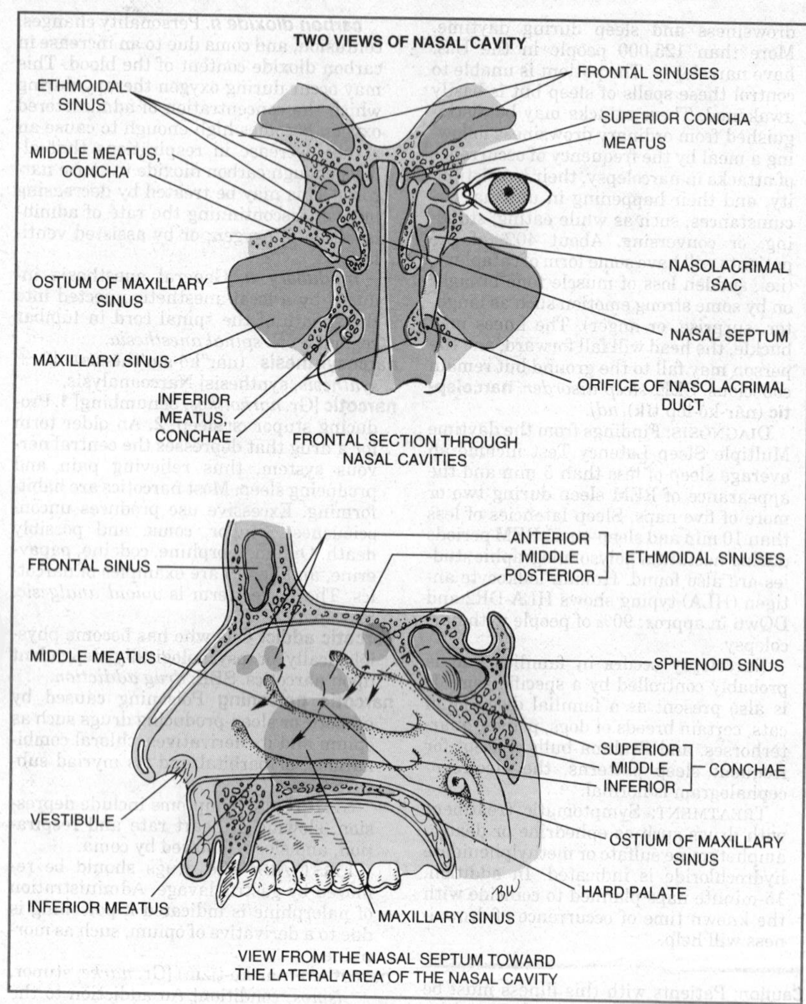


**nasal** (nā′zl) [L. *nasus,* nose] **1.** Pert. to the nose. **2.** Uttered through the nose. **3.** A nasal bone.

**nasal bleeding** Epistaxis.

**nasal bone** Either of the two small bones forming the arch of the nose.

**nasal cartilage** Any of the cartilages forming the principal portion of the subcutaneous framework of the external nose.

**nasal cavity** One of two cavities between the floor of the cranium and the roof of the mouth, opening to the nose anteriorly and the nasopharynx posteriorly. Its lining of ciliated epithelium warms and moistens inhaled air, and traps dust and pathogens on mucus that is then swept toward the pharynx. The nasal septum (ethmoid and vomer) separates the nasal cavities, and the olfactory receptors are in the upper part of each cavity. The paranasal sinuses (frontal, maxillary, sphenoidal, and ethmoidal) open into the meatus below the conchae. The orifices of the frontal, anterior ethmoidal, and maxillary sinuses are in the middle meatus. The orifices of the posterior ethmoidal and sphenoidal sinuses are in the superior meatus. The nasal mucosa is highly vascular; blood is supplied by the maxillary arteries from the external carotid arteries, and by the ethmoidal arteries from the internal carotid arteries. SEE: illus.; *nose.*

**nasal concha** SEE: under *concha.*

**nasal douche** SEE: under *douche.*

**nasal feeding** SEE: *feeding, tube.*

**nasal flaring** Intermittent outward movement of the nostrils with each inspiratory effort; indicates an increase in the work of breathing.

**nasal fossa** SEE: under *fossa.*

**nasal gavage** SEE: *feeding, tube.*
**nasal hemorrhage** Epistaxis.
**nasal height** Distance between the lower border of the nasal aperture and the nasion.
**nasal index** The greatest width of the nasal aperture in relation to a line from the lower edge of the nasal aperture to the nasion.
**nasal line** A line from lower edge of the ala nasi curving to outer side of the orbicularis oris muscle.
**nasal meatus** SEE: *meatus.*
**nasal obstruction** Blockage of the nasal passages. Common causes of nasal obstruction in adults are irregular septum, enlarged turbinates, and nasal polyps. In children, the commonest cause is a foreign body, such as food, buttons, or pins. Complications such as infections, sinusitis, and otitis may develop.

TREATMENT: Depending upon the cause of the obstruction, nasal douches, inhalations, or operative care, including resection of septum, turbinectomy, removal of polypi, opening and draining sinuses, or removal of foreign body.
**nasal polyp** A pedunculated polyp of the nasal mucosa. SEE: illus.
**nasal reflex** Sneezing resulting from irritation of nasal mucosa.
**nasal septum** SEE: *septum, nasal.*
**nasal sinuses, accessory** SEE: *sinuses, accessory nasal.*
**nasal width** The maximum width of the nasal aperture.
**nascent** (năs′ĕnt; nā′sĕnt) [L. *nascens,* born] **1.** Just born; incipient or beginning. **2.** Pert. to a substance being set free from a compound.
**nasioiniac** (nā″zē-ō-ĭn′ē-ăk) [L. *nasus,* nose, + Gr. *inion,* back of the head] Concerning the nasion and inion.
**nasion** (nā′zē-ōn) [L. *nasus,* nose] The point at which the nasofrontal suture is cut across by the median anteroposterior plane.
**Nasmyth's membrane** (năz′mĭths) [Alexander Nasmyth, Scottish dental surgeon, d. 1847] A thin cuticle consisting of the cellular remnants of the enamel organ and the mucopolysaccharide basement membrane that attaches them to the enamel surface. This covering is very friable and usually lost after eruption of the tooth into the oral cavity; however, it may persist in protected areas, such as the labial surface of maxillary incisors. SYN: *enamel membrane.*
**naso-** [L. *nasus,* nose] Combining form denoting *nose.*
**nasoantral** (nā″zō-ăn′trăl) [″ + Gr. *antrum,* cavity] Concerning the nose and maxillary antrum (sinus).
**nasoantritis** (nā″zō-ăn-trī′tĭs) [″ + ″ + *itis,* inflammation] Inflammation of the nose and antrum of Highmore.
**nasociliary** (nā″zō-sĭl′ē-ār-ē) Pert. to the nose, eyebrow, and eyes. Applied esp. to the nerve supplying these structures.
**nasofrontal** [″ + *frontalis,* forehead] Pert. to nasal and frontal bones.
**nasogastric** (nā″zō-găs′trĭk) [″ + Gr. *gaster,* belly] Pert. to the nasal passages and the

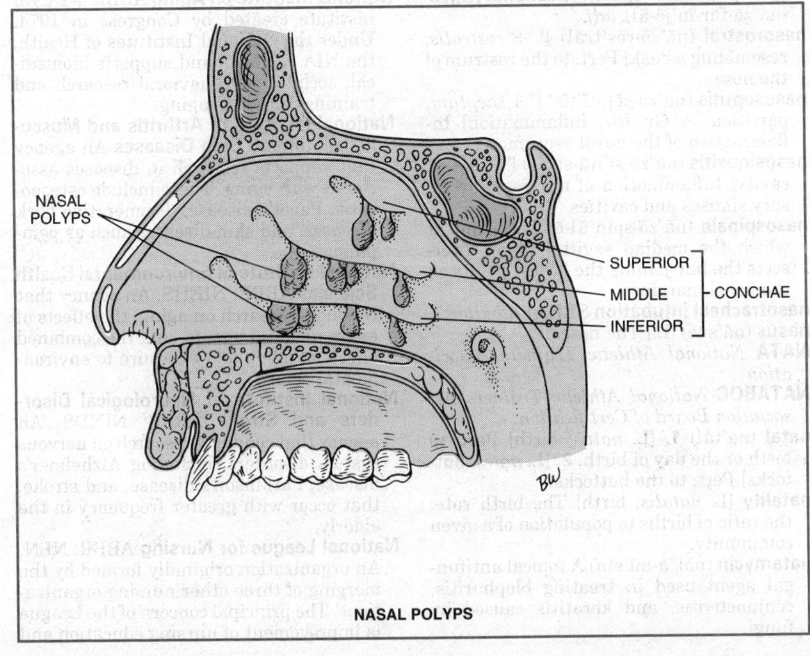

NASAL POLYPS

stomach, esp. relating to intubation.

**nasolabial** [" + *labium,* lip] Pert. to the nose and lip.

**nasolacrimal** (nā"zō-lăk'rĭm-ăl) [" + *lacrima,* tear] Pert. to the nose and lacrimal apparatus.

**nasology** (nā-zŏl'ō-jē) [" + Gr. *logos,* word, reason] Study of the nose and its diseases.

**nasomental** (nā"zō-mĕn'tăl) [" + *mentum,* chin] Pert. to the nose and chin.

**nasomental reflex** Contraction of mentalis muscle with elevation of lower lip and wrinkling of skin of chin. The reflex is elicited by percussion of the side of the nose.

**naso-oral** (nā"zō-ō'răl) [" + *oralis,* pert. to the mouth] Pert. to the nose and oral cavity.

**nasopalatine** (nā"zō-păl'ă-tĭn) [L. *nasus,* nose, + *palatum,* palate] Pert. to the nose and palate.

**nasopharyngeal airway, maintenance of** By means of a flexible tube that is inserted into the nose of an unresponsive patient and rests above the hypopharynx, the airway is maintained. Used in patients with intact gag reflexes to prevent retching during attempt to maintain an air passage.

**nasopharyngitis** (nā"zō-făr-ĭn-jī'tĭs) [" + Gr. *pharynx,* throat + *itis,* inflammation] Inflammation of the nasopharynx.

**nasopharyngography** Radiographic examination of the nasopharynx.

**nasopharyngoscope** Device used to visualize the nasal passage and pharynx.

**nasopharynx** (nā"zō-făr'ĭnks) [L. *nasus,* nose, + Gr. *pharynx,* throat] The part of the pharynx situated above the soft palate (postnasal space). **nasopharyngeal** (nā"zō-făr-ĭn'jē-ăl), *adj.*

**nasorostral** (nā"zō-rŏs'trăl) [" + *rostralis,* resembling a beak] Pert. to the rostrum of the nose.

**nasoseptitis** (nā"zō-sĕp-tī'tĭs) [" + *saeptum,* partition, + Gr. *itis,* inflammation] Inflammation of the nasal septum.

**nasosinusitis** (nā"zō-sī"nū-sī'tĭs) [" + *sinus,* cavity] Inflammation of the nasal accessory sinuses and cavities.

**nasospinale** (nā"zō-spīn'ăl-ē) The point at which the median sagittal plane intersects the line joining the lowest points on the nasal margins.

**nasotracheal intubation** SEE: *intubation.*

**nasus** (nā'sŭs) [L.] The nose.

**NATA** *National Athletic Trainers Association.*

**NATABOC** *National Athletic Trainers Association Board of Certification.*

**natal** (nā'tăl) **1.** [L. *natus,* birth] Pert. to birth or the day of birth. **2.** [L. *nates,* buttocks] Pert. to the buttocks.

**natality** [L. *natalis,* birth] The birth rate; the ratio of births to population of a given community.

**natamycin** (năt"ă-mī'sĭn) A topical antifungal agent used in treating blepharitis, conjunctivitis, and keratitis caused by fungi.

**nates** (nā'tēz) *sing.,* **natis** [L.] **1.** The buttocks. **2.** The anterior, superior, or upper two corpora quadrigemina.

**natimortality** (nā"tĭ-mor-tăl'ĭ-tē) [L. *natus,* birth, + *mortalitas,* death] Rate of stillbirths in proportion to birth rate.

**National Board for Respiratory Care** ABBR: NBRC. The national accrediting agency for pulmonary function technologists and respiratory care practitioners.

**National Council Licensure Examination–Practical Nurse** ABBR: NCLEX–PN. Computer-administered standardized tests taken by new applicants for state licensure as practical nurses that attempt to determine the candidate's minimum competence for safe practice. The examinations are available in all states and are administered by the National Council of State Boards of Nursing.

**National Council Licensure Examination–Registered Nurse** ABBR: NCLEX–RN. Computer-administered standardized tests taken by new applicants for state licensure as registered nurses that attempt to determine the candidate's minimum competence for safe practice. The examinations are available in all states and are administered by the National Council of State Boards of Nursing.

**National Formulary** ABBR: NF. Collection of officially recognized drug names originally issued by the American Pharmaceutical Association, but now published by the U.S. Pharmacopeial Convention. Included in the NF are drugs of established usefulness that are not listed in the U.S. Pharmacopeia.

**National Institute on Aging** ABBR: NIA. An institute created by Congress in 1974. Under the National Institutes of Health, the NIA conducts and supports biomedical, social, and behavioral research and training related to aging.

**National Institute of Arthritis and Musculoskeletal and Skin Diseases** An agency that supports research in diseases associated with aging. These include osteoporosis, Paget's disease, degenerative back diseases, and skin diseases such as pemphigus.

**National Institute of Environmental Health Sciences** ABBR: NIEHS. An agency that conducts research on aging, the effects of environmental agents, and the combined effects of aging and exposure to environmental agents.

**National Institute of Neurological Disorders and Stroke** ABBR: NINDS. An agency that conducts research on nervous system disorders, including Alzheimer's disease, Parkinson's disease, and stroke, that occur with greater frequency in the elderly.

**National League for Nursing** ABBR: NLN. An organization originally formed by the merging of three other nursing organizations. The principal concern of the League is improvement of nursing education and service.

**National Practitioner Data Bank** ABBR: NPDB. The computerized information system containing the mandatory reporting of all payments by or on behalf of physicians as a result of medical malpractice settlements or judgments in the U.S. The NPDB collects information regarding the professional conduct and competence of physicians (MD and DO), dentists, and in some cases other licensed health care professionals. The data are collected from a medical malpractice payment report (MMPR) that the physician or insurance company must submit within 30 days from the date payment is made. If a physician pays a patient in response to the patient's oral demand for money, the MMPR is not prepared.

**Nationally Registered Emergency Medical Technician** ABBR: N.R.E.M.T. The designation awarded after successful completion of written and practical examination administered by the National Registry of Emergency Medical Technicians.

**National Marrow Donor Program** ABBR: NMDP. The coordinating center for bone marrow donors. Phone 1-800-654-1247.

**National Organization for Rare Disorders** ABBR: NORD. An organization created by a group of voluntary agencies, medical researchers, and individuals concerned about orphan diseases and orphan drugs. Orphan diseases are rare, debilitating illnesses that strike small numbers of people. Orphan drugs are therapies that alleviate symptoms of some rare diseases, but have not been developed by the pharmaceutical industry because they are unprofitable.

NORD's address is P.O. Box 8423, New Fairfield, CT 06812, phone (203) 746-6518.

**native** (nā'tĭv) [L. *nativus*] **1.** Born with; inherent. **2.** Natural, normal. **3.** Belonging to, as place of one's birth. SYN: *indigenous.*

**natremia** (nă-trē'mē-ă) [L. *natrium,* sodium, + Gr. *haima,* blood] Sodium in the blood.

**natrium** (nā'trē-ŭm) [L.] SYMB: Na. Sodium.

**natriuresis** (nā"trē-ū-rē'sĭs) [" + Gr. *ouresis,* make water] The excretion of abnormal amounts of sodium in the urine. SEE: *aldosterone.*

**natriuretic** (nā"trē-ūr-ĕt'ĭk) A drug that increases rate of excretion of sodium in the urine. SEE: *diuretic.*

**natural** [L. *natura,* nature] Not abnormal or artificial.

**natural childbirth** SEE: under *childbirth.*

**natural killer cells** SEE: under *cell.*

**natural selection** SEE: *selection, natural.*

**nature and nurture** The combination of an individual's genetic constitution and the environmental conditions to which he or she is exposed. The interplay of these effects produces physical and mental characteristics that make each human being different from another. In many cases, it is not readily apparent which of these effects is the more important in producing a particular characteristic.

**naturopath** (nā'tūr-ō-păth) [" + Gr. *pathos,* disease, suffering] One who practices naturopathy.

**naturopathy** (nā"tūr-ŏp'ă-thē) A drugless therapeutic system that employs natural forces such as light, heat, air, water, and massage.

**nausea** (naw'sē-ă) [Gr. *nausia,* seasickness] An unpleasant sensation usually preceding vomiting. Nausea may be precipitated by motion sickness, early pregnancy, diseases of the central nervous system, certain gallbladder disturbances. It may be due to the sight or odor of obnoxious matter or conditions or to mental images of same. SEE: *vomitus.*

NURSING IMPLICATIONS: Remove any materials or environmental factors that precipitate the nausea. Note frequency, time, amount, and characteristics of emesis. Test vomitus for blood when indicated. Record and report any pertinent factors to physician. Provide oral hygiene and comfort measures to patient.

***n. gravidarum*** Morning sickness. SEE: *hyperemesis gravidarum.*

**nauseant** (naw'shē-ănt, naw'sē-ănt) **1.** Provoking nausea. **2.** An agent that causes nausea.

**nauseate** (naw'shē-āt, naw'sē-āt) To cause nausea.

**nauseous** (naw'shŭs, naw'shē-ŭs) **1.** Producing nausea, disgust, or loathing. **2.** Affected with nausea.

**navel** (nā'vĕl) [AS. *nafela*] Umbilicus.

**navicula** (nă-vĭk'ū-lă) [L. *navicula,* boat] Navicular fossa.

**navicular** (nă-vĭk'ū-lăr) **1.** Shaped like a boat. **2.** Scaphoid bones in the carpus (wrist) and in the tarsus (ankle). SEE: *skeleton.*

**navicular fossa** SEE: under *fossa.*

**Nb** Symbol for the element niobium.

**nCi** *nanocurie.*

**N.C.I.** *National Cancer Institute.*

**NCLEX–PN** *National Council Licensure Examination–Practical Nurse.*

**NCLEX–RN** *National Council Licensure Examination–Registered Nurse.*

**Nd** Symbol for the element neodymium.

**N.D.A.** *National Dental Association.*

**NDDK** *National Institute of Diabetes and Digestive and Kidney Diseases.*

**Ne** Symbol for the element neon.

**near-death experience** ABBR: NDE. The belief held by certain individuals that they have glimpsed an afterlife while actually coming close to death. These perceptions may reveal more about psychological events than death. SEE: *out-of-body experience.*

**near-drowning** The survival of someone in an immersion incident that could have been fatal. SEE: *drowning.*

**near point** ABBR: n.p. Closest point of distinct vision with maximum accommodation. This point becomes more distant with age, varying from about 3 in. (7.62 cm) at age 2 to 40 in. (101.60 cm) at age 60. SYN: *punctum proximum*.

**nearsighted** Able to see clearly only those objects held close to the eye. SYN: *myopic*. SEE: *myopia*.

**nearsightedness** Myopia.

**nearthrosis** (nē″ăr-thrō′sĭs) [Gr. *neos,* new, + *arthron,* joint, + *osis,* condition] A false joint or abnormal articulation, as one developing after a fracture that has not united. SYN: *neoarthrosis; pseudarthrosis*.

**nebula** (nĕb′ū-lă) *pl.* **nebulae** [L., mist, cloud] **1.** Slight haziness on the cornea. **2.** Cloudiness in urine. **3.** Aqueous or oily substance for use in an atomizer.

**nebulization** Production of particles such as a spray or mist from liquid. The size of particles produced depends upon the method used. SEE: *nebulizer*.

**nebulizer** (nĕb′ū-lī″zĕr) [L. *nebula,* mist] An apparatus for producing a fine spray or mist. This may be done by rapidly passing air through a liquid or by vibrating a liquid at a high frequency so that the particles produced are extremely small. SEE: *aerosol; atomizer; vaporizer*.

***ultrasonic n.*** An aerosol produced by the action of a vibrating ultrasonic transducer under water.

**NEC** *necrotizing enterocolitis*.

**Necator** (nē-kā′tor) [L., murderer] A genus of parasitic hookworms belonging to the family Ancylostomidae.

***N. americanus*** A species of hookworm commonly found in parts of the southern United States, and Central and South America, where the effects of tropical or semitropical climate and poor sanitation bring infected feces in contact with bare skin, usually the skin of the foot. SYN: *hookworm disease*. SEE: illus.

When the hookworm eggs hatch, the larvae enter through the host's skin, causing inflammation, itching, and sometimes allergic reactions. They pass from the skin to the venous circulation, where they migrate to the lungs and respiratory tree. If larvae are numerous, they may cause eosinophilic pneumonia. They travel up the bronchi and are finally swallowed, thus gaining entry to the intestinal tract. Larvae mature in the intestines, where they attach to the mucous membrane and suck blood from the host. They secrete an anticoagulant, which causes additional bleeding; the loss of blood leads to anemia. Nausea, colicky pains, and diarrhea may also result. In children, normal mental and physical growth is retarded. If untreated, larvae may live in the intestinal tract for as long as 5 years. However, most individuals lose the infection within 2 years.

TREATMENT: In severe cases it may be necessary to treat the severe anemia prior to ridding the patient of the parasites. Mebendazole, albendazole, levamisole, and pyrantel pamoate are the drugs of choice for *Necator* infection. The latter has the advantage of single-dose administration. A nutritional supplement with iron will be needed when anemia is severe. In some severe cases in children, blood transfusion may be needed.

**necatoriasis** (nē-kā″tō-rī′ă-sĭs) Infestation by *Necator americanus*. SEE: *ancylostomiasis*.

**neck** [AS. *hnecca,* nape] **1.** The part of the body between the head and shoulders. SEE: illus.; *muscle* for illus. **2.** The constricted portion of an organ, or that resembling a neck. **3.** The region between

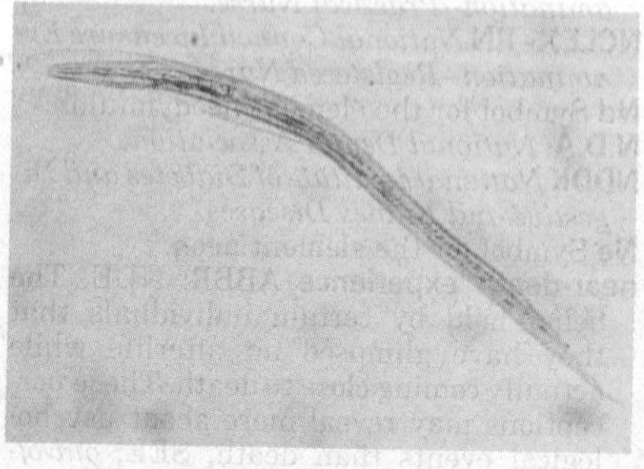

NECATOR
INFECTIVE FILARIFORM LARVA
(ORIG. MAG. ×100)

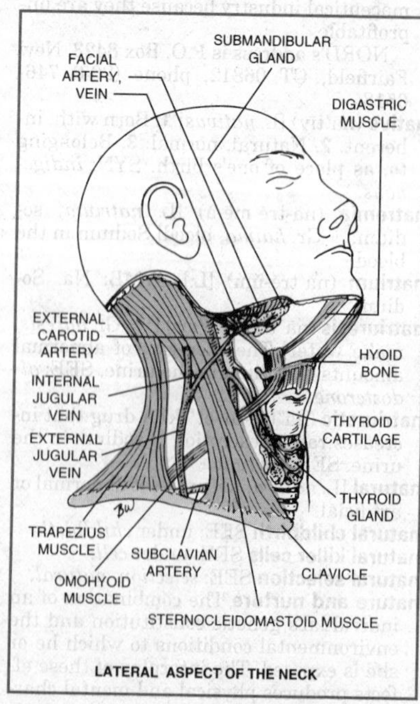


LATERAL ASPECT OF THE NECK

the crown and the root of a tooth.

***anatomical n. of the humerus*** The constriction just below the head of the humerus.

***n. of the femur*** The heavy column of bone that connects the head of the femur to the shaft.

***Madelung's n.*** Madelung's disease.

***n. of the mandible*** The constricted area below the articular condyle; the area of attachment for the articular capsule and the lateral pterygoid muscle.

***surgical n. of the humerus*** The narrow part of the humerus below the tuberosity. Fracture is common at this location.

***n. of the tooth*** The constricted area that connects the crown of a tooth to the root of a tooth.

***n. of the uterus*** Cervix uteri.

***webbed n.*** A broad neck as seen anteriorly or posteriorly. The breadth is due to a fold of skin that extends from the clavicle to the head. Webbed neck is present in Turner's syndrome.

***wry n.*** Torticollis.

**neck conformer** A splint, usually fabricated of thermoplastic material, that positions the neck to prevent flexion contractures due to burns of the anterior neck.

**neck-righting reflex** SEE: under *reflex*.

**necr-** SEE: *necro-*.

**necrectomy, necronectomy** (nĕ-krĕk′tō-mē, nĕk-rō-nĕk′tō-mē) [Gr. *nekros*, corpse, + *ektome*, excision] Surgical removal of necrotic tissue.

**necro-, necr-** [Gr. *nekros*, corpse] Combining form meaning *death, necrosis*.

**necrobiosis** (nĕk-rō-bī-ō′sĭs) [″ + *biosis*, life] Gradual degeneration and swelling of collagen bundles in the dermis. SEE: *necrosis*. **necrobiotic** (nĕ″krō-bī-ŏt′ĭk), *adj*.

***n. lipoidica diabeticorum*** A skin disease marked by necrobiosis of connective and elastic tissue. The lesions have a central yellowish area surrounded by a brownish border and are usually present on the anterior surface of the legs. The disease is commonly found in diabetics.

**necrocytotoxin** (nĕk″rō-sī″tō-tŏks′ĭn) A toxin that causes the death of cells.

**necrogenic, necrogenous** (nĕ-krō-jĕn′ĭk, -krŏj′ĕn-ŭs) [″ + *gennan*, to produce] Caused by, pert. to, or originating in dead matter.

**necrology** (nĕk-rŏl′ō-jē) The study of mortality statistics.

**necrolysis** (nĕ-krŏl′ĭ-sĭs) [″ + *lysis*, dissolution] Necrosis and dissolution of tissue.

**necromania** (nĕk-rō-mā′nē-ă) [″ + *mania*, madness] Abnormal interest in dead bodies or in death.

**necroparasite** (nĕk″rō-păr′ă-sīt) [″ + *para*, beside, + *sitos*, food] Saprophyte.

**necrophagous** (nĕ-krŏf′ă-gŭs) [″ + *phagein*, to eat] Feeding on dead flesh.

**necrophile** (nĕk′rō-fĭl) [″ + *philein*, to love] One who is affected with necrophilia.

**necrophilia** (nĕk″rō-fĭl′ē-ă) [″ + *philein*, to love] **1.** Abnormal interest in corpses. **2.** Sexual intercourse with a dead body.

**necrophilic** (nĕk″rō-fĭl′ĭk) [″ + *philein*, to love] **1.** Concerning necrophilia. **2.** Descriptive of bacteria that prefer dead tissue.

**necrophobia** (nĕk-rō-fō′bē-ă) [″ + *phobos*, fear] **1.** Abnormal aversion to dead bodies. **2.** Insane dread of death. SYN: *thanatophobia*.

**necropneumonia** (nĕk″rō-nū-mō′nē-ă) [″ + *pneumon*, lung] Pulmonary gangrene.

**necropsy** (nĕk′rŏp-sē) [″ + *opsis*, view] Autopsy.

**necrosadism** (nĕk″rō-sā′dĭzm) [″ + *sadism*] Sexual gratification derived from the mutilation of dead bodies.

**necroscopy** (nĕ-krŏs′kō-pē) [″ + *skopein*, to examine] Autopsy.

**necrose** (nĕk-rōs′) [Gr. *nekroun*, to make dead] To cause or to undergo necrosis.

**necrosis** (nĕ-krō′sĭs) *pl.* **necroses** [Gr. *nekrosis*, state of death] The death of areas of tissue or bone surrounded by healthy parts. SEE: *gangrene; mortification*. **necrotizing** (nĕk′rō-tīz″ĭng), *adj*.

The causes of necrosis include insufficient blood supply, physical agents such as trauma or radiant energy (electricity, infrared, ultraviolet, roentgen, and radium rays), chemical agents acting locally, acting internally following absorption, or placed into the wrong tissue (e.g., some medicines cause necrosis if injected into the tissues rather than the vein, and iron dextran causes necrosis if injected into areas other than deep muscle or vein).

***anemic n.*** Necrosis caused by disturbed blood circulation in a body part.

***aseptic n.*** Necrosis occurring without infection.

***Balser's fatty n.*** SEE: *Balser's fatty necrosis*.

***caseous n.*** Necrosis with soft, dry, cheeselike formation, usually seen in tuberculosis or syphilis. SYN: *cheesy n.*

***central n.*** Necrosis that affects only the center of a body part.

***cheesy n.*** Caseous n.

***coagulation n.*** Necrosis occurring esp. in infarcts. Coagulation occurs in the necrotic area, converting it into a homogenous mass and depriving the organ or tissue of blood. SYN: *fibrinous n.; ischemic n.*

***colliquative n.*** Necrosis caused by liquefaction of tissue due to autolysis or bacterial putrefaction. SYN: *liquefactive n.*

***dry n.*** Dry gangrene.

***embolic n.*** Necrosis resulting from an embolic occlusion of an artery.

***fat n.*** Necrosis in small scattered areas of the fatty tissue.

***fibrinous n.*** Coagulation n.

***focal n.*** Necrosis in small scattered areas, often seen in infection.

***gummatous n.*** Necrosis forming a dry rubbery mass, resulting from syphilis.

***ischemic n.*** Coagulation n.

***liquefactive n.*** Colliquative n.

***medial n.*** Necrosis of cells in the tunica media of an artery.

***moist n.*** Necrosis with softening and wetness of the dead tissue.

***postpartum pituitary n.*** Necrosis of the pituitary gland following childbirth. SEE: *Sheehan's syndrome.*

***putrefactive n.*** Necrosis caused by bacterial decomposition.

***radiation n.*** Necrosis caused by radiation exposure.

***subcutaneous fat n. of newborn*** An inflammatory disorder of fat tissue that may occur in the newborn at the site of application of forceps during delivery, and occasionally in premature infants. The cause is unknown.

***superficial n.*** Necrosis affecting only the outer layers of bone or any tissue.

***thrombotic n.*** Necrosis due to thrombus formation.

***total n.*** Necrosis affecting an entire organ or body part.

***Zenker's n.*** SEE: *Zenker's degeneration.*

**necrotic** [Gr. *nekrosis,* state of death] Relating to death of a portion of tissue.

**necrotomy** (nĕ-krŏt′ō-mē) [″ + *tome,* incision] **1.** Dissection of a cadaver. **2.** Excision of a sequestrum or other necrotic tissue.

**need** Something required or essential. Certain elements are essential for the physical and mental health of humans. Included in physical needs are oxygen, water, food, shelter, freedom from fear and physical harm. Most human beings seem to need some form of physical exercise over and above that required for ordinary daily living. Mental health needs include some form of human (loving) relationship and the feeling of self-worth. Not an absolute need, but highly desirable, is that each individual have some goal, no matter how trivial or grandiose, and the feeling that the goal is socially acceptable and is being attained.

**needle** [AS. *naedl*] A pointed instrument for stitching, ligaturing, or puncturing. It may be straight, half-curved, full-curved, semicircular, double-curved (sometimes called "S-" or sigmoid-shaped), or double-ended. Cutting edge and round point are the two classifications of needles. Cutting edge needles are used in skin and dense tissue, while round point needles are used for more delicate operations, esp. on soft tissues.

***aneurysm n.*** A blunt, curved needle with an eye in the tip used for passing a suture around a vessel.

***aspirating n.*** A long, hollow needle, usually fitted to a syringe, for withdrawing fluids from a cavity.

***atraumatic n.*** A needle of smaller diameter than the suture material. Use of this type of needle causes minimal damage to the tissue being sutured.

***cataract n.*** A needle used in removing a cataract.

***discission n.*** A special cataract needle for making multiple cuts into the lens capsule.

***Hagedorn n.*** A curved, flattened needle with a cutting edge near the end.

***hypodermic n.*** A hollow needle used for administration of hypodermic solutions.

***knife n.*** A narrow needle-pointed knife.

***ligature n.*** Aneurysm n.

***obturator n.*** A device that fits into the lumen of a needle to prevent blockage during the puncture procedure.

***Reverdin's n.*** A needle used to carry a suture. It has an eye at the tip that can be opened and closed by a lever.

***scalp vein n.*** A specially designed needle with a flat flange on each side to facilitate anchoring it after its placement in a small vein.

***stop n.*** A needle with an eye at its tip, with a flange or shelf extending out from its shank end that prevents the needle being inserted farther than the shelf.

**needle-stick injury** Accidental puncturing of the skin with an unsterilized needle. Health care workers are esp. at risk for injury while handling needles. Prevention of needle-stick injury is essential because of the danger of exposure of those involved to infection from diseases transmitted by blood (e.g., AIDS, hepatitis B). SEE: *sharps; Universal Precautions Appendix.*

**NEFA** *nonesterified fatty acids.*

**negation** (nē-gā′shŭn) [L. *negare,* to deny] Denial.

**negative** (nĕg′ă-tĭv) [L. *negare,* to deny] **1.** Possessing a numerical value that is less than zero. **2.** Lacking results or indicating an absence, as in a test result. **3.** Marked by resistance or retreat.

**negative sign** Minus sign (−) used in subtraction and to indicate a lack.

**negative study** Investigation in which only negative results are obtained. Such studies may be important in disproving myths or contrary evidence about a drug or therapy.

**negativism** A behavior peculiarity marked by not performing suggested actions (passive negativism) or in doing the opposite (active negativism), as seen in some forms of mental illness. A patient may refuse to respond to suggestions because of sluggish mental reflexes or from fear. Retardation may be slow, or sudden and intense, as in manic-depressive insanity.

**neglect, altitudinal** Unilateral visual inattention.

**neglect, hemispatial** Unilateral visual inattention.

**negligence** In forensic medicine, the failure to act as a reasonably prudent person with the same knowledge, experience, and background would do under similar circumstances; this failure to act causes injury or damage to a person. There are four elements of negligence: duty owed, breach of duty or standard of care, proximate cause or causal connection (between the breach and damages), and damages or injuries. Nurses are legally liable for their own negligence, as well as the negligence of others of which they have knowledge but do not report.

**Negri bodies** (nā'grē) [Adelchi Negri, It. physician, 1876–1912] Inclusion bodies found in the cells of the central nervous system of animals infected with rabies. They are acidophilic masses appearing in large ganglion cells or in cells of the brain, esp. those of the hippocampus and cerebellum. Their presence is considered conclusive proof of rabies.

**NEI** *National Eye Institute.*

**Neisseria** (nī-sē'rē-ă) [Albert Neisser, Ger. physician, 1855–1916] A genus of bacteria belonging to the family Neisseriaceae. They are gram-negative cocci and usually occur in pairs with flattened sides but may occur singly or in irregular groups. The two species most often associated with disease in humans are meningococcus (*Neisseria meningitidis*) and gonococcus (*Neisseria gonorrhoeae.*)

***N. catarrhalis*** A nonpathogenic species found in the upper respiratory tract. It may be mistaken for meningococci.

***N. gonorrhoeae*** The species causing gonorrhea. SYN: *gonococcus.* SEE: illus.; *gonorrhea.*

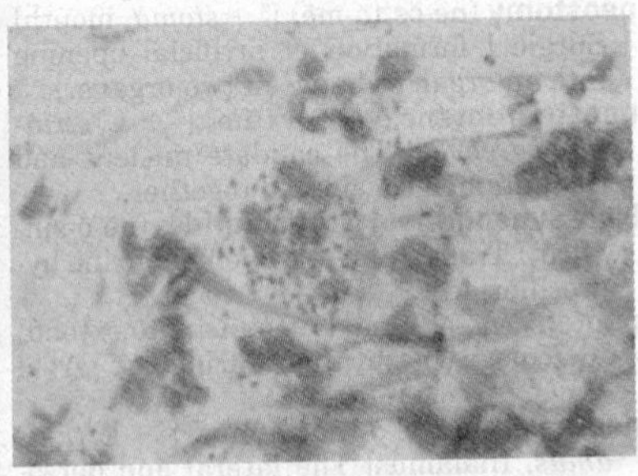

NEISSERIA GONORRHOEAE WITHIN A NEUTROPHIL (CENTER) (ORIG. MAG. ×500)

***N. meningitidis*** The species causing epidemic cerebrospinal meningitis. SEE: *meningitis.*

***N. sicca*** Species found in mucous membrane of respiratory tract. Occasionally, this species may cause bacterial endocarditis.

**Neisseriaceae** (nīs-sē"rē-ā'sē-ē) A family of bacteria that are spherical, gram-negative, and nonmotile.

**Nélaton's line** (nā-lă-tŏnz') [Auguste Nélaton, Fr. surgeon, 1807–1873] Line from the anterior superior spine of the ilium to tuberosity of the ischium.

**nemathelminth** (nĕm"ă-thĕl'mĭnth) [Gr. *nema,* thread, + *helmins,* worm] A roundworm belonging to the phylum Nemathelminthes.

**Nemathelminthes** (nĕm"ă-thĕl-mĭn'thēz) The phylum of the roundworm.

**nematocide** (nĕm'ă-tō-sīd") [Gr. *nema,* thread, + L. *caedere,* to kill] An agent that kills nematodes.

**nematocyst** (nĕm'ă-tō-sĭst) [" + *kystis,* bladder] The small stinging barb present in jellyfish and some other coelenterates. It can penetrate the skin upon contact and inflict painful lesions. In some cases, multiple contact can be fatal.

**Nematoda** (nĕm"ă-tō'dă) [" + *eidos,* form, shape] A class of the phylum Nemathelminthes that includes the true roundworms or threadworms, many species of which are parasitic. They are cylindrical or spindle-shaped worms that possess a resistant cuticle, have a complete alimentary canal, and lack a true coelom. The sexes usually separate, and development usually is direct and simple.

**nematode** (nĕm'ă-tōd) [Gr. *nema,* thread, + *eidos,* form, shape] A member of the class Nematoda.

**nematodiasis** (nĕm"ă-tō-dī'ă-sĭs) [" + " + *-iasis,* condition] Infestation by a parasite belonging to the class Nematoda.

**nematoid** (nĕm'ă-toyd) Threadlike, like a nematode.

**nematology** (nĕm"ă-tŏl'ō-jē) The division of parasitology that deals with worms belonging to the class Nematoda.

**Nembutal** (nĕm'bū-tăl) Trade name for pentobarbital sodium. It is a short-acting drug used as a preanesthetic, sedative, and hypnotic.

**neo-** [Gr. *neos*] Combining form meaning *new, recent.*

**neoadjuvant therapy** In treating cancer, the use of chemotherapy before therapy such as radiation or surgery.

**neoantigen** (nē"ō-ăn'tĭ-jĕn) [" + *anti,* against, + *gennan,* to produce] A nonspecific term for various tumor antigens.

**neoarthrosis** (nē"ō-ăr-thrō'sĭs) [" + *arthron,* joint, + *osis,* condition] Nearthrosis.

**neoblastic** [" + *blastos,* germ] Pert. to or constituting a new growth of tissue.

**neocerebellum** (nē"ō-sĕr-ĕ-bĕl'ŭm) [Gr. *neos,* new, + L. *cerebellum,* little brain] The portion of the corpus cerebelli of the cerebellum that lies between the primary and prepyramidal fissures and consists principally of the ansiform lobules. Phylogenetically, it develops last, in conjunction with cerebral cortex, and is concerned with the integration of voluntary movements. It is the posterior lobe of the cerebellum.

**neocortex** (nē"ō-kor'tĕks) Isocortex.

**neodymium** (nē"ō-dĭm'ē-ŭm) SYMB: Nd. A shiny, silvery, rare-earth chemical element, atomic weight 144.24, atomic number 60.

**neofetus** (nē-ō-fē'tŭs) [" + L. *foetus,* offspring] The embryo during eighth or ninth week of intrauterine life.

**neoformation** (nē"ō-for-mā'shŭn) [" + L. *formatio,* a shaping] **1.** Regeneration. **2.** A neoplasm or new growth.

**neogenesis** (nē-ō-jĕn′ĕ-sĭs) [″ + *genesis,* generation, birth] Regeneration; reformation, as of tissue. **neogenetic** (nē″ō-jĕn-ĕt′ĭk), *adj.*

**neokinetic** (nē″ō-kĭ-nĕt′ĭk) [″ + *kinetikos,* pert. to movement] Concerning the portion of the nervous system that regulates voluntary muscular control.

**neolalism** (nē″ō-lăl′ĭzm) [″ + *laleo,* to chatter] The use of neologisms in speech, esp. that associated with schizophrenia.

**neologism** (nē-ŏl′ō-jĭzm) [″ + *logos,* word, reason, + *-ismos,* state] A mental condition in which the patient coins new words that are meaningless or words to which he or she gives special significance without being aware of their normal significance.

**neomembrane** (nē-ō-mĕm′brān) [″ + L. *membrana,* membrane] Pseudomembrane.

**neomorph** (nē′ō-morf) [″ + *morphe,* form] A new formation or development that is not inherited from a similar structure in an ancestor.

**neomycin sulfate** (nē″ō-mī′sĭn) [″ + *mykes,* fungus] An antibiotic from a species of *Streptomyces,* isolated from soil. Active against gram-positive and gram-negative bacteria, as well as streptomycin-resistant strains of *Mycobacterium tuberculosis.* It is toxic to kidneys and to the eighth nerve and may cause hearing difficulties.

**neon** (nē′ŏn) [Gr. *neos,* new] SYMB: Ne. A rare, inert, gaseous element in the air. Only 18 parts per million parts of air are neon. Neon's atomic weight is 20.183, and its atomic number is 10.

***n. gas*** A colorless gas that makes a reddish-orange glow when an electric charge strikes it.

**neonatal** (nē″ō-nā′tăl) [″ + L. *natus,* born] Concerning the first 28 days after birth.

**neonatal mortality rate** SEE: under *rate.*

**neonate** (nē′ō-nāt) A newborn infant up to 1 month of age. SEE: *Nursing Diagnoses Appendix.*

**neonate, killing of a** SEE: *infanticide.*

**neonatologist** (nē″ō-nā-tŏl′ō-jĭst) [″ + ″ + Gr. *logos,* word, reason] A physician who specializes in the study, care, and treatment of neonates.

**neonatology** (nē″ō-nā-tŏl′ō-jē) The study, care, and treatment of neonates.

**neopallium** (nē″ō-păl′ē-ŭm) [Gr. *neos,* new, + L. *pallium,* cloak] Isocortex.

**neophilism** (nē-ŏf′ĭl-ĭzm) [″ + *philein,* to love, + *-ismos,* condition] Abnormal love of novelty and new persons and scenes.

**neophobia** (nē″ō-fō′bē-ă) [″ + *phobos,* fear] Fear of new scenes or novelties; aversion to all that is unknown or not understood. SYN: *kainophobia.*

**neoplasia** (nē″ō-plā′zē-ă) [″ + *plassein,* to form] The development of neoplasms.

**neoplasia, cervical intraepithelial** SEE: *cervical intraepithelial neoplasia.*

**neoplasm** (nē′ō-plăzm) [″ + LL. *plasma,* form, mold] A new and abnormal formation of tissue, as a tumor or growth. It serves no useful function, but grows at the expense of the healthy organism. **neoplastic** (nē″ō-plăs′tĭk), *adj.*

***benign n.*** Growth not spreading by metastases or infiltration of tissue.

***histoid n.*** Neoplasm in which structure resembles the tissues and elements that surround it.

***malignant n.*** Growth that infiltrates tissue, metastasizes, and often recurs after attempts at surgical removal. SYN: *cancer.*

***mixed n.*** Neoplasm composed of tissues from two of the germinal layers.

***noninvasive n.*** A tumor that has not spread or does not spread.

***organoid n.*** Neoplasm in which the structure is similar to some organ of the body.

**neoplasty** (nē′ō-plăs-tē) [″ + *plassein,* to form] Surgical formation or restoration of parts.

**neostigmine** (nē-ō-stĭg′mĭn) A cholinergic drug used clinically in the form of a bromide or methylsulfate.

***n. bromide*** A preparation of neostigmine used for oral administration in the treatment of myasthenia gravis. Ophthalmic solution used for glaucoma.

***n. methylsulfate*** A preparation of neostigmine used for parenteral administration in treatment of myasthenia gravis.

**neostomy** (nē-ŏs′tō-mē) [″ + *stoma,* mouth] Surgical formation of artificial opening into an organ or between two organs.

**neostriatum** (nē″ō-strī-ā′tŭm) [″ + L. *striatum,* grooved] The caudate nucleus and the putamen considered together.

**Neo-Synephrine Hydrochloride** (nē″ō-sĭn-ĕf′rĭn) Trade name for phenylephrine hydrochloride.

**neoteny** (nē-ŏt′ĕ-nē) [″ + *teinein,* to extend] In zoology, maturation during the larval stage.

**neothalamus** (nē″ō-thăl′ă-mŭs) [″ + L. *thalamus,* thalamus] The lateral and dorsomedial nuclei of the thalamus.

**nephelometer** (nĕf″ĕl-ŏm′ĕ-ter) [Gr. *nephele,* mist, + *metron,* measure] A device used in nephelometry to measure the number of particles in a solution. For example, it is used to measure the turbidity of a fluid and also may be used to estimate the degree of contamination of air by particulate matter.

**nephelometry** (nĕf″ĕl-ŏm′ĕ-trē) An analytical technique that measures the number of particles in a colloidal solution by quantitating the light scattered by the particles. SEE: *nephelometer.*

**nephelopia** (nĕf″ĕ-lō′pē-ă) [Gr. *nephele,* mist, + *ops,* eye] Dim or cloudy vision from lessened transparency of the ocular media.

**nephr-** [Gr. *nephros,* kidney] SEE: *nephro-.*

**nephradenoma** (nĕf″răd-ĕ-nō′mă) [Gr. *nephros,* kidney, + *aden,* gland, + *oma,* tumor] Renal adenoma.

**nephralgia** (nĕ-frăl′jē-ă) [″ + *algos,* pain] Renal pain. **nephralgic** (nĕ-frăl′jĭk), *adj.*

**nephrapostasis** (nĕf″ră-pŏs′tă-sĭs) [″ + *apostasis,* suppuration] Renal abscess or purulent inflammation of the kidney.

**nephrectasia, nephrectasis, nephrectasy** (nĕf-rĕk-tā′zē-ă, -rĕk′tă-sĭs, -tă-sē) [Gr. *nephros,* kidney, + *ektasis,* distention] Distention of the kidney.

**nephrectomize** (nĕ-frĕk′tō-mīz) [″ + *ektome,* excision] To remove surgically one or both kidneys.

**nephrectomy** (nĕ-frĕk′tō-mē) [″ + *ektome,* excision] Surgical removal of a kidney. Complications include spontaneous pneumothorax and secondary hemorrhage. SEE: *Nursing Diagnoses Appendix.*

NURSING IMPLICATIONS: Adequate preoperative and postoperative instruction is provided. The nurse physically prepares the patient according to protocol, including skin preparation, laboratory studies, and administration of preoperative medications. Activities are provided that are interesting but not tiring. Fluid and electrolyte imbalances are prevented, and daily weight obtained. The nurse encourages the patient to verbalize feelings and concerns and provides support and reassurance. Vital signs are checked every 2 to 4 hr. Analgesics and other medications are administered as prescribed. Any excessive bleeding is recorded and reported. The nurse turns the patient frequently, observing the operative site and dressing and changing the dressing as necessary. Frequent position changes also help to prevent complications of immobility. The nurse assists the patient with deep-breathing and coughing exercises. Range-of-motion exercises are instituted. Drainage tubes are checked frequently for patency. Intake and output are monitored and recorded. Frequent mouth care is provided while the patient takes nothing by mouth. A progressive diet is encouraged on return of normal bowel sounds. Discharge teaching focuses on diet; activities, particularly those that could injure the remaining kidney; incision care; and medications.

***abdominal n.*** Nephrectomy through an incision in the abdominal wall.

***paraperitoneal n.*** Removal of a kidney through an extraperitoneal incision.

**nephrelcosis** (nĕf-rĕl-kō′sĭs) [Gr. *nephros,* kidney, + *helkosis,* ulceration] Ulceration of the mucosa of the kidney.

**nephrelcus** (nĕf-rĕl′kŭs) Renal ulcer.

**nephremphraxis** (nĕf″rĕm-frăks′ĭs) [″ + *emphraxis,* obstruction] Obstruction in the renal vessels.

**nephric** (nĕf′rĭk) [Gr. *nephros,* kidney] Pert. to the kidney or kidneys. SYN: *renal.*

**nephridium** (nĕ-frĭd′ē-ŭm) [Gr. *nephridios,* pert. to the kidney] A segmented excretory tubule present in many invertebrates.

**nephritic** (nĕ-frĭt′ĭk) **1.** Relating to the kidney. **2.** Pert. to nephritis. **3.** An agent used in nephritis.

**nephritis** (nĕf-rī′tĭs) *pl.* **nephritides** [Gr. *nephros,* kidney, + *itis,* inflammation] Inflammation of the kidney due to bacteria or their toxins, streptococcal infections, diphtheria, septicemia, or toxic substances (e.g., mercury, arsenic, alcohol). The glomeruli, tubules, and interstitial tissue may be affected. The condition may be either acute or chronic.

NURSING IMPLICATIONS: Renal function is assessed, and signs of renal failure (oliguria, azotemia, acidosis) are reported. Hemoglobin, hematocrit, and electrolyte levels are monitored. Aseptic technique is used in handling catheters. The nurse observes, records, and reports hematuria and monitors blood pressure using the same cuff, arm, and position each time. The nurse also observes or questions the patient concerning headache, restlessness, lethargy, convulsions, tachycardia, and arrhythmias. Antihypertensive drugs are administered as prescribed. The patient is encouraged to maintain adequate hydration and follow the prescribed dietary restrictions. Intravenous fluid intake is monitored. Complications of hypertension are anticipated and prevented.

***acute n.*** An inflammatory form of nephritis involving the glomeruli, the tubules, or the entire kidney. It may be called degenerative, diffuse, suppurative, hemorrhagic, interstitial, or parenchymatous, depending upon the portion of the kidney involved.

***analgesic n.*** Chronic nephritis caused by excess intake of almost any of the anti-inflammatory analgesics (e.g., salicylates, acetaminophen, nonsteroidal anti-inflammatory agents).

***chronic n.*** A progressive form of nephritis in which the entire structure of kidney or only the glomerular or tubular processes may be affected. One variety of nephritis may merge with another, causing a diffuse nephritis. Symptoms depend upon the tissues involved.

***glomerular n.*** Glomerulonephritis.

***interstitial n.*** Nephritis associated with pathological changes in the renal interstitial tissue that in turn may be primary or due to a toxic agent such as a drug or chemical. The end result is the destruction of the nephrons and serious impairment of renal function.

***scarlatinal n.*** Acute glomerulonephritis complicating scarlet fever.

***suppurative n.*** Nephritis associated with abscesses in the kidney.

***transfusion n.*** Renal failure and tubular disease caused by transfusion of incompatible blood.

**nephritogenic** (nĕ-frĭt″ō-jĕn′ĭk) [″ + *gennan,* to produce] Causing nephritis.

**nephro-, nephr-** [Gr. *nephros,* kidney] Combining form meaning *kidney.*

**nephroabdominal** (nĕf″rō-ăb-dŏm′ĭ-năl) [″ + L. *abdominalis,* abdomen] Concerning the kidney and abdomen.

**nephroblastoma** (nĕf″rō-blăs-tō′mă) [″ + *blastos,* germ, + *oma,* tumor] Wilms' tumor.

**nephrocalcinosis** (nĕf-rō″kăl″sĭn-ō′sĭs) [″ + L. *calx,* lime, + Gr. *osis,* condition] Calcinosis of the kidney characterized by deposits of calcium phosphate in renal tubules.

**nephrocapsectomy** (nĕf″rō-kăp-sĕk′tō-mē) [″+ L. *capsula,* capsule, + Gr. *ektome,* excision] Excision of the renal capsule.

**nephrocardiac** (nĕf″rō-kăr′dē-ăk) [″ + *kardia,* heart] Concerning the kidney and the heart.

**nephrocele** (nĕf′rō-sēl) [″ + *kele,* tumor, swelling] Renal hernia.

**nephrocolic** (nĕf″rō-kŏl′ĭk) [Gr. *nephros,* kidney, + *kolikos,* colic] **1.** Renal colic. **2.** Concerning the kidney and the colon.

**nephrocolopexy** (nĕf″rō-kŏl′ō-pĕks″ē) [″ + *kolon,* colon, + *pexis,* fixation] Surgical suspension of the kidney and the colon using the nephrocolic ligament.

**nephrocoloptosis** (nĕf″rō-kō″lŏp-tō′sĭs) [″ + ″ + *ptosis,* a dropping] Condition in which the kidney and the colon are displaced downward.

**nephrocystanastomosis** (nĕf″rō-sĭst-ă-năs″tō-mō′sĭs) [″ + *kystis,* bladder, + *anastomosis,* outlet] Surgical formation of an artificial connection between the kidney and the bladder where there is permanent ureteral obstruction.

**nephrocystitis** (nĕf″rō-sĭs-tī′tĭs) [″ + ″ + *itis,* inflammation] Inflammation of the kidneys and the bladder.

**nephrocystosis** (nĕf″rō-sĭs-tō′sĭs) [″ + ″ + *osis,* condition] Formation of renal cysts.

**nephrogenetic** (nĕf″rō-jĕn-ĕt′ĭk) [″ + *gennan,* to produce] Arising in or from the renal organs; capable of giving rise to kidney tissue.

**nephrography** (nĕ-frŏg′ră-fē) [″ + *graphein,* to write] Radiography of the kidneys, usually after intravenous injection of a contrast medium.

**nephrohypertrophy** (nĕf″rō-hī-pĕr′trō-fē) [″ + *hyper,* over, + *trophe,* nourishment] Increased size of kidneys.

**nephroid** (nĕf′royd) [″ + *eidos,* form, shape] Resembling a kidney; kidney-shaped. SYN: *reniform.*

**nephrolithiasis** (nĕf″rō-lĭth-ī′ă-sĭs) The presence of calculi in the kidney. SEE: *calculus, renal.*

**nephrolithotomy** (nĕf″rō-lĭth-ŏt′ō-mē) [″ + *lithos,* stone, + *tome,* incision] Renal incision for removal of calculus.

**nephrology** (nĕ-frŏl′ō-jē) [″ + *logos,* word, reason] The branch of medical science concerned with the structure and function of the kidneys.

**nephrolysis** (nĕ-frŏl′ĭ-sĭs) [″ + *lysis,* dissolution] **1.** Surgical detachment of an inflamed kidney from paranephric adhesions. **2.** Destruction of kidney tissue by the action of a nephrotoxin.

**nephroma** (nĕ-frō′mă) [″ + *oma,* tumor] Renal tumor.

**nephromalacia** (nĕf″rō-mă-lā′sē-ă) [″ + *malakia,* softening] Abnormal renal softness or softening.

**nephromegaly** (nĕf″rō-mĕg′ă-lē) [″ + *megas,* great] Extreme enlargement of a kidney.

**nephromere** (nĕf′rō-mēr) [″ + *meros,* part] The intermediate mesoderm in an embryo from which the kidney develops. SYN: *nephrotome.*

**nephron** (nĕf′rŏn) [Gr. *nephros,* kidney] The structural and functional unit of the kidney, consisting of a renal (malpighian) corpuscle (a glomerulus enclosed within Bowman's capsule), the proximal convoluted tubule, the loop of Henle, and the distal convoluted tubule. These connect by arched collecting tubules with straight collecting tubules. Urine is formed by filtration in renal corpuscles; selective reabsorption and secretion is performed by the cells of the renal tubule. There are approx. one million nephrons in each kidney. SEE: *kidney* for illus.; *malpighian capsule; urine.*

**nephropathy** (nĕ-frŏp′ă-thē) [″ + *pathos,* disease, suffering] Disease of the kidney. This term includes inflammatory (nephritis), degenerative (nephrosis), and sclerotic (arteriosclerotic) lesions of the kidney.

***analgesic n.*** Nephritis.

***hypercalcemic n.*** Renal damage due to hypercalcemia. It is usually caused by hyperparathyroidism, sarcoidosis, excess vitamin D intake, excess ingestion of milk and alkali, multiple myeloma, malignant disease, and, occasionally, by immobilization or Paget's disease. Correction of the primary disease is indicated. If the underlying cause is allowed to persist, the damage to the renal tubules may be permanent.

***hypokalemic n.*** Renal damage due to abnormal depletion of potassium, regardless of the basic cause of the electrolyte abnormality. Characteristically, there are multiple vacuoles in microscopic sections of the renal tubular epithelium. Clinically, the patient is unable to concentrate urine. Therapy for the primary cause of the hypokalemia may allow the kidney lesions to become completely reversed.

***membranous n.*** A glomerular disease of unknown etiology that produces nephrotic syndrome. It may be distinguished from lipoid nephrosis by the use of immunofluorescence and electron microscopy. SEE: *glomerular disease; nephrotic syndrome.*

TREATMENT: Treatment consists of a high-protein diet and diuretics. Adrenocortical hormones may be of benefit in young patients.

***radiocontrast-induced n.*** Nephropathy caused by the use of radio contrast media.

In normal patients, use of such agents rarely causes nephropathy. However, in some individuals, esp. those with conditions that cause diminished renal blood flow, diabetic renal failure, jaundice, or multiple myeloma, acute renal failure may result.

**nephropexy** (nĕf′rō-pĕks-ē) [″ + *pexis,* fixation] Surgical fixation of a floating kidney.

**nephrophthisis** (nĕ-frŏf′thĭ-sĭs) [″ + *phthisis,* a wasting] **1.** Tuberculosis of the kidney with caseous degeneration. **2.** Suppurative nephritis with wasting of the kidney substance.

**nephroptosis** (nĕf″rŏp-tō′sĭs) [″ + *ptosis,* a dropping] Downward displacement of the kidney.

**nephropyelitis** (nĕf″rō-pī-ĕl-ī′tĭs) [″ + *pyelos,* pelvis, + *itis,* inflammation] Pyelonephritis.

**nephropyelography** (nĕf″rō-pī″ĕ-lŏg′ră-fē) [″ + *pyelos,* pelvis, + *graphein,* to write] Radiography of the kidney and renal pelvis after injection of a contrast medium.

**nephropyeloplasty** (nĕf″rō-pī′ĕ-lō-plăs″tē) [″ + ″ + *plassein,* to form] Plastic surgery on the kidney and renal pelvis.

**nephropyosis** (nĕf″rō-pī-ō′sĭs) [″ + *pyosis,* suppuration] Purulence of a kidney.

**nephrorrhagia** (nĕf-ror-ā′jē-ă) [″ + *rhegnynai,* to burst forth] Renal hemorrhage into the pelvis and tubules.

**nephrorrhaphy** (nĕf-ror′ă-fē) [″ + *rhaphe,* seam, ridge] Surgical procedure of suturing the kidney.

**nephros** (nĕf′rŏs) [Gr.] The kidney.

**nephrosclerosis** (nĕf″rō-sklĕ-rō′sĭs) [″ + *sklerosis,* a hardening] Renal sclerosis or hardening.

***arterial n.*** Arteriosclerosis of the renal arteries resulting in ischemia, atrophy of parenchyma, and fibrosis of the kidney.

***arteriolar n.*** Sclerosis of the smaller renal arterioles, esp. the afferent glomerular arterioles with resulting fibrosis, ischemic necrosis, and glomerular degeneration and failure. This type of nephrosclerosis occurs in most cases of essential hypertension.

***malignant n.*** Nephrosclerosis that develops rapidly in patients with severe hypertension. SEE: *hypertension.*

**nephrosis** (nĕf-rō′sĭs) *pl.* **nephroses** [Gr. *nephros,* kidney, + *osis,* condition] **1.** Condition in which there are degenerative changes in the kidneys, esp. the renal tubules, without the occurrence of inflammation. **2.** Clinical classification of kidney disease in which protein loss is so extensive that edema and hypoproteinemia are produced. SEE: *nephrotic syndrome.*

***lipoid n.*** Idiopathic nephrotic syndrome.

**nephrosonephritis** (nĕ-frō″sō-nĕ-frī′tĭs) [″ + *osis,* condition, + *nephros,* kidney, + *itis,* inflammation] Renal disease with characteristics of nephritis and nephrosis.

**nephrostoma** (nĕ-frŏs′tō-mă) [″ + *stoma,* mouth] The internal orifice of a wolffian tubule, connected with the coelom in the human embryo.

**nephrostomy** (nĕ-frŏs′tō-mē) The formation of an artificial fistula into the renal pelvis.

***percutaneous n.*** The placement of a catheter into the renal pelvis from the posterolateral aspect of the body below the 11th rib by using ultrasound or fluoroscopy. This technique is used to alleviate sepsis due to ureteral obstruction or in patients with disseminated cancer.

**nephrotic** (nĕ-frŏt′ĭk) [Gr. *nephros,* kidney] Relating to, or caused by, nephrosis.

**nephrotic syndrome** ABBR: NS. The end result of a variety of diseases that damage the capillaries of the glomerulus. Clinically, this leads to loss of a large amount of protein in the urine, which in turn results in hypoalbuminemia and edema. Hyperlipidemia also develops in many cases. Factors causing NS include any disorder that may affect the glomerulus, immunologic disorders, toxic injury to the kidneys, neoplasms, metabolic abnormalities, biochemical defects, multisystem diseases, infections, and diseases of the vascular system.

Idiopathic NS is diagnosed when the known causes of NS have been excluded. It is usually diagnosed in adults by use of renal biopsy. Causes are classified according to the changes found in the capillaries of the glomerulus when examined by use of electron microscopy. SEE: *Nursing Diagnoses Appendix.*

TREATMENT: Management of this condition and the complication of venous and arterial thromboembolism requires use of diuretics and medicines to reduce the lipid levels in the blood. Long-term use of anticoagulants may be needed for the complication of chronic renal vein thrombosis. If NS is secondary to a specific disease, infection, certain forms of cancer, specific drugs, or any of the other diseases known to be associated with NS, then those are treated appropriately. Adrenal cortical steroid hormones have a dramatic, immediate effect on the condition, but their use does not alter the survival rate.

Idiopathic NS is treated with the use of corticosteroids and therapy for associated conditions or complications. Depending on severity of NS and the cellular changes in the glomerulus, 5% to 50% of cases of idiopathic NS may be treated without the need for renal dialysis or transplantation.

NURSING IMPLICATIONS: Symptoms of proteinuria and fluid and electrolyte balance are monitored (intake and input, weight). Adequate nutritional intake is encouraged. The nurse assists the patient with skin care and prevents trauma, plans activities to provide periods of rest and to prevent fatigue and weakness, and protects the patient from infection. Support is offered to the patient experiencing grief and difficulties in coping with changes in body image and self-concept.

**nephrotome** (něf′rō-tōm) [″ + *tome,* incision] The embryonic bridge of cells connecting primitive segments along neural tube to the somatic and splanchnic mesoderm from which arises the urogenital system. SYN: *mesomere; nephromere.*

**nephrotomogram** (něf″rō-tō′mō-grăm) A tomogram of the kidney.

**nephrotomography** (něf″rō-tō-mŏg′ră-fē) [″ + ″ + *graphein,* to write] Tomograph of the kidney after the intravenous injection of a radiopaque contrast medium that is excreted by the kidney.

**nephrotomy** (nĕ-frŏt′ō-mē) [″ + *tome,* incision] Surgical incision of the kidney.

**nephrotoxin** (něf″rō-tŏk′sĭn) [″ + *toxikon,* poison] A toxic substance that damages kidney tissues.

**nephrotropic** (něf″rō-trŏp′ĭk) [″ + *tropos,* turning] **1.** Affecting the kidneys. **2.** An agent or drug that exerts its effect principally on the kidney or renal function.

**nephrotuberculosis** (něf″rō-tū-bĕr″kū-lō′sĭs) [″ + *tuberculum,* a little swelling, + *osis,* condition] Infection of the kidney due to *Mycobacterium tuberculosis.*

**nephroureterectomy** (něf″rō-ū-rē″tĕr-ĕk′tō-mē) [″ + *oureter,* ureter, + *ektome,* excision] Surgical excision of the kidney with all or part of the ureter.

**nephrydrosis** (něf″rĭ-drō′sĭs) [″ + *hydor,* water, + *osis,* condition] Hydronephrosis.

**neptunium** [planet Neptune] SYMB: Np. An element obtained by bombarding uranium with neutrons. Its atomic weight is 237 and its atomic number is 93.

**nerve** [L. *nervus,* sinew; Gr. *neuron,* sinew] A bundle of nerve fibers outside the central nervous system (CNS) that connect the brain and spinal cord with various parts of the body. Afferent nerves conduct sensory impulses from receptors to the CNS; efferent nerves conduct motor impulses from the CNS to effector organs and tissues. The fibers of peripheral nerves are the axons and dendrites of neurons whose cell bodies are located within the brain, the spinal cord, or ganglia. A bundle of nerve fibers is called a fasciculus. The fibers within a fasciculus are surrounded and held together by delicate connective tissue fibers forming the endoneurium. Each fasciculus is surrounded by a sheath of connective tissue (perineurium). The entire nerve is enclosed in a thick sheath of connective tissue (epineurium), which may contain numerous fat cells. Small nerves may lack an epineurium. SYN: *nervus.* SEE: *cell* and *nerve cell* for illus.; *Nerves Appendix.*

*Test for loss of function:* It is important to know the extent of peripheral nerve damage and to follow the course of healing. This may be done for injury of nerves of the hand by observing the wrinkling of the hand when it is soaked in warm water for 30 minutes. If the nerve supply is intact, skin of the fingers shows characteristic wrinkling; however, the fingers remain unwrinkled over the area in which the nerve supply is absent. SEE: *test, wrinkle.*

***accelerator n.*** A sympathetic nerve to the heart that carries impulses that speed the heart rate.

***acoustic n.*** The eighth cranial nerve. SEE: *vestibulocochlear nerve* for illus.

***adrenergic n.*** A sympathetic nerve that liberates norepinephrine at a synapse when it transmits a stimulus.

***afferent n.*** Any nerve that transmits impulses from receptors to the central nervous system. SYN: *sensory nerve.*

***autonomic n.*** SEE: *autonomic nervous system.*

***cerebrospinal n.*** A nerve originating from the brain or spinal cord.

***cholinergic n.*** A parasympathetic nerve that liberates acetylcholine when it transmits a stimulus.

***cranial n.*** One of the 12 pairs of nerves arising from the brain. They exit through the foramina of the cranium. SEE: *cranial nerves; Cranial Nerve Appendix.*

***depressor n.*** Any afferent nerve whose stimulation depresses the activity of an organ or nerve center.

***efferent n.*** A nerve that transmits impulses from the central nervous system to an effector. SYN: *motor nerve.*

***excitatory n.*** A nerve that transmits impulses that stimulate function.

***excitoreflex n.*** A visceral nerve whose stimulation causes reflex action.

***facial n.*** The seventh cranial nerve. SEE: *facial nerve.*

***gangliated n.*** Any nerve of the sympathetic nervous system.

***glossopharyngeal n.*** The ninth cranial nerve. SEE: *glossopharyngeal nerve.*

***inhibitory n.*** A nerve whose stimulation lessens activity in a body part.

***lumbar n.'s*** The five pairs of spinal nerves, corresponding with the lumbar vertebrae.

***median n.*** A combined motor and sensory nerve of the arm having its origin in the brachial plexus.

***mixed n.*** A nerve containing both afferent (sensory) and efferent (motor) fibers.

***motor n.*** A nerve that transmits impulses from the central nervous system to an effector. SYN: *efferent nerve.*

***olfactory n.'s*** The first pair of cranial nerves. SEE: *olfactory nerves.*

***optic n.*** The second cranial nerve. SEE: *optic nerve.*

***parasympathetic n.*** SEE: *parasympathetic nervous system.*

***peripheral n.*** Any nerve that connects the brain or spinal cord with peripheral receptors or effectors. SEE: illus.

***phrenic n.*** A nerve arising in the cervical plexus, entering the thorax, and passing to the diaphragm; a motor nerve to the diaphragm with sensory fibers to the pericardium.

PERIPHERAL CUTANEOUS NERVES

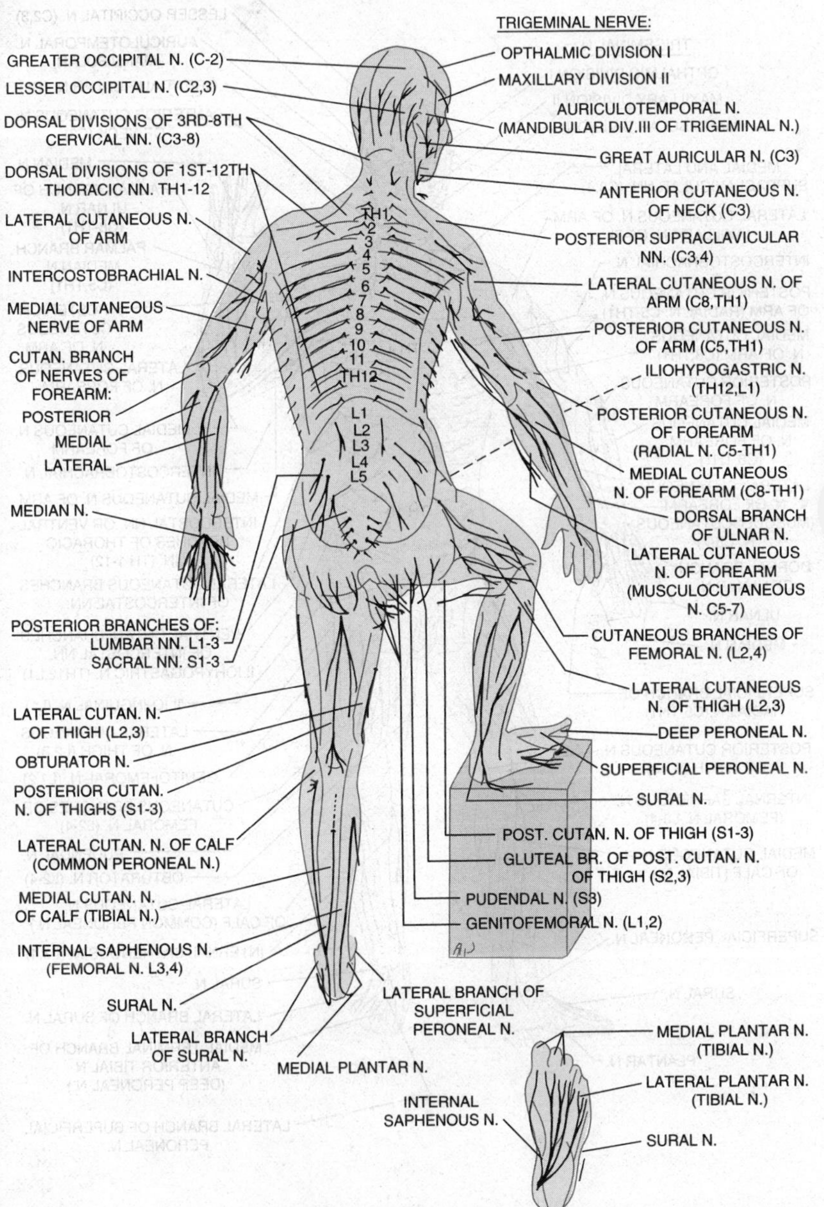


POSTERIOR VIEW

PERIPHERAL CUTANEOUS NERVES

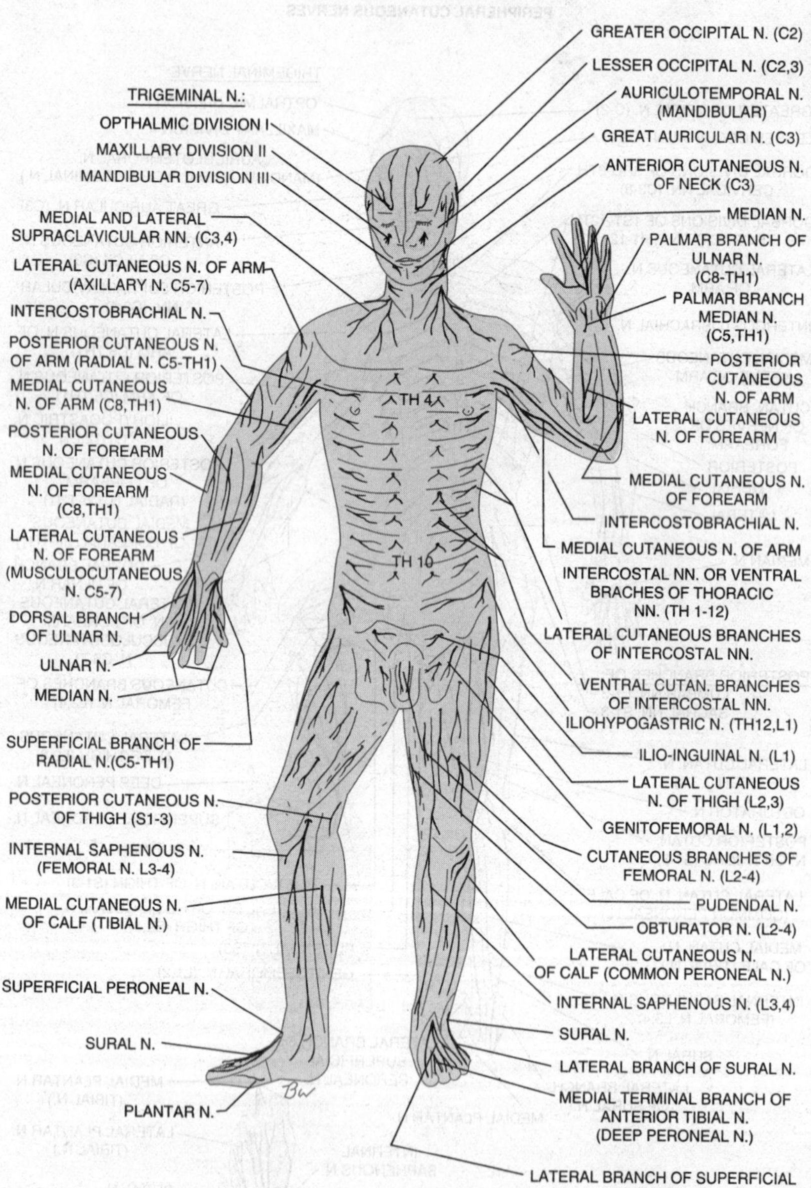


ANTERIOR VIEW

***pilomotor n.*** A nerve that innervates the arrectores pilorum muscles of hair follicles.

***pressor n.*** An afferent nerve whose stimulation excites the vasoconstrictor center, thus increasing the blood pressure.

***secretory n.*** A nerve whose stimulation excites secretion in a gland or a tissue.

***sensory n.*** A nerve conveying impulses from receptors to the central nervous system, or one composed of sensory neurons. SYN: *afferent nerve.*

***somatic n.*** A nerve that innervates somatic structures. These include skeletal muscle (motor nerves) and receptors in skin, joints, and skeletal muscle (sensory nerves).

***spinal n.*** One of 31 pairs of peripheral nerves that connect with the spinal cord. Includes 8 cervical, 12 thoracic, 5 lumbar, 5 sacral, 1 coccygeal. SEE: *spinal nerves.*

***splanchnic n.*** Any of the nerves from the thoracic sympathetic ganglia that supply the visceral organs.

***sudomotor n.*** One of the nerves that supply sweat glands.

***sympathetic n.*** Nerve of the sympathetic division of the autonomic nervous system. SEE: *autonomic nervous system.*

***thoracic n.'s*** The 12 pairs of spinal nerves that emerge from the foramina between the thoracic vertebrae. All are mixed nerves (sensory and motor).

***trigeminal n.*** The fifth cranial and the most important sensory and motor nerve of the oral area. SEE: *cranial nerves; trigeminal nerve.*

***trophic n.*** Any nerve involved in regulating the nutrition of tissues.

***vagus n.*** The tenth cranial nerve. SEE: *vagus* for illus.

***vasoconstrictor n.*** A nerve conducting impulses that bring about constriction of a blood vessel.

***vasodilator n.*** A nerve conducting impulses that bring about dilation of a blood vessel.

***vasomotor n.*** A nerve that controls the caliber of a blood vessel; a vasoconstrictor or vasodilator nerve.

***vasosensory n.*** Any nerve providing sensory fibers for a vessel.

**nerve block** SEE: *block, nerve.*

**nerve cell** Neuron. The nerve cell consists of a cell body and its processes (an axon and one or more dendrites) extending from the cell body. The axon transmits nerve impulses and the dendrite(s) receives impulses and transmits them to the cell body. SEE: illus.

**nerve ending** The termination of a nerve fiber (axon or dendrite) in a peripheral structure. It may be sensory (receptor) or motor (effector). Sensory endings can be nonencapsulated (e.g., free nerve endings, peritrichal endings, or tactile corpuscles of Merkel) or they can be encapsulated (e.g., end-bulbs of Krause, Meissner's cor-

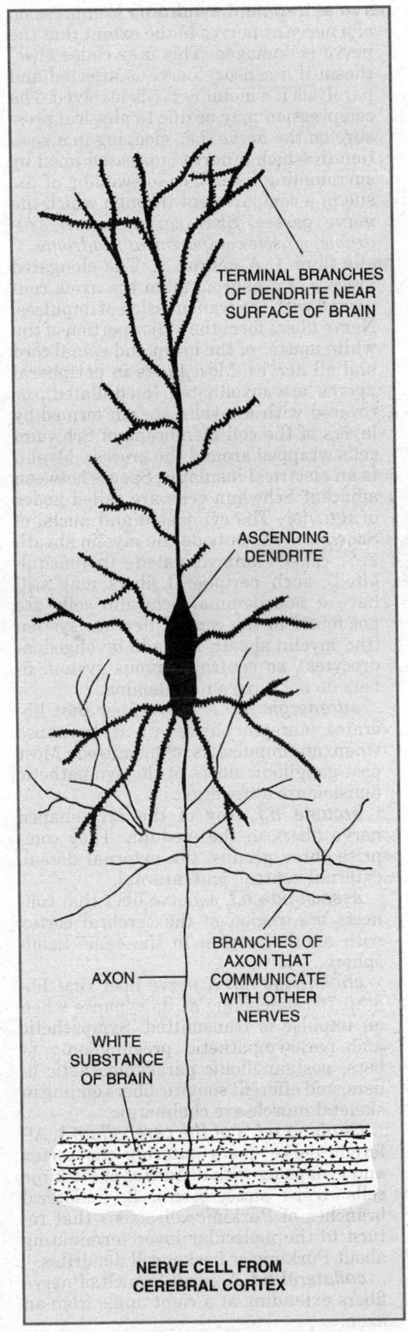

NERVE CELL FROM CEREBRAL CORTEX

puscles, Vater-Pacini corpuscles, or neuromuscular and neurotendinous spindles).

**nerve entrapment syndrome** Compression of a nerve or nerves to the extent that the nerve is damaged. This may cause anesthesia if a sensory nerve is affected and paralysis if a motor nerve is involved. The compression may be due to physical pressure on the nerve (i.e., sleeping in a position in which a nerve is pressed upon by surrounding tissue), or to swelling of tissue in a compartment through which the nerve passes. SEE: *carpal tunnel syndrome; muscle compartment syndrome.*

**nerve fiber 1.** A neuron. **2.** The elongated process of a neuron, often the axon, concerned with the transmission of impulses. Nerve fibers form the major portion of the white matter of the brain and spinal cord and all nerves. Most fibers in peripheral nerves are myelinated (medullated), or covered with a myelin sheath formed by layers of the cell membrane of Schwann cells wrapped around the process. Myelin is an electrical insulator. Spaces between adjacent Schwann cells are called nodes of Ranvier. The cytoplasm and nuclei of Schwann cells outside the myelin sheath are called unmyelinated (nonmedullated); such peripheral fibers may still have a neurilemma. Schwann cells are not found in the central nervous system (the myelin sheath is made by oligodendrocytes), so central nervous system fibers do not have a neurilemma.

***adrenergic n.f.*** A nerve fiber that liberates norepinephrine at its synapse when an impulse is transmitted. Most post-ganglionic fibers of the sympathetic division are adrenergic.

***arcuate n.f.*** Any of the arch-shaped nerve fibers in the medulla. They comprise three groups, the external dorsal, external ventral, and internal.

***association n.f.*** A nerve fiber that connects one region of the cerebral cortex with another region in the same hemisphere.

***cholinergic n.f.*** A nerve fiber that liberates acetylcholine at its synapse when an impulse is transmitted. Sympathetic and parasympathetic preganglionic fibers, postganglionic parasympathetic fibers, and efferent somatic fibers ending in skeletal muscle are cholinergic.

***climbing n.f.'s of the cerebellum*** **1.** Afferent nerve fibers entering the cortex and synapsing with dendrites of Purkinje cells. SYN: *mossy fibers.* **2.** Collateral branches of Purkinje cell axons that return to the molecular layer terminating about Purkinje or basket cell dendrites.

***collateral n.f.*** A small branch of nerve fibers extending at a right angle from an axon.

***commissural n.f.*** A nerve fiber that passes from one cerebral hemisphere to the other.

***medullated n.f.*** A nerve fiber possessing a myelin sheath. SYN: *myelinated nerve fiber.*

***myelinated n.f.*** Medullated n.f.

***nonmedullated n.f.*** A nerve fiber lacking a myelin sheath.

***postganglionic n.f.*** A nerve fiber of the autonomic nervous system that terminates in smooth or cardiac muscle or in a gland. Its cell body lies in an autonomic ganglion.

***preganglionic n.f.*** A nerve fiber of the autonomic nervous system that terminates and synapses in one of the autonomic ganglia. Its cell body lies in the brain or spinal cord.

***projection n.f.*** **1.** A nerve fiber arising in the diencephalon and passing to the cerebral cortex. **2.** A nerve fiber arising in the cerebral cortex and terminating in lower portions of the brain or in the spinal cord.

**nerve fibril** Neurofibril.

**nerve gas** Gaseous materials used in chemical warfare. The agents may actually be in liquid form but are aerosolized at the time of use. These chemicals are readily absorbed through the skin. Some forms (organophosphates that inhibit acetylcholinesterase) cause copious secretions from the nose, eyes, mouth, lungs, and intestines. Muscle fasiculations, twitching, and miosis will result from exposure. A large dose may cause sudden unconsciousness, convulsions, flaccid paralysis, apnea, and death. With some agents, only a few breaths of the vapor may cause death.

PROTECTION: Charcoal-lined suits offer the only protection. The agents will penetrate ordinary clothing worn with a gas mask.

TREATMENT: Pretreatment with pyridostigmine and concurrent treatment at the time of exposure with atropine, pralidoxime, and diazepam may be life-saving. Artificial respiration is mandatory. The skin should be decontaminated with household bleach diluted with water at a ratio of 1:10, or with soap and water, and the eyes should be irrigated with plain water. Military personnel carry small towels impregnated with chloramine, hydroxide, and phenol.

---

Caution: Gas masks should cover face and eyes and be proven to be adequately effective. Persons treating patients must protect themselves from the nerve agents.

---

**nerve growth factor** ABBR: NGF. A protein necessary for the growth and maintenance of sympathetic and certain sensory neurons.

**nerve impulse** SEE: *impulse, nerve.*

**nerve plexus** SEE: under *plexus.*

**nerve trunk** The main stem of a peripheral nerve.

**nervimotor** (nĕr″vĭ-mō′tor) [″ + *motus,* moving] Pert. to a motor nerve.

**nervone** A cerebroside present in brain tissue. It contains nervonic acid.

**nervous** [L. *nervosus*] **1.** Anxious. **2.** Characterized by excitability. **3.** Pert. to the nerves.

***n. breakdown*** A lay term for any mental illness, esp. one with acute onset, that interferes with normal function, thought, or action.

***n. debility*** Nervous fatigue with resultant physical exhaustion. SYN: *neurasthenia.*

***n. prostration*** Neurasthenia.

***n. tissue*** Tissue that makes up the nervous system, including the nervous elements proper (neurons) and the interstitial tissue (neuroglia, neurilemma cells, and satellite cells).

**nervousness** The state of being nervous.

**nervous system** One of the regulatory systems, made of millions of neurons in precise pathways to transmit electrochemical impulses, and of neuroglial cells that have several functions, including formation of myelin sheaths of neurons. It consists of the brain and spinal cord (central nervous system [CNS]) and the cranial nerves and spinal nerves (peripheral nervous system), which include the nerves of the autonomic nervous system and its ganglia. SEE: *autonomic nervous system; central nervous system; parasympathetic nervous system; sympathetic nervous system.*

FUNCTION: Receptors detect external and internal changes and transmit impulses along sensory nerves to the CNS. Receptors are found in the skin, muscles and joints, viscera, and the organs of special sense: the eye, the ear, and the organs of taste and smell. The CNS uses this sensory information to initiate appropriate responses to changes; reflexes involving muscle contraction or glandular secretion, or voluntary movement, all mediated by motor nerves. A function specific to the brain is the integration, analysis, and storage of information for possible later use; this function is learning and memory.

**nervus** [L.] Nerve. SEE: *Nerves Appendix.*

***n. erigens*** A bundle of parasympathetic autonomic fibers originating from the 2nd to 4th sacral nerves and passing to terminal ganglia from which postganglionic fibers pass to the pelvic organs (bladder, colon, rectum, prostate gland, seminal vesicles, external genitalia).

***n. intermedius*** A branch of the facial nerve consisting principally of sensory fibers.

***nervi nervorum*** Nerve fibers that innervate sheaths of nerves.

***n. terminales*** A terminal nerve accompanying the olfactory nerve to the brain and consisting principally of sensory fibers from the mucosa of the nasal septum.

***nervi vasorum*** Nerve fibers that innervate the walls of blood vessels.

**nesidioblastoma** (nē-sĭd″ē-ō-blăs-tō′mă) [″ + *blastos,* germ, + *oma,* tumor] Islet-cell tumor of the pancreas.

**nest** A small mass of cells that resembles a bird's nest and is alien to the surrounding tissue.

***cancer n.*** A mass of cells extending from a common center seen in cancerous growths.

***cell n.*** A mass of epithelial cells set apart from surrounding cells by connective tissue.

**nesteostomy** (nĕs″tē-ŏs′tō-mē) [Gr. *nestis,* jejunum, + *stoma,* mouth] Jejunostomy.

**n. et m.** *nocte et mane,* night and morning.

**net reproductive rate** ABBR: NRR. A measure of whether a population is reproducing at a greater or lesser rate than needed for its replacement. It is determined by calculating the average number of surviving daughters born to the women in that population during their reproductive years. An NRR of 1 indicates that each woman in the population has one surviving daughter during her lifetime.

**ne tr. s. num.** *ne tradas sine nummo,* do not deliver unless paid.

**nettle** [AS. *netel*] Any plant of the genus *Urtica.* A nettle's sawtoothed leaves contain hairs that secrete a fluid that irritates the skin.

***n. rash*** A skin rash with intense itching, resembling the condition produced by stinging with nettles. SYN: *hives; urticaria.*

**network** [AS. *net,* net, + *wyrcan,* to work] Fiber arrangement in a structure resembling a net. SYN: *rete; reticulum.*

***artificial neural n.*** A group of interconnected mathematic equations that accept input data and that calculate an output based on this input. This system has been used to predict both the presence and the absence of acute myocardial infarction.

**Neuman, Betty** Nursing educator, born 1924, who developed Neuman's systems model, a conceptual model of nursing. SEE: *Nursing Theory Appendix.*

***N.'s systems model*** A conceptual model of nursing developed by Betty Neuman in which individuals and groups are considered client systems made up of physiological, psychological, sociocultural, developmental, and spiritual variables. The goal of nursing is to facilitate optimal wellness through retention, attainment, or maintenance of client system stability.

**Neumann's disease** (noy′mănz) [Isidor Neumann, Austrian dermatologist, 1832–1906] Pemphigus vegetans.

**neur-, neuri-, neuro-** Combining form denoting *nerve, nervous system.*

**neurad** (nū′răd) [Gr. *neuron,* nerve, sinew, + L. *-ad,* toward] Toward a nerve or its axis.

**neuragmia** (nū-răg′mē-ă) [Gr. *neuron,*

nerve, sinew, + *agmos,* break] The tearing or rupturing of a nerve trunk.

**neural** (nū'răl) [L. *neuralis*] Pert. to nerves or connected with the nervous system.

***n. crest*** A band of cells extending longitudinally along the neural tube of an embryo from which cells forming cranial, spinal, and autonomic ganglia arise, as well as to cells (ectomesenchyme) that migrate into the forming facial region and become odontoblasts, which form the dentin of the teeth.

***n. fold*** One of two longitudinal elevations of the neural plate of an embryo that unite to form the neural tube.

***n. grafting*** An experimental procedure for transplanting tissue into the brain and spinal cord. Possible sources of material to be used include human fetal tissue, cultured and genetically engineered cells, and tissues from the patient's own body.

***n. plate*** A thickened band of ectoderm along the dorsal surface of an embryo. The nervous system develops from this tissue.

***n. spine*** Spinous process of vertebrae.

**neuralgia** (nū-răl'jē-ă) [Gr. *neuron,* nerve, sinew, + *algos,* pain] Severe sharp pain occurring along the course of a nerve. It is caused by pressure on nerve trunks, faulty nerve nutrition, toxins, or inflammation. Usually, no morphologic changes can be detected. SYN: *neurodynia.* SEE: *sciatica.* **neuralgic** (nū-răl'jĭk), *adj.*

***cardiac n.*** Angina pectoris.

***degenerative n.*** Neuralgia occurring in the elderly, caused by degenerative changes in the nerves or nerve cells.

***facial n.*** Trigeminal n.

***geniculate n.*** Neuralgia characterized by pain over all or any area supplied by sensory fibers of the facial nerve. The pain may be deep in facial muscles, within the ear, or in pharynx. SYN: *Hunt's n.*

***glossopharyngeal n.*** Neuralgia along the course of the glossopharyngeal nerve, characterized by severe pain in back of the throat, tonsils, and middle ear.

***hallucinatory n.*** An impression of local pain without an actual stimulus to cause the pain.

***Hunt's n.*** Geniculate n.

***idiopathic n.*** Neuralgia without structural lesion or pressure from a lesion.

***intercostal n.*** Neuralgia in which pain follows the course of the intercostal nerves, frequently associated with eruption of herpes zoster. There are spots of tenderness near the vertebral column, in the middle of the nerve, and near the sternum. SYN: *pleuralgia.*

***mammary n.*** Neuralgia of the breast. SYN: *mastodynia.*

***Morton's n.*** Neuralgia of the joint of the third and fourth toes. SYN: *metatarsalgia.*

***nasociliary n.*** Neuralgia of the eyes, brows, and root of the nose.

***occipital n.*** Neuralgia involving the upper cervical nerves. A spot of tenderness is found between the mastoid process and the upper cervical vertebrae. It may be due to spinal caries.

***otic n.*** Geniculate n.

***postherpetic n.*** Neuralgia following an attack of herpes zoster (shingles). It is caused by irritation of the nerve roots of the spinal cord. SEE: *herpes zoster.*

***reminiscent n.*** Continued mental perception of pain after neuralgia has ceased.

***sphenopalatine n.*** Neuralgia of the sphenopalatine ganglion, causing pain in the area of the upper jawbone and radiating into the neck and shoulders. There is pain on one side of face radiating to the eyeball, ear, and occipital and mastoid areas of the skull, and sometimes to the nose, upper teeth, and shoulder on the same side.

***stump n.*** Neuralgia due to irritation of nerves at the site of an amputation.

***symptomatic n.*** Neuralgia not primarily involving the nerve structure but occurring as a symptom of local or systemic disease.

***trifacial n.*** Former term for trigeminal neuralgia.

***trigeminal n.*** Neuralgia involving the gasserian ganglion or one or more branches of the trigeminal nerve. SEE: *Nursing Diagnoses Appendix.*

SYMPTOMS: Symptoms include tender points corresponding to supraorbital, infraorbital, and mental foramina, and often violent spasm of muscles. In long-standing cases, the hair on the affected side sometimes becomes coarse and bleached.

ETIOLOGY: The cause of this type of neuralgia is unknown. Attacks are often precipitated by obvious stimuli on certain hypersensitive areas (trigger points or trigger zones) on the face, lips, or tongue.

TREATMENT: Drugs such as phenytoin or dibenzazepine have been useful in suppressing or shortening attacks. Their use for temporary relief may permit spontaneous remission. If the syndrome persists, the nerve is injected with alcohol or phenol, or it is surgically sectioned. SYN: *facial n.; Fothergill's neuralgia; tic douloureux.*

**neuralgiform** (nū-răl'jĭ-form) [" + " + L. *forma,* form] Similar to neuralgia.

**neural tube** Tube formed from fusion of the neural folds from which the brain and spinal cord arise.

***n.t. defect*** ABBR: NTD. A defective closure of the neural tube during early embryogenesis. Included are fetal anencephaly, spina bifida, lumbar meningomyelocele, and meningocele. The tendency for this condition to be present may be inherited. The overall incidence is 1 to 2 in every 1000 live births. If the defect is of the type with an open tube, the levels of maternal and fetal serum alpha-fetoprotein (AFP) are elevated. The alleged association of NTD with vitamin use around the time of conception has not been validated. Folic acid during pregnancy helps to prevent NTDs in the embryo.

An adequate intake of folic acid during pregnancy is an important factor in reducing the risk of fetal NTDs. Thus the U.S. Public Health Service recommends that all women of childbearing age in the U.S. who are capable of becoming pregnant should consume 0.4 mg of folic acid per day to reduce the risk of having a child affected with spina bifida or other NTDs.

**neuraminidase** (nūr-ăm′ĭn-ĭ-dās″) An enzyme present on the surface of influenza virus particles. The activity of this enzyme enables the virus particle to separate itself from cells. Persons with increased levels of antibodies against neuraminidase in their serum may have increased resistance to influenza infection.

**neurapophysis** (nū″ră-pŏf′ĭ-sĭs) [″ + *apo,* from, + *physis,* growth] Either of the two sides of a vertebra that unite to form the neural arch.

**neurarchy** (nū′răr-kē) [″ + *arche,* rule] The domination of the nervous system over the body.

**neurarthropathy** (nū″răr-thrŏp′ă-thē) [″ + *arthron,* joint, + *pathos,* disease, suffering] Neuroarthropathy.

**neurasthenia** (nū″răs-thē′nē-ă) [″ + *astheneia,* weakness] A term previously used for persons with unexplained chronic fatigue and lassitude. Accompanying these symptoms were usually nervousness, irritability, anxiety, depression, headache, insomnia, and sexual disorders. Those individuals are now diagnosed according to their total condition, such as some form of psychiatric illness, esp. anxiety neurosis or tension state.

**neurasthenic** (nū-răs-thē′nĭk) **1.** Individual suffering from neurasthenia. **2.** Suffering from or concerning neurasthenia.

**neuraxis** (nū-răk′sĭs) [″ + L. *axon,* axis] The cerebrospinal axis.

**neuraxon, neuraxone** (nū-răks′ōn) The axis cylinder process of a nerve cell. SYN: *axon.* SEE: *nerve fiber.*

**neurectasia, neurectasis, neurectasy** (nū″rĕk-tā′sē-ă, -rĕk′tă-sĭs, -rĕk′tă-sē) [″ + *ektasis,* a stretching] Surgical stretching of a nerve. SYN: *neurotension.*

**neurectomy** (nū-rĕk′tō-mē) [″ + *ektome,* excision] Partial or total excision or resection of a nerve.

***presacral n.*** Surgical procedure for removing the hypogastric (presacral) nerve plexus. This is done to treat conditions such as dysmenorrhea and chronic idiopathic pelvic pain.

**neurectopia, neurectopy** (nū-rĕk-tō′pē-ă, nūr-ĕk′tō-pē) [″ + *ek,* out, + *topos,* place] Displacement or abnormal position of a nerve.

**neurenteric** (nū-rĕn-tĕr′ĭk) [″ + *enteron,* intestine] Relating to the neural canal and intestinal tube of the embryo.

***n. canal*** A temporary canal in the vertebrate embryo between the neural and intestinal tubes. In human development, the temporary communication between cavities of the yolk sac and the amnion.

**neurepithelium** (nūr″ĕp-ĭ-thē′lē-ŭm) [″ + *epi,* upon, + *thele,* nipple] Neuroepithelium.

**neurexeresis** (nūr″ĕks-ĕr′ĕ-sĭs) [″ + *exairein,* to draw out] The tearing out of a nerve to relieve neuralgia.

**neurilemma** (nū′rĭ-lĕm″mă) [″+ *lemma,* husk] In the peripheral nervous system, the cytoplasm and nuclei of Schwann cells wrapped around the myelin sheath or the unmyelinated processes of nerve fibers. This contributes to regeneration of damaged nerve fibers by producing growth factors and serving as a tunnel or guide for regrowth. SYN: *neurolemma; Schwann's sheath.* SEE: *nerve fiber; neuron* for illus.

**neurilemmitis** (nū″rĭ-lĕm-mī′tĭs) [″ + ″ + *itis,* inflammation] Inflammation of a neurilemma.

**neurilemmoma, neurilemoma** (nū″rĭ-lĕm-ō′mă) [″ + *eilema,* tight sheath, + *oma,* tumor] A firm, encapsulated fibrillar tumor of a peripheral nerve. SYN: *neurinoma; neurofibroma; schwannoma.*

**neurilemmosarcoma** (nū″rĭ-lĕm″ō-săr-kō′mă) A malignant neurilemoma.

**neurimotor** [″ + L. *motor,* a mover] Concerning a motor nerve.

**neurinoma** (nū-rĭ-nō′mă) [″ + *oma,* tumor] Neurilemmoma.

**neurinomatosis** (nū″rĭ-nō-mă-tō′sĭs) [″ + ″ + *osis,* condition] Neurofibromatosis.

**neurite** (nū′rīt) [Gr. *neuron,* nerve, sinew] Neuraxon.

**neuritis** (nū-rī′tĭs) [″ + *itis,* inflammation] Inflammation of a nerve, usually associated with a degenerative process. SEE: *Guillain-Barré syndrome; polyneuritis; Nursing Diagnoses Appendix.*

SYMPTOMS: There are many forms of neuritis, which produce a variety of symptoms, including neuralgia in part affected, hyperesthesia, paresthesia, dysesthesia, hypesthesia, anesthesia, muscular atrophy of the body part supplied by the affected nerve, paralysis, and lack of reflexes.

ETIOLOGY: Neuritis may be caused by mechanical factors, such as compression or contusion of the nerve, or localized infection involving direct infection of a nerve. It may accompany diseases such as leprosy, tetanus, tuberculosis, malaria, or measles. Toxins, esp. poisoning by heavy metals (arsenic, lead, mercury), alcohol, or carbon tetrachloride may be the causative factor. Neuritis may accompany thiamine deficiency, gastrointestinal dysfunction, diabetes, toxemias of pregnancy, or peripheral vascular disease.

NURSING IMPLICATIONS: Changes in motor and sensory function are monitored. Correct positioning and prescribed analgesic drugs are used to relieve pain. Rest is provided, and affected extremities are rested by limiting their use and by using supportive appliances. Passive range-of-motion exercises are performed to help prevent contracture formation. Skin care is provided, and proper nutrition and dietary therapy are prescribed for metabolic disorders. The nurse removes causative factors or counsels the patient about their avoidance. After pain subsides, the nurse supports prescribed activities, such as massage, electrostimulation, and exercise.

**adventitial n.** Inflammation of a nerve sheath.

**ascending n.** Neuritis moving upward along a nerve trunk away from the periphery.

**axial n.** Inflammation of the inner portion of a nerve.

**degenerative n.** Neuritis with rapid degeneration of a nerve.

**descending n.** Neuritis that leads away from the central nervous system toward the periphery.

**diphtheritic n.** Neuritis following diphtheria.

**disseminated n.** Neuritis involving a large group of nerves.

**interstitial n.** Neuritis involving the connective tissue of a nerve.

**intraocular n.** Neuritis of the retinal fibers of the optic nerve causing disturbed vision, contracted field, enlarged blind spot, and fundus findings such as exudates, hemorrhages, and abnormal condition of the blood vessels. Treatment depends on the etiology (e.g., brain tumor, meningitis, syphilis, nephritis, diabetes).

**n. migrans** Ascending or descending neuritis that passes along a nerve trunk, affecting one area and then another.

**multiple n.** Simultaneous impairment of a number of peripheral nerves. SYN: *polyneuritis*.

SYMPTOMS: Symptoms are related to the suddenness of onset and severity. Usually, lower limbs are affected first, with weakness that may progress until the entire body is affected. Muscle strength, deep tendon reflexes, sensory nerves, and autonomic nerves become involved.

ETIOLOGY: Causes include infectious diseases (e.g., diphtheria), metabolic disorders (e.g., alcoholism, diabetes, pellagra, beriberi, sprue), and various poisons, including lead. In some instances, the disease arises without apparent cause.

TREATMENT: Causative factors should be removed, if possible. Treatment includes skilled nursing, with particular care taken to prevent bedsores, and dietary therapy (depending upon the etiology).

**n. nodosa** Neuritis with formation of nodes on nerves.

**optic n.** Neuritis of the optic nerve.

**parenchymatous n.** Neuritis of nerve fiber substance.

**peripheral n.** Neuritis of terminal nerves or end organs.

**retrobulbar n.** Neuritis of the portion of the optic nerve behind the eyeball.

SYMPTOMS: The main symptom is acute loss of vision in one or both eyes. Pain may be absent or it may be unbearable, lasting for only a brief period or for days.

ETIOLOGY: This type of neuralgia may be caused by a variety of illnesses, but in adults it is most frequently associated with multiple sclerosis.

**rheumatic n.** Neuritis with symptoms of rheumatism.

**sciatic n.** Inflammation of the sciatic nerve. SEE: *sciatica*.

**segmental n.** Neuritis affecting segments of a nerve interspersed with healthy segments.

**senile n.** Neuritis in the elderly, usually affecting the extremities.

**sympathetic n.** Neuritis of the opposite nerve without attack of the nerve center.

**tabetic n.** Neuritis in locomotor ataxia caused by syphilis.

**toxic n.** Neuritis resulting from metallic poisons (e.g., arsenic, mercury, and thallium) or nonmetallic poisons, such as various hydrocarbons and organic solvents.

**traumatic n.** Neuritis following an injury.

**neuro-** [Gr. *neuron,* nerve, sinew] Combining form denoting *nerve, nervous tissue, nervous system*.

**neuroablation** The destruction or inactivation of nerve tissue. This may be done by several means including surgery, cautery, injection of sterile ethyl alcohol, use of lasers, or cryotherapy. An early example is prefrontal lobotomy, formerly used to treat certain types of mental illness. Freezing of part of the brain was done experimentally to treat parkinsonism; the technique is being reexamined using better tools. Neuroablation is also used to remove abnormal nerve tissue from the atrium of the heart, where it may cause cardiac arrhythmia.

**neuroanastomosis** (nū″rō-ă-năs″tō-mō′sĭs) [″ + *anastomosis,* opening] Surgical attachment of one end of a severed nerve to the other end.

**neuroanatomy** (nū″rō-ăn-ăt′ō-mē) The anatomy of the nervous system.

**neuroarthropathy** (nū″rō-ăr-thrŏp′ă-thē) [″ + ″ + *pathos,* disease, suffering] Disease of a joint combined with disease of the central nervous system.

**neuroastrocytoma** (nū″rō-ăs″trō-sī-tō′mă) [″ + *kytos,* cell, + *oma,* tumor] A tumor of the central nervous system composed of neurons and glial cells.

**neuroaugmentation** Any method used to increase the function of a nerve, esp. in managing pain. Transcutaneous electrical nerve stimulation has been used for this purpose.

**neurobiology** (nū″rō-bī-ŏl′ō-jē) [″ + *bios,* life, + *logos,* word, reason] Biology of the nervous system.

**neurobiotaxis** (nū″rō-bī-ō-tăk′sĭs) [″ + *bios,* life, + *taxis,* order] The phenomenon involving the growth of dendrites and the migration of nerve-cell bodies during development toward the region from which their dominant impulses are initiated.

**neuroblast** (nū′rō-blăst) [″ + *blastos,* germ] An embryonic cell derived from the neural tube or neural crest, giving rise to a neuron.

**neuroblastoma** (nū″rō-blăs-tō′mă) [″ + ″ + *oma,* tumor] A malignant hemorrhagic tumor composed principally of cells resembling neuroblasts that give rise to cells of the sympathetic system, esp. adrenal medulla. This condition occurs chiefly in infants and children. The primary sites are in the mediastinal and retroperitoneal regions.

**neurocanal** (nū″rō-kă-năl′) [″ + L. *canalis,* passage] The central canal of the spinal cord.

**neurocardiac** (nū″rō-kăr′dē-ăk) [″ + *kardia,* heart] **1.** Pert. to the nerves supplying the heart or nervous system and the heart. **2.** Concerning a cardiac neurosis.

**neurocardiogenic syncope** SEE: *syncope, vasodepressor.*

**neurocentral** (nū″rō-sĕn′trăl) [″ + *kentron,* center] Pert. to the centrum of a vertebra and the neural arch.

**neurocentrum** (nū″rō-sĕn′trŭm) The body of a vertebra.

**neurochemistry** (nū″rō-kĕm′ĭs-trē) Physiological chemistry dealing with nervous tissue.

**neurochorioretinitis** (nū″rō-kō″rē-ō-rĕ″tĭn-ī′tĭs) [Gr. *neuron,* nerve, sinew, + *chorion,* skin, + L. *retina,* retina, + Gr. *itis,* inflammation] Inflammation of choroid and retina combined with optic neuritis.

**neurochoroiditis** (nū″rō-kō-roy-dī′tĭs) [″ + ″ + *eidos,* form, shape, + *itis,* inflammation] Inflammation of the choroid coat and optic nerve.

**neurocirculatory** (nū″rō-sŭr′kū-lă-tō″rē) [″ + L. *circulatio,* circulation] Pert. to circulation and the nervous system.

**neurocirculatory asthenia** SEE: *asthenia.*

**neurocladism** (nū-rŏk′lă-dĭzm) [″ + *klados,* a young branch, + *-ismos,* condition] Phenomenon occurring after a nerve is severed, where an outgrowth of fibrils closes the gap and begins the process of nerve repair. SYN: *odogenesis.*

**neuroclonic** (nū″rō-klŏn′ĭk) [″+ *klonos,* spasm] Marked by spasms of neural origin.

**neurocranium** (nū″rō-krā′nē-ŭm) [″ + *kranion,* skull] The part of the skull enclosing the brain.

**neurocrine** (nū′rō-krĭn) [″ + *krinein,* to secrete] **1.** Indicating an endocrine influence on nerves or the influence of nerves on endocrine tissue. **2.** A chemical transmitter.

**neurocutaneous** (nū″rō-kū-tā′nē-ŭs) [″ + L. *cutis,* skin] Pert. to the nervous system and skin.

**neurocyte** (nū′rō-sīt) [″ + *kytos,* cell] A nerve cell. SYN: *neuron.*

**neurocytolysis** (nū″rō-sī-tŏl′ĭ-sĭs) [″ + *kytos,* cell, + *lysis,* dissolution] Dissolution or destruction of nerve cells.

**neurocytoma** (nū″rō-sī-tō′mă) [″ + ″ + *oma,* tumor] A tumor formed of cells of nervous origin (usually ganglionic). SEE: *neuroma.*

**neurodealgia** (nū-rō″dē-ăl′jē-ă) [Gr. *neurodes,* retina, + *algos,* pain] Pain in the retina.

**neurodegenerative** Concerning degeneration of tissue of the nervous system.

**neurodendrite, neurodendron** (nū″rō-dĕn′drīt, -drŏn) [Gr. *neuron,* nerve, sinew, + *dendron,* tree] Protoplasmic branched process of a nerve cell. SYN: *dendrite; dendron.* SEE: *dendrite* for illus.

**neurodermatitis** (nū″rō-dĕr-mă-tī′tĭs) [″ + *derma,* skin, + *itis,* inflammation] Cutaneous inflammation with itching that is associated with, but not entirely due to, emotional stress. After an initial irritant, scratching becomes a habit and prolongs the condition. Treatment is corticosteroid ointment or cream. Circumscribed neurodermatitis is used as a synonym for lichen simplex chronicus. SEE: illus.

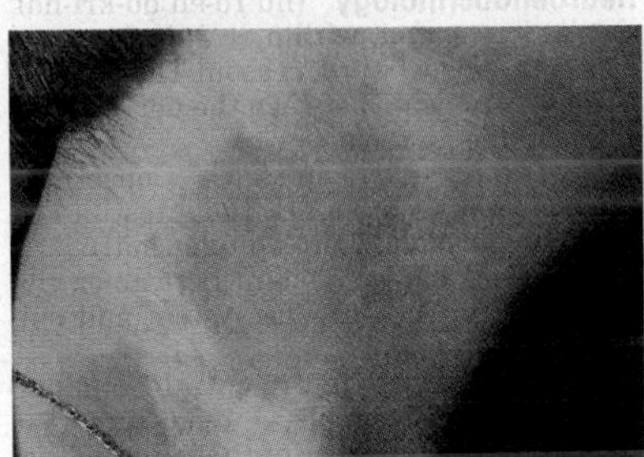

NEURODERMATITIS ON NECK

***disseminated n.*** Chronic superficial inflammation of the skin characterized by thickening, excoriation, and lichenification, usually beginning in infancy. It is common in families with a high incidence of allergic diseases. SYN: *atopic dermatitis.*

**neurodermatosis** (nū″rō-dĕr-mă-tō′sĭs) [″ + ″ + *osis,* condition] Any skin disease of neural origin, including neurofibromatosis, von Hippel-Lindau disease, Sturge-Weber syndrome, and tuberous sclerosis. SYN: *phacomatosis.*

**neurodermatrophia** (nū″rō-dĕrm″ă-trōf′ē-ă)

Atrophy of the skin from nervous disease.

**neurodevelopmental treatment** ABBR: NDT. A rehabilitation treatment approach for cerebral palsy, hemiplegia, and other central nervous system deficits that emphasizes the use of carefully considered handling to inhibit abnormal reflexes and movement patterns and facilitate higher level reactions and patterns in order to attain normal movement. This method was developed by Karel and Bertha Bobath, contemporary German physiotherapists working in England.

**neurodiagnosis** (nū″rō-dī-ăg-nō′sĭs) Diagnosis of nervous disorders.

**neurodynamic** (nū″rō-dī-năm′ĭk) Pert. to nervous energy.

**neurodynia** (nū″rō-dĭn′ē-ă) [Gr. *neuron,* nerve, + *odyne,* pain] Pain in a nerve. SYN: *neuralgia.*

**neuroectoderm** (nū″rō-ĕk′tō-dĕrm) [″ + *ektos,* outside, + *derma,* skin] The embryonic tissue that gives rise to nerve tissue.

**neuroencephalomyelopathy** (nū″rō-ĕn-sĕf″ă-lō-mī″ĕ-lŏp′ă-thē) [″ + *enkephalos,* brain, + *myelos,* marrow, + *pathos,* disease, suffering] Disease of the brain, spinal cord, and nerves.

**neuroendocrine** (nū″rō-ĕn′dō-krĭn) Pert. to the nervous and endocrine systems as an integrated functioning mechanism.

***n. carcinoma*** A diverse group of tumors, such as carcinoid, islet cell tumors, neuroblastoma, and small-cell carcinomas of the lung. All have dense core granules and produce polypeptides that can be identified by immunochemical methods.

**neuroendocrinology** (nū″rō-ĕn″dō-krĭ-nŏl′ō-jē) [″ + *endon,* within, + *krinein,* to secrete, + *logos,* word, reason] The study of the relationship between the nervous and endocrine systems.

**neuroenteric** (nū″rō-ĕn-tĕr′ĭk) Concerning the nervous system and the intestines.

**neuroepidermal** (nū″rō-ĕp-ĭ-dĕr′măl) [″ + *epi,* upon, + *derma,* skin] Pert. to or giving rise to the nervous system and epidermis.

**neuroepithelioma** (nū″rō-ĕp″ĭ-thē-lē-ō′mă) [″ + ″ + *thele,* nipple, + *oma,* tumor] A relatively rare tumor of the neuroepithelium in a nerve of special sense.

**neuroepithelium** (nū″rō-ĕp″ĭ-thē′lē-ŭm) **1.** A specialized epithelial structure forming the termination of a nerve of special sense, including gustatory cells, olfactory cells, hair cells of the inner ear, and the rods and cones of the retina. **2.** The embryonic layer of the epiblast from which the cerebrospinal axis is developed. SYN: *neurepithelium.*

**neurofibril, neurofibrilla** (nū-rō-fī′brĭl, -fī-brĭl′ă) [″ + L. *fibrilla,* a small fiber] Any of the many tiny fibrils that extend in every direction in the cytoplasm of the nerve cell body. They extend into the axon and dendrites of the cell. SEE: *neuron.*

**neurofibroma** (nū″rō-fī-brō′mă) *pl.* **neurofibromata, -mas** [Gr. *neuron,* nerve, + L. *fibra,* fiber, + Gr. *oma,* tumor] A tumor of the connective tissue (esp. Schwann cells) of a nerve. SYN: *fibroneuroma.*

**neurofibromatosis** (nū″rō-fī-brō″mă-tō′sĭs) [″ + ″ + ″ + *osis,* condition] A genetic disorder that affects the cell growth of neural tissues. For those persons with affected family members, genetic assessment and counseling of parents may be indicated. Genetic assessment and counseling can identify the parents' risk of being a gene carrier and passing the disease on to subsequent offspring. SYN: *Recklinghausen's disease.*

***Type 1 n.*** ABBR: NF-1. A genetic disorder that affects about 1 in 4000 persons. Clinically, there are multiple hyperpigmented areas. These appear shortly after birth and may be present any place on the body. Multiple cutaneous and subcutaneous tumors appear in late childhood (there may be only a few or thousands). When the tumors are pressed, they pass through a small opening in the skin, leaving the space previously occupied vacant. This characteristic, called buttonholing, helps to distinguish these tumors from lipomas. In about 2% to 5% of cases, the tumors become malignant. No cure has yet been found. Tumors that give rise to symptoms or those that become malignant should be excised; however, if the tumor is on a vital nerve, excision may be impossible. Radiation therapy and surgery are of benefit.

***Type 2 n.*** ABBR: NF-2. A genetic disorder that affects 1 in 50,000 persons. Most tumors form in the 8th cranial nerve, but may also be present in other intracranial and intraspinal locations. These tumors are treated by the use of microsurgery, in an attempt to remove them and preserve hearing.

**neurofibrosarcoma** (nū″rō-fī″brō-săr-kō′mă) [″ + ″ + Gr. *sarx,* flesh, + *oma,* tumor] A malignant neurofibroma.

**neurofibrositis** (nū″rō-fī″brō-sī′tĭs) [″ + ″ + Gr. *itis,* inflammation] Inflammation of nerve fibers and sensory nerve fibers in muscular tissue.

**neurogangliitis** (nū″rō-găn-glē-ī′tĭs) [″ + *ganglion,* knot, + *itis,* inflammation] Inflammation of a neuroganglion.

**neuroganglion** (nū″rō-găn′glē-ŏn) A group of neuron cell bodies outside the central nervous system.

**neurogastric** (nū″rō-găs′trĭk) [″ + *gaster,* belly] Concerning the nerves of the stomach.

**neurogenesis** (nū″rō-jĕn′ĕ-sĭs) [″ + *genesis,* generation, birth] **1.** Growth or development of nerves. **2.** Development from nervous tissue. **neurogenetic** (nū″rō-jĕn-ĕt′ĭk), *adj.*

**neurogenic, neurogenous** (nū-rō-jĕn′ĭk, -rŏj′ĕn-ŭs) **1.** Originating from nervous tissue. **2.** Due to or resulting from nervous impulses.

**neuroglia** (nū-rŏg′lē-ă) [″ + *glia,* glue] The

tissue that forms the interstitial or supporting elements (cells and fibers) of the nervous system. Neuroglia (also called glia) includes astrocytes, oligodendroglias, microglia (mesoglia), ependyma, neurilemma sheath cells of nerve fibers (cells of Schwann), and satellite (capsule) cells surrounding cranial and spinal ganglia. All except the microglia are of ectodermal origin. Neuroglia acts as connective or supporting tissue and also plays an important role in the reaction of the nervous system to injury or infection. **neuroglial** (nū-rŏg'lē-ăl), *adj.*

**neurogliacyte** (nū-rŏg'lē-ă-sīt) [" + " + *kytos,* cell] Any of the cells found in neuroglial tissue. SYN: *glia cell.*

**neuroglioma** (nū"rō-glī-ō'mă) [Gr. *neuron,* nerve, + *glia,* glue, + *oma,* tumor] A tumor composed of neuroglial tissue. SYN: *glioma.*

***n. ganglionare*** A glioma containing ganglion cells. SYN: *ganglioneuroma.*

**neurogliomatosis** (nū"rō-glī"ō-mă-tō'sĭs) [" + " + " + *osis,* condition] Multiple glioma formation in the nervous system.

**neurogliosis** (nū-rŏg"lē-ō'sĭs) [" + " + *osis,* condition] Development of numerous neurogliomas.

**neuroglycopenia** Hypoglycemia of sufficient duration and degree to interfere with normal brain metabolism. Patients with an insulinoma or hypoglycemia due to an insulin overdose may have this condition. If prolonged, permanent brain damage may result.

**neurohistology** (nū"rō-hĭs-tŏl'ō-jē) [" + *histos,* tissue, + *logos,* study] Branch of histology concerned with the study of the microscopic anatomy of nervous tissue.

**neurohypophysis** (nū"rō-hī-pŏf'ĭs-ĭs) [" + *hypo,* under, + *physis,* growth] Posterior portion (pars nervosa) of the pituitary gland.

**neurokeratin** (nū"rō-kĕr'ă-tĭn) [" + *keras,* horn] The type of keratin found in myelinated nerve fibers.

**neurolemma** Neurilemma.

**neurolemmitis** (nū"rō-lĕ-mī'tĭs) [" + *lemma,* husk, + *itis,* inflammation] Neurilemmitis.

**neurolemmoma** (nū"rō-lĕ-mō'mă) [" + " + *oma,* tumor] Neurilemmoma.

**neuroleptanesthesia** (nū"rō-lĕp"tăn-ĕs-thē'zē-ă) [" + *leptos,* slender, + *-an,* not, + *aisthesis,* sensation] General anesthesia involving intravenous administration of a neuroleptic drug and an analgesic.

**neuroleptic** (nū"rō-lĕp'tĭk) [" + *lepsis,* a taking hold] **1.** An agent or drug that modifies psychotic behavior. In general, the term is synonymous with antipsychotic. **2.** A condition produced by a neuroleptic agent.

***n. anesthesia*** SEE: *anesthesia, neuroleptic.*

***n. drug*** Any drug that produces symptoms resembling those of diseases of the nervous system.

***n. malignant syndrome*** ABBR: NMS. The combination of catatonic rigidity, stupor, unstable blood pressure, hyperthermia, profuse sweating, dyspnea, and incontinence that sometimes occurs as a toxic reaction to the use of potent neuroleptic (antipsychotic) agents in therapeutic doses. The condition lasts 5 to 10 days after discontinuation of the drug. The mortality rate may be as high as 20%. Bromocriptine and dantrolene have been used to treat NMS, if the usual treatment for hyperthermia is ineffective. Drug withdrawal is mandatory. SEE: *hyperpyrexia, malignant.*

**neurologist** (nū-rŏl'ō-jĭst) A specialist in diseases of the nervous system.

**neurology** (nū-rŏl'ō-jē) [" + *logos,* word, reason] The branch of medicine that deals with the nervous system and its diseases. **neurologic, neurological** (nū-rō-lŏj'ĭk, -ĭ-kăl), *adj.*

***clinical n.*** The branch of medicine concerned with the study and treatment of diseases of the nervous system.

**neurolymphomatosis** (nū"rō-lĭm"fō-mă-tō'sĭs) [" + L. *lympha,* lymph, + Gr. *oma,* tumor, + *osis,* condition] Malignant lymphoma involving the nervous system.

**neurolysin** (nū-rŏl'ĭs-ĭn) [" + *lysis,* dissolution] A substance that destroys nerve cells.

**neurolysis** (nū-rŏl'ĭs-ĭs) **1.** The stretching of a nerve to relieve pain. **2.** The loosening of adhesions surrounding a nerve. **3.** The disintegration or destruction of nerve tissue. **neurolytic** (nū-rō-lĭt'ĭk), *adj.*

**neuroma** (nū-rō'mă) [" + *oma,* tumor] Former term for any type of tumor composed of nerve cells. Classification is now made with respect to the specific portion of the nerve involved. SEE: *ganglioneuroma; neurilemmoma.* **neuromatous** (nū-rō'mă-tŭs), *adj.*

***acoustic n.*** A benign tumor of the eighth cranial nerve. The symptoms may include hearing loss, balance disturbances, pain, headache, and tinnitus.

***amputation n.*** Neuroma occurring on the nerves of a stump after amputation.

***amyelinic n.*** Neuroma composed principally of unmyelinated nerve fibers.

***appendiceal n.*** Neuroma found in the mucosa and submucosa of the appendix.

***n. cutis*** Neuroma in the skin.

***cystic n.*** Neuroma with cystic formations.

***false n.*** A tumor arising from the connective tissue of nerves, including the myelin sheath. SYN: *neurofibroma; pseudoneuroma.*

***ganglionated n.*** Neuroma composed of true nerve cells.

***multiple n.*** Neurofibromatosis.

***myelinic n.*** Neuroma composed of medullated nerve fibers.

***plexiform n.*** Neuroma of nerve trunks that appear to be twisted.

***n. telangiectodes*** Neuroma containing

an abundance of blood vessels.

***traumatic n.*** An unorganized mass of nerve fibers occurring in wounds or on an amputation stump, resulting after accidental or intentional incision of the nerve.

**neuromalacia** (nū″rō-măl-ā′sē-ă) [″ + *malakia,* softening] Pathological softening of neural tissue.

**neuromatosis** (nū-rō″mă-tō′sĭs) [″ + *oma,* tumor, + *osis,* condition] A condition characterized by the occurrence of multiple neuromas in the body.

**neuromere** (nū′rō-mēr) [″ + *meros,* part] One of a series of segmental elevations on the ventrolateral surface of the rhombencephalon. SYN: *rhombomere.*

**neuromodulator** Biologically active substances produced by neurons that enhance or diminish the effects of neurotransmitters. Some neuromodulators are substance P, cholecystokinin, and somatostatin. SEE: *neuron; neurotransmitter.*

**neuromuscular** (nū″rō-mŭs′kū-lăr) [″ + L. *musculus,* a muscle] Concerning both nerves and muscles.

***n. blocking agent*** A drug that causes muscle paralysis by blocking the transmission of nerve stimuli to muscles. It is esp. useful as an adjunct to anesthesia to induce skeletal muscle relaxation, to facilitate the management of patients undergoing mechanical ventilation, and to facilitate tracheal intubation. It is also used to treat status epilepticus and to reduce metabolic demands by preventing shivering or muscle rigidity.

---

Caution: This drug may cause respiratory depression and should be administered only by those experienced in artificial respiration and administration of oxygen under positive pressure.

---

**neuromyasthenia** (nū″rō-mī″ăs-thē′nē-ă) [″ + *mys,* muscle, + *astheneia,* weakness] Muscular weakness usually due to an emotional disorder.

**neuromyelitis** (nū″rō-mī-ĕl-ī′tĭs) [″ + *myelos,* marrow, + *itis,* inflammation] Inflammation of nerves and the spinal cord.

***n. optica*** A syndrome resulting from demyelinization occurring in the spinal cord, optic nerves, and chiasma. The cause of this condition is unknown, but it may be a variant form of multiple sclerosis.

**neuromyopathy** (nū″rō-mī-ŏp′ă-thē) [″ + *mys,* muscle, + *pathos,* disease, suffering] Pert. to pathological conditions involving both muscles and nerves.

**neuromyositis** (nū″rō-mī″ō-sī′tĭs) [″ + ″ + *itis,* inflammation] Neuritis complicated by inflammation of muscles that come in contact with the affected nerves.

**neuron** (nū′rŏn) [Gr. *neuron,* nerve, sinew] A nerve cell, the structural and functional unit of the nervous system. A neuron consists of a cell body (perikaryon) and its processes, an axon and one or more dendrites. Neurons function in initiation and conduction of impulses. They transmit impulses to other neurons or cells by releasing neurotransmitters at synapses. Alternatively, a neuron may release neurohormones into the bloodstream. SYN: *nerve cell.* SEE: illus. **neuronal** (nū′rō-năl), *adj.*

***afferent n.*** A neuron that conducts sensory impulses toward the brain or spinal cord.

***associative n.*** A neuron that mediates impulses between a sensory and a motor neuron.

***bipolar n.*** **1.** A neuron that bears two processes. **2.** A neuron of the retina that receives impulses from the rods and cones and transmits them to a ganglion neuron. SEE: *retina* for illus.

***central n.*** A neuron confined entirely to the central nervous system.

***commissural n.*** A neuron whose axon crosses to the opposite side of the brain or spinal cord.

***efferent n.*** A neuron that conducts motor impulses away from the brain or spinal cord.

***ganglion n.*** A neuron of the retina that receives impulses from bipolar neurons. Axons of ganglion neurons converge at the optic disk to form the optic nerve. SEE: *retina* for illus.

***internuncial n.*** Interneuron.

***lower motor n.*** A neuron whose cell body lies in the anterior gray column of spinal cord. Its axon innervates striated muscle fibers.

***motor n.*** A neuron that conveys impulses initiating muscle contraction or glandular secretion. SYN: *motoneuron.*

***multipolar n.*** A neuron with one axon and many dendrites.

***peripheral n.*** A neuron whose process constitutes a part of the peripheral nervous system (cranial, spinal, or autonomic nerves).

***postganglionic n.*** A neuron whose cell body lies in an autonomic ganglion and whose axon terminates in an effector organ (smooth or cardiac muscle or glands).

***preganglionic n.*** A neuron of the autonomic nervous system whose cell body lies in the central nervous system and whose axon terminates in peripheral ganglia.

***sensory n.*** An afferent neuron that carries impulses from receptors to the central nervous system.

***unipolar n.*** A neuron whose cell body bears one process.

***upper motor n.*** A neuron whose cell body lies in the motor area of the cerebral cortex. Its axon passes down the spinal cord and synapses with the lower motor neurons.

**neuronephric** (nū″rō-nĕf′rĭk) [″ + *nephros,* kidney] Concerning the nervous and renal systems.

**neuronevus** (nū″rō-nē′vŭs) An intradermal

nevus.

**neuronitis** (nū-rō-nī′tĭs) [Gr. *neuron,* nerve, + *itis,* inflammation] Inflammation or degenerative inflammation of nerve cells.

**neuronophage** (nū-rŏn′ō-fāj) [″ + *phagein,* to eat] A phagocyte that destroys tissue in the nervous system.

**neuronophagia, neuronophagy** (nū-rŏn″ō-fā′jē-ă, -ŏf′ă-jē) Destruction of nerve cells by phagocytes.

**neuro-ophthalmology** (nū″rō-ŏf″thăl-mŏl′ŏ-jē) [″ + *ophthalmos,* eye, + *logos,* word, reason] The branch of ophthalmology concerned with the neurology of the visual system.

**neuro-optic** (nū″rō-ŏp′tĭk) [″ + *optikos,* pert. to vision] Concerning the central nervous system and the eye.

**neuropacemaker** An implantable device for electrical stimulation of the spinal cord. The electrical energy is provided in pulses at an appropriate rate in order to inhibit

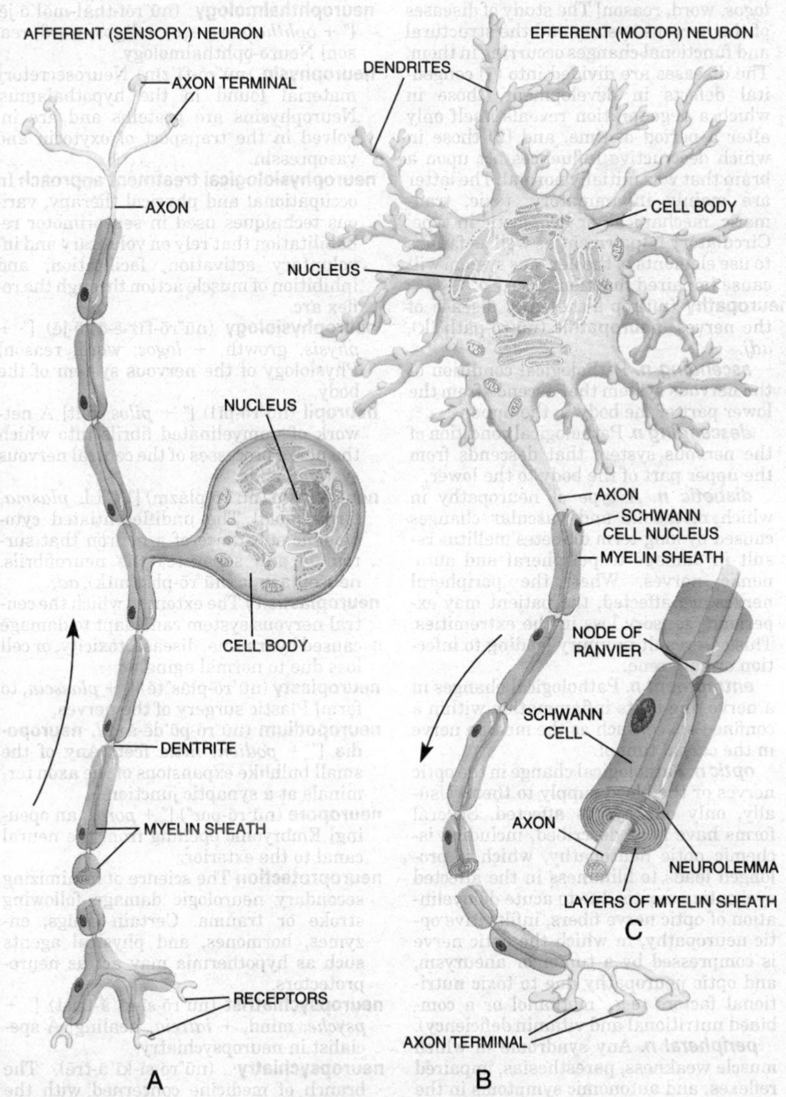


**NEURON STRUCTURE**

**(A)** SENSORY NEURON **(B)** MOTOR NEURON (ARROWS INDICATE DIRECTION OF IMPULSE TRANSMISSION) **(C)** MYELIN SHEATH AND NEUROLEMMA FORMED BY SCHWANN CELLS

the perception of pain.

**neuropapillitis** (nū″rō-păp″ĭ-lī′tĭs) [″ + L. *papilla,* nipple, + Gr. *itis,* inflammation] Optic neuritis.

**neuropathogenesis** (nū″rō-păth″ō-jĕn′ĕ-sĭs) [″ + *pathos,* disease, suffering, + *genesis,* generation, birth] The origin and development of a neural disease.

**neuropathogenicity** (nū″rō-păth″ō-jĕ-nĭs′ĭ-tē) [″ + *pathos,* disease, suffering, + *gennan,* to produce] The ability to cause pathological changes in nerves.

**neuropathology** (nū″rō-pă-thŏl′ō-jē) [″ + ″ + *logos,* word, reason] The study of diseases of the nervous system and the structural and functional changes occurring in them. The diseases are divided into (1) congenital defects in development, those in which a degeneration reveals itself only after a period of time, and (2) those in which destructive influences act upon a brain that was initially normal. The latter are mainly inflammatory, toxic, traumatic, mechanical, or neoplastic in type. Circulatory impairment as well as failure to use elements of the nervous system will cause impaired function.

**neuropathy** (nū-rŏp′ă-thē) Any disease of the nerves. **neuropathic** (nū-rō-păth′ĭk), *adj.*

***ascending n.*** Pathological condition of the nervous system that ascends from the lower part of the body to the upper.

***descending n.*** Pathological condition of the nervous system that descends from the upper part of the body to the lower.

***diabetic n.*** A type of neuropathy in which metabolic and vascular changes caused by long-term diabetes mellitus result in damage to peripheral and autonomic nerves. When the peripheral nerves are affected, the patient may experience sensory loss in the extremities. This can result in injury leading to infection or gangrene.

***entrapment n.*** Pathological changes in a nerve due to its inflammation within a confined space, such as the median nerve in the carpal tunnel.

***optic n.*** Pathological change in the optic nerves or the blood supply to them. Usually, only one eye is affected. Several forms have been described, including ischemic optic neuropathy, which if prolonged leads to blindness in the affected eye, optic neuritis due to acute demyelination of optic nerve fibers, infiltrative optic neuropathy, in which the optic nerve is compressed by a tumor or aneurysm, and optic neuropathy due to toxic nutritional factors (e.g., methanol or a combined nutritional and vitamin deficiency).

***peripheral n.*** Any syndrome in which muscle weakness, paresthesias, impaired reflexes, and autonomic symptoms in the hands and feet are common. This syndrome occurs in patients with diabetes mellitus, renal or hepatic failure, alcoholism, or certain medications such as phenytoin and isoniazid. Also called *polyneuritis*; *polyneuropathy*.

**neuropharmacology** (nū″rō-făr″mă-kŏl′ō-jē) [″ + *pharmakon,* drug, + *logos,* word, reason] The branch of pharmacology concerned with the effects of drugs on the nervous system.

**neurophilic** (nū″rō-fĭl′ĭk) [″ + *philos,* fond] Having an affinity for nervous tissue.

**neurophonia** (nū″rō-fō′nē-ă) [Gr. *neuron,* nerve, + *phone,* voice] A tic or spasm of the muscles of speech resulting in an involuntary cry or sound.

**neurophthalmology** (nū″rŏf-thăl-mŏl′ō-jē) [″ + *ophthalmos,* eye, + *logos,* word, reason] Neuro-ophthalmology.

**neurophysin** (nū″rō-fī′zĭn) Neurosecretory material found in the hypothalamus. Neurophysins are proteins and are involved in the transport of oxytocin and vasopressin.

**neurophysiological treatment approach** In occupational and physical therapy, various techniques used in sensorimotor rehabilitation that rely on voluntary and involuntary activation, facilitation, and inhibition of muscle action through the reflex arc.

**neurophysiology** (nū″rō-fĭz-ē-ŏl′ō-jē) [″ + *physis,* growth, + *logos,* word, reason] Physiology of the nervous system of the body.

**neuropil** (nū′rō-pĭl) [″ + *pilos,* felt] A network of unmyelinated fibrils into which the nerve processes of the central nervous system divide.

**neuroplasm** (nū′rō-plăzm) [″ + LL. *plasma,* form, mold] The undifferentiated cytoplasmic substance of a neuron that surrounds and separates the neurofibrils. **neuroplasmic** (nū″rō-plăz′mĭk), *adj.*

**neuroplasticity** The extent to which the central nervous system can adapt to damage caused by trauma, disease, toxicity, or cell loss due to normal aging.

**neuroplasty** (nū′rō-plăs″tē) [″ + *plassein,* to form] Plastic surgery of the nerves.

**neuropodium** (nū″rō-pō′dē-ă) *pl.* **neuropodia** [″ + *podion,* little feet] Any of the small bulblike expansions of the axon terminals at a synaptic junction.

**neuropore** (nū′rō-por″) [″ + *poros,* an opening] Embryonic opening from the neural canal to the exterior.

**neuroprotection** The science of minimizing secondary neurologic damage following stroke or trauma. Certain drugs, enzymes, hormones, and physical agents such as hypothermia may act as neuroprotectors.

**neuropsychiatrist** (nū″rō-sī-kī′ă-trĭst) [″ + *psyche,* mind, + *iatreia,* healing] A specialist in neuropsychiatry.

**neuropsychiatry** (nū″rō-sī-kī′ă-trē) The branch of medicine concerned with the study and treatment of both nervous and mental diseases.

**neuropsychopharmacology** (nū″rō-sī″kō-făr″mă-kŏl′ō-jē) [″ + ″+ *pharmakon,* drug, + *logos,* word, reason] The study of the effects of drugs on mental illness.

**neuroradiography** (nū″rō-rā″dē-ŏg′ră-fē) [″ + L. *radius,* ray, + Gr. *graphein,* to write] Radiography of the structures of the nervous system.

**neuroradiology** (nū″rō-rā″dē-ŏl′ō-jē) [″ + ″ + Gr. *logos,* word, reason] The branch of medicine that utilizes radiography for diagnosis of pathology of the nervous system.

**neuroretinitis** (nū″rō-rĕt″ĭn-ī′tĭs) [″ + L. *retina,* retina, + Gr. *itis,* inflammation] Inflammation of the optic nerve and retina.

**neuroretinopathy** (nū″rō-rĕt″ĭ-nŏp′ă-thē) [″ + ″ + Gr. *pathos,* disease, suffering] Pathology of the retina and optic nerve.

**neurorrhaphy** (nū-ror′ă-fē) [″ + *rhaphe,* seam, ridge] The suturing of the ends of a severed nerve.

**neurosarcocleisis** (nū″rō-săr″kō-klī′sĭs) [″ + *sarx,* flesh, + *kleisis,* closure] Operation for the relief of neuralgia by resection of a wall of the osseous canal carrying a nerve and transplanting the nerve to soft tissues.

**neurosarcoma** (nū″rō-săr-kō′mă) [″ + ″ + *oma,* tumor] A sarcoma containing neuromatous components.

**neuroscience** (nū″rō-sī′ĕns) Any one of the various branches of science (e.g., embryology, anatomy, physiology, histopathology, biochemistry, pharmacology) concerned with the growth, development, and function of the nervous system.

**neurosclerosis** (nū″rō-sklĕ-rō′sĭs) [″ + *sklerosis,* a hardening] Hardening of nervous tissue.

**neurosecretion** (nū″rō-sē-krē′shŭn) [″ + L. *secretio,* separation] The elaboration and discharge of a chemical substance by a neuron, such as the secretion of hormones by cells of the hypothalamus.

**neurosensory** (nū″rō-sĕn′sō-rē) [″ + L. *sensorius,* pert. to a sensation] Concerning a sensory nerve.

**neurosis** (nū-rō′sĭs) *pl.* **neuroses** [″ + *osis,* condition] The definition of this term is controversial. Some feel its use should be limited to describing an unpleasant mental symptom in an individual with intact reality testing; others would have it apply to the etiological process, i.e., unconscious conflict that arouses anxiety and leads to maladaptive use of defensive mechanisms that result in symptom formation. Alternatively, some consider the neuroses to have a physical basis. To further confuse the picture, some would entirely abandon the terms neurosis and psychoneurosis and replace them with anxiety disorders (panic states, phobias, and obsessive-compulsive neuroses) and somatoform disorders (hysteria, conversion symptoms, and hypochondriasis). The various neuroses listed below are of both the descriptive and etiological types. SYN: *psychoneurosis.* SEE: *neurotic disorder.*

TREATMENT: Psychotherapy, tranquilizers, and sedatives. It must be remembered that in general, a symptom due to a neurotic reaction to a situation is just as real to the patient as if it were due to organic disease. Usually such a symptom is much more difficult to treat than it would be if due to organic disease.

***anxiety n.*** Neurosis marked by excessive anxiety or apprehension that is not restricted to specific situations or objects, unlike the normal anxiety occurring in genuinely threatening situations. Anxiety neurosis is often associated with somatic symptoms, such as palpitation, heart pain, dyspepsia, constriction of the throat, bandlike pressure about the head, or cold, sweaty, tremulous extremities, manifesting in an individual free of organic disease, during clear consciousness. SEE: *effort syndrome.*

***cardiac n.*** Neurocirculatory asthenia.

***compensation n.*** A form of malingering that develops subsequent to an injury in the belief that financial or other forms of compensation can be obtained or will be continued by being ill. SYN: *pension neurosis.* SEE: *factitious disorders.*

***compulsion n.*** A neurosis marked by the overpowering impulse to perform certain acts or rituals repetitively (e.g., hand-washing, counting, touching).

***expectation n.*** Condition in which anticipation of an event produces nervous symptoms.

***hysterical n.*** An outmoded term. SEE: *somatization disorder.*

***obsessional n.*** Neurosis in which recurrent and persistent thoughts dominate the victim's behavior, such as reluctance to shake hands for fear of contamination.

***war n.*** Neurosis brought on by conditions of war, seen in soldiers.

**neuroskeleton** (nū″rō-skĕl′ĕ-tŏn) [Gr. *neuron,* nerve, + *skeleton,* a dried-up body] That portion of the skeleton that surrounds and protects the nervous system, i.e., the cranium, and spinal column. **neuroskeletal** (-tăl), *adj.*

**neurosome** (nū′rō-sōm) [″ + *soma,* body] **1.** The body of a neuron. **2.** One of the minute granules in the protoplasm of nerve cells.

**neurospasm** (nū′rō-spăzm) [″ + *spasmos,* a convulsion] Spasmodic muscular twitching due to a nervous disorder.

**neurosplanchnic** (nū″rō-splăngk′nĭk) [″ + *splanchnikos,* pert. to the viscera] Concerning the sympathetic and parasympathetic nervous system.

**neurospongioma** (nū″rō-spŏn″jē-ō′mă) [″ + *spongos,* sponge, + *oma,* tumor] Spongioblastoma.

**Neurospora** (nū-rŏs′pō-ră) Genus of fungi belonging to the Ascomycetes class. It includes certain bread molds.

**neurosurgeon** (nū″rō-sŭr′jŭn) A physician specializing in surgery of the nervous system.

**neurosurgery** [Gr. *neuron,* nerve, sinew, +

L. *chirurgia,* hand, + *ergon,* work] Surgery of the nervous system.

**neurosyphilis** (nū″rō-sĭf′ĭ-lĭs) Syphilis affecting the nervous structures. SEE: *dementia paralytica.*

***asymptomatic n.*** Neurosyphilis showing no symptoms. It is diagnosed by changes in spinal fluid.

***meningovascular n.*** A form of neurosyphilis involving the meninges and vascular structures in the brain or spinal cord, or in both.

***paretic n.*** Dementia paralytica.

***tabetic n.*** Tabes dorsalis.

**neurotendinous** (nū″rō-tĕn′dĭ-nŭs) [″ + L. *tendinosus,* tendinous] Concerning a nerve and tendon.

**neurotension** (nū″rō-tĕn′shŭn) [″ + L. *tensio,* a stretching] Surgical stretching of a nerve. SYN: *neurectasia.*

**neurothecitis** (nū″rō-thē-sī′tĭs) [″ + *theke,* sheath, + *itis,* inflammation] Inflammation of a nerve sheath.

**neurothele** (nū″rō-thē′lē) [″ + *thele,* nipple] A nerve papilla.

**neurotic** (nū-rŏt′ĭk) [Gr. *neuron,* nerve, sinew] **1.** One suffering from a neurosis. **2.** Pert. to neurosis. **3.** Nervous.

**neurotic disorder** A mental disorder in which the predominant disturbance is a symptom or group of symptoms that is distressing to the individual and is recognized by that person as being unacceptable, undesirable, and alien (ego-dystonic). Reality testing is grossly intact and behavior is socially acceptable. This disorder is chronic unless treated. This term does not imply that there is a special etiological process. SEE: *neurosis.*

**neuroticism** (nū-rŏt′ĭ-sĭzm) [″ + *-ismos,* condition] A condition or trait of neurosis.

**neurotization** (nū″rŏt-ĭ-zā′shŭn) [Gr. *neuron,* nerve, sinew] **1.** Regeneration of a nerve after division. **2.** Surgical introduction of a nerve into a paralyzed muscle.

**neurotmesis** (nū″rŏt-mē′sĭs) [″ + *tmesis,* cutting] Nerve injury with complete loss of function of the nerve even though there is little apparent anatomic damage.

**neurotology** (nū″rŏ-tŏl′ō-jē) [″ + *ous,* ear, + *logos,* word, reason] Otoneurology.

**neurotome** (nū′rō-tōm) A fine knife used in the division of a nerve.

**neurotomy** (nū-rŏt′ō-mē) [″ + *tome,* an incision] Division or dissection of a nerve.

**neurotonic** (nū″rō-tŏn′ĭk) [″ + *tonos,* tension] **1.** Concerning neural stretching. **2.** Having a stimulating effect upon nerves or the nervous system.

**neurotony** (nū-rŏt′ō-nē) Nerve stretching, usually to ease pain.

**neurotoxicity** (nū″rō-tŏk-sĭs′ĭ-tē) [″ + *toxikon,* poison] Having the capability of harming nerve tissue.

**neurotoxin** (nū″rō-tŏks′ĭn) A substance that attacks nerve cells. SYN: *neurolysin.* **neurotoxic** (-ĭk), *adj.*

**neurotransmitter** (nū″rō-trăns′mĭt-ĕr) Substance (e.g., norepinephrine, acetylcholine, or dopamine) that is released when the axon terminal of a presynaptic neuron is excited. The substance then travels across the synapse to act on the target cell to either inhibit or excite it. Disorders in the brain physiology of neurotransmitters have been implicated in the pathogenesis of a variety of psychiatric illnesses. SEE: *substance P.*

**neurotrauma** (nū-rō-traw′mă) [″ + *trauma,* wound] Injury of a nerve.

**neurotripsy** (nū″rō-trĭp′sē) [″ + *tripsis,* a rubbing] Surgical crushing of a nerve.

**neurotubule** (nū″rō-too′būl) [″ + L. *tubulus,* a tubule] A microtubule in nerve cells, dendrites, and axons, that may be seen by use of electron microscopy.

**neurovaccine** (nū″rō-văk′sĭn) A standardized vaccine virus of specific strength, usually prepared by cultivation in a rabbit's brain.

**neurovascular** (nū″rō-văs′kū-lăr) [″ + L. *vasculus,* a small vessel] Concerning both the nervous and vascular systems.

**neurovegetative** (nū″rō-vĕj′ĕ-tā″tĭv) Concerning the autonomic nervous system.

**neurovirus** (nū″rō-vī′rŭs) Virus that has been modified by its growth in nervous tissue and used in preparing vaccines.

**neurovisceral** (nū″rō-vĭs′ĕr-ăl) [″ + L. *viscera,* body organs] Neurosplanchnic.

**neurula** (nū′roo-lă) The stage in the development of an embryo (esp. amphibian embryos) during which the neural plate develops and axial embryonic nervous structures are elaborated.

**neurulation** (nū″roo-lā′shŭn) Formation of the neural plate in the embryo and the development and closure of the neural tube.

**neutral** (nū′trăl) [L. *neutralis,* neither] **1.** Neither alkaline nor acid. **2.** Indifferent; having no positive qualities or opinions. **3.** Pert. to electrical charges that are neither positive nor negative.

***n. fat*** SEE: *fat.*

***n. point*** A point on the pH scale (pH 7.0) that represents neutrality, i.e., the solution is neither acid or alkaline in reaction.

***n. red*** SEE: *red.*

**neutralization** (nū″trăl-ĭ-zā′shŭn) **1.** The opposing of one force or condition with an opposite force or condition to such degree as to cause counteraction that permits neither to dominate. **2.** In chemistry, the process of destroying the peculiar properties or effect of a substance (e.g., the neutralization of an acid with a base or vice versa). **3.** In medicine, the process of checking or counteracting the effects of any agent that produces a morbid effect.

**neutralize** (nū′trăl-īz) **1.** To counteract and make ineffective. **2.** In chemistry, to destroy peculiar properties or effect; to make inert.

**neutrino** (nū-trē′nō) In physics, a subatomic particle at rest, with no mass and no electric charge. These particles are constantly flowing through the universe and are not known to affect the matter through which they pass.

**neutroclusion** (nū″trŏ-kloo′zhŭn) [L. *neuter,* neither, + *occludo,* to close] A state in which the anteroposterior occlusal positions of the teeth or the mesiodistal positions are normal but malocclusion of other teeth exists.

**neutron** (nū′trŏn) [L. *neuter,* neither] A subatomic particle equal in mass to a proton but without an electric charge. It is believed to be a particle of all nuclei of mass number greater than one. As a free particle, it has an average life of about 12 minutes.

**neutron capture analysis** The use of the ability of a neutron to be absorbed (captured) by an atomic nucleus to detect the presence of various substances.

**neutropenia** (nū-trō-pē′nē-ă) [″ + Gr. *penia,* lack] The presence of an abnormally small number of neutrophil cells in the blood.

***malignant n.*** Agranulocytosis.

**neutrophil, neutrophile** (nū′trō-fĭl, -fīl) [″ + Gr. *philein,* to love] A granular white blood cell (WBC), the most common type (55% to 70%) of WBC. Neutrophils are responsible for much of the body's protection against infection. They play a primary role in inflammation, are readily attracted to foreign antigens (chemotaxis), and destroy them by phagocytosis. Neutrophils killed during inflammation release an enzyme that dissolves all cells in the immediate area, resulting in the formation of pus. An inadequate number of neutrophils (neutropenia) leaves the body at high risk for infection from many sources and requires protective precautions on the part of health care workers. Leukemia patients receiving chemotherapy, which destroys all leukocytes, must be carefully protected from infections during the course of therapy and until the bone marrow produces additional leukocytes.

As part of a severe inflammatory response or autoimmune disorder, neutrophils may begin attacking normal cells and cause tissue damage. This occurs in adult respiratory distress syndrome, inflammatory bowel disease, myocarditis, and rheumatoid arthritis. Corticosteroids are the most commonly used drugs to minimize the damage caused by severe inflammation. SYN: *polymorphonuclear leukocyte.* SEE: illus.; *blood* for illus.

**neutrophilia** (nū″trō-fĭl′ē-ă) Increase in the number of neutrophilic leukocytes in the blood.

**neutrophilic, neutrophilous** (nū-trō-fĭl′ĭk, -trŏf′ĭ-lŭs) [″ + Gr. *philein,* to love] Staining readily with neutral dyes.

**neutrotaxis** (nū″trō-tăk′sĭs) [*neutrophil* + Gr. *taxis,* arrangement] The phenomenon in which neutrophils are repelled by or attracted to a substance.

**nevocarcinoma** (nē″vō-kăr″sĭ-nō′mă) [L. *naevus,* birthmark, + Gr. *karkinos,* crab, + *oma,* tumor] Malignant melanoma.

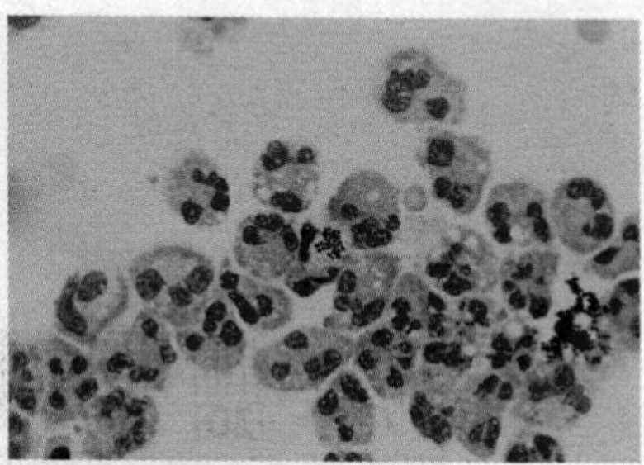

NEUTROPHILS (ORIG. MAG. ×1000) (WITH INGESTED BACTERIA)

**nevoid** (nē′voyd) [″ + Gr. *eidos,* form, shape] Resembling a nevus.

**nevolipoma** (nē″vō-lĭ-pō′mă) [″+ Gr. *lipos,* fat, + *oma,* tumor] Nevus lipomatodes.

**nevose** (nē′vōs) [L. *naevus,* birthmark] Spotted or marked with nevi. SEE: *nevus.*

**nevoxanthoendothelioma** (nē″vō-zăn″thō-ĕn″dō-thē″lē-ō′mă) [″ + Gr. *xanthos,* yellow, + *endon,* within, + *thele,* nipple, + *oma,* tumor] Juvenile xanthogranuloma. SEE: *xanthogranuloma.*

**nevus** (nē′vŭs) *pl.* **nevi** [L. *naevus,* birthmark] **1.** A congenital discoloration of a circumscribed area of the skin due to pigmentation. SYN: *birthmark; mole.* **2.** A circumscribed vascular tumor of the skin, usually congenital, due to hyperplasia of the blood vessels. SEE: *angioma.*

***n. araneus*** Acquired or congenital dilatation of the capillaries, marked by red lines radiating from a central red dot. SYN: *spider nevus.*

***blue n.*** A dark blue nevus covered by smooth skin. It is composed of melanin-pigmented spindle cells in the mid-dermis.

***blue rubber bleb n.*** An erectile, easily compressable, bluish, cavernous hemangioma that is present in the skin and gastrointestinal tract.

***capillary n.*** A nevus of dilated capillary vessels elevated above the skin. It is usually treated by ligature and excision.

***n. comedonicus*** A horny nevus that contains a hard plug of keratin. It is caused by failure of the pilosebaceous follicles to develop normally.

***connective tissue n.*** A nevus composed of collagenous tissue.

***cutaneous n.*** A nevus formation on the skin.

***epidermal n.*** Raised lesions present at birth. They may be hyperkeratotic and widely distributed.

***n. flammeus*** A large reddish-purple discoloration of the face or neck, usually not elevated above the skin. It is considered a serious deformity due to its large

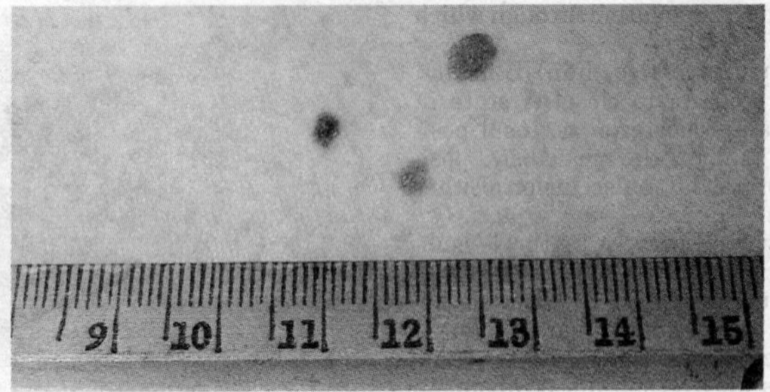


JUNCTION NEVI

size and color. In children, these have been treated with the flashlamp-pulsed tunable dye laser. SYN: *port-wine stain.*

***hairy n.*** A nevus covered by a heavy growth of hair. It is usually darkly pigmented. SYN: *nevus pilosus.*

***halo n.*** A papular brown nevus with an oval halo occurring in the first three decades of life. This type of nevus is usually benign, but should be evaluated for malignancy.

***intradermal n.*** A nevus in which the melanocytes are found in nests in the dermis and have no connection with the deeper layers from which they were formed.

***Ito's n.*** Mongolian spot–like cutaneous lesion over the shoulders, supraclavicular areas, sides of the neck, scapula areas, and upper arms. It is present at birth and tends to disappear with time, usually by age 4 or 5. Although cosmetically undesirable, the lesion is benign.

***junction n.*** A nevus in the basal cell zone at the junction of the epidermis and dermis. It is slightly raised, pigmented, and does not contain hair. This type of nevus may become malignant. SEE: illus.

***n. lipomatodes*** A tumor composed of fatty connective tissue. It is probably a degenerated nevus containing numerous blood vessels. SYN: *nevolipoma.*

***melanocytic n.*** Any nevus that contains melanocytes.

***nevocytic n.*** A common mole. Moles may appear at any age. They are classified according to their stage of growth and whether or not they are still growing.

***Ota's n.*** A lesion resembling a mongolian spot in the skin surrounding the eye and on the face. Some infants with this condition will have bluish discoloration of the sclera of the eye on the affected side. SEE: *mongolian spot.*

***n. pigmentosus*** A congenital pigment spot varying in color from light yellow to black. Intradermal or nevocytic nevi are benign. Other types of nevi may become malignant.

TREATMENT: Malignant or suspicious lesions should be treated by wide surgical excision. Benign lesions do not require treatment except when located at sites of friction causing bleeding or ulceration. Some nevi are removed for cosmetic reasons.

***sebaceous n.*** An epidermal nevus containing sebaceous gland tissue.

***spider n.*** N. araneus.

***n. spilus*** A pigmented nevus with a smooth, unraised surface.

***n. spongiosus albus mucosae*** A white, spongy nevus that may occur in the mouth, labia, vagina, or rectum. SYN: *white sponge n.*

***strawberry n.*** N. vascularis.

***telangiectatic n.*** A nevus containing dilated capillaries.

***n. unius lateris*** A congenital nevus that occurs in streaks or linear bands on one side of the body. They usually occur between the neurotomes of the lumbar or sacral area.

***n. vascularis*** A nevus in which superficial blood vessels are enlarged. Nevi of this type are usually congenital. They are of variable size and shape, slightly elevated, and red or purple in color. They generally appear on the face, head, neck, and arms, though no region is exempt. The nevi usually disappear spontaneously, but wrinkling, pigmentation, and scarring are sometimes seen. SYN: *strawberry mark.*

***n. venosus*** A nevus formed of dilated venules.

***n. verrucosus*** A nevus with a raised, wartlike surface.

***white sponge n.*** N. spongiosus albus mucosae.

**newborn 1.** Born recently. **2.** A term applied to human infants less than 28 days old. SYN: *neonate.*

**Newcastle disease** (nū′kăs-ĕl) [Newcastle, England] An acute viral disease of birds, particularly chickens. It occasionally produces accidental infections in humans, usually in the form of a mild conjunctivitis.

**Newman, Margaret** Nursing educator, born 1933, who developed the Theory of Health as Expanding Consciousness. SEE: *Nurs-*

*ing Theory Appendix.*

**newton** SYMB: N. The name of a measure of force derived from the base units used in SI units of measurement. It is equal to the force that will accelerate one kilogram a meter per second squared, $10^5$ dynes. SEE: *SI Units Appendix.*

**newton meter** SYMB: Nm. In SI units, one newton per square meter. This is called one pascal (Pa). Thus 1 Pa = 1N/M$^2$.

**nexus** (nĕk′sŭs) *pl.* **nexus** [L., bond] A connection or link; a binding together. It is used to designate a bond between components of a group.

**NF** *National Formulary.*

**N.F.L.P.N.** *National Federation of Licensed Practical Nurses.*

**NFPA** *National Fire Protection Association.*

**ng** *nanogram.*

**NG tube** *nasogastric* tube.

**$NH_3$** Ammonia.

**$NH_4^+$** The univalent ammonium radical.

**$NH_4Br$** Ammonium bromide.

**$NH_4Cl$** Ammonium chloride.

**N.H.I.** *National Heart Institute.*

**NHL** *non-Hodgkin's lymphoma.*

**N.H.L.I.** *National Heart and Lung Institute.*

**$NH_4NO_3$** Ammonium nitrate.

**$NH_4OH$** Ammonium hydroxide.

**Ni** Symbol for the element nickel.

**NIA** *National Institute on Aging.*

**NIAAA** *National Institute on Alcohol Abuse and Alcoholism.*

**niacin** (nī′ă-sĭn) The antipellagra factor of vitamin B complex, occuring naturally in liver, yeast, milk, cheese, and cereals. Niacin is used orally or parenterally for treatment of pellagra. Niacin is part of NAD and NADP, coenzymes that are essential for metabolic processes in each cell of the body. Thus a deficiency decreases cellular function throughout the body. Trade names are Nicobid, Nicocap, and Nicolar. SYN: *nicotinic acid.*

Caution: Niacin has been used as a self-medication by persons seeking to control hypercholesterolemia. Taken in excess, niacin can cause hyperglycemia, dry skin, itching, flushing, and abnormal liver function tests.

**niacinamide** (nī″ă-sĭn-ăm′īd) Nicotinamide.

**N.I.A.I.D.** *National Institute of Allergy and Infectious Diseases.*

**N.I.A.M.D.** *National Institute of Arthritis and Metabolic Diseases.*

**NIAMSD** *National Institute of Arthritis and Musculoskeletal and Skin Diseases.*

**nib** (nĭb) In dentistry, the smooth or serrated blade of a condensing instrument that contacts the restorative material placed in a cavity preparation.

**nicardipine** A calcium channel blocker.

**niche** (nĭch) [Fr.] A depression or recess on a smooth surface, esp. an erosion in the wall of a hollow organ, detected by radiography.

***enamel n.*** One of two depressions that develop between the dental lamina and the enamel organ.

**N.I.C.H.H.D.** *National Institute of Child Health and Human Development.*

**nickel** SYMB: Ni. A metallic element with an atomic weight of 58.70 and an atomic number of 28.

***n. carbonyl*** $Ni(CO)_4$. An industrial chemical used in plating metals. It is toxic when inhaled, causing pulmonary edema.

**nicking 1.** Compression of the retinal vessels of the eye at the point where a vein and an artery cross, seen in hypertensive cardiovascular disease. **2.** To notch a tissue.

**niclosamide** (nĭ-klō′să-mīd) An anthelminthic esp. effective against the cestodes that infect humans.

**Nicolas-Favre disease** (nē″kō-lă-făv′r) [Josef Nicolas, b. 1868, and M. Favre, 1876–1954, Fr. physicians] Lymphogranuloma venereum.

**nicotinamide** (nĭk″ō-tĭn′ă-mīd) A basic amide that is a member of the vitamin B complex, used in the prophylaxis and treatment of pellagra. The peripheral flush that often accompanies therapy with nicotinic acid is avoided with nicotinamide. SYN: *niacinamide.*

***n. adenine dinucleotide*** ABBR: NAD. An enzyme that is important in accepting electrons in the course of metabolic reactions. In its oxydized form, $NAD^+$ gives up its electron and is converted to the reduced form, NADH.

***n. adenine dinucleotide-dehydrogenase*** SEE: *nicotinamide adenine dinucleotide phosphate.*

***n. adenine dinucleotide phosphate*** ABBR: NADP. A coenzyme that contains adenosine, nicotinamide, and phosphoric acid. When in its oxydized form ($NADP^+$), it serves as an electron carrier in catabolic and anabolic reactions. In its reduced form (NADPH or NADPH-diaphorase), it is important in reducing the ferric iron ($Fe^{+++}$) to its ferrous ($Fe^{++}$) form, thus converting methemoglobin (which is unable to transport oxygen) to hemoglobin (which can transport oxygen). Deficiency of NADPH-diaphorase causes congenital methemoglobinemia. SYN: *methemoglobin reductase.*

**nicotine** (nĭk′ō-tēn, -tĭn) [L. *nicotiana,* tobacco] A poisonous alkaloid found in all parts of the tobacco plant, but esp. in the leaves. When pure, it is a colorless oily fluid with little odor but a sharp burning taste. On exposure to air or in crude materials, it becomes deep brown with the characteristic tobacco-like smell. Nicotine is one of the most toxic and addictive of all poisons. Cigarette tobacco contains varying amounts of nicotine per cigarette. The absolute amount of nicotine in each cigarette is 8 to 9 mg and represents 1.5% to 2.5 % of the weight. The blood nicotine level rises within 10 to 15 sec after each puff. A smoker's average daily nicotine intake varies with the depth of inhalation, how much of each cigarette is smoked, and the total number of cigarettes smoked. Cigarette filters decrease exposure to tar but not to nicotine. Smokers experience withdrawal symptoms when their daily nicotine levels fall below 5 mg.

Smoking during pregnancy is associated with high risk for low-birth-weight infants, prematurity, and perinatal respiratory infections. SEE: *cancer, lung; cotinine; nicotine chewing gum; nicotine poisoning, acute; patch, nicotine; smokeless tobacco.*

**nicotine chewing gum** The incorporation of nicotine in a chewing gum, for use as an aid to stop smoking. Although the success rate is low unless the product is used in conjunction with a smoking cessation program, some individuals who wish to discontinue the use of tobacco products use it alone. Trade name is Nicorette. SEE: *tobacco.*

**nicotine patch** SEE: under *patch.*

**nicotine poisoning, acute** Nicotine is an extremely toxic substance that acts as swiftly as cyanide. The fatal dose for an adult is estimated to be less than 5 mg/kg body weight. SEE: *Poisons and Poisoning Appendix.*

SYMPTOMS: Nausea, salivation, abdominal pain, vomiting, diarrhea, sweating, dizziness, and mental confusion. If dose is sufficient, the patient will collapse, develop shock, convulse, and die of respiratory failure due to paralysis of respiratory muscles.

TREATMENT: If patient is conscious, oral administration of universal antidote, tannic acid, activated charcoal, or strong tea, followed by gastric lavage or an emetic. If patient is unconscious, use gastric lavage. Keep patient warm with external heat and maintain the airway. Artificial or mechanical respiration and oxygen therapy if necessary. If convulsions are severe or persist, intravenous barbiturates in small doses are indicated.

**nicotinic** Pert. to the stimulating effect of acetycholine on the parasympathetic and sympathetic ganglionic or somatic skeletal muscle receptors.

**nicotinic acid** SEE: *niacin.*

**nicotinism** (nĭk′ō-tĭn-ĭzm) Poisoning from excessive use of tobacco or nicotine.

**nictitate** (nĭk′tĭ-tāt) To wink.

**nictitating** (nĭk′tĭ-tāt-ĭng) Winking.

***n. membrane*** SEE: *membrane, nictitating.*

***n. spasm*** Clonic spasm of the eyelid with continuous winking.

**NICU** *neonatal intensive care unit.*

**nidation** (nī-dā′shŭn) The implantation of the fertilized ovum in the lining of the uterus (endometrium) in pregnancy.

**NIDA** *National Institute on Drug Abuse.*

**NIDDM** *non-insulin dependent diabetes mellitus.*

**N.I.D.R.** *National Institute of Dental Research.*

**N.I.D.R.R.** *National Institute of Disability and Rehabilitation Research.*

**nidus** (nī′dŭs) *pl.* **nidi** [L., nest] **1.** A nestlike structure. **2.** Focus of infection. **3.** A nucleus or origin of a nerve. **nidal** (nī′dăl), *adj.*

***n. avis cerebelli*** A deep sulcus on each side of the inferior vermis, separating it from the adjacent lobes of the hemispheres.

***n. hirundinis*** Cerebral depression between the uvula and the posterior velum. SYN: *swallow's nest.*

**Niemann-Pick cell** A foamy, lipid-filled cell present in the spleen and bone marrow in Niemann-Pick disease.

**Niemann-Pick disease** (nē′măn-pĭk) [Albert Niemann, Ger. pediatrician, 1880–1921; Ludwig Pick, Ger. physician, 1868–1944] A disturbance of sphingolipid metabolism characterized by enlargement of liver and spleen (hepatosplenomegaly), anemia, lymphadenopathy, and progressive mental and physical deterioration. It is a hereditary disease, with its onset in early infancy and death usually occurring before the third year. A typical cell, having a foamy appearance and filled with a lipoid believed to be sphingomyelin, can be found in the bone marrow, spleen, or lymph nodes, and aids in establishing the diagnosis.

**night blindness** Decreased ability to see at night. It is caused by lack of visual purple in the rod cells of the retina, or by its slowness to adjust after exposure to light. Night blindness may result from vitamin A deficiency or hereditary factors. SYN: *nyctalopia* (1). SEE: *night vision.*

**nightguard** A dental prosthesis worn at night to prevent traumatic grinding of the teeth during sleep. SEE: *bruxism; occlusal guard.*

**Nightingale, Florence** (nīt′ĭn-gāl) A British philanthropist, 1820–1910, who is considered the founder of nursing as a profession, a formidable statistician, and a pioneering hospital reformer. She was one of many trained nurses to serve in Crimea and dramatically lowered the death rate in the British army by advocating cleanliness and reform of sanitary conditions in hospitals at the battle front. The astonishing decrease in morbidity and mortality at the front riveted the public both in Britain and in the rest of the West, and the Nightingale Fund gained large contributions from donors around the world. The fund was used to establish a school of nursing at St. Thomas' Hospital in London, England, in 1860. The school became a model for nursing schools around the world, and the first nursing school based on the Nightingale model to be established in the U.S. was at Bellevue Hospital in New York.

**Nightingale Pledge** An oath used by nurses on graduation as a pledge of commitment and integrity. The pledge was formulated by a committee of the Farrand School of Nursing, Harper Hospital, Detroit, Michigan, of which Lystra Gretter was the chairperson, and was first administered to the graduating class in 1893.

"I solemnly pledge myself before God and in the presence of this assembly to pass my life in purity and to practice my profession faithfully. I will abstain from whatever is deleterious and mischievous, and will not take or knowingly administer any harmful drug. I will do all in my power to maintain and elevate the standard of my profession, and will hold in confidence all personal matters committed to my keeping and all family affairs coming to my knowledge in the practice of my calling. With loyalty will I endeavor to aid the physician in his work, and devote myself to the welfare of those committed to my care." SEE: *Declaration of Hawaii; Declaration of Geneva; Hippocratic Oath; Prayer of Maimonides.*

**nightmare** (nīt′mār) [AS. *nyht,* night, + *mara,* a demon] A frightening dream accompanied by great fear. SYN: *incubus; oneirodynia.* SEE: *sleep disorder.*

**nightshade** (nīt′shād) [AS. *nihtscada*] Any of several of the plants of the genus *Solanum.*

***deadly n.*** Belladonna.

**night sweat** [AS. *nyht,* night, + *swat,* sweat] Profuse sweating during sleep at night. Often it is an early sign of disease, esp. with intermittent fever. In children, it occurs in rickets and in debilitated states. In perimenopausal women, it is a common vasomotor response to fluctuating hormone levels. The patient should be rubbed down, sponged, and changed into dry clothing.

**night terrors** [″ + L. *terrere,* to frighten] A form of nightmare in children causing them to awaken screaming in terror. The fear continues for a period after the return to consciousness. SYN: *pavor nocturnus.* SEE: *sleep disorder.*

**night vision** The ability to see at night or in light of low intensity. It results from dark adaptation in which the pupil dilates, visual purple increases, and the intensity threshold of the retina is lowered. Any decrease in the oxygen content of the blood is accompanied by some loss of night vision. Thus, smoking cigarettes or being in an atmosphere with decreased oxygen content decreases night vision. SYN: *scotopic vision.*

**nightwalking** Sleepwalking; somnambulism. SEE: *sleep disorder.*

**night work, maladaption to** Difficulty in adapting to sleeping during the day and working at night. In the U.S. about 7.3 million people work at night. Thus, they are forced to attempt to readjust their day-night schedule for working and sleeping. Adaptation may be facilitated by making the work space as light as possible and scheduling the sleep period (8 hours) in a totally dark environment. SEE: *clock, biological; shift work.*

**N.I.G.M.S.** *National Institute of General Medical Sciences.* A division of the National Institutes of Health of the U.S. Department of Health and Human Services.

**nigra** (nī′gră) [L., black] Substantia nigra.

**nigricans** (nī′grĭ-kăns) Blackened.

**nigrities** (nī-grĭsh′ĭ-ēz) Blackness; black pigmentation.

***n. linguae*** A black pigmentation of the tongue.

**nigrostriatal** (nī″grō-strī-ā′tăl) Concerning a bundle of nerve fibers that connect the substantia nigra of the brain to the corpus striatum.

**NIH** *National Institutes of Health* (of the U.S. Department of Health and Human Services).

**nihilism** (nī′ĭ-lĭzm) [L. *nihil,* nothing, + Gr. *-ismos,* condition] **1.** Disbelief in efficacy of medical therapy. **2.** In psychiatry, a delusion in which everything is unreal or does not exist. **nihilistic,** *adj.*

**nikethamide** (nĭ-kĕth′ă-mīd) A drug that is supposed to selectively stimulate central respiratory centers. When used for this purpose in treating respiratory depression due to poisoning from sedative-hypnotic drugs, it is ineffective. Trade name is Coramine.

**Nikolsky's sign** (nĭ-kŏl′skēz) [Pyotr Nikolsky, Russ. dermatologist, 1855–1940] A condition seen in pemphigus, where the external layer of the skin can be detached from the basal layer and rubbed off by slight friction or injury.

**N.I.M.H.** *National Institute of Mental Health,* a division of the National Institutes of Health of the U.S. Department of Health and Human Services.

**NINCDS** *National Institute of Neurological and Communicative Disorders and Stroke.*

**N.I.N.D.B.** *National Institute of Neurological Diseases and Blindness,* a division of the National Institutes of Health of the U.S. Department of Health and Human Services.

**ninth cranial nerve** Glossopharyngeal nerve. SEE: *Cranial Nerves Appendix.*

**niobium** (nī-ō′bē-um) [Mythological Gr. woman, Niobe, who was turned into stone] SYMB: Nb. A chemical element, formerly called columbium, with an atomic number of 41 and an atomic weight of 92.906.

**niphotyphlosis** (nĭf″ō-tĭf-lō′sĭs) [Gr. *nipha,* snow, + *typhlosis,* blindness] Snow blindness.

**nipple** (nĭp′l) [AS. *neble,* a little protuberance] **1.** The protuberance at the tip of each breast from which the lactiferous ducts discharge. The nipple contains erectile tissue and is surrounded by a pigmented area called the areola. The areola may be darker in those women who have borne children. It is supplied with a row of small sebaceous glands (Montgomery's glands) around its base, called areolar glands, which secrete an oily substance to keep it supple. SYN: *mammilla; papilla mamma; teat.* SEE: *breast* for illus. **2.** An artificial substitute for a female nipple to be used on a nursing bottle.

NURSING IMPLICATIONS: *Postpartum:* Nipples are washed with warm water and patted dry, and a nonalcoholic lubricant, such as lanolin or liquid petrolatum, is gently massaged into the nipples and allowed to air dry for 20 to 30 min. The nurse instructs the mother to position the nipple and areola in the infant's mouth properly and to limit the length of early feeding periods to prevent trauma. Cracked or eroded nipples require further intervention and maternal support if breast-feeding is to be successful.

***crater n.*** Retracted n.

***retracted n.*** A nipple whose tip lies below the level of the surrounding skin. Retraction is caused by deficiency of muscle tissue or the flattening of erectile tissue.

***n. shield*** A device consisting of an artificial nipple used by some nursing mothers to protect the natural nipple.

**Nissl body** (nĭs'l) [Franz Nissl, Ger. neurologist, 1860–1919] A large granular body found in nerve cells. They can be demonstrated by selective staining. They are rough endoplasmic reticulum (with ribosomes) and are the site of protein synthesis. Nissl bodies show changes under various physiological conditions, and in pathological conditions they may dissolve and disappear (chromatolysis). SYN: *Nissl granules; tigroid bodies.*

**nit** (nĭt) [AS. *hnitu*] The egg of a louse or any other parasitic insect. SEE: *Pediculus.*

**nitr-** [Gr. *nitron,* salt] Combining form denoting combination with nitrogen or presence of the group $NO_2$.

**nitrate** (nī'trāt) [L. *nitratum*] A salt of nitric acid.

**nitrated** Combined with nitric acid or a nitrate.

**nitration** Combination with nitric acid or a nitrate.

**nitremia** (nī-trē'mē-ă) Azotemia.

**nitric acid** $HNO_3$. A colorless, corrosive, poisonous liquid in concentrated form, employed as a caustic. It is widely used in industry and in chemical laboratories.

***fuming n.a.*** Concentrated nitric acid that emits toxic fumes that cause choking if inhaled. SEE: *fumes.*

***n.a. poisoning*** Injury sustained from contact with nitric acid. Symptoms include pain, burning, vomiting, thirst, and shock.

TREATMENT: Emergency measures include oral administration of magnesium oxide, milk of magnesia, milk, or egg white in large amounts, as well as large volumes of water. Emetics and stomach tubes should be avoided because they may cause rupture of the esophagus or stomach.

**nitric oxide** ABBR: NO. A gas that is normally produced in the human body and is present in expired air at a concentration of about 10 parts per billion. A vasodilator produced by vascular endothelium originally referred to as endothelium-derived-relaxing factor (ERDF) is now known to be nitric oxide. Endogenously synthesized from L-arginine NO is important in regulating vascular tone. It also inhibits the adhesion, activation, and aggregation of platelets and thus confers an important antithrombotic property on endothelial cells. Conditions for which NO is being investigated include adult respiratory distress syndrome, persistent pulmonary hypertension of the newborn, and pulmonary hypertension in adults. The role of NO in immunity, mediating septic hypotension, and as a factor in penile erection are all subjects of research.

---

Caution: Administration of NO by inhalation must be carefully controlled and monitored.

---

**nitride** (nī'trīd) A binary compound formed by direct combination of nitrogen with another element (e.g., lithium nitride [$Li_3N$]), formed from nitrogen and lithium.

**nitrification** (nī"trĭ-fĭ-kā'shŭn) The process by which the nitrogen of ammonia or other compounds is oxidized to nitric or nitrous acid or their salts (nitrates, nitrites). This process takes place continually in the soil through the action of nitrifying bacteria.

**nitrifying bacteria** Bacteria that induce nitrification, including the nitrite bacteria of the genus *Nitrosomonas,* which convert ammonia to nitrites, and nitrate bacteria of the genus *Nitrobacter,* which convert nitrites to nitrates.

**nitrile** (nī'trĭl) An organic compound in which trivalent nitrogen is attached to a carbon atom.

**nitrite** (nī'trīt) [Gr. *nitron,* salt] A salt of nitrous acid. Nitrites dilate blood vessels, reduce blood pressure, depress motor centers of the spinal cord, and act as antispasmodics.

**nitritoid crisis** A syndrome characterized by symptoms resembling those produced by the use of a nitrite, and usually occurring after arsphenamine injection.

**nitrituria** (nī-trĭ-tū'rē-ă) [" + *ouron,* urine] Nitrites present in the urine.

**nitro-** [Gr. *nitron,* salt] Combining form denoting combination with nitrogen or presence of the group $NO_2$.

**nitrobenzene** (nī"trō-bĕn'zēn) A toxic derivative of benzene used esp. in making aniline.

**nitroblue tetrazolium test** A test of the ability of leukocytes to transform nitroblue tetrazolium from a colorless state to deep blue. Failure to produce this reaction indicates that the leukocytes do not have the capability of reacting in a normal manner to the ingestion of the particular bacteria used in the test.

**nitrocellulose** (nī″trō-sĕl′ū-lōs) Pyroxylin.

**nitrofurantoin** (nī″trō-fū-răn′tō-ĭn) An antibacterial drug used in treating certain urinary tract infections.

**nitrofurazone** (nī″trō-fū′ră-zōn) An antibacterial agent used topically.

**nitrogen** (nī′trō-jĕn) [Fr. *nitrogene*] SYMB: N. A colorless, odorless, tasteless, gaseous element occurring free in the atmosphere, forming approx. 80% of its volume. Its atomic number is 7 and its atomic weight is 14.0067. SYN: *azote*.

A component of all proteins, nitrogen is essential to plant and animal life for tissue building. Generally it is found organically only in the form of compounds such as ammonia, nitrites, and nitrates. These are transformed by plants into proteins and, being consumed by animals, are converted into animal proteins of the blood and tissues.

***n. balance*** The difference between the amount of nitrogen ingested and that excreted each day. If intake is greater, a positive balance exists; if less, there is a negative balance.

***n. cycle*** A natural cycle in which nitrogen is discharged from animal life into the soil; it is then taken up from soil into plants for their nourishment; and in turn nitrogen returns to animal life through plants eaten.

***n. equilibrium*** Condition during which nitrogen excreted in the urine, feces, and sweat equals amount taken in by the body in food.

***n. fixation*** The conversion of atmospheric nitrogen into nitrates through the action of bacteria in the soil.

***n. lag*** The extent of time required after a given protein is ingested before an amount of nitrogen equal to that in the protein has been excreted.

***n. monoxide*** Nitrous oxide.

***n. mustards*** **1.** A term that includes certain therapeutic mustard compounds that act as alkylating agents and therefore have the ability to disturb cell growth during a cell's growth phase. Nitrogen mustards are used to destroy lymphoid tissue in Hodgkin's disease. They are also used in treating lymphosarcoma, giant follicular lymphoblastoma, chronic lymphoid myeloid leukemia, rheumatoid arthritis, and nephritis. Nitrogen mustards include mechlorethamine, cyclophosphamide, uracil mustard, melphalan, and chlorambucil. **2.** Gases used in chemical warfare (e.g., mustard gas, vesicant gas).

***n. narcosis*** A condition of euphoria, impaired judgment, and decreased coordination and motor ability seen in persons exposed to high air pressure (e.g., divers and submariners). The effects, caused by the increased concentration of nitrogen gas in body tissues (including the brain), are similar to those produced by alcoholic intoxication.

***nonprotein n.*** **1.** A nitrogenous constituent of blood that is not a protein. **2.** Sum of all nonprotein nitrogen in the blood.

**nitrogenase** (nī′trō-jĕn-ās) [*nitrogen* + *-ase,* enzyme] An enzyme that catalyzes the reduction of nitrogen to ammonia.

**nitrogenous** (nī-trŏj′ĕn-ŭs) Pert. to or containing nitrogen. Foods that contain nitrogen are the proteins; those that do not contain nitrogen are the fats and carbohydrates. The retention of nitrogenous waste products such as urea in the blood indicates kidney disease.

**nitroglycerin** (nī″trō-glĭs′ĕr-ĭn) [Gr. *nitron,* salt, + *glycerin*] Any nitrate of glycerol, but specifically the trinitrate—a heavy, oily, explosive, colorless liquid obtained by treating glycerol with nitric and sulfuric acids. Well-known as the explosive constituent of dynamite, in medicine it has the action of nitrites and is a vasodilator, used esp. in angina pectoris.

Nitroglycerin tablets must be stored in a tightly sealed dark-tinted glass (not plastic) container without a cotton plug. Nitroglycerin ointment (2%) is esp. helpful in the prophylactic treatment of angina. It is rubbed into the chest wall. A long-term transdermal delivery system is also available for nitroglycerin.

**nitroglycerin tablets** A standardized preparation of nitroglycerin. The previously used name was glyceryl trinitrate.

**nitromersol** (nī″trō-mĕr′sŏl) An organic mercurial antiseptic used topically. It penetrates poorly, and the mercury is fixed by tissues so that its bacteriostatic action is prevented.

**Nitrosomonas** A genus of gram-negative, aerobic bacteria that oxidize ammonia to nitrate.

**nitrous** (nī′trŭs) [Gr. *nitron,* salt] Containing nitrogen in its lowest valency.

**nitrous acid** $HNO_2$. A chemical reagent used in biological laboratories.

**nitrous oxide** $N_2O$. A colorless, odorless, sweet-tasting gas that causes temporary general anesthesia when inhaled in proper concentration. It is given in various amounts with oxygen and is used as an adjuvant with other anesthetic agents. It should not be used as the sole anesthetic agent because the concentration required to produce anesthesia is close to the concentration that would also lead to hypoxia. Its action as an anesthetic can be potentiated by other classes of drugs—barbiturates, narcotics, and tranquilizers. Nitrous oxide is not flammable, but it will support combustion when it is present in proper concentration with a flammable anesthetic. SYN: *laughing gas*.

Nitrous oxide has little or no effect on body temperature, metabolism, blood pressure, volume, or composition, or the genitourinary system. Diaphoresis, increased muscle tone, or both may occur with induction of anesthesia with nitrous oxide.

Asphyxiation may occur if it is not administered properly. Prolonged administration of nitrous oxide will cause depression of bone marrow.

SYMPTOMS: Signs of deep nitrous oxide anesthesia include a slight increase in respirations and some dyspnea. The eyeballs become fixed in a dilated form (upward or downward), and there is muscular rigidity and cyanosis that increases to a grayish pallor.

TREATMENT: The patient who suffers from an overdose should be resuscitated and given oxygen under pressure.

**NK cells** *natural killer cells.*

**N.L.N.** *National League for Nursing.*

**nm** *nanometer.*

**N.M.D.P.** *National Marrow Donor Program.*

**NMRI** *Naval Medical Research Institute* (U.S. Navy); *nuclear magnetic resonance imaging.*

**NMR spectroscopy** *nuclear magnetic resonance spectroscopy.*

**N.M.S.S.** *National Multiple Sclerosis Society.*

**N.N.D.** *New and Nonofficial Drugs,* a former publication of the American Medical Association, which described new drugs that had not been admitted to the U.S. Pharmacopeia.

**NO** Nitric oxide.

**$N_2O$** Nitrous oxide.

**$N_2O_3$** Nitrogen trioxide.

**$N_2O_5$** Nitrogen pentoxide.

**No** Symbol for the element nobelium.

**no** [L. *numero*] Abbreviation meaning *to the number of.*

**nobelium** (nō-bē′lē-ŭm) [Named for Nobel Institute, where it was first isolated] SYMB: No. An element obtained from the bombardment of curium. Its atomic number is 102. The atomic weight of the most stable isotope of nobelium is 254; other isotopes vary in weight from 252 through 256.

**Nobel Prize** [Alfred B. Nobel, Swedish chemist and philanthropist who developed nitroglycerin, 1833–1896, whose will provided funds for awarding the annual prizes] Awards consisting of a medal and monetary prize of over $250,000, usually awarded annually to those honored for peace efforts and excellence in such fields as chemistry, literature, economics, medicine, physics, and physiology. The first prizes were awarded in 1901.

**Nocardia** [Edmund I. E. Nocard, Fr. veterinary pathologist, 1850–1903] A genus of gram-positive aerobic bacilli that often appear in filaments. Some species are acid-fast and thus may be confused with the causative organism for tuberculosis when stained. A species pathogenic for humans causes the disease nocardiosis.

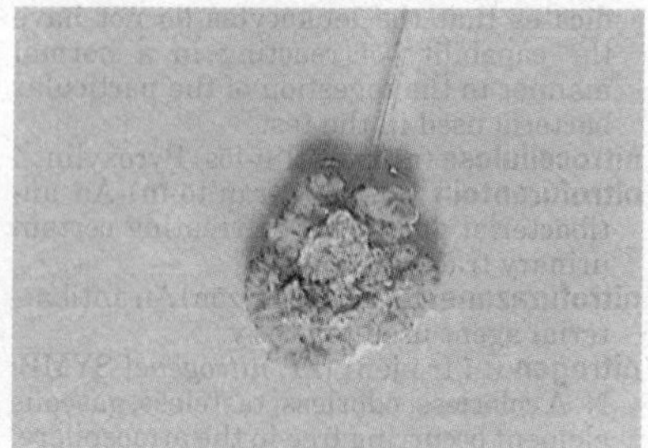

NOCARDIA ASTEROIDES IN CULTURE

**nocardial** (nō-kăr′dē-ăl), *adj.*

***N. asteroides*** A species pathogenic for humans in which abscesses called mycetomas arise in the skin. The invasion site may be the lungs or skin. SEE: illus.

***N. brasiliensis*** A species pathogenic for humans in which chronic subcutaneous abscesses are formed.

**nocardiosis** A pathological condition resulting from infection by any species of *Nocardia.* It may occur as a pulmonary infection that spreads, resulting in abscesses in the skin, brain, or other areas, and it may also give rise to tumors that occur most frequently in lower extremities, esp. the foot, in which case it is called maduromycosis or Madura foot. Nocardiosis is distinguishable from actinomycosis by identification of the organism. It is treated with sulfadiazine daily for several months. SEE: illus.

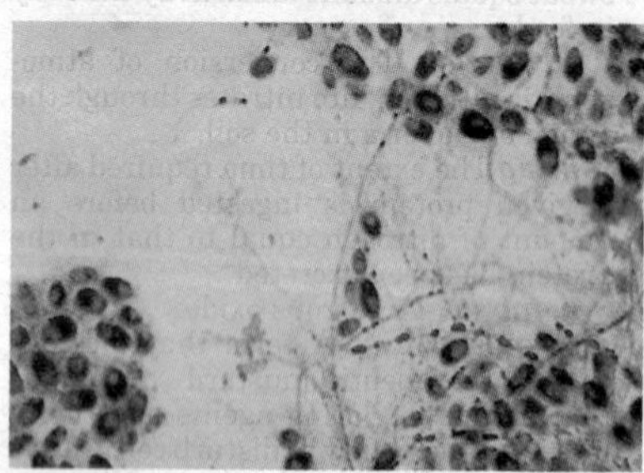

NOCARDIOSIS

NOCARDIA (CHAINS OF BACILLI) IN TISSUE (ORIG. MAG. ×500)

**nocebo** [L., I will harm] The concept that if a test subject is told a procedure or therapy will be harmful it will be, even though no harmful treatment or procedure was done. The nocebo effect can be contagious as in cases of mass hysteria. SEE: *placebo.*

**noci-** (nō′sē) [L. *nocere,* to injure] Combining form indicating *pain, injury.*

**nociassociation** (nō″sē-ă-sō″sē-ā′shŭn) [″ + *ad,* to, + *socius,* companion] The involuntary release of nervous energy during surgical shock or following trauma.

**nociceptive impulse** Impulse giving rise to sensations of pain.

**nociceptor** (nō″sē-sĕp′tor) [″ + *receptor*, receiver] A free nerve ending that is a receptor for painful stimuli. **nociceptive** (nō″sĭ-sĕp′tĭv), *adj*.

**nociperception** (nō″sĭ-pĕr-sĕp′shŭn) [″ + *perceptio*, apprehension] The perception by the nerve centers of injurious influences or painful stimuli.

**"no code" orders** An indication on the chart of a terminally ill patient that he or she does not want heroic and life-saving measures to be instituted at the time when death is imminent.

**noct** L. *nocte*, night.

**noctiphobia** (nŏk″tĭ-fō′bē-ă) [L. *nocte*, at night, + Gr. *phobos*, fear] Abnormal fear of the night and darkness. SYN: *nyctophobia; scotophobia*.

**nocturia** (nŏk-tū′rē-ă) [″ + Gr. *ouron*, urine] Excessive urination during the night, possibly due to excessive fluid intake before going to bed, prostatic disease, urinary tract infection, or impaired renal function that results in excretion of urine with a low specific gravity. SYN: *nycturia*. SEE: *enuresis*.

NURSING IMPLICATIONS: Safety is emphasized for patients who need to get up to go to the bathroom at night because they may not be fully awake or alert. Specific recommendations include strategic placement and use of night lights and removal of objects blocking the route from the bedroom to bathroom, because these may cause the patient to trip or fall.

**nocturnal** [L. *nocturnus*, at night] Pert. to or occurring in the night. Opposed to diurnal. SEE: words beginning with *nyct-*.

***n. emission*** Harmless involuntary discharge of semen during sleep, usually occurring in conjunction with an erotic dream. SYN: *wet dream*.

***n. enuresis*** SEE: under *enuresis*.

***n. myoclonus*** SEE: under *myoclonus*.

***n. penile tumescence*** ABBR: NPT. Erection occurring during sleep. In the normal male, these erections occur beginning in early childhood and continuing to at least the eighth decade. The total time of NPT averages 100 minutes per night. In evaluating impotence, confirmation of the occurrence of NPT usually indicates that the cause of the impotence is due to a psychiatric disorder.

**nocuous** (nŏk′ū-ŭs) [L. *nocuus*] Noxious, injurious, harmful, poisonous.

**nodal** (nō′dăl) [L. *nodus*, knot] Pert. to a protuberance.

***n. rhythm*** Cardiac rhythm with origin at atrioventricular node.

**nodding** (nŏd′ĭng) Involuntary motion of the head downward, as when momentarily dozing. SYN: *nutation* (1).

**nodding spasm** SEE: *spasm, nodding*.

**node** (nōd) [L. *nodus*, knot] **1.** A knot, knob, protuberance, or swelling. **2.** A constricted region. **3.** A small rounded organ or structure.

***Aschoff's n.*** Atrioventricular n.

***atrioventricular n.*** Specialized cardiac muscle fibers in the lower interatrial septum that receive impulses from the sinoatrial node and transmit them to the bundle of His. SEE: *bundle, atrioventricular; heart, conduction system of* for illus.

***A-V n.*** Atrioventricular n.

***Bouchard's n.*** In rheumatoid arthritis, bony enlargement of the proximal interphalangeal joints.

***Haygarth's n.'s*** Joint swelling seen in rheumatoid arthritis.

***Heberden's n.'s*** SEE: *Heberden's nodes*.

***hemal n.*** A lymphoid structure in which blood sinuses are present instead of lymph sinuses. These structures occur in animals but most probably not in humans.

***Hensen's n.*** A mass of rapidly proliferating cells at the anterior end of the primitive streak of the embryo.

***lymph n.*** SEE: *lymph node*.

***Meynet's n.'s*** SEE: *Meynet's nodes*.

***neurofibril n.*** Ranvier's node.

***Osler's n.'s*** SEE: *Osler's nodes*.

***Parrot's n.'s*** SEE: *Parrot's nodes*.

***piedric n.*** A node on the hair shaft seen in piedra.

***Ranvier's n.*** SEE: *Ranvier's node*.

***Schmorl's n.*** Node seen in radiographs of the spine. It is caused by prolapse of the nucleus pulposus into the end-plate of the vertebra.

***sentinel n.*** Signal n.

***signal n.*** Enlargement of one of the supraclavicular lymph nodes; usually indicative of primary carcinoma of thoracic or abdominal organs. SYN: *sentinel n*.

***singer's n.*** SEE: *chorditis nodosa*.

***sinoatrial n.*** ABBR: SA node. A specialized group of cardiac muscle cells in the wall of the right atrium at the entrance of the superior vena cava. These cells depolarize spontaneously and rhythmically to initiate normal heartbeats. SYN: *pacemaker* (2); *sinus n*.

***sinus n.*** Sinoatrial n.

***syphilitic n.*** Circumscribed swelling at end of long bones due to congenital syphilis. The nodes are sensitive and painful during inflammation, esp. at night. SEE: *Parrot's nodes*.

***Troisier's n.*** SEE: *signal n*.

***Virchow n.*** SEE: *signal n*.

**no diagnosis** The condition existing when a patient is studied extensively but no evidence of mental or physical disease can be established.

**nodose** (nō′dōs) [L. *nodosus*, knotted] Swollen or knotlike at intervals; marked by nodes or projections.

**nodosity** (nō-dŏs′ĭ-tē) [L. *nodositas*, a knot] **1.** A protuberance or knot. **2.** Condition of having nodes.

**nodular** (nŏd′ū-lăr) Containing or resembling nodules.

***n. elastosis*** A severe form of elastosis caused by prolonged exposure to the sun. Elastotic material accumulates in the skin and forms cysts and comedones around the face. This condition occurs almost exclusively in white males of middle age or older.

TREATMENT: Treatment consists of removal of cysts and evacuation of comedones, followed by nightly application of retinoic acid cream to the area for 6 to 8 weeks. Patient should avoid sun exposure to prevent recurrence.

**nodule** (nŏd′ūl) [L. *nodulus,* little knot] **1.** A small node. **2.** A small cluster of cells.

***aggregate n.'s*** A group of solitary lymph nodules, such as Peyer's patches of the small intestine.

***Albini's n.'s*** SEE: *Albini's nodules.*

***apple jelly n.*** The jelly-like lesion of lupus vulgaris.

***Arantius' n.*** SEE: *Arantius' body, nodule.*

***Aschoff's n.'s*** SEE: *Aschoff's nodules.*

***cortical n.'s*** Lymph nodules located in the cortex of a lymph node.

***lymph n., lymphatic n.*** A mass of compact, densely staining lymphocytes forming the structural unit of lymphatic tissue. These nodules may occur singly, in groups (as in Peyer's patches), or in encapsulated organs as lymph nodes. Each contains a lighter-staining germinal center where new lymphocytes are formed.

***milker's n.'s*** Painless smooth or warty lesions due to a poxvirus that is transmitted from the udders of infected cows to the hands of milkers. SEE: *paravaccinia.*

***n. of the semilunar valve*** SEE: *Arantius' body, nodule.*

***rheumatic n.'s*** Subcutaneous nodes of fibrous tissue that may be present in patients with rheumatic fever.

***Schmorl's n.*** Schmorl's node.

***siderotic n.'s*** Small brown nodules seen in the spleen and other organs and consisting of necrotic tissue encrusted by iron salts.

***solitary n.*** An isolated nodule of lymphatic tissue such as occurs in mucous membranes.

***subcutaneous n.'s*** Small, nontender swellings resembling Aschoff's bodies and found over the bony prominences on the hands and feet in persons with rheumatic fever.

***surfer's n.'s*** Nodular swelling and possible bone changes of the area of the lower leg and foot exposed to pressure and trauma while on a surfboard. The nodules may be painful. SYN: *surfer's knots.*

***typhoid n.'s*** Nodules characteristic of typhoid fever and found in the liver.

***typhus n.'s*** Small nodules of the skin seen in typhus. They are composed of mononuclear cell infiltration around vessels.

**nodulus** (nŏd′ū-lŭs) *pl.* **noduli** [L.] **1.** Nodule. **2.** The anterior portion of the vermis of the cerebellum.

**nodus** (nō′dŭs) *pl.* **nodi** [L.] **1.** Node. **2.** Anatomically, a small circumscribed mass of undifferentiated tissue.

**noesis** (nō-ē′sĭs) [Gr. *noesis,* thought] The act of thinking; cognition.

**Noguchia** (nō-goo′chē-ă) [Hideyo Noguchi, Japanese bacteriologist in U.S., 1876–1928] A genus of microorganisms of the family Brucellaceae. They are slim, gram-negative, flagellated rods present in the conjunctiva of humans and animals with follicular conjunctivitis.

**noise** [O. Fr. *noise,* strife, brawl] **1.** Sound of any sort, including that which is loud, harsh, confused, or senseless. SEE: table; *acoustic trauma; pollution, noise.* **2.** In electronics or physics, any electronic disturbance that interferes with the signal being recorded or monitored. In electrocardiography, the 60-cycle alternating current used to power the machine may be inadvertently recorded. This obscures

**Typical Noise Levels in Decibels and Their Effect**

| Situation | Level Decibels | Effect |
|---|---|---|
| Jet engine (close by)* | 140 | Harmful to hearing |
| Jet takeoff* | 130 | |
| Propeller aircraft* | 120 | |
| Live rock band | 110 | Risk of hearing loss |
| Jackhammer | 100 | |
| Heavy-duty truck | 90 | |
| Private car; business office | 70 | Probably no risk of permanent damage to hearing |
| Wooded residential area | 50 | No harm |
| Whisper | 30 | No harm |
| Rustle of leaf | 10 | No harm |

* Outside aircraft

the signal from the electrical activity of the heart. **3.** Unwanted information on a radiograph caused by fogging, or scattered radiation.

***n. pollution*** A level of environmental noise of such nature or intensity as to cause mental or physical discomfort or damage to the hearing system.

**noli me tangere** (nō″lē mē tăn′jĕ-rē) [L., touch me not] A cancerous ulcer, generally of the face, that eats away bone and soft tissue. SYN: *rodent ulcer.*

**noma** (nō′mă) [Gr. *nome,* a spreading] A gangrenous, progressive condition generally found in undernourished children that spreads rapidly from the mucous membrane of the cheek or gum to the cutaneous surface. SYN: *cancrum oris; gangrenous stomatitis.* SEE: *gingivitis, acute necrotizing ulcerative.*

***n. pudendi*** An ulcerative condition affecting the labia majora, esp. in young children.

**nomadism** [Gr. *nomas,* roaming about] Impulse to wander about aimlessly; restlessness.

**nomenclature** (nō′mĕn-klā″chūr) [L. *nomen,* name, + *calare,* to call] A classified system of technical or scientific names. SYN: *terminology.*

***binomial n.*** The system of classifying living organisms by the use of two Latin-derived words to indicate the genus and species.

**Nomina Anatomica** (nō′mĭ-nă ăn-ă-tŏm′ĭ-kă) [″ + Gr. *anatome,* dissection] ABBR: NA. The collected anatomical terminology adopted as official by the International Congress of Anatomists at meetings held periodically since 1955.

**nomogram** (nŏm′ō-grăm) [Gr. *nomos,* law, + *gramma,* something written] Representation by graphs, diagrams, or charts of the relationship between numerical variables.

**nomography** (nō-mŏg′ră-fē) [″ + *graphein,* to write] The construction of a nomogram.

**nonabandonment** The ethical obligation of a health care provider to remain in a continuous caring partnership with his or her patient. This partnership remains in place during periods of health and illness and is particularly important when the patient has a chronic or life-threatening disease. Several aspects of modern medical care, in which the patient's choice of physician may be limited and disrupt the continuity of the physician-patient relationship, make carrying out this obligation difficult. SEE: *abandonment.*

**noncompliance** The failure or refusal of a patient to cooperate by carrying out that portion of the medical care plan under his or her control (e.g., not taking prescribed medicines or not adhering to the diet or rehabilitation procedures ordered). SEE: *Nursing Diagnoses Appendix.*

**non compos mentis** (nŏn kŏm′pŏs mĕn′tĭs) [L.] Not of sound mind; mentally incompetent to handle one's affairs.

**nonconductor** [L. *non,* not, + *con,* with, + *ductor,* a leader] Any substance that does not transmit heat, sound, or electricity or that conducts it with difficulty. Strictly speaking, there is no perfect nonconductor. On the application of a sufficiently high voltage, current may be caused to flow through materials usually spoken of as nonconductors. SEE: *insulator.*

**nondisclosure** The act of withholding relevant information. Health care providers have a legal and an ethical obligation to ensure that patients have access to information regarding their health and health management. Failure to provide data concerning diagnosis, prognosis, or treatment options and implications, and the projected consequences of choices denies the patient the right to make an informed decision.

**nondisjunction** The failure of a pair of chromosomes to separate at meiosis, allowing one daughter cell to have two chromosomes and the other to have none.

**nonelectrolyte** [″ + Gr. *elektron,* amber, + *lytos,* dissolved] A solution that will not conduct electricity because its chemical constituents are not sufficiently dissociated into ions.

**nongonococcal urethritis** SEE: under *urethritis.*

**non-Hodgkin's lymphoma** SEE: under *lymphoma.*

**nonigravida** (nō″nĭ-gră′vĭ-dă) [L. *nonus,* ninth, + *gravida,* pregnant] A woman pregnant for the ninth time. Written gravida IX. SEE: *nonipara.*

**noninvasive 1.** Not tending to spread, as certain tumors. **2.** A device or procedure that does not require entering the body including puncturing the skin.

**nonipara** (nō-nĭp′ăr-ă) [″ + *parere,* to bring forth, to bear] A woman who has given birth nine times. Written para IX.

**nonlaxative diet** A low-residue diet containing boiled milk and toasted crackers. No strained oatmeal, vegetable juice, or fruit juice is given. Fats and concentrated sweets are restricted.

**nonmedullated** (nŏn-mĕd′ū-lāt″ĕd) [L. *non,* not, + *medulla,* marrow] Nonmyelinated.

**nonmyelinated** (nŏn-mī′ĕ-lĭ-nāt″ĕd) [″ + Gr. *myelos,* marrow] Containing no myelin.

**nonnucleated** (nŏn-nū′klē-āt″ĕd) [″ + *nucleatus,* having a kernel] Containing no nucleus.

**nonocclusion** (nŏn″ŏ-kloo′zhŭn) [″ + *occlusio,* occlusion] A type of malocclusion in which the teeth fail to make contact.

**nonopaque** (nŏn″ō-pāk′) Not opaque, esp. to x-rays.

**nonose** (nŏn′ōs) [L. *nonus,* ninth] A nine-carbon carbohydrate.

**nonoxynol** (nō-nŏks′ĭ-nŏl) A general class of surface-active agents with the basic formula of $C_{15}H_{24}O(C_2H_4O)_n$, named with respect to the value of *n.* Nonoxynol 9 is a spermicide.

**nonpolar** [" + *polus,* a pole] Not having separate poles; sharing electrons.

***n. compound*** A compound formed by the sharing of electrons.

**nonproprietary name** The name of a drug other than its trademarked (proprietary) name. The nonproprietary name for a new drug is usually the same as that selected by the United States Adopted Name (USAN) Council. The official names for older drugs may differ from the nonproprietary names. In some cases, the generic name is the same as the nonproprietary name. Drugs also have chemical names; in most cases those names are too long and complex to permit their use. Thus the use of a USAN-selected name simplifies and standardizes drug nomenclature. SYN: *generic drugs.* SEE: *proprietary medicine.*

**nonprotein** [L. *non,* not, + Gr. *protos,* first] Any substance not derived from protein.

**nonprotein nitrogen** SEE: *nitrogen.*

**non rep** [L. *non repetatur*] Abbreviation meaning *do not repeat.*

**nonresectable** Not removable by surgery.

**nonresponder 1.** An individual who does not achieve an immunological response to a vaccine. **2.** A person who does not respond in the expected way to therapy, particularly medication.

**nonrestraint** (nŏn″rē-strānt′) [L. *non,* not, + *re,* back, + *stringere,* to bind back] Treatment of the insane without using mechanical restraints.

**nonrotation** (nŏn″rō-tā′shŭn) [" + *rotare,* to turn] Failure of a part or organ to rotate, esp. during embryological development.

***n. of the intestine*** In embryonic development, the intestines fail to rotate, so that the descending colon is on the left side of the abdominal cavity instead of the right.

**nonsecretor** (nŏn″sē-krē′tor) [" + *secretio,* separation] An individual whose saliva and other body fluids do not contain the ABO blood antigens.

**nonseptate** (nŏn-sĕp′tāt) [" + *septum,* a partition] Having no dividing walls.

**nonsexual** (nŏn-sĕk′shū-ăl) Asexual.

**nonspecific** Term used in reference to the cause of a disease when the exact organism or agent has not been identified.

**nonsteroidal anti-inflammatory drug** ABBR: NSAID. A drug that has analgesic, anti-inflammatory, and antipyretic action. Drugs of this type have been used extensively in treating arthritis, dysmenorrhea, and general inflammation. Even though effective as analgesics and in moderating inflammation, there is no evidence that NSAIDs alter the pathological progression of a disease such as rheumatoid arthritis. As many as 10% to 15% of patients using NSAIDs will experience side effects, esp. gastrointestinal irritation and hemorrhage of such severity as to require discontinuing the use of NSAIDs. A complication of long-term NSAID use is acute renal failure. Hepatotoxicity is a rare but important undesired side effect of NSAID use. SEE: *nephritis, analgesic.*

NURSING IMPLICATIONS: Patients who are sensitive to NSAID therapy are told to inform caregivers so they will not be given NSAIDs. Patients are instructed to watch for adverse effects when taking a drug of this category, report any gastrointestinal pain or discomfort, and seek immediate medical attention for any coughing or vomiting of blood. The nurse cautions the patient not to take NSAIDs on an empty stomach.

**nontoxic** (nŏn-tŏk′sĭk) [L. *non,* not, + Gr. *toxikon,* poison] Not poisonous or productive of poison.

**nontoxic substances** Any substance characteristic of being nonpoisonous as ordinarily encountered. For those involved in patient care, it is important to know that some of the common materials that children and adults can accidentally ingest are not toxic. A list of substances considered generally nontoxic is provided in the Appendix.

**nonunion** (nŏn-ūn′yŭn) [" + *unio,* oneness] Failure to unite, as a fractured bone that fails to heal completely. Diagnosis of nonunion is established when a minimum of 9 months has elapsed since the injury and the fracture site shows no progressive signs of healing for a minimum of 3 months and is not complicated by a synovial pseudoarthrosis. SEE: *bone fracture, nonunion, electrical stimulation for.*

**nonus** [L.] **1.** Ninth. **2.** Hypoglossal nerve, formerly regarded as ninth cranial nerve.

**nonviable** (nŏn-vī′ă-b′l) [L. *non,* not, + *via,* life] Incapable of life or of living. This term is frequently used to indicate a fetus that has died in utero, born prior to 20th week of gestation.

**nonyl** $CH_3(CH_2)_8$. A univalent radical that contains nine carbon atoms.

**nookleptia** (nō-ō-klĕp′tē-ă) [Gr. *nous,* mind, + *kleptein,* to steal] An obsession that one's thoughts are being stolen by others.

**Noonan's syndrome** [Jacqueline A. Noonan, U.S. cardiologist, b. 1921] The male equivalent of Turner's syndrome. Clinically, there are low-set ears, webbing of the neck, congenital heart disease, cubitum valgum, and sometimes severe mental retardation.

**noopsyche** (nō′ō-sī″kē) [Gr. *nous,* mind, + *psyche,* soul] Mental processes.

**NORD** *National Organization for Rare Disorders.*

**norepinephrine** (nor-ĕp″ĭ-nĕf′rĭn) **1.** A hormone produced by the adrenal medulla, similar in chemical and pharmacological properties to epinephrine, but chiefly a vasoconstrictor with little effect on cardiac output. **2.** A neurotransmitter released by most sympathetic postganglionic neurons and by some neurons of the brain. A disturbance in its metabolism at important brain sites has been implicated in affective disorders.

***n. bitartrate*** A standardized preparation of norepinephrine. The former name was levarterenol bitartrate.

**norethindrone** (nor-ĕth′ĭn-drōn) A steroid hormone that is similar in action to progesterone and that is used in progestational agents for birth control.

**norethynodrel** (nor″ĕ-thī′nō-drĕl) A progestational agent used in certain birth control pills.

**norflurane** (nor-floor′ān) An inhalation anesthetic.

**norgestrel** (nor-jĕs′trĕl) A progestational agent used in certain birth control pills.

**norm** [L. *norma,* rule] **1.** A standard or ideal for a specific group. **2.** Normal.

**norma** [L., rule] A view or aspect, esp. with reference to the skull.

***anterior n.*** N. frontalis.

***n. basilaris*** N. ventralis.

***n. facialis*** N. frontalis.

***n. frontalis*** The outline of the skull viewed from the front. SYN: *anterior n.; n. facialis.*

***inferior n.*** N. ventralis.

***n. lateralis*** A view of the skull as seen from the side; a profile view.

***n. occipitalis*** A view of the skull as seen from behind.

***n. sagittalis*** A view of the skull as seen in sagittal section.

***superior n.*** N. verticalis.

***n. ventralis*** A view of the inferior surface of skull. SYN: *n. basilaris; inferior n.*

***n. verticalis*** A view of the skull as seen from above. SYN: *superior n.*

**normal** (nor′măl) [L. *normalis,* according to pattern] **1.** Standard; performing proper functions; natural; regular. **2.** In biology, not affected by experimental treatment; occurring naturally and not because of disease or experimentation. **3.** In psychology, free from mental disorder; of average development or intelligence.

***n. distribution*** SEE: under *distribution.*

***n. salt*** SEE: under *salt.*

***n. solution*** A solution in which 1 L contains 1 g equivalent of the solute.

**normalization** (nor″măl-ī-zā′shŭn) [L. *normalis,* according to pattern] Modification or reduction to the normal standard.

**normergic** (nor-mĕr′jĭk) Reacting, or pert. to that which reacts, in a normal manner.

**normetanephrine** (nor-mĕt″ă-nĕf′rĭn) A metabolite of epinephrine.

**normo-** [L. *norma,* rule] Combining form indicating *normal, usual.*

**normoblast** (nor′mō-blăst) [″ + Gr. *blastos,* germ] An immature nucleated red blood cell similar in size to a mature erythrocyte, usually found in the red bone marrow. **normoblastic** (-blăs-tĭk), *adj.*

**normoblastosis** (nor″mō-blăs-tō′sĭs) [″ + ″ + *osis,* condition] Increased production and circulation of normoblasts. This indicates a need for greater oxygen-carrying capacity of the blood, as when mature erythrocytes are being rapidly destroyed.

**normocalcemia** (nor″mō-kăl-sē′mē-ă) Normal level of blood calcium.

**normocapnia** (nor″mō-kăp′nē-ă) The presence of a normal concentration of carbon dioxide in the blood and serum. **normocapnic** (-kăp′nĭk), *adj.*

**normocholesterolemia** (nor″mō-kō-lĕs″tĕr-ō-lē′mē-ă) The presence of a normal concentration of cholesterol in the blood.

**normochromasia** (nor″mō-krō-mā′zē-ă) [″ + Gr. *chroma,* color] Average staining capacity in a cell or tissue.

**normocyte** (nor′mō-sīt) [″ + Gr. *kytos,* cell] An average-sized red blood corpuscle. SYN: *erythrocyte.*

**normoglycemia** (nor″mō-glī-sē′mē-ă) [″ + Gr. *glykys,* sweet, + *haima,* blood] Normal sugar content of the blood. **normoglycemic** (-sē′mĭk), *adj.*

**normokalemia** (nor″mō-kă-lē′mē-ă) Normal level of blood potassium.

**normospermic** (nor″mō-spĕr′mĭk) [″ + Gr. *sperma,* seed] Producing normal spermatozoa.

**normosthenuria** (nor″mō-sthĕn-ū′rē-ă) [″ + Gr. *sthenos,* strength, + *ouron,* urine] Urination which is of a normal amount and specific gravity.

**normotensive** (nor″mō-tĕn′sĭv) **1.** Normal blood pressure. **2.** A person with normal blood pressure.

**normothermia** (nor″mō-thĕr′mē-ă) [″ + Gr. *therme,* heat] Normal body temperature.

**normotopia** (nor″mō-tō′pē-ă) [″ + Gr. *topos,* place] Situation in the normal place. **normotopic** (nor″mō-tŏp′ĭk), *adj.*

**normovolemia** (nor″mō-vō-lē′mē-ă) [″ + *volumen,* volume, + Gr. *haima,* blood] Normal blood volume.

**Norplant** Trade name for a contraceptive system that prevents pregnancy for up to 5 yr. Six matchstick-sized sillicone plastic capsules containing levonorgestrel are inserted in a fanlike pattern just under the skin of a woman's arm. The procedure takes approx. 15 min and is performed in a physician's office under a local anesthetic. When the implant is removed, fertility is restored.

Norplant, like all drugs, is not free of side effects. Some users report amenorrhea, menstrual irregularities, weight change, mood swings, and headache. Some of these side effects are the same as would serve to identify early pregnancy. Thus, tests should be performed whenever pregnancy is suspected.

**Norrie's disease** [Gordon Norrie, Danish ophthalmologist, 1855–1941] A rare form of sex-linked hereditary blindness due to retinal malformation. Also present are peripheral vascular pathology, vitreous opacities, microphthalmia, and sometimes mental retardation and loss of hearing.

**nortriptyline hydrochloride** (nor-trĭp′tĭ-lēn) An antidepressant drug of the tricyclic class.

**Norwalk agent** [virus first identified in Norwalk, Ohio, U.S.A.] A calicivirus that is the causative organism in over half of the reported cases of epidemic viral gastroenteropathy. The incubation period ranges from 18 to 72 hr. The outbreaks are usually self-limiting and the intestinal signs and symptoms last for 24 to 48 hr. Treatment, if required, is supportive and directed to maintaining hydration and electrolyte balance. SEE: *Calicivirus.*

**Norwegian itch** SEE: *scabies, Norwegian.*

**nose** [AS. *nosw*] The specialized projection in the center of the face that serves as the organ of smell and the entrance to the nasal cavities that warms, moistens, and filters inhaled air as it passes through to the respiratory tract. The nose is a triangle composed of and bounded by bone and cartilage covered with skin and lined with mucous membrane. SYN: *nasus; organum olfactus.*

EXAMINATION: Note the shape, size, color, and state of the alae nasi, and any discharge, interference with respiration, evidence of injury, deflected or perforated septum, enlarged turbinates, and tenderness over frontal and maxillary sinuses.

DIAGNOSIS: *Chronic red nose:* Dilated capillaries as a result of alcoholism, lupus erythematosus, acne rosacea, pustules, and boils. *Superficial ulceration:* Tuberculous ulcer, epithelioma, syphilis. *Broad and coarse:* Cretinism, myxedema, acromegaly. *Sunken:* Syphilis or injury. *Pinched with small nares:* Hypertrophied adenoid tissue or chronic obstructions; tumors. *Inoffensive watery discharge:* Nasal catarrh, early stages of measles, hay fever, acute irritation of lining membranes. *Offensive discharge:* Nasopharyngeal diphtheria, lupus, local infection, impacted foreign bodies, caries, rhinitis, glanders, syphilitic infection.

***bridge of the n.*** The superior portion of the external nose formed by the union of the two nasal bones.

***foreign body in the n.*** Presence of material in the nasal cavity that was either inhaled or accidentally placed there. A child may place a foreign object in his or her own or another child's nose.

SYMPTOMS: Irritation of the nose resulting in coughing or watery or purulent discharge; occasionally pain and obstruction of nose. If not recognized immediately, the foreign body often causes a foul discharge on the affected side of the nose. There may be obstruction to breathing in one nostril. If the foreign body is very small, symptoms may be absent.

TREATMENT: The patient should be taken to a physician. Vigorous nose blowing should be discouraged because it may spread infection to the various cavities and sinuses about the nose or to the middle ear. Attempts to dislodge the foreign body should be avoided because doing so may cause it to slip further into the nose or down the throat and into the bronchus.

***hammer n.*** Rhinophyma.

***saddle n.*** A nose with a depressed bridge due to congenital absence of bony or cartilaginous support, to a disease such as leprosy or congenital syphilis, or to postoperative complications of suppuration and destruction of the supporting framework.

**nosebleed** Hemorrhage from the nose. SEE: illus.; *epistaxis; Kiesselbach's area.*

**Nosema** (nō-sē′mă) A genus of parasites of the order Microsporidia. SEE: *microsporidiosis.*

**nosepiece** (nōz′pēs) The portion of a microscope to which the objective lenses attach.

**nose springs** A springlike device applied to the bridge of the nose that pulls the nostrils open slightly. The device may reduce nasal airway resistance, thereby improving sleep quality and decreasing snoring. The trade name of the device, which is available over-the-counter, is Breathe Right.

**noso-** [Gr. *nosos,* disease] Combining form denoting *disease.*

**nosochthonography** (nŏs″ŏk-thō-nŏg′ră-fē) [″ + *chthon,* earth, + *graphein,* to write] Study of geographical distribution of diseases. SYN: *geomedicine.*

**nosocomial** (nŏs″ō-kō′mē-ăl) [Gr. *nosokomos,* one who tends the sick] Pert. to or occurring in a hospital or infirmary.

**nosocomial infection** Infection acquired in a hospital.

**nosology** (nō-sŏl′ō-jē) [″ + *logos,* word, reason] The science of description or classification of diseases.

**nosomycosis** (nŏs″ō-mī-kō′sĭs) [″ + *mykes,* fungus, + *osis,* condition] Any disease caused by a parasitic fungus or schizomycete.

**nosophobia** (nō″sō-fō′bē-ă) [″ + *phobos,* fear] An abnormal aversion to illness or to a particular disease.

**nosophyte** (nŏs′ō-fīt) [″ + *phyton,* plant] A disease-causing plant microorganism.

**Nosopsyllus** (nŏs″ō-sĭl′ŭs) [″ + *psylla,* flea] A genus of fleas belonging to the order Siphonaptera.

***N. fasciatus*** A species of rat fleas responsible for transmission of murine typhus and possibly plague.

**nostalgia** (nŏs-tăl′jē-ă) [Gr. *nostos,* a return home, + *algos,* pain] Homesickness; longing to return home.

**nostril** [AS. *nosu,* nose, + *thyrel,* a hole] One of the external apertures of the nose. SYN: *naris.* SEE: *nose.*

***n. reflex*** Reduction of the opening of the naris on the affected side in lung disease in proportion to lessened alveolar air capacity on the affected side.

**nostrum** (nŏs′trŭm) [L., our] A patent, secret, or quack remedy.

**notalgia** (nō-tăl′jē-ă) [Gr. *noton,* back, + *algos,* pain] Pain in the back. SYN: *dorsalgia.*

**notancephalia** (nō″tăn-sĕ-fā′lē-ă) [″ + *-an*, not, + *kephale*, head] Congenital absence of the back of the skull.

**notanencephalia** (nō″tăn-ĕn-sĕ-fā′lē-ă) [″ + ″ + *enkephalos*, brain] Absence of the cerebellum.

**notch** (nŏch) A deep indentation or narrow gap in the edge of a structure. SYN: *incisure*.

***acetabular n.*** The notch in the inferior border of the acetabulum. SYN: *cotyloid notch*.

***antigonial n.*** A depression in the inferior border of the mandible at the anterior edge of the insertion of the masseter muscle.

***aortic n.*** The notch in a sphygmogram caused by rebound at aortic valve closure.

***cardiac n.*** The concavity on the anterior border of the left lung into which the

TECHNIQUE FOR CONTROL OF HEMORRHAGE FROM POSTERIOR NASAL CAVITY

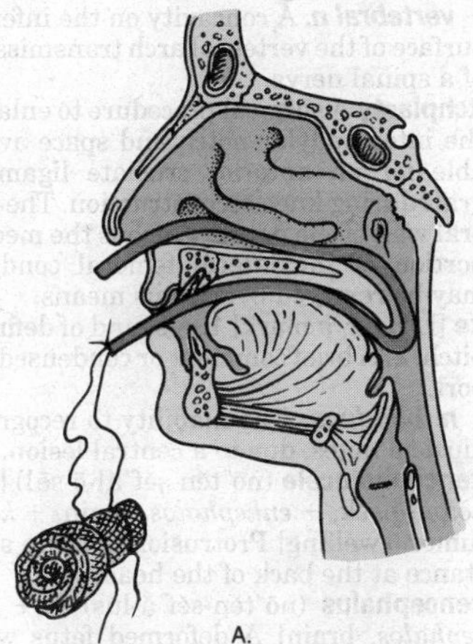

A.
INSERT SOFT FLEXIBLE CATHETER INTO NOSE AND BRING DISTAL TIP OUT THROUGH THE MOUTH. ATTACH MOISTENED PACK TO CATHETER

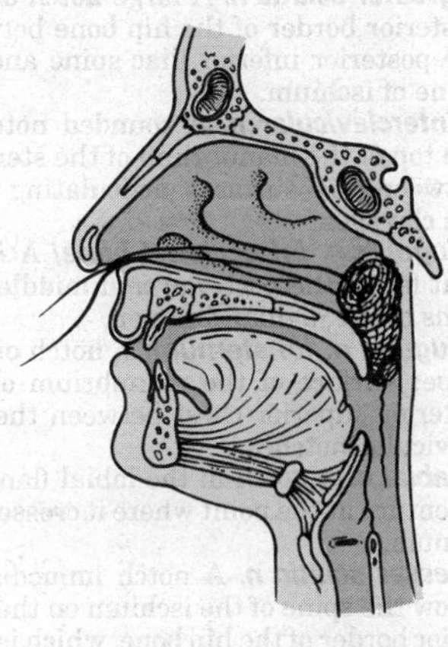

B.
BY PULLING ON CATHETER DRAW PACK IN PLACE SO IT IS PLACED SECURELY IN POSTERIOR NASAL CAVITY

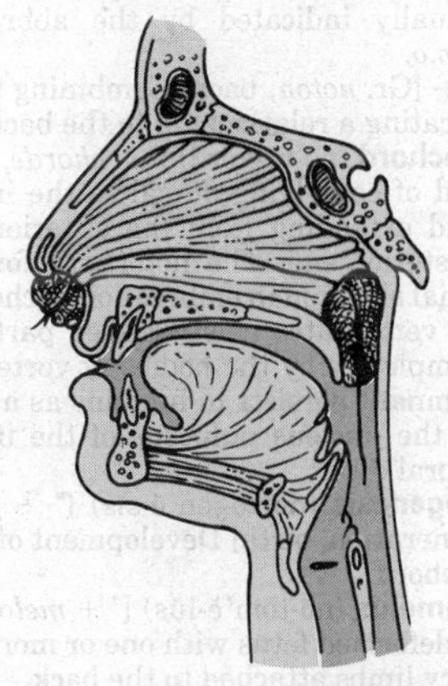

C.
REMOVE CATHETER AND USE STRING TO ATTACH TO A SOFT CUSHION OF SUFFICIENT SIZE TO PREVENT ITS PASSING INTO THE NOSTRIL

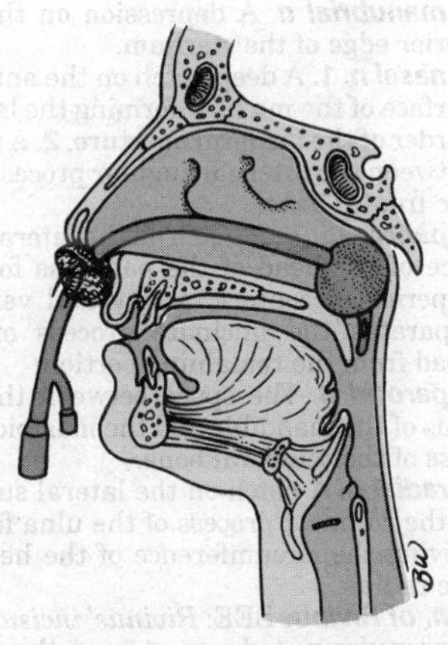

D.
ALTERNATIVELY, A FOLEY CATHETER MAY BE USED. THE INFLATED TIP IS HELD SECURELY IN PLACE AS IN PREVIOUS ILLUSTRATIONS

heart projects.

***cerebellar n.*** Either of two deep notches (anterior and posterior) separating the hemispheres of the cerebellum.

***clavicular n.*** A notch at the upper angle of the sternum with which the clavicle articulates.

***costal n.*** Any of seven pairs of indentations on the lateral surfaces of the sternum, for articulation with costal cartilages.

***ethmoidal n.*** The notch separating the two orbital portions of the frontal bone.

***frontal n.*** The notch on the supraorbital arch that transmits the frontal artery and nerve.

***greater sciatic n.*** A large notch on the posterior border of the hip bone between the posterior inferior iliac spine and the spine of ischium.

***interclavicular n.*** A rounded notch at the top of the manubrium of the sternum between the surfaces articulating with the clavicles.

***jugular n. (of occipital bone)*** A notch that forms the posterior and middle portions of the jugular foramen.

***jugular n. (of sternum)*** A notch on the upper surface of the manubrium of the anterior superior chest between the two clavicular notches.

***labial n.*** A notch in the labial flange of a denture at the point where it crosses the frenum.

***lesser sciatic n.*** A notch immediately below the spine of the ischium on the posterior border of the hip bone, which is converted into a foramen by the sacrotuberous ligament.

***mandibular n.*** A notch on the superior border of the ramus of the mandible separating the coronoid and condyloid processes.

***manubrial n.*** A depression on the superior edge of the sternum.

***nasal n.*** **1.** A deep notch on the anterior surface of the maxilla, forming the lateral border of the piriform aperture. **2.** A notch between the internal angular processes of the frontal bone.

***pancreatic n.*** A notch on the lateral surface of the head of the pancreas for the superior mesenteric artery and vein. It separates the uncinate process of the head from the remaining portion.

***parotid n.*** The space between the ramus of the mandible and the mastoid process of the temporal bone.

***radial n.*** A notch on the lateral surface of the coronoid process of the ulna for receiving the circumference of the head of the radius.

***n. of Rivinus*** SEE: *Rivinus' incisure.*

***scapular n.*** A deep notch on the superior border of the scapula that transmits the suprascapular nerve.

***semilunar n.*** A notch on the anterior aspect of the proximal end of the ulna for articulation with the trochlea of the humerus.

***sphenopalatine n.*** A notch between the orbital and sphenoidal processes of the palatine bone.

***tentorial n.*** An arched cavity in the free border of the tentorium cerebelli through which the brainstem passes.

***thyroid n.*** A deep notch on the superior border of the thyroid cartilage of the larynx that separates the two laminae.

***tympanic n.*** SEE: *Rivinus' incisure.*

***ulnar n.*** The notch on the distal end of the radius that receives the head of the ulna.

***umbilical n.*** A notch on the anterior border of the liver where it is crossed by the falciform ligament.

***vertebral n.*** A concavity on the inferior surface of the vertebral arch transmission of a spinal nerve.

**notchplasty** A surgical procedure to enlarge the intercondylar notch and space available for an anterior cruciate ligament graft during knee reconstruction. The lateral wall of the notch, which is the medial portion of the lateral femoral condyle, may be removed by various means.

**note** [L. *nota,* a mark] **1.** A sound of definite pitch. **2.** A brief comment or condensed report.

***n. blindness*** The inability to recognize musical notes, due to a central lesion.

**notencephalocele** (nō″tĕn-sĕf′ăl-ō-sēl) [Gr. *noton,* back, + *enkephalos,* brain, + *kele,* tumor, swelling] Protrusion of brain substance at the back of the head.

**notencephalus** (nō″tĕn-sĕf′ă-lŭs) [″ + *enkephalos,* brain] A deformed fetus with notencephalocele.

**nothing by mouth** An instruction used in patient care to indicate that the patient is not to take or receive food, liquid, or medicine (i.e., *nothing*) orally. This order is usually indicated by the abbreviation *n.p.o.*

**noto-** [Gr. *noton,* back] Combining form indicating a relationship to the back.

**notochord** (nō′tō-kord) [″ + *chorde,* cord] A rod of cells lying dorsal to the intestine and extending from the anterior to the posterior end. The notochord forms the axial skeleton in embryos of all chordates. In vertebrates it is replaced partially or completely by the bodies of vertebrae. A remnant persists in humans as a portion of the nucleus pulposus of the intervertebral disk.

**notogenesis** (nō″tō-jĕn′ĕ-sĭs) [″ + *genesis,* generation, birth] Development of the notochord.

**notomelus** (nō-tŏm′ĕ-lŭs) [″ + *melos,* limb] A deformed fetus with one or more accessory limbs attached to the back.

**noumenon** (nū′mē-nŏn) [Gr. *nooumenon,* a thing perceived] That which one knows or perceives by intellectual intuition alone, as distinguished from something perceived through sensory perception. **noumenal** (nū′mē-năl), *adj.*

**nourishment** [L. *nutrire,* to nurse] **1.** Sustenance; nutriment; food. **2.** The act of nourishing or of being nourished. SEE: *trophic.*

**noxa** (nŏk'să) *pl.* **noxae** [L., injury] Anything harmful to health.

**noxious** (nŏk'shŭs) [L. *noxius,* injurious] Harmful; not wholesome.

**NP** *nucleoprotein; nurse practitioner; nursing practice; nursing procedure; neuropsychiatrist; neuropsychiatry.*

**Np** Symbol for the element neptunium.

**NPC** *nodal premature complex.*

**NPDB** *National Practitioner Data Bank.*

**NPH insulin** *neutral protamine Hagedorn* insulin.

**NPN** *nonprotein nitrogen.*

**NPO, n.p.o.** [L.] *non per os,* nothing by mouth.

**NPT** *normal pressure and temperature; nocturnal penile tumescence.*

**NREM** *nonrapid eye movement.* SEE: under *sleep.*

**N.R.E.M.T.** *Nationally Registered Emergency Medical Technician.*

**N.R.M.S.** *National Registry of Medical Secretaries.*

**ns 1.** *nanosecond.* **2.** *nonsignificant.*

**NSA** *Neurosurgical Society of America.*

**NSAID** *nonsteroidal anti-inflammatory drug.*

**NSCC** *National Society for Crippled Children.*

**NSD in ret** *nominal standard dose* in *r*adiation *e*quivalent *t*herapy. SEE: *ret.*

**nsec** *nanosecond.*

**N.S.N.A.** *National Student Nurses' Association.*

**NSPB** *National Society for the Prevention of Blindness.*

**NSR** *normal sinus rhythm.*

**nth** (ĕnth) Used in medical statistics to indicate the continuation of data or subjects to large numbers in a progression or series. Thus, one would indicate patients numbered P1, P2, P3, and so forth through Pnth. Pnth would be the last patient indicated.

**nubile** (nū'bĭl) [L. *nubere,* to marry] Of marriageable age; pert. to a girl who has attained puberty.

**nucha** (nū'kă) [L.] The nape (back) of the neck. **nuchal** (nū'kăl), *adj.*

**Nuck's canal** (nŭks) [Anton Nuck, Dutch anatomist, 1650–1692] A persistent peritoneal pouch that accompanies the round ligament of the uterus through the inguinal canal.

**nuclear** (nū'klē-ăr) [L. *nucleus,* a kernel] Resembling or concerning a nucleus.

***n. antigen*** An antigen present in the cells of patients with certain types of connective tissue disorders. Corticosteroids are very helpful in treating patients with high concentrations of extractable nuclear antigen.

***n. arc*** Spiral patterns on the surface of the lens due to a concentric pattern of fiber growth.

***n. envelope*** SEE: under *envelope.*

***n. family*** The basic family unit consisting of parents and their children.

***n. magnetic resonance imaging*** ABBR: NMRI. SEE: *magnetic resonance imaging.*

***n. medicine*** SEE: under *medicine.*

***n. medicine scanning test*** Any of the tests involving the use of radioactive substances to diagnose certain conditions. The substances are either injected into the body or inhaled, the dose of radiation is minimal, and the substances used either lose their radioactivity in a short time or are excreted. This technique, called a "scan," may be used to diagnose tumors, biliary disease, gastrointestinal emptying or bleeding, coronary artery disease, valvular heart disease, red blood cell survival time, renal dysfunction, deep vein thrombosis, and thyroid function. Examples of nuclear medicine scanning tests include positron emission tomography and single photon emission computed tomography.

**nuclease** (nū'klē-ās) [L. *nucleus,* kernel, + *-ase,* enzyme] Any enzyme in animals or plants that facilitates hydrolysis of nuclein and nucleic acids.

**nucleate** (nū'klē-āt) [L. *nucleatus,* having a kernel] **1.** Having a nucleus. **2.** To form a nucleus.

**nucleic acid** Any one of a group of high-molecular-weight substances found in the cells of all living things. They have a complex chemical structure formed of sugars (pentoses), phosphoric acid, and nitrogen bases (purines and pyrimidines). Most important are ribonucleic acid (RNA) and deoxyribonucleic acid (DNA). SEE: illus.

**nuclein** (nū'klē-ĭn) [L. *nucleus,* a kernel] A normal chemical constituent of a cell nucleus that is a colorless, shapeless substance obtained by hydrolysis of nucleoproteins to form nucleic acid and proteins.

**nuclein base** Any of the bases formed from decomposition of nuclein, such as adenine, guanine, xanthine, hypoxanthine.

**nucleo-** [L. *nucleus,* kernal] Pert. to a nucleus.

**nucleocapsid** (nū″klē-ō-kăp'sĭd) In a virus, the protein coat and the viral nucleic acid.

**nucleofugal** (nū-klē-ŏf'ū-găl) [″ + *fugere,* to flee] Directed or moving away from a nucleus.

**nucleohistone** (nū″klē-ō-hĭs'tŏn, -tōn) [″ + Gr. *histos,* tissue] A substance composed of nuclein and histone, found in sperm of various animals.

**nucleoid** (nū'klē-oyd) [″ + Gr. *eidos,* form, shape] Resembling a nucleus.

**nucleoliform** (nū-klē-ō'lĭ-form) [L. *nucleolus,* a little kernel, + *forma,* shape] Like a nucleolus.

**nucleoloid** (nū'klē-ō-loyd) Similar to a nucleus.

**nucleolonema** (nū″klē-ō″lō-nē'mă) [″ + Gr. *nema,* thread] A fine network in the nucleolus of a cell.

**nucleolus** (nū-klē'ō-lŭs) *pl.* **nucleoli** [L., lit-

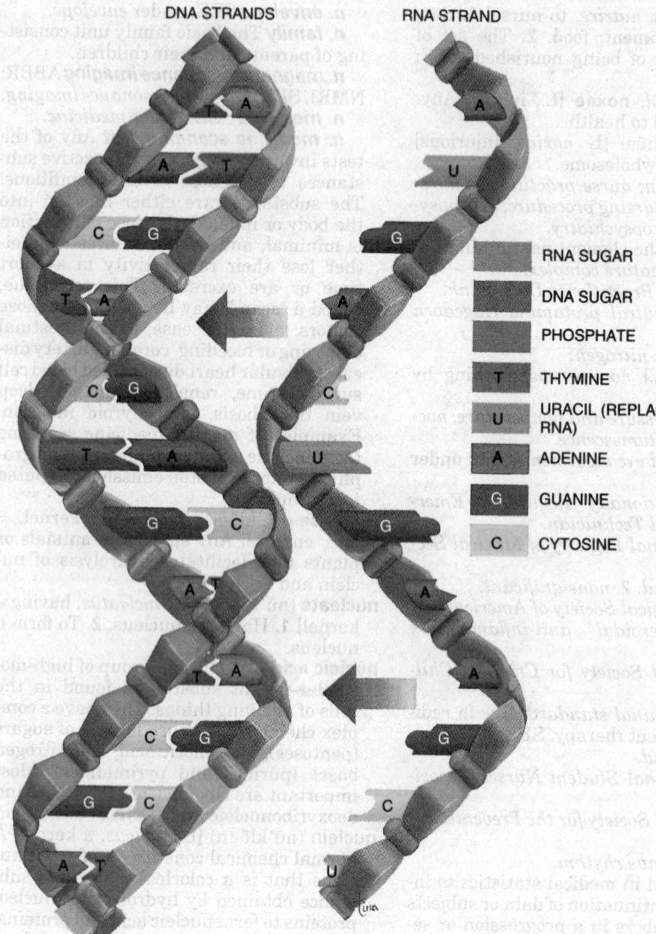


NUCLEIC ACID
DNA AND RNA

tle kernel] A spherical structure in the nucleus of a cell made of DNA, RNA, and protein. It is the site of synthesis of ribosomal RNA (rRNA); a cell may have more than one. Embryonic cells and those in malignancies actively synthesize rRNA. Therefore they are much larger than cells that do not require increased amounts of rRNA. **nucleolar** (nū-klē′ō-lăr), *adj.*

**nucleomicrosome** (nū″klē-ō-mī′krō-sōm) [L. *nucleus,* kernel, + Gr. *mikros,* tiny, + *soma,* body] Any one of the minute granules that make up nuclear fibers.

**nucleon** (nū′klē-ŏn) Any of the particles that collectively make up the nucleus of an atom.

**nucleopetal** (nū-klē-ŏp′ĕ-tăl) [L. *nucleus,* kernel, + *petere,* to seek] Seeking or moving toward the nucleus.

**nucleophilic** (nū″klē-ō-fĭl′ĭk) [″ + Gr. *philein,* to love] Having an attraction to nuclei.

**nucleoplasm** (nū′klē-ō-plăzm″) [″ + LL. *plasma,* form, mold] The protoplasm of a cell nucleus. **nucleoplasmic,** *adj.*

**nucleoprotein** (nū″klē-ō-prō′tē-ĭn) [″ + Gr. *protos,* first] The combination of one of the proteins with nucleic acid to form a conjugated protein found in cell nuclei.

**nucleoreticulum** (nū″klē-ō-rē-tĭk′ū-lŭm) [″ + *reticulum,* network] Any mesh framework in a nucleus.

**nucleosidase** (nū″klē-ō-sī′dās) An enzyme that catalyzes the hydrolysis of nucleosides.

**nucleoside** A glycoside formed by the union of a purine or pyrimidine base with a sugar (pentose).

**nucleosome** The combination of positively charged histone proteins and negatively charged DNA; the first step in the folding of DNA into chromatin.

**nucleospindle** (nū″klē-ō-spĭn′d′l) A spindle-shaped body occurring in karyokinesis.

**nucleotidase** (nū″klē-ŏt′ĭ-dās) An enzyme (nucleophosphatase) that splits phosphoric acid from nucleotides, leaving a nucleoside.

**5′-nucleotidase** An enzyme present in serum. Its serum level is increased in carcinoma of the pancreas when there is common bile duct obstruction or metastasis to the liver.

**nucleotide** (nū′klē-ō-tīd) [L. *nucleus,* kernel] A compound formed of phosphoric acid, a pentose sugar, and a base (purine or pyrimidine), all of which constitute the structural unit of nucleic acid. SYN: *mononucleotide.*

**nucleotidyl** (nū″klē-ō-tīd′ĭl) The residue of a nucleotide.

**nucleotidyltransferase** (nū″klē-ō-tīd″ĭl-trăns′fĕr-ās) An enzyme that transfers nucleotidyls from nucleosides into dimer or polymer forms.

**nucleotoxin** [″ + Gr. *toxikon,* poison] A toxin acting upon or produced by cell nuclei.

**nucleus** (nū′klē-ŭs) *pl.* **nuclei** [L., kernel] **1.** A central point about which matter is gathered, as in a calculus. **2.** The structure within a cell that contains the chromosomes. It is responsible for the cell's metabolism, growth, and reproduction. SEE: *cell.* **3.** A group of nerve cells or mass of gray matter in the central nervous system, esp. the brain. **4.** In chemistry, a heavy central atomic particle in which most of the mass and total positive electric charge are concentrated.

***n. abducens*** A gray nucleus, the origin of the abducens nerve, on the floor of the 4th ventricle, behind the trigeminal nucleus.

***ambiguous n.*** The nucleus of the glossopharyngeal and vagus nerves in the medulla oblongata. It lies in the lateral half of the reticular formation.

***amygdaloid n.*** A nucleus projecting into the inferior cornua of the lateral ventricle. It constitutes part of the basal ganglia.

***angular n.*** The superior vestibular nucleus. SYN: *Bechterew's n.* SEE: *vestibular n.*

***anterior n. of the thalamus*** A nucleus located in the rostral part of the thalamus. It receives the fibers of the mamillothalamic tract.

***arcuate n.*** **1.** The nucleus located on the basal aspect of the pyramid of the medulla. **2.** The posteromedial ventral nucleus of the thalamus.

***atomic n.*** The central part of an atom, which contains protons and electrons.

***auditory n.*** A nest of nerve cells where the auditory nerves arise.

***Bechterew's n., Bekhterev's n.*** Angular n.

***n. of Burdach*** Cuneate n.

***caudate n.*** A comma-shaped mass of gray matter forming part of the corpus striatum. It constitutes part of the basal ganglia. SYN: *intraventricular nucleus.*

***central n. of the thalamus*** A group of nuclei in the middle part of the thalamus. SYN: *centromedian nucleus.*

***centromedian n.*** Central n. of the thalamus.

***cerebellar n.*** One of the nuclei of the cerebellum.

***cornucommissural n. posterior*** A column of cells that extends the entire length of the spinal cord and lies along the medial border of the posterior column near the posterior gray commissure.

***cuneate n.*** A nucleus in the inferior portion of the medulla oblongata in which fibers of the fasciculus cuneatus terminate. SYN: *n. of Burdach.*

***Deiters' n.*** The lateral vestibular nucleus. SEE: *vestibular n.*

***dentate n.*** A large convoluted mass of gray matter in the lateral portion of the cerebellum. It is folded so as to enclose some of the central white matter and gives rise to the fibers of the superior cerebellar peduncle.

***diploid n.*** A nucleus containing the normal double complement of chromosomes.

***dorsal cochlear n.*** The nucleus in the medulla oblongata lying dorsal to the restiform body and receiving fibers from the cochlear nerve.

***dorsal motor n. of vagus*** A column of cells in the medulla oblongata lying lateral to the hypoglossal nucleus. Its cells give rise to most of the efferent fibers of the vagus nerve.

***dorsal sensory n. of vagus*** A nucleus lying lateral to the dorsal motor nucleus of the vagus. It receives the fibers of the solitary tract.

***dorsal n. of the spinal cord*** A column of gray matter lying at the base of the dorsal horn of the gray matter and extending from the seventh cervical to the third lumbar segments. These cells give rise to fibers of the dorsal spinocerebellar tract. SYN: *Clarke's column.*

***ectoblastic n.*** A nucleus in the cells of the epiblast.

***Edinger-Westphal n.*** A nucleus of the midbrain located dorsomedially to the oculomotor nucleus. It gives rise to the visceral efferent fibers terminating in the ciliary ganglion, the axons from which innervate the ciliary muscle and the sphincter iridis of the eye.

***emboliform n.*** A nucleus of the cerebellum lying between the dentate and globose nuclei. It receives the axons of Purkinje cells and sends efferent fibers into the brachium conjunctivum.

***facial motor n.*** A nucleus in the medulla oblongata in the floor of the fourth ventricle giving rise to efferent fibers of the facial nerve.

***fastigial n.*** A nucleus in the medullary portion of the cerebellum that receives afferent fibers from the vestibular nerve and superior vestibular nucleus. The afferent fibers form the fasciculus uncinatus and the fastigiobulbar tract.

***fertilization n.*** A nucleus produced by the joining of the male and female nuclei in the fertilization of the ovum.

***free n.*** A nucleus that is no longer surrounded by the other cellular elements.

***n. funiculi gracilis*** An elongated mass of gray matter in the dorsal pyramid of the medulla oblongata of the brain. SYN: *postpyramidal n.*

***germinal n.*** A nucleus resulting from the union of male and female pronuclei.

***globose n.*** A nucleus of the cerebellum located medial to the emboliform nucleus.

***gonad n.*** Micronucleus (2).

***n. gracilis*** A nucleus in the medulla oblongata in which fibers of the fasciculus gracilis terminate.

***habenular n.*** A nucleus of the diencephalon located in the habenular trigone. It functions as an olfactory correlation center.

***haploid n.*** A cell nucleus with half the normal number of chromosomes, as in germ cells (ova and sperm) following the normal reduction divisions in gametogenesis.

***hypoglossal n.*** An elongated mass of gray matter in the medulla oblongata in the floor of the fourth ventricle, giving rise to the motor fibers of the hypoglossal nerve.

***hypothalamic n.*** One of the nuclei occurring in four groups found in the hypothalamus. Hypothalamic nuclei include the dorsomedial, intercalatus, lateral, mamillary (lateral and medial), paraventricular, posterior, supraoptic, tuberal, and ventromedial. The cells of these nuclei, esp. the supraoptic and paraventricular, in addition to serving a neural function, are secretory and produce the vasopressor oxytocin, as well as antidiuretic principles of the hypophysis. These hormones pass through the efferent fibers of the infundibular stalk to the pars nervosa (posterior lobe) of the hypophysis, where they are stored and liberated. SYN: *subthalamic n.*

***inferior olivary n.*** A large convoluted mass of cells lying in the ventral part of the medulla oblongata and forming part of the reticular system. It gives rise to fibers of the olivocerebellar tract.

***inferior salivatory n.*** A nucleus located in the pons near the level of the dorsal motor nucleus of the vagus. It gives rise to preganglionic parasympathetic fibers that pass to the otic ganglion via the hypoglossal nerve. Impulses regulate secretions of the parotid gland.

***interpeduncular n.*** A nucleus of the midbrain near the superior border of the pons. It receives fibers of the habenulopeduncular tract.

***interstitial n. of Cajal*** A nucleus in the superior portion of the midbrain. It receives fibers from the vestibular nuclei, basal ganglia, and occipital regions of cerebral cortex. The efferent fibers pass to the ipsilateral and contralateral fasciculi and the interstitiospinal tracts.

***intraventricular n.*** Caudate n.

***lenticular n.*** One of the nuclei forming part of the basal ganglia of the cerebrum, consisting of the globus pallidus and putamen. With the caudate nucleus, it forms the corpus striatum.

***n. lentis*** The core or inner dense section of the crystalline lens.

***masticatory n.*** Motor n. of the trigeminal nerve.

***mesencephalic tract n.*** The only site of primary sensory neurons within the central nervous system for proprioceptive impulses from the trigeminal nerve.

***mother n.*** A nucleus that divides into two or more parts to form daughter nuclei.

***motor n.*** A nucleus giving rise to the motor fibers of a nerve.

***motor n. of the trigeminal nerve*** A nucleus in the medulla oblongata near the first margin of the superior part of the 4th ventricle. It gives rise to the motor fibers of the trigeminal nerve, which innervates the muscles of mastication, tensor tympani, tensor palatini, and the anterior digastric muscle. SYN: *masticatory nucleus.*

***oculomotor n.*** A nucleus in the central gray matter of the midbrain lying below the rostral end of the cerebral aqueduct.

***n. of origin*** Any of the collection of nerve cells giving rise to the fibers of a nerve or nerve tract.

***paraventricular n.*** A nucleus of the hypothalamus lying in the supraoptic portion. Its axons with those of the supraoptic nucleus form the supraopticohypophyseal tract. SEE: *hypothalamic n.*

***pontine n.*** One of several groups of nerve cells located in the pons. It receives afferent fibers from the cerebral cortex; efferent fibers pass through the brachium pontis to the cerebellum.

***postpyramidal n.*** N. funiculi gracilis.

***principal trigeminal sensory n.*** The site of sensory neurons of the trigeminal nerve associated with discriminatory touch. It is located in the pons.

***n. pulposus*** The center cushioning gelatinous mass lying within an intervertebral disk; the remains of the notochord.

***pyramidal n.*** A band of gray matter near the olivary nucleus in the medulla.

***red n.*** A large, oval, pigmented mass in the upper portion of the midbrain extending upward into the subthalamus. It receives fibers from the cerebral cortex and cerebellum; the efferent fibers give rise to the rubrospinal tracts. SYN: *nucleus ruber.*

***reproductive n.*** Micronucleus (2).

***reticular n.*** A column of neurons in the spinal cord, brainstem, and thalamus affecting local reflex activity, muscle tone, and wakefulness.

***n. ruber*** Red n.

***segmentation n.*** The nucleus of a zygote formed by fusion of the male and female pronuclei.

***sensory n.*** The nucleus of termination of the afferent fibers of a peripheral nerve.

***sensory n. of the trigeminal nerve*** A group of nuclei in the pons and medulla oblongata consisting of the spinal nucleus, which extends inferiorly into the spinal cord, the main nucleus, which lies dorsal and lateral to the motor nucleus, and the mesencephalic nucleus, which lies in the lateral wall of the 4th ventricle.

***sperm n.*** The head of the spermatozoon.

***subthalamic n.*** Hypothalamic n.

***superior olivary n.*** A small nucleus located in the mid-lateral tegmental region of the pons. It receives fibers from the ventral cochlear nucleus.

***superior salivatory n.*** An ill-defined nucleus in the pons lying dorsomedial to the facial nucleus. It gives rise to preganglionic parasympathetic fibers passing through the chorda tympani and lingual nerve to the submaxillary ganglion. Impulses regulate secretions of the submaxillary and sublingual glands.

***supraoptic n.*** The nucleus of the hypothalamus lying above the rostral ends of the optic tracts and lateral to the optic chiasma. SEE: *hypothalamic n.*

***n. of termination*** Any of the clusters of cells in the brain and medulla in which fibers of a nerve or nerve tract terminate.

***thalamic n.*** Any of the nuclei of the thalamus, including a large number belonging to the anterior, intralaminar, lateral, and medial thalamic nuclei groups.

***thoracic n.*** A column of large neurons in the posterior gray column of the spinal cord. These cells give rise to the dorsal spinocerebellar tract on the same side.

***trigeminal spinal n.*** The site of sensory neurons of the trigeminal nerve associated with pain, temperature, and light touch. It is located in the pons and upper spinal tract.

***ventral cochlear n.*** The nucleus in the medulla oblongata lying anterior and lateral to the restiform body and receiving fibers from the cochlear nerve.

***vesicular n.*** A nucleus having a deeply staining membrane and a pale center.

***vestibular n.*** One of four nuclei in the medulla oblongata in which fibers of the vestibular nerve terminate. These four nuclei are the medial (Schwalbe's), superior (Bechterew's), lateral (Deiters'), and inferior nuclei.

***vitelline n.*** Nucleus formed by union of male and female pronuclei within the vitellus; a part of the cytoplasm of an ovum in which the initial process of accumulation of food supplies is probably located. SYN: *yolk n.*

***white n.*** The central white substance of the corpus dentatum of the olive.

***yolk n.*** Vitelline n.

**nuclide** (nū′klīd) An atomic nucleus identified by its atomic number, mass, and energy state.

**nude** [L. *nudus,* naked] **1.** Bare; naked; unclothed. **2.** An unclothed body.

**nude mouse** SEE: under *mouse.*

**nudism 1.** In psychiatry, morbid desire to remove clothing. **2.** The cult or practice of living in a nude condition.

**nudomania** (nū″dō-mā′nē-ă) [L. *nudus,* naked + Gr. *mania,* madness] Abnormal desire to be naked.

**nudophobia** (nū″dō-fō′bē-ă) [″ + Gr. *phobos,* fear] Abnormal fear of being naked. SEE: *gymnophobia.*

**Nuel's space** (nū′ĕlz) [Jean-Pierre Nuel, Belg. physician, 1847–1920] The space in the organ of Corti between the outer pillar and the outer phalangeal cells (Deiters' cells).

**NUG** *necrotizing ulcerative gingivitis.*

**Nuhn's glands** (noonz) [Anton Nuhn, Ger. anatomist, 1814–1889] Blandin's glands.

**null cell** SEE: under *cell.*

**null hypothesis** SEE: under *hypothesis.*

**nulligravida** A woman who has never conceived a child.

**nullipara** (nŭl-ĭp′ă-ră) [L. *nullus,* none, + *parere,* to bear] A woman who has never produced a viable offspring.

**nulliparity** (nŭl″ĭ-păr′ĭ-tē) Condition of not having given birth to a child.

**nulliparous** (nŭl-lĭp′ăr-ŭs) Never having borne a child.

**numb** (nŭm) **1.** Insensible; lacking in feeling. **2.** Deadened or lacking in the power to move.

**number** [L. *numerus,* number] **1.** A total of units. **2.** A symbol graphically representing an arithmetical sum.

***atomic n.*** The number indicating the number of negatively charged electrons in an uncharged atom, or the number of protons in the nucleus. This number determines the position of elements in the periodic table of elements.

***Avogadro's n.*** SEE: *Avogadro's number.*

***hardness n.*** A number on a calibrated scale indicating the relative hardness as determined by a particular system of testing (e.g., Knoop, Mohs, Rockwell, Vickers hardness tests). A steel ball or diamond point is applied with a known variable load for a determined period of time to produce an indent whose depth or diameter can be measured.

***mass n.*** The mass of the atom of a specific isotope relative to the mass of hydrogen. In general, this number is equal to the total of the protons and neutrons in the atomic nucleus of that specific isotope.

**numbness** Lack of sensation in a part, esp.

from cold. SEE: *narcohypnia.*

**numeral** (nū′mĕr-ăl) [L. *numerus,* number] **1.** Denoting or pert. to a number. **2.** A conventional symbol expressing a number.

**nummiform** (nŭm′mĭ-form) [L. *nummus,* a coin, + *forma,* shape] **1.** Coin-shaped, said of some mucous sputum. **2.** Arranged like a stack of coins.

**nummular** (nŭm′ū-lăr) [L. *nummus,* coin] **1.** Coin-shaped. **2.** Stacked like coins, as in a rouleau of red blood cells.

**nunnation** (nŭn-ā′shŭn) [Heb. *nun,* letter N] The frequent and abnormal use of the "n" sound.

**Nuremberg Code** A set of principles established after World War II to protect the rights of research participants (subjects).

**nurse** [L. *nutrix,* nurse] **1.** An individual who provides health care. The extent of participation varies from simple patient care tasks to the most expert professional techniques necessary in acute life-threatening situations. The ability of a nurse to function in making self-directed judgments and to act independently will depend on his or her professional background, motivation, and opportunity for professional development. The health care team includes the technical nurse, who is technique-oriented, deals with commonly recurring nursing problems, and knows standardized procedures and medically delegated techniques. Also included is the professional nurse, who is prepared to assume responsibility for the care of individuals and groups through a colleague relationship with a physician. The roles of nurses constantly change in response to the growth of biomedical knowledge, changes in patterns of demand for health services, and the evolution of professional relationships among nurses, physicians, and other health care professionals. **2.** To feed an infant at the breast. **3.** To perform the duties of caring for an invalid. **4.** To care for a young child.

***advanced practice n.*** A registered nurse with additional education, skill, and specialization in various fields of medicine. SEE: *n. anesthetist; clinical n. specialist; n. midwife; n. practitioner.*

***n. anesthetist*** ABBR: CRNA. A registered nurse who administers anesthesia to patients in the operating room and delivery room. The knowledge and skill required to provide this service are attained through an organized program of study recognized by the American Association of Nurse Anesthetists.

***charge n.*** A nurse who is responsible for supervising the nursing staff on a hospital or nursing home unit. This nurse reports to the nurse manager.

***clinical n. specialist*** A nurse with particular competence in certain areas such as intensive care, cardiology, oncology, obstetrics, or psychiatry. A clinical nurse specialist holds a master's degree in nursing, preferably with emphasis in clinical nursing.

***n. clinician*** A registered nurse with preparation in a specialized educational program. At present this preparation may be in the context of a formal continuing education program, a baccalaureate nursing program, or an advanced-degree nursing program. The nurse clinician is capable of working independently in solving patient-care problems and is able to teach and work successfully with others on the medical care team. The term was first used by Frances Reiter, R.N., M.A., Dean, Graduate School of Nursing, New York Medical College.

***community health n.*** A nurse who combines the principles and practices of nursing and public health to provide care to the people in a community rather than in an institution.

***dental n.*** A dental auxiliary trained to provide oral hygiene instruction and dental health care to school children. Formerly, the term applied to dental hygienists, but now it refers to persons trained according to a program developed in New Zealand.

***epidemiologist n.*** A registered nurse with special training and certification in the prevention of hospital-acquired infections in patients. SEE: *infection control n.*

***flight n.*** A nurse who cares for patients being transported in an aircraft.

***general duty n.*** A nurse not specializing in a particular field but available for any nursing duty.

***graduate n.*** A nurse who is a graduate of a state-approved school of nursing but has not yet passed the National Council Licensure Examination.

***head n.*** Outdated term for nurse manager.

***health n.*** A community or visiting nurse whose duty is to give information on hygiene and prevention of disease. SEE: *community health n.*

***home health n.*** A nurse who visits patients in their homes to provide skilled nursing services, such as assessment and patient and family teaching.

***infection control n.*** A registered nurse employed by an agency to monitor the rate and causes of nosocomial infections and to promote measures to prevent such infections.

***licensed practical n.*** ABBR: L.P.N. A graduate of a school of practical nursing who has passed the practical nursing state board examination and is licensed to administer care, usually working under direction of a licensed physician or a registered nurse.

***licensed vocational n.*** ABBR: L.V.N. Licensed practical n.

***n. manager*** A nurse who has responsibility for a unit within a hospital, nursing home, or ambulatory care setting. The nurse manager supervises staff performance and patient care.

***n. midwife*** A registered nurse who has completed specialized theory and clinical courses in obstetrics and gynecology and is certified by the American College of Nurse Midwives. This person provides primary care to women who are experiencing normal, uncomplicated pregnancies and deliveries.

***n. practitioner*** ABBR: NP. A licensed registered nurse who has had advanced preparation for practice that includes 9 to 24 months of supervised clinical experience in the diagnosis and treatment of illness. The NP concept was developed in 1965 by Henry Silver, M.D., and Loretta Ford, R.N. Most contemporary NP programs are at the master's degree level; graduates are prepared for primary care practice in family medicine, women's health, neonatology, pediatrics, school health, geriatrics, or mental health. NPs may work in collaborative practice with physicians or independently in private practice or in nursing clinics. Depending upon state laws, NPs may be allowed to write prescriptions for medications. SEE: *n. clinician; n. midwife; nursing, advanced practice.*

***prescribing n.*** A nurse who is allowed to prescribe drugs. Certain states in the U.S. permit nurses to prescribe only certain types and classes of drugs; most states require that prescribing nurses work with a supervising or collaborating physician; and approval for prescribing is granted only to nurse practitioners.

***private duty n.*** A nurse who cares for a patient on a fee-for-service basis, usually in an institution. The nurse is not a staff member of the institution.

***probationer n.*** A student nurse who is on probation until the instructors have had sufficient time to determine his or her suitability for the nursing profession.

***psychiatric n. practitioner*** A registered nurse with advanced preparation who combines medical and nursing skills in the care and treatment of psychiatric or mental health patients.

***public health n.*** Community health n.

***registered n.*** ABBR: RN. A nurse who has graduated from a state-approved school of nursing, has passed the professional nursing state board examination, and has been granted a license to practice within a given state.

***school n.*** A nurse working in a school or college who is responsible for the health of children, adolescents, and young adults in school.

***scrub n.*** An operating room nurse who directly assists the surgeon, primarily by passing instruments and supplies.

***special n.*** Private duty n.

***specialist n.*** Clinical n. specialist.

***visiting n.*** Community health n.

***wet n.*** A woman who breast-feeds a child that is not her own.

**nursery** A hospital department in which the newborn are cared for.

***day n.*** SEE: *day care center.*

**nurse's aide** An individual who assists nurses by performing the patient-care procedures that do not require special technical training, such as feeding and bathing patients.

**nursing 1.** The care and nurturing of healthy and ill people, individually or in groups and communities. The American Nurses Association identifies four essential features of contemporary nursing practice: attention to the full range of human experiences and responses to health and illness without restriction to a problem-focused orientation; integration of objective data with knowledge gained from an understanding of the patient or group's subjective experience; application of scientific knowledge to the processes of diagnosis and treatment; and provision of a caring relationship that facilitates health and healing. SEE: *nurse.* **2.** Breastfeeding.

***advanced practice n.*** Primary medical care provided by nurses who have been prepared as practitioners and are competent to provide that level of care. These practitioners may act independently or under the supervision of a physician.

**nursing assessment** In the nursing process, the systematic collection of all data and information relevant to the patients, and their problems and needs. The initial step of the assessment consists of obtaining a careful and complete history from the patient. If this cannot be done because the mental or physical condition of the patient makes communication impossible, the nursing history is obtained from those who have information about the patient and the reason(s) for his or her need of medical and nursing care. Obtaining an accurate and comprehensive history requires skill in communicating with individuals who are ill and who may feel that obtaining a history of their illness is not what they need at that time. The skilled nurse will be able to obtain the essential information despite resistance. Next in the assessment is the physical examination of the patient in order to determine how the disease has altered physical and mental status. To do this requires that the nurse be capable of performing visual and tactile inspection, palpation, percussion, and auscultation and have knowledge of what represents deviation from the norm and how disease and trauma alter the physical and mental condition of a patient. After these two steps have been completed, the nurse will be able to establish a nursing diagnosis. SEE: illus.; *evaluation; nursing process.*

**nursing assistant** ABBR: N.A. An unlicensed nursing staff member who assists with basic patient care such as giving baths, checking vital signs, bedmaking, and positioning. Nursing assistants usu-

## NURSING ASSESSMENT TOOL (Medical/Surgical)

This is a suggested tool for development by an individual or institution to create a data base reflecting Diagnostic Divisions of Nursing Diagnoses. Although the divisions are alphabetized for ease of presentation, they can be prioritized or rearranged to meet individual needs.

### GENERAL INFORMATION

Name: ______

Age: ______ DOB: ______ Sex: ______ Race: ______

Admission date: ______ Time: ______ From: ______

Source of information: ______ Reliability (1–4 with 4 = very reliable): ______

### ACTIVITY/REST

**Reports (Subjective)**

Occupation: ______ Usual activities/hobbies: ______

Leisure time activities: ______

Feelings of boredom/dissatisfaction: ______

Limitations imposed by condition: ______

Sleep: Hours: ______ Naps: ______ Aids: ______

Insomnia: ______ Related to: ______

Rested upon awakening: ______

Other: ______

**Exhibits (Objective)**

Observed response to activity: Cardiovascular: ______

Respiratory: ______

Mental status (i.e., withdrawn/lethargic): ______

Neuromuscular assessment: ______

Muscle mass/tone: ______

Posture: ______ Tremors: ______

ROM: ______ Strength: ______

Deformity: ______

### CIRCULATION

**Reports (Subjective)**

History of: Hypertension: ______ Heart trouble: ______

Rheumatic fever: ______ Ankle/leg edema: ______

Phlebitis: ______ Slow healing: ______

Claudication: ______

Extremities: Numbness: ______ Tingling: ______

Cough/hemoptysis: ______

Change in frequency/amount of urine: ______

**Exhibits (Objective)**

BP: R and L: Lying/sitting/standing: ______

Pulse pressure: ______ Auscultatory gap: ______

Pulse (palpation): Carotid: ______ Temporal: ______

Jugular: ______ Radial: ______

Femoral: ______ Popliteal: ______

Posttibial: ______ Dorsalis pedis: ______

Cardiac (palpation): ______

Thrill: ______ Heaves: ______

SOURCE: Doenges, Marilynn E, et al: Nursing Care Plans: Guidelines for Planning and Documenting Patient Care, ed. 3. FA Davis, Philadelphia, 1993.

## NURSING ASSESSMENT TOOL (Medical/Surgical)—continued

Heart sounds: Rate: ______ Rhythm: ______ Quality: ______
Friction rub: ______ Murmur: ______
Breath sounds: Vascular bruit: ______ Jugular vein distention: ______
Extremities: Temperature: ______ Color: ______
Capillary refill: ______
Homan's sign: ______ Varicosities: ______
Nail abnormalities: ______
Distribution/quality of hair: ______
Color: ______ Mucous membranes: ______ Lips: ______
Nail beds: ______ Conjunctiva: ______ Sclera: ______
Diaphoresis: ______

### EGO INTEGRITY

#### Reports (Subjective)

Stress factors: ______
Ways of handling stress: ______
Financial concerns: ______
Relationship status: ______
Cultural factors: ______
Religion: ______ Practicing: ______
Lifestyle: ______ Recent changes: ______
Feelings: Helplessness: ______ Hopelessness: ______
Powerlessness: ______

#### Exhibits (Objective)

Emotional status (check those that apply):
Calm: ______ Anxious: ______ Angry: ______
Withdrawn: ______ Fearful: ______ Irritable: ______
Restive: ______ Euphoric: ______
Observed physiologic response(s): ______

### ELIMINATION

#### Reports (Subjective)

Usual bowel pattern: ______ Laxative use: ______
Character of stool: ______ Last bowel movement: ______
History of bleeding: ______ Hemorrhoids: ______
Constipation: ______ Diarrhea: ______
Usual voiding pattern: ______ Incontinence/when: ______
Urgency: ______ Frequency: ______ Retention: ______
Character of urine: ______
Pain/burning/difficulty voiding: ______
History of kidney/bladder disease: ______
Diuretic use: ______

#### Exhibits (Objective)

Abdomen: Tender: ______ Soft/firm: ______
Palpable mass: ______ Size/girth: ______
Bowel sounds: ______
Hemorrhoids: ______
Bladder palpable: ______ Overflow voiding: ______

### FOOD/FLUID

#### Reports (Subjective)

Usual diet (type): ______ Number of meals daily: ______

## NURSING ASSESSMENT TOOL (Medical/Surgical)—continued

Last meal/intake: ______ Dietary pattern: ______
Loss of appetite: ______ Nausea/vomiting: ______
Heartburn/indigestion: ______ Related to: ______ Relieved by: ______
Allergy/Food intolerance: ______
Mastication/swallowing problems: ______
Dentures: ______
Usual weight: ______ Changes in weight: ______
Diuretic use: ______

**Exhibits (Objective)**

Current weight: ______ Height: ______ Body build: ______
Skin turgor: ______ Mucous membranes moist/dry: ______
Edema: General: ______ Dependent: ______
Periorbital: ______ Ascites: ______
Jugular vein distention: ______
Thyroid enlarged: ______ Hernia/masses: ______ Halitosis: ______
Condition of teeth/gums: ______
Appearance of tongue: ______
Mucous membranes: ______
Bowel sounds: ______
Breath sounds: ______
Urine S/A or Chemstix: ______

### HYGIENE

**Reports (Subjective)**

Activities of daily living: Independent/dependent: ______
Mobility: ______ Feeding: ______
Hygiene: ______ Dressing: ______
Toileting: ______
Preferred time of bath: ______
Equipment/prosthetic devices required: ______
Assistance provided by: ______

**Exhibits (Objective)**

General appearance: ______
Manner of dress: ______ Personal habits: ______
Body odor: ______ Condition of scalp: ______
Presence of vermin: ______

### NEUROSENSORY

**Reports (Subjective)**

Fainting spells/dizziness: ______
Headaches: Pain location: ______ Frequency: ______
Tingling/numbness/weakness (location): ______
Stroke (residual effects): ______
Seizures: ______ Type: ______ Aura: ______ Frequency: ______
Postical state: ______ How controlled: ______
Eyes: Vision loss: ______ Last examination: ______
Glaucoma: ______ Cataract: ______
Ears: Hearing loss: ______ Last examination: ______
Epistaxis: ______ Sense of smell: ______

**Exhibits (Objective)**

Mental status: ______
Oriented/disoriented: Time: ______

## NURSING ASSESSMENT TOOL (Medical/Surgical)—continued

Place: ____________

Person: ____________

Alert: ____________ Drowsy: ____________ Lethargic: ____________

Stuporous: ____________ Comatose: ____________

Cooperative: ____________ Combative: ____________ Delusions: ____________

Hallucinations: ____________ Affect (describe): ____________

Memory: Recent: ____________ Remote: ____________

Glasses: ____________ Contacts: ____________ Hearing aids: ____________

Pupil size/reaction: R/L: ____________

Facial droop: ____________ Swallowing: ____________

Handgrasp/release: R/L: ____________ Posturing: ____________

Deep tendon reflexes: ____________ Paralysis: ____________

### PAIN/DISCOMFORT

**Reports (Subjective)**

Location: ____________ Intensity (1–10 with 10 most severe): ____________ Frequency: ____________

Quality: ____________ Duration: ____________ Radiation: ____________

Precipitating factors: ____________

How relieved, associated factors: ____________

**Exhibits (Objective)**

Facial grimacing: ____________ Guarding affected area: ____________

Emotional response: ____________ Narrowed focus: ____________

### RESPIRATION

**Reports (Subjective)**

Dyspnea, related to cough/sputum:

History of bronchitis: ____________ Asthma: ____________

Tuberculosis: ____________ Emphysema: ____________

Recurrent pneumonia: ____________

Exposure to noxious fumes: ____________

Smoker: ____________ Pack/d: ____________ Number of years: ____________

Use of respiratory aids: ____________ Oxygen: ____________

**Exhibits (Objective)**

Respiratory: Rate: ____________ Depth: ____________ Symmetry: ____________

Use of accessory muscles: ____________ Nasal flaring: ____________

Fremitis: ____________

Breath sounds: ____________

Egophony: ____________

Cyanosis: ____________ Clubbing of fingers: ____________

Sputum characteristics: ____________

Mentation/restlessness: ____________

### SAFETY

**Reports (Subjective)**

Allergies/sensitivity: ____________ Reaction: ____________

Previous alteration of immune system: ____________ Cause: ____________

History of sexually transmitted disease (date/type): ____________

High-risk behaviors: ____________ Testing: ____________

Blood transfusion/number: ____________ When: ____________

## NURSING ASSESSMENT TOOL (Medical/Surgical)—continued

Reaction described: ____
History of accidental injuries: ____
Fractures/dislocations: ____
Arthritis/unstable joints: ____
Back problems: ____
Changes in moles: ____ Enlarged nodes: ____
Impaired vision, hearing: ____
Prosthesis: ____ Ambulatory devices: ____

**Exhibits (Objective)**

Temperature: ____ Diaphoresis: ____
Skin integrity: ____
Scars: ____ Rashes: ____
Lacerations: ____ Ulcerations: ____
Ecchymosis: ____ Blisters: ____
Burns: (degree/percent): ____ Drainage: ____
Mark location of above on diagram:

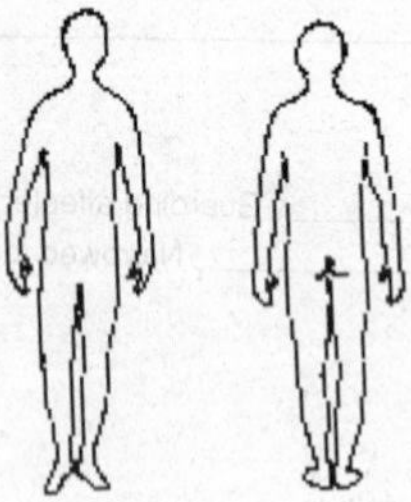

General strength: ____ Muscle tone: ____
Gait: ____ Range of motion: ____
Paresthesia/paralysis: ____
Results of cultures, immune system testing: ____

**SEXUALITY: (Component of Social Interaction)**

Sexually active: ____ Use of condoms: ____ Sexual concerns/difficulties: ____ Recent change in frequency/interest: ____

**Female**

**Reports (Subjective)**

Age at menarche: ____ Length of cycle: ____ Duration: ____
Last menstrual period: ____ Menopause: ____
Vaginal discharge: ____ Bleeding between periods: ____
Practices breast self-examination/mammogram: ____ Last PAP smear: ____

**Exhibits (Objective)**

Breast examination: ____
Genital warts/lesions: ____

**Male**

**Reports (Subjective)**

Penile discharge: ____ Prostate disorder: ____
Circumcised: ____ Vasectomy: ____
Practices self-examination: ____ Breast/testicles: ____
Last proctoscopic/prostate examination: ____

## NURSING ASSESSMENT TOOL (Medical/Surgical)—continued

**Exhibits (Objective)**

Examination: ______ Breast/penis/testicles: ______

Genital warts/lesions: ______

### SOCIAL INTERACTIONS

**Reports (Subjective)**

Marital status: ______ Years in relationship: ______

Living with: ______

Concerns/stresses: ______

Extended family: ______

Other support person(s): ______

Role within family structure: ______

Problems related to illness/condition: ______

Change in speech: Use of communication aids: ______

Laryngectomy present: ______

**Exhibits (Objective)**

Speech: Clear: ______ Slurred: ______

Unintelligible: ______ Aphasic: ______

Unusual speech pattern/impairment: ______

Use of speech aids: ______

Verbal/nonverbal communication with family/SO(s): ______

Family interaction (behavioral) pattern: ______

### TEACHING/LEARNING

**Reports (Subjective)**

Dominant language (specify): ______ Literate: ______

Education level: ______

Learning disabilities (specify): ______

Cognitive limitations: ______

Health beliefs/practices: ______

Special health care concerns (e.g., impact of religious/cultural practices): ______

Familial risk factors (indicate relationship): ______

Diabetes: ______ Tuberculosis: ______

Heart disease: ______ Strokes: ______

High BP: ______ Epilepsy: ______

Kidney disease: ______ Cancer: ______

Mental illness: ______ Other: ______

Prescribed medications (circle last dose):

| *Drug* | *Dose* | *Times* | *Take regularly* | *Purpose* |
|---|---|---|---|---|
| | | | | |
| | | | | |
| | | | | |

Nonprescription drugs: OTC drugs: ______

Street drugs: ______ Tobacco: ______ Smokeless tobacco: ______

Use of alcohol (amount/frequency): ______

Admitting diagnosis per physician: ______

Reason for hospitalization per patient: ______

History of current complaint: ______

Patient expectations of this hospitalization: ______

Previous illnesses and/or hospitalizations/surgeries: ______

## NURSING ASSESSMENT TOOL (Medical/Surgical)—continued

Evidence of failure to improve: ____________

Last complete physical examination: ____________

**Discharge Plan Considerations**

DRG projected mean length of stay: ____________

Date information obtained: ____________

1. Anticipated date of discharge: ____________
2. Resources available: Persons: ____________
   Financial: ____________
3. Anticipated changes in living situation after discharge: ____________
4. Areas that may require alteration/assistance: ____________

Food preparation: ____________ Shopping: ____________

Transportation: ____________ Ambulation: ____________

Medication/IV therapy: ____________ Treatments: ____________

Wound care: ____________ Supplies: ____________

Self-care assistance (specify): ____________

Physical layout of home (specify): ____________

Homemaker/maintenance assistance (specify): ____________

Living facility other than home (specify): ____________

ally must complete a training course, including classroom instruction and clinical practice under supervision. Each state regulates nursing assistant practice.

**nursing audit** A procedure to evaluate the quality of nursing care provided for a patient. Established criteria for care are the yardstick for the evaluation. SEE: *nursing process; problem-oriented medical record.*

**nursing care plan** SEE: under *plan*.

**nursing diagnosis** The patient problem identified by the nurse for nursing intervention by analysis of assessment findings in comparison with what is considered to be normal. Nurses, esp. those involved in patient care, are in virtually constant need to make decisions and diagnoses based on their clinical experience and judgment. In many instances, that process dictates a course of action for the nurse that is of vital importance to the patient. As the nursing profession evolves and develops, nursing diagnosis will be defined and specified in accordance with the specialized training and experience of nurses, particularly for nurse practitioners and clinical nurse specialists. SEE: *nursing process; planning.*

**nursing goal** A specific expected outcome of nursing intervention as related to the established nursing diagnosis. A goal is stated in terms of a desired, measurable change in patient status or behavior. Nursing goals provide direction for selection of appropriate nursing interventions and evaluation of patient progress.

**nursing history** The first step of the assessment stage of the nursing process that leads to development of a nursing care plan. Valuable information can be obtained from this history, and reactions to previous hospitalization can be recorded and utilized in managing the patient's care during the current stay.

**nursing home** An extended-care facility for persons who need medical attention of the type and complexity not requiring hospitalization. Nursing homes provide 24-hr nursing supervision, rehabilitation services, activity and social services, a restraint-appropriate environment, careful attention to nutritional needs, and measures to prevent complications of decreased mobility. In addition, some nursing homes have specialty units for patients with dementia, chronic ventilator support, or head injuries. Some nursing homes provide subacute units for patients who are not as medically stable as patients in the typical nursing home setting.

Most nursing homes are licensed and certified to provide an intermediate or skilled level of care or both. Medicare reimbursement is available for patients receiving skilled care in a skilled nursing facility.

In 1990, it was estimated that 43% of all Americans who turn 65 will use a nursing home at least once before they die. Of those, 55% will stay at least 1 year, and 21% will stay 5 years or longer. It is estimated that 1.5 million Americans live in nursing homes and that by the year 2030, the number will be 5 million. The cost of nursing home care in 1990 was $53 billion, and is estimated to exceed $700 billion by the year 2030.

**nursing intervention** In the nursing process, the step after planning. This step involves all aspects of actual caring for the patient and requires full knowledge of the assessment and planning stages of the nursing process. The goals of nursing intervention will have been stated in the planning step of the nursing process. Included in this step are patient care in the areas of hygiene and mental and physical comfort, including assistance in feeding and elimination, controlling the physical aspects of the patient's environment, and instructing the patient about the factors important to his or her care and what actions to take to facilitate recovery. After the patient's acute and immediate needs are met, he or she should be instructed concerning actions that could be taken to help prevent a recurrence of the condition. SEE: *nursing process; planning; problem-oriented medical record.*

**Nursing Minimum Data Set** ABBR: NMDS. An abstracting system designed to collect minimal, comparable standardized nursing care information. It may be used in different settings and for different types of patients. Among its purposes are to identify trends and emerging needs in nursing care, to guide nursing research, and to use statistics to influence decisions in health care policy. It provides data for multiple users in the health care system. SEE: *Minimum Data Set.*

**nursing model** SEE: under *model.*

**nursing process** An orderly, logical approach to administering nursing care so that the patient's needs for such care are met comprehensively and effectively. The objective of health care is to provide total, comprehensive care of patients. Nursing has always been dedicated to this concept and, from the holistic viewpoint, has formalized the scientific processes that contribute to the prevention of illness as well as restoration and maintenance of health. In so doing, the traditional approaches used in problem solving have been used. Therefore the nurse needs skills in the following five areas to provide comprehensive care of patients: (1) *Assessment:* The systemic collection of all data and information relevant to the patients, their problems, and needs. (2) *Problem identification:* The interpretation of the information obtained during assessment that establishes the nursing diagnosis. (3) *Planning:* The use of skills to determine individualized patient-centered goals and the optimum course of action to solve the problem. (4) *Implementation or intervention:* The process of putting the plan into action. (5) *Evaluation:* The ongoing process of assessing the effectiveness of the plan and altering it as the need arises. SEE: *evaluation; nursing assessment; nursing intervention; planning; problem-oriented medical record.*

**nursing protocol** A specific written procedure that prescribes nursing actions in a given situation. Health agencies and physicians establish protocols to ensure consistency and quality of care. A protocol may describe mandatory nursing assessments, behaviors, and documentation for establishing and maintaining invasive appliances; methods of administering specific drugs; special-care modalities for patients with certain disorders; other components of patient care; lines of authority; or channels of communication under particular circumstances.

**nursing standards** The criteria established by professional nursing organizations that describe peer expectations for safe, competent, ethical performance of professional responsibilities. Documents such as the American Nurses' Association Standards of Clinical Practice and Standards of Professional Performance describe general behaviors expected of all professional nurses. Criteria established by specialty nursing organizations, such as the Standards for the Nursing Care of Women and Newborns developed by the Associaton of Women's Health, Obstetric, and Neonatal Nurses, contain both universal and specialty-specific expectations. Standards are used to develop nursing curricula and job descriptions and to evaluate nursing effectiveness and accountability. SEE: *standard of care; standards of practice.*

**nursing student** An individual enrolled in a school of nursing.

**nursing supervisor** A substitute for the director or vice president of nursing. This position is seen most commonly, but not exclusively, in nursing home settings. Also called *house supervisor.*

**nursing theorist** An individual who develops theories regarding the purpose, meaning, structure, and functions of the profession and discipline of nursing. SEE: under *theory.*

**nursing theory** SEE: under *theory.*

**nutation** (nū-tā′shŭn) [L. *nutare,* to nod] **1.** Nodding, as of the head. SEE: *nodding.* **2.** A complex movement of the sacrum.

**nutgall** (nŭt′gawl) A growth on certain oak trees produced by insect eggs and larvae. Gallic and tannic acids are obtained from these growths.

**nutrient** (nū′trē-ĕnt) [L. *nutriens*] **1.** Food or any substance that supplies the body with elements necessary for metabolism. **2.** Nourishing; supplying nutriment.

Certain nutrients (carbohydrates, fats, and proteins) provide energy; other nutrients (water, electrolytes, minerals, and vitamins) are essential to the metabolic process. Those containing carbon are organic food nutrients. Organic food nutrients may or may not contain nitrogen.

**nutrilite** (nū′trĭ-līt) Any essential nutrient, esp. ones that are required by bacteria in only trace quantities.

**nutriment** (nū′trĭ-mĕnt) [L. *nutrimentum,* nourishment] That which nourishes; nutritious substance; food.

**nutrition** (nū-trĭ′shŭn) [L. *nutritio,* nourish]

All the processes involved in the taking in and utilization of food substances by which growth, repair, and maintenance of activities in the body as a whole or in any of its parts are accomplished. These processes include ingestion, digestion, absorption, and metabolism. Some nutrients are capable of being stored by the body in various forms and drawn upon when the food intake is not sufficient. Vitamin C is an example of a nutrient that is not stored. **nutritional** (nū-trĭsh′ŭn-ăl), *adj.*

***n., altered: less than body requirements*** The state in which an individual has an intake of nutrients insufficient to meet metabolic needs. SEE: *Nursing Diagnoses Appendix.*

***n., altered: more than body requirements*** The state in which an individual has an intake of nutrients which exceeds metabolic needs. SEE: *Nursing Diagnoses Appendix.*

***n., altered: risk for more than body requirements*** The state in which an individual is at risk of experiencing an intake of nutrients that exceeds metabolic needs. SEE: *Nursing Diagnoses Appendix.*

***enteral n.*** Nutrition provided by introducing nutritional substances into the intestines. This is usually done via a nasogastric tube, but oral insertion is required for intubated patients.

**nutritional adequacy** The relationship between intake of nutrients and individual requirements.

**nutritious** (nū-trĭsh′ŭs) [L. *nutritius*] Affording nourishment.

**nutritive** (nū′trĭ-tĭv) **1.** Pert. to the process of assimilating food. **2.** Having the property of nourishing.

**nux vomica** (nŭks vŏm′ĭ-kă) The poisonous seed from an East Indian tree that contains several alkaloids, the principal ones being brucine and strychnine.

**nyct-** SEE: *nycto-*.

**nyctalbuminuria** (nĭk″tăl-bū″mĭn-ū′rē-ă) [Gr. *nyx,* night, + L. *albus,* white, + Gr. *ouron,* urine] A cyclic albuminuria occurring at night.

**nyctalgia** (nĭk-tăl′jē-ă) [″ + *algos,* pain] Pain occurring at night.

**nyctalopia** (nĭk-tă-lō′pē-ă) [″ + *alaos,* blind, + *ops,* eye] **1.** Inability to see well in a faint light or at night. This condition occurs in retinitis pigmentosa and choroidoretinitis, or it may be due to vitamin A deficiency. Smoking tobacco may impair the ability to see at night. Hypoxia associated with being above sea level in an aircraft will also decrease night vision. SYN: *night blindness.* **2.** Incorrectly used to indicate the ability to see better at night or in semidarkness than by day.

**nyctamblyopia** (nĭk″tăm-blē-ō′pē-ă) [Gr. *nyx,* night, + *amblyopia,* poor sight] Reduction or dimness of vision at night without visible eye changes.

**nyctaphonia, nyctophonia** (nĭk″tă-fō′nē-ă, nĭk″tō-fō′nē-ă) [″ + *a,* not, + *phone,* voice] Loss of voice during the night.

**nycterine** (nĭk′tĕr-īn) [Gr. *nykterinos,* by night] **1.** Nocturnal. **2.** Obscure.

**nycto-, nyct-** (nĭk′tō) [Gr. *nyx,* night] Combining form indicating *night, darkness.*

**nyctohemeral, nycthemerus** (nĭk″tō-hĕm′ĕr-ăl, nĭk-thĕm′ĕ-rŭs) Relating to both day and night.

**nyctophilia** (nĭk″tō-fĭl′ē-ă) [Gr. *nyx,* night, + *philein,* to love] A preference for darkness or night.

**nyctophobia** (nĭk″tō-fō′bē-ă) [″ + *phobos,* fear] Abnormal dread of the night or of darkness. SYN: *scotophobia.*

**nyctotyphlosis** (nĭk″tō-tĭf-lō′sĭs) [″ + *typhlosis,* blindness] Nyctalopia.

**nycturia** (nĭk-tū′rē-ă) [″ + *ouron,* urine] Nocturia.

**nylidrin hydrochloride** (nĭl′ĭ-drĭn) A drug used to produce peripheral vasodilation.

**nymph** (nĭmf) [Gr. *nymphe,* a maiden] The immature stage of insect development in which wings and genitalia have not fully developed.

**nympha** [Gr. *nymphe,* a maiden] One of the labia minora; the small folds of mucous membrane forming the inner lips of the vulva. SYN: *labium minus pudendi.*

**nymphectomy** (nĭm-fĕk′tō-mē) [″ + *ektome,* excision] Excision of hypertrophied nymphae.

**nymphitis** (nĭm-fī′tĭs) [″ + *itis,* inflammation] Inflammation of the nymphae.

**nympholepsy** (nĭm′fō-lĕp″sē) [Gr. *nymphe,* a maiden, + *lepsis,* a seizure] **1.** Frenzied ecstasy, usually erotic in nature. **2.** Obsession for something that is unattainable.

**nymphomania** (nĭm″fō-mā′nē-ă) [″ + *mania,* madness] Abnormally excessive sexual desire in a female. SYN: *furor femininus.* SEE: *satyriasis.*

**nymphomaniac** (nĭm″fō-mā′nē-ăk) [″ + *mania,* madness] **1.** One who is afflicted with excessive sexual desire. **2.** Affected with or characterized by excessive sexual desire.

**nymphoncus** (nĭm-fŏn′kŭs) [″ + *onkos,* a swelling] Swelling or tumor of the nymphae.

**nymphotomy** (nĭm-fŏt′ō-mē) [″ + *tome,* incision] **1.** Removal of the nymphae. SYN: *nymphectomy.* **2.** Incision into a nympha or clitoris.

**nystagmic** (nĭs-tăg′mĭk) [Gr. *nystagmos,* to nod] Relating to or suffering from nystagmus.

**nystagmiform** (nĭs-tăg′mĭ-form) [″ + L. *forma,* shape] Resembling nystagmus. SYN: *nystagmoid.*

**nystagmograph** (nĭs-tăg′mō-grăf) [″ + *graphein,* to write] An apparatus for recording the oscillations of the eyeball in nystagmus.

**nystagmoid** (nĭs-tăg′moyd) [″ + *eidos,* form, shape] Resembling nystagmus.

**nystagmus** (nĭs-tăg′mŭs) [Gr. *nystagmos,* to nod] Constant, involuntary, cyclical movement of the eyeball. The movement may be in any direction. The condition may be congenital and inapparent to the patient, or it may be the result of occupational hazards. Nystagmus is seen in bilateral amblyopia, labyrinthine irritability, and neurologic diseases. SEE: *saccades.*

***aural n.*** Nystagmus due to a disorder in the labyrinth of the ear. Eye movement is spasmodic.

***Cheyne's n.*** Rhythmic nystagmus that resembles the rhythm of Cheyne-Stokes breathing.

***convergence n.*** Slow abduction of eyes followed by rapid adduction. This type of nystagmus usually accompanies other types.

***dissociated n.*** Nystagmus in one eye that is not synchronized with that in the other eye.

***end-position n.*** Nystagmus that occurs when eyes are turned to extreme positions. It may occur normally in debilitation or fatigue, or it may be due to pathology of the subcortical centers for conjugate gaze.

***fixation n.*** Nystagmus that occurs only when the eyes gaze at an object.

***gaze-evoked n.*** Nystagmus upon holding the eyes in an eccentric position. It is due to dysfunction of the brainstem, or it may be caused by drugs such as sedatives or anticonvulsants. The direction of the nystagmus may change when the individual is fatigued or returns fixation to the primary position. This is called *rebound nystagmus.*

***jerk n.*** Rhythmic n.

***labyrinthine n.*** Nystagmus due to disease of the labyrinthine vestibular apparatus.

***latent n.*** Nystagmus that occurs only when one eye is covered.

***lateral n.*** Horizontal movement of the eyes from side to side.

***miner's n.*** Nystagmus occurring in those who work in comparative darkness for long periods.

***opticokinetic n.*** A rhythmic jerk nystagmus occurring when one is looking at constantly moving objects (e.g., viewing telephone poles from a moving car or train).

***pendular n.*** Nystagmus characterized by movement that is approx. equal in both directions. It is usually seen in those who have bilateral congenital absence of central vision or who lost it prior to the age of two.

***postrotatory n.*** A form of vestibular nystagmus that occurs when the body is rotated and then the rotation is stopped. If, while sitting upright in a chair that can be swiveled, the body is rapidly rotated to the right, the nystagmus during rotation has its slow component to the left. When the rotation stops, the slow component is to the right. Stimulation of the semicircular canals causes this type of nystagmus, and it is a normal reaction.

***rebound n.*** SEE: *gaze-evoked n.*

***retraction n.*** Nystagmus associated with the drawing of the eye backward into the orbit. SYN: *nystagmus retractorius.*

***rhythmic n.*** Nystagmus in which the eyes move slowly in one direction and then are jerked back rapidly. SYN: *jerk n.*

***rotatory n.*** Nystagmus in which eyes rotate about the visual axis.

***seesaw n.*** Nystagmus in which the inturning eye moves up and the opposite eye moves down, and then both eyes move in the opposite direction.

***vertical n.*** Involuntary up-and-down ocular movements.

***vestibular n.*** Nystagmus caused by disease of the vestibular apparatus of the ear, or due to normal stimuli produced when the semicircular canals are tested by rotating the body. SEE: *postrotatory n.*

***voluntary n.*** A rare type of pendular nystagmus in persons who have learned to oscillate their eyes rapidly, usually by extreme convergence.

**nystatin** (nĭs′tă-tĭn) An antifungal agent.

**nystaxis** (nĭs-tăk′sĭs) [Gr.] Nystagmus.

**Nysten's law** (nē-stănz′) [Pierre Hubert Nysten, Fr. pediatrician, 1774–1817] A law stating that rigor mortis begins with the muscles of mastication and progresses from the head down the body, affecting the legs and feet last.

**nyxis** (nĭk′sĭs) [Gr.] Puncture or piercing. SYN: *paracentesis.*

**NZB mouse** SEE: under *mouse.*

# O

**ω** Omega, the twenty-fourth letter in the Greek alphabet.

**Ω** Capital of the Greek letter omega. Symbol for ohm.

**O 1.** Symbol for the element oxygen. **2.** *oculus,* eye. **3.** Symbol for a particular blood type.

**o-** *ortho-.*

**$O_2$** Symbol for the molecular formula for oxygen.

**$O_3$** Symbol for ozone.

**O.A.** *anterior.*

**OAF** *osteoclast activating factor.*

**OAM** *Office of Alternative Medicine.*

**oarialgia** (ō″ăr-ē-ăl′jē-ă) [Gr. *oarion,* little egg, + *algos,* pain] Ovaralgia.

**oasis** (ō-ā′sĭs) *pl.* **oases** [Gr., a fertile area in an arid region] An area of healthy tissue surrounded by a diseased portion.

**oasthouse urine disease** Methionine malabsorption syndrome, which is associated with mental retardation, diarrhea, convulsions, phenylketonuria, and a peculiar odor. The odor is due to the absorption from the intestinal tract of fermentation products of methionine. SYN: *Smith-Strang disease.*

**oat** [AS. *ate,* oat] Grain or seed of a cereal grass used as food.

**oath** [AS. *ooth*] A solemn attestation or affirmation. SEE: *Hippocratic oath; Nightingale Pledge.*

**oatmeal** [AS. *ate,* oat, + *mele,* meal] A meal made from oats. Oatmeal is sometimes used in a tepid bath to soothe inflamed or irritated skin.

**OB** *obstetrics.*

**obelion** (ō-bē′lē-ŏn) [Gr. *obelos,* a spit] A craniometric point on the sagittal suture between the two parietal foramina.

**Ober test** A clinical test for tightness of the iliotibial band. The patient lies on the uninvolved side and abducts the hip maximally in neutral flexion. The examiner stands behind the patient, with the patient's foot resting on the examiner's arms with the thigh supported. The thigh is then released. The result is negative if the abducted knee falls into adduction. It is positive if the knee does not fall into adduction.

**obese** (ō-bēs′) [L. *obesus*] Extremely fat. SYN: *corpulent.*

**obesity** (ō-bē′sĭ-tē) [L. *obesitas,* corpulence] Abnormal amount of fat on the body. The term is usually not employed unless the individual is from 20% to 30% over average weight for his or her age, sex, and height. SYN: *adiposity; corpulence; overweight.* SEE: *body mass index; weight* for table; *weight, set point; Recommended Daily Dietary Allowances Appendix; Nursing Diagnoses Appendix.*

Obesity is the most common metabolic disease in the U.S.; more than 30% of the population is obese. It is more likely to exist in women, minority groups, and in the poor. Obese individuals have an increased risk of developing chronic disease such as diabetes mellitus, hypertension, and some types of cancer. In addition, obesity is associated with increased risk of developing osteoarthritis of the knees. Obesity, including its cause and treatment, is poorly understood. What is clear is that the obese may not be in control of the factors that contribute to their being obese. The stigmata that can accompany obesity include ridicule by persons who assume weight could be lost if the individual really wanted to, failure to obtain admission to college, employment, or advancement in a job when competing with the nonobese, being asked by one's children to not attend school functions, or the refusal of some practitioners to provide medical or surgical care.

An accepted technical definition of obesity in adults is a body mass index of greater than 27.8 $kg/m^2$ in males and greater than 27.3 $kg/m^2$ in females.

ETIOLOGY: Obesity is the result of an imbalance between food eaten and energy expended, but the underlying causes are often quite complex and difficult to diagnose and treat.

Comprehensive studies have demonstrated that when obese individuals and persons who have never been obese lose weight, they experience a compensatory decrease in energy expenditure both in the resting and nonresting state. The obese decrease their energy expenditure much less than the nonobese. This, of course, makes loss of weight and maintenance of the loss more difficult for the obese individual. Some obese persons who have maintained weight loss have symptoms of chronic starvation in that they feel cold, are always hungry, and are obsessed with food; women in this group may stop menstruating. These symptoms make remaining nonobese almost impossible for most persons.

TREATMENT: In general, the efforts of obese individuals to establish and maintain loss of weight have been unsuccessful. This does not mean that an obese individual will not be able to lose weight and to maintain normal weight, but for most obese persons this has not been the case. SEE: *gastroplasty; liposuction.*

DIET: Caloric intake should be less than maintenance requirements, but all other essential nutrients must be included. Maintenance requirements are based on what the average or desired weight should be. A slow reduction regimen, depending on ideal body weight considerations, is 1200 to 1600 calories per day; intake of 1000 to 1200 calories will provide a more rapid loss of weight.

The average basic reducing diet is about 9 Cal per pound of ideal body weight per day. Thus, a 160-pound (72.6-kg) person whose ideal weight is 135 pounds (61.2 kg) should maintain a diet of about 1200 Cal a day. These calories should be obtained from foods that would provide adequate protein, carbohydrates, fats, minerals, and vitamins, and not from a fad diet. Adherence to this diet should cause the person to lose the excess weight. After that the diet is adjusted so that caloric intake is just equal to total energy required. Obviously this is different for each individual.

Losing weight by fasting is effective but is not recommended unless done under strict medical and nursing supervision. Death has occurred in persons fasting without medical care.

***abdominal o.*** A condition in which excessive adipose tissue is prevalent in the abdominal area. The risk of cardiovascular disease, hypertension, and diabetes is greater than the risk associated with gluteal-femoral obesity. SYN: *android o.*

***adult-onset o.*** Obesity first appearing in the adult years.

***android o.*** Abdominal o.

***endogenous o.*** Obesity associated with some metabolic or endocrine abnormality within the body.

***exogenous o.*** Obesity due to an excessive intake of food.

***gluteal-femoral o.*** Obesity in which fat deposits are located primarily below the waist in the hips and thighs. The health risk is not thought to be as great as with abdominal obesity. SYN: *gynecoid o.*

***gynecoid o.*** Gluteal-femoral o.

***hypothalamic o.*** Obesity resulting from dysfunction of the hypothalamus, esp. the appetite-regulating center.

***juvenile o.*** Obesity that occurs before adulthood.

***morbid o.*** Obesity of such degree as to interfere with normal activities, including respiration. SEE: *pickwickian syndrome.*

**obex** (ō′bĕks) [L., a band] A thin, crescent-shaped band of tissue covering the calamus scriptorius at the point of convergence of nervous tissue at the caudal end of the fourth ventricle of the brain.

**obfuscation** (ŏb-fŭs-kā′shŭn) [L. *obfuscare,* to darken] **1.** The act of making obscure or confusing. **2.** Mental confusion.

**OB/GYN, OB-GYN** *obstetrics* and *gynecology.*

**object** [L. *objectus*] That which is visible or tangible to the senses.

**object, sex 1.** An individual regarded as being of little interest except for providing sexual pleasure. **2.** A person to whom one is sexually attracted.

**objective** (ŏb-jĕk′tĭv) **1.** Perceptible to other persons, said of symptoms. Opposite of subjective. **2.** Directed toward external things. **3.** The lens of a microscope that is closest to the object.

***achromatic o.*** A microscope objective in which chromatic aberration is corrected for red and blue light.

***apochromatic o.*** A microscope objective in which chromatic aberration is corrected for red, blue, and green light.

***immersion o.*** A microscope objective designed so that the space between the objective lens and the specimen is filled with oil or water.

**objective sign** SEE: under *sign.*

**objective symptom** SEE: under *symptom.*

**object permanence** The thought process, first described by Piaget, whereby infants perceive that objects have constancy. This process normally develops by 6 to 12 months.

**object relations** Emotional attachment for other persons or objects.

**object span test** A test of the temporal-sequential organization of a child. The child is asked to point to or tap a series of objects in the order demonstrated by the examiner. SEE: *digit span test; temporal-sequential organization.*

**obligate** (ŏb′lĭ-gāt) [L. *obligatus*] Necessary or required; without alternative. SEE: under *anaerobe.*

**oblique** (ō-blēk′, ō-blīk′) [L. *obliquus*] Slanting, diagonal.

**obliquimeter** (ŏb″lĭ-kwĭm′ĕt-ĕr) [″ + Gr. *metron,* measure] An apparatus for determining the angle of the pelvic brim with the upright body.

**obliquity** (ŏb-lĭk′wĭ-tē) [L. *obliquus,* slanting] The state of being oblique or slanting.

***Litzmann's o.*** SEE: *Litzmann's obliquity.*

***Naegele's o.*** SEE: *Naegele's obliquity.*

***o. of the pelvis*** Inclination of pelvis.

***Roederer's o.*** Presentation of the fetal head with the occiput at the pelvic brim.

**obliquus reflex** SEE: under *reflex.*

**obliteration** (ŏb-lĭt″ĕr-ā′shŭn) [L. *obliterare,* to remove] Extinction or complete occlusion of a part or a reflex by degeneration, disease, or surgery.

**Oblomov syndrome** [After Ilya Ilych Oblomov, a character in Ivan Goncharov's 19th century novel who would not get out of bed] Refusal to resume normal activity after an illness or during depression.

**oblongata** (ŏb″lŏng-gă′tă) [L. *oblongus,* long] Medulla oblongata.

**obscure** (ŏb-skūr′) [L. *obscurus,* hide] **1.** Hidden, indistinct, as the cause of a condition. **2.** To make less distinct or to hide.

**observerscope** (ŏb-zĕr′vĕr-skōp) A type of endoscope designed so that two persons can view the image simultaneously.

**obsession** [L. *obsessus,* besiege] A neurotic mental state in which an individual has an uncontrollable desire to dwell on an idea or an emotion. The individual is usually aware of the abnormality and attempts to resist these thoughts. SEE: *obsessive-compulsive disorder.*

**obsessive-compulsive disorder** ABBR: OCD. A disorder characterized by recurrent obsessions or compulsions that are severe enough to be time consuming or cause marked distress or significant impairment. The person recognizes that the obsessions or compulsions are excessive or unreasonable. The most common obsessions are repeated thoughts about being contaminated as could occur with shaking hands, repeated doubts concerning having failed to lock a door or having hurt someone in a traffic accident, the need to have things in a particular order, aggressive or horrific impulses, and sexual imagery. These obsessions are unlikely to be related to a real-life problem. Compulsions are repetitive behavior (e.g., hand washing, ordering, checking) or mental acts (e.g., praying, counting, repeating words silently) the goal of which is to prevent or reduce anxiety or distress, not to provide pleasure or gratification. This diagnosis is established if distress is present, the acts are time consuming (i.e., take more than an hour a day), or the illness significantly interferes with the individual's normal routine, occupation, or social activities. In the general population, the lifetime prevalence of this disorder is approximately 2.5%. It is estimated to be present in 35% to 50% of patients with Tourette's syndrome. SEE: *Tourette's syndrome; personality disorder, obsessive-compulsive; trichotillomania.*

TREATMENT: Drugs such as clomipramine and fluoxetine have been used to treat OCD. In addition, behavior therapy has been found to be effective. The patient is exposed to a feared object or idea and then discouraged or prevented from carrying out the usual compulsive response. If successful, repeated sessions gradually decrease the anxiety and the patient may be able to refrain from the compulsive actions.

**obstetrician** (ŏb-stĕ-trĭsh′ăn) A physician who treats women during pregnancy and parturition and delivers infants.

**obstetrics** (ŏb-stĕt′rĭks) [L. *obstetrix,* midwife] The branch of medicine that concerns management of women during pregnancy, childbirth, and the puerperium. **obstetric** (ŏb-stĕt′rĭk), *adj.*

**obstruction** (ŏb-strŭk′shŭn) **1.** Blockage of a structure that prevents it from functioning normally. **2.** A thing that impedes; an obstacle.

***aortic o.*** Blockage of the aorta, thereby preventing the flow of blood.

***foreign body airway o.*** Blockage of the free passage of air from the mouth and nose to the lungs by any object accidentally inhaled into the bronchus or pharynx. Common causes of this type of obstruction are red meat, hard candy, hot dogs, coins, and marbles. SEE: *Heimlich maneuver.*

***intestinal o.*** A partial or complete blockage of the lumen of the large or small intestine.

*Acute:* The small intestine is usually involved. This condition may be due to intussusception, strangulation, volvulus (twists), foreign bodies, adhesions, tumors, stricture, and gallstones in the intestines. Auscultation of the abdomen may reveal a high-pitched tinkle or no sound at all. SEE: *Nursing Diagnoses Appendix.*

SYMPTOMS: Characteristic of intestinal obstruction are pain, localized and intense; temperature, subnormal or normal; vomiting; constipation; and abdominal distention.

TREATMENT: Intestinal and gastric distention is relieved by use of gastric and intestinal suction tubes. Fluid balance must be maintained. Surgical exploration may be necessary to determine the cause. Parenteral antibodies are indicated for peritonitis.

*Chronic:* This type involves the large intestine and may be due to stricture, inflammation, abscesses, tumors, fecal matter, or chronic peritonitis. Gallstones also may obstruct feces. Constipation gradually develops, with pain becoming more severe in a few days. Acute symptoms follow.

**obstructive lung disease, chronic** ABBR: COLD. Increased resistance to the passage of air in and out of the lung due to narrowing of the bronchial tree. It is diagnosed by determining that the amount of air forcibly expired from the lung in one second is less than normal. The disease process may be caused by a number of irritants or diseases that damage the bronchial tree, including pulmonary tuberculosis, cigarette smoking, and silicosis. SYN: *chronic obstructive pulmonary disease.*

NURSING IMPLICATIONS: The nurse teaches breathing and coughing exercises and postural drainage to strengthen respiratory muscles and to mobilize secretions. Participation in a pulmonary rehabilitation program is encouraged, as well as smoking cessation and avoidance of other respiratory irritants. Patients are instructed to avoid contact with other persons with respiratory infections and taught the use of prescribed prophylactic antibiotics and bronchodilator therapy. The rationale for using low-concentration oxygen therapy is explained. Frequent small meals and adequate fluid intake are encouraged. The patient's schedule alternates periods of activity with rest. The nurse assists the patient and family with disease-related lifestyle changes and encourages them to express their feelings and concerns.

**obstruent** (ŏb′stroo-ĕnt) [L. *obstruens*] **1.** Blocking up. **2.** That which closes a normal passage in the body. **3.** Any agent or agency causing obstruction.

**obtund** (ŏb-tŭnd′) [L. *obtundere,* to beat against] To dull or blunt, as sensitivity or pain. SEE: *consciousness, levels of.*

**obtundent** (ŏb-tŭn′dĕnt) [L. *obtundens*] **1.** Having the capacity to deaden sensibility of a part or reduce irritability. **2.** A soothing agent.

**obturation** (ŏb-tūr-ā′shŭn) [L. *obturare,* to stop up] Closure of a passage or opening, as in intestinal obstruction.

**obturator** (ŏb′tū-rā″tor) **1.** Anything that obstructs or closes a cavity or opening. **2.** Relating to the obturator membrane. **3.** A prosthetic bridge used for spanning the gap in a cleft palate.

**obturator foramen** SEE: under *foramen.*

**obturator membrane** SEE: under *membrane.*

**obturator muscles** SEE: under *muscle.*

**obturator sign** Pain on inward rotation of the hip so that the obturator internus muscle is stretched. This test result may be positive in acute appendicitis.

**obtuse** (ŏb-tūs′) [L. *obtusus*] **1.** Not pointed or acute; dull or blunt. **2.** Of dull mentality.

**obtusion** (ŏb-tū′zhŭn) Blunting or weakening of normal sensation, as in certain diseases.

**O.C.** *oral contraceptive.*

**Occam's razor** (ŏck′hăms) [William of Occam, or Ockham, Brit. Franciscan and philosopher, c. 1285–1349] The concept that entities do not have to be proved beyond the point of proof; or "what can be done with fewer (assumptions) is done in vain with more."

**occipital** (ŏk-sĭp′ĭ-tăl) [L. *occipitalis*] Concerning the back part of the head.

**occipital bone** A bone in the lower back part of the skull between the parietal and temporal bones.

**occipitalis** (ŏk-sĭp″ĭ-tā′lĭs) [L.] The posterior portion of the occipitofrontalis muscle at the back of the head.

**occipitalization** (ŏk-sĭp″ĭ-tăl-ī-zā′shŭn) Fusion of the atlas and occipital bones.

**occipital lobe** SEE: under *lobe.*

**occipito-** [L. *occiput*] Combining form denoting *occiput.*

**occipitoatloid** (ŏk-sĭp″ĭ-tō-ăt′loyd) Concerning the occipital and atlas bones.

**occipitoaxoid** (ŏk-sĭp″ĭ-tō-ăk′soyd) Concerning the occipital and axis bones.

**occipitobregmatic** (ŏk-sĭp″ĭ-tō-brĕg-măt′ĭk) Concerning the occiput and the bregma.

**occipitocervical** (ŏk-sĭp″ĭ-tō-sĕr′vĭ-kăl) Concerning the occiput and the neck.

**occipitofacial** (ŏk-sĭp″ĭ-tō-fā′shăl) Concerning the occiput and the face.

**occipitofrontal** (ŏk-sĭp″ĭ-tō-frŏn′tăl) Concerning the occiput and the forehead.

**occipitomastoid** (ŏk-sĭp″ĭ-tō-măs′toyd) Concerning the occiput and the mastoid process.

**occipitomental** (ŏk-sĭp″ĭ-tō-mĕn′tăl) Concerning the occiput and the chin.

**occipitoparietal** (ŏk-sĭp″ĭ-tō-pă-rī′ĕ-tăl) Concerning the occipital and parietal bones or lobes of the brain.

**occipitotemporal** (ŏk-sĭp″ĭ-tō-tĕm′pō-răl) Concerning the occipital and temporal bones.

**occipitothalamic** (ŏk-sĭp″ĭ-tō-thă-lăm′ĭk) Concerning the occiput and the thalamus.

**occiput** (ŏk′sĭ-pŭt) [L.] The back part of the skull. On the fetal head, it is used to determine the position of cephalic presentations in relation to the maternal pelvis.

***persistent o. posterior*** A fetal malposition; a cephalic presentation with the occiput directed toward the mother's sacrum. Labor often is longer and the woman complains of back pain.

**occlude** (ŏ-klūd′) [L. *occludere,* to shut up] To close up, obstruct, or join together, as bringing the biting surfaces of opposing teeth together.

**occlusal** (ŏ-kloo′zăl) Pert. to the closure of an opening.

***o. adjustment*** Reshaping the occlusal surface of teeth by grinding to create a harmonious contact relationship between upper and lower teeth. This is done to equalize the stress of occlusal forces on the supporting tissues of the teeth, thereby eliminating pain, root resorption, and periodontal problems.

***o. equilibration*** The modification of the occlusal forms of teeth by grinding with the intent of equalizing occlusal forces or producing simultaneous occlusal contacts and harmonious cuspal relations.

***o. guard*** A removable dental appliance that covers one or both arches and is designed to minimize the damaging effects of bruxism, jaw and head trauma during contact sports, or any occlusal habits that are detrimental.

***o. plane*** SEE: under *plane.*

***o. surface*** The masticating surface of the premolar and molar teeth.

***o. wear*** The attritional loss of substance on opposing occlusal surfaces in natural or artificial teeth; the modification of tooth cusps, ridges, and grooves by functional use.

**occlusion** (ŏ-kloo′zhŭn) [L. *occlusio*] **1.** The acquired or congenital closure, or state of being closed, of a passage. SYN: *imperforation.* **2.** Alignment of the mandibular and maxillary teeth when the jaw is closed or in functional contact, i.e., dental occlusion. SEE: *malocclusion.*

***abnormal o.*** Malocclusion of the teeth.

***adjusted o.*** The alteration of occlusal contacts by dental restorations in order to achieve a balanced or functional occlusion.

***anatomical o.*** A dental occlusion in which the posterior teeth of a denture have masticatory surfaces that resemble natural, healthy dentition and articulate with the surfaces of similar or opposing teeth. The opposing teeth may be artificial or natural.

***arterial o.*** A blockage of the lumen of an artery that prevents adequate blood flow and oxygenation. It may be acute or chronic and occurs most often in peripheral arteries and their branches. Patient with acute arterial occlusion have severe pain in the affected extremity, decreased or absent pulse, and mottled skin. The occlusion is removed to prevent gangrene or loss of the extremity.

***balanced o.*** The ideal and equal contact of the teeth of the working side of the jaw by the complementary contact of the teeth on the opposite side of the jaw. SYN: *balanced bite.*

***centric o.*** The position of the mandible, vertically and horizontally, that produces maximal interdigitation of the cusps of the maxillary and mandibular teeth. This is the ideal position or type of occlusion. It is also described as intercuspal position, tooth-to-tooth position, habitual centric, or acquired centric.

***coronary o.*** Complete or partial obstruction of a coronary vessel by thrombosis or as a result of spasm. SYN: *coronary thrombosis.* SEE: *myocardial infarction.*

***eccentric o.*** Any dental occlusion other than centric.

***habitual o.*** The usual relationship between the teeth of the maxilla and mandible that represents the maximum contact; this varies from individual to individual and is seldom ideal or true centric occlusion.

***traumatic o.*** Injury to the tissues that support the teeth due to malocclusion, missing teeth, improper chewing habits, or a pathological condition that causes an individual to chew in an abnormal way.

***working o.*** The usual method of contact of teeth as the mandible is moved to one side during chewing. SYN: *working bite.*

**occlusive** (ŏ-kloo′sĭv) Concerning occlusion.

**occlusive dressing** SEE: under *dressing.*

**occlusometer** (ŏk″loo-sŏm′ĕ-tĕr) Gnathodynamometer.

**occult** (ŭ-kŭlt′) [L. *occultus*] Obscure; not easily understood; mysterious; concealed, as a hemorrhage.

***o. blood*** Blood in such minute quantity that it can be recognized only by microscopic examination or by chemical means.

***o. blood test*** A chemical test or microscopic examination for blood, esp. in feces, that is not apparent on visual inspection.

NURSING IMPLICATIONS: The importance of the test in identifying gastrointestinal bleeding is explained. Because the patient often must collect a specimen at home, instruction is given in specimen collection. The patient should place plastic wrap or some other means of collection over the toilet bowl and use the wooden spatula enclosed with the specimen receptacles to obtain a feces sample from the middle of the specimen. The nurse explains that specimens are collected 3 days in succession and should be returned to the laboratory as soon as possible after collection.

**occupation** An ordinary, everyday goal-directed pursuit. Although the term is often used interchangeably with "vocation," the latter is the preferred term for paid employment.

**occupational** Relating to source of income or livelihood.

***certified o. therapy assistant*** ABBR: COTA. An occupational therapy assistant who has passed the national certification examination. SEE: *o. therapy assistant.*

***o. illness*** A disorder associated with or caused by an individual's occupation. The disorder may be acute or chronic due to exposure to chemicals. SEE: *lead poisoning, chronic.*

***o. medicine*** SEE: under *medicine.*

***o. neurosis*** SEE: under *neurosis.*

***o. performance*** A term used by occupational therapists to refer to a person's ability to perform the required activities, tasks, and roles of living.

***o. science*** The systematic study of the occupational nature of humans. Its goal is to understand how and why people select, organize, perform, and derive meaning from everyday occupations or pursuits.

***o. therapist*** SEE: under *therapist.*

***o. therapy assistant*** ABBR: OTA. One who works under the supervision of an occupational therapist to assist with patient or client assessment and intervention. The degree and scope of supervision required depends on practice statutes and the levels of competency the assistant is able to provide. SEE: *certified o. therapy assistant.*

**occupational therapy** SEE: under *therapy.*

**occupational therapy aide** An individual with on-the-job training or experience in occupational therapy who performs routine tasks under the direction of an occupational therapist.

**ochlophobia** (ŏk″lō-fō′bē-ă) [Gr. *ochlos,* crowd, + *phobos,* fear] Abnormal fear of crowds or populated places. SYN: *agoraphobia.*

**ochronosis** (ō-krō-nō′sĭs) [″ + *nosos,* disease] A rare condition marked by dark pigmentation of the ligaments, cartilage, fibrous tissues, skin, and urine. This condition is often associated with alkaptonuria, an inborn error of metabolism, or may be the result of chronic phenol poisoning.

**OCT** *oxytocin challenge test.*

**octa-, octo-** [Gr. *okto,* L. *octo*] Combining form meaning *eight.*

**octahedron** (ŏk-tă-hē′drŏn) An eight-sided solid figure.

**octan** (ŏk′tăn) [L. *octo,* eight] Reappearing

every eighth day, as a fever.

**octane** (ŏk′tān) $C_8H_{18}$. A hydrocarbon of the paraffin series.

**octapeptide** (ŏk″tă-pĕp′tĭd) A peptide that contains eight amino acids.

**octaploid** (ŏk′tă-ployd) **1.** Concerning octaploidy. **2.** Having eight pairs of chromosomes.

**octaploidy** (ŏk′tă-ploy″dē) The condition of having eight sets or pairs of chromosomes.

**octavalent** (ŏk″tă-vā′lĕnt) [L. *octo,* eight, + *valeo,* to have power] Having a valency of eight.

**octigravida** (ŏk″tĭ-grăv′ĭ-dă) [″ + *gravida,* pregnant] A woman who has been pregnant eight times.

**octipara** (ŏk-tĭp′ă-ră) [″ + L. *parere,* to bring forth, to bear] A woman who has given birth to eight children.

**octogenarian** (ŏk″tō-jĕn-ĕr′ē-ĕn) [L. *octogenarius,* containing eighty] A person who is 80 to 89 years old.

**octreotide acetate** A synthetic drug that mimics the action of somatostatin and is used in treating acromegaly, carcinoid tumors, and vasoactive intestinal peptide tumors.

**ocular** (ŏk′ū-lăr) [L. *oculus,* eye] **1.** Concerning the eye or vision. **2.** The eyepiece of a microscope.

**ocularist** An allied health specialist who is prepared by training and experience to make and fit artificial eyes.

**oculi** (ŏk′ū-lī) Pl. of oculus.

**oculist** (ŏk′ū-lĭst) Obsolete term for ophthalmologist, a physician who is a specialist in diseases of the eye.

**oculo-** (ŏk′ū-lō) [L. *oculus,* eye] Combining form denoting *eye.*

**oculocerebrorenal syndrome** A sex-linked hereditary condition characterized by hydrophthalmia, cataracts, mental retardation, aminoaciduria, impaired renal ammonia production, and vitamin D-resistant rickets.

**oculocutaneous** (ŏk″ū-lō-kū-tā′nē-ŭs) Concerning the eyes and the skin.

**oculofacial** (ŏk″ū-lō-fā′shē-ăl) Concerning the eyes and the face.

**oculogyration** (ŏk″ū-lō-jī-rā′shŭn) [″ + Gr. *gyros,* circle] The circular motion of the eyeball around its anterior-posterior axis. SEE: *nystagmus.*

**oculogyria** (ŏk″ū-lō-jī′rē-ă) The limits of rotation of the eyeballs.

**oculogyric** (ŏk″ū-lō-jī′rĭk) Producing or concerning movements of the eye. SYN: *oculomotor.*

**oculogyric crisis** A spasmodic attack of involuntary deviation and fixation of the eyeballs, usually upward. It may last for only several minutes or for hours. This condition may be seen with postencephalitic parkinsonism or encephalitis lethargica.

**oculomotor** (ŏk″ū-lō-mō′tor) [″ + *motor,* mover] Relating to eye movements. SYN: *oculogyric.*

**oculomotor nerve** The cranial nerve that originates in the medial surface of the cerebral peduncle of the midbrain and consists of general somatic efferent, general visceral efferent, and general somatic afferent fibers. It is distributed through all extrinsic muscles of the eye except the exterior rectus and superior oblique, through the levator palpebrae superioris of the eyelid, through the ciliary muscle, and through the sphincter muscle of the iris. Its function is primarily motor, but it also contains proprioceptive fibers. SYN: *third cranial nerve.* SEE: *Cranial Nerves Appendix.*

**oculomycosis** (ŏk″ū-lō-mī-kō′sĭs) [″ + Gr. *mykes,* fungus, + *osis,* condition] Any disease of the eye or its parts caused by fungus.

**oculonasal** (ŏk″ū-lō-nā′săl) [″ + *nasus,* nose] Concerning the eyes and the nose.

**oculopupillary** (ŏk″ū-lō-pū′pĭ-lăr-ē) Concerning the pupil of the eye.

**oculoreaction** (ŏk″ū-lō-rē-ăk′shŭn) [L. *oculus,* eye, + *re,* back, + *actus,* acting] Calmette's reaction.

**oculovestibular test** Caloric test.

**oculozygomatic** (ŏk″ū-lō-zī″gō-măt′ĭk) [″ + Gr. *zygon,* yoke] Pert. to the eye and the zygoma.

***o. line*** A line appearing between the inner canthus of the eye and the cheek, supposedly indicative of neural disorders.

**oculus** (ŏk′ū-lŭs) *pl.* **oculi** [L.] Eye; the organ of vision made up of the eyeball and optic nerve.

***o. dexter*** ABBR: O.D. The right eye.

***o. sinister*** ABBR: O.S. The left eye.

***o. uterque*** Each eye.

**O.D.** *Doctor of Optometry; overdose;* [L.] *oculus dexter,* right eye.

**OD'd** Slang term for a death due to a drug overdose, esp. a drug of abuse.

**odaxesmus** (ō″dăk-sĕz′mŭs) [Gr. *odaxesmos,* an irritation] The biting of the tongue, lip, or cheek during an epileptic attack.

**odaxetic** (ō″dăk-sĕt′ĭk) Producing a stinging or itching sensation.

**Oddi's sphincter** (ŏd′ēz) [Ruggero Oddi, It. physician, 1864–1913] A contracted region at the opening of the common bile duct into the duodenum at the papilla of Vater. It is commonly referred to as the sphincter of Oddi.

**odditis** (ŏd-dī′tĭs) [*Oddi* + Gr. *itis,* inflammation] Inflammation of the sphincter of Oddi.

**odogenesis** (ŏ″dō-jĕn′ĕ-sĭs) [Gr. *hodos,* pathway, + *genesis,* generation, birth] Neurocladism.

**odont-, odonto-** [Gr. *odous,* tooth] Combining form denoting *tooth, teeth.*

**odontagra** (ō-dŏn-tă′gră) [Gr. *odous,* tooth, + *agra,* seizure] Toothache, esp. when originating from gout.

**odontalgia** (ō-dŏn-tăl′jē-ă) [″ + *algos,* pain] Toothache. SYN: *odontia; odontodynia.*

***phantom o.*** Pain felt in the area from

which a tooth has been pulled.

**odontatrophy** (ō″dŏn-tăt′rō-fē) [″ + *atrophia,* atrophy] Imperfect development of the teeth.

**odontectomy** (ō-dŏn-tĕk′tō-mē) [″ + *ektome,* excision] Surgical removal of a tooth.

**odonterism** (ō-dŏn′tĕr-ĭzm) [″ + *erismos,* quarrel] Chattering of the teeth.

**odontia** (ō-dŏn′shē-ă) [Gr. *odous,* tooth] **1.** Pain in a tooth. SYN: *odontalgia; odontodynia.* **2.** Condition or abnormality of the teeth.

**odontic** (ō-dŏn′tĭk) [Gr. *odous,* tooth] Concerning the teeth.

**odontitis** (ō″dŏn-tī′tĭs) [″ + *itis,* inflammation] Inflammation of a tooth.

**odontoblast** (ō-dŏn′tō-blăst) [″ + *blastos,* germ] One of the cells forming the surface layer of the dental papilla that is responsible for the formation of the dentin of a tooth. After a tooth is formed, the odontoblasts line the pulp cavity and continue to produce dentin for years after the tooth has erupted.

**odontoblastoma** [″ + ″ + *oma,* tumor] A tumor composed principally of odontoblasts.

**odontobothritis** [″ + ″ + *itis,* inflammation] Inflammation of alveolar process of the tooth.

**odontocele** (ō-dŏn′tō-sēl) [″ + *kele,* tumor, swelling] An alveolodental cyst.

**odontochirurgical** (ō-dŏn″tō-kĭ-rŭr′jĭ-kăl) [″ + *chirurgia,* surgery] Pert. to dental surgery.

**odontoclasis** (ō″dŏn-tŏk′lă-sĭs) [″ + *klasis,* fracture] The breaking or fracture of a tooth.

**odontodynia** (ō-dŏn″tō-dĭn′ē-ă) [″ + *odyne,* pain] Toothache. SYN: *odontalgia; odontia.*

**odontogenesis, odontogeny** (ō-dŏn″tō-jĕn′ĕ-sĭs, -tŏj′ĕn-ē) [″ + *genesis,* generation, birth] The origin and formation of the teeth.

***o. imperfecta*** A congenital anomaly of the developing teeth in which there is deficient production of enamel and dentin in affected teeth, producing decreased density and enlarged pulp chambers.

**odontograph** (ō-dŏn′tō-grăf) [″ + *graphein,* to write] Device for determining the degree of uneven surface of tooth enamel.

**odontography** (ō-dŏn-tŏg′ră-fē) Descriptive anatomy of the teeth.

**odontoid** (ō-dŏn′toyd) [″ + *eidos,* form, shape] Toothlike.

***o. process*** SEE: under *process.*

**odontolith** (ō-dŏn′tō-lĭth) [″ + *lithos,* stone] Tartar.

**odontolysis** (ō-dŏn-tŏl′ĭ-sĭs) [″ + *lysis,* dissolution] Loss of calcium from a tooth.

**odontoma** (ō″dŏn-tō′mă) [″ + *oma,* tumor] A tumor originating in the dental tissue.

***ameloblastic o.*** A neoplasm that contains enamel, dentin, and odontogenic tissue that does not develop to form enamel.

***composite o.*** A tumor in which the epithelial and mesenchymal cells are completely differentiated. This causes enamel and dentin to be formed in an abnormal manner.

***coronary o.*** A bony tumor at the crown of a tooth.

***follicular o.*** A bony shell in the gums below the tooth margin, usually appearing after the second dentition. It is due to an excessive number of dental follicles. The tumor often involves one or more teeth and is crepitating to pressure. SYN: *dentigerous cyst.*

***radicular o.*** Odontoma close to or on the root of a tooth.

**odontonecrosis** (ō-dŏn″tō-nĕ-krō′sĭs) [″ + *nekros,* corpse, + *osis,* condition] Extensive decay of a tooth.

**odontonomy** (ō″dŏn-tŏn′ō-mē) [″ + *onoma,* name] Dental nomenclature.

**odontophobia** (ō-dŏn″tō-fō′bē-ă) [″ + *phobos,* fear] Abnormal fear of teeth.

**odontoprisis** (ō-dŏn″tō-prī′sĭs) [″ + *prisis,* sawing] Bruxism.

**odontorrhagia** (ō-dŏn″tō-rā′jē-ă) [″ + *rhegnynai,* to burst forth] Hemorrhage from a tooth socket following extraction.

**odontoschism** (ō-dŏn′tō-skĭzm) [″ + *schisma,* cleft] Fissure of a tooth.

**odontoscopy** (ō″dŏn-tŏs′kō-pē) [″ + *skopein,* to examine] **1.** Examination of the teeth and oral cavity by use of an odontoscope. **2.** An impression made of the biting marks made by teeth. These are used as a means of identification.

**odontosis** (ō-dŏn-tō′sĭs) [″ + *osis,* condition] The development or eruption of the teeth.

**odontotherapy** (ō-dŏn″tō-thĕr′ă-pē) [″ + *therapeia,* treatment] The care of diseased teeth.

**odor** (ō′dĕr) [L.] That quality of a substance that renders it perceptible to the sense of smell.

Each odoriferous substance causes its own sensations, the description of which is complex and subjective. Odors have been classed as (1) pure, (2) those mixed with sensations from the mucous membrane, and (3) those mixed with the sensation of taste. A suggested classification of odors includes aromatic, burning, fragrant, fetid, nauseating, and repulsive. Another classification is spicy, flowery, fruity, resinous, foul, and scorched. Although classification attempts are useful, it is important to realize that most complex substances do not produce a single odor.

Body and breath odor in certain disease conditions can be of assistance in establishing a diagnosis. Examples are a "mousy" odor present in the breath of patients with liver failure (liver breath); an odor of stale urine (uremic breath) in uremia, and the sweet smell of acetone in diabetic acidosis. The characteristic smell of some alcoholic beverages can be detected in the breath. Within an hour after eating asparagus, a characteristic odor will be present in the urine. Following intercourse, semen absorbed from the vagina may produce a distinct breath odor. In some hospitals, the employees and staff who work in the presence of patients are asked to refrain from wearing scented substances such as perfumes, hair sprays, underarm deodorants, or after-shave lotions. This is done to prevent olfactory discomfort to patients. Individuals who have just returned from surgery, or who have asthma or other respiratory problems are particularly sensitive to odors. Electronic devices for detecting and characterizing odors have been developed. SEE: *breath; odorimetry; pheromone.*

**odorant** (ō′dor-ănt) Something that stimulates the sense of smell.

**odoriferous** (ō″dor-ĭf′ĕ-rŭs) [L. *odor,* smell, + *ferre,* to bear] Bearing an odor; fragrant; perfumed.

**odorimetry** The measurement of the ability of a substance to induce olfactory sensations.

**odoriphore** (ō-dor′ĭ-for) [″ + Gr. *phoros,* bearing] The portion of a molecule that imparts odor to the substance.

**odorography** (ō″dor-ŏg′ră-fē) [″ + Gr. *graphein,* to write] A description of odors.

**odorous** [L. *odor,* smell] Having an odor, scent, or fragrance.

**odynacusis** (ō″dĭn-ă-kū′sĭs) [Gr. *odyne,* pain, + *akousis,* hearing] A condition in which noise causes pain in the ear.

**-odynia, odyno-** (ō-dĭn′ē-ă, ō-dĭn′ō) [Gr. *odyne,* pain] Combining form denoting *pain.*

**odynometer** (ō″dĭn-om′ĕt-ĕr) [″ + *metron,* measure] A device for measuring pain.

**odynophagia** (ŏd″ĭn-ō-fā′jē-ă) [″ + *phagein,* to eat] Pain upon swallowing.

**odynophobia** (ŏd″ĭn-ō-fō′bē-ă) [″ + *phobos,* fear] Abnormal fear of pain.

**Oedipus complex** (ĕd′ĭ-pŭs) [Oedipus, a character in Gr. tragedy who unwittingly killed his father and married his mother] Abnormally intense love of the child for the parent of the opposite sex. This love continues in adulthood, and usually involves jealous dislike of the other parent. Most commonly, it is the love of a son for his mother. SEE: *Electra complex; Jocasta complex.*

**oersted** (ĕr′stĕd) [Hans Christian Oersted, Danish physicist, 1777–1851] A unit of magnetic field intensity. An oersted is the magnetism that exerts a force of one dyne on a unit magnetic pole. This term has largely been replaced by the SI unit amperes per meter.

**oesophagostomiasis** (ē-sŏf″ă-gō-stō-mī′ă-sĭs) [Gr. *oisophagos,* esophagus, + *stoma,* mouth, + *-iasis,* state] Infection with the nematode of the genus *Oesophagostomum.*

**Oesophagostomum** (ē-sŏf″ă-gŏs′tō-mŭm) [Gr. *oisophagos,* esophagus, + *stoma,* mouth] A genus of nematodes belonging to the suborder Strongylata that is parasitic in the intestinal walls of animals and humans.

***O. apiostomum*** The nodular nematode worm parasitic to monkeys that occasionally infests humans.

**oestrus** Estrus.

**Oestrus ovis** A botfly that may cause ocular myiasis in humans.

**OFD** *object-film distance.* Distance from the radiographic film to the object being radiographed.

**Office of Alternative Medicine** ABBR: OAM. An office established at the National Institutes of Health in 1992 to investigate the scientific merits of alternative medicine. SEE: *alternative medicine.*

**official** Said of medicines authorized as standard in the U.S. Pharmacopeia and in the National Formulary.

**off-label drug use 1.** The use of a drug in the treatment of a condition for which it has not been approved. **2.** In cancer treatment, the prescribing of drugs that lack sufficient evidence of effectiveness for Food and Drug Administration approval. The oncologists who prescribe such drugs feel that the drugs are effective and that the long approval process makes it necessary to use the drugs without delay. In the U.S., some states have passed laws requiring coverage of off-label uses of FDA-approved cancer drugs when the off-label use is recognized as safe and effective for treatment of specific types of cancer.

**Ogilvie's syndrome** [Sir William Heneage Ogilvie, Brit. physician, 1887–1971] Acute intestinal pseudo-obstruction due to intestinal dilatation, mostly of the colon. An individual displaying this syndrome has usually undergone recent severe surgical or medical stress (e.g., myocardial infarction, sepsis, or respiratory failure), may be on a respirator, may have metabolic and electrolyte disturbances, and may have received narcotics.

TREATMENT: Treatment consists of therapy for the underlying disease, correction of electrolyte disturbances, avoidance of drugs that inhibit intestinal motility, and intubation of small intestine for decompression. Cecostomy may be required in order to avoid ischemic necrosis and perforation of the bowel.

**Oguchi's disease** (ō-goot′chēz) [Chuta Oguchi, Japanese ophthalmologist, 1875–1945] Hereditary night blindness with onset in infancy. Commonly found in Japan, the disease is rare in the U.S.

**$OH^-$** Symbol for the hydroxyl ion.

**ohm** (ōm) The unit of electrical resistance equal to that of a conductor in which a current of one ampere is produced by a potential of one volt across the terminals. SEE: *electromotive force.*

**ohmammeter** (ōm′ăm-mē″tĕr) A combined ohmmeter and ammeter.

**Ohm's law** [Georg S. Ohm, Ger. physicist, 1789–1854] The strength of an electric current, expressed in amperes, is equal to the electromotive force, expressed in volts, divided by the resistance, expressed in ohms. SEE: *electricity.*

**ohmmeter** (ōm′mē-tĕr) A device for determining the electrical resistance of a conductor.

**-oid** [Gr. *eidos,* form, shape] Suffix indicating resemblance to the item designated in the first part of the word.

**oikofugic** (oy″kō-fū′jĭk) [Gr. *oikos,* house, + L. *fugere,* to flee] Having a compulsion to leave home.

**oikomania** (oy″kō-mā′nē-ă) [″ + *mania,* madness] A nervous disorder induced by unhappy home surroundings.

**oikophobia** (oy″kō-fō′bē-ă) Morbid dislike of the home.

**oil** (oyl) [L. *oleum*] A greasy liquid not miscible with water, usually obtained from and classified as mineral, vegetable, or animal. According to character, oils are subdivided principally as fixed (fatty) and volatile (essential).

Examples of fixed oils are castor oil, olive oil, and cod liver oil. Examples of volatile oils are oils of mustard, peppermint, and rose.

***essential o.*** Volatile oil, esp. one that has an odor and produces taste sensations, obtained from certain plants by various means of extraction. Some of these oils have been used since antiquity as preservatives and antiseptics (e.g., thymol and eugenol); some are used in flavorings, perfumes, and medicines. They are usually complex chemicals that are difficult to purify.

***fixed o.'s*** Oils in plants and animals that are glyceryl esters of fatty acids. These oils serve as food reserves in animals. They are nonvolatile and contain no acid.

***halibut liver o.*** An oil obtained from the liver of the halibut fish that is rich in vitamins A and D.

***medium-chain triglyceride o.*** A cooking oil of medium-chain triglycerides, used therapeutically as a source of calories and fatty acids. These triglycerides are more readily absorbed from the gut than are most long-chain triglycerides.

***peanut o.*** A refined oil obtained from the seed kernels of one or more of the cultivated varieties of *Arachis hypogaea;* may be used as a solvent for some medicines that are injected intramuscularly.

***volatile o.*** Essential o.

**ointment** (oynt′mĕnt) [Fr. *oignement*] A soft, medicated, fatty substance for external application to the body, having antiseptic, cosmetic, or healing properties. Usually, its base is petroleum jelly or lanolin to which the medicament is added. These forms are not water soluble; however, some ointments are composed of ingredients that are water soluble. SYN: *salve; unguent.*

***hydrophilic o.*** An oil-in-water emulsion in the form of a standardized ointment preparation used topically as an emollient.

***white o.*** Ointment containing white wax and white petrolatum.

***yellow o.*** Ointment containing yellow wax and petrolatum.

**O.L.** L. *oculus laevus,* left eye.

**ol** L. *oleum,* oil.

**O.L.A.** L. *occipitolaeva anterior* (fetal presentation). SYN: *L.O.A.* SEE: *position.*

**olea** (ō′lē-ă) [L.] **1.** Olive. **2.** Pl. of oleum.

**oleaginous** (ō-lē-ăj′ĭ-nŭs) [L. *oleaginus*] Greasy; oily; unctuous.

**oleander** (ō″lē-ăn′dĕr) A poisonous ornamental evergreen shrub, *Nerium oleander.*

**oleate** (ō′lē-āt) [L. *oleatum*] **1.** Any salt of oleic acid. **2.** A salt of oleic acid dissolved in an excess of the acid and used as an ointment.

**oleatum** (ō-lē-ā′tŭm) [L.] Preparation made by dissolving metallic salts or alkaloids in oleic acid. SYN: *oleate* (2).

**olecranarthritis** (ō-lĕk″răn-ăr-thrī′tĭs) [Gr. *olekranon,* elbow, + *arthron,* joint, + *itis,* inflammation] Inflammation of the elbow joint.

**olecranarthrocace** (ō-lĕk″răn-ăr-thrŏk′ă-sē) [″ + ″ + *kake,* badness] Tuberculous ulceration of the elbow joint.

**olecranarthropathy** (ō-lĕk″răn-ăr-thrŏp′ă-thē) [″ + ″ + *pathos,* disease, suffering] Any disease of the elbow joint.

**olecranoid** (ō-lĕk′ră-noyd) [″ + *eidos,* form, shape] Similar to the olecranon.

**olecranon** (ō-lĕk′răn-ŏn) [Gr., elbow] A large process of the ulna projecting behind the elbow joint and forming the bony prominence of the elbow. In treating a fracture of the olecranon, it is important to prevent spasm of triceps muscle (to avoid separation of the fracture fragments) by placing the arm in a sling or bandaging the arm to the side. The fragments may have to be wired. SEE: *elbow; skeleton; ulna.* **olecranal** (ō-lĕk′răn-ăl), *adj.*

**oleic** (ō-lē′ĭk) [L. *oleum,* oil] Derived from or pert. to oil.

**olein** (ō′lē-ĭn) [L. *oleum,* oil] An oleate of glyceryl found in nearly all fixed oils and fats; an important part of oils. SYN: *triolein.*

**oleo-** [L. *oleum,* oil] Combining form meaning *oil.*

**oleogranuloma** (ō″lē-ō-grăn″ū-lō′mă) [″ + L. *granulum,* little grain, + Gr. *oma,* tumor] A granuloma caused by continuous contact with oil, or at sites of subcutaneous injection of oily substances.

**oleoresin** (ō″lē-ō-rĕz′ĭn) [″ + *resina,* resin] An extract of a plant containing a resinous substance and oil, which is prepared by dissolving the crude extract in ether, acetone, or alcohol.

**oleosaccharum** (ō-lē-ō-săk′ă-rŭm) [″ + *saccharum,* sugar] A compound of sugar and volatile oil used to mitigate the bad taste of some drugs.

**oleotherapy** (ō″lē-ō-thĕr′ă-pē) [L. *oleum,* oil, + Gr. *therapeia,* treatment] The therapeutic injection of oil.

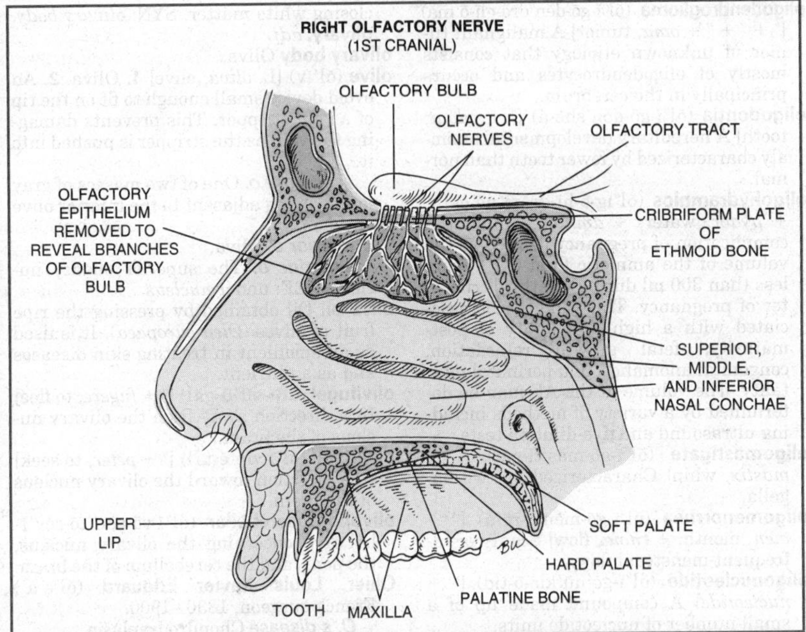


**oleothorax** (ō-lē-ō-thō′răks) [″ + Gr. *thorax,* chest] The therapeutic injection of oil into the pleural cavity, as in pulmonary tuberculosis.

**oleovitamin** (ō″lē-ō-vī′tă-mĭn) A vitamin preparation in an edible oil.

***o. A and D*** A standardized preparation of vitamins A and D.

**Olestra** Trade name for a synthetic mixture of sugar and vegetable oil that passes through the digestive tract without being absorbed. This fat replacement has been approved for use in food; however, it can interfere with utilization of fat-soluble vitamins, such as A, D, E, and K.

**oleum** (ō′lē-ŭm) *pl.* **olea** [L.] Oil.

***o. morrhuae*** Cod liver oil.

***o. olivea*** Olive oil.

***o. percomorphum*** A mixture of oils obtained from the livers of various fish of the order Percomorphi. This oil is more potent in vitamins A and D than cod liver oil.

***o. ricini*** Castor oil.

**olfaction** (ŏl-făk′shŭn) [L. *olfacere,* to smell] **1.** The sense of smell. **2.** The act of smelling.

**olfactometer** (ŏl″făk-tŏm′ĕt-ĕr) [″ + Gr. *metron,* measure] Apparatus for testing the power of the sense of smell.

**olfactory** (ŏl-făk′tō-rē) Pert. to smell.

***o. esthesioneuroma*** A slowly growing malignant tumor of the nasal fossa, developing from epithelial and neural tissues of the olfactory mucosa.

***o. membrane*** SEE: under *membrane.*

***o. nasal sulcus*** An anterior-posterior groove in the wall of the nasal cavity. It passes from the anterior area to the lamina cribrosa.

***o. nerve*** Any of the nerves supplying the nasal olfactory mucosa. These nerves consist of delicate bundles of unmyelinated fibers (fila olfactoria) that pass through cribriform plate and terminate in olfactory glomeruli of olfactory bulb. The fila are central processes of bipolar receptor neurons of olfactory mucous membrane. SEE: illus.; *cranial nerves.*

***o. organ*** The nose.

**olig-** SEE: *oligo-.*

**oligo-, olig-** [Gr. *oligos,* little] Combining form meaning *small, few.*

**oligodactylia** (ŏl-ĭ-gō-dăk-tĭl′ē-ă) [″ + *daktylos,* digit] Subnormal number of fingers or toes.

**oligodendroblast** (ŏl″ĭ-gō-dĕn′drō-blăst) [″ + Gr. *dendron,* tree, + *blastos,* germ] A primitive precursor cell of the oligodendrocyte.

**oligodendroblastoma** (ŏl″ĭ-gō-dĕn″drō-blăs-tō′mă) [″ + ″ + ″ + *oma,* tumor] A neoplasm derived from oligodendroblasts.

**oligodendrocyte** [″ + ″ + *kytos,* cell] Neuroglial cells having few and delicate processes. SEE: *oligodendroglia.*

**oligodendroglia** (ŏl″ĭ-gō-dĕn-drŏg′lē-ă) [″ + ″ + *glia,* glue] A neuroglial cell of ectodermal origin that functions in the central nervous system to form or maintain the myelin sheath of neural processes. This type of cell has long, slender processes and is often found associated with nerve cells or satellites.

**oligodendroglioma** (ŏl″ĭ-gō-dĕn″drō-glī-ō′mă) [″ + ″ + ″ + *oma,* tumor] A malignant tumor of unknown etiology that consists mostly of oligodendrocytes and occurs principally in the cerebrum.

**oligodontia** (ŏl″ĭ-gō-dŏn′shē-ă) [″ + *odont,* tooth] A hereditary developmental anomaly characterized by fewer teeth than normal.

**oligohydramnios** (ŏl″ĭg-ō-hī-drăm′nē-ōs) [″ + *hydor,* water, + *amnion,* amnion] A complication of pregnancy defined as the volume of the amniotic fluid (AF) being less than 300 ml during the third trimester of pregnancy. This condition is associated with a high probability of postmaturity, fetal growth retardation, congenital anomalies, and perinatal mortality. The volume of the AF may be determined by a variety of methods including ultrasound and dye-dilution tests.

**oligomastigate** (ŏl″ĭ-gō-măs′tĭ-gāt) [″ + *mastix,* whip] Characterized by two flagella.

**oligomenorrhea** (ŏl″ĭ-gō-mĕn″ō-rē′ă) [″ + *men,* month, + *rhoia,* flow] Scanty or infrequent menstrual flow.

**oligonucleotide** (ŏl″ĭ-gō-nū′klē-ō-tīd) [″ + *nucleotide*] A compound made up of a small number of nucleotide units.

**oligopnea** (ŏl-ĭ-gŏp′nē-ă) [″ + *pnoia,* breath] Infrequent or shallow respiration, with a rate as slow as 6 to 10 per minute. This condition is usually accompanied by slow pulse, although high in some conditions.

ETIOLOGY: Oligopnea may be due to increased intracranial pressure, meningeal or pontine hemorrhage, cerebral or cerebellar tumors, abscess, gumma of meninges, osteoma of cranium, some forms of meningitis, trauma of brain, drug poisoning, or shock.

**oligoptyalism** (ŏl-ĭ-gō-tī′ă-lĭzm) [″ + *ptyalon,* saliva] Insufficient secretion of saliva.

**oligosaccharide** (ŏl″ĭ-gō-săk′ă-rīd) A compound made up of a small number of monosaccharide units. Some are found on the outer surface of the cell membranes as part of antigens.

**oligospermia, oligozoospermatism** (ŏl″ĭ-gō-spĕr′mē-ă, -zō″ō-spĕr′mă-tĭzm) [″ + *sperma,* seed] A temporary or permanent deficiency of spermatozoa in seminal fluid.

**oligotrichia** (ŏl″ĭ-gō-trĭk′ē-ă) [″ + *thrix,* hair] Congenital scantiness of hair.

**oliguria** (ŏl-ĭg-ū′rē-ă) [″ + *ouron,* urine] Diminished urination. This condition is seen after profuse perspiration, bleeding, diarrhea, and renal failure due to any disease. It may also be caused by retention of urine due to disease of the central nervous system, shock, drug poisoning, deep coma, or hypertrophy of the prostate.

**oliva** (ō-lī′vă) *pl.* **olivae** [L., olive] An oval body located behind the anterior pyramid of the medulla oblongata and consisting of a convoluted sheet of gray matter enclosing white matter. SYN: *olivary body.*
**olivary,** *adj.*

**olivary body** Oliva.

**olive** (ŏl′ĭv) [L. *oliva,* olive] **1.** Oliva. **2.** An ovoid device small enough to fit on the tip of a vein stripper. This prevents damaging the vein as the stripper is pushed into it.

***accessory o.*** One of two masses of gray matter lying adjacent to the inferior olive of the brain.

***inferior o.*** Oliva.

***superior o.*** The superior olivary nucleus. SEE: under *nucleus.*

**olive oil** Oil obtained by pressing the ripe fruit of olives (*Olea europaea*). It is used as an emollient in treating skin diseases and as a nutrient.

**olivifugal** (ŏl″ĭ-vĭf′ū-găl) [″ + *fugere,* to flee] In a direction away from the olivary nucleus of the brain.

**olivipetal** (ŏl″ĭ-vĭp′ĕ-tăl) [″ + *peter,* to seek] In a direction toward the olivary nucleus of the brain.

**olivopontocerebellar** (ŏl″ĭ-vō-pŏn″tō-sĕr″ĕ-bĕl′ăr) Concerning the olivary nucleus, the pons, and the cerebellum of the brain.

**Ollier, Louis Xavier Edouard** (ŏl″ē-ā′) French surgeon, 1830–1900.

***O.'s disease*** Chondrodysplasia.

***O. layer*** The innermost layer of the periosteum. The osteoblasts are found in this layer.

***O. graft*** A split-thickness skin graft that is quite thin.

**-ology** [Gr. *logos,* word, reason] Suffix meaning *study of, knowledge of, science of* the subject noted in the body of the word.

**O.L.P.** L. *occipitolaeva posterior* (fetal presentation). SYN: *L.O.P.* SEE: *position.*

**olsalazine** A drug used to treat ulcerative colitis. It is esp. useful in treating adult patients who cannot tolerate sulfasalazine.

**o.m.** L. *omni mane,* every morning.

**-oma** [Gr.] Suffix meaning *tumor.*

**omagra** (ō-mă′gră) [Gr. *omos,* shoulder, + *agra,* seizure] Gout in the shoulder.

**omalgia** (ō-măl′jē-ă) [″ + *algos,* pain] Neuralgia of the shoulder.

**ombrophobia** (ŏm-brō-fō′bē-ă) [Gr. *ombros,* rain, + *phobos,* fear] Fear and anxiety induced by storms or rain.

**ombudsman** In medicine, an advocate, esp. for the elderly in a nursing home; a volunteer trained by the state to receive complaints from nursing home residents. The ombudsman verifies complaints and advocates for their resolution. SEE: *Patient's Bill of Rights.*

**omega-3 ($\omega$3) fatty acids** SEE: under *acid.*

**omental** (ō-mĕn′tăl) [L. *omentum,* covering] Pert. to the omentum.

**omentectomy** (ō-mĕn-tĕk′tō-mē) [″ + Gr. *ektome,* excision] Surgical removal of a portion of the omentum.

**omentitis** (ō-mĕn-tī′tĭs) [″ + Gr. *itis,* inflammation] Inflammation of the omentum.

**omentopexy** (ō-mĕn′tō-pĕks″ē) [″ + Gr.

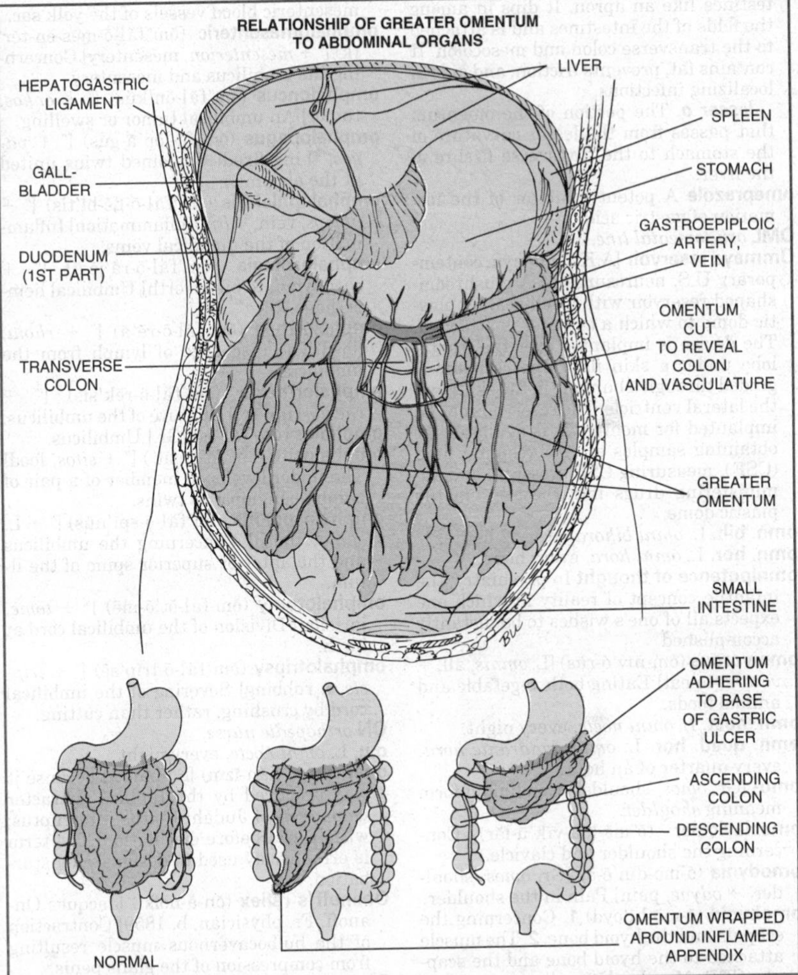


*pexis,* fixation] Fixation of the omentum to the abdominal wall or adjacent organ.

**omentoplasty** (ō-mĕn′tō-plăs″tē) [L. *omentum,* covering, + Gr. *plassein,* to form] The use of tissue from the greater omentum as a graft in rejoining tissues.

**omentorrhaphy** (ō-mĕn-tor′ră-fē) [″ + Gr. *rhaphe,* seam, ridge] Suturing of the omentum.

**omentosplenopexy** (ō-mĕn″tō-splē′nō-pĕks-ē) [″ + Gr. *splen,* spleen, + *pexis,* fixation] Fixation of the spleen and omentum. Combined omentopexy and splenopexy.

**omentotomy** (ō-mĕn-tŏt′ō-mē) [″ + Gr. *tome,* incision] Surgical incision of the omentum.

**omentovolvulus** (ō-mĕn″tō-vŏl′vū-lŭs) [″ + *volvere,* to roll] Twisting of the omentum.

**omentum** (ō-mĕn′tŭm) *pl.* **omenta** [L., a covering] A double fold of peritoneum attached to the stomach and connecting it with certain of the abdominal viscera. It contains a cavity, the omental bursa (lesser peritoneal cavity). SEE: illus.

PALPATION: Infiltration of the omentum by any kind of new growth, either inflammatory or malignant, can be distinguished by the fact that upon palpation the changes found are limited to the omentum and thus do not extend to the posterior portion of the abdominal cavity, but extend across the abdomen, cannot be traced backward, do not ascend behind the ribs, and are rough, hard, and uneven.

**omental** (ō-mĕn′tăl), *adj.*

***gastrocolic o.*** Greater o.

***gastrohepatic o.*** Lesser o.

***greater o.*** The portion of the omentum that is suspended from the greater curvature of the stomach and covers the intestines like an apron. It dips in among the folds of the intestines and is attached to the transverse colon and mesocolon. It contains fat, prevents friction, and aids in localizing infections.

***lesser o.*** The portion of the omentum that passes from the lesser curvature of the stomach to the transverse fissure of the liver.

**omeprazole** A potent inhibitor of the formation of gastric acid.

**OML** *orbitomeatal line.*

**Ommaya reservoir** [A.K. Ommaya, contemporary U.S. neurosurgeon] A mushroom-shaped reservoir with a self-sealing plastic dome to which a catheter is attached. The device is implanted over the frontal lobe under a skin flap. The catheter is guided through a bur hole in the skull into the lateral ventricle. The reservoir may be implanted for months. It is available for obtaining samples of cerebrospinal fluid (CSF), measuring CSF pressure, and administering drugs intrathecally via the plastic dome.

**omn. bih.** L. *omni bihora,* every 2 hours.

**omn. hor.** L. *omni hora,* every hour.

**omnipotence of thought** In psychiatry, the infantile concept of reality in which one expects all of one's wishes to be instantly accomplished.

**omnivorous** (ŏm-nĭv′ō-rŭs) [L. *omnis,* all, + *vorare,* to eat] Eating both vegetable and animal foods.

**omn. noct.** L. *omni nocte,* every night.

**omn. quad. hor.** L. *omni quadrante hora,* every quarter of an hour.

**omo-** [Gr. *omos,* shoulder] Combining form meaning *shoulder.*

**omoclavicular** (ō″mō-klă-vĭk′ū-lăr) Concerning the shoulder and clavicle.

**omodynia** (ō-mō-dĭn′ē-ă) [Gr. *omos,* shoulder, + *odyne,* pain] Pain in the shoulder.

**omohyoid** (ō-mō-hī′oyd) **1.** Concerning the scapula and the hyoid bone. **2.** The muscle attached to the hyoid bone and the scapula. SEE: *Muscles Appendix.*

**omophagia** (ō-mō-fā′jē-ă) [Gr. *omos,* raw, + *phagein,* to eat] The custom of eating raw foods, esp. raw flesh.

**omphal-** SEE: *omphalo-.*

**omphalectomy** (ŏm-făl-ĕk′tō-mē) [Gr. *omphalos,* navel, + *ektome,* excision] Surgical removal of the umbilicus.

**omphalic** (ŏm-făl′ĭk) [Gr. *omphalos,* navel] Concerning the umbilicus.

**omphalitis** (ŏm-făl-ī′tĭs) [″+ *itis,* inflammation] Inflammation of the umbilicus.

**omphalo-, omphal-** [Gr. *omphalos,* navel] Combining form denoting *navel.*

**omphaloangiopagus** (ŏm″fă-lō-ăn″jē-ŏp′ă-gŭs) [″+ *angeion,* vessel, + *pagos,* thing fixed] Conjoined twins united by the vessels of the umbilical cord.

**omphalocele** (ŏm-făl′ō-sēl) [″+ *kele,* tumor, swelling] Congenital hernia of the umbilicus. SEE: *hernia.*

**omphalochorion** (ŏm″fă-lō-kō′rē-ŏn) A chorion supplied with blood by the omphalomesenteric blood vessels of the yolk sac.

**omphalomesenteric** (ŏm″făl-ō-mĕs-ĕn-tĕr′ĭk) [″ + *mesenterion,* mesentery] Concerning the umbilicus and mesentery.

**omphaloncus** (ŏm″făl-ŏn′kŭs) [″ + *onkos,* tumor] An umbilical tumor or swelling.

**omphalopagus** (ŏm″fă-lŏp′ă-gŭs) [″ + *pagos,* thing fixed] Conjoined twins united at the abdomen.

**omphalophlebitis** (ŏm″făl-ō-flē-bī′tis) [″ + *phleps,* vein, + *itis,* inflammation] Inflammation of the umbilical veins.

**omphalorrhagia** (ŏm″făl-ō-rā′jē-ă) [″ + *rhegnynai,* to burst forth] Umbilical hemorrhage.

**omphalorrhea** (ŏm″făl-ō-rē′ă) [″ + *rhoia,* flow] The discharge of lymph from the umbilicus.

**omphalorrhexis** (ŏm″făl-ō-rĕk′sĭs) [″ + *rhexis,* rupture] Rupture of the umbilicus.

**omphalos** (ŏm′făl-ŏs) [Gr.] Umbilicus.

**omphalosite** (ŏm′fă-lō-sīt″) [″ + *sitos,* food] The underdeveloped member of a pair of omphaloangiopagus twins.

**omphalospinous** (ŏm″făl-ō-spī′nŭs) [″ + L. *spina,* thorn] Concerning the umbilicus and the anterior superior spine of the ilium.

**omphalotomy** (ŏm-făl-ŏt′ō-mē) [″ + *tome,* incision] Division of the umbilical cord at birth.

**omphalotripsy** (ŏm″făl-ō-trĭp′sē) [″ + *tripsis,* a rubbing] Severing of the umbilical cord by crushing, rather than cutting.

**ON** *orthopedic nurse.*

**o.n.** L. *omni nocte,* every night.

**onanism** (ō′năn-ĭzm) [So named because it was practiced by the Biblical character Onan, son of Judah] Coitus interruptus; withdrawal before ejaculation. The term is erroneously used to designate masturbation.

**Onanoff's reflex** (ŏn-ă-nŏfs′) [Jacques Onanoff, Fr. physician, b. 1859] Contraction of the bulbocavernous muscle resulting from compression of the glans penis.

**Onchocerca** (ŏng″kō-sĕr′kă) [Gr. *onkos,* hook, + *kerkos,* tail] A genus of filarial worms that live in the subcutaneous and connective tissues of their hosts, usually

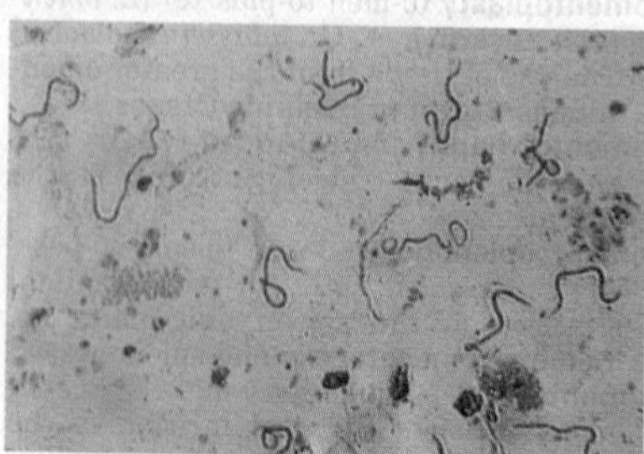


**ONCHOCERCA VOLVULUS** IN SKIN NODULE (ORIG. MAG. ×100)

enclosed in fibrous cysts or nodules.

***O. volvulus*** A species of *Onchocerca* that infests humans, frequently invading the tissues of the eye. The parasites are transmitted by species of the black fly *Simulium* and *Eusimulium*. SEE: illus.

**onchocerciasis** (ŏng″kō-sĕr-kī′ă-sĭs) [″ + ″ + *iasis,* infestation] A condition produced by infestation with one of the filarial worms of the genus *Onchocerca*. It is marked by a nodular swelling over the coiled parasite. The microfilariae present in the nodules eventually affect the eyes and cause blindness. The disease is spread by the bites of black flies of the genus *Simulium*. In some areas of Africa, half or more of the middle-aged men are blind from this disease. Treatment includes a single annual dose of Ivermectin. SYN: *river blindness*. SEE: illus.

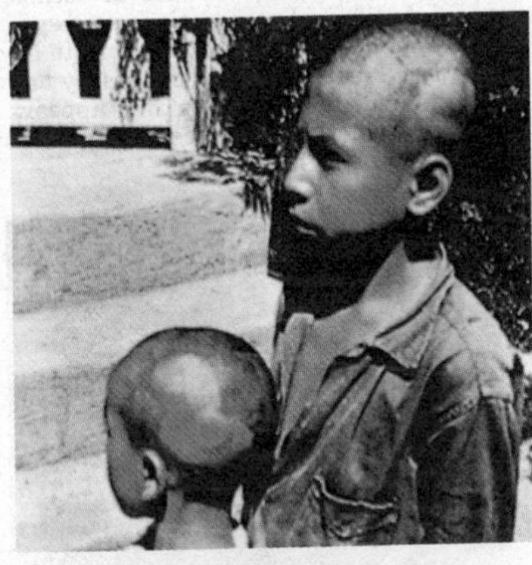

CUTANEOUS NODULES OF ONCHOCERCIASIS

**onco-** [Gr. *onkos,* bulk, mass] Combining form meaning *tumor, swelling, mass.*

**Oncocerca** *Onchocerca*.

**oncocercosis** Onchocerciasis.

**oncocyte** (ŏn′kō-sīt) [″ + *kytos,* cell] A large columnar cell with granular, acidophilic cytoplasm and a large number of mitochondria. They may become neoplastic.

**oncocytoma** (ŏng″kō-sī-tō′mă) [″ + ″ + *oma,* tumor] A benign adenoma composed of eosinophilic epithelial cells, esp. one of the salivary or parathyroid glands.

**oncofetal** (ŏng″kō-fē′tăl) Concerning tumors in the fetus.

**oncogene** (ŏng′kō-jēn) [″ + *gennan,* to produce] A gene in a virus that has the ability to induce a cell to become malignant. Oncogenes have been identified in human tumors. In addition to genes that can induce tumor formation, there are anti-oncogenes that suppress tumors.

**oncogenesis** (ŏng″kō-jĕn′ĕ-sĭs) [″ + *genesis,* generation, birth] Tumor formation and development. **oncogenic** (-jĕn′ĭk), *adj.*

**oncoides** (ŏng-koy′dēz) [″ + *eidos,* form, shape] Turgescence.

**oncologist** [Gr. *onkos,* bulk, + *logos,* word] A specialist in oncology.

**oncology** (ŏng-kŏl′ō-jē) [″ + *logos,* word, reason] The branch of medicine dealing with tumors.

**oncolysis** (ŏng-kŏl′ĭ-sĭs) [″ + *lysis,* dissolution] The absorption or dissolution of tumor cells.

**oncolytic** (ŏng″kō-lĭt′ĭk) Destructive to tumor cells.

**oncometry** The measurement of variations in size of internal organs.

**oncornaviruses** A group of RNA viruses that can cause cancer in humans or animals.

**oncosphere** (ŏng′kō-sfēr) [″ + *sphaira,* sphere] The embryonic stage of a tapeworm in which it has hooks.

**oncotherapy** (ŏng″kō-thĕr′ă-pē) [″ + *therapeia,* treatment] The treatment of tumors.

**oncothlipsis** (ŏng″kō-thlĭp′sĭs) [″ + *thlipsis,* pressure] The pressure caused by the presence of a tumor.

**oncotic** (ŏng-kŏt′ĭk) [Gr. *onkos,* bulk, mass] Concerning, caused, or marked by swelling.

**oncotomy** (ŏng-kŏt′ō-mē) [″ + *tome,* incision] The incision of a tumor, abscess, or boil.

**oncovirus** (ŏn′kō-vī″rŭs) [″ + *virus*] Any virus that causes malignant neoplasms.

**Ondine's curse** [Fr. Undine, mythical water nymph whose human lover was cursed to continuous sleep] **1.** Primary alveolar hypoventilation caused by reduced responsiveness of the respiratory center to carbon dioxide. **2.** Loss of automatic respiratory function owing to a lesion in the cervical portion of the spinal cord.

**oneiric** (ō-nī′rĭk) [Gr. *oneiros,* dream] Resembling, relating to, or accompanied by dreams.

**oneirism** (ō-nī′rĭzm) [″ + *-ismos,* state of] A dreamlike hallucination in a waking state.

**oneirodynia** (ō-nī″rō-dĭn′ē-ă) [″ + *odyne,* pain] Painful dreaming; nightmare.

**oneirology** (ō″nī-rŏl′ō-jē) [Gr. *oneiros,* dream, + *logos,* word, reason] The scientific study of dreams.

**oniomania** (ō″nē-ō-mā′nē-ă) [Gr. *onios,* for sale, + *mania,* madness] A psychoneurotic urge to spend money.

**onion** (ŭn′yŭn) [AS. *oignon*] The edible bulb of the onion plant, cultivated as a vegetable. Latin name for the common onion is *Allium cepa*. The characteristic odor of onions is due to several volatile chemicals, some of which contain sulfur. The ability of onions to cause persons who peel them to shed tears is probably caused by the chemical propanethial *S*-oxide. When this material comes in contact with tears, sulfuric acid is formed.

**onlay 1.** A graft applied to the surface of a tissue, esp. a bone graft applied to bone. **2.** In dentistry, a cast metal restoration that overlays the cusps of the tooth, thereby providing additional strength to the restored tooth.

**onomatology** (ŏn″ō-mă-tŏl′ō-jē) [Gr. *onoma,* name, + *logos,* word, reason] The science of names. SYN: *nomenclature; terminology.*

**onomatomania** (ŏn″ō-mă″tō-mā′nē-ă) [″ + *mania,* madness] A mental illness characterized by an abnormal impulse to dwell upon or repeat certain words or by attaching significance to their imagined hidden meanings.

**onomatophobia** (ŏn″ō-mă″tō-fō′bē-ă) [″ + *phobos,* fear] An abnormal fear of hearing a certain name or word because of an imagined dreadful meaning attached to it.

**onomatopoiesis** (ŏn″ō-mă″tō-poy-ē′sĭs) [Gr. *onoma,* name, + *poiein,* to make] **1.** The formation of words that imitate the sounds with which they are associated (e.g., hiss, buzz). **2.** In psychiatry, imitative words and sounds created by patients with schizophrenia.

**ontogeny** (ŏn-tŏj′ĕn-ē) [Gr. *on,* being, + *gennan,* to produce] The history of the development of an individual.

**onych-** SEE: *onycho-.*

**onychalgia** (ŏn″ĭ-kăl′jē-ă) [Gr. *onyx,* nail, + *algos,* pain] Pain in the nails.

***o. nervosa*** Extreme sensitivity of the nails.

**onychatrophia** (ō″nĭk-ă-trō′fē-ă) [″ + *trophe,* nourishment] Atrophy of the nails.

**onychauxis** (ŏn″ĭ-kawk′sĭs) [″ + *auxein,* to increase] Overgrowth of the nails.

**onychectomy** (ŏn″ĭ-kĕk′tō-mē) [″ + *ektome,* to cut] Surgical removal of the nail of a finger or toe.

**onychia** (ō-nĭk′ē-ă) [Gr. *onyx,* nail] Inflammation of the nailbed with possible suppuration and loss of the nail. SYN: *matrixitis; onychitis; onyxitis.* SEE: *paronychia.*

**onychitis** (ŏn″ĭ-kī′tĭs) [″ + *itis,* inflammation] Onychia.

**onycho-, onych-** [Gr. *onyx,* nail] Combining form meaning *fingernail, toenail.*

**onychodystrophy** (ŏn″ĭ-kō-dĭs′trō-fē) [″ + *dys,* bad, + *trophe,* nutrition] Any maldevelopment of a nail.

**onychogenic** (ŏn″ĭ-kō-jĕn′ĭk) [″ + *gennan,* to produce] Concerning nail formation.

**onychograph** (ŏn-ĭk′ō-grăf) [″ + *graphein,* to write] A device used for making a record of capillary pulse under the fingernails.

**onychogryposis** (ŏn″ĭ-kō-grĭ-pō′sĭs) [″ + *gryposis,* a curving] Abnormal overgrowth of the nails with inward curvature.

**onychoheterotopia** (ŏn″ĭ-kō-hĕt″ĕr-ō-tō′pē-ă) [″ + *heteros,* other, + *topos,* place] Abnormally located nails.

**onychoid** (ŏn′ĭ-koyd) [″ + *eidos,* form, shape] Similar to a nail, esp. a fingernail.

**onycholysis** (ŏn″ĭ-kŏl′ĭ-sĭs) [″ + *lysis,* dissolution] Loosening or detachment of the nail from the nailbed. SEE: *photo-onycholysis.*

**onychoma** (ŏn-ĭ-kō′mă) [″ + *oma,* tumor] A tumor of the nail or nailbed.

**onychomadesis** (ŏn′ĭ-kō-mă-dē′sĭs) [Gr. *onyx,* nail, + *madesis,* loss of hair] The complete loss of the nails.

**onychomalacia** (ŏn″ĭ-kō-mă-lā′sē-ă) [″ + *malakia,* softening] Abnormal softening of the nails. SYN: *hapalonychia.*

**onychomycosis** (ŏn″ĭ-kō-mī-kō′sĭs) [″ + *mykes,* fungus, + *osis,* condition] A disease of the nails (esp. the toenails) caused by a parasitic fungus. Because the fungus invades the nail, it is extremely difficult to treat. The nails may turn yellow, gray, brown, or black depending on the type of fungus involved. Factors that favor development of this condition include excessive perspiration; wearing socks that do not absorb foot perspiration; wearing shoes with impermeable soles that do not allow ventilation; and walking barefoot in public swimming pools, showers or locker rooms. Antifungal preparations used systemically may take a year or more to be effective. Treatment is not necessary unless the nails are painful or their appearance is cosmetically unacceptable. SYN: *tinea unguium.* SEE: illus.

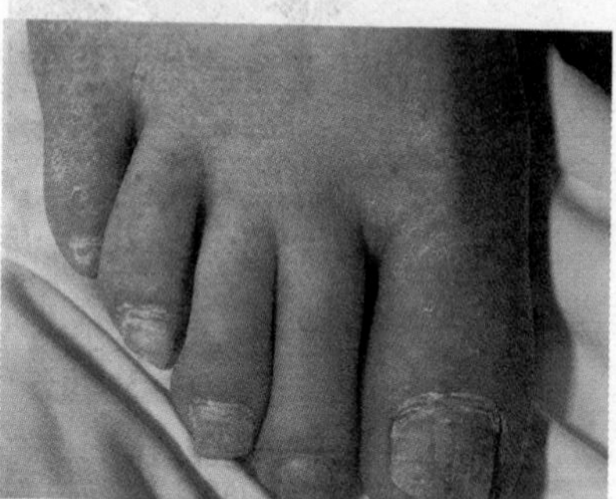

ONYCHOMYCOSIS

**onycho-osteodysplasia** (ŏn″ĭ-kō-ŏs″tē-ō-dĭs-plā′zē-ă) A genetic disease involving ectodermal and mesodermal tissues. The nails and patellae may be absent; other bones and joints are affected. SYN: *nail-patella syndrome.*

**onychopathology** (ŏn″ĭ-kō-pă-thŏl′ō-jē) [″ + *pathos,* disease, suffering, + *logos,* word, reason] The study of diseases of the nails.

**onychopathy** (ŏn-ĭ-kŏp′ăth-ē) [″ + *pathos,* disease, suffering] Any disease of the nails. SYN: *onychosis.*

**onychophagy** (ŏn-ĭ-kŏf′ă-jē) [″ + *phagein,* to eat] Nail biting.

**onychophosis** (ŏn″ĭk-ō-fō′sĭs) An accumulation of horny layers of epidermis under the toenail.

**onychophyma** (ŏn″ĭ-kō-fī′mă) [″ + *phyma,* a growth] Painful degeneration of the nail with hypertrophy.

**onychoptosis** (ŏn″ĭk-ŏp-tō′sĭs) [″ + *ptosis,* a dropping] Dropping off of the nails.

**onychorrhexis** (ŏn″ĭ-kō-rĕk′sĭs) [″ + *rhexis,*

a rupture] Abnormal brittleness and splitting of the nails.

**onychoschizia** (ŏn″ĭ-kō-skĭz′ē-ă) [″ + *schizein,* to split] Loosening and eventual separation of the nail from its bed.

**onychosis** (ŏn-ĭ-kō′sĭs) [″ + *osis,* disease] Onychopathy.

**onychotillomania** (ŏn″ĭ-kō-tĭl″ō-mā′nē-ă) [″ + *tillein,* to pluck, + *mania,* insanity] A neurotic tendency to pick at the nails.

**onychotomy** (ŏn″ĭ-kŏt′ō-mē) [″ + *tome,* incision] Surgical incision of a fingernail or toenail.

**onychotrophy** (ŏn-ĭ-kŏt′rō-fē) [″ + *trophe,* nourishment] Nourishment of the nails.

**onyx** (ŏn′ĭks) [Gr., nail] **1.** A fingernail or toenail. **2.** Pus collection between the corneal layers of the eye. SYN: *hypopyon.*

**onyxitis** (ŏn-ĭk-sī′tĭs) [Gr. *onyx,* nail, + *itis,* inflammation] Onychia.

**oo-** (ō-ō) [Gr. *oon,* egg] Combining form meaning *egg* or *ovary*. SEE: words beginning with *ovo-*.

**ooblast** (ō′ō-blăst) [″ + *blastos,* germ] The primitive cell from which the ovum is developed.

**oocyesis** (ō″ō-sī-ē′sĭs) [″ + *kyesis,* pregnancy] Ectopic pregnancy in an ovary.

**oocyst** (ō′ō-sĭst) [Gr. *oon,* egg, + *kystis,* bladder] The encysted form of a fertilized gamete (zygote) occurring in certain sporozoa. SEE: *ookinete.*

**oocyte** (ō′ō-sīt) [″ + *kytos,* cell] The early or primitive ovum before it has developed completely.

***primary o.*** An oocyte at end of the growth period of the oogonium and before the first maturation division has occurred.

***secondary o.*** The larger of two oocytes resulting from the first maturation division. SEE: *body, polar.*

**oogenesis** (ō″ō-jĕn′ĕ-sĭs) [″ + *genesis,* generation, birth] Meiosis for the formation of the ovum. SYN: *ovigenesis.* SEE: illus.; *meiosis.* **oogenetic** (-jĕ-nĕt′ĭk), *adj.*

**oogonium** (ō″ō-gō′nē-ŭm) *pl.* **oogonia** [″ + *gone,* seed] **1.** The primordial cell from

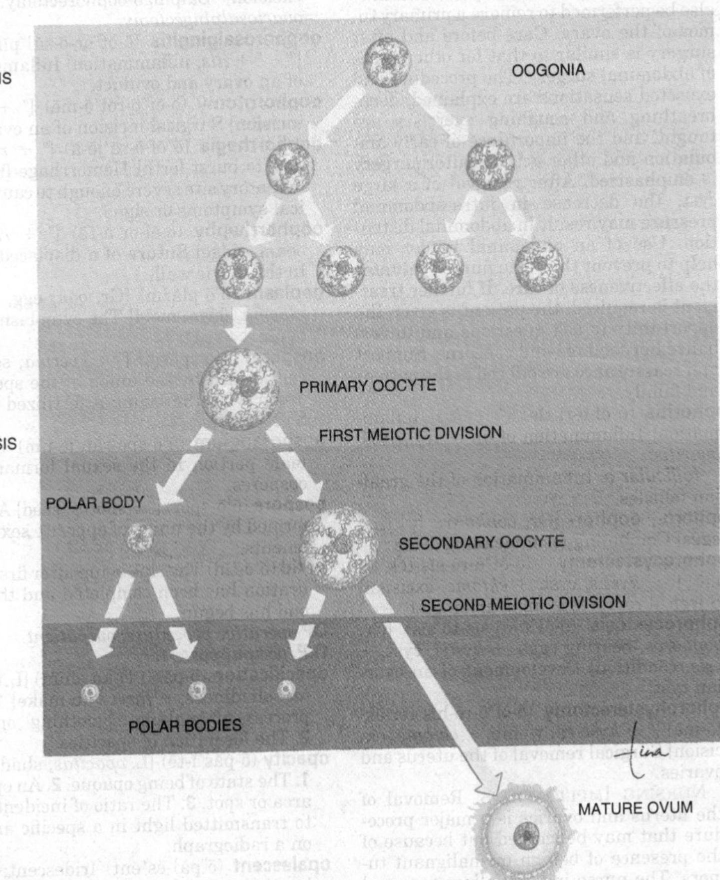


**OOGENESIS**

which an oocyte originates. **2.** A descendant of the primordial cell from which the oocyte arises.

**ookinesis** (ō″ō-kĭn-ē′sĭs) [″ + *kinesis,* movement] The mitosis of oogonia in the embryonic ovary to form primary oocytes.

**ookinete** (ō″ō-kĭ-nēt′) [″ + *kinetos,* motile] An elongated motile zygote occurring in the life cycle of certain sporozoan parasites, esp. those of the genus *Plasmodium.* It penetrates the stomach wall of a mosquito and gives rise to an oocyst.

**oolemma** (ō″ō-lĕm′ă) [″ + *lemma,* sheath] The plasma membrane of the oocyte.

**oophagy** (ō-ŏf′ă-jē) [″ + *phagein,* to eat] Eating of eggs.

**oophor-** SEE: *oophoro-.*

**oophorectomy** (ō″ŏf-ō-rĕk′tō-mē) [Gr. *oophoros,* bearing eggs, + *ektome,* excision] Excision of an ovary. SYN: *ovariectomy.*

Nursing Implications: The nurse individualizes teaching according to the reason for removal of the ovary. Most commonly, the procedure is carried out to remove a benign ovarian cyst, but it may also be performed to remove a primary tumor of the ovary. Care before and after surgery is similar to that for other types of abdominal surgery. The procedure and expected sensations are explained, deep-breathing and coughing exercises are taught, and the importance of early ambulation and other activity after surgery is emphasized. After removal of a large cyst, the decrease in intra-abdominal pressure may result in abdominal distention. Use of an abdominal binder may help to prevent this. The nurse evaluates the effectiveness of care. If further treatment is required, the patient is given the opportunity to ask questions and to verbalize her feelings and concerns. Support and reassurance are offered to the patient and family.

**oophoritis** (ō″ŏf-ō-rī′tĭs) [″ + *itis,* inflammation] Inflammation of an ovary. SYN: *ovaritis.*

***follicular o.*** Inflammation of the graafian follicles.

**oophoro-, oophor-** [Gr. *oophoros,* bearing eggs] Combining form meaning *ovary.*

**oophorocystectomy** (ō-ŏf″ō-rō-sĭs-tĕk′tō-mē) [″ + *kystis,* cyst, + *ektome,* excision] Surgical removal of an ovarian cyst.

**oophorocystosis** (ō-ŏf″ō-rō-sĭs-tō′sĭs) [Gr. *oophoros,* bearing eggs, + *kystis,* cyst, + *osis,* condition] Development of an ovarian cyst.

**oophorohysterectomy** (ō-ŏf″ō-rō-hĭs″tĕr-ĕk′tō-mē) [″ + *hystera,* womb, + *ektome,* excision] Surgical removal of the uterus and ovaries.

Nursing Implications: Removal of the uterus and ovaries is a major procedure that may be carried out because of the presence of benign or malignant tumors. The nurse individualizes care and teaching on this basis. Care before and after surgery is similar to that for other types of abdominal surgery. The procedure and expected sensations are explained, deep-breathing and coughing exercises are taught, and the importance of early ambulation and other activity after surgery is emphasized. Pain control measures are discussed, and the patient is advised to seek pain relief in the early postoperative period before pain becomes severe. The nurse evaluates the effectiveness of care. If further treatment is required, the patient is given the opportunity to ask questions and to verbalize feelings and concerns. Support and reassurance are offered to the patient and family.

**oophoroma** (ō-ŏf″ō-rō′mă) [″ + *oma,* tumor] A malignant ovarian tumor.

**oophoropexy** (ō-ŏf″ō-rō-pĕk′sē) [″ + *pexis,* fixation] Fixation of a displaced ovary.

**oophoroplasty** (ō-ŏf′ō-rō-plăs″tē) [″ + *plassein,* to form] Plastic surgery on an ovary.

**oophorosalpingectomy** (ō-ŏf″ō-rō-săl-pĭn-jĕk′tō-mē) [″ + *salpinx,* tube, + *ektome,* excision] Salpingo-oophorectomy. SYN: *ovariosalpingectomy.*

**oophorosalpingitis** (ō-ŏf″or-ō-săl″pĭn-jī′tĭs) [″ + ″ + *itis,* inflammation] Inflammation of an ovary and oviduct.

**oophorotomy** (ō-ŏf″ō-rŏt′ō-mē) [″ + *tome,* incision] Surgical incision of an ovary.

**oophorrhagia** (ō″ŏf-ō-rā′jē-ă) [″ + *rhegnynai,* to burst forth] Hemorrhage from an ovulatory site severe enough to cause clinical symptoms or signs.

**oophorrhaphy** (ō-ŏf-or′ă-fē) [″ + *rhaphe,* seam, ridge] Suture of a displaced ovary to the pelvic wall.

**ooplasm** (ō′ō-plăzm) [Gr. *oon,* egg, + LL. *plasma,* form, mold] The cytoplasm of an ovum.

**oosperm** (ō′ō-spĕrm) [″ + *sperma,* seed] A cell formed by the union of the spermatozoon with the ovum; a fertilized ovum. SYN: *zygote.*

**oosporangium** (ō″ō-spō-răn′jē-ŭm) The female portion in the sexual formation of oospores.

**oospore** (ō′ō-spor) [″ + *sporos,* seed] A spore formed by the union of opposite sexual elements.

**ootid** (ō′ō-tĭd) The ripe ovum after first maturation has been completed and the second has begun.

**OP** *operative procedure; outpatient.*

**O.P.** *occiput posterior.*

**opacification** (ō-păs″ĭ-fĭ-kā′shŭn) [L. *opacitas,* shadiness, + *facere,* to make] **1.** The process of making something opaque. **2.** The formation of opacities.

**opacity** (ō-păs′ĭ-tē) [L. *opacitas,* shadiness] **1.** The state of being opaque. **2.** An opaque area or spot. **3.** The ratio of incident light to transmitted light in a specific area or on a radiograph.

**opalescent** (ō″păl-ĕs′ĕnt) Iridescent; similar to an opal with respect to the colors produced.

**opaque** (ō-pāk′) [L. *opacus,* dark] **1.** Impenetrable by visible light rays or by other forms of radiant energy such as x-rays. **2.** Not transparent or translucent.

**OPC** *outpatient clinic.*

**OPD** *outpatient department.*

**open** [AS.] **1.** Not closed. **2.** Uncovered or exposed, as a wound to air. **3.** To puncture, as to open a boil. **4.** Interrupted, as in an electric circuit when current cannot pass because a switch is open.

**opening 1.** The act of making or becoming open. **2.** A hole, aperture, entrance, or open space.

***aortic o.*** The opening in the diaphragm through which the aorta passes.

***cardiac o.*** The opening of the esophagus into the cardiac end of the stomach.

***pyloric o.*** The opening between the stomach and duodenum.

**opening snap** An abnormal early diastolic extra heart sound usually associated with stenosis of one of the atrioventricular valves. Most commonly, the sound reflects mitral valve stenosis. The brief, high-pitched snapping sound is unaffected by respiration and is heard best between the apex and the lower left sternal border.

**open-label study** An experimental study involving the use of a medicine, the identity of which is known to the patient.

**operable** (ŏp′ĕr-ă-bl) [L. *operor,* to work] **1.** Practicable. **2.** Subject to treatment by surgery with reasonable expectation of cure.

**operant** Producing effects.

**operant conditioning** SEE: under *conditioning.*

**operate** (ŏp′ĕr-āt) [L. *operatus,* worked] **1.** To perform an excision or incision, or to make a suture on the body or any of its organs or parts to restore health. **2.** To produce an effect, as a drug.

**operation** (ŏp-ĕr-ā′shŭn) [L. *operatio,* a working] **1.** The act of operating. **2.** A surgical procedure. **3.** The effect or method of action of any type of therapy. SEE: *surgery.*

Preoperative shaving of the skin over the surgical site may be unnecessary insofar as bacterial considerations are concerned; nevertheless, it is still used to facilitate access to the operative site.

**operative** (ŏp′ĕr-ă-tĭv) [L. *operativus,* working] **1.** Effective, active. **2.** Pert. to or brought about by an operation.

**operative dentistry** SEE: under *dentistry.*

**operculitis** (ō-pĕr″kū-lī′tĭs) [L. *operculum,* a cover, + Gr. *itis,* inflammation] Inflammation of the gingiva over a partially erupted tooth.

**operculum** (ō-pĕr′kū-lŭm) *pl.* **opercula** [L., a cover] **1.** Any lid or covering. **2.** The narrow opening at the top of the thoracic cage bordered by the sternum and first ribs. **3.** The plug of mucus that fills the opening of the cervix on impregnation. **4.** The convolutions of the cerebrum, the margins of which are separated by the lateral cerebral (sylvian) fissure. The opercula cover the insula. **opercular** (ō-pĕr′kū-lăr), *adj.*

***dental o.*** The soft tissue overlying the crown of a partially erupted tooth.

***trophoblastic o.*** The plug of fibrin that covers the opening in the endometrium made by the implanting ovum.

**operon** (ŏp′ĕr-ŏn) A group of linked genes and regulatory elements that produces a messenger RNA molecule during transcription in response to a change in the intracellular environment.

**ophiasis** (ō-fī′ă-sĭs) [Gr. *ophis,* snake] Baldness occurring in winding streaks across the head.

**ophidiophobia** (ō-fĭd″ē-ō-fō′bē-ă) [Gr. *ophidion,* snake, + *phobos,* fear] Abnormal fear of snakes.

**ophidism** (ō′fĭd-ĭzm) [″ + *-ismos,* condition] Poisoning from snake bite.

**ophritis, ophryitis** (ŏf-rī′tĭs, -rē-ī′tĭs) [Gr. *ophrys,* eyebrow, + *itis,* inflammation] Inflammation of the eyebrow.

**ophryon** (ŏf′rē-ŏn) The meeting point of the facial median line with a transverse line across the forehead's narrowest portion.

**ophryosis** (ŏf″rē-ō′sĭs) [″ + *osis,* condition] Eyebrow spasm.

**ophthalm-** SEE: *ophthalmo-.*

**ophthalmagra** (ŏf″thăl-măg′ră) [Gr. *ophthalmos,* eye, + *agra,* seizure] Sudden development of eye pain.

**ophthalmalgia** (ŏf″thăl-măl′jē-ă) [″ + *algos,* pain] Pain in the eye. SYN: *ophthalmodynia.*

**ophthalmatrophy** (ŏf-thăl-măt′rō-fē) [″ + *atrophia,* a wasting] Atrophy of the eyeball.

**ophthalmectomy** (ŏf-thăl-mĕk′tō-mē) [″ + *ektome,* excision] Surgical excision of an eye.

**ophthalmencephalon** (ŏf″thăl-mĕn-sĕf′ă-lŏn) [″ + *enkephalos,* brain] The vision apparatus from the retina to the optic nerves, optic chiasm, optic tract, and the visual centers of the brain.

**ophthalmia** (ŏf-thăl′mē-ă) [Gr. *ophthalmos,* eye] Severe inflammation of the eye, usually including the conjunctiva.

***catarrhal o.*** Conjunctivitis of a severe, frequently purulent, form.

***Egyptian o.*** Trachoma.

***electric o.*** Ophthalmia marked by eye pain, intolerance to light, and tearing (lacrimation). The condition occurs following prolonged exposure to intense light such as that encountered in arc welding.

***gonorrheal o.*** Severe purulent conjunctivitis due to infection with gonococcus.

***granular o.*** Trachoma.

***metastatic o.*** Sympathetic inflammation of the choroid due to pyemia or metastasis.

***o. neonatorum*** Severe purulent conjunctivitis in the newborn.

ETIOLOGY: Infection of the birth canal at the time of delivery. *Neisseria gonorrhoeae* and *Chlamydia trachomatis* are responsible for the great majority of cases. Symptoms are present 12 to 48 hr after birth when due to gonorrhea and 1 week or more after birth for chlamydia infections.

PROPHYLAXIS: Erythromycin ophthalmic ointment is introduced into the conjunctival sac of each eye of the newborn to prevent gonorrheal or chlamydial conjunctivitis. SEE: *Credé's method* (2).

***neuroparalytic o.*** Ophthalmia resulting from injury or disease involving the semilunar ganglion or the branches of the trigeminal nerve supplying the affected eyeball.

***phlyctenular o.*** Vesicular formations on the epithelium of the conjunctiva or cornea.

***purulent o.*** Purulent inflammation of the eye, usually due to gonococcus.

***spring o.*** Conjunctivitis occurring in the spring, usually due to an allergic reaction to pollen. SYN: *vernal conjunctivitis.*

***sympathetic o.*** A rare bilateral granulomatous inflammation of the entire uveal tract of both eyes. The condition occurs in the untraumatized eye following perforation of the globe of the other eye.

SYMPTOMS: Photophobia, lacrimation, pain, blurring of vision, eyeball tenderness, and deposits on posterior surface of cornea are present. Exudate appears in pupillary area with posterior synechia, seclusio pupillae, and secondary atrophy with blindness.

TREATMENT: Mydriatics, analgesics, and topical and systemic corticosteroids are used to treat this condition. Enucleation of the traumatized eye may reduce the chances of developing this condition. However, if sympathetic ophthalmia does occur, enucleation may be beneficial regardless of the time elapsed since injury.

***varicose o.*** Inflammation that accompanies varicosities of the conjunctival veins.

**ophthalmic** (ŏf-thăl′mĭk) Pert. to the eye.

***o. nerve*** A branch of the trigeminal (5th cranial) nerve. It is sensory and has lacrimal, frontal, and nasociliary branches.

**ophthalmic reaction** Calmette's reaction.

**ophthalmitis** (ŏf″thăl-mī′tĭs) [″ + *itis,* inflammation] Inflammation of the eye.

**ophthalmo-, ophthalm-** [Gr. *ophthalmos,* eye] Combining form meaning *eye.*

**ophthalmoblennorrhea** (ŏf-thăl″mō-blĕn″ō-rē′ă) [″ + *blenna,* mucus, + *rhoia,* flow] Purulent inflammation of the eye or conjunctiva, usually due to gonococcus.

**ophthalmocopia** (ŏf-thăl″mō-kō′pē-ă) [″ + *kopos,* fatigue] Asthenopia.

**ophthalmodesmitis** (ŏf-thăl″mō-dĕs-mī′tĭs) [″ + *desmos,* ligament, + *itis,* inflammation] Inflammation of the tendons of the eye.

**ophthalmodiaphanoscope** (ŏf-thăl″mō-dī-ă-făn′ō-skōp) [″ + ″ + *phainein,* to appear, + *skopein,* to examine] A device for examining the retina by transillumination.

**ophthalmodonesis** (ŏf-thăl″mō-dō-nē′sĭs) [″ + *donesis,* trembling] Tremor or oscillatory movement of the eye.

**ophthalmodynamometer** (ŏf-thăl″mō-dī″nă-mŏm′ĕ-tĕr) [″ + *dynamis,* power, + *metron,* measure] An instrument for determining the pressure in the ophthalmic arteries. The device is placed against the conjunctiva of the eye. If the pressure is higher on one side than on the other, appropriate studies to attempt to define the cause are indicated.

**ophthalmodynamometry** (ŏf-thăl″mō-dī″nă-mŏm′ĕ-trē) Determination of pressure in the ophthalmic artery by use of an instrument that produces pressure on the eyeball until pulsations in the ophthalmic artery are seen through the ophthalmoscope, indicating the diastolic pressure. As the pressure is increased, the vessel collapses and the systolic pressure is obtained.

**ophthalmodynia** (ŏf-thăl″mō-dĭn′ē-ă) [″ + *odyne,* pain] Pain in the eye. SYN: *ophthalmalgia.*

**ophthalmoeikonometer** (ŏf-thăl″mō-ī″kō-nŏm′ĕ-tĕr) [″ + *eikon,* image, + *metron,* measure] A device for measuring the relative size of the two ocular images.

**ophthalmofundoscope** (ŏf-thăl″mō-fŭn′dō-skōp) [″ + L. *fundus,* base, + Gr. *skopein,* to examine] An apparatus used in examining the fundus of the eye.

**ophthalmography** (ŏf″thăl-mŏg′ră-fē) [″ + *graphein,* to write] Description of the eye.

**ophthalmolith** (ŏf-thăl′mō-lĭth) [″ + *lithos,* stone] A calculus of the lacrimal duct.

**ophthalmologist** (ŏf-thăl-mŏl′ō-jĭst) [″ + *logos,* word, reason] A physician who specializes in the treatment of disorders of the eye. SEE: *optician; optometrist.*

**ophthalmology** (ŏf-thăl-mŏl′ō-jē) [″ + *logos,* word, reason] The health science dealing with the eye and its diseases.

**ophthalmomalacia** (ŏf-thăl″mō-măl-ā′sē-ă) [″ + *malakia,* softening] Abnormal shrinkage or softening of the eyeball.

**ophthalmometer** (ŏf-thăl-mŏm′ĕt-ĕr) [″ + *metron,* measure] **1.** An instrument for measuring errors of eye refraction. **2.** An instrument for measuring the volume of various chambers of the eye. **3.** An instrument for measuring the anterior curvatures of the eye. **4.** An instrument for measuring the size of the eye.

**ophthalmomycosis** (ŏf-thăl″mō-mī-kō′sĭs) [″ + *mykes,* fungus, + *osis,* condition] Any fungus disease of the eye.

**ophthalmomyiasis** (ŏf-thăl″mō-mī-ī′yă-sĭs) [Gr. *ophthalmos,* eye, + *myia,* a fly, + *-iasis,* condition] Infestation of the eye by larvae of the fly *Oestrus ovis.*

**ophthalmomyitis** (ŏf-thăl″mō-mī-ī′tĭs) [″ + *mys,* muscle, + *itis,* inflammation] Inflammation of the ocular muscles.

**ophthalmomyotomy** (ŏf-thăl″mō-mī-ŏt′ō-mē) [″ + *mys,* muscle, + *tome,* incision] Surgical section of the muscles of the eyes.

**ophthalmoneuritis** (ŏf-thăl″mō-nū-rī′tĭs) [″

+ *neuron,* sinew, + *itis,* inflammation] Inflammation of the optic nerve.

**ophthalmopathy** Any disease of the eye.

**ophthalmophlebotomy** (ŏf-thăl″mō-flĕ-bŏt′ō-mē) [″ + *phleps,* vein, + *tome,* incision] Incision of the conjunctiva of the eye to overcome congestion of conjunctival veins.

**ophthalmoplasty** (ŏf-thăl′mō-plăs″tē) [″ + *plassein,* to form] Ocular plastic surgery.

**ophthalmoplegia** (ŏf-thăl″mō-plē′jē-ă) [″ + *plege,* stroke] Paralysis of ocular muscles.

***o. externa*** Paralysis of extraocular muscles.

***o. interna*** Paralysis of the iris and ciliary muscle.

***nuclear o.*** Paralysis due to a lesion of the nuclei of the ocular motor nerves.

***Parinaud's o.*** SEE: *Parinaud's ophthalmoplegia syndrome.*

***o. partialis, partial o.*** Incomplete paralysis involving only one or two of the ocular muscles.

***o. progressiva, progressive o.*** Ocular muscle paralysis in which all the muscles become involved slowly, due to deterioration of the motor nerve nuclei.

***o. totalis, total o.*** Paralysis that affects both internal and external ocular muscles.

**ophthalmorrhagia** (ŏf-thăl″mō-rā′jē-ă) [″ + *rhegnynai,* to burst forth] Ocular hemorrhage.

**ophthalmorrhea** (ŏf-thăl″mō-rē′ă) [″ + *rhoia,* flow] Discharge from the eye.

**ophthalmorrhexis** (ŏf-thăl″mō-rĕk′sĭs) [″ + *rhexis,* rupture] Rupture of an eyeball.

**ophthalmoscope** (ŏf-thăl′mō-skōp) [″ + *skopein,* to examine] An instrument used for examining the interior of the eye, esp. the retina.

**ophthalmoscopy** (ŏf-thăl-mŏs′kō-pē) Examination of the interior of the eye.

***medical o.*** The use of ophthalmoscopy to diagnose systemic disease.

***metric o.*** **1.** The use of ophthalmoscopy to determine the refractive error of the lens of the eye. **2.** The use of ophthalmoscopy to measure the height of the head of the optic nerve in cases of papilledema.

**ophthalmospasm** (ŏf-thăl′mō-spăsm) Spasm of the ocular muscles.

**ophthalmostat** (ŏf-thăl′mō-stăt) [″ + *statikos,* standing] An instrument used to hold the eye still during surgery.

**ophthalmostatometer** (ŏf-thăl″mō-stăt-ŏm′ĕ-tĕr) [″ + ″ + *metron,* measure] An instrument used for determining the presence or absence of exophthalmos.

**ophthalmosynchysis** (ŏf-thăl″mō-sĭn′kĭ-sĭs) [″ + *synchisis,* a mixing] Effusion into one of the cavities of the eye.

**ophthalmotomy** (ŏf″thăl-mŏt′ō-mē) [″ + *tome,* incision] Surgical incision of the eyeball.

**ophthalmotonometer** (ŏf-thăl″mō-tō-nŏm′ĕ-tĕr) [″ + *tonos,* tension, + *metron,* measure] An instrument used for determining tension within the eye.

**ophthalmotoxin** (ŏf-thăl″mō-tŏk′sĭn) [″ + *toxikon,* poison] Any substance that has a toxic effect on the eyes.

**ophthalmotropometer** (ŏf-thăl″mō-trō-pŏm′ĕ-tĕr) [″ + ″ + *metron,* measure] An instrument used for measuring the movements of the eye.

**ophthalmovascular** (ŏf-thăl″mō-văs′kū-lăr) [″ + L. *vasculum,* a small vessel] Pert. to the blood vessels of the eye.

**ophthalmoxyster** (ŏf-thăl″mŏks-ĭs′tĕr) [″ + *xyster,* scraper] An instrument used to scrape the conjunctiva.

**-opia** Suffix denoting *vision.*

**opiate** (ō′pē-ăt) Any drug containing or derived from opium.

**opiate abstinence syndrome** The group of symptoms that the opiate-dependent individual will experience upon withdrawal of the drug. The symptoms range from restlessness, depression, and mild disturbances in function of the autonomic nervous system, to chills, nausea, vomiting, and diarrhea. Emotional reactions may be pronounced.

**opiate poisoning** The toxic reaction to an overdose of an opium-derived drug.

SYMPTOMS: Acute poisoning causes euphoria, flushing, itching of the skin, miosis, drowsiness, decreased respiratory rate and depth, bradycardia, hypotension, and a decrease in body temperature. If the condition is untreated, death may be the outcome. SEE: *morphine* in *Poisons and Poisoning Appendix.*

**opiate receptor** A specific site on a cell surface that interacts in a highly selective fashion with opiate drugs. These receptors mediate the major known pharmacological actions of opiates and the physiologic functions of the endogenous opiate-like substances—endorphins and enkephalins.

**opioid** (ō′pē-oyd) [L. *opium,* opium, + Gr. *eidos,* form, shape] **1.** Any synthetic narcotic not derived from opium. **2.** Indicating substances such as enkephalins or endorphins occurring naturally in the body that act on the brain to decrease the sensation of pain.

**opioid peptide, endogenous** Any of a group of more than 15 substances present in the brain, certain endocrine glands, and the gastrointestinal tract. They have morphine-like analgesic properties, behavioral effects, and neurotransmitter and neuromodulator functions. Included in this group of chemicals are endorphins, enkephalins, and dynorphin.

**opisthenar** (ō-pĭs′thē-năr) [Gr. *opisthen,* behind, in the rear, + *thenar,* palm] The back (dorsum) of the hand.

**opisthiobasial** (ō-pĭs″thē-ō-bā′sē-ăl) Concerning the opisthion and basion of the skull.

**opisthion** (ō-pĭs′thē-ŏn) [NL. fr. Gr. *opisthen,* back, in the rear] The craniometric point at the middle of the lower border of the foramen magnum.

**opisthionasial** (ō-pĭs″thē-ō-nā′zē-ăl) Concerning the opisthion and nasion of the skull.

**opistho-, opisth-** [Gr. *opisthen,* behind, in the rear] Combining form meaning *backward, behind.*

**opisthognathism** (ō″pĭs-thō′nă-thĭzm) [″+ *gnathos,* jaw, + *-ismos,* state of] A skull abnormality marked by a receding lower jaw.

**opisthoporeia** (ō-pĭs″thō-pō-rē′ă) [″ + *poreia,* walk] Involuntary walking backward. SYN: *retropulsion* (2).

**opisthorchiasis** (ō″pĭs-thor-kī′ă-sĭs) Infestation of the liver by flukes of the genus *Opisthorchis.*

**Opisthorchis** (ō″pĭs-thor′kĭs) [″ + *orchis,* testicle] A genus of parasitic flukes characterized by having testicles near the posterior end of the tapered body.

***O. felineus*** A species of liver flukes found in cats and other mammals, including humans. Infestation occurs through ingesting raw or partially cooked fish.

***O. sinensis*** A common liver fluke found in humans, esp. in the Far East. It develops in those who eat inadequately cooked fish infected with the larval form of the fluke.

**opisthotic** (ō″pĭs-thŏt′ĭk) [Gr. *opisthen,* behind, in the rear, + *ous,* ear] Located behind the ear.

**opisthotonos** (ō″pĭs-thŏt′ō-nŏs) [″ + *tonos,* tension] A tetanic spasm in which head and heels are bent backward and body is bowed forward. This type of spasm is seen in strychnine poisoning, tetanus, hysteria, epilepsy, the convulsions of rabies, and in severe cases of meningitis. In the latter case, the patient's neck is rigid and the head retracted, seeming to press into the pillow. SEE: illus.; *emprosthotonos; pleurothotonos.* **opisthotonic,** *adj.*

**opium** (ō′pē-ŭm) [L.] **1.** The substance obtained by air-drying the juice from the unripe capsule of the poppy, *Papaver somniferum.* It contains a number of important alkaloids, such as morphine, codeine, heroin, and papaverine. The growing and transportation of the poppy as well as the manufacture of drugs from the juice are controlled by national and international laws. **2.** A standardized preparation of the air-dried milky exudate from unripe capsules of the poppy, *Papaver somniferum* or *P. album.* It contains not less than 9.5% anhydrous morphine.

**opium poisoning** SEE: *morphine* in *Poisons and Poisoning Appendix.*

**opo- 1.** [Gr. *opos,* juice] Prefix meaning *juice;* used in trade names of some organic extracts. **2.** [Gr. *ops,* face] Prefix denoting *face.*

**opocephalus** (ō″pō-sĕf′ă-lŭs) [Gr. *ops,* face, + *kephale,* head] A congenitally deformed fetus without nose or mouth, fused at the ears. There is either a single orbit or two orbits very close together.

**opodidymus** (ō″pō-dĭd′ĭ-mŭs) [″ + *didymos,* twin] Congenitally deformed twins in which there is a single body, two fused heads, and partial fusion of the sense organs.

**Oppenheim, Hermann** (ŏp′ĕn-hīm) German neurologist, 1858–1919.

***O.'s disease*** Myotonia congenita.

***O.'s gait*** Manner of walking in which there is a wide swinging motion of the head, body, and extremities. It is a variation of the gait seen in multiple sclerosis.

**opponens** (ō-pō′nĕns) [L.] Opposing, a term applied to muscles of hand or foot by which one of the lateral digits may be opposed to one of the other digits. SEE: *Muscles Appendix.*

**opportunistic infection** SEE: under *infection.*

**opposition** The ability to move the thumb into contact with the other fingers.

**opsialgia** (ŏp″sē-ăl′jē-ă) [Gr. *ops,* face, + *algos,* pain] Neuralgic pain of the face.

**opsin** (ŏp′sĭn) The protein portion of the rhodopsin molecule in the retina of the eye.

**opsinogen** (ŏp-sĭn′ō-jĕn) An antigen that causes the production of opsonins.

**opsoclonus** Conjugate irregular and nonrhythmical jerking movements of the eyes. The eyes move in any linear or rotating direction at a rate of up to 10 times per second. Any one of several areas of the brain, including the cerebellum and brainstem, may be diseased and cause this condition.

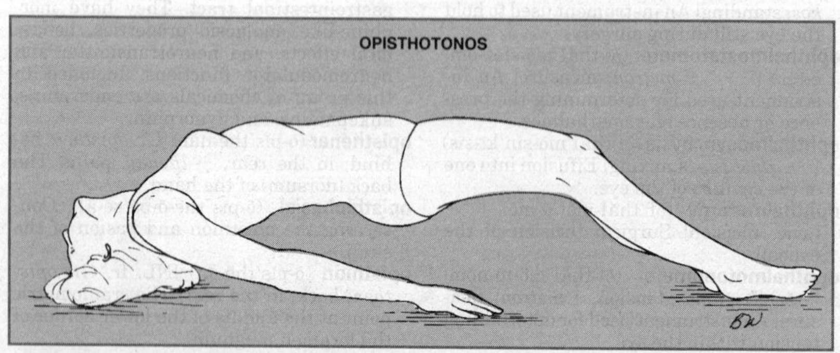
OPISTHOTONOS

**opsomania** (ŏp″sō-mā′nē-ă) [Gr. *opson,* food, + *mania,* madness] Craving for some special type of food.
**opsonification** (ŏp-sŏn″ĭ-fī-kā′shŭn) Opsonization.
**opsonin** (ŏp-sō′nĭn) [Gr. *opsonein,* to purchase food] A substance that coats foreign antigens, making them more susceptible to macrophages and other leukocytes, thus increasing phagocytosis of the organism. Complement and antibodies are the two main opsonins in human blood. **opsonic** (-sŏn′ĭk), *adj.*
***immune o.*** Opsonin formed after stimulation by a specific antigen.
**opsonization** (ŏp″sō-nī-zā′shŭn) The action of opsonins to facilitate phagocytosis. SYN: *opsonification.*
**opsonocytophagic** (ŏp″sŏn-ō-sī″tō-fā′jĭk) [″ + *kytos,* cell, + *phagein,* to eat] Pert. to the phagocytic action of the blood when serum opsonins are present.
**opsonophilia** (ŏp″sō-nō-fĭl′ē-ă) [″ + *philein,* to love] Affinity for opsonins. **opsonophilic,** *adj.*
**opsonotherapy** (ŏp″sō-nō-thĕr′ă-pē) Treatment by stimulation of a specific opsonin with bacterial vaccines. SEE: *vaccine.*
**Optacon II** Acronym for *Op*tical to *Ta*ctile *Con*verter, a proprietary name of a portable electronic reading device for use by the blind. It translates printed material to patterns of raised pins under the user's fingers. It is manufactured by TeleSensory, Inc., 455 N. Bernardo Ave., Mountain View, CA, 94043; (800) 227-8418 or (415) 960-0920.
**optic** (ŏp′tĭk) [Gr. *optikos*] Pert. to the eye or to sight.
**optical** (ŏp′tĭ-kăl) [Gr. *optikos;* L. *opticus*] Pert. to vision, the eye, or optics.
***o. tweezers*** A laser device used to alter or manipulate microorganisms, molecules, or living cells.
**optical activity** SEE: under *activity.*
**optic chiasm** SEE: under *chiasm.*
**optic disk** SEE: under *disk.*
**optic foramen** SEE: under *foramen.*
**optician** (ŏp-tĭsh′ăn) One who is a specialist in filling prescriptions for corrective lenses for eyeglasses and contact lenses.
**optic nerve** Second cranial nerve.
**optic neuropathy** SEE: under *neuropathy.*
**optico-** [Gr. *optikos*] Combining form denoting *eye, vision.*
**opticociliary** (ŏp″tĭ-kō-sĭl′ē-ăr-ē) Concerning the optic and ciliary nerves.
**opticokinetic** (ŏp″tĭ-kō-kĭ-nĕt′ĭk) [Gr. *optikos,* of or for sight, + *kinesis,* movement] Concerning the movement of the eye.
**opticonasion** (ŏp″tĭ-kō-nā′sē-ŏn) The length of an imaginary line drawn from the posterior edge of the optic foramen to the nasion.
**opticopupillary** (ŏp″tĭ-kō-pū′pĭl-ĕr″ē) Concerning the optic nerve and the pupil.
**optics** (ŏp′tĭks) [Gr. *optikos,* pert. to vision] The science dealing with light and its relationship to vision.
**optic tract** SEE: under *tract.*
**optimism** The characteristic of regarding only the bright side of a condition or event. SEE: *pessimism.*
**optimum** (ŏp′tĭ-mŭm) *pl.* **optima** [L. *optimus,* best] Most conducive to a function.
***o. temperature*** The temperature that is most suitable for a procedure or operation, esp. the development of bacterial cultures.
**opto-** [Gr. *optos,* seen] Combining form meaning *vision, eye.*
**optogram** (ŏp′tō-grăm) [Gr. *optos,* seen, + *gramma,* something written] The image of an external object that is fixed on the retina by the photochemical bleaching action of light on the visual purple.
**optokinetic** (ŏp″tō-kĭ-nĕt′ĭk) [″ + *kinesis,* movement] Concerning the appearance of a twitching movement of the eyes, as in nystagmus when the eyes gaze at moving objects.
**optometer** (ŏp-tŏm′ĕ-tĕr) [″ + *metron,* measure] An instrument used to measure the eye's refractive power.
**optometrist** (ŏp-tŏm′ĕ-trĭst) A doctor of optometry (O.D.); a primary health care provider who practices optometry, as regulated and permitted by state laws. Most states permit optometrists to prescribe drugs for the treatment of certain eye diseases. SEE: *optometry.*
**optometry** (ŏp-tŏm′ĕ-trē) The science of diagnosing, managing, and treating conditions and diseases of the human eye and visual system as permitted by state laws.
**optomyometer** (ŏp″tō-mī-ŏm′ĕ-tĕr) [″ + *mys,* muscle, + *metron,* a measure] An instrument used for determining the strength of the muscles of the eye.
**optophone** (ŏp′tō-fōn) [″ + *phone,* voice] A scanning instrument that converts light energy into sound waves, thereby enabling the blind to read.
**optostriate** (ŏp-tō-strī′āt) [″ + L. *striatus,* grooved] Concerning the optic thalamus and the corpus striatum.
**optotype** (ŏp′tō-tīp) The variable-sized type used in testing visual acuity.
**OPV** *oral poliovirus vaccine.*
**OR** *operating room.*
**ora** (ō′ră) [L.] **1.** Plural of os. **2.** *pl.* **orae** A border or margin.
***o. serrata retinae*** Notched anterior edge of sensory portion of retina.
**orad** (ō′răd) [L. *oris,* mouth, + *ad,* toward] Toward the mouth or oral region.
**oral** (or′ăl) [L. *oralis*] **1.** Concerning the mouth. **2.** In dental anatomy, describes the surface of the tooth towards the oral cavity or tongue and the opposite of the buccal or facial tooth surface.
**oral contraceptive** SEE: *contraceptive.*
**oral diagnosis** SEE: under *diagnosis.*
**orale** (ō-rā′lē) The point on the hard palate where lines drawn tangent to the lingual margins of the alveoli of the medial incisor teeth intersect the midsagittal plane.
**oral hygiene** SEE: under *hygiene.*

**orality** (ō-răl′ĭ-tē) The oral stage of psychosexual development, which involves sucking or chewing on objects other than food.

**oral mucous membrane, altered** The state in which the individual experiences disruptions in the tissue layers of the oral cavity. SEE: *Nursing Diagnoses Appendix.*

**oral rehydration solution** ABBR: ORS. A solution used in oral rehydration therapy. The World Health Organization recommends that the solution contain 3.5 g sodium chloride; 2.9 g potassium chloride; 2.9 g trisodium citrate; and 1.5 g glucose dissolved in each liter (approx. 1 qt) of drinking water.

**oral rehydration therapy** ABBR: ORT. The administration by mouth of a solution of electrolytes in sufficient quantity to correct the deficits produced by dehydration due to diarrhea. The earlier this therapy is begun, the more effective it is (i.e., the fluid should be started before the infant is dehydrated). Because this therapy is simple, is economical, and can be supervised by nonprofessionals, it has been extremely effective in treating infantile diarrhea in countries lacking economic resources and health care professionals.

In many parts of the world, commercially prepared ORT solutions are not available or are too expensive. In these areas, very inexpensive and effective solutions can be prepared from sources such as cooled water from a pot in which rice is boiled or two pinches of salt and one ounce of molasses added to a quart of water. SEE: *oral rehydration solution; viral gastroenteritis.*

**orb** [L. *orbis,* circle, disk] A spherical body, esp. the eyeball.

**orbicular** (or-bĭk′ū-lăr) [L. *orbiculus,* a small circle] Circular.

***o. bone*** The rounded end of the long process of the incus, a middle ear ossicle. It probably represents a secondary ossification center in the long or lenticular process. SYN: *orbiculare.*

***o. muscle*** Muscle encircling an opening.

***o. sign*** SEE: *wink.*

***o. process*** Lenticular process.

**orbiculus** (or-bĭk′ū-lŭs) *pl.* **orbiculi** [L., little circle] Muscle surrounding an orifice; a sphincter muscle.

***o. ciliaris*** The portion of the ciliary body consisting of a bandlike zone lying directly anterior to the ora serrata. SYN: *ciliary ring.*

***o. oris*** The circular muscle surrounding the mouth.

**orbit** (or′bĭt) [L. *orbita,* track] The bony pyramid-shaped cavity of the skull that contains and protects the eyeball. It is pierced posteriorly by the optic foramen (which transmits the optic nerve and ophthalmic artery), the superior and inferior orbital fissures, and several foramina. It is formed by the frontal, malar, ethmoid, maxillary, lacrimal, sphenoid, and palatine bones. **orbital** (-bĭ-tăl), *adj.*

**orbitale** An anthropometric landmark, being the lowest point along the inferior margin of the orbit. It is one of two landmarks (the other is the porion) used to establish the Frankfort horizontal plane, most frequently in positioning the head for radiographs or measurements.

**orbitonasal** (or″bĭ-tō-nā′zăl) Concerning the orbit and nasal cavity of the skull.

**orbitopagus** (or″bĭ-tŏp′ă-gŭs) [L. *orbita,* track, + Gr. *pagos,* thing fixed] Conjoined twins in which the smaller fetus is attached to the orbit of the larger fetus.

**orbitotomy** (or-bĭ-tŏt′ō-mē) [″+ Gr. *tome,* incision] Surgical incision into the orbit.

**orcein** (or-sī′ĭn) A chemical used as a histological stain.

**orchectomy** (or-kĕk′tō-mē) [Gr. *orchis,* testicle, + *ektome,* excision] Orchiectomy.

**orcheoplasty** (or′kē-ō-plăs″tē) [″ + *plassein,* to form] Orchioplasty.

**orchi-** SEE: *orchio-.*

**orchialgia** (or-kē-ăl′jē-ă) [″ + *algos,* pain] Pain in the testes. SYN: *orchiodynia.*

**orchio-, orchi-** Combining form meaning *testicle.*

**orchichorea** (or″kĭ-kō-rē′ă) [″ + *choreia,* a dance] Involuntary jerking movements of the testicles.

**orchid-** SEE: *orchido-.*

**orchidectomy** (or″kĭ-dĕk′tō-mē) [″ + *ektome,* excision] Orchiectomy.

**orchidic** (or-kĭd′ĭk) Concerning or relating to the testes.

**orchiditis** (or″kĭ-dī′tĭs) [″ + *itis,* inflammation] Orchitis.

**orchido-, orchid-** [Gr. *orchidion*] Combining form meaning *testicle.* SEE: words beginning with *orchio-.*

**orchidoncus** (or-kĭ-dŏng′kŭs) [″ + *onkos,* bulk, mass] Orchioncus.

**orchidopexy** (or′kĭd-ō-pĕk″sē) [″ + *pexis,* fixation] Orchiopexy.

**orchidoplasty** (or′kĭd-ō-plăs″tē) [″ + *plassein,* to form] Orchioplasty.

**orchidoptosis** (or″kĭd-ŏp-tō′sĭs) [″ + *ptosis,* a dropping] Downward displacement of the testes.

**orchidorrhaphy** (or″kĭ-dor′ă-fē) [″ + *rhaphe,* seam, ridge] Orchiopexy.

**orchidotomy** (or-kĭd-ŏt′ō-mē) [″+ *tome,* incision] Orchiotomy.

**orchiectomy** (or″kē-ĕk′tō-mē) [Gr. *orchis,* testicle, + *ektome,* excision] Surgical excision of a testicle. SYN: *castration, male; orchectomy; orchidectomy.*

Nursing Implications: The nurse explains the plan of care and expected outcome of the surgery and provides information about placing oblate spheroidal prostheses in the scrotum. Patient teaching is modified according to the extent of surgery. Deep-breathing and coughing exercises are taught, and the importance of early ambulation and activity after surgery is emphasized. Pain control measures are discussed, and the patient is advised to seek pain relief in the postoperative period before pain becomes severe. If only one testicle is removed and the other one is healthy, impotence does not occur. Support and reassurance are offered to the patient and family.

**orchiepididymitis** (or″kē-ĕp″ĭ-dĭd″ĭ-mī′tĭs) [″ + *epi,* upon, + *didymos,* testis, + *itis,* inflammation] Inflammation of a testicle and epididymis.

**orchilytic** (or″kĭ-lĭt′ĭk) [″ + *lysis,* dissolution] Destructive to testicular tissue. SYN: *orchitolytic.*

**orchio-, orchi-** Combining form meaning *testicle.*

**orchiodynia** (or″kē-ō-dĭn′ē-ă) [″ + *odyne,* pain] Orchialgia.

**orchioncus** (or″kē-ŏng′kŭs) [″ + *onkos,* bulk, mass] A neoplasm of the testicle. SYN: *orchidoncus.*

**orchiopathy** (or″kē-ŏp′ăth-ē) [″ + *pathos,* disease, suffering] Any disease of the testes.

**orchiopexy** (or″kē-ō-pĕk′sē) [″ + *pexis,* fixation] The suturing of an undescended testicle to fix it in the scrotum. SYN: *orchidopexy; orchiorrhaphy.*

**orchioplasty** (or′kē-ō-plăs″tē) [″ + *plassein,* to form] Plastic repair of the testicle.

**orchiorrhaphy** (or″kē-or′ră-fē) [″ + *rhaphe,* seam, ridge] Orchiopexy.

**orchioscheocele** (or″kē-ŏs′kē-ō-sēl) [″ + *oscheon,* scrotum, + *kele,* tumor, swelling] A scrotal hernia with enlargement or tumor of the testicle.

**orchioscirrhus** (or″kē-ō-skĭr′rŭs) [″ + *skirros,* hard] Testicular hardening due to tumor formation.

**orchiotomy** (or″kē-ŏt′ō-mē) [″ + *tome,* incision] Surgical incision of a testicle. SYN: *orchidotomy; orchotomy.*

**orchis** (or′kĭs) [Gr.] Testis.

**orchitis** (or-kī′tĭs) [Gr. *orchis,* testicle, + *itis,* inflammation] Inflammation of a testis due to trauma, metastasis, mumps, or infection elsewhere in the body.

SYMPTOMS: The symptoms of orchitis include swelling, severe pain, chills, fever, vomiting, hiccough, and delirium. Atrophy of the organ may be an end result.

TREATMENT: The patient is confined to bed for the first eight days with the organ immobilized. An ice bag is applied. **orchitic** (-kĭt′ĭk), *adj.*

***gonorrheal o.*** Orchitis due to gonococcus.

***metastatic o.*** Orchitis due to infection by organisms in the bloodstream.

***syphilitic o.*** Orchitis due to syphilis. This type of orchitis usually begins painlessly in the body of the gland and is apt to be bilateral. It causes dense, irregular, knotty induration but little enlargement in size.

***tuberculous o.*** A form of orchitis generally arising in the epididymis. It may be accompanied by formation of chronic sinuses, and destruction of tissues.

SYMPTOMS: There is little or no pain. It begins with hard, irregular enlargement at the lower and posterior aspects of the gland that gradually increases and sometimes extends along the vas deferens. Later, the whole gland undergoes caseous degeneration.

**orchitolytic** (or″kĭt-ō-lĭt′ĭk) [″ + *lysis,* dissolution] Orchilytic.

**orchotomy** (or-kŏt′ō-mē) [″ + *tome,* incision] Orchiotomy.

**orcin, orcinol** (or′sĭn, -ŏl) A white, crystalline substance derived from lichens and used as a reagent.

**order** [L. *ordo,* a row, series] **1.** An arrangement or sequence of events; rules; regulations; procedures. **2.** In biological classification, the main division under class, superior to family.

**orderly** (or′dĕr-lē) An attendant in a hospital who does general work to assist nurses. Orderlies are responsible for lifting and transporting patients and preparing them for surgery (e.g., shaving, catheterizing, or administering enemas).

**ordinate** (or′dĭ-năt) The vertical line parallel to the y-axis in a graph in which horizontal and perpendicular lines are crossed in order to provide a frame of reference. The abscissa is the horizontal line parallel to the x-axis. SEE: *abscissa* for illus.

**ordure** (or′dūr) Feces or other excrement.

**Orem, Dorothea** Nursing educator, born 1914, who developed the Self-Care Framework, also known as the Self-Care Deficit Theory of Nursing. SEE: *Nursing Theory Appendix.*

**oreximania** (ō-rĕk″sĭ-mā′nē-ă) [″ + *mania,* madness] Abnormal desire for food because of the fear of losing weight.

**orf** A contagious pustular dermatitis caused by the orf virus, a DNA virus of the *Parapoxvirus* genus, which is related to the vaccinia-variola subgroup of poxviruses. Orf mainly affects lambs and occurs in the spring. The disease rarely occurs in humans. When it does, it is usually confined to a single pustular lesion on a finger, which encrusts and finally heals. Antibiotics are not indicated except for secondary bacterial infections.

**organ** (or′găn) [Gr. *organon;* L. *organum*] A part of the body having a special function. Many organs occur in pairs. In such pairs, one organ may be extirpated and the remaining one can perform all necessary functions peculiar to it. One third to two fifths of some organs may be removed without loss of function necessary to support life. SEE: table.

***accessory o.*** An organ that has a subordinate function.

***acoustic o.*** Organ of Corti.

***o. of Corti*** SEE: under *Corti.*

***o. donation*** Making a postmortem anatomical gift of transplantable organs (e.g., heart, lung, kidney, cornea) to persons who will most probably die if transplantation is not performed. The United

## Size, Weight, and Capacity of Various Organs and Parts of the Adult Body
## ♂ Male ♀ Female

| Description | Size | Weight | Capacity |
|---|---|---|---|
| Adrenal gland | 5 cm high<br>3 cm across<br>1 cm thick | 5 g | |
| Bladder | 12 cm in diameter | | 500 ml (when moderately full) |
| Blood volume | | | ♂ 4–6 L<br>♀ 3–5 L |
| Brain | | ♂ 1240–1680 g<br>♀ 1130–1570 g | |
| Ear, external canal | 2.5 cm long (from concha) | | |
| Esophagus | 23–25 cm | | |
| Eye | 23.5 mm vertical diameter<br>24 mm anteroposterior diameter | | |
| Fallopian tube | 10 cm | | |
| Gallbladder | 7–10 cm long<br>3 cm wide | | 30–50 ml |
| Heart | 12 × 8–9 × 6 cm | ♂ 280–340 g<br>♀ 230–280 g | |
| Intestines—small | Variable<br>6–7 m long | | |
| Intestines—large | 1.5 m long | | |
| Intestines—vermiform appendix | 2–20 cm long<br>Average 9 cm | | |
| Intestines—rectum | 12 cm long | | |
| Kidney | 11 cm long<br>6 cm broad<br>3 cm thick | ♂ 150 g<br>♀ 135 g | |
| Larynx | ♂ 44 × 43 × 36 mm<br>♀ 36 × 41 × 26 mm | | |
| Liver | | ♂ 1.4–1.8 kg<br>♀ 1.0–2.5 kg | 6500 cc |
| Lung | | Right 625 g<br>Left 565 g | |
| Ovaries | 3 × 1.5 × 1 m | 2–3.5 g | |
| Pancreas | 15 cm long | ♂ 74–106 g<br>♀ 70–100 g | |
| Parathyroid | 6 × 3–4 × 1–2 mm | 50 mg | |
| Pharynx | 12.5 cm long | | |
| Prostate | 2 × 4 × 3 cm | 8 g | |
| Skeleton | | Average adult male, 4957 g | |
| Skull | | Average (without teeth), 642 g | Variable<br>♂ 406 ml<br>♀ 207 ml |
| Spinal cord | 42–45 cm long | 30 g | |
| Spleen | 12 × 7 × 3–4 cm | 150 g<br>80–300 g<br>Decreases with age | |
| Stomach | Variable<br>25 cm long<br>10 cm wide | | Variable<br>1500 ml |
| Testes | 4–5 × 2.5 × 3 cm | 10.5–14 g | |
| Thoracic duct | 38–45 cm long | | |

**Size, Weight, and Capacity of Various Organs and Parts of the Adult Body ♂ Male ♀ Female** (Continued)

| Description | Size | Weight | Capacity |
|---|---|---|---|
| Thymus | | Newborn, 10.9 g<br>10–15 yr, 29.5 g<br>20–25 yr, 18.6 g | |
| Thyroid | Each lobe 5 × 3 × 2 cm | 30 g total | |
| Trachea | 11 cm long<br>2–2.5 cm in diameter | | |
| Ureter | 28–34 cm long | | |
| Urethra | ♂ 17.5–20 cm long<br>♀ 4 cm long | | |
| Uterus | 7.5 × 5.0 × 2.5 cm | 30–40 g (nonpregnant) | |
| Vagina | Anterior wall length 7.5 cm<br>Posterior wall length 9.0 cm | | |

SOURCE: Adapted from Gray's Anatomy, ed 27. Lea & Febiger Philadelphia, 1959; Gray's Anatomy, ed 37. Churchill Livingstone, London, 1987; Growth. Federation of American Societies for Experimental Biology, Washington, DC, 1962; Jandl, JH, Blood. Little, Brown and Co., Boston, 1987.

Network for Organ Transplantation (UNOS) maintains a list of patients waiting for organ transplantation and a registry of patients who have received organs. Donor organs were received by 18,251 patients in 1994. In 1995, over 40,000 patients were waiting for donor organs.

***enamel o.*** A cup-shaped structure that forms on the dental lamina of an embryo. It produces the enamel and serves as a mold for the remainder of the tooth. SEE: *morphogenesis.*

***end o.*** SEE: *end organ.*

***excretory o.*** An organ that is concerned with the excretion of waste products from the body. SEE: *excretion.*

***o. of Giraldés*** Paradidymis.

***Golgi tendon o.*** SEE: *Golgi tendon organ.*

***gustatory o.*** The organ of taste; a taste bud. SYN: *organum gustus.*

***o. of Jacobson*** A blind tubular sac that develops in the medial wall of the nasal cavity, becoming a functional olfactory organ in lower animals, but degenerating or remaining rudimentary in humans. SYN: *vomeronasal o.*

***lymphatic o.*** A structure composed principally of lymphatic tissue. It includes the lymph nodes, spleen, tonsils, and thymus.

***reproductive o.*** Any organ concerned with the production of offspring. These include the primary organs (testes and ovaries) and accessory structures (penis and spermatic cord in the male and fallopian tubes, uterus, and vagina in the female). SYN: *sex o.*

***o. of Ruffini*** SEE: *Ruffini's corpuscles.*

***sense o.*** A sensory receptor; a structure consisting of specialized sensory nerve endings that are capable of reacting to a stimulus (an external or internal change) by generating nerve impulses that pass through afferent nerves to the central nervous system. These impulses may give rise to sensations or reflexly bring about responses in the body.

***sex o.*** Reproductive o.

***special sense o.'s*** The organs of smell, taste, sight, and hearing.

***spiral o.*** Organ of Corti.

***target o.*** An organ upon which a chemical or hormone acts.

***vestigial o.*** An organ that is immature or underdeveloped in humans but is fully functional in some animals.

***vomeronasal o.*** O. of Jacobson.

***Weber's o.*** [Moritz I. Weber, Ger. anatomist, 1795–1875] The residual prostatic pouch in the male, the remains of the müllerian ducts.

***o.'s of Zuckerkandl*** [Emil Zuckerkandl, Hungarian anatomist working in Germany, 1849–1910] A pair of organs containing chromaffin tissue present in the embryo and persisting until shortly after birth. They are located adjacent to the anterior surface of the abdominal aorta. The cells secrete epinephrine. SYN: *corpora para-aortica.*

**organelle** (or″găn-ĕl′) A specialized part of a cell that performs a distinctive function.

**organic** (or-găn′ĭk) [Gr. *organikos*] **1.** Pert. to an organ or organs. **2.** Structural. **3.** Pert. to or derived from animal or vegetable forms of life. **4.** Denoting chemical substances containing carbon.

**organic brain syndrome** Any of a large group of acute and chronic mental disorders associated with brain damage or impaired cerebral function.

SYMPTOMS: The clinical characteristics vary not only with the nature and severity of the underlying organic disorder but also occasionally between individuals. Consciousness, orientation, memory, intellect, judgment and insight, and thought content may be impaired (e.g., hallucinations, illusions).

ETIOLOGY: Any acute or chronic disease or injury that interferes with cerebral function may trigger symptoms. Possible causes include infection, intoxication, trauma, circulatory disturbance, epilepsy, metabolic and endocrine diseases, or intracranial trauma or neoplasms.

DIAGNOSIS: Difficulty in diagnosis may be encountered because of the possibility of attributing all of the signs and symptoms to a psychiatric disorder, thereby ignoring the possibility of organic disease.

TREATMENT: Treatment of the basic organic disease and provision of psychiatric care are indicated.

**organic chemistry** SEE: under *chemistry*.

**organic disease** SEE: under *disease*.

**organic dust toxic syndrome** ABBR: ODTS. A nonallergenic, noninfectious, respiratory disorder caused by inhalation of organic dusts. The most important sources are cotton dust, which causes byssinosis; grain dust; and exposure to moldy hay, called "farmer's lung." SEE: *byssinosis; pneumonitis, hypersensitivity*.

**organic psychosis** SEE: under *psychosis*.

**organism** (or′găn-ĭzm) [Gr. *organon,* organ, + *-ismos,* condition] Any living thing, plant or animal. An organism may be unicellular (bacteria, yeasts, protozoa) or multicellular (all complex organisms including humans).

***fastidious o.*** In microbiology, an organism that has precise nutritional and environmental requirements for growth and survival.

**organization** (or″găn-ĭ-zā′shŭn) **1.** The process of becoming organized. **2.** Systematic arrangement. **3.** That which is organized; an organism.

***o. center*** **1.** An embryonic group of cells that induces the development of another structure. **2.** A region in an ovum that is responsible for the mode of development of the fertilized ovum.

**organize** (or′găn-īz) To develop from an amorphous state to that having structure and form.

**organo-** (or′gă-nō) A combining form meaning *organ*.

**organoferric** (or″gă-nō-fĕr′ĭk) Concerning iron and an organic molecule.

**organogel** (or-găn′ō-jĕl) A gel in which the continuous phase is an organic liquid instead of water.

**organogenesis** (or″găn-ō-jĕn′ĕ-sĭs) [″ + *genesis,* generation, birth] The formation and development of body organs from embryonic tissues.

It is important that a fetus not be exposed to harmful chemicals, particularly during organogenesis. The first critical period for the effects of teratogenic drugs on the human fetus is between the 13th and 56th days of gestation. The second period of high risk is during the last trimester when metabolic enzyme systems are beginning to be defined.

**organoid** [″ + *eidos,* form, shape] **1.** Resembling an organ. **2.** An organelle.

**organoleptic** (or″găn-ō-lĕp′tĭk) [″ + *lepsis,* a seizure] **1.** Affecting an organ, esp. the organs of special sense. **2.** Susceptible to sensory impressions.

**organoma** (or-gă-nō′mă) [″ + *oma,* tumor] A neoplasm containing cellular elements that can be definitely identified as being specific to certain tissues and organs.

**organomegaly** (or″gă-nō-mĕg′ă-lē) [″ + *megas,* large] The enlargement of visceral organs.

**organometallic** (or-gă-nō-mĕ-tăl′ĭk) A compound containing a metal combined with an organic molecule.

**organonomy** (or″gă-nŏn′ō-mē) [″ + *nomos,* law] The laws regulating the biological processes of living organisms.

**organopexy** (or′găn-ō-pĕk″sē) [″+ *pexis,* fixation] The surgical fixation of an organ that is detached from its proper position.

**organotherapy** (or″găn-ō-thĕr′ă-pē) [″ + *therapeia,* treatment] The treatment of disease by preparations of the endocrine glands of animals or by extracts made from them.

**organotrope, organotropic** (or-găn′ō-trōp, -găn-ō-trŏp′ĭk) [″ + *tropos,* turning] Having affinity for tissues or certain organs.

**organotropism** (or″gă-nŏt′rō-pĭzm) [″ + *trope,* a turn, + *-ismos,* condition] The attraction or affinity of chemicals or biological agents for body organs or tissues.

**organ perfusion system** A mechanical device equipped to supply metabolic, oxygen, and electrolyte needs to an organ obtained from a cadaver or donor in order to keep it viable for transplantation. The organ and the perfusion solution pumped through it can be kept at the ideal temperature for organ survival. They can be transported together by any means required to deliver the organ to the recipient.

**organ-specific** (or′găn-spĕ-sĭf′ĭk) Originating in a single organ or affecting only one specific organ.

**organum** [L.] An organ.

***o. auditus*** O. vestibulocochleare.

***o. gustus*** The organ of taste.

***o. olfactus*** The organ of smell; the olfactory region in the nasal cavity.

***o. spirale*** Organ of Corti.

***o. vestibulocochleare*** The organ of hearing. SYN: *o. auditus*. SEE: *ear*.

***o. visus*** The organ of sight; the eye and

its adnexa.

***o. vomeronasale*** The canal opening into the nasal septum. SYN: *organ of Jacobson.*

**orgasm** (or′găzm) [Gr. *orgasmos,* swelling] A state of physical and emotional excitement that occurs at the climax of sexual intercourse. In the male it is accompanied by the ejaculation of semen. SYN: *climax.*

**Oriental sore** Cutaneous leishmaniasis. SYN: *Aleppo boil.* SEE: *leishmaniasis.*

**orientation** (or″ē-ĕn-tā′shŭn) [L. *oriens,* to arise] The ability to comprehend and to adjust oneself in an environment with regard to time, location, and identity of persons. This ability is partially or completely absent in some psychoses.

**orifice** (or′ĭ-fĭs) [L. *orificium,* outlet] The mouth, entrance, or outlet of any anatomical structure. **orificial** (-fĭ′shăl), *adj.*

***anal o.*** The anus.

***atrioventricular o.*** The opening between the atrium and the ventricle on each side of the heart.

***cardiac o.*** The opening of the esophagus into the stomach.

***external urethral o.*** The exterior opening of the urethra. In the male, it is located at the tip of the glans penis; in the female, it is located anterior and cephalad to the vaginal opening.

***internal urethral o.*** The opening from which the urethra makes its exit from the bladder.

***mitral o.*** The opening between the left atrium and the left ventricle.

***oral o.*** The aperture of the mouth. SYN: *rima oris.*

***pyloric o.*** Pylorus.

***ureteric o.*** The opening of the ureter into the bladder.

**origin** (or′ĭ-jĭn) [L. *origo,* beginning] **1.** The source of anything; a starting point. **2.** The beginning of a nerve. **3.** The more fixed attachment of a muscle.

***deep o.*** The region within the brain where the fibers that make up a cranial nerve terminate.

***superficial o.*** The point where a cranial nerve exits from the brain.

**Orlando, Ida Jean** Nursing educator, born 1926, who developed the Theory of the Deliberative Nursing Process. SEE: *Nursing Theory Appendix.*

**Ormond's disease** [U.S. physician, b. 1886] Retroperitoneal fibrosis.

**ornithine** (or′nĭ-thĭn) An amino acid formed when arginase hydrolyzes arginine. It is not present in proteins.

**Ornithodoros** (or″nĭ-thŏd′ō-rōs) A genus of ticks (family Argasidae) that infests mammals, including humans. Several species serve as transmitters of the causative agents of disease, including spotted fever, tick fever, Q fever, tularemia, Russian encephalitis, and relapsing fever.

**ornithosis** (or″nĭ-thō′sĭs) [Gr. *ornithos,* bird, + *osis,* condition] An acute, generalized, infectious disease of birds and domesticated fowls sometimes communicated to humans. SEE: *Chlamydia psittaci.*

**oro-** Combining form meaning *mouth.*

**orodiagnosis** (or″ō-dī-ăg-nō′sĭs) [Gr. *oros,* serum, + *dia,* through, + *gnosis,* knowledge] Serodiagnosis.

**orofacial** (or″ō-fā′shē-ăl) [L. *oris,* mouth, + *facies,* face] Concerning the mouth and face.

**orofaciodigital syndrome** An inherited disorder characterized by mental retardation and deformities of the mouth, tongue, fingers, and sometimes the face.

**orolingual** (or″ō-lĭng′gwăl) [L. *oris,* mouth, + *lingua,* tongue] Concerning the mouth and tongue.

**oronasal** (or″ō-nā′zăl) [″ + *nasus,* nose] Concerning the mouth and nose.

**oropharyngeal airway** SEE: under *airway.*

**oropharynx** (or″ō-făr′ĭnks) [″ + Gr. *pharynx,* throat] The central portion of the pharynx lying between the soft palate and the upper portion of the epiglottis.

**orosomucoid** (or″ŏ-sō-mū′koyd) An alpha 1-globulin in blood plasma.

**orotic aciduria** SEE: under *aciduria.*

**orotracheal** Pert. to the passageway between the mouth and the trachea.

**Oroya fever** [Oroya, a region of Peru] The first clinical stage of bartonellosis. An acute infectious disease endemic in Peru and other South American countries and characterized by intermittent fever, lymphadenopathy, severe anemia, and pains in the joints and long bones. SEE: *bartonellosis.*

**orphan** [L. *orphanus,* destitute, without parents] A child whose parents have died or are unknown.

***o. disease*** A type of illness that, because of its rarity, has received minimal attention from medical researchers. SEE: *National Organization for Rare Disorders.*

***o. drug*** Any drug that is effective for certain illnesses but, for a variety of reasons, is not profitable for manufacturers to produce. SEE: *National Organization for Rare Disorders.*

**orphenadrine citrate** (or-fĕn′ă-drēn) An antiparkinsonism drug.

**orrhomeningitis** (or″ō-mĕn″ĭn-jī′tĭs) [″ + *meninx,* membrane, + *itis,* inflammation] Inflammation of a serous membrane.

**orris root** (or′ĭs) The powder made from the root of certain varieties of iris. It is used in making some types of cosmetics. It may be a sensitizer by contact or inhalation.

**ORS** *oral rehydration solution.*

**ORT** *oral rehydration therapy.*

**orth-** SEE: *ortho-.*

**ortho-, orth-** [Gr. *orthos,* straight] Combining form meaning *straight, correct, normal, in proper order;* commonly used in chemical terminology.

**orthoacid** (or″thō-ăs′ĭd) An acid with as many hydroxyl groups as the number of valences of the acid-forming portion of the molecule.

**orthobiosis** (or″thō-bī-ō′sĭs) [″ + *bios,* life] Right living; a term used by Metchnikoff to encompass all the factors that may affect longevity and well-being.

**orthocephalic** (or″thō-sĕ-făl′ĭk) [″ + *kephale,* head] Having a well-proportioned head with a cephalic index between 70 and 75.

**orthochorea** (or″thō-kō-rē′ă) [″ + *choreia,* dance] A type of chorea in which attacks appear mainly when the person is in an erect position.

**orthochromatic** (or″thō-krō-măt′ĭk) [″ + *chroma,* color] Having normal color or staining normally.

**orthochromophil** (or″thō-krō′mō-fĭl) [″ + ″ + *philein,* to love] Staining normally with neutral dyes.

**orthodentin** (or″thō-dĕn′tĭn) Tubular dentin, as seen in human teeth.

**orthodeoxia** Decreased arterial oxygen concentration while in an upright position. The condition improves when the patient assumes the supine position. SEE: *syndrome, hepatopulmonary.*

**orthodiagraph** (or″thō-dī′ă-grăf) [″ + *dia,* through, + *graphein,* to write] An instrument for accurate recording of the outlines and positions of organs or foreign bodies as seen by radiographic apparatus.

**orthodigita** (or″thō-dĭj′ĭ-tă) [″ + L. *digitus,* finger] **1.** The division of podiatry that deals with the correction of deviated toes. **2.** The prevention and correction of deformities of the fingers or toes.

**orthodontia, orthodontics** (or″thō-dŏn′shē-ă, -dŏn′tĭks) [″ + *odous,* tooth] The division of dentistry dealing with the prevention and correction of abnormally positioned or aligned teeth.

**orthodontist** A dentist who is a specialist in orthodontia.

**orthodromic** (or″thō-drŏm′ĭk) [Gr. *orthodromein,* to run straight forward] Denoting nerve impulses moving in the normal direction. SEE: *antidromic.*

**orthogenesis** (or″thō-jĕn′ĕ-sĭs) [Gr. *orthos,* straight, + *genesis,* generation, birth] A biological principle that the evolution of an animal species is in a given direction, governed by intrinsic factors, and independent of external factors.

**orthogenic** Pert. to, or related to, the correction, treatment, or rehabilitation of children with mental or emotional difficulties.

**orthogenics** (or″thō-jĕn′ĭks) Eugenics.

**orthograde** (or′thō-grād) [″ + L. *gradi,* to walk] Walking with the body vertical or upright; pert. to bipeds, esp. humans. Opposite of pronograde.

**orthokeratology** Use of special hard contact lenses to treat myopia by altering the curvature of the cornea. The lens presses on the center of the cornea, thus decreasing the protrusion.

**orthokinetics** Various tactile stimulation techniques used to stimulate the proprioceptors of muscles and tendons and thereby enhance motor performance in rehabilitation.

**orthomelic** (or″thō-mē′lĭk) [″ + *melos,* limb] Correcting deformed arms and legs.

**orthomolecular** (or″thō-mō-lĕk′ū-lăr) Indicating the normal chemical constituents of the body or the restoration of those constituents to normal.

**orthomyxovirus** (or″thō-mĭk″sō-vī′rŭs) Any of the family of viruses including the viruses of influenza.

**orthopantograph** A panoramic radiographic device that images the entire dentition, alveolar bone, and other contiguous structures on a single extraoral film.

**orthopedic, orthopaedic** (or″thō-pē′dĭk) Concerning orthopedics; concerning the prevention or correction of musculoskeletal deformities.

**orthopedics, orthopaedics** (or″thō-pē′dĭks) [″ + *pais,* child] The branch of medical science that deals with prevention or correction of disorders involving locomotor structures of the body, esp. the skeleton, joints, muscles, fascia, and other supporting structures such as ligaments and cartilage.

**orthopedist, orthopaedist** (or″thō-pē′dĭst) A specialist in orthopedics.

**orthopercussion** (or″thō-pĕr-kŭsh′ŭn) [″ + L. *percussio,* a striking] Percussion with the distal phalanx of the percussing finger held perpendicularly to the surface percussed.

**orthophoria** (or″thō-fō′rē-ă) [″ + *pherein,* to bear] Parallelism of visual axes, the normal eye muscle balance.

**orthopnea** (or″thŏp′nē-ă) [″ + *pnoia,* breath] Respiratory condition in which there is breathing difficulty in any but an erect sitting or standing position.

SYMPTOMS: The respiratory rate may be either slow or rapid with the muscles of respiration forcibly used in the struggle to inhale and exhale. A sitting or standing posture is necessary to ease breathing. Patients often feel the necessity to brace themselves in order to breathe. There is a characteristic anxious expression and the face is cyanosed.

ETIOLOGY: Orthopnea is seen in heart failure, bronchial and cardiac asthma, pulmonary edema, severe emphysema, pneumonia, angina pectoris, and spasmodic cough.

**orthopneic position** (or″thŏp-nē′ĭk) The upright or nearly upright position of the upper trunk of a patient in a bed or chair. It facilitates breathing in those with congestive heart failure and some forms of pulmonary disease.

**Orthopoxvirus** A genus of virus that includes the virus causing smallpox (variola) and monkeypox.

**orthopraxis** (or″thō-prăk′sĭs) [″ + *prassein,* to make] The mechanical correction of deformities.

**orthopsychiatry** (or″thō-sī-kī′ă-trē) [″ + *psyche,* soul, + *iatreia,* treatment] The

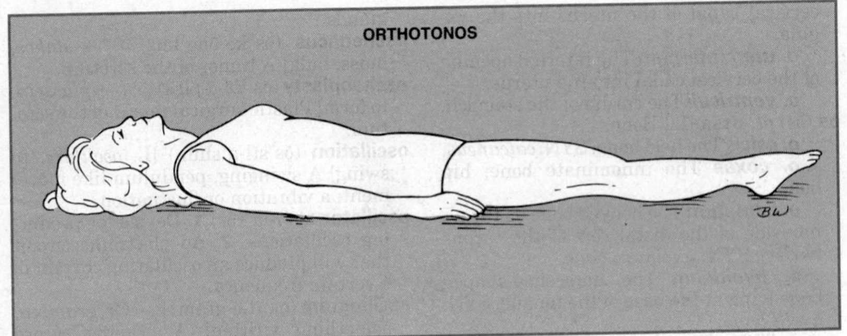

ORTHOTONOS

branch of psychiatry concerned with mental and emotional development. It encompasses child psychiatry and mental hygiene.

**orthoptic** (or-thŏp′tĭk) [″ + *optikos,* pert. to vision] Pert. to or producing normal binocular vision.

**orthoptics 1.** The science of correcting defects in binocular vision resulting from defects in optic musculature. **2.** The technique of eye exercises for correcting faulty eye coordination affecting binocular vision. The technique is also referred to as orthoptic training.

**orthoroentgenography** (or″thō-rĕnt-gĕn-ŏg′ră-fē) A technique for obtaining accurate measurement of the size and position of the internal organs using radiographic apparatus. A radiographic procedure used for the accurate measurement of long bones. SEE: *orthodiagraph.*

**orthoscopic** (or″thō-skŏp′ĭk) **1.** Having correct and undistorted vision. **2.** Made to correct optical distortion.

**orthoscopy** (or-thŏs′kō-pē) Ocular examination with an orthoscope.

**orthosis** [Gr., straightening] Any device added to the body to stabilize or immobilize a body part, prevent deformity, protect against injury, or assist with function. Orthotic devices range from arm slings to corsets and finger splints. They may be made from a variety of materials, including rubber, leather, canvas, rubber synthetics, and plastic. **orthotic,** *adj.*

***balanced forearm o.*** Mobile arm support.

**orthostatic** (or″thō-stăt′ĭk) [Gr. *orthos,* straight, + *statikos,* causing to stand] Concerning or caused by an erect position.

***o. hypotension*** SEE: under *hypotension.*

***o. vital signs determination*** The measurement of blood pressure and pulse rate in supine and erect positions. A significant change in vital signs signifies hypovolemia or dehydration. A positive test occurs if the patient becomes dizzy, has a pulse increase of 20 or more beats per minute, or a systolic blood pressure decrease of 20 or more mmHg (millimeters of mercury). Also known as tilt test or postural vital signs.

**orthotast** (or′thō-tăst) [″ + *tassein,* to arrange] An instrument used for straightening bone curvatures.

**orthotic** [Gr. *orthosis,* straightening] Relating to orthosis.

**orthotics** (or-thŏt′ĭks) **1.** The science pert. to mechanical appliances for orthopedic use. **2.** The use of orthopedic appliances.

**orthotist** (or′thō-tĭst) [Gr. *orthosis,* straightening] One skilled in orthotics.

**orthotonos, orthotonus** (or-thŏt′ō-nŏs, -nŭs) [″ + *tonos,* tension] Tetanic spasm marked by rigidity of the body in a straight line. SEE: illus.

**orthotopic** (or″thō-tŏp′ĭk) **1.** In the correct place. **2.** Pert. to a tissue graft to a site where that tissue would normally be present.

**orthovoltage** (or″thō-vŏl′tĭj) The median voltage used in x-ray therapy, approx. 250 kilovolts.

**orthropsia** (or-thrŏp′sē-ă) [Gr. *orthros,* time near dawn, + *opsis,* sight] A characteristic of human vision by which sight is better at dawn or dusk than in bright sunlight.

**Ortolani's maneuver** [Marius Ortolani, 20th century Italian orthopedic surgeon] The assessment maneuver designed to detect congenital subluxation or dislocation of the hip. The examiner places the infant on the back with hips and knees flexed while abducting and lifting the femurs. A palpable click is felt as the femur enters the dysplastic joint.

**O.S., o.s.** L. *oculus sinister,* left eye. SEE: *o.d.*

**Os** Symbol for the element osmium.

**os** (ōs) *pl.* **ora** [L.] Mouth, opening.

***incompetent cervical o.*** A uterine cervix that cannot maintain a diameter small enough to support the increasing weight of the fetus. This condition usually results in early second trimester abortion. The cause is a congenital structural defect or previous trauma to the cervix. It is treated with a purse-string ligature that encircles, encloses, and reinforces the cervix.

***o. uteri*** The mouth of the uterus.

***o. uteri externum*** The opening of the

cervical canal of the uterus into the vagina.

***o. uteri internum*** The internal opening of the cervical canal into the uterus.

***o. ventriculi*** The cardia of the stomach.

**os** (ŏs) *pl.* **ossa** [L.] Bone.

***o. calcis*** The heel bone. SYN: *calcaneus.*

***o. coxae*** The innominate bone; hip bone.

***o. hamatum*** The hooked bone on the ulnar side of the distal row of the carpus (wrist). SYN: *unciform bone.*

***o. hyoideum*** The horseshoe-shaped bone lying at the base of the tongue. SYN: *hyoid bone.*

***o. ilii*** The ilium.

***o. innominatum*** The innominate (hip) bone.

***o. magnum*** The third bone in the second distal row of the carpus. SYN: *capitatum.*

***o. orbiculare*** The tiny bone in the ear that becomes attached to the incus, forming the lenticular process.

***o. peroneum*** A bone occasionally found in the tendon of the peroneus longus muscle.

***o. planum*** **1.** Flat bone; any bone that has only a slight thickness. **2.** The orbital plate of the ethmoid bone.

***o. pubis*** The pubic bone; the anteroinferior part of the hip bone. In the adult, it unites the innominate bone with the ilium and ischium to form the pelvis. It is irregular in shape, divided into a horizontal, ascending, and descending ramus. The outer extremity constitutes approx. one fifth of the acetabulum. The inner ramus forms the symphysis pubis.

***o. scaphoideum*** A proximal boat-shaped bone of the carpus or the tarsus. SYN: *scaphoid.*

***o. temporale*** Temporal bone.

***o. trigonum*** A bone of the foot that develops from an extra center of ossification along the posterior surface of the talus.

***o. unguis*** Lacrimal bone.

***o. vesalianum*** A bone that develops from the ossification of the posterior tubercle of the fifth metatarsal.

**osazone** (ō′sā-zōn) Any of a series of compounds resulting from heating sugars with acetic acid and phenylhydrazine.

**oscheal** (ŏs′kē-ăl) [Gr. *oscheon,* scrotum] Scrotal.

**oscheitis** (ŏs-kē-ī′tĭs) [″ + *itis,* inflammation] Inflammation of the scrotum.

**oschelephantiasis** (ŏsk″ĕl-ĕ-făn-tī′ă-sĭs) Elephantiasis of the scrotum.

**oscheo-** [Gr. *oscheon*] Combining form meaning *scrotum.*

**oscheocele** (ŏs′kē-ō-sēl) [″ + *kele,* tumor, swelling] A scrotal swelling or tumor.

**oscheohydrocele** (ŏs″kē-ō-hī′drō-sēl) [″ + *hydor,* water, + *kele,* tumor, swelling] Scrotal hydrocele; collection of fluids in the sac of a scrotal hernia.

**oscheolith** (ŏs′kē-ō-lĭth) [″ + *lithos,* stone] A concretion in the scrotal sebaceous glands.

**oscheoncus** (ŏs″kē-ŏng′kŭs) [″ + *onkos,* mass, bulk] A tumor of the scrotum.

**oscheoplasty** (ŏs′kē-ō-plăs″tē) [″ + *plassein,* to form] Plastic surgical repair of the scrotum.

**oscillation** (ŏs″sĭl-ā′shŭn) [L. *oscillare,* to swing] A swinging, pendulum-like movement; a vibration or fluctuation.

**oscillator** (ŏs′ĭ-lā″tor) **1.** Device for producing oscillations. **2.** An electronic circuit that will produce an oscillating current of a certain frequency.

**oscillogram** (ŏs′ĭl-ō-grăm) [″ + Gr. *gramma,* something written] A graphic record made by the oscillograph.

**oscillograph** (ŏs′ĭl-ō-grăf) [″ + Gr. *graphein,* to write] An electronic device used for detecting, displaying, and recording variations in electrical phenomena. In medicine, it is used for recording electrical activity of the brain, the heart, and other muscular tissues. Electrocardiographs and electroencephalographs are examples of the application of this technique. SEE: *oscilloscope.*

**oscillometer** (ŏs-ĭl-ŏm′ĕ-tĕr) [″ + Gr. *metron,* measure] A machine used to measure oscillations, esp. those of the bloodstream.

**oscillometry** (ŏs-ĭl-ŏm′ĕ-trē) The measurement of oscillations with an instrument.

**oscillopsia** The sensation of oscillation or swinging of the visual field. It is illusory and may be associated with a severe form of labyrinthine nystagmus.

**oscilloscope** (ŏ-sĭl′ō-skōp) [L. *oscillare,* to swing, + Gr. *skopein,* to examine] An instrument that makes visible the presence, nature, and form of oscillations or irregularities of an electric current. SEE: *oscillograph.*

**Oscinidae** The eye flies. A family of small hairless flies that includes the genera *Hippelates, Siphunculina,* and *Oscinis.* They are serious pests and transmit a number of infectious diseases.

**osculation** [L. *osculum,* little mouth, kiss] **1.** The union of two vessels or structures by their mouths. **2.** Kissing.

**osculum** (ŏs′kū-lŭm) *pl.* **oscula** [L.] A tiny aperture or pore.

**-ose** **1.** Chemical suffix indicating that a substance is a carbohydrate, such as glucose. **2.** Suffix indicating a primary alteration product of a protein, such as proteose.

**Osgood-Schlatter disease** (ŏz-good-shlăt′ĕr) [Robert B. Osgood, U.S. orthopedist, 1873–1956; Carl Schlatter, Swiss surgeon, 1864–1934] Osteochondritis of the epiphysis of the tibial tuberosity.

**OSHA** *Occupational Safety and Health Administration.* A U.S. governmental regulatory agency concerned with the health and safety of workers.

**-osis** [Gr.] Suffix indicating *condition, status, process,* sometimes denoting an abnormal increase. SEE: *-asis; -sis.*

**Osler, Sir William** (ŏs′lĕr) Canadian-born

physician, 1849–1919. During his career he was associated with McGill, Johns Hopkins, and Oxford Universities, where he prepared a number of editions of his monumental *The Principles and Practice of Medicine.*

***O.'s disease*** **1.** Polycythemia vera. **2.** Hereditary hemorrhagic telangiectasia.

***O.'s maneuver*** An attempt to compress the radial artery sufficiently to prevent palpation of the radial pulse past the point of compression. If this pulse is still palpable, then the artery is sclerosed. This could lead to the diagnosis of hypertension when, in fact, the blood pressure could be normal.

***O.'s nodes*** Small, tender cutaneous nodes, usually present in the fingers and toes, that may be seen in subacute bacterial endocarditis. The nodes are due to infected emboli from the heart.

**osmatic** (ŏz-măt'ĭk) [Gr. *osmasthai,* to smell] Pert. to, or having, a keen sense of smell.

**osmesis** (ŏz-mē'sĭs) [Gr. *osmesis,* smelling] **1.** The sense of smell. **2.** The act of smelling. SYN: *olfaction.*

**osmesthesia** (ŏz"mĕs-thē'zē-ă) [Gr. *osme,* odor, + *aisthesis,* sensation] Olfactory sensibility; the power of perceiving and distinguishing odors.

**osmic acid** (ŏz'mĭk) $OsO_4$. A volatile, colorless compound formed by heating osmium in air. It is used as a caustic, a stain for fats, and a tissue fixative for electron microscopy. SYN: *osmium tetroxide.*

Caution: Vapors are extremely toxic to the eyes, skin, and respiratory tract. The container must not be opened without safeguarding the eyes from vapors released from uncapping and possible spilling.

**osmicate** (ŏz'mĭ-kāt) To impregnate or stain with osmic acid.

**osmidrosis** (ŏz-mĭ-drō'sĭs) [" + *hidros,* sweat] Bromidrosis.

**osmiophilic** (ŏz"mē-ō-fĭl'ĭk) Having an affinity for the staining material osmium tetroxide.

**osmiophobic** (ŏz"mē-ō-fō'bĭk) Having resistance to the staining material osmium tetroxide.

**osmium** (ŏz'mē-ŭm) [Gr. *osme,* smell] SYMB: Os. A metallic element with an atomic weight of 190.2 and the atomic number 76.

***o. tetroxide*** $OsO_4$. Osmic acid.

**osmo- 1.** [Gr. *osme,* odor] A combining form indicating *odor, smell.* **2.** [Gr. *osmos,* impulse] A combining form meaning *a thrusting forth.* **3.** [Gr. *osmos,* impulse] Pert. to osmosis.

**osmol, osmole** The standard unit of osmotic pressure based on a one molal concentration of an ion in a solution.

**osmodysphoria** (ŏz-mō-dĭs-fō'rē-ă) [Gr. *osme,* odor, + *dys,* bad, + *pherein,* to bear] A deep-seated and abnormal dislike of certain odors.

**osmolagnia** (ŏz"mō-lăg'nē-ă) [" + *lagneia,* lust] Erotic excitement derived from odors, usually of the body. SYN: *osphresiolagnia.*

**osmolality** (ŏs"mō-lăl'ĭ-tē) Osmotic concentration; the characteristic of a solution determined by the ionic concentration of the dissolved substances per unit of solvent.

***plasma o.*** The osmotic concentration of plasma. Normally the ionic concentration in the plasma is maintained within a narrow range: 275 to 295 mOsm/kg. When plasma osmolality increases above normal, antidiuretic hormone (ADH, also called vasopressin) is released. ADH prevents loss of water by the kidney and thus decreases plasma osmolality. An increase in plasma osmolality also produces the sensation of thirst, which stimulates the person to drink fluids; this, too, serves to decrease plasma osmolality.

***serum o.*** The osmotic concentration of the serum.

***urine o.*** The osmotic concentration of the urine.

**osmolar** (ŏz-mō'lăr) Concerning the osmotic concentration of a solution.

**osmolarity** (os"mō-lăr'ĭ-tē) The concentration of osmotically active particles in solution.

**osmology** (ŏz-mŏl'ō-jē) **1.** [Gr. *osme,* odor, + *logos,* word, reason] The study of odors. SYN: *osphresiology.* **2.** [Gr. *osmos,* impulse, + *logos,* word, reason] The study of osmosis.

**osmometer** (ŏz-mŏm'ĕt-ĕr) **1.** [Gr. *osme,* odor, + *metron,* measure] A device for measuring the acuity of the sense of smell. **2.** [Gr. *osmos,* impulse, + *metron,* measure] A device for measuring osmotic pressure either directly or indirectly. It is used clinically to assess the extent of dehydration or blood loss.

**osmometry 1.** The study of osmosis. **2.** The measurement of osmotic forces using an osmometer.

**osmonosology** (ŏz"mō-nō-sŏl'ō-jē) [Gr. *osme,* odor, + *nosos,* disease, + *logos,* word, reason] The branch of medicine dealing with diseases and disorders of the organs of smell.

**osmophore** (ŏz'mō-for) [Gr. *osme,* odor, + *phoros,* bearing] The portion of a chemical responsible for the odor of the compound.

**osmoreceptor** (ŏz"mō-rē-sĕp'tor) **1.** A receptor in the hypothalamus that is sensitive to the osmotic pressure of the serum. **2.** A receptor in the brain that is sensitive to olfactory stimuli.

**osmoregulation** (ŏz"mō-rĕg"ū-lā'shŭn) The regulation of osmotic pressure.

**osmose** (ŏz'mōs) [Gr. *osmos,* impulse] **1.** To subject to osmosis. **2.** To undergo osmosis.

**osmosis** (ŏz-mō'sĭs) [Gr. *osmos,* impulse, + *osis,* condition] The passage of solvent through a semipermeable membrane that separates solutions of different concentra-

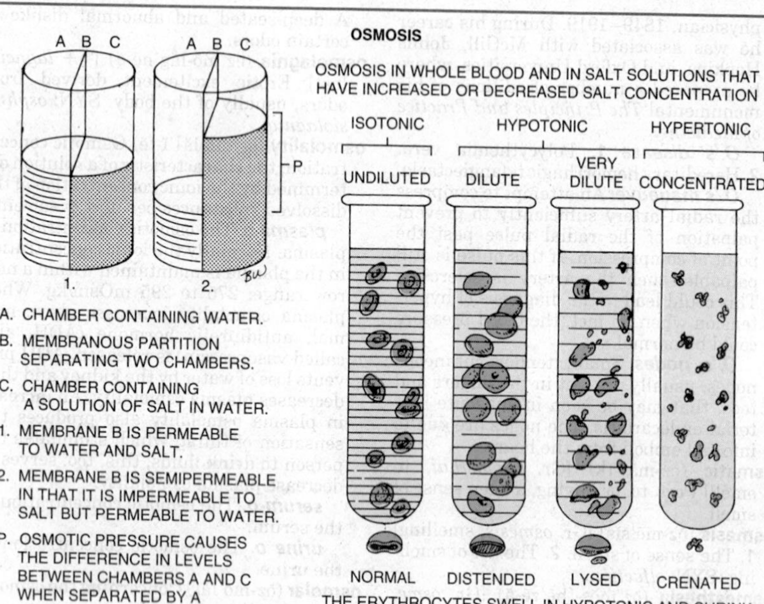

OSMOSIS

tions. The solvent, usually water, passes through the membrane from the region of lower concentration of solute to that of a higher concentration of solute, thus tending to equalize the concentrations of the two solutions. The rate of osmosis is dependent primarily upon the difference in osmotic pressures of the solutions on the two sides of a membrane, the permeability of the membrane, and the electric potential across the membrane and the charge upon the walls of the pores in it. SEE: illus. **osmotic** (-mŏt′ĭk), *adj.*

**osmostat** The area in the anterior region of the hypothalamus that contains cells that control osmolality.

**osmotherapy** (ŏz″mō-thĕr′ă-pē) [″ + *therapeia,* treatment] Intravenous administration of hypertonic solutions in order to increase the osmolar concentration of the serum. This therapy is used in treating cerebral edema.

**osmotic pressure 1.** Pressure that develops when two solutions of different concentrations are separated by a semipermeable membrane. **2.** Pressure that would develop if a solution were enclosed in a membrane impermeable to all solutes present and surrounded by pure solvent. Osmotic pressure varies with concentration of the solution and with temperature increase. Animal cells have an osmotic pressure approx. equal to that of the circulating fluid, the blood. Solutions exerting this osmotic pressure are said to be isotonic or isosmotic; stronger solutions that cause cells to shrink are hypertonic; weaker solutions that cause cells to swell are hypotonic.

**osphresiolagnia** (ŏs-frē″zē-ō-lăg′nē-ă) [Gr. *osphresis,* smell, + *lagneia,* lust] Erotic excitement produced by odors. SYN: *osmolagnia.*

**osphresiology** (ŏs″frē-zē-ŏl′ō-jē) [″ + *logos,* word, reason] Science of odors and the sense of smell. SYN: *osmology* (1).

**osphresiometer** (ŏs″frē-zē-ŏm′ĕ-tĕr) [″ + *metron,* measure] An apparatus for measuring the acuteness of the sense of smell. SYN: *osmometer* (1).

**osphresis** (ŏs-frē′sĭs) [Gr.] The sense of smell. SYN: *olfaction.* **osphretic** (-frĕt′ĭk), *adj.*

**osphyalgia** (ŏs-fē-ăl′jē-ă) [Gr. *osphys,* loin, + *algos,* pain] Pain in the hips. SEE: *lumbago; sciatica.*

**osphyitis** (ŏs-fē-ī′tĭs) [″ + *itis,* inflammation] Inflammation of the lumbar region.

**osphyomyelitis** (ŏs″fē-ō-mī″ĕl-ī′tĭs) [″ + *myelos,* marrow, + *itis,* inflammation] Inflammation of the lumbar region of the spinal cord.

**ossa** (ŏs′ă) [L., bones] Pl. of os.

**ossein** (ŏs′ē-ĭn) [L. *ossa,* bones] The collagen of bone. It forms the framework of bone.

**osseocartilaginous** (ŏs″ē-ō-kăr″tĭ-lăj′ĭ-nŭs) Concerning bone and cartilage.

**osseofibrous** (ŏs″ē-ō-fī′brŭs) [″ + *fibra,* fiber] Composed of bone and fibrous tissue.

**osseointegration** A stable, compatible interface between a dental implant and the bone. It is devoid of fibrous connective tissue. The interface is created by the growth of living bone into direct contact and potential bonding with the implant.

**osseous** (ŏs′ē-ŭs) [L. *osseus,* bony] Bonelike; concerning bones. SYN: *bony.*

**ossicle** (ŏs′ĭ-kl) [L. *ossiculum,* little bone] Any small bone, esp. one of the three bones of the ear.

***auditory o.*** One of the three bones of the inner ear: malleus, incus, and stapes. SEE: *ear* for illus.

**ossicula** (ŏ-sĭk′ū-lă) [L.] Pl. of ossiculum.

**ossiculectomy** (ŏs″ĭk-ū-lĕk′tō-mē) [L. *ossiculum,* little bone, + Gr. *ektome,* excision] Excision of an ossicle, esp. one of the ear.

**ossiculotomy** (ŏ″sĭk-ū-lŏt′ō-mē) [″ + Gr. *tome,* incision] Surgical incision of one or more of the ossicles of the ear.

**ossiculum** (ŏ-sĭk′ū-lŭm) *pl.* **ossicula** [L.] Tiny bone, esp. one of the three in the middle ear.

**ossific** (ŏs-if′ĭk) [″ + *facere,* to make] Producing or becoming bone.

**ossification** (ŏs″ĭ-fĭ-kā′shŭn) [″ + *facere,* to make] **1.** The formation of bone substance. **2.** The conversion of other tissue into bone. SYN: *osteogenesis.*

***endochondral o.*** The formation of bone in cartilage, as in the formation of long bones, involving the destruction and removal of cartilage and the formation of osseous tissue in the space formerly occupied by the cartilage. SEE: illus.

***intramembranous o.*** The formation of

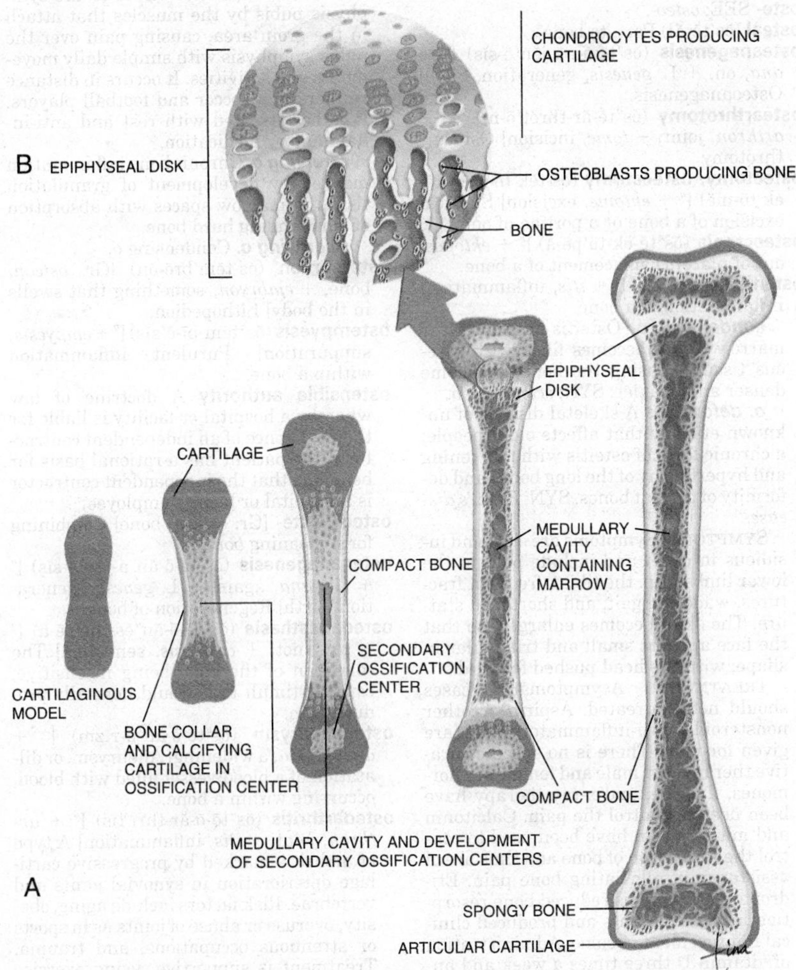


**ENDOCHONDRAL OSSIFICATION**

THE OSSIFICATION PROCESS IN A LONG BONE. **(A)** PROGRESSION FROM EMBRYO TO YOUNG ADULT, **(B)** MICROSCOPIC VIEW OF AN EPIPHYSEAL DISK

bone in or underneath a fibrous membrane, such as occurs in the formation of the cranial bones.

***pathologic o.*** The formation of bone in abnormal sites or abnormal development of bone.

***periosteal o.*** The formation of successive thin layers of bone by osteoblasts between the underlying bone or cartilage and the cellular and fibrous layer that covers the forming bone. Also called subperiosteal ossification.

**ossiform** (ŏs′ĭ-form) Resembling bone. SYN: *osteoid* (1).

**ossify** (ŏs′ĭ-fī) [″ + *facere,* to make] To turn into bone.

**ostalgia** (ŏs-tăl′jē-ă) [Gr. *osteon,* bone, + *algos,* pain] Pain in a bone.

**oste-** SEE: *osteo-*.

**osteal** (ŏs′tē-ăl) Pert. to bone.

**osteanagenesis** (ŏs″tē-ăn-ă-jĕn′ĕ-sĭs) [″ + *ana,* on, + L. *genesis,* generation, birth] Osteoanagenesis.

**ostearthrotomy** (ŏs″tē-ăr-thrŏt′ō-mē) [″ + *arthron,* joint, + *tome,* incision] Osteoarthrotomy.

**ostectomy, osteectomy** (ŏs-tĕk′tō-mē, -tē-ĕk′tō-mē) [″ + *ektome,* excision] Surgical excision of a bone or a portion of one.

**osteectopia** (ŏs″tē-ĕk-tō′pē-ă) [″ + *ektopos,* out of place] Displacement of a bone.

**osteitis** (ŏs-tē-ī′tĭs) [″ + *itis,* inflammation] Inflammation of a bone.

***condensing o.*** Osteitis in which the marrow cavity becomes filled with osseous tissue, causing the bone to become denser and heavier. SYN: *sclerosing o.*

***o. deformans*** A skeletal disease of unknown etiology that affects older people; a chronic form of osteitis with thickening and hypertrophy of the long bones and deformity of the flat bones. SYN: *Paget's disease.*

SYMPTOMS: Symptoms are slow and insidious in onset and include pain in the lower limbs (esp. the tibia), frequent fractures, waddling gait, and shortened stature. The skull becomes enlarged, so that the face appears small and triangular in shape, with the head pushed forward.

TREATMENT: Asymptomatic cases should not be treated. Aspirin or other nonsteroidal anti-inflammatory drugs are given for pain. There is no specific curative therapy, but male and female sex hormones, fluoride, and x-ray therapy have been used to control the pain. Calcitonin and mithramycin have been used to control the resorption of bone and thus are of assistance in alleviating bone pain. Etidronate sodium has reduced bone resorption in most patients and produced clinical improvement in some. Administration of vitamin D three times a week and anabolic hormones may be of help in treating osteoporosis.

***o. fibrosa cystica generalisata*** A condition resulting from overactivity of the parathyroid glands with resulting disturbances in calcium and phosphorus metabolism. It is characterized by decalcification and softening of bone, nephrolithiasis, elevation of blood calcium, and lowering of blood phosphorus. Cysts form and tumors may develop. SEE: *hyperparathyroidism.*

***o. fragilitans*** Osteogenesis imperfecta.

***gummatous o.*** Chronic osteitis associated with syphilis and characterized by the formation of gummas.

***localized alveolar o.*** A localized inflammation of a tooth socket following extraction. Destruction of the primary clot results in denuded bone surfaces. SYN: *dry socket.*

***pubis o.*** A chronic inflammatory process due to repetitive stress to the symphysis pubis by the muscles that attach in the groin area, causing pain over the pubis symphysis with simple daily movements and activities. It occurs in distance runners and soccer and football players. It is best treated with rest and anti-inflammatory medication.

***rarefying o.*** Chronic bone inflammation marked by development of granulation tissue in marrow spaces with absorption of surrounding hard bone.

***sclerosing o.*** Condensing o.

**ostembryon** (ŏs-tĕm′brē-ŏn) [Gr. *osteon,* bone, + *embryon,* something that swells in the body] Lithopedion.

**ostempyesis** (ŏs″tĕm-pī-ē′sĭs) [″ + *empyesis,* suppuration] Purulent inflammation within a bone.

**ostensible authority** A doctrine of law whereby a hospital or facility is liable for the negligence of an independent contractor if the patient has a rational basis for believing that the independent contractor is a hospital or facility employee.

**osteo-, oste-** [Gr. *osteon,* bone] Combining form meaning *bone.*

**osteoanagenesis** (ŏs″tē-ō-ăn″ă-jĕn′ĕ-sĭs) [″ + Gr. *ana,* again, + L. *genesis,* generation, birth] Regeneration of bone.

**osteoanesthesia** (ŏs″tē-ō-ăn″ĕs-thē′zē-ă) [″ + *an-*, not, + *aisthesis,* sensation] The condition of the bone being insensitive, esp. to stimuli that would normally produce pain.

**osteoaneurysm** (ŏs″tē-ō-ăn′ū-rĭzm) [″ + *aneurysma,* a widening] Aneurysm, or dilatation of a blood vessel filled with blood, occurring within a bone.

**osteoarthritis** (ŏs″tē-ō-ăr-thrī′tĭs) [″ + *arthron,* joint, + *itis,* inflammation] A type of arthritis marked by progressive cartilage deterioration in synovial joints and vertebrae. Risk factors include aging, obesity, overuse or abuse of joints as in sports or strenuous occupations, and trauma. Treatment is supportive, using exercise balanced with rest, heat, weight reduction if needed, and analgesics. If these measures are unsuccessful in controlling pain, a joint replacement may be necessary. SYN: *degenerative joint disease.*

SEE: *Nursing Diagnoses Appendix.*

NURSING IMPLICATIONS: Activities are paced to prevent excessive fatigue or irritation to the joints, and rest is provided after activity. Support is offered to assist the patient to cope with mobility limitations. The nurse teaches the patient about exercise and treatments for affected joints including applications of moist heat, range-of-motion exercises to the limit of pain, maintenance of correct body weight and posture, use of supportive appliances and devices, and home safety measures as ordered.

**osteoarthropathy** (ŏs″tē-ō-ăr-thrŏp′ă-thē) [″ + ″ + *pathos,* disease, suffering] Any disease involving the joints and bones.

***hypertrophic pulmonary o.*** A disorder characterized by enlargement of the distal phalanges of the fingers and toes and a thickening of their distal ends, accompanied by a peculiar longitudinal curving of nails. The wrists and interphalangeal joints may become enlarged, as may the distal ends of the tibia, the fibula, and the jaw. This condition may be associated with emphysema, pulmonary tuberculosis, chronic bronchitis, bronchiectasis, and congenital heart disease.

**osteoarthrotomy** (ŏs″tē-ō-ăr-thrŏt′ō-mē) [″ + ″ + *tome,* incision] Surgical excision of the articular end of a bone. SYN: *ostearthrotomy.*

**osteoblast** (ŏs′tē-ō-blăst) [Gr. *osteon,* bone, + *blastos,* germ] A cell of mesodermal origin concerned with the formation of bone.

**osteoblastoma** (ŏs″tē-ō-blăs-tō′mă) [″ + ″ + *oma,* tumor] A large, benign tumor of osteoblasts in a patchy osteoid matrix. It occurs mostly in the vertebral columns of young people.

**osteocampsia** (ŏs″tē-ō-kămp′sē-ă) [″ + *kamptein,* to bend] Curvature of a bone, as in osteomalacia.

**osteocarcinoma** (ŏs″tē-ō-kăr-sĭn-ō′mă) [″ + *karkinos,* cancer, + *oma,* tumor] **1.** Combined osteoma and carcinoma. **2.** Carcinoma of a bone.

**osteocartilaginous** (ŏs″tē-ō-kăr″tĭ-lăj′ĭ-nŭs) Concerning bone and cartilage.

**osteocele** (ŏs′tē-ō-sēl) [″ + *kele,* tumor, swelling] **1.** A testicular or scrotal tumor that contains bony tissue. **2.** A bone-containing hernia.

**osteochondral** (ŏs″tē-ō-kŏn′drăl) Concerning bone and cartilage.

**osteochondritis** (ŏs″tē-ō-kŏn-drī′tĭs) [″ + *chondros,* cartilage, + *itis,* inflammation] Inflammation of bone and cartilage.

***o. deformans juvenilis*** Chronic inflammation of the head of the femur in children, resulting in atrophy and shortening of the neck of femur with a wide flat head. SYN: *Perthes' disease; Waldenström's disease.*

***o. dissecans*** A condition affecting a joint in which a fragment of cartilage and its underlying bone become detached from articular surface. It commonly occurs in the knee joint.

**osteochondrodystrophy** (ŏs″tē-ō-kŏn″drō-dĭs′trō-fē) [″ + ″ + *dys,* bad, + *trephein,* to nourish] A disorder of skeletal growth resulting from bone and cartilage malformation. The condition produces a form of dwarfism. SYN: *Morquio's syndrome.*

***familial o.*** Morquio's syndrome. SEE: *mucopolysaccharidosis IV.*

**osteochondrolysis** (ŏs″tē-ō-kŏn-drŏl′ĭ-sĭs) [″ + ″ + *lysis,* dissolution] Osteochondritis dissecans.

**osteochondroma** (ŏs″tē-ō-kŏn-drō′mă) [″ + ″ + *oma,* tumor] A tumor composed of both cartilaginous and bony substance.

**osteochondromatosis** (ŏs″tē-ō-kŏn″drō-mă-tō′sĭs) [″ + ″ + ″ + *osis,* condition] A disease in which there are multiple osteochondromata.

**osteochondrosarcoma** (ŏs″tē-ō-kŏn″drō-săr-kō′mă) [″ + ″ + *sarx,* flesh, + *oma,* tumor] Chondrosarcoma occurring in bone.

**osteochondrosis** (ŏs″tē-ō-kŏn-drō′sĭs) [″ + ″ + *osis,* condition] A disease causing degenerative changes in the ossification centers of the epiphyses of bones, particularly during periods of rapid growth in children. The process continues to the stage of avascular and aseptic necrosis and then there is slow healing and repair.

NURSING IMPLICATIONS: Bedrest is encouraged, and support is offered through disruption of normal activity. The nurse teaches the correct use of crutches. Neurocirculatory function distal to supportive device (splint, elastic support, or cast) is evaluated. Joint mobility and limitation of motion are assessed daily.

***o. deformans tibiae*** Degeneration or aseptic necrosis of the medial condyle of the tibia.

**osteochondrous** (ŏs″tē-ō-kŏn′drŭs) Concerning bone and cartilage.

**osteoclasia, osteoclasis** (ŏs″tē-ō-klā′zē-ă, -ŏk′lă-sĭs) [″ + *klasis,* a breaking] **1.** Surgical fracture of a bone in order to remedy a deformity. SYN: *diaclasis.* **2.** Bony tissue absorption and destruction.

**osteoclast** (ŏs′tē-ō-klăst) [″ + *klan,* to break] **1.** A device for fracturing bones for therapeutic purposes. **2.** A giant multinuclear cell formed in the bone marrow of growing bones. Osteoclasts are found in depressions (called Howship's lacunae) on the surface of the bone. It aids in absorbing and removing excess bone tissue as in the remodeling of growing bones, or damaged bone in the repair of fractures. SEE: illus. **osteoclastic** (-klăs′tĭk), *adj.*

**osteoclast activating factor** ABBR: OAF. A lymphokine produced in certain conditions associated with resorption of bone, including periodontal disease and lymphoid proliferative diseases such as multiple myeloma and malignant lymphoma. Interleukin-1 is an OAF, as are other substances produced by T lymphocytes and prostaglandins.

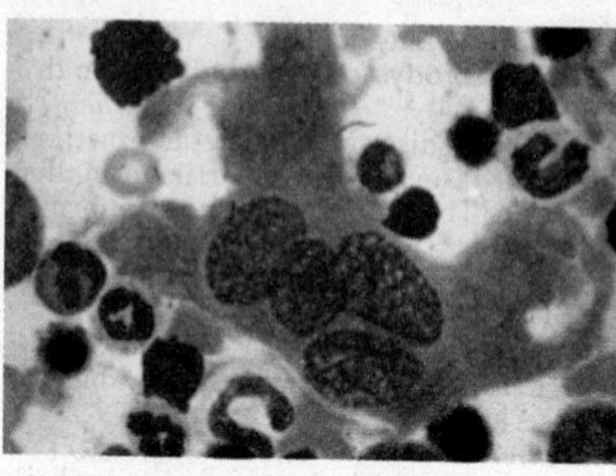

**OSTEOCLAST** WITH MULTIPLE NUCLEI (ORIG. MAG. ×640)

**osteoclastoma** (ŏs″tē-ō-klăs-tō′mă) [″ + ″ + *oma,* tumor] Giant cell tumor of bone.

**osteocope** (ŏs′tē-ō-kōp) [″ + *kopos,* pain] Extreme pain in the bones, esp. in syphilitic bone disease. **osteocopic** (-kŏp′ĭk), *adj.*

**osteocranium** (ŏs″tē-ō-krā′nē-ŭm) [″ + *kranion,* skull] The portion of the cranium formed of membrane bones in contrast to that formed of cartilage (chondrocranium).

**osteocystoma** (ŏs″tē-ō-sĭs-tō′mă) [″ + *kystis,* sac, bladder, + *oma,* tumor] Cystic tumor of a bone.

**osteocyte** (ŏs′tē-ō-sīt″) [″ + *kytos,* cell] A mesodermal bone-forming cell that has become entrapped within the bone matrix. It lies within a lacuna with processes extending outward through canaliculi and, by its metabolic activity, helps to maintain bone as a living tissue.

**osteodensitometer** A device used for determining the density of bones.

**osteodentin** Dentin that forms very rapidly or in response to severe trauma so that cells and blood vessels are incorporated, resembling bone.

**osteodermia** (ŏs″tē-ō-dĕr′mē-ă) [″ + *derma,* skin] The formation of bony deposits in the skin.

**osteodesmosis** (ŏs″tē-ō-dĕs-mō′sĭs) [″ + *desmos,* tendon, + *osis,* condition] The transformation of tendon into bone.

**osteodiastasis** (ŏs″tē-ō-dī-ăs′tă-sĭs) [″ + *diastasis,* separation] The separation of two adjacent bones.

**osteodynia** (ŏs″tē-ō-dĭn′ē-ă) [″ + *odyne,* pain] Ostalgia.

**osteodystrophy** (ŏs″tē-ō-dĭs′trō-fē) [″ + *dys,* ill, + *trophe,* nourishment] Defective bone development.

***renal o.*** A condition marked by generalized pathological changes in bone with a resemblance to osteitis fibrosa cystica, osteomalacia, and osteoporosis. These changes are associated with renal failure. The serum phosphorus level is elevated, the calcium level is low or normal, and there is increased parathyroid gland activity.

**osteoepiphysis** (ŏs″tē-ō-ē-pĭf′ĭs-ĭs) [″ + *epi,* upon, + *physis,* growth] A small piece of bone that is separated in childhood from a larger bone by cartilage; during later growth, the two bones join.

**osteofibroma** (ŏs″tē-ō-fī-brō′mă) [″ + L. *fibra,* fiber, + Gr. *oma,* tumor] A tumor composed of bony and fibrous tissues. SYN: *fibro-osteoma.*

**osteogen** (ŏs′tē-ō-jĕn) [″ + *gennan,* to produce] The substance of the inner periosteal layer from which bone is formed.

**osteogenesis, osteogeny** (ŏs″tē-ō-jĕn′ĕ-sĭs, -ŏj′ĕ-nē) The formation and development of bone taking place in connective tissue or in cartilage. SYN: *ossification.* **osteogenic,** *adj.*

***o. imperfecta*** An inherited disorder of the connective tissue characterized by defective bone matrix with calcification occurring normally on whatever matrix is present. Clinical findings are multiple fractures with minimal trauma, blue sclerae, early deafness, opalescent teeth, a tendency to capillary bleeding, translucent skin, and joint instability. Although the disease is heterogeneous, two different classifications of osteogenesis imperfecta are still used for clinical distinction. *Osteogenesis imperfecta congenita* manifests in utero or at birth. *Osteogenesis imperfecta tarda* occurs later in childhood with delayed onset of fracturing and much milder manifestations. The healing of bone fractures progresses normally. Later in life, the tendency to fracture decreases and often disappears. The vast majority of cases are inherited as an autosomal dominant trait, although a small percentage of congenital cases are transmitted as an autosomal recessive. There is no known cure for osteogenesis imperfecta; therefore, treatment is supportive and palliative. Definition provided by the American Brittle Bone Society, Inc.

**osteogenic** Pert. to osteogenesis.

**osteography** (ŏs″tē-ŏg′răf-ē) [Gr. *osteon,* bone, + *graphein,* to write] A descriptive treatise of the bones.

**osteohalisteresis** (ŏs″tē-ō-hăl-ĭs″tĕr-ē′sĭs) [″ + *hals,* salt, + *sterein,* to deprive] Softening of the bones caused by a deficiency of mineral constituents of the bone.

**osteoid** (ŏs′tē-oyd) [″ + *eidos,* form, shape] **1.** Resembling bone. SYN: *ossiform.* **2.** The noncalcified matrix of young bone. Also called prebone.

**osteokinematics** The branch of biomechanics concerned with the description of bone movement when a bone swings through a range of motion around the axis in a joint, such as with flexion, extension, abduction, adduction, or rotation.

**osteolipochondroma** (ŏs″tē-ō-lĭ-pō″kŏn-drō′mă) [″ + *lipos,* fat, + *chondros,* cartilage, + *oma,* tumor] A cartilaginous tumor containing fatty and bony tissue.

**osteologist** (ŏs″tē-ŏl′ō-jĭst) [″ + *logos,* word, reason] A specialist in the study of the bones.

**osteology** (ŏs-tē-ŏl′ō-jē) [″ + *logos,* word, reason] The science concerned with the structure and function of bones.

**osteolysis** (ŏs″tē-ŏl′ĭ-sĭs) [″ + *lysis,* dissolution] A softening and destruction of bone without osteoclastic activity. Osteolysis occurs within compact bone and results from a breakdown of the organic matrix and subsequent leaching out of the inorganic fraction. The condition is probably caused by localized metabolic disturbances, vascular changes, or the release of hydrolytic enzymes by osteocytes.

**osteolytic** (ŏs″tē-ō-lĭt′ĭk) Causing osteolysis.

**osteoma** (ŏs-tē-ō′mă) *pl.* **osteomata, osteomas** [″ + *oma,* tumor] A benign bony tumor; a bonelike structure that develops on a bone or at other sites. SYN: *exostosis.*

***cancellous o.*** A soft and spongy tumor. Its thin and delicate trabeculae enclose large medullary spaces similar to that in cancellous bone.

***cavalryman's o.*** A bony outgrowth of the femur at the insertion of the adductor femoris longus.

***o. cutis*** A benign formation of bone nodules in the skin.

***dental o.*** A bony outgrowth of the root of a tooth.

***o. durum, o. eburneum*** A very hard osteoma in which the bone is ivorylike.

***o. medullare*** A bony tumor containing medullary spaces.

***osteoid o.*** A rare benign bone tumor composed of sheets of osteoid tissue that is partially calcified and ossified. The condition occurs esp. in the bones of the extremities of the young.

***o. spongiosum*** A spongy tumor in the bone. SYN: *osteospongioma.*

**osteomalacia** (ŏs″tē-ō-măl-ā′shē-ă) [Gr. *osteon,* bone, + *malakia,* softening] A disease marked by increasing softness of the bones, so that they become flexible and brittle, thus causing deformities. Osteomalacia is the adult form of rickets.

SYMPTOMS: Clinical findings are rheumatic pains in the limbs, spine, thorax, and pelvis, anemia, signs of deficiency disease, and progressive weakness.

ETIOLOGY: Osteomalacia is due to a deficiency of vitamin D, resulting in a shortage or loss of calcium salts.

TREATMENT: If the diet contains an adequate amount of calcium and phosphorus, a 1600 I.U. dose of vitamin D taken daily for about a month will produce great improvement. The dose can then be gradually decreased to the normal daily requirement for vitamin D. **osteomalacic** (-măl-ā′sĭk), *adj.*

**osteomatosis** (ŏs″tē-ō″mă-tō′sĭs) [″ + ″ + *osis,* condition] The formation of multiple osteomas.

**osteomere** (ŏs′tē-ō-mēr) [″ + *meros,* part] One in a series of similar bony segments, such as the vertebrae.

**osteometry** (ŏs-tē-ŏm′ĕt-rē) [″ + *metron,* measure] The study of the measurement of parts of the skeletal system.

**osteomyelitis** (ŏs″tē-ō-mī″ĕl-ī′tĭs) [″ + *myelos,* marrow, + *itis,* inflammation] Inflammation of bone, esp. the marrow, caused by a pathogenic organism. SEE: *Nursing Diagnoses Appendix.*

SYMPTOMS: Clinical findings are pain in the affected part, fever, sweats, leukocytosis, rigid overlying muscles, inflamed skin, and pain on pressure over affected part. Suppuration may also occur.

TREATMENT: Prompt and adequate doses of antibiotics should be given, along with sedation for pain and anxiety, aspiration of the abscess, and immobilization of the affected extremity. Surgery may be necessary if the abscess persists. SEE: *bone scan.*

NURSING IMPLICATIONS: The patient is instructed to obtain adequate bedrest; complete rest of the affected part may be indicated. The nurse is careful in positioning the affected part, and once positioned, the part is kept still to maintain proper muscle condition and to prevent additional pain due to tenderness. Extreme care is exercised in handling and disposing of drainage. If the patient remains at home, the nurse teaches family members proper positioning of the affected part, measures to dispose of drainage, and the importance of frequent handwashing before and after caring for the patient. The importance of taking antibiotic medication as prescribed and of keeping follow-up appointments is stressed.

**osteomyelodysplasia** (ŏs″tē-ō-mī″ĕ-lō-dĭs-plā′sē-ă) [″ + ″ + *dys,* bad, + *plassein,* to form] A condition characterized by an increase in the marrow space of the bones, thinning of the bony tissue, leukopenia, and fever.

**osteon** (ŏs′tē-ŏn) [Gr., bone] The microscopic unit of compact bone, consisting of a haversian canal and the surrounding lamellae.

**osteonecrosis** (ŏs″tē-ō-nē-krō′sĭs) [″ + *nekrosis,* state of death] The death of a segment of bone. Onset is usually associated with interference with blood supply to the affected portion of bone which in turn causes necrosis at that site. This is a relatively common disorder and an estimated 10% of total joint replacements are for osteonecrosis. From 5% to 25% of patients receiving prolonged therapy with corticosteroids will develop this condition. Treatment is symptomatic, but in some cases of osteonecrosis of the knee or hip joint, prosthetic replacement is required.

**osteonectin** A glycoprotein present in the noncollagenous portion of the matrix of bone.

**osteoneuralgia** (ŏs″tē-ō-nū-răl′jē-ă) [″ + *neuron,* nerve, + *algos,* pain] Bone pain.

**osteopath** (ŏs′tē-ō-păth) [″ + *pathos,* disease] A practitioner of osteopathy.

**osteopathic** (ŏs″tē-ō-păth′ĭk) Concerning

osteopathy.

**osteopathology** (ŏs″tē-ō-păth-ŏl′ō-jē) [″ + *pathos,* disease, + *logos,* word, reason] **1.** Any bone disease. SYN: *osteopathy* (1). **2.** The study of bone diseases.

**osteopathy** (ŏs-tē-ŏp′ă-thē) [″ + *pathos,* disease, suffering] **1.** Any bone disease. **2.** A system of medicine founded by Dr. Andrew Taylor Still (1828–1917). It is based upon the theory that the normal body is a vital organism in which structural and functional states are of equal importance and that the body is able to rectify toxic conditions when it has favorable environmental circumstances and satisfactory nourishment.

Although manipulation is the primary method used to restore structural and functional balance, osteopaths also rely upon physical, medicinal, and surgical methods. Osteopathy is recognized as a standard method or system of medical and surgical care. Physicians with a degree in osteopathy use the designation D.O.

**osteopedion** (ŏs″tē-ō-pē′dē-ŏn) [″ + *paidion,* child] Lithopedion.

**osteopenia** (ŏs″tē-ō-pē′nē-ă) [″ + *penia,* lack] **1.** Any decrease in the amount of bone tissue, regardless of the cause. **2.** Decreased bone density caused by failure of the rate of osteoid tissue synthesis to keep up with the normal rate of bone lysis. SEE: *osteoporosis.*

**osteoperiosteal** (ŏs″tē-ō-pĕr″ē-ŏs′tē-ăl) [″ + *peri,* around, + *osteon,* bone] Concerning bone and its periosteum.

**osteoperiostitis** (ŏs″tē-ō-pĕr″ē-ŏs-tī′tĭs) [″ + ″ + ″ + *itis,* inflammation] Inflammation of a bone and its periosteum.

**osteopetrosis** (ŏs″tē-ō-pĕ-trō′sĭs) [″ + *petra,* stone, + *osis,* condition] A rare hereditary bone disorder of two types: the infantile (malignant) form, which is transmitted as an autosomal recessive trait, and the adult (benign) form, which is transmitted as an autosomal dominant trait. In both types of osteopetrosis, normal bone metabolism is disrupted. Although bone continues to be formed, normal resorption diminishes; the result is that bones become increasingly dense. Radiographs reveal the spotted, marblelike appearance of abnormally calcified bone. In severe cases, this process leads to cranial nerve entrapment, bone marrow failure, and recurrent fractures. SYN: *Albers-Schönberg disease; marble bone disease.*

PROGNOSIS: If untreated, the infantile form is usually fatal during the first decade of life.

TREATMENT: Some infants have responded to bone marrow transplants. Children who are not candidates for bone marrow transplants have improved considerably with long-term administration of interferon gamma-1b. Therapy for the adult type is symptomatic.

**osteophage** (ŏs′tē-ō-fāj) [″+ *phagein,* to eat] A large multinuclear cell that causes absorption of bone. SEE: *osteoclast.*

**osteophlebitis** (ŏs″tē-ō-flē-bī′tĭs) [″ + *phleps, phleb-,* vein, + *itis,* inflammation] Inflammation of the veins of a bone.

**osteophone** (ŏs′tē-ō-fōn″) [Gr. *osteon,* bone, + *phone,* voice] A device used by the deaf for conducting sound through facial bones.

**osteophony** (ŏs″tē-ŏf′ō-nē) Bone conduction of sound.

**osteophore** (ŏs′tē-ō-for) [″ + *pherein,* to carry] A forceps for crushing bone.

**osteophyte** (ŏs′tē-ō-fīt) [″ + *phyton,* plant] A bony excrescence or outgrowth, usually branched in shape.

**osteoplaque** (ŏs′tē-ō-plăk) Any layer of bone.

**osteoplast** (ŏs′tē-ō-plăst) [″ + *plastos,* formed] Osteoblast.

**osteoplastic** (ŏs″tē-ō-plăs′tĭk) [″ + *plastikos,* formed] **1.** Pert. to bone repair by plastic surgery or grafting. **2.** Concerning bone formation.

**osteopoikilosis** (ŏs″tē-ō-poy″kĭ-lō′sĭs) [″ + *poikilos,* spotted] A benign, hereditary disease of the bones marked by excessive calcification in spots less than 1 cm in diameter.

**osteoporosis** (ŏs″tē-ō-por-ō′sĭs) [″ + *poros,* a passage, + *osis,* condition] A general term describing any disease process that results in reduction in the mass of bone per unit of volume. The reduction is sufficient to interfere with the mechanical support function of bone. This term does not indicate a specific etiological agent; many conditions and diseases may be involved in the process. The condition becomes apparent when the osteoporosis has progressed to the stage at which a bone fractures in a situation that would not normally damage the skeleton (i.e., a pathological fracture). The bones most frequently involved are the vertebrae of the lower dorsal and lumbar areas. Osteoporosis may affect any bone, including those of the jaw. *Involutional osteoporosis* is seen in women aged 51 to 70 and is caused by factors related to menopause. It affects mainly trabecular bone. *Senile osteoporosis* is seen mainly after age 70 in both men and women. It affects both trabecular and cortical bone and results in both vertebral and hip fractures. SEE: illus.; *bone scan; hip, fracture of; hormone replacement therapy; Nursing Diagnoses Appendix.* **osteoporotic** (-por-ŏt′ĭk), *adj.*

ETIOLOGY: Osteoporosis can be caused by a number of factors. Bone loss is a universal concomitant of advanced age, but it proceeds faster in women, esp. following menopause, and is more likely to occur in sedentary individuals. SEE: table.

TREATMENT: Supplemental calcium and vitamin D are indicated and may help to stop the rate of bone loss. In menopausal women, therapy with estrogen decreases the rate of bone resorption, but

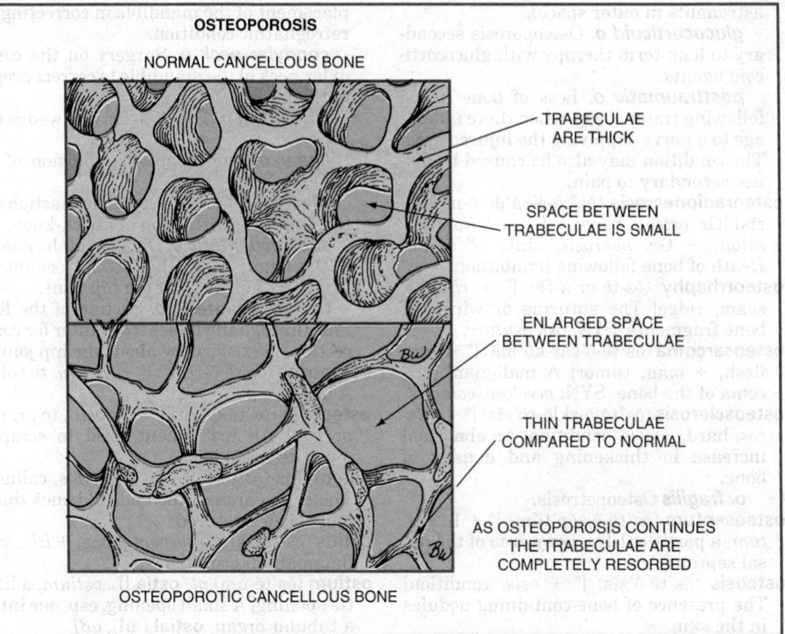


bone formation does not increase; thus, skeletal mass is not increased. Prevention of osteoporosis should begin prior to bone loss, because there has been little success in therapy aimed at restoring bone. Regular exercise, which helps to prevent bone loss, has been shown to reduce the risk of hip fracture by about one half. Patients who smoke should be encouraged to stop. The decrease in estrogen that is a normal aspect of menopause contributes to the development of osteoporosis. This can be treated, preferably at the beginning of menopause, with estrogen. The drug alendronate, a bone resorption inhibitor, produces progressive increase in bone mineral density when given to postmenopausal women with osteoporosis. This therapy can reduce the risk of vertebral fractures, the progression of vertebral deformities, and height loss in postmenopausal women. The treament of osteoporosis in men is similar to that of women with the exception that estrogen is not used.

NURSING IMPLICATIONS: The nurse recommends participation in an exercise program including proper body mechanics and range-of-motion exercises. The patient is taught to use a firm mattress and assistive safety devices at home. A diet high in vitamin C, calcium, and protein to prevent further bone loss is encouraged. The patient is instructed to seek regular gynecological follow-up examinations if maintained on estrogen therapy, to maintain good nutrition and an adequate weight, and to engage in moderate exercise throughout her life.

***o. circumscripta cranii*** Localized osteoporosis of the skull associated with Paget's disease.

***o. of disuse*** Osteoporosis due to the lack of normal functional stress on the bones. It may occur during a prolonged period of bedrest or as the result of being exposed to periods of weightlessness (e.g.,

**Risk Factors for Osteoporosis**

| |
|---|
| Female |
| Advanced age |
| White or Asian |
| Thin, small-framed body |
| Positive family history |
| Low calcium intake |
| Early menopause (before age 45) |
| Sedentary lifestyle |
| Nulliparity |
| Smoking |
| Excessive alcohol or caffeine |
| High protein intake |
| High phosphate intake |
| Certain medications, when taken for a long time (high doses of glucocorticoid, phenytoin, thyroid medication more than 2 grains) |
| Endocrine diseases (hyperthyroidism, Cushing's disease, acromegaly, hypogonadism, hyperparathyroidism |

SOURCE: Stanley, M and Beare, PG: Gerontological Nursing, FA Davis, Philadelphia, 1995.

astronauts in outer space).

***glucocorticoid o.*** Osteoporosis secondary to long-term therapy with glucocorticoid agents.

***posttraumatic o.*** Loss of bone tissue following trauma, esp. when there is damage to a nerve supplying the injured area. The condition may also be caused by disuse secondary to pain.

**osteoradionecrosis** (ŏs″tē-ō-rā″dē-ō-nē-krō′sĭs) [Gr. *osteon,* bone, + L. *radiatio,* radiation, + Gr. *nekrosis,* state of death] Death of bone following irradiation.

**osteorrhaphy** (ŏs-tē-or′ă-fē) [″ + *rhaphe,* seam, ridge] The suturing or wiring of bone fragments. SYN: *osteosuture.*

**osteosarcoma** (ŏs″tē-ō-săr-kō′mă) [″ + *sarx,* flesh, + *oma,* tumor] A malignant sarcoma of the bone. SYN: *myelosarcoma.*

**osteosclerosis** (ŏs″tē-ō-sklē-rō′sĭs) [″ + *skleros,* hard, + *osis,* condition] An abnormal increase in thickening and density of bone.

***o. fragilis*** Osteopetrosis.

**osteoseptum** (ŏs″tē-ō-sĕp′tŭm) [″ + L. *septum,* a partition] The bony area of the nasal septum.

**osteosis** (ŏs″tē-ō′sĭs) [″ + *osis,* condition] The presence of bone-containing nodules in the skin.

***o. cutis*** The formation of bone tissue in skin and subcutaneous tissue.

**osteospongioma** (ŏs″tē-ō-spŏn″jē-ō′mă) [″ + *spongos,* sponge, + *oma,* tumor] A spongy tumor in bone. SYN: *osteoma spongiosum.*

**osteosteatoma** (ŏs″tē-ō-stē″ă-tō′mă) [″ + *stear,* fat, + *oma,* tumor] A benign fatty tumor with bony elements.

**osteosuture** (ŏs″tē-ō-sū′chŭr) [″ + L. *sutura,* a stitch] Osteorrhaphy.

**osteosynovitis** (ŏs″tē-ō-sĭn″ō-vī′tĭs) [″ + *syn,* with, + *oon,* egg, + *itis,* inflammation] Inflammation of a synovial membrane and the surrounding bones.

**osteosynthesis** (ŏs″tē-ō-sĭn′thĕ-sĭs) [″ + *synthesis,* a joining] Surgical fastening of the ends of a fractured bone by mechanical means, such as a screw or plate.

**osteotelangiectasia** (ŏs″tē-ō-tĕl-ăn″jē-ĕk-tā′zē-ă) [″ + *telos,* end, + *angeion,* vessel, + *ektasis,* a stretching] A sarcomatous, heavily vascularized tumor of the bone.

**osteothrombosis** (ŏs″tē-ō-thrŏm-bō′sĭs) [″ + *thrombosis,* a clotting] The formation of a blood clot in the veins of a bone.

**osteotome** (ŏs′tē-ō-tōm) [″ + *tome,* incision] A chisel beveled on both sides for cutting through bones.

**osteotomoclasis** (ŏs″tē-ō-tō-mŏk′lă-sĭs) [Gr. *osteon,* bone, + *tomos,* section, + *klasis,* breaking] Correction of a pathologically curved bone by bending it after a wedge has been chiseled out of it by use of an osteotome.

**osteotomy** (ŏs-tē-ŏt′ō-mē) [″ + *tome,* incision] The operation for cutting through a bone.

***C-form o.*** A C-shaped cut through the ramus of the mandible to allow forward placement of the mandible in correcting a retrognathic condition.

***condylar neck o.*** Surgery on the condylar neck of the mandible to correct prognathism.

***cuneiform o.*** The excision of a wedge of bone.

***linear o.*** The lengthwise division of a bone.

***Macewen's o.*** Supracondylar section of the femur for correction of knock-knee.

***subtrochanteric o.*** Division of the shaft of the femur below the lesser trochanter to correct ankylosis of the hip joint.

***transtrochanteric o.*** Section of the femur through the lesser trochanter for correction of a deformity about the hip joint.

**osteotribe** (ŏs′tē-ō-trīb″) [″ + *tribein,* to rub] A bone rasp.

**osteotrite** (ŏs′tē-ō-trīt) [″ + *tribein,* to grind or rub] An instrument used to scrape away diseased bone.

**osteotylus** (ŏs″tē-ŏt′ĭ-lŭs) [″ + *tylos,* callus] The callus around the ends of bones that have been fractured.

**ostitis** (ŏs-tī′tĭs) [Gr. *osteon,* bone, + *itis,* inflammation] Osteitis.

**ostium** (ŏs′tē-ŭm) *pl.* **ostia** [L. *ostium,* a little opening] A small opening, esp. one into a tubular organ. **ostial** (-ăl), *adj.*

***o. abdominale tubae uterinae*** The fimbriated end of fallopian tube.

***o. arteriosum*** The arterial orifice of the ventricle of the heart into the aorta or pulmonary artery.

***o. internum*** The uterine end of a fallopian tube.

***o. pharyngeum*** The pharyngeal opening of the auditory (eustachian) tube.

***o. primum*** The primary opening in the lower part of the septum of the atria of the embryonic heart. This closes shortly after birth.

***o. primum defect*** An atrial septal defect located low in the septum.

***o. secundum*** An opening in the higher part of the septum of the atria of the embryonic heart. This closes shortly after birth.

***o. secundum defect*** An atrial septal defect located high in the septal wall.

***o. tympanicum*** The tympanic opening of the auditory (eustachian) tube.

***o. urethrae externum*** The external opening of the urethra.

***o. uteri*** The opening from the uterus to the vagina. SYN: *cervical os.*

***o. uterinum tubae*** The opening of the uterine tube into the uterus.

***o. vaginae*** The external opening of the vagina.

**ostomate** (ŏs′tō-māt) [L. *ostium,* little opening] One who has a surgically formed fistula connecting the bowel or intestine to the outside, usually through the abdominal wall. SEE: *colostomy; ileostomy.*

**ostomy** (ŏs′tō-mē) The surgically formed artificial opening that serves as the exit site for connections that the surgeon has made from the bowel or intestine to the outside of the body. SEE: *colostomy; ileostomy.*

OSTOMY CARE: Whether the ostomy is temporary or permanent, the patient should be assured that it will be possible to carry on normal activities with a minimum of inconvenience. Prior to being discharged from the hospital, the patient should be provided full explanation and demonstration of ostomy care. It is esp. important to have the patient and family become involved in ostomy care as soon as possible. This will promote confidence that a normal life will be possible. Consultation with another patient who has become competent in ostomy care will be esp. helpful. Those individuals may be contacted through ostomy clubs that have been organized in various cities. The patient should be provided with precise directions concerning places that sell ostomy care equipment. Detailed instructions for care and use of ostomy devices are included in the package.

Specific care involves the stoma (enterostomal care) and irrigation of the bowel leading from the stoma. In caring for a double-barrel colostomy, it is important to irrigate only the proximal stoma.

STOMA CARE: The character of the material excreted through the stoma will depend on the portion of the bowel to which it is attached. Excretions from the ileum will be fluid and quite irritating to skin, those from the upper right colon will be semifluid, those from the upper left colon are mushy, and those from the sigmoid colon will tend to be solid. Care of the stoma, whether for ileostomy or colostomy, is directed toward maintaining the peristomal skin and mucosa of the stoma in a healthy condition. This is more difficult to achieve with an ileostomy than with a lower colon colostomy. The skin surrounding the stoma can be protected by use of commercially available discs (washers) made of karaya gum or hypoallergenic skin shields. The collecting bag or pouch can be attached to the karaya gum washer or skin shield so that a watertight seal is made. The karaya gum washers can be used on weeping skin, but the skin shields cannot. New skin will grow beneath the karaya gum. The stoma may require only a gauze pad covering in the case of a sigmoid colostomy that is being irrigated daily or every other day. If a plastic bag is used for collecting drainage, it will need to be emptied periodically and changed as directed. At each change of the bag, meticulous but gentle skin care will be given. The stoma should not be manually dilated except by those experienced in enterostomal care.

IRRIGATION OF COLOSTOMY: Many individuals will be able to regulate the character of their diet so that the feces may be removed from the colon at planned intervals. The stoma is attached to a plastic bag held in place with a self-adhering collar or a belt. The irrigating fluid, tap water or saline solution (1 tsp or 4 g salt to 1 pint or 500 ml of water) at 40°C (104°F), is introduced slowly through a soft rubber catheter. The catheter is inserted about 10 to 15 cm, and the irrigating fluid container is hung at height that will allow fluid to flow slowly. The return from the irrigation may be collected in a closed or open-ended bag. The latter will allow the return to empty into a basin or toilet. The return of fluid and feces should be completed in less than one-half hour after irrigating fluid has entered the bowel.

At the completion of the irrigating process, the skin and stoma should be carefully cleaned and the dressing or pouch replaced. The equipment should be cleaned thoroughly and stored in a dry, well-ventilated space. When irrigation of an ostomy is provided for a hospitalized patient, charting is done on the amount and kind of fluid instilled, the amount and character of return, the care provided for the stoma, the condition of the stoma, and if a pouch or bag is replaced.

MISCELLANEOUS CONSIDERATIONS: Odor may be controlled by avoiding foods that the individual finds to cause undesirable odors. Gas may be controlled by avoiding foods known to produce gas, which will vary from patient to patient. The diet should be planned to provide a stool consistency that will be neither hard and constipating nor loose and watery. The patient may learn this by trial and error and by consulting with nutritionists and ostomy club members. Daily physical activity, sexual relations, and swimming are all possible.

**ostosis** (ŏs-tō′sĭs) Osteogenesis.

**ostraceous** (ŏs-trā′shŭs) Shaped like an oyster shell.

**ostreotoxism** (ŏs″trē-ō-tŏks′ĭzm) [Gr. *ostreon,* oyster, + *toxikon,* poison] Poisoning from eating oysters containing toxic microorganisms.

**O.T.** *occupational therapy.*

**ot-** SEE: *oto-.*

**otacoustic** (ō″tă-koo′stĭk) [Gr. *otakousteo,* to listen] **1.** Aiding or concerning the hearing. **2.** A device to aid hearing; an ear trumpet.

**otalgia** (ō-tăl′jē-ă) [Gr.] Pain in the ear. SYN: *earache; otodynia.*

TREATMENT: Local treatment consists of application of heat in the form of compresses or a hot water bottle, or instillation of warm glycerin in the affected ear. Generally, nasal astringents help maintain the patency of the eustachian tube, and appropriate systemic antibiotics may be used if there is an infection.

---

Caution: Medicines should not be placed in the external auditory canal unless the eardrum is intact.

---

**otantritis** (ō″tăn-trī′tĭs) [Gr. *otos,* ear, + L. *antrum,* sinus, + Gr. *itis,* inflammation] Inflammation of the mastoid antrum.

**O.T.(C)** *occupational therapist (Canada);* one who is a member of the Canadian Association of Occupational Therapists.

**O.T.C.** *over the counter;* refers to drugs and devices available without a prescription.

**OTD** *organ tolerance dose;* the maximum amount of radiation tolerated by specific tissues.

**otectomy** (ō-tĕk′tō-mē) [Gr. *otos,* ear, + *ektome,* excision] Surgical excision of the contents of the middle ear.

**othematoma** (ōt″hē-mă-tō′mă) [″ + *haima,* blood, + *oma,* tumor] Hematoma auris.

**otic** (ō′tĭk) [Gr. *otikos*] Concerning the ear.

**otitis** (ō-tī′tĭs) [Gr. *otos,* ear, + *itis,* inflammation] Inflammation of the ear. It is differentiated as externa, media, and interna, depending upon which portion of the ear is inflamed. **otitic** (ō-tĭt′ĭk), *adj.*

***acute o. media*** The presence of fluid in the middle ear accompanied by signs and symptoms of intense local or systemic infection.

SYMPTOMS: There may be pain in the ear, drainage of fluid from the ear canal, and hearing loss. The systemic signs include fever, irritability, headache, lethargy, anorexia, and vomiting.

TREATMENT: Nasal decongestants and antihistamines may provide some comfort for patients with upper respiratory congestion, but will not alter the course of the disease. Tympanocentesis is done in order to obtain fluid for bacteriological examination. The results of that study will help to determine appropriate antibiotic therapy. The effectiveness of therapy should be apparent within 24 to 72 hr. Pain is treated symptomatically. It usually subsides within 8 to 24 hr after institution of antibiotics. SEE: *tympanocentesis.*

---

Caution: The routine use of grommets, also called ventilation tubes, as part of the initial therapy for otitis media is not advised. It is felt that their use should be reserved for persistent or recurrent infections that have failed to respond to appropriate therapy. SEE: *grommet.*

---

NURSING IMPLICATIONS: Because some children are prone to recurrences, the nurse teaches the parents to recognize signs of otitis media and to seek medical assistance when their child complains of pain or they observe the child experiencing pain to prevent spontaneous rupture of the eardrum. Failure to treat acute and chronic ear infections may lead to temporary or permanent hearing loss in children; therefore, parents must understand the importance of proper medical follow-up.

***allergic o. media*** O. media with effusion.

***o. externa*** Inflammation of the external auditory canal.

***furuncular o.*** A furuncle formation in the external meatus of the ear.

***o. interna*** Labyrinthitis.

***o. labyrinthica*** Inflammation of the labyrinth of the ear.

***o. mastoidea*** Inflammation of the middle ear, involving the mastoid spaces.

***o. media*** Acute o. media.

***o. media with effusion*** The presence of fluid in the middle ear without signs or symptoms of acute infection. This causes retraction of the eardrum. Upon examination, a level of air fluid may be seen through the tympanic membrane. The cause of the obstruction may be enlarged adenoid tissue in the pharynx, inflammation in the pharynx, tumors in the pharyngeal area, or allergy. SYN: *allergic otitis media; nonsuppurative otitis media; secretory otitis media; serous otitis media.*

TREATMENT: Nasal decongestants may afford symptomatic relief. The use of antibiotics is controversial. Adenoidectomy and bilateral myringotomy may be necessary if conservative measures, including insertion of a ventilation or tympanostomy tube, are not effective. Adenoidectomy is not advisable in children under 4 years of age. SEE: *tympanocentesis; tympanostomy tubes.*

---

Caution: The routine use of grommets, also called ventilation tubes, as part of the initial therapy for otitis media is not advised. It is felt that their use should be reserved for persistent or recurrent infections that have failed to respond to appropriate therapy. SEE: *grommet.*

---

***o. mycotica*** Inflammation of the ear caused by a fungal infection.

***nonsuppurative o. media*** O. media with effusion.

***o. parasitica*** Inflammation of the ear caused by a parasite.

***o. sclerotica*** Inflammation of the inner ear accompanied by hardening of the aural structures.

***secretory o. media*** O. media with effusion.

***serous o. media*** O. media with effusion.

**oto-, ot-** [Gr. *otos,* ear] Combining form meaning *ear.*

**otoantritis** (ō″tō-ăn-trī′tĭs) [″ + *antron,* cavity, + *itis,* inflammation] Inflammation of the mastoid antrum and tympanic attic.

**otocephalus** (ō″tō-sĕf′ă-lŭs) One with otocephaly.

**otocephaly** (ō″tō-sĕf′ă-lē) [″ + *kephale,* head] A congenital absence of the lower jaw and fusion or near fusion of the ears on the front of the neck.

**otocyst** (ō′tō-sĭst) [″ + *kystis,* sac, bladder] A primordial chamber from which arises the membranous labyrinth.

**otodynia** (ō″tō-dĭn′ē-ă) [″ + *odyne,* pain] Otalgia.

**otogenic, otogenous** (ō″tō-jĕn′ĭk, ō-tŏj′ĕn-ŭs) [″ + *gennan,* to produce] Originating in the ear.

**otolaryngologist** (ō″tō-lar″ĭn-gŏl′ō-jĭst) [″ + *larynx,* larynx, + *logos,* word, reason] A specialist in otolaryngology.

**otolaryngology** (ō″tō-lar″ĭn-gŏl′ō-jē) The division of medical science that includes otology, rhinology, and laryngology.

**otological** (ō″tō-lŏj′ĭ-kăl) [″ + *logos,* word, reason] Relating to study of diseases of the ear.

**otologist** (ō-tŏl′ō-jĭst) One knowledgeable in the anatomy, physiology, and pathology of the ear; a specialist in diseases of the ear.

**otology** (ō-tŏl′ō-jē) [Gr. *otos,* ear, + *logos,* word, reason] The science dealing with the ear, its function, and its diseases.

**otomassage** [″ + *massein,* to knead] Massage of the tympanic membrane and bones of the middle ear by means such as sound waves, puffs of air in the ear canal, or vibratory percussion of the tympanic membrane.

**otomucormycosis** (ō″tō-mū″kor-mī-kō′sĭs) [″ + L. *mucor,* mold, + Gr. *mykes,* fungus, + *osis,* condition] Mucormycosis of the ear.

**otomyces** (ō″tō-mī′sēz) [″ + *mykes,* fungus] Any fungus infection of the ear.

**otomycosis** (ō″tō-mī-kō′sĭs) [″ + ″ + *osis,* condition] An infection of the external auditory meatus of the ear caused by a fungus infestation. SYN: *myringomycosis; otitis mycotica.*

**otoncus** (ō-tŏng′kŭs) [″ + *onkos,* tumor] A tumor of the ear.

**otonecrectomy, otonecronectomy** (ō″tō-nē-krĕk′tō-mē, ō″tō-nē″krō-nĕk′tō-mē) [″ + *nekros,* corpse, + *ektome,* excision] Excision of necrosed areas from the ear.

**otoneurasthenia** (ō″tō-nū″răs-thē′nē-ă) [″ + ″ + *astheneia,* weakness] Neurasthenia caused by ear disease.

**otoneurology** (ō″tō-nū-rŏl′ō-jē) [″ + ″ + *logos,* word, reason] The division of otology that deals with the inner ear, esp. its nerve supply, nerve connections with the brain, and auditory and labyrinthine pathways and centers within the brain. SYN: *neurotology.*

**otopharyngeal** (ō″tō-făr-ĭn′jē-ăl) [″ + *pharynx,* throat] Concerning the ear and pharynx.

**otoplasty** (ō′tō-plăs″tē) [″ + *plassein,* to form] Plastic surgery of the ear to correct defects and deformities.

**otorhinolaryngology** (ō″tō-rī″nō-lăr″ĭn-gŏl′ō-jē) [″ + *rhis,* nose, + *larynx,* larynx, + *logos,* word, reason] The science of the ear, nose, and larynx, and their functions and diseases.

**otorhinology** (ō″tō-rī-nŏl′ō-jē) [″ + ″ + *logos,* word, reason] The branch of medicine dealing with the ear and nose and their diseases.

**otorrhea** (ō″tō-rē′ă) [″ + *rhein,* flow] Inflammation of ear with purulent discharge. SEE: *otitis.*

**otoscleronectomy** (ō″tō-sklē″rō-nĕk′tō-mē) [″ + *skleros,* hard, + *ektome,* excision] Surgical excision of sclerosed and ankylosed ear ossicles.

**otosclerosis** (ō″tō-sklē-rō′sĭs) [″ + *sklerosis,* hardening] A condition characterized by chronic progressive deafness, esp. for low tones. It is caused by the formation of spongy bone, esp. around the oval window, with resulting ankylosis of the stapes. In the late stages of this condition, atrophy of the organ of Corti may occur. The cause of this condition is unknown; however, it may be familial. It is more common in women, and may be made worse by pregnancy.

TREATMENT: Various surgical procedures, including stapedectomy, have been used with considerable improvement in hearing. Because the three bones of the middle ear become fused, patients with this condition cannot normally transmit sound to inner ear from the vibrations of the tympanic membrane. The excellent results achieved from removing the stapes and inserting a stapes implant to allow the bones to function normally again makes identification of children and adults who could benefit from this procedure especially important.

**otoscope** (ō′tō-skōp) [″ + *skopein,* to examine] A device for examination of the ear.

**otoscopy** (ō-tŏs′kō-pē) The use of the otoscope in examining the ear.

**otosteal** (ō-tŏs′tē-ăl) [″ + *osteon,* bone] Concerning the bones or ossicles of the ear.

**ototomy** (ō-tŏt′ō-mē) [″ + *tome,* incision] Incision or dissection of the ear.

**ototoxic** (ō″tō-tŏk′sĭk) [″ + *toxikon,* poison] Having a detrimental effect on the eighth nerve or the organs of hearing.

**O.T.R.** *Occupational Therapist, Registered.*

**Otrivin Hydrochloride** Trade name for xylometazoline hydrochloride.

**OTR/L** *Licensed Occupational Therapist.*

**Otto pelvis** (ŏt′ō) [Adolph W. Otto, Ger. surgeon, 1786–1845] The protrusion of the acetabulum into the pelvic cavity. This condition may occur in association with severe osteoarthritis of the hip.

**O.U., o.u.** L. *oculus uterque,* each eye.

**ouabain** (wă-bā′ĭn) A glycoside prepared from *Strophanthus gratus.* Its action is similar to that of digitalis.

**oulitis** (oo-lī′tĭs) [Gr. *oulon,* gum, + *itis,* inflammation] Inflammation of the gums.

**oulorrhagia** (oo-lō-rā′jē-ă) [″ + *rhegnynai,* to burst forth] Hemorrhage from the gums.

**-ous 1.** Suffix meaning *possessing, full of.* **2.** Suffix meaning *pertaining to.*

**outbreak** The sudden increase in the incidence of a disease or condition in a specific area.

**outcome** The result of an action.

***o. criteria*** Quality assurance program guidelines in which the adequacy of the program is judged by the achievement of predetermined goals.

***functional o.*** In rehabilitation therapy, a long-term goal toward which a therapeutic program is directed to help a patient return to or achieve a specific activity level.

**outflow** In neurology, the passage of impulses outwardly from the central nervous system.

***craniosacral o.*** Impulses passing through parasympathetic nerves.

***thoracolumbar o.*** Impulses passing through sympathetic nerves.

**outlet** A vent or opening through which something can escape.

***pelvic o.*** The lower pelvic opening between the tip of the coccyx, the ischial tuberosities, and the lower margin of the symphysis pubis.

***quick-connect o.*** A device that allows a compressed gas container to be quickly connected to and disconnected from the delivery unit.

**out-of-body experience** The perception of being away from and overlooking oneself; the feeling that the mind and soul have separated from the body.

**outpatient** One who receives treatment at a hospital, clinic, or dispensary but is not hospitalized.

**outpocketing** Evagination.

**output** (owt′poot) That which is produced, ejected, or expelled.

***cardiac o.*** The volume of blood pumped into the arterial system per unit of time. The stroke volume multiplied by the heart rate per minute gives the cardiac output. The normal cardiac output value in healthy adults is 2.5 to 6.0 liters per minute.

***energy o.*** The work expended by the body per unit of time.

***stroke o.*** The amount of blood pumped in a single heartbeat.

***urinary o.*** The amount of urine produced by the kidneys.

**outrigger** An attachment for hand splints that permits the fingers to be placed in elastic traction.

**outsourcing** A method in which services usually provided by the health care agency are now allocated to an outside firm or agency.

**ova** (ō′vă) [L. *ovum,* egg] Pl. of ovum.

**oval** (ō′văl) [L. *ovalis,* egg shaped] **1.** Concerning an ovum, the reproductive cell of the female. **2.** Having an elliptical shape like an egg.

**ovalbumin** (ō″văl-bū′mĭn) [″ + *albumen,* white of egg] Albumin occurring in egg white.

**ovalocyte** (ō′văl-ō-sīt″) [″ + Gr. *kytos,* cell] An elliptical red blood corpuscle.

**ovalocytosis** (ō-văl″ō-sī-tō′sĭs) [″ + ″ + *osis,* condition] An abnormally large amount of elliptical red blood corpuscles in the blood.

**oval window** An oval-shaped aperture in the middle ear into which fits the base of the stapes.

**ovaralgia, ovarialgia** (ō″văr-ăl′jē-ă, -ē-ăl′jē-ă) [LL. *ovarium,* ovary, + Gr. *algos,* pain] Ovarian pain. SYN: *oarialgia.*

**ovari-** SEE: *ovario-.*

**ovarian** (ō-vā′rē-ăn) [LL. *ovarium,* ovary] Concerning or resembling the ovary.

**ovarian cyst** A sac that develops in the ovary proper. It consists of one or more chambers containing fluid. These loculi, or chambers, may contain an enormous amount of fluid. Although nonmalignant, the cyst may have to be removed surgically because of twisting of the pedicle, which causes gangrene, or because of pressure. SEE: *polycystic ovary syndrome.*

**ovariectomy** (ō″vā-rē-ĕk′tō-mē) [″ + Gr. *ektome,* excision] The partial or complete excision of an ovary. SYN: *oophorectomy.*

**ovario-, ovari-** [LL. *ovarium,* ovary] Combining form meaning *ovary.*

**ovariocele** (ō-vā′rē-ō-sēl) [″ + Gr. *kele,* tumor, swelling] An ovarian tumor or hernia.

**ovariocentesis** (ō-vā″rē-ō-sĕn-tē′sĭs) [″ + Gr. *kentesis,* puncture] Surgical puncture and drainage of an ovarian cyst.

**ovariocyesis** (ō-vā″rē-ō-sī-ē′sĭs) [″ + Gr. *kyesis,* pregnancy] An ectopic pregnancy in an ovary. SEE: *gestation, ectopic.*

**ovariogenic** (ō-vā″rē-ō-jĕn′ĭk) [″ + *gennan,* to produce] Originating in the ovary.

**ovariopexy** (ō-vā″rē-ō-pĕk′sē) [″ + *pexis,* fixation] Surgical fixation of the ovary to the abdominal wall.

**ovariorrhexis** (ō-vā″rē-ō-rĕk′sĭs) [″ + Gr. *rhexis,* a rupture] Rupture of an ovary.

**ovariosalpingectomy** (ō-vā″rē-ō-săl″pĭn-jĕk′tō-mē) [″ + Gr. *salpinx,* tube, + *ektome,* excision] Salpingo-oophorectomy.

**ovariostomy** (ō-vā″rē-ŏs′tō-mē) [″ + Gr. *stoma,* mouth] The creation of an opening in an ovarian cyst for the purpose of drainage.

**ovariotomy** (ō-vā″rē-ŏt′ō-mē) [LL. *ovarium,* ovary, + Gr. *tome,* incision] **1.** The incision or removal of an ovary. **2.** The removal of a tumor of the ovary.

**ovariotubal** (ō-vā″rē-ō-tū′băl) [″ + *tuba,* a narrow duct] Concerning the ovary and oviducts.

**ovariprival** (ō-vā″rĭ-prī′văl) [″ + *privare,* to remove] Resulting from loss of the ovaries.

**ovaritis** (ō″vă-rī′tĭs) [″ + Gr. *itis,* inflammation] The acute or chronic inflammation of an ovary, usually secondary to inflammation of the oviducts or pelvic peritoneum. It may involve the substance of the organ (oophoritis) or its surface (perioophoritis).

**ovarium** (ō-vā′rē-ŭm) *pl.* **ovaria** [LL.] The ovary.

**ovary** (ō′vă-rē) [LL. *ovarium,* ovary] One of

two glands in the female that produce the reproductive cell, the ovum, and two known hormones. The ovaries are almond-shaped bodies lying in the fossa ovarica on either side of the pelvic cavity, attached to the uterus by the utero-ovarian ligament, and lying close to the fimbria ovarica of the fallopian tube. Each ovary is about 4 cm long, 2 cm wide, and 8 mm thick, and is attached to the broad ligament by the mesovarium and to the side of the pelvis by the suspensory ligament. In early life, the surface of the ovary is smooth; in later life, it is markedly pitted as an end result of the rupture and atrophy of the corpora lutea.

Each ovary consists of two parts. The outer portion (cortex) encloses a central medulla, which consists of a stroma of connective tissue containing nerves, blood, and lymphatic vessels, and some smooth muscle tissue at region of hilus. The cortex consists principally of follicles in various stages of development (primary, growing, and mature or graafian). Its surface is covered by a single layer of cells, the germinal epithelium, beneath which is a layer of dense connective tissue, the tunica albuginea. Each of the 400,000 follicles present in the ovaries at birth has the potential for maturity but fewer than 400 mature during the reproductive period. Other structures (corpus luteum, corpus albicans) may be present. The blood supply is mainly derived from the ovarian artery, which reaches the ovary through the infundibulopelvic ligament. SEE: *fertilization* for illus.; *oogenesis* for illus.

PHYSIOLOGY: The two functions of the ovaries are the production of ova and hormones. The hormones produced are estrogen, secreted by the follicles, and progesterone, secreted by the corpus luteum. These hormones are responsible for development and maintenance of secondary sexual characteristics, preparation of uterus for pregnancy, and development of the mammary gland.

The functional activity of the ovary is controlled primarily by gonadotropins of the hypophysis, esp. the follicle-stimulating hormone (FSH) and luteinizing hormone (LH).

**overbite** The vertical extension of the incisal ridges of the upper teeth over the incisal ridges of the lower anterior teeth when the jaws are in occlusion.

**overclosure** A form of defective bite in which the mandible closes too far before the teeth make contact.

**overcompensation** The process by which a person substitutes an opposite trait or exerts effort in excess of that needed to compensate for, or conceal, a psychological feeling of guilt, inadequacy, or inferiority. May lead to maladjustment.

**overcorrection** The use of too powerful a lens to correct a defect in the refractive power of the eye.

**overdenture** A denture supported by the soft tissue and whatever natural teeth remain. These have been altered so the denture will fit over them.

**overdetermination** The idea in psychoanalysis that every symptom and dream may have several meanings, being determined by more than a single association.

**overdose** ABBR: OD. A dose of a drug, esp. a drug of abuse, sufficient to cause an acute reaction such as coma, mania, hysteria, or even death.

**overeruption** A condition in which the occluding surface of a tooth projects beyond the line of occlusion.

**overexertion** Physical exertion to a state of abnormal exhaustion.

**overextension 1.** Extension beyond that which usually occurs. SYN: *hyperextension*. **2.** In dentistry, the assessment of the vertical extent of a root canal filling, denoting an extrusion beyond the apical foramen.

**overflow** The continuous escape of fluid from a vessel or viscus, as of urine or tears.

**overgrowth 1.** Excessive growth. SYN: *hyperplasia; hypertrophy*. **2.** In bacteriology, the growth of one type of microorganism on a culture plate so that it covers and obscures the growth of other types.

**overhang** The undesirable extension beyond the margins of a cavity of the excess filling material used.

**overhydration** An excess of fluids in the body.

**overjet** Horizontal overlap of the teeth.

**overlap** Something that covers the tissue or object but also extends past the border.

**overlay 1.** An addition superimposed upon an already existing state. **2.** In dentistry, a cast restoration for the occlusal surface of one or more cusps of a tooth but not a three-quarter- or full-cast crown.

***psychogenic o.*** The emotional component of a symptom or illness that has an organic basis.

**overmedication** The practice of taking more medicines than are needed. This is esp. prevalent in elderly patients who have several conditions that require medication. The patient may forget which pill to take and at what frequency. Often this is complicated by the patient's being under the care of two or more physicians who do not coordinate their management of the patient and the drugs prescribed. Drug interaction, both with prescribed and over-the-counter drugs, is another possibility in any patient taking a variety of drugs. Therefore, it is important that one individual have full knowledge of all of the medicines a patient is taking.

**overpressure** A force applied passively to a joint and surrounding soft tissue at the end of the range of motion in order to determine the end feel of the tissues.

**overproduction** Excessive output of an organic element during the reparative process, as excessive callous development after a bone fracture. SEE: *keloid.*

**overresponse** An abnormally intense reaction to a stimulus; an inappropriate degree of response.

**overriding** The slipping of one end of a fractured bone past the other part.

**overshoot** A response to a stimulus that is greater than would normally be expected.

**overtoe** Hallux varus of the great toe to the extent that it rests over the other toes.

**overtone** In music and acoustics, a harmonic.

**overuse syndrome** An injury to musculoskeletal tissues typically affecting the upper extremity or cervical spine, resulting from repeated movement, temperature extremes, overuse, incorrect posture, or sustained force or vibration. Resulting disorders include carpal tunnel syndrome, tenosynovitis, tendinitis, pronator syndrome, peritendinitis, thoracic outlet syndrome, and cervical syndrome, each of which often results from demands of the work environment. Treatment for these conditions often involves surgery or immobilization. There is a growing awareness of the importance of prevention through education, task modification, and workplace design based on ergonomic principles. SYN: *cumulative trauma syndrome; repetitive motion injury; repetitive strain injury.* SEE: *ergonomics.*

**overvalued idea** An unreasonable and strongly held belief or idea. Such a belief is beyond the norm of beliefs held or accepted by other members of the person's culture or subculture.

**ovi-** [L. *ovum,* egg] Combining form meaning *egg.*

**ovi albumin** (ō″vē-ăl-bū′mĭn) [L.] Ovalbumin.

**ovicide** (ō′vĭ-sīd) [L. *ovum,* egg, + *caedere,* to kill] An agent destructive to ova.

**oviduct** (ō′vĭ-dŭkt) [″+ *ductus,* a path] In the human female, one of two tubes extending laterally from the superior angles of the uterus and conveying the ovum from the ovary to the uterus. Each oviduct consists of the infundibulum, an expanded portion surrounding the ostium or opening through which the ovum enters, bearing many fingerlike processes called fimbriae; the ampulla, the tube itself; and the isthmus, a straight narrow portion that connects with the uterus. Each oviduct is a tube consisting of three layers: mucosa, muscle, and serosa. The mucosa consists of columnar epithelial cells, some ciliated, others glandular. In addition to conveying the ovum, the oviduct provides a passageway through which sperm travel from the uterus toward the ovary. It is the usual site of fertilization of the ovum. SYN: *fallopian tube; uterine tube.*

**oviferous** (ō-vĭf′ĕr-ŭs) [″ + *ferre,* to bear] Containing or producing ova.

**oviform** (ō′vĭ-form) [″+ *forma,* shape] **1.** Having the shape of an egg. SYN: *ovoid.* **2.** Resembling an ovum.

**ovigenesis** [″ + Gr. *gennan,* to produce] Oogenesis.

**ovigerm** (ō′vĭ-jĕrm) [″ + *germen,* a bud] The cell that produces or develops into an ovum.

**ovination** (ō″vĭ-nā′shŭn) [L. *ovinus,* of a sheep] Inoculation with the sheep-pox virus.

**ovine** (ō′vīn) [L. *ovinus,* of a sheep] Concerning sheep.

**oviparity** (ō″vĭ-păr′ĭ-tē) The quality of being oviparous.

**oviparous** (ō-vĭp′ăr-ŭs) [L. *ovum,* egg, + *parere,* to produce] Producing eggs that are hatched outside the body; egg laying; the opposite of ovoviviparous.

**oviposition** [″ + *ponere,* to place] The laying of eggs as in oviparous reproduction.

**ovipositor** (ō″vĭ-pŏs′ĭ-tor) A specialized tubular structure found in many female insects, through which they lay their eggs in plants or soil.

**ovisac** (ō′vĭ-săk) The graafian follicle.

**ovo-** [L. *ovum,* egg] Combining form meaning *egg.*

**ovocenter** The centrosome of a fertilized ovum.

**ovocyte** (ō′vō-sīt) [″ + *kytos,* cell] Oocyte.

**ovoflavin** (ō″vō-flā′vĭn) [″+ *flavus,* yellow] A flavin derived from eggs; identical to riboflavin.

**ovogenesis** (ō″vō-jĕn′ĕ-sĭs) [″ + Gr. *genesis,* generation, birth] Production of ova. SYN: *oogenesis.*

**ovoglobulin** (ō″vō-glŏb′ū-lĭn) [″ + *globulus,* globule] The globulin found in egg white. SEE: *albumin; protein, simple.*

**ovoid** (ō′voyd) [L. *ovum,* egg, + Gr. *eidos,* form, shape] **1.** Shaped like an egg. SYN: *oviform.* **2.** A cylindrical apparatus attached to a handle, used as a pair to hold a radioactive source during brachytherapy of the cervix.

**ovomucin** (ō″vō-mū′sĭn) A glycoprotein in the white of an egg.

**ovomucoid** (ō″vō-mū′koyd) [″+ *mucus,* mucus, + Gr. *eidos,* form, shape] A glycoprotein principle derived from egg white.

**ovoplasm** (ō′vō-plăzm) [″+ LL. *plasma,* form, mold] The protoplasm of an unfertilized egg. SEE: *ooplasm.*

**ovotestis** (ō″vō-tĕs′tĭs) A gonad that contains both testicular and ovarian tissue.

**ovovitellin** (ō″vō-vī-tĕl′ĭn) [″ + *vitellus,* yolk] A protein found in an egg yolk.

**ovoviviparous** (ō″vō-vī-vĭp′ă-rŭs) [″ + *vivus,* alive, + *parere,* to bring forth, to bear] Reproducing by eggs that have a well-developed membrane and that hatch inside the maternal organism; opposite of oviparous.

**ovular** (ō′vū-lăr) [L. *ovulum,* little egg] Concerning an ovule or ovum.

**ovulation** (ŏv″ū-lā′shŭn) [L. *ovulum,* little egg] The periodic ripening and rupture of the mature graafian follicle and the discharge of the ovum from the cortex of the ovary. Ovulation occurs approx. 14 days before the next menstrual period. It is virtually impossible to determine when ovulation will occur by counting from the first day of the preceding menstrual period. Following ovulation, a corpus luteum develops within the collapsed follicle. The ovum, being liberated from the follicle, enters the fallopian tube and is transported slowly toward the uterus. If sperm are present, the ovum may become fertilized; if not, it degenerates within the oviduct and is passed out of the body with the menstrual flow.

**ovulation induction** Stimulating ovulation by the use of drugs such as clomiphene citrate, bromocriptine, human menopausal gonadotropin, or gonadotropin-releasing hormone. SEE: *fertilization, in vitro; syndrome, ovarian hyperstimulation.*

**ovulatory** (ŏv′ū-lă-tō″rē) Concerning ovulation.

**ovule** (ō′vūl) [L. *ovulum*] **1.** The ovum in the graafian follicle. **2.** A small egg.

**ovulogenous** (ō-vū-lŏj′ĕn-ŭs) **1.** Giving rise to ovules or ova. **2.** Originating from an ovule or ovum.

**ovum** (ō′vŭm) *pl.* **ova** [L., egg] The female reproductive or germ cell; a cell that is capable of developing into a new organism of the same species. Usually fertilization by a spermatozoon is necessary, although in some lower animals ova develop without fertilization (parthenogenesis).

The various parts of the ovum are the protoplasm, known as the vitellus or yolk and its outermost layer referred to as the ectoplasm; the zona pellucida or zona radiata, the inner layer (cell membrane), known as the vitelline membrane; the nucleus, called the germinal vesicle; and the nucleolus, the germinal spot.

The cellular layers proliferate, becoming cuboid, and a clear albuminous fluid (liquor folliculi) forms in the center. The follicular cells surrounding the fluid-filled cavity are known as the membrana granulosa. The layer surrounding the egg cell, or oocyte, is known as the discus proligerus or cumulus oophorus.

As the follicular layer enlarges to form the graafian follicle, the term for the developed ovum before it leaves the ovary, there is a slight protrusion of the ovarian surface. Rupture through the ovarian surface frees the ovum, which then proceeds through the fallopian tube and into the uterus. This process is known as ovulation. It usually takes the ovum from 5 to 7 days to go from the ovary to the uterus. Normally, only one graafian follicle matures each month, not necessarily in alternate ovaries. SEE: illus.; *conception; fertilization; menstrual cycle; menstruation.*

***alecithal o.*** An ovum with a small yolk portion that is distributed throughout the protoplasm. SYN: *isolecithal o.*

***centrolecithal o.*** An ovum having a large central food yolk, as in a bird's egg.

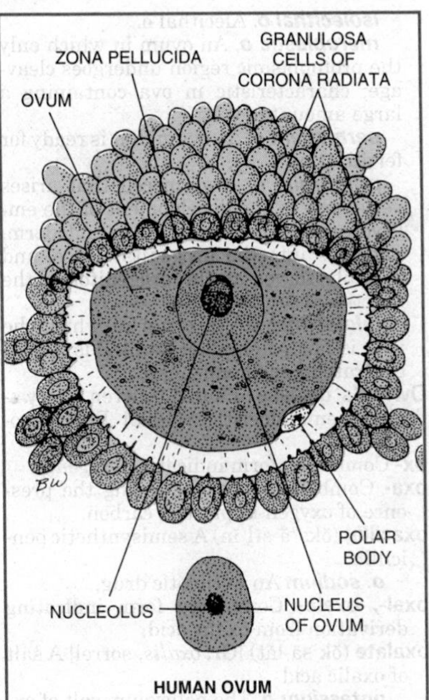

HUMAN OVUM

***holoblastic o.*** An ovum that undergoes complete cleavage, as opposed to partial or meroblastic cleavage.

***human o.*** The female reproductive cell that develops within the graafian follicle of the ovary. It develops from an oogonium that undergoes a process of maturation (oogenesis), during which primary and secondary oocytes are produced, finally giving rise to the mature ovum. During this process, the number of chromosomes is reduced from 46 to 23 and the egg is prepared for fertilization. SEE: *cleavage; conception; embryo, development of; fertilization; follicle; menstruation; ovulation; spermatozoon.*

A mature ovum is approx. 0.130 to 0.140 mm (0.0051 to 0.0055 in.) in diameter. Each contains a spherical nucleus, bounded by a nuclear membrane, enclosing chromatin material and one or more nucleoli. The cytoplasm is granular and contains yolk granules or deuteroplasm and other characteristic organoids of cells. Its surface layer is the vitelline membrane. When liberated from the ovary as a primary oocyte, it is surrounded by a clear layer, zona pellucida, and several layers of adhering follicular cells, the latter constituting the corona radiata.

The length of time a human ovum retains its ability to be fertilized and develop is not known precisely, but it is probably at least 48 hours. If fertilized, it undergoes development. If not fertilized, it degenerates.

***isolecithal o.*** Alecithal o.

***meroblastic o.*** An ovum in which only the protoplasmic region undergoes cleavage; characteristic in ova containing a large amount of yolk.

***permanent o.*** An ovum that is ready for fertilization.

***primordial o.*** A germ cell that arises very early in the development of the embryo, usually in the yolk sac endoderm, migrates into the urogenital ridge, and possibly serves as the progenitor of the functional sex cell.

***telolecithal o.*** An ovum in which the yolk is fairly abundant and tends to concentrate in one hemisphere.

**Owren's disease** [Paul A. Owren, Norwegian hematologist, b. 1905] Parahemophilia.

**ox-** Combining form indicating *oxygen.*

**oxa-** Combining form indicating the presence of oxygen in place of carbon.

**oxacillin** (ŏks″ă-sĭl′ĭn) A semisynthetic penicillin.

***o. sodium*** An antibiotic drug.

**oxal-, oxalo-** Combining form indicating derivation from oxalic acid.

**oxalate** (ŏk′să-lāt) [Gr. *oxalis,* sorrel] A salt of oxalic acid.

***potassium o.*** The potassium salt of oxalic acid.

**oxalemia** (ŏk″să-lē′mē-ă) [″ + *haima,* blood] Excess oxalates in the blood.

**oxalism** (ŏks′ăl-ĭzm) [Gr. *oxalis,* sorrel, + *-ismos,* condition] Poisoning from oxalic acid or an oxalate.

**oxaloacetic acid** (ŏks″ă-lō-ă-sē′tĭk) A product of carbohydrate metabolism $HOOC \cdot CH_2 \cdot CO \cdot COOH$ resulting from oxidation of malic acid during the Krebs cycle. May be derived from other sources.

**oxalosis** An autosomal recessive hereditary disease due to faulty metabolism of glyoxylic acid. Oxalic acid is elevated in the urine because of the increased production of oxalic acid. Calcium oxalate is deposited in body tissues, esp. in the kidneys.

**oxaluria** (ŏk-să-lū′rē-ă) [″ + *ouron,* urine] Excess excretion of oxalates in the urine, esp. calcium oxalate.

**oxalylurea** (ŏk″săl-ĭl-ū-rē′ă) An oxidation product of uric acid.

**oxandrolone** (ŏk-săn′drō-lōn) An anabolic steroid.

**oxazepam** (ŏks-ăz′ĕ-păm) A short-acting, benzodiazepine, antianxiety drug.

**oxidant** (ŏk′sĭ-dănt) In oxidation-reduction reactions, the acceptor of an electron.

**oxidase** (ŏk′sĭ-dās) [Gr. *oxys,* sharp] A class of enzymes present in animal and vegetable life that catalyzes an oxidation reaction; a respiratory enzyme.

***cytochrome o.*** An enzyme present in most cells that oxidizes reduced cytochrome back to cytochrome.

**oxidation** (ŏk′sĭ-dā′shŭn) [Gr. *oxys,* sharp] **1.** The process of a substance combining with oxygen. **2.** The loss of electrons in an atom with an accompanying increase in positive valence. SEE: *reduce* (2).

**oxidation-reduction reaction** A chemical interaction in which one substance is oxidized and loses electrons, and thus is increased in positive valence, while another substance gains an equal number of electrons by being reduced. This is called a redox system or reaction.

**oxide** (ŏk′sīd) Any chemical compound in which oxygen is the negative radical.

**oxidize** (ŏk′sĭ-dīz) **1.** To combine with oxygen. **2.** To increase the positive valence, or to decrease the negative valence, by bringing about a loss of electrons. SYN: *oxygenize.* SEE: *oxidation-reduction reaction.*

**oxidoreductase** (ŏk″sĭ-dō-rē-dŭk′tās) An enzyme that catalyzes oxidation-reduction reactions.

**oxim, oxime** (ŏk′sĭm) Any compound produced by the action of hydroxylamine on an aldehyde or ketone. When an aldehyde is involved, the general formula $RCH = NOH$ is produced. When a ketone is acted upon, $R_2CH = NOH$ is produced.

**oximeter** (ŏk-sĭm′ĕ-tĕr) [Gr. *oxys,* sharp, + *metron,* measure] An electronic device for determining the oxygen concentration in arterial blood. The oximeter may be attached to the bridge of the nose, the forehead, an ear lobe, or to the tip of a finger, preferably the index, middle, or ring finger. Also an oximeter may be attached to a toe if there is adequate circulation to the foot.

---

Caution: The oximeter should not be so tight that it prevents circulation to the finger, toe, or ear lobe.

---

***ear o.*** An oximeter that attaches to the pinna of the ear to determine the degree of oxygen saturation of blood flowing through the ear.

***finger o.*** A pulse oximeter that attaches to the finger.

***pulse o.*** Finger o.

**oximmetry** The use of an oximeter to determine the oxygen saturation of blood.

**oxisensor** A noninvasive device used to determine the oxygen saturation. It is usually applied to a readily accessible site such as the nose, earlobe, toe, or finger. SEE: *oximeter.*

**oxtriphylline** (ŏks-trĭf′ĭ-lēn) A drug that resembles theophylline in its actions.

**oxy-** [Gr. *oxys*] **1.** Combining form indicating *sharp, keen, acute, acid, pungent.* **2.** Combining form indicating the presence of oxygen in a compound. **3.** Combining form indicating the presence of a hydroxyl group.

**oxyacusis** (ŏk″sē-ă-kū′sĭs) [Gr. *oxys,* sharp, + *akousis,* hearing] Hyperacusis.

**oxybenzene** (ŏk″sē-bĕn′zēn) Phenol.

**oxyblepsia** (ŏk″sē-blĕp′sē-ă) [Gr. *oxys,* sharp, + *blepsis,* vision] Extraordinary acuteness of vision.

**oxybutyria** (ŏk″sē-bū-tĭr′ē-ă) Oxybutyric acid in the urine.

**oxycalcium** (ŏk″sē-kăl′sē-ŭm) Of or pert. to oxygen and calcium.

**oxycellulose** Cellulose that has undergone oxidation.

**oxycephalous** (ŏk-sē-sĕf′ă-lŭs) [Gr. *oxys,* sharp, + *kephale,* head] Denoting a head that is pointed and conelike.

**oxycephaly** (ŏk″sē-sĕf′ă-lē) Acrocephaly.

**oxychloride** (ŏk″sē-klō′rīd) [Gr. *oxys,* sharp, + *chloros,* green] A compound consisting of an element or radical combined with oxygen and chlorine or the hydroxyl radical (OH) and chlorine.

**oxychromatic** (ŏk″sē-krō-măt′ĭk) [″ + *chroma,* color] Staining readily with acid dyes.

**oxychromatin** (ŏk″sē-krō′mă-tĭn) The part of chromatin that stains readily with acid dyes.

**oxyecoia** (ŏk″sē-ē-koy′ă) [″ + *akoe,* hearing] Abnormal sensitivity to noises.

**oxyesthesia** (ŏk″sē-ĕs-thē′zē-ă) [″ + *aisthesis,* sensation] Abnormal acuteness of sensation. SYN: *algesia; hyperesthesia.*

**oxygen** (ŏk′sĭ-jĕn) [Gr. *oxys,* sharp, + *gennan,* to produce] **1.** A standardized preparation of oxygen used as a medicinal gas. **2.** SYMB: O. A nonmetallic element occurring free in the atmosphere (approx. 21%) as a colorless, odorless, tasteless gas; atomic weight 15.9994; atomic number 8. It is a constituent of animal, vegetable, and mineral substances. Oxygen is essential to respiration for most living organisms and is the most important and abundant element. At sea level, it represents 10% to 16% of venous blood and 17% to 21% of arterial blood.

Oxygen is absorbed in the free state by most living organisms. It is produced by green plants from carbon dioxide and water during photosynthesis; carbohydrates such as glucose and starch are also produced by this process. When oxygen is used in cell respiration, the end products are water and carbon dioxide, the latter of which is returned to the atmosphere. Thus, the balance of oxygen and carbon dioxide in the atmosphere is maintained.

When oxygen combines with another substance, the process is called oxidation. When combination takes place rapidly enough to produce light and heat, the process is called burning or combustion. Oxygen combines readily with other elements to form oxides.

USES: Oxygen is used in cases where there is insufficient oxygen carried by the blood to the tissues (e.g., severe anemia, shock or circulatory collapse, pulmonary edema, pneumonia) or by mountain climbers, astronauts, or aviators when at heights where the amount of oxygen present in the atmosphere is insufficient to support life.

Frequently oxygen is employed with agents used for the induction of general anesthesia. Following extensive surgery, oxygen reduces reactions to the anesthetic. It is also employed to treat septicemia, gas gangrene, peritonitis, and intestinal obstruction.

ADMINISTRATION: Oxygen is administered by mask, nasal tube, tent, or in an airtight chamber in which pressure may be increased. No matter how much oxygen is given, it is important to have it adequately humidified. It is desirable to administer oxygen at whatever rate is necessary to increase the oxygen content of inspired air to 50%. SEE: *hypoxia.*

---

Caution: Inhalation of high concentrations of oxygen, esp. at pressures of more than one atmosphere, may produce deleterious effects such as irritation of respiratory tract, reduced vital capacity, and sometimes neurological symptoms. Serious eye defects may result if premature infants are exposed to a high concentration of oxygen as part of their therapy. SEE: *retrolental fibroplasia.*

Because oxygen provides a perfect environment for combustion, it should not be used in the presence of oil, lighted cigarettes or open flames, or where there is the possibility of electrical or spark hazards.

---

***hyperbaric o.*** Oxygen under greater pressure than at normal atmospheric pressure. It is usually at 1½ to 3 times absolute atmospheric pressure. SEE: *hyperbaric oxygenation.*

***singlet o.*** A highly active form of oxygen produced during reactions of hydrogen peroxide with superoxide and hypochlorite ions. It is believed that this free radical is bactericidal.

***transtracheal o.*** The delivery of oxygen to the lungs via a transtracheal tube. SEE: *transtracheal oxygenation.*

**oxygenase** (ŏk′sĭ-jĕn-ās″) [Gr. *oxys,* sharp, + *gennan,* to produce, + *-ase,* enzyme] An enzyme that enables an organism to use atmospheric oxygen in respiration.

**oxygenate** (ŏk′sĭ-jĕn-āt) To combine or supply with oxygen.

**oxygenation** (ŏk″sĭ-jĕn-ā′shŭn) Saturation or combination with oxygen, as the aeration of the blood in the lungs.

***hyperbaric o.*** Administration of oxygen under increased pressure while the patient is in an airtight chamber. Pressure chambers in which the oxygen is hyperbaric have been used to treat carbon monoxide poisoning, anaerobic infections such as gas gangrene, necrotizing fasciitis, crush injuries with acute ischemia of tissues, compromised skin grafts and flaps, mixed soft tissue reactions, burns, smoke inhalation, carbon monoxide poisoning, soft tissue radiation necrosis, chronic refractory osteomyelitis, decompression sickness (bends) and gas embolism.

Consultation at any hour concerning treatment of patients in a hyperbaric chamber is available from Divers Alert Network coordinated by Duke University Medical Center, (919) 684-8111.

Caution: Hyperbaric oxygenation should not be used in untreated pneumothorax or premature infants.

***tissue o.*** The oxygen level in tissues. Measurement of the oxygen concentration in body fluids is not as important as knowing the oxygen level in the tissues themselves. Determining the gastrointestinal interstitial pH provides an indication of the adequacy of tissue oxygenation. Decreased oxygen supply leads to anaerobic metabolism in cells, which produces a fall in pH. Thus the tissue pH serves as a marker for the adequacy of oxygen supply in the tissues.

***transtracheal o.*** The application of oxygen via a catheter system inserted into the trachea.

**oxygenator** (ŏk″sĭ-jĕ-nā′tor) A device for mechanically oxygenating anything, but esp. blood. When used to oxygenate blood, it is usually used during thoracic surgery or open-heart surgery.

***bubble o.*** A device for bubbling oxygen through the blood during extracorporeal circulation.

***rotating disk o.*** A device for oxygenating blood during extracorporeal circulation. A thin film of blood attaches to a disk as it dips into the blood flow. The portion of the disk not in the blood is rotating in an atmosphere of oxygen.

***screen o.*** A device for oxygenating blood during extracorporeal circulation. The blood passes over a series of screens that are in an oxygen atmosphere. Oxygen is exchanged in the thin film of blood on the screens.

**oxygen capacity** The maximum amount of oxygen expressed in volume percent (cc per 100 ml) that a given amount of blood will absorb. For normal blood it is about 20 cc.

**oxygen concentrator** A device used for home oxygen therapy that removes most of the nitrogen from room air and delivers the oxygen at a low flow rate. SYN: *oxygen enricher.*

**oxygen content** The amount of oxygen in volume percent that is present in the blood at any one moment.

**oxygen debt** After strenuous (i.e., anaerobic) physical activity, the oxygen required in the recovery period, in addition to that required while resting, to oxidize the excess lactic acid produced and to replenish the depleted stores of adenosine triphosphate and phosphocreatinase.

**oxygen-derived free radical** SEE: *oxygen radical; superoxide.*

**oxygen enricher** Oxygen concentrator.

**oxygenic** (ŏk″sĭ-jĕn′ĭk) [″ + *gennan,* to produce] Concerning, resembling, containing, or consisting of oxygen.

**oxygenize** Oxidize.

**oxygen radical** Hydrogen peroxide ($H_2O_2$) or the superoxide radical ($O_2^-$) produced by the incomplete reduction of oxygen. Oxygen free radicals are released during the "respiratory burst" phase of phagocytosis by neutrophils and macrophages during the inflammatory process. They cause direct cell damage, increase vascular permeability through damage to the capillary endothelium, and promote chemotaxis. Oxygen free radicals are normally contained by antioxidant protective measures; however, with severe inflammation they cause significant damage. They are believed to be responsible for much of the cellular damage involved in adult respiratory distress syndrome (ARDS), in which massive neutrophil aggregation and phagocytosis occur. SEE: *oxygen, singlet.*

**oxygen therapy** The administration of oxygen for the treatment of conditions resulting from oxygen deficiency. It is used to combat acute arterial hypoxemia that may result from pneumonia, pulmonary edema, or obstruction to breathing. It is also employed in congestive heart failure, coronary thrombosis, and following surgery. It may be administered by nasal cannula, mask (oronasal or tracheostomy), oxygen tent, or special oxygen chamber, usually at a concentration of 100% and at a metered rate. The oxygen is humidified by bubbling it through water. This will prevent drying of the mucosal epithelium of the upper respiratory tract. Supplemental oxygen is available through a method called molecular sieve, in which a device removes nitrogen from room air. The oxygen remaining is available for use just as if it were stored in a cylinder. SEE: *hyperbaric oxygen; oximeter.*

Caution: When administering supplemental oxygen, particularly at high concentrations, it is important to monitor the levels of oxygen and carbon dioxide in the blood. An increase in carbon dioxide (hypercapnia) may lead to carbon dioxide narcosis. SEE: *narcosis, carbon dioxide.*

Because oxygen provides a perfect environment for combustion, it should not be used in the presence of oil, lighted cigarettes or open flames, or where there is the possibility of electrical or spark hazards.

***transtracheal o.t.*** The delivery of oxygen via a small plastic cannula inserted directly into the trachea. SEE: illus.

**oxygen toxicity** Progressive respiratory failure that develops when high oxygen concentrations (more than 60%) are breathed for a prolonged period. Respiratory failure leads to decreased oxygen tension in the blood.

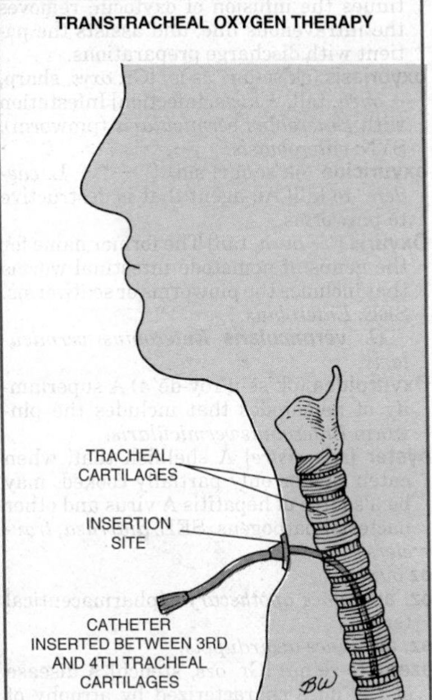


Prolonged exposure to a high oxygen concentration can cause blindness or damage to lung tissue in a preterm newborn.

**oxygeusia** (ŏk″sē-gū′sē-ă) [Gr. *oxys,* sharp, + *geusis,* taste] Abnormally keen sense of taste.

**oxyhematin** (ŏk″sē-hĕm′ă-tĭn) An iron compound that constitutes the coloring matter in oxyhemoglobin. When oxidized, it yields hematinic acid; when reduced, hematoporphyrin.

**oxyhematoporphyrin** (ŏk″sē-hĕm″ă-tō-por′fĭ-rĭn) A derivative of hematoporphyrin sometimes present in urine.

**oxyhemoglobin** (ŏk″sē-hē″mō-glō′bĭn) [″ + *haima,* blood, + L. *globus,* a sphere] The combined form of hemoglobin and oxygen. Hemoglobin with oxygen is found in arterial blood and is the oxygen carrier to the body tissues.

**oxyhemoglobin dissociation curve** A curve that shows the relationship between the partial pressure of oxygen and the percentage of saturation of hemoglobin with oxygen (i.e., the proportion of oxyhemoglobin to reduced hemoglobin). Factors that favor a shift of the curve to the right, accelerating the decomposition of hemoglobin, are a rise in temperature and an increase of H ions that results from liberation of $CO_2$ and formation of lactic acid. SEE: illus.

**oxyhemoglobinometer** (ŏk″sē-hē″mō-glō″bĭn-ŏm′ĕ-tĕr) [″ + ″ + ″ + Gr. *metron,* measure] An apparatus for measurement of the amount of oxygen in the blood.

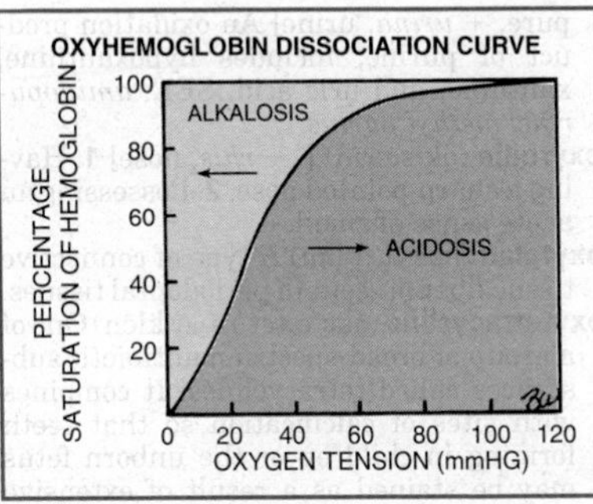


**oxyhydrocephalus** (ŏk″sē-hī-drō-sĕf′ăl-ŭs) [″ + *hydor,* water, + *kephale,* brain] A type of hydrocephalus in which the head has a pointed shape.

**oxyiodide** (ŏk″sē-ī′ō-dīd) [″ + *ioeides,* violet colored] A compound of iodine and oxygen with an element or radical.

**oxylalia** (ŏk″sē-lā′lē-ă) [″ + *lalein,* to speak] Abnormal rapidity of speech.

**oxymetazoline hydrochloride** (ŏk″sē-mĕt-ăz′ō-lēn) A vasoconstrictor drug used topically for nasal decongestion.

**oxymetholone** (ŏk″sē-mĕth′ō-lōn) An anabolic steroid.

**oxymorphone hydrochloride** (ŏk″sē-mor′fōn) A semisynthetic analgesic narcotic similar in action to morphine.

**oxymyoglobin** (ŏk″sē-mī″ō-glō′bĭn) The compound formed when myoglobin is exposed to oxygen.

**oxyntic** (ŏk-sĭn′tĭk) [Gr. *oxynein,* to make acid] Producing or secreting acid.

**oxyopia** (ŏk″sē-ō′pē-ă) [Gr. *oxys,* sharp, + *ops,* sight] Abnormal acuteness of vision.

**oxyopter** (ŏk″sē-ŏp′tĕr) A unit of measuring visual acuity; the reciprocal of the visual angle expressed in degrees.

**oxyosmia** (ŏk″sē-ŏz′mē-ă) [″ + *osme,* odor] Unusual acuity of the sense of smell.

**oxyosphresia** (ŏk″sē-ŏs-frē′zē-ă) [″ + *osphresis,* smell] Abnormal acuity of the sense of smell.

**oxypathia, oxypathy** (ŏk″sē-păth′ē-ă, -sĭp′ă-thē) [″ + *pathos,* disease, suffering] **1.** Unusual acuity of sensation. **2.** An acute condition. **3.** A condition in which the body is unable to eliminate unoxidizable acids, which combine with fixed alkalies of the tissues and harm the organism.

**oxyperitoneum** (ŏk″sĭ-pĕr-ĭ-tō-nē′ŭm) [″ + *peritonaion,* peritoneum] The introduction of oxygen into the peritoneal cavity.

**oxyphencyclimine hydrochloride** (ŏk″sē-fĕn-sī′klĭ-mēn) A belladonna-like drug.

**oxyphil(e)** (ŏk′sē-fĭl, -fīl) [″ + *philein,* to love] **1.** Staining readily with acid dyes. **2.** A cell that stains readily with acid dyes.

**oxyphonia** (ŏk″sē-fō′nē-ă) An abnormally sharp or shrill pitch to the voice.

**oxypurine** (ŏk″sē-pū′rēn) [″ + L. *purus,*

pure, + *urina,* urine] An oxidation product of purine; includes hypoxanthine, xanthine, and uric acid. SEE: *aminopurine; methyl purine.*

**oxyrhine** (ŏk′sē-rīn) [″ + *rhis,* nose] **1.** Having a sharp-pointed nose. **2.** Possessing an acute sense of smell.

**oxytalan** (ŏks-ĭt′ă-lăn) A type of connective tissue fiber present in periodontal tissues.

**oxytetracycline** (ŏks″ē-tĕt″ră-sī′klēn) One of a group of broad-spectrum antibiotic substances called tetracyclines. It combines with sites of calcification so that teeth forming in children or the unborn fetus may be stained as a result of extensive medication with this group of antibiotics. Originally obtained from a strain of *Streptomyces,* it is now prepared synthetically.

**oxytocic** (ŏk″sē-tō′sĭk) **1.** Agent that stimulates uterine contractions. **2.** Accelerating childbirth.

**oxytocin [injection]** (ŏk″sē-tō′sĭn) A pituitary hormone that stimulates the uterus to contract, thus inducing parturition. It also acts on the mammary gland to stimulate the release of milk.

**oxytocin challenge test** ABBR: OCT. The intravenous infusion of 10 very small doses of oxytocin in order to determine whether contraction of the uterus in response to the oxytocin will cause signs of fetal distress. The results of the test provide a basis of making a decision concerning continuation of high-risk pregnancies. Uterine contractions can also be induced by manual stimulation of the nipple. This process stimulates the hypothalamus, which causes the posterior lobe of the pituitary to release oxytocin. SYN: *contraction stress test.*

*Criteria for Interpretation: Negative result:* The monitor records a minimum of three uterine contractions and an absence of late decelerations within 10 min. The fetal heart rate exhibits average baseline variablity and acceleration associated with movement. *Positive result:* The monitor records late decelerations with more than 50% of uterine contractions. *Suspicious result:* The monitor records late decelerations associated with fewer than 50% contractions. *Hyperstimulation:* The monitor records uterine hypertonus and uterine contractions occurring more often than every 2 min or lasting longer than 90 sec.

NURSING IMPLICATIONS: The nurse explains the test and supports the patient through the procedure. Oxytocin solution is piggybacked into the tubing of the main intravenous line and delivered via infusion pump or controller to ensure accurate dosing. Uterine contractions and fetal heart rate are monitored until three uterine contractions occur in a 30-min period. The fetal heart rate pattern is then interpreted for the absence or presence of late decelerations. The nurse then discontinues the infusion of oxytocin, removes the intravenous line, and assists the patient with discharge preparations.

**oxyuriasis** (ŏk″sē-ū-rī′ăs-ĭs) [Gr. *oxys,* sharp, + *oura,* tall, + *iasis,* infection] Infestation with *Enterobius vermicularis* (pinworm). SYN: *enterobiasis.*

**oxyuricide** (ŏk″sē-ū′rĭ-sīd) [″ + ″ + L. *caedere,* to kill] An agent that is destructive to pinworms.

**Oxyuris** [″ + *oura,* tail] The former name for the genus of nematode intestinal worms that includes the pinworms or seatworms. SEE: *Enterobius.*

***O. vermicularis*** *Enterobius vermicularis.*

**Oxyuroidea** (ŏk″sē-ū″roy-dē′ă) A superfamily of nematodes that includes the pinworm *Enterobius vermicularis.*

**oyster** [AS. *oistre*] A shellfish that, when eaten raw or only partially cooked, may be a source of hepatitis A virus and other bacterial pathogens. SEE: *diarrhea, travelers'.*

**oz** *ounce.*

**oz. ap.** *ounce apothecary's* (pharmaceutical term).

**oz. av.** *ounce avoirdupois.*

**ozena** (ō-zē′nă) [Gr. *oze,* stench] A disease of the nose characterized by atrophy of the turbinates and mucous membrane accompanied by considerable crusting, discharge, and a very offensive odor. It is present in various forms of rhinitis.

**ozone** (ō′zōn) [Gr. *ozein,* to smell] A form of oxygen, present in the stratosphere, in which three atoms of the element combine to form the molecule $O_3$. Depletion of the ozone in the stratosphere permits increased exposure to ultraviolet light. This favors the development of skin cancers and cataracts, and may impair cellular immunity.

Persons exposed to arc welding, flour bleaching, fumes from copying equipment, or photochemical air pollutants may be in contact with toxic levels of ozone. The signs and symptoms include asthma, mucous membrane irritation, pulmonary hemorrhage and edema, and transient reduced pulmonary function when exposed to summer haze.

**ozonization** (ō″zō-nĭ-zā′shŭn) The act of converting to, or impregnating with, ozone.

**ozonize** (ō′zō-nīz) [Gr. *ozein,* to smell] **1.** To convert oxygen to ozone. **2.** To impregnate the air of a substance with ozone.

**ozonometer** (ō″zō-nŏm′ĕ-tĕr) [Gr. *oze,* stench, + *metron,* measure] An apparatus for estimating the quantity of ozone in the atmosphere.

**ozonoscope** (ō-zō′nō-skōp) [″ + *skopein,* to examine] A device for showing the presence or amount of ozone.

**ozostomia** (ō″zō-stō′mē-ă) [″+ *stoma,* mouth] Fetid breath; halitosis.

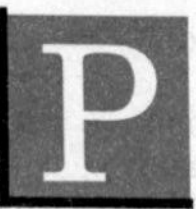

**P** **1.** *position; posterior; postpartum; pressure; pulse; pupil.* **2.** Symbol for the element phosphorus.

**p** *page; probability* (in statistics); *pupil.*

**p-** *para-* in chemical formulas.

**p̄** *after-* or *post-*.

**$P_1$** *first parental generation* (in genetics); *first pulmonic heart sound.*

**$P_2$** *pulmonic second sound.*

**$^{32}P$** Symbol for radioactive isotope of phosphorus.

**p53** A protein, produced by a tumor-suppressor gene, that is believed to play an important role in the birth and death of cells.

**PA** *pulmonary artery.*

**P.A.** *physician's assistant.*

**Pa** **1.** Symbol for the element protactinium. **2.** Pascal.

**P-A, p-a** *posteroanterior.*

**P & A** *percussion and auscultation.*

**$P(A\text{-}a)O_2$** The oxygen pressure gradient between the alveoli and the arterial blood.

**pabular** (păb′ū-lăr) [L. *pabulum,* food] Pert. to nourishment.

**pabulum** (păb′ū-lŭm) [L.] Food; nourishment.

**PAC** *premature atrial contraction.*

**PA catheter** Intravenous catheter with the tip in the pulmonary artery.

**pacchionian body** SEE: *arachnoid villus.*

**pacchionian depressions** Small pits produced on the inner surface of the skull by protuberance of the pacchionian bodies.

**PACE** *Patient Advise and Consent Encounter.*

**pacemaker** (pās′māk-ĕr) [L. *passus,* a step, + AS. *macian,* to make] **1.** Anything that influences the rate and rhythm of occurrence of some activity or process. **2.** In cardiology, a specialized cell or group of cells that automatically generates impulses that may spread to other regions of the heart. The normal cardiac pacemaker is the sinoatrial node, a group of cells in the atrium near the entrance of the superior vena cava into the right atrium. **3.** A generally accepted term for artificial cardiac pacemaker.

***artificial cardiac p.*** An electrical device that can substitute for a defective natural pacemaker and control the beating of the heart by a series of rhythmic electrical discharges. If the electrodes that deliver the discharges to the heart are placed on the outside of the chest, the device is called a transcutaneous pacemaker. If the pacemaker is placed within the body, the device is called an internal pacemaker. Artificial pacemakers were first used more than 30 years ago. Since that time, more than a million have been implanted to prolong life.

These devices are powered by batteries that last 10 years or longer. Internal pacemakers are usually installed under local anesthesia. The functional status of a pacemaker and the strength of its battery can be monitored by telephone. While the patient is at home, the signal from the patient's pacemaker can be transmitted by use of a modem to a receiving unit in the physician's office. At the same time, the patient's electrocardiogram can be transmitted and recorded. An individual with an implanted pacemaker can carry on his or her usual activities. Modern pacemakers are shielded from interference from ordinary household and office electronic devices. Patients should avoid being close to strong magnetic fields from arc welding machines and magnetic resonance imaging diagnostic devices. SEE: *defibrillator, implantable cardioverter; pacemaker syndrome; pacing code; sick sinus syndrome.*

NURSING IMPLICATIONS: *Preoperative:* The nurse should monitor the cardiac rate and rhythm for evidence of failure of the heart's pacemaker, and treat using the hospital protocol; teach the patient and family about cardiac function and pacemaker insertion and function; encourage verbalization of fears and concerns, answer questions, and dispel myths and correct misconceptions; and provide routine preoperative preparation.

*Postoperative:* The nurse should ascertain the type of pacemaker employed and expectations for its function; monitor the cardiac rate and rhythm for evidence of pacemaker function; assess the patient for evidence of pacemaker failure or noncapture (vertigo, loss of consciousness, hypotension, chest discomfort, dyspnea) and evaluate the patient for effects on cardiac output; teach the patient technique and rationale for monitoring own pulse rate, and care and protection of insertion site; counsel concerning telephone monitoring check-up, battery replacement, medication regimen, physical activity, and follow-up care. The nurse should encourage the patient to wear or carry medical identification and information indicating the presence and type of pacemaker implanted, along with an electrocardiogram rhythm strip showing pacemaker activity and capture. Pacemaker patients who travel extensively should be cautioned to have spare batteries available.

***breathing p.*** A device that stimulates breathing by delivering electrical pulses to both phrenic nerves from an external radio transmitter to an implanted receiver. It is used in patients with quadriplegia or sleep apnea.

***DDD p.*** A rate-adaptive implanted pacing device. It senses and paces both atrial and ventricular events, triggering the atrioventricular (AV) interval so that AV synchrony is maintained over a wide range of sinus rhythm rates. This type of pacing has reduced the incidence of pacemaker syndrome. It is the most versatile pacing device used. SEE: *pacemaker syndrome.*

***DDI p.*** An implanted pacing device that senses both atrial and ventricular events but can inhibit only atrial impulses. This type of pacing is used only when atrioventricular conduction is intact. It may be suitable when frequent atrial tachyarrhythmias cause rapid ventricular rates.

***demand p.*** An implanted pacemaker that is designed to permit its electrical output to be inhibited by the heart's electrical impulses. This decreases the chances for the pacemaker to induce ventricular fibrillation.

***dual-chamber p.*** A pacemaker that is also known as an atrioventricular sequential pacemaker because it stimulates both atria and ventricles sequentially.

***ectopic p.*** Any endogenous cardiac pacemaker other than the sinoatrial node.

***failure of artificial p.*** A defect in a pacemaker device caused by either a failure to sense the patient's intrinsic beat or a failure to pace. Failure to pace can be caused by a worn-out battery, fracture or displacement of the electrode, or pulse generator defect.

***fixed rate p.*** An artificial pacemaker that stimulates the heart at a fixed rate.

***internal p.*** A cardiac pacemaker placed within the body.

***permanent p.*** An electronic device for permanent cardiac pacing. The leads are usually inserted transvenously through the subclavian or cephalic veins with leads positioned in the right atrium for atrial pacing or in the right ventricular apex for ventricular pacing. The leads are connected to the pulse generator, which is implanted in a subcutaneous pocket below the clavicle.

***programmable p.*** An electronic permanent pacemaker in which one or more settings can be changed from outside the patient by use of an electronic device.

***rate-responsive p., rate-adaptive p.*** An electronic pacemaker that senses changes in the body's need for adjustment of the cardiac rate as can occur in sleeping, waking, sitting, walking, or running. The device alters cardiac rate by sensing body motion, changes in breathing, or slight changes in blood temperature. This permits a more nearly normal lifestyle.

***temporary p.*** An electronic device for temporary cardiac pacing. This is usually done by transvenous insertion of an electrode catheter in the right ventricular apex that receives impulses from an external generator.

***transcutaneous p.*** An artificial cardiac pacemaker that is located outside the body. The electrodes for delivering the stimulus are located on the chest wall.

***transthoracic p.*** A cardiac pacemaker connected to electrodes passed through the chest wall, usually used only in emergency situations, on a temporary basis.

***uterine p.*** One or more areas in the uterus that stimulate contraction of the myometrium.

***wandering p.*** A cardiac arrhythmia in which the site of origin of the pacemaker stimulus shifts from one site to another, usually from the atrioventricular node to some other part of the atrium.

**pacemaker syndrome** A group of symptoms associated with ventricular pacing. Included are syncope or presyncope, weakness, lightheadedness, orthopnea, paroxysmal nocturnal dyspnea, dizziness, and pulmonary edema. DDD pacing has reduced the incidence of this condition by allowing restoration of atrioventricular synchrony.

**pacer** Pacemaker.

**pachy-, pach-** [Gr. *pachys*, thick] Combining form meaning *thick*.

**pachyblepharosis** (păk″ē-blĕf″ă-rō′sĭs) Chronic thickening of the eyelid.

**pachycephalic** (păk″ē-sĕ-făl′ĭk) [″ + *kephale,* brain] Possessing an abnormally thick skull.

**pachycheilia** (păk″ē-kī′lē-ă) [″ + *cheilos,* lip] Unusual thickness of the lips.

**pachychromatic** (păk″ē-krō-măt′ĭk) [″ + *chroma,* color] Possessing a coarse chromatin network.

**pachydactylia, pachydactyly** (păk″ē-dăk-tĭl′ē-ă, -dăk′tĭ-lē) [″ + *daktylos,* digit] A condition marked by unusually large fingers and toes.

**pachyderma** (păk-ē-dĕr′mă) [″ + *derma,* skin] Unusual thickness of the skin. SEE: *elephantiasis.*

***p. lymphangiectatica*** A diffuse form of skin thickening caused by blocked or defective lymph drainage.

***occipital p.*** A disease in which the skin of the scalp, esp. in the occipital region, falls into thickened folds.

**pachydermatocele** (păk″ē-dĕr-măt′ō-sēl) [″ + ″ + *kele,* tumor, swelling] **1.** A pendulous state of the skin with thickening. SYN: *cutis laxa; dermatolysis.* **2.** Huge neurofibroma.

**pachydermoperiostosis** (păk″ē-dĕr″mō-pĕr″ē-ŏs-tō′sĭs) A hereditary form of osteoarthropathy of unknown origin marked by thickening of the skin over the face and extremities. If associated with an underlying disease, treatment of the disease may cause the symptoms and signs of this condition to disappear.

**pachyglossia** (păk″ē-glŏs′sē-ă) [″ + *glossa,* tongue] Unusual thickness of the tongue.

**pachygnathous** (pă-kĭg′năth-ŭs) [″ + *gnathos,* jaw] Having a thick or large jaw.

**pachygyria** (păk-ē-jī′rē-ă) [″ + *gyros,* a circle] Flat, broad formation of the cerebral convolutions.

**pachyleptomeningitis** (păk-ē-lĕp″tō-mĕn″ĭn-jī′tĭs) [″ + *leptos,* thin, + *meninx,* membrane, + *itis,* inflammation] Inflammation of the pia and dura of the brain and spinal cord.

**pachymenia** (păk-ē-mē′nē-ă) [″ + *hymen,* membrane] A thickening of the skin or membranes.

**pachymeningitis** (păk-ē-mĕn″ĭn-jī′tĭs) [″ + *meninx,* membrane, + *itis,* inflammation] Inflammation of the dura mater. Inflammation of any of three membranes—the pia, dura, or arachnoid—is sure to extend to one or both of the other two membranes, and the consequence in any form is suppuration, abscess, effusion into the ventricles, and softening of cerebral tissue if brain is involved. SYN: *perimeningitis.*

***external p.*** Inflammation of the outer layer of the dura mater.

***hemorrhagic p.*** Circumscribed effusion of blood on the inner surface of the dura with inflammation.

SYMPTOMS: Symptoms include intermittent headache, choked optic disks, hemiparesis, dilated pupils, and unconsciousness.

ETIOLOGY: This condition is usually the result of trauma, such as a blow, resulting in a venous tear. Blood oozes into subdural space, and a blood clot is formed, becomes encysted, and gives rise to a hematoma. SEE: *hematoma, subdural.*

***internal p.*** Inflammation of the inner layer of the dura mater.

***spinal p.*** Inflammation of the dura of the spinal cord.

**pachymeningopathy** (păk″ē-mĕn″ĭn-gŏp′ă-thē) [″ + ″ + *pathos,* disease] Any noninflammatory disease of the dura mater.

**pachymeninx** (păk-ē-mē′nĭnks) [″ + *meninx,* membrane] The dura mater.

**pachymeter** [″ + *metron,* to measure] A device to determine the thickness of a material or object.

**pachyonychia** (păk″ē-ō-nĭk′ē-ă) [Gr. *pachys,* thick, + *onyx,* nail] Abnormal thickening of the fingernails or toenails.

***p. congenita*** A congenital condition characterized by thickening of the nails, thickening of the skin on the palms of the hands and the soles of the feet, follicular keratosis at the knees and elbows, and corneal dyskeratosis.

**pachyostosis** (păk″ē-ŏs-tō′sĭs) [″ + *osteon,* bone, + *osis,* condition] A benign condition of thickening of the bones.

**pachyotia** (păk-ē-ō′shē-ă) [″ + *ous,* ear] Abnormal thickness of the ears.

**pachypelviperitonitis** (păk″ē-pĕl″vĭ-pĕr″ĭ-tō-nī′tĭs) [″ + L. *pelvis,* basin, + Gr. *peritonaion,* peritoneum, + *itis,* inflammation] Inflammation of the pelvic and peritoneal membranes with hypertrophy and thickening of their surfaces.

**pachyperiostitis** (păk″ē-pĕr″ē-ŏs-tī′tĭs) [″ + *periosteon,* periosteum, + *itis,* inflammation] Thickening of the periosteum caused by inflammation.

**pachyperitonitis** (păk″ē-pĕr″ĭ-tō-nī′tĭs) [″ + ″ + *itis,* inflammation] Inflammation of the peritoneum with thickening of the membrane.

**pachypleuritis** (păk-ē-plū-rī′tĭs) [″ + *pleura,* side, + *itis,* inflammation] Inflammation of the pleura with thickening.

**pachypodous** (pă-kĭp′ō-dŭs) [″ + *pous,* foot] Having abnormally thick feet.

**pachyrhinic** (păk″ē-rī′nĭk) [″ + *rhis,* nose] Having a thick, flat nose.

**pachytene** (păk′ē-tēn) [″ + *tainia,* band] The stage in meiosis, or cell division, in which the paired homologous chromosomes contract due to their becoming intertwined in a spiral fashion and then become much thicker than in the preceding leptotene and zygotene stages.

**pachytrichous** Presence of enlarged hair fibers.

**pachyvaginalitis** (păk″ē-văj″ĭn-ă-lī′tĭs) [″ + L. *vagina,* sheath, + Gr. *itis,* inflammation] Inflammation of the tunica vaginalis of the testes.

**pachyvaginitis** (păk″ē-văj″ĭn-ī′tĭs) Chronic inflammation of the vagina with thickening of the vaginal walls.

**pacifier** An artificial nipple, usually made of plastic, provided for infants to satisfy their need to suck.

**pacing** (pās′ĭng) [L. *passus,* a step] Setting the rate or pace of an event, esp. the heartbeat. SEE: *pacemaker.*

***transcutaneous p.*** The application of an electrical current between electrodes placed on the skin to stimulate the heart to beat. Typically, the electrodes are placed on the anterior and posterior chest, or to the right of the sternum and below the clavicle and on the midaxillary line at the level of the sixth to seventh ribs. Also called *external pacing, noninvasive pacing, external thoracic pacing,* and *transchest pacing.*

**pacing code** A code of 3 to 5 letters used for describing pacemaker type and function. The first letter indicates the chamber or chambers paced: V for ventricle, A for atrium, or D (dual) for pacing of both chambers. The second letter, which may also be V, A, or D, indicates the chamber from which electrical activity is sensed. The third letter indicates the response to the sensed electrical activity. O indicates no response to the electrical activity sensed; I, inhibition of the pacing action; T, triggering of the pacemaker function; and D, that a dual response of spontaneous atrial and ventricular activity will inhibit atrial and ventricular pacing. The fourth letter, previously used to describe programmable functions, is now used to designate variability of the pace rate with metabolic need. A fifth letter may indicate antitachycardia-pacing capability, but this is more usually incorporated into automatic implantable defibrillators. SEE: *pacemaker; pacemaker, cardiac, artificial.*

**pacing wire** Pacemaker electrode.

**pacinian corpuscles** (pă-sĭn′ē-ăn) [Filippo Pacini, It. anatomist, 1812–1883] Encapsulated sensory nerve endings found in subcutaneous tissue and many other parts of the body (pancreas, penis, clitoris, nipple). These corpuscles are sensitive to deep or heavy pressure. SYN: *Vater's corpuscles.*

**pack** (păk) [AS. *pak*] **1.** A dry or moist, hot or cold blanket or sheet wrapped around a patient and used for treatment. **2.** To fill up a cavity with cotton, gauze, or a similar substance.

***cold p.*** A physiological sedative and hypnotic employed for relief of restlessness and insomnia; used extensively in psychiatric conditions. The patient is wrapped in two or more sheets that have been placed in cold water and wrung out before application, and then in heavy blankets to prevent loss of cooling and evaporation of moisture.

***dry p.*** A procedure used in combination with a hot bath to induce perspiration. When leaving the hot bath, the patient is placed in a dry warm sheet and wrapped in several warm blankets.

***full p.*** Any pack that enwraps the entire body.

***half p.*** A wet-sheet pack extending from the axillae to below the knees.

***hot p.*** A type of superficial moist heat applied to reduce pain and promote muscle relaxation. The pack usually has a canvas cover and is filled with a silicon dioxide gel. The pack is heated to 65° to 90°C in hot water.

***ice p.*** A substitute for an ice bag; a local cold application made by folding a soft towel so that it will fit the area and filling it with crushed ice.

***partial p.*** A wet pack that covers a portion of the body.

***periodontal p.*** A surgical dressing applied over an area involved in periodontal surgery to enhance healing and tissue recovery. Components may include eugenol, resin zinc oxide, tannic acid, cocoa butter, paraffin, olive oil, and an antibiotic.

***posterior nasal p.*** SEE: *epistaxis.*

***umbrella p.*** Pack inserted through the abdominal incision following hysterectomy to stop arterial bleeding. The pack itself consists of a piece of absorbent cloth about 24 in. (61 cm) square into the middle of which is placed about 60 ft (18.28 m) of 2-in. (5-cm) gauze. The tails of the pack are pulled through the vagina from below, and the corners of the cloth are brought together to form the tail of the pack. After placement, the tail is pulled firmly, and the bolus of gauze in the cloth exerts enough pressure against the blood vessels to stop arterial bleeding. In Greece it is known as the Logothetopulos tampon, named after the physician who developed it in 1926.

***wet-dry p.*** A pack placed in a healing area, esp. an ulcer, to facilitate débridement. The pack, which may contain a topical antiseptic, is moistened, placed in the ulcer, and changed when it becomes dry. SYN: *wet-dry dressing.*

***wet-sheet p.*** The envelopment of a patient in one, two, or three linen or soft cotton sheets that have been wrung out of water. They are held against the body by large woolen blankets. The temperature of the water used for the sheets varies, depending on the purpose.

**package insert** An informational leaflet placed inside the container or package of prescription drugs. The Food and Drug Administration requires that the drug's generic name, indications, contraindications, adverse effects, dosage, and route of administration be described in the leaflet.

**packed cells** Red blood cells that have been separated from the plasma, used in treating conditions that require red blood cells but not the liquid components of whole blood. This prevents excess hydration of the vascular system.

**packer** (păk′ĕr) A device for packing a cavity or a wound.

**packing** (păk′ĭng) **1.** The process of filling a cavity or wound with gauze sponges or gauze strips. **2.** Material used to fill a cavity or wound.

**$PaCO_2$** Partial pressure of carbon dioxide in the arterial blood; arterial carbon dioxide concentration or tension. It is usually expressed in millimeters of mercury (mm Hg).

**pad** (păd) **1.** A cushion of soft material, usually cotton or rayon, used to apply pressure, relieve pressure, or support an organ or part. **2.** A fleshlike or fatty mass.

***abdominal p.*** A dressing for absorbing discharges from surgical wounds of the abdomen.

***dinner p.*** A pad placed on the stomach before application of a plaster cast. The pad is then removed, leaving space for abdominal distention after meals.

***fat p.*** **1.** Sucking p. **2.** The pad of fat behind and below the patella.

***kidney p.*** An air or water pad fixed on an abdominal belt for compression over a movable kidney.

***knuckle p.'s*** A congenital condition in which small nodules appear on the dorsal side of fingers.

***Malgaigne's p.*** [Joseph François Malgaigne, Fr. physician, 1806–1865] A mass of fat in the knee joint on either side of the patella's upper end.

***perineal p.*** A pad covering the perineum; used to cover a wound or to absorb the menstrual flow.

***sucking p.*** A pad of fat inside the cheeks of infants. SYN: *fat p.* (1).

***surgical p.*** A soft rubber pad with an

apron and inflatable rim for drainage of escaping fluids; used in surgery and obstetrics.

**paed-, paedo-** SEE: words beginning with *ped-, pedia-, pedo-*.

**PAF** *platelet aggregating factor.*

**Paget, Sir James** (păj′ĕt) British surgeon, 1814–1899.

***extramammary P.'s disease*** A plaque with a definite margin found in the anogenital area and in the axilla. It is a rare malignant disease and is treated by surgical excision.

***mammary P.'s disease*** Carcinoma of the mammary ducts.

***P.'s disease*** Osteitis deformans.

**pagetoid** (paj′ĕ-toyd) [*Paget* + Gr. *eidos,* form, shape] Similar to Paget's disease.

**page turner** An adaptive device for persons with limited or absent upper extremity movement; used to turn the pages of a book.

**pagophagia** [Gr. *pagos,* frost, + *phagein,* to eat] A form of pica characterized by the deliberate eating of large quantities of ice. This condition may be associated with iron-deficiency anemia.

**-pagus** [Gr. *pagos,* thing fixed] A terminal combining form indicating twins joined together at the site indicated in the initial part of the word. SEE: *craniopagus.*

**PAH, PAHA** *para-aminohippuric acid.*

**pain** (pān) [L. *poena,* a fine, a penalty, punishment] As defined by the International Association for the Study of Pain, an unpleasant sensory and emotional experience arising from actual or potential tissue damage or described in terms of such damage. Pain includes not only the perception of an uncomfortable stimulus but also the response to that perception. Approx. one half of the persons who seek medical help do so because of the primary complaint of pain. In the U.S. each year 155 million persons experience at least one episode of acute pain, and one third of that number report pain that is severe. An estimated 700 million workdays, at a cost of $60 billion, are lost annually in the U.S. because of chronic pain.

Experiencing pain is influenced by a great number of dynamic and ever-changing interacting physical, mental, biochemical, physiological, psychological, social, cultural, and emotional factors. Thus, the pain that is perceived to be of a certain intensity at one time may, at another time, be perceived as being either less or more intense, even though all other factors appear to be the same.

Acute pain is to be distinguished from chronic pain. Acute pain warns the patient that something is wrong, but persistent acute pain may interfere with the healing and recovery process. Thus, the pain of myocardial infarction or postoperative pain may cause a series of autonomic reflexes that prevent optimum function of the heart and lungs as well as other essential body systems.

The signs of pain include increased heart rate and output, increased blood pressure, pupillary dilatation, palmar sweating, hyperventilation, hypermotility, escape behavior, and anxiety state.

Acute pain is managed by diagnosing the underlying cause and attempting to remove it or decrease its intensity; use of drugs appropriate for the severity and type of pain; use of noninvasive measures such as application of heat, cold, manipulation, or splint; transcutaneous electrical nerve stimulation (TENS); relaxation therapy; and biofeedback to attempt to prevent the development of chronic pain at this stage.

In treating pain, it is not unusual for analgesics to be administered strictly in accordance with the time specified to have elapsed between doses. This practice is neither humane nor merciful. It stems from an obsession with the possibility of causing addiction to the drug. Investigators have reported that creation of physical dependence requires the regular routine administration of therapeutic doses of opioids four to six times a day for 6 wk. Also, the incidence of addiction has been found to be 1 per 4000 hospitalized patients who have received opioids. SEE: table; *endorphins; mercy; patient-controlled analgesia; substance P; TENS; trigger point.*

When pain persists beyond the expected time required for healing of an injury or after the expected course of an acute disease, it is considered chronic. Because the cause may not be apparent, chronic pain is considered to be a separate disease entity.

With respect to chronic intractable pain, there are known causes, including carcinomatosis; invasion or compression syndromes due to cancer; mental illness; neurological disorders such as neuralgias, phantom limb pain, nerve entrapment syndromes, spinal cord damage, myofascial syndromes, or thalamic syndrome pain. The signs of chronic pain include sleep disturbance, irritability, appetite disturbance, constipation, psychomotor retardation, decreased pain tolerance, social withdrawal, and mental depression. The management of chronic pain is similar to that of acute pain, but the goal is to decrease the use of analgesics. The patient should be encouraged concerning the eventual success of the therapy, but at the same time realistic therapeutic goals should be set. The patient should be informed also that some pain is likely to continue.

It is important for those responsible for treating neonates to be aware that the mechanism for pain perception is fully developed and functioning by the time the fetus is born. Thus, the decision to use analgesics and local anesthesia or general

### Usual Adult Doses and Intervals of Drugs for Relief of Pain

**Nonopioid Analgesics**

| Generic Name | Dose, mg* | Interval | Comments |
|---|---|---|---|
| Acetylsalicylic acid | 650 | 4 hr | Enteric-coated preparations available |
| Acetaminophen | 650 | 4 hr | Side effects uncommon |
| Ibuprofen | 400 | 4–6 hr | Available without prescription |
| Indomethacin | 25–50 | 8 hr | Gastrointestinal side effects common |
| Naproxen | 250–500 | 12 hr | Delayed effects may be due to long half-life |
| Ketorolac | 15–60 IM | 4–6 hr | Similar to ibuprofen but more potent |

**Opioid Analgesics**

| Generic Name | Parenteral Dose (mg) | PO Dose (mg) | Comments |
|---|---|---|---|
| Codeine | 30–60 every 4 hr | 30–60 every 4 hr | Nausea common |
| Hydromorphone | 1–2 every 4 hr | 2–4 every 4 hr | Shorter acting than morphine sulfate |
| Levorphanol | 2 every 6–8 hr | 4 every 6 hr | Longer acting than morphine sulfate; absorbed well PO |
| Methadone | 10 every 6–8 hr | 20 every 6–8 hr | Delayed sedation due to long half-life |
| Meperidine | 75–100 every 3–4 hr | 300 every 4 hr | Poorly absorbed PO; normeperidine is a toxic metabolite |
| Morphine | 10 every 4 hr | 60 every 4 hr | |
| Morphine, sustained release | 90 every 12 hr | 60–180 2 or 3 times daily | |
| Oxycodone | — | 5–10 every 4–6 hr | Usually available with acetaminophen or aspirin |

SOURCE: Adapted from Isselbacher, K.J., et al.: Harrison's Principles of Internal Medicine, ed 13. McGraw-Hill, New York, 1994.

* By mouth unless indicated otherwise.

PO—by mouth

anesthesia should be based on the same principles as those used in decisions involving adult patients.

NURSING IMPLICATIONS: Pain characteristics should be evaluated to determine the location and radiation, quality, severity (on a scale of 1 to 10), temporal qualities (onset and duration), any associated symptoms experienced, any known exacerbators, and treatments the person has used to obtain relief. The nurse should believe that the patient's pain exists, because pain is a subjective phenomenon and only the individual experiencing it can know its characteristics. The nurse must remember that there is a time lag before prescribed medications become effective and provide relief. SEE: *Nursing Diagnoses Appendix.*

***abdominal p.*** Pain in the abdomen that usually increases with respiration. Experienced in a great variety of conditions including appendicitis; broken ribs; intercostal neuralgia; wounds; herpes zoster; pleurisy; pleurodynia; myalgia; periostitis; acute peritonitis; sickle cell anemia crisis; colic; hepatic, gastric, or renal ulcer; gallbladder disorders; carcinoma in late stages; and syphilitic gummata of this region.

***aching p.*** Generalized aching that may accompany infectious disease such as influenza, smallpox, or rheumatic fever. It is also found in myalgia and headaches.

***acute p.*** **1.** A short, sharp, cutting pain; usually associated with inflammation, esp. of serous membranes. SYN: *lancinating p.* **2.** Sudden or slow onset of any intensity from mild to severe with an anticipated or predictable end and a duration of less than 6 months. SEE: *Nursing Diagnoses Appendix.*

***adnexal p.*** Pain arising from the fallopian tubes and ovaries; most commonly due to infection of those structures.

***agonizing p.*** Intense, torturing pain of mind or body; may be due to coronary thrombosis, angina pectoris, aortic aneurysm, or mediastinitis. It may occur in a milder form in asthma or tracheobronchitis, or it may be caused by referred pain from gallbladder disorders, intestinal obstruction, diaphragmatic hernia, pancreatitis, or a perforated ulcer.

***angina pectoris p.*** Severe paroxysmal pain due to decreased blood supply to the myocardium, radiating through the shoulder down the arm, or rarely from the heart to the abdomen, ear, or back. At the same time, the patient may experience a feeling that the chest is being crushed or compressed. This pain lasts from a few seconds to several minutes. SEE: *angina pectoris.*

**appendicitis p.** Acute, usually severe pain, generally in the abdomen, followed by localization of pain in the lower right quadrant of the abdomen, with tenderness over the right rectus muscle with rigidity. Rebound pain at McBurney's point is a classic symptom. SEE: *appendicitis.*

**bearing-down p.'s** Pain and pressure of the second stage of labor that causes the female to strain or bear down as one does to defecate.

**boring p.** Pain deep in the tissues that gives the sensation of being produced by a boring instrument.

**Brodie's p.** Pain caused near a joint affected with neuralgia when the skin is folded near it.

**burning p.** Pain experienced in heat burns, superficial skin lesions, herpes zoster, and circumscribed neuralgias.

**causalgic p.** Spontaneous pain, esp. burning in character, when associated with anesthesia or hyperesthesia in a given nerve. SYN: *causalgia.*

**central p.** Pain due to a lesion in the central nervous system.

**chest p.** Severe pain in the chest from exercise; may be due to heart disease. If due to pleurisy, it is associated with breathing. If pain accompanies a stiff shoulder or neck, it may be due to arthritis or fibrositis. If it comes when the patient is bending over after a meal, it may be due to diaphragmatic or hiatal hernia.

**chronic p.** Sudden or slow onset of any intensity from mild to severe, constant or recurring without anticipated or predictable end and a duration greater than 6 months. SEE: *acute p.; Nursing Diagnoses Appendix.*

**chronic intractable p.** Chronic pain due to a known cause, such as malignancy, mental illness, or a neurological disorder.

**constant rectal p.** Pain in the rectal area; usually aggravated by defecation. It may be due to ischiorectal abscess, anal abscess, inflamed or strangulated hemorrhoids, carcinoma, periproctitis, prostatic abscess, seminal vesiculitis, fecal impaction, acute salpingitis, tabes dorsalis, irritation from diarrhea, foreign bodies, fissures, rectal polyps, or adenoma. Pain during defecation may result from anal fissure, ulcer, hemorrhoids, anal abscess, stenosis, stricture, dysentery, impaction, foreign body, or any inflammation. SEE: *proctalgia fugax.*

**cramplike p.** Muscular spasm such as epigastric pain, the significance of which depends on the location of the pain. Menstrual pain is often cramplike. SEE: *cramp; muscle cramps.*

**dental p.** Pain in the oral area, which, in general, may be of two origins. Soft tissue pain may be acute or chronic, and a burning pain is due to surface lesions and usually can be discretely localized; pulpal pain or tooth pain varies according to whether it is acute or chronic, but it is often difficult to localize.

**dilating p.'s** Rhythmic pains occurring during the first stage of labor accompanying dilatation of the cervix.

**dull p.** Continuous mild throbbing.

**eccentric p.** Pain occurring in peripheral structures owing to a lesion involving the posterior roots of the spinal nerves.

**epigastric p.** Severe pain occurring in paroxysms in gastric disorders. In general, it may accompany any gastric or intestinal disorder, as well as some pleural and cardiac disorders. SYN: *gastralgic p.* SEE: *cardialgia.*

**expulsive p.'s** Pains associated with uterine contractions in the second and third stages of labor.

**false p.** Pain mistaken for a true labor pain; an ineffective pain of labor. Braxton Hicks contractions are often confused with labor, particularly by the woman experiencing her first pregnancy. SEE: *Braxton Hicks sign.*

**fulgurant p.** Lightning p.

**gallbladder p.** Pain in the upper right abdominal quadrant, dull pain just below the last rib in infection, or sharp pain in same area radiating to the back and up under the right shoulder, esp. if calculi are present.

**gas p.** Pain in the intestines caused by an accumulation of gas therein.

**gastralgic p.** Epigastric p.

**girdle p.** Pain resembling the sensation of a constricting cord around the waist, occurring in spinal cord disease.

**growing p.'s** Pains felt in the joints or limbs of growing children; may be rheumatic; an imprecise term indicating ill-defined pains in the muscular system of young persons. There is no evidence that the pains are related to rapid growth.

**head p.** Headache.

**heterotopic p.** Referred p.

**homotopic p.** Pain felt at the point of injury.

**hunger p.** Pain due to need for food; coincides with powerful contractions of the stomach. It may be indicative of gastric disorder. SEE: *hunger.*

**hypogastric p.** Pain in the area below the umbilicus.

**inflammatory p.** Pain in the presence of inflammation that is increased by pressure.

**intermenstrual p.** Pelvic pain arising during the cycle between the menses; may accompany ovulation. SEE: *mittelschmerz.*

**intractable p.** Pain that cannot be easily relieved, as that occurring from certain neoplastic invasions.

***labor p.'s*** Rhythmical uterine contractions at childbirth; increasing in frequency and intensity, climaxing in vaginal delivery.

***lancinating p.*** Acute p.

***lightning p.*** A sudden brief pain that may be repetitive, usually in the legs but may be at any location. It is associated with tabes dorsalis. SYN: *fulgurant p.*

***lingual p.*** Pain in the tongue that may be due to local lesions, glossitis, fissures, or pernicious anemia. SYN: *tongue p.*

***lung p.*** Sharp pain in the region of the lungs.

***menstrual p.*** Dysmenorrhea.

***mental p.*** Pain of psychic origin such as mental distress or grief. If persistent, it may cause true physical pain.

***middle p.*** Intermenstrual p.

***migraine p.*** SEE: *migraine.*

***mind p.*** Pain of mental origin or occurring subsequent to mental effort, noted esp. in melancholia.

***mobile p.*** Pain that moves from one area to another.

***movement p.*** Kinesalgia.

***neuralgic p.*** Pain, frequently paroxysmal, occurring along the branches of a nerve. It may be rheumatic in origin and is temporarily relieved by heat or pressure.

***night p.*** Musculoskeletal pain that awakens the patient at night or interferes with sleep; may be due to infection, inflammation, neurovascular compromise, or severe structural damage. Night pain is a frequent occurrence in patients with arthritis or bursitis of the shoulder.

***noise p.*** Odynacusis.

***objective p.*** Pain induced by some external or internal irritant, by inflammation, or by injury to nerves, organs, or other tissues that interferes with the function, nutrition, or circulation of the affected part. It is usually traceable to a definite pathologic process.

***paresthesic p.*** A stinging or tingling sensation manifested in central and peripheral nerve lesions. SEE: *paresthesia.*

***periodontal p.*** A discrete, well-localized pain caused by inflammation of tissues surrounding a tooth. This may be contrasted with the throbbing, nonlocalized pain typical of a toothache or pulpal pain.

***phantom p.*** SEE: *sensation, phantom.*

***postprandial p.*** Abdominal pain after eating.

***precordial p.*** The sensation of pain over the heart.

***premonitory p.*** Ineffective contractions of the uterus before the beginning of true labor.

***pseudomyelic p.*** The false sensation of movement in a paralyzed limb or of no movement in a moving limb; not a true pain.

***psychogenic p.*** Pain having mental, as opposed to organic, origin.

***referred p.*** Pain seeming to arise in an area other than its origin, as pain from appendicitis, which often seems to occur in areas other than that of the appendix. It may be caused by visceral pain or by proximal or deep musculoskeletal injury and is usually referred to areas distant from the source of the problem. Pain from the heart, angina pectoris, may be referred to either arm, but most commonly the left, or to the ear, jaw, back, or teeth. SYN: *heterotopic p.; sympathetic p.; synalgia.*

***remittent p.*** Pain with temporary abatements in severity; characteristic of neuralgia and colic.

***rest p.*** Pain due to ischemia that comes on when sitting or lying.

***root p.*** Cutaneous pain caused by disease of the sensory nerve roots.

***shooting p.*** Pain that seems to travel like lightning from one place to another.

***spot p.*** A pain that seems to be located in a patch of skin.

***standards for p. relief*** Standards for the Relief of Acute Pain and Cancer Pain developed by the American Pain Society in 1991. These are summarized as follows:

1. Acute pain and cancer pain are recognized and effectively treated. Essential to this process is the development of a clinically useful and easy-to-use scale for rating pain and its relief. Patients will be evaluated according to the scales and the results recorded as frequently as needed.
2. Information about analgesics is readily available. This includes data concerning the effectiveness of various agents in controlling pain and the availability of equianalgesic charts wherever drugs are used for pain.
3. Patients are informed on admission of the availability of methods of relieving pain, and that they must communicate the presence and persistence of pain to the health care staff.
4. Explicit policies for use of advanced analgesic technologies are defined. These advances include patient-controlled analgesia, epidural analgesia, and regional analgesia. Specific instructions concerning use of these techniques must be available for the health care staff.
5. Adherence to standards is monitored by an interdisciplinary committee. The committee is responsible for overseeing the activities related to implementing and evaluating the effectiveness of these pain standards.

***starting p.*** A pain accompanied by muscular spasm during the early stages of sleep.

***subdiaphragmatic p.*** A sharp stitchlike pain occurring during breathing. When the breath is held, the pain ceases. Pressure against the lower rib cage eases the pain.

***subjective p.*** Pain with no apparent physical basis for its existence. It may be found among highly imaginative neurotic individuals in whom mild sensations are perceived as pain.

***sympathetic p.*** Referred p.

***tenesmic p.*** Pain accompanying urination or defecation. SEE: *tenesmus.*

***terebrant p.*** A boring or piercing type of pain.

***thalamic p.*** SEE: *thalamic syndrome.*

***thermalgesic p.*** Pain caused by heat.

***thoracic p.*** Sharp pain over the sternum, primarily in the chest or thoracic region, often running down the arm to the elbow. It may indicate angina pectoris but must not be confused with pain from gastric pressure in the region of the heart, caused by an accumulation of gas. It increases with respiration and is associated with broken ribs; intercostal neuralgia; wounds; herpes zoster; pleurisy; pleurodynia; myalgia; periostitis; acute peritonitis; colic; hepatic, gastric, or renal ulcer; gallbladder disorders; or carcinoma in late stages.

***throbbing p.*** Pain found in dental caries, headache, and localized inflammation.

***tongue p.*** Lingual p.

***tracheal p.*** Trachealgia.

***wandering p.*** Pain that changes its location repeatedly.

**painful arc** During active movement of an extremity, a portion of the range of motion in which pain is perceived. Pain is usually due to pinching of soft tissues at only a specific portion of the range of motion. A painful arc may be caused by tendinitis or bursitis.

**painful fat syndrome** Lipidemia.

**paint** (pānt) **1.** A solution of medication for application to the skin. **2.** To apply a medicated liquid to the skin.

**painters' colic** Colic accompanying lead poisoning. SEE: *lead* in *Poisons and Poisoning Appendix.*

**pair** Two of anything similar in shape, size, and conformation.

***base p.*** A pair of nucleotides, one a purine and the other a pyrimidine, joined by hydrogen bonds. These pairs make up deoxyribonucleic acid (DNA).

***ion p.*** Two particles of opposite charge, usually an electron and the positive atom residue from the interaction of ionizing radiation with the orbital electron of an atom.

**PAL** *posterior axillary line.*

**palatable** (păl′ăt-ă-b'l) [L. *palatum,* palate] Pleasing to the palate or taste, as food.

**palatal** (păl′ă-tăl) Pert. to the roof of the mouth, the palate.

**palate** (păl′ăt) [L. *palatum,* palate] The horizontal structure separating the mouth and the nasal cavity; the roof of the mouth. SEE: *mouth* for illus.

DIFFERENTIAL DIAGNOSIS: *Koplik's spots:* This rash is frequently seen on the palate in measles. *Secondary syphilis:* This is indicated by mucous patches on the palate. *Herpes of the throat:* This is characterized by vesicles in the circles on the pharyngeal walls and soft palate. *Swelling of uvula:* This is noted in inflammations of pharynx and tonsil, in nephritis, severe anemia, angioneurotic edema, and general debility. In diphtheria and Vincent's angina, a membranous exudate appears. In purpura hemorrhagica and some hemorrhagic diatheses, bloody extravasation appears. *Kaposi's sarcoma:* Dark purplish-red lesions may be found on the hard and soft palate. *Paralysis:* This may result from diphtheria, bulbar paralysis, neuritis, basal meningitis, or a tumor at the base of the brain. *Anesthesia:* This is seen in pathological conditions of the second division of the fifth nerve.

***artificial p.*** A prosthetic device molded to fill a cleft in the palate.

***bony p.*** Hard p.

***cleft p.*** A palate with a congenital opening.

***gothic p.*** An excessively high palatal arch.

***hard p.*** The anterior part of the palate supported by the maxillary and palatine bones. SYN: *bony p.*

***pendulous p.*** Uvula.

***primary p.*** In the embryo, the partition between the nasal cavities and mouth.

***secondary p.*** In the embryo, the palate formed from the maxillary arches and frontonasal process.

***soft p.*** The posterior musculomembranous fold partly separating the mouth and pharynx. SYN: *velum palatinum.*

**palate bone** Palatine bone.

**palatiform** (pă-lăt′ĭ-form) [L. *palatum,* palate, + *forma,* form] Resembling the palate.

**palatine** (păl′ă-tīn) [L. *palatinus*] **1.** Concerning the palate. **2.** The palate bones.

**palatine arches** Two archlike folds of mucous membrane (glossopalatine and pharyngopalatine arches) that form the lateral margins of faucial and pharyngeal isthmuses. They are continuous above with the soft palate.

**palatine artery, greater** The branch of the maxillary artery that supplies the palate, upper pharynx, and pharyngotympanic tube.

**palatine bone** One of the bones forming the posterior part of the hard palate and lateral nasal wall between the interior pterygoid plate of the sphenoid bone and maxilla. SYN: *palate bone.*

**palatitis** (păl-ăt-ī′tĭs) [L. *palatum,* palate, + Gr. *itis,* inflammation] Inflammation of the palate.

**palatoglossal** (păl″ă-tō-glŏs′ăl) Concerning the palate and tongue.

**palatoglossus** (păl″ă-tō-glŏs′ŭs) [″ + Gr. *glossa,* tongue] The muscle arising from the sides and undersurface of the tongue. Fibers pass upward through glossopalatine arch and are inserted in palatine aponeurosis. It constricts the faucial isthmus by raising the root of the tongue and drawing the sides of the soft palate downward.

**palatognathous** (păl″ă-tŏg′nă-thŭs) [″ + Gr. *gnathos,* jaw] Having a congenital cleft in the palate.

**palatography** (păl″ă-tŏg′ră-fē) [″ + Gr. *graphein,* to write] **1.** Recording of the movements of the palate in speech. **2.** Radiographical examination of the soft palate after injection of a contrast medium.

**palatomaxillary** (păl″ă-tō-măk′sĭ-lĕr″ē) Concerning the palate and maxilla.

**palatopharyngeal** (păl″ă-tō-fă-rĭn′jē-ăl) Concerning the palate and pharynx.

**palatopharyngeus** (păl″ăt-ō-fă″rĭn′jē-ŭs) [″ + Gr. *pharynx,* throat] The muscle arising from thyroid cartilage and pharyngeal wall, extending upward in posterior pillar, and inserting into aponeurosis of soft palate. It constricts the pharyngeal isthmus, raises the larynx, and depresses the soft palate.

**palatopharyngoplasty** Plastic surgical procedure for decreasing the size of the opening of the nasopharyngeal passageway. It has been used to treat chronic snoring.

**palatoplasty** (păl′ăt-ō-plăs″tē) [″ + Gr. *plassein,* to form] Plastic surgery of the palate, usually to correct a cleft. SEE: *staphylorrhaphy.*

**palatoplegia** (păl″ă-tō-plē′jē-ă) [″ + Gr. *plege,* stroke] Paralysis of muscles of the soft palate. SEE: *palate.*

**palatorrhaphy** (păl-ă-tor′ă-fē) [″ + Gr. *rhaphe,* seam, ridge] An operation for uniting a cleft palate. SYN: *staphylorrhaphy.*

**palatosalpingeus** (păl″ă-tō-săl-pĭn′jē-ŭs) [″ + Gr. *salpinx,* tube] The tensor veli palatini muscle.

**palatoschisis** (păl-ă-tŏs′kĭ-sĭs) [″ + *schisis,* a splitting] Palate with a cleft in it.

**palatum** (păl-ă′tŭm) *pl.* **palata** [L.] The palate.

**paleencephalon, paleoencephalon** (pā″lē-ĕn-sĕf′ă-lŏn, -ō-ĕn-sĕf′ă-lŏn) [Gr. *palaios,* old, + *enkephalos,* brain] The phylogenetically older portion of the brain; includes all of it except the cerebral cortex and its allied structures.

**paleocerebellum** (păl″ē-ō-sĕr″ĕ-bĕl′ŭm) [Gr. *palaios,* old, + L. *cerebellum,* little brain] Phylogenetically, the older portion of the cerebellum including the flocculi, certain parts of the vermis (lingula, nodulus, uvula), and the lobulus centralis (culmen, pyramis, uvula, and simple lobule). These parts are concerned primarily with equilibrium and movements of locomotion.

**paleogenesis** (pā″lē-ō-jĕn′ĕ-sĭs) [″ + *genesis,* generation, birth] Atavism.

**paleogenetic** (pā″lē-ō-jĕn-ĕt′ĭk) [″ + *gennan,* to produce] Originating in a previous generation.

**paleokinetic** (pā″lē-ō-kĭ-nĕt′ĭk) [″ + *kinetikos,* concerning movement] Regarding a peripheral motor nervous system controlling automatic associated movements. It is older phylogenetically than the system controlling voluntary movement.

**paleontology** (pā″lē-ŏn-tŏl′ō-jē) [″ + *onta,* existing things, + *logos,* word, reason] The branch of biology dealing with ancient plant and animal life of the earth.

**paleopathology** (pā″lē-ō-pă-thŏl′ō-jē) [″ + *pathos,* disease, + *logos,* word, reason] The study of diseases in the remains of bodies and fossils of ancient times.

**paleostriatal** (pā″lē-ō-strī-ā′tăl) [″+ L. *striatus,* ridged] Concerning the primitive portion of the corpus striatum.

**paleostriatum** (pā″lē-ō-strī-ā′tŭm) The primitive portion of corpus striatum, the globus pallidus. SEE: *neostriatum.*

**paleothalamus** (pā″lē-ō-thăl′ă-mŭs) [″ + *thalamos,* chamber] The medial portion of the thalamus (the medullary or noncortical part), which is older phylogenetically. SEE: *thalamus.*

**pali-, palin-** [Gr. *palin,* backward, again] Prefix meaning *recurrence, repetition.*

**palilalia** (păl-ĭ-lā′lē-ă) [″ + *lalein,* to speak] A pathological condition characterized by coherent speech in which certain words and phrases are repeated frequently and with increasing rapidity.

**palindromia** (păl-ĭn-drō′mē-ă) [″ + *dromos,* a running] The recurrence of a disease or a relapse.

**palindromic** (păl-ĭn-drŏm′ĭk) Relapsing.

**palinesthesia** (păl″ĭn-ĕs-thē′zē-ă) [Gr. *palin,* again, + *aisthesis,* sensation] The return of the power of sensation, as after recovery from anesthesia or coma.

**palingenesis** (păl″ĭn-jĕn′ĕ-sĭs) [″ + *genesis,* generation, birth] **1.** Regeneration or restoration of an organism or part of one. **2.** Atavism.

**palingraphia** (păl″ĭn-grăf′ē-ă) [″ + *graphein,* to write] Pathologic repetition of words or phrases in writing.

**palinopsia** [″ + *opsis,* vision] Persistence of a visual image after the object has been removed. It may be associated with a lesion in the occipital lobe of the brain. SEE: *afterimage.*

**palladium** (pă-lā′dē-ŭm) [L.] SYMB: Pd. A metallic element used in dentistry and surgical instruments; atomic weight 106.4; atomic number 46.

**pallesthesia** (păl-ĕs-thē′zē-ă) [Gr. *pallein,* to shake, + *aisthesis,* sensation] The sensation of vibration felt in the skin or bones, as that produced by a tuning fork held against the body.

**palliate** (păl′ē-āt) [L. *palliatus,* cloaked] To ease or reduce effect or intensity, esp. of a disease; to allay temporarily, as pain, without curing.

**palliative** (păl′ē-ā″tĭv) **1.** Relieving or alleviating without curing. **2.** An agent that alleviates or eases a painful or uncomfortable condition.

**pallid** (păl′ĭd) [L. *pallidus,* pale] Lacking color, pale, wan.

**pallidal** (păl′ĭ-dăl) Concerning the pallidum

of the brain.

**pallidectomy** (păl″ĭ-dĕk′tō-mē) [L. *pallidum,* pallidum, + Gr. *ektome,* excision] Surgical, chemical, electrical, or cryogenic removal or inactivation of the globus pallidus of the brain.

**pallidoansotomy** (păl″ĭ-dō-ăn-sŏt′ō-mē) [″ + *ansa,* a handle, + Gr. *tome,* incision] Production of lesions in the globus pallidus and ansa lenticularis of the brain.

**pallidotomy** (păl″ĭ-dŏt′ō-mē) [″ + Gr. *tome,* incision] Surgical destruction of the globus pallidus done to treat involuntary movements or muscular rigidity. The procedure is used experimentally in treating patients with Parkinson's disease.

**pallidum** (păl′ĭ-dŭm) [L.] The globus pallidus of the lenticular nucleus in the corpus striatum.

**pallium** (păl′ē-ŭm) [L., cloak] The cerebral cortex with its adjacent white substance, considered as a cover for the rest of the brain.

**pallor** (păl′or) [L.] Lack of color; paleness. SEE: *skin.*

**palm** [L. *palma,* hand] The anterior or flexor surface of the hand from the wrist to the fingers. SYN: *palma; vola manus.* SEE: *antithenar; thenar.*

**palma** (păl′mă) [L.] The palm.

**palmar** (păl′măr) Concerning the palm of the hand.

***p. cuff*** SEE: *universal cuff.*

**palmaris** (păl-mā′rĭs) One of two muscles, palmaris brevis and palmaris longus. SEE: *Muscles Appendix.*

**palmature** (păl′mă-tūr) [L. *palma,* hand] A pathological condition in which the fingers are joined or united.

**palm-chin reflex** A contraction of the superficial muscles of the eye and chin produced on the same side as the palmar area that is stimulated. This reflex is initiated when the thenar eminence is scratched with a sharp object.

**palmitin** (păl′mĭ-tĭn) An ester of glycerol and palmitic acid, derived from fat of both animal and vegetable origin.

**palmomental reflex** Palm-chin reflex.

**palmoplantar** (păl″mō-plăn′tăr) Pert. to the palms of the hands and soles of the feet.

**palmus** (păl′mŭs) [Gr. *palmos,* pulsation, quivering] **1.** Palpitation; a throb. **2.** Jerking; a disease with convulsive nervous twitching of the leg muscles, similar to jumping. **3.** Heartbeat.

**palpable** (păl′pă-b′l) [L. *palpabilis,* stroke, touch] Perceptible, esp. by touch.

**palpate** (păl′pāt) [L. *palpare,* to touch] To examine by touch; to feel.

**palpation** (păl-pā′shŭn) [L. *palpatio*] **1.** Examination by application of the hands or fingers to the external surface of the body to detect evidence of disease or abnormalities in the various organs. **2.** In obstetrics, a technique used to evaluate pelvic diameters, fetal presentation, position, and station, and cervical effacement and dilation.

***light-touch p.*** The process of determining the outline of abdominal organs by lightly palpating the abdominal wall with the fingers.

**palpatopercussion** (păl″pă-tō-pĕr-kŭsh′ŭn) Palpation combined with percussion.

**palpebra** (păl′pĕ-bră) *pl.* **palpebrae** [L.] An eyelid.

***p. inferior*** The lower eyelid.

***p. superior*** The upper eyelid.

**palpebral** (păl′pĕ-brăl) Concerning an eyelid.

**palpebral cartilage** One of the thin plates of connective tissue resembling cartilage that form the framework of the eyelid. SYN: *tarsal cartilage.*

**palpebral commissure** The union of the eyelids at each end of the palpebral fissure.

**palpebral muscles 1.** Palpebral portion of musculus orbicularis oculi. **2.** Levator palpebrae superioris.

**palpitant** (păl′pĭ-tănt) [L. *palpitare,* to quiver] Throbbing; trembling.

**palpitate** (păl′pĭ-tāt) [L. *palpitatus,* throbbing] **1.** To cause to throb. **2.** To throb or beat intensely or rapidly, usually said of the heart.

**palpitation** (păl-pĭ-tā′shŭn) A rapid, violent, or throbbing pulsation, as an abnormally rapid throbbing or fluttering of the heart. The palpitation is perceptible to the patient. SEE: *heart.*

***arterial p.*** Palpitation felt in the course of an artery.

**PALS** *pediatric advanced life support.*

**palsy** (pawl′zē) [ME. *palesie,* from L. *paralysis*] Paralysis.

***birth p.*** Palsy arising from an injury received at birth.

***brachial p.*** Partial or complete paralysis of one of the arms of a newborn. The cause is an injury to the brachial nerve plexus resulting from traction during a difficult vaginal delivery.

***bulbar p.*** Palsy caused by degeneration of the nuclear cells of the lower cranial nerves. This causes progressive muscular paralysis.

***cerebral p.*** SEE: *cerebral palsy.*

***crutch p.*** Paralysis resulting from pressure on nerves in the axilla from use of a crutch.

***diver's p.*** Paralysis caused by decompression illness. SEE: *bends; caisson disease.*

***Erb's p.*** Erb's paralysis.

***facial p.*** Bell's palsy.

***lead p.*** Paralysis of the extremities in lead poisoning.

***mercurial p.*** Paralysis induced by mercury poisoning.

***night p.*** A form of paresthesia characterized by numbness, esp. at night.

***pressure p.*** Temporary paralysis due to pressure on a nerve trunk.

***progressive supranuclear p.*** A chronic progressive degenerative disease of the central nervous system that has its onset in middle age. Conjugate ocular palsies, dystonia of the neck, and widespread rigidity occur.

***Saturday night p.*** Musculospiral paralysis.

***scrivener's p.*** Writer's cramp.

***shaking p.*** Parkinson's disease.

***wasting p.*** Progressive muscular atrophy.

**palynology** [Gr. *palumein,* to sprinkle, + *logos,* word, reason] The study of pollens, spores, or microscopic segments of organisms present in sediments.

**pamidronate disodium** A drug used to treat hypercalcemia associated with malignancy, with or without bone metastases, and moderate to severe Paget's disease. In the U.S., it is approved for intravenous use.

Caution: This drug should not be mixed with calcium-containing infusion solutions such as Ringer's solution.

**pampiniform** (păm-pĭn′ĭ-form) [L. *pampinus,* tendril, + *forma,* shape] Convoluted like a tendril.

**pan-** [Gr.] Combining form indicating *all.*

**panacea** (păn-ă-sē′ă) [Gr. *panakeia,* universal remedy] A remedy for all ills; a cure-all.

**panagglutinable** (păn″ă-gloo′tĭ-nă-b'l) [Gr. *pan,* all, + L. *agglutinare,* to glue to] Referring to blood cells that are agglutinable by every blood group serum of the species.

**panagglutinin** (păn″ă-glū′tĭn-ĭn) [Gr. *pan,* all, + L. *agglutinare,* to glue to] A substance capable of agglutinizing corpuscles of every blood group.

**panangiitis** (păn″ăn-jē-ī′tĭs) [″ + *angeion,* vessel, + *itis,* inflammation] Inflammation of all the coats of a blood vessel.

**panaris** (păn′ă-rĭs) [L. *panaricium,* disease of the fingernail] Paronychia.

**panarteritis** (păn″ăr-tĕ-rī′tĭs) [Gr. *pan,* all, + *arteria,* artery, + *itis,* inflammation] Inflammation of all the coats of an artery.

**panarthritis** (păn″ăr-thrī′tĭs) [″ + *arthron,* joint, + *itis,* inflammation] **1.** Inflammation of all parts of a joint. **2.** Inflammation of all the joints of the body.

**panasthenia** (păn″ăs-thē′nē-ă) [″ + *astheneia,* weakness] Neurasthenia.

**panatrophy** (păn-ăt′rō-fē) [″ + *a-,* not, + *trophe,* nourishment] Wasting away of an entire structure; generalized wasting away of the body.

**panblastic** (păn-blăs′tĭk) [″ + *blastos,* germ] Concerning all the layers of the blastoderm.

**pancarditis** (păn-kăr-dī′tĭs) [″ + *kardia,* heart, + *itis,* inflammation] Inflammation of all the structures of the heart.

**Pancoast syndrome** [Henry Khunrath Pancoast, U.S. physician, 1875–1939] Production of Horner's syndrome by a malignant neoplasm of the cervical area with involvement of the brachial plexus and cervical sympathetic nerves. The neoplasm is called Pancoast's tumor.

**pancolectomy** (păn″kō-lĕk′tō-mē) [Gr. *pan,* all, + *kolon,* colon, + *ektome,* excision] Surgical excision of the entire colon.

**pancreas** (păn′krē-ăs) *pl.* **pancreata** [″ + *kreas,* flesh] Both an exocrine and endocrine organ; a compound acinotubular gland situated behind the stomach in front of the first and second lumbar vertebrae in a horizontal position, its head attached to the duodenum and its tail reaching to the spleen. The portion between the head and the tail constitutes the body. The exocrine glands of the pancreas are acini, each with its own duct; these ducts anastomose to form the main pancreatic duct or duct of Wirsung, which joins the common bile duct and empties into the duodenum at the hepatopancreatic ampulla. An accessory pancreatic duct or duct of Santorini frequently is often present and opens into the duodenum directly. Scattered throughout the exocrine glandular tissue are masses of cells called islets of Langerhans, endocrine glands that secrete hormones. SEE: illus.

FUNCTION: The exocrine secretion of the pancreas is called pancreatic juice and contributes to digestion of all foods in the small intestine. It contains sodium bicarbonate, and the enzymes trypsinogen, chymotrypsinogen, amylase, and lipase. SEE: *pancreatic juice.*

The islets of Langerhans contain alpha, beta, and delta cells. Alpha cells secrete glucagon, which raises blood glucose; beta cells secrete insulin, which lowers blood glucose; delta cells secrete somatostatin, which inhibits the secretion of insulin, glucagon, growth hormone from the anterior pituitary, and gastrin from the stomach. SEE: *somatostatin.*

Diminished secretion of insulin by the islets of Langerhans results in diabetes mellitus. In this disease there are disturbances in the metabolism of carbohydrates and fats resulting in the elevation of blood glucose, cholesterol, and ketone bodies. Excessive secretion of insulin, called hyperinsulinism, may sometimes occur. This results in marked lowering of blood sugar (hypoglycemia). SEE: *diabetes mellitus; insulin; pancreatic function tests.*

***accessory p.*** A small mass of pancreatic tissue close to the pancreas but detached from it.

***annular p.*** An anomalous condition in which a portion of the pancreas encircles the duodenum.

***p. divisum*** A congenital anomaly in which the two portions of the embryonic pancreas fail to unite.

***dorsal p.*** A dorsal outpocketing of the embryonic gut that gives rise to the body and tail of the adult pancreas.

***lesser p.*** The semidetached lobular part of the posterior surface of a head of the

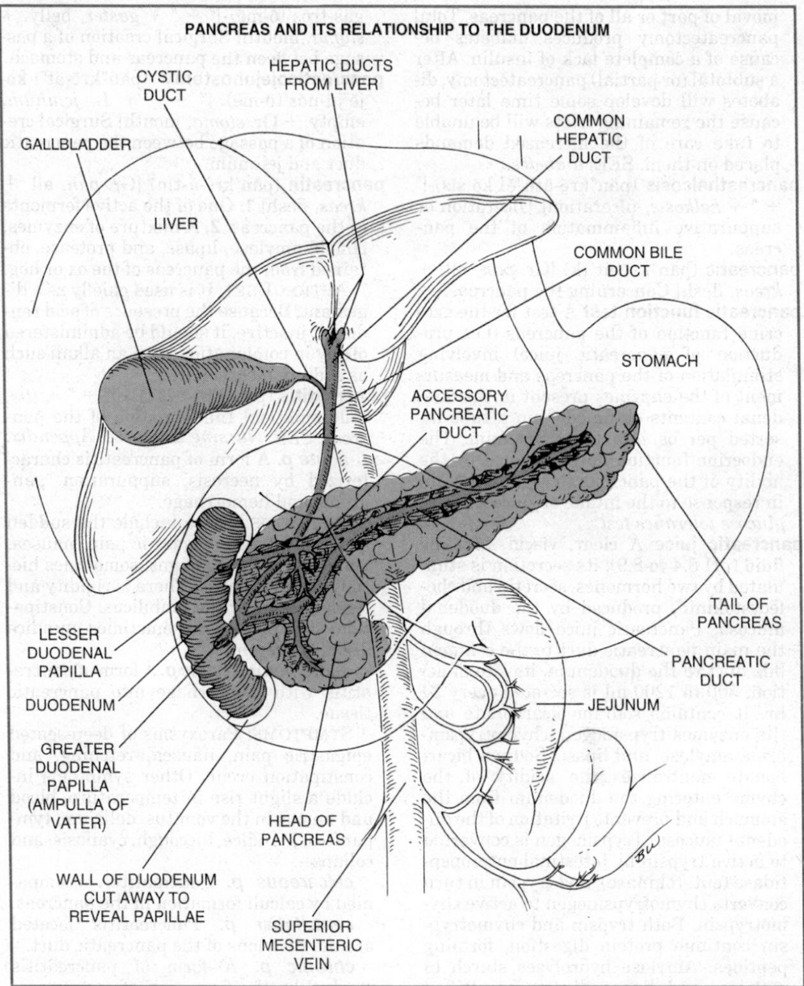


pancreas, sometimes having a separate duct opening into the principal one. SYN: *Willis' p.*

***transplantation of the p.*** The implantation of a part of the pancreas or the entire gland from a donor into a patient whose own pancreas is no longer functioning. The survival rate of the transplanted tissue for 1 year is about 50%. Transplantation of islet cells is being actively investigated.

***ventral p.*** An outgrowth at the angle of the hepatic diverticulum and the embryonic gut that migrates and fuses with the dorsal pancreas. It forms the head of the definitive organ.

***Willis' p.*** Lesser p.

**pancreas, carcinoma of** Cancer of the pancreas. This cancer accounts for 22% of deaths from gastrointestinal cancer. The prognosis is extremely poor, as only 3% of patients are alive 5 years after the diagnosis is made. The cause of this cancer, which occurs more frequently in men than in women, is unknown, but two risk factors are important: cigarette smoking and a high intake of fat, meat, or both. Also, a history of gastric cancer or peptic ulcer surgery increases the risk of developing this type of cancer. There is no statistically significant association between coffee consumption and pancreatic cancer. A variety of therapeutic approaches have been used, including surgery, radiation, chemotherapy, and endocrine therapy.

**pancreatalgia** (păn″krē-ă-tăl′jē-ă) [″ + *kreas,* flesh, + *algos,* pain] Pain in the pancreas.

**pancreatectomy** (păn″krē-ă-tĕk′tō-mē) [″ + ″ + *ektome,* excision] An operation for removal of part or all of the pancreas. Total pancreatectomy produces diabetes because of a complete lack of insulin. After a subtotal (or partial) pancreatectomy, diabetes will develop some time later because the remaining islets will be unable to take care of the increased demands placed on them. SEE: *diabetes.*

**pancreathelcosis** (păn″krē-ăth″ĕl-kō′sĭs) [″ + ″ + *helkosis,* ulceration] Ulceration or suppurative inflammation of the pancreas.

**pancreatic** (păn″krē-ăt′ĭk) [Gr. *pan,* all, + *kreas,* flesh] Concerning the pancreas.

**pancreatic function test** A test for the exocrine function of the pancreas (i.e., production of pancreatic juice) involving stimulation of the pancreas and measurment of the enzymes present in the duodenal contents obtained from a tube inserted per os into the duodenum. The endocrine function may be tested by the ability of the pancreas to secrete insulin in response to the intake of glucose. SEE: *glucose tolerance test.*

**pancreatic juice** A clear, viscid, alkaline fluid (pH 8.4 to 8.9); its secretion is stimulated by two hormones, secretin and cholecystokinin, produced by the duodenal mucosa. Pancreatic juice flows through the main pancreatic duct to the common bile duct to the duodenum, its site of action; 500 to 1200 ml is secreted every 24 hr. It contains sodium bicarbonate and the enzymes trypsinogen, chymotrypsinogen, amylase, and lipase. Sodium bicarbonate neutralizes the acidity of the chyme entering the duodenum from the stomach and prevents irritation of the duodenal mucosa. Trypsinogen is converted to active trypsin by intestinal enteropeptidase (enterokinase), and trypsin in turn converts chymotrypsinogen to active chymotrypsin. Both trypsin and chymotrypsin continue protein digestion, forming peptides. Amylase hydrolyzes starch to maltose, and lipase digests emulsified fats to fatty acids and glycerol. SEE: *enzyme; pancreas; secretion.*

**pancreaticocholecystostomy** (păn″krēăt″ĭ-kō-kō″lē-sĭs-tŏs′tō-mē) [Gr. *pan,* all, + *kreas,* flesh, + *chole,* bile, + *kystis,* bladder, + *stoma,* mouth] The surgical creation of a passage between the gallbladder and pancreas.

**pancreaticoduodenal** (păn″krē-ăt″ĭ-kō-dū-ō-dē′năl) [″ + ″+ L. *duodeni,* twelve] Concerning the duodenum and pancreas.

**pancreaticoduodenostomy** (păn″krē-ăt″ĭ-kō-dū″ō-dē-nŏs′tō-mē) [″ + ″ + ″ + Gr. *stoma,* mouth] Surgical creation of an artificial passage between the pancreas and duodenum.

**pancreaticoenterostomy** (păn″krē-ăt″ĭ-kō-ĕn″tĕr-ŏs′tō-mē) [″+ ″+ *enteron,* intestine, + *stoma,* mouth] Surgical creation of a passage between the pancreatic duct and intestine.

**pancreaticogastrostomy** (păn″krē-ăt″ĭ-kō-găs-trŏs′tō-mē) [″ + ″ + *gaster,* belly, + *stoma,* mouth] Surgical creation of a passage between the pancreas and stomach.

**pancreaticojejunostomy** (păn″krē-ăt″ĭ-kō-jĕ″jū-nŏs′tō-mē) [″ + ″ + L. *jejunum,* empty, + Gr. *stoma,* mouth] Surgical creation of a passage between the pancreatic duct and jejunum.

**pancreatin** (păn′krē-ă-tĭn) [Gr. *pan,* all, + *kreas,* flesh] **1.** One of the active ferments of the pancreas. **2.** A mixture of enzymes, chiefly amylase, lipase, and protease, obtained from the pancreas of the ox or hog.

ACTION/USES: It is used chiefly as a digestant. Because the presence of acid renders it inactive, it should be administered orally in combination with an alkali such as sodium bicarbonate.

**pancreatitis** (păn″krē-ă-tī′tĭs) [″ + ″ + *itis,* inflammation] Inflammation of the pancreas. SEE: *Nursing Diagnoses Appendix.*

***acute p.*** A form of pancreatitis characterized by necrosis, suppuration, gangrene, and hemorrhage.

SYMPTOMS: These include the sudden onset of intense epigastric pain, nausea, vomiting, belching of gas, sometimes hiccough, and collapse. There is rigidity and tenderness over the umbilicus. Constipation, slow pulse, and sometimes jaundice are also present.

***acute hemorrhagic p.*** A form of pancreatitis with hemorrhage into pancreatic tissue.

SYMPTOMS: Paroxysms of deep-seated epigastric pain, nausea, retching, and constipation occur. Other symptoms include a slight rise in temperature, blood and mucus in the vomitus, delirium, tympanites, jaundice, hiccough, cyanosis, and collapse.

***calcareous p.*** Pancreatitis accompanied by calculi formation in the pancreas.

***centrilobar p.*** Pancreatitis located around divisions of the pancreatic duct.

***chronic p.*** A form of pancreatitis marked by the formation of scar tissue, which leads to malfunction of the pancreas.

SYMPTOMS: The pain may be mild or severe, tending to radiate to the back. Jaundice, weakness, emaciation, and diarrhea are present.

***interstitial p.*** Pancreatitis with overgrowth of interacinar and intra-acinar connective tissue.

***perilobar p.*** Fibrosis of the pancreas between acinous groups.

***purulent p.*** Pancreatitis with suppuration.

***suppurative p.*** A form of pancreatitis marked by the development of many small abscesses. Symptoms may be those of the acute or the chronic form of pancreatitis.

**pancreatoduodenectomy** (păn″krē-ă-tō-dū″ō-dē-nĕk′tō-mē) [Gr. *pan,* all, + *kreas,* flesh, + L. *duodeni,* twelve, + Gr. *ektome,* excision] Excision of the head of the pancreas and the adjacent portion of the duodenum.

**pancreatoduodenostomy** (păn″krē-ă-tō-dū″ō-dĕ-nŏs′tō-mē) [″ + ″ + ″ + *stoma,* mouth] Surgical anastomosis of the pancreatic duct, or a pancreatic fistula, to the duodenum.

**pancreatogenic, pancreatogenous** (păn″krē-ă-tō-jĕn′ĭk, -tŏj′ĕ-nŭs) [″ + ″ + *gennan,* to produce] Produced in or by the pancreas; originating in the pancreas.

**pancreatography** (păn″krē-ă-tŏg′ră-fē) [″ + ″ + *graphein,* to write] Endoscopic and radiological examination of the pancreas after injection of a radiopaque contrast medium through the duct of Wirsung.

**pancreatolith** (păn″krē-ăt′ō-lĭth) [″ + ″ + *lithos,* stone] A calculus in the pancreas.

**pancreatolithectomy** (păn″krē-ăt-ō-lĭth-ĕk′tō-mē) [″ + ″ + ″ + *ektome,* excision] Removal of a calculus from the pancreas.

**pancreatolithiasis** (păn″krē-ă-tō-lĭ-thī′ă-sĭs) [″ + ″ + ″ + *-iasis,* condition] Calculi in the duct system of the pancreas.

**pancreatolithotomy** (păn″krē-ăt-ō-lĭ-thŏt′ō-mē) [″ + ″ + ″ + *tome,* incision] Incision of the pancreas for removal of a calculus. SYN: *pancreolithotomy.*

**pancreatolysis** (păn″krē-ă-tŏl′ĭ-sĭs) [″ + ″ + *lysis,* dissolution] Destruction of the pancreatic substance by pancreatic enzymes.

**pancreatolytic** (păn″krē-ăt-ō-lĭt′ĭk) Destructive to pancreatic tissues.

**pancreatomy** (păn-krē-ăt′ō-mē) [″ + ″ + *tome,* incision] Pancreatotomy.

**pancreatoncus** (păn-krē-ăt-ŏng′kŭs) [″ + ″ + *onkos,* tumor] A pancreatic tumor.

**pancreatopathy** (păn″krē-ă-tŏp′ă-thē) [″ + ″ + *pathos,* disease, suffering] Any pathologic state of the pancreas. SYN: *pancreopathy.*

**pancreatotomy** (păn″krē-ă-tŏt′ō-mē) [″ + ″ + *tome,* incision] Surgical incision into the pancreas. SYN: *pancreatomy.*

**pancreatotropic** (păn-krē″ă-tō-trŏp′ĭk) [″ + ″ + *tropikos,* turning] Having an affinity for or action on the pancreas.

**pancreectomy** (păn″krē-ĕk′tō-mē) [″ + ″ + *ektome,* excision] Partial or total excision of the pancreas.

**pancrelipase** (păn″krē-lī′pās) A standardized preparation of enzymes, principally lipase, with amylase and protease, obtained from the pancreas of the hog. It is used in treating conditions associated with deficient secretion from the pancreas.

**pancreolithotomy** (păn″krē-ō-lĭ-thŏt′ō-mē) [″ + *kreas,* flesh, + *lithos,* stone, + *tome,* incision] Pancreatolithotomy.

**pancreolysis** (păn″krē-ŏl′ĭ-sĭs) [″ + ″ + *lysis,* dissolution] Enzymatic destruction of the pancreas.

**pancreopathy** (păn″krē-ŏp′ă-thē) [″ + ″ + *pathos,* disease, suffering] Pancreatopathy.

**pancreoprivic** (păn″krē-ō-prĭv′ĭk) Having no pancreas.

**pancuronium bromide** (păn″kū-rō′nē-ŭm) A neuromuscular blocking agent.

**pancytopenia** (păn″sī-tō-pē′nē-ă) [″ + *kytos,* cell, + *penia,* poverty] A reduction in all cellular elements of the blood. SEE: *anemia, aplastic.*

**pandemic** (păn-dĕm′ĭk) A disease affecting the majority of the population of a large region, such as dental caries or periodontal disease, or one that is epidemic at the same time in many different parts of the world.

**pandiculation** (păn″dĭk-ū-lā′shŭn) [L. *pandiculari,* to stretch one's self] Stretching of the limbs and yawning, as on awakening from normal sleep.

**panel 1.** A number of patients or normal subjects who participate in medical investigations, esp. studies in which new drugs, devices, or procedures are tested. SEE: *informed consent; institutional review board.* **2.** The list of patients who obtain their primary medical care from the physician to whom they are assigned. This system is used in some health care plans.

**panencephalitis** (păn″ĕn-sĕf″ă-lī′tĭs) [Gr. *pan,* all, + *enkephalos,* brain, + *itis,* inflammation] A diffuse inflammation of the brain.

***subacute sclerosing p.*** ABBR: SSPE. A cerebral degenerative disease thought to be secondary to entrance of the measles virus into the brain. The first signs are a progressive decrease in higher cerebral functions, usually manifested as failure to progress in school. There are personality changes, emotional instability, and generalized myoclonic jerks. In late stages, dementia and generalized rigidity occur. There is no treatment, and most patients die of the disease.

**panendoscope** (păn-ĕn′dō-skōp) [″ + *endon,* within, + *skopein,* to view] A cystoscope that gives a wide view of the bladder.

**Paneth, cells of** (pă′nāt) [Josef Paneth, Ger. physician, 1857–1890] Large secretory cells containing coarse granules, found at the blind end of the crypts of Lieberkühn (the intestinal glands).

**pang 1.** A paroxysm of extreme agony. **2.** A sudden attack of any emotion.

**pangenesis** (păn″jĕn′ĕ-sĭs) [Gr. *pan,* all, + *genesis,* generation, birth] The discredited hypothesis that each cell of the parent is represented by a particle in the reproductive cell, and thus each part of the organism reproduces itself in the progeny.

**panhypopituitarism** (păn-hī″pō-pĭ-tū′ĭ-tăr-ĭzm) [″ + *hypo,* under, + L. *pituita,* mucus, + Gr. *-ismos,* condition] Defective or absent function of the entire pituitary gland. SEE: *Simmonds' disease.*

**panhysterectomy** (păn″hĭs-tĕr-ĕk′tō-mē) [″ + *hystera,* womb, + *ektome,* excision] Excision of the entire uterus including the cervix uteri. SEE: *hysterectomy.*

**panhysterocolpectomy** (păn-hĭs″tĕr-ō-kŏl-pĕk′tō-mē) [″ + ″ + *kolpos,* vagina, + *ektome,* excision] Total excision of the uterus and vagina.

**panhystero-oophorectomy** (păn-hĭs″tĕr-ō-ō-ŏf-ō-rĕk′tō-mē) [″ + ″ + *oophoros,* bearing eggs, + *ektome,* excision] Excision of the uterus, cervix, and one or both ovaries.

**panhysterosalpingectomy** (păn-hĭs″tĕr-ō-săl″pĭn-jĕk′tō-mē) [″ + ″ + *salpinx,* tube, + *ektome,* excision] Surgical removal of the uterus, cervix, and fallopian tubes.

**panhysterosalpingo-oophorectomy** (păn-hĭs″tĕr-ō-săl″pĭng-gō-ō-ŏf-ō-rĕk′tō-mē) [″ + ″ + ″ + *oophoros,* bearing eggs, + *ektome,* excision] Excision of the entire uterus, including the cervix, ovaries, and uterine tubes.

**panic** (păn′ĭk) Acute anxiety, terror, or fright that is usually of sudden onset, may be uncontrollable, and may require sedation. Because the cause of this reaction is often unknown, it is quite difficult to evaluate the response. If hyperventilation and tetany are present, the patient should breathe with the mouth closed and one nostril held closed, which alleviates the symptoms in a short time.

***p. attack*** A discrete period of intense fear or discomfort that is accompanied by at least 4 of the following symptoms: palpitations, sweating, trembling or shaking, sensations of shortness of breath or smothering, feeling of choking, chest pain or discomfort, nausea or abdominal distress, dizziness or light headedness, feeling of unreality or being detached from oneself, feeling of losing control or going crazy, fear of dying, paresthesias (numbness or tingling sensations), and chills or hot flushes. The onset is sudden and builds to a peak usually in 10 min or less and may include a sense of imminent danger or impending doom and an urge to escape.

NURSING IMPLICATIONS: The nurse allows the patient to release energy and express feelings of anxiety. Precautions are taken to ensure the patient's safety. A calm, quiet, and reassuring environment helps the patient to overcome feelings of anxiety.

***p. disorder*** An anxiety disorder characterized by panic attacks (e.g., agoraphobia with panic attacks).

***homosexual p.*** An acute anxiety syndrome caused by unconscious homosexual conflicts. Symptoms include fear, paranoid ideas, and excitement, and sometimes hallucinations and combative behavior.

**panmyeloid** (păn-mī′ĕ-loyd) [Gr. *pan,* all, + *myelos,* marrow, + *eidos,* form, shape] Concerning all of the elements of the bone marrow.

**panneuritis** (păn″ū-rī′tĭs) [″ + *neuron,* sinew, + *itis,* inflammation] Generalized neuritis.

***p. epidemica*** Beriberi.

**panniculitis** (păn-ĭk″ū-lī′tĭs) [L. *panniculus,* a small piece of cloth, + *itis,* inflammation] Inflammation of a layer of fatty connective tissue in the anterior wall of the abdomen. Patients experience pain, tenderness, and hypertrophy of tissue in parts where fat is the thickest.

***nodular nonsuppurative p.*** Weber-Christian disease.

**panniculus** (păn-ĭk′ū-lŭs) [L., a small piece of cloth] Any clothlike sheet or layer of tissue.

***p. adiposus*** The subcutaneous layer of fat, esp. where fat is abundant; the superficial fascia that is heavily laden with fat cells.

***p. carnosus*** The thin layer of muscular tissue in the superficial fascia. SEE: *platysma myoides.*

**pannus** (păn′nŭs) [L., cloth] **1.** Newly formed superficial vascular invasion of the cornea. The area is cloudy, and its surface is uneven because it is infiltrated with a film of new capillary blood vessels. This condition may be seen in trachoma, acne rosacea, eczema, and as a result of irritation in granular conjunctivitis. SEE: *micropannus.* **2.** Inflamed synovial granulation tissue seen in chronic rheumatoid arthritis.

***corneal p.*** An overgrowth of vascular tissue in the periphery of the cornea, occurring in response to inflammation of the cornea, esp. in trachoma.

***p. crassus*** Pannus that is highly vascularized, thick, and opaque.

***phlyctenular p.*** Pannus that occurs in conjunction with phlyctenular conjunctivitis.

***p. siccus*** Pannus accompanying xerophthalmia. It is composed principally of connective tissue that is dry and poorly vascularized.

***p. tenuis*** Pannus that is thin, poorly vascularized, and slightly opaque.

**panodic** (pă-nŏd′ĭk) Radiating in all directions, esp. said of a nerve impulse.

**panography** (păn-nŏg′ră-fē) A radiographical procedure that provides a panoramic view of an entire dental arch on one film.

**panophobia** (păn-ō-fō′bē-ă) [Gr. *pan,* all, + *phobos,* fear] Morbid groundless fear of some unknown evil or of everything in general; general apprehension. SYN: *pantophobia.*

**panophthalmia, panophthalmitis** (păn-ŏf-thăl′mē-ă, -thăl-mī′tĭs) [″ + *ophthalmos,* eye, + *itis,* inflammation] Inflammation of the entire eye.

**panoptic** (păn-ŏp′tĭk) [″ + *optikos,* vision] Making every part visible.

**panoptosis** (păn-ŏp-tō′sĭs) [″ + *ptosis,* a dropping] General prolapse of the abdominal organs.

**panphobia** (păn-fō′bē-ă) [″ + *phobos,* fear] Panophobia.

**panplegia** (păn-plē′jē-ă) [″ + *plege,* stroke] Total paralysis.

**pansclerosis** (păn″sklē-rō′sĭs) [″ + *sklerosis,* hardening] Hardening of an entire organ.

**pansinusitis** (păn″sī-nŭs-ī′tĭs) [″ + L. *sinus,*

curve, hollow, + *itis,* inflammation] Inflammation of all of the paranasal sinuses.

**pansphygmograph** (păn-sfĭg′mō-grăf) [″ + *sphygmos,* pulse, + *graphein,* to write] An apparatus for registering cardiac movements, the pulse wave, and chest movements at the same time.

**Panstrongylus** (păn-strŏn′jĭ-lŭs) A genus of insects belonging to the order Hemiptera, family Reduviidae. This species may serve as the vector for *Trypanosoma cruzi,* the causative agent of Chagas′ disease.

**pansystolic** Occurring throughout systole of the heart; used to describe that type of cardiac murmur.

**pant** [ME. *panten*] **1.** To gasp for breath. **2.** A short and shallow breath. Panting is produced by physical overexertion, as in running, or from fear.

**pant-, panto-** [Gr. *pantos,* all] Combining form indicating *all, whole.*

**pantanencephaly** (păn″tăn-ĕn-sĕf′ă-lē) [″ + *an-,* not, + *enkephalos,* brain] Complete absence of the brain in the fetus.

**pantankyloblepharon** (păn-tăng″kĭ-lō-blĕf′ă-rŏn) [″ + *ankyle,* noose, + *blepharon,* lid] Generalized adhesion of the eyelids to the eyeball.

**pantetheine** (păn-tĕ-thē′ĭn) The naturally occurring amide of pantothenic acid. It is a growth factor for *Lactobacillus bulgaricus.*

**panting** (pănt′ĭng) [ME. *panten*] Short, shallow, rapid respirations. SYN: *polypnea.*

**pantograph** (păn′tō-grăf) [Gr. *pantos,* all, + *graphein,* to write] A device that will reproduce, through a system of levers connected to a stylus, a duplicate of whatever figure or drawing is being copied by the device.

**pantomography** (păn″tō-mŏg′ră-fē) SEE: *panoramic radiograph.*

**pantomorphia** (păn″tō-mor′fē-ă) [″ + *morphe,* form] **1.** The state of being symmetrical. **2.** Able to assume any shape.

**pantophobia** (păn-tō-fō′bē-ă) [″ + *phobos,* fear] Panophobia.

**pantothenate** (păn-tō′thĕn-āt) A salt of pantothenic acid.

**pantothenic acid** (păn-tō-thĕn′ĭk) $C_9H_{17}NO_5$. A vitamin of the B-complex group widely distributed in nature, occurring naturally in yeast, liver, heart, salmon, eggs, and various grains. It was synthesized in 1940. It is part of coenzyme A, which is necessary for the Krebs cycle and for conversion of amino acids and lipids to carbohydrates.

**panturbinate** (păn-tŭr′bĭ-nāt) [″ + L. *turbinatus,* shaped like a top] All of the turbinate structures of the nose; the nasal conchae.

**Panwarfin** Trade name for warfarin sodium.

**panzootic** (păn″zō-ŏt′ĭk) [″ + *zoon,* animal] Any animal disease that is widespread.

**$PaO_2$** The partial pressure of oxygen in arterial blood; arterial oxygen concentration, or tension; usually expressed in millimeters of mercury (mm Hg).

**pap** (păp) [L. *pappa,* infant′s sound for food] Any soft, semiliquid food.

**papain** (pă-pā′ĭn) Proteolytic enzyme obtained from the fruit of the papaya, *Carica papaya;* used to tenderize meat.

**Papanicolaou test** [George Nicholas Papanicolaou, Gr.-born U.S. scientist, 1883–1962] ABBR: Pap test. A study for early detection of cancer cells. It involves collecting material from areas of the body that shed cells or in which shed cells collect, esp. the cervix and vagina. This material is then prepared for microscopic study by special staining. Analysis of the cells is extremely helpful in diagnosing cancer. The cells may be obtained by using a spatula and cotton swab, or a combination of a spatula and a special brush (Cytobrush), or the brush alone. SYN: *Pap smear.*

Because of the use of the Pap test, death from cervical cancer has declined by 70% since the test was developed in the 1940s. Although interpretation of the test is subject to human error, a variety of developments have improved test accuracy, including use of computer-generated procedures for detection and examination of abnormal cells and mandated reexamination of sample batches to test quality control.

A woman may augment the accuracy and value of the Pap test by following these guidelines: Asking her physician about the quality of the laboratory evaluating the results; having an annual Pap test beginning at age 18; scheduling the test 2 weeks after the end of a menstrual period; abstaining from sexual activity for 48 hr before the test; providing a detailed medical history, including use of birth control pills or hormones and results of past Pap tests; and requesting a second opinion on the Pap test if she is at risk for cancer of the reproductive tract.

---

Caution: As with any test, it is possible that human errors may cause an incorrect interpretation of the slides. It is important that the quality of performance of the technicians and physicians be periodically reviewed by persons not employed by the laboratory or hospital.

---

**papaverine hydrochloride** (pă-păv′ĕr-ēn) [L., poppy] The salt of an alkaloid obtained from opium; used as a smooth muscle relaxant, esp. in gastric and intestinal distress and in bronchial spasm.

**papaya** (pă-pă′yă) [Sp. Amerind.] **1.** A tropical tree, *Carica papaya.* **2.** Large, oblong, edible fruit from that tree; the source of papain.

**paper** [L. *papyrus,* paper] **1.** Cellulose pulp prepared in thin sheets from fibers of wood, rags, and other substances. **2.** Charta. **3.** A thin sheet of cellulosic material impregnated with specific chemicals that react in a definite manner when exposed to certain solutions. This permits use of these papers for testing purposes.

***articulating p.*** Paper coated on both sides with a pigment that marks the teeth when their occlusal surfaces contact the paper. This allows the contact points of the teeth to be demonstrated.

***bibulous p.*** Paper that absorbs water readily.

***filter p.*** A porous, unglazed paper used for filtration.

***indicator p.*** Paper saturated with an indicator solution of known strength and then dried; used for testing the pH (acidity or alkalinity) of a solution.

***litmus p.*** An indicator paper impregnated with litmus, which turns blue in alkaline solutions and red in acidic solutions.

***test p.*** Paper impregnated with a substance that will change color when exposed to solutions of a certain pH or to specific chemicals.

**papilla** (pă-pĭl′ă) *pl.* **papillae** [L.] A small, nipple-like protuberance or elevation.

***acoustic p.*** The spiral organ of the ear.

***Bergmeister's p.*** A veil in front of the retina of the eye. It is made of a conical mass of glial elements that are the developmental tissue of the eye that has not been reabsorbed.

***circumvallate p.*** One of the large papillae near the base on the dorsal aspect of the tongue, arranged in a V-shape. The taste buds are located in the epithelium of the trench surrounding the papilla.

***clavate p.*** Fungiform p.

***conical p.*** **1.** Papillae on the dorsum of the tongue. **2.** Papillae in the ridgelike projections in the corium of the surface of the skin. SYN: *p. of corium.*

***p. of corium*** Conical p. (2).

***dental p.*** A mass of connective tissue that becomes enclosed by the developing enamel organ. It gives rise to dentin and dental pulp.

***dermal p.*** Small elevations of the corium that indent the inner surface of the epidermis.

***duodenal p.*** P. of Vater.

***filiform p.*** One of the very slender papillae at the tip of the tongue.

***foliate p.*** Folds, which are rudimentary papillae, in the sides of the tongue.

***fungiform p.*** One of the broad flat papillae resembling a fungus, chiefly found on the dorsal central area of the tongue. SYN: *clavate p.*

***gingival p.*** The gingiva that fills the space between adjacent teeth.

***gustatory p.*** Taste papilla of tongue; one of those possessing a taste bud. SYN: *taste p.*

***p. of hair*** A conical process of the corium that projects into undersurface of a hair bulb. It contains capillaries through which a hair receives its nourishment. SYN: *p. pili.*

***incisive p.*** Projection on the anterior portion of the raphe of the palate. SYN: *palantine p.*

***interdental p.*** The triangular part of the gingivae that fits between adjacent teeth, including both free gingiva and attached gingiva.

***interproximal p.*** The gingival papillae between adjacent teeth. These include the projections seen from the lingual, buccal, or labial sides.

***lacrimal p.*** An elevation in the medial edge of each eyelid, in the center of which is the opening of the lacrimal duct.

***lenticular p.*** A small rounded elevation underlying lymphatic nodules in the mucosa of the root of the tongue.

***lingual p.*** Any one of the tiny eminences covering the anterior two thirds of the tongue, including circumvallate, filiform, fungiform, and conical papillae.

***mammae p.*** The nipple of the mammary gland.

***optic p.*** Blind spot (1).

***palatine p.*** Incisive p.

***parotid p.*** The projections around the opening of the parotid duct into the mouth.

***p. pili*** P. of hair.

***renal p.*** The apex of a malpighian pyramid in the kidney.

***tactile p.*** A dermal papilla that contains a sensory end organ for touch.

***taste p.*** Gustatory p.

***urethral p.*** The small projection in the vestibule of the vagina at the entrance of the urethra.

***vallate p.*** Circumvallate p.

***p. of Vater*** The duodenal end of the drainage systems of the pancreatic and common bile ducts; commonly, but inaccurately, called the ampulla of Vater. SYN: *duodenal p.; hepatopancreatic ampulla.*

**papillary** (păp′ĭ-lăr-ē) [L. *papilla,* nipple] **1.** Concerning a nipple or papilla. **2.** Resembling or composed of papillae.

***p. ducts of Bellini*** Short ducts that open on the tip of the renal papillae. They are formed by the union of the straight collecting tubules.

***p. layer*** The layer of the corium that adjoins the epidermis. SYN: *stratum papillare.*

***p. tumor*** Neoplasm composed of or resembling enlarged papillae. SEE: *papilloma.*

**papillate** (păp′ĭ-lāt) [L. *papilla,* nipple] Having nipple-like growths on the surface, as a culture in bacteriology.

**papillectomy** (păp″ĭ-lĕk′tō-mē) [″ + Gr. *ektome,* excision] Excision of any papilla or papillae.

**papilledema** (păp″ĭl-ĕ-dē′mă) [″ + Gr. *oidema,* swelling] Edema and inflammation of the optic nerve at its point of entrance into the eyeball. It is caused by increased intracranial pressure, often due to a tumor of the brain pressing on the optic nerve. Blindness may result very rapidly unless relieved. SYN: *choked disk; papillitis.*

**papilliferous** (păp″ĭ-lĭf′ĕr-ŭs) [″ + *ferre,* to carry] Having or containing papillae.

**papilliform** (pă-pĭl′ĭ-form) [″ + *forma,* shape] Having the characteristics or appearance of papillae.

**papillitis** (păp-ĭ-lī′tĭs) [″ + Gr. *itis,* inflammation] Papilledema.

**papilloadenocystoma** (păp″ĭl-ō-ăd″ē-nō-sĭs-tō′mă) [″ + Gr. *aden,* gland, + *kystis,* a cyst, + *oma,* tumor] A tumor composed of elements of papilloma, adenoma, and cystoma.

**papillocarcinoma** (păp″ĭl-ō-kăr-sĭ-nō′mă) [″ + Gr. *karkinos,* crab, + *oma,* tumor] **1.** A malignant tumor of hypertrophied papillae. **2.** Carcinoma with papillary growths.

**papilloma** (păp-ĭ-lō′mă) [″ + Gr. *oma,* tumor] **1.** A benign epithelial tumor. **2.** Epithelial tumor of skin or mucous membrane consisting of hypertrophied papillae covered by a layer of epithelium. Included in this group are warts, condylomas, and polyps. SEE: *acanthoma; papillomavirus.*

***p. durum*** A hardened papilloma, as a wart or corn.

***fibroepithelial p.*** A skin tag containing fibrous tissue.

***hard p.*** Papilloma that develops from squamous epithelium.

***Hopmann's p.*** [Carl Melchior Hopmann, Ger. physician, 1849–1925] Papillomatous overgrowth of the nasal mucosa.

***intracystic p.*** Papilloma within a cystic adenoma.

***intraductal p.*** A solitary neoplasm of the breast that occurs in the large, lactiferous ducts. A distinct neoplasm that displays a papillary histological pattern.

***p. molle*** Condyloma.

***soft p.*** Papilloma formed from columnar epithelium; applies to any small, soft growth.

***villous p.*** Papilloma with thin, long excrescences present in the urinary bladder, breast, intestinal tract, or choroid plexus of the cerebral ventricles.

**papillomatosis** (păp″ĭ-lō-mă-tō′sĭs) [″+ Gr. *oma,* tumor, + *osis,* condition] **1.** Widespread formation of papillomas. **2.** The condition of being afflicted with many papillomas.

**papillomavirus** Any of a group of viruses that cause papillomas or warts in humans and animals. They belong to the papovavirus family or group. SEE: *wart, genital.*

***human p.*** ABBR: HPV. A papillomavirus that is specific to humans. HPVs cause three types of cutaneous infections: common warts, plantar warts, and juvenile or flat warts. A fourth type of infection, condyloma acuminata or genital warts, is a common viral sexually transmitted disease in the U.S. Also a number of HPV types, esp. numbers 16 and 18, are believed to be important in the pathogenisis of cancer of the uterine cervix. A direct epidemiological link between HPV infection and cervical cancer has been difficult to establish; however, HPV has been implicated as a major factor in the development of some vaginal, vulvar, anal, and penile squamous cell cancers. SEE: *wart, genital.*

TREATMENT: There is no universally effective systemic therapy for HPV infection. Most commonly, small external warts are treated with topical podophyllin. Because podophyllin has teratogenic properties and should not be used during pregnancy, other therapeutic agents such as trichloroacetic acid or 5-fluorouracil have been used when treating pregnant women or for recurrent lesions. Cervical HPV lesions may be removed by loop electrosurgical excision procedure. Cryotherapy and laser surgery also may be used in treatment.

**papilloretinitis** (păp″ĭ-lō-rĕt-ĭn-ī′tĭs) [″ + *rete,* net, + Gr. *itis,* inflammation] Inflammation of the papilla and retina, extending to the optic disk. SYN: *retinopapillitis.*

**papovavirus** (păp″ō-vă-vī′rŭs) [*pa*pilloma, + *po*lyoma, + *va*cuolating agent + *virus*] Any of a group of viruses important in investigating viral carcinogenesis; including polyoma virus, simian virus 40 (SV 40), and papillomaviruses.

**pappataci fever** Sandfly fever.

**pappose** (păp′pōs) [L. *pappus,* down] Covered with fine, downy hair.

**pappus** [L.] The first growth of beard hair appearing on the cheeks and chin as fine, downy hair.

**Pap smear, Pap test** Papanicolaou test.

**papula** (păp′ū-lă) [L.] Papule.

**papular** (păp′ū-lĕr) Concerning an eruption of the nature of papules.

**papule** (păp′ūl) [L. *papula,* pimple] A small, red, elevated area on the skin, solid and circumscribed; a pimple. Papules often precede vesicular or pustular formation and may appear in erythema multiforme, eczema papulosum, prurigo, syphilis, measles, and smallpox, and they may develop after use of bromides, iodides, or coal tar preparations. SEE: illus.

DIFFERENTIAL DIAGNOSIS: In measles, they are small and run together. In smallpox, they are hard and feel like pellets, terminating in umbilicated vesicles that itch. In prurigo, they are small, pale, deep-seated, and accompanied by intense itching. In syphilis, they are dark and widely distributed, esp. on the trunk and surfaces of the extremities; they do not cause itching. In eczema, they are small, are often associated with pustules and vesicles, and are closely aggregated; there is intense itching and the skin is thickened. In erythema multiforme, they are

PAPULES OF MILIARIA

found with macules and tubercles and are bright red or purple and flat, appearing esp. on the extremities; they do not suppurate or cause itching.

***dry p.*** Chancre.

***moist p.*** Condyloma latum.

***pearly penile p.*** An asymptomatic white papule with a pink, white, or pearly surface on the dorsum of the penis of blacks and uncircumcised men. No treatment is indicated, just reassurance.

***piezogenic pedal p.*** (pī-ē′zō-jĕn″ĭk) [Gr. *piezein,* to squeeze, + *gennan,* to produce] A soft painful skin-colored papule present on the non–weight-bearing portion of the heel. It disappears when weight is taken off the foot and heel. This papule is caused by herniation of fat through connective tissue defects.

***split p.'s*** Fissures at the corners of the mouth; seen in some cases of secondary syphilis.

**papuliferous** (păp″ū-lĭf′ĕr-ŭs) [L. *papula,* pimple, + *ferre,* to bear] Having papules or pimples.

**papulo-** [L. *papula,* pimple] Combining form indicating *pimple, papule.*

**papuloerythematous** (păp″ū-lō-ĕr″ĕ-thĕm′ă-tŭs) [″ + Gr. *erythema,* redness] Denoting the occurrence of papules on an erythematous surface.

**papulopustular** (păp″ū-lō-pŭs′tū-lăr) [″ + *pustula,* blister] Denoting the presence of both pustules and papules.

**papulosis** (păp-ū-lō′sĭs) [″ + Gr. *osis,* condition] The presence of numerous and generalized papules.

**papulosquamous** (păp″ū-lō-skwā′mŭs) [″ + *squamosus,* scalelike] Denoting the presence of both papules and scales.

**papulovesicular** (păp″ū-lō-vē-sĭk′ū-lăr) [″ + *vesicula,* tiny bladder] Denoting the presence of both papules and vesicles.

**papyraceous** (păp-ĭ-rā′shŭs) [L.] Parchment-like; in obstetrics, denoting a fetus that is retained in the uterus beyond natural term and appears mummified.

**par** [L., equal] A pair, esp. a pair of cranial nerves.

**para** [L. *parere,* to bring forth, to bear] A woman who has produced a viable infant (weighing at least 500 g or of more than 20 weeks' gestation) regardless of whether the infant is alive at birth. A multiple birth is considered to be a single parous experience. SEE: *gravida; multipara.*

**para-** [Gr. *para,* beyond; L. *par,* equal, pair] Prefix meaning *near, beside, past, beyond, opposite, abnormal, irregular, two like parts.*

**-para** Suffix meaning *to bear forth* (offspring).

**para-aminobenzoic acid** (păr″ă-ăm″ĭ-nō-bĕn-zō′ĭk) ABBR: PABA. Previously used name for aminobenzoic acid.

**para-aminohippuric acid** ABBR: PAHA. A derivative of aminobenzoic acid. The salt, para-aminohippurate, is used to test the excretory capacity of the renal tubules.

**para-aminosalicylic acid** (păr″ă-ăm″ĭ-nō-săl″ĭ-sĭl′ĭk) ABBR: PAS. $C_7H_7NO_3$. A white or nearly white and practically odorless powder that darkens when exposed to air or light. It is an antituberculosis drug, and its effectiveness is greatly enhanced when used in combination with streptomycin and isoniazid; it is believed to delay development of bacterial resistance. SYN: *aminosalicylic acid.*

**para-aortic body** One of the small masses of chromaffin tissue along the abdominal aorta that secrete epinephrine.

**parabionts** (păr-ăb′ē-ŏnts) [″ + *bioun,* to live] Two individuals living in the condition of parabiosis.

**parabiosis** (păr″ă-bī-ō′sĭs) [″ + *biosis,* living] **1.** The joining together of two individuals. It may occur congenitally as with conjoined twins or may be produced surgically for experimentation in animals. **2.** The temporary suppression of the excitability of a nerve. **parabiotic** (-ŏt′ĭk), *adj.*

**parablepsia, parablepsis** (păr″ă-blĕp′sē-ă, -sĭs) [Gr. *para,* beside, + *blepsis,* vision] Abnormality of vision (e.g., visual hallucinations).

**paracanthoma** (păr″ă-kăn-thō′mă) [Gr. *para,* beside, + *akantha,* thorn, + *oma,* tumor] A tumor involving the prickle-cell layer of the epidermis.

**paracasein** (păr-ă-kā′sē-ĭn) A substance formed when rennin or pepsin acts on the casein of milk. In the presence of calcium ions, an insoluble protein is formed, resulting in the curdling of milk.

**Paracelsus** (păr-ă-sĕl′sŭs) [Philippus Aureolus Theophrastus Bombastus von Hohenheim, 1493–1541] Swiss alchemist and physician who introduced several chemicals (lead, sulfur, iron, and arsenic) into pharmaceutical chemistry. He is remembered for his independent spirit, observant mind, and fearlessness in breaking with traditional practice.

**paracentesis** (păr″ă-sĕn-tē′sĭs) [Gr. *para,* beside, + *kentesis,* a puncture] The puncture of a cavity with removal of fluid, as in pleural effusion or ascites. **paracentetic** (-tĕt′ĭk), *adj.*

NURSING IMPLICATIONS: The nurse

explains the procedure to the patient and has the patient void before treatment. Emotional support is offered during the procedure, and the patient is encouraged to express feelings. The patient is positioned as directed by the physician. The nurse assists the physician during the procedure. Vital signs are monitored, and the patient is observed for signs of shock. The amount of fluid removed is measured and recorded, and its appearance, color, odor, specific gravity, and tendency to clot when the patient stands are described. The puncture site is observed and redressed as necessary. Specimens are sent to laboratories as directed. The nurse documents the procedure and the patient's response and continues to monitor the patient for several hours after the procedure.

***abdominal p.*** Paracentesis of the abdominal cavity.

***p. pulmonis*** Removal of fluid from a lung.

***p. thoracis*** Drainage of fluid from the cavity of the chest. SEE: *aspiration*.

***p. tympani*** Drainage or irrigation through incision of the tympanic membrane.

***p. vesicae*** Puncture of the wall of the urinary bladder.

**paracentral** (păr″ă-sĕn′trăl) [″ + L. *centralis*, center] Located near the center.

**paracentral lobule** A cerebral convolution on the mesial surface joining the upper terminations of the ascending parietal and frontal convolutions.

**paracephalus** (păr″ă-sĕf′ă-lŭs) [″ + *kephale*, head] A parasitic placental twin with a small rudimentary head.

**parachlorophenol** (păr″ă-klō″rō-fē′nŏl) A drug that has the same actions and uses as phenol.

***camphorated p.*** A mixture of parachlorophenol and camphor. Its activity as a topical antiseptic in root canal therapy is markedly decreased by blood and necrotic tissue.

**paracholera** (păr″ă-kŏl′ĕr-ă) [″ + L. *cholera*, cholera] A disease resembling cholera but caused by vibriones other than true *Vibrio cholerae*.

**parachordal** (păr-ă-kor′dăl) [Gr. *para*, beside, + *chorde*, cord] Lying alongside the anterior portion of the notochord in the embryo.

**parachordal cartilage** One of a pair of cartilages in the cephalic portion of the notochord of the embryo that unite in humans to form a single basal plate that is the forerunner of the occipital bone.

**parachromatism** (păr″ă-krō′mă-tĭzm) [″ + *chroma*, color, + *-ismos*, condition] Incorrect perception of colors but not true color blindness.

**parachromatopsia** (păr″ă-krō-mă-tŏp′sē-ă) [″ + ″ + *opsis*, vision] Color blindness.

**paracinesia, paracinesis** (păr″ă-sī-nē′zē-ă, -sĭs) [″ + *kinesis*, movement] A condition in which motor powers are perverted; motor abnormality.

**Paracoccidioides** (păr″ă-kŏk-sĭd″ē-oy′dēz) A genus of yeastlike fungi.

***P. brasiliensis*** Blastomyces brasiliensis.

**paracoccidioidomycosis** (păr″ă-kŏk-sĭd″ē-ŏy″dō-mī-kō′sĭs) A chronic granulomatous disease of the skin caused by *Paracoccidioides brasiliensis*. SYN: *South American blastomycosis*.

**paracolitis** (păr″ă-kō-lī′tĭs) Inflammation of the tissue surrounding the colon.

**paracolpitis** (păr″ă-kŏl-pī′tĭs) [″ + *kolpos*, vagina, + *itis*, inflammation] Inflammation of tissues surrounding the vagina.

**paracone** (păr′ă-kōn) [″ + *konos*, cone] The mesiobuccal cusp of an upper molar tooth.

**paraconid** (păr″ă-kō′nĭd) The mesiobuccal cusp of a lower molar tooth.

**paracrine** Secretion of a hormone from a source other than an endocrine gland.

***p. control*** A general form of bioregulation in which one cell type in a tissue selectively influences the activity of an adjacent cell type by secreting chemicals that diffuse into the tissue and act specifically on cells in that area. SEE: *autocrine factor*.

**paracusia, paracusis** (păr″ă-kū′sē-ă, -kū′sĭs) [″ + *akousis*, hearing] Any abnormality or disorder of the sense of hearing.

***p. loci*** Difficulty in locating the direction of sound.

***p. willisiana*** An apparent ability to hear better in a noisy place, found in deafness due to stapes fixation and adhesive processes. SEE: *otosclerosis*.

**paracystitis** (păr″ă-sĭs-tī′tĭs) [″ + ″ + *itis*, inflammation] Inflammation of connective tissues and other structures around the urinary bladder.

**paracytic** (păr″ă-sĭt′ĭk) [″ + *kytos*, cell] Concerning cells other than those normally present in a specific location.

**paradenitis** (păr″ăd-ĕn-ī′tĭs) [″ + *aden*, gland, + *itis*, inflammation] Inflammation of tissues around a gland.

**paradental** (păr″ă-dĕn′tăl) [″ + L. *dens*, tooth] **1.** Concerning the practice of dentistry. **2.** Periodontal.

**paradentium** (păr″ă-dĕn′shē-ŭm) Periodontium.

**paradidymal** (păr″ă-dĭd′ĭ-măl) [″ + *didymos*, testicle] **1.** Concerning the paradidymis. **2.** Adjacent to the testis.

**paradidymis** (păr-ă-dĭd′ĭ-mĭs) [″ + *didymos*, testicle] The atrophic remnants of the tubules of the wolffian body, situated on the spermatic cord above the epididymis. SYN: *organ of Giraldès*.

**paradigm** An example that serves as a model.

**paradox** [Gr. *paradoxos*, conflicting with expectation] Something that seems untrue, and even absurd and inconsistent with a logical explanation of the true condition, but in fact is actually true.

***Weber's p.*** Paradox that states that a

muscle loaded beyond its ability to contract may elongate.

**paradoxic, paradoxical** (păr″ă-dŏk′sĭk, -sĭ-kăl) Seemingly contradictory but demonstrably true.

**paraffin** (păr′ă-fĭn) [L. *parum,* too little, + *affinis,* neighboring] **1.** A waxy, white, tasteless, odorless mixture of solid hydrocarbons obtained from petroleum; used as an ointment base or wound dressing. SEE: *petrolatum.* **2.** One of a series of saturated aliphatic hydrocarbons having the formula $C_nH_{2n+2}$. Paraffins constitute the methane or paraffin series. **3.** A series of solid waxes prepared according to their melting point, to be used to infiltrate and embed tissues for sectioning in the preparation of microscope slides.

***hard p.*** Solid paraffin with a melting point between 45°C and 60°C.

***liquid p.*** Liquid petrolatum.

***soft p.*** Petrolatum.

***white soft p.*** White petrolatum.

***yellow soft p.*** Petrolatum.

**paraffinoma** (păr″ă-fĭn-ō′mă) [″ + ″ + Gr. *oma,* tumor] A tumor that arises at the site of an injection of paraffin.

**paraformaldehyde** (păr″ă-for-măl′dĕ-hīd) A white, powdered antiseptic and disinfectant, a polymer of formaldehyde.

**paragammacism** (păr″ă-găm′mă-sĭzm) [Gr. *para,* beside, + *gamma,* Gr. letter G, + *-ismos,* condition] An inability to pronounce "g," "k," and "ch" sounds, with substitution of other consonants such as "d" or "t."

**paraganglia** (păr″ă-găng′lē-ă) *sing.* **paraganglion** [″ + *ganglion,* knot] Groups of chromaffin cells, similar in staining reaction to cells of the adrenal medulla, associated anatomically and embryologically with the sympathetic system. They are located in various organs and parts of the body.

**paraganglioma** (păr″ă-găng-lē-ō′mă) [″ + ″ + *oma,* tumor] A tumor derived from chromaffin cells; including tumors of the adrenal medulla and the paraganglia. SYN: *chemodectoma.* SEE: *pheochromocytoma.*

**paraganglion** (păr″ă-găng′lē-ŏn) [″ + *ganglion,* knot] Sing. of paraganglia.

**parageusia, parageusis** (păr-ă-gū′sē-ă, -sĭs) [″ + *geusis,* taste] Disorder or abnormality of the sense of taste. Intravenous fluid therapy, esp. postoperatively, may create temporary parageusia and parosmia.

**paragnathus** (păr-ăg′nă-thŭs) [″ + *gnathos,* jaw] **1.** A congenital deformity in which there is an accessory jaw. **2.** A parasitic fetus attached to the outer part of the jaw of the autosite.

**paragonimiasis** (păr″ă-gŏn″ĭ-mī′ă-sĭs) [*Paragonimus* + *-iasis,* condition] Infection with worms of genus *Paragonimus.* The clinical signs depend on the path the worm takes in migrating through the body, after the larvae contained in partially cooked freshwater crabs or crayfish are eaten. The larvae migrate from the duodenum to various organs, including the lungs, intestinal wall, lymph nodes, brain, subcutaneous tissues, and genitourinary tract. When the lungs are involved, the symptoms are cough and hemoptysis. In peritoneal infections, there may be an abdominal mass, pain, and dysentery. When the larvae invade the brain, paralysis, epilepsy, homonymous hemianopsia, optic atrophy, and papilledema are common. In some cases, the infected person may appear to be well. This infection is treated by administration of praziquantel.

**Paragonimus** (păr″ă-gŏn′ĭ-mŭs) A genus of trematode worms.

***P. westermani*** The lung fluke, a common parasite of certain mammals including humans, dogs, cats, pigs, and minks. Human infestation occurs through eating partially cooked crabs or crayfish, the second intermediate host. This infestation is endemic in certain parts of Asia. SEE: illus.

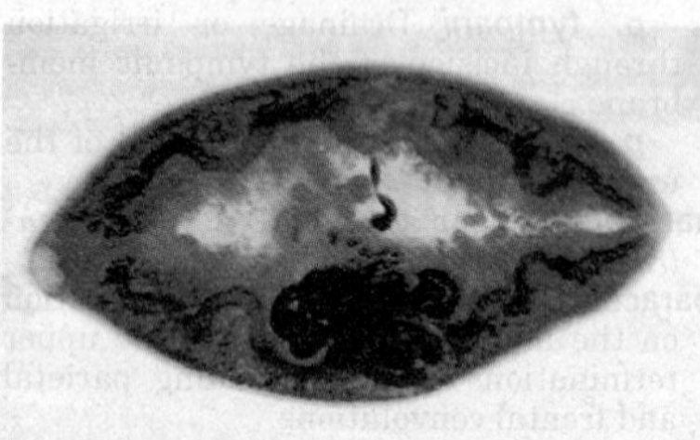

PARAGONIMUS WESTERMANI
(ORIG. MAG. ×4)

**paragrammatism** A speech defect characterized by improper use of words and inability to arrange them grammatically.

**paragranuloma** (păr″ă-grăn″ū-lō′mă) [Gr. *para,* beside, + L. *granulum,* little grain, + Gr. *oma,* tumor] A benign form of Hodgkin's disease usually limited to lymph nodes.

**paragraphia** (păr-ă-grăf′ē-ă) [″ + *graphein,* to write] The writing of letters or words other than those intended.

**parahepatic** (păr″ă-hē-păt′ĭk) [″ + *hepar,* liver] Adjacent to the liver.

**parahypnosis** [″ + *hypnos,* sleep] Abnormal or disordered sleep.

**parahypophysis** (păr″ă-hī-pŏf′ĭ-sĭs) [″ + *hypophysis,* an undergrowth] Accessory to the pituitary tissue.

**parainfluenza viruses** A group of viruses that cause acute respiratory infections in humans, esp. in children. Virtually all children in the U.S. have been infected by age 6.

**parakeratosis** (păr″ă-kĕr″ă-tō′sĭs) [″ + *keras,* horn, + *osis,* condition] The persistence of nuclei within the keratinocytes of the stratum corneum of epidermis or mucosal layers, which indicates a partial keratinization process; a general term applied to disorders of the keratinized layer of the skin.

***p. ostracea*** P. scutularis.

***p. psoriasiformis*** Scab formation resembling that of psoriasis.

***p. scutularis*** A scalp disease with hairs encircled by epidermic crust formation.

**paralalia** (păr″ă-lā′lē-ă) [″ + *lalein,* to babble] Any speech defect characterized by sound distortion.

***p. literalis*** Stammering.

**paralambdacism** (păr″ă-lăm′dă-sĭzm) [″ + *lambda,* Gr. letter L, + *-ismos,* condition] An inability to sound the letter "l" correctly, substituting some other letter for it.

**paraldehyde** (păr-ăl′dĕ-hīd) $C_6H_{12}O_3$; a liquid polymer of acetaldehyde that is colorless, has an unpleasant taste, and has a characteristic odor. It is made by the action of hydrochloric acid on acetic aldehyde. Trade name is Paral.

ACTION/USES: The agent is used as a hypnotic, having low toxicity and prompt action as a sedative. It is useful in treating acute alcoholism and delirium tremens and is sometimes used as an analgesic in obstetrics, esp. in combination with rectal ether.

---

Caution: Paraldehyde should not be dispensed from a bottle that has been open for longer than 24 hr. In partially filled containers, oxidation occurs, forming acetic acid.

---

**paraldehyde poisoning** Poisoning in which symptoms resemble those of chloral hydrate poisoning: cardiac and respiratory depression, dizziness, and collapse with partial or complete anesthesia. Odor on the breath is a constant distinct sign.

FIRST AID: Airway and physiological responses are maintained by use of tracheostomy, artificial ventilation, and oxygen. If poisoning is mild, vomiting should be induced. Because of the danger of asphyxiation, gastric lavage is dangerous unless the airway is protected.

**paralepsy** (păr′ă-lĕp″sē) [″ + *lepsis,* seizure] A temporary attack of mental inertia and hopelessness, or sudden alteration in mood or mental tension.

**paralexia** (păr″ă-lĕk′sē-ă) [″ + *lexis,* speech] An inability to comprehend printed words or sentences, together with substitution of meaningless combinations of words.

**paralgia** (păr-ăl′jē-ă) [″ + *algos,* pain] An abnormal sensation that is painful.

**paralipophobia** Fear of omitting or neglecting a duty.

**parallagma** (păr″ăl-ăg′mă) [Gr., alternation] Overlapping or displacement of the fragments of a fractured bone.

**parallax** (păr′ă-lăks) [Gr. *parallaxis,* change of position] The apparent movement or displacement of objects caused by change in the observer's position or by movement of the head or eyes.

***binocular p.*** The basis of stereoscopic vision; the difference in the angles formed by the lines of sight to two objects at different distances from the eyes. This is important in depth perception.

***heteronymous p.*** Parallax in which, when one eye is closed, the object viewed appears to move closer to the closed eye.

***homonymous p.*** Parallax in which, when one eye is covered, the object viewed appears to move closer to the uncovered eye.

**parallelometer** (păr″ă-lĕl-ŏm′ĕ-tĕr) A device used in dentistry to determine whether or not lines and tooth surfaces are parallel to each other.

**parallel play** The stage in social development in which a child plays alongside, but not with, other children; characteristic of toddlers.

**parallergy** (păr-ăl′ĕr-jē) The condition of being allergic to nonspecific stimuli after having been sensitized with a specific allergen. **parallergic** (păr″ă-lĕr′jĭk), *adj.*

**paralogia** (păr″ă-lō′jē-ă) [Gr. *para,* beside, + *logos,* word, reason] A disorder of the reasoning.

***benign p.*** Disordered thinking and communication of thought in which delusions, bizarre thoughts, hallucinations, and regressive behavior are absent. The patient is not severely incapacitated and should not be considered to have schizophrenia.

**paralysis** (pă-răl′ĭ-sĭs) *pl.* **paralyses** [Gr. *paralyein,* to disable] Temporary suspension or permanent loss of function, esp. loss of sensation or voluntary motion.

Any voluntary movement depends on the integrity of two types of motor neurons: the upper motor neurons, arising in the motor cortex, coursing through the brainstem, and ending in the anterior gray horn of the spinal cord; and the lower neurons, arising in the anterior horn cell and passing to the muscle. If the latter are destroyed, the muscle loses tone, atrophies (withers away), and shows reaction of degeneration (RD).

The flaccidity and absent muscular reflexes reveal the loss of tonus. If the upper neuron is paralyzed, the patient is equally unable to move the affected part, but the intact lower neuron may permit other motor centers to act on the muscle. In addition, tone is increased, there is no RD, and there is no atrophy except that of disuse. So-called pathologic reflexes may appear in addition to the increase of normal deep reflexes.

Paralyses are divided into two groups: *spastic* when due to lesion of upper motor neuron and *flaccid* when due to lesion of lower motor neuron. Psychic inhibition of motor function occurs most characteristically in hysteria, but the evidence of organic disease is always lacking in these hysterical paralyses.

NURSING IMPLICATIONS: Referral is made to the physical therapy department for evaluation of the patient's motor and sensory capabilities (muscle size, tone and strength, involuntary movement, response to touch or to painful stimuli). The patient is positioned to prevent deformities, and the extremities are put through their range of motion to prevent contractures. The patient is repositioned frequently to prevent pressure sores. Massage or electrical stimulation is given as prescribed. Local and systemic responses, including fatigue, are evaluated. The nurse assesses and attends to any self-care deficits the patient may have. Support is offered to the patient and family to assist them in dealing with psychological concerns and the grief and loss response. Assistance is provided to help the patient in achieving optimal level of function and in adapting to the disability.

***p. of accommodation*** Inability of the eye to adjust itself to various distances owing to paralysis of ciliary muscles.

***acoustic p.*** Deafness.

***p. agitans*** Parkinson's disease.

***alcoholic p.*** Paralysis caused by the toxic effect of alcohol on nerve tissue.

***anesthesia p.*** Paralysis that develops following administration of anesthesia.

***arsenical p.*** Paralysis caused by the toxic effect of arsenic.

***Bell's p.*** Bell's palsy.

***birth p.*** Paralysis caused by injury received at birth. SYN: *obstetrical p.*

***brachial p.*** Paralysis of one or both arms.

***brachiofacial p.*** Paralysis of the face and an arm.

***bulbar p.*** Paralysis caused by changes in the motor centers of the medulla oblongata. SYN: *progressive bulbar p.*

***complete p.*** Paralysis in which there is total loss of function and sensation.

***compression p.*** Paralysis due to prolonged pressure on a nerve, as by improper use of a crutch or during sleep.

***conjugate p.*** Paralysis of the conjugate movement of the eyes in all directions even though the fixation axis remains parallel.

***crossed p.*** Paralysis affecting one side of the face and limbs of the opposite side of the body.

***crutch p.*** Paralysis due to pressure on nerves in the axilla caused by improper use of a crutch.

***decubitus p.*** Paralysis due to pressure on a nerve from lying in one position for a long time, as in sleep or while in a coma.

***diphtheritic p.*** Paralysis of the muscles of the palate, eyes, limbs, diaphragm, and intercostal muscles that occurs as a complication of diphtheria. It is caused by a toxin produced by the diphtheria bacillus. SYN: *postdiphtheritic p.*

***diver's p.*** Bends.

***Duchenne-Erb p.*** Paralysis of the muscles of the upper arm due to injury of the upper nerves, the fifth and sixth cervical roots, of the brachial plexus. The hand muscles are unaffected.

***facial p.*** Bell's palsy.

***flaccid p.*** Paralysis in which there is loss of muscle tone, loss or reduction of tendon reflexes, atrophy and degeneration of muscles, and reaction of degeneration; caused by lesions of lower motor neurons of spinal cord.

***general p.*** Paresis.

***ginger p.*** Jamaica ginger p.

***glossolabial p.*** Paralysis of the tongue and lips; occurs in bulbar paralysis.

***Gubler's p.*** A form of alternate hemiplegia in which a brainstem lesion causes paralysis of the cranial nerves on one side and of the body on the opposite side.

***histrionic p.*** Paralysis of certain facial muscles, producing a fixed facial expression of a certain emotion.

***hyperkalemic p.*** A rare form of periodic paralysis characterized by brief, 1- to 2-hr attacks of limb weakness. In some cases, respiratory muscles are involved. The term "hyperkalemic" is misleading in that the potassium levels may be normal. However, because an attack is precipitated by the administration of potassium, this form of paralysis should be termed "potassium-sensitive periodic paralysis."

TREATMENT: Emergency treatment is seldom necessary. Oral glucose hastens recovery. In addition, attacks may be prevented by use of acetazolamide or thiazide diuretics.

***hypokalemic periodic p.*** A form of periodic paralysis with onset usually prior to adulthood. An attack typically comes on during sleep, after strenuous exercise during the day. The weakness may be so pronounced as to prevent the patient from being able to call for help. The attack may last from several hours to a day or more. The diagnosis is established by determining that the serum potassium level is decreased during an attack.

TREATMENT: Administration of oral potassium salts improves the paralysis. If the patient is too weak to swallow, intravenous potassium salts are required. Attacks may be prevented by oral administration of 5 to 10 g of potassium chloride daily.

***hysterical p.*** Apparent loss of movement with no organic cause that may simulate any form of paralysis. SEE: *Hoover sign.*

***immunological p.*** The inability to form antibodies after exposure to large doses of an antigen.

***incomplete p.*** Partial paralysis of the body or a part.

***infantile p.*** Poliomyelitis.

***infantile cerebral ataxic p.*** SEE: *palsy, cerebral.*

***ischemic p.*** Volkmann's contracture.

***Jamaica ginger p.*** Paralysis due to polyneuropathy that affects the muscles of the distal portions of the limbs. It is caused by drinking an alcoholic beverage called Jamaica ginger that contains the toxic substance triorthocresylphosphate.

***Klumpke's p.*** Wasting paralysis of the arms and hands, often resulting from birth injury.

***Landry's p.*** Flaccid paralysis that begins in the lower extremities and rapidly ascends to the trunk.

***lead p.*** Paralysis due to lead poisoning.

***local p.*** Paralysis of a single muscle or one group of muscles.

***mimetic p.*** Paralysis of the facial muscles.

***mixed p.*** Paralysis of motor and sensory nerves.

***muscular p.*** Loss of the capacity of muscles to contract; may be due to a structural or functional disorder in the muscle at the myoneural junction, in efferent nerve fibers, in cell bodies of nuclei of origin of brain or gray matter of spinal cord, in conducting pathways of brain or spinal cord, or in motor centers of the brain.

***musculospiral p.*** Paralysis due to prolonged ischemia of the musculospiral nerve incident to compressing an arm against a hard edge. It occurs if the patient has been comatose or in a stupor or has fallen asleep with the arm hanging over the edge of a bed or chair. Sometimes called "Saturday night paralysis" because in some cultures individuals traditionally become intoxicated on Saturday night; while stuporous, they may remain in a position that allows the nerve to be compressed. SYN: *radial p.; Saturday night p.*

***nuclear p.*** Paralysis caused by lesion of nuclei in the central nervous system.

***obstetrical p.*** Birth p.

***ocular p.*** Paralysis of the extraocular and intraocular muscles.

***postdiphtheritic p.*** Diphtheritic p.

***posticus p.*** Paralysis of the posterior cricothyroid muscles.

***Pott's p.*** Paralysis of the lower part of the body owing to tuberculosis of the spine (Pott's disease).

***pressure p.*** Paralysis due to pressure on the spinal cord or a nerve.This may be caused by injury, tumor, or gummata.

***primary periodic p.*** The occurrence of intermittent weakness, usually following rest or sleep, and almost never during vigorous activity. The condition usually begins in early life and rarely has its onset after age 25. The attacks may last from a few hours to a day or more. The patient is alert during an attack.

The causes include hypokalemia, hyperkalemia, thyrotoxicosis, and a form of paramyotonia. Both forms of the disease in which potassium regulation is a factor respond to acetazolamide; the thyrotoxicosis-related disorder is treated by correcting the underlying thyrotoxicosis. In cases of paramyotonia congenita with periodic paralysis, the treatment is spironolactone.

***progressive bulbar p.*** Bulbar p.

***pseudobulbar p.*** Paralysis caused by cerebral center lesions, simulating the bulbar types of paralysis.

***pseudohypertrophic muscular p.*** SEE: *dystrophy, pseudohypertrophic muscular.*

***radial p.*** Musculospiral p.

***Saturday night p.*** Musculospiral p.

***sensory p.*** Loss of sensation; may be due to a structural or functional disorder of the sensory end organs, sensory nerves, conducting pathways of spinal cord or brain, or sensory centers in the brain.

***sleep p.*** SEE: *sleep, disorders of.*

***spastic p.*** Paralysis usually involving groups of muscles; characterized by excessive tone and spasticity of muscles, exaggeration of tendon reflexes but loss of superficial reflexes, positive Babinski's reflex, no atrophy or wasting except from prolonged disuse, and absence of reaction of degeneration. This form of paralysis is due to lesions of the upper motor neurons or the cerebrum.

***spinal p.*** Paralysis due to injury or disease of the spinal cord.

***supranuclear p.*** Paralysis resulting from disorders in pathways or centers above the nuclei of origin.

***tick-bite p.*** Paralysis resulting from bites of certain species of ticks, esp. of the genera *Ixodes* and *Dermacentor,* due to a toxin in tick saliva. It affects domestic animals and humans, esp. children, and causes a progressive ascending, flaccid, motor paralysis. Recovery usually occurs after removal of the ticks.

***tourniquet p.*** Paralysis, esp. of the arm, resulting from a tourniquet being applied for too long a time.

***vasomotor p.*** Paralysis of the vasomotor centers, resulting in lack of tone and dilation of the blood vessels.

***vocal p.*** Paralysis of the vocal cords.

***Volkmann's p.*** Volkmann's contracture.

***wasting p.*** Progressive muscular atrophy.

**paralytic** (păr″ă-lĭt′ĭk) [Gr. *paralyein,* to disable] **1.** Concerning paralysis. **2.** One afflicted with paralysis.

**paralytic dementia** Paresis.

**paralytic ileus** Paralysis of the intestines, usually temporary, with distention and symptoms of acute obstruction; may occur after any abdominal surgery. It can be a rare anticholinergic side effect of certain psychotropic drugs.

**paralyzant** (păr′ă-līz″ănt) [Fr. *paralyser,* paralyze] **1.** Causing paralysis. **2.** A drug or other agent that induces paralysis.

**paralyze** (păr′ă-līz) [Fr. *paralyse*] **1.** To cause temporary or permanent loss of muscular power or sensation. **2.** To render ineffective.

**paralyzer** (păr′ă-līz″ĕr) **1.** That which causes paralysis. **2.** A substance that inhibits a chemical reaction.

**paramagnetic** (păr″ă-măg-nĕt′ĭk) Anything that is attracted by the poles of a magnet and becomes parallel to the lines of magnetic force.

**paramania** (păr″ă-mā′nē-ă) [Gr. *para,* beside, + *mania,* madness] A type of emotional disturbance in which the individual derives pleasure from complaining.

**paramastigote** (păr″ă-măs′tĭ-gōt) [″ + *mastix,* lash] Having a small supernumerary flagellum next to a larger one.

**paramastitis** (păr″ă-măs-tī′tĭs) [″ + *mastos,* breast, + *itis,* inflammation] Inflammation around the breast.

**paramastoid** (păr″ă-măs′toyd) [″ + ″ + *eidos,* form, shape] Next to the mastoid.

**paramedian** (păr″ă-mē′dē-ăn) [″ + L. *medianus,* median] Close to the midline. SYN: *paramesial.*

**paramedian incision** A surgical incision, esp. of the abdominal wall, close to the midline.

**paramedic** (păr″ă-mĕd′ĭk) [Gr. *para,* beside, + L. *medicus,* doctor] A health care professional trained in the emergency care of patients who suffer from sudden illnesses or injuries. Paramedics typically function in the prehospital environment, under the medical direction of a physician. SEE: *emergency medical technician.*

**paramedical** Supplementing the work of medical personnel in related fields: social work; physical, occupational, and speech therapy.

**paramedical personnel** Health care workers who are not physicians or nurses. These include medical technicians, emergency medical technicians, and physician's assistants. SEE: *allied health professional.*

**paramesial** (păr″ă-mē′sē-ăl) [″ + *mesos,* middle] Paramedian.

**parameter** (păr-ăm′ĕ-tĕr) [″ + *metron,* measure] **1.** In mathematics, an arbitrary constant, each value of which determines the specific form of the equation in which it appears; often misused to indicate a variable. **2.** In biostatistics, a measurement taken on a population, which consists of all the subjects in a defined group.

**paramethadione** (păr″ă-mĕth″ă-dī′ōn) Anticonvulsive drug used in treating absence seizures.

**paramethasone acetate** (păr″ă-mĕth′ă-sōn) A glucocorticosteroid drug.

**parametric** (păr″ă-mĕt′rĭk) [Gr. *para,* beside, + *metra,* uterus] **1.** Concerning the area near the uterus. **2.** Rel. to the parametrium, the tissue surrounding the uterus. **3.** [Gr. *para,* beside, + *metron,* measure] Adjectival form of parameter.

**parametric statistics** The class of statistics based on the assumption that the samples measured are from normally distributed populations.

**parametritic** (păr″ă-mĕ-trĭt′ĭk) Concerning parametritis.

**parametritis** (păr″ă-mĕ-trī′tĭs) [″ + *metra,* uterus, + *itis,* inflammation] An inflammation of the parametrium, the cellular tissue adjacent to the uterus. It may occur in puerperal fever or septic conditions of the uterus and appendages. SYN: *pelvic cellulitis.*

**parametrium** (păr-ă-mē′trē-ŭm) [″ + *metra,* uterus] Loose connective tissue around the uterus.

**paramimia** (păr″ă-mĭm′ē-ă) [″ + *mimeisthai,* to imitate] The use of gestures that are inappropriate to the spoken words that they accompany.

**paramnesia** (păr″ăm-nē′zē-ă) [″ + *amnesia,* loss of memory] **1.** Use of words without meaning. **2.** Distortion of memory in which there is inability to distinguish imaginary or suggested experiences from those that have actually occurred. **3.** Seeming recall of events that never have occurred.

**paramolar** (păr″ă-mō′lăr) A supernumerary tooth close to a molar.

**paramucin** (păr″ă-mū′sĭn) A glycoprotein found in ovarian and some other cysts.

**paramusia** (păr″ă-mū′zē-ă) [″ + *mousa,* music] A form of aphasia in which the ability to render music correctly is lost.

**paramyloidosis** (păr-ăm″ĭ-loy-dō′sĭs) [″ + L. *amylum,* starch, + Gr. *eidos,* form, shape, + *osis,* condition] The presence and buildup of atypical amyloid in tissues.

**paramyoclonus multiplex** (păr-ă-mī-ŏk′lō-nŭs mŭl′tĭ-plĕks) [″ + *mys,* muscle, + *klonos,* tumult] Sudden and frequent shocklike contractions usually affecting the muscles of both legs, and particularly the trunk muscles. The contractions, which disappear during sleep and motion, may occur 10 to 50 times each minute. Usually the condition develops spontaneously, but it has been known to follow fright, trauma, infectious diseases, and poliomyelitis. SYN: *polymyoclonus.*

**paramyosinogen** (păr″ă-mī″ō-sĭn′ō-jĕn) [Gr. *para,* beside, + *myosin,* protein globin of muscle, + *gennan,* to produce] Protein derived from muscle plasma.

**paramyotonia** (păr″ă-mī″ō-tō′nē-ă) [″ + *mys,* muscle, + *tonos,* tone] A disorder marked by muscular spasms and abnormal muscular tonicity.

***ataxic p.*** Tonic muscular spasm with slight ataxia or paresis during any attempt at movement.

***p. congenita*** A congenital condition of tonic muscular spasms when body is exposed to cold. SYN: *Eulenburg's disease.*

***symptomatic p.*** Temporary muscular rigidity when one first tries to walk, as in paralysis agitans.

**paramyxovirus** Any virus of a subgroup of the myxoviruses that are similar in physical, chemical, and biological characteristics, even though they are quite different pathogenetically. The group includes parainfluenza, measles, mumps, Newcastle disease, and respiratory syncytial viruses.

**paranasal** (păr″ă-nā′săl) [″ + L. *nasalis,* pert. to the nose] Situated near or along the nasal cavities.

**paraneoplastic syndromes** Indirect effects of neoplasms that may be so severe as to be the actual cause of death, rather than the tumor itself being the cause. These include endocrine effects of neoplasms of the lungs or kidneys and various neoplasms of the endocrine glands.

**paranephric** (păr″ă-nĕf′rĭk) [″ + *nephros,* kidney] **1.** Close to the kidney. **2.** Concerning the adrenal glands.

**paranephros** (păr-ă-nĕf′rŏs) A suprarenal or adrenal capsule.

**paranesthesia** (păr″ăn-ĕs-thē′zē-ă) [″ + *an-,* not, + *aisthesis,* sensation] Para-anesthesia.

**paraneural** (păr″ă-nū′răl) [″ + *neuron,* nerve] Adjacent to a nerve.

**paranoia** (păr″ă-noy′ă) [Gr. *para,* beside, + *nous,* mind] A condition in which patients show persistent persecutory delusions or delusional jealousy, with emotion and behavior appropriate to the content of the delusional system. The disorder must have been present at least 1 week. The condition also is characterized by symptoms of schizophrenia such as bizarre delusions or incoherence. There are no prominent hallucinations and a full depressive or manic syndrome is either not present or is of brief duration. The illness is not due to organic disease of the brain.

This disorder, which usually occurs in middle or late adult life and may be chronic, often includes resentment and anger that may lead to violence. These patients rarely seek medical attention but are brought for care by associates or relatives.

***erotomanic type p.*** A form of paranoid delusion that one is loved by another. The delusion is more nearly one of romantic or spiritual love, rather than physical. The object is usually someone who is of a higher status or who is famous, but may be a complete stranger.

***jealous type p.*** The unfounded conviction that the patient's spouse or lover is unfaithful.

***litigious p.*** Paranoia in which the patient institutes or threatens to institute legal action because of the imagined persecution.

***somatic p.*** The delusion that one's body is malodorous, or is infested with an internal or external parasite, or that the body is physically misshapen or unduly ugly.

**paranoiac** (păr-ă-noy′ăk) **1.** Concerning or afflicted with paranoia. **2.** One suffering from paranoia.

**paranoid** (păr′ă-noyd) [″ + *nous,* mind, + *eidos,* form, shape] **1.** Resembling paranoia. **2.** A person afflicted with paranoia.

**paranoid disorder** SEE: *Nursing Diagnoses Appendix; personality disorder, paranoid.*

**paranoid ideation** Suspicious thinking that is persecutory, accompanied by feelings that one is being harassed, treated wrongly, or being judged critically.

**paranoid reaction type** An individual who has fixed systematized delusions, is suspicious, has a persecution complex, is resentful and bitter, and is a megalomaniac. Many states approach true paranoia and resemble it but lack one or more of its distinguishing features. Some of these are transitory paranoid states caused by toxic conditions, a paranoid type of schizophrenia, and paranoid states due to alcoholism.

**paranomia** (păr″ă-nō′mē-ă) [″ + *onoma,* name] Form of aphasia in which there is an inability to remember correct names of objects shortly after seeing or using them.

**paranormal 1.** Pert. to claimed experiences that are not within the range of normal experiences or are not scientifically explainable. SEE: *extrasensory perception; psychokinesis.* **2.** Moderately abnormal.

**paranuclear** (păr″ă-nū′klē-ăr) Adjacent to the nucleus of a cell.

**paranucleolus** (păr″ă-nū-klē′ō-lŭs) A small basophil body in the sac enclosing the nucleus.

**paranucleus** (păr″ă-nū′klē-ŭs) [Gr. *para,* beside, + L. *nucleus,* a kernel] A small body lying close to a cell nucleus.

**paraoperative** (păr″ă-ŏp′ĕr-ă-tĭv) [″ + L. *operari,* to work] Concerning all the details and accessories of surgery and preparation of the patient.

**parapancreatic** (păr″ă-păn″krē-ăt′ĭk) [″ + *pan,* all, + *kreas,* flesh] Located close to the pancreas.

**paraparesis** (păr″ă-păr-ē′sĭs, -păr′ĕ-sĭs) [″ + *parienai,* to let fall] Partial paralysis affecting the lower limbs.

**parapeptone** (păr″ă-pĕp′tōn) [″ + *peptein,* to digest] Intermediate digestion product of albumin. SEE: *peptone.*

**paraperitoneal** (păr″ă-pĕr″ĭ-tō-nē′ăl) [″ + *peritonaion,* peritoneum] Near the peritoneum.

**paraphasia** (păr-ă-fā′zē-ă) [″ + *aphasis,* speech loss] The misuse of spoken words or word combinations; a form of aphasia. SEE: *paraphrasia.*

**paraphemia** (păr″ă-fē′mē-ă) [″ + *pheme,* speech] A disorder marked by consistent use of the wrong words or by mispronunciation of words.

**paraphilia** [″ + *philein,* to love] A psychosexual disorder in which unusual or bizarre imagery or acts are necessary for realization of sexual excitement. Included in this disorder are bestiality, fetishism, transvestism, zoophilia, pedophilia, exhibitionism, voyeurism, sexual masochism, and sexual sadism.

**paraphimosis** (păr″ă-fī-mō′sĭs) [″ + *phimoun,* to muzzle, + *osis,* condition] Strangulation of the glans penis due to retraction of a narrowed or inflamed foreskin.

***p. oculi*** Retraction of the eyelid behind a protruding eyeball.

**paraphobia** (păr″ă-fō′bē-ă) [″ + *phobos,* fear] A mild form of phobia.

**paraphrasia** (păr-ă-frā′zē-ă) [Gr. *para,* beside, + *phrasis,* speech] A condition characterized by loss of ability to use words correctly and coherently. The words spoken are so jumbled and misused as to make speech unintelligible.

**paraphrenitis** (păr″ă-frē-nī′tĭs) [″ + *phren,* diaphragm, + *itis,* inflammation] Inflammation of the tissues around the diaphragm.

**paraphysis** (pă-răf′ĭ-sĭs) [Gr., offshoot] The vestigial structure that originates from the roof plate of the telencephalon. Presumably the colloid cyst of the third ventricle arises from it. It is also a midline organ that develops from the roof plate of the diencephalon of some lower vertebrates.

**paraplasm** (păr′ă-plăzm) [Gr. *para,* beside, + LL. *plasma,* form, mold] **1.** Any abnormal new formation or malformation. **2.** Hyaloplasm.

**paraplastic** (păr″ă-plăs′tĭk) [″ + *plastikos,* formed] **1.** Misshapen; deformed. **2.** Pert. to the fluid portion of the protoplasm.

**paraplegia** (păr-ă-plē′jē-ă) [Gr. *paraplegia,* stroke on one side] Paralysis of the lower portion of the body and of both legs. It is caused by a lesion involving the spinal cord that may be due to maldevelopment, epidural abscess, hematomyelia, acute transverse myelitis, spinal neoplasms, multiple sclerosis, syringomyelia, or trauma. SEE: *Nursing Diagnoses Appendix.*

***alcoholic p.*** Paraplegia of spinal origin due to excessive use of alcohol.

***ataxic p.*** Lateral and posterior sclerosis of the spinal cord characterized by slowly progressing ataxia and paresis.

***cerebral p.*** Paraplegia from a bilateral cerebral lesion.

***congenital spastic p.*** Infantile spastic p.

***p. dolorosa*** Paraplegia due to pressure of a neoplasm on the posterior spinal cord and nerve roots; extremely painful despite paralysis.

***infantile spastic p.*** Spastic paraplegia that occurs in infants, usually due to birth injury. SYN: *congenital spastic p.* SEE: *spastic p.*

***peripheral p.*** Paraplegia due to pressure on, injury to, or disease of peripheral nerves.

***Pott's p.*** Paraplegia associated with tuberculosis of the spine.

***primary spastic p.*** Paraplegia from degeneration in corticospinal tracts.

***senile p.*** Paraplegia resulting from sclerosis of arteries supplying spinal cord.

***spastic p.*** Paraplegia characterized by increased muscular tone and accentuated tendon reflexes; seen in multiple sclerosis and other conditions involving the corticospinal tracts. SYN: *tetanoid p.*

***superior p.*** Paralysis of both arms.

***tetanoid p.*** Spastic p.

**paraplegic** (păr-ă-plē′jĭk) [Gr. *paraplegia,* stroke on one side] Pert. to, or afflicted with, paraplegia.

**paraplegiform** (păr″ă-plĕj′ĭ-form) [″ + L. *forma,* form] Similar to paraplegia.

**parapleuritis** (păr″ă-plū-rī′tĭs) [Gr. *para,* beside, + *pleura,* side, + *itis,* inflammation] **1.** Inflammation in the thoracic wall. **2.** Mild inflammation of the pleura. **3.** Pleurodynia.

**parapoplexy** (păr-ăp′ō-plĕk″sē) [″ + *apoplessein,* to cripple by a stroke] A mild or slight apoplexy with partial stupor; a stupor resembling apoplexy. SYN: *pseudoapoplexy.*

**parapraxia** (păr-ă-prăk′sē-ă) [″ + *praxis,* doing] Disturbed mental processes producing inaccuracy, forgetfulness, and tendency to misplace things and make slips of speech or pen.

**paraproctitis** (păr″ă-prŏk-tī′tĭs) [Gr. *para,* beside, + *proktos,* anus, + *itis,* inflammation] Inflammation of the tissues near the rectum.

**paraproctium** (păr″ă-prŏk′shē-ŭm) [″ + *proktos,* anus] The connective tissue around the anus and rectum.

**paraprostatitis** (păr″ă-prŏs″tă-tī′tĭs) [″ + *prostates,* prostate, + *itis,* inflammation] Inflammation of the tissues around the prostate.

**paraprotein** (păr″ă-prō′tē-ĭn) An abnormal plasma protein, such as a macroglobulin, cryoglobulin, or the protein present in myeloma.

**paraproteinemia** The presence of abnormal immunoglobulins or antibodies in the serum or urine of patients with various disease states which, as a group, are called plasma cell dyscrasias. Paraproteinemias include various forms of lymphoid malignancies, amyloidosis, and benign disorders associated with drug administration. SEE: *Bence Jones protein.*

**parapsoriasis** (păr″ă-sō-rī′ă-sĭs) [″ + *psoriasis,* an itching] A chronic disorder of the skin marked by scaly red lesions.

***p. en plaque*** A form of parapsoriasis that is often the precursor of mycosis fungoides.

***p. lichenoides chronica*** A form of parapsoriasis that forms a widespread network over the extremities and trunk that is red to blue, sometimes resembling psoriasis or lichen planus.

**parapsychology** (păr″ă-sī-kŏl′ō-jē) The division of psychology that deals with extrasensory perception, telepathy, psychokinesis, clairvoyance, and associated phenomena.

**paraquat** (păr′ă-kwăt) A toxic chemical used in agriculture to kill certain weeds. It damages the skin on contact and if ingested may cause liver, renal, and pulmonary disease. This chemical is sometimes present as a contaminant in marijuana.

***p. poisoning*** Poisoning due to ingestion of paraquat. The substance should be removed from the stomach and gastrointestinal tract by emesis, gastric lavage, and catharsis. A slurry of clay and charcoal should be administered to absorb the poison. Intravenous cortisone and hemodialysis are helpful.

**pararectal** (păr″ă-rĕk′tăl) [″ + L. *rectum,* straight] Close to the rectum.

**parareflexia** (păr″ă-rē-flĕk′sē-ă) An abnormal condition of the reflexes.

**pararenal** (păr″ă-rē′năl) [″ + L. *ren,* kidney] Near the kidneys.

**pararhotacism** (păr″ă-rō′tă-sĭzm) [″ + *rho,* Gr. letter R, + *-ismos,* condition] Constant erroneous use of the letter "r" or the placing of undue emphasis on letter "r."

**pararthria** (păr-ăr′thrē-ă) [″ + *arthron,* articulation] A speech disorder characterized by difficulty in uttering sounds.

**parasacral** (păr″ă-sā′krăl) [″ + L. *sacrum,* sacred] Close to the sacrum.

**parasalpingitis** (păr″ă-săl-pĭn-jī′tĭs) [″ + *salpinx,* tube, + *itis,* inflammation] Inflammation of the tissues around an oviduct or a eustachian tube.

**parasecretion** (păr″ă-sē-krē′shŭn) [″ + L. *secretio,* secretion] **1.** An abnormality in secretion. **2.** A substance abnormally secreted.

**parasexuality** (păr″ă-sĕks″ū-ăl′ĭ-tē) [″ + L. *sexus,* sex] Any sexually deviant act.

**parasigmatism** (păr″ă-sĭg′mă-tĭzm) [″ + *sigma,* Gr. letter S, + *-ismos,* condition] Lisping.

**parasinoidal** (păr″ă-sī-noy′dăl) [″ + L. *sinus,* a curve] Close to a sinus.

**parasite** (păr′ă-sīt) [″ + *sitos,* food] **1.** An organism that lives within, upon, or at the expense of another organism (the host) without contributing to its survival. **2.** The smaller or incomplete element of conjoined twins that is attached to and dependent on the more nearly normal twin (autosite).

***accidental p.*** A parasite infesting a host that is not its normal host. SYN: *incidental p.*

***external p.*** A parasite that lives on the outer surface of its hosts, such as fleas, lice, mites, or ticks. SYN: *ectoparasite.*

***facultative p.*** A parasite capable of living independently of its host at times; the opposite of an obligate parasite.

***incidental p.*** Accidental p.

***intermittent p.*** A parasite that visits its host at intervals for nourishment. SYN: *occasional p.*

***internal p.*** A parasite such as a protozoon or worm that lives within the body of the host, occupying the digestive tract or body cavities, or living within body organs, blood, tissues, or even cells.

***malarial p.*** Any one of the four species of *Plasmodium* that can cause malaria. SEE: *malaria.*

***obligate p.*** A parasite completely dependent on its host; the opposite of a facultative parasite.

***occasional p.*** Intermittent p.

***periodic p.*** A parasite that lives on the host for short periods of time.

***permanent p.*** A parasite, such as a fluke or an itch mite, that lives on its host until maturity or spends its entire life on its host.

***specific p.*** A parasite that requires a specific host in order to complete its life cycle.

***temporary p.*** A parasite that is free-living during a part of its life cycle.

**parasitemia** (păr″ă-sī-tē′mē-ă) [″ + ″ + *haima,* blood] The presence of parasites in the blood.

**parasitic** (păr″ă-sĭt′ĭk) [Gr. *para,* beside, + *sitos,* food] Resembling, caused by, or concerning a parasite.

**parasiticide** (păr″ă-sĭt′ĭ-sīd) [″ + ″ + L. *caedere,* to kill] **1.** Destructive to parasites. **2.** An agent that kills parasites.

**parasitism** (păr′ă-sīt″ĭzm) [″ + ″ + *-ismos,* condition] **1.** The state or condition of being infected or infested with parasites. **2.** The behavior of a parasite.

**parasitize** (păr′ă-sĭt-īz″, -sĭt-īz″) To infest or infect with a parasite.

**parasitogenic** (păr″ă-sī″tō-jĕn′ĭk) [″ + ″ + *gennan,* to produce] **1.** Caused by parasites. **2.** Favoring parasitic development.

**parasitologist** (păr″ă-sī-tŏl′ō-jĭst) [″ + ″ + *logos,* word, reason] One who specializes in the science of parasitology.

**parasitology** (păr″ă-sī-tŏl′ō-jē) [″ + ″ + *logos,* word, reason] The study of parasites and parasitism.

**parasitophobia** (păr″ă-sī″tō-fō′bē-ă) [″ + ″ + *phobos,* fear] An unusual fear of parasites.

**parasitosis** (păr″ă-sī-tō′sĭs) [″ + ″ + *osis,* condition] A disease or condition resulting from parasitism.

**parasitotropic** (păr″ă-sī″tō-trŏp′ĭk) [″ + ″ + *tropos,* turning] Having an attraction for parasites, esp. certain drugs that act chiefly on parasites in the body.

**parasitotropism** (păr″ă-sī-tŏt′rō-pĭzm) [″ + ″ + ″ + *-ismos,* condition] The special affinity of drugs or other agents for parasites.

**parasitotropy** (păr″ă-sī-tŏt′rō-pē) Parasitotropism.

**parasomnias** (păr″ă-sŏm′nē-ăz) [″ + L. *somnus,* sleep] An abnormal event that occurs during sleep. SEE: *sleep disorder.*

**paraspadia** (păr-ă-spā′dē-ă) [Gr. *paraspadein,* to draw aside] A condition in which the urethra has an opening through one side of the penis.

**paraspasm** (păr′ă-spăzm) [L. *paraspasmus*] **1.** Muscular spasm of the lower extremities. **2.** Spastic paralysis of the lower extremities.

**parasteatosis** (păr″ă-stē″ă-tō′sĭs) [Gr. *para,* beside, + *steatos,* fat, + *osis,* condition] Any disordered condition of the sebaceous secretions.

**parasternal** (păr-ă-stĕrn′ăl) [″ + *sternon,*

chest] Beside the sternum.

***p. region*** The area between the sternal margin and parasternal line.

**parasympathetic** (păr″ă-sĭm″pă-thĕt′ĭk) [″ + *sympathetikos,* sympathetic nerve] Of or pert. to the craniosacral division of the autonomic nervous system.

***parasympathetic nervous system*** The craniosacral division of the autonomic nervous system. Preganglionic fibers originate from nuclei in the midbrain, medulla, and sacral portion of the spinal cord. They pass through the third, seventh, ninth, and tenth cranial nerves and the second, third, and fourth sacral nerves, and synapse with postganglionic neurons located in autonomic (terminal) ganglia that lie in the walls of or near the organ innervated.

Some effects of parasympathetic stimulation are constriction of the pupil, contraction of the smooth muscle of the alimentary canal, constriction of the bronchioles, slowing of the heart rate, and increased secretion by the glands, except the sweat glands.

**parasympathicotonia** (păr″ă-sĭm-păth″ĭk-ō-tō′nē-ă) [″ + *sympathetikos,* sympathetic nerve, + *tonos,* tension] A condition in which there is an imbalance in functioning of the autonomic nervous system, the parasympathetic division dominating over the sympathetic. SYN: *vagotonia.*

**parasympatholytic** (păr″ă-sĭm″pă-thō-lĭt′ĭk) [″ + ″ + *lytikos,* dissolving] Having a destructive effect on or blocking parasympathetic nerve fibers.

**parasympathomimetic** (păr″ă-sĭm″pă-thō-mĭm-ĕt′ĭk) [″ + ″ + *mimetikos,* imitative] Producing effects similar to those resulting from stimulation of parasympathetic nervous system.

**parasynovitis** (păr″ă-sĭn″ō-vī′tĭs) [″ + *syn,* with, + *oon,* egg, + *itis,* inflammation] Inflammation of tissues around a synovial sac.

**parasystole** (păr-ă-sĭs′tō-lē) [″ + *systole,* contraction] An ectopically originating cardiac rhythm independent of the normal sinus rhythm.

**paratarsium** (păr-ă-tăr′sē-ŭm) [″ + *tarsos,* tarsus] The covering and connective tissues of the tarsus of the feet.

**paratenon** (păr″ă-tĕn′ŏn) [″ + *tenon,* tendon] Fatty and areolar tissue that surrounds the tendon and fills the spaces around the tendon.

**paratereseomania** (păr″ă-tĕr-ē″sē-ō-mā′nē-ă) [Gr. *parateresis,* observation, + *mania,* madness] The insane desire to investigate new scenes and subjects.

**parathion** (păr″ă-thī′ŏn) An agricultural insecticide that is highly toxic to humans and animals.

***p. poisoning*** Poisoning contracted by accidental inhalation or ingestion while working with the pesticide or because of the inadvertent contamination of food products eaten. Shortly after exposure, headache, sweating, salivation, lacrimation, vomiting, diarrhea, muscular twitching, convulsions, dyspnea, and blurred vision occur. SEE: *Poisons and Poisoning Appendix.*

**parathormone** (păr″ă-thor′mōn) [Gr. *para,* beside, + *thyreos,* shield, + *eidos,* form, shape, + *hormaein,* to excite] Parathyroid hormone.

**parathyroid** (păr-ă-thī′royd) [″ + *thyreos,* shield, + *eidos,* form, shape] **1.** Located close to the thyroid gland. **2.** One of four small endocrine glands about 6 mm long by 3 to 4 mm broad on the back of and at lower edge of the thyroid gland, or embedded within its substance. These glands secrete a hormone, parathyroid hormone (parathormone), that regulates calcium and phosphorus metabolism. SEE: *calcitonin* for illus.

ABNORMALITIES: Hypoparathyroidism or hyposecretion results in neuromuscular hyperexcitability manifested by convulsions and tetany, carpopedal spasm, wheezing, muscle cramps, urinary frequency, mood changes, and lassitude. Blood calcium falls and blood phosphorus rises. Other symptoms include blurring of vision caused by cataracts, poorly formed teeth if onset was in childhood, maldevelopment of hair and nails, and dry and scaly skin. Hyperparathyroidism or hypersecretion results in a rise in blood calcium and fall in blood phosphorus. Calcium is removed from bones, resulting in increased fragility. Muscular weakness, reduced muscular tone, and general neuromuscular hypoexcitability occur. Generalized osteitis fibrosa, or osteitis fibrosa cystica, is a clinical entity associated with hyperplasia and resulting hypersecretion of the parathyroids. Parathormone secreted by these glands, contains the active principle or principles.

***p. injection*** A standard preparation of the water-soluble hormone obtained from the parathyroid glands of mammals used for food by humans. It increases the calcium content of the blood.

**parathyroidectomy** (păr″ă-thī-royd-ĕk′tō-mē) [″ + ″ + ″ + *ektome,* excision] Excision of one or more of the parathyroid glands. SEE: *Nursing Diagnoses Appendix.*

NURSING IMPLICATIONS: The patient's understanding of the procedure and postoperative care is assessed, and the nurse provides additional information and answers questions. Deep-breathing exercises and coughing are taught, and the importance of early ambulation and activity after surgery is explained. The patient's bed should be slightly elevated, and vital signs monitored regularly. The patient is observed for signs of calcium deficiency, and serum electrolyte levels are monitored. The patient is instructed to report immediately hoarseness or loss of voice. Pain is monitored, and pain relief provided. When moving the patient, the nurse supports the patient's neck to protect the incision. Before discharge, the nurse teaches the patient the importance of recognizing and seeking medical attention for signs of calcium deficiency. Instruction is provided in incisional care. The importance of early ambulation and activity is emphasized.

**parathyroprivia** (păr″ă-thī″rō-prĭ′vē-ă) [″ + ″ + L. *privus,* deprived of] A condition that results when the parathyroids are removed or cease functioning.

**parathyrotropic** (păr″ă-thī-rō-trŏp′ĭk) [″ + ″ + *tropikos,* turning] Having an affinity for the parathyroid gland.

**paratonsillar** (păr″ă-tŏn′sĭl-ăr) [″ + L. *tonsillaris,* pert. to tonsil] Near or about the tonsil.

**paratope** (păr′ă-tōp) [″ + *topos,* a place] The site on an antibody to which an antigen attaches. SEE: *epitope.*

**paratrichosis** (păr″ă-trĭ-kō′sĭs) [″ + *trichosis,* being hairy] An abnormality of the hair or of its location.

**paratripsis** (păr″ă-trĭp′sĭs) [″ + *tribein,* to rub] Rubbing, chafing.

**paratrophic** (păr″ă-trō′fĭk) [″+ *trophe,* nourishment] **1.** Requiring living substances for food; parasitic. **2.** Pert. to abnormal nutrition.

**paratyphlitis** (păr″ă-tĭf-lī′tĭs) [″ + *typhlos,* blind, + *itis,* inflammation] An inflammation of the connective tissue close to the cecum.

**paratyphoid fever** An infectious fever resembling typhoid.

SYMPTOMS: Fever with gastroenteritis characterizes this disease. The incubation period may be less than in typhoid. Usually the patient's condition is less severe than that found in typhoid fever, but symptoms vary from a mild transient diarrhea to those quite similar to typhoid fever.

ETIOLOGY: Although the disease is caused by bacteria of the genus *Salmonella,* esp. the species *S. paratyphi* (A and B strains) and *S. schottmülleri,* any species of *Salmonella* pathogenic to humans may cause a similar disease.

**paratypic** (păr″ă-tĭp′ĭk) [″ + *typos,* type] Diverging from a type.

**paraumbilical** (păr″ă-ŭm-bĭl′ĭk-ăl) [″ + L. *umbilicus,* navel] Located close to the navel.

**paraurethral** (păr″ă-ū-rē′thrăl) [″ + *ourethra,* urethra] Located close to the urethra.

**parauterine** (păr″ă-ū′tĕr-ĭn) [″ + L. *uterus,* womb] Located close to or around the uterus.

**paravaccinia** (păr″ă-văk-sĭn′ē-ă) A viral disease that affects the udders of cows and may be transmitted to humans. In humans, the virus produces painless smooth or warty lesions, called "milker's nodules," on the hands and arms. SEE: *milker's nodules.*

**paravaginal** (păr″ă-văj′ĭn-ăl) [″ + *vagina,* sheath] Located close to or around the vagina.

**paravaginitis** (păr″ă-văj-ĭn-ī′tĭs) [″ + ″ + *itis,* inflammation] Inflammation of the tissue surrounding the vagina.

**paravenous** (păr″ă-vē′nŭs) [″ + L. *vena,* vein] Located close to a vein.

**paravertebral** (păr″ă-vĕr′tē-brăl) [″ + L. *vertebralis,* pert. to vertebrae] Alongside or near the vertebral column.

**paravertebral anesthesia** Injection of a local anesthetic at the roots of spinal nerves.

**paravesical** (păr″ă-vĕs′ĭk-ăl) [″ + L. *vesica,* bladder] Near the urinary bladder.

**paraxial** (păr-ăk′sē-ăl) [″ + L. *axis,* axis] On either side of the axis of the body or one of its parts.

**paraxon** (păr-ăk′sŏn) [″ + *axon,* axis] A collateral branch of an axon.

**parazoon** (păr″ă-zō′ŏn) [″ + *zoon,* animal] An animal that lives as a parasite on another animal.

**parched** [ME. *parchen*] Extremely dry.

**Paré, Ambroise** (păr-ā′) French surgeon, 1510–1590, who instituted certain refined techniques into surgery and obstetrics.

**parectasia, parectasis** (păr″ĕk-tā′sē-ă, -tă-sĭs) [Gr. *para,* beside, + *ektasis,* stretching] Excessive dilatation or stretching of a structure.

**parectropia** (păr″ĕk-trō′pē-ă) [″ + *ek,* out, + *trope,* a turn] Apraxia.

**paregoric** (păr-ĕ-gor′ĭk) [L. *paregoricus,* soothing] **1.** Camphorated tincture of opium, a narcotic-containing drug that in large doses is poisonous; used in the symptomatic treatment of diarrhea. **2.** Soothing.

***p. poisoning*** SEE: *morphine poisoning.*

**parelectronomic** (păr″ē-lĕk″trō-nŏm′ĭk) [Gr. *para,* beside, + *elektron,* amber, + *nomos,* law] Not subject to electric stimulus.

**parencephalia** (păr″ĕn-sĕ-fā′lē-ă) [″ + *enkephalos,* brain] A congenital defect of the brain.

**parencephalocele** (păr″ĕn-sĕf′ă-lō-sēl) [″ + ″ + *kele,* tumor, swelling] Herniation of the cerebellum through a defect in the cranium.

**parencephalous** (păr″ĕn-sĕf′ă-lŭs) [″ + *enkephalos,* brain] A fetus with imperfect development of the cranium.

**parenchyma** (păr-ĕn′kĭ-mă) [Gr. *parenkheim,* to pour in beside] The essential parts of an organ that are concerned with its function in contradistinction to its framework.

***p. testis*** The functional portion of the testis, including the seminiferous tubules within the lobules.

**parenchymatitis** (păr″ĕn-kĭm″ă-tī′tĭs) [″ + *itis,* inflammation] Inflammation of the parenchyma or substance of a gland.

**parenchymatous** (păr″ĕn-kĭm′ă-tŭs) Concerning the essential substances of an organ.

**parent** [L. *parens*] A father or a mother; one who begets offspring.

**parentage, determination of** SEE: *paternity test.*

**parental leave** The policy of allowing one or both parents to have leave from work following the birth of their child.

**parental role conflict** The state in which a parent experiences role confusion and conflict in response to crisis. SEE: *Nursing Diagnoses Appendix.*

**parenteral** (păr-ĕn′tĕr-ăl) [Gr. *para,* beside, + *enteron,* intestine] Denoting any medication route other than the alimentary canal, such as intravenous, subcutaneous, intramuscular, or mucosal. SEE: *medication routes.*

***p. digestion*** The digestion of foreign substances by body cells as opposed to enteral digestion, which occurs in the alimentary canal.

***p. nutrition*** SEE: *total parenteral nutrition.*

**parent/infant/child attachment, altered, risk for** Disruption of the interactive process between parent/significant other and infant that fosters the development of a protective and nurturing reciprocal relationship. SEE: *Nursing Diagnoses Appendix.*

**parenting 1.** Caring for and raising a child or children. **2.** Producing offspring.

***altered p.*** The state in which a nurturing figure(s) experiences an inability to create an environment that promotes the optimum growth and development of another human being. SEE: *Nursing Diagnoses Appendix.*

***altered p., risk for*** The state in which a nurturing figure(s) is at risk to experience an inability to create an environment that promotes the optimum growth and development of another human being. SEE: *Nursing Diagnoses Appendix.*

***surrogate p.*** An alternative method of childbearing for an infertile couple in which the wife is unable to bear a child. The surrogate mother agrees to be artificially inseminated by the husband's sperm and to relinquish the baby to the couple. Another approach is to retrieve eggs from the infertile wife and have them impregnated in vitro by her husband. The fertilized ovum is then implanted in the surrogate mother. SEE: *fertilization, in vitro; GIFT; surrogate parenting.*

**parepithymia** (păr″ĕp-ĭ-thī′mē-ă) [″ + *epithymia,* desire] An abnormal desire or craving.

**paresis** (păr′ĕ-sĭs, pă-rē′sĭs) [Gr. *parienai,* to let fall] **1.** Partial or incomplete paralysis. SEE: *paralysis.* **2.** An organic mental disease with somatic, irritative, and paralytic focal symptoms and signs running a slow, chronic, progressive course. SYN: *dementia paralytica; paralytic dementia.*

SYMPTOMS: The symptoms may include pupillary changes, facial tremors, tremors of the lips and tongue, and speech disturbances. Usually the patient exhibits Argyll Robertson pupils, impaired vision, headache, and slurred speech, with letters and syllables often omitted. As the disease progresses, the patient demonstrates a disregard for social convention and moral standards. Memory is defective, and depression and dementia are present, as are epileptic convulsions and unequal exaggeration of the reflexes. Always present is a positive serological test for syphilis (spinal fluid) with increases of protein and lymphocytes.

ETIOLOGY: The cause of this condition is diffuse and focal involvement of the brain and spinal cord owing to syphilis, usually occurring 5 to 15 years after the primary infection.

PATHOLOGY: Pathologically, it is a diffuse meningoencephalitis with degenerative changes dependent on vascular and toxic factors.

TREATMENT: This condition is treated with intravenous penicillin G, given every 4 hr for 10 to 14 days. An alternative therapy is a daily intramuscular dose of penicillin G and oral probenecid given 4 times a day for 10 to 14 days.

***juvenile p.*** General paresis due to congenital syphilis; seen in children.

**paresthesia** (păr″ĕs-thē′zē-ă) [Gr. *para,* beside, + *aisthesis,* sensation] A sensation of numbness, prickling, or tingling; heightened sensitivity; experienced in central and peripheral nerve lesions and in locomotor ataxia.

***Berger's p.*** Paresthesia of the legs that occurs in young people.

**paretic** (pă-rĕt′ĭk, pă-rē′tĭk) [Gr. *parienai,* to let fall] Afflicted with or concerning paresis.

**pareunia** [Gr. *pareunos,* lying beside] Sexual intercourse. SEE: *dyspareunia.*

**pargyline hydrochloride** (păr′gĭ-lēn) An antihypertensive drug.

**parhidrosis** (păr″hĭ-drō′sĭs) [Gr. *para,* beside, + *hidrosis,* sweat] Any disordered secretion of perspiration.

**paries** (pā′rē-ēs) *pl.* **parietes** [L., a wall] The enveloping wall of any structure; applied esp. to hollow organs.

**parietal** (pă-rī′ĕ-tăl) [L. *parietalis*] **1.** Pert. to, or forming, the wall of a cavity. **2.** Pert. to the parietal bone.

***p. bone*** One of two bones that together form the roof and sides of the skull.

***p. cell*** A large cell on the margin of the peptic glands of the stomach that secretes hydrochloric acid and the intrinsic factor. SYN: *oxyntic cell.* SEE: *achlorhydria; anemia, pernicious; intrinsic factor.*

**parietofrontal** (pă-rī″ĕ-tō-frŏn′tăl) Concerning the parietal or frontal bones or lobes.

**parietography** (pă-rī″ĕ-tŏg′ră-fē) [″ + Gr. *graphein,* to write] A radiographical study of the walls of an organ.

**parieto-occipital** (pă-rī″ĕ-tō-ŏk-sĭp′ĭ-tăl) Concerning the parietal and occipital bones or lobes.

**parietosquamosal** (pă-rī″ĕ-tō-skwă-mō′săl) Concerning the parietal bone and squamous part of the temporal bone.

**parietotemporal** (pă-rī″ĕ-tō-tĕm′pō-răl) Concerning the parietal and temporal bones or lobes.

**parietovisceral** (pă-rī″ĕ-tō-vĭs′ĕr-ăl) Concerning the wall of a body cavity and the viscera within.

**Parinaud, Henri** (pă-rĭ-nō′) French ophthalmologist, 1844–1905.

***P.'s oculoglandular syndrome*** Conjunctivitis with palpable preauricular lymph nodes.

***P.'s ophthalmoplegia syndrome*** Palsy of vertical gaze that may or may not be associated with pupillary or oculomotor nerve paresis. It is caused by a lesion at the level of the anterior corpora quadrigemina of the brain.

**pari passu** (păr′ē-păs′ū) [L., with equal speed] Occurring at the same time or at the same rate; side by side.

**parity** (păr′ĭ-tē) **1.** [L. *par,* equal] Equality, similarity. **2.** [L. *parere,* to bring forth, to bear] The condition of having carried a pregnancy to a point of viability (500 g birth weight or 20 weeks' gestation), regardless of the outcome. SEE: *multiparity; nulliparity.*

**Parkinson, James** British physician, 1755–1824.

***P.'s disease*** A chronic nervous disease characterized by a fine, slowly spreading tremor, muscular weakness and rigidity, and a peculiar gait. SYN: *paralysis agitans; parkinsonism; shaking palsy.* SEE: *Nursing Diagnoses Appendix.*

SYMPTOMS: The onset may be abrupt, but is usually insidious. Early changes may include aching, fatigue, and malaise. However, in over half the cases, the first symptoms are rigidity and immobility of the hands, followed by a fine tremor (pill-rolling tremor) beginning in the hand or the foot that may spread until it involves all the members. At first the tremor is paroxysmal but becomes almost continuous. The face becomes expressionless and fixed. Infrequent eye blinking is often an early sign. The speech becomes slow and measured, and later generalized muscular rigidity occurs. The head becomes bowed, the body bent forward, the arms flexed, the thumbs turned in toward the palms, the knees slightly bent. The gait (festination) is characteristic by this time: steps grow faster and faster, and the body inclines more and more forward until the patient begins to fall and seeks some support. Occasionally, a tendency to fall backwards (retropulsion) replaces festination. Numbness, tingling, and a sensation of heat may be present. Drooling, due to failure to swallow rather than increased saliva production, may become troublesome. It is not known whether the dementia that occurs in approx. 30% of patients is a normal manifestation of the disease or is the coincidental development of Alzheimer's disease. SEE: illus.; *positron emission tomography* for illus. of normal PET scan.

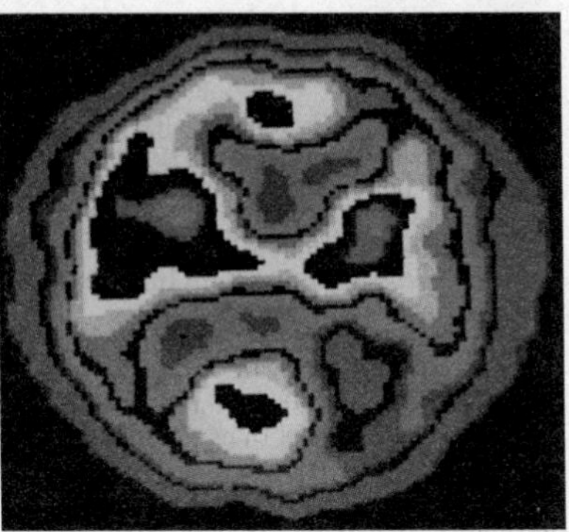

PARKINSON'S DISEASE

PET SCAN OF BRAIN IN PARKINSON'S DEMENTIA SHOWING WIDESPREAD REDUCED METABOLISM (BLUE AND GREEN)

TREATMENT: Treatment is generally supportive. Additionally, medicines are used to combat muscle rigidity and lethargy. These include anticholinergics, antidepressants, antihistamines, dopa inhibitor combined with levodopa (Sinemet), dopamine agonists such as bromocriptine or pergolide, monoamine oxidase-B inhibitor (deprenyl), and antivirals such as amantidine. Patients often benefit from referral to occupational or physical therapy, or both. Recovery rarely, if ever, occurs, and duration is indefinite.

NURSING IMPLICATIONS: Prescribed drugs are administered and evaluated for desired effects and any adverse reactions, and the patient is instructed in their use and potential side effects so that the dosage can be adjusted to minimize these effects. The nurse teaches the patient and family about safety measures to prevent injury; about drug-related dietary restrictions; and about provision of needed fluids, calories, and dietary bulk by frequent small feedings. The patient should plan daily activities to prevent fatigue. Physical and occupational therapy consultations are recommended. The patient is also referred to national organizations for further information.

***P.'s facies*** The immobile, masklike facies characteristic of Parkinson's disease.

***P.'s mask*** Expressionless appearance of the face. The eyebrows are raised, wrinkles are smoothed out, and there is immobility of the facial muscles. A typical symptom seen in Parkinson's disease and in postencephalitic states.

**parkinsonian** (păr″kĭn-sōn′ē-ăn) Concerning parkinsonism.

**parkinsonism** (păr′kĭn-sŏn-ĭzm″) Parkinson's disease.

**PAR nurse** *Postanesthesia recovery room nurse.*

**paroccipital** (păr-ŏk-sĭp′ĭt-ăl) [Gr. *para,* beside, + L. *occiput,* occiput] **1.** Close to the occipital bone. **2.** The paramastoid process.

**parodontitis** (păr″ō-dŏn-tī′tĭs) [″ + *odous,* tooth, + *itis,* inflammation] Inflammation of the tissues around a tooth.

**parodontium** (păr″ō-dŏn′shē-ŭm) Periodontium.

**parole** [Fr. *parole,* short for *parole d'honneur,* word of honor] In psychiatry, the release of a patient from the hospital on a trial basis.

**parolivary** (păr-ŏl′ĭ-vă″rē) [Gr. *para,* beside, + L. *oliva,* olive] Situated close to the olivary body.

***p. bodies*** Nuclei in medulla oblongata, lying close to the olivary bodies.

**paromomycin sulfate** (păr′ō-mō-mī″sĭn) An aminoglycoside antibiotic used in treating intestinal amebiasis and various tapeworms. It is not effective against extraintestinal infections with amebae.

**paromphalocele** (păr″ŏm-făl′ō-sēl″) [″ + *omphalos,* navel, + *kele,* tumor, swelling] A hernia or tumor close to the umbilicus.

**paroniria** (păr-ō-nī′rē-ă) [″ + *oneiros,* dream] Abnormal or terrifying dreams.

**paronychia** (păr-ō-nĭk′ē-ă) [″ + *onyx,* nail] An acute or chronic infection of the marginal structures about the nail. SYN: *felon; panaris; runaround; whitlow.* SEE: illus.

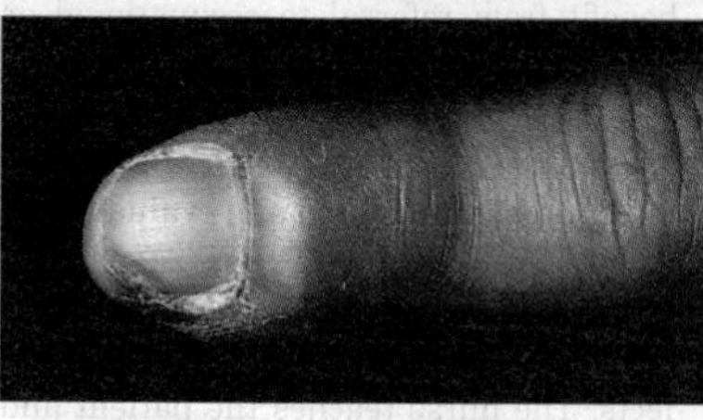

PARONYCHIA

SYMPTOMS: Redness, swelling, and suppuration around the nail edge occur.

TREATMENT: Therapy involves application of heat to the area unless there is inadequate blood supply. Surgery is required in severe cases.

***p. tendinosa*** Inflammation of the sheath of a digital tendon owing to sepsis.

**paronychomycosis** (păr″ō-nĭk″ō-mī-kō′sĭs) [″ + ″ + *mykes,* fungus, + *osis,* condition] A fungus infection about the nails.

**paronychosis** (păr-ō-nĭ-kō′sĭs) Growth of a nail in an abnormal position.

**paroophoritis** (păr″ō-ŏf-ō-rī′tĭs) [″ + *oophoros,* bearing eggs, + *itis,* inflammation] Inflammation of the tissues around the ovary.

**paroophoron** (păr-ō-ŏf′ō-rŏn) [″ + *oophoros,* bearing eggs] A group of minute tubules located in the mesosalpinx between the uterus and ovary. It is a vestigial structure consisting of the remains of the caudal group of mesonephric tubules and is a homologue of the paradidymis of the male.

**parophthalmia** (păr-ŏf-thăl′mē-ă) [″ + *ophthalmos,* eye] Inflammation of the tissue around the eye.

**parophthalmoncus** (păr″ŏf-thăl-mŏn′kŭs) [″ + ″ + *onkos,* mass] A tumor located near the eye.

**parorchidium** (păr-or-kĭd′ē-ŭm) [″ + *orchis,* testicle] Abnormal position, or nondescent, of a testicle. SYN: *ectopia testis.*

**parorexia** (păr-ō-rĕk′sē-ă) [″ + *orexis,* appetite] An abnormal or perverted craving for special or strange foods. SEE: *appetite, perverted; taste.*

**parosmia** (păr-ŏz′mē-ă) [″ + *osme,* odor] Any disorder or perversion of the sense of smell; a false sense of odors or perception of those that do not exist. Agreeable odors are considered offensive, and disagreeable ones pleasant. Intravenous fluid therapy, esp. postoperatively, may create temporary parageusia and parosmia. SYN: *parosphresia.* SEE: *cacosmia.*

**parosphresia, parosphresis** (păr″ŏs-frē′zē-ă, -sĭs) [″ + *osphresis,* smell] Parosmia.

**parosteal** (păr-ŏs′tē-ăl) Concerning the outermost layer of the periosteum.

**parosteitis, parostitis** (păr-ŏs-tē-ī′tĭs, -tī′tĭs) [Gr. *para,* beside, + *osteon,* bone, + *itis,* inflammation] Inflammation of tissues next to the bone.

**parosteosis, parostosis** (păr″ŏs-tē-ō′sĭs, -tō′sĭs) [″ + *osteon,* bone, + *osis,* condition] **1.** Bone formation outside of the periosteum. **2.** Bone development in an unusual location.

**parotic** (pă-rŏt′ĭk) [″ + *ous,* ear] Near the ear.

**parotid** (pă-rŏt′ĭd) Located near the ear; esp. the parotid gland.

**parotidectomy** (pă-rŏt″ĭ-dĕk′tō-mē) [″ + *ous,* ear, + *ektome,* excision] Excision of the parotid gland. This procedure is most often performed to excise a malignancy and less often to remove a calculus that cannot be extracted from the duct in the mouth.

NURSING IMPLICATIONS: The patient's understanding of the procedure and postoperative care is assessed, including suctioning and nasogastric tube for drainage. The patient is encouraged to express feelings and anxiety about the surgery and alterations in body image. After surgery, the nurse asks the patient to perform facial movements such as smiling, frowning, and exposing teeth to observe for possible damage to the facial nerve. Drainage should be observed for excessive bleeding. A patent airway is maintained, and good oral hygiene and nutrition are encouraged.

**parotidoscirrhus** (pă-rŏt″ĭd-ō-skĭr′ŭs) [″ + ″

+ *skirrhos,* hardness] **1.** Hardening of the parotid gland. **2.** A scirrhous cancer of the parotid area.

**parotitis** (păr″rō-tī′tĭs) [″ + *ous,* ear, + *itis,* inflammation] Inflammation of the parotid gland.

**parous** (păr′ŭs) [L. *pario,* to bear] Parturient; fruitful; having borne at least one child.

**parovarian** (păr-ō-vā′rē-ăn) [Gr. *para,* beside, + LL. *ovarium,* ovary] **1.** Situated near or beside the ovary. **2.** Pert. to the parovarium, a residual structure in the broad ligament.

**parovariotomy** (păr″ō-vā″rē-ŏt′ō-mē) [″ + ″ + Gr. *tome,* incision] Removal of a parovarian cyst.

**parovaritis** (păr″ō-vă-rī′tĭs) [″ + LL. *ovarium,* ovary, + Gr. *itis,* inflammation] Inflammation of the epoophoron.

**parovarium** (păr″ō-vā′rē-ŭm) Epoophoron.

**paroxysm** (păr′ŏk-sĭzm) [Gr. *paroxysmos,* irritation] **1.** A sudden, periodic attack or recurrence of symptoms of a disease; an exacerbation of the symptoms of a disease. **2.** A sudden spasm or convulsion of any kind. **3.** A sudden emotional state, as of fear, grief, or joy.

**paroxysmal** (păr″ŏk-sĭz′măl) **1.** Occurring in or concerning paroxysms. **2.** Of the nature of a paroxysm.

***p. cold hemoglobinuria*** ABBR: PCH. A rare form of an acquired hemolytic syndrome that occurs idiopathically, in association with syphilis, or following viral or presumed viral diseases such as measles, mumps, chickenpox, infectious mononucleosis, and influenza.

SYMPTOMS: The syndrome is characterized by acute onset of back and extremity pain and abdominal cramps following chilling. Hemoglobinuria occurs if enough red blood cells have been destroyed. The fever may be as high as 40°C (104°F).

TREATMENT: The primary disease should be treated; otherwise, protection from the cold is the only practical therapy in the idiopathic form. In general, once the cold exposure terminates, therapy is not needed.

**paroxysmal nocturnal dyspnea** SEE: *dyspnea, paroxysmal nocturnal.*

**Parrot, Joseph Marie Jules** (păr-ō′) French physician, 1829–1883.

***P.'s disease*** **1.** Osteochondritis that occurs in infants with congenital syphilis. **2.** A form of dwarfism that is transmitted as an autosomal dominant.

***P.'s nodes*** Bony nodules on the skull of infants with congenital syphilis. SYN: *P.'s sign.*

***P.'s pseudoparalysis*** Pseudoparalysis caused by syphilitic osteochondritis.

***P.'s sign*** P.'s nodes.

***P.'s ulcer*** Lesions seen in thrush or stomatitis.

**parrot fever** Psittacosis.

**Parry's disease** (păr′ēz) [Caleb H. Parry, Brit. physician, 1755–1822] Hyperthyroidism.

**pars** (părz) *pl.* **partes** [L.] A part; portion of a larger structure.

***p. basilaris ossis occipitalis*** The basilar process of the occipital bone.

***p. buccalis hypophyseos*** A developmental protrusion in the primitive buccal cavity of the anterior lobe of the hypophysis.

***p. caeca oculi*** The optic disk.

***p. caeca retinae*** The parts of the retina not sensitive to light (pars ciliaris retinae and pars iridica retinae).

***p. cephalica et cervicalis systematis autonomici*** The cranial and cervical portions of the autonomic nervous system.

***p. ciliaris retinae*** The portion of the retina situated in front of the ora serrata and covering the ciliary body.

***p. distalis adenohypophyseos*** The part of the hypophysis forming the major portion of the anterior lobe. SEE: *pituitary gland.*

***p. flaccida membranae tympani*** The portion of the membrane of the eardrum that fills the notch of Rivinus. This portion of the drum is not taut. SYN: *Shrapnell's membrane.*

***p. interarticularis*** The region between the superior and inferior articulating facets of a vertebra; the region where fracture frequently occurs with spondylolysis.

***p. intermedia adenohypophyseos*** The intermediate lobe of the hypophysis cerebri. SEE: *pituitary gland.*

***p. iridica retinae*** The portion of the retina on the posterior surface of the iris.

***p. mastoidea ossis temporalis*** The mastoid portion of the temporal bone.

***p. membranacea urethrae masculinae*** The membranous portion of the urethra. It extends from the prostate to the bulb of the penis. SEE: *p. spongiosa urethrae masculinae.*

***p. nervosa hypophyseos*** The posterior lobe of the pituitary gland.

***p. optica hypothalami*** The optic chiasm.

***p. optica retinae*** The sensory portion of the retina, extending from the optic disk to the ora serrata.

***p. petrosa ossis temporalis*** The petrous portion of the temporal bone.

***p. plana corporis ciliaris*** The ciliary ring of the eye.

***p. radiata lobuli corticalis renis*** SEE: *ray, medullary.*

***p. spongiosa urethrae masculinae*** The portion of the male urethra included from the point of entrance to the bulb of the penis to its termination at the end of the penis. The bulbourethral glands empty into it via their ducts just after the urethra passes the perineal membrane.

***p. squamosa ossis temporalis*** The flat portion of the temporal bone that forms part of the lateral wall of the skull.

***p. tensa membranae tympani*** The larger portion of the tympanic membrane, a tightly stretched membrane lying inferior to the malleolar folds. SEE: *p. flaccida membranae tympani.*

***p. tuberalis adenohypophyseos*** The portion of the anterior lobe of the hypophysis cerebri that invests the infundibular stalk.

***p. tympanica ossis temporalis*** The tympanic portion of the temporal bone.

**Parse, Rosemarie** A nursing educator who developed the Theory of Human Becoming. SEE: *Nursing Theory Appendix.*

**pars planitis** (părs plā-nī'tĭs) Inflammation of the peripheral retina characterized by aggregations of inflammatory cells on the anterior inferior retina. These are called "snowbanks." This chronic condition, which occurs mostly in the young, is of unknown etiology. It may cause loss of vision. Corticosteroids are administered systemically or by injection behind the eye to treat this condition.

**part, presenting** Before delivery, the fetal anatomical structure nearest the internal cervical os, identified by sonogram or palpation during vaginal examination. SEE: *presentation* for illus.

**part. aeq.** *partes aequales,* in equal parts.

**partes** (păr'tēs) Pl. of pars.

**parthenogenesis** (păr"thĕn-ō-jĕn'ĕ-sĭs) [Gr. *parthenos,* virgin, + *genesis,* generation, birth] Reproduction arising from a female egg that has not been fertilized by the male; unisexual reproduction.

**parthenophobia** (păr"thĕ-nō-fō'bē-ă) [" + *phobos,* fear] Fear of virgins or girls.

**participant observation** A method of field research whereby the investigator observes and records information about the characteristics of a setting through his or her experiences as a participant in that setting.

**particle** [L. *particula*] **1.** A very small piece or part of matter; a tiny fragment or trace. **2.** One of several subatomic components of the nuclei of radioactive elements, such as alpha and beta particles. **3.** Attraction particle or centriole of the nucleus of a cell. **4.** Virion.

***alpha p.*** A charged particle emitted from a radioactive substance made up of a helium nucleus consisting of two protons and two electrons. The particle has very low penetrability.

***beta p.*** A high-speed electron emitted during the decay of an atom.

***Dane p.*** A very small, round particle present in the serum of some patients with viral hepatitis.

***elementary p.*** The subatomic parts of the atomic nucleus.

***elementary p. of the mitochondria*** A surface particle on the mitochondrial cristae.

**particulate** (păr-tĭk'ū-lāt) Made up of particles.

**parts per million** ABBR: PPM; ppm. Phrase used with a number to indicate the concentration of one substance with respect to another. For example, a chemical substance may be said to be present in air at a level of 50 parts per million (parts of air). The units also may be expressed as weight of one substance to the weight of another. This is called weight-to-weight comparison, or the concentration may be expressed as volume-to-volume.

**parturient** (păr-tū'rē-ĕnt) [L. *parturiens,* in labor] Concerning childbirth or parturition; giving birth.

**parturifacient** (păr-tū-rĭ-fā'shĕnt) [" + *facere,* to make] **1.** Inducing or accelerating labor. **2.** A drug used to cause or hasten delivery of the fetus.

**parturiphobia** [" + Gr. *phobos,* fear] Fear of childbirth.

**parturition** (păr-tū-rĭsh'ŭn) [L. *parturitio*] The act of giving birth to young. SYN: *childbirth.*

**part. vic.** *partitis vicibus,* in divided doses.

**parulis** (păr-ū'lĭs) [Gr. *para,* beside, + *oulon,* gum] Gumboil.

**parumbilical** (păr"ŭm-bĭl'ĭ-kăl) [" + L. *umbilicus,* navel] Close to the navel.

**parvovirus** (păr"vō-vī'rŭs) [" + *virus,* poison] A group of viruses similar to adeno-associated viruses. They are pathogenic in animals and humans.

***p. B-19*** A type of parvovirus that causes erythema infectiosum (fifth disease), a usually benign, nonfebrile disease. However, intrauterine infection may produce fetal anemia with hydrops fetalis and death. Infection of immunocompromised patients may cause aplastic anemia, and complications may lead to death.

**parvule** (păr'vūl) [L. *parvulus,* very small] A small pill, pellet, or granule.

**PAS, PASA** *para-aminosalicylic acid.*

**pascal** A unit of pressure equal to the force of one newton acting uniformly over 1 $m^2$. SEE: *newton; SI Units Appendix.*

**Paschen bodies** (pă'shĕn) [Enrique Paschen, Ger. pathologist, 1860–1936] Particles thought to be the pathogenic virus of vaccinia and variola found in great numbers in skin exanthemas.

**PASG** *pneumatic anti-shock garment.* SEE: *MAST.*

**passage** (păs'ăj) [ME., to pass] **1.** A channel between cavities and body structures or with the external surface of an organ. **2.** The act of passing. **3.** An evacuation of the bowels. **4.** Introduction of a probe or catheter. **5.** Incubation of a pathogenic organism, esp. a virus, in one or a series of tissue cultures or living organisms.

**passion** (păsh'ŭn) [L. *passio,* suffering] **1.** Suffering. **2.** Great emotion or zeal; frequently associated with sexual excitement.

**passive** (păs'ĭv) [L. *passivus,* capable of suffering] Submissive; not active.

**passivism** (păs'ĭ-vĭzm) [" + Gr. *-ismos,* condition] **1.** Passive behavior or character. **2.** Sexual perversion with subjugation of the will to another.

**passivity** (păs-sĭv'ĭ-tē) [L. *passivus,* capable

of suffering] In psychiatry, the condition of being dependent on others and a reluctance to be assertive or responsible.

**Pasteur, Louis** (păs-tĕr′) French chemist and bacteriologist, 1822–1895, who founded the science of microbiology. His greatest accomplishments were in the fields of bacteriology and immunology. He developed the technique of immunization and produced vaccines.

***P. effect*** The inhibition of fermentation by bacteria when oxygen is abundant.

***P. treatment*** A procedure used for the prevention of rabies, consisting of a daily injection of increasingly virulent suspensions prepared from the brains or spinal cords of rabbits that have died of rabies. The treatment is continued for 21 days. The suspension is treated so as to kill or inactivate the virus. This treatment is no longer used but is presented for historical purposes. SEE: *rabies*.

**Pasteurella** (păs-tĕr-ĕl′ă) [Louis Pasteur] A genus of bacteria that at one time included the species *P. pestis, P. tularensis, P. multocida,* and *P. pseudotuberculosis. P. pestis,* the organism that causes plague, is now classed as *Yersinia pestis. P. tularensis,* the causative organism of tularemia, is now classed as *Francisella tularensis. P. pseudotuberculosis,* which can cause acute mesenteric lymphadenitis or enterocolitis, is now classed as *Yersinia pseudotuberculosis.*

***P. canis*** Previous name for *P. multocida.*

***P. multocida*** A small nonmotile gram-negative coccobacillus that can cause disease in animals and humans. The infection may be transmitted to humans by animal bites. In other cases the organism can cause cellulitis, abscesses, osteomyelitis, pneumonia, peritonitis, or meningitis. Penicillin is used to treat this infection; chlortetracycline or cephalosporin are also effective.

**pasteurellosis** (păs″tĕr-ĕ-lō′sĭs) A disease caused by infection with bacteria of the genus *Pasteurella.*

**pasteurization** (păs″tūr-ī-zā′shŭn) [Louis Pasteur] The process of heating a fluid at a moderate temperature for a definite period of time to destroy undesirable bacteria without changing to any extent the chemical composition. In pasteurization of milk, pathogenic bacteria are destroyed by heating at 62°C for 30 min, or by "flash" heating to higher temperatures for less than 1 min. The pasteurization process, reducing total bacterial count of the milk by 97% to 99%, is effective because the common milk-borne pathogens (tubercle bacillus, and *Salmonella, Streptococcus,* and *Brucella* organisms) do not form spores and are quite sensitive to heat. However, pasteurization should not be considered a substitute for hygienic practices in milk production. SEE: *milk.*

**pastille** (păs-tēl′, -tĭl′) [L. *pastillus,* a little roll] **1.** A medicated disk used for local action on the mucosa of the throat and mouth. SYN: *lozenge; troche.* **2.** A small cone used to fumigate or scent the air of a room.

**past-pointing** The inability to place a finger or some other part of the body accurately on a selected point; seen in certain neurological disorders.

**PAT** *paroxysmal atrial tachycardia.*

**patagia** (pă-tā′jē-ă) [L.] Pl. of patagium.

**patagium** (pă-tā′jē-ŭm) *pl.* **patagia** [L.] A weblike membrane. SEE: *pterygium.*

**patch** (păch) [ME. *pacche*] A small circumscribed area distinct from the surrounding surface in character and appearance.

***cotton-wool p.*** The appearance of exudative areas in the retina; usually seen in connection with hypertensive retinopathy.

***herald p.*** A solitary oval patch of efflorescence showing before the general eruption of pityriasis rosea, often several days before.

***Hutchinson's p.*** SEE: *Hutchinson's patch.*

***mucous p.*** A syphilitic eruption having an eroded, moist surface; usually on the mucous membrane of the mouth or external genitals, or on a surface subject to moisture and heat.

***nicotine p.*** A patch containing nicotine. When the patch is applied to the skin the nicotine is absorbed. It is used to assist in overcoming addiction to the nicotine in tobacco products. SEE: *cancer, lung; cotinine; nicotine; nicotine chewing gum.*

***Peyer's p.*** SEE: *Peyer's patch.*

***salmon p.*** A salmon-colored area of the cornea seen in interstitial keratitis caused by syphilis.

***smoker's p.*** Leukoplakia of the oral mucosa.

***white p.*** A white, thickened area of oral mucosa that will not rub off and represents a benign hyperkeratosis. SEE: *leukoplakia.*

**patella** (pă-tĕl′ă) *pl.* **patellae** [L., a small pan] A lens-shaped sesamoid bone situated in front of the knee in the tendon of the quadriceps femoris muscle. SYN: *kneecap.* SEE: *osteochondritis dissecans.*

***p. alta*** A high-riding patella (high positioning of patella). When a person is standing, the patella rests in a more superior position than normal.

***p. baja*** A low-riding patella (low positioning of patella). When a person is standing, the patella rests in a more inferior position than normal.

***bipartite p.*** The developing patella that matures from two centers rather than one. This usually congenital condition causes no symptoms but may be mistaken for a fracture.

***floating p.*** A patella that rides up from the condyles owing to a large effusion in the knee.

***fracture of p.*** A break in the continuity

of the kneecap. Treatment consists of suturing the bone fragments. A plaster cast is applied from the toes to the groin, remaining on for 6 to 8 weeks. Following removal of the cast, gradual exercise may be started and weight placed on the leg for a few weeks, after which the patient may walk.

***rider's painful p.*** Tenderness and pain in the patella from horseback riding.

***squinting p.*** A disorder in which the patella appears to be pointing inward when the patient is standing; caused by excessive femoral anteversion.

**patellapexy** (pă-tĕl′ă-pĕk″sē) [L. *patella,* small pan, + Gr. *pexis,* fixation] Fixation of the patella to the lower end of the femur to stabilize the joint.

**patellar** (pă-tĕl′ăr) Concerning the patella.

**patellectomy** (păt″ĕ-lĕk′tō-mē) [″ + Gr. *ektome,* excision] Surgical removal of the patella.

**patelliform** (pă-tĕl′ĭ-form) [″ + *forma,* shape] Shaped like the patella.

**patellofemoral** (pă-tĕl″ō-fĕm′ō-răl) Concerning the patella and femur.

**patency** (pā′tĕn-sē) [L. *patens,* open] The state of being freely open.

***p. of tear duct*** The open and functional state of a lacrimal duct. The patency of a tear duct can be tested by placing several drops of a weak solution of sugar in the eye. If the person detects a sweet taste in the mouth, then the duct is patent.

**patent** (păt′ĕnt, pā′tĕnt) Wide open; evident; accessible.

**patent ductus arteriosus** Persistence of a communication between the main pulmonary artery and the aorta, after birth. The condition of patent and persistent ductus arteriosus in preterm infants has been treated successfully by using drugs, such as indomethacin, that inhibit prostaglandin synthesis. SEE: *prostaglandins.*

**paternal** (pă-tĕr′năl) [L. *paternis,* fatherly] Of, pert. to, or inherited from the father.

**paternalism** A unilateral and sometimes unreasonable decision by health care providers that implies they know what is best, regardless of the patient's wishes.

**paternity test** A test to determine the father of a child. Because paternity is a clinical estimate, there is the need to have tests to determine whether it would be possible for an individual to have fathered a specific child. At one time, the tests used to prove or exclude the possibility of paternity used blood type data from the child and the suspected father. Tests involving the technique of molecular genetic fingerprinting and of determining genetic markers are available and have the ability to exclude almost all except the father. Use of these techniques makes it possible to distinguish differences between the genotype of all individuals except identical twins.

**path** A particular course that is followed or traversed. SEE: *pathway.*

***p. of closure*** The path traversed by the mandible as it closes when its neuromuscular mechanisms are in a balanced functional state.

***condyle p.*** The path traversed by the condyle during various mandibular movements.

***incisor p.*** An arc described by the incisal edge of the lower incisors when the mandible closes to normal occlusion.

**path-** SEE: *patho-.*

**pathetic** (pă-thĕt′ĭk) [L. *patheticus*] **1.** Pert. to, or arousing, the emotions of pity, sympathy, or tenderness. **2.** Pert. to the trochlear nerve.

**pathfinder** [AS. *paeth,* road, + *findan,* to locate] **1.** An instrument for locating stricture of the urethra. **2.** A dental instrument for tracing the course of root canals.

**patho-, path-** [Gr. *pathos,* disease, suffering] Combining form meaning *disease.* SEE: *-pathy.*

**pathoanatomy** (păth″ō-ă-năt′ō-mē) Anatomic pathology.

**pathobiology** (păth″ō-bī-ŏl′ō-jē) Pathology.

**pathodontia** (păth″ō-dŏn′shē-ă) [″ + *odous* tooth] The science of dental pathology.

**pathogen** (păth′ō-jĕn) [″+ *gennan,* to produce] A microorganism or substance capable of producing a disease.

***bloodborne p.*** A pathogen present in blood that can be transmitted to an individual who is exposed to the blood or body fluids of an infected individual. The most significant bloodborne pathogens are hepatitis B and human immunodeficiency virus 1 (HIV-1). SEE: *hepatitis B; human immunodeficiency virus; Universal Precautions Appendix.*

***opportunistic p.*** SEE: *opportunistic infections.*

**pathogenesis** (păth″ō-jĕn′ĕ-sĭs) The origin and development of a disease. SYN: *pathogeny.*

***bacterial p.*** The development of a bacterial disease. There are three stages: entry and colonization in the host, bacterial invasion and growth with the production of toxic substances, and the response of the host. The mere presence of an organism in the body does not necessarily mean that disease will follow. This progression of the infection will depend upon a number of interacting factors, including the virulence and number of invading organisms and the ability of the host to respond.

**pathogenetic, pathogenic** (păth″ō-jĕn-ĕt′ĭk, -jĕn′ĭk) Productive of disease. SYN: *morbific.*

**pathogenicity** (păth″ō-jĕ-nĭs′ĭ-tē) [″ + *gennan,* to produce] The state of producing or being able to produce pathological changes and disease.

**pathogeny** (păth-ŏj′ĕn-ē) Pathogenesis.

**pathognomonic** (păth″ŏg-nō-mŏn′ĭk) [Gr. *pathognomonikos,* skilled in diagnosing] Indicative of a disease, esp. its characteristic symptoms.

**pathognomy** (păth-ŏg′nō-mē) [Gr. *pathos,* disease, suffering, + *gnome,* a means of knowing] Diagnosing the cause of an illness after careful study of the signs and symptoms of a disease.

**pathologic, pathological** (păth-ō-lŏj′ĭk, -ĭ-kăl) [Gr. *pathos,* disease, suffering, + *logos,* word, reason] **1.** Concerning pathology. **2.** Diseased; due to a disease. SYN: *morbid.*

**pathologist** (pă-thŏl′ō-jĭst) [″ + *logos,* word, reason] A specialist in diagnosing the abnormal changes in tissues removed at operations and postmortem examinations.

**pathology** (pă-thŏl′ō-jē) [Gr. *pathos,* disease, suffering, + *logos,* word, reason] **1.** The study of the nature and cause of disease, which involves changes in structure and function. **2.** A condition produced by disease.

***anatomic p.*** The field of pathology that deals with structural changes in disease.

***cellular p.*** Pathology based on microscopic changes in body cells produced by disease.

***chemical p.*** The study of chemical changes that occur in disease.

***clinical p.*** Pathology that uses clinical analysis and other laboratory procedures in the diagnosis and treatment of disease.

***comparative p.*** The observation of pathological condition, spontaneous or artificial, in the lower animals or in vegetable organisms as compared with those of the human body.

***dental p.*** The science of diseases of the mouth. SYN: *oral p.*

***experimental p.*** The study of diseases induced artificially and intentionally, esp. in animals.

***functional p.*** The study of alterations of functions that occur in disease processes without associated structural changes.

***geographical p.*** Pathology in its relationship to climate and geography.

***humoral p.*** Pathology of the fluids of the body.

***medical p.*** Pathology of disorders that are not accessible for surgical procedures.

***molecular p.*** The study of the pathological effects of specific molecules.

***oral p.*** Dental p.

***special p.*** Pathology of particular diseases or organs.

***surgical p.*** The application of pathological procedures and techniques for investigating tissues removed surgically.

**pathomimesis** (păth″ō-mĭm-ē′sĭs) [Gr. *pathos,* disease, suffering, + *mimesis,* imitation] Intentional (conscious or unconscious) imitation of a disease. SYN: *pathomimicry.*

**pathomimicry** (păth″ō-mĭm′ĭ-krē) Pathomimesis.

**pathophobia** (păth-ō-fō′bē-ă) [″ + *phobos,* fear] Morbid fear of disease.

**pathophysiology** (păth″ō-fĭz″ē-ŏl′ō-jē) [″ + *physis,* nature, + *logos,* word, reason] The study of how normal physiological processes are altered by disease.

**pathopsychology** (păth″ō-sī-kŏl′ō-jē) [″ + *psyche,* soul, + *logos,* word, reason] The branch of psychology dealing with mental processes during disease.

**pathway 1.** A path or a course; more specifically, a pathway formed by neurons (cell bodies and their processes) over which impulses pass from their point of origin to their destination. **2.** A chemical or metabolic pathway; the various chemical reactions that occur in metabolism as specific substances are absorbed, metabolized, and altered as they undergo biotransformation in the body.

***afferent p.*** The pathway leading from a receptor to the spinal cord, the brain, or both.

***biosynthetic p.*** The chemical and metabolic events that lead to the formation of substances in the body.

***central p.*** A pathway within the brain or spinal cord.

***clinical p.*** A guide that outlines the optimum sequencing for interdisciplinary patient care to ensure consistency and continuity. Clinical pathways are typically developed for patients with high-risk, high-cost, high-volume, problem-prone medical diagnoses, procedures, or symptoms. They are valuable communication tools in case management. Also called *critical pathway, care map, anticipated recovery path, plan of care.*

***complement alternative p.*** A complement cascade initiated by a foreign protein, usually a bacterium. SEE: *complement.*

***complement classic p.*** A first complement cascade initiated by an antibody-antigen reaction that activates complement factor 1 (C1). SEE: *complement.*

***conduction p.*** A group of fibers in a nerve, spinal cord, or brain over which impulses are conducted.

***critical p.*** Clinical p.

***efferent p.*** A pathway from the central nervous system to an effector.

***Embden-Myerhof p.*** The anaerobic series of enzymatic reactions involved in glucose metabolism to form pyruvic acid or lactic acid, and to produce adenosine triphosphate, which releases energy for muscular and other cellular activity.

***metabolic p.*** The sequence of chemical reactions that occur as a substance is metabolized.

***motor p.*** A pathway over which motor impulses are conveyed via nerves from a motor center to muscles.

***p. of incidence*** The path of a penetrating foreign object from the point of entry into the body to the point where it stops (e.g., the path of a bullet from where it enters the body to where it lodges).

***pentose phosphate p.*** The pathway of glucose metabolism in tissues during which five-carbon sugars are formed.

***sensory p.*** A pathway over which sensory impulses are conveyed from sense organs or receptors to sensory or reflex centers of the spinal cord or brain.

**-pathy** Combining form indicating *disease.*

**patient** (pā′shĕnt) [L. *patiens*] **1.** One who is sick with, or being treated for, an illness or injury. **2.** An individual receiving medical care, including those with no demonstrable illness who are being investigated for signs of insidious pathology such as altered blood chemical values or physical changes such as asymptomatic cardiovascular abnormalities.

***p. advocate*** A person who ensures that a patient is served adequately by the health care system.

***p. autonomy*** The right of an informed patient to choose to accept or to refuse therapy. SEE: *advance directive; informed consent; living will; quality of life.*

***p. day*** The basic time unit for calculating the cost of keeping a patient in a hospital for one day.

***p. delay*** Delay on the part of the patient in seeking medical attention or in taking prescribed medicines or advice.

***p. mix*** The numbers and types of patients served by a hospital or other health program.

***surrogate p.*** A normal, healthy individual who is employed to be examined and perhaps interviewed by health-care students. The purpose is to provide students with the opportunity to examine an individual in a less stressful setting than would be the case if the person being examined were indeed sick. This also prevents persons who are ill from being subjected to multiple examinations by students. In some cases, the surrogate patient is an actor who has been instructed to pretend to be sick, injured, disabled, or hostile.

**Patient Advise and Consent Encounter** ABBR: PACE. An interactive computer program to assist a patient to understand certain medical and surgical procedures and their risks. The program uses touchscreen technology, animation, and an actor-doctor narrator to communicate with the patient. At the end of each program, the patient may take an interactive quiz that evaluates understanding of the presentation. A printout of the entire session is available for the patient and the physician.

**patient outcomes research team** ABBR: PORT. Those involved in investigating the outcome of disease interventions and comparing the benefit or lack of benefit of various therapeutic measures.

**Patient's Bill of Rights** A declaration of the entitlements of hospital patients, compiled by the American Hospital Association. First published in 1973 and revised in 1992, it emphasizes the responsibilities of hospitals and patients and the need for communication and collaboration between them. The patient is entitled to consideration and respect while receiving care; accurate, understandable information about the condition and treatment; privacy and confidentiality; an appropriate response to the request for treatment; and continued care as necessary after leaving the hospital. The patient may also have an advance directive regarding treatment; designate a surrogate to make decisions; review his or her medical records; be informed of hospital policies or business relationships that may affect care; and agree or refuse to participate in research studies. Patient responsibilities include providing any information (e.g., an advance directive) that may influence treatment; providing the needed information for insurance claims; and understanding how lifestyle affects health. The full text of the Patient's Bill of Rights is available from the American Hospital Association, One North Franklin, Chicago, IL 60606. SEE: *ombudsman.*

**Patient Self-Determination Act** ABBR: PSDA. A 1991 act of the U.S. Congress that preserves individual rights to decisions related to personal survival. There are several methods for preserving autonomy: filing appropriate forms for durable power of attorney for health care, making a living will, or giving a directive to the physician.

**patricide** (păt′rĭ-sīd) [L. *patricida*] The murdering of one's own parent or a close relative.

**Patrick's test** (păt′rĭks) [Hugh Talbot Patrick, U.S. neurologist, 1860–1939] A test for arthritis of the hip. The thigh and knee of the supine patient are flexed, and the external malleolus of the ankle is placed over the patella of the opposite leg. The test result is positive if depression of the knee produces pain.

**patrilineal** (păt-rē-lĭn′ē-ăl) [L. *pater,* father, + *linea,* line] Tracing descent through the father.

**patten** (păt′ĕn) [Fr. *patin,* wooden shoe] A support applied under one shoe as part of the treatment for hip disease or unequal length of the legs. The device may be attached to a leg caliper.

**pattern 1.** A design, figure, model, or example. **2.** In psychology, a set or arrangement of ideas or behavior reactions.

***capsular p.*** In a joint, the proportional loss or limitation of passive range of motion that suggests arthritis in that joint (e.g., the capsular pattern of the glenohumeral joint, in order of most restriction, is lateral rotation, abduction, and medial rotation).

***cephalocaudal p. of development*** The principle of maturation that states motor development, control, and coordination progress from the head to the feet.

***functional health p.*** Collective features of an individual's health history used to assess, plan, diagnose, intervene, and evaluate appropriate nursing care. The term is associated with Margery Gordon. SEE: *Nursing Diagnoses Appendix.*

***occlusal p.*** The appearance and anatomical location of the occluding surfaces of teeth.

***sinusoidal p.*** An abnormal fetal heart rate finding in which the monitor records a consistent rhythmic, uniform, undulating wave. Although the number of beats per minute is within normal limits and the recording shows long-term variability, beat-to-beat variability is absent and no accelerations in heart rate occur with fetal movement.

***synergy p.*** Primitive movements that dominate reflex and voluntary effort when spasticity is present following a cerebrovascular accident. They interfere with coordinated volitional movement such as eating, dressing, walking, and isolated movement. *Flexion synergy patterns* include scapular retraction, shoulder abduction and external rotation, elbow flexion, forearm supination, and wrist and finger flexion in the upper extremity; and hip flexion, abduction and external rotation, knee flexion, and ankle dorsiflexion in the lower extremity. *Extension synergy patterns* include scapular protraction, shoulder adduction and internal rotation, elbow extension, forearm pronation, and wrist and finger flexion in the upper extremity; and hip extension, adduction and internal rotation, knee extension, ankle plantar flexion and inversion, and toe flexion in the lower extremity.

***trabecular p.*** The arrangement of the trabeculae of bone in relation to marrow spaces.

***wax p.*** A molded or carved pattern in wax used extensively in dentistry and jewelry-making whereby casts are made using the lost wax technique.

***wear p.*** The location of tooth wear as determined by the wear characteristics of the facets of the teeth.

**patterning** A therapeutic method used in treating children and adults with brain damage. The patient is guided through movements such as creeping or crawling, based on the theory that undamaged sections of the brain will develop the ability to perform these functions.

**patulous** (păt′ū-lŭs) [L. *patulus*] Patent.

**pauciarticular** A classification of juvenile rheumatoid arthritis that indicates that four or fewer joints are affected at the time of onset of the disease.

**Paul-Bunnell test** [John R. Paul, U.S. physician, 1893–1971; Walls W. Bunnell, U.S. physician, b. 1902] A test for heterophil antibodies in the serum of patients thought to have infectious mononucleosis.

**pause** [ME.] An interruption; a temporary cessation of activity.

***compensatory p.*** The long interval following an extrasystole, so called because its duration is such that the next beat occurs at the exact time of the succeeding normal beat.

**pavementing** A condition occurring during inflammation in which leukocytes adhere to the linings of capillaries.

**Pavlik harness** A device used to stabilize the hip in neonates with congenital hip dislocation.

**Pavlov, Ivan Petrovich** (păv′lŏv) Russian physiologist, 1849–1936; winner of Nobel prize in medicine in 1904. He is remembered particularly for his work on conditioned response. SEE: *reflex, conditioned.*

**pavor** (pā′vor) [L.] Anxiety, dread.

***p. diurnus*** Attacks of terror or fright during the day, esp. in children.

***p. nocturnus*** Night terror during sleep in children and the aged.

**PAWP** *pulmonary artery wedge pressure.*

**P.B.** *Pharmacopoeia Britannica,* British pharmacopeia.

**Pb** [L. *plumbum*] Symbol for the element lead.

**PBI** *protein-bound iodine.*

**P.B.W.** *posterior bitewing* in dentistry.

**PBZ** *pyribenzamine.*

**p.c.** L. *post cibum,* after a meal.

**PCG** *phonocardiogram.*

**pCi** *picocurie.*

**$pCO_2$** Symbol for *partial pressure of carbon dioxide.*

**PCP** *Pneumocystis carinii pneumonia.*

**PCR** *polymerase chain reaction.*

**PCV** *packed cell volume.*

**PCWP** *pulmonary capillary wedge pressure.*

**Pd** Symbol for the element palladium.

**p.d.** *prism diopter; pupilla diameter; pupillary distance.*

**PDA** *patent ductus arteriosus.*

**PDR** *Physicians' Desk Reference.*

**pearl** [ME. *perle*] **1.** A small, tough mass in the sputum in asthma. **2.** A small capsule containing a medicinal fluid for inhalation. The capsule is crushed in a handkerchief and inhaled. **3.** A small mass of cells.

***enamel p.'s*** Small rounded globules of highly mineralized material seen near or attached to the enamel margin or furcation of the tooth roots. These are formed by aberrant ameloblasts and hypermineralization.

***epithelial p.*** Concentric squamous epithelial cells in carcinoma.

***gouty p.*** Sodium urate concretion on the cartilage of the ear seen in people with gout.

**peau d'orange** (pō″dō-rănj′) [Fr., orange skin] A dimpled skin condition that resembles an orange; seen in lymphatic edema and possibly over an area of carcinoma of the breast.

**peccant** (pĕk′ănt) [L. *peccans,* sinning] **1.** Corrupt; producing disease. **2.** Sinning, or violating a law. SYN: *morbid; pathogenic.*

**peccatiphobia** (pĕk″ăt-ĭ-fō′bē-ă) [″ + Gr. *phobos,* fear] Abnormal fear of sinning.

**pecilo-** SEE: words beginning with *poikilo-*.

**pecten** (pĕk′tĕn) *pl.* **pectines** [L., comb] **1.** A comblike organ. **2.** The pubic bone. **3.** The middle portion of the anal canal.

***p. ossis pubis*** A sharp ridge on the superior ramus of the pubis that forms the pubic portion of the terminal (iliopectineal) line.

**pectic acid** (pĕk′tĭk) [Gr. *pektos,* congealed] An acid derived from pectin by hydrolyzing the methyl ester group and found in many fruits.

**pectin** (pĕk′tĭn) [Gr. *pektos,* congealed] A purified carbohydrate obtained from peel of citrus fruits, or from apple pulp. When pectin is cooked with sugar at the proper pH, a gel forms. SEE: *pectose.*

**pectinase** (pĕk′tĭ-nās) An enzyme that catalyzes the formation of sugars and galacturonic acid from pectin.

**pectinate** (pĕk′tĭ-nāt) [L. *pecten,* comb] Having teeth like a comb. SYN: *pectiniform.*

**pectineal** (pĕk-tĭn′ē-ăl) Relating to the os pubis or the pectineal muscle.

**pectineus** (pĕk-tĭn-ē′ŭs) [L. *pecten,* comb] A flat quadrangular muscle at the upper and inner part of the thigh, arising from the superior ramus of pubis and inserted between the lesser trochanter and linea aspera of the femur, which flexes and adducts the thigh. SEE: *Muscles Appendix.*

**pectiniform** (pĕk-tĭn′ĭ-form) [″ + *forma,* shape] Pectinate.

**pectization** (pĕk-tī-zā′shŭn) [Gr. *pektos,* congealed] In colloidal chemistry, the conversion of a substance from sol to gel state.

**pectora** (pĕk′tor-ă) [L.] Pl. of pectus.

**pectoral** (pĕk′tō-răl) [L. *pectoralis*] **1.** Concerning the chest. **2.** Efficacious in relieving chest conditions, as a cough.

**pectoralgia** (pĕk″tō-răl′jē-ă) [L. *pectoralis,* chest, + Gr. *algos,* pain] Neuralgic pain in the chest.

**pectoralis** (pĕk″tō-rā′lĭs) [L.] **1.** Pert. to the breast or chest. **2.** One of the four muscles of the anterior upper portion of the chest.

***p. major*** A large triangular muscle that extends from the sternum to the humerus and functions to flex, horizontally adduct, and internally rotate the arm, and aids in chest expansion when the upper extremities are stabilized.

***p. minor*** A muscle beneath the pectoralis major, attached to the coracoid process of the scapula that depresses as well as causes anterior tipping of the scapula.

**pectoriloquy** (pĕk″tō-rĭl′ō-kwē) [L. *pectoralis,* chest, + *loqui,* to speak] The distinct transmission of vocal sounds to the ear through the chest wall in auscultation. The words seem to emanate from the spot that is auscultated. This is heard over cavities that communicate with a bronchus and areas of consolidation near a large bronchus, over pneumothorax when the opening in the lung is patulous, and over some pleural effusions. SYN: *pectorophony.* SEE: *chest.*

***aphonic p.*** In auscultation, a whispered sound heard over a lung with a cavity or pleural effusion.

***whispering p.*** A sound heard in auscultation of the chest over a lung with a cavity of limited extent when the patient whispers.

**pectorophony** (pĕk″tō-rŏf′ō-nē) [″ + Gr. *phone,* voice] Pectoriloquy.

**pectose** (pĕk′tōs) [Gr. *pektos,* congealed] A substance found in some fruits and vegetables. It yields pectin when boiled.

**pectunculus** (pĕk-tŭn′kū-lŭs) [L., little comb] One of the tiny longitudinal ridges on the sylvian aqueduct of the brain.

**pectus** (pĕk′tŭs) *pl.* **pectora** [L.] The chest, breast, or thorax.

***p. carinatum*** Pigeon breast.

***p. excavatum*** A congenital condition in which the sternum is abnormally depressed. SYN: *funnel breast; p. recurvatum.*

***p. recurvatum*** P. excavatum.

**ped-** SEE: *pedo-.*

**pedal** (pĕd′l) [L. *pedalis*] Concerning the foot.

**pedal spasm** Involuntary contractions of the muscles of the feet.

**pedarthrocace** (pē″dăr-thrŏk′ă-sē) [Gr. *paidos,* child, + *arthron,* joint, + *kakos,* bad] A carious condition of the joints of children.

**pedatrophy** (pē-dăt′rō-fē) [Gr. *pais,* child, + *atrophia,* want of nourishment] **1.** Marasmus. **2.** Any wasting disease in children. **3.** Tabes mesenterica.

**pederast** (pĕd′ĕr-ăst) [Gr. *paiderastes,* a lover of boys] A man who indulges in anal intercourse with young boys.

**pederasty** (pĕd′ĕr-ăs″tē) Anal intercourse between a man and a young boy.

**pedesis** (pē-dē′sĭs) [Gr., leaping] Brownian movement.

**pedi-** SEE: *pedo-.*

**pedia-** [Gr. *pais,* child] Combining form denoting *child.*

**pedialgia** (pĕd-ē-ăl′jē-ă, pē-dē-) [Gr. *pedion,* foot, + *algos,* pain] Pain of the foot.

**Pediamycin** Trade name for erythromycin ethylsuccinate.

**pediatric** (pē-dē-ăt′rĭk) [Gr. *pais,* child, + *iatreia,* treatment] Concerning the treatment of children.

**pediatric advanced life support** ABBR: PALS. The treatment measures, including basic and advanced life support, needed to stabilize a critically ill or injured child.

**pediatrician** (pē-dē-ă-trĭsh′ăn) [″ + *iatrikos,* healing] A specialist in the treatment of children's diseases.

**Pediatric Nurse Practitioner** ABBR: P.N.P. A registered nurse who provides primary health care to children (e.g., Jane Grey, R.N., P.N.P). Special preparation is required.

**pediatrics** (pē-dē-ăt′rĭks) [Gr. *pais,* child, + *iatreia,* treatment] The medical science relating to the care of children and treatment of their diseases.

**pediatric trauma score** ABBR: PTS. A method for scoring and quantifying the severity of trauma in pediatric patients. SYN: *revised trauma score.*

**pedicel** (pĕd'ĭ-sĕl) **1.** Foot process or footplate. **2.** A secondary process of a podocyte that in conjunction with other podocytes forms the inner layer of Bowman's capsule of a renal corpuscle.

**pedicellation** (pĕd"ĭ-sĕl-ā'shŭn) [L. *pediculus,* a little foot; stalk] The formation and development of a pedicle.

**pedicle** (pĕd'ĭ-k'l) **1.** The stem that attaches a new growth. SYN: *peduncle* (1). **2.** The bony process that projects backward from the body of a vertebra, connecting with the lamina on each side. It forms the root of the vertebral arch.

**pedicle flap** In plastic surgery, a type of flap that is attached by a pedicle to its source of blood supply. The other end may be attached to a site from which a new blood supply will develop. This permits the eventual severance of the original pedicle, so the flap may be moved step by step to where it is needed in the plastic surgical procedure.

**pedicterus** (pē-dĭk'tĕr-ŭs) [Gr. *pais,* child, + *ikteros,* jaundice] Icterus neonatorum.

**pedicular** (pē-dĭk'ū-lar) **1.** [L. *pediculus,* a louse] Infested with or concerning lice. **2.** [L. *pediculus,* a little foot] Concerning a stalk or stem.

**pediculate** (pē-dĭk'ū-lāt) [L. *pediculus,* a little foot] Pedunculate.

**pediculation** (pē-dĭk"ū-lā'shŭn) [L. *pediculatio*] **1.** Infestation with lice. **2.** Development of a pedicle.

**pediculicide** (pē-dĭk'ū-lĭ-sīd) [L. *pediculus,* a louse, + *caedere,* to kill] Destroying, or that which destroys, lice.

**Pediculidae** A family of lice belonging to the order Anoplura. It includes the species parasitic on primates including humans. SEE: *Pediculus.*

**pediculophobia** (pē-dĭk"ū-lō-fō'bē-ă) [" + Gr. *phobein,* to fear] Abnormal dread of lice.

**pediculosis** (pē-dĭk"ū-lō'sĭs) [" + Gr. *osis,* condition] Lousiness; infestation with lice. SEE: *Pediculus.*

NURSING IMPLICATIONS: The patient and family are taught how to apply medication to dry hair for lice and are warned that the eyes should be immediately flushed with copious amounts of water if the medication accidentally contacts them. The nurse informs the patient and family members about minimizing the spread of infection by washing or dry cleaning all clothing and linen used in the home, keeping combs and brushes separate, and using the medicinal shampoo if there has been contact with the patient.

***p. capitis*** Pediculosis due to infestation with the head louse, *Pediculus humanus capitis.* Transmission is by personal contact or common use of brushes, combs, or headgear. SEE: illus.

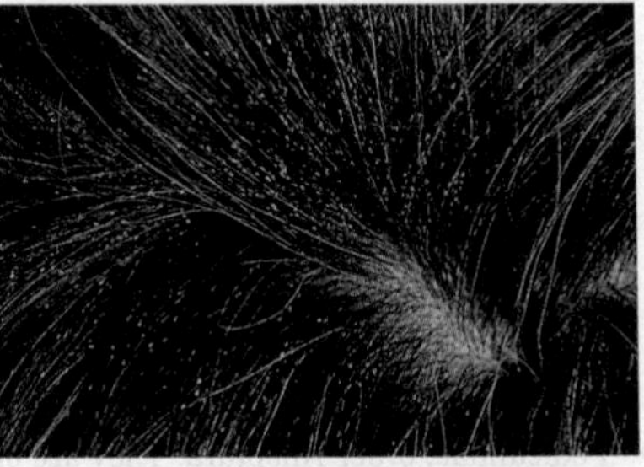

PEDICULOSIS CAPITIS

SYMPTOMS: Itching and eczematous dermatitis. In long-standing, neglected cases, scratching may result in marked inflammation. Secondary infection by bacteria may occur, with formation of pustules, crusts, and suppuration. Hair may become matted and malodorous.

TREATMENT: The individual should shampoo the hair, dry it, and apply 1% permethrin cream, 25 to 50 ml or enough to wet the hair and scalp. This is left on the head for 10 min, and rinsed off with clear water. Alternatively, 1% gamma benzene hexachloride may be applied to the scalp or affected areas once each day for 2 days. This is repeated in 10 days to destroy nits that may have survived. All possible sources of infection should be examined and treated if necessary. Headgear, combs, and brushes should be disinfected by solutions or heat. If lice have infested the eyelashes and eyelids, the lice will have to be removed with forceps.

***p. corporis*** Pediculosis due to infestation with body louse, *Pediculus humanus corporis.* It is transmitted by direct contact or use of infested wearing apparel and occurs as a result of crowding or unhygienic conditions.

SYMPTOMS: Intense itching characterizes this condition. In heavy infestations there is generalized red skin eruption, mild fever, tiredness, irritability, and in severe cases, weakness and debility.

TREATMENT: Treatment is as for pediculosis capitis. In addition, clothing and bedding should be sterilized by dry heat (140°F or 60°C for 5 min), by hot water (150°F or 65.6°C for 5 min), or by dry cleaning.

***p. palpebrarum*** Infestation by lice of the eyebrows and eyelashes.

***p. pubis*** Pediculosis caused by infestation with the crab louse, *Phthirus pubis.* It is generally confined to hairs of the genital region but hair of the axilla, eyebrows, eyelashes, beard, and, in hairy individuals, body surface may be involved. Lice may be acquired through personal contact, by wearing contaminated clothing, from toilet seats, or from bed clothes. SEE: *p. capitis* for treatment.

SYMPTOMS: This condition is characterized by itching and irritation of the external genital area (not introital), esp. the mons. The pubic louse bite produces in light-skinned individuals blue- or slate-colored macules that do not blanch when pressure is applied.

**pediculous** (pĕ-dĭk′ū-lŭs) Infested with lice.

**Pediculus** (pē-dĭk′ū-lŭs) A genus of parasitic insects commonly called lice that infest humans and other primates. Lice are sucking insects belonging to the family Pediculidae, order Anoplura. They are of medical importance in that they are the vectors of the causative organisms of epidemic typhus, trench fever, and relapsing fever.

***P. humanus capitis*** The head louse that lives in the fine hair of the head, although the beard and eyebrows may also be infested. Its eggs, commonly called nits, are glued to hairs and frequently form nests in the vicinity of the ears. This organism is the cause of pediculosis capitis.

***P. humanus corporis*** The body louse that inhabits the seams of clothing worn next to the body and feeds on regions of the body covered by that clothing. Eggs are attached to fibers of the clothing. This organism is the cause of pediculosis corporis.

**pediculus** (pē-dĭk′ū-lŭs) *pl.* **pediculi** [L.] **1.** A little foot. **2.** Louse. SEE: *Pediculus.*

**pedicure** (pĕd′ĭ-kūr) [L. *pes,* foot, + *cura,* care] **1.** Care of the feet. **2.** Cosmetic care of the feet and toenails. **3.** A podiatrist.

**pediform** (pĕd′ĭ-form) [″ + *forma,* shape] Having the shape of a foot.

**pedigree** A chart, diagram, or table of an individual's ancestors used in human genetics in the analysis of mendelian inheritance.

**pedionalgia** (pē″dē-ō-năl′jē-ă) [Gr. *pedion,* metatarsus, + *algos,* pain] Neuralgic pain in the sole of the foot.

**pediophobia** (pē″dē-ō-fō′bē-ă) [Gr. *pais,* child, + *phobos,* fear] An unnatural dread of young children or of dolls.

**pediphalanx** (pĕd″ĭ-fā′lănks) [L. *pes,* foot, + Gr. *phalanx,* closely knit row] A phalanx of the foot. SEE: *maniphalanx.*

**pedo-, pedi-, ped-** [L. *pes,* foot] Combining form meaning *foot.*

**pedobaromacrometer** (pē″dō-băr″ō-mă-krŏm′ĕ-tĕr) [Gr. *pais,* child, + *baros,* weight, + *makros,* long, + *metron,* measure] An apparatus for determining the measurement and weight of infants.

**pedodontia, pedodontics** (pē″dō-dŏn′shē-ă, -tĭks) [Gr. *pais,* child, + *odous,* tooth] The phase of dentistry dealing with care of children's teeth.

**pedodontist** (pē″dō-dŏn′tĭst) A dentist who specializes in care of children's teeth.

**pedodynamometer** (pĕd″ō-dī-nă-mŏm′ĕ-tĕr) [L. *pes,* foot, + Gr. *dynamis,* power, + *metron,* measure] A device for measuring the strength of the leg muscles.

**pedograph** (pĕd′ō-grăf) [″ + Gr. *graphein,* to write] An imprint of the foot on paper.

**pedometer** **1.** (pē-dŏm′ĕ-tĕr) [Gr. *pais,* child, + *metron,* measure] A device for the measurement of infants. **2.** (pĕd-ŏm′ĕ-tĕr) [L. *pes,* foot, + Gr. *metron,* measurement] An instrument that indicates the number of steps taken while walking.

**pedomorphism** (pē″dō-mor′fĭzm) [Gr. *pais,* child, + *morphe,* form, + *-ismos,* condition] The retention of juvenile characteristics in the adult.

**pedophilia** (pē″dō-fĭl′ē-ă) [″ + *philein,* to love] **1.** Fondness for children. **2.** In psychology, an unnatural desire for sexual relations with children.

**peduncle** (pĕ-dŭn′kl) [L. *pedunculus,* a little foot] **1.** Pedicle (1). **2.** A brachium of the brain; a band connecting parts of the brain. SYN: *pedunculus.* SEE: *cimbia; crus; sessile.*

***cerebral p.*** A pair of white bundles from the upper part of the pons to the cerebrum. It constitutes the ventral portion of the midbrain. SYN: *crus cerebri.*

***p. of flocculus*** A band of fibers connecting the flocculus of the cerebellum with the vermis.

***inferior cerebellar p.*** A band of fibers running along the lateral border of the fourth ventricle, connecting the spinal cord and medulla with the cerebellum. SYN: *restiform body.*

***mamillary p.*** A band of fibers extending from the tegmentum of the midbrain to the mamillary body.

***middle cerebellar p.*** A band of fibers connecting the cerebellum with the basilar portion of the pons. SYN: *brachium pontis.*

***olfactory p.*** The long stalk of the olfactory bulb.

***pineal p.*** A band from either side of the pineal gland to the anterior pillars of the fornix.

***superior cerebellar p.*** A band of fibers connecting the cerebellum with the midbrain. SYN: *brachium conjunctivum.*

***p. of superior olive*** A slender band of fibers extending from the superior olivary nucleus in the medulla to the nucleus of the abducens nerve.

***thalamic p.*** One of four groups of fibers known as thalamic radiations that connect the thalamus with the cerebral cortex. SEE: *radiation, thalamic.*

**peduncular** (pĕ-dŭn′kū-lăr) [L. *pedunculus,* a little foot] Concerning a peduncle.

**pedunculate, pedunculated** (pĕ-dŭn′kū-lāt, -ĕd) Possessing a stalk or peduncle. SYN: *pediculate.*

**pedunculotomy** (pĕ-dŭng″kū-lŏt′ō-mē) [″ + Gr. *tome,* incision] Surgical section of a cerebral peduncle. This is done in treating involuntary movement disorders.

**peeling** [ME. *pelen,* to peel] Shedding of the surface layer of the skin. SYN: *desquamation.*

***chemical p.*** Chemicals applied to skin to produce a mild, superficial burn; done to remove wrinkles.

**PEEP** *positive end-expiratory pressure.*

**peer** (pēr) [ME.] One who has an equal standing with another in age, class, or rank.

***p. review*** The evaluation of the quality of the work effort of an individual by his or her peers. It could involve evaluation of articles submitted for publication or the quality of medical care administered by an individual, group, or hospital.

**PEG** *percutaneous endoscopic gastrostomy.*

**peg, rete** SEE: *rete ridge.*

**peg tooth** An abnormally shaped tooth of genetic origin. Usually noted as a maxillary lateral incisor with a smaller cone-shaped crown.

**PEJ** *percutaneous endoscopic jejunostomy.*

**pejorative** (pĭ-jor′ă-tĭv, pē″jă-rā′tĭv) [L. *pejor,* worse] **1.** Tending to become or make worse. **2.** Being disparaging or belittling (e.g., in making a less than flattering remark about something or someone). SEE: *honorific.*

**PEL** *permissible exposure limits.*

**pelade** (pĕl-ăd′) [Fr., to remove hair] Alopecia areata.

**pelage** (pĕl′ĭj) [Fr.] The collective hair of the body.

**Pel-Ebstein fever** [Pieter K. Pel, Dutch physician, 1852–1919; Wilhelm Ebstein, Ger. physician, 1836–1912] Cyclic fever occurring in Hodgkin's disease in which periods of fever lasting from 3 to 10 days are separated by an afebrile period of about the same length.

**Pelger-Huët anomaly** (pĕl″jĕr hū′ĕt) [Karel Pelger, Dutch physician, 1885–1931; Gauthier Jean Huët, Dutch physician, 1879–1970] Granulocytes of the blood with rodlike, dumbbell, peanut-shaped, and spectacle-like nuclei. The chromatin of the nuclei is unusually coarse. The condition is inherited as a non–sex-linked dominant. The cells function normally and carriers have no demonstrably lowered resistance to infection.

**pelioma** (pē-lē-ō′mă) [Gr.] Ecchymosis.

**peliosis** (pē-lē-ō′sĭs) [Gr.] Purpura.

***bacillary p.*** A complication of an infection due to *Bartonella henselae* and *B. quintana,* esp. in immunocompromised patients. The lesions are in the viscera, liver, and spleen, and cause nonspecific symptoms. The prognosis in immunocompromised patients who are not treated is gradual decline and death. If bacteremia is present, the treatment consists of oral doxycycline or erythromycin for 4 weeks. SEE: *Bartonella quintana.*

***p. hepatis*** Multiple, cystic, blood-filled spaces in the liver associated with dilatation of the sinusoids. These cause enlargement of and pain in the liver. These lesions are associated with use of oral contraceptives, certain types of anabolic steroids, and infections with *Bartonella* organisms. If the condition is due to infection, treatment consists of parenteral doxycycline for several weeks followed by several months of oral therapy. SEE: *angiomatosis, bacillary; cat scratch disease.*

**pellagra** (pĕl-ă′gră, pĕ-lăg′ră) [L. *pellis,* skin, + Gr. *agra,* rough] A deficiency disease or syndrome endemic in certain parts of the world, characterized by cutaneous, gastrointestinal, mucosal, neurological, and mental symptoms.

SYMPTOMS: In advanced cases, scarlet stomatitis and glossitis, diarrhea, dermatitis, and central nervous system involvement occur. Cutaneous lesions include erythema followed by vesiculation, crusting, and desquamation. The skin may become dry, scaly, and atrophic. The mucous membranes of the mouth, esophagus, and vagina may atrophy, and ulcers and cysts may develop. Anemia is common. Nausea, vomiting, and diarrhea occur, the last being characteristic. Involvement of the central nervous system is first manifested by neurasthenia, followed by organic psychosis characterized by disorientation, memory impairment, and confusion. Later, delirium and clouding of consciousness may occur.

ETIOLOGY: This condition is due to deficiency in the diet or failure of the body to absorb niacin (nicotinic acid) or its amide (niacinamide, nicotinamide). Usually it is associated with a deficiency of tryptophan-containing proteins, such as occurs in a high-corn diet. Pellagra may occur secondary to gastrointestinal diseases or alcoholism.

TREATMENT: The disease is treated by following a diet adequate in all vitamins, minerals, and amino acids supplemented by 500 to 1000 mg of niacinamide given orally three times daily. If there is any doubt about the ability of the intestinal tract to absorb vitamins, the vitamins should be given parenterally.

**pellagrazein** (pĕl-ă-grā′zē-ĭn) A poisonous substance in decomposed cornmeal. At one time it was regarded erroneously as the cause of pellagra.

**pellagrin** (pĕ-lā′grĭn, -lăg′rĭn) A person afflicted with pellagra.

**pellagroid** (pĕ-lāg′royd, -lăg′royd) [L. *pellis,* skin, + Gr. *agra,* rough, + *eidos,* form, shape] Resembling pellagra.

**Pellegrini's disease, Pellegrini-Stieda disease** (pĕl″ā-grē′nē-stē′dă) [Augusto Pellegrini, It. surgeon, b. 1877; Alfred Stieda, Ger. surgeon, 1869–1945] Following trauma, ossification of the superior portion of the medial collateral ligament of the knee.

**pellet** (pĕl′ĕt) [Fr. *pelote,* a ball] A tiny pill or small ball of medicine or food.

***cotton p.*** A small rolled cottonball, less than ⅜ in. (about 1 cm) in diameter, used for desiccation or topical application of medicaments, particularly in dentistry; also called pledgets.

***foil p.*** Loosely rolled gold foil used for

direct filling in dental restoration. SEE: *foil.*

**pellicle** (pĕl′ĭ-k'l) [L. *pellicula,* a little skin] **1.** A thin piece of cuticle or skin. **2.** Film or surface on a liquid. **3.** Scum.

***salivary p.*** The thin layer of salivary proteins and glycoproteins that quickly adhere to the tooth surface after the tooth has been cleaned; this amorphous, bacteria-free layer may serve as an attachment medium for bacteria, which in turn form plaque.

**pellucid** (pĕl-lū′sĭd) [L. *pellucidus*] Clear.

**pellucid zone** Zona pellucida.

**pelotherapy** (pĕ″lō-thĕr′ă-pē) [Gr. *pelos,* mud, + *therapeia,* treatment] The therapeutic use of mud, peat, moss, or clay applied to all or part of the body.

**pelvic** (pĕl′vĭk) [L. *pelvis,* basin] Pert. to a pelvis, usually the bony pelvis.

**pelvicephalography** (pĕl″vē-sĕf″ă-lŏg′ră-fē) [″ + Gr. *kephale,* head, + *graphein,* to write] Radiographical study and measurement of the fetal head and the maternal pelvic outlet.

**pelvicephalometry** (pĕl″vē-sĕf″ă-lŏm′ĕ-trē) [″ + ″ + *metron,* measure] Measurement of the diameters of the fetal head and comparison of these with the diameters of the maternal pelvis.

**pelvic inflammatory disease** ABBR: PID. Infection of the uterus, fallopian tubes, and adjacent pelvic structures that is not associated with surgery or pregnancy. It is usually an ascending infection in which pathogenic microorganisms spread from the vagina and cervix to the upper portions of the reproductive tract. Almost any bacterium may cause PID, but the most frequent agents are *Neisseria gonorrhoeae* and *Chlamydia trachomatis.* In most cases of PID, more than one organism is involved. SEE: *Nursing Diagnoses Appendix.*

SYMPTOMS: A mucopurulent vaginal discharge is present, caused by cervicitis. There may be associated dysuria caused by urethritis. Anorectal pain and bleeding due to proctitis are sometimes present. The abdominal pain may be in the midline or bilateral in the lower abdominal area. When salpingitis is present, the pain and tenderness are severe and usually accompanied by nausea and vomiting. Infertility due to tubal occlusion is the most troubling long-term complication.

DIAGNOSIS: Diagnosis of PID involves a history of previous PID or of sexual intercourse with a man with urethritis, abortion, childbirth, fever, and increased white blood cell count. Risk factors include multiple sexual partners and the use of an intrauterine device for contraception, esp. in the first few months after insertion. Cigarette smoking and vaginal douching may also be risk factors. There is severe pain during pelvic examination when the cervix or the adnexa are moved. Lower genital tract infection is evidenced by the preponderance of white blood cells in the vaginal fluid. Despite these signs and symptoms, it is difficult to establish a diagnosis from the clinical findings. Ultrasonographic, endometrial biopsy and laparoscopy are of considerable help in making the diagnosis of PID. Vaginal and cervical cultures may be helpful in identifying the causative organism. PID must be distinguished from ectopic pregnancy and other pelvic disease, esp. surgical emergencies such as acute appendicitis. All patients suspected of having PID should have a test for syphilis and should be offered a test for antibodies to HIV.

PREVENTION: Barrier methods of contraception and oral contraceptive agents protect against upper genital tract infections.

TREATMENT: Multiple antibiotics effective against gonococci, chlamydiae, facultative gram-negative rods, and anaerobes are usually used to treat PID. Early therapy with appropriate antibiotics is important if subsequent infertility with occlusion of the fallopian tubes by adhesions is to be prevented. Pelvic and tubal abscesses may need to be drained but may subside with conservative therapy. All sexual partners should be examined for evidence of sexually transmitted diseases and, if test results are positive, treated with an appropriate antibiotic. PID patients should be followed for several days after discontinuation of therapy to be certain that they are cured, as judged by culture of the cervix and vagina. SEE: *safe sex* for prevention.

NURSING IMPLICATIONS: Because this disease can result in infertility and cause damage to pelvic organs, the nurse should stay alert for signs and symptoms that might indicate this condition in a patient. Most organisms causing PID can be sexually transmitted, and therefore woman should seek treatment for any infection of the reproductive organs. After childbirth and surgery, strict asepsis should be maintained in women with this condition to minimize the risk of infections.

**pelvic pain, chronic idiopathic** ABBR: CIPP. Unexplained pelvic pain in a woman, that has lasted 6 months or longer. A complete medical, social, and sexual history must be obtained. In an experimental study, women with this illness reported more sexual partners, significantly more spontaneous abortions, and previous nongynecological surgery. These women were more likely to have experienced previous significant psychosexual trauma.

TREATMENT: It is important to stop clinical investigations when it is clear that there are no positive findings including those from laparoscopy. If pain continues or becomes worse and there is no explanation for its cause, treatment is symptomatic. Medroxyprogesterone acetate, oral contraceptives, presacral neurectomy, hypnosis, and hysterectomy have been tried with varying degrees of success.

**pelvic rock** An exercise to strengthen the abdominal muscles and reduce the risk of backache during pregnancy. The woman kneels on her hands and knees, hollows her back and pushes out her abdomen while inhaling, and arches her back like a cat and contracts the abdominal, gluteal, and levator muscles while exhaling. The exercise can be done while standing with the hands on the knees. The effects are maximized by concurrent abdominal breathing. SEE: *pelvic tilt.*

**pelvic tilt** An exercise to strengthen the abdominal muscles and reduce the risk of backache during pregnancy. The woman assumes a supine position and flattens the hollow of her back against the floor. The abdominal, gluteal, and levator muscles are contracted with each exhalation and relaxed with each inhalation. The effects are maximized by concurrent abdominal breathing. SEE: *pelvic rock.*

**pelvilithotomy** (pĕl″vĭ-lĭ-thŏt′ō-mē) [″ + Gr. *lithos,* stone, + *tome,* incision] Pyelolithotomy.

**pelvimeter** (pĕl-vĭm′ĕ-tĕr) [″ + Gr. *metron,* measure] A device for measuring the pelvis.

**pelvimetry** (pĕl-vĭm′ĕ-trē) Measurement of the pelvic dimensions or proportions, which helps determine whether or not it will be possible to deliver a fetus through the normal route. This is done by various methods including manual or x-ray. SEE: *pelvis.*

**pelviolithotomy** (pĕl″vē-ō-lĭ-thŏt′ō-mē) [L. *pelvis,* basin, + Gr. *lithos,* stone, + *tome,* incision] Pyelolithotomy.

**pelvioplasty** (pĕl′vē-ō-plăs″tē) [″ + Gr. *plassein,* to form] **1.** Enlargement of the pelvic outlet to facilitate childbirth. SYN: *pelviotomy* (1); *pubiotomy; symphysiotomy.* **2.** Plastic surgical procedure on the pelvis of the kidney.

**pelvioscopy** (pĕl″vē-ŏs′kō-pē) [L. *pelvis,* basin, + Gr. *skopein,* to examine] Inspection of the pelvis.

**pelviotomy** (pĕl-vē-ŏt′ō-mē) [″ + Gr. *tome,* incision] **1.** Enlargement of the pelvic outlet to facilitate childbirth. **2.** Incision of the renal pelvis; usually done in order to remove a calculus.

**pelviperitonitis** (pĕl″vĭ-pĕr-ĭ-tō-nī′tĭs) [″ + Gr. *peritonaion,* peritoneum, + *itis,* inflammation] Inflammation of the peritoneum lining the pelvic cavity.

**pelvirectal** (pĕl″vē-rĕk′tăl) [″ + *rectum,* straight] Concerning the pelvis and rectum.

**pelvis** (pĕl′vĭs) *pl.* **pelves** [L., basin] **1.** Any basin-shaped structure or cavity. **2.** The bony structure formed by the innominate bones, the sacrum, the coccyx, and the ligaments uniting them. The structure serves as a support for the vertebral column and for articulation with the lower limbs. SEE: illus. **3.** The cavity included within the innominate bones, the sacrum, and the coccyx.

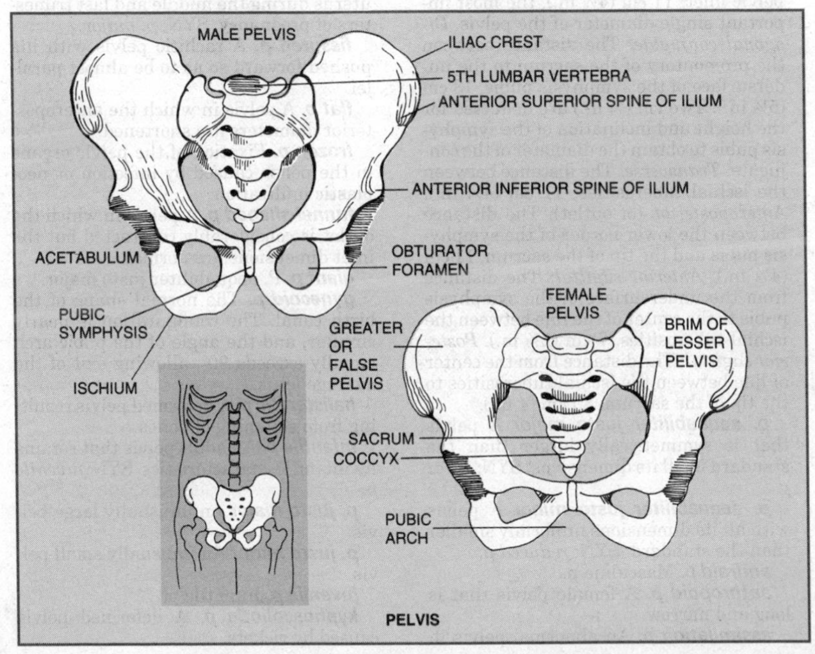

PELVIS

ANATOMY: The pelvis is separated into a false or superior pelvis and a true or inferior pelvis by the iliopectineal line and the upper margin of the symphysis pubis. The circumference of this area constitutes the inlet of the true pelvis. The lower border of the true pelvis, termed the outlet, is formed by the coccyx, the protuberances of the ischia, the ascending rami of the ischia, and the descending rami of the ossa pubis and the sacrosciatic ligaments. The floor of the pelvis is formed by the perineal fascia, the levator ani, and the coccygeus muscles. All diameters normally are larger in the female than in the male.

EXTERNAL DIAMETERS: *Interspinous:* The distance between the outer edges of the anterosuperior iliac spines, the diameter normally measuring 26 cm (10¼ in.). *Intercristal:* The distance between the outer edges of the most prominent portion of the iliac crests, the diameter normally being 28 cm (11 in.). *Intertrochanteric:* The distance between the most prominent points of the femoral trochanters, 32 cm (12½ in.). *Oblique* (right and left): The distance from one posterosuperior iliac spine to the opposite anterosuperior iliac spine, 22 cm (8½ in.), the right being slightly greater than the left. *External conjugate:* The distance from the undersurface of the spinous process of the last lumbar vertebra to the upper margin of the anterior surface of the symphysis pubis, 20 cm (7⅞ in.). SYN: *Baudelocque's diameter.*

INTERNAL DIAMETERS: *True conjugate:* The anteroposterior diameter of the pelvic inlet, 11 cm (4¼ in.), the most important single diameter of the pelvis. *Diagonal conjugate:* The distance between the promontory of the sacrum to the undersurface of the symphysis pubis, 13 cm (5⅛ in.). Two cm (¾ in.) are deducted for the height and inclination of the symphysis pubis to obtain the diameter of the conjugate. *Transverse:* The distance between the ischial tuberosities, 11 cm (4¼ in.). *Anteroposterior* (of outlet): The distance between the lower border of the symphysis pubis and the tip of the sacrum, 11 cm (4¼ in.). *Anterior sagittal:* The distance from the undersurface of the symphysis pubis to the center of the line between the ischial tuberosities, 7 cm (2¾ in.). *Posterior sagittal:* The distance from the center of line between the ischial tuberosities to the tip of the sacrum, 10 cm (4 in.).

**p. aequabiliter justo major** A pelvis that is symmetrically larger than the standard in all its dimensions. SYN: *giant p.*

**p. aequabiliter justo minor** A pelvis with all its dimensions uniformly smaller than the standard. SYN: *reduced p.*

**android p.** Masculine p.

**anthropoid p.** A female pelvis that is long and narrow.

**assimilation p.** An abnormal pelvis in which the transverse processes of the last lumbar vertebra are fused with the sacrum, or the last sacral vertebra is fused with the coccyx.

**beaked p.** A pelvis with the pelvic bones laterally compressed and pushed forward so that the outlet is narrow and long. SYN: *rostrate p.; triradiate p.*

**brachypellic p.** An oval pelvis in which the transverse diameter is at least 1 cm longer, but no more than 3 cm longer, than the anteroposterior diameter of the pelvis.

**brim of the p.** Inlet of the pelvis. SEE: *brim* (2).

**contracted p.** A pelvis in which one or more of the principal diameters is reduced to a degree that parturition is impeded.

**cordate p.** A pelvis possessing a heart-shaped inlet.

**coxalgic p.** A pelvis deformed subsequent to hip joint disease.

**dolichopellic p.** An abnormal pelvis in which the anteroposterior diameter is greater than the transverse diameter.

**dwarf p.** An aequabiliter justo minor pelvis, reduced in all its diameters and resembling an infantile pelvis. The bones are usually united by cartilage.

**elastic p.** Osteomalacic p.

**extrarenal p.** A renal pelvis located outside the kidney. This occurs when there is obstruction of the uteropelvic junction of the ureter.

**false p.** The portion of the pelvic cavity that lies above the pelvic brim, bounded by the linea terminalis and the iliac fossae. It supports the weight of the growing uterus during the middle and last trimesters of pregnancy. SYN: *p. major.*

**fissured p.** A rachitic pelvis with ilia pushed forward so as to be almost parallel.

**flat p.** A pelvis in which the anteroposterior diameters are shortened.

**frozen p.** Fixation of the pelvic organs in the pelvis caused by infection or neoplastic infiltration.

**funnel-shaped p.** A pelvis in which the outlet is considerably contracted but the inlet dimensions are normal.

**giant p.** P. aequabiliter justo major.

**gynecoid p.** The normal shape of the birth canal. The configuration is nearly circular, and the angle of the pubic arch usually exceeds 90°, allowing exit of the average fetus.

**halisteretic p.** A deformed pelvis resulting from softening of bones.

**infantile p.** An adult pelvis that retains its infantile characteristics. SYN: *juvenile p.*

**p. justo major** An unusually large pelvis.

**p. justo minor** An unusually small pelvis.

**juvenile p.** Infantile p.

**kyphoscoliotic p.** A deformed pelvis caused by rickets.

***kyphotic p.*** A deformed pelvis characterized by an increase of the conjugate diameter at the brim with reduction of the transverse diameter at the outlet.

***large p.*** P. justo major.

***lordotic p.*** A deformed pelvis in which the spinal column has an anterior curvature in the lumbar region.

***p. major*** False p.

***malacosteon p.*** Rachitic p.

***masculine p.*** A female pelvis that resembles a male pelvis, esp. in that it is narrower, more conical, and heavier-boned and has a heart-shaped inlet. SYN: *android p.*

***p. minor*** P. justo minor.

***p. obtecta*** A deformed pelvis in which the vertebral column extends across the pelvic inlet.

***osteomalacic p.*** A pelvis distorted because of osteomalacia. SYN: *elastic p.*

***Otto p.*** SEE: *Otto pelvis.*

***platypellic p., platypelloid p.*** A pelvis in which there are short anteroposterior and wide transverse diameters.

***pseudo-osteomalacic p.*** A rachitic pelvis similar to that of a person with osteomalacia.

***rachitic p.*** A pelvis deformed from rickets. SYN: *malacosteon p.*

***reduced p.*** P. aequabiliter justo minor.

***renal p.*** The expanded proximal end of the ureter. It lies within the renal sinus of the kidney and receives the urine through the major calyces.

***reniform p.*** A pelvis shaped like a kidney.

***Robert's p.*** SEE: *Robert's pelvis.*

***rostrate p.*** Beaked p.

***p. rotunda*** A tympanic depression in the inner wall, at the bottom of which is the fenestra rotunda.

***round p.*** A pelvis with a circular inlet.

***scoliotic p.*** A deformed pelvis resulting from spinal curvature.

***simple flat p.*** A pelvis with a shortened anteroposterior diameter.

***small p.*** P. justo minor.

***p. spinosa*** A rachitic pelvis with a pointed pubic crest.

***split p.*** A pelvis with a congenital division at the symphysis pubis.

***spondylolisthetic p.*** A pelvis in which the last lumbar vertebra is dislocated in front of the sacrum, causing occlusion of the brim.

***triangular p.*** A pelvis whose inlet is triangular.

***triradiate p.*** Beaked p.

***true p.*** The part of the pelvis below the iliopectineal line.

**pelvitherm** (pĕl′vĭ-thĕrm) [L. *pelvis,* basin, + Gr. *therme,* heat] A device for applying heat to the pelvis through the vagina.

**pelvoscopy** (pĕl-vŏs′kō-pē) [″ + Gr. *skopein,* to examine] Inspection of the pelvis.

**pelvospondylitis** (pĕl″vō-spŏn″dĭ-lī′tĭs) [″ + Gr. *spondylos,* vertebra, + *itis,* inflammation] Inflammation of the pelvic portion of the spine.

***p. ossificans*** Rheumatoid spondylitis.

**pemoline** (pĕm′ō-lĕn) A central nervous system–stimulating drug that is used in treating children with hyperkinesis and minimal brain damage. Trade name is Cylert.

**pemphigoid** (pĕm′fĭ-goyd) [Gr. *pemphigodes,* breaking out in blisters] A skin condition similar to pemphigus.

***bullous p.*** A blistering disease found almost exclusively in the elderly. Large, tense bullae filled with clear serum form on normal and urticarial skin. Lesions predominate in the flexural aspects of the limbs and abdomen. This condition is treated with corticosteroids and immunosuppressive agents, such as azathioprine or cyclophosphamide.

**pemphigus** (pĕm′fĭ-gŭs) [Gr. *pemphix,* a blister] An acute or chronic autoimmune disease principally of adults but sometimes found in children, characterized by occurrence of successive crops of bullae that appear suddenly on apparently normal skin and disappear, leaving pigmented spots. A characteristic sign is a positive Nikolsky's sign: when pressure is applied to an area as if trying to push the skin parallel to the surface, the skin will detach from the lower layers.

***erythematous p.*** Scaling, erythematous macules and blebs of the scalp, face, and trunk. The lesions have a "butterfly" distribution over the face. The disease resembles pemphigus foliaceus.

***p. foliaceus*** Pemphigus with a chronic course and in which bullous lesions may be absent. Once lesions develop, they may spread to the entire body and mimic generalized exfoliative dermatitis. The positive Nikolsky's sign helps to make the correct diagnosis. The condition is treated with systemic corticosteroids.

***p. vegetans*** A form of pemphigus vulgaris characterized by pustules instead of bullae. Pustules are followed by warty vegetations. Prognosis is good, even prior to therapy with corticosteroids.

***p. vulgaris*** The most common form of pemphigus. Lesions develop suddenly and are round or oval, thin-walled, tense, and translucent with contents bilateral in distribution. The lesions have little tendency to heal, and bleed easily when they burst. Since the introduction of corticosteroids, the prognosis is favorable, but the mortality rate is still high. Immunosuppressive agents, such as azathioprine or cyclophosphamide, are used with corticosteroid therapy. SEE: *photochemotherapy.*

**pencil** A material rolled into cylindrical form; may contain a caustic substance or a therapeutic paste or ointment.

**pendular** (pĕn′dū-lĕr) [L. *pendulus*] Hanging so as to swing by an attached part; oscillating like a pendulum.

**pendulous** (pĕn′dū-lŭs) Swinging freely like

a pendulum; hanging.

**penectomy** Surgical or traumatic removal of the penis.

**penetrance 1.** The frequency of manifestation of a hereditary condition in individuals. In theory, if the genotype is present, penetrance should be 100%. That is not usually the case, and the cause is attributed to the modifying effects of other genes. **2.** The extent to which something enters an object.

**penetrate** (pĕn′ĕ-trāt) [L. *penetrare*] To enter or force into the interior; pierce.

**penetrating** (pĕn′ĕ-trāt-ĭng) Entering beyond the exterior.

***p. power*** The penetrating capacity of a lens.

***p. wound*** A wound entering the interior of an organ or cavity.

**penetration** (pĕn″ĕ-trā′shŭn) [L. *penetrare,* to go within] **1.** The process of entering within a part. **2.** The capacity to enter within a part. **3.** The power of a lens to give a clear focus at varying depths. **4.** The ability of radiation to pass through a substance.

**penetrometer** (pĕn″ĕ-trŏm′ĕ-tĕr) [″ + Gr. *metron,* measure] An instrument that compares roughly the comparative absorption of roentgen rays in various metals, esp. silver, lead, and aluminum; hence, it gives a rough estimation of the ability of x-rays to penetrate tissues. SYN: *qualimeter.*

**-penia** (pē′nē-ă) [Gr. *penia,* lack] Combining form indicating *decrease, deficiency.*

**penicillamine** (pĕn″ĭ-sĭl′ă-mēn) A hydrolytic degradation product of penicillin. It is used to treat copper, mercury, zinc, or lead poisoning. It promotes the urinary excretion of these metals.

**penicillic acid** $C_8H_{10}O_4$. An antibiotic produced by some species of *Penicillium.*

**penicillin** (pĕn-ĭ-sĭl′ĭn) One of a group of antibiotics biosynthesized by several species of molds, esp. *Penicillium notatum* and *P. chrysogenum.* Penicillin is bactericidal, inhibiting the growth of most gram-positive bacteria and certain gram-negative forms. It is effective also against certain molds, spirochetes, and rickettsiae. There are many different penicillins, including synthetic ones, and their effectiveness varies for different organisms. SEE: *penicillin allergy.*

***beta-lactamase resistant p.*** Synthetic penicillins that resist the action of the enzyme beta-lactamase, produced by some organisms. Bacteria that produce the enzyme are not susceptible to the action of non–beta-lactamase resistant penicillins.

***p. G benzathine*** An antibiotic of the penicillin class available in a variety of dosage forms, used orally and parenterally.

***penicillinase-resistant p.*** Any of a group of penicillins that are not inactivated by the enzyme penicillinase. These penicillins retain their effectiveness as antibiotics used for infections caused by bacteria that produce penicillinase. SEE: *bacterial resistance; beta-lactamase resistance; Staphylococcus aureus, methicillin-resistant.*

***p. V potassium*** An antibiotic of the penicillin class. It is relatively stable in an acid medium and is therefore not inactivated by gastric acid when taken orally.

**penicillin allergy** An allergy caused by penicillin. If anaphylaxis occurs, immediate therapy with subcutaneous epinephrine is indicated. If the allergic response is not acute and penicillin therapy is needed to treat infection with a life-threatening organism for which no alternative antibiotic is available, it is possible to desensitize the patient by giving very small doses by mouth in gradually increasing doses. This should be done by a clinician experienced in this technique and with the equipment and medicines needed to treat anaphylaxis.

**penicillinase** (pĕn-ĭ-sĭl′ĭ-nās) A bacterial enzyme that inactivates most but not all penicillins.

**penicillinase-producing Neisseria gonorrhoeae** ABBR: PPNG. Penicillin-resistant strains of *Neisseria gonorrhoeae.*

**penicilliosis** (pĕn″ĭ-sĭl″ē-ō′sĭs) [L. *penicillum,* brush, + *osis,* condition] Infection with the fungi of the genus *Penicillium.*

**Penicillium** (pĕn″ĭ-sĭl′ē-ŭm) [L. *penicillum,* brush] A genus of molds belonging to the Ascomycetes (sac fungi). They form the blue molds that grow on fruits, bread, and cheese. A number of species *(P. chrysogenum, P. notatum)* are the source of penicillin. Occasionally in humans they produce infections of the external ear, skin, or respiratory passageways. They are common allergens. SEE: illus.

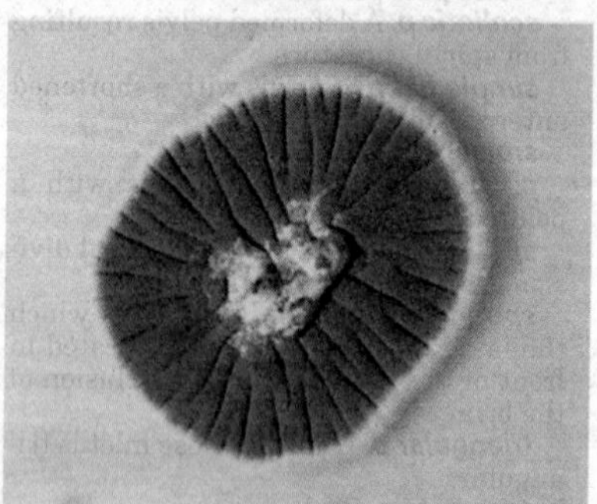

**PENICILLIUM** SP. IN CULTURE

**penicilloyl-polylysine** (pĕn″ĭ-sĭl′oyl-pŏl″ē-lī′sēn) A substance used to determine sensitivity to some forms of penicillin. When it is injected intradermally into a sensitive individual, a wheal appears within 20 minutes.

**penicillus** (pĕn″ĭ-sĭl′ŭs) *pl.* **penicilli** [L.,

paint brush] A group of the branches of arteries in the spleen that are arranged like the bristles of a brush. Each consists of successive portions: the pulp arteries, sheathed arteries, and terminal arteries.

**penile** (pē′nĭl, -nīl) [L. *penis*, penis] Pert. to the penis. SEE: *penile prosthesis*.

**penile ring** A ring made of metal, plastic, or leather. When placed around the flaccid penis, it is small enough to prevent venous return. Use of the device assists in causing and maintaining erection of the penis and in delaying orgasm. In practice the ring is removed prior to the penis becoming so large that it is impossible to remove. If this is not done, the ring has to be cut off to prevent gangrene of the penis.

**penis** (pē′nĭs) *pl.* **penises, penes** [L.] The male organ of copulation and, in mammals, of urination. It is a cylindrical pendulous organ suspended from the front and sides of the pubic arch. It is homologous to the clitoris in the female. Contrary to popular myths, the size of the normal penis has no physical bearing on the male's or female's enjoyment of sexual intercourse. SEE: illus.; *circumcision; pearly penile papules; penile prosthesis; Peyronie's disease; priapism.*

ANATOMY: The penis is composed mainly of erectile tissue arranged in three columns, the whole being covered with skin. The two lateral columns are the corpora cavernosa penis. The third or median column, known as the corpus spongiosum, contains the urethra. The body is attached to the descending portion of the pubic bone by the crura of the penis. The cone-shaped head of the penis, the glans penis, contains the urethral orifice. It is covered with a movable hood known as the foreskin or prepuce, under which is secreted the substance called smegma.

Hyperemia of the genitals fills the corpora cavernosa with blood as the result of sexual excitement or stimulation, thus causing an erection. The hyperemia subsides following orgasm and ejaculation of the seminal fluid. The organ then returns to its flaccid condition. The size of the flaccid penis does not necessarily correlate with that of the erect penis.

***p. captivus*** During sexual intercourse, the locking of a couple together owing to the penis being entrapped in the vagina. Even though this is quite common in dogs, the evidence that it occurs in human beings for more than a few moments, if ever, is lacking.

***clubbed p.*** The condition in which the penis is curved during erection.

***double p.*** A congenital deformity in which the penis in the embryo is completely divided by the urethral groove.

***p. envy*** In psychoanalysis, the female's desire to have a penis. The validity of this concept is controversial.

***p. lunatus*** Chordee.

***p. palmatus*** A penis enclosed by the scrotum. SYN: *webbed p.*

***webbed p.*** P. palmatus.

**penischisis** (pĕ-nĭs′kĭ-sĭs) [L. *penis*, penis, + Gr. *schisis*, a splitting] Epispadias, hypospadias, paraspadias, or any fissured con-

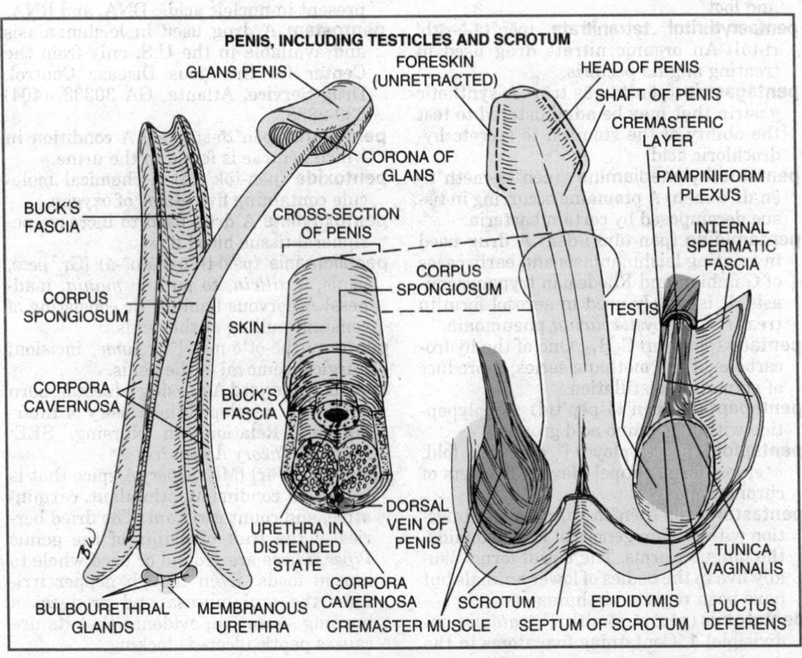

dition of the penis.

**penitis** (pĕ-nī'tĭs) [" + Gr. *itis,* inflammation] Inflammation of the penis.

**pennate** (pĕn'āt) [L. *penna,* feather] An object in which parts extend at an angle from a central portion, as do the barbs from a feather.

**penniform** (pĕn'ĭ-form) [" + *forma,* shape] Feather-shaped.

**pennyroyal** (pĕn"ĭ-roy'ăl) Name for various plants, esp. those of the genera *Hedeoma* and *Mentha,* that yield commercial oil used as a carminative and stimulant.

**pennyweight** Troy weight containing 24 gr or 1/20 of a troy ounce; equal to 1.555 g. This unit of measure was previously used for describing the quantities of precious metals, as the amount of gold needed for dental restorations.

**penoscrotal** (pē"nō-skrō'tăl) Concerning the penis and scrotum.

**pent-, penta-** [Gr. *pente,* five] Combining form meaning *five.*

**pentabasic** (pĕn"tă-bā'sĭk) **1.** A compound that contains five replaceable hydrogen atoms. **2.** An alcohol that contains five hydroxyl groups.

**pentachlorophenol** $C_6HCl_5O$. A chemical previously used as a wood preservative for termite control and as a defoliant. It is extremely toxic on its own, but some grades are additionally contaminated with dioxin.

**pentad** (pĕn'tăd) [Gr. *pente,* five] **1.** A radical or element with a valence of five. **2.** A group of five.

**pentadactyl** (pĕn"tă-dăk'tĭl) [" + *daktylos,* finger] Having five digits on each hand and foot.

**pentaerythritol tetranitrate** (pĕn"tă-ĕ-rĭth'rĭ-tōl) An organic nitrate drug used in treating angina pectoris.

**pentagastrin** (pĕn"tă-găs'trĭn) A synthetic gastrin that may be administered to test the ability of the stomach to secrete hydrochloric acid.

**pentamethylenediamine** (pĕn"tă-mĕth"ĭl-ĕn-dī'ă-mĕn) A ptomaine occurring in tissue decomposed by certain bacteria.

**pentamidine** (pĕn-tăm'ĭ-dĕn) A drug used in treating leishmaniasis and early cases of Gambian and Rhodesian trypanosomiasis. It is widely used in aerosol form to treat *Pneumocystis carinii* pneumonia.

**pentane** (pĕn'tān) $C_5H_{12}$. One of the hydrocarbons of the methane series; a product of petroleum distillation.

**pentapeptide** (pĕn"tă-pĕp'tĭd) A polypeptide with five amino acid groups.

**pentaploid** (pĕn'tă-ployd) [" + *ploos,* a fold, + *eidos,* form, shape] Having five sets of chromosomes.

**pentastomiasis** (pĕn"tă-stō-mī'ă-sĭs) Infection with certain genera of Pentastomida, the tongue worms. The larval forms usually live in the bodies of lower animals but have been reported in humans.

**pentatomic** (pĕn"tă-tŏm'ĭk) [" + *atomos,* indivisible] **1.** Containing five atoms in the molecule. **2.** An alcohol with five hydroxyl groups.

**pentavalent** (pĕn"tă-vā'lĕnt, -tăv'ă-lĕnt) [Gr. *pente,* five, + L. *valens,* having power] Having a chemical valence of five.

**pentazocine** (pĕn-tăz'ō-sēn) An analgesic drug that is effective orally and parenterally. Although originally thought to be nonaddicting, it is potentially addicting. Prolonged use of the drug may cause a woody sclerosis of the skin and subcutaneous tissues around injection sites. The lesions may appear on other areas of the skin also. Ulcers surrounded by areas of hyperpigmentation may develop. Skin changes do not develop in short-term users of the drug.

**Pentids** Trade name for penicillin G potassium.

**pentobarbital** (pĕn"tō-băr'bĭ-tăl) A hypnotic sedative drug of the barbiturate class.

***p. sodium*** A barbituric acid derivative used as an oral or intravenous hypnotic agent in preanesthetic medication; used in labor with or without scopolamine.

**pentosazon** (pĕn"tō-sā'zŏn) A crystalline compound formed when a pentose is treated with phenylhydrazine. It is not normally present in urine.

**pentose** (pĕn'tōs) [Gr. *pente,* five] $C_5H_{10}O_5$; a monosaccharide containing five carbon atoms.

**pentosemia** (pĕn"tō-sē'mē-ă) Pentose in the blood.

**pentoside** (pĕn'tō-sīd) Pentose combined with some other substance. Pentoses combined with purine or pyrimidine bases are present in nucleic acids, DNA, and RNA.

**pentostam** A drug used in leishmaniasis and available in the U.S. only from the Center for Infectious Disease Control, Drug Service, Atlanta, GA 30333, (404) 639-2888.

**pentosuria** (pĕn"tō-sū'rē-ă) A condition in which pentose is found in the urine.

**pentoxide** (pĕn-tŏk'sīd) A chemical molecule containing five atoms of oxygen.

**pentoxifylline** A drug used to increase peripheral tissue blood flow.

**peotillomania** (pē"ō-tĭl"ō-mā'nē-ă) [Gr. *peos,* penis, + *tillein,* to pull, + *mania,* madness] A nervous habit or tic consisting of constant pulling at the penis.

**peotomy** (pē-ŏt'ō-mē) [" + *tome,* incision] Surgical removal of the penis.

**Peplau, Hildegard** A nursing educator, born 1909, who developed the Theory of Interpersonal Relations in Nursing. SEE: *Nursing Theory Appendix.*

**pepper** (pĕp'ĕr) [ME. *peper*] A spice that is used as a condiment, stimulant, carminative, and counterirritant. The dried berries of the fruit of plants of the genus *Piper.* These are ground or used whole to season foods. Even though pepper irritates the oral mucosa and produces a burning sensation, evidence that its use causes peptic ulcers is lacking.

A scale (Scoville scale) for judging the amount of material in pepper which causes it to be hot has been developed. Using this scale, the hottest peppers have a rating of 250,000 to 400,000 units. Gloves should be worn when preparing peppers that are hot and care should be taken to protect the eyes while handling peppers. All peppers should be kept away from children.

**peppermint spirit** The leaves and tops of the plant *Mentha piperita,* from which oil of peppermint is derived. It is used as an aromatic stimulant, carminative, and flavoring agent.

**pepsic** (pĕp'sĭk) [Gr. *peptein,* to digest] Peptic.

**pepsin** (pĕp'sĭn) [Gr. *pepsis,* digestion] The chief enzyme of gastric juice, which converts proteins into proteoses and peptones. It is formed by the chief cells of gastric glands and produces its maximum activity at a pH of 1.5 to 2. It is obtainable in granular form. In the presence of hydrochloric acid, it digests proteins in vitro.

**pepsinogen** (pĕp-sĭn'ō-jĕn) [" + *gennan,* to produce] The antecedent of pepsin existing in the form of granules in the chief cells of gastric glands.

**pepsinuria** (pĕp"sĭ-nū'rē-ă) [" + *ouron,* urine] Excretion of pepsin in the urine.

**peptic** (pĕp'tĭk) [Gr. *peptikos*] **1.** Concerning digestion. **2.** Concerning pepsin. SYN: *pepsic.*

**peptic ulcer** An ulcer occurring in the lower end of the esophagus; in the stomach usually along the lesser curvature; in the duodenum; or on the jejunal side of a gastrojejunostomy. SEE: *Nursing Diagnoses Appendix.*

SYMPTOMS: Pain is the most characteristic symptom, tending to be of uniform quality and usually described as "gnawing." It is localized in the epigastrium and exhibits a rhythmicity and periodicity usually appearing 1 to 3 hours after a meal. It is usually absent before breakfast but may occur during the night. Usually, but not always, the pain is relieved by food and alkalies. The pain lasts for minutes rather than hours, and the clusters of pain may be present for days or weeks followed by long symptom-free periods.

Other symptoms include dyspepsia, heartburn, acid eructations, nausea, vomiting, and anorexia. In some cases, physical signs may be absent, the first indication of the condition being hemorrhage or perforation.

ETIOLOGY: The usual but not the only cause is the action of gastric acid and peptic activity on the mucosa of the esophagus, stomach, or duodenum. Ulcers may form in other situations where the mucosal defenses are overcome by forces that can damage the mucosa. It is believed that most peptic ulcers are caused by colonization with the bacterium *Helicobacter pylori.* SEE: *ulcer, Curling's; ulcer, stress; Zollinger-Ellison syndrome.*

TREATMENT: *Medical therapy* consists of giving antibiotics such as amoxocillin combined with agents that block production of hydrochloric acid or an antisecretory such as omperazole.

*Diet* has not proven to be as effective in treating peptic ulcer as previously thought. Cessation of tobacco and alcohol use is beneficial in treating peptic ulcer. Because some analgesics can cause peptic ulcers, their use should be discontinued. SEE: *nonsteroidal anti-inflammatory agents.*

*Surgical therapy* including vagotomy and subtotal gastric resection may be needed if hemorrhage, perforation or intractable bleeding occurs.

NURSING IMPLICATIONS: The patient is instructed to reduce emotional stress, rest, and take prescribed medications to control gastric acidity. In the acute state, vomitus and stool are tested for blood. The nurse observes for complications such as perforation or hemorrhage. Steps are taken to prevent injuries due to drowsiness associated with tranquilizer and sedative use. The nurse assists the patient to develop coping mechanisms to relieve anxiety. All activities should be performed in moderation. Patient teaching should cover prescribed medications, drugs to avoid because they cause gastric irritation, discontinuation or decrease of smoking, and importance of follow-up care.

**peptidase** An enzyme that converts peptides to amino acids.

**peptide** (pĕp'tīd) [Gr. *peptein,* to digest] A compound formed by hydrolytic cleavage of peptones and containing two or more amino acids. A class of substances prepared by synthesis from amino acids and intermediate in molecular weight and chemical properties between the amino acids, which can be made artificially, and the proteins, which cannot.

**peptidoglycan** The dense material consisting of cross-linked polysaccharide chains that make up the cell wall of most bacteria. This membrane is much thicker in gram-positive bacteria than it is in gram-negative organisms.

**peptidolytic** (pĕp"tĭ-dō-lĭt'ĭk) [" + *lytikos,* dissolving] Causing the splitting up or digestion of peptides.

**peptinotoxin** (pĕp"tĭn-ō-tŏk'sĭn) [" + *toxikon,* poison] Poisonous ptomaine found in the body as a result of disordered or defective digestion.

**peptization** (pĕp"tĭ-zā'shŭn) [Gr. *peptein,* to digest] In the chemistry of colloids, the process of making a colloidal solution more stable; conversion of a gel to a sol.

**Peptococcaceae** A family of bacteria that includes the genus *Peptococcus.* These gram-positive anaerobic cocci may be normal or pathologic inhabitants of the respiratory and intestinal tracts.

**Peptococcus** (pĕp″tō-kŏk′ŭs) Strictly anaerobic gram-positive cocci that are normally present in the oral cavity, on the skin, and in the intestinal and urinary tracts. They are usually associated with infections, in which they act synergistically with other organisms.

**peptogenic, peptogenous** (pĕp-tō-jĕn′ĭk, -tŏj′ĕn-ŭs) [″+ *gennan,* to produce] **1.** Producing peptones and pepsin. **2.** Promoting digestion.

**peptone** (pĕp′tōn) [Gr. *pepton,* digesting] A secondary protein formed by the action of proteolytic enzymes, acids, or alkalies on certain proteins. Peptones are nitrogenous compounds soluble in water; they are not coagulated by boiling.

**peptonization** (pĕp″tō-nĭ-zā′shŭn) [Gr. *pepton,* digesting] The process of changing protein substance into peptones by action of proteolytic enzymes.

**peptonize** To convert into peptones; to predigest with pepsin.

**peptonuria** (pĕp″tō-nū′rē-ă) [″ + *ouron,* urine] Excretion of peptones in the urine.

**Peptostreptococcus** (pĕp″tō-strĕp″tō-kŏk′ŭs) A genus of gram-positive anaerobic cocci of the Peptococcaceae family. They may be normal or pathogenic inhabitants of the intestinal and respiratory tracts. They are also important as opportunistic pathogens.

**peptotoxin** (pĕp″tō-tŏk′sĭn) [″ + *toxikon,* poison] Any toxin produced from a peptone.

**per** [L. *per,* through] **1.** Through, by, by means of. **2.** In chemistry, the highest valence of an element. **3.** For each unit or entity (e.g., milligrams per kilogram, usually written as *mg/kg).*

**per-** A prefix indicating *throughout, through, utterly, intense.*

**peracephalus** (pĕr″ă-sĕf′ă-lŭs) [″+ Gr. *a-,* not, + *kephale,* head] A parasitic placental twin. It does not contain a head or arms, and the thorax is malformed.

**peracid** (pĕr-ăs′ĭd) **1.** An acid that contains the highest valence possible. **2.** An acid containing the peroxide group, O—OH.

**peracidity** (pĕr″ă-sĭd′ĭ-tē) [L. *per,* through, + *acidus,* sour] Abnormal acidity.

**peracute** (pĕr″ă-kūt′) [″ + *acutus,* keen] Very acute or violent.

**per anum** (pĕr ā′nŭm) [L.] Through or by way of the anus.

**perarticulation** (pĕr″ăr-tĭk″ū-lā′shŭn) [L. *per,* through, + *articulatio,* joint] Diarthrosis.

**percent** Per hundred; for or out of each hundred. Its symbol, %, is used to indicate that the preceding number is a percentage.

**percentile** (pĕr-sĕn′tĭl) One of 100 equal divisions of a series of items or data. Thus if a value such as a test score is higher than 92% of all the other test scores, that result is above the 92nd percentile of the range of scores.

**percept** (pĕr′sĕpt) The mental image of an object seen.

**perception** (pĕr-sĕp′shŭn) [L. *percepitio,* perceive] **1.** The process of being aware of objects; consciousness. **2.** The process of receiving sensory impressions. **3.** The elaboration of a sensory impression; the ideational association modifying, defining, and usually completing the primary impression or stimulus. Vague or inadequate association occurs in confused and depressed states.

***depth p.*** A term used in evaluating visual function; the ability to recognize that an object has depth as well as height and width. It is generally believed that both eyes must function normally for a person to have normal ability to perceive depth. Sometimes this is true, but most persons with the use of only one eye learn to judge depth quite accurately.

***extrasensory p.*** ABBR: ESP. Perception not through the recognized senses.

***stereognostic p.*** The recognition of objects by touch.

**perceptivity** (pĕr-sĕp-tĭv′ĭ-tē) The power to receive sense impressions.

**percolate** (pĕr′kō-lāt) [L. *percolare,* to strain through] **1.** To allow a liquid to seep through a powdered substance. **2.** Any fluid that has been filtered or percolated. **3.** To strain a fluid through powdered substances in order to impregnate it with soluble principles of such substances.

**percolation** (pĕr″kō-lā′shŭn) [L. *percolatio*] **1.** Filtration. **2.** The process of extracting soluble portions of a drug of powdered composition by filtering a liquid solvent through it.

**percolator** (pĕr′kō-lā″tor) An apparatus used for extraction of a drug with a liquid solvent.

**per contiguum** (pĕr kŏn-tĭg′ū-ŭm) [L.] Touching, as in the spread of an inflammation from one part to an adjacent structure.

**per continuum** (pĕr kŏn-tĭn′ū-ŭm) [L.] Continuous, as in the spread of an inflammation from part to part.

**percuss** (pĕr-kŭs′) [L. *percutere*] To tap parts of the body to aid diagnosis by sound emitted.

**percussion** (pĕr-kŭsh′ŭn) [L. *percussio,* a striking] **1.** The use of the fingertips to tap the body lightly but sharply to determine position, size, and consistency of an underlying structure and the presence of fluid or pus in a cavity. These conditions are established by alterations felt and heard in resonance and pitch of the sound emitted, vibration elicited, or resistance encountered. **2.** A technique used with postural drainage to mobilize secretions by mechanically dislodging viscous or adherent secretions in the lungs by manually cupping over the chest wall. SEE: *cystic fibrosis.*

***auscultatory p.*** Percussion combined with auscultation.

***bimanual p.*** Mediate p.

***deep p.*** Forceful percussion used to elicit a note from a deeply seated tissue or organ.

***direct p.*** Immediate p.

***finger p.*** Striking of the examiner's finger as it rests upon the patient's body with a finger of the examiner's other hand.

***immediate p.*** Percussion performed by striking the surface directly with the fingers. SYN: *direct p.*

***indirect p.*** Mediate p.

***mediate p.*** Percussion performed by using the fingers of one hand as a plexor and those of the opposite hand as a pleximeter. SYN: *bimanual p.; indirect p.*

***palpation p.*** Percussion in which the examiner's fingers perceive the tactile impression rather than the examiner relying on the sounds produced.

***threshold p.*** Percussing lightly with the fingers on a glass-rod pleximeter, the far end of which is covered with a rubber cap. The cap is usually placed on an intercostal space. This technique is used to confine the percussion to a very small area.

**percussor** (pĕr-kŭs′or) [L., striker] A device used for diagnosis by percussion, consisting of a hammer with a rubber or metal head.

**percutaneous** (pĕr″kū-tā′nē-ŭs) [L. *per,* through, + *cutis,* skin] Effected through the skin; describes the application of a medicated ointment by friction, or the removal or injection of a fluid by needle.

**per diem cost** Hospital or other inpatient institutional cost per day.

**perencephaly** (pĕr″ĕn-sĕf′ă-lē) [Gr. *pera,* pouch, + *enkephalos,* brain] Porencephalia.

**perfectionism** (pĕr-fĕk′shŭn-ĭzm) A type of neurosis in which the individual attempts to achieve goals of behavior or performance that are unrealistic or unnecessary.

**perflation** (pĕr-flā′shŭn) [L. *perflatio*] The process of blowing air into a cavity to expand its walls or to force out secretions or other matter.

**perforans** (pĕr′fō-răns) [L.] Perforating or penetrating, as a nerve or muscle.

**perforate** (pĕr′fō-rāt) [L. *perforatus,* pierced with holes] **1.** To puncture or to make holes. **2.** Pierced with holes.

**perforation** (pĕr″fō-rā′shŭn) **1.** The act or process of making a hole, such as that caused by ulceration. **2.** The hole made through a substance or part.

***Bezold's p.*** [Friedrich Bezold, Ger. physician, 1842–1908] A perforation on the inner surface of the mastoid bone.

***tooth p.*** An opening through the wall of a tooth, produced by pathologic processes or accidentally, thereby exposing the dental pulp. It is also called pulp exposure.

**perforation of stomach or intestine** Abdominal crisis due to escape of contents of the perforated viscus into the peritoneal cavity. Peritonitis is certain to develop unless there is immediate surgical intervention. SEE: *intestinal perforation; peritonitis.*

SYMPTOMS: The onset is accompanied by acute pain, beginning over the perforated area and spreading all over the abdomen, which has become rigid. The patient's face is anxious, with beads of perspiration on it. Nausea and vomiting occur. The pulse is rapid and feeble, and respiration is rapid and shallow. The body temperature drops, but then rises as peritonitis sets in, at which time the pulse becomes stronger.

TREATMENT: Surgical treatment is necessary. Pending operation, the patient is given no fluids. Complete rest is needed.

**perforator** (pĕr′fō-rā-tor) [L., a piercing device] An instrument for piercing the skull and other bones.

***tympanum p.*** An instrument for perforating the tympanum.

**perforatorium** (pĕr″fō-ră-tō′rē-ŭm) The pointed tip of the acrosome of the spermatozoa.

**performance** The act of performing (i.e., the undertaking and completing of) mental or physical work. Thus, a person's performance is observed and measured in order to determine functional capability.

**perfusate** (pĕr-fū′zāt) The fluid used to perfuse a tissue or organ.

**perfusion** (pĕr-fū′zhŭn) [L. *perfundere,* to pour through] **1.** Passing of a fluid through spaces. **2.** Pouring of a fluid. **3.** Supplying of an organ or tissue with nutrients and oxygen by injecting blood or a suitable fluid into an artery.

***coronary p.*** The passage of blood through the arteries of the heart. When the heart is unable to do this naturally, an external device may be used to keep blood flowing through these vessels.

**perfusionist** An individual who assists the physician in all aspects of managing the equipment and techniques used during extracorporeal circulation. A perfusionist may also be involved in inducing prescribed hypothermia.

**perhydrocyclopentanophenanthrene** (pĕr-hī″drō-sī″klō-pĕn-tăn″ō-phĕn-ăn′thrēn) The name of the ring structure of the chemical nucleus of the steroids. SEE: *steroid hormones* for illus.

**peri-** [Gr.] Prefix meaning *around, about.*

**periadenitis** (pĕr″ē-ă″dĕ-nī′tĭs) [″ + *aden,* gland, + *itis,* inflammation] Inflammation of the tissues surrounding a gland.

***p. mucosa necrotica recurrens*** Recurring necrotic or ulcerative lesions on the buccal and pharyngeal mucosa. These start as small hard nodules that ulcerate and leave a deep crater. These may be associated with Behçet's syndrome.

**perianal** (pĕr″ē-ā′năl) [″ + L. *anus,* anus] Around or close to the anus.

**periangiitis** (pĕr″ē-ăn″jē-ī′tĭs) [″ + *angeion,* vessel, + *itis,* inflammation] Inflammation of tissue around a blood or lymphatic vessel.

**periangiocholitis** (pĕr″ē-ăn″jē-ō-kō-lī′tĭs) [″ + ″ + *chole,* bile, + *itis,* inflammation] Pericholangitis.

**periaortic** (pĕr″ē-ā-or′tĭk) [″ + *aorte,* aorta] Around the aorta.

**periaortitis** (pĕr″ē-ā-or-tī′tĭs) [″ + *aorte,* aorta, + *itis,* inflammation] Inflammation of adventitia and tissues around the aorta.

**periapex** (pĕr″ē-ā′pĕks) [″ + L. *apex,* tip] The area around the apex of a tooth.

**periapical** (pĕr″ē-ăp′ĭ-kăl) [″ + L. *apex,* tip] Around the apex of the root of a tooth.

**periappendicitis** (pĕr″ē-ă-pĕn″dĭ-sī′tĭs) [″ + L. *appendix,* appendage, + Gr. *itis,* inflammation] Inflammation of the appendix and its surrounding tissues.

***p. decidualis*** A condition in which decidual cells exist in the peritoneum of the appendix vermiformis in cases of tubal pregnancy owing to adhesions between fallopian tubes and the appendix.

**periappendicular** (pĕr″ē-ăp″ĕn-dĭk′ū-lăr) [″ + L. *appendix,* appendage] Surrounding an appendix.

**periarterial** (pĕr″ē-ăr-tē′rē-ăl) [″ + *arteria,* artery] Placed around an artery.

**periarteritis** (pĕr″ē-ăr-tĕr-ī′tĭs) [″ + ″ + *itis,* inflammation] Inflammation of the external coat of an artery.

***p. gummosa*** Gummas in the blood vessels in syphilis.

***p. nodosa*** Polyarteritis nodosa. SEE: *Nursing Diagnoses Appendix.*

**periarthric** (pĕr″ē-ăr′thrĭk) Circumarticular.

**periarthritis** (pĕr″ē-ăr-thrī′tĭs) [″ + ″ + *itis,* inflammation] Inflammation of the area around a joint.

**periarticular** (pĕr″ē-ăr-tĭk′ū-lăr) Circumarticular.

**periatrial** (pĕr″ē-ā′trē-ăl) [″ + L. *atrium,* corridor] Around the atria, or auricles, of the heart.

**periauricular** Around the ear.

**periaxial** (pĕr-ē-ăk′sē-ăl) [″ + *axon,* axis] Located around an axis.

**periaxillary** (pĕr″ē-ăk′sĭl-ĕ″rē) [″ + L. *axilla,* armpit] Occurring around the axilla.

**periaxonal** (pĕr″ē-ăk′sō-năl) [″ + *axon,* axis] Around an axon.

**peribronchial** (pĕr″ĭ-brŏng′kē-ăl) [″ + *bronchos,* windpipe] Surrounding a bronchus.

**peribronchiolar** (pĕr″ĭ-brŏng-kī′ō-lăr) [″ + L. *bronchiolus,* bronchiole] Surrounding a bronchiole.

**peribronchiolitis** (pĕr″ĭ-brŏng″kē-ō-lī′tĭs) [″ + ″ + Gr. *itis,* inflammation] Inflammation of the area around the bronchioles.

**peribulbar** (pĕr″ĭ-bŭl′băr) [″ + L. *bulbus,* bulbous root] Surrounding a bulb, esp. the bulb of the eye.

**peribursal** (pĕr″ĭ-bĕr′săl) [″ + *bursa,* leather sack] Around a bursa.

**pericanalicular** (pĕr″ĭ-kăn″ă-lĭk′ū-lăr) [″ + L. *canaliculus,* small canal] Around a canaliculus.

**pericardiac, pericardial** (pĕr-ĭ-kăr′dē-ăk, -ăl) [″ + *kardia,* heart] Concerning the pericardium.

**pericardicentesis, pericardiocentesis** (pĕr″ĭ-kăr″dĭ-sĕn-tē′sĭs, -kăr″dē-ō-sĕn-tē′sĭs) [″ + ″ + *kentesis,* puncture] Surgical perforation of the pericardium.

**pericardiectomy** (pĕr″ĭ-kăr-dē-ĕk′tō-mē) [″ + ″ + *ektome,* excision] Excision of part or all of the pericardium.

**pericardiolysis** (pĕr″ĭ-kăr″dē-ŏl′ĭ-sĭs) [″ + ″ + *lysis,* dissolution] Separation of adhesions between the visceral and parietal pericardium.

**pericardiomediastinitis** (pĕr″ĭ-kăr″dē-ō-mē-dē-ăs″tĭ-nī′tĭs) [″ + ″ + L. *mediastinum,* + Gr. *itis,* inflammation] Inflammation of the pericardium and mediastinum.

**pericardiopexy** [″ + ″ + *pexis,* fixation] A surgical procedure designed to increase the blood supply to the heart by joining the pericardium to an adjacent tissue.

**pericardiophrenic** (pĕr-ĭ-kăr″dē-ō-frĕn′ĭk) [″ + *kardia,* heart, + *phren,* diaphragm] Concerning the pericardium and diaphragm.

**pericardiopleural** (pĕr″ĭ-kăr″dē-ō-ploo′răl) [″ + ″ + *pleura,* rib] Concerning the pericardium and pleura.

**pericardiorrhaphy** (pĕr″ĭ-kăr″dē-or′ă-fē) [″ + ″ + *rhaphe,* seam, ridge] Suture of a wound in the pericardium.

**pericardiostomy** (pĕr″ĭ-kăr″dē-ŏs′tō-mē) [″ + *kardia,* heart, + *stoma,* mouth] Formation of an opening into the pericardium for drainage.

**pericardiosymphysis** (pĕr″ĭ-kăr″dē-ō-sĭm′fĭ-sĭs) [″ + ″ + *symphysis,* a joining] Adhesion between the layers of the pericardium.

**pericardiotomy** (pĕr″ĭ-kăr-dē-ŏt′ō-mē) [″ + ″ + *tome,* incision] Incision of the pericardial sac around the heart.

**pericarditic** (pĕr″ĭ-kăr-dĭt′ĭk) Concerning the pericardium.

**pericarditis** (pĕr-ĭ-kăr-dī′tĭs) [″ + *kardia,* heart, + *itis,* inflammation] Inflammation of the pericardium. SEE: *Nursing Diagnoses Appendix.*

SYMPTOMS: Moderate fever, precordial pain and tenderness, dry cough, dyspnea, and palpitation are present. The pulse is at first rapid and forcible, then weak and irregular.

*First stage:* Auscultation reveals to-and-fro friction sound heard over the fourth left intercostal space near sternum. Inspection and palpation sometimes reveal a diffuse apex beat. Friction rub may sometimes be palpated.

*Second stage:* Serofibrinous effusion is present, and there is bulging of the precordium. There is an increased area of dullness, triangular, with the base down. Heart sounds are muffled, distant, and feeble. Purulent effusion yields similar signs, but in addition high, irregular fever; sweats; chills; and progressive pallor are present. Sometimes edema exists over the precordium.

ETIOLOGY: This condition may be caused by tuberculosis, mycoses, infection by pyogenic organisms, collagen disease, uremia, myocardial infarction, neoplasms, or trauma.

TREATMENT: General treatment involves absolute bedrest and a light diet. For relief of pain an ice bag is applied over the precordium or pain-relieving drugs are given, depending on the intensity. Specific treatment involves giving the appropriate antibiotic for specific organisms involved. If purulent effusion occurs, aspiration or surgical drainage are employed. If gallop rhythm or signs of heart failure occur, fluids and salt are restricted. For chronic constrictive pericarditis, resection of the pericardium is performed.

PROGNOSIS: Prognosis is fair in the early stages but extremely grave in the purulent and fibrinous stages.

NURSING IMPLICATIONS: The patient is observed for severity of symptoms of cardiac tamponade, such as weak or absent peripheral pulses and point of maximal impulse, distended neck veins, decreased blood pressure, and narrowing pulse pressure. Medications are administered as prescribed. In the convalescent phase, the nurse teaches the patient about importance of taking prescribed medications, their purposes, and any potentially recurring symptoms to report.

***acute fibrinous p.*** Pericarditis characterized by fibrinous exudation.

***acute nonspecific p.*** A disease of unknown etiology that usually follows respiratory infections. SYN: *idiopathic p.*

***adhesive p.*** A form of pericarditis in which the layers of pericardium adhere.

***constrictive p.*** Pericarditis in which adhesions form between the visceral and parietal layers of the pericardium.

***external p.*** Inflammation of the exterior surface of the pericardium.

***fibrinous p.*** Pericarditis in which the membrane is covered with a butter-like exudate that organizes and unites the pericardial surfaces.

SYMPTOMS: The condition is characterized by precordial bulging, a weak apex beat with loud sounds, a systolic retraction at the apex and over a large part of the precordium, a peculiar diastolic collapse of the jugular veins, and a feeble apex beat with a forcible impulse over the body of the heart. Signs of heart failure (e.g., dyspnea, generalized edema, cyanosis) are present.

***hemorrhagic p.*** Pericarditis in which the exudate contains blood.

***idiopathic p.*** Acute nonspecific p.

***ischemic p.*** Pericarditis resulting from myocardial infarction.

***neoplastic p.*** Pericarditis due to invasion of the pericardium by malignant tumors of adjoining structures.

***p. obliterans*** Pericardial inflammation causing adhesions and obliteration of the pericardial cavity.

***serofibrinous p.*** Pericarditis in which there is a considerable quantity of serous exudate but little fibrin.

***uremic p.*** Pericarditis caused by uremia.

**pericardium** (pĕr″ĭ-kăr′dē-ŭm) [Gr. *peri*, around, + *kardia*, heart] The membranous fibroserous sac enclosing the heart and the bases of the great vessels. The three layers are the fibrous pericardium (the outer layer); the parietal pericardium, a serous membrane that lines the fibrous pericardium; and the visceral pericardium (epicardium), a serous membrane on the surface of the myocardium. The space between the two serous layers is the pericardial cavity, a potential space filled with serous fluid that reduces friction as the heart beats. Its base is attached to the diaphragm, its apex extending upward as far as the first subdivision of the great blood vessels. It is attached in front to the sternum, laterally to the mediastinal pleura, and posteriorly to the esophagus, trachea, and principal bronchi. SEE: illus.

***adherent p.*** A condition in which fibrous bands form between the two serous layers of the pericardium, obliterating the

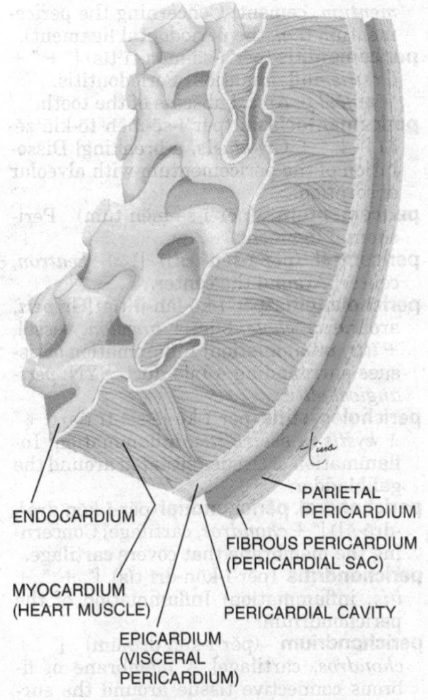


**PERICARDIUM**

LAYERS OF THE HEART WALL

pericardial cavity. SEE: *pericarditis, constrictive.*

***bread-and-butter p.*** A condition seen in fibrinous pericarditis, in which the pericardium has a peculiar appearance as a result of fibrinous deposits on the two opposing surfaces.

***p. externum*** The outer fibrous layer of the pericardium.

***fibrous p.*** Strong fibrous tissue on the outer surface of the pericardial sac.

***p. internum*** The inner serous layer of the pericardium. SYN: *visceral p.; epicardium.*

***parietal p.*** The middle serous layer of the pericardial sac, lining the fibrous layer.

***serous p.*** The parietal and visceral pericardial membranes.

***shaggy p.*** A condition occurring in fibrinous pericarditis in which loose shaggy deposits of fibrin are seen on the surfaces of the pericardium.

***visceral p.*** P. internum.

**pericardotomy** (pĕr″ĭ-kăr-dŏt′ō-mē) [Gr. *peri,* around, + *kardia,* heart, + *tome,* incision] Incision of the pericardium.

**pericecal** (pĕr″ĭ-sē′kăl) [″ + L. *caecum,* blind] Situated around the cecum.

**pericecitis** (pĕr″ĭ-sē-sī′tĭs) [″ + ″ + Gr. *itis,* inflammation] Inflammation of the area around the cecum.

**pericellular** (pĕr″ĭ-sĕl′ū-lăr) [″ + L. *cellula, cell*] Around a cell.

**pericemental** (pĕr″ĭ-sē-mĕn′tăl) [″ + L. *caementum,* cement] Concerning the pericementum (i.e., the periodontal ligament).

**pericementitis** (pĕr″ĭ-sē-mĕn-tī′tĭs) [″ + ″ + Gr. *itis,* inflammation] Periodontitis.

***apical p.*** Apical abscess of the tooth.

**pericementoclasia** (pĕr″ĭ-sē-mĕn″tō-klā′zē-ă) [″ + ″ + Gr. *klasis,* a breaking] Dissolution of the pericementum with alveolar absorption.

**pericementum** (pĕr″ĭ-sē-mĕn′tŭm) Periodontal ligament.

**pericentral** (pĕr″ĭ-sĕn′trăl) [″ + *kentron,* center] Around the center.

**pericholangitis** (pĕr″ĭ-kō-lăn-jī′tĭs) [Gr. *peri,* around, + *chole,* bile, + *angeion,* vessel, + *itis,* inflammation] Inflammation of tissues surrounding a bile duct. SYN: *periangiocholitis.*

**pericholecystitis** (pĕr″ĭ-kō-lē-sĭs-tī′tĭs) [″ + ″ + *kystis,* a sac, + *itis,* inflammation] Inflammation of tissues situated around the gallbladder.

**perichondral, perichondrial** (pĕr-ĭ-kŏn′drăl, -drē-ăl) [″ + *chondros,* cartilage] Concerning the membrane that covers cartilage.

**perichondritis** (pĕr-ĭ-kŏn-drī′tĭs) [″ + ″ + *itis,* inflammation] Inflammation of the perichondrium.

**perichondrium** (pĕr-ĭ-kŏn′drē-ŭm) [″ + *chondros,* cartilage] A membrane of fibrous connective tissue around the surface of cartilage.

**perichondroma** (pĕr″ĭ-kŏn-drō′mă) [″ + ″ + *oma,* tumor] A tumor arising from fibrous tissue that covers cartilage.

**perichord** (pĕr′ĭ-kord) [″ + *chorde,* cord] The sheath of the notochord.

**perichordal** (pĕr-ĭ-kor′dăl) [″ + *chorde,* cord] Placed around the notochord.

**perichorioidal, perichoroidal** (pĕr″ĭ-kō-rē-oy′dăl, -roy′dăl) [″ + *chorioeides,* skinlike] Situated around the choroid coat.

**pericolic** (pĕr-ĭ-kō′lĭk) [″ + *kolon,* colon] Around or encircling the colon.

**pericolitis** (pĕr″ĭ-kō-lī′tĭs) [″ + ″ + *itis,* inflammation] Inflammation of an area around the colon.

**pericolpitis** (pĕr″ĭ-kŏl-pī′tĭs) [Gr. *peri,* around, + *kolpos,* vagina, + *itis,* inflammation] Inflammation of connective tissues surrounding the vagina.

**periconchal** (pĕr-ĭ-kŏng′kăl) [″ + *konche,* concha] Around the concha of the ear.

**pericorneal** (pĕr″ĭ-kor′nē-ăl) [″ + L. *cornu,* horn] Placed around the cornea.

**pericoronal** (pĕr″ĭ-kor′ō-năl) [″ + *korone,* crown] Around the crown of a tooth.

**pericoronitis** (pĕr″ĭ-kor″ō-nī′tĭs) [″ + ″ + *itis,* inflammation] Inflammation around the crown of a tooth.

**pericranial** (pĕr″ĭ-krā′nē-ăl) [″ + *kranion,* skull] Pert. to the periosteum of the skull.

**pericranitis** (pĕr″ĭ-krā-nī′tĭs) [″ + ″ + *itis,* inflammation] Inflammation of the pericranium.

**pericranium** (pĕr″ĭ-krā′nē-ŭm) The fibrous membrane surrounding the cranium; periosteum of the skull.

***p. internum*** The lining surface of the cranium. SYN: *endocranium.*

**pericystic** (pĕr″ĭ-sĭs′tĭk) [″ + *kystis,* bladder] Surrounding a cyst.

**pericystitis** (pĕr″ĭ-sĭs-tī′tĭs) [″ + ″ + *itis,* inflammation] Inflammation of the tissues about the bladder.

**pericystium** (pĕr″ĭ-sĭs′tē-ŭm) [″ + *kystis,* bladder] **1.** The vascular wall surrounding a cyst. **2.** The tissues around the urinary bladder or gallbladder.

**pericyte** (pĕr′ĭ-sīt) [″ + *kytos,* cell] A flat, undifferentiated, contractile connective tissue cell around the capillary walls.

**pericytial** (pĕr-ĭ-sĭsh′ăl) [″ + *kytos,* cell] Placed around a cell.

**peridendritic** (pĕr″ĭ-dĕn-drĭt′ĭk) [″ + *dendron,* a tree] Surrounding a dendrite of a nerve cell.

**peridens** (pĕr′ĭ-dĕns) [″ + L. *dens,* tooth] A supernumerary tooth not situated in the dental arch.

**peridental** (pĕr″ĭ-dĕn′tăl) [″ + L. *dens,* tooth] Surrounding a tooth or part of one. SYN: *periodontal.*

**peridentitis** [″ + ″ + *itis,* inflammation] Inflammation of tissues surrounding a tooth. SYN: *periodontoclasia.*

**peridentium** (pĕr″ĭ-dĕn′tē-ŭm) [″ + L. *dens,* tooth] Periodontium.

**periderm** [″ + *derma,* skin] A thin layer of flattened cells forming a transient layer of embryonic epidermis. SYN: *epitrichial layer; epitrichium.*

**peridesmitis** (pĕr″ĭ-dĕz-mī′tĭs) [″ + *desmion,*

band, + *itis,* inflammation] Inflammation of the areolar tissue around a ligament.
**peridesmium** (pĕr″ĭ-dĕz′mē-ŭm) The connective tissue membrane sheathing a ligament.
**perididymis** (pĕr″ĭ-dĭd′ĭ-mĭs) [″ + *didymos,* testicle] The tunica vaginalis of the testicle.
**perididymitis** (pĕr″ĭ-dĭd″ĭ-mī′tĭs) [″ + ″ + *itis,* inflammation] Inflammation of the perididymis.
**peridiverticulitis** (pĕr″ĭ-dī″vĕr-tĭk″ū-lī′tĭs) [″ + L. *diverticulare,* to turn aside, + Gr. *itis,* inflammation] Inflammation of tissues situated around an intestinal diverticulum.
**periductal** (pĕr-ĭ-dŭk′tăl) [″ + L. *ductus,* a passage] Situated around a duct.
**periduodenitis** (pĕr″ĭ-dū″ō-dĕ-nī′tĭs) [″ + L. *duodeni,* twelve, + Gr. *itis,* inflammation] Inflammation around the duodenum, often causing adhesions attaching it to the peritoneum.
**peridural** (pĕr″ĭ-dū′răl) [″ + L. *durus,* hard] Outside the dura mater of the spinal cord.
**periencephalitis** (pĕr″ē-ĕn-sĕf″ă-lī′tĭs) [″ + *enkephalos,* brain, + *itis,* inflammation] Inflammation of the surface of the brain.
**periencephalomeningitis** (pĕr″ē-ĕn-sĕf″ă-lō-mĕn″ĭn-jī′tĭs) [″ + ″ + *meninx,* membrane, + *itis,* inflammation] Inflammation of the cerebral cortex and meninges.
**periendothelioma** (pĕr″ē-ĕn″dō-thē″lē-ō′mă) [″ + *endon,* within, + *thele,* nipple, + *oma,* tumor] A tumor arising from the endothelium of the lymphatics and the perithelium of blood vessels.
**perienteric** (pĕr″ē-ĕn-tĕr′ĭk) [Gr. *peri,* around, + *enteron,* intestine] Around the intestines.
**perienteritis** (pĕr″ē-ĕn″tĕr-ī′tĭs) [″ + ″ + *itis,* inflammation] Inflammation of the intestinal peritoneum.
**perienteron** (pĕr″ē-ĕn′tĕr-ŏn) [″ + *enteron,* intestine] The peritoneal cavity of the embryo.
**periependymal** (pĕr″ē-ĕp-ĕn′dĭ-măl) [″ + *ependyma,* an upper garment] Around the ependyma.
**periesophagitis** (pĕr″ē-ĕ-sŏf″ă-jī′tĭs) [″ + *oisophagos,* esophagus, + *itis,* inflammation] Inflammation of the tissues around the esophagus.
**perifistular** (pĕr-ĭ-fĭs′tū-lĕr) [″ + L. *fistula,* pipe] Located around a fistula.
**perifocal** (pĕr″ĭ-fō′kăl) [″ + L. *focus,* hearth] Around a focus, esp. around an infected focus.
**perifollicular** (pĕr″ĭ-fŏl-lĭk′ū-lăr) [″ + L. *folliculus,* a little sac] Around a follicle.
**perifolliculitis** (pĕr″ĭ-fō-lĭk″ū-lī′tĭs) [″ + ″ + Gr. *itis,* inflammation] Inflammation of an area around the hair follicles.
**perigangliitis** (pĕr″ĭ-găng″lē-ī′tĭs) [″ + *ganglion,* knot, + *itis,* inflammation] Inflammation of the region around a ganglion.
**periganglionic** (pĕr″ĭ-găng″glē-ŏn′ĭk) [″ + *ganglion,* knot] Around a ganglion.
**perigastric** (pĕr″ĭ-găs′trĭk) [″ + *gaster,* belly] Around the stomach.
**perigastritis** (pĕr″ĭ-găs-trī′tĭs) [″ + ″ + *itis,* inflammation] Inflammation of the peritoneal covering of the stomach.
**perigemmal** (pĕr″ĭ-jĕm′ăl) [″ + L. *gemma,* bud] Around any bud, esp. a taste bud.
**periglandulitis** (pĕr″ĭ-glăn″dū-lī′tĭs) [″ + L. *glandula,* small gland, + Gr. *itis,* inflammation] Inflammation of tissues around a gland.
**periglottic** (pĕr″ĭ-glŏt′ĭk) [″ + *glotta,* tongue] Around the base of the tongue and epiglottis.
**perihepatic** (pĕr″ĭ-hē-păt′ĭk) [Gr. *peri,* around, + *hepar,* liver] Around the liver.
**perihepatitis** (pĕr″ĭ-hĕp-ă-tī′tĭs) [″ + ″ + *itis,* inflammation] Inflammation of the peritoneal covering of the liver, usually occurring in circumscribed areas.
**perihernial** (pĕr″ĭ-hĕr′nē-ăl) [″ + L. *hernia,* rupture] Around a hernia.
**perijejunitis** (pĕr″ĭ-jē-jū-nī′tĭs) [″ + L. *jejunum,* empty, + Gr. *itis,* inflammation] Inflammation of tissues around the jejunum.
**perikaryon** (pĕr″ĭ-kăr′ē-ŏn) [″ + *karyon,* nucleus] The cell body of a neuron.
**perikeratic** (pĕr″ĭ-kĕr-ă′tĭk) [″ + *keras,* horn] About the cornea. SYN: *pericorneal.*
**perikymata** (pĕr″ĭ-kī′mă-tă) [″ + *kyma,* wave] The transverse wavelike grooves most apparent in the surface enamel of newly erupted anterior teeth; they are more pronounced at eruption and are reduced in depth with wear in advancing age.
**perilabyrinthitis** (pĕr″ĭ-lăb″ĭr-ĭn-thī′tĭs) [″ + *labyrinthos,* a maze of canals, + *itis,* inflammation] Inflammation of tissues around the labyrinth.
**perilaryngeal** (pĕr″ĭ-lă-rĭn′jē-ăl) [″ + *larynx,* larynx] Around the larynx.
**perilaryngitis** (pĕr″ĭ-lăr″ĭn-jī′tĭs) [″ + ″ + *itis,* inflammation] Inflammation of tissues around the larynx.
**perilenticular** (pĕr″ĭ-lĕn-tĭk′ū-lăr) [″ + L. *lenticularis,* pert. to a lens] Around the lens of the eye.
**periligamentous** (pĕr″ĭ-lĭg″ă-mĕn′tŭs) [″ + L. *ligamentum,* a band] Around a ligament.
**perilymph, perilympha** (pĕr′ĭ-lĭmf, pĕr″ĭ-lĭm′fă) [″ + L. *lympha,* serum] The pale, transparent fluid within the bony (not the membranous) labyrinth of the inner ear.
**perilymphangeal** (pĕr″ĭ-lĭm-făn′jē-ăl) [″ + ″ + Gr. *angeion,* vessel] Around a lymphatic vessel.
**perilymphangitis** (pĕr″ĭ-lĭmf-ăn-jī′tĭs) [″ + ″ + ″ + *itis,* inflammation] Inflammation of tissues around a lymphatic vessel.
**perimastitis** (pĕr″ĭ-măs-tī′tĭs) [″ + *mastos,* breast, + *itis,* inflammation] Inflammation of the fibrous tissue around a breast.
**perimeningitis** (pĕr″ĭ-mĕn″ĭn-jī′tĭs) [Gr. *peri,* around, + *meninx,* membrane, + *itis,* inflammation] Pachymeningitis.
**perimenopause** The phase prior to the onset of menopause, during which the

woman with regular menses changes, perhaps abruptly, to a pattern of irregular cycles and increased periods of amenorrhea. For epidemiological investigations, the inception of perimenopause is characterized by 3 to 11 months of amenorrhea or, for those without amenorrhea, increased menstrual irregularity. While menopause has a clear and accepted definition, perimenopause does not.

**perimeter** (pĕr-ĭm′ĕ-tĕr) [″ + *metron,* measure] **1.** The outer edge or periphery of a body or measure of the same. **2.** A device for determining the extent of the field of vision. SEE: *perimetry.*

**perimetric** (pĕr″ĭ-mĕt′rĭk) **1.** [″ + *metron,* measure] Concerning perimetry. **2.** [″ + *metra,* uterus] Around the uterus.

**perimetritic** (pĕr″ĭ-mē-trĭt′ĭk) [″ + *metra,* uterus, + *itis,* inflammation] Concerning perimetritis.

**perimetritis** (pĕr″ĭ-mē-trī′tĭs) [″ + ″ + *itis,* inflammation] Inflammation of the peritoneal covering of the uterus; may be associated with parametritis.

**perimetrium** (pĕr-ĭ-mē′trē-ŭm) The serous layer of the uterus.

**perimetry** (pĕr-ĭm′ĕ-trē) [″ + *metron,* measure] **1.** Circumference; edge; border of a body. **2.** Measurement of the scope of the field of vision with a perimeter.

**perimyelitis** (pĕr″ĭ-mī″ĕ-lī′tĭs) [″ + ″ + *itis,* inflammation] **1.** Inflammation of the pia mater and arachnoid of the brain or spinal cord. SYN: *leptomeningitis.* **2.** Inflammation of the endosteum or membrane around medullary cavity of a bone.

**perimyelography** (pĕr″ĭ-mī″ĕ-lŏg′ră-fē) [″ + ″ + *graphein,* to write] Radiological examination of the area around the spinal cord.

**perimyoendocarditis** (pĕr″ĭ-mī″ō-ĕn″dō-kăr-dī′tĭs) [″ + *mys,* muscle, + *endon,* within, + *kardia,* heart, + *itis,* inflammation] Inflammation of the muscular wall of the heart, its endothelial lining, and the pericardium.

**perimyositis** (pĕr″ĭ-mī″ō-sī′tĭs) [″ + ″ + *itis,* inflammation] Inflammation of the connective tissue around a muscle.

**perimysia** (pĕr″ĭ-mĭs′ē-ă) Pl. of perimysium.

**perimysial** (pĕr-ĭ-mĭs′ē-ăl) Concerning, or of the nature of, the fibrous sheath of a muscle.

**perimysiitis** (pĕr″ĭ-mĭs″ē-ī′tĭs) [″ + *mys,* muscle, + *itis,* inflammation] Inflammation of the sheath surrounding a muscle.

**perimysium** (pĕr″ĭ-mĭs′ē-ŭm) *pl.* **perimysia** A connective tissue sheath that envelops each primary bundle of muscle fibers; sometimes called perimysium internum.

***p. externum*** The epimysium.

**perinatal** (pĕr″ĭ-nā′tăl) [Gr. *peri,* around, + L. *natalis,* birth] Concerning the period beginning after the 28th week of pregnancy and ending 28 days after birth.

**perinatology** The study of the fetus and infant during the perinatal period. SEE: *perinatal.*

**perineal** (pĕr″ĭ-nē′ăl) [Gr. *perinaion,* perineum] Concerning, or situated on, the perineum.

**perineo-** [Gr. *perinaion*] Combining form meaning *perineum.*

**perineocele** (pĕr″ĭ-nē′ō-sēl) [Gr. *perinaion,* perineum, + *kele,* tumor, swelling] A hernia in the region of the perineum, between the rectum and vagina or between the rectum and prostate. SYN: *perineal hernia.*

**perineocolporectomyomectomy** (pĕr″ĭ-nē-ō-kŏl″pō-rĕk″tō-mī″ō-mĕk′tō-mē) [″ + *kolpos,* vagina, + L. *rectus,* straight, + Gr. *mys,* muscle, + *oma,* tumor, + *ektome,* excision] Excision of a myoma by incising the perineum, vagina, and rectum.

**perineometer** (pĕr″ĭ-nē-ŏm′ĕ-ter) [Gr. *perinaion,* perineum, + *metron,* measure] An apparatus for measuring the pressure or force that is produced in the vagina when the pubococcygeus and levator ani muscles are contracted voluntarily. SEE: *Kegel exercises.*

**perineoplasty** (pĕr″ĭ-nē′ō-plăs″tē) [″ + *plassein,* to form] Reparative surgery on the perineum.

**perineorrhaphy** (pĕr″ĭ-nē-or′ă-fē) [″ + *rhaphe,* a sewing] Suture of the perineum to repair a laceration that occurs or is made surgically during the delivery of the fetus.

NURSING IMPLICATIONS: Infections are prevented by thorough irrigation of the perineum with warm, sterile saline after urination and defecation. The nurse should ensure that the washing solution drains down toward the anal area and should blot the area dry with sterile cotton. Sutures are kept clean and dry. The perineum is assessed daily for signs of infection. A heat lamp is used several times a day to dry area and to promote healing. Application of an ice bag so that weight is on the bed and not on the vulva and perineum may help to relieve pain. Ambulation is encouraged. The patient is assessed daily for bowel movement, and diet and fluid intake are adjusted to prevent constipation. The nurse should provide support and reassurance because the patient may experience anxiety about the ability to resume normal physical functions and sexual activity and should provide opportunities for the patient to express feelings and to ask questions.

***anterior p.*** Surgical repair of anterior perineum and vaginal wall to correct a cystocele.

***posterior p.*** The removal and repair of a rectocele.

**perineoscrotal** (pĕr″ĭ-nē-ō-skrō′tăl) [″ + L. *scrotum,* a bag] Concerning the perineum and scrotum.

**perineotomy** (pĕr″ĭ-nē-ŏt′ō-mē) [″ + *tome,* incision] Surgical incision into the perineum. SYN: *perineal section.*

**perineovaginal** (pĕr″ĭ-nē″ō-văj′ĭn-ăl) [″ + L. *vagina,* sheath] Concerning the perineum and vagina.

**perinephrial** (pĕr″ĭ-nĕf′rē-ăl) Concerning the perinephrium.

**perinephric** (pĕr″ĭ-nĕf′rĭk) [Gr. *peri,* around, + *nephros,* kidney] Located or occurring around the kidney.

**perinephritis** (pĕr″ĭ-nĕ-frī′tĭs) [″ + ″ + *itis,* inflammation] Inflammation of peritoneal tissues around the kidney. SYN: *paranephritis* (2).

**perinephrium** (pĕr″ĭ-nĕf′rē-ŭm) The connective and fatty tissue surrounding the kidney.

**perineum** (pĕr″ĭ-nē′ŭm) [Gr. *perinaion*] **1.** The structures occupying the pelvic outlet and constituting the pelvic floor. **2.** The external region between the vulva and anus in a female or between the scrotum and anus in a male. It is made up of skin, muscle, and fasciae. The muscles of the perineum are the anterior portion of the intact levator ani muscle, the transverse perineal muscle, and the pubococcygeus muscle. SEE: illus.; *body, perineal.*

***tears of the p.*** Laceration of the perineum during delivery. There are four degrees of severity caused by overstretching of the vagina and perineum during delivery. Fetal malposition increases the chance of tears occurring.

A first-degree tear involves superficial tissues of the perineum and vaginal mucosa but does not injure muscular tissue. A second-degree tear involves those tissues included in a first-degree tear and the muscles of the perineum but not the muscles of the anal sphincter. A third-degree tear involves all of the tissues of the second-degree tear and the muscles of the anal sphincter. A fourth-degree tear extends completely through the perineal skin, vaginal mucosa, perineal body, anal sphincter muscles, and the rectal mucosa.

Complications include hemorrhage, infection, cystocele, rectocele, descent of uterus, and perhaps loss of bowel control. Surgery is necessary to treat this condition.

PERINEUM
LABIA MAJORA
PREPUCE OF CLITORIS
LABIA MINORA
CLITORIS
VESTIBULE OF ENTRANCE TO VAGINA
ANUS
URETHRAL ORIFICE
HYMEN
POSTERIOR LABIAL COMMISSURE
VAGINAL ORIFICE

**perineural** (pĕr″ĭ-nū′răl) [Gr. *peri,* around, + *neuron,* nerve] Around a nerve.

**perineurial** (pĕr″ĭ-nū′rē-ăl) [″ + *neuron,* sinew] Concerning the perineurium, the sheath around a bundle of nerve fibers.

**perineuritis** (pĕr″ĭ-nū-rī′tĭs) [″ + ″ + *itis,* inflammation] Inflammation of the sheath enveloping nerve fibers.

**perineurium** (pĕr″ĭ-nū′rē-ŭm) [″ + *neuron,* sinew] A connective tissue sheath investing a fasciculus or bundle of nerve fibers.

**perinuclear** (pĕr″ĭ-nū′klē-ăr) [″ + L. *nucleus,* a kernel] Around a nucleus.

**periocular** (pĕr″ē-ŏk′ū-lăr) [″ + L. *oculus,* eye] Located around the eye. SYN: *circumocular.*

**period** [L. *periodus*] **1.** The interval of time between two successive occurrences of any regularly recurring phenomenon or event; a cycle. **2.** The menses. **3.** Time occupied by a disease in running its course, or by a stage of a disease, such as an incubation period.

***absolute refractory p.*** Following contraction of a muscle or transmission of a nerve impulse by a neuron, the period in which a stimulus, no matter how strong, will not elicit a response.

***childbearing p.*** The period in the female during which she is capable of procreation; puberty to the menopause.

***critical p.*** **1.** The phase of the life cycle during which cells are responsive to certain regulators. **2.** The time during gestation when important organ systems are being formed and the fetus is most vulnerable to environmental factors that may cause deformities.

***effective refractory p.*** Used in electrocardiography; the interval during which a second action potential cannot occur in an excitable fiber unless the stimulus is much stronger than usual; the membrane is still in the repolarization phase of the previous action potential.

***ejection p.*** Sphygmic p.

***fertile p.*** The time during the menstrual cycle when the ovum can be fertilized.

***gestation p.*** The period of pregnancy from conception to parturition. Average length is 10 lunar months or 280 days, measured from the onset of the last menstrual period, but length varies from 250 to 310 days. SEE: *gestation; pregnancy* for table.

***incubation p.*** The time from the moment of infection to the appearance of the first symptom.

***isoelectric p.*** In an occurrence that normally produces an electric force, such as a muscle contraction, the time or point when no electric energy is produced. In an electrocardiogram, the period when the electrical tracing is at zero and is neither positive nor negative.

***isometric p.*** Postsphygmic p.

***last menstrual p.*** ABBR: LMP. The date of the first day of menstruation before the advent of pregnancy-related anemorrhea; used in estimating the expected date of delivery. SEE: *Naegele's rule*.

***latency p.*** The time from the stimulus to the response of the tissue stimulated.

***latent p.*** **1.** The time between stimulation and the resulting response. SYN: *lag phase*. **2.** The time during which a disease is supposed to be existent without manifesting itself; period of incubation. **3.** The time from exposure to ionizing radiation to the first visible sign of the effects.

***menstrual p.*** Menstruation.

***missed p.*** Menstruation not occurring at the time it was expected.

***monthly p.*** The time of menstrual flow.

***neonatal p.*** The first 30 days of infant life.

***patent p.*** The time in a parasitic disease during which organisms are demonstrable in the body.

***postsphygmic p.*** The short period in diastole when the ventricles are relaxed and no blood is entering. This lasts until the atrioventricular valves open. SYN: *isometric p.*

***presphygmic p.*** The short period in systole beginning with closing of the atrioventricular valves and ending with opening of the valves connecting the right and left ventricles to the pulmonary artery and aorta, respectively.

***puerperal p.*** The interval of time from the birth of a child to approx. 6 weeks later, at which time complete involution of the uterus has occurred.

***p. of reactivity*** In obstetrics, an initial episode of activity, alertness, and responsiveness to interaction, characteristic of newborn physiological and social response to stimuli. The first period of reactivity begins with birth, lasts approx. 30 min, and ends when the infant falls into a deep sleep. Common assessment findings include transient tachypnea, nasal flaring, sternal retraction, crackles, tachycardia, and irregular heart rhythms. The second period of reactivity begins when the infant awakens and usually lasts 4 to 6 hr. Common assessment findings include signs of excessive respiratory and gastric mucus, hunger, apneic episodes, and the passing of a meconium stool.

***relative refractory p.*** The period after activation of a nerve or muscle, during recovery, when it can be excited only by a stronger-than-normal stimulus.

***safe p.*** The time during the menstrual cycle when conception is allegedly not possible. Because of the great variability of the menstrual cycle, it is either extremely difficult or impossible to predict the portion of the cycle in which intercourse may take place and be "safe" from conception.

***silent p.*** **1.** The time in the course of a disease in which the signs and symptoms are so mild as to be difficult to detect. **2.** A pause in normally continuous electrical events such as an ECG or EEG.

***sphygmic p.*** The period in the cardiac cycle when the blood is being ejected into the arterial system. SYN: *ejection p.*

**periodic** (pēr-ē-ŏd′ĭk) [Gr. *periodikos*] Recurring after definite intervals.

**periodic health examination** A health screening examination done according to a regular schedule. The effectiveness of providing a periodic health examination for healthy individuals is controversial. This is not the case for individuals who have a family history of a potentially lethal disease such as colorectal cancer.

As medical progress occurs and techniques employed in this type of examination are refined and have greater degrees of sensitivity and specificity, the periodic health examination will have greater importance.

**periodicity** (pēr″ē-ō-dĭs′ĭ-tē) **1.** The state of being regularly recurrent. **2.** The rate of rise and fall or interruption of a unidirectional current in physical therapy.

**periodic leg movements** Leg movements, originally called nocturnal myoclonus, that consist of repetitive movements occurring every 20 to 40 sec during sleep. Movements usually include extension of the great toe, sometimes followed by flexion of the hip, knee, or ankle. These movements may not be apparent to the patient, yet they are associated with a variety of sleep disturbances. They are not the same as the gross jerks that occur in some normal patients at the time they are falling asleep. Many patients with the restless legs syndrome also have periodic leg movements.

**periodic table** A chart with the chemical elements arranged by their atomic numbers according to the periodic law. SEE: *law, periodic*.

**periodontal** (pĕr″ē-ō-dŏn′tăl) [Gr. *peri*, around, + *odous*, tooth] Located around a tooth. SYN: *peridental*.

***p. disease*** A disease of the supporting structures of the teeth, the periodontium, including alveolar bone to which the teeth are anchored. The most common symptom is bleeding gums, but loosening of the teeth, receding gums, abscesses in pockets between the gums and the teeth, and necrotizing ulcerative gingivitis may be present as the disease process continues. Proper dental hygiene, including proper brushing of the teeth, use of dental floss, and periodic removal of plaque by a dentist or dental hygienist, will help to prevent periodontal disease.

TREATMENT: In the early stages of the disease, curettage of the irritating material—plaque and calculus (tartar)—from the crown and root surfaces of the teeth may be the only treatment required. In more advanced stages, procedures such as gingivectomy, gingivoplasty, and correction of the bony architecture of the teeth may be required. Adjustment of the occlusion of the teeth and orthodontic treatment may be used in order to help prevent recurrences. SEE: *plaque; teeth; tooth; toothbrushing.*

NURSING IMPLICATIONS: The nurse teaches the patient about the importance of proper dental care, including brushing, flossing, and regular dental examinations and prophylaxis. Patients should consult a dentist if recession of teeth from gums, any drainage from gums, or bleeding gums occur, because these symptoms may indicate periodontal disease.

**periodontia** (pĕr″ē-ō-dŏn′shē-ă) [Gr. *peri,* around, + *odous,* tooth] **1.** Plural of periodontium. **2.** The study and treatment of diseases of the periodontal tissues. SYN: *periodontology.*

**periodontics** (pĕr″ē-ō-dŏn′tĭks) [″ + *odous,* tooth] Periodontia (2).

**periodontitis** (pĕr″ē-ō-dŏn-tī′tĭs) [″ + ″ + *itis,* inflammation] Inflammation or degeneration, or both, of the dental periosteum, alveolar bone, cementum, and adjacent gingiva. Suppuration usually occurs, supporting bone is resorbed, teeth become loose, and recession of gingivae occurs. This condition usually follows chronic gingivitis, Vincent's infection, or poor dental hygiene. Systemic factors may predispose one to this condition. SYN: *pyorrhea alveolaris; Riggs' disease.*

***apical p.*** Periodontitis of the periapical region usually leading to formation of periapical abscess.

**periodontium** (pĕr-ē-ō-dŏn′shē-ŭm) The structures that support the teeth, cushion the shock of chewing, and keep the teeth firmly anchored in the bone. These structures are the gingivae, periodontal membrane or ligament, cementum, and alveolar bone.

**periodontoclasia** (pĕr″ē-ō-dŏn″tō-klā′zē-ă) [″ + *odous,* tooth, + *klasis,* breaking] A condition characterized by inflammation accompanied by degenerative and retrogressive changes in the periodontium. SYN: *peridentitis.*

**periodontology** (pĕr″ē-ō-dŏn-tŏl′ō-jē) [″ + ″ + *logos,* word, reason] The branch of dentistry dealing with treatment of diseases of the tissues around the teeth.

**periodontosis** (pĕr″ē-ō-dŏn-tō′sĭs) [″ + ″ + *osis,* condition] Any degenerative disease of the periodontal tissues.

**periodoscope** (pĕr″ē-ŏd′ō-skōp) [LL. *periodus,* interval of time, + *skopein,* to examine] A table or dial for the calculation of the expected date of delivery. SEE: *pregnancy* for table.

**periomphalic** (pĕr″ē-ŏm-făl′ĭk) [Gr. *peri,* around, + *omphalos,* navel] Located around or near the umbilicus.

**perionychia** (pĕr″ē-ō-nĭk′ē-ă) [″ + *onyx,* nail] Inflammation around a nail.

**perionychium** (pĕr″ē-ō-nĭk′ē-ŭm) The epidermis surrounding a nail.

**perionyx** (pĕr″ē-ō′nĭks) [″ + *onyx,* nail] The remnant of the eponychium that persists as a band across the root of the nail.

**perionyxis** (pĕr″ē-ō-nĭk′sĭs) Inflammation of the epidermis surrounding a nail.

**perioophoritis** (pĕr″ē-ō-ŏf″ō-rī′tĭs) [″ + *oophoron,* ovary, + *itis,* inflammation] Inflammation of the surface membrane of the ovary. SYN: *perioothecitis; periovaritis.*

**perioophorosalpingitis** (pĕr″ē-ō-ŏf″ō-rō-săl″pĭn-jī′tĭs) [″ + ″ + *salpinx,* tube, + *itis,* inflammation] Inflammation of the tissues around an ovary and oviduct. SYN: *perioothecosalpingitis; perisalpingoovaritis.*

**perioothecitis** (pĕr″ē-ō″ō-thē-sī′tĭs) [″ + *oon,* egg, + *theke,* box, + *itis,* inflammation] Perioophoritis.

**perioothecosalpingitis** (pĕr″ē-ō″ō-thē″kō-săl-pĭn-jī′tĭs) [″+ ″ + ″ + *salpinx,* tube, + *itis,* inflammation] Perioophorosalpingitis.

**perioperative** Occurring in the period immediately before, during, and immediately after surgery.

**perioperative positioning injury, risk for** A state in which the client is at risk for injury as a result of the environmental conditions found in the perioperative setting. SEE: *Nursing Diagnoses Appendix.*

**periophthalmic** (pĕr″ē-ŏf-thăl′mĭk) [″ + *ophthalmos,* eye] Around the eye.

**perioral** (pĕr″ē-or′ăl) [″ + L. *oralis,* mouth] Surrounding the mouth. SYN: *circumoral.*

**periorbita** (pĕr″ē-or′bĭ-tă) [″ + L. *orbita,* orbit] Connective tissue covering the socket of the eye.

**periorbital** (pĕr″ē-or′bĭ-tăl) Surrounding the socket of the eye. SYN: *circumorbital.*

**periorbititis** (pĕr″ē-or″bĭ-tī′tĭs) [″+ L. *orbita,* orbit, + Gr. *itis,* inflammation] Inflammation of the periorbita.

**periorchitis** (pĕr″ē-or-kī′tĭs) [″ + *orchis,* testicle, + *itis,* inflammation] Inflammation of the tissues investing a testicle.

***p. hemorrhagica*** A chronic hematocele of the tunica vaginalis coat of the testis.

**periosteal** (pĕr-ē-ŏs′tē-ăl) [″+ *osteon,* bone] Concerning the periosteum. SYN: *periosteous.*

**periosteitis** (pĕr″ē-ŏs″tē-ī′tĭs) [″ + ″ + *itis,* inflammation] Periostitis.

**periosteoedema** (pĕr″ē-ŏs″tē-ō-ĕ-dē′mă) [Gr. *peri,* around, + *osteon,* bone, + *oidema,* swelling] Edema of the periosteum, the membrane surrounding a bone.

**periosteoma** (pĕr″ē-ŏs-tē-ō′mă) [″ + ″ + *oma,* tumor] **1.** An abnormal growth surrounding a bone. **2.** A tumor of the periosteum, the tissue surrounding a bone.

**periosteomyelitis** (pĕr″ē-ŏs″tē-ō-mī″ĕ-lī′tĭs) [″ + ″ + *myelos,* marrow, + *itis,* inflammation] Inflammation of bone, including the periosteum and marrow. SYN: *periostomedullitis.*

**periosteophyte** (pĕr″ē-ŏs′tē-ō-fīt) [″ + *osteon,* bone, + *phyton,* growth] An abnormal bony growth on the periosteum, or arising from it.

**periosteorrhaphy** (pĕr″ē-ŏs″tē-or′ă-fē) [″ + ″ + *rhaphe,* seam, ridge] Joining by suture the margins of a severed periosteum.

**periosteotome** (pĕr″ē-ŏs′tē-ō-tōm) [″+ *osteon,* bone, + *tome,* incision] An instrument for cutting the periosteum or removing it from the bone.

**periosteotomy** (pĕr″ē-ŏs-tē-ŏt′ō-mē) Incision into the periosteum.

**periosteous** (pĕr″ē-ŏs′tē-ŭs) [″ + *osteon,* bone] Periosteal.

**periosteum** (pĕr-ē-ŏs′tē-ŭm) [Gr. *periosteon*] The fibrous membrane that forms the investing covering of bones except at their articular surfaces; consists of a dense external layer containing numerous blood vessels and an inner layer of connective tissue cells that function as osteoblasts when the bone is injured and then participate in new bone formation. Periosteum serves as a supporting structure for blood vessels nourishing bone and for attachment of muscles, tendons, and ligaments. It extends over the whole surface except at the cartilaginous articulations.

***alveolar p.*** The periodontal ligament.

***p. externum*** Periosteum covering external surfaces of bones.

***p. internum*** Interior periosteum lining the medullary canal of a bone.

**periostitis** (pĕr″ē-ŏs-tī′tĭs) [″ + *itis,* inflammation] Inflammation of the periosteum, the membrane investing a bone. Symptoms include pain over the affected part, esp. under pressure; fever; sweats; leukocytosis; skin inflammation, and rigidity of overlying muscles. Infectious diseases, esp. syphilis, and trauma cause this condition. SYN: *periosteitis.*

***albuminous p.*** Periostitis with albuminous serous fluid exudate beneath the membrane affected.

***alveolar p.*** Periodontitis.

***diffuse p.*** Periostitis of the long bones.

***hemorrhagic p.*** Periostitis with extravasation of blood under the periosteum.

**periostoma** (pĕr″ē-ŏs-tō′mă) [Gr. *peri,* around, + *osteon,* bone, + *oma,* tumor] A bony neoplasm around a bone or arising from its membranous sheath.

**periostomedullitis** (pĕr″ē-ŏs″tō-mĕd-ū-lī′tĭs) [″ + ″ + L. *medulla,* marrow, + Gr. *itis,* inflammation] Periosteomyelitis.

**periostosis** (pĕr″ē-ŏs-tō′sĭs) [″ + ″ + *osis,* condition] A bony neoplasm around a bone or arising from it.

**periostosteitis** (pĕr″ē-ŏs-tŏs″tē-ī′tĭs) [″ + ″ + *osteon,* bone, + *itis,* inflammation] Osteoperiostitis.

**periostotome** (pĕr″ē-ŏs′tō-tōm) [″ + ″ + *tome,* incision] Periosteotome.

**periostotomy** (pĕr″ē-ŏs-tŏt′ō-mē) [″ + ″ + *tome,* incision] Periosteotomy.

**periotic** (pĕr-ē-ō′tĭk) [″ + *ous,* ear] Situated around the ear, esp. the internal ear.

***p. bone*** The mastoid and petrous portions of the temporal bone.

**periovaritis** (pĕr″ē-ō″vă-rī′tĭs) [″ + L. *ovarium,* ovary, + Gr. *itis,* inflammation] Perioophoritis.

**periovular** (pĕr″ē-ō′vū-lăr) [″ + L. *ovulum,* little egg] Around an ovum.

**peripachymeningitis** (pĕr″ĭ-pak″ē-mĕn″ĭn-jī′tĭs) [″ + *pachys,* thick, + *meninx,* membrane, + *itis,* inflammation] Inflammation of the connective tissue between the dura mater and the bone that encloses the central nervous system.

**peripancreatitis** (pĕr″ĭ-păn″krē-ă-tī′tĭs) [″ + *pankreas,* pancreas, + *itis,* inflammation] Inflammation of the tissues around the pancreas.

**peripapillary** (pĕr″ĭ-păp′ĭ-lĕr″ē) [″ + L. *papilla,* nipple] Around a papilla.

**peripatetic** (pĕr″ĭ-pă-tĕt′ĭk) [L. *peripateticus,* to walk about while teaching] Moving from place to place.

**peripenial** (pĕr″ĭ-pē′nē-ăl) [Gr. *peri,* around, + L. *penis,* penis] Around the penis.

**periphacitis** (pĕr-ĭ-fă-sī′tĭs) [″ + *phakos,* lens, + *itis,* inflammation] Inflammation of the capsule of the lens of the eye.

**periphakus** (pĕr″ĭ-fā′kŭs) The elastic capsule surrounding the lens of the eye.

**peripharyngeal** (pĕr″ĭ-fă-rĭn′jē-ăl) [″ + *pharynx,* throat] Around the pharynx.

**peripherad** (pĕr-ĭf′ĕr-ăd) [″ + *pherein,* to bear, + L. *ad,* to] In the direction of the periphery.

**peripheral** (pĕr-ĭf′ĕr-ăl) Located at, or pert. to, the periphery; occurring away from the center.

**peripheral nervous system** ABBR: PNS. The portion of the nervous system outside the central nervous system: the 12 pairs of cranial nerves and 31 pairs of spinal nerves. These nerves contain sensory and somatic motor fibers and the motor fibers of the autonomic nervous system.

**peripheral neurovascular dysfunction, risk for** A state for which an individual is at risk of experiencing a disruption in circulation, sensation, or motion of an extremity. SEE: *Nursing Diagnoses Appendix.*

**peripheral vascular disease** ABBR: PVD. An imprecise term indicating diseases of the arteries and veins of the extremities, esp. those conditions that interfere with adequate flow of blood to or from the extremities, such as atherosclerosis with narrowing of the arterial lumen. SEE: *Nursing Diagnoses Appendix.*

**peripheraphose** (pĕr-ĭf′ĕr-ă-fōs) A subjective sensation of darkness or shadow that originates in the peripheral optic structures (optic nerve or eyeball).

**peripherocentral** (pĕ-rĭf″ĕr-ō-sĕn′trăl) [″ +

*pherein,* to bear, + *kentron,* center] Concerning both the periphery and central part of an organ.

**peripherophose** (per-ĭf'ĕr-ō-fōs) A subjective sensation of light or color that originates in the peripheral optic structures (optic nerve or eyeball).

**periphery** (pĕr-ĭf'ĕ-rē) [Gr. *periphereia*] The outer part or surface of a body; the part away from the center.

**periphlebitis** (pĕr"ĭ-flĕ-bī'tĭs) [Gr. *peri,* around, + *phleps,* vein, + *itis,* inflammation] Inflammation of the external coat of a vein or tissues around it.

**periphoria** (pĕr-ĭ-fō'rē-ă) [" + *phoros,* bearing] The tendency of the axis of the eye to deviate from the normal owing to weakness of oblique muscles. SYN: *cyclophoria.*

**periphrastic** (pĕr"ĭ-frăs'tĭk) [Gr. *periphrastikos*] Relating to the use of superfluous words in expressing a thought; which appears in the writings and speech of some schizophrenics.

**periphrenitis** (pĕr"ĭ-frē-nī'tĭs) [Gr. *peri,* around, + *phren,* diaphragm, + *itis,* inflammation] Inflammation of the structures around the diaphragm.

**Periplaneta** (pĕr"ĭ-plă-nē'tă) A genus of cockroaches belonging to the order Orthoptera. Roaches contaminate food by mechanically transporting disease-producing bacteria, ova, and protozoa to the food.

***P. americana*** The American cockroach.

***P. australasiae*** The Austrialian cockroach.

**periplast** (pĕr'ĭ-plăst) [" + *plassein,* to form] The peripheral protoplasm of a cell exclusive of the nucleus.

**peripleural** (pĕr"ĭ-plū'răl) [" + *pleura,* rib] Encircling the pleura.

**peripleuritis** (pĕr-ĭ-plū-rī'tĭs) [" + " + *itis,* inflammation] Inflammation of the connective tissues between the pleura and wall of the chest.

**peripolar** (pĕr"ĭ-pō'lăr) [" + L. *polus,* pole] Around a pole.

**peripolesis** (pĕr"ĭ-pō-lē'sĭs) [Gr., a going about] In tissue culture, the collecting of lymphocytes around macrophages.

**periporitis** (pĕr"ĭ-por-ī'tĭs) [Gr. *peri,* around, + L. *porus,* pore, + Gr. *itis*] Multiple abscesses around sweat glands, esp. as a complication of malaria in children.

**periportal** (pĕr"ĭ-por'tăl) [" + L. *porta,* gate] Around the portal vein and its branches.

**periproctic** (pĕr"ĭ-prŏk'tĭk) [" + *proktos,* anus] Around the anus.

**periproctitis** (pĕr"ĭ-prŏk-tī'tĭs) [" + " + *itis,* inflammation] Inflammation of the areolar tissues in the region of the rectum and anus. SYN: *perirectitis.*

**periprostatic** (pĕr"ĭ-prŏs-tăt'ĭk) [" + *prostates,* prostate] Surrounding or occurring about the prostate.

**periprostatitis** (pĕr"ĭ-prŏs-tă-tī'tĭs) [" + " + *itis,* inflammation] Inflammation of the tissues surrounding the prostate.

**peripylephlebitis** (pĕr"ĭ-pī"lē-flĕ-bī'tĭs) [" + *pyle,* gate, + *phlebos,* vein, + *itis,* inflammation] Inflammation of tissues about the portal vein.

**peripyloric** (pĕr"ĭ-pī-lor'ĭk) [" + *pyloros,* pylorus] Extending around the pylorus.

**periradicular** Around a root or a rootlike process, esp. relating to a tooth.

**perirectal** (pĕr"ĭ-rĕk'tăl) [" + L. *rectus,* straight] Extending around the rectum.

**perirectitis** (pĕr"ĭ-rĕk-tī'tĭs) [" + " + Gr. *itis,* inflammation] Periproctitis.

**perirenal** (pĕr"ĭ-rē'năl) [" + L. *ren,* kidney] Extending around the kidney. SYN: *circumrenal; perinephric.*

**perirhinal** (pĕr"ĭ-rī'năl) [" + *rhis,* nose] Located about the nose or nasal fossae.

**perirhizoclasia** (pĕr"ĭ-rī"zō-klā'zē-ă) [" + *rhiza,* root, + *klasis,* destruction] Inflammation and destruction of tissues extending around the roots of a tooth.

**perisalpingitis** (pĕr"ĭ-săl"pĭn-jī'tĭs) [" + *salpinx,* tube, + *itis,* inflammation] Inflammation of peritoneal coat about the oviduct.

**perisalpingoovaritis** (pĕr"ĭ-săl-pĭn"gō-ō"văr-ī'tĭs) [" + " + L. *ovarium,* ovary, + Gr. *itis,* inflammation] Perioophorosalpingitis.

**perisalpinx** (pĕr"ĭ-săl'pĭnks) [" + *salpinx,* tube] The peritoneum covering the upper borders of the uterine tubes.

**perisclerium** (pĕr"ĭ-sklē'rē-ŭm) [" + *skleros,* hard] Fibrous tissue encircling ossifying cartilage.

**periscopic** (pĕr"ĭ-skŏp'ĭk) [" + *skopein,* to examine] Viewing on all sides; providing a wide range of vision.

**perisigmoiditis** (pĕr"ĭ-sĭg"moy-dī'tĭs) [Gr. *peri,* around, + *sigma,* Gr. letter S, + *eidos,* form, shape, + *itis,* inflammation] Inflammation of peritoneal tissues around the sigmoid flexure of the colon.

**perisinuous** Adjacent to or around a sinus.

**perisinusitis** (pĕr"ĭ-sī"nŭ-sī'tĭs) [" + L. *sinus,* cavity, + Gr. *itis,* inflammation] Inflammation of membranes about a sinus, esp. a venous sinus of the dura mater.

**perispermatitis** (pĕr"ĭ-spĕr"mă-tī'tĭs) [" + *sperma,* seed, + *itis,* inflammation] Inflammation of tissues about the spermatic cord.

***p. serosa*** Hydrocele of the spermatic cord.

**perisplanchnic** (pĕr"ĭ-splănk'nĭk) [" + *splanchnon,* viscus] Extending around a viscus or the viscera.

**perisplanchnitis** (pĕr"ĭ-splănk-nī'tĭs) [" + " + *itis,* inflammation] Perivisceritis.

**perisplenic** (pĕr"ĭ-splĕn'ĭk) [" + *splen,* spleen] Near or around the spleen.

**perisplenitis** (pĕr"ĭ-splĕ-nī'tĭs) [" + " + *itis,* inflammation] Inflammation of the peritoneal coat of the spleen, the splenic capsule.

***p. cartilaginea*** Inflammation of the capsule of the spleen resulting in thickening and hardening.

**perispondylic** (pĕr"ĭ-spŏn-dĭl'ĭk) [Gr. *peri,* around, + *spondylos,* vertebra] Around a vertebra.

**perispondylitis** (pĕr″ĭ-spŏn-dĭl-ī′tĭs) [″ + ″ + *itis,* inflammation] Inflammation of the parts around a vertebra.

**perissodactylous** (pĕr-ĭs″sō-dăk′tĭ-lŭs) [Gr. *perissos,* odd, + *daktylos,* digit] Having an odd number of digits on a hand or foot. SYN: *imparidigitate.*

**peristalsis** (pĕr-ĭ-stăl′sĭs) [Gr. *peri,* around, + *stalsis,* contraction] A progressive wavelike movement that occurs involuntarily in hollow tubes of the body, esp. the alimentary canal. It is characteristic of tubes possessing longitudinal and circular layers of smooth muscle fibers.

Peristalsis is induced reflexly by distention of the walls of the tube. The wave consists of contraction of the circular muscle above the distention with relaxation of the region immediately distal to the distended portion. The simultaneous contraction and relaxation progresses slowly for a short distance as a wave that causes the contents of the tube to be forced onward.

***mass p.*** Forced peristaltic movements of short duration in which contents are moved from one section of the colon to another, occurring three or four times daily.

***reverse p.*** Peristalsis in a direction opposite to the normal direction. SYN: *antiperistalsis.*

**peristaltic** (pĕr″ĭ-stăl′tĭk) Concerning, or of the nature of, peristalsis.

**peristaphyline** (pĕr″ĭ-stăf′ĭ-lĭn) [″ + *staphyle,* uvula] About the uvula.

**peristasis** (pĕr-rĭs′tă-sĭs) [″ + *stasis,* standing] **1.** In the early stage of inflammation, the decrease in blood flow in the affected area. **2.** Environment.

**peristomatous** (pĕr″ĭ-stŏm′ă-tŭs) [″ + *stoma,* mouth] Around the mouth.

**peristome** (pĕr′ĭ-stōm) [″ + *stoma,* mouth] The channel leading to the cytosome or mouth in certain types of protozoa.

**peristrumitis** (pĕr″ĭ-stroo-mī′tĭs) [″ + L. *struma,* goiter, + *itis,* inflammation] Perithyroiditis.

**peristrumous** (pĕr″ĭ-stroo′mŭs) [″ + L. *struma,* goiter] Around a goiter.

**perisynovial** (pĕr″ĭ-sĭ-nō′vē-ăl) [Gr. *peri,* around, + L. *synovia,* joint fluid] Extending around a synovial structure.

**perisystole** (pĕr″ĭ-sĭs′tō-lē) [″ + *systole,* contraction] Presystole.

**peritectomy** (pĕr″ĭ-tĕk′tō-mē) [″ + *ektome,* excision] Surgical removal of a ring of conjunctiva around the cornea.

**peritendineum** (pĕr″ĭ-tĕn-dĭn′ē-ŭm) [″ + L. *tendo,* tendon] A sheath of fibrous connective tissue investing a fiber bundle of a tendon.

**peritendinitis, peritenonitis** (pĕr″ĭ-tĕn″dĭ-nī′tĭs, -tĕn″ō-nī′tĭs) [″ + ″ + Gr. *itis,* inflammation] Tenosynovitis.

***p. calcarea*** The deposition of calcareous material in tendons and associated regions, characterized by pain, tenderness, and limitation of motion.

***p. serosa*** Peritendinitis with effusion into the sheath.

**peritenon** (pĕr″ĭ-tē′nŏn) [″ + *tenon,* tendon] **1.** The sheath of a tendon. **2.** Peritendineum.

**perithelioma** (pĕr″ĭ-thē-lē-ō′mă) [″ + *thele,* nipple, + *oma,* tumor] A tumor derived from the perithelial layer of the blood vessels.

**perithelium** (pĕr″ĭ-thē′lē-ŭm) The fibrous outer layer of the smaller blood vessels and capillaries.

***Eberth's p.*** An incomplete layer of cells covering capillaries.

**perithoracic** (pĕr″ĭ-thō-răs′ĭk) [″ + *thorax,* chest] Around the thorax.

**perithyroiditis** (pĕr″ĭ-thī-roy-dī′tĭs) [″ + *thyreos,* shield, + *eidos,* form, shape, + *itis,* inflammation] Inflammation of capsule or tissues sheathing the thyroid gland. SYN: *peristrumitis.*

**peritomy** (pĕr-ĭt′ō-mē) [″ + *tome,* incision] **1.** Excision of a narrow strip of conjunctiva around the cornea in the treatment of pannus. SYN: *syndectomy.* **2.** Circumcision.

**peritoneal** (pĕr″ĭ-tō-nē′ăl) [Gr. *peritonaion,* peritoneum] Concerning the peritoneum.

***p. fluid*** The clear straw-colored serous fluid secreted by the cells of the peritoneum. The few milliliters present in the peritoneal cavity moisten the surfaces of the viscera and allow them to glide over each other as the intestinal tract changes shape during the process of digestion and absorption. In certain disease states the amount of peritoneal fluid is increased. If this is not due to inflammation, the fluid is called ascitic fluid. SEE: illus.; *ascites.*

**peritonealize** During abdominal surgery, to cover a tissue with peritoneum.

**peritoneo-** Combining form meaning *peritoneum.*

**peritoneocentesis** (pĕr″ĭ-tō″nē-ō-sĕn-tē′sĭs) [Gr. *peritonaion,* peritoneum, + *kentesis,* puncture] Piercing of the peritoneal cavity to obtain fluid. SEE: *paracentesis.*

**peritoneoclysis** (pĕr″ĭ-tō″nē-ō-klī′sĭs) [″ + *klysis,* a washing out] Introduction of fluid into the peritoneal cavity.

**peritoneopericardial** (pĕr″ĭ-tō-nē″ō-pĕr″ĭ-kăr′dē-ăl) [″ + *peri,* around, + *kardia,* heart] Concerning the peritoneum and pericardium.

**peritoneopexy** (pĕr″ĭ-tō′nē-ō-pĕks″ē) [Gr. *peritonaion,* peritoneum, + *pexis,* fixation] Fixation of the uterus via the vagina.

**peritoneoplasty** (per″ĭ-tō′nē-ō-plăs″tē) [″ + *plassein,* to form] Reparative surgery to prevent the re-formation of loosened adhesions.

**peritoneoscope** (pĕr″ĭ-tō′nē-ō-skōp″) [Gr. *peritonaion,* peritoneum, + *skopein,* to examine] A long, slender periscope or telescope device with a light at one end and an eyepiece at the other; used to inspect the peritoneal and abdominal cavities through a small incision in the abdominal wall.

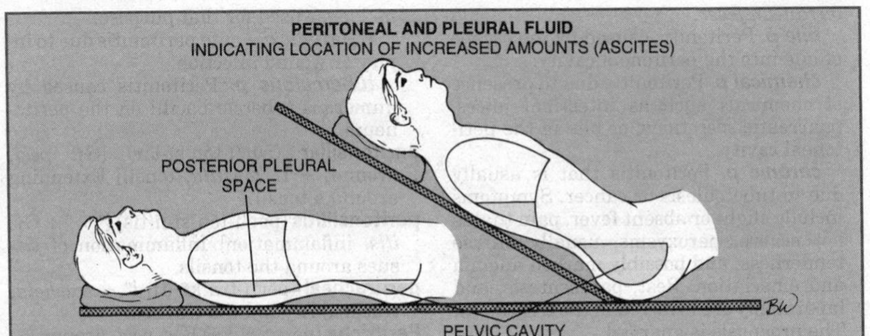


**peritoneoscopy** (pĕr″ĭ-tō″nē-ŏs′kō-pē) Examination of the peritoneal cavity with a peritoneoscope.

**peritoneotomy** (pĕr″ĭ-tō″nē-ŏt′ō-mē) The process of incising the peritoneum.

**peritoneum** (pĕr″ĭ-tō-nē′ŭm) [LL., Gr. *peritonaion*] The serous membrane reflected over the viscera and lining the abdominal cavity.

PALPATION: If the palmar surface of the hand is applied to the side of the abdomen at the level of the liquid in ascites and light percussion is performed on the opposite side, a sense of fluctuation will be communicated to the hand.

***parietal p.*** Peritoneum lining the abdominal and pelvic walls and the undersurface of the diaphragm.

***visceral p.*** Peritoneum that invests the abdominal organs. The peritoneum holds the viscera in place by its folds, which are called the *mesentery*.

**peritonism** (pĕr′ĭ-tō-nĭzm) [Gr. *peritonaion*, peritoneum, + *-ismos*, condition] A condition having the clinical signs of shock and peritonitis but without inflammation of the peritoneum.

**peritonitic** (pĕr″ĭ-tō-nĭt′ĭk) [″ + *itis*, inflammation] Affected with or concerning peritonitis.

**peritonitis** (pĕr″ĭ-tō-nī′tĭs) [″ + *itis*, inflammation] Inflammation of the peritoneum, the serous membrane lining the abdominal cavity and covering the viscera. This condition is caused by infectious organisms that gain access by way of rupture or perforation of viscera or associated structures, via the female genital tract, by piercing of abdominal wall, via the bloodstream or lymphatic vessels, via surgical incisions, and by failure to practice aseptic techniques during surgery. Prophylactic measures to prevent the development of peritonitis are of utmost importance in the care of all patients. Patients who develop peritonitis are treated with antibiotic therapy. The prognosis is guarded. SEE: *Nursing Diagnoses Appendix*.

NURSING IMPLICATIONS: Patients who might have undergone rupture or perforation of structures in the abdominal cavity are observed for symptoms of peritonitis. Because such information is crucial to proper diagnosis, assessment includes any history of symptoms before seeking treatment. Because this condition can have serious outcomes, immediate medical attention is imperative; surgery may be required if the appendix or other abdominal structures are about to rupture or perforate or if either has already occurred. Medications are administered as prescribed, and proper nutrition and a high-protein diet are provided. Support and reassurance are offered to both patient and family, and opportunities are provided for questions and discussion of concerns.

***acute diffuse p.*** Generalized peritonitis of a large area.

SYMPTOMS: Symptoms include chill; fever, 102° to 103°F (38.9° to 39.4°C); rapid pulse rate; and abdominal pain and tenderness so intense that abdominal respiration and bodily movement are inhibited. The patient lies on the back with thighs flexed; facial features are pinched and anxious; vomiting is persistent; bowels are usually constipated; hiccough and abdominal distention are present.

ETIOLOGY: This condition results from rupture of an intra-abdominal viscus, such as the appendix or stomach. Infection may take place directly from an adjacent organ that is inflamed or from the bloodstream in patients with septicemia.

TREATMENT: Surgical intervention is needed. Absolute bedrest is required. Sips of water are permitted. Saline or glucose solution, blood, or plasma are administered parenterally; analgesics are given for pain. Suction of the gastrointestinal tract and antibiotic therapy are also necessary.

***adhesive p.*** Peritonitis in which the visceral and parietal layers stick together by means of adhesions.

***aseptic p.*** Peritonitis due to causes other than bacterial infection, such as trauma, presence of chemicals produced naturally or introduced from without, or irradiation.

***benign paroxysmal p.*** Familial paroxysmal polyserositis. SEE: *familial Medi-*

*terranean fever.*

***bile p.*** Peritonitis caused by the escape of bile into the peritoneal cavity.

***chemical p.*** Peritonitis due to presence of chemicals such as intestinal juices, pancreatic secretions, or bile in the peritoneal cavity.

***chronic p.*** Peritonitis that is usually due to tuberculosis or cancer. Symptoms include slight or absent fever, pain that is not severe, paroxysms, usually diffuse tenderness, and possibly marked anemia and emaciation. Rest, paracentesis, and laparotomy are involved in the treatment. The prognosis is guarded

***circumscribed p.*** Localized p.

***p. deformans*** Chronic peritonitis with a thickened membrane and adhesions contracting and causing retraction of the intestines.

***diaphragmatic p.*** Peritonitis in which the peritoneal surface of the diaphragm is mainly affected.

***diffuse p.*** Peritonitis that is widespread, involving most of the peritoneum. SYN: *generalized p.*

***p. encapsulans*** A localized abscess in the peritoneal cavity, which may occur after generalized peritonitis has subsided.

***fibrocaseous p.*** Peritonitis with fibrosis and caseation; usually caused by tuberculosis.

***gas p.*** Peritonitis in which gas is present in the peritoneal cavity.

***generalized p.*** Diffuse p.

***localized p.*** Peritonitis in which only a small area is involved. SYN: *circumscribed p.*

***meconium p.*** Peritonitis in the newborn caused by perforation of the gastrointestinal tract in utero. Neonatal intestinal obstruction may be present. In boys a soft hydrocele or scrotal mass may be found.

***pelvic p.*** Peritonitis involving the peritoneum of the pelvic region, usually the sequela of uterine tube infection in women.

***periodic p.*** Familial Mediterranean fever.

***primary p.*** Peritonitis resulting from infectious organisms transmitted through blood or lymph.

***puerperal p.*** Peritonitis that develops following childbirth.

***secondary p.*** Peritonitis resulting from extension of infection from adjoining structures, rupture of a viscus, abscess, or trauma.

***septic p.*** Peritonitis caused by a pyogenic bacterium.

***serous p.*** Peritonitis in which there is copious liquid exudation.

***silent p.*** Peritonitis in which there are no signs or symptoms.

***talc p.*** Peritonitis due to particles of talcum powder in the peritoneal cavity. Talc was present because of having been used as a powder on surgeon's gloves. Talc is no longer used for that purpose.

***traumatic p.*** Acute peritonitis due to injury or wound infection.

***tuberculous p.*** Peritonitis caused by numerous tubercle bacilli on the peritoneum.

**peritonsillar** (pĕr″ĭ-tŏn′sĭ-lăr) [Gr. *peri,* around, + L. *tonsilla,* tonsil] Extending around a tonsil.

**peritonsillitis** (pĕr″ĭ-tŏn″sĭ-lī′tĭs) [″ + ″ + Gr. *itis,* inflammation] Inflammation of tissues around the tonsils.

**peritracheal** (pĕr″ĭ-trā′kē-ăl) [″ + *tracheia,* trachea] Around the trachea.

**Peritricha** (pĕr-ĭt′rĭ-kă) [Gr. *peri,* around, + *thrix,* hair] A group of protozoa having flagella over the entire surface.

**peritrichal, peritrichic** (pĕ-rĭt′rĭ-kăl, pĕr″ē-trĭk′ĭk) [″ + *thrix,* hair] Peritrichous.

**peritrichous** (pĕ-rĭt′rĭk-ŭs) [″ + *thrix,* hair] Indicating microorganisms that have cilia or flagella covering the entire surface of a bacterial cell. SYN: *peritrichal; peritrichic.*

**peritrochanteric** (pĕr″ĭ-trō″kăn-tĕr′ĭk) [″ + *trokhanter,* runner] Around a trochanter.

**perityphlic** (pĕr″ĭ-tĭf′lĭk) [″ + *typhlon,* cecum] Around the cecum.

**perityphlitis** (pĕr″ĭ-tĭf-lī′tĭs) [″ + ″ + *itis,* inflammation] Appendicitis.

**periumbilical** (pĕr″ē-ŭm-bĭl′ĭ-kăl) [″ + L. *umbilicus,* a pit] Around the navel (i.e., umbilicus).

**periungual** (pĕr″ē-ŭng′gwăl) [″ + L. *unguis,* nail] Around a nail.

**periureteral** (pĕr″ē-ū-rē′tĕr-ăl) [″ + *oureter,* ureter] Around a ureter.

**periureteritis** (pĕr″ē-ū-rē″tĕr-ī′tĭs) [″ + ″ + *itis,* inflammation] Inflammation of parts about the ureter.

**periurethral** (pĕr″ē-ū-rē′thrăl) [″ + *ourethra,* urethra] Located about the urethra.

**periurethritis** (pĕr″ē-ū″rē-thrī′tĭs) [″ + ″ + *itis,* inflammation] Inflammation of the tissues around the urethra.

**periuterine** (pĕr″ē-ū′tĕr-ĭn) [″ + L. *uterus,* womb] Located about the uterus. SYN: *perimetric.*

**periuvular** (pĕr″ē-ū′vū-lăr) [″ + L. *uvula,* little grape] Around the uvula.

**perivaginal** (pĕr″ĭ-văj′ĭ-năl) [″ + L. *vagina,* sheath] Around the vagina.

**perivaginitis** (pĕr″ĭ-văj″ĭ-nī′tĭs) [″ + ″ + Gr. *itis,* inflammation] Inflammation of the region around the vagina. SYN: *pericolpitis.*

**perivascular** (pĕr″ĭ-văs′kū-lăr) [″ + L. *vasculus,* a little vessel] Located around a vessel, esp. a blood vessel.

**perivasculitis** (pĕr″ĭ-văs″kū-lī′tĭs) [″ + ″ + Gr. *itis,* inflammation] Inflammation of the tissues surrounding a blood vessel. SYN: *periangiitis.*

**perivenous** (pĕr″ĭ-vē′nŭs) [″ + L. *vena,* vein] Surrounding or occurring around a vein.

**perivertebral** (pĕr″ĭ-vĕr′tĕ-brăl) [″ + L. *vertebra,* vertebra] Around a vertebra.

**perivesical** (pĕr″ĭ-vĕs′ĭ-kăl) [″ + L. *vesicula,* little bladder] Around the urinary bladder.

**perivesiculitis** (pĕr″ĭ-vĕ-sĭk″ū-lī′tĭs) [″ + ″ + Gr. *itis,* inflammation] Inflammation of tissues around a seminal vesicle.

**perivisceral** (pĕr″ĭ-vĭs′ĕr-ăl) [″ + L. *viscera,* internal organs] Around the viscera or a seminal vesicle.

**perivisceritis** (pĕr″ĭ-vĭs″ĕr-ī′tĭs) [″ + ″ + Gr. *itis,* inflammation] Inflammation of the tissues surrounding the viscera. SYN: *perisplanchnitis.*

**perivitelline** (pĕr″ĭ-vī-tĕl′ēn) [″ + L. *vitellus,* yolk] Around a vitellus or yolk.

**perixenitis** (pĕr″ĭ-zĕ-nī′tĭs) [″ + *xenos,* strange, + *itis,* inflammation] Noninfection inflammation occurring around a foreign body in a tissue or organ.

**perle** (pĕrl) [Fr., pearl] A soft capsule containing medicine.

**perlèche** (pĕr-lĕsh′) [Fr.] A disorder marked by fissures and epithelial desquamation at the corners of the mouth, esp. seen in children. The condition may be due to oral candidiasis or may be a symptom of dietary deficiency, esp. riboflavin deficiency.

**perlingual** (pĕr-lĭng′gwăl) [L. *per,* through, + *lingua,* tongue] By way of the tongue; a method of administering medicines.

**permanent** (pĕr′mă-nĕnt) [″ + *manere,* to remain] Enduring; without change.

**permanganate** (pĕr-măn′gă-nāt) Any one of the salts of permanganic acid.

**permeability** (pĕr″mē-ă-bĭl′ĭ-tē) [LL. *permeabilis*] The quality of being permeable; that which may be traversed.

***capillary p.*** The condition of the capillary wall that enables substances in the blood to diffuse into tissue spaces or into cells, or vice versa.

**permeable** (pĕr′mē-ă-b′l) Capable of allowing the passage of fluids or substances in solution. SYN: *pervious* (1).

**permeation** (pĕr″mē-ā′shŭn) [L. *permeare,* permeate] Penetration of and spreading throughout an organ, tissue, or space.

**permethrin** A pediculocide used in treating head lice.

**permissible exposure limits** The limits, usually expressed as a combination of time and concentration, to which humans may be safely exposed to physical agents, ionizing radiations, or chemical substances in the environment in general and in work areas specifically. SEE: *hazardous material; health hazard; maximum allowable concentration; right-to-know law; toxic substance.*

**permutation** (pĕr″mū-tā′shŭn) [L. *per,* completely, + *mutare,* to change] Transformation; complete change; act of altering objects in a group.

**pernicious** (pĕr-nĭsh′ŭs) [L. *perniciosus,* destructive] Destructive; fatal; harmful.

***p. trend*** In psychology, an abnormal departure from conventional ideas and social interests.

**pernio** (pĕr′nē-ō) [L.] Chilblain; congestion and swelling of the skin because of cold.

SYMPTOMS: Severe burning or itching accompanies this condition. Ulceration may result from vesicles and bullae that sometimes form.

**pero-** [Gr. *peros,* maimed] Combining form meaning *deformed.*

**perobrachius** (pē″rō-brā′kē-ŭs) [″ + *brachion,* arm] An individual with congenitally deformed forearms and hands.

**perocephalus** (pē″rō-sĕf′ă-lŭs) [″ + *kephale,* head] An individual with a congenitally deformed head.

**perochirus** (pē″rō-kī′rŭs) [″ + *cheir,* hand] An individual with congenitally deformed hands.

**perocormus** (pē″rō-kor′mŭs) [″ + *kormos,* trunk] An individual with a congenitally deformed trunk.

**perodactylus** (pē″rō-dăk′tĭ-lŭs) [″ + *daktylos,* finger] An individual with congenitally deformed fingers or toes.

**peromelia** (pē″rō-mē′lē-ă) [″ + *melos,* limb] A birth defect with absence or deformity of the terminal part of a limb or limbs.

**peromelus** (pē-rŏm′ĕ-lŭs) [″ + *melos,* limb] An individual with congenital malformation of the extremities, including absence of a hand or foot.

**perone** (pĕr-ō′nē) [Gr. *perone,* pin] The fibula.

**peroneal** (pĕr″ō-nē′ăl) [Gr. *perone,* pin] Concerning the fibula.

***p. sign*** In patients with tetany, eversion and dorsiflexion of the foot caused by tapping on the fibular side over the peroneal nerve.

**peroneo-** [Gr. *perone,* pin] Combining form meaning *fibula.*

**peroneotibial** (pĕr″ō-nē″ō-tĭb′ē-ăl) [″ + L. *tibia,* shinbone] Concerning the fibula and tibia.

**peroneus** (pĕr″ō-nē′ŭs) [Gr. *perone,* pin] One of several muscles of the leg that act to move the foot.

**peropus** (pē′rō-pŭs) [″ + *pous,* foot] An individual with congenitally deformed feet.

**peroral** (pĕr-or′ăl) [L. *per,* through, + *oris,* mouth] Administered through the mouth.

**per os** [L.] By mouth.

**perosomus** (pē″rō-sō′mŭs) [Gr. *peros,* maimed, + *soma,* body] An individual with a congenitally defective body.

**perosplanchnia** (pē″rō-splănk′nē-ă) [″ + *splanchnon,* viscus] Congenital malformation of the viscera.

**perosseous** (pĕr-ŏs′ē-ŭs) [L. *per,* through, + *os,* bone] Through bone.

**peroxidase** (pĕr-ŏk′sĭ-dās) [″ + Gr. *oxys,* acid, + *-ase,* enzyme] An enzyme that hastens the transfer of oxygen from peroxide to a tissue that requires oxygen. This process is essential to intracellular respiration.

**peroxide** (pĕr-ŏk′sīd) In chemistry, a compound containing more oxygen than the other oxides of the element in question.

**peroxisome** (pĕ-rŏks′ĭ-sōm) A class of single-membrane-bound vesicles that contain a variety of enzymes including catalase. They are present in most human cells but are concentrated in the liver. The absence of functional peroxisomes is involved in a number of diseases; the most severe is Zellweger's syndrome, which affects newborns and is usually fatal before one year of age. This syndrome consists of cirrhosis of the liver and congenital malformations of the central nervous system and skeleton.

**perphenazine** (pĕr-fĕn′ă-zēn) An antipsychotic drug that is also used as an antiemetic and in treating intractable hiccoughs.

**perplication** (pĕr-plĭ-kā′shŭn) [″ + *plicare,* to fold] Inserting the cut end of an artery through an incision in its own wall to arrest bleeding.

**per primam intentionem** (pĕr prī′măm ĭn-tĕn-shē-ō′nĕm) [L.] By first intention. SEE: *healing.*

**per rectum** (pĕr rĕk′tŭm) [L.] By the rectum; through the rectum.

**PERRLA** *pupils equal, regular, react to light and accommodation.*

**persalt** (pĕr′sawlt) In chemistry, a salt containing the largest possible amount of an acid radical.

**per secundam intentionem** (pĕr sē-kŭn′dăm) [L.] By second intention. SEE: *healing.*

**perseveration** (pĕr-sĕv″ĕr-ā′shŭn) [L. *perseverare,* to persist] Continued repetition of a meaningless word or phrase, or repetition of answers that are not related to successive questions asked.

**person** A human being.

**persona** (pĕr-sō′nă) [L., mask] The outer attitude or appearance a person presents to others.

**personal emergency system** A device consisting of a portable battery-powered help button and a machine that automatically dials a monitoring station. The device is connected to the individual's telephone or to a phone jack. When the system is activated, it either allows a two-way communication between the monitoring station and the individual or alerts the station personnel to phone the individual. In the latter case, if there is no response the station may call a neighbor or family member or dispatch emergency medical technicians to the person's home.

**personal equation** A personal bias or peculiarity that may explain a difference in approach or interpretation.

**personal identity disturbance** Inability to distinguish between self and nonself. SEE: *Nursing Diagnoses Appendix.*

**personality** [LL. *personalitas*] The unique organization of traits, characteristics, and modes of behavior of an individual, setting the individual apart from others and at the same time determining how others react to the individual. Personality refers to the mental aspects of an individual, in contrast to the person's physique. SEE: *personality testing.*

***alternating p.*** Multiple p.

***borderline p.*** Personality disorder in which individuals have difficulty maintaining a consistent stable mood and self-image. This manifests as unpredictable and impulsive behavior, outbursts of anger, irritability, sadness, and fear. Self-mutilation or suicidal behavior may be present. Some of these individuals have a chronic feeling of emptiness or boredom. SEE: *Nursing Diagnoses Appendix.*

***compulsive p.*** SEE: *obsessive-compulsive disorder.*

***extroverted p.*** A personality type in which activities or libido is directed to other individuals or the environment.

***inadequate p.*** A personality type in which the individual is ineffective and is physically and emotionally unstable to the extent of being unable to cope with the normal stress of living.

***introverted p.*** A personality type in which activities or libido are directed to the individual himself or herself.

***multiple p.*** A state in which two or more personalities alternate in the same individual, usually with each personality unaware of the others. SEE: *dissociation of personality; Nursing Diagnoses Appendix.*

***obsessive-compulsive p.*** SEE: *compulsive p.*

***paranoid p.*** SEE: *paranoid personality disorder.*

***psychopathic p.*** SEE: *antisocial personality disorder.*

***type A p.*** SEE: under *behavior.*

***type B p.*** SEE: under *behavior.*

**personality disorder** A pathological disturbance of the patterns of perception, communication, and thinking. Personality disorders are manifested in at least two of the following areas: cognition, affectivity, interpersonal functioning, or impulse control. Generally, the disorder is of long duration and its onset can be traced to early adolescence.

TREATMENT: Psychotherapy, psychopharmacological drugs, or some combination of these approaches, are used in treating these disorders. SEE: *coping.*

***antisocial p.d.*** A type of personality disorder characterized by disregard of the rights of others. It usually begins prior to age 15. In early childhood there are lying, stealing, fighting, truancy, and disregard of authority. In adolescence there are usually aggressive sexual behavior, excessive use of alcohol, and use of drugs of abuse. In adulthood these behavior patterns continue with the addition of poor work performance, inability to function responsibly as a parent, and inability to accept normal restrictions imposed by laws. These individuals may repeatedly perform illegal acts (e.g., destroying property, harassing others, or stealing) or pursue illegal occupations. They disregard the safety, wishes, rights, and feelings of others. This type of personality disorder is not due to mental retardation, schizophrenia, or manic episodes. It is much more common in males than females. This condition has been referred to as psychopathy, sociopathy, or dyssocial personality disorder.

***avoidant p.d.*** A personality disorder marked by a pervasive pattern of social inhibition, feelings of inadequacy, and hypersensitivity to criticism. This begins by early adulthood and is present in various situations such as school, work or activities involving contact with others. Individuals with this disorder desire affection, security, certainty, and acceptance and may fantasize about idealized relationships with others.

***borderline p.d.*** A personality disorder in which there is difficulty in maintaining stable interpersonal relationships and self-image. This manifests as unpredictable and impulsive behavior, outbursts of anger, irritability, sadness, and fear. Self-mutilation or suicidal behavior may be present. Sometimes there is a chronic feeling of emptiness or boredom. SEE: *Nursing Diagnoses Appendix.*

***histrionic p.d.*** A personality disorder marked by excessive emotionalism and attention-seeking. The individual is active, dramatic, prone to exaggerate, and subject to irrational, angry outbursts or tantrums. He or she expresses boredom with normal routines and craves novelty and excitement. Although usually attractive and productive, behavior in interpersonal relationships is shallow, vain, demanding, and dependent.

***obsessive-compulsive p.d.*** A disorder characterized by a pervasive pattern of preoccupation with orderliness, perfectionism, and mental and interpersonal control at the expense of flexibility, openness, and efficiency. These symptoms begin by early adulthood and are manifested in various contexts. Four or more of the following criteria must be present: preoccupation with details, rules, lists, order, organization, or schedules to the extent that the major point of the activity is lost; perfectionism interfering with task completion because the person's own overly strict standards are not met; excessive devotion to work and productivity to the exclusion of leisure activities and friendships (not accounted for by obvious economic necessity); overconscientiousness, scrupulousness, and inflexibility about matters of morality, ethics, or values (not accounted for by cultural or religious identification); inability to discard worn-out or worthless objects even when they have no sentimental value; reluctance to delegate tasks or to work with others unless they submit to exactly the person's way of doing things; adoption of a miserly spending style toward both self and others, and a view of money as something to be hoarded for future catastrophes; and showing rigidity and stubbornness.

Even though obsessive-compulsive disorder and obsessive-compulsive personality disorder have similar names, they are usually easily distinguished by the presence of true obsessions and compulsions in the former. Obsessive-compulsive disorder should be considered esp. when hoarding is extreme. When the diagnostic criteria for both disorders are met, both diagnoses should be recorded.

***narcissistic p.d.*** A personality disorder marked by a grandiose sense of self-importance and preoccupation with fantasies of unlimited success, power, brilliance, or beauty. The individual believes that his or her problems are unique and can only be understood by other "special" people. There is an exhibitionistic need for admiration and attention, a lack of empathy, and an inability to understand how others feel.

***paranoid p.d.*** A personality disorder characterized by unwarranted suspiciousness and mistrust of others, hypervigilance directed at hidden motives or intent to harm, hypersensitivity to criticism, tendency to hold grudges and to be easily offended, and reluctance to confide in others. SEE: paranoid disorder in *Nursing Diagnoses Appendix.*

***passive-aggressive p.d.*** A personality disorder marked by indirect resistance to demands for adequate occupational or social performance through procrastination, dawdling, stubbornness, inefficiency, or forgetfulness. The disorder begins in early childhood and may manifest as refusal to complete routine tasks, complaints of being misunderstood or unappreciated, sullen or argumentative attitude, pronounced envy of others, and behavior that alternates between hostile defiance and contrition.

***schizoid p.d.*** A personality disorder characterized by shyness, oversensitivity, seclusiveness, dissociation from close interpersonal or competitive relationships, eccentricity, daydreaming, preference for solitary activities, and inability to express anger in situations that would call for such a reaction.

**personality testing** Testing that attempts to evaluate an individual's personality dysfunction and stress. A test that has been found to be useful in the fields of mental health, medicine, education, job placement, and counseling is the copyrighted Minnesota Multiphasic Personality Inventory (MMPI). It contains 550 statements that describe a wide variety of thoughts, feelings, attributes, and life experiences. The test requires the individual to answer "true" or "false" to each statement. The responses are measured against those of "normal" adults or adolescents.

**personnel, unlicensed assistive** ABBR:

UAP. Any unlicensed health care personnel who work under the direction of a registered nurse. In addition to delivering direct patient care, they may take blood samples, provide respiratory treatments, or keep track of medical records. Some UAPs are multiskilled—they can perform a variety of tasks. Each state regulates UAP practice.

**persons in need of supervision** ABBR: PINS. A legal term for children who, because of behavioral problems, require supervision, usually in an institution.

**person-years of life lost** A calculation of the impact of a disease on society owing to premature death from the specific disease; that is, the number of years the person would have been alive if the disease had not occurred. SEE: *cancer, person-years of life lost due to.*

**perspiration** (pĕr″spĭr-ā′shŭn) [L. *perspirare,* breathe through] **1.** The secretion of the sudoriparous glands of the skin; sweating. **2.** The salty fluid secreted through the sweat glands of the skin; sweat. Essentially, the fluid is a weak solution of sodium chloride, but it also contains potassium, lactate, and urea.

Perspiration is a means of removing heat from the body. This is best accomplished by sweat evaporating from the skin rather than dripping off. Evaporation of 1 L of sweat removes 580 kcal of heat from the body. Sweat loss varies from 100 to 1000 ml/hr but may exceed those amounts in a hot climate.

Perspiration is increased by temperature and humidity of the atmosphere, exercises, pain, nausea, nervousness, mental excitement, dyspnea, diaphoretics, and shock. It is decreased by cold, diarrhea, voiding large quantities of urine, and using certain drugs.

***insensible p.*** Evaporation of water vapor from the body without appearing as moisture on the skin.

***sensible p.*** Perspiration that forms moisture on the skin.

**perspire** (pĕr-spīr′) [L. *perspirare,* breathe through] To secrete fluid through the pores of the skin. SYN: *sweat* (3).

**persuasion** (pĕr-swā′zhŭn) In psychiatry, the attempt to influence behavior by authority, reason, or argument.

**persulfate** (pĕr-sŭl′fāt) One of a series of sulfates containing more sulfuric acid than the others in the same series.

**per tertiam intentionem** (pĕr tĕr′shē-ăm ĭn-tĕn-shē-ō′nĕm) [L.] By third intention. SEE: *healing.*

**Perthes' disease** (pĕr′tēz) [Georg C. Perthes, Ger. surgeon, 1869–1927] Osteochondritis deformans juvenilis.

**Pertofrane** Trade name for desipramine hydrochloride.

**per tubam** (pĕr tū′băm) [L.] Through a tube.

**perturbation** (pĕr″tĕr-bā′shŭn) [L. *perturbare,* thoroughly disordered] The state of being greatly disturbed or agitated; uneasiness of mind.

**pertussis** (pĕr-tŭs′ĭs) [L. *per,* through, + *tussis,* cough] An acute, infectious disease characterized by a catarrhal stage, followed by a peculiar paroxysmal cough, ending in a whooping inspiration. Pertussis may be prevented by immunization of infants beginning at 3 months of age. The disease is caused by a small, nonmotile, gram-negative bacillus, *Bordetella pertussis.* The incubation period is 7 to 10 days. Treatment is symptomatic and supportive. Antibiotics are given to prevent secondary bacterial pneumonia, esp. in infants and young children. SYN: *whooping cough.*

SYMPTOMS: The signs of this disease include elevated white blood count with marked lymphocytosis, possibly in excess of 30,000/mm³. Pertussis is often divided into the following three stages:

*Catarrhal:* At this stage the symptoms are chiefly suggestive of the common cold—slight elevation of fever, sneezing, rhinitis, dry cough, irritability, and loss of appetite.

*Paroxysmal:* This stage sets in after approx. 2 weeks. The cough is more violent and consists of a series of several short coughs, followed by a long drawn inspiration during which the typical whoop is heard, this being occasioned by the spasmodic contraction of the glottis. Often with the beginning of each paroxysm, the patient assumes a worried expression, sometimes even one of terror. The face becomes cyanosed, eyes injected, veins distended. With the conclusion of the paroxysm, vomiting is common. Also at this time there may be epistaxis, subconjunctival hemorrhages, or hemorrhages in other portions of the body. The number of paroxysms in 24 hr may vary from 3 or 4 to 40 or 50. The cough is precipitated by eating, drinking, or pressing on the trachea, and may be followed by vomiting.

*Decline:* This stage begins after an indefinite period of several weeks. Paroxysms grow less frequent and less violent. The child's nutrition improves, and after a period that may be prolonged for several months, the cough finally ceases.

NURSING IMPLICATIONS: The nurse advises the parents that immunization prevents pertussis in children younger than 7 years, except for those children with a history of known allergy. For those children who contract the disease (mainly nonimmunized children), precautions are taken to prevent spread after onset of symptoms. Bedrest, isolation, and a quiet environment are provided. Because cough may be severe and debilitating, both patient and family may require support. The nurse provides comfort measures as indicated.

**pertussis immune globulin** A sterile solution of globulins derived from the blood of adults who have been immunized with pertussis vaccine; used to produce passive immunity to pertussis.

**pertussis vaccine** Sterile bacterial fraction of killed pertussis bacilli; used for active immunization against pertussis.

**pertussoid** (pĕr-tŭs′oyd) [L. *per,* through, + *tussis,* cough, + Gr. *eidos,* form, shape] **1.** Of the nature of whooping cough. **2.** A cough generally similar to that of whooping cough.

**per vaginam** (pĕr vă-jī′năm) [L.] Through the vagina.

**perversion** (pĕr-vĕr′zhŭn) [L. *perversus,* perverted] Deviation from the normal path, whether it be in the area of one's intellect, emotions, actions, or reactions. SEE: *paraphilia.*

***sexual p.*** Maladjustment of sexual life in which satisfaction is sought in ways deviating from the accepted norm. In judging the sexual actions of individuals, it is important to remember that what is normal behavior in one society may be regarded as grossly abnormal or perverted in another.

**pervert** [L. *pervetere,* to turn the wrong way] **1.** (pĕr-vĕrt′) To turn from the normal; to misuse. **2.** (pĕr′vĕrt) One who has turned from the normal or socially acceptable path, esp. sexually.

**per vias naturales** (pĕr vē′ăs năt″ū-ră′lēz) [L.] Through natural ways.

**pervious** (pĕr′vē-ŭs) [L. *pervius*] **1.** Permeable. **2.** Penetrating.

**pes** (pĕs) *pl.* **pedes** [L.] The foot or a footlike structure.

***p. abductus*** Talipes valgus.

***p. adductus*** Talipes varus.

***p. anserinus*** **1.** The three primary branches of the facial nerve after leaving the stylomastoid foramen. **2.** The tendinous expansions of the sartorius, gracilis, and semitendinosus muscles at the medial border of the tibial tuberosity.

***p. cavus*** An abnormal hollowness or concavity of the sole of the foot; an excessively high longitudinal arch in the foot.

***p. contortus*** Talipes equinovarus.

***p. equinovalgus*** A condition in which the heel is elevated and turned laterally.

***p. equinovarus*** A condition in which the heel is turned inward and the foot is plantar flexed.

***p. equinus*** A deformity marked by walking without touching the heel to the ground. SYN: *talipes equinus.*

***p. gigas*** Macropodia.

***p. hippocampi*** The lower portion of the hippocampus major.

***infraorbital p.*** Terminal radiating branches of the infraorbital nerve after exit from the infraorbital canal.

***p. planus*** Flatfoot.

***p. valgus*** Talipes valgus.

***p. varus*** Talipes varus.

**pessary** (pĕs′ă-rē) [L. *pessarium*] A device inserted into the vagina to function as a supportive structure for the uterus.

***cup p.*** Pessary that has a cup-shaped hollow that fits over the os uteri.

***diaphragm p.*** A cup-shaped rubber pessary used as a contraceptive device.

***Hodge's p.*** A pessary used to correct retrodeviations of the uterus.

***ring p.*** A round pessary.

**pessimism** The characteristic of regarding events and situations from the darkest possible aspect. SEE: *optimism.*

***therapeutic p.*** The tendency not to believe in the effectiveness of therapeutic measures, esp. of drugs.

**pest** (pĕst) [L. *pestis,* plague] **1.** A fatal epidemic disease, esp. plague. **2.** A noxious, destructive insect.

**pesticemia** (pĕs″tĭ-sē′mē-ă) [″ + Gr. *haima,* blood] The presence of plague organisms in the blood.

**pesticide** (pĕs′tĭ-sīd) [″ + *cida,* killer] Any chemical used to kill pests, esp. rodents and insects.

***p. residue*** The amount of any pesticide remaining on or in food or beverages intended for human consumption.

**pestiferous** (pĕs-tĭf′ĕr-ŭs) [L. *pestiferus*] Producing a pestilence; carrying infection. SYN: *pestilential.*

**pestilence** (pĕs′tĭl-ĕns) [L. *pestilentia*] **1.** An epidemic contagious disease. **2.** An epidemic caused by such a disease.

**pestilential** (pĕs-tĭ-lĕn′shăl) Pestiferous.

**pestis** (pĕs′tĭs) [L.] Plague.

***p. ambulans*** Ambulatory plague.

***p. fulminans*** The most severe form of plague.

**pestle** (pĕs′l) [L. *pistillum*] A device for macerating drugs in a mortar.

**PET** *positron emission tomography.*

**petechiae** (pē-tē′kē-ē) *sing.* **petechia** [It. *petecchia,* skin spot] **1.** Small, purplish, hemorrhagic spots on the skin that appear in certain severe fevers and are indicative of great prostration, as in typhus. They may be due to an abnormality of the blood-clotting mechanism. This term is also applied to similar spots occurring on the mucous membranes or serous surfaces. **2.** Red spots from the bite of a flea.

**petechial** (pē-tē′kē-ăl) Marked by the presence of petechiae.

**Peter Pan syndrome** The reluctance of an adult to adopt traditional male adult behavior.

**pethidine hydrochloride** (pĕth′ĭ-dĭn) The international nonproprietary name for meperidine hydrochloride.

**petiole** (pĕt′ē-ōl) [LL. *petiolus*] A slender stalk or stem, as petiole of the epiglottic cartilage.

**petiolus** (pĕ-tī′ō-lŭs) [LL.] The stalk or stem of a fruit; a pedicle.

***p. epiglottidis*** The pedicle of the cartilage of the epiglottis. It is attached to the superior notch of the thyroid cartilage.

**Petit, François Pourfour du** (pĕt-ē′) French anatomist and surgeon, 1664–1741.

***P.'s canal*** A space or cleft encircling the lens between the points of attachment of fibers of suspensory ligament. SYN: *zon-*

*ular spaces.*

***P.'s sinuses*** Hollows in the aortic and pulmonary arteries behind the semilunar valves.

**Petit, Jean Louis** (pĕt-ē′) French surgeon, 1674–1750.

***P.'s ligament*** A thickened portion of the pelvic fascia between the cervix and vagina. It passes posteriorly in the rectouterine fold to attach to the anterior surface of the sacrum.

***P.'s triangle*** The area on the lateral abdominal wall bounded by the crest of the ilium, the posterior margin of the external oblique muscle, and the lateral margin of the latissimus dorsi muscle. SYN: *trigonum lumbale.*

**petit mal** SEE: *epilepsy.*

**Petri dish** (pā′trē) [Julius Petri, Ger. bacteriologist, 1852–1921] A shallow covered dish made of plastic or glass, used to hold solid media for culturing bacteria.

**petrifaction** (pĕt-rĭ-făk′shŭn) [L. *petra,* stone, + *facere,* to make] The process of changing into stone or hard substance.

**petrified** (pĕt′rĭ-fīd) Changed into stone; rigid.

**petrify** (pĕt′rĭ-fī) To convert into stone; make rigid.

**pétrissage** (pā″trē-săzh′) [Fr.] A kneading movement in massage; performed generally by the tips of the thumbs, with the index finger and thumb, or with the palm of the hand. It is used principally on the extremities. The operator picks up a special muscle or tendon and, placing one finger on each side of the part, proceeds in centripetal motion with a firm pressure. SYN: *kneading.*

**petro-** [L. *petra,* stone] Combining form meaning *stone;* pert. to the petrous portion of the temporal bone.

**petrolatoma** (pĕt″rō-lă-tō′mă) [L. *petrolatum,* petroleum] A tumor or swelling caused by the introduction of liquid petrolatum under the skin.

**petrolatum** (pĕt″rō-lā′tŭm) [L.] A purified semisolid mixture of hydrocarbons obtained from petroleum. This substance is used as a base for ointments but is not suitable for use as a vaginal lubricant because it is not miscible in body secretions. SYN: *soft paraffin.*

***liquid p.*** A mixture of liquid hydrocarbons obtained from petroleum. This mixture is used as a vehicle for medicinal substances for local applications. Light petrolatum is employed as a topical spray, whereas heavy petrolatum is given internally to treat constipation. SYN: *mineral oil.*

***white p.*** A purified mixture of semisolid hydrocarbons obtained from petroleum. It is decolorized and may contain a suitable stabilizer.

**petroleum** (pĕ-trō′lē-ŭm) [L. *petra,* stone, + *oleum,* oil] An oily inflammable liquid found in the upper strata of the earth; a hydrocarbon mixture.

**petromastoid** (pĕt″rō-măs′toyd) Pert. to the petrous and mastoid portions of the temporal and occipital bones.

**petro-occipital** (pĕt″rō-ŏk-sĭp′ĭ-tăl) [″ + *occipitalis,* occipital] Concerning the petrous portion of the temporal bone and the occipital bone.

**petropharyngeus** (pĕt″rō-făr-rĭn′jē-ŭs) [″ + Gr. *pharynx,* throat] A small muscle joining the lower surface of the petrous portion of the temporal bone and the pharynx. It helps to constrict the pharynx.

**petrosa** (pĕ-trō′să) [L. *petrosus,* stony] The petrous part of the temporal bone.

**petrosal** (pĕt-rō′săl) [L. *petrosus,* stony] Of, pert. to, or situated near the petrous portion of the temporal bone.

**petrosalpingostaphylinus** (pĕt″rō-săl-pĭng″gō-stăf″ĭ-lī′nŭs) [L. *petra,* stone, + Gr. *salpinx,* tube, + *staphyle,* uvula] Musculus levator veli palatini.

**petrositis** (pĕt″rō-sī′tĭs) [″ + Gr. *itis,* inflammation] Inflammation of the petrous region of the temporal bone.

**petrosomastoid** (pĕ-trō″sō-măs′toyd) [″ + Gr. *mastos,* breast, + *eidos,* form, shape] Concerning the petrous portion of the temporal bone and its mastoid process.

**petrosphenoid** (pĕt″rō-sfē′noyd) [″ + Gr. *sphen,* wedge, + *eidos,* form, shape] Pert. to the petrous portion on the temporal and sphenoid bones.

**petrosquamous** (pĕt″rō-skwā′mŭs) [″ + *squamosus,* scaly] Pert. to the petrous and squamous portions of the temporal bones.

**petrostaphylinus** (pĕt″rō-stăf″ĭ-lī′nŭs) [″ + Gr. *staphyle,* uvula] Musculus levator veli palatini.

**petrous** (pĕt′rŭs) [L. *petrosus*] **1.** Resembling stone. **2.** Relating to the petrous portion of the temporal bone. SYN: *petrosal.*

**Peutz-Jeghers syndrome** (pūtz-jā′kĕrs) [Johannes Laurentius Augustinus Peutz, Dutch physician, 1886–1957; Harold J. Jeghers, U.S. physician, b. 1904] An inherited disorder characterized by the presence of polyps of the small intestine and melanin pigmentation of the lips, mucosa, fingers, and toes. Anemia due to bleeding from the intestinal polyps is a common finding.

**pexin** (pĕk′sĭn) Rennet.

**pexis** [Gr., fixation] Fixation of material in the tissue.

**-pexy** [Gr. *pexis,* fixation] A combining form used as a suffix meaning *fixation,* usually surgical.

**Peyer's patch** (pī′ĕrz) [Johann Conrad Peyer, Swiss anatomist, 1653–1712] An aggregation of lymph nodules found chiefly in the ileum near its junction with the colon. They are circular or oval, about 1 cm wide, and 2 to 3 cm long. They lie in the mucosal and submucosal layers and always occur on the side of the intestine opposite to the attachment of the mesentery. In typhoid fever, they undergo hyperplasia and often become ulcerated. SYN: *aggregated follicles.*

**peyote** (pā-ō′tē) **1.** The cactus plant, *Lophophora williamsii,* from which the hallucinogen mescaline is obtained. **2.** The drug from the flowering heads, buttons, of *L. williamsii,* used by some Native Americans to produce altered states of consciousness. In certain tribes the buttons are used in religious ceremonies. For that reason, members of that tribe are permitted to use this substance even though the drug is classed as a narcotic and its use is otherwise restricted to research.

**Peyronie's disease** (pā-rō-nēz′) [François de la Peyronie, Fr. surgeon, 1678–1747] Hardening of the corpora cavernosa of the penis. This condition, which may be painful, causes distortion and curvature of the penis, esp. when erect.

TREATMENT: The disease is self-limiting in many instances. Persistence or progression of the penile deformity requires therapy, but of the several medical, surgical, and radiological approaches, none seem to be completely effective. There are devices that assist individuals with the disease to participate in sexual intercourse. SEE: *penile prosthesis.*

**Pfeiffer, Emil** (fī′fĕr) German physician, 1846–1921.

***P.'s disease*** Infectious mononucleosis.

**Pfeiffer, Richard F** (fī′fĕr) German bacteriologist, 1858–1945.

***P.'s bacillus*** *Haemophilus influenzae.*

***P.'s phenomenon*** A discovery announced in 1894 stating that serum of guinea pigs immunized with cholera vibrios destroyed cholera organisms in peritoneal cavity of immune and nonimmune guinea pigs and that the same reaction occurred in vitro. Also, that same lytic reaction occurred with typhoid and colon bacteria.

**PFT** *pulmonary function test.*

**PG** *prostaglandin.*

**pg** *picogram.*

**PGA** *pteroylglutamic acid.*

**Ph 1.** *Pharmacopoeia.* **2.** Symbol for phenyl.

**pH** *potential of hydrogen.* In chemistry, the degrees of acidity or alkalinity of a substance are expressed in pH values. The neutral point, where a solution would be neither acid nor alkaline, is pH 7. Increasing acidity is expressed as a number less than 7, and increasing alkalinity as a number greater than 7. Maximum acidity is pH 0 and maximum alkalinity is pH 14. Because each unit on the scale represents a logarithm, there is a 10-fold difference between each unit. For example, pH 5 is 10 times as acid as pH 6 and pH 4 is 100 times as acid as pH 6. Expressed mathematically, pH is logarithm of the hydrogen ion concentration divided into one. The pH of a solution may be determined electrically by a pH meter or colorimetrically by the use of indicators. A list of indicators and the pH range registered by each is given under indicator. SEE: illus.; table; *indicator.*

### pH of Some Fluids

| Material | pH |
|---|---|
| Decinormal HCl | 1.0 |
| Gastric juice | 1.0–5.0 |
| Thousandth-normal HCl | 3.0 |
| Pure water (neutral) at 25°C | 7.0 |
| Blood plasma | 7.35–7.45 |
| Pancreatic juice | 8.4–8.9 |
| Thousandth-normal NaOH | 11.0 |
| Decinormal NaOH | 13.0 |

HCl—hydrochloric acid; NaOH—sodium hydroxide

**PHA** *phytohemagglutinin.*

**phacitis** (fă-sī′tĭs) [Gr. *phakos,* lens, + *itis,* inflammation] Phakitis.

**phaco-** [Gr. *phakos*] Combining form denoting *lens.*

**phacoanaphylaxis** (făk″ō-ăn″ă-fī-lăk′sĭs) [Gr. *phakos,* lens, + *ana,* excessive, + *phylaxis,* protection] Hypersensitivity to protein of the crystalline lens.

**phacocele** (făk′ō-sēl) [″ + *kele,* tumor, swelling] Displacement of the crystalline lens into the interior chamber of the eye. SYN: *phacometachoresis.*

**phacocyst** (făk′ō-sĭst) [Gr. *phakos,* lens, + *kystis,* a sac] The capsule of the crystalline lens.

**phacocystectomy** (făk″ō-sĭs-tĕk′tō-mē) [″ + ″ + *ektome,* excision] Surgical excision of part of the crystalline lens capsule for treatment of cataract.

**phacocystitis** (făk″ō-sĭs-tī′tĭs) [″ + ″ + *itis,* inflammation] Inflammation of the capsule of the lens of the eye. SYN: *phacohymenitis.*

**phacoemulsification** (făk″ō-ē-mŭl′sĭ-fĭ-kā″shŭn) A method of treating cataracts of the lens of the eye. An ultrasonic device is used to disintegrate the cataract, which is then aspirated and removed.

**phacoerysis** (făk″ō-ĕr-ē′sĭs) [″ + *eresis,* removal] Removal of the lens of the eye by attaching a suction device, an erysiphake, to it. SEE: *erysiphake.*

**phacoglaucoma** (făk″ō-glaw-kō′mă) [″ + *glaukos,* green, + *oma,* tumor] Glaucoma and the changes it induces in the crystalline lens. SEE: *glaucoma.*

**phacohymenitis** (făk″ō-hī″mĕn-ī′tĭs) [″ + *hymen,* membrane, + *itis,* inflammation] Phacocystitis.

**phacoid** (făk′oyd) [″ + *eidos,* form, shape] Lentil- or lens-shaped.

**phacoiditis** (făk″oy-dī′tĭs) [″ + ″ + *itis,* inflammation] Phakitis.

**phacoidoscope** (fă-koyd′ō-skōp) [″ + ″ + *skopein,* to examine] Phacoscope.

**phacolysis** (făk-ŏl′ĭ-sĭs) [″ + *lysis,* dissolution] **1.** Dissection and removal of the lens of the eye in treatment of cataract. **2.** Any dissolution or disintegration of the crystalline lens. SYN: *phakolysis.*

**phacoma** (fă-kō′mă) [″ + *oma,* tumor] Pha-

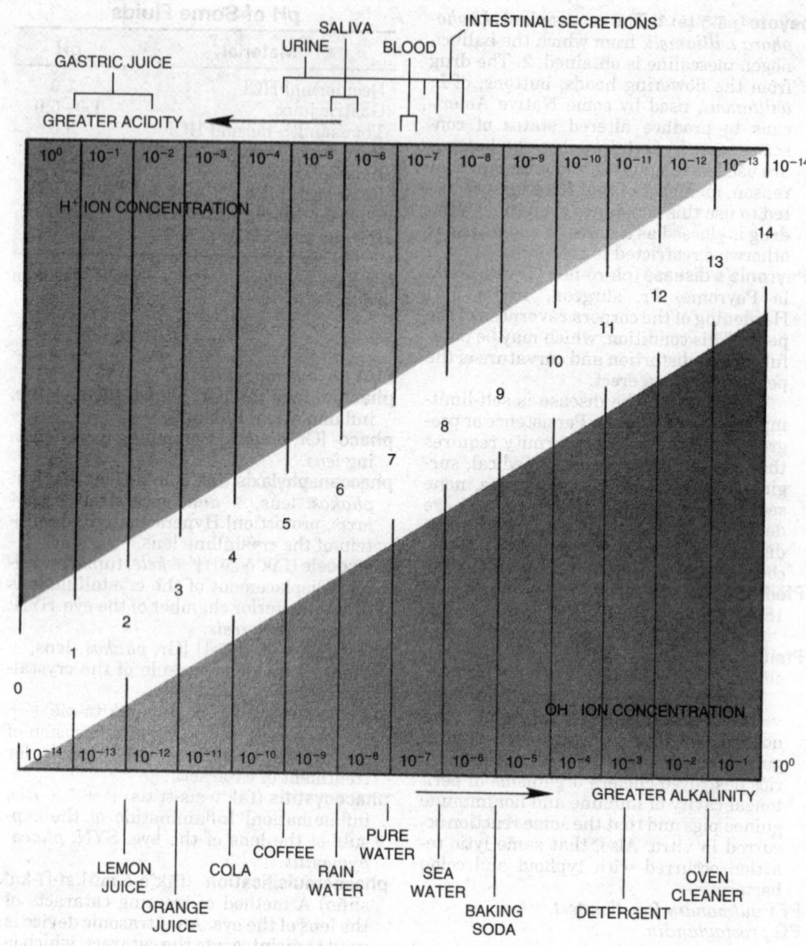


**pH SCALE**

VALUES OF BODY FLUIDS AND SOME FAMILIAR SOLUTIONS

koma.

**phacomalacia** (făk″ō-mă-lā′shē-ă) [″ + *malakia,* softening] A softening of the lens, usually resulting from a soft cataract.

**phacomatosis** Phakomatosis.

**phacometachoresis** (făk″ō-mĕt″ă-kō-rē′ sĭs) [″ + *metachoresis,* displacement] Phacocele.

**phacometer** (făk-ŏm′ĕ-tĕr) [Gr. *phakos,* lens, + *metron,* measure] A device for ascertaining the refractive power of a lens.

**phacoplanesis** (făk″ō-plăn-ē′sĭs) [″ + *planesis,* wandering] Abnormal mobility of the crystalline lens.

**phacosclerosis** (făk″ō-sklĕr-ō′sĭs) [″ + *sklerosis,* a hardening] A hardening of the crystalline lens of the eye.

**phacoscope** (făk′ō-skōp) [″ + *skopein,* to examine] An instrument for observing change of curvature of the lens of the eye during accommodation.

**phacoscotasmus** (făk″ō-skō-tăs′mŭs) [″ + *skotasmos,* clouding] A clouding of the lens of the eye.

**phacotoxic** (făk″ō-tŏk′sĭk) [″ + *toxikon,* poison] Concerning the toxicity of material in the lens of the eye.

**Phaedra complex** [Wife of King Theseus of Athens] The love and attraction between a stepparent and a stepchild; so named because of Phaedra's tragic love for the son (Hippolytus) of her husband by a previous marriage.

**phag-** SEE: *phago-*.

**phage** (fāj) [Gr. *phagein,* to eat] Bacteriophage.

**phagedena** (făj-ĕ-dē′nă) [Gr. *phagedaina*] A sloughing ulcer that spreads rapidly.

***sloughing p.*** Hospital gangrene; bedsores.

**phagedenic** (făj-ĕ-dĕn′ĭk) Concerning, or of the nature of, phagedena.

**phago-, phag-** [Gr. *phagein,* to eat] Combining form meaning *eating, ingestion, devouring.*

**phagocyte** (făg′ō-sīt) [Gr. *phagein,* to eat, + *kytos,* cell] A cell (such as a leukocyte or macrophage) having the ability to ingest and destroy particulate substances such as bacteria, protozoa, cells and cell debris, dust particles, and colloids. SEE: *cytokine; endocytosis; histiocyte; macrophage; phagosome; pinocytosis; reticuloendothelial system.*

**phagocytic** (făg″ō-sĭt′ĭk) Concerning phagocytes or phagocytosis.

**phagocytize** (făg′ō-sīt″īz) To ingest bacteria and foreign particles by phagocytosis.

**phagocytoblast** (făg″ō-sī′tō-blăst) [″ + ″ + *blastos,* germ] A cell that develops into a phagocyte.

**phagocytolysis** (făg″ō-sī-tŏl′ĭ-sĭs) [″ + *kytos,* cell, + *lysis,* dissolution] Destruction or disintegration of phagocytes. SYN: *phagolysis.*

**phagocytolytic** (făg″ō-sī″tō-lĭt′ĭk) Destroying phagocytes.

**phagocytose** (făg″ō-sī′tōs) [″ + *kytos,* cell] Phagocytize.

**phagocytosis** (făg″ō-sī-tō′sĭs) [″ + ″ + *osis,* condition] Ingestion and digestion of bacteria and particles by phagocytes. SEE: illus.; *autophagocytosis; endocytosis; heterophagocytosis; phagolysome; phagosome; pinocytosis.*

***induced p.*** Phagocytosis that is aided or stimulated by the effect of serum opsonins or bacteria.

***spontaneous p.*** Phagocytosis occurring in an indifferent medium such as physiological salt solution.

**phagodynamometer** (făg″ō-dī″nă-mŏm′ĕ-tĕr) [″ + *dynamis,* power, + *metron,* measure] A device that measures energy expended in chewing food.

**phagokaryosis** (făg″ō-kăr″ē-ō′sĭs) [″ + *karyon,* nucleus, + *osis,* condition] Phagocytic action that is performed by a cell nucleus.

**phagolysis** (făg-ŏl′ĭ-sĭs) [″ + *lysis,* dissolution] Phagocytolysis.

**phagolysosome** (făg″ō-lī′sō-sōm) [″ + *lysis,* dissolution, + *soma,* body] The body formed when the membrane-bound phagosome inside a macrophage fuses with a lysosome. SEE: *phagosome.*

**phagophobia** (făg″ō-fō′bē-ă) [″ + *phobos,* fear] Fear of eating.

**phagosome** (făg′ō-sōm) [″ + *soma,* body] A membrane-bound vacuole inside a phagocyte that contains material waiting to be digested. Digestion is facilitated by the fusion of the vacuole with the lysosome. The phagosome is then called a phagolysosome or a secondary lysosome. SEE: *phagocytosis.*

**phagotype** (făg′ō-tīp) [″ + *typos,* mark] The classification of bacteria by their sensitivity to phage types.

**phakitis** (făk-ī′tĭs) [Gr. *phakos,* lens, + *itis,* inflammation] Inflammation of the crystalline lens of the eye. SYN: *phacitis; lentitis.*

**phakolysis** (făk-ŏl′ĭ-sĭs) [″ + *lysis,* dissolution] Disintegration or removal of the crystalline lens of the eye. SYN: *phacolysis* (2).

**phakoma** (fă-kō′mă) [″ + *oma,* tumor] **1.** A microscopic gray white tumor present in the retina in tuberous sclerosis. **2.** An area of myelinated nerve fibers rarely seen in the retina in association with neurofibromatosis. SYN: *phacoma.*

**phakomatosis** (fă″kō-mă-tō′sĭs) [Gr. *phakos,* lens, + *oma,* tumor, + *osis,* condition] Any of a group of congenital and probably hereditary neurocutaneous disorders spread unevenly throughout body tissues. SYN: *phacomatosis.* SEE: *Hippel's disease; neurofibromatosis; sclerosis, tuberous; Sturge-Weber syndrome.*

**phalangeal** (fă-lăn′jē-ăl) [Gr. *phalanx,* closely knit row] Concerning a phalanx.

**phalangectomy** (făl-ăn-jĕk′tō-mē) [″ + *ektome,* excision] Excision of one or more phalanges.

**phalanges** (fă-lăn′jēz) Pl. of phalanx.

**phalangette** (făl″ăn-jĕt′) The distal phalanx of a digit.

***drop p.*** Falling of the distal phalanx of a digit with loss of power to extend it when the hand is prone. This is due to trauma or overstretching of the extensor tendon.

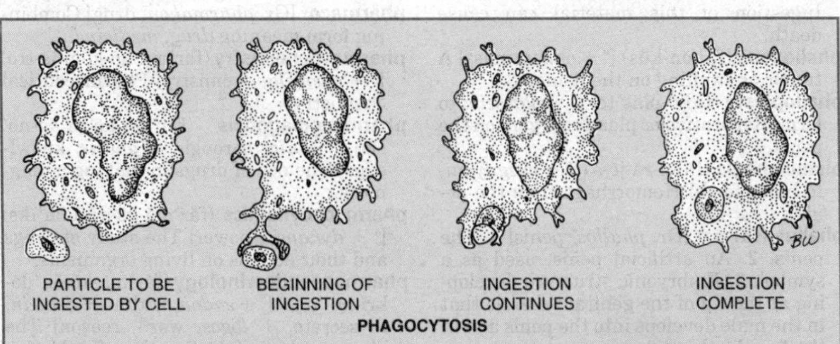


PHAGOCYTOSIS

**phalangitis** (făl″ăn-jī′tĭs) [Gr. *phalanx,* closely knit row, + *itis,* inflammation] Inflammation of one or more phalanges.

**phalanx** (fāl′ănks) *pl.* **phalanges** [Gr., closely knit row] **1.** Any one of the bones of the fingers or toes. SEE: *skeleton.* **2.** One of a set of plates formed of phalangeal cells (inner and outer) forming the reticular membrane of the organ of Corti.

***distal p.*** The phalanx most remote from the metacarpus or metatarsus. SYN: *terminal p.; ungual p.*

***metacarpal p.*** Any phalanx that articulates with a metacarpal bone. SEE: *proximal p.*

***metatarsal p.*** Any phalanx that articulates with a metatarsal bone. SEE: *proximal p.*

***middle p.*** When there are three phalanges, the phalanx intermediate between distal and proximal phalanges.

***proximal p.*** Any phalanx that articulates with a metacarpal or metatarsal bone.

***terminal p.*** Distal p.

***ungual p.*** Distal p.

**Phalen's test** A physical test involving flexion of the fully extended hand at the wrist to aid in the diagnosis of carpal tunnel syndrome.

**phall-** [Gr. *phallos,* penis] Combining form indicating *penis.*

**phallalgia** (făl-ăl′jē-ă) [Gr. *phallos,* penis, + *algos,* pain] Pain in the penis.

**phallectomy** (făl-ĕk′tō-mē) [″ + *ektome,* excision] Surgical removal of the penis.

**phallic** (făl′ĭk) Concerning the penis.

**phalliform** (făl′ĭ-form) [″ + L. *forma,* form] Shaped like a penis.

**phallitis** (făl-ī′tĭs) [″ + *itis,* inflammation] Inflammation of the penis.

**phallocampsis** (făl-ō-kămp′sĭs) [″ + *kampsis,* a bending] Painful downward curvature of the penis when erect.

**phallocrypsis** (făl″ō-krĭp′sĭs) [″ + *krypsis,* hiding] Contraction of the penis so that it is almost invisible.

**phallodynia** (făl-ō-dĭn′ē-ă) [″ + *odyne,* pain] Pain in the penis. SYN: *phallalgia.*

**phalloid** (făl′oyd) [″ + *eidos,* form, shape] Similar to a penis.

**phalloidin** (fă-loyd′ĭn) A poisonous peptide from the mushroom *Amanita phalloides.* Ingestion of this material can cause death.

**phalloncus** (făl-ŏn′kŭs) [″ + *onkos,* mass] A tumor or swelling on the penis.

**phalloplasty** (făl′ō-plăs″tē) [″ + *plassein,* to form] Reparative or plastic surgery on the penis.

**phallorrhagia** (făl-ō-rā′jē-ă) [″ + *rhegnynai,* to burst forth] Hemorrhage from the penis.

**phallus** (făl′ŭs) [Gr. *phallos,* penis] **1.** The penis. **2.** An artificial penis, used as a symbol. **3.** Embryonic structure developing at the tip of the genital tubercle that in the male develops into the penis and in the female, the clitoris.

**phanero-, phaner-** [Gr. *phaneros,* visible] Combining form meaning *evident, visible.*

**phanerogenic** (făn″ĕr-ō-jĕn′ĭk) [″ + *gennan,* to produce] Indicating a disease with a known cause.

**phaneromania** (făn″ĕr-ō-mā′nē-ă) [″ + *mania,* madness] An abnormal tendency to bite the nails or pick, scratch, or pull a pimple, wart, hair, beard, or mustache.

**phanerosis** (făn″ĕr-ō′sĭs) [Gr.] The process of becoming visible.

**phanic** (făn′ĭk) [Gr. *phainein,* to show] Manifest; apparent.

**phantasia** (făn-tā′zē-ă) [Gr.] An appearance that is imaginary.

**phantasm** (făn′tăzm) [Gr. *phantasma*] An optical illusion; an apparition, or illusion of something that does not exist.

**phantasmagoria** [Gr. *phantasma,* an appearance, + *agora,* assembly, gathering] A series of phantasms, deceptive illusions, either imagined or remembered from a dream.

**phantasmology** (făn″tăz-mŏl′ō-jē) [″ + *logos,* word, reason] The study of dreams, phantoms, and spiritually derived apparitions.

**phantasy** (făn′tă-sē) [Gr. *phantasia,* imagination] A daydream. Phantasy-thinking is a form of wish fulfillment, a disregard for reality, from which one would escape through reveling in imaginative possibilities.

**phantogeusia** (făn-tō-gū′sē-ă) [″ + *geusis,* taste] An intermittent or persistent taste sensation in the mouth not produced by an external stimulus.

**phantom** (făn′tŭm) [Gr. *phantasma,* an appearance] **1.** An apparition. **2.** A model of the body or of one of its parts.

**phantosmia** (făn-tŏs′mē-ă) [″ + *osme,* smell] An intermittent or persistent perception of odor when no odor is inhaled.

**pharmacal** (făr′mă-kăl) [Gr. *pharmakon,* drug] Concerning pharmacy.

**pharmaceutical** (făr-mă-sū′tĭ-kăl) [Gr. *pharmakeutikos*] Concerning drugs or pharmacy.

**pharmaceutics** (făr-mă-sū′tĭks) Pharmacy (1).

**pharmacist** (făr′mă-sĭst) [Gr. *pharmakon,* drug] A druggist; one licensed to prepare and dispense drugs. SYN: *apothecary.*

**pharmaco-** [Gr. *pharmakon,* drug] Combining form meaning *drug, medicine.*

**pharmacochemistry** (făr″mă-kō-kĕm′ĭs-trē) [″ + *chemeia,* chemistry] Pharmaceutical chemistry.

**pharmacodiagnosis** (făr″mă-kō-dī″ăg-nō′sĭs) [″ + *dia,* through, + *gnosis,* knowledge] The use of drugs in making a diagnosis.

**pharmacodynamics** (făr″mă-kō-dī-năm′ĭks) [″ + *dynamis,* power] The study of drugs and their actions on living organisms.

**pharmacoendocrinology** (făr″mă-kō-ĕn″dō-krĭ-nŏl′ō-jē) [″ + *endon,* within, + *krinein,* to secrete, + *logos,* word, reason] The pharmacology of the function of endocrine glands.

**pharmacoepidemiology** The application of the science of epidemiology to the study of the effects of drugs, desired and undesired, and uses of drugs in human populations.

**pharmacogenetics** (făr″mă-kō-jĕn-ĕt′ĭks) [″ + *genesis,* generation, birth] The study of the influence of hereditary factors on the response of individual organisms to drugs.

**pharmacogeriatrics** The study of the dynamics of medication use in the elderly.

**pharmacokinetics** (făr″mă-kō-kī-nĕt′ĭks) The study of the metabolism and action of drugs with particular emphasis on the time required for absorption, duration of action, distribution in the body, and method of excretion.

**pharmacologist** (făr″mă-kŏl′ō-jĭst) An individual who by training and experience is a specialist in pharmacology.

**pharmacology** (făr″mă-kŏl′ō-jē) [″ + *logos,* word, reason] The study of drugs and their origin, nature, properties, and effects upon living organisms.

**pharmacomania** (făr″mă-kō-mā′nē-ă) [″ + *mania,* madness] An abnormal desire to give or take medicines.

**pharmacopedia** (făr″mă-kō-pē′dē-ă) [″ + *paideia,* education] Information concerning drugs and their preparation.

**pharmacopeia** (făr″mă-kō-pē′ă) [Gr. *pharmakopoeia,* preparation of drugs] An authorized treatise on drugs and their preparation, esp. a book containing formulas and information that provide a standard for preparation and dispensation of drugs.

**Pharmacopeia, United States** ABBR: USP. A pharmacopeia issued every 5 years, but with periodic supplements, prepared under the supervision of a national committee of pharmacists, pharmacologists, physicians, chemists, biologists, and other scientific and allied personnel. The U.S. Pharmacopeia was adopted as standard in 1906. Beginning with the U.S. Pharmacopeia XIX, 1975, the National Formulary has been included in that publication.

**pharmacophobia** (făr″mă-kō-fō′bē-ă) [″ + *phobos,* fear] An abnormal fear of taking medicines.

**pharmacophore** (făr′mă-kō-for) [″ + *phoros,* bearing] The particular group or arrangement of atoms in a molecule that gives the material its medicinal activity.

**pharmacotherapy** (făr″mă-kō-thĕr′ă-pē) [″ + *therapeia,* treatment] The use of medicine in treatment of disease.

**pharmacy** (făr′mă-sē) [Gr. *pharmakon,* drug] **1.** The practice of compounding and dispensing medicinal preparations. **2.** A drugstore.

**Pharm.D.** *Doctor of Pharmacy.*

**pharyng-** SEE: *pharyngo-.*

**pharyngalgia** (făr″ĭn-găl′jē-ă) [Gr. *pharynx,* throat, + *algos,* pain] Pain in the pharynx.

**pharyngeal** (făr-ĭn′jē-ăl) [L. *pharyngeus*] Concerning the pharynx.

**pharyngectomy** (făr-ĭn-jĕk′tō-mē) [Gr. *pharynx,* throat, + *ektome,* excision] Partial excision of the pharynx to remove growths or abscesses.

**pharyngismus** (făr″ĭn-jĭz′mŭs) [″ + *-ismos,* condition] Spasm of the muscles in the pharynx. SYN: *pharyngospasm.*

**pharyngitis** (făr″ĭn-jī′tĭs) [″ + *itis,* inflammation] Inflammation of the pharynx.

***acute p.*** Inflammation of the pharynx with pain in the throat.

SYMPTOMS: Symptoms include malaise, fever, dysphagia, throat pain, and postnasal secretion.

TREATMENT: Local treatment includes gargles, lozenges, and topical application to the oral pharynx. General treatment involves bedrest, adequate fluids, and analgesics. An appropriate antibiotic should be given after material has been taken for bacterial study, esp. for beta-hemolytic streptococci.

***atrophic p.*** A chronic form of pharyngitis with some atrophy of mucous glands and abnormal secretion.

***chronic p.*** Pharyngitis associated with pathology in the nose and sinuses, mouth breathing, excessive smoking, and chronic tonsillitis. Dryness and irritation of the throat and a cough characterize this condition. Intranasal medication and removal of pathological factors in sinuses and tonsillectomy are the treatment choices.

***diphtheritic p.*** Sore throat with general symptoms of diphtheria and formation of a true membrane.

***gangrenous p.*** Gangrenous inflammation of the mucous membrane of the pharynx. SYN: *angina maligna.*

***granular p.*** Chronic pharyngitis with granulations seen on the pharynx.

***p. herpetica*** Pharyngitis characterized by formation of vesicles and ulcers.

***hypertrophic p.*** Chronic pharyngitis with thickened red mucous membrane on each side with a glazed central portion.

***membranous p.*** Pharyngitis in which a membranous exudate forms a false membrane.

***p. ulcerosa*** Pharyngitis with fever, pain, and the formation of ulcerations.

**pharyngo-, pharyng-** [Gr. *pharynx,* throat] Combining form meaning *throat.*

**pharyngoamygdalitis** (fă-rĭn″gō-ă-mĭg″dăl-ī′tĭs) [″ + *amygdale,* tonsil, + *itis,* inflammation] Inflammation of the pharynx and tonsil.

**pharyngocele** (făr-ĭn′gō-sēl) [″ + *kele,* tumor, swelling] Hernia through the pharyngeal wall.

**pharyngoconjunctival fever, acute** ABBR: APC. An acute disease consisting of fever, pharyngitis, and conjunctivitis. This disease is caused by adenovirus type 3. It is particularly predisposed to occur in children in summer camp and may temporarily disable more than half of the campers in a few weeks. Treatment is symptomatic.

**pharyngoepiglottic, pharyngoepiglottidean** (fă-rĭng″gō-ĕp″ĭ-glŏt′ĭk, -glŏ-tĭd′ē-ăn) [″ + *epi,* upon, + *glottis,* glottis] Concerning the pharynx and glottis.

**pharyngoesophageal** (fă-rĭng″gō-ē-sŏf′ă-jē″ăl) [″ + *oisophagos,* esophagus] Concerning the pharynx and esophagus.

**pharyngoglossal** (fă-rĭng″gō-glŏs′ăl) [″ + *glossa,* tongue] Concerning the pharynx and tongue.

**pharyngography** Radiographical examination of the pharynx after ingestion of a contrast medium.

**pharyngokeratosis** (făr-ĭn″gō-kĕr″ă-tō′sĭs) [″ + *keras,* horn, + *osis,* condition] Thickening and hardening of the mucous lining of the pharynx.

**pharyngolaryngeal** (fă-rĭng″gō-lă-rĭn′jē-ăl) [″ + *larynx,* larynx] Concerning the pharynx and larynx.

**pharyngolith** (făr-ĭn′gō-lĭth) [″ + *lithos,* stone] A concretion in pharyngeal walls.

**pharyngology** (făr″ĭn-gŏl′ō-jē) [″ + *logos,* word, reason] The branch of medicine dealing with the pharynx.

**pharyngomaxillary** (fă-rĭng″gō-măk′sĭ-lĕr″ē) [″ + L. *maxilla,* jawbone] Concerning the pharynx and maxillae.

**pharyngomycosis** (făr-ĭn″gō-mī-kō′sĭs) [″ + *mykes,* fungus, + *osis,* condition] Disease of the pharynx caused by fungi.

**pharyngonasal** (fă-rĭng″gō-nā′săl) [″ + L. *nasus,* nose] Concerning the pharynx and nose.

**pharyngo-oral** (fă-rĭng″gō-or′ăl) [″ + L. *os,* mouth] Concerning the pharynx and mouth.

**pharyngopalatine** (fă-rĭng″gō-păl′ă-tīn) [″ + L. *palatum,* palate] Concerning the pharynx and palate.

**pharyngoparalysis** (făr-ĭn″gō-păr-ăl′ĭ-sĭs) [″ + *paralysis,* a loosening at the side] Paralysis of the muscles of the pharynx.

**pharyngopathy** (făr″ĭn-gŏp′ă-thē) [″ + *pathos,* disease, suffering] Any disorder of the pharynx.

**pharyngoperistole** (făr-ĭn″gō-pĕr-ĭs′tō-lē) [″ + *peristole,* contracture] Narrowing or stricture of the lumen of the pharynx.

**pharyngoplasty** (făr-ĭn′gō-plăs″tē) [″ + *plassein,* to form] Reparative surgery of the pharynx.

**pharyngorhinitis** (făr-ĭn″gō-rī-nī′tĭs) [″ + *rhis,* nose, + *itis,* inflammation] Inflammation of the nasopharynx.

**pharyngorhinoscopy** (făr-ĭn″gō-rī-nŏs′kō-pē) [″ + ″ + *skopein,* to examine] Inspection of the nasopharynx and posterior nares.

**pharyngorrhea** (făr″ĭn-gō-rē′ă) [″ + *rhoia,* flow] Discharge of mucus from the pharynx.

**pharyngoscleroma** (făr-rĭng″gō-sklē-rō′mă) [″ + *skleroma,* induration] An indurated patch, or scleroma, in the pharynx.

**pharyngoscope** (făr-ĭn′gō-skōp) [″ + *skopein,* to examine] An instrument for visual examination of the pharynx.

**pharyngoscopy** (făr″ĭn-gŏs′kō-pē) Visual examination of the pharynx.

**pharyngospasm** (făr-ĭn′gō-spăzm) [″ + *spasmos,* a convulsion] Pharyngismus.

**pharyngostenosis** (fă-rĭng″gō-stē-nō′sĭs) [″ + *stenosis,* narrowing] Narrowing or stricture of the pharynx.

**pharyngotherapy** (făr-ĭn″gō-thĕr′ă-pē) [″ + *therapeia,* treatment] Treatment of pharyngeal disturbances or diseases.

**pharyngotome** (făr-ĭn′gō-tōm) [″ + *tome,* incision] An instrument for incision of the pharynx.

**pharyngotomy** (făr-ĭn-gŏt′ō-mē) Incision of the pharynx.

**pharyngotonsillitis** (fă-rĭng″gō-tŏn″sĭ-lī′tĭs) [″ + L. *tonsilla,* almond, + Gr. *itis,* inflammation] Inflammation of the pharynx and tonsils.

**pharyngoxerosis** (fă-rĭng″gō-zē-rō′sĭs) [″ + *xerosis,* dryness] Dryness of the pharynx.

**pharynx** (făr′ĭnks) *pl.* **pharynges** [Gr.] The passageway for air from the nasal cavity to the larynx and for food from the mouth to the esophagus. It also acts as a resonating cavity. SEE: *mouth* for illus.

ANATOMY: The pharynx is a musculomembranous tube extending from base of skull to level of the sixth cervical vertebra, where it becomes continuous with the esophagus. The upper portion, the nasopharynx, is above the soft palate, lined with pseudostratified ciliated epithelium, and has openings to the posterior nares and eustachian tubes. The middle part, the oropharynx, is lined with stratified squamous epithelium and has an opening to the oral cavity. The lowest part, the laryngopharynx, is also lined with stratified squamous epithelium and opens inferiorly to the larynx anteriorly and the esophagus posteriorly.

The pharynx communicates with the posterior nares, eustachian tube, mouth, esophagus, and larynx. The nasopharynx is the section above the palate; the oropharynx lies between the palate and the hyoid bone; and the laryngopharynx is below the hyoid bone.

The nerve supply is from the autonomic nervous system and from the vagus and glossopharyngeal nerves. Blood vessels branch from the exterior carotid artery. Veins form an extensive pharyngeal plexus and drain into the interior jugular vein.

**phase** (fāz) [Gr. *phasis,* an appearance] **1.** A stage of development. **2.** A transitory appearance. **3.** The state of a component of a heterogeneous system, as when oil is mixed with water, which is homogeneous throughout itself and bounded by an interface with other phases of the system.

***aqueous p.*** The water portion of a mixture of liquids and solids.

***continuous p.*** The state of a substance in a heterogeneous system in which particles are continuous (e.g., the water particles in which oil has been dispersed).

***disperse p.*** The state of a substance in a heterogeneous system in which particles are separated from each other (e.g., oil particles in water).

***lag p.*** Lag (2).

**phasic** (fā'sĭk) Of, or pert. to, a phase.

**phatnorrhagia** (făt"nō-rā'jē-ă) [Gr., socket of a tooth, + *rhegnynai,* to burst forth] Hemorrhage from the socket of a tooth.

**Ph.D.** *Doctor of Philosophy.*

**phenacemide** (fĕ-năs'ĕ-mīd) An anticonvulsive drug. Serious adverse side effects limit its usefulness.

**phenakistoscope** (fē"nă-kĭs'tō-skōp) [Gr. *phenakistos,* deceiver, + *skopein,* to view] A device that produces a stroboscopic-like view of the figures seen through slits that revolve in the same direction. The figures are seen in a mirror, and they appear to move.

**phenanthrene** (fē-năn'thrēn) $C_{14}H_{10}$. A coal tar derivative that is carcinogenic.

**phenate** (fē'nāt) A salt of phenic acid (phenol).

**phenazopyridine hydrochloride** (fĕn"ă-zō-pēr'ĭ-dēn) A drug with analgesic action on the urinary tract. It causes the urine to turn red or orange.

**phencyclidine hydrochloride** An anesthetic used in veterinary medicine. It is also used illegally as a hallucinogen, referred to as PCP or angel dust. Moderate doses cause elevated blood pressure, rapid pulse, increased skeletal muscle tone and sometimes, myoclonic jerks. Large doses can cause seizures, ataxia, nystagmus, respiratory depression, and death. Pupils are usually of normal size or small.

TREATMENT: For agitation caused by acute intoxication, diazepam is indicated. After initial therapy the patient should be observed in a quiet room. Efforts to "talk down" the patient are contraindicated.

**phenelzine sulfate** (fĕn'ĕl-zēn) An antidepressant drug.

**pheniramine maleate** (fĕn-ĭr'ă-mēn) An antihistamine drug.

**phenmetrazine hydrochloride** (fĕn-mĕt'ră-zēn) A sympathomimetic drug. Its effectiveness in treating obesity is unpredictable.

**phenobarbital** (fē"nō-băr'bĭ-tăl) Phenylethylbarbituric acid, a white crystalline substance soluble in alcohol.

ACTION/USES: This drug is used as a hypnotic, long-acting sedative, and anticonvulsant. Often in combination with diphenylhydantoin sodium, it is used in the treatment of epilepsy because it has a depressive effect on motor areas of the cerebral cortex.

***sodium p.*** Soluble phenobarbital; more rapidly absorbed than phenobarbital but with the same uses.

**phenocopy** (fē'nō-kŏp"ē) [Gr. *phainein,* to show, + *copy*] An individual with a biochemical or physical characteristic that resembles that produced by a genetic mutation but is instead due to an environmental condition.

**phenol** (fē'nōl) **1.** $C_6H_5OH$. A crystalline, colorless or light pink solid, melting at 43°C, obtained from the distillation of coal tar. It has a characteristic odor and is dangerous because of its rapid corrosive action on tissues. SYN: *carbolic acid.* **2.** Any of the aromatic derivatives of benzene with one or more hydroxyl groups attached.

***p. poisoning*** Poisoning caused by skin absorption or ingestion of phenol. SEE: *Poisons and Poisoning Appendix.*

SYMPTOMS: Strong solutions cause burning pain and, later, anesthesia. The skin and mucous membrane first become pale, then gray-white, opalescent, and finally brown to black. Even a 1% solution may cause local gangrene. It is absorbed from intact skin wounds and mucous membrane to cause general effects, including collapse and coma. When taken by mouth, it causes a whitish discoloration of the mucous membranes, intense burning, nausea and rarely vomiting, followed shortly by faintness, weakness, and collapse. The pulse is slow and weak and hypothermia with respiratory arrest may be present. Perspiration is increased and there is renal damage. Profound coma may occur within 30 min of exposure of the skin to phenol.

PROGNOSIS: A guarded prognosis should always be given because, although the patient may improve at first, damage to the mucous membrane and absorption of phenol may lead to serious complications later.

NURSING IMPLICATIONS: Poison should be removed from stomach as soon as possible. While waiting to do this, the nurse administers 5 to 6 tsp (25 to 30 ml) of activated charcoal in water and turns the patient from side to side to ensure that all portions of the stomach come in contact with the charcoal.

A well-lubricated gastric tube should be used with caution. Extensive lavage is performed with charcoal. If charcoal is not available, olive oil should be used and some should be left in stomach. If olive oil is not available, cottonseed oil or water should be used. Ethyl alcohol should not be used as lavage fluid because it speeds absorption of phenol. Demulcents, such as egg whites or milk, may be left in the stomach when lavage is finished.

Contaminated clothing is removed instantly, and external burns are washed with copious amounts of water or with olive oil. External heat, oxygen therapy, and morphine are used as required. The nurse explains all procedures and activities to the patient and provides reassurance and support.

***p. red*** An indicator used in determining hydrogen ion concentration.

**phenolemia** (fē″nō-lē′mē-ă) [*phenol* + Gr. *haima,* blood] The presence of phenol in the blood.

**phenology** (fē-nŏl′ō-jē) [Gr. *phainesthai,* to appear, + *logos,* word, reason] The study of the effects of climate on living things.

**phenolphthalein** (fē″nŏl-thăl′ē-ĭn, fē″nŏl-thăl′ēn) A white or yellow crystallized powder, produced by the interaction of phenol and phthalic anhydride. It is used as a laxative.

Sometimes this drug is self-administered to induce diarrhea. This occurs more frequently in women. If this is suspected, it may be validated by the pink color of a stool specimen that has been made alkaline.

**phenolsulfonphthalein** (fē″nŏl-sŭl″fōn-thăl′ē-ĭn) A dye that is given parenterally to test renal function. It is also an indicator of pH, being yellow at pH 6.8 and red at 8.4.

**phenoluria** (fē″nŏl-ū′rē-ă) Presence of phenols in the urine.

**phenomenology** (fĕ-nŏm″ĕ-nŏl′ō-jē) [Gr. *phainomenon,* appearing, + *logos,* word, reason] **1.** The study and classification of phenomena. **2.** The science of the subjective processes by which phenomena are presented, with emphasis on mental processes and essential elements of experiences. A phenomenological study emphasizes a person's descriptions of and feelings about experienced events.

**phenomenon** (fĕ-nŏm′ĕ-nŏn) *pl.* **phenomena** [Gr. *phainomenon,* appearing] A change, perceivable by the senses, that occurs in an organ or vital function; an objective symptom.

***breakaway p.*** Persons flying in outer space may experience the sensation of losing contact with all other human beings. SYN: *breakoff p.*

***breakoff p.*** Breakaway p.

***déjà vu p.*** SEE: *déjà vu.*

**phenothiazine** (fē″nō-thī′ă-zēn) An organic compound used in manufacturing a certain class of tranquilizers and in the production of insecticides, anthelmintics for livestock, and dyes. SEE: *chlorpromazine in Poisons and Poisoning Appendix.*

---

Caution: Overdose may cause severe postural hypotension, drowsiness, tachycardia, nausea, drying of the mouth, ataxia, fever, tremor, blurring of vision, and occasionally paralytic ileus.

---

TREATMENT: Symptomatic therapy is required. The drug should be removed from the stomach by gastric lavage.

**phenotype** (fē′nō-tīp) [Gr. *phainein,* to show, + *typos,* type] The expression of the genes present in an individual. This may be directly observable (e.g., eye color) or apparent only with specific tests (e.g., blood type). Some phenotypes, such as the blood groups, are completely determined by heredity, while others are readily altered by environmental agents. SEE: *genotype.*

**phenoxybenzamine hydrochloride** (fĕ-nŏk″sē-bĕn′ză-mēn) An alpha-adrenergic blocking agent used to produce peripheral vasodilation.

**phenozygous** (fē-nŏz′ĭ-gŭs) [″ + *zygon,* yoke] Possessing a cranium much narrower than the face.

**phensuximide** (fĕn-sŭk′sĭ-mīd) An anticonvulsant drug used in treating absence seizures.

**phentermine** (fĕn′tĕr-mēn) A sympathomimetic drug used as an anorexic.

**phentolamine hydrochloride** (fĕn-tŏl′ă-mēn) An $\alpha$-adrenergic blocking agent used in diagnosing pheochromocytoma.

**phenyl** (fĕn′ĭl, fē′nĭl) The univalent radical of phenol, $C_6H_5$.

**phenylalanine** (fĕn″ĭl-ăl′ă-nīn) An essential amino acid formed from protein.

**phenylamine** $C_6H_7N$. The simplest aromatic amine, an oily liquid derived from benzene; used in manufacture of dyes for medical and industrial purposes. SYN: *aminobenzene.*

**phenylbutazone** (fĕn″ĭl-bū′tă-zōn) An antiarthritic and anti-inflammatory drug originally developed for use in various forms of arthritis. Because of the possibility of serious side effects, the drug is used only when it is possible to supervise the patient carefully. Its long-term unsupervised use is contraindicated.

**phenylephrine hydrochloride** An adrenergic compound used in a suitably weak concentration to produce nasal decongestion; may also be used in ophthalmic solutions.

**phenylethyl alcohol** An antibacterial agent that has been used as a preservative in ophthalmic solutions.

**phenylhydrazine** (fĕn″ĭl-hī′dră-zēn) An oily nitrogenous base used as a test for the presence of sugar in the urine.

**phenylketonuria** (fĕn″ĭl-kē″tō-nū′rē-ă) ABBR: PKU. **1.** Phenylpyruvic acid in the urine. **2.** A recessive hereditary disease caused by the body's failure to oxidize an amino acid (phenylalanine) to tyrosine, because of a defective enzyme. If the disease is not treated early, brain damage may occur, causing severe mental retardation. A test for phenylketonuria should be made at birth; some states require it. The disease is seen equally in the sexes, and in the United States the incidence is approx. 1 : 14,000 births. Tremor, spasticity, convulsions, hyperactivity, mental deficiency, eczema, unusual hand posturing, and offensive odor of the urine and sweat characterize this disease.

Treatment consists of a low-phenylalanine diet. Prognosis is excellent if treatment is started early postnatally. If started after age 3 years, no improvement will occur because of brain damage.

Adult women who have PKU, plan to become pregnant and have an elevated level of phenylalanine should start a low-phenylalanine diet prior to pregnancy. The level of phenylalanine should be kept below 10 mg/dl throughout pregnancy.

NURSING IMPLICATIONS: Testing of babies for the disease is primarily a nursing responsibility and is normally carried out at birth so that affected children may be put on a low-phenylalanine diet to prevent brain damage. The nurse teaches parents the importance of a low-phenylalanine diet for their child and foods to avoid.

**phenylmercuric acetate** (fĕn″ĭl-mĕr-kū′rĭk) A bacteriostatic agent that also acts as a fungicide and herbicide.

**phenylpropanolamine hydrochloride** (fĕn″ĭl-prō″pă-nŏl′ă-mēn) A sympathomimetic drug used to produce bronchodilation.

**phenylpyruvic acid** (fĕn″ĭl-pī-roo′vĭk) A metabolic derivative of phenylalanine.

**phenylpyruvic acid oligophrenia** A form of inherited mental deficiency resulting from phenylketonuria.

**phenylthiocarbamide** (fĕn″ĭl-thī″ō-kăr′bă-mīd) ABBR: PTC. A chemical used in studying medical genetics to detect the presence of a marker gene. About 70% of the population inherit the ability to note the taste of phenylthiocarbamide to be extremely bitter. To the remainder of the population, it is tasteless. The gene for tasting is dominant and is expressed in both homozygous and heterozygous individuals. SYN: *phenylthiourea.*

**phenylthiourea** (fĕn″ĭl-thī″ō-ū-rē′ă) Phenylthiocarbamide.

**phenytoin** (fĕn′ĭ-tō-ĭn) An anticonvulsant drug. A very small number of patients using this anticonvulsant will develop benign pseudolymphoma that may resemble Hodgkin's disease. SYN: *diphenylhydantoin.* SEE: *Dupuytren's contracture.*

**pheochrome** (fē′ō-krōm) [Gr. *phaios,* dusky, + *chroma,* color] Staining darkly with chrome salts.

**pheochromoblast** (fē″ō-krō′mō-blăst) [″ + ″ + *blastos,* germ] Embryonic cells that develop into pheochromocytes.

**pheochromoblastoma** (fē″ō-krō″mō-blăs-tō′mă) [″ + ″ + ″ + *oma,* tumor] Pheochromocytoma.

**pheochromocyte** (fē″ō-krō′mō-sīt) [″ + ″ + *kytos,* cell] A chromaffin cell, such as one of those in the adrenal medulla, that gives a positive chromaffin reaction, that is, it yields a yellowish reaction with chrome salts.

**pheochromocytoma** (fē-ō-krō″mō-sī-tō′mă) [″ + ″ + ″ + *oma,* tumor] A chromaffin cell tumor of the sympathoadrenal system that produces catecholamines (i.e., norepinephrine and epinephrine). Although the tumor usually is benign, it produces hypertension that may be paroxysmal in about half the patients. The patient will complain of attacks of pounding headaches, sweating, palpitation, apprehension, flushing of the face, nausea and vomiting, and tingling of the extremities. The tumor should be removed surgically. SYN: *paraganglioma; pheochromoblastoma.* SEE: *Nursing Diagnoses Appendix.*

NURSING IMPLICATIONS: The patient is prepared for diagnostic tests and surgery if indicated. Patients should limit activities because they may initiate paroxysms. If crisis occurs, intensive monitoring of cardiac and neurological status is necessary. Vital functions are monitored on a continuous basis postoperatively, and fluid and electrolyte balance is watched closely. Medications are administered as prescribed, and the need for hormonal therapy is explained to patient. Strict aseptic technique is maintained, and incisional healing is monitored because wound healing is sometimes poor and complicated by infections. The nurse should provide reassurance to the patient and family throughout because the symptoms of this condition are frightening and distressing.

**pheomelanins** (fē-ō-mĕl′ă-nĭnz) [″ + Gr. *melas,* black] Yellow-brown, sulfur-containing pigments present as the pigment in human red hair.

**pheresis** Removal of blood from the individual, separating certain elements (e.g., cells such as platelets or red blood cells) and reintroducing the remaining components into the patient. SYN: *apheresis.* SEE: *leukapheresis; plateletpheresis; plasmapheresis.*

**pheromone** (fĕr′ō-mōn) A substance that provides chemical means of communication between animals, and between certain insects, of the same species. It is probably detected by smell and may affect the development, reproduction, or behavior of other individuals.

**Ph.G.** *German Pharmacopeia; Graduate in Pharmacy.*

**phial** (fī′ăl) [Gr. *phiale,* a bowl] A small vessel for medicine; a vial.

**Philadelphia collar** A lightweight orthosis for the head and neck to restrict cervical movement.

**-philia, -phil, -philic** (fĭl′ē-ă) [Gr. *philein,* to love] Combining form used as a suffix meaning *love for, tendency toward, craving for.*

**philtrum** The median groove on the external surface of the upper lip.

**phimosis** (fī-mō′sĭs) [Gr., a muzzling] Stenosis or narrowness of the preputial orifice so that the foreskin cannot be pushed back over the glans penis. The condition is treated by circumcision.

***p. vaginalis*** Narrowness or closure of the vaginal orifice.

**pHisoHex** (fī′sō-hĕks) Trade name for an antibacterial skin cleanser containing hexachlorophene as the main ingredient.

**phlebalgia** (flĕ-băl′jē-ă) [Gr. *phlebos,* vein, + *algos,* pain] Pain arising from a vein.

**phlebangioma** (flĕb″ăn-jē-ō′mă) [″ + *angeion,* vessel, + *oma,* tumor] An aneurysm occurring in a vein.

**phlebarteriectasia** (flĕb″ăr-tē″rē-ĕk-tā′zē-ă) [″ + *arteria,* artery, + *ektasis,* dilatation] Dilatation of blood vessels.

**phlebarteriodialysis** (flĕb″ăr-tē″rē-ō-dī-ăl′ĭ-sĭs) [″ + ″ + *dialysis,* separation] Arteriovenous aneurysm.

**phlebectasia, phlebectasis** (flĕb-ĕk-tā′zē-ă, -ĕk′tă-sĭs) [″+ *ektasis,* dilatation] Varicosity.

**phlebectomy** (flĕb-ĕk′tō-mē) [″ + *ektome,* excision] Surgical removal of a vein or part of a vein.

**phlebectopia** (flĕb″ĕk-tō′pē-ă) [″ + *ek,* out, + *topos,* place] Abnormal position of a vein.

**phlebitis** (flĕ-bī′tĭs) [″ + *itis,* inflammation] Inflammation of a vein. SYN: *milk leg; phlegmasia alba dolens; thrombophlebitis.* SEE: *Nursing Diagnoses Appendix.*

SYMPTOMS: There are pain and tenderness along the course of the vein, discoloration of the skin, inflammatory swelling and acute edema below the obstruction, rapid pulse, mild elevation of temperature, and pain in the joints.

ETIOLOGY: The cause is unknown. It may occur in acute or chronic infections or following operations or childbirth.

NURSING IMPLICATIONS: In the acute phase, direct efforts toward reducing inflammation and preventing emboli by ensuring rest, elevation of affected limb, and use of antiembolic stockings. Administer analgesics and anticoagulants as ordered. Observe patient carefully for bleeding in nose, gums, urine, and feces.

*Prevention:* Teach individual to avoid long periods of standing or sitting with little body movement; also avoid pressure behind the knees such as that produced by crossing the legs. If oral anticoagulants are being taken, advise discussion with physician relative to contraindicated medications such as aspirin. Advise against smoking because of negative effects on cardiovascular system. Encourage use of elastic stockings if indicated. Reinforce long-term medical follow-up if patient has had episodes of phlebitis.

***adhesive p.*** Phlebitis in which the vein tends to become obliterated.

***migrating p.*** A transitory phlebitis that appears in a portion of a vein and then clears up, only to reappear later in another location.

***p. nodularis necrotisans*** Circumscribed inflammation of cutaneous veins resulting in nodules that ulcerate.

***obliterative p.*** Phlebitis in which the lumen of a vein becomes permanently closed.

***puerperal p.*** Venous inflammation following childbirth.

***sclerosing p.*** Phlebitis in which the veins become obstructed and hardened.

***sinus p.*** Inflammation of a sinus of the cerebrum.

***suppurative p.*** Phlebitis characterized by the formation of pus.

**phlebo-** [Gr. *phleps, phlebos*] Combining form meaning *vein.*

**phlebogram** (flĕb′ō-grăm) [Gr. *phlebos,* vein, + *gramma,* something written] A tracing of the venous pulse.

**phlebography** (flĕ-bŏg′ră-fē) [″ + *graphein,* to write] A study of the structure and function of the veins.

**phlebolith, phlebolite** (flĕb′ō-lĭth, -līt) [″ + *lithos,* a stone] A calcareous concretion in a vein.

**phlebolithiasis** (flĕb″ō-lĭ-thī′ă-sĭs) [″ + *lithiasis,* forming stones] The formation of phleboliths in veins.

**phlebology** (flĕb-ŏl′ō-jē) [″ + *logos,* word, reason] The science of veins and their diseases.

**phlebomanometer** (flĕb″ō-mă-nŏm′ĕ-tĕr) [″ + *manos,* thin, + *metron,* measure] A device for the direct measurement of venous pressure.

**phlebometritis** (flĕb″ō-mĕ-trī′tĭs) [″ + *metra,* uterus, + *itis,* inflammation] Inflammation of uterine veins.

**phlebomyomatosis** (flĕb″ō-mī″ō-mă-tō′sĭs) [″ + *mys,* muscle, + *oma,* tumor, + *osis,* condition] Thickening of the tissue of a vein from an overgrowth of muscular fibers.

**phlebopexy** (flĕb′ō-pĕk″sē) [″ + *peksis,* fixation] Extraserous transplantation of the testes for varicocele, with preservation of the venous network.

**phlebophlebostomy** (flĕb″ō-flĕ-bŏs′tō-mē) [″ + *phlebos,* vein, + *stoma,* mouth] Surgical anastomosis of veins.

**phleboplasty** (flĕb′ō-plăs″tē) [″ + *plassein,* to form] Plastic repair of an injured vein.

**phleborrhagia** (flĕb″ō-rā′jē-ă) [″ + *rhegnynai,* to burst forth] Bleeding from a vein.

**phleborrhaphy** (flĕb-or′ă-fē) [″ + *rhaphe,* seam, ridge] Suturing of a vein.

**phleborrhexis** (flĕb″ō-rĕk′sĭs) [″ + *rhexis,* rupture] Rupture of a vein.

**phlebosclerosis** (flĕb″ō-sklē-rō′sĭs) [″ + *sklerosis,* hardening] Fibrous hardening of a vein's walls.

**phlebostasia, phlebostasis** (flĕb-ō-stā′zē-ă, -ŏs′tă-sĭs) [″ + *stasis,* stoppage] Compression of veins temporarily to restrict an amount of blood from the general circulation. SYN: *bloodless phlebotomy.*

**phlebostenosis** (flĕb″ō-stĕ-nō′sĭs) [″ + *stenosis,* narrowing] Constriction of a vein.

**phlebothrombosis** (flĕb″ō-thrŏm-bō′sĭs) [″ + *thrombos,* a clot] Clotting in a vein; phlebitis with secondary thrombosis.

**phlebotomist** (flĕ-bŏt′ō-mĭst) [″ + *tome,* incision] One who practices venesection (i.e., draws blood by use of a syringe and needle).

**phlebotomize** (flĕ-bŏt′ō-mīz) To take blood from a person.

**Phlebotomus** (flĕ-bŏt′ō-mŭs) [″ + *tome,* incision] A genus of insects, the sandflies, belonging to the family Psychodidae, order Diptera. The bloodsucking insects are annoying and transmit various forms of leishmaniasis, sandfly (pappataci) fever, and Oroya fever.

***P. argentipes*** In India, the transmitter of *Leishmania donovani,* causative agent of kala-azar.

***P. chinensis*** Transmitter of kala-azar in China.

***P. papatasii*** Transmitter of the causative agent of sandfly fever. The virus is capable of being transmitted through the offspring of flies.

***P. sergenti*** Transmitter of kala-azar in Middle East and India.

***P. verrucarum*** The transmitter of *Bartonella bacilliformis,* causative agent of Oroya fever (Carrion's disease), in South America.

**phlebotomy** (flĕ-bŏt′ō-mē) [″ + *tome,* incision] The surgical opening of a vein to withdraw blood. SYN: *venesection.*

***bloodless p.*** Phlebostasia.

**phlegm** (flĕm) [Gr. *phlegma*] **1.** Thick mucus, esp. that from the respiratory passages. **2.** One of the four "humors" of early physiology.

**phlegmasia** (flĕg-mā′zē-ă) [Gr. *phlegmasia*] Inflammation.

***p. alba dolens*** Acute edema, esp. of the leg, from venous obstruction, usually a thrombosis. SYN: *milk leg; white leg.*

SYMPTOMS: This condition usually begins with slight fever, esp. in women who have recently given birth. Pain in the lower part of the abdomen follows, extends to the hips and back, passes under Poupart's ligament, then down the thigh and into the calf of the leg. Sometimes it proceeds from the calf upward. The whole extremity becomes excessively swollen, hot, and painful, but not red; hence the name.

Tenderness on pressure is most marked along course of the femoral vein, and veins of the affected region together with associated lymphatics may feel hard and cordlike. Sometimes the condition is marked by a faint red line over the vein. Progress is rapid, frequently doubling the size of the limb in 24 hr or less. Often, evacuation of the bladder and rectum becomes difficult, glands in the groin sometimes swell and suppurate, and abscesses may form in different parts of the limb.

TREATMENT: The limb should be elevated and protected with a cradle. Heat should be applied. Anticoagulants are necessary to prevent clot formation. Vasodilator drugs and paracervical block may be used to combat vasospasm. Ligation of the main venous channel proximal to the thrombus may be done to prevent embolus.

NURSING IMPLICATIONS: Strict bedrest is maintained, and the affected limb is elevated and immobilized. A leg and foot cradle is used to protect the limb from pressure by bed linens. Pneumatic or antiembolism devices are applied as prescribed to the affected limb. Intermittent or continuous warm, moist compresses are applied to affected limb as prescribed to resolve inflammation. Anticoagulant and analgesic drug therapies are administered as prescribed, and patient and laboratory studies are evaluated for desired responses. The nurse assesses for embolic complications and teaches the patient about the importance of bedrest in preventing immobilization of thrombi; about concerns pertaining to oral birth control pills; about the importance of walking rather than standing; and about long-term use of oral anticoagulant drugs and antiembolism stockings in preventing recurrence.

***cellulitic p.*** Septic inflammation of the connective tissue of the leg following childbirth.

***p. cerulea dolens*** A deep venous thrombosis in which blood may stagnate in the veins and become very dark red due to deoxygenation. This gives a cyanotic hue to the area.

**phlegmatic** (flĕg-măt′ĭk) [Gr. *phlegmatikos*] Of sluggish or dull temperament; apathetic.

**phlegmon** (flĕg′mŏn) [Gr. *phlegmone,* inflammation] Acute suppurative inflammation of subcutaneous connective tissue, esp. a pyogenic inflammation that spreads along fascial planes or other natural barriers.

***diffuse p.*** Diffuse inflammation of subcutaneous tissues with sepsis.

***gas p.*** Gas gangrene.

**phlegmonous** (flĕg′mŏn-ŭs) Pert. to inflammation of subcutaneous tissues.

**phlogogenic, phlogogenous** (flō-gō-jĕn′ĭk, -gŏj′ĕn-ŭs) [Gr. *phlogosis,* inflammation, + *gennan,* to produce] Producing inflammation.

**phlorhizin** (flō-rī′zĭn) A glycoside present in the bark of some fruit trees. It is a powerful inhibitor of sugar transport in some animals.

**phlyctena** (flĭk-tē′nă) *pl.* **phlyctenae** [Gr. *phlyktaina*] A vesicle, esp. one of many after a first-degree burn.

**phlyctenar** (flĭk′tĕ-năr) Concerning a vesicle.

**phlyctenula** (flĭk-tĕn′ū-lă) *pl.* **phlyctenulae** [L.] A tiny vesicle or pustule, esp. that seen on the cornea.

**phlyctenular** (flĭk-tĕn′ū-lăr) Resembling or pert. to vesicles or pustules.

**phlyctenule** (flĭk′tĕn-ūl) [Gr. *phlyktaina,* a blister; L. *phlyctenula*] A small vesicle or blister, as on the cornea or conjunctiva.

**phobia** (fō′bē-ă) [Gr. *phobos,* fear] Any persistent and irrational fear of a specific object, activity, or situation that results in a compelling desire to avoid the feared or phobic stimulus. SEE: *Nursing Diagnoses Appendix; Phobias Appendix.*

***social p.*** Avoidance of social situations in which the individual would be noticed or would attract attention to himself or herself (e.g., speaking or lecturing in public).

**-phobia** [Gr.] Combining form used as a suffix indicating *fear, aversion.*

**phobic** (fō′bĭk) [Gr. *phobos,* fear] Concerning a phobia.

**phobophobia** (fō″bō-fō′bē-ă) [″ + *phobos,* fear] The morbid fear of acquiring a phobia.

**phocomelia** (fō″kō-mē′lē-ă) [Gr. *phoke,* seal, + *melos,* limb] A congenital malformation in which the proximal portions of the extremities are poorly developed or absent. Thus the hands and feet are attached to the trunk directly or by means of a poorly formed bone. In some cases this condition was due to the the pregnant woman taking thalidomide, a sleeping pill, during early pregnancy. That drug is no longer approved for such use. SYN: *amelia.*

**phocomelus** (fō-kŏm′ĕ-lŭs) A person with phocomelia.

**phon-** SEE: *phono-.*

**phonacoscope** (fō-năk′ō-skōp) [Gr. *phone,* voice, + *skopein,* to examine] A device for amplifying the percussion note or voice sounds.

**phonacoscopy** (fō-nă-kŏs′kō-pē) Examination of the chest with a phonacoscope.

**phonal** (fō′năl) [Gr. *phone,* voice] Concerning the voice.

**phonasthenia** (fōn-ăs-thē′nē-ă) [″ + *asthenia,* weakness] Vocal weakness or hoarseness caused by straining the voice.

**phonation** (fō-nā′shŭn) The process of uttering vocal sounds.

**phone** (fōn) [Gr. *phone,* voice] An element of speech; a single speech sound.

**phoneme** (fō′nēm) [Gr. *phonema,* an utterance] In linguistics, the smallest unit of speech that distinguishes one sound from another.

**phonendoscope** (fō-nĕn′dō-skōp) [Gr. *phone,* voice, + *endon,* within, + *skopein,* to examine] A stethoscope that intensifies sounds.

**phonetics** (fō-nĕt′ĭks) [Gr. *phonetikos,* spoken] The science of speech and pronunciation. SYN: *phonology.*

**phoniatrics** (fō″nē-ăt′rĭks) [Gr. *phone,* voice, + *iatrikos,* treatment] The study of the voice and treatment of its disorders.

**phonic** (fŏ′nĭk) Concerning the voice or sound.

**phonism** (fō′nĭzm) [″ + *-ismos,* condition] An auditory sensation occurring when another sense is stimulated. SEE: *synesthesia.*

**phono-** [Gr. *phone,* voice] Combining form indicating *sound, voice.*

**phonocardiogram** (fō″nō-kăr′dē-ō-grăm) [″ + *kardia,* heart, + *gramma,* something written] A graphic recording of the heart sounds.

**phonocardiography** (fō″nō-kăr″dē-ŏg′ră-fē) [″ + ″ + *graphein,* to write] The mechanical or electronic registration of heart sounds.

**phonocatheter** (fō″nō-kăth′ĕ-tĕr) [″ + *katheter,* something inserted] A catheter with a microphone at its end.

**phonogram** (fō′nō-grăm) [″ + *gramma,* something written] A graphic curve indicating the intensity and duration of a sound.

**phonograph** (fō′nō-grăf) [″ + *graphein,* to write] An instrument used for the reproduction of recorded sounds.

**phonology** (fō-nŏl′ō-jē) [″ + *logos,* word, reason] Phonetics.

**phonomassage** (fō″nō-mă-sahzh′) [Gr. *phone,* voice, + *massein,* to knead] Exciting movements of the ossicles of the ear by means of noise or alternating suction and pressure directed through the external auditory meatus.

**phonometer** (fō-nŏm′ĕ-tĕr) [″ + *metron,* measure] A device for determining the intensity of vocal sounds.

**phonomyoclonus** (fō″nō-mī-ŏk′lō-nŭs) [″ + *mys,* muscle, + *klonos,* a contraction] Invisible fibrillary muscular contractions revealed by auscultation.

**phonomyogram** (fō″nō-mī′ō-grăm) [″ + ″ + *gramma,* something written] A recording of sound produced by the action of a muscle.

**phonomyography** (fō″nō-mī-ŏg′ră-fē) [″ + ″ + *graphein,* to write] The recording of sounds made by contracting muscular tissue.

**phonopathy** (fō-nŏp′ă-thē) [″ + *pathos,* disease, suffering] Any disease of organs affecting speech.

**phonophobia** (fō″nō-fō′bē-ă) [″ + *phobos,* fear] **1.** A morbid fear of sound or noise. **2.** A fear of speaking or hearing one's own voice.

**phonophoresis** The use of ultrasound to introduce medication into a tissue. This has been used in treating injuries to soft tissues. Not all medicines are suitable for application using this technique.

Caution: The use of phonophoresis should be supervised by persons skilled in using the technique.

**phonopsia** (fō-nŏp′sē-ă) [″ + *opsis,* vision] The subjective perception of sensations upon hearing certain sounds.

**phonoreceptor** A receptor for sound waves.

**phonorenogram** (fō″nō-rē′nō-grăm) [″+ L. *ren,* kidney, + Gr. *gramma,* something written] A recording of the pulse in the renal artery.

**phonoscope** (fō′nō-skōp) [″ + *skopein,* to examine] A device for recording heart sounds.

**phonoscopy** (fō-nŏs′kō-pē) A recording made by use of a phonoscope.

**-phoresis** (fō-rē′sĭs) [Gr. *phoresis,* being borne] Suffix indicating transmission, as *electrophoresis, cataphoresis, anaphoresis.*

**-phoria** [Gr. *phoresis,* being borne] In ophthalmology, a combining form meaning *a turning,* with reference to the visual axis, such as cyclophoria.

**Phormia** (for′mē-ă) A genus of blowflies belonging to the family Calliphoridae. Their larvae normally live in decaying flesh of dead animals, but they may infest neglected wounds or sores, giving rise to myiasis.

**phorozoon** (fō″rō-zō′ŏn) [Gr. *phoros,* fruitful, + *zoon,* animal] The nonsexual stage of an animal that in its life cycle passes through several stages.

**phose** (fōz) [Gr. *phos,* light] A subjective sensation of light or color. SEE: *chromophose; erythrophose.*

**phosgene** (fŏs′jēn) [″ + *genes,* born] Carbonyl chloride, $COCl_2$, a poisonous gas that causes nausea and suffocation when inhaled; used in chemical warfare.

**phosphagen** (fŏs′fă-jĕn) Several chemicals, including phosphocreatine, that release energy when split. They are high-energy phosphate compounds.

**phosphatase** (fŏs′fă-tās) One of a group of enzymes that catalyze the hydrolysis of phosphoric acid esters. They are of importance in absorption and metabolism of carbohydrates, nucleotides, and phospholipids and are essential in the calcification of bone.

***acid p.*** A phosphatase whose optimum pH is between 4.0 and 5.4. It is present in kidney, semen, serum, and prostate gland, and particularly in osteoclasts or odontoclasts in which it is associated with demineralization or resorption of bone and teeth.

***alkaline p.*** A phosphatase whose optimum pH is about 9.0 and which functions in the mineralization process of bone. It is present in teeth, developing bone, plasma, kidney, and intestine. Because it is excreted by the liver, its blood level increases in obstructive jaundice. It is also elevated in diseases of the pancreas, lung, and bone, in some malignancies without metastases, and in pregnancy. In the first month of life, it may be as high as six times the normal level in adults. The level gradually decreases during childhood and puberty. By use of special techniques alkaline phosphatase can be separated into bone, intestinal, and placental fractions.

**phosphate** (fŏs′fāt) [Gr. *phosphas*] Any salt of phosphoric acid containing the radical $PO_4$. Phosphates are important in the maintenance of the acid-base balance of the blood, the principal ones being monosodium and disodium phosphate. The former is acid, the latter alkaline. In the blood, because of their low concentration, they exert a minor buffering action. In the formation of urine, through alteration of the proportions of acid and alkaline phosphates, an acid urine is formed, and the body's fixed base, chiefly sodium but also potassium, magnesium, and calcium, is conserved.

Decreased phosphate excretion in the urine occurs when the alkaline reserve is high and in nephritis, tetany (hypoparathyroidism), adrenal cortical deficiency, and certain bone diseases.

Increased phosphate excretion in the urine occurs when the alkali reserve is low and in starvation, hyperparathyroidism, high-protein diet, and extreme muscular exercise.

***acid p.*** A phosphate in which only one or two hydrogen atoms of phosphoric acid have been replaced by a metal.

***calcium p.*** Any one of three salts of calcium and phosphate; used as an antacid and dietary supplement.

***creatine p.*** Phosphocreatine.

***normal p.*** A phosphate in which all three hydrogen atoms of phosphoric acid have been replaced by metals.

***triple p.*** Calcium, ammonium, and magnesium phosphate.

**phosphate-bond energy** Energy derived from phosphorylated compounds such as adenosine triphosphate (ATP) and creatine phosphate.

**phosphatemia** (fŏs″fă-tē′mē-ă) [Gr. *phosphas,* phosphate, + *haima,* blood] Phosphates in the blood.

**phosphatide** (fŏs′fă-tīd) Phospholipid.

**phosphatidyl glycerol** ABBR: PG. A phospholipid found in amniotic fluid, pulmonary effluent, and semen. It first appears in amniotic fluid during week 36 of pregnancy, confirms fetal gestational age, and is an accurate predictor of fetal lung maturity.

**phosphaturia** (fŏs″fă-tū′rē-ă) [″ + *ouron,* urine] An excessive amount of phosphates in the urine; often causing renal calculi. SYN: *phosphoruria; phosphuria.*

SYMPTOMS: This condition is characterized by cloudy, opaque, and pale urine; alkaline reaction; and pearly or pink-white deposits of phosphates in standing urine.

**phosphene** (fŏs′fēn) [Gr. *phos,* light, + *phainein,* to show] A subjective sensation of light caused by pressure on the eyeball.

***accommodation p.*** Phosphene resulting from contraction of the ciliary muscles in accommodation. This is seen esp. in the dark.

**phosphide** (fŏs′fīd) [″ + *phorein,* to carry] A binary compound of phosphorus with an element or radical.

**phosphite** (fŏs′fīt) A salt of phosphoric acid.

**phosphoamidase** (fŏs″fō-ăm′ĭ-dās) An enzyme that catalyzes the conversion of phosphocreatine to creatine and orthophosphate.

**phosphocreatine** (fŏs″fō-krē′ă-tĭn) A compound found in muscle. It is important as an energy source, yielding phosphate and creatine in this process, and releasing energy that is used to synthesize adenosine triphosphate.

**phosphodiesterase** An enzyme critical for the breakdown of cyclic adenosine monophosphate.

**phosphofructokinase** (fŏs″fō-frŭk″tō-kī′nās)

A glycolytic enzyme that catalyzes phosphorylation of fructose-6-phosphate by adenosine triphosphate.

**phospholipase** (fŏs″fō-lĭp′ās) An enzyme that catalyzes hydrolysis of a phospholipid.

**phospholipid** (fŏs″fō-lĭp′ĭd) [Gr. *phos,* light, + *phorein,* to carry, + *lipos,* fat] A lipoid substance containing phosphorus and fatty acids, as lecithen. The lipid portion of cell membranes is primarily phospholipids. SYN: *phosphatide; phospholipin.*

**phospholipin** (fŏs″fō-lĭp′ĭn) Phospholipid.

**phosphonecrosis** (fŏs″fō-nĕ-krō′sĭs) [″ + *phorein,* to carry, + *nekros,* dead, + *osis,* condition] Necrosis of the alveolar process in persons working with phosphorus.

**phosphonuclease** (fŏs″fō-nū′klē-ās) An enzyme that catalyzes the hydrolysis of nucleotides to nucleosides and phosphoric acid.

**phosphopenia** (fŏs″fō-pē′nē-ă) [″ + *phorein,* to carry, + *penia,* lack] A deficiency of phosphorus in the body.

**phosphoprotein** (fŏs″fō-prō′tē-ĭn) [″ + ″ + *protos,* first] One of a group of proteins in which the protein is combined with a phosphorus-containing compound. Caseinogen and vitellin are examples. Phosphoprotein was formerly called nucleoalbumin.

**phosphor** A substance in the fluoroscopic image intensifier that converts photons of energy into light.

***rare earth p.*** An element such as yttrium, gadolinium, or lanthanum, that is used for ultra-high-speed radiographic intensification screens.

**phosphorated** (fŏs′fō-rā″tĕd) [″ + *phorein,* to carry] Impregnated with phosphorus.

**phosphorescence** (fŏs-fō-rĕs′ĕns) The induced luminescence that persists after cessation of the irradiation that caused it; the emission of light without appreciable heat.

**phosphoribosyltransferase** (fŏs″fō-rī″bō-sĭl-trăns′fĕr-ās) An enzyme that catalyzes reconversion to the ribonucleotide stage of the purine bases, hypoxanthine and guanine. The deficiency is inherited as an X chromosome–linked trait.

**phosphorism** (fŏs′for-ĭzm) [″ + ″ + *-ismos,* condition] Chronic poisoning from phosphorus.

**phosphorolysis** (fŏs″fō-rŏl′ĭ-sĭs) The chemical reaction of incorporating phosphoric acid into a molecule.

**phosphorous acid** (fŏs-fō′rŭs, fŏs′for-ŭs) [″ + *phoros,* carrying] $H_3PO_3$. Crystalline acid formed when phosphorus is oxidized in moist air.

**phosphoruria** (fŏs″for-ū′rē-ă) [″ + *phorein,* to carry, + *ouron,* urine] Phosphaturia.

**phosphorus** (fŏs′fō-rŭs) [Gr. *phos,* light, + *phoros,* carrying] SYMB: P. A nonmetallic element not found in a free state but in combination with alkalies; atomic weight 30.9738; atomic number 15. The normal serum value of phosphorus is 2.5 to 4.5 mg/dl. Normally, plasma concentrations of phosphorus and calcium have a reciprocal relationship; as one increases, the other decreases.

The adult body contains from 600 to 900 g of phosphorus in various forms: 70% to 80% in bones and teeth, principally combined with calcium; 10% in muscle; and 1% in nerve tissue. Minimum daily requirement is approx. 800 mg. This amount should be increased during pregnancy and lactation. Vitamin D is important in the absorption and metabolism of phosphorus. Excess phosphorus is excreted by the kidneys and intestines, about 60% being excreted in urine principally as phosphates. Perverted appetite, retarded growth, loss of weight, weakness, rickets, and imperfect bone and teeth development characterize the deficiency of this element.

Phosphorus compounds are found in the nucleic acids DNA and RNA; in adenosine triphosphate, the principal energy source in cells; and in phosphocreatine, a secondary energy source for muscle contraction.

EXCESS: An excess of phosphorus is caused most often by renal disease. Few direct problems result from hyperphosphatemia, but the patient may have an associated hypocalcemia. Treatment is directed at the cause and at managing the hypocalcemia.

SOURCES: Phosphorus is found in many foods. Excellent sources are almonds, beans, barley, bran, cheese, cocoa, chocolate, eggs, lentils, liver, milk, oatmeal, peanuts, peas, rye, walnuts, and whole wheat. Good sources are asparagus, beef, cabbage, carrots, celery, cauliflower, chard, chicken, clams, corn, cream, cucumbers, eggplant, fish, figs, meat, prunes, pineapples, pumpkin, raisins, and string beans.

***p. poisoning*** Poisoning caused by the ingestion of substances containing yellow phosphorus, such as rat and roach poison. Before the introduction of safety matches (which contain no yellow phosphorus), phosphorus poisoning was quite common. Yellow phosphorus is also used in manufacturing fireworks and fertilizers. SEE: *Poisons and Poisoning Appendix.*

SYMPTOMS: In this type of poisoning acute irritation of gastrointestinal tract is followed by symptoms resembling acute yellow atrophy of the liver and marked blood changes. Bloody vomitus, garlic odor of breath, cramps, headache, and liver and kidney damage also occur. Other symptoms include profound weakness, hemorrhage, and heart failure. Occasionally nervous system symptoms predominate.

NURSING IMPLICATIONS: Gastric lavage is preferred to induce emesis if phosphorus was swallowed. The airway is protected by cuffed endotracheal intubation or left lateral decubitus position. Charcoal slurry and a cathartic drug are administered. The patient requires close monitoring for delayed effects for at least 24 hr.

**phosphoryl** (fŏs′for-ĭl) The radical [PO]≡.

**phosphorylase** (fŏs-for′ĭ-lās) An enzyme that catalyzes the formation of glucose-1-phosphate from glycogen.

**phosphorylation** (fŏs″for-ĭ-lā′shŭn) The combining of a phosphate with an organic compound.

**phosphuria** (fŏs-fū′rē-ă) [Gr. *phos,* light, + *phoros,* a bearer, + *ouron,* urine] Phosphaturia.

**phot** (fōt) [Gr. *photos,* light] ABBR: ph. The unit of photochemical energy equal to 1 lumen/cm² or about 929 foot-candles.

**phot-** SEE: words beginning with *photo-*.

**photalgia** (fō-tăl′jē-ă) [Gr. *photos,* light, + *algos,* pain] Pain produced by light.

**photaugiaphobia** (fō-taw″jē-ă-fō′bē-ă) [Gr. *photaugeia,* glare, + *phobos,* fear] Intolerance of bright light.

**photic** (fō′tĭk) **1.** Concerning light. **2.** In biology, pert. to the production of light by certain organisms.

***p. driving*** In neurology, altering the electroencephalogram by intermittently flashing light into the eyes.

***p. sneezing*** Sneezing initiated or hastened in its onset by light stimulus. It is sometimes due to light causing tears, which, upon draining into the nasal area, cause sneezing. SYN: *photoptarmosis.*

**photism** (fō′tĭzm) [″ + *-ismos,* condition] A subjective sensation of color or light produced by a stimulus of another sense, such as smell, hearing, taste, or touch. SEE: *synesthesia.*

**photo-** [Gr. *photos*] Combining form indicating *light.*

**photoactinic** (fō″tō-ăk-tĭn′ĭk) Emitting both luminous and actinic rays.

**photoallergy** (fō″tō-ăl′ĕr-jē) [Gr. *photos,* light, + *allos,* other, + *ergon,* work] An immunological reaction produced by the interaction of light rays and certain chemicals. It is a form of contact allergic reaction in which light is necessary to cause the sensitivity reaction. Some of the photocontact allergens are phenothiazine, sulfonamides, hexachlorophene, sunscreen agents, optical bleaches, and topical antihistamines. SEE: *persistent light reaction; photosensitivity; phototoxic.*

**photobiology** (fō″tō-bī-ŏl′ō-jē) [″ + *bios,* life, + *logos,* word, reason] The study of the effect of light on living things.

**photobiotic** (fō″tō-bī-ŏt′ĭk) [″ + *bios,* life] Capable of living only in the light.

**photochemistry** (fō″tō-kĕm′ĭs-trē) [″ + *chemeia,* chemistry] The branch of chemistry concerned with the effects of light rays.

**photochemotherapy** The use of light and chemicals together to treat certain conditions.

***extracorporeal p.*** Administering drugs in the usual manner, exposing drawn blood to ultraviolet A radiation, then returning the blood to the body. The combination of 8-methoxypsoralen and light has been used in treating drug-resistant pemphigus vulgaris.

**photochromogen** [″ + *chroma,* color, + *gennan,* to produce] Certain microorganisms in which a pigment develops when it is grown in the presence of light, such as *Mycobacterium kansasii.*

**photocoagulation** Alteration of proteins in tissue by the use of light energy in the form of ordinary light rays or a laser beam; used esp. in treating retinal detachments or bleeding from the retina.

**photodermatitis** (fō″tō-dĕr-mă-tī′tĭs) [″ + *dermatos,* skin, + *itis,* inflammation] Sensitivity of the epithelium to light; may be due to photoallergy or to phototoxic reaction.

**photodynamic** (fō″tō-dī-năm′ĭk) [″ + *dynamis,* force] Pert. to the energy or force effected by light on organisms.

***p. action*** Action exerted by certain dyes, such as methylene blue and eosin, on certain biological systems when subjected to light.

***p. therapy*** The administration of drugs to make tumors sensitive to light. The lesions are then subject to light, which kills cancer cells. SYN: *photoradiotherapy.*

**photodysphoria** (fō″tō-dĭs-for′ē-ă) [″ + *dysphoria,* distress] Photophobia.

**photoelectricity** (fō″tō-ē-lĕk-trĭ′sĭ-tē) [″ + *elektron,* amber] Electricity formed by the action of light.

**photoelectron** (fō″tō-ē-lĕk′trŏn) [″ + *elektron,* amber] An electron that is ejected from its orbit around the nucleus of an atom by interaction with a photon of energy (light, x-radiation, and so on).

**photoerythema** (fō″tō-ĕr″ĭ-thē′mă) [″ + *erythema,* redness] Erythema of the skin caused by light.

**photofluorography** (fō″tō-flū″ĕr-ŏg′ră-fē) Photographing the images seen during fluoroscopic examination.

**photogastroscope** (fō″tō-găs′trō-skōp) [″ + *gaster,* belly, + *skopein,* to view] A device for viewing and taking photographs of the interior of the stomach.

**photogenic, photogenous** (fō″tō-jĕn′ĭk, -tŏj′ĕn-ŭs) Induced by, or inducing, light.

**photokinetic** (fō″tō-kĭn-ĕt′ĭk) [″ + *kinetikos,* motion] Reacting with motion to stimulus of light.

**photokymograph** (fō″tō-kī′mō-grăf) [″ + *kyma,* wave, + *graphein,* to write] A device for making continuous photographs of a physiological event.

**photolabile** The characteristic of being destroyed or inactivated by light.

**photoluminescence** (fō″tō-lū-mĭ-nĕs′ĕns) [″ + L. *lumen,* light] The power of an object to become luminescent when acted on by light.

**photolysis** (fō-tŏl′ĭ-sĭs) [″ + *lysis,* dissolution] Dissolution or disintegration under stimulus of light rays.

**photolytic** (fō″tō-lĭt′ĭk) Dissolved by stimulus of light rays.

**photomania** (fō″tō-mā′nē-ă) [″ + *mania,* madness] **1.** A psychosis produced by prolonged exposure to intense light. **2.** A psychotic desire for light.

**photomedicine** The use of light to treat certain conditions. SEE: *hemolytic disease of the newborn; phototherapy; psoriasis.*

**photometer** (fō-tŏm′ĕ-tĕr) [″ + *metron,* measure] A device for measuring the intensity of light.

**photometry** (fō-tŏm′ĕ-trē) Measurement of light rays.

**photomicrograph** (fō″tō-mī′krō-grăf) [″ + *mikros,* small, + *graphein,* to write] A photograph of an object under a microscope.

**photon** (fō′tŏn) [Gr. *photos,* light] A light quantum or unit of energy of a light ray or other form of radiant energy. It is generally considered to be a discrete particle having zero mass, no electric charge, and indefinitely long life.

**photo-onycholysis** Separation of the nail from the distal nailbed in conjunction with sun exposure and simultaneous use of drugs such as antibiotics.

**photo-ophthalmia, photophthalmia** (fō″tō-ŏf-thăl′mē-ă, fō″tŏf-thăl′mē-ă) [″ + *ophthalmos,* eye] Keratoconjunctivitis produced by excess exposure to intense light rays.

**photoperceptive** (fō″tō-pĕr-sĕp′tĭv) [″ + L. *percipere,* to receive] Capable of perceiving light.

**photoperiod** (fō″tō-pĕr′ē-ŏd) [″ + L. *periodus,* period] The daily duration of exposure to light of a living thing.

**photoperiodism** (fō″tō-pĕr′ē-ō-dĭzm) [″ + ″ + Gr. *-ismos,* condition] The periodic occurrence of biological phenomena in relationship to the presence or absence of light. In most animals, the sleep-wake cycle is a form of photoperiodism.

**photophilic** (fō-tō-fĭl′ĭk) [″ + *philein,* to love] Seeking, or fond of, light.

**photophobia** (fō″tō-fō′bē-ă) [″ + *phobos,* fear] Unusual intolerance of light, occurring in measles, rubella, meningitis, and inflammation of the eyes. SYN: *photodysphoria.*

**photophoresis** A technique used in treating cutaneous T-cell lymphoma. It incorporates exposure of a lymphocyte-enriched blood fraction, obtained by use of apheresis to ultraviolet A light after the patient has ingested the cytotoxic agent 8-methoxypsoralen. SYN: *extracorporeal photochemotherapy.*

**photopia** Adjustment of the eye for vision in bright light; the opposite of scotopia.

**photopsia, photopsy** (fō-tŏp′sē-ă, fō-tŏp′sē) [Gr. *photos,* light, + *opsis,* vision] The subjective sensation of sparks or flashes of light in retinal, optic, or brain diseases.

**photopsin** (fō-tŏp′sĭn) The protein portion (opsin) of the photopigments in the cones of the retina.

**photoptarmosis** (fō″tō-tăr-mō′sĭs) [″ + *ptarmosis,* sneezing] Photic sneezing.

**photoptometer** (fō-tŏp-tŏm′ĕ-tĕr) [″ + *opsis,* vision, + *metron,* measure] A device for determining the smallest amount of light that will make an object visible.

**photoradiometer** (fō″tō-rā″dē-ŏm′ĕ-tĕr) [″ + L. *radius,* ray, + Gr. *metron,* measure] A device for determining the ability of ionizing radiation to penetrate substances.

**photoradiotherapy** Photodynamic therapy.

**photoreaction** (fō″tō-rē-ăk′shŭn) [″ + LL. *reactus,* reacted] A chemical reaction produced or influenced by light.

**photoreactivation** (fō″tō-rē-ăk″tĭ-vā′shŭn) Enzymatic repair of lesions such as can be produced in DNA by ultraviolet light.

**photoreception** (fō″tō-rē-sĕp′shŭn) [″ + L. *recipere,* to receive] The perception of light rays in the visible light spectrum.

**photoreceptor** (fō″tō-rē-sĕp′tor) Sensory nerve endings or cells that are capable of being stimulated by light. In humans, these include the rods and cones of the retina.

**photoretinitis** (fō″tō-rĕt″ĭ-nī′tĭs) [Gr. *photos,* light, + L. *retina,* retina, + Gr. *itis,* inflammation] Damage to the macula of the eye owing to exposure to intense light. SEE: *blindness, eclipse.*

**photoscan** A representation of the concentration of a radioisotope outlining an organ in the body. The map is printed on photographic paper. SEE: *scintiscan.*

**photosensitivity** [″ + L. *sensitivus,* feeling] Sensitivity to light. Many medications and other agents contain ingredients that may cause a chemically induced change in the skin that makes an individual unusually sensitive to light. Photosensitive individuals may develop a rash, sunburn, or other adverse effect from exposure to light of an intensity or duration that would normally not have affected them. Exposure to ultraviolet light in combination with certain medications may result in skin cancer, premature skin aging, skin and eye burns, allergic reactions, cataracts, and altered immunity. Medications associated with photosensitizing reactions include antihistamines, coal tar derivatives, estrogens and progestins, nonsteroidal anti-inflammatory drugs, phenothiazines, psoralens, sulfonamides, sulfonylureas (oral hypoglycemic agents), thiazide diuretics, tetracyclines, and tricyclic antidepressants. Persons known to have increased sensitivity to light caused by the medications they are taking should avoid exposure to sunlight or, when in the sun, should use sunscreens or clothing to cover exposed areas of the skin. SEE: *photoallergy.*

**photosensitization** (fō″tō-sĕn″sĭ-tĭ-zā′shŭn) A condition in which the skin reacts abnormally to light, esp. ultraviolet radiations or sunlight. It is due to the presence of drugs, hormones, or heavy metals in the system. SEE: *photoallergy.*

**photosensitizer** (fō″tō-sĕn′sĭ-tī″zĕr) A substance that, in combination with light, will cause a sensitivity reaction in the substance or organism.
**photosensor** A device that detects light.
**photostable** (fō′tō-stā″b′l) [″ + L. *stabilis,* stable] Uninfluenced by exposure to light.
**photosynthesis** (fō″tō-sĭn′thĕ-sĭs) [″ + *synthesis,* placing together] The process by which plants are able to manufacture carbohydrates by combining carbon dioxide and water, using light energy in the presence of chlorophyll.
**phototaxis** (fō″tō-tăk′sĭs) [Gr. *photos,* light, + *taxis,* arrangement] The reaction and movement of cells and microorganisms under the stimulus of light.
**phototherapy** (fō″tō-thĕr′ă-pē) [″ + *therapeia,* treatment] **1.** Exposure to sunlight or artificial light for therapeutic purposes. **2.** The use of light to treat hyperbilirubinemia in newborns. Hemolytic jaundice of the newborn is treated with exchange transfusion or phototherapy, or both. Phototherapy is used by exposing the jaundiced newborn to either natural sunlight or fluorescent light (blue light). The exposure is continuous; the infant is turned frequently for maximal exposure to the light. The use of phototherapy has decreased the need for exchange transfusion in infants with hemolytic disease of the newborn. SEE: *exchange transfusion; hemolytic disease of the newborn; icterus neonatorum; kernicterus; photomedicine; psoriasis.*

Caution: The infant's eyes must be protected from the light, but the pressure from the eye bandage should not be so tight as to prevent opening of the eyes under the bandage. Also, the infant should be shielded from bulb breakage and the temperature should be monitored. The dose of light must be known and kept within the limits prescribed.

**photothermal** (fō″tō-thĕr′măl) [″ + *therme,* heat] Concerning heat produced by light.
**photothermolysis, selective** The use of short pulses of light to treat skin conditions. This method causes less damage to normal tissue than do continuous beam lasers. SEE: *laser.*
**phototimer** SEE: *control, automatic exposure.*
**phototoxic** (fō″tō-tŏk′sĭk) [″ + *toxikon,* poison] Pert. to the harmful reaction produced by light energy, esp. that produced in the skin. Simple sunburn of the skin is an example of phototoxicity.
**phototrophic** (fō″tō-trŏf′ĭk) [″ + *trophe,* nutrition] Concerning the ability to use light in metabolism.
**phototropism** (fō-tŏt′rō-pĭzm) [″ + *tropos,* turning, + *-ismos,* condition] A tendency exhibited by green plants and some microorganisms to turn toward or grow toward light.
**photuria** (fō-tū′rē-ă) [″ + *ouron,* urine] Excretion of phosphorescent urine.
**phren-** SEE: *phreno-.*
**phrenalgia** (frē-năl′jē-ă) **1.** [Gr. *phren,* mind, + *algos,* pain] Pain of hysterical origin. **2.** [Gr. *phren,* diaphragm, + *algos,* pain] Pain in the diaphragm.
**phrenectomy** (frē-nĕk′tō-mē) [Gr. *phren,* diaphragm, + *ektome,* excision] **1.** Surgical excision of all or part of the diaphragm. **2.** Surgical resection of part of the phrenic nerve.
**phrenemphraxis** (frĕn″ĕm-frăk′sĭs) [″ + *emphraxis,* stoppage] Crushing of the phrenic nerve in order to induce temporary paralysis of the diaphragm, a therapeutic measure that was previously employed in treatment of pulmonary tuberculosis.
**phrenetic** (frĕn-ĕt′ĭk) [Gr. *phren,* mind] **1.** Maniacal; frenzied. **2.** A maniac.
**-phrenia** Combining form indicating *mental disorder.*
**phrenic** (frĕn′ĭk) **1.** [Gr. *phren,* diaphragm] Concerning the diaphragm, as the phrenic nerve. **2.** [Gr. *phren,* mind] Concerning the mind.
**phrenicectomy** (frĕn-ĭ-sĕk′tō-mē) [Gr. *phren,* diaphragm, + *ektome,* excision] Resection of a part of the phrenic nerve; used to collapse the lung on one side by paralyzing the diaphragm.
**phreniconeurectomy** (frĕn″ĭ-kō-nū-rĕk′tō-mē) [″ + *neuron,* nerve, + *ektome,* excision] Excision of part of the phrenic nerve.
**phrenicotomy** (frĕn″ĭ-kŏt′ō-mē) [″ + *tome,* incision] Cutting of the phrenic nerve to immobilize a lung by inducing paralysis of one side. This causes the diaphragm to rise, compressing the lung and diminishing respiratory movement, thus resting the lung on that side.
**phreno-, phren-** [Gr. *phren,* mind; L. *phrenicus,* diaphragm] **1.** Combining form meaning *mind.* **2.** Combining form meaning *diaphragm.*
**phrenocolopexy** (frĕn″ō-kō′lō-pĕk″sē) [″ + *kolon,* colon, + *pexis,* fixation] Suture of the transverse colon to the diaphragm.
**phrenodynia** (frĕn″ō-dĭn′ē-ă) [″ + *odyne,* pain] Pain in the diaphragm.
**phrenogastric** (frĕn″ō-găs′trĭk) [″ + *gaster,* belly] Concerning the diaphragm and stomach.
**phrenohepatic** (frĕn″ō-hĕ-păt′ĭk) [″ + *hepar,* liver] Concerning the diaphragm and liver.
**phrenopericarditis** (frē″nō-pĕr″ĭ-kăr-dī′tĭs) [Gr. *phren,* diaphragm, + *peri,* around, + *kardia,* heart, + *itis,* inflammation] Attachment of the heart by adhesions to the diaphragm.
**phrenoplegia** (frĕn-ō-plē′jē-ă) **1.** [Gr. *phren,* mind, + *plege,* stroke] A sudden attack of mental illness. **2.** [Gr. *phren,* diaphragm, + Gr. *plege,* stroke] Paralysis of the diaphragm.
**phrenoptosis** (frĕn″ŏp-tō′sĭs) [Gr. *phren,* diaphragm, + *ptosis,* a dropping] Down-

ward displacement of the diaphragm.

**phrenospasm** (frĕn′ō-spăzm) [″ + *spasmos,* a convulsion] Spasm of the diaphragm.

**phrenosplenic** (frĕn″ō-splĕn′ĭk) [″ + *splen,* spleen] Concerning the diaphragm and spleen.

**Phthirus** (thĭr′ŭs) [Gr. *phtheir,* louse] A genus of sucking lice belonging to the order Anoplura.

***P. pubis*** The crab louse. It infests primarily the pubic region but it may also be found in armpits, beard, eyebrows, and eyelashes. SEE: *pediculosis pubis.*

**phyco-** [Gr. *phykos,* seaweed] Combining form meaning *seaweed.*

**phycology** (fī-kŏl′ō-jē) [Gr. *phykos,* seaweed, + *logos,* word, reason] The study of algae.

**Phycomycetes** (fī″kō-mī-sē′tēz) [″ + *mykes,* fungus] A class of fungi, several genera of which consist of organisms that occasionally cause disease in humans.

**phylactic** (fī-lăk′tĭk) [Gr. *phylaktikos,* preservative] Concerning or producing phylaxis.

**phylaxis** (fī-lăk′sĭs) [Gr., protection] The active defense of the body against infection.

**phyletic** (fī-lĕt′ĭk) [Gr. *phyletikos*] Phylogenetic.

**phylloquinone** (fĭl″ō-kwĭn′ōn) Phytonadione.

**phylogenesis** (fī″lō-jĕn′ĕ-sĭs) [Gr. *phyle,* tribe, + *genesis,* generation, birth] The evolutionary development of a group, race, or species. SEE: *phylogeny.*

**phylogenetic** (fī″lō-jĕ-nĕt′ĭk) Concerning the development of a race or phylum. SYN: *phyletic.*

**phylogeny** (fī-lŏj′ĕ-nē) Development and growth of a race or group of animals. SEE: *ontogeny.*

**phylum** (fī′lŭm) *pl.* **phyla** [Gr. *phylon,* tribe] In taxonomy, one of the primary divisions of a kingdom, one division higher than a class.

**physaliform, physalliform** (fĭ-săl′ĭ-form) [Gr. *physallis,* bubble, + L. *forma,* shape] Resembling a bleb or bubble.

**physaliphorous** (fĭs″ă-lĭf′ō-rŭs) Pert. to a highly vacuolated cell present in a chordoma.

**physalis** (fĭs′ă-lĭs) [Gr. *physallis,* bubble] A large vacuole present in the cell of certain malignancies such as a chondroma.

**Physaloptera** (fĭs″ă-lŏp′tĕr-ă) [″ + *pteron,* wing] A genus of nematode worms belonging to the suborder Spiruata.

***P. caucasica*** A species that occurs in and damages the upper gastrointestinal tract.

**physiatrics** (fĭz″ē-ăt′rĭks) [Gr. *physis,* nature, + *iatrikos,* treatment] The curing of disease by natural methods, esp. physical therapy.

**physiatrist** (fĭz″ē-ăt′rĭst) A physician who specializes in physical medicine.

**physic** (fĭz′ĭk) [Gr. *physikos,* natural] **1.** The art of medicine and healing. **2.** A medicine, esp. a cathartic.

**physical** (fĭz′ĭ-kăl) **1.** Of or pert. to nature or material things. **2.** Concerning or pert. to the body; bodily.

***p. activity and exercise*** A general term for any sort of muscular effort but esp. the kind intended to train, condition, or increase flexibility of the muscular and skeletal systems of the body.

***p. examination*** Examination of the body by auscultation, palpation, percussion, inspection, and smelling.

***p. fitness*** The ability to carry out daily tasks with vigor and alertness, without undue fatigue, and with ample energy to enjoy leisure-time pursuits and meet unforeseen emergencies. It is the ability to withstand stress and persevere under difficult circumstances in which an unfit person would quit. Implied in this is more than lack of illness; it is a positive quality that everyone has to some degree. Physical fitness is minimal in the severely ill and maximal in the highly trained athlete. Persons who maintain a high level of fitness may have increased longevity as compared to those who are sedentary. In addition, the quality of life is enhanced in those who are fit.

**physical mobility, impaired** A state in which the individual has limited ability for independent movement. SEE: *Nursing Diagnoses Appendix.*

**physical therapy** Rehabilitation concerned with the restoration of function and the prevention of disability following disease, injury, or loss of a body part. The therapeutic properties of exercise, heat, cold, electricity, ultraviolet radiation, and massage are used to improve circulation, strengthen muscles, encourage return of motion, and train or retrain an individual to perform the activities of daily living. SYN: *physiotherapy.*

**physical therapy assistant** A technical health care worker trained to use and apply physical therapy procedures such as exercise and physical agents under the supervision of a physical therapist.

**physical therapy diagnosis** Decisions regarding appropriate treatment for patients requiring rehabilitation and education made by physical therapists. As the physical therapy profession evolves and develops, physical therapy diagnoses are becoming accepted in accordance with specialized training and experience. Frequently, functional definitions of problems can be used as diagnostic statements for specific physical therapy intervention. This is not meant to replace or supersede medical or pathologic diagnosis.

**physician** (fĭ-zĭsh′ŭn) [O. Fr. *physicien*] A person who has successfully completed the prescribed course of studies in medicine in a medical school officially recognized by the country in which it is located, and who has acquired the requisite qualifications for licensure in the practice of medicine.

***attending p.*** A physician who is on the staff of a hospital and regularly cares for patients therein.

***family p.*** SEE: *primary care p.*

***primary care p.*** A physician to whom a family or individual goes initially when ill or for a periodic health check. This physician assumes medical coordination of care with other physicians for the patient with multiple health concerns.

***resident p.*** A physician who works full or part time in a hospital to continue training after internship; commonly called a resident.

**Physicians' Desk Reference** ABBR: PDR. An annual compendium of information concerning drugs, primarily prescription and diagnostic products. The information is largely that included by the manufacturer in the labeling or package insert as required by the Food and Drug Administration: indications for use, effects, dosages, administration, warnings, hazards, contraindications, drug interactions, side effects, and precautions.

**physician shortage area** An area with an inadequate supply of physicians, usually with a physician-to-population ratio less than 1:4000.

**physicist** (fĭz'ĭ-sĭst) [L. *physics,* natural sciences] A specialist in the science of physics.

**physico-** [Gr. *physikos*] Combining form meaning *physical, natural.*

**physicochemical** (fĭz″ĭ-kō-kĕm'ĭ-kăl) [″ + *chemeia,* chemistry] Concerning the application of the laws of physics to chemical reactions.

**physics** (fĭz'ĭks) [Gr. *physis,* nature] The study of the laws of matter and their interactions with energy. Included are the fields of acoustics, optics, mechanics, electricity, and thermodynamics, and ionizing radiation.

**physio-** [Gr. *physis*] Combining form denoting *nature.*

**physiochemical** (fĭz″ē-ō-kĕm'ĭ-kăl) [Gr. *physis,* nature, + *chemeia,* chemistry] Concerning clinical chemistry.

**physiocogenic** (fĭz″ē-ō-kō-jĕn'ĭk) [″ + *gennan,* to produce] Originating from physical causes.

**physiocopyrexia** (fĭz″ē-ō-kō″pī-rĕk'sē-ă) [″ + *pyressein,* feverish] Fever produced artificially by physical means.

**physiognomy** (fĭz″ē-ŏg'nō-mē) [Gr. *physis,* nature, + *gnomon,* a judge] **1.** The countenance. **2.** Assumed ability to diagnose a disease or illness based on the appearance and expression(s) on the face.

**physiognosis** (fĭz″ē-ŏg-nō'sĭs) [″ + *gnosis,* knowledge] Diagnosis determined from one's facial expression and appearance.

**physiological** (fĭz″ē-ō-lŏj'ĭ-kăl) [Gr. *physis,* nature, + *logos,* word, reason] Concerning body function.

**physiologicoanatomical** (fĭz″ē-ō-lŏj″ĭ-kō-ăn″ă-tŏm'ĭ-kăl) [″ + ″ + *anatome,* dissection] Concerning physiology and anatomy.

**physiologist** (fĭz″ē-ŏl'ō-jĭst) A person trained in and capable in the field of physiology.

**physiology** (fĭz″ē-ŏl'ō-jē) [Gr. *physis,* nature, + *logos,* study] The science of the functions of the living organism and its components and of the chemical and physical processes involved.

***cell p.*** The physiology of cells.

***comparative p.*** The study and comparison of the physiology of different species.

***general p.*** The broad scientific basis of physiology.

***pathologic p.*** The physiological explanation of pathologic events.

***special p.*** The physiology of special organs or systems.

**physiopathologic** (fĭz″ē-ō-păth″ō-lŏj'ĭk) [″ + *pathos,* disease, suffering, + *logos,* word, reason] **1.** Concerning physiology and pathology. **2.** Pert. to a pathologic alteration in a normal function.

**physiotherapy** (fĭz″ē-ō-thĕr'ă-pē) [″ + *therapeia,* treatment] Physical therapy.

**physique** (fĭ-zēk') [Fr.] Body build; the structure and organization of the body.

**physo-** [Gr. *physa,* air] Combining form indicating *air, gas.*

**physocele** (fī'sō-sēl) [Gr. *physa,* air, + *kele,* tumor, swelling] **1.** A tumor filled with gas or circumscribed swelling due to gas. **2.** A gas-distended hernial sac.

**physometra** (fī″sō-mē'tră) [″ + *metra,* uterus] Air or gas in the uterine cavity.

**physopyosalpinx** (fī″sō-pī″ō-săl'pĭnks) [″ + *pyon,* pus, + *salpinx,* tube] Pus and gas in a fallopian tube.

**physostigmine salicylate** (fī″sō-stĭg'mēn săl-ĭs'ĭl-āt) The salicylate of an alkaloid usually obtained from the dried ripe seed of *Physostigma venenosum.*

ACTION/USES: This substance is a cholinergic. It inactivates cholinesterase, thus prolonging and intensifying the action of acetylcholine. It improves the tone and action of skeletal muscle; increases intestinal peristalsis through its effects on the parasympathetic nervous system; and acts as a miotic in the eye. It is used in tetanus and strychnine poisoning and in the treatment of myasthenia gravis.

**phytalbumose** (fī-tăl'bū-mōs) [Gr. *phyton,* plant, + L. *albumen,* white of egg] An albumose found in plants and vegetables.

**phytase** (fī'tās) [″ + *ase,* enzyme] An enzyme found in grains and present in the kidneys; important in splitting phytin or phytic acid into inositol and phosphoric acid.

**phytin** (fī'tĭn) A calcium or magnesium salt of inositol and hexaphosphoric acid, present in cereals. SEE: *inositol.*

**phyto-, phyt-** [Gr. *phyton*] Combining form indicating *plant, that which grows.*

**phytoagglutinin** (fī″tō-ă-gloo'tĭ-nĭn) [Gr. *phyton,* plant, + L. *agglutinans,* gluing] A lectin that agglutinates red blood cells and leukocytes.

**phytobezoar** (fī″tō-bē'zor) [″ + Arabic *ba-*

*zahr,* protecting against poison] A mass composed of vegetable matter found in the stomach. SYN: *food ball.* SEE: *bezoar.*

**phytochemical** Any of the hundreds of natural chemical substances present in plants. Many have nutritional value; others are protective (e.g., antioxidants) or cause cell damage (e.g., free radicals). Important phytochemicals include indole, isothiocyanate, phytosterol, polyphenol, saponin, phenolic acids, protease inhibitors, carotenoids, monoterpene, capsaicin, lignans, and triterpenoids.

**phytochemistry** (fī″tō-kĕm′ĭs-trē) [″ + *chemeia,* chemistry] The study of plant chemistry.

**phytogenous** (fī-tŏj′ĕ-nŭs) [″ + *gennan,* to produce] Arising in or caused by plants.

**phytohemagglutinin** (fī″tō-hĕm-ă-glū′tĭ-nĭn) [″ + *haima,* blood, + L. *agglutinare,* to glue to] ABBR: PHA. A substance derived from red kidney beans that agglutinates red blood cells and is a mitogen that stimulates T lymphocytes.

**phytoid** (fī′toyd) [″ + *eidos,* form, shape] Plantlike.

**phytomenadione** (fī″tō-mĕn″ă-dī′ōn) Phytonadione.

**phytonadione** (fī″tō-nă-dī′ōn) **1.** Synthetic vitamin $K_1$; used as a prothrombogenic agent. **2.** An anticoagulant drug that is little used because of its toxicity. SYN: *phytomenadione.*

**phytopharmacology** (fī″tō-făr″mă-kŏl′ō-jē) [″ + *pharmakon,* drug, + *logos,* word, reason] The study of the effects of drugs and chemicals on plants.

**phytophotodermatitis** (fī″tō-fō″tō-dĕr″mă-tī′tĭs) [″ + *photos,* light, + *derma,* skin, + *itis,* inflammation] A dermatitis produced by exposure to certain plants and then sunlight.

**phytoplankton** (fī″tō-plănk′tŏn) [″ + *planktos,* wandering] Plant life consisting of the millions of microscopic organisms present in each cubic meter of sea water near the surface.

**phytoprecipitin** (fī″tō-prē-sĭp′ĭ-tĭn) A precipitin produced by immunization with a plant protein.

**phytosis** (fī-tō′sĭs) [″ + *osis,* condition] **1.** A disease caused by a vegetable parasite. **2.** The presence of vegetable parasites.

**phytosterol** (fī″tō-stē′rŏl) Any sterol present in vegetable oil or fat.

**phytotoxin** (fī″tō-tŏk′sĭn) [Gr. *phyton,* plant, + *toxikon,* a poison] A toxin produced by or derived from a plant. SEE: *ricin.*

**pI** The pH of the isoelectric point of a substance in solution.

**pia** (pē′ă) [L.] Tender, soft.

**pia-arachnitis** (pē″ă-ăr″ăk-nī′tĭs) Piarachnitis.

**pia-arachnoid** Piarachnoid.

**Piaget, Jean** Swiss philosopher and psychologist, 1896–1980, whose work provided understanding of how children's thinking differs from adults' and of how children learn. Concerning education, he explained, "The goal of education is not to increase the amount of knowledge but to create the possibilities for a child to invent and discover, to create men who are capable of doing new things."

**pial** (pī′ăl) Concerning the pia mater.

**pia mater** (pē′ă mā′tĕr) [L. *pia,* soft, + *mater,* mother] A thin vascular membrane closely investing the brain and spinal cord and proximal portions of the nerves. It is the innermost of the three meninges. The other portions of the covering are the dura mater and the arachnoid. SEE: *meninges.*

**pian** (pē-ăn′) [Fr.] A contagious skin disease of the tropics. SYN: *yaws.*

**piarachnitis** (pī″ăr-ăk-nī′tĭs) [L. *pia,* tender, + Gr. *arachne,* spider, + *itis,* inflammation] Inflammation of the arachnoid and pia mater. SYN: *leptomeningitis; pia-arachnitis.*

**piarachnoid** (pī″ăr-ăk′noyd) [″ + ″ + *eidos,* form, shape] The pia mater and arachnoid membranes when regarded as one structure. SYN: *leptomeninges; pia-arachnoid.*

**piblokto, pibloktog** [Inuit] A syndrome, apparently culturally specific for Eskimo women, in which the individual screams, removes or tears off her clothes, and runs naked in the snow. She has no memory of these events.

**pica** (pī′kă) [L., magpie] An eating disorder manifested by a craving to ingest any material not fit for food, including starch, clay, ashes, toy balloons, crayons, cotton, grass, cigarette butts, soap, twigs, wood, paper, metal, or plaster. This condition is seen in pregnancy, chlorosis, hysteria, helminthiasis, and certain psychoses. It may also be associated with iron-deficiency anemia. The importance of this condition, the etiology of which is unknown, stems from the toxicity of ingested material (e.g., paint that contains lead) or from ingesting materials in place of essential nutrients. The inclusion of compulsive ingestion of nonfood and food items such as licorice, croutons, chewing gum, coffee grounds, or oyster shells as examples of pica is controversial. SEE: *appetite; geophagia; taste.*

**pick 1.** A sharp, pointed, curved dental instrument used to explore tooth surfaces and restorations for defects. **2.** To remove bits of food from teeth.

**Pick, Arnold** Czechoslovakian physician, 1851–1924.

***P.'s disease*** A form of presenile dementia due to atrophy of the frontal and temporal lobes. It usually occurs between the ages of 40 and 60, more often in women than in men. The disease involves progressive, irreversible loss of memory, deterioration of intellectual functions, disordered emotions, apathy, speech disturbances, and disorientation. The course may take from a few months to 4 or 5 years to progress to complete loss of intellectual function. SEE: *Alzheimer's* *disease*.

**Pick, Friedel** Czechoslovakian physician, 1867–1926.

***P.'s disease*** Nonrheumatic chronic pericarditis of unknown etiology.

**Pick, Ludwig** German physician, 1868–1944.

***P.'s cell*** A foamy, lipid-filled cell present in the spleen and bone marrow in Niemann-Pick disease. SYN: *Niemann-Pick cell*.

***P.'s disease*** Niemann-Pick disease.

**pickling 1.** A method of preserving and flavoring food in which the food is soaked in a solution of salt and vinegar. **2.** The use of a chemical solution to remove scales and oxides from metals after casting or before plating them.

**pickwickian syndrome** [Inspired by Joe, an obese character in Pickwick Papers by Charles Dickens. The term was applied to this syndrome in 1956 by Charles S. Burwell, M.D.] Obesity, decreased pulmonary function, and polycythemia.

**pico-** Combining form used to indicate a unit of measurement that is one trillionth of the basic unit.

**picocurie** ABBR: pCi. An amount of radiation equal to $10^{-12}$ curies. SEE: *becquerel*.

**picogram** ABBR: pg. $1 \times 10^{-12}$ g or 1 trillionth of a gram.

**picornavirus** (pī-kor″nă-vī′rŭs) [″ + *RNA*, ribonucleic acid, + L. *virus*, virus] Any of a group of very small ether-resistant viruses that includes enteroviruses and rhinoviruses.

**picrate** (pĭk′răt) A salt of picric acid.

**picro-, picr-** [Gr. *pikros*, bitter] Combining form meaning *bitter*.

**picrotoxin** (pĭk″rō-tŏk′sĭn) [″ + *toxikon*, poison] A stimulant to the central nervous system, no longer used as such, obtained from the seed of *Anamirta cocculus*, a shrub.

**pictograph** (pĭk′tō-grăf) A set of test pictures used for testing vision in children and illiterate adults.

**PID** *pelvic inflammatory disease*.

**piedra** (pē-ā′dră) [Sp., stone] Sheathlike nodular masses in the hair of the beard and mustache from growth of either *Piedraia hortai*, which causes black piedra, or *Trichosporon beigelii*, which causes white piedra. The masses surround the hairs, which become brittle; hairs may be penetrated by fungus and thus split. SYN: *tinea nodosa*. SEE: illus.

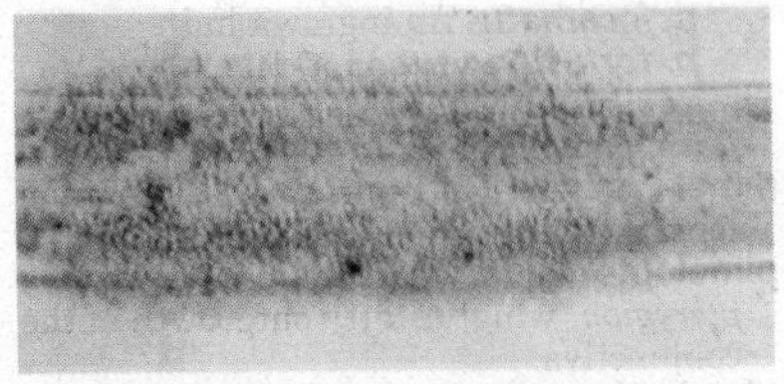

WHITE **PIEDRA** ON HAIR (ORIG. MAG. ×200)

**Pierre Robin syndrome** [Pierre Robin, French physician, 1867–1950] Unusual smallness of the jaw combined with cleft palate, downward displacement of the tongue, and an absent gag reflex.

**piesesthesia** (pī-ē″zĕs-thē′zē-ă) [Gr. *piesis*, pressure, + *aisthesis*, sensation] Sensitivity to pressure.

**piesimeter, piesometer** (pī″ĕ-sĭm′ĕ-tĕr, -sŏm′ĕ-tĕr) [″ + *metron*, measure] A device for measurement of the skin's sensitivity to pressure.

**-piesis** Combining form used as a suffix meaning *pressure*.

**piezoelectricity** [″ + *elektron*, amber] Production of an electric current by application of pressure to certain crystals such as mica, quartz, or Rochelle salt. SEE: *triboluminescence*.

**PIF** *proliferation inhibiting factor*. SEE: *factor, proliferation inhibiting*.

**pigeon breeder's disease** Bird breeder's lung.

**pigeon-toed** With feet turned inward.

**pigment** (pĭg′mĕnt) [L. *pigmentum*, paint] Any organic coloring matter in the body. SEE: *albino;* words beginning with *chrom-*.

***bile p.*** A complex, highly colored substance found in bile derived from the hemoglobin of old red blood cells and imparting brown color to intestinal contents and feces. Included are bilirubin, biliverdin, and their derivatives (urobilinogen, urobilin, bilicyanin, and bilifuscin). SYN: *hepatogenous p.*

***blood p.*** A pigment in blood (hemoglobin) or a derivative of it (hematin, hemin, methemoglobin, hemosiderin).

***endogenous p.*** A pigment produced within the human body, as melanin.

***exogenous p.*** A pigment produced outside the human body.

***hematogenous p.*** A pigment from hemoglobin of the erythrocytes.

***hepatogenous p.*** Bile p.

***respiratory p.*** Any pigment such as hemoglobin, myoglobin, or cytochrome that has a part in metabolic processes of the body.

***skin p.*** Melanin, melanoid, and carotene.

***urinary p.*** Urochrome and sometimes urobilin.

***uveal p.*** Melanin in the choroid layer of the eye, the ciliary processes, and the posterior surface of the iris; absorbs light within the eyeball to prevent glare.

**pigmentary** (pĭg′mĕn-tĕr″ē) [L. *pigmentum*, paint] Concerning, or like, a pigment.

**pigmentation** (pĭg″mĕn-tā′shŭn) Coloration caused by deposition of pigments. SEE: *albinism; carotenemia;* words beginning with *chrom-*.

***hematogenous p.*** Pigmentation produced by the collection of hemoglobin, or pigment carried to a site through the blood.

**pigmented** (pĭg′mĕnt-ĕd) Colored by a pigment.

**pigmentolysin** (pĭg″mĕn-tŏl′ĭ-sĭn) [″ + Gr. *lysis,* dissolution] A substance that destroys a pigment.

**pigmentophore** (pĭg-mĕn′tō-for) [″ + Gr. *phorein,* to carry] A cell that carries pigment.

**pigmentum nigrum** (pĭg-mĕn′tŭm nī′grŭm) [L., black paint] The black pigment of the lamina vitrea of the choroid of the eye.

**piitis** (pī-ī′tĭs) [L. *pia,* tender, + Gr. *itis,* inflammation] Inflammation of the pia mater.

**pil** L. *pilula,* pill, or *pilulae,* pills.

**pila** (pī′lă) *pl.* **pilae** [L., pillar] A pillar-like structure in spongy bone.

**pilar, pilary** (pī′lăr, pĭl′ă-rē) [L. *pilaris*] Concerning, or covered with, hair.

**pile** [L. *pila,* a ball, a pillar] **1.** A single hemorrhoid. SEE: *piles.* **2.** The hair. **3.** A battery for production of electricity. **4.** An apparatus for producing and regulating a nuclear chain-reaction fission process.

***sentinel p.*** A localized thickening of the mucous membrane at the distal end of an anal fissure.

**pileous** (pī′lē-ŭs) [L. *pilus,* hair] Hirsute.

**piles** (pīls) [L. *pila,* a mass] Hemorrhoids.

**pileum** (pī′lē-ŭm) [L., a cap] Caul.

**pileus** (pī′lē-ŭs) [L., a cap] Caul.

**pili** (pī′lē) *sing.* **pilus** Hairs; in bacteria, filamentous appendages of which there may be hundreds on a single cell. One function of pili is to attach the bacterium to cells of the host; another to propel the bacterial cell.

***p. incarnati*** The condition of ingrowing hair, esp. in the beard area.

***p. tactiles*** Sensitive or tactile hairs.

***p. torti*** A condition in which hairs are broken and twisted.

**piliation** (pī-lē-ā′shŭn) [L. *pilus,* hair] The formation and development of hair.

**piliform** (pī′lĭ-form) [″ + *forma,* shape] Hairlike.

**pill** (pĭl) [L. *pilula,* small mass] **1.** Medicine in the form of a tiny solid mass or pellet to be swallowed or chewed; may be coated. **2.** Birth control pill.

***morning-after p.*** A pill containing an estrogen or synthetic estrogen that can be taken after intercourse to prevent pregnancy.

**pillar** (pĭl′ĕr) [L. *pila,* a column] An upright support, column, or structure resembling a column.

***anterior p. of the fornix*** One of two diverging columns extending downward from anterior extremity of body of the fornix of cerebrum.

***p. cell*** One of two groups of cells (inner and outer) resting on basement membrane of organ of Corti in which elongated bodies (pillars) develop. These enclose the inner tunnel (Corti's tunnel).

***p.'s of Corti*** One of two layers resting on membrana basilaris in the ear. SYN: *rods of Corti.*

***p.'s of the diaphragm*** Crura of the diaphragm, two bundles of muscle fibers extending from the lumbar vertebrae to the central tendon and forming the sides of the hiatus aorticus.

***p.'s of the fauces*** Folds of mucous membrane, one on each side of the fauces and between which is situated the tonsil. SYN: *glossopalatine arches; pharyngopalatine arches.*

**pillion** (pĭl′yŭn) [L. *pellis,* skin] A temporary form of artificial leg, esp. a peg-leg type of stump.

**pilo-** [L. *pilus*] Combining form indicating *hair.*

**pilobezoar** (pī″lō-bē′zor) [″ + Arabic *bazahr,* protecting against poison] Trichobezoar.

**pilocarpine hydrochloride** (pī″lō-kăr′pĭn) $C_{11}H_{16}N_2O_2 \cdot HCl$. Hydrochloride of an alkaloid obtained from leaflets of *Pilocarpus jaborandi* and *P. microphyllus.*

ACTION/USES: It is used as a cholinergic. Because it causes contraction of the pupil, it is used topically as a miotic, esp. in glaucoma.

**pilocarpine nitrate** A nitrate of the alkaloid obtained from leaves of the jaborandi tree. Uses are the same as for pilocarpine hydrochloride.

**pilocystic** (pī″lō-sĭs′tĭk) [L. *pilus,* hair, + Gr. *kystis,* bladder] Encysted and containing hair, said of a dermoid cyst.

**piloerection** A skin reaction caused by erection of the hair follicles, as from cold or shock due to contraction of the arrector pili muscles. This causes transient roughness of the skin. SYN: *cutis anserina; goose flesh; horripilation.*

**pilojection** [″ + *jacere,* to throw] Introduction of hairs, by use of a pneumatic gun, into an aneurysm to induce clotting in the aneurysmal sac. It has been used in treating intracranial aneurysms.

**pilomotor** (pī″lō-mō′tor) [″ + *motor,* mover] Causing movements of hairs, as the arrectores pilorum.

**pilonidal** (pī″lō-nī′dăl) [″ + *nidus,* nest] Containing hairs in a dermoid cyst in nest formation.

**pilosebaceous** (pī″lō-sē-bā′shŭs) [″ + *sebaceus,* fatty] Concerning the hair and sebaceous glands.

**Piltz's reflex** (pĭlts′ĕz) [Jan Piltz, Polish neurologist, 1870–1931] Change in the size of the pupil on sudden fixation of attention. SYN: *pupillary reflex.*

**pilus** (pī′lŭs) *pl.* **pili** [L.] A hair.

***p. cuniculatus*** A hair that burrows into the skin.

***p. incarnatus*** An ingrown hair.

***p. tortus*** A twisted hair.

**PImax** *maximum inspiratory pressure.* SEE: *force, maximum inspiratory.*

**pimel-, pimelo** [Gr. *pimele,* fat] Combining form meaning *fat* or *fatty.*

**pimelopterygium** (pĭm″ĕ-lō-tĕ-rĭj′ē-ŭm) [″ + *pterygion,* wing] A fatty outgrowth of the conjunctiva.

**pimelorthopnea** (pĭm″ĕl-or″thŏp′nē-ă) [″ + *orthos,* straight, + *pnoia,* breath] Difficulty in breathing when lying down, due to obesity.

**pimelosis** (pĭm″ĕ-lō′sĭs) [″ + *osis*, condition] **1.** Conversion into fat. **2.** Fatty degeneration of any tissue. **3.** Obesity.

**pimple** (pĭm′pl) [ME. *pinple*] A papule or pustule of the skin, sometimes going on to suppuration; often seen in clusters on skin of the adolescent with acne. Patients should be warned not to pick at pimples because infection may result.

**pin** A short, slim piece of wire, plastic, or metal. It may have one end blunt and the other sharp.

***endodontic p.*** A straight or threaded pin that is passed through the root canal to the alveolar bone beyond the apex of the tooth root.

***self-threading p.*** A pin screwed through a small hole into dentin.

***sprue p.*** In dentistry, a wax, plastic, or metal pattern used to make the channel or channels through which molten metal flows into a mold to make a casting. Also called *sprue former*.

**pincement** (păns-mŏn′) [Fr.] Pinching or nipping of the flesh in massage.

**pinch** A type of hand prehension. The pinch of the human hand is achieved principally through holding objects between the thumb and index finger or the index and long fingers.

Hand pinch is classified according to the anatomical parts involved, as follows:

*Pinch, fingertip*—pinch using the tips of strongly arched digits, primarily the thumb and index finger; used to pick up very small objects such as pins and needles.

*Pinch, palmar tripod or three-jaw chuck* – pinch using the palmar pads of the thumb and index and long fingers.

*Pinch, lateral*—pinch accomplished by clamping the palmar surface of the distal portion of the thumb against the side of the index finger.

**pinch meter** A device for objectively measuring the strength of hand pinch in grams or pounds.

**pindolol** (pĭn′dō-lōl) A $\beta$-adrenergic blocking agent.

**pineal** (pĭn′ē-ăl) [Fr., pine cone] **1.** Shaped like a pine cone. **2.** Pert. to the pineal gland.

**pinealectomy** (pĭn″ē-ăl-ĕk′tō-mē) [L. *pineus*, of the pine, + Gr. *ektome*, excision] Removal of the pineal gland.

**pineal gland** SEE: *gland, pineal*.

**pinealoblastoma** (pĭn″ē-ă-lō-blăs-tō′mă) [″ + Gr. *blastos*, germ, + *oma*, tumor] Pineoblastoma.

**pinealocyte** (pĭn′ē-ă-lō-sīt″) [″ + Gr. *kytos*, cell] The principal cell of the pineal gland. It contains pale-staining cytoplasm and has long processes that terminate in bulbous expansions.

**pinealoma** (pĭn″ē-ă-lō′mă) [″ + Gr. *oma*, tumor] A tumor of the pineal gland, usually encapsulated; often associated with precocious puberty.

**pinealopathy** (pĭn″ē-ă-lŏp′ă-thē) [″ + Gr. *pathos*, disease, suffering] Any disorder of the pineal gland.

**Pinel, Philippe** (pē-nĕl′) French psychologist, 1745–1826, who developed a method or system of treating the mentally ill without the use of restraint, at a time when use of restraint was the accepted form of therapy.

**pineoblastoma** (pĭn″ē-ō-blăs-tō′mă) [L. *pineus*, of the pine, + Gr. *blastos*, germ, + *oma*, tumor] A malignant tumor of the pineal gland that may occur in childhood and early adulthood. SYN: *pinealoblastoma.*

**pineocytoma** A malignant tumor of the pineal gland of the brain.

**ping-ponging** The transmission of an infectious disease, esp. a sexually transmitted one, between two people. After the first person has been cured, the second person reinfects the first.

**pinguecula** (pĭn-gwĕk′ū-lă) [L. *pinguiculus*, fatty] A yellow triangular thickening of the bulbar conjunctiva on the inner and outer margins of the cornea. The base of the triangle is toward the limbus. The yellow color is due to an increase in elastic fibers.

**pinhole** (pĭn′hōl) [AS. *pinn*, pin, + *hol*, hole] A small perforation made by, or size of that made by, a pin.

***p. os*** A very small opening to the uterus from the vagina. It may be present in very young women.

**piniform** (pĭn′ĭ-form) [L. *pinea*, pine cone, + *forma*, shape] Conical; shaped like a pine cone.

**pink disease** Acrodynia.

**pinkeye** [D. *pinck oog*] Acute conjunctivitis caused by various organisms. It is treated with local application of ointment or drops containing an appropriate antibiotic. Systemic therapy may be needed.

**pinna** (pĭn′ă) *pl.* **pinnae** [L., feather] **1.** The auricle or projected part of the exterior ear. It collects and directs sound waves into the external acoustic meatus and then to the tympanic membrane. **2.** A feather, fin, wing, or similar appendage.

***p. nasi*** A protruding cartilaginous extension on each nostril. SYN: *ala nasi*.

**pinnal** (pĭn′ăl) Concerning pinna.

**pinocyte** (pī′nō-sīt) [Gr. *pinein*, to drink, + *kytos*, cell] A cell that exhibits pinocytosis.

**pinocytosis** (pī″nō-sī-tō′sĭs) [″ + ″ + *osis*, condition] The process by which cells absorb or ingest nutrients and fluid. A hollowed-out portion of the cell membrane is filled with liquid, and the area closes to form a small sac or vacuole. The nutrient, now inside, is available for use in the cell's metabolism. SEE: illus.

**pinosome** (pī′nō-, pĭn′ō-sōm) [″ + *soma*, body] The fluid-filled vacuole formed during pinocytosis.

**PINS** *persons in need of supervision.*

**Pins' sign** [Emil Pins, Aust. physician,

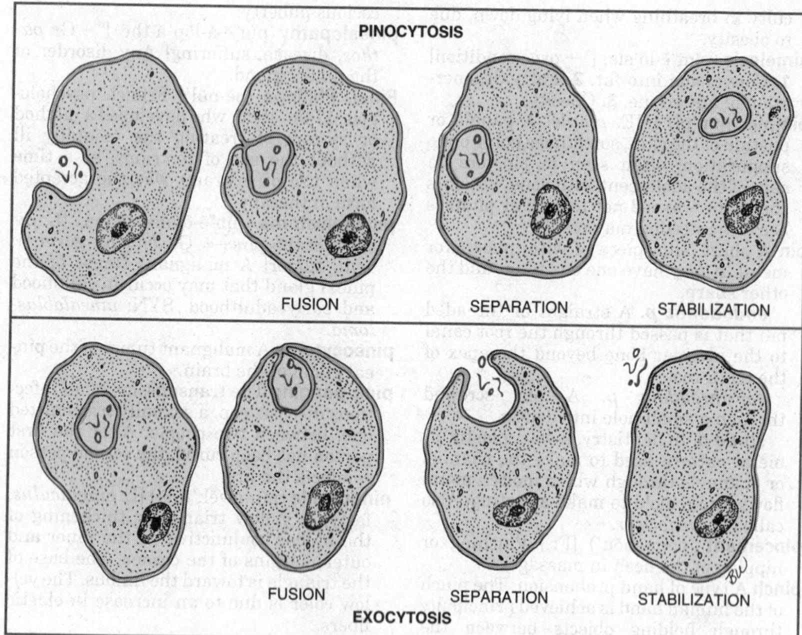


1845–1913] In pericarditis, the disappearance of symptoms of pleurisy when the patient assumes knee-chest position.

**pint** (pīnt) [ME. *pinte*] ABBR: pt. In the U.S. a measure of capacity equal to ½ qt.; 16 fl. oz; 473.2 ml. SEE: *Weights and Measures Appendix.*

**pinta** (pēn′tă) [Sp., paint] A nonvenereal disease spread by body contact, caused by the spirochete *Treponema carateum.* It is manifested by depigmented spots or patches. The treatment is administration of penicillin.

**pintid** (pĭn′tĭd) A flat red skin lesion present in the second stage of pinta.

**pinus** (pī′nŭs) [L., pine] Pert. to the pineal gland.

**pinworm** A parasitic nematode, *Enterobius vermicularis,* causing enterobiasis, infection of the intestines and rectum. SEE: *Enterobius vermicularis* for illus.

**pioepithelium** (pī″ō-ĕp″ĭ-thē′lē-ŭm) [Gr. *pion,* fat, + *epi,* upon, + *thele,* nipple] Epithelium that contains fat globules.

**pion therapy** Experimental use of the subatomic particle, the pion, in treating cancer.

**Piper** (pī′pĕr) [L.] Genus of plants that produce pepper.

**piperazine** (pī-pĕr′ă-zēn) A white crystalline powder used in the treatment of ascariasis and enterobiasis.

**piperoxan** (pī″pĕr-ŏks′ăn) An alpha-adrenergic blocking agent effective in inhibiting the response to catecholamines.

**pipet, pipette** (pī-pĕt′) [Fr. *pipette,* tiny pipe] Narrow glass tube with both ends open for transferring and measuring liquids by suctioning them into the tube.

**pipobroman** (pī″pō-brō′măn) A cytotoxic drug that has been used in treating certain blood diseases.

**piriform, pyriform** (pĭr′ĭ-form) [L. *pirum,* pear, + *forma,* shape] Pear-shaped.

**piriformis syndrome** A condition marked by pain in the hip and buttock that radiates up into the lower back and down the leg. In women, the pain may occur during sexual intercourse. This is caused by entrapment of the sciatic nerve as it passes through the piriformis muscle in the buttock. Because the symptoms mimic those caused by a herniated lumbar disk, the syndrome may be confused with that disease. Treatment includes physical therapy to relieve pressure, ultrasound to reduce muscle spasm, and anti-inflammatory medicines. Surgical therapy to free the entrapped nerve may be necessary. SEE: *sciatica.*

**Pirogoff's amputation** (pĭr″ō-gŏfs′) [Nikolai Ivanovich Pirogoff, Russ. surgeon, 1810–1881] Foot amputation at the ankle, removing a portion of the os calcis.

**Pirquet's test** (pĕr-kāz′) [Clemens Peter Johann von Pirquet, Austrian pediatrician, 1874–1929] A test for tuberculosis by means of a skin reaction, used esp. in children.

**piscicide** (pĭs′ĭ-sīd) [L. *piscis,* fish, + *caedere,* to kill] An agent that kills fish.

**pisiform** (pī′sĭ-form) [L. *pisum,* pea, + *forma,* shape] **1.** Pea-shaped. **2.** The smallest carpal bone, located in the flexor carpi ulnaris tendon as a sesamoid bone, on the ulnar side in the proximal row of carpals.

**pit** (pĭt) [ME. *pitt,* hole] **1.** A tiny hollow or pocket. SYN: *depression; fossa.* **2.** To be or become marked with a shallow depression; to cause a depression on pressure in edema. **3.** A small depression in the enamel surface of a tooth often connected with one or more developmental grooves. It contributes to pit and fissure caries. SYN: *occlusal p.*

***anal p.*** Proctodeum.

***auditory p.*** A pit that develops in the auditory placode.

***costal p.*** The inferior facet on the body of a thoracic vertebra. It articulates with the head of a rib.

***gastric p.*** One of many minute depressions (foveolae) in gastric mucosa into which the gastric glands open.

***lens p.*** The depression on the skin of the embryonic head where the lens of the eye will develop.

***nasal p.*** One of two horseshoe-shaped depressions on the ventrolateral surface of the head bounded by lateral and median nasal processes. It give rise to nostrils and a portion of the nasal fossa. SYN: *olfactory p.*

***occlusal p.*** Pit (3).

***olfactory p.*** Nasal p.

***primitive p.*** A minute depression at the anterior end of the primitive groove or streak and immediately posterior to the primitive knot.

***p. of the stomach*** **1.** The depression at the end of the ensiform process. **2.** The center of the abdominal region above the navel. SYN: *scrobiculus cordis.*

**pitch** (pĭch) [ME. *picchen,* to fix] **1.** That quality of the sensation of sound that enables one to classify it in a scale from high to low. It is dependent principally on frequency of vibrations. **2.** Residue obtained from distillation of coal or wood tar.

**pitchblende** (pĭch′blĕnd) Uraninite, the principal source of uranium. It is a mineral that resembles pitch.

**pith** (pĭth) **1.** The center of a hair or the soft material in the stalk of a plant. **2.** Destruction of a part of the central nervous system of an animal being prepared for certain experiments. A blunt probe is inserted in the brain through a foramen.

**pithing** (pĭth′ĭng) [ME. *pithe*] Destruction of the central nervous system by the piercing of brain or spinal cord, as in vivisection. This is done on experimental animals to render them insensible to pain and to inhibit controlling effects of the central nervous system during research and experimentation. SEE: *decerebration.*

**pithode** (pī′thōd) [Gr. *pithose,* wine cask, + *eidos,* form, shape] The barrel-shaped spindle formed during karyokinesis.

**Pitres' section** (pē-trĕs′) [Jean A. Pitres, Fr. physician, 1848–1927] Any of the series of six coronal vertical sections of the brain for study. The sections are prefrontal, pediculofrontal, frontal, parietal, pediculoparietal, and occipital.

**Pitressin** (pĭt-rĕs′ĭn) Trade name for vasopressin, a product obtained from the posterior lobe of the pituitary gland. It contains pressor and antidiuretic principles and is used for increasing blood pressure, increasing the muscular contraction of the intestinal tract, and diminishing urinary output in diabetes insipidus. SEE: *principle, antidiuretic; vasopressin.*

**pitting** (pĭt′ĭng) [ME. *pitt,* hole] **1.** The formation of pits, depressions, or scars, as in smallpox. **2.** In the spleen, removal of the remains of red blood cells that have completed their lifespan or have been injured. Nucleated red blood cells are also removed from circulating blood in this pitting function. SEE: *culling.* **3.** In dentistry, the formation of depressions in the materials used in restoring teeth. **4.** In radiography, the imperfections created on the face of the x-ray tube anode by overloading current limits.

**pituicyte** (pĭ-tū′ĭ-sīt) [L. *pituita,* phlegm, + Gr. *kytos,* cell] A modified branched neuroglia cell characteristic of pars nervosa of the posterior lobe of the pituitary gland; also present in the infundibular stalk.

**pituitary** (pĭ-tū′ĭ-tār″ē) [L. *pituitarius,* phlegm] The pituitary body or gland. SYN: *hypophysis.* SEE: *hormone, releasing; hormone, inhibiting; pituitary gland.*

***anterior p.*** A preparation consisting of dried, defatted, powdered anterior lobe of the pituitary gland of domestic animals.

***posterior p.*** The dried, powdered posterior lobe of the pituitary gland of animals used as food by humans.

***whole p.*** The dried, defatted, powdered entire pituitary gland of domestic animals.

**pituitary gland** A small, gray, rounded gland that develops from ingrown oral epithelium (Rathke's pouch) and is attached to the lower surface of the hypothalamus by the infundibular stalk. The Rathke's pouch portion forms the anterior lobe and an intermediate area; the neural tissue of the infundibular stalk forms the posterior lobe. The pituitary gland averages 1.3 × 1.0 × 0.5 cm in size and weighs 0.55 to 0.6 g. SYN: *hypophysis cerebri.* SEE: illus. (Pituitary Gland and Hypothalamus).

FUNCTION: The pituitary is an endocrine gland secreting a number of hormones that regulate many bodily processes including growth, reproduction, and various metabolic activities. It is often referred to as the "master gland of the body." SEE: illus. (Pituitary Hormones and Target Organs).

Hormones are secreted in the following lobes: *Intermediate lobe:* In cold-blooded animals, intermedin is secreted, influencing the activity of pigment cells (chromatophores) of fishes, amphibians, and reptiles. In warm-blooded animals, no effects are known.

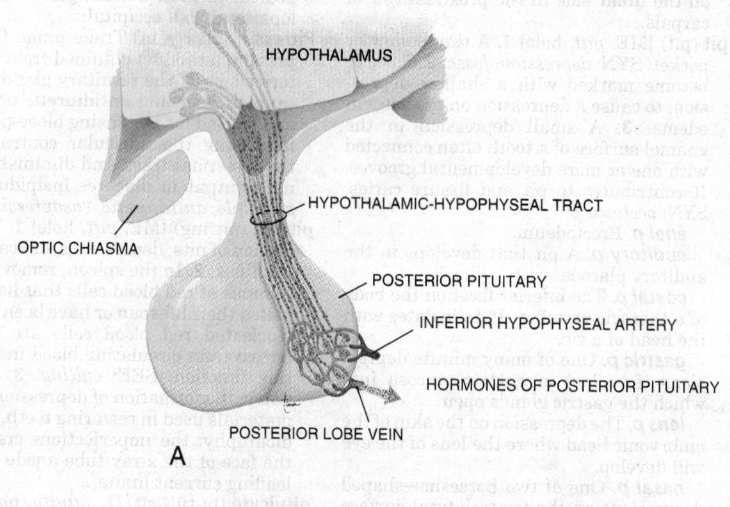


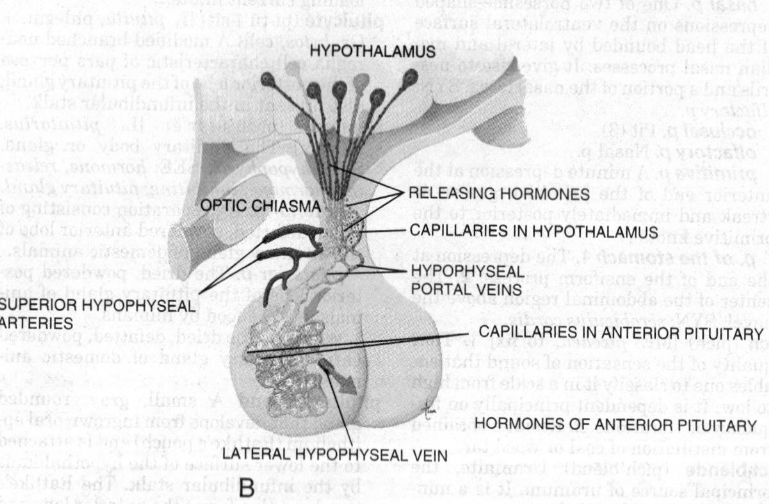


**PITUITARY GLAND** AND HYPOTHALAMUS, **(A)** POSTERIOR AND **(B)** ANTERIOR

*Anterior lobe:* Secretions here are the somatotropic, or growth, hormone (STH or GH), which regulates cell division and protein synthesis for growth; adrenocorticotropic hormone (ACTH), which regulates functional activity of the adrenal cortex; thyrotropic hormone (TTH or TSH), which regulates functional activity of the thyroid gland; and the following gonadotrophic hormones: Follicle-stimulating hormone (FSH) stimulates development of ovarian follicles and spermatogenesis in the testis. In women, luteinizing hormone (LH) stimulates ovulation and formation of the corpus luteum and its secretion of estrogen and progesterone. In men LH, also called interstitial cell–stimulating hormone (ICSH), stimulates testosterone secretion. Prolactin, also called lactogenic hormone, induces secretion of milk in the adult female.

*Posterior lobe:* Hormones are secreted by the neurosecretory cells of the hypothalamus and pass through fibers of the supraopticohypophyseal tracts in the infundibular stalk to the neurohypophysis, where they are stored. Secretions here are oxytocin, which acts specifically on smooth muscle of the uterus, increasing tone and contractility; and antidiuretic hormone (ADH), which increases reabsorption of water by the kidney tubules. ADH also has a vasopressor effect and also is called vasopressin.

DISORDERS: *Hypersecretion of anterior lobe* causes gigantism, acromegaly, and

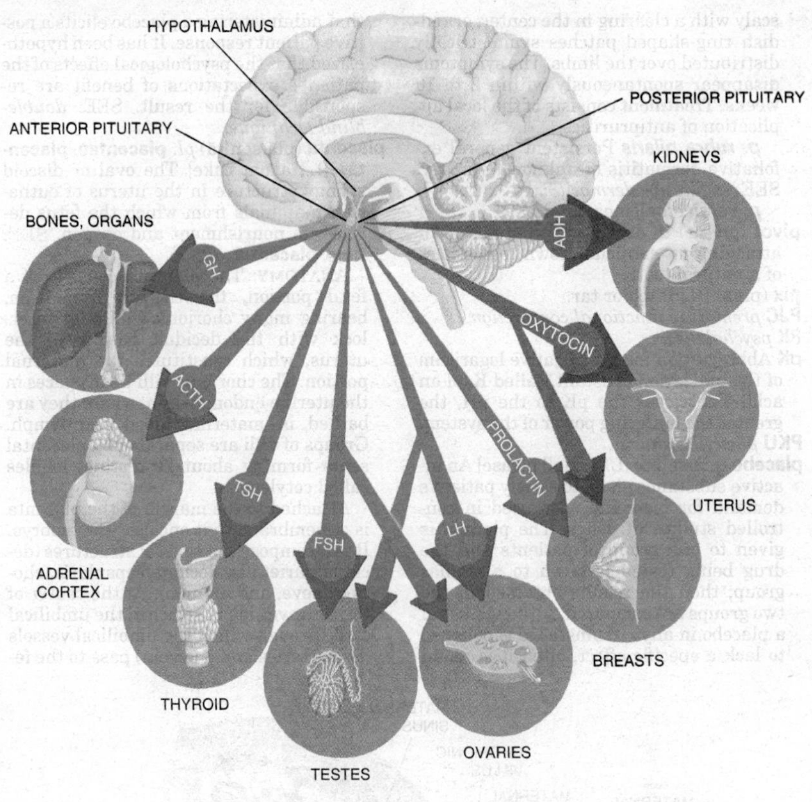


PITUITARY GLAND

PITUITARY HORMONES AND TARGET ORGANS

pituitary basophilism (Cushing's disease). *Hyposecretion of anterior lobe* causes dwarfism, pituitary cachexia (Simmonds' disease), Sheehan's syndrome, acromicria, eunuchoidism or hypogonadism. *Posterior lobe deficiency* or *hypothalamic lesion* causes diabetes insipidus. *Anterior and posterior lobe deficiency* and *hypothalamic lesion* cause Frohlich's syndrome (adiposogenital dystrophy) and pituitary obesity.

**pituitary (injection), posterior** Antidiuretic hormone.

**pityriasis** (pĭt″ĭ-rī′ă-sĭs) [Gr. *pityron,* bran, + *-iasis,* disease] A skin disease characterized by branny scales.

***p. alba*** A form of decreased melanin in the skin. Patches of round or oval macular skin lesions with fine adherent scales. They are commonly seen in the facial areas of children. The lesions are virtually painless and usually require no therapy. They may disappear spontaneously. The etiology is unknown, but the disease is regarded as a mild form of eczema.

***p. capitis*** Dandruff.

***p. lichenoides, acute*** A skin disorder characterized by development of an edematous pink papule that undergoes central vesiculation and hemorrhagic necrosis. The lesions clear spontaneously after weeks or months but leave scars.

***p. linguae*** Transitory benign plaques of the tongue. SYN: *geographical tongue.*

***p. nigra*** Tinea nigra.

***p. rosea*** An acute inflammatory skin disease of unknown etiology, marked by a macular eruption on the trunk, obliquely to the ribs, and on the upper extremities. The initial (herald) patch appears in more than half of the cases. In a few days it enlarges to several centimeters. Then, within 2 to 21 days, secondary eruptions occur. They are rose-red and somewhat scaly with a clearing in the center, or reddish ring-shaped patches symmetrically distributed over the limbs. The symptoms disappear spontaneously within 2 to 10 weeks. Treatment consists of the local application of antipruritics.

***p. rubra pilaris*** Persistent general exfoliative dermatitis of unknown etiology. SEE: *exfoliative dermatitis.*

***p. versicolor*** Tinea versicolor.

**pivot** (pĭv′ŭt) In dentistry, a part used for attaching an artificial crown to the base of a natural tooth.

**pix** (pĭks) [L.] Pitch or tar.

**PJC** *premature junctional contraction.*

**PK** *psychokinesis.*

**pK** Abbreviation for the negative logarithm of the ionization constant, called K, of an acid. The closer the pK to the pH, the greater the buffering power of the system.

**PKU** *phenylketonuria.*

**placebo** (plă-sē′bō) [L., I shall please] An inactive substance given to satisfy patient's demand for medicine; also used in controlled studies of drugs. The placebo is given to one group of patients and the drug being tested is given to a similar group; then the results obtained in the two groups are compared. Although use of a placebo in any circumstance is believed to lack a specific effect, often it is found that administering a placebo elicits a positive patient response. It has been hypothesized that the psychological effects of the patient's expectations of benefit are responsible for the result. SEE: *double-blind technique.*

**placenta** (plă-sĕn′tă) *pl.* **placentae, placentas** [L., a flat cake] The oval or discoid spongy structure in the uterus of eutherian mammals from which the fetus derives its nourishment and oxygen. SEE: illus. **placental,** *adj.*

ANATOMY: The placenta consists of a fetal portion, the chorion frondosum, bearing many chorionic villi that interlock with the decidua basalis of the uterus, which constitutes the maternal portion. The chorionic villi lie in spaces in the uterine endometrium, where they are bathed in maternal blood and lymph. Groups of villi are separated by placental septa forming about 20 distinct lobules called cotyledons.

Attached to the margin of the placenta is a membrane that encloses the embryo. It is a composite of several structures (decidua parietalis, decidua capsularis, chorion laeve, and amnion). At the center of the concave side is attached the umbilical cord through which the umbilical vessels (two arteries and one vein) pass to the fe-

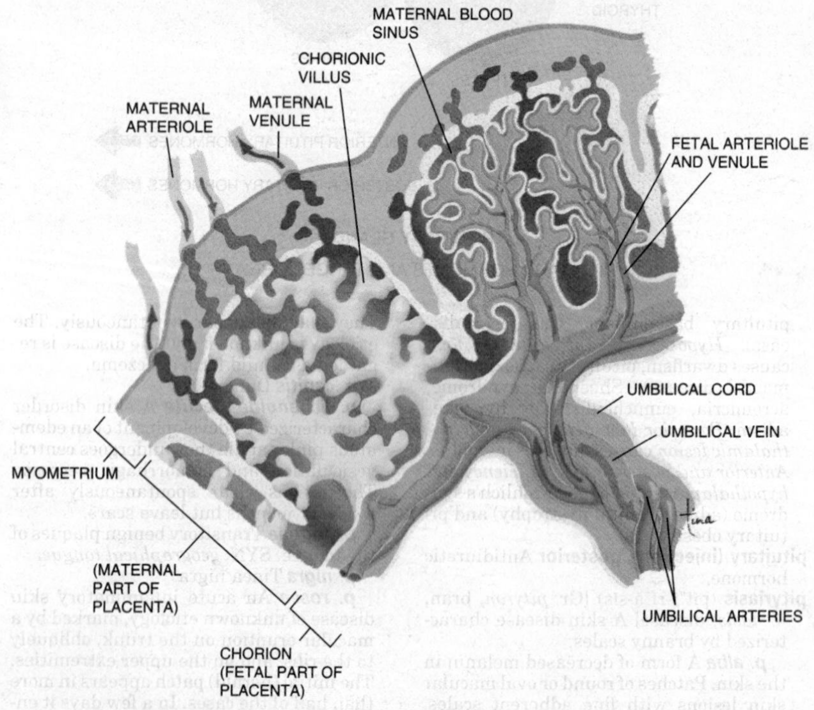


**PLACENTA**
MATERNAL AND FETAL PORTIONS

tus. The cord is approx. 50 cm long at full term.

The mature placenta is 15 to 18 cm (6 to 7 in.) in diameter and weighs about 450 gm (approx. 1 lb). When expelled following parturition, it is known as the afterbirth.

Maternal blood enters the intervillous spaces of the placenta through spiral arteries, branches of the uterine arteries. It bathes the chorionic villi and flows peripherally to the marginal sinus, which leads to uterine veins. Food substances, oxygen, and antibodies pass into fetal blood of the villi; metabolic waste products pass from fetal blood into the mother's blood. Normally, there is no admixture of fetal and maternal blood. The placenta also serves as an endocrine organ. It produces chorionic gonadotropins, the presence of which in urine is the basis of one type of pregnancy test. Estrogen and progesterone are also secreted by the placenta.

***abruption of p.*** Abruptio placentae.

***accessory p.*** A placenta separate from the main placenta.

***p. accreta*** A placenta in which the cotyledons have invaded the uterine musculature, resulting in difficult or impossible separation of the placenta.

***adherent p.*** A placenta that remains adherent to the uterine wall after normal period following childbirth.

***annular p.*** A placenta that extends like a belt around the interior of the uterus. SYN: *zonary p.*

***battledore p.*** A form of insertion of the umbilical cord into the margin of the placenta in which it spreads out to resemble a paddle or battledore.

***bidiscoidal p.*** The presence of two discoidal masses. This is normal in some primates.

***bilobate p.*** A placenta consisting of two lobes. SYN: *dimidiate p.*

***bipartite p.*** A placenta divided into two separate parts.

***chorioallantoic p.*** A placenta in which the allantoic mesoderm and vessels fuse with the inner face of the serosa to form the chorion.

***circinate p.*** A cup-shaped placenta.

***p. circumvallata*** A cup-shaped placenta with raised edges that exposes an area of fetal surface encircling the site of umbilical cord insertion.

***circumvallate p.*** P. circumvallata.

***cirsoid p.*** A placenta with appearance of varicose veins.

***cordiform p.*** A placenta having a marginal indentation, giving it a heart shape.

***deciduate p.*** A placenta of which the maternal part escapes with delivery.

***dimidiate p.*** Bilobate p.

***discoid p.*** A placenta that constitutes practically one circumscribed and circular mass.

***double p.*** A placental mass of the two placentae of a twin gestation.

***endotheliochorial p.*** A placenta in which the syncytial trophoblasts of the chorion penetrate to the blood vessels of the uterus.

***epitheliochorial p.*** A placenta in which the chorion is next to the lining of the uterus but does not invade or erode the lining.

***p. fenestrata*** A placenta in which a portion of the placental tissue is thinning or absent.

***fetal p.*** That part of the placenta formed by aggregation of chorionic villi in which the umbilical vein and arteries ramify.

***fundal p.*** A placenta attached to the uterine wall within the fundal zone.

***hemochorial p.*** A placenta in which the maternal blood is in direct contact with the chorion. The human placenta is of this type.

***hemoendothelial p.*** A placenta in which the maternal blood is in contact with the endothelium of the chorionic vessels.

***horseshoe p.*** A formation in which the two placentae of a twin gestation are united.

***incarcerated p.*** A placenta retained in the uterus by irregular uterine contractions after delivery.

***p. increta*** A form of placenta accreta in which the chorionic villi invade the myometrium.

***lateral p.*** A placenta attached to the lateral wall of the uterus.

***maternal p.*** A portion of the placenta that develops from the decidua basalis of the uterus.

***membranous p.*** Thinning of the placenta from atrophy.

***multilobate p.*** A placenta with more than three lobes.

***nondeciduate p.*** A placenta that does not shed the maternal portion.

***p. percreta*** A type of placenta accreta in which the myometrium is invaded to the serosa of the peritoneum covering the uterus. This may cause rupture of the uterus.

***p. previa*** A placenta that is implanted in the lower uterine segment. There are three types: centralis, lateralis, and marginalis. Placenta previa centralis is the condition in which the placenta has been implanted in the lower uterine segment and has grown to completely cover the internal cervical os. Placenta previa lateralis is the condition in which the placenta lies just within the lower uterine segment. Placenta previa marginalis is the condition in which the placenta partially covers the internal cervical os. SEE: *Nursing Diagnoses Appendix.*

SYMPTOMS: Slight hemorrhage, recurrent with greater severity, appears in the seventh or eighth month of pregnancy. Gradual anemia, pallor, rapid weak pulse, air hunger, and low blood pressure occur.

DIAGNOSIS: Painless bleeding during last 3 months and a placenta found in the lower portion of the uterus are diagnostic.

TREATMENT: The blood supply before and during delivery should be conserved. Postpartum hemorrhage should be prevented or controlled. Anemia should be treated before and after labor. Prevention of sepsis is necessary.

PROGNOSIS: The prognosis depends on the control of hemorrhage and prevention of sepsis.

***p. previa partialis*** A placenta that only partially covers the internal os of the uterus.

***p. reflexa*** An abnormal placenta in which the margin is thickened and appears to turn back on itself.

***reniform p.*** A kidney-shaped placenta.

***retained p.*** A placenta not expelled within two hours after completion of the second stage of labor.

***p. spuria*** An outlying portion of the placenta that has not maintained its vascular connection with the decidua vera.

***succenturiate p.*** An accessory placenta that has a vascular connection to the main part of the placenta.

***trilobate p.*** A placenta with three lobes.

***tripartite p.*** A three-lobed placenta attached to a single fetus.

***triple p.*** A placental mass of three lobes in a triple gestation.

***p. uterina*** The uterine part of the placenta.

***velamentous p.*** A placenta with the umbilical cord attached to the membrane a short distance from the placenta, the vessels entering the placenta at its margin.

***villous p.*** A placenta in which the chorion forms villi.

***zonary p.*** Annular p.

**placental** (plă-sĕn′tăl) [L. *placenta,* a flat cake] Rel. to the placenta.

**placentation** (plă″sĕn-tā′shŭn) The process of formation and attachment of the placenta.

**placentitis** (plă″sĕn-tī′tĭs) [″ + Gr. *itis,* inflammation] Inflammation of the placenta.

**placentography** (plă″sĕn-tŏg′ră-fē) [″ + Gr. *graphein,* to write] Examination of the placenta by radiography.

***indirect p.*** Measurement of the space between the placenta and the head of the fetus by means of radiographical examination. It is done to diagnose placenta previa.

**placentolysin** (plă″sĕn-tŏl′ĭ-sĭn) [″ + Gr. *lysis,* dissolution] A lysin obtained by injecting placental tissue into an animal, the serum thus obtained being destructive to placental cells of the species of animal from which the placenta was originally taken.

**Placido's disk** (plă-sē′dōz) [Antonio Placido, Portuguese ophthalmologist, 1848–1916] A disk marked with black and white circles used in determining the amount and character of corneal astigmatism.

**placode** (plăk′ōd) [Gr. *plax,* plate, + *eidos,* form, shape] In embryology, a platelike thickening of epithelium, usually the ectoderm, that serves as the anlage of an organ or structure.

***auditory p.*** A dorsolateral placode located alongside the hindbrain that gives rise to the otocyst, which in turn develops into the internal ear.

***lens p.*** A placode developing in the ectoderm directly overlying the optic vesicle. It forms the lens vesicle, which becomes enclosed in the optic cup and eventually becomes the lens of the eye.

***olfactory p.*** A placode that gives rise to the olfactory pit and finally the major portion of the nasal cavity.

**placoid** (plăk′oyd) [″ + *eidos,* form, shape] Platelike.

**pladaroma** (plăd-ă-rō′mă) [Gr. *pladaros,* damp, + *oma,* tumor] A soft growth like a wart on the eyelid.

**pladarosis** (plăd-ă-rō′sĭs) [″ + *osis,* condition] The condition of pladaroma.

**plagio-** [Gr. *plagios,* slanting or sideways] Combining form meaning *slanting, oblique.*

**plagiocephaly** (plā″jē-ō-sĕf′ă-lē) A malformation of the skull producing the appearance of a twisted and lopsided head; caused by irregular closure of the cranial sutures.

**plague** (plāg) [ME., calamity] **1.** Any widespread contagious disease associated with a high death rate. **2.** A highly fatal disease caused by *Yersinia pestis* (previously classed as *Pasteurella pestis*) infection. This disease is characterized by high fever, restlessness, staggering gait, mental confusion, prostration, delirium, shock, and coma. It exists in several forms. The pneumonic form may be spread from person to person. Streptomycin, gentamicin, tetracyclines, and chloramphenicol are effective in treating plague.

***ambulatory p.*** A mild form of bubonic plague.

***black p.*** An acute, severe infection appearing in a bubonic or pneumonic form. This term was applied to the condition in the Middle Ages when massive epidemics occurred in Europe.

***bubonic p.*** The most common form of plague marked by the formation of buboes.

***hemorrhagic p.*** A severe form of bubonic plague in which there is hemorrhage into the skin.

***murine p.*** A plague infecting rats.

***pneumonic p.*** A highly virulent form of plague with extensive involvement of the lungs. It occurs as a sequela of bubonic plague or as a primary infection.

***septicemic p.*** A plague characterized by septicemia before the formation of buboes.

***sylvatic p.*** A plague infecting various species of rodents.

***white p.*** Tuberculosis.

**plaintiff** The person or party who sues or brings a legal action against another and seeks damages or other legal relief. SEE: *defendant.*

**plan** The conscious design of desired future states and of the goals, objectives, and activities required.

***birth p.*** Written specifications for the management of labor, delivery, and recovery as desired by the expectant mother or couple and approved by the physician or midwife. Components usually include pain management techniques, method of delivery, and family participation. SEE: *Lamaze technique or method; Leboyer method.*

***dental care p.*** **1.** The statement of the goals, objectives, and procedures related to the dentist's care for the patient, based on the medical history, oral examination, and oral radiographs. **2.** Third-party insurance that covers part or all of the cost for regular dental care. SYN: *dental health insurance.*

***Individualized Family Service p.*** ABBR: IFSP. A written document, developed collaboratively by parents of young children with disabilities and related service personnel, that describes plans for intervention and educational placement. Twenty-five percent of occupational therapists now practice in school settings with the purpose of meeting the legislated mandate for public schools to provide related services for children with disabilities.

***medical care p.*** The goals and objectives of the physician's care and the treatment instituted to accomplish them.

***nursing care p.*** The statement of the goals and objectives of the nursing care provided for the patient and the activities or tasks required to accomplish the plan, including the criteria to be used to evaluate the effectiveness and appropriateness of the plan.

**planaria** (plă-năr′ē-ă) Free-living flatworms of the Turbellaria class. They are used extensively in studying regeneration.

**planchet** (plăn′chĕt) A small flat container or dish on which a radioactive sample is placed.

**plane** (plān) [L. *planus*] **1.** A flat or relatively smooth surface. SYN: *planum.* **2.** A flat surface formed by making a cut, imaginary or real, through the body or a part of it. Planes are used as points of reference by which positions of parts of the body are indicated. In the human subject, all planes are based on the body being in an upright anatomical position. SEE: illus.; *position, anatomic.* **3.** A certain stage, as in levels of anesthesia. **4.** To smooth a surface or rub away.

***Addison's p.*** [Christopher Addison, Brit. anatomist, 1869–1951] One of the planes used as landmarks in thoracoabdominal topography.

***Aeby's p.*** [Christopher T. Aeby, Swiss anatomist, 1835–1885] A plane perpendicular to the median plane of the cranium through the basion and nasion.

***alveolocondylar p.*** A plane tangent to the alveolar point with most prominent points on lower aspects of condyles of the occipital bone.

***axiolabiolingual p.*** A plane that passes through an incisor or canine tooth parallel to the long axis of the tooth and in a labiolingual direction.

***axiomesiodistal p.*** A plane that passes through a tooth parallel to the axis and in a mesiodistal direction.

***Baer's p.*** A plane through the upper border of the zygomatic arches.

***bite p.*** A plane formed by the biting surfaces of the teeth.

***coccygeal p.*** The fourth parallel plane of the pelvis.

***coronal p.*** A vertical plane at right angles to a sagittal plane. It divides the body into anterior and posterior portions. SYN: *frontal p.*

***datum p.*** An assumed horizontal plane from which craniometric measurements are taken.

***Daubenton's p.*** [Louis Jean Marie Daubenton, Fr. physician, 1716–1800] A plane passing through the opisthion and inferior bones of the orbits.

***focal p.*** One of two planes through the anterior and posterior principal foci of a dioptric system and perpendicular to the line connecting the two.

***Frankfort horizontal p.*** The cephalometric plane joining the porion and orbitale, the upper part of the ear openings and the lowest margin of the orbit, to establish a reproducible position of the head for radiographical and cephalometric studies.

***frontal p.*** Coronal p.

***Hodge's p.*** [Hugh Lennox Hodge, U.S. physician, 1796–1873] A plane running parallel to the pelvic inlet and passing through the second sacral vertebra and the upper border of the os pubis.

***horizontal p.*** A transverse plane at right angles to the vertical axis of the body. SYN: *transverse p.*

***inclined p.'s of the pelvis*** Anterior and posterior inclined planes of the pelvic cavity, two unequal sections divided by the sciatic spines. In the larger, anterior section, the lateral walls slope toward the symphysis and arch of the pubes; and the posterior walls slope in the direction of the sacrum and coccyx. The anterior inclined planes are the declivities over which rotation of the occiput takes place in the mechanism of normal labor.

***inclined p. of a tooth*** Any sloping surface of the cusp of a tooth.

***intertubercular p.*** A horizontal plane

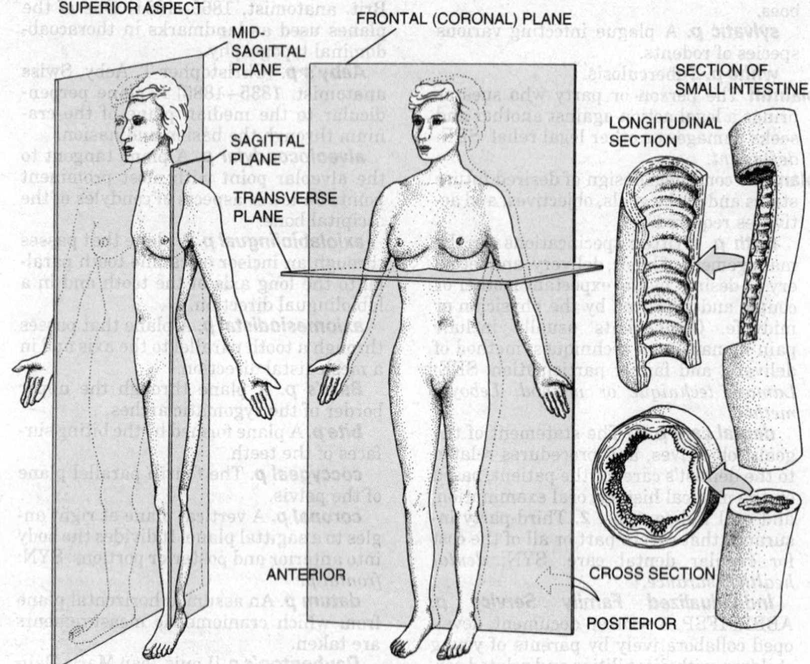


BODY **PLANES** AND SECTIONS

passing through the tubercles of the crests of the ilia; lies approx. at the level of the fifth lumbar vertebra.

***Listing's p.*** [Johann Benedict Listing, Ger. physiologist, 1808–1882] A transverse vertical plane lying perpendicular to the anteroposterior axis of the eye and containing the center of motion of the eyes. In it also lie the transverse and vertical axes of voluntary ocular rotation.

***Meckel's p.*** A plane through the auricular and alveolar points.

***median p.*** A vertical plane through the trunk and head dividing the body into right and left halves. SYN: *midsagittal plane*. SEE: *plane* for illus.

***midsagittal p.*** Median p.

***Morton's p.*** A plane passing through the most projecting points of the parietal and occipital protuberances.

***occlusal p.*** An imaginary plane extending from the incisal edge of the incisors along the tips of the cusps of the posterior teeth to contact the cranium. Although not a true plane, it represents the mean of the curvature of the occlusal surface.

***parallel p.'s of the pelvis*** The planes intersecting the axis of the pelvic canal at right angles. The first plane is that of the superior strait; the second that extending from the middle of the sacral vertebra to the level of the subpubic ligament. The third plane is at the level of the spines of the ischia, and the fourth plane is at the outlet.

***p.'s of the pelvis*** Imaginary planes touching the same parts of the pelvic canal on both sides.

***p. of refraction*** A plane passing through a refracted ray of light and drawn perpendicular to the surface at which refraction takes place.

***p. of regard*** A plane through the fovea of the eye; fixation point.

***sagittal p.*** A vertical plane parallel to the midsagittal plane. It divides the body into right and left portions.

***subcostal p.*** A horizontal plane passing through the lowest points of the 10th costal cartilages. It lies approx. at level of third lumbar vertebra.

***transverse p.*** Horizontal p.

***treatment p.*** A plane in the concave joint surface that defines the direction of joint mobilization techniques. The plane is perpendicular to a line drawn from the axis of rotation in the convex joint surface to the center of the concave surface. Joint distraction techniques are applied perpendicular to, and gliding techniques parallel to, the treatment plane.

***vertical p.*** Any body plane perpendicular to a horizontal plane.

***visual p.*** A plane passing the visual axis of the eye.

**planigraphy** (plă-nĭg′ră-fē) [″ + Gr. *graphein,* to write] Body section radiography.

**planimeter** (plā-nĭm′ĕ-tĕr) [″ + Gr. *metron,* measure] An apparatus used to measure the area of a plane figure by passing a tracer around the boundaries.

**planing** (plā′nĭng) **1.** Dermabrasion. **2.** In dentistry, a meticulous deep scaling procedure designed to remove calculus, diseased cementum or dentin, microbial flora, and bacterial toxins on the root surface of a tooth or in a gingival pocket. The smooth, healthy root facilitates reattachment of the soft tissues of the peridontium. SYN: *root planing.*

**plankton** (plănk′tŏn) [Gr. *planktos,* wandering] Free-floating marine life including diatoms, other algae, copepods, and some crustacea, protozoa, and worms.

**planned parenthood** The concept that a couple or a woman may choose when to conceive and give birth. This is, of course, accomplished only by the careful and proper use of some form of birth control.

**planning** In the nursing process, the step following nursing diagnosis. After the nursing diagnoses have been established, the next action is planning for the actual nursing care of the patient. This is done by noting the priority of the diagnoses and indicating the actions that will accomplish the immediate and long-range goals of the nursing process. Specific nursing interventions are indicated, and the expected outcome of these actions are recorded on the chart. This portion of the nursing process is dynamic and will need to be altered as the patient's course evolves. The evaluation of the effectiveness of the nursing process will be essential to restating the plan for administering nursing care. SEE: *nursing process; nursing assessment; evaluation; nursing intervention; problem-oriented medical record.*

**planocellular** (plā″nō-sĕl′ū-lăr) [L. *planus,* plane, + *cellula,* cell] Composed of flat cells.

**planoconcave** (plā″nō-kŏn′kāv) [″ + *concavus,* hollow] An optical lens that is flat on one side and concave on the other.

**planoconvex** (plā″nō-kŏn′vĕks) [″ + L. *convexus,* arched] An optical lens that is flat on one side and convex on the other.

**planomania** (plā″nō-mā′nē-ă) [Gr. *plane,* wandering, + Gr. *mania,* madness] The morbid desire to wander and be free of social restraints.

**Planorbis** (plăn-or′bĭs) A genus of freshwater snails serving as intermediate hosts for certain species of blood flukes *(Schistosoma).*

**planotopokinesia** (plā″nō-tŏp″ō-kī-nē′zē-ă) [″ + *topos,* place, + *kinesis,* movement] Loss of orientation in space.

**plant** (plănt) [L. *planta,* a sprout] An organism that contains chlorophyll and synthesizes carbohydrates and oxygen from carbon dioxide and water. Plants make up one of the five kingdoms of living things. SEE: *chlorophyll.*

**planta pedis** (plăn′tă pē′dŭs) *pl.* **plantae** [L.] The sole of the foot.

**plantago seed** (plăn-tā′gō) The cleaned, dried, ripe seed of *Plantago psyllium* or *P. indica.* It is used as a cathartic, but usually in a powdered form rather than in the form of whole seeds.

**plantalgia** (plăn-tăl′jē-ă) [L. *planta,* sole of the foot, + Gr. *algos,* pain] Pain in the sole of the foot.

**plantar** (plăn′tăr) Concerning the sole of the foot.

**plantar flexion** Extension of the foot so that the forepart is depressed with respect to the position of the ankle. SEE: *dorsiflexion.*

**plantaris** (plăn-tăr′ĭs) [L.] A long slim muscle of the calf between the gastrocnemius and soleus. It is sometimes double and at other times missing.

**plantation** (plăn-tā′shŭn) [L. *plantare,* to plant] Insertion of a tooth into the bony socket from which it may have been removed by accident; or transplantation of a tooth into the socket from which a tooth has just been removed. The transplanted tooth may come from the patient or a donor.

**plantigrade** [L. *planta,* sole of the foot, + *gradi,* to walk] A type of foot posture in which the entire sole of the foot is placed on the ground in walking, as in the bear, rabbit, or human.

**planula** (plăn′ū-lă) The larval stage of a coelenterate.

**planum** (plā′nŭm) *pl.* **plana** [L.] A flat or relatively smooth surface; a plane.

***nuchal p.*** The outer surface of the occipital bone between the foramen magnum and superior nuchal line.

***occipital p.*** The outer surface of the occipital bone lying above the superior nuchal line.

***orbital p.*** The portion of the maxilla that forms the greater part of the floor of the orbit.

***popliteal p.*** A smooth triangular area on posterior surface of distal end of femur. It is bordered by the medial and lateral supracondylar lines and forms the floor of the popliteal fossa.

***sternal p.*** The anterior or ventral surface of the sternum.

***temporal p.*** The depressed area on the side of the skull below the inferior temporal line; underlies the temporal fossa.

**planuria** (plā-nū′rē-ă) [Gr. *plane,* wandering, + *ouron,* urine] The voiding of urine from an abnormal passage of the body.

**plaque** (plăk) [Fr., a plate] A patch on the skin or on a mucous surface.

***atheromatous p.*** A yellow swollen area of the lining of an artery. It is formed by deposition of lipid in the area.

***bacterial p.*** Dental p.

***dental p.*** A gummy mass of microorganisms that grows on the crowns and spreads along the roots of teeth. It usually is too small to be seen and is both colorless and transparent. Dental plaques are the forerunners of dental caries and periodontal disease. They may be prevented by proper daily self-care of the teeth. SYN: *bacterial p.* SEE: *caries; periodontal disease; periodontitis; pyorrhea alveolaris; tooth; toothbrushing; teeth.*

***Hollenhorst p.*** Orange-yellow emboli in the retinal vessels.

***mucous p.*** Condyloma latum.

**-plasia** [Gr. *plasis,* molding] Combining form used as a suffix indicating *formation, growth, proliferation.*

**plasm** (plăzm) [LL. *plasma,* form, mold] Plasma.

**plasm-** [Gr. *plasma,* anything formed] Combining form meaning *living substance, tissue.*

**plasma** (plăz′mă) [LL. *plasma,* form, mold] **1.** Protoplasm; cell substance outside the nucleus. **2.** An ointment base of glycerol and starch. **3.** The liquid part of the lymph and of the blood. SEE: *blood.*

In the blood, corpuscles and platelets are suspended in plasma. The plasma consists of serum, protein, and chemical substances in aqueous solution. The aqueous solution also contains solids and dissolved gases. Among the chemical materials are electrolytes, glucose, proteins including enzymes and hormones, fats, bile pigments, and bilirubin.

Plasma serves as the medium for transporting the substances previously mentioned to various structures and, at the same time, transports waste products to various sites of clearance (i.e., lungs, liver, kidneys, and spleen).

Different constituents of plasma have specific functions within the blood. Proteins, bicarbonates, carbon dioxide, chlorides, phosphates, and ammonia serve to keep the acid-base equilibrium of the blood constant when acid or base substances are added to it. Proteins, esp. albumin, by virtue of their osmotic pressure, tend to prevent undue leakage of fluids out of the capillaries and to maintain a proper exchange of fluid between capillaries and tissues.

Normal plasma is thin and colorless when free of corpuscles; it may have a faint yellow tinge when seen in thick layers.

After clotting of the blood, the liquid squeezed out by the clot is called blood serum. If whole blood is prevented from clotting either by chilling it or by adding anticoagulants, such as sodium citrate, it can be centrifuged. The clear fluid that then occupies the upper half of the centrifuge tube is called plasma.

***antihemophilic factor p.*** Human plasma in which the antihemophilic globulin has been preserved; used to correct temporarily the bleeding tendency in some forms of hemophilia. SEE: *antihemophilic factor.*

***blood p.*** Fluid in which cellular elements of the blood are suspended.

***fresh frozen p.*** ABBR: FFP. The fluid portion of one unit of human blood that has been centrifuged, separated, and frozen solid within 6 hours of collection. SEE: *blood component therapy.*

***hyperimmune p.*** Plasma with a high titer of a specific antibody, administered to create passive immunity to the antigen.

***lymph p.*** Lymph without its corpuscles.

***normal human p.*** Pooled plasma from a number of human donors. The plasma is sterile and the donors are free from diseases that could be transmitted by transfusion.

**plasmablast** (plăz′mă-blăst) [LL. *plasma,* form, mold, + Gr. *blastos,* germ] The undifferentiated cell that will mature into a B lymphocyte and ultimately into a plasma cell.

**plasmacyte** (plăz′mă-sīt) [″ + Gr. *kytos,* cell] A plasma cell.

**plasmacytoma** (plăz″mă-sī′tō′mă) [″ + ″ + *oma,* tumor] A plasma cell myeloma occurring in bone marrow. SEE: *myeloma, multiple.*

**plasmacytosis** (plăz″mă-sī-tō′sĭs) [″ + ″ + *osis,* condition] An excess of plasma cells in the blood.

**plasma exchange therapy** Removal of several liters of plasma from a patient and replacement with normal plasma. This is used experimentally to treat certain diseases, esp. neurological and immunological ones. SEE: *plasmapheresis.*

**plasmagel** (plăz′mă-jĕl″) [″ + L. *gelare,* to congeal] The peripheral portion of the endoplasm of a cell, such as in an ameba. It is immobile and has the consistency of a gel.

**plasmagene** (plăz′mă-jēn″) [″ + Gr. *gennan,* to produce] A cytoplasmic hereditary determiner.

**plasmalemma** (plăz″mă-lĕm′ă) [″ + Gr. *lemma,* husk] Plasma, or cell, membrane.

**plasmapheresis** (plăz″mă-fĕr-ē′sĭs) [″ + Gr. *aphairesis,* separation] A procedure in which blood is removed from the body, the cellular components evacuated by use of an automatic blood cell separator device, and the plasma returned to the body by infusion. In addition to the cellular components, various other substances such as antibodies, immune complexes, and protein-bound toxins are removed. The technique is used in treating hyperviscosity of the blood, Guillain-Barré syndrome, and thrombotic thrombocytopenic purpura.

**plasma protein fraction** A standard sterile preparation of serum albumin and globulin obtained by fractionating blood, serum, or plasma from healthy human donors and testing for absence of hepatitis B surface antigen. It is used as a blood volume expander.

**plasmasome** (plăz′mă-sōm) [″ + Gr. *soma,* body] A leukocyte granule; nucleolar substance (nonchromatin-staining) in the cytoplasm.

**plasmatherapy** (plăz″mă-thĕr′ă-pē) [″ + Gr. *therapeia,* service] The use of blood plasma for therapeutic purposes, as injection in treatment of shock.

**plasmatic** (plăz-măt′ĭk) **1.** Relating to plasma. **2.** Formative or plastic.

**plasmatogamy** (plăz″mă-tŏg′ă-mē) [″ + Gr. *gamos,* marriage] The union of the cytoplasm of two or more cells without joining of the nuclei.

**plasmatorrhexis** (plăz″mă-tō-rĕk′sĭs) [″+ Gr. *rhexis,* rupture] The rupture of a cell with loss of its contents, resulting from internal pressure caused by swelling.

**plasma volume extender** A nontoxic substance composed of high–molecular-weight compounds in a solution suitable for intravenous use. The materials, such as dextran or certain proteins, are used in treating shock caused by loss of blood volume.

**plasmid** A diverse group of extrachromosomal genetic elements. They are circular double-stringed DNA molecules present intracellularly and symbiotically in most bacteria. They reproduce inside the bacterial cell but are not essential to its viability. Plasmids can influence a great number of bacterial functions including resistance to antibiotics, production of enzymes that produce some antibiotics; the ability of the cell to detoxify harmful materials; and production of bacteriocins. Plasmids are gained or lost depending on their value to the bacterial cell in a specific circumstance. SEE: *bacteriocin; transposon.*

**plasmin** (plăz′mĭn) A fibrinolytic enzyme derived from its precursor plasminogen.

**plasminogen** (plăz-mĭn′ō-jĕn) A protein found in many tissues and body fluids; important in preventing fibrin clot formation.

**plasmocyte** (plăz′mō-sīt) [″ + Gr. *kytos,* cell] Cells found in bone marrow, connective tissue, and sometimes in blood plasma; considered by some to be abnormal leukocytes. They are numerous in plasma cell myeloma.

**plasmodesmata** (plăz″mō-dĕz′mă-tă) *sing.* **plasmodesma** [″ + Gr. *desmos,* bond] Tunnels in plant cells. These facilitate communication between cells.

**plasmodial** (plăz-mō′dē-ăl) Concerning *Plasmodia.*

**plasmodicidal** (plăz″mō-dĭ-sī′dăl) [″ + Gr. *eidos,* form, shape, + L. *caedere,* to kill] Lethal to plasmodia.

**Plasmodium** (plăz-mō′dē-ŭm) A genus of protozoa belonging to subphylum Sporozoa, class Telosporidia; includes causative agents of malaria in humans and lower animals. SEE: illus.; *malaria; mosquito.*

***P. falciparum*** The causative agent of malignant tertian (estivoautumnal) malaria. SEE: illus.

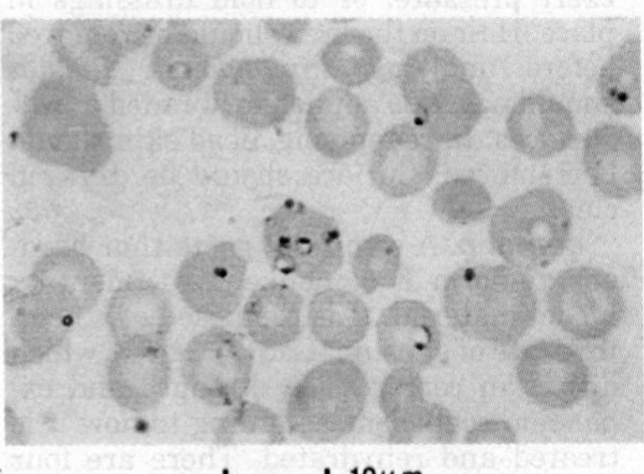


**PLASMODIUM FALCIPARUM**

SPOROZOITE RING FORMS IN RED BLOOD CELLS (ORIG. MAG. ×1000)

***P. malariae*** The causative agent of quartan malaria.

***P. ovale*** The causative agent of benign tertian or ovale malaria.

***P. vivax*** The causative agent of benign tertian or vivax malaria.

**plasmodium** (plăz-mō′dē-ŭm) *pl.* **plasmodia** [LL. *plasma,* form, mold, + Gr. *eidos,* form, shape] **1.** A multinucleate mass of naked protoplasm, occurring commonly among slime molds. **2.** An organism in the genus *Plasmodium.*

**plasmogamy** (plăs-mŏg′ă-mē) [″ + Gr. *gamos,* marriage] The fusion of cells.

**plasmolysis** (plăz-mŏl′ĭ-sĭs) [″ + Gr. *lysis,* dissolution] Shrinking of cytoplasm in a living cell caused by loss of water by osmosis.

**plasmoma** (plăz-mō′mă) [″ + Gr. *oma,* tumor] **1.** A collection of plasma cells. **2.** Plasmacytoma.

**plasmoptysis** (plăz-mŏp′tĭ-sĭs) [″ + Gr. *ptyein,* to spit] Escape of cytoplasm from a cell.

**plasmorrhexis** (plăz″mō-rĕk′sĭs) [″ + Gr. *rhexis,* rupture] The rupture of a cell with loss of its contents. SYN: *erythrocytorrhexis; plasmatorrhexis.*

**plasmotomy** (plăz-mŏt′ō-mē) [″ + Gr. *tome,* incision] Mitosis in which the cytoplasm divides into two or more masses.

**plastein** (plăs′tē-ĭn) Proteins or polypeptides synthesized by proteolytic enzymes following the peptic digestion of proteins.

**plaster** [Gr. *emplastron*] **1.** A material, usually plaster of Paris, that is applied to a part and allowed to harden in order to immobilize the part or to make an impression. **2.** A topical preparation in which the constituents are formed into a tenacious mass of substance harder than an ointment and spread upon muslin, linen, skin, or paper.

***adhesive p.*** Plaster made of a strong cloth coated on one side with an adhesive substance; used to immobilize a part, to relieve pressure upon sutures, to protect wounds, to secure traction in fractures, to exert pressure, or to hold dressings in place. Hair on the area should be removed before applying any plaster. Plaster should never be applied to abraded or raw surfaces. In reapplying, dead skin should be removed. Surface should be dry and clean.

***dental p.*** A semisolid paste that hardens to form a stonelike investment or model material. It is composed of a hemihydrate of gypsum ($CaSO_4 \cdot 2H_2O$), which differs in compression strength and expansion coefficient according to how it is treated and rehydrated. There are four classes of dental plaster, with differing uses as materials for casts, impressions, or stone models, based on the differences of characteristics.

***mustard p.*** Sinapism.

***p. of Paris*** Gypsum cement, hemihydrated calcium sulfate ($CaSO_4 \cdot 2H_2O$), mixed with water to form a paste that sets rapidly; used to make casts and stiff bandages.

***salicylic acid p.*** A uniform mixture of salicylic acid spread on an appropriate base such as paper, cotton, or fabric. It is applied topically for use as a keratolytic agent.

**plaster cast** Rigid dressing made of gauze impregnated with plaster of Paris, used to immobilize an injured part, esp. in bone fractures.

NURSING IMPLICATIONS: Neurovascular status of the casted part is monitored hourly for 24 hr, then every 4 hr, and patient is taught about assessment concerns. The patient is assessed for pressure areas and skin irritation at least daily and for indications of infection. Once the cast is dry, unfinished edges may be covered with adhesive tape or mole-skin strips to prevent irritation. If the patient complains of discomfort not relieved by repositioning or comfort measures, this should be reported immediately; cast removal, bivalving, or windowing may be necessary. Physical mobility is encouraged as permitted or prescribed, and preventive measures pertaining to immobility hazards and safety measures are taught to prevent further injury. The patient should never insert anything under the cast to relieve itching, because further irritation or infection may result. The nurse assists the patient with self-care as required and teaches measures to avoid wetting or soiling the cast. Respiratory, nutritional, and elimination status is monitored, and respiratory toilet is provided. The nurse prepares the patient for cast removal and for the appearance of the casted area. If the patient is sent home with a cast, the importance of either returning to the hospital or of calling the physician to report any pain is emphasized, particularly in the 24 to 48 hr after cast application. If pain occurs, the patient should be instructed to cut the cast immediately to avoid permanent damage to the part, then call the hospital or physician.

**plastic** (plăs′tĭk) [Gr. *plastikos,* fit for molding] **1.** Capable of being molded. **2.** Contributing to building tissues.

**plasticity** (plăs-tĭs′ĭ-tē) The ability to be molded.

**plastid** (plăs′tĭd) [Gr. *plastos,* formed] A cytoplasmic organoid found in plant cells. It includes chloroplasts (which contain chlorophyll), leukoplasts (colorless), chromoplasts (which contain pigment), and amyloplasts (which store starch). Plastids are centers of chemical activity involved in cell metabolism.

**plastron** [Fr., breastplate] The sternum and attached cartilages.

**-plasty** [Gr. *plastos,* formed] A word ending meaning *molding, surgically forming.*

**plate** (plāt) [Gr. *plate,* flat] **1.** A thin flattened part or portion, such as a flattened process of a bone. SYN: *lamella; lamina.* **2.** An incorrect reference to a full denture. **3.** A shallow covered dish for culturing microorganisms. **4.** To inoculate and culture microorganisms in a culture plate.

***auditory p.*** The bony roof of the external auditory meatus.

***axial p.*** The primitive streak of the embryo.

***bite p.*** In dentistry, a plate made of some suitable plastic material into which the patient bites in order to have a record of the relationship between the upper and lower jaws. The device may be reinforced with wire and used as a splint in the mouth or to treat temporomandibular joint difficulties.

***bone p.*** A flat, round or oval, decalcified bone or metal disk, employed in pairs, used in approximation.

***cortical p.*** The compact layers of bone forming the surfaces of the alveolar processes of the mandible and maxilla.

***cribriform p.*** The thin, perforated, medial portion of the horizontal plate of the ethmoid bone; also, a synonym for alveolar bone proper, the sievelike layer of bone that makes up the wall of the socket and supports the tooth.

***deck p.*** The roof plate of the embryonic neural tube.

***dental p.*** An old term for the denture base of metal or acrylic material that rests on the oral mucosa and to which artificial teeth are attached; by extension, *incorrectly* used to mean the complete denture.

***dorsal p.*** One of two prominences of the notochord in the embryo.

***epiphyseal p.*** The thin layer of cartilage between the epiphysis and the shaft of a bone. Growth in length of the bone occurs at this layer.

***equatorial p.*** The platelike mass of

chromosomes at the equator of the spindle in cell division.

***floor p.*** The floor of the embryonic neural tube. SYN: *ventral p.*

***medullary p.*** The central portion of the ectoderm in the embryo developing into the neural canal. SYN: *neural p.*

***muscle p.*** In the somite, the myotome from which the striated muscles are formed.

***neural p.*** Medullary p.

***palate p.*** Part of the palate bone forming the dorsal half of the roof of the mouth.

***polar p.*** In some cells, the flattened platelike bodies seen at the end of the spindle during mitosis.

***pterygoid p.*** Either of a pair of thin, bony processes that arise from the sphenoid bone. They are termed medial and lateral pterygoid plates on each side and serve to bound the infratemporal fossa and give origin to muscles of mastication.

***tarsal p.*** The dense connective tissue structure that supports the eyelid. It was formerly called *tarsal cartilage*; however, it is not true cartilage.

***tympanic p.*** The bony plate between the anterior wall of the external auditory meatus and the tympanum.

***ventral p.*** Floor p.

**plateau 1.** An elevated and usually flat area; a steady and consistent fever appears as a plateau on the patient's chart of vital signs. **2.** The stage in training or skill acquisition when progress occurs at a very slow or flat rate in comparison with earlier phases.

***ventricular p.*** The flat portion of the record of intraventricular pressure during the end of the ejection phase of ventricular systole.

**platelet** (plăt′lĕt) [Gr. *plate,* flat] A round or oval disk, 2 to 4 $\mu$m in diameter, found in the blood of vertebrates. Platelets number 130,000 to 400,000/mm$^3$. They are fragments of megakaryocytes, large cells found in the bone marrow. SYN: *thrombocyte.* SEE: illus.; *blood* for illus.; *megakaryocyte* for illus.; *thrombopoietin.*

FUNCTION: Platelets play an important role in blood coagulation, hemostasis, and blood thrombus formation. When a small vessel is injured, platelets adhere to each other and the edges of the injury and form a plug that covers the area. This leads to enhancement of the coagulation mechanism and deposition of fibrin. The plug or blood clot formed soon retracts and stops the loss of blood. The actions of platelets, though quite beneficial in initiating the reaction to injury, may actually be harmful in conditions such as coronary occlusion. In that case, platelet function may delay reperfusion and help to cause reocclusion of the vessel.

DISORDERS: Thrombocytopenia (reduced platelet count) occurs in acute infections, anaphylactic shock, and certain hemorrhagic diseases and anemias. Thrombocytosis (increased platelet count) occurs after operations, esp. splenectomy, and after violent exercise and tissue injury.

**platelet concentrate** Platelets prepared from a single unit of whole blood or plasma and suspended in a specific volume of the original plasma. This blood fraction must be used before the expiration date shown on its label. Platelets are stored at room temperature (22°C) either in plasma or in a concentrated form as platelet-rich plasma.

**plateletpheresis** The process of treating donor blood to remove platelets and then returning the remaining blood to the donor.

**plating** In bacteriology, inoculation of liquefiable, solid media (gelatin or agar) with microorganisms and pouring of medium into a shallow flat dish.

**platinic** (plă-tĭn′ĭk) Pert. to a compound containing quadrivalent platinum.

**platinosis** Cutaneous and respiratory allergic reactions to exposure to complex salts of platinum.

**platinous** (plăt′ĭ-nŭs) A compound containing divalent platinum.

**platinum** (plăt′ĭ-nŭm) [Sp. *platina*] SYMB: Pt. A heavy silver-white metal; atomic weight 195.09; atomic number 78; specific gravity 21.45.

**platy-** [Gr. *platys,* broad] Combining form meaning *broad.*

**platybasia** (plăt″ē-bā′sē-ă) A developmental defect of the skull in which the floor of the posterior fossa of the skull around the foramen magnum protrudes upward.

**platycelous** (plăt-ē-sē′lŭs) [Gr. *platys,* broad, + *koilos,* hollow] Concave ventrally and convex dorsally, said of vertebrae.

**platycephalic, platycephalous** (plăt″ē-sē-făl′ĭk, -sĕf′ă-lŭs) [″ + *kephale,* head] Having a wide skull with a vertical index less than 70.

**platycephaly** (plăt″ē-sĕf′ă-lē) Flattening of the skull. SYN: *platycrania.*

**platycnemia** (plăt-ĭk-nē′mē-ă) [″ + *kneme,* leg] **1.** The condition of having an unusually broad tibia. **2.** A broad-legged condition.

**platycoria, platycoriasis** (plăt″ē-kor-ē′ă, -kor-ī′ă-sĭs) [″ + *kore,* pupil] Mydriasis.

**platycrania** (plăt″ē-krā′nē-ă) [″ + *kranion,* skull] Platycephaly.

**platyglossal** (plăt″ē-glŏs′ăl) [Gr. *platys,* broad, + *glossa,* tongue] Having a broad, flat tongue.

**platyhelminth** (plăt″ē-hĕl′mĭnth) The common name for any flatworm.

**Platyhelminthes** (plăt″ē-hĕl-mĭn′thēz) [″ + *helmins,* worm] A phylum of flatworms including the classes Turbellaria, Trematoda (flukes), and Cestoidea (tapeworms). The last two are parasitic and include many species of medical importance. SEE: *Cestoda; Cestoidea; fluke; tapeworm; trematode.*

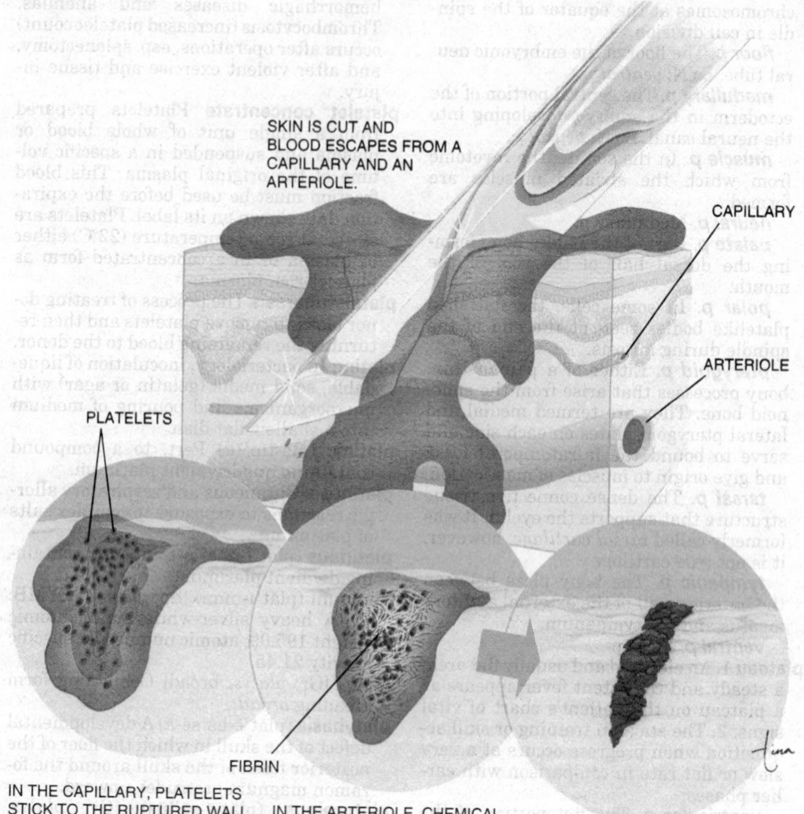


**PLATELET** PLUG FORMATION AND CLOTTING

**platyhieric** (plăt″ē-hī-ĕr′ĭk) [″ + *hieron*, sacrum] Having a broad sacrum with a sacral index over 100.

**platymeric** (plăt″ē-mē′rĭk) [″ + *meros*, thigh] Having an unusually broad femur.

**platymorphia** (plăt″ē-mor′fē-ă) [″ + *morphe*, form] Having an eye with a shortened anteroposterior diameter, which results in hyperopia.

**platyopia** (plăt″ē-ō′pē-ă) [″ + *ops*, face] Having a very broad face, with a nasomalar index of less than 107.5.

**platyopic** (plăt″ē-ŏp′ĭk) Having a broad, flattened face.

**platypellic, platypelvic, platypelloid** (plăt″ē-pĕl′ĭk, -vĭk, -oyd) [″ + *pella*, a basin] Having a broad pelvis. SEE: under *pelvis*.

**platypnea** (plă″tĭp′nē-ă) [″ + *pnoia*, breath] Shortness of breath, dyspnea, only when the patient is upright or seated. SEE: *orthopnea*.

**platyrrhine** (plăt′ĭr-īn) [″ + *rhis*, nose] **1.** Having a very wide nose in proportion to length. **2.** Pert. to a skull with a nasal index between 51.1 and 58.

**platysma myoides** (plă-tĭz′mă mī-oy′dēz) [Gr. *platysma*, plate, + *mys*, muscle, + *eidos*, form, shape] A broad, thin, platelike layer of muscle that extends from the fascia of both sides of the neck to the jaw and muscles around the mouth. It acts to wrinkle the skin of the neck and depress the jaw.

**platyspondylia** (plăt″ē-spŏn-dĭl′ē-ă) Flatness of the vertebral bodies.

**platystencephaly** (plăt″ĭ-stĕn-sĕf′ă-lē) [″ + *kephale*, head] Having a skull wide at the occiput.

**play** Involvement in a sport, amusement, or any form of recreation, esp. an activity other than that in which one is usually engaged as an occupation. What is play to one individual might be considered work to another. From the medical standpoint, it is important that the recreational activity be enjoyable and that participation in it be safe and satisfactory. From the medical aspect, the value of engaging in a sport or recreation that causes frustration, anger, or uncontrolled stress to the extent that the activity is no longer fun is questionable.

**pleasure** [L. *placere,* to please] The feeling of being delighted or pleased.

**pleasure principle** Hedonism.

**pledget** (plĕj′ĕt) [origin uncertain] **1.** A small, flat compress, usually of gauze or absorbent cotton, used to apply or absorb fluid, to protect, or to exclude air. **2.** A small spherical mass of cotton about ⅛ in. (3 mm) in diameter that is used with forceps for topical application of medicinal substances, particularly in dentistry.

**plegaphonia** (plĕg″ă-fō′nē-ă) [Gr. *plege,* stroke, + *a-,* not, + *phone,* voice] A sound produced in percussion of the larynx when the glottis is open during auscultation of the chest.

**-plegia** (plē′jē-ă) [Gr. *plege,* stroke] Combining form used as a suffix meaning *paralysis, stroke.*

**pleio-, pleo-, plio-** Combining form meaning *more.*

**pleiotropia** (plī″ō-trō′pē-ă) [Gr. *pleion,* more, + *trope,* turn] The ability of a gene to have many effects. SYN: *pleiotropism.*

**pleiotropism** (plī-ŏt′rō-pĭzm) [″ + ″ + *-ismos,* condition] Pleiotropia.

**Pleistophora** A genus of microsporidia. SEE: *microsporidiosis.*

**pleochroic** (plē″ō-krō′ĭk) [Gr. *pleon,* more, + *chroia,* color] Pleochromatic.

**pleochroism** (plē-ŏk′rō-ĭzm) [″ + ″ + *-ismos,* condition] The property of a crystal that produces different colors when light passes through it at different angles.

**pleochromatic** (plē″ō-krō-măt′ĭk) [″ + *chroma,* color] Pert. to the property of crystals and some other bodies that show different colors when seen from different axes. SYN: *pleochroic.*

**pleocytosis** (plē″ō-sī-tō′sĭs) [″ + *kytos,* cell, + *osis,* condition] An increased number of lymphocytes in the cerebrospinal fluid.

**pleomorphic** (plē-ō-mor′fĭk) [″ + *morphe,* form] Having many shapes.

**pleomorphism** (plē-ō-mor′fĭzm) [″ + ″ + *-ismos,* condition] Polymorphism.

**pleomorphous** (plē-ō-mor′fŭs) Having many shapes or crystallizing into several forms.

**pleonasm** (plē′ō-năzm) [Gr. *pleonasmos,* exaggeration] **1.** The state of having more than the normal number of organs or parts. **2.** The use of more words than necessary to express an idea.

**pleonexia** (plē″ō-nĕk′sē-ă) [Gr.] Having a morbid desire for possession of material things; greediness.

**pleonosteosis** (plē″ŏn-ŏs″tē-ō′sĭs) [Gr. *pleon,* more, + *osteon,* bone, + *osis,* condition] Premature and excessive ossification of bones.

**pleoptics** (plē-ŏp′tĭks) [″ + *optikos,* sight] A method of eye exercises created to stimulate and train an amblyopic eye.

**plerocercoid** The solid wormlike larva of certain tapeworms. Plerocercoids develop in secondary hosts.

**plesiomorphism** (plē″sē-ō-mor′fĭzm) [Gr. *plesios,* close, + *morphe,* form, + *-ismos,* condition] Similarity of form.

**plesiopia** (plē″sē-ō′pē-ă) [″ + *ops,* eye] An increase in the convexity of the lens of the eye.

**plessesthesia** (plĕs″ĕs-thē′zē-ă) [Gr. *plessein,* to strike, + *aisthesis,* sensation] Palpatory percussion with the left middle finger pressed against the body and the right index finger percussing in contact with the left finger.

**plessimeter** (plĕs-sĭm′ĕ-tĕr) [″ + *metron,* measure] Pleximeter.

**plessor** (plĕs′or) [Gr. *plessein,* to strike] Plexor.

**plethora** (plĕth′ō-ră) [Gr. *plethore,* fullness] **1.** Overfullness of blood vessels or of the total quantity of any fluid in the body. SEE: *sanguine.* **2.** Congestion causing distention of the blood vessels.

**plethoric** (plĕ-thor′ĭk, plĕth′ō-rĭk) Pert. to, or characterized by, plethora; overfull.

**plethysmograph** (plē-thĭz′mō-grăf) [Gr. *plethysmos,* to increase, + *graphein,* to write] A device for finding variations in the size of a part owing to variations in the amount of blood passing through or contained in the part.

***body p.*** A body box used to measure lung volume and pressure.

***impedance p.*** A device that uses gas-to-tissue ratio to set an alarm or measure a volume.

**plethysmography** (plĕth″ĭz-mŏg′ră-fē) The use of a plethysmograph to record the changes in volume of an organ or extremity.

**pleur-, pleuro-** [Gr. *pleura,* rib, side] Combining form meaning *pleura, side, rib.*

**pleura** (ploo′ră) *pl.* **pleurae** [Gr., side] A serous membrane that enfolds both lungs and is reflected upon the walls of the thorax and diaphragm. The pleurae are moistened with a serous secretion that reduces friction during respiratory movements of the lungs. SEE: *effusion, pleural; mediastinum; thorax.*

***costal p.*** Parietal p.

***p. diaphragmatica*** The part of the pleura covering the upper surface of the diaphragm.

***mediastinal p.*** The portion of the parietal pleura that extends to cover the mediastinum.

***parietal p.*** The portion of the pleura that extends from the mediastinal roots of the lungs and covers the sides of the pericardium to the chest wall and backward to the spine. The visceral and parietal pleural layers are separated only by a lubricating secretion. These layers may become adherent or separated by fluid or air in diseased conditions. SYN: *costal p.*

***p. pericardiaca*** The portion of the pleura covering the pericardium.

***p. pulmonalis*** The pleura investing the

lungs and fissures between the lobes.

***visceral p.*** The pleura that covers the lungs and enters into and lines the interlobar fissures. It is loose at the base and at sternal and vertebral borders to allow for lung expansion.

**pleuracotomy** (ploor″ă-kŏt′ō-mē) [″ + *tome,* incision] Incision into the pleura through the chest wall.

**pleural** (ploo′răl) [Gr. *pleura,* side] Concerning the pleura.

***p. fibrosis*** A condition occurring in pulmonary tuberculosis in which the pleura becomes thickened and the pleural cavity often is obliterated.

**pleuralgia** (ploo-răl′jē-ă) [″ + *algos,* pain] Pain in the pleura, or in the side. SYN: *intercostal neuralgia.*

**pleurapophysis** (ploo-ră-pŏf′ĭ-sĭs) [″ + *apo,* from, + *physis,* a growth] A rib or a vertebral lateral process.

**pleurectomy** (ploo-rĕk′tō-mē) [″ + *ektome,* excision] Excision of part of the pleura.

**pleurisy** (ploo′rĭs-ē) [Gr. *pleuritis*] Inflammation of the pleura. It may be primary or secondary; unilateral, bilateral, or local; acute or chronic; fibrinous, serofibrinous, or purulent. SYN: *pleuritis.* SEE: *Nursing Diagnoses Appendix.*

NURSING IMPLICATIONS: Respiratory function is monitored by percussion, auscultation, and arterial blood gas values. The patient is positioned in the high Fowler position to facilitate chest expansion. Deep breathing and coughing are encouraged every 1 to 2 hr to prevent atelectasis. During coughing, the nurse should splint the chest as necessary and administer analgesic drugs and use noninvasive measures, such as local application of warm or cool compresses, to reduce pain. Respiratory toilet is provided and antitussives are avoided if secretions are present. Rest is recommended. Prescribed medical regimens are carried out, and the patient's responses evaluated.

***acute p.*** A type of pleurisy characterized by chilliness and a stabbing pain or stitch in the affected side, which is intensified by coughing or deep breathing. There is a fever of 101° to 103°F (38.3° to 39.4°C); a short, dry, partially suppressed cough; and a pale, anxious face. The patient usually lies on the affected side. An effusion of fluid that remains unabsorbed in the pleural space characterizes chronic pleurisy.

***adhesive p.*** Pleurisy in which the exudate causes the parietal pleura to adhere to the visceral. If this is extensive, the pleural space is obliterated.

***diaphragmatic p.*** Inflammation of the diaphragmatic pleura. Symptoms include intense pain under the margin of the ribs, sometimes referred into the abdomen, with tenderness upon pressure; thoracic breathing; tenderness over the phrenic nerve referred to the supraclavicular region in the neck on the same side; hiccough; and extreme dyspnea.

***dry p.*** A condition in which the pleural membrane is covered with a fibrinous exudate. It clings together, causing pain during respiration. There is slight pain when the apical pleura is inflamed, but there is acute stabbing pain in costal or diaphragmatic pleural inflammation.

***p. with effusion*** Serous p.

***encysted p.*** Pleurisy with effusion limited by adhesions.

***fibrinous p.*** Pleurisy with severe and continuous pain. Aspiration gives negative results, and later much retraction of the affected side.

***hemorrhagic p.*** Pleurisy with hemorrhage.

***interlobar p.*** Pleurisy in interlobar spaces.

***pulmonary p.*** Inflammation of the pleura covering the lung.

***purulent p.*** Pleurisy with high, irregular fever; sweats; chills; anemia; and purulent effusion found on aspiration. SYN: *empyema.*

***sacculated p.*** Pleurisy in which there are inflammatory areas, sealed off and filled with fluid.

***serofibrinous p.*** Pleurisy with fibrinous exudate and serous effusion.

***serous p.*** Pleurisy with a serous effusion. SYN: *wet p.; p. with effusion.*

***tuberculous p.*** Inflammation of the pleura as a result of tuberculosis. The effusion may be bloody.

***typhoid p.*** Pleurisy with symptoms of typhoid.

***wet p.*** Serous p.

**pleuritic** (ploo-rĭt′ĭk) [Gr. *pleuritis,* pleurisy] Relating to, or resembling, pleurisy.

**pleuritis** (ploo-rī′tĭs) [Gr.] Pleurisy.

**pleuritogenous** (ploor″ĭ-tŏj′ĕ-nŭs) [″ + *gennan,* to produce] Causing pleurisy.

**pleurocele** (ploo′rō-sēl) [Gr. *pleura,* side, + *kele,* tumor, swelling] **1.** Hernia of the lungs or pleura. **2.** A serous pleural effusion.

**pleurocentesis** (ploo″rō-sĕn-tē′sĭs) [″ + *kentesis,* a piercing] Thoracentesis.

**pleurocentrum** (ploo″rō-sĕn′trŭm) *pl.* **pleurocentra** [″ + *kentron,* center] The lateral half of the centrum of a vertebra.

**pleurocholecystitis** (ploo″rō-kō″lē-sĭst-ī′tĭs) [″ + *chole,* bile, + *kystis,* bladder, + *itis,* inflammation] Inflammation of the pleura and gallbladder.

**pleuroclysis** (ploo-rŏk′lĭ-sĭs) [″ + *klysis,* a washing] Injection and removal of fluid into the pleural cavity to wash it out.

**pleurodesis** (ploo″rō-dē′sĭs) [″ + *desis,* binding] Production of adhesions between the parietal and visceral pleura; usually done surgically. This method is useful in treating recurrent pneumothorax.

**pleurodynia** (ploo″rō-dĭn′ē-ă) [″ + *odyne,* pain] Pain of sharp intensity in the intercostal muscles due to chronic inflammatory changes in the chest fasciae; pain of the pleural nerves.

***epidemic p.*** Bornholm disease.

**pleurogenic, pleurogenous** (ploo-rŏj′ĕn-ŭs) Arising in the pleura.

**pleurography** (ploo-rŏg′ră-fē) [″ + *graphein,* to write] Radiographical examination of the lungs and pleura.

**pleurohepatitis** (ploo″rō-hĕp″ă-tī′tĭs) [″ + *hepatos,* liver, + *itis,* inflammation] Inflammation of the pleura and liver.

**pleurolith** (ploo′rō-lĭth) [″ + *lithos,* stone] A calculus in the pleura.

**pleurolysis** (ploo-rŏl′ĭ-sĭs) [″ + *lysis,* dissolution] Loosening of parietal pleura from intrathoracic fascia to facilitate contraction of the lung or artificial pneumothorax.

**pleuromelus** (ploor″ō-mē′lŭs) [″ + *melos,* limb] A congenital anomaly in which an accessory limb arises from the thorax or flank.

**pleuroparietopexy** (ploo″rō-păr-ī′ĕt-ō-pĕk″sē) [″ + L. *parietalis,* wall, + Gr. *pexis,* fixation] Fastening of the lung to the wall of the chest by binding the visceral pleura to the wall of its cavity.

**pleuropericardial** (ploor″ō-pĕr-ĭ-kăr′dē-ăl) [″ + *peri,* around, + *kardia,* heart] Concerning the pleura and pericardium.

**pleuropericarditis** (ploo″rō-pĕr″ĭ-kăr-dī′tĭs) [″ + ″ + ″ + *itis,* inflammation] Pleuritis accompanied by pericarditis.

**pleuroperitoneal** (ploo″rō-pĕr″ĭ-tō-nē′ăl) [″ + *peritonaion,* peritoneum] Concerning the pleura and peritoneum.

***p. cavity*** The ventral body cavity. SEE: *coelom.*

**pleuropneumonia** (ploo″rō-nū-mō′nē-ă) [″ + *pneumon,* lung] Pleurisy accompanied by pneumonia.

**pleuropneumonia-like organisms** ABBR: PPLO. The name once given organisms that are now called mycoplasmas.

**pleuropneumonolysis** (ploo″rō-nū″mōn-ŏl′ĭ-sĭs) [Gr. *pleura,* side, + *pneumon,* lung, + *lysis,* a loosening] Resection of one or more ribs from one side to collapse the lung in unilateral pulmonary tuberculosis. This procedure is rarely necessary.

**pleuropulmonary** (ploor″ō-pŭl′mō-nĕr″ē) [″ + L. *pulmo,* lung] Concerning the pleura and lung.

**pleurorrhea** (ploor″ō-rē′ă) [″ + *rhoia,* flow] Effusion of fluid into the pleura.

**pleuroscopy** (ploo-rŏs′kō-pē) [″ + *skopein,* to examine] Inspection of the pleural cavity through an incision into the thorax.

**pleurosoma** (ploor″ō-sō′mă) [″ + *soma,* body] A fetus with a cleft in the abdominal wall and thorax with protrusion of the contents of the thoracic and abdominal cavities.

**pleurothotonos** (ploo″rō-thŏt′ō-nŏs) [Gr. *pleurothen,* from the side, + *tonos,* tension] A tetanic spasm in which the body is arched to one side.

**pleurotomy** (ploo-rŏt′ō-mē) [Gr. *pleura,* side, + *tome,* incision] Incision of the pleura.

**pleurotyphoid** (ploo″rō-tī′foyd) [″ + *typhos,* fever, + *eidos,* form, shape] Typhoid fever with pleural involvement.

**pleurovisceral** (ploo″rō-vĭs′ĕr-ăl) [″ + L. *viscera,* viscera] Concerning the pleura and viscera.

**plexal** (plĕk′săl) [L. *plexus,* a braid] Pert. to, or of the nature of, a plexus.

**plexectomy** (plĕk-sĕk′tō-mē) [″ + Gr. *ektome,* excision] Surgical removal of a plexus.

**plexiform** (plĕk′sĭ-form) [″ + *forma,* shape] Resembling a network or plexus.

**pleximeter** (plĕks-ĭm′ĕ-tĕr) [Gr. *plexis,* stroke, + *metron,* measure] A device for receiving the blow of the percussion hammer, consisting of a disk that is struck in mediate percussion while being held over the surface of the body. SYN: *plessimeter; plexometer.*

**plexitis** (plĕk-sī′tĭs) [L. *plexus,* a braid, + Gr. *itis,* inflammation] Inflammation of a nerve plexus.

**plexometer** (plĕk-sŏm′ĕ-tĕr) Pleximeter.

**plexopathy** A disorder of either the brachial or lumbosacral plexus. This may be caused by trauma, infiltration by malignant cells, or radiation therapy.

**plexor** (plĕks′or) A hammer or other device for striking on the pleximeter in percussion. SYN: *plessor.*

**plexus** (plĕks′ŭs) *pl.* **plexus, plexuses** [L., a braid] A network of nerves or of blood or lymphatic vessels. SEE: *rete; Nerve Plexus Appendix.*

***autonomic p.*** An extensive network of nerve fibers and neuron cell bodies belonging to the sympathetic or parasympathetic nervous system. SEE: *Nerve Plexus Appendix.*

***cavernous p.*** Plexus of a cavernous part of the body. The following are included: Of the nose: a venous plexus in the mucosa covering the superior and middle conchae. Of the penis: a nerve plexus at the base of the penis giving rise to large and small cavernous nerves. Of the clitoris: nerve plexus at the base of the clitoris, formed of fibers from the uterovaginal plexus. Of the cavernous sinus: a sympathetic plexus that supplies fibers to the internal carotid artery and its branches within the cranium.

***celiac p.*** A sympathetic plexus lying near the origin of thest celiac artery. SEE: *Nerve Plexus Appendix.*

***choroid p.*** A capillary network located in each of the four ventricles of the brain (two lateral, the third, and the fourth) that produces cerebrospinal fluid by filtration and secretion.

***dental p.*** A network of sensory nerve fibers that are distributed to the teeth. The inferior alveolar nerve is distributed to the mandibular teeth; the anterior, middle, and posterior superior alveolar nerves contribute fibers to innervate the maxillary teeth.

***enteric p.*** One of two plexuses of nerve fibers and ganglion cells that lie in the wall of the alimentary canal. These are the myenteric (Auerbach's) and submucosal (Meissner's) plexuses.

***lumbar p.*** A nerve plexus formed by the ventral branches of the first four lumbar nerves.

***lumbosacral p.*** The lumbar plexus and sacral plexus, considered as one.

***myenteric p.*** Auerbach's plexus.

***nerve p.*** Plexus made of nerve fibers. SEE: *Nerve Plexus Appendix.*

***pampiniform p.*** In the male, a complicated network of veins lying in the spermatic cord and draining the testis. In the female, a network of veins lying in the mesovarium and draining the ovary.

***prevertebral p.*** One of three plexuses of autonomic nerve division that lie in body cavities. These are the cardiac, celiac, and hypogastric (pelvic) plexuses. SEE: *Nerve Plexus Appendix.*

**pliability** (plī″ă-bĭl′ĭ-tē) [O. Fr. *pliant,* bend, + L. *abilis,* able] Capacity of being bent or twisted easily.

**plica** (plī′kă) *pl.* **plicae** [L.] A fold. SEE: *fold.*

***circular p.*** One of the transverse folds of the mucosa and submucosa of the small intestine. Collectively they resemble accordion pleats, do not disappear with distention of the intestine, and increase the surface area for absorption. SYN: *Kerckring's folds; valvulae conniventes.*

***epiglottic p.*** One of three folds of mucosa between the tongue and the epiglottis.

***lacrimal p.*** A mucosal fold at the lower orifice of the nasolacrimal duct.

***palmate p.*** A radiating fold in the uterine mucosa on the anterior and posterior walls of the cervical canal.

***semilunar p. of the colon*** The transverse fold of mucosa of the large intestine lying between sacculations.

***semilunar p. of the conjunctiva*** The mucosal fold at the inner canthus of the eye.

***synovial p.*** A fold of synovial membrane that projects into a joint cavity.

***transverse p. of the rectum*** One of the mucosal folds in the rectum.

**plicamycin** An antineoplastic agent that has been used in treating Paget's disease of the bone.

**plicate** (plī′kāt) [L. *plicatus*] Braided or folded.

**plication** (plī-kā′shŭn) [L. *plicare,* to fold] The stitching of folds or tucks in an organ's walls to reduce its size.

***p. of the stomach*** The surgical creation of tucks in the wall of the stomach. This technique has been used experimentally in treating obesity.

**plicotomy** (plī-kŏt′ō-mē) [″ + Gr. *tome,* incision] Section of the posterior fold of the tympanic membrane.

**pliers 1.** Commonly, a scissor-action, pointed-jawed tool for bending or cutting metal wires or grasping small objects. **2.** In dentistry, a variety of instruments that have been shaped or adapted for special uses such as cutting arch wires or metal clasps, shaping metal crown details, applying cotton pledgets or rolls, carrying metal foils, tying ligatures, and placing or removing matrix bands.

**plinth** [Gr. *plinthos,* tile] A table, seat, or apparatus on which a patient lies or sits while doing remedial exercise.

**-ploid** [Gr. *ploos,* fold] Combining form used as a suffix indicating the number of chromosome pairs of the root word to which it is added.

**ploidy** (ploy′dē) [Gr. *ploos,* a fold, + *eidos,* form, shape] The number of chromosome sets in a cell (e.g., haploidy, diploidy, and triploidy for one, two, and three sets, respectively, of chromosomes).

**plombage** (plŏm-băzh′) [Fr. *plomber,* to plug] A method of collapsing the apex of the lung by stripping the parietal pleura from the chest wall at the site of desired collapse and packing the space between the lung and the chest wall with an inert substance such as small balls made of certain plastic materials.

**plototoxin** (plō″tō-tŏk′sĭn) A toxic substance present in catfish, *Plotosus lineatus.*

**plug** (plŭg) [MD. *plugge*] A mass obstructing a hole or intended for closing a hole.

***epithelial p.*** A mass of epithelial cells temporarily plugging an orifice in the embryo, esp. the nasal openings.

***mucous p.*** A mass of cells and mucus that closes the cervical canal of the uterus during pregnancy and between menstrual periods.

***vaginal p.*** A closed tube for maintaining patency of the vagina following operation for fistula.

**plugger** A hand- or machine-operated device for condensing amalgam, or gold foil, in the cavity of a tooth.

***automatic p.*** A plugger that is run by a machine rather than by hand.

***back-action p.*** A plugger with a bent shank so that the pressure applied is back toward the operator.

***foot p.*** A plugger having a broad, foot-shaped tip.

**plumbic** (plŭm′bĭk) [L. *plumbicus,* leaden] Pert. to, or containing, lead.

**plumbism** (plŭm′bĭzm) [L. *plumbum,* lead, + Gr. *-ismos,* condition] Poisoning from lead.

**plumbum** (plŭm′bŭm) [L.] Lead; a bluish-white metal. SEE: *lead.*

**Plummer-Vinson syndrome** (plŭm′ĕr-vĭn′sŏn) [Henry S. Plummer, U.S. physician, 1874–1937; Porter P. Vinson, U.S. surgeon, 1890–1959] Iron-deficiency anemia, associated with dysphagia, gastric achlorhydria, splenomegaly, and spooning of the nails due to an esophageal web. It occurs most commonly in premenopausal women. Treatment consists of disrupting the web. SEE: *esophageal web.*

**plumose** (plū′mōs) [L. *plumosus*] Having a delicate, feathery growth.

**plumper** (plŭm′pĕr) [Middle Low Ger. *plump,* to fill] A pad for filling out sunken cheeks, sometimes in the form of a flange or extension from artificial dentures.

**pluri-** [L. *plus,* more] Prefix meaning *several, more.*

**pluriceptor** (ploo″rĭ-sĕp′tor) [L. *plus,* more, + *ceptor,* a receiver] A receptor that has more than two groups uniting with the complement.

**pluriglandular** (ploo″rĭ-glănd′ū-lăr) [″ + *glandula,* gland] Polyglandular.

**plurigravida** (ploo″rĭ-grăv′ĭ-dă) [″ + *gravida,* pregnant] A pregnant woman who has had three or more pregnancies.

**plurilocular** (ploo″rĭ-lŏk′ū-lăr) [″ + *loculus,* a cell] Multilocular.

**plurinuclear** (ploor″ĭ-nū′klē-ăr) [″ + *nucleus,* kernel] Having a number of nuclei.

**pluripara** (ploo-rĭp′ă-ră) [″ + *parere,* to bring forth, to bear] A woman who has given birth three or more times.

**pluriparity** (ploo″rĭ-păr′ĭ-tē) The condition of having three or more pregnancies that have reached a point of viability regardless of the outcome.

**pluripotent, pluripotential** (ploo-rĭp′ō-tĕnt, ploor″ĭ-pō-tĕn′shăl) [″ + *potentia,* power] **1.** Concerning an embryonic cell that can form different kinds of cells. **2.** Having a number of different actions.

**pluriresistant** (ploor″ĭ-rē-zĭs′tănt) [″ + *resistens,* standing back] Resistant to several drugs, esp. antibiotics.

**plutonium** (ploo-tō′nē-ŭm) [Named after the planet Pluto] SYMB: Pu. A chemical element obtained from neptunium, which in turn is obtained from uranium; atomic weight of the most stable isotope is 244; atomic number 94.

**plyometrics** A stretching and shortening exercise technique that combines strength with speed to achieve maximum power in functional movements. This regimen combines eccentric training of muscles with concentric contraction.

**Pm** Symbol for the element promethium.

**PML** *progressive multifocal leukoencephalopathy.*

**PMS** *premenstrual syndrome.*

**PMSG** *pregnant mare serum gonadotropin.* SEE: *gonadotropin, human chorionic.*

**PMT** *photomultiplier tube*; *premenstrual tension.*

**PNC** *premature nodal contraction* or *complex.*

**pneo-** (nē′ō) [Gr. *pnein,* to breathe] Combining form meaning *breath, breathing.* SEE: *pneumo-.*

**pneum-, pneuma-, pneumato-** [Gr. *pneuma, pneumatos,* air, breath] Combining form meaning *air, gas, respiration.*

**pneumarthrogram** (nū-măr′thrō-grăm) [Gr. *pneuma,* air, + *arthron,* joint, + *gramma,* something written] A radiograph of a synovial joint after injection of a radiolucent contrast medium, usually air.

**pneumarthrography** (nū″măr-thrŏg′ră-fē) [″ + ″ + *graphein,* to write] Radiography of a synovial joint after injection of a radiolucent contrast medium, usually air. SYN: *pneumoarthrography.*

**pneumarthrosis** (nū-măr-thrō′sĭs) [″ + ″ + *osis,* condition] Accumulation of gas or air in a joint.

**pneumatic** (nū-măt′ĭk) [Gr. *pneumatikos,* pert. to air] **1.** Concerning gas or air. **2.** Relating to respiration. **3.** Relating to rarefied or compressed air.

**pneumatics** (nū-măt′ĭks) The branch of physics that is concerned with the physical and mechanical properties of gases and air.

**pneumatinuria** (nū″măt-ĭn-ū′rē-ă) [″ + *ouron,* urine] Pneumaturia.

**pneumatization** (nū″mă-tī-zā′shŭn) The formation of air-filled cells or cavities, usually in bone (e.g., the paranasal sinuses and mastoid processes).

**pneumatocardia** (nū″măt-ō-kăr′dē-ă) [″ + *kardia,* heart] Air or gas in the heart chambers.

**pneumatocele** (nū-măt′ō-sēl) [″ + *kele,* tumor, swelling] **1.** A hernia protuberance of the lung tissue. **2.** A swelling containing gas or air, esp. a swelling of the scrotum. SYN: *pneumonocele.*

***extracranial p.*** A collection of gas under the scalp, caused by a fracture of the skull that communicates with a paranasal sinus.

***intracranial p.*** A collection of gas within the skull.

**pneumatodyspnea** (nū″măt-ō-dĭsp′nē-ă) [″ + *dys,* bad, + *pneia,* breath] Dyspnea caused by pulmonary emphysema.

**pneumatology** (nū″mă-tŏl′ō-jē) [″ + *logos,* word, reason] The science of gases and air and their chemical properties and use in treatment.

**pneumatosis** (nū″mă-tō′sĭs) [Gr. *pneumatosis*] The presence of air or gas in an abnormal location in the body.

***p. cystoides intestinalis*** The presence of thin-walled gas-filled cysts in the intestines. The cause is unknown. The cysts usually disappear but occasionally rupture and cause pneumoperitoneum.

**pneumatotherapy** (nū″măt-ō-thĕr′ă-pē) [Gr. *pneumatos,* air, + *therapeia,* treatment] Pneumotherapy.

**pneumaturia** (nū″măt-ū′rē-ă) [Gr. *pneuma,* air, + *ouron,* urine] Excretion of urine containing free gas. SYN: *pneumatinuria.*

**pneumatype** (nū′mă-tīp) [″ + *typos,* type] The deposit of moisture on glass from the breath exhaled through the nostrils with the mouth closed for purpose of comparing the airflow through the nostrils.

**pneumectomy** (nū-mĕk′tō-mē) [Gr. *pneumon,* lung, + *ektome,* excision] Excision of all or part of a lung.

**pneumo-, pneumono-** [Gr. *pneumon,* lung] Combining form meaning *air, lung.*

**pneumoangiography** (nū″mō-ăn″jē-ŏg′ră-fē) [Gr. *pneumon,* lung, + *angeion,* vessel, + *graphein,* to write] A radiographical study of the vessels of the lungs; usually performed using a contrast medium.

**pneumoarthrography** (nū″mō-ăr-thrŏg′ră-fē) [″ + *arthron,* joint, + *graphein,* to write] Pneumarthrography.

**pneumobulbar** (nū″mō-bŭl′băr) [″ + L. *bulbus,* bulbous root] Concerning the lungs and respiratory center in the medulla oblongata of the brain.

**pneumocentesis** (nū″mō-sĕn-tē′sĭs) [″ + *kentesis,* a piercing] Paracentesis or surgical puncture of a lung to evacuate a cavity. SYN: *pneumonocentesis.*

**pneumocephalus** (nū″mō-sĕf′ă-lŭs) [Gr. *pneuma,* air, + *kephale,* head] Gas or air in the cavity of the cranium. SYN: *pneumocranium.*

**pneumocholecystitis** (nū″mō-kō″lē-sĭs-tī′tĭs) [″ + *chole,* bile, + *kystis,* bladder, + *itis,* inflammation] Cholecystitis with gas in the gallbladder.

**pneumococcal** (nū″mō-kŏk′ăl) [″ + *kokkos,* berry] Concerning or caused by pneumococci.

**pneumococcemia** (nū″mō-kŏk-sē′mē-ă) The presence of pneumococci in the blood.

**pneumococci** (nū″mō-kŏk′sī) Pl. of pneumococcus.

**pneumococcidal** (nū″mō-kŏk-sī′dăl) [″ + ″ + L. *cidus,* killing] Killing pneumococci.

**pneumococcolysis** (nū″mō-kŏk-ŏl′ĭ-sĭs) [″ + *kokkos,* berry, + *lysis,* dissolution] Destruction or lysis of pneumococci.

**pneumococcus** (nū″mō-kŏk′ŭs) *pl.* **pneumococci** [″ + *kokkos,* berry] An oval-shaped, encapsulated, non–spore-forming, gram-positive organism occurring usually in pairs (diplococcus) and having lancet-shaped ends. There are more than 80 serological types of pneumococci. Beside causing pneumonia, pneumococci cause otitis media, mastoiditis, meningitis, bronchitis, bloodstream infections, keratitis, and conjunctivitis. A pneumococcal vaccine is available. Pneumococcal infections are usually treated effectively with penicillin, although resistant strains have emerged. Erythromycin may be used if the patient is allergic to penicillin. SYN: *Streptococcus pneumoniae.* SEE: *pneumonia; vaccine, pneumococcal polyvalent.*

**pneumocolon** (nū″mō-kō′lŏn) [″ + *kolon,* colon] Air in the colon. This may be introduced as an aid in radiological diagnosis.

**pneumoconiosis** (nū″mō-kō″nē-ō′sĭs) [″ + *konis,* dust, + *osis,* condition] A condition of the respiratory tract owing to inhalation of dust particles; an occupational disorder such as that caused by mining or stonecutting. SYN: *pneumonoconiosis.* SEE: *bituminosis.*

**pneumocranium** (nū″mō-krā′nē-ŭm) [″ + *kranion,* skull] Pneumocephalus.

**Pneumocystis carinii** (nū″mō-sĭs′tĭs kă-rī′nē-ī) The causative organism of *Pneumocystis carinii* pneumonia. SEE: illus.; *AIDS.*

**pneumocystography** (nū″mō-sĭs-tŏg′ră-fē) [Gr. *pneuma,* air, + *kystis,* bladder, + *graphein,* to write] A cystogram done after air has been introduced into the urinary bladder.

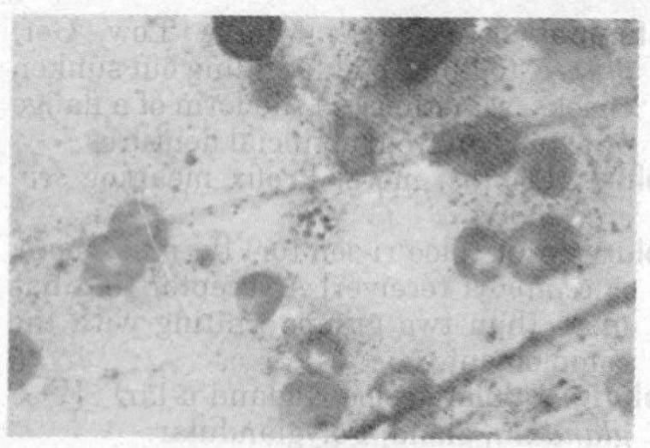

PNEUMOCYSTIS CARINII
(ORIG. MAG. ×1000)

**pneumocystosis** (nū″mō-sĭs-tō′sĭs) *Pneumocystis carinii* pneumonia.

**pneumocyte** Either of the two types of cells that form the alveoli of the lung. Type I cells are simple squamous epithelium that permit exchange. Type II cells are rounded and produce surfactant.

**pneumoderma** (nū″mō-dĕr′mă) [″ + *derma,* skin] Emphysema under the skin.

**pneumodynamics** (nū″mō-dī-năm′ĭks) [″ + *dynamis,* force] The branch of science dealing with force employed in respiration.

**pneumoempyema** (nū″mō-ĕm-pī-ē′mă) [″ + *en,* in + *pyon,* pus] Empyema accompanied by an accumulation of gas.

**pneumoencephalitis** (nū″mō-ĕn-sĕf″ă-lī′tĭs) [″ + *enkephalos,* brain, + *itis,* inflammation] Newcastle disease.

**pneumoencephalogram** (nū″mō-ĕn-sĕf′ă-lō-grăm) [″ + ″ + *gramma,* something written] A radiograph of the subarachnoid space and ventricular system of the brain during pneumoencephalography.

**pneumoencephalography** (nū″mō-ĕn-sĕf″ă-lŏg′ră-fē) [″ + ″ + *graphein,* to write] Radiography of the ventricles and subarachnoid spaces of the brain following withdrawal of cerebrospinal fluid and injection of air or gas via lumbar puncture. This technique has been replaced by computed tomography and magnetic resonance imaging.

**pneumofasciogram** (nū″mō-făs′ē-ō-grăm) [″ + L. *fascia,* a band, + Gr. *gramma,* something written] A radiograph of fascial tissues and spaces after air has been injected in the fascia.

**pneumogalactocele** (nū″mō-găl-ăk′tō-sēl) [″ + *gala,* milk, + *kele,* tumor, swelling] A breast tumor containing milk and gas.

**pneumogastric** (nū″mō-găs′trĭk) [Gr. *pneumon,* lung, + *gaster,* stomach] Pert. to the lungs and stomach.

**pneumogastric nerve** Term formerly used for the vagus nerve.

**pneumogastrography** (nū″mō-găs-trŏg′ră-fē) [Gr. *pneuma,* air, + *gaster,* stomach, + *graphein,* to write] A radiographical study of the stomach after air has been introduced into it.

**pneumogram** (nū′mō-grăm) [″ + *gramma,* something written] **1.** A record of respiratory movements. **2.** A radiograph following injection of air.

**pneumograph** (nū′mō-grăf) [″ + *graphein,* to write] A device for recording the frequency and intensity of respiration.

**pneumography** (nū-mŏg′ră-fē) **1.** An anatomical description or illustration of the lung. **2.** The recording of respiratory movements on a graph. **3.** Radiography of a part or organ after injection of air.

***pelvic p.*** Radiography of the pelvis after injection of carbon dioxide into the peritoneal cavity.

**pneumohemopericardium** (nū″mō-hēm″ō-pĕr-ĭ-kăr′dē-ŭm) [Gr. *pneumon,* lung, + *haima,* blood, + *peri,* around, + *kardia,* heart] The accumulation of air and blood in the pericardium.

**pneumohemorrhagica** (nū″mō-hēm-ō-rā′jĭ-kă) [″ + ″ + *rhegnynai,* to burst forth] Hemorrhage into pulmonary air cells; apoplexy of the lungs.

**pneumohemothorax** (nū″mō-hēm″ō-thō′răks) [″ + ″ + *thorax,* chest] Gas or air and blood collected in the pleural cavity.

**pneumohydrometra** (nū″mō-hī″drō-mē′tră) [″ + *hydor,* water, + *metra,* uterus] The accumulation of gas and fluid in the uterus.

**pneumohydropericardium** (nū″mō-hī″drō-pĕr-ĭ-kăr′dē-ŭm) [″ + *hydor,* water, + *peri,* around, + *kardia,* heart] Air and fluid accumulated in the pericardium.

**pneumohydrothorax** (nū″mō-hī″drō-thō′răks) [″ + ″ + *thorax,* chest] Gas or air and fluid in the pleural cavity.

**pneumohypoderma** (nū″mō-hī″pō-dĕr′mă) [″ + *hypo,* under, + *derma,* skin] Air in the tissues under the skin.

**pneumokidney** (nū″mō-kĭd′nē) [″ + ME. *kidenei,* kidney] Air in the pelvis of the kidney.

**pneumolith** (nū′mō-lĭth) [″ + *lithos,* stone] A pulmonary calculus.

**pneumolithiasis** (nū″mō-lĭth-ī′ăs-ĭs) [″ + ″ + *-iasis,* condition] Formation of concretions in the lungs.

**pneumolysin** (nū-mŏl′ĭ-sĭn) A hemolytic toxin produced by pneumococci.

**pneumomalacia** (nū″mō-mă-lā′shē-ă) [″ + *malakia,* a softening] Abnormal softening of the lung.

**pneumomassage** (nū″mō-mă-săzh′) [Gr. *pneuma,* air, + *massein,* to knead] Massage of the tympanum with air to cause movement of the ossicles of the inner ear.

**pneumomediastinum** (nū″mō-mē″dē-ăs-tī′nŭm) [″ + L. *mediastinum,* in the middle] The presence of air or gas in the mediastinal tissues, either owing to disease or following injection of air into the area for diagnostic purposes.

**pneumomelanosis** (nū″mō-mĕl-ăn-ō′sĭs) [Gr. *pneumon,* lung, + *melano,* black, + *osis,* condition] Pigmentation of the lung seen in pneumoconiosis. SYN: *pneumonomelanosis.*

**pneumometer** (nū-mŏm′ĕt-ĕr) [Gr. *pneuma,* air, + *metron,* measure] Spirometer.

**pneumomycosis** (nū″mō-mī-kō′sĭs) [Gr. *pneumon,* lung, + *mykes,* fungus, + *osis,* condition] A fungal pulmonary disease. SYN: *pneumonomycosis.*

**pneumomyelography** (nū″mō-mī-ĕl-ŏg′ră-fē) [Gr. *pneuma,* air + *myelos,* marrow, + *graphein,* to write] A radiographical study of the spinal canal following injection of air or other gas.

**pneumonectasia, pneumonectasis** (nū″mŏn-ĕk-tā′zē-ă, -ĕk′tă-sĭs) [″ + *ektasis,* dilatation] Distention of the lungs with air.

**pneumonectomy** (nū″mŏn-ĕk′tō-mē) [Gr. *pneumon,* lung, + *ektome,* excision] Pneumectomy.

**pneumonia** (nū-mō′nē-ă) [Gr.] An inflammation of the alveoli, interstitial tissue, and bronchioles of the lungs due to infection by bacteria, viruses, or other pathogenic organisms, or to irritation by chemicals or other agents (e.g., oil, radiation, drugs). Current estimates for the U.S. are that pneumonia occurs in 4 million persons each year. It is the sixth leading cause of death in the U.S. and is the most common cause of death due to infectious disease. It has many causes and is associated with a wide range of acute and chronic disorders. Clinically, the term *pneumonia* usually indicates an infectious cause; pulmonary inflammation due to other causes is generally called *pneumonitis.* SEE: *Nursing Diagnoses Appendix.*

PATHOLOGY: Pneumonia occurs when an organism overcomes the body's defenses in the respiratory tract: mucous and cilia in the upper airways that trap pathogens, alveolar macrophages, and neutrophils drawn to the tissues as needed. Smoking, general anesthesia, chronic bronchitis, immobility, and endotracheal intubation can inhibit the mucociliary system, enabling pathogens to reach the alveoli and overwhelm the phagocytic cells. Also, some organisms release enzymes or toxins that disable the mucociliary or macrophage defenses. Aspiration of gastric contents, inhalation of smoke or toxic gases, physical trauma, and some chronic diseases destroy cells in the bronchial epithelium or alveoli, creating significant inflammation that makes it easier for pathogens to gain entry. Septicemia may bring pathogens from other sites to the pulmonary capillaries, where they cross into interstitial tissue. Following all of these events, inflammation and the specific immune response cause alveolar edema and white blood cell aggregation, producing congestion that inhibits gas exchange and causes hypoxemia. SEE: *immune response; inflammation.*

Pneumonia is categorized by site and cause. Lobar pneumonia affects most of an entire lobe; bronchopneumonia involves smaller areas in several lobes, particularly in the periphery of the lung. Interstitial pneumonia involves tissues surrounding the alveoli and bronchi.

ETIOLOGY: Many pathogenic microorganisms cause pneumonia. Common bacteria include *Streptococcus pneumoniae* (pneumococcus), *Haemophilus influenzae*, and *Staphylococcus aureus*; *Klebsiella pneumoniae* and *Legionella pneumophila* often cause pneumonia in patients with chronic disease. Adenovirus and influenza viruses can cause a mild atypical pneumonia often referred to as "walking pneumonia"; respiratory syncytial virus can cause severe pneumonia, particularly in children. In addition, viral upper respiratory infections damage the bronchial epithelium, enhancing bacterial infection. *Mycoplasma pneumoniae*, a tiny organism similar to bacteria, causes another type of atypical pneumonia that is becoming increasingly common. Immunosuppressed patients are susceptible to pneumonia from fungi (e.g., *Candida albicans* and *Aspergillus fumigatus*) and other organisms that are not usually pathogenic in the lung. SEE: *bacteria; fungi; infection, opportunistic; virus.*

SYMPTOMS: Bacterial pneumonias tend to have an abrupt onset, whereas others develop more slowly. High fevers with shaking chills, pain on inspiration, crackles, rhonchi and decreased breath sounds on auscultation, elevated white blood cell count, and cough producing purulent sputum characterize bacterial pneumonias. Patients with atypical pneumonia generally have lower temperatures, a nonproductive cough, and systemic symptoms (myalgia, headache, sore throat). Chest x-rays show white infiltrates in the affected areas. NOTE: The possibility of tuberculosis should be considered in all patients with radiographic changes.

TREATMENT: Erythromycin, ceftriaxone, or other broad-spectrum antibiotics are given until the causative organism can be identified on culture. Pneumococcal vaccine (Pneumovax) is recommended for all persons over 65 years of age; those with chronic respiratory, cardiac, or neuromuscular disease; those with diabetes; and those who have had a splenectomy, including children, because the spleen is a major component of the immune system. Pneumonia remains a significant cause of death in the elderly, chronically ill, and patients who are immunosuppressed as the result of disease or drug therapy. SEE: *vaccine, polyvalent pneumococcal.*

NURSING IMPLICATIONS: Patients at risk for pneumonia are identified. Immunization is recommended for older persons and those persons with chronic illnesses, because research shows that this is one of the most effective interventions for these groups. Supportive care is provided for the patient with pneumonia to reduce oxygen demand, to remove secretions, and to improve gas exchange; such care includes position changes; deep-breathing and coughing exercises and respiratory toilet; active and passive limb exercises; and assistance with self-care. Respiratory status is monitored by chest assessment and arterial blood gas studies for indications of respiratory failure (e.g., hypoxemia, hypercapnia, deteriorating level of consciousness), and the patient is assessed for sepsis and shock. Prescribed analgesics are administered. The prescribed medical regimen is carried out, and the patient's response is evaluated. The nurse encourages the patient to verbalize concerns, explains diagnostic studies and therapeutic measures, and teaches the patient about the importance of follow-up care.

***abortive p.*** Mild pneumonia with a brief course.

***acute lobar p.*** Lobar p.

***p. alba*** A pneumonia seen in stillborn infants; it is caused by congenital syphilis.

***aspiration p.*** Pneumonia caused by inhalation of gastric contents, food, or other substances. A frequent cause is loss of the gag reflex in patients with central nervous system depression or damage or alcoholic intoxication with stupor and vomiting. This condition also occurs in newborns who inhale infected amniotic fluid, meconium, or vaginal secretions during delivery.

***atypical p.*** Pneumonia caused by a virus or *Mycoplasma pneumoniae.* The symptoms are low fever, nonproductive cough, pharyngitis, myalgia, and minimal adventitious lung sounds. SYN: *mycoplasma pneumonitis.*

***desquamative interstitial p.*** Pneumonia of unknown etiology accompanied by cellular infiltration or fibrosis in the pulmonary interstitium. Progressive dyspnea and a nonproductive cough are symptoms characterizing this disease. Clubbing of the fingers is a common finding. Diffusion of oxygen and carbon dioxide is abnormal. Diagnosis is made by lung biopsy. The condition is treated by corticosteroids.

***double p.*** Pneumonia that involves both lungs.

***embolic p.*** Pneumonia following embolization of a pulmonary blood vessel.

***eosinophilic p.*** Inflammation of the lung associated with an elevation in eosinophils. The cause in unclear, but is believed to be a hypersensitivity or allergic reaction to drugs, parasites, or fungi. It is usually accompanied by asthma.

***fibrous p.*** Pneumonia followed by formation of scar tissue.

***Friedländer's p.*** A form of lobar pneumonia caused by the specific organism *Klebsiella pneumoniae*.

***gangrenous p.*** Pulmonary gangrene.

***giant cell p.*** An interstitial pneumonitis of infancy and childhood. The lung tissue contains multinucleated giant cells. The disease often occurs in connection with measles.

***hypostatic p.*** Pneumonia occurring in elderly or bed-ridden patients who remain constantly in the same position. Ventilation is greatest in dependent areas; remaining in one position causes hypoventilation in many areas, causing alveolar collapse (atelectasis) and creating a pulmonary environment that supports the growth of bacteria or other organisms. Development of this condition is prevented by having the patient change positions and take deep breaths to inflate peripheral alveoli. SEE: *pneumonia*.

NURSING IMPLICATIONS: Prevention is the most important factor, esp. in elderly and immobile persons. Patients should be moved and turned frequently at least every 1 to 2 hr. The nurse should encourage the patient to engage in active movement and to perform deep-breathing coughing exercises frequently and regularly.

***intrauterine p.*** Pneumonia contracted in utero.

***Legionella p.*** SEE: *Legionnaires' disease*.

***lipoid p.*** Chronic damage to pulmonary tissue due to long-term use of oily substances which trickle down the bronchus from the oropharynx to the lungs. The oil is not metabolized or phagocytized. It remains in the lung and interferes with gas exchange.

***lobar p.*** Pneumonia infecting one or more lobes of the lung, usually caused by *Streptococcus pneumoniae*. The pathologic changes are, in order, congestion; redness and firmness due to exudate and red blood cells in the alveoli; and, finally, gray hepatization as the exudate degenerates and is absorbed. SYN: *acute lobar p.*

***Pneumocystis carinii p.*** ABBR: PCP. An acute interstitial plasma cell pneumonia marked by slight if any fever, nonproductive cough, tachypnea, and dyspnea. It is caused by *Pneumocystis carinii*, an organism formerly thought to be a protozoan but now tentatively categorized as a fungus. This disease is seen in marasmic and otherwise debilitated children and in immunodeficient adults; it is one of the defining opportunistic infections of acquired immunodeficiency syndrome (AIDS). SEE: *AIDS; infection, opportunistic*.

DIAGNOSIS: Symptoms are fever, fatigue, nonproductive cough, dyspnea and hypoxemia with exercise, and interstitial infiltrates on radiograph. The organism can be visualized in sputum, bronchial lavage fluid, or tissue obtained via biopsy. SEE: illus.

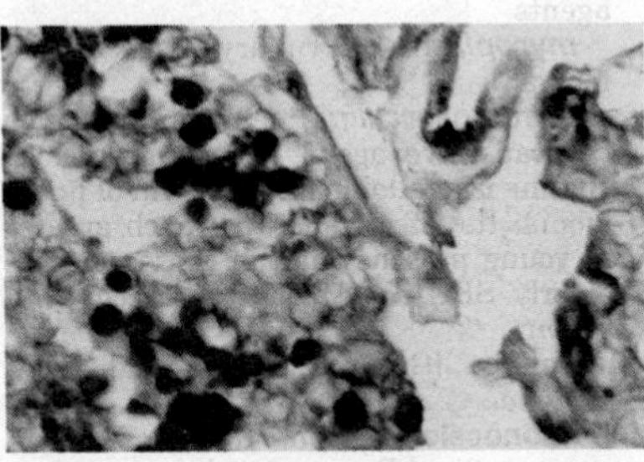


PNEUMOCYSTIS CARINII PNEUMONIA
DARKLY STAINED CYSTS IN LUNG TISSUE
(ORIG. MAG. ×400)

TREATMENT: Trimethoprim-sulfamethoxazole (Bactrim) taken orally three times a week is an effective prophylactic agent against PCP and is used to prevent recurrence after an acute episode. The same drug is given intravenously with prednisone for severe infection. Pentamidine, clindamycin, or primaquine is used if for any reason other drugs are unsuitable. Even with treatment, PCP is a major cause of death in persons with AIDS.

***secondary p.*** Pneumonia that occurs in connection with a specific systemic disease such as typhoid, diphtheria, or plague.

***tuberculous p.*** Pneumonia caused by the tubercle bacilli, which may result in rapid and widespread inflammatory exudation. If untreated, it may run a malignant course, ending fatally, or may subside and become chronic.

***tularemic p.*** Pneumonia caused by *Francisella tularensis*. It may be primary or associated with tularemia.

***woolsorter's p.*** Pulmonary anthrax.

**pneumonic** (nū-mŏn′ĭk) [Gr. *pneumon*, lung] Concerning the lungs or pneumonia.

**pneumonitis** (nū″mō-nī′tĭs) [″ + *itis*, inflammation] Inflammation of the lung, usually due to hypersensitivity (allergic) reactions to organic dusts, such as wheat or other grains, or chemicals.

***hypersensitivity p.*** Immunologically induced inflammation of the lungs of a susceptible host caused by repeated inhalation of a variety of substances including organic dusts. Included are molds and other fungi from sources such as cheese, vegetables, mushrooms, flour, mushroom compost, bark of trees, detergents, and contaminated humidification systems. In the acute stage, patients may present with cough, fever, chills, malaise, and shortness of breath. In the subacute and chronic forms, the onset of symptoms is gradual and prolonged. Treatment includes identifying and avoiding causative agents.

***mycoplasma p.*** Primary atypical pneumonia.

***pneumococcal p.*** Pneumonia in which the causative agent is pneumococci. A vaccine is available for this form of pneumonia. Its effectiveness is much greater in young persons than in those who are elderly. SEE: *vaccine, pneumococcal polyvalent.*

**pneumono-** [Gr. *pneumon,* lung] SEE: *pneumo-.*

**pneumonocele** (nū-mōn′ō-sēl) [″ + *kele,* tumor, swelling] Pneumatocele.

**pneumonocentesis** (nū-mō″nō-sĕn-tē′sĭs) [″ + *kentesis,* a piercing] Pneumocentesis.

**pneumonoconiosis** (nū-mō″nō-kō″nē-ō′sĭs) [″ + *konis,* dust, + *osis,* condition] Pneumoconiosis.

**pneumonocyte** A term for the three types of cells of the alveoli of the lungs: type I and II alveolar cells and alveolar macrophages.

**pneumonolysis** (nū″mŏ-nŏl′ĭ-sĭs) [″ + *lysis,* dissolution] The loosening and separation of an adherent lung from the costal pleura to induce a collapse of the lung. SYN: *pneumolysis.*

***extrapleural p.*** Separation of the parietal pleura from the chest wall. SEE: *apicolysis.*

***intrapleural p.*** Separation of adhering visceral and parietal layers of pleura.

**pneumonomelanosis** (nū″mō-nō-mĕl″ăn-ō′sĭs) [″ + *melano,* black, + *osis,* condition] Pneumomelanosis.

**pneumonomycosis** (nū-mōn″ō-mī-kō′sĭs) [″ + *mykes,* fungus, + *osis,* condition] Pneumomycosis.

**pneumonopathy** (nū″mō-nŏp′ăth-ē) [″ + *pathos,* disease, suffering] Any diseased condition of the lung.

**pneumonoperitonitis** (nū″mō-nō-pĕr″ĭ-tō-nī′tĭs) [″ + *peritonaion,* peritoneum, + *itis,* inflammation] Peritonitis with gas in the peritoneal cavity.

**pneumonopexy** (nū-mō″nō-pĕk′sē) [″ + *pexis,* fixation] Surgical attachment of the lung to the chest wall. SYN: *pneumopexy.*

**pneumonopleuritis** (nū-mō″nō-ploo-rī′tĭs) [Gr. *pneumon,* lung, + *pleura,* side, + *itis,* inflammation] Pneumopleuritis.

**pneumonorrhapy** (nū″mō-nor′ă-fē) [″ + *rhaphe,* seam, ridge] Suture of a lung.

**pneumonotherapy** Pneumotherapy.

**pneumonotomy** (nū-mō-nŏt′ō-mē) [″ + *tome,* incision] Incision into the lung. SYN: *pneumotomy.*

**pneumopericardium** (nū″mō-pĕr-ĭ-kăr′dē-ŭm) [Gr. *pneuma,* air, + *peri,* around, + *kardia,* heart] Air or gas in the pericardial sac; caused by trauma or pathological communication between the esophagus, stomach, or lungs and the pericardium. It is characterized by unusual metallic heart sounds and tympany over the precordial area.

**pneumoperitoneography** Radiographical examination of the peritoneum and internal organs after introduction of sterile air into the peritoneal cavity.

**pneumoperitoneum** (nū″mō-pĕr-ĭ-tō-nē′ŭm) [″ + *peritonaion,* peritoneum] A condition in which air or gas is collected in the peritoneal cavity; may be artificially induced to treat tuberculous peritonitis.

**pneumoperitonitis** (nū″mō-pĕr-ĭ-tō-nī′tĭs) [″ + *peritonaion,* peritoneum, + *itis,* inflammation] Peritonitis with gas accumulation.

**pneumopexy** (nū′mō-pĕks″ē) [Gr. *pneumon,* lung, + *pexis,* fixation] Pneumonopexy.

**pneumopleuritis** (nū″mō-ploo-rī′tĭs) [″ + *pleura,* a side, + *itis,* inflammation] Inflammation of the lungs and pleura.

**pneumopleuroparietopexy** (nū″mō-ploo″rō-pă-rī″ĕt-ō-pĕk″sē) [″ + ″ + L. *paries,* wall, + Gr. *pexis,* fixation] The operation of attaching the lung with its parietal pleura to the border of the thoracic wound.

**pneumopyelography** (nū″mō-pī-ĕ-lŏg′ră-fē) [Gr. *pneuma,* air, + *pyelos,* pelvis, + *graphein,* to write] A radiographical examination of the renal pelvis and ureters after they are injected with oxygen.

**pneumopyopericardium** (nū″mō-pī″ō-pĕr-ĭ-kar′dē-ŭm) [″ + *pyon,* pus, + *peri,* around, + *kardia,* heart] Air, gas, and pus collected in the pericardial sac.

**pneumopyothorax** (nū″mō-pī″ō-thō′răks) [″ + ″ + *thorax,* chest] Air and pus collected in the pleural cavity.

**pneumoradiography** (nū″mō-rā-dē-ŏg′ră-fē) [″ + L. *radius,* ray, + Gr. *graphein,* to write] Injection of air into a part for the purpose of x-ray examination.

**pneumoretroperitoneum** (nū″mō-rĕt″rō-pĕr″ĭ-tō-nē′ŭm) [″+ L. *retro,* backwards, + Gr. *peritonaion,* peritoneum] Air or gas in the retroperitoneal space.

**pneumorrhachis** (nū″mō-rā′kĭs) [Gr. *pneumon,* lung, + *rhachis,* spine] Gas accumulation in the spinal canal.

**pneumorrhagia** (nū″mō-rā′jē-ă) [Gr. *pneumon,* lung, + *rhegnynai,* to burst forth] Lung hemorrhage. SEE: *hemoptysis.*

**pneumoserothorax** (nū″mō-sē-rō-thō′răks) [Gr. *pneuma,* air, + L. *serum,* whey, + Gr. *thorax,* chest] Air or gas and serum collected in the pleural cavity.

**pneumosilicosis** (nū″mō-sĭl″ĭ-kō′sĭs) [Gr. *pneumon,* lung, + L. *silex,* flint, + Gr. *osis,* condition] Silicosis.

**pneumotaxic** (nū″mō-tăk′sĭk) [″ + *taxis,* arrangement] Concerning the regulation of breathing.

**pneumotherapy** (nū-mō-thĕr′ă-pē) **1.** [Gr. *pneumon,* lung, + *therapeia,* treatment] The treatment of diseases of the lungs. **2.** [Gr. *pneuma,* air, + *therapeia,* treatment] The treatment of diseases by the use of rarefied or condensed gases. SYN: *pneumatotherapy; pneumonotherapy.*

**pneumothorax** (nū-mō-thō′răks) [″ + *tho-*

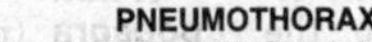

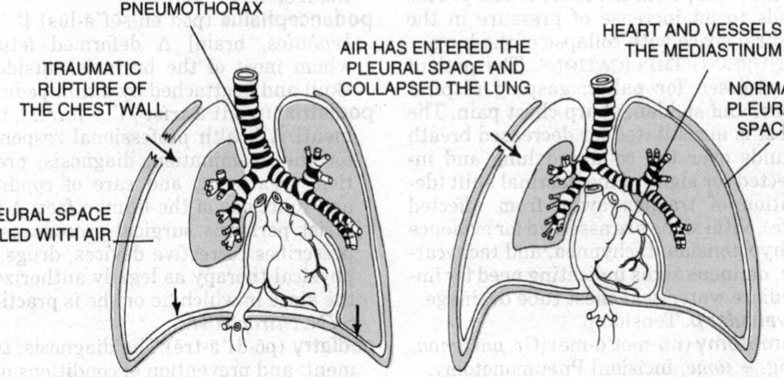


*rax*, chest] A collection of air or gas in the pleural cavity. The gas enters as the result of a perforation through the chest wall or the pleura covering the lung (visceral pleura). This perforation may be the result of an injury or of the rupture of an emphysematous bleb or superficial lung abscess. The most common cause of the latter is a tuberculous abscess in the presence of pulmonary tuberculosis. SYN: *aeropleura; aerothorax; pneumatothorax*. SEE: illus.; *Nursing Diagnoses Appendix*.

SYMPTOMS: The onset is sudden, usually with a severe sharp pain in the side and marked dyspnea. Fluid very frequently is found, developing within 48 hr (hydropneumothorax). The physical signs are those of a distended unilateral chest, tympanitic resonance, absence of breath sounds, and, if fluid is present, a splashing sound on succussion (or shaking) of the patient.

NURSING IMPLICATIONS: The nurse explains the procedure for chest tube insertion and assists as necessary. Vital signs, breath sounds, chest expansion, chest tube site, drainage, and blood gas analysis are assessed. Oxygen is administered as prescribed. Coughing and deep-breathing exercises and chest physical therapy are carried out. The patient is placed in the semi-Fowler position to promote drainage, comfort, and ease of breathing. Adequate rest periods are provided. Range-of-motion exercises and activity are encouraged as tolerated. Medications are administered as prescribed (analgesics, antibiotics, expectorants). Intake and output are monitored. The patient should maintain adequate nutrition and fluid intake to promote tissue healing and repair and to maintain proper hydration. The catheter site is observed daily and redressed as necessary. The patient should avoid excessive exercise and smoking. The nurse stresses the importance of follow-up examination and teaches care of the insertion site.

***artificial p.*** A pneumothorax induced intentionally by artificial means, used to treat pulmonary tuberculosis or pneumonia. Pneumothorax allows the diseased lung to rest temporarily. The lung collapses when the air enters the pleural space.

Scattered adhesions may afford only a partial collapse. Effusion may occur in about one third of the cases. Hazards are minimal.

***extrapleural p.*** The formation of a pneumothorax by introducing air into the space between the pleura and the inside of the rib cage.

***open p.*** A pneumothorax in which the pleural cavity is exposed to the atmosphere through an open wound in the chest wall.

***spontaneous p.*** The spontaneous entrance of air into the pleural cavity. The pressure may collapse the lung and displace the mediastinum away from the side of the lesion.

SYMPTOMS: Sudden sharp pain, dyspnea, and cough characterize this condition although it may be asymptomatic (silent). Pain may be referred to the shoulder. The majority of cases are mild and require only rest. Rarely shock and collapse occur.

***tension p.*** A type of pneumothorax in which air can enter the pleural space but cannot escape via the route of entry. This leads to an increase of pressure in the pleural space with collapse of the lung.

NURSING IMPLICATIONS: The patient is assessed for pallor; gasping respirations; and sudden, sharp chest pain. The chest is auscultated for decreased breath sounds over the collapsed lung and inspected for signs of mediastinal shift (deviation of trachea away from affected side). Vital signs are assessed for evidence of hypotension, tachypnea, and tachycardia, ominous signs indicating need for immediate water-seal chest tube drainage.

***valvular p.*** Tension p.

**pneumotomy** (nū-mŏt′ō-mē) [Gr. *pneumon,* lung, + *tome,* incision] Pneumonotomy.

**pneumotoxin** (nū″mō-tŏks′ĭn) [″ + *toxikon,* poison] A toxin produced by pneumococcus.

**pneumotyphus** (nū″mō-tī′fŭs) [″ + *typhos,* fever] **1.** Typhoid fever with pneumonia at onset. **2.** The development of pneumonia during typhoid fever.

**pneumoventricle** (nū″mō-vĕn′trĭ-k′l) [″ + L. *ventriculus,* little belly] Air accumulation in the cerebral ventricles.

**pneumoventriculography** (nū″mō-vĕn-trĭk″ū-lŏg′ră-fē) [″ + ″ + Gr. *graphein,* to write] Radiography of the ventricles of the brain after the injection of air.

**pnigophobia** (nī″gō-fō′bē-ă) [Gr. *pnigos,* choking, + *phobos,* fear] Morbid fear of choking; sometimes experienced in angina pectoris.

**Po** Symbol for the element polonium.

**$Po_2$** Abbr. for *partial pressure of oxygen.*

**p.o.** L. *per os,* by mouth.

**pock** (pŏk) [AS. *poc,* pustule] A pustule of an eruptive fever, esp. of smallpox.

**pocket** (pŏk′ĕt) [ME. *poket,* pouch] A saclike cavity.

***gingival p.*** Periodontal p.

***periodontal p.*** A gingival sulcus enlarged beyond normal limits as a result of poor oral hygiene; the space bordered on one side by the tooth and the other side by ulcerated sulcular epithelium. It will be several millimeters deep when probed and limited at its apex by attachment epithelium.

**pocketing** A method of treating the pedicle in ovariotomy by enclosing it within the edges of the wound.

**pockmarked** Pitted or marked with cicatrices from healed pustules, esp. those due to smallpox.

**poculum diogenis** (pŏk′ū-lŭm dī-ŏj′ĕ-nĭs) [L. *poculum,* cup, + Diogenes, Gr. philosopher, 4th century B.C.] The concavity formed by contracting the muscles of the hand so the palm becomes cupped instead of flat.

**podagra** (pō-dăg′ră) [Gr. *podos,* foot, + *agra,* seizure] Gout, esp. of the joints of the foot or of the great toe.

**podalgia** (pō-dăl′jē-ă) [″ + *algos,* pain] Pain in the feet.

**podalic** (pō-dăl′ĭk) [Gr. *podos,* foot] Pert. to the feet.

**podencephalus** (pŏd″ĕn-sĕf′ă-lŭs) [″ + *enkephalos,* brain] A deformed fetus in whom most of the brain is outside the skull and is attached by a thin pedicle.

**podiatrist** (pō-dī′ă-trĭst″) [″ + *iatreia,* treatment] A health professional responsible for the examination, diagnosis, prevention, treatment, and care of conditions and functions of the human foot. A podiatrist performs surgical procedures and prescribes corrective devices, drugs, and physical therapy as legally authorized in the state in which he or she is practicing. SYN: *chiropodist.*

**podiatry** (pō-dī′ă-trē) The diagnosis, treatment, and prevention of conditions of human feet. SYN: *chiropody.*

**podium** (pō′dē-ŭm) [Gr. *podos,* foot] A footlike projection.

**podo-, pod-** [Gr. *pous, podos,* foot] Combining form meaning *foot.*

**podobromidrosis** (pŏd″ō-brō″mĭ-drō′sĭs) [″ + *bromos,* stench, + *hidros,* sweat] Offensive perspiration of the feet.

**podocyte** (pŏd′ō-sīt) [″ + *kytos,* cell] A special epithelial cell with numerous footplates (pedicels). These form the inner layer of Bowman's capsule of the renal corpuscle and have spaces for the passage of renal filtrate from the glomerulus.

**pododynamometer** (pŏd″ō-dī″nă-mŏm′ĕ-tĕr) [″ + *dynamis,* force, + *metron,* measure] A device for testing the strength of the leg and foot muscles.

**podophyllum** (pŏd-ō-fĭl′ŭm) [″ + *phyllon,* leaf] The dried rhizome and roots of *Podophyllum peltatum;* used for treating, by direct application, certain papillomas such as verruca acuminata. SEE: *verruca acuminata.*

**podophyllum resin** (pŏd″ō-fĭl′ŭm) The resinous extract from podophyllum.

**POEMS** An acronym for *p*olyneuropathy, *o*rganomegaly, *e*ndocrinopathy, *m*onoclonal gammopathy, and *s*kin changes.

**pogoniasis** (pō″gō-nī′ă-sĭs) [Gr. *pogon,* beard, + *-iasis,* disorder] **1.** Excessive growth of the beard. **2.** Growth of a beard in a woman.

**pogonion** (pō-gō′nē-ŏn) Mental point.

**-poiesis** [Gr.] Combining form used as a suffix meaning *formation, production.*

**poikilo-** Combining form meaning *irregular, varied.*

**poikilocyte** A teardrop or pear-shaped red blood cell, seen in myelofibrosis and certain anemias. SEE: illus.

**poikilocytosis** (poy″kĭl-ō-sī-tō′sĭs) [″ + ″ + *osis,* condition] A term used to describe variations in shape of red blood corpuscles (e.g., elliptocytes, spherocytes, dacryo-

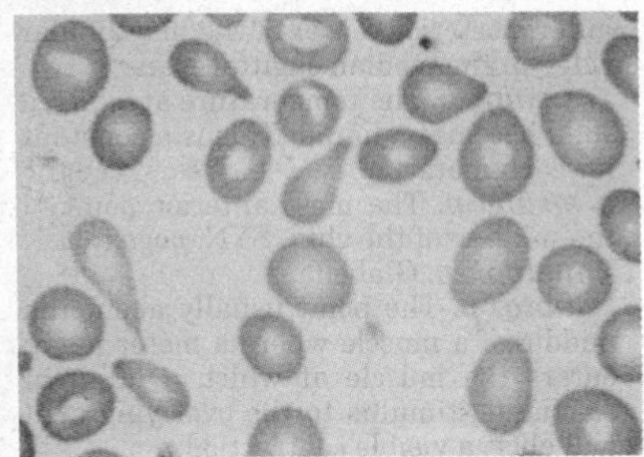

TEARDROP **POIKILOCYTES** IN PERIPHERAL BLOOD (ORIG. MAG. ×640)

cytes, sickle cells, schizocytes, echinocytes, and acanthocytes).

**poikilodentosis** (poy″kĭ-lō-dĕn-tō′sĭs) [″ + L. *dens,* tooth, + Gr. *osis,* condition] Mottling of the teeth usually caused by an excess of fluoride in the drinking water.

**poikiloderma** (poy-kĭl-ō-dĕr′mă) [″ + *derma,* skin] A skin disorder characterized by pigmentation, telangiectasia, purpura, pruritus, and atrophy.

***p. atrophicans vasculare*** A generalized dermatitis of unknown cause. It is symmetrical and occurs almost exclusively in adults. There is widespread telangiectasia, pigmentation, and atrophy of the skin.

***p. of Civatte*** Reticulated pigmentation and telangiectasia of the sides of the face and neck; seen quite commonly in middle-aged women.

**poikilonymy** (poy″kĭ-lŏn′ĭ-mē) [″ + *onoma,* name] The use of terms from several nomenclature systems.

**poikilotherm** (poy-kĭl′ō-thĕrm) [″ + *therme,* heat] An animal whose body temperature varies according to the temperature of the environment. SYN: *allotherm.* SEE: *homotherm.*

**poikilothermal, poikilothermic** (poy″kĭ-lō-thĕr′măl, -mĭk) Concerning poikilothermy.

**poikilothermy** (poy″kĭ-lō-thĕr′mē) The condition of having the temperature of the organism or animal match the temperature of the environment. Reptiles have this property. SEE: *homoiotherm.*

**poikilothrombocyte** (poy-kĭl″ō-thrŏm′bō-sīt) [″ + *thrombos,* clot, + *kytos,* cell] A blood platelet of abnormal shape.

**point** (poynt) [O.Fr., a prick, a dot] **1.** The sharp end of any object. **2.** The stage at which the surface of an abscess is about to rupture. **3.** A minute spot. **4.** A position in space, time, or degree.

***absorbent p.*** A cone of paper used in drying or in keeping liquid medicines in a root canal of a tooth.

***acupuncture p.*** Any specific anatomical location where needles are inserted and stimulated to achieve anesthesia or pain relief by the acupuncture method.

***auricular p.*** The center of the external orifice of the auditory canal. SYN: *Broca's p.*

***Boas' p.*** [Ismar Isador Boas, Ger. physician, 1858–1938] A tender spot left of the 12th thoracic vertebra in patients with gastric ulcer.

***boiling p.*** The temperature at which a liquid will boil.

***Broca's p.*** Auricular p.

***Capuron's p.*** One of four fixed points in the pelvic inlet, the two iliopectineal eminences and the two sacroiliac joints. SYN: *cardinal p.* (2).

***cardinal p.*** **1.** One of six points determining the direction of light rays emerging from and entering the eye. SEE: *nodal p.; principal p.* **2.** Capuron's p.

***cold rigor p.*** The temperature at which cell activity ceases.

***contact p.*** The point on a tooth that touches an opposed tooth.

***convergence p.*** **1.** The point to which rays of light converge. **2.** The closest point to the patient on which the eyes can converge as the object is moved closer and closer.

***corresponding p.*** The point in the retina of each eye that, when stimulated simultaneously, results in a single visual sensation.

***craniometric p.*** One of the fixed points of the skull used in craniometry.

***critical p. of gases*** The temperature at or above which a gas is no longer liquefied by pressure.

***critical p. of liquids*** The temperature above which no pressure may retain a substance in a liquid form.

***deaf p. of the ear*** One of several points or areas close to the external auditory meatus where a vibrating tuning fork is not heard.

***dew p.*** The temperature at which moisture begins to be condensed and deposited as dew.

***disparate p.'s*** Points on the retinas that are unequally paired.

***end p.*** The point or time at which a reaction or activity is completed.

***external orbital p.*** The prominent point at the outer edge of the orbit above the frontomalar suture.

***far p.*** Point (normally 20 ft [6.1 m] or more) at which distinct vision is possible without aid of the muscles of accommodation. It may be nearer than 20 ft (6.1 m) according to the degree of myopia. There is no far point in the hypermetropic eye.

***fixation p.*** The point at which the two visual axes converge.

***flash p.*** The lowest temperature at which a volatile liquid will ignite.

***focal p.*** The point at which a group of light rays converge.

***freezing p.*** The temperature at which liquids become solid.

***fusion p.*** Melting p.

***Guéneau de Mussy's p.*** The point located at the junction of a line extending down from the left border of the sternum with a horizontal line at the level of the bony part of the anterior portion of the tenth rib. Pressure on this point causes pain in cases of diaphragmatic pleurisy.

***gutta-percha p.*** A cone made of gutta-percha combined with other material that is used in filling root canals of teeth.

***Halle's p.*** [Adrien Joseph Marie Nöel Halle, Fr. physician, 1859–1947] The point at the intersection of a horizontal line drawn from the anterior superior iliac spines and an angled line extending up from the pubic spine. At that point, the ureter is palpable as it crosses the pelvic brim.

***hot p.*** A spot on the skin that perceives hot but not cold stimuli.

***hysterogenic p.*** One of the circumscribed areas of the body that produce symptoms of a hysterical aura, and eventually a hysterical attack, when rubbed or pressed.

***ice p.*** The temperature at which there is equilibrium between ice and air-saturated water at one atmosphere of pressure.

***identical retinal p.'s*** The points in the two retinas upon which the images are seen as one.

***isoelectric p.*** The particular pH of a solution of an amphoteric electrolyte such as an amino acid or protein in which the charged molecules do not migrate to either electrode. Proteins are least soluble at this point. Thus at the appropriate pH, proteins may be precipitated.

***isoionic p.*** The pH at which a solution of ionized material has as many negative as positive ions.

***jugal p.*** The posterior border of the frontal process of the malar bone where bisected by a line tangent to the upper border of the zygoma.

***lacrimal p.*** The outlet of the lacrimal canaliculus. SYN: *punctum lacrimale.*

***Lanz's p.*** [Otto Lanz, Swiss surgeon in the Netherlands, 1865–1935] The point on the line between the two anterior superior iliac spines, one third of the distance from the right spine, indicating the origin of the vermiform appendix.

***Lian's p.*** The point at the junction of the outer and middle thirds of a line from the umbilicus to the anterior superior spine of the ilium where a trocar may be introduced safely for paracentesis.

***malar p.*** The most prominent point on the external tubercle of the malar bone.

***p. of maximal impulse*** ABBR: P.M.I. The point on the chest wall over the heart at which the contraction of the heart is best seen or felt; normally at the fourth to fifth intercostal space in the midclavicular line.

***maximum occipital p.*** The point on the occipital bone farthest from the glabella.

***median mandibular p.*** The point on the anteroposterior center of the mandibular ridge in the median sagittal plane.

***melting p.*** The temperature at which a solid becomes a liquid. This is a constant for each material.

***mental p.*** The most anterior point of the midline of the chin. SYN: *pogonion.*

***metopic p.*** Glabella.

***motor p.*** The point usually about the middle of a muscle where a motor nerve enters the muscle at which a minimal electrical stimulus to the overlying skin will elicit a visible contraction.

***Munro's p.*** [John Cummings Munro, U.S. surgeon, 1858–1910] The point halfway between the left anterior iliac spine and the umbilicus.

***nasal p.*** Nasion.

***near p.*** The nearest point at which the eye can accommodate for distinct vision.

***nodal p.*** Either of a pair of points situated on the axis of an optical system so that any incident ray sent through one will produce a parallel emergent ray sent through the other.

***p. of no return*** An unofficial term describing a critical biochemical event that indicates lethal, irreversible changes in cells following ischemic cell injury.

***occipital p.*** The most posterior point on the occipital bone.

***painful p.'s*** Valleix's p.'s.

***preauricular p.*** The point immediately in front of the auricular point.

***pressure p.*** **1.** A point on the skin that, when stimulated, gives rise to a sensation of pressure. **2.** A point where an artery comes near the surface and at which pressure may be applied to stop arterial bleeding.

***principal p.*** One of two points so situated that the optical axis is cut by the two principal planes.

***p. of regard*** The point at which the eye is looking.

***silver p.*** An elongated, tapered silver plug used to fill the root canal in the endodontic treatment of teeth.

***spinal p.*** Subnasal p.

***subnasal p.*** The center of the root of the anterior nasal spine. SYN: *spinal p.*

***supra-auricular p.*** The point on the skull on the posterior root of the zygomatic process of the temporal bone, directly above the auricular point.

***supranasal p.*** Supraorbital p.

***supraorbital p.*** **1.** The point on the skull in the midline of the forehead, just above the glabella. SYN: *ophryon.* **2.** A neuralgic point just above the supraorbital notch.

***tender p.*** One of the clinical signs used to identify fibromyalgia. The deep diffuse muscular pain is localized to a number of possible tender areas when palpated. Tender points differ from trigger points in that pain does not radiate to referred areas. SEE: *fibromyalgia* for table.

***thermal death p.*** The temperature required to kill all of the organisms in a culture in a specified time.

***trigger p.*** A spot at which the application of pressure will cause pain. The pain is not necessarily in the area of the pressure.

***triple p.*** The temperature and pressure that allow the solid, liquid, and vapor forms of a substance to exist in equilibrium.

***Trousseau's apophysiary p.'s*** Sensitive points over the dorsal and lumbar vertebrae in neuralgia.

***Valleix's p.'s*** Tender spots upon pressure over the course of a nerve in neuralgia. SYN: *painful p.'s.*

***vital p.*** The point in the medulla oblongata close to the floor of the fourth ventricle, the puncture of which causes instant death owing to destruction of the respiratory center.

***Voillemier's p.*** The point on the linea alba of the abdominal wall about 6 to 7 cm below a line connecting the anterior superior iliac spines. Suprapubic puncture of the bladder may be made at this point in obese or edematous individuals.

**pointer, light** A head-mounted input device to enable computer use by persons with paralysis or limited movement. These devices typically operate through visible or invisible light sources at the tip of the pointer, which transmits a signal to a computer-mounted light sensor or receiver.

**pointillage** (pwăn″tĭ-yăzh′) [Fr.] Massage with the fingertips.

**pointing** Reaching a point.

**poise** (poyz) [J. M. Poiseuille] The unit of viscosity; the tangential shearing force required to be applied to an area of 1 $cm^2$ between two parallel planes of 1 $cm^2$ in area and 1 cm apart in order to produce a velocity of flow of the liquid of 1 cm/sec.

**Poiseuille's law** (pwă-zŭ′yĕz) [Jean Marie Poiseuille, Fr. physiologist, 1799–1869] A law that states that the rapidity of the capillary current is directly proportional to the fourth power of the radius of the capillary tube, the pressure on the fluid, and inversely proportional to the viscosity of the liquid and the length of the tube.

**Poiseuille's space** The inert capillary current in which leukocytes close to the wall of the vessel move slowly; the erythrocytes travel more rapidly in the middle current.

**POISINDEX™** A computerized database, revised quarterly, on over 300,000 commercial compounds. For information, contact Micromedex, Inc., 600 Grant St., Denver, CO 80203; (800) 525-9083.

**poison** (poy′zn) [L. *potio,* a poisonous draft] Any substance taken into the body by ingestion, inhalation, injection, or absorption that interferes with normal physiological functions. Virtually any substance can be poisonous if consumed in sufficient quantity; therefore the term poison more often implies an excessive degree of dosage rather than a specific group of substances. Aspirin is not usually thought of as a poison, but overdoses of this drug kill more children accidentally each year than any of the traditional poisons. Because the list of poisonous substances is infinite, it defies classification in any simple way. For a list of commonly encountered hazardous substances in the home, SEE: *Poisons and Poisoning Appendix.*

***cellular p.*** Anything that damages or kills cells.

***p. ivy*** A climbing vine, *Rhus toxicodendron,* which on contact may produce a severe form of dermatitis. *Rhus* species contain urushiol, an extremely irritating oily resin. Urushiol may also be a potent sensitizer since in many cases subsequent contacts produce increasingly severe reactions. SEE: illus. (Poison Ivy–Poison Oak Poison Sumac; Poison Ivy Dermatitis).

***p. oak*** A climbing vine, *Rhus radicans* or *R. diversiloba,* closely related to poison ivy and containing the same active toxic principle. The symptoms and treatment of poison oak dermatitis are identical to those for poison ivy dermatitis. SEE: illus.

***pesticidal p.*** Chemicals whose toxic properties are commercially exploited in agriculture, industry, or commerce to increase quantity, improve quality, or generally promote consumer acceptability of a variety of products. Common types include insecticides, rodenticides, herbicides, defoliants, fungicides, insect repellants, molluscicides, and some kinds of food additives. The wide variety of poi-

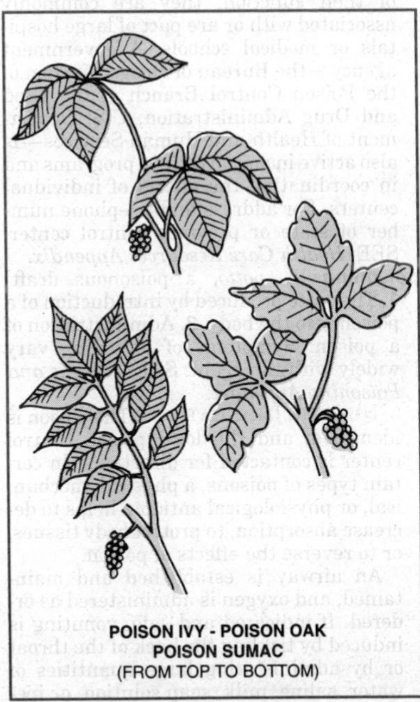

POISON IVY - POISON OAK
POISON SUMAC
(FROM TOP TO BOTTOM)

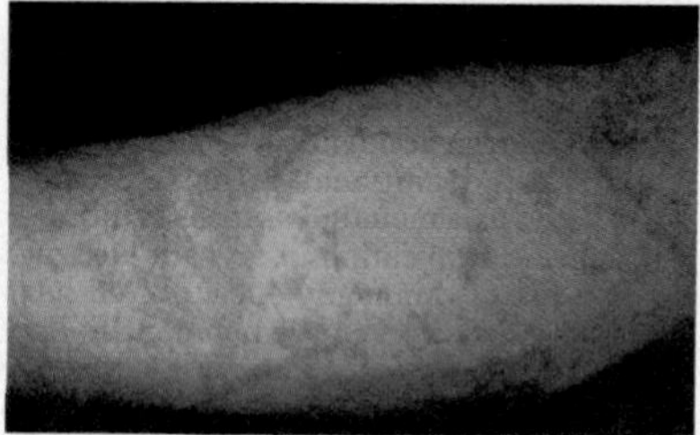

POISON IVY DERMATITIS

sons commonly found in and around the home constitutes an important source of accidental poisonings. SEE: *Poisons and Poisoning Appendix.*

***p. sumac*** A shrublike plant, *Toxicodendron vernix,* widely distributed in the U.S. Because it contains the same active toxic principle as poison ivy, the symptoms and treatment of poison sumac dermatitis are the same as for poison ivy dermatitis. SEE: illus.

**poison control center** A facility meeting the staffing and equipment standards of the American Association of Poison Control Centers and recognized to be able to give information on, or treatment to patients suffering from, poisoning. A poison information center consists only of a reference library and does not have treatment facilities. More than 400 poison centers of these two types are scattered throughout the U.S. Staffed largely by volunteer personnel, they offer 24-hr service. By virtue of their function, they are commonly associated with or are part of large hospitals or medical schools. A government agency—the Bureau of Drugs Division of the Poison Control Branch of the Food and Drug Administration, U.S. Department of Health and Human Services—is also active in poison control programs and in coordinating the efforts of individual centers. For address and telephone number of state or province control center, SEE: *Health Care Resources Appendix.*

**poisoning** [L. *potio,* a poisonous draft] **1.** The state produced by introduction of a poison into the body. **2.** Administration of a poison. Symptoms of poisoning vary widely with the agent. SEE: *Poisons and Poisoning Appendix.*

NURSING IMPLICATIONS: The poison is identified, and the local poison control center is contacted for directions. In certain types of poisons, a physical, mechanical, or physiological antidote helps to decrease absorption, to protect body tissues, or to reverse the effects of poison.

An airway is established and maintained, and oxygen is administered as ordered. If indicated and safe, vomiting is induced by tickling the back of the throat or by administering large quantities of water, saline, milk, soap solution, or ipecac syrup.

The nurse supports the patient physically and emotionally. The patient is hospitalized for treatment and close observation. Shock is treated, and the patient is kept warm. Appropriate nursing measures are provided for the convulsing patient to prevent injury. Intake and output are monitored. Fluid and electrolyte balance is monitored. Cool or alcohol sponge baths and antipyretics are used to reduce elevated temperature. The nurse assists with medical procedures such as dialysis.

The nurse teaches the patient and family methods to avoid food contamination, to place toxic substances in a safe place out of children's reach, and to keep the poison control center number with the list of emergency numbers. Ipecac syrup should also be kept on hand in the home.

NOTE: The nurse should not hastily conclude that patient has been poisoned, because many other conditions mimic the symptoms of poisoning. Cerebral hemorrhage, epilepsy, overdose of insulin, diabetic coma, meningitis, thrombosis, and uremia may simulate poisoning. Acute indigestion, appendicitis, gastritis, renal colic, or peptic ulcer may mimic poisoning by corrosive substances.

***arsenic p.*** Poisoning by arsenic. In acute poisoning, symptoms may appear in a few minutes. When the arsenic is ingested with solid food, symptoms may not appear for many hours. Symptoms are metallic taste and odor of garlic on breath, burning pain throughout gastrointestinal tract, vomiting and purging, dehydration, shock syndrome, coma, convulsions, paralysis, and death.

FIRST AID: The stomach should be lavaged with copious amounts of water. If this cannot be done, vomiting should be induced. Dimercaprol (British antilewisite) should be given.

TREATMENT: After first aid, fluid and electrolyte balance must be maintained. Morphine should be given for pain. The patient is treated for shock and pulmonary edema. Blood transfusion may be required. SEE: arsenic in *Poisons and Poisoning Appendix.*

***blood p.*** Septicemia.

***convulsant p.*** Poisoning by one of the toxic substances that cause the person affected to experience convulsions. The common poisons are strychnine and other drugs of the nux vomica group, and various infrequently used drugs such as picrotoxin.

SYMPTOMS: These poisons produce a sense of suffocation, dyspnea, and then muscular rigidity. There are powerful tetanic contractions that may be very painful. These spasms may be brought on by trivial stimuli, such as touching the patient, or they may come on spontaneously and involuntarily at intervals of from 3 to 30 min. Convulsions last from 1 to 5 min.

Trismus, cyanosis, and tachycardia are frequent accompaniments. Death results from asphyxia or exhaustion.

TREATMENT: Appropriate therapy depends on the substance that caused the convulsion. General measures for emptying the stomach or attempting to neutralize the drug may be indicated. Sedatives may be ordered by the physician. Oxygen and artificial respiration may be indicated.

***corrosive p.*** Poisoning by strong acids, alkalies, strong antiseptics including bichloride of mercury, carbolic acid (phenol), Lysol, cresol compounds, tincture of iodine, and arsenic compounds. These are destructive and cause tissue damage similar to that caused by burns. If the substances have been swallowed, any part of the alimentary canal may be affected. Tissues involved are easily perforated. Death comes very shortly from shock or swelling of the throat and pharynx, which causes choking, or by closure of the esophagus, causing slow starvation if not treated. SEE: individual poisons in *Poisons and Poisoning Appendix*.

SYMPTOMS: This type of poisoning is marked by intense burning about the mouth, throat, pharynx, and abdomen; abdominal cramping, retching, nausea, and vomiting, and often collapse. There may be bloody vomitus (hematemesis) and diarrhea; the stools are watery, mucoid, bloody, and possibly stained with the poison or its products, resulting from its action on the contents of the alimentary tract. Stains about the lips, cheeks, tongue, mouth, or pharynx are often a characteristic brown; stains on the mucous membranes may be violet or black. Carbolic acid (phenol) leaves white or gray stains resembling boiled meat, hydrochloric acid stains are grayish, nitric acid leaves yellow stains, and sulfuric acid leaves tan or dark burns.

TREATMENT: Immediate treatment, preferably in a hospital, is mandatory. It is also important to attempt to discover the chemical substance ingested. For this reason, all materials such as food, bottles, jars, or containers that may help to answer this question should be saved. This is essential if the patient is either comatose or an infant.

---

Caution: In treating corrosive poisoning, vomiting must be induced; gastric lavage must not be attempted; and no attempt should be made to neutralize the corrosive substance.

---

Vomiting will increase the severity of damage to the esophagus by renewing contact with the corrosive substance. Gastric lavage may cause the esophagus or stomach to perforate. If the trachea has been damaged, tracheostomy may be needed. Emergency surgery must be considered if there are signs of possible esophageal perforation or perforation of abdominal viscera. Opiates will be needed to control pain. For esophageal burns, broad-spectrum antibiotic and corticosteroid therapy should be started. Intravenous fluids will be required if esophageal or gastric damage prevents ingestion of liquids. Long-range therapy will be directed toward preventing or treating esophageal scars and strictures.

***fish p.*** A form of food poisoning caused by eating fish that are inherently poisonous or that are poisonous because they had decomposed, become infected, or been feeding on other poisonous life forms.

*Ciguatera poisoning:* Poisoning due to eating certain types of bottom-dwelling shore fish. These include grouper, red snapper, and barracuda. The toxin, ciguatoxin, is present in fish that feed on dinoflagellates. It acts within 5 hr of ingestion, and symptoms may persist for 8 days or longer. Symptoms include abdominal cramps, nausea, vomiting, diarrhea, paresthesia, hypotension, and respiratory paralysis. Treatment is supportive.

*Scromboid fish poisoning:* Poisoning due to eating fish that have spoiled and are infested with bacteria, usually *Proteus morganii,* that degrade the protein in fish to produce scrombotoxin.

SYMPTOMS: About 30 min to 2 hr after eating the fish, a peppery sensation of the tongue develops, followed by a rash, pruritus, headache, dizziness, periorbital edema, thirst, nausea, vomiting, diarrhea, and abdominal cramps. These symptoms last about 12 to 24 hr.

TREATMENT: Treatment is symptomatic, but antihistamines may be of benefit. If the stomach has not been emptied by vomiting, gastric lavage should be used. SEE: *shellfish p.*

***food p.*** Illness resulting from ingestion of foods containing poisonous substances. These include mushrooms; shellfish; foods contaminated with pesticides, lead, or mercury; milk from cows that have fed on poisonous plants; or foods that have putrefied or decomposed due to bacterial action.

***heavy metal p.*** Toxicity caused by ingestion, inhalation, or absorption of any heavy metal, esp. lead or mercury. Symptoms are determined by the type and duration of exposure and may include pulmonary, neurological, integumentary, or gastrointestinal disorders.

***ink p.*** Poisonings caused by contact with ink. Many are forms of dermatitis caused by several types of materials. Ordinary ink may cause irritation because of its composition or because of a person's sensitivity to certain ingredients in the ink. Sometimes cleaning materials used to remove ink stains are toxic. Symptoms of ink poisoning include redness, occasionally small pustules, and cracking of the skin.

FIRST AID: The area should be washed with alcohol, soap, and water. It then should be rinsed carefully and covered with a bland dressing such as cold cream.

***iodine p.*** An acute condition caused by the accidental ingestion of iodine or its compounds. This condition is characterized by brown stains on the lips and mouth; burning pain in the mouth, throat, and stomach; vomiting (blue vomitus if stomach contained starches, otherwise yellow vomitus); bloody diarrhea. SEE: *Poisons and Poisoning Appendix.*

FIRST AID: The patient should be given immediately by mouth a cornstarch or flour solution, 15 g in 500 ml (2 cups) of water. Lavage should be performed, with starch solution or 2% sodium thiosulfate solution. Morphine may be given for pain, as well as mild stimulants as indicated. After this therapy, catharsis should be promoted, using 30 g of sodium sulfate and 15 g of starch in 250 ml (1 cup) of water.

***iron p.*** Acute poisoning usually caused by the accidental ingestion by infants or small children of iron-containing medications intended for use by adults.

SYMPTOMS: The victim vomits, usually within an hour of taking the iron. Vomiting of blood and melena may occur. If untreated, restlessness, hypotension, rapid respirations, and cyanosis may develop, followed within a few hours by coma and death.

FIRST AID: The stomach should be emptied promptly, either by digital stimulation of the pharynx if done in the home or by gastric lavage if done in the emergency room. Administration of warm solution of baking soda may help to induce vomiting, and the bicarbonate helps to prevent absorption of the iron. Gastric lavage with a solution containing 4 g of sodium bicarbonate per 100 ml is done, leaving 60 ml of the bicarbonate solution in the stomach. Deferoxamine may be administered intramuscularly in an initial dose of 50 mg/kg up to 2 g. This dose may be repeated intramuscularly in 4 to 8 hr and then at 12-hr intervals if needed. Acidosis is treated with intravenous sodium bicarbonate solution. If the patient is in shock, the shock should be treated using the usual methods.

***lead p.*** Ingestion or inhalation of substances containing lead. Symptoms of acute poisoning include a metallic taste in mouth, burns in throat and pharynx, and later abdominal cramps and prostration. Chronic lead poisoning is characterized by anorexia, nausea, vomiting, excess salivation, anemia, a lead line on the gums, abdominal pains, muscle cramps, and pains in the joints.

TREATMENT: Seizures are treated with diazepam. Fluid and electrolyte balance is maintained. Cerebral edema is treated with mannitol and dexamethasone. The blood lead level is determined. If it is above 50 to 60 $\mu$g/dl, the lead is removed from the body with a chelator (e.g., edetate calcium disodium, dimercaprol, D-penicillamine, or succimer). Succimer has the advantage of being orally active and is esp. helpful in treating children. The effect of treatment is monitored closely and may have to be continued for a week or longer or repeated if the lead level rebounds.

***mercury p.*** Mercury per se (i.e., mass of mercury) is not poisonous, but elemental mercury vapor is toxic when inhaled. The bivalent salt, mercuric chloride ($HgCl_2$), is highly poisonous. Symptoms of acute poisoning include severe gastrointestinal irritation with pain, cramping, constriction of the throat, vomiting, and a metallic taste in the mouth. A stronger solution causes a white coating due to coagulation. Abdominal pain is very severe, bloody diarrhea and vomitus appear, and urine flow is scanty. Prostration, convulsions, unconsciousness, and death occur. Chronic poisoning is characterized by bad breath, loosening of teeth, fever, urinary difficulties, nausea, diarrhea, sore tongue, paralysis, weakness, and death.

FIRST AID: The stomach should be evacuated and washed out with milk or with a solution of 1 tsp of sodium bicarbonate dissolved in 6 oz (177 ml) of water. Treatment with the chelators dimercaprol (British antilewisite) and D-penicillamine should be instituted immediately. Fluid and electrolyte balance should be maintained. If renal function declines while chelators are being used, hemodialysis may be necessary. Chelators are removed by dialysis and can, therefore, be continued. SEE: mercuric chloride in *Poisons and Poisoning Appendix.*

***mushroom p.*** Poisoning caused by ingestion of mushrooms such as *Amanita muscaria,* which contains muscarine, or species that contain phalloidin, a component of the amanita toxin. The nearest poison control center should be called for emergency treatment. SEE: amanita in *Poisons and Poisoning Appendix.*

***oxalic acid p.*** Acute poisoning occurring when oxalic acid is accidentally ingested or when large quantities of foods rich in oxalic acid are eaten. Ingestion of 5 g of oxalic acid may be fatal. Chronic poisoning may result from inhalation of vapors. SEE: *Poisons and Poisoning Appendix.*

SYMPTOMS: Signs and symptoms include a corrosive action on the mucosa of the mouth, esophagus, and stomach; a sour taste; burning in the mouth, throat, and stomach; great thirst; bloody vomitus; collapse; and sometimes convulsions and coma.

TREATMENT: Prompt treatment with

any soluble calcium salt such as powdered chalk in water or milk, lime water, or calcium lactate should be given. This procedure inactivates the acid by precipitating it as an insoluble calcium salt. Careful gastric lavage is done using dilute lime water. Vomiting should not be induced. Intravenous calcium gluconate or calcium chloride may be given to treat tetany. Morphine may be required for pain.

***pokeroot p.*** Poisoning resulting from ingestion of pokeroot. Nausea, vomiting, drowsiness, vertigo, and possibly convulsions and respiratory paralysis characterize this type of poisoning. Treatment includes administration of an emetic or performance of lavage.

***potato p.*** Poisoning due to ingestion of potatoes that contain excess amounts of solanine. This toxic substance is present in the potato peel and in the green sprouts. Potatoes usually contain about 7 mg of solanine per 100 g; the toxic dose of solanine is about 20 to 25 g. Boiling but not baking removes most of the solanine from the potato. Symptoms of poisoning include headache, vomiting, abdominal pain, diarrhea, and fever. Neurological disturbances include apathy, restlessness, drowsiness, confusion, stupor, hallucinations, and visual disturbances. There is no specific therapy. With appropriate supportive and symptomatic therapy, prognosis is good.

***risk for p.*** Accentuated risk of accidental exposure to or ingestion of drugs or dangerous products in doses sufficient to cause poisoning. SEE: *Nursing Diagnoses Appendix.*

***shellfish p.*** Poisoning produced when humans ingest shellfish that have themselves ingested toxic phytoplankton. Symptoms of shellfish poisoning include muscular weakness, dysphonia, paresthesias of the face and extremities, nausea and vomiting, and occasionally paralysis and respiratory distress. Treatment is symptomatic. Spontaneous recovery usually takes place in 24 hr. SEE: *fish p.*

***p. by unknown substances*** Cases in which there is no information concerning the nature of the poison taken, and the signs and symptoms are not recognized as being due to any particular substance. Specific antidotes cannot be given in this situation. There are, however, certain agents that act in a general manner and may be efficacious.

One of these is activated charcoal, which is available from many sources. Although a slurry of this in water is messy and offensive to the patient, it is a highly effective adsorbent for certain kinds of poisons. Another substance is referred to as the universal antidote. It consists of a mixture of 2 parts activated charcoal, 1 part magnesium oxide, and 1 part tannic acid. The universal antidote has been used empirically for a number of years and prepackaged units are now available commercially. It is doubtful if this mixture offers any real advantage over activated charcoal alone, which has a proven effectiveness against many substances. Each of these materials may be given as a slurry made from several heaping teaspoonsful in a glass of water. Because the ingredients are essentially harmless and the efficiency is increased by increasing the amount of adsorbent relative to the amount of poison, the dose may be repeated several times.

**poisonous** (poy′zŏn-ŭs) [L. *potio,* a poisonous draft] Having the properties or qualities of a poison. SYN: *toxic; venomous.*

**poisonous plants** Plants containing a poisonous substance that may be fatal if ingested, including azalea, castor bean, chinaberry, European bittersweet, wild or black cherry, oleander, berries of holly and mistletoe, dieffenbachia, horse chestnuts, poison hemlock, laurel, death cup, black nightshade or deadly nightshade, rhododendron, choke cherry, Japanese yew, unripe fruit of akee, cassava roots, betel nut, seeds and pods of bird-of-paradise, belladonna, angels trumpet, fava bean (if eaten by a person with glucose-6-phosphate deficiency), foxglove, bulb of hyacinth, Indian tobacco, iris root, poinsettia, pokeroot, apricot kernals, apple seeds, green tubers and new sprouts of potatoes, privet, rhubarb leaves, wild tomatoes, skunk cabbage, and jimsonweed; and plants containing irritating substances, such as poison ivy, poison oak, and poison sumac.

**poker back** Stiffness of the spine; may result from spondylitis or rheumatoid arthritis. SEE: *arthritis, rheumatoid.*

**pokeroot** (pōk′root) An herb, *Phytolacca americana,* with white flowers and purple berries. The root is poisonous. Also called *pokeweed.*

**polar** [L. *polaris*] Concerning a pole.

**polarimeter** (pō″lăr-ĭm′ĕ-tĕr) [″ + Gr. *metron,* measure] An instrument for measuring amount of polarization of light or rotation of polarized light.

**polarimetry** (pō″lăr-ĭm′ĕ-trē) The measurement of the amount and rotation of polarized light.

**polariscope** (pō-lăr′ĭ-skōp) [L. *polaris,* pole, + Gr. *skopein,* to examine] An apparatus used in the measurement of polarized light.

**polariscopy** (pō″lăr-ĭs′kō-pē) The study of polarized light by the use of a polariscope.

**polarity** (pō-lăr′ĭ-tē) **1.** The quality of having poles. **2.** The exhibition of opposite effects at the two extremities in physical therapy. **3.** The positive or negative state of an electrical battery. **4.** In cell division, the relation of cell constituents to the poles of the cell.

**polarization** (pō″lăr-ī-zā′shŭn) [L. *polaris,* pole] **1.** A condition in a ray of light in which vibrations occur in only one plane.

**2.** In a galvanic battery, collection of hydrogen bubbles on negative plate and oxygen on the positive plate, whereby generation of current is impeded. **3.** The electrical state that exists at the cell membrane of an excitable cell at rest; the inside is negatively charged in relation to the outside. The difference is created by the distribution of ions within the cell and in the extracellular fluid. SYN: *potential, resting*. SEE: *depolarization* for illus.

**polarizer** (pō'lă-rīz"ĕr) The part of a polariscope that polarizes light.

**pole** (pōl) [L. *polus*] **1.** The extremity of any axis about which forces acting on it are symmetrically disposed. SYN: *polus*. **2.** One of two points in a magnet, cell, or battery having opposite physical qualities.

***animal p.*** The pole opposite the yolk in an ovum. At this point, polar bodies are formed and pinched off and protoplasm is concentrated and has its greatest activity.

***p.'s of the eye*** The anterior and posterior extremities of the optic axis.

***frontal p.*** The farthest projecting part of the anterior extremity of both cerebral hemispheres.

***germinal p.*** The pole of an ovum at which the development begins.

***p.'s of the kidney*** The upper and lower extremities of the kidney.

***occipital p.*** The posterior extremity of the occipital lobe.

***pelvic p.*** The breech of a fetus.

***placental p. of the chorion*** The spot at which the domelike placenta is situated.

***temporal p.*** The anterior extremity of the temporal lobe.

***p.'s of the testicle*** The upper and lower extremities of a testicle.

***vegetal p.*** The part of the egg containing the food yolk.

**polio** *acute anterior poliomyelitis*.

**polio-** Combining form indicating *gray*.

**polioclastic** (pōl"ē-ō-klăs'tĭk) [Gr. *polios*, gray, + *klastos*, breaking] Destructive to the gray matter of the nervous system.

**polioencephalitis** (pōl"ē-ō-ĕn-sĕf"ă-lī'tĭs) [" + *enkephalos*, brain, + *itis*, inflammation] A condition characterized by inflammatory lesions of the gray matter of the brain.

***anterior superior p.*** A disease involving necrotic changes in the gray matter around the third ventricle, the anterior portion of the fourth ventricle, and the aqueduct of Sylvius. It is characterized by ocular abnormalities, mental disturbances, and ataxia. The origin of the disease is nutritional, probably thiamine (vitamin $B_1$) deficiency.

***p. hemorrhagica*** Polioencephalitis accompanied by hemorrhagic lesions.

***posterior p.*** Polioencephalitis involving the gray matter around the fourth ventricle.

**polioencephalomeningomyelitis** (pōl"ē-ō-ĕn-sĕf"ăl-ō-mĕn-ĭn"gō-mī-ĕl-ī'tĭs) [" + " + *meninx*, membrane, + *myelos*, marrow, + *itis*, inflammation] Inflammation of the gray matter of the brain and spinal cord and their meninges.

**polioencephalomyelitis** (pōl"ē-ō-ĕn-sĕf"ăl-ō-mī"ĕl-ī'tĭs) Inflammation of the gray matter of the brain and spinal cord.

**polioencephalopathy** (pōl"ē-ō-ĕn-sĕf"ăl-ŏp'ă-thē) [Gr. *polios*, gray, + *enkephalos*, brain, + *pathos*, disease, suffering] Disease of the gray matter of the brain.

**poliomyelencephalitis** (pōl"ē-ō-mī"ĕl-ĕn-sĕf"ăl-ī'tĭs) [" + *myelos*, marrow, + *enkephalos*, brain, + *itis*, inflammation] Poliomyelitis with polioencephalitis.

**poliomyelitis** (pōl"ē-ō-mī"ĕl-ī'tĭs) [" + " + *itis*, inflammation] Inflammation of the gray matter of the spinal cord. It is an acute viral disease characterized by fever, sore throat, headache, vomiting, and often stiffness of the neck and back. There may also be subsequent atrophy of groups of muscles ending in contraction and permanent deformity.

***abortive p.*** Poliomyelitis in which the illness is mild with no involvement of the central nervous system.

***acute anterior p.*** An acute infectious inflammation of the anterior horns of the gray matter of the spinal cord. In this acute, systemic, infectious disease, paralysis may or may not occur. In the majority of patients, the disease is mild, being limited to respiratory and gastrointestinal symptoms, such constituting the minor illness or the abortive type, which lasts only a few days. In the major illness, muscle paralysis or weakness occurs with loss of superficial and deep reflexes. In such cases characteristic lesions are found in the gray matter of the spinal cord, medulla, motor area of cerebral cortex, and cerebellum.

SYMPTOMS: The onset often is abrupt, although the ordinary manifestations of a severe cold or some gastrointestinal disturbances may come on gradually, accompanied by slight elevation of temperature, frequently enduring for not more than 3 days. At the end of this period, paralysis may or may not develop. The extent of any paralysis necessarily depends on the degree of nerve involvement. Consequently, paralysis may be confined to one small group of muscles or affect one or all extremities. When the respiratory muscles also are involved, death is likely to ensue. In the average paralytic case it is the extensor muscles in particular that are affected.

ETIOLOGY: The causative agent is a virus consisting of particles from 270 to 300 angstrom units in diameter. The virus that is excreted in the feces is resistant and stable, remaining viable for months outside the body. Three immunological types exist. The incubation period ranges from 5 to 35 days but is usually 7 to 12 days.

DIFFERENTIAL DIAGNOSIS: Among the diseases confused with this infection are the various types of meningitis, postinfection encephalomyelitis, and hysteria.

PROPHYLAXIS: Active immunization with either poliovirus vaccine live oral or poliovirus vaccine inactivated has greatly reduced the incidence of paralytic poliomyelitis. The oral vaccine containing all three types of the virus should be given to young infants beginning at age 6 to 12 weeks, with a second dose about 2 months later and then a third dose 8 to 12 months later. Older children who have not been previously immunized with trivalent oral poliovirus vaccine should be given two doses at 8-week intervals and a third dose 6 months to 1 year later. SEE: *poliovirus vaccine, inactivated.*

COMPLICATIONS: Paralysis, atrophy of muscles, and ultimate deformities constitute the complications of this disease. Aside from bronchopneumonia, which may develop in very severe cases, other complications are surprisingly few.

PROGNOSIS: Ordinarily the outcome as to life is good. It is only the bulbar and respiratory types in which death is likely to occur. These two types constitute nearly all of the fatal cases. Even when paralysis develops, 50% of the patients make a full recovery and about 25% have mild permanent paralysis.

Progressive paralysis may occur years after the acute attack. This recently described syndrome may be due to a combination of aging and atrophy of anterior horn cells. SEE: *postpoliomyelitis muscular atrophy; post-polio syndrome.*

INCIDENCE: Poliomyelitis is endemic throughout the world but occurs in epidemics in certain countries. Polio no longer occurs in epidemics in the U.S. Virtually all cases for the last several years have been vaccine-associated. In countries where polio vaccine has not been used extensively, epidemics are seasonal, occurring in summer and fall. Children are more susceptible than adults. Infection is spread by direct contact, the virus probably entering the body via the mouth. It reaches the central nervous system through the blood.

PREDISPOSING CAUSES: Tonsillectomy and other nose and throat operations, routine immunizations, excessive physical strain, and fatigue can predispose individuals to this disease. Pregnant women are esp. susceptible during epidemics.

TREATMENT: Treatment is supportive. A respirator is used for patients whose respiratory muscles are paralyzed. Physical therapy is used to attain maximum function and prevent deformities that are late manifestations of the disease.

NURSING IMPLICATIONS: The nurse enforces strict isolation with concurrent disinfection of throat discharge and feces to prevent transmission of polio virus. The nurse maintains a calm, reassuring manner. A patent airway is maintained, the patient is observed closely for signs of respiratory distress, oxygen is administered as necessary, and a tracheostomy tray kept at bedside.

The patient should maintain strict bedrest during the acute phase. Gentle passive range-of-motion exercises and application of hot moist packs at 20-min intervals, or tub baths for children, help to alleviate muscle pain. Proper body alignment is maintained, and the patient turned frequently to prevent deformity and decubiti. A mild sedative or analgesic is administered to decrease pain and anxiety and to promote rest. The patient is observed for distended bladder due to transitory paralysis. The nurse promotes personal hygiene and provides oral hygiene. Appetizing food is offered because anorexia is common. Antipyretics are administered to reduce fever. Fluid and electrolyte balance and elimination are monitored closely. A foot board is used to prevent footdrop. Emotional support is provided to assist the patient to cope with loss of body function and paralysis.

***anterior p.*** Inflammation of the anterior horns of the spinal cord.

***ascending p.*** Poliomyelitis in which paralysis begins in the lower extremities and progresses up the legs, thighs, and trunk, and finally involves the respiratory muscles.

***bulbar p.*** Poliomyelitis in which the gray matter of the medulla oblongata is involved, resulting in paralysis and usually respiratory failure.

***chronic anterior p.*** Progressive wasting of the muscles; myelopathic progressive muscular atrophy.

***nonparalytic p.*** Pain and stiffness in the muscles of the axial skeleton, esp. of the neck and back; mild fever; increased proteins and leukocytes in the cerebrospinal fluid. Diagnosis depends on the isolation of the virus and serological reactions.

***paralytic p.*** Poliomyelitis with a variable combination of signs of damage of the central nervous system. These include weakness, incoordination, muscle tenderness and spasms, flaccid paralysis, and disturbance of consciousness.

***provocative p.*** During an epidemic of poliomyelitis, the onset of paralysis in the area close to the site of an invasive procedure. Thus an injection in muscle increases the risk of paralysis of the side of the body injected; and tonsillectomy and adenoidectomy increases the risk that poliomyelitis will affect the brain stem.

**poliosis** (pŏl″ē-ō′sĭs) [Gr. *polios,* gray, + *osis,* condition] Whiteness of the hair, esp. when due to a hereditary condition or as a result of infection. SYN: *canities.*

**poliovirus** (pō″lē-ō-vī′rŭs) The etiological

agent of poliomyelitis, separable into three serotypes based on the specificity of the neutralizing antibody. The three serotypes are types I, II, and III. A virus found worldwide, it spreads directly or indirectly from infected persons or convalescent carriers. Epidemics of poliomyelitis that were characteristic of infections with this virus have been virtually eliminated by the poliovirus vaccine. SEE: *poliovirus vaccine, inactivated.*

**poliovirus vaccine, inactivated** ABBR: IPV. A poliovirus vaccine recommended for the prevention of paralytic poliomyelitis. The vaccine, which contains inactivated types I, II, and III polioviruses, is suitable for parenteral administration to all infants and children.

Infants should be given three doses, the first at 2 months of age, followed by two more doses at 8-week intervals. A fourth dose should be given at age 18 months unless poliomyelitis is endemic in the area, in which case the fourth dose is given 6 to 12 months after the third. Additional doses are recommended prior to school entry and then every 5 years until age 18.

**poliovirus vaccine, live oral** ABBR: OPV. A standard preparation of one type or a combination of the three types of live, attenuated polioviruses. It is suitable for immunizing children and adults against all three types of poliovirus, but the inactivated poliovirus vaccine is preferred for adults because of the slightly high risk of vaccine-associated paralysis. The schedule for infants is first dose at 6 to 12 weeks, the second about 2 months later, a third 8 to 12 months after the second. No additional "boosters" are recommended. For children and adolescents not previously immunized prior to age 18, two doses are given 8 weeks apart and a third dose is given 6 to 12 months later. Trade name is Orimune.

**polishing** (pŏl′ĭsh-ĭng) Producing a smooth, glossy finish on a denture or a dental restoration.

**Politzer bag** (pŏl′ĭt-zĕr) [Adam Politzer, Hungarian otologist, 1835–1920] A soft rubber bag with a rubber tip for inflating the middle ear by increasing the pressure in the nasopharynx. SEE: *aerotitis.*

**politzerization** (pŏl″ĭt-sĕr-ĭ-zā′shŭn) The inflation of the middle ear by means of a Politzer bag.

**pollen** (pŏl′ĕn) [L., dust] The microspores of a seed plant that develop in the anther at the tip of the stamen. Each pollen grain develops a pollen tube and constitutes the male gametophyte. Within it develops a tube nucleus and two sperm nuclei, the latter constituting the male reproductive elements. Many airborne pollens are allergens. SEE: *hay fever.*

**pollenogenic** (pŏl″ĕn-ō-jĕn′ĭk) [″ + Gr. *gennan,* to produce] Caused by the pollen of plants, or producing plant pollen.

**pollex** (pŏl′ĕks) *pl.* **pollices** [L.] The thumb.

***p. extensus*** Backward deviation of the thumb.

***p. flexus*** Permanent flexion of the thumb.

***p. valgus*** Abnormal deviation of the thumb toward the ulnar side.

***p. varus*** Abnormal deviation of the thumb toward the radial side.

**pollicization** (pŏl″ĭs-ī-zā′shŭn) [L. *pollex,* thumb] The plastic surgical procedure of constructing a thumb from adjacent tissues.

**pollinosis** (pŏl-ĭn-ō′sĭs) [L. *pollen,* dust, + Gr. *osis,* disease] Hay fever.

**pollution** (pŭ-loo′shŭn) [ME. *polluten*] The state of making impure or defiling.

**polocyte** (pō′lō-sīt) [Gr. *polos,* pole, + *kytos,* cell] Polar body.

**polonium** (pō-lō′nē-ŭm) [L. *Polonia,* Poland, native country of its discoverers, the Curies] SYMB: Po. A radioactive element isolated from pitchblende; atomic weight 210; atomic number 84.

**polus** (pō′lŭs) *pl.* **poli** [L.] Pole (1).

**poly** (pŏl′ē) *polymorphonuclear leukocyte.*

**poly-** [Gr. *polys,* many] Combining form indicating *many, much.*

**polyacid** (pŏl″ē-ăs′ĭd) An alcohol or a base with two or more hydroxyl groups that will combine with an acid.

**polyadenitis** (pŏl″ē-ăd″ĕ-nī′tĭs) [″ + Gr. *aden,* gland, + *itis,* inflammation] Inflammation of the lymph nodes, esp. the cervical lymph nodes.

**polyadenomatosis** (pŏl″ē-ăd″ĕ-nō-mă-tō′sĭs) [″ + ″ + *oma,* tumor, + *osis,* condition] Adenomas in many glands.

**polyadenopathy** (pŏl″ē-ăd″ĕ-nŏp′ă-thē) [″ + ″ + *pathos,* disease, suffering] Any disease in which many glands are involved.

**polyadenous** (pŏl″ē-ăd′ĕ-nŭs) Involving or relating to many glands.

**polyagglutination** Red cells that are agglutinated by a large proportion of adult human sera regardless of blood group.

**polyalgesia** (pŏl″ē-ăl-jē′zē-ă) [″ + *algesis,* sense of pain] A single stimulus of a part, producing sensation in many parts.

**polyandry** (pŏl″ē-ăn′drē) [Gr. *polyandria*] The practice of having more than one husband at the same time. SEE: *polygamy.*

**polyangiitis** (pŏl″ē-ăn″jē-ī′tĭs) [Gr. *polys,* many, + *angeion,* vessel, + *itis,* inflammation] Inflammation of a number of blood vessels.

**polyarteritis nodosa** (pŏl″ē-ăr″tĕr-ī′tĭs) [″ + *arteria,* artery, + *itis,* inflammation] ABBR: PAN. A disease of medium and small arteries, particularly at the point of bifurcation and branching. Segmental inflammation, infiltration with fibrinoid, and necrosis of the vessel lining and walls lead to a diminished flow of blood to the areas normally supplied by these arteries. Signs and symptoms depend on the location of the affected vessels and may affect any organ or body system. SYN: *periarteritis nodosa.* SEE: *Nursing Diagnoses Appendix.*

ETIOLOGY: The cause is unknown, but the disease is associated with hypersensitivity. Drug therapy, vaccines, and bacterial and viral infections have been associated with the onset of polyarteritis.

TREATMENT: Prednisone and cyclophosphamide are effective. General supportive therapy including control of hypertension is required.

PROGNOSIS: Without therapy, only one person in eight will live 5 years. Death is due to failure of a function of a vital organ such as the heart or kidney; hemorrhage from the gastrointestinal tract; or a ruptured aneurysm.

**polyarthritis** (pŏl-ē-ăr-thrī′tĭs) [″ + *arthron,* joint + *itis,* inflammation] Inflammation of more than one joint. The role of infection in this disease is being investigated.

**polyarthric** (pŏl″ē-ăr′thrĭk), *adj.*

***acute p. rheumatica*** Acute rheumatic fever.

***chronic villous p.*** Chronic inflammation of the synovial membrane of several joints.

**polyarticular** (pŏl″ē-ăr-tĭk′ū-lăr) [″ + L. *articulus,* a joint] Concerning, having, or affecting many joints. SYN: *multiarticular.*

**polyatomic** (pŏl″ē-ă-tŏm′ĭk) [″ + *atomon,* atom] **1.** Having several atoms. **2.** Having more than two replaceable hydrogen atoms.

**polyavitaminosis** (pŏl″ē-ā-vī″tă-mĭn-ō′sĭs) [″ + *a-,* not, + L. *vita,* life, + *amine* + Gr. *osis,* condition] A deficiency of more than one vitamin.

**polybasic** (pŏl″ē-bā′sĭk) [Gr. *polys,* many, + *basis,* base] Pert. to an acid with two or more hydrogen ions that will combine with a base.

**polyblast** (pŏl′ē-blăst) [″ + *blastos,* a germ] A large mononuclear phagocyte that is derived from an embryonic wandering cell and is present in inflammation.

**polyblennia** (pŏl″ē-blĕ′nē-ă) [″ + *blennos,* mucus] Secretion of an abnormal amount of mucus.

**polycarbophil** (pŏl″ē-kăr′bō-fĭl) A hydrophilic substance that is used as a bulk-forming laxative.

**polycentric** (pŏl″ē-sĕn′trĭk) [″ + *kentron,* center] The condition of having many centers.

**polycheiria** (pŏl″ē-kī′rē-ă) [″ + *cheir,* hand] Having more than two hands.

**polychemotherapy** (pŏl″ē-kē″mō-thĕr′ă-pē) [″ + *chemeia,* chemistry, + *therapeia,* treatment] Treatment with several chemotherapeutic agents at once.

**polychlorinated biphenyls** ABBR: PCBs. A group of complex chemicals classed as chlorinated aromatic hydrocarbons. They were widely used in industry as a component of transformers and capacitors; in paints and hydraulic systems; and in carbonless NCR paper. Because of their extremely low rate of biodegradation, accumulation in animal tissues (particularly in adipose tissue), and their potential for chronic or delayed toxic effects, the manufacture of PCBs was discontinued in the U.S. in 1977. PCBs were sold in the U.S. under the trade name Aroclor.

**polychondritis** (pŏl″ē-kŏn-drī′tĭs) [″ + *chondros,* cartilage, + *itis,* inflammation] Inflammation of several cartilages of the body.

***chronic atrophic relapsing p.*** A degenerative disease of cartilage associated with polyarthritis, involvement of the cartilage of the nose, ears, joints, bronchi, and trachea. It is most common between the ages of 40 and 60 years but may occur at any time. The cause is unknown. Because of the collapse of the bronchial walls, repeated infections of the lungs will occur, and death may result from these infections.

TREATMENT: Prednisone is the treatment of choice. Immunosuppressive drugs such as cyclophosphamide or azathioprine are used if patients fail to respond to prednisone. Heart valve replacement or repair of aortic aneurysm may be necessary.

**polychromasia** (pŏl″ē-krō-mā′zē-ă) [″ + *chroma,* color] The quality of having many colors.

**polychromatic** (pŏl″ē-krō-măt′ĭk) Multicolored.

**polychromatocyte** (pŏl″ē-krō-măt′ō-sīt) [″ + ″ + *kytos,* cell] A cell that has an affinity for various stains. SEE: *polychromatophilia* (1).

**polychromatophil(e)** (pŏl″ē-krō-măt′ō-fĭl) [Gr. *polys,* many, + *chroma,* color, + *philein,* to love] A cell, esp. an erythrocyte, that is stainable with more than one kind of stain.

**polychromatophilia** (pŏl″ē-krō-măt″ō-fĭl′ē-ă) **1.** The quality of being stainable with more than one stain. **2.** An excess of polychromatophils in the blood.

**polychylia** (pŏl″ē-kī′lē-ă) [″ + *chylos,* juice] Excessive secretion of chyle.

**Polycillin-N** Trade name for ampicillin sodium.

**polyclinic** (pŏl″ē-klĭn′ĭk) [″ + *kline,* bed] A hospital or clinic treating patients with various medical and surgical conditions; a general hospital.

**polyclonal** (pŏl″ē-klōn′ăl) Arising from different cell lines.

**polycoria** (pŏl″ē-kō′rē-ă) [″ + *kore,* pupil] The state of having more than one pupil in one eye.

**polycrotic** (pŏl″ē-krŏt′ĭk) [″ + *krotos,* beat] Having several pulse waves for each heartbeat.

**polycrotism** (pŏl-ĭk′rō-tĭzm) [″ + ″ + *-ismos,* condition] The condition of having several pulse waves for each heartbeat.

**polycystic** (pŏl″ē-sĭs′tĭk) [″ + *kystis,* cyst] Composed of many cysts.

**polycystic ovary syndrome** Stein-Leventhal syndrome.

**polycythemia** (pŏl″ē-sī-thē′mē-ă) [″ + *kytos,* cell, + *haima,* blood] An excess of red blood cells. In a newborn, it may reflect hemoconcentration due to hypovolemia or prolonged intrauterine hypoxia, or hypervolemia due to intrauterine twin-to-twin transfusion or placental transfusion resulting in delayed clamping of the umbilical cord. SYN: *erythrocytosis*. SEE: *twin-to-twin transfusion*.

***relative p.*** A relative increase in the number of erythrocytes that occurs in hemoconcentration.

***secondary p.*** Polycythemia resulting from some physiological condition that stimulates erythropoiesis, such as lowered oxygen tension in blood.

***p. vera*** A chronic, life-shortening myeloproliferative disorder of unknown etiology involving all bone marrow elements; characterized by an increase in red blood cell mass and hemoglobin concentration. SYN: *erythremia*. SEE: *Nursing Diagnoses Appendix*.

SYMPTOMS: Weakness, fatigue, vertigo, tinnitus, irritability, enlarged spleen, flushing of face, redness and pain of extremities, and black-and-blue spots. The bone marrow shows increased cellularity.

TREATMENT: Permanent cure cannot be achieved today, but remissions of many years can be produced. Phlebotomy and radioactive phosphorus ($^{32}P$) are effective. Phlebotomy followed by chemotherapy with cyclophosphamide or melphalan has been used but requires much closer follow-up than phlebotomy and use of $^{32}P$.

NURSING IMPLICATIONS: The nurse explains the symptoms and the need to seek medical attention when signs and symptoms of bleeding and thrombus formation occur. Rest should be balanced with exercise. Limbs should be protected from injury due to heat, cold, and pressure, and safety precautions, including use of a soft toothbrush, should be instituted to prevent injury. Reassurance and support are provided to the patient family, and opportunities are provided for questions and discussion of concerns.

**polydactylism** (pŏl″ē-dăk′tĭ-lĭzm) [Gr. *polys*, many, + *daktylos*, digit, + *-ismos*, condition] The state of having supernumerary fingers or toes.

**polydactyly** (pŏl″ē-dăk′tĭ-lē) [″ + *daktylos*, finger] The condition of having more than the normal number of fingers and toes.

**polydipsia** (pŏl″ē-dĭp′sē-ă) [″ + *dipsa*, thirst] Excessive thirst.

**polydrug use** In drug abusers, the practice of concurrent use of several dissimilar drugs. Thus, alcohol, cocaine, opiates, and other drugs may be used at the same time. The toxic potential of multiple drug use is increased as compared with use of a single drug.

**polydysplasia** (pŏl″ē-dĭs-plā′zē-ă) [″ + *dys*, bad, + *plassein*, to form] The condition of having multiple developmental abnormalities.

**polydystrophic** (pŏl″ē-dĭs-trō′fĭk) Concerning or having polydystrophy.

**polydystrophy** (pŏl″ē-dĭs′trō-fē) [″ + ″ + *trophe*, nourishment] The condition of having multiple congenital anomalies of the connective tissues.

**polyendocrine deficiency syndromes** *Type I:* A disease that begins at about age 12, characterized by hypoparathyroidism, primary adrenal insufficiency, and mucocutaneous candidiasis. Alopecia, pernicious anemia, malabsorption, and chronic hepatitis may also be present. *Type II:* A disease for which the average age of onset is about 30 years and which is characterized by primary adrenal insufficiency, autoimmune thyroid disease, and insulin-dependent diabetes mellitus.

**polyene** (pŏl-ē′ēn) An organic compound containing alternating, or conjugate, double bonds. An example is butadiene, $CH_2{=}CHCH{=}CH_2$.

**polyesthesia** (pŏl″ē-ĕs-thē′zē-ă) [″ + *aisthesis*, sensation] An abnormal sensation of touch in which a single stimulus is felt at two or more places.

**polyesthetic** (pŏl″ē-ĕs-thĕt′ĭk) **1.** Pert. to polyesthesia. **2.** Pert. to several senses or sensations.

**polyestrous** (pŏl″ē-ĕs′trŭs) [″ + *oistros*, mad desire] Having two or more estrous cycles in each mating season.

**polyethylene** (pŏl″ē-ĕth′ĭ-lēn) A polymerized resin of ethylene; used to make a wide variety of products, including tubing used in intravenous sets.

***p. glycol 400*** A polymer consisting of ethylene oxide and water. The formula is $H(OCH_2CH_2)_nOH$, in which the value of n is from 8.2 to 9.1. It is used as a water-soluble ointment base.

***p. glycol 4000*** A polymer consisting of ethylene oxide and water. The formula is $H(OCH_2CH_2)_nOH$, in which the value of n is from 68 to 84. It is used as a water-soluble ointment base.

***p. glycol electrolyte for gastrointestinal lavage solution*** A white powder added to water to make a volume of 4 L. An isosmotic solution for oral administration, it contains 236 g of polyethylene glycol 3350; 23.74 g of sodium sulfate; 6.74 g of sodium bicarbonate; 5.86 g of sodium chloride; and 2.97 g of potassium chloride. For adults the 4 L are given at the rate of 8 oz (240 ml) every 10 min until completed. This solution is given before colonoscopy and barium enema examinations. The bowel will be cleansed within 3 to 4 hr. Trade name is Golytely.

**polygalactia** (pŏl″ē-gă-lăk′shē-ă) [Gr. *polys*, many, + *gala*, milk] Excessive secretion or flow of milk.

**polygamy** (pō-lĭg′ă-mē) [″ + *gamos*, marriage] The practice of having several wives, husbands, or mates at the same time. SEE: *polyandry; polygyny*.

**polyganglionic** (pŏl″ē-găng″glē-ŏn′ĭk) [″ + *ganglion*, ganglion] **1.** Concerning many ganglia. **2.** Affecting many glands.

**polygastria** (pŏl″ē-găs′trē-ă) [″ + *gaster,* stomach] Excessive secretion or flow of gastric juice.

**polygen** (pŏl′ĕ-jĕn) **1.** An element that has more than one valency and that can form more than one series of compounds. **2.** An antigen that will cause the formation of two or more specific antibodies.

**polygenic** (pŏl″ē-jĕn′ĭk) [″ + *gennan,* to produce] Pert. to or caused by several genes.

**polyglandular** (pŏl″ē-glăn′dū-lăr) [″ + L. *glandula,* a little kernel] Pert. to or affecting many glands. SYN: *pluriglandular.*

**polyglycolic acid** A polymer of glycolic acid anhydride units. It is used in manufacturing surgical sutures.

**polygnathus** (pō-lĭg′nă-thŭs) [″ + *gnathos,* jaw] Conjoined twins of unequal size in which the smaller is attached to the jaw of the larger.

**polygram** (pŏl′ē-grăm) [″ + *gramma,* something written] A tracing or record made by a polygraph.

**polygraph** (pŏl′ē-grăf) [″ + *graphein,* to write] An instrument for determining minor physiological changes assumed to occur under the stress of lying (or any other emotion). Variations in respiratory rhythm, pulse rate, blood pressure, and sweating of the hands are among the functions that are monitored. Increased perspiration lessens resistance to passage of electrical current. The test has popular appeal among law enforcement departments, but results obtained are presumptive and not absolute; nevertheless, interpretations of polygraph data have been admitted as evidence in some legal proceedings. The advisability of accepting the results of polygraph tests is controversial. SYN: *sphygmograph.*

**polygyny** The practice of having more than one female mate at a time. SEE: *polygamy.*

**polygyria** (pŏl″ē-jī′rē-ă) [″ + *gyros,* circle] Excess of the normal number of convolutions in the brain.

**polyhedral** (pŏl″ē-hē′drăl) [Gr. *polys,* many, + *hedra,* base] Having many surfaces.

**polyhistor** (pŏl″ē-hĭs′tŭr) [″ + *histor,* learned] A scholar or physician who has great and varied abilities and knowledge (e.g., Hippocrates, Galen, Paracelsus, Leonardo da Vinci, Boerhaave, Sir William Osler, Richard Mead, and Thomas Jefferson). SYN: *polymath.*

**polyhybrid** (pŏl″ē-hī′brĭd) [″ + L. *hybrida,* mongrel] The offspring of parents that are different with respect to three or more characteristics.

**polyhydramnios** (pŏl″ē-hī-drăm′nē-ŏs) [″ + *hydor,* water, + *amnion,* amnion] An excess of amniotic fluid in the bag of waters in pregnancy. SEE: *amnion.*

**polyhydric** (pŏl″ē-hī′drĭk) Containing more than two hydroxyl groups.

**polyhydruria** (pŏl″ē-hī-droo′rē-ă) [″ + ″ + *ouron,* urine] An excessive amount of water in the urine.

**polyhypermenorrhea** (pŏl″ē-hī″pĕr-mĕn″ō-rē′ă) [″ + *hyper,* over, + *men,* month, + *rhoia,* flow] Frequent menstruation with excessive discharge.

**polyhypomenorrhea** (pŏl″ē-hī″pō-mĕn″ō-rē′ă) [″ + *hypo,* under, + *men,* month, + *rhoia,* flow] Frequent menstruation with scanty discharge.

**Poly I:C** A complex of synthetic polyriboinosinic and polyribocytidylic acids. They are a form of double-stranded ribonucleic acids that may help to induce resistance to virus infection. Poly I:C stimulates production of interferon.

**polyidrosis** (pŏl″ē-ĭd-rō′sĭs) [″ + *hidrosis,* sweat] Hyperhidrosis.

**polyinfection** (pŏl″ē-ĭn-fĕk′shŭn) [″ + ME. *infecten,* infect] Infection with two or more microorganisms. SYN: *multi-infection.*

**polykaryocyte** (pŏl″ē-kăr′ē-ō-sīt) [″ + *karyon,* nucleus, + *kytos,* cell] A cell possessing several nuclei.

**polylysine** (pŏl″ē-lī′sĭn) A polypeptide in which two lysine molecules are joined by a peptide linkage.

**polymastia** (pŏl″ē-măs′tē-ă) [Gr. *polys,* many, + *mastos,* breast] The condition of having more than two breasts. SYN: *multimammae; polymazia.*

**polymastigote** (pŏl″ē-măs′tĭ-gōt) [″ + *mastix,* whip] Possessing several flagella.

**polymath** Polyhistor.

**polymazia** [″ + *mazos,* breast] Polymastia.

**polymelia** (pŏl″ē-mē′lē-ă) [″ + *melos,* limb] A congenital abnormality in which there are supernumerary limbs.

**polymelus** (pō-lĭm′ĕ-lŭs) [″+ *melos,* limb] One having polymelia.

**polymenorrhea** (pŏl″ē-mĕn-ō-rē′ă) [″ + ″ + *rhoia,* to flow] Menstrual periods occurring with abnormal frequency.

**polymer** (pŏl′ĭ-mĕr) [″ + *meros,* a part] A natural or synthetic substance formed by a combination of two or more molecules (and up to millions) of the same substance.

**polymerase** (pŏl-ĭm′ĕr-ās) An enzyme that catalyzes polymerization of nucleotides to form DNA molecules before cell division, or RNA molecules before protein synthesis.

***p. chain reaction*** ABBR: PCR. A process that permits making, in vitro, unlimited numbers of copies of genes. This is done beginning with a single molecule of the genetic material DNA. One hundred billion similar molecules can be generated within a few hours. The practical importance of this method of investigating genetic material is enormous. Thus, the technique can be used in investigating and diagnosing bacterial diseases, viruses associated with cancer, genetic diseases such as diabetes mellitus, human immunodeficiency virus (HIV), pemphigus vulgaris, and various diseases of the blood (e.g., sickle cell anemia) and of muscles.

***RNA p.*** Transcriptase.

**polymer fume fever** Condition resulting from breathing fumes produced by certain polymers when they are heated to 300° to 700°C or higher. Symptoms include a tight gripping sensation of the chest associated with shivering, sore throat, fever, and weakness. Treatment consists of discontinuance of exposure to fumes. SEE: *metal fume fever.*

**polymeria** (pŏl-ĭ-mē′rē-ă) The condition of having more than normal number of parts. SYN: *polymerism.*

**polymeric** (pŏl″ĭ-mĕr′ĭk) **1.** Having the characteristics of a polymer. **2.** Muscles derived from more than one myotome.

**polymerid** (pō-lĭm′ĕr-ĭd) A polymer.

**polymerism** (pŏl′ĭ-mĕr″ĭzm, pō-lĭm′ĕr-ĭzm) [″ + *meros,* part, + *-ismos,* condition] Polymeria.

**polymerization** (pŏl″ĭ-mĕr″ĭ-zā′shŭn) The process of changing a simple chemical substance or substances into another compound having the same elements usually in the same proportions but with a higher molecular weight.

**polymerize** (pŏl′ĭ-mĕr-īz) To cause polymerization.

**polymicrobial** (pŏl″ē-mī-krō′bē-ăl) [Gr. *polys,* many, + *mikros,* small, + *bios,* life] Concerning a number of species of microorganisms.

**polymicrobic infections** Bacterial infections caused by two or more different microorganisms.

**polymicrogyria** (pŏl″ē-mī″krō-jī′rē-ă) [″ + ″ + *gyros,* convolution] A malformed brain in which multiple small convolutions have developed.

**polymorph** (pŏl′ē-morf) [″ + *morphe,* form] A polymorphonuclear leukocyte.

**polymorphic** Occurring in more than one form. SYN: *multiform; polymorphous.*

**polymorphism** [″ + *morphe,* form, + *-ismos,* condition] **1.** The property of crystallizing into two or more different forms. **2.** The occurrence of more than one form in a life cycle. SYN: *pleomorphism.*

**polymorphocellular** (pŏl″ē-mor″fō-sĕl′ū-lăr) [″ + ″ + L. *cellula,* a small chamber] Composed of cells of many forms.

**polymorphonuclear** (pŏl″ē-mor″fō-nū′klē-ăr) [″ + ″ + L. *nucleus,* a kernel] Possessing a nucleus consisting of several parts or lobes connected by fine strands.

**polymorphous** (pŏl″ē-mor′fŭs) Polymorphic.

**polymyalgia arteritica** (pŏl″ē-mī-ăl′jē-ă) [″ + *mys,* muscle, + *algos,* pain] Polymyalgia rheumatica.

**polymyalgia rheumatica** ABBR: PMR. A poorly understood condition almost always found in patients over 50 years of age and found four times more frequently in women than in men. It is marked by the following: pain and weakness in the shoulder muscles and pelvic girdle; marked elevation of erythrocyte sedimentation rate; morning stiffness, and jelling after prolonged sitting; absence of evidence of inflammatory arthritis of any kind; absence of signs of muscle disease such as atrophy, weakness, or fibrillation; and prompt and dramatic response to low doses of corticosteroid therapy. SYN: *polymyalgia arteritica.*

Corticosteroids relieve symptoms and the sedimentation rate approaches normal. Temporal and cranial arteritis may be associated with this disease.

**polymyoclonus** (pŏl″ē-mī-ŏk′lō-nŭs) [″ + ″ + *klonos,* tumult] Paramyoclonus multiplex.

**polymyositis** (pŏl″ē-mī″ō-sī′tĭs) [″ + ″ + *itis,* inflammation] A rare, inflammatory disease of the skeletal muscle tissue characterized by symmetric weakness of proximal muscles of the limbs, neck and pharynx. Some patients have various connective tissue disorders such as rheumatoid arthritis and lupus erythematosus.

TREATMENT: Treatment consists of supportive therapy plus prednisone, which may be needed for years. Prednisone combined with a cytotoxic drug such as azathioprine allows a lower dose of prednisone to be used.

**polymyxin** (pŏl″ē-mĭks′ĭn) One of several closely related antibiotics isolated from various strains of *Bacillus polymyxa* and designated polymyxins A, B, C, D, and E. Most polymyxins cause renal toxicity.

***p. B sulfate*** The least toxic of the antibiotic fractions of polymyxin, and the only one used therapeutically for treating infection.

**polyneural** (pŏl″ē-nū′răl) [″ + *neuron,* nerve, sinew] Pert. to, innervated, or supplied by many nerves.

**polyneuralgia** (pŏl″ē-nū-răl′jē-ă) [″ + ″ + *algos,* pain] Neuralgia in several nerves.

**polyneuritic** (pŏl″ē-nū-rĭt′ĭk) [″ + ″ + *itis,* inflammation] Inflammation of several nerves at once.

**polyneuritis** (pŏl″ē-nū-rī′tĭs) [″ + ″ + *itis,* inflammation] Multiple neuritis.

***acute idiopathic p.*** Guillain-Barré syndrome.

***diabetic p.*** Diabetic polyneuropathy.

***Jamaica ginger p.*** Polyneuritis, esp. of the nerves of the extremities following ingestion of Jamaica ginger beverage. SYN: *Jamaica ginger paralysis.*

***metabolic p.*** Polyneuritis resulting from metabolic disorders such as nutritional deficiency, esp. the lack of thiamine; gastrointestinal disorders; or pathologic conditions such as diabetes, pernicious anemia, and toxemias of pregnancy.

***toxic p.*** Polyneuritis resulting from poisons such as heavy metals, alcohol, carbon monoxide, or various organic compounds.

**polyneuromyositis** (pŏl″ē-nū″rō-mī″ō-sī′tĭs) [″ + ″ + *mys,* muscle, + *itis,* inflammation] A disease in which polyneuritis and polymyositis occur together.

**polyneuropathy** (pŏl″ē-nū-rŏp′ă-thē) [Gr.

*polys,* many, + *neuron,* nerve, sinew, + *pathos,* disease, suffering] Multiple neuritis.

***acute inflammatory p.*** Guillain-Barré syndrome.

***amyloid p.*** Polyneuropathy characterized by deposition of amyloid in nerves.

***chronic inflammatory demyelinating p.*** ABBR: CIDP. A gradually progressing autoimmune muscle weakness in arms and legs caused by inflammation of the myelin sheath covering peripheral nerve axons. Myelin destruction (demyelination) slows or blocks conduction of impulses to muscles. Numbness and paresthesia may accompany or precede loss of motor function, which varies from mild to severe. Other signs include elevated protein levels in the cerebrospinal fluid. The disorder is marked by remissions and exacerbations. The inflammatory damage involves not only phagocytes (neutrophils and macrophages), but also immune complexes and complement activation by myelin autoantigens. Patients are treated with prednisone to suppress the immune response. If prednisone is not effective, a 3-month course of azathioprine is recommended. Plasmapheresis has been used to remove circulating autoantibodies.

***diabetic p.*** The most common disabling chronic complication of diabetes mellitus, affecting up to 50% of patients with either type of diabetes. The neuropathy may be symmetrical or asymmetrical and affects peripheral nerves as well as the autonomic nervous system and cranial nerves. Clinically, neuropathic ulcers may develop, esp. on the feet. Thus, patients should be instructed to examine their feet daily for evidence of trauma, callous formation, and blisters. Treatment is supportive, with emphasis on preventing tissue damage. SYN: *diabetic polyneuritis.*

***porphyric p.*** Polyneuropathy resulting from acute porphyria, characterized by pains and paresthesias in the extremities and by flaccid paralysis.

***progressive hypertrophic p.*** A rare familial disease beginning in childhood and characterized by increased size of peripheral nerves owing to multiplication and hypertrophy of cells of the sheath of Schwann.

**polyneuroradiculitis** (pŏl″ē-nū″rō-ră-dĭk″ū-lī′tĭs) [″ + ″ + *radix,* root, + *itis,* inflammation] Inflammation of the nerve roots, the peripheral nerves, and spinal ganglia.

**polynuclear, polynucleate** (pŏl″ē-nū′klē-ăr, -āt) [″ + L. *nucleus,* a kernel] Possessing more than one nucleus. SYN: *multinuclear; multinucleate.*

**polynucleotidase** (pŏl″ē-nū″klē-ō′tĭ-dās) An enzyme present in intestinal mucosa and intestinal juice that catalyzes the breakdown of nucleic acid to nucleotides.

**polynucleotide** (pŏl″ē-nū′klē-ō-tīd) Nucleic acid composed of two or more nucleotides.

**polyodontia** (pŏl″ē-ō-dŏn′shē-ă) [″ + *odous,* tooth] The state of having supernumerary teeth.

**polyomavirus** (pŏl″ē-ō-mă-vī′rŭs) A virus of the papovavirus family that produces malignancies in lower animals.

**polyonychia** (pŏl″ē-ō-nĭk′ē-ă) [″ + *onyx,* nail] Having supernumerary nails.

**polyopia, polyopsia** (pŏl″ē-ō′pē-ă, -ŏp′sē-ă) [″ + *opsis,* vision] Multiple vision; perception of more than one image of the same object.

**polyorchidism** (pŏl″ē-or′kĭ-dĭzm) [″ + *orchis,* testicle, + *-ismos,* condition] The condition of having more than two testicles.

**polyorchis** (pŏl″ē-or′kĭs) An individual with more than two testicles.

**polyostotic** (pŏl″ē-ŏs-tŏt′ĭk) [″ + *osteon,* bone] Concerning many bones.

**polyotia** (pŏl″ē-ō′shē-ă) [″ + *ous,* ear] The state of having more than two ears.

**polyovulatory** (pŏl″ē-ŏv′ū-lă-tō″rē) [″ + L. *ovulum,* little egg] Releasing several ova in a single ovulatory cycle.

**polyoxyl stearate** (pŏl″ē-ŏks′ĭl) Any of several polyoxyethylene stearates. They have varying lengths of the polymer chain (e.g., polyoxyl 8 stearate and polyoxyl 40 stearate [trade name Myrj 52] have polymer lengths of 8 and 40, respectively). They are nonionic surface-active agents that are useful emulsifiers.

**polyp** (pŏl′ĭp) [Gr. *polypous,* many-footed] A tumor with a pedicle; commonly found in vascular organs such as the nose, uterus, colon, and rectum. Polyps bleed easily; if there is a possibility that they will become malignant, they should be removed surgically. SYN: *polypus.*

***adenomatous p.*** Benign neoplastic tissue originating in the glandular epithelium.

***aural p.*** Polypoid granulation tissue in the external canal of the ear attached to the tympanic membrane or middle ear structures.

***bleeding p.*** An angioma of the nasal mucous membrane.

***cardiac p.*** A pedunculated tumor attached to the inside of the heart. If situated close to a valve, it may cause blockage of the valve intermittently.

***cervical p.*** A fibrous or mucous polyp of the cervical mucosa.

***choanal p.*** A nasal polyp that extends into the pharynx.

***colonic p.*** A polyp of the colon. It is usually benign but may undergo malignant transformation.

***fibrinous p.*** A polyp containing fibrin and blood, located in the uterine cavity.

***fibroepithelial p.*** A smooth-surfaced polyp of the oral mucosa, usually developing after trauma to the area. SEE: *acrochordon.*

***fleshy p.*** A submucous myoma in the uterus.

***gelatinous p.*** **1.** A polyp made up of loose swollen edematous tissue. **2.** A myxoma.

***Hopmann's p.*** A papillary growth of the nasal mucosa.

***hydatid p.*** A cystic polyp.

***juvenile p.*** A benign rounded mucosal hamartoma of the large bowel. This type of polyp may be present in large numbers in infants and are commonly associated with rectal bleeding. SYN: *retention p.*

***laryngeal p.*** A polyp attached to the vocal cords and extending to the air passageway.

***lymphoid p.*** A benign lymphoma of the rectum.

***mucous p.*** A polyp of soft or jelly-like consistency and exhibiting mucoid degeneration.

***placental p.*** A polyp composed of retained placental tissue.

***retention p.*** Juvenile p.

***vascular p.*** A pedunculated angioma.

**polypapilloma** (pŏl″ē-păp″ĭ-lō′mă) [Gr. *polys,* many, + L. *papilla,* nipple, + Gr. *oma,* tumor] Yaws.

**polypectomy** (pŏl″ĭ-pĕk′tō-mē) [″ + *pous,* foot, + *ektome,* excision] The surgical removal of a polyp.

**polypeptidase** (pŏl″ē-pĕp′tĭ-dās) An enzyme that catalyzes the hydrolysis of peptides.

**polypeptide** (pŏl″ē-pĕp′tīd) [″ + *peptein,* to digest] A union of two or more amino acids. SEE: *peptide.*

**polypeptidorrhachia** (pŏl″ē-pĕp″tĭ-dō-ră′kē-ă) [″+ ″+ *rhachis,* spine] The presence of polypeptides in the cerebrospinal fluid.

**polyphagia** (pŏl″ē-fā′jē-ă) [Gr. *polys,* many, + *phagein,* to eat] Eating abnormally large amounts of food; gluttony.

**polyphalangism** (pŏl″ē-fă-lăn′jĭzm) [″ + *phalanx,* closely knit row, + *-ismos,* condition] Hyperphalangism.

**polypharmacy** (pŏl″ē-făr′mă-sē) [″ + *pharmakon,* drug] **1.** Multiple drug therapy in which there is concurrent use of a number of drugs. In many illnesses, this is unavoidable and apt to happen when a patient is in the care of a number of physicians who are unaware of what medicines have been prescribed by the others. This situation is esp. liable to occur when the elderly with multiple diseases and complaints are treated by several physicians. In addition the patient may forget to inform each of the treating physicians about the over-the-counter drugs and herbal extracts he or she is using. For several reasons, including increased chance of medication errors and adverse drug interactions, the health and welfare of the patient may be in danger as long as polypharmacy continues. Any person taking more than one drug should keep a careful record of all of the drugs being taken, how often they are taken, and by whom they were prescribed, and share that information with all health care providers. The information on the patient's chart should be shown at each office visit to all of those involved in administering medicines to the patient. **2.** Excessive use of drugs.

**polyphenoloxidase** (pŏl″ē-fē″nŏl-ŏk′sĭ-dās) An enzyme present in bacteria, fungi, and some plants that catalyzes the oxidation of polyphenols, but not monophenols such as tyrosine, to quinones.

**polyphobia** (pŏl″ē-fō′bē-ă) [Gr. *polys,* many, + *phobos,* fear] Excessive or abnormal fear of a number of things.

**polyphrasia** (pŏl″ē-frā′zē-ă) [″ + *phrasis,* speech] Excessive talkativeness, a manifestation of mental illness.

**polyphyletic** (pŏl″ē-fī-lĕt′ĭk) [″ + *phyle,* tribe] Having more than one origin; opposite of monophyletic.

**polyphyodont** (pŏl″ē-fī′ō-dŏnt) [″ + *phyein,* to produce, + *odous,* tooth] Developing more than two sets of teeth at intervals during a lifetime.

**polypiform** (pō-lĭp′ĭ-form) [″ + *pous,* foot, + L. *forma,* form] Resembling a polyp.

**polyplastic** (pŏl″ē-plăs′tĭk) [″ + *plastos,* formed] **1.** Having had many evolutionary modifications. **2.** Having many substances in the cellular composition.

**polyplegia** (pŏl″ē-plē′jē-ă) [″ + *plege,* stroke] Paralysis affecting several muscles.

**polyploid** (pŏl′ē-ployd) **1.** Characterized by polyploidy. **2.** An individual in which the chromosome number is two or more times the normal haploid number.

**polyploidy** (pŏl′ē-ploy″dē) A condition in which the chromosome number is two or more times the normal haploid number found in gametes.

**polypnea** (pŏl″ĭp-nē′ă) [″ + *pnoia,* breath] Panting.

**polypodia** (pŏl″ē-pō′dē-ă) [″+ *pous,* foot] Possession of more than the normal number of feet.

**polypoid** (pŏl′ē-poyd) [″+ ″+ *eidos,* form, shape] Like a polyp.

**polyporous** (pŏl-ĭp′ō-rŭs) [″ + *poros,* pore] Possessing many small openings or pores.

**polyposia** (pŏl″ē-pō′zē-ă) [″ + *posis,* drinking] The sustained ingestion of large amounts of fluid.

**polyposis** (pŏl″ē-pō′sĭs) [″ + *pous,* foot, + *osis,* condition] The presence of numerous polyps.

***p. coli*** Polyposis of the large intestine.

***familial p.*** A rare familial condition in which the mucosa of the colon is covered with polyps. This causes rectal bleeding and the passage of polyps that come loose. These may become infected and cause chronic intussusception of the colon. The polyps may become malignant.

***multiple intestinal p.*** Polyps or tumors that are derived from mucous membrane and are scattered throughout the intestine and rectum. They may undergo degeneration.

***p. ventriculi*** The presence of numerous polyps in the stomach, sometimes involving the entire mucosa, accompanied by chronic atrophic gastritis.

**polypotrite** (pō-lĭp′ō-trīt) [″ + ″ + L. *terere,* to crush] A device for crushing polyps.

**polyptychial** (pŏl″ē-tī′kē-ăl) [″ + *ptyche,* fold] Arranged in several layers, as is the case in some glands.

**polypus** (pŏl′ĭ-pŭs) *pl.* **polypi** [L.] A polyp.

**polyradiculitis** (pŏl″ē-ră-dĭk′ū-lī′tĭs) [″ + L. *radix,* root, + Gr. *itis,* inflammation] Inflammation of nerve roots, esp. the roots of spinal nerves. SEE: *Nursing Diagnoses Appendix.*

**polyradiculoneuritis** (pŏl″ē-ră-dĭk″ū-lō-nū-rī′tĭs) [″ + ″ + Gr. *neuron,* nerve, + *itis,* inflammation] Inflammation of the peripheral nerves and spinal ganglia.

**polyradiculopathy, acute inflammatory** Guillain-Barré syndrome.

**polyribosome** (pŏl″ē-rī′bō-sōm) A cluster or group of ribosomes. They are the site of attachment for mRNA in the cytoplasm and the translation of genetic information into the synthesis of specific proteins. SYN: *polysome.*

**polyrrhea, polyrrhoea** (pōl″ē-rē′ă) [″ + *rhoia,* flow] The excessive secretion of fluid.

**polysaccharide** (pŏl″ē-săk′ă-rīd) [″ + Sanskrit *sarkara,* sugar] One of a group of carbohydrates that, upon hydrolysis, yield more than 20 monosaccharide molecules. They are complex carbohydrates of high molecular weight, usually insoluble in water, but when soluble, they form colloidal solutions. Their basic formula is $(C_6H_{12}O_6)_n$. They include two groups: starch (e.g., starch, inulin, glycogen, dextrin) and cellulose (e.g., cellulose and hemicelluloses). The hemicelluloses include the pentosans (e.g., gum arabic), hexosans (e.g., agar-agar), and hexopentosans (e.g., pectin). SEE: *carbohydrates; disaccharide; monosaccharide.*

***immune p.'s*** Polysaccharides in bacteria, esp. in the cell wall, that are antigenic.

**polysaccharose** (pŏl″ē-săk′ă-rōs) A polysaccharide.

**polyscelia** (pŏl″ē-sē′lē-ă) [″ + *skelos,* leg] The condition of having more than the normal number of legs.

**polyscelus** (pŏ-lĭs′ĕ-lŭs) One having polyscelia.

**polyserositis** (pŏl″ē-sē-rō-sī′tĭs) [″ + L. *serum,* whey, + *itis,* inflammation] Inflammation of several serous membranes simultaneously. SYN: *Concato's disease.*

***recurrent p.*** Familial Mediterranean fever.

**polysinusitis, polysinuitis** (pŏl″ē-sī″nŭs-ī′tĭs, -nū-ī′tĭs) [″ + L. *sinus,* a hollow, + Gr. *itis,* inflammation] Inflammation of several sinuses simultaneously.

**polysomaty** (pŏl″ē-sō′mă-tē) [″ + *soma,* body] Having reduplicated chromatin in the nucleus.

**polysome** Polyribosome.

**polysomia** (pŏl″ē-sō′mē-ă) [″+ *soma,* body] Having more than one body, as in the doubling of the body of a fetus.

**polysomnography** Continuous measurement and recording of physiological activity during sleep.

**polysorbates** (pŏl″ē-sor′bāts) Nonionic surface-active agents composed of polyoxyethylene esters of sorbitol. They usually contain associated fatty acids. The series includes polysorbates 20, 40, 60, and 80, which are used in preparing pharmaceuticals. These polysorbates have the trade names of Tween 20, Tween 40, and so forth.

**polyspermia** (pŏl″ē-spĕr′mē-ă) [Gr. *polys,* many, + *sperma,* seed] **1.** The excessive secretion of seminal fluid. **2.** The entrance of several spermatozoa into one ovum. SYN: *polyspermism.*

**polyspermism** (pŏl″ē-spĕrm′ĭzm) Polyspermia.

**polyspermy** (pŏl″ē-spĕr′mē) The fertilization of an ovum by multiple spermatozoa.

**polystichia** (pŏl″ē-stĭk′ē-ă) [″ + *stichos,* a row] A condition in which there are two or more rows of eyelashes.

**polystomatous** (pŏl″ē-stō′mă-tŭs) [″+ *stoma,* mouth] Possessing many mouths or openings.

**polystyrene** (pŏl″ē-stī′rēn) A synthetic resin produced by the polymerization of styrene from ethylene and benzene. The formula is $(CH_2CHC_6H_5)_n$. It is used in the plastics industry.

**polysynaptic** (pŏl″ē-sī-năp′tĭk) [″ + *synapsis,* point of contact] Pert. to nerve pathways involving multiple synapses.

**polysyndactyly** (pŏl″ē-sĭn-dăk′tĭl-ē) [″ + *syn,* together, + *daktylos,* finger] Multiple syndactyly.

**polytendinitis** (pŏl″ē-tĕn″dĭ-nī′tĭs) [″ + L. *tendo,* tendon, + Gr. *itis,* inflammation] Inflammation of several tendons.

**polytene** (pŏl′ĕ-tēn) [″ + *tainia,* band] Composed of many filaments of chromatin.

**polyteny** (pŏl″ĕ-tē′nē) [″ + *tainia,* band] Multiple lateral duplication of the chromosome. This produces a giant chromosome.

**polytetrafluoroethylene** ABBR: PTFE. A synthetic polymer that has slippery, nonsticking properties. It is used in a variety of products, including frying pan coatings and, in manufacturing, the fabric known by its trade name, Gore-Tex. The expanded form has the property of becoming "fatter" when it is stretched, rather than thinner. Trade name is Teflon.

**polythelia** (pŏl″ē-thē′lē-ă) [″ + *thele,* nipple, + *-ismos,* condition] The presence of more than one nipple on a mamma.

**polythiazide** (pŏl″ē-thī′ă-zīd) A diuretic drug.

**polytrichia** (pŏl″ē-trĭk′ē-ă) [″ + *thrix,* hair] Hypertrichosis.

**polytrichosis** (pŏl″ē-trĭ-kō′sĭs) [″ + ″ + *osis,* condition] Hypertrichosis.

**polytropic** (pŏl″ē-trŏp′ĭk) [″ + *trope,* a turning] Affecting more than one type of cell, said of viruses, or affecting more than one type of tissue, said of certain poisons.

**polyunguia** (pŏl″ē-ŭng′gwē-ă) [″ + L. *unguis,* nail] Polyonychia.

**polyunsaturated** In chemistry, relating to long-chain carbon compounds, esp. fats that have many carbon atoms joined by double or triple bonds.

**polyuria** (pŏl″ē-ū′rē-ă) [″ + *ouron,* urine] Excessive secretion and discharge of urine. The urine does not, as a rule, contain abnormal constituents. Several liters in excess of normal may be voided each day. The urine is virtually colorless. Specific gravity is 1.000 to 1.002 and higher in diabetes. Polyuria occurs in diabetes insipidus; diabetes mellitus; chronic nephritis; nephrosclerosis; hyperthyroidism; following edematous states, esp. those induced by heart failure treated with diuretics; and following excessive intake of liquids.

**polyvalent** (pŏl″ē-vā′lĕnt, pō-lĭv′ă-lĕnt) [″ + L. *valere,* to be strong] Multivalent; having a combining power of more than two atoms of hydrogen.

**polyvinyl alcohol** (pŏl″ē-vī′nĭl) A water-soluble synthetic resin used in preparing medicines, esp. ophthalmic solutions.

**polyvinyl chloride** ABBR: PVC. A thermoplastic polymer formed from vinyl chloride, used in the manufacture of many products such as rainwear, garden hoses, and floor tiles.

NOTE: Exposure to toxic fumes of PVC can cause respiratory arrest owing to oxygen deprivation. The reaction to PVC is delayed for 6 to 24 hr after exposure. Patients with suspected exposure should be closely monitored.

**polyvinylpyrrolidone** (pŏl″ē-vī″nĭl-pĕr-rŏl′ĭ-dōn) ABBR: PVP. Previously used name for povidone.

**pomatum** (pō-mā′tŭm) A medicinal ointment, esp. one used on the hair.

**Pompe's disease** Glycogen storage disease type II.

**pompholyx** Deep-seated vesicles of the hands and feet, esp. the palms and soles. The condition may be chronic and produce itching. The cause is unknown, but it may be associated with contact allergy or a fungal infection. This condition is treated with cortisone combined with diiodohydroxyquin ointment applied under an occlusive dressing, which is worn at night. Although pompholyx is often considered to be due to dyshidrosis, sweating may be normal, decreased, or increased. SEE: illus.; *hyperhidrosis.*

**pomphus** (pŏm′fŭs) *pl.* **pomphi** [L.] A blister or a circumscribed elevation on the skin; a wheal.

**POMR** *problem-oriented medical record.*

**pomum** (pō′mŭm) [L.] An apple.

***p. adami*** A prominence in the middle line of the throat, caused by junction of two lateral wings of the thyroid cartilage. SYN: *Adam's apple.*

**ponderal** (pŏn′dĕr-ăl) [L. *pondus,* weight] Relating to weight.

**ponderal index** The ratio of an individual's height to the cube root of his or her weight; used to determine body mass. SEE: *Quatelet index.*

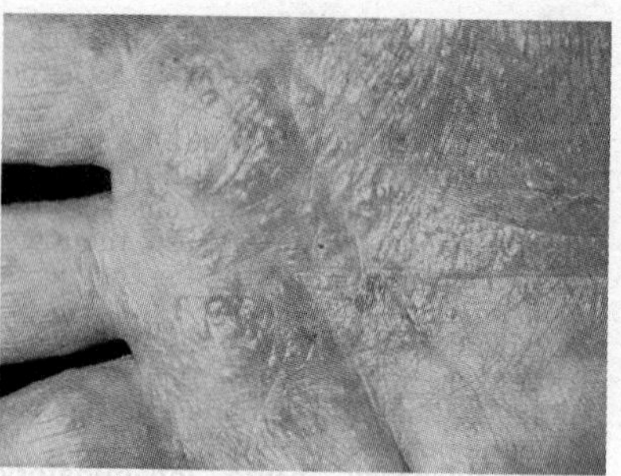

POMPHOLYX

**ponophobia** (pŏ″nō-fō′bē-ă) [Gr. *ponos,* pain, + *phobos,* fear] **1.** An abnormal distaste for exerting oneself. **2.** A dread of pain.

**pons** (pŏnz) *pl.* **pontes** [L., bridge] **1.** A process of tissue connecting two or more parts. **2.** P. varolii.

***p. cerebelli*** P. varolii.

***p. hepatis*** The part of the liver sometimes present that extends from the quadrate lobe to the left lobe across the umbilical fissure.

***p. varolii*** A rounded eminence on the ventral surface of the brain stem. It lies between the medulla and cerebral peduncles, and appears externally as a broad band of transverse fibers. It is connected to the cerebellum by the midcerebellar peduncle, or brachium pontis. It contains fiber tracts connecting the medulla oblongata and cerebellum with the upper portions of the brain, and contains two respiratory centers that work with those in the medulla.The origins of the abducens, facial, trigeminal, and cochlear divisions of the eighth (vestibulocochlear) nerve are at the borders of the pons. SYN: *pons* (2); *p. cerebelli.*

**pontic** (pŏn′tĭk) [L. *pons, pontis,* bridge] An artificial tooth set in a bridge.

**pontile** (pŏn′tēl) Pert. to the pons varolii.

**pontile nuclei** The gray matter in the pons.

**pontine** (pŏn′tēn) Pert. to the pons varolii.

**pontobulbar** (pŏn″tō-bŭl′bar) Pert. to the pons and medulla oblongata.

**Pontocaine Hydrochloride** (pŏn′tō-kān) Trade name for tetracaine hydrochloride; available in several forms for use as a topical or spinal anesthetic.

**pool 1.** To mix blood from several donors. **2.** The accumulation of blood in a body site.

***abdominal p.*** The accumulation of blood in the visceral organs of the abdominal cavity. This may occur during shock.

***amino acid p.*** A variety of amino acids stored in the liver and awaiting protein synthesis.

***gene p.*** The sum of the genetic material in the members of a specified population.

***metabolic p.*** All of the chemical compounds included in metabolic processes in the body.

***vaginal p.*** The mucus and cells that are present in the posterior fornix of the vagina when the patient is in a supine position. Material obtained from this site is used in cancer detection and in evaluating the character of the vaginal fluid in investigating infertility problems.

**poples** (pŏp′lēz) [L., ham of the knee] The popliteal or posterior region of the knee.

**popliteus** (pŏp-lĭt′ē-ŭs, -lĭt-ē′ŭs) [L. *poples,* ham of the knee] Muscle located in hind part of the knee joint that flexes the leg and aids it in rotating. SEE: *Muscles Appendix.* **popliteal** (pŏp″lĭt-ē′ăl, pŏp-lĭt′ē-ăl), *adj.*

**poppy** Any of the several plants of the genus *Papaver.* Opium is obtained from the juice of the unripe pods of *Papaver somniferum.*

**POR** *problem-oriented record.*

**poradenitis** (por″ăd-ĕ-nī′tĭs) [Gr. *poros,* passage, + *aden,* gland, + *itis,* inflammation] The formation of small abscesses in the iliac glands.

**porcelain** (por′sĕ-lĭn) A hard, translucent ceramic made by fusing clay and colored by glazing with fusible pigments. It is used in dentistry.

**porcelaneous, porcelanous** (por″sĕ-lā′nē-ŭs, -sĕl′ăn-ŭs) [Fr. *porcelaine*] Translucent or white like porcelain, as the skin.

**porcine** (por′sīn) [L. *porcus,* pig] Relating to or concerning swine.

**pore** (por) [Gr. *poros,* passage.] **1.** A minute opening, esp. one on an epithelial surface. SYN: *porus.* **2.** The opening of the secretory duct of a sweat gland. SEE: *skin; stoma; sweat glands.*

***alveolar p.*** A minute opening that is thought to exist between adjacent alveoli of the lung.

***gustatory p.*** Taste p.

***taste p.*** The external opening of a taste bud. SYN: *gustatory p.* SEE: *taste.*

**porencephalia, porencephaly** (por″ĕn-sĕf-ā′lē-ă, por″ĕn-sĕf′ă-lē) [″ + *enkephalos,* brain] An anomalous condition in which the ventricles of the brain are connected with the subarachnoid space.

**porencephalitis** (por″ĕn-sĕf″ă-lī′tĭs) [″ + ″ + *itis,* inflammation] Inflammation of the brain with development of cavities communicating with the subarachnoid space.

**pores of Kohn** [Hans Kohn, Ger. pathologist, b. 1866] A passageway for gas from one alveolus of the lung to an adjacent one. These may be of assistance in preventing atelectasis.

**pori** Pl. of porus.

**poriomania** [Gr. *poreia,* walking, + *mania,* madness] The morbid desire to wander from home.

**porion** (pō′rē-ŏn) [Gr. *poros,* passage] The midpoint of the upper margin of the auditory meatus.

**porocele** (pō′rō-sēl) [Gr. *poros,* passage, + *kele,* tumor, swelling] A herniation into the scrotal sac. This causes hardening and thickening of the scrotum.

**porocephaliasis, porocephalosis** (pō″rō-sĕf″ă-lī′ă-sĭs, -lō′sĭs) [″ + *kephale,* head, + *-iasis,* state or condition of] Infection with a species of *Porocephalus.*

**Porocephalus** (pō″rō-sĕf′ă-lŭs) A genus of wormlike arthropods found commonly in snakes. The young sometimes infest mammals, including humans.

**porokeratosis** (pō″rō-kĕr″ă-tō′sĭs) [″ + *keras,* horn, + *osis,* condition] A rare skin disease marked by thickening of the stratum corneum in a linear arrangement, followed by its atrophy. Porokeratosis appears on smooth areas. It is irregular in form and size with a circumscribed outline and affects the hands and feet, forearms and legs, the face, neck, and scalp.

**poroma** (pō-rō′mă) [Gr.] **1.** A callosity. **2.** A tumor of cells lining the opening of the sweat glands.

***cerebral p.*** At postmortem examination, the presence of cavities in the brain substance caused by gas-forming bacteria.

***eccrine p.*** A tumor arising from the duct of an eccrine gland; usually occurring on the palm or sole.

**porosis** (pō-rō′sĭs) [Gr. *poros,* passage, + *osis,* condition] Callus formation in repair of fractured bone. SEE: *callus.*

**porosity** (pō-rŏs′ĭ-tē) [Gr. *poros,* passage] The state of being porous.

**porous** (pō′rŭs) Full of pores; able to admit passage of a liquid.

**porphin** (por′fĭn) The basic ring structure forming the framework of all porphyrins. Consisting of four pyrrole rings united by methene couplings.

**porphobilinogen** (por″fō-bī-lĭn′ō-jĕn) An intermediate product in heme synthesis sometimes found in the urine of patients with acute porphyria. The urine may appear normal when fresh but will change to a burgundy wine color or even to black when heated with dilute hydrochloric acid to 100°C.

**porphyria** (por-fī′rē-ă, por-fĭr′ē-ă) [Gr. *porphyra,* purple] A group of disorders that result from a disturbance in porphyrin metabolism, causing increased formation and excretion of porphyrin or its precursors.

***acute intermittent p.*** A rare metabolic disorder inherited as an autosomal dominant trait. It is characterized by excessive excretion of porphyrins, acute abdominal pain, sensitivity to light, and neurological disturbances. The disorder is sometimes precipitated by the excessive use of sulfonamides, barbiturates, or other drugs.

***congenital erythropoietic p.*** A rare condition inherited as an autosomal recessive trait. It is characterized by severe skin lesions, hemolytic anemia, and splenomegaly.

***p. cutanea tarda hereditaria*** Porphyria

inherited as an autosomal dominant characteristic. The onset of symptoms usually occurs between the ages of 10 and 30.

***p. erythropoietica*** A mild form of porphyria characterized by cutaneous lesions and excess protoporphyrin in the erythrocytes and feces.

***p. hepatica*** Porphyria caused by a disturbance in liver metabolism such as occurs following hepatitis, poisoning by heavy metals, certain anemias, and other conditions.

***South African genetic p.*** Variegate p.

***variegate p.*** A form of hepatic porphyria in which there are recurrent episodes of abdominal pain and neuropathy. The skin is esp. fragile. SYN: *South African genetic p.*

**porphyrin** (por′fĭ-rĭn) [Gr. *porphyra,* purple] Any of a group of nitrogen-containing organic compounds that occur in protoplasm and form the basis of animal and plant respiratory pigments; obtained from hemoglobin and chlorophyll.

**porphyrinuria** (por″fĭ-rĭ-nū′rē-ă) [″ + *ouron,* urine] Excretion of an increased amount of porphyrin in the urine. SYN: *porphyruria.*

**porphyruria** (por″fĭr-ū′rē-ă) [″ + *ouron,* urine] Porphyrinuria.

**Porro's operation** (por′ōz) [Eduardo Porro, It. obstetrician, 1842–1902] Cesarean section followed by removal of the uterus, the ovaries, and fallopian tubes. SYN: *cesarean hysterectomy.*

**PORT** *patient outcomes research team.*

**porta** [L., gate] The point of entry of nerves and vessels into an organ or part.

***p. hepatis*** The fissure of the liver where the portal vein and hepatic artery enter and the hepatic duct leaves.

***p. lienis*** The hilus of the spleen where vessels enter and leave.

***p. pulmonis*** A pulmonary hilus for the entry and exit of the bronchi, nerves, and vessels.

***p. renis*** The hilus of the kidney; the site of entry and exit of vessels. SYN: *hilum renalis.*

**portacaval** (por″tă-kā′văl) Concerning the portal vein and the vena cava.

**portal** [L. *porta,* gate] **1.** An entryway. **2.** Concerning a porta or entrance to an organ, esp. that through which the blood is carried to the liver.

***p. of entry*** The avenue by which infectious organisms gain access to the body.

***p. of exit*** The pathway by which pathogens leave the body of a host (e.g., respiratory droplets, feces, urine, blood).

***intestinal p.*** The opening of the midgut or yolk sac into the foregut or hindgut of an embryo.

***p. vein*** Vein formed by the veins of the splanchnic area that conveys its blood into the liver. It is made of the combined superior and inferior mesenteric, splenic, gastric, and cystic veins.

**portio** (por′shē-ō) *pl.* **portiones** [L.] A part. In anatomy, it designates a certain portion of a structure or organ.

***p. dura*** The facial nerve.

***p. intermedia*** Nervus intermedius.

***p. vaginalis*** The part of the cervix within the vagina.

**portoenterostomy, hepatic** A surgical procedure performed to establish bile flow in an infant who has external biliary atresia associated with absence of the extrahepatic biliary system. A section of the jejunum is attached to the liver at the normal exit site of the hepatic duct to allow bile drainage into the small intestine. The jejunal segment may be looped to form a cutaneous double-barreled ostomy. Postoperatively, liver function continues to deteriorate in most children, and liver transplantation is often needed. SYN: *Kasai procedure.*

**portogram** (por′tō-grăm) [L. *porta,* gate, + Gr. *gramma,* something written] A radiograph of the portal vein after injection of a contrast medium.

**portography** (por-tŏg′ră-fē) [″ + Gr. *graphein,* to write] Radiography of the portal vein after injection of a radiopaque contrast medium.

***portal p.*** Portography after injection of opaque material into the superior mesenteric vein. This is usually done during laparotomy.

***splenic p.*** Radiography of the splenic and portal veins after injection of a contrast medium into the splenic artery.

**portosystemic** (por″tō-sĭs-tĕm′ĭk) Joining the portal and systemic venous circulation.

**Portuguese man-of-war** A type of jellyfish, *Physalia physalis,* whose tentacles contain a neurotoxin that produces a burning sensation on contact. SEE: *bite.*

**port-wine stain** Nevus flammeus.

**porus** (pō′rŭs) *pl.* **pori** [L.] A meatus or foramen; a tiny aperture in a structure; a pore.

***p. acusticus externus*** The outer opening of the external acoustic meatus.

***p. acusticus internus*** The opening of the internal acoustic meatus into the cranial cavity.

***p. gustatorius*** The small taste pore openings in the taste buds of the tongue.

***p. lactiferous*** The opening of a lactiferous duct on the tip of the nipple of the mammary gland.

***p. opticus*** The opening in the center of the optic disk through which retinal vessels (central artery and vein) reach the retina through the lamina cribrosa of the sclera.

***p. sudoriferus*** The opening of a sweat gland.

**position** (pō-zĭsh′ŭn) [L. *positio*] **1.** The place or arrangement in which a thing is put. **2.** The manner in which a body is arranged, as by the nurse or physician for examination. **3.** In obstetrics, the relationship of a selected fetal landmark to the maternal front or back, and on the right or left side. SEE: table; *presentation* for illus.

***anatomical p.*** The position assumed when a person is standing erect with arms at the sides, palms forward. SYN: *orthograde p.*

***anteroposterior p.*** A radiographical examination position in which the central ray enters the front of the body and exits from the back.

***axial p.*** A radiographical examination position in which an image is obtained with the central ray entering the body at an angle.

***Bonnet's p.*** In inflammation of the hip joint, the flexion, abduction, and outward rotation of the thigh, which produces relief.

***Bozeman's p.*** The knee-elbow position in which the patient is strapped to supports.

***Brickner p.*** A method of obtaining traction, abduction, and external rotation of the shoulder by tying the patient's wrists to the head of the bed.

***centric p.*** The most posterior position of the mandible in relation to the maxilla.

***decubitus p.*** The position of the patient on a flat surface. The exact position is indicated by which surface of the body is closest to the flat surface (i.e., in left or right lateral decubitus, the patient is flat on the left or right side, respectively; in dorsal or ventral decubitus, the patient is on the back or abdomen, respectively).

***dorsal p.*** A position in which the patient lies on the back. SYN: *supine.*

***dorsal elevated p.*** A position in which the patient lies on the back with the head and shoulders elevated at an angle of 30° or more. It is employed in digital examination of genitalia and in bimanual examination of the vagina.

***dorsal recumbent p.*** A position in which the patient lies on the back with the lower extremities moderately flexed and rotated outward. It is employed in the application of obstetrical forceps, repair of lesions following parturition, vaginal examination, and bimanual palpation. SEE: illus.

***dorsosacral p.*** Lithotomy p. SEE: *dorsal recumbent p.* for illus.

***Edebohls' p.*** Simon's position.

***Elliot's p.*** A position in which supports are placed under the small of the patient's back so that the patient is in a posture resembling a double inclined plane.

***en face p.*** In obstetrics, a position in which the mother and infant are face to face. This position encourages eye contact and is conducive to attachment.

***English p.*** Left lateral recumbent p.

***fetal p.*** The relationship of a specified bony landmark on the fetal presenting part to the quadrants of the maternal pelvis.

***Fowler's p.*** SEE: *dorsal recumbent p.* for illus.; *Fowler's position.*

***genucubital p.*** A position with the patient on the knees, thighs upright, body resting on elbows, head down on hands. Employed when it is not possible to use the classic knee-chest position. SYN: *knee-elbow position.*

***genupectoral p.*** A position with the patient on the knees, thighs upright, the head and upper part of the chest resting on the table, arms crossed above the head. It is employed in displacement of a prolapsed fundus, dislodgment of the impacted head of a fetus, management of transverse presentation, replacement of a retroverted uterus or displaced ovary, or flushing of the intestinal canal. SYN: *knee-chest p.* SEE: *dorsal recumbent p.* for illus.

***horizontal p.*** A position in which the patient lies supine with feet extended. It is used in palpation, in auscultation of fetal heart, and in operative procedures.

***horizontal abdominal p.*** A position in which the patient lies flat on the abdomen, feet extended; employed in examination of the back and spinal column.

***jackknife p.*** A position in which the patient lies on the back, shoulders elevated,

## Positions of Fetus in Utero

| | |
|---|---|
| **Vertex Presentation (point of designation – occiput)** | |
| Left occiput anterior | LOA |
| Right occiput posterior | ROP |
| Right occiput anterior | ROA |
| Left occiput posterior | LOP |
| Right occiput posterior | ROT |
| Occiput anterior | OA |
| Occiput posterior | OP |
| **Breech Presentation (point of designation – sacrum)** | |
| Left sacroanterior | LSA |
| Right sacroposterior | RSP |
| Right sacroanterior | RSA |
| Left sacroposterior | LSP |
| Sacroanterior | SA |
| Sacroposterior | SP |
| Left sacrotransverse | LST |
| Right sacrotransverse | RST |
| **Face Presentation (point of designation – chin [mentum])** | |
| Left mentoanterior | LMA |
| Right mentoposterior | RMP |
| Right mentoanterior | RMA |
| Left mentoposterior | LMP |
| Mentoposterior | MP |
| Mentoanterior | MA |
| Left mentotransverse | LMT |
| Right mentotransverse | RMT |
| **Transverse Presentation (point of designation – scapula of presenting shoulder)** | |
| Left acromiodorso-anterior | LADA |
| Right acromiodorso-posterior | RADP |
| Right acromiodorso-anterior | RADA |
| Left acromiodorso-posterior | LADP |

POSITIONS

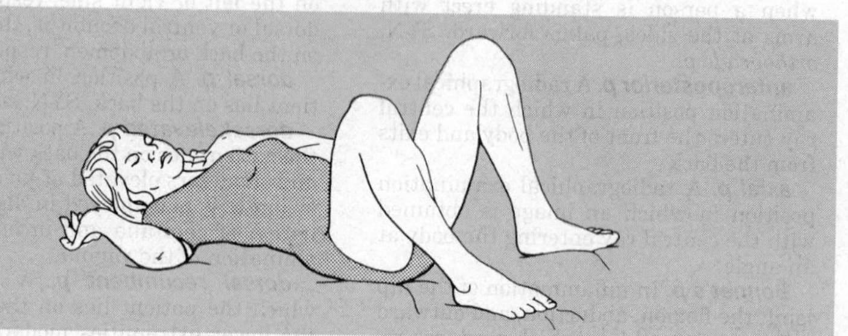
DORSAL RECUMBENT POSITION

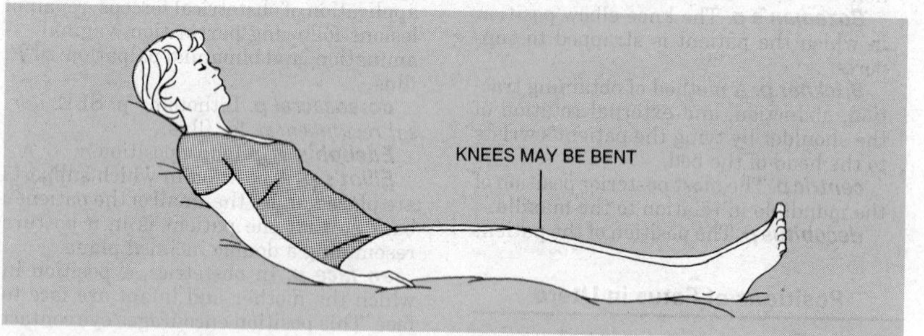

FOWLER'S POSITION

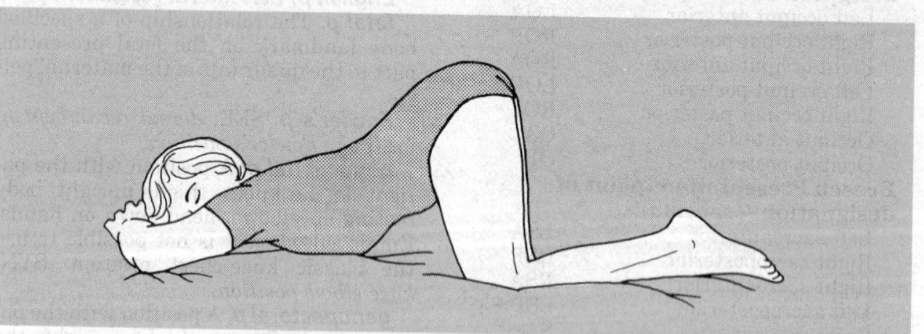
KNEE-CHEST OR GENUPECTORAL POSITION

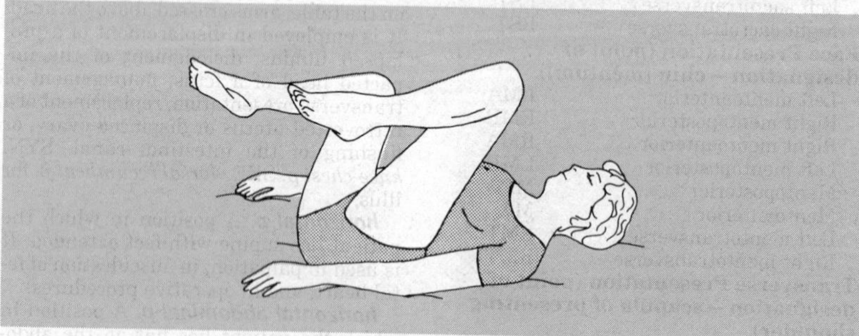
LITHOTOMY OR DORSOSACRAL POSITION

POSITIONS

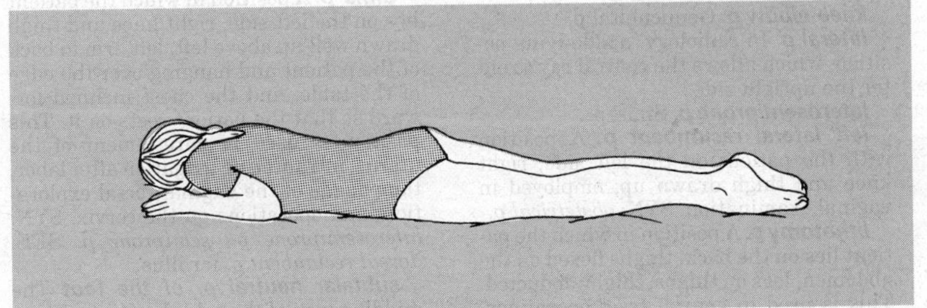

PRONE POSITION

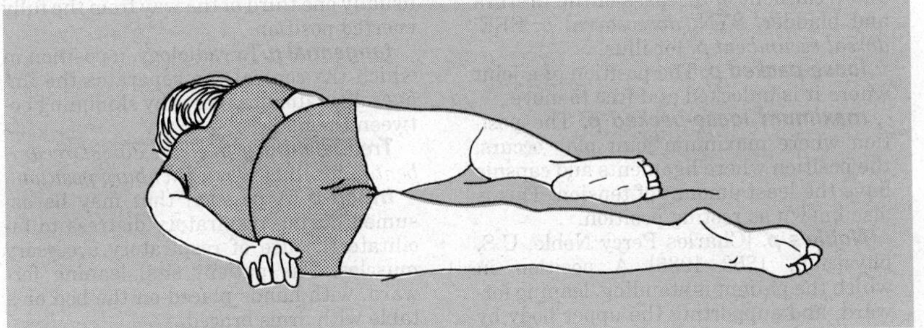

SIMS' POSITION

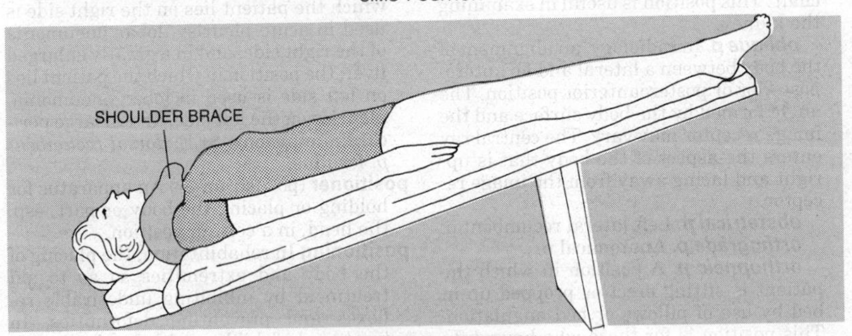


TRENDELENBURG POSITION

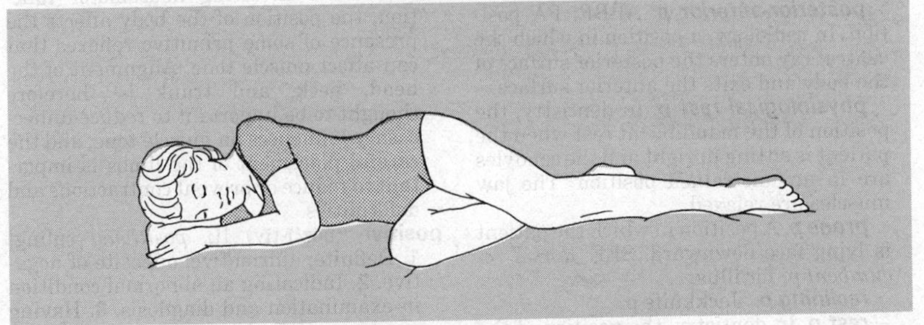

RIGHT LATERAL RECUMBENT POSITION

legs flexed on thighs, thighs at right angles to the abdomen. It is employed when passing urethral sound. SYN: *reclining p.*

***knee-chest p.*** Genupectoral p. SEE: *dorsal recumbent p.* for illus.

***knee-elbow p.*** Genucubital p.

***lateral p.*** In radiology, a side-lying position, which allows the central ray to enter the upright side.

***laterosemiprone p.*** Sims' p.

***left lateral recumbent p.*** A position with the patient on the left side, right knee and thigh drawn up; employed in vaginal examination. SYN: *obstetrical p.*

***lithotomy p.*** A position in which the patient lies on the back, thighs flexed on the abdomen, legs on thighs, thighs abducted. This is used in genital tract operations, vaginal hysterectomy, and the diagnosis and treatment of diseases of the urethra and bladder. SYN: *dorsosacral p.* SEE: *dorsal recumbent p.* for illus.

***loose-packed p.*** The position of a joint where it is unlocked and free to move.

***maximum loose-packed p.*** The position where maximum joint play occurs; the position where ligaments and capsule have the least amount of tension. This is also known as resting position.

***Noble's p.*** [Charles Percy Noble, U.S. physician, 1863–1935] A position in which the patient is standing, leaning forward, and supporting the upper body by bracing the arms against the wall or a chair. This position is useful in examining the kidney.

***oblique p.*** In radiology, an alignment of the body between a lateral and an anteroposterior or posteroanterior position. The angle formed by the body surface and the image receptor may vary. The central ray enters the aspect of the body that is upright and facing away from the image receptor.

***obstetrical p.*** Left lateral recumbent p.

***orthograde p.*** Anatomical p.

***orthopneic p.*** A position in which the patient is sitting erect or propped up in bed by use of pillows or bed angulation. This position is for those who have difficulty breathing.

***posterior-anterior p.*** ABBR: PA position. In radiology, a position in which the central ray enters the posterior surface of the body and exits the anterior surface.

***physiological rest p.*** In dentistry, the position of the mandible at rest when the patient is sitting upright and the condyles are in an unstrained position. The jaw muscles are relaxed.

***prone p.*** A position in which the patient is lying face downward. SEE: *dorsal recumbent p.* for illus.

***reclining p.*** Jackknife p.

***rest p.*** In dentistry, the position of the mandible when the jaws are at rest. The masticatory musculature is relaxed, and the teeth are slightly separated.

***semi-Fowler's p.*** A position in which the patient lies on the back with the trunk elevated at an approximate 45-degree angle.

***semiprone p.*** Sims' p.

***Sims' p.*** A position in which the patient lies on the left side, right knee and thigh drawn well up above left, left arm in back of the patient and hanging over the edge of the table, and the chest inclined forward so that the patient rests on it. This position is used in curettement of the uterus, intrauterine irrigation after labor, tamponade of the vagina, rectal exploration, and operations on the cervix. SYN: *laterosemiprone p.; semiprone p.* SEE: *dorsal recumbent p.* for illus.

***subtalar neutral p. of the foot*** The middle range of the subtalar joint with no pronation or supination measured. It is usually one third of the way from the fully everted position.

***tangential p.*** In radiology, a position in which the central ray separates the images of anatomical parts by skimming between them.

***Trendelenburg p.*** SEE: *dorsal recumbent p.* for illus.; *Trendelenburg position.*

***tripod p.*** A position that may be assumed during respiratory distress to facilitate the use of respiratory accessory muscles. The patient sits, leaning forward, with hands placed on the bed or a table with arms braced.

***unilateral recumbent p.*** The position in which the patient lies on the right side is used in acute pleurisy, lobar pneumonia of the right side, and in a greatly enlarged liver; the position in which the patient lies on left side is used in lobar pneumonia, pleurisy on the left side, and in large pericardial effusions. SEE: *dorsal recumbent p.* for illus.

**positioner** (pō-zĭsh′ŭn-ĕr) An apparatus for holding or placing the body or part, esp. the head, in a certain position.

**positioning** In rehabilitation, the placing of the body and extremities so as to aid treatment by inhibiting undesirable reflexes and preventing deformities. In treatment of children with developmental disabilities involving neuromotor function, the position of the body affects the presence of some primitive reflexes that can affect muscle tone. Alignment of the head, neck, and trunk is therefore thought to be important to reduce unnecessary influences on muscle tone, and the careful placement of the limbs is important to reduce or prevent contractions and deformities.

**positive** (pŏz′ĭ-tĭv) [L. *positivus,* ruling] **1.** Definite; affirmative; opposite of negative. **2.** Indicating an abnormal condition in examination and diagnosis. **3.** Having a value greater than zero.

Often in laboratory findings and mathematical expressions, positive is indicated by a plus (+) sign.

**positron** (pŏz′ĭ-trŏn) A particle having the

same mass as a negative electron but possessing a positive charge.

**Possum** (pŏs′ŭm) [*p*atient *o*perated *s*elector *m*echanis*m*] A device that permits a disabled individual to control and operate various machines such as switches, telephones, and typewriters by breathing into the master control of the apparatus.

**post** In dentistry, a dowel or pin anchored in an upright position in a tooth or bone for the attachment of a dental crown or prosthesis.

**post-** [L.] A prefix meaning *behind, after, posterior*.

**postabortal** (pōst″ă-bor′tăl) [L. *post,* behind, after, + *abortus,* abortion] Happening subsequent to abortion.

**postacetabular** (pōst″ăs-ĕ-tăb′ū-lăr) [″ + *acetabulum,* a little saucer for vinegar] Behind the acetabulum.

**postadolescent** (pōst″ăd-ō-lĕs′ĕnt) [″ + *adolescens,* to grow up] An individual who has passed adolescence.

**postanal** (pōst-ā′năl) [″ + *anus,* anus] Located behind the anus.

**postanesthesia recovery room nurse** ABBR: PAR nurse. A nurse who has received special training in caring for patients who have come from surgery and are recovering from the effects of anesthesia.

**postanesthetic** (pōst″ăn-ĕs-thĕt′ĭk) [″ + Gr. *an-,* not, + *aisthesis,* sensation] Pert. to the period following anesthesia.

**postapoplectic** (pōst″ăp-ō-plĕk′tĭk) [″ + Gr. *apoplessein,* to cripple by a stroke] Pert. to the period immediately following a stroke or apoplexy.

**postaxial** (pōst-ăk′sē-ăl) [″ + Gr. *axon,* axis] Situated or happening behind an axis.

**postbrachial** (pōst-brā′kē-ăl) [″ + *brachiolis,* arm] Pert. to the posterior portion of the upper arm.

**postcapillary** (pōst-kăp′ĭl-lā-rē) Venous capillary.

**postcardial** (pōst-kăr′dē-ăl) [″ + Gr. *kardia,* heart] Behind the heart.

**postcardiotomy** (pōst-kăr″dē-ŏt′ō-mē) [″ + ″ + *tome,* incision] The period after open-heart surgery.

**postcaval** Concerning the postcava, the ascending or inferior vena cava.

**postcentral** (pōst-sĕn′trăl) [″ + Gr. *kentron,* center] **1.** Situated or happening behind a center. **2.** Located behind the fissure of Rolando.

**postcibal** (pōst-sī′băl) [″ + *cibum,* food] ABBR: pc. Occurring after meals.

**postclavicular** (pōst″klă-vĭk′ū-lăr) [″ + *clavicula,* a little key] Located or occurring behind the clavicle.

**postclimacteric** (pōst″klī-măk-tĕr′ĭk, -măk′tĕr-ĭk) [″ + Gr. *klimakter,* rung of a ladder] Occurring after menopause.

**postcoital** (pōst-kō′ĭt-ăl) [″ + *coitio,* a coming together] Subsequent to sexual intercourse.

**postconnubial** (pōst″kŏn-ū′bē-ăl) [″ + *connubium,* marriage] Occurring after marriage.

**postconvulsive** (pōst″kŏn-vŭl′sĭv) [″ + *convulsus,* pull violently] Occurring after a convulsion.

**postdiastolic** (pōst″dī-ăs-tŏl′ĭk) [″ + Gr. *diastole,* expansion] Occurring after the cardiac diastole.

**postdicrotic** (pōst″dī-krŏt′ĭk) [″ + Gr. *dikrotos,* beating double] Occurring after the dicrotic pulse wave.

***p. wave*** A recoil or second wave (not always present) in a sphygmographic tracing.

**postdiphtheritic** (pōst″dĭf-thĕr-ĭt′ĭk) Following diphtheria.

**postencephalitis** (pōst″ĕn-sĕf-ă-lī′tĭs) [″ + Gr. *enkephalos,* brain, + *itis,* inflammation] Occurring after encephalitis; an abnormal state remaining after the acute stage of encephalitis has passed.

**postepileptic** (pōst″ĕp-ĭ-lĕp′tĭk) [″ + Gr. *epi,* upon, + *lepsis,* a seizure] Following an epileptic seizure. SEE: *postictal*.

**posterior** (pŏs-tē′rē-or) [L. *posterus,* behind] **1.** Toward the rear or caudal end; opposite of anterior. **2.** In humans, toward the back; dorsal. **3.** Situated behind; coming after.

**posterior pituitary injection** A standard preparation of the polypeptide hormones obtained from the posterior lobe of the pituitary body of healthy domestic animals used for food by humans. Trade name is Pituitrin.

**postero-** (pŏs′tĕr-ō) [L.] Prefix indicating *posterior, situated behind, toward the back*.

**posteroanterior** (pŏs″tĕr-ō-ăn-tēr′ē-or) [L. *posterus,* behind, + *anterior,* anterior] Indicating the flow or movement from back to front.

**posteroexternal** (pŏs″tĕr-ō-ĕks-tĕr′năl) [″ + *externus,* outer] Toward the back and outer side.

**posteroinferior** (pŏs″tĕr-ō-ĭn-fēr′ē-or) [″ + *inferus,* below] Posterior and inferior.

**posterointernal** [″ + *internus,* inner] Toward the back and inner side.

**posterolateral** [″ + *lateralis,* side] Located behind and at the side of a part.

**posteromedial** (pŏs″tĕr-ō-mē′dē-ăl) [″ + *medius,* middle] Toward the back and toward the median plane.

**posteromedian** Situated posteriorly and in the median plane.

**posteroparietal** (pŏs″tĕr-ō-pă-rī′ĕ-tăl) [″ + *paries,* a wall] Located at the back of the parietal bone.

**posterosuperior** (pŏs″tĕr-ō-sū-pē′rē-or) [″ + *superior,* upper] Located behind and above a part.

**posterotemporal** (pŏs″tĕr-ō-tĕm′pō-răl) [″ + *temporalis,* temporal] Located at the back of the temporal bone.

**posteruption** Referring to the stage of tooth eruption in which the tooth has reached the occlusal plane and is functional, but continues to erupt to compensate for loss of tooth substance because of wear. SEE:

*eruption; pre-eruption.*

**postesophageal** (pōst″ē-sŏf″ă-jē′ăl) [L. *post,* behind, after, + Gr. *oisophagos,* gullet] Located behind the esophagus.

**postethmoid** (pōst-ĕth′moyd) [″ + Gr. *ethmos,* sieve, + *eidos,* form, shape] Located behind the ethmoid bone.

**postfebrile** (pōst-fē′brĭl) [″ + *febris,* fever] Occurring after a fever.

**postganglionic** (pōst″găn-glē-ŏn′ĭk) [″ + Gr. *ganglion,* knot] Situated posterior or distal to a ganglion.

**posthemiplegic** (pōst″hĕm-ĭ-plē′jĭk) [″ + Gr. *hemi,* half, + *plege,* a stroke] Occurring after hemiplegia.

**posthemorrhagic** (pōst-hĕm″ō-răj′ĭk) [″ + Gr. *haima,* blood, + *rhegnynai,* to burst forth] Occurring after hemorrhage.

**posthepatitic** (pōst″hĕp-ă-tĭt′ĭk) [″ + Gr. *hepar,* liver, + *itis,* inflammation] Occurring after hepatitis.

**posthioplasty** (pŏs′thē-ō-plăs″tē) [″ + *plastos,* formed] Plastic surgery of the prepuce or foreskin.

**posthitis** (pŏs-thī′tĭs) [″ + *itis,* inflammation] Inflammation of the foreskin. SYN: *acroposthitis.*

**posthumous** (pŏs′tū-mŭs) [L. *postumus,* last] **1.** Occurring after death. **2.** Born after the death of the father. **3.** Said of a child taken by cesarean section after the death of the mother.

**posthypnotic** (pōst″hĭp-nŏt′ĭk) [L. *post,* behind, after, + Gr. *hypnos,* sleep] Occurring or performed subsequent to the hypnotic state.

***p. suggestion*** A suggestion given during the hypnotic state influencing a later action when an individual returns to a normal state.

**posthypoxia syndrome** One of several syndromes occurring after an individual has experienced severe hypoxia including persistent coma or stupor, dementia, visual agnosia, parkinsonism, choreoathetosis, cerebral ataxia, inattention or action myoclonus, and amnesic state. SEE: *hypoxia.*

**postictal** (pōst-ĭk′tăl) [″ + *ictus,* a blow or stroke] Occurring after a sudden attack or stroke, as an epileptic seizure or apoplexy.

***p. confusion*** Confusion that follows a seizure. After a minor seizure, it lasts only a few seconds; after a major seizure it usually resolves in an hour unless complicated by head injury, hypoxia, or status epilepticus. SEE: *epilepsy.*

**posticteric** (pōst″ĭk-tĕr′ĭk) [″ + Gr. *ikteros,* jaundice] Occurring after jaundice.

**postmalarial** (pōst″mă-lā′rē-ăl) [″ + It. *malaria,* bad air] Occurring after malaria.

**postmature** (pōst″mă-tūr′) [″+ *maturus,* ripe] **1.** Pert. to an infant born after the calculated due date. **2.** Pert. to an infant born after 42 weeks of gestation.

**postmaturity** SEE: *syndrome, postmaturity.*

**postmediastinal** (pōst″mē-dē-ăs′tĭ-năl) [″ + *mediastinum,* in the middle] Behind the mediastinum.

**postmenopausal** (pōst″mĕn-ō-paw′zăl) [″ + Gr. *men,* month, + *pausis,* cessation] Occurring after menopause.

**postmortem** [L.] **1.** Occurring or performed after death. **2.** Autopsy.

**postmyocardial infarction syndrome** A syndrome described in France originally in 1953 and again in 1958. Chest pain similar to that of pericarditis appears in the second week after the onset of myocardial infarction. The pain is aggravated by deep breathing, swallowing, and change in body position. Usually present are fever and a pericardial friction rub. The white blood cell count and sedimentation rate may be elevated. SYN: *Dressler's syndrome.*

ETIOLOGY: The cause is unknown but thought to be due to an autoimmune response.

TREATMENT: This syndrome usually responds to salicylates or other mild analgesics.

**postnasal** (pōst-nā′zăl) [L. *post,* behind, after, + *nasus,* nose] Located behind the nose.

**postnatal** [″ + *natus,* birth] Occurring after birth.

**postnecrotic** (pōst″nĕ-krŏt′ĭk) [″ + Gr. *nekros,* corpse] Occurring after the death of a tissue or a part.

**postneuritic** (pōst″nū-rĭt′ĭk) [″ + Gr. *neuron,* nerve, + *itis,* inflammation] Occurring after neuritis.

**postocular** (pōst-ŏk′ū-lar) [″ + *oculus,* eye] Behind the eye.

**postocular neuritis** Inflammation of the optic nerve behind the eyeball.

**postolivary** (pōst-ŏl′ĭ-vā-rē) [″ + *oliva,* olive] Behind the olivary body; the back of the anterior pyramid of the medulla.

**postoperative care** [″ + *operatus,* work] Care after or following a surgical operation. SEE: *Nursing Diagnoses Appendix.*

NURSING IMPLICATIONS: Before discharge from the recovery room, the patient should meet the following criteria: recovery from the effects of anesthesia, presence of stable vital signs, no evidence of excessive drainage from any site or body cavity, maintenance of satisfactory level of consciousness, and demonstration of adequate urine output (30 ml/hr). In addition, the nurse should have completed all essential orders and notified the receiving unit regarding the patient's status and essential equipment needed for the patient's care.

Common problems associated with postoperative discomfort that require monitoring and care include nausea, vomiting, headache, sore throat, confusion or disorientation esp. in the elderly, paresthesias, atelectasis, abdominal gas, muscle aches, and urinary retention.

Throughout the postoperative period, the nurse monitors vital signs at prescribed intervals, obtains necessary equipment and supplies, observes the patient for adequate circulatory function, provides for adequate nutrition and elimination, maintains fluid and electrolyte balance, checks wounds and tubes for drainage, administers analgesics as prescribed, and provides comfort by properly positioning the patient. The nurse also ensures that guard rails are in place, if these are required, and that electrical devices are properly grounded. In addition to these duties, the nurse provides adequate rest periods, performs wound care, establishes range-of-motion exercises progressing to ambulation, prevents and recognizes postoperative complications, and prepares patient and family for discharge and provides adequate discharge instruction.

**postoperculum** (pōst-ō-pŭr'kū-lŭm) [" + *operculum,* a covering] The fold covering the insula that is formed of part of the superior temporal gyrus of the brain.

**postoral** (pōst-or'ăl) [" + *os,* mouth] Behind, or in the posterior part of, the mouth.

**postorbital** (pōst-or'bĭ-tăl) [" + *orbita,* track] Behind the orbit of the eye.

**postpalatine** (pōst-păl'ă-tĭn) [" + *palatum,* palate] Behind the palate.

**postpallium** (pōst-păl'ē-ŭm) [" + *pallium,* cloak] That part of the cerebral cortex behind the fissure of Rolando.

**postpaludal** (pōst-păl'ū-dăl) [" + *palus,* swamp] Occurring after a malarial attack.

**postparalytic** (pōst"păr-ă-lĭt'ĭk) [" + *para,* beside, + *lyein,* to loosen] Subsequent to an attack of paralysis.

**postpartal period** The time following childbirth. Some women experience postpartum blues during this time. SEE: *Nursing Diagnoses Appendix.*

**postpartum** (pōst-păr'tŭm) [L. *post,* after, + *partus,* birth] Occurring after childbirth.

***p. blues*** The "let-down" feeling experienced during the postpartum period for no apparent reason. The mother becomes tearful and irritable, loses her appetite, and finds sleeping difficult. This temporary state may occur during the hospital stay or after. It is thought to be due to hormonal changes as well as emotional needs during this period. This occurs in 70% to 80% of mothers.

***p. pituitary necrosis*** Sheehan's syndrome.

**postpharyngeal** (pōst-fă-rĭn'jē-ăl) [L. *post,* after, + Gr. *pharynx,* throat] Behind the pharynx.

**postpneumonic** (pōst"nū-mŏn'ĭk) [" + Gr. *pneumon,* lung] Occurring after pneumonia.

**postpoliomyelitis muscular atrophy** ABBR: PPMA. The development of new neuromuscular symptoms, including muscle weakness, many years after recovery from acute paralytic poliomyelitis. This may occur in muscles that were previously affected by polio and recovered or in muscles that were clinically unaffected by the acute disease. There is no treatment for this slowly progressing atrophy, but the unaffected muscles remain strong. The disease is not thought to be related to amyotrophic lateral sclerosis. SEE: *poliomyelitis, acute anterior.*

**postpolio syndrome** A variety of musculoskeletal symptoms and muscular atrophy that create new difficulties with activities of daily living 25 to 30 years after the original attack of acute paralytic poliomyelitis.

**postpontile** (pōst-pŏn'tĭl) [" + *pons,* bridge] Situated behind the pons varolii.

**postprandial** (pōst-prăn'dē-ăl) Following a meal.

***p. dumping syndrome*** Dumping syndrome.

***p. (reactive) hypoglycemia syndrome*** A disorder in which the symptoms of weakness, nausea, hunger, sweating, and difficulty concentrating are not correlated with detectable hypoglycemia. Use of a glucose tolerance test is of little diagnostic benefit.

**postpuberty** (pōst-pū'bĕr-tē) [" + *pubertas,* puberty] The period after puberty. **postpubertal** (-tăl), *adj.*

**postpubescent** (pōst"pū-bĕs'ĕnt) [" + *pubescens,* becoming hairy] Following puberty.

**postpyramidal** (pōst-pĭ-răm'ĭd-ăl) Behind a pyramidal tract.

**postradiation** (pōst"rā-dē-ā'shŭn) Occurring after exposure to ionizing radiation.

**postsacral** (pōst-sā'krăl) [" + *sacrum,* sacred] Below the sacrum.

**postscapular** (pōst-skăp'ū-lăr) [" + *scapula,* shoulder blade] Below or behind the scapula.

**postscarlatinal** (pōst"skăr-lă-tī'năl) [" + *scarlatina,* scarlet fever] Following scarlet fever.

**postsphygmic** (pōst-sfĭg'mĭk) [" + Gr. *sphygmos,* pulse] Following the pulse wave.

**postsplenic** (pōst-splĕn'ĭk) [" + Gr. *splen,* spleen] Behind the spleen.

**poststenotic** (pōst"stĕ-nŏt'ĭk) [" + Gr. *stenosis,* act of narrowing] Distal to a stenosed or constricted area, esp. of an artery.

**postsynaptic** (pōst"sĭ-năp'tĭk) [" + Gr. *synapsis,* point of contact] Located distal to a synapse.

**post-tarsal** (pōst-tăr'săl) [" + Gr. *tarsos,* a broad, flat surface] Behind the tarsus.

**post-term pregnancy** Pregnancy continuing beyond the beginning of the 42nd week (294 days) of gestation, as counted from the first day of the last normal menstrual period. This occurs in an estimated 3% to 12% of pregnancies. Complications include oligohydramnios, meconium passage, macrosomatia, and dysmaturity, all of which may lead to poor pregnancy outcome. The fetus should be delivered if any sign of fetal distress is detected. SEE: *syndrome, postmaturity.*

**post-tibial** (pōst-tĭb′ē-ăl) [″ + *tibia,* shinbone] Behind the tibia.

**post-transfusion syndrome** A condition consisting of fever, splenomegaly, atypical lymphocytes, abnormal liver function tests, and occasionally a skin rash that develops following blood transfusion or perfusion of an organ during surgery. The syndrome appears 3 to 5 weeks after transfusion or perfusion with fresh (less than 24 hr old) blood, usually in large quantities. The causative agent is thought to be cytomegalovirus.

**post-trauma response** The state of an individual's experiencing a sustained painful response to an overwhelming traumatic event. SEE: *Nursing Diagnoses Appendix.*

**post-traumatic** (pōst″traw-măt′ĭk) [″ + Gr. *traumatikos,* traumatic] Following an injury or traumatic event.

**post-traumatic stress disorder** ABBR: PTSD. The development of characteristic symptoms after a psychologically traumatic event that is generally outside the range of usual human experience. It is important to remember that the reaction to stress is highly individualized; and, because of that, the stress that would cause this syndrome in one individual might have little if any effect on another.

The symptoms include re-experiencing the traumatic event; avoiding stimuli associated with the trauma; numbing of general responsiveness; and experiencing symptoms related to increased arousal, including insomnia, recurrent nightmares, and hypervigilance; exhibiting an exaggerated startle response; and experiencing changes in aggression.

The disorder may last for decades. It is estimated that 15% of male and 9% of female Vietnam combat veterans have PTSD. SEE: *Nursing Diagnoses Appendix.*

**postulate** (pŏs′tū-lāt) [L. *postulare,* to request] A supposition or view, usually self-evident, that is assumed without proof. SEE: *Koch's law.*

**postural** (pŏs′tū-răl) [L. *postura,* position] Pert. to or affected by posture.

**postural drainage** Drainage of secretions from the bronchi or a cavity in the lung by having the patient positioned so that gravity will allow drainage of the particular lobe or lobes of the lung involved. This is used in bronchiectasis and before operation for lobectomy. The position aggravates coughing, resulting in expectoration of much sputum, 5 to 10 oz (148 to 296 ml) in severe cases. Five to 10 min morning and evening is recommended. A high-protein diet is required to replace the protein lost. SEE: illus.

NURSING IMPLICATIONS: Physical tolerance to the procedure is evaluated. The nurse teaches and assists the patient in the procedure, as ordered, by positioning the patient for effective drainage and by encouraging the patient to mechanically remove secretions with forceful cough. To prevent aspiration, the patient should not perform the procedure after meals.

**postural hypotension** A decrease in blood pressure upon assuming erect posture. This is normal but may be of such degree as to cause fainting, esp. in persons who first stand up after having been flat in bed for several days. Persons with this condition may treat the dizziness by crossing their legs or squatting at the time of onset. SYN: *orthostatic hypotension.* SEE: *blackout; syncope, vasodepressor.*

**posture** (pŏs′tŭr) [L. *postura*] Attitude or position of the body.

***coiled p.*** Posture in which the body is on one side with legs drawn up to meet the trunk noted in cerebral diseases and in hepatic, intestinal, and renal colic.

***dorsal rigid p.*** Posture in which the patient lies on the back with both legs drawn up; seen in peritonitis, meningitis, ascites, tympanites. In appendicitis the right leg is drawn up. This also occurs in pelvic inflammation or peritonitis of right side, renal calculus in right ureter, and in psoas abscess.

***kyphosis-lordosis p.*** A stance in which the pelvis is tilted forward, causing hip flexion, increased lumbar lordosis, and thoracic kyphosis.

***orthopnea p.*** Posture in which the patient sits upright, hands or elbows resting upon some support; seen in asthma, emphysema, dyspnea, ascites, effusions into the pleural and pericardial cavities, and in late stages of heart disease.

***orthotonos p.*** Posture in which the neck and trunk are extended rigidly in a straight line; seen in tetanus, strychnine poisoning, rabies, and meningitis.

***prone p.*** Posture assumed after abdominal colic or because of tuberculosis of the spine, eroded vertebrae, abdominal pain, or gastric ulcer.

***semireclining p.*** Posture used for patients with heart diseases and interference with respiration in asthma and pleural effusions.

***standard p.*** The skeletal alignment accepted as normal; used for evaluating posture. There is equilibrium around the line of gravity and the least amount of stress and strain on supporting muscles, joints, and ligaments. From either the front or the back, a plumb bob would bisect the body equally. From the side, a plumb bob would be anterior to the lateral malleolus and the axis of the knee, posterior to the axis of the hip and the apex of the coronal suture, and through the bodies of the lumbar vertebrae, the tip of the shoulder, the bodies of the cervical vertebrae, and the external auditory meatus.

***swayback p.*** A relaxed stance in which the pelvis is shifted forward, resulting in hip extension, and the thorax is shifted backward, resulting in an increased tho-

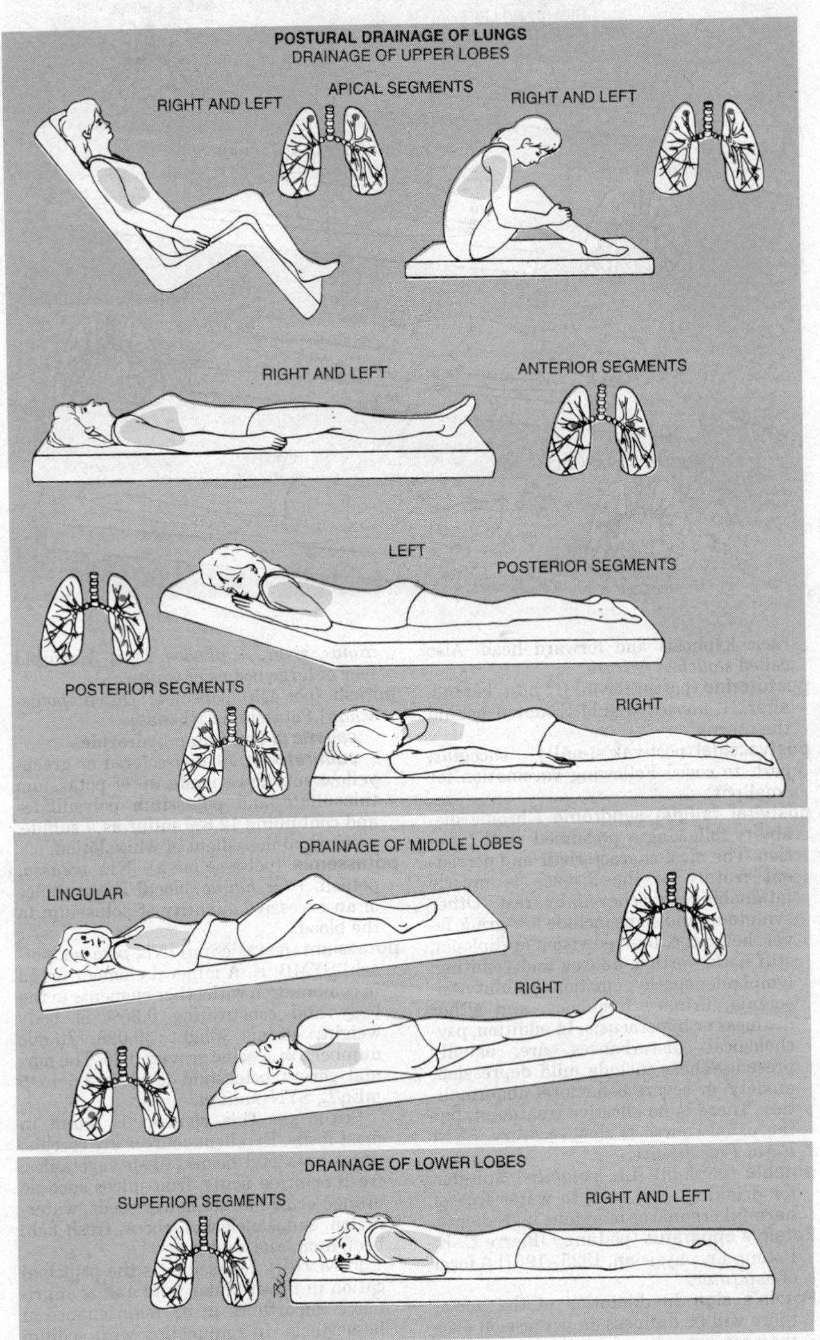


*(see following page)*

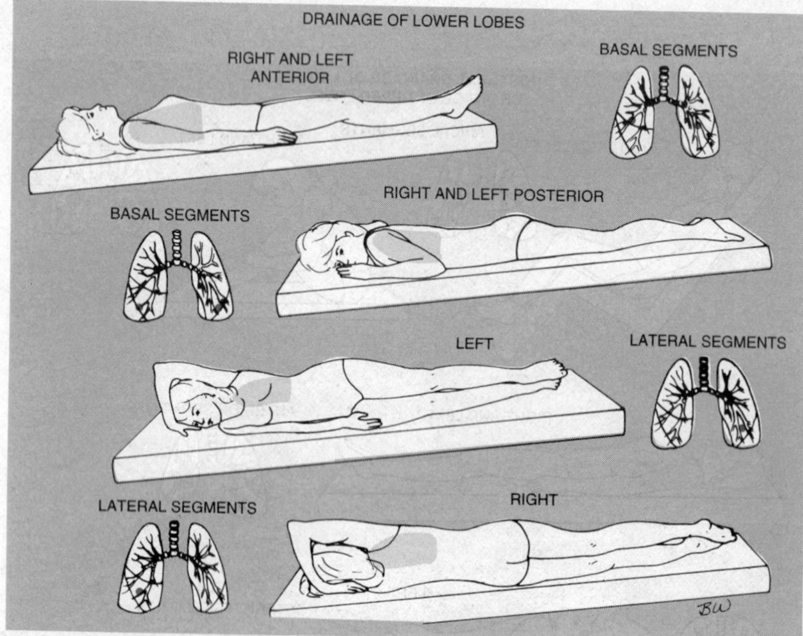


racic kyphosis and forward head. Also called *slouched posture*.

**postuterine** (pōst-ū′tĕr-ĭn) [L. *post,* behind, after, + *uterus,* womb] Situated behind the uterus.

**postvaccinal** (pōst-văk′sĭ-năl) [″ + *vaccinus,* pert. to cows] Following vaccination for smallpox.

**postviral fatigue syndrome** Chronic disability following a presumed viral infection. The most characteristic and persistent feature of the disease is muscle fatiguability unrelieved by rest. Other symptoms and signs include low-grade fever, headache, blurred vision or diplopia, stiff neck, vertigo, nausea and vomiting, lymphadenopathy, emotional lability, insomnia, urinary frequency, and either deafness or hyperacusis. In addition, psychological disturbances are usually present. These include mild depression, anxiety, or severe behavioral abnormalities. There is no effective treatment, but the usual course is slow recovery. SYN: *Royal Free disease*.

**potable** (pō′tă-bl) [LL. *potabilis*] Suitable for drinking, esp. pert. to water free of harmful organic or inorganic ingredients.

**Potain's apparatus** (pō-tānz′) [Pierre C. E. Potain, Fr. physician, 1825–1901] A form of aspirator.

**Potain's sign** In dilatation of the aorta, there will be dullness on percussion over the area extending from the manubrium sterni toward the third costal cartilage on the right, and to the base of the sternum.

**potamophobia** (pŏt″ă-mō-fō′bē-ă) [Gr. *potamos,* river, + *phobos,* fear] A morbid fear of large bodies of water.

**potash** (pŏt′ăsh) [Obsolete Dutch, *potasschan*] Potassium carbonate.

***caustic p.*** Potassium hydroxide.

***sulfurated p.*** A liver-colored or green-yellow substance made up of potassium thiosulfate and potassium polysulfides and containing 12.8% sulfur as a sulfide; a principal ingredient of white lotion.

**potassemia** (pŏt-ă-sē′mē-ă) [NL. *potassa,* potash, + Gr. *haima,* blood] The presence of an excessive quantity of potassium in the blood.

**potassium** (pō-tăs′ē-ŭm) [NL. *potassa,* potash] SYMB: K. A mineral element found in combination with other elements in the body and constituting 0.35% of body weight; atomic weight 39.098; atomic number 19; specific gravity 0.86. The normal serum potassium level is 3.5 to 5 mEq/L. SYN: *kalium*.

SOURCES: This element is found in most foods. Excellent sources are cereals, dried peas and beans, fresh vegetables, fresh or dried fruits, fruit juices such as orange or prune, sunflower seeds, watermelon, nuts, molasses, cocoa, fresh fish, beef, ham, and poultry.

FUNCTION: Potassium is the principal cation in intracellular fluid and is of primary importance in its maintenance of hemostasis. In conjunction with sodium and chloride, it aids in regulation of osmotic pressure and acid-base balance. A proper balance of potassium, calcium, and magnesium ions is essential for normal excitability of muscle tissue, esp. cardiac muscle, and plays a role in the conduction of nerve impulses.

The usual intake of potassium is 50 to 150 mEq/day. Intake must be monitored carefully to be certain it is adequate in prolonged intravenous feeding, in severe diarrhea or diabetic acidosis, and in patients receiving diuretics. In these conditions an intake of 1 to 3 mEq/kg/day usually is adequate.

DEFICIENCY: Muscle weakness, dizziness, thirst, mental confusion, and changes in the electrocardiogram characterize deficiency of this mineral.

EXCESS: Extracellular potassium is increased in renal failure; in destruction of cells with release of intracellular potassium in burns, crushing injuries, or severe infection; in adrenal insufficiency; in overtreatment with potassium salts; and in metabolic acidosis. This causes weakness and paralysis, impaired electrical conduction in the heart, and eventually ventricular fibrillation and death. Hyperkalemia can be treated by withholding potassium, by using drugs such as sodium polystyrene sulfonate, a cation exchange resin, to lower the potassium concentration in cells, and by using calcium gluconate to counteract the effects on the heart.

Caution: Rapid infusion of potassium intravenously may cause severe hyperkalemia and cardiac arrest.

***p. acetate*** $C_2H_3KO_2$. A white powder or crystalline flakes; used to replenish potassium.

***p. alum*** Aluminum potassium sulfate; strongly astringent, used topically as a styptic. SEE: *alum*.

***p. aminosalicylate*** Para-aminosalicylic acid.

***p. arsenite solution*** Fowler's solution.

***p. bicarbonate*** $KHCO_3$. White crystals or powder; used to neutralize acid of the stomach and to treat acid-base imbalance. Trade name is K-Lyte.

***p. bitartrate*** $C_4H_5KO_6$. White powder or crystalline salt, used as a dusting powder in place of starch for surgical gloves. SYN: *cream of tartar*.

***p. bromide*** White cubical crystals of powder, used as a sedative.

***p. carbonate*** $K_2CO_3$. A white crystalline powder used in pharmaceutical and chemical preparations. SYN: *potash*.

***p. chlorate*** $KClO_3$. An explosive white crystalline salt, soluble in water; formerly used internally in treatment of pharyngitis and stomatitis but its use has been discontinued because of destructive effect on red blood cells.

***p. chloride*** KCl. A white crystalline salt, soluble in water; one of the three chlorides used in preparation of Ringer's solution. It is used in the treatment of potassium deficiencies and digitalis intoxication.

***p. chromate*** $K_2CrO_4$. Lemon-yellow crystals used as a dye and furniture stain, in manufacture of batteries, in photography, and in laboratories to preserve tissue.

***p. citrate*** $C_6H_5K_3O_7 \cdot H_2O$. Transparent prismatic crystals; used as an alkalizer. It is incompatible with caffeine sodium benzoate.

***p. cyanide*** KCN. A highly poisonous compound used as a fumigant.

***dibasic p. phosphate*** $K_2HPO_4$. A drug used to treat calcium imbalance.

***p. gluconate*** $C_6H_{11}KO_7$. A drug used orally to replenish loss of potassium ion.

***p. guaiacolsulfonate*** An expectorant.

***p. hydroxide*** KOH. A gray-white compound used in the preparation of soap and as a chemical reagent. SYN: *caustic potash*.

***p. iodide*** KI. Colorless or white crystals having a faint odor of iodine; used as an expectorant. This form of potassium is recommended for use following exposure to radioactive iodides downwind from a nuclear reactor accident. The rationale is that it blocks the uptake of radioactive iodides by the thyroid gland, thus preventing or decreasing the chance of developing cancer of the thyroid many years later.

***p. nitrite*** $KNO_2$. A medicine formerly used as a diuretic.

***p. permanganate*** $KMnO_4$. Crystals of dark purple prisms, sweet and odorless; used as a topical astringent and antiseptic, as an oxidizing agent, and as an antidote in phosphorus poisoning. Concentrated solutions irritate and even corrode the skin and, when swallowed, induce gastroenteritis. The solutions have considerable power as disinfectants because their oxidizing ability destroys bacteria. They fail to penetrate deeply in an active form, which renders them of less value than many other disinfectants, except for use in very superficial infections.

***p. sodium tartrate*** $C_4H_4KNaO_6 \cdot 4H_2O$. A saline cathartic.

***p. sulfate*** $K_2SO_4$. A substance that has been used as a laxative but, because of its irritant qualities, is not recommended.

***p. tartrate*** $C_4H_4K_2O_6$. A medicine used as a cathartic.

**potassium chlorate poisoning** Poisoning by potassium chlorate, large doses of which cause abdominal discomfort, vomiting, diarrhea, hematuria with nephritis, and disturbances of the blood. Gastric lavage should be used to empty the stomach. Other treatment is symptomatic.

Caution: Vomiting should not be induced.

**potassium chromate poisoning** Poisoning by potassium chromate, possibly contracted by inhalation or from touching the nose with contaminated fingers, causing deep indolent ulcers.

SYMPTOMS: When taken by mouth potassium chromate has a disagreeable taste; causes cramping, pain, vomiting, diarrhea, slow respiration; and may affect the liver and kidneys.

Caution: Vomiting should not be induced.

NURSING IMPLICATIONS: For ingestion, the nurse should treat the patient as if poisoned with a strong acid. Dilute with water and milk. Bronchoalveolar lavage or penicillamine may be used.

**potassium hydroxide poisoning** Poisoning by potassium hydroxide, characterized by nausea, soapy taste, and burning pain in mouth; bloody, slimy vomitus; abdominal cramping; bloody purging and prostration.

Caution: Vomiting should not be induced.

NURSING IMPLICATIONS: The patient requires hospitalization, morphine for pain, and most probably treatment for shock. If airway has been burned, tracheostomy may be required. Corticosteroids and antibiotics may be given.

**potbelly** Slang term for the selective deposition of adipose tissue in the abdominal subcutaneous tissue. This condition usually occurs in middle-aged persons who have sedentary occupations. It is accentuated by weakening of the anterior abdominal musculature and lumbar lordosis. Weight reduction, exercises to strengthen the abdominal muscles, and therapy for lordosis are the treatment for this condition.

**potency** (pō′tĕn-sē) [L. *potentia,* power] **1.** Strength; force; power. **2.** Strength of a medicine. **3.** The ability of a man to perform coitus.

**potent** (pō′tĕnt) [L. *potens,* powerful] **1.** Powerful. **2.** Highly effective medicinally. **3.** Having the power of procreation.

**potentia coeundi** (pō-tĕn′shē-ă kō-ē-ŭn′dī) [L.] The ability to perform sexual intercourse in a normal manner.

**potential 1.** Latent; existing in possibility. **2.** In electricity, voltage or electrical pressure; a condition in which a state of tension or pressure, capable of doing work, exists. When two electrically charged bodies of different potentials are brought together, an electric current passes from the body of high potential to that of low.

***action p.*** ABBR: A.P. The change in electrical potential of nerve or muscle fiber when it is stimulated; depolarization followed by repolarization.

***after p.*** The period occurring subsequent to the spike potential.

***demarcation p.*** The difference in potential between an intact longitudinal surface and the injured end of a muscle or nerve. SYN: *injury p.*

***injury p.*** Demarcation p.

***liquid junction p.*** The potential that develops at the liquid junction of a potentiometric measurement system, An example is a pH reference electrode.

***membrane p.*** The electrical charge or potential difference between the inside and outside of a cell membrane.

***resting p.*** Polarization (3).

***spike p.*** A change in potential that occurs when a cell membrane is stimulated.

**potentiate** (pō-tĕn′shē-āt) To increase the potency or action.

**potentiation** (pō-tĕn″shē-ā′shŭn) The synergistic action of two substances, such as hormones or drugs, in which the total effects are greater than the sum of the independent effects of the two substances.

**potentiometer** (pō-tĕn″shē-ŏm′ĕ-tĕr) A voltmeter.

***calibration p.*** A mechanically adjusted resistance used as a calibration control on many instruments. It adjusts a voltage or current within the device.

**potion** (pō′shŭn) [L. *potio,* draft] A drink or draft; a dose of poison or liquid medicine.

**Pott, Sir Percivall** British surgeon, 1714–1788. He pioneered research into chemical carcinogenesis by describing scrotal cancer in chimney sweeps.

**Pott's disease** Caries or osteitis of the vertebrae, usually of tuberculous origin; tubercular inflammation of bodies of the vertebrae. The disease occurs primarily in children and in adults up to age 40. Destruction and compression of the affected vertebrae often causes kyphosis, with resulting compression of the spinal cord and nerves. The condition often spreads to paravertebral tissues, giving rise to paravertebral abscesses. SYN: *tuberculous spondylitis.* SEE: *kyphosis.*

SYMPTOMS: The patient will complain of pain in the region supplied by the nerves arising from the affected segment of the cord. If the disease is lumbar, the pains are abdominal and apt to be associated with vesical irritability; if dorsal, the pains are epigastric or intercostal, and respiration is sometimes irregular and hurried from failure of the respiratory muscles to function adequately; if cervical, there is neuralgic pain or numbness in the hands, a tickling cough, and difficult swallowing. Pains apt to be symmetrical.

Pain that increases on jumping, flexing, or rotating the spine is extremely significant. If the patient can jump painlessly from a step to the floor, it is almost certain that inflammation of the body of a vertebra is not present. If the vertebrae are compressed by pressure on the head or shoulders while the patient sits or stands or while he or she lies face downward across the knees of the surgeon, pain is increased. If the patient is placed in traction to elongate the spine, relief is obtained.

Involuntary immobilization of the spine, as a result of pain on movement, gives an exaggerated characteristic military posture (i.e., stiff and straight). If asked to look at something behind him or her, the patient turns the whole trunk. If requested to pick up something from the floor, he or she stoops by bending the trunk on the thighs and the knees on the thighs, never by flexing the spinal column in the usual way.

In walking, the patient moves as if on ice, sliding or shuffling along so as to avoid the jar of successive steps. In standing, he or she fixes the upper portion of the spinal column by the aid of the trapezii and other scapular muscles, the action of which at the same time raises the shoulders and throws the arms out from the sides. In standing or sitting, there is an involuntary transfer of the weight of the head and shoulders and parts above the diseased area to the pelvis, by means of the upper extremities. Hands are placed on the hips, and the arm muscles are tense. In walking about the room, the patient holds onto furniture for aid. Spinal abscess occurs later, with the location varying according to the seat of the caries. Paralysis may occur, always motor at first, not affecting sensation at all.

TREATMENT: Resolution of the tuberculous osteitis should be made if possible. Tissue destruction and resulting deformity should be limited. Ankylosis should be promoted if indicated. Abscesses should be evacuated. A sequestrum or the focus of carious bone should be removed. The patient should rest in bed in a recumbent position. Adequate diet and exercise help prevent development of decubitus ulcers. Chemotherapy is given as for pulmonary tuberculosis.

**Pott's fracture** Fracture of the lower end of the fibula and medial malleolus of the tibia, with dislocation of the foot outward and backward. After reduction, foot and leg are put in a cast in which a walking iron is incorporated. The patient is able to walk, and the cast is removed in about 6 weeks.

**pouch** (powch) [ME. *pouche*] Any pocket or sac.

***branchial p.*** Pharyngeal p.

***Broca's p.*** A sac in the tissues of the labia majora.

***p. of Douglas*** Rectouterine p.

***Heidenhain p.*** A small, surgically constructed pouch of the stomach that is denervated and separated from the stomach and drained to the outside of the body. It is used to study the physiology of the stomach.

***laryngeal p.*** A blind pouch of mucosa entering the ventral portion of the ventricle of the larynx.

***Pavlov p.*** A stomach pouch formed surgically for the experimental study of gastric secretion. A section of the stomach is separated from the main stomach except for the vagal nerves. This pouch is named after I. P. Pavlov, who devised it to investigate gastric function and conditioned reflexes.

***perianal p.*** A pouch device applied to cover the anal and perianal area. It is used to collect feces from incontinent patients. The pouch is held in place with an adhesive skin barrier.

***pharyngeal p.*** One of a series of five pairs of entodermal outpocketings that develop in lateral walls of the pharynx of the embryo. SYN: *branchial p.*

***Prussak's p.*** The anterior recess of the tympanic membrane.

***Rathke's p.*** An outpocketing of the roof of embryonic stomodeum. It gives rise to the anterior lobe of the hypophysis cerebri.

***rectouterine p.*** The pouch between the anterior rectal wall and the posterior uterine wall. SYN: *p. of Douglas; cul-de-sac.*

***rectovesical p.*** A fold of peritoneum that in men extends downward between the bladder and rectum.

**pouchitis** Acute inflammation of the surgically produced pouch used in restorative proctocolectomy.

**poudrage** (pū-drăzh′) [Fr.] Application of an irritating, but otherwise nontoxic, powder to the pleural space of the lung in order to produce pleural adhesions.

**poultice** (pōl′tĭs) [L. *pultes,* thick paste] A hot, moist mass of linseed, mustard, or soap and oil between two pieces of muslin applied to the skin to relieve congestion or pain, to stimulate absorption of inflammatory products, and to act as a counterirritant. SEE: *plaster*.

**pound** (pownd) [L. *pondus,* weight] SYMB: lb. A measure of weight of the avoirdupois and the apothecaries' systems that is equal to 16 oz. SEE: *Weights and Measures Appendix.*

***avoirdupois p.*** Sixteen ounces, equal to 453.59 g.

***foot p.*** Work expended when 1 lb is moved a distance of 1 ft in the direction of the force.

***troy p.*** Twelve ounces, 5760 gr, equal to 373.242 g.

**Poupart's ligament** (pū-părz′) [François Poupart, Fr. anatomist, 1661–1708] The ligament forming the lower border of aponeurosis of external oblique muscle between the anterosuperior spine of the ilium and spine of the pubis. SYN: *inguinal ligament.*

**poverty** The condition of having an inadequate supply of money, resources, or means of subsistence.

***p. of thought*** The mental state of being devoid of thought and having a feeling of emptiness.

**povidone** (pō′vĭ-dōn) A synthetic polymer used as a dispersing and suspending agent in manufacturing drugs.

**povidone-iodine** A complex of iodine with povidone. It contains not less than 9% and not more than 12% available iodine. This iodophor is used in dilute concentration as a surgical scrub, in aerosol spray, in vaginal douche solutions, and in ointments and gels.

**powder** [ME. *poudre*] **1.** An aggregation of fine particles of one or more substances that may be passed through fine meshes. **2.** A dose of such a powder, contained in a paper.

**power** [ME. *power*] **1.** The rate at which work is done. Power may be calculated by multiplying force times velocity. The metric unit for power is the watt. One watt equals one newton meter per second, or 0.7376 foot pound per second. Sometimes power is measured in horsepower. A horsepower unit equals 745.7 watts or 550 foot pounds per second. **2.** The capacity for action. **3.** In optics, the degree to which a lens or optical instrument magnifies. **4.** In microscopy, the number of times the diameter of an object is magnified, indicated by placing an × after the number (e.g., 10× indicates magnification of 10 times). **5.** In mathematics and in scientific nomenclature, the number of times a value is to be multiplied by itself (i.e., $10^2 = 10 \times 10 = 100$; $10^3 = 10 \times 10 \times 10 = 1000$). A negative power (e.g., $10^{-2}$) indicates the reciprocal of that value. For example, $10^{-2} = 1/10^2 = 1/100$. **6.** In statistics, the probability that a planned investigation will yield a statistically significant result. This is done by calculating how many individuals had to be randomly assigned to each group studied and how many would have to demonstrate improvement after receiving therapy in order to be able to conclude that the information will permit a statistically valid statement that one form of therapy is or is not more effective than another.

**power of attorney** ABBR: POA. A legal document by which a person identifies someone to make financial decisions if he or she is unable to perform this task independently. SEE: *power of attorney, durable, for health care.*

**power of attorney, durable, for health care** An advance directive that designates another person to make health care decisions regarding how aggressive treatment should be if the patient becomes incompetent or unable to make decisions in the future, for example, in the case of coma or a persistent vegetative state. The document also lists medical treatments that the person would not want to have. Durable power of attorney goes into effect when the document is signed. The Patient Self-Determination Act, enacted in 1991, mandates the responsibility of health care providers to develop written materials concerning advance directives. Also called *health care proxy*. SEE: *advance directive; living will.*

**powerlessness** Perception that one's own action will not significantly affect an outcome; a perceived lack of control over a current situation or immediate happening. SEE: *helplessness; Nursing Diagnoses Appendix.*

**pox** (pŏks) [ME. *pokkes,* pits] **1.** An eruptive, contagious disease. **2.** A papular eruption that becomes pustular. SEE: *chickenpox; smallpox.*

**poxvirus** (pŏks′vī-rŭs) One of a group of DNA viruses that produce characteristic spreading vesicular lesions, often called pocks. It is the largest of the true viruses and includes viruses responsible for smallpox, vaccinia, molluscum contagiosum, and orf. Lower animals are also susceptible to the poxvirus.

**p.p.** *punctum proximum,* the near point of accommodation (in vision).

**ppb** *parts per billion.*

**P.P.D.** *purified protein derivative,* the substance used in an intradermal test for tuberculosis.

**PPLO** *pleuropneumonia-like organisms,* now called mycoplasmas.

**ppm** *parts per million.*

**ppt** *parts per trillion; precipitate; prepared.*

**Pr 1.** *presbyopia.* **2.** Symbol for the element praseodymium.

**p.r.** L. *punctum remotum,* the far point of visual accommodation.

**practice** (prăk′tĭs) [Gr. *praxis,* practice] **1.** The use, by a health care professional, of knowledge and skill to provide a service in the prevention, diagnosis, and treatment of illness and in the maintenance of health. **2.** The continuing and repetitive effort to become proficient and to excel or at least to improve one's skill in the practice of medicine.

**practitioner** (prăk-tĭsh′ŭn-ĕr) One who has met the professional and legal requirements necessary to provide a health care service, such as a physician, nurse, dentist, dental hygientist, or physical therapist.

***adult nurse p.*** ABBR: ANP. A nurse practitioner who is licensed to treat people over 18 years of age.

***advanced nurse p.*** An umbrella term that includes the following health care workers: Certified Midwife, Certified Registered Nurse Anesthetist, Clinical Nurse Specialist, and Nurse Practitioner.

***family nurse p.*** ABBR: FNP. A nurse practitioner who is licensed to treat people of any age. SEE: *adult nurse p.*

***nurse p.*** SEE: *nurse practitioner.*

**Practitioners' Reporting Network, USP** ABBR: USP-PRN. Three separate programs designed to collect practitioners' experience with unreliable drug products, defective medical devices, drug problems with radiopharmaceuticals, and medication errors. Practitioners and pharmacists report their experience to the United States Pharmacopeia, 12601 Twinbrook Parkway, Rockville, MD 20852. The USP receives the reports and publishes the results. Drug problem reports and medical device and laboratory product problem reports may be made by calling (800) 638-6725; medication errors may be reported by calling (800) 23ERROR.

**prae-** SEE: *pre-*.

**praecox** (prē′kŏks) [L.] Early.

**praevia, praevius** (prē′vē-ă, prē′vē-ŭs) [L.] Going before in time or place.

**pragmatagnosia** (prăg″măt-ăg-nō′zē-ă) [Gr. *pragma,* object, + *agnosia,* lack of recognition] Inability to recognize once familiar objects.

**pragmatamnesia** (prăg″măt-ăm-nē′zē-ă) [″ + *amnesia,* forgetfulness] The inability to recall the appearance of an object.

***visual p.*** The mental condition making possible pragmatamnesia.

**pragmatism** (prăg′mă-tĭzm) [Gr. *pragma,* a thing done, + *-ismos,* condition] The belief that the practical application of a principle should be the determining factor. **pragmatic** (prăg-măt′ĭk), *adj.*

**pragmatist** (prăg′mă-tĭst) A person whose goals are achieved or attempted from a practical concept, action or approach; a practical person.

**pralidoxime chloride** (prăl″ĭ-dŏks′ēm) A cholinesterase reactivator used in treating poisoning due to certain pesticides or drugs with anticholinesterase activity.

**pramoxine hydrochloride** (prăm-ŏk′sēn) A topical anesthetic. It should not be used on mucous membranes.

**prandial** (prăn′dē-ăl) [L. *prandium,* breakfast] Relating to a meal.

**praseodymium** (prā″sē-ō-dĭm′ē-ŭm) [Gr. *prasios,* leek-green, + *didymium*] SYMB: Pr. A metallic element obtained from rare earth; atomic weight 140.907; atomic number 59.

**Prausnitz-Küstner reaction** (prows′nĭts-kĭst′nĕr) [Carl Willi Prausnitz, Ger. bacteriologist, b. 1876; Heinz Küstner, Ger. gynecologist, b. 1897] The intracutaneous injection of a hypersensitive patient's serum into a nonallergic person followed, 24 to 48 hr later, by the application of the suspected antigen to the injection site. If a wheal and flare occur, there is evidence that the suspected antigen is causing the hypersensitivity. Because of the danger of transmitting viral hepatitis and AIDS, this test is no longer used.

**praxinoscope** (prăk-sĭn′ō-skōp) [Gr. *praxis,* action, + *skopein,* to examine] A device for studying the larynx.

**praxiology** (prăk″sē-ŏl′ō-jē) [″ + *logos,* word, reason] The study of behavior.

**praxis** (prăk′sĭs) [Gr., action] The ability to plan and execute coordinated movement.

**-praxis** [Gr., action] Combining form indicating *act, activity, practice, use.*

**Prayer of Maimonides** [Rabbi Moses ben Maimon, Jewish philosopher and physician in Egypt, 1135–1204] A prayer used at graduation ceremonies by some medical schools. SEE: *Declaration of Geneva; Declaration of Hawaii; Hippocratic oath; Nightingale Pledge.*

"Thy eternal providence has appointed me to watch over the life and health of Thy creatures. May the love for my art actuate me at all times; may neither avarice nor miserliness, nor thirst for glory, or for a great reputation engage my mind; for the enemies of truth and philanthropy could easily deceive me and make me forgetful of my lofty aim of doing good to Thy children.

"May I never see in the patient anything but a fellow creature in pain.

"Grant me strength, time, opportunity always to correct what I have acquired, always to extend its domain; for knowledge is immense and the spirit of man can extend indefinitely to enrich itself daily with new requirements.

"Today he can discover his errors of yesterday and tomorrow he can obtain a new light on what he thinks himself sure of today. Oh, God, Thou has appointed me to watch over the life and death of Thy creatures; here am I ready for my vocation and now I turn unto my calling."

**praziquantel** A broad-spectrum antischistosomal drug that is useful in treating infections with helminths such as *Hymenolepis nana* and *Taenia saginata.* It is also effective in treating infections with *Diphyllobothrium latum.*

**prazosin hydrochloride** A drug used in treating hypertension. It acts as an alpha-adrenergic receptor blocker.

**pre-** [L. *prae,* before] Prefix indicating *before, in front of.* SEE: *anti-; pro-.*

**preadmission certification** A review of the need for proposed inpatient services before admission to an institution.

**preagonal** (prē-ăg′ō-năl) [L. *prae,* before, in front of, + Gr. *agonia,* agony] Pert. to the condition immediately before death agony.

**preanal** (prē-ā′năl) [″ + *anus,* anus] In front of the anus.

**preanesthesia** (prē″ăn-ĕs-thē′zē-ă) A light anesthesia produced by a medication given before the anesthesia.

**preanesthetic** (prē″ăn-ĕs-thĕt′ĭk) [″ + Gr. *anaisthesia,* lack of sensation] A preliminary drug given to facilitate induction of general anesthesia.

**preantiseptic** (prē″ăn-tĭ-sĕp′tĭk) [″ + Gr. *anti,* against, + *sepsis,* putrefaction] Before the adoption of antisepsis in surgery.

**preaortic** (prē″ā-or′tĭk) [″ + Gr. *aorte,* aorta] Located in front of the aorta.

**preataxic** (prē-ă-tăk′sĭk) [″ + Gr. *ataxia,* lack of order] Before the onset of ataxia.

**preauricular** (prē″aw-rĭk′ū-lăr) [″ + *auricula,* little ear] Located in front of the ear.

**preaxial** (prē-ăk′sē-ăl) [″ + Gr. *axon,* axis] In front of the axis of a limb or of the body.

**precancer** (prē′kăn-sĕr) [″ + *cancer,* crab] A

condition that tends to become malignant.

**precancerous** (prē-kăn′sĕr-ŭs) [″ + *cancer,* crab] Said of a growth that is not yet, but probably will become, cancerous.

**precapillary** [″ + *capillaris,* hairlike] An arterial capillary; one that branches from an arteriole or venule. SYN: *metarteriole.*

**precautions, universal** SEE: *Universal Precautions Appendix.*

**precava** (prē-kā′vă) [″ + *cavus,* hollow] The descending or superior vena cava. SEE: *vena cava superior.*

**precentral** (prē-sĕn′trăl) [″ + Gr. *kentron,* center] In front of a center, as the central fissure of the brain.

**precentral convolution** The ascending frontal convolution of the brain.

**prechordal** (prē-kor′dăl) [″ + Gr. *chorde,* cord] In front of the notochord.

**precipitable** (prē-sĭp′ĭ-tă-b′l) Capable of being precipitated.

**precipitant** (prē-sĭp′ĭ-tănt) [L. *praecipitare,* to cast down] A substance bringing about precipitation.

**precipitate** (prē-sĭp′ĭ-tāt) **1.** A deposit separated from a suspension or solution by precipitation, the reaction of a reagent that causes the deposit to fall to the bottom or float near the top. **2.** To separate as a precipitate. **3.** Occurring suddenly or unexpectedly.

**precipitation** (prē-sĭp″ĭ-tā′shŭn) [L. *praecipitatio*] **1.** The process of a substance being separated from a solution by the action of a reagent so that a precipitate forms. **2.** The sudden and unprepared-for delivery of an infant. SEE: *delivery, precipitate.*

**precipitation test** A test in which a positive reaction is indicated by formation of a precipitate in the solution being tested.

**precipitin** (prē-sĭp′ĭ-tĭn) An antibody formed in the blood serum of an animal owing to the presence of a soluble antigen, usually a protein. When added to a solution of the antigen, it brings about precipitation. The injected protein is called the antigen, and the antibody produced is the precipitin. It was originally thought that these antibodies were members of a unique class, but most antibodies are capable of precipitating when combined with their antigens. SEE: *autoprecipitin; precipitinogen.*

**precipitinogen** (prē-sĭp″ĭ-tĭn′ō-jĕn) Any protein that, acting as an antigen, stimulates the production of a specific precipitin.

**precipitinoid** (prĕ-sĭp′ĭt-ĭn-oyd) A precipitin that can no longer cause precipitation when mixed with its antigen but that retains its affinity to the antigen.

**precipitin test** A test in which a precipitate forms in a solution containing a soluble antigen upon addition of serum containing the specific precipitin. The reaction is specific. The test is used for identification of unknown proteins; determination of types of pneumococci and meningococci; and determination of types of blood stains, whether human or animal.

**precipitophore** (prē-sĭp′ĭt-ō-for″) The part of a precipitin that produces the actual precipitation.

**precipitum** (prē-sĭp′ĭ-tŭm) The precipitate produced by action of a precipitin.

**preclinical** (prē-klĭn′ĭ-kăl) [L. *prae,* before, in front of, + Gr. *klinike,* medical treatment in bed] Occurring before diagnosis of a definite disease is possible.

**preclinical dental training** Study and mastery of the theory and techniques related to the various dental procedures required prior to treating human patients.

**preclinical technique** In dentistry, the use of manikins, mechanical articulator, artificial or extracted teeth, and the variety of dental instruments and materials to study and master the techniques necessary to do clinical dentistry.

**preclival** (prē-klī′văl) [″ + *clivus,* slope] In front of the cerebellar clivus.

**precocious** (prē-kō′shŭs) [L. *praecox,* ripening early] Mental or physical development earlier than would be expected.

**precocity** (prē-kŏs′ĭ-tē) Premature development of physical or mental traits.

***sexual p.*** Premature genital maturation; precocious sexual maturity.

**precognition** (prē″kŏg-nĭsh′ŭn) [L. *prae,* before, in front of, + *cognoscere,* to know] Prior knowledge that an event will occur even though there is no rational explanation of why one would have that knowledge.

**precoital** (prē-kō′ĭ-tăl) [″ + *coitio,* a going together] Prior to sexual intercourse.

**precoma** (prē-kō′mă) [″ + Gr. *koma,* a deep sleep] The mental state immediately before a coma.

**preconscious** (prē-kŏn′shŭs) [″ + *conscius,* aware] Not present in consciousness but able to be recalled as desired.

**preconvulsive** (prē″kŏn-vŭl′sĭv) [″ + *convulsio,* pulling together] Before a convulsion.

**precordia** (prē-kor′dē-ă) [L. *praecordia*] The precordium.

**precordial** (prē-kor′dē-ăl) Pert. to the precordium or epigastrium.

**precordium** (prē-kor′dē-ŭm) The area on the anterior surface of the body overlying the heart and lower part of the thorax. SYN: *antecardium; precordia.*

**precornu** (prē-kor′nū) [L. *prae,* before, in front of, + *cornu,* horn] The anterior horn of the lateral ventricle of the brain.

**precostal** (prē-kŏs′tăl) [″ + Gr. *costa,* rib] In front of the ribs.

**precuneus** (prē-kū′nē-ŭs) [″ + *cuneus,* wedge] The division of the mesial surface of a cerebral hemisphere between the cuneus and the paracentral lobule.

**precursor** A substance that precedes another substance, or a substance from which another is synthesized.

**predentin** Uncalcified dentinal matrix.

**prediabetes** (prē-dī″ă-bē′tēz) [″ + Gr. *diabetes,* passing through] The condition before the development of clinical diabetes.

**prediastole** (prē″dī-ăs′tō-lē) [″ + Gr. *dias-*

*tellein,* to expand] The period in the cardiac cycle immediately before diastole.

**prediastolic** (prē″dī-ă-stŏl′ĭk) [″ + Gr. *diastole,* expansion] Before the diastole, or interval in the cardiac cycle that precedes it.

**predicrotic** (prē″dī-krŏt′ĭk) [″ + Gr. *dikrotos,* beating double] Preceding the dicrotic wave of the sphygmographic tracing.

**prediction rules** Identifying predictive factors important in establishing a diagnosis and giving each a certain "weight," in order to establish the probability of various diagnoses being present.

**predigestion** (prē″dĭ-jĕs′chŭn) [″ + *digestio,* carrying apart] Artificial proteolysis or digestion of proteins and amylolysis of starches before ingestion.

**predisposing** (prē″dĭs-pōz′ĭng) [″ + *disponere,* to dispose] Indicating a tendency to, or susceptibility to, disease.

**predisposition** (prē″dĭs-pō-zĭsh′ŭn) The potential to develop a certain disease or condition in the presence of specific environmental stimuli.

**prednisolone** (prĕd-nĭs′ō-lōn) A glucocorticosteroid drug, available in a variety of dosage forms. It is similar in action to cortisone.

**prednisone** (prĕd′nĭ-sōn) A glucocorticosteroid with the same effects as cortisone.

**pre-eclampsia** (prē″ē-klămp′sē-ă) [″ + Gr. *ek,* out, + *lampein,* to flash] A complication of pregnancy characterized by increasing hypertension, proteinuria, and edema. The condition may progress rapidly from mild to severe and, if untreated, to eclampsia. It is the leading cause of fetal and maternal morbidity and death, esp. in underdeveloped countries. SYN: *pregnancy-induced hypertension.* SEE: *eclampsia; syndrome, HELLP; Nursing Diagnoses Appendix.*

ETIOLOGY: The cause is unknown; however, the incidence is higher among adolescent and older primigravidas, diabetic patients, and in multiple pregnancy. Pathophysiology associated with pre-eclampsia includes generalized vasospasm, damage to the glomerular membranes, and hypovolemia and hemoconcentration due to a fluid shift from intravascular to interstitial compartments.

SYMPTOMS: The condition develops between the 20th week of gestation and the end of the first postpartum week; however, most commonly it occurs during the last trimester. Characteristic complaints include sudden weight gain, severe headaches, and visual disturbances. Indications of increasing severity include complaints of epigastric or abdominal pain; generalized, presacral, and facial edema; oliguria; and hyperreflexia.

TREATMENT: Treatment includes bedrest; high-protein diet; and medications including mild sedatives, antihypertensives, and, if indicated, intravenous anticonvulsants. Magnesium sulfate is the drug of choice.

**pre-embryo** The morula and blastocyst stages produced by the division of the zygote until the formation of the embryo proper at the appearance of the primitive streak about 14 days after fertilization.

**pre-eruption** (prē″ē-rŭp′shŭn) [″ + *eruptio,* a breaking out] **1.** Before an eruption. **2.** The stage of tooth eruption when the tooth bud is in the bony socket prior to root formation. SEE: *eruptive stage.*

**pre-excitation, ventricular** (prē-ĕk″sī-tā′shŭn) [″ + *excitare,* to arouse] Premature excitation of the ventricle by an impulse that traveled a path other than through the atrioventricular node. This produces a short P-R interval. SEE: *Wolff-Parkinson-White syndrome.*

**pre-existing condition** Any injury, disease, or physical condition occurring prior to an arbitrary date; usually used in reference to the issuance of a health insurance policy. This often results in an exclusion from coverage for costs resulting from the injury, disease, or condition.

**preferred provider organization** ABBR: PPO. A form of health-care delivery in which a group of health providers agrees to supply services to a defined group of patients at an agreed-upon fee-for-service rate.

**prefrontal** (prē-frŏn′tăl) [″ + *frons,* front] **1.** The middle portion of the ethmoid bone. **2.** In the anterior part of the frontal lobe of the brain.

**preganglionic** (prē″găng-lē-ŏn′ĭk) [″ + Gr. *ganglion,* knot] Situated in front of or anterior to a ganglion.

**preganglionic fiber** The axon of a preganglionic neuron.

**preganglionic neuron** The first of a series of two efferent neurons that transmit impulses to visceral effectors. Its cell body lies in the central nervous system. Its axon terminates in an autonomic ganglion.

**pregenital** (prē-jĕn′ĭ-tăl) [″ + *genitalia,* genitals] In psychology, relating to that period when erotic interest in the reproductive organs and functions is not yet organized.

**pregnancy** (prĕg′năn-sē) [L. *praegnans*] The condition of carrying an embryo in the uterus. SEE: table; *prenatal care; prenatal diagnosis; Nursing Diagnoses Appendix.*

SYMPTOMS: Probable signs are alterations in uterine shape, size, and abdominal location, softening of the cervix and lower uterine segment, ballotement, a palpable embryonic outline, and Braxton Hicks contractions.

Positive signs are hearing and counting the embryonic heartbeat, detection of movements of the embryo, and use of ultrasound to detect the embryonic outline. The various immunodiagnostic tests for pregnancy are 90% to 95% accurate. These tests are based on various methods

**Pregnancy Table for Expected Date of Delivery**

| Jan. | 1 | 2 | 3 | 4 | 5 | 6 | 7 | 8 | 9 | 10 | 11 | 12 | 13 | 14 | 15 | 16 | 17 | 18 | 19 | 20 | 21 | 22 | 23 | 24 | 25 | 26 | 27 | 28 | 29 | 30 | 31 | |
|---|---|---|---|---|---|---|---|---|---|---|---|---|---|---|---|---|---|---|---|---|---|---|---|---|---|---|---|---|---|---|---|---|
| Oct. | **8** | **9** | **10** | **11** | **12** | **13** | **14** | **15** | **16** | **17** | **18** | **19** | **20** | **21** | **22** | **23** | **24** | **25** | **26** | **27** | **28** | **29** | **30** | **31** | **1** | **2** | **3** | **4** | **5** | **6** | **7** | **Nov.** |
| Feb. | 1 | 2 | 3 | 4 | 5 | 6 | 7 | 8 | 9 | 10 | 11 | 12 | 13 | 14 | 15 | 16 | 17 | 18 | 19 | 20 | 21 | 22 | 23 | 24 | 25 | 26 | 27 | 28 | | | | |
| Nov. | **8** | **9** | **10** | **11** | **12** | **13** | **14** | **15** | **16** | **17** | **18** | **19** | **20** | **21** | **22** | **23** | **24** | **25** | **26** | **27** | **28** | **29** | **30** | **1** | **2** | **3** | **4** | **5** | | | | **Dec.** |
| Mar. | 1 | 2 | 3 | 4 | 5 | 6 | 7 | 8 | 9 | 10 | 11 | 12 | 13 | 14 | 15 | 16 | 17 | 18 | 19 | 20 | 21 | 22 | 23 | 24 | 25 | 26 | 27 | 28 | 29 | 30 | 31 | |
| Dec. | **6** | **7** | **8** | **9** | **10** | **11** | **12** | **13** | **14** | **15** | **16** | **17** | **18** | **19** | **20** | **21** | **22** | **23** | **24** | **25** | **26** | **27** | **28** | **29** | **30** | **31** | **1** | **2** | **3** | **4** | **5** | **Jan.** |
| April | 1 | 2 | 3 | 4 | 5 | 6 | 7 | 8 | 9 | 10 | 11 | 12 | 13 | 14 | 15 | 16 | 17 | 18 | 19 | 20 | 21 | 22 | 23 | 24 | 25 | 26 | 27 | 28 | 29 | 30 | | |
| Jan. | **6** | **7** | **8** | **9** | **10** | **11** | **12** | **13** | **14** | **15** | **16** | **17** | **18** | **19** | **20** | **21** | **22** | **23** | **24** | **25** | **26** | **27** | **28** | **29** | **30** | **31** | **1** | **2** | **3** | **4** | | **Feb.** |
| May | 1 | 2 | 3 | 4 | 5 | 6 | 7 | 8 | 9 | 10 | 11 | 12 | 13 | 14 | 15 | 16 | 17 | 18 | 19 | 20 | 21 | 22 | 23 | 24 | 25 | 26 | 27 | 28 | 29 | 30 | 31 | |
| Feb. | **5** | **6** | **7** | **8** | **9** | **10** | **11** | **12** | **13** | **14** | **15** | **16** | **17** | **18** | **19** | **20** | **21** | **22** | **23** | **24** | **25** | **26** | **27** | **28** | **1** | **2** | **3** | **4** | **5** | **6** | **7** | **Mar.** |
| June | 1 | 2 | 3 | 4 | 5 | 6 | 7 | 8 | 9 | 10 | 11 | 12 | 13 | 14 | 15 | 16 | 17 | 18 | 19 | 20 | 21 | 22 | 23 | 24 | 25 | 26 | 27 | 28 | 29 | 30 | | |
| Mar | **8** | **9** | **10** | **11** | **12** | **13** | **14** | **15** | **16** | **17** | **18** | **19** | **20** | **21** | **22** | **23** | **24** | **25** | **26** | **27** | **28** | **29** | **30** | **31** | **1** | **2** | **3** | **4** | **5** | **6** | | **April** |
| July | 1 | 2 | 3 | 4 | 5 | 6 | 7 | 8 | 9 | 10 | 11 | 12 | 13 | 14 | 15 | 16 | 17 | 18 | 19 | 20 | 21 | 22 | 23 | 24 | 25 | 26 | 27 | 28 | 29 | 30 | 31 | |
| April | **7** | **8** | **9** | **10** | **11** | **12** | **13** | **14** | **15** | **16** | **17** | **18** | **19** | **20** | **21** | **22** | **23** | **24** | **25** | **26** | **27** | **28** | **29** | **30** | **1** | **2** | **3** | **4** | **5** | **6** | **7** | **May** |
| Aug. | 1 | 2 | 3 | 4 | 5 | 6 | 7 | 8 | 9 | 10 | 11 | 12 | 13 | 14 | 15 | 16 | 17 | 18 | 19 | 20 | 21 | 22 | 23 | 24 | 25 | 26 | 27 | 28 | 29 | 30 | 31 | |
| May | **8** | **9** | **10** | **11** | **12** | **13** | **14** | **15** | **16** | **17** | **18** | **19** | **20** | **21** | **22** | **23** | **24** | **25** | **26** | **27** | **28** | **29** | **30** | **31** | **1** | **2** | **3** | **4** | **5** | **6** | **7** | **June** |
| Sept. | 1 | 2 | 3 | 4 | 5 | 6 | 7 | 8 | 9 | 10 | 11 | 12 | 13 | 14 | 15 | 16 | 17 | 18 | 19 | 20 | 21 | 22 | 23 | 24 | 25 | 26 | 27 | 28 | 29 | 30 | | |
| June | **8** | **9** | **10** | **11** | **12** | **13** | **14** | **15** | **16** | **17** | **18** | **19** | **20** | **21** | **22** | **23** | **24** | **25** | **26** | **27** | **28** | **29** | **30** | **1** | **2** | **3** | **4** | **5** | **6** | **7** | | **July** |
| Oct. | 1 | 2 | 3 | 4 | 5 | 6 | 7 | 8 | 9 | 10 | 11 | 12 | 13 | 14 | 15 | 16 | 17 | 18 | 19 | 20 | 21 | 22 | 23 | 24 | 25 | 26 | 27 | 28 | 29 | 30 | 31 | |
| July | **8** | **9** | **10** | **11** | **12** | **13** | **14** | **15** | **16** | **17** | **18** | **19** | **20** | **21** | **22** | **23** | **24** | **25** | **26** | **27** | **28** | **29** | **30** | **31** | **1** | **2** | **3** | **4** | **5** | **6** | **7** | **Aug.** |
| Nov. | 1 | 2 | 3 | 4 | 5 | 6 | 7 | 8 | 9 | 10 | 11 | 12 | 13 | 14 | 15 | 16 | 17 | 18 | 19 | 20 | 21 | 22 | 23 | 24 | 25 | 26 | 27 | 28 | 29 | 30 | | |
| Aug. | **8** | **9** | **10** | **11** | **12** | **13** | **14** | **15** | **16** | **17** | **18** | **19** | **20** | **21** | **22** | **23** | **24** | **25** | **26** | **27** | **28** | **29** | **30** | **31** | **1** | **2** | **3** | **4** | **5** | **6** | | **Sept.** |
| Dec. | 1 | 2 | 3 | 4 | 5 | 6 | 7 | 8 | 9 | 10 | 11 | 12 | 13 | 14 | 15 | 16 | 17 | 18 | 19 | 20 | 21 | 22 | 23 | 24 | 25 | 26 | 27 | 28 | 29 | 30 | 31 | |
| Sept. | **7** | **8** | **9** | **10** | **11** | **12** | **13** | **14** | **15** | **16** | **17** | **18** | **19** | **20** | **21** | **22** | **23** | **24** | **25** | **26** | **27** | **28** | **29** | **30** | **1** | **2** | **3** | **4** | **5** | **6** | **7** | **Oct.** |

The date of the last menstrual period is in the top line (light-face type) of the pair of lines. The dark number (bold-face type) in the line below will be the expected day of delivery.

of detecting human chorionic gonadotropin (HCG) in the urine or serum.

The duration of pregnancy is approx. 280 days. To estimate the day of delivery, one should count back 3 months from the day of onset of the last menstrual period and then add 7 days. For example, if the last menstrual period began June 10, subtracting 3 months leaves March 10, and adding 7 days indicates the expected day of delivery would be March 17 of the next year. This method assumes all months have the same number of days; thus the date determined will not agree exactly with that found by using the Pregnancy table.

PHYSICAL CHANGES: The *uterus* changes shape, size, and consistency; the lining undergoes changes, the peritoneal covering enlarges, and the muscle mass increases enormously. The cervix and lower uterine segment become softer. SEE: *Goodell's sign; Hegar's sign.*

The *vaginal canal* elongates because of rising of the uterus in the pelvis; the mucosa thickens; secretions increase; vascularity and elasticity increase; and the cervix, vagina, and vulva become softer. SEE: *Chadwick's sign.*

The *abdomen* reveals a growing distention and flattened navel, as well as striae gravidarum.

The *breasts* become enlarged and tender; the skin thins and grows sensitive; the nipples become erectile and the areolas become enlarged and darker; colostrum escapes; a tingling sensation is felt.

*Endocrine Glands:* The thyroid increases in size and activity; the parathyroids enlarge and secretion increases; the pituitary increases its activity; and the placenta produces hormones which affects the ovaries and corpus luteum.

In the *circulatory system* there are increased activity and increased blood volume and coagulability. Blood pressure should be normal; varicose veins may be present.

*Skeletal System:* The pelvic joints soften and become more flexible. The bones and teeth are also affected.

*Respiratory System:* Full ventilation of the lungs may be diminished in late pregnancy and breathing is more frequent.

In the *digestive tract,* nausea and vomiting occur in early pregnancy; the appetite affected; there may be weight loss in early pregnancy; metabolism is increased in later pregnancy; constipation occurs frequently.

The *liver* is displaced in late pregnancy.

*Skin:* The sudoriparous and sebaceous glands are very active. There may be a deposit of brown pigment on the face (mask of pregnancy). Linea nigra may occur.

*Weight:* In normal-sized individuals, the expected first-trimester weight gain is 2 to 5 lb (1 to 2.3 kg) per month of pregnancy. During the second and third trimesters, the weekly weight gain approximates 1 lb (0.4 kg). Deviations should be explored to rule out pregnancy-related health problems common to the particular point in gestation.

The *posture* changes as enlargement of abdomen advances; the sacroiliac joints and symphysis pubis become more movable; there may be painful locomotion and back pain; the gait may be altered.

*Urinary Tract:* Kidney activity increases; kidney failure produces nephritic toxemia; ureters, esp. the right one, are dilated; and there is pressure on the bladder; frequent urination is common in late pregnancy; when the bladder is lifted into the abdomen the pressure diminishes. The bladder is later pressed on by the presenting part; urinary output varies; the presence of albumin is abnormal.

DISORDERS: *Nausea and vomiting* may occur when the stomach is empty at any time. Having four or five small meals per day, instead of three larger ones, may control this.

*Constipation and flatulence* may be caused by the pressure of the uterus on the intestines. Stool softeners and an increase in fiber content of diet may help. Intestinal stasis may cause flatulence. Gas-forming foods should be avoided.

*Muscular cramps* may be avoided by resting between periods of standing. Tetany may ensue because of deficient calcium supply. Calcium and vitamin D supplements are indicated.

*Pressure edema* may occur at the end of pregnancy, with the condition better in the morning and worse at the end of the day. Frequent rest and elevation of the limbs are indicated. The condition may be due to calcium deficiency, and toxemia must also be considered as a cause. The blood pressure and weight should be recorded, and a urinalysis done at each prenatal visit. All of these will help to alert the physician to the possible development of toxemia of pregnancy.

*Headache* may be caused by sinusitis or toxemia.

*Toothache* may be due to caries induced by deficient calcium. Frequent dental examinations are desirable.

*Back pain* can result from abnormal balance caused by the protruding abdomen. Proper shoes are indicated. Intra-abdominal pressure may also be a cause. Flatulence aggravates the back pain; thus, enemas may help.

*Dyspnea* occurs from pressure of the uterus upward on the transverse colon and stomach. It is aggravated by flatulence, esp. when lying down. Alkalies may help. Pillows under the head and shoulders are indicated. Re-examination of the heart is indicated as well.

*Vaginal discharge:* Routine perineal hygiene is recommended, but douches are not indicated. Foul, blood-tinged, or profuse discharge should be reported.

*Pruritus* may develop on the breasts, abdomen, and vulva, caused by the stretching of the abdominal skin. If general, a toxic or nervous origin may be cause. Diabetes mellitus may cause pruritus of vulva.

*Heartburn* may be the result of hyperacidity or nervous tension. Sedation, taking frequent small meals, and avoiding highly seasoned foods may help.

*Varicose veins* are aggravated by pregnancy. These may occur in the pelvis, vulva, and legs. One should avoid tight garters, tight clothing, and standing. Rest and the use of support stockings are indicated, with elevation of the lower limbs while sleeping. One should lie in Sims' position, with a pillow under the hips to shift the uterus.

*Hemorrhoids* are aggravated by constipation, which should be avoided. Ointments, wet compresses, Sitz baths, and suppositories on physician's orders are indicated, and surgical therapy may be required.

NUTRITION: A woman's nutritional status before and during pregnancy is an important factor that affects both her health and that of her unborn child. Nutritional assessment is an essential part of antepartal care. In addition, the presence of pre-existing and coexisting disorders, such as anemia, diabetes mellitus, chronic renal disease, and phenylketonuria, may affect dietary recommendations. Substance abuse increases the risk of inadequate nutrition, low maternal weight gain, low-birth-weight infants, and perinatal mortality.

Dietary recommendations emphasize a high-quality, well-balanced diet. Increased amounts of essential nutrients (i.e., protein, calcium, magnesium, zinc, and selenium, B vitamins, vitamin C, folate, and iron) are necessary to meet nutritional needs of both mother and fetus. Most nutritional and metabolic needs can be met by eating a balanced daily diet containing approximately 35 kcal for each kilogram of optimal body weight plus an additional 300 kcal/day during the second and third trimesters. Vitamin supplements are not required if the woman adheres to the dietary recommendations; however, daily iron supplements are recommended.

Weight gain goals are individualized and influenced by the woman's weight when becoming pregnant; caloric recommendations may be modified to achieve the desired outcome. The anticipated average weight gain for a woman who exhibits the standard weight for height and age ranges between 25 and 35 lb (11.5 to 15.9 kg). For women who are underweight on entering pregnancy, an optimal weight gain ranges between 28 and 40 lb (12.5 to 18 kg). For obese women who become pregnant, dieting is not recommended during pregnancy; the recommended weight gain is between 15 and 25 lb (7 to 11.5 kg). For markedly obese women (i.e., those who weigh more than 20% above the recommended prepregnancy weight), the risk of perinatal mortality begins to increase when they gain more than 15 lb (6.8 kg).

RISK FACTORS: *Teenage and adolescent pregnancy:* Pregnancy in this age group is more likely to be associated with being single, having poor prenatal care, being of a low socioeconomic group, and having poor social support. Many of these pregnancies would be classed as high risk and have an increased risk of adverse embryonic outcome. In 1992, 12.7% of all live births were to mothers less than 20 years of age. Of the more than 1 million pregnancies in girls and women under the age of 20, 14% resulted in miscarriages and 35% in induced abortions. Most teenage pregnancies (81.7% among 15 to 19 year olds in 1987) were unintended, and over half of these unintended pregnancies ended in abortions. Adolescents are considered to be at high risk for complications during pregnancy. A higher incidence of nutritional anemia, pregnancy-induced hypertension, preterm labor, low-birth-weight infants, and cephalopelvic disproportion has been identified. The rising incidence of substance abuse and sexually transmitted diseases, including AIDS, among teenagers is of serious concern. SEE: *high-risk pregnancy; Nursing Diagnoses Appendix.*

*Pregnancy after menopause:* Some women past the age of menopause have become pregnant as a result of having received an embryo donation, and the pregnancy continued until the birth of a child at term. Prior to undergoing this procedure, the women had been taking hormone replacement therapy. Previously, it had been assumed that the postmenopausal uterus would not be capable of supporting the growth and development of an embryo. Pregnancies in mature women are considered to be high risk. Some women may not be candidates for assisted conception because of coexisting medical disorders. Those who are successful in achieving pregnancy usually are monitored closely through the pregnancy.

CONSIDERATIONS: *Travel and pregnancy:* Preparing for travel during pregnancy will depend upon the number of weeks gestation, the duration of the travel, and the method (i.e., auto, boat, bus, train, airplane). Safety belts, preferably the combined lap and shoulder type, should be worn. If nausea and vomiting of pregnancy is a factor, travel by sea isn't advisable. If antimotion medication is used, it should be approved for use during pregnancy. Travel during the last part of pregnancy isn't advised unless obstetrical care is available at the destination(s). It is important to have a copy of current medical records along when traveling. Travel abroad should be discussed with the obstetrician so that appropriate immunizations can be given. If traveling in an area known to be endemic for malaria, certain drugs will be needed for prophylaxis.

Caution: Not all antimalarials are safe for use during pregnancy. Live virus immunization should not be administered during pregnancy.

*Working during pregnancy:* For the normal, healthy, pregnant woman working in a job that presents no more risks than those found in daily life there is no contraindication to work and it may be continued until shortly prior to delivery. Persons involved in heavy lifting, climbing, or working in locations in which balance is required will need to alter their work habits and location. Pregnant women should not be exposed either at work or in the home to toxic substances. Chemicals in the workplace known to harm the fetus include chemotherapeutic agents such as methotrexate, lead, and ionizing radiation.

*Exercise during pregnancy:* If both the mother and the fetus are normal, exercise may and should be continued. The amount and type of exercise is an individual matter. A woman who has exercised regularly before her pregnancy should experience no difficulty with continuing; however, a previously sedentary woman should not attempt to institute a vigorous exercise program such as long-distance running or jogging during her pregnancy. No matter what the type of exercise, it is important to remember that, with the progress of pregnancy, the center of gravity will change and probably prevent participation at the same level and skill as before pregnancy. Sports to avoid include water skiing, horseback riding, and scuba diving. In water skiing, high-speed falls could cause miscarriage due to an inadvertent, forceful vaginal douche. In horseback riding, in addition to the possibility of falling from the horse, the repeated bouncing may lead to bruising of the perianal area. Scuba diving may lead to decompression sickness and bends and to intravascular air embolism in the fetus. Women who breast-feed their children can continue exercising if they maintain hydration and adequate breast support.

*Tests during pregnancy:* Common tests include blood tests for nutritional or sickle cell anemia, type and Rh factor, Rh and rubella titers, syphilis, and serum alpha-fetoprotein for the presence of neural tube defects such spina bifida. Ultrasound may be used to determine age, rate of growth, position, some birth defects, and fetal sex. Chorionic villus sampling is done early in pregnancy if the family history indicates potential for genetic diseases. Second trimester amniocentesis may be used to detect chromosomal abnormalities, genetic disorders, and fetal sex. Additional testing may include determining HIV status and hepatitis immunity. In late pregnancy, nonstress tests, contraction stress tests, and fetal biophysical profiles may be done; amniocentesis may be done to evaluate fetal lung maturity.

***abdominal p.*** Ectopic gestation in which the embryo develops in the peritoneal cavity. SYN: *abdominocysesis*. SEE: *ectopic pregnancy*.

***ampullar p.*** Pregnancy occurring in the ampulla of the uterine tube.

***bigeminal p.*** Pregnancy with twins in utero.

***cervical p.*** Pregnancy with implantation of the embryo in the cervical canal.

***coitus during p.*** Sexual intercourse during pregnancy. There is no evidence that this has adverse effects on the pregnancy or the embryo (i.e., perinatal mortality). Also, sexual intercourse does not initiate labor.

***cornual p.*** Pregnancy occurring in an ill-developed cornu of a bicornuate uterus.

***ectopic p.*** Pregnancy in which the embryo develops outside the uterus. SEE: *ectopic pregnancy* for illus.

***extrauterine p.*** Ectopic p.

***false p.*** Pseudocyesis.

***heterotopic p.*** Combined intrauterine and extrauterine pregnancies.

***high-risk p.*** Pregnancy involving factors such as diabetes, hypertension, kidney disease, viral infections, vaginal bleeding, multiple pregnancies, and certain lifestyle and environmental factors such as drug, alcohol, or cigarette abuse or exposure to toxic chemicals. Pregnancy in association with these conditions produces a greater risk to the mother's health, the health of the embryo, or both. SEE: *teenage p.*

***hydatid p.*** Pregnancy giving rise to a hydatidiform mole. SEE: *hydatid mole*.

***interstitial p.*** Pregnancy in which the embryo is developed in a portion of the fallopian tube that traverses the wall of the uterus. SYN: *mural p.*

***intraligamentary p.*** Pregnancy that occurs within the broad ligament.

***mask of p.*** Chloasma gravidarum.

***membranous p.*** Pregnancy in which the amniotic sac ruptures and the embryo comes to lie in direct contact with the uterine wall.

***mesenteric p.*** Tuboligamentary p.

***molar p.*** Pregnancy in which, instead of the ovum developing into an embryo, it develops into a mole.

***multiple p.*** The presence of two or more embryos in the uterus. The incidence of this in the U.S. is about 1.5% of all births. Up to 40% of twin gestations are undiagnosed before labor and delivery. When twins are diagnosed by ultrasound early in the first trimester, in about half of these cases one twin will silently abort, and this may or may not be accompanied by bleeding. This has been termed the vanishing twin. The incidence of birth defects in each embryo of a twin pregnancy is twice that in singular pregnancies.

***mural p.*** Interstitial p.

***ovarian p.*** Implantation of the embryo in the substance of the ovary.

***phantom p.*** Pseudocyesis.

***postdate p.*** Pregnancy that extends beyond 42 wk of gestation. An average of 10% of normal pregnancies are so classified.

***surrogate p.*** SEE: *surrogate mother*.

***tubal p.*** A form of ectopic pregnancy in which the embryo develops in the fallopian tube.

***tuboabdominal p.*** Extrauterine pregnancy in which the embryonic sac is formed partly in the abdominal extremity of the oviduct and partly in the abdominal cavity.

***tuboligamentary p.*** Pregnancy occurring in the uterine tube and extending into the broad ligament. SYN: *mesenteric p.*

***tubo-ovarian p.*** Extrauterine pregnancy in which the embryonic sac is partly in the ovary and partly in the abdominal end of the fallopian tube.

***uteroabdominal p.*** Twin pregnancy with one embryo in the uterus and the other in the abdominal cavity.

**pregnancy-induced hypertension** SEE: *hypertension, pregnancy-induced.*

**pregnancy-specific $\beta_1$ glycoprotein** A protein found in 97% of women who have been pregnant for 6 to 8 weeks and in 100% of those at later stages of pregnancy. The function of this protein is not known, but it may be useful in estimating the quality of placental function.

**pregnancy test** In addition to the clinical signs and symptoms of pregnancy, almost none of which are reliable within the first several weeks of pregnancy, chemical tests done in the physician's office are quite accurate by as early as the time the first menstrual period is missed. There are also test kits available for purchase without a prescription. If that type of test is used, it is very important to follow the directions carefully.

A major class of pregnancy tests is those using immunodiagnostic procedures. They are the hemagglutination inhibition test, which requires a sample of urine; radioreceptor assay, which requires blood from the patient; radioimmunoassay, which requires a blood sample; and monoclonal antibody determination, which requires a sample of urine. In general, these tests are accurate beginning the 40th day following the first day of the last menstrual period; the monoclonal antibody test is somewhat more sensitive. The reliability of the test methods increases as pregnancy continues.

**pregnane** (prĕg′nān) The organic compound that is a precursor of two series of steroid hormones: the progesterones and several adrenal cortical hormones.

**pregnanediol** (prĕg″nān-dī′ŏl) $C_{21}H_{36}O_2$. The inactive end product of metabolism of progesterone present in the urine. The amount in the urine increases during the premenstrual or luteal phase of the menstrual cycle and during pregnancy.

**pregnanetriol** (prĕg″nān-trī′ŏl) A metabolite of progesterone. Its presence in the urine is increased in those who have congenital adrenal hyperplasia.

**pregnant** (prĕg′nănt) [L. *praegnans*] Having conceived; with child. SYN: *gravid.*

**pregnene** (prĕg′nēn) A steroid that forms the nucleus of progesterone.

**pregneninolone** (prĕg″nēn-ĭn′ō-lōn) A progestin, ethisterone.

**pregnenolone** (prĕg-nĕn′ō-lōn) A synthetic corticosteroid hormone produced from progesterone.

**pregravidic** (prē-gră-vĭd′ĭk) [L. *prae,* before, in front of, + *gravida,* pregnant] Before pregnancy.

**prehallux** (prē-hăl′ŭks) [″ + *hallux,* the great toe] A supernumerary bone, accessory naviculare pedis, or sometimes a prolongation inward of it on the foot.

**prehemiplegic** (prē″hĕm-ĭ-plē′jĭk) [″ + Gr. *hemi,* half, + *plege,* a stroke] Occurring before an attack of hemiplegia.

**prehensile** (prē-hĕn′sĭl) [L. *prehendere,* to seize] Adapted for grasping or holding, esp. by encircling an object.

**prehension** (prē-hĕn′shŭn) [L. *prehensio*] The primary function of the hand; includes pinching, grasping, and seizing.

**prehormone** A precursor of a hormone.

**prehospital care** The care a patient receives from emergency medical service before arriving at the hospital. This is usually done by emergency medical technicians and paramedics.

**prehospital provider** A medical technician who provides care to emergency patients before they arrive at a hospital.

**prehyoid** (prē-hī′oyd) [L. *prae,* before, in front of, + Gr. *hyoeides,* U-shaped] In front of the hyoid bone.

**prehypophysis** (prē″hī-pŏf′ĭ-sĭs) [″ + Gr. *hypophysis,* an undergrowth] The anterior lobe of the pituitary gland.

**preictal** (prē-ĭk′tăl) [″ + *ictus,* stroke] The period just prior to a stroke or convulsion.

**preicteric** (prē-ĭk-tĕr′ĭk) [″ + *ikteros,* jaundice] In liver disease, the period prior to the appearance of jaundice.

**preimmunization** (prē-ĭm″ū-nĭ-zā′shŭn) [″ + *immunis,* safe] Immunization produced artificially in very young infants.

**preinvasive** (prē″ĭn-vā′sĭv) [″ + *in,* into, + *vadere,* to go] Referring to a stage of development of a malignancy in which the neoplastic cells have not metastasized.

**Preiser's disease** (prī'zĕrz) [Georg K.F. Preiser, Ger. orthopedic surgeon, 1879–1913] Osteoporosis caused by trauma and affecting the scaphoid bone of the wrist.

**prekallikrein** A cofactor in blood coagulation. SEE: *coagulation, blood.*

**preleukemia** A group of nondiagnostic physical and blood abnormalities that may indicate leukemia will develop later. They include unexplained anemia, purpura, susceptibility to infections, or slow healing of skin and mucous membrane lesions. Possible laboratory findings are anemia, neutropenia, sometimes a relative lymphopenia, and marked monocytosis. The diagnosis of preleukemia is usually made in retrospect because all of the findings and signs may be reversible abnormalities that occur in patients with various other illnesses.

**preload** In cardiac physiology, the end-diastolic stretch of the muscle fiber. In the intact ventricle, this is approx. equal to the end-diastolic volume or pressure. SEE: *afterload.*

**premaniacal** (prē"mā-nī'ă-kăl) [L. *prae,* before, in front of, + Gr. *mania,* madness] Prior to an attack of mania.

**premature** (prē-mă-chūr') [L. *praematurus,* ripening early] Not mature; before term or full development.

**premature infant** SEE: under *infant.*

**premature rupture of membranes** ABBR: PROM. In pregnancy, rupture of the amniotic membrane prior to the time labor was expected. This occurs in about 10% of patients. PROM is the single most common diagnosis leading to admission of the newborn to intensive care nursing.

PROM is more common in women of poor socioeconomic groups, teenagers, single women, smokers, and women who have a sexually transmitted organism cultured from the cervix or vagina in the first half of pregnancy. PROM increases the risk of intrauterine infection.

***preterm p.r.m.*** ABBR: PPROM. Rupture of the fetal membranes before completion of week 37 of pregnancy. SEE: *prematurity.*

**premature ventricular contraction** ABBR: PVC. The contraction of the cardiac ventricle prior to the normal time, caused by an electrical impulse to the ventricle arising from a site other than the sinoatrial node. The PVC may be a single event or occur several times in a minute or in pairs or strings. PVCs of such duration as to cause ventricular tachycardia may lead to death.

**prematurity** The state of an infant born any time prior to completion of the 37th week of gestation. The normal gestation period for the human being is 40 weeks. Because of the difficulty of obtaining accurate and objective data on the exact length of gestation, a birth weight of 2500 g (5.5 lb) or less has been accepted internationally as the clinical criterion of prematurity regardless of the period of gestation. Other measures suggestive of prematurity are crown-heel length (47 cm or less), crown-rump length (32 cm or less), occipitofrontal circumference (33 cm or less), occipitofrontal diameter (11.5 cm or less), and ratio of the thorax circumference to the head circumference (less than 93%).

The use of a single-criterion measure (birth weight) imposes limitations in accurately identifying those infants born before adequate development of body organs and systems has been achieved. It can easily include mature infants who are of low birth weight for reasons other than a shortened gestation period. The Expert Committee on Prematurity of the World Health Organization (1961) recommended that the concept of prematurity in the international definition be replaced by that of low birth weight. This term, low birth weight, more accurately describes infants weighing less than 2500 g at birth than does the term prematurity. The latter term should be reserved for those neonates within the low birth weight group with evidence of incomplete development.

In the United States approx. 7.1% white liveborn and 13.4% nonwhite liveborn infants weigh 2500 g or less. Chances of survival depend on the degree of maturity achieved, general medical condition, and quality of care received.

Prematurity is the leading cause of death in the neonatal period. Mortality among infants weighing less than 2500 g at birth is 17 times greater than among infants with birth weight above 2500 g. Chief causes of mortality are abnormal pulmonary ventilation, infection, intracranial hemorrhage, abnormal blood conditions, and congenital anomalies.

ETIOLOGY: The incidence of neonates of low birth weight is more frequent among the female sex, nonwhite races, plural births, and the first- and fifth- (and over) born infants. Delivery of infants of low birth weight is reported to be more frequent among women with one or more of the following characteristics: having their children at either a very young age or between ages 45 and 49; being unmarried; having children closely spaced (i.e., less than 2 to 4 years between births); and living in a large urban area.

Another factor associated with low birth weight is the socioeconomic status of the family as measured by the mother's educational attainment. The proportion of infants of low birth weight born to mothers with 16 years or more of education was half of that of infants born to mothers with less than 9 years of education. Low birth weight is also associated with generally elevated risk of infant mortality, congenital malformations, mental retardation, and various other physical and neurological impairments.

COMPLICATIONS: Frequently, premature infants are handicapped by a number of anatomical and physiological limitations. These limitations vary in direct proportion to the degree of immaturity present. Limitations include weakness of the sucking and swallowing reflexes, small capacity of stomach, impairment of renal function, incomplete development of capillaries of the lungs, immature alveoli of the lungs, weakness of the cough and gag reflexes, weakness of the thoracic cage muscles and other muscles used in respiration, inadequate regulation of body temperature, incomplete or poorly developed enzyme systems, hepatic immaturity, and deficient placental transfer and antenatal storage of minerals, vitamins, and immune substances. SEE: *intrauterine growth retardation; premature rupture of membranes.*

NURSING IMPLICATIONS: A physical assessment correlated with the expected maturation for fetal age is performed. The nurse performs a neurological evaluation, obtains an Apgar score, ensures proper environmental temperature, provides proper fluid and caloric intake, ensures parental bonding and support, assesses laboratory reports, monitors intake and output, notifies the nursery of the premature birth, weighs infant daily at the same time without clothing and on the same scale, monitors oxygen concentration at frequent intervals, holds and cuddles the infant during feedings, covers the infant when removing from isolette, and provides adequate time for feeding.

*Care of low-birth-weight infants:* Care of low-birth-weight infants should be individualized and reflect the needs of the developing infant with regard to anatomical and physiological handicaps. Evaluation for degree of immaturity and identification of special problems after birth dictates care required by these infants. In general, care centers on prevention of infection, stabilization of body temperature, maintenance of respiration, and provision of adequate nutrition and hydration.

Aseptic technique is required. An incubator or heated bed provides a suitable environment for maintenance of body temperature. A high-humidity environment may be of value for infants with respiratory difficulties. Gentle nasal and pharyngeal suctioning aid in keeping airways clear. Use of oxygen should be restricted to the minimal amounts required for survival of the infant. Because of the danger of retrolental fibroplasia, the oxygen concentration should not exceed 30%.

Depending on the infant's sucking and swallowing abilities, gavage feeding may be necessary. Some of these infants may not be given anything by mouth for as long as 72 hr after birth. Caloric and fluid intakes are gradually increased until 100 to 120 cal/kg and 140 to 150 ml/kg, respectively, in 24 hr are reached. The time required to achieve these intake levels depends on the condition of the newborn. The infant may require small, frequent feedings to cope with the small capacity of the stomach, to prevent vomiting and distention, and to meet caloric and fluid requirements of the body. Overfeeding should be avoided. During the early days of life, clyses are sometimes administered to maintain adequate hydration.

The nurse should not allow the infant to become fatigued from excessive handling, prolonged feeding procedures, or too much crying. Body position should be changed every 2 to 4 hr. Gentle handling should be practiced. The newborn and infant should receive cuddling several times a day.

Because of the possibility of retinal damage, premature infants should not exposed to bright light.

**premaxilla** (prē″măk-sĭl′ă) [L. *prae,* before, in front of, + *maxilla,* jawbone] A separate element, derived from the median nasal process embryologically, that fuses with the maxilla in humans; formerly called the incisive bone.

**premaxillary** (prē-măk′sĭ-lĕr″ē) Located before the maxilla.

**premedication** (prē″mĕd-ĭ-kā′shŭn) [″ + *medicari,* to heal] **1.** Administration of drugs before treatment to enhance the therapeutic effect and safety of a given procedure. **2.** Induction of unconsciousness by drugs prior to administration of inhalation anesthesia. SYN: *prenarcosis.*

**premenarchal** (prē″mĕ-năr′kăl) [″ + Gr. *men,* mouth, + *arche,* beginning] The time prior to the first menstrual period (i.e., prior to menarche).

**premenstrual** (prē-mĕn′stroo-ăl) [″ + *menstruare,* to discharge the menses] Before menstruation.

**premenstrual dysphoric disorder** A disorder characterized by symptoms such as markedly depressed mood, marked anxiety, marked affective lability, and decreased interest in activities. It is the current term, according to *DSM-IV,* for what was previously known as premenstrual tension syndrome.

SYMPTOMS: In patients with this disease, the symptoms occur regularly during the last week of the luteal phase in most menstrual cycles during the year preceding diagnosis. These symptoms begin to remit within a few days of the onset of the menses (the follicular phase) and are always absent the week following menses.

DIAGNOSIS: For diagnosis, five or more of the following must be present most of the time during the last week of the luteal phase, with at least one of the symptoms being one of the first four: feeling sad, hopeless, or self-deprecating; feeling tense, anxious, or "on edge"; marked lability of mood interspersed with frequent tearfulness; persistent irritability, anger, and increased interpersonal conflicts; decreased interest in usual activities, which may be associated with withdrawal from social relationships; difficulty concentrating; feeling fatigued, lethargic, or lacking in energy; marked changes in appetite, which may be associated with binge eating or craving certain foods; hypersomnia or insomnia; a subjective feeling of being overwhelmed or out of control; and physical symptoms such as breast tenderness or swelling, headaches, or sensation of "bloating" or weight gain, with tightness of fit of clothing, shoes or rings. There may also be joint or muscle pain. The symptoms may be accompanied by suicidal thoughts.

The pattern of symptoms must have occurred most months for the previous 12 months. The symptoms disappear completely shortly after the onset of menstruation. In atypical cases, some women also have symptoms for a few days around ovulation; and a few women with short cycles might, therefore, be symptom free for only 1 week per cycle. Women commonly report that their symptoms worsen with age until relieved by the onset of menopause.

TREATMENT: Therapy depends on the severity of symptoms. Mild analgesics may be helpful. Fluoxetine is also beneficial in treating this disorder. The patient should limit intake of salt, refined sugars, caffeine, and animal fats but increase intake of leafy green vegetables, whole-grain cereals, and complex carbohydrates. Use of a diuretic to control fluid retention is indicated. Therapy to prevent ovulation may be necessary if symptoms are severe. A regular exercise program may help to relieve discomfort.

NURSING IMPLICATIONS: Support and reassurance are offered, and the woman is encouraged to develop her own resources to help her cope with the syndrome.

**premenstrual tension syndrome** ABBR: PMS. Premenstrual dysphoric disorder. SEE: *Nursing Diagnoses Appendix.*

**premenstruum** (prē-mĕn′stroo-ŭm) [″ + *menstruus,* menstrual fluid] The period of time prior to menstruation.

**premolar** (prē-mō′lĕr) [″ + *moles,* a mass] One of the permanent teeth that erupt to replace the deciduous molars. They are often called bicuspid teeth, for the maxillary premolars have two cusps, whereas the mandibular premolars may have from one to three cusps. They are located between the canine and first molar of each quadrant of the dental arches. SEE: *dentition.*

**premonition** (prĕm″ĕ-, prē-mĕ-nĭsh′ŭn) [L. *praemonere,* to warn beforehand] A feeling of an impending event.

**premonitory** (prē-mŏn′ĭ-tō-rē) [LL. *praemonitorius*] Giving a warning, as an early symptom.

**premonocyte** (prē-mŏn′ō-sīt) [L. *prae,* before, in front of, + Gr. *monos,* alone, + *kytos,* cell] An embryonic cell transitional in development prior to a monocyte.

**premorbid** (prē-mor′bĭd) [″ + *morbidus,* sick] Prior to the development of disease.

**premyeloblast** (prē-mī′ĕ-lō-blăst) [″ + Gr. *myelos,* marrow, + *blastos,* germ] A precursor of the mature myeloblast.

**premyelocyte** (prē-mī′ĕl-ō-sīt) [″ + ″ + *kytos,* cell] The cell that is the immediate precursor of a myelocyte.

**prenarcosis** (prē-năr-kō′sĭs) [″ + Gr. *narkosis,* a benumbing] Premedication.

**prenatal** (prē-nā′tl) [″ + *natalis,* birth] Before birth.

**prenatal care** Care of the woman during the period of gestation. It consists of periodic examinations for determination of blood pressure, weight, changes in the size of the uterus, and the condition of the fetus; urinalysis; instruction in nutritional requirements, preparation for labor and delivery, care of the newborn; and provision of suggestions and support to deal with the discomforts of pregnancy.

Comprehensive care during pregnancy is based on a careful review of the patient's medical, surgical, obstetric and gynecologic, nutritional, and social history. The family history is reviewed for indications of genetic or other risk factors. Findings of laboratory tests provide important data describing current status and indications for treatment or anticipatory guidance. Patient teaching is important to enable active participation in care; emphasis is given to dietary counseling, preparation for childbirth, and basic care of the newborn. SEE: *pregnancy; prenatal diagnosis.*

**prenatal diagnosis** Diagnosis of disease or developmental defects while the infant is in utero. A great number of pathologic conditions can be diagnosed prenatally by use of tests such as ultrasound, amniocentesis, chorionic villus sampling, embryoscopy, and fetoscopy. Thus the sex of the child and information provided by study of the physical and chemical characteristics of the placenta, fetus, and inherited characteristics can be determined in the early months of pregnancy. If the results of these tests indicate the presence of a treatable disease, the indicated therapy can sometimes be instituted prenatally and, if needed, on the first day of life. If the tests indicate an incurable condition, genetic counseling is advisable. SEE: *prenatal surgery.*

**prenatal surgery** Intrauterine surgical procedures. These techniques have been used to repair heart defects and anatomical defects of other organs. SEE: *prenatal diagnosis.*

**preoperative care** (prē-ŏp′ĕr-ă-tĭv) [″ + *operatus,* work] Care preceding an operation.

NURSING IMPLICATIONS: The nurse should allow for time to discuss the meaning of procedure with the patient and to allow the patient to express concerns and fears. The patient should be instructed to cough, breathe deeply (splinting incision as necessary), turn, and exercise the extremities at frequent intervals. The nurse should prepare the operative site as prescribed; prepare the gastrointestinal tract as indicated (restrict food and fluids as ordered); promote rest and sleep; review laboratory results; and administer preoperative medications as prescribed after the patient has voided. The patient should perform oral hygiene; remove dentures, if present, as well as jewelry and make-up; and dress in a gown. The nurse should verify proper identification on the patient identification bracelet. If the patient is menstruating, the type of menstrual protection used should be noted on the chart. The patient's tampons or pads should be changed, at least every 4 to 6 hr in the case of tampons.

The nurse should counsel the patient concerning the timing of prescribed activities, including when to return to work and athletic endeavors, when sexual activity may be resumed, and whether or not there will be postoperative restriction on driving automobiles.

**preoptic area** The anterior portion of the hypothalamus. It is above the optic chiasma and on the sides of the third ventricle.

**preoral** (prē-ō′răl) [L. *prae,* before, in front of, + *os,* mouth] In front of the mouth.

**preoxygenation** Breathing of 100% oxygen via a face mask by the fully conscious patient prior to induction of anesthesia. Duration is 2 to 7 min. In that time, the nitrogen is washed out of the lungs and oxygen replaces it.

This same procedure is used for a longer period of time in persons prior to exposure to very low atmospheric pressure (e.g., aviators prior to flying to high altitudes) or to very high atmospheric pressure (e.g., divers descending to a great depth in water). In both cases, the goal is to rid the body of nitrogen to prevent bends.

**prep** (prĕp) [*prepare; preparation*] Used esp. when referring to preparation for surgery. SEE: *preoperative care.*

**prepalatal** (prē-păl′ă-tăl) [L. *prae,* before, in front of, + *palatum,* plate] Located in front of the teeth.

**preparalytic** (prē″păr-ă-lĭt′ĭk) [″ + Gr. *para,* at the side, + *lyein,* to loosen] Before the appearance of paralysis.

**preparation** (prĕp-ă-rā′shŭn) [L. *praeparatio*] **1.** The making ready, esp. of a medicine for use. **2.** A specimen set up for demonstration in anatomy, pathology, or histology. **3.** A medicine made ready for use.

***cavity p.*** The preparation of an artificial hole in a tooth so that the tooth can be restored by use of appropriate dental materials.

***chlorine p.*** A preparation used for disinfecting. Compounds (hypochlorites) such as Dakin's solution or Javelle water are very effective as germicides. As a disinfecting agent in washing dishes and utensils used by infected patients, $\frac{1}{10}$ of 1% solution should be used; the dishes should then be washed well in soap and hot water and rinsed thoroughly, or boiled and then washed well.

To disinfect the stools of patients, 5% or even stronger solutions may be used for ½ hr or longer. The covered container is set aside while the solution acts. Dakin's solution is nonirritating and is used as a wound disinfectant, but it must be carefully prepared daily and used only when fresh.

***corrosion p.*** In anatomical and pathology investigations, hollow organs and structures such as vessels are filled with a liquid substance that hardens. Then the surrounding tissues are dissolved by use of suitable chemicals. This leaves a cast of the structures.

***heart-lung p.*** In animal studies and in open-heart surgery, the use of devices that take over the function of the heart and lungs while those organs are being treated or possibly replaced.

**prepatellar** (prē″pă-tĕl′ăr) [L. *prae,* before, in front of, + *patella,* pan] In front of the patella.

**prepatellar bursitis** Inflammation of the bursa in front of the patella. SYN: *housemaid's knee.* SEE: *bursitis.*

**prepatent** Before becoming evident or manifest.

**prepatent period** The period between the time of introduction of parasitic organisms into the body and their appearance in the blood or tissues.

**preperception** (prē″pĕr-sĕp′shŭn) [″ + *percepitio,* to perceive] The anticipation of a perception. This intensifies the response to the perception.

**preperitoneal** (prē″pĕr-ĭ-tō-nē′ăl) [″ + Gr. *peritonaion,* peritoneum] Located in front of the peritoneum.

**preplacental** (prē″plă-sĕn′tăl) [″ + *placenta,* a flat cake] Occurring prior to formation of the placenta.

**prepotent** (prē-pō′tĕnt) [″ + *potentia,* power] Pert. to the greater power of one parent to transmit inherited characteristics to the offspring.

**preprandial** (prē-prăn′dē-ăl) [″ + *prandium,* breakfast] Before a meal.

**prepuberal, prepubertal** (prē-pū′bĕr-ăl, -tăl) [″ + *pubertas,* puberty] Before puberty.

**prepubescent** (prē″pū-bĕs′ĕnt) [″ + *pubescens,* becoming hairy] Pert. to the period just before puberty.

**prepuce** (prē′pūs) [L. *praeputium,* prepuce] Foreskin.

***p. of the clitoris*** A fold of the labia minora that covers the clitoris. SEE: *clitoris*.

**preputial** (prē-pū′shăl) Concerning the prepuce.

**preputial gland** Tyson's gland.

**preputiotomy** (prē-pū″shē-ŏt′ō-mē) [″ + Gr. *tome*, incision] Incision of the prepuce of the penis to relieve phimosis.

**preputium** (prē-pū′shē-ŭm) *pl.* **preputia** Prepuce.

***p. clitoridis*** The prepuce of the clitoris.

***p. penis*** Foreskin.

**prepyloric** (prē″pī-lor′ĭk) Anterior to, or preceding, the pylorus of the stomach.

**prerectal** (prē-rĕk′tăl) [L. *prae*, before, + *rectus*, straight] Located in front of the rectum.

**prerenal** (prē-rē′năl) [″ + *ren*, kidney] **1.** Located in front of the kidney. **2.** Occurring prior to reaching the kidney, such as changes in consistency of the blood prior to its flow to the kidney.

**preretinal** (prē-rĕt′ĭ-năl) [″ + *retina*, retina] In front of the retina of the eye.

**presacral** (prē-sā′krăl) [″ + *sacrum*, sacred] In front of the sacrum.

**presby-** Combining form meaning *old*.

**presbyacusia, presbyacousia** (prĕz″bē-ă-kū′sē-ă) [Gr. *presbys*, old, + *akousis*, hearing] The progressive loss of hearing ability due to the normal aging process. SYN: *presbycusis*.

**presbyatrics, presbyatry** (prĕz-bē-ăt′rĭks, prĕz′bē-ăt-rē) [″ + *iatrikos*, healing] Geriatrics.

**presbycardia** (prĕz-bĭ-kăr′dē-ă) [″ + *kardia*, heart] Disease or decreased functional capacity of the heart associated with aging.

**presbycusis, presbykousis** (prĕz-bĭ-kū′sĭs) [″ + *akousis*, hearing] Presbyacusia.

**presbyope** (prĕs′bē-ōp) [″ + *ops*, eye] A person who is presbyopic.

**presbyopia** (prĕz-bē-ō′pē-ă) [″ + *ops*, eye] A defect of vision in advancing age involving loss of accommodation or recession of near point. It is caused by a loss of elasticity of the crystalline lens. The onset usually occurs between 40 and 45 years of age. SEE: *farsightedness*.

**presbyopic** (prĕs″bē-ŏp′ĭk) Concerning presbyopia.

**presbytiatrics** (prĕz″bĭ-tē-ăt′rĭks) [″ + *iatrikos*, healing] Geriatrics.

**prescribe** (prē-skrīb′) [L. *praescriptio*, prescription] To indicate the medicine to be administered. This can be done orally but is usually done by writing a prescription or an order in the patient's hospital chart.

**prescribing error** An error in prescribing medications. Included are incorrect dose or medicine, duplicate therapy, incorrect route of administration, or wrong patient. In one extensive study of prescriptions written by physicians in a tertiary-care teaching hospital, 0.3% were erroneous and more than half of these were rated as having the potential for adverse consequences. Monitoring of medications and patients is thought to be helpful in limiting these errors.

**prescription** (prē-skrĭp′shŭn) [L. *praescriptio*] A written direction or order for dispensing and administering drugs. It is signed by a physician, dentist, or other practitioner licensed by law to prescribe such a drug. Historically, a prescription consists of four main parts.

*Superscription:* Represented by the symbol ℞, which signifies Recipe, from the Latin *recipere*, meaning to take.

*Inscription:* Containing the ingredients. This is generally constructed of four parts: the basis or principal drug; the adjuvant, which assists the action of the basis; the corrective, which diminishes unpleasant taste or pain or griping, and so on; and the vehicle to hold the drugs in either solution or suspension.

*Subscription:* Directions to the dispenser as to the manner of preparation of the drugs.

*Signature:* Directions to the patient with regard to the manner of taking dosage and the physician's signature, address, telephone number, date, and whether or not the prescription may be refilled. When applicable, the physician's narcotics registry number must be included. Also, some states require that the prescriber indicate on the prescription whether or not a generic drug may be substituted for the trade name equivalent.

---

Caution: Unused prescription pads should be kept in a secure place in order to prevent their being misused or stolen. Each prescription should be numbered consecutively. One should never sign a prescription blank in advance. The prescriber should use ink to prevent changes being made and not use prescription pads for writing notes or memos.

---

***p. drug*** A drug available to the public only upon prescription written by a physician, dentist, or other practitioner licensed to do so.

***shotgun p.*** An indiscriminate prescription for a large number of drugs in the hope that at least one of them will be of benefit.

**prescription writing** Modern practice is to write prescriptions entirely in the language of the country in which written (as English in the United States) and to use few, if any, abbreviations. All drug quantities should be shown by using the metric system of weights and measures (e.g., grams, milligrams, liters, milliliters). SEE: *Prescription Writing in Abbreviations Appendix*.

The following classic presentation of the art of prescription writing is included primarily for its historical interest: An official Latin name is in the nominative case. Drugs are written in the genitive case because the prescription is an order, meaning "take thou." The word "of" is not written in Latin but is indicated by the ending of a word: *quinina* means *quinine,* but changing the termination to "ae," we have *quininae,* meaning *of quinine.*

ALKALOIDS: Written the same as in English, except that the final "e" is changed to "a" to form the nominative case, as *quinina,* for the English quinine. To form the genitive case, the final "e" is changed to "ae," as *quininae.*

ACTIVE PRINCIPLES: These, such as glucosides, resinoids, and others, add "um" to the nominative and "i" to the genitive, so that strophanthin becomes *strophanthinum* to form the Latin nominative, and *strophanthini,* to form the Latin genitive.

ACIDS: The names of these are formed in the same way as those of alkaloids, except that the adjective is formed in the same way and follows the nominative, as *acidum hydrochloricum,* or the genitive, *acidi hydrochlorici.*

METALS: Latin names of metals, except those of a few known to the ancients, are the same as English forms ending in "um," as in *sodium,* forming the Latin nominative, but ending in "i" to form the genitive, *sodii.*

SALTS: These are written first with the name of the base in its genitive form, next the acid radical in the nominative, followed by the qualitative adjective in the nominative, as *ferri sulfas exsiccatus,* exsiccated sulfate of iron.

NAMES OF PREPARATIONS: For these, the class to which the preparation belongs is shown first, the name of the ingredient next, and the qualifying adjective last, as *syrupus scillae compositus* (compound syrup of squills). First and last words are in nominative case and middle one in genitive.

DRUGS WITH TWO NAMES: Both should be in the genitive, as *liquor potassi arsenitis.* (-ate endings): The Latin nominative ends in "as," as *sulfas,* for sulfate; and the genitive in "atis," as *sulfatis.* (-ite endings): If the English word ends in "ite," as *sulfite,* the Latin nominative ends in "is," as *sulfis,* and the genitive in "itis," as *sulfitis.* (-ide endings): If an English word has this ending, as "bromide," the Latin nominative ends in "um," dropping the final "e" in the English form, as *bromidum;* the genitive dropping the "um" to add "i," as *bromidi.* (-a, -us, -um endings): English words with these endings are the same in the Latin nominative, but the genitive is formed by changing "a" to "ae," or the "us" or "um" to "i." (-in endings): An English word having this ending adds "um" (usually) to form the Latin nominative as benzoin and *benzoinum,* the genitive being formed by merely adding "i," as *benzoini.* (-ol endings): The Latin nominative is the same as the English, as in phenol, but "is" is added to form the genitive, as *phenolis.* (-al endings): To form the Latin nominative, "um" is added, as chloral and *chloralum.* To form the genitive, "i" is added to the English form, as *chlorali.*

There are, of course, exceptions to the foregoing. Many Latin words have the same form as in English.

**prescriptive authority** The limited authority to prescribe certain medications according to established protocol.

**presenile** (prē-sē′nīl) [L. *prae,* before, in front of, + *senilis,* old] Pert. to premature old age as judged by mental or physical condition but usually the former. Dementia may appear as early as age 40 to 45 and is characterized by personality disintegration as well as loss of intellectual functioning. Alzheimer's disease, Pick's disease, and Creutzfeldt-Jakob disease are characterized as presenile dementias.

**presenium** (prē-sē′nē-ŭm) [″ + *senium,* old age] Just prior to the onset of senility.

**present** [L. *praesent,* to be present before others] The presence of the patient for examination.

**presentation** (prē″zĕn-tā′shŭn) [L. *praesentatio*] **1.** In obstetrics, the position of the fetus presenting itself to the examining finger in the vagina or rectum (e.g., longitudinal or normal and transverse or pathologic presentation). **2.** The relationship of the long axis of fetus to that of the mother; also called *lie.* SEE: illus.; *position* for table. **3.** The fetal body part that first enters the maternal pelvis. SEE: *position* for table.

***breech p.*** Presentation in which the buttocks of the fetus present. Breech presentation is of three types: complete breech, when the thighs of the fetus are flexed on the abdomen and the legs flexed upon the thighs; frank breech, when the legs of the fetus are extended over the anterior surface of the body; and footling, when a foot or feet present. Footling can be single, double, or, if the leg remains flexed, knee presentation. SYN: *pelvic p.*

***brow p.*** Presentation in which the brow or face of the infant comes first during labor, making vaginal delivery almost impossible. Cesarean section may be needed if the presentation cannot be altered.

***cephalic p.*** Presentation of the head of the fetus in any position.

***compound p.*** Presentation in which a prolapsed limb is alongside the main presenting part.

***face p.*** Presentation in which the head of the fetus is sharply extended so that the face presents.

***footling p.*** Presentation in which the feet present. SEE: *breech p.*

***funic p., funis p.*** Appearance of the umbilical cord during labor.

***longitudinal p.*** Presentation in which the long axis of the fetus is parallel to the long axis of the mother.

## PRESENTATIONS OF FETUS

### ATTITUDES OF THE FETUS

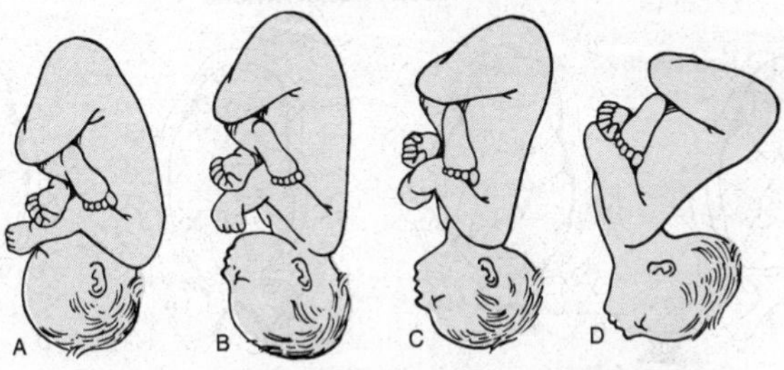


A—VERTEX PRESENTATION; B—SINCIPUT PRESENTATION; C—BROW PRESENTATION; D—FACE PRESENTATION*

### BROW PRESENTATION

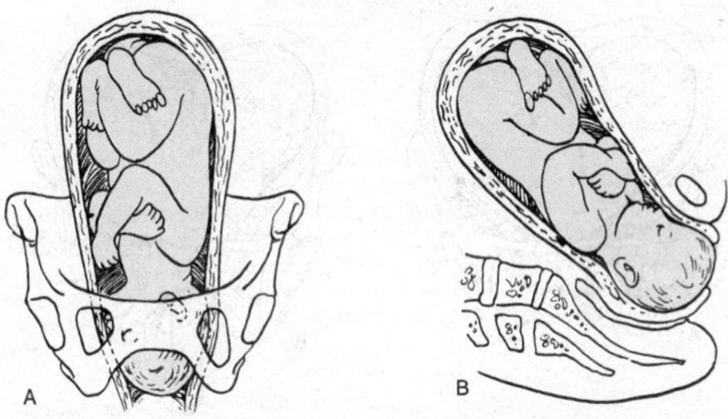


A—ANTERIOR VIEW; B—SAGITTAL VIEW*

### FACE PRESENTATIONS

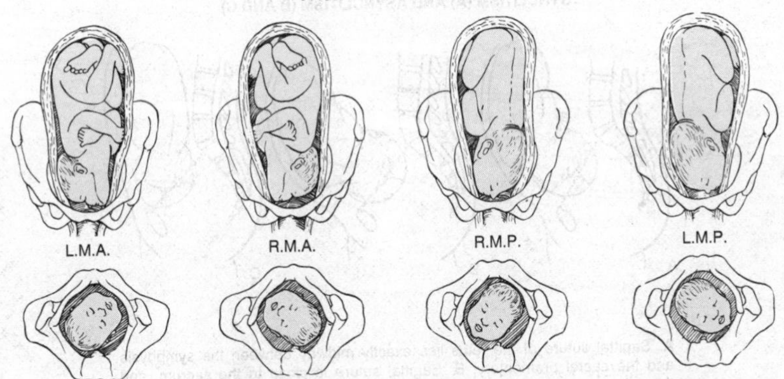


LEFT MENTOANTERIOR (L.M.A.); RIGHT MENTOANTERIOR (R.M.A.); RIGHT MENTOPOSTERIOR (R.M.P.); LEFT MENTOPOSTERIOR (L.M.P.)*

*Reproduced with permission from Bonica, J.: *Principles and Practice of Obstetric Analgesia and Anesthesia.* F.A. Davis, Philadelphia, 1972.

*(see following page)*

## PRESENTATIONS OF FETUS

### TYPES OF BREECH PRESENTATIONS

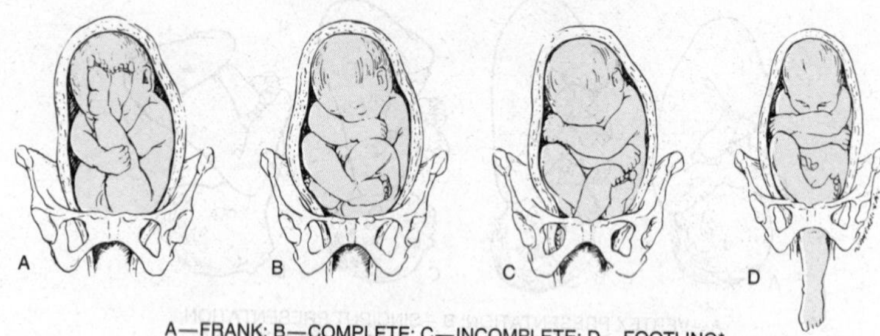


A—FRANK; B—COMPLETE; C—INCOMPLETE; D—FOOTLING*

### TRANSVERSE PRESENTATION

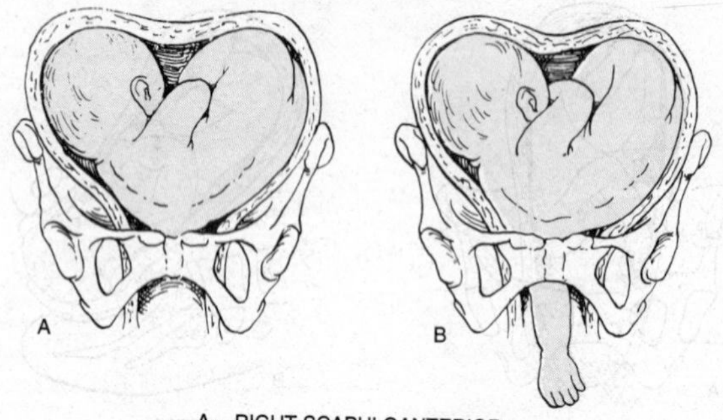


A—RIGHT SCAPULOANTERIOR;
B—PROLAPSE OF AN ARM IN TRANSVERSE LIE*

### SYNCLITISM (A) AND ASYNCLITISM (B AND C)

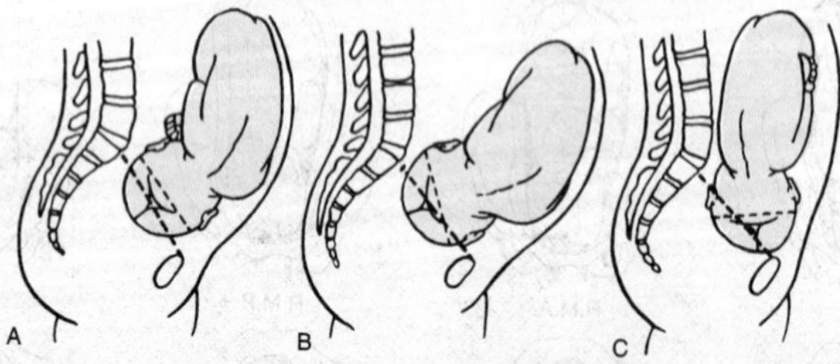


A. Sagittal suture of the fetus lies exactly midway between the symphysis and the sacral promontory. B. Sagittal suture is close to the sacrum, and the anterior parietal bone is felt by the examining finger (anterior asynclitism of Nägele's obliquity). C. Posterior parietal presentation of posterior asynclitism (Litzmann's obliquity).*

*Reproduced with permission from Bonica, J.: *Priniciples and Practice of Obstetric Analgesia and Anesthesia.* F.A. Davis, Philadelphia, 1972.

***oblique p.*** Presentation in which the long axis of the fetus is oblique to that of the mother.

***pelvic p.*** Breech p.

***placental p.*** Placenta previa.

***shoulder p.*** Presentation in which the shoulder of the fetus is the presenting part.

***transverse p.*** Presentation with the fetus lying crosswise.

***vertex p.*** Presentation of the upper and back part of the fetal head.

**preservative** (prē-zĕr′vă-tĭv) [L. *prae,* before, in front of, + *servare,* to keep] A substance added to medicines or foods to prevent them from spoiling. It may act by interfering with certain chemical reactions or with the growth of molds, fungi, bacteria, or parasites. Some common preservatives are sugar, salt, vinegar, ethyl alcohol, sulfur dioxide, and benzoic acid.

**presomite** (prē-sō′mīt) [″ + Gr. *soma,* body] The embryonic stage prior to the formation of somites.

**presphenoid** (prē-sfē′noyd) [″ + Gr. *sphen,* wedge, + *eidos,* form, shape] The anterior region of the body on the sphenoid bone.

**presphygmic** (prē-sfĭg′mĭk) [″ + Gr. *sphygmos,* pulse] Pert. to the period preceding the pulse wave.

**prespinal** (prē-spī′năl) [″ + *spina,* thorn] In front of the spine, or ventral to it.

**prespondylolisthesis** (prē-spŏn″dĭl-ō-lĭs-thē′sĭs) [″ + Gr. *spondylos,* vertebra, + *olisthanein,* to slip] A congenital defect of both pedicles of the fifth lumbar vertebra without displacement, predisposing the individual to spondylolisthesis.

**pressor** (prĕs′or) [O. Fr. *presser,* to press] **1.** Stimulating, increasing the activity of a function, esp. of vasomotor activity, as a nerve. **2.** Inducing an elevation in blood pressure.

***p. base*** One of several amines or nitrogenous bases of plant or animal origin that, when injected, have the ability to increase blood pressure.

**pressoreceptive** (prĕs″ō-rē-sĕp′tĭv) Sensitive to pressure stimuli. SYN: *pressosensitive.*

**pressoreceptor** (prĕs″ō-rē-sĕp′tor) A sensory nerve ending, such as those in the aorta and carotid sinus, that is stimulated by changes in blood pressure. SYN: *baroreceptor.*

**pressosensitive** (prĕs″ō-sĕn′sĭ-tĭv) Pressoreceptive.

**pressure** (prĕsh′ŭr) [L. *pressura*] **1.** A compression. **2.** Stress or force exerted on a body, as by tension, weight, or pulling. **3.** In psychology, the quality of sensation aroused by moderate compression of the skin. **4.** In physics, the quotient obtained by dividing a force by the area of the surface on which it acts.

***alveolar p.*** Air pressure in the alveoli and bronchial tree. It fluctuates below and above atmospheric pressure during breathing; this causes air to enter or leave the lungs. SYN: *intrapulmonic p.*

***arterial p.*** The pressure of the blood in the arteries. For a normal young person at physical and mental rest and in sitting position, systolic blood pressure averages about 120 mm Hg; diastolic pressure about 80 mm Hg. A wide range of normal variation is due to constitutional, physical, and psychic factors. For women, the figures are slightly lower. For older people, they are higher. Normally there is little difference in the blood pressure recorded in the two arms. SEE: *blood pressure.*

***atmospheric p.*** The pressure of the weight of the atmosphere; at sea level it averages about 760 mm Hg.

***back p.*** The pressure resulting from interference in flow of blood from the ventricles, such as occurs in valvular disorders. It results in reduced venous return to the heart and consequent venous engorgement.

***bilevel positive airway p.*** ABBR: BiPAP A type of continuous positive airway pressure in which both inspiratory and expiratory pressure are set.

***biting p.*** The pressure exerted on the teeth during biting. SYN: *occlusal p.*

***blood p.*** SEE: *blood pressure.*

***capillary p.*** The blood pressure in the capillaries.

***central venous p.*** The pressure in the right atrium of the heart. It is determined by inserting a catheter into the heart via a vein, usually in the arm. The catheter is attached to a manometer.

***cerebrospinal p.*** The pressure of the cerebrospinal fluid. This varies with body position.

***critical p.*** The pressure exerted by a vapor at its critical temperature in an evacuated container.

***diastolic p.*** Arterial pressure during diastole or dilatation of the heart chambers.

***effective osmotic p.*** That portion of the total osmotic pressure of a solution that determines the tendency of the solvent to pass through a membrane, usually one that is semipermeable. The tendency is for the solvent to pass from a solution containing a high concentration of the solute to the side of the membrane with the low concentration.

***end-diastolic p.*** Blood pressure in a ventricle of the heart at the end of diastole.

***endocardiac p.*** Blood pressure within the heart.

***hydrostatic p.*** The pressure exerted by a fluid within a closed system.

***intra-abdominal p.*** Pressure within the abdominal cavity, such as that caused by descent of the diaphragm.

***intracranial p.*** The pressure of the cerebrospinal fluid in the subarachnoid space between the skull and the brain. The pressure is normally the same as that found during lumbar puncture.

***intraocular p.*** Normal tension within the eyeball, equal to approx. 12 to 20 mm Hg.

***intrapleural p.*** The pressure between the two pleural membranes. It is normally always lower than atmospheric pressure and therefore sometimes called a negative pressure. SYN: *intrathoracic p.*

***intrapulmonic p.*** Alveolar p.

***intrathoracic p.*** Intrapleural p.

***intraventricular p.*** The pressure within the ventricles of the heart during different phases of diastole and systole.

***negative p.*** Any pressure less than that of the atmosphere, or less than that pressure to which the initial pressure is being compared.

***occlusal p.*** Biting p.

***oncotic p.*** Osmotic pressure exerted by colloids in a solution.

***osmotic p.*** The force with which a solvent, usually water, passes through a semipermeable membrane separating solutions of different concentrations. It is measured by determining the hydrostatic (mechanical) pressure that must be opposed to the osmotic force to bring the passage to a standstill.

***partial p.*** In a gas containing several different components, the pressure exerted by each component.

***positive p.*** Pressure greater than atmospheric or greater than the pressure to which the initial pressure is being compared.

***positive end-expiratory p.*** ABBR: PEEP. In respiratory medicine, a method of holding alveoli open during expiration. This is done by gradually increasing the expiratory pressure. When PEEP is used, it is important that pulmonary capillary wedge pressure be monitored by use of a Swan-Ganz catheter in the pulmonary artery. The goal is to achieve adequate arterial oxygenation without using toxic levels of inspired oxygen, and without compromising cardiac output.

Caution: The patient must be carefully monitored during the therapy to ensure compliance and to allow observation for undesired side effects such as pneumomediastinum, subcutaneous emphysema, and pneumothorax.

***positive end-expiratory p., auto*** ABBR: auto-PEEP. A complication of mechanical ventilation in which the device does not permit the patient sufficient time to exhale. This causes air to be trapped in the lungs, particularly the alveoli. If continued, auto-PEEP causes respiratory muscle fatigue and can cause rupture of the lung (i.e., pneumothorax). Auto-PEEP may be corrected by increasing exhalation time, decreasing the ventilator rate, or switching the ventilation mode so that the patient's spontaneous respiratory pattern governs the inspiratory and expiratory times.

***posterior cricoid p.*** Pressure applied by firmly placing the thumb and index finger on the lateral aspects of a patient's cricoid ring to occlude the esophagus. SYN: *Sellick's maneuver.*

***preload filling p.*** The amount of pressure or volume in the ventricle at end diastole, measured by central venous pressure (right ventricular end-diastolic pressure) or pulmonary capillary wedge pressure (left ventricular end-diastolic pressure).

***pulse p.*** The difference between systolic and diastolic pressures. It characterizes the tone of the arterial walls. The systolic pressure is normally about 40 points greater than the diastolic. A pulse pressure over 50 points or under 30 points is considered abnormal.

***solution p.*** Pressure that tends to dissolve a solid present in a solution.

***static p.*** The pressure existing in all points in the circulation when the heart is stopped. It provides a measure of how well the circulatory bed is filled with blood.

***systolic p.*** Arterial pressure at the time of the contraction of the ventricles, or the ventricular systole.

***venous p.*** The pressure of the blood within the veins. It is highest near the periphery, diminishing progressively from capillaries to the heart. Near the heart the venous pressure may be below zero (negative pressure) owing to negative intrathoracic pressure.

***wedge p.*** Pressure determined by use of a fluid-filled catheter wedged in the distal end of a branch of the pulmonary artery. This provides an indirect measurement of the pressure in the left atrium of the heart.

**pressure of speech** Loud and emphatic speech that is increased in amount, accelerated, and usually difficult or impossible to interrupt. The speech is not in response to a stimulus and may continue even though no one is listening. It may be present in manic episodes, organic brain disease, depression with agitation, psychotic disorders, and sometimes as an acute reaction to stress.

**pressure point** An area that can be used for exerting pressure to control bleeding. For control of hemorrhage, pressure above the bleeding point when an artery passes over a bone may be sufficient. SEE: *bleeding* for table.

TECHNIQUE: Principal pressure points and the type of pressure that should be exerted follow: *Common carotid artery,* 2 in. (5 cm) above the clavicle, pressing backward against the spine. *Temporal artery,* at the side of the face in front of the ear. *Occipital artery,* behind the mastoid process. *Subclavian artery,* behind the clavicle, pressing down onto the first rib. *Axillary artery,* by compression in the axilla. *Brachial artery,* compressed by pressure at the inner edge of the biceps muscle halfway down the arm and also above the bend of the elbow before the artery divides into the radial and ulnar arteries. *Radial artery,* pressure on the thumb side of the wrist against the radius. *Ulnar artery,* pressure on the little finger side of the wrist against the ulna. *Deep palmar arch,* in the thumb opposite the root of the abducted thumb. *Abdominal artery,* compression against the lumbar vertebrae to the left of the middle line when the patient lies on the back. *Femoral artery,* by abduction and external rotation of thigh, bringing the head of femur forward into groin and compressing the artery against it. *Popliteal artery,* in the popliteal space over the artery. *Anterior tibial artery,* at the front of the bend of the ankle. *Posterior tibial artery,* behind the internal malleolus as it passes into foot.

***equal p. p.*** During forced exhalation, the point at an airway where the pressure inside the wall equals the intrapleural pressure. The pleural pressure is greater than the pressure inside the airway, tending to cause bronchiolar collapse.

**pressure sore** A sore caused by pressure from a splint or other appliance, or from the body itself when it has remained immobile in bed for extended periods of time. The likelihood of a patient developing a pressure sore is increased if urinary incontinence is present. In actual practice, the tendency is to speak of decubitus ulcers as being synonymous with pressure sores. However, the latter is due to pressure on the skin, even when the patient is not lying down. Nevertheless, the operative force is pressure, leading to inadequate blood supply of the area and, if continued, to a sore or ulcer. SYN: *decubitus ulcer.* SEE: *Nursing Diagnoses Appendix.*

**presternum** (prē-stĕr′nŭm) [L. *prae,* before, in front of, + Gr. *sternon,* chest] The upper part of the sternum. SYN: *manubrium sterni.*

**presuppurative** (prē-sŭp′ū-rā″tĭv) [″ + *sub,* under, + *puris,* pus] Relating to the period of inflammation before suppuration.

**presylvian fissure** (prē-sĭl′vē-ăn) The anterior division of the sylvian fissure.

**presymptomatic** (prē″sĭmp-tō-măt′ĭk) The state of health prior to the clinical appearance of the signs and symptoms of a disease.

**presynaptic** (prē″sĭ-năp′tĭk) [″ + Gr. *synapsis,* point of contact] Located before the nerve synapse.

**presyncope** Faintness.

**presystole** (prē-sĭs′tō-lē) [L. *prae,* before, in front of, + Gr. *systole,* contraction] The period in the heart's cycle just before the systole. SYN: *perisystole.*

**presystolic** (prē-sĭs-tŏl′ĭk) Before the systole of the heart.

**pretarsal** (prē-tăr′săl) [″ + Gr. *tarsos,* a broad flat surface] In front of the tarsus.

**preterm** In obstetrics, occurring prior to the 37th week of gestation. SYN: *premature.*

**preterm birth** Delivery occurring between 20 and 38 weeks' gestation. Despite intensive study of causes and methods of preventing preterm birth, progress has been slow. In the U.S., preterm birth occurs in about 10% of all births. Neonatal morbidity is high and physiologic immaturity is a major factor in about three fourths of all neonatal deaths not associated with congenital malformations. Preterm neonates are at high risk for developing respiratory distress syndrome, intraventricular hemorrhage, sepsis, patent ductus arteriosis, retinopathy of prematurity, and necrotizing enterocolitis. SEE: *prematurity.*

TREATMENT: When there is a risk of birth occurring between 24 and 34 weeks' gestation, corticosteroid therapy to stimulate fetal lung maturation and production of pulmonary surfactant should be considered; however, birth must occur in no less than 24 hr after administration. Therapy should be repeated weekly until 34 weeks' gestation. There is no evidence that this treatment is harmful to fetuses of either gender.

CONTRAINDICATIONS: Corticosteroid therapy should not be administered if the mother has chorioamnionitis or if there is evidence that the drug will have an adverse effect on the mother. Caution is recommended in women who have diabetes mellitus and/or hypertension.

**preterm labor** SEE: under *labor.*

**pretibial** (prē-tĭb′ē-ăl) [″ + *tibia,* shinbone] In front of the tibia.

**pretibial fever** A form of leptospirosis caused by one of the several serotypes of the autumnalis serogroup. It is characterized by fever, a rash on the legs, prostration, splenomegaly, and respiratory disturbances. SYN: *Fort Bragg fever.*

**pretympanic** (prē″tĭm-păn′ĭk) [″ + *tympanon,* drum] Located in front of the tympanic membrane.

**preurethritis** (prē″ū-rē-thrī′tĭs) [″ + Gr. *ourethra,* urethra, + *itis,* inflammation] Inflammation around the urethral orifice of the vaginal vestibule.

**prevalence** (prĕv′ă-lĕns) [L. *praevalens,* prevail] The number of cases of a disease present in a specified population at a given time. SEE: *incidence.*

**preventive** (prē-vĕn′tĭv) [ME. *preventen,* to anticipate] Hindering the occurrence of something, esp. disease. SYN: *prophylactic* (1).

**preventive medicine** The branch of medicine concerned with preventing the occurrence of both mental and physical illness and disease. There are three levels of preventive effort. Primary preventive medicine is concerned with preventing the development of disease in a susceptible or potentially susceptible population. These efforts include general promotion of health and specific protection such as immunization. Secondary preventive medicine involves early diagnosis and prompt therapy to shorten duration of illness, reduce the severity of disease, reduce the possibility of contagion, and limit sequelae. Tertiary preventive medicine is important in limiting the degree of disability and promoting rehabilitation in chronic and irreversible diseases. SEE: *preventive nursing; public health.*

**preventive nursing** The branch of nursing concerned with preventing the occurrence of both mental and physical illness and disease. The nurse is an essential part of the health care team and has the opportunity to emphasize and indeed implement health care services to promote health and prevent disease. Nursing expertise and general professional competence can also be used in supporting community action at all levels for promoting public health measures. There are three levels of preventive nursing:

*A. Primary.* Nursing care aimed at general health promotion. This includes whatever intervention is required to provide a health-promoting environment at home, in the schools, in public places, and in the workplace by ensuring good nutrition, adequate clothing and shelter, rest and recreation, and health education (including sex education and, for the aging, realistic plans for retirement). Areas of emphasis are specific protective measures such as immunizations, environmental sanitation, accident prevention, and protection from occupational hazards. Changes in lifestyle through behavior therapy, though difficult, must be attempted with respect to those areas known to represent major health risk factors (i.e., smoking, obesity, sedentary lifestyle, improper diet, alcohol and drug abuse, sexual promiscuity and not practicing safe sex, and falls). Major efforts must be made to prevent automobile accidents.

*B. Secondary.* Nursing care aimed at early recognition and treatment of disease. It includes general nursing interventions and teaching of early signs of disease conditions. Infectious diseases, glaucoma, obesity, and cancer fall into this category.

*C. Tertiary.* Nursing care for patients with incurable diseases, and patient instruction concerning how to manage those conditions and diseases. Parkinson's disease, multiple sclerosis, and diabetes are conditions that lend themselves to tertiary prevention. The goal is to prevent further deterioration of physical and mental function, and to have the patient use whatever residual function is available for maximum enjoyment of and participation in life's activities. Rehabilitation is of course an essential part of tertiary prevention. SEE: *preventive medicine; public health.*

**prevertebral** (prē-vĕr′tē-brăl) [L. *prae,* before, in front of, + *vertebra,* vertebra] In front of a vertebra.

**prevertebral ganglion** Any of the ganglia of the sympathetic division of the autonomic nervous system, located near origins of the celiac and mesenteric arteries. These include the celiac and mesenteric ganglia. SYN: *ganglion, collateral.*

**prevertiginous** (prē-vĕr-tĭj′ĭ-nŭs) [″ + *vertigo,* a turning round] Having a tendency to fall forward.

**prevesical** (prē-vĕs′ĭ-kl) [″ + *vesica,* bladder] Located in front of the bladder.

**previa, praevia** (prē′vē-ă) [L.] Appearing before or in front of.

**previable** Pert. to a fetus not sufficiently mature to survive outside the uterus.

**prevocational evaluation** In rehabilitation, the assessment of those interests, aptitudes, abilities, and behavioral traits that are necessary for developing or performing specific job skills.

**prezonular** Pert. to the posterior chamber of the eye, the space between the iris and ciliary zonule (suspensory ligament).

**prezygotic** (prē-zī-gŏt′ĭk) [″ + *zygotos,* yoked] Happening prior to fertilization of the ovum.

**priapism** (prī′ă-pĭzm) [LL. *priapismus*] Abnormal, painful, and continued erection of the penis caused by disease, occurring usually without sexual desire. SEE: *erection; gonorrhea.*

ETIOLOGY: It may be due to lesions of the cord above the lumbar region; turgescence of the corpora cavernosa without erection may exist. It may be reflex from peripheral sensory irritants, from organic irritation of nerve tracts or nerve centers when libido may be lacking. It is sometimes seen in patients with acute leukemia. It can also be due to medicines injected into the penis to promote erection.

***stuttering p.*** Painful, recurrent attacks of priapism that last 2 to 6 hr. The condition is seen in some patients with homozygous sickle cell disease.

**priapitis** (prī-ă-pī′tĭs) [Gr. *priapos,* phallus, + *itis,* inflammation] Inflammation of the penis.

**priapus** (prī′ă-pŭs) [Gr. *priapos*] The penis.

**prickly heat** Miliaria.

**prilocaine hydrochloride** (prĭl′ō-kān) A local anesthetic. It may cause methemoglobinemia.

**primal scene** In psychiatry, the term for a child's first observation of sexual intercourse, real or imagined.

**primaquine phosphate** (prĭm′ă-kwĭn) An antimalarial drug.

**primary** (prī′mă-rē) [L. *primarius,* principal] First in time or order. SYN: *principal.*

**primary bubo** An inflamed lymph node that represents the initial lesion following exposure to a venereal disease, esp. to syphilis. Also called *bubon d'emblée.*

**primary care** Integrated, accessible health care provided by clinicians who are responsible for most of a patient's personal health care needs and who work in a sustained partnership with their patients. The primary health care provider assumes ongoing responsibility for health maintenance and therapy for illness, including consultation with specialists.

**primary cell** In physical therapy, a device consisting of a container, two solid conducting elements, and an electrolyte for the production of electric current by chemical energy.

**primary health care** An approach to providing health care that was articulated at a conference of the World Health Organization in 1978 at Alma Ata, Russia. The goal of health for all by the year 2000 is the principal aim of primary health care. Each member country identified ways in which it would institute primary health care to meet this goal.

**primary nursing** The nursing practice system in which the entire nursing care of a patient is managed and coordinated by one nurse for a 24-hr period. The nurse is involved in, manages, and coordinates all aspects of the patient's case in that period. This includes scheduling of activities, tests, and procedures.

**primary radiation** That radiation being emitted directly to the patient from the x-ray source.

**primary sore** The initial sore or hard chancre of syphilis.

**primate** (prī′māt) [L. *primus,* first] A member of the order Primates.

**Primates** (prī-mā′tēz) An order of vertebrates belonging to the class Mammalia, subclass Theria, including the lemurs, tarsiers, monkeys, apes, and humans. This order is most highly developed with respect to the brain and nervous system.

**prime** (prīm) [L. *primus,* first] **1.** The period of greatest health and strength. **2.** To give an initial treatment in preparation for either a larger dose of the same medicine, or a different medicine.

**primidone** (prĭm′ĭ-dōn) An anticonvulsive drug used in treating epilepsy.

**primigravida** (prī-mĭ-grăv′ĭ-dă) [″ + *gravida,* pregnant] A woman during her first pregnancy.

***elderly p.*** A woman who is 35 years of age or older and pregnant for the first time. In the past, women were informed that delaying childbearing until age 35 or more would greatly increase the chance of an adverse outcome of pregnancy. A well-controlled study of the outcome of first pregnancy in this age group indicates little, if any, increased risk of adverse fetal outcome. The women themselves had significantly more antepartum and intrapartum complications than younger women. The women studied were private patients who were predominantly white, college educated, married, nonsmoking, and had had excellent prenatal care.

**primipara** (prī-mĭp′ă-ră) [″ + *parere,* to bring forth, to bear] A woman who has been delivered of one infant of 500 g (or of 20 weeks' gestation), regardless of its viability.

**primiparous** (prī-mĭp′ă-rŭs) Pert. to a primipara.

**primitiae** (prī-mĭsh′ē-ē) [L. *primus,* first] Liquor amnii appearing just before the birth of the fetus. SEE: *amnion; bag of waters; labor; liquor amnii.*

**primitive** (prĭm′ĭ-tĭv) [L. *primitivus*] Original; early in point of time; embryonic.

**primitive streak** In embryology, the initial band of cells from which the embryo begins to develop. These cells are at the caudal end of the embryonic disc. It is present at about 15 days after fertilization.

**primordial** (prī-mor′dē-ăl) [L. *primordialis*] **1.** Existing first. **2.** Existing in an undeveloped, primitive, or early form.

**primordium** (prī-mor′dē-ŭm) *pl.* **primordia** [L., origin] The first accumulation of cells in an embryo that constitutes the beginning of a future tissue, organ, or part. SYN: *anlage.*

**primum non nocere** (prī″mŭm nōn nō′sĕ-rā) [L.] "First do no harm." No one's condition should be made worse because of having visited a physician. This is an idealistic but virtually unattainable goal, because there is no medical procedure, operation, or drug that does not have the potential for harm. SEE: *risk-benefit analysis.*

**princeps** (prĭn′sĕps) [L., chief] **1.** Original; first. **2.** The name of certain arteries (e.g., princeps cervicis). **3.** Chief, principal.

**principal** (prĭn′sĭ-păl) **1.** Chief. **2.** Outstanding.

**principal fibers of the periodontal ligament** ABBR: PDL. The oriented bundles of collagen fibers that, by their attachments and position within the periodontal ligament space, are recognized as specific parts of the alveolodental ligament. Bundles of PDL fibers are named according to orientation and attachment.

**principle** (prĭn′sĭ-pl) [L. *principium,* foundation] **1.** A constituent of a compound representing its essential properties. **2.** A fundamental truth. **3.** An established rule of action.

***active p.*** The portion of a pharmaceutical preparation that produces the therapeutic action.

***antianemic p.*** A substance stored in the liver that is essential for the normal development of red blood cells in the bone marrow. It is formed in the stomach and intestine by the interaction of an extrinsic factor, vitamin $B_{12}$, and an intrinsic factor present in gastric juice. It is used in the treatment of pernicious anemia. SYN: *antianemic factor.*

***antidiuretic p.*** The antidiuretic hormone (ADH) present in extracts of the posterior lobe of the pituitary gland.

***gastrointestinal p.*** Any of the substances, secreted by the mucosa of the stomach and intestine, that are absorbed by the blood and act as hormones. SEE: *cholecystokinin-pancreozymin; gastrin; secretin.*

***oxytocic p.*** A hormone in extracts of the posterior lobe of the hypophysis that stimulates contraction of the uterine muscle.

***pleasure p.*** In psychoanalysis, the idea that unconsciously the individual is striving to attain pleasure and avoid painful situations.

***proximate p.*** A substance that may be extracted from its complex form without destroying or altering its chemical properties.

***purpura-producing p.*** A toxic substance produced when pneumococci are autolyzed. This causes dermal and internal hemorrhages when injected into rabbits.

***reality p.*** In psychoanalysis, the idea that the striving for pleasure is balanced by the situations produced by the real world.

**Prinzmetal's angina** [Myron Prinzmetal, U.S. cardiologist, b. 1908] An atypical form of angina pectoris thought to be due to vasospasm of otherwise normal coronary arteries. Pain is experienced at rest and sometimes while in bed rather than during activity. The electrocardiogram taken during an attack will indicate S–T segment elevation rather than depression. Nitroglycerin and drugs that influence calcium metabolism by the myocardium are of benefit. SYN: *variant angina.*

**prion** (prē′ŏn) [*pro*teinaceous *in*fection particle] A small proteinaceous infection particle that is resistant to most procedures that modify nucleic acid.

**prion disease** Any disease caused by a proteinaceous infectious particle (prion). These particles, which are not viruses, are responsible for human transmissible neurodegenerative diseases including kuru, Creutzfeldt-Jacob disease, Gerstmann-Strüssler-Scheinker syndrome, and fatal familial insomnia. Prions may be responsible for transmissible and inherited disorders of proteins. How they alter normal cellular proteins is unknown. The possibility that prion diseases are somehow related to Alzheimer's disease, amyotrophic lateral sclerosis, and Parkinson's disease is being investigated. SEE: *insomnia, fatal familial; syndrome, Gerstmann-Strüssler-Scheinker.*

**prism** (prĭzm) [Gr. *prisma*] A transparent solid, three sides of which are parallelograms. The bases, perpendicular to the three sides, are triangles, and a transverse section of the solid is a triangle. Light rays going through a prism are deflected toward the base of the triangle and at the same time are split into the primary colors.

***enamel p.*** A minute rod of calcareous material deposited at the end of an ameloblast in the formation of the enamel of a tooth.

***Maddox p.*** Two base-together prisms used in testing for cyclophoria or torsion of the eyeball.

***Nicol p.*** A prism made by splitting a prism of Icelandic spar and rejoining the cut surfaces. This causes the light passing through to be split. Ordinary light rays are reflected by the joined surfaces, and polarized light is transmitted.

***Risley's rotary p.*** A prism mounted in a device that allows it to be rotated. This is used in testing eye muscle imbalance.

**prismatic** (prĭz-măt′ĭk) **1.** Shaped like a prism. **2.** Produced by a prism.

**prismoid** (prĭz′moyd) [″ + *eidos,* form, shape] Resembling a prism.

**prismoptometer** (prĭz-mŏp-tŏm′ĕ-tĕr) [″ + *opsis,* vision, + *metron,* measure] A device for estimating abnormal refraction of the eye by using prisms.

**privacy** In the medical context, the rights of a patient to control the distribution and release of data concerning his or her illness. This includes information the patient has provided to the health care professionals and all additional information contained in the chart, medical records, and laboratory data. Failure to observe this aspect of a patient's rights is classed as an invasion of privacy. SEE: *Hippocratic oath.*

**private patient** A patient whose care is the responsibility of one identifiable health care professional, usually a physician or dentist. The health care professional is paid directly, either by the patient or by the patient's insurer.

**private practice** The practice by a health care professional, usually a physician or dentist, in a setting in which the practice and the practitioner are independent of external policy control other than ethics of the professional and state licensing laws.

**privileged communication** Confidential information furnished (to facilitate diagnosis and treatment) by the patient to a professional authorized by law to provide. In some states, the person who has received this communication cannot be made to divulge it. When this is the case, communication between the patient and the recipient is classed as privileged.

Information given by the patient with the family present may not be considered privileged.

**p.r.n.** L. *pro re nata,* as circumstance may require; as necessary. Frequently used in prescription and order writing.

**pro-** [L., Gr. *pro,* before] Prefix indicating *for, in front of, before, from, in behalf of, on account of.* SEE: also *ante-; pre-.*

**proaccelerin** The fifth factor (factor V) in blood coagulation. SEE: *coagulation factors.*

**proagglutinoid** (prō″ă-gloo′tĭ-noyd) An agglutinoid having a greater affinity for the agglutinogen than that possessed by the agglutinin.

**proal** (prō′ăl) [Gr. *pro,* before] Concerning forward movement.

**proamnion** (prō-ăm′nē-ŏn) [Gr. *pro,* before, + *amnion,* amnion] A region anterior to the head in a vertebrate embryo in which mesoderm is lacking.

**proantithrombin** (prō″ăn-tĭ-thrŏm′bĭn) A substance present in blood plasma or serum which, through the action of heparin, is converted into antithrombin.

**proarrhythmia** A situation with the potential for development of an arrhythmia. For example, a drug may be proarrhythmic and thus should not be given to a patient (or should be monitored closely if given) who is at risk for that arrhythmia.

**proatlas** (prō-ăt′lăs) [″ + *atlas,* a support] A rudimentary vertebra in front of the atlas of small animals. It may be present as an anomaly in the understructure of the occipital bone in humans.

**probability** The ratio that expresses the likelihood of the occurrence of a specific event. The probability of a tossed coin landing head side up is one-half or 50%, as is the probability of the tail side landing up. This 50% probability remains the same each time a coin is tossed. Probability ratios based on sophisticated techniques are used for estimating the chance of occurrence of diseases in a population and in projecting vital statistics such as birth and death rates.

**proband** [L. *probare,* to test] The initial subject presenting a mental or physical disorder, who causes a study of his or her heredity in order to determine if other members of the family have had the same disease or carry it. SYN: *index case; propositus.*

**probang** (prō′băng) A slim, flexible rod with a sponge or similar material attached to the end; used for determining the location of strictures in the larynx or esophagus and for removing objects from the trachea. Medicines may also be applied to these areas by use of this device.

**probationer** (prō-bā′shŭn-ĕr) A person working during a trial period, as a student nurse just after entering training.

**probe** (prōb) [L. *probare,* to test] An instrument, usually flexible, for exploring the depth and direction of a wound or sinus.

***dental p.*** A sharp, pointed hand instrument used to examine the surface features of teeth and dental restorations for irregularities, cracks, and soft or carious enamel. SYN: *dental explorer.*

***Florida p.*** A periodontal probe connected to a computer that measures the depth of periodontal pockets automatically.

***periodontal p.*** A fine-caliber probe, calibrated in millimeters, designed and used to measure the depth and extent of the gingival sulcus and periodontal pockets present.

**probenecid** A benzoic acid derivative useful in treating gout. In large doses it prevents reabsorption of uric acid by the kidney and retards the excretion of penicillin in the urine.

**problem-oriented medical record** ABBR: POMR. Method of establishing and maintaining the patient's medical record so that problems are clearly stated, usually in order of importance, and a rational plan for dealing with them is stated. These data are kept at the front of the chart and are evaluated as frequently as indicated with respect to recording changes in the patient's problems as well as progress made in solving the problems. Use of this system may bring a degree of comprehensiveness to total patient care that might not be possible with conventional medical records.

**problem-oriented record** ABBR: POR. SEE: *problem-oriented medical record.*

**probucol** (prō′bū-kōl) An antihypercholesteremic drug.

**procainamide hydrochloride** A drug used in treating cardiac arrhythmias, particularly those that originate in the ventricle.

**procaine hydrochloride** (prō′kān) A white, colorless, crystalline compound; a safe, local anesthetic, less toxic than cocaine. It is used in infiltration anesthesia, nerve block, and spinal anesthesia. Its effect is prolonged by simultaneous injection of epinephrine. Trade name is Novocain.

**procarbazine hydrochloride** (prō-kăr′bă-zēn) A cytotoxic drug used in treating Hodgkin's disease and certain other neoplastic diseases.

**procarboxypeptidase** (prō″kăr-bŏk″sē-pĕp′tĭ-dās) The inactive precursor of carboxypeptidase. Trypsin activates it.

**procaryote** (prō-kăr′ē-ōt) [Gr. *pro,* before, + *karyon,* nucleus] Prokaryote.

**procedure** (prō-sē′dūr) [L. *procedere,* to proceed] A particular way of accomplishing a desired result.

**procentriole** (prō-sĕn′trē-ōl) The early form of the centrioles and ciliary basal bodies in the cell. SEE: *centriole.*

**procephalic** (prō″sē-făl′ĭk) [″ + *kephale,* head] Of, or relating to, the anterior part of the head.

**procercoid** (prō-sĕr′koyd) The first larval stage in the development of certain cestodes belonging to the order Pseudophyllidea. It is an elongated structure that develops in crustaceans.

**procerus muscle** A muscle that arises in the skin over the nose and is connected to the forehead. It acts to draw the eyebrows down.

**process** (prŏs′ĕs) [L. *processus,* going before] **1.** A method of action. **2.** The state of progress of a disease. **3.** A projection or outgrowth of bone or tissue. SYN: *processus.* **4.** A series of steps or events that lead to achievement of specific results.

***acromion p.*** The acromion.

***alar p.*** The process of the cribriform plate of the ethmoid bone that articulates with the frontal bone.

***alveolar p.*** **1.** The inferior border of the maxilla containing sockets for upper teeth. **2.** The superior border of the body of the mandible containing sockets for the lower teeth.

***articular p. of vertebra*** One of four processes (two superior and two inferior) by which vertebrae articulate with each other.

***basilar p.*** The narrow part of the base of the occipital bone, in front of the foramen magnum, articulating with the sphenoid bone. SYN: *pars basilaris ossis occipitalis.*

***caudate p.*** The process of the caudate lobe of the liver extending under the right lobe.

***ciliary p.*** One of about 70 prominent meridional ridges projecting from the corona ciliaris of the choroid coat of the eye to which the suspensory ligament of the lens is attached. These have the same structure as the rest of the choroid and secrete nutrient fluids that nourish neighboring parts, as cornea, lens, and vitreous body.

***clinoid p.*** One of the three processes of the sphenoid bone: anterior, middle, and posterior clinoid.

***condyloid p.*** A posterior process on the superior border of the ramus of the mandible consisting of a capitulum and neck. It articulates with the mandibular fossa of the temporal bone.

***coracoid p.*** A beak-shaped process extending upward and laterally from the neck of the scapula.

***coronoid p.*** **1.** The process on the proximal end of the ulna that forms the anterior portion of the semilunar notch. **2.** The process on the anterior upper end of the ramus of the mandible that serves for attachment of the temporalis muscle.

***ensiform p.*** Xiphoid p.

***ethmoidal p.*** A small process on the superior border of the inferior concha that articulates with the uncinate process of the ethmoid.

***falciform p.*** An extension of the posterior edge of the sacrotuberous ligament to the ramus of the ischium.

***frontal p.*** An upward projection of the maxilla that articulates with the frontal bone; forms part of the orbit and nasal fossa.

***frontonasal p.*** In the area of the primitive mouth of the embryo, a median swelling that is the anlage of the nose, upper lip, and front part of the palate.

***frontosphenoidal p.*** The upward-projecting process of the zygomatic bone.

***head p.*** An axial strand of cells in vertebrate embryos extending forward from the primitive knot. It forms a primitive axis about which the embryo differentiates.

***horizontal p.*** The part of the palatine bone that fuses with its counterpart at the midline to form the dorsal extension of the bony hard palate.

***infraorbital p.*** The medially-projecting process of the zygomatic bone that articulates with the maxilla. It forms inferior lateral margin of orbit.

***jugal p.*** A temporal bone process forming the zygomatic arch. SYN: *zygomatic p.*

***jugular p.*** A process of the occipital bone lying lateral to the occipital condyle.

***lacrimal p.*** A short process of the inferior concha that articulates with the lacrimal bone.

***lenticular p.*** A knob on the malleus in the middle ear that articulates with the stapes.

***malar p.*** A projection from the maxilla that articulates with the zygomatic bone.

***mandibular p.*** The posterior portion of the first branchial arch from which the lower jaw develops.

***mastoid p.*** A projection of the mastoid portion of the temporal bone.

***maxillary p.*** **1.** The anterior portion of the first branchial arch, which, with medial nasal processes, forms the upper jaw. **2.** The process of the inferior nasal concha extending laterally and covering the orifice of the antrum. **3.** A process on the anterior border of the perpendicular portion of the palatine bone.

***nursing p.*** SEE: *nursing process.*

***odontoid p.*** A toothlike process extending upward from the axis and about which the atlas rotates. SYN: *dens.*

***olecranon p.*** The olecranon, an extension at the proximal end of the ulna.

***orbital p.*** **1.** The process at the tip of the perpendicular portion of the palatine bone directed upward and backward. **2.** The process of the zygomatic bone that forms the anterior boundary of the temporal fossa.

***palatine p.*** A process extending transversely from the medial surface of the maxilla. With the corresponding process from the other side, it forms the major portion of the hard palate.

***postglenoid p.*** The process of the temporal bone separating the mandibular fossa from the external acoustic meatus.

***pterygoid p.*** The process of the sphenoid bone extending downward from the junction of the body and great wing. It consists of the lateral and medial pterygoid plates.

***spinous p. of vertebrae*** The posteriormost part of a vertebra. This spine projects back and serves as a point of attachment for muscles of the back.

***styloid p.*** **1.** A pointed process of the temporal bone, projecting downward, and to which some of the muscles of the tongue are attached. **2.** A pointed projection behind the head of the fibula. **3.** A protuberance on the outer portion of the distal end of the radius. **4.** An ulnar projection on the inner side of the distal end.

***transverse p.*** The process extending laterally and dorsally from the arch of a vertebra.

***uncinate p. of the ethmoid bone*** A sickle-shaped bony process on the medial wall of the ethmoidal labyrinth below the concha.

***vermiform p.*** Vermiform appendix.

***vocal p.*** The process of the arytenoid cartilage that serves for attachment of the vocal ligament.

***xiphoid p.*** A thin, elongated process extending caudally from the body of the sternum. SYN: *ensiform p.*

***zygomatic p.*** **1.** A thin projection from the temporal bone bounding its squamous portion. **2.** A part of the malar bone helping to form the zygoma.

**processing** In radiology, the use of a developer, fixer, washer, and dryer to change a latent film image or electrical impulses to a visible image for interpretation.

***daylight p.*** The use of an automatic system that accepts radiographic film, inserts it into the processor, and refills the cassette without the need for a darkroom.

***extended p.*** In mammography, extension of the development time or developer temperature to enhance image contrast and lower the patient dose.

**processor** In radiology, an automatic machine that helps to convert the latent image to a visible image. It consists of a transporter, electrical system, temperature control, circulation system, and dryer.

**processus** (prō-sĕs′ŭs) *pl.* **processus** [L.] Process or processes.

***p. cochleariformis*** The curved portion of a thin plate of bone separating the eustachian tube from the canal for the tensor tympani muscle over which the tendon of the muscle passes before insertion into the manubrium of the malleus.

***p. retromandibularis*** The wedge-shaped portion of the parotid gland that projects medially toward the pharynx.

***p. uncinatus*** **1.** The curved process of the ethmoid labyrinth projecting from the lateral wall of the middle meatus that forms the inferior border of hiatus semilunaris. **2.** A hooklike portion of the head of the pancreas that curves around the superior mesenteric vessels.

**procheilon** (prō-kī′lŏn) [Gr. *pro,* before, + *cheilon,* lip] A prominence in the central portion of the upper lip.

**prochlorperazine** (prō″klor-pĕr′ă-zēn) A phenothiazine-type drug used in treating nausea and vomiting.

**prochondral** (prō-kŏn′drăl) [″ + *chondros,* cartilage] Preceding the formation of cartilage.

**prochordal** (prō-kor′dăl) [″ + *chorde,* cord] In front of the notochord.

**procidentia** (prō″sĭ-dĕn′shē-ă) [L.] A complete prolapse, esp. of the uterus, to such an extent that the uterus lies outside of the vulva with everted vaginal walls. This is generally due to relaxation of the tissues that provide support for the pelvic organs. SYN: *hysteroptosia.*

**procoagulant factor** A lymphokine that can assume the role of factor VIII, antihemolytic factor, in coagulation cascade.

**procollagen** (prō-kŏl′ă-jĕn) [″ + *kolla,* glue, + *gennan,* to produce] Precursor of collagen.

**proconvertin** (prō″kŏn-vĕr′tĭn) Coagulation factor VII.

**procreate** [L. *procreare*] To beget; to be the parents of an infant.

**procreation** (prō″krē-ā′shŭn) The act or state of conceiving and giving birth to an infant. SYN: *reproduction.*

**proct-** SEE: *procto-.*

**proctagra** (prŏk-tăg′ră) [Gr. *proktos,* anus, + *agra,* seizure] Sudden rectal pain.

**proctalgia** (prŏk-tăl′jē-ă) [″+ *algos,* pain] Pain in or around the anus and rectum.

***p. fugax*** Rectal pain that occurs usually nocturnally. The pain is usually of short duration, and even though its cause is unknown, it is not considered to be due to organic disease. In some individuals, having an orgasm or a bowel movement will alleviate the pain.

**proctatresia** (prŏk″tă-trē′zē-ă) [″ + *atresis,* imperforation] Imperforation of the anus.

**proctectasia** (prŏk″tĕk-tā′sē-ă) [″ + *ektasis,* dilatation] Dilatation of the anus or rectum.

**proctectomy** (prŏk-tĕk′tō-mē) [″ + *ektome,* excision] Excision of the rectum or anus.

**proctenclisis** (prŏk″tĕn-klī′sĭs) [″ + *enkleiein,* to shut in] Stricture of the anus or rectum.

**procteurynter** (prŏk′tū-rĭn″tĕr) [″ + *euryein,* to widen] An instrument for dilation of the anus or rectum.

**proctitis** [″ + *itis,* inflammation] Inflammation of rectum and anus. It may be acute or chronic with rectal discomfort and repeated urge to evacuate the rectum accompanied by inability to pass feces. Mucus, blood, or pus may be present in the stools and there may be tenesmus. The condition may be caused by infectious organisms; trauma; radiation injury; drugs, esp. broad-spectrum antibiotics; or allergy. SYN: *rectitis.*

***diphtheritic p.*** Proctitis in which a diphtheritic and albuminous membrane forms over the surface of mucous membrane. The condition is characterized by headache with roaring in the ears; constipation, gas, and bloating; and neurasthenia.

***dysenteric p.*** Proctitis resulting from ordinary diarrhea. It may produce ulcers and scarring of the rectum and anus.

***gonorrheal p.*** Gonorrheal infection around the rectum and anus.

***traumatic p.*** Proctitis with pain, pressure as if bowels were going to move; irritation; and red, eroded mucous membrane. Surface tissues are sensitive to the touch, and chronic constipation develops.

**procto-, proct-** Combining form meaning *anus, rectum.*

**proctocele** (prŏk′tō-sēl) [Gr. *proktos,* anus, + *kele,* tumor, swelling] A protrusion of the rectal mucosa into the vagina. SYN: *rectocele.*

**proctoclysis** (prŏk-tŏk′lĭ-sĭs) [″ + *klysis,* a washing] A continuous infusion into the rectum and colon. SEE: *enteroclysis.*

THERAPEUTIC EFFECT: This procedure has the following therapeutic effects: to supply fluid in postoperative cases when fluids cannot be taken otherwise; to supply the body with fluid as in hemorrhage, vomiting, or diarrhea; to relieve thirst as in persistent vomiting; and to lower body temperature by giving ice water enemas.

SOLUTIONS: The fluid usually consists of a normal saline solution, a sodium bicarbonate solution, or plain tap water at body temperature. Normal salt solution at half strength frequently is used. This need not be a sterile solution unless so ordered. Sodium bicarbonate of 2% to 5% strength or a glucose solution of 2% to 5%, but no stronger, may be used. A combination of these may also be ordered as a normal saline with glucose and sodium bicarbonate, 5% and 2%, respectively, or other combinations may be used.

NURSING IMPLICATIONS: The nurse administers a cleansing enema before beginning proctoclysis. When the bowel is completely evacuate, fluid at body temperature is introduced through a lubricated rectal catheter inserted to approximately 4 in. (10 cm). The liquid is given at a rate of 40 to 60 drops/min. If the fluid is given faster, the bowel will be stimulated. No more than 6 oz (180 ml) of fluid should be given in a single continuous proctoclysis. The nurse should turn the patient frequently during the treatment. If rectal gas needs to be passed, clamp the tube temporarily. If pain or distention develops, treatment should be discontinued.

**proctococcypexia, proctococcypexy** (prŏk″tō-kŏk-sĭ-pĕk′sē-ă, -kŏk′sĭ-pĕk″sē) [″ + *kokkyx,* coccyx, + *pexis,* fixation] Suture of the rectum to the coccyx.

**proctocolitis** (prŏk″tō-kō-lī′tĭs) [″ + *kolon,* colon, + *itis,* inflammation] Inflammation of the colon and rectum.

**proctocolonoscopy** (prŏk″tō-kō″lŏn-ŏs′kō-pē) [″ + ″ + *skopein,* to examine] Examination of the interior of the rectum and lower colon.

**proctocystoplasty** (prŏk″tō-sĭs′tō-plăs″tē) [Gr. *proktos,* anus, + *kystis,* bladder, + *plastos,* formed] Plastic surgery involving the rectum and bladder.

**proctocystotomy** (prŏk″tō-sĭs-tŏt′ō-mē) [″ + *kystis,* bladder, + *tome,* incision] Incision into the bladder through the rectum.

**proctodeum** (prŏk-tō-dē′ŭm) [″ + *hodaios,* a way] An ectodermal depression located caudally that, upon rupture of the cloacal membrane, forms the anal canal.

**proctodynia** (prŏk″tō-dĭn′ē-ă) [″ + *odyne,* pain] Pain in the rectum or around the anus.

**proctologic** (prŏk″tō-lŏj′ĭk) [″ + *logos,* word, reason] Concerning proctology.

**proctologist** (prŏk-tŏl′ō-jĭst) [″ + *logos,* word, reason] One who specializes in diseases of the colon, rectum, and anus.

**proctology** (prŏk-tŏl′ō-jē) The phase of medicine dealing with treatment of diseases of the colon, rectum, and anus.

**proctoparalysis** (prŏk″tō-păr-ăl′ĭ-sĭs) [″ + *para,* at the side, + *lyein,* to loosen] Paralysis of the anal sphincter muscle.

**proctoperineoplasty** (prŏk″tō-pĕr″ĭ-nē′ō-plăs″tē) [″ + *perinaion,* perineum, + *plassein,* to form] Plastic surgery of the anus and rectum. SYN: *proctoperineorrhaphy.*

**proctoperineorrhaphy** (prŏk″tō-pĕr″ĭ-nē-or′ă-fē) [″ + ″ + *rhaphe,* seam, ridge] Proctoperineoplasty.

**proctopexia, proctopexy** (prŏk-tō-pĕk′sē-ă, prŏk′tō-pĕk″sē) [″ + *pexis,* fixation] Suture of the rectum to some other part.

**proctophobia** (prŏk″tō-fō′bē-ă) [″ + *phobos,* fear] Abnormal apprehension in those suffering from rectal disease.

**proctoplasty** (prŏk′tō-plăs″tē) [″ + *plastos,* formed] Plastic surgery of the anus or rectum.

**proctopolypus** (prŏk″tō-pŏl′ĭ-pŭs) [″ + *polys,* many, + *pous,* foot] Polyp of the rectum.

**proctoptosis** (prŏk″tŏp-tō′sĭs) [″ + *ptosis,* a dropping] Prolapse of the anus and rectum. SEE: *procidentia.*

**proctorrhagia** (prŏk″tō-rā′jē-ă) [″ + *rhegnynai,* to burst forth] Bleeding from the rectum.

**proctorrhaphy** (prŏk-tor′ă-fē) [″ + *rhaphe,* seam, ridge] Suturing of the rectum or anus.

**proctorrhea** (prŏk-tōr-ē′ă) [″ + *rhoia,* flow] Mucous discharge from the anus.

**proctoscope** [″ + *skopein,* to examine] An instrument for inspection of the rectum.

**proctoscopy** (prŏk-tŏs′kō-pē) Inspection of the rectum with a proctoscope.

**proctosigmoidectomy** (prŏk″tō-sĭg″moy-dĕk′tō-mē) [″ + *sigma,* Gr. letter S, + *eidos,* form, shape, + *ektome,* excision] Surgical removal of the anus, rectum, and sigmoid flexure of the colon.

**proctosigmoiditis** (prŏk″tō-sĭg″moyd-ī′tĭs) [″ + ″ + *eidos,* form, shape, + *itis,* inflammation] Inflammation of the rectum and sigmoid.

**proctosigmoidoscopy** (prŏk″tō-sĭg-moyd-ŏs′kō-pē) Visual examination of the rectum and sigmoid colon by use of a sigmoidoscope.

**proctospasm** [″ + *spasmos,* a convulsion] Rectal spasm.

**proctostasis** (prŏk″tō-stā′sĭs) [″ + *stasis,* stoppage] Constipation resulting from failure of the rectum to respond to defecation stimulus.

**proctostenosis** (prŏk″tō-stĕn-ō′sĭs) [″ + *stenosis,* act of narrowing] Stricture of the anus or rectum.

**proctostomy** (prŏk-tŏs'tō-mē) [" + *stoma,* mouth] Surgical creation of a permanent opening into the rectum.

**proctotome** (prŏk'tō-tōm) [" + *tome,* incision] A knife for incision into the rectum.

**proctotomy** (prŏk-tŏt'ō-mē) Incision of the rectum or anus.

NURSING IMPLICATIONS: The nurse assesses the dressing frequently and records the presence and amount of bleeding and drainage. Dressings should be changed or reinforced as prescribed by the physician. A T binder (female patients) or split T binder (male patients) is advantageous to ensure proper placement of dressing.

**proctotresia** (prŏk-tō-trē'sē-ă) [" + *tresis,* a perforation] Surgical correction of an imperforate anus.

**proctovalvotomy** (prŏk"tō-văl-vŏt'ō-mē) [" + L. *valva,* leaf of a folding door, + Gr. *tome,* incision] Incision of the rectal valves.

**procumbent** [L. *procumbens,* lying down] Prone.

**procursive** (prō-kŭr'sĭv) [L. *procursivus*] Having an involuntary tendency to run forward.

**procurvation** (prō"kŭr-vā'shŭn) [L. *procurvare,* to bend forward] A bending forward.

**procyclidine hydrochloride** (prō-sī'klĭ-dēn) An antiparkinsonism drug.

**prodromal** (prō-drō'măl) [Gr. *prodromos,* running before] Pert. to the initial stage of a disease; the interval between the earliest symptoms and the appearance of a rash or fever.

**prodromal rash** A rash that precedes the true rash of an infectious disease.

**prodrome** *pl.* **prodromes, prodromata** A symptom indicative of an approaching disease.

**prodrug** An inert drug that becomes active after biotransformation.

**product** (prŏd'ŭkt) [L. *productum*] Anything that is made; also, the resulting compound after the reaction of two chemical substances.

**production** (prō-dŭk'shŭn) Development or formation of a substance.

**productive** (prō-dŭk'tĭv) Forming, esp. new tissue.

**productive inflammation** An inflammation producing new tissue with or without an exudate.

**proencephalus** (prō"ĕn-sĕf'ă-lŭs) [Gr. *pro,* before, + *enkephalos,* brain] A deformed fetus in which the brain protrudes through a fissure in the frontal area of the skull.

**proenzyme** (prō-ĕn'zīm) [" + *en,* in, + *zyme,* a leaven] The inactive form of an enzyme found within a cell, which, upon leaving the cell, is converted into the active form, such as pepsinogen, which is converted to pepsin.

**proerythroblast** (prō"ĕ-rĭth'rō-blăst) [" + *erythros,* red, + *blastos,* germ] The earliest cell that shows differentiation in the direction of erythrocyte formation.

**proestrus** (prō-ĕs'trŭs) The period preceding estrus in females, characterized by development of ovarian follicles and uterine endometrium.

**professional** (prō-fĕsh'ŭn-ăl) [ME. *profession,* sacred vow] Pert. to a profession.

**professional liability** The obligation of health care providers or their insurers to pay for damages resulting from the providers' acts of omission or commission in treating patients.

**professional liability insurance** A type of insurance contract that provides compensation for a person or party injured by a professional's acts or omissions. Two common types of policies are as follows: (1) *Claims made.* The claim for damages by the injured party must be made during the policy coverage period in order for the professional to be covered and represented by the insurance company. (2) *Occurrence basis.* The claim for damages by the injured party is covered by the insurance company as long as the act of professional liability occurs during the policy coverage period, even though the claim is filed after the coverage period ends.

**Professional Standards Review Organization** ABBR: PSRO. Peer review at the local level required by Public Law 92-603 of the U.S. for the services provided under the Medicare, Medicaid, and maternal and child health programs funded by the federal government.

**profibrinolysin** (prō"fī-brĭ-nō-lī'sĭn) [Gr. *pro,* before, + L. *fibra,* fiber, + Gr. *lysis,* dissolution] The inactive precursor of the proteolytic enzyme fibrinolysin.

**profile** (prō'fīl) [L. *pro,* forward, + *filare,* to draw a line] **1.** An outline of the side view of an object, esp. the human head. **2.** A summary, graph, or table presenting a subject's most notable characteristics and achievements.

***biophysical p.*** ABBR: BPP. An estimate of fetal status determined by analysis of five variables via ultrasound and nonstress testing. Fetal breathing movements, gross body movement, and tone (active extension and flexion, volume of amniotic fluid, and heart rate activity) are compared with specific criteria. Each expected normal finding is rated as 2; each abnormal finding is rated as 0. A score of 8 to 10 with normal amniotic fluid voume indicates satisfactory fetal status. A score of 6 with normal amniotic fluid volume requires reassessment of a preterm fetus within 24 hr of delivery. A score below 6 indicates fetal compromise and the need for prompt delivery. SEE: *Apgar score.*

***practice p.*** In theory, a performance-based method of assessing individual practitioners. This is usually done by companies who use information about a physician's patients including process of care, outcome, and comparing those data with what are felt to be normative or community standards of quality of care, use of services, and cost. The profile of an individual practitioner's performance could provide information such as the number of pneumonia patients who recovered or died, the number of diagnostic procedures done, and whether the practitioner's patients differ in the frequency of certain outcomes from the accepted standard or community norm. Individual physicians who received this practice profile information privately could use it to further their education and to provide guidance for their future patterns of care. That same information could be used for certifying and recertifying physicians; and for making decisions about hiring, firing, disciplining, and paying physicians. Unfortunately, the profiling procedures may not reflect what physicians do, may erroneously list the physician of record, or may misclassify the episode of care. When this happens, the result would be an inaccurate profile. The outcome of establishing practice profiles could, if done correctly, help to increase the quality medical care and to provide patients the opportunity of evaluating physicians. The methods used at this time to profile practice may be inadequate.

***PULSES p.*** One of the first formal, widely used scales to assess daily living skills. PULSES is an acronym formed by the domains measured: *P*hysical condition, *U*pper extremity function, *L*ower extremity function, *S*ensory, *E*xcretory, and psychosocial *S*tatus. SEE: *activities of daily living.*

**profluvium** (prō-floo'vē-ŭm) [L.] An excessive flow or discharge; a flux.

***p. seminis*** The flow from the vagina of semen deposited during coition.

**profunda** [L.] Deep seated; term applied to certain deeply located blood vessels.

**profundus** (prō-fŭn'dŭs) [L.] Located deeper than the indicated reference point.

**progastrin** (prō-găs'trĭn) The inactive precursor of gastrin.

**progenitor** (prō-jĕn'ĭ-tor) [L.] An ancestor.

**progeny** (prŏj'ĕ-nē) [ME. *progenie*] Offspring.

**progeria** (prō-jē'rē-ă) [Gr. *pro,* before, + *geras,* old age] The syndrome of premature aging, which may be an inherited disorder that is transmitted as an autosomal dominant trait. The incidence appears higher in children of older fathers. Onset is from birth to 18 months of age and the average age at death is 12 to 13 years.

SYMPTOMS: The child has an aged and wizened appearance. In addition there is small stature, slightness of build, alopecia, thick and inelastic skin that has brownish spots on it, delayed dentition, high-pitched voice, prominent eyes, and infantile sex organs.

**progestational** (prō"jĕs-tā'shŭn-ăl) Concerned with the luteal phase of the menstrual cycle, at which time, by the action of the hormone progesterone, the endometrium is further prepared for implantation of the fertilized ovum.

**progestational agent** Progestin (1).

**progesterone** (prō-jĕs'tĕr-ōn) $C_{21}H_{30}O_2$. A steroid hormone obtained from the corpus luteum and placenta. It is responsible for changes in the endometrium in the second half of the menstrual cycle preparatory to implantation of the blastocyst, development of the maternal placenta after implantation, and development of the mammary glands. It is used to treat menstrual disorders (secondary amenorrhea, abnormal uterine bleeding, luteal phase deficiency) and renal or endometrial carcinoma. It is also used in combination with estrogen for contraception and for treatment of postmenopausal syndrome. SYN: *progestin* (1).

**progestin** (prō-jĕs'tĭn) **1.** A corpus luteum hormone that prepares the endometrium for implantation of the fertilized ovum. SYN: *progesterone.* **2.** A term used to cover a large group of synthetic drugs that have a progesterone-like effect on the uterus.

**progestogen** (prō-jĕs'tō-jĕn) Any natural or synthetic hormonal substance that produces effects similar to those due to progesterone.

**proglossis** (prō-glŏs'ĭs) [Gr.] The tip of the tongue.

**proglottid** Proglottis.

**proglottis** (prō-glŏt'tĭs) *pl.* **proglottides** [Gr. *pro,* before, + *glossa,* tongue] A segment of a tapeworm, containing both male and female reproductive organs. SEE: *Cestoda; tapeworm.*

**prognathic** (prŏg-nā'thĭk) [" + *gnathos,* jaw] Prognathous.

**prognathism** (prŏg'nă-thĭzm) [" + *gnathos,* jaw + *-ismos,* condition] Projection of the jaws beyond projection of the forehead.

**prognathous** (prŏg'nă-thŭs) Having jaws projecting forward beyond the rest of the face.

**prognose** (prŏg-nōs') To predict the course of a disease.

**prognosis** (prŏg-nō'sĭs) [Gr., foreknowledge] Prediction of the course and end of a disease, and the estimate of chance for recovery.

**prognosticate** (prŏg-nŏs'tĭ-kāt) [Gr. *prognostikon,* knowing before] To make a statement on the probable outcome of an illness.

**program** A plan or system, usually printed, outlining procedures or actions to be followed.

***Individualized Education P.*** ABBR: IEP. A documented program of intervention mandated for each child provided education-related rehabilitation services under federal legislation. The program guarantees a free and appropriate public education for children with disabilities.

***preprosthetic p.*** Postsurgical intervention following amputation during which the patient is taught stump care, positioning, sitting tolerance, transfer techniques, and other skills that are necessary before prosthetic training can begin.

***prosthetic training p.*** Systematic education and training provided to persons with amputations following fitting of a prosthetic device.

**progranulocyte** (prō-grăn′ū-lō-sīt) [″ + L. *granula,* granule, + Gr. *kytos,* cell] A promyelocyte.

**progravid** (prō-grăv′ĭd) [″ + L. *gravidus,* pregnant] Preceding pregnancy.

**progress** [L. *progressus,* a going forward] The ongoing sequence of events of an illness.

**progression** (prō-grĕsh′ŭn) [L. *progressus*] An advancing or moving forward.

**progressive** (prō-grĕs′ĭv) Advancing, as a disease from bad to worse.

**progressive lens** An eyeglass lens that gradually changes prescription strength from the top of the lens, which is used for viewing distance, to the bottom of the lens, which is used for seeing objects that are nearby. Progressive lenses enable the eyes to adjust from one distance to another (e.g., when looking up from a book) without the "image jump" associated with bifocals, lenses that require the eye to shift between two separate prescriptions.

**progressive ossifying myositis** A tendency to bony deposits in the muscles with chronic inflammation.

**progressive resistive exercise** ABBR: PRE. A form of active resistive exercise based on a principle of gradual increase in the amount of resistance in order to achieve maximum strength.

**progress notes** Notes made on the chart by those involved in caring for a patient. Physicians, nurses, consultants, and therapists may record their notes concerning the progress or lack of progress made by the patient in the interim between the previous note and the time of the most recent note. In patients who are not critically ill, a note concerning progress might be made daily or less frequently; in critical care situations, notes could be made hourly. It is important that each note be signed and written clearly, and the date and time recorded.

**progress report** The written or verbal account of a patient's present condition, esp. as compared with the previous state.

**prohormone** (prō-hor′mōn) Precursor of a hormone.

**proinsulin** Precursor of insulin produced in the beta cells of the pancreas.

**projection** (prō″jĕk′shŭn) [Gr. *pro,* before, + *jacere,* to throw] **1.** The act of throwing forward. **2.** A part extending beyond the level of its surroundings. **3.** The mental process by which sensations are referred to the sense organs or receptors stimulated, or outside the body to the object that is the stimulus. **4.** The distortion of a perception as a result of its repression, resulting in such a phenomenon as hating without cause one who has been dearly loved, or attributing to others one's own undesirable traits. These are characteristics of the paranoid reaction. **5.** In radiology, the path of the x-ray photon beam. In an anteroposterior projection, for example, the beam enters the anterior surface of the body and exits the posterior surface.

***isometric p.*** A projection of an x-ray photon beam that yields an image having the same dimensions as the object being examined.

**projective technique** Any one of several forms of psychological assessment or evaluation. Using ambiguous activities and tasks which encourage self-expression, the products or results and the individual's verbalizations about them are evaluated and interpreted to determine indications of unconscious needs, thoughts, or concerns.

**prokaryon** (prō-kăr′ē-ŏn) [″ + *karyon,* nucleus] **1.** Nuclear material that is spread throughout the cell cytoplasm and is not bounded by a membrane. **2.** Prokaryote.

**Prokaryotae** In taxonomy, the kingdom of organisms with prokaryotic cell structure, that is, they lack membrane-bound cell organelles and a nuclear membrane around the chromosome. Included are the bacteria and cyanobacteria (formerly the blue-green algae). SYN: *Monera.*

**prokaryote** (prō-kăr′ē-ōt) [″ + *karyon,* nucleus] An organism of the kingdom Monera with a single, circular chromosome, without a nuclear membrane, or membrane-bound organelles (i.e., mitochondria and lysosomes). Included in this classification are bacteria and cyanobacteria (formerly the blue-green algae). SYN: *procaryote; prokaryon* (2). SEE: *eukaryote.*

**prolabium** (prō-lā′bē-ŭm) [″ + *labium,* lip] The entire central portion of the upper lip.

**prolactin** (prō-lăk′tĭn) [″ + *lac,* milk] A hormone produced by the pituitary gland. In humans, prolactin in association with estrogen and progesterone stimulates breast development and the formation of milk during pregnancy. The act of sucking is an important stimulus for the production of prolactin in the postpartum period. Some of the metabolic effects of prolactin resemble those of growth hormone. In the female this includes amenorrhea, galactorrhea, and infertility. In the male it may cause impotence. Hyperprolactinemia may be associated with amenorrhea in women and reduced sexual potency in men. Thyrotropin-releasing hormone and stress of all kinds can stimulate prolactin release.

**prolactinoma** An adenoma of the pituitary that produces prolactin. The excess prolactin secreted may be treated by the use of a dopamine agonist, bromocriptine. In some cases, surgical removal of the tumor may be necessary.

**prolapse** (prō-lăps′) [L. *prolapsus*] A falling or dropping down of an organ or internal part, such as the uterus or rectum. SEE: *procidentia; ptosis.*

***p. of the anus*** Protrusion of the lower portion of the digestive tract through the external sphincter of the anus.

***p. of the iris*** Protrusion of the iris through an injury in the cornea.

***pelvic organ p.*** Protrusion of the pelvic organs into or through the vaginal canal. This condition is usually due to direct or indirect damage to the vagina and its pelvic support system. The damage may be related to stretching or laceration of the vaginal wall, hypoestrogenic atrophy, or injury to the nerves of the pelvic support structures.

SYMPTOMS: Symptoms include a sensation of pelvic pressure, groin pain, coital difficulty, sacral backache, bloody vaginal discharge, difficult bowel movents, and urinary frequency, urgency, or incontinence.

PROPHYLAXIS: Preventive measures include treatment of chronic respiratory disorders or constipation, estrogen replacement for menopausal women, weight control, smoking cessation, avoidance of strenuous occupational or recreational stresses to the pelvic support system, and pelvic muscle exercise to strengthen the pelvic diaphragm.

TREATMENT: Treatment may be nonsurgical (e.g., use of a vaginal pessary) or surgical, including reconstructive operations, vaginal hysterectomy, and cystocele or rectocele repair.

***p. of the rectum*** Protrusion of the rectal mucosa through the anus.

***p. of the umbilical cord*** Premature expulsion of the umbilical cord in labor before the fetus is delivered. SEE: *labor.*

***p. of the uterus*** Downward displacement of the uterus, the cervix sometimes protruding from the vaginal orifice. The causes include age with weakening of pelvic musculature, traumatic vaginal delivery, chronic straining in association with coughing or difficult bowel movements, and pelvic tumors that push the uterus down. SEE: *Kegel exercises.*

**prolapsus** [L.] Prolapse.

**prolepsis** [Gr. *pro,* before, + *lepsis,* a seizure] The return of paroxysmal attacks at successively shorter intervals.

**proleptic** Recurring before the time expected, said of paroxysms.

**proleukocyte** (prō-lū′kō-sīt) [″ + *leukos,* white, + *kytos,* cell] An undeveloped leukocyte.

**proliferate** (prō-lĭf′ĕr-āt) [L. *proles,* offspring, + *ferre,* to bear] To increase by reproduction of similar forms.

**proliferation** (prō-lĭf″ĕr-ā′shŭn) **1.** Rapid and repeated reproduction of new parts, as by cell division. **2.** The process or result of rapid reproduction.

**proliferous 1.** Multiplying, as by formation of new tissue cells. **2.** Bearing offspring.

**prolific** [L. *prolificus*] Fruitful; reproductive. SYN: *fertile.*

**prolinase** An enzyme that is found in animal tissues and yeast and that hydrolyzes proline peptides to simpler peptids and proline.

**proline** (prō′lēn) $C_4H_8NCOOH$. An important amino acid formed by digestion of protein.

**prolymphocyte** (prō″lĭmf′ō-sīt) [″ + L. *lympha,* lymph, + Gr. *kytos,* cell] A cell intermediate between a lymphoblast and lymphocyte.

**PROM** *premature rupture of membranes.*

**promazine hydrochloride** (prō′mă-zēn) An antipsychotic drug.

**promegakaryocyte** (prō-mĕg″ă-kăr′ē-ō-sīt) [″ + *megas,* big, + *karyon,* nucleus, + *kytos,* cell] A cell from which a megakaryocyte develops.

**promegaloblast** (prō-mĕg′ă-lō-blast″) [″ + ″ + *blastos,* germ] A cell of the erythrocyte series preceding the megaloblast.

**prometaphase** (prō-mĕt′ă-fāz) [″ + *meta,* change, + *phasis,* to appear] The stage of mitosis in which the nuclear membrane disintegrates, and the chromosomes move toward the equatorial plate.

**promethazine hydrochloride** (prō-mĕth′ă-zēn) An antihistamine drug used as an antiemetic and anticough medicine.

**promethium** (prō-mē′thē-ŭm) SYMB: Pm. A radioactive element of the rare earth series; atomic weight 144.9128; atomic number 61.

**prominence** (prŏm′ĭ-nĕns) [L. *prominens,* project] A projection or protrusion.

**prominentia** (prŏm″ĭ-nĕn′shē-ă) *pl.* **prominentiae** [L.] A projection.

***p. laryngea*** The laryngeal prominence; Adam's apple.

***p. spiralis*** A small ridge extending entire length of the cochlea located on the inner surface of the spiral ligament. It projects slightly into the cochlear canal and contains blood vessels, including the vas prominens.

**promonocyte** (prō-mŏn′ō-sīt) [Gr. *pro,* before, + *monos,* single, + *kytos,* cell] In the development of white blood cells, the precursor of the monocyte. It is between the monoblast and monocyte.

**promontory** (prŏm′ŏn-tor″ē) [L. *promontorium*] A projecting process or part.

***p. of the sacrum*** The anterior projecting portion of the pelvic surface of the base of the sacrum. With the fifth lumbar vertebra, it forms the sacrovertebral angle.

***p. of the tympanic cavity*** The projection on the medial wall of the tympanic cavity produced by the first turn of the cochlea.

**promoter** (prō-mō′tĕr) A substance that assists a catalyst to act.

**prompt** Assistance, reinforcement, or feedback given during the acquisition or relearning of skills necessary for task completion.

**promyelocyte** (prō-mī'ĕl-ō-sīt) [Gr. *pro,* before, + *myelos,* marrow, + *kytos,* cell] **1.** A large mononuclear myeloid cell seen in the blood in leukemia. **2.** Cell development between a myeloblast and a myelocyte, resembling a myeloblast. SEE: illus.

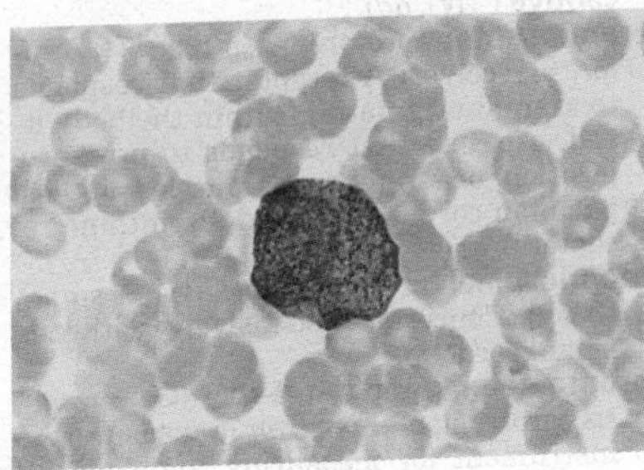

**PROMYELOCYTE** (ORIG. MAG. ×600)

**pronate** (prō'nāt) To place in a prone position. SEE: *supinate.*

**pronation** (prō-nā'shŭn) [L. *pronus,* prone] **1.** The act of lying prone or face downward. **2.** The act of turning the hand so that the palm faces downward or backward. SEE: *supination.*

**pronator** A muscle that pronates. SEE: *Muscles Appendix.*

**pronator syndrome** A neurological disorder caused by entrapment of the median nerve at the elbow. Symptoms and signs include aching pain in the wrist with a subjective feeling of poor coordination; paresthesias extending into the hand; paresis of the thumb muscles; pain on pronation of the forearm and flexion of the wrist against resistance; and tenderness in the proximal thenar muscles. A positive Tinel's sign over the pronator teres muscles may be present. The disease usually affects the dominant arm in men. Corticosteroid injection into the site is usually effective.

**pronaus, pronaeus** (prō-nā'ŭs) [Gr. *pro,* before, + *naos,* temple] The vagina or vestibule of the vagina.

**prone** (prōn) [ME.] **1.** Horizontal with the face downward. **2.** Denoting the hand with the palm turned downward. It is the opposite of supine.

**pronephric** (prō-nĕf'rĭk) [Gr. *pro,* before, + *nephros,* kidney] Pert. to the pronephros.

**pronephric duct** A duct that connects posteriorly to the cloaca and to which pronephric tubules are connected.

**pronephric tubule** Any of several pairs of segmentally arranged tubules that open into the cranial portion of the pronephric duct. They communicate with coelom through a ciliated funnel-shaped nephrostome. They are vestigial in higher vertebrates.

**pronephros, pronephron** (prō-nĕf'rŏs, -rŏn) The earliest and simplest type of excretory organ of vertebrates, functional in simpler forms (cyclostomes), and serving as a provisional kidney in some fishes and amphibians. In reptiles, birds, and mammals, it appears in the embryo as a temporary, functionless structure.

**prong** (prŏng) A cone-shaped body such as the root of a tooth.

**pronograde** (prō'nō-grād) [L. *pronus,* prone, + *gradus,* a step] In animals, walking on the hands and feet or resting with the body in a horizontal position. It is the opposite of orthograde.

**pronometer** (prō-nŏm'ĕ-tĕr) [" + Gr. *metron,* measure] A device for showing the amount of pronation or supination of the forearm.

**pronormoblast** (prō-nor'mō-blăst) [Gr. *pro,* before, + L. *norma,* rule, + Gr. *blastos,* germ] An early precursor of the red blood cell.

**pronucleus** (prō-nū'klē-ŭs) [Gr. *pro,* before, + *nucleus,* little kernel] The nucleus of the ovum (the female pronucleus) or of the spermatozoon (the male pronucleus) after fertilization of the ovum.

**prootic** (prō-ŏt'ĭk, -ō'tĭk) [" + *ous,* ear] In front of the ear.

**prop** A device of sturdy material used to support or hold something in place.

***mouth p.*** A metal or rubber device inserted between the jaws to maintain the mouth in an open position. SYN: *bite block; jaw brace.*

**propagation** (prŏp-ă-gā'shŭn) [L.] The act of reproducing or giving birth. SYN: *generation; reproduction.*

**propagative** (prŏp'ă-gā"tĭv) Pert. to or taking part in reproduction.

**propalinal** (prō-păl'ĭ-năl) [Gr. *pro,* before, + *palin,* back] Applied to a backward and forward movement, as of the jaws.

**propane** (prō'pān) $C_3H_8$. An inflammable odorless, colorless hydrocarbon that is present in natural gas. When it is to be used in dwellings, as a fuel, to produce heat, or in hot air balloons, an odoriferous substance is added so that a leak that could go undetected would be obvious because of the odor.

**propantheline bromide** (prō-păn'thĕ-lēn) An anticholinergic drug that acts like belladonna.

**proparacaine hydrochloride** (prō-păr'ă-kān) A topical anesthetic drug used in ophthalmology.

**propepsin** (prō-pĕp'sĭn) Pepsinogen.

**propeptone** (prō-pĕp'tōn) [" + *peptein,* to digest] An intermediate product in the digestive conversion of protein into peptone. SYN: *hemialbumose.*

**propeptonuria** (prō"pĕp-tō-nū'rē-ă) [" + " + *ouron,* urine] Excretion of propeptone in the urine. SYN: *hemialbumosuria.*

**properdin** (prō-pĕrd'ĭn) A serum protein that, in the presence of magnesium ions and complement, has the ability to help destroy various bacteria and viruses. SEE: *complement.*

**prophase** (prō′făz) [″ + *phasis,* an appearance] The first stage of indirect cell division. SEE: *cell division* for illus.; *centriole; metaphase; mitosis.*

**prophylactic** (prō-fī-lăk′tĭk) [Gr. *prophylaktikos,* guarding] **1.** Any agent or regimen that contributes to the prevention of infection and disease. **2.** A popular term for a condom.

**prophylaxis** (prō-fī-lăk′sĭs, prō-fĭl-ăks′ĭs) [Gr. *prophylassein,* to guard against] Observance of rules necessary to prevent disease.

***oral p.*** The removal of calculus and stains from the exposed and unexposed surfaces of the teeth by scaling and polishing as a preventive measure for the control of local irritational factors.

**propiolactone** (prō″pē-ō-lăk′tōn) A disinfectant used in preparing certain viral and bacterial vaccines.

**propiomazine hydrochloride** (prō″pē-ō-mā′zēn) A sedative drug.

**propionic acid** $C_2H_5COOH$, methylacetic acid, which is present in sweat.

**Propionibacterium acnes** A gram-positive rod bacterium that may be part of the normal skin flora, but can also be pathogenic in wounds and infected prosthetic devices. It was formerly called *Corynebacterium acnes.*

**proplasmacyte** (prō-plăz′mă-sīt) [Gr. *pro,* before, + LL. *plasma,* form, mold, + Gr. *kytos,* cell] The precursor of the plasma cell.

**proplastid** (prō-plăs′tĭd) The cytoplasmic body from which a plastid is formed.

**Proplex** Trade name for factor IX complex.

**propolis** [Gr. *pro,* before, + *polis,* city] A sticky resin present in the buds and bark of certain trees and plants. It is collected by bees for the purpose of repairing combs, filling cracks, and making the entrance to the hive waterproof. There is anecdotal evidence that propolis may be of benefit in treating certain diseases. Scientific in vitro investigations indicate that the material inhibits the reproduction of certain viruses. These studies employed propolis as well as the resin obtained from poplar trees and then refined.

**propositus** (prō-pŏz′ĭ-tŭs) [L. *proponere,* to put on view] Proband.

**propoxycaine hydrochloride** (prō-pŏk′sē-kān) A local anesthetic drug.

**propoxyphene hydrochloride** (prō-pŏk′sē-fēn) An analgesic drug available in a variety of dosage forms and combinations.

**propranolol hydrochloride** A beta-adrenergic blocking agent used in treating hypertension; for prevention of angina pectoris; and for treating certain cardiac arrhythmias, esp. those caused by overdose of digitalis.

Caution: Persons with asthma should not be treated with this drug.

**proprioception** (prō″prē-ō-sĕp′shŭn) [L. *proprius,* one's own, + *capio,* to take] The awareness of posture, movement, and changes in equilibrium and the knowledge of position, weight, and resistance of objects in relation to the body. **proprioceptive** (-tĭv), *adj.*

**proprioceptor** (prō″prē-ō-sĕp′tor) [″ + *ceptor,* a receiver] A receptor that responds to stimuli originating within the body itself, esp. one that responds to pressure, position, or stretch (e.g., muscle spindles, pacinian corpuscles, and labyrinthine receptors).

**propriospinal** (prō″prē-ō-spī′năl) [″ + *spina,* thorn] Concerned exclusively with the spinal cord.

**proptometer** (prŏp-tŏm′ĕ-tĕr) [Gr. *proptosis,* protrusion, + *metron,* a measure] An instrument for measuring the extent of exophthalmos.

**proptosis** (prŏp-tō′sĭs) A downward displacement such as the uterus or the eyeball in exophthalmic goiter or in inflammatory conditions of the orbit.

**propulsion** (prō-pŭl′shŭn) [L. *propulsus,* driven forward] **1.** A tendency to push or fall forward in walking. **2.** A condition seen in paralysis agitans. SEE: *festination.*

**propyl** (prō′pĭl) The radical of propyl alcohol or propane, $CH_3—CH_2—CH_2—$.

**propylene glycol** (prŏp′ĭ-lēn) A demulcent agent used as a solvent for medicines, and in cosmetics.

**propylhexedrine** (prō″pĭl-hĕk′sĕ-drēn) A sympathomimetic drug usually dispensed in an inhaler to produce nasal decongestion.

**propyliodone** (prō″pĭl-ī′ō-dōn) A radiopaque dye used in radiographical studies of the bronchi.

**propylparaben** (prō″pĭl-păr′ă-bĕn) Propyl *p*-hydroxybenzoate, $C_{10}H_{12}O_3$, a chemical used as an antifungal agent and as a preservative in pharmaceuticals.

**propylthiouracil** (prō″pĭl-thī″ō-ū′ră-sĭl) An antithyroid drug used in treatment of hyperthyroidism, thyroiditis, and thyrotoxicosis. It is also employed for preoperative therapy and in cases in which surgery is contraindicated.

**pro re nata** (prō rē nā′tă) [L.] ABBR: p.r.n. According to the circumstances; as necessary.

**prorrhaphy** (prō′ră-fē) [Gr. *pro,* before, + *rhaphe,* seam, ridge] Surgical movement of a muscle or tendon insertion to a point farther away; done to change the action of a muscle. SYN: *advancement.*

**prorsad** (pror′săd) In a forward direction.

**prorubricyte** (prō-roo′brĭ-sīt) A basophilic normoblast.

**proscription** Behavior that is forbidden by religious or cultural tenet or belief. SEE: *taboo.*

**prosecretin** (prō″sē-krē′tĭn) [″ + *secretio,* separation] A substance present in the duodenal mucosa that, when acted on by hydrochloric acid in chyme, is converted into secretin. SEE: *secretin.*

**prosection** (prō-sĕk′shŭn) [″ + L. *sectio,* a cutting] Dissection for the purpose of demonstrating anatomical structure.

**prosector** (prō-sĕk′tor) [L.] One who prepares cadavers for dissection or dissects for demonstration.

**prosencephalon** (prŏs″ĕn-sĕf′ă-lŏn) [Gr. *proso,* before, + *enkephalos,* brain] The embryonic forebrain, which gives rise to the telencephalon and diencephalon.

**proso-** [Gr. *proso,* forward] Combining form indicating *forward, anterior.*

**prosodemic** (prŏs″ō-dĕm′ĭk) [″ + *demos,* people] Spread by individual contact; said of a disease. SEE: *epidemic.*

**prosody** (prŏs′ă-dē) [L. *prosodia,* accent of a syllable] The normal rhythm, melody, and articulation of speech.

**prosopagnosia** (prŏs″ō-păg-nō′sē-ă) [Gr. *prosopon,* face, + *a-,* not, + *gnosis,* recognition] An inability to recognize faces, even one's own face.

**prosopalgia** (prŏs″ō-păl′jē-ă) [″ + *algos,* pain] Tic douloureux.

**prosopectasia** (prŏs″ō-pĕk-tā′zē-ă) [″ + *ektasis,* dilatation] Abnormal enlargement of the face.

**prosopic** (prō″sŏp′ĭk) Pert. to a face or facial skeleton that is convex anteriorly.

**prosoplasia** (prŏs″ō-plā′sē-ă) [Gr. *proso,* forward, + *plassein,* to form] Progressive transformation of cells until they develop into cells with a higher degree of function.

**prosopoanoschisis** (prŏs″ō-pō″ă-nŏs′kĭ-sĭs) [Gr. *prosopon,* face, + *ana,* up, + *schisis,* a splitting] An oblique facial cleft, a slanting furrow extending from mouth to eye.

**prosopodiplegia** (prŏs″ō-pō-dī-plē′jē-ă) [″ + *dis,* twice, + *plege,* a stroke] Paralysis on both sides of the face.

**prosopodynia** (prŏs″ō-pō-dĭn′ē-ă) [″ + *odyne,* pain] Tic douloureux.

**prosoponeuralgia** (prŏs″ō-pō-nū-răl′jē-ă) [″ + *neuron,* sinew, + *algos,* pain] Tic douloureux.

**prosopopagus** (prŏs″ō-pŏp′ă-gŭs) [″ + *pagos,* a thing fixed] Unequal conjoined twins in which the parasite is attached to some part of the face other than the jaw.

**prosopoplegia** (prŏs″ō-pō-plē′jē-ă) [″ + *plege,* stroke] Facial paralysis.

**prosoposchisis** (prŏs-ō-pŏs′kĭ-sĭs) [Gr. *prosopon,* face, + *schisis,* a splitting] A congenital cleft of the face.

**prosopospasm** (prŏs′ō-pō-spăzm) [″ + *spasmos,* a convulsion] Facial spasm.

**prosopothoracopagus** (prŏs″ō-pō-thō″ră-kŏp′ă-gŭs) [″ + *thorax,* chest, + *pagos,* a thing fixed] Conjoined twins joined in the frontal area between the face and the chest.

**prosopotocia** (prŏs″ō-pō-tō′shē-ă) [″ + *tokos,* birth] Presentation of the face in parturition.

**prosopus varus** (prŏs′ō-pŭs vā′rŭs) [Gr. *prosopon,* face, + L. *varus,* crooked] Congenital obliquity of the face caused by atrophy of one side of the head.

**prospective payment system** A reimbursement method used in which a fixed, predetermined amount is allocated for treating patients with a specific diagnosis when an individual is hospitalized. It was originally developed for use with Medicare recipients. It is also referred to as payment-by-diagnosis.

**prospective study** A clinical or epidemiological investigation of patients or health subjects with respect to the medical, social, and environmental factors encountered from the time of the beginning of the study until the investigation is terminated. SEE: *retrospective study.*

**prostacyclin** Prostaglandin $GI_2$.

**prostaglandin $GI_2$** ABBR: $PGI_2$. A compound formed from the metabolism of arachidonic acid. It is a potent vasodilator and inhibitor of platelet aggregation.

**prostaglandin inhibitor** A substance that inhibits the production of prostaglandins. Nonsteroidal and steroid anti-inflammatory agents are two major categories that inhibit prostaglandins.

**prostaglandin** (prŏs′tă-glănd-ĭn) ABBR: PG. Any of a large group of biologically active, carbon-20, unsaturated fatty acids that represent some of the metabolites of arachidonic acid. They are local short-range autacoids that are formed rapidly, exert their effects locally, and then decay or are destroyed enzymatically. Some of the physiologically important are $PGD_2$, $PGE_2$, $PGF_{2\alpha}$, and $PGI_1$. The PGs have a wide assortment of biological effects that are not mediated via the plasma, but they act as local intercellular or intracellular modulators of the biochemical activity of the tissues in which they are formed. Therefore they are classed as autacoids rather than hormones.

Some physiological actions influenced by PGs include lipolysis, fluid balance, platelet aggregation, blood flow, gastrointestinal function and activity, neurotransmission, pancreatic endocrine function, and corpus luteum regression. Increased production of PGs is important in causing bone resorption and dysmenorrhea and in influencing glucose metabolism. The normal closure of the patent ductus arteriosus is inhibited if endogenous PG production is enhanced. In some types of congenital heart disease, it is important to maintain the patency of the ductus until the appropriate surgical procedure can be performed. Conversely, if the heart is normal except for delayed closure of the patent ductus, PG inhibitors may be given to hasten the closing.

In obstetrics, $PGE_2$ gel is used to ripen the cervix before induction of labor. SEE: *arachidonic acid; nonsteroidal anti-inflammatory drugs; patent ductus arteri-*

*osus.*

**prostanoids** The name of the end products of the cyclo-oxygenase pathway of the metabolism of arachidonic acid. These are prostaglandins and thromboxanes. SEE: *eicosanoid; prostaglandins; thromboxane* $A_2$.

**prostatalgia** (prŏs-tă-tăl′jē-ă) [Gr. *prostates,* prostate, + *algos,* pain] Prostatodynia.

**prostate** (prŏs′tāt) [Gr. *prostates*] A gland, consisting of a median lobe and two lateral lobes, that surrounds the neck of the bladder and the urethra in the male. It is partly muscular and partly glandular, with ducts opening into the prostatic portion of the urethra. About 2 × 4 × 3 cm, and weighing about 20 g, it is enclosed in a fibrous capsule containing smooth muscle fibers in its inner layer. Muscle fibers also separate the glandular tissue and encircle the urethra. The gland secretes a thin, opalescent, slightly alkaline fluid that forms part of the seminal fluid.

PATHOLOGY: Inflammation of the prostate may occur, often the result of gonorrheal urethritis. Enlargement of the prostate is common, esp. after middle age. This results in urethral obstruction, impeding urination and sometimes leading to retention. Benign and malignant tumors, calculi, and nodular hyperplasia are common, particularly in men past 60. SEE: *benign prostatic hypertrophy; prostate cancer.*

***balloon dilatation of the p.*** SEE: *benign prostatic hypertrophy.*

***transrectal ultrasonography of the p.*** The use of an ultrasonic detection device placed in the rectum in order to guide biopsy of the prostate.

**prostate cancer** Malignant neoplasm, usually adenocarcinoma, of the prostate gland. It is the most frequent cause of cancer in men and the second leading cause of death in men. In 1995, it was estimated that 244,000 men were diagnosed as having prostate cancer and 40,000 died. Because there may be no early clinical signs or symptoms of cancer of the prostate, the task of early detection when the disease could be effectively treated is difficult. Tests include blood analysis for prostate specific antigen (PSA), periodic digital rectal exam (DRE), and use of transurethral ultrasound (TRUS) to provide information about the size and shape of the prostate. The first two exams should be done annually on all men beginning when they attain age 40. Use of TRUS as a routine screening procedure on healthy men over age 50 is controversial. However, if the DRE and PSA are abnormal, then TRUS should be done and tissue for pathological examination obtained. The TRUS study may be done with or without anesthesia. If the tests are positive and the cancer cells are believed to be confined to the prostate, several options are available. Depending on several factors (e.g., the age of the patient and his general health status), the treatment options include watchful waiting, radical prostatectomy, and radiation therapy. Watchful waiting has been advised in patients who are 70 years or older. The rationale is that the results of radical prostatectomy are no more beneficial than doing nothing because in both cases the life expectancy is no more than 10 or 11 years. The chances that urinary incontinence and impotency will develop are possible with either surgery or radiation. Radiation may cause injury to the colon and bladder. Radical prostatectomy has become a more attractive option since the nerve-sparing technique has become available. This type of surgery attempts to spare the nerves important to sexual potency. Patients with prostate cancer that has spread beyond the prostate are treated with hormone therapy. SEE: *benign prostatic hypertrophy; brachytherapy; prostatectomy.*

**prostatectomy** (prŏs″tă-tĕk′tō-mē) [Gr. *prostates,* prostate, + *ektome,* excision] Excision of part or all of the prostate gland. The operation may be performed through an incision in the perineum (perineal prostatectomy), into the bladder (suprapubic prostatectomy), or through the urethra (transurethral prostatectomy, TUP). After prostatectomy the libido is unaffected, but during ejaculation sperm enters the bladder rather than the urethra. In the past, about 90% of patients who had prostatectomy became impotent. New surgical techniques, however, have made it possible to preserve the autonomic nerves to the corpora cavernosa of the penis. Radical prostatectomy in which the nerves important to potency are not removed or traumatized (nerve-sparing technique) has improved the chances that impotency or incontinence will not persist after the initial recovery period. Up to 70% of men having surgery done by urologists who do not use the nerve-sparing procedure will have impotency and up to 30% will have incontinence. Of patients whose surgeons use the nerve-sparing technique, 20% to 30% will be impotent and 4% to 7% or less will have mild incontinence. Complications include retention or incontinence of urine, impotence, hematuria, cystitis, infection of kidney, pyelitis, infective nephritis, and renal failure. SEE: *Nursing Diagnoses Appendix.*

NURSING IMPLICATIONS: *Preoperative:* To prepare the patient for surgery and postoperative recovery, the nurse explains the type of procedure planned and expected results, as well as the process of retrograde ejaculation. The patient is encouraged to verbalize feelings and concerns (the patient may fear loss of erectile function more than he fears cancer). The patient is prepared physically for the procedure according to the urologist's protocol.

*Postoperative:* Vital signs are monitored closely for indications of hemorrhage or shock. The nurse manages any dressings and drainage tubes, protects skin from excoriation, and assesses incisions or tube insertion wounds for signs of infection. If a suprapubic tube is present, patency and drainage are monitored; drainage fluid should be amber to pink tinged. Urinary catheter patency is monitored, and intermittent or continuous bladder irrigation is maintained as prescribed, usually via a three-channel indwelling catheter. Irrigation rate should be fast enough to limit drainage color change to amber to pink tinged, rather than red; rate should be increased if color deepens or clots appear. Volume of irrigant and amount of drainage are carefully tracked, and the former is subtracted from the latter to determine urinary output. This figure is then compared with intake to assess fluid balance. Findings are documented, and any abnormalities in drainage color, output volume, or patient's response to surgery are reported. If bleeding increases, traction may be applied to the catheter as directed to provide tamponade. Medicines are administered as prescribed to reduce bladder spasms and pain. Sitz baths also may be used to relieve pain and discomfort.

When the catheter is removed, the patient should void every 2 hr, and the nurse should monitor serial urines for color, time, and amount of each voiding. Fluid intake of 2 to 3 L/day (unless restricted by cardiac or renal deficits), mainly as water, is encouraged; caffeine is avoided. The patient may experience urinary frequency temporarily and dribbling, but he can regain control of urinary function with Kegel exercises. Urine may be blood tinged for a few weeks, but any bright red bleeding and fever, chills, or other signs of infection should be reported. The patient should avoid straining at stool (stool softeners are often prescribed) and lifting objects of more than 10 lb, long automobile trips, and strenuous exercise for several weeks. Walking is usually considered acceptable exercise. Sexual intercourse should be delayed until the patient has been evaluated by the physician at the follow-up visit and has the physician's permission to begin such activity. The patient should also continue prescribed medications at least until the follow-up visit and should have an annual prostatic examination if prostate removal was partial.

**prostatic** (prŏs-tăt′ĭk) [Gr. *prostates,* prostate] Concerning the prostate gland.

**prostatic calculus** A stone in the prostate.

**prostatic plexus 1.** The veins around the base and neck of the bladder and prostate gland. **2.** The nerves from the pelvic plexus to the prostate gland, erectile tissue of the penis, and the seminal vesicles.

**prostatic syncope** Fainting during examination of the prostate. It is a rare occurrence that usually can be avoided by examining the patient in the lateral recumbent position.

**prostatic urethra** That part of the urethra surrounded by the prostate gland.

**prostatism** (prŏs′tă-tĭzm) [″ + *-ismos,* condition] Any condition of the prostate gland that interferes with the flow of urine from the bladder. The condition is characterized by frequent uncomfortable urination and nocturia. Retention of urine may occur with development of uremia. Causes include benign hypertrophy, carcinoma, prostatitis, and nodular hyperplasia.

**prostatitis** (prŏs″tă-tī′tĭs) [″ + *itis,* inflammation] Inflammation of the prostate gland. It may be a complication of gonorrheal infection.

***acute p.*** Inflammation of the prostate characterized by discomfort and pain in the perineal area; frequent urination; and, later, retention of urine. If severe, marked malaise, rise of temperature, constipation, chills, and vomiting occur.

***chronic p.*** Inflammation of the prostate characterized by dull, aching pain in the perineal region and discharge from the penis.

***chronic bacterial p.*** ABBR: CBP. Inflammation of the prostate caused by a long-standing bacterial infection. Clinical symptoms of fever, pain, and dysuria may be relatively mild as compared with the acute infection. Therapy depends on the causative organism and, in addition to antibiotics, may involve treatment of prostatic hypertrophy.

**prostatocystitis** (prŏs″tă-tō-sĭs-tī′tĭs) [Gr. *prostates,* prostate, + *kystis,* bladder, + *itis,* inflammation] Inflammation of the prostatic urethra involving the bladder.

**prostatocystotomy** (prŏs″tă-tō-sĭs-tŏt′ō-mē) [″ + ″ + *tome,* incision] Surgical incision of the prostate and bladder.

**prostatodynia** (prŏs″tă-tō-dĭn′ē-ă) [″ + *odyne,* pain] The condition of having the symptoms and signs of prostatitis but no evidence of inflammation of the prostate, with negative urine culture. Use of antibiotics in patients with prostatodynia is unnecessary. SYN: *proctalgia fugax; prostatalgia.*

**prostatolith** (prŏs-tăt′ō-lĭth) [″ + *lithos,* stone] A calculus of the prostate gland.

**prostatolithotomy** (prŏs-tăt″ō-lĭ-thŏt′ō-mē) [″ + ″ + *tome,* incision] Incision of the prostate in order to remove a calculus.

**prostatomegaly** (prŏs″tă-tō-mĕg′ă-lē) [″ + *megas,* large] Enlargement of the prostate gland.

**prostatomy, prostatotomy** (prŏs-tăt′ō-mē, prŏs″tă-tŏt′ō-mē) [″ + *tome,* incision] Incision into the prostate.

**prostatomyomectomy** (prŏs″tă-tō-mī″ō-mĕk′tō-mē) [″ + *mys,* muscle, + *ektome,* excision] Surgical excision of a prostatic myoma.

**prostatorrhea** (prŏs″tă-tō-rē′ă) [″ + *rhoia,* flow] Abnormal discharge from the prostate gland.

**prostatovesiculectomy** (prŏs″tă-tō-vē-sĭk″ ū-lĕk′tō-mē) [Gr. *prostates,* prostate, + L. *vesiculus,* a little sac, + Gr. *ektome,* excision] Removal of the prostate gland and seminal vesicles.

**prostatovesiculitis** (prŏs″tă-tō-vē-sĭk″ū-lī′ tĭs) [″ + ″ + Gr. *itis,* inflammation] Inflammation of the seminal vesicles and prostate gland.

**prosternation** (prō″stĕr-nā′shŭn) [Gr. *pro,* before, + *sternon,* chest] Camptocormia.

**prostheon** (prŏs′thē-ŏn) [Gr. *prosthios,* foremost] The alveolar point; the midpoint of the lower border of the upper alveolar arch of the jaw.

**prosthesis** (prŏs′thē-sĭs) *pl.* **prostheses** [Gr. *prosthesis,* an addition] **1.** Replacement of a missing part by an artificial substitute, such as an artificial extremity. **2.** An artificial organ or part. Advances in bioengineering have enabled scientists to develop artificial extremities, including arms, hands, and portions of legs. SEE: *Boston arm.* **3.** A device to augment performance of a natural function, such as a hearing aid.

***dental p.*** The replacement of a tooth or of a section of teeth by partial or full dentures.

***expansion p.*** A prosthesis that expands the lateral segment of the maxilla; used in clefts of the soft and hard palates and alveolar processes.

***maxillofacial p.*** The repair and artificial replacement of the face and jaw missing because of disease or injury.

***myoelectric p.*** An advanced prosthetic device operated by battery-powered electric motors that are activated through electrodes by the myoelectric potentials provided by muscles.

***penile p.*** A device implanted in the penis that assists it to become erect. The device is used in patients with impotence due to such organic causes as trauma, prostatectomy, or diabetes. It is usually in the form of inflatable plastic cylinders implanted in each corpus cavernosum of the penis. These cylinders are attached to a pump embedded in the scrotal pouch. A reservoir for the fluid used to fill the cylinders is implanted behind the rectus muscle. This system allows the cylinders to be filled when an erection is desired and the fluid to be drained back into the reservoir when the need for the erection has passed. In most patients, this device permits the attaining of a nearly physiological erection. SEE: *Peyronie's disease.*

**prosthetic group** (prŏs-thĕt′ĭk) The nonamino acid component of a conjugated protein; usually the portion of an enzyme that is not an amino acid. SEE: *apoenzyme; holoenzyme.*

**prosthetics** (prŏs-thĕt′ĭks) The branch of surgery dealing with replacement of missing parts.

***externally powered p.*** Any prosthesis in which a small electric motor has been incorporated for the purpose of providing force to control various functions.

**prosthetist** (prŏs′thĕ-tĭst) **1.** A specialist in artificial dentures. **2.** A maker of artificial limbs.

**prosthetosclerokeratoplasty** (prŏs″thĕ-tō-sklē″rō-kĕr′ă-tō-plăs″tē) The surgical procedure for replacement of diseased scleral and corneal tissue with a transparent prosthesis.

**prosthion** (prŏs′thē-ŏn) [Gr. *prosthios,* foremost] The lowest point on the alveolar process of the maxilla.

**prosthodontics** (prŏs″thō-dŏn′tĭks) [″ + *odous,* tooth] The branch of dentistry dealing with construction of artificial appliances for the mouth.

**prosthodontist** (prŏs″thō-dŏn′tĭst) A dentist who specializes in the mechanics of making and fitting artificial teeth.

**prosthokeratoplasty** (prŏs″thō-kĕr′ă-tō-plăs″tē) [″ + *keras,* horn, + *plassein,* to form] Surgical replacement of diseased or scarred corneal tissue with a transparent prosthesis.

**Prostin/15M** Trade name for carboprost tromethamine.

**prostitute** (prŏs′tĭ-tūt) [L. *prostituere,* to prostitute] **1.** A person who solicits or accepts payment for sexual relations. **2.** To sell oneself basely, such as to prostitute one's talents.

**prostitution** (prŏs″tĭ-tū′shŭn) The act or practice of prostituting. Prostitution is a major cause of the spread of venereal disease and is a common mode of transmission of AIDS.

**prostrate** (prŏs′trāt) [Gr. *pro,* before, + L. *sternere,* stretch out] **1.** Lying with the body extended. **2.** To deprive of strength or to exhaust.

**prostrated** Depleted of strength; exhausted.

**prostration** (prŏs-trā′shŭn) Absolute exhaustion.

***heat p.*** Exhaustion resulting from exposure to excessive heat.

***nervous p.*** General physical and nervous exhaustion. SYN: *neurasthenia.*

**protactinium** (prō″tăk-tĭn′ē-ŭm) SYMB: Pa. A radioactive element; atomic weight 231; atomic number 91.

**protal** (prō′tăl) [Gr. *protos,* first] Congenital.

**protamine** (prō′tă-mĭn) **1.** One of a class of simple proteins that are strongly basic, noncoagulable in heat, and yield diamino acids when hydrolyzed. **2.** An amine, $C_{16}H_{32}O_2N_9$, isolated from spermatozoa and the spawn of fish, and named for the fish from which it is derived. SEE: *salmin(e); sturine.*

***p. insulin*** Preparations of insulin that are more slowly dissolved and absorbed by body tissues than ordinary insulin.

They are longer-acting than ordinary insulin and lower the blood sugar for 20 to 24 hr. Examples are NPH (isophane) insulin and protamine zinc insulin.

***p. sulfate*** A purified form of protamine used to neutralize the anticoagulant action of heparin.

**protanope** (prō′tă-nōp) [Gr. *protos,* first, + *an-,* not, + *opsis,* vision] A person with protanopia.

**protanopia** (prō-tăn-ō′pē-ă) [″ + ″ + *opsis,* vision] Red blindness; color blindness in which there is a defect in the perception of red. SEE: *color blindness.*

**protean** (prō′tē-ăn) [Gr. *Proteus,* a god who could change his form] Having the ability to change form, as the ameba; variable.

**protease inhibitor** A substance that inhibits the action of enzymes.

**proteases** (prō′tē-ās-ĕs) [Gr. *protos,* first, + *-ase,* enzyme] A class of enzymes that break down, or hydrolyze, the peptide bonds that join the amino acids in a protein. The protein is broken down into its basic building blocks (i.e., amino acids). SEE: *digestion.*

**protection, altered** The state in which an individual experiences a decrease in the ability to guard the self from internal or external threats such as illness or injury. SEE: *Nursing Diagnoses Appendix.*

**protective** (prō-tĕk′tĭv) [L. *protectus,* shielding] **1.** Covering, preventing infection, providing immunity. **2.** Dressing.

**proteidogenous** (prō″tē-ĭd-ŏj′ĕn-ŭs) Producing proteins.

**protein** (prō′tēn, prō′tē-ĭn) [Gr. *protos,* first] One of a class of complex nitrogenous compounds that are synthesized by all living organisms and yield amino acids when hydrolyzed. Proteins provide the amino acids essential for the growth and repair of animal tissue.

COMPOSITION: Proteins, composed of carbon, hydrogen, oxygen, nitrogen, phosphorus, sulfur, and iron, make up the greater part of plant and animal tissue. Amino acids represent the basic structure of proteins. Foods containing protein consist of different numbers and kinds of amino acids. A complete protein is one that contains all the essential amino acids (tryptophan, lysine, methionine, valine, leucine, isoleucine, phenylalanine, threonine, arginine, and histidine). In humans, they are necessary for growth and maintenance of body weight.

SOURCES: Milk, eggs, cheese, meat, fish, and some vegetables such as soybeans are the best sources. Proteins are found in both vegetable and animal sources of food. Many "incomplete" proteins are found in vegetables; they contain some of the essential amino acids. A vegetarian diet can make up for this by combining vegetable groups that complement each other in their basic amino acid groups. This provides the body with complete protein.

Principal animal proteins are lactalbumin and lactoglobulin in milk; ovalbumin and ovoglobulin in eggs; serum albumin in serum; myosin and actin in striated muscle tissue; fibrinogen in blood; serum globulin in serum; thyroglobulin in thyroid; globin in blood; thymus histones in thymus; collagen and gelatin in connective tissue; collagen and elastin in connective tissue; and keratin in the epidermis. Chondroprotein is found in tendons and cartilage; mucin and mucoids are found in various secreting glands and animal mucilaginous substances; caseinogen in milk; vitellin in egg yolk; hemoglobin in red blood cells; and lecithoprotein in the blood, brain, and bile.

FUNCTION: Ingested proteins are a source of amino acids needed to synthesize the body's own proteins, which are essential for the growth of new tissue or the repair of damaged tissue; proteins are part of all cell membranes. Excess amino acids in the diet may be changed to simple carbohydrates and oxidized to produce adenosine triphosphate and heat; 1 g supplies 4 kcal of heat.

Infants and children require from 2 to 2.2 g of protein per kilogram of body weight per day. This should be calculated on the basis of the ideal, rather than the actual, weight of the child. Age also is a factor in determining protein requirements, the amount decreasing with age. Physical work, menstruation, pregnancy, lactation, and convalescence require increased protein intake. Excess protein in the diet results in increased nitrogen excretion in the urine.

***acute phase p.*** Any of the antimicrobial proteins released into the blood by the liver during inflammation as the result of stimulation of interleukins 1 and 6 and tumor necrosis factor. They include C-reactive protein and complement factor C3. Their specific role in fighting pathogens is unclear, but they are known to influence the erythrocyte sedimentation rate.

***blood p.*** A protein present in the blood, including hemoglobin in red blood cells and serum proteins. Normal values are hemoglobin, 13 to18 g/dl in men and 12 to 16 g/dl in women; albumin, 3.5 to 5.0 g/dl of serum; globulin, 2.3 to 3.5 g/dl of serum. The amount of albumin in relation to the amount of globulin is referred to as the albumin-globulin (A/G) ratio, which is normally 1.5 : 1 to 2.5 : 1.

***carrier p.*** A protein that elicits an immune response when coupled with a hapten.

***complete p.*** A protein containing all the essential amino acids.

***conjugated p.*** A protein containing the protein molecule with some other molecule(s). Included are chromoproteins (e.g., hemoglobin); glycoproteins (e.g., mucin); lecithoproteins, nucleoproteins, and phosphoproteins (e.g., casein).

***C-reactive p.*** SEE: *C-reactive protein.*

***denatured p.*** A protein in which the amino acid composition and stereochemical structure have been altered by physical or chemical means.

***derived p.*** A derivative of protein molecules obtained by the action of chemical alteration or a physical agent such as heat.

***G p.*** A protein that determines the activation of a physiologic event. It acts at the cell surface to couple receptors for neurotransmitters such as epinephrine, hormones, odorants, and light photons.

***immune p.*** An antibody or immunoglobulin produced by plasma cells that label foreign antigens and initiate their destruction.

***incomplete p.*** A protein lacking one or more of the essential amino acids. SEE: *amino acid, essential.*

***native p.*** A protein in its natural state; one that has not been denatured.

***plasma p.*** A protein present in blood plasma, such as albumin or globulin.

***serum p.*** A protein present in the serum part of the blood.

***simple p.*** Any of the proteins that produce alpha amino acids on hydrolysis (e.g., albumins, albuminoids, globulins, glutelins, histones, prolamines, and protamines).

**proteinaceous** (prō″tē-ĭn-ā′shŭs) Concerning or resembling proteins.

**proteinase** (prō′tē-ĭn-ās) [Gr. *protos,* first, + *lase,* enzyme] A proteolytic enzyme; an enzyme that catalyzes the breakdown of native proteins.

**protein balance** Equilibrium between protein intake and anabolism, and protein catabolism and elimination of nitrogenous products. SEE: *nitrogen equilibrium.*

**protein C** A plasma protein that inhibits coagulation factors V and XIII, preventing excessive clotting. Deficiency of this protein causes thrombosis.

**protein-calorie malnutrition** Malnutrition usually seen in infants and young children whose diets are deficient in both proteins and calories. Clinically the condition may be precipitated by other factors such as infection or intestinal parasites. SEE: *kwashiorkor.*

**protein hydrolysate injection** A sterile solution of amino acids and short-chain peptides. They represent the approximate nutritive equivalent of casein, lactalbumin, plasma, fibrin, or other suitable proteins from which the hydrolysate is derived by acid, enzymatic, or other method of hydrolysis. It may contain alcohol, dextrose, or other carbohydrates suitable for intravenous infusion. It is used intravenously in the treatment of hypoproteinemia in patients who are unable to eat or absorb food.

**protein kinase** One of several enzymes that are part of the immune reaction and after activation by cytokines mediate cellular processes such as motility and secretion.

**protein-losing enteropathy** The abnormal loss of protein into the gastrointestinal tract. It may be due to any disease that causes extensive ulceration of the intestinal mucosa.

**proteinogenous** (prō″tē-ĭn-ŏj′ĕn-ŭs) [″ + *gennan,* to produce] Developing from a protein.

**proteinophobia** (prō″tē-ĭn-ō-fō′bē-ă) [″ + *phobos,* fear] An aversion to foods containing protein.

**proteinosis** (prō″tē-ĭn-ō′sĭs) [″ + *osis,* condition] Accumulation of excess proteins in the tissues.

***lipoid p., lipid p.*** A rare hereditary condition resulting from an undefined metabolic defect. Yellow deposits of a mixture of protein and lipoid occur, esp. on the mucous surface of the mouth and tongue. Nodules may appear on the face, extremities, and on the epiglottis and vocal cords, the latter producing hoarseness.

***pulmonary alveolar p.*** A disease of unknown cause in which eosinophilic material is deposited in the alveoli. The principal symptom is dyspnea. Death from pulmonary insufficiency may occur, but complete recovery has been observed. There is no specific treatment, but general supportive measures including antibiotics and bronchopulmonary lavage have helped. In about 25% of cases, the disease clears spontaneously, but in most untreated cases the disease is progressive and leads to respiratory failure. SEE: *bronchoalveolar lavage.*

**protein sparer** A substance in the diet such as carbohydrate or fat that prevents the use of protein for energy needs.

**proteinuria** (prō″tē-ĭn-ū′rē-ă) [″ + *ouron,* urine] Protein, usually albumin, in the urine. This finding may be transient and entirely benign or a sign of severe renal disease. SYN: *albuminuria.*

***orthostatic p.*** Protein in the urine when the patient has been standing but not while reclining.

***postural p.*** Protein in the urine in relation to bodily position.

**proteolipid** (prō″tē-ō-lĭp′ĭd) A lipid-protein complex that is insoluble in water. It is found principally in the brain.

**proteolysin** (prō″tē-ŏl′ĭ-sĭn) [″ + *lysis,* dissolution] A specific substance causing decomposition of proteins.

**proteolysis** (prō″tē-ŏl′ĭ-sĭs) The hydrolysis of proteins, usually by enzyme action, into simpler substances.

**proteolytic** (prō″tē-ō-lĭt′ĭk) Hastening the hydrolysis of proteins.

**proteometabolism** (prō″tē-ō-mĕ-tăb′ō-lĭzm) [″ + *metabole,* change, + *-ismos,* condition] Digestion, absorption, and assimilation of proteins.

**proteopepsis** (prō″tē-ō-pĕp′sĭs) [″ + *peptein,* to digest] The digestion of proteins.

**proteopeptic** (prō″tē-ō-pĕp′tĭk) [″ + *peptein,*

to digest] Pert. to the digestion of protein.

**proteopexy** (prō″tē-ō-pĕks′ē) [″ + *pexis,* fixation] The fixation of proteins within the body. **proteopexic** (prō-tē-ō-pĕks′ĭk), *adj.*

**proteose** (prō′tē-ōs) [Gr. *protos,* first] One of the class of intermediate products of proteolysis between protein and peptone.

***primary p.*** The first products formed during proteolysis of proteins.

***secondary p.*** The protein resulting from further hydrolysis of primary proteoses.

**proteosuria** (prō″tē-ōs-ū′rē-ă) [″ + *ouron,* urine] Proteose in urine.

**Proteus** (prō′tē-ŭs) [Gr. *Proteus,* a god who could change his form] A genus of gram-negative enteric bacilli, found in intestines and decaying material, causing protein decomposition.

***P. mirabilis*** A species abundant in nature but only rarely a human pathogen.

***P. morganii*** Previous name of *Morganella morganii.*

***P. vulgaris*** An essentially saprophytic species that may produce urinary tract infections.

**prothrombin** A plasma protein coagulation factor synthesized by the liver (vitamin K is necessary) that is converted to thrombin by prothrombinase and thrombokinase (activated factor X) in the presence of calcium ions. SEE: *coagulation factors.*

**prothrombinase** An enzyme important in blood coagulation. In a reaction with activated factors X (Xa) and V (Va) in the presence of calcium and platelets, prothrombinase catalyzes the conversion of prothrombin to thrombin.

**prothrombinemia** (prō-thrŏm″bĭn-ē′mē-ă) [Gr. *pro,* before, + *thrombos,* clot, + *haima,* blood] The presence of prothrombin in the blood.

**prothrombinogenic** (prō-thrŏm″bĭ-nō-jĕn′ĭk) [″ + ″ + *gennan,* to produce] Promoting the formation of prothrombin.

**prothrombinopenia** (prō-thrŏm″bĭ-nō-pē′nē-ă) [″ + ″ + *penia,* lack] A deficiency of prothrombin in the blood. SYN: *hypoprothrombinemia.*

**prothrombin time** The time it takes for clotting to occur after thromboplastin and calcium are added to decalcified plasma. This test is used to evaluate the effect of administration of anticoagulant drugs.

**prothymocyte** A precursor cell that matures and differentiates into a functioning T cell in the thymus gland. SEE: *T cell.*

**protide** (prō′tīd) Protein.

**protist** (prō′tĭst) Any member of the Protista kingdom.

**Protista** (prō-tĭs′tă) [LL., simplest organisms] In taxonomy, a kingdom of organisms that includes the protozoa, unicellular and multicellular algae, and the slime molds. The cells are eukaryotic. SEE: Protozoa for illus.; *eukaryote; prokaryote.*

**protistologist** (prō-tĭs-tŏl′ō-jĭst) [″ + *logos,* word, reason] One who studies the Protista, the unicellular organisms.

**protium** (prō-tē-ŭm) Hydrogen with an atomic weight of one.

**proto-** **1.** Combining form meaning *first.* **2.** Prefix indicating the lowest of a series of compounds having the same elements.

**protobiology** (prō″tō-bī-ŏl′ō-jē) [Gr. *protos,* first, + *bios,* life, + *logos,* word, reason] The phase of science dealing with life forms more minute than bacteria (i.e., the ultraviruses and bacteriophages).

**protocol** (prō′tō-kŏl) [Gr. *protokollon,* first notes glued to manuscript] **1.** A clinical report from the first notes taken. **2.** The minutes of a meeting. **3.** A description of the steps to be taken in an experiment.

***therapist-driven p.*** A patient care plan initiated and carried out by a respiratory care practitioner with the approval of the hospital medical staff.

**protodiastole** (prō″tō-dī-ăs′tō-lē) [Gr. *protos,* first, + *diastole,* expansion] The first of four phases of ventricular diastole characterized by a drop in intraventricular pressure and the closure of the semilunar valves. This occurs immediately after the second heart sound.

**protoduodenum** (prō″tō-dū-ō-dē′nŭm) [″ + L. *duodeni,* twelve] The upper half of the duodenum. It is derived from the embryonic foregut.

**protogaster** (prō″tō-găs′tĕr) [″ + *gaster,* belly] The archenteron or gastrocele; the cavity in a gastrula or developing embryo from which the digestive tract develops.

**protoleukocyte** (prō″tō-lū′kō-sīt) [″ + *leukos,* white, + *kytos,* cell] A minute lymphoid cell in the red bone marrow and spleen.

**Protomastigida** (prō″tō-măst-ĭj′ĭ-dă) [″ + *mastix,* whip, + *eidos,* form, shape] An order of flagellate protozoa. It contains several pathogenic genera including *Leishmania* and *Trypanosoma.*

**proton** (prō′tŏn) [Gr. *protos,* first] A positively charged particle forming the nucleus of hydrogen and present in the nuclei of all elements, the atomic number of the element indicating the number of protons present. Its mass is 1836 times that of an electron. SEE: *atom; atomic theory; electron; element.*

**protoneuron** (prō″tō-nū′rŏn) [″ + *neuron,* nerve] The initial neuron in a reflex arc.

**protopathic** [″ + *pathos,* disease, suffering] Primitive, undiscriminating, esp. with respect to sensing and localizing pain stimuli. SEE: *sensibility.*

**protoplasia** (prō-tō-plā′zē-ă) [″ + *plassein,* to form] The primary formation of tissue.

**protoplasm** (prō′tō-plăzm) [″ + LL. *plasma,* form, mold] A thick, viscous colloidal substance that constitutes the physical basis of all living activities, exhibiting the properties of assimilation, growth, motility, secretion, irritability, and reproduction. It is a complex mixture of heterogeneous substances surrounded by a chemically active membrane that regulates the interchange of substances with the surrounding medium. It possesses the physical properties of a colloidal mass, the medium of dispersion being water.

Protoplasm consists of inorganic substances (water, mineral compounds) and organic substances (proteins, carbohydrates, and lipids). The principal elements present are oxygen, carbon, hydrogen, nitrogen, calcium, and phosphorus, which constitute about 99% of protoplasm. Others present in small amounts are potassium, sulfur, chlorine, sodium, magnesium, and iron, together with trace elements (copper, cobalt, manganese, zinc, and others). SEE: *cell; cytoplasm; nucleus.* **protoplasmic** (prō-tō-plăz′mĭk), *adj.*

**protoplast** (prō′tō-plăst) [″ + *plassein,* to form] In bacteriology, the sphere remaining after gram-positive bacteria have had their cell contents lysed. The bacterial cell wall constituents are absent. In gram-negative organisms these spheres retain an outer wall layer and are called spheroplasts.

**protoporphyria** (prō″tō-por-fĭr′ē-ă) Porphyria erythropoietica.

**protoporphyrin** (prō″tō-por′fĭ-rĭn) A derivative of hemoglobin containing four pyrrole nuclei; $C_{34}H_{34}N_4O_4$. It occurs naturally and is formed from heme (ferriprotoporphyrin) by deletion of an atom of iron.

**protoporphyrinuria** (prō″tō-por″fĭ-rĭn-ū′rē-ă) Protoporphyrin in the urine.

**protoproteose** (prō″tō-prō′tē-ōz) A primary proteose that, upon further digestion, is converted to deuteroproteose.

**protospasm** (prō′tō-spăzm) [Gr. *protos,* first, + *spasmos,* a convulsion] A spasm beginning in one area and extending to other parts.

**prototype** (prō″tō-tīp) An original or initial model or type from which subsequent types arise.

**protovertebra** (prō″tō-vĕr′tĕ-bră) [″ + L. *vertebra,* vertebra] Primitive vertebra in the notochord.

**Protozoa** [″ + *zoon,* animal] The phylum that includes the smallest known members of the animal kingdom. Protozoa are single-celled parasitic organisms with flexible membranes and the ability to move. Most protozoa are saprophytes, living in the soil and obtaining nourishment from dead or decaying organic material. Most protozoa infect only humans without adequate immunological defenses, although a few infect immunocompetent persons. Infections are spread by the fecal-oral route, through ingestion of food or water contaminated with cysts or spores, or by the bite of a mosquito or other insect that has previously bitten an infected person. Common protozoan infections include malaria (*Plasmodium vivax*, *P. malariae*); gastroenteritis (*Entamoeba histolytica*, *Giardia lamblia*); Leishmaniasis, an inflammatory skin disease (*Leishmania* species); sleeping sickness (*Trypanosoma gambiense*); and vaginal infections (*Trichomonas vaginalis*). *Pneumocystis carinii*, previously classified as a protozoon, is now categorized as a fungus. Opportunistic protozoan infections caused by *Cryptosporidium parvum* and *Toxoplasma gondii* are seen in patients who are immunosuppressed by disease or drug therapy. SEE: illus.; table.

**protozoa** Pl. of protozoon.

**protozoacide** (prō-tō-zō′ă-sīd) [″ + *zoon,* animal, + L. *cidus,* kill] Destructive to, or that which kills, protozoa.

**protozoal** (prō″tō-zō′ăl) Pert. to protozoa, unicellular organisms.

**protozoal disease** A disease produced by single-celled organisms, such as amebic dysentery, sleeping sickness, and malaria.

**protozoan** (prō″tō-zō′ăn) [″ + *zoon,* animal] Concerning protozoa.

**protozoology** (prō″tō-zō-ŏl′ō-jē) [Gr. *protos,* first, + *zoon,* animal, + *logos,* word, reason] The branch of science dealing with the study of protozoa.

**protozoon** *pl.* **protozoa** Unicellular organism. SEE: *Protozoa.*

**protozoophage** (prō″tō-zō′ō-făj) [″ + *zoon,* animal, + *phagein,* to eat] A phagocyte that ingests protozoa.

**protraction** (prō-trăk′shŭn) [″ + L. *protractus,* dragged out] The extension forward or drawing forward of a part of the body such as the mandible.

**protractor** (prō-trăk′tor) [L. *protractus,* dragged out] **1.** An instrument for removing foreign bodies from wounds. **2.** A muscle that draws a part forward; the opposite of retractor.

**protriptyline hydrochloride** (prō-trĭp′tĭ-lēn) An antidepressant drug.

**protrude** [L. *protrudere*] To project; to extend beyond a border or limit.

**protrusion** (prō-troo′zhŭn) The state or condition of being thrust forward or projecting. In dentistry, particularly related to the position of the mandible, as opposed to retrusion.

**protuberance** (prō-tū′bĕr-ăns) [Gr. *pro,* before, + L. *tuber,* bulge] A part that is prominent beyond a surface, like a knob.

**protuberantia** (prō-tū″bĕr-ăn′shē-ă) A protuberance, eminence, or projection.

**proud flesh** A mass of excessive granulation formed when a wound shows no other sign of healing or tendency to cicatrization.

**provertebra** (prō-vĕr′tĕ-bră) Protovertebra.

**provirus** (prō-vī′rŭs) The precursor of a virus.

**provisional** (prō-vĭzh′ŭn-ăl) [L. *provisio,* provision] Serving a temporary use pending permanent arrangements.

**provitamin** (prō-vī′tă-mĭn) [L. *pro,* before, + *vita,* life, + *amine*] An inactive substance that can be transformed in the body to a corresponding active vitamin and thus function as a vitamin.

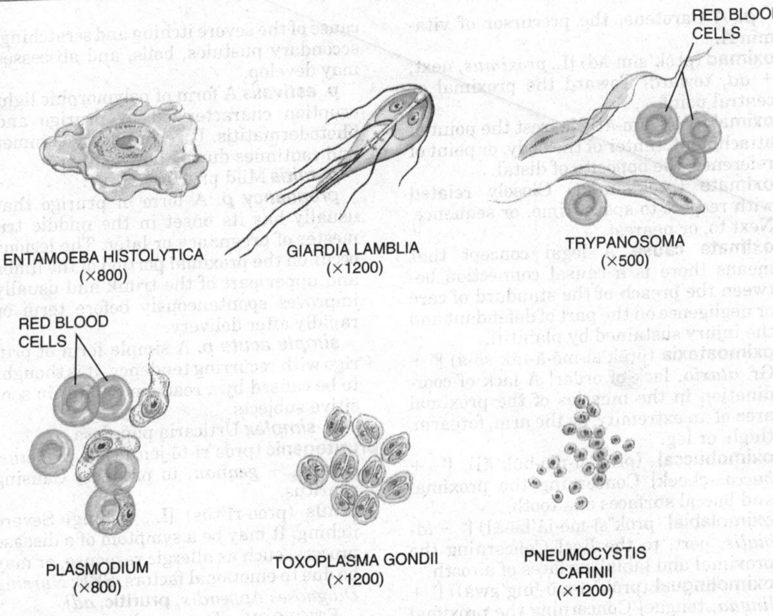


**PROTOZOA**

## Table of Pathogenic Protozoa

| Subphylum | Genus and Species | Disease Caused |
|---|---|---|
| Zoomastigophora (Mastigophora) Locomotion by flagella | *Giardia lamblia* | Gastroenteritis |
| | *Leishmania donovani* | Kala-azar |
| | *Leishmania braziliensis* | American leishmaniasis |
| | *Leishmania tropica* | Oriental sore |
| | *Trichomonas vaginalis* | Trichomoniasis |
| | *Trypanosoma gambiense* | Sleeping sickness |
| | *Trypanosoma rhodesiense* | Sleeping sickness |
| | *Trypanosoma cruzi* | Chagas' disease |
| Rhizopoda (Sarcodine) Locomotion by pseudopodia | *Acanthamoeba castellani* | Amebic meningoencephalitis |
| | *A. culbertsonii* | |
| | *A. astromyxis* | |
| | *Dientamoeba fragilis* | Diarrhea, fever |
| | *Entamoeba histolytica* | Amebic dysentery |
| | *Naegleria fowleri* | Amebic meningoencephalitis |
| Apicomplexa (Sporozoa) No locomotion in adult stage | *Babesia microti, B. divergens* | Babesiosis |
| | *Isospora belli* | Diarrhea |
| | *Cryptosporidium parvum* | Cryptosporidiosis |
| | *Toxoplasma gondii* | Toxoplasmosis |
| | *Plasmodium malariae* | Quartan malaria |
| | *Plasmodium falcipurum* | Malignant tertian malaria |
| | *Plasmodium vivax* | Tertian malaria |
| | *Plasmodium ovale* | Tertian malaria |
| Ciliophora Possession of cilia in some stage of life cycle | *Balantidium coli* | Balantidiasis |

***p. A*** Carotene, the precursor of vitamin A.

**proximad** (prŏk′sĭm-ăd) [L. *proximus,* next, + *ad,* toward] Toward the proximal or central point.

**proximal** (prŏk′sĭm-ăl) Nearest the point of attachment, center of the body, or point of reference; the opposite of distal.

**proximate** (prŏk′sĭm-āt) Closely related with respect to space, time, or sequence. Next to, or nearest.

**proximate cause** A legal concept that means there is a causal connection between the breach of the standard of care or negligence on the part of defendant and the injury sustained by plaintiff.

**proximoataxia** (prōk″sĭ-mō-ă-tăk′sē-ă) [″ + Gr. *ataxia,* lack of order] A lack of coordination in the muscles of the proximal area of an extremity, as the arm, forearm, thigh, or leg.

**proximobuccal** (prŏk″sĭ-mō-bŭk′ăl) [″ + *bucca,* cheek] Concerning the proximal and buccal surfaces of a tooth.

**proximolabial** (prŏk″sĭ-mō-lā′bē-ăl) [″ + *labialis,* pert. to the lips] Concerning the proximal and labial surfaces of a tooth.

**proximolingual** (prŏk″sĭ-mō-lĭng′gwăl) [″ + *lingua,* tongue] Concerning the proximal and lingual surfaces of a tooth.

**prozone** That portion of the low dilution range of a homologous serum that fails to agglutinate bacteria that are agglutinated by the same serum in a higher dilution.

**prozymogen** (prō-zī′mō-jĕn) [Gr. *pro,* before, + *zyme,* leaven, + *gennan,* to produce] An intranuclear substance that is a precursor of zymogen.

**prune** (proon) [L. *pruna*] A dried plum, rich in carbohydrate, that contains a substance that is useful in stimulating the bowel, esp. for those who suffer from chronic constipation. The ability of prunes and prune juice to exert a laxative effect is due to the presence of dihydroxyphenyl isatin.

**prune-belly defect** A nonstandard, but descriptive, term for children with congenital absence of one or more layers of abdominal muscles.

**pruriginous** (proo-rĭj′ĭ-nŭs) [L. *prurigo,* itch] Pert. to, or of the nature of, prurigo.

**prurigo** (proo-rī′gō) [L., the itch] A chronic skin disease of unknown etiology, marked by constantly recurring, discrete, pale, deep-seated, intensely itchy papules on extensor surfaces of limbs. Superimposed exanthematous manifestations may mask the true nature. This term is used by dermatologists throughout the world, but it has not received a universally acceptable definition. Treatment is constitutional and local, with antipruritics given locally. Prurigo begins in childhood and may last a lifetime.

***p. agria*** A severe type of prurigo that starts in childhood and persists. The skin becomes thickened and pigmented. Because of the severe itching and scratching, secondary pustules, boils, and abscesses may develop.

***p. estivalis*** A form of polymorphic light eruption characterized by prurigo and photodermatitis. It recurs every summer and continues during hot weather.

***p. mitis*** Mild prurigo.

***pregnancy p.*** A form of prurigo that usually has its onset in the middle trimester of pregnancy or later. The lesions occur on the proximal portion of the limbs and upper part of the trunk and usually improves spontaneously before term or rapidly after delivery.

***simple acute p.*** A simple form of prurigo with recurring tendency. It is thought to be caused by a reaction to bites in sensitive subjects.

***p. simplex*** Urticaria papulosa.

**pruritogenic** (proo″rĭ-tō-jĕn′ĭk) [L. *pruritus,* itching, + *gennan,* to produce] Causing pruritus.

**pruritus** (proo-rī′tŭs) [L., itching] Severe itching. It may be a symptom of a disease process, such as allergic response, or may be due to emotional factors. SEE: *Nursing Diagnoses Appendix.* **pruritic,** *adj.*

ETIOLOGY: The predisposing factor is cutaneous hyperesthesia. Localized causes are present in pruritus ani, pruritus vulvae, intestinal parasites (pinworms), and mycotic infection.

TREATMENT: The exciting or contributory cause should be located and removed. Hygienic regimen should be followed. Patients with anal or vulvar pruritus should be examined by a competent gynecologist or proctologist before cutaneous therapy is instituted. In the bath, too sudden changes of temperature should be avoided. For dry skin, frequent soap and water bathing should be avoided. Soft, nonirritating underclothing and soothing lotions are of benefit.

***p. ani*** Itching around the anus. This may be due to poor perineal hygiene; perianal skin damage caused by scratching, or abrasion due to use of harsh, dry paper; excess moisture caused by wearing tight, nonporous clothing; decreased resistance to fungi and yeasts during steroid therapy; ingestion of dietary irritants; pinworms; anal fistula or hemorrhoids; or contact with soap or detergents that remain in underclothing following improper washing.

TREATMENT: The primary cause should be removed or avoided. The anus should be kept scrupulously clean by use of a mild soap, and applications of drugs that produce sensitivity and irritation should be avoided. It is not possible to adequately cleanse the anal area by use of toilet tissue. SEE: *bidet.*

***aquagenic p.*** Pruritus produced by contact with water.

***emperor of p.*** SEE: *emperor of pruritus.*

***essential p.*** Pruritus without apparent

skin lesion.

*p. estivalis* Pruritus with prickly heat occurring in hot weather.

*p. hiemalis* Pruritus that occurs in cold weather and is provoked by cooling of the skin.

*p. senilis* Pruritus in the aged with degenerative skin changes.

*vulvar p.* A disorder marked by severe itching of the external female genitalia. Other conditions that may be associated are diabetes mellitus, vulvovaginitis, hepatic disease, psoriasis, polycythemia, anemia, leukemia, Hodgkins' disease, pinworms, body lice, scabies, fat malabsorption, allergic response to antimicrobials such as penicillin and sulfonamides, and any disease that causes generalized itching. Irritation from soaps, deodorants, douche solutions, spermicides, and wearing underclothes made of synthetic materials may be important factors in causing or aggravating the itching. SEE: *vulvodynia.*

**Prussak's space** (proo'săks) [Alexander Prussak, Russ. otologist, 1839–1897] The tiny space in the middle ear between Shrapnell's membrane laterally and the neck of the malleus medially.

**PSA** *Prostate-specific antigen.*

**psalterium** (săl-tē'rē-ŭm) [Gr. *psalterion,* harp] **1.** Omasum. **2.** Commissure of the fornix of the brain.

**psammoma** (săm-ō'mă) [Gr. *psammos,* sand, + *oma,* tumor] A small tumor of the brain, the choroid plexus, and other areas, containing calcareous particles.

**psammosarcoma** (săm"ō-săr-kō'mă) [" + *sarx,* flesh, + *oma,* tumor] A sarcoma in which psammoma bodies are present.

**psammotherapy** (săm"ō-thĕr'ă-pē) [" + *therapeia,* treatment] The application of sand baths in treatment.

**psammous** (săm'ŭs) Sandy, gritty.

**psellism, psellismus** (sĕl'ĭzm, sĕl-ĭz'mŭs) [Gr. *psellisma,* stammer] Defective pronunciation, stuttering, or stammering.

*p. mercurialis* Jerking, hurried, unintelligible speech present as part of the tremor that accompanies mercury poisoning.

**pseudacousma** (soo"dă-kooz'mă) [Gr. *pseudes,* false, + *akousma,* a thing heard] A condition in which all sounds are heard falsely, seeming to be altered in quality of pitch, or imaginary sounds are heard. SYN: *pseudacusis.*

**pseudacusis** (soo"dă-kū'sĭs) Pseudacousma.

**pseudagraphia** (soo"dă-grăf'ē-ă) [" + *a-,* not, + *graphein,* to write] A form of agraphia in which a person is unable to write independently, but is able to copy words or letters. SYN: *pseudoagraphia.*

**pseudarthritis** (soo"dăr-thrī'tĭs) [" + *arthron,* joint, + *itis,* inflammation] A condition that imitates arthritis.

**pseudarthrosis** (soo"dăr-thrō'sĭs) [" + *arthron,* joint, + *osis,* condition] A false joint or abnormal articulation, as one developing after a fracture that has not united. SYN: *nearthrosis.*

**pseudencephalus** (soo"dĕn-sĕf'ă-lŭs) [" + *enkephalos,* brain] A congenital deformity in which the cranium is open and contains poorly organized vascular tissue.

**pseudesthesia** (soo"dĕs-thē'zē-ă) [" + *aisthesis,* sensation] **1.** An imaginary or false sensation, as that felt in the lost part after amputation. **2.** A sense of feeling not caused by external stimulation. SYN: *pseudoesthesia.*

**pseudo-** (soo'dō) [Gr. *pseudes,* false] Combining form meaning *false.*

**pseudoacanthosis nigricans** (soo"dō-ăk"ăn-thō'sĭs) [" + *akantha,* thorn, + *osis,* condition] A velvety, pigmented thickening of the flexural surfaces, occurring in dark-skinned obese persons.

**pseudoacephalus** (soo"dō-ā-sĕf'ă-lŭs) [" + *a-,* not, + *kephale,* head] A parasitic twin that has a rudimentary cranium.

**pseudoagglutination** (soo"dō-ă-glū"tĭ-nā'shŭn) The clumping together of red blood cells as in the formation of rouleaux, but differing from true agglutination in that they can be dispersed by shaking.

**pseudoagraphia** Pseudagraphia.

**pseudoalbinism** (soo"dō-ăl'bĭ-nĭzm) [" + L. *albus,* white, + Gr. *-ismos,* condition] Loss of pigment of the skin, as occurs in leukopathia or vitiligo.

**pseudoalleles** (soo"dō-ă-lēlz') [" + *allelon,* of one another] A set of genes that seem to be present in the same locus in certain conditions and in closely situated loci in other conditions.

**pseudoanemia** (soo"dō-ă-nē'mē-ă) [" + *an-,* not, + *haima,* blood] Pallor of mucous membranes and skin without other signs of true anemia.

*p. of pregnancy* A drop in hematocrit during pregnancy. The increase in circulating blood volume reflects an altered ratio of serum to red blood cells; plasma volume increases by 50%, whereas the red blood cell count increases by 30%.

**pseudoaneurysm** (soo"dō-ăn'ū-rĭzm) [" + *aneurysma,* a widening] A dilation or tortuosity in a vessel that gives the impression of an aneurysm.

**pseudoangina** (soo"dō-ăn'jĭ-nă, -ăn-jī'nă) [" + L. *angina,* a choking] False symptoms of nervous origin, resembling angina pectoris. Symptoms include functional attacks of pain in the cardiac region but not associated with any disease of the heart or its vessels.

**pseudoankylosis** (soo"dō-ăng"kĭ-lō'sĭs) [" + *ankyle,* stiff joint, + *osis,* condition] A false joint.

**pseudoapoplexy** (soo"dō-ăp'ŏ-plĕk"sē) A mild condition simulating apoplexy but not accompanied by cerebral hemorrhage. SYN: *parapoplexy.* SEE: *transient ischemic attack.*

**pseudoarthrosis** The failure of spinal fusion to occur following surgery. This judgment is not made until 1 year following surgery.

**pseudoataxia** (soo″dō-ă-tăk′sē-ă) [″ + *ataxia,* lack of order] A condition resembling ataxia but not due to tabes dorsalis.

**pseudoblepsia, pseudoblepsis** (soo″dō-blĕp′sē-ă, -sĭs) [″ + *blepsis,* sight] False or imaginary vision. SYN: *parablepsia; pseudopsia.*

**pseudocartilaginous** (soo″dō-kăr″tĭ-lăj′ĭ-nŭs) [″ + L. *cartilago,* gristle] Pert. to, or formed of, a substance resembling cartilage.

**pseudocast** (soo′dō-kăst) [″ + ME. *casten,* to carry] A sediment in urine composed of epithelial cells and resembling a true cast; a false cast. Alkaline urine tends to dissolve pseudocasts.

**pseudocele** (soo′dō-sēl) [″ + *koilos,* hollow] The cavity of the septum pellucidum, the so-called fifth ventricle. SYN: *pseudocoele.* SEE: *cavum septi pellucidi.*

**pseudocholesteatoma** (soo″dō-kō″lĕs-tē-ă-tō′mă) [″ + *chole,* bile, + *steatos,* fat, + *oma,* tumor] Hard epithelium present as a mass in the tympanic cavity in association with chronic inflammation of the middle ear.

**pseudocholinesterase** (soo″dō-kō″lĭn-ĕs′tĕr-ās) A nonspecific cholinesterase that hydrolyzes noncholine esters as well as acetylcholine. It is found in the blood serum and pancreatic tissue.

**pseudochorea** (soo″dō-kō-rē′ă) [″ + *choreia,* dance] A hysterical state resembling chorea.

**pseudochromesthesia** (soo″dō-krō″mĕs-thē′zē-ă) [″ + *chroma,* color, + *aisthesis,* sensation] A condition in which sounds, esp. of the vowels, seem to induce a sensation of a distinct visual color. SEE: *phonism; photism; synesthesia.*

**pseudochromidrosis** (soo″dō-krō″mĭd-rō′sĭs) [″ + ″ + *hidros,* sweat, + *osis,* condition] The appearance of colored sweat, in which the sweat acquires its color after it is excreted.

**pseudocirrhosis** (soo″dō-sĭr-ō′sĭs) [″ + *kirrhos,* orange yellow, + *osis,* disease] A condition with symptoms of cirrhosis of the liver, caused by any process that causes obstruction of venous flow from the liver. Constrictive pericarditis can cause this condition. Cyanosis, ascites, and dyspnea characterize this condition.

**pseudocoele** (soo′dō-sēl) [″ + *koilos,* hollow] Pseudocele.

**pseudocolloid** (soo″dō-kŏl′oyd) [″ + *kollodes,* glutinous] A mucoid substance present in various locations and in ovarian cysts.

**pseudocoloboma** (soo″dō-kŏl-ō-bō′mă) [″ + *koloboma,* a mutilation] A scarcely noticeable scar on the iris from an embryonic fissure.

**pseudocoma** Locked-in syndrome.

**pseudocoxalgia** (soo″dō-kŏk-săl′jē-ă) [″ + L. *coxa,* hip, + Gr. *algos,* pain] Legg-Calvé-Perthes disease.

**pseudocrisis** (soo-dō-krī′sĭs) [″ + *krisis,* turning point] A false crisis; a temporary fall of body temperature, which may be followed by a rise.

**pseudocroup** (soo-dō-kroop′) False croup. SYN: *laryngismus stridulus.*

**pseudocyesis** (soo″dō-sī-ē′sĭs) [″ + *kyesis,* pregnancy] A condition in which a patient has nearly all of the usual signs and symptoms of pregnancy, such as enlargement of the abdomen, weight gain, cessation of menses, and morning sickness, but is not pregnant. It is usually seen in women who either are very desirous of having children or wish to avoid pregnancy. Treatment usually is done by psychiatric means. Pseudocyesis also occurs in men. SYN: *phantom pregnancy; pseudopregnancy* (2).

**pseudocylindroid** (soo″dō-sĭ-lĭn′droyd) [″ + *kylindros,* cylinder, + *eidos,* form, shape] A shred of mucus in the urine that resembles a cast.

**pseudocyst** (soo′dō-sĭst) [″ + *kystis,* bladder] A dilatation resembling a cyst.

**pseudodementia** (soo″dō-dē-mĕn′shē-ă) [″ + L. *dementare,* to make insane] An exaggerated indifference to the environment without disorientation or impairment of mental capacity. The symptoms mimic those of dementia and are sometimes evident in older, depressed individuals. Perseveration and confabulation, often seen in true dementia, are absent.

**pseudodiphtheria** (soo″dō-dĭf-thē′rē-ă) [″ + *diphthera,* membrane] A condition resembling diphtheria but not due to *Corynebacterium diphtheriae.*

**pseudoedema** (soo″dō-ē-dē′mă) [″ + *oidema,* a swelling] A puffy condition of the skin simulating edema.

**pseudoemphysema** (soo″dō-ĕm-fĭ-zē′mă) [″ + *emphysema,* an inflation] A bronchial condition simulating emphysema, caused by temporary blockage of the bronchi.

**pseudoencephalitis** (soo″dō-ĕn-sĕf″ă-lī′tĭs) [″+ *enkephalos,* brain, + *itis,* inflammation] A false encephalitis due to profuse diarrhea.

**pseudoephedrine hydrochloride** (soo″dō-ĕ-fĕd′rĭn) A sympathomimetic drug, an isomer of ephedrine, that has actions similar to those of ephedrine. Trade names are Sudafed and Novafed.

**pseudoerysipelas** (soo″dō-ĕr-ĭ-sĭp′ĕ-lăs) [″ + *erythros,* red, + *pella,* skin] An inflammation of subcutaneous cellular tissue simulating erysipelas.

**pseudoesthesia** (soo″dō-ĕs-thē′zē-ă) [″ + *aisthesis,* sensation] Pseudesthesia.

**pseudofolliculitis barbae** Inflammation of beard follicles when tightly coiled hairs become ingrown. The only sure prevention is not shaving. SEE: illus.

**pseudofracture** (soo″dō-frăk′chūr) A ribbonlike zone of decalcification seen in certain types of osteomalacia.

**pseudoganglion** (soo″dō-găn′glē-ŏn) [″ + *ganglion,* knot] A slight thickening of a nerve, resembling a ganglion.

**pseudogeusesthesia** (soo″dō-gūs″ĕs-thē′

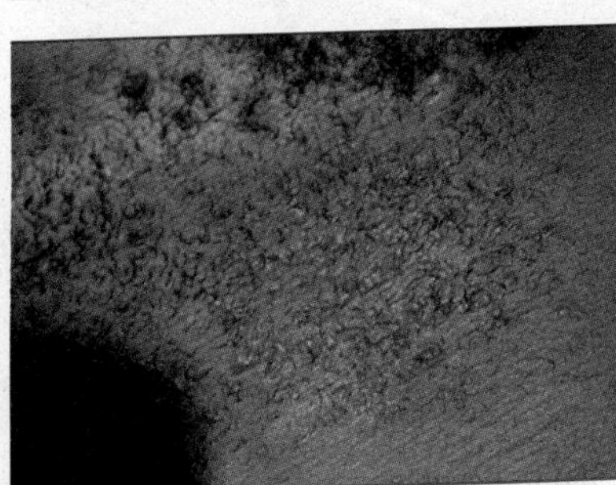

PSEUDOFOLLICULITIS BARBAE

zē-ă) [″ + *geusis,* taste, + *aisthesis,* sensation] A sense of taste stimulated by one of the other senses.

**pseudogeusia** (soo″dō-gū′sē-ă) A subjective sensation of taste not produced by external stimulus.

**pseudoglioma** (soo″dō-glī-ō′mă) [″ + *glia,* glue, + *oma,* tumor] Inflammatory changes occurring in the vitreous body that simulate glioma of retina but are due to iridochoroiditis.

**pseudoglobulin** (soo″dō-glŏb′ū-lĭn) [″ + L. *globulus,* little globe] One of a class of globulins characterized by being soluble in salt-free water. SEE: *euglobulin.*

**pseudoglottis** (soo″dō-glŏt′ĭs) [″ + *glottis,* back of tongue] The area between the false vocal cords.

**pseudogout** (soo′dō-gowt″) Chronic recurrent arthritis clinically similar to gout. The crystals found in synovial fluid are calcium pyrophosphate dihydrate (CPPD) and not urate crystals. Also, the most commonly involved joint is the knee. Multiple joints are involved in at least two thirds of patients. This condition is treated by joint aspiration, nonsteroidal anti-inflammatory agents, or intra-articular injection of glucocorticoid salts. SYN: *chondrocalcinosis.*

**pseudogynecomastia** (soo″dō-jĭn″ĕ-kō-măs′tē-ă) [Gr. *pseudes,* false, + *gyne,* woman, + *mastos,* breast] Excess adipose tissue in the male breast but with no increase in glandular tissue.

**pseudohematuria** (soo″dō-hē″mă-tū′rē-ă) [″ + *haima,* blood, + *ouron,* urine] A red pigment in the urine that makes the urine appear to have blood in it.

**pseudohemophilia** (soo″dō-hē″mō-fĭl′ē-ă) [″ + ″ + *philos,* to love] Von Willebrand's disease.

**pseudohemoptysis** (soo″dō-hē-mŏp′tĭ-sĭs) [″ + *haima,* blood, + *ptyein,* to spit] Spitting of blood that does not arise from the bronchi or the lungs.

**pseudohermaphrodite** (soo″dō-hĕr-măf′rō-dīt) An individual having the sex glands of only one sex but having some of the physical appearances of an individual of the opposite sex.

**pseudohermaphroditism** (soo″dō-hĕr-măf′rō-dīt″ĭzm) [″ + *Hermaphroditos,* mythical two-sexed god, + *-ismos,* condition] A congenital abnormality of the external genitalia and of the body in which one possesses sex glands of one sex but genitalia of the opposite sex. SYN: *false hermaphroditism.* SEE: *intersex.*

***female p.*** A condition in a female marked by a large clitoris, resembling the penis, and hypertrophied labia majora, resembling the scrotum, thus producing a resemblance to male genitalia. This condition can be caused by disease of the adrenal gland.

***male p.*** A condition in a male marked by a small penis, perineal hypospadias, and scrotum without testes, thereby resembling the vulva. This condition can be due to disease of the adrenal gland or a feminizing tumor of the undescended testis.

**pseudohernia** (soo″dō-hĕr′nē-ă) [″ + L. *hernia,* rupture] Inflammation in the scrotal area resembling a hernia.

**pseudohypertension** The observation of elevated blood pressure when taken by conventional means (i.e., sphygmomanometer), that is in reality not elevated when compared with the actual pressure in the artery when determined by more nearly accurate methods. True blood pressure may be obtained directly by use of either an intra-arterial catheter or an infrasonic recorder, the latter being almost as accurate as the former. Pseudohypertension is more likely to be found in elderly patients. SEE: *blood pressure, indirect measurement of; hypertension; infrasonic recorder.*

**pseudohypertrophy** (soo″dō-hī-pĕr′trō-fē) [″ + *hyper,* above, + *trophe,* nourishment] The increase in size of an organ or structure owing to hypertrophy or hyperplasia of tissue other than parenchyma. It often is accompanied by diminution of function. **pseudohypertrophic** (-trō′fĭk), *adj.*

**pseudohypoparathyroidism** (soo″dō-hī″pō-păr″ă-thī′royd-ĭzm) A hereditary disease resembling hypoparathyroidism but caused by an inadequate response to parathyroid hormone rather than a deficiency of the hormone. Some of these patients are obese with short, stocky build and a moonface. Mental deficiency may be present along with cataracts, strabismus, tetany, stridor, convulsions, and muscular cramps.

**pseudoicterus** (soo″dō-ĭk′tĕr-ŭs) [″ + *ikteros,* jaundice] Pseudojaundice.

**pseudoisochromatic** (soo″dō-ī″sō-krō-măt′ĭk) [″ + *isos,* equal, + *chroma,* color] Seemingly of the same color; colors used in charts testing for color blindness.

**pseudojaundice** (soo″dō-jawn′dĭs) [″ + Fr. *jaune,* yellow] Pigment in the skin, such as in carotenemia, that resembles jaundice, but is not due to jaundice. SYN: *pseudoicterus.* SEE: *carotenemia.*

**pseudologia** (soo-dō-lō′jē-ă) [″ + *logos,*

word, reason] Falsification in writing or in speech, a form of pathological lying.

*p. fantastica* Pathological lying; one of the forms of the psychopathic state.

**pseudomania** (soo-dō-mā′nē-ă) [″ + *mania,* madness] **1.** A psychosis in which patients falsely accuse themselves of crimes that they think they have committed. **2.** Pathological lying.

**pseudomasturbation** (soo″dō-măs-tŭr-bā′shŭn) [″ + L. *manus,* hand, + *stuprare,* to rape] Peotillomania.

**pseudomelanosis** (soo″dō-mĕl-ă-nō′sĭs) [″ + *melas,* black, + *osis,* condition] Discoloration of the tissues after death.

**pseudomembrane** (soo″dō-mĕm′brān) [″ + L. *membrana,* membrane] A false membrane, as in diphtheria.

**pseudomembranous** (soo″dō-mĕm′bră-nŭs) Pert. to, or marked by, false membranes.

**pseudomeningitis** (soo″dō-mĕn-ĭn-jī′tĭs) [″ + *meninx,* membrane, + *itis,* inflammation] A condition resembling the symptoms of meningitis without the lesions of meningeal inflammation.

**pseudomenstruation** (soo″dō-mĕn″strū-ā′shŭn) [″ + L. *menstruare,* menstruate] Bleeding from the uterus not accompanied by the usual changes in the endometrium.

*p. of the newborn* Withdrawal bleeding after birth, a scant vaginal discharge that reflects the physiological response of some female infants to an exposure to high levels of maternal hormones in utero.

**pseudomnesia** (soo″dŏm-nē′zē-ă) [″ + *mnesis,* memory] A memory perversion in which the patient remembers that which never occurred.

**Pseudomonas** (soo-dō-mō′năs) [″ + *monas,* single] A genus of small, motile, gram-negative bacilli with polar flagella. Most are saprophytic, living in soil and decomposing organic matter. Some produce blue and yellow pigments.

*P. aeruginosa* A species that is sometimes pathogenic for humans. It may cause urinary tract infections, otitis externa, or folliculitis, including the inflammation that may follow use of a "hot tub." It is a serious, potentially life-threatening pathogen for those with cystic fibrosis or extensive third-degree burns.

*P. cepacia* A strain of *Pseudomonas* that has emerged as a frequent cause of pneumonia and septicemia in patients with cystic fibrosis.

*P. mallei* A species that causes glanders in horses.

*P. maltophilia* A species potentially pathogenic for humans. It is found in plants, soil, water, sewage, and raw milk.

*P. pseudomallei* A species that causes melioidosis in humans and animals.

**pseudomucin** (soo-dō-mū′sĭn) [″ + L. *mucus,* mucus] A variety of mucin found in ovarian cysts.

**pseudomyopia** (soo″dō-mī-ō′pē-ă) [″ + *myein,* to shut, + *ops,* eye] A condition in which defective vision causes persons to hold objects close in order to see them, even though myopia is not present.

**pseudomyxoma** (soo″dō-mĭk-sō′mă) [″ + *myxa,* mucus, + *oma,* tumor] A peritoneal tumor resembling a myxoma and containing a thick viscid fluid.

*p. peritonei* A type of tumor that develops in the peritoneum from implantation metastases resulting from rupture of ovarian cystadenoma or cells escaping during surgical removal. Numerous papillomas develop, attached to the abdominal wall and intestine, and the peritoneal cavity becomes filled with mucus-like fluid.

**pseudoneoplasm** (soo-dō-nē′ō-plăsm) [″ + *neos,* new, + LL. *plasma,* form, mold] A false or phantom tumor; a temporary swelling, usually of an inflammatory nature, that simulates a tumor.

**pseudoneuritis** (soo″dō-nū-rī′tĭs) [″ + *neuron,* nerve, + *itis,* inflammation] Reddening and blurring of the optic disk, which resembles optic neuritis.

**pseudoneuroma** (soo″dō-nū-rō′mă) [″ + ″ + *oma,* tumor] A mass of interlacing, coiled fibers, cells of Schwann, and fibrous tissue forming a mass at end of amputation stump. Also called amputation or traumatic neuroma, this is not a true neuroma.

**pseudonucleolus** (soo″dō-nū″klē-ō′l′ŭs) [″ + L. *nucleus,* a nut] The false nucleolus or karyosome.

**pseudopapilledema** (soo″dō-păp″ĭ-lĕ-dē′mă) [″ + *papilla,* nipple, + *oidema,* swelling] A swelling of the optic nerve head that is not caused by optic neuritis.

**pseudoparalysis** (soo″dō-pă-răl′ĭ-sĭs) [″ + *para,* at the side, + *lyein,* to loosen] The loss of muscular power not caused by a lesion of the nervous system and of hysterical origin.

**pseudoparaplegia** (soo″dō-păr-ă-plē′jē-ă) [″ + ″ + *plege,* a stroke] A seeming paralysis of the lower extremities without impairment of the reflexes.

**pseudoparasite** (soo″dō-păr′ă-sīt) [″ + ″ + *sitos,* food] **1.** Anything resembling a parasite. **2.** An organism that can live as a parasite, although it is normally not one. SEE: *parasite, facultative.*

**Pseudophyllidea** (soo″dō-fĭ-lĭd′ē-ă) An order belonging to the class Cestoidea, subclass Cestoda. It includes tapeworms with scolices bearing two lateral (or one terminal) sucking grooves (bothria) and includes *Diphyllobothrium latum,* the fish tapeworm of humans.

**pseudopocket** A pocket that results from gingival inflammation with edema that produces an apparent abnormal depth of the gingival sulcus without apical movement of the bottom of the sulcus; a false pocket. SEE: *gingivitis.*

**pseudopod** (soo′dō-pŏd) [″ + *pous,* foot] Pseudopodium (1).

**pseudopodium** (soo″dō-pō′dē-ŭm) *pl.* **pseu-**

dopodia **1.** A temporary protruding process of a protozoan or ameboid cell, such as a leukocyte, that aids in locomotion and the engulfing of food particles or foreign substances, as in phagocytosis. SYN: *pseudopod.* **2.** An irregular projection at the edge of a wheal.

**pseudopolyp** (soo″dō-pŏl′ĭp) [″ + *polys,* many, + *pous,* foot] A hypertrophied area of mucous membrane resembling a polyp.

**pseudopolyposis** (soo″dō-pŏl″ĭ-pō′sĭs) [″ + ″ + ″ + *osis,* condition] A large number of pseudopolyps in the colon due to chronic inflammation.

**pseudopregnancy** (soo″dō-prĕg′năn-sē) [Gr. *pseudes,* false, + L. *praegnans,* with child] **1.** A condition in lower animals following sterile matings in which anatomical and physiological changes occur, similar to those of pregnancy. **2.** Pseudocyesis.

**pseudopuberty, precocious** Feminization of a young girl due to enhanced estrogen production, but ovulation and cyclic menstruation are absent. Estrogen-secreting tumors of the ovary are the usual cause. Treatment is removal of the tumor.

**pseudo-pseudohypoparathyroidism** (soo″dō-soo″dō-hī″pō-păr″ă-thī′royd-ĭzm) [″ + *pseudes,* false, + *hypo,* under, + *para,* beside, + *thyreos,* shield, + *eidos,* form, shape + *-ismos,* condition] Pseudohypoparathyroidism in which most of the clinical but none of the biochemical changes are present.

**pseudopsia** (soo-dŏp′sē-ă) [″ + *opsis,* vision] Visual hallucinations or false perceptions. SYN: *parablepsia; pseudoblepsia.*

**pseudopterygium** (soo″dō-tĕr-ĭj′ē-ŭm) [″ + *pterygion,* wing] A scar on the conjunctiva of the eye that is firmly attached to the underlying tissue.

**pseudoptosis** (soo-dō-tō′sĭs) [″ + *ptosis,* a dropping] Apparent ptosis of the eyelid, resulting from a fold of skin or fat projecting below the edge of the eyelid.

**pseudorabies** (soo″dō-rā′bēz) [″ + L. *rabere,* to rage] A rabies-like disease in animals that is due to a type of herpesvirus. It causes death within several days.

**pseudoreaction** (soo″dō-rē-ăk′shŭn) A false reaction; a response to injection of a test substance into the tissues owing to the presence of an allergen other than one for which test is made.

**pseudorickets** (soo″dō-rĭk′ĕts) Renal rickets.

**pseudoscarlatina** (soo″dō-skăr-lă-tē′nă) A septic febrile condition with a rash resembling scarlatina.

**pseudosclerosis** (soo″dō-sklē-rō′sĭs) [″ + *sklerosis,* a hardening] A condition with the symptoms, but without the lesions, of multiple sclerosis of the nervous system.

**pseudosmia** (soo-dŏz′mē-ă) [″ + *osme,* smell] An olfactory hallucination or perversion of the sense of smell.

**pseudostoma** (soo-dŏs′tō-mă) [″ + *stoma,* mouth] An apparent aperture between endothelial cells that have been stained.

**pseudostratified** (soo-dō-străt′ĭ-fīd) [″ + L. *stratificare,* to arrange in layers] Apparently composed of layers.

**pseudosyphilis** (soo″dō-sĭf′ĭ-lĭs) A nonspecific condition resembling syphilis.

**pseudotabes** (soo″dō-tā′bēz) [Gr. *pseudes,* false, + L. *tabes,* wasting away] A neural disease simulating tabes dorsalis.

**pseudotetanus** (soo″dō-tĕt′ă-nŭs) [″ + *tetanos,* stretched] Persistent muscular contractions resembling tetanus.

**pseudotruncus arteriosus** (soo″dō-trŭnk′ŭs ăr-tē″rē-ō′sŭs) The severest form of tetralogy of Fallot.

**pseudotuberculosis** (soo″dō-tū-ber″kū-lō′sĭs) [″ + L. *tuberculus,* tubercle, + Gr. *osis,* condition] A group of diseases that resemble tuberculosis but are due to an organism other than the tubercle bacillus. In humans the most common cause is *Yersinia pseudotuberculosis,* a gram-negative organism.

**pseudotumor cerebri** (soo″dō-tū′mor sĕr′ĕ-brī) Benign intracranial hypertension. This diagnosis is made after exclusion of tumors, obstruction of the ventricles, intracranial infection, and vascular hypertensive encephalopathy. The cause may be a variety of disorders but in most cases is unknown. The prognosis is for spontaneous recovery.

**pseudotympany** (soo″dō-tĭm′pă-nē) [″ + *tympanon,* drum] Flattening of the arch of the diaphragm and a swelling of the abdomen with increased respiration. It disappears under anesthesia and is of purely nervous origin.

**pseudoxanthoma** (soo″dō-zăn-thō′mă) [″ + *xanthos,* yellow, + *oma,* tumor] A condition resembling xanthoma.

***p. elasticum*** A chronic degenerative cutaneous disease marked by yellow patches and stretching of the skin. It is associated with hypertension and degeneration of the elastic coat of the arteries. Angioid streaks in the retina are common.

**p.s.i.** *pounds per square inch.*

**psilocin** (sī′lō-sĭn) A hallucinogen similar to psilocybin.

**psilocybin** (sī″lō-sī′bĭn) A hallucinogen obtained from a particular mushroom.

**psi phenomena** Occurrences, events, or actions that have no logical explanation (e.g., extrasensory perception, clairvoyance, precognition, psychokinesis, and telepathy).

**psittacosis** (sĭt-ă-kō′sĭs) [Gr. *psittakos,* parrot, + *osis,* condition] An infectious disease, caused by *Chlamydia psittaci,* of parrots and other birds that may be transmitted to humans. Symptoms may include headache, epistaxis, chill followed by fever, constipation, anorexia, myalgia, sore throat, nausea, vomiting, and sometimes pneumonia. Tetracyclines, erythromycin, or penicillin are effective in treatment. SYN: *ornithosis; parrot fever.* SEE: *Chlamydia.*

**psoas** (sō′ăs) [Gr. *psoa*] One of two muscles

of the loins. SEE: *Muscles Appendix*.

**psoitis** (sō-ī′tĭs) [Gr. *psoa*, muscle of the loin, + *itis*, inflammation] Inflammation of the psoas muscles or of the area of the loins.

**psomophagia** (sō″mō-fā′jē-ă) [Gr. *psomos*, morsel, + *phagein*, to eat] The habit of swallowing food without thoroughly chewing it. SEE: *fletcherism*.

**psoralen** One of a group of substances derived from plants, some of which can cause a phototoxic dermatitis when applied to the skin and exposed to sunlight or artificial ultraviolet wavelengths. Methoxsalen is a psoralen, and trioxsalen is a synthetic psoralen. SEE: *psoriasis; PUVA therapy; vitiligo*.

**psorelcosis** (sō″rĕl-kō′sĭs) [″ + *helkosis*, ulceration] Ulceration occurring as a result of scabies.

**psoriasis** (sō-rī′ă-sĭs) [Gr., an itching] A common, chronic disease of the skin consisting of erythematous papules that coalesce to form plaques with distinct borders. If the disease progresses and is untreated, a silvery, yellow-white scale develops. New lesions tend to appear at sites of trauma. They may be in any location but frequently are located on the scalp, knees, elbows, umbilicus, and genitalia. SEE: illus.

The clinical course is variable but fewer than one half of the patients followed for a prolonged period will have prolonged remissions. Severity may range from a minimal cosmetic problem to a life-threatening emergency. In about 5% of psoriasis patients, arthritis will develop, and in most of these, joint involvement will occur after the onset of the skin lesions. The course of the arthritis is usually mild, affecting only a few joints, and spontaneous remissions occur. Most of the skin changes, with the exception of inflammation, may be explained by the rapid turnover of the epidermis. Normal skin produces about 1250 cells a day for each square centimeter, and these come from 27,000 cells; psoriatic skin produces 35,000 new cells each day for each square centimeter, and these come from 52,000 cells. The normal duration of the cell cycle of skin is 311 hr, but is reduced to 36 hr for psoriatic skin. SEE: *Nursing Diagnoses Appendix*.

ETIOLOGY: The cause of psoriasis is unknown, but a genetic factor is present. Certain conditions (e.g., infection, some drugs, climate, and perhaps hormonal factors and smoking) may trigger attacks.

TREATMENT: Therapy includes general care, including explanation of what is known about the course and treatment of the disease, and reassurance. Topical glucocorticoids are used with a keratolytic agent such as salicylic acid, which removes surface scales and enhances penetration of the glucocorticoid. Calcipotriene ointment is available for treating psoriasis. It inhibits proliferation of keratinocytes. Long-wave ultraviolet light (330 to 360 nm) combined with topical psoralens has been effective. For severe,

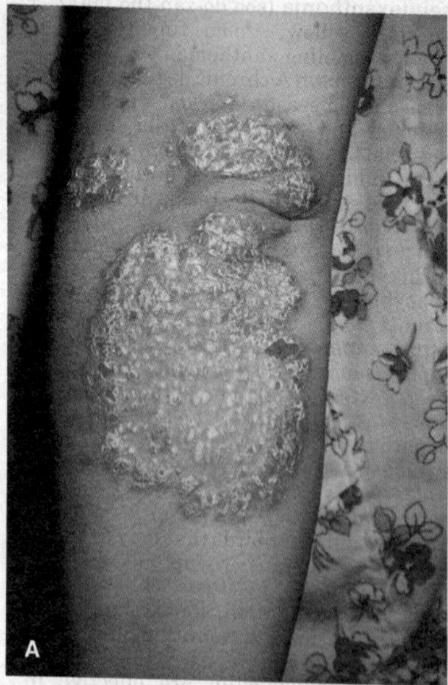


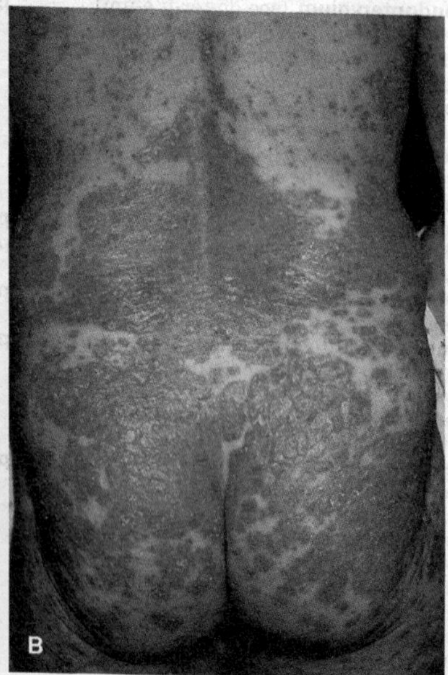


**PSORIASIS**

**(A)** TYPICAL SCALY PLAQUE AT ELBOW, **(B)** EXTENSIVE PSORIASIS ON TRUNK life-threatening cases that have failed to respond to other treatment, the systemic drugs methotrexate or etretinate are effective; however, etretinate is a potent teratogen with a long half-life, so it should not be used by women of childbearing age.

Caution: The use of ultraviolet light is contraindicated in patients with a history of cancer of the skin. All male psoriasis patients treated with ultraviolet light should be protected in the genital area from the ultraviolet light. The use of methotrexate requires that the patient be carefully monitored for renal, hematological, or hepatic changes.

NURSING IMPLICATIONS: The nurse teaches the patient about the prescribed therapy, to soften and remove scales, to relieve pruritus, to reduce pain and discomfort, to retard rapid cell proliferation, and to help induce remission and monitors for adverse reactions. Assistance is provided to help the patient gain confidence in managing these largely palliative treatments, many of which require special instructions for application and removal. The patient should protect against and minimize trauma. The patient's ability to manage therapies and their results are evaluated. The patient learns to identify stressors that exacerbate the condition, such as cold weather, emotional stress, infection, and to avoid and reduce these as much as possible. If the patient smokes cigarettes, participation in a smoking cessation program is recommended. The nurse helps the young patient (aged 20 to 30) to deal with body image changes and effects on self-esteem, encourages the patient to verbalize feelings, and supports the patient through loss of body image and associated grief. Referral for psychological counseling or cosmetic concealment therapy may be necessary.

***p. annularis*** Circular or ringlike lesions of psoriasis.

***p. arthropica*** Psoriasis associated with arthritis. SYN: *psoriatic arthropathy.*

***p. buccalis*** Leukoplakia of the oral mucosa.

***elephantine p.*** A rare but persistent psoriasis that occurs on the back, thighs, and hips in thick scaling plaques.

***guttate p.*** Psoriasis characterized by small distinct lesions that generally occur over the body. The lesions appear particularly in the young after acute streptococcal infections. SEE: illus.

***nummular p.*** The most common form of psoriasis with discs and plaques of varying sizes on the extremities and trunk. There may be a great number of lesions or a solitary lesion.

***pustular p.*** Psoriasis in which small sterile pustules form, dry up, and then

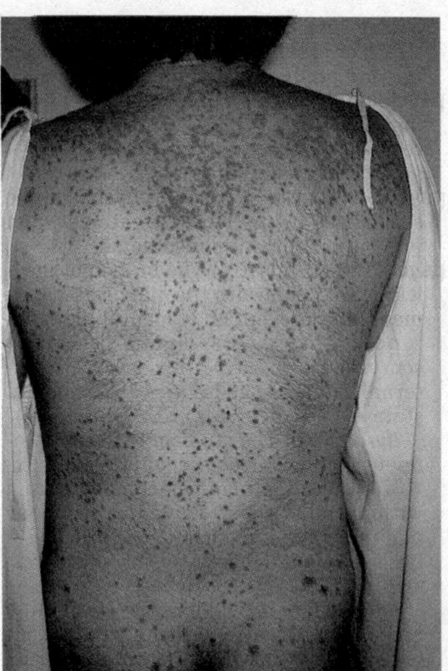

GUTTATE PSORIASIS

form a scab.

***rupioid p.*** Psoriasis with hyperkeratotic lesions on the feet.

***p. universalis*** Severe generalized psoriasis.

**psorophthalmia** (sō″rŏf-thăl′mē-ă) [Gr.] Marginal inflammation of the eyelids with ulceration.

**psorous** (sō′rŭs) [Gr. *psoros*] Relating to, or affected with, itch.

**P.S.P.** *phenolsulfonphthalein;* a substance used to test kidney function.

**PSRO** *Professional Standards Review Organization.*

**PSV** *pressure support ventilation.*

**PSVT** *paroxysmal supraventricular tachycardia.*

**psych-, psycho-** Combining form meaning *mind, mental processes.*

**psychalgia** (sī-kăl′jē-ă) [″ + *algos,* pain] **1.** Pain of hysterical origin. **2.** Mental distress marked by auditory and visual hallucinations, often associated with melancholia.

**psychataxia** (sī″kă-tăk′sē-ă) [″ + *ataxia,* lack of order] Disordered power of concentration.

**psychauditory** (sīk-aw′dĭ-tor-ē) [″+ L. *auditorius,* hearing] Pert. to the perception and interpretation of sounds.

**psyche** (sī′kē) [Gr. *psyche,* soul, mind] All that constitutes the mind and its processes.

**psychedelic** (sī″kĕ-dĕl′ĭk) [″ + *delos,* manifest] Originally used in 1963 to mean mind-manifesting and now used by lay persons to describe some of the subjective aspects of intoxication, particularly with a drug such as lysergic acid diethylamide (LSD) or other drugs that are mind-altering and produce visual hallucinations.

**psychiatric** (sī-kē-ă′trĭk) [″ + *iatrikos,* healing] Pert. to psychiatry, the science concerned with the study, diagnosis, and prevention of mental illness.

**psychiatrist** (sī-kī′ă-trĭst) A physician who specializes in the study, treatment, and prevention of mental disorders.

**psychiatry** (sī-kī′ă-trē) The branch of medicine that deals with the diagnosis, treatment, and prevention of mental illness.

***descriptive p.*** A system of psychiatry concerned with the readily observable external factors that influence the mental state of an individual. SEE: *dynamic p.*

***dynamic p.*** The study of the origin, influence, and control of emotions. This involves investigating the factors both from within and without that alter emotions and motivation. Such analysis provides a basis for judging regression or progression.

***emergency p.*** The emergency therapy and intervention in patients who are suicidal, homicidal, or perpetrators or victims of child abuse, spouse abuse, or incest. Most of these individuals see a physician within hours or days of their violent or abusive act. Many physician training programs fail to prepare a student for managing patients who need this emergency service.

***forensic p.*** The use of psychiatry in legal matters, esp. in determining social adaptability of an individual suspected of insanity; or the presence or absence of insanity, esp. at the time the individual committed a crime.

***orthomolecular p.*** The concept that mental illness is due to biochemical abnormalities resulting in increased requirements for specific substances, such as vitamins and minerals.

**psychic** (sī′kĭk) [Gr. *psychikos*] **1.** Concerning the mind or psyche. **2.** An individual said to be endowed with semisupernatural powers, such as the ability to read the minds of others or to foresee coming events; one apparently sensitive to nonphysical forces.

***p. determinism*** The theory that mental processes are determined by conscious or unconscious motives and are never irrelevant.

***p. force*** Force generated apart from physical energy.

**psychoactive** (sī″kō-ăk′tĭv) [″ + L. *actio,* action] Affecting the mental state, such as a drug that has that action.

**psychoanaleptic** (sī″kō-ăn″ă-lĕp′tĭk) [″ + *analepsis,* a taking up] Having a stimulating effect on the mind.

**psychoanalysis** (sī″kō-ă-năl′ĭ-sĭs) [″ + *analysis,* a dissolving] A method of obtaining a detailed account of past and present mental and emotional experiences and repressions in order to determine the source and to eliminate or diminish the undesirable effects of unconscious conflicts by making patients aware of their existence, origin, and inappropriate expression in emotions and behavior. It is largely a system created by Sigmund Freud that was originally the outgrowth of his observations of neurotics. Frequently the term is used synonymously with freudianism, but more commonly it is used for a more extensive system of psychological fact and theory applying both to normal and abnormal groups.

Psychoanalysis is based on the theory that abnormal phenomena are caused by repression of painful or undesirable past experiences that, although totally forgotten, later manifest themselves in various abnormal ways. Psychoanalysis includes a study of the ego in relationship to reality and the conflicting goals so created. This conflict is solved by repressing one component. This repressed or censored emotion-laden complex of ideas exists in the subconscious, manifesting itself in the hidden content of dreams, neuroses, and tension states. Angry outbursts, rationalization of unfair attitudes, or slips of the tongue occur because the patient is unaware of the influence of the subconscious.

Repressed material is largely sexual, and the peculiar conditioning of the patient is determined chiefly by emotional experiences of earlier years. Reactions of inferiority may result in a compensatory reaction of goodness or ambition. Sublimation is the escape of creative interest on levels not socially taboo. Therefore, psychoanalysis makes an effort to bring forgotten memories into the conscious mind. The patient thus is enabled to view the occurrence in its true perspective and to minimize its harm.

In addition to the freudian method, other schools of thought used in psychoanalysis include analytical psychology (Jung), psychobiology (Meyer), and individual psychology (Adler).

**psychoanalyst** (sī″kō-ăn′ă-lĭst) [Gr. *psyche,* mind, + *analysis,* a dissolving] One who practices psychoanalysis.

**psychobiology** (sī″kō-bī-ŏl′ō-jē) [″ + *bios,* life, + *logos,* word, reason] **1.** The study of the biology of the psyche, including the anatomy, physiology, and pathology of the mind. SYN: *biopsychology.* **2.** A method of psychoanalysis employing distributive analysis, which includes a study of all mental and physical factors involved in an individual's growth and development.

***objective p.*** Psychobiology in which special emphasis is placed on the relationship of the individual to his or her environment.

**psychocatharsis** (sī″kō-kă-thăr′sĭs) [″ + *katharsis,* purification] The bringing of so-called traumatic experiences and their affective associations into consciousness by interview, hypnosis, or use of drugs such as sodium amytal. SEE: *catharsis*.

**psychochrome** (sī′kō-krōm) [″ + *chroma*, color] Color impression resulting from sensory stimulation of a part other than the visual organ.

**psychochromesthesia** (sī″kō-krōm″ĕs-thē′zē-ă) [″ + ″ + *aisthesis*, sensation] Color sensation produced by the stimulus of a sense organ other than that of vision. SEE: *pseudochromesthesia*.

**psychocoma** (sī″kō-kō′mă) [″ + *koma*, a deep sleep] The condition of mental stupor.

**psychocortical** (sī″kō-kor′tĭ-kăl) [″ + L. *cortex*, rind] Pert. to the cerebral cortex as the seat of sensory, motor, and psychic functions.

**psychodiagnosis** (sī″kō-dī″ăg-nō′sĭs) [″ + *diagignoskein*, to discern] The use of psychological tests to assist in diagnosing diseases, esp. mental illness.

**psychodiagnostics** (sī″kō-dī″ăg-nŏs′tĭks) The use of psychological testing as an aid in diagnosing mental disorders.

**Psychodidae** (sī″kŏd′ĭ-dē) A family of the order Diptera, characterized by minute size, long legs, and hairy bodies and wings. It includes moth flies, owl midges, and sandflies. SEE: *Phlebotomus*.

**psychodrama** (sī″kō-drăm′ă) [″ + L. *drama*, drama] A form of group psychotherapy. Patients act out assigned roles and, in so doing, are able to gain insight into their own mental disturbances.

**psychodynamics** (sī″kō-dī-năm′ĭks) [″ + *dynamis*, power] The scientific study of mental action or force.

**psychogalvanometer** (sī″kō-găl″vă-nŏm′ĕ-tĕr) [″ + *galvanism* + Gr. *metron*, measure] A device for determining the changes in the electrical resistance of the skin in response to emotional stimuli.

**psychogenesis** (sī″kō-jĕn′ĕ-sĭs) [″ + *genesis*, generation, birth] **1.** The origin and development of mind; the formation of mental traits. **2.** Origin within the mind or psyche.

**psychogenetic** (sī″kō-jĕn-ĕt′ĭk) **1.** Originating in the mind, as a disease. **2.** Concerning formation of mental traits.

**psychogenic** (sī-kō-jĕn′ĭk) [″ + *gennan*, to produce] **1.** Of mental origin. **2.** Concerning the development of the mind. SYN: *psychogenetic*.

**psychogeriatric** Concerning elderly patients who have a psychiatric disorder.

**psychogeusic** (sī″kō-gū′sĭk) [″ + *geusis*, taste] Pert. to perception of taste.

**psychograph** (sī′kō-grăf) [″ + *graphein*, to write] **1.** A chart that lists personality traits. **2.** A history of the personality of an individual.

**psychokinesis** (sī″kō-kĭ-nē′sĭs) [″ + *kinesis*, movement] **1.** Explosive or impulsive maniacal action caused by defective inhibition. **2.** In parapsychology, claimed or alleged influence exerted on a physical object by a subject without any intermediate physical energy or instrumentation. SEE: *paranormal; psi phenomena*.

**psycholagny** (sī″kō-lăg′nē) [″ + *lagneia*, lust] Sexual excitation brought about by mental imagery; psychic or mental masturbation.

**psycholinguistics** (sī″kō-lĭng-gwĭs′tĭks) The study of linguistics as it relates to human behavior.

**psychological** (sī″kō-lŏj′ĭ-kăl) [″ + *logos*, word, reason] Pert. to the study of the mind in all of its relationships, normal and abnormal.

**psychologist** (sī-kŏl′ō-jĭst) One who is trained in methods of psychological analysis, therapy, and research.

**psychology** (sī-kŏl′ō-jē) [″ + *logos*, word, reason] The science dealing with mental processes, both normal and abnormal, and their effects upon behavior. There are two main approaches to the study: introspective, looking inward or self-examination of one's own mental processes; and objective studying of the minds of others. SEE: words beginning with *psych-*.

***abnormal p.*** The study of deviant behavior and the associated mental phenomena.

***analytic p.*** Psychoanalysis based on the concepts of Carl Jung, de-emphasizing sexual factors in motivation and emphasizing the "collective unconscious" and "psychological types" (introvert and extrovert).

***animal p.*** The study of animal behavior.

***applied p.*** The application of the principles of psychology to special fields, such as clinical, industrial, educational, nursing, or pastoral applications.

***clinical p.*** The branch of psychology concerned with diagnosing and treating mental disorders.

***criminal p.*** The branch of psychology concerned with the behavior and therapy of criminals.

***dynamic p.*** Psychology of motivation; that which seeks the causes of mental phenomena.

***experimental p.*** The study of mental acts by tests and experiments.

***genetic p.*** The branch of psychology concerned with the evolution of and inheritance of psychological characteristics.

***gestalt p.*** Psychology that emphasizes the wholeness of psychological processes and behavior, maintaining that such cannot be adequately explained by breaking down into constituent parts.

***individual p.*** A system of psychological thinking developed by Alfred Adler in which an individual is regarded as having three life goals: physical security, sexual satisfaction, and social integration. Self-evaluations lead to feelings of inferiority and inadequacy, which often lead to overcompensation or a striving for superiority.

***physiological p.*** Psychology that deals with the structure and function of the nervous system and other bodily organs and their relationship to behavior.

*social p.* The branch of psychology concerned with the study of groups and their influence on the individual's actions and mental processes.

**psychometrician** (sī″kō-mĕ-trĭsh′ăn) [Gr. *psyche,* mind, + *metron,* measure] **1.** A person skilled in psychometry. **2.** A person skilled in the application of statistical analysis to psychological data.

**psychometry** (sī-kŏm′ĕ-trē) [″ + *metron,* measure] The measurement of psychological variables, such as intelligence, aptitude, behavior, and emotional reactions.

**psychomotor** (sī″kō-mō′tor) [″ + L. *motor,* a mover] Concerning or causing physical activity associated with mental processes.

**psychomotor and physical development of infant** The physical growth of an infant and the effect of mental activity on motor skills. It is important that all concerned with the care of the newborn through infancy have guidelines for comparing the growth and development of an individual with normal standards. Certain activities of infants serve as general indicators of normal psychomotor development. The average ages for certain of these activities are shown in the accompanying table. SEE: table; *arousal level.*

**Psychomotor and Physical Development: Birth to 1 Year**

| ***Physical Development*** | | | | | |
|---|---|---|---|---|---|
| | | **Length Range** | | **Weight Range** | |
| | | **In.** | **Cm** | **Lb** | **Kg** |
| Birth | boys | 18¼–21½ | 46.4–54.4 | 5½–9¼ | 2.54–4.15 |
| | girls | 17¾–20¾ | 45.4–52.9 | 5¼–8½ | 2.36–3.81 |
| 1 Month | boys | 19¾–23 | 50.4–58.6 | 7–11¾ | 3.16–5.38 |
| | girls | 19¼–22½ | 49.2–56.9 | 6½–10¾ | 2.97–4.92 |
| 3 Months | boys | 22¼–25¾ | 56.7–65.4 | 9¾–16¼ | 4.43–7.37 |
| | girls | 21¾–25 | 55.4–63.4 | 9¼–14¾ | 4.18–6.74 |
| 6 Months | boys | 25–28½ | 63.4–72.3 | 13¾–20¾ | 6.20–9.46 |
| | girls | 24¼–27¾ | 61.8–70.2 | 12¾–19¼ | 5.79–8.73 |
| 9 Months | boys | 26¾–30¼ | 68.0–77.1 | 16½–24 | 7.52–10.93 |
| | girls | 26–29½ | 66.1–75.0 | 15½–22½ | 7.0–10.17 |
| 12 Months | boys | 28¼–32 | 71.7–81.2 | 18½–26½ | 8.43–11.99 |
| | girls | 27½–31¼ | 69.8–79.1 | 17¼–24¾ | 7.84–11.24 |

| ***Psychomotor Development*** | |
|---|---|
| Birth through 1st Month | Ability to suck, swallow, gag, cry, and maintain eye contact with a person. Head needs to be supported. Loud noises may cause a startle reflex. |
| 2nd Month | May turn to either side when on their backs; will follow moving objects; able to lift head but not for a sustained period; begin to smile, frown, and turn away. |
| 3rd Month | Greater movement and vocal response to stimuli; notice own hands and suck on them; head steady while supported. |
| 4th and 5th Months | Able to lift head higher when lying on stomach; will reach for objects and may be able to encircle a bottle with both hands; may drool a lot; attempt to put all kinds of objects in mouth. |
| 6th–9th Month | Develop ability to grasp and pick up food; are able to pull up to a sitting position and eventually will crawl; begin to make noises that sound like words and to recognize certain words; will play peek-a-boo. |
| 9th–11th Month | Develop ability to handle food and to drink from a cup; may imitate sounds and say certain words; crawl by pulling body along with arms, and pull themselves to a standing position; they will point at objects and throw things; they want to feed themselves and to help with dressing and undressing; they will walk while holding a person's hand. |
| 12th Month | Can eat food alone and drink from a cup with assistance; able to move around easily and crawl up stairs and out of crib. |

*Appearance and loss of certain reflexes and reactions:* The Moro reflex is present at birth and disappears by 3 months; the stepping and placing reflexes are present at birth and are no longer obtainable by 6 weeks; the tonic neck reflex is usually present at 2 months and is gone by 6 months; neck righting appears at 4 to 6 months and is gone by 24 months; the parachute reaction is present at 9 months and persists; sucking and rooting are present at birth and are usually gone by 4 months if tested while awake and by 7 months if tested while the infant is asleep; palmar grasp is present from birth to 6 months; plantar grasp is present from birth to 10 months.

**psychomotor epilepsy** Temporal lobe epilepsy.

**psychomotor retardation** A generalized slowing of physical and mental reactions; seen frequently in depression.

**psychoneuroimmunology** The study of the relationships that exist among the central nervous system, autonomic nervous system, endocrine system, and immune system. Social scientists use the data gathered from studies as they examine the impact of psychosocial stressors and the psychophysiological stress response on the development of disease.

**psychoneurosis** (sī″kō-nū-rō′sĭs) [″ + *neuron,* sinew, + *osis,* condition] Emotional maladaptation due to unresolved unconscious conflicts. This leads to disturbances in thought, feelings, attitudes, and behavior. There is little, if any, loss of contact with reality, but the patient's effectiveness in performing his or her usual responsibilities is handicapped. Psychoneurosis is a major category in mental illness and is classified according to the symptoms that predominate. The patient usually recognizes that the altered thoughts and feelings are abnormal and indeed unwelcome. This is in contrast to the patient with a psychosis or character disorder. SYN: *neurosis.*

***anxiety reaction p.*** Anxiety with apprehension out of proportion to any obvious external cause. SEE: *neurosis, anxiety.*

***conversion reaction p.*** Psychoneurosis in which unacceptable unconscious impulses are converted into hysterical somatic symptoms. Although the symptoms have a specific symbolic meaning to the patient, their interpretation is different in each individual.

***depressive reaction p.*** Psychoneurosis marked by depression out of proportion to any obvious cause.

***dissociated reaction p.*** Psychoneurosis characterized by dissociated behavior such as amnesia, fugue, sleepwalking, and dream states. It is important to differentiate this from schizophrenia.

***obsessive-compulsive reaction p.*** Psychoneurosis consisting of persistent, repetitive impulses to perform certain acts or rituals, such as handwashing, touching something, or counting. SEE: *obsessive-compulsive disorder.*

***phobic reaction p.*** Irrational fear of any of a variety of situations, persons, or objects.

**psychoneurotic** (sī″kō-nū-rŏt′ĭk) [Gr. *psyche,* mind, + *neuron,* sinew] **1.** Pert. to a functional disorder of mental origin. **2.** A person suffering from a psychoneurosis.

**psychopath** (sī′kō-păth) [″ + *pathos,* disease, suffering] An individual with a psychopathic personality. SEE: *personality, psychopathic.*

**psychopathic** (sī″kō-păth′ĭk) **1.** Concerning or characterized by a mental disorder. **2.** Concerning the treatment of mental disorders. **3.** Abnormal.

**psychopathology** (sī″kō-păth-ŏl′ō-jē) [″ + *pathos,* disease, suffering + *logos,* word, reason] The study of the causes and nature of mental disease or abnormal behavior.

**psychopathy** (sī-kŏp′ă-thē) Any mental disease, esp. one associated with defective character or personality. SEE: *personality, psychopathic.*

**psychopharmacology** (sī″kō-făr″mă-kŏl′ō-jē) The science of drugs having an effect on psychomotor behavior and emotional states.

**psychophysical** (sī″kō-fĭz′ĭ-kăl) [″ + *physikos,* natural] Concerning the relationship of the physical and the mental. SEE: *childbirth, natural; psychoprophylactic childbirth.*

**psychophysics** (sī″kō-fĭz′ĭks) **1.** The study of mental processes in relationship to physical processes. **2.** The study of stimuli in relationship to the effects they produce.

**psychophysiological** (sī″kō-fĭz-ē-ō-lŏj′ĭ-kăl) Pert. to psychophysiology.

**psychophysiological disorder** One of a large number of disorders of the organs and viscera innervated by the autonomic nervous system in which emotional factors are a primary contributing factor. It was formerly called psychosomatic disease or disorder.

**psychophysiology** (sī″kō-fĭz″ē-ŏl′ō-jē) Physiology of the mind; science of the correlation of body and mind.

**psychoplegic** (sī″kō-plē′jĭk) [″ + *plege,* a stroke] An agent reducing excitability of the mental processes.

**psychoprophylactic preparation for childbirth** Mental and physical training of the mother in preparation for delivery. The goals of the preparation are the dispelling of the fear of pain and the delivery of a healthy child. SEE: *childbirth, natural; childbirth, prepared; Lamaze technique or method.*

**psychoprophylaxis** (sī″kō-prō″fĭ-lăk′sĭs) In obstetrics, a method of mental and physical preparation for natural childbirth. SEE: *childbirth, natural; Lamaze technique or method.*

**psychosensory** (sī″kō-sĕn′sō-rē) [″ + L. *sen-*

*sorius,* organ of sensation] **1.** Understanding and interpreting sensory stimuli. **2.** Concerning perceptions not arising in sensory organs, as hallucinations.

**psychosexual** (sī″kō-sĕks′ū-ăl) [Gr. *psyche,* soul, mind, + L. *sexus,* sex] Concerning the emotional components of sexual instinct.

**psychosexual development** Evolution of personality through infantile and pregenital periods to sexual maturity.

**psychosexual disorder** A disorder of sexual function not due to organic causes. Included are gender identity disorders, transsexualism, paraphilias, transvestism, zoophilia, pedophilia, exhibitionism, voyeurism, and sexual sadism.

**psychosis** (sī-kō′sĭs) *pl.* **psychoses** [″ + *osis,* condition] A term formerly applied to any mental disorder but now generally restricted to those disturbances of such magnitude that there is personality disintegration and loss of contact with reality. The disturbances are of psychogenic origin or are without clearly defined physical cause or structural change in the brain. They usually are characterized by delusions and hallucination, and hospitalization generally is required.

This condition is manifest in the behavior, emotional reaction, and ideation of the patient, who fails to mirror reality as it is, reacts erroneously to it, and builds up false concepts regarding it. Behavior responses are peculiar, abnormal, inefficient, or definitely antisocial.

All this does not include amentia because defective intelligence merely lessens comprehension of reality but does not distort it.

***alcoholic p.*** Psychosis resulting from chronic alcoholism. SEE: *delirium tremens; Korsakoff's syndrome.*

***depressive p.*** Psychosis characterized by extreme depression, melancholia, and feelings of unworthiness.

***drug p.*** Psychosis caused by ingestion of a drug.

***exhaustion p.*** An acute state of confusion and delirium that occurs in relation to extreme fatigue, chronic illness, prolonged sleeplessness, or tension.

***functional p.*** Psychosis that is not due to an organic disease.

***gestational p.*** Psychosis that occurs during pregnancy.

***involutional p.*** Psychosis occurring during involutional period of bodily and intellectual decline.

***manic-depressive p.*** Ordinarily a series of periods of psychotic depression or excessive well-being, appearing in any sequence and alternating with longer periods of relative normalcy. Though intensity may vary greatly, the manic shows an elated though unstable mood, a flight of ideas, and great physical activity. In primary depression, the victim finds all exertion exhausting; there is difficulty in thinking or acting, and the victim is very unhappy. SYN: *bipolar affective disorder.*

***organic p.*** Psychosis induced by structural brain changes. A character change is generally manifested in behavior and disposition. Emotional instability, irritability, and angry outbursts become frequent. Attention fluctuates widely and gradually the patient deteriorates. At any time in the course of the disease, memory, comprehension, ideation, and orientation may become defective. Possible causes include alcohol, narcotics, trauma, syphilis, drugs, poisons, chronic infections, encephalitis, and brain tumors, among many others.

***polyneuritic p.*** Korsakoff's syndrome.

***postinfectious p.*** A psychosis following an infectious disease such as meningitis, pneumonia, or typhoid fever.

***postpartum p.*** A psychosis that develops during the 6 mo following childbirth, the highest incidence being in the third to sixth day after delivery through the first month postpartum. The symptoms and signs include hallucinations, delusions, preoccupation with death, self-multilation, infanticide, distorted reality, extreme dependency, and a demanding attitude. This psychosis may become a chronic condition, but for most women it is an isolated event in their lives. SYN: *puerperal p.*

***puerperal p.*** Postpartum p.

***senile p.*** Psychosis in which onset occurs in an aged individual.

***situational p.*** Psychosis due to excessive stress in an unbearable environmental situation.

***toxic p.*** Psychosis resulting from toxic agents.

***traumatic p.*** Psychosis resulting from head injuries and belonging to the organic group.

**psychosocial** (sī″kō-sō′shăl) Related to both psychological and social factors.

**psychosomatic** (sī″kō-sō-măt′ĭk) [Gr. *psyche,* mind, + *soma,* body] Pertaining to the relationship of the mind and body; pert. to disorders that have a physiological component but are thought to originate in the emotional state of the patient. When so used, the impression is created that the mind and body are separate entities and that a disease may be purely somatic in its effect or entirely emotional. This partitioning of the human being is not possible; thus no disease is limited to only the mind or the body. A complex interaction is always present even though in specific instances a disease might on superficial examination appear to involve only the body or the mind. SEE: *psychophysiological disorders.*

**psychosurgery** (sī″kō-sur′jĕr-ē) [″ + L. *chirurgia,* surgery] Surgical intervention for mental disorders, esp. for certain types of violent or antisocial behavior.

**psychotechnics** (sī″kō-tĕk′nĭks) [″ + *techne,*

art] The use of psychological methods in the study of economic and social problems.

**psychotherapeutic drug** A drug that is used because of its effects in ameliorating the principal symptoms that occur in mentally disturbed persons, such as anxiety, depression, and psychosis.

**psychotherapy** (sī-kō-thĕr′ă-pē) [Gr. *psyche,* mind, + *therapeia,* treatment] A method of treating disease, esp. nervous disorders, by mental rather than physical means (e.g., suggestion, re-education, hypnotism, and psychoanalysis).

**psychotic** (sī-kŏt′ĭk) Pert. to or affected by psychosis.

**psychotogenic** (sī-kŏt″ō-jĕn′ĭk) [″ + *gennan,* to produce] Producing a psychosis, usually temporary and due to certain powerful drugs.

**psychotomimetic** (sī-kŏt″ō-mī-mĕ′tĭk) [″ + *mimetikos,* imitative] Relating to or producing a state resembling psychosis.

**psychotropic drug** [″ + *trope,* a turning] A drug that affects psychic function, behavior, or experience. Many drugs can be classed as being intentionally psychotropic, but many other drugs also occasionally may produce undesired psychotropic side effects.

**psychro-** Combining form meaning *cold.* SEE: also *cryo-.*

**psychroalgia** (sī″krō-ăl′jē-ă) [Gr. *psychros,* cold, + *algos,* pain] A painful sensation of cold.

**psychroesthesia** (sī″krō-ĕs-thē′zē-ă) [″ + *aisthesis,* sensation] A sensation of cold in a part of the body, even though it is warm.

**psychrometer** (sī-krŏm′ĕ-tĕr) [″ + *metron,* measure] A device for measuring relative humidity of the atmosphere. Calculations are made using the readings of two thermometers, one with a dry bulb and one with a wet bulb.

**psychrophilic** (sī-krō-fĭl′ĭk) [″ + *philein,* to love] Preferring cold, as bacteria that thrive at low temperatures, between 0° and 30°C (32° and 86°F).

**psychrophobia** (sī-krō-fō′bē-ă) [″ + *phobos,* fear] Abnormal aversion or sensitiveness to cold.

**psychrophore** (sī′krō-for) [″ + *phorein,* to carry] A double-lumen catheter for applying cold to the urethra or any canal.

**psychrotherapy** (sī″krō-thĕr′ă-pē) [″ + *therapeia,* treatment] The treatment of disease by the use of cold.

**psyllium seed** (sĭl′ē-ŭm) The dried ripe seed of the psyllium plant, grown in France, Spain, and India; used as a mild laxative. It is also used in symptomatic treatment of diarrhea. It enhances stool consistency by absorbing water from the bowel contents.

**PT** *prothrombin time; physical therapist.*

**Pt** Symbol for the element platinum.

**pt** *pint.*

**PTA** *plasma thromboplastin antecedent; physical therapy assistant.*

**ptarmic** (tăr′mĭk) [Gr. *ptarmikos,* causing to sneeze] **1.** Causing sneezing. **2.** An agent that causes sneezing. SYN: *sternutatory.*

**ptarmus** (tar′mŭs) Spasmodic sneezing.

**PTC** *percutaneous transhepatic cholangiography; phenylthiocarbamide; plasma thromboplastin component.*

**PTCA** *percutaneous transluminal coronary angioplasty.*

**pterion** (tē′rē-ŏn) [Gr. *pteron,* wing] Point of suture of frontal, parietal, temporal, and sphenoid bones.

**pternalgia** (tĕr-năl′jē-ă) [Gr. *pterna,* heel, + *algos,* pain] Pain in the heel.

**pterygium** (tĕr-ĭj′ē-ŭm) [Gr. *pterygion,* wing] Triangular thickening of the bulbar conjunctiva extending from the inner canthus to the border of the cornea with the apex toward the pupil.

***p. colli*** A congenital band of fascia extending from the mastoid process of the temporal bone to the clavicle.

***progressive p.*** A stage in which the growth extends toward the center of the cornea.

**pterygoid** (tĕr′ĭ-goyd) [Gr. *pterygoeides*] Wing-shaped. SYN: *alate.*

***p. hamulus*** A small bony projection, just medial to the pterygoid process, that serves as an attachment for the tensor veli palatini muscle.

**pterygomandibular** (tĕr″ĭ-gō-măn-dĭb′ū-lăr) [″ + L. *mandibula,* lower jawbone] Concerning the pterygoid process of the sphenoid bone and mandible.

**pterygomaxillary** (tĕr″ĭ-gō-măk′sĭ-lĕr″ē) [″ + L. *maxillaris,* upper jaw] Concerning the pterygoid process and upper jaw.

**pterygopalatine** (tĕr″ĭ-gō-păl′ă-tĭn) [″+ L. *palatinus,* palate] Relating to the pterygoid process and the palate bone.

**PTFE** *polytetrafluoroethylene* (Teflon).

**PTH** *parathyroid hormone.*

**ptilosis** (tī-lō′sĭs) [Gr.] Loss of eyelashes.

**ptomaine** (tō′mān, tō-mān′) [Gr. *ptoma,* dead body] One of a class of nitrogenous organic bases formed in the action of putrefactive bacteria on proteins and amino acids.

**ptosed** (tōst) Having ptosis.

**ptosis** (tō′sĭs) [Gr. *ptosis,* a dropping] Dropping or drooping of an organ or part, as the upper eyelid from paralysis, or the visceral organs from weakness of the abdominal muscles. **ptotic** (tŏt′ĭk), *adj.*

***abdominal p.*** Sagging of the transverse colon, sometimes almost to the pelvic floor. This is caused by obesity or lack of abdominal muscle tone.

TREATMENT: A properly adjusted abdominal belt may help. This is contraindicated if the patient shows dependence on the belt instead of exercising and developing the abdominal muscles.

***morning p.*** Difficulty in raising the eyelids upon awakening.

***waking p.*** Morning p.

**PTT** *partial thromboplastin time.*

**ptyalagogue** (tī-ăl′ă-gŏg) [Gr. *ptyalon,* saliva, + *agogos,* leading] Causing, or something that causes, a flow of saliva. SYN: *sialogogue.*

**ptyalectasis** (tī″ă-lĕk′tă-sĭs) [″ + *ektasis,* dilation] Surgical dilation of a salivary duct.

**ptyalin** (tī′ă-lĭn) A salivary enzyme that hydrolyzes starch and glycogen to maltose and a small amount of glucose. The optimum pH for ptyalin activity is 6.9. SYN: *amylase, salivary.* SEE: *enzyme; ptyalism; saliva.*

**ptyalism** (tī′ă-lĭzm) [″ + *-ismos,* condition] Excessive secretion of saliva. This may be due to pregnancy, stomatitis, rabies, exophthalmic goiter, menstruation, epilepsy, hysteria, nervous conditions, and gastrointestinal disorders and may be induced by mercury, iodides, pilocarpine, and other drugs. SYN: *salivation.* SEE: *xerostomia.*

**ptyalith** (tī′ă-lĭth) [″ + *lithos,* stone] A calculus in a salivary gland.

**ptyalocele** (tī-ăl′ō-sēl) [″ + *kele,* tumor, swelling] A salivary cystic tumor or cystic dilatation of a salivary duct.

**ptyalogenic** (tī″ăl-ō-jĕn′ĭk) [Gr. *ptyalon,* saliva, + *gennan,* to produce] Of salivary origin.

**ptyalogogue** (tī″ăl′ō-gŏg) [″ + *agogos,* leading] An agent that causes the flow of saliva. SYN: *sialogogue.*

**ptyalography** (tī-ăl-ŏg′ră-fē) [″ + *graphein,* to write] SEE: *sialography.*

**ptyalolith** (tī′ă-lō-lĭth) [″ + *lithos,* stone] A salivary concretion.

**ptyalolithiasis** (tī″ă-lō-lĭ-thī′ă-sĭs) The presence of a concretion in a salivary gland or duct.

**ptyalolithotomy** (tī″ăl-ō-lĭ-thŏt′ō-mē) [Gr. *ptyalon,* saliva, + *lithos,* stone, + *tome,* incision] The surgical removal of a concretion from a salivary duct or gland.

**ptyaloreaction** (tī″ă-lō-rē-ăk′shŭn) A reaction occurring in saliva.

**ptyalorrhea** (tī″ă-lō-rē′ă) [″ + *rhoia,* flow] An excessive flow of saliva.

**ptyocrinous** (tī-ŏk′rĭ-nŭs) A type of glandular secretion in which the contents of the cell are discharged.

**ptysis** (tī′sĭs) [Gr.] Spitting; the ejection of saliva from the mouth.

**Pu** Symbol for the element plutonium.

**pubarche** (pū-băr′kē) [L. *puber,* grown up, + Gr. *arche,* beginning] **1.** The beginning of puberty. **2.** Beginning development of pubic hair. SEE: *semenarche; thelarche.*

**puber** (pū′bĕr) [L., grown up] One at the onset of puberty.

**puberal** (pū′bĕr-ăl) [L. *pubertas,* puberty] Pubertal.

**pubertal** Pert. to puberty.

**pubertas** (pū′bĕr-tăs) [L.] Puberty.

***p. praecox*** Precocious puberty or puberty at an early age.

**puberty** (pū′bĕr-tē) The stage in life at which members of both sexes become functionally capable of reproduction. A period of rapid change occurs between the ages of 13 and 15 in boys and 9 to 16 in girls, ending in the attainment of sexual maturity. There is evidence that the onset of puberty is related to a decrease in secretion of the pineal gland.

***onset of p.*** *Boys:* Between the ages of 13 and 15, a relatively rapid increase in height and weight occurs with broadening of the shoulders and increase in size of the penis and testicles. Pubic hair and the beard begin to grow. Endocrine and sebaceous gland activity is increased. Nocturnal emissions usually occur. Young boys should be assured that the size of the penis is not related to the degree of masculinity and is not an important factor in experiencing or providing sexual gratification.

*Girls:* Between the ages of 9 and 16, a marked increase in growth is accompanied by breast enlargement and appearance of pubic hair. Within 1 to 2 years after these changes, underarm hair grows and the normal whitish vaginal secretion (physiological leukorrhea) characteristic of the adult female is noticed. Several months later the first menstrual period (menarche) occurs. Each individual will vary somewhat from this schedule. The young girl should be told prior to puberty about menstruation and the technique of menstrual protection through use of perineal pads or tampons. In addition, she should be told that a certain amount of intermenstrual vaginal discharge (leukorrhea) is normal but if the secretion is malodorous or causes irritation of the vulva, a physician should be consulted. SEE: *menstruation.*

***precocious p.*** The appearance of secondary sex characteristics before 8 years of age in girls and 9 years of age in boys. The pituitary and hypothalamus glands may be involved, or the condition may result from premature secretion of sex hormones not caused by pituitary or hypothalamic action. Gonadotropin-releasing hormone (GnRH) has been used to treat this condition.

**pubes** (pū′bēz) *sing.* **pubis** [L., grown up] **1.** The anterior part of the innominate bone. SYN: *os pubis.* **2.** The pubic region. **3.** The pubic hair.

**pubescence** (pū-bĕs′ĕns) [L. *pubescens,* becoming hairy] **1.** Puberty or its approach. **2.** A covering of fine, soft hairs on the body. SYN: *lanugo.*

**pubescent** (pū-bĕs′ĕnt) **1.** Reaching puberty. **2.** Covered with downy hair.

**pubetrotomy** (pū″bĕ-trŏt′ō-mē) [NL. *(os) pubis,* bone of the groin, + Gr. *etron,* belly, + *tome,* incision] Section through the os pubis and lower abdominal wall.

**pubic** (pū′bĭk) [L. *pubes,* pubic hair] Concerning the pubes.

**pubic bone** The lower anterior part of the innominate bone. SYN: *os pubis.*

**pubic hair** Hair over the pubes, which appears at onset of sexual maturity. The distribution is somewhat different in men than in women.

**pubio-, pubo-** Combining form meaning *pubic bone, pubic region.*

**pubiotomy** (pū-bē-ŏt′ō-mē) [L. *pubes,* pubic region, + *tome,* incision] Incision across the pubis in order to enlarge the pelvic passage, facilitating the delivery of the fetus when the pelvis is malformed. SYN: *hebotomy.*

**pubis** (pū′bĭs) *pl.* **pubes** [NL. *(os) pubis,* bone of the groin] Pubic bone.

**public health** The discipline concerned with preventive measures intended to improve the health of an entire community. These programs include but are not limited to ones that protect communities from epidemics or toxic exposures, predict environmental disasters, and enforce the laws that provide a safe supply of water and food. Various government agencies such as the Centers for Disease Control and Prevention, Food and Drug Administration, and National Institute of Health are active in maintaining the public health, and there are an estimated 2800 local health departments, 62% of which employ a full or part-time physician. Each of the 50 states has a health department in which at least one physician is the public health official. SEE: *preventive medicine; preventive nursing.*

**Public Health Service Act** One of the principal laws of Congress giving the authority for federal health activities. First enacted July 1, 1944, it provided a complete codification of all the federal public health laws. Many of the health laws since 1944 have actually been amendments to the Public Health Service act that have revised, extended, or given new authority to the act.

**Public Law 94-142** ABBR: PL-142. A law enacted in the U.S. in 1975 stating that disabled children from 3 to 21 years of age are entitled to an appropriate, tax-supported education.

**pubococcygeal** (pū″bō-kŏk-sĭj′ē-ăl) [″ + Gr. *kokkyx,* coccyx] Concerning the pubis and coccyx.

**pubofemoral** (pū″bō-fĕm′or-ăl) [″ + *femur,* thigh bone] Pert. to the os pubis and femur.

**pubomadesis** [L. *pubes,* pubic hair, + Gr. *madesis,* baldness] Loss of or absent pubic hair.

**puboprostatic** (pū″bō-prŏs-tăt′ĭk) [″+ Gr. *prostates,* prostate] Relating to the os pubis and prostate gland.

**puborectal** (pū″bō-rĕk′tăl) [″ + *rectus,* straight] Concerning the pubis and rectum.

**pubovaginal device** An apparatus that is fitted for use in the vagina to help prevent urinary incontinence.

**pubovesical** (pū″bō-vĕs′ĭ-kl) [″ + *vesiculus,* a little sac] Pert. to the os pubis and bladder.

**pudenda** (pū-dĕn′dă) *sing.* **pudendum** [L.] Vulva.

**pudendagra** (pū″dĕn-dăg′ră) [″ + Gr. *agra,* seizure] Pain in the external genitals.

**pudendal** (pū-dĕn′dăl) [L. *pudenda,* external genitals] Relating to the external genitals of the female.

**pudendum** (pū-dĕn′dŭm) *pl.* **pudenda** [L.] Vulva.

***p. femininum*** Vulva.

***p. muliebre*** External genitals of the female.

**puerile** (pū′ĕ-rĭl) [L. *puerilis*] Concerning a child; childlike.

**puerilism** (pū′ĕr-ĭl-ĭzm) [″ + Gr. *-ismos,* condition] Childishness; second childhood.

**puerperal** (pū-ĕr′pĕr-ăl) [L. *puerperalis*] Concerning the puerperium.

**puerperal eclampsia** Convulsions and eclampsia during puerperium.

**puerperal fever** Septicemia following childbirth. SYN: *childbed fever; puerperal sepsis.*

**puerperalism** (pū-ĕr′pĕr-ăl-ĭzm) [L. *puer,* child, + *parere,* to bring forth, to bear, + Gr. *-ismos,* condition] A pathologic condition accompanying childbirth.

**puerperant** (pū-ĕr′pĕr-ănt) A woman in labor, or one who has recently given birth.

**puerperium** (pū″ĕr-pē′rē-ŭm) [L.] The period of 42 days following childbirth and expulsion of the placenta and membranes. The generative organs usually return to normal during this time.

**PUFA** *polyunsaturated fatty acids.* SEE: *acid, fatty.*

**puff** A soft, short, blowing sound heard on auscultation.

**Pulex** (pū′lĕks) [L., flea] A genus of fleas belonging to the order Siphonaptera.

***P. irritans*** The human flea, which also infests dogs, hogs, and other mammals. It may serve as an intermediate host of the tapeworms *Dipylidium caninum* and *Hymenolepis diminuta.* SEE: *flea.*

**pulicatio** (pū″lĭ-kā′tē-ō) Infested with fleas.

**Pulicidae** (pū-lĭs′ĭ-dē) A family of fleas belonging to the order Siphonaptera. Pulicidae includes the genera *Pulex, Echidnophaga, Ctenocephalides,* and *Xenopsylla.* SEE: *flea.*

**pulicide** (pū′lĭ-sīd) [L. *pulex,* flea, + *caedere,* to kill] An agent that kills fleas.

**pullulate** (pŭl″ū-lāt) [L. *pullulare,* to sprout] To bud or germinate.

**pullulation** (pŭl″ū-lā′shŭn) The act of budding or germinating, as seen in the yeast plant.

**pulmo-** (pŭl′mō-, pool′mō-) Combining form meaning *lung.*

**pulmoaortic** (pŭl″mō-ā-or′tĭk) [L. *pulmo,* lung, + Gr. *aorte,* aorta] **1.** Concerning the lungs and the aorta. **2.** Relating to the pulmonary artery and aorta.

**pulmometry** (pūl-mŏm′ĕ-trē) Determination of capacity of the lungs.

**pulmonary** (pŭl′mō-nĕ-rē) [L. *pulmonarius*] Concerning or involving the lungs.

**pulmonary arterial web** A weblike deformity seen in pulmonary angiograms at the site of previous pulmonary thromboembolism.

**pulmonary artery** The artery leading from the right ventricle of the heart to the lungs.

**pulmonary artery wedge pressure** ABBR: PAWP. Pressure measured in the pulmonary artery at its capillary end. The catheter is positioned in the pulmonary artery, and the distal portion of the catheter is isolated from pressure behind it in the artery by inflating a balloon with air. This allows the catheter to float into a wedged position, and permits sensing of transmission of pressures ahead of the catheter (in the pulmonary capillary bed) by the transducer. Because no valve is present between this location and the left atrium, the measurement reflects left atrial pressure, and, in the presence of a competent mitral valve, the measurement provides an indication of left ventricular end-diastolic pressure. The balloon is then passively deflated, allowing the catheter to drift back into the main pulmonary artery where it measures pulmonary artery forward pressure. SYN: *wedge pressure.* SEE: *Swan-Ganz catheter.*

NURSING IMPLICATIONS: The nurse prepares and sets up the transducer equipment to monitor pulmonary artery pressure and PAWP alternately according to institutional protocol and manufacturer's instructions. The transducer is balanced and calibrated as required (every 4 to 8 hr). Hemodynamic status is monitored, and findings are documented, including pulmonary artery pressure (normally 20 to 30 mm Hg systolic and 8 to 12 mm Hg diastolic) every hour as directed. To measure PAWP every 1 to 4 hr as directed, the nurse inflates the balloon with 0.75 to 1.5 cc of air depending on balloon size (balloon with fluid is never inflated) while watching for change in waveform indicating wedging and assessing for balloon rupture (lack of resistance on inflation, with absence of wedging). If this occurs, the wedging procedure is discontinued (because of concern for air embolism), and therapy is managed based on pulmonary artery diastolic pressures. Pulmonary artery wedge pressure is read, documented (normally 4 to 12 mm Hg), and correlated to clinical findings and other hemodynamic values, and any abnormal findings are reported. The nurse then removes the syringe and permits passive deflation of the balloon while observing for reappearance of pulmonary artery pressure waveform. If the balloon remains inflated, the patient is at risk for pulmonary artery necrosis. The patient should be positioned on the right side and encourage to take deep breaths and to cough as the nurse mobilizes the right arm. If balloon remains wedged, the physician should be notified. Fluid and diuretic therapy are adjusted based on PAWP and other values as prescribed.

**pulmonary function test** One of a number of different tests used to determine the ability of the lungs to exchange oxygen and carbon dioxide. These are done by measuring the amount of air that can be maximally exhaled after a maximum inspiration and the time required for that expiration; and by determining the ability of the alveolar capillary membrane to transport oxygen into the blood and carbon dioxide from the blood into the expired air. SEE: illus.; *$FEV_1$*.

**pulmonary mucociliary clearance** The removal of inhaled particles, endogenous cellular debris, and excessive secretions from the tracheobronchial tree by the action of the ciliated cells that live in the respiratory tract. The cilia of these cells beat and are therefore able to propel mucus and debris upward and out of the tracheobronchial tree. This action is one of the most important defenses of the respiratory tract.

**pulmonary vein** One of the four veins draining the lungs and returning the blood to the left atrium of the heart.

**pulmonectomy** (pŭl″mō-nĕk′tō-mē) [L. *pulmonis,* lung, + Gr. *ektome,* excision] Pneumectomy.

**pulmonic** (pŭl-mŏn′ĭk) **1.** Concerning the lungs. **2.** Concerning the pulmonary artery.

**pulmonitis** (pŭl-mō-nī′tĭs) [″ + Gr. *itis,* inflammation] Pneumonia.

**pulmonologist** A physician trained and certified to treat pulmonary diseases.

**pulmotor** (pŭl′mō-tor) [″ + *motor,* mover] An apparatus for inducing artificial respiration by forcing air or oxygen into the lungs.

**pulp** [L. *pulpa,* flesh] **1.** The soft part of fruit. **2.** The soft part of an organ. **3.** A mass of partly digested food passed from stomach to duodenum. SYN: *chyme.* **4.** The soft vascular portion of the center of a tooth.

***p. amputation*** The technique of removing the coronal portion of an exposed or involved vital pulp in an effort to retain the radicular pulp in a healthy, vital condition. SYN: *pulpotomy.*

***p. capping*** The technique and material for covering and protecting from external conditions a vital, exposed pulp while the pulp heals and secondary or tertiary dentin forms to cover it.

***coronal p.*** The portion of dental pulp in the crown of the pulp cavity.

***dead p.*** Devitalized or necrotic dental pulp.

***dental p.*** The connective tissues that fill the pulp cavity enclosed by dentin of the tooth; it includes a vascular and nerve network, a peripheral layer of odontoblasts involved with dentin formation, and other cellular and fibrous components.

***devitalized p.*** A dead or necrotic dental pulp as indicated by a vitalometer used

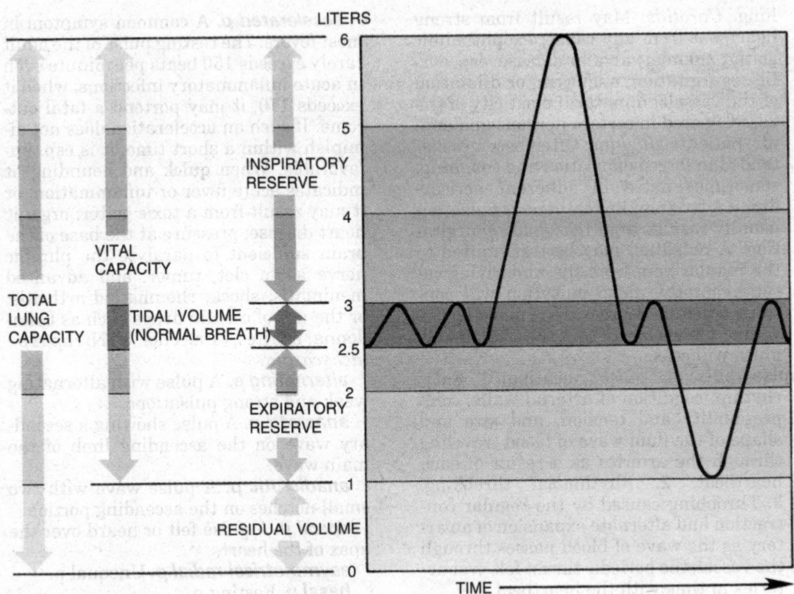


PULMONARY FUNCTION TEST

PULMONARY VOLUMES

for pulp testing.

***digital p.*** The elastic, soft prominence on the palmar or plantar surface of the last phalanx of a finger or toe.

***enamel p.*** Cells forming a stellate reticulum lying between outer and inner layers of the enamel organ of a tooth.

***exposed p.*** Pulp that, due to disease, is exposed to the air and saliva in the mouth.

***p. extirpation*** The complete removal of the pulp tissue from the pulp chamber and root canal, irrespective of the state of health of the pulp. SYN: *pulpectomy.*

***putrescent p.*** Dead pulp that has a foul odor because of the action of putrefactive bacteria.

***radicular p.*** Pulp that is in the root canal of a tooth.

***red p.*** The portion of splenic pulp consisting of venous sinuses plus pulp cords.

***splenic p.*** The soft spongelike tissue-forming substance of the spleen.

***tooth p.*** SEE: *tooth.*

***vertebral p.*** Nucleus pulposus of the intervertebral disk.

***vital p.*** Dental pulp that is alive and thus normal.

***white p.*** The portion of splenic pulp consisting of a compact type of lymphatic tissue that forms a sheath about certain arteries in the spleen.

***wood p.*** A soft form of cellulose, derived from wood or cotton, used as a food additive.

**pulpa** (pŭl′pă) [L., flesh] Pulp.

**pulpal** (pŭl′păl) Relating to pulp.

**pulpalgia** (pŭl-păl′jē-ă) [″ + Gr. *algos,* pain] Pain in the pulp of a tooth.

**pulpectomy** (pŭl-pĕk′tō-mē) [″ + Gr. *ektome,* excision] Pulp extirpation.

**pulpefaction** (pŭl-pĭ-făk′shŭn) [L. *pulpa,* pulp, + *facere,* to make] Conversion into a pulpy substance.

**pulpitis** (pŭl-pī′tĭs) *pl.* **pulpitides** [″ + *itis,* inflammation] Inflammation of the pulp of a tooth.

**pulpotomy** (pŭl-pŏt′ō-mē) [″ + Gr. *tome,* incision] Pulp amputation.

**pulpy** (pŭl′pē) Resembling pulp; flabby.

**pulsate** (pŭl′sāt) [L. *pulsare*] To throb or beat in rhythm.

**pulsatile** (pŭl′să-tĭl) Pulsating; characterized by a rhythmic beat. SYN: *throbbing.*

**pulsation** (pŭl-sā′shŭn) [L. *pulsatio,* a beating] The rhythmic beat, as of the heart and blood vessels; a throbbing. SEE: *pulse.*

ABNORMAL CENTERS OF PULSATION: *Epigastric:* May result from forceful action of heart from any cause; enlargement of right ventricle; pulsating aorta noted in certain anxious persons and in anemic patients; aortic aneurysm; tumors of left lobe of liver resting on the aorta. *Left axillary region:* May result from enlargement of heart; a tense purulent effusion in left pleural sac (pulsating empyema); aneurysm; chronic disease of left lung and pleura associated with retraction of the lung. *Carotids:* May result from strong heartbeat from any cause; exophthalmic goiter; anemia; valvular disease, esp. aortic regurgitation; aneurysm or dilatation of the vessels; unnatural elasticity of the vessels noted in certain nervous and anemic patients. *Jugular:* Often becomes distended in forced expiration and coughing; sometimes noted in adherent pericardium. A true rhythmical venous pulsation usually results from tricuspid regurgitation. A pulsation may be transmitted to the jugular vein from the underlying carotid, but this false pulsation will continue when light pressure is made on the vein of the neck, whereas the true venous pulse will cease.

**pulse** (pŭls) [L. *pulsus,* beating] **1.** Rate, rhythm, condition of arterial walls, compressibility and tension, and size and shape of the fluid wave of blood traveling through the arteries as a result of each heartbeat. **2.** Rhythmical throbbing. **3.** Throbbing caused by the regular contraction and alternate expansion of an artery as the wave of blood passes through the vessel; the periodic thrust felt over arteries in time with the heartbeat.

A tracing of this is called a sphygmogram and consists of a series of waves in which the upstroke is called the anacrotic limb, and the downstroke (on which is normally seen the dicrotic notch), the catacrotic limb.

The normal pulse rate of the adult is about 72 in men and 80 in women. It is usually felt in the radial artery of the wrist.

POINTS TO BE OBSERVED: The hour, frequency, pressure, regularity, and force of the pulse should be observed. Temperature and respiration are of clinical importance to the physician. Right and left radial arteries are usually tested and differences, if any, or absence of either pulse should be noted. If pressure of finger on artery is too great, the vessel will be collapsed and the pulse will not be discernible. The thumb should not be used because the examiner may be counting the pulse in his or her own thumb rather than in the patient's. The pulse should be counted for at least half a minute.

The rate of the pulse depends upon sex, age, exertion, position of body, and state of general health. It is higher in children and increases with very old age. It is slower in tall persons than it is in short persons. It is about 10 to 12 beats more frequent during standing than during sitting. Physical exertion will increase it normally to as much as 200 beats per minute in young healthy persons. Eating and drinking also increase heart action. Pulse rate decreases during sleep, relaxation, and rest.

***abdominal p.*** A palpable pulse in the abdominal area. This is produced by the pulse of the abdominal aorta.

***accelerated p.*** A common symptom in most fevers. The resting pulse of the adult rarely exceeds 150 beats per minute even in acute inflammatory infections; when it exceeds 170, it may portend a fatal outcome. If such an acceleration does not diminish within a short time, it is esp. unfavorable. When quick and bounding, it indicates acute fever or inflammation, or it may result from a toxic goiter; organic heart disease; pressure at the base of the brain sufficient to paralyze the phrenic nerve as in clot, tumor, and advanced meningitis; shock; rheumatoid arthritis; or the use of certain drugs such as belladonna, nitrites, or alcohol. SYN: *rapid p.; tachycardia.*

***alternating p.*** A pulse with alternating weak and strong pulsations.

***anacrotic p.*** A pulse showing a secondary wave on the ascending limb of the main wave.

***anadicrotic p.*** A pulse wave with two small notches on the ascending portion.

***apical p.*** A pulse felt or heard over the apex of the heart.

***asymmetrical radial p.*** Unequal p.

***basal p.*** Resting p.

***bigeminal p.*** A pulse in which two regular beats are followed by a longer pause. It has the same significance as an irregular pulse. SYN: *coupled p.*

***bisferiens p.*** A pulse marked by two systolic peaks on the pulse waveform. It is characteristic of aortic regurgitation (with or without aortic stenosis) and hypertrophic cardiomyopathy.

***bounding p.*** A pulse that reaches a higher intensity than normal, then disappears quickly. Best detected when the arm is held aloft, this pulse is due to shortened ventricular systole and reduced peripheral pressure. SYN: *collapsing p.*

***brachial p.*** A pulse felt in the brachial artery.

***capillary p.*** Alternating redness and pallor of a capillary region, as in the matrices beneath the nails, occurring chiefly where an excessive cardiac impulse coincides with general arterial narrowing. SYN: *Quincke's pulse.*

***carotid p.*** A pulse felt in the carotid artery.

***catacrotic p.*** A pulse showing one or more secondary waves on the descending limb of the main wave.

***catadicrotic p.*** A pulse wave with two small notches on the descending portion.

***central p.*** A pulse recorded near the origin of the carotid or subclavian arteries.

***collapsing p.*** Bounding p.

***coupled p.*** Bigeminal p.

***deficit p.*** A condition in which the number of pulse beats counted at the wrist is less than those counted in the same period of time at the heart. This is seen in atrial fibrillation.

***dicrotic p.*** A pulse with a double beat,

one heartbeat for two arterial pulsations, or a seemingly weak wave between the usual heartbeats. This weak wave should not be counted as a regular beat. It is indicative of low arterial tension and is noted in fevers.

***dorsalis pedis p.*** A pulse felt over the dorsalis pedis artery of the foot.

***entoptic p.*** Intermittent subjective sensations of light that accompany the heartbeat.

***febrile p.*** A full, bounding pulse at the onset of fever, becoming feeble and weak when the fever subsides.

***femoral p.*** A pulse felt over the femoral artery.

***filiform p.*** Thready p.

***full p.*** A distended pulse in an artery, giving a tense feeling; observed in inflammation.

***hard p.*** A pulse with a sensation of hardness caused by changes in the arterial wall or to vascular distention.

***hepatic p.*** A pulse due to expansion of veins of the liver at each ventricular contraction.

***high-tension p.*** A pulse in which the force of the beat is relatively increased. The force may be roughly estimated by noting the amount of pressure of the fingers that is required to arrest the beat. It is observed in many conditions: cardiac diseases, such as hypertrophy; chronic nephritis; cerebral affections; high fever; irritation of the vasomotor center as in apoplexy, tumors, and beginning meningitis; after the use of certain drugs such as digitalis, ergot, and alcoholic stimulants; chills; angina pectoris; epileptic and hysterical seizures; gout; and uremia.

***intermediate p.*** A pulse recorded in the proximal portions of the carotid, femoral, and brachial arteries.

***intermittent p.*** A pulse in which occasional beats are skipped, caused by an apparent drop of a heartbeat. It is not inconsistent with health, yet it is commonly an indication of disease, frequently from gastric, hepatic, uterine, and renal causes. It is common in fatty degeneration of the heart and is habitual in certain people after exercise, eating, or excitement.

***irregular p.*** A pulse with a variation in force and frequency; having the same significance as an intermittent pulse. It is common in myocarditis and valvular diseases, esp. in mitral regurgitation. Heart trouble may be noted by long-continued irregular pulse.

***jerky p.*** A pulse characteristic of aortic regurgitation, because from a state of emptiness, the artery is suddenly filled with blood.

***jugular p.*** A venous pulse felt in the jugular vein.

***Kussmaul's p.*** Paradoxical p.

***long p.*** A pulse in which the duration of the systolic wave is comparatively long.

***low-tension p.*** A pulse with sudden onset, short duration, and rapid decline, esp. noted in heart failure, collapse, debility, and fevers.

***monocrotic p.*** A pulse in which the sphygmogram shows a simple ascending and descending uninterrupted line and no dicrotism.

***nail p.*** A visible pulsation in the capillaries under the nails.

***paradoxical p.*** A pulse that is more or less suppressed at the close of each full inspiration, frequently noted in adherent pericarditis. It is thought to be due to compression of the great vessels by inflammatory adhesions, the latter being stretched during act of inspiration. SYN: *Kussmaul's p.*

***p. parvus*** A weak, small pulse, present in patients with diminished left ventricular stroke volume, narrow pulse pressure, and increased peripheral vascular resistance.

***peripheral p.*** A pulse recorded in the arteries (radial or pedal) in the distal portion of the limbs.

***pistol-shot p.*** A pulse resulting from rapid distention and collapse of an artery as occurs in aortic regurgitation.

***plateau p.*** A pulse associated with an increase in pressure that slowly rises but is maintained.

***popliteal p.*** A pulse felt over the popliteal artery.

***radial p.*** A pulse felt over the radial artery.

***rapid p.*** Accelerated p.

***regular p.*** A pulse felt when the force and frequency are the same (i.e., when the length of beat and number of beats per minute and the strength are the same).

***respiratory p.*** Alternate dilatation and contraction of the large veins of the neck occurring simultaneously with inspiration and expiration.

***resting p.*** A pulse rate obtained while an individual is at rest and calm.

***Riegel's p.*** A diminution of the pulse during expiration.

***running p.*** A weak, rapid pulse with one wave continuing into the next.

***senile p.*** A pulse characteristic of the aged. The sphygmogram shows a high position of the secondary waves in descent with increased amplitude of the first secondary wave as compared with the second.

***short p.*** A pulse with a short, quick systolic wave.

***slow p.*** A very slow pulse, fully accentuated, often found among the aged. It is a habitual rate among those inclined to be slow and easy in their actions and is found in the highly conditioned athlete. Such a pulse rate ranges between 40 and 60 beats per minute.

***small p.*** SEE: *pulse parvus.*

***soft p.*** A pulse that may be stopped by moderate digital compression.

***tense p.*** A full but not bounding pulse.

***thready p.*** A fine, scarcely perceptible pulse. SYN: *filiform p.*

***tremulous p.*** A pulse in which a series of oscillations is felt with each beat.

***tricrotic p.*** A pulse with three separate expansions during each heartbeat.

***trigeminal p.*** A pulse in which a pause follows three regular beats.

***triphammer p.*** Waterhammer p.

***undulating p.*** A pulse that seems to have several successive waves.

***unequal p.*** A pulse in which beats vary in force. SYN: *asymmetrical radial p.*

***vagus p.*** A slow pulse resulting from vagus inhibition of the heart.

***venous p.*** A pulse in a vein, esp. one of the large veins near the heart, such as the internal or external jugular. Normally it is undulating and scarcely palpable. In conditions such as tricuspid regurgitation, it is pronounced.

***vermicular p.*** A small, frequent pulse with a wormlike feeling.

***waterhammer p.*** A pulse characterized by a short, powerful, jerky beat that suddenly collapses. The peculiar pulsation may be distinctly visible, not only in the carotids but throughout the brachial artery. It is diagnostic of aortic regurgitation during the period of compensation, and its force is due to excessive ventricular hypertrophy and to the large amount of blood expelled with each systole; its sudden recession is due to the incompetent valves failing to support the column of blood. SYN: *triphammer p.; Corrigan's pulse.*

***wiry p.*** A tense pulse that feels like a wire or firm cord.

**pulseless disease** Takayasu's arteritis.

**pulseless electrical activity** The continuation of electrical activity in the heart not accompanied by a palpable pulse.

**pulsing electromagnetic field** ABBR: PEMF. The production of a pulsing electromagnetic field applied to a fractured bone in order to induce healing. The electric field is applied externally to the affected leg and does not involve invasion of the tissue. This treatment is esp. useful in treating fractures that have previously failed to heal. Direct-current stimulation has also been used in treating these conditions.

**pulsion** (pŭl′shŭn) Driving or propelling in any direction.

***lateral p.*** Movement, particularly walking as if pulled to one side.

**pulsus** (pŭl′sŭs) [L.] Pulse.

***p. alternans*** A weak pulse alternating with a strong one.

***p. bigeminus*** Bigeminal pulse.

***p. celer*** A quick pulse that rises and falls suddenly.

***p. differens*** A condition in which the pulses on either side of the body are of unequal intensity.

***p. paradoxus*** Paradoxical pulse.

***p. parvus et tardus*** A pulse that is small and rises and falls slowly.

***p. tardus*** An abnormally slow pulse.

**pulv** L. *pulvis,* powder.

**pulverization** (pŭl″vĕr-ī-zā′shŭn) [L. *pulvis,* powder] The crushing of any substance to powder or tiny particles.

**pulverulent** (pŭl-vĕr′ū-lĕnt) Of the nature of, or resembling, powder.

**pulvinar** (pŭl-vī′năr) [L., cushioned seat] The part of the thalamus comprising a portion of the posterior nuclei. It projects posteriorly and medially, partially overlying the midbrain.

**pulvinate** (pŭl′vĭ-nāt) [L. *pulvinus,* cushion] Convex; shaped like a cushion.

**pulvis** [L.] Powder.

**pumice** (pŭm′ĭs) A substance derived from volcanic material. It contains chiefly complex silicates of aluminum, potassium, and sodium. Used as an abrasive, esp. in dental prophylaxis.

**pump** [ME. *pumpe*] **1.** An apparatus that transfers fluids or gases by pressure or suction. **2.** To force air or fluid along a certain pathway, as when the heart pumps blood.

***air p.*** A device for forcing air in or out of a chamber.

***blood p.*** A device for pumping blood. It is attached to an extracorporeal circulation system.

***breast p.*** An apparatus for removing milk from the breasts.

***dental p.*** An apparatus for removing saliva from the mouth during operation on teeth or jaws.

***insulin p.*** SEE: under *insulin.*

***lymphedema p.*** A pneumatic compression device for application to an edematous limb. It works best when combined with elevation of the limb and manual massage. The device, which may be single-chambered or multichambered, is designed to provide calibrated, sequential pressure to the extremity. This action "milks" edema fluid from the extremity. It is essential that the device be used in the early phase of the development of lymphedema. If the affected lymph vessels develop fibrotic changes (i.e., scar tissue), then pneumatic compression devices are of questionable benefit.

***sodium p.*** The active transport mechanism that moves sodium ions across a membrane to their area of greater concentration. In neurons and muscle cells, this is outside the cell. In many cells, the sodium pump is linked with the potassium pump that transports potassium ions into the cell, also against a concentration gradient, and may be called the *sodium-potassium pump.* In neurons and muscle fibers, this pump maintains the polarization of the membrane.

***stomach p.*** An apparatus for removing contents from the stomach.

**pump-oxygenator** A device that pumps and

oxygenates blood.

**punch** An instrument for making a small circular hole in material or tissue, esp. the skin.

**punchdrunk** **1.** A concussion syndrome present in persons who have boxed and experienced multiple episodes of trauma to the head. If severe, both the cognitive and memory functions of the brain are affected. Symptoms may resemble those of Parkinson's disease. At autopsy, there is evidence of multiple scars of the cerebral tissue. SYN: *dementia pugilistica.* **2.** One who is punchdrunk.

**punched out** Appearing as if holes have been made; used to describe appearance of bones (as seen on x-ray film) in certain pathologic states.

**puncta** (pŭnk′tă) *sing.* **punctum** [L.] Points.

**punctate** (pŭnk′tāt) [L. *punctum,* point] Having pinpoint punctures or depressions on the surface; marked with dots.

***p. keratoses*** Discrete yellow-to-brown firm keratotic papules of the palms and soles, most probably due to the performing of manual labor.

***p. pits*** Depressed areas of the skin, esp. of the palmar creases of the hands and soles.

***p. rash*** A rash with minute red points.

**punctiform** (pŭnk′tĭ-form) [″ + *forma,* shape] **1.** Formed like a point. **2.** In bacteriology, referring to pinpoint colonies of less than 1 mm in diameter.

**punctio** (pŭnk′shē-ō) [L. *punctura,* a point] The act of puncturing or pricking.

**punctum** (pŭnk′tŭm) *pl.* **puncta** [L.] Point.

***p. caecum*** Blind spot (1).

***puncta dolorosa*** Painful points in the course of, or at the exit of, nerves affected by neuralgia.

***p. lacrimale*** The outlet of a lacrimal canaliculus.

***p. nasale inferius*** Rhinion.

***p. proximum*** ABBR: P.P. Visual accommodation near-point.

***p. remotum*** ABBR: P.R. Visual accommodation far-point.

***p. saliens*** The first trace of the embryonic heart.

***puncta vasculosa*** Minute red areas that mark the cut surface of white central substance of the brain, caused by blood escaping from divided blood vessels.

**puncture** (pŭnk′chūr) [L. *punctura,* prick] **1.** A hole or wound made by a sharp pointed instrument. **2.** To make a hole with such an instrument.

***cisternal p.*** A spinal puncture with a hollow needle between the cervical vertebrae, through the dura mater, and into the cisterna at the base of the brain. This is done to inject a drug or a serum as in cerebral meningitis or cerebral syphilis, to remove spinal fluid for diagnostic purposes, or to reduce intracranial pressure. It should be used as a source of spinal fluid only if fluid cannot be obtained by lumbar puncture. SEE: *cerebrospinal fluid; spinal puncture.*

---

Caution: This procedure may be lethal if not done by one skilled in this technique.

---

***diabetic p.*** Puncture in the floor of the fourth ventricle, which results in glycosuria. This lesion was produced experimentally by the French physiologist Claude Bernard.

***exploratory p.*** Piercing of a cavity or cyst for the purpose of examining the fluid or pus removed.

***lumbar p.*** SEE: *lumbar puncture.*

***Quincke's p.*** Lumbar puncture.

***spinal p.*** SEE: *spinal puncture.*

***sternal p.*** Puncture of the manubrium sternum by use of a needle, the purpose of which is to obtain a bone marrow specimen.

***ventricular p.*** Puncture of a ventricle of the brain for purpose of withdrawing fluid or introducing air for ventriculography.

**pungency** (pŭn′jĕn-sē) [L. *pungens,* prick] The quality of being sharp, strong, or bitter, as an odor or taste.

**pungent** (pŭn′jĕnt) Acrid or sharp, as applied to an odor or taste.

**punitive damages** Compensation awarded in an amount intended to punish the defendant (the person committing the tort) for the obvious and preventable harmful act. The defendant's actions must be willful and wanton, and the damages are not based on the plaintiff's actual monetary loss. SEE: *tort.*

**P.U.O.** *pyrexia of unknown origin.*

**pupa** (pū′pă) [L., girl] The stage in complete metamorphosis of an insect that follows the larva and precedes the adult or imago. The insect does not feed during this stage and usually is inactive.

**pupil** (pū′pĭl) [L. *pupilla*] The contractile opening at the center of the iris of the eye. It contracts when exposed to strong light and when the focus is on a near object; dilates in the dark and when the focus is on a distant object. Average diameter is 4 to 5 mm. The pupils should be equal. SYN: *pupilla.*

DIFFERENTIAL DIAGNOSIS: Constriction of the pupil occurs in old age and in photophobia. It is induced by morphine, pilocarpine, physostigmine, eserine, and other miotic drugs.

Dilation of the pupil may occur in blindness or deficient sight from any cause; from intracranial trauma; from distress or strong emotion; in fevers, comatose states, oculomotor nerve paralysis, and glaucoma. It may be induced by belladonna (atropine), cocaine, homatropine, hyoscine (scopolamine), and other mydriatic drugs.

***Adie's p.*** Tonic p. SEE: *Adie's syn-*

*drome.*

***artificial p.*** A pupil made by iridectomy when the normal pupil is occluded.

***bounding p.*** Rapid dilatation of a pupil, alternating with contraction.

***Bumke's p.*** Dilatation of the pupil owing to psychic stimulus.

***cat's-eye p.*** A pupil that is narrow and slitlike.

***cornpicker's p.'s*** Dilated pupils found in agricultural workers who are exposed to dust from jimsonweed. The dust contains stramonium, a mydriatic.

***fixed p.*** A pupil that does not react to stimuli.

***keyhole p.*** A pupil with an artificial coloboma at the pupillary margin.

***occlusion of the p.*** A pupil with an opaque membrane shutting off the pupillary area.

***pinhole p.*** A pupil of minute size; one excessively constricted; seen after use of miotics, in opium poisoning, and in certain brain disorders.

***stiff p.*** Argyll Robertson pupil.

***tonic p.*** A pupil that reacts slowly in accommodation-convergence reflexes.

**pupilla** (pū-pĭl′ă) [L., pupil] The pupil of the eye.

**pupillary** (pū′pĭ-lĕr-ē) [L. *pupilla,* pupil] Concerning the pupil.

**pupillography** Recording movements of the pupil of the eye.

**pupillometer** (pū-pĭl-ŏm′ĕ-tĕr) [″ + Gr. *metron,* measure] A device for measuring the diameter of a pupil.

**pupillometry** (pū-pĭl-lŏm′ĕ-trē) [″ + *metron,* measure] Measurement of the diameter of the pupil.

**pupillomotor reflex** Purkinje phenomenon.

**pupilloplegia** (pū″pĭ-lō-plē′jē-ă) [″ + *plege,* stroke] Slow reaction of the pupil of the eye.

**pupilloscopy** (pū-pĭl-ŏs′kō-pē) [″ + Gr. *skopein,* to examine] **1.** Retinoscopy. **2.** Examination of the pupil.

**pupillostatometer** (pū″pĭl-ō-stă-tŏm′ĕ-tĕr) [″+ Gr. *statos,* placed, + *metron,* measure] A device for measuring the distance between the centers of the pupils.

**Purdue Pegboard Test** A standardized test of manual dexterity for adults and children.

**pure** (pūr) [ME.] Free from pollution; uncontaminated.

**pure line 1.** The progeny of a single homozygous individual obtained by self-fertilization. **2.** The progeny of an individual reproducing asexually by simple fission, or by buds, runners, stolons, and so on. **3.** The progeny of two homozygous individuals reproducing sexually.

**purgation** (pŭr-gā′shŭn) [L. *purgatio*] **1.** Cleansing. **2.** Evacuation of the bowels by the action of a purgative medicine. SYN: *catharsis.*

**purgative** (pŭr′gă-tĭv) [L. *purgativus*] **1.** Cleansing. **2.** An agent that will stimulate the production of bowel movements. SEE: *catharsis; cathartic.*

***cholagogue p.*** A purgative that stimulates the flow of bile, producing green stools.

***drastic p.*** A purgative that produces violent bowel movements.

***saline p.*** A purgative that produces copious watery discharges.

**purgative enema** A strong, high colonic purgative that is used when other enemas fail. SEE: *enema.*

**purge** (pŭrj) [L. *purgare,* to cleanse] **1.** To evacuate the bowels by means of a cathartic. **2.** A drug that causes evacuation of the bowels. **3.** Removal of malignant or other pathologic cells from bone marrow that has been removed from a patient so that it could be purged and then reinfused in the same patient. This technique is experimental. SEE: *bone marrow transplant, autologous; magnetic microspheres.*

**puriform** (pū′rĭ-form) [L. *pus,* pus, + *forma,* shape] Resembling pus. SYN: *puruloid.*

**purinase** (pū′rĭ-nās) An enzyme that catalyzes purine metabolism.

**purine** (pū′rēn″) [L. *purum,* pure, + *uricus,* uric acid] Parent compound of purine bases, as adenine, guanine, xanthine, caffeine, and uric acid. Purines are the end products of nucleoprotein digestion. They may be synthesized in the body. They break down to form uric acid. SEE: *aminopurine; oxypurine; methyl purine.*

***endogenous p.*** Purine originating from nucleoproteins within the tissues.

***exogenous p.*** Purine present in, or derived from, foods. SEE: table.

**purine base** Xanthine base.

**purinemia** (pū″rĭ-nē′mē-ă) [*purine,* + Gr. *haima,* blood] Purine in the blood.

**purity** [L. *puris,* clean, pure, unmixed] The state of being clean and free of contamination.

**Purkinje, Johannes E. von** (pŭr-kĭn′jē) Bohemian anatomist and physiologist, 1787–1869.

***P. cell*** A large neuron that has dendrites extending to the molecular layer of the cerebellar cortex and into the white matter of the cerebellum.

***P. fiber*** A cardiac muscle cell beneath the endocardium of the ventricles of the heart. These extend from the bundle branches to the ventricular myocardium and form the last part of the cardiac conduction system.

***P. figures*** Shadows of blood vessels perceived when light is projected out of focus or obliquely onto the retina.

***P. layer*** A single row of large flask-shaped cells (Purkinje cells) lying between molecular and granular layers of the cerebellar cortex.

***P. network*** A network of Purkinje fibers found in cardiac muscle.

***P. phenomenon*** A phenomenon of adjustment of the pupil of the eye to light intensity. When the eye adapts from light

**Purines in Food**

| | |
|---|---|
| ***Group A: High Concentration (150–1000 mg/100 g)*** | |
| Liver | Sardines (in oil) |
| Kidney | Meat extracts |
| Sweetbreads | Consommé |
| Brains | Gravies |
| Heart | Fish roes |
| Anchovies | Herring |
| ***Group B: Moderate Amounts (50–150 mg/100 g)*** | |
| Meat, game, and fish other than those mentioned in Group A | |
| Fowl | Asparagus |
| Lentils | Cauliflower |
| Whole-grain cereals | Mushrooms |
| Beans | Spinach |
| Peas | |
| ***Group C: Very Small Amounts: Need Not be Restricted in Diet of Persons with Gout*** | |
| Vegetables other than those mentioned above | |
| Fruits of all kinds | Coffee |
| Milk | Tea |
| Cheese | Chocolate |
| Eggs | Carbonated beverages |
| Refined cereals, spaghetti, macaroni | Tapioca |
| | Yeast |
| Butter, fats, nuts, peanut butter* | |
| Sugars and sweets | |
| Vegetable soups | |

* Fats interfere with the urinary excretion of urates and thus should be limited if the objective is to promote excretion of uric acid.

to dark conditions, the maximum pupillary movement is caused by green instead of yellow light. SYN: *pupillomotor reflex.*

***P.-Sanson images*** Three images of the same object, produced by reflections from the surface of the cornea and the anterior and posterior surfaces of the lens of the eye. For the most part, the viewer adapts to this phenomenon and ignores these "extra" images.

***P. vesicle*** The nuclear portion of an ovum. SYN: *germinal vesicle.*

**purohepatitis** (pū″rō-hĕp″ă-tī′tĭs) [L. *pus,* pus + Gr. *hepar,* liver, + *itis,* inflammation] Purulent inflammation of the liver.

**puromucous** (pū″rō-mū′kŭs) [″ + *mucus,* mucus] Mucopurulent, containing both mucus and pus.

**purple** A color formed by mixing red with blue.

***visual p.*** Rhodopsin.

**purposeful movement** Motor activity requiring the planned and consciously directed involvement of the patient. It is hypothesized that evoking cortical involvement in movement patterns during sensorimotor rehabilitation will enhance the development of coordination and voluntary control.

**purpura** (pŭr′pū-ră) [L., purple] A condition with various manifestations and diverse causes, characterized by hemorrhages into the skin, mucous membranes, internal organs, and other tissues. Hemorrhage into the skin shows red, darkening into purple, then brownish-yellow and finally disappearing in 2 to 3 weeks. Areas of discoloration do not disappear under pressure. SEE: illus.

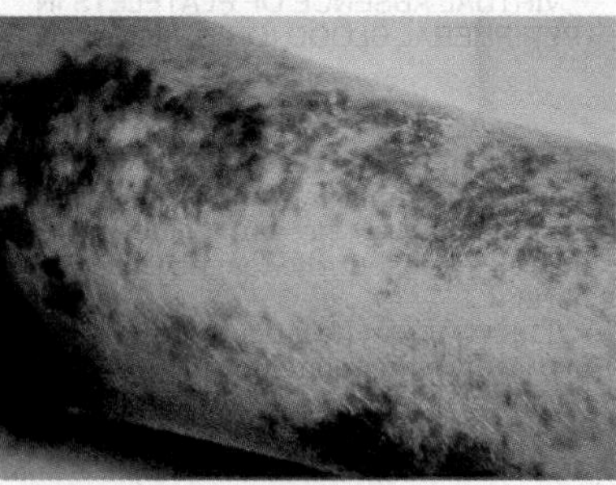

PURPURA

***allergic p.*** Any of a group of purpuras caused by a variety of agents, including bacteria, drugs, and food. SYN: *nonthrombocytopenic p.*

***anaphylactoid p.*** Schönlein-Henoch p.

***p. annularis telangiectodes*** Majocchi's disease.

***fibrinolytic p.*** Purpura resulting from excess fibrinolytic activity of the blood.

***p. fulminans*** A rapidly progressing form of purpura occurring principally in children; of short duration and frequently fatal.

***hemorrhagic p.*** Idiopathic thrombocytopenic p.

***Henoch p.*** Schönlein-Henoch purpura with acute vomiting, diarrhea, and renal colic, but without joint involvement.

***idiopathic thrombocytopenic p.*** ABBR: ITP. A hemorrhagic autoimmune disease in which there is a pronounced reduction in circulating blood platelets, caused by the presence in the blood plasma of a substance that agglutinates platelets. This condition occurs in individuals, esp. children, with drug sensitivities, serum sickness, and other allergic disorders. It is usually accompanied by pains in the joints and abdomen. SYN: *thrombocytopenic p.; thrombopenic p.; Schönlein's disease.* SEE: illus.; *Nursing Diagnoses Appendix.*

SYMPTOMS: Symptoms include bleeding from mouth and skin upon slight injury. Bleeding may also occur from the mucous membranes, in serous mem-

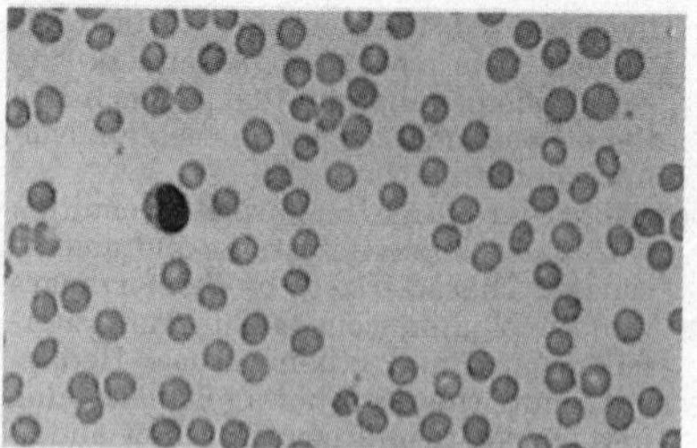

IDIOPATHIC THROMBOCYTOPENIC PURPURA

VIRTUAL ABSENCE OF PLATELETS IN PERIPHERAL BLOOD (ORIG. MAG. ×400)

branes, and sometimes into the brain. Increased bleeding time and reduced platelet count are present. The clot is nonretractile, but the coagulation time is normal.

TREATMENT: If patients are asymptomatic and the platelet count is above 50,000 per cubic mm, treatment is unnecessary. For symptomatic patients, prednisone is the initial therapy. Episodes of severe bleeding are treated with platelet transfusion. Intravenous immune globulin is valuable in managing acute bleeding and in preparing a patient for blood loss, as in delivery of a baby. Splenectomy is effective in producing a remission in two thirds of patients. Cytotoxic drug therapy has been successful, although its mechanism is unclear.

NURSING IMPLICATIONS: Platelet count is monitored daily. The patient is observed for bleeding (petechiae, ecchymoses, epistaxis, oral mucous membrane or G.I. bleeding, hematuria, menorrhagia) and stools, urine, and vomitus are tested for occult blood. The amount of bleeding or size of ecchymoses is measured at least every 24 hr. Any complications of ITP are monitored. The patient is educated about the disorder, prescribed treatments, importance of reporting bleeding (such as epistaxis, gingival, urinary tract, or uterine or rectal bleeding) and signs of internal bleeding (such as tarry stools or coffee-ground vomitus). The patient should avoid straining during defecation or coughing because both can lead to increased intracranial pressure, possible causing cerebral hemorrhage. Stool softeners are provided as necessary to prevent tearing of the rectal mucosa and bleeding due to passage of constipated or hard stools. The purpose, procedure, and expected sensations of each diagnostic test are explained. The role of platelets and the way in which the results of platelet counts can help to identify symptoms of abnormal bleeding are also explained. The lower the platelet count falls, the more precautions the patient will need to take; in severe thrombocytopenia, even minor bumps or scrapes can result in bleeding. The nurse guards against bleeding by taking the following precautions to protect the patient from trauma: keeping the side rails of the bed raised and padded, promoting use of a soft toothbrush or sponge-stick and an electric razor, and avoiding invasive procedures if possible. When venipuncture is unavoidable, pressure is exerted on the puncture site for at least 20 min or until the bleeding stops. During active bleeding, the patient maintains strict bedrest, with the head of the bed elevated to prevent gravity-related intracranial pressure increases, possibly leading to intracranial bleeding. All areas of petechiae and ecchymoses are protected from further injury. Rest periods are provided between activities if the patient tires easily. Both patient and family are encouraged to discuss their concerns about the disease and its treatment, and emotional support is provided and questions answered honestly. The nurse reassures the patient that areas of petechiae and ecchymoses will heal as the disease resolves. The patient should avoid taking aspirin in any form as well as any other drugs that impair coagulation including nonsteroidal anti-inflammatory drugs listed on the labels of nonprescription remedies. If the patient experiences frequent nosebleeds, the patient should use a humidifier at night and should moisten the inner nostrils twice a day with an anti-infective ointment. The nurse teaches the patient to monitor the condition by examining the skin for petechiae and ecchymoses and demonstrates the correct method to test stools for occult blood. If the patient is receiving corticosteroid therapy, fluid and electrolyte balance is monitored and the patient is assessed for signs of infection, pathological fractures, and mood changes. If the patient is receiving blood or blood components, they are administered according to protocol; vital signs are monitored before, during, and after the transfusion, and the patient is observed closely for adverse reactions. If the patient is receiving immunosuppressants, the patient is monitored closely for signs of bone marrow depression, opportunistic infections, mucositis, G.I. tract ulceration, and severe diarrhea or vomiting. If the patient is scheduled for a splenectomy, the nurse determines the patient's understanding of the procedure, corrects misinformation, administers prescribed blood transfusions, explains postoperative care and expected activities and sensations, ensures that a signed informed consent has been obtained, and prepares the patient physically (according to institutional or surgeon's protocol) and emotionally for the surgery. The patient with chronic ITP should wear or carry a medical identification device.

***p. nervosa*** Henoch p.

***nonthrombocytopenic p.*** Allergic p.

***p. rheumatica*** Purpura with joint pain, colic, bloody stools, and vomiting of blood.

***Schönlein-Henoch p.*** Purpura due to vasculitis. It was first described by William Heberden prior to 1800, by Schönlein in 1830, and by Henoch in the 1870s. The skin lesions are obvious, but the visceral lesions are difficult to diagnose and are very serious. The cause is unknown, but allergy or drug sensitivity is important in some cases. There is no specific treatment unless a specific allergen can be identified and then removed. SYN: *anaphylactoid p.* SEE: illus.

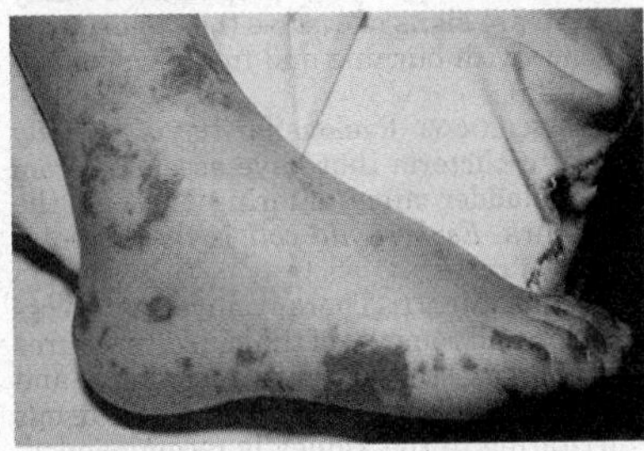

SCHÖNLEIN-HENOCH PURPURA

***senile p.*** Purpura occurring in debilitated and aged persons with ecchymoses and petechiae on the legs.

***p. simplex*** Purpura that is not associated with systemic illness.

***thrombocytopenic p.*** Idiopathic thrombocytopenic p.

***thrombopenic p.*** Idiopathic thrombocytopenic p.

***thrombotic thrombocytopenic p.*** A rare disease characterized by embolism and thrombosis of the small blood vessels of the brain. Shifting neurological signs such as aphasia, blindness, and convulsions are present. Therapy has been of little value, but adrenal corticosteroids in large doses have been tried. Exchange transfusions have been of some help in treating this disease.

**purpureaglycosides A and B** (pŭr-pū″rē-ă-glī′kō-sīds) True cardiac glycosides present in the leaves of *Digitalis purpurea,* foxglove.

**purpuric** (pŭr-pū′rĭk) [L. *purpura,* purple] Pert. to, resembling, or suffering from purpura.

**purring thrill** A vibration, like a cat's purring, due to mitral stenosis, aneurysm, or valvular disease of the heart; felt by palpation over the precordium.

**purulence** (pūr′ū-lĕns) [L. *purulentus,* full of pus] The state of containing pus. SYN: *suppuration.*

**purulency** (pūr′ū-lĕn″sē) Purulence.

**purulent** (pūr′ū-lĕnt) [L. *purulentus,* full of pus] Suppurative; forming or containing pus. SEE: *sputum.*

**puruloid** (pūr′ū-loyd) [L. *pus,* pus, + Gr. *eidos,* form, shape] Like pus. SYN: *puriform.*

**pus** (pŭs) [L.] The liquid product of inflammation composed of albuminous substances, a thin fluid, and leukocytes; generally yellow in color. If red, it suggests rupture of small vessels. If blue or green, it indicates the presence of *Pseudomonas aeruginosa.* Streptococci, staphylococci, gonococci, pneumococci, and other species of bacteria cause the formation of pus.

***blue p.*** Purulence with a blue tint; usually associated with infection due to *Pseudomonas aeruginosa.*

***cheesy p.*** Very thick pus.

***ichorous p.*** Pus that is thin with shreds of sloughing tissue. It may have a fetid odor.

**pustula** (pŭs′tū-lă) [L., blister] Pustule.

**pustulant** (pŭs′tū-lănt) [L. *pustula,* blister] **1.** Causing pustules. **2.** An agent that produces the formation of pustules.

**pustular** (pŭs′tū-lĕr) Pert. to, or characterized by, pustules.

**pustulation** (pŭs″tū-lā′shŭn) The development of pustules.

**pustule** (pŭs′tūl) [L. *pustula,* blister] A small elevation of the skin filled with lymph or pus. Pustules may be circumscribed, flat, rounded, or umbilicated. They occur in eczema pustulosum, acne vulgaris, dermatitis herpetiformis, impetigo simplex, ecthyma, varicella, syphilis, and smallpox. SEE: *pus.*

**pustulocrustaceous** (pŭs″tū-lō-krŭs-tā′shŭs) [″ + *crusta,* shell] Characterized by formation of pustules and crusts.

**pustulosis** (pŭs″tū-lō′sĭs) [″ + Gr. *osis,* condition] A generalized eruption of pustules.

**putamen** (pū-tā′mĕn) [L., shell] The darker outer layer of the lenticular nucleus.

**Putnam-Dana syndrome** (pŭt′năm-dā′nă) [James J. Putnam, U.S. neurologist, 1846–1918; Charles L. Dana, U.S. neurologist, 1852–1935] Subacute combined degeneration of the spinal cord that may be present in patients with untreated pernicious anemia.

**putrefaction** (pū″trē-făk′shŭn) [L. *putrefactio*] Decomposition of animal matter, esp. protein associated with malodorous and poisonous products such as the ptomaines, mercaptans, and hydrogen sulfide, caused by certain kinds of bacteria and fungi. Decomposition occurring spontaneously in sterile tissue after death is called autolysis. SEE: *sepsis.*

***intestinal p.*** The chemical changes by bacteria in the intestine, forming indole, skatole, paracresol, phenol, phenylpropionic acid, phenylacetic acid, paraoxyphenylacetic acid, hydroparacumaric acid, fatty acids, carbon dioxide, hydrogen, methane, methylmercaptan, and sulfurated hydrogen.

**putrefactive** (pū″trĕ-făk′tĭv) [L. *putrefacere,* to putrefy] **1.** Causing, or pert. to, putrefaction. **2.** Agent promoting putrefaction.

**putrefy** (pū′trĕ-fī) [L. *putrefacere,* to putrefy] To undergo putrefaction.

**putrescence** (pū-trĕs′ĕns) [L. *putrescens,* grow rotten] Decay; rottenness.

**putrescine** (pū-trĕs′ĭn) A poisonous polyamine formed by bacterial action on the amino acid arginine.

**putrid** (pū′trĭd) [L. *putridus*] Decayed; rotten; foul.

**PUVA therapy** [*p*soralen + *u*ltra*v*iolet *A*] Treatment of psoriasis by the use of a psoralen and high-intensity long-wave ultraviolet light. SEE: *psoralen; psoriasis.*

**PVC** *polyvinyl chloride; premature ventricular contraction.*

**P$\bar{v}O_2$** *partial pressure of oxygen in mixed venous blood.*

**PVP** *polyvinylpyrrolidone.*

**PVP-iodine** *povidone-iodine.*

**PWA** *person with AIDS.*

**PWB** *partial weight bearing.*

**pyarthrosis** (pī″ăr-thrō′sĭs) [Gr. *pyon,* pus, + *arthron,* joint, + *osis,* condition] Pus in the cavity of a joint.

**pycno-, pycn-** (pĭk′nō) [Gr. *pyknos,* thick] Combining form meaning *dense, thick, compact, frequent.* SEE: also *pykno-.*

**pyecchysis** (pī-ĕk′ĭ-sĭs) [Gr. *pyon,* pus, + *ek,* out, + *chein,* to pour] An effusion of pus.

**pyelectasia, pyelectasis** (pī″ĕ-lĕk-tā′zē-ă, -lĕk′tăs-ĭs) [Gr. *pyelos,* pelvis, + *ektasis,* dilatation] Dilatation of the renal pelvis.

**pyelitic** (pī″ĕ-lĭt′ĭk) Relating to, or affected with, pyelitis.

**pyelitis** (pī″ĕ-lī′tĭs) [Gr. *pyelos,* pelvis, + *itis,* inflammation] Inflammation of the pelvis of the kidney and its calices.

***calculous p.*** Pyelitis resulting from a calculus.

***p. cystica*** Pyelitis associated with multiple small cysts in the mucosa of the renal pelvis.

**pyelo-** [Gr. *pyelos,* pelvis] Combining form meaning *pelvis.*

**pyelocaliectasis** (pī″ĕ-lō-kăl″ē-ĕk′tă-sĭs) [″ + *kalyx,* cup, + *ektasis,* dilation] Dilation of the pelvis and calices of the kidney.

**pyelocystitis** (pī″ĕ-lō-sĭs-tī′tĭs) [″ + *kystis,* bladder, + *itis,* inflammation] Inflammation of the renal pelvis and bladder.

**pyelocystostomosis** (pī″ĕ-lō-sĭs″tō-stō-mō′sĭs) [″ + ″ + *stoma,* mouth, + *osis,* condition] The surgical establishment of communication between the kidney and bladder.

**pyelogram** (pī′ĕ-lō-grăm) [Gr. *pyelos,* pelvis, + *gramma,* something written] A radiograph of the ureter and renal pelvis.

***intravenous p.*** ABBR: I.V.P. A pyelogram in which a radiopaque material is given intravenously. Multiple radiographs of the urinary tract taken while the material is excreted provide important information about the structure and function of the kidney, ureter, and bladder. Any blockage along this tract is readily detected by this examination.

**pyelography** (pī″ĕ-lŏg′ră-fē) [″ + *graphein,* to write] Radiography of the renal pelvis and ureter after injection of a radiopaque contrast medium.

**pyelolithotomy** (pī″ĕ-lō-lĭth-ŏt′ō-mē) [″ + *lithos,* stone, + *tome,* incision] The removal of calculus from the pelvis of a kidney through an incision.

**pyelonephritis** (pī″ĕ-lō-nĕ-frī′tĭs) [″ + *nephros,* kidney, + *itis,* inflammation] Inflammation of kidney and renal pelvis. SEE: *Nursing Diagnoses Appendix.*

SYMPTOMS: This condition is characterized by the sudden onset of chills and fever with dull pain in the flank over either or both kidneys. There is tenderness when the kidney is palpated. Usually there are signs of cystitis (i.e., pyuria, urgency with burning and frequency of urination).

ETIOLOGY: Pyelonephritis is usually due to bacteria that have ascended from the bladder after entering through the urethra. *Escherichia coli* is the cause in 85% of cases.

TREATMENT: Therapy involves recognition and removal of the cause, measures to increase the patient's resistance, and bedrest. Avoidance of alcohol and drugs irritating to the kidney is recommended. Heat should be applied to flanks and antipyretic drugs and an appropriate antibiotic given. If there is urinary tract obstruction, surgery may be indicated.

PROGNOSIS: The outcome depends on the character and virulence of the infection, accessory etiological factors, drainage of the kidney, presence or absence of complications, and general physical condition of the patient. SEE: *glomerulonephritis.*

NURSING IMPLICATIONS: Antibiotics and antipyretics are administered as prescribed. The patient is encouraged to complete the full course of antibiotics and drink 2 to 3 L of fluids per day to prevent urinary stasis and to flush byproducts of the inflammatory process. The nurse teaches the patient the proper technique for collecting clean-catch urine specimens, including refrigerating them within 30 min of collection. Weight is monitored, and any significant gain is reported. The patient should report any signs of infection and seek immediate follow-up care. Emotional support is provided to the patient and family.

**pyelonephrosis** (pī″ĕ-lō-nĕ-frō′sĭs) [″ + ″ + *osis,* condition] Any disease of the pelvis of the kidney. SYN: *pyelopathy.*

**pyelopathy** (pī″ĕ-lŏp′ăth-ē) [″ + *pathos,* disease, suffering] Pyelonephrosis.

**pyeloplasty** (pī′ĕ-lō-plăs″tē) [″ + *plastos,* formed] Reparative surgery on the pelvis of the kidney.

**pyeloplication** (pī″ĕ-lō-plĭ-kā′shŭn) [″ + L. *plicare,* to fold] Shortening of the wall of a dilated renal pelvis by taking tucks in it.

**pyelostomy** (pī″ĕ-lŏs′tō-mē) [″ + *stoma,* mouth] Creation of an opening into the renal pelvis.

**pyelotomy** (pī″ĕ-lŏt′ō-mē) [″ + *tome,* incision] Incision of the renal pelvis.

NURSING IMPLICATIONS: All catheters should be secured to the patient to prevent dislodgement. The nurse should assess and record the appearance of the urine, including color, consistency, and amount. Catheter drainage tubing must be kept free of kinks. Catheters should never be clamped. The nurse should monitor and record intake and output. After removal of the catheter, a stoma-bag collection device should be used to collect any drainage and maintain skin integrity while the wound heals.

**pyeloureterectasis** Dilatation of the pelvis of the kidney and ureter.

**pyemia** (pī-ē′mē-ă) [″ + *haima,* blood] A form of septicemia due to the presence of pus-forming organisms in the blood, manifested by formation of multiple abscesses of a metastatic nature.

SYMPTOMS: The disease is characterized by intermittent high temperature with recurrent chills; metastatic processes in various parts of the body, esp. in lungs; septic pneumonia, empyema. It may be fatal.

TREATMENT: Antibiotics are effective. Prophylactic treatment consists in prevention of suppuration.

***arterial p.*** Pyemia resulting from dissemination of emboli from a thrombus in cardiac vessels.

***cryptogenic p.*** Pyemia of an origin that is hidden in the deeper tissues.

***metastatic p.*** Multiple abscesses resulting from infected pyemic thrombi.

***portal p.*** Suppurative inflammation of the portal vein.

**pyemic** (pī-ē′mĭk) [Gr. *pyon,* pus, + *haima,* blood] Relating to, or affected with, septicemia.

**Pyemotes** (pī-ĕ-mō′tēz) A genus of mites parasitic on the larvae of insects.

***P. ventricosus*** A mite present in the straw of some cereals, contact with which causes a vesiculopapular dermatitis in humans. This is called grain itch.

**pyencephalus** (pī″ĕn-sĕf′ă-lŭs) [″ + *enkephalos,* brain] A brain abscess with suppuration within the cranium. SYN: *pyocephalus.*

**pyg-** SEE: *pygo-.*

**pygal** (pī′găl) [Gr. *pyge,* rump] Concerning the buttocks. SEE: *steatopygia.*

**pygalgia** (pī-găl′jē-ă) [″ + *algos,* pain] Pain in the buttocks.

**pygmalionism** (pĭg-mā′lē-ŏn-ĭzm) [named for Pygmalion, a sculptor and king in Gr. mythology, who fell in love with a figure he carved] The psychopathic condition of falling in love with one's own creation.

**pygmy** (pĭg′mē) A very small person, a dwarf.

**pygo-, pyg-** Combining form meaning *buttocks.*

**pygoamorphus** (pī″gō-ă-mor′fŭs) [Gr. *pyge,* rump, + *a-,* not, + *morphe,* form] Conjoined twins in which the parasite, joined to the buttocks, is an amorphous mass of tissue, or a teratoma.

**pygodidymus** (pī″gō-dĭd′ĭ-mŭs) [″ + *didymos,* twin] Conjoined twins with fusion of the cephalothoracic area, but with doubling of the pelvis and extremities.

**pygomelus** (pī-gŏm′ĕ-lŭs) [″ + *melos,* limb] Unequal conjoined twins with the parasite represented by an accessory limb attached to the pelvic area.

**pykn-** SEE: *pykno-.*

**pyknic** (pĭk′nĭk) [Gr. *pyknos,* thick] Pert. to a body type characterized by roundness of the extremities, stockiness, large chest and abdomen, and tendency to obesity.

**pykno-, pykn-** [Gr. *pyknos,* thick] Combining form meaning *thick, compact, dense, frequent.* SEE: also *pycno-.*

**pyknocyte** (pĭk′nō-sīt) [″ + *kytos,* cell] A form of spiculed red cell. SEE: *spiculed red cell.*

**pyknodysostosis** (pĭk″nō-dĭs″ŏs-tō′sĭs) [″ + *dys,* bad, + *osteon,* bone, + *osis,* condition] An autosomal recessive disease that affects bones and resembles osteopetrosis, but the disease is mild and not associated with hematological or neurological abnormalities. The children have short stature, open fontanels, frontal bossing, hypoplastic facial bones, blue sclerae, and dental abnormalities. There may be double rows of malformed teeth. Despite the multiple abnormalities, life span is unaffected. The patient usually seeks medical care because of frequent fractures. The only treatment is surgical correction of deformities and fractures.

**pyknomorphous** (pĭk″nō-morf′ŭs) [″ + *morphe,* form] Characterized by compact arrangement of the stainable portions, said esp. of certain nerve cells.

**pyknophrasia** (pĭk″nō-frā′zē-ă) [″ + *phrasis,* speech] Thickness of words uttered in speech.

**pyknosis** (pĭk-nō′sĭs) [″ + *osis,* condition] Thickness, esp. shrinking of cells through degeneration. SYN: *inspissation.*

**pyle-** [Gr. *pyle,* gate] Combining form meaning *orifice,* esp. that of the portal vein.

**pylemphraxis** (pī″lĕm-frăk′sĭs) [″ + *emphraxis,* stoppage] Occlusion of the portal vein.

**pylephlebectasia, pylephlebectasis** (pī″lē-flē-bĕk-tā′zē-ă, -bĕk′tă-sĭs) [″ + *phleps,* vein, + *ektasis,* dilatation] Distention of the portal vein.

**pylephlebitis** (pī″lē-flē-bī′tĭs) [″ + ″ + *itis,* inflammation] Inflammation of the portal vein, generally suppurative.

***adhesive p.*** Thrombosis of the portal vein.

***p. obturans*** Pylephlebitis with obstructed flow in the portal vein.

**pylethrombophlebitis** (pī″lē-thrŏm″bō-flē-bī′tĭs) [″ + *thrombos,* clot, + *phleps,* vein, + *itis,* inflammation] Thrombosis and inflammation of the portal vein.

**pylethrombosis** (pī″lē-thrŏm-bō′sĭs) [Gr. *pyle,* gate, + *thrombos,* clot, + *osis,* condition] Occlusion of the portal vein by a thrombus.

**pylon** (pī′lŏn) A temporary artificial leg.

**pylorectomy** (pī″lō-rĕk′tō-mē) [″ + *ektome,* excision] Surgical removal of the pylorus.

**pyloric** (pī-lor′ĭk) [Gr. *pyloros,* gatekeeper] Pert. to the distal portion of the stomach or to the opening between the stomach and duodenum.

**pyloric canal** The narrow constricted region of the pyloric portion of the stomach that opens through the pylorus into the duodenum.

**pyloric cap** The first part of the duodenum.

**pyloric obstruction and dilatation** Blockage of the lower orifice of the stomach with consequent hypertrophy and dilatation. Pyloric obstruction increases the resistance offered to the expulsion of food from the stomach. The causes of dilatation are pyloric obstruction, laxness of walls from simple atony, or excessive ingestion of food or drink.

SYMPTOMS: The general symptoms are dyspepsia and the following symptoms relating to vomiting. Vomiting occurs long after eating, sometimes several hours or days. The amount is often excessive, sometimes several quarts; it is sour and fermented, and on standing it separates into a sediment of undigested food and a turbid, frothy liquid. Ejected fluid is rich in torulae and sarcinae, forms of bacteria. Obstinate constipation is present. There is bulging over the epigastrium. In thin subjects, the outline of the stomach may be visible. Palpation gives a splashing fremitus. In percussion there is an increased area of gastric tympany. In auscultation, splashing sounds often are audible at some distance.

TREATMENT: Therapy involves a light, nutritious, not bulky diet that should be given in small amounts at frequent intervals.

PROGNOSIS: The outcome is guarded, depending on the cause, and is more favorable in dilatation without obstruction.

**pyloric sphincter** The thickened circular smooth muscle around the pyloric orifice at the junction of the stomach and duodenum. The sphincter is usually contracted but relaxes at intervals (when gastric pressure exceeds duodenal pressure) to permit acid chyme to enter the duodenum. It then contracts to prevent backup of chyme to the stomach.

**pyloric stenosis** Narrowing of the pyloric orifice, which may be due to excessive thickening of the pyloric sphincter (hypertrophic pyloric stenosis) or hypertrophy and hyperplasia of mucosa and submucosa. Treatment involves surgical section of the thickened muscle around the pyloric orifice.

NURSING IMPLICATIONS: *Preoperative:* The nurse positions the infant to prevent aspiration, feeds and observes the infant after feeding, obtains accurate daily weights, records vomitus, provides pacifier as needed, monitors and records administration of parenteral fluids, charts intake and output, and instructs parents concerning surgery.

*Postoperative:* Parenteral fluids are administered as prescribed, and a nothing by mouth restriction is continued for 12 to 24 hr. Parents are instructed about deep-breathing exercises, and the infant is turned and positioned at scheduled intervals. Oral feedings are increased gradually, and the infant is positioned in the upright position for 1 hr after feeding to prevent aspiration. The nurse instructs the parents in care of the infant and provides visual stimulation. Before discharge, the parents learn how to meet the infant's needs at home, and a schedule for follow-up is established.

**pyloristenosis** (pī-lor″ĭ-stĕn-ō′sĭs) [Gr. *pyloros,* gatekeeper, + *stenos,* narrow] Constriction of the pylorus.

**pyloritis** (pī″lō-rī′tĭs) [″ + *itis,* inflammation] Inflammation of the pylorus.

**pyloro-** Combining form meaning *gatekeeper,* applied to the pylorus.

**pylorodiosis** (pī-lō″rō-dī-ō′sĭs) [Gr. *pyloros,* gatekeeper, + *diosis,* pushing under] Dilation of the pylorus of the stomach.

**pyloroduodenitis** (pī-lor″ō-dū″ō-dē-nī′tĭs) [″ + L. *duodeni,* twelve, + Gr. *itis,* inflammation] Inflammation of the mucosa of the pyloric outlet of the stomach and duodenum.

**pylorogastrectomy** (pī-lor″ō-găs-trĕk′tō-mē) [″ + *gaster,* belly, + *ektome,* excision] Excision of pyloric portion of the stomach.

**pyloromyotomy** (pī-lor″ō-mī-ŏt′ō-mē) [″ + *mys,* muscle, + *tome,* incision] Incision and suture of the pyloric sphincter.

**pyloroplasty** (pī-lor′ō-plăs″tē) [″ + *plassein,* to form] Operation to repair the pylorus, esp. one to increase the caliber of the pyloric opening by stretching.

***Finney p.*** Surgical procedure for enlarging the opening from the stomach to the duodenum.

**pyloroscopy** (pī-lō-rŏs′kō-pē) [Gr. *pyloros,* gatekeeper, + *skopein,* to examine] Fluoroscopic examination of the pylorus.

**pylorospasm** (pī-lor′ō-spăzm) [″ + *spasmos,* a convulsion] Spasmodic contraction of the pyloric orifice. The usual cause is a disturbance in the motor innervation of the pyloric sphincter. It may occur secondary to lesions of the stomach or duodenum near the pyloric orifice.

**pylorostenosis** (pī-lor″ō-stĕn-ō′sĭs) [″ + *stenos,* narrow] Abnormal narrowing or stricture of the pyloric orifice. SEE: *pyloric stenosis.*

**pylorostomy** (pī-lor-ŏs′tō-mē) [″ + *stoma,*

mouth] Formation of an opening through the abdominal wall into the pylorus.

**pylorotomy** (pī-lor-ŏt′ō-mē) [″ + *tome,* incision] Incision of the pyloric submucosa to relieve hypertrophic stenosis.

**pylorus** (pī-lor′ŭs) [Gr. *pyloros,* gatekeeper] **1.** The lower portion of the stomach that opens into the duodenum, consisting of the pyloric antrum and pyloric canal. **2.** In older texts, a term that may be used for the pyloric orifice or the pyloric sphincter. **pyloric,** *adj.*

**pyo-, py-** [Gr. *pyon,* pus] Combining form meaning *pus.*

**pyocele** (pī′ō-sēl) [Gr. *pyon,* pus, + *kele,* tumor, swelling] A hernia or distended cavity containing pus.

**pyocephalus** (pī″ō-sĕf′ă-lŭs) [″ + *kephale,* head] Effusion of purulent nature within the cranium.

**pyococcus** (pī″ō-kŏk′ŭs) [″ + *kokkos,* berry] A micrococcus that causes pus formation, such as *Streptococcus pyogenes.*

**pyocolpocele** (pī″ō-kŏl′pō-sēl) [″ + *kolpos,* vagina, + *kele,* tumor, swelling] A vaginal tumor containing pus. SEE: *pyocolpos.*

**pyocolpos** (pī″ō-kŭl′pōs) Accumulation of pus in the vagina.

**pyocyanic** (pī″ō-sī-ăn′ĭk) [″ + *kyanos,* dark blue] Pert. to pyocyanin or blue pus.

**pyocyst** (pī′ō-sĭst) [″ + *kystis,* sac] A cyst containing pus.

**pyoderma** (pī-ō-dĕr′mă) [″ + *derma,* skin] Any acute, inflammatory, purulent bacterial dermatitis.

***p. gangrenosum*** Pyoderma usually associated with ulcerative colitis or any severe chronic disease that leads to wasting; occurs principally on the trunk.

**pyodermatitis** (pī″ō-dĕr″mă-tī′tĭs) [″ + ″ + *itis,* inflammation] Pyogenic infection of the skin causing a dermatitis.

**pyodermia** (pī″ō-dĕr′mē-ă) Any suppurative skin disease.

**pyogenesis** (pī″ō-jĕn′ĕ-sĭs) [″ + *genesis,* generation, birth] The formation of pus. SYN: *suppuration.*

**pyogenic** (pī-ō-jĕn′ĭk) [″ + *gennan,* to produce] Producing pus.

**pyogenic microorganism** A microorganism that forms pus. The principal ones are *Staphylococcus aureus, Staphylococcus epidermidis, Streptococcus hemolyticus, Bacillus anthracis, Bacillus subtilis, Clostridium perfringens, Pseudomonas aeruginosa,* and *Neisseria gonorrhoeae.* These pathogens also stimulate a huge influx of neutrophils to the site. The pus is formed from dead organisms, white blood cells, and other cells destroyed during the immune response.

**pyohemothorax** (pī″ō-hē″mō-thō′răks) [″ + *haima,* blood, + *thorax,* chest] Pus and blood in the pleural cavity.

**pyoid** (pī′oyd) [″ + *eidos,* form, shape] Resembling pus.

**pyolabyrinthitis** (pī″ō-lăb″ĭ-rĭn-thī′tĭs) [″ + *labyrinthos,* maze, + *itis,* inflammation] Inflammation with suppuration of the labyrinth of the ear.

**pyometra** (pī″ō-mē′tră) [″ + *metra,* uterus] Retained pus accumulation in the uterine cavity.

**pyometritis** (pī″ō-mē-trī′tĭs) [″ + ″ + *itis,* inflammation] Inflammation of the uterus with purulent exudate.

**pyonephritis** (pī″ō-nĕf-rī′tĭs) [″ + *nephros,* kidney, + *itis,* inflammation] Inflammation of the kidney, suppurative in character.

**pyonephrolithiasis** (pī″ō-nĕf″rō-lĭth-ī′ă-sĭs) [″ + ″ + *lithos,* stone, + *-iasis,* condition] Pus and calculi in the kidney.

**pyonephrosis** (pī″ō-nĕf-rō′sĭs) [″ + ″ + *osis,* condition] Pus accumulation in the pelvis of the kidney.

**pyoovarium** (pī″ō-ō-vā′rē-ŭm) [″ + LL. *ovarium,* ovary] Abscess formation in an ovary.

**pyopericarditis** (pī″ō-pĕr″ĭ-kăr-dī′tĭs) [″ + *peri,* around, + *kardia,* heart, + *itis,* inflammation] Pericarditis with suppuration.

**pyopericardium** (pī″ō-pĕr″ĭ-kăr′dē-ŭm) Pus formation in the pericardium.

**pyoperitoneum** (pī″ō-pĕr″ĭ-tō-nē′ŭm) [Gr. *pyon,* pus, + *peritonaion,* peritoneum] Pus formation in the peritoneal cavity.

**pyoperitonitis** (pī″ō-pĕr″ĭ-tō-nī′tĭs) [″ + ″ + *itis,* inflammation] Purulent inflammation of the lining of peritoneum.

**pyophthalmia** (pī″ŏf-thăl′mē-ă) [″ + *ophthalmos,* eye] Pyophthalmitis.

**pyophthalmitis** (pī″ŏf-thăl-mī′tĭs) [″ + ″ + *itis,* inflammation] Suppurative inflammation of the eye. SYN: *pyophthalmia.*

**pyophysometra** (pī″ō-fī″sō-mē′tră) [″ + *physa,* air, + *metra,* uterus] Pus and gas accumulation in the uterus.

**pyopneumocholecystitis** (pī″ō-nū″mō-kō-lē-sĭs-tī′tĭs) [″ + *pneuma,* air, + *chole,* bile, + *kystis,* sac, + *itis,* inflammation] Distention of the gallbladder with air and pus.

**pyopneumocyst** (pī″ō-nū′mō-sĭst) [″ + ″ + *kystis,* bladder] A cyst enclosing pus and gas.

**pyopneumohepatitis** (pī″ō-nū″mō-hĕp″ă-tī′tĭs) [″ + *pneuma,* air, + *hepar,* liver, + *itis,* inflammation] A liver abscess with gas in the abscess cavity.

**pyopneumopericardium** (pī″ō-nū″mō-pĕr″ĭ-kăr′dē-ŭm) [″ + ″ + *peri,* around, + *kardia,* heart] Pus and air or gas in the pericardium.

**pyopneumoperitoneum** (pī″ō-nū″mō-pĕr″ĭ-tō-nē′ŭm) [″ + ″ + *peritonaion,* peritoneum] Peritonitis with gas and pus in the peritoneal cavity.

**pyopneumoperitonitis** (pī″ō-nū″mō-pĕr″ĭ-tō-nī′tĭs) [″ + ″ + ″ + *itis,* inflammation] Pus and air in the peritoneal cavity complicating peritonitis.

**pyopneumothorax** (pī″ō-nū″mō-thō′răks) [″ + ″ + *thorax,* chest] The presence of pus and gas in the pleural cavity.

**pyoptysis** (pī-ŏp′tĭ-sĭs) [″ + *ptysis,* spitting] Spitting of pus.

**pyopyelectasis** (pī″ō-pī″ĕ-lĕk′tă-sĭs) [″ +

*pyelos*, pelvis, + *ektasis*, dilation] Purulent fluid in the dilated renal pelvis.

**pyorrhea** (pī″ō-rē′ă) [″ + *rhoia*, flow] A discharge of purulent matter.

**pyosalpingitis** (pī″ō-săl″pĭn-jī′tĭs) [Gr. *pyon*, pus, + *salpinx*, tube, + *itis*, inflammation] Retained pus in the oviduct with inflammation.

**pyosalpingo-oophoritis** (pī″ō-săl-pĭn″gō-ō″ŏf-ō-rī′tĭs) [″ + ″ + *oon*, ovum, + *phoros*, a bearer, + *itis*, inflammation] Inflammation of the ovary and oviduct, with suppuration.

**pyosalpinx** (pī″ō-săl′pĭnks) Pus in the fallopian tube.

**pyosemia** (pī″ō-sē′mē-ă) [Gr. *pyon*, pus, + L. *semen*, seed] Pus in the semen.

**pyostatic** (pī″ō-stăt′ĭk) [″ + *statikos*, standing] **1.** Preventing pus formation. **2.** An agent preventing the development of pus.

**pyothorax** (pī″ō-thō′răks) [″ + *thorax*, chest] Empyema.

**pyotorrhea** (pī″ō-tō-rē′ă) [″ + *ous*, ear, + *rhoia*, flow] Purulent discharge from the ear.

**pyourachus** (pī″ō-ū′ră-kŭs) [″ + *ourachos*, fetal urinary canal] Accumulation of pus in the urachus.

**pyoureter** (pī″ō-ū-rē′tĕr) [″ + *oureter*, ureter] Pus collection in the ureter.

**pyovesiculosis** (pī″ō-vĕ-sĭk″ū-lō′sĭs) [″ + L. *vesiculus*, a small vessel, + Gr. *osis*, condition] Pus collection in the seminal vesicles.

**pyoxanthin(e)** (pī″ō-zăn′thĭn) [″ + *xanthos*, yellow] A yellow pigment resulting from oxidation of pyocyanin, sometimes present in pus.

**pyramid** (pĭr′ă-mĭd) [Gr. *pyramis*, a pyramid] **1.** A solid on the base with three or more triangular sides that meet at an apex. **2.** Any part of the body resembling a pyramid. **3.** A compact bundle of nerve fibers in the medulla oblongata. **4.** The petrous portion of the temporal bone. SYN: *pyramis*.

***p. of the cerebellum*** A median ventral projection of the vermis of the cerebellum lying between the tuber and uvula.

***p. of light*** The triangular light reflex from the typanic membrane of the ear.

***malpighian p.*** Renal p.

***p. of the medulla*** One of a pair of elongated tapering prominences on the anterior surface of the medulla oblongata, composed of descending corticospinal fibers.

***renal p.*** One of a number of cone-shaped structures making up the medulla of the kidney along with renal columns. Each pyramid has its base adjacent to the renal cortex, with the apex projecting as a renal papilla into a calyx of the renal pelvis. Parts of the nephron found in a pyramid are the loops of Henle and collecting tubules; a papillary duct terminates at the apex and empties urine into the renal pelvis. The pyramids converge. SYN: *malpighian p.*

***p. of the temporal bone*** The pyramis or petrous portion of the temporal bone.

***p. of the thyroid*** A conical process sometimes present, extending cephalad from the isthmus of the thyroid gland.

***p. of the tympanum*** A hollow projection on the inner wall of the middle ear through which passes the stapedius muscle.

**pyramidal** (pĭ-răm′ĭ-dăl) [L. *pyramidalis*] In the shape of a pyramid.

**pyramidalis** (pĭ-răm″ĭ-dăl′ĭs) [L.] The muscle that arises from the crest of the pubis and is inserted into the linea alba upward about halfway to the navel.

***p. auriculae*** A small muscle inserted into the auricle of the ear. It is often absent.

**pyramidotomy** (pĭ-răm-ĭ-dŏt′ō-mē) [Gr. *pyramis*, a pyramid, + *tome*, incision] Excision of the pyramidal tracts of the spinal cord in order to alleviate involuntary muscular movements.

**pyran** (pī′răn) The compound $C_5H_6O$, the ring structure of which consists of five carbon atoms and one oxygen atom.

**pyranose** (pī′ră-nōs) A cyclic sugar or glycoside with a structure similar to a pyran.

**pyrantel pamoate** (pĭ-răn′tĕl) A drug used in treating the parasitic diseases ascariasis and enterobiasis, as well as those caused by *Ancylostoma*, *Necator americanus*, and *Trichostrongylus*.

**pyrazinamide** (pī″ră-zĭn′ă-mīd) A drug used in treating tuberculosis. It is used in treating persons who are resistant to usually effective agents.

**pyrectic** (pī-rĕk′tĭk) Concerning fever.

**pyrenemia** (pī″rĕ-nē′mē-ă) [Gr. *pyren*, fruit stone, + *haima*, blood] A condition in which there are nucleated red cells in the blood.

**pyretherapy** (pī″rĕ-thĕr′ă-pē) [Gr. *pyr*, fever, + *therapeia*, treatment] Treatment by artificially raising the patient's temperature.

**pyrethrins** (pī-rē′thrĭnz) The general name given to substances derived from pyrethrum flowers (chrysanthemums); used as insecticides.

**pyretic** (pī-rĕt′ĭk) [Gr. *pyretos*, fever] Concerning fever.

**pyreto-** (pī-rĕt′ō) Prefix indicating *fever*.

**pyretogenesia, pyretogenesis** (pī″rĕ-tō-jĕn-ē′zē-ă, -jĕn′ĕ-sĭs) [″ + *genesis*, generation, birth] Origin and production of fever.

**pyretogenic bacteria** Pathogenic bacteria causing fever.

**pyretolysis** (pī″rĕ-tŏl′ĭ-sĭs) [″ + *lysis*, dissolution] **1.** Reduction of fever. **2.** Lysis of symptoms of a disease process that is accelerated by fever.

**pyretotyphosis** (pī″rĕ-tō-tī-fō′sĭs) [″ + *typhosis*, delirium] The delirious or stuporous condition characteristic of high fever.

**pyrexia** (pī-rĕk′sē-ă) [Gr. *pyressein*, to be feverish] Fever.

**pyrexin** (pī′rĕks′ĭn) A substance extracted from inflammatory exudates that induces fever.

**pyridine** (pēr′ĭ-dēn) A colorless, volatile liquid with a charred odor. It is obtained by dry distillation of nitrogen-containing organic matter. It is used as an industrial solvent.

**pyridostigmine bromide** (pēr″ĭ-dō-stĭg′mēn) An anticholinesterase drug used in treating myasthenia gravis.

**pyridoxal 5-phosphate** A derivative of pyridoxine. It serves as a coenzyme of certain amino-acid decarboxylases in bacteria, and in animal tissues of 3,4-dihydroxyphenylalanine (dopa) decarboxylase.

**pyridoxamine** (pĭr″ĭ-dŏks′ă-mīn) One of the vitamin $B_6$ group; a 4-aminoethyl analog of pyridoxine.

**4-pyridoxic acid** (pĭr″ĭ-dŏks′ĭk) The principal end product of pyridoxine metabolism excreted in human urine.

**pyridoxine hydrochloride** (pĭ-rĭ-dŏks′ēn) One of a group of substances, including pyridoxal and pyridoxamine, that make up vitamin $B_6$. SEE: *vitamin* $B_6$ in *Vitamins Appendix.*

**pyriform** (pĭr′ĭ-form) [L. *pirum,* pear, + *forma,* shape] Shaped like a pear. Also spelled piriform.

**pyrilamine maleate** (pĭ-rĭl′ă-mēn) A histamine antagonist drug used in treating certain allergic diseases.

**pyrimethamine** (pĭr-ĭ-mĕth′ă-mēn) An antimalarial drug used in prophylaxis against malaria rather than in treatment of an acute attack. Trade name is Daraprim.

**pyrimidine** (pĭ-rĭm′ĭd-ĭn) The parent of a group of heterocyclic nitrogen compounds, $C_4H_4N_2$, including uracil, cytosine, and thymine, some of which are components of nucleic acid.

**pyrithiamine** (pĭr″ĭ-thī′ă-mĭn) A synthetic analog of thiamine that acts as an antithiamine substance. When administered, it produces many of the symptoms of thiamine deficiency.

**pyro-** (pī′rō) [Gr. *pyr,* fire] Prefix meaning *heat, fire.*

**pyrogallol** (pī″rō-găl′ōl) $C_6H_6O_3$. A toxic chemical derived from gallic acid.

**pyrogen** (pī′rō-jĕn) [Gr. *pyr,* fire, + *gennan,* to produce] Any agent that causes fever. These substances may be exogenous, such as bacteria or viruses, or endogenous, produced in the body. The latter are usually in response to stimuli accompanying infection or inflammation.

Caution: A fluid that has been opened previously and allowed to stand should not be given intravenously, even though the top may have been closed tightly, because pyrogens will have formed.

***leukocytic p.*** A substance found in the blood during a fever that acts upon the thermoregulatory centers of the hypothalamus.

**pyrogenic** (pī″rō-jĕn′ĭk) [Gr. *pyr,* fire, + *gennan,* to produce] Producing fever.

**pyroglobulinemia** (pī″rō-glŏb″ū-lĭ-nē′mē-ă) [″ + *globulus,* globule, + *haima,* blood] The presence of an abnormal globulin in the blood of patients with multiple myeloma and certain other diseases. The globulin is irreversibly precipitated when heated to 56°C.

**pyrolysis** (pī-rŏl′ĭ-sĭs) [″ + *lysis,* dissolution] The decomposition of organic matter when there is a rise in temperature.

**pyromania** (pī″rō-mā′nē-ă) [″ + *mania,* madness] Fire madness; a mania for setting fires or seeing them.

**pyrometer** (pī-rŏm′ĕ-tĕr) [″ + *metron,* measure] A device for measuring temperature.

**pyronine** (pī′rō-nĭn) A histological stain used to demonstrate the presence of RNA and DNA.

**pyronyxis** (pī″rō-nĭk′sĭs) [″ + *nyxis,* a piercing] Treatment or cauterization by puncturing a part with hot needles.

**pyrophobia** (pī″rō-fō′bē-ă) [″ + *phobos,* fear] Abnormal fear of fire.

**pyrophosphatase** (pī″rō-fŏs′fă-tās) An enzyme that catalyzes splitting of phosphoric groups.

**pyrophosphate** (pī″rō-fŏs′fāt) Any salt of phosphoric acid.

**pyroptothymia** (pī″rŏp-tō-thī′mē-ă) [″ + *ptoein,* to scare, + *thymos,* mind] A psychosis in which one imagines himself or herself surrounded by flames.

**pyropuncture** (pī″rō-pŭnk′chūr) [″ + L. *punctura,* piercing] Treatment by puncture of a part with hot needles. SEE: *counterirritation.*

**pyrosis** (pī-rō′sĭs) [Gr. *pyrosis,* burning] Heartburn.

NURSING IMPLICATIONS: The nurse assesses the meaning of this term to the patient and determines the exact location, timing, and duration of discomfort. If position changes exaggerate discomfort, precipitating factors (such as type and amount of food), method of relief, and factors that aggravate the discomfort are determined.

**pyrotic** (pī-rŏt′ĭk) [Gr. *pyrotikos*] **1.** Caustic; burning. **2.** Pert. to pyrosis.

**pyrotoxin** (pī″rō-tŏk′sĭn) [Gr. *pyr,* fire, + *toxikon,* poison] A toxin produced during a febrile disease.

**pyroxylin** (pī-rŏk′sĭ-lĭn) A substance obtained by the action of a mixture of nitric and sulfuric acids on cotton. It consists chiefly of cellulose tetranitrate and is combined with ether and alcohol to form collodion.

Caution: Pyroxylin and collodion are exceedingly flammable.

**pyrrobutamine phosphate** (pēr″rō-bū′tă-mēn) An antihistamine drug.

**pyrrole** (pēr′ŏl) A heterocyclic substance

that provides the building blocks for a large number of vital compounds such as hemoglobin, chlorophyll, and bile acids. It is a colorless liquid with the odor of chloroform.

**pyrrolidine** (pĭ-rŏl′ĭ-dĭn) Tetramethylamine, $(CH_2)_4NH$. It may be obtained from pyrrole or tobacco, which contains pyrrole.

**pyruvate** (pī′roo-vāt) A salt or ester of pyruvic acid.

**pyrvinium pamoate** (pĭr-vĭn′ē-ŭm) A cyanine dye drug used in treating pinworms.

**pythogenesis** (pī″thō-jĕn′ĕ-sĭs) [Gr. *pythein,* to rot, + *genesis,* generation, birth] Originating in decaying matter.

**pyuria** (pī-ū′rē-ă) [Gr. *pyon,* pus, + *ouron,* urine] Pus in the urine; evidence of renal disease; a condition in which there are more than the normal number of pus or white blood cells in the urine. Freshly passed urine may be cloudy due to the presence of phosphates or pus. If the former are present, the addition of acid will cause it to clear; if the latter, it will not clear but may become gelatinous. The etiology includes lesion of the urethra, ureters, bladder, or kidneys, and infection.

**PZI** *protamine zinc insulin.* SEE: *insulin.*

**Q 1.** *quantity*. **2.** Symbol for coulomb.

**q** Symbol for long arm of a chromosome.

**Q angle** The acute angle formed by a line from the anterior superior iliac spine of the pelvis through the center of the patella and a line from the tibial tubercle through the patella. The angle describes the tracking of the patella in the trochlear groove of the femur. The normal angle is around 15 degrees. It is usually greater in females.

**$Qco_2$** The number of microliters of $CO_2$ given off per milligram of dry weight of tissue per hour.

**q.d.** L. *quaque die,* every day.

**Q fever** [Q is for *query* because its etiology was unknown] An acute infectious disease characterized by headache, fever, severe sweating, malaise, myalgia, and anorexia. Q fever is caused by the rickettsial organism, *Coxiella burnetii,* and is contracted by inhaling infected dusts, drinking unpasteurized milk from infected animals, or handling infected animals such as goats, cows, or sheep. Transmission by human contact is rare but has occurred. An effective vaccine is available for the prevention of infection in persons who have a good chance of being exposed to the disease. Tetracyclines and chloramphenocol are effective in treating Q fever.

**q.h.** L. *quaque hora,* every hour.

**q.i.d.** L. *quater in die,* four times a day.

**q.l.** L. *quantum libet,* as much as one pleases.

**Q law** As temperature decreases, chemical activity decreases.

**$Qo_2$** The number of microliters of $O_2$ taken up per milligram of dry weight of tissue per hour.

**q.q.h.** L. *quaque quarta hora,* every four hours.

**QRS complex** The Q, R, and S waves or deflections of an electrocardiogram produced during the transmission of the excitation wave through the conductile tissue of the heart. In the anterior cardiac leads, the complex consists of an initial downward deflection (Q wave), a large upward deflection (R wave), and a second downward deflection (S wave) that represents the spread of the electrical impulse from the Purkinje fibers to the ventricular muscle, initiating ventricular depolarization. Normal duration is 0.06 to 0.08 sec.

**QRST complex** The Q, R, S, and T waves of an electrocardiogram. The duration is approx. the same as that of mechanical systole. The T wave, which follows the QRS complex, reflects ventricular repolarization. During the T wave, the ventricles are in their recovery period. Between the QRS complex and the T wave is the ST segment, which represents the completion of depolarization and the beginning of repolarization of the ventricles; this being the time of ventricular contraction. SEE: *electrocardiogram* for illus.

**q.s.** L. *quantum sufficit,* as much as suffices.

**qt** *quart.*

**Q-T segment** The portion of the cardiac complex on the electrocardiogram that extends from the beginning of the Q wave to the end of the T wave.

**Quaalude** Trade name for methaqualone hydrochloride. Because of the illegal use and abuse of this drug, it is no longer distributed in the United States.

**quack** (kwăk) [D. *kwaksalven,* to peddle salve] One who pretends to have knowledge or skill in medicine. SYN: *charlatan.*

**quad** Medical "shorthand" for quadriceps, quadrilateral, quadrant, quadriplegia.

**quadrangular** (kwŏd-răng′ū-lĕr) [L. *quadri,* four, + *angulus,* angle] Having four angles.

**quadrangular lobe** A region forming the superior portion of each cerebellar hemisphere.

**quadrant** (kwŏd′rănt) [L. *quadrans,* a fourth] **1.** One quarter or fourth of a circle. **2.** One of four corresponding regions, as of the abdomen, divided for descriptive and diagnostic purposes.

***dental q.*** One quarter of the mouth. Each arch is divided in half so that one can easily describe the location of teeth or soft tissue observations. Quadrants are labeled as maxillary right and left or mandibular right and left and are shown in diagram form for dental records.

**quadrantanopia** (kwŏd″rănt-ă-nō′pē-ă) [″ + Gr. *an-,* not, + *opsis,* vision] Blindness or diminished visual acuity in one fourth of the visual field.

**quadrantanopsia** (kwŏd″rănt-ăn-ŏp′sē-ă) [″ + ″ + *opsis,* vision] Loss of sight in approx. one fourth of the visual field.

**quadrate** (kwŏd′rāt) [L. *quadratus,* squared] Square, or having four equal sides.

**quadrate lobe** A small lobe of liver located on the visceral surface and lying in contact with the pylorus and duodenum.

**quadrate lobule** The square lobule of the upper surface of the cerebellum.

**quadri-, quadr-** Combining form meaning *four.*

**quadribasic** (kwŏd″rĭ-bā′sĭk) [L. *quattuor,* four + basic] Having four replaceable atoms of hydrogen.

**quadriceps** (kwŏd′rĭ-sĕps) [″ + *caput,* head] Four-headed, as a quadriceps muscle.

**quadriceps femoris** A large muscle on the

anterior surface of the thigh composed of the rectus femoris, vastus lateralis, vastus medialis, and vastus intermedius muscles. These muscles are inserted by a common tendon on the tuberosity of the tibia. The quadriceps femoris is an extensor of the leg. SEE: *Muscles Appendix.*

**quadricepsplasty** (kwŏd″rĭ-sĕps′plăs-tē) [″ + ″ + Gr. *plassein,* to form] Plastic surgery to repair adhesions and scars around the quadriceps femoris muscle in order to restore function.

**quadricuspid** (kwŏd″rĭ-kŭs′pĭd) [″ + *cuspis,* point] Having four cusps, as a heart valve or a tooth.

**quadridigitate** (kwŏd″rĭ-dĭj′ĭ-tāt) Having only four fingers on a hand or four toes on a foot.

**quadrigemina** (kwŏd″rĭ-jĕm′ĭn-ă) [″ + *geminus,* twin] The corpora quadrigemina. SEE: *colliculus inferior; colliculus superior.*

**quadrigeminal** (kwŏd″rĭ-jĕm′ĭn-ăl) Fourfold; having four symmetrical parts; pert. to the corpora quadrigemina.

**quadrigeminum** (kwŏd″rĭ-jĕm′ĭ-nŭm) One of the four quadrigeminal bodies of the brain.

**quadrigeminus** (kwŏd″rĭ-jĕm′ĭ-nŭs) Composed of four parts.

**quadrilateral** (kwŏd″rĭ-lăt′ĕr-ăl) [″ + *latus,* side] Having four sides.

**quadrilocular** (kwŏd″rĭ-lŏk′ū-lăr) [″ + *loculus,* a small space] Having four chambers, cavities, or spaces.

**quadripara** (kwŏd-rĭp′ă-ră) [″ + *parere,* to bring forth, to bear] A woman who has had four pregnancies that have continued beyond the 20th week of gestation. SYN: *quartipara.* SEE: *para.*

**quadripartite** (kwŏd″rĭ-păr′tīt) [″ + *partire,* to divide] Divided into four parts.

**quadriplegia** (kwŏd″rĭ-plē′jē-ă) [″ + Gr. *plege,* stroke] Paralysis of all four extremities and usually the trunk caused by injury to the spinal cord in the cervical spine. The higher the injury, the less function is available in the arms. Injury above the third cervical vertebra requires a mechanical respiratory device to maintain life. SEE: *Nursing Diagnoses Appendix.*

EMERGENCY MEASURES: When a fracture of a cervical vertebra is suspected, the injured patient's head and neck should be stabilized during transportation.

TREATMENT: Initial treatment includes administration of glucocorticoids, immobilization with the use of Crutchfield tongs, and antibiotic therapy. When the fracture has healed, physical and occupational therapy are instituted.

NURSING IMPLICATIONS: The patient's neck is immobilized according to established procedures. A patent airway is established and maintained, and respiratory status is monitored for signs of insufficiency (hypoxemia, hypercapnia, and acidemia). Bowel sounds are assessed for development of paralytic ileus. Antithromboembolic devices are applied to the leg. When positioning the patient upright, the nurse should monitor blood pressure for evidence of orthostatic hypotension. If the condition is present, an abdominal binder may help. If injury is above T-4, the nurse should assess for hypertension, a sign of autonomic dysreflexia. Assistance is provided with self-care deficits, including skin and oral care, feeding and nutrition, elimination, respiratory toilet, positioning, and exercise. The patency of the urinary catheter is checked, and a bulk diet is provided to prevent impaction. Both patient and family are encouraged to verbalize their concerns, and support is offered to help them cope with their grief and loss. Assistance is provided to help the family set realistic plans for the future in view of the patient's functional abilities, body image, and self-concept. The patient is urged to participate in a rehabilitation program as soon as stabilized.

**quadripolar** (kwŏd″rĭ-pō′lăr) Pert. to a cell having four poles.

**quadrisect** (kwŏd′rĭ-sĕkt) [″ + *sectio,* a cutting] To divide into four parts.

**quadrisection** (kwŏd″rĭ-sĕk′shŭn) Dividing into four sections or parts.

**quadritubercular** (kwŏd″rĭ-tū-bĕr′kū-lĕr) [″ + *tuberculum,* a little swelling] Having four tubercles or cusps.

**quadrivalent** (kwŏd″rĭ-vā′lĕnt) [″ + *valens,* powerful] Having the ability to replace four atoms of hydrogen in a compound (i.e., a chemical valence of four).

**quadruped** (kwŏd′roo-pĕd″) [″ + *pes,* foot] **1.** A four-footed animal. **2.** Assuming a position with hands and feet on floor.

**quadrupedal reflex** (kwŏd-roop′ĕd-ăl) Extension of the flexed arm on assuming a quadrupedal posture.

**quadruplet** (kwŏd′roo-plĕt, kwŏ-droo′plĕt) [L. *quadruplus,* fourfold] One of four children born of the same mother in the same confinement. SEE: *Hellin's law.*

**quail poisoning** Acute myoglobinuria following ingestion of quail. It is postulated that the actual cause of the poisoning is a toxic substance the quail has ingested, perhaps hemlock. Fatigued persons who presumably have an enzymatic abnormality in their muscular tissue are susceptible to this type of poisoning. It has been suggested that this type of poisoning accounts for a plague associated with eating quails mentioned in the Holy Bible (Numbers 11:31-35).

**quale** (kwā′lē) [L. *qualis,* of what kind] The quality of anything, esp. of a sensation.

**qualimeter** (kwŏl-ĭm′ĕt-ĕr) [″ + Gr. *metron,* measure] A device for measuring the quality of x-ray photons. SEE: *penetrometer.*

**qualitative** (kwŏl′ĭ-tā″tĭv) [L. *qualitativus*] Referring to the quality of anything. SEE: *quantitative.*

**quality** (kwŏl'ĭ-tē) [L. *qualitas,* quality] **1.** That which constitutes or characterizes a thing; the natural character. **2.** In radiology, the energy or penetrating power of the x-ray beam.

**quality-adjusted life-years** ABBR: QALY. In economic analyses, a numerical description of the value of a medical procedure or service to groups of patients with similar medical conditions. This attempt to quantify the outcome of medical procedures is predicated on a number of difficult-to-measure assumptions. The validity and, therefore, the usefulness of this concept is controversial.

**quality assurance** Activities and programs designed to achieve a desired degree or grade of care in a defined medical, nursing, or health-care setting or program. The quality assurance program must include evaluation and educational components to identify and correct problems. Such programs are required for funding by the Public Health Act.

The Quality Assurance Program for Medical Care in the Hospital (QAP) is a guide developed by the American Hospital Association for development of such programs by hospital administrators and medical staffs.

**quality of life** A concept that differs for each person and may vary for the same individual as that person's life situation changes. The holistic treatment of a patient requires that the health-care team assess what is most important to that individual. In some cases, it is not possible to establish a situation in which there is complete freedom from the signs and symptoms of disease. In those cases, the goal is to have the quality of life be as good as possible despite the disease. Also, in persons who have suffered disabilities or loss of mental or physical skills, it is important to emphasize the positive features of their remaining capabilities rather than to dwell on the negative aspects of what has been lost. A variety of methods have been used to attempt to quantify an individual's quality of life. Whether these tests and questionnaires do indeed measure the quality of life is being investigated.

**quanta** (kwŏn'tă) [L.] Pl. of quantum.

**quantimeter** (kwŏn-tĭm'ĕt-ĕr) [L. *quantus,* how great, + Gr. *metron,* measure] A device for measuring the amount of x-ray photons given during an exposure.

**quanti-Pirquet** (kwŏn″tĭ-pēr-kā') [Clemens Peter Johann von Pirquet, Austrian pediatrician, 1874–1929] A quantitative cutaneous test of sensitivity to tuberculin by the use of graduated dilutions.

**quantitative** (kwŏn″tĭ-tā'tĭv) [LL. *quantitativus*] Concerning quantity. SEE: *qualitative.*

**quantity** (kwŏn'tĭ-tē) [L. *quantitas,* quantity] Amount; portion.

**quantivalence** The number of hydrogen atoms with which an element or radical will combine.

**quantum** (kwŏn'tŭm) *pl.* **quanta** [L., how much] **1.** A definite amount. **2.** A unit of radiant energy.

**quantum libet** (kwŏn'tŭm lī'bĕt) [L.] ABBR: q.l. As much as desired.

**quantum mottle** A variation in the number of x-ray photons that strike the radiographic film during an exposure. This phenomenon causes a non-uniform intensity over the areas of similar densities on the film.

**quantum sufficit** (kwŏn'tŭm sŭf'fĭ-sĭt) [L.] ABBR: q.s. As much as suffices.

**quarantine** (kwor'ăn-tēn″) [It. *quarantina,* 40 days] **1.** The period during which entry to a country is prohibited or the period of isolation of persons exposed to infectious diseases—formerly 40 days. **2.** The period of isolation from public communication following onset of a contagious disease. Complete quarantine is the limitation of the freedom of movement of healthy persons or domestic animals that have been exposed to a communicable disease for a period of time equal to the longest incubation period of the disease, in such a manner as to prevent effective contact with those not so exposed. SEE: *contagious; isolation; reportable disease.*

**quart** (kwort) [L. *quartus,* a fourth] ABBR: qt. A unit of fluid equal to one fourth of a gallon, or 2 pints, or 946 ml; in dry measure, one eighth of a peck.

**quartan** (kwor'tăn) [L. *quartana,* of the fourth] Occurring every fourth day. SEE: *malaria.*

**quartile** (kwor'tĭl) [L. *quartus,* a fourth] One of the two middle values of each half of a series of variables.

**quartipara** (kwor-tĭp'ă-ră) [″ + *parere,* to bring forth, to bear] Quadripara.

**quartz** (kwărts) [Ger. *quarz*] Silicon dioxide, the principal ingredient of sandstone (crystallized silica; rock crystal). When crystal is clear and colorless, it permits the passage of large amounts of ultraviolet radiations.

***q. applicator*** A quartz rod containing various shapes and angles used to conduct, by total internal reflection, ultraviolet radiation from a water-cooled mercury arc quartz lamp.

***q. glass*** Crystalline quartz used for prisms and lenses; fused quartz used for windows, through which ultraviolet radiations are freely transmitted.

**Quatelet index** Body mass index.

**quater in die** (kwŏ'tĕr ĭn dē'ă) [L.] ABBR: q.i.d. Four times a day.

**quaternary** (kwŏ-tĕr'nă-rē) [L. *quaternarius,* of four] **1.** The fourth in order. **2.** Composed of four elements.

**Queckenstedt's sign** (kwĕk'ĕn-stĕts) [Hans Queckenstedt, Ger. physician, 1876–1918] In vertebral canal block, the cerebrospinal fluid pressure is scarcely affected by compression of the veins of the neck, unilaterally or bilaterally. In healthy persons, the pressure rises rapidly on compression, then disappears when the compression is released.

**quenching** (kwĕnch′ĭng) **1.** Cooling something that is hot; or decreasing the radioactive energy released. **2.** In toxicology, the ability of a material to decrease the toxicity of some of the chemical or chemicals in the compound.

***fluorescence q.*** A technique for investigating antigen-antibody reactions by measuring the light absorbed by an antigen mixed with a fluorescent-labeled antibody.

**querulent** (kwĕr′ū-lĕnt) [L. *querulus,* complaining] **1.** Complaining; fretful. **2.** One who is dissatisfied, complaining, and suspicious.

**Quervain's disease** (kār′vănz) [Fritz de Quervain, Swiss surgeon, 1868–1940] Chronic tenosynovitis of the abductor pollicis longus and extensor pollicis brevis muscles. Also called *de Quervain's tenosynovitis*.

**questionnaire** A list of questions submitted to a patient or research subject in order to obtain data for analysis.

**quick** (kwĭk) [ME. *quicke,* alive] **1.** A part susceptible to keen feeling, esp. the part of a finger or toe to which the nail is attached. **2.** Pregnant and experiencing fetal movements.

**quickening** (kwĭk′ĕn-ĭng) The first movements of the fetus felt in utero, usually occurring by the 18th to 20th week of pregnancy. Movements have been felt as early as the tenth week and in rare cases are not felt during the entire pregnancy.

**quicklime** CaO. Calcium oxide, unslaked lime. It forms calcium hydroxide when water is added to it.

**Quick Neurological Screening Test** ABBR: QNST. A standardized test of neurological function for persons 5 years of age or older. It assesses various areas, including attention, balance, motor planning, coordination, and spatial organization.

**quicksilver** [ME. *quicke,* alive, + *silver,* silver] The metal mercury.

**Quick's test** (kwĭks) [Armand James Quick, U.S. physician, 1894–1978] **1.** A liver function test that measures the amount of hippuric acid excreted after a dose of sodium benzoate is given. **2.** A test for the amount of prothrombin present in blood plasma.

**quiescent** The condition of being inactive or at rest. SYN: *dormant; latent.*

**quinacrine hydrochloride** An agent used in the treatment of malaria. It is also used in infestations of *Giardia lamblia,* a parasite.

**Quincke's disease** (kwĭnk′ēz) [Heinrich I. Quincke, Ger. physician, 1842–1922] Angioedema.

**Quincke's pulse** Alternating redness and pallor seen under the fingernails; a sign of aortic insufficiency. SYN: *capillary pulse.*

**Quincke's puncture** Lumbar puncture to determine the tension of the spinal fluid, or to remove some of the spinal fluid.

**quinestrol** (kwĭn-ĕs′trōl) An estrogen.

**quinethazone** (kwĭn-ĕth′ă-zōn) A diuretic.

**quinic acid** A substance present in some plants, including cinchona bark, and berries.

**quinidine sulfate** (kwĭn′ĭ-dēn) The sulfate of an alkaloid obtained from cinchona bark; a white, crystalline substance with a bitter taste. It is used to regulate heart rhythm, esp. to prevent fibrillation.

**quinine** (kwī′nīn″, kwĭ-nēn′) [Sp. *quina*] A bitter white crystalline alkaloid derived from cinchona bark and used as an antimalarial. It is usually administered in the form of its salts.

***q. bisulfate*** The acid sulfate of quinine; used similarly as quinine sulfate, but has greater solubility.

***q. dihydrochloride*** The dihydrochloride of quinine, freely soluble in water, 1 gm dissolving in 0.6 ml of water. It is suitable for intravenous injection.

***q. hydrochloride*** The hydrochloride of quinine; used in treatment of malaria.

***q. sulfate*** The sulfate of an alkaloid obtained from cinchona; used to treat malaria.

**quinine and urea hydrochloride** The combination used, in dilute solutions, as a sclerosing agent for injection treatment of hemorrhoids and varicose veins.

**quininism** (kwī′nīn-ĭzm, kwĭ-nēn′ĭzm) Cinchonism.

**quinolone** Any of a general class of broad-spectrum antibiotics that are readily absorbed from the gastrointestinal tract and have a low incidence of adverse reactions.

**quinone** (kwĭn′ōn) **1.** A yellow crystalline oxidation product of quinic acid. **2.** A class of organic compounds in which two atoms of hydrogen are replaced by two oxygen atoms.

**quinqu-** Combining form meaning *five.*

**Quinquaud's disease** (kăn-kōz′) [Charles E. Quinquaud, Fr. physician, 1841–1894] Purulent inflammation of the hair follicles of the scalp, resulting in bald patches. SEE: *folliculitis.*

**quinquetubercular** (kwĭn″kwē-tū-bĕr′kū-lăr) [L. *quinque,* five] Having five cusps or tubercles.

**quinquevalent** (kwĭng″kwĕ-vā′lĕnt) Pert. to a radical or element with a valence of five.

**quinquina** (kwĭn-kwī′nă, kĭn-kē′nă) Cinchona.

**quintan** (kwĭn′tăn) [L. *quintanus,* of a fifth] **1.** Occurring every fifth day. **2.** Trench fever.

**quinti-** [L. *quintus,* fifth] Combining form meaning *fifth.*

**quintipara** (kwĭn-tĭp′ă-ră) [″ + *parere,* to bear] A woman who has had five pregnancies that have continued beyond the 20th week of gestation. SEE: *para.*

**quintuplet** (kwĭn′tū-plĕt, kwĭn-tŭp′lĕt) [LL.

*quintuplex,* fivefold] One of five children born of one mother during the same confinement. SEE: *Hellin's law.*

**quotidian** (kwō-tĭd′ē-ăn) [L. *quotidianus,* daily] Occurring daily.

**quotient** (kwō′shĕnt) [L. *quotiens,* how many times] The number of times one number is contained in another.

***achievement q.*** A percentile rating of a child's score on a test with respect to age, level of education, and peer performance.

***intelligence q.*** ABBR: IQ. An index of relative intelligence determined through the subject's answers to arbitrarily chosen questions. IQ is merely a standard score that places an individual in reference to the scores of others within the same age group. The IQ test may not be an accurate indicator of an individual's skills or potential in creative, artistic, or motor skills areas. SEE: *intelligence; mental retardation; test, intelligence.*

***respiratory q.*** The result of dividing the amount of carbon dioxide in expired air by the oxygen inhaled, normally 0.9.

**q.v.** L. *quantum vis,* as much as you please; *quod vide,* which see.

**Q wave** A downward or negative wave of an electrocardiogram following the P wave. It is usually not prominent and may be absent without significance.

# R

**R 1.** *respiration; right; roentgen.* **2.** In chemistry, a radical.

**R–** Abbr. used in organic chemistry to indicate part of a molecule.

**–R** Rinne negative. SEE: *Rinne test.*

**+R** Rinne positive. SEE: *Rinne test.*

**℞** Symbol for L. *recipe,* take. SEE: *prescription.*

**RA** *rheumatoid arthritis; right atrium.*

**Ra** Symbol for the element radium.

**rabbetting** (răb′ĕt-ĭng) [Fr. *raboter,* to plane] Interlocking of the jagged edges of a fractured bone.

**rabbit fever** Tularemia.

**rabbitpox** An acute viral disease of laboratory rabbits.

**rabiate** (rā′bē-āt) [L. *rabies,* rage] Rabid.

**rabic** (răb′ĭk) Pert. to rabies.

**rabicidal** (răb-ĭ-sī′dăl) [L. *rabies,* rage, + *cidus,* kill] Destructive to the virus causing rabies.

**rabid** (răb′ĭd) Pert. to or affected with rabies. SYN: *rabiate.*

**rabies** (rā′bēz) [L. *rabere,* to rage] An acute infectious disease of warm-blooded mammals, esp. carnivores, caused by a neurotropic virus present in the saliva of infected animals. Wildlife, esp. bats, skunks, foxes, and raccoons, have been found to have rabies; dogs, cats, and cattle are the domestic animals particularly susceptible. Rabbits, squirrels, chipmunks, rats, and mice are rarely infected. If untreated, the disease is marked by involvement of the central nervous system, resulting in paralysis and finally death. The virus may be communicated to humans through the bite of a rabid animal. It can also be transmitted from bats to humans or other animals without a direct bite. This mode of transmission, which is rare, is assumed to occur through inhalation of infectious aerosols. The virus can be transmitted if the conjunctiva, mucous membranes, or scratches are contaminated with saliva from a rabid animal. SYN: *hydrophobia; lyssa.* SEE: *Nursing Diagnoses Appendix.*

Symptoms: Early symptoms are usually nonspecific and may mimic a respiratory or abdominal infection. Symptoms include malaise, fatigue, headache, anorexia, fever, cough, chills, sore throat, abdominal pain, nausea, vomiting, and diarrhea. In approx. half the patients, the site of the bite is painful, tingles, and is sensitive to changes in temperature. Attempts to drink water produce laryngeal spasm. Behavior is restless and abnormal, and sensory stimuli may produce convulsions. Fever, muscle twitches, hyperventilation, and excess saliva may be present during an acute attack.

Diagnosis: No tests are available to diagnose rabies in humans before the onset of clinical disease. The rapid fluorescent focus inhibition test (RFFIT) is used to measure rabies-neutralizing antibodies in serum. This test has the advantage of providing results within 48 hr.

Incubation: During the incubation period, the patient is well except for symptoms related to local wound healing. The incubation period is usually 20 to 90 days but has been as short as 4 days and as long as 1 year or more; it is 25 to 48 days shorter when the bite is on the head and longer, 46 to 78 days, when the wound is on an extremity. The virus moves along nerve axons passively at about 3 mm/hr. It is not known how the virus remains viable or where it is located during prolonged incubation periods.

Prevention: The most important preventive measure is to provide rabies vaccination for domestic animals, esp. house pets. When rabies is known to be present in an area, it is important to prevent exposure of domestic dogs and cats to wild animals. Garbage containers should be designed to prevent attracting wild animals such as raccoons. Rabid domestic or wild animals should be reported to the proper authorities. Unvaccinated dogs or cats bitten by known rabid animals should be destroyed immediately. If it is decided to detain the animal, it should be vaccinated and held in an approved pound or kennel for at least 6 months under veterinary supervision and vaccinated again 30 days before release. Immunization of a person who has been exposed to rabies should be started as soon as possible because it is ineffective once the clinical symptoms develop. The vaccine should be given in the deltoid muscle where it will be more readily absorbed than if given in the gluteal region. If it is proven that the animal who bit the patient is free of rabies, the immunization schedule can be discontinued.

---

Caution: Individuals treating patients exposed to rabies must take precautions to prevent coming in contact with either the clothes worn by the victim or the wound. SEE: *Universal Precautions Appendix.*

---

Treatment: If the patient develops rabies, aggressive management of respiratory, circulatory, and central nervous system involvement is essential. All bites or scratches made by any animal should be treated without delay by thorough and vigorous cleaning of the area to the depth of the wound with a 20% solution of soap. Deep puncture wounds should be opened to permit access of the solution. The wound should be infiltrated with human rabies immune globulin (HRIG). The wound should be sutured only if this is absolutely required. Tetanus prophylaxis is included in the treatment, as is the use of antibiotics when indicated.

PROGNOSIS: To date, in only three well-documented cases of rabies has recovery been reported in the U.S.

NURSING IMPLICATIONS: The rabies vaccine is administered as prescribed, and local erythema, pruritus, or pain are treated symptomatically. Antibiotics and other drug therapy are administered as prescribed. Wounds are assessed, cleansed, and redressed as needed. If rabies develops, the patient is isolated in a dark, quiet room. Universal precautions are used to handle saliva and salvia-contaminated articles. Cardiac and pulmonary function is monitored and supported. Psychological support is provided to the patient and family regarding impending death. Public education focuses on the need to vaccinate pets to prevent the spread of rabies. Persons should also avoid contact with wild animals because they may have rabies.

**rabies immune globulin, human rabies immune globulin** ABBR: RIG, HRIG. A standardized preparation of globulins derived from blood plasma or serum from selected human donors who have been immunized with rabies vaccine and have developed high titers of rabies antibody. It is used to produce passive immunity in persons bitten by animals. Trade name is Hyperab. SEE: *rabies.*

**rabies virus group** A genus of viruses whose official designation is *Lyssavirus*. The virus that causes human rabies is included in this group.

**rabiform** (rā'bĭ-form) [" + *forma,* shape] Resembling rabies.

**raccoon sign** [raccoons have distinctive periorbital coloration] Periorbital ecchymosis, which may be present in patients who have a basilar skull fracture.

**race** (rās) [Fr.] **1.** A distinct ethnic group characterized by traits that are transmitted through the offspring. **2.** A group of individuals with the same characteristics who originated from a common ancestor. **3.** A taxonomic classification of individuals within the same species who show distinct genetic characteristics.

**racemase** (rā'sē-mās) An enzyme that catalyzes racemization (i.e., the production of an optically active compound).

**racemate** (rā'sē-māt) A racemic compound.

**racemic** (rā-sē'mĭk) Optically inactive; used of compounds.

**racemization** (rā"sē-mī-zā'shŭn) The production of a racemic form of an optically active compound.

**racemose** (răs'ĕ-mōs) [L. *racemosus,* full of clusters] Resembling a clustered bunch of grapes, as a gland; divided and subdivided; ending in a bunch of follicles.

**rachi-, rachio-** [Gr. *rhachis,* spine] Combining form meaning *spine.*

**rachial** (rā'kē-ăl) [Gr. *rhachis,* spine] Spinal.

**rachicele** (rā'kĭ-sēl) [" + *kele,* tumor, swelling] Protrusion of the contents of the spinal canal in spina bifida cystica.

**rachidial** (ră-kĭd'ē-ăl) Spinal.

**rachidian** (ră-kĭd'ē-ăn) Pert. to the spinal column.

**rachilysis** (rā-kĭl'ĭ-sĭs) [" + *lysis,* dissolution] The mechanical treatment of lateral curvature of the spine through traction and pressure.

**rachiometer** (rā-kē-ŏm'ĕ-tĕr) [" + *metron,* measure] An instrument for measuring a spinal curvature.

**rachiopagus** (rā"kē-ŏp'ă-gŭs) [" + *pagos,* thing fixed] A conjoined twin deformity in which the two are joined at the vertebral column.

**rachiotome** (rā'kē-ō-tōm") [" + *tome,* incision] An instrument for dividing the vertebrae.

**rachis** (rā'kĭs) *pl.* **rachises** [Gr. *rhachis*] The spinal column.

**rachischisis** (ră-kĭs'kĭ-sĭs) [" + *schisis,* a splitting] A congenital spinal column fissure (e.g., spina bifida).

***posterior r.*** Spina bifida.

**rachitic** (ră-kĭt'ĭk) Pert. to or affected with rickets.

***r. rosary*** SEE: *beads, rachitic.*

**rachitis** (ră-kī'tĭs) [" + *itis,* inflammatory] **1.** Inflammation of the spine. **2.** Rickets.

***r. fetalis annularis*** Congenital enlargement of the epiphyses of the long bones.

***r. fetalis micromelica*** Congenital shortness of the bones.

**rachitome** (răk'ĭ-tōm") [" + *tome,* incision] An instrument used to open the spinal canal.

**rachitomy** (ră-kĭt'ō-mē) [" + *tome,* incision] Surgical cutting of the vertebral column.

**raclage** (ră-klŏzh') [Fr.] The destruction and removal of a soft growth by scraping or rubbing. SEE: *curettage.*

**rad** *radiation absorbed dose.*

**radectomy** (rā-dĕk'tō-mē) [L. *radix,* root, + Gr. *ektome,* excision] Surgical removal of all or a portion of a dental root.

**radiability** (rā"dē-ă-bĭl'ĭ-tē) [L. *radius,* ray, + *habilitas,* able] The capability of being penetrated readily by x-ray photons or any other ionizing radiation. **radiable** (rā'dē-ă-băl), *adj.*

**radiad** (rā'dē-ăd) [L. *radialis,* radial, + *ad,* toward] In the direction of the radial side.

**radial** (rā'dē-ăl) **1.** Radiating out from a given center. **2.** Pert. to the radius.

**radialis** (rā"dē-ā'lĭs) [L.] Pert. to the radius bone.

**radial reflex** Flexion of forearm resulting when the lower end of the radius is percussed.

**radian** (rā′dē-ăn) **1.** A unit of angular measurement equivalent to 57.295 degrees. It is subtended at the center of a circle by an arc the length of the radius of the circle. **2.** In ophthalmometry, a lens of 1 radian would have one plane surface equal in length to the radius of curvature of the curved surface.

**radiant** (rā′dē-ănt) [L. *radians,* radiate] **1.** Emitting beams of light. **2.** Transmitted by radiation. **3.** Emanating from a common center. SEE: *energy; heat; radiation.*

**radiate** (rā′dē-āt) [L. *radiatre,* to emit rays] To spread from a common center.

**radiatio** (rā-dē-ā′shē-ō) [L.] An anatomical structure, esp. a neurological one, that forms interconnections between parts by means of radiating fibers.

**radiation** (rā-dē-ā′shŭn) [L. *radiatio,* to radiate] **1.** The process by which energy is propagated through space or matter. **2.** The emission of rays in all directions from a common center. **3.** Ionizing rays used for diagnostic or therapeutic purposes. Two types of radiation therapy are commonly used for patients with cancer: teletherapy and brachytherapy. SEE: *brachytherapy.* **4.** A general term for any form of radiant energy emission or divergence, as of energy in all directions from luminous bodies, radiographical tubes, particle accelerators, radioactive elements, and fluorescent substances. **5.** In neurology, a group of fibers that diverge from a common origin.

***acoustic r.*** Auditory r.

***actinic r.*** Ionizing radiation that can cause photochemical changes, such as the production of a latent image in film emulsion by visible light or x-ray photons.

***auditory r.*** A band of fibers that connect auditory areas of the cerebral cortex with the medial geniculate body of the thalamus. SYN: *acoustic r.*

***Bremsstrahlung r.*** Diagnostic radiation produced at the target of the anode. An electron from the filament interacts with the nuclear field of a target atom, changing direction and losing energy in the form of radiation. The result is a heterogenous beam.

***characteristic r.*** In radiology, the production of radiation in an anode caused by an interaction between an electron from the electron stream and an inner-shell electron of the target material. The result is an ejected electron, a positive atom, and radiation characteristic of the difference in binding energies between the atomic shells.

***r. of corpus callosum*** All of the fibers radiating from the corpus callosum into each cerebral hemisphere.

***corpuscular r.*** Radiation composed of discrete elements or particles such as elements of atomic nuclei (i.e., alpha, beta, neutron, positron, or proton particles).

***cosmic r.*** Ionizing radiation from the sun and other extraterrestrial sources. It accounts for about one tenth of the yearly total of ionizing radiation exposure for each person. SEE: *radiation.*

***electromagnetic r.*** Rays that travel at the speed of light. They exhibit both magnetic and electrical properties. SEE: *electromagnetic spectrum* for table.

***heterogeneous r.*** Radiation containing waves of various wavelengths.

***homogeneous r.*** Radiation containing waves of only one wavelength.

***infrared r.*** Invisible heat rays beyond the red end of the spectrum. Near or short infrared rays extend from 7,200 to 14,000 angstrom units (A.U.); far or long infrared rays extend from 15,000 to 120,000 A.U. SEE: *infrared ray.*

***interstitial r.*** Radiation treatment accomplished by inserting sealed sources of a particle emitter directly into tissues.

***ionizing r.*** Radiation that either directly or indirectly induces ionization of radiation-absorbing material. SEE: *radiation injury, ionizing.*

***irritative r.*** An overdose of ultraviolet irradiation resulting in erythema and, in exceptional cases, blister formation.

***low-level r.*** Radiation, usually nonionizing, emitted by the magnetic fields produced by electric currents, including power lines and appliances such as electric blankets, television sets, and computer terminals. Although evidence that these levels of radiation are harmful is controversial, it would be prudent to avoid exposure to these sources of radiation as much as possible.

***nonionizing r.*** ABBR: NIR. SEE: *low-level r.*

***optic r.*** A system of fibers extending from the lateral geniculate body of the thalamus through the sublenticular portion of the internal capsule to the calcarine occipital cortex (striate area). SYN: *geniculocalcarine tract.*

***photochemical r.*** Light rays that penetrate tissues only fractions of a millimeter, are absorbed by protoplasm, and cause physical and biological changes. This type of radiation does not penetrate the skin but causes surface heating. A heating pad provides photothermal (i.e., infrared) heat.

***photothermal r.*** Radiation of heat by a source of light, as that from an electric bulb.

***pyramidal r.*** The radiation of fibers from the cerebral cortex to the pyramidal tract.

***solar r.*** Radiation of the sun; 60% is infrared and 40% is visible and ultraviolet.

***striatomesencephalic r.*** Fibers originating in the corpus striatum and terminating principally in the substantia nigra of the midbrain.

***striatosubthalamic r.*** A system of fibers consisting of three groups that emerge from the medial aspect of the lentiform nucleus and enter the subthalamic region, most terminating there but some continuing into the midbrain. SYN: *ansa lenticularis.*

***striatothalamic r.*** Groups of fibers connecting the corpus striatum with the thalamus and subthalamus.

***thalamic r.*** Groups of fibers connecting the thalamus with the cerebral hemispheres. These include frontal, centroparietal, occipital, and optic radiations.

***ultraviolet r.*** Radiant energy extending from 3900 to 200 angstrom units (A.U.) Divided into near ultraviolet, which extends from 3900 to 2900 A.U., and far ultraviolet, which extends from 2900 to 200 A.U.

***visible r.*** The radiation of the visible spectrum, which may be broken up into different wavelengths representing different colors:

Violet, 3900–4550 angstrom units (A.U.)
Blue, 4550–4920 A.U.
Green, 4920–5770 A.U.
Yellow, 5770–5970 A.U.
Orange, 5970–6220 A.U.
Red, 6220–7700 A.U.

SEE: *heliotherapy; spectrum.*

**radiation absorbed dose** ABBR: rad. The quantity of ionizing radiation, measured in rad or gray (Gy), absorbed by any material per unit mass of matter. One Gy equals 100 rad.

**radiation accidents, emergency handling of** The plan of action for managing accidental contamination by radioactive materials. As the field of nuclear energy expands into industry, medicine, and university studies, a rise in contamination accidents is to be expected.

The U.S. Energy Research and Development Administration has regional offices for information and assistance on radiological emergencies. Contacts may be made in person or by telephone.

Emergency handling of radiation exposure or radioactive contamination cases should not be feared. It involves common sense, cleanliness, and good housekeeping. Radiation accident problems have parallels in other conditions handled frequently by emergency rooms and rescue squads.

Radiation can be detected and measured by a simple instrument, a survey meter. The following information provides management techniques for various types of radiation accidents.

There are four types of radiation accident patients. The first type has received whole or partial external body radiation and may have received a lethal dose, but is no hazard to attendants, other patients, or the environment. This patient is no different from the radiation therapy or diagnostic x-ray patient.

The second type of patient has received internal contamination by inhalation or ingestion. This patient also is no hazard to attendants, other patients, or the environment. After cleaning to remove minor amounts of contaminated material deposited on the body surface during airborne exposure, this individual is similar to the patient with chemical poisoning, such as lead poisoning. Body wastes should be collected and saved for measurements of nuclides to assist in determination of appropriate therapy.

The third type of patient has received external contamination of body surface and clothing by liquids or dirt particles. This patient is associated with problems similar to those of someone with vermin infestation. Surgical isolation technique to protect attendants and cleaning to protect other patients and the hospital environment are necessary to confine and remove a potential hazard.

In the fourth type of patient, external contamination is complicated by a wound. Care must be taken not to cross-contaminate surrounding surfaces from the wound and vice versa. The wound and surrounding surfaces should be cleaned separately and then sealed off. When crushed, dirty tissue is involved, early preliminary wet debridement following wound irrigation may be indicated. Further debridement and more definitive therapy can await sophisticated measurement and consultant guidance.

*Standing Orders for Emergency Handling:* If the ambulance or rescue squad that picks up the radiation accident case has a radio or telephone, the crew should alert the Emergency Room to expect a patient who may have had radiation exposure or radioactive contamination.

After being notified of the impending arrival of a patient with radiation exposure or contamination, the senior person (nurse or physician) on duty in the hospital Emergency Room must take the following steps:

1. Notify the responsible staff physician or nurse and aides (trained health physicists or technologists from the nuclear medicine or radiology department).
2. Get an appropriate survey meter if one is available in the hospital. If the hospital has no meter, the hospital administrator or responsible hospital official should be notified so that a survey meter and other pertinent equipment may be obtained from the police department.
3. Notify the hospital administrator so he or she can seek expert professional consultation for technical management of the case.
4. Prepare a separate space if contamination is suspected, using either an isolation room or a cubicle. Some hospitals use the morgue because the autopsy table lends itself to washing. The morgue entrance rather than the Emergency Room entrance would be used, and the patient and family must be reassured as to why

that space is being used. If no separate space is available, a floor area immediately adjacent to the Emergency Room entrance should be covered with absorbent paper. The area should be adequate for a stretcher-cart, disposal hampers, and working space for professional attendants. This area must be marked and closed off. If dust is involved, the air-circulation system may need to be cut off to prevent the spread of contamination.

When the ambulance arrives, the responsible physician or nurse in the Emergency Room should:

5. Check the patient on the stretcher for contamination (preferably as the stretcher is removed from the ambulance) by use of a survey meter.

6. If the patient is seriously injured, give emergency lifesaving assistance immediately.

7. Handle the contaminated patient and wound as in a surgical procedure, with gown, gloves, cap, and mask.

8. If possible external contamination is involved, save all clothing and bedding from the ambulance, as well as blood, urine, stool, vomitus, and all metal objects (such as jewelry, belt buckles, dental plates). These should be labeled with the patient's name, body location, and the time and date. Each object should be saved in an appropriate container; the containers should be clearly marked, "Radioactive—Do Not Discard."

9. If physical status permits, start decontamination by cleaning and scrubbing the area of highest contamination. If an extremity alone is involved, clothing may serve as an effective barrier and the affected limb alone may be scrubbed and cleaned. Initial cleaning should be done with soap and warm water. If the entire body is involved or clothing is generally permeated by contaminated material, showering and scrubbing will be necessary. Special attention must be paid to hair-covered areas, body orifices, and body folds. The radiation contamination level should be remeasured and the measurement recorded after each washing or showering.

If a wound is involved, it should be prepared and covered with self-adhering disposable surgical drape. Neighboring skin surfaces should be cleaned and then sealed off with self-adhering disposable surgical drape. The wound covering should be removed and the wound irrigated with sterile water. The irrigating fluid should be collected in a basin or can to be marked and handled as described in rule 4. The containers should be securely covered to prevent spill while being moved or stored. Each step in the decontamination should be preceded and followed by monitoring and recording of the location and extent of contamination.

10. Save physicians', nurses', and attendants' scrub or protective clothing, as described in rule 8 for the patient's clothing. Physicians, nurses, and attendants must follow the same monitoring and decontamination routine as the patient.

11. Be prepared to do a preliminary simple wet debridement if there is a grossly contaminated wound with dirt particles and crushed tissue. Further measurements may necessitate sophisticated wound-counting detection instruments supplied by the consultant, who will advise if further definitive debridement is necessary.

When the accident has occurred at a plant, university, or medical center regularly working with nuclear material, the health physicist, supervisor, coworker, and patient should be able to inform the rescue squad of the nature of the accident, the type of radiation exposure or radioactive contamination involved, and possible body areas that may be affected.

**radiation biology** The scientific study of the effects of radiation on living organisms.

**radiation injury, ionizing** Injury to cell life caused by therapeutic radiation. Ionizing radiation can penetrate cells and deposit energy within them at random, unaffected by the usual cellular barriers. This form of energy, when sufficiently intense, kills cells by inhibiting their division. The sensitivity of cells to ionizing radiation varies considerably in different stages of cell life. Because ionizing radiation has this effect, the amount of exposure to all forms of it, including x-rays, radioisotopes, and other radioactive sources, is limited to a certain amount each year and to a specific total lifetime dose. In sufficient dosage, radiation damages DNA and can inhibit the cells' capacity to divide. When the dose is experienced during fetal development, selective cell killing leads to the teratogenic and somatic effects of radiation. SEE: *radiation accidents, emergency handling of; radiation, low-level.*

**radiation protection** Prophylaxis against injury from ionizing radiation. The only effective preventive measures are shielding the source and the operator, handlers, and patients; maintaining appropriate distance from the source; and limiting the time and amount of exposure. In general, the use of drugs to protect against radiation is not practical because of their toxicity. An exception is the use of orally administered potassium iodide to protect the thyroid from radioactive iodine.

**radiation sickness** Radiation syndrome.

**radiation symbol** A universal symbol used to indicate radioactive sources, containers for radioactive materials, and areas where radioactive materials are stored and used. The presence of the symbol denotes the need for caution to avoid contamination with or undue exposure to atomic radiation. The symbol consists of

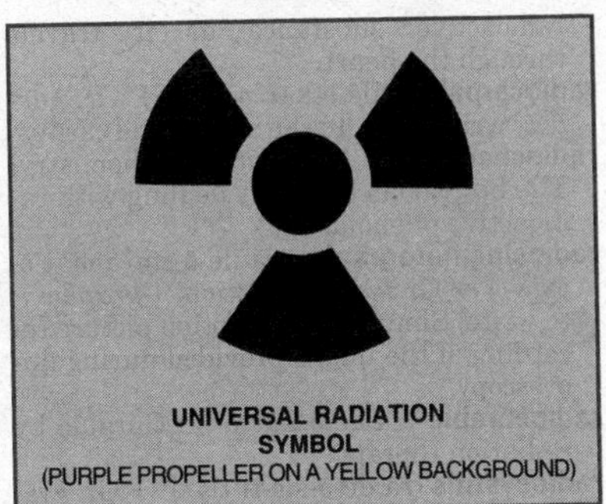


a purple propeller on a yellow field. SEE: illus.

**radiation syndrome** 1. Illness resulting from exposure of body tissue to ionizing radiations from radioactive substances (radium, radon) or x-ray photons. Mild acute illness is manifested by anorexia, headache, nausea, vomiting, and diarrhea. Delayed effects resulting from repeated or prolonged exposure may result in amenorrhea, sterility, disturbances in blood cell formation, cataract formation, carcinogenesis, and leukemia. 2. Illness resulting from the effects of an atomic bomb explosion. Effects include destruction of lymphatic tissue, extensive hemorrhages, aplastic bone marrow, prolonged clotting and bleeding times, loss of hair and teeth, and possible genetic changes. In massive exposure, such as would occur in persons close to the center of an atomic bomb explosion, death may occur within several weeks among individuals who do not die immediately from the physical effects of the explosion. SYN: *radiation sickness.*

**radiation therapy** The branch of medicine that uses ionizing radiation and particles in the treatment of malignant neoplasms. The goal of therapy is to deliver the therapeutic dose to the area, usually a malignancy, and at the same time to minimize radiation damage to healthy tissues surrounding the area being treated. Sophisticated electronic techniques have been developed to deliver the radiation at one angle and then to rotate the source so that the dose to the overlying and adjacent normal tissues is minimized. If the target site is irregular, the intensity of the radiation dose can be adjusted to conform to the irregularity of the site or organ being treated. This approach, which uses a multileaf collimator, allows precise focusing of the proper dose on the target. Another method of delivering radiation to a target is brachytherapy, in which radioactive sources are implanted in a tumor. Accurate guiding of the implant into the tumor may be done using ultrasound.

**radiator** (rā′dē-ā″tor) [LL. *radiatus,* radiate] A device for radiating heat or light.

***infrared r.*** A device for transmitting infrared rays.

**radical** (răd′ĭ-kăl) [LL. *radicalis,* having roots] 1. In chemistry, a group of atoms acting as a single unit, passing without change from one compound to another, but unable to exist in a free state. 2. Oriented toward the origin or root. 3. A foundation or principle.

***acid r.*** The electronegative portion of a molecule when the acid hydrogen is removed.

***alcohol r.*** The portion of an alcohol molecule left when the hydrogen of the OH group is removed.

***color r.*** Any group that when introduced into an organic compound causes it to become colored.

***free r.*** SEE: *free radical.*

**radical treatment** A treatment that seeks an absolute cure, as radical surgery; not palliative. This is the opposite of conservative treatment.

**radices** (răd′ĭ-sēz) [L.] Pl. of radix.

**radiciform** Resembling a root.

**radicle** (răd′ĭ-kl) [L. *radicula,* little root] A structure resembling a rootlet, as a radicle of a nerve or vein. SYN: *radicula.*

**radicotomy** (răd″ĭ-kŏt′ō-mē) [L. *radix,* root, + Gr. *tome,* incision] Rhizotomy. SEE: *radiculectomy.*

**radicula** (ră-dĭk′ū-lă) [L.] Radicle.

**radiculalgia** (ră-dĭk″ū-lăl′jē-ă) [L. *radix,* root, + Gr. *algos,* pain] Neuralgia of nerve roots.

**radicular** (ră-dĭk′ū-lăr) [L. *radix,* root] 1. Pert. to a root or radicle. 2. Pert. to the tissues on or around a tooth root (e.g., radicular dentin, radicular bone).

**radiculectomy** (ră-dĭk″ū-lĕk′tō-mē) [″ + Gr. *ektome,* excision] 1. Excision of a spinal nerve root. 2. Resection of a posterior spinal nerve root. SEE: *rhizotomy.*

**radiculitis** (ră-dĭk″ū-lī′tĭs) [L. *radicula,* little root, + Gr. *itis,* inflammation] Inflammation of the spinal nerve roots, accompanied by pain and hyperesthesia.

**radiculoganglionitis** (ră-dĭk″ū-lō-găng″glē-ō-nī′tĭs) [″ + Gr. *ganglion,* knot, + *itis,* inflammation] Inflammation of the posterior spinal roots and their ganglia.

**radiculomedullary** (ră-dĭk″ū-lō-mĕd′ū-lĕr″ē) [″ + *medullaris,* marrow] Pert. to the nerve roots and the spinal cord.

**radiculomeningomyelitis** (ră-dĭk″ū-lō-mĕ-nĭn″gō-mī-ĕl-ī′tĭs) [″ + Gr. *meninx,* membrane, + *myelos,* marrow, + *itis,* inflammation] Inflammation of the nerve roots, meninges, and spinal cord.

**radiculoneuritis** (rā-dĭk″ū-lō″nū-rī′tĭs) [L. *radicula,* little root, + Gr. *neuron,* sinew, + *itis,* inflammation] Inflammation of the spinal nerve roots.

**radiculoneuropathy** (ră-dĭk″ū-lō-nū-rŏp′ă-thē) [″ + ″ + *pathos,* disease, suffering] A pathological condition of the nerve roots and nerve.

**radiectomy** (rā″dē-ĕk′tō-mē) [L. *radix,* root, + Gr. *ektome,* excision] Surgical removal of the root of a tooth.

**radii** (rā′dē-ī) [L.] Pl. of radius.

**radio-** [L. *radius,* ray] **1.** Combining form indicating *radiant energy, radioactive substances.* **2.** Combining form used as a prefix indicating *radioactive isotope.*

**radioactinium** (rā″dē-ō-ăk-tĭn′ē-ŭm) A radioactive product formed from disintegration of the element actinium.

**radioactive** (rā″dē-ō-ăk′tĭv) [L. *radius,* ray, + *activus,* acting] Capable of emitting radiant energy.

**radioactive patient** An individual who originally was treated or accidentally contaminated with radioactive materials and who continues to be radioactive. If still emitting radiation when discharged from the hospital, the patient should be told how long to avoid close contact with children and pregnant women. SEE: *radiation accidents, emergency handling of.*

**radioactivity** (rā″dē-ō-ăk″tĭv′ĭ-tē) The ability of a substance to emit rays or particles (alpha, beta, or gamma) from its nucleus.

***artificial r.*** Radioactivity resulting from bombardment of a substance with high-energy particles in a cyclotron, betatron, or other apparatus.

***induced r.*** Temporary radioactivity of a substance that has been exposed to a radioactive element.

***natural r.*** Radioactivity possessed by numerous elements that are continuously disintegrating and emitting alpha particles (helium nuclei) or beta particles (electrons) atom by atom. Radium is an example.

**radioallergosorbent test** (rā″dē-ō-ăl″ĕr-gō-sor′bĕnt) ABBR: RAST. A blood test for allergy that measures minute quantities of immunoglobulin E in blood. Persons who are allergic to foreign substances develop antibodies that can be detected through this test.

**radioautograph** (rā″dē-ō-aw′tō-grăf) [″ + ″ + *graphein,* to write] A photograph of a histologic section of a tissue showing the distribution of radioactive substances in the tissue.

**radiobicipital** (rā″dē-ō-bī-sĭp′ĭ-tăl) Pert. to the radius and biceps muscle of the arm.

**radiobiology** (rā″dē-ō-bī-ŏl′ō-jē) The branch of biology that deals with the effects of ionizing radiations on living organisms.

**radiocalcium** (rā″dē-ō-kăl′sē-ŭm) A radioisotope of calcium; $^{45}$Ca and $^{47}$Ca are used in medical studies.

**radiocarbon** (rā″dē-ō-kăr′bŏn) A radioisotope of carbon; $^{11}$C and $^{14}$C are used in medical studies.

**radiocardiogram** (rā″dē-ō-kăr′dē-ō-grăm) [L. *radius,* ray, + Gr. *kardia,* heart, + *gramma,* something written] The record or film obtained during radiocardiography.

**radiocardiography** (rā″dē-ō-kăr″dē-ŏg′ră-fē) [″ + ″ + *graphein,* to write] The investigation of the anatomy and function of the heart by obtaining a record or film of a radioactive substance as it travels through the heart.

**radiocarpal** (rā″dē-ō-kăr′păl) [″ + Gr. *karpos,* wrist] Pert. to the radius and carpus.

**radiochemistry** [″ + Gr. *chemeia,* chemistry] The branch of chemistry dealing with radioactive phenomena.

**radiocinematograph** (rā″dē-ō-sĭn″ĕ-măt′ō-grăf) [″ + Gr. *kinema,* motion, + *graphein,* to write] Simultaneous motion picture recording of the image provided during fluoroscopy.

**radiocurable** (rā″dē-ō-kūr′ă-bl) Curable by radiation therapy.

**radiocystitis** (rā″dē-ō-sĭs-tī′tĭs) [″ + Gr. *kystis,* bladder, + *itis,* inflammation] Inflammation of the bladder following radiation therapy.

**radiodensity** The property of certain substances that does not allow the passage of x-rays. SYN: *radiopacity.*

**radiodermatitis** (rā″dē-ō-dĕr″mă-tī′tĭs) [″ + Gr. *derma,* skin, + *osis,* condition] Inflammation of the skin caused by exposure to x-ray photons or emissions from radioactive particles. SYN: *radioepidermitis.*

**radiodiagnosis** (rā″dē-ō-dī″ăg-nō′sĭs) [″ + Gr. *dia,* through, + *gnosis,* knowledge] Diagnosis by using a radiological imaging modality.

**radiodigital** (rā″dē-ō-dĭg′ĭ-tăl) Pert. to the radius and the fingers.

**radiodontia** (rā″dē-ō-dŏn′shē-ă) [″ + Gr. *odous,* tooth] Radiography of the teeth.

**radioecology** (rā″dē-ō-ē-kŏl′ō-jē) [″ + Gr. *oikos,* house, + *logos,* word, reason] Investigation of the effect of radiation on the living organisms in the environment.

**radioelectrocardiogram** (rā″dē-ō-ē-lĕk″trō-kăr′dē-ō-grăm) The record obtained by radioelectrocardiography.

**radioelectrocardiography** (rā″dē-ō-ē-lĕk″trō-kăr″dē-ŏg′ră-fē) [L. *radius,* ray, + Gr. *elektron,* amber, + *kardia,* heart, + *graphein,* to write] Recording of changes in heartbeats by radio wave from subject to receiver without direct attachment of the apparatus. Thus, recordings can be made during normal life activities of the patient. SEE: *telemetry.*

**radioelement** (rā″dē-ō-ĕl′ĕ-mĕnt) [″ + *elementum,* a rudiment] Any of the radioactive elements.

**radioencephalogram** (rā″dē-ō-ĕn-sĕf′ă-lō-grăm″) [″ + Gr. *enkephalos,* brain, + *gramma,* something written] The record obtained when a radioactive tracer passes through the cerebral blood vessels.

**radioencephalography** (rā″dē-ō-ĕn-sĕf″ă-lŏg′ră-fē) [″ + ″ + *graphein,* to write] The recording of radio waves transmitted from the brain to a receiver but without electrodes being placed on the scalp.

**radioepidermitis** (rā″dē-ō-ĕp″ĭ-dĕr-mī′tĭs) [″ + Gr. *epi,* upon, + *derma,* skin, + *itis,* inflammation] Radiodermatitis.

**radioepithelitis** (rā″dē-ō-ĕp″ĭ-thē-lī′tĭs) [″ + ″ + *thele,* nipple, + *itis,* inflammation] Disintegration of the epithelium due to exposure to radiation.

**radiofrequency electrophrenic respiration** A method of stimulating respiration in cases of respiratory paralysis from spinal cord injury at the cervical level. Intermittent electrical stimuli to the phrenic nerves are supplied by a radiofrequency transmitter implanted subcutaneously. The diaphragmatic muscles contract in response to these stimuli.

**radiogenic** (rā″dē-ō-jĕn′ĭk) [″ + *gennan,* to produce] **1.** Producing radiation. **2.** Caused by radiation. SYN: *actinogenic.*

**radiogold** (rā′dē-ō-gōld) A radioisotope of gold.

**radiograph** (rā′dē-ō-grăf) [″ + Gr. *graphein,* to write] **1.** The film on which an image is produced through exposure to x-rays. SYN: *roentgenogram.* **2.** To make a radiograph.

***bitewing r.*** SEE: *bitewing radiograph.*

***body section r.*** SEE: *tomography.*

***bregma-menton r.*** A radiograph taken in the submental-vertex plane, from below the chin to the top of the skull. It shows the contour of the zygomatic arches and the lateral separation of the mandibular condyles, coronoid processes, or both.

***cephalogram r.*** A radiograph of the jaws and skull on which anatomical points, planes, and angles may be drawn to assist in measurement.

***dental r.*** Periapical r.

***interproximal r.*** Bitewing radiograph.

***lateral cephalometric r.*** A film of the entire head, taken from the side with the head in a known, fixed position for the purpose of making definitive observations or measurements.

***lateral oblique r.*** A radiograph used to examine the body of the mandible and the ramus. Projections may be performed with conventional dental radiographical film and cover a broader area than a typical periapical radiograph. Also called *lateral jaw survey.*

***lateral skull r.*** A radiograph of the sinuses and lateral aspects of the cranial skeleton.

***maxillary sinus r.*** A frontal radiograph of the maxillary sinuses and the zygomas that allows direct comparison of both sides.

***panoramic r.*** A type of extraoral curved-surface radiograph that shows the entire upper and lower jaws in a continuous single film.

***periapical r.*** An intraoral film that depicts the tooth and surrounding tissues extending to the apical region. SYN: *dental r.*

***posteroanterior r.*** A frontal radiograph of the skull; used to examine the skull for disease, trauma, and developmental abnormalities.

***rotational r.*** Panoramic r.

***transcranial r.*** A radiograph of the temporomandibular articulation.

**radiographer** A health care professional who operates radiological equipment and performs related duties under the supervision of a radiologist.

**radiography** (rā-dē-ŏg′ră-fē) The process of obtaining an image for diagnosis using a radiological modality.

**radiohumeral** (rā″dē-ō-hū′mĕr-ăl) [″ + *humerus,* upper arm] Pert. to the radius and humerus.

**radioimmunity** (rā″dē-ō-ĭ-mū′nĭ-tē) [″ + *immunitas,* immunity] Apparent decreased sensitivity to radiation that may follow repeated radiation therapy.

**radioimmunoassay** (rā″dē-ō-ĭm″ū-nō-ăs′ā) ABBR: RIA. A very sensitive method of determining the concentration of a substance, particularly a protein-bound hormone, in blood plasma. The procedure is based on the competitive inhibition of binding of radioactively labeled hormones to a specific antibody. Protein concentrations in the picogram ($10^{-12}$ g) range can be measured by this technique.

**radioimmunodiffusion** (rā″dē-ō-ĭm″ū-nō-dĭf-fū′zhŭn) [″ + ″ + *dis,* apart, + *fundere,* to pour] A method of studying antigen-antibody interaction by use of radioisotope-labeled antigens or antibodies diffused through a gel.

**radioimmunoelectrophoresis** (rā″dē-ō-ĭm″ū-nō-ē-lĕk″trō-fō-rē′sĭs) [″ + ″ + Gr. *elektron,* amber, + *phoresis,* bearing] Electrophoresis involving the use of a radioisotope-labeled antigen or antibody. An autoradiograph is taken of the electrophoretic pattern produced.

**radioiodine** (rā″dē-ō-ī′ō-dīn) A radioactive isotope of iodine, used in the diagnosis and treatment of thyroid disorders. The most commonly used isotope is $^{131}$I.

**radioiron** (rā″dē-ō-ī′ĕrn) A radioactive isotope of iron; $^{55}$Fe and $^{59}$Fe are used in medical studies.

**radioisotope** (rā″dē-ō-ī′sō-tōp) A radioactive form of an element.

**radiolead** (rā″dē-ō-lĕd′) A radioactive isotope of lead.

**radiolesion** (rā″dē-ō-lē′zhŭn) A lesion or injury caused by radiation.

**radioligand** (rā″dē-ō-lī′gănd, răd″dē-ō-lĭg′ănd) A molecule, esp. an antigen or antibody, with a radioactive tracer attached to it.

**radiological emergency assistance** SEE: *radiation accidents, emergency handling of.*

**radiologist** (rā-dē-ŏl′ō-jĭst) [L. *radius,* ray, + Gr. *logos,* word, reason] A physician who uses x-rays or other sources of radiation for diagnosis and treatment.

***dental r.*** A dentist whose specialty is the production of radiographs and their use in diagnosing dental and oral diseases.

**radiology** (rā-dē-ŏl′ō-jē) The branch of medicine concerned with radioactive substances, including x-rays, radioactive isotopes, and ionizing radiations, and the application of this information to prevention, diagnosis, and treatment of disease.

**radiolucency** (rā″dē-ō-lū′sĕn-sē) [″ + *lucere,* to shine] The property of being partly or wholly penetrable by radiant energy.

**radiolucent** (rā″dē-ō-lū′sĕnt) [″ + *lucere,* to shine] Allowing x-rays to pass through. A dark area appears on the radiograph.

**radiolus** (rā-dē′ō-lŭs) [L., a little ray] A sound or probe.

**radiometer** (rā-dē-ŏm′ĕ-tĕr) [″ + Gr. *metron,* measure] An instrument for measuring the intensity of radiation.

***photographic r.*** An instrument containing a half-tone color index for strips of photographic paper after exposure to roentgen rays; after development, it is used to estimate the quantity of roentgen rays received by the area.

**radiomicrometer** (rā″dē-ō-mī-krŏm′ĕ-tĕr) [″ + Gr. *mikros,* small, + *metron,* measure] An instrument for measuring small changes in radiation.

**radiomimetic** (rā″dē-ō-mĭm-ĕt′ĭk) [″ + Gr. *mimetikos,* imitation] Imitating the biological effects of radiation. Alkylating agents are examples of substances with this property. SEE: *alkylating agent.*

**radiomuscular** (rā″dē-ō-mŭs′kū-lăr) Pert. to the radius or radial artery and the muscles of the arm.

**radiomutation** The permanent alteration of the genetic material of a cell caused by the effects of ionizing radiation.

**radionecrosis** (rā″dē-ō-nĕ-krō′sĭs) [″ + Gr. *nekrosis,* state of death] The disintegration of tissue resulting from exposure to radiant energy.

**radioneuritis** (rā″dē-ō-nū-rī′tĭs) [″ + Gr. *neuron,* sinew, + *itis,* inflammation] Inflammation of a nerve caused by exposure to a radioactive substance.

**radionitrogen** (rā″dē-ō-nī′trō-jĕn) A radioisotope of nitrogen.

**radionuclide** (rā″dē-ō-nū′klīd) An atom that disintegrates by emitting electromagnetic radiation.

**radiopacity** (rā″dē-ō-păs′ĭ-tē) Radiodensity.

**radiopaque** (rā-dē-ō-pāk′) [″ + *opacus,* dark] Impenetrable to x-rays or other forms of radiation. A light area appears on the radiograph.

**radioparency** (rā″dē-ō-păr′ĕn-sē) Condition of being radiolucent or radioparent.

**radioparent** (rā″dē-ō-păr′ĕnt) [″ + *parere,* to appear] Penetrable by radioactive rays.

**radiopathology** (rā″dē-ō-pă-thŏl′ō-jē) [″ + Gr. *pathos,* disease, suffering, + *logos,* word, reason] The study of pathological changes induced by radiation.

**radiopelvimetry** (rā″dē-ō-pĕl-vĭm′ĕt-rē) [″ + *pelvis,* basin, + Gr. *metron,* measure] Measurement of the pelvis by use of x-rays.

**radiopharmaceutical** (rā″dē-ō-fărm″ă-sū′tĭ-kăl) A radioactive chemical, occurring either as an individual element or as an element attached to another substance called a carrier. It is used in testing the location, size, outline, or function of tissues, organs, vessels, or body fluids. The presence and location of radiopharmaceuticals in the body are detected by special methods or devices that record the radioactivity being emitted. These compounds may also be used to treat certain diseases.

---

Caution: Radiopharmaceuticals must be handled in accordance with prescribed methods to prevent the patient or those treating the patient from being exposed to unnecessary ionizing radiation.

---

**radiophobia** (rā″dē-ō-fō′bē-ă) [″ + Gr. *phobos,* fear] An abnormal fear of x-rays and radiation.

**radiophosphorus** (rā″dē-ō-fŏs′fō-rŭs) A radioactive isotope of phosphorus. $^{32}P$ is used in medical studies.

**radiopotassium** (rā″dē-ō-pō-tăs′ē-ŭm) A radioactive isotope of potassium. $^{42}K$ is used in medical studies.

**radiopotentiation** (rā″dē-ō-pō-tĕn″shē-ā′shŭn) [″ + *potentia,* power] The augmentation of the effect of radiation. This may be produced by certain drugs and by oxygen.

**radioprotective drug** A drug that protects humans against the damaging or lethal effects of ionizing radiation. For example, Lugol's solution or a saturated solution of potassium iodide blocks the uptake of inhaled or ingested radioactive iodine by the thyroid.

**radiopulmonography** (rā″dē-ō-pŭl″mō-nŏg′ră-fē) [″ + *pulmo,* lung, + Gr. *graphein,* to write] The use of radioactive materials to measure the flow, or lack of flow, of gases through the lung during respiration.

**radioreaction** (rā″dē-ō-rē-ăk′shŭn) The reaction of the body to radiation.

**radioreceptor** (rā″dē-ō-rē-sĕp′tor) Something that receives radiant energy such as light, heat, or x-rays.

**radioresistant** Resistant to the action of radiation; used esp. of a tumor that cannot be destroyed by radiation treatment.

**radioresponsive** (rā″dē-ō-rē-spŏn′sĭv) Radiosensitive.

**radioscopy** (rā-dē-ŏs′kō-pē) [L. *radius,* ray, + Gr. *skopein,* to examine] Inspection and examination of the inner structures of the body by fluoroscopic procedures. SYN: *fluoroscopy.*

**radiosensibility** Radiosensitivity.

**radiosensitive** (rā″dē-ō-sĕn′sĭ-tĭv) Reactive or responsive to radiation, as a cell.

**radiosensitivity** (rā″dē-ō-sĕn″sĭ-tĭv′ĭ-tē) Reactiveness or responsiveness of a cell to radiation. SYN: *radiosensibility.*

**radiosodium** (rā″dē-ō-sō′dē-ŭm) A radioisotope of sodium. $^{24}Na$ and $^{22}Na$ are used in medical studies.

**radiostrontium** (rā″dē-ō-strŏn′shē-ŭm) A radioisotope of strontium.

**radiosulfur** (rā″dē-ō-sŭl′fŭr) A radioisotope

of sulfur.

**radiosurgery** (rā″dē-ō-sŭr′jĕr-ē) [″ + Gr. *cheirurgia,* handwork] The use of high-energy protons and alpha particles in the form of beams as an "atomic knife" in treating diseases such as cancer or in selectively destroying an overactive endocrine gland.

**radiotelemetry** (rā″dē-ō-tĕl-ĕm′ĕ-trē) [″ + Gr. *tele,* distant, + *metron,* measure] The transmission of data, including biological data, by radio from a patient to a remote monitor or recording device for storage, analysis, and interpretation.

**radiotherapeutics** (rā″dē-ō-thĕr″ă-pū′tĭks) **1.** Radiotherapy. **2.** The study of radiotherapeutic agents.

**radiotherapist** (rā″dē-ō-thĕr′ă-pĭst) [″ + Gr. *therapeia,* treatment] Someone trained in use of radiant energy for therapeutic purposes.

**radiotherapy** (rā″dē-ō-thĕr′ă-pē) The treatment of disease by particle application, as of x-ray photons, nuclear disintegrations, or ultraviolet radiation.

**radiothermy** (rā″dē-ō-thĕr′mē) [″ + Gr. *therme,* heat] **1.** The use of radiant heat or heat from radioactive substances for therapeutic purposes. **2.** Short-wave diathermy.

**radiothorium** (rā″dē-ō-thō′rē-ŭm) A radioisotope of thorium.

**radiotoxemia** (rā″dē-ō-tŏk-sē′mē-ă) [″+ Gr. *toxikon,* poison, + *haima,* blood] Toxemia produced by exposure to a radioactive substance. SEE: *radiation syndrome.*

**radiotransparent** (rā″dē-ō-trăns-păr′ĕnt) [″ + *trans,* across, + *parere,* to appear] Penetrable by radiation.

**radioulnar** (rā″dē-ō-ŭl′năr) [″ + *ulna,* arm] Concerning the radius and ulna.

**radium** (rā′dē-ŭm) [L. *radius,* ray] SYMB: Ra. A metallic element found in very small quantities in uranium ores such as pitchblende; atomic number 88, atomic weight 226, half-life 1622 years. It is radioactive and fluorescent. Radon is produced by the breakdown of radium. Of the more than a dozen isotopes, radium is the most common. The most stable isotope, $^{226}$Ra, has been used as a source of radioactivity in medical research and therapy. SEE: *actin-.*

**radium needle** A slender container for radium. It is inserted into tissue to kill malignant cells.

**radium therapy** [″ + Gr. *therapeia,* treatment] Radiotherapy.

**radius** [L., ray] **1.** A line extending from a circle's center point to its circumference. **2.** The outer and shorter bone of the forearm. It revolves partially about the ulna. Its head articulates with the capitulum of the humerus and with the radial notch on the ulna and is encircled by the annular ligament. Its lower portion articulates with the ulna by the ulnar notch, and by another articulation with the navicular (scaphoid) and lunate bones of the wrist.

**radial,** *adj.*

***fracture of r.*** A break in the radius. A common fracture of the lower end of the radius is a Colles' fracture, caused by falling on the outstretched hand. Fractures also occur along the shaft or at the upper end frequently involving the radial head. SEE: under *fracture.*

**radix** (rā′dĭks) *pl.* **radices** [L., root] **1.** The root portion of a cranial or spinal nerve. **2.** The root of a plant.

**radon** (rā′dŏn) [L. *radius,* ray] SYMB: Rn. A radioactive gaseous element resulting from the disintegration of isotopes of radium; atomic weight 222, atomic number 86. Because radium is present in the earth's crust, radon and its disintegration products accumulate in caves, mines, houses (particularly those that are energy efficient), and any space not freely exchanging the air contained in it with the outside air. The level of radon in a house may be measured, and if it exceeds acceptable limits, steps should be taken to reduce it. Radon exposure is estimated to cause 5% to 10% of the lung cancers occurring in the general population.

***radon seed*** A small container made of biocompatible material that is used to contain radon. It is placed in malignant tissue to provide a source of radioactive material to that area.

**raffinose** (răf′ĭ-nōs) A trisaccharide, melitose, present in certain plants, cereals, and fungi. Hydrolysis yields fructose and melibiose.

**rage** (rāj′) [ME.] Violent anger.

***sham r.*** A rage reaction produced by stimuli in decorticated animals.

**ragsorter's disease** A febrile pulmonary disease that may occur in people who sort paper and rags. It is caused by the anthrax bacillus.

**ragweed** One of several species of the genus *Ambrosia,* whose pollen is an important allergen. The pollen-producing period of grasses in temperate zones is from the middle of August to the first hard frost, usually the middle of October. SEE: *allergy.*

**Raillietina** (rī″lē-ĕ-tī′nă) A genus of tapeworms belonging to the family Davaineidae.

***R. demerariensis*** A species that infests humans, reported from several South American countries, esp. Ecuador.

**Raimiste's phenomenon, Raimiste's sign** An associated reaction in hemiplegia in which resistance to hip abduction or adduction in the noninvolved extremity evokes the same motion in the involved extremity.

**raised** (rāzd) [ME. *reisen,* to rise] In bacteriology, when a colony grown on a culture medium is elevated above the surface.

**rale** SEE: *crackle.*

**ramal** (rā′măl) [L. *ramus,* branch] Pert. to a ramus.

**rami** (rā′mī) [L.] Pl. of ramus.

**ramicotomy** (răm″ĭ-kŏt′ō-mē) [L. *ramus,* branch, + Gr. *tome,* incision] Ramisection.

**ramification** (răm″ĭ-fĭ-kā′shŭn) [L. *ramificare,* to make branches] **1.** The process of branching. **2.** A branch. **3.** Arrangement in branches.

**ramify** (răm′ĭ-fī) To branch; to spread out in different directions.

**ramisection** (răm′ĭ-sĕk″shŭn) [L. *ramus,* branch, + *sectio,* a cutting] The surgical division of a ramus communicans between a spinal nerve and a ganglion of the sympathetic trunk.

**ramisectomy** (răm-ĭs-ĕk′tō-mē) [″ + Gr. *ektome,* excision] Excision of a ramus, specifically a ramus communicans. SEE: *ramisection.*

**ramitis** (răm-ī′tĭs) [″ + Gr. *itis,* inflammation] Inflammation of a ramus.

**ramose** (rā′mōs) [L. *ramus,* branch] Branching; having many branches.

**Ramsay Hunt syndrome** A condition caused by herpes zoster of the geniculate ganglion of the brain or neuritis of the facial nerve and characterized by severe facial palsy and vesicular eruption in the pharynx, external ear canal, tongue, and occipital area. Deafness, tinnitus, and vertigo may be present.

**ramulus** [L.] A small branch or ramus.

**ramus** (rā′mŭs) *pl.* **rami** [L., branch] A branch; one of the divisions of a forked structure. **ramal** (-măl), *adj.*

***anterior r.*** A primary division of a spinal nerve that supplies the lateral and ventral portions of the body wall, limbs, and perineum.

***bronchial r.*** One of the collateral branches of each primary bronchus.

***r. communicans*** One of the primary branches of a spinal nerve that connects with a sympathetic ganglion. Each consists of a white portion (white ramus communicans) composed of myelinated preganglionic sympathetic fibers and a gray portion (gray ramus communicans) composed of unmyelinated postganglionic fibers.

***mandibular r.*** The vertical portion of the mandible.

***meningeal r.*** One of the primary branches of a spinal nerve that reenters the vertebral foramen and supplies the meninges and vertebral column.

***posterior r.*** One of the primary branches of a spinal nerve that supplies the muscles and skin of the back.

**Rancho Los Amigos Guide to Cognitive Levels** A scale widely used to classify a neurological patient's level of cognitive dysfunction according to behavior. This scale provides eight levels with descriptors, progressing from level I (no response) to level VIII (purposeful and appropriate response), as follows:

I. No response: is unresponsive to any stimuli.

II. Generalized response: exhibits limited, inconsistent, nonpurposeful responses, often to pain only.

III. Localized response: displays purposeful responses; may follow simple commands; may focus on presented object.

IV. Confused, agitated: demonstrates heightened state of activity; confusion, disorientation; aggressive behavior; inability to perform self-care; unawareness of present events; agitation, which appears as internal confusion.

V. Confused, inappropriate: is nonagitated; appears alert; responds to commands; is distractible; does not concentrate on task; demonstrates agitated responses to external stimuli; is verbally inappropriate; does not learn new information.

VI. Confused, appropriate: demonstrates goal-directed behavior, needs cueing; can relearn old skills, such as activities of daily living; displays serious memory problems; exhibits some awareness of self and others.

VII. Automatic, appropriate: appears appropriate, oriented; frequently acts robot-like in daily routine; has minimal or no confusion; demonstrates shallow recall; exhibits increased awareness of self, interaction in environment; lacks insight into condition; shows decreased judgment and problem solving ability; lacks realistic planning for future.

VIII. Purposeful, appropriate: is alert, oriented; recalls and integrates past events; learns new activities and can continue without supervision; is independent in home and living skills; is capable of driving; demonstrates defects in stress tolerance, judgment, abstract reasoning; possibly functions at reduced levels in society.

**rancid** (răn′sĭd) [L. *rancidus,* stink] Offensive; having a disagreeable smell or taste from partial decomposition, esp. of a fatty substance.

**rancidify** (răn-sĭd′ĭ-fī) To make rancid.

**rancidity** (răn-sĭd′ĭ-tē) The condition of being rancid.

**random controlled trial** An experimental study to assess the effects of a particular variable (such as a drug or treatment) in which subjects are assigned randomly to either an experimental or a control group. The experimental group receives the drug or procedure; the control group may receive a placebo or nothing. Laboratory tests or clinical evaluations are performed on both groups (usually using the double-blind technique) to determine the effects of the drug or procedure.

**randomization** In research, a method used to assign subjects to experimental groups. Before this step every attempt is made to ensure that the subjects are as nearly equivalent as possible. Then by some random method, such as a coin toss or a list of numbers, each subject is assigned to either a treatment or a nontreatment group. Use of this technique helps to prevent inadvertent selection bias in the study. SEE: *clinical trial; double-blind technique.*

**random sample** In experimental medicine and in epidemiology, the selection of samples from a population or some other grouping, so that each individual or item in the group has the same opportunity of being selected in the sample.

**range** [ME., series] The difference between the highest and lowest in a set of variables or in a series of values or observations.

***r. of accommodation*** The difference between the least and the greatest distance of distinct vision. SEE: *accommodation.*

***r. of motion*** ABBR: ROM. The range on which a joint can move. SEE: *goniometer.*

***continuous passive r. of motion*** Continuous passive motion.

**ranine** (rā′nīn) [L. *rana,* a frog] **1.** Pert. to a ranula, or the region beneath the tip of the tongue. **2.** The branch of the lingual artery supplying that area. **3.** Pert. to frogs.

**ranula** (răn′ū-lă) [L., little frog] A large cystic tumor seen on the underside of the tongue on either side of the frenum; a retention cyst of the submandibular or sublingual ducts. The swelling may be small or large.

SYMPTOMS: The tumor is semitranslucent, with soft, large, dilated veins coursing over it. The patient experiences fullness and discomfort, but usually no pain. The tumor contains clear glairy fluid owing to dilatation of the salivary glands and obstruction of the sublingual mucous glands.

TREATMENT: Periodic emptying of the sac by careful needle aspiration provides temporary relief. Surgical intervention is required for complete removal.

***pancreatic r.*** Cystic disease of the pancreas caused by obstruction of its ducts.

**Ranvier's node** (rŏn-vē-āz′) [Louis A. Ranvier, Fr. pathologist, 1835–1922] A space between adjacent Schwann cells along a nerve fiber; no myelin sheath is present. SYN: *neurofibril node.* SEE: *nerve fiber; neuron* for illus.; *Schwann cell.*

**RAO** *right anterior oblique* position.

**rape** (rāp) [L. *rapere,* to seize] Heterosexual or homosexual intercourse against the will of the victim. Rape involves an attempt at or actual penetration of the vagina or another body orifice by a penis, finger, or inanimate object. Complete penetration by the penis or emission of seminal fluid is not necessary to constitute rape. Most rapes include force or violence, but acquiescence because of verbal threats does not indicate consent. It is accepted that rape is a violent criminal act that happens to be associated with sexual activity. In many cases in which a man is the rapist, there is no evidence that orgasm occurred. In 1991 the reported annual incidence of sexual assault was 80 per 100,000 women. The peak incidence is among women 16 to 19 years of age in the U.S. Nevertheless, more than 60,000 rapes of women older than 50 years of age are reported annually. SEE: *rape and sexual assault prevention; rape-trauma syndrome; sexual abuse; Nursing Diagnoses Appendix.*

TREATMENT: The medical care of the rape victim must include appropriate antibiotic prophylactic treatment for sexually transmitted diseases, and prophylaxis against hepatitis B, which will require administration of hepatitis B immune globulin (0.06 ml/kg of body weight). This should be given within 24 hr of exposure. The importance of HIV testing while in the treatment center and scheduling of repeat tests at monthly intervals for at least 6 months should be stressed. In cases where semen entered the vagina, medication to prevent pregnancy may be given.

NURSING IMPLICATIONS: The nurse provides sensitive care, esp. psychological support, by remaining with the patient and by encouraging verbalization of feelings. State regulations regarding reporting of rape should be followed. The nurse explains and assists with the physical, pelvic, and rectal examinations and diagnostic tests. Directions should be followed exactly in collecting rape evidence such as head and pubic hair combings, nail scrapings, and so forth for police investigation. The patient should be allowed as much control as possible throughout examination, treatment, and interview procedures. An assault and sexual history is obtained, including whether the female rape victim was menstruating and, if so, the type of menstrual protection used.

Prescribed treatments of associated injuries are performed. Prescribed prophylactic medications for venereal disease are administered. Crisis intervention services are offered to assist the patient with emotional expression. Information regarding antipregnancy measures is provided. If the patient desires, cleansing measures are also provided. Assistance is offered to help the patient explain the rape to family. Follow-up services and written and verbal instructions for prescribed medications, including drug actions and possible side effects, are provided. The nurse arranges for someone to escort the patient home.

***date r.*** Rape occurring while the individual raped was involved socially with the rapist. The individual may have been an intimate friend, but the sexual assault at that time was unsolicited and unwelcome.

***gang r.*** Forcible sexual intercourse or other sexual activity committed on an individual by several persons. SEE: *rape.*

***male r.*** Sexual assault, usually penetrative, of a man by a man. Estimating the prevalence of male rape is difficult because it often is not reported. Anyone involved in male rape should be tested for infection with human immunodeficiency virus (HIV) because the anal trauma incident to the assault favors the spread of HIV infection.

***marital r.*** Forcible sexual assault by a spouse at a time when the sexual encounter was neither solicited nor welcome.

***prison r.*** Rape that occurs when the victim is assaulted by another prisoner or by a prison employee.

***statutory r.*** Sexual intercourse with an individual younger than the legal age of consent.

**rape and sexual assault prevention** The precautions taken to decrease the chances of one's being raped or sexually assaulted. Attempting to reason with one's attacker, who may be irrational, may or may not effectively prevent a rape. A rapist may fit any description; many are neither "crazy" nor "macho," but in fact quite ordinary. Many of these individuals are persons with low self-esteem who lack control over their lives. Most rapes are committed by persons known by the victim, and the act usually occurs in the home of either the victim or the attacker. Rape by a complete stranger does occur, but this is not the usual situation. Because alcohol consumption is a related factor in many rapes, it is advisable to keep alcohol intake to a minimum and not allow a companion who is intoxicated into one's home. In the following suggestions, it is assumed that the potential victim is a woman who is being forced to have sexual intercourse or participate in other sexual acts.

As much as possible, preventive measures should be directed at remaining in a well-secured area and being close to persons who can be called for assistance day or night. If the latter is not possible, emergency police and fire department telephone numbers should be kept readily available. Help should be summoned without delay if it is suspected that one's apartment or home is being illegally entered.

When preparing to enter a car, one should be constantly alert for the presence of a stranger hidden either in the dark or behind, under, or within a car. Before leaving a well-lighted and populated area, one should have the car keys in hand and ready for quick use. It is advisable to leave one arm free of packages, handbag, or other items. Individual keys placed firmly between the fingers like claws can be a useful weapon. One should walk quickly and with assurance to the car, and look under and inside it before unlocking the door. Once it has been ascertained that entrance is safe, one should enter quickly and not fumble with keys. It is important to lock the car doors and close any open windows immediately.

When preparing to enter the home, one should be alert to any outward signs of danger (i.e., nonfunctioning hall light, unfamiliar noises or odors in the hallways, barking of a normally quiet resident dog, unlatched or ajar hall door that is normally secure, unfamiliar persons loitering outside or standing at or inside the hall door). Often, even the sense of danger can be a useful warning. If the situation does not "feel" familiarly safe, one should not attempt to enter or brush by a stranger, but should leave, go to a secure telephone, and call a neighbor who might assist in safe entry.

If possible, one should never enter one's residence when no one else is home. If this is unavoidable, before closing the door, one should immediately turn on a light and then speak aloud as if a friend is present. Holding the keys in one hand and spread through the fingers, one should walk through the entire dwelling from front to back, checking in closets, behind open doors, in the shower, and any other places where an intruder might hide. At least one possible exit should always remain available before safety is ascertained and the door closed. One may also enlist the assistance of a known neighbor, law enforcement officer, or friend to search the home.

Once one is safely inside, the door should be locked securely. If a stranger comes to the door, a security chain should be kept on and a peephole preferably used for communication until proper identification has been presented. If doubt exists about the credentials or demeanor of the stranger, admission should be refused and help summoned immediately.

When on the street, one should avoid unlighted or dimly lighted streets, parks, and parking lots. If traffic permits, one should walk in the street. Otherwise, the middle or street side of the sidewalk should be used to avoid dark alleyways or doors. One should always walk quickly and with assurance.

It is not possible to provide advice that applies to all situations and guarantees rape and injury prevention. Even if it seems advisable to attempt resistance, the attacker usually has the advantage of being stronger than the victim. Nevertheless, if the victim is certain that persons are close by who would both hear a cry and be willing to help, a loud scream might be beneficial. A repeated loud cry of "fire" may more readily bring assistance than a cry of "help." However, even this approach could lead to injury or death if the attacker has a gun or other weapon ready to use at the first sign of resistance.

If raped, one should attempt to remember as many details as possible about the attacker: clothes, size, race, accent, hair color, identifying marks and scars, facial hair, vehicle, and evidence of drug or alcohol use.

**rape counseling** The provision of advice, comfort, and sources of therapy for victims of sexual assault. The emotional reaction and sequelae of rape may be devastating to the mental well-being of the victim. It is therefore important that the victim be reassured about what to expect from both internal feelings and the potential reactions of society. Historically, law enforcement officers have been less than sympathetic to rape victims, but now most police departments have officers trained in rape investigation who are sensitive to the emotional and physical trauma the victim has experienced. Various services are available to the victim, including advocate groups and health care professionals experienced in counseling rape victims.

**rapeseed** [L. *rapa,* turnip] The seed of *Brassica campestris* and other *Brassica* species. Rapeseed oil, which is used in foods and industry, is obtained from this seed.

**rape-trauma syndrome** The trauma syndrome that develops from rape or attempted rape of a male or female. SEE: *rape; Nursing Diagnoses Appendix.*

Like other post-traumatic stress disorders, this condition initially causes an acute phase of disorganization and involves a long-term reorganization of lifestyle. Sequelae may include marked changes in lifestyle and a variety of phobias.

*Acute phase:* Profound emotional responses mark the acute phase (i.e., fear, shame, and feelings of humiliation; self-blame and self-degradation; and anger and desire for revenge). Most commonly, rape victims exhibit crying, trembling, talkativeness, statements of disbelief, and emotogenic shock. Some may exhibit overt signs of hostility, which reflect their anger and feelings of powerlessness. Later, patient complaints of sleep pattern disturbances, gastrointestinal irritability, and genitourinary discomforts reflect physical responses to emotional trauma. Some women may appear quiet, dispassionate, and smiling; however, these behaviors should not be misinterpreted as indicating a lack of concern; rather, they may represent an avoidance reaction.

*Long-term phase:* Many rape victims experience one or more of the following: nightmares; chronic suspicion, inability to trust, and altered interpersonal relationships; anxiety, aversion to men, and avoidance of sex; depression; and phobias. Paradoxically, patients express feelings of guilt and shame because they feel that either they invited the attack, should have prevented the episode, or that they deserved being punished.

NURSING IMPLICATIONS: The nurse exhibits empathy and understanding and ensures privacy and a quiet supportive environment. The patient is encouraged to verbalize feelings, fears, and concerns. Positive self-perception and self-esteem are promoted and supported. The nurse emphasizes that rape usually is an expression of the rapist's overwhelming feelings of psychosocial impotence and anger and that the act conveys a sense of power over others; the woman was a victim of the rapist's inability to contain a violent personal rage that is not related to her or to sex. The patient is referred to community resources (support groups).

**raphania** (ră-fā′nē-ă) [Gr. *rhaphanos,* radish] A spasmodic disease caused by eating seeds of the wild radish; allied to ergotism. SYN: *rhaphania.*

**raphe** (rā′fē) [Gr. *rhaphe*] A crease, ridge, or seam denoting union of the halves of a part. SYN: *rhaphe.*

***abdominal r.*** Linea alba.

***buccal r.*** A raphe on the cheek indicating the line of fusion of the maxillary and mandibular processes.

***lateral r.*** A ridge along the lateral margin of the erector spinae muscles formed by the aponeurosis of the latissimus dorsi internal oblique and transversus abdominis muscles and the layers of the thoracolumbar fascia.

***palatine r.*** A line or ridge in the median line of the palate.

***r. of penis*** A median ridge on the posterior surface of the penis, a continuation of the raphe of the scrotum.

***perineal r.*** A line or ridge in the midline of the perineum.

***pterygomandibular r.*** A tendinous line of fusion between the buccinator and superior pharyngeal constrictor muscles that passes between the pterygoid process and the mandible, serving as an important landmark in dental anesthesia.

***r. of scrotum*** A ridge in the midline of the scrotum.

***r. of tongue*** A median groove on the dorsum of the tongue.

**rapport** (ră-por′) [Fr. *rapporter,* to bring back] A relationship of mutual trust and understanding, esp. between the patient and physician, nurse, or other health care provider.

**rapture** A state of great joy, delight, or ecstasy.

**rarefaction** (răr″ĕ-făk′shŭn) [L. *rarefacere,* to make thin] The process of decreasing in density and weight, as of air. The farther from the surface of the earth, the less dense the atmosphere becomes.

***r. of bone*** The process by which bone becomes more porous because of absorption of mineral substances. This may be caused by a disturbed calcium-phosphorus metabolism possibly resulting from excess parathyroid hormone. SEE: *osteo-*

*porosis; parathyroid.*

**rarefy** (rār′ĕ-fī) To make less dense; to increase the porosity of something.

**RAS** *reticular activating system.*

**rash** (răsh) [O. Fr. *rasche*] A general term applied to any eruption of the skin, esp. one associated with a communicable disease. It is usually temporary and a shade of red that varies with disease. A rash is difficult to see in persons with darkly pigmented skin. SYN: *exanthem.* SEE: *eruption; lesion; roseola.*

NURSING IMPLICATIONS: The nurse assesses the location and characteristics of the lesion, such as color; size (height and diameter); pattern, whether discrete or coalesced; and any secondary changes (crusting, scaling, lichenification). Associated symptoms such as pruritus or discomfort, temporal elements, history of known allergies, drugs used, and contacts with communicable diseases during prior 2-week period are also assessed. Suspected drugs are discontinued, and the potential communicable disease patient is isolated until the physician can be contacted. Cool compresses are applied to relieve itching. Topical preparations and dressings are applied and systemic medications administered as prescribed. The nurse instructs the patient to keep hands clean and nails short and even, and to avoid touching the rash. The nurse also teaches the patient about the treatment regimen, its actions, and its side effects and evaluates for desired effects and side effects.

***butterfly r.*** A rash on both cheeks joined by an extension across the bridge of the nose. It is seen in systemic lupus erythematosus, esp. after the patient's face has been exposed to sunlight, and in seborrheic dermatitis, tuberous sclerosis, and dermatomyositis. SEE: *discoid lupus erythematosus.*

***diaper r.*** Irritant contact dermatitis as a reaction to friction, maceration, and prolonged contact with urine, feces, soap retained in diapers, and topical preparations. A persistent diaper rash may be colonized by yeast or bacteria. SYN: *diaper dermatitis.* SEE: illus.

TREATMENT: Treatment is symptomatic. Diapers should be changed frequently. If washable cloth diapers are used, they should be thoroughly washed and rinsed; occlusive plastic pants should not be used over diaper; the perianal and genital areas should be washed with warm water and mild, nonperfumed soap. If these measures and application of a bland protective agent (e.g., zinc oxide paste), do not promote healing, then a small amount of 0.5% to 1% topical hydrocortisone cream should be applied to the area after each diaper change. This should be done for several days.

***drug r.*** Dermatitis medicamentosa.

***ecchymotic r.*** Hemorrhagic r.

***gum r.*** A red, papular eruption of an infant's chin and anterior chest area seen during teething. A form of miliaria due to excess saliva coming in contact with the skin. SYN: *red r.; tooth r.; strophulus.*

***heat r.*** Miliaria.

***hemorrhagic r.*** A rash consisting chiefly of hemorrhages or ecchymoses. SYN: *ecchymotic r.*

***macular r.*** A rash in which the lesions are flat and level with the surrounding skin.

***maculopapular r.*** A rash in which there are discrete macular and papular lesions or a combination of both.

***mercurial r.*** A rash caused by local application of mercurial preparations.

***mulberry r.*** A dusky rash seen in typhus fever.

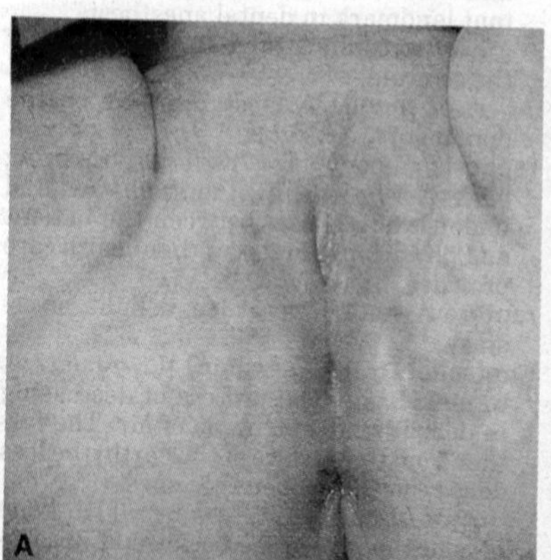


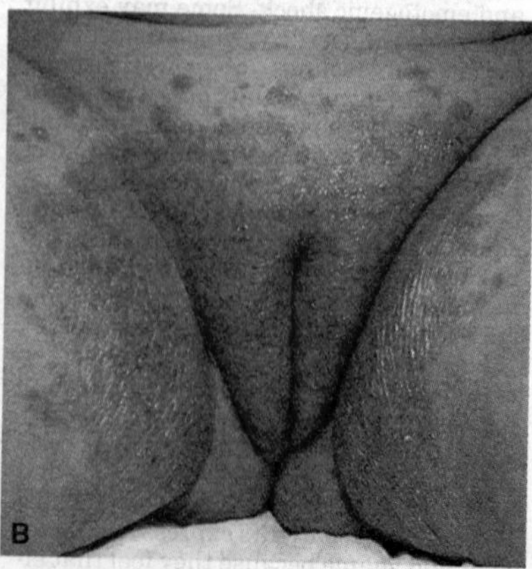


**DIAPER RASH**

**(A)** MILD DIAPER RASH, **(B)** SEVERE YEAST INFECTION IN DIAPER AREA

***nettle r.*** Urticaria.

***red r.*** Gum r.

***rose r.*** Any rose-colored rash.

***serum r.*** A rash accompanying serum sickness resulting from injection of a foreign serum. SEE: *serum sickness.*

***sunburn-like r.*** A macular rash resembling the reddened skin characteristic of a severe sunburn. It may be associated with circulating bacterial toxins. SEE: *toxic shock syndrome.*

***tooth r.*** Gum r.

***wandering r.*** Geographic tongue.

**Rashkind procedure** Balloon atrial septostomy.

**rasion** (rā′zhŭn) [L. *rasio*] The grating of drugs by use of a file.

**raspatory** (răs′pă-tō″rē) [L. *raspatorium*] A file used in surgery, esp. for trimming bone surfaces. SYN: *xyster.*

**RAST** *radioallergosorbent test.*

**Rastafarian cult** A religious cult that originated in Jamaica in the 1930s and has members in the Caribbean, Europe, Canada, and the U.S. It is of medical importance because cult members' dietary practices may lead to vitamin $B_{12}$ deficiency with subsequent neurological disease, megaloblastic anemia, or both.

**rasura** (ră-sū′ră) [L. *rasura,* a scraping] **1.** The process of scraping or shaving. **2.** Scrapings or filings.

**rat** [ME] A rodent of the genus *Rattus,* found in and around human habitations. In addition to causing economic loss from crop destruction, rats are of primary importance in the spread of human and animal diseases. They are hosts of various protozoans, flukes, tapeworms, and threadworms, and reservoirs of amebiasis, murine and scrub typhus, and bubonic plague. Typhus and plague are transmitted to people mainly by the rat flea. Rats also transmit rat-bite fever. SEE: *flea; vector.*

**rat-bite fever** Either of two infectious diseases transmitted by the bite of a rat. One is caused by *Streptobacillus moniliformis* and is marked by skin inflammation, fever, chills, headache, vomiting, and back and joint pain. The other is caused by *Spirillum minus* and is associated with ulceration, rash, and recurrent fever. The latter disease is rare in the U.S. SYN: *sodokosis; sodoku.*

Treatment: Both diseases are treated with penicillin. Therapy is most effective when penicillin is given intravenously for 1 week, then orally for 1 week. Tetanus prophylaxis is also administered.

**rate** (rāt) [L. *rata,* calculated] The speed or frequency of occurrence of an event, usually expressed with respect to time or some other known standard.

***attack r.*** The rate of occurrence of new cases of a disease.

***basal metabolic r.*** SEE: *basal metabolic rate.*

***birth r.*** The number of live births per 1000 in the population in a given year.

***case r.*** Morbidity r.

***case fatality r.*** The ratio of the number of deaths caused by a disease to the total number of people who contract the disease.

***death r.*** The number of deaths in a specified population, usually expressed per 100,000 population, over a given period, usually 1 year. SYN: *mortality r.*

***DMF r.*** An expression pert. to dental caries in school children. It is noted how many teeth are decayed (D), missing or requiring extraction (M), and filled or with restorations (F). SEE: *DMF index.*

***dose r.*** The quantity of medicine administered per unit of time.

***erythrocyte sedimentation r.*** ABBR: ESR. SEE: *sedimentation r.*

***false-negative r.*** The rate of occurrence of negative test results in individuals who actually have the attribute or disease for which they are being tested.

***false-positive r.*** The rate of occurrence of positive test results in individuals who actually do not have the attribute or disease for which they are being tested.

***fertility r.*** The number of births per year per 1000 women between ages 15 and 44 in a given population.

***fetal heart r.*** ABBR: FHR. The number of fetal heartbeats per minute. Normal findings range between 120 and 160 bpm.

***glomerular filtration r.*** ABBR: GFR. The rate of filtrate formation as the blood passes through the glomeruli of the kidneys.

***growth r.*** The rate at which an individual, tissue, or organ grows. It may be expressed per arbitrary unit of time such as hours, days, months, or years.

***heart r.*** The number of heart contractions per unit of time, usually expressed or written as number per minute. SEE: *sinus bradycardia; sinus tachycardia.*

***infant mortality r.*** The number of deaths per year of live-born infants less than 1 year of age divided by the number of live births in the same year. This value is usually expressed as deaths per 100,000 live births. SEE: *neonatal mortality r.; perinatal mortality r.*

***maternal mortality r.*** The number of maternal deaths in 1 year from puerperal causes (i.e., those associated with pregnancy, childbirth, and the puerperium) within 42 days after delivery divided by the number of live births in that same year. This value is usually expressed as deaths per 100,000 live births.

***morbidity r.*** The number of cases per year of certain diseases in relation to the population in which they occur. SYN: *case r.*

***mortality r.*** Death r.

***neonatal mortality r.*** The number of deaths in 1 year of infants aged 0 to 28 days divided by the number of live births in that same year. SEE: *maternal mortal-*

*ity r.; perinatal mortality r.*

***peak expiratory flow r.*** The maximum rate of exhalation during a forced expiration, measured in liters per second or liters per minute. It is used in testing for airway obstruction.

***perinatal mortality r.*** The number of stillbirths (in which the gestation period was 28 weeks or more) in the first 7 days of life divided by the number of live births plus stillbirths in the same year. This value is usually expressed as deaths per 100,000 live births plus stillbirths. SEE: *infant mortality r.; neonatal mortality r.*

***periodontal disease r.*** SEE: *periodontal index.*

***pulse r.*** The number of heart contractions per unit of time that can be detected by palpating a peripheral artery.

***respiration r.*** The number of breaths per unit of time.

***sedimentation r.*** ABBR: ESR (erythrocyte sedimentation rate). A nonspecific laboratory test of the speed at which erythrocytes settle out of unclotted blood. In this test, blood to which an anticoagulant has been added is placed in a long, narrow tube, and the distance the red cells fall in 1 hr is the ESR. Normally, it is less than 10 mm/hr in men and slightly higher in women.

The speed at which the cells settle depends on how many red blood cells clump together. Clumping is increased by the presence of acute-phase proteins, released during inflammation. Therefore, the sedimentation rate indicates the presence of inflammation and is used to track the onset and progress of inflammatory disorders. An elevated ESR helps to differentiate an acute myocardial infarction from angina pectoris because no inflammation is present in the latter state.

**Rathke's pouch** (răth'kĕz) [Martin H. Rathke, Ger. anatomist, 1793–1860] A depression in the mouth of the embryo just anterior to the buccopharyngeal membrane. The anterior lobe of the pituitary arises from this structure.

**ratio** (rā'shē-ō) [L., computation] The relationship in degree or number between two things.

***a:A r.*** The ratio of arterial oxygen partial pressure ($PaO_2$) to alveolar oxygen partial pressure ($PAO_2$), a measure of oxygen transfer across the lung. This figure is normally greater than 0.9.

***A/G r.*** Abbreviation for albumin-globulin r.

***albumin-globulin r.*** ABBR: A/G r. The ratio of albumin to globulin in blood plasma or serum. Normally this value is 1.3:1 to 3.0:1.

***arm r.*** In chromosomes, the relation of the length of the long arm of the mitotic chromosome to that of the short arm.

***body weight r.*** Body weight in grams divided by body height in centimeters.

***cardiothoracic r.*** The relation of the overall diameter of the heart to the widest part of the inside of the thoracic cavity. Usually the heart diameter is half or less than half that of the thoracic cavity.

***common mode rejection r.*** ABBR: CMRR. The ability of an amplifier to amplify a signal in the presence of electrical noise. The higher the number, the better the amplification.

***curative r.*** Therapeutic r.

***dextrose-nitrogen r.*** The ratio of dextrose to nitrogen in urine.

***grid r.*** In a radiographical grid, the ratio of the height of the lead strips to the distance of the interspace. High ratios indicate increased ability of the grid to remove scatter.

***I:E r.*** In respiratory therapy or mechanical ventilation, the ratio of a patient's inspiratory to expiratory time.

***international normalized r.*** ABBR: INR. In anticoagulant therapy, the ratio used to standardize reporting of prothrombin time (PT) in order to provide consistent regulation of coagulation. The ratio is calculated from the patient's PT divided by the mean control PT of that laboratory, and the result is transformed exponentially by an amount equal to the international sensitivity index (ISI) provided by the manufacturer of the thromboplastin in the package insert. In the U.S., the ISI of thromboplastins varies from 1.0 to 2.8. The recommended INR range is 2.0 to 3.0 for all conditions in which anticoagulant therapy is used except mechanical prosthetic cardiac valves, for which a slightly higher INR is necessary.

***lecithin-sphingomyelin r.*** ABBR: L/S ratio. The ratio of lecithin to sphingomyelin in the amniotic fluid. This ratio is used to determine fetal maturity. The ratio increases as the pregnancy approaches term, so that by the time of delivery it is at least 2:1.

***odds r.*** In epidemiological case-control studies, a relative measure of disease occurrence. The odds in favor of a particular disease occurring in an exposed group are divided by the odds in favor of its occurring in an unexposed group. If the condition being studied is rare, the odds ratio is a close approximation to the relative risk. SEE: *relative risk.*

***P:F r.*** The ratio of arterial partial pressure of oxygen to inspired fractional concentration of oxygen; used to measure oxygen transfer.

***sex r.*** The ratio of males to females in a given population, usually expressed as the number of males per 100 females.

***therapeutic r.*** The ratio obtained by dividing the effective therapeutic dose by the minimum lethal dose. SYN: *curative r.*

**ration** (rā'shŭn) A fixed allowance of food and drink for a certain period.

**rational** (răsh'ŭn-ăl) [L. *rationalis,* reason]

**1.** Of sound mind. SYN: *sane.* **2.** Reasonable or logical; employing treatments based on reasoning or general principles; opposed to empiric.

**rationale** (răsh″ŭn-ăl′) [L.] The logical or fundamental reason for a course of action or procedure.

**rationalization** (răsh″ŭn-ăl-ĭ-zā′shŭn) In psychology, a justification for an unreasonable or illogical act or idea to make it appear reasonable.

**rattle** (răt′l) [ME. *ratelen,* to rattle] A sound or crackle heard on auscultation.

***death r.*** A gurgling sound or subcrepitant crackle heard in the trachea of the dying.

**rattlesnake** A poisonous snake of the genus *Crotalus.* Articulated cuticular extensions at the tip of the tail produce a characteristic rattle. SEE: *snake.*

**raucous** (raw′kŭs) [L. *raucus, hoarse*] Hoarse, harsh, as the sound of a voice.

**Rauscher leukemia virus** [Frank J. Rauscher, U.S. virologist, b. 1931] A virus known to cause leukemia in mice.

**rauwolfia serpentina** (raw-wŏlf′ē-ă) [Leonhard Rauwolf, Ger. botanist, 1535–1596] The dried roots of *Rauwolfia serpentina,* the extracts from which are potent hypotensive agents and sedatives with low toxicity. Derivatives are serpentine, serpentinine, and reserpine.

**rave** (rāv) [ME. *raven,* to be delirious] To talk irrationally, as in delirium.

**raving 1.** Irrational utterance. **2.** Talking irrationally.

**ray** (rā) [L. *radius,* ray] **1.** One of several lines diverging from a common center. **2.** A line of propagation of any form of radiant energy, esp. light or heat; loosely, any narrow beam of light.

***actinic r.*** A solar ray of the spectrum, capable of producing chemical changes. SYN: *chemical r.*

***alpha r.*** A ray composed of positively charged helium particles derived from atomic disintegration of radioactive elements. Its velocity is one tenth the speed of light. Alpha rays are completely absorbed by a thin sheet of paper and possess powerful fluorescent, photographic, and ionizing properties. They are less penetrative than beta rays.

***beta r.*** A ray composed of negatively charged electrons expelled from atoms of disintegrating radioactive elements.

***border r.*** Grenz r.

***cathode r.*** A ray composed of negatively charged electrons discharged by a cathode through a vacuum, moving in a straight line and producing x-ray photons on hitting solid matter.

***central r.*** The theoretical center of an x-ray beam. The term designates the direction of the x-ray photons as projected from the focal spot of the x-ray tube to the radiographical film.

***characteristic r.*** A secondary photon produced by an electron giving up energy as it changes location from an outer to a more inner shell in an atom. The wavelengths are characteristic of the difference in binding energies.

***chemical r.*** Actinic r.

***cosmic r.'s*** Electromagnetic waves (radiation) coming from sources in outer space. Cosmic rays have a short wavelength and exceptionally high velocity and penetrative power.

***delta r.'s*** Highly penetrative waves given off by radioactive substances.

***erythema-producing r.*** A ray between 1800 and 4000 A.U., the spectrum that produces erythema, with those around 2540 and between 2050 and 3100 A.U. being the most effective.

***gamma r.'s*** Heterogeneous vibrations caused by electronic disturbance in atoms of radioactive elements during their disintegration. They appear identical with x-rays except that the wavelengths range from about 1.4 to 0.01 A.U. and the rays derive from the nucleus rather than the orbit of the element. They have high velocity and penetrative power.

***grenz r.*** A low-energy x-ray photon with an average wavelength of 2 A.U. (range from 1 to 3 A.U.); obtained with peak voltage of less than 10 kV. Grenz rays lie between ultraviolet and x-rays. SYN: *border r.*

***hard r.*** An x-ray photon of short wavelength and great penetrative power.

***heat r.*** A visible ray from 3,900 to 7,700 A.U. or an infrared ray from 7,700 to 14,000 A.U. The heating effect of visible rays on deeper tissue is proportionately stronger than that of infrared rays because the visible rays have greater penetrating power. SEE: *heat.*

***infrared r.*** An invisible heat ray from beyond the red end of the spectrum. Infrared wavelengths range from 7700 angstrom units (A.U.) to 1 mm. Long-wave infrared rays (15,000 to 150,000 A.U.) are emitted by all heated bodies and exclusively by bodies of low temperature such as hot water bottles and electric heating pads; short-wave infrared rays (7,200 to 15,000 A.U.) are emitted by all incandescent heaters. The sun, electric arcs, incandescent globes, and so-called infrared burners are sources of infrared rays.

USES: Infrared ray energy is transformed into heat in a superficial layer of the tissues. It is used therapeutically to stimulate local and general circulation and to relieve pain. The infrared thermograph, a device for detecting and photographing infrared rays, has been useful in studying the heat of tissues. This device has many applications such as in investigation of the rate of blood flow through a part. SEE: *radiation; thermography.*

***luminous r.*** One of the visible rays of the spectrum.

***medullary r.*** In the kidney, one of many

slender processes composed of straight tubules that project into the cortex from the bases of renal pyramids. SYN: *pars radiata lobuli corticalis renis.*

***monochromatic r.*** A ray characterized by a definite wavelength, as a secondary ray.

***pigment-producing r.*** A ray between 2540 and 3100 A.U. that is most effective in stimulating pigment production in the skin. This is due to a local response to irritation of cutaneous prickle cells.

***positive r.*** A ray composed of positively charged ions that in a discharge tube moves from the anode toward the cathode.

***primary r.*** A ray discharged directly from a radioactive substance, as the alpha, beta, and gamma rays.

***roentgen r.*** X-ray photon.

***scattered r.*** An x-ray photon or gamma ray that has been deflected in its passage through a substance and changed by an increase in wavelength.

***secondary r.'s*** X-ray photons produced after the incoming, primary x-ray photons remove an inner-shell electron from the atom. They are of lower energy than the primary radiation and usually are absorbed in matter.

***ultraviolet r.*** An invisible ray of the spectrum beyond the violet rays. The wavelengths of ultraviolet rays vary. They may be refracted, reflected, and polarized, but will not traverse many substances impervious to the rays of the visible spectrum. They rapidly destroy the vitality of bacteria, and are able to produce photochemical and photographic effects.

**Raynaud, Maurice** (rā-nōz′) French physician, 1834–1881.

***R.'s disease*** A peripheral vascular disorder found most frequently in women between 18 and 30 years of age. It is marked by abnormal vasoconstriction of the extremities on exposure to cold or emotional stress. A history of symptoms for at least 2 years is necessary for diagnosis.

SYMPTOMS: Patients have intermittent attacks of pallor or cyanosis of the digits (usually fingers) associated with cold or emotional disturbance, pallor or cyanosis that is bilateral or symmetrical, and normal radial and ulnar pulses. No evidence of occlusive disease is present; gangrene may occur but is limited to the skin of the tips of the digits.

TREATMENT: Persons with this disease should maintain warmth in the extremities by wearing wool gloves and socks. Contact with cold materials and tobacco use should be avoided. Vasodilators and tranquilizers may be helpful.

PROGNOSIS: The attacks persist but can be controlled. No serious disability develops, but this condition is sometimes associated with the development of rheumatoid arthritis or scleroderma.

***R.'s phenomenon*** Intermittent attacks of pallor followed by cyanosis, then redness of the digits, before a return to normal. It is initiated by exposure to cold or emotional disturbance. Numbness, tingling, and burning may occur during the attacks. This condition may occur secondary to such conditions as occlusive arterial disease, systemic scleroderma, thoracic outlet syndrome, pulmonary hypertension, myxedema, and trauma. Therapy is based on recognition and treatment of the underlying condition. SEE: *Nursing Diagnoses Appendix.*

**rayon, purified** A fibrous form of regenerated cellulose manufactured by the viscose process, desulfured, washed, and bleached. It is used in surgical dressings and bandages.

**Rb** Symbol for the element rubidium.

**RBBB** *right bundle branch block.*

**RBC, rbc** *red blood cell; red blood count.*

**R.B.E.** *relative biological effectiveness.*

**RBRVS** *resource-based relative value scale.*

**R.C.D.** *relative cardiac dullness.*

**R.C.P.** *Royal College of Physicians; Respiratory Care Practitioner.*

**R.C.S.** *Royal College of Surgeons.*

**RD** *Registered Dietitian.*

**R.D.A.** *right dorsoanterior,* presentation position of the fetus; *recommended dietary allowance.*

**R.D.D.A.** *recommended daily dietary allowance.*

**R.D.H.** *registered dental hygienist.*

**RDMS** *registered diagnostic medical sonographer.*

**R.D.P.** *right dorsoposterior,* presentation position of the fetus.

**RDS** *respiratory distress syndrome.*

**R.E.** *radium emanation; right eye; reticuloendothelium.*

**Re** Symbol for the element rhenium.

**re-** [L.] Prefix meaning *back, again.*

**reabsorb** (rē″ăb-sorb′) To absorb again.

**reabsorption** (rē″ăb-sorp′shŭn) The process of absorbing again. It occurs in the kidney when some of the materials filtered out of the blood by the glomerulus are reabsorbed as the filtrate passes through the nephron.

**reacher** A type of extension device for assisting persons with limited reach to grasp and manipulate objects in the performance of everyday tasks.

**react** (rē-ăkt′) [L. *re,* again, + *agere,* to act] **1.** To respond to a stimulus. **2.** To participate in a chemical reaction.

**reactant** (rē-ăk′tănt) A chemical or substance taking part in a chemical reaction.

***acute phase r.*** Any one of several serum proteins that increase or decrease in response to the progress or decline of inflammation.

**reaction** (rē-ăk′shŭn) [LL. *reactus,* reacted] **1.** The response of an organism, or part of it, to a stimulus. **2.** In chemistry, a chemical process or change; transformation of one substance into another in response to a stimulus. **3.** An opposing action or counteraction. **4.** An emotional and mental state created by a situation.

***alarm r.*** The first stage in the general adaptation syndrome, which includes changes occurring in the body when subjected to stressful stimuli. Physiological changes that occur are direct results of damage, shock, or both, or reactions of the body to defend itself against shock.

***allergic r.*** A reaction resulting from hypersensitivity to an antigen.

***anamnestic r.*** The reappearance of antibodies that may occur when an antigen is injected a considerable time after the first injection.

***anaphylactic r.*** Anaphylaxis.

***antigen-antibody r.*** The combination of molecules of an antigen with one or more molecules of its specific antibody.

***anxiety r.*** In current psychiatric terminology, this condition is classed as an anxiety disorder.

***Arias-Stella r.*** A reaction marked by decidual changes in the endometrial epithelium. These changes consist of hyperchromatic cells with large nuclei; they may be associated with ectopic pregnancy.

***automatic movement r.*** Automatic r.

***automatic r.*** A category of reflexes that includes righting and equilibrium reactions. SYN: *automatic movement r.*

***biuret r.*** **1.** A test for measuring proteins in serum. **2.** A chemical test for urea.

***chain r.*** A self-renewing reaction in which the initial stage causes the next reaction, which in turn causes the next, and so on.

***complement-fixation r.*** A reaction seen when the complement enters into combinations formed between soluble or particulate antigens and antibody. It is used for diagnosis of certain diseases, esp. syphilis. SEE: *complement; fixation, complement.*

***consensual r.*** **1.** An involuntary action. **2.** A crossed reflex.

***conversion r.*** A type of hysterical neurosis in which loss or alteration of physical functioning suggests a physical disorder but instead expresses a psychological conflict or need. The disturbance is not under voluntary control and cannot be explained by a disease process; it is not limited to pain or sexual dysfunction. SEE: *somatoform disorder.*

***cross r.*** A reaction between an antibody and an antigen that is not specific for the antibody but is closely allied to the antigen that is.

***defense r.*** A mental response whose purpose is to protect the ego.

***r. of degeneration*** A change in muscle reactivity to electricity, seen in lower motor neuron paralysis.

***delayed r.*** A reaction occurring a considerable time after a stimulus, esp. a reaction such as a skin inflammation occurring hours or days after exposure to the allergen.

***dissociative r.*** A sudden, temporary alteration in the normal functions of consciousness, identity, or motor behavior. These individuals may temporarily forget their identity or important personal events, or they may wander as if in a dream state.

***false-negative r.*** A test result that is negative in an individual with the attribute or disease being tested for.

***false-positive r.*** A positive reaction in a test, esp. for syphilis, that is due to faulty technique or the presence of another disease.

***foreign body r.*** A localized inflammatory response elicited by the presence of foreign material.

***hemianopic r.*** A reaction in which the pupils of both eyes fail to react to a thin pencil of light from the blind side but react normally to light from the normal side. It is seen in some forms of homonymous hemianopia.

***hemiopic pupillary r.*** A reaction in which light from one side causes the iris to contract but light from the other side does not cause the contraction. It is seen in certain cases of hemianopia.

***hypersensitivity r.*** Allergy.

***immune-mediated inflammatory r.*** The process by which the immune system constantly and silently destroys, dilutes, or walls off injurious agents and injured tissue. The local reaction is to dilate small blood vessels and to increase their permeability. This increases blood flow and permits exudation of plasma and leucocytes to accumulate at the site of the inflammation. The cells arriving from the blood include monocytes, neutrophils, basophils, and lymphocytes; those of local origin include endothelial cells, mast cells, tissue fibroblasts, and macrophages. Local immune response includes the generation of cytokines and neuropeptides. All of these events may be undetectable but the inflammation can progress and produce symptoms and signs.

***immune r.*** A reaction that demonstrates the presence of antibodies in the blood. It indicates a high degree of immunity.

***intracutaneous r.*** A reaction following the injection of a substance into the skin. SYN: *intradermal r.*

***intradermal r.*** Intracutaneous r.

***leukemic r., leukemoid r.*** A change in the peripheral blood that is consistent with a change occurring in leukemia. This may occur in patients with an infection or tumor who do not have leukemia.

***local r.*** A reaction occurring at the point of stimulation or injection of exciting substances.

***myasthenic r.*** A gradual decrease and eventual cessation of muscle contractions when a muscle is stimulated repeatedly by direct current.

***neutral r.*** In chemistry, a reaction indicating the absence of acid or alkaline properties; expressed as pH 7.0.

***ophthalmic r.*** Calmette's reaction.

***persistent light r.*** A persistent, intense sensitivity to light that afflicts some patients with photoallergy even after contact with the photoallergen has been eliminated. This persistent light reaction may be debilitating for years.

***Prausnitz-Küstner r.*** SEE: *Prausnitz-Küstner reaction.*

***quellung r.*** The swelling of capsules of bacteria when they are mixed with their specific immune serum.

***transfusion r.*** A reaction that follows transfusion of incompatible blood, which causes agglutination and hemolysis of the recipient's or donor's red blood cells or both.

***wheal and flare r.*** The response within 10 to 15 min to an antigen injected into the skin. The area demonstrates an elevated, blanched irregular wheal surrounded by erythema.

**reactivate** To make active again, esp., to return activity to immune serum that has lost its potency by the addition of fresh normal serum. This process restores the complement, which had become inactive through age, heat, or other factors.

**reactivation** (rē-ăk″tĭ-vā′shŭn) The process of making something active again.

**reactivity** (rē″ăk-tĭv′ĭ-tē) **1.** The action of reacting to a stimulus. **2.** In measurement of function or behavior, the influence that the presence of the examiner and the assessment process may have on performance and therefore on the outcome or finding.

**Read method** [Grantley Dick-Read, Brit. physician, 1890–1959] The original psychoprophylactic method of prepared childbirth, based on the premise that fear causes tension, which generates or increases pain during labor. Women are taught to control the response to each uterine contraction with slow abdominal breathing. Each breath is evenly divided between inhalation and exhalation.

**reading** Interpreting or perusing written or printed characters or material. Reading may or may not include comprehension of the material.

***lip r.*** Interpretation of what is being spoken by watching the movements of the speaker's lips.

**reading disorder** A condition that interferes with or prevents comprehension of written or printed material; used esp. in reference to children. In some adults, the condition may have developed from a brain injury or may have persisted from infancy. SEE: *dyslexia.*

**reading machine for the blind** An electronic device that converts printed matter into speech. Several machines for home use are available. Information may be obtained from the Lighthouse National Center for Vision and Aging at (800) 334-5497 or the American Foundation for the Blind at (800) 232-5463.

**reagent** (rē-ā′jĕnt) [L. *reagere,* to react] **1.** A substance involved in a chemical reaction. **2.** A substance used to detect the presence of another substance. **3.** A subject of a psychological experiment, esp. one reacting to a stimulus.

**reagin** (rē′ă-jĭn) A type of immunoglobulin E (IgE) present in the serum of atopic individuals that mediates hypersensitivity reactions. Reagin does not cross the placental barrier. **reaginic** (rē-ă-jĭn′ĭk), *adj.*

**reality** The quality of being genuine or actual.

**reality orientation** An intervention intended to orient persons with early dementia or delirium. It involves repetition of verbal and nonverbal information. The environment remains constant and the person is reminded and reviewed about names, dates, weather, and other pertinent information.

**reality principle** (rē-ăl′ĭ-tē) Awareness of external demands and adjustment in a manner that meets these demands, yet assures continued self-gratification.

**reality testing** The attempt by the individual to evaluate and understand the real world and his or her relation to it.

**reality therapy** A psychiatric treatment based on the concept that some patients deny the reality of the world around them. Therapy is directed to assist such patients in recognizing and accepting the present situation. The main technique is confrontation; the therapist consistently confronts the client with the reality of the situation. Illness or pathology is viewed as a defense against the real world. The purpose of the confrontation is to minimize distortion.

**reamer** (rē′mĕr) A small instrument used in dentistry for enlarging the root canal of a tooth.

**reanastomosis, surgical** The surgical procedure for rejoining structures, esp. vessels or tubes, that had been previously ligated.

**reanimate** (rē-ăn′ĭ-māt) [L. *re,* again, + *animare,* fill with life] To reactivate, restore to life, revive, or resuscitate.

**reapers' keratitis** (rēp′ĕrs kĕr-ă-tī′tĭs) A corneal inflammation caused by dust from grain. SEE: *keratitis.*

**reasonable care** In law, the degree of care that an ordinarily prudent person or professional would exercise under given circumstances.

**reasonable cost** The amount a third party (usually the medical insurer) will actually reimburse for health care. This amount is based on the cost to the provider for delivering that service.

**reattachment** (rē″ă-tăch′mĕnt) **1.** Recementing of a dental crown. **2.** Re-embedding of periodontal ligament fibers into the cementum of a tooth that has become dislodged. **3.** Rejoining of parts that have been separated, as a finger that has been traumatically detached.

**rebase** (rē-bās′) To refit a denture by replacing the base material without altering the occlusal characteristics.

**rebound** [ME. *rebounden,* to leap back] A reflex response in which sudden withdrawal of a stimulus is followed by fresh activity, such as a strong contraction following a moderate one, marked relaxation following moderate relaxation, or contraction replacing inhibition.

**rebound phenomenon** A symptom indicating a cerebellar lesion. When a limb or part is acting against a resistance and the resistance is suddenly removed, the limb moves forcibly in the direction toward which effort was being directed.

**rebreathing** The inhalation of gases that had been previously exhaled.

**Rebuck skin window test** An in vivo method of assessing inflammation. A superficial abrasion is made in the skin and a glass coverslip applied to the area. Leukocytes accumulate at the site and adhere to the coverslip.

**recalcification** (rē″kăl-sĭ-fĭ-kā′shŭn) [L. *re,* again, + *calx,* lime, + *facere,* to make] The restoration of calcium salts to tissues from which they have been withdrawn.

**recall** [″ + AS. *ceallian,* to call] The act of bringing back to mind something previously learned or experienced.

***24-hr dietary r.*** A dietary assessment form listing everything eaten in the previous 24 hr.

**recanalization** Re-establishment of an opening through a vessel that had been previously occluded.

**receiver** (rē-sēv′ĕr) [″ + *capere,* to take] **1.** A container for holding a gas or a distillate. **2.** An apparatus for receiving electric waves or current, such as a radio receiver.

**receptaculum** (rē″sĕp-tăk′ū-lŭm) *pl.* **receptacula** [L.] A vessel or cavity in which a fluid is contained.

***r. chyli*** Inferior, pear-shaped, expanded portion of the lower end of the thoracic duct, near the first and second lumbar vertebrae, into which the right and left lumbar trunks, an intestinal trunk, and some thoracic vessels empty. SYN: *cisterna chyli.*

**receptor** (rē-sĕp′tor) [L., a receiver] **1.** In pharmacology, a cell component that combines with a drug, hormone, or chemical mediator to alter the function of the cell. SEE: *Ehrlich's side-chain theory.* **2.** A sensory nerve ending. SYN: *ceptor.*

***accessory r.'s*** Proteins on the surface of T lymphocytes that enhance the response of the T-cell receptor to foreign antigens and stimulate signals from the receptor to the cytoplasm. SEE: *cell, antigen-presenting; receptor, T-cell.*

***adrenergic r.*** The area in certain cells that is thought to be the site of action of adrenergic stimulation, whether produced by the body or by drugs. There are two types of adrenergic receptors. Some act in response to sympathomimetic or adrenergic stimuli or drugs. These are called alpha-adrenergic receptors. Some inhibit the action of sympathomimetic or adrenergic stimuli. These are called beta-adrenergic receptors. Epinephrine is a powerful activator of alpha-adrenergic receptors; isoproterenol is a powerful activator of beta-adrenergic receptors.

***antigen r.*** In immunology, the site in or on a cell with which an antigen combines to influence cell function.

***auditory r.*** One of the hair cells in the organ of Corti in the cochlea of the ear.

***cell r.*** SEE: *drug r.*

***cholinergic r.*** A site in a nerve synapse or effector cell that responds to the effect of acetylcholine.

***complement r.*** ABBR: CR. A receptor on phagocytes, neutrophils, and macrophages that allows complement factors to bind, thus stimulating inflammation, phagocytosis, and cell destruction.

***contact r.*** A receptor that produces a sensation such as touch, temperature, or pain that can be localized in or on the surface of the body.

***cutaneous r.*** A receptor located in the skin.

***distance r.*** Teleceptor.

***drug r.*** Cell constituents, including chemicals, protein, and portions of a membrane, that sense extracellular signals and translate them into intracellular physiological or metabolic events. In the case of drugs, the receptors sense the presence of the pharmacologically active agent and produce the effects of the drug on the cell. There may be thousands of such receptors in *each* cell. SYN: *cell r.*

***gravity r.*** A macular hair cell of the utricle and saccule. It responds to changes in position of the head and linear acceleration.

***immunologic r.*** A receptor on the surface of white blood cells that identifies the type of cell and links with monokines, lymphokines, or other chemical mediators during the immune response.

***olfactory r.*** One of the bipolar nerve cells found in olfactory epithelium whose axons form olfactory nerve fibers.

***optic r.*** A rod or cone cell of the retina.

***proprioceptive r.*** A muscle or tendon spindle. These are the receptors of muscle or kinesthetic stimuli.

***rotary r.*** One of the hair cells in the cristae of the ampulla of the semicircular ducts of the ear. It is stimulated by angular acceleration or rotation.

***sensory r.*** A sensory nerve ending, a cell or group of cells, or a sense organ that when stimulated produces an afferent or sensory impulse.

CLASSIFICATION: *Exteroreceptors* are receptors located on or near the surface that respond to stimuli from the outside world. They include eye and ear receptors (for remote stimuli) and touch, temperature, and pain receptors (for contact). *Interoceptors* are those in the mucous linings of the alimentary and digestive tracts that respond to internal stimuli; also called visceroceptors. *Proprioceptors* are those responding to stimuli arising within body tissues.

Receptors also are classified according to the nature of stimuli to which they respond. This type includes *chemoreceptors,* which respond to chemical substances (taste buds, olfactory cells, receptors in aortic and carotid bodies); *pressoreceptors,* which respond to pressure (receptors in the aortic arch and carotid sinus); *photoreceptors,* which respond to light (rods and cones); and *tactile receptors,* which respond to touch (Meissner's corpuscle).

***stretch r.*** One of the neuromuscular and neurotendinar spindles and organs of Golgi, which are stimulated by stretch. SEE: *proprioceptor.*

***taste r.*** A gustatory cell of a taste bud.

***temperature r.*** A Krause's end-bulb (a cold receptor) or a Ruffini's corpuscle (a warmth receptor).

***touch r.*** A Merkel's disk, a Meissner's corpuscle, or a nerve plexus around a hair root.

**receptosome** Endosome.

**recess** (rē′sĕs) [L. *recessus,* receded] A small indentation, depression, or cavity. SYN: *recessus.*

***cochlear r.*** A small concavity, lying between the two limbs of the vestibular crest in the vestibule of the ear, that lodges the beginning of the cochlear duct.

***elliptical r.*** A small concavity lying superiorly and posteriorly on the medial wall of the vestibule that lodges the utricle of the ear.

***epitympanic r.*** Attic.

***infundibular r.*** A small projection of the third ventricle that extends into the infundibular stalk of the hypophysis.

***lateral r. of fourth ventricle*** One of two lateral extensions of the fourth ventricle, forming narrow pockets on each side and around the upper portions of the restiform bodies.

***nasopalatine r.*** A small depression on the floor of the nasal cavity near the nasal septum, lying immediately over the incisive foramen.

***omental r.*** One of three pocket-like extensions of the omental bursa. The superior recess extends upward behind the caudate lobe of the liver, the inferior recess extends downward into the great omentum, and the lineal recess extends laterally to the hilus of the spleen.

***optic r.*** A pocket of the third ventricle lying anterior to the infundibular recess. It is bound inferiorly by the optic chiasma.

***pharyngeal r.*** A recess in the lateral wall of the nasopharynx lying above and behind the opening to the auditory tube. SYN: *Rosenmüller's fossa.*

***pineal r.*** Recess of the roof of the third ventricle extending into the stalk of the pineal body.

***piriform r.*** A deep depression in the wall of the laryngeal pharynx lying lateral to the orifice of the larynx. It is bounded laterally by the thyroid cartilage and medially by the cricoid and arytenoid cartilages. It is a common site for lodgment of foreign objects.

***sphenoethmoidal r.*** A small space in the nasal fossa above the superior concha. It lies between the ethmoid bone and the anterior surface of the body of the sphenoid bone and posteriorly receives the opening of the sphenoidal sinus.

***spherical r.*** A recess on the medial wall of the vestibule of the inner ear that accommodates the saccule.

***suprapineal r.*** A posterior extension of the roof of the third ventricle forming a small cavity above the pineal body.

***tympanic membrane r.*** One of two pouches of tympanic mucous membrane (anterior and posterior) lying between the tympanic membrane and anterior and posterior malleolar folds.

***umbilical r.*** A dilatation on the left main branch of the portal vein that marks the position where the umbilical vein was originally attached.

**recession** (rē-sĕsh′ŭn) [L. *recessus,* recess] The withdrawal of a part from its normal position.

***gingival r.*** The complete or partial loss of the gingiva covering the root of the tooth, a condition resulting from poor oral hygiene. SEE: *gingivitis.*

**recessive** Tending to recede or go back; lacking control; not dominant.

**recessus** (rē-sĕs′ŭs) [L.] Recess.

**recidivation** (rē-sĭd″ĭ-vā′shŭn) [L. *recidivus,* falling back] **1.** The relapse of a disease or recurrence of a symptom. **2.** The return to criminal activity.

**recidivism** Habitual criminality; the repetition of antisocial acts.

**recidivist 1.** A confirmed criminal. **2.** A patient, esp. one with mental illness, who has repeated relapses into behavior marked by antisocial acts.

**recidivity** Tendency to relapse, or to return to a former condition.

**recipe** (rĕs′ĭ-pē) [L., take] **1.** Take, indicated by the sign ℞. **2.** A prescription or formula for a medicine. SEE: *prescription.*

**recipient** (rĭ-sĭp′ē-ĕnt) [L. *recipiens,* receiving] One who receives something, esp. blood, tissues, or an organ, provided by a donor, as in a blood transfusion or kidney transplant. SEE: *donor.*

**reciprocal** (rĭ-sĭp′rō-kăl) [L. *reciprocus,* alternate] Interchangeable.

**reciprocal inhibition 1.** The inhibition of muscles antagonistic to those being facilitated; this is essential for coordinated movement. **2.** Inhibition of a complementary nerve center by the one being stimulated (e.g., the inspiration center in the medulla generates impulses to the respiratory muscles to bring about inhalation, and inhibits the expiration center at the same time).

**reciprocation** (rĭ-sĭp″rō-kā′shŭn) [L. *reciprocare,* to move backward and forward] The countering of a reaction by an action. In dentistry, the action of one part of a dental device to counter the effect of another part.

**reciprocity** The recognition by one state of the license to practice granted to a health care professional by another state.

**Recklinghausen, Friedrich D. von** (rĕk′lĭng-how″zĕn) German pathologist, 1833–1910.

***R.'s canals*** Rootlets of the lymphatics, minute spaces in connective tissue. SYN: *von Recklinghausen's canals.*

***R.'s disease*** Type 1 neurofibromatosis.

***R.'s tumor*** An adenoleiomyofibroma on the wall of the fallopian tube or the posterior uterine wall. SYN: *von Recklinghausen's tumor.*

**reclination** (rĕk″lĭ-nā′shŭn) [L. *reclinatio,* lean back] The turning of a cataract-covered lens over into the vitreous to remove it from the line of vision.

**recline** (rē-klīn′) [L. *reclinare*] To be in recumbent position; to lie down.

**Reclus' disease** (rā-klooz′) [Paul Reclus, Fr. surgeon, 1847–1914] Multiple benign cystic growths in the breast.

**recombinant** In genetics and molecular biology, pert. to genetic material combined from different sources.

**recombinant DNA** Artificial manipulation of segments of DNA from one organism into the DNA of another organism. Using a technique known as gene splicing, it is possible to join genetic material of unrelated species. When the host's genetic material is reproduced, the transplanted genetic material is also copied. This technique permits isolating and examining the properties and action of specific genes. SEE: *plasmid; gene splicing.*

Studies in this area must be done in a carefully controlled environment. Levels of need for containment have been defined and are designated P-1 for the lowest level and P-4 for the highest. Level P-4 is for experiments involving animal virus DNA that contains potentially lethal genes. Experiments using DNA from pathogenic organisms, cancer-causing viruses, and viruses associated with certain toxins are prohibited in the U.S.

**recombinant TPA** SEE: *tissue plasminogen activator.*

**recombination** (rē″kŏm-bĭ-nā′shŭn) **1.** Joining again. **2.** In genetics, the joining of gene combinations in the offspring that were not present in the parents.

**recomposition** [L. *re,* again, + *composer,* to place together] The recombination of constituents or parts.

**recompression** [″ + LL. *compressare,* press together] The resubjection of a person to increased atmospheric pressure, a procedure used in the treatment of caisson disease (bends).

**reconcentration** The process of repeated concentration.

**reconstitution** (rē″kŏn-stĭ-tū′shŭn) The return of a substance previously altered for preservation and storage to its approximate original state, as is done with dried blood plasma.

**reconstruction** Surgical repair of a missing part or organ.

***r. of the knee*** Procedures to re-establish knee stability following injury, usually to the anterior or posterior cruciate ligaments or both.

***neovaginal r.*** Construction of an artificial vagina after the vagina has been removed because of cancer, or trauma of the pelvic area. The tissue used may be obtained from muscle and skin tissue from the abdomen. Normal sexual function is possible after the area has healed.

**record** (rĕk′ord) **1.** A written account of something. SEE: *problem-oriented medical record.* **2.** In dentistry, a registration of jaw relations in a malleable material or on a device.

***functional chew-in r.*** A record of the natural chewing action of the mandible made on an occlusion rim by the teeth or scribing studs.

***interocclusal r.*** A record of the positional relationship of the teeth or jaws to each other. A plastic material that hardens is placed between the teeth, and the patient bites down on it.

**recover** (rĭ-kŭv′ĕr) [O. Fr. *recoverer*] **1.** To regain health after illness; to regain a former state of health. **2.** To regain a normal state, as to recover from fright.

**recovery** (rĭ-kŭv′ĕr-ē) The process or act of becoming well or returning to a state of health.

**recovery position** The position in which the patient is placed on the left side with the left arm moved aside and supported to allow for lung expansion and the right leg crossed over the left. This position affords the unconscious, breathing patient the best protection from airway occlusion or aspiration of fluids into the lungs.

**recovery room** An area provided with equipment and nurses needed to care for patients who have just come from surgery. Patients remain there until they regain consciousness and are no longer drowsy and stuporous from the effects of the anesthesia. SEE: *postoperative care.*

**recreation** Literally, to create anew; participation in an endeavor that refreshes, provides mental or physical relaxation, or both. What one individual would consider work might well be a form of recreation to another.

**recredentialing** The process whereby an individual certified in a profession completes the current requirements for certification in that profession.

**recrement** (rĕk′rē-mĕnt) [L. *recrementum,* sifted again] A secretion, such as saliva or part of the bile, that is reabsorbed by the body.

**recrudescence** (rē″kroo-dĕs′ĕns) Relapse.

**recrudescent** (rē″kroo-dĕs′ĕnt) Assuming renewed activity after a dormant or inactive period.

**recruitment** (rĭ-kroot′mĕnt) [O. Fr. *recrute,* new growth] **1.** A condition in which response in a reflex action increases to a maximum when a stimulus is prolonged, even though the strength of the stimulus is unchanged. It is due to activation of increasingly greater numbers of motor neurons. For example, if, during a patellar reflex test, the normal patient clasps his or her hands together and attempts to pull them apart, the intensity of the reflex response increases. SEE: *Jendrassik's maneuver.* **2.** In audiology, an increase in the perceived intensity of a sound out of proportion to the actual increase in the sound level.

***r. of end organs*** An increase in discharge from sensory end organs, resulting from an increase in the number of end organs discharging and an increase in frequency of discharge from each.

**rectal** (rĕk′tăl) [L. *rectus,* straight] Pert. to the rectum.

**rectal anesthesia** Introduction of anesthetic into rectum for local desensitization, used esp. in labor.

**rectal crisis** Tenesmus and rectal pain in locomotor ataxia.

**rectalgia** (rĕk-tăl′jē-ă) [L. *rectus,* straight, + Gr. *algos,* pain] Pain in the rectum.

**rectal reflex** The normal desire to evacuate feces present in the rectum.

**rectification** (rĕk″tĭ-fĭ-kā′shŭn) [″ + *facere,* to make] **1.** The process of refining or purifying a substance. **2.** The act of straightening or correcting. **3.** The process of changing an alternating current into a pulsating direct current.

**rectified** (rĕk′tĭ-fīd) Made pure or straight; set right.

**rectifier** (rĕk′tĭ-fī″ĕr) [L. *rectum,* straight, + *-ficare,* to make] In electricity, a device for transforming an alternating current into a pulsating direct current.

**rectitis** (rĕk-tī′tĭs) Proctitis.

**recto-** Combining form meaning *straight.*

**rectoabdominal** (rĕk″tō-ăb-dŏm′ĭ-năl) [L. *rectus,* straight, + *abdomen,* belly] Pert. to the rectum and abdomen.

**rectocele** (rĕk′tō-sēl) [″ + Gr. *kele,* tumor, swelling] Protrusion or herniation of the posterior vaginal wall with the anterior wall of the rectum through the vagina. SEE: *cystocele.*

**rectoclysis** (rĕk-tŏk′lĭ-sĭs) [″ + Gr. *klysis,* a washing] The slow introduction of fluid into the rectum.

**rectococcygeal** (rĕk-tō-kŏk-sĭj′ē-ăl) [″ + Gr. *kokkyx,* coccyx] Pert. to the rectum and coccyx.

**rectococcypexia** (rĕk″tō-kŏk-sĭ-pĕks′sē-ă) [″ + ″ + *pexis,* fixation] Fixation of the rectum by suturing it to the coccyx.

**rectocolitis** (rĕk″tō-kō-lī′tĭs) Proctocolitis.

**rectocystotomy** (rĕk″tō-sĭs-tŏt′ō-mē) [″ + Gr. *kystis,* bladder, + *tome,* incision] An incision of the bladder through the rectum, usually to remove a calculus.

**rectolabial** (rĕk″tō-lā′bē-ăl) [″ + *labium,* lip] Pert. to the rectum and a labium of the vaginal introitus.

**rectoperineorrhaphy** (rĕk″tō-pĕr″ĭ-nē-or′ă-fē) Proctoperineoplasty.

**rectopexy** (rĕk′tō-pĕk-sē) Proctopexy.

**rectophobia** (rĕk″tō-fō′bē-ă) [″ + Gr. *phobos,* fear] Acute anxiety in patients with rectal disease concerning the possibility of having cancer.

**rectoplasty** (rĕk′tō-plăs″tē) Proctoplasty.

**rectorrhaphy** (rĕk-tor′ă-fē) Proctorrhaphy.

**rectoscope** (rĕk′tō-skōp) [″ + Gr. *skopein,* to examine] Proctoscope.

**rectoscopy** (rĕk-tŏs′kō-pē) Proctoscopy.

**rectosigmoid** (rĕk″tō-sĭg′moyd) [″ + Gr. *sigma,* letter S, + *eidos,* form, shape] The upper part of the rectum and the adjoining portion of the sigmoid colon.

**rectosigmoidectomy** (rĕk″tō-sĭg″moy-dĕk′tō-mē) [″ + ″ + *ektome,* excision] Surgical removal of the rectum and sigmoid colon.

**rectostenosis** (rĕk″tō-stĕn-ō′sĭs) [″ + Gr. *stenos,* narrow] Stricture of the rectum.

**rectostomy** (rĕk-tŏs′tō-mē) Proctostomy.

**rectotomy** (rĕk-tŏt′ō-mē) Proctotomy.

**rectourethral** (rĕk″tō-ū-rē′thrăl) [″ + Gr. *ourethra,* urethra] Pert. to the rectum and urethra.

**rectouterine** (rĕk″tō-ū′tĕr-ĭn) [″ + *uterus,* womb] Pert. to the rectum and uterus.

**rectovaginal** (rĕk″tō-văj′ĭ-năl) [″ + *vagina,* sheath] Pert. to the rectum and vagina.

**rectovesical** (rĕk″tō-vĕs′ĭ-kăl) [″ + *vesica,* bladder] Pert. to the rectum and bladder.

**rectovestibular** (rĕk″tō-vĕs-tĭb′ū-lăr) [″ + *vestibulum,* vestibule] Pert. to the rectum and vestibule of the vagina.

**rectovulvar** (rĕk″tō-vŭl′văr) [″ + *vulva,* covering] Pert. to the rectum and vulva.

**rectum** (rĕk′tŭm) [L., straight] The lower part of the large intestine, about 5 in. (12.7 cm) long, between the sigmoid colon and the anal canal. The centers for the defecation reflex are in the second, third, and fourth sacral segments. SEE: *colon* for illus.

**rectus** (rĕk′tŭs) [L.] Straight; not crooked.

**rectus muscle 1.** One of two external abdominal muscles on either side, from the pubic bone to the ensiform cartilage and the fifth, sixth, and seventh ribs. **2.** One of the four short muscles of the eye: exterior, interior, superior, and inferior.

**recumbency** (rĭ-kŭm′bĕn-sē) [L. *recumbens,* lying down] The condition of leaning or reclining.

**recumbent 1.** Lying down. SEE: *position, left lateral recumbent; position, unilateral recumbent; prone.* **2.** Inactive, idle.

***dorsal r.*** Lying on one's back. SYN: *su-*

*pine* (1).

***lateral r.*** Lying on one's side.

***ventral r.*** Lying with one's anterior side down. SYN: *prone* (1).

**recuperation** (rĭ-kū″pĕr-ā′shŭn) [L. *recuperare,* to recover] The process of returning to normal health following an illness.

**recurrence** (rĭ-kŭr′ĕns) Relapse. **recurrent** (-ĕnt), *adj.*

**recurvation** (rĭ″kŭr-vā′shŭn) [L. *recurvus,* bent back] The act of bending backward.

**recurvatum** Backward bowing. At the knee, it is called genu recurvatum or back knee.

**recurve** (rē-kŭrv′) To bend backward.

**red** (rĕd) [AS. *read*] A primary color of the spectrum.

***Congo r.*** An odorless red-brown powder used in testing for amyloid. In polarized light, amyloid treated with Congo red produces a green fluorescence.

***cresol r.*** An indicator of pH. It is yellow below pH 7.4 and red above 9.0.

***methyl r.*** An indicator of pH. It is red at pH 4.4 and yellow at 6.2.

***neutral r.*** An indicator of pH. It is red at pH 6.8 and yellow at 8.0.

***phenol r.*** Phenolsulfonphthalein.

***scarlet r.*** An azo dye used in staining tissues for microscopic examination.

***vital r.*** A stain used in preparing tissues for microscopic examination.

**red bag** Term used to describe infectious material or the placement of that material in a special red container. SEE: *Universal Precautions Appendix.*

**red bag waste** Infectious material placed in a special container to prevent its being the source of infection to anyone exposed to it. SEE: *Universal Precautions Appendix.*

**red blindness** Inability to see red hues. The most frequent type of color blindness.

**red blood cell** Erythrocyte.

***spiculed r.b.c.*** Spiculed red cell.

**redbug** Chigger.

**red cross** A red cross on a white background; an internationally recognized sign of a medical installation or of medical personnel. It is also the emblem of the American Red Cross.

**redia** (rē′dē-ă) *pl.* **rediae** [Francesco Redi, It. naturalist, 1626–1698] The stage in the life cycle of a trematode that follows the sporocyst stage. Rediae are saclike structures possessing an oral sucker and a blind gut. They arise parthenogenetically from germ masses within the sporocyst and in turn produce second- or third-generation rediae or cercaria.

**redifferentiation** (rē″dĭf-ĕr-ĕn″shē-ā′shŭn) The resuming of the characteristics of mature cells by malignant cells.

**red. in pulv.** [L., *reductus in pulverum*] Let it be reduced to powder.

**redintegration** (rĕd-ĭn″tĕ-grā′shŭn) [L. *redintegratio*] **1.** Restitution of a part. **2.** Restoration to health. **3.** Recall by mental association.

**redistribution** The matching of health care personnel resources to the population's site of care. Generally, the term is used in discussing the maldistribution of in-hospital personnel compared with in-community personnel.

**red lead** $Pb_3O_4$. Lead tetroxide.

**red man (neck) syndrome** An adverse anaphylactoid reaction to vancomycin therapy causing pruritus, flushing, and erythema of the head and upper body. The condition is caused by release of histamine.

**red nucleus** SEE: under *nucleus.*

**red-out** (rĕd′owt) A term used in aerospace medicine to describe what happens to the vision and central nervous system (i.e., seeing red and perhaps experiencing unconsciousness) when the aircraft is doing part or all of an outside loop at high speed, or any other maneuver that causes the pilot to experience a negative force of gravity. The condition is due to engorgement of the vessels of the head including those of the retina.

**redox** Combined form indicating oxidation-reduction system or reaction.

**red precipitate** Red mercuric oxide. Poisoning symptoms are similar to those of mercuric chloride.

**red tide** Seasonal proliferation of certain dinoflagellates in coastal waters. These blooms change the color of the water to red, green, or brown and produce a potent neurotoxin that kills fish and contaminates shellfish. SEE: *poisoning, shellfish.*

**reduce** (rĭ-dūs′) [L. *re,* again, + *ducere,* to lead] **1.** To restore to usual relationship, as the ends of a fractured bone. **2.** To weaken, as a solution. **3.** To diminish, as bulk or weight.

**reducible** (rĭ-dūs′ĭ-bl) Capable of being replaced in a normal position, as a dislocated bone or a hernia.

**reducing agent** A substance that loses electrons easily and therefore causes other substances to be reduced (e.g., hydrogen sulfide, sulfur dioxide).

**reductant** (rĭ-dŭk′tănt) The atom that is oxidized in an oxidation-reduction reaction.

**reductase** (rĭ-dŭk′tās) [″ + *ducere,* to lead, + *ase,* enzyme] An enzyme that accelerates the reduction process of chemical compounds.

**reduction** (rĭ-dŭk′shŭn) [L. *reductio,* leading back] **1.** Restoration to a normal position, as a fractured bone or a hernia. **2.** In chemistry, a type of reaction in which a substance gains electrons and positive valence is decreased. SEE: *oxidation.*

***closed r. of fractures*** The treatment of bone fractures by placing the bones in their proper position (i.e., reducing the fragments without surgery).

***open r. of fractures*** The treatment of bone fractures by the use of surgery to place the bones in their proper position (i.e., reducing the fragments).

**reduction division** Meiosis.

**redundant** (rĭ-dŭn′dĕnt) [L. *redundare,* to overflow] More than necessary.

**reduplicated** (rĭ-dū′plĭ-kā″tĕd) [L. *re,* again, + *duplicare,* to double] **1.** Doubled. **2.** Bent backward on itself, as a fold.

**reduplication** (rĭ-dū″plĭ-kā′shŭn) **1.** A doubling, as of the heart sounds in some morbid conditions. **2.** A fold.

**Reduviidae** (rē″dū-vī′ĭ-dē) A family of the order Hemiptera, including the assassin bugs.

**Reduvius** (rē-dū′vē-ŭs) A genus of true bugs belonging to the family Reduviidae.

***R. personatus*** A species that normally feeds on other insects but sometimes attacks humans, inflicting painful bites about the face. In some individuals, these bites may cause severe allergic symptoms. SYN: *kissing bug.*

**Reed-Sternberg cell** [Dorothy Reed, U.S. pathologist, 1874–1964; Karl Sternberg, Aust. pathologist, 1872–1935] A giant connective tissue cell with one or two large nuclei that is characteristic of Hodgkin's disease. SEE: illus.

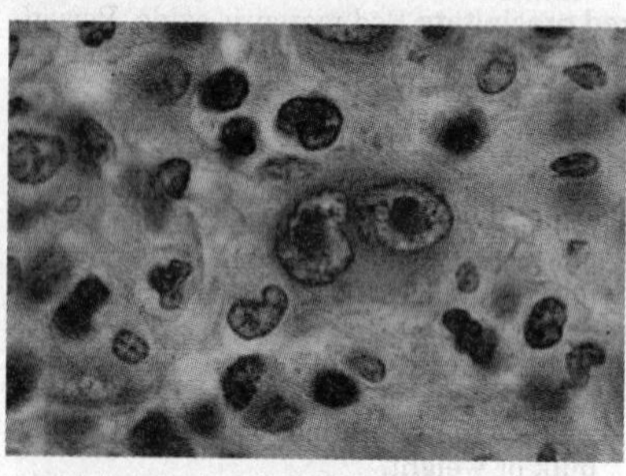

REED-STERNBERG CELL (CENTER)
(ORIG. MAG. ×600)

**re-education** (rē″ĕd-ū-kā′shŭn) [L. *re,* again, + *educare,* to educate] **1.** Training to develop partial competence in a disabled or mentally ill person. **2.** A physical means of restoring muscular tone and activity.

***sensory r.*** A rehabilitation regimen used after sensation is impaired by peripheral nerve injuries or surgery to the hand. The purpose is to relearn the interpretation of sensory information related to pain, temperature, and object identification.

**reef** (rēf) A fold or tuck, usually taken in redundant tissue.

**re-entry** (rē-ĕn′trē) In cardiology, the diversion of a repolarization wave from a direction in which it is blocked to another in which it is not blocked. The wave then goes back up the original pathway to produce a contraction. This leads to a continuing series of premature beats.

**refection** (rē-fĕk′shŭn) [L. *reficere,* to refresh] **1.** The act of restoring. **2.** In laboratory rats, recovery from symptoms of vitamin B-complex deficiency on a diet deficient in vitamin B. It is thought to be due to vitamin synthesis by intestinal bacteria.

**reference man** A concept used in nutritional investigation and surveys; a man 22 years of age, weighing 70 kg, living in an environment with a mean temperature of 20°C, wearing clothing compatible with thermal comfort, engaged in light physical activity, and with an estimated caloric intake of 2800 kcal/day.

**reference woman** A hypothetical model used in nutritional references, described the same as reference man, except in weight (58 kg) and caloric intake (2000 kcal/day).

**referral** The practice of sending a patient to another practitioner or specialty program for consultation or service. Such a practice involves a delegation of responsibility for patient care, which should be followed up to ensure satisfactory care.

**refine** (rē-fīn′) [L. *re,* again, + ME. *fin,* finished] To purify or render free from foreign material.

**reflectance** The fraction of total light reflected after it hits a surface, and the angle at which it is reflected.

***diffuse r.*** The reflectance of light from a rough or nonpolished surface in which the radiant energy tends to go in all directions. The angle of reflectance does not equal the angle of incidence.

***r. photometer*** An instrument used to measure reflectance; used clinically in chemical analyzers, glucometers, and dip stick readers, such as the Ames serolyzer.

***spectral r.*** The reflectance of light from a polished surface in which the angle of reflectance equals the angle of incidence.

**reflection** (rĭ-flĕk′shŭn) [L. *reflexio,* a bending back] **1.** The condition of being turned back on itself, as when the peritoneum passes from the wall of a body cavity to and around an organ and back to the body wall. **2.** The throwing back of a ray of radiant energy from a surface not penetrated. **3.** Mental consideration of something previously considered.

***diffuse r.*** The reflection of a light ray by a rough surface in which the angle of reflection is NOT equal to the angle of incidence. As opposed to *specular* reflection by a smooth surface in which the angle of reflection equals the angle of incidence. Employed in the analytical technique of reflectometry.

**reflectometer** An instrument that measures the light reflected by a surface. Reflectometers are used clinically in urinalysis and chemistry.

**reflector** (rĭ-flĕk′tor) [L. *re,* again, + *flectere,* to bend] A device or surface that reflects waves, radiant energy, or sound.

**reflex** (rē′flĕks) [L. *reflexus,* bend back] An involuntary response to a stimulus; an involuntary action. Reflexes are specific and predictable and are usually purposeful and adaptive. They depend on an intact neural pathway between the stimulation point and a responding organ (a muscle or gland). This pathway is called the reflex arc. In a simple reflex this includes a sensory receptor, afferent or sensory neuron, reflex center in the brain or spinal cord, one or more efferent neurons, and an effector organ (a muscle or gland). Most reflexes, however, are more complicated and include internuncial or associative neurons intercalated between afferent and efferent neurons. SEE: *arc, reflex* for illus.

***abdominal r.*** SEE: *abdominal reflexes.*

***abdominocardiac r.*** A change in heart rate, usually a slowing, resulting from mechanical stimulation of abdominal viscera.

***accommodation r.*** One of the changes that take place when the eye adjusts to bring light rays from an object to focus on the retina. This involves a change in the size of the pupil, convergence or divergence of the eyes, and either a decrease or an increase in the convexity of the lens depending on the previous condition of the lens.

***Achilles r.*** SEE: *Achilles tendon reflex.*

***acquired r.*** Conditioned r.

***allied r.'s*** Reflexes initiated by several stimuli originating in widely separated receptors whose impulses follow the final common path to the effector organ and reinforce one another.

***anal r.*** SEE: *anal reflex.*

***ankle r.*** SEE: *ankle jerk.*

***antagonistic r.'s*** Two or more reflexes initiated simultaneously in different receptors that involve the same motor center but produce opposite effects. The most important or adaptive response takes place.

***asymmetrical tonic neck r.*** In an infant, extension of one or both extremities on the side to which the head is forcibly turned. Flexion of the extremities occurs on the other side.

***auditory r.*** SEE: *auditory reflex.*

***autonomic r.*** Any reflex involving the response of a visceral effector (cardiac muscle, smooth muscle, or gland). Such reflexes always involve two efferent neurons (preganglionic and postganglionic).

***axon r.*** A reflex that does not involve a complete reflex arc and hence is not a true reflex. Its afferent and efferent limbs are branches of a single nerve fiber, the axon (axon-like dendrite) of a sensory neuron. An example is vasodilation resulting from stimulation of the skin.

***Babinski's r.*** SEE: *Babinski's reflex.*

***Bainbridge r.*** An increase in heart rate caused by an increase in blood pressure or distention of the heart. SYN: *Bainbridge effect.*

***biceps r.*** Flexion of the forearm on percussion of the tendon of the biceps brachii.

***brachioradial r.*** Supinator longus r.

***Brain's r.*** SEE: *Brain's reflex.*

***carotid sinus r.*** Slowing of the heart due to pressure in the area of the neck over the carotid sinus.

***cat's eye r.*** In children, a pupillary flash or reflection from the eye that may be momentary; may be white, yellow, or pink; and is best seen under diminished natural illumination. This reflex, which may be noticed first by a parent, may be caused by various conditions, the most important of which is retinoblastoma. It is also observed in tuberous sclerosis, inflammatory eye diseases, and certain congenital malformations of the eye. SEE: *retinoblastoma.*

***Chaddock's r.*** SEE: *Chaddock's reflex.*

***chain r.*** A reflex initiated by several separate serial reflexes, each activated by the preceding one.

***chin r.*** A clonic movement resulting from percussion or stroking of the lower jaw.

***ciliary r.*** The normal contraction of the pupil in accommodation of vision from distant to near.

***ciliospinal r.*** Dilation of the pupil following stimulation of the skin of the neck by pinching or scratching.

***clasp-knife r.*** Quick inhibition of the stretch reflex when extensor muscles are forcibly stretched by flexing the limb. SYN: *lengthening reaction.*

***conditioned r.*** A reflex acquired as a result of training in which the cerebral cortex is an essential part of the neural mechanism; any reflex not inborn or inherited. SYN: *acquired r.*

***conjunctival r.*** SEE: *conjunctival reflex.*

***consensual r.*** Crossed r.

***convulsive r.*** A reflex induced by a weak stimulus and causing widespread uncoordinated and purposeless muscle contractions; seen in strychnine poisoning.

***corneal r.*** SEE: *corneal reflex.*

***cough r.*** SEE: *cough reflex.*

***cranial r.*** Any reflex whose origin is in the brain.

***cremasteric r.*** Retraction of the testis when the skin is stroked on the front inner side of the thigh.

***crossed r.*** A reflex in which stimulation of one side of the body results in response on the opposite side. SYN: *consensual r.; indirect r.*

***crossed extension r.*** An extension of the lower extremity on the opposite side when a painful stimulus is applied to the skin.

***deep r.*** A reflex caused by stimulation of parts beneath skin, such as tendons or bones. Examples include the jaw, elbow, wrist, triceps, knee, and ankle jerk reflexes.

***delayed r.*** A reflex that does not occur until several seconds after the application of a stimulus.

***digital r.*** SEE: *digital reflex.*

***diving r.*** Slowing of the heart rate when the head is immersed in water. This reflex helps to protect a person from drowning, esp. during immersion in cold water. SEE: *drowning.*

***elbow r.*** Triceps r.

***elementary r.*** A typical reflex common to all vertebrates; includes the postural, flexion, stretch, and extensor thrust reflexes.

***embrace r.*** SEE: *Moro reflex.*

***extensor thrust r.*** A quick and brief extension of a limb on application of pressure to the plantar surface.

***flexor withdrawal r.*** Flexion of a body part in response to a painful stimulus. SYN: *withdrawal r.*

***gag r.*** Gagging and vomiting resulting from irritation of the throat or pharynx.

***gastrocolic r.*** Peristaltic wave in the colon induced by entrance of food into the stomach.

***gastroileal r.*** The physiological relaxation of the ileocecal valve resulting from food in the stomach.

***Gault's r.*** SEE: *Gault's reflex.*

***Geigel's r.*** SEE: *Geigel's reflex.*

***gluteal r.*** Contraction of the gluteal muscles from stimulation of the overlying skin.

***grasp r.*** The grasping reaction of the fingers and toes when stimulated.

***Grünfelder's r.*** SEE: *Grünfelder's reflex.*

***heart r.*** Any reflex in which the stimulation of a sensory nerve causes the heart rate to increase or decrease. An example is the Bainbridge reflex, in which stimulation of sensory receptors in the right atrium by increased venous return results in an increase in heart rate.

***Hering-Breuer r.*** SEE: *Hering-Breuer reflex.*

***Hoffmann's r.*** A reflex that occurs when the tip of the nail of the ring, middle, or index finger is flicked, producing flexion of the terminal phalanx of the thumb and the second and third phalanges of another finger.

***hung-up r.*** Slowness of the relaxation phase of deep tendon reflexes; present in hypothyroidism.

***hypochondrial r.*** Sudden inspiration resulting from abrupt pressure below the costal border.

***inborn r.*** An unconditioned reflex; an innate or inherited reflex.

***indirect r.*** Crossed r.

***inhibition of r.*** The prevention of a reflex action, as inhibiting a sneeze by pressure on a facial nerve as it passes just under the upper lip.

***interscapular r.*** A scapular muscular contraction following percussion or stimulus between the scapulae.

***intersegmental r.*** A reflex involving several segments of the spinal cord. SYN: *long r.*

***intestinal r.*** Myenteric r.

***intrasegmental r.*** Reflex that involves only a single segment of the spinal cord.

***irradiation of r.'s*** The spreading of reflexes through the central nervous system whereby impulses entering the cord in one segment activate motor neurons located in many segments.

***jaw r.*** Chin r.

***kinetic r.*** Labyrinthine righting r.

***Kisch's r.*** SEE: *Kisch's reflex.*

***knee-jerk r.*** Extension of the leg resulting from percussion of the patellar tendon. This is one of the myotatic or stretch reflexes important in maintaining posture. The reflex is diminished or abolished in lesions of the nerve supplying the muscle and tendon, posterior root lesions involving a sensory pathway as in tabes dorsalis, anterior root lesions involving motor pathways, or lower motor neuron lesions in the anterior horns of the gray matter of the spinal cord, as in poliomyelitis. If, however, the upper motor neuron is destroyed, muscle tone and motor response are greatly increased. So-called pathologic reflex may appear under these conditions. Reflexes are also modified by higher centers; for example, emotional tension increases the knee jerk (and muscle tension generally). SYN: *patellar r.* SEE: *Babinski's reflex; Jendrassik's maneuver.*

***labyrinthine righting r.*** A reflex, esp. a postural reflex, resulting from stimulation of receptors in the semicircular ducts, utricle, and saccule of the inner ear. This reflex helps orient the head in space and to the rest of the body. SYN: *kinetic r.; optical righting r.*

***lacrimal r.*** Secretion of fluid resulting from irritation of the corneal conjunctiva.

***laryngeal r.*** Coughing as a result of irritation of the larynx or fauces.

***letdown r.*** The movement of breast milk from the alveoli into the lactiferous ducts in response to oxytocin-stimulated contractions. The reflex may be stimulated by suckling or by infant crying. Stimulation of the nipple increases the secretion of oxytocin and this technique may be used to stimulate contraction of the postpartum uterus.

***lid r.*** Closure of eyelids resulting from direct corneal stimulation. SYN: *corneal reflex.*

***light r.*** Constriction of the pupil when light is flashed into the eye.

***lip r.*** The reflex movement of the lips when the angle of the mouth is suddenly and lightly tapped during sleep.

***local r.*** A reflex that does not involve the central nervous system (e.g., the myenteric reflex, which occurs even when extrinsic nerves to the intestine have been cut).

***long r.*** Intersegmental r.

***lumbar r.*** An irritation of the skin over the erector spinae muscles, causing contraction of the back muscles.

***Magnus-de Kleijn r.*** In decerebrate rigidity, extension of the limbs on the side to which the chin is turned by rotating the head. There is flexion of the limbs on the opposite side.

***mandibular r.*** Clonic movement resulting from percussing or stroking the lower jaw.

***mass r.*** A condition following spinal cord section in which a weak stimulus through radiation causes widespread responses due to release of higher cortical centers from inhibition.

***Mayer's r.*** Opposition and adduction of the thumb, flexion at the metacarpophalangeal joint, and extension at the interphalangeal joint in response to downward pressure on the index finger.

***Mendel-Bekhterev r.*** Plantar flexion of the toes in response to percussion of the dorsum of the foot.

***monosynaptic r.*** A reflex involving only two neurons, an afferent and an efferent.

***Moro r.*** SEE: *Moro reflex.*

***myenteric r.*** Reflex caused by distention of the intestine, resulting in contraction above the point of stimulation and relaxation below it. SYN: *intestinal r.*

***myotatic r.*** Stretch r.

***near r.*** Accommodation r.

***neck-righting r.*** In a supine infant, rotation of the trunk in the same direction as that in which the head is turned. This reflex appears at age 4 to 6 months and is no longer obtainable by age 2 years.

***nociceptive r.*** A reflex initiated by a painful stimulus.

***obliquus r.*** Contraction of the entire external obliquus muscle on application of stimulus to the skin of the thigh below Poupart's ligament.

***oculocardiac r.*** SEE: *Aschner's phenomenon.*

***oculocephalic r.*** The deviation of a neonate's eyes to the opposite side when the head is rotated. SYN: *doll's eye reflex.*

***optical righting r.*** Labyrinthine righting r.

***palatal r.*** Swallowing induced by stimulation of the soft palate.

***palmar grasp r.*** A reflex in which the lightly stimulated palm grasps the stimulating object. This reflex is present at birth and is gone by age 6 months.

***palm-chin r.*** Vigorous stroking or scratching of the thenar eminence, producing contraction of the skin and lower lip muscles on the same side.

***parachute r. (response)*** Extension of the arms, hands, and fingers when the infant is suspended in the prone position and dropped a short distance onto a soft surface. This reaction appears at age 9 months and persists. An asymmetrical response indicates a motor nerve abnormality.

***paradoxical r.*** A response to a stimulus that is unexpected and may be the opposite of what would be considered normal.

***patellar r.*** Knee-jerk r.

***pathological r.*** An abnormal reflex due to disease; the reflex is seen as one of the symptoms of the disease.

***penile r.*** **1.** Sudden downward movement of the penis when the prepuce or gland of a completely relaxed penis is pulled upward. **2.** Contraction of the bulbocavernous muscle on percussing the dorsum of the penis. **3.** Contraction of the bulbocavernous muscle resulting from compression of the glans penis.

***pharyngeal r.*** An attempt to swallow following any application of stimulus to the pharynx.

***pilomotor r.*** Piloerection when skin is cooled or as a result of emotional reaction.

***placing r.*** Flexion and then extension of an infant's leg that occurs when an infant is held erect and the dorsum of one foot is dragged along the underedge of a table top. This reflex lasts from birth until age 6 weeks.

***plantar r.*** SEE: *Babinski's reflex; plantar reflex.*

***plantar grasp r.*** A grasp reflex resulting from light stimulation of the sole of the foot. This reflex lasts from birth until age 10 months.

***platysmal r.*** Dilation of the pupil resulting from sharp pinching of the platysma myoides.

***pneocardiac r.*** A change in the rate and rhythm of the heart and blood pressure when an irritant vapor is inhaled.

***pneopneic r.*** A change in respiratory depth and rate, coughing, suffocation, and pulmonary edema when an irritant vapor is inhaled.

***postural r.*** Any reflex that is concerned with maintaining posture.

***pressor r.*** A reflex in which the response to stimulation is an increase in blood pressure brought about by constriction of arterioles.

***proprioceptive r.*** A reflex initiated by body movement to maintain the position of the moved part; any reflex initiated by stimulation of a proprioceptor.

***psychogalvanic r.*** Decreased electric resistance of the skin in response to emotional stress or stimuli.

***pupillary r.*** **1.** Constriction of the pupil upon stimulation of the retina by light. **2.** Constriction of the pupil upon accommodation for near vision, and dilatation upon accommodation for far vision. **3.** Constriction of the pupil of one eye in response to stimulation of the other by light. **4.** Constriction of the pupil upon attempted closure of eyelids that are held apart.

***quadriceps r.*** Knee-jerk r.

***quadrupedal extensor r.*** Brain's reflex.

***red r.*** The red light reflection seen in ophthalmoscopic examination of the eye.

***righting r.*** Any of the reflexes that enable an animal to maintain the body in a definite relationship to the head and thus maintain its body right side up.

***rooting r.*** The turning of an infant's mouth toward the stimulus when the infant's cheek is stroked. This reflex is present at birth; by age 4 months it is gone when the infant is awake; by age 7 months it is gone when the infant is asleep.

***Rossolimo's r.*** SEE: *Rossolimo's reflex.*

***scapular r.*** Muscular contraction following percussion or stimulus between the scapulae.

***scapulohumeral r.*** A reflex in which the upper arm is adducted and rotated outward when the vertebral border of the scapula is percussed.

***scrotal r.*** Slow vermicular contraction of the scrotal muscle when the perineum is stroked or cold is applied.

***segmental r.*** A reflex action in which afferent impulses enter the cord in the same segment or segments from which the efferent impulses emerge.

***sexual r.*** A reflex concerned with sexual activities, esp. erection and ejaculation, which results from direct genital stimulation or indirectly from emotion, whether the individual is asleep or awake.

***short r.*** A reflex involving one or a few segments of spinal cord.

***simple r.*** A reflex in which only two or possibly three neurons are interposed between receptor and effector organs.

***solar sneeze r.*** A sneeze that occurs following exposure to bright sunlight. This benign condition may affect a great number of normal persons, and it may also be associated with rhinitis. The mechanism of the cause of this type of sneeze reflex is unknown.

***sole r.*** Plantar reflex.

***somatic r.*** A reflex induced by stimulation of somatic sensory nerve endings.

***spinal r.*** A reflex whose center is in the spinal cord.

***startle r.*** Moro reflex.

***static r.*** A reflex concerned with establishing and maintaining posture when the body is at rest.

***statokinetic r.*** A reflex that occurs when the body is moving (e.g., walking or running).

***stepping r.*** Movements of progression elicited by holding an infant upright, inclined forward, and touching the soles of the feet to a flat surface. This reflex lasts from birth to age 6 weeks.

***stretch r.*** The contraction of a muscle as a result of quickly stretching the same muscle. Stretch reflexes are of primary importance in the maintenance of posture. SYN: *myotatic r.*

***sucking r.*** A sucking movement of an infant's mouth produced by stroking the lips. A primitive form of this reflex is present in the fetus by the 16th week of gestation; it is fully developed by the time of birth.

***superficial r.*** A cutaneous reflex caused by irritation of the skin or areas depending on the spinal cord as a motor center (e.g., the scapular, epigastric, abdominal, cremasteric, gluteal, and plantar reflexes) or on centers in the medulla (e.g., the conjunctival, pupillary, and palatal reflexes). This reflex is induced by a very light stimulus, such as stroking the skin lightly with a soft cotton wad.

***supinator longus r.*** Flexion of the forearm caused by tapping of the tendon of the supinator longus. SYN: *brachioradial r.*

***supraorbital r.*** A contraction of orbicularis oculi muscle with closure of lids resulting from percussion above the supraorbital nerve.

***suprapubic r.*** Deflection of the linea alba toward the stroked side when the abdomen is stroked above Poupart's ligament.

***swallowing r.*** The production of successive reflexes and muscular activity concerned with swallowing when the palate is stimulated by food.

***symmetrical tonic neck r.*** In an infant, flexion or extension of the arms in response to flexion and extension, respectively, of the neck.

***tendon r.*** A deep reflex obtained by sharply tapping the skin over the tendon of a muscle. It is exaggerated in upper neuron disease and diminished or lost in lower neuron disease.

***tonic neck r.*** A general term used to denote either the asymmetrical or symmetrical tonic neck reflexes seen in infants. The presence of these reflexes suggests that head movements cause reflexive movements of the upper extremities.

***tonic vibration r.*** ABBR: T.V.R. A polysynaptic reflex believed to depend on spinal and supraspinal pathyways.

***triceps r.*** Sharp extension of the forearm resulting from tapping of the triceps tendon while the arm is held loosely in a bent position. SYN: *elbow r.*

***triceps surae r.*** Achilles tendon reflex.

***true autonomic r.*** A visceral response in which afferent impulses do not pass through the central nervous system, but instead enter prevertebral ganglia where connections are made with efferent neurons.

***unconditioned r.*** A natural or inherited reflex action; one not acquired.

***urinary r.*** The spinal cord reflex, initiated by accumulated urine stretching the bladder and the resulting contraction of the bladder to expel urine.

***vascular r.*** Vasomotor r.

***vasomotor r.*** The constriction or dilatation of a blood vessel in response to a stimulus, as in becoming pale from fright. SYN: *vascular r.*

***visceral r.*** Any reflex induced by stimulation of the visceral nerves.

***visceromotor r.*** Contraction or tenseness of the skeletal muscles resulting from painful stimuli originating in visceral organs.

***withdrawal r.*** Flexor withdrawal r.

**reflexogenic** (rĭ-flĕks″ō-jĕn′ĭk) [L. *reflexus,* bend back, + Gr. *gennan,* to produce] Causing a reflex action.

**reflexogenous** (rĭ″flĕks-ŏj′ĕ-nŭs) Reflexogenic.

**reflexograph** (rĭ-flĕks′ō-grăf) [″ + Gr. *graphein,* to write] A device for recording and graphing a reflex, esp. one produced by muscular activity.

**reflexology** (rē″flĕk-sŏl′ō-jē) [″ + Gr. *logos,* word, reason] **1.** The study of the anatomy and physiology of reflexes. **2.** A system of massage in which the feet and sometimes the hands are massaged in an attempt to favorably influence other body functions.

**reflexometer** (rē″flĕks-ŏm′ĕ-tĕr) [″ + Gr. *metron,* measure] An instrument that measures the force of the tap required to produce a reflex.

**reflexophil** (rē-flĕks′ō-fĭl) [″ + Gr. *philein,* to love] Marked by reflex activity or by exaggerated reflexes.

**reflexotherapy** (rē-flĕks″ō-thĕr′ă-pē) [″ + Gr. *therapeia,* treatment] Treatment by manipulating, anesthetizing, or cauterizing an area distant from the location of the disorder. SEE: *spondylotherapy.*

**reflex sympathetic dystrophy** An excessive or abnormal response of the sympathetic nervous system following injury to the face, shoulder, or extremity. Treatment includes pharmacological or surgical sympathectomy. SEE: *Nursing Diagnoses Appendix.*

ETIOLOGY: The variable complex of symptoms may be due to multiple underlying etiological mechanisms including immobilization of a part to avoid significant pain; self-inflicted injury as part of a factitious disorder with secondary gain, as in Munchausen's syndrome or malingering; or a set of neuropathic events occurring in the context of nerve injury or absence.

SYMPTOMS: There is long-standing, severe, burning pain of the face, and a hypersensitive painful reaction to all types of stimuli. In addition, there may be cyanosis, pallor, coldness, or swelling of the area. A symptom ascribed to RSD is abnormal response of the sympathetic nervous system to injury of the shoulder, arm, or leg. This ill-defined condition has been referred to as *shoulder-hand syndrome* and *Sudek's atrophy.*

**reflux** (rē′flŭks) [L. *re,* back, + *fluxus,* flow] A return or backward flow. SEE: *regurgitation.*

***hepatojugular r.*** Increased cervical venous pressure caused by pressure on the liver in patients with congestive heart failure.

***vesicoureteral r.*** A reflux of urine up the ureter during urination.

**reflux disease** The illness produced when gastric contents reflux into the esophagus. The symptoms are heartburn, regurgitation of acid, peptic ulcer-like pain, and difficulty swallowing. If the symptoms cannot be controlled by medical therapy, surgery is needed.

**refract** (rĭ-frăkt′) [L. *refractus,* broken off] **1.** To turn back; to deflect. **2.** To detect and correct refractive errors in the eyes.

**refracta dosi** (rē-frăk′tă dō′sē) [L.] In divided doses, denoting a definite amount of drug taken within a given time in a number of fractional equal parts.

**refraction** (rĭ-frăk′shŭn) [LL. *refractio,* break back] **1.** Deflection from a straight path, as of light rays as they pass through media of different densities; the change in direction of a ray when it passes from one medium to another of a different density. **2.** Determination of the amount of ocular refractive errors and their correction.

***angle of r.*** The angle formed by a refracted ray of light with a line perpendicular to the surface at the refraction point.

***coefficient of r.*** The quotient of the sine of the angle of incidence divided by the sine of the angle of refraction.

***double r.*** Possession of more than one refractive index, resulting in a double image. SEE: *birefractive; birefringence.*

***dynamic r.*** The static refraction of the eye plus that accomplished by accommodation; the reciprocal of the near-point distance.

***error of r.*** Ametropia.

***r. of eye*** The refraction brought about by the refractive media of the eye (cornea, aqueous humor, crystalline lens, vitreous body). SYN: *ocular r.*

***index of r.*** **1.** The ratio of the angle made by the incident ray with the perpendicular (angle of incidence) to that made by the emergent ray (angle of refraction). **2.** The ratio of the speed of light in air to its speed in another medium. The refractive index of water is 1.33; that of the crystalline lens of the eye is 1.413.

***ocular r.*** R. of eye.

***static r.*** Refraction of the eye when accommodation is at rest or paralyzed.

**refractionist** (rĭ-frăk′shŭn-ĭst) [LL. *refractio,* break back] A person skilled in determining and correcting ocular refractive errors by the use of appropriate glass lenses.

**refractive** (rĭ-frăk′tĭv) [L. *refractus,* broken off] Concerning refraction. SYN: *refringent.*

**refractive power** The degree to which a transparent body deflects a ray of light from a straight path. SEE: *diopter.*

**refractivity** (rē″frăk-tĭv′ĭ-tē) The quality of being refractive; the ability to refract.

**refractometer** (rē-frăk-tŏm′ĕt-ĕr) [″ + Gr. *metron,* measure] A device for measuring refractive power, as of the eye.

**refractometry** (rē″frăk-tŏm′ĕ-trē) Measurement of the refractive power of lenses.

**refractory** (rē-frăk′tō-rē) [L. *refractarius*] **1.** Obstinate; stubborn. **2.** Resistant to ordinary treatment. **3.** Resistant to stimulation; used of muscle or nerve.

**refractory period, absolute** The brief period during depolarization of a neuron or muscle fiber when the cell does not respond to any stimulus, no matter how strong.

**refractory period, relative** The brief period during repolarization of a neuron or muscle fiber when excitability is depressed. If stimulated, the cell may respond, but a stronger than usual stimulus is required.

**refracture** (rē-frăk′chūr) [L. *refractus,* broken off] **1.** To break again, as a bone set wrongly. **2.** Rebreaking of a fracture united in a malaligned or incorrect position.

**refrangible** (rē-frăn′jĭ-bl) [L. *re,* again, + ME. *frangible,* breakable] Capable of being refracted.

**refresh** (rĭ-frĕsh′) [O. Fr. *refreschir,* to renew] **1.** To restore strength; to relieve from fatigue; to renew; to revive. **2.** To scrape epithelial covering from two opposing surfaces of a wound to facilitate healing and joining together.

**refrigerant** (rĭ-frĭj′ĕr-ănt) [L. *refrigerans,* making cold] **1.** Cooling. **2.** An agent that produces coolness or reduces fever. SYN: *algefacient.*

**refrigerant gas** One of several gases used in ordinary household refrigerators. Poisoning may be caused by leaks, faulty connections or breakage, or gas dissipated into the atmosphere.

**refrigeration** (rĭ-frĭj″ĕr-ā′shŭn) [L. *refrigeratio,* make cold] Cooling; reduction of heat.

**refringent** Refractive.

**Refsum's disease** (rĕf′soomz) [Sigvald Bernhard Refsum, Norwegian physician, b. 1907] An inherited metabolic disease caused by the inability to metabolize phytanic acid. Clinical symptoms include visual disturbances, ataxia, and heart disease. Diets low in animal fat and milk products may relieve some of the symptoms.

**regainer** (rē-gān′ĕr) **1.** A device that ameliorates or restores something that was lost. **2.** A device that applies pressure between teeth on either side of the space left by a missing tooth. This is done to push the teeth toward the edentulous space.

**regeneration** (rē-jĕn″ĕr-ā′shŭn) [L. *re,* again, + *generare,* to produce] Repair, regrowth, or restoration of a part, such as tissues. Opposite of degeneration.

**regimen** (rĕj′ĭ-mĕn) [L., rule] A systematic plan of activities and regulation of diet, sleep, and exercise designed to improve or maintain health or to keep a certain condition under control.

**regio** (rē′jē-ō) [L.] Region.

**region** (rē′jŭn) [L. *regio,* boundary] A portion of the body with natural or arbitrary boundaries. SYN: *regio.* **regional** (-ăl), *adj.*

**register** [LL. *regesta,* list] **1.** An official recording of names or facts. **2.** The compass or range of a voice. **3.** A series of tones of like quality or character, as low or high register, chest or head register.

**registered nurse** SEE: under *nurse.*

**registered record administrator** ABBR: R.R.A. A person in charge of medical records who has been certified as an R.R.A. after passing the examination given by the American Medical Record Association.

**registrant** (rĕj′ĭs-trănt) [L. *registrans,* registering] A nurse named on the books of a registry as being "on call" or available to be called for duty.

**registrar** (rĕj′ĭs-trăr) [O. Fr. *registreur*] The official manager of a registry.

**registration** [L. *registratio*] The recording of information such as births or deaths; the recording of those who are registered or licensed to practice within a state.

**registry** (rĕj′ĭs-trē) [LL. *regesta,* list] An office or book cotaining a list of nurses ready for duty; a placement bureau for nurses.

**regression** (rĭ-grĕsh′ŭn) [L. *regressio,* go back] **1.** A turning back or return to a former state. **2.** A return of symptoms. **3.** Retrogression. **4.** In psychology, an abnormal return to an earlier reaction, characterized by a mental state and behavior inappropriate to the situation. Regression may occur as a result of frustration or in states of fatigue, dreams, hypnosis, intoxication, illness, and certain psychoses (e.g., schizophrenia). **5.** In statistics, a procedure used to predict one variable on the basis of data about one or more other variables. **regressive** (-grĕs′ĭv), *adj.*

**regressive resistive exercise** ABBR: RRE. A form of active resistive exercise that advocates gradual reduction in the amount of resistance as muscles fatigue.

**regular** (rĕg′ū-lăr) [L. *regula,* rule] **1.** Conforming to a rule or custom. **2.** Methodical, steady in course, as a pulse. SEE: *normal; typical.*

**regulation 1.** The condition of being controlled or directed. **2.** The ability of an organism, such as a developing embryo, to develop normally despite experimental modifications. **regulative,** *adj.*

**regulation development** In embryology, the condition in which a single blastomere or a portion of an embryo can give rise to a whole embryo; the opposite of mosaic development.

**regulator** A device for adjusting or controlling the rate of flow or administration of fluids, oxygen, or blood.

**regurgitant** (rē-gŭr′jĭ-tănt) [L. *re,* again, + *gurgitare,* to flood] Throwing back or flowing in a direction opposite to the normal.

**regurgitation** (rē-gŭr″jĭ-tā′shŭn) A backward flowing, as in the return of solids or fluids to the mouth from the stomach or the backflow of blood through a defective heart valve.

***aortic r.*** A backflow of blood into the left ventricle as a result of an incompetent aortic valve.

***cardiac r.*** A backflow of blood through the aortic, mitral, or tricuspid valves owing to incomplete closure.

***duodenal r.*** A return flow of chyme from the duodenum to the stomach.

***functional r.*** Regurgitation caused not by valvular disorder but by dilatation of ventricles, the great vessels, or valve rings.

***mitral r.*** A backflow of blood from the left ventricle into the left atrium, resulting from imperfect closure of the mitral or bicuspid valve.

***pulmonic r.*** A backflow of blood from the pulmonary artery into the right ventricle.

***tricuspid r.*** A backflow of blood from the right ventricle into the right atrium.

***valvular r.*** A backflow of blood through a valve, esp. a heart valve, that is not completely closed as it would normally be.

**REHABDATA** A computerized bibliographical database of rehabilitation information supplied by the National Rehabilitation Information Center (NARIC). For information, contact National Rehabilitation Information Center, 8455 Colesville Road, Suite 935, Silver Spring, MD 20910-3319. (800) 34-NARIC.

**rehabilitation** (rē″hă-bĭl″ĭ-tā′shŭn) [L. *rehabilitare*] **1.** The processes of treatment and education that help disabled individuals to attain maximum function, a sense of well-being, and a personally satisfying level of independence. Rehabilitation may be necessitated by any disease or injury that causes mental or physical impairment serious enough to result in disability. The postmyocardial infarction patient, the posttrauma patient, and the postsurgical patient need and can benefit from rehabilitation efforts. The individual who is recovering from a mental disorder also needs rehabilitative support. The combined efforts of the individual, family, friends, medical, nursing, and allied health personnel, and community resources are essential to making rehabilitation possible. **2.** In dentistry, the methods used to restore dentition to its optimal functional condition. It may involve restoration of teeth by fillings, crowns, or bridgework; adjustment of occlusal surfaces by selective grinding; orthodontic realignment of teeth; or surgical correction of diseased or malaligned parts. It may be done to provide masticatory function, an acceptable aesthetic appearance of the face and teeth, improved phonetics, and preservation of the dentition and supporting tissues. Also called *occlusorehabilitation* and *mouth,* or *oral, rehabilitation.*

***cardiac r.*** A structured, interdisciplinary program of supervised activity, progressive exercise, psychological support, and patient education to enable attainment of maximum functional capacity by patients who have experienced a myocardial infarction.

***pulmonary r.*** A system of retraining and relaxation exercises in breathing, designed to return patients with pulmonary disease to optimal function.

**rehabilitee** (rē″hă-bĭl′ĭ-tē) A person who has been rehabilitated.

**rehalation** (rē″hă-lā′shŭn) [L. *re,* again, + *halare,* to breathe] A rebreathing process occasionally used in anesthesia.

**rehydration** (rē″hī-drā′shŭn) [″ + Gr. *hydor,* water] The restoration of fluid volume in a person who has been dehydrated, replenishing fluids orally or parenterally.

**Reichert's cartilage** (rī′kĕrts) [Karl Bogislaus Reichert, Ger. anatomist, 1811–1883] The second branchial arch of the embryo, which gives rise to the stapes, styloid process, stylohyoid ligament, and lesser cornua to the hyoid bone.

**Reid's base line** (rēdz) [Robert William Reid, Scottish anatomist, 1851–1939] The line extending from the lower edge of the orbit to the center of the aperture of the external auditory canal and backward to the center of the occipital bone.

**Reil's island** (rīlz) Island of Reil.

**reimplantation** (rē″ĭm-plăn-tā′shŭn) [L. *re,* again, + *in,* into, + *plantare,* to set] Replantation.

**reinfection** (rē″ĭn-fĕk′shŭn) [″ + ME. *infecten,* infect] A second infection by the same organism. SEE: *superinfection.*

**reinforcement** (rē″ĭn-fors′mĕnt) [″ + *inforce,* enforce] Strengthening; an augmentation of force; part of the fundamental learning process, along with motivation, stimulation, and action. Reinforcement is the reward for the appropriate response in a learning situation.

**reinforcement of reflex** Strengthening of the response to one stimulus by concurrent action of another; the exaggeration of a reflex by nervous activity elsewhere. Thus, during the raising of a heavy weight, the knee jerk is stronger. SEE: *Jendrassik's maneuver.*

**reinforcer** (rē″ĭn-fors′ĕr) Something that produces reinforcement.

**reinfusion** (rē″ĭn-fū′zhŭn) [″ + *infusio,* to pour in] The reinjection of blood serum or cerebrospinal fluid.

**reinnervation** (rē″ĭn-ĕr-vā′shŭn) [″ + *in,* into, + *nervus,* nerve] **1.** Anastomosis of a paralyzed part with a living nerve. **2.** Grafting of a fresh nerve for restoration of function in a paralyzed muscle.

**reinoculation** (rē″ĭn-ŏk″ū-lā′shŭn) [″ + *in,* into, + *oculus,* bud] A second inoculation with the same virus or organism. SEE: *reinfection.*

**reintegration** In psychology, the resumption of normal behavior and mental functioning following disintegration of personality in mental illness.

**reinversion** (rē″ĭn-vĕr′shŭn) [″ + *in,* into, + *versio,* turning] Correction of an inverted organ.

**Reissner's membrane** (rīs′nĕrz) [Ernst

Reissner, Ger. anatomist, 1824–1878] A delicate membrane separating the cochlear canal from the scala vestibuli.

**Reiter's syndrome** (rī′tĕrz) [Hans Conrad Julius Reiter, Ger. physician, 1881–1969] ABBR: RS. A syndrome consisting of urethritis, which usually occurs first; arthritis; and conjunctivitis. It occurs mainly in young men. *Chlamydia* is the organism most frequently associated with RS. The prognosis is generally good; however, recurrences are common.

TREATMENT: There is no specific therapy. Tetracycline or erythromycin is used for urethritis. The sexual partner should be treated if RS was transmitted sexually. Arthritis and conjunctivitis are treated symptomatically.

**rejection** [L. *rejicere,* to throw back] **1.** Refusal to accept or to show affection for. In lower animals the young may be ignored or driven away by their mother. **2.** In tissue and organ transplantation, destruction of transplanted material at the cellular level by the host's immune mechanism. Transplant rejection is controlled primarily by T cells, but macrophages and B lymphocytes are also involved. Increased use of testing for HLA matching has lowered the incidence of organ transplant rejection. Immunosuppressant drugs, such as cyclosporine and corticosteroids, inhibit T-cell function and reduce the possibility of rejection.

***acute r.*** The early destruction of grafted or transplanted material, usually beginning a week after implantation. It may be reversed by increased use of immunosuppressive agents.

***chronic r.*** The slow destruction of grafted or transplanted material, a process that may occur over months or years.

***hyperacute r.*** Immediate, intense, and irreversible destruction of grafted material due to preformed antibodies.

***parental r.*** The refusal of a parent to accept or show affection for a son or daughter.

**rejuvenation** (rĭ-jū″vē-nā′shŭn) [L. *re,* again, + *juvenis,* young] A return to a youthful condition or to the normal.

**rejuvenescence** (rĭ-jū″vē-nĕs′ĕns) [″ + *juvenescere,* to become young] The renewal of youth; the return to an earlier stage of existence.

**relapse** (rē-lăps′) [L. *relapsus*] The recurrence of a disease or symptoms after apparent recovery.

**relapsing** Recurring after apparent recovery.

**relation** (rĭ-lā′shŭn) [L. *relatio,* a carrying back] The condition, connection, or state of one thing compared with another.

***jaw r.*** Any relation of the position of the maxilla to that of the mandible.

***occlusal jaw r.*** The relation of the mandibular teeth to the maxillary teeth when the teeth are in contact.

***unstrained jaw r.*** The position of the jaw during normal tonus of all the jaw muscles.

**relative biological effect** The effectiveness of types of radiation compared with that of x-rays or gamma rays.

**relative value scale** ABBR: RVS. A proposal for setting the amount paid for medical services. It is based on the concept that payment rates for medical services should, as with other purchased services and goods, reflect the costs of producing those services.

**relax** [L. *relaxare,* to loosen] To decrease tension or intensity; to be rid of strain, anxiety, and nervousness.

**relaxant** (rĭ-lăk′sănt) **1.** Pert. to or producing relaxation. **2.** A drug that reduces tension. **3.** A laxative.

***muscle r.*** A drug or therapeutic treatment that specifically relieves muscular tension.

***neuromuscular r.*** A drug (e.g., succinylcholine) that prevents transmission of stimuli to muscle tissue, esp. striated muscle.

***smooth muscle r.*** A drug that reduces the tension of smooth muscles such as those in the intestinal tract or bronchi.

**relaxation** (rē-lăk-sā′shŭn) **1.** A lessening of tension or activity in a part. **2.** A phase or period in a single muscle twitch following contraction in which tension decreases, fibers lengthen, and the muscle returns to a resting position. **3.** In magnetic resonance imaging, the return of an excited atom to alignment with the applied magnetic field.

***general r.*** Relaxation of the entire body.

***local r.*** Relaxation limited to a particular muscle group or to a certain part.

***pelvic r.*** Diminished support of the pelvic tissues and organs, esp. in women; it is usually due to childbirth or aging. The organs affected and the pathological conditions associated with the relaxation are bladder and cystocele; rectum and rectocele; uterus and uterine prolapse; small intestine with production of enterocele; urethra with protrusion of urethra into the vagina. Symptoms are related to the organ(s) affected. Treatment is determined by the severity of the relaxation. Surgery may be required.

**relaxation response** The physiological reaction sought and produced by sitting quietly and alone in a quiet place with the eyes closed and the arms and hands relaxed, paying careful attention to respiration, and repeating a brief word or phrase at each respiratory cycle. This is done for 15 to 30 min at a time, twice daily. This approach to quiet meditation is found in the practices of many religions and in transcendental meditation. It has been used by some physicians to produce therapeutic alteration in stress control, as indicated by a reduction in blood pressure in hypertensive patients.

**relaxed movement** Passive exercise.

**relaxin** (rĭ-lăk′sĭn) A polypeptide hormone secreted in the corpus luteum during pregnancy. It is obtained commercially from the ovaries of pregnant sows. In certain rodents, it relaxes the symphysis, inhibits uterine contractions, and softens the cervix.

**relearning** Acquiring a skill or ability that had been previously present but was lost or removed as a result of physical damage to the muscles or brain.

**release** A document that, if signed by the patient or the patient's legal representative in the case of a minor, permits the treating physician to perform certain procedures (e.g., surgery, anesthesia, blood transfusion, removal of tissues or fluids for analysis). In addition to being signed by the patient, the release should also be signed by a witness. Most releases have a notation indicating the applicable time of the release.

***myofascial r.*** ABBR: MFR. The manipulation of soft tissue, usually in the vertebral region, to improve posture and motor control. These benefits are thought to occur through the reduction (release) of adhesions that restrict movement.

**reliability 1.** The condition of being dependable, accurate, and honest. **2.** In statistics, the ability of the measuring method or device to produce reproducible data or information.

**relief** (rĭ-lēf′) [ME.] The alleviation or removal of a distressing or painful symptom.

**relieve** [L. *relevare,* to raise] To provide relief.

**reline** (rē-līn′) To replace or resurface the lining of a denture.

**relinquishment, infant** The psychological process experienced by a birth mother during adoption of her child by others.

**relocation stress syndrome** Physiological and/or psychosocial disturbances as a result of transfer from one environment to another. SEE: *Nursing Diagnoses Appendix.*

**REM** *rapid eye movements.* Cyclic movement of the closed eyes observed or recorded during sleep. SEE: *sleep.*

**rem** *roentgen equivalent* (in) *man.*

**Remak, Robert** (ră′māk) German neurologist, 1815–1865.

***R.'s axis cylinder*** The conducting part of a nerve.

***R.'s band*** The axis cylinder of a neuron.

***R.'s fibers*** The nonmedullated nerve fibers.

***R. ganglion*** A group of nerve cells in coronary sinus near its entry into the right atrium.

**Remak's sign** [Ernest Julius Remak, Ger. neurologist, 1849–1911] A sign or symptom pert. to perception of stimuli. It can be one of two types: a single stimulus may be perceived as if it were several stimuli applied in separate locations (polyesthesia), or there may be a delay in perception of stimuli. Both types are seen in tabes dorsalis.

**remedial** (rĭ-mē′dē-ăl) [L. *remedialis*] Curative; intended as a remedy.

**remedy** (rĕm′ĕd-ē) [L. *remedium,* medicine] **1.** To cure or relieve a disease. **2.** Anything that relieves or cures a disease.

***herbal r.*** Plant leaves, roots, seeds, or extracts used to prevent or treat human ailments. Historically, plants have been the source of therapeutic drugs used to treat human disorders (e.g., digitalis). Although many herbs contain potent chemicals that have important known therapeutic properties, others have equally important toxic actions. Herbal remedies are established therapeutic agents in some cultures. Problems may arise due to the lack of uniformity of the ingredients; variation of the concentration of the herb in a given preparation; toxicity due to prolonged therapy with an herb that might be helpful when taken in small doses over a brief period; inadvertent or intentional adulteration by individuals who are unqualified to dispense medicines; misidentification of the herbs; and misuse. SEE: *alternative medicine.*

Caution: Herbal preparations of unknown potency and ingredients should not be taken during pregnancy or while nursing. Further, they should not be given to newborns. In addition, persons who decide to use herbs for medical purposes should be advised to purchase only preparations that list the plants they contain. If the herbs are to be taken during a serious illness, blood, kidney, and hepatic studies should be done before initiating herbal therapy.

***local r.*** An agent used to relieve a local condition such as a sore.

***systemic r.*** An agent used to relieve or cure a disease affecting the entire organism.

**remineralization** (rē-mĭn″ĕr-ăl-ī-zā′shŭn) Therapeutic replacement of the mineral content of the body after it has been disrupted by disease or improper diet.

**reminiscence therapy** A type of supportive talk therapy prescribed by health care professionals for patients who are aged and experiencing loss. Reminiscence therapy assists patients to review and highlight the meaningful components of their past. This is thought to increase self-esteem and life satisfaction. It can be conducted in groups or individually.

**remission** (rĭ-mĭsh′ŭn) [L. *remissio,* remit] **1.** A lessening of severity or an abatement of symptoms. **2.** The period during which symptoms abate.

**remittance** (rē-mĭt′ĕns) A temporary abatement of symptoms.

**remittent** (rē-mĭt′ĕnt) [L. *remittere,* to send back] Alternately abating and returning at certain intervals. SEE: *fever.*

**remittent fever** A fever alternately abating and returning, without intervals of afebrility. SEE: *malaria.*

**remnant** Something that remains or is left over.

**remnant radiation** Ionizing radiation that passes through the part being examined to make the radiographical image.

**remodeling 1.** The reshaping or reconstruction of a part or area. **2.** Bone change or growth that is the net effect of all appositional growth and bone resorption and that continues throughout life to adapt the skeletal elements to the changing forces of growth, muscular activity, gravity, or mechanical pressures.

***temporomandibular joint r.*** The slow changes in the articular surfaces of the temporomandibular joint as it adapts to changing occlusal forces, resulting in shape changes or irregularities of the condyle or articular eminence.

**Remsed** Trade name for promethazine hydrochloride.

**ren** (rĕn) *pl.* **renes** [L.] The kidney.

**renal** (rē′năl) [LL. *renalis,* kidney] **1.** Pert. to the kidney. SYN: *nephric.* SEE: *kidney* for illus. **2.** Shaped like a kidney.

**renal biopsy, percutaneous** Obtaining of renal tissue for analysis by use of a needle inserted through the skin. This is usually done after the kidney has been localized by ultrasound, computed tomography, or angiography. The major complication is hematuria. This technique is used to establish a diagnosis of renal dysfunction, determine prognosis in patients with renal disease, evaluate the extent of renal injury, and determine appropriate therapy.

**renal clearance test** One of several kidney function tests based on the kidney's ability to eliminate a given substance in a standard time. Urea, phenolsulfonphthalein (PSP), iodopyracet, and other substances are employed.

**renal failure, acute** Acute failure of the kidney to perform its essential functions. It may be due to trauma; any condition that impairs the flow of blood to the kidneys; certain toxic substances such as mercury compounds, carbon tetrachloride, or ethylene glycol; bacterial toxins; glomerulonephritis; or acute obstruction of the urinary tract. The treatment consists of specific therapy for the primary condition and either peritoneal dialysis or hemodialysis. SEE: *dialysis; Nursing Diagnoses Appendix.*

NURSING IMPLICATIONS: The cause is identified and removed. The nurse instructs the patient regarding dietary and fluid restrictions and implements these restrictions, promotes infection prevention, and advises the patient about activity restrictions due to metabolic alterations.

Complications of immobility are prevented by respiratory toilet, position changes, and range-of-motion exercises. Neurological status is assessed, and safety measures are instituted. Intake and output are monitored, as well as acid-base and electrolyte balance, particularly for signs and symptoms of hyperkalemia, and daily weights. The patient is assessed for G.I. and cutaneous bleeding and anemia, and blood components are replaced or erythropoietin therapy is administered as prescribed. Vital signs are assessed for signs of pericarditis or hypotension, and findings are recorded.

If this condition is not reversed but progresses to chronic (end-stage) renal failure, follow-up care is arranged, and evaluation and teaching are provided for possible dialysis. Referral is made for vocational, sexual, or other counseling as needed.

**renal papillary necrosis** Destruction of the papillae of the kidney. It may be caused by several conditions including diabetes mellitus, acute pyelonephritis, urinary obstruction, sickle cell trait, and repeated use of phenacetin. Management consists of ureteral catheter irrigation of the renal pelvis to remove obstruction, appropriate antibiotics, and adequate hydration.

**renal scanning** A method of determining renal function and shape. A radioactive substance that concentrates in the kidney is given intravenously. The radiation emitted from the substance as it accumulates in the kidneys is recorded on a suitable photographic film.

**renal transplantation** The surgical implantation of a donor kidney to replace one removed from a patient. SEE: *Nursing Diagnoses Appendix.*

**renal tubular acidosis** ABBR: RTA. A group of four disorders. Types I and II are hereditary; type III, a combination of types I and II, is rare; and type IV is acquired. In all types, the excretion rate of bicarbonate is excessive. In addition, the kidneys resorb chloride in an excessive amount. This results in hyperchloremic acidosis.

Type I is marked by hypercalciuria, calcium phosphate stones, and nephrocalcinosis. In children, rickets develops and growth is stunted. Adults with this condition have osteomalacia. Treatment consists of administration of sodium bicarbonate and Shohl's solution.

Type II may be a transient disorder of proximal tubular function. Treatment, if required, consists of bicarbonate given in large amounts each day in combination with potassium supplements.

Type IV is usually associated with hypoaldosteronism due to diabetic nephropathy, or nephrosclerosis associated with hypertension, or chronic nephropathy. These patients have high serum potassium levels and low urine ammonia excretion. They do not have renal calculi. The hyperkalemia may be managed by administration of mineralocorticoids in combination with furosemide.

**Rendu-Osler-Weber syndrome** Hereditary hemorrhagic telangiectasia.

**reniculus** (rĕ-nĭk′ū-lŭs) [L.] A lobule of the kidney.

**renifleur** (rā-nĭ-flŭr′) [Fr.] One stimulated sexually by certain odors, esp. that of the the urine of others.

**reniform** (rĕn′ĭ-form) [L. *ren,* kidney, + *forma,* shape] Shaped like a kidney. SYN: *nephroid.*

**renin** (rĕn′ĭn) An enzyme produced by the kidney that splits angiotensinogen to form angiotensin I, which is then transformed to angiotensin II, which stimulates vasoconstriction and secretion of aldosterone. The blood renin level is elevated in some forms of hypertension.

**renin substrate** Hypertensinogen.

**renipelvic** (rĕn″ĭ-pĕl′vĭk) [″ + *pelvis,* basin] Pert. to the renal pelvis.

**reniportal** (rĕn″ĭ-por′tăl) [″ + *porta,* gate] **1.** Pert. to the "hilum" of the kidney. **2.** Pert. to the renal and portal circulations.

**renipuncture** (rĕn″ĭ-pŭnk′chūr) [″ + *punctura,* a piercing] Surgical puncture of the renal capsule.

**rennet** (rĕn′ĕt) [ME.] **1.** The lining of the fourth stomach of a calf. **2.** A fluid containing rennin (chymosin), a coagulating enzyme, used for making junket or cheese.

**rennin** (rĕn′ĭn) Chymosin.

**renninogen** (rĕn-ĭn′ō-jĕn) [ME. *rennet,* rennet, + Gr. *gennan,* to produce] The antecedent or zymogen from which rennin is formed; the inactive form of rennin.

**reno-, ren-** Combining form meaning *kidney.* SEE: *nephro-.*

**renocutaneous** (rē″nō-kū-tā′nē-ŭs) [″ + *cutis,* skin] Pert. to the kidneys and skin.

**renogastric** (rē″nō-găs′trĭk) [L. *ren,* kidney, + Gr. *gaster,* belly] Pert. to the kidneys and stomach.

**renogram** (rē′nō-grăm) [″+ Gr. *gramma,* something written] A record of the rate of removal of an intravenously injected dose of radioactive iodine ($^{131}I$) from the blood by the kidneys.

**renography** (rē-nŏg′ră-fē) [″ + Gr. *graphein,* to write] Radiography of the kidney.

**renointestinal** (rē″nō-ĭn-tĕs′tĭn-ăl) [″ + *intestinum,* intestine] Pert. to the kidneys and intestine.

**renoprival** (rē″nō-prī′văl) Pert. to loss of kidney function.

**renovascular** Pert. to the vascular supply of the kidney.

**Renshaw cell** (rĕn′shaw) [B. Renshaw, U.S. neurophysiologist, 1911–1948] A small cell with a short axon that connects motor nerve axons with each other. The process inhibits motor neurons.

**reovirus** (rē″ō-vī′rŭs) [*r*espiratory *e*nteric *o*rphan *virus*] One of the viruses found in the respiratory and digestive tracts of apparently healthy persons. Their exact importance in producing disease is not known. This group of viruses was formerly classed as ECHO virus, type 10.

**rep** [L., *repetatur*] Let it be repeated.

**repair** (rĭ-păr′) [L. *reparare,* to prepare again] To remedy, replace, or heal, as in a wound or a lost part.

***plastic r.*** Use of plastic surgery to repair tissue.

***tooth r.*** Recovery from pathological changes, involving the reduction of inflammation and the production of tertiary or reparative cementum. This is usually accompanied by improved health of the gingiva and the periodontal ligament.

**repellent** [L. *repellere,* to drive back] An agent that repels noxious organisms such as insects, ticks, and mites. Repellents may be applied to the surface of the body as a liquid, spray, or dust, or they may be used to impregnate clothing.

***insect r.*** A commercial preparation effective in repelling insects. Many insect repellents contain diethyltoluamide. When applying insect repellent, do not allow it to contact the eyes and use only as necessary, esp. on children.

**repercolation** (rē″pĕr-kō-lā′shŭn) [L. *re,* again, + *percolare,* to filter] Repeated percolation using the same materials.

**repercussion** (rē-pĕr-kŭsh′ŭn) [L. *repercussio,* rebound] **1.** A reciprocal action. **2.** An action involved in causing the subsidence of a swelling, tumor, or eruption. **3.** Ballottement.

**repercussive** (rē″pĕr-kŭs′ĭv) **1.** Causing repercussion. **2.** An agent that repels; a repellent.

**reperfusion** [L. *re,* back, + *perfundere,* to pour through] **1.** The reinstitution of blood flow to a previously ischemic area; in cardiology, the return of blood supply to a portion of the heart muscle that had become ischemic owing to myocardial infarction. This is done by the use of thrombolytic agents such as streptokinase, or tissue plasminogen activator (TPA). The use of such agents has reduced in-hospital mortality for myocardial infarction by up to 50% when administered within the first hour following the onset of symptoms. **2.** The reinstitution of blood flow to tissues that have been traumatized, esp. by a long period of crushing. This may damage other organs because of the material released from the traumatized tissues into the circulation. SEE: *crush syndrome; rhabdomyolysis.*

***r. injury*** Tissue changes following reperfusion after periods of ischemia.

**repetitive motion injury** Tissue damage caused by repeated trauma, usually associated with writing, painting, typing, or use of vibrating tools or hand tools. Almost any form of activity that produces repeated trauma to a particular area of soft tissue, including tendons and synovial sheaths, may cause this type of injury. Carpal tunnel syndrome, may be, but is not always, caused by repetitive wrist motion. SYN: *cumulative trauma syndrome; repetitive strain injury; overuse syndrome.*

**replacement** The act of putting back or of restoring something to its original position.

**replantation** [L. *re,* again, + *planto,* to plant] Surgical reimplantation of something removed from the body, esp. the surgical procedure of rejoining a hand, arm, or leg to the body after its accidental detachment. In dentistry, replantaton is the replacement of a tooth that has been removed from its socket.

**repletion** (rē-plē′shŭn) [L. *repletio,* a filling up] The condition of being full or satisfied.

**replication** (rĕp″lĭ-kā′shŭn) **1.** A doubling back of tissue. **2.** In medical investigations, the repetition of an experiment. **3.** In genetics, the duplication process of genetic material.

**replicon** (rĕp′lĭ-kŏn) Any genetic element that behaves as an autonomous unit of DNA replication. The element can replicate under its own control.

**repolarization** Restoration of the polarized state at a cell membrane (negative inside in relation to the outside) following depolarization as in muscle or nerve fibers.

**report** The account, usually verbal, that the nursing staff going off duty gives to the oncoming staff. The purpose is to provide continuity of care despite the change in staff. Obviously the information provided is of the utmost importance in caring for critically ill patients.

**reportable disease** A disease that must be reported to the health authorities by the physician. The communicable diseases required by International Health Regulations to be reported universally are the internationally quarantinable diseases: plague, cholera, and yellow fever. Other diseases that must be reported are those under surveillance by the World Health Organization. They are louse-borne typhus fever, relapsing fever, paralytic poliomyelitis, malaria, and influenza. Special notification is required of all outbreaks or epidemics of diseases not listed here. Even a single case of a communicable disease long absent from a population or not previously recognized in that area requires immediate reporting and institution of a full field investigation. SEE: *privacy; quarantine.*

**reposition** (rē″pō-zĭsh′ŭn) [L. *repositio,* a replacing] Restoration of an organ or tissue to its correct or original position.

**repositioning** (rē″pō-zĭsh′ŭn-ĭng) Placement of a part in its original place.

***jaw r.*** Changing of the position of the mandible in relation to the maxilla by altering the occlusion of the teeth.

***muscle r.*** Surgical placement of a muscle to another attachment point to enhance function.

**repositor** An instrument for restoring a tissue or an organ to its normal position.

***inversion r.*** An instrument for replacing an inverted uterus.

***uterine r.*** A lever for replacing the uterus when it is out of normal position.

**repression** (rē-prĕsh′ŭn) [L. *repressus,* press back] In psychology, the refusal to entertain distressing or painful ideas. As a result they are submerged in the unconscious, where they continue to influence the individual. Psychoanalysis seeks to discover and release repressions.

***coordinate r.*** Simultaneous reduction of the enzyme levels of a metabolic pathway.

***enzyme r.*** Interference with enzyme synthesis by a metabolic product.

**repressor** (rē-prĕs′or) [L. *repressus,* press back] Something, esp. an enzyme, that inhibits or interferes with the initiation of protein synthesis by genetic material.

**reproducibility** A quality control test of radiographical output for multiple exposures using the same exposure factors. These factors must not vary by more than ±5%.

**reproduction** (rē-prō-dŭk′shŭn) [L. *re,* again, + *productio,* production] **1.** The process by which plants and animals produce offspring. SEE: *ovary* for illus. **2.** The creation of a similar structure or situation; the act of duplicating.

***asexual r.*** Reproduction in which sex cells are not involved, as by fission or budding.

***cytogenic r.*** Reproduction by means of asexual single germ cells.

***sexual r.*** Reproduction by means of sexual or germ cells. Usually a male cell (spermatozoon) fuses with a female cell (egg or ovum). SYN: *syngamy.* SEE: *parthenogenesis.*

***somatic r.*** Asexual reproduction by budding of somatic cells.

**reproductive** (rē″prō-dŭk′tĭv) Pert. to or employed in reproduction.

**repulsion** (rĭ-pŭl′shŭn) [L. *repulsio,* a thrusting back] **1.** The act of driving back. **2.** The force exerted by one body on another to cause separation; the opposite of attraction.

**request for production of documents and objects** A demand by a plaintiff or defendant for documents or objects from the other party that may lead to discoverable information and pertain to the issues of a lawsuit.

In medical negligence cases, requests for medical records, office records, and hospital policies and procedures can be made by using this discovery technique.

**required service** A service that must be included in a health program for it to qualify for federal funds.

**RES** *reticuloendothelial system.*

**rescinnamine** (rē-sĭn′ă-mĭn) An antihypertensive drug derived from species of *Rauwolfia.*

**rescue tool** A piece of equipment used by

rescuers in emergency medical service to free trapped victims. Rescue tools include a *come-a-long,* a hand-operated winch used to gain forceful entry during a rescue; *cutting tools,* used to cut open vehicles and metal to gain access to a patient; a *hydraulic jack,* a hand-operated jack used to lift objects away from patients; and a *power chisel,* a pressure-operated device used to cut into heavy metal. The trade name of one rescue tool is Jaws of Life.

**research** (rĭ-sĕrch′, rē′sĕrch) [O. Fr. *recerche,* research] Scientific and diligent study, investigation, or experimentation to establish facts and analyze their significance. Inherent in such study is an orderly approach with accurate record keeping. A hallmark of acceptable research is that its conduct and description provide other scientists with enough information concerning the design and methods that they can repeat it.

***clinical r.*** Research based mainly on bedside observation of the patient rather than on laboratory work.

***laboratory r.*** Research done principally in the laboratory.

***medical r.*** Research concerned with any phase of medical science.

***preembryo r.*** Research involving the use of the fertilized egg from its unicellular zygote stage until the embryo stage (i.e., to the 14th day following fertilization). The ethical questions concerning this subject have been difficult to resolve.

**resect** (rē-sĕkt′) [L. *resectus,* cut off] To cut off or cut out a portion of a structure or organ, as to cut off the end of a bone or to remove a segment of the intestine.

**resectable** (rē-sĕk′tă-bl) Able to be removed, esp. by surgery; usually used in reference to malignant growths that can be removed completely by surgery.

**resection** (rē-sĕk′shŭn) [L. *resectio,* a cutting off] Partial excision of a bone or other structure.

***gastric r.*** Surgical resection of a part of the stomach.

***transurethral r.*** Surgical removal of the prostate using an instrument introduced through the urethra.

***wedge r.*** Surgical removal of a wedge-shaped piece of tissue, esp. from the ovary as a means of treating polycystic ovaries. SEE: *polycystic ovary syndrome.*

***window r.*** Resection of a portion of the nasal septum after reflection of a flap of mucous membrane.

**resectoscope** (rē-sĕk′tō-skōp) [L. *resectus,* cut off, + Gr. *skopein,* to examine] An instrument for resection of the prostate gland through the urethra.

**resectoscopy** (rē″sĕk-tŏs′kō-pē) Resection of the prostate through the urethra.

**reserpine** (rĭ-sĕr′pĭn) A chemically pure derivative of the plant *Rauwolfia serpentina,* a folk medicine used in India for centuries for snake bite, mental illness, and anxiety states. It lowers blood pressure and acts as a tranquilizer.

**reserve** (rē-zĕrv′) [L. *reservare,* to keep back] **1.** Something held back for future use. **2.** Self-control of one's feelings and thoughts.

***alkali r.*** The alkali content of the body available for neutralizing acid.

***cardiac r.*** The ability of the heart to increase cardiac output to meet the needs of increased energy output.

**reservoir** (rĕz′ĕr-vwor) [Fr.] A place or cavity for storage of fluids.

***r. of infectious agents*** Any person, animal, arthropod, plant, soil, or substance in which an infectious agent normally lives and multiplies, on which it depends primarily for survival, and where it reproduces itself in a way that allows transmission to a susceptible host.

**residency** A period of at least 1 year and often 3 to 4 years of on-the-job training, usually postgraduate, that is part of the formal educational program for health care professionals.

**resident** A physician obtaining further clinical training after internship, usually as a member of the house staff of a hospital.

**residual** (rĭ-zĭd′ū-ăl) [L. *residuum,* residue] **1.** Pert. to something left as a residue. **2.** In psychology, any aftereffect of experience influencing later behavior.

**residual air** SEE: under *air.*

**residual function** The functional capacity remaining after an illness or injury.

**residual urine** Urine left in the bladder after urination, an abnormal occurrence that may accompany enlargement of the prostate.

**residue** (rĕz′ĭ-dū) The remainder of something after a part is removed.

**residue-free diet** A diet without cellulose or roughage. Semisolid and bland foods are included.

**residuum** (rē-zĭd′ū-ŭm) *pl.* **residua** [L.] Residue.

**resilience** (rē-zĭl′ē-ĕns) [L. *resiliens,* leaping back] **1.** Elasticity. **2.** The ability to endure mental or physical stress and return to normal, even in situations that might be thought overwhelming.

**resilient** (rē-zĭl′ē-ĕnt) Elastic.

**resin** (rĕz′ĭn) [L. *resina,* fr. Gr. *rhetine,* resin of the pine] **1.** An amorphous, nonvolatile solid or soft-solid substance, a natural exudation from plants. It is practically insoluble in water but dissolves in alcohol. SEE: *rosin.* **2.** Any of a class of solid or soft organic compounds of natural or synthetic origin. They are usually of high molecular weight and most are polymers. Included are polyvinyl, polyethylene, and polystyrene. These are combined with chemicals such as epoxides, plasticizers, pigments, fillers, and stabilizers to form plastics.

***acrylic r.*** Quick-cure r.

***anion-exchange r.*** SEE: *ion-exchange r.*

***cation-exchange r.*** SEE: *ion-exchange r.*

***cold-cure r.*** Quick-cure r.

***ion-exchange r.*** An ionizable synthetic substance, which may be acid or basic, used accordingly to remove either acid or basic ions from solutions. Anion-exchange resins are used to absorb acid in the stomach, and cation-exchange resins are used to remove basic (alkaline) ions from solutions.

***quick-cure r.*** An autopolymer resin that can be polymerized by an activator and catalyst without the use of external heat. It is used in many dental procedures. SYN: *acrylic r.; cold-cure r.; self-curing r.*

***self-curing r.*** Quick-cure r.

**resinoid** (rĕz′ĭ-noyd) [″ + Gr. *eidos,* form, shape] Resembling a resin.

**resinous** (rĕz′ĭ-nŭs) Having the nature of or pert. to resin.

**res ipsa loquitur** [L.] Literally, "the thing speaks for itself." In malpractice this concept is used for cases in which an injury occurs to the plaintiff in a situation solely under the control of the defendant. If the injury would not have occurred had the defendant exercised due care, the defendant is judged negligent. In medicine the classic example of this situation is the leaving of an object such as a sponge or clamp in a patient's body after a surgical procedure, or the inadvertent removal of a healthy organ or extremity.

**resistance** (rĭ-zĭs′tăns) [L. *resistens,* standing back] **1.** Opposition to, or the ability to oppose, something. Examples include the power of a fluid to retard something passing through it or the ability of the body to oppose the passage of an electric current. **2.** The sum total of body mechanisms that oppose the progress of invasion, multiplication of infectious agents, or damage by their toxic products. Immunity is resistance associated with the presence of antibodies having a specific action on infectious microorganisms. Inherent resistance is the ability to resist disease independently of antibodies. **3.** The force exerted to penetrate the unconscious or to submerge memories in the unconscious. **4.** In psychoanalysis, a condition in which the ego avoids bringing into consciousness conflicts and unpleasant events responsible for neurosis; the reluctance of a patient to give up old patterns of thought and behavior. It may take various forms such as silence, failure to remember dreams, forgetfulness, and undue annoyance with trivial aspects of the treatment situation. **5.** Force applied to a body part by weights, machinery, or another person to load muscles as an exercise to increase muscle strength.

***airway r.*** The inherent resistance of the flow of air into the pulmonary tract.

***antibiotic r.*** The ability of microorganisms to develop mechanisms that block the action of antibiotics. These mechanisms have been developed in part because of excessive public demand for antibiotics, often for viral infections that do not respond to them, as well as unnecessary prescription of antibiotics by physicians. An organism such as *Staphylococcus aureus* may be exposed to an antibiotic so often that it creates a defense against it. For example, bacteria have developed the ability to produce enzymes that inactivate penicillin, amoxicillin, or the aminoglycosides. Others have learned to change the site on their surface to which antibiotics bind, or to create new enzymes, previously blocked by drugs, for essential cell functions. Experts in infectious disease warn that indiscriminate use of antibiotics will create bacteria for which researchers can find no effective antibiotic. SYN: *bacterial resistance.* SEE: *enterococcus, vancomycin-resistant; resistance transfer factor; Staphylococcus aureus, methicillin-resistant.*

---

Caution: The most effective, and frequently ignored, measure to reduce the spread of many organisms is *careful handwashing with antimicrobial soap* after contact with *all* patients.

---

***drug r.*** SEE: *resistance transfer factor.*

***expiratory r.*** The use of a restricted orifice, or flow resistor, during positive-pressure ventilation to retard the flow of exhaled gases.

***insulin r.*** A cellular-level phenomenon that prevents insulin from exerting its effect on glucose metabolism.

***multidrug r.*** ABBR: MDR. The genetic abilities of an increasing number of microorganisms to withstand treatment and remain unaffected by a number of antibiotics. The continued and sometimes inappropriate use of antibiotics to treat infectious diseases has resulted in some organisms becoming resistant to antibiotics to which they had been sensitive. SEE: *bacterial resistance; transfer factor.*

***peripheral r.*** The resistance of the arterial vascular system, esp. the arterioles and capillaries, to the flow of blood.

***systemic vascular r.*** ABBR: SVR. The amount of resistance to the flow of blood through vessels. It increases as the vessel constricts. Any change in lumen diameter or vessel elasticity can influence the amount of resistance.

***threshold r.*** The amount of pressure necessary in overcoming resistance to flow.

***transthoracic r.*** The amount of resistance to the flow of electrical energy across the chest. This is an important factor to consider when electrical therapies such as defibrillation, cardioversion, and transthoracic pacing are used to treat abnormal cardiac rhythms.

***viscous r.*** Nonelastic opposition of tissue to ventilation due to the energy required to displace the thorax and airways.

**resistance exercise** Exercise in which an

outside force is applied to a muscle, requiring it to develop greater tension. This is done to increase strength. If the resistance is applied by using weights, it is called mechanical resistance; if applied by a therapist, it is called manual resistance.

**resistance transfer factor** A genetic factor in bacteria that controls resistance to certain antibiotic drugs. The factor may be passed from one bacterium to another. This makes it possible for nonpathogenic bacteria to become resistant to antibiotics and to transfer that resistance to pathogens, thereby establishing a potential source for an epidemic. SEE: *plasmid*.

**resolution** (rĕz-ō-lū′shŭn) [L. *resolutio,* a relaxing] **1.** Decomposition; absorption or breaking down of the products of inflammation. **2.** Cessation of inflammation without suppuration; a return to normal. **3.** The ability of the eye or a series of lenses to distinguish fine detail. **4.** In radiology, the ability to record small images placed very close together as separate images.

**resolve** (rē-zŏlv′) [L. *resolvere,* to release] **1.** To return to normal as after a pathological process. **2.** To separate into component parts.

**resonance** (rĕz′ō-năns) [L. *resonantia,* resound] **1.** The quality or act of resounding. **2.** The quality of the sound heard on percussion of a hollow structure such as the chest or abdomen. An absence of resonance is termed *flatness;* diminished resonance, *dullness.* **3.** In physics, the modification of sound caused by vibrations of a body that are set up by waves from another vibrating body. **4.** In electricity, a state in which two electrical circuits are in tune with each other.

***amphoric r.*** A sound similar to that produced by blowing across the mouth of an empty bottle.

***bandbox r.*** The pulmonary resonance heard during chest percussion in patients with emphysema.

***bell-metal r.*** The sound heard in pneumothorax on auscultation when a coin is held against the chest wall and struck by another coin.

***cracked-pot r.*** The peculiar clinking sound sometimes heard on chest percussion in cases of advanced tuberculosis when cavities are present.

***electron spin r.*** ABBR: ESR. A technique used in medical imaging that identifies atoms by their electron spin characteristics.

***normal r.*** Vesicular r.

***skodaic r.*** An increased percussion sound over the upper lung when there is a pleural effusion in the lower part.

***tympanic r.*** A low-pitched, drumlike sound heard on percussion over a large air-containing space.

***tympanitic r.*** The resonance obtained by percussion of a hollow structure, such as the stomach or colon, when it is moderately distended with air.

***vesicular r.*** The resonance obtained by percussion of normal lungs. SYN: *normal r.*

***vocal r.*** In auscultation, the vibrations of the voice transmitted to the examiner's ear, normally more marked over the right apex of the lung. These vibrations are abnormally increased in pneumonic consolidation, in lungs infiltrated with tuberculosis, or in cavities that communicate freely with a bronchus.

Vocal resonance is diminished or absent in pleural effusion (air, pus, serum, lymph, or blood); emphysema; pulmonary collapse; pulmonary edema; and egophony, a modified bronchophony characterized by a trembling, bleating sound usually heard above the upper border of dullness of pleural effusions and occasionally heard in beginning pneumonia.

***whispering r.*** The auscultation sound heard when a patient whispers.

**resonant** (rĕz′ō-nănt) Producing a vibrating sound on percussion.

**resonating** [L. *resonantia,* resound] Vibrating sympathetically with a source of sound or electrical oscillations.

**resonating cavities** The resonator of the human voice, including the upper portion of the larynx, pharynx, nasal cavity, paranasal sinuses, and oral cavity.

**resonator** (rĕz′ō-nā″tĕr) **1.** A structure that can be set into sympathetic vibration when sound waves of the same frequency from another vibrating body strike it. **2.** In electricity, an apparatus consisting of an electric circuit in which oscillations of a certain frequency are set up by oscillations of the same frequency in another circuit.

**resorb** (rē-sorb′, rē-zorb′) [L. *resorbere,* to suck in] **1.** To undergo resorption. **2.** To absorb again.

**resorbent** (rē-sor′bĕnt) [L. *resorbens,* sucking in] An agent that promotes the absorption of abnormal matters, as exudates or blood clots (e.g., potassium iodide, ammonium chloride).

**resorcin** (rĕ-zor′sĭn) Resorcinol.

**resorcinol** (rĕ-zor′sĭ-nŏl) An agent with keratolytic, fungicidal, and bactericidal actions, used in treating certain skin diseases. SYN: *resorcin.*

**resorcinolphthalein** (rē-zor″sĭ-nŏl-thăl′ē-ĭn) Fluorescein sodium.

**resorption** (rē-sorp′shŭn) [L. *resorbere,* to suck in] **1.** Removal by absorption, as of an exudate or pus. **2.** The removal of enamel and other calcific portions of a tooth as a result of lysis and other pathological processes. It often results from pressure or vascular changes as in root resorption of deciduous teeth prior to shedding, or bone resorption on the pressure side during tooth movement.

***bone r.*** The removal of bone tissue by resorption.

**resource-based relative value scale** ABBR:

RBRVS. A measuring tool developed to increase payment to nonsurgeons for cognitive services (i.e., evaluation and management of patients). The scale is based on the total work required for a given service and on other considerations, including the cost of the physician's practice, the income lost during training, and the relative cost of liability insurance. This method of calculating medical care services was implemented by law in January 1992. SEE: *managed care; managed competition.*

**respirable** (rē-spīr'ă-bl, rĕs'pĕr-ă-bl) [L. *respirare,* breathe again] Fit or adapted for respiration.

**respiration** (rĕs-pĭr-ā'shŭn) [L. *respiratio,* breathing] **1.** The interchange of gases between an organism and the medium in which it lives; more specifically, the taking in of oxygen, its use in the tissues, and the giving off of carbon dioxide. **2.** The act of breathing (i.e., inhaling and exhaling) during which the lungs are provided with air through inhaling and the carbon dioxide is removed through exhaling. Normal respiratory exchange of oxygen and carbon dioxide in the lungs is, of course, impossible unless the pulmonary tissue is adequately perfused with blood. Normally the inspiratory phase of respiration lasts longer than the expiratory phase. There are various abnormal forms of respiration: jerking, spasmodic, stertorous, stridulous, whistling, wavy, uneven, abdominal, and thoracic. SEE: *diaphragm* for illus.; *lung; ventilation.*

SOUNDS: *Friction:* This sound is produced by the rubbing together of roughened pleural surfaces. It may be heard in both inspiration and expiration. Friction often resembles subcrepitant crackles, but is more superficial and localized than the latter and is not modified by cough or deep inspiration.

*Metallic tinkling:* A silvery bell-like sound heard at intervals over a hydropneumothorax or large cavity. Speaking, coughing, and deep breathing usually induces this sound. It must not be confused with a similar sound produced by liquids in the stomach.

*Crackles:* Abnormal bubbling sounds heard in air cells or bronchial tubes.

*Succussion-splash or hippocratic succussion:* A splashing sound produced by the presence of air and liquid in the chest. It may be elicited by gently shaking the patient during auscultation. This sound nearly always indicates either a hydropneumothorax or a pyopneumothorax, although it has also been detected over very large cavities. The presence of air and liquid in the stomach produces similar sounds.

AUSCULTATION: *Normal breath sounds:* In the healthy person, breath sounds are low-pitched and have a frequency of 200 to 400 cycles per second (cps); frequency rarely exceeds 500 cps. These sounds are called vesicular breath sounds when heard over the lungs, as is normal. They are produced by air passing in and out of the airways.

*Bronchial and tracheal breath sounds:* These are higher-pitched and louder than vesicular sounds, and are produced by air passing over the walls of the bronchi and trachea. These sounds are normally heard only over the bronchi and trachea.

*Amphoric and cavernous breathing:* These two nearly identical sounds are loud, with a prolonged, hollow expiration. The pitch of amphoric breathing is slightly higher than that of the cavernous type, and may be imitated by blowing over the mouth of an empty jar. It is heard in bronchiectatic cavities or pneumothorax when the opening to the lung is patulous; in the consolidation area near a large bronchus; and sometimes over a lung compressed by a moderate effusion.

METHOD OF COUNTING: The examiner places his or her hand in the same position as when taking a pulse. The examiner then watches the patient's chest, without the patient's knowledge if possible because although breathing is a reflex, the rate or rhythm can be changed voluntarily. Each inspiration and expiration is counted as one breath. The examiner watches the rise and fall of the patient's chest or upper abdomen for a full minute. When the movements are scarcely perceptible, the examiner places the hand gently but firmly on the patient's chest or back and counts in this manner. The hour, frequency, and any abnormal condition, such as pain associated with breathing, should be recorded. SEE: table.

*Total lung capacity (TLC):* In normal men, depending on their size, TLC ranges from 3.6 to 9.4 L; in women, from 2.5 to 6.9 L.

***abdominal r.*** Respiration in which chiefly the diaphragm exerts itself while the chest walls are nearly at rest; used in normal, quiet breathing, esp. by men, and in pathological conditions such as pleurisy, pericarditis, and rib fracture. SYN: *diaphragmatic r.*

***absent r.*** Respiration in which respiratory sounds are suppressed.

***accelerated r.*** Respiration occurring at

**Rate of Respiration**
**(breaths/min)**

| | |
|---|---|
| Premature infant | 40–90 |
| Newborn | 30–60 |
| 1st yr | 20–40 |
| 2nd yr | 20–30 |
| 5th yr | 20–25 |
| 15th yr | 15–20 |
| Adult | 12–20 |

a faster rate than normal, considered accelerated when it exceeds 25 per minute in adults. Increased frequency may result from exercise, physical exertion, excitement, fear, exposure to high altitudes, or mental disturbances, and frequently occurs in disease. It is present in many lung disorders, such as pneumonia, bronchiectasis, advanced pulmonary tuberculosis, consolidation or compression of a lobe or of the entire lung, congestion, asthma, emphysema, abscess, tumors, aneurysms, diseases of the chest wall, hernia of the diaphragm, and partial obstruction to the entrance of air into the lungs. It may be seen in blood diseases, such as the anemias; kidney disease; febrile disease; and heart disease; it may also result from drugs or nervous conditions such as anxiety, panic, and hysteria.

***aerobic r.*** Respiration in which oxygen is used in the production of energy.

***amphoric r.*** Respiration having amphoric resonance. SEE: *resonance, amphoric.*

***anaerobic r.*** Respiration in which energy is obtained from chemical reactions that do not involve free oxygen.

***apneustic r.*** Breathing marked by prolonged inspiration unrelieved by attempts to exhale. Seen in patients who have had the upper part of the pons of the brain removed or damaged.

***artificial r.*** Artificial methods to restore respiration in cases of suspended breathing. For specific methods, SEE: *artificial respiration; cardiopulmonary resuscitation.*

***Biot's r.*** SEE: *Biot's breathing.*

***cell r.*** The gradual breakdown of food molecules in the presence of oxygen within cells, resulting in the formation of carbon dioxide and water and the release of energy. In many intermediary reactions, substances other than oxygen act as oxidizing agents (i.e., hydrogen or electron acceptors). Reactions are catalyzed by respiratory enzymes, which include the flavoproteins, cytochromes, and other enzymes. Certain vitamins (nicotinamide, riboflavin, thiamine, pyridoxine, and pantothenic acid) are essential in the formation of components of various intracellular enzyme systems.

***Cheyne-Stokes r.*** A common and bizarre breathing pattern marked by a period of apnea lasting 10 to 60 sec, followed by gradually increasing depth and frequency of respirations. It accompanies frontal lobe depression and diencephalic dysfunction. This condition may be present as a normal finding in children. SEE: illus.

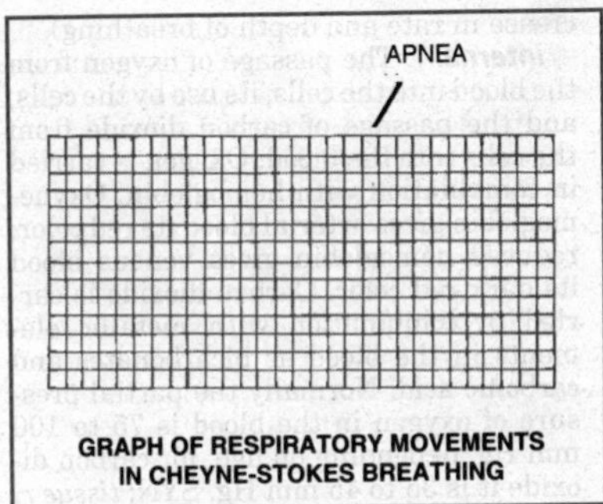

GRAPH OF RESPIRATORY MOVEMENTS IN CHEYNE-STOKES BREATHING

***cogwheel r.*** Interrupted r.

***costal r.*** Respiration in which the chest cavity is enlarged by raising the ribs.

***decreased r.*** Respiration at less than a normal rate for the individual's age. It occurs in uremia, diabetic coma, most conditions that increase intracranial pressure, shock, hysteria, stenosis of the larynx, poisoning with opium or its derivatives, and approaching death.

***diaphragmatic r.*** Abdominal r.

***direct r.*** Respiration in which an organism, such as a one-celled ameba, secures its oxygen and gives up carbon dioxide directly to the surrounding medium.

***electrophrenic r.*** The application of intermittent electrical stimuli to cutaneous electrodes over the phrenic nerves in the neck to stimulate respiration rhythmically. This method is used in patients whose respiratory center has been damaged. SEE: *radiofrequency electrophrenic respiration.*

***external r.*** The processes involved in ventilating the lungs (breathing) and the exchange of gases (oxygen and carbon dioxide) between the air in lungs and the blood within capillaries in the walls of alveoli.

Inspiration, or the drawing in of air, is accomplished by expansion of the thoracic cavity. This is brought about by contraction of the diaphragm and raising of the ribs and sternum. Expiration, or the expulsion of air, may be active or passive. In ordinary breathing it is passive, no muscular effort being needed to bring the chest wall back to normal position. In forced or labored respiration, muscular effort is involved.

When the aspiration of air is accomplished chiefly by contraction of the diaphragm, the abdomen bulges with each inspiration because the diaphragm, forming both the floor of the thorax and the roof of the abdominal cavity, is dome-shaped with its concavity downward. In contracting, it pushes the abdominal viscera down. This type of respiration is called diaphragmatic or abdominal. Its opposite is the thoracic type, in which the ribs and sternum must be raised. It is seen when the abdomen is confined by tight clothing.

***fetal r.*** Gas exchange in the placenta between the fetal and maternal blood. SYN: *placental r.*

***forced r.*** Voluntary hyperpnea (increase in rate and depth of breathing).

***internal r.*** The passage of oxygen from the blood into the cells, its use by the cells, and the passage of carbon dioxide from the cells into the blood. Oxygen is carried in combination with hemoglobin. Oxyhemoglobin gives arterial blood its red color; reduced hemoglobin gives venous blood its dark red color. Carbon dioxide is carried in combination with metallic elements in the blood as bicarbonates and carbonic acid. Normally the partial pressure of oxygen in the blood is 75 to 100 mm Hg, depending on age; for carbon dioxide it is 35 to 45 mm Hg. SYN: *tissue r.* SEE: *cell r.*

***interrupted r.*** Respiration in which inspiratory or expiratory sounds are not continuous. SYN: *cogwheel r.*

***intrauterine r.*** Respiration by the fetus before birth. SEE: *fetal respiration.*

***Kussmaul's r.*** SEE: *Kussmaul's breathing.*

***labored r.*** Dyspnea or difficult breathing; respiration that involves active participation of accessory inspiratory and expiratory muscles.

***muscles of r.*** *Inspiration:* diaphragm and external intercostals. *Forced inspiration* (assist in elevating ribs and sternum): scaleni, levatores costorum, sternocleidomastoideus, pectoralis major, platysma myoides, and serratus posterior superior. *Expiration* (voluntary deep breathing or forced expiration): rectus abdominis, external and internal oblique, transverse abdominis. SEE: *diaphragm; expiration; inspiration.*

The following accessory muscles may assist in depressing the ribs: internal intercostals, serratus posterior inferior, quadratus lumborum.

***paradoxical r.*** **1.** Respiration occurring in patients with chest trauma and multiple rib fractures in which a portion of the chest wall sinks inward with each spontaneous inspiratory effort. **2.** A condition seen in paralysis of the diaphragm in which the diaphragm ascends during inspiration.

***periodic r.*** SEE: *breathing, periodic.*

***placental r.*** Fetal r.

***slow r.*** Breathing at a rate of fewer than 12 respirations each minute. Generally this is the result of some structural or functional derangement of the nervous system. It has been observed in apoplexy, increased intracranial pressure and hemorrhage, uremia, and most of the circumstances that occasion coma. It may be induced by carbon monoxide or opium or its derivatives.

***stertorous r.*** Respiration marked by rattling or bubbling sounds.

***stridulous r.*** Respiration marked by high-pitched crowing or barking sound heard on inspiration, caused by an obstruction near the glottis or in the respiratory passageway.

***thoracic r.*** Respiration performed entirely by expansion of the chest when the abdomen does not move. It is seen when the peritoneum or diaphragm is inflamed, when the abdominal cavity is restricted by tight bandages or clothes, or during abdominal surgery.

***tissue r.*** Internal r.

**respirator** (rĕs′pĭ-rā″tor) [L. *respirare,* to breathe] A machine for prolonged artificial respiration. Mechanical methods of assisting respiration usually include the capability of producing either intermittent or continuous positive pressure in the lungs. SEE: *Drinker respirator; ventilation, continuous positive-pressure; ventilation, intermittent positive-pressure.*

***abdominal belt r.*** A device used for noninvasive ventilatory assistance by patients with chronic respiratory failure, consisting of an inflatable rubber bladder held over the abdomen that inflates and deflates to assist diaphragm movement and ventilation. It may be used in the home.

**respiratory** (rĕs-pīr′ă-tō-rē, rĕs′pĭ-ră-tō″rē) [L. *respiratio,* breathing] Pert. to respiration.

**respiratory anemometer** A form of respirometer used in investigating pulmonary function. The passage of air through the mask or mouthpiece drives a vane so that it rotates. This motion is recorded by use of a clockwise mechanism that permits measurement of the amount of air passed through the system.

**respiratory center** A region in the medulla oblongata of the brainstem that regulates movements of respiration. This area consists of an inspiratory center, located in the rostral half of the reticular formation overlying the olivary nuclei, and an expiratory center, located dorsal to the inspiratory center. The pons contains the apneustic center, which prolongs inhalation, and the pneumotaxic center, which helps bring about exhalation.

**respiratory defense function** The cellular resistance of the lungs to invading microorganisms and inhaled particles such as nuisance dust. In addition to providing for oxygen and carbon dioxide exchange in the blood, the respiratory tract warms and humidifies the inspired air and provides the mucous secretions that protect the epithelium of the airway. Ciliated cells, each containing about 275 cilia that beat 1000 times a minute, move the mucus with trapped dust and pathogens toward the pharynx at the rate of 10 mm/min in the trachea. Inhaled bacteria or pollutants that reach the alveoli are engulfed and destroyed by the alveolar macrophages. SEE: *lung.*

**respiratory distress syndrome of the preterm infant** ABBR: RDS. Severe impairment of respiratory function in a preterm newborn, caused by immaturity of the enzymatic system essential to pulmonary surfactant production. This condition is rarely present in a newborn of more than 37 weeks' gestation or in one weighing at least 2.2 kg (5 lb). RDS is the leading cause of death in prematurely born infants in the U.S. SYN: *hyaline membrane disease.* SEE: *acute respiratory distress syndrome; Nursing Diagnoses Appendix.*

SYMPTOMS: Shortly after birth the preterm infant with RDS has a low Apgar score, and develops signs of acute respiratory distress owing to atelectasis of the lung, impaired blood perfusion of the lung, and reduced pulmonary compliance. Tachypnea, tachycardia, retraction of the rib cage during inspiration, cyanosis, and grunting during expiration are present. In addition to these signs and symptoms, blood gas studies reflect the impaired ventilatory function and radiographical examination of the lung is typical for generalized atelectasis.

TREATMENT: Preterm infants with RDS require treatment in a specially staffed and equipped neonatal intensive care unit. Therapy is supportive to ensure adequate hydration and electrolyte control. Every attempt should be made to reduce oxygen requirements by reducing any fever and minimizing activity. Supplemental oxygen is given. If necessary, assisted ventilation is used with great care to prevent the traumatic formation of pulmonary air leaks that could cause pulmonary emphysema and tension pneumothorax. Instillation of surfactant into the respiratory tract is essential in managing this condition.

**respiratory failure, acute** A clinical condition in which the patient's arterial oxygen concentration drops markedly with or without an increase in carbon dioxide concentration. In all cases, the diagnosis is made by comparing the previous "normal" baseline for the blood gas values with those in the acute situation. A drop in $PaO_2$ of 10 to 15 mm Hg or more indicates acute failure. With respect to $PaCO_2$, an acute decrease in arterial pH in the absence of metabolic acidemia is diagnostic of hypercapnia and acute respiratory failure.

TREATMENT: If the respiratory failure is due to obstruction, the condition causing the obstruction should be treated. If it is due to impaired gas exchange, positive-pressure ventilation is indicated. If the combination of ventilation and lung perfusion does not maintain the arterial oxygen concentration ($PaO_2$) at 50 to 55 mm Hg or greater, supplemental oxygen is required.

**respiratory failure, chronic** Chronic inability of the respiratory system to maintain the function of oxygenating blood and remove carbon dioxide from the lungs. Any disease process that interferes with ventilation and perfusion of the lungs will cause various degrees of pulmonary insufficiency, depending on the severity and duration of the disease. Many diseases can cause chronic pulmonary insufficiency, including asthmatic airway obstruction, emphysema, chronic bronchitis, and cystic fibrosis; and chronic pulmonary interstitial tissue diseases such as sarcoidosis, pneumoconiosis, idiopathic pulmonary fibrosis, disseminated carcinoma, radiation sickness, and leukemia.

**respiratory function monitoring** The use of various techniques to provide alarms that alert a patient's attendants to a change in the ability of the lungs to perform their functions. These techniques include noninvasive devices for measuring the oxygen content of the blood (e.g., pulse oximetry); methods of monitoring respiratory muscle function and breathing pattern; and a device for monitoring the carbon dioxide content of expired air (i.e., capnography). SEE: *apnea monitoring.*

**respiratory myoclonus** Leeuwenhoek's disease.

**respiratory therapy** Treatment to preserve or improve pulmonary function.

**respire** To breathe and to consume oxygen and release carbon dioxide.

**respirometer** (rĕs″pĭr-ŏm′ĕt-ĕr) [L. *respirare,* to breathe, + Gr. *metron,* a measure] An instrument to ascertain the character of respirations. Several devices are available for measuring specific respiratory qualities such as minute and tidal volume. SEE: *respiratory anemometer.*

**respite** Short-term, intermittent care, often for persons with chronic or debilitating conditions. One of the goals is to provide rest for family members or caregivers from the burden of sustained caregiving.

**respondeat superior** [L., *let the master answer*] The law stating that the employer is responsible for the employee's negligence in causing injury to a patient while in the "course and scope of employment." The term has been handed down from English common law.

**response** [L. *respondere,* to reply] **1.** A reaction, such as contraction of a muscle or secretion of a gland, resulting from a stimulus. SEE: *reaction.* **2.** The sum total of an individual's reactions to specific conditions, such as the response (favorable or unfavorable) of a patient to a certain treatment or to a challenge to the immune system.

***acute phase r.*** Acute phase reaction.

***anamnestic r.*** The rapid response by T and B lymphocytes following a second exposure to a specific foreign antigen. SYN: *secondary immune response.*

***conditioned r.*** SEE: *reflex, conditioned.*

***galvanic skin r.*** The measurement of the change in the electrical resistance of the skin in response to emotional stimuli.

***immune r.*** SEE: *immune response.*

***inflammatory r.*** A localized protective response elicited by the injury or destruction of tissue. Histologically, it involves the dilatation and increased permeability of small blood vessels, which result in migration and accumulation of leukocytes and exudation of plasma proteins into the area. The result dilutes, destroys, or walls off the injurious agent and injured tissue and is marked by the classic signs of inflammation: pain (dolor), heat (calor), redness (rubor), swelling (tumor), and loss of function (functio laesa). SEE: *leukotrienes.*

***physiological stress r.*** Stress r.

***reticulocyte r.*** An increase in reticulocyte production in response to the administration of a hematinic agent.

***stress r.*** The predictable physiological response that occurs in humans as a result of injury, surgery, shock, ischemia, or sepsis. SYN: *physiological stress r.*

This response is hormonally mediated and is divided into three distinct phases: *Ebb phase (lag phase):* For 12 to 36 hr after the precipitating event, the body attempts to conserve its resources. Vital signs (heart, respiration, temperature) are less than normal. *Flow phase (hypermetabolic phase):* This stage peaks in 3 to 4 days and lasts 9 to 14 days, depending on the extent of the injury or infection and the person's physical and nutritional status. Carbohydrate, protein, and fat are mobilized from tissue stores and catabolized to meet the energy needs of an increased metabolic rate (hypermetabolism). Serum levels of glucose and electrolytes such as potassium can increase dramatically. If this stage is not controlled by removal of the cause or activator, multiple system organ failure or death can result. *Anabolic phase (recovery):* The anabolic, or healing, phase occurs as the catabolism declines, and electrolyte balances are restored. Often, aggressive nutritional support is necessary to promote a positive nitrogen balance.

***triple r.*** The three phases of vasomotor reactions that occur when a pointed instrument is drawn across the skin. In order of appearance, these are red reaction, flare or spreading flush, and wheal.

***unconditioned r.*** An inherent response rather than one that is learned. SEE: *reflex, conditioned.*

**rest** (rĕst) [AS. *raest*] **1.** Repose of the body caused by sleep. **2.** Freedom from activity, as of mind or body. **3.** To lie down; to cease voluntary motion. **4.** A remnant of embryonic tissue that persists in the adult.

**restenosis** (rē″stĕ-nō′sĭs) [L. *re,* again, + Gr. *stenos,* narrow] The recurrence of a stenotic condition as in a heart valve or vessel.

**restiform** (rĕs′tĭ-form) [L. *restis,* rope, + *forma,* shape] Ropelike; rope-shaped.

**resting** Inactive, motionless, at rest.

**resting cell 1.** A cell not in the process of dividing. SEE: *interphase.* **2.** A cell that is not performing its normal function (i.e., a nerve cell that is not conducting an impulse or a muscle cell that is not contracting).

**resting pan splint** Splint designed to position fingers and stabilize hand in a functional position with the fingers held in opposition. Also called *resting hand splint.*

**restitutio ad integrum** (rĕs″tĭ-tū′shē-ō ăd ĭn-tĕ′grŭm) [L.] Complete restoration to health.

**restitution** (rĕs″tĭ-tū′shŭn) [L. *restitutio*] **1.** The return to a former status. **2.** The act of making amends. **3.** The turning of a fetal head to the right or left after it has completely emerged through the vagina.

**restless legs syndrome** A condition of unknown etiology marked by an intolerable creeping and internal itching sensation occurring in the lower extremities and causing an almost irresistible urge to move the legs. The symptoms are worse at the end of the day when the patient is either seated or in bed. This syndrome is sometimes associated with the onset of renal colic caused by the attempt to pass or the actual passage of a renal stone. Sometimes it is a side effect of psychotropic drugs. About 10% of pregnant women and 25% of people with iron-deficiency anemia experience this condition. Also, the condition may be associated with intake of caffeine. Patients should stop caffeine intake. Clonazine or diazepam may also be beneficial. SYN: *Ekbom's syndrome.*

**restoration** (rĕs″tō-rā′shŭn) [L. *restaurare,* to fix] **1.** The return of something to its previous state. **2.** In dentistry, any treatment, material, or device that restores a tooth surface, or replaces a tooth or all of the teeth and adjacent tissues.

***temporary r.*** A temporary filling of a tooth cavity made from zinc oxide and eugenol or some plastic material.

**restorative** (rĭ-stor′ă-tĭv) [L. *restaurare,* to fix] **1.** Pert. to restoration. **2.** An agent that is effective in the regaining of health and strength.

**restraint** (rĭ-strānt′) [O. Fr. *restrainte*] **1.** The process of refraining from any action, mental or physical. **2.** The condition of being hindered. **3.** In medicine, the use of major tranquilizers or physical means to prevent patients from harming themselves or others. In nursing homes, restraints are used in 36% to 85% of patients; in acute care hospitals, between 7.4% and 17% of patients will be restrained.

The Food and Drug Administration, which regulates medical devices, has defined restraint as "a device, usually a wristlet, anklet, or other type of strap intended for medical purposes and that limits a patient's movements to the extent necessary for treatment, examination, or protection of the patient." Protective devices include safety vests, hand mitts, lap and wheelchair belts, body holders, strait-jackets, and protection nets.

Restraints should be fitted properly (i.e., neither too loose nor too tight). They should be applied in a manner that will protect the patient from accidental self-injury, such as strangling or smothering themselves by slipping down in a bed, wheelchair, or chair.

Caregivers are legally and ethically responsible for the safety and well-being of patients in their care; however, when patient protection or achieving the therapeutic goal appears to require physical or pharmacological restraint, health care providers must consider that such action limits the patient's legal rights to autonomy and self-determination. Decisions to institute physical or pharmacological restraint must be based on a clear, identifiable, documented need for their use (i.e., that protecting the patient from harm or achievement of the therapeutic goals cannot be met in any other manner.

With many patients, effective alternatives to physical restraint include providing companionship and close supervision of activities; explaining procedures to reduce anxiety; when possible, removing indwelling tubes, drains, and catheters to reduce discomfort and the potential for displacement; providing good lighting, ensuring that pathways are clear, and that furniture is adequately secured to minimize potential environmental hazards; ensuring that the call button is easily accessible to facilitate patient requests for assistance with ambulation; reducing unwelcome distractions (e.g., background noise), and enabling patient access to diversions such as music and video movies to encourage relaxation; and encouraging ambulation and exercise to meet patient needs for mobility.

---

Caution: Informed consent must be obtained from the patient or guardian prior to use of restraints. Restraints should not be used without a specific order from the treating physician. Almost any type of restraint has the potential for harming the patient, thus it is extremely important to monitor use and be certain that it is applied correctly and removed periodically.

---

NURSING IMPLICATIONS: The nurse records and reports patient behaviors that demonstrate a need for restraint to ensure safety and achievement of therapeutic goals; describes nursing actions designed to achieve care objectives without resort to restraint and their effects; suggests the minimum amount of restraint required to achieve the objectives of care (i.e., restriction of mobility only to the degree necessary); secures or reviews physician orders for specific types of restraints; validates informed consent; explains the use of the specific type of restraint to the patient and family members as a "reminder"needed for protection; and encourages verbalization of feelings and concerns and provides emotional support.

The nurse follows these general guidelines for application of restraints: the device that is most appropriate for the purpose is selected (e.g., padded mitts protect against patient removal of intravenous or other invasive tubing by limiting the ability to manipulate equipment with fingers but do not elicit the restlessness and frustration that occurs when the hands are tied down with wrist restraints). The status of tissues is assessed and documented before application. Bony prominences that will be in contact with the restraining devices are padded before application of such restraints. Restraints are applied to maintain a comfortable normal anatomic position, and mobility is limited only as much as is necessary to protect the patient (i.e., the nurse may change the position without defeating the objectives of the restraint). The nurse anchors restraint devices securely and ensures that they do not interfere with blood flow to the limbs or trunk; ensures that the restraints can be released quickly in the event of emergency; documents application and evaluation of current status; assesses and records the effects of the restraint on patient behavior, and on the neurovascular status distal to the site of the restraint at frequent intervals (e.g., every 30 min); reports signs of increased agitation promptly; releases restraints (one at a time if the patient is unreliable or combative) and allows or provides range-of-motion exercises two to four times each shift; and evaluates the need for continuing restraint at least once each shift, discontinuing the devices as soon as the patient's status permits.

***r. in bed*** The therapeutic use of physical means to prevent limb or body motion in bed. If a proper bed is not available, the following may provide a makeshift alternative. With the bed against the wall, straight-backed chairs are placed along the open side of the bed. They are tied into place by interlacing them with rope and then tying the rope to the foot and head of the bed. Another method is to place a wide board the length of the bed on either side and to fasten it through three or four holes bored near the ends of the boards. A sheet is folded lengthwise to a 1-ft width, placed under the patient's back, and crossed in front below the armpits. The hem ends are secured at the side to the side bar or the bedsprings. This allows some freedom for turning from side to side. The patient's hands and feet may be restrained by a clove hitch of wide bandage around the wrists and ankles and tied to the side or foot of the bed.

NURSING IMPLICATIONS: The nurse

follows general guidelines for restraint application. The nurse never ties restraints to bed siderails; rather, the restraint is anchored to a part of the bed that moves when the head is lowered or elevated; the nurse uses a clove hitch to secure restraints so they will not tighten if tension is applied and so that they can be released rapidly if an emergency arises. A simple body restraint can be made by folding a sheet lengthwise to a 1-ft width. This restraint is placed under the patient's back and crossed in front below the armpits. The ends are secured to the side bar of the bed. This prevents some freedom in side-to-side movement.

***clove hitch r.*** A device used to restrain a person's arm or leg. Gauze or other soft material is placed on a flat surface in a figure-8 configuration. The loops are then lifted from the underside and the tops brought together. The extremity is placed through both loops at once and the loose ends of the material are tied to an immobile surface. It is important to check circulation regularly in any extremity restrained by this device.

***r. of lower extremities*** The use of physical means to restrict movement of the legs and feet. A sheet is tied across the knees and the feet are tied together with a figure-of-eight bandage. The correct method is to start the loop under the ankles, cross it between the feet, bring the ends around the feet, and tie them on top.

---

Caution: The restraint should not interfere with blood circulation to an extremity.

---

***mechanical r.*** Restraint by physical devices, esp. restraint of the mentally ill.

***medicinal r.*** Restraint of combative or violent patients through use of narcotics or sedatives.

**Resusci-Anne™** A manikin used in cardiopulmonary resuscitation training.

**resuscitation** (rĭ-sŭs″ĭ-tā′shŭn) [L. *resuscitatio*] Revival after apparent death; also called *anabiosis*. SEE: *artificial respiration.*

***cardiopulmonary r.*** SEE: *cardiopulmonary resuscitation.*

***heart-lung r.*** SEE: *cardiopulmonary resuscitation.*

***mouth-to-mouth r.*** SEE: *cardiopulmonary resuscitation.*

***oral r.*** SEE: *artificial respiration.*

**resuscitator** (rĭ-sŭs′ĭ-tā″tor) [L. *resuscitare,* to revive] An automatic breathing-assist machine that forces oxygen into the lungs under pressure of 4 oz/sq in. (1.4 mm Hg) when back pressure of 3 oz/sq in. (about 1 mm Hg) trips the machine for exhalation.

***manual r.*** A device, usually a hand-held mask with bag attached, that permits air to be forced into the lungs each time it is squeezed. A patent airway is essential. The goal is to deliver at least 800 cc of air every 5 sec. The device may or may not have provisions for adding supplemental oxygen to the bag.

**ret** *roentgen equivalent therapy*. It is analogous to rem, used in describing radiation protection or exposure.

**retainer** (rĭ-tān′ĕr) **1.** Any device or attachment for keeping something in place. **2.** In dentistry, a device used in orthodontia for maintaining the teeth and jaws in position.

**retardate** (rĭ-tăr′dāt) [L. *retardare,* to delay] One who is mentally retarded.

**retardation** (rē″tăr-dā′shŭn) [L. *retardare,* to delay] **1.** A holding back or slowing down; a delay. **2.** Delayed mental or physical response resulting from pathological conditions. SEE: *mental retardation.*

***mental r.*** SEE: *mental retardation.*

**retarder** A substance used in dentistry to slow the hardening of a material.

**retch** (rĕch) [AS. *hraecan,* to cough up phlegm] To make an involuntary attempt to vomit.

**retching** (rĕch′ĭng) Intense rhythmic contraction of the respiratory and abdominal muscles that may precede or accompany vomiting.

**rete** (rē′tē) *pl.* **retia** [L.] A network; a plexus of nerves or blood vessels.

***arterial r., arteriosum r.*** A vascular arterial network just before the point where arteries become capillaries.

***articular r.*** A rete about a joint, esp. a deep anastomosis at the knee joint.

***r. cutaneum*** A network of blood vessels at the junction of the corium and superficial fascia.

***malpighian r.*** Stratum germinativum.

***r. mirabile*** A plexus formed by the sudden division of a vessel into small twigs that reunite to form one vessel, as in the glomeruli of the kidneys.

***r. olecrani*** A network of vessels at the back of the elbow formed by divisions of the recurrent ulnar arteries.

***r. ovarii*** A layer of cells lying in the broad ligament and mesovarium of the ovary. It is homologous to rete testes in men.

***r. patellae*** A superficial network of vessels lying about the patella; formed by branches of genicular arteries.

***r. subpapillare*** A network of vessels between the papillary and reticular layers of the dermis.

***r. testis*** A network of tubules in the mediastinum testis that receives sperm through the tubuli recti from the seminiferous tubules. From the rete testis, efferent ducts convey sperm to the epididymis. The rete testis is homologous to the rete ovarii in women.

***r. venosum*** Venous network.

***vertebral r.*** One of two plexuses within the vertebral canal that extends from the foramen magnum to the coccyx. These retia lie posteriorly and laterally to the dura and between the dura and the arches of the vertebrae.

**retention** (rĭ-tĕn′shŭn) [L. *retentio,* a holding back] **1.** The act or process of keeping in possession or of holding in place. **2.** The persistent keeping within the body of materials normally excreted, such as urine, feces, or perspiration. **3.** In dentistry, any of several procedures or materials used to keep a dental device or dentures in place.

***urinary r.*** The inability to empty the bladder. Causes of this condition include loss of muscle tone of the bladder from anemia, old age, exposure to cold, or a prolonged operation; lesions involving nervous pathways to and from the bladder; lesions involving reflex centers in the brain and spinal cord; urethral obstruction, which may result from inflammation, stricture, stones, diverticula, cysts, tumors, or pressure from outside as in cases of prostatic hypertrophy; psychogenic factors; and medication such as morphine or certain antihistamines.

**retention defect** The inability to recall a name, number, or fact shortly after being requested to remember it.

**retention with overflow** A spasm of the sphincter, causing failure to empty the bladder at one voiding, with only overflow dribbling away. It results from the same causes as urinary retention.

**rete ridge** One of the downgrowths of epithelium surrounding the connective tissue papillae in the irregular internal surface of the epidermis. Microscopic sections often appear as single downgrowths when in fact the epithelium is in a series of interconnecting ridges at the dermis-epidermis interface. SYN: *rete peg.*

**retia** (rē′tē-ă) [L.] Pl. of rete.

**retial** (rē′tē-ăl) Pert. to a rete.

**reticula** (rē-tĭk′ū-lă) [L.] Pl. of reticulum.

**reticular** (rĭ-tĭk′ū-lăr) [L. *reticula,* net] Meshed; in the form of a network. SYN: *retiform.*

**reticular activating system** ABBR: RAS. The alerting system of the brain consisting of the reticular formation, subthalamus, hypothalamus, and medial thalamus. It extends from the central core of the brainstem to all parts of the cerebral cortex. This system is essential in initiating and maintaining wakefulness and introspection and in directing attention. Some of the tranquilizing drugs depress this system.

**reticular fiber** One of the extremely fine argyrophilic (silver-staining) fibers found in reticular tissue.

**reticular membrane** The membrane formed by the cuticular plates of the distal ends of supporting cells in the organ of Corti.

**reticulate substance** Reticular formation.

**reticulation** (rē-tĭk″ū-lā′shŭn) The formation of a network mass.

**reticulin** (rē-tĭk′ū-lĭn) [L. *reticula,* net] An albuminoid or scleroprotein substance in the connective tissue framework of reticular tissue.

**reticulo-** Combining form meaning *network.*

**reticulocyte** (rĕ-tĭk′ū-lō-sīt) [″ + Gr. *kytos,* cell] The last immature stage of a red blood cell. Its darkly staining granules are fragments of the endoplasmic reticulum. Reticulocytes normally constitute about 1% of the circulating red blood cells. SEE: illus.

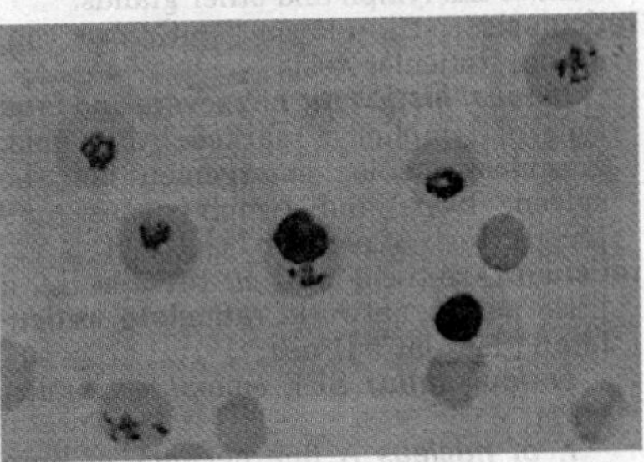

RETICULOCYTES IN PERIPHERAL BLOOD (ORIG. MAG ×600)

**reticulocytopenia** (rē-tĭk″ū-lō-sī″tō-pē′nē-ă) [″ + ″ + *penia,* poverty] A decreased number of the reticulocytes of the blood.

**reticulocytosis** (rē-tĭk″ū-lō-sī-tō′sĭs) [″ + ″ + *osis,* condition] An increased number of reticulocytes in the circulating blood. This condition indicates active erythropoiesis in the red bone marrow and the need for greater oxygen-carrying capacity of the blood. It occurs after hemorrhage, during acclimatization to high altitude, during any pulmonary disorder that induces hypoxia, and in all types of anemia.

**reticuloendothelial** (rē-tĭk″ū-lō-ĕn″dō-thē′lē-ăl) [″ + Gr. *endon,* within, + *thele,* nipple] Pert. to the reticuloendothelial system.

**reticuloendothelioma** (rĕ-tĭk″ū-lō-ĕn″dō-thē-lē-ō′mă) [″ + ″ + ″ + *oma,* tumor] A neoplasm composed of reticuloendothelial tissue.

**reticuloendotheliosis** (rĕ-tĭk″ū-lō-ĕn″dō-thē-lē-ō′sĭs) [″ + ″ + *thele,* nipple, + *osis,* condition] Hyperplasia of reticuloendothelium.

**reticuloendothelium** (rĕ-tĭk″ū-lō-ĕn″dō-thē′lē-ŭm) The tissue of the reticuloendothelial system. SYN: *retothelium.*

**reticulohistiocytoma** (rĕ-tĭk″ū-lō-hĭs″tē-ō-sī-tō′mă) [L. *reticula,* net, + Gr. *histion,* little web, + *kytos,* cell, + *oma,* tumor] A giant-cell granulomacytosis involving the skin, mucous membranes, and synovial membranes of the long bones.

**reticulohistiocytosis** (rĕ-tĭk″ū-lō-hĭs″tē-ō-sī-tō′sĭs) [″ + ″ + ″ + *osis,* condition] Reticuloendotheliosis.

**reticuloid** (rĕ-tĭk′ū-loyd) [″ + Gr. *eidos,* form, shape] Resembling reticulosis.

**reticuloma** (rĕ-tĭk″ū-lō′mă) [″ + Gr. *oma,* tumor] A neoplasm composed of reticuloendothelial cells.

**reticulopenia** (rĕ-tĭk″ū-lō-pē′nē-ă) [″ + Gr.

*penia,* lack] A decreased number of reticulocytes in the blood.

**reticulopodium** (rĕ-tĭk″ū-lō-pō′dē-ŭm) Rhizopodium.

**reticulosarcoma** (rĕ-tĭk″ū-lō-săr-kō′mă) [″ + Gr. *sarx,* flesh, + *oma,* tumor] A neoplasm composed of large monocytic cells that originated in the reticuloendothelium of the lymph and other glands.

**reticulosis** (rĕ-tĭk-ū-lō′sĭs) [″ + Gr. *osis,* condition] Reticulocytosis.

***familial histiocytic r.*** A severe and fatal type of lymphoma marked by anemia; granulocytopenia; enlargement of the spleen, liver, and lymph nodes; and phagocytosis of red blood cells.

**reticulum** (rĕ-tĭk′ū-lŭm) *pl.* **reticula** [L., a little net] A network. **reticulate, reticulated** (-lāt, -lāt″ĕd), *adj.*

***endoplasmic r.*** SEE: *endoplasmic reticulum.*

***r. of nucleus*** A fine network of linin threads on which masses of chromatin are arranged.

***sarcoplasmic r.*** The endoplasmic reticulum of striated muscle cells, surrounding the sarcomeres. In response to an action potential, it releases calcium ions to induce contraction, then reabsorbs calcium ions to induce relaxation.

***stellate r.*** The enamel pulp of a developing tooth, consisting of stellate cells lying between the inner and outer epithelial layers of the enamel organ.

**retiform** (rĕt′ĭ-form) [L. *rete,* net, + *forma,* shape] Reticular.

**retina** (rĕt′ĭ-nă) *pl.* **retinae** [L.] The innermost layer of the eye, which receives images transmitted through the lens and contains the receptors for vision, the rods and cones. SEE: illus. (Retina of Right Eye).

The retina is a light-sensitive structure on which light rays come to a focus. It extends from the entrance point of the optic nerve anteriorly to the margin of the pupil, completely lining the interior of the eye. It consists of three parts. The pars optica, the nervous or sensory portion, extends from the optic disk forward to the ora serrata, a wavy line immediately behind the ciliary process; the pars ciliaris lines the inner surface of the ciliary process; and the pars iridica forms the posterior surface of the iris. Slightly lateral to the posterior pole of the eye is a small, oval, yellowish spot, the macula lutea, in the center of which is a depression, the fovea centralis. This region contains only cones and is the region of the most acute vision. About 3.5 mm nasally from the fovea is the optic papilla (optic disk), where nerve fibers from the retina make their exit and form the optic nerve. This region is devoid of rods and cones and is insensitive to light; hence it is named the blind spot.

The layers of the retina, in the order light strikes them, are the optic nerve fi-

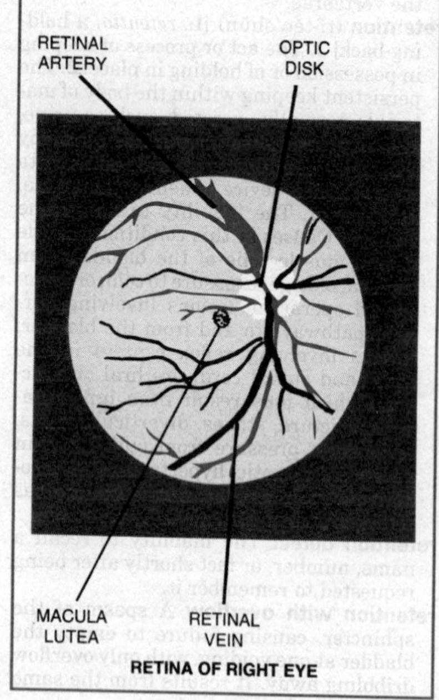

RETINA OF RIGHT EYE

ber layer, ganglion cell layer, inner synaptic layer, bipolar cell layer, outer synaptic layer, layer of rods and cones, and pigment epithelium. SEE: illus. (Retina).

COLOR: The retina is normally red, reflecting blood flow, and is pale in anemia or ischemia.

VESSELS: The arteries are branches of a single central artery, a branch of the ophthalmic artery. The central artery enters at the center of the optic papilla and supplies the inner layers of the retina. The outer layers, including rods and cones, are nourished by capillaries of the choroid layer. The veins lack muscular coats. They parallel the arteries; blood leaves by a central vein that leads to the superior ophthalmic vein. **retinal** (-năl), *adj.*

***coarctate r.*** A condition in which there is an effusion of fluid between the retina and choroid, giving the retina a funnel shape.

***shot-silk r.*** A retina having an opalescent appearance, sometimes seen in young persons.

***tigroid r.*** A retina having a spotted or striped appearance, seen in retinitis pigmentosa.

**retinaculum** (rĕt″ĭ-năk′ū-lŭm) *pl.* **retinacula** [L., halter] A band or membrane holding any organ or part in its place. Thickenings of the deep fascia in distal portions of limbs that hold tendons in position when muscles contract are called retinaculum tendinum.

***r. cutis*** A fibrous band connecting the

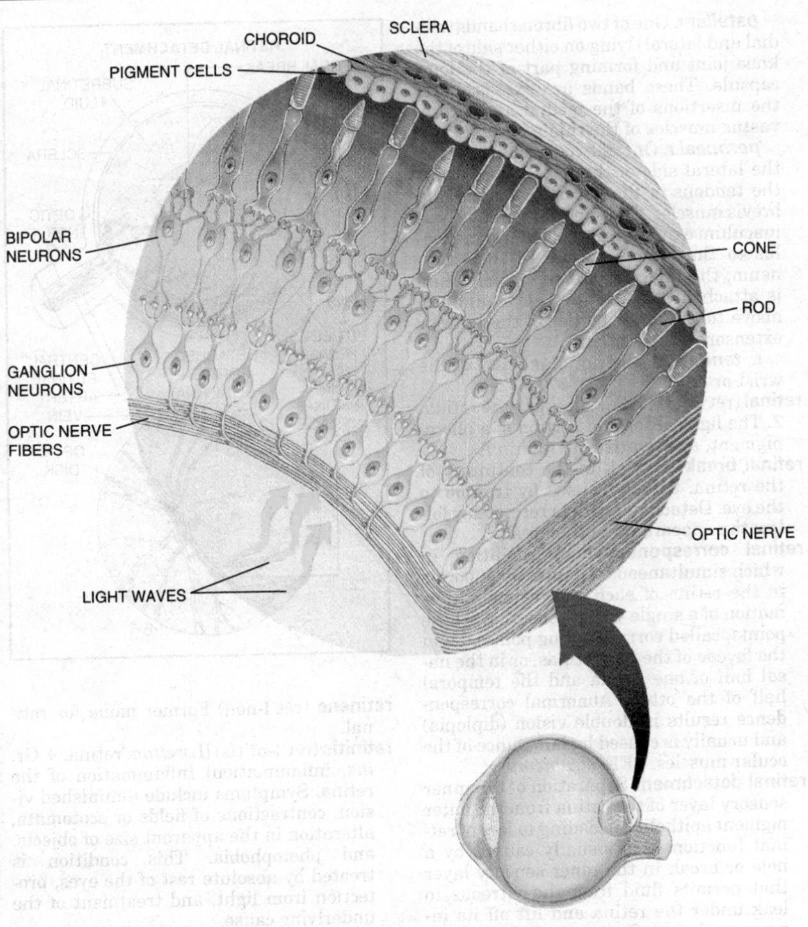


RETINA

MICROSCOPIC STRUCTURE OF OPTIC DISK AREA

corium with underlying fascia.

***extensor r. of ankle*** **1.** The superior extensor retinaculum, a band crossing the extensor tendons of the foot and attached to the lower portion of the tibia and fibula. **2.** The inferior extensor retinaculum, a band located on the dorsum of the foot. It consists of two limbs having a common origin on the lateral surface of the calcaneum. The upper limb is attached to the medial malleolus; the lower limb curves around the instep and is attached to the fascia of the abductor hallucis on the medial side of the foot.

***extensor r. of wrist*** An oblique band attached medially to the styloid process of the ulna, the hammate bone, and the medial ligament of the wrist joint. Laterally it is attached to the anterior border of the radius. It contains six separate compartments for passage of the extensor tendons to the hand.

***flexor r. of ankle*** The retinaculum extending from the medial malleolus to the medial tubercle of the calcaneum.

***flexor r. of hand*** The fascial band that holds down the flexor tendons of the digits.

***flexor r. of wrist*** The retinaculum extending from the trapezium and scaphoid bones laterally to the hammate and pisiform bones medially.

***r. of hip joint*** Any of three flat bands lying along the neck of the femur and continuous with the capsule of the hip joint.

***r. mammae*** Strands of connective tissue in the mammary gland extending from glandular tissue through fat toward the skin, where they are attached to deep fascia. Over the cephalic portion of the mammae, they are well developed and are called suspensory ligaments of Cooper.

***patellar r.*** One of two fibrous bands (medial and lateral) lying on either side of the knee joint and forming part of the joint capsule. These bands are extensions of the insertions of the medial and lateral vastus muscles of the thigh.

***peroneal r.*** One of two fibrous bands on the lateral side of the foot that contains the tendons of the peroneus longus and brevis muscles. The superior peroneal retinaculum extends from the lateral malleolus to the lateral surface of the calcaneum; the inferior peroneal retinaculum is attached below to the calcaneum and above to the lower border of the inferior extensor retinaculum.

***r. tendinum*** The annular band of the wrist or ankle.

**retinal** (rĕt′ĭ-năl) **1.** Pertaining to the retina. **2.** The light-absorbing portion of a photopigment, a derivative of vitamin A.

**retinal break** A break in the continuity of the retina, usually caused by trauma to the eye. Detachment of the retina may follow the appearance of the break.

**retinal correspondence** A condition in which simultaneous stimulation of points in the retina of each eye results in formation of a single visual sensation. These points, called corresponding points, lie in the foveae of the two retinas, or in the nasal half of one retina and the temporal half of the other. Abnormal correspondence results in double vision (diplopia) and usually is caused by imbalance of the ocular muscles. SEE: *strabismus.*

**retinal detachment** Separation of the inner sensory layer of the retina from the outer pigment epithelium, leading to loss of retinal function. It is usually caused by a hole or break in the inner sensory layer that permits fluid from the vitreous to leak under the retina and lift off its innermost layer. Causes include trauma and any disease that causes retinopathy, such as diabetes or sickle cell disease. Symptoms are blurred vision, flashes of light, vitreous floaters, and loss of visual acuity. The location of holes must be determined so that they can be repaired by laser therapy (i.e., photocoagulation). SEE: illus.; *Nursing Diagnoses Appendix.*

TREATMENT: Experimental treatments include injection of silicone oil into the eye to hold the detached area in place. Reattachment may require a year. Another experimental treatment is pneumatic retinopexy, in which a bubble of gas is instilled into the vitreous. As the bubble attains equilibrium with body gases, it expands and forces the detached area back into place; then, cryotherapy or photocoagulation is used to reattach the retina permanently.

**retinal isomerase** The enzyme in rods and cones that converts *trans*-retinal to *cis*-retinal, which then combines with the opsin present to form a photopigment responsive to light.

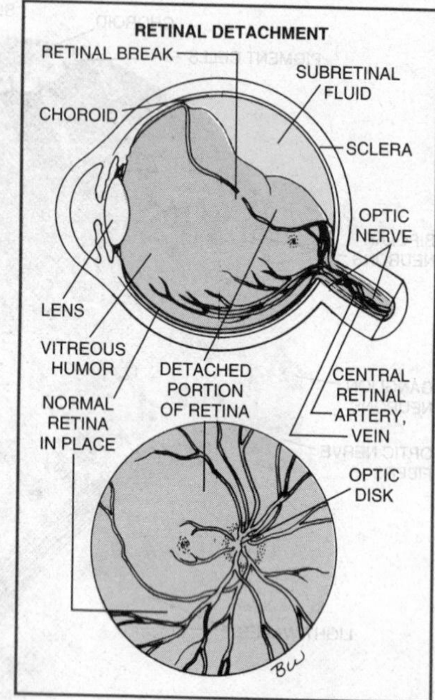


**retinene** (rĕt′ĭ-nēn) Former name for retinal.

**retinitis** (rĕt-ĭ-nī′tĭs) [L. *retina,* retina, + Gr. *itis,* inflammation] Inflammation of the retina. Symptoms include diminished vision, contractions of fields or scotomata, alteration in the apparent size of objects, and photophobia. This condition is treated by absolute rest of the eyes, protection from light, and treatment of the underlying cause.

***actinic r.*** Retinitis caused by exposure to intense light or other forms of radiant energy.

***albuminuric r.*** Retinitis associated with chronic kidney disease and malignant hypertension. The general signs of retinitis are present. This type of retinitis is distinguished by white patches in the fundus, esp. surrounding the papilla and in the macular region.

***apoplectic r.*** Retinitis associated with hemorrhaging of the retinal vessels.

***circinate r.*** Retinitis marked by a circle of white spots about the macula.

***circumpapillar r.*** Retinitis marked by a proliferation of the outer layers of retina about the optic disk.

***diabetic r.*** Retinitis occurring in diabetes, esp. that of long duration. It is marked by aneurysmal dilatation of the blood vessels, hemorrhages, and waxy and cottonwool exudates.

***disciform r.*** Retinitis accompanied by degeneration of the retina in the macular region.

***exogenous purulent r.*** Retinitis following the introduction of infectious organisms into the eye as a result of a perforating wound or ulcer.

***external exudative r.*** Retinitis in which large masses of white and yellow crystals occur beneath the retina due to organization of hemorrhages.

***exudative r.*** Chronic retinitis with elevated areas around the optic disk.

***hemorrhagic r.*** Retinitis with pronounced hemorrhage into the retina.

***metastatic r.*** Acute purulent retinitis resulting from the presence of infective emboli in retinal vessels.

***r. of prematurity*** SEE: *retrolental fibroplasia.*

***r. pigmentosa*** A chronic progressive disease that has its onset in early childhood. It is marked by degeneration of the retinal epithelium, esp. the rods, without inflammation; atrophy of the optic nerve; and widespread pigmentary changes in the retina. An early symptom is defective night vision followed by a constricted field of vision. The cause is unknown, but a hereditary tendency is suspected.

TREATMENT: No specific therapy is available, but professional and vocational guidance and genetic counseling can be provided. Family members should be examined to determine whether their vision is affected.

***r. proliferans*** Retinitis marked by vascularized masses of connective tissue that project from the retina into the vitreous; the end result of recurrent hemorrhage from the retina into the vitreous.

***r. punctata albescens*** A nonprogressive, degenerative familial disease in which innumerable minute white spots are scattered over entire retina. There are no pigmentary changes. The disease usually starts early in life.

***punctate r.*** Retinitis marked by numerous white or yellow spots in the fundus of the eye.

***solar r.*** Retinitis resulting from exposure of the retina to the rays of the sun. SEE: *scotoma, eclipse.*

***stellate r.*** Retinitis marked by exudates, hemorrhages, blurring of the optic disk, and formation of a star-shaped figure around the macula.

***suppurative r.*** Retinitis associated with septicemia resulting from pyogenic organisms.

***syphilitic r.*** Retinitis resulting from or associated with syphilis. It may also involve the optic nerve (syphilitic neuroretinitis).

**retinoblastoma** (rĕt″ĭ-nō-blăs-tō′mă) [L. *retina,* retina, + Gr. *blastos,* germ, + *oma,* tumor] A malignant glioma of the retina, usually unilateral, that occurs in young children and usually is hereditary. The initial diagnostic finding is usually a yellow or white light reflex seen at the pupil (cat's eye reflex). Several treatment options are available depending on the size and extent of the tumor, whether both eyes are involved, and the general health of the patient. Included are enucleation, radiation, scleral plaque irradiation, cryotherapy, photocoagulation, and chemotherapy.

**retinochoroid** (rĕt″ĭ-nō-kō′royd) [″ + Gr. *chorioeides,* skinlike] Pert. to the retina and choroid. SYN: *chorioretinal.*

**retinochoroiditis** (rĕt″ĭ-nō-kō-royd-ī′tĭs) [″ + ″ + *itis,* inflammation] Inflammation of the retina and choroid. SYN: *chorioretinitis; choroidoretinitis.*

***r. juxtapapillaris*** Retinochoroiditis close to the optic nerve.

**retinocystoma** (rĕt″ĭ-nō-sĭs-tō′mă) [″ + Gr. *kysis,* sac, + *oma,* tumor] Glioma of the retina.

**retinodialysis** (rĕt″ĭ-nō-dī-ăl′ĭ-sĭs) [″ + Gr. *dialysis,* separation] Detachment of the retina at its periphery. SYN: *disinsertion.*

**retinoic acid** A metabolite of vitamin A used in the treatment of cystic acne.

**retinol** (rĕt′ĭ-nŏl) A form of vitamin A. This 20-carbon alcohol is present in liver, egg yolk, chicken, whole milk, butter, and breakfast cereals. Vitamin A activity in foods is expressed as retinol equivalents (RE).

**retinopapillitis** (rĕt″ĭ-nō-pă″pĭl-ī′tĭs) [L. *retina,* retina, + *papilla,* nipple, + Gr. *itis,* inflammation] Inflammation of the retina and optic papilla extending to the optic disk. SYN: *papilloretinitis.*

**retinopathy** (rĕt″ĭn-ŏp′ă-thē) [″ + Gr. *pathos,* disease, suffering] Any disorder of the retina.

***arteriosclerotic r.*** Retinopathy accompanying generalized arteriosclerosis and moderate hypertension.

***circinate r.*** A ring of degenerated white exudative area of the retina around the macula.

***diabetic r.*** Retinopathy occurring in diabetics.

***hypertensive r.*** Retinopathy associated with hypertension, toxemia of pregnancy, or glomerulonephritis.

***r. of prematurity*** ABBR: ROP. A bilateral disease of the retinal vessels in preterm infants, some of whom have been exposed to prolonged periods of high postnatal oxygen concentrations. High oxygen concentration used in treating preterm infants, esp. those weighing less than 1500 g, causes vasoconstriction of the immature retinal vessels and eventually occlusion of the vessels. This may be followed by fibrous proliferation and invasion of the vitreous. Retinal detachment may occur at that time or many years later. Blindness develops within several weeks. Other factors can have an important role in the pathogenesis of ROP. Apnea, asphyxia, sepsis, nutritional deficiencies, and many blood transfusions given over a short period have all been related to ROP. SYN: *retrolental fibroplasia.*

In treating preterm infants, it is possible to prevent ROP by using only the lowest possible effective oxygen concentration that will not endanger the life of the infant. Monitoring arterial blood oxygen levels is essential in preventing ROP. Too severe oxygen restriction, however, increases the likelihood of hyaline membrane disease and neurological disorders. All preterm infants treated with supplemental oxygen should be examined carefully by an ophthalmologist before discharge from the hospital. Once blindness develops, there is no effective treatment.

***solar r.*** Pathological changes in the retina after looking directly at the sun. This condition is seen frequently following an eclipse of the sun. SEE: *scotoma, eclipse.*

***syphilitic r.*** Retinopathy occurring in the later stages of syphilis.

**retinopexy** [" + Gr. *pexis,* fixation] In the treatment of retinal detachment, the formation of adhesions between the detached portion and the underlying tissue.

***pneumatic r.*** An experimental treatment for retinal detachment, in which a bubble of gas is instilled into the vitreous. As the bubble attains equilibrium with body gases, it expands and forces the detached area back into place; then, cryotherapy or photocoagulation is used to reattach the retina permanently. SEE: *retinal detachment.*

**retinoschisis** (rĕt″ĭ-nŏs′kĭ-sĭs) [" + Gr. *schisis,* a splitting] A splitting of the retina into two layers with cyst formation between the layers.

**retinoscope** (rĕt′ĭ-nō-skōp) [" + Gr. *skopein,* to examine] An instrument used in performing retinoscopy.

**retinoscopy** (rĕt″ĭn-ŏs′kō-pē) An objective method of determining refractive errors of the eye. The examiner projects light into the eyes and judges error of refraction by the movement of reflected light rays. SYN: *skiascopy* (1).

**retinosis** (rĕt″ĭ-nŏ′sĭs) [" + Gr. *osis,* condition] Any degenerative process of the retina not associated with inflammation.

**retire 1.** To discontinue formal employment or work at a specific place or task. In the past, in many industries, educational institutions, and public service, retirement was mandated when an employee had attained a specified age. This practice has lost its attractiveness to a large segment of the work force, esp. among those who enjoy work. SEE: *recreation.* **2.** To go to bed.

**retisolution** (rĕt″ĭ-sō-lū′shŭn) [L. *rete,* net, + *solutio,* dissolution] Dissolution of the Golgi structures.

**retispersion** (rĕt″ĭ-spĕr′zhŭn) [" + *spersio,* a scattering] Transference of Golgi structures to the periphery of the cell.

**retoperithelium** (rē″tō-pĕr″ĭ-thē′lē-ŭm) [L. *rete,* net, + Gr. *peri,* around, + *thele,* nipple] Epithelium covering a reticulum.

**retort** (rē-tort′) [L. *retortus,* bent back] A flasklike, long-necked vessel used in distillation.

**retothelium** (rē″tō-thē′lē-ŭm) Reticuloendothelium.

**retract** (rĭ-trăkt′) [L. *retractus*] To draw back.

**retractile** (rĭ-trăkt′ĭl) [L. *retractilis*] Capable of being drawn back or in.

**retraction** (rĭ-trăk′shŭn) A shortening; the act of drawing backward or the condition of being drawn back.

***clot r.*** **1.** The shrinking of the clot that forms when blood is allowed to stand, due to the fibrin network formed in the clot. **2.** The platelet-mediated folding of fibrin threads in a formed clot, which diminishes the size of the damaged area.

***uterine r.*** The process by which the muscular fibers of the uterus remain permanently shortened to a small degree following each contraction or labor pain.

**retraction ring** A ridge sometimes felt on the uterus above the pubes, marking the line of separation between the upper contractile and lower dilatable segments of the uterus. SEE: *Bandl's ring.*

**retractor 1.** An instrument for holding back the margins of a wound. **2.** A muscle that draws in any organ or part.

**retrad** (rē′trăd) [L. *retro,* backward] Toward the posterior part of the body.

**retrain** To instruct a person in a skill or trade different from the person's previous work.

**retreat** (rĭ-trēt′) [ME. *retret,* draw back] The act of retiring or withdrawing from difficult life situations. This may be direct, as in physical flight, or indirect, as in malingering, illness, abnormal preoccupation, and self-deception.

**retrenchment** [Fr. *retrenchier,* to cut back] A procedure used in plastic surgery to remove excess tissue.

**retrieval** (rĭ-trē′văl) In psychology, the process of bringing remembered information back to the conscious level.

**retro-** [L.] Prefix meaning *backward, back, behind.*

**retroaction** (rĕt″rō-ăk′shŭn) Action in a reverse direction.

**retroauricular** (rĕt″rō-aw-rĭk′ū-lăr) [L. *retro,* behind, + *auricula,* ear] Behind the auricle or ear.

**retrobuccal** (rĕt″rō-bŭk′ăl) [L. *retro,* back, + *bucca,* cheek] Pert. to the back part of the mouth or the area behind the mouth.

**retrobulbar** (rĕt″rō-bŭl′băr) [L. *retro,* behind, + Gr. *bulbus,* bulb] **1.** Behind the eyeball. **2.** Posterior to the medulla oblongata.

**retrocecal** (rĕt″rō-sē′kăl) [L. *retro,* back, + *caecum,* cecum] Behind or pert. to the area posterior to the cecum.

**retrocedent** (rĕt″rō-sē′dĕnt) [L. *retrocedere*] Going backward, returning.

**retrocervical** (rĕt″rō-sĕr′vĭ-kăl) [L. *retro,* back, + *cervix,* neck] Posterior to the cervix uteri.

**retrocession** (rĕt″rō-sĕsh′ŭn) [L. *retrocessio,*

going back] **1.** A going back; a relapse. **2.** Metastasis from the surface to an internal organ. **3.** Backward displacement of the uterus.

**retroclusion** (rĕt″rō-kloo′zhŭn) [″ + *claudere,* to close] A method of stopping arterial bleeding. A needle is placed through the tissues over a severed artery and then turned around and down so that it is passed back through the tissues under the artery. This compresses the vessel.

**retrocolic** (rĕt″rō-kŏl′ĭk) [L. *retro,* back, + Gr. *kolon,* colon] Posterior to the colon.

**retrocollic** (rĕt″rō-kŏl′ĭk) [″ + *collum,* neck] Pert. to the back of the neck.

**retrocollic spasm** Torticollis with spasms affecting the posterior neck muscles.

**retrocollis** (rĕt″rō-kŏl′ĭs) A spasm of the posterior neck muscles with drawing of the head backward. SEE: *torticollis.*

**retrocursive** (rĕt″rō-kŭr′sĭv) [L. *retro,* back, + *curro,* to run] Stepping or turning backward.

**retrodeviation** (rĕt″rō-dē″vē-ā′shŭn) [″ + *deviare,* to turn aside] Backward displacement, as of an organ.

**retrodisplacement** (rĕt″rō-dĭs-plās′mĕnt) [″ + Fr. *desplacer,* displace] Backward displacement of a part.

**retroesophageal** (rĕt″rō-ē-sŏf″ă-jē′ăl) [L. *retro,* behind, + Gr. *oisophagos,* gullet] Behind the esophagus.

**retrofilling** (rĕt″rō-fĭl′ĭng) The placement of filling material in a root canal through an opening made in the apex of the tooth.

**retroflexed** (rĕt′rō-flĕkst″) [L. *retro,* backward, + *flexus,* bent] Bent backward.

**retroflexion** (rĕt″rō-flĕk′shŭn) A bending or flexing backward.

***r. of uterus*** A condition in which the body of the uterus is bent backward at an angle with the cervix, whose position usually remains unchanged.

**retrogasserian** (rĕt″rō-găs-sē′rē-ăn) Pert. to the posterior root of the gasserian ganglion.

**retrognathia** (rĕt″rō-năth′ē-ă) [L. *retro,* back, + Gr. *gnathos,* jaw] Location of the mandible behind the frontal plane of the maxilla.

**retrognathism** (rĕt″rō-năth′ĭzm) [″ + Gr. *gnathos,* jaw] The condition of having retrognathia.

**retrograde** (rĕt′rō-grād) [L. *retro,* backward, + *gradi,* to step] Moving backward; degenerating from a better to a worse state.

**retrograde flow** The flow of fluid in a direction opposite to that considered normal.

**retrograde pyelography** A surgical procedure in which an endoscope is placed through the urethra into the urinary bladder and a catheter is placed into the ureter for instillation of a contrast medium to visualize the renal pelvis and ureter.

**retrography** (rĕt″rŏg′ră-fē) [″ + Gr. *graphein,* to write] Mirror writing, a symptom of certain brain diseases. It also may be present in persons with dyslexia.

**retrogression** (rĕt″rō-grĕsh′ŭn) [L. *retrogressus,* go backward] A going backward, as in the involution, degeneration, or atrophy of a tissue or structure.

**retroinfection** (rĕt″rō-ĭn-fĕk′shŭn) [L. *retro,* backward, + *infectio,* infection] An infection communicated by the fetus in utero to the mother.

**retroinsular** (rĕt″rō-ĭn′sū-lăr) [″ + *insula,* island] Located behind the island of Reil in the brain.

**retroiridian** (rĕt″rō-ī-rĭd′ē-ăn) [L. *retro,* behind, + Gr. *iridos,* colored circle] Posterior to the iris.

**retrojection** (rĕt″rō-jĕk′shŭn) [″ + *jacio,* throw] Washing out a cavity from within by injection of a fluid.

**retrolabyrinthine** (rĕt″rō-lăb″ĭ-rĭn′thĭn) [L. *retro,* behind + Gr. *labyrinthos,* a maze] Located behind the labyrinth of the ear.

**retrolental** Behind the crystalline lens. SYN: *retrolenticular.*

**retrolenticular** (rĕt″rō-lĕn-tĭk′ū-lăr) Retrolental.

**retrolingual** (rĕt″rō-lĭng′gwăl) [L. *retro,* behind, + *lingua,* tongue] Behind the tongue.

**retromammary** (rĕt″rō-măm′mă-rē) [″ + *mamma,* breast] Behind the mammary gland.

**retromandibular** (rĕt″rō-măn-dĭb′ū-lăr) [″ + *mandibulum,* jaw] Behind the lower jaw.

**retromastoid** (rĕt″rō-măs′toyd) [″ + Gr. *mastos,* breast, + *eidos,* form, shape] Behind the mastoid process.

**retromorphosis** (rĕt″rō-mor′fō-sĭs) [″ + Gr. *morphe,* form, + *osis,* condition] **1.** A change in shape accompanying a transition from a higher to a lower type of structure. **2.** Retrogressive changes within cells or tissues. SYN: *catabolism.*

**retronasal** (rĕt″rō-nā′zăl) [L. *retro,* back, + *nasus,* nose] Pert. to or situated at the back part of the nose.

**retro-ocular** (rĕt″rō-ŏk′ū-lar) [L. *retro,* behind, + *oculus,* eye] Behind the eye.

**retroparotid** (rĕt″rō-pă-rŏt′ĭd) [″ + Gr. *para,* beside, + *ous,* ear] Behind the parotid gland.

**retroperitoneal** (rĕt″rō-pĕr″ĭ-tō-nē′ăl) [″ + Gr. *peritonaion,* peritoneum] Behind the peritoneum and outside the peritoneal cavity (e.g., the kidneys).

**retroperitoneal fibrosis** Development of a mass of fibrotic tissue in the retroperitoneal space. This may lead to physical compression of the ureters, and even the vena cava and aorta. This disease may be associated with taking methysergide for migraine, and with other drugs. SYN: *Ormond's disease.*

**retroperitoneum** (rĕt″rō-pĕr-ĭ-tō-nē′ŭm) The space behind the peritoneum.

**retroperitonitis** (rĕt″rō-pĕr″ĭ-tō-nī′tĭs) Inflammation behind the peritoneum.

**retropharyngeal** (rĕt″rō-făr-ĭn′jē-ăl) [L. *retro,* behind, + Gr. *pharynx,* throat] Behind the pharynx.

**retropharyngitis** (rĕt″rō-făr″ĭn-jī′tĭs) [″ + ″ +

*itis,* inflammation] Inflammation of the retropharyngeal tissue.

**retropharynx** (rĕt″rō-făr′ĭnks) [″ + Gr. *pharynx,* throat] The posterior portion of the pharynx.

**retroplacental** (rĕt″rō-plă-sĕn′tăl) [″ + *placenta,* a flat cake] Behind the placenta, or behind both the placenta and the uterine wall.

**retroplasia** (rĕt″rō-plā′zē-ă) [″ + Gr. *plassein,* to form] The degenerative change of a cell or tissue into a more primitive form.

**retroposed** (rĕt-rō-pōsd′) [L. *retro,* backward, + *positus,* placed] Displaced backward.

**retroposition** (rĕt″rō-pō-zĭsh′ŭn) The backward displacement of a tissue or organ.

**retropulsion** (rĕt″rō-pŭl′shŭn) [″ + *pulsio,* a thrusting] **1.** The pushing back of any part, as of the fetal head in labor. **2.** Walking or running backward involuntarily, seen in some nervous system disorders.

**retrorunning** The practice of running backward. In addition to being dangerous, this practice can cause muscle and joint pain.

**retrospective study** A clinical study in which patients or their records are investigated after the patients have experienced the disease or condition. SEE: *prospective study.*

**retrospondylolisthesis** (rĕt″rō-spŏn″dĭ-lō-lĭs-thē′sĭs) [L. *retro,* behind + Gr. *spondylos,* vertebra, + *olisthesis,* a slipping] The posterior displacement of a vertebra.

**retrosternal** (rĕt″rō-stĕr′năl) [″ + Gr. *sternon,* chest] Behind the sternum.

**retrosternal pulse** A venous pulse felt over the suprasternal notch.

**retrotarsal** (rĕt″rō-tăr′săl) [″+ Gr. *tarsos,* a broad, flat surface] Behind the tarsus of the eye.

**retrouterine** (rĕt″rō-ū′tĕr-ĭn) [L. *retro,* backward,+ *uterus,* womb] Behind the uterus.

**retroversioflexion** (rĕt″rō-vĕr″sē-ō-flĕk′shŭn) [″ + *versio,* a turning, + *flexio,* flexion] Retroversion and retroflexion of the uterus.

**retroversion** (rĕt″rō-vĕr′shŭn) [L. *retro,* back, + *versio,* a turning] A turning, or a state of being turned back; esp., the tipping of an entire organ.

***femoral r.*** A decrease in the head-neck angle of the femur, causing outward rotation of the shaft of the bone when the person is standing.

***r. of uterus*** Backward displacement of the uterus with the cervix pointing forward toward the symphysis pubis. Normally the cervix points toward the lower end of the sacrum with the fundus toward the suprapubic region.

**Retrovir** Trade name for zidovudine, an antiviral drug.

**retroviruses** (rĕt″rō-vī′rŭs-ĕs) The common name for the family of Retroviridae. Some of these RNA-containing tumor viruses are oncogenic and induce sarcomas, leukemias, lymphomas, and mammary carcinomas in lower animals. These viruses contain reverse transcriptase, which is essential for reverse transcription (i.e., the production of a DNA molecule from an RNA model).

**retrude** (rĭ-trood′) [L. *re,* back, + *trudere,* to shove] To force inward or backward.

**retrusion** (rĭ-troo′shŭn) **1.** The process of forcing backward, esp. with reference to the teeth. **2.** A condition in which teeth are retroposed.

**Rett's syndrome** [Andreas Rett, contemporary Austrian physician] A multiple-deficit developmental disorder marked by hand-wringing or hand-washing movements; it occurs almost exclusively in girls beginning at 6 to 18 months of age. In addition, there may be breath holding and hyperventilation, seizures, and loss of communication skills. There is a general decline in motor and cognitive function. Head growth decelerates, hand skills are lost, interest in social environment diminishes, and retardation ensues. The course of the disease often leads to severe retardation. The patients may survive into adulthood. The cause is unknown, and no specific therapy is available.

**Retzius, lines of** (rĕt′zē-ŭs) [Gustav Magnus Retzius, Swedish anatomist, 1842–1919] Brownish incremental lines seen in microscopic sections of tooth enamel. They appear as concentric lines in transverse sections through the enamel crown.

**Retzius, Anders Adolf** Swedish anatomist, 1796–1860.

***space of R.*** An area in the lower portion of the abdomen between the bladder and pubic bones and bounded superiorly by the peritoneum. It contains areolar tissue, fat, and a plexus of veins.

***veins of R.*** The veins that communicate between the mesenteric veins and the inferior vena cava.

**reunient** (rē-ūn′yĕnt) [L. *re,* again, + *unire,* to unite] **1.** Connecting or uniting tissue. **2.** Ductus reuniens.

**Reuss's color charts** (roys) [August R. von Reuss, Austrian ophthalmologist, 1841–1924] Colored letters printed on colored backgrounds to test color vision. A color-blind person sees the letters as being the same color as the background.

**revaccination** (rē″văk-sĭ-nā′shŭn) Subsequent vaccination after the initial one.

**revascularization** (rē-văs″kū-lăr-ĭ-zā′shŭn) Restoration of blood flow to a part. This may be done surgically or by removing or dissolving thrombi occluding arteries, esp. coronary or renal arteries.

**reverberation** (rĭ″vĕr-bĕr-ā′shŭn) [L. *reverberare,* to cause to rebound] **1.** The process by which closed chains of neurons, when excited by a single impulse, continue to discharge impulses from collaterals of their cells. **2.** The repeated echoing of a sound.

**Reverdin's needle** (rā-vĕr-dănz′) [Jacques L. Reverdin, Swiss surgeon, 1842–1929] A special needle with an eye at the tip that can be opened and closed by a lever.

**reversal** (rĭ-vĕr′săl) [L. *reversus*, revert] **1.** A change or turning in the opposite direction. **2.** In psychology, a change in an instinct or emotion to its opposite, as from love to hate.

***sex r.*** The process of changing an individual's sexual identity to that of the opposite sex. SEE: *sexual reassignment*.

**reversible** (rĭ-vĕr′sĭ-bl) Able to change back and forth.

**reversion** (rĭ-vĕr′zhŭn) **1.** A return to a previously existing condition. **2.** In genetics, the appearance of traits possessed by a remote ancestor. SEE: *atavism*.

**revertant** An organism that has reverted to a less advanced type by mutation.

**review of systems** ABBR: ROS. The process of asking questions concerning each organ and region of the body during the examination of a patient, esp. one not previously seen or examined. A physician who fails to do this may overlook something in the history that is essential to the diagnosis of a disease. This review is done in an orderly and systematic manner and is recorded. In general, if the examining person's findings are not recorded in the chart, they might as well have not been done in that they are not available to others involved in the patient's care.

In asking questions, the examiner should keep in mind any possible differences with respect to economic values, social and cultural mores, language, and life experiences. Hence questions concerning areas generally considered personal, private, and confidential, such as neuropsychiatric, sexual, and marital history, must be tactful and asked in a nonjudgmental manner. Also important for the examiner is constant awareness that the patient's vocabulary probably does not include complex or abstruse medical, anatomical, and chemical terms. Many individuals who know slang terms for urine, feces, and sexual intercourse may be unaware of the usual medical terms. It is sometimes useful to do the ROS during the physical examination. The ROS outline that follows should not be used slavishly for each patient. Obviously the questions asked of an adolescent will reasonably be less detailed than those asked of an elderly patient.

The systems and regions and questions include, but are not restricted to, the following.

*General*. The examiner should determine any history of fatigue, weight loss, travel to other climates or countries, recent weight change, chills, fever, and lifestyle change in the patient. Has the individual ever been refused for life insurance or military service? How many persons occupy the patient's dwelling? What is the patient's relationship to the persons with whom he or she lives? Is it a happy home? What are the patient's hobbies and outside interests. A history of exercise and athletic activity should be recorded. Is the patient involved in any religious activities? The examiner should get the patient's history of exposure to pets and the health of those animals; of military service and occupational record (including locations, and sources of income); and of the health of the patient's spouse and sex partners. What is the highest level of education attained by the patient? Does he or she have a criminal record?

*Skin*. Is the patient experiencing any rash, itching, sunburn, change in the size of moles, vesicles, or hair loss?

*Head, face, and neck*. Does the patient have headaches, migraine, vertigo, stiffness, pain, or swelling? Has there been trauma to this area?

*Eyes*. Are glasses worn and when were the eyes last examined for visual acuity and glaucoma? Is the patient experiencing pain, diplopia, scotomata, itch, discharge, redness, or infection?

*Ears*. Does the patient have acute or chronic hearing loss, pain, discharge, tinnitus, or vertigo? Does earwax collect and periodically need to be removed? Is there a history of failure to adjust to descent from a high altitude?

*Nose*. Is there any dryness, crust formation, bleeding, pain, discharge, obstruction, malodor, or sneezing? How acute is the patient's sense of smell? Do nose hairs have to be trimmed to prevent irritation?

*Mouth and teeth*. The patient should be asked about any soreness, ulcers, pain, dryness, infection, hoarseness, bleeding gums, swallowing difficulty, bruxism, or temporomandibular syndrome. What is the condition of the patient's teeth (real or false)?

*Breasts*. Has the patient had any pain, swelling, tenderness, lumps, bleeding from the nipple, infection, or change in the ability of the nipples to become erect? Has plastic surgery been done, and if so, were implants used?

*Respiratory*. Has there been any cough, pain, sputum production (including character of sputum), hemoptysis, or exposure to persons with contagious diseases such as tuberculosis? Is there a history of occupational or other exposure to asbestos, silica, chickens, parrots, or a dusty environment? The presence of dyspnea, cyanosis, tuberculosis, pneumonia, and pleurisy should be determined. If pulmonary function tests were done, the date or dates should be recorded. The extent and duration of all forms of tobacco use should be determined.

*Cardiac*. The following should be determined: angina, dyspnea, orthopnea, palpitations, heart murmur, heart failure, cardiac infarction, surgical procedures on coronary arteries or heart valves, history of stress test results and how recently they were done, hypertension, rheumatic fever, cardiac arrhythmias, exercise tolerance, history of athletic participation (including jogging and running) and if these are current activities, the dates of electrocardiograms if they were ever taken.

*Vascular*. Has the patient experienced claudication, cold intolerance (esp. of the extremities), frostbite, phlebitis, or ulcers (esp. of the extremities) due to poor blood supply?

*Gastrointestinal*. The examiner should assess the patient's appetite, history of recent weight gain or loss, and whether the patient has been following a particular diet for gaining or losing weight. Is the patient a vegetarian? Has he or she had any difficulty in swallowing? Anorexia, nausea, vomiting (including the character of the vomitus), diarrhea and its possible explanation (such as foreign travel or food poisoning), belching, constipation, change in bowel habits, melena, hemorrhoids and history of surgery for this condition, use of laxatives or antacids, jaundice, hepatitis, other liver disease, and use of injected "street" drugs should be determined.

*Renal; urinary and genital tract*. The examiner should take a history of kidney or bladder stones and date of last occurrence, dysuria, hematuria, pyuria, nocturia, incontinence, urgency, antibiotics used for urinary tract infections, bedwetting, sexually transmitted diseases, libido, sexual preference, penile or urethral discharge, marital history, and frequency of sexual activity.

Women should be questioned regarding any vulval pruritus, vaginal discharge, vaginal malodor, history of menarche, frequency and duration of menstrual periods, amount of flow, type of menstrual protection used, type or types of contraception and douches used, and the total number of pregnancies, abortions, miscarriages, and normal deliveries. The number, sex, age, and health status of living children, and the cause of death of children who died, should be determined. Vaginal, cervical, and uterine infections; pelvic inflammatory disease; tubal ligation; dilation and curettement; hysterectomy; and dyspareunia should be recorded. Any history of the mother's use of diethylstilbestrol while pregnant with the patient should be determined.

Men should be asked about vasectomy, "wet dreams," scrotal pain or swelling, and prostate trouble.

*Musculoskeletal*. The examiner should ask about muscle twitches, pain, heat, tenderness, swelling, loss of range of motion or strength, cramps, sprains, strains, trauma, fractures, stiffness, back pain, osteoporosis, and character regarding time of day of onset and duration (esp. with respect to the effect of exercise, back pain, and osteoporosis).

*Hematological*. A history of anemia, bleeding, bruising, hemarthrosis, hemophilia, sickle cell disease or trait, recent blood loss, transfusions received, and blood donation should be recorded. Was a transfusion received at a time when blood was not being screened for AIDS? Was the patient ever turned down as a blood donor?

*Endocrine*. The patient should be questioned about sexual maturation and development or their lack, weight change, tolerance to heat or cold (esp. with respect to other persons in the same environment), dryness of hair and skin, hair loss, and voice change. Any change in the rate of beard growth in men, development of facial hair in women, increase in or loss of libido, polyuria, polydipsia, polyphagia, pruritus, diabetes, exophthalmos, goiter, unexplained flushing, and sweating should be noted.

*Nervous system*. Has the patient experienced any recent change in ability to control muscular activity, or any syncope, stroke ("shock"), seizures, tremor, coordination, sensory disturbance, falls, pain, change in memory, dizziness, or head trauma?

*Emotional and psychological status*. Has there been a history of psychiatric illness, anxiety, depression, overactivity, mania, lassitude, change in sleep pattern, insomnia, hypersomnia, nightmares, sleepwalking, hallucinations, feeling of unreality, paranoia, phobias, obsessions, compulsions, criminal behavior, increase in or loss of libido, satyriasis, nymphomania, or suicidal thoughts? Is the patient satisfied with his or her occupation and life in general? What is his or her marital and divorce record? Has there been family discord? Does the patient attend church? The patient's employment history and any recent job changes, educational history and achievement, and self-image should be assessed. Has the patient abused drugs and shared needles? If it is appropriate, the examiner should ask the patient if he or she is happy and in love.

**Révilliod sign** SEE: *wink*.

**revised trauma score** ABBR: RTS. Pediatric trauma score.

**revivification** (rē-vĭv″ĭ-fĭ-kā′shŭn) [L. *re*, again, + *vivere*, to live, + *facere*, to make] **1.** An attempt to restore life to those apparently dead; restoration to life or consciousness; also the restoration of life in local parts, as a limb after freezing. **2.** The pairing of surfaces to facilitate healing, as in a wound.

**revulsant** (rĭ-vŭl′sănt) [L. *revulsio*, pulling back] **1.** Causing transfer of disease or blood from one part of the body to another. **2.** A counterirritant that increases blood flow to an inflamed part.

**revulsion** (rĭ-vŭl′shŭn) **1.** The act of driving

backward, as diverting disease from one part to another by a quick withdrawal of blood from that part. **2.** In physical therapy, circulatory changes obtained by sudden and intense reactions to heat and cold. SEE: *counterirritation.*

**revulsive** (rĭ-vŭl′sĭv) **1.** Causing revulsion. **2.** A counterirritant.

**reward** Something given to an individual as recognition of a good performance or of having achieved a certain level of competence in a field of endeavor.

**rewarming** The process of warming the body of an individual whose body temperature has dropped to a subnormal level. It is usually accomplished by providing a warm environment; one way of doing this is to immerse the hypothermic person in warm water.

**Reye's syndrome** (rīz) [R. D. K. Reye, Australian pathologist, 1912–1977] A syndrome first recognized in 1963, marked by acute encephalopathy and fatty infiltration of the liver and possibly of the pancreas, heart, kidney, spleen, and lymph nodes. It is seen in children under age 15 after an acute viral infection. The mortality rate depends on the severity of the central nervous system involvement but may be as high as 80%. The cause of the disease is unknown, but association with increased use of aspirin is evident from epidemiological studies. SEE: *Nursing Diagnoses Appendix.*

SYMPTOMS: The patient experiences a viral upper respiratory infection followed in about 6 days by pernicious nausea and vomiting, a change in mental status (disorientation, agitation, coma, seizures), and hepatomegaly without jaundice in 40% of cases. The disease should be suspected in any child with acute onset of encephalopathy and altered liver function.

Caution: Aspirin should not be used as an antipyretic or for any reason in treating children with viral infections.

TREATMENT: Supportive care includes intravenous administration of fluids and electrolytes. The blood electrolytes should be controlled carefully.

NURSING IMPLICATIONS: Neurological assessment is performed at frequent intervals. Temperature is monitored, and prescribed measures to alleviate hyperthermia are instituted. Seizure precautions are also instituted. Intake and output are monitored carefully. The patient is observed for evidence of impaired hepatic function, such as signs of bleeding. The nurse instructs the parent or guardian not to administer aspirin to children experiencing chickenpox or influenza, because use of aspirin in children with these conditions may induce Reye's syndrome.

**RF, Rf** *rheumatoid factor.*

**R.F.A.** *right frontoanterior* fetal position.

**R factor** *Resistance transfer factor*.

**R.F.P.** *right frontoposterior* fetal position.

**R.F.T.** *right frontotransverse* fetal position.

**RH** *releasing hormone.*

**Rh 1.** Symbol for the element rhodium. **2.** *Rhesus,* a monkey (*Macaca rhesus*) in which the Rh factor was first identified.

**Rhabditis** (răb-dī′tĭs) [Gr. *rhabdos,* rod] A genus of small nematode worms, some of which are parasitic.

**rhabdo-** Combining form meaning *rod.*

**rhabdoid** (răb′doyd) [Gr. *rhabdos,* rod, + *eidos,* form, shape] Resembling a rod.

**rhabdomyoblastoma** (răb″dō-mī″ō-blăs-tō′mă) Rhabdomyosarcoma.

**rhabdomyolysis** (răb″dō-mī-ŏl′ĭ-sĭs) [″ + ″ + *lysis,* dissolution] An acute, sometimes fatal disease marked by destruction of skeletal muscle. Rarely, this may occur following strenuous exercise and in association with use of drugs that can cause coma, such as alcohol, heroin, or cocaine. Renal damage manifested by acute tubular necrosis may result if myoglobinuria is accompanied by acute dehydration or anoxia. SEE: *reperfusion.*

***traumatic r.*** SEE: *crush syndrome; reperfusion* (2).

**rhabdomyoma** (răb″dō-mī-ō′mă) [″ + ″ + *oma,* tumor] A striated muscular tissue tumor. SYN: *myoma striocellulare.*

**rhabdomyosarcoma** (răb″dō-mī″ō-săr-kō′mă) [″ + ″ + *sarx,* flesh, + *oma,* tumor] An extremely malignant neoplasm originating in skeletal muscle. SYN: *rhabdomyoblastoma.*

**rhabdophobia** (răb-dō-fō′bē-ă) [″ + *phobos,* fear] An abnormal fear of being hit or beaten with a stick or rod.

**rhabdovirus** (răb″dō-vī′rŭs) [″ + L. *virus,* poison] Any of a group of rod-shaped RNA viruses with one important member, the rabies virus, being pathogenic to humans. The virus has a predilection for the tissue of mucus-secreting glands and the central nervous system. All warm-blooded animals are susceptible to infection with these viruses.

**rhachialgia** (rā″kē-ăl′jē-ă) [Gr. *rhachis,* spine, + *algos,* pain] Pain in the spine.

**rhachiocampsis** (rā″kē-ō-kămp′sĭs) [″ + *kampsis,* a bending] Curvature of the spine.

**rhachioplegia** (rā″kē-ō-plē′jē-ă) [″ + *plege,* stroke] Spinal paralysis.

**rhachioscoliosis** (rā″kē-ō-skō″lē-ō′sĭs) [″ + *skoliosis,* curvature] Curvature of the spine laterally.

**rhachis** (rā′kĭs) [Gr.] The spinal column.

**rhachischisis** (ră-kĭs′kĭ-sĭs) [″ + *schisis,* a splitting] A congenital cleft in the spinal column. SYN: *spondyloschisis.*

**rhagades** (răg′ă-dēz) [Gr., tears] Linear fissures appearing in the skin, esp. at the corner of the mouth or anus, causing pain. If due to syphilis, they form a radiating scar on healing.

**rhagadiform** (rā-găd′ĭ-form) [Gr. *rhagas,* tear, + L. *forma,* shape] Fissured; having cracks.

**-rhage, -rhagia** SEE: *-rrhage; -rrhagia.*

**Rh antiserum** Human serum that contains Rh antibodies.

**rhaphania** (ră-fā′nē-ă) Raphania.

**rhaphe** (rā′fē) Raphe.

**-rhaphy** SEE: *-rrhaphy.*

**Rh blood group** A system of antigens discovered on the surface of red blood cells of the rhesus monkey. It is present to a variable degree in human populations. When the Rh factor (an antigen often called D) is present, an individual's blood type is designated $Rh^+$ (Rh positive); when the Rh antigen is absent, the blood type is $Rh^-$ (Rh negative). If an individual with $Rh^-$ blood receives a transfusion of $Rh^+$ blood, it causes the formation of anti-Rh agglutinin. Subsequent transfusions of $Rh^+$ blood may result in serious transfusion reactions (agglutination and hemolysis of red blood cells). A pregnant woman who is $Rh^-$ may become sensitized by blood of an $Rh^+$ fetus. In subsequent pregnancies, if the fetus is $Rh^+$, Rh antibodies produced in maternal blood may cross the placenta and destroy fetal cells, causing erythroblastosis fetalis. SEE: *immune globulin, $Rh_o$ (D).*

**-rhea** SEE: *-rrhea.*

**rhenium** (rē′nē-ŭm) SYMB: Re. A metallic element similar to manganese; atomic weight 186.2, atomic number 75.

**rheo-** [Gr. *rheos,* current] Combining form meaning *current, stream, flow.*

**rheobase** (rē′ō-bās) [″ + *basis,* base] In unipolar testing with the galvanic current using the negative as the active pole, the minimal voltage required to produce a stimulated response. Also called *threshold of excitation.* SEE: *chronaxie.*

**rheobasic** (rē″ō-bā′sĭk) Concerning the rheobase.

**rheology** (rē-ŏl′ō-jē) [″ + *logos,* word, reason] The study of the deformation and flow of materials.

**rheostat** (rē′ō-stăt) [″ + *statos,* standing] A device maintaining fixed or variable resistance for controlling the amount of electric current entering a circuit.

**rheostosis** (rē-ŏs-tō′sĭs) [″ + *osteon,* bone] A hypertrophying and condensing osteitis occurring in streaks, involving the long bones.

**rheotaxis** (rē″ō-tăk′sĭs) [″ + *taxis,* arrangement] A reaction to a current of fluid, causing the part acted on to move against the current.

**rheum, rheuma** (room, room′ă) [Gr. *rheuma,* discharge] Any catarrhal or watery discharge.

**rheumatic** (roo-măt′ĭk) [Gr. *rheumatikos*] Pert. to rheumatism.

**rheumatic disease, functional class** Classifications created by The American Rheumatism Association that define the capacity level at which a patient with rheumatic disease is capable of functioning. Class I is complete functional capacity with ability to carry on all usual duties without handicaps; class II is functional capacity adequate to conduct normal activities despite handicap or discomfort or limited mobility of one or more joints; class III is functional capacity adequate to perform only a few or none of the duties of usual occupations or of self-care; and class IV indicates a patient who is largely or wholly incapacitated and is bedridden or confined to a wheelchair, permitting little or no self-care.

**rheumatic fever** A systemic, febrile disease that is an inflammatory and nonsuppurative complication that may follow infection with group A streptococci that have the capacity to produce clinical infection of the upper respiratory tract. It is frequently followed by serious heart or kidney disease. SEE: *Nursing Diagnoses Appendix.*

SYMPTOMS: Following a pharyngeal infection with group A streptococci, some patients experience sudden fever and joint pain; this is the most common type of onset. Other symptoms include fever, migratory polyarthritis, pain on motion, abdominal pain, chorea, and cardiac involvement (pericarditis, myocarditis, and endocarditis). Precordial discomfort and heart murmurs develop suddenly. Skin manifestations include erythema marginatum or circinatum and the development of subcutaneous nodules. Epistaxis is common.

Rheumatic fever may occur without any sign or symptom of joint involvement. Two major manifestations (carditis, polyarthritis, chorea, erythema marginatum, subcutaneous nodules) or one major and two minor criteria (fever, arthralgia, previous rheumatic fever, elevated erythrocyte sedimentation rate or positive C-reactive protein, prolonged P-R interval) are required to establish the diagnosis of acute rheumatic fever.

ETIOLOGY: The onset follows a preceding infection with a strain of group A streptococci. Rheumatic fever is believed to be an autoimmune response in which immune complexes (antibodies and complement) damage the heart valves or heart muscle. It usually occurs between the ages of 5 and 15 years, but may occur at any age; an individual is susceptible to recurrences.

PROPHYLAXIS: Prompt and adequate treatment of streptococcal infections with oral penicillin or cephalosporin is given for at least 10 days. Erythromycin is substituted in patients with penicillin allergy.

Patients known to have carditis who must undergo dental or surgical procedures (esp. those involving instrumentation of the urinary tract, rectum, or colon) should receive additional antibiotic coverage on the day of the procedure and for several days thereafter.

To prevent streptococcal reinfection and possible recurrence of rheumatic fever, monthly injections of long-acting benzathine penicillin G are given for at least 5 years. Those who do not tolerate penicillin may be given oral sulfisoxazole for the same period of time.

TREATMENT: The treatment involves enforced bedrest until the signs of active rheumatic fever have disappeared. Salicylates may be given for symptomatic relief. Complications, esp. those involving the heart, require special treatment.

NURSING IMPLICATIONS: The patient maintains bedrest. Temperature is monitored frequently for elevation, and appropriate nursing measures are instituted for fever reduction. Pulse is also monitored, and the physician is notified of any arrhythmia. The nurse instructs the patient about lifestyle and activity modifications and about the prescribed bland, high-protein and high-carbohydrate diet. Fluids are forced unless cardiac status contraindicates this practice, in which case the diet should include salt restriction. Rheumatic fever is a known sequela of streptococcal pharyngitis. Parents should know about the importance of prescribed prophylactic administration of penicillin for such infection.

**rheumatid** (roo′mă-tĭd) A skin lesion associated with rheumatic disease.

**rheumatism** (roo′mă-tĭzm) [Gr. *rheumatismos*] A general term for acute and chronic conditions characterized by inflammation, muscle soreness and stiffness, and pain in joints and associated structures. It includes arthritis (infectious, rheumatoid, gouty), arthritis due to rheumatic fever or trauma, degenerative joint disease, neurogenic arthropathy, hydroarthrosis, myositis, bursitis, fibromyositis, and many other conditions. SEE: *arthritis; rheumatic fever*.

***acute articular r.*** Rheumatic fever.

***chronic r.*** Rheumatism associated with a joint disorder, such as rheumatoid arthritis, gout, or degenerative joint disease, usually resulting in deformity of the joint.

***gonorrheal r.*** Arthritis resulting from gonorrheal infection. SEE: *gonorrhea*.

***inflammatory r.*** Rheumatism caused by rheumatic fever.

***muscular r.*** One of several muscular conditions marked by tenderness, soreness, pain, and local spasm, including fibromyositis, myositis, myalgia, and torticollis.

***palindromic r.*** Intermittent joint pain with tenderness, heat, and swelling that lasts from a few hours to as long as a week. The knee is most often involved, but the disease does not necessarily return to the same joint or joints. Between attacks there is no evidence of the disease. The cause is unknown, and there is no specific treatment.

***psychogenic r.*** Rheumatism of psychic origin, esp. that occurring under emotional stress.

***soft tissue r.*** Any of several localized and generalized conditions that cause pain around joints but are not related to or caused by joint disease (e.g., bursitis, tennis elbow, tendinitis, perichondritis, stiff man syndrome, Tietze's disease).

**rheumatoid** (roo′mă-toyd) [Gr. *rheuma*, discharge, + *eidos*, form, shape] Of the nature of rheumatism; resembling rheumatism.

**rheumatoid factor** An immunoglobulin present in the serum of 50% to 95% of adults with rheumatoid arthritis. This factor, although not specific for rheumatoid arthritis, is helpful in diagnosing and investigating the disease.

**rheumatologist** (roo″mă-tŏl′ō-jĭst) A physician who specializes in rheumatic diseases.

**rheumatology** (roo″mă-tŏl′ō-jē) The division of medicine concerned with rheumatic diseases.

**rhexis** (rĕk′sĭs) [Gr., rupture] The rupture of any organ, blood vessel, or tissue.

**Rh factor** Rh antigen. SEE: *Rh blood group*.

**Rh gene** Any of eight allelic genes that are responsible for the various Rh blood types. They have been designated by A. S. Wiener as $R^1$, $R^2$, $R^0$, $R^z$, r, r′, r″, and $r_y$. Genes represented by small r's are responsible for the Rh-negative ($Rh^-$) blood type; those by capital R's, for the Rh-positive ($Rh^+$) blood type.

**rhigosis** (rī-gō′sĭs) [Gr., shivering] Perception of cold.

**rhinal** (rī′năl) Nasal.

**rhinalgia** (rī-năl′jē-ă) [″ + *algos*, pain] Pain in the nose; nasal neuralgia.

**rhinedema** (rī″nĕ-dē′mă) [″ + *oidema*, swelling] Edema of the nose.

**rhinencephalon** (rī-nĕn-sĕf′ă-lŏn) [″ + *enkephalos*, brain] The portion of brain concerned with receiving and integrating olfactory impulses. It includes the olfactory bulb, olfactory tract and striae, intermediate olfactory area, pyriform area, paraterminal area, hippocampal formation, and fornix, and constitutes the paleopallium and archipallium.

**rhinencephalus** (rī″nĕn-sĕf′ă-lŭs) [″ + *enkephalos*, brain] Rhinocephalus.

**rhinenchysis** [″ + Gr. *enchein*, to pour in] A nasal douche using a medicated or nonmedicated solution.

**rhinesthesia** (rī-nĕs-thē′zē-ă) [″ + *aisthesis*, sensation] The sense of smell.

**rhineurynter** (rĭn″ū-rĭn′tĕr) [″ + *eurynein*, to dilate] An elastic bag used for dilating the nostrils.

**rhinion** (rĭn′ē-ŏn) [Gr.] The lower end of the suture between the nasal bones; a craniometric point. SYN: *punctum nasale inferius*.

**rhinism** (rī′nĭzm) Rhinolalia.

**rhinitis** (rī-nī′tĭs) [″ + *itis*, inflammation] Inflammation of the nasal mucosa. Symptoms include nasal congestion, rhinorrhea, sneezing, and itching of the nose. Children with this condition may have a characteristic way of rubbing their noses with an upward movement of their hands. This is called the "allergic salute." SEE: *ozena*.

***acute r.*** Acute nasal congestion with increased mucus secretion. This condition is the usual manifestation of the common cold.

TREATMENT: No specific treatment is known. General measures include rest, adequate fluids, and a well-balanced diet. Analgesics and antipyretics may be used to make the patient comfortable. Sulfonamides and other antibiotics are of no value and should not be administered. Antihistamines may relieve early symptoms but do not abort or alter the course. Vasoconstrictors in the form of inhalants, nasal sprays, or drops may give temporary relief. Their use helps prevent the development of middle ear infections by helping to maintain the patency of the eustachian tubes. SYN: *coryza*.

***allergic r.*** Hay fever.

***atrophic r.*** Chronic inflammation with marked atrophy of the mucous membrane and with considerable dry crusting and disturbance in the sense of smell; usually accompanied by ozena. The throat is dry and usually contains crusts. A husky voice or hoarseness is common.

TREATMENT: The nose should be irrigated using warm alkalinized saline solution twice daily. General hygienic measures should be followed and any associated disorders corrected. Surgery is seldom helpful.

***r. caseosa*** Rhinitis characterized by the accumulation of offensive cheeselike masses in the nose and sinuses and accompanied by a seropurulent discharge.

***chronic hyperplastic r.*** Chronic inflammation of the nasal mucous membrane accompanied by polypoid formation and underlying sinus pathology. SEE: *sinus*.

***chronic hypertrophic r.*** Inflammation of the nasal mucous membrane marked by hypertrophy of the mucous membrane of the turbinates and the septum. The symptoms are those of nasal obstruction, postnasal discharge, and recurrent head colds. The treatment is surgical removal of the hypertrophic or mulberry ends of the inferior turbinates and cauterization of the mucosa of the inferior turbinates and septum.

***fibrinous r.*** Rhinitis marked by the formation of a false membrane in the nasal cavities. SYN: *pseudomembranous r.*

***hypertrophic r.*** Rhinitis marked by thickening and swelling of the nasal mucosa.

***infectious r.*** Rhinitis due to infections of the nasal mucosa.

***membranous r.*** Chronic rhinitis accompanied by a fibrinous exudate.

***perennial r.*** Nonseasonal rhinitis that continues indefinitely with variations in severity.

***pseudomembranous r.*** Fibrinous r.

***purulent r.*** Chronic rhinitis accompanied by pus formation.

***vasomotor r.*** Rhinitis with rhinorrhea due to increased secretion of mucus from the nasal mucosa. This may be caused by allergy or neurovascular imbalance.

**rhino-** [Gr. *rhis*] Combining form meaning *nose*. SEE: *naso-*.

**rhinoanemometer** (rī″nō-ăn″ĕ-mŏm′ĕ-tĕr) A device that determines the presence of nasal obstruction by measuring the rate of air flow through the nasal passages.

**rhinoantritis** (rī″nō-ăn-trī′tĭs) [″ + *antron*, cavity, + *itis*, inflammation] Inflammation of the nasal cavities and one or both maxillary antra.

**rhinocanthectomy** (rī″nō-kăn-thĕk′tō-mē) [Gr. *rhis*, nose, + *kanthos*, canthus, + *ektome*, excision] Surgical excision of the inner corner of the eye. SYN: *rhinommectomy*.

**rhinocele** (rī′nō-sēl) [″ + *koilia*, cavity] The ventricle or hollow of the olfactory lobe or rhinoencephalon.

**rhinocephalus** (rī″nō-sĕf′ă-lŭs) [″ + *kephale*, head] An individual with rhinocephaly. SYN: *rhinencephalus*.

**rhinocephaly** (rī″nō-sĕf′ă-lē) [″ + *kephale*, head] A congenital deformity in which the eyes are fused and the nose is present as a fleshy protuberance above the eyes.

**rhinocheiloplasty** (rī″nō-kī′lō-plăs″tē) [″ + *cheilos*, lip, + *plastos*, formed] Plastic surgery of the nose and upper lip.

**rhinodacryolith** (rī″nō-dăk′rē-ō-lĭth) [″ + *dakryon*, tear, + *lithos*, stone] A calculus in the nasolacrimal duct.

**Rhinoestrus** (rī-nĕs′trŭs) A genus of flies belonging to the family Oestridae. Larvae may be deposited in eye or in the nasal or buccal cavity of mammals.

***R. purpureus*** The Russian gadfly, whose larvae sometimes cause nasomyiasis and ophthalmomyiasis in humans.

**rhinogenous** (rī-nŏj′ĕn-ŭs) [″ + *gennan*, to produce] Originating in the nose.

**rhinokyphosis** (rī″nō-kī-fō′sĭs) [″ + *kyphos*, hump, + *osis*, condition] A deformity of the bridge of the nose.

**rhinolalia** (rī″nō-lā′lē-ă) [″ + *lalia*, speech] A nasal quality of the voice. SYN: *rhinosis*. SEE: *whinolalia*.

***r. aperta*** Rhinolalia caused by undue patency of the posterior nares.

***r. clausa*** Rhinolalia caused by closure of the nasal passages.

**rhinolaryngitis** (rī″nō-lăr″ĭn-jī′tĭs) [″ + *larynx*, larynx, + *itis*, inflammation] Simultaneous inflammation of the mucosa of the nose and larynx.

**rhinolith** (rī′nō-lĭth) [″ + *lithos*, stone] A nasal concretion.

**rhinolithiasis** (rī″nō-lĭth-ī′ă-sĭs) The formation of nasal calculi.

**rhinologist** (rī-nŏl′ō-jĭst) [″ + *logos*, word,

reason] A specialist in diseases of the nose.

**rhinology** (rī-nŏl′ō-jē) The science of the nose and its diseases.

**rhinomanometry** (rī″nō-mă-nŏm′ĕ-trē) The measurement of air flow through and air pressure in the nose.

**rhinometer** (rī-nŏm′ĕt-ĕr) A device for measuring the nose or its cavities.

**rhinomiosis** (rī″nō-mī-ō′sĭs) [″ + *meiosis,* a lessening] Surgical reduction in the size of the nose.

**rhinommectomy** (rī″nŏm-mĕk′tō-mē) [″ + *omma,* eye, + *ektome,* excision] Rhinocanthectomy.

**rhinomycosis** (rī″nō-mī-kō′sĭs) [″ + *mykes,* fungus, + *osis,* condition] Fungi in the mucous membranes and secretions of the nose.

**rhinonecrosis** (rī″nō-nē-krō′sĭs) [″ + *nekrosis,* state of death] Necrosis of the nasal bones.

**rhinopathy** (rī-nŏp′ă-thē) [″ + *pathos,* disease] Any nasal disease.

**rhinopharyngeal** (rī″nō-fă-rĭn′jē-ăl) Pert. to the nasopharynx.

**rhinopharyngitis** (rī″nō-făr-ĭn-jī′tĭs) [″ + *pharynx,* throat, + *itis,* inflammation] Inflammation of the nasopharynx.

**rhinopharyngocele** (rī″nō-făr-ĭn′gō-sēl) [″ + ″ + *kele,* tumor, swelling] A nasopharyngeal tumor.

**rhinopharyngolith** (rī″nō-făr-ĭn′gō-lĭth) [″ + ″ + *lithos,* stone] A concretion in the nasal pharynx.

**rhinopharynx** (rī″nō-făr′ĭnks) Nasopharynx.

**rhinophonia** (rī″nō-fō′nē-ă) Rhinolalia.

**rhinophycomycosis** (rī″nō-fī″kō-mī-kō′sĭs) [″ + *phykos,* seaweed, + *mykes,* fungus, + *osis,* condition] A fungal infection that may occur in humans or animals. It affects the nasal and paranasal sinuses and may spread to the brain. It is caused by the phycomycete *Entomophthora coronata.*

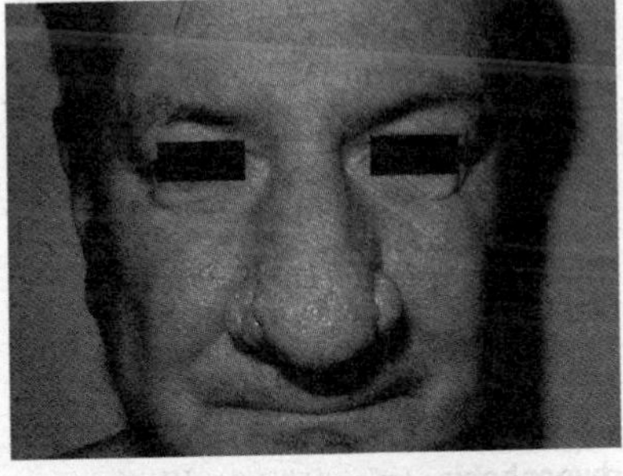

RHINOPHYMA AND ROSACEA

**rhinophyma** (rī-nō-fī′mă) [″ + *phyma,* growth] Nodular swelling and congestion of the nose associated with advanced acne rosacea. SEE: illus.; *rosacea.*

**rhinoplasty** (rī′nō-plăs″tē) [″ + *plastos,* formed] Plastic surgery of the nose.

**rhinopneumonitis** (rī″nō-nū″mō-nī′tĭs) [Gr. *rhis,* nose, + *pneumon,* lung, + *itis,* inflammation] Inflammation of the nasal and pulmonary mucous membranes.

**rhinopolypus** (rī″nō-pŏl′ĭ-pŭs) [″ + *polys,* many, + *pous,* foot] A nasal polyp.

**rhinorrhagia** (rī″nō-rā′jē-ă) Epistaxis.

**rhinorrhea** (rī″nō-rē′ă) [″ + *rhoia,* flow] A thin watery discharge from the nose.

***cerebrospinal r.*** A discharge of spinal fluid from the nose caused by a defect in or trauma to the cribriform plate.

***gustatory r.*** A flow of thin watery material from the nose while one is eating.

**rhinosalpingitis** (rī″nō-săl″pĭn-jī′tĭs) [″ + *salpinx,* tube, + *itis,* inflammation] Inflammation of the mucosa of the nose and eustachian tube.

**rhinoscleroma** (rī″nō-sklē-rō′mă) [″ + *skleros,* hard, + *oma,* tumor] A chronic infectious disease in which growths of almost stony hardness develop in the nose and the upper portions of the respiratory tract, sometimes leading to marked deformity. The disease is caused by *Klebsiella rhinoscleromatis,* a gram-negative encapsulated bacillus. Surgical debridement is combined with prolonged antimicrobial therapy.

SYMPTOMS: The disease presents a hard, nodular growth, which usually begins at the anterior end of the nose and spreads to the lower respiratory tract. There usually is no pain and no tendency to ulceration.

**rhinoscope** (rī′nō-skōp) [″ + *skopein,* to examine] An instrument for examining the nose.

**rhinoscopy** (rī-nŏs′kō-pē) Examination of nasal passages. **rhinoscopic** (rī″nō-skŏp′ĭk), *adj.*

***anterior r.*** Examination through the anterior nares.

***posterior r.*** Examination through the posterior nares, usually with a small mirror in the nasopharynx.

**rhinosporidiosis** (rī″nō-spō-rĭd″ē-ō′sĭs) [″ + *sporidion,* little seed, + *osis,* condition] A condition caused by a fungus, *Rhinosporidium seeberi,* and marked by development of pedunculated polyps on the mucous membranes of the nose, larynx, eyes, penis, vagina, and sometimes skin of various parts of the body. The disease is contracted from cattle and is found in India, Sri Lanka, and other parts of the world.

**Rhinosporidium** (rī″nō-spō-rĭd′ē-ŭm) A genus of fungi that are pathogenic to humans.

***R. seeberi*** The causative agent of rhinosporidiosis.

**rhinostenosis** (rī″nō-stĕn-ō-′sĭs) [″ + *stenos,* narrow, + *osis,* condition] Obstruction of the nasal passages.

**rhinotomy** (rī-nŏt′ō-mē) [″ + *tome,* incision] Incision of the nose for drainage purposes.

**rhinotracheitis** (rī″nō-trā″kē-ī′tĭs) [″ + *tracheia,* rough, + *itis,* inflammation] Inflammation of the nasal mucous membranes and the trachea.

**rhinovirus** (rī″nō-vī′rŭs) One of a species of picornaviruses, that causes the common cold in humans. Probably more than 100 rhinoviruses exist and occur worldwide. There is no specific therapy. Viruses other than rhinoviruses also cause the syndrome diagnosed as a cold. These include the A21 coxsackievirus and coronaviruses.

**Rhipicephalus** (rī″pĭ-sĕf′ă-lŭs) [Gr. *rhipis,* fan, + *kephale,* head] A genus of ticks belonging to the family Ixodidae. Several species, esp. *R. sanguineus,* are vectors for the organisms of spotted fever, boutonneuse fever, and other rickettsial diseases.

**rhitidectomy** (rĭt″ĭ-dĕk′tō-mē) Rhytidectomy.

**rhitidosis** (rĭt-ĭ-dō′sĭs) Rhytidosis.

**rhizo-** [Gr. *rhiza*] Combining form meaning *root.*

**rhizodontropy** (rī″zō-dŏn′trō-pē) [Gr. *rhiza,* root, + *odous,* tooth, + *trope,* a turning] The process of attaching an artificial crown onto the root of a tooth.

**rhizodontrypy** (rī″zō-dŏn′trĭ-pē) [″ + ″ + *trype,* a hole] The puncture of the root of a tooth.

**rhizoid** (rī′zoyd) [″ + *eidos,* form, shape] **1.** Rootlike. **2.** A rootlike structure, usually one-celled, occurring in lower forms of plant life. **3.** In bacteriology, a colony showing an irregular rootlike system of branching.

**rhizome** (rī′zōm) [Gr. *rhizoma,* mass of roots] A rootlike stem growing horizontally along or below the ground and sending out roots and shoots.

**rhizomelic** (rī″zō-mĕl′ĭk) [Gr. *rhiza,* root, + *melos,* limb] Concerning the hip joint and the shoulder joint.

**rhizomeningomyelitis** (rī″zō-mĕ-nĭn″gō-mī″ĕ-lī′tĭs) Radiculomeningomyelitis.

**Rhizopoda** (rī-zŏp′ō-dă) [″ + *pous,* foot] A phylum of the kingdom Protista; unicellular amoebas with pseudopod locomotion. It includes free-living and pathogenic species such as *Entamoeba histolytica.*

**rhizotomy** (rī-zŏt′ō-mē) [″ + *tome,* incision] Surgical section of a nerve root (e.g., the root of a spinal or dental nerve) to relieve pain or reduce spasticity.

***anterior r.*** Surgical section of the ventral root of the spinal nerve.

***posterior r.*** Surgical section of the dorsal root of the spinal nerve.

**rhodium** (rō′dē-ŭm) SYMB: Rh. A rare metallic element; atomic weight 102.905, atomic number 45.

**rhodo-** (rō′dō) Combining form meaning *red.*

**rhodogenesis** (rō″dō-jĕn′ĕ-sĭs) [Gr. *rhodon,* rose, + *genesis,* generation, birth] Regeneration of visual purple that has been bleached by light.

**rhodophane** (rō′dō-fān) [″ + *phainein,* to show] A red pigment found in the retinal cones of birds and fish.

**rhodophylaxis** (rō″dō-fī-lăk′sĭs) [″ + *phylaxis,* protection] The ability of the retinal epithelium to regenerate visual purple that has been bleached by light.

**rhodopsin** (rō-dŏp′sĭn) [″ + *opsis,* vision] The glycoprotein opsin of the rods of the retina; combines with retinal to form a functional photopigment responsive to light. Formerly called visual purple.

**RhoGAM** Trade name for $Rh_o$(D) immune globulin.

**rhombencephalon** (rŏm″bĕn-sĕf′ă-lŏn) Hindbrain.

**rhombocele** (rŏm′bō-sēl) [″ + *koilos,* a hollow] The cavity of the rhombencephalon.

**rhomboid** (rŏm′boyd) [″ + *eidos,* form, shape] An oblique parallelogram.

**rhomboideus** (rŏm-bō-ĭd′ē-ŭs) [L.] One of two muscles beneath the trapezius muscle. SEE: *muscle* for illus.; *Muscles Appendix.*

**rhomboid fossa** The fourth ventricle of the brain.

**rhombomere** (rŏm′bō-mēr) Neuromere.

**rhoncal, rhonchial** (rŏng′kăl, rŏng′kē-ăl) [Gr. *rhonchos,* a snore] Pert. to or produced by a rattle in the throat.

**rhonchi** Pl. of rhonchus.

**rhonchus** (rŏng′kŭs) *pl.* **rhonchi** An adventitious or abnormal sound heard when listening to the chest as the person breathes. Wheezing noises are heard during inspiration, expiration, or both. They are present when an airway is partially obstructed owing to secretions, mucosal swelling, or tumor tissue pressing on the passage.

**rhopheocytosis** (rō″fē-ō-sī-tō′sĭs) [Gr. *rhophein,* gulp down, + *kytos,* cell, + *osis,* condition] The mechanism by which ferritin is transferred from macrophages in the bone marrow to normoblasts. SEE: *pinocytosis.*

**rhotacism** (rō′tă-sĭzm) [Gr. *rhotakizein,* to overuse letter "r"] Overuse or improper utterance of "r" sounds, with too much emphasis on this sound.

**rhubarb** (roo′bărb) [ME. *rubarbe*] An extract made from the roots and rhizome of *Rheum officinale, R. palmatum,* and other species, used as a cathartic and astringent. It is high in oxalic acid. The stems are used as food.

**rHuEPO** *recombinant human erythropoietin.*

**Rhus** (rŭs) [L.] A genus of trees and shrubs, some of which are poisonous and produce a severe dermatitis, such as poison ivy *(R. toxicodendron)* and poison sumac *(R. venenata).*

**rhypophobia** (rī″pō-fō′bē-ă) [Gr. *rhypos,* filth, + *phobos,* fear] An abnormal disgust at the act of defecation, feces, or filth. SYN: *rupophobia.*

**rhythm** (rĭth′ŭm) [Gr. *rhythmos,* measured motion] **1.** A measured time or movement; regularity of occurrence of action or function. **2.** In electroencephalography, the regular occurrence of an impulse. **rhyth-**

mic (-mĭk), *adj.*

***alpha r.*** In electroencephalography, oscillations in electric potential occurring at a rate of 8½ to 12 per second.

***atrioventricular r.*** The rhythmic discharges of impulses from the atrioventricular node that occur when the activity of the sinoatrial node is depressed or abolished. SYN: *nodal r.*

***beta r.*** In electroencephalography, waves ranging in frequency from 15 to 30 per second and of lower voltage than alpha waves. This rhythm is more pronounced in the frontomotor leads.

***bigeminal r.*** The coupling of extrasystoles with previously normal beats of the heart. SEE: *pulse, bigeminal.*

***biological r.*** The regular occurrence of certain phenomena in living organisms. SEE: *circadian r.; clock, biological.*

***cantering r.*** Gallop r.

***cardiac r.*** The nature of the cyclical activity of the heart. It may be determined by obtaining the pulse rate or electronically by using the electrocardiograph. SEE: *cardiac cycle; electrocardiogram; heart, conduction system of.*

***circadian r.*** The recurrence of certain biological activities approx. every 24 hr regardless of environmental influences. SYN: *diurnal r.*

***coupled r.*** A rhythm in which every other heartbeat produces no pulse at the wrist.

***delta r.*** In electroencephalography, slow waves with a frequency of 4 or fewer per second and of relatively high voltage (20 to 200 $\mu$V). It may be found over the area of a gross lesion such as a tumor or hemorrhage.

***diurnal r.*** Circadian r.

***ectopic r.*** A heart rhythm originating outside the sinoatrial node.

***escape r.*** The heart rhythm when the supraventricular rate set by the sinoatrial node rhythm is completely blocked.

***gallop r.*** An abnormal heart rhythm with three sounds in each cycle, resembling the gallop of a horse. SYN: *cantering r.*

***gamma r.*** The 50-per-second rhythm seen in the electroencephalogram.

***idioventricular r.*** The rhythm of the ventricles occurring in heart block resulting from establishment of a new center of rhythmicity in the ventricular myocardium, usually in the bundle of His.

***junctional r.*** An electrocardiographic rhythm arising in the atrioventricular junction. It appears as a narrow QRS complex that lacks an upright P wave preceding it.

***nodal r.*** Atrioventricular r.

***normal sinus r.*** The normal heart rhythm. The stimulus arises in the sinoatrial node. It is marked by regularity, a ventricular rate of 60 to 100, an upright P wave in lead II, a P-R interval of 0.12 to 0.20 sec, and one P wave preceding each QRS complex.

***nyctohemeral r.*** Day and night rhythm.

***pendulum r.*** A rhythm with the two heart sounds alike, similar to the sound of a ticking clock.

***sinus r.*** The normal heart rhythm proceeding from the sinoatrial node.

***theta r.*** The 4 to 7 per second rhythm seen in the electroencephalogram.

***tic-tac r.*** Embryocardia.

***ventricular r.*** Very slow ventricular contractions in heart block.

**rhythmicity** (rĭth-mĭs′ĭ-tē) The condition of being rhythmic.

**rhythm method of birth control** SEE: *contraception.*

**rhytidectomy** (rĭt″ĭ-dĕk′tō-mē) [Gr. *rhytis,* wrinkle, + *ektome,* excision] The excision of wrinkles by plastic surgery; often called a "face-lift." SYN: *rhitidectomy.*

**rhytidoplasty** (rĭt′ĭ-dō-plăs″tē) [″ + *plassein,* to form] The elimination of facial wrinkles by plastic surgery.

**rhytidosis** (rĭt″ĭ-dō′sĭs) [″ + *osis,* condition] Wrinkling of the cornea, which occurs when tension in the eyeball is greatly diminished, particularly after the escape of aqueous or vitreous humor; usually a sign of impending death. SYN: *rhitidosis.*

**RIA** *radioimmunoassay.*

**rib** (rĭb) [AS. *ribb*] One of a series of 12 pairs of narrow, curved bones extending laterally and anteriorly from the sides of the thoracic vertebrae and forming a part of the skeletal thorax. With the exception of the floating ribs, they are connected to the sternum by costal cartilages. SEE: illus.

***abdominal r.*** False r.

***asternal r.*** False r.

***bicipital r.*** An irregular condition resulting from the fusion of two ribs, usually involving the first rib.

***cervical r.*** A supernumerary rib sometimes developing in connection with a cervical vertebra, usually the lowest.

***false r.*** Ribs 8 through 10 on each side, indirectly attached to the sternum. SYN: *abdominal r.; asternal r.*

***floating r.*** Ribs 11 and 12 on each side, not attached to the sternum. SYN: *vertebral r.*

***lumbar r.*** A rudimentary rib that develops in relation to a lumbar vertebra.

***slipping r.*** A rib in which the costal cartilage dislocates repeatedly.

***sternal r.*** True r.

***true r.*** Any of the upper seven ribs on each side, which join the sternum by separate cartilages. SYN: *sternal r.; vertebrosternal r.*

***vertebral r.*** Floating r.

***vertebrocostal r.*** Any of the upper three false ribs on each side.

***vertebrosternal r.*** True r.

**ribbon** (rĭb′ŭn) A long, thin, band-shaped structure.

**riboflavin** (rī″bō-flā′vĭn) $C_{17}H_{20}N_4O_6$. A water-soluble vitamin of the B complex group. It is an orange-yellow crystalline

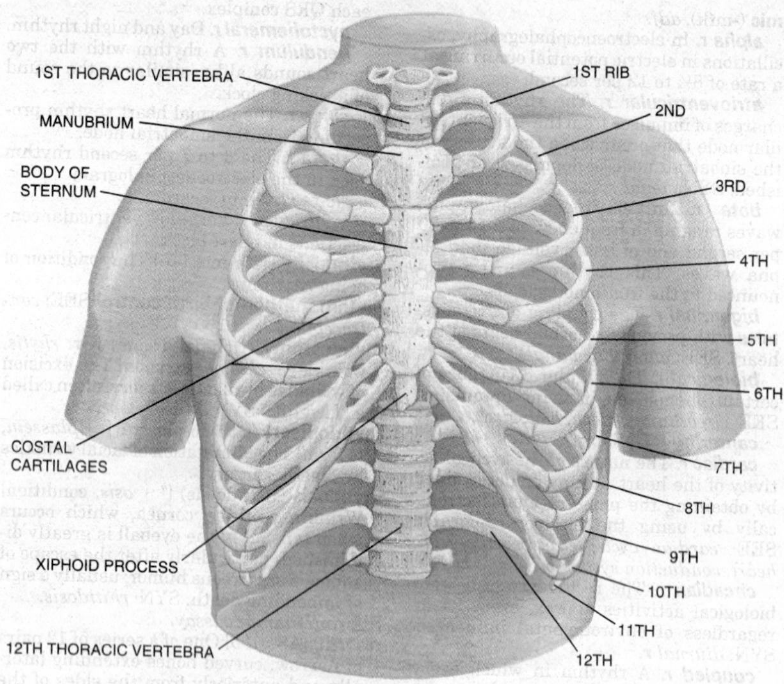


RIB CAGE
(ANTERIOR VEIW)

powder that is comparatively stable to heat and air but unstable to light. Symptoms of riboflavin deficiency are eye disorders, cheilosis, glossitis, and seborrheic dermatitis, esp. of the face and scalp. SYN: *vitamin $B_2$*.

FUNCTION: Riboflavin is a constituent of certain flavoproteins that function as coenzymes in cellular oxidations. It is essential for tissue repair.

SOURCES: Riboflavin is found in milk and milk products, leafy green vegetables, liver, beef, fish, and dry yeast. It is also synthesized by bacteria in the body.

DAILY REQUIREMENT: Adults require 0.6 mg/1000 kcal of food intake. Infants, children, and pregnant and lactating women require increased amounts.

**ribonuclease** (rī″bō-nū′klē-ās) ABBR: RNase. An enzyme that catalyzes the depolymerization of ribonucleic acid (RNA) with formation of mononucleotides.

**ribonucleic acid** (rī″bō-nū″klē′ĭk) ABBR: RNA. A nucleic acid that controls protein synthesis in all living cells and takes the place of DNA in certain viruses. It differs from DNA in that its sugar is ribose and the pyrimidine uracil rather than thymine is present. RNA occurs in several forms that are determined by the number of nucleotides. SEE: illus.; *deoxyribonucleic acid.*

Messenger RNA (mRNA) carries the code for specific amino acid sequences from the DNA to the cytoplasm for protein synthesis.

Transfer RNA (tRNA) carries the amino acid groups to the ribosome for protein synthesis.

Ribosomal RNA exists within the ribosomes and is thought to assist in protein synthesis.

**ribonucleoprotein** (rī″bō-nū″klē-ō-prō′tē-ĭn) A compound containing both protein and ribonucleic acid.

**ribonucleotide** (rī″bō-nū′klē-ō-tīd) A nucleotide in which the sugar ribose is combined with the purine or pyrimidine base.

**ribose** (rī′bōs) $C_5H_{10}O_5$, a pentose sugar present in ribonucleic acids, riboflavin, and some nucleotides.

**ribosome** (rī′bō-sōm) A cell organelle made of ribosomal RNA and protein. Ribosomes may exist singly, in clusters called polyribosomes, or on the surface of rough endoplasmic reticulum. In protein synthesis, they are the site of messenger RNA attachment and amino acid assembly in the sequence ordered by the genetic code carried by mRNA.

**ribosyl** (rī′bō-sĭl) The compound glycosyl, $C_5H_9O_4$, formed from ribose.

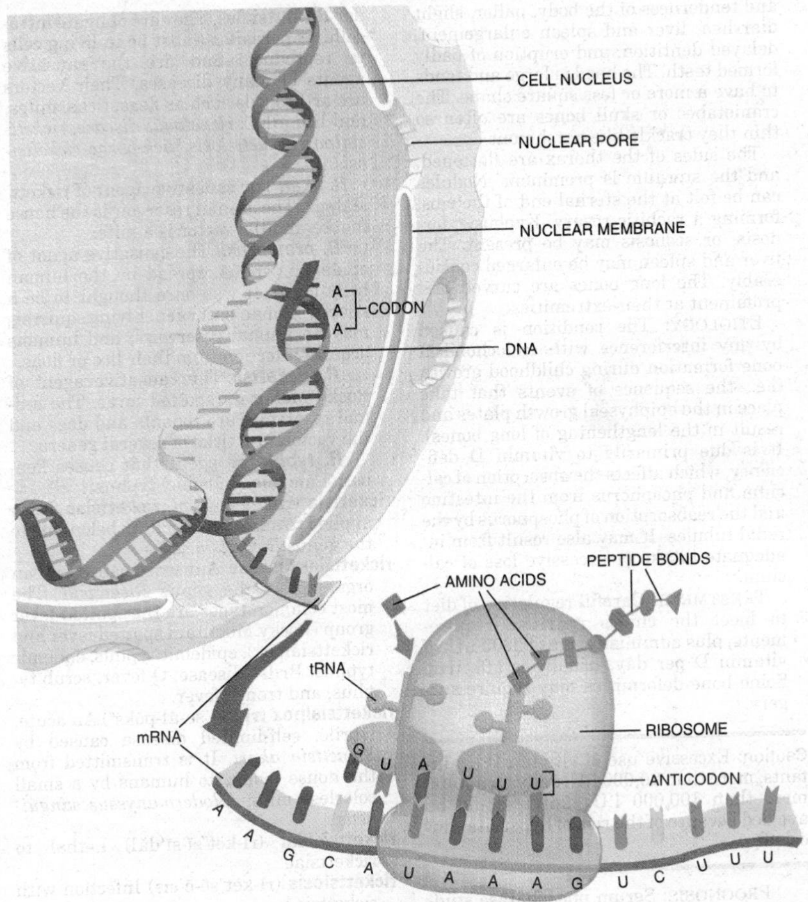


RIBONUCLEIC ACID

ROLES IN PROTEIN SYNTHESIS

**RICE** Acronym for *r*est, *i*ce, *c*ompression, and *e*levation, the elements of management of soft tissue stress or trauma, esp. sports injuries.

**rice, polished** Rice that has been milled to produce the white product commercially available in Western countries. This treatment removes the hull, which contains most of the vitamin $B_1$.

**rice water, boiled** The water remaining after rice has been cooked in it and removed. It is useful as an oral rehydration agent, esp. for children with diarrhea. SEE: *oral rehydration therapy.*

**ricin** (rī′sĭn) A white, amorphous, highly toxic protein (albumin) present in the seed of the castor bean, *Ricinus communis.*

**ricinine** (rĭs′ĭn-ĕn, -ĭn) A poisonous alkaloid present in the leaves and seeds of the castor bean plant, *Ricinus communis.*

**ricinoleic acid** 12-hydroxy-9-octadecenoic acid; an unsaturated hydroxy acid comprising about 80% of fatty acids in the glycerides of castor oil. It has a strong laxative action.

**rickets** (rĭk′ĕts) A vitamin D deficiency in children that results in inadequate deposition of lime salts in developing cartilage and newly formed bone, causing abnormalities in the shape and structure of bones. This condition may be prevented by exposure to ultraviolet light (sunlight or artificial light) and administration of vitamin D in quantities that provide 400 I.U. of vitamin D activity per day. SYN: *osteomalacia; rachitis* (2). SEE: *osteomalacia; Nursing Diagnoses Appendix.*

SYMPTOMS: Patients experience restlessness and slight fever at night (101°F to 102°F or 38.3°C to 38.9°C), free perspiration about the head, diffuse soreness and tenderness of the body, pallor, slight diarrhea, liver and spleen enlargement, delayed dentition, and eruption of badly formed teeth. The head is large and tends to have a more or less square shape. The craniotabes or skull bones are often so thin they crackle like parchment.

The sides of the thorax are flattened, and the sternum is prominent. Nodules can be felt at the sternal end of the ribs, forming a rachitic rosary. Kyphosis, lordosis, or scoliosis may be present. The liver and spleen may be enlarged considerably. The long bones are curved and prominent at their extremities.

ETIOLOGY: The condition is caused by any interference with endochondral bone formation during childhood growth (i.e., the sequence of events that take place in the epiphyseal growth plates and result in the lengthening of long bones). It is due primarily to vitamin D deficiency, which affects the absorption of calcium and phosphorus from the intestine and the reabsorption of phosphorus by the renal tubules. It may also result from inadequate intake or excessive loss of calcium.

TREATMENT: Careful regulation of diet to meet the child's nutritive requirements, plus administration of 2200 I.U. of vitamin D per day, usually is effective. Some bone deformities may require surgery.

---

Caution: Excessive use of vitamin D (in infants, more than 20,000 I.U. daily; in adults, more than 100,000 I.U. daily) should be avoided because of the risk of hypervitaminosis D.

---

PROGNOSIS: Serum phosphatase studies are helpful in making the diagnosis and determining the prognosis, which is usually favorable. The deformity disappears in 90% of cases treated early.

***adult r.*** Osteomalacia.

***late r.*** Rickets that has its onset in older children.

***renal r.*** A disturbance in epiphyseal growth during childhood due to severe chronic renal insufficiency resulting in persistent acidosis. Dwarfism and failure of gonadal development result. The prognosis is poor.

TREATMENT: Renal rickets is treated with a diet low in meat, milk, cheese, and egg yolk. Calcium lactate or calcium gluconate is given in large doses.

***vitamin D–resistant r.*** A defect of renal tubular function that causes an excessive loss of phosphorus and results in rickets that responds poorly to vitamin D therapy. Also called *type II vitamin D–dependent rickets.*

**Rickettsia** (rĭ-kĕt′sē-ă) [Howard T. Ricketts, U.S. pathologist, 1871–1910] A genus of bacteria of the family Rickettsiaceae, order Rickettsiales. They are obligate intracellular parasites (must be in living cells to reproduce) and are the causative agents of many diseases. Their vectors are arthropods such as fleas, ticks, mites, and lice. SEE: *rickettsial disease; rickettsialpox; rickettsiosis; tick-borne rickettsiosis.*

***R. akari*** The causative agent of rickettsialpox. The animal reservoir is the house mouse and the vector is a mite.

***R. prowazekii*** The causative agent of epidemic typhus, spread by the human body louse. It was once thought to be a strictly human pathogen. Flying squirrels may be animal reservoirs; and humans acquire infection from their lice or fleas.

***R. rickettsii*** The causative agent of Rocky Mountain spotted fever. The animal reservoirs are rodents and dogs and the vectors are ticks of several genera.

***R. typhi*** The agent that causes flea-borne murine (endemic) typhus.

**rickettsia** (rĭ-kĕt′sē-ă) *pl.* **rickettsiae** Term applied to any of the bacteria belonging to the genus *Rickettsia.*

**rickettsial disease** A disease caused by an organism of the genus *Rickettsia.* The most common types are the spotted-fever group (Rocky Mountain spotted fever and rickettsialpox), epidemic typhus, endemic typhus, Brill's disease, Q fever, scrub typhus, and trench fever.

**rickettsialpox** (rĭ-kĕt′sē-ăl-pŏks″) An acute, febrile, self-limited disease caused by *Rickettsia akari.* It is transmitted from the house mouse to humans by a small colorless mite, *Allodermanyssus sanguineus.*

**rickettsicidal** (rĭ-kĕt″sĭ-sī′dăl) Lethal to rickettsiae.

**rickettsiosis** (rĭ-kĕt″sē-ō′sĭs) Infection with rickettsiae.

**rickettsiostatic** (rĭ-kĕt″sē-ō-stăt′ĭk) Preventing or slowing the growth of rickettsiae.

**rider's bone** A bony formation in the adductor muscle of the leg (adductor magnus femoris), seen sometimes in people who ride horses extensively. SYN: *cavalry bone.*

**ridge** (rĭj) [ME. *rigge*] An elongated projecting structure or crest.

***alveolar r.*** The bony process of the maxilla or mandible that contains the alveoli or tooth sockets; the alveolar process without teeth present.

***carotid r.*** The sharp ridge between the carotid canal and the jugular fossa.

***dental r.*** Any elevation on the crown of a tooth.

***dermal r.*** One of the ridges on the surface of the fingers that make up the fingerprints; also called *crista cutis.*

***epicondylic r.*** One of two ridges for muscular attachments on the humerus.

***external oblique r.*** An anatomical landmark that is a continuation of the anterior border of the mandibular ramus and extends obliquely to the region of the first molar. It serves as an attachment of the buccinator muscle and appears superior to the mylohyoid ridge on a dental radiograph.

***gastrocnemial r.*** A ridge on the posterior femoral surface for attachment of the gastrocnemius muscles.

***genital r.*** A ridge that develops on the ventromedial surface of the urogenital ridge and gives rise to the gonads.

***gluteal r.*** A ridge extending obliquely downward from the great trochanter of the femur for attachment of the gluteus maximus muscle.

***interosseous r.*** A ridge on the fibula for attachment of the interosseous membrane.

***interureteric r.*** A ridge between the openings of the ureters in the bladder.

***mammary r.*** In mammal embryos, a ridge extending from the axilla to the groin. The breasts arise from this ridge. In humans, only one breast normally remains on each side. SYN: *milk line.*

***mesonephric r.*** A ridge that develops on the lateral surface of the urogenital ridge and gives rise to the mesonephros. SYN: *wolffian r.*

***mylohyoid r.*** The line of attachment on the medial aspect of the body of the mandible for the mylohyoid muscle, which forms the floor of the mouth.

***pronator r.*** An oblique ridge on the anterior surface of the ulna for attachment of the pronator quadratus.

***pterygoid r.*** A ridge at the angle of junction of the temporal and infratemporal surfaces of the great wing of the sphenoid bone.

***superciliary r.*** A curved ridge of the frontal bone over the supraorbital arch.

***supracondylar r.*** One of two ridges (lateral and medial) on the distal end of the humerus, extending upward from the lateral to the medial epicondyles.

***tentorial r.*** A ridge on the upper inner surface of the cranium to which the tentorium is attached.

***trapezoid r.*** An oblique ridge on the upper surface of the clavicle for attachment of the trapezoid ligament.

***urogenital r.*** A ridge on the dorsal wall of the coelom that gives rise to the genital and mesonephric ridges. SYN: *urogenital fold.* SEE: *genital r.; mesonephric r.*

***wolffian r.*** Mesonephric r.

**ridgel** (rĭj′ĕl) A male animal, esp. a horse, with only one testicle, or only one descended testicle.

**Riedel's lobe** (rē′dĕlz) [Bernhard M. C. L. Riedel, Ger. surgeon, 1846–1916] A tongue-shaped process of the liver that often protrudes over the gallbladder in cases of chronic cholecystitis.

**Rieder cell** A myeloblast that may be present in acute leukemia, possessing a lobulated or double nucleus.

**rifampin** (rĭf′ăm-pĭn) An antibiotic synthesized from rifamycin B, which in turn is produced by fermentation of *Streptomyces mediterranei.* It is used in treating *Mycobacterium tuberculosis* and carriers of *Neisseria meningitidis.*

**rifamycin** (rĭf″ă-mī′sĭn) An antibiotic produced by certain strains of *Streptomyces mediterranei.*

**Riga-Fede's disease** (rē′gă fā′dāz) [Antonio Riga, It. physician, 1832–1919; Francesco Fede, It. physician, 1832–1913] Ulceration of the frenum of the tongue with membrane formation. It occurs after abrasion by the lower central incisors.

**Riggs' disease** [John M. Riggs, U.S. dentist, 1810–1885] Periodontitis.

**right** (rīt) [AS. *riht*] ABBR: R; rt. Pert. to the dextral side of the body (the side away from the heart), which in most persons is the stronger or preferred. SYN: *dexter.*

**right-handedness** The condition of greater adeptness in using the right hand. SYN: *dextrality.* SEE: *sinistrality.*

**right to die** Literally, the right of an individual to die on his or her terms. Many ethical and legal dilemmas surround issues related to biomedical interference with patient autonomy and control over the length and quality of life. Contemporary biomedical technology often enables health care providers to prolong life in circumstances where, in the natural course of biologic events, it would end. The ability to postpone death has generated philosophical questions regarding a person's acknowledged right to life and the validity of an equivalent right to die. Thus, conflicts arise over the patient's right to determine whether artificial means should be used to postpone death, whether assistance in terminating life should be granted, and the comparative personal and professional merits and values of life and death. Of particular concern is who should make those decisions if patients have not made their wishes known previously and their current cognitive status precludes communicating that decision to health care providers. SEE: *assisted suicide; euthanasia; suicide.*

**right-to-know law** A law that dictates that employers must inform their employees of the health effects and chemical hazards of the toxic substances used in each workplace. The employer must provide information concerning the generic and chemical names of the substances used; the level at which the exposure is hazardous; the effects of exposure at hazardous levels; the symptoms of such effects; the potential for flammability, explosion, and reactivity of the substances; the appropriate emergency treatment; proper conditions for safe use and exposure to the substances; and procedures for cleanup of leaks and spills. The law provides that an employee may refuse to work with a toxic substance until he or she has received information concerning its potential for hazard. SEE: *hazardous material; health hazard; material safety data sheet; permissible exposure limits; toxic substance.*

**rigid** (rĭ'jĭd) [L. *rigidus*] Stiff, hard, unyielding.

**rigidity** (rĭ-jĭd'ĭ-tē) **1.** Tenseness; immovability; stiffness; inability to bend or be bent. **2.** In psychiatry, an excessive resistance to change.

***cadaveric r.*** Rigor mortis.

***cerebellar r.*** Stiffness of the body and extremities resulting from a lesion of the middle lobe of the cerebellum.

***clasp-knife r.*** A condition in which passive flexion of the joint causes increased resistance of the extensors. This gives way abruptly if the pressure to produce flexion is continued.

***cogwheel r.*** Jerky resistance on passive stretching of a hypertonic muscle.

***decerebrate r.*** Sustained contraction of the extensor muscles of the limbs resulting from a lesion in the brainstem between the superior colliculi and the vestibular nuclei.

***lead-pipe r.*** The generalized muscular rigidity seen in parkinsonism.

**rigor** (rĭg'or) [L. *rigor,* stiffness] **1.** A sudden paroxysmal chill with high temperature, called the cold stage, followed by a sense of heat and profuse perspiration, called the hot stage. **2.** A state of hardness and stiffness, as in a muscle.

***r. mortis*** The stiffness that occurs in dead bodies. SYN: *cadaveric rigidity.* SEE: *Nysten's law.*

**rim** An edge or border.

***bite r.*** Occlusion r.

***occlusion r.*** The biting surfaces built on denture bases to make maxillomandibular relation records and to arrange teeth. SYN: *bite r.*

**rima** (rī'mă) *pl.* **rimae** [L., a slit] A slit, fissure, or crack.

***r. cornealis*** A groove in the sclera holding edge of the cornea.

***r. glottidis*** An elongated slit between the vocal folds. SYN: *r. vocalis.*

***r. oris*** The aperture of the mouth.

***r. palpebrarum*** The slit between the eyelids.

***r. pudendi*** The space between the labia majora, through which the urethra and vagina open.

***r. respiratoria*** The space behind the arytenoid cartilages.

***r. vestibuli*** The space between the false vocal cords.

***r. vocalis*** R. glottidis.

**rimantadine hydrochloride** An antiviral drug given orally to treat influenza A.

**rimose** (rī'mōs, rī-mōs') [L. *rimosus*] Fissured or marked by cracks.

**rimula** (rĭm'ū-lă) *pl.* **rimulae** [L.] A minute fissure or slit, esp. of the spinal cord or brain.

**rind** (rīnd) [AS.] A thick or firm outer coating of an organ, plant, or animal.

**ring** (rĭng) [AS. *hring*] **1.** Any round area, organ, or band around a circular opening. SEE: *annulus.* **2.** In chemistry, a collection of atoms chemically bound in a circle.

***abdominal r.*** SEE: *abdominal ring.*

***abdominal inguinal r.*** The internal opening of the inguinal canal. SEE: *abdominal inguinal ring; abdominal ring.*

***Albl's r.*** A curved thin shadow seen on roentgenogram of an intracranial aneurysm.

***Bandl's r.*** SEE: *Bandl's ring.*

***benzene r.*** The closed ring of six carbon atoms.

***Cannon's r.*** A contracted band of muscles in the transverse colon near the hepatic flexure.

***ciliary r.*** Orbiculus ciliaris.

***conjunctival r.*** A narrow ring at the junction of the edge of the cornea with the conjunctiva; also called *anulus conjunctiva.*

***constriction r.*** A stricture of the body of the uterus; a circular area of the uterus that contracts around a part of the fetus.

***deep inguinal r.*** The opening of the inguinal canal deep inside the abdominal wall.

***femoral r.*** The superior aperture of the femoral canal.

***lymphoid r.*** A ringlike arrangement of lymphoid tonsillar tissue around the oronasal region of the pharynx. It consists of the palatine, pharyngeal, and lingual tonsils and provides protection against invading bacteria, viruses, and other foreign protein. SYN: *Waldeyer's ring.*

***pathologic retraction r.*** During delivery, a prolonged contraction of the ring formed by the junction of the body and isthmus of the uterus.

***physiologic retraction r.*** A normal contraction of the ring formed by the junction of the body and isthmus of the uterus.

***Schatzki r.*** SEE: *Schatzki ring.*

***subcutaneous inguinal r.*** The external opening of the inguinal canal. SEE: *abdominal ring.*

***superficial inguinal r.*** The opening of the superficial end of the inguinal canal.

***tympanic r.*** A band of bone formed by three elements (squamous, petromastoid, and tympanic) that develops into the tympanic plate.

***umbilical r.*** The opening in the linea alba of the embryo through which the umbilical vessels pass.

***vascular r.*** An anomalous ring of vascular structures around the trachea and esophagus.

***Waldeyer's r.*** SEE: *lymphoid r.*

**ring, removal from swollen finger** A technique for the removal of a ring from an injured or swollen finger. One end of a length of string is passed under the ring. The ring is pushed as far from the swollen area toward the hand as possible; the string is wrapped on the side of the swollen area around the finger for about a dozen turns. The end of the string that extends under the ring is grasped. While being held firmly, the string is unwound from the hand side of the ring. This moves the ring toward the free end of the finger. This procedure should be continued until the ring is free. If this technique fails, the ring must be cut from the finger.

**Ringer, Sydney** (rĭng′ĕr) British physiologist, 1835–1910.

***lactated R.'s injection*** A sterile solution of specified amounts of calcium chloride, potassium chloride, sodium chloride, and sodium lactate in water for injection. It is used intravenously to replace electrolytes.

***R.'s irrigation*** A solution of recently boiled distilled water containing 8.6 g sodium chloride, 0.3 g potassium chloride, and 0.33 g calcium chloride per liter; for topical use only. The previously used name was *Ringer's solution.*

**ringworm** (rĭng′wŭrm) The popular term for dermatomycosis caused by various species of fungi belonging to the genera *Microsporum* and *Trichophyton*. Ringworm of the scalp is called tinea capitis; of the body, tinea corporis; of the beard, tinea barbae; of the nails, tinea unguium; and of the feet, athlete's foot. The condition is marked by a red-ringed patch of vesicles, with itching, pain, and scaling. SEE: illus.; *tinea; Nursing Diagnoses Appendix.*

TREATMENT: Griseofulvin may be helpful in certain types of ringworm. At the same time, treatment with topical fungistatic preparations is important.

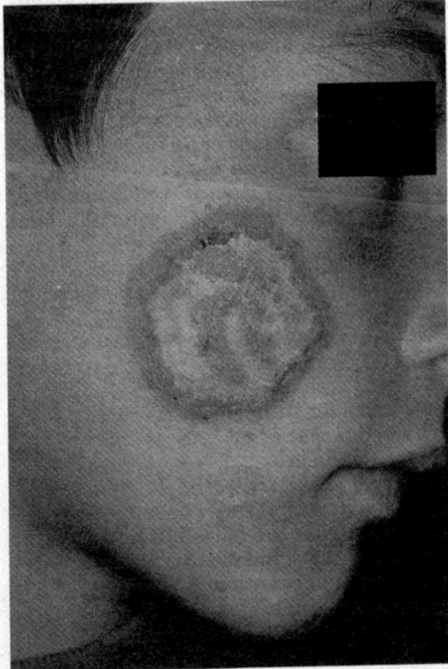

RINGWORM

**Rinne test** (rĭn′ē) [Heinrich Adolf Rinne, Ger. otologist, 1819–1868] The use of a tuning fork to compare bone conduction hearing with air conduction. The vibrating fork is held by its stem on the mastoid process of the ear until the patient no longer hears it. Then it is held close to the external auditory meatus. If the subject still hears the vibrations, the result is a positive Rinne test. If the fork is not heard by air conduction the test is repeated, but first air conduction is tested until the sound is no longer heard, and then the stem of the fork is placed on the mastoid process. If the sound is still heard, the result is negative. SEE: *Weber test.*

**rinse 1.** To wash lightly. **2.** A solution or water used to rinse.

***mouth r.*** A flavored, sometimes mildly antiseptic solution used to help cleanse the mouth or improve breath odor.

***sodium fluoride r.*** A 0.05% aqueous solution of sodium fluoride also containing coloring and flavoring agents, used as a mouth rinse to help prevent dental caries.

**Riolan** (rē″ō-lănz′) Jean, French anatomist, 1577–1657.

***R.'s arch*** The arch formed by the mesentery of the transverse colon.

***R.'s bouquet*** The two ligaments and three muscles attached to the styloid process of the temporal bone.

***R.'s muscle*** The ciliary portion of the orbicularis oculi.

**Riopan** Trade name for magaldrate.

**ripa** (rī′pă) [L., bank] Any reflection line of the ependyma of the brain from the ventricular wall to the choroid plexus.

**Ripault's sign** (rē-pōz′) [Louis H. A. Ripault, Fr. physician, 1807–1856] A change in the shape of the pupil produced by unilateral (external) pressure on the eyeball.

**ripening 1.** Softening and dilatation of the uterine cervix during labor. **2.** Maturation of a cataract.

**risk** [origin obscure] The probability that something harmful will occur.

***r. assessment*** Quantitation of the risks to which people are exposed by compilation of morbidity and mortality data over specified periods of time.

***attributable r.*** The portion of the risk of developing a condition that can be traced to each known risk factor (e.g., persons exposed to asbestos have a certain risk of developing lung cancer, and if they also smoke tobacco, they are also at risk from that factor). These risks may be estimated from cohort studies.

***material r.*** A significant risk that a reasonable patient would want to consider when deciding whether to undergo medical treatment.

***relative r.*** In epidemiological studies, a method of measuring the relative amount of disease occurring in different populations; the ratio of incidence rate in the exposed group to that in the unexposed group. SEE: *ratio, odds.*

**risk-benefit analysis** Examination of the potential positive and negative results of undertaking a specific therapeutic course of action. An example would be the risk of dying from a surgical procedure versus the outcome if the procedure were successful and the course of the disease if the procedure were not done. SEE: *primum non nocere.*

**risk factor** An element in the environment, or a chemical, psychological, physiological, or genetic element, thought to predispose an individual to the development of a disease. For example, the known risk factors for coronary artery disease include hypertension, high circulating blood lipids and cholesterol, obesity, cigarette smoking, diabetes mellitus, inability to cope with stress, physical inactivity, and a family history of atherosclerosis. SEE: *ratio, odds; risk, relative.*

**risk management** A subspecialty in the health care field that addresses the prevention and containment of liability by careful and objective investigation and documentation of critical or unusual patient care incidents. In psychiatry, risk management may be concerned with preventing suicide and patient-related violence and its associated liability.

**risk-taker** An individual who willfully exposes himself or herself to a risk (one who engages in activities that others regard as hazardous).

**risorius** (rī-sŏ′rē-ŭs) [L., laughing] The muscular fibrous band arising over the masseter muscle and inserted into the tissues at the corner of the mouth. SEE: *Muscles Appendix.*

**RIST** *radioimmunosorbent test.*

**ristocetin** (rĭs″tō-sē′tĭn) An antibiotic obtained from cultures of *Nocardia lurida.*

**risus** (rī′sŭs) [L.] Laughter; a laugh.

***r. sardonicus*** A peculiar grin, as seen in tetanus, caused by acute facial spasm.

**Ritalin Hydrochloride** Trade name for methylphenidate hydrochloride.

**Ritgen's maneuver** A manual method of controlling the delivery of the fetal head. The nondominant hand exerts pressure against the fetal chin through the perineum. At the same time, the dominant hand exerts pressure against the fetal occiput. The maneuver should be performed slowly and between contractions to avoid perineal lacerations.

**Ritter's disease** (rĭt′ĕrz) [Gottfried Ritter von Rittershain, Ger. physician, 1820–1883] A generalized form of impetigo of the newborn.

**ritual** (rĭch′ū-ăl) **1.** A routine that the individual feels is essential and must be carried out. **2.** In psychiatry, any activity that is performed compulsively in an attempt to relieve anxiety.

**ritualistic surgery** Surgical procedures without scientific justification, performed in primitive societies without the purpose of treating or preventing disease. Included are alterations of the skin, ears, lips, teeth, genitalia, and head. In some cases, even in nonprimitive societies, surgical procedures without rational justification are considered ritualistic. SEE: *circumcision.*

**rivalry** (rī′văl-rē) Competition between two or more individuals, groups, or systems seeking to attain the same goal.

***binocular r.*** The continuous alternation in the conscious perception of visual stimuli to the two eyes.

***retinal r.*** Binocular r.

***sibling r.*** The competition between children for attention and affection from others, esp. their parents.

**rivalry strife** Alternate sensations of color and shape when the fields of vision of the two eyes cannot combine in one visual image.

**Rivinus, August Quirinus** (rē-vē′nŭs) German anatomist, 1652–1723.

***R.'s canal*** Any duct of the sublingual glands.

***R.'s gland*** A sublingual gland.

***R.'s incisure*** The tympanic notch in the upper part of the tympanic portion of the temporal bone. It extends from the lesser to the greater tympanic spines and is occupied by the pars flaccida of the tympanic membrane. SYN: *notch of Rivinus.*

***R.'s ligament*** The small portion of the tympanic membrane in Rivinus' incisure. SYN: *Shrapnell's membrane.*

**rivus lacrimalis** (rī′vŭs) [L. *rivus,* little stream, + *lacrima,* tear] The pathway under the eyelids through which tears travel from their source in the lacrimal glands to the punctum lacrimale.

**riziform** (rĭz′ĭ-form) [Fr. *riz,* rice, + L. *forma,* form] Resembling rice grains.

**R.L.E.** *right lower extremity.*

**RLF** *retrolental fibroplasia.*

**R.L.L.** *right lower lobe* of the lung.

**RLQ** *right lower quadrant* (of abdomen).

**R.M.A.** *registered medical assistant; right mentoanterior presentation* (of the fetal face).

**RML** *right middle lobe* (of the lung).

**R.M.P.** *right mentoposterior presentation* (of the fetal face).

**RMS** *rhabdomyosarcoma.*

**R.M.T.** *right mentotransverse* fetal position.

**R.N.** *registered nurse.*

**Rn** Symbol for the element radon.

**RNA** *ribonucleic acid.*

**RNase** *ribonuclease.*

**RNC** *registered nurse certified.*

**R.O.A.** *right occipitoanterior* fetal position.

**Robert's pelvis** (rō′bārts) [Heinrich L. F. Robert, Ger. gynecologist, 1814–1874] A transverse contraction of the pelvis caused by osteoarthritis of the sacroiliac joints.

**Robertson's pupil** Argyll Robertson pupil.

**Rochalimaea** Former name for the genus *Bartonella.*

***R. quintana*** SEE: *Bartonella quintana.*

**Rochelle salt** (rō-shĕl′) Potassium sodium tartrate, a colorless, transparent powder having a cooling and saline taste and used as a saline cathartic.

**rocker board** A board with rockers or a partial sphere on the undersurface so that a rocking motion occurs when a person stands on it. It is for proprioception and balance training, esp. in lower-extremity injuries and central nervous system disturbances. Also called *balance board*; *wobble board*.

**rocker knife** An adapted device for persons with limited upper-extremity function. It allows one-handed stabilization and cutting of food.

**rocking** A technique in neurodevelopmental rehabilitation designed to increase muscle tone in hypotonic patients through vestibular stimulation.

**Rocky Mountain spotted fever** An infectious disease caused by the bacterium *Rickettsia ricketsii* and transmitted by the wood tick *Dermacentor andersoni* or *D. variabilis*. Originally thought to exist only in the western U.S., it can occur anywhere that the tick vector is present.

The organism causes vasculitis, producing fever, headache, myalgia, and a characteristic rash. The rash appears several days after the other symptoms, first erupting on the wrists and ankles, then on the palms and soles. It is nonpruritic and macular and spreads to the legs, arms, trunk, and face. Disseminated intravascular coagulation or pneumonia may be serious complications. Tetracycline is the drug of choice for treating this disease.

Persons living in areas with wood ticks should wear clothing that covers much of their bodies, including the neck, to prevent ticks carrying the disease from burrowing under the skin. Persons who live in or travel to areas where ticks flourish should examine their scalps, skin, and clothing for ticks two or three times per day. Tick repellent can be applied to exposed parts of the body and to clothing. Ticks should be removed carefully with tweezers by grasping close to attachment to the body. Ticks can also be covered with gasoline or heavy lubricant to attempt removal. Hands need to be washed after tick removal. Pets should be examined regularly for ticks.

**rod** (rŏd) [AS. *rodd,* club] **1.** A slender, straight bar. **2.** One of the slender, long sensory bodies in the retina, which respond to faint light. **3.** A bacterium shaped like a rod.

***Corti's r.*** Pillar cell.

***enamel r.*** One of the minute calcareous rods or prisms laid down by ameloblasts and forming tooth enamel.

***retinal r.*** A receptor in the retina that responds to dim light. SEE: *retina* for illus.

**rodent** Any mammal of the Rodentia order, such as mice, rats, and squirrels.

**rodenticide** (rō-dĕn′tĭ-sīd) [L. *rodens,* gnawing, + *caedere,* to kill] An agent that kills rodents.

**rodent ulcer** [″ + *ulcus,* ulcer] A slowly growing, gnawing cancer that slowly destroys soft tissues and bones, causing great destruction. The usual sites are the outer angle of the eye, near the side and on the tip of the nose, and the edges of the scalp. SYN: *Jacob's ulcer*.

**rods and cones** The photoreceptor cells of the retina. They are between the pigment epithelium and the bipolar layer of neurons. The rods contain rhodopsin, which is stimulated by dim light; the cones contain one of three other photopigments, which are stimulated by various wavelengths of visible light (colors). SEE: *cone, ocular; night vision*.

**Roentgen, Wilhelm Konrad** (rĕnt′gĕn) German physicist, 1845–1923, who discovered roentgen rays (x-rays) in 1895. He won the Nobel Prize in physics in 1901.

**roentgen** (rĕnt′gĕn) ABBR: R. A unit for describing the exposure dose of x-rays or gamma rays. One unit can liberate enough electrons and positrons to produce emissions of either charge of one electrostatic unit of electricity per 0.001293 g of air (the weight of 1 $cm^3$ of dry air at 0°C and at 760 mm Hg).

**roentgenocinematography** (rĕnt″gĕn-ō-sĭn″ĕ-mă-tŏg′ră-fē) [″ + Gr. *kinema,* motion, + *graphein,* to write] Moving picture photography of x-ray studies.

**roentgenogram** (rĕnt-gĕn′ō-grăm, rĕnt′gĕn-ō-grăm″) Radiograph.

**roentgenography** (rĕnt″gĕn-ŏg′ră-fē) Radiography.

***body section r.*** Tomography.

***mucosal relief r.*** An x-ray examination of the intestinal mucosa after ingested barium has been removed and air under slight pressure has been injected. This leaves a light coat of barium on the mucosa and permits x-ray pictures of the fine detail of the mucosa.

***serial r.*** Repeated x-ray pictures taken of an area at defined but arbitrary intervals.

***spot-film r.*** An x-ray picture taken of a small area during fluoroscopy.

**roentgenology** (rĕnt″gĕn-ŏl′ō-jē) Radiology.

**roentgenometer** (rĕnt″gĕ-nŏm′ĕ-tĕr) Radiometer.

**roentgenotherapy, roentgentherapy** (rĕnt″gĕn-ō-thĕr′ăp-ē) Radiotherapy.

**roentgen ray** X-ray photon.

**roeteln, roetheln** (rĕt′ĕln) [Ger.] Rubella.

**Roger's disease** (rō-zhāz′) [Henri L. Roger, Fr. physician, 1809–1891] Ventricular septal defect.

**Rogers, Martha** A nursing educator, born 1914, who developed the Science of Unitary Human Beings. SEE: *Nursing Theory Appendix*.

**Rokitansky's disease** (rō″kĭ-tăn′skēz) [Karl

Freiherr von Rokitansky, Austrian pathologist, 1804–1878] Acute yellow atrophy of liver.

**Rolando's area** (rō-lăn′dōz) [Luigi Rolando, It. anatomist, 1773–1831] A motor area in the cerebral cortex, situated in the anterior central convolution in front of Rolando's fissure in each hemisphere.

**Rolando's fissure** Sulcus centralis.

**role** (rōl) [O. Fr. *rolle,* roll of paper on which a part is written] The characteristic social behavior of an individual in relationship to the group.

***gender r.*** SEE: *gender role.*

**role model** Someone who serves as an example for others by demonstrating the behavior associated with a particular position or profession.

**role performance, altered** Disruption in the way one perceives one's role performance. SEE: *Nursing Diagnoses Appendix.*

**role playing** The assignment and acting out of a role in a treatment setting to provide individuals an opportunity for people to see themselves as others see them. It is also used to teach such skills as interviewing, history taking, and doing a physical examination.

**Rolfing** [Ida P. Rolf, U.S. biochemist, 1897–1979] A therapy designed to realign the body with gravity through fascial manipulation.

**rolitetracycline** (rō″lē-tĕt″ră-sī′klēn) An antibiotic drug. Trade name is Syntetrin.

**roll** An usually solid, cylindrical structure.

***cotton r.*** A cylindrical mass of purified and sterilized cotton used as packing or absorbent material in various dental procedures.

***ilial r.*** A sausage-shaped mass in the left iliac fossa. It is due to a collection of feces in or induration of the walls of the sigmoid colon.

***scleral r.*** SEE: *spur, scleral.*

**roller** (rōl′ĕr) [O. Fr., roll] **1.** A strip of muslin or other cloth rolled up in cylinder form for surgical use. **2.** A roller bandage. SEE: *bandage.*

**ROM** *read-only memory; rupture of membranes.*

**R.O.M.** *range of motion.*

**roman numeral** One of the letters used by the ancient Romans for numeration, as distinct from the arabic numerals that we now use. In roman notation, values are changed either by adding one or more symbols to the initial symbol or by subtracting a symbol to the right of it. For example, V is 5, IV is 4, and VI is 6. Hence, because X is 10, IX is 9 and XI is 11. SEE: roman numerals in *Latin and Greek Nomenclature Appendix.*

**romanopexy** (rō-măn′ō-pĕk″sē) Sigmoidopexy.

**romanoscope** (rō-măn′ō-skōp) Sigmoidoscope.

**rombergism** (rŏm′bĕrg-ĭzm) The tendency to fall from a standing position when the eyes are closed and the feet are close together. SEE: *Romberg's sign.*

**Romberg's sign** (rŏm′bĕrgs) [Moritz Heinrich Romberg, Ger. physician, 1795–1873] The inability to maintain body balance when the eyes are shut and the feet are close together. The sign is positive if the patient sways and falls when the eyes are closed. This is seen in sensory ataxia.

**rongeur** (rŏn-zhŭr′) [Fr., to gnaw] An instrument for removing small amounts of tissue, particularly bone; also called *bone nippers.* A rongeur is a spring-loaded forceps with a sharp blade that may be either end cutting or side cutting.

**roof nucleus** A small mass of gray matter in the white substance of the vermis of the cerebellum.

**room** [AS. *rum*] An area or space in a building, partitioned off for occupancy or available for specific procedures.

***clean r.*** A room, particularly one housing delicate electronic medical instruments, that is constructed to be isolated from the free entry of air. Only filtered air enters, and personnel wear special clothing so that particles from their bodies do not become freely dispersed in the room.

***delivery r.*** A room to which an obstetric patient is taken for childbirth.

***dust-free r.*** A type of room designed to eliminate or reduce circulating particulate matter, including airborne microorganisms. This kind of room is useful for housing burn patients, removing allergens from the air, providing an environment for transplantation surgery, and preparing drugs and solutions for intravenous use.

***intensive therapy r.*** An intensive care room in which patients who need close medical attention and use of various medical devices such as resuscitation equipment are treated.

***labor r.*** A room in which an obstetric patient is placed during the first stage of labor, prior to being taken to the delivery room.

***operating r.*** A hospital room used for surgical procedures.

***recovery r.*** SEE: *recovery room.*

**rooming-in** The practice of placing an infant in the same hospital room as the mother, beginning immediately after birth.

**root** (rūt) [AS. *rot*] **1.** The underground part of a plant. **2.** The proximal end of a nerve. **3.** A portion of an organ implanted in tissues. SYN: *radix.* **4.** The part of the human tooth covered by cementum; designated by location (mesial, distal, buccal, lingual).

***anterior r.*** One of the two roots by which a spinal nerve is attached to the spinal cord; contains efferent nerve fibers.

***dorsal r.*** The radix dorsalis or sensory root of each spinal nerve. SYN: *sensory r.*

***motor r.*** The anterior root of a spinal nerve. SYN: *ventral r.*

***posterior r.*** One of the two roots by

which a spinal nerve is attached to the spinal cord; contains afferent nerve fibers.

***sensory r.*** Dorsal r.

***ventral r.*** Motor r.

**root artery** An artery accompanying a nerve root into the spinal cord.

**root formation** The development of tooth roots by Hertwig's root sheath and the epithelial diaphragm. It involves the formation of root dentin with a covering of cementum essential for the attachment of the tooth to the surrounding bony tissues. Root formation or development continues for months or years after the tooth has erupted into the mouth.

**root pick** A dental instrument for retrieving root fragments resulting from tooth extraction; also called *apical elevator*.

**root planing** Planing (2).

**root resorption of teeth** A condition of tooth roots caused by endocrine imbalance or excessive pressure of orthodontic appliances. Radiographs demonstrate roots that appear to be sawed off or shortened.

**root zone** Fasciculus cuneatus.

**R.O.P.** *right occipitoposterior*. In this fetal presentation, the occiput of the fetus is in relationship to the right sacroiliac joint of the mother.

**Rorschach test** (ror'shăk) [Hermann Rorschach, Swiss pyschiatrist, 1884–1922] A psychological test consisting of 10 different inkblot designs. The subject is asked to interpret each design individually. This may reveal personality disturbances.

**rosa** (rō'ză) [L.] Rose.

**rosacea** (rō-zā'sē-ă) [L. *rosaceus,* rosy] A chronic disease of the skin of the face usually occurring in middle-aged and older persons. The cause is unknown. It is marked by varying degrees of papules, pustules, erythema, telangectasia, and hyperplasia (rhinophyma) of the soft tissues of the nose. The onset is usually between 30 and 50 years of age, but may be as early as 10 or may occur first in old age. In adults, it occurs three times as often in men as in women. SYN: *acne rosacea.* SEE: illus.; *rhinophyma* for illus.

TREATMENT: The treatment is symptomatic, with systemic antimicrobials and topical metronidazole. Isotretinoin and topical metronidazole are also effective. Rhinophyma may be treated by laser therapy to remove the excess tissue.

***steroid r.*** Acne caused by systemic or topical use of corticosteroid drugs. SEE: illus.

**rosaniline** (rō-zăn'ĭ-lĭn) A basic dye used in preparing other dyes.

**rosary** (rō'ză-rē) Something that resembles a string of beads.

***rachitic r.*** Palpable areas at the juncture of the ribs with their cartilages. This is seen in conjunction with rickets.

**Rose's position** (rōz) [Frank A. Rose, Brit. surgeon, 1873–1935] A fully extended position in which the patient's head is allowed to hang over the end of the operating room table to prevent aspiration of blood during surgery on the mouth and lips.

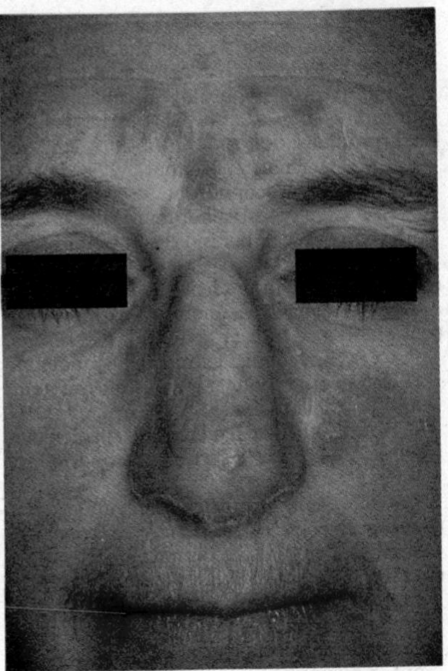

ROSACEA

**rose bengal sodium I 131** A standardized preparation of radioactive iodine and rose bengal used in photoscanning the liver and testing liver function.

**rose fever** Hay fever of early summer attributed to inhaling rose pollen. SEE: *hay fever*.

**Rosenbach, Ottomar** (rō'zĕn-bŏk) German physician, 1851–1907.

***R.'s sign*** **1.** A fine, rapid tremor of the closed eyelids, seen in hyperthyroidism. **2.** In hysteria, the inability to obey a command to close the eyes. **3.** The absence of an abdominal skin reflex in intestinal inflammation or hemiplegia.

***R.'s test*** A test for bile in the urine.

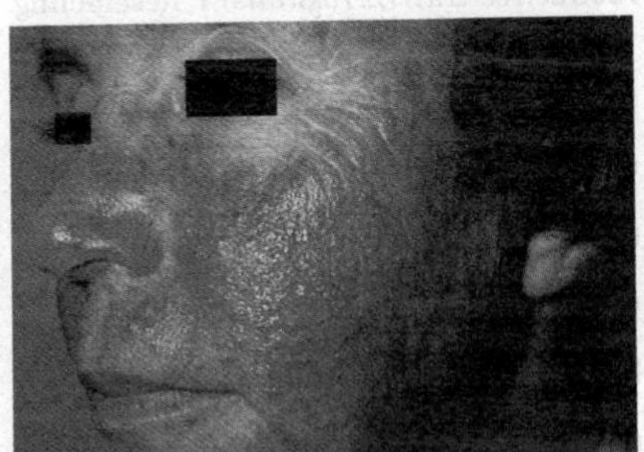

STEROID ROSACEA

Urine is passed several times through the same filter paper. After the paper has dried, a drop of nitric acid is added to it. If bile is present, a play of colors is produced.

**Rosenmüller, Johann Christian** (rō′zĕn-mül″ĕr) German anatomist, 1771–1820.

***R.'s body*** Epoophoron.

***R.'s cavity*** A slitlike depression in the pharyngeal wall behind the opening of the eustachian tube.

**roseo-** **1.** Combining form meaning *rose-colored.* **2.** A prefix in chemical terms.

**roseola** (rō-zē′ō-lă, rō″zē-ō′lă) [L. *roseus,* rosy] A skin condition marked by maculae or red spots of varying sizes on the skin; any rose-colored rash.

***r. idiopathica*** A macular eruption not associated with any well-defined symptoms.

***r. infantum*** Exanthem subitum.

**roseolous** (rō-zē′ō-lŭs) [L. *roseus,* rosy] Resembling or pert. to roseola.

**rosette** [Fr., small rose] **1.** Something resembling a rose. **2.** A spherical group of fine red vacuoles surrounding the cytocentrum of a monocyte. **3.** A mature schizont. SYN: *segmenter.*

**rose water** A saturated aqueous solution of rose oil, used to impart agreeable odor to lotions.

**rose water ointment** An emollient used to soften the skin. It contains waxes, almond oil, sodium borate, rose water, rose oil, and purified water.

**rosin** (rŏz′ĭn) [L. *resina*] A substance distilled from species of pine and used as a stiffening agent in preparing plasters.

**Ross' body** [Edward Halford Ross, Brit. pathologist, 1875–1928] A copper-colored, round body, showing dark granules, that is found in blood and tissue fluids in syphilis. Sometimes these exhibit ameboid movements.

**Rossolimo's reflex** (rŏs″ō-lē′mōz) [Gregoriy I. Rossolimo, Russian neurologist, 1860–1928] Plantar flexion of the second to fifth toes in response to percussion of the plantar surface of the toes.

**rostellum** (rŏs-tĕl′lŭm) *pl.* **rostella** [L., little beak] A fleshy protrusion on the anterior end of the scolex of a tapeworm, bearing one or more rows of spines or hooks.

**rostral** (rŏs′trăl) [L. *rostralis*] **1.** Resembling a beak. **2.** Toward the front or cephalic end of the body.

**rostrate** (rŏs′trāt) [L. *rostratus,* beaked] Having a beak or hook formation.

**rostriform** (rŏs′trĭ-form) [″ + *forma,* shape] Shaped like a beak.

**rostrum** (rŏs′trŭm) *pl.* **rostrums, rostra** [L., beak] Any hooked or beaked structure.

**rosulate** (rŏs′ū-lāt) [L. *rosulatus,* like a rose] Shaped like a rosette.

**R.O.T.** *right occipitotransverse* fetal position.

**rot** (rŏt) [ME. *roten*] To decay or decompose.

***jungle r.*** The common term for certain fungal skin diseases that occur in the tropics.

**rotameter** (rō-tăm′ĕ-tĕr) A device for measuring the flow of a gas or liquid.

**rotate** (rō-tāt) [L. *rotare,* to turn] To twist or revolve.

**rotation** (rō-tā′shŭn) [L. *rotatio,* a turning] The process of turning on an axis.

***fetal r.*** Twisting of the fetal head as it follows the curves of the birth canal downward.

***optical r.*** SEE: *activity, optical.*

***tooth r.*** The repositioning of a tooth by turning it on its long axis to a more normal occlusal position.

**rotator** (rō-tā′tor) *pl.* **rotatores** A muscle revolving a part on its axis.

**rotaviruses** (rō′tă-vī″rŭs-ĕs) [L. *rota,* wheel, + *virus,* poison] A group of viruses that are a major cause of sporadic acute enteritis in infants and small children and of epidemic acute gastroenteritis.

**röteln, rötheln** (rĕt′ĕln) Rubella.

**rotenone** (rō′tĕn-nōn) A poisonous chemical, $C_{23}H_{22}O_6$, used as an insecticide.

**Roth's spots** [Moritz Roth, Swiss physician and pathologist, 1839–1914] Small white spots in the retina close to the optic disk, often surrounded by areas of hemorrhage. The condition is caused by a systemic infection, particularly acute infective endocarditis.

**Rotor syndrome** An inherited liver disorder that is transmitted as an autosomal recessive trait; it is similar to but genetically distinct from Dubin-Johnson syndrome. A distinguishing characteristic is that there is no abnormal pigment in the liver cells.

**rototome** A device for cutting tissue, used in arthroscopic surgery.

**rotoxamine** (rō-tŏks′ă-mēn) An antihistaminic drug.

**Rouget's cells** (roo-zhāz′) [Charles M. B. Rouget, Fr. physiologist, 1824–1904] Contractile cells that surround the capillaries, observed in frogs and salamanders.

**rough** (rŭf) Not smooth.

**roughage** SEE: *cellulose; fiber, dietary.*

**rouleau** (roo-lō′) *pl.* **rouleaux** [Fr., roll] A group of red blood corpuscles that are stuck together, resembling a roll of coins.

**round** (rownd) [O. Fr. *ronde*] **1.** Circular. **2.** Spherical, globular.

**roundworm** Any member of the phylum Nemathelminthes (Aschelminthes), esp. one belonging to the class Nematoda. SEE: *threadworm.*

**Roux-en-Y** An anastomosis of the distal divided end of the small bowel to another organ such as the stomach or esophagus. The proximal end is anastomosed to the small bowel below the anastomosis.

**Roven's IMDC** [Milton D. Roven, contemporary U.S. podiatrist] A new procedure for *i*ntra*m*edullary *m*etatarsal *d*ecompression performed through a small dorsal incision. It is less traumatic than previous procedures, allowing immediate ambulation and minimal postoperative pain and edema.

**Roy Adaptation Model** A conceptual model of nursing developed by Callista Roy. Individuals and groups are adaptive systems with physiological, self-concept, role function, and interdependence modes of response to focal, contextual, and residual environmental stimuli. The goal of nursing is promotion of adaptation through increasing decreasing, maintaining, removing, altering, or changing environmental stimuli. SEE: *Nursing Theory Appendix.*

**Royal Free disease** [After Royal Free Hospital, London, from which cases were reported in 1955] Postviral fatigue syndrome.

**Roy, Callista** A nursing educator, born 1939, who developed the Roy Adaptation Model of Nursing. SEE: *Nursing Theory Appendix.*

**RPF** *renal plasma flow.*

**RPFT** *Registered Pulmonary Function Technician.*

**R.Ph.** *Registered Pharmacist.*

**rpm** *revolutions per minute.*

**RPO** *right posterior oblique* position.

**RPS** *renal pressor substance.* SEE: *renin.*

**R.Q.** *respiratory quotient.*

**R.R.A.** *registered record administrator.*

**-rrhage, -rhage** Combining form used as a suffix meaning *rupture, profuse fluid discharge,* as in hemorrhage.

**-rrhagia, -rhagia** (rā′jē-ă) [Gr. *rhegnynai,* to burst forth] Combining form used as a suffix meaning *rupture, profuse fluid discharge.*

**-rrhaphy, -rhaphy** [Gr. *raphe,* suture] Combining form used as a suffix meaning *suture, surgical repair.*

**-rrhea, -rhea** [Gr. *rhoia,* flow] Combining form used as a suffix denoting *flow, discharge.*

**-rrhexis, -rhexis** [Gr. *rhexis,* a breaking, bursting] Combining form used as a suffix meaning *rupture.*

**rRNA** *ribosomal RNA.*

**RRT** *Registered Respiratory Therapist.*

**R.S.A.** *right sacroanterior* fetal position.

**R.Sc.A.** *right scapuloanterior* fetal position.

**R.Sc.P.** *right scapuloposterior* fetal position.

**R.S.P.** *right sacroposterior* fetal position.

**R.S.T.** *right sacrotransverse* fetal position.

**R.S.V.** *respiratory syncytial virus; Rous sarcoma virus.*

**R.T.** *radiation therapy; reading test; registered technologist.*

**R.T.(N.)** *registered technologist – nuclear medicine.*

**R.T.(R.)** *registered technologist radiographer.*

**R.T.(T.)** *registered technologist – radiation therapy.*

**R.U.** *rat unit.*

**RU 486** An abortifacient used in some countries. It is not used more than 47 days after the last menstrual period. A prostaglandin is administered by injection or as a suppository as an adjunct to RU 486.

**Ru** Symbol for the element ruthenium.

**rub** Friction of one surface moving over another. In auscultation, a roughened surface moving over another causes a characteristic sound.

***pericardial r.*** The sound heard by means of auscultation with each heartbeat when the inflamed pericardial surface moves over the heart.

***pleural friction r.*** The friction rub caused by inflammation of the pleural space.

**rubber dam** SEE: *dam.*

**rubbing alcohol** A preparation containing not less than 68.5% and not more than 71.5% dehydrated alcohol by volume. The remainder consists of water and denaturants and may or may not contain color additives and perfume oils. It is used as a rubefacient. Rubbing alcohol is packaged, labeled, and sold in accordance with the regulations issued by the U.S. Treasury Department, Bureau of Alcohol, Tobacco, and Firearms.

---

Caution: Because of the added denaturant, it is poisonous if taken internally.

---

**rubedo** [L. *ruber,* red] Redness of the skin that may be temporary.

**rubefacient** (roo″bĕ-fā′shĕnt) [L. *rubefaciens,* making red] **1.** Causing redness, as of the skin. **2.** An agent that reddens the skin, producing a local congestion, with dilated vessels and an increased blood supply. Rubefacients include mustard, turpentine, capsicum, flaxseed, arnica, rubbing alcohol, and liniments.

**rubella** (roo-bĕl′lă) [L. *rubellus,* reddish] A mild, febrile, highly infectious viral disease historically common in childhood prior to the advent of an effective vaccine. SYN: *German measles; roeteln; röteln.* SEE: *Nursing Diagnoses Appendix.*

SYMPTOMS: A variable 1- to 5-day prodromal period of drowsiness, mild temperature elevation, slight sore throat, Forschheimer spots (pinpoint reddish areas on the palate), and postauricular, postcervical, and occipital lymphadenopathy commonly precedes the rash eruption. The rash resembles that of measles or scarlet fever, begins on the forehead and face, spreads downward to the trunk and extremities, and lasts about 3 days. The rash appears in only about 50% of infections.

INCUBATION: Infection occurs approx. 14 to 23 days before the advent of symptoms.

COMPLICATIONS: Complications include generalized lymphadenopathy and splenomegaly. A transient polyarthritis (inflammation of the wrist, finger, knee, toe, and ankle joints) may occur within 5 days of the rash, but usually lasts less than 2 weeks. Encephalomyelitis is rare and usually self-limiting. The disease is most important because of its ability to produce defects in the developing fetus. Rubella infection during the first timester of pregnancy is of concern; transplacental transmission to the fetus may result in several types of congenital anomalies. SEE: *congenital r. syndrome.*

PREVENTION: Prophylaxis consists of childhood immunization with a combination measles, mumps, rubella (MMR) vaccine.

---

Caution: Administration of live virus vaccines is contraindicated during pregnancy.

---

***congenital r. syndrome*** Transplacental transmission of the rubella virus to a fetus resulting in spontaneous abortion, stillbirth, or major birth defects of the heart, eyes, or central nervous system, including deafness. Women who become pregnant and have not received rubella immunization should be advised of the risk of fetal development of congenital rubella syndrome (CRS). For unimmunized women who develop rubella in the first trimester of pregnancy, there is a 90% possibility that the fetus will be infected with the rubella virus. Fetal infection can be determined by serial studies of the immunoglobulin gamma M and immunoglobulin gamma G rubella antibodies. Prevention of CRS consists of active immunization of all children and women of childbearing age.

---

Caution: Immunization is contraindicated during pregnancy, and it is recommended that women avoid pregnancy during the 3-month period after immunization. Infants with CRS are considered to be contagious. Only health care workers known to be immune to rubella (seropositive) should be permitted to care for infants with CRS.

---

**rubella titer** A serology test to determine a person's immune status to rubella.

**rubella virus vaccine, live** SEE: under *vaccine.*

**rubeola** (roo-bē'ō-lă, roo"bē-ō'lă) [L. *rubeolus,* reddish] **1.** Measles. **2.** Term occasionally applied to an acute infectious disease with mild symptoms and a rose-colored macular eruption.

**rubeosis iridis** A condition in which new blood vessels form on the anterior surface of the iris. It is associated with vascular disease that affects the retinal vein of the eye and is seen most frequently in diabetics, although not limited to these patients. It leads to painful, hemorrhagic glaucoma.

**ruber** (roo'bĕr) [L.] Red.

**rubescent** (roo-bĕs'ĕnt) [L. *rubescere,* to grow red] Growing red; flushing.

**rubidium** (roo-bĭd'ē-ŭm) [L. *rubidus,* red] SYMB: Rb. A soft, silvery metal that decomposes water with violence and bursts into flame spontaneously in air; atomic weight 85.47, atomic number 37. Its salts are used medicinally.

**rubiginous** (roo-bĭj'ĭ-nŭs) [L. *rubiginosus*] Rusty.

**rubigo** (roo-bī'gō) [L., rust] Rust; mildew.

**Rubin, Reva** A nursing educator who developed the Theory of Clinical Nursing. SEE: *Nursing Theory Appendix.*

**Rubin's test** (roo'bĭns) [Isidor Clinton Rubin, U.S. physician, 1883–1958] Transuterine insufflation of the fallopian tubes with carbon dioxide to test their patency. SYN: *tubal insufflation.* SEE: *sterility.*

**Rubner's test** (roob'nĕrz) [Max Rubner, Ger. physiologist, 1854–1932] **1.** A test for lactose or glucose in urine. **2.** A test for carbon monoxide in blood.

**rubor** (roo'bor) [L.] Discoloration or redness caused by inflammation. It is one of the four classic symptoms of inflammation. The others are calor (heat), dolor (pain), and tumor (swelling).

**rubriblast** (roo'brĭ-blăst) Pronormoblast.

**rubric** (roo'brĭk) [L. *ruber,* red] **1.** Concerning or being red. **2.** An established procedure or protocol.

**rubricyte** (roo'brĭ-sīt) [L. *ruber,* red, + Gr. *kytos,* cell] A polychromatic normoblast.

**rubrospinal** (roo"brō-spī'năl) [" + *spina,* thorn] Pert. to a descending tract that consists of a small bundle of nerve fibers in the lateral funiculus of the spinal cord. Fibers arise in the cells of the red nucleus of the midbrain and terminate in the ventral horn of the gray matter.

**rubrothalamic** (roo"brō-thăl-lăm'ĭk) [" + Gr. *thalamos,* chamber] Pert. to the red nucleus of the brain and thalamus.

**rubrum** (roo'brŭm) [L., red] The red nucleus of the gray matter in the crus cerebri near the optic thalamus.

***r. scarlatinum*** Scarlet red, a substance used as a stain.

**rudiment** (roo'dĭ-mĕnt) [L. *rudimentum,* beginning] **1.** Something undeveloped. **2.** In biology, a part just beginning to develop. **3.** The remains of a part that was functional at an earlier stage of one's development or in one's ancestors. SYN: *rudimentum.*

**rudimentary** (roo"dĭ-mĕn'tă-rē) **1.** Elementary. **2.** Undeveloped; not fully formed; remaining from an earlier stage. SYN: *vestigial.*

**rudimentum** (roo"dĭ-mĕn'tŭm) [L., beginning] Rudiment.

**Ruffini's corpuscle** (roo-fē'nēz) [Angelo Ruffini, It. anatomist, 1864–1929] One of the encapsulated sensory nerve endings found in the dermis and subcutaneous tissue, thought to mediate the sense of warmth. SYN: *organ of Ruffini.*

**rufous** (roo'fŭs) [L. *rufus,* red] Ruddy; having a ruddy complexion and reddish hair.

**ruga** (roo'gă) *pl.* **rugae** [L.] A fold or crease,

esp. one of the folds of mucous membrane on the internal surface of the stomach.

***palatal r.*** A fold or crease, esp. one of the folds of mucous membrane on the internal surface of the stomach. SYN: *palatine r.*

***palatine r.*** Palatal r.

***r. of vagina*** One of the small ridges on the inner surface of the vagina extending laterally and upward from the columna rugarum (long ridges on the anterior and posterior walls).

**Ruggeri's reflex** [Ruggero Ruggeri, It. physician, d. 1905] The increase in pulse rate that occurs when the eyes are strongly converged on a near object.

**rugine** (roo-zhēn') **1.** Periosteal elevator. **2.** A raspatory.

**rugose, rugous** (roo'gōs, -gŭs) [L. *rugosus,* wrinkled] Having many wrinkles or creases; used in describing microbiological colonies. SEE: illus.

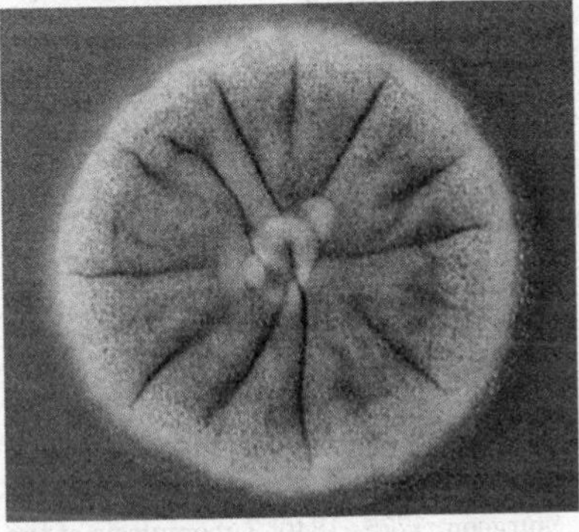

RUGOSE APPEARANCE OF ASPERGILLUS CULTURE

**rugosity** (rū-gŏs'ĭ-tē) [L. *rugositas*] **1.** The condition of being folded or wrinkled. **2.** A ridge or wrinkle.

**R.U.L.** *right upper lobe* of lung.

**rule** (rool) [ME. *riule*] A guide or principle based on experience or observation.

***buccal object r.*** A radiographical technique used to identify the position of an object within a three-dimensional area. A reference radiograph is taken. The projection angle is changed and the resulting radiograph compared with the reference radiograph. If the image remains in the same position, the object is located buccal to the reference object. If the image changes position, the object is lingual to the reference object. Also called *Clark's rule; Clark's technique; tube shift technique.*

***r. of nines*** A formula for estimating percentage of body surface areas, particularly helpful in judging the portion of skin that has been burned. The head represents 9%; each upper extremity 9%; the back of the trunk 18%, and the front 18%; each lower extremity 18%; and the perineum the remaining 1%. SEE: illus.

***r. of ten*** The criteria used to judge the readiness of an infant for surgical repair of a cleft lip. The infant must weigh 10 lb, be 10 weeks old, have a hemoglobin value of 10 g, and have a white blood cell count less than 10,000.

**rum** [origin obscure] **1.** An alcoholic beverage prepared from fermented sugar cane juice. **2.** Colloquially, any alcoholic beverage.

**rum fits** Epileptiform convulsions associated with withdrawal from chronic inebriation due to alcohol abuse. Most occur during the 7- to 48-hr period following abstinence. There may be a single seizure, but most occur in bursts of two to six. These seizures do not represent latent epilepsy.

**ruminant** (roo'mĭ-nănt) An animal that regurgitates food in order to chew it again. This is called chewing the cud.

**rumination** (roo"mĭ-nā'shŭn) [L. *ruminatio*] **1.** Regurgitation, esp. with rechewing, of previously swallowed food. This condition may be present in otherwise normal individuals, in emotionally deprived or mentally retarded infants, or in mentally retarded adults. **2.** In psychiatry, an obsessional preoccupation by a single idea or a set of thoughts, with an inability to dismiss or dislodge them. Also called *merycism.*

**rump** (rŭmp) [ME. *rumpe*] The posterior end of the back, the gluteal region, or the buttocks.

**Rumpf's symptom** (roompfs) [Heinrich Theodor Rumpf, Ger. physician, 1851–1923] **1.** In neurasthenia, a quickening of the pulse when pressure is exerted over a painful spot. **2.** Twitching after strong faradization, in traumatic neuroses.

**run** [AS. *rinnan,* run] To exude pus or mucus.

**runaround, runround** Whitlow.

**runners' high** The euphoric feelings experienced by many persons who participate in an intensive exercise program, such as running. After achieving a new level of physical fitness, they experience a feeling of elation and euphoria as they continue to run or exercise, and at the completion of a session. The relation of this to the stimulation of endorphin production by the exercise is unknown. SEE: *endorphin.*

**rupia** (roo'pē-ă) [Gr. *rhypos,* filth] A cutaneous eruption, usually of tertiary syphilis, first manifested by large elevations of the epidermis filled with a clear or blood-stained serum, soon becoming turbid and purulent. The bulla bursts and allows some fluid to escape. As it desiccates, it is covered with a crust that dries, accumulates new layers, and becomes covered with greenish-brown scales, sometimes to a depth of ½ in. (13 mm). It is the thickest

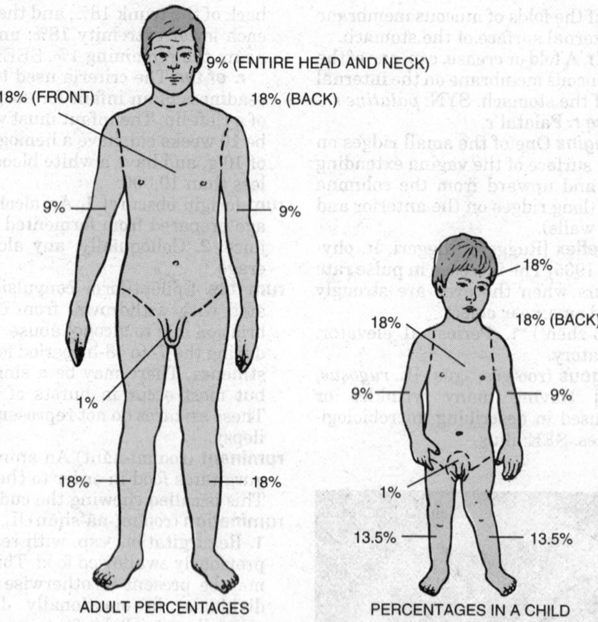


RULE OF NINES

of all syphilides and presents the most extensive ulcerations. The condition is treated with antisyphilitic antibiotics.

**rupioid** (roo′pē-oyd) [″ + *eidos,* form, shape] Resembling rupia.

**rupophobia** (roo″pō-fō′bē-ă) Rhypophobia.

**rupture** (rŭp′chūr) [L. *ruptura,* breaking] **1.** A breaking apart of an organ or tissue. **2.** Hernia.

***r. of membranes*** The rupture of the amniotic sac as a normal result of dilation of the cervix uteri in labor. Preterm premature rupture (before week 37 of pregnancy) increases the risk of intrauterine infection. SEE: *premature rupture of membranes, preterm.*

***r. of perineum*** A rupture of the perineum in labor, occurring more frequently in primiparas. It can be prevented by episiotomy.

***r. of tubes*** A rupture of a fallopian tube, a serious event in extrauterine pregnancy. This may occur without the woman's knowledge of her pregnancy.

***r. of uterus*** Uterine rupture due to unrelieved obstructed labor. This condition is rare.

**RUQ** *right upper quadrant* of abdomen.

**rush 1.** A strong contraction wave that moves down the small intestine. **2.** The first surge of pleasure produced by a drug, esp. a narcotic drug.

**Russell body** (rŭs′ĕl) [William Russell, Scot. physician, 1852–1940] A small spherical hyaline body found in cancerous and simple inflammatory growths.

**Russell's viper venom** (rŭs′ĕlz) [Patrick Russell, Irish physician who worked in India, 1727–1805] The toxin from Russell's viper. It is used in investigating defective blood coagulation caused by a deficiency of factor X.

**Rust's disease** (rŭsts) [Johann N. Rust, Ger. surgeon, 1775–1840] Tuberculosis of the cervical vertebrae and their articulations.

**rust** One of several members of an order of parasitic fungi (Uredinales), all of which are parasitic on plants. Many of these are allergens.

**rusty** (rŭst′ē) [AS. *rustig*] Reddish; resembling or containing rust. SYN: *rubiginous.*

**rut-formation** In psychology, a loss of interest in the environment, the fixation on a single object, and the narrowing of concentration of emotional or other interests.

**ruthenium** (roo-thē′nē-ŭm) SYMB: Ru. A hard, brittle, metallic element of the platinum group; atomic weight 101.07, atomic number 44.

**rutherford** [Ernest Rutherford, Brit. physicist, 1871–1937] ABBR: rd. A unit of radioactivity representing $10^6$ disintegrations per second.

**rutidosis** (roo″tĭ-dō′sĭs) Rhytidosis.

**rutilism** (roo′tĭl-ĭzm) [L. *rutilis,* red, + Gr. *-ismos,* condition] Having red or auburn hair.

**rutin** (roo′tĭn) A crystalline glucoside of quercetin, closely related to hesperidin. It is derived from buckwheat but is present in many plants.

**Ruysch's membrane** [Frederik Ruysch,

Dutch anatomist, 1638-1731] Lamina choriocapillaris.

**RV** *residual volume; right ventricle.*

**rye** (rī) [AS. *ryge*] A cereal grass that produces a grain used in food and beverage production. When rye grain is infected with a certain fungus, ergot is produced.

**rytidosis** (rĭt″ĭ-dō′sĭs) Rhytidosis.

# S

**σ** Sigma, the 18th letter of the Greek alphabet. In statistics, this is the symbol for standard deviation.

**Σ** The capital of the Greek letter sigma. In statistics, this is the symbol for summation.

**S** L. *signa,* mark, or let it be written. **1.** In prescription writing, the symbol indicating the instructions to the patient that the pharmacist will place on the dispensed medicine. **2.** *Smooth,* in reference to bacterial colonies. **3.** *Spherical* or *spherical lens.* **4.** *Subject* (pl. *Ss*); a participant in an experiment. **5.** Symbol for the element sulfur. **6.** Symbol for siemens.

**s** L. *semis,* half; *sinister,* left.

**s̄, s** Symbol for [L.] *sine,* without; used as a form of shorthand in hospital charts and clinical records.

**S1, S2, etc** *first sacral nerve, second sacral nerve,*and so forth.

**$S_1$, $S_2$** Normal first and second heart sounds.

**$S_3$** Ventricular gallop, an abnormal heart sound.

**$S_4$** Atrial gallop, an abnormal heart sound.

**S-A, SA, S.A.** *sinoatrial.*

**SAARD** *slow-acting antirheumatic drug.*

**Sabiá virus** An arenavirus that causes Brazilian hemorrhagic fever, a potentially fatal acute febrile disease. The reservoir for the virus is unknown. Several cases have been reported in laboratory personnel working with the virus. Persons with the disease are not believed to be infectious. Ribavirin, which is effective against Lassa fever, also caused by an arenavirus, may be effective in this illness.

**Sabin vaccine** [Albert Bruce Sabin, Russ.-born U.S. virologist, 1906–1993] A live oral vaccine for poliomyelitis. SEE: *live oral poliomyelitis vaccine.*

**sabulous** (săb'ū-lŭs) [L. *sabulosus,* sand] Gritty; sandy.

**sac** (săk) [L. *saccus,* sack, bag] A baglike part of an organ, a cavity or pouch, sometimes containing fluid. SYN: *saccus.* SEE: *cyst.*

***air s.*** An alveolus in the lung; made of simple squamous epithelium. SEE: *alveolar s.*

***allantoic s.*** The expanded end of the allantois, well developed in birds and reptiles.

***alveolar s.*** The terminal portion of an air passageway within the lung. Its wall is made of simple squamous epithelium and is surrounded by pulmonary capillaries. This is the site of gas exchange. Each alveolar sac is connected to a respiratory bronchiole by an alveolar duct.

***amniotic s.*** Amnion.

***chorionic s.*** A saclike structure, consisting of chorion, that encloses the developing embryo.

***conjunctival s.*** The cavity, lined with conjunctiva, that lies between the eyelids and the anterior surface of the eye.

***dental s.*** The mesenchymal tissue surrounding a developing tooth.

***endolymphatic s.*** The expanded distal end of the endolymphatic duct. SYN: *saccus endolymphaticus.*

***heart s.*** The pericardium.

***hernial s.*** In the peritoneum, a saclike protrusion containing a herniated organ. SEE: *hernia.*

***lacrimal s.*** The upper dilated portion of the nasolacrimal duct situated in the groove of the lacrimal bone. The upper part is behind the internal tarsal ligament. It is 12 to 15 mm long. SYN: *saccus lacrimalis.*

***lesser peritoneal s.*** Omental bursa.

***vitelline s.*** Yolk s.

***yolk s.*** In mammals, the embryonic membrane that is the site of formation of the first red blood cells and the cells that will become oogonia or spermatogonia. SYN: *vitelline s.* SEE: *embryo* for illus.

**saccades** (să-kāds') [Fr. *saccade,* jerk] Fast, involuntary movements of the eyes as they change from one point of gaze to another.

**saccadic** (să-kăd'ĭk) [Fr. *saccade,* jerk] Pert. to rapid intermittent movements, esp. of the eye. This type of eye movement is important when the fovea follows a moving target. SEE: *nystagmus; vergence.*

**saccate** (săk'āt) [NL. *saccatus,* baglike] **1.** Encysted. **2.** In bacteriology, making a sac shape, as in a type of liquefaction.

**saccharase** (săk'ă-rās) [Sanskrit *sarkara,* sugar] An enzyme that catalyzes the breakdown of disaccharides to monosaccharides, esp. the hydrolysis of sucrose to dextrose (e.g., sucrase, invertase).

**saccharated** (săk'ă-rāt"ĕd) Containing sugar.

**saccharide** (săk'ă-rīd) A group of carbohydrates including sugars. It is divided into the following classifications: monosaccharides, disaccharides, oligosaccharides, and polysaccharides.

**saccharin** (săk'ă-rĭn) $C_7H_5NO_3S$; a sweet, white, powdered, synthetic product derived from coal tar, 300 to 500 times sweeter than sugar, used as an artificial sweetener. Its use is now restricted because of its ability to cause cancer in experimental animals.

**saccharine** (săk'ă-rĭn, -rīn) [L. *saccharum,* sugar] Of the nature of, or having the quality of, sugar. SYN: *sweet.*

**saccharo-** Combining form meaning *sugar.*

**saccharogalactorrhea** (săk″ă-rō-gă-lăk″tō-rē′ă) [Sanskrit *sarkara,* sugar, + Gr. *gala,* milk, + *rhoia,* flow] Excessive lactose secreted in milk.
**saccharolytic** (săk″ă-rō-lĭt′ĭk) [″ + Gr. *lysis,* dissolution] Able to split up sugar.
**Saccharomyces** (săk″ă-rō-mī′sēz) [Sanskrit *sarkara,* sugar, + Gr. *mykes,* fungus] Yeast (1).
**saccharomycosis** (săk″ă-rō-mī-kō′sĭs) [″ + ″ + *osis,* condition] Any disease or pathologic condition caused by yeasts (saccharomycetes).
**saccharum** (săk′ă-rŭm) [L.] Sugar.
**sacciform** (săk′sĭ-form) [L. *saccus,* sack, bag, + *forma,* shape] Bag-shaped or saclike. SYN: *encysted.*
**saccular** (săk′ū-lăr) [NL. *sacculus,* small bag] Sac-shaped or saclike.
**sacculated** (săk′ū-lāt″ĕd) [NL. *sacculus,* small bag] Consisting of small sacs or saccules.
**sacculation** (săk″ū-lā′shŭn) **1.** Formation into a sac or sacs. **2.** Group of sacs, collectively.
**saccule** (săk′ūl) [NL. *sacculus,* small bag] **1.** A small sac. SYN: *sacculus.* **2.** The smaller of two sacs comprising the portion of the membranous labyrinth occupying the vestibule of the inner ear. It communicates with the utricle, cochlear duct, and endolymphatic duct, all of which are filled with endolymph. In its wall is the macula sacculi, a sensory area containing hair cells that respond to gravity or bodily movement. SEE: *labyrinth* for illus.
 ***laryngeal s.*** A small diverticulum extending ventrally from the laryngeal ventricle lying between the ventricular fold and the thyroarytenoid muscle. SYN: *sacculus laryngis; ventricular appendix.*
**sacculocochlear** (săk″ū-lō-kŏk′lē-ăr) [″ + Gr. *kokhlos,* land snail] Concerning the saccule and cochlea of the ear.
**sacculus** (săk′ū-lŭs) *pl.* **sacculi** [NL., small bag] Saccule.
 ***s. laryngis*** Laryngeal saccule.
**saccus** (săk′ŭs) *pl.* **sacci** [L., sack, bag] Sac.
 ***s. endolymphaticus*** Endolymphatic sac.
 ***s. lacrimalis*** Lacrimal sac.
**SACH foot** *Solid ankle cushion heel* foot; a prosthetic (artificial) foot that has no definite ankle joint but is designed to absorb shock and allow movement of the shank over the foot during ambulation.
**sacrad** (sā′krăd) [L. *sacrum,* sacred, + *ad,* toward] Toward the sacrum.
**sacral** (sā′krăl) [L. *sacralis*] Relating to the sacrum.
**sacral bone** Sacrum.
**sacral flexure** Rectal curve in front of the sacrum.
**sacralgia** (sā-krăl′jē-ă) [L. *sacrum,* sacred, + Gr. *algos,* pain] Pain in the sacrum.
**sacral index** Sacral breadth multiplied by 100 and divided by sacral length.
**sacralization** (sā″krăl-ĭ-zā′shŭn) Fusion of the sacrum and the fifth lumbar vertebra.
**sacral nerves** Five pairs of spinal nerves, the upper four of which emerge through the posterior sacral foramina, the fifth pair through the sacral hiatus (termination of the sacral canal). All are mixed nerves (motor and sensory).
**sacral plexus** A nerve plexus formed by the ventral branches of the fourth and fifth lumbar nerves and the first four sacral nerves, from which the sciatic nerve originates.
**sacral vertebra** One of the fused vertebrae forming the sacrum.
**sacrectomy** (sā-krĕk′tō-mē) [L. *sacrum,* sacred, + Gr. *ektome,* excision] Excision of part of the sacrum.
**sacro-** (sā′krō) Combining form meaning *sacrum.*
**sacroanterior** (sā″krō-ăn-tē′rē-or) [L. *sacrum,* sacred, + *anterior,* before] Denoting intrauterine fetal position in which the fetal sacrum is directed anteriorly.
**sacrococcygeal** (sā″krō-kŏk-sĭj′ē-ăl) [″ + Gr. *kokkyx,* coccyx] Concerning the sacrum and coccyx.
**sacrococcygeus** (sāk″rō-kŏk-sĭj′ē-ŭs) One of two small muscles (anterior and posterior) extending from the sacrum to the coccyx.
**sacrocoxalgia** (sā″krō-kŏks-ăl′jē-ă) [″ + *coxa,* hip, + Gr. *algos,* pain] Pain in the sacroiliac joint, usually owing to inflammation. SEE: *sacrocoxitis.*
**sacrocoxitis** (sā″krō-kŏks-ī′tĭs) [″ + ″ + Gr. *itis,* inflammation] Inflammation of the sacroiliac joint. SEE: *sacrocoxalgia.*
**sacrodynia** (sā″krō-dĭn′ē-ă) [″ + *odyne,* pain] Pain in the region of the sacrum.
**sacroiliac** (sā″krō-ĭl′ē-ăk) [″ + *iliacus,* hipbone] Of, or pert. to, the sacrum and ilium.
**sacroiliac joint** The articulation between the sacrum and the innominate bone of the pelvis. Joint movement is limited because of interlocking of the articular surfaces.
**sacroiliitis** (sā″krō-ĭl″ē-ī′tĭs) [″ + ″ + Gr. *itis,* inflammation] Inflammation of the sacroiliac joint.
**sacrolisthesis** (sā″krō-lĭs-thē′sĭs) [″ + Gr. *olisthesis,* a slipping] A deformity in which the sacrum is in front of the last lumbar vertebra. SEE: *spondylolisthesis.*
**sacrolumbar** (sā″krō-lŭm′băr) [″ + *lumbus,* loin] Of, or concerning, the sacrum and lumbar area.
**sacrolumbar angle** The angle formed by articulation of the last lumbar vertebra and the sacrum.
**sacroposterior** (sā″krō-pŏs-tē′rē-or) [″ + *posterus,* behind] Denoting intrauterine fetal position in which the fetal sacrum is directed posteriorly.
**sacrosciatic** (sā″krō-sī-ăt′ĭk) [″ + *sciaticus,* hip joint] Concerning the sacrum and ischium.
**sacrospinal** (sā″krō-spī′năl) [″ + *spina,* thorn] Concerning the sacrum and spine.
**sacrospinalis** [″ + *spina,* thorn] A large

muscle lying on either side of the vertebral column extending from the sacrum to the head. Its two chief components are the iliocostalis and longissimus muscles. SEE: *Muscles Appendix*.

**sacrotomy** (sā-krŏt′ō-mē) [″ + Gr. *tome*, incision] Surgical excision of the lower part of the sacrum.

**sacrouterine** (sā″krō-ū′tĕr-ĭn) [″ + *uterus*, womb] Concerning the sacrum and the uterus.

**sacrovertebral** (sā″krō-vĕr′tĕ-brăl) [″ + *vertebra*, vertebra] Concerning the sacrum and the spinal column.

**sacrovertebral angle** The angle formed by the base of the sacrum and the fifth lumbar vertebra.

**sacrum** (sā′krŭm) [L., sacred] The triangular bone situated dorsal and caudal from the two ilia between the fifth lumbar vertebra and the coccyx. It is formed of five united vertebrae and is wedged between the two innominate bones, its articulations forming the sacroiliac joints. It forms the base of the vertebral column and, with the coccyx, forms the posterior boundary of the true pelvis. The male sacrum is narrower and more curved than the female sacrum. SYN: *sacral bone; vertebra magnum*. SEE: illus.

**sactosalpinx** (săk″tō-săl′pĭnks) [Gr. *saktos*, stuffed, + *salpinx*, tube] A dilated fallopian tube owing to retention of secretions, as in pyosalpinx or hydrosalpinx.

**SAD** *seasonal affective disorder; source-to-axis distance*.

**saddle** A surface or structure that resembles a seat used to ride a horse. The base of artificial dentures is often referred to as a saddle.

***s. area*** The portion of the buttocks, perineum, and thighs that comes in contact with the seat of the saddle when one rides a horse.

***s. back*** Lordosis.

***s. block anesthesia*** SEE: under *anesthesia*.

**sadism** (sā′dĭzm, săd′ĭzm) [Comte Donatien Alphonse François de Sade, Marquis de Sade, 1740–1814] Conscious or unconscious sexual pleasure derived from inflicting mental or physical pain on others. SEE: *algolagnia; masochism*.

**sadist** (sā′dĭst, săd′ĭst) One who practices sadism.

**sadness** A normal emotional feeling of dejection or melancholy that one may experience after an unhappy event.

**sadomasochism** (sā″dō-măs′ĕ-kĭzm, săd″ō-măs′ĕ-kĭzm) Sexual pleasure related to both sadism and masochism.

**sadomasochist** (sā″dō-măs′ĕ-kĭst) One whose personality includes sadistic and masochistic elements.

**Saemisch's ulcer** (sā′mĭsh-ĕs) [Edwin Theodor Saemisch, Ger. ophthalmologist, 1833–1909] Serpiginous infectious ulcer of the cornea.

**safelight** A darkroom device that emits a light of a specified wavelength that causes less fogging of undeveloped film than white light does.

**safe sex** The practice of protecting oneself and one's partner from sexually transmit-

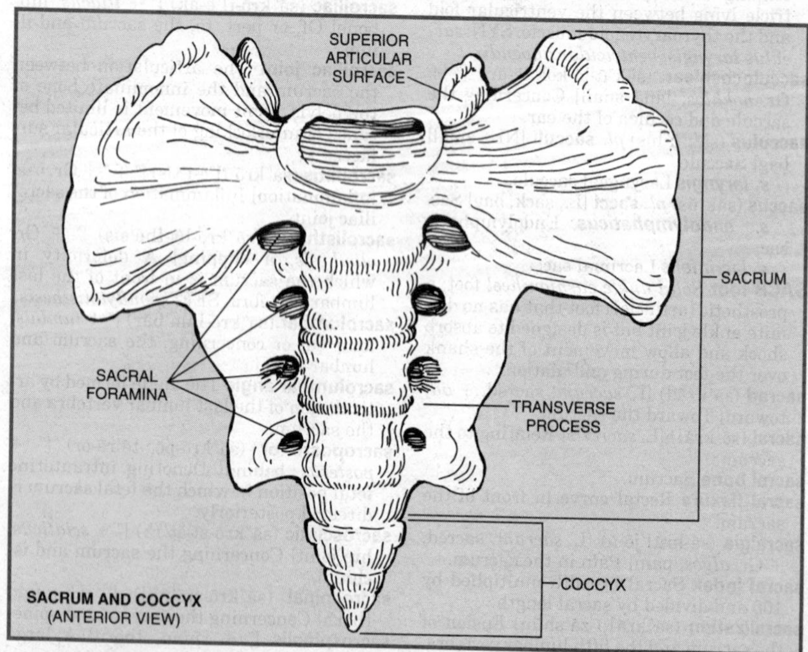

SACRUM AND COCCYX
(ANTERIOR VIEW)

ted diseases (STDs) including AIDS. The only absolutely safe sexual practices are celibacy and masturbation. However, steps can be taken to reduce the risk of contracting or transmitting STDs when performing other sexual activities. If both partners have no clinical or laboratory evidence of AIDS, and neither partner has outside sexual partners or other AIDS risk factors, then the main concern is that effective birth control measures be employed. However, the consistent use of condoms is strongly advised because behavior and circumstances change. If either partner has evidence of infection with HIV (human immunodeficiency virus), condoms should always be used. Any person having casual sexual contacts should avoid anal intercourse and should use condoms for all other sexual activity in which orgasm could lead to semen contacting the skin or mucosa of the partner. A single negative laboratory test for AIDS may be deceiving because an AIDS test may not show positive results until years after infection.

With respect to the possibility of transmission of the human immunodeficiency virus (HIV), the risks may be classified as follows: *Safe:* dry kissing; masturbation of a partner on healthy, intact skin; oral sex with use of a condom; touching; external sexual activities involving urine; fantasy. *Possibly Safe:* condom-protected vaginal or anal intercourse. *Risky:* Wet kissing, oral sex on a woman (without a dental dam or latex or plastic barrier), oral sex on a man not wearing a condom, masturbation of a woman without a latex barrier or use of latex gloves, and masturbation on open or broken skin.

Caution: Alcohol may impair one's judgment regarding the practice of safe sex, resulting in engagement in risky sexual activities.

*Dangerous:* vaginal or anal intercourse without a condom; fisting (insertion of the entire hand into the rectum or vagina); sexual activities involving urine entering another person's body; anal stimulation with the tongue or mouth. SEE: *AIDS; condom, instructions for use; sexually transmitted disease.*

**safflower oil** The oil expressed from the seeds of the safflower plant, *Carthamus tinctorius*. It is high in linoleic acid and low in saturated fatty acids.

**sagittal** (săj′ĭ-tăl) [L. *sagittalis*] Arrow-like; in an anteroposterior direction. SYN: *sagittalis*.

**sagittalis** (săj″ĭ-tā′lĭs) [L.] Sagittal.

**sagittal plane** A vertical plane through the longitudinal axis of the trunk dividing the body into two portions. If it is through the anteroposterior midaxis and divides the body into right and left halves, it is called a *median* or *midsagittal plane*.

**sagittal sulcus** A groove on the inner surface of the parietal bones, forming a channel for the superior sagittal sinus.

**sago** (sā′gō) [Malay *sagu*] A substance prepared from various palms, consisting principally of starches; used as a demulcent and as a food with little residue.

**St. Joseph's Cough Syrup for Children.** Trade name for dextromethorphan hydrobromide.

**Saint Vitus' dance** Sydenham's chorea.

**sal** (săl) [L.] Salt or a saltlike substance.

***s. ammoniac*** Chloride of ammonia.

***s. soda*** Sodium carbonate.

**salaam convulsion** (sŭ-lŏm′) [Arabic *salam*, peace] Nodding spasm.

**salacious** (sĕ-lā′shŭs) [L. *salax*, lustful] Lustful or inciting to lust.

**Salem sump tube** A double-lumen nasogastric tube with an air vent, used to rest the gastrointestinal tract or drain gastric secretions. The vent protects against damage to the gastric mucosa.

**salicylamide** (săl″ĭ-sĭl-ăm′ĭd) The amide of salicylic acid, $C_7H_7NO_2$. An analgesic drug.

**salicylanilide** (săl″ĭ-sĭl-ăn′ĭ-lĭd) An antifungal drug.

**salicylate** (săl″ĭ-sĭl′āt, săl-ĭs′ĭl-āt) Any salt of salicylic acid.

***methyl s.*** The principal constituent of oil of wintergreen. It is applied externally as a counterirritant.

***sodium s.*** A white crystalline substance with a disagreeable, even nauseating, taste; used to reduce pain and temperature. SEE: *acetylsalicylic acid*.

**salicylated** (săl-ĭs′ĭl-āt-ĕd) Impregnated with salicylic acid.

**salicylate poisoning** SEE: *aspirin poisoning*.

**salicylic acid** (săl″ĭ-sĭl′ĭk) $C_7H_6O_3$. A white crystalline acid derived from phenol used to make aspirin; as a preservative and flavoring agent; and in topical treatment of certain skin conditions.

**salicylism** (săl′ĭ-sĭl″ĭzm) A toxic condition caused by an overdose of salicylic acid or its derivatives.

**salicyluric acid** (săl″ĭ-sĭ-lū′rĭk) Acid found in the urine after an individual takes salicylic acid or its derivatives.

**salient** [L. *salio*, to spring, jump] Prominent, conspicuous.

**saline** (sā′lĭn, sā′lēn) [L. *salinus*, of salt] Containing or pert. to salt; salty.

***s. cathartic*** A salt, such as epsom salts, used to produce evacuation of the bowel.

***hypertonic s.*** An aqueous solution of sodium chloride of greater than 0.85%.

***hypotonic s.*** An aqueous solution of sodium chloride of less than 0.85%.

**saline enema** An enema consisting of a salt solution, used to induce peristalsis and evacuation. The salt solutions most frequently used are physiological saline; 1 tsp (4 g) table salt (sodium chloride) dissolved in 1 pt (500 ml) of warm water (115°F or 46.1°C); and epsom salts (magnesium sulfate) 15 to 113 g in a sufficient quantity of warm water to dissolve the salt.

**saline solution** A solution of sodium chloride and distilled water. A 0.9% solution of sodium chloride is considered isotonic to the body. A normal saline solution (one having an osmolality similar to that of blood serum) consists of 0.85% salt solution, which is necessary to maintain osmotic pressure and the stimulation and regulation of muscular activity.

**salinometer** (săl″ĭ-nŏm′ĕ-tĕr) [L. *salinus,* of salt, + *metron,* measure] An instrument for determining the salt content of a solution.

**saliva** (să-lī′vă) [L., spittle] Salivary gland and oral mucous gland fluid; the secretion that begins the process of digesting food. Saliva moistens food for tasting, chewing, and swallowing; initiates digestion of starches, moistens and lubricates mouth parts; and acts as a solvent for excretion of waste products. SYN: *spit* (1); *spittle.*

CHARACTERISTICS: It is normally tasteless, clear, odorless, viscid, and weakly alkaline, being neutralized after being acted on by gastric acid in the stomach. Its specific gravity is 1.002 to 1.006. The amount secreted in 24 hr is estimated to be 1500 ml. The flow varies from 0.2 ml/min from resting glands to 4.0 ml/min with maximum secretion.

COMPOSITION: Inorganic substances in saliva include 99.5% water; salts (chlorides, carbonates, phosphates, sulfates); gases in solution; and sometimes abnormal substances being excreted from the body (e.g., acetone). Organic substances include enzymes (amylase, lysozyme); proteins (serum albumin and globulin, mucin); and small amounts of urea, uric acid, creatine, and amino acids. Cellular elements include epithelial cells and leukocytes.

***artificial s.*** A solution that is useful in treating excessive dryness of the mouth (xerostomia). One such formula is 20 ml of a 4% solution of methylcellulose, 10 ml of glycerin, sufficient normal saline to make 90 ml, and one drop of lemon oil.

**saliva ejector** A device used during dental work to remove saliva.

**salivant** (săl′ĭ-vănt) [L. *saliva,* spittle] Something that stimulates the flow of saliva.

**salivary** (săl′ĭ-vĕr-ē) [L. *salivarius,* slimy] Pert. to, producing, or formed from saliva.

**salivary corpuscle** One of the nucleated spherical bodies in saliva, thought to be modified leukocytes from lymphatic tissue.

**salivary digestion** Digestion occurring in the mouth as a result of the action of salivary enzymes. Salivary amylase (ptyalin) is an enzyme that initiates the breakdown of starch and glycogen. Oral digestion is limited because of the short time that food remains in the mouth, but digestion continues in the stomach until the food becomes acidified by gastric juice. The optimum pH for amylase activity is 6.9. SEE: *digestion.*

**salivary gland** A gland of the oral cavity that secretes saliva. The major glands are paired and include the parotid, below the ear and inside the ramus of the mandible; the sublingual, below the tongue in the anterior floor of the mouth; and the submandibular, below the posterior floor of the mouth, medial to the body of the mandible. Minor salivary glands are numerous in the oral cavity and are named according to their locations: lingual, sublingual, palatal, buccal, labial, and glossopharyngeal. SEE: illus.

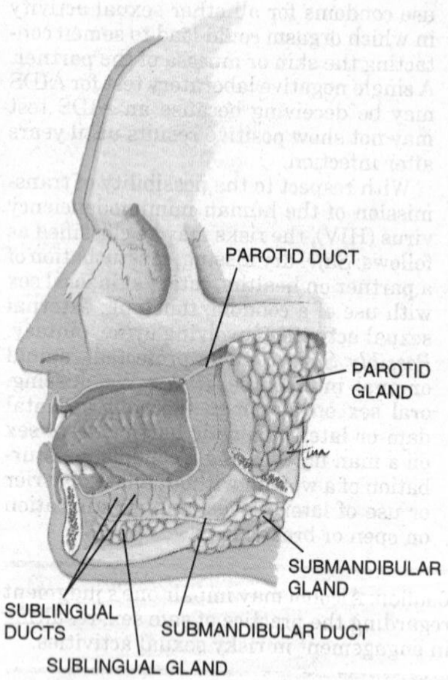


SALIVARY GLANDS

Salivary secretion is under nervous control, being reflexly initiated by mechanical, chemical, or radiant stimuli acting on gustatory receptors (taste buds) in the mouth, olfactory receptors, visual receptors (eyes), or other sense organs. Secretion may also occur as a result of conditioned reflexes, as when one thinks about food or hears a dinner bell. The nerve supply of the salivary glands is from the facial and glossopharyngeal nerves, which are parasympathetic and increase secretion, and from the sympathetic nerves, which decrease secretion. The blood supply is from branches of the external carotid artery.

**salivation** (săl″ĭ-vā′shŭn) [LL. *salivatio,* to spit out] **1.** The act of secreting saliva. **2.** Excessive secretion of saliva. SYN: *pty-*

*alism.*

**salivatory** (săl′ĭ-vă-tor″ē) Producing the secretion of saliva.

**salivolithiasis** (să-lī″vō-lĭ-thī′ă-sĭs) [L. *saliva,* spittle, + Gr. *lithos,* stone, + *-iasis,* condition] Sialolithiasis.

**Salk vaccine** (sŏlk) [Jonas E. Salk, U.S. microbiologist, b. 1914-1995] The first successful poliomyelitis vaccine. It contains three types of formalin-inactivated poliomyelitis viruses and induces immunity against the disease. SEE: *poliomyelitis.*

**sallow** (săl′ō) [AS. *salo*] A sickly yellow, color, usually describing complexion or skin color.

**salmin(e)** (săl′mēn, -mĭn) [L. *salmo,* salmon] $C_{30}H_{57}N_{14}O_6$; a toxic protamine obtained from the spermatozoa of salmon. SEE: *protamine; protein.*

**Salmonella** (săl″mō-nĕl′ă) [Daniel Elmer Salmon, U.S. veterinarian, 1850–1914] A genus of bacteria belonging to the family Enterobacteriaceae. Salmonella are gram-negative, usually motile, rods. More than 1400 species have been classified. Several species are pathogenic, some producing mild gastroenteritis and others a severe and often fatal food poisoning. Those persons preparing food should cook all foods from animal sources thoroughly, refrigerate leftover cooked foods during storage, and wash hands before and after handling foods. Persons should avoid ingesting raw eggs in any form and using cracked eggs. SEE: *egg, raw; salmonellosis.*

NURSING IMPLICATIONS: Patients who have contracted salmonella should drink clear fluids until abdominal pain has subsided. Fluid and electrolyte balance is monitored, and supportive therapy is maintained as indicated. Enteric precautions are used until infection has subsided.

***S. arizonae*** A species that may be isolated from animals and humans. In humans, it may cause gastroenteritis, urinary tract infection, bacteremia, meningitis, osteomyelitis, and brain abscess.

***S. choleraesuis*** A species often found to be the cause of septicemia.

***S. enteritidis*** A species causing gastroenteritis and food poisoning in humans.

***S. paratyphi*** A group of organisms of *Salmonella,* types A, B, and C, that cause paratyphoid fever.

***S. typhi*** A species causing typhoid fever in humans.

***S. typhimurium*** A species frequently isolated from persons having acute gastroenteritis.

**salmonellosis** (săl-mō-nĕ-lō′sĭs) Infestation with bacteria of the genus *Salmonella.* Three forms of salmonella infection occur in humans: enteric fever (typhoid fever); septicemia, which usually is caused by *S. choleraesuis;* and acute gastroenteritis, which can be caused by a variety of species of *Salmonella.*

Outbreaks of gastroenteritis associated with eating undercooked eggs have been found to be related to contamination of the eggs with *Salmonella enteritidis.* The incubation period may be as long as 48 hr; symptoms are nausea, vomiting, chills, diarrhea, fever, and abdominal cramping. The illness is usually self-limiting and lasts from 4 to 10 days. If the diarrhea persists for longer than 10 days another cause should be considered. SEE: *egg, raw.*

TREATMENT: Supportive therapy including fluid replacement is needed. Antibiotics should not be used routinely in treating this condition. Because of the development of bacterial resistance to antibiotics, patients with a severe infection should be given more than one class of antibiotic until the sensitivity of the organism is known.

PREVENTION: Eggs should be stored at 45°F (7.2°C) or less but not frozen. When preparing foods, hands should be washed thoroughly, and only clean, intact eggs and clean equipment should be used. The eggs should be cooked thoroughly (i.e., they should not be "runny"). Cold egg dishes should be stored below 40°F (4.4°C); hot egg dishes should be held above 140°F (60°C). Egg dishes should not be kept at room temperature for more than one hour.

**salpingectomy** (săl″pĭn-jĕk′tō-mē) [Gr. *salpinx,* tube, + *ektome,* excision] The surgical removal of a fallopian tube.

**salpingemphraxis** (săl″pĭn-jĕm-frăk′sĭs) [″ + *emphraxis,* a stoppage] An obstruction of the eustachian tube.

**salpingian** (săl-pĭn′jē-ăn) Concerning the eustachian tube or a fallopian tube.

**salpingion** (săl-pĭn′jē-ŏn) A point at the inferior surface of the apex of the petrous portion of the temporal bone.

**salpingitis** (săl″pĭn-jī′tĭs) [Gr. *salpinx,* tube, + *itis,* inflammation] Inflammation of a fallopian tube. The condition may be acute, subacute, or chronic.

ETIOLOGY: The organisms most often associated with salpingitis are the gonococcus, staphylococcus, streptococcus, chlamydia, colon bacillus, and tubercle bacillus.

***eustachian s.*** Eustachitis.

***gonococcal s.*** Salpingitis due to gonococci.

**salpingo-** Combining form indicating *tube.*

**salpingocatheterism** (săl-pĭng″gō-kăth′ĕt-ĕr-ĭzm) [Gr. *salpinx,* tube, + *katheter,* something inserted, + *-ismos,* condition] Catheterization of the eustachian tube.

**salpingocele** (săl-pĭng′gō-sēl) [″ + *kele,* tumor, swelling] The hernial protrusion of a fallopian tube.

**salpingocyesis** (săl-pĭng″ō-sī-ē′sĭs) [″ + *kyesis,* pregnancy] Tubal pregnancy.

**salpingography** (săl″pĭng-gŏg′ră-fē) [″ + *graphein,* to write] Radiography of the fallopian tubes after the introduction of a radiopaque contrast medium; used in testing for patency of the tubes in investigating infertility.

**salpingolithiasis** (săl-pĭng″gō-lĭ-thī′ă-sĭs) [″+ *lithos,* stone, + *iasis,* condition] The presence of calculi in a fallopian tube.

**salpingolysis** (săl″pĭng-gŏl′ĭ-sĭs) [″ + *lysis,* dissolution] The surgical disruption of adhesions in a fallopian tube.

**salpingo-oophorectomy** (săl-pĭng″gō-ō″ŏf-ō-rĕk′tō-mē) [″ + *oon,* egg, + *phoros,* a bearer, + *ektome,* excision] Excision of an ovary and a fallopian tube. SYN: *oophorosalpingectomy; ovariosalpingectomy; salpingo-ovariectomy.*

**salpingo-oophoritis** (săl-pĭng″ō-ō″ŏf-ō-rī′tĭs) [″ + ″ + ″ + *itis,* inflammation] Inflammation of a fallopian tube and an ovary. SYN: *salpingo-oothecitis.*

**salpingo-oophorocele** (săl-pĭng″gō-ō-ŏf′or-ō-sēl) [Gr. *salpinx,* tube, + *oon,* egg, + *phoros,* a bearer, + *kele,* tumor, swelling] A hernia enclosing an ovary and a fallopian tube.

**salpingo-oothecitis** (săl-pĭng″gō-ō″ō-thē-sī′tĭs) [″ + *ootheke,* ovary, + *itis,* inflammation] Salpingo-oophoritis.

**salpingo-oothecocele** (săl-pĭng″gō-ō″ō-thē′kō-sēl) [″+ ″ + *kele,* tumor, swelling] A hernia of an ovary and a fallopian tube.

**salpingo-ovariectomy** (săl-pĭng″gō-ō″văr-ē-ĕk′tō-mē) [″+ LL. *ovarium,* ovary, + Gr. *ektome,* excision] Salpingo-oophorectomy.

**salpingoperitonitis** (săl-pĭng″gō-pĕr″ĭ-tō-nī′tĭs) [″ + *peritonaion,* peritoneum, + *itis,* inflammation] Inflammation of the serosal covering of the fallopian tubes.

**salpingopexy** (săl-pĭng′ō-pĕk″sē) [″ + *pexis,* fixation] Fixation of a fallopian tube.

**salpingopharyngeal** (săl-pĭng″gō-fă-rĭn′jē-ăl) [″ + *pharynx,* throat] Concerning the eustachian tube and the pharynx.

**salpingopharyngeus** (săl-pĭng″gō-făr-ĭn′jē-ŭs) [″ + *pharynx,* throat] The muscle near the opening of the eustachian tube that raises the nasopharynx.

**salpingoplasty** (săl-pĭng′gō-plăs″tē) [″ + *plassein,* to form] Plastic surgery of a fallopian tube; used in treating female infertility. SYN: *tuboplasty.*

**salpingorrhaphy** (săl″pĭng-gor′ă-fē) [″ + *rhaphe,* seam, ridge] Suture of a fallopian tube.

**salpingosalpingostomy** (săl-pĭng″gō-săl″pĭng-gŏs′tō-mē) [″ + *salpinx,* tube, + *stoma,* mouth] The operation of attaching one fallopian tube to the other.

**salpingoscope** (săl-pĭng′gō-skōp″) [″ + *skopein,* to examine] A device for examining the nasopharynx and the eustachian tube.

**salpingostenochoria** (săl-pĭng″gō-stĕn″ō-kor′ē-ă) [″ + *stenos,* narrow, + *choreia,* dance] A stenosis or stricture of the eustachian tube.

**salpingostomatomy** (săl-pĭng″gō-stō-măt′ō-mē) [″ + *stoma,* mouth, + *tome,* incision] The creation of an artificial opening in a fallopian tube after it has been occluded as a result of inflammation and scarring.

**salpingostomy** (săl-pĭng-ŏs′tō-mē) The surgical opening of a fallopian tube that has been occluded, or for drainage purposes.

**salpingotomy** (săl-pĭng-ŏt′ō-mē) [″ + *tome,* incision] Incision of a fallopian tube.

**salpingo-ureterostomy** (săl-pĭng″gō-ūr-ēt″ĕr-ŏs′tō-mē) [″ + *oureter,* ureter, + *stoma,* mouth] A surgical connection of the ureter and a fallopian tube.

**salpinx** (săl′pĭnks) *pl.* **salpinges** [Gr., tube] A fallopian tube or the eustachian tube.

**salt** [AS. *sealt*] **1.** White crystalline compound occurring in nature, known chemically as sodium chloride, NaCl. **2.** Containing or treated with salt. **3.** To treat with salt. **4.** In the plural, any mineral salt or saline mixture used as an aperient or cathartic, esp. epsom salts or Glauber's salt. **5.** In chemistry, a compound consisting of a positive ion other than hydrogen and a negative ion other than hydroxyl. **6.** A chemical compound resulting from the interaction of an acid and a base.

Salts and water are the inorganic or mineral constituents of the body. They play specific roles in the functions of cells and are indispensable for life. The principal salts are chlorides, carbonates, bicarbonates, sulfates, and phosphates, combined with sodium, potassium, calcium, or magnesium.

In general, salts serve the following roles in the body: maintenance of proper osmotic conditions; maintenance of water balance and regulation of blood volume; maintenance of proper acid-base balance; provision for essential constituents of tissue, esp. bones and teeth; maintenance of normal irritability of muscle and nerve cells; maintenance of condition for coagulation of the blood; provision for essential components of certain enzyme systems, respiratory pigments, and hormones; and regulation of cell membrane and capillary permeability. SEE: *sodium chloride.*

***acid s.*** A salt in which one or more hydrogen atoms remain unreplaced by the hydroxyl (OH) radical.

***basic s.*** A salt retaining the ability to react with an acid radical.

***bile s.*** A salt of glycocholic and taurocholic acid present in bile.

***buffer s.*** A salt that fixes excess amounts of acid or alkali without a change in hydrogen ion concentration.

***double s.*** Any salt formed from two other salts.

***epsom s.*** Magnesium sulfate.

***Glauber's s.*** SEE: *Glauber's salt.*

***glow s.*** Rubbing of the entire body with moist salt for stimulation.

***haloid s.*** A salt made up of a base and a halogen (i.e., chloride, iodide, bromide, fluorine, or astatine).

***hypochlorite s.*** A salt of hypochlorous acid used in household bleach and as an oxidizer, deodorant, and disinfectant.

***iodized s.*** A salt containing 1 part sodium or potassium iodide to 10,000 parts of sodium chloride. It is an important source of iodine in the diet. Its use prevents goiter due to iodine deficiency.

***neutral s.*** Normal s.

***normal s.*** An ionic compound containing no replaceable hydrogen or hydroxyl ions. SYN: *neutral salt.*

***Rochelle s.*** SEE: *Rochelle salt.*

***rock s.*** Natural sodium chloride.

***sea s.*** Sodium chloride obtained from sea water.

***smelling s.*** Aromatized ammonium carbonate.

***substitute s.*** A substance that has a flavor similar to that of salt but is low in sodium content. It is used by individuals whose medical condition requires limited salt intake.

**saltation** (săl-tā′shŭn) [L. *saltatio,* leaping] Act of leaping or dancing, as in chorea.

**saltatory** (săl′tă-tō″rē) Marked by dancing or leaping.

**saltatory conduction** The transmission of a nerve impulse along a myelinated nerve fiber. The action potential occurs only at the nodes of Ranvier, making velocity faster than along unmyelinated fibers.

**salt-free diet** A low-sodium diet that allows 500 mg (0.5 g) or less of salt per day (a diet absolutely free of sodium chloride is impractical). On this diet, table salt should not be added to food, and the salt content of commonly used beverages such as beer should be noted. In some areas, drinking water contains a large amount of sodium. Some medicines (e.g., sodium salicylate) also are quite high in sodium. To help regulate sodium consumption, sodium-containing medicines should be avoided. SEE: *salt.*

**salting out** A method of separating a specific protein from a mixture of proteins by the addition of a salt (e.g., ammonium sulfate).

**salt-losing syndrome** The condition of greatly increased sodium loss from the body as a result of renal disease, adrenocortical insufficiency, or gastrointestinal disease.

**saltpeter, saltpetre** (sawlt-pē′tĕr) [L. *sal,* salt, + *petra,* rock] A common name for potassium nitrate.

***Chile s.*** A common name for sodium nitrate, $NaNO_3$; a crystalline powder, saline in taste and soluble in water.

**salubrious** (să-lū′brē-ŭs) [L. *salubris,* healthful] Promoting or favorable to health; wholesome.

**Saluron** Trade name for hydroflumethiazide.

**salutary** (săl′ū-tā″rē) [L. *salutaris,* health] Healthful; promoting health; curative.

**Salvarsan** (săl′văr-săn) [L. *salvus,* safe, + Gr. *arsen,* arsenic] An arsenical, yellow powder preparation developed by Paul Ehrlich for treatment of syphilis. Since the development of penicillin, there has been little need for Salvarsan. SYN: *arsphenamine.*

**salve** (săv) [AS. *sealf*] **1.** An ointment applied to wounds. **2.** In pharmacology, any ointment or cerate made with a base of a fat, oil, petrolatum, or resin.

**samarium** (să-mā′rē-ŭm) SYMB: Sm. A very rare metallic element. Atomic weight 150.35; atomic number 62; specific gravity approx. 7.50.

**sample 1.** A piece or portion of a whole that demonstrates the characteristics or quality of the whole, such as a specimen of blood. **2.** In research, a portion of a population selected to represent the entire population.

***biased s.*** In epidemiology or medical research, a sample of a group that is not equally represented by the members of that group.

***fetal blood s.*** A small amount of blood drawn from a fetal scalp vein to assess acid-base status. The normal fetal blood pH level is 7.25. Levels between 7.20 and 7.24 reflect a preacidotic state; levels below 7.20 indicate acidosis and fetal jeopardy.

**sampling** The process of selecting a portion or part to represent the whole.

***random s.*** A method of selecting a sample population using a table of random numbers to select the sample from a listing of the population.

**sanatorium** (săn″ă-tō′rē-ŭm) [L. *sanatorius,* healing] Sanitarium.

**sand** (sănd) [AS.] Fine grains of disintegrated rock.

***auditory s.*** Crystals of calcium carbonate in the utricle and saccule of the inner ear. SYN: *ear dust; otoconium; otolith.*

***brain s.*** Concretion of matter near the base of the pineal gland. SYN: *acervulus cerebri.*

**sandflies** Flies of the order Diptera belonging to the genus *Phlebotomus.* They transmit sandfly fever, Oroya fever, and various types of leishmaniasis.

**sandfly fever** A mild viral disease that clinically resembles influenza, except for the absence of respiratory symptoms. The causative organism, any one of three species of arboviruses, is transmitted by the common sandfly *Phlebotomus papatasii,* a small, hairy, blood-sucking midge that bites at night and has a limited flight range. The disease occurs in tropical and subtropical areas that experience long periods of hot, dry weather. There is no specific therapy. SYN: *pappataci fever; phlebotomus fever.*

**Sandhoff's disease** A rare form of Tay-Sachs disease in which two essential enzymes (hexosaminidase A and B) for metabolizing gangliosides are absent. In Tay-Sachs disease only one enzyme, hexosaminidase A, is absent.

**Sandril** Trade name for reserpine.

**Sandwith's bald tongue** (sănd′wĭths) [Fleming M. Sandwith, Brit. physician,

1777–1843] An abnormally clean tongue seen in the late stages of pellagra.

**SANE** *Sexual Assault Nurse Examiner.*

**sane** (sān) [L. *sanus,* healthy] Sound of mind; mentally normal.

**Sanfilippo's disease** [S. J. Sanfilippo, contemporary U.S. pediatrician] Mucopolysaccharidosis III.

**sanguicolous** (săng-gwĭk′ō-lŭs) [L. *sanguis,* blood, + *colere,* to dwell] Inhabiting the blood, as a parasite.

**sanguiferous** (săng-gwĭf′ĕr-ŭs) [″ + *ferre,* to carry] Conducting or containing blood, as the circulatory organs.

**sanguine** (săng′gwĭn) [L. *sanguineus,* bloody] **1.** Optimistic; cheerful. **2.** Plethoric, bloody; marked by abundant and active blood circulation, particularly a ruddy complexion. **3.** Pert. to, or consisting of, blood.

**sanguineous** (săng-gwĭn′ē-ŭs) [L. *sanguineus,* bloody] **1.** Bloody; relating to blood. **2.** Having an abundance of blood. SYN: *plethoric.*

**sanguinopurulent** (săng″gwĭ-nō-pū′rū-lĕnt) [″ + *purulentus,* full of pus] Concerning or containing blood and pus.

**sanguirenal** (săng″gwĭ-rē′năl) [L. *sanguis,* blood, + *ren,* kidney] Pert. to the blood supply of the kidneys.

**sanguis** (săng′gwĭs) [L.] Blood.

**sanguisuga** (săng-gwĭ-sū′gă) [″ + *sugere,* to suck] A leech or bloodsucker. SEE: *Hirudo.*

**sanies** (sā′nē-ēz) [L., thin, fetid pus] A thin, fetid, greenish discharge from a wound or ulcer, appearing as pus tinged with blood.

**saniopurulent** (sā″nē-ō-pū′roo-lĕnt) [L. *sanies,* thin, fetid pus, + *purulentus,* full of pus] Having characteristics of sanies and pus; pert. to a fetid, serous, blood-tinged discharge containing pus.

**sanitarian** (săn″ĭ-tā′rē-ăn) [L. *sanitas,* health] A person who by training and experience is skilled in sanitation and public health.

**sanitarium** (săn-ĭ-tā′rē-ŭm) [L. *sanitas,* health] An institution for the treatment and recuperation of persons having physical or mental disorders. SYN: *sanatorium.*

**sanitary** (săn′ĭ-tā″rē) [L. *sanitas,* health] **1.** Promoting or pert. to conditions that are conducive to good health. **2.** Clean, free of dirt.

**sanitary napkin** Perineal pad, esp. one used for absorbing menstrual fluid. SEE: *menstrual tampon; menstruation.*

**sanitation** (săn″ĭ-tā′shŭn) [L. *sanitas,* health] The formulation and application of measures to promote and establish conditions favorable to health, esp. public health. SEE: *hygiene.*

**sanitization** (săn″ĭ-tī-zā′shŭn) [L. *sanitas,* health] The act of making sanitary.

**sanitize** (săn′ĭ-tīz) **1.** To make sanitary. **2.** In food processing and preparation, to inactivate microorganisms on equipment and surfaces. Chemicals, heat, and ionizing radiation can be used as sanitizing agents.

**sanitizer** An agent that reduces the number of bacterial contaminants to safe levels as judged by public health requirements. Usually used to describe agents applied to eating and drinking utensils and dairy equipment. All chemicals are removed from equipment and surfaces before food preparation or processing.

**sanity** (săn′ĭ-tē) Soundness of health or mind; mentally normal.

**San Joaquin valley fever** Coccidioidomycosis.

**SA node** Sinoatrial node of the heart.

**santonin** (săn′tō-nĭn) A colorless, crystalline substance obtained from the unexpanded flower heads of plants of the genus *Artemisia cina.*

ACTION/USES: This vermifuge against the roundworm is not used because of its toxicity.

**$SaO_2$** The saturation of the arterial blood with oxygen, expressed as a percentage. $SaO_2$ can be monitored noninvasively with a pulse oximeter. It is normally greater than 96%.

**sap** (săp) [AS. *saep*] **1.** Any fluid essential to the life and vitality of a living structure. **2.** To cause gradual exhaustion or weakness, as to sap one's strength.

***cell s.*** Hyaloplasm.

***nuclear s.*** Karyolymph.

**saphena** (să-fē′nă) *pl.* **saphenae** [Gr. *saphenes,* manifest] A saphenous vein.

**saphenectomy** (săf″ĕ-nĕk′tō-mē) [″ + *ektome,* excision] The surgical removal of a saphenous vein.

**saphenous** (să-fē′nŭs) Pert. to, or associated with, a saphenous vein or nerve in the leg.

**saphenous nerve** A deep branch of the femoral nerve. In the lower leg, it follows the long saphenous vein that supplies the medial side of the leg, ankle, and foot.

**saphenous opening** An oval aperture in the fascia in the inner and upper part of the thigh, transmitting the saphenous vein below Poupart's ligament. SYN: *fossa ovalis.*

**saphenous vein** One of two superficial veins, the great and small, passing up the leg. The great saphenous vein extends from the foot to the saphenous opening; the small vein runs behind the outer malleolus up the back of the leg, joining the popliteal vein. SYN: *saphena.*

**saponification** (să-pŏn″ĭ-fĭ-kā′shŭn) [L. *sapo,* soap, + *facere,* to make] **1.** Conversion into soap; chemically, the hydrolysis or the splitting of fat by an alkali yielding glycerol and three molecules of alkali salt of the fatty acid, the soap. **2.** In chemistry, hydrolysis of an ester into its corresponding alcohol and acid (free or in the form of a salt).

***s. number*** In analysis of fats, the number of milligrams of potassium hydroxide needed to saponify 1 g of oil or fat.

**saponify** (să-pŏn′ĭ-fī) To convert into a soap, as when fats are treated with an alkali to produce a free alcohol plus the salt of the fatty acid. Thus, stearin, saponified with sodium hydroxide, yields the alcohol glycerol plus the soap sodium stearate.

**saponin** (săp′ō-nĭn) [Fr. *saponine,* soap] An unabsorbable glucoside contained in the roots of some plants that forms a lather in an aqueous solution. Saponins cause hemolysis of red blood cells even in high dilutions. When taken orally, they may cause diarrhea and vomiting.

**sapophore** (săp′ō-for) [L. *sapor,* taste, + Gr. *phoros,* bearing] The component of a molecule that gives a substance its taste.

**saporific** (săp″ō-rĭf′ĭk) [NL. *saporificus,* producing taste] Imparting a taste or flavor.

**sapphism** (săf′ĭzm) [Sappho, Gr. poetess, 7th-century B.C.] Lesbianism.

**sapro-** Combining form meaning *putrid, rotten.*

**saprobes** (să′prōbs) [Gr. *sapros,* putrid, + *bios,* life] Organisms such as fungi that live as parasites because they do not possess photosynthetic pigments.

**saprogenic** (săp″rō-jĕn′ĭk) Causing putrefaction, or resulting from it.

**saprophilous** (săp-rŏf′ĭl-ŭs) [Gr. *sapros,* putrid, + *philein,* to love] Living on decaying or dead substances, as a microorganism. SYN: *saprophytic.*

**saprophyte** (săp′rō-fīt) [″ + *phyton,* plant] Any organism living on decaying or dead organic matter. Most of the higher fungi are saprophytes. SEE: *parasite.* **saprophytic** (-t′ĭk), *adj.*

**saquinavir** A protease inhibitor used in treating HIV infection in combination with other antiviral drugs, such as zidovudine.

**Sarcina** (săr′sĭ-nă) [L., bundle] A genus of spherical saprophytic bacteria of the family Micrococcaceae. The individual organisms remain adherent to each other after splitting in three planes. This process yields square tetrads or cubical packets.

**sarcina** (săr′sĭ-nă) *pl.* **sarcinas, sarcinae** Any organism of the genus *Sarcina.* SEE: *bacteria* for illus.

**sarcitis** (săr-sī′tĭs) [Gr. *sarx,* flesh, + *itis,* inflammation] Inflammation of muscle tissue. SYN: *myositis.*

**sarco-** Combining form meaning *flesh.*

**sarcoadenoma** (săr″kō-ăd″ĕn-ō′mă) [Gr. *sarx,* flesh, + *aden,* gland, + *oma,* tumor] A fleshy tumor of a gland. SYN: *adenosarcoma.*

**sarcocarcinoma** (săr″kō-kăr″sĭn-ō′mă) [″ + *karkinos,* crab, + *oma,* tumor] A malignant tumor of sarcomatous and carcinomatous types.

**sarcocele** (săr′kō-sēl) [″ + *kele,* tumor, swelling] A fleshy tumor of the testicle.

**sarcocyst** (săr′kō-sĭst) [″ + *kystis,* bladder] An elongated tubular body produced by *Sarcocystis.*

**Sarcocystis** (săr″kō-sĭs′tĭs) [″ + *kystis,* bladder] A genus of sporozoa found in the muscles of higher vertebrates (reptiles, birds, and mammals).

***S. lindemanni*** A species infesting the muscles of humans, causing myositis, eosinophilia, and fever.

**Sarcodina** (săr-kō-dī′nă) [″ + *eidos,* form, shape] A subphylum of protozoa that includes the order Amoebida. It is characterized by pseudopod locomotion.

**sarcoid** (săr′koyd) [″ + *eidos,* form, shape] **1.** Resembling flesh. **2.** A small epithelioid tubercle-like lesion characteristic of sarcoidosis.

**sarcoidosis** (săr″koyd-ō′sĭs) [″ + ″ + *osis,* condition] A chronic multisystem disease of unknown etiology characterized by infiltration of the affected organs by T lymphocytes, mononuclear phagocytes, and granulomas that alter the tissue architecture.

SYMPTOMS: The clinical symptoms may be generalized or focused on the affected organs. The lungs are usually involved and this causes dyspnea on exertion and, rarely, wheezing. There may be lymphadenopathy, esp. in the intrathoracic area. Skin changes, including erythema nodosum, plaques, maculopapular eruptions, and subcutaneous nodules, occur in approx. 25% of the cases. Almost any other organ system may be involved.

DIAGNOSIS: Diagnosis is made by a combination of clinical, radiographic, and histologic findings.

TREATMENT: Glucocorticoids are the first choice for therapy. If these can't be used then methotrexate, chloroquine, azathioprine, or oxyphenbutazone should be tried.

PROGNOSIS: Prognosis is generally good; however, fatalities occur in approx. 10% of patients.

**sarcolemma** (săr″kō-lĕm′ă) [″ + *lemma,* husk] The cell membrane of a muscle cell. Invaginations called transverse tubules (T-tubules) penetrate the cytoplasm adjacent to the myofibrils and carry the action potential to the interior of the muscle cell.

**sarcology** (săr-kŏl′ō-jē) [″ + *logos,* word, reason] The branch of medicine dealing with study of the soft tissues of the body.

**sarcolysis** (săr-kŏl′ĭ-sĭs) [″ + *lysis,* dissolution] Decomposition of the soft tissues or flesh.

**sarcoma** (săr-kō′mă) *pl.* **sarcomata** [″ + *oma,* tumor] A cancer arising from connective tissue such as muscle or bone, which may affect the bones, bladder, kidneys, liver, lungs, parotids, and spleen.

***alveolar soft part s.*** A malignant neoplasm composed of a reticular stroma of connective tissue surrounding clumps of large round cells.

***botryoid s.*** A sarcoma of the uterus composed of a polypoid mass of soft edematous tissues. This type of cancer is most often seen in infants and children.

***endometrial s.*** A malignant neoplasm

of the endometrial stroma.

***giant-cell s.*** A sarcoma from cancellous bone tissue with large cells with many nuclei. A special type called an epulis is seen in the jaw.

***osteogenic s.*** A sarcoma composed of osseous tissue containing variously shaped cells.

***reticulum cell s.*** A variety of malignant lymphoma involving the lymph nodes and other lymphatic tissue.

***spindle cell s.*** A sarcoma consisting of small and large spindle-shaped cells.

**sarcomatoid** (sar-kō′mă-toyd) [Gr. *sarx,* flesh, + *oma,* tumor, + *eidos,* form, shape] Resembling a sarcoma.

**sarcomatosis** (săr″kō-mă-tō′sĭs) [″ + ″ + *osis,* condition] A condition marked by the presence and spread of a sarcoma; sarcomatous degeneration.

**sarcomatous** (săr-kō′mă-tŭs) Of the nature of, or like, a sarcoma.

**sarcomere** (săr′kō-mēr) [″ + *meros,* a part] The contraction unit of the myofibrils of muscle tissue, made of myosin and actin filaments arranged between two Z disks.

**sarcomphalocele** (săr″kŏm-făl′ō-sēl) [″ + *omphalos,* umbilicus, + *kele,* tumor, swelling] A fleshy tumor of the umbilicus.

**Sarcophagidae** (săr″kō-făj′ĭ-dē) [Gr. *sarx,* flesh, + *phagein,* to eat] The family of the order Diptera that includes the flesh flies. Females deposit their eggs or larvae on the decaying flesh of dead animals. Larvae of two genera, *Sarcophaga* and *Wohlfahrtia,* frequently infest open sores and wounds of humans, giving rise to cutaneous myiasis.

**sarcoplasm** (săr′kō-plăzm) [″ + LL. *plasma,* form, mold] The cytoplasm of muscle cells, esp. striated muscle cells.

**sarcoplasmic** (săr″kō-plăz′mĭk) Concerning or containing sarcoplasm.

**Sarcoptes** (săr-kŏp′tēz) A genus of Acarina that includes the mites that infest humans and animals. *Sarcoptes scabiei* causes scabies in humans. SEE: illus.

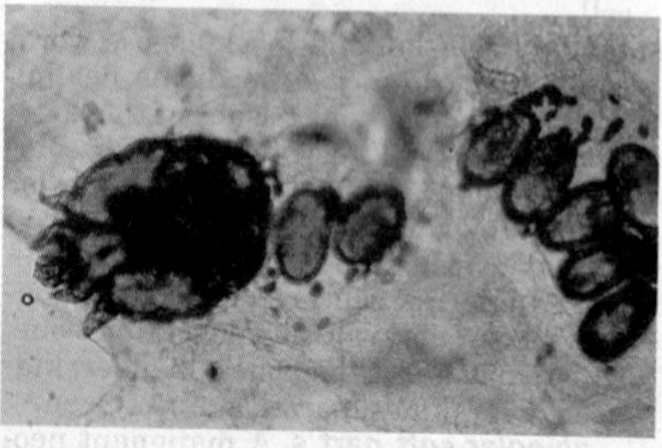

SARCOPTES

ADULT, EGGS, AND FECES IN SKIN SPECIMEN (ORIG. MAG. ×100)

**Sarcoptidae** (săr-kŏp′tĭ-dē) A family of mites of the order Acarina, class Arachnida, that includes *Sarcoptes scabiei,* the causative agent of scabies or itch in humans and of mange and scab in other animals.

**sarcosis** (săr-kō′sĭs) [″ + *osis,* condition] Abnormal formation of flesh.

**sarcosome** (săr′kō-sōm) [″ + *soma,* body] Former term for *mitochondria,* particularly of muscle cells.

**Sarcosporidia** (săr″kō-spō-rĭd′ē-ă) [″ + *sporos,* a seed] An order of protozoa that belong to the class Sporozoa and are parasitic in the muscles of higher vertebrates. It includes the genus *Sarcocystis.*

**sarcosporidiosis** (săr″kō-spō-rĭd″ē-ō′sĭs) [″ + ″ + *osis,* condition] Infestation with organisms of the order Sarcosporidia or the condition produced by them.

**sarcostosis** (săr″kŏs-tō′sĭs) [″ + *osteon,* bone, + *osis,* condition] Ossification of fleshy or muscular tissue.

**sarcostyle** (săr′kō-stīl) [″ + *stylos,* a column] Any one of the fine longitudinal fibrillae of a striated muscle fiber.

**sarcotubule** (săr″kō-tū′būl) Term previously used for the sarcoplasmic reticulum of striated muscle cells.

**sarcous** (săr′kŭs) [Gr. *sarko,* flesh] Concerning flesh or muscle.

**sarin (GB)** Isopropylmethylphosphonofluoridate. An extremely toxic nerve gas.

**SART** *Sexual Assault Response Team.*

**sartorius** (săr-tō′rē-ŭs) [L. *sartor,* tailor] A long, ribbon-shaped muscle in the leg that functions to flex, abduct, and laterally rotate the thigh. This muscle, the longest in the body, enables the crossing of the legs in the tailor's position, the function for which it is named. It also aids in the flexing of the knee. SEE: *Muscles Appendix.*

**sashimi** A general term for a food made of raw fish that can be the source of infections of human tissues.

**sat** *saturated.*

**satellite** (săt′l-īt) [L. *satelles,* attendant] A small structure attached to a larger one, esp. a minute body attached to a chromosome by a slender chromatin filament.

***bacterial s.*** A bacterial colony that grows best when close to a colony of another microorganism.

**satellitosis** (săt″l-ī-tō′sĭs) [″ + Gr. *osis,* condition] The accumulation of neuroglial cells about neurons of the central nervous system. This condition is seen in certain degenerative and inflammatory conditions.

**satiety** (să-tī′ĕt-ē) [L. *satietas,* enough] Being full to satisfaction, esp. with food.

***center s.*** An area in the hypothalamus that, following a meal, senses a feeling of satiety and thus inhibits the urge to eat by acting on the feeding center, also located in the hypothalamus.

**saturated** (săt′ū-rā″tĕd) [L. *saturare,* to fill] Holding all that can be absorbed, received, or combined, as a solution in which no more of a substance can be dissolved. This term is applied to hydrocarbons in which the maximum number of hydrogen atoms is present and there are no double or triple bonds between the carbon atoms.

**saturated compound** An organic compound with all carbon bonds filled. It does not contain double or triple bonds. SEE: *unsaturated compound.*

**saturated hydrocarbon** A carbon-hydrogen compound with all carbon bonds filled so there are no double or triple bonds. SEE: *polyunsaturated.*

**saturation** (săt″ū-rā′shŭn) **1.** State in which all of a substance that can be dissolved in a solution is dissolved. Adding more of the substance will not increase the concentration. **2.** In organic chemistry, to have all available carbon atom valences satisfied so that there are no double or triple bonds between the carbon atoms.

**saturation index** In hematology, the amount of hemoglobin present in a known volume of blood compared with the normal.

**saturation oxygen** The ratio of amount of oxygen present in a known volume of blood to amount of oxygen that could be carried by that volume of blood.

**saturation time** The time required for the arterial blood of a person inhaling pure oxygen to become saturated.

**saturnine** (săt′ŭr-nīn) [L. *saturnus,* lead] Concerning or produced by lead.

**saturnine breath** Sweet breath produced by lead poisoning.

**saturnism** (săt′ŭr-nĭzm) [″ + Gr. *-ismos,* condition] Lead poisoning. SYN: *plumbism.*

**satyriasis** (săt-ĭ-rī′ă-sĭs) [LL.] An excessive, and often uncontrollable, sexual drive in men. SYN: *satyromania.* SEE: *nymphomania.*

**satyromania** (săt″ĭ-rō-mā′nē-ă) Satyriasis.

**saucerization** (saw″sĕr-ĭ-zā′shŭn) The creation of a shallow area in tissue either surgically or owing to trauma.

**sauna** An enclosure in which a person is exposed to moderate to very high temperatures and high humidity, produced by water poured on heated stones. A stay in the sauna may be followed by a cool bath or shower. Sauna water is not sterile and may contain harmful microorganisms, including yeasts and molds. Even though the sauna has no proven benefits in preventing illnesses or promoting fitness, the regimen does help to promote relaxation, relieve aches and pains, and loosen stiff joints.

---

Caution: Saunas are not advised for those with fever, those who are dehydrated, or those who are unable to sweat. Those who have recently used alcohol or have participated in strenuous exercise should not use a sauna. If soft tissue has been traumatized in the past 24 to 48 hr, the sauna should not be used. Prolonged exposure to the sauna may be dangerous due to induced hyperpyrexia, dehydration, and renal failure.

---

**saw** [AS. *sagu*] A cutting instrument with an edge of sharp toothlike projections; used esp. for cutting bone in surgery.

**saxifragant** (săks-ĭf′ră-gănt) [L. *saxum,* rock, + *frangere,* to break] Dissolving or breaking calculi, esp. in the bladder.

**saxitoxin** (săk″sĭ-tŏk′sĭn) A toxin obtained from some forms of marine life, including mussels, clams, and plankton. It is the active ingredient in paralytic shellfish poisoning. If ingested, saxitoxin can produce death in hours; if inhaled, it can be lethal in minutes.

**Sayre's jacket** (sārz) [Lewis Albert Sayre, U.S. surgeon, 1820–1900] A jacket of plaster of paris worn to support the spine in vertebral diseases.

**Sb** Symbol for the element antimony.

**$SbCl_3$** Antimony trichloride.

**SBE** *subacute bacterial endocarditis.*

**$Sb_2O_5$** Antimonic oxide; antimony pentoxide.

**$Sb_4O_6$** Antimonious oxide.

**Sc** Symbol for the element scandium.

**s.c.** *subcutaneously.*

**scab** (skăb) [ME. *scabbe*] **1.** Crust of a cutaneous sore, wound, ulcer, or pustule formed by drying of the discharge. **2.** To become covered with a crust.

**scabicide** (skā′bĭ-sīd) An agent that kills mites, esp. the causative agent of scabies. SYN: *scabieticide.*

**scabies** (skā′bēz) [L. *scabies,* itch] A highly communicable skin disease caused by an arachnid, *Sarcoptes scabiei,* variety *hominis,* the itch mite. The impregnated females live in burrows that appear as slightly discolored lines several millimeters to several centimeters in length. The eggs are deposited within the tunnel hatch within 3 to 5 days. The larvae molt into nymphs on the skin surface and mature in 2 to 3 weeks. Mature insects mate, and the gravid female invades the skin to begin a new cycle. Scabies is transmitted by direct contact with infected persons, and rarely by fomites. SYN: *itch* (2). SEE: illus.; *Nursing Diagnoses Appendix*. **scabietic** (-ĕt′ĭk), *adj.*

SYMPTOMS: Scabies manifests as papules, vesicles, pustules, and burrows, and causes intense itching resulting in eczema. The body parts most commonly affected are the hands, between the fingers, the wrists, axillae, genitalia, beneath the breasts, and the inner aspect of the thighs.

DIAGNOSIS: Mites are identified in tissue scraped from burrows, lesions, or fresh papules.The clinical appearance is also usually diagnostic.

TREATMENT: The treatment of choice for children 2 months and older is permethrin 5% cream applied once to the entire skin area, avoiding the eyes, nose, and mouth. The cream is thoroughly

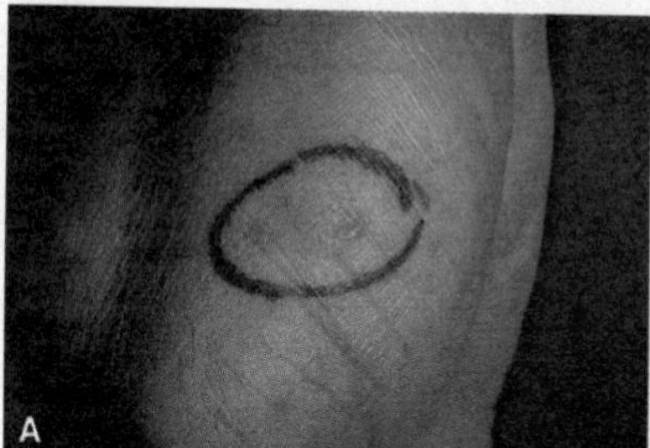


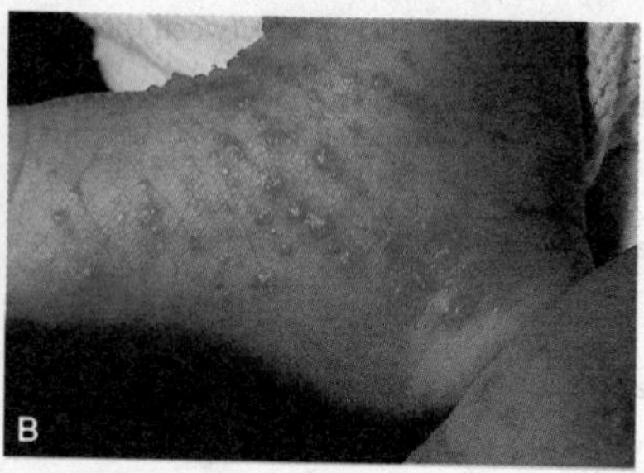


SCABIES

(A) BURROW ON PALM, (B) VESICULAR ERUPTION ON INFANT'S FOOT

washed off after 8 to 10 hr. The fingernails should be trimmed to prevent the harboring of mites. If the hands are washed, the cream must be reapplied. For adults, permethrin 5% cream or lindane 1% lotion is applied and left on overnight for 8 to 14 hr before being thoroughly washed off. Pregnant women and infants under 2 months of age should be treated with 6% to 10% precipitated sulfur in petrolatum daily for 3 days. Patients should be warned that itching may be present for up to 3 weeks after successful therapy.

***Norwegian s.*** A rare form of scabies in which the mites are present in great number.

**scabieticide** (skā″bē-ĕt′ĭ-sīd) [″ + *cidus,* killing] Scabicide.

**scabiphobia** (skă″bĭ-fō′bē-ă) [″ + Gr. *phobos,* fear] An abnormal fear of acquiring scabies.

**scabrities** (skā-brĭsh′ē-ēz) [L. *scaber,* rough] A scaly, roughened condition of the skin.

***s. unguium*** Morbid degeneration of the nails, making them rough, thick, distorted, and separated from the flesh at the root; symptomatic of syphilis and leprosy.

**scala** (skā′lă) [L. *scala,* staircase] Any one of the three spiral passages of the cochlea of the inner ear.

***s. media*** The cochlear duct that lies between the scala tympani and scala vestibuli. Its floor contains the spiral organ of Corti. It extends from the saccule to the tip of the cochlea and is filled with endolymph.

***s. tympani*** The cochlear duct filled with perilymph lying below the spiral lamina. It extends from the tip of the cochlea to the round cochlear window.

***s. vestibuli*** The cochlear duct forming the upper portion of the osseous canal. It lies above the spiral lamina and extends from the oval window to the tip of the cochlea, where it communicates with the scala tympani through an aperture, the helicotrema.

**scald** (skŏld) [ME. *scalden,* to burn with hot liquid] **1.** A burn to the skin or flesh caused by moist heat and hot vapors, as steam. **2.** To cause a burn with hot liquid or steam.

When the heat applied is approx. equivalent, a scald is deeper than a burn from dry heat and should be treated as a burn. Healing is slower and scar formation greater in scalds. Emergency treatment of a scalded area should be the immediate application of cold in the most readily available form, (i.e., ice packs or immersion of the part in very cold water). This should be continued for at least 1 hr.

**scalded skin syndrome, staphylococcal** Necrosis of the epidermal layer of the skin with very little damage to the underlying dermis. Initially, there is an upper body and facial rash, fever, and extremely tender skin. Then bullae, filled with clear fluid, form. As much as 80% of the skin may be affected. The syndrome is caused by an exotoxin produced by one of several phage types of staphylococci.

TREATMENT: Beta-lactamase–resistant synthetic penicillin is given. The bullae and denuded skin should be treated symptomatically. Uncomplicated lesions heal without scarring.

**scale** (skāl) **1.** [O. Fr. *escale,* husk] A small, thin, dry exfoliation shed from the upper layers of skin. Shedding of scales from the skin in small amounts is normal. More shedding is seen in cutaneous disorders such as squamous eczema, seborrhea sicca, psoriasis, ichthyosis, syphilis, lupus erythematosus, pityriasis rosea, and tinea tonsurans. SEE: *macule; rash.* **2.** A film of tartar encrusting the teeth. **3.** To remove a film of tartar from the teeth. **4.** To form a scale on. **5.** To shed scales. **6.** [ME. *scole,* balance] An instrument for weighing. **7.** [L. *scala,* staircase] A graduated or proportioned measure, a series of tests, or an instrument for measuring quantities or for rating some individual intelligence characteristics.

***absolute s.*** Scale used for indicating low temperatures based on absolute zero. SEE: *absolute temperature; absolute zero.*

***centigrade s.*** Celsius scale.

***s. of contrast*** The range of densities on a radiograph; the number of tonal grays that are visible.

***hydrogen ion s.*** A scale used to express the degree of acidity or alkalinity of a solution. It extends from 0.00 (total acidity) to 14 (total alkalinity), the numbers running in inverse order of hydrogen ion concentration. The pH value is the negative logarithm of the hydrogen ion concentration of a solution, expressed in moles per liter.

As the hydrogen ion concentration decreases, a change of 1 pH unit means a 10-fold decrease in hydrogen ion concentration. Thus a solution with a pH of 1.0 is 10 times more acid than one with a pH of 2.0 and 100 times more acid than one with a pH of 3.0. A pH of 7.0 indicates neutrality.

As the hydrogen ion concentration varies in a definite reciprocal manner with the hydroxyl ion ($OH^-$) concentration, a pH reading above 7.0 indicates alkalinity. The arterial blood is slightly alkaline, having a normal pH range of 7.35 to 7.45. SEE: *pH.*

**scalene** (skā-lēn′) [Gr. *skalenos,* uneven] **1.** Having unequal sides and angles, said of a triangle. **2.** Designating a scalenus muscle.

***s. tubercle*** Lisfranc's tubercle.

**scalenectomy** (skā″lĕ-nĕk′tō-mē) [″ + *ektome,* excision] Resection of any of the scalenus muscles.

**scaleniotomy** (skā-lēn″ē-ŏt′ō-mē) [″ + *tome,* incision] Incision of scalenus muscles near their insertion to check expansive movements in tuberculosis of the apex of the lung.

**scalenotomy** (skā″lĕ-nŏt′ō-mē) [″ + *tome,* incision] Surgical division of one or more of the scalenus muscles.

**scalenus** (skā-lē′nŭs) [L., uneven] One of three deeply situated muscles on each side of the neck, extending from the tubercles of the transverse processes of the third through sixth cervical vertebrae to the first or second rib. The three muscles are the scalenus anterior (anticus), medius, and posterior. SEE: *Muscles Appendix.*

**scalenus syndrome** A symptom complex characterized by brachial neuritis with or without vascular or vasomotor disturbance in the upper extremities. Also called *scalenus anticus syndrome.*

SYMPTOMS: The symptoms are not clearly defined, but pain, tingling, and numbness may occur anywhere from the shoulder to the fingers. Small muscles of the hand or even the deltoid or other muscles of the arm atrophy.

TREATMENT: The posture should be corrected, and sometimes the arm and shoulder are immobilized. When relief is not obtained, surgical correction may be required.

**scaler** (skā′lĕr) [O. Fr. *escale,* husk] **1.** A dental instrument used in the procedure of removing calculus from the teeth. **2.** A device for counting pulses detected by a radiation detector.

***ultrasonic s.*** A device that uses high-frequency vibration to remove stains and adherent deposits on the teeth.

**scaling** (skāl′ĭng) [O. Fr. *escale,* husk] The removal of calculus from the teeth.

**scall** (skawl) [Norse *skalli,* baldhead] Dermatitis of the scalp producing a crusted scabby eruption.

**scalp** (skălp) [ME., sheath] The hairy integument of the head. In anatomy, this includes the skin, dense subcutaneous tissue, occipitofrontalis muscle with the galea aponeurotica, loose subaponeurotic tissue, and cranial periosteum.

**scalpel** (skăl′pĕl) [L. *scalpellum,* knife] A small, straight surgical knife with a convex edge and thin keen blade. SEE: illus.

**scalpriform** (skăl′prĭ-form) [L. *scalprum,* knife, + *forma,* shape] Shaped like a chisel.

**scalprum** (skăl′prŭm) *pl.* **scalpra** [L., knife] **1.** A toothed instrument for removal of carious bone or for trephining. **2.** A large scalpel. **3.** The cutting edge of an incisor tooth.

**scalp tourniquet** A tourniquet applied to the scalp during I.V. administration of antineoplastic drugs to restrict blood flow to the hair-bearing portion of the scalp. This procedure helps prevent the cranial alopecia that may accompany the chemotherapy used to treat certain types of cancer.

**scaly** (skā′lē) [O. Fr. *escale,* husk] Resembling or characterized by scales.

**scan 1.** Scintiscan. **2.** An image obtained from computed tomography, ultrasound, or magnetic resonance imaging.

**scandium** [L. *Scandia,* Scandinavia] SYMB: Sc. A rare metal belonging to the aluminum group; atomic weight 44.956; atomic number 21.

**scanning 1.** Recording on a photographic plate the emission of radioactive waves from a specific substance injected into the body. The radioactive agent selected is concentrated in a specific tissue, such as thyroid, brain, or liver. **2.** The process of obtaining different images of a specified anatomical part through computed tomography, ultrasound, or magnetic resonance imaging.

***s. electron microscope*** ABBR: SEM. An electron microscope that scans an image point by point and displays the image on a photographic film or television screen. The SEM, unlike other types of microscopes, allows a three-dimensional view of the tissues, and tissues do not need to be extensively handled and prepared to be visualized. The magnification ranges from 20 to 100,000 times.

***radioisotope s.*** Recording of radioisotope emanations from tissues into which the radioactive substances have been injected. The scanner can be moved around the site and a multiview picture obtained.

**scanty** (skăn′tē) [ME. from O. Norse, *skamt,*

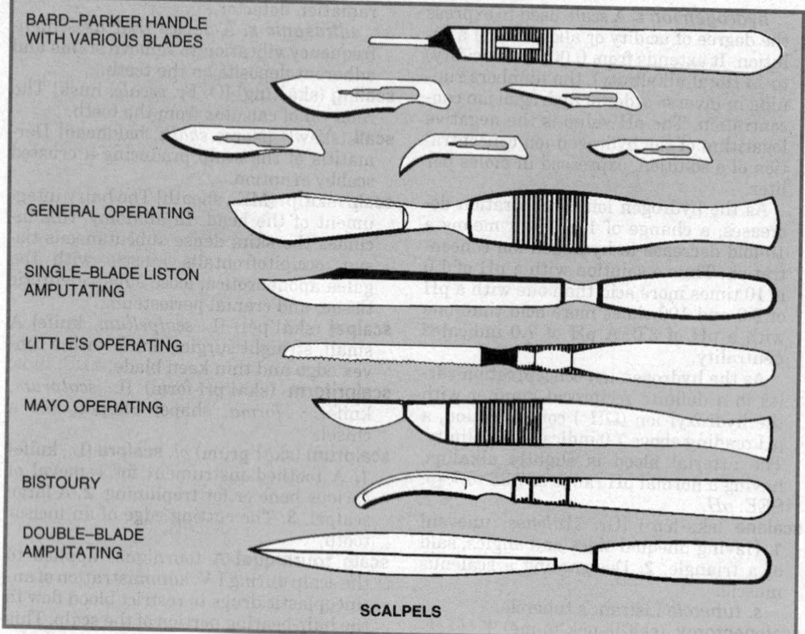


short] Not abundant; insufficient, as a secretion.

**scapha** (skā′fă) [NL., skiff] An elongated depression of the ear between the helix and antihelix. SYN: *scaphoid fossa.*

**scapho-** Combining form meaning *boat-shaped.*

**scaphocephalism** (skăf″ō-sĕf′ăl-ĭzm) [″ + ″ + *-ismos,* condition] Condition of having a deformed head, projecting like the keel of a boat. **scaphocephalic,** *adj.* (-ăl′ĭk) SYN: scaphocephaly

**scaphocephalous** (skăf″ō-sĕf′ă-lŭs) [″ + *kephale,* head] Scaphocephalic.

**scaphocephaly** (skăf″ō-sĕf′ă-lē) [″ + *kephale,* head] Scaphocephalism.

**scaphohydrocephaly** (skăf″ō-hī″drō-sĕf′ă-lē) [″+ *hydor,* water, + *kephale,* head] Hydrocephalus combined with scaphocephalism.

**scaphoid** (skăf′oyd) [″ + *eidos,* form, shape] **1.** Boat-shaped, navicular, hollowed. **2.** A proximal boat-shaped bone of the carpus or the tarsus. SYN: *os scaphoideum.*

**scaphoid fossa** Scapha.

**scaphoiditis** (skăf″oyd-ī′tĭs) [″ + ″ + *itis,* inflammation] Inflammation of the scaphoid bone.

**scapula** [L., shoulder blade] The large, flat, triangular bone that forms the posterior part of the shoulder. It articulates with the clavicle and the humerus. SYN: *shoulder blade.* SEE: illus.; *triceps.*

***plane of s.*** The angle of the scapula in its resting position, normally 30° to 45° forward from the frontal plane toward the sagittal plane. Movement of the humerus in this plane is less restricted than in the frontal or sagittal planes because the capsule is not twisted.

***tipped s.*** A condition in which the inferior angle of the scapula is prominent, usually the result of faulty posture and a tight pectoralis minor muscle. Tipping is a normal motion when a person reaches with the hand behind the back.

***winged s.*** Condition in which the medial border of the scapula is prominent, usually the result of paralysis of the serratus anterior or trapezius muscles. SYN: *angel's wing.*

**scapular** (skăp′ū-lăr) Of, or pert. to, the shoulder blade.

**scapulary** (skăp′ū-lā-rē) A shoulder bandage for keeping a body bandage in place. A broad roller bandage is split in half. The undivided section of the roller bandage is fastened in front with the two ends passing over the shoulders and attached to the back of the body bandage.

**scapulectomy** (skăp″ū-lĕk′tō-mē) [L. *scapula,* shoulder blade, + Gr. *ektome,* excision] Surgical excision of the scapula.

**scapulo-** Combining form meaning *shoulder.*

**scapuloclavicular** (skăp″ū-lō-klă-vĭk′ū-lar) [L. *scapula,* shoulder blade, + *clavicula,* little key] Concerning the scapula and clavicle.

**scapulodynia** (skăp″ū-lō-dĭn′ē-ă) [″ + *odyne,* pain] Inflammation and pain in the shoulder muscles.

**scapulohumeral** (skăp″ū-lō-hū′mĕr-ăl) [″ + *humerus,* upper arm] Concerning the

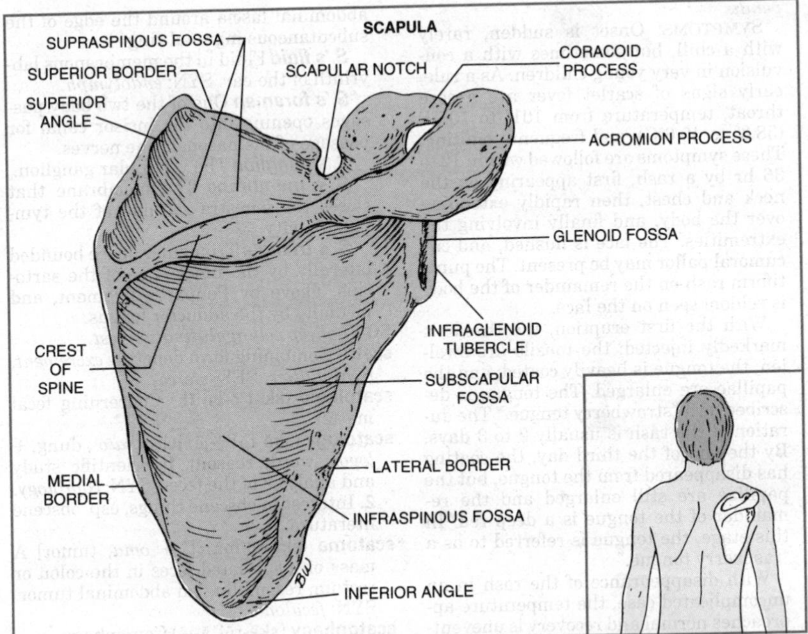


scapula and humerus.

**scapulopexy** (skăp″ū-lō-pĕk′sē) [″ + Gr. *pexis*, fixation] Fixation of the scapula to the ribs.

**scapulothoracic** (skăp″ū-lō-thō-răs′ĭk) [″ + Gr. *thorax*, chest] Concerning the scapula and thorax.

**scapus** (skā′pŭs) *pl.* **scapi** [L. *scapus*, stalk] A shaft or stem.

***s. penis*** The shaft of the penis.

***s. pili*** Hair shaft.

**scar** (skăr) [Gr. *eskhara*, scab] A mark left in the skin or an internal organ by the healing of a wound, sore, or injury because of replacement by connective tissue of the injured tissue. Scars may result from wounds that have healed, lesions of diseases, or surgical operations. When it first develops, a scar is red or purple, and later becomes white and glistening. SYN: *cicatrix*. SEE: *keloid*.

***cicatricial s.*** A scar with considerable contraction. It may be necessary to divide the scar and then graft on new skin, as done for burns. SEE: *Z-plasty*.

***keloid s.*** A red, raised, smooth scar containing blood vessels. This type of scar is often irritable. SEE: *keloid*.

***painful s.*** A scar that is painful because of involvement of a nerve during healing. The end of the nerve may become bulbous. The condition is treated by dissection of the scar or excision of the nerve.

**scarabiasis** (skăr″ă-bī′ă-sĭs) [L. *scarabaeus*, beetle, + Gr. *-iasis*, condition] A condition in which the intestine is invaded by the dung beetle. It occurs principally in children.

**Scarf sign** A newborn assessment finding in which the infant's elbow crosses the body midline without resistance as the examiner draws the arm across the chest to the opposite shoulder. This is characteristic of preterm infants born before 30 weeks gestation.

**scarification** (skăr″ĭ-fĭ-kā′shŭn) [Gr. *skariphismos*, scratching up] The making of numerous superficial incisions in the skin.

**scarificator** (skăr′if-ĭ-kā″tor) An instrument used for making small incisions in the skin. SYN: *scarifier*.

**scarifier** Scarificator.

**scarlatina** (skăr″lă-tē′nă) [NL., red] Scarlet fever. **scarlatinal** (-năl), *adj.*

***s. anginosa*** A severe form of scarlatina with extensive necrosis and ulceration of the pharynx, and in some cases peritonsillar abscess.

***s. hemorrhagica*** Scarlatina with hemorrhage into the skin and mucous membranes.

***s. maligna*** A fulminant and usually lethal form of scarlatina.

**scarlatiniform** (skăr-lă-tĭn′ĭ-form) [L. *scarlatina*, red, + *forma*, shape] Resembling scarlatina or its rash.

**scarlatinoid** (skăr-lăt′ĭ-noyd) [″ + Gr. *eidos*, form, shape] Resembling scarlet fever.

**scarlet fever** [L. *scarlatum*, red] An acute contagious disease characterized by sore throat, strawberry tongue, fever, punctiform scarlet rash, and rapid pulse. SYN: *scarlatina*. SEE: *Nursing Diagnoses Ap-*

*pendix.*

SYMPTOMS: Onset is sudden, rarely with a chill, but sometimes with a convulsion in very young children. As a rule, early signs of scarlet fever are a sore throat, temperature from 101° to 105°F (38.3° to 40.6°C), and frequent vomiting. These symptoms are followed within 12 to 36 hr by a rash, first appearing on the neck and chest, then rapidly extending over the body, and finally involving the extremities. The face is flushed, and circumoral pallor may be present. The punctiform rash on the remainder of the body is seldom seen on the face.

With the first eruption, the throat is markedly injected; the tonsils are swollen; the tongue is heavily coated; and the papillae are enlarged. The tongue is described as a "strawberry tongue." The duration of the rash is usually 2 to 3 days. By the end of the third day, the coating has disappeared from the tongue, but the papillae are still enlarged and the remainder of the tongue is a deep red. In this stage, the tongue is referred to as a "raspberry tongue."

With disappearance of the rash in an uncomplicated case, the temperature approaches normal and recovery is uneventful. Extremely mild cases occur in which the rash is very faint and of very short duration, possibly not exceeding 24 hr. Scarlet fever may actually occur without any rash whatsoever. In any form, a leukocytosis is to be expected in the average case. The number of leukocytes may range from 10,000 to 20,000, with 75% to 90% neutrophils.

ETIOLOGY: The disease is caused by many strains (more than 40) of group A, $\beta$-hemolytic streptococci that elaborate an erythrogenic toxin. The toxin was discovered by George and Gladys Dick (1924–1925). SEE: *Dick method.*

INCUBATION: The incubation period is probably never less than 24 hr. It may be 1 to 3 days, and rarely longer.

TREATMENT: Penicillin is the agent of choice. It should be given for a minimum of 10 days, no matter how mild the infection, to prevent the subsequent development of complications such as rheumatic fever, carditis, or acute glomerulonephritis.

Patients are isolated from the time of diagnosis until 1 day after beginning antibiotic therapy. Patients with uncomplicated scarlet fever should be kept in bed during the acute phase of the illness.

**scarlet rash** A rose-colored rash, specifically that of German measles.

**scarlet red** A red azo dye used to stimulate healing of indolent ulcers, burns, wounds, and so on; in histology, used as a stain. SYN: *rubrum scarlatinum.*

**Scarpa, Antonio** (skăr′păs) Italian anatomist, 1752–1832.

***S.'s fascia*** The deep layer of superficial abdominal fascia around the edge of the subcutaneous inguinal ring.

***S.'s fluid*** Fluid in the membranous labyrinth of the ear. SYN: *endolymph.*

***S.'s foramen*** One of the two bony passages opening into the incisor canal for passage of the nasopalatine nerves.

***S.'s ganglion*** The vestibular ganglion.

***S.'s membrane*** The membrane that closes the fenestra rotunda of the tympanic cavity.

***S.'s triangle*** Triangular space bounded laterally by the inner edge of the sartorius, above by Poupart's ligament, and medially by the adductor longus.

**SCAT** *sheep cell agglutination test.*

**scato-** Combining form denoting *excrement, fecal matter.* SEE: *sterco-.*

**scatologic** (skăt″ō-lŏj′ĭk) Concerning fecal matter.

**scatology** (skă-tŏl′ō-jē) [Gr. *skato-*, dung, + *logos,* word, reason] **1.** Scientific study and analysis of the feces. SYN: *coprology.* **2.** Interest in obscene things, esp. obscene literature.

**scatoma** (skă-tō′mă) [″ + *oma,* tumor] A mass of inspissated feces in the colon or rectum, resembling an abdominal tumor. SYN: *fecaloma.*

**scatophagy** (skă-tŏf′ă-jē) Coprophagy.

**scatoscopy** (skă-tŏs′kō-pē) [″ + *skopein,* to examine] The examination of feces for diagnostic purposes.

**scatter** (skăt′ĕr) The diffusion of x-rays when they strike an object.

***coherent s.*** An interaction between x-rays and matter in which the incoming photon is absorbed by the atom and leaves with the same energy in a different direction. Fewer than 5% of the interactions between x-rays and matter are of this type.

**scattered radiation** X-rays that have changed direction because of a collision with matter.

**scattergram** (skăt′ĕr-grăm) **1.** A display of data on a chart so that each value is indicated by a symbol. The symbols are not connected by a line. **2.** A graphic interpretation of blood cell populations generated by some types of hematology blood cell analyzers.

**scavenger cell** (skăv′ĕn-jĕr) [ME. *skawager,* toll collector] A phagocytic cell, such as a macrophage or a neutrophil leukocyte, that functions in the removal of disintegrating tissues.

**Sc.D.** *Doctor of Science* (degree).

**SCE** *saturated calomel electrode.*

**scent** (sĕnt) An emanation from living or dead tissues, or materials that stimulate the olfactory sense.

**Schäffer's reflex** (shā′fĕrs) [Max Schäffer, Ger. neurologist, 1852–1923] Dorsiflexion of the toes and flexion of the foot resulting when the middle portion of the Achilles tendon is pinched.

**Schatzki ring** [Richard Schatzki, U.S. radiologist, 1901–1992] A lower esophageal mucosal ring composed of an annular, thin, weblike tissue located at the squamocolumnar junction at or near the border of the lower esophageal sphincter. When the diameter of the ring is less than 1.3 cm, dysphagia is present. The treatment involves stretching the ring with dilators.

**schedule** A timetable, usually written; a plan for action to achieve a certain goal.

**Scheie's syndrome** [Harold Glendon Scheie, U.S. ophthalmologist, 1909–1990] Mucopolysaccharidosis IS.

**schema** (skē′mă) [Gr., shape] Shape, plan, or outline.

**schematic** (skē-măt′ĭk) [NL. *schematicus,* shape, figure] Pert. to a diagram or model; showing part for part in a diagram.

**scheroma** (shē-rō′mă) Xerophthalmia.

**Scheuermann's disease** [Holger W. Scheuermann, Danish physician, 1877–1960] A spinal deformity that occurs most commonly in teenaged boys. It is characterized by thoracic or thoracolumbar kyphosis. Treatment of an individual who is still growing involves the use of a brace. Symptomatic treatment includes nonsteroidal anti-inflammatory drugs, rest, and activity modification.

**Schick test** (shĭk) [Béla Schick, Hungarian-born U.S. pediatrician, 1877–1967] A test to determine the degree of immunity to diphtheria, involving the injection intradermally of 0.1 ml of dilute diphtheria toxin, 1⁄50 MLD. (MLD: minimum lethal dose, the amount of diphtheria toxin that would kill a small guinea pig in 4 days.) Results are obtained 3 to 4 days later. Susceptibility (positive test result) is indicated by the development of a red inflamed area at the point of injection, which slowly disappears after a few days. A negative test result (little or no reaction) indicates the presence of antibodies sufficient to neutralize the toxin; hence, the person is immune. SEE: *diphtheria*.

**Schick test control** Inactivated diphtheria toxin for the Schick test. It is used in the Schick test as a control.

**Schilder's disease** (shĭl′dĕrs) [Paul Ferdinand Schilder, Austrian-U.S. neurologist, 1886–1940] A rare but invariably fatal disease of the central nervous system characterized by adrenal atrophy and diffuse cerebral demyelination. This leads to mental deterioration and blindness. SYN: *adrenoleukodystrophy*.

**Schiller's test** (shĭl′ĕrs) [Walter Schiller, Austrian-U.S. pathologist, 1887–1960] A test for superficial cancer, esp. of the cervix uteri. The tissue is painted with an iodine solution. Cells lacking glycogen fail to stain, and their presence may indicate a malignant change.

**Schilling's classification** [Victor Schilling, Ger. hematologist, 1883–1960] A method of classifying polymorphonuclear neutrophils into four categories according to the number and arrangement of the nuclei in the cells.

**Schilling test** [Robert F. Schilling, U.S. hematologist, b. 1919] A test, using radioactive vitamin $B_{12}$, that assesses the gastrointestinal absorption of vitamin $B_{12}$ in order to diagnose primary pernicious anemia.

**schindylesis** (skĭn″dĭ-lē′sĭs) [Gr. *schindylesis,* a splitting] A form of wedge and groove suture in which a crest of one bone fits into a groove of another.

**Schiötz tonometer** [Hjalamar Schiötz, Norwegian physician, 1850-1927] An instrument for measuring intraocular pressure by the degree of indentation produced by pressure on the cornea.

**Schirmer's test** [Rudolph Schirmer, Ger. ophthalmologist, 1831–1896] The use of a piece of absorbent paper placed so that it hangs out of the conjunctival sac of the eye. The rate and amount of wetting of the paper provide an estimate of tear production.

**schisto-** (skĭs′tō) Combining form meaning *split, cleft*.

**schistocelia** (skĭs″tō-sē′lē-ă) [Gr. *schistos,* divided, + *koilia,* belly] A congenital abdominal fissure.

**schistocephalus** (skĭs″tō-sĕf′ă-lŭs) [″ + *kephale,* head] A fetus with a cleft head.

**schistocormia** (skĭs″tō-kor′mē-ă) [″ + *kormos,* trunk] A fetus with a cleft trunk.

**schistocystis** (skĭs″tō-sĭs′tĭs) [″ + *kystis,* bladder] A fissure of the bladder.

**schistocyte** (skĭs′tō-sīt) [″ + *kytos,* cell] Fragmented red blood cells that appear in a variety of shapes, from small triangular forms to round cells with irregular surfaces. SYN: *schizocyte*. SEE: illus.

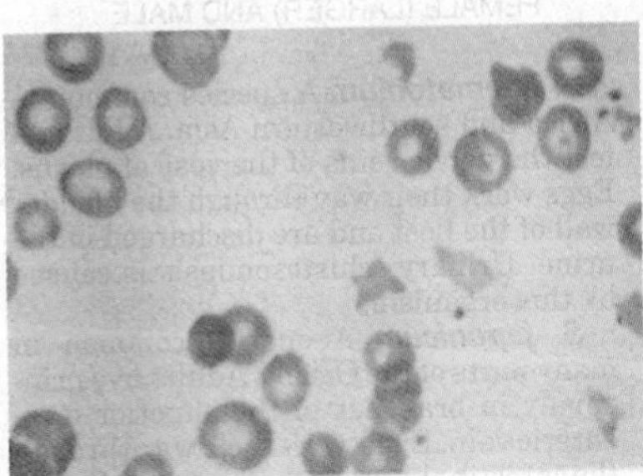

**SCHISTOCYTES** IN PERIPHERAL BLOOD (ORIG. MAG. ×600)

**schistocytosis** (skĭs″tō-sī-tō′sĭs) [″ + ″ + *osis,* condition] Schistocytes in the blood. SYN: *schizocytosis*.

**schistoglossia** (skĭs″tō-glŏs′ē-ă) [″ + *glossa,* tongue] A cleft tongue.

**schistomelus** (skĭs-tŏm′ĕ-lŭs) [″ + *melos,* limb] A fetus with a cleft in a limb.

**schistoprosopia** (skĭs″tō-prō-sō′pē-ă) [″ + *prosopon,* face] A congenital fissure of the face.

**schistorachis** (skĭs-tor′ă-kĭs) [″ + *rhachis,*

spine] Protrusion of membranes through a congenital cleft in the lower vertebral column. SYN: *spina bifida cystica; rachischisis.*

**Schistosoma** (skĭs″tō-sō′mă) [″ + *soma,* body] A genus of blood flukes belonging to the family Schistosomatidae, class Trematoda. Adults live in blood vessels of visceral organs. Eggs make their way into the bladder or intestine of the host and are discharged in the urine or feces. Eggs hatch into miracidia, which enter snails and transform into sporocysts. These develop daughter sporocysts, which give rise to fork-tailed cercariae. These leave the snail and enter the final host directly through the skin or mucous membrane. SEE: illus.

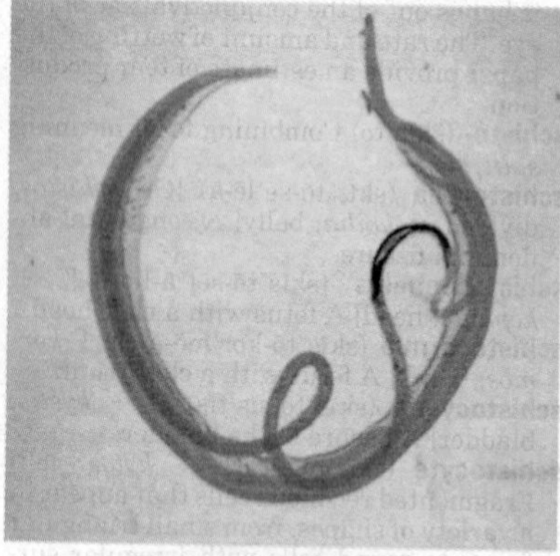

SCHISTOSOMA

FEMALE (LARGER) AND MALE

***S. haematobium*** A species common in Africa and southwestern Asia. Adults infest the pelvic veins of the vesical plexus. Eggs work their way through the bladder wall of the host and are discharged in the urine. Urinary schistosomiasis is caused by this organism.

***S. japonicum*** A species common in many parts of the Orient. Adults live principally in branches of the superior mesenteric vein. Eggs work their way through the intestinal wall of the host into the lumen and are discharged with feces. Oriental schistosomiasis is caused by this species.

***S. mansoni*** A species occurring in many parts of Africa and tropical America, including the West Indies. Adults live in branches of the inferior mesenteric veins. Eggs are discharged through either the host's intestine or bladder. This species causes bilharzial dysentery or Manson's intestinal schistosomiasis.

**schistosome dermatitis** (skĭs′tō-sōm) Dermatitis resulting from penetration of the skin of humans by cercariae of nonhuman blood flukes. This is common in the lake region of the northern U.S. It is not associated with visceral schistosomiasis. SYN: *swimmer's itch.*

**schistosomia** (skĭs″tō-sō′mē-ă) [″ + *soma,* body] A deformed fetus with a fissure in the abdomen. The limbs are rudimentary if present.

**schistosomiasis** (skĭs″tō-sō-mī′ăs-ĭs) [Gr. *schistos,* divided, + *soma,* body, + *-iasis,* infection] A parasitic disease due to infestation with blood flukes belonging to the genus *Schistosoma.* The disease is endemic throughout Asia, Africa, and South America, as well as some Carribean islands. Infestation occurs by wading or bathing in water containing cercariae that have issued from snails. SYN: *bilharziasis.*

**schistosomicide** (skĭs″tō-sō′mĭ-sīd) [″ + ″ + L. *cidus,* killing] Something that destroys schistosomes.

**schistosternia** (skĭs″tō-stĕr′nē-ă) [″ + *sternon,* chest] Schistothorax.

**schistothorax** (skĭs″tō-thō′răks) [″ + *thorax,* chest] A fissure of the thorax. SYN: *schistosternia.*

**schistotrachelus** (skĭs″tō-tră-kē′lŭs) A fetus with a cleft in the neck.

**schizamnion** (skĭz-ăm′nē-ŏn) [Gr. *schizein,* to divide, + *amnion,* lamb] An amnion formed by development of a cavity in the inner cell mass.

**schizaxon** (skĭz-ăk′sŏn) [″ + *axon,* axle] An axon that divides in two equal, or nearly equal, branches.

**schizencephaly** (skĭz″ĕn-sĕf′ă-lē) [″ + *enkephalos,* brain] A deformed fetus with a longitudinal cleft in the skull.

**schizo-** (skĭz′ō) Combining form indicating *division.*

**schizoblepharia** (skĭz″ō-blĕf′ă-rē″ă) [Gr. *schizein,* to split, + *blepharon,* eyelid] A fissure of an eyelid.

**schizocyte** (skĭz′ō-sīt) [″ + *kytos,* cell] Schistocyte.

**schizocytosis** (skĭz″ō-sī-tō′sĭs) [″ + ″ + *osis,* condition] Schistocytosis.

**schizogenesis** (skĭz″ō-jĕn′ĕs-ĭs) [″ + *genesis,* generation, birth] Reproduction by fission.

**schizogony** (skĭz-ŏg′ō-nē) [″ + *gone,* seed] Reproduction by multiple asexual fission characteristic of sporozoa, esp. the life cycle of the malarial parasite.

**schizogyria** (skĭz″ō-jī′rē-ă) [″ + *gyros,* a circle] A cleft in the cerebral convolutions.

**schizoid** (skĭz′oyd) [″ + *eidos,* form, shape] Resembling schizophrenia.

**schizoid personality disorder** A personality disorder marked by a persistent indifference to social interaction and a limited range of emotional experience and expression. It begins in early adulthood. These persons neither seek nor enjoy close relationships, and have no desire to be part of a family. They lead lonely lives and have no close friends or confidants; sexual interests and participation in pleasurable activities are almost nonexistent;

rarely do they experience strong emotions such as anger and joy. They appear cold and aloof and rarely reciprocate gestures or facial expressions such as smiles or nods.

**schizomycete** (skĭz″ō-mī-sēt′) [″ + *mykes,* fungus] Any organism belonging to the class Schizomycetes.

**Schizomycetes** (skĭz″ō-mī-sē′tēz) [″ + *mykes,* fungus] A class of plant microorganisms or fungi that multiply by fission; it includes the bacteria.

**schizont** (skĭz′ŏnt) [″ + *ontos,* being] **1.** A stage appearing in the life cycle of a sporozoan protozoon resulting from multiple division or schizogony. **2.** A stage in the asexual phase of the life cycle of *Plasmodium* organisms found in red blood cells. By schizogony, each gives rise to 12 to 24 or more merozoites. An early schizont is called a *presegmenter*; a mature schizont is called a *rosette* or *segmenter*.

**schizonticide** (skĭ-zŏn′tĭ-sīd) [″ + ″ + L. *cidus,* killing] Something that destroys schizonts.

**schizonychia** (skĭz″ō-nĭk′ē-ă) [″ + *onyx,* nail] A split condition of the nails.

**schizophasia** (skĭz″ō-fā′zē-ă) [″ + *phasis,* speech] The muttered and incomprehensible speech of the schizophrenic.

**schizophrenia** (skĭz″ō-frĕn′ē-ă) [Gr. *schizein,* to divide, + *phren,* mind] A disorder that alters perception, inferential thinking, language and communication, behavior, affect, volition and drive, social functioning, and attention. Characteristic symptoms may be both positive and negative. Positive symptoms such as delusions, hallucinations, and disorganized speech and behavior reflect an excess of normal function; negative symptoms such as flat affect, alogia, and avolition reflect a loss of normal function. Schizophrenia involves dysfunction in one or more areas such as interpersonal relations, work or education, or self-care. Associated features include inappropriate affect, anhedonia, dysphoric mood, abnormal psychomotor activity, cognitive dysfunction, confusion, lack of insight, and depersonalization. Abnormal neurological findings may show a broad range of dysfunction including slow reaction time, poor coordination, abnormalities in eye tracking, and impaired sensory gating. Some individuals drink excessive amounts of water (water intoxication) and develop abnormalities in urine specific gravity or electrolyte imbalance. Because none of its clinical features are diagnostic, schizophrenia remains a diagnosis of exclusion. It is important to exclude psychoses with known organic causes such as temporal-lobe epilepsy, metabolic disturbances, toxic substances, or psychoactive drugs.

The onset of schizophrenia typically occurs between the late teens and the mid-30s; onset prior to adolescence is rare. Gender differences suggest that women are more likely to have a later onset, more prominent mood symptoms, and a better prognosis. Hospital-based studies show a higher rate of schizophrenia in men, whereas community-based studies suggest an equal sex ratio. The onset of symptoms usually occurs between the ages of 17 and 30 years in men and between 20 and 40 in women. The worldwide lifetime prevalence is about 0.85%. The annual direct and indirect costs of schizophrenia in the U.S. in 1990 were estimated to be $33 billion. Although complete remission is not common, the prognosis is variable. SEE: *Nursing Diagnoses Appendix.* **schizophrenic** (-ĭk), *adj.*

ETIOLOGY: Etiology is unknown but the origin is thought to be related to altered development of the central nervous system and may be genetic.

TREATMENT: Treatment is focused on control of symptoms, prevention of relapse, and social and occupational rehabilitation. Medications used to control the symptoms almost invariably have the potential for causing undesired side effects. Clozapine has few side effects but may cause agranulocytosis. Persons taking clozapine should have their white blood count monitored weekly; the drug should not be given intravenously. Risperidone is also useful and its use is not associated with an increased risk of developing agranulocytosis. Supportive psychotherapy should be provided for the patient and the family.

***catatonic* s.** A schizophrenic disorder marked by motor immobility or stupor; excessive, purposeless motor activity; extreme negativism or mutism; echolalia or echopraxia; and peculiar voluntary movements such as posturing.

***paranoid* s.** A type of schizophrenic disorder characterized by delusions of persecution, grandiosity, jealousy, or hallucinations with persecutory or grandiose content.

***residual* s.** A schizophrenic disorder marked by continuing evidence of flat affect, impoverished or disorganized speech, and eccentric or odd behavior, but showing no evidence of delusions, hallucinations, or disorganized speech.

**schizoprosopia** (skĭz″ō-prō-sō′pē-ă) [″ + *prosopon,* face] Fissure of the face, such as harelip or cleft palate.

**schizotrichia** (skĭz″ō-trĭk′ē-ă) [″ + *thrix,* hair] Splitting of the tips of the hair.

**schizozoite** (skĭz″ō-zō′ĭt) [″ + *zoon,* animal] Merozoite.

**Schlatter-Osgood disease** (shlăt′ĕr-ŏz′good) Osgood-Schlatter disease.

**Schlemm, canal of** (shlĕm) [Friedrich S. Schlemm, Ger. anatomist, 1795–1858] A permeable venous sinus at the junction of the cornea and the iris; the site of reabsorption of aqueous humor from the anterior chamber of the eye. SYN: *scleral venous sinus.*

**Schmorl's disease** [Christian G. Schmorl, Ger. pathologist, 1861–1932] Herniation of the nucleus pulposus through a cracked vertebral end plate into the vertebral body. The resulting bone necrosis is detectable on radiograph and is called *Schmorl's nodes*.

**Schmorl's nodes** SEE: *Schmorl's disease*.

**schneiderian membrane** (shnī-dē'rē-ăn) [Conrad Viktor Schneider, Ger. anatomist, 1614–1680] The nasal mucosa.

**Schönlein's disease** (shān'līnz) [Johann Lukas Schönlein, Ger. physician, 1793–1864] Idiopathic thrombocytopenic purpura.

**Schönlein-Henoch purpura** SEE: *Henoch-Schönlein purpura*.

**school phobia** A child's refusal to go to school because of fear.

**Schüffner's dots** (shĭf'nĕrz) [Wilhelm P. A. Schüffner, Ger. pathologist, 1867–1949] Minute granules present in the red blood cells when they are infected by *Plasmodium vivax*.

**Schüller's disease** SEE: *Hand-Schüller-Christian disease*.

**Schultze's bundle, Schultze's tract** (shooltz'ĕs) [Max Johann Schultze, Ger. biologist, 1825–1874] A longitudinal, comma-shaped mass of descending fibers in the fasciculus cuneatus of the spinal cord.

**Schultze's cell** Olfactory cell.

**Schultz reaction** [Werner Schultz, Ger. physician, 1878–1947] A test that demonstrates the ability of muscle tissues from an animal that has been made anaphylactic to contract when re-exposed to the antigen. Guinea pig uterine muscles or intestines are used. The test is very specific, as unrelated antigens will not cause the sensitized muscle to contract. Sir Henry Dale demonstrated the same phenomenon independent of Schultz's work. Also called *Schultz-Dale reaction*. SYN: *Dale reaction*.

**Schulze mechanism** Placental expulsion with the fetal surface presenting. This indicates placental separation progressed from the inside to the outer margins. SEE: *mechanism, Duncan's*.

**Schwabach test** (shvă'băk) [Dagobert Schwabach, Ger. otologist, 1846–1920] A test for hearing using five tuning forks, each of a different tone.

**Schwalbe's ring** (shvăl'bĕz) [Gustav Albert Schwalbe, Ger. anatomist, 1844–1916] The thickened peripheral margin of the Descemet's membrane of the cornea of the eye; it is formed by a circular bundle of connective tissue. Also called *Schwalbe's line*.

**Schwann cell** (shvŏn) [Theodor Schwann, Ger. anatomist, 1810–1882] One of the cells of the peripheral nervous system that form the myelin sheath and neurilemma of peripheral nerve fibers. In the embryo, the Schwann cells grow around the nerve fiber, forming concentric layers of cell membrane (the myelin sheath). The cytoplasm and nuclei of the Schwann cells, external to the myelin sheath, form the neurilemma. SEE: *neuron* for illus.

**schwannoma** (shwŏn-nō'mă) A benign tumor of the neurilemma of a nerve.

**schwannosis** (shwŏn-nō'sĭs) Hypertrophy of the neurolemma of a nerve.

**Schwann's sheath** Neurilemma.

**Schwann's white substance** Myelin of a medullated nerve fiber.

**sciage** (sē-ăzh') [Fr., a sawing] A movement of the hand used in massage resembling that used in sawing.

**sciatic** (sī-ăt'ĭk) [L. *sciaticus*] **1.** Pert. to the hip or ischium. **2.** Pert. to, due to, or afflicted with sciatica. SYN: *ischiac; ischiatic*. SEE: *sciatica*.

**sciatica** (sī-ăt'ĭ-kă) [L.] Severe pain in the leg along the course of the sciatic nerve felt at the back of the thigh and running down the inside of the leg.

This symptom, which is usually self-limiting, costs patients at least $16 million each year. About 40% of the population will experience sciatica at some time during their lives. Recovery follows treatment in the majority of cases. SEE: *meralgia; piriformis syndrome; sciatic nerve; Nursing Diagnoses Appendix*.

SYMPTOMS: This condition may begin abruptly or gradually and is characterized by a sharp shooting pain running down the back of the thigh. Movement of the limb generally intensifies the suffering. Pain may be uniformly distributed along the limb, but frequently there are certain spots where it is more intense. Numbness and tingling may be present, and the nerve may be extremely sensitive to touch.

ETIOLOGY: The condition may be caused by compression or trauma of the sciatic nerve or its roots, esp. that resulting from a ruptured intervertebral disk or osteoarthrosis of the lumbosacral vertebrae; inflammation of the sciatic nerve resulting from metabolic, toxic, or infectious disorders; or pain referred to distribution of the sciatic nerve from other sources.

TREATMENT: The cause of the symptoms should be determined if possible and treated with appropriate intervention. If the nerve is being compromised, surgery may be indicated. Because more than 50% of patients with sciatica recover in 6 weeks, surgical therapy should be delayed to provide time for recovery. In the acute stage, rest is essential. Heat may give temporary relief from pain. Medication depends on the diagnosis. Morphine or meperidine may be required to control pain, but the danger of habituation must be kept in mind. In arthritic patients, full doses of salicylates or other nonsteroidal anti-inflammatory drugs are useful. Early intervention with appropriate physical therapy may be indicated if mechanical positioning, traction, or stabilization decreases the symptoms. Ultimately, a therapeutic exercise program to develop stabilizing strength and endurance in the trunk musculature should be considered for functional recovery.

**sciatic nerve** The largest nerve in the body, arising from the sacral plexus on either side, passing from the pelvis through the greater sciatic foramen, and down the back of the thigh, where it divides into the tibial and peroneal nerves. Lesions cause paralysis of flexion and extension of the toes, abduction and adduction of the toes, rotation inward and adduction of the foot, plantar flexion and lowering of the ball of the foot; anesthesia in cutaneous distribution (external popliteal nerve); paralysis of dorsiflexion and adduction of the foot; and paralysis of the rotation of the ball of the foot outward and of raising the external border of the foot and of extension of the toes. Lesions also cause anesthesia in cutaneous distribution. SEE: *Nerves Appendix.*

**sciatic nerve, small** The posterior femoral cutaneous nerve, a cutaneous nerve supplying the skin of the buttocks, perineum, popliteal region, and the back of the thigh and the leg.

**science** (sī′ĕns) [L. *scientia,* knowledge] The intellectual process using all available mental and physical resources to better understand, explain, quantitate, and predict normal as well as unusual natural phenomena. Thus, the scientific approach to understanding anything involves observation, measurement of entities that can be quantitated, the accumulation of data, and analysis of the findings as distinguished from an intuitive approach.

***life s.'s*** All of the scientific disciplines concerned with living things; included are biology, zoology, medicine, dentistry, surgery, nursing, and psychology.

**Science of Unitary Human Beings** A conceptual model of nursing developed by Martha Rogers. The human being and the environment are unitary, patterned, open, pandimensional energy fields. The goal of nursing is to help human beings to achieve maximum well-being through pattern manifestation appraisal and deliberative mutual patterning that promotes helicy, integrality, and resonancy. SEE: *Nursing Theory Appendix.*

**scieropia** (sī-ĕr-ō′pē-ă) [Gr. *skieros,* shadow, + *opsis,* vision] Abnormal vision in which things appear to be in a shadow.

**scintigram** (sĭn′tĭ-grăm) The record produced by a scintiscan.

**scintillascope** (sĭn-tĭl′ă-skōp) [L. *scintilla,* spark, + Gr. *skopein,* to examine] A device for viewing the effect of ionizing radiation, alpha particles, on a fluorescent screen.

**scintillation** (sĭn″tĭ-lā′shŭn) [L. *scintillatio*] **1.** Sparkling; a subjective sensation, as of seeing sparks. **2.** The emissions that come from radioactive substances.

**scintiphotography** (sĭn″tĭ-fō-tŏg′ră-fē) Photographing the scintillations emitted by radioactive substances injected into the body; used to determine the outline and function of organs and tissues in which the radioactive substance collects or is secreted.

**scintiscan** (sĭn′tĭ-skăn) The use of scintiphotography to create a map of scintillations produced when a radioactive substance is introduced into the body. The intensity of the record indicates the differential accumulation of a substance in the various parts of the body.

**scintiscanner** (sĭn″tĭ-skăn′ĕr) The device used in doing a scintiscan.

**scirrho-** A combining form meaning *hard.*

**scirrhoid** (skĭr′oyd) [Gr. *skirrhos,* hard, + *eidos,* form, shape] Pert. to, or like, a hard carcinoma.

**scirrhoma** (skĭr-ō′mă) [″ + *oma,* tumor] A hard carcinoma.

**scirrhosarca** (skĭr″ō-săr′kă) [″ + *sarx,* flesh] Scleroderma neonatorum.

**scirrhous** (skĭr′rŭs) [NL. *scirrhosus,* hard] Hard, like a scirrhus.

**scirrhus** (skĭr′ŭs) [Gr. *skirrhos,* hard tumor] A hard, cancerous tumor caused by an overgrowth of fibrous tissue.

**scission** (sĭzh′ŭn) [L. *scindere,* to split] Dividing, cutting, or splitting.

**scissors** (sĭz′ors) [LL. *cisorium*] A cutting instrument composed of two opposed cutting blades with handles, held together by a central pin. This allows the cutting edge to be opened and closed.

**scissura** (sĭ-sū′ră) *pl.* **scissurae** [L., to split] A fissure or cleft; a splitting.

**sclera** (sklĕr′ă) *pl.* **sclerae** [Gr. *skleros,* hard] The outer layer of the eyeball made of fibrous connective tissue. At the front of the eye, it is visible as the white of the eye and ends at the cornea, which is transparent. SYN: *sclerotica.* **scleral,** *adj.*

***blue s.*** An abnormal degree of blueness of the sclera. It may be a sign of osteogenesis imperfecta.

**scleradenitis** (sklĕ″răd-ĕn-ī′tĭs) [″ + *aden,* gland, + *itis,* inflammation] Inflammation and induration of a gland.

**scleratogenous** (sklĕ″ră-tŏj′ĕ-nŭs) Sclerogenous.

**sclerectasia** (sklĕ″rĕk-tā′zē-ă) [″ + *ektasis,* dilatation] Protrusion of the sclera.

**sclerectoiridectomy** (sklĕ-rĕk″tō-ĭr″ĭ-dĕk′tō-mē) [″ + *iris,* colored circle, + *ektome,* excision] Formation of a filtering cicatrix in glaucoma by combined sclerectomy and iridectomy.

**sclerectoiridodialysis** (sklĕ-rĕk″tō-ĭr″ĭd-ō-dī-ăl′ĭ-sĭs) [″ + ″ + *dialysis,* loosening] Sclerectomy and iridodialysis for the relief of glaucoma.

**sclerectomy** (sklĕ-rĕk′tō-mē) [″ + *ektome,* excision] **1.** Excision of a portion of the sclera. SYN: *scleroticectomy.* **2.** Removal of adhesions in chronic otitis media.

**scleredema** (sklĕr″ĕ-dē′mă) [″ + *oidema,* swelling] A condition usually following an acute infection characterized by edema and induration of the skin. It is a benign self-limited disease occurring more frequently in woman than in men. It is often confused with scleroderma.

*s. adultorum* Buschke's scleredema.

*s. neonatorum* Scleroderma neonatorum.

**sclerema** (sklĕ-rē′mă) [Gr. *skleros,* hard] Scleroderma.

*s. adiposum* Scleroderma neonatorum.

*s. adultorum* Scleroderma.

*s. neonatorum* Scleroderma neonatorum.

**sclerencephalia** (sklĕ″rĕn-sĕ-fā′lē-ă) [″ + *enkephalos,* brain] Sclerosis of the brain.

**scleriasis** (sklĕ-rī′ă-sĭs) [Gr. *skleriasis*] **1.** Progressive hardening of the skin. **2.** Hardening of the eyelid.

**scleriritomy** (sklĕ-rĭ-rĭt′ō-mē) [″ + *iris,* colored circle, + *tome,* incision] Incision of the iris and sclera.

**scleritis** (sklĕ-rī′tĭs) [″ + *itis,* inflammation] Superficial and deep inflammation of the sclera. SYN: *sclerotitis.* SEE: *episcleritis.*

*annular s.* Inflammation limited to the area surrounding the limbus of the cornea. A complete ring is formed.

*anterior s.* Scleritis of the area adjacent to the limbus of the cornea.

*posterior s.* Scleritis limited to the posterior half of the globe of the eye.

**scleroblastema** (sklĕ″rō-blăs-tē′mă) [Gr. *skleros,* hard, + *blastema,* sprout] The embryonic tissue from which formation of bone takes place.

**scleroblastemic** (sklĕ″rō-blăs-tĕm′ĭk) Relating to or derived from scleroblastema.

**sclerochoroiditis** (sklĕ″rō-kō″royd-ī′tĭs) [″ + *chorioeides,* skinlike, + *itis,* inflammation] Inflammation of the sclera and choroid coat of the eye. SYN: *scleroticochoroiditis.*

*posterior s.* Posterior staphyloma.

**scleroconjunctival** (sklĕ″rō-kŏn″jŭnk-tī′văl) [″ + L. *conjunctivus,* to bind together] Pert. to the sclera and conjunctiva.

**sclerocornea** (sklĕ″rō-kor′nē-ă) [″ + L. *corneus,* horny] The sclera and cornea together considered as one coat.

**sclerodactylia** (sklĕr″ō-dăk-tĭl′ē-ă) [″ + *daktylos,* a finger] Induration of the skin of the fingers and toes. SYN: *acroscleroderma.*

**scleroderma** (sklĕr″ă-dĕr′mă) [Gr. *skleros,* hard, + *derma,* skin] A chronic manifestation of progressive systemic sclerosis in which the skin is taut, firm, and edematous, limiting movement. SEE: *sclerosis, progressive systemic; Nursing Diagnoses Appendix.*

*circumscribed s.* Localized patches of linear sclerosis of the skin. There is no systemic involvement, and the course of the disease is usually benign.

*s. neonatorum* Hardness and tightness of the skin in early infancy; usually fatal. SYN: *sclerema adiposum; sclerema neonatorum; scirrhosarca.*

**sclerodermatitis** (sklĕ″rō-dĕr-mă-tī′tĭs) [Gr. *skleros,* hard, + *derma,* skin, + *itis,* inflammation] Inflammation of the skin accompanied by thickening and hardening.

**sclerodermatous** (sklĕ″rō-dĕr′mă-tŭs) [″ + *derma,* skin] Concerning scleroderma.

**sclerogenic** (sklĕ″rō-jĕn′ĭk) [″ + *gennan,* to produce] Sclerogenous.

**sclerogenous** (sklĕ-rŏj′ĕ-nŭs) [″ + *gennan,* to produce] Causing sclerosis or hardening of tissue. SYN: *sclerogenic.*

**scleroid** (sklĕ′rŏyd) [″ + *eidos,* form, shape] Having a hard or firm texture.

**scleroiritis** (sklĕ″rō-ī-rī′tĭs) [″ + *iris,* colored circle + *itis,* inflammation] Inflammation of both the sclera and iris.

**sclerokeratitis** (sklĕr″ō-kĕr-ă-tī′tĭs) [″ + *keras,* horn, + *itis,* inflammation] Cellular infiltration with inflammation of the sclera and cornea. SYN: *sclerokeratosis.*

**sclerokeratoiritis** (sklĕ″rō-kĕr″ă-tō-ī-rī′tĭs) [″ + ″ + *iris,* colored circle, + *itis,* inflammation] Inflammation of the sclera, cornea, and iris.

**sclerokeratosis** (sklĕr″ō-kĕr″ă-tō′sĭs) [″ + ″ + *osis,* condition] Sclerokeratitis.

**scleroma** (sklĕ-rō′mă) [″ + *oma,* tumor] Indurated, circumscribed area of granulation tissue in the mucous membrane or skin. SEE: *sclerosis.*

**scleromalacia** (sklĕ″rō-mă-lā′sē-ă) [Gr. *skleros,* hard, + *malakia,* softening] A softening of the sclera.

*s. perforans* Scleromalacia accompanied by perforation.

**scleromere** (sklĕr′ō-mēr) [″ + *meros,* a part] **1.** Any segment of the metamere of the skeleton. **2.** The caudal half of a sclerotome.

**scleromyxedema** (sklĕr″ō-mĭk″sē-dē′mă) [″ + *myxa,* mucus, + *oidema,* swelling] A type of lichen myxedematosus in which the skin under the papules is greatly thickened.

**scleronychia** (sklĕ″rō-nĭk′ē-ă) [″ + *onyx,* nail] Thickening and hardening of the nails.

**scleronyxis** (sklĕ-rō-nĭk′sĭs) [Gr. *skleros,* hard, + *nyxis,* a piercing] Surgical puncture of the sclera. SYN: *scleroticonyxis; scleroticopuncture.*

**sclero-oophoritis** (sklĕ″rō-ō-ŏf″ō-rī′tĭs) [″ + *oophoros,* bearing eggs, + *itis,* inflammation] Induration and inflammation of the ovary.

**sclerophthalmia** (sklĕ″rŏf-thăl′mē-ă) [″ + *ophthalmos,* eye] A congenital condition in which opacity of the sclera advances over the cornea.

**scleroplasty** (sklĕ′rō-plăs″tē) [″ + *plassein,* to form] Plastic surgery of the sclera.

**scleroprotein** (sklĕ″rō-prō′tē-ĭn) [″ + *protos,* first] A group of proteins noted for their insolubility in most chemicals; found in skeletal tissue, cartilage, hair, and nails, and in animal claws and horns.

**sclerosal** (sklĕ-rō′săl) Sclerous.

**sclerosant** (sklĕ-rō′sănt) [Gr. *skleros,* hard] Something that produces sclerosis.

**sclerose** (sklĕ-rōs′) [Gr. *skleros,* hard] To become hardened.

**sclerosed** (sklĕ-rōsd′, sklē′rōsd) [Gr. *skleros,* hard] Having sclerosis; hardened. SYN: *indurated.*

**sclerosing** (sklĕ-rōs′ĭng) Causing or developing sclerosis.

**sclerosis** (sklĕ-rō′sĭs) [Gr. *sklerosis,* to harden] **1.** A hardening or induration of an organ or tissue, esp. that due to excessive growth of fibrous tissue. **2.** A hardening within the nervous system, esp. of the brain and spinal cord, resulting from degeneration of nervous elements, as the myelin sheath. SYN: *cerebrosclerosis.* **3.** Thickening and hardening of the layers in the wall of an artery. SEE: *arteriosclerosis; atherosclerosis.*

***amyotrophic lateral s.*** Progressive muscular atrophy resulting from disease conditions, degenerative in nature, involving anterior horn cells and the corticospinal tracts. It is rapidly progressive, usually ending in bulbar paralysis. Also called *Lou Gehrig's disease.*

***annular s.*** Sclerosis in which a hardened substance forms a band about the spinal cord.

***arterial s.*** Arteriosclerosis. SEE: *vascular s.*

***arteriolar s.*** Sclerosis of the arterioles.

***diffuse s.*** Sclerosis affecting large areas of the brain and spinal cord.

***hyperplastic s.*** Medial s.

***insular s.*** Multiple s.

***intimal s.*** Atherosclerosis.

***lateral s.*** Sclerosis of the lateral column of the spinal cord. SEE: *amyotrophic lateral s.*

***lobar s.*** Sclerosis of the cerebrum resulting in mental disturbances.

***medial s.*** Sclerosis involving the tunica media of arteries, usually the result of involutional changes accompanying aging. SYN: *hyperplastic s.*

***multiple s.*** ABBR: MS. A chronic autoimmune inflammatory disease of the central nervous system marked by intermittent damage to the myelin sheath that covers nerve cell axons. Visual changes and muscle weakness occur often and have no consistent pattern; as the disease progresses, different nerves may be affected at different times, exacerbating current symptoms or creating new problems. The disease may progress steadily, or acute attacks may be followed by partial or complete temporary remission of symptoms. Most patients live a relatively normal lifespan. SYN: *insular s.* SEE: *Nursing Diagnoses Appendix.*

ETIOLOGY: The current theory is that an autoimmune process involving T lymphocytes and macrophages begins in the periphery and somehow breaks through the blood-brain barrier, producing inflammation in the myelin sheath. The damaged areas of myelin, called plagues, contain B cells and macrophages that release cytokines, proteolytic enzymes, and immunoglobulin G autoantibodies, which increase inflammatory damage. The initial cause of the T-cell autoimmune response in unclear. There may be abnormalities in the CD8+ and CD4+ T cells that normally help regulate the immune response, and the strong association between MS and histocompatibility antigens HLA-DR2 and HLA-DQw1 indicates a genetic susceptibility. This susceptibility may be age-related; MS rarely occurs before puberty and most often begins between ages 20 and 40. The disease is more common in colder climates than in the tropics.

SYMPTOMS: Because the damage is in the central nervous system, signs of nerve damage appear in many locations. Blurred vision with blind spots (signs of optic neuritis) and muscle weakness with paresthesia in the extremities are usually the initial symptoms. Urinary retention, diplopia, tremors, and spasticity are common. Cognitive deficits and mood disorders develop in some patients.

TREATMENT: Until recently, symptomatic management was the only treatment available. Beta interferon is the first drug that actually influences the disease itself; it slows its progression by preventing or minimizing new plaque formation. Another drug, Copolymer 1 (Copaxone) is also available. Researchers are still investigating the use of methotrexate, a cytotoxic drug that has been effective in treating other autoimmune disorders. Human beta interferon has been used to treat patients aged 18 to 50 who are ambulatory without assistance and who have a relapsing-remitting course. It is not recommended for those with a chronic progressive course.

NURSING IMPLICATIONS: The nurse provides support to patients with multiple sclerosis and their families. The patient is advised to avoid fatigue, overexertion, exposure to extreme heat or cold, and stressful situations, and is encouraged to follow a regular plan of daily activity and exercise. The nurse teaches the patient about symptoms that may occur during excerbations of the disease and the need to adapt the plan of care to changing needs, as well as about the administration of prescribed medications. Both patient and family are encouraged to promote safety in the home and the work environment.

***neural s.*** Sclerosis with chronic inflammation of a nerve trunk with branches.

***progressive systemic s.*** ABBR: PSS. A chronic disease of unknown etiology that occurs four times as frequently in women than in men. It causes sclerosis of the skin and certain organs including the gastrointestinal tract, lungs, heart, and kidneys. The skin is taut, firm, and edematous and is firmly bound to subcutaneous tissue, which often causes limitation of the range of motion; it feels tough and leathery, may itch, and later becomes hyperpigmented. The skin changes usually precede the development of signs of visceral involvement. For a limited period, the only findings may be the CREST syndrome: calcinosis, Raynaud's phenomenon, esophageal dysfunction, sclerodactyly, and telangiectasia. SEE: *collagen diseases; scleroderma.*

TREATMENT: There is no specific therapy. General supportive therapy is indicated. A great number of drugs including corticosteroids, vasodilators, D-penicillamine, and immunosuppressive agents have been tried. Physical therapy will help maintain range of motion and muscular strength but will not influence the course of joint disease.

PROGNOSIS: The prognosis is variable and unpredictable with respect to the rate of pathologic changes.

***renal s.*** Nephrosclerosis.

***systemic s.*** Progressive systemic s.

***tuberous s.*** ABBR: TS. A syndrome manifested by convulsive seizures, progressive mental disorder, adenoma sebaceum, and tumors of the kidneys and brain with projections into the cerebral ventricles.

***vascular s.*** Sclerosis of the walls of blood vessels; arterial and venous sclerosis.

***venous s.*** Phlebosclerosis. SEE: *vascular s.*

**scleroskeleton** (sklĕr″ō-skĕl′ĕ-tŏn) [Gr. *skleros,* hard, + *skeleton,* a dried-up body] Skeletal changes resulting from ossification of fibrous structures, such as ligaments, fasciae, and tendons.

**sclerostenosis** (sklĕr″ō-stĕ-nō′sĭs) [″ + *stenosis,* act of narrowing] Contraction and induration of tissues, esp. those about an orifice.

***s. cutanea*** Scleroderma.

**sclerostomy** (sklĕ-rŏs′tō-mē) [″ + *stoma,* mouth] The surgical formation of an opening in the sclera.

**sclerotherapy** (sklĕr″ō-thĕr′ă-pē) [″ + *therapeia,* treatment] The use of sclerosing agents injected into varices such as varicose veins in the extremities, hemorrhoids, and for superficial varicosities of the skin.

**sclerothrix** (sklĕr′ō-thrĭks) [″ + *thrix,* hair] Brittleness of the hair.

**sclerotic** (sklĕ-rŏt′ĭk) [L. *scleroticus,* hard] Pert. to or affected with sclerosis.

**sclerotica** (sklĕ-rŏt′ĭ-kă) [L. *scleroticus,* hard] Sclera.

**sclerotic acid** An amorphous, brown powder from ergot; a hemostatic and oxytocic.

**sclerotic dentin** Areas of dentin where the tubules have been filled by mineralization, producing a more dense, radiopaque dentin; it is often produced in response to caries, attrition, and abrasion.

**scleroticectomy** (sklĕ-rŏt″ĭ-sĕk′tō-mē) [″ + Gr. *ektome,* excision] Excision of a part of the sclera. SYN: *sclerectomy.*

**scleroticochoroiditis** (sklĕ-rŏt″ĭ-kō-kō″roy-dī′tĭs) [″ + Gr. *chorioeides,* skinlike, + *itis,* inflammation] Inflammation of sclerotic and choroid coats of the eye. SYN: *sclerochoroiditis.*

**scleroticonyxis** (sklĕ-rŏt″ĭ-kō-nĭk′sĭs) [″ + Gr. *nyxis,* a piercing] Surgical puncture of the sclera. SYN: *scleronyxis; scleroticopuncture.*

**scleroticopuncture** (sklĕ-rŏt″ĭ-kō-pŭnk′tūr) [″ + *punctura,* a piercing] Surgical puncture of the sclera. SYN: *scleronyxis; scleroticonyxis.*

**scleroticotomy** (sklĕ-rŏt″ĭ-kŏt′ō-mē) [″ + Gr. *tome,* incision] Sclerotomy.

**sclerotic teeth** Teeth that are hard and highly resistant to caries.

**sclerotitis** (sklĕr-ō-tī′tĭs) [Gr. *skleros,* hard, + *itis,* inflammation] Inflammation of the sclera. SYN: *scleritis.*

**sclerotium** (sklĕ-rō′shē-ŭm) A hardened mass formed by the growth of certain fungi. The sclerotium formed by ergot on rye is of medical importance due to its toxicity.

**sclerotome** (sklĕr′ō-tōm) [″ + *tome,* incision] **1.** A knife used in incision of the sclera. **2.** One of a series of segmentally arranged masses of mesenchymal tissue lying on either side of the notochord. They give rise to the vertebrae and ribs.

**sclerotomy** (sklĕ-rŏt′ō-mē) Surgical incision of the sclera. SYN: *scleroticotomy.*

***anterior s.*** An incision made at the angle of the anterior chamber of the eye in glaucoma.

***posterior s.*** An incision through the sclera into the vitreous for treatment of a detached retina or removal of a foreign body.

**sclerotrichia** (sklĕ-rō-trĭk′ē-ă) [Gr. *sclerosis,* hard, + *thrix,* hair] Hardness and brittleness of the hair.

**sclerous** (sklĕr′ŭs) Hard; indurated. SYN: *sclerosal.*

**scobinate** (skō′bĭn-āt) [L. *scobina,* rasp] Having a rough, uneven, nodular surface.

**scoleciasis** (skō-lē-sī′ă-sĭs) [Gr. *skolex,* worm, + *-iasis,* condition] The presence of larval forms of butterflies or moths in the body.

**scoleciform** (skō-lĕs′ĭ-form) [″ + L. *forma,* form] Resembling a scolex.

**scolecoid** (skō′lĕ-koyd) [″ + *eidos,* form, shape] Resembling a worm.

**scolex** (skō′lĕks) *pl.* **scolices** [Gr. *skolex,* worm] The portion of a tapeworm, the so-called head, by which it attaches itself to the wall of the intestine. Scolices usually possess organs such as hooks, suckers, or grooves (bothria) for attachment.

**scoliokyphosis** (skō″lē-ō-kī-fō′sĭs) [Gr. *skolios,* twisted, + *kyphosis,* humpback] A condition combining scoliosis and kyphosis.

**scoliometer** (skō″lē-ŏm′ĕt-ĕr) [″ + *metron,* measure] A device for measuring curves, esp. the lateral ones of the spine.

**scoliorachitic** (skō″lē-ō-ră-kĭt′ĭk) [″ + *rhachis,* spine] Pert. to, or afflicted with, spinal curvature from rickets.

**scoliosis** (skō″lē-ō′sĭs) [Gr. *skoliosis,* crookedness] A lateral curvature of the spine. It usually consists of two curves, the original abnormal curve and a compensatory curve in the opposite direction. SEE: *Nursing Diagnoses Appendix.*

NURSING IMPLICATIONS: Provisions are made to assist the adolescent and family to meet the psychosocial needs associated with the illness. The nurse teaches the patient and family about treatment (cast brace, traction, or electrical stimulation), exercises, activity level, skin care, prevention of complications, and breathing exercises. When necessary, preoperative teaching is provided, including preanesthesia breathing exercises, postoperative apparatus (such as Stryker frame or Circ-O-Lectric bed), and prescribed exercises and diet. Socialization with peers is encouraged, and every effort is made to help the adolescent feel accepted and worthwhile. Educational and support resources are discussed with the patient and family.

***cicatricial s.*** Scoliosis due to cicatricial contraction resulting from necrosis.

***congenital s.*** Scoliosis present at birth, usually the result of defective embryonic development of the spine.

***coxitic s.*** Scoliosis in the lumbar spine caused by tilting of the pelvis in hip disease.

***empyematic s.*** Scoliosis following empyema and retraction of one side of the chest.

***functional s.*** Scoliosis that is not caused by actual spinal deformity but by another condition such as unequal leg lengths.

***habit s.*** Scoliosis due to habitually assumed improper posture or position.

***idiopathic s.*** Scoliosis due to unknown causes.

***inflammatory s.*** Scoliosis due to disease of the vertebrae.

***ischiatic s.*** Scoliosis due to hip disease.

***myopathic s.*** Scoliosis due to weakening of the spinal muscles.

***neuropathic s.*** A structural scoliosis caused by congenital or acquired neurological disorders.

***ocular s.*** Scoliosis from tilting of the head because of visual defects or extraocular muscle imbalance.

***osteopathic s.*** Scoliosis caused by bony deformity of the spine.

***paralytic s.*** Scoliosis due to paralysis of muscles.

***protective s.*** An acute side shifting of the lumbar spine, usually away from the side of pathology. The body is attempting to move a nerve root away from a bulging intervertebral disk herniation.

***rachitic s.*** Scoliosis due to rickets.

***sciatic s.*** Scoliosis due to sciatica.

***static s.*** Scoliosis due to a difference in the length of the legs.

***structural s.*** An irreversible lateral spinal curvature that has a fixed rotation. The vertebral bodies rotate toward the convexity of the curve; the rotation results in a posterior rib hump in the thoracic region on the convex side of the curve. In structural scoliosis, the spine does not straighten when the patient bends.

**scoliosometry** (skō″lē-ō-sŏm′ĕt-rē) [″ + *metron,* measure] Measurement of the degree of spinal curvature.

**scoliotic** (skō-lē-ŏt′ĭk) Suffering from, or related to, scoliosis.

**scombrine** (skŏm′brĭn) A protamine present in mackerel sperm.

**scombroid** Fish of the suborder Scombroidea, including mackerel, tuna, bonitos, albacores, and skipjacks.

**scombroid fish poisoning** Intoxication due to eating raw or inadequately cooked fish of the suborder Scombroidea, such as tuna and mackerel, as well as certain nonscombroid fish, such as amberjack, mahimahi, and bluefish. Certain bacteria act on the fish after they are caught to produce a histamine-like toxin. Therefore, these fish should be either properly cooked and eaten shortly after being caught or refrigerated immediately.

SYMPTOMS: This type of poisoning is characterized by nausea, vomiting, abdominal cramps, diarrhea, flushing, headache, urticaria, and a burning sensation and metallic taste in the mouth. The incubation period varies from 15 min to 3 hr, with an average of 45 min. Symptoms last less than 1 day.

TREATMENT: There is no specific therapy, but ingested fish should be removed by gastric lavage or emesis.

**scoop** (skoop) [ME., a ladle] A spoon-shaped surgical instrument.

***bone s.*** An instrument for scraping or removing necrosed bone or the contents of suppurative tracts.

***bullet s.*** An instrument for dislodging bullets.

***cataract s.*** An instrument for removing fluids or foreign growths.

***ear s.*** Instrument for removing middle ear granulations.

***lithotomy s.*** An instrument for dislodging encysted calculi or removing stones, debris, and so forth.

***mastoid s.*** An instrument used in mastoid operations.

***renal s.*** An instrument used to dislodge or remove small stones from the pelvis of a kidney.

**scoparius** (skō-pā′rē-ŭs) The fresh or dried tops of broom, *Cytisus scoparius.* It has been used as a diuretic and emetic.

**-scope** [Gr. *skopein,* to examine] Combining form, used as a suffix, meaning *to view, to examine.*

**scopolamine hydrobromide** (skō-pŏl′ă-mēn hī″drō-brō′mīd) The hydrobromide of alkaloids obtained from plants of the nightshade family. SYN: *hyoscine hydrobromide.*

ACTION/USES: The drug is useful as a sedative; locally as a mydriatic; and with morphine and pentobarbital in labor to produce "twilight" sleep.

***transdermal s.*** A method of delivering scopolamine by applying a patch containing the drug to the skin. The medicine is slowly absorbed over a period of several days. It is esp. useful in treating vertigo and motion sickness. In the latter condition, the medicine is effective if applied several hours before the individual is exposed to the motion. The drug should be used cautiously in elderly patients because it may cause confusion, memory loss, and hallucinations.

**scopometer** (skō-pŏm′ĕ-tĕr) [Gr. *skopein,* to examine, + *metron,* measure] An instrument for measuring the density of a suspension.

**scopophilia** (skō″pō-fĭl′ē-ă) [″ + *philein,* to love] The derivation of sexual pleasure from visual sources such as nudity and obscene pictures.

***active s.*** Voyeurism.

***passive s.*** Sexual pleasure derived from being observed by others.

**scopophobia** (skō″pō-fō′bē-ă) [″ + *phobos,* fear] An abnormal fear of being seen.

**-scopy** [Gr. *skopein,* to examine] Combining form meaning *examination.*

**scorbutic** (skor-bū′tĭk) [NL. *scorbuticus,* scurvy] Concerning or affected with scurvy.

**scorbutigenic** (skor-bū″tĭ-jĕn′ĭk) [LL. *scorbutus,* scurvy, + Gr. *gennan,* to produce] Something that causes scurvy.

**scorbutus** (skor-bū′tŭs) [LL., scurvy] Scurvy.

**scordinema** (skor-dĭ-nē′mă) [Gr. *skordinema,* yawning] Yawning and stretching accompanied by fatigue and heaviness of the head. This may be a prodromal symptom of an infectious disease.

**score** (skor) **1.** A rating or grade as compared with a standard of other individuals, esp. in a competitive event. **2.** To mark the skin with lines in order to have landmarks available, as in plastic surgery. **3.** In dentistry, a rating that represents some assessment of the oral health or history of the individual. For example, a DMF score or index represents decayed-missing-filled teeth; a periodontal score, or periodontal disease index, represents the relative health of the soft tissue of the mouth. SEE: *index, DMF; index, periodontal.*

***C.R.O.P. s.*** A critical care assessment score that measures compliance, respiratory rate, oxygenation, and pressure values.

**scorpion** (skor′pē-ŏn) [Gr. *skorpios,* to cut off] An insect of the class Arachnida and order Scorpionida. It varies in length from less than 2 in. (5 cm) for the small bark scorpions of Arizona to 8 in. (20 cm) for some African scorpions. Most scorpions are nocturnal and reclusive, and are most active when the night temperatures remain above 70°F (21°C). The tail of the scorpion contains two venom glands connected to the tip of the stinger.

***s. sting*** Injury resulting from scorpion venom. The stings of most species in the U.S. seldom produce severe toxic reactions, but because of the difficulty of distinguishing one species of scorpion from another, each scorpion sting should be treated as if it had been inflicted by a species capable of delivering a very toxic dose of venom. The stings may vary in severity from only a local tissue reaction consisting of swelling at the puncture site to a severe neurotoxic reaction that produces intense, aching pain and numbness radiating from the site of the bite, paralysis, and convulsions. Also present could be a rapid weak pulse, shock, excessive salivation, extreme thirst, and dysuria. The venom capable of causing the latter type reaction contains hemolysins, lytic enzymes, and neurotoxins. Death can occur, particularly in very young children.

TREATMENT: For mild reactions, application of cold compresses to the area will lessen the pain and may inhibit spread of the venom to the general circulation. In these cases, the symptoms usually subside within 4 hr. For severe reactions, cold compresses should be applied to the affected area, the shock treated, and appropriate therapy provided for convulsions. Analgesics should be given for pain.

Caution: The use of morphine and its derivatives is contraindicated because they act synergistically to increase the toxic effects of the venom.

Antivenins are available. Sources for those may be obtained by contacting the Arizona Poison Control Center at (520) 626-6016 or the Oklahoma Poison Control Center at (405) 271-5854.

**scoto-** (skō′tō) Combining form meaning *darkness.*

**scotodinia** (skō″tō-dĭn′ē-ă) [″ + *dinos,* whirling] Vertigo with black spots before the eyes and faintness of vision.

**scotogram, scotograph** (skō′tō-grăm, -grăf) [″ + *gramma,* something written; ″ + *graphein,* to write] Any radiation effect recorded in the dark on a photographic plate.

**scotoma** (skō-tō′mă) *pl.* **scotomata** [Gr. *skotoma,* to darken] An island-like blind gap in the visual field.

***absolute s.*** An area in the visual field in which there is absolute blindness.

***annular s.*** A scotomatous zone that encircles the point of fixation like a ring, not always completely closed, but leaving the fixation point intact. SYN: *ring s.*

***arcuate s.*** An arc-shaped scotoma near the blind spot of the eye. It is caused by a nerve bundle defect on the temporal side of the optic disk.

***central s.*** An area of depressed vision involving the point of fixation, seen in lesions of the macula.

***centrocecal s.*** A defect in vision that is oval-shaped and includes the fixation point and the blind spot of the eye.

***color s.*** Color blindness in a limited portion of the visual field.

***eclipse s.*** An area of blindness in the visual field caused by looking directly at a solar eclipse.

***flittering s.*** Scintillating s.

***negative s.*** A scotoma not perceptible by the patient.

***peripheral s.*** A defect in vision removed from the point of fixation of the vision.

***physiological s.*** A blind spot caused by an absence of rods and cones where the optic nerve enters the retina.

***positive s.*** An area in the visual field that is perceived by the patient as a dark spot.

***relative s.*** A scotoma that causes the perception of an object to be impaired but not completely lost.

***ring s.*** Annular s.

***scintillating s.*** An irregular outline around a luminous patch in the visual field that occurs following mental or physical labor, eyestrain, or during a migraine. SYN: *flittering s.*

**scotometer** (skō-tŏm′ĕt-ĕr) [″ + *metron,* a measure] A device for detecting and measuring scotomata in the visual field.

**scotometry** (skō-tŏm′ĕ-trē) The locating and measurement of scotomata.

**scotophobia** (skō″tō-fō′bē-ă) [″ + *phobos,* fear] An abnormal dread of darkness. SYN: *noctiphobia; nyctophobia.*

**scotopia** (skō-tō′pē-ă) [″ + *ops,* eye] Adjustment of the eye for vision in dim light; the opposite of photopia. **scotopic** (-tŏp′ĭk), *adj.*

**scotopsin** (skō-tŏp′sĭn) The protein portion of the rods of the retina of the eye. It combines with 11-*cis*-retinal to form rhodopsin.

**scotoscopy** (skō-tŏs′kō-pē) [Gr. *skotos,* darkness, + *skopein,* to examine] Fluoroscopy.

**scout film** In radiology, an x-ray film, esp. of the abdomen, for detecting abnormalities. These films assist in excluding or including certain diseases being considered as diagnostic possibilities.

**scr** *scruple.*

**scratch** (skrăch) [ME. *cracchen,* to scratch] **1.** A mark or superficial injury produced by scraping with the nails on a rough surface. **2.** To make a thin, shallow cut with a sharp instrument. **3.** To rub the skin, esp. with the fingernails, to relieve itching. Scratching temporarily relieves itching by soothing the cutaneous nerves, but in the long run, it may worsen the condition that caused the itching. SEE: *pruritus.*

**scratch test** Placement of an appropriate dilution of a test material, suspected of being an allergen, in a lightly scratched area of the skin. If the material is an allergen, a wheal will develop within 15 min.

**screen** [O. Fr. *escren*] **1.** A flat area on which movies or slides are viewed. **2.** To examine, using physical and mental examinations and laboratory tests, to determine the presence of a certain disease or characteristics. **3.** A structure or substance used to protect, guard, or shield from a damaging influence such as x-rays or sun rays. **4.** A system used to select or reject personnel. **5.** In psychiatry, the blocking of one memory with another.

***intensifying s.*** A thin sheet of celluloid or other substance evenly coated with a fine layer of crystals that fluoresce when exposed to x-rays. These screens line the inside of the cassette and are in direct contact with x-ray film. The crystals intensify the effect of x-rays, decreasing the patient dose but also the detail on the radiograph. SYN: *fluorescent screen.*

***tangent s.*** Bjerrum screen.

**screening test 1.** Various methods used to attempt to determine disease or the potential for developing an illness. The screening is usually done on a large number of persons who are thought to be at risk for disease. Examples of screening tests include Pap tests (for women older than age 40), tests for elevated prostate specific antigen and digital rectal examination of the prostate (for men older than age 40), fecal occult blood tests, tests for determining blood cholesterol level (for adults), mammography examinations (done periodically in women older than age 40), and special blood tests such as for sickle cell trait or Rh status (done during pregnancy). **2.** In psychiatry, the initial examination to determine the mental status of an individual and the appropriate initial therapy.

***multiphasic s.t.*** A battery of tests used to attempt to determine the presence of one or more diseases.

**screw, expansion** A mechanical device set into a removable or fixed appliance to enlarge the dental arch.

**Scribner shunt** [Belding Scribner, U.S. physician, b. 1921] A tube, usually made of synthetic material, used to connect an artery to a vein. It is used in patients requiring frequent venipuncture as in hemodialysis. This type of device helps simplify the care of patients requiring hemodialysis. However, the shunts may develop complications such as infection, thrombosis, and release of septic emboli.

**scrobiculate** (skrō-bĭk′ū-lāt) [L. *scrobiculus,* little trench] Having shallow depressions; pitted.

**scrobiculus** (skrō-bĭk′ū-lŭs) [L., little trench] A small groove or pit.

**scrofula** (skrŏf'ū-lă) [L., breeding sow] A variety of tuberculous adenitis of the cervical lymph nodes due to a localized hematogenous spread from a pulmonary lesion. It is most common in childhood. This condition responds to specific antituberculosis chemotherapy. SEE: *lymphadenitis, tuberculous.*

**scrotectomy** (skrō-tĕk'tō-mē) [" + Gr. *ektome,* excision] Excision of part of the scrotum.

**scrotitis** [" + Gr. *itis,* inflammation] Inflammation of the scrotum.

**scrotocele** (skrō'tō-sēl) [" + Gr. *kele,* tumor, swelling] Hernia in the scrotum.

**scrotoplasty** (skrō'tō-plăs"tē) [" + Gr. *plassein,* to form] Plastic surgery on the scrotum.

**scrotum** (skrō'tŭm) *pl.* **scrota, -ums** [L., a bag] The pouch found in most male mammals that contains the testicles and part of the spermatic cord. Constituent parts of the scrotum are skin; a network of nonstriated muscular fibers called dartos; cremasteric, spermatic, and infundibuliform fasciae; cremasteric muscle; and tunica vaginalis. **scrotal** (-tăl), *adj.*

**scrubbing** [MD. *schrubben*] A term applied to washing the hands, fingernails, and lower arms in preparation for performing surgery. The precise procedure to follow usually is posted in a special area where the washing is done. The method to follow entails scrubbing the hands with soap, water, and a nail brush; immersing the hands in a mild germicidal solution; and wearing sterilized rubber gloves, as well as a cap, gown, and mask.

**scrub typhus** An acute febrile illness caused by *Rickettsia tsutsugamushi* transmitted by several species of mites, including *Trombicula akamushi* and *T. deliensis.* It is common in the Asiatic-Pacific area. If untreated, the fever lasts about 14 days. Tetracycline or chloramphenicol should be given. Mortality rate varies in untreated cases from 1% to 4%. SYN: *tsutsugamushi disease.*

**scruple** (skrū'pl) [L. *scrupulus,* small, sharp stone] ABBR: scr. Twenty grains in apothecaries' weight; 1.296 g.

**SCUBA** *self-contained underwater breathing apparatus.*

**Scultetus binder** SEE: *binder, Scultetus.*

**Scultetus position** Position in which the head is low and the body is on an inclined plane.

**scum** (skŭm) [ME. *scume*] Slimy floating islands of bacteria or impurities on the surface of a culture; an interrupted pellicle of bacterial growth.

**scurf** [AS. *scurf*] A branny desquamation of the epidermis, esp. on the scalp. SEE: *dandruff.*

**scurvy** (skŭr'vē) [L. *scorbutus*] A deficiency disease characterized by hemorrhagic manifestations and the abnormal formation of bones and teeth. It is caused by a deficiency of vitamin C, usually resulting from a lack of fresh fruits and vegetables in the diet. Prognosis is favorable in the early stages.

SYMPTOMS: Scurvy is preceded by a period of ill health characterized by sallow complexion; loss of energy; and pains in the extremities and joints. Anemia; great weakness; spongy, bleeding gums; fetor of breath; loosening of teeth; subcutaneous hemorrhages and hemorrhages from mucous membranes; and painful, brawny indurations of muscles characterize overt symptoms.

TREATMENT: Treatment for infants is 300 mg of vitamin C (ascorbic acid) daily for 1 week, then 150 mg daily for 1 month, or 4 to 8 oz (52 to 104 ml) of orange juice or 12 to 24 oz (155 to 311 ml) of tomato juice daily. For adults, treatment involves 300 to 500 mg of ascorbic acid daily until symptoms have disappeared.

***infantile s.*** A form of scurvy that sometimes follows the prolonged use of condensed milk, sterilized milk, or proprietary foods that do not contain supplementary vitamin C.

SYMPTOMS: This condition is characterized by anemia, immobility of the legs, pseudoparalysis, extreme tenderness, swelling without pitting, thickening of the bones from subperiosteal hemorrhage, ecchymoses, and tendency toward fractures of the epiphyses. SYN: *Barlow's disease.*

***rebound s.*** Ascorbic acid deficiency symptoms caused by discontinuation of megadoses of vitamin C.

**scute** (skūt) [L. *scutum,* shield] **1.** A thin plate or scale, esp. the horny plates found on the carapace of a turtle. **2.** Formerly the term for the tegmen tympani.

**scutiform** (skū'tĭ-form) [" + *forma,* shape] Shield-shaped.

**scutulum** (skū'tū-lŭm) *pl.* **scutula** [L., a little shield] A lesion of the scalp caused by the fungus *Trichophyton schoenleinii.* The lesion appears as a yellow cup-shaped crust consisting of a dense mass of mycelia and epithelial debris. The cup faces up, and its center is pierced by the hair around which it has developed. **scutular** (-lăr), *adj.* SEE: *favus.*

**scutum** (skū'tŭm) [L., shield] A plate of bone resembling a shield.

**scybalous** (sĭb'ă-lŭs) [Gr. *skybalon,* dung] Of the nature of hard fecal matter.

**scybalum** (sĭb'ă-lŭm) *pl.* **scybala** A hard rounded fecal mass.

**scyphoid** (sī'foyd) [Gr. *skyphos,* cup, + *eidos,* form, shape] Cup-shaped.

**S.D. 1.** *skin dose.* **2.** *standard deviation.*

**SDA 1.** *specific dynamic action.* **2.** Abbr. for Latin *sacrodextra anterior,* the right sacroanterior fetal position.

**SDMS** *Society of Diagnostic Medical Sonographers.*

**S.E.** *standard error.*

**Se** Symbol for the element selenium.

**seabather's eruption** Itching red papules that may appear on the skin within a few hours of swimming in the sea. The lesions progress to form crusted papules and disappear spontaneously in 7 to 10 days. Treatment is symptomatic. This condition may be caused by the larvae of thimble jellyfish, *Linuche unguiculata,* or the larval form of the sea anemone, *Edwardsiella lineata.* The 0.5 mm, virtually invisible larvae release a toxin when trapped between the swimming suit and the skin. Therapy is symptomatic, with oral and topical antipruritic drugs, and topical glucocorticoids. The patient should remove the swimming suit and not reuse it until it has been washed. The larvae can survive in the suit.

**seal 1.** To close firmly. **2.** A material such as an adhesive or wax used to make an airtight closure.

***border s.*** The edge of a denture that contacts the tissues in order to close the area under the denture to entrance by food, air, or liquids.

***posterior palatal s.*** A seal at the posterior border of a denture.

***velopharyngeal s.*** A seal between the oral and nasopharyngeal cavities.

**sealant** A substance applied to prevent leakage into or out of an area.

***dental s.*** A type of resin that bonds to the etched enamel of a tooth and forms a protective coating resistant to chemical or physical breakdown.

***pit and fissure s.*** A method of helping to prevent dental caries by applying adhesive resins to teeth to fill the deep pits and fissures of the occlusal surfaces. This prevents accumulation of debris or decay-producing bacteria from entering these vulnerable areas.

**seal finger** An infection of the finger owing to a bite from a seal. The infectious agent has not been identified, but it is carried in the blood of the seal. The infection is sensitive to tetracycline. Tetanus prophylaxis should be given.

**searcher** (sĕrch′ĕr) [ME. *serchen*] An instrument for locating the opening of the ureter previous to inserting a catheter or exploring the sinuses, and esp. for detecting stones in the bladder. SYN: *sound.*

**seasickness** [AS. *sae,* sea, + *seocness,* illness] A disorder due to the motion of a boat. This condition produces giddiness, vomiting, headache, nausea, and often extreme drowsiness, and prostration. Prevention involves selecting a position in the craft where up-and-down motion is least; avoidance of dietary and alcoholic excesses; avoidance of reading or unusual visual stimuli; and the assumption of a supine or recumbent position. SEE: *motion sickness.*

ETIOLOGY: Motion affects the inner ear, and the vomiting center in the medulla is stimulated. There is wide individual variation in susceptibility.

TREATMENT: Fifty milligrams of Dramamine (dimenhydrinate) should be given every 4 hr as necessary. This medicine causes some people to experience drowsiness; those individuals should not operate a motor vehicle or dangerous machinery when taking Dramamine. Sedatives and supportive therapy, such as intravenous fluids, may be required in severe and prolonged cases. Generally, antinausea pills should not be given to pregnant women during early pregnancy. Transdermal scopolamine is effective in preventing seasickness if it is given several hours before the individual is exposed to the motion. This drug should be used cautiously in elderly patients because it may cause confusion, memory loss, and hallucinations.

**seasonal affective disorder** ABBR: SAD. A mood disorder characterized by mental depression related to a certain season of the year, esp. winter. Symptoms include daytime drowsiness, fatigue, and diminished concentration. Symptoms usually begin during adulthood. It is four times more common in women than in men. The decreased amount of sunlight during the winter is believed to be an important etiological factor. Treatment consists of light therapy along with antidepressants such as fluoxetine, stress management, and exercise.

**seat** The structure on which another structure rests or is supported.

***basal s.*** Tissues in the mouth that support a denture.

***elevated toilet s.*** Raised toilet s.

***raised toilet s.*** A device for raising the height of a toilet to facilitate use by persons with limited strength or movement. SYN: *elevated toilet s.*

***rest s.*** An area on which a denture or restoration rests.

**Seattle foot** [after the city Seattle, Washington, U.S., where it was developed] An artificial foot that has a spring-back quality that makes it feel like a real foot. The use of this device allows single- or double-foot amputees to run and engage in other physical activities, such as sports.

**seatworm** A pinworm.

**sebaceous** (sē-bā′shŭs) [L. *sebaceus,* made of tallow] Containing, or pert. to, sebum, an oily, fatty matter secreted by the sebaceous glands.

**sebaceous cyst** A cyst filled with sebum from a distended sebaceous gland. These cysts are sometimes known as wens. They frequently form on the scalp and consist of a small sac, containing sebaceous matter, that may grow large. They may result from impairment of localized circulation and closure of sebaceous glands or ducts. Drainage does not remove them permanently because they will recur unless entirely extirpated. Extirpation should be done with an electric current or cutting knife. One should never attempt to drain such a cyst without taking every precaution against infection.

**sebaceous gland** An oil-secreting gland of the skin. The glands are simple or branched alveolar glands, most of which open into hair follicles. They are holocrine glands; their secretion, known as sebum, arises from the disintegration of cells filling the alveoli. Most sebaceous glands have a hair follicle associated with them. Some aberrant glands are found in the cheeks or lips of the oral cavity, well separated from hair follicles. SEE: *Fordyce's disease.*

**sebiparous** (sē-bĭp′ă-rŭs) [″ + *parere,* to produce] Producing sebum or sebaceous matter.

**sebo-** Combining form meaning *fat, tallow.*

**sebolite, sebolith** (sĕb′ō-līt, -lĭth) [L. *sebum,* grease, tallow, + Gr. *lithos,* a stone] A concretion in a sebaceous gland.

**seborrhea** (sĕb-or-ē′ă) [″ + Gr. *rhoia,* flow] A functional disease of the sebaceous glands marked by an increase in the amount, and often an alteration of the quality, of the sebaceous secretion.

TREATMENT: Mild dandruff, a type of seborrhea, may be treated with a shampoo containing selenium sulfide or sulfur. If severe, a lotion or cream containing corticosteroids, preferably in the form of hydrocortisone, is rubbed into the affected areas two or three times a day.

***s. capiti*** Seborrhea of the scalp.

***s. corporis*** Dermatitis seborrheica.

***s. faciei*** Seborrhea of the face.

***s. furfuracea*** Dermatitis seborrheica.

***s. nigricans*** Seborrhea with pigmented crusts.

***s. oleosa*** Seborrhea in which fat elements predominate, characterized by shiny skin with widely dilated follicular orifices, many of which contain comedones.

***s. sicca*** Seborrhea with gray-brown or yellow scale and crust formation in addition to abnormal oiliness. Differentiation from seborrheic dermatitis is difficult. This form is most frequently observed on the scalp and constitutes what is commonly called dandruff. Examination reveals an encrustation composed of thin yellowish-gray scales. In uncomplicated cases, the skin is pale but often becomes hyperemic or inflamed from irritation. When allowed to continue, the nutrition of the hair is interfered with, and baldness results. SYN: *dermatitis seborrheica.*

On the body, seborrhea sicca appears as yellowish-gray, slightly elevated patches covered with greasy scales. Outlets of follicles are often dilated. There is generally more or less redness of the skin from hyperemia (seborrheal eczema).

**seborrheic** (sĕb″ō-rē′ĭk) [L. *sebum,* tallow, + Gr. *rhoia,* flow] Afflicted with or like seborrhea.

**seborrheid** (sĕb″ō-rē′ĭd) [″ + Gr. *rhoia,* flow] Dermatitis seborrheica.

**sebum** (sē′bŭm) [L., tallow] A fatty secretion of the sebaceous glands of the skin. It varies in different parts of the body. Sebum from the ears is called *cerumen;* that from the foreskin is called *smegma.*

***s. palpebrale*** Lema.

**seclusion of pupil** Annular synechia.

**secobarbital** A barbiturate used for its sedative and hypnotic effects.

***s. sodium*** A hypnotic and sedative drug.

**secodont** (sē′kō-dŏnt) [L. *secare,* to cut, + Gr. *odous,* tooth] Having molar teeth with cutting edges on the cusps.

**secondary 1.** Next to or following; second in order. **2.** Produced by a primary cause.

**secondary nursing care** Nursing care aimed at early recognition and treatment of disease. It includes general nursing intervention and teaching of early signs of disease conditions so that prompt medical care can be obtained.

**secondary radiation** X-rays produced by the interaction between primary radiation and the substance being radiated.

**second cranial nerve** The nerve carrying impulses for the sense of sight. It originates in the lateral geniculate body of the thalamus and travels by the optic tract and optic chiasma, where it enters the retina through the optic disk. SYN: *optic nerve.* SEE: *cranial nerves; Cranial Nerves Appendix.*

**second intention** Healing by granulation or indirect union. Granulation tissue is formed to fill the gap between the edges of the wound with a thin layer of fibrinous exudate. It bars bacteria and aids in checking bleeding by the coagulation of the blood. Connective tissue cells support the new capillaries. This form of healing is slower than that by first intention, and its grayish-red surface may become pale and flabby if the healing is too long delayed. If the granulations show above the surface, they may have to be removed with caustics. If the granulations first form at the top instead of the bottom of the wound, the wound may have to be kept open with drainage. SEE: *resolution.*

**secreta** (sē-krē′tă) [L.] The products of secretion.

**secretagogue** (sē-krē′tă-gŏg) [L. *secretum,* secretion, + Gr. *agogos,* leading] **1.** That which stimulates secreting organs. **2.** An agent that causes secretion. SYN: *secretogogue.*

**secrete** (sē-krēt′) [L. *secretio,* separation] **1.** To separate from the blood, a living organism, or a gland. **2.** More specifically, to form a secretion.

**secretin** (sē-krē′tĭn) A hormone secreted by the duodenal mucosa that stimulates sodium bicarbonate secretion by the pancreas and bile secretion by the liver. It decreases gastrointestinal peristalsis and motility. SEE: *cholecystokinin-pancreozymin; motilin.*

**secretinase** (sē-krē′tĭ-năs) An enzyme in blood that inactivates secretin.

**secretion** [L. *secretio,* separation] **1.** The

process whereby cells of glandular organs produce certain materials from the blood. **2.** The substance produced by glandular organs. If the material leaves the gland through a duct (e.g., saliva), it is called an exocrine secretion; if it enters the blood or lymph (e.g., insulin), it is called an endocrine secretion.

FLUIDS OF BODY: *Blood:* A secretion composed of 52% to 62% plasma and 38% to 48% cells. *Bile:* A secretion that emulsifies fats and precipitates soluble peptones, producing 20 to 24 oz (259 to 311 ml) daily; specific gravity 1.026 to 1.032. The reaction is alkaline. *Chyle:* A secretion that is absorbed by lacteals, the lymphatics of the small intestines; containing fat absorbed from food. *Chyme:* Food that has undergone gastric digestion only. *Gastric juice:* A clear, acid, watery secretion of the glands of the stomach; whose principal ingredients are hydrochloric acid, mucus, and pepsin. *Intestinal juice:* A secretion that has the combined action of saliva and gastric and pancreatic juices. Starch and complex sugars are converted into monosaccharides. The reaction is alkaline. *Lymph:* A secretion whose characteristics vary with the site of origin. If derived from a limb, it may be clear and have less than 1 g of protein/100 ml. If derived from the gut, protein is increased and fluid may have a milky appearance. *Menstrual:* Menstrual flow; an average of 80 ml during each period; consists of blood, cellular tissue, and mucus. Blood clots are not usually abnormal. *Pancreatic juice:* A secretion that contains enzymes that act on fats, proteins or products of protein digestion, and carbohydrates; approx. 2000 ml of a fluid of pH 7.5 to 8.0 is secreted daily. *Perspiration:* The secretion of sweat glands; from 100 to 1000 ml/day under normal conditions but possibly many times that amount in extremely hot and dry conditions. *Saliva:* A secretion whose composition varies with particular glands, being watery if from parotid and viscous if from submandibular glands; approx. 1500 ml/day. It serves to lubricate food and break down starch and glycogen. *Urine:* 1000 to 2500 ml/24 hr, but highly variable; specific gravity 1.003 to 1.025. The reaction is acid. It contains 50 to 70 g of solids, 12 to 20 g/day of urea nitrogen, and chlorides 110 to 250 nmol/L depending upon chloride intake. SEE: *urine*.

***apocrine s.*** A secretion in which the apical end of a secreting cell is broken off and its contents extruded, as in the mammary gland.

***external s.*** A secretion that passes through a duct and is discharged upon an epithelial surface, either internal or external. Also called *exocrine secretion*.

***holocrine s.*** A secretion in which the entire cell and its contents are extruded as a part of the secretory product, as in sebaceous glands.

***internal s.*** A secretion of the ductless glands, which, entering the bloodstream, activates other glands and organs. SYN: *hormones*. SEE: *ductless glands; endocrine; hormone*.

***merocrine s.*** A secretion in which the product is elaborated within cells and discharged through the cell membrane, the cell itself remaining intact.

***paralytic s.*** The continuous abundant watery secretion from a gland after section of its secretory nerves.

**secretogogue** (sē-krē'tō-gŏg) [L. *secretio,* separation, + Gr. *agogos,* leading] Secretagogue.

**secretoinhibitory** (sē-krē"tō-ĭn-hĭb'ĭ-tō"rē) Inhibiting secretion.

**secretomotor** (sē-krē"tō-mō'tor) Something, esp. a nerve, that stimulates secretion.

**secretor** (sē-krē'tor) [L. *secretio,* separation] A person who secretes ABO blood group substances into mucous secretions such as saliva, gastric juice, or semen.

**secretory** (sē-krē'tō-rē, sē'krē-tō"rē) Pert. to or promoting secretion; secreting.

**secretory capillaries** Very small canaliculi receiving secretion discharged from gland cells.

**secretory fiber** A peripheral motor nerve fiber that innervates glands and stimulates secretion.

**sectarian** (sĕk-tā'rē-ăn) [L. *sectus,* having cut] A medical practitioner who follows a dogma, tenet, or principle based on some unscientific belief.

**sectile** (sĕk'tĭl) [L. *sectilis*] Capable of being cut.

**sectio** (sĕk'shē-ō) [L., a cutting] Section or cut.

**section** [L. *sectio,* a cutting] **1.** Process of cutting. **2.** A division or segment of a part. SEE: *plane* for illus. **3.** A surface made by cutting.

***abdominal s.*** Laparotomy.

***cesarean s.*** SEE: *cesarean section*.

***coronal s.*** Frontal s.

***cross s.*** A section perpendicular to the long axis of an organ.

***frontal s.*** A section dividing the body into two parts, dorsal and ventral. SYN: *coronal s*.

***frozen s.*** A thin section of the body, an organ, or a piece of tissue that has been frozen before being sectioned and then studied microscopically.

***ground s.*** A section of bone or tooth prepared for histological study by polishing until thin enough for microscope viewing.

***longitudinal s.*** A section parallel to the long axis of an organ.

***midsagittal s.*** A section that divides the body into right and left halves.

***paraffin s.*** A section of a tissue that has been infiltrated with paraffin.

***perineal s.*** An external incision into the urethra to relieve stricture.

***sagittal s.*** A section cut parallel to the

median plane of the body.

***serial s.*** One of the microscopic sections made and arranged in consecutive order.

***vaginal s.*** Incision into the abdominal cavity through the vagina.

**sectioning** [L. *sectio,* a cutting] The slicing of thin sections of tissue for examination under the microscope. SEE: *microtome.*

***ultrathin s.*** The cutting of sections extraordinarily thin (less than 1 $\mu$m thick), esp. for use in electron microscopy.

**sector** (sĕk′tor) [L., cutter] The area of a circle included between two radii and an arc.

**sectorial** (sĕk-tō′rē-ăl) Having cutting edges, as teeth.

**secundigravida** (sē-kŭn″dĭ-grăv′ĭd-ă) [L. *secundus,* second, + *gravida,* pregnant] A woman in her second pregnancy.

**secundines** (sĕk′ŭn-dīnz, sĭ-kŭn′dīnz) [LL. *secundinae*] Afterbirth; the placenta and its membranes.

**secundipara** (sē″kŭn-dĭp′ă-ră) [L. *secundus,* second, + *parere,* to bring forth, to bear] A woman who has produced two infants at separate times that have weighed 500 g or more, regardless of their viability. SEE: *gravida; para.*

**secundiparity** (sē-kŭn″dĭ-păr′ĭ-tē) The condition of being a secundipara.

**S.E.D.** *skin erythema dose.*

**sedation** (sē-dā′shŭn) [L. *sedatio,* from *sedare,* to calm] **1.** The process of allaying nervous excitement. **2.** The state of being calmed.

***conscious s.*** A minimally depressed level of consciousness during which the patient retains the ability to maintain a patent airway and respond appropriately to physical or verbal commands. This is accomplished by the use of appropriate analgesics and sedatives. This type of sedation is used for a variety of procedures including changing of wound or burn dressings and endoscopic examinations.

---

Caution: Although this method is effective, it must be used carefully to prevent loss of consciousness. The health care team must be ready to recognize and respond to complications that require airway management, intubation, and resuscitation. Drugs to reverse the effects of opioids and antidepressants may need to be used. Naloxone is effective for opioids and flumazenil is used for benzodiazepines.

---

**sedative** (sĕd′ă-tĭv) [L. *sedativus,* calming] **1.** Quieting. **2.** An agent that exerts a soothing or tranquilizing effect. Sedatives may be general, local, nervous, or vascular.

**sedentary** (sĕd′ĕn-tā′rē) [L. *sedentarius*] **1.** Sitting. **2.** Pert. to an occupation or mode of living requiring minimal physical exercise.

***s. lifestyle*** A lifestyle involving little exercise, even of the least strenuous type. Increasing evidence indicates that this lifestyle is not conducive to maximum enjoyment of life, to health, or to longevity. SEE: *physical fitness; risk factors.*

**sediment** (sĕd′ĭ-mĕnt) [L. *sedimentum,* a settling] The substance settling at the bottom of a liquid. SEE: *precipitate.*

***urinary s.*** Substances present in urine (i.e., bacteria, mucus, phosphates, uric acid, calcium oxalate, calcium carbonate, calcium phosphate, magnesium and ammonium phosphate; more rarely, cystine, tyrosine, xanthine, hippuric acid, hematoidin) that separate and accumulate at the bottom of a container of urine. This process may be accelerated by centrifuging the urine specimen.

**sedimentation** (sĕd″ĭ-mĕn-tā′shŭn) Formation or depositing of sediment.

**seed** (sēd) [AS. *saed*] **1.** The ripened ovule of a spermatophyte plant usually consisting of the embryo (germ) and a supply of nutrient material enclosed within the seed coats. It is a resting sporophyte. **2.** Sperm; semen. **3.** Capsule containing radon or radium for use in the treatment of cancer. **4.** To introduce microorganisms into a culture medium.

**seeker, bone** An ion or compound that localizes preferentially in bone (e.g., strontium).

**Seessel's pouch** (zā′sĕlz) [Albert Seessel, U.S. embryologist and neurologist, 1850–1910] In the embryo, a small ectodermal diverticulum of the foregut close to the buccopharyngeal membrane. It disappears in humans.

**segment** (sĕg′mĕnt) [L. *segmentum,* a portion] **1.** A part or section, esp. a natural one, of an organ or body. **2.** One of the serial divisions of an animal.

***bronchopulmonary s.*** A small subdivision of the lobes of the lung.

***hepatic s.*** A subdivision of the lobes of the liver.

***interannular s.*** The portion of a neuron between the two nodes of Ranvier.

***mesodermal s.*** A somite.

***uterine s.*** One of the segments of the uterus during labor. The upper portion becomes thicker and the lower segment is thinned out.

**segmental** (sĕg-mĕn′tăl) Pert. to, resembling, or composed of segments.

**segmental static reaction** A postural reflex in which the movement of one extremity results in a movement in an opposite extremity.

**segmentation** (sĕg″mĕn-tā′shŭn) Cleavage.

**segmenter** A stage in the development of the malarial organism (of the genus *Plasmodium*) in which the organism undergoes schizogony.

**segregation** [L. *segregare,* to separate] **1.** Setting apart, separating. **2.** In genetics, the process that takes place in the formation of germ cells (gametogenesis) in which each gamete (egg or sperm) receives only one of each pair of genes.

**segregator** An instrument composed of two

ureteral catheters for securing urine from each kidney separately.

**Séguin's signal symptom** (sā-gănz') [Edouard Séguin, French psychiatrist in U.S., 1812–1880] The involuntary contractions of the muscles just before an epileptic attack.

**SeHCAT** Selenium-75 labeled artificial bile salt; homologue to taurocholate.

**Seidlitz powder** (sĕd'lĭts, sīd'lĭtz) [Seidlitz, village in Bohemia] An effervescent cathartic composed of tartaric acid, sodium bicarbonate, and sodium and potassium tartrate.

**seismesthesia** (sīz"mĕs-thē'zē-ă) [Gr. *seismos,* a shaking, + *aisthesis,* sensation] The perception of vibrations.

**seizure** (sē'zhūr) [O. Fr. *seisir,* to take possession of] A sudden attack of pain, a disease, or certain symptoms.

***absence s.*** SEE: *epilepsy.*

***convulsive s.*** **1.** A convulsion. **2.** An attack of epilepsy. SEE: *epilepsy.*

***grand mal s.*** SEE: *epilepsy.*

***jacksonian s.*** SEE: *jacksonian epilepsy.*

***petit mal s.*** SEE: *epilepsy.*

**Seldinger technique** [Sven I. Seldinger, Swedish physician, b. 1921] A method of percutaneous introduction of a catheter into a vessel. The vessel is located and a needle is inserted. Once a good blood flow is obtained, a wire is threaded through the needle well into the vessel; the needle is then removed and the catheter threaded over the wire into the vessel. The wire assists in inserting the catheter and guiding it into the appropriate vessel. Once the catheter is positioned in the desired intravascular area, the wire is removed. Sterile technique is imperative.

**selection** [L. *selectus,* having chosen] **1.** Choice; the process of choosing or selecting. **2.** In biology, the factors that determine the reproductive ability of a certain genotype.

***artificial s.*** A process by which humans select desirable characteristics in animals and breed them for these phenotypes.

***clonal s.*** **1.** The process by which T lymphocytes with receptors that react to self-antigens are destroyed in the thymus. **2.** The increase of particular B or T lymphocyte clones that recognize a specific antigen. When a particular microorganism invades the body, only the clones that recognize it multiply. SEE: *negative s.; clone.*

***natural s.*** A mechanism of evolution proposed by Darwin stating that the genotypes best adapted to their environment have a tendency to survive and reproduce.

***negative s.*** The process by which immature T lymphocytes (thymocytes) with receptors for self-antigens are destroyed in the thymus. This is part of the process of autoimmunity. SEE: *autoimmunity.*

***sexual s.*** A theory originated to account for differences in secondary sex characteristics between men and women. It assumes that individuals preferentially mate with individuals of the opposite sex who possess these characteristics.

**selenium** (sē-lē'nē-ŭm) [Gr. *selene,* moon] SYMB: Se. A chemical element resembling sulfur; atomic weight 78.96; atomic number 34. Toxicity can occur when an excessive amount is ingested, characterized by a sour breath odor, nausea, vomiting, abdominal pain, restlessness, hypersalivation, and muscle spasms.

***s. sulfide*** A drug used in treating dandruff and tinea versicolor.

**selenoid cell** Achromocyte. SYN: *crescent body.*

**selenomethionine Se 75 injection** (sĕl" ĕn-ō-mĕ-thī'ō-nēn) Radioactive L-selenomethionine in which the sulfur atom in the methionine has been replaced by selenium. The compound is used intravenously to investigate methionine metabolism.

**self** **1.** In psychology, the sum of mind and body that constitutes the identity of a person. **2.** In immunology, an individual's own antigenic makeup.

**self-acceptance** Being realistic about oneself and at the same time comfortable with that personal assessment.

**self-care** **1.** A concept central to Dorothea Orem's theory of nursing that includes actions directed toward the self and toward the environment with the specific purpose of regulating one's functioning and well-being. The nurse's central function is to enhance the self-care of patients through the nursing process of assessment, planning, intervention, and evaluation. **2.** In rehabilitation, the subset of activities of daily living that includes eating, dressing, grooming, bathing, and toileting. SYN: *personal care.*

***s.-c. deficit*** A deficit of thinking, action, emotion, or resources within a patient's environment that impedes successful self-care (e.g., feeding, bathing, toileting, dressing, and grooming) and necessitates the services of a nurse on a temporary, permanent, or progressing basis. Self-care also may be expanded to include the practices used by the client to promote health, the individual responsibility for self, or a way of thinking. SEE: *health maintenance, altered; home maintenance management, impaired; Nursing Diagnoses Appendix.*

**Self-Care Framework** A conceptual model of nursing, also known as the Self-Care Deficit Theory of Nursing, developed by Dorothea Orem. The person is a self-care agent who has a therapeutic self-care demand made up of universal, developmental, and health deviation self-care requisites. The goal of nursing is to help people to meet their therapeutic self-care demands. SEE: *Nursing Theory Appendix.*

**self-concept** An individual's perception of self in relation to others and the environment. SEE: *self-esteem.*

**self-conscious** Being aware of oneself, esp. overly aware of appearance and actions, and thus being ill at ease.

**self-contained underwater breathing apparatus** ABBR: SCUBA. A device used by swimmers and divers that enables them to breathe underwater. The mask worn is watertight and is connected to a tank of compressed air. SEE: *bends.*

**self-differentiation** The differentiation of a structure or tissues due to intrinsic factors.

**self-digestion** Destruction or disintegration of a cell or tissue by its own juice, as that of the walls of the stomach by the gastric juice occurring in certain diseases of that organ. SYN: *autodigestion.*

**self-efficacy** An aspect of self-perception postulated by Albert Bandura that pertains to one's belief in his or her ability to perform a given task or behavior.

**self-esteem** One's personal evaluation or view of self, generally thought to influence feelings and behaviors. One's personal successes, expectations, and appraisals of the views others hold toward oneself are thought to influence this personal appraisal. SYN: *self-concept.*

***chronic low s.-e.*** Longstanding negative feelings about self or capabilities. SEE: *situational low s.-e.; Nursing Diagnoses Appendix.*

***s.-e. disturbance*** Negative self-evaluation/feelings about self or self-capabilities that may be directly or indirectly expressed. SEE: *Nursing Diagnoses Appendix.*

***situational low s.-e.*** Episodic feelings about self or capabilities which develop in response to a loss or change. SEE: *chronic low s.-e.; Nursing Diagnoses Appendix.*

**self-governance** A model of nursing management where the power base for decisions of patient care is decentralized. The responsibility and accountability for patient care rests directly with all levels of nurses through self-direction, self-regulation, and self-management. Advisory committees reflecting a cross section of nurses (new graduates, experienced nurses, faculty, and managers) maintain final decision-making authority within the work setting. SEE: *shared governance.*

**self-hypnosis** Hypnotizing oneself.

**self-limited disease** Disease that, without treatment, runs a definite course within a limited time.

**self-mutilation, risk for** A state in which an individual is at high risk to perform a deliberate act upon the self with the intent to injure, not kill, which produces immediate tissue damage to the body. SEE: *Nursing Diagnoses Appendix.*

**self-ranging** Patient-administered passive range of motion following stroke. By using their unaffected arms and specific techniques, patients with hemiplegia can be taught to prevent contractures by moving their paralyzed extremities through full range of motion at the shoulder, elbow, wrist, and finger joints. Care should be used to prevent injury, esp. at the shoulder.

**self-tolerance** In immunology, tolerance to self-antigens.

**Seligmann's disease** Alpha heavy chain disease.

**sellar** (sĕl′ăr) Concerning the sella turcica.

**sella turcica** (sĕl′ă tŭr′sĭ-kă) [NL., Turkish saddle] A concavity on the superior surface of the body of the sphenoid bone that houses the hypophysis cerebri (pituitary gland). SEE: *empty-sella syndrome.*

**Sellick's maneuver** [Brian A. Sellick, contemporary Brit. anesthetist] The application of digital pressure to the cricoid cartilage in the neck in an unconscious patient to reduce gastric distention and passive regurgitation during positive pressure ventilation, and to permit visualization of the glottic opening during endotracheal intubation.

**seltzer water 1.** Naturally occurring water with a high mineral and carbon dioxide content. **2.** Water that has been artificially charged with carbon dioxide.

**semantics** (sē-măn′tĭks) [Gr. *semantikos,* significant] The study of meanings; a branch of semiotics.

**semen** (sē′mĕn) *pl.* **semina** [L., seed] A thick, opalescent, viscid secretion discharged from the urethra of the male at the climax of sexual excitement (orgasm). Semen is the mixed product of various glands (prostate and bulbourethral) plus the spermatozoa, which, having been produced in the testicles, are stored in the seminal vesicles.

Normal values for the seminal fluid ejaculate are as follows: volume, 2 to 5 ml; pH, 7.8 to 8.0; leukocytes, absent or only an occasional one seen per high-power field; sperm count, 60 to 150 million/ml; motility, 80% or more should be motile; morphology, 80% to 90% should be normal.

***frozen s.*** Semen stored in a bank for future use in insemination. It offers a supply of donors in small communities where it would be impossible to maintain anonymity of local donors. However, in artificial insemination the number of successful pregnancies is lower with frozen semen than with fresh.

**semenarche** (sē′mĕn-ăr″kē) [″ + *arche,* beginning] During puberty, the beginning of the production of semen. SEE: *pubarche; thelarche.*

**semenuria** (sē″mĕn-ū′rē-ă) [L. *semen,* seed, + Gr. *ouron,* urine] The excretion of semen in the urine. SYN: *seminuria; spermaturia.*

**semi-** Prefix meaning *half.*

**semicanal** (sĕm″ē-kăn-ăl′) [L. *semis,* half, + *canalis,* channel] A duct open on one side.

**semicanalis** (sĕm″ē-kă-nā′lĭs) [L., semi-canal] A channel open on one side.

***s. musculi tensoris tympani*** The semicanal of the tensor tympani muscle in the temporal bone.

***s. tubae auditivae*** The semicanal of the auditory tube.

**semicartilaginous** (sĕm″ē-kăr″tĭ-lăj′ĭ-nŭs) [″ + *cartilago,* gristle] Partially cartilaginous.

**semicircular** (sĕm″ē-sŭr′kū-lăr) [″+ *circulus,* a ring] In the form of a half circle.

**semicircular canal** One of the superior, posterior, and inferior passages of the inner ear, concerned with detecting motion. SEE: *ear; labyrinth* for illus.

**semicoma** (sĕm″ē-kō′mă) [″+ Gr. *koma,* a deep sleep] Mild degree of impaired consciousness from which it is possible to arouse the patient.

**semicomatose** (sĕm″ē-kō′măt-ōs) In a condition of impaired consciousness from which the patient may be aroused. SEE: *consciousness.*

**semiconscious** Half-conscious or not fully conscious. SEE: *Glasgow Coma Scale.*

**semicrista** (sĕm″ē-krĭs′tă) [L.] A small or rudimentary crest.

***s. incisiva*** The nasal crest of the maxilla.

**semidecussation** (sĕm″ē-dē″kŭs-sā′shŭn) [″ + *decussare,* to make an X] Incomplete crossing of nerve fibers.

**semierection** (sĕm″ē-ĕ-rĕk′shŭn) [″ + *erigere,* to erect] An incomplete erection.

**semiflexion** (sĕm″ē-flĕk′shŭn) [″+ *flexio,* bending] Halfway between flexion and extension of a limb.

**semilunar** (sĕm″ē-lū′năr) [L. *semis,* half, + *luna,* moon] Shaped like a crescent.

**semilunar bone** Crescent-shaped bone of the carpus. Also called the *lunate bone.* SYN: *semilunare.*

**semilunar cusp** One of the three segments of the aorta, or of the pulmonary valve between the right ventricle and the pulmonary artery.

**semilunare** (sĕm″ē-lū-nā′rē) [L.] Semilunar bone.

**semilunar lobe** A lobe on the upper surface of the cerebellum.

**semiluxation** (sĕm″ē-lŭk-sā′shŭn) [″ + *luxatio,* dislocation] Subluxation.

**semimembranosus** (sĕm″ē-mĕm″brăn-ō′ sŭs) [L.] A large muscle of the inner and back part of the thigh. SEE: *Muscles Appendix.*

**semimembranous** (sĕm″ē-mĕm′bră-nŭs) [″ + L. *membrana,* membrane] Composed partly of a membrane.

**seminal** (sĕm′ĭ-năl) [L. *seminalis*] Concerning the semen or seed.

**seminal duct** Any duct that conveys sperm, esp. the ductus deferens and the ejaculatory duct. SYN: *spermatic duct.*

**seminal emission** Discharge of semen.

**seminal vesicle** One of two saclike structures in the male, lying behind the bladder close to the prostate and connected to the ductus deferens on each side. These vesicles secrete a thick alkaline fluid that forms a part of the semen.

**semination** (sĕm-ĭ-nā′shŭn) [L. *seminatio,* a begetting] Insemination.

***artificial s.*** Artificial insemination.

**seminiferous** (sĕm-ĭn-ĭf′ĕr-ŭs) [L. *semen,* seed, + *ferre,* to produce] Producing or conducting semen, as the tubules of the testes.

**seminoma** (sĕm″ĭ-nō′mă) [″ + Gr. *oma,* tumor] A tumor of the testis.

**seminormal** (sĕm″ē-nor′măl) [L. *semis,* half, + *norma,* rule] One-half the normal standard.

**seminose** (sĕm′ĭ-nōs) Mannose.

**seminuria** (sē″mĭn-ū′rē-ă) [L. *semen,* seed, + Gr. *ouron,* urine] Semen in the urine. SYN: *semenuria; spermaturia.*

**semiorbicular** (sĕm″ē-or-bĭk′ū-lăr) [L. *semis,* half, + *orbiculus,* a small circle] Semicircular.

**semiotics** (sē″mī-ŏt′ĭks) The philosophy of the function of signs and symbols in language.

**semipermeable** (sĕm″ē-per′mē-ă-bl) [″ + *per,* through, + *meare,* to pass] Half-permeable; said of a membrane that will allow fluids, but not the dissolved substance, to pass through it. SEE: *membrane; osmosis.*

**semipronation** (sĕm″ē-prō-nā′shŭn) [″ + *pronus,* prone] **1.** A semiprone position. **2.** The act of assuming a semiprone position.

**semiprone** (sĕm-ē-prōn′) [″+ *pronus,* prone] In a position on left side and chest, with both thighs flexed on abdomen, the right higher than the left, and left arm back. SYN: *Sims' position.*

**semirecumbent** (sĕm″ē-rē-kŭm′bĕnt) [″ + *recumbere,* to lie down] Reclining, but not fully recumbent.

**semis** (sē′mĭs) [L.] ABBR: ss. Half.

**semispinalis** (sĕm″ē-spī-năl′ĭs) [L.] The deep layer of muscle of the back on either side of the spinal colum. It is divided into the following three parts: the semispinalis capitis, semispinalis cervicis, and semispinalis thoracis. SEE: *Muscles Appendix.*

**semisulcus** (sĕm″ē-sŭl′kŭs) [L. *semis,* half, + *sulcus,* groove] A small sulcus or channel in a structure. It usually joins with another small channel to form a complete sulcus.

**semisupination** (sĕm″ē-sū-pĭn-ā′shŭn) [″+ *supinus,* lying on the back] A position halfway between supination and pronation.

**semisupine** (sĕm″ē-sū′pīn) [″+ *supinus,* lying on the back] Not completely supine.

**semisynthetic** (sĕm″ē-sĭn-thĕt′ĭk) [″+ Gr. *synthetikos,* synthetic] The chemical alteration of a portion of a natural substance.

**semitendinosus** (sĕm″ē-tĕn″dĭn-ō′sŭs) [L.] The fusiform muscle of the posterior and inner part of the thigh. SEE: *Muscles Appendix.*

**semitendinous** (sĕm″ē-tĕn′dĭ-nŭs) [L. *semis,* half, + *tendinosus,* tendinous] Being partially tendinous.

**Semmelweiss, Ignaz Phillip** Hungarian physician, 1818–1865, the discoverer of the mode of transmission of childbed fever (puerperal sepsis) in the 19th century. Semmelweiss noted the significantly lower incidence of this condition in women who were attended by midwives who used chlorinated lime solution as a disinfectant hand rinse to prevent transfer of organisms to the birth canal during delivery.

**senescence** (sē-nĕs′ĕns) [L. *senescens,* growing old] **1.** The process of growing old. **2.** The period of old age.

**Sengstaken-Blakemore tube** (sĕngz′tā-kĕn-blāk′mor) [Robert W. Sengstaken, U.S. neurosurgeon, b. 1923; Arthur H. Blakemore, U.S. surgeon, 1897–1970] A three-lumen tube used to treat bleeding esophageal varices. One lumen leads to the stomach; another leads to a balloon at the gastric end—it is used to inflate the balloon after the tube is in place; the third lumen leads to an inflatable cuff around a portion of the entire tube. This third lumen allows the cuff to be inflated and provide pressure against the varices. The gastric balloon permits the cuff to resist being inadvertently removed and serves to keep the entire tube in place.

**senile** (sē′nīl, sĕn′īl) [L. *senilis,* old] Pert. to growing old and the mental or physical weakness with which it is sometimes associated.

**senilism** (sē′nĭl-ĭzm, -nĭl-ĭzm) [″ + Gr. *ismos,* condition] Old age, particularly when premature. SEE: *progeria.*

**senility** (sē-nĭl′ĭ-tē) [L. *senilis,* old] Mental or physical weakness that may be associated with old age.

***premature s.*** Onset of senile characteristics before old age, as early as 40 years of age.

***psychosis of s.*** Mental disorder in old age.

**senium** (sē′nē-ŭm) [L.] Old age, esp. its debility.

**senna** (sĕn′ă) [Arabic *sana*] The dried leaves of the plants *Cassia acutifolia* and *C. angustifolia;* used as a cathartic.

**sennosides** (sĕn′ō-sīdz) Anthraquinone glucosides present in senna that are used as cathartics.

**senopia** (sĕn-ō′pē-ă, sē-nō′-) [L. *senilis,* old, + Gr. *ops,* eye] Improvement in near vision of old people. Usually precedes the development of nuclear cataract. SYN: *sight, second.*

**sensate** Perceived by the senses.

**sensate focus** An area, such as an erogenous zone, that is particularly sensitive to tactile stimulation.

**sensation** (sĕn-sā′shŭn) [L. *sensatio*] A feeling or awareness of conditions within or without the body resulting from the stimulation of sensory receptors.

***cincture s.*** Girdle s.

***cutaneous s.*** A sensation arising from the receptors of the skin.

***delayed s.*** A sensation not experienced immediately following a stimulus.

***epigastric s.*** A sinking feeling in the stomach.

***external s.*** The effect upon the mind of stimuli produced from a source outside the body.

***girdle s.*** A painful sensation, as a bandage tightened about a limb or the trunk, as in spinal disease. SYN: *cincture s.; zonesthesia.*

***gnostic s.*** One of the more finely developed senses such as touch, tactile discrimination, position sense, and vibration.

***internal s.*** Subjective s.

***palmesthetic s.*** A sensation felt in the skin from vibration.

***phantom s.*** The experience of sensation in the missing part or limb following amputation. The perceived sensation may resemble the actual presence of the limb (phantom limb) or may be experienced as tingling, gripping, or clenching. Burning or cramping (phantom pain) may also occur. These sensory changes are thought to be caused by sensory representations from the missing limb that remain in the brain. Severe phantom pain can lead to difficulties in prosthetic training.

***primary s.*** A sensation that results from a direct stimulus.

***proprioceptive s.*** Sensation of the position or location of the body or a part of the body. This is usually subconscious but is essential for coordination.

***referred s.*** A sensation that seems to arise from a source other than the actual one. SYN: *reflex s.*

***reflex s.*** Referred s.

***somesthetic s.*** A sense; proprioception.

***subjective s.*** A sensation that does not result from any external stimulus and is perceptible only by the subject. SYN: *internal s.*

***tactile s.*** A sensation produced through the sense of touch.

**sense** (sĕns) [L. *sensus,* a feeling] **1.** To perceive through a sense organ. **2.** The general faculty by which conditions outside or inside the body are perceived. **3.** Any special faculty of sensation connected with a particular organ. **4.** Normal power of understanding.

The most important of the senses are sight, hearing, smell, taste, touch and pressure, temperature, weight, resistance and tension (muscle sense), pain, position, proprioception, visceral and sexual sensations, equilibrium, and hunger and thirst.

***color s.*** The ability to distinguish differences in color; one of the three parts of visual function.

***form s.*** The ability to recognize shapes; one of the three parts of visual function.

***kinesthetic s.*** Muscular s.

***light s.*** The ability to distinguish degrees of light intensity; one of the three parts of the visual function.

***muscular s.*** A consciousness of the muscular movement required in a given act. SYN: *kinesthetic s.*

***posture s.*** Proprioception.

***pressure s.*** The ability to feel various degrees of pressure on the body surface. SYN: *baresthesia.*

***proprioceptive s.*** The correlation of unconscious sensations from the skin, muscles, and joints that allows a conscious appreciation of the position of the body and its parts.

***sixth s.*** A general feeling of normal functioning of the body. SYN: *cenesthesia.*

***space s.*** The sense by which people recognize objects in space, their relationship, and their dimensions.

***special s.'s*** The five senses of sight, hearing, smell, touch, and taste.

***static s.*** The sense that makes it possible to maintain equilibrium.

***stereognostic s.*** The ability to judge the consistency and shape of objects held in the fingers.

***temperature s.*** The ability to detect differences of temperature.

***time s.*** The ability to detect differences in time intervals.

***tone s.*** The ability to distinguish between different tones.

***visceral s.*** The subjective perception of the sensations of the internal organs.

**sensibility** (sĕn″sĭ-bĭl′ĭ-tē) [L. *sensibilitas*] The capacity to receive and respond to stimuli.

***deep s.*** **1.** The sensibility existing after an area of the skin is made anesthetic. **2.** The sensation by which the position of a limb and estimation of difference in weight and tension are apparent.

***palmesthetic s.*** The sensibility of the skin to vibration.

**sensibilization** (sĕn″sĭ-bĭl-ĭz-ā′shŭn) **1.** Sensitization. **2.** Production of hypersusceptibility to a foreign substance by injecting it into the body. SYN: *sensitization.*

**sensible** (sĕn′sĭ-bl) [L. *sensibilis,* capable of being perceived] **1.** Capable of being perceived by the senses; perceptible. **2.** Having reason.

**sensiferous** (sĕn-sĭf′ĕr-ŭs) [L. *sensus,* a feeling, + *ferre,* to bear] Causing, conducting, or transmitting sensations.

**sensimeter** (sĕn-sĭm′ĕ-tĕr) [″ + Gr. *metron,* measure] A machine for recording the degree of sensitiveness of various areas of the body.

**sensitinogen** (sĕn″sĭ-tĭn′ō-jĕn) [″ + Gr. *gennan,* to produce] The collective of antigens that sensitize the body.

**sensitive** (sĕn′sĭ-tĭv) [L. *sensitivus,* of sensation] **1.** Capable of perceiving a sensation. **2.** Able to feel a sensation. SYN: *sentient.* **3.** Subject to destructive action of a complement. **4.** Susceptible to suggestions, as a hypnotic. **5.** Abnormally susceptible to a substance, as a drug or foreign protein. SEE: *allergy.*

**sensitivity** In assessing the value of a diagnostic test, procedure, or clinical observation, the proportion of people who truly have a specific disease and are so identified by the test. SEE: *specificity, diagnostic.*

**sensitivity test, antimicrobial** A laboratory method of determining the susceptibility of a patient's bacterial infection to antibiotics or antibacterials. The specimen obtained from the patient is cultured in various liquid dilutions of the drugs or on solid media containing various concentrations of the drugs in disks placed on the surface of the media. The disk-type test is not completely reliable. Also called *culture and sensitivity test.* SEE: illus.

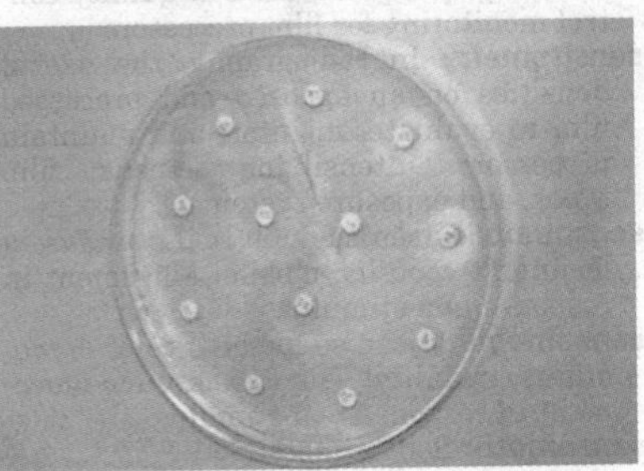

ANTIMICROBIAL SENSITIVITY TEST

ZONES OF INHIBITED BACTERIAL GROWTH AROUND ANTIBIOTIC DISKS

**sensitivity training** A form of group therapy in which individuals are given the opportunity to relate verbally and physically with complete candor and honesty with other members of the group. The goals of therapy are to increase self-awareness, learn constructive ways of dealing with conflicts, establish a better sense of inner direction, and relate to persons with feelings of warmth and affection.

**sensitization** (sĕn″sĭ-tĭ-zā′shŭn) **1.** A condition of being made sensitive to a specific substance (i.e., antigen) such as a protein or pollen. **2.** The process of making a person susceptible to a substance by repeated injections of it. SYN: *sensibilization.*

***active s.*** Sensitization produced by injecting an antigen into a susceptible person.

***autoerythrocyte s.*** A syndrome characterized by the spontaneous appearance of painful ecchymoses, usually at the site of a bruise. The areas itch and burn. The condition is commonly associated with headache, nausea, vomiting, and occasionally with intracranial, genitourinary, and gastrointestinal bleeding. With few exceptions, the disorder affects women of middle age. The cause is assumed to be autosensitivity to a component of the red blood cell membrane. There is no specific therapy.

***passive s.*** Sensitization produced in a healthy person by injecting the person with the serum from a sensitized animal or human.

***protein s.*** Sensitization as a result of previous injection of a foreign protein into the body.

**sensitized** (sĕn′sĭ-tīzd) Made susceptible to a specific substance.

**sensitizer** (sĕn′sĭ-tī″zĕr) [L. *sensitivus,* of sensation] In allergy and dermatology, a substance that makes the susceptible individual react to the same or other irritants.

**sensitometer** A calibrated instrument with an optical step wedge and light source that puts a graduated set of densities on a radiographic film; used in quality control monitoring for film processors.

**sensitometry** In radiography, the use of densities on an exposed and processed film to evaluate, monitor, and maintain processors, intensifying screens, film types, and exposure systems.

**sensomobile** (sĕn″sō-mō′bĭl) [L. *sensus,* a feeling, + *mobilis,* mobile] Movement in response to a stimulus.

**sensomobility** (sĕn″sō-mō-bĭl′ĭ-tē) [″ + *mobilitas,* mobility] The capacity for movement in response to a stimulus.

**sensomotor** Sensorimotor.

**sensor 1.** A sense organ. **2.** A device sensitive to light, heat, radiation, sound, or mechanical or other physical stimuli. These devices may be equipped to record the phenomena being detected and to sound an alarm if the value falls below or rises above a certain level.

**sensoriglandular** (sĕn″sō-rē-glănd′dū-lăr) [L. *sensus,* a feeling, + *glandula,* little acorn] Concerning glandular excretion in response to stimulation of a nerve.

**sensorimetabolism** (sĕn″sō-rē-mĕ-tăb′ō-lĭzm) [″ + Gr. *metaballein,* to alter, + *-ismos,* condition] Metabolic activity in response to sensory nerve stimulation.

**sensorimotor** (sĕn″sō-rē-mō′tor) [L. *sensus,* a feeling, + *motus,* moving] Both sensory and motor. SYN: *sensomotor.*

**sensorimuscular** (sĕn″sō-rē-mŭs′kū-lăr) [″ + *muscularis,* muscular] Muscular activity in response to a sensory stimulus.

**sensorineural** (sĕn″sō-rē-nū′răl) [″ + *neuralis,* neural] Concerning a sensory nerve.

**sensorium** (sĕn-sor′ē-ŭm) *pl.* **sensoriums, sensoria** [L., organ of sensation] **1.** That portion of the brain that functions as a center of sensations. **2.** The sensory apparatus of the body taken as a whole. **sensorial** (-sō′rē-ăl), *adj.*

**sensorivasomotor** (sĕn″sō-rē-văs″ō-mō′tor) [L. *sensus,* a feeling, + *vas,* vessel, + *motor,* a mover] Vascular changes induced by sensory nerve stimulation.

**sensory** (sĕn′sō-rē) [L. *sensorius*] **1.** Conveying impulses from sense organs to the reflex or higher centers. SYN: *afferent.* **2.** Pert. to sensation.

**sensory area** Any area of the cerebral cortex in which sensations are perceived.

***somesthetic s.a.*** An area in the postcentral gyrus of the parietal lobes and extending into adjacent areas in which sensations of general somatic sensibility are perceived; the area for the cutaneous senses and conscious proprioceptive sense.

**sensory deprivation** The enforced absence of usual and accustomed sensory stimuli (e.g., patients whose eyes are bandaged for extended periods following eye surgery, patients in respirators, astronauts, a sailor adrift alone at sea, or those imprisoned in completely dark, soundproof cells). The absence of normal stimuli will, if continued, lead to severe mental changes including auditory and visual hallucinations, anxiety, depression, and insanity.

In psychological experimentation, sensory deprivation may be achieved by confining a volunteer wearing gloves, an eye mask, and ear muffs in a small soundproof room or by immersing an individual equipped for underwater breathing in a tank of water that is devoid of stimuli except for the sound of breathing.

NURSING IMPLICATIONS: The patient's usual response to prolonged quiet or isolation is assessed. Patients who require more environmental stimuli (radio, TV noise, people) suffer more (and more quickly) than do those who prefer quiet. Stimulation is provided to replace those stimuli which the patient is deprived of. The nurse tells those patients who cannot see or whose visual field is limited by position or equipment about weather, time of day, and surrounding colors. The nurse also describes equipment, locations, food, and anything else the patient wants to know that cannot be visualized, allowing touch to help replace vision. For the patient whose hearing is reduced by location or equipment (or by effects of drug therapy), devices are used that assist hearing-impaired persons to understand speech. Sensory-deprived patients are encouraged to use radio or TV as desired, and the nurse makes frequent visits to prevent these patients from feeling abandoned. Therapies are related to time of day (before breakfast, after dinner, at bedtime, etc.), and a clock and calendar are provided to assist with time orientation. Reported auditory or visual hallucinations should be investigated thoroughly and a source sought that could simulate the sound or sight reported by the patient (e.g., linen cart may sound like truck going by, curtain moving may look like ghost). The nurse validates reality for the patient by changing lighting or altering external noises to eliminate confusion.

**sensory ending** A termination of an afferent

nerve fiber that upon stimulation gives rise to a sensation. SEE: *receptor, sensory.*

**sensory epilepsy** Disturbances of sensation without convulsions.

**sensory integration** Skill and performance required in the development and coordination of sensory input, motor output, and sensory feedback. It includes sensory awareness, visual spatial awareness, body integration, balance, bilateral motor coordination, visuomotor integration, praxis, and other components.

**sensory overload** The condition in which sensory stimuli are received at a rate and intensity beyond the level that the patient can handle. This stressful situation can lead to confusion, anxiety, mental distress, and panic.

**sensory-perceptual alterations** Changes that an individual experiences in the amount or patterning of incoming stimuli accompanied by a diminished, exaggerated, distorted, or impaired response to such stimuli (visual, auditory, kinesthetic, gustatory, tactile, and olfactory). SEE: *Nursing Diagnoses Appendix.*

**sensory registration** The brain's ability to receive input and select that which will receive attention and that which will be inhibited from conscious attention.

**sensory unit** A single sensory nerve fiber with all its branches and their terminal nerve endings.

**sensual** (sĕn′shū-ăl) [L. *sensus,* a feeling] Concerning or consisting in the gratification of the senses; indulgence of the appetites; not spiritual or intellectual; carnal, worldly.

**sensualism** (sĕn′shū-ăl-ĭzm) The state of being sensual, in which one's actions are dominated by the emotions.

**sensuous** (sĕn′shū-ŭs) [L. *sensus,* a feeling] **1.** Pert. to or affecting the senses. **2.** Susceptible to influence through the senses.

**sentient** (sĕn′shē-ĕnt) [L. *sentiens,* perceive] Capable of perceiving sensation. SYN: *sensitive.*

**sentiment** (sĕn′tĭ-mĕnt) [L. *sentio,* to feel] Feeling, sensibility, esp. susceptibility to tender feelings; an emotional attitude toward an object or a group of objects.

**separation** The process of disconnecting, disuniting, or severing.

***acromioclavicular s.*** A sprain to the acromioclavicular and coracoclavicular ligaments, commonly caused by a fall or a blow directly to the shoulder (shoulder separation).

**separator** [LL. *separator*] **1.** Anything that prevents two substances from mingling. **2.** Any device or instrument used for separating two substances such as cream from milk.

**separatorium** (sĕp″ă-rā-tō′rē-ŭm) [L.] An instrument for separating the pericranium from the skull.

**sepsis** (sĕp′sĭs) [Gr., putrefaction] The spread of an infection from its initial site to the bloodstream, initiating a systemic response that adversely affects bloodflow to vital organs. Bacterial infections are the most common source of initial infection, but sepsis also occurs with fungal, parasitic, and mycobacterial infections, particularly in immunocompromised patients. The number of patients with moderate to severe sepsis has increased significantly over the past 20 years.

PATHOLOGY: Organisms that enter the body through skin or the respiratory, genitourinary, or gastrointestinal tracts damage local cells and stimulate both the inflammatory and cell-mediated immune responses, resulting in the release of cytokines, which enhance immune defenses. When the organism overwhelms local defenses and enters the bloodstream, the resulting condition is called *septicemia.* Depending on the organism involved, septicemia may be referred to as bacteremia, fungemia, or viremia.

As organisms circulate, more and more phagocytes and lymphocytes are drawn into the body's defense, and more cytokines, particularly interleukins 1 and 2, tumor necrosis factors, and gamma interferon and other chemical mediators such as leukotrienes, kinin, and complement are released or activated. It is these regulatory proteins, affecting the cardiovascular, central nervous system, bone marrow, and other organ systems, that produce systemic signs and symptoms. Antigenic factors associated with the organisms, such as gram-negative bacterial endotoxin, also stimulate cytokine release.

Pathogens leave the bloodstream or are deposited on blood vessel walls as part of immune complexes, initiating inflammation at other body sites. The extent of local and systemic tissue damage depends on the virulence of the organism, the quality of the host's defenses, and the effectiveness of antimicrobial and supportive therapy. At times, sepsis may inhibit immune responses, particularly when it is caused by viral infections. If host defenses continue to be overwhelmed and blood flow to organ systems is disrupted, septic shock, also known as sepsis syndrome, occurs. SEE: *cytokine; disseminated intravascular coagulation; infection; interferon; interleukin; tumor necrosis factor.*

SYMPTOMS: Symptoms of sepsis are a white blood cell count greater than 12,000 cells/mm$^3$ or less than 4000 cells/mm$^3$, with increased bands (immature neutrophils); temperature greater than 38°C; rapid respiration; hypotension; and tachycardia. Blood, body fluid, and infection site cultures are often negative. Blood cultures are most likely to grow the causative organism if obtained when the patient's temperature is elevated because fever is the result of interleukin-1 release by macrophages when the organism is in the bloodstream.

TREATMENT: Broad-spectrum antibiotic therapy is used initially. An extended-spectrum penicillin (e.g., piperacillin) or third-generation cephalosporin (e.g., cefotaxime) plus an aminoglycoside (e.g., gentamycin) is administered until the results of blood, urine, sputum, or wound cultures indicate the causative organism and its sensitivity to specific antimicrobial drugs.

***puerperal s.*** Any infection of the genital tract occurring during the puerperium or as a complication of abortion. This disease is presumed to be present when the temperature is 38°C (100.4°F) on any two consecutive days, exclusive of the first 24 hr postpartum, if no other causes of fever are apparent. This is a polymicrobial infection caused by a wide variety of bacteria. The establishment of careful techniques of asepsis and hygiene in maternity wards has effectively reduced the importance of this disease as a cause of death in the puerperium. Although this complication of childbirth has been reduced dramatically with an understanding of asepsis and the use of antibiotics to treat infections, the dangers still exist. In home births, a trend particularly popular among many young women, the same aseptic precautions must apply as do in hospitals and birthing centers. Although licensed midwives are educated in aseptic techniques, sometimes attendants engaged by parents to attend home births are not professionally prepared and may not understand the problems and complications that may arise. SYN: *childbed fever.* SEE: *Nursing Diagnoses Appendix.*

DIAGNOSIS: Diagnosis is made on the basis of clinical findings consistent with infection of the genital tract, including fever and pain and tenderness of the lower abdominal area and genital tract.

SYMPTOMS: The onset may be gradual or sudden. The patient begins to have general malaise, headache, chilly sensations or shaking chills, and a rise in temperature. The uterus is tender, and there is some abdominal distention.

PATHOLOGY: In minor cases of ulceration, the vaginal tract is covered by a dirty membrane. In streptococcal and staphylococcal infections, the endometrium is smooth and the lymphatics are congested with the invading organisms. As a rule, the uterine cavity is filled with very little lochia. The uterus shows poor involution. If the infection extends farther beyond the uterus, the parametrium or cellular tissues show edema, inflammation, and in some cases purulent infiltration. Extension of the process to the veins produces infectious thrombi, which in turn produce localized abscesses in other parts of the body.

TREATMENT: Treatment includes appropriate antibiotic, incision and drainage if abscess forms, and supportive therapy.

**septan** (sĕp′tăn) [L. *septem,* seven] Recurring every seventh day, as the paroxysms of malarial fever.

**septate** (sĕp′tāt) [L. *saeptum,* a partition] Having a dividing wall.

**septectomy** (sĕp-tĕk′tō-mē) [″ + Gr. *ektome,* excision] Excision of a septum, esp. the nasal septum or a part of it.

**septi-** Combining form meaning *seven.*

**septic** (sĕp′tĭk) [Gr. *septikos,* putrefying] **1.** Pert. to sepsis. **2.** Pert. to pathogenic organisms or their toxins.

**septicemia** (sĕp-tĭ-sē′mē-ă) [″ + *haima,* blood] The presence of pathogenic microorganisms in the blood. SEE: *sepsis; Nursing Diagnoses Appendix.* **septicemic** (-ĭk), *adj.*

**septicophlebitis** (sĕp″tĭ-kō-flē-bī′tĭs) [Gr. *septikos,* putrefying, + *phleps,* vein, + *itis,* inflammation] Septic inflammation of a vein.

**septic shock** Sepsis syndrome.

**septigravida** (sĕp″tĭ-grăv′ĭ-dă) [L. *septem,* seven, + *gravida,* pregnant] A woman pregnant for the seventh time.

**septimetritis** (sĕp″tĭ-mē-trī′tĭs) [Gr. *septos,* putrid, + *metra,* uterus, + *itis,* inflammation] An inflammation of the uterus caused by sepsis.

**septipara** (sĕp-tĭp′ă-ră) [L. *septem,* seven, + *parere,* to bring forth] A woman who has had seven pregnancies, each of which produced an infant, alive or dead, weighing 500 g or more.

**septivalent** (sĕp-tĭ-vā′lĕnt, -tĭv′ă-lĕnt) [″ + *valere,* to be strong] Having a valence of seven or combining with or replacing seven hydrogen atoms.

**septomarginal** (sĕp″tō-măr′jĭ-năl) [L. *saeptum,* a partition, + *marginalis,* border] Pert. to the margin or the border of a septum.

**septometer** (sĕp-tŏm′ĕ-ter) **1.** [L. *saeptum,* a partition, + Gr. *metron,* measure] Calipers for measuring the width of the nasal septum. **2.** [Gr. *sepsis,* putrefaction, + *metron,* measure] A device for determining bacterial contamination of air.

**septonasal** (sĕp-tō-nā′zăl) [L. *saeptum,* a partition, + *nasus,* nose] Concerning the nasal septum.

**septoplasty** (sĕp″tō-plăs′tē) [″ + Gr. *plassein,* to form] Plastic surgery of the nasal septum.

**septostomy** (sĕp-tŏs′tō-mē) [″ + Gr. *stoma,* mouth] Surgical formation of an opening in a septum.

***balloon atrial s.*** The surgical enlargement of an opening between the cardiac atria for palliative relief of congestive heart failure in newborns with certain heart defects. A deflated balloon is inserted into a vein, passed through the foramen ovale, and then inflated and pulled vigorously through the atrial septum to enlarge the opening and improve oxygenation of the blood. SYN: *Rashkind procedure.*

**septotome** (sĕp′tō-tōm) [″ + Gr. *tome,* incision] An instrument for cutting or removing a section of the nasal septum.

**septotomy** (sĕp-tŏt′ō-mē) [″ + Gr. *tome,* incision] Incision of a septum, esp. the nasal septum.

**septula testis** The thin partition extending inward from the mediastinum testis and separating the testis into the lobuli testis.

**septulum** (sĕp′tū-lŭm) *pl.* **septula** [L.] A small partition or septum.

**septum** (sĕp′tŭm) *pl.* **septa** [L. *saeptum,* a partition] A wall dividing two cavities. **septal** (-tăl), *adj.*

***atrial s.*** S. atriorum cordis.

***s. atriorum cordis*** A wall between the atria of the heart. SYN: *atrial s.; interatrial s.*

***atrioventricular s.*** The septum that separates the right and left atria of the heart from the respective ventricles.

***crural s.*** Femoral s.

***femoral s.*** Connective tissue that closes the femoral ring. SYN: *crural s.*

***interatrial s.*** S. atriorum cordis.

***interdental s.*** The bony partition across the alveolar process between adjacent teeth that forms part of the tooth sockets.

***intermuscular s.*** **1.** A connective tissue septum that separates two muscles, esp. one from which muscles may take their origin. **2.** One of two connective tissue septa that separate the muscles of the leg into anterior, posterior, and lateral groups.

***interradicular s.*** One of the thin bony partitions between the roots of a multirooted tooth that forms part of the walls of the tooth socket.

***interventricular s.*** Ventricular s.

***lingual s.*** A sheet of connective tissue separating the halves of the tongue.

***s. lucidum*** S. pellucidum.

***mediastinal s.*** A mediastinum.

***nasal s.*** The partition that divides the nasal cavity into two nasal fossae. The bony portion is formed by the perpendicular plate of ethmoid and the vomer bone. The cartilaginous portion is formed by septal and vomeronasal cartilages and medial crura of greater alar cartilages.

***orbital s.*** A fibrous sheet extending partially across the anterior opening of the orbit and partially closing it.

***s. pectiniforme*** Comblike partition that separates the corpora cavernosa.

***s. pellucidum*** A thin, translucent, triangular sheet of nervous tissue consisting of two laminae attached to the corpus callosum above and the fornix below. It forms the medial wall and interior boundary of the lateral ventricles of the brain. SYN: *s. lucidum.*

***s. primum*** In the primitive, embryonic heart, a septum between the right and left chambers.

***rectovaginal s.*** The partition between the rectum and the vagina.

***rectovesical s.*** The membranous septum between the rectum and the urinary bladder.

***s. scroti*** The partition dividing the left and right sides of the scrotum.

***ventricular s.*** The partition between the ventricles of the heart. SYN: *interventricular s.*

**septuplet** (sĕp′tŭ-plĕt) [L. *septuplus,* sevenfold] One of seven children born from the same gestation.

**sequel** (sē′kwĕl) [L. *sequela,* sequel] Sequela.

**sequela** (sē-kwē′lă) *pl.* **sequelae** [L., sequel] A condition following and resulting from a disease.

**sequence** (sē′kwĕns) [L.] The order or occurrence of a series of related events.

**sequential** Occurring in order (i.e., one after another).

**sequester** (sē-kwĕs′tĕr) [L. *sequestrare,* to separate] **1.** To isolate. **2.** Sequestrum.

**sequestration** (sē″kwĕs-trā′shŭn) [L. *sequestratio,* a separation] **1.** The formation of sequestrum. **2.** The isolation of a patient for treatment or quarantine. **3.** Reduction of hemorrhage of the head or trunk by temporarily stopping the return of blood from the extremities by applying tourniquets to the thighs and arms. **4.** Fragment of nucleus pulposus of the intervertebral disk separating and freely floating in the spinal canal.

***pulmonary s.*** A nonfunctioning area of the lung that receives its blood supply from the systemic circulation.

**sequestrectomy** (sē″kwĕs-trĕk′tō-mē) [″ + Gr. *ektome,* excision] Excision of a necrosed piece of bone. SYN: *sequestrotomy.*

**sequestrotomy** (sē″kwĕs-trŏt′ō-mē) [″ + Gr. *tome,* incision] Operation for removal of a sequestrum, a fragment of necrosed bone. SYN: *sequestrectomy.*

**sequestrum** (sē-kwĕs′trŭm) *pl.* **sequestra** [L., something set aside] A fragment of a necrosed bone that has become separated from the surrounding tissue. It is designated *primary* if the piece is entirely detached, *secondary* if it is still loosely attached, and *tertiary* if it is partially detached but still remaining in place. SYN: *sequester.* **sequestral** (-ăl), *adj.*

**seralbumin** (sĕr-ăl-bū′mĭn) [L. *serum,* whey, + *albumen,* white of egg] Albumin of the blood.

**serendipity** (sĕr″ĕn-dĭp′ĭ-tē) The gift of finding, by chance and wisdom, valuable or agreeable things not sought for. In medical research, an unexpected reaction or result may produce new insights into some area totally unrelated to that which prompted the investigation.

**serial** (sē′rē-ăl) [L. *series,* row, chain] In numerical order, in continuity or in sequence, as in a series.

**serial sevens test** A test of mental status. The patient is asked to subtract seven from 100 and to take seven from that value and continue serially. The number of correct responses out of the 14 possible is the score.

**series** (sēr′ēz) [L. *series*, row, chain] **1.** Arrangement of objects in succession or in order. **2.** In electricity, batteries or mode of arranging the parts of a circuit by connecting them successively end to end to form a single path for the current. The parts so arranged are said to be "in series."

***acute abdomen s.*** In radiology, an erect kidney, ureter, and bladder (KUB) projection, a recumbent KUB projection, and a posteroanterior projection of the chest to assess free air, infections, or obstructions.

***aliphatic s.*** Chemical compounds with a structure of an open chain of carbon atoms.

***aromatic s.*** Any series of organic compounds containing the benzene ring.

***erythrocytic s.*** The group of immature cells that develop into mature erythrocytes.

***fatty s.*** Aliphatic series, esp. those similar to methane.

***granulocytic s.*** The immature cells in the bone marrow that develop into mature granular leukocytes. SYN: *leukocytic s.*

***homologous s.*** In chemistry, compounds that proceed from one to the next by some constant such as a $CH_2$ group.

***leukocytic s.*** Granulocytic s.

***monocytic s.*** The immature cells that proceed to develop into the mature monocyte.

***thrombocytic s.*** The immature cells that proceed to develop into platelets.

***upper GI s.*** Radiographical and fluoroscopic examinations of the stomach and duodenum after the ingestion of a contrast medium.

**serine** 2-amino-3-hydroxypropionic acid; an amino acid present in many proteins including casein, vitellin, and others. It is found in the urine of healthy human beings.

**serine protease inhibitor** ABBR: SERPIN. Any of the compounds that inhibit platelet function and coagulation. SERPINs have been used to reduce deposition of microemboli in cases of disseminated intravascular coagulation associated with sepsis.

**seriscission** (sĕr-ĭ-sĕsh′ŭn) [L. *sericum*, silk, + *scindere*, to cut] The division of soft tissues, as a pedicle, by tying a silk ligature around it.

**sero-** [L.] Combining form meaning *serum*.

**seroalbuminuria** (sē″rō-ăl-bū″mĭn-ū′rē-ă) [L. *serum*, whey, + *albumen*, white of egg, + Gr. *ouron*, urine] Serum albumin in the urine.

**serocolitis** (sē″rō-kō-lī′tĭs) [″ + Gr. *kolon*, colon, + *itis*, inflammation] Inflammation of the serous layer of the colon. SYN: *pericolitis*.

**seroconversion** The development of evidence of antibody response to a disease or vaccine.

**seroculture** (sē′rō-kŭl-chūr) [L. *serum*, whey, + *cultura*, tillage] A bacterial culture on blood serum.

**serocystic** (sē″rō-sĭs′tĭk) [″ + Gr. *kystis*, bladder, sac] Composed of cysts containing serous fluid.

**serodermatosis** (sē″rō-der-mă-tō′sĭs) [″ + Gr. *derma*, skin, + *osis*, condition] Skin disease with serous effusion into tissues of the epidermis.

**serodiagnosis** (sē″rō-dī-ăg-nō′sĭs) [″ + Gr. *dia*, through, + *gnosis*, knowledge] Diagnosis by observing the reactions of blood serum.

**seroenteritis** (sē″rō-ĕn-tĕr-ī′tĭs) [″ + Gr. *enteron*, intestine, + *itis*, inflammation] An inflammation of the serous covering of the intestine.

**seroepidemiology** (sē-rō-ĕp″ĭ-dē-mē-ŏl′ō-jē) [″ + *epi*, upon, + *demos*, people, + *logos*, word, reason] Study of the epidemiology of a pathologic condition by investigating the presence of a diagnostic characteristic in the serum.

**serofast** (sē′rō-făst″) Serum-fast.

**serofibrinous** (sē″rō-fī′brĭn-ŭs) [″ + *fibra*, fiber] **1.** Composed of both serum and fibrin. **2.** Denoting a serofibrinous exudate.

**serofibrous** (sē″rō-fī′brŭs) [″ + *fibra*, fiber] Concerning serous and fibrous surfaces.

**seroflocculation** (sē″rō-flŏk″ū-lā′shŭn) [″ + *flocculus*, little tuft] Flocculation produced in serum by an antigen.

**seroimmunity** (sē″rō-ĭ-mū′nĭ-tē) [″ + *immunitas*, immunity] Immunity produced by the administration of an antiserum.

**serologist** (sē-rŏl′ō-jĭst) [″ + Gr. *logos*, word, reason] One who has special knowledge and ability in serology.

**serology** (sē-rŏl′ō-jē) [″ + Gr. *logos*, word, reason] The scientific study of serums and their reactions. SYN: *orrhology*. **serologic, serological** (-rō-lŏj′ĭk, -rō-lŏj′ĭk-ăl), *adj.*

**serolysin** (sē-rŏl′ĭs-ĭn) [″ + Gr. *lysis*, dissolution] A bactericidal substance or lysin found in the blood serum.

**seromembranous** (sē″rō-mĕm′brăn-ŭs) [″ + *membrana*, membrane] **1.** Both serous and membranous. **2.** Relating to a serous membrane.

**seromucoid** Concerning a secretion that is part serous and part mucous.

**seromucous** (sē″rō-mū′kŭs) [″ + *mucus*, mucus] Pert. to or composed of both serum and mucus.

**seromuscular** (sē″rō-mŭs′kū-lăr) [″ + *muscularis*, muscular] Concerning the serous and muscular layers of the intestinal wall.

**seronegative** (sē″rō-nĕg′ă-tĭv) Producing a negative reaction to serological tests.

**seroperitoneum** (sē″rō-pĕr″ĭ-tō-nē′ŭm) [″ + Gr. *peritonaion*, peritoneum] Ascites.

**seropositive** (sē″rō-pŏz′ĭ-tĭv) Producing a positive reaction to serological tests.

**seroprevention** Seroprophylaxis.

**seroprognosis** (sē″rō-prŏg-nō′sĭs) [″+ Gr.

*pro,* before, + *gnosis,* knowledge] Prognosis of disease determined by seroreactions.

**seroprophylaxis** (sē″rō-prō-fĭ-lăks′ĭs) [″ + Gr. *prophylatikos,* guarding] Prevention of a disease by injection of serum. SYN: *seroprevention.*

**seropurulent** (sē″rō-pū′roo-lĕnt) [″ + *purulentus,* full of pus] Composed of serum and pus, as an exudate.

**seroreaction** (sē″rō-rē-ăk′shŭn) [″ + *re,* back, + *actio,* action] **1.** Any reaction taking place in or involving serum. **2.** A reaction to an injection of serum marked by rash, fever, pain, and so on.

**seroresistance** (sē″rō-rē-zĭs′tăns) Failure of a serum reaction to become negative or be reduced in titer following treatment.

**seroresistant** (sē″rō-rē-zĭs′tănt) Concerning seroresistance.

**serosa** (sē-rō′să) [L. *serum,* whey] A serous membrane (e.g., the peritoneum, pleura, and pericardium).

**serosanguineous** (sē″rō-săn-gwĭn′ē-ŭs) [L. *serum,* whey, + *sanguineus,* bloody] Containing or of the nature of serum and blood.

**seroserous** (sē″rō-sē′rŭs) [L. *serosus,* serous, + *serum,* whey] Pert. to two serous surfaces.

**serositis** (sē″rō-sī′tĭs) *pl.* **serositides** [″ + Gr. *itis,* inflammation] An inflammation of a serous membrane.

**serosity** (sē-rŏs′ĭ-tē) [Fr. *serosite*] The quality of being serous.

**serosynovial** (sē″rō-sĭ-nō′vē-ăl) [L. *serum,* whey, + *synovia,* joint fluid] Concerning serous and synovial material.

**serosynovitis** (sē″rō-sĭn″ō-vī′tĭs) [″ + *synovia,* joint fluid, + Gr. *itis,* inflammation] Synovitis with an increase of synovial fluid.

**serotonergic neuron** A neural pathway that uses serotonin as a neurotransmitter.

**serotonin** (sĕr″ō-tōn′ĭn) A chemical, 5-hydroxytryptamine (5-HT), present in platelets, gastrointestinal mucosa, mast cells, and carcinoid tumors. Serotonin is a potent vasoconstrictor. It is also a neurotransmitter in the central nervous system and is important in sleep-waking cycles. SEE: *carcinoid syndrome.*

***s. reuptake inhibitor*** Any one of a class of drugs that interferes with serotonin transport, used in treating depression.

**serotype** (sē′rō-tīp) In microbiology, a microorganism determined by the kinds and combinations of constituent antigens present in the cells.

**serous** (sĕr′ŭs) [L. *serosus*] **1.** Having the nature of serum. **2.** Producing a serous secretion, or containing serum or a serum-like substance.

**serous cell** A cell that secretes a thin, watery, albuminous secretion.

**serous effusion** The escape of serum into tissues or a body cavity.

**serous exudate** An exudate consisting mostly of serum.

**serovaccination** A process with combined injection of serum, to secure immediate passive immunity, and bacterial vaccine, to acquire subsequent active immunity.

**serovar** [*sero*logical *var*iation] Variants within a species defined by variation in serological reactions. SEE: *biovar; morphovar.*

**serozymogenic** (sē″rō-zī″mō-jĕn′ĭk) [L. *serum,* whey, + Gr. *zyme,* ferment, + *gennan,* to produce] Pert. to a serous fluid and enzymes.

**serpiginous** (sĕr-pĭj′ĭ-nŭs) [L. *serpere,* to creep] Creeping from one part to another.

**serrate** (sĕr′āt) [L. *serratus,* toothed] Dentate.

**Serratia** (sĕr-ā′shē-ă) [Serafino Serrati, 18th-century Italian physicist] A genus of bacteria of the family Enterobacteriaceae. It is a gram-negative rod.

***S. marcescens*** A species formerly called *Chromobacterium prodigiosum* and erroneously believed to be nonpathogenic to humans. It causes septicemia and pulmonary disease, esp. in immunocompromised patients, and is found in water, soil, milk, and stools. In the proper environment, the organism will grow on food and produce the red pigment prodigiosin.

**serration** (sĕr-ā′shŭn) [L. *serratio,* a notching] **1.** A formation with sharp projections like the teeth of a saw. **2.** A single tooth or notch in a serrated edge.

**serratus muscle** Any of several muscles arising from the ribs or vertebrae by separate slips. SEE: *Muscles Appendix.*

**serrefine** (sār-fēn′) [Fr.] A small wire-spring forceps for compressing bleeding vessels.

**serrenoeud** (sār-nŭd′) [Fr. *serrer,* to squeeze, + *noeud,* knot] A device for tightening ligatures, esp. those placed on vessels in a deep cavity out of reach of the fingers.

**serrulate** (sĕr′ū-lāt) [L. *serrulatus*] Finely notched or serrated.

**Sertoli cell** (sĕr-tō′lēz) [Enrico Sertoli, Italian histologist, 1842–1910] One of the supporting elongated cells of the seminiferous tubules of the testes to which spermatids attach to be nourished until they become mature spermatozoa. Sertoli cells produce the hormone inhibin. Also called *sustentacular cell.*

**serum** (sē′rŭm) *pl.* **serums, sera** [L., whey] **1.** Any serous fluid, esp. the fluid that moistens the surfaces of serous membranes. **2.** The watery portion of the blood after coagulation; a fluid found when clotted blood is left standing long enough for the clot to shrink. **3.** Serum from an animal rendered immune against a pathogenic organism, to be injected into a patient with the disease resulting from the same organism. It consists of plasma minus fibrinogen.

***s. albumin*** A protein found in blood serum. SEE: *blood; protein, simple.*

***antitetanic s.*** Serum given to counteract tetanus toxin.

***antitoxic s.*** Antitoxin.

***bactericidal s.*** Serum having no effect on toxins but destructive to bacteria.

***bacteriolytic s.*** Serum containing a lysin that destroys certain bacteria.

***blood s.*** The clear liquid portion of blood without its fibrin and corpuscles. SEE: *plasma.*

***convalescent s.*** Blood serum from a person convalescing from an infection, to be used in treating others having the same disease.

***foreign s.*** Serum from one animal injected into one of another species or into a human.

***grouping s.*** A serum used for determining the blood group to which unknown cells belong. The grouping serums commonly used are human serums secured from donors and rabbit antiserums prepared commercially.

***immune s.*** Serum containing antibodies for specific antigens.

***polyvalent s.*** Serum containing antibodies to several types of the same bacterial species.

***pooled s.*** Mixed blood serum from several persons.

***pregnancy s.*** Blood serum from pregnant women.

***pregnant mare's s.*** Serum derived from the blood of pregnant mares; source of hormones, esp. chorionic gonadotropin.

**serum bank** A place for long-term storage of samples of serum because of their potential future use in studying disease. Specimens are stored frozen or after lyophilization. The storage of such specimens permits investigation of a newly discovered disease (e.g., AIDS) in persons whose serum was collected many years earlier.

**serum-fast** Capable of resisting the destructive forces present in serum. SYN: *serofast.*

**serum glutamic-oxaloacetic transaminase** ABBR: SGOT. Aspartate aminotransferase.

**serum glutamic pyruvic transaminase** ABBR: SGPT. Alanine aminotransferase.

**serum hepatitis** SEE: under *hepatitis.*

**serum protein** Any protein in the blood serum. Serum protein forms weak acids mixed with alkali salts; this increases the buffer effects of the blood but to a lesser extent than does cell protein.

**serum rash** A rash first seen at the site of an injection of serum. It remains thickest there but may spread to other parts of the body. It resembles a combination of urticarial, morbilliform, and scarlatiniform rashes. The patient experiences severe irritation; marked swelling of the skin, esp. of the face; malaise; and constitutional symptoms.

**serum sickness** An adverse (type III hypersensitivity) immune response following administration of antitoxins derived from horses or other animals used for passive immunization against snake venom or rabies and occasionally following administration of penicillin or sulfonamides. The inflammatory response that results produces fever, myalgia, arthritis, urticaria, and an enlarged spleen and lymph nodes 7 to 14 days after exposure. Treatment is symptomatic; adrenal cortical hormones may be given if needed. SEE: *hypersensitivity; Nursing Diagnoses Appendix.*

**servomechanism** (sŭr″vō-mĕk′ă-nĭzm) In biology and physiology, a control mechanism that operates by negative or positive feedback. For example, when in the normal person the blood glucose level rises, the pancreas responds by releasing insulin, which enables the glucose to be metabolized. The level of hormones is also regulated by this mechanism when the anterior pituitary responds to the levels of hormones circulating in the blood.

**SES** *socioeconomic status.*

**sesame oil** Oil obtained from the seeds of *Sesamum indicum,* used as a pharmaceutical aid and as a cooking oil.

**sesamoid** (sĕs′ă-moyd) [L. *sesamoides*] Resembling a grain of sesame in size or shape.

**sesamoid bone** An oval nodule of bone or fibrocartilage in a tendon playing over a bony surface. The patella is the largest one.

**sesamoid cartilage** One or more small cartilage plates present in fibrous tissue between the lateral nasal and greater alar cartilages of the nose.

**sesamoiditis** (sĕs″ă-moy-dī′tĭs) [″ + Gr. *itis,* inflammation] Inflammation of a sesamoid bone.

**sesqui-** [L.] Prefix meaning *one and one-half.*

**sesquihora** (sĕs″kwĭ-hō′ră) [L.] Every 1½ hr.

**sessile** (sĕs′l) [L. *sessilis,* low] Having no peduncle but attached directly by a broad base.

**set 1.** To fix firmly in place, as to set a bone in reduction of a fracture. **2.** To allow an amalgam or plaster to harden. **3.** In psychology, a group of conditions or attitudes that favor the occurrence of a certain response. **4.** In resistance exercise, a grouping of repetitions of a specific exercise.

**seta** (sē′tă) *pl.* **setae** [L., bristle] A stiff, bristle-like structure. SEE: *vibrissae.*

**setaceous** (sē-tā′shŭs) [L. *setaceus*] Bristly, hairy; resembling a bristle.

**Setchenov phenomenon** [I.M. Setchenov, Russ. scientist] The more rapid recovery of a limb if the opposite limb is exercised during the rest period.

**Setchenow's inhibitory centers** (sĕtch′en-ŏfs) [Ivan M. Setchenow, Russian neurologist, 1829–1905] Centers in the spinal cord and medulla oblongata involved in reflex inhibition of muscular and visceral activity.

**setiferous** (sē-tĭf′ĕr-ŭs) [L. *seta,* bristle, +

*ferre,* to bear] Having bristles.

**seton** (sē″tŏn) [L. *seta,* bristle] A thread or threads drawn through a fold of skin to act as a counterirritant or as a guide for instruments.

**setose** (sē′tōs) Having bristle-like appendages.

**set-point** The concept that homeostatic mechanisms maintain variables such as body temperature, body weight, blood glucose level, and hormone levels within a certain physiological range compatible with optimal function. SEE: *homeostasis.*

**setup** The arrangement of teeth on a trial denture base.

**severe combined immunodeficiency disease** ABBR: SCID. A syndrome marked by gross functional impairment of both humoral and cell-mediated immunity and by susceptibility to fungal, bacterial, and viral infections. Although the disorder may occur sporadically, most commonly it is inherited and transmitted as an X-linked or autosomal recessive trait. If untreated, infants rarely survive beyond one year. It is important that the disease be recognized early and that patients not be given live viral vaccines or blood transfusions. The immunologic defects may be repaired by transplantation of bone marrow or fetal liver as a source of stem cells.

**Severinghaus electrode** SEE: *electrode, carbon dioxide.*

**Sever's disease** [James W. Sever, U.S. orthopedist, 1878–1964] Apophysitis of the calcaneus in adolescent children who are actively engaged in sports. This overuse syndrome is best treated with icing, Achilles tendon stretching, anti-inflammatory medication, and rest from weight bearing. Heel lifts are usually used unless the child has pronated feet, in which case medial heel wedges are indicated.

**sewer gas** A gas produced by the biodegradation of sewage; containing methane and hydrogen sulfide. It may be used for fuel. SEE: *carbon monoxide.*

**sex** [L. *sexus*] The characteristics that differentiate males and females in most plants and animals.

***chromosomal s.*** Sex as determined by the presence of the female XX or male XY genotype in somatic cells.

***morphological s.*** The sex of an individual as determined by the form of the external genitalia.

***nuclear s.*** The genetic sex of an individual determined by the absence or presence of sex chromatin in the body cells, particularly blood cells.

***psychological s.*** The individual's self-image of his or her gender, which may be at variance with the morphological sex.

**sex chromatin** A mass seen within the nuclei of normal female somatic cells. According to the Lyon hypothesis, one of the two X chromosomes in each somatic cell of the female is genetically inactivated. The sex chromatin represents the inactivated X chromosome. SYN: *Barr body.*

**sex clinic** A clinic for the diagnosis and treatment of an individual or couple with sexual problems.

**sex determination** The concept that a couple may choose the sex of their offspring. To date, all efforts to make this a reality have been in vain. This concept should not be confused with determining the sexual identity of the fetus by analysis of cells obtained by amniocentesis or chorionic villus sampling.

**sexdigital** (sĕks-dĭj′ĭ-tăl) [L. *sex,* six, + *digitus,* digit] Having six fingers and toes.

**sex drive** Motivation, both psychological and physiological, for behavior associated with procreation and erotic pleasure.

**sexduction** (sĕks-dŭk′shŭn) The process of transfer of bacterial genes from one cell to another by means of the sex factors within which they are incorporated.

**sexism** All of the actions and attitudes that relegate individuals of either sex to a secondary and inferior status in society.

**sexivalent** (sĕks″ĭ-vă′lĕnt, -ĭv′ăl-ĕnt) [″ + *valere,* to be strong] Capable of combining with six atoms of hydrogen.

**sex-limited** The expression of a genetic character or trait in one sex only.

**sex-linked** A character that is controlled by genes on the sex chromosomes.

**sexology** [L. *sexus,* sex, + Gr. *logos,* word, reason] Scientific study of sexuality.

**sex ratio** The ratio of females to males, used in defining the proportion of births of the two sexes or in the representation by sexual distribution in certain diseases.

**sex surrogate** In sex therapy, a person serving as a surrogate sexual partner to assist in the therapeutic process.

**sextan** (sĕks′tăn) [L. *sextanus,* of the sixth] Occurring every sixth day.

**sex test** A test to determine an individual's chromosomal sex. This has been done to attempt to prevent athletes from masquerading as a person of the opposite sex, that is, to prevent a chromosomal male from competing as a female.

**sex therapy** A form of psychotherapy involving sexual guidance for partners in whom one or both have psychogenic impotence.

**sextigravida** (sĕks″tĭ-grăv′ĭd-ă) [L. *sextus,* six, + *gravida,* a pregnant woman] A woman pregnant for the sixth time.

**sextipara** (sĕks-tĭp′ă-ră) [″ + *parere,* to bear a child] A woman who has had six pregnancies that produced infants of 500 g (or 20 weeks' gestation) regardless of their viability.

**sextuplet** (sĕks′tū-plĕt) [L. *sextus,* six] One of six children born of a single gestation.

**sexual** (sĕks′ū-ăl) [L. *sexualis*] **1.** Pert. to sex. **2.** Having sex.

**sexual abuse** Rape, sexual assault, or sexual molestation. The abuser may be a male or female adult or child, and the abused person may be of the same sex as the abuser or of the opposite sex. SEE: *in-*

*cest; rape.*

**sexual activity depressant** Anything that suppresses libido, potency, or orgasmic ability. Drugs with this effect include those used to control high blood pressure or cholesterol, some contraceptives, and recreational drugs including alcohol and marijuana, which may decrease inhibitions, but impair sexual performance. Fatigue, mental depression, anxiety, excess use of tobacco products, starvation, and stress all have the potential for depressing sexual desire and activity. SEE: *sexual stimulant.*

**Sexual Assault Response Team** ABBR: SART. A group of health care professionals who have had special preparation in the examination of rape victims. The training includes techniques for collecting, labeling, and storing evidence so it may be used in court proceedings concerning the person accused of rape and in psychological approaches to reduce the emotional trauma. SEE: *rape.*

**sexual dysfunction** Inadequate enjoyment or failure to enjoy sexual activity. The areas of importance are desire, arousal, orgasm, satisfaction, and pain. The dependence of most of these phases on the mental attitude of the partners is considerable, as is the hormonal balance of the patient(s). A careful history and physical examination will help to determine the possible pathological aspects of the various phases. Is desire absent, overactive, or is there aversion? Is arousal sufficient to maintain desire and, in men, to attain erection? Does orgasm occur, and if so, is it delayed or premature? Do the partners experience satisfaction at the completion of orgasm? Is pain present at any stage of the sexual activity?

A great number of physical and mental forces interact to culminate in enjoyable and fulfilling sexual activity. It is therefore important to keep this in mind in evaluating patients; and to realize that a great number of drugs have the undesired side effect of causing sexual dysfunction. Aging does not necessarily cause sexual dysfunction or obliteration of sexual capability.

Many commonly used drugs can cause sexual dysfunction in men and women (e.g., some antihypertensive agents, histamine-$H_2$-receptor antagonists, antipsychotic drugs, central nervous system depressants, and anticancer drugs). The physical or mental factors that are involved should be treated and, if possible, alternate drugs should be substituted for those that appear to cause the disorder. SEE: *Nursing Diagnoses Appendix.*

**sexual harassment** Unsolicited and unprovoked mental or physical sexually-oriented advances or innuendo, esp. between employers and employees. In many instances, compliance with a harasser's wishes is a condition of continued employment or advancement.

**sexual health** The World Health Organization has defined three elements of sexual health: a capacity to enjoy and control sexual behavior in accordance with a social and personal ethic; freedom from fear, shame, guilt, false beliefs, and other psychological factors inhibiting sexual response and impairing sexual relationships; and freedom from organic disorder, disease, and deficiencies that interfere with sexual and reproductive functions. Medical studies of human sexual function and activity have provided no evidence that having attained a certain age is, of itself, reason to discontinue participating in and enjoying sexual intercourse. SEE: *sexually transmitted disease.*

**sexual intercourse** Sexual union between a man and a woman. SYN: *coition; coitus; copulation.*

***homosexual s.i.*** Sexual union between persons of the same sex.

**sexuality** (sĕks-ū-ăl′ĭ-tē) [L. *sexus,* sex] **1.** The state of having sex; the collective characteristics that mark the differences between the male and the female. **2.** The constitution and life of an individual as related to sex; all the dispositions related to intimacy, whether associated with the sex organs or not.

**sexuality patterns, altered** The state in which an individual expresses concern regarding his or her sexuality. SEE: *Nursing Diagnoses Appendix.*

**sexually transmitted disease** ABBR: STD. Disease acquired as a result of sexual intercourse with an infected individual. A more inclusive term than venereal disease, STDs include syphilis, gonorrhea, AIDS, lymphogranuloma venereum, chancroid, granuloma inguinale, chlamydiosis, viral hepatitis, pelvic inflammatory disease, and other conditions such as trichomoniasis, genital candidiasis, genital herpes, genital warts, amebiasis, viral hepatitis, scabies, crab lice, cervical dysplasia, and bacterial vaginitis. While some of these conditions are specifically STDs, others may be contracted through nonsexual means. SEE: *AIDS; Reiter's syndrome; venereal disease; Nursing Diagnoses Appendix.*

**sexual maturity rating** The order and extent of the development of a patient's primary and secondary sexual characteristics as compared with the established norms for chronological age. In both sexes, the changes leading to puberty are the result of major hormonal changes that, although somewhat variable in age of occurrence, proceed in a predictable sequence. Assessing the degree of age-related sexual maturity enables the health care provider to detect abnormalities and to provide anticipatory guidance for the patient and family. An important and easily identified development in a girl is the onset of menstruation. There is no definitive and easily recognized marker for male maturation during puberty. Physical changes in the male such as voice change, facial hair growth, and testicular and penile growth are obvious but occur over a prolonged period.

**sexual preference** The sexual orientation one prefers in choosing his or her sex partners.

**sexual reassignment** The legal, surgical, or social action or decision to assign the appropriate sexuality to an individual who has been considered previously to be of the opposite (or ambiguous) sex.

**sexual stimulant** A pharmacological agent that enhances sexual arousal. Few, if any, are both available and free of side effects. No doubt some drugs that are thought to be effective have obtained that reputation because of the placebo effect. The mind is the primary source of sexual arousal. In both men and women, a powerful stimulant is produced in the anticipation, challenge, and excitement of sexual activity. Nonpharmacologic sexual stimulants include exercise, fantasy, romantic music, perfume, wine in moderation, candlelight, and both partners being free of stress. SEE: *impotence; sexual activity depressant.*

**Sézary cell** [A. Sézary, Fr. dermatologist, 1880–1956] A T-cell lymphocyte, that contains an abundance of vacuoles filled with a mucopolysaccharide; present in the blood of patients with Sézary syndrome. SEE: illus.

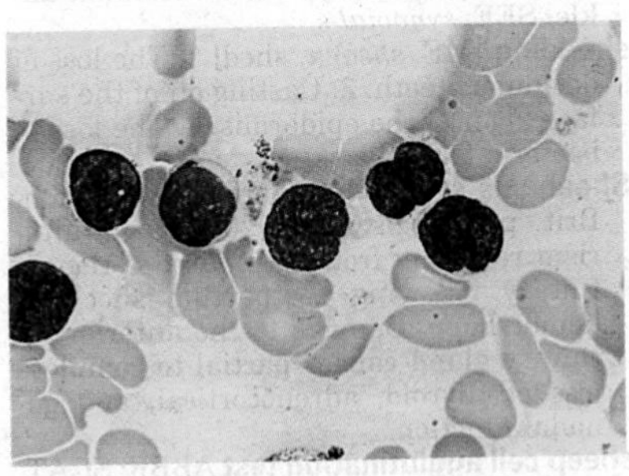

**SÉZARY CELLS** IN PERIPHERAL BLOOD (ORIG. MAG. ×1000)

**Sézary syndrome** A form of cutaneous T-cell lymphoma in which there is cutaneous and systemic involvement. SEE: *lymphoma, cutaneous T-cell; mycosis fungoides.*

**SGA** *small for gestational age.*

**S.G.O.** *Surgeon-General's Office.*

**SGOT** *serum glutamic-oxaloacetic transaminase.*

**SGPT** *serum glutamic pyruvic transaminase.*

**SH** *serum hepatitis.*

**shadow** [AS. *sceaduwe*] Ghost corpuscle.

**shadow-casting** A technique to increase the definition of the material being examined by use of electron microscopy. The object is sprayed from an oblique angle with a heavy metal.

**shaft** [AS. *sceaft*] **1.** The principal portion of any cylindrical body. **2.** The diaphysis of a long bone.

***hair s.*** The keratinized portion of a hair that extends from a hair follicle beyond the surface of the epidermis. SEE: *hair.*

**shaken baby syndrome** A syndrome seen in abused infants and children. The patient has been subjected to violent, whiplash-type shaking injuries inflicted by the abuser. This may cause coma, convulsions, and increased intracranial pressure due to tearing of the cerebral veins with consequent bleeding into the subdural space. Retinal hemorrhages are usually present, as well as bruises on the arms or trunk where the patient was forcefully grabbed. In domestic situations in which a child is abused, it is important to examine other children and infants living in the same home because about 20% of them will have signs of physical abuse. That examination should be done without delay in order to attempt to prevent further abuse of children in that place of residence. SEE: *battered child syndrome; child abuse.*

**shakes** (shāks) [AS. *sceacen*] **1.** Shivering caused by a chill, esp. in intermittent fever. **2.** Colloquial term for state of tremulousness and extreme irritability often seen in chronic alcoholics. SYN: *jitters.*

**shaking** A passive movement in Swedish massage.

**shaman** (shā′mŭn, shŏ′-) [Russ., ascetic] A traditional healer who, while in a trance, uses spirits, rather than techniques of Western medicine, to heal. Shamans have multifaceted holistic roles in their societies, which include judge, psychotherapist, magician, holder of the mores and traditions of the group, as well as medicine man or woman. SYN: *medicine man.* SEE: *shamanism.*

**shamanism** (shā′mŭn-ĭsm, shŏ′-) **1.** Primitive religion of certain peoples of northern Asia who believe good and evil spirits pervade the world and can be influenced only by shamans acting as mediums. **2.** Any similar form of primitive spiritualism, such as that practiced among American Indian tribes.

**shank** (shăngk) [AS. *sceanca*] **1.** Shin. **2.** The tapered portion of a dental hand instrument between the handle and the blade or nub. It may be straight or angled to provide better access or leverage in its use.

**shape** (shāp) [AS. *sceapan*] **1.** To mold to a particular form. **2.** Outward form; contour.

**shared decision** The practice of the physician and patient discussing the approach to the medical care proposed for the patient. The success of this sharing is, of course, dependent on both the physician and patient being rational and competent.

**shared governance** A model of nursing management in which the staff nurse shares responsibility and accountability for patient care with the hospital management. Shared governance assumes a participatory style of management and is aimed at quality patient care and a professional nursing practice. Shared governance is in contrast to self-governance and the traditional bureaucratic model of management. SEE: *self-governance.*

**sharkskin** A condition seen in pellagra (nicotinic acid deficiency) in which openings of sebaceous glands become plugged with a dry yellowish material.

**Sharpey, William** Scottish physiologist, 1802–1880.

***S.'s intercrossing fibers*** The fibers forming the lamellae constituting the walls of the haversian canals in bone.

***S.'s perforating fibers*** **1.** The fibers extending from the periosteum into the lamellae of bone. **2.** The fibers extending from the periodontal ligament into the cementum of a tooth.

**sharps** Medical articles that may cause punctures or cuts to those handling them, including all broken medical glassware, syringes, needles, scalpel blades, suture needles, and disposable razors. SEE: *AIDS; medical waste; Universal Precautions Appendix.*

**shear** (shēr) A force applied parallel to the planes of an object but opposite in direction to whatever force was present.

**sheath** (shēth) [AS. *sceath*] **1.** A covering structure of connective tissue, usually of an elongated part, such as the membrane covering a muscle. **2.** An instrument introduced into a vessel during angiographic procedures when multiple catheter changes are anticipated. It facilitates ease of change and decreases morbidity at the puncture site.

***arachnoid s.*** The delicate partition between the pial sheath and the dural sheath of the optic nerve.

***axon s.*** A myelin sheath or a neurilemma. SEE: *myelin s.*

***carotid s.*** The portion of cervical or pretracheal fascia enclosing the carotid artery, interior jugular vein, and vagus nerve.

***crural s.*** The fascial covering of femoral vessels.

***dural s.*** A fibrous membrane or external investment of the optic nerve.

***femoral s.*** The fascial covering of femoral vessels.

***s. of Henle*** SEE: *Henle's sheath.*

***s. of Hertwig*** SEE: *Hertwig's root sheath.*

***s. of Key and Retzius*** Henle's sheath.

***lamellar s.*** A connective tissue sheath covering a bundle of nerve fibers. SYN: *nerve s.; perineurium.*

***medullary s.*** Myelin s.

***myelin s.*** Layers of the cell membrane of Schwann cells (peripheral nervous system) or oligodendrocytes (central nervous system) that wrap nerve fibers, providing electrical insulation and increasing the velocity of impulse transmission. SYN: *medullary s.* SEE: *nerve fiber; neuron.*

***nerve s.*** Lamellar s.

***s. of Schweigger-Seidel*** The thickened wall of a sheathed artery of the spleen.

***pial s.*** An extension of the pia that closely invests the surface of the optic nerve.

***root s.*** **1.** One of the layers of a hair follicle derived from the epidermis. It includes the outer root sheath, which is a continuation of the stratum germinativum, and the inner root sheath, which consists of three layers of cells that closely invest the root of the hair. SEE: *hair.* **2.** The epithelial covering that induces root formation in teeth. Also called *Hertwig's root sheath.*

***synovial s.*** A double-walled tubelike bursa that encloses a tendon. It consists of an inner visceral layer lying on and adhering to a tendon and an outer parietal layer; the two layers are separated by a space filled with synovial fluid. This sheath is found esp. in the hands and feet where tendons are confined to osteofibrous canals or pass over bony surfaces.

***tendon s.*** A dense fibrous sheath that confines a tendon to an osseous groove, converting it into an osteofibrous canal. It is found principally in the wrist and ankle. SEE: *synovial s.*

**shedding** [ME. *sheden,* shed] **1.** The loss of deciduous teeth. **2.** Casting off of the surface layer of the epidermis. **3.** The loss of bacteria from the skin.

**Sheehan's syndrome** [Harold L. Sheehan, Brit. pathologist, b. 1920] Hypopituitarism resulting from an infarct of the pituitary following postpartum shock or hemorrhage. Damage to the anterior pituitary gland causes partial to complete loss of thyroid, adrenocortical, and gonadal function.

**sheep cell agglutination test** ABBR: SCAT. A test for rheumatoid factor in serum. Sheep erythrocytes sensitized with rabbit antisheep erythrocyte immune globulin will be agglutinated if serum containing the rheumatoid factor is added.

**sheet** (shēt) [AS. *sciete,* cloth] **1.** A linen or cotton bedcovering. **2.** Something that resembles a sheet (e.g., a sheet of connective tissue).

***draw s.*** A sheet folded under a patient so that it may be withdrawn without lifting the patient. This is accomplished by turning the patient to the side of the bed to allow one side of the sheet to be removed and replaced with a clean one. The patient is then turned to the other side of the bed. The soiled sheet is removed and replaced with a clean one. In many hospitals, draw sheets have been replaced by paper and plastic pads that resemble disposable diapers.

***lift s.*** Sheet folded under a patient over the bottom sheet to assist with moving the patient up in bed.

**shelf** Any shelflike structure.

***dental s.*** SYN: *dental lamina.*

**shelf-life** **1.** The time a food may be kept on a store shelf and still be considered safe to eat. **2.** The length of time a substance, preparation, or medication can be kept without separation or chemical changes of its component parts.

**shell** A hard covering, as that for an egg or turtle.

**shellac** (shĕ-lăk′) A refined resinous substance obtained from plants that contain the secretions of certain insects. It is used in paints, varnishes, and as a coating for pills.

**shell shock** An obsolete term used during World War I to designate a wide variety of psychotic and neurotic disorders associated with the stress of combat. SEE: *hysteria; post-traumatic stress disorder.*

**Shenton's line** (shĕn′tŏnz) [Thomas Shenton, Brit. radiologist, 1872–1955] A radiographical line used to determine the relationship of the head of the femur to the acetabulum. The line follows the inferior border of the ramus of the pubic bone and continued outward follows the curve down the medial border of the neck of the femur.

**shiatsu, shiatzu** [Chinese, finger + pressure] Japanese massage method used in treating disease. It incorporates acupressure.

**shield** (shēld) [AS. *scild,* shield] **1.** Any protecting device. **2.** In biology, a protective plate or hard outer covering.

***embryonic s.*** The two-layered blastoderm or blastodisk from which a mammalian embryo develops. SYN: *embryonic disk.*

***gonadal s.*** A lead device that is placed over the gonadal area to help protect it during radiation exposure.

***nipple s.*** A cover to protect the sore nipples of a nursing woman.

***phallic s.*** An antiseptic covering for the male genitals during operations.

**shift** [AS. *sciftan,* to arrange] A change in position or direction.

***antigenic s.*** SEE: *antigenic drift.*

***chloride s.*** The shift of chloride ions from the plasma into the red blood cells upon the addition of carbon dioxide from the tissues, and the reverse movement when carbon dioxide is released in the lungs. It is a mechanism for maintaining constant pH of the blood.

***s. to the left*** **1.** In hematology, an increase in the number of young polymorphonuclear leukocytes in the blood. SEE: *Arneth's classification of neutrophils.* **2.** In acid-base physiology, a left-shifted oxyhemoglobin dissociation level, indicating an increased affinity of hemoglobin for oxygen.

***s. to the right*** In hematology, an increase in the number of older polymorphonuclear leukocytes in the blood. SEE: *Arneth's classification of neutrophils.*

**shift work** Work for a specific time period, esp. working a certain time of the day for a week or two and then shifting to a period either 8 hr before or after the original work period. This changing schedule every several weeks continues as long as one is on shift work rather than working the same period of time each day. SEE: *circadian; clock, biological; night work, maladaption to; sleep.*

A great number of persons work regularly at night, either on a permanent or rotating schedule. In most of these workers, adaptation to the altered work schedule is inadequate. This leads to disturbed daytime sleep, decreased alertness and performance while at work, and an increased safety hazard. In addition, the general health of shift workers may be impaired.

Shift changes should be clockwise and should occur no more frequently than every 2 to 3 weeks. The number of consecutive days worked at night should be decreased to four or five.

**Shiga's bacillus** (shē′găs) [Kiyoshi Shiga, Japanese physician, 1870–1957] Shigella dysenteriae.

**Shigella** (shĭ-gĕl′lă) [Kiyoshi Shiga] A genus of non–lactose-fermenting, nonmotile, gram-negative rods belonging to the family Enterobacteriaceae. It contains a number of species that cause digestive disturbance ranging from mild diarrhea to a severe and often fatal dysentery. SEE: *dysentery, bacillary.*

***S. boydii*** A species that causes acute diarrhea in humans. Also called *group C dysentery bacilli.*

***S. dysenteriae*** Shiga's bacillus, a virulent form isolated during a severe epidemic of dysentery in Japan in 1896. Also called *group A dysentery bacilli.*

***S. flexneri*** A species that is a frequent cause of acute diarrhea in humans. Also called *group B dysentery bacilli.*

***S. sonnei*** A species that is a frequent cause of bacillary dysentery. Also called *group D dysentery bacilli.*

**shigellosis** (shĭ″gĕl-lō′sĭs) [*Shigella* + *osis,* condition] The disease produced by infection with *Shigella* organisms.

**shin** (shĭn) [AS. *scinu,* shin] The anterior edge of the tibia, the portion of the leg between the ankle and knee. SYN: *shank.*

***saber s.*** A condition seen in congenital syphilis in which the anterior edge of the tibia is extremely sharp.

**shingles** (shĭng′lz) [L. *cingulus,* a girdle] An acute infectious viral disease. SEE: illus.; *herpes zoster.*

**shinsplints** Pain in the anterior, posterior, or posterolateral compartment of the

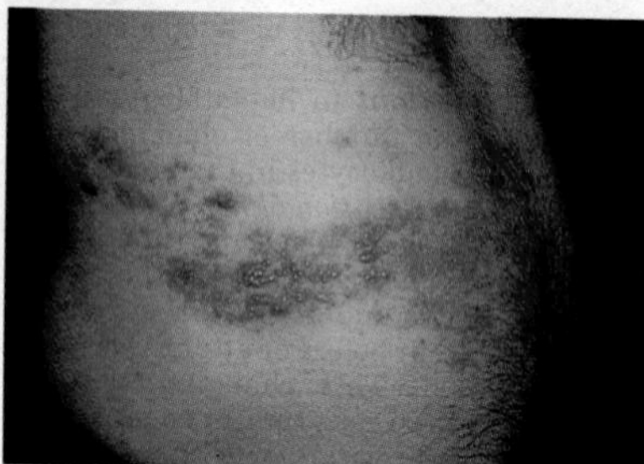

SHINGLES

tibia. It usually follows strenuous or repetitive exercise and is often related to faulty foot mechanics such as pes planus or pes cavus. The cause may be ischemia of the muscles in the compartment, minute tears in the tissues, or partial avulsion from the periosteum of the tibial or peroneal muscles. Proper shoes and foot orthotics may help to prevent onset of the condition. Treatment consists of ice massage, nonsteroidal anti-inflammatory drugs, decrease in intensity of exercise, and avoidance of hills and hard surfaces when running. SYN: *medial tibial syndrome.*

**shin spots** Hyperpigmented and retracted scars of the skin on the anterior lower legs. This condition is usually, but not always, associated with diabetes.

**Shirodkar operation** [Shirodkar, Indian physician, 1900–1971] The surgical placement of a purse-string suture around an incompetent cervical os to attempt to prevent the premature onset of labor. The suture material used for this cerclage procedure is nonabsorbable and must be removed before delivery.

**shiver** (shĭv′ĕr) [ME. *chiveren*] **1.** Involuntary increased muscle activity in response to fear, onset of fever, or exposure to cold. The activity leads to increased heat production. **2.** To tremble or shake.

**shock** (shŏk) [ME. *schokke*] A clinical syndrome in which the peripheral blood flow is inadequate to return sufficient blood to the heart for normal function, particularly transport of oxygen to all organs and tissues. Shock may be caused by a variety of conditions including hemorrhage, anoxia, infection, drug reaction, trauma, poisoning, myocardial infarction, and dehydration. Every injury is accompanied by some degree of shock and should be treated promptly. Syncope is caused by an insufficient supply of blood to the brain, and the clinical picture resembles shock. SEE: *catalepsy; Nursing Diagnoses Appendix.*

SYMPTOMS: The most outstanding symptoms are marked paleness of the skin and evidence of decreased oxygenation of the skin as shown by cyanosis as the process continues. The face is pinched and without expression. There may be a staring of the eyes, which often lose their characteristic luster, and the pupils may be dilated. The pulse is weak and rapid, the breathing rate increased and shallow. The blood pressure is decreased and may be unobtainable. There may be urinary retention and incontinence of feces. Occasionally the patient is unusually restless or excited; very often there is extreme thirst. If conscious, the patient seems quite uninterested in the surroundings and complains little of pain even though he or she may be groaning.

FIRST AID: First aid for shock depends on the diagnosis. In general, one should treat specific etiological factors and maintain body heat by warm, rather than hot, blankets or water bottles. The patient should remain either flat or with the head lower than the feet. The patient should not be moved except for transport to a medical care facility. Fluids are given sparingly but, when head injuries are present or internal bleeding is suspected, stimulants should never be given. A physician should be called immediately.

TREATMENT: Circulation is maintained by keeping the patient lying down with the head lower than the body. The lower extremities can be slightly elevated by placing the lower half of the body on pillows or by elevating the foot of the bed. The patient should be kept comfortably warm, but application of external heat is not advisable. Unnecessary questions and noises should be avoided. It is important to provide constant encouragement and perform all procedures with extreme gentleness.The patient should not be moved unnecessarily.

Even though thirst is present, fluids should be given by mouth sparingly to reduce the possibility of vomiting and aspiration. If bleeding is present, it should be controlled. If internal hemorrhage is suspected or head injuries are present, no stimulants are permissible.

The use of intramuscular and intravenous injections such as norepinephrine, dopamine, or dobutamine may be recommended by the physician. Supplemental oxygen may be necessary. Blood transfusion or even artificial respiration may be required, depending on the seriousness of the condition.

Splints, posture, supporting bandages, and drugs such as morphine are used to relieve pain. Blood transfusions may be lifesaving. If blood is not available, artificial substances for increasing plasma volume may be used. Respiration may be aided by administration of oxygen preferably mixed with 4% to 10% carbon dioxide as a respiratory stimulant.

---

Caution: The shock syndrome is a serious

life-endangering medical emergency and requires very careful therapy and monitoring. If the patient does not respond at once, treatment and monitoring in the best facility available (e.g., intensive care unit) is essential. It is important that the ECG; arterial and central venous blood pressures; blood gases; core and skin temperatures; pulse rate; blood volume; blood glucose; hematocrit; cardiac output; urine flow rate; changes in size, shape, and reaction of pupils; and mental state be monitored as frequently as needed. An electroencephalogram may be required.

---

***anaphylactic*** **s.** SEE: *anaphylactic shock.*

***anesthesia s.*** Shock due to an overdose of a general anesthetic. This calls for the immediate cessation of anesthesia. Artificial respiration, oxygen, and appropriate stimulants should be given at once. The condition is manifested by a weak rapid pulse, a fall or drop in blood pressure, cold clammy skin, and shallow respirations.

***cardiogenic s.*** Shock resulting from failure to maintain the blood supply to the circulatory system and tissues because of inadequate cardiac output. SEE: *Nursing Diagnoses Appendix.*

NURSING IMPLICATIONS: The patient is assessed for a history of any cardiac disorder that severely decreases left ventricular function and for anginal pain, and urinary output is measured (usually less than 20 ml/hr). The skin is inspected for pallor, decreased sensorium, and rapid shallow respirations. Peripheral pulses are palpated for evidence of a rapid, thready pulse, and the skin for a cold, clammy feeling. Blood pressure is auscultated for a mean arterial pressure of less than 60 mm Hg and a narrowing pulse pressure. Heart sounds are auscultated for a gallop rhythm, faint heart sounds, and possibly a holosystolic murmur (related to rupture of the ventricular septum or papillary muscles).

The patient should be moved to the intensive care unit (ICU). There vital signs and peripheral pulses are monitored every 1 to 5 min until treatment stabilizes the patient. Hemodynamic pressure readings are obtained every 15 min, cardiac rhythm is monitored continuously, and a urinary catheter is inserted and urine output measured hourly. Arterial blood gas values and electrolyte levels are also monitored. Prescribed intravenous fluids are administered via a large-bore intravenous catheter (14 G to 18 G) according to hemodynamic patterns and urine output. Oxygen is administered by face mask or artificial airway to ensure adequate tissue oxygenation. Skin color and temperature are continually assessed, and any changes documented. Prescribed inotropic agents and vasopressors are administered and evaluated for desired effects and any adverse reactions.

The nurse assists with insertion of an intra-aortic balloon pump (IABP), a mechanical assist device that can improve coronary artery perfusion and decrease cardiac workload. During use of the IABP, pedal pulses, skin temperature, and color are assessed to ensure adequate peripheral circulation, and the dressing over the insertion site is checked frequently to detect bleeding and changed according to protocol. When the patient is on the IABP, unnecessary patient movement should be avoided, esp. flexing the involved leg or placing the patient in a sitting position. As the patient becomes more hemodynamically stable, the frequency of balloon inflation is gradually reduced, and the patient is weaned from the IABP as prescribed. During weaning, the patient is observed closely for ECG changes, chest pain, and other signs of recurrent cardiac ischemia, as well as for shock.

The ICU setting, special procedures, and equipment are explained to the patient and family to reduce their anxiety; a calm environment with as much privacy as possible and frequent rest periods provided; and frequent family visits permitted. The family is prepared for the possibility of a fatal outcome and assisted to find effective coping strategies.

***compensated s.*** The early phase of shock in which the body's compensatory mechanisms (e.g., increased heart rate, vasoconstriction, increased respiratory rate) are able to maintain tissue perfusion. Typically, the patient is normotensive in compensated shock.

***decompensated s.*** The late phase of shock in which the body's compensatory mechanisms (e.g., increased heart rate, vasoconstriction, increased respiratory rate) are unable to maintain tissue perfusion. Typically, the patient is hypotensive in decompensated shock.

***deferred s.*** Late manifestation of shock following injury or burns. It may appear in 3 to 30 hr and may be due to transportation, emotional stress, hemorrhage, dehydration, acidosis, or toxemia. SYN: *secondary s.*

***distributive s.*** Shock in which there is a marked decrease in peripheral vascular resistance and consequent hypotension. Examples are septic shock, neurogenic shock, and anaphylactic shock.

***electric s.*** Shock resulting from the passage of electric current through any part of the body.

***endotoxin s.*** Septic shock due to toxins from gram-negative bacteria. SEE: *septic shock.*

***epigastric s.*** Shock resulting from a blow or other trauma (surgery) in upper abdomen.

***hemorrhagic s.*** Shock due to loss of

blood. SEE: *Nursing Diagnoses Appendix.*

***hypoglycemic s.*** Shock produced by induction of hypoglycemia by intramuscular insulin administration during treatment of schizophrenia.

***hypovolemic s.*** A condition occurring when there is an insufficient amount of blood in the circulatory system. Usually, this is due to trauma that causes blood loss into a body cavity or frank external hemorrhage. SYN: *oligemic s.*

***insulin s.*** A condition resulting from an overdose of insulin resulting in reduction of the blood sugar level below normal (hypoglycemia). SEE: *Nursing Diagnoses Appendix.*

SYMPTOMS: This form of shock is characterized by a rapid bounding pulse, pale moist skin, weakness, and coma. Acetone odor on breath is not present.

TREATMENT: The patient should be given sugar or candy, orange juice, glucose, or other carbohydrates. A strong glucose solution should be given intravenously if the patient is unconscious. Epinephrine is of great but transient value. SEE: *Medic Alert.*

---

Caution: Persons taking insulin should wear an easily seen bracelet or necklace indicating that they have diabetes and take insulin. This will facilitate diagnosis and treatment in case of coma due to insulin.

---

***irreversible s.*** Shock of such intensity that even heroic therapy cannot prevent death.

***mental s.*** Shock due to emotional stress or to seeing an injury or accident. SEE: *psychic s.*

***neurogenic s.*** A form of distributive shock due to decreased peripheral vascular resistance. Damage to either the brain or the spinal cord inhibits transmission of neural stimuli to the arteries and arterioles, which reduces vasomotor tone. The decreased peripheral resistence results in vasodilation and hypotension; cardiac output diminishes due to the altered distribution of blood volume.

***oligemic s.*** Hypovolemic s.

***protein s.*** Shock reaction resulting from parenteral administration of a protein.

***psychic s.*** Shock due to excessive fear, joy, anger, grief. SEE: *mental s.*

***secondary s.*** Deferred s.

***septic s.*** SEE: *septic shock.*

***serum s.*** Shock occurring as part of a reaction to the injection of serum. SEE: *anaphylactic shock.*

***spinal s.*** Immediate flaccid paralysis and loss of all sensation and voluntary and involuntary reflex activity below the level of injury in acute transverse spinal cord injury. Arterial hypotension may be present in this condition.

***surgical s.*** Shock following operations and including traumatic shock. SEE: *traumatic s.*

***toxic s. syndrome*** SEE: *toxic shock syndrome.*

***traumatic s.*** Shock due to injury or surgery. It may occur as the result of abdominal injury from any cause. The shock is proportional to the extent of injury. It is esp. severe in the upper abdomen and more marked when viscera are damaged. If prolonged, it indicates hemorrhage, peritonitis, or both. In addition to abdominal injury, traumatic shock may be caused by any of the following:

*Cerebral injury:* Shock from concussion of brain or skull fracture. It may come on immediately or later from edema or intracranial hemorrhage. *Chemical injury:* Shock due to pain from the effect of chemicals, esp. corrosives. *Crushing injury:* Shock caused by a crushing injury. The greater the extent of injury, the more severe the degree of shock. *Fracture: (esp. compound fracture):* Shock accompanied often by extensive blood loss into tissues, thereby impairing circulation. *Heart damage:* Shock caused by angina pectoris, myocardial infarction, pericarditis, or myocarditis. *Inflammation:* Shock caused by acute general peritonitis of fulminating sepsis anywhere in the body. *Intestinal obstruction:* Shock that is present when obstruction is acute. *Nerve injury:* Shock caused by contusion of highly sensitive parts, such as a testicle, solar plexus, eye, urethra. *Operations:* Shock that may occur even after minor operations, as paracentesis and catheterization. *Perforation or rupture of viscera:* Shock resulting from acute pneumothorax, ruptured aneurysm, perforated peptic ulcer, perforation in appendicitis, or ectopic pregnancy. *Strangulation:* Shock from hernia, intussusception, or volvulus. *Thermal injury:* Shock caused by burns, frostbite, or heat exhaustion. *Torsion of viscera:* Shock caused by torsion of an ovary or a testicle.

**shock-collapse** A hypotonic-hyporesponsive vascular collapse, possibly evidenced by signs or symptoms such as a decrease in or loss of muscle tone, paralysis (partial or complete), hemiplegia, hemiparesis, skin pallor, unresponsiveness to environmental stimuli, depression of or loss of consciousness, prolonged sleeping with difficulty arousing, or cardiovascular or respiratory arrest. SEE: *disseminated intravascular coagulation; septic shock.*

**shock therapy** Electroconvulsive therapy.

**shoemakers' cramp** A spasm of the muscles of the hand and arm occurring in shoemakers.

**short bowel syndrome** Inadequate absorption of ingested nutrients resulting from a surgical procedure in which a considerable length of the intestinal tract has been removed or bypassed. SEE: *total parenteral nutrition.*

**shortness of breath** SEE: *breathlessness.*

**shortsightedness** (short-sīt′ĕd-nĕs) Myopia.

**shot** A hypodermic injection.

**shotgun prescription** A prescription containing many drugs, given with the hope that one of them may prove effective; not a recommended approach to the treatment of disease.

**shoulder** (shōl′dĕr) [AS. *sculdor*] The region of the proximal humerus, clavicle, and scapula; a part of the shoulder girdle complex. SEE: *scapula.*

***adhesive capsulitis of s.*** A condition that causes shoulder pain, with restricted movement even though there is no obvious intrinsic shoulder disease. This may follow bursitis or tendonitis of the shoulder or may be associated with systemic conditions such as chronic pulmonary disease, myocardial infarction, or diabetes mellitus. Prolonged immobility of the arm favors development of adhesive capsulitis. The condition is more common in women after age 50. It may resolve spontaneously 12 to 18 months after onset or may result in permanent restriction of movement. Treatment includes injection of glucocorticoids; use of nonsteroidal anti-inflammatory agents and physical therapy may provide symptomatic relief; early range-of-motion exercises following an injury may prevent development of the disease; manipulation of the shoulder while the patient is anesthetized may be of benefit. SYN: *frozen shoulder*.

***dislocation of s.*** A condition in which the head of the humerus is displaced beyond the boundaries of the glenoid fossa. Because dislocation of the shoulder is frequently accompanied by a fracture, surgeons advise making an x-ray examination of affected bones. Attempting to reduce dislocations without knowledge of the presence of fractures is very dangerous and sometimes results in paralysis of the entire upper extremity or grave damage to the large blood vessels in the armpit.

ETIOLOGY: The most common cause is from trauma with the arm in external rotation with abduction, causing the head of the humerus to sublux anteriorly; a posterior subluxation may occur from a fall on an outstretched arm. It is very common among athletes, esp. football and basketball players. A patient with a dislocated shoulder usually has a hollow in place of the normal bulge of the shoulder, as well as a slight depression at the outer end of the clavicle. Such patients cannot place their hand at their opposite shoulder while their elbow is on their chest. Both sides should always be compared. An inferior dislocation may occur from poor muscle tone as with hemiplegia and from the weight of the arm pulling the humerus downward.

FIRST AID: A physician should be consulted as soon as possible. The patient should be placed on his or her back, with a pillow (or folded pad) between the shoulders. A large, soft pad should be placed under the elbow on the affected side, and the forearm bound horizontally across the chest using an open sling that is reinforced by a broad cravat bandage. Cold should be applied to the affected shoulder. The patient should be treated for shock, if present.

***s. separation*** SEE: *acromioclavicular separation.*

**shoulder blade** The scapula.

**shoulder girdle** The two scapulae and two clavicles attaching the bones of the upper extremities to the axial skeleton (i.e., the vertebrae of the backbone).

**shoulder joint** A joint formed by the humerus and the glenoid cavity of the scapula.

**show** (shō) [AS. *scewian*, to look at] The sanguinoserous discharge from the vagina during the first stage of labor or just preceding menstruation. Also called *bloody show.*

**Shrapnell's membrane** (shrăp′nĕls) [Henry J. Shrapnell, British anatomist, 1761–1841] A small triangular portion of the tympanic membrane lying above the malleolar folds. It is thin and lax and attached directly to the petrous bone at the tympanic notch (notch of Rivinus). SYN: *pars flaccida membranae tympani; Rivinus' ligament.*

**shreds** (shrĕds) [AS. *screade*] Slender strands of mucus seen in freshly voided urine, indicative of inflammation of the urinary tract or associated organs.

**shrink 1.** To reduce in size. **2.** Slang term for psychiatrist [from *headshrinker*].

**shudder** [ME. *shuddren*] A temporary convulsive tremor resulting from fright, horror, or aversion.

**shunt** (shŭnt) [ME. *shunten,* to avoid] **1.** To turn away from; to divert. **2.** An anomalous passage or one artificially constructed to divert flow from one main route to another. **3.** An electric conductor connecting two points in a circuit to form a parallel circuit through which a portion of the current may pass.

***anatomical s.*** A normal or abnormal direct connection between arterial and venous circulation. An example of a normal anatomical shunt is the bronchial and thebesian vein connection.

***arteriovenous s.*** An abnormal connection between an artery and the venous system.

***cardiovascular s.*** An abnormal connection between the cavities of the heart or between the systemic and pulmonary vessels.

***dialysis s.*** An arteriovenous shunt created for use during renal dialysis.

***left-to-right s.*** The passage of blood from the left side of the heart to the right side through an abnormal opening, as in patent ductus arteriosus.

***physiological s.*** The route by which pulmonary blood perfuses unventilated alveoli. This process is caused by an imbalance in ventilation perfusion.

***portacaval s.*** Surgical creation of a connection between the portal vein and the vena cava. SYN: *postcaval s.*

***postcaval s.*** Portacaval s.

***reversed s.*** Right-to-left s.

***right-to-left s.*** The passage of blood from the right to the left side of the heart through some abnormal opening such as a septal defect. The shunted blood has no opportunity to become oxygenated because of having failed to pass through the lungs. SYN: *reversed s.*

**Shy-Drager syndrome** [George Milton Shy, U.S. neurologist, 1919–1967; G. A. Drager, U.S. physician, 1917–1967] Chronic orthostatic hypotension resulting from a primary autonomic nervous system insufficiency.

**shyness** The feeling of being timid, esp. in an unfamiliar setting or when encountering strangers. This feeling is so common that it cannot be classed as abnormal unless it interferes with activities essential to employment or interpersonal relations.

**SI** *Système International;* International System of Measurement. SEE: *SI Units Appendix.*

**Si** Symbol for the element silicon.

**SIADH** *syndrome of inappropriate antidiuretic hormone.*

**siagonantritis** (sī″ăg-ōn-ăn-trī′tĭs) [Gr. *siagon,* jawbone, + *antron,* cavity, + *itis,* inflammation] Inflammation of the maxillary sinus.

**sialo-, sial-** (sī′ă-lō) Combining form meaning *saliva.*

**sialadenitis** (sī″ăl-ăd″ĕ-nī′tĭs) [″ + ″ + *itis,* inflammation] Inflammation of a salivary gland. SYN: *sialitis.*

**sialadenoncus** (sī″ăl-ăd″ĕ-nŏng′kŭs) [″ + ″ + *onkos,* tumor] A tumor of a salivary gland.

**sialogram** A radiograph of the ductal system of a salivary gland. A radiopaque fluid is instilled into the major duct to determine the presence or absence of calcareous deposits or other pathological changes.

**sialagogue, sialogogue** (sī-ăl′ă-gŏg, sī-ăl′ō-gŏg) [″ + *agogos,* leading] **1.** An agent increasing the flow of saliva. **2.** Producing or promoting the secretion of saliva. SYN: *ptyalagogue.*

**sialectasia, sialectasis** (sī″ăl-ĕk-tā′sē-ă, sī″a-lĕk′tă-sĭs) [″ + *ektasis,* dilatation] Hypertrophy or swelling of the salivary glands.

**sialemesis** (sī″ăl-ĕm′ĕs-ĭs) [″ + *emein,* to vomit] The vomiting of saliva or vomiting caused by an excessive secretion of saliva.

**sialic** (sī-ăl′ĭk) Concerning or resembling saliva.

**sialine** (sī′ă-līn) [Gr. *sialon,* saliva] Concerning saliva.

**sialism, sialismus** (sī′ăl-ĭzm, sī-ăl-ĭz′mŭs) [″ + *-ismos,* condition] Ptyalism.

**sialitis** (sī″ă-līt′tĭs) [″ + *itis,* inflammation] Sialadenitis.

**sialoadenitis** (sī″ă-lō-ăd″ĕ-nī′tĭs) [″ + *aden,* gland, + *itis,* inflammation] Sialadenitis.

**sialoadenotomy** (sī″ă-lō-ăd″ĕ-nŏt′ō-mē) [″ + ″ + *tome,* incision] Incision of a salivary gland.

**sialoaerophagy** (sī″ă-lō-ĕr″ŏf′ă-jē) [″ + *aer,* air, + *phagein,* to eat] Constant swallowing, thus taking saliva and air into the stomach.

**sialoangiectasis** (sī″ă-lō-ăn″jē-ĕk′tă-sĭs) [Gr. *sialon,* saliva, + *angeion,* vessel, + *ektasis,* dilatation] Dilation of a salivary duct.

**sialoangiography** (sī″ă-lō-ăn″jē-ŏg′ră-fē) [″ + ″ + *graphein,* to write] Sialography.

**sialoangitis, sialoangiitis** (sī″ă-lō-ăn-jī′tĭs, -ăn″jē-ī′tĭs) [″ + ″ + *itis,* inflammation] Inflammation of the salivary ducts. SYN: *sialodochitis.*

**sialocele** (sī′ă-lō-sēl) [″ + *kele,* tumor, swelling] Cyst or tumor of a salivary gland.

**sialodochitis** (sī″ă-lō-dō-kī′tĭs) [″ + *doche,* receptacle, + *itis,* inflammation] Sialoangitis.

***s. fibrinosa*** Sialodochitis with the duct obstructed by a fibrinous exudate.

**sialodochoplasty** (sī″ă-lō-dō′kō-plăs″tē) [″ + ″ + *plassein,* to form] Plastic surgery of a salivary gland.

**sialoductitis** (sī″ă-lō-dŭk-tī′tĭs) [″ + L. *ductus,* duct, + Gr. *itis,* inflammation] Inflammation of Stensen's duct.

**sialogenous** (sī″ă-lŏj′ĕ-nŭs) [″ + *gennan,* to produce] Forming saliva.

**sialogogic** (sī″ă-lō-gŏj′ĭk) Producing or promoting a secretion of saliva.

**sialogram** (sī-ăl′ō-grăm) [″ + *gramma,* something written] A radiographical record of sialography.

**sialography** (sī″ă-lŏg′ră-fē) [″ + *graphein,* to write] Radiography of the salivary glands and ducts after injection of a radiopaque contrast medium. SYN: *ptyalography; sialoangiography.*

**sialolith** (sī-ăl′ō-lĭth) [″ + *lithos,* stone] A salivary concretion or calculus.

**sialolithiasis** (sī″ă-lō-lĭ-thī′ă-sĭs) The presence of salivary calculi. SYN: *salivolithiasis.*

**sialolithotomy** (sī″ă-lō-lĭ-thŏt′ō-mē) [Gr. *sialon,* saliva, + *lithos,* stone, + *tome,* incision] The removal of a calculus from a salivary gland or duct.

**sialoncus** (sī″ă-lŏng′kŭs) [″ + *onkos,* bulk, mass] A tumor under the tongue caused by obstruction of a salivary gland or duct.

**sialorrhea** (sī″ă-lō-rē′ă) [″ + *rhoia,* a flow] Ptyalism.

**sialoschesis** (sī″ă-lŏs′kĕ-sĭs) [″ + *schesis,* suppression] Suppression or retention of saliva.

**sialosemeiology** (sī″ă-lō-sē″mī-ŏl′ŏ-jē) [″ + *semeion,* sign, + *logos,* word, reason] Diagnosis based on examination of saliva.

**sialosis** (sī-ă-lō′sĭs) [″ + *osis,* condition] The flow of saliva.

**sialostenosis** (sī″ă-lō-stĕ-nō′sĭs) [″ + *steno-*

*sis,* act of narrowing] Closure of a salivary duct.

**sialosyrinx** (sī″ă-lō-sī′rĭnks) [″ + *syrinx,* a pipe] **1.** A fistula into the salivary gland. **2.** A syringe for washing out salivary ducts. **3.** A drainage tube for a salivary duct.

**sialotic** (sī″ă-lŏt′ĭk) [Gr. *sialon,* saliva] Concerning the flow of saliva.

**Siamese twins** (sī-ă-mēz′) [After Chang and Eng (1811–1874), joined Chinese twins born in Siam] Congenitally united twins. In some cases, the individuals are joined in a small area and are capable of activity, but the extent of union may be so great that survival is impossible. Nevertheless, modern surgical techniques have made it possible to separate infants who in the past would not have been expected to survive and who now have a good prognosis. SEE: *twin.*

**sib** [AS. *sibb,* kin] **1.** Sibling. **2.** A blood relative.

**sibilant** (sĭb′ĭ-lănt) [L. *sibilans,* hissing] Hissing or whistling, as a sound heard in a certain rale.

**sibilation** Pronunciation in which the hissing sound is predominant.

**sibilismus** A hissing sound.

***s. aurium*** Tinnitus.

**sibilus** (sĭb′ĭ-lŭs) [L. *sibilans,* hissing] A hissing rale.

**sibling** (sĭb′lĭng) [AS. *sibb,* kin, + *-ling,* having the quality of] One of two or more children of the same parents; a brother or sister. SYN: *sib.*

***half s.*** A half brother or sister.

**sibship** Brothers and sisters of a single family.

**siccant** (sĭk′ănt) [L. *siccus,* dry] Siccative.

**siccative** (sĭk′ă-tĭv) [L. *siccativus,* drying] Drying or that which dries. SYN: *siccant.*

**siccolabile** (sĭk″ō-lā′bĭl) [L. *siccus,* dry, + *labilis,* unstable] Altered or destroyed by drying.

**siccostabile** (sĭk″ō-stā′bĭl) [″ + *stabilis,* stable] Resistant to drying.

**siccus** (sĭk′ŭs) [L.] Dry.

**sick** (sĭk) [AS *seoc,* ill] **1.** Not well. SYN: *ill.* **2.** Mentally ill or disturbed. **3.** Nauseated.

**sick building syndrome** An excess of work-related irritations of the skin and mucous membranes and other symptoms, including headache, fatigue, and difficulty concentrating, reported by workers in modern office buildings. The cause of this syndrome is unknown.

**sickle cell crisis** A condition in sickle cell anemia in which the sickled cells interfere with oxygen transport, obstruct capillary blood flow, and cause fever and severe pain in the joints and abdomen. The abdominal pain may simulate that caused by appendicitis or other indications for surgical intervention. The cause of the onset of symptoms is usually unknown, but a crisis may be precipitated by decreased ambient oxygen as can occur during flying at high altitude without the use of supplemental oxygen. Also, acidosis and dehydration may precipitate a crisis.

**sickle cell trait** The condition of being heterozygous with respect to hemoglobin. The gene for sickle cell anemia is hemoglobin S. Thus each red blood cell has both normal hemoglobin A and abnormal hemoglobin S. These cells will not become sickled until extremely low concentrations of oxygen occur. SEE: *hemoglobin S.*

**sicklemia** (sĭk-lē′mē-ă) [AS. *sicol,* sickle, + Gr. *haima,* blood] Sickle cells in the blood.

**sickling** The tendency of red blood cells to be sickle-shaped. SEE: *sickle cell anemia.*

**sickness** [AS. *seoc,* ill] A state of being unwell. SYN: *illness.*

***balloon s.*** Discomfort or illness due to ascent in a balloon to an altitude sufficient to cause symptoms of anoxia.

***bleeding s.*** Hemophilia.

***car s.*** Motion s.

***morning s.*** Nausea of early pregnancy.

***motion s.*** Nausea and vomiting caused by a variety of motions, such as those experienced on boats, airplanes, trains, automobiles, or amusement park rides.

***mountain s.*** Nausea and dyspnea caused by insufficient oxygen at high altitudes.

***sea s.*** Sickness caused by motion of a vessel while at sea.

***serum s.*** Sickness following injection of serum.

***sleeping s.*** **1.** Trypanosomiasis. **2.** Encephalitis lethargica.

**sick sinus syndrome** ABBR: SSS. Several electrocardiographical abnormalities caused by a malfunction of the sinoatrial node of the heart. They may include persistent sinus bradycardia that may alternate with tachyarrhythmias; sinoatrial block; and sinus arrest for brief or prolonged periods. Symptoms include lightheadedness, dizziness, fainting, dyspnea, fatigue, and angina pectoris. SEE: *Nursing Diagnoses Appendix.*

TREATMENT: A pacemaker should be inserted. Anticoagulant therapy may be required to prevent thromboembolism.

**SICU** *surgical intensive care unit.*

**SID** *source-to-image receptor distance.*

**S.I.D** *Society for Investigative Dermatology.*

**side** (sīd) [AS. *side*] **1.** The left or right part of the trunk of the body. **2.** An outer portion considered as facing in a particular direction.

**side effect** An action or effect of a drug other than that desired. Commonly it is an undesirable effect such as nausea, headache, insomnia, acute toxic reaction, or drug interaction.

**side-lyer** A device for positioning the patient with central nervous system dysfunction in the side-lying position in order to reduce decerebrate posturing and counteract the effects of the tonic labyrinthine (supine) reflex.

**side-lying** A lateral recumbent position in which the individual rests on either the right or left side, usually with the knees slightly bent. This position is useful in persons with multiple disabilities resulting from damage to the central nervous system and allows relaxation while requiring minimal postural control.

**sidero-** (sĭd′ĕr-ō) Combining form meaning *iron.*

**sideroblast** (sĭd′ĕr-ō-blăst″) [Gr. *sideros,* iron, + *blastos,* germ] A ferritin-containing normoblast in the bone marrow. Sideroblasts constitute from 20% to 90% of normoblasts in the marrow. The ferritin gives a positive Prussian-blue reaction, indicating the iron is ionized and not bound to the heme protein.

**siderocyte** (sĭd′ĕr-ō-sīt) [″ + *kytos,* cell] A red blood cell containing iron in a form other than hematin.

**siderofibrosis** (sĭd″ĕr-ō-fī-brō′sĭs) [″ + L. *fibra,* fiber, + Gr. *osis,* condition] Fibrosis associated with iron deposits.

**siderogenous** (sĭd″ĕr-ŏj′ĕ-nŭs) [″ + *gennan,* to produce] Producing or forming iron.

**sideropenia** (sĭd″ĕr-ō-pē′nē-ă) [″ + *penia,* poverty] Iron deficiency in the blood.

**sideropenic** (sĭd″ĕr-ō-pē′nĭk) Characterized by deficiency of iron in the blood.

**siderophil** (sĭd′ĕr-ō-fĭl) A cell that has an affinity for iron.

**siderophilous** (sĭd″ĕr-ŏf′ĭ-lŭs) [″ + *philein,* to love] Having a tendency to absorb iron, as the red blood corpuscles.

**siderophone** (sĭd′ĕr-ō-fōn) A telephone-like device used to detect intraocular, iron-containing foreign bodies.

**siderophore** (sĭd′ĕr-ō-for) [″ + *phoros,* bearing] A macrophage that contains hemosiderin.

**sideroscope** (sĭd′ĕr-ō-skōp) [″ + *skopein,* to examine] An instrument for finding particles of iron in the eye.

**siderosis** (sĭd″ĕr-ō′sĭs) [″ + *osis,* condition] A form of pneumoconiosis resulting from inhalation of dust or fumes containing iron particles. SYN: *arc-welder's disease.* SEE: *hemosiderosis.*

***hepatic s.*** Accumulation of an abnormal amount of iron in the liver.

***urinary s.*** Hemosiderin granules in the urine.

**siderosome** (sĭd″ĕr-ō-sōm′) [″ + *soma,* body] A reticulocyte in which iron-containing granules are present.

**siderotic** (sĭd″ĕr-ŏt′ĭk) Concerning siderosis.

**SIDS** *sudden infant death syndrome.*

**SIECUS** *Sex Information and Education Council of the U.S.*

**siemens** (sē′mĕnz) A unit of conductance derived from SI units. It is the reciprocal of the resistance in ohms. SYN: *mho.*

**Siemens' syndrome** [Hermann Werner Siemens, German physician, 1891–1969] Harlequin fetus.

**sieve** (sĭv) A device consisting of a mesh with holes of uniform size. It is used to separate particles above a certain size from solutions or powders.

***molecular s.*** A type of sieve in which the molecular material present in the gel or crystal will adsorb molecules of a certain kind and let others pass.

**sievert** [Rolf Maximillian Sievert, Swedish radiologist, 1896–1966] ABBR: Sv. A unit of absorbed radiation energy derived from SI units. One sievert is equal to 1 J/kg or 100 rem.

**sig** *Signa.*

**Sigault's operation** (sē-gōz′) [Jean René Sigault, French obstetrician, b. 1740] Division of the symphysis pubis to facilitate childbirth by enlarging the pelvic outlet. SYN: *symphysiotomy.*

**sigh** [AS. *sican*] A deep inspiration followed by a slow audible expiration.

**sight** (sīt) [AS. *sihth*] **1.** The power or faculty of seeing. **2.** Range of sight. **3.** A thing or view seen. SYN: *vision.*

***blind s.*** The ability to see that occurs in persons who are blind because of a brain lesion rather than damage to the eye. It is manifested by their being able to reach for and track an object. These individuals apparently do not know they can see.

***day s.*** Night blindness.

***far s.*** Hyperopia.

***near s.*** Myopia.

***night s.*** Day blindness.

***old s.*** Presbyopia.

***second s.*** Senopia.

**sigma** (sĭg′mă) The 18th letter, Σ or σ, in the Greek alphabet.

**Sigma Theta Tau** ABBR: STT. The international honor society of nursing, founded in 1922 by six students and one alumna of Indiana University Training School. There are 346 chapters in the U.S., Taiwan, Australia, Canada, and Korea. The national headquarters is at Indiana University in Indianapolis.

**sigmatism** (sĭg′mă-tĭzm) [Gr. *sigma,* letter S, + *-ismos,* condition] Excessive or defective use of "s" sounds in speech.

**sigmoid** (sĭg′moyd) [Gr. *sigmoeides*] **1.** Shaped like the capital Greek letter sigma, Σ. **2.** Pert. to the sigmoid colon.

**sigmoid colon** The part of the colon that turns medially at the left iliac crest, between the descending colon and the rectum; shaped like the letter S.

**sigmoidectomy** (sĭg″moyd-ĕk′tō-mē) [″ + *ektome,* excision] Removal of all or part of the sigmoid colon.

**sigmoiditis** (sĭg″moyd-ī′tĭs) [″ + *itis,* inflammation] Inflammation of the sigmoid colon.

**sigmoidopexy** (sig-moy′dō-pĕk″sē) [″ + *pexis,* fixation] Fixation of the sigmoid to an abdominal incision for prolapse of the rectum. SYN: *romanopexy.*

**sigmoidoproctostomy** (sĭg-moy″dō-prŏk-tŏs′tō-mē) [Gr. *sigmoeides,* shaped like Gr. letter S, + *proktos,* anus, + *stoma,* mouth] The establishment of an artificial passage by anastomosis of the sigmoid flexure with the rectum.

**sigmoidorectostomy** (sĭg-moy″dō-rĕk-tŏs′

tō-mē) [″ + L. *rectus,* straight, + Gr. *stoma,* mouth] Anastomosis of the sigmoid colon with the rectum to establish an artificial passage. SYN: *sigmoidoproctostomy.*

**sigmoidoscope** (sĭg-moy′dō-skōp) [″ + *skopein,* to examine] A tubular speculum for examination of the sigmoid colon.

***flexible s.*** A sigmoidoscope that uses fiberoptics. This permits the tubular extension to flex, enabling the examiner to visualize a greater portion of the colon than would be possible with a rigid sigmoidoscope.

**sigmoidoscopy** (sĭg″moy-dŏs′kō-pē) [″+ *skopein,* to examine] Use of a sigmoidoscope to inspect the sigmoid colon.

**sigmoidosigmoidostomy** (sĭg-moy″dō-sĭg-moy-dŏs′tō-mē) [″ + *sigmoeides,* sigmoid, + *stoma,* mouth] Surgical creation of a connection between two segments of the sigmoid colon.

**sigmoidostomy** (sĭg-moyd-ŏs′tō-mē) [″ + *stoma,* mouth] Creation of an artificial anus in the sigmoid colon.

**sigmoidotomy** (sĭg-moyd-ŏt′ō-mē) [″ + *tome,* incision] Incision of the sigmoid.

**sigmoidovesical** (sĭg-moy″dō-vĕs′ĭ-kăl) [″ + L. *vesica,* bladder] Concerning a connection between the sigmoid colon and the urinary bladder.

**sign** (sīn) [L. *signum*] **1.** Symbol or abbreviation, esp. one used in pharmacy. **2.** Any objective evidence or manifestation of an illness or disordered function of the body. Signs are more or less definitive and obvious, and apart from the patient's impressions, in contrast to symptoms, which are subjective. SEE: *symptom.* **3.** To use sign language to communicate.

***jump s.*** During physical examination, an involuntary reaction to stimulation of a tender area or trigger point. This may take the form of wincing or sudden jerking of the part being examined, of adjacent areas, or even of the entire body. This sign should not be confused with the startle reaction seen in Jumping Frenchmen of Maine.

***objective s.*** In physical diagnosis, a sign that can be seen, heard, measured, or felt by the diagnostician. Finding of such sign(s) can be used to confirm or deny the diagnostician's impressions of the disease suspected of being present. SYN: *physical s.*

***physical s.*** Objective s.

***positive s.'s of pregnancy*** Assessment findings present only during pregnancy: fetal heart tones, fetal movements felt by the examiner, and visualization by sonogram.

***presumptive s.'s of pregnancy*** Signs and symptoms commonly associated with pregnancy that may be present in other conditions. SEE: *pregnancy.*

***probable s.'s of pregnancy*** Objective assessment findings that strongly suggest but do not confirm pregnancy. SEE: *pregnancy.*

***vital s.'s*** Those physical signs concerning functions essential to life (i.e., pulse, rate of respiration, blood pressure, and temperature).

**signa** (sĭg′nă) [L.] ABBR: S or sig. A term used in writing prescriptions meaning to label the subscription according to the dose, route of administration, and frequency of medication.

**signal** Any form of communication that provides information. It is usually visual, verbal, or written, or it could be transmitted by electronic means (i.e., telephone, TV, radio, laser, or via optical fibers).

**signature** (sĭg′nă-tūr) [L. *signatura,* to mark] **1.** The part of a prescription giving instructions to the patient. **2.** The act of writing one's name on a document to certify its validity; the written name on the document.

**significance, statistical** SEE: *statistical significance.*

**significant** (sĭg-nĭf′ĭ-kănt) Important. In statistics, a difference is said to be statistically significant if the analysis indicates that the results have little probability of having occurred owing to chance.

**significant other** A person with whom a patient has a close relationship, which may or may not include relatives or a spouse.

**signing** The use of sign language to communicate with hearing-impaired persons.

**sign language** Representing words by signs made with the position and movement of the fingers and hand. SEE: *American Sign Language.*

**silent** Free from noise; mute; still.

**silent disease** A disease that produces no clinically obvious symptoms or signs.

**silent period** A period in a tendon reflex that immediately follows the contraction of the responding muscles during which the motor neurons do not respond to afferent impulses entering the reflex center.

**silica** (sĭl′ĭ-kă) [L. *silex,* flint] $SiO_2$. Silicon dioxide. SEE: *silicon.*

**silicate** (sĭl′ĭ-kāt) [L. *silicus,* flintlike] A salt of silicic acid.

**siliceous, silicious** (sĭ-lĭsh′ŭs) Containing silica.

**silicic** (sĭl-ĭs′ĭk) Pert. to silica or silicon.

**silicoanthracosis** (sĭl″ĭ-kō-ăn″thră-kō′sĭs) [L. *silex,* flint, + Gr. *anthrax,* coal, + *osis,* condition] Silicosis combined with anthracosis, in coal miners.

**silicofluoride** (sĭl″ĭ-kō-floo′ō-rīd) A compound of silicon, fluorine, and the fluoride of a metal.

**silicon** (sĭl′ĭ-kŏn) [L. *silex,* flint] SYMB: Si. A nonmetallic element found in the soil; atomic weight 28.086; atomic number 14; specific gravity 2.33. Silicon makes up approx. 25% of the earth's crust, being exceeded only by oxygen. It occurs in traces in skeletal structures (bones and teeth).

Silicon is commonly combined with oxygen to form silicon dioxide, $SiO_2$, which occurs in many forms, both crystalline and amorphous. In a pure state, it forms quartz or rock crystal. It is present in many abrasive materials and is the principal constituent of glass.

**silicone** (sĭl′ĭ-kōn″) **1.** An organic compound in which carbon has been replaced by silicon. **2.** Any of a group of polymeric organic silicon compounds; used in adhesives, lubricants, synthetic rubber, and prostheses.

***injectable s.*** Medical-grade silicone compounds suitable for implantation in the body; used in plastic surgery. The use of non–medical-grade silicone for cosmetic breast augmentation has produced a foreign body response to the implanted material. SEE: *breast implant.*

**silicosiderosis** (sĭl″ĭ-kō-sĭd″ĕr-ō′sĭs) [″ + Gr. *sideros,* iron, + *osis,* condition] A type of pneumonoconiosis in which the inhaled particles contain silicates and iron.

**silicosis** (sĭl-ĭ-kō′sĭs) [″ + Gr. *osis,* condition] A form of pneumonoconiosis resulting from inhalation of silica (quartz) dust, characterized by the formation of small discrete nodules. In advanced cases, a dense fibrosis and emphysema with impairment of respiratory function may develop.

**silicotic** (sĭl-ĭ-kŏt′ĭk) **1.** Relating to silicosis. **2.** One affected with silicosis.

**silicotuberculosis** (sĭl″ĭ-kō-tū-bĕr-kū-lō′sĭs) [″ + *tuberculum,* a little swelling, + Gr. *osis,* condition] Silicosis associated with pulmonary tuberculosis.

**siliqua olivae** (sĭl′ĭ-kwē ŏl′ĭ-vē) [L.] Fibers that appear to encircle the olive of the brain.

**siliquose** (sĭl′ĭ-kwōs) [L. *siliqua,* pod] Resembling a two-valve capsule or a pod.

**siliquose cataract** A cataract with a dry, wrinkled capsule.

**siliquose desquamation** Shedding of dried vesicles from the skin.

**silo-filler's disease** Damage to the lungs produced in silo workers when they are exposed to nitrogen dioxide ($NO_2$), the highly toxic gas produced by the fermenting organic matter in the silo. If the concentration of $NO_2$ is high enough to cause immediate symptoms (i.e., irritation of the eyes and pharynx), the person becomes unconscious. Unless the individual is removed from the site, death is the usual outcome. If the exposure is to low concentrations that do not cause immediate symptoms, delayed injury to the lungs may result.

PREVENTION: No one should enter a silo until 7 to 10 days after it is filled. Good ventilation above the base of a silo should be maintained during the 7- to 10-day period. The area should be fenced in, to prevent children or animals from straying into the space surrounding a silo. The blower fan should always be activated before a person enters a silo.

**silver** (sĭl′vĕr) [AS. *siolfor*] SYMB: Ag. A white, soft, ductile malleable metal, its salts being widely used in medicine for their caustic, astringent, and antiseptic effects. Its atomic weight is 107.870; atomic number is 47; and specific gravity is 10.5. In dentistry, silver is used in prosthetic devices, as an alloy with copper or mercury, as silver solder, and as tapering points to obliterate root canals in the endodontic treatment of teeth. Silver nitrate has been used as a germicidal astringent with the treatment of caries, root canals, tooth sensitivity, and gingival diseases. SEE: *argyria.*

***s. amalgam*** An alloy of silver with varying amounts of tin or copper, using mercury as a major component to produce a silvery, malleable restorative material used in dentistry. It is mixed and condensed, then placed in the space left after removal of the decayed area of the tooth, where it hardens into a solid mass that can be shaped to the desired tooth form.

***s. chloride*** SYMB: AgCl. An insoluble salt of silver.

***colloidal s.*** Silver preparations in which the particles of silver or silver proteinate are suspended in the solution rather than being dissolved in it.

***s. halide*** The active ingredient in a radiographical film emulsion that, when exposed to radiant energy and developed, forms the image on the film.

***s. nitrate*** $AgNO_3$. A toxic preparation made from silver. Most of its former uses have passed out of vogue, but it remains important as a germicide and local astringent. It is incompatible with aspirin and sodium chloride. SEE: *silver nitrate poisoning.*

***s. nitrate, toughened*** A mixture of silver nitrate and silver chloride used as a caustic on wounds and granulation tissue, and in treating warts.

***s. picrate*** A compound of silver and picric acid, containing 30% silver. It is useful as an antiseptic, as are other preparations of silver.

***s. protein*** A combination of silver and protein, containing from 7.5% to 8.5% (strong) silver.

***s. sulfadiazine*** A topical medicine composed of silver and sulfadiazine. It is the treatment of choice in preventing infections associated with burns of the skin.

**silverfish** An insect about ½ in. (13 mm) long that is fast, slick, and silver. It is carrot-shaped and has long antennae. The common variety, *Lepisma saccharina,* is not harmful but is destructive because it eats sugar, starch, glue, book bindings, and stamps, as well as food-stained linen, rayon, and cotton. It may be controlled by use of insecticides.

**silver fork deformity** A deformity in the Colles' fracture of the wrist and hand resembling the curve on the back of a fork.

**silver nitrate poisoning** Toxicity caused by excessive ingestion or absorption of silver nitrate. SEE: *silver salts, nitrate, and* *other soluble salts in Poisons and Poisoning Appendix.*

SYMPTOMS: There is burning in the throat and stomach, and rather prompt vomiting. When small amounts of silver are taken over a long period, as in nose drops or eye drops, the patient develops argyria, a peculiar bluish discoloration of all the exposed tissues of the body, including the gingiva.

FIRST AID: Large volumes of ordinary table salt in water precipitate the silver as a slightly soluble chloride. This should be followed with egg whites, oils, and other demulcents.

**simethicone** (sī-měth'ĭ-kōn) A mixture of liquid demethylpolysiloxanes that because of its antifoaming properties is used in treating intestinal gas.

**simian crease** A crease on the palm of the hand, so termed because of its similarity to the transverse flexion crease found in some monkeys. Normally the palm of the hand at birth contains several flexion creases, two of which are separate and approx. transverse. When these two appear to fuse and thus form a single transverse crease, it is termed a simian crease. The crease may be present in a variety of developmental abnormalities including Down syndrome, rubella syndrome, Turner's syndrome, Klinefelter's syndrome, pseudohypoparathyroidism, and gonadal dysgenesis. SEE: illus.

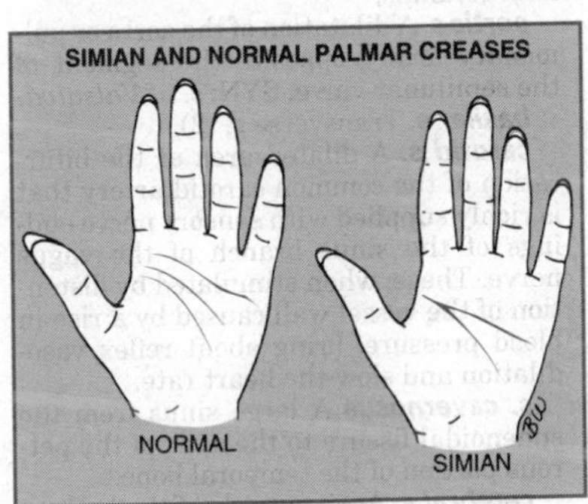

SIMIAN AND NORMAL PALMAR CREASES

**similia similibus curantur** (sī-mĭl'ē-ă sī-mĭl'ĭ-bŭs kū-răn'tūr) [L., likes are cured by likes] The homeopathic doctrine that a drug producing pathological symptoms in those who are well will cure such symptoms in disease states.

**similimum** (sĭ-mĭl'ĭ-mŭm) [L., most like] A medicine that causes a symptom quite similar to that produced by the disease. This therapeutic concept and practice is used in homeopathic medicine.

**Simmonds' disease** (sĭm'mŏnds) [Morris Simmonds, German physician, 1855–1925] A condition in which complete atrophy of the pituitary gland causes loss of function of the thyroid, adrenals, and gonads, premature senility, psychic symptoms, and cachexia. SYN: *cachexia, pituitary.*

**Simon's position** (zē'mŏns) [Gustav Simon, German surgeon, 1824–1876] An exaggerated lithotomy position in which the hips are somewhat elevated and the thighs are strongly abducted. It is used in operations on the vagina. SYN: *Edebohls' position.*

**simple** (sĭm'pl) [L. *simplex*] **1.** Not complex; not compound. **2.** A medicinal plant.

**simple inflammation** Inflammation without pus or other inflammatory exudates.

**Simplesse** Trade name for a low-calorie fat replacement. SEE: *fat replacement.*

**Sims' position** (sĭmz) [James Marion Sims, U.S. gynecologist, 1813–1883] A semiprone position with the patient on the left side, right knee and thigh drawn well up, left arm along the patient's back, and chest inclined forward so patient rests upon it. It is the position of choice for administering enemas, because the sigmoid and descending colon are located on the left side of the body and fluid is readily accepted in this position. It is also employed in curettement of the uterus, intrauterine irrigation after labor, and rectal examination.

**simul** (sī'mŭl, sĭm'ŭl) [L.] At once or at the same time; term used in signature of prescription.

**simulation** (sĭm-ū-lā'shŭn) [L. *simulatio,* imitation] **1.** Pretense of having a disease; feigning of illness. SEE: *malingerer; Munchausen syndrome.* **2.** The imitation of symptoms of one disease by another.

**simulator** (sĭm″ū-lā'tor) Any situation or device that creates a condition or situation similar to one that might be encountered. This technique is useful in teaching.

**Simulium** (sī-mū'lē-ŭm) A genus of insects of the order Diptera that includes the black flies (buffalo gnats). The females are blood suckers.

***S. damnosum*** A species that serves as the intermediate host of a filarial worm *Onchocerca volvulus.*

***S. venustum*** A species common in North America.

**simultanagnosia** The failure to perceive simultaneously all the elements of a scene.

**SIMV** *synchronized intermittent mandatory ventilation.*

**Sinapis** (sĭn-ā'pĭs) [Gr. *sinapi,* mustard] A genus of plants commonly known as mustard plants.

**sinapism** (sĭn'ă-pĭzm) [Gr. *sinapismos*] A mustard plaster used to produce counterirritation by applying it to the skin. Enough water is added to flour to make a paste in these proportions: *adult:* 3 to 4 parts wheat flour to 1 part mustard flour; *child:* 8 to 10 parts wheat flour to 1 part mustard flour; and *infant:* 10 to 12 parts wheat flour to 1 part mustard flour.

**sincipital** (sĭn-sĭp'ĭ-tăl) [L. *sinciput,* half a head] Concerning the sinciput.

**sinciput** (sĭn′sĭp-ŭt) [L., half a head] **1.** The fore and upper part of the cranium. **2.** The upper half of the skull. SYN: *calvaria.*

**Sinding-Larsen Johansson disease** Anterior knee pain caused by persistent traction on an immature inferior patellar pole. There is point tenderness at the patellar-patellar tendon junction, and Osgood-Schlatter disease may be present. The adult equivalent of this disease is patellar tendinitis. This condition occurs commonly in boys 10 to 12 years of age who are actively involved in running and jumping sports. It resolves eventually but can be treated with activity modification, a patella-stabilizing knee brace, ice, and nonsteroidal anti-inflammatory drugs.

**sinew** (sĭn′ū) [AS. *sinu*] A tendon.

***weeping s.*** A ganglion cyst that contains synovial fluid.

**sing** [L., *singulorum*] Of each; used in writing prescriptions.

**singer's node** Chorditis nodosa.

**singleton** One of something described, esp. a single infant rather than a twin.

**singultation** (sĭng″gŭl-tā′shŭn) [L. *singultus,* a hiccup] Hiccupping.

**singultus** (sĭng-gŭl′tŭs) [L.] Hiccup.

**sinister** (sĭn-ĭs′tĕr) [L.] In anatomy, left; or present on the left side of the body.

**sinistrad** (sĭn′ĭs-trăd) [L. *sinister,* left, + *ad,* toward] Toward the left.

**sinistral** (sĭn′ĭs-trăl) [L.] **1.** Pert. to or showing preference for the left hand, eye, or foot in certain actions. **2.** On the left side.

**sinistrality** (sĭn″ĭs-trăl′ĭ-tē) Left-handedness.

**sinistraural** (sĭn-ĭs-traw′răl) [″ + *auris,* ear] Having better hearing with the left ear.

**sinistro-** (sĭn′ĭs-trō) Combining form meaning *left.*

**sinistrocardia** (sĭn″ĭs-trō-kăr′dē-ă) [L. *sinister,* left, + Gr. *kardia,* heart] Displacement of the heart to left of the medial line; the opposite of dextrocardia.

**sinistrocerebral** (sĭn″ĭs-trō-sĕr′ĕ-brăl) [″ + *cerebrum,* brain] Located in the left cerebral hemisphere.

**sinistrocular** (sĭn-ĭs-trŏk′ū-lar) [″ + *oculus,* eye] Having stronger vision in the left eye.

**sinistrocularity** (sĭn″ĭs-trŏk″ū-lăr′ĭ-tē) Condition in which the left eye is dominant.

**sinistrogyration** (sĭn″ĭs-trō-jī-rā′shŭn) [″ + Gr. *gyros,* a circle] Inclination to the left.

**sinistromanual** (sĭn″ĭs-trō-măn′ū-ăl) [″ + *manus,* hand] Left-handed.

**sinistropedal** (sĭn-ĭs-trŏp′ĕd-ăl) [″ + *pes,* foot] Left-footed.

**sinistrotorsion** (sĭn″ĭs-trō-tor′shŭn) [″ + *torsio,* a twisting] A twisting or turning toward the left.

**sinistrous** (sĭn′ĭs-trŭs) Awkward, clumsy, unskilled; the opposite of dextrous.

**sinoatrial** (sīn″ō-ā′trē-ăl) Pert. to the sinus venosus and atrium. SYN: *sinoauricular.*

**sinoauricular** (sī″nō-aw-rĭk′ū-lar) Sinoatrial.

**sinobronchitis** (sī″nō-brŏng-kī′tĭs) [L. *sinus,* curve, + *bronchos,* windpipe, + Gr. *itis,* inflammation] Paranasal sinusitis with bronchitis.

**sinogram** (sī′nō-grăm″) [L. *sinus,* curve, + Gr. *gramma,* something written] A radiograph of a sinus tract filled with a radiopaque contrast medium to determine the range and course of the tract.

**sinter** (sĭn′tĕr) **1.** The calcium or silica deposits formed from water obtained from mineral springs. **2.** To reduce material to a solid form by heating without melting.

**sinuous** (sĭn′ū-ŭs) [L. *sinuosus,* winding] Winding; wavy; tortuous.

**sinus** (sī′nŭs) *pl.* **sinuses, sinus** [L., curve, hollow] **1.** A cavity within a bone. **2.** A dilated channel for venous blood. **3.** A canal or passage leading to an abscess. **4.** Any cavity having a relatively narrow opening.

***accessory nasal s.*** One of the paranasal sinuses: frontal, maxillary, ethmoidal, and sphenoidal. The anterior group consists of the frontal, maxillary, and anterior ethmoids; the posterior group includes the posterior ethmoids and sphenoid. These sinuses develop embryologically from nasal cavities, are lined with the same type of epithelium, are filled with air, and communicate with nasal cavities through their various ostia. They lighten the skull, being lighter than dense bone, and act as resonating chambers for the voice.

***anal s.*** The saclike recesses behind the anal columns.

***aortic s.*** A dilatation of the aorta or pulmonary artery opposite the segment of the semilunar valve. SYN: *s. of Valsalva.*

***basilar s.*** Transverse s. (2).

***carotid s.*** A dilated area at the bifurcation of the common carotid artery that is richly supplied with sensory nerve endings of the sinus branch of the vagus nerve. These, when stimulated by distention of the vessel wall caused by a rise in blood pressure, bring about reflex vasodilation and slow the heart rate.

***s. cavernosus*** A large sinus from the sphenoidal fissure to the apex of the petrous portion of the temporal bone.

***cerebral s.*** Any ventricle of the brain.

***circular s.*** A venous sinus around the pituitary body, communicating on each side with the cavernous sinus.

***coccygeal s.*** A sinus in the midline of the nasal cleft just over the coccyx.

***coronary s. of heart*** A vein in the transverse groove between the left cardiac atrium and ventricle.

***cranial s.*** One of the venous canals between the folds of the dura.

***dermal s.*** A congenital sinus tract connecting the surface of the body with the spinal canal.

***draining s.*** An abnormal passageway leading from inside the body to the outside. This is usually due to an infectious process.

***ethmoidal s.*** One of the air cavities in

the ethmoid bone.

***frontal s.*** An irregular cavity in the frontal bone on each side of the midline above the nasal bridge. One may be larger than the other. A duct carries secretions to the upper part of the nasal cavity.

***genitourinary s.*** Urogenital s.

***hair s.*** The sinus formed when hair is embedded in the skin and acts as a foreign body.

***inferior longitudinal s.*** Inferior sagittal s.

***inferior petrosal s.*** A large venous sinus from the cavernous sinus, running along the lower margin of the petrous portion of the temporal bone.

***inferior sagittal s.*** A venous sinus in the inferior margin of the falx cerebri. SYN: *inferior longitudinal s.*

***intercavernous s.*** One of the anterior and posterior halves of the circular sinus.

***lateral s.*** One of two large venous sinuses in the inner side of the skull passing near the mastoid antrum and emptying into the jugular vein.

***lymph s.*** One of the small spaces throughout the parenchyma of a lymphatic gland.

***marginal s.*** **1.** A large venous sinus around part of the margin of the placenta. **2.** One of the small bilateral venous sinuses of the dura mater at the edge of the foramen magnum. **3.** A venous sinus around a portion of the white pulp of the spleen.

***maxillary s.*** A cavity in the maxillary bone communicating with the middle meatus of the nasal cavity. SYN: *antrum of Highmore.*

***occipital s.*** A small venous sinus in the attached margin of the falx cerebelli extending to the margin of the foramen magnum.

***paranasal s.*** Any of the anterior accessory nasal sinuses that open into the nasal cavities. They are the frontal, ethmoidal, sphenoidal, and maxillary. All are lined with a ciliated mucous membrane continuous with that of the nasal cavities. SEE: illus.

***pilonidal s.*** Pilonidal fistula.

***pleural s.*** One of the spaces in the pleural sac along the lower and inferior portions of the lung that the lung does not occupy.

***s. pocularis*** A lacuna in the prostatic part of the urethra. SYN: *s. prostaticus.*

***s. prostaticus*** S. pocularis.

***s. of the pulmonary trunk*** One of the dilatations in the pulmonary trunk, across from a cusp of the pulmonary valve of the heart.

***s. rectus*** A venous sinus at the junction of the falx cerebri and the cerebellar tentorium. SYN: *straight s.*

***renal s.*** The area in the kidney composed of the renal pelvis, renal calices, vessels, nerves, and fatty tissue.

***rhomboid s.*** The fourth cranial ventricle.

***scleral venous s.*** Schlemm's canal.

***sigmoid s.*** The continuation, on both sides, of the transverse sinuses down along the posterior border of the petrous part of the temporal bone to the jugular foramen and jugular veins.

***sphenoidal s.*** One of the air sinuses that occupy the body of the sphenoid bone and connect with the nasal cavity.

***sphenoparietal s.*** **1.** A venous sinus uniting the cavernous sinus and a meningeal vein. **2.** The portion of the cavernous sinus below the ensiform process.

***s. of spleen*** A venous sinusoid in the reticulum of the spleen.

***straight s.*** S. rectus.

***superior longitudinal s.*** Superior sagittal s.

***superior petrosal s.*** A venous canal running in a groove in the petrous portion of the temporal bone.

***superior sagittal s.*** A large venous sinus along the attached border of the falx cerebri from the crista galli to the internal occipital protuberance where it joins either the right or left transverse sinuses or both. SYN: *superior longitudinal s.*

***tarsal s.*** A tunnel between the calcaneus and talus of the ankle.

***tentorial s.*** SEE: *s. rectus.*

***terminal s.*** A vein encircling the vascular area of the blastoderm.

***transverse s.*** **1.** A sinus that unites the two inferior petrosal sinuses of the cranium. **2.** Venous network in the dura over the basilar process of the occipital bone. SYN: *basilar s.*

***transverse s. of the dura mater*** One of the large, bilateral venous sinuses along the attached margin of the cerebellar tentorium. They receive the superior sagittal and straight sinuses and drain into the sigmoid sinuses and then into the jugular veins.

***transverse s. of the pericardium*** A channel posterior to the aorta and the pulmonary trunk but in front of the atria.

***tympanic s.*** A deep recess in the labyrinthine wall of the tympanic cavity. It opens into the fenestra of the cochlea.

***urogenital s.*** **1.** A duct into which, in the embryo, the wolffian ducts and bladder empty; it opens into the cloaca. **2.** The common receptacle of the genital and urinary ducts. SYN: *genitourinary s.*

***uterine s.*** One of the venous channels in the walls of the uterus during pregnancy.

***uteroplacental s.*** One of the slanting venous channels from the placenta serving to convey the maternal blood from the intervillous lacunae back into the uterine veins.

***s. of Valsalva*** Aortic s.

***s. of venal canal, s. venarum cavarum*** The portion of the right atrium of the heart posterior, and to the left of the crista terminalis. The inferior and supe-

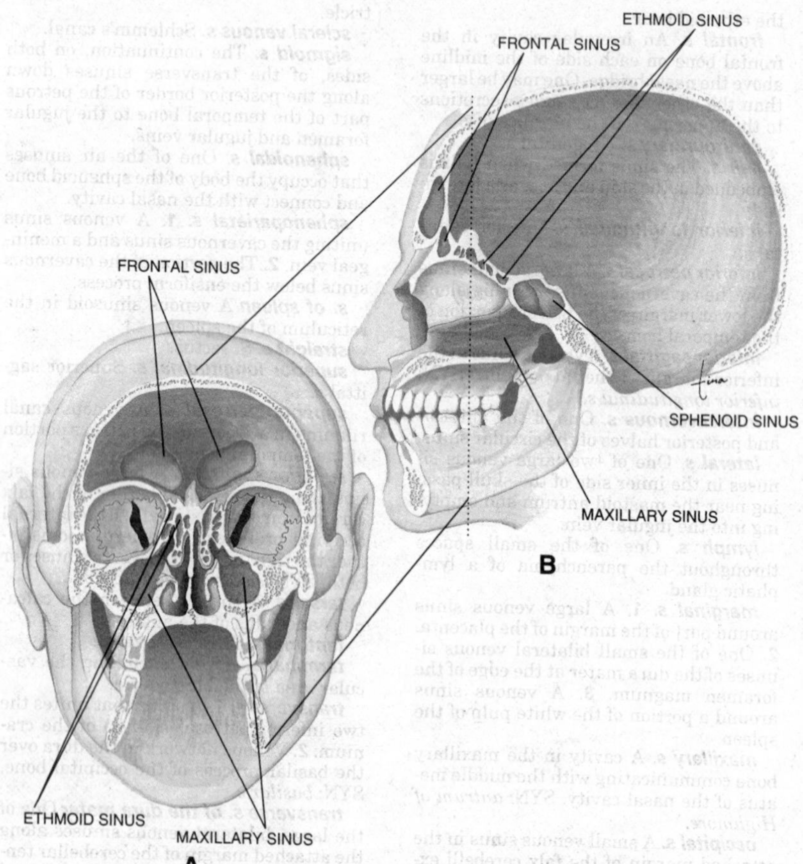


PARANASAL SINUSES, (A) ANTERIOR (B) LEFT LATERAL

rior vena caval veins empty into it.

***venous s.*** A sinus conveying venous blood.

***venous s. of the dura mater*** One of the venous channels between the two layers of the dura mater. They drain the venous blood from the brain.

***venous s. of sclera*** Sceral venous s.

**sinus arrhythmia** Cardiac irregularity characterized by an increased heart rate during inspiration and a decrease in heart rate on expiration. This arrhythmia has no clinical significance except in older patients, in whom it may occur in coronary artery disease.

**sinus bradycardia** Heart rate of 50 beats per minute or less. SEE: *sinus tachycardia.*

**sinusitis** (sī-nŭs-ī′tĭs) [L. *sinus,* curve, hollow, + Gr. *itis,* inflammation] Inflammation of a sinus, esp. a paranasal sinus. It may be caused by various agents, including viruses, bacteria, or allergy. Predisposing factors include inadequate drainage, which may result from presence of polyps, enlarged turbinates, or deviated septum; chronic rhinitis; general debility; or dental abscess in maxillary bone.

***acute suppurative s.*** Purulent inflammation with symptoms of pain over the sinus, fever, chills, and headache.

TREATMENT: Therapy is conservative. Shrinkage in the nasal mucosa is useful to facilitate ventilation and drainage of the sinus. The patient should rest in bed, force fluids, take decongestants, and apply hot packs. If inflammation is due to bacterial infection, antibiotic therapy is indicated. Cefaclor, a cephalosporin, is effective against a great number of the organisms that can cause acute sinusitis.

***chronic hyperplastic s.*** Polyps present in sinuses and nose and underlying osteitis of sinus walls.

TREATMENT: This condition is treated surgically. Conservative surgery involves the removal of polyps and intranasal opening into sinuses for adequate ventilation and drainage. Radical surgery would involve the complete removal of sinus mucosa through either the external or the intranasal route.

**sinusoid** (sī'nŭs-oyd) [" + Gr. *eidos,* form, shape] **1.** Resembling a sinus. **2.** A large, permeable capillary, often lined with macrophages, found in organs such as the liver, spleen, bone marrow, and adrenal glands. Their permeability allows cells or large proteins to easily enter or leave the blood.

**sinusoidal** (sī-nŭs-oyd'ăl) Pert. to a sinusoid.

**sinusoidal current** Alternating induced electric current, the two strokes of which are equal.

**sinusoidalization** (sī"nŭ-soy"dăl-ĭ-zā'shŭn) [L. *sinus,* hollow, curve, + Gr. *eidos,* form, shape] The use of a sinusoidal current.

**sinusotomy** (sī-nŭs-ŏt'ō-mē) [" + Gr. *tome,* incision] The incising of a sinus.

**sinus rhythm** The normal cardiac rhythm the stimulus for which begins at the sinoatrial node.

**sinus tachycardia** A heart rate of 90 beats per min or more. SEE: *sinus bradycardia.*

**$SiO_2$** Silicon dioxide.

**si op sit** [L., *si opus sit*] If needed; used in writing prescriptions.

**siphon** (sī'fŭn) [Gr. *siphon,* tube] A tube bent at an angle to form two unequal lengths for transferring liquids from one container to another by atmospheric pressure. One container must be higher than the other for this to work.

**siphonage** (sī'fŭn-ĭj) Use of a siphon to drain a body cavity such as the stomach or bladder.

**Siphonaptera** (sī"fō-năp'tĕr-ă) [" + *apteros,* wingless] An order of insects commonly called fleas. They are wingless, undergo complete metamorphosis, and have piercing and sucking mouth parts. The body is compressed laterally, and the legs are adapted for leaping. Fleas feed on the blood of birds and mammals. They transmit the causative organisms of several diseases (bubonic plague, endemic or murine typhus, and among rodents, tularemia) and also serve as intermediate hosts of certain tapeworms. SEE: *flea.*

**siphonoma** (sī-fŏn-ō'mă) [" + *oma,* tumor] A tumor made up of fine tubes.

**Sipple syndrome** [John H. Sipple, U.S. physician, b. 1930] Multiple endocrine neoplasia type III. SEE: *multiple endocrine neoplasia.*

**sirenomelia** (sī"rĕn-ŏm-ē'lē-ă) [Gr. *seiren,* mermaid, + *melos,* limb] A congenital anomaly in which the lower extremities are fused.

**-sis** [Gr.] Suffix meaning *condition, state.* Depending on the preceding vowel, it may appear in the form of *-asis, -esis, -iasis,* or *-osis.*

**sister** A term used by the British for nurse, esp. a senior or head nurse.

**Sister Mary Joseph nodule** A hard, periumbilical lymph node sometimes present when pelvic or gastrointestinal tumors have metastasized.

**site** [L. *situs,* place] Position or location.

***active s.*** The active portion of a chemical substance, esp. a catalyst or enzyme, which binds to the material it is acting upon.

***binding s.*** The particular location on a cell surface or chemical to which other chemical substances bind or attach.

***receptor s.*** The particular component of a cell surface that has the ability to react with certain molecules such as proteins, or a virus.

**sitio-, sito-** Combining form meaning *bread, made from grain, food.*

**sitophobia** (sī"tō-fō'bē-ă) [Gr. *sition, sitos,* food, + *phobos,* fear] Psychoneurotic abhorrence of food, or morbid dread of or repugnance to food, whether generally or only to specific dishes.

**sitosterols** (sī-tŏs'tĕr-ŏls) A group of similar organic compounds that occur in plants. They contain the steroid nucleus, perhydrocyclopentanophenanthrene.

**sitotherapy** (sī"tō-thĕr'ă-pē) [" + *therapeia,* treatment] The therapeutic use of food.

**sitotoxin** (sī"tō-tŏk'sĭn) [" + *toxikon,* poison] Any poison developed in food, esp. one produced by bacteria growing in a cereal or grain product.

**sitotoxism** (sī"tō-tŏks'ĭzm) [" + " + *-ismos,* condition] Poisoning by vegetable foods infested with molds or bacteria. SEE: *aflatoxin.*

**situation 1.** A set of circumstances. **2.** The location of an entity in relation to other objects.

**situs** (sī'tŭs) [L.] A position.

***s. inversus viscerum*** The abnormal relation and displacement of viscera to the opposite side of the body.

***s. perversus*** Malposition of any visceral structure.

**sitz bath** (sĭtz) A bath to sit in with water above and covering the hips. The water may be warm and contain medication. The tub or fixture is usually shaped to allow the legs to be out of the water.

**SI units** SEE: tables; *International System of Units; SI Units Appendix.*

**Sjögren's syndrome** ABBR: SS. A chronic, slowly progressive autoimmune disorder characterized by dryness of the eyes and mouth and recurrent salivary gland enlargement. This is called the sicca complex and is diagnostic. The disease may be seen alone or in association with other autoimmune diseases such as rheumatoid arthritis, systemic lupus erythematosis, or scleroderma. Treatment is symptomatic, including application of medicines to replace deficient tears. Some assistance has been provided by use of a device placed in the mouth to stimulate secretion from the salivary gland. SEE: *Schirmer test.*

### Units of the International System of Units (SI units)

| Basic Quantity | Basic Unit | Symbol |
|---|---|---|
| Length | meter | m |
| Mass | kilogram | kg |
| Time | second | s |
| Electric current | ampere | A |
| Thermodynamic temperature | kelvin | K |
| Luminous intensity | candela | cd |
| Amount of substance | mole | mol |

**skateboard** A therapeutic device used for upper or lower extremity rehabilitation. It consists of a platform mounted on ball-bearing rollers. It assists the patient in making coordinated movements.

**skatol(e)** (skăt′ōl) [Gr. *skatos,* dung] $C_9H_9N$. Beta-methyl indole, a malodorous, solid, heterocyclic nitrogen compound found in feces, formed by protein decomposition in the intestines and giving them their odor.

**skatoxyl** (skă-tŏk′sĭl) A derivative of skatole.

**skein** (skān) A continuous tangled thread.

**skeletal** (skĕl′ĕ-tăl) [Gr. *skeleton,* a dried-up body] Pert. to the skeleton.

**skeletal muscle** Muscle fibers that with few exceptions are attached to parts of the skeleton and involved primarily in movements of the parts of the body. SYN: *striated muscle; voluntary muscle.*

**skeletal survey** A procedure in which entire skeleton is radiographed to determine the presence of pathology.

**skeletal traction** A pulling force applied directly to the bone through surgically applied pins and tongs.

NURSING IMPLICATIONS: The patient in traction is placed on a firm mattress in the prescribed position. Ropes, weights, and pulleys are assessed daily for wear, chafe, and improper position. Care must be taken to keep the skin insertion points of pins and tongs clean and free of infection. Infection at insertion sites can lead to osteomyelitis. Assessing the area for odor and other signs of infection and cleansing the area and then applying prescribed medication and sterile dressing can help to prevent osteomyelitis; aseptic technique is used to perform these procedures. Daily skin inspection for signs of pressure or friction is performed, and appropriate nursing measures are instituted to alleviate any pressure or friction. Proper traction alignment should be maintained at all times, and adjusted as necessary. An exercise regimen is established for the unaffected extremities. The nurse should respond to any patient complaint without delay. Respiratory toilet is provided to prevent pulmonary complications. Analgesics are administered as prescribed. Adequate nutrition and fluid intake promotes tissue healing and repair. Dietary and medical management helps to prevent constipation and fecal impaction. The affected extremity is assessed daily or more frequently if necessary for complications such as phlebitis and nerve or circulatory impairment, and the lower extremity, for footdrop. Social and diversional activities are promoted. The nurse teaches the patient the use of a trapeze, exercises, and activity limitations and establishes discharge plans and follow-up care.

**skeletization** (skĕl″ĕt-ĭ-zā′shŭn) Excessive emaciation.

**skeleto-** Combining form meaning *skeleton.*

**skeletogenous** (skĕl-ĕ-tŏj′ĕ-nŭs) [Gr. *skeleton,* a dried-up body, + *gennan,* to produce] Forming skeletal structures or tissues.

**skeletology** (skĕl″ĕ-tŏl′ō-jē) [″ + *logos,* word, reason] The special division of anatomy and biomechanics concerned with the skeleton.

**skeleton** (skĕl′ĕt-ŏn) [Gr., a dried-up body]

### Prefixes and Their Symbols Used to Designate Decimal Multiples and Submultiples in SI Units

| Prefix | Symbol | Factor |
|---|---|---|
| tera | T | $10^{12}$ = 1 000 000 000 000 |
| giga | G | $10^{9}$ = 1 000 000 000 |
| mega | M | $10^{6}$ = 1 000 000 |
| kilo | k | $10^{3}$ = 1 000 |
| hecto | h | $10^{2}$ = 100 |
| deka | da | $10^{1}$ = 10 |
| deci | d | $10^{-1}$ = 0.1 |
| centi | c | $10^{-2}$ = 0.01 |
| milli | m | $10^{-3}$ = 0.001 |
| micro | μ | $10^{-6}$ = 0.000 001 |
| nano | n | $10^{-9}$ = 0.000 000 001 |
| pico | p | $10^{-12}$ = 0.000 000 000 001 |
| femto | f | $10^{-15}$ = 0.000 000 000 000 001 |
| atto | a | $10^{-18}$ = 0.000 000 000 000 000 001 |

The bony framework of the body consisting of 206 bones: 80 axial or trunk and 126 of the limbs (appendicular). This number does not include teeth or sesamoid bones other than the patella. SEE: illus.; table.

***appendicular s.*** Bones of the appendages and their supporting pectoral and pelvic girdles.

***axial s.*** Bones of the head and trunk.

***cartilaginous s.*** The part of the skeleton formed by cartilage; it serves as support and protection but is more flexible and resistant to resorption due to pressure than bone.

**Skene's glands** (skēns) [Alexander Johnston Chalmers Skene, Scot.-born U.S. gynecologist, 1837–1900] Glands lying just inside of and on the posterior area of

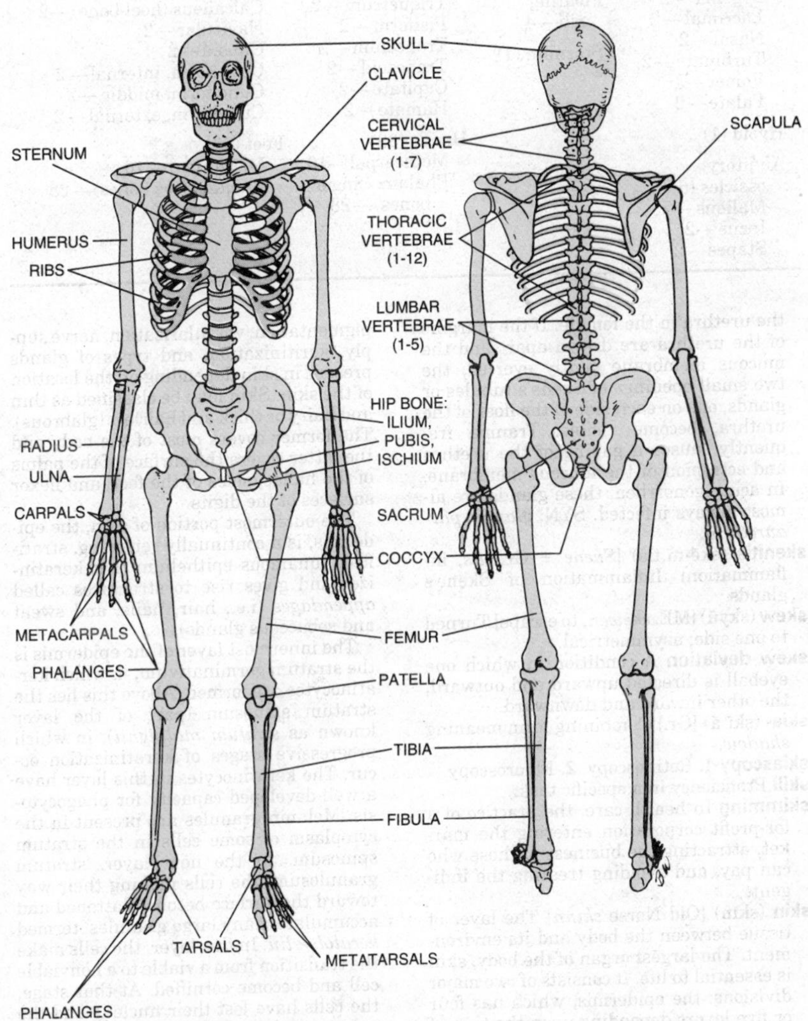

## Bones of the Human Skeleton

| Axial (80 bones) | | Appendicular (126 bones) | |
|---|---|---|---|
| **Head (29 bones)** | **Trunk (51 bones)** | **Upper Extremities (64 bones)** | **Lower Extremities (62 bones)** |
| Cranial (8)<br>Frontal—1<br>Parietal—2<br>Occipital—1<br>Temporal—2<br>Sphenoid—1<br>Ethmoid—1 | Vertebrae (26)<br>Cervical—7<br>Thoracic—12<br>Lumbar—5<br>Sacrum—1<br>Coccyx—1 | Arms and shoulders (10)<br>Clavicle—2<br>Scapula—2<br>Humerus—2<br>Radius—2<br>Ulna—2 | Legs and hips (10)<br>Innominate or hip bone (fusion of the ilium, ischium, and pubis)—2<br>Femur—2<br>Tibia—2<br>Fibula—2<br>Patella (kneecap)—2 |
| Facial (14)<br>Maxilla—2<br>Mandible—1<br>Zygoma—2<br>Lacrimal—2<br>Nasal—2<br>Turbinate—2<br>Vomer—1<br>Palate—2 | Ribs (24)<br>True rib—14<br>False rib—6<br>Floating rib—4<br><br>Sternum (1) | Wrists (16)<br>Scaphoid—2<br>Lunate—2<br>Triquetrum—2<br>Pisiform—2<br>Trapezium—2<br>Trapezoid—2<br>Capitate—2<br>Hamate—2 | Ankles (14)<br>Talus—2<br>Calcaneus (heel bone)—2<br>Navicular—2<br>Cuboid—2<br>Cuneiform, internal—2<br>Cuneiform, middle—2<br>Cuneiform, external—2 |
| Hyoid (1)<br><br>Auditory ossicles (6)<br>Malleus—2<br>Incus—2<br>Stapes—2 | | Hands (38)<br>Metacarpal—10<br>Phalanx (finger bones)—28 | Feet (38)<br>Metatarsal—10<br>Phalanx (toe bones)—28 |

the urethra in the female. If the margins of the urethra are drawn apart and the mucous membrane gently everted, the two small openings of Skene's tubules or glands, one on each side of the floor of the urethra, become visible. Trauma frequently causes a gaping of the urethra and ectropion of the mucous membrane. In acute gonorrhea, these glands are almost always infected. SYN: *glands, paraurethral.*

**skenitis** (skē-nī′tĭs) [*Skene* + Gr. *itis,* inflammation] Inflammation of Skene's glands.

**skew** (skyū) [ME. *skewen,* to escape] Turned to one side; asymmetrical.

**skew deviation** A condition in which one eyeball is directed upward and outward, the other inward and downward.

**skia-** (skī′ă) [Gr.] Combining form meaning *shadow.*

**skiascopy 1.** Retinoscopy. **2.** Fluoroscopy.

**skill** Proficiency in a specific task.

**skimming** In health care, the practice of a for-profit corporation entering the market, attracting the business of those who can pay, and avoiding treating the indigent.

**skin** (skĭn) [Old Norse *skinn*] The layer of tissue between the body and its environment. The largest organ of the body, skin is essential to life. It consists of two major divisions: the epidermis, which has four or five layers depending upon the type of skin present in specific locations, and the dermis. There is considerable variation in the thickness, strength, number of hairs, pigmentation, vascularization, nerve supply, keritinization, and types of glands present in skin depending on the location of the skin. Skin may be classified as thin and hairy or thick and hairless (glabrous). The former covers most of the body and the latter covers the surface of the palms of the hands, soles of the feet, and flexor surfaces of the digits.

The outermost portion of skin, the epidermis, is a continually renewing, stratified, squamous epithelium that keratinizes and gives rise to structures called *appendages* (i.e., hair, nails, and sweat and sebaceous glands).

The innermost layer of the epidermis is the stratum germinativum, in which keratinocytes are formed. Above this lies the stratum spinosum (part of the layer known as *stratum malpighii*), in which progressive stages of keratinization occur. The keratinocytes in this layer have a well-developed capacity for phagocytosis. Melanin granules are present in the cytoplasm of some cells in the stratum spinosum. In the next layer, stratum granulosum, the cells making their way toward the surface become flattened and accumulate many large granules, termed *keratohyalin.* In this layer, the cells make the transition from a viable to a nonviable cell and become cornified. At that stage, the cells have lost their nucleus and the only material remaining is filaments of keratin. Above this layer is the stratum lucidum, a hyalinized layer containing eleidin. Its cells have indistinct bounda-

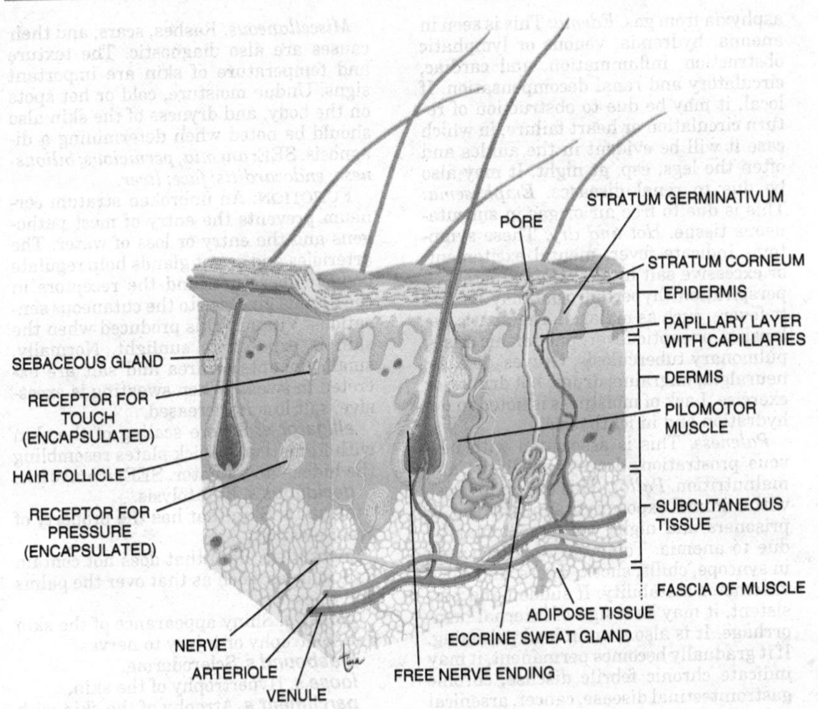


SKIN SECTION

ries and appear similar to those of the next layer. It is seen best in thick, glabrous skin, being represented by only a few cell layers in thin skin. The outermost layer, the stratum corneum, is composed of closely packed cornified, or horny, flattened cells that are the dead keratinocytes, called *squames*. This layer in the scalp may be only a few cells deep, but in thick skin may be 50 cells deep. Eventually, these cells separate from one another and become detached from the surface of the epidermis, a process called desquamation.

The time required for a newly formed keratinocyte to pass from the deepest layer to the surface and be shed has been estimated to be from 45 to 75 days. SEE: illus.; *hair* for illus; *melanin; nails; photoaging; tanning salon.*

DIFFERENTIAL DIAGNOSIS: *Abnormal dryness:* This may indicate abnormal deficiency of thyroid function, diabetes, ichthyosis, or continued exposure to a hot, dry environment. *Ashy:* This is associated with malignant diseases, severe anemia, cancer, tuberculosis, and chronic interstitial nephritis. *Bronzing:* This indicates Addison's disease, poisoning with certain dyes or metals, or early stages of pellagra. *Brownish-yellow spots* (liver spots): These may be due to aging; noted in pregnancy (chloasma uterinum), in exophthalmic goiter, and uterine and liver malignancies; also may be due to freckles, sunburn, cosmetics, turpentine, and other irritants.

*Cherry red:* This indicates carbon monoxide poisoning. *Cold sweats:* This indicates great prostration, fear, anxiety, or depression.

*Cyanosis:* This may be congenital; if acquired, may be due to asthma, pulmonary tuberculosis, whooping cough, advanced emphysema, croup, tracheal obstruction, aneurysm, goiter, flushing (hyperemia), emotion, febrile disorders, pulmonary tuberculosis, convulsions, large ovarian tumor, plethora, polycythemia. *Cyanosis alternating with pallor:* This indicates a lack of oxygen and excess of carbon dioxide in the blood. It may be noted in the lips, mucous membranes, fingertips, and external ear. In extreme cases, the entire body shows a dusky, leaden tint. These symptoms are associated with cerebrospinal diseases, typhoid, vasomotor disturbances, or argyria associated with ingestion of silver salts. They may be due to inflammation or abscess of the pharynx and larynx, Ludwig's angina, croup, and disorders affecting respiration, or to overdose of drugs or asphyxiation by gas.

*Discolorations:* These are seen in icterus, chlorosis, leprosy, application of silver nitrate, jaundice, carotenemia, vitiligo, albinism, malignant diseases, and asphyxia from gas. *Edema:* This is seen in anemia, hydremia, venous or lymphatic obstruction, inflammation, and cardiac, circulatory and renal decompensation. If local, it may be due to obstruction of return circulation or heart failure, in which case it will be evident in the ankles and often the legs, esp. at night. It may also be due to renal diseases. *Emphysema:* This is due to free air or gas in subcutaneous tissue. *Hot and dry:* These symptoms indicate fever, mental excitement, or excessive salt intake. *Moist:* Increased perspiration (hyperhidrosis) may be due to fevers, such as malarial, rheumatic, relapsing, or septic fever; pneumonic crisis; pulmonary tuberculosis; Graves' disease; neuralgia; migraine; drugs; hot drinks; or exercise. Lack of moistness is noted in dehydration and in ichthyosis.

*Paleness:* This is associated with nervous prostration, dropsy, paralysis, and malnutrition. *Pallor:* This occurs in those with minimal exposure to sunlight, esp. in prisoners and night workers. It may be due to anemia. Temporary pallor occurs in syncope, chills, shock, rigors, and some vasomotor instability. If sudden and persistent, it may be a sign of internal hemorrhage. It is also seen in lead poisoning. If it gradually becomes permanent, it may indicate chronic febrile disease, chronic gastrointestinal disease, cancer, arsenical poisoning, chronic suppuration, chronic mercurial poisoning, hemorrhages, leukemia, cachexia, nephrosis, nephritis, syphilis, parasitic diseases, tuberculosis, or malaria. *Purplish:* This indicates an interference of circulation common in asthma and typhus.

*Rashes:* Local redness is seen in inflammation, skin diseases, chronic alcoholism, vasomotor disturbances, and pyrexia. Local redness with pain indicates inflammation as in sunburn (actinic dermatitis). *Sallowness:* This is seen in cachexia, syphilis, chronic gallbladder disease, arthritis deformans, constipation, and some anemias. It is also associated with gastric, pancreatic, enteric, or hepatic disorders.

*Temperature:* The skin temperature usually correlates with the body's internal temperature, unless it is raised by local applications of heat or exposure to cold. Generally, cold skin may be due to poor circulation or obstruction of blood flow (esp. to extremities), vasomotor spasms, venous or arterial thrombosis, or exposure to cold. Generally, abnormally hot skin is seen in febrile disorders, although in some patients, the skin is cold and clammy. *Wrinkling:* Permanent wrinkling may be associated with aging; temporary wrinkling is due to prolonged immersion in water or dehydration. *Yellow:* This may be due to increased carotene intake, jaundice, or liver disease. It should be noted if the skin is jaundiced, plethoric, hyperemic, or pigmented.

*Miscellaneous:* Rashes, scars, and their causes are also diagnostic. The texture and temperature of skin are important signs. Undue moisture, cold or hot spots on the body, and dryness of the skin also should be noted when determining a diagnosis. SEE: *anemia, pernicious; biliousness; endocarditis; face; liver.*

FUNCTION: An unbroken stratum corneum prevents the entry of most pathogens and the entry or loss of water. The arterioles and sweat glands help regulate body temperature, and the receptors in the dermis give rise to the cutaneous sensations. Vitamin D is produced when the skin is exposed to sunlight. Normally, small amounts of urea and salt are excreted in sweat. When sweating is excessive, salt loss is increased.

**alligator s.** Severe scaling of the skin with formation of thick plates resembling the hide of an alligator. SEE: *ichthyosis.*

**deciduous s.** Keratolysis.

**elastic s.** Skin that has the property of great elasticity.

**glabrous s.** Skin that does not contain hair follicles, such as that over the palms and soles.

**glossy s.** Shiny appearance of the skin due to atrophy or injury to nerves.

**hidebound s.** Scleroderma.

**loose s.** Hypertrophy of the skin.

**parchment s.** Atrophy of the skin with stretching.

**photoaged s.** Skin changes caused by chronic sun exposure. This condition has been treated with topical tretinoin. SYN: *photodamaged skin.* SEE: *dermatoheliosis.*

**photodamaged s.** Photoaged s.

**piebald s.** Vitiligo.

**scarf s.** The cuticle, epidermis; the outer layer of the skin.

**true s.** The corium or inner layer of the skin.

**skin, chemical peel of** The use of chemicals to erode superficial skin layers; used to treat acne, wrinkles, and blemishes. SEE: *dermabrasion; Retin-A.*

Caution: This technique can be dangerous. It must be done under the supervision of a person skilled in this type of therapy.

**skin, tenting of** When normal skin and subcutaneous tissue are lightly pinched, raised up, and released, it returns to the flat position without delay. Return to the flat position is delayed when the individual is dehydrated. The return becomes progressively slower as the skin ages and subcutaneous elastic tissue decreases. Thus, the test for tenting can be used as a rough index of the aging process. SEE: *dehydration.*

**skin cancer** Cancer that may arise on the

surface of the body and manifest as a small ulcer, pimple, or mole. It may be red, brown, black, or white, according to the type. It may occur singly or in a group, and may be open or ulcerated. It may be localized or invade the blood vessels, lymph glands, and connecting ducts.

**skinfold tenderness** Tenderness elicited by the examiner's rolling the skin and subcutaneous tissues over the upper border of the trapezius muscle. Normally, this produces minor discomfort, but in patients with nonarticular rheumatic disorders, this rolling of the skin consistently produces pain.

**skinfold thickness** Measurement with calibrated calipers of the thickness of a fold of skin at a selected body site. The sites usually are the upper arm or triceps, subscapular region, and upper abdomen. The measurements are used in evaluating nutritional status by estimating the amount of subcutaneous fat.

**skin integrity, impaired** A state in which the individual's skin is adversely altered; an interruption in the integumentary system, the largest, multifunctional organ of the body. SEE: *Nursing Diagnoses Appendix.*

**skin integrity, impaired, risk for** A state in which the individual's skin is at risk of being adversely altered. SEE: *Nursing Diagnoses Appendix.*

**skin marking** The application of nontoxic, temporary paints or dyes to the skin to provide landmarks during plastic surgery, to permit accurate alignment of wound edges at the time the skin is closed, or to align the treament beam accurately during radiotherapy.

**Skinner box** (skĭn'ĕr) [Burrhus Frederic Skinner, U.S. psychologist, 1904–1990] A device used in experimental psychology. It is designed so that an animal presses a lever or button and is rewarded by receiving food. This is termed programmed learning.

**skin rash** A usually temporary eruption of the skin covering a small area, a portion of the body, or the entire body. The rash may consist of macules, papules, vesicles, or pustules and is usually red or red-blue. It may be itchy. A rash is often indicative of a systemic disease such as measles or lupus, or it may indicate a local irritation such as contact dermatitis or diaper rash.

**skin tag** Acrochordon.

**skin test** Any test in which a suspected allergen or sensitizer is applied to the skin. A variety of tests have been developed to detect an individual's sensitivity to specific allergens. The most commonly used tests are the intradermal test, the prick or puncture test, and the scratch test. The intensity of the response is determined by the wheal-and-flare reaction 20 min after the suspected allergen is applied. Positive and negative controls are used to verify normal skin reactivity. Histamine is the positive control and the diluent used for the allergen is the negative control.

***PPD s.t.*** SEE: *PPD; tuberculin test.*

**skin tightening** A loss of normal skin folds and pliability due to various sclerosing disorders. This may be generalized or localized and may occur over any part of the body. The skin is taut, bound down to the underlying tissue, and may be thickened or indurated. In severe cases, the skin may be so tight as to interfere with function of the fingers and toes. Flexion contractions of the mouth may decrease the patient's ability to open the mouth. Skin tightening due to edema is not included in this classification.

**sklero-** SEE: words beginning with *sclero-*.

**skodaic** (skō-dā'ĭk) Concerning Josef Skoda. SEE: *Skoda, Josef.*

**Skoda, Josef** (skō'dă) Austrian physician, 1805–1881.

***S.'s crackles*** Bronchial crackles heard through consolidated tissue of the lungs in pneumonia.

***S.'s resonance*** Tympanic resonance above the line of fluid in pleuritic effusion, or above consolidation in pneumonia.

**skull** (skŭl) [ME. *skulle,* bowl] The bony framework of the head, composed of 8 cranial bones, the 14 bones of the face, and the teeth. SYN: *calvaria; cranium.* SEE: illus.; *skeleton.*

***fracture of s.*** Loss of the integrity of one or more bones of the cranium. A fracture is classified according to whether it is in the vault or the base but, from the point of view of treatment, a more useful classification is differentiating between a *simple fracture* (uncommon) and a *compound frature.* When a compound fracture occurs in the vault of the skull, the bone is depressed and driven inward, possibly damaging the brain. Treatment is operative. SEE: *fracture.*

**skullcap** The upper round portion of the skull covering the brain. Also called *calvaria.*

**slant** A tube of solid culture medium that is slanted to increase the surface area of the medium; used in culturing bacteria. SYN: *slope.*

**slave** A device that allows the body movements to be transferred to a machine either directly or by remote control (e.g., an apparatus for lifting, squeezing, and turning laboratory equipment containing radioactive materials). The remote "hands" are controlled by the operator from a sufficient distance, and proper shielding is used to prevent the operator from being exposed to radiation or other highly toxic materials. Artificial arms and legs equipped to respond to physical or electrical stimulation have been developed.

**SLE** *systemic lupus erythematosus.*

**sleep** (slēp) [AS. *slaep*] A periodic state of rest accompanied by varying degrees of unconsciousness and relative inactivity. Although sleep is thought of as something

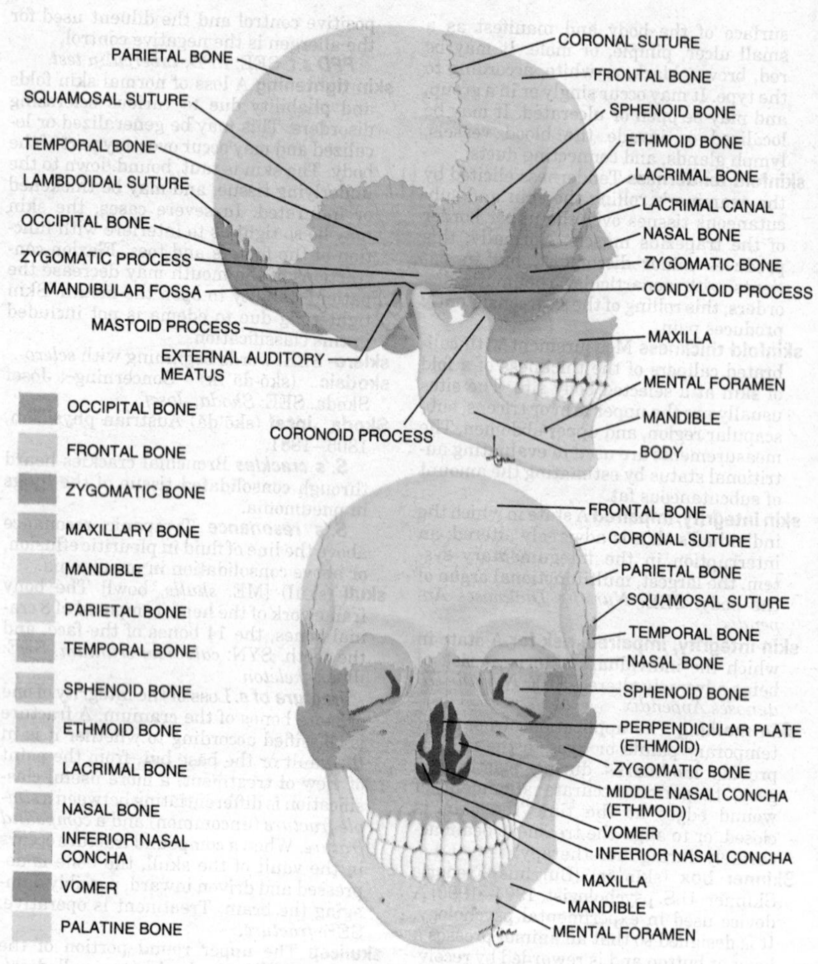


**SKULL**

**(RIGHT LATERAL AND ANTERIOR VIEWS)**

that occurs once each 24-hr period, at least half of the world's population has an afternoon nap or siesta as part of their lifelong sleep-wake pattern. The need for and value of sleep is obvious, yet the explanation of why it is so effective in providing a daily renewal of a feeling of health and well-being is lacking.

The sleep-wake cycle varies in relation to the age and gender of the individual. The newborn may sleep as much as 20 hr each day; a child, 8 to 14 hr depending on age; adults, 3 to 12 hr with a mean of 7 to 8 hr, and this may decrease to 6.5 hr in the elderly. Women past age 35 tend to sleep more than men. There is great individual variation in the amount and depth of sleep.

Sleep has been found to have two states: one with no rapid eye movements (NREM or synchronized sleep, which involves four stages) and one with rapid eye movements (REM or dreaming sleep). NREM and REM sleep alternate during the night; each cycle requires 90 to 100 min. NREM sleep composes approx. 75% of the sleep cycle and REM sleep approx. 25%, with variations among individuals.

Persons deprived of sleep for several days or more become irritable, fatigued, unable to concentrate, and usually disoriented. Performance of mental and physical tasks deteriorates. Some individuals experience paranoid thoughts and auditory, visual, and tactile illusions or hallucinations. Deprivation of REM sleep may cause anxiety, overeating, and hypersexuality. The effects of sleep depri-

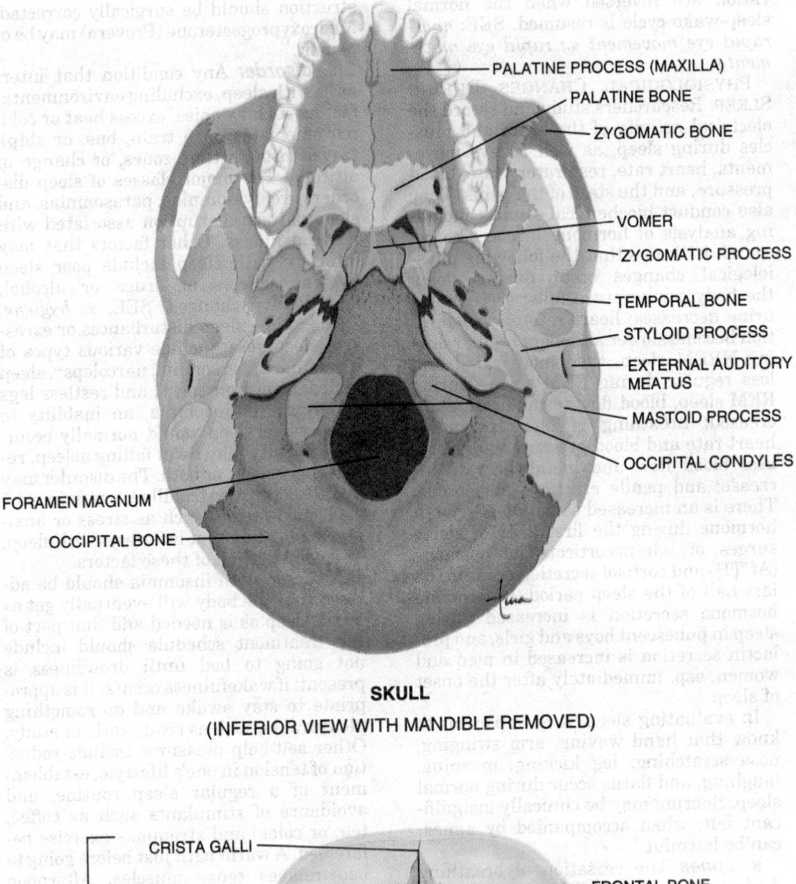

PALATINE PROCESS (MAXILLA)
PALATINE BONE
ZYGOMATIC BONE
VOMER
ZYGOMATIC PROCESS
TEMPORAL BONE
STYLOID PROCESS
EXTERNAL AUDITORY MEATUS
MASTOID PROCESS
OCCIPITAL CONDYLES
FORAMEN MAGNUM
OCCIPITAL BONE

**SKULL**
**(INFERIOR VIEW WITH MANDIBLE REMOVED)**

ETHMOID BONE
CRISTA GALLI
CRIBRIFORM PLATE
OLFACTORY FORAMINA
GREATER WING
FRONTAL BONE
SPHENOID BONE
SELLA TURCICA
SQUAMOSAL SUTURE
TEMPORAL BONE
PARIETAL BONE
FORAMEN MAGNUM
LAMBDOIDAL SUTURE
OCCIPITAL BONE

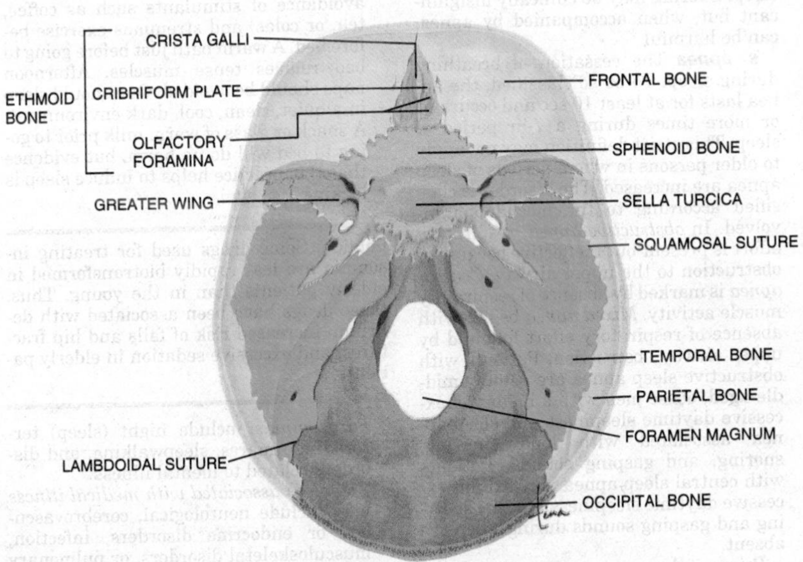

**SKULL**
**(SUPERIOR VIEW WITH TOP OF CRANIUM REMOVED)**

vation are reversed when the normal sleep-wake cycle is resumed. SEE: *non-rapid eye movement s.; rapid eye movement s.*

PHYSIOLOGICAL CHANGES DURING SLEEP: Researchers study and record the electrical activity of the brain and muscles during sleep, as well as eye movements, heart rate, respiratory rate, blood pressure, and the state of the penis. They also conduct biochemical studies including analysis of hormone levels. The research indicates that the following physiological changes occur during sleep: the body temperature falls; secretion of urine decreases; heart rate and respiration become slower and more regular during NREM sleep, then more rapid and less regular during REM sleep. During REM sleep, blood flow to the brain is increased; breathing is more irregular; heart rate and blood pressure vary; cerebral blood flow and metabolic rate increase; and penile erections may occur. There is an increased secretion of growth hormone during the first 2 hr of sleep; surges of adrenocorticotropic hormone (ACTH) and cortisol secretion occur in the last half of the sleep period. Luteinizing hormone secretion is increased during sleep in pubescent boys and girls, and prolactin secretion is increased in men and women, esp. immediately after the onset of sleep.

In evaluating sleep, it is important to know that hand waving, arm swinging, nose scratching, leg kicking, moaning, laughing, and flatus occur during normal sleep. Snoring may be clinically insignificant but, when accompanied by apnea, can be harmful.

***s. apnea*** The cessation of breathing during sleep. To be so classified, the apnea lasts for at least 10 sec and occurs 30 or more times during a 7-hr period of sleep. This strict definition may not apply to older persons in whom periods of sleep apnea are increased. The disorder is classified according to the mechanism involved. In *obstructive apnea,* respiratory effort is present but ineffective because of obstruction to the upper airway. *Central apnea* is marked by absence of respiratory muscle activity. *Mixed apnea* begins with absence of respiratory effort followed by upper airway obstruction. Patients with obstructive sleep apnea are usually middle-aged, obese men with a history of excessive daytime sleepiness and sleep apnea associated with loud snorting, snoring, and gasping sounds. Patients with central sleep apnea may exhibit excessive daytime sleepiness, but the snorting and gasping sounds during sleep are absent.

Primary therapy is to assist breathing with continuous positive airway pressure. The underlying disease of obesity, if present, should be corrected. Palatal obstruction should be surgically corrected. Medroxyprogesterone (Provera) may be of benefit.

***s. disorder*** Any condition that interferes with sleep, excluding environmental factors such as noise, excess heat or cold, movement (as on a train, bus, or ship), travel through time zones, or change in altitude. The major classes of sleep disorders are dyssomnias, parasomnias, and sleep pattern disruption associated with medical illness. Other factors that may interfere with sleep include poor sleep hygiene, effects of drugs or alcohol, and dietary changes. SEE: *s. hygiene.* *Dyssomnias*, sleep disturbances or excessive sleepiness, include various types of insomnia, hypersomnia, narcolepsy, sleep apnea, brief limb jerks, and restless legs syndrome. In insomnia, an inability to sleep when sleep would normally occur, the difficulty may be in falling asleep, remaining asleep, or both. The disorder may be caused by physical illness or pain, psychological factors such as stress or anxiety, medication that interferes with sleep, or a combination of these factors.

A person with insomnia should be advised that the body will eventually get as much sleep as is needed and that part of the treatment schedule should include not going to bed until drowsiness is present; if wakefulness occurs, it is appropriate to stay awake and do something pleasurable, such as read, work, or study. Other self-help measures include reduction of tension in one's lifestyle, establishment of a regular sleep routine, and avoidance of stimulants such as coffee, tea, or colas) and strenuous exercise before bed. A warm bath just before going to bed relaxes tense muscles. Afternoon naps should be avoided. One should sleep in a quiet, clean, cool, dark environment. A snack or glass of warm milk prior to going to bed will do no harm, but evidence that this practice helps to induce sleep is lacking.

---

Caution: Some drugs used for treating insomnia are less rapidly biotransformed in elderly patients than in the young. Thus, these drugs have been associated with delirium, increased risk of falls and hip fractures, and excessive sedation in elderly patients.

---

*Parasomnias* include night (sleep) terrors, nightmares, sleepwalking, and disorders related to mental illness.

*Factors associated with medical illness* may include neurological, cerebrovascular, or endocrine disorders, infection, musculoskeletal disorders, or pulmonary disease.

***s. drunkenness*** The condition present in persons who require a long period of time to become fully alert upon awakening from deep sleep. During this transition period, they may become ataxic, disoriented, or aggressive. Persons whose usual awakening sequence includes sleep drunkenness should not attempt to make decisions until they are fully alert and awake.

***s. hygiene*** The influence of behavioral patterns or sleeping environment on the quality and quantity of sleep. Persons with insomnia not caused by a known disease may find that the following may assist in obtaining a good night's sleep: establishing a routine time to go to bed; avoiding trying to sleep; using practices that assist in going to sleep such as reading, watching television, or listening to music; sleeping in a dark room, free of noise; and avoiding caffeine and excessive food or drink before bedtime.

***hypnotic s.*** **1.** Sleep induced by hypnotic suggestion. **2.** Sleep induced by the use of medicines classified as hypnotics.

***non–rapid eye movement s.*** ABBR: NREM sleep. Sleep during which non–rapid eye movements occur. In NREM stage 1, the transition from wakefulness to sleep occurs. Eye movements are slow, and an electroencephalogram (EEG) shows low brain wave activity. In stage 2, EEG activity is increased, with the appearance of spikes called K complexes. Eye movement ceases in stage 3; wave frequency is reduced and amplitude increased. In stage 4, the EEG is dominated by large spikes, or delta activity. Stages 3 and 4 are considered deep sleep. SEE: *rapid eye movement s.; sleep.*

***pathological s.*** A term used in encephalitis lethargica, in which sleep is excessive.

***rapid eye movement s.*** ABBR: REM sleep. Sleep during which rapid eye movements occur. In REM sleep, which follows stage 4 of non–rapid eye movement (NREM) sleep, electroencephalographic activity is similar to that of NREM stage 1, and muscle paralysis occurs. SEE: *non–rapid eye movement s.; sleep.*

***twilight s.*** The injection of scopolamine and morphine to abolish the subsequent memory of pain without completely abolishing pain at the time. At one time this was widely used during labor and delivery.

**sleeping sickness 1.** Encephalitis lethargica. **2.** African trypanosomiasis caused by a protozoon introduced into the blood and cerebrospinal fluid by the bite of a tsetse fly; characterized by fever, protracted lethargy, weakness, tremors, and wasting.

**sleep pattern disturbance** A disruption of sleep time that causes the patient discomfort or interferes with his or her desired lifestyle. SEE: *Nursing Diagnoses Appendix.*

**sleep-phase syndrome disorder** A condition in which the person sleeps well and for a normal amount of time but not at the usual bedtime hours. Those with the delayed type of syndrome may function best if they go to sleep about the time most people are awakening. Those with the advanced type of syndrome do best when they go to sleep in late afternoon or early evening and arise about midnight. When allowed to sleep at these hours, persons with this disease function normally.

**sleep-wake cycle** The amount of time spent asleep and awake and the cycle of that schedule from day to day.

**sleepwalking** Autonomic actions performed during sleep. This condition occurs mostly in children, each episode lasting less than 10 min. The eyes are open and the facial expression is blank. The patient appears to awaken, sits on the edge of the bed, and may walk or talk. Some patients may even leave the bedroom. Activity may cause trauma to the patient and others. The principal aim is to prevent injury by removing objects that could be dangerous, locking doors and windows, and preventing the person from falling down stairs. Night terrors may accompany sleepwalking. There is little or no recollection of the event the next day. Children usually outgrow this condition. SYN: *somnambulism.*

**slide 1.** A thin glass plate on which an object is placed for microscopic examination. **2.** A photograph prepared so that it may be used in a film slide projector. **3.** To move along a smooth surface in continuous contact, as the movement in dentistry of the mandibular teeth toward a centric position with the teeth in contact before closing completely in occlusion.

**slimy** (slī′mē) [AS. *slim,* smooth] Resembling slime or a viscid substance; regarding a growth, the ability to adhere to a needle so it can be drawn out as a long thread.

**sling** (slĭng) [AS. *slingan,* to wind] A support for an injured upper extremity. SEE: *triangular bandage* for illus.; *bandage.*

Caution: Prolonged skin-to-skin contact should be avoided while a sling is in use.

***clove-hitch s.*** A sling made by placing a clove hitch in the center of a roller bandage, fitting it to the hand, and carrying the ends over the shoulder. The sling is tied beside the neck with a square knot, making longer ends. These may be carried over and behind the shoulders, brought under each axilla, and tied over the chest.

***counterbalanced s.*** A rehabilitation device to assist upper extremity motion; it suspends the arm by way of an overhead frame and a pulley and weight system. SYN: *suspension s.; deltoid aid.*

***cravat s.*** A sling made by placing the center of the cravat under the wrist or forearm with the ends tied around the neck.

***folded cravat s.*** A lower-arm sling made by placing a broad fold of cloth in position on the chest with one end over the affected shoulder and the other hanging down in front of the chest. The arm is flexed as desired across the sling. The lower end is brought up over the uninjured shoulder and secured with a knot located where it will not press on the affected shoulder.

***open s.*** A sling made by placing the point of a triangular cloth at the tip of the elbow. The ends are brought around at the back of the neck and tied. The point should be brought forward and pinned or tied in a single knot, forming a cup to prevent the elbow from slipping out.

***reversed triangular s.*** A sling made as follows: A triangular bandage is applied with one end over the injured shoulder, point toward the sound side, the base vertical under the injured elbow. The arm is flexed acutely over the triangle. The lower end is brought upward over the front of the arm and over the sound shoulder. The ends are pulled taut and tied over the sound shoulder. The point is pulled taut over the forearm and fixed to the anterior and posterior layers between the forearm and arm. This sling holds the elbow more acutely flexed—the weight is supported by the elbow.

***simple figure-of-eight roller arm s.*** A sling made as follows: The arm is flexed on the chest in the desired position, then a bandage is fixed with a single turn toward the uninjured side around the arm and chest, crossing the elbow just above the external epicondyle of the humerus. A second turn is made, overlapping two thirds of the first, and the bandage is brought forward under the tip of the elbow, then upward along the flexed forearm to the root of the neck of the sound side. Then it is brought downward over the scapula, crossing the chest and arm horizontally, overlapping, turning above, and continued as in a progressive figure-of-eight.

***suspension s.*** Counterbalanced s.

***swathe arm s., cravat s.*** A sling for support of the arm that is made as follows: The center of a folded cloth band is placed under the acutely flexed elbow. One end of the sling is then carried to the front and upward across the forearm and over the affected shoulder. Then it is brought obliquely across the back to the sound axilla. Next, the other end of the sling is brought around the front of the arm and across the body to the sound axilla, where it is pinned to the first end of the sling and then continued around the back to the part of the sling surrounding the affected elbow, where it is pinned again.

***triangular s.*** A sling for the arm that is made with suspension from the uninjured side. The triangle is placed on the chest with one end over the sound shoulder, the point under the affected extremity, and the base folded. The injured arm is flexed outside of the triangle. The lower end is carried upward under the axilla of the injured side, back of the shoulder, and tied with the upper end behind the back. The point of the triangle is brought anteriorly and medially around the back of the elbow, and fastened to the body of the bandage. This bandage changes the point of carrying and also relieves the clavicle on the injured side of the load. SEE: *triangular bandage* for illus.

**slit** [ME. *slitte*] A narrow opening.

***vestibular s.*** The opening between the left and right ventricular folds of the larynx.

**slope 1.** An inclined plane or surface. **2.** A tube of solid culture medium that is slanted to increase the surface area of the medium; used in culturing bacteria. SYN: *slant*.

***lower ridge s.*** The slope of the crest of the mandibular residual ridge from the third molar forward as viewed in profile.

**slough** (slŭf) [ME. *slughe,* a skin] **1.** Dead matter or necrosed tissue separated from living tissue or an ulceration. **2.** To separate in the form of dead or necrosed parts from living tissue. **3.** To cast off, as dead tissue. SEE: *escharotic*.

**sloughing** (slŭf′ĭng) The formation of a slough; separation of dead from living tissue.

**slow** (slō) [AS. *slaw,* dull] **1.** Mentally dull. **2.** Exhibiting retarded speed, as the pulse. **3.** Said of a morbid condition or of a fever when it is not acute.

**slow-acting antirheumatic drug** ABBR: SAARD. A drug used to treat rheumatoid arthritis that acts slowly as compared to nonsteroidal anti-inflammatory drugs (NSAIDs). Included are hydroxychloroquine, intramuscular gold preparations, D-penicillamine, methotrexate, and azathioprine. To date, these drugs have only been used after a course of NSAIDs has been completed; however, it is believed by some investigators that earlier use may be of benefit.

**slow-reacting substance of anaphylaxis** ABBR: SRS-A. A substance released by certain tissues, including the lungs, during anaphylaxis. It causes slow contraction of smooth muscle tissue and may be of major importance in allergic bronchospasm.

**slows** (slōz) A condition resulting from ingestion of plants such as snakeroot *(Eupatorium urticaefolium)* or jimmyweed *(Haplopappus heterophyllus)*. It is common in domestic animals and may occur in humans as a result of ingesting the plants or, more commonly, from drinking milk or eating the meat of poisoned animals. Symptoms are weakness, anorexia, nausea and vomiting, prostration, and possibly death. SYN: *trembles.*

**slow virus infection** An infection caused by a virus that remains dormant in the body for a prolonged period before causing signs and symptoms of illness. Such viruses may require years to incubate before causing such diseases as scrapie in sheep or kuru in humans. Chronic degenerative diseases that are now suspected to be due to slow viruses include subacute sclerosing panencephalitis and progressive multifocal leukoencephalopathy. SEE: *Creutzfeldt-Jakob disease; prion.*

**sludge** (slŭjh) Under the Resource Conservation and Recovery Act of 1976, sludge is defined as any solid, semisolid, or liquid waste generated from a municipal, commercial, or industrial wastewater treatment plant, or air pollution control facility, or any such waste having similar characteristics or effects.

**sludged blood** A condition of the blood in certain abnormal states, such as tissue injury, sepsis syndrome, multiple organ failure, acute respiratory distress syndrome, or shock, in which the volume of plasma is reduced and the cells show a pronounced tendency to agglutinate and form large clumps or masses that move slowly through the vessels and sometimes clog the smaller vessels.

**slurry** (slŭr′ē) [ME. *slory*] A thin, watery mixture.

**Sm** Symbol for the element samarium.

**SMA-12** Trade name of a device that does 12 blood chemistry tests on a single blood sample.

**small for gestational age** ABBR: SGA. Term describing an infant whose birth weight is less than would be considered normal for the length of the calculated gestation period.

**smallpox** (smawl′pŏks) [AS. *smael,* tiny, + *poc,* pustule] Variola.

**smallpox vaccine** A standardized preparation of the living virus of vaccinia. It was used in immunizing against smallpox but is no longer thought to be necessary, as smallpox is considered to have been eradicated worldwide.

**smear** (smēr) [AS. *smerian,* to anoint] **1.** In bacteriology, material spread on a surface, as a microscopic slide or a culture medium. **2.** Material obtained from infected matter spread over solid culture media.

***blood s.*** A thin film of blood on a glass slide. Blood is prepared in this manner for staining and microscopic examination.

***buccal s.*** A sample of cells taken from the mucosa lining the cheek for chromosomal studies.

***Pap s., Papanicolaou s.*** SEE: *Papanicolaou test.*

**smegma** (smĕg′mă) [Gr. *smegma,* soap] Secretion of sebaceous glands, specifically, the thick, cheesy, odoriferous secretion found under the labia minora about the glans clitoridis or under the male prepuce. **smegmatic** (-măt′ĭk), *adj.*

**smegmolith** (smĕg′mō-lĭth) [Gr. *smegma,* soap, + *lithos,* a stone] A calcareous mass in the smegma.

**smell** (smĕl) [ME. *smellen,* to reek] **1.** To perceive by stimulation of the olfactory nerves. **2.** To emit an odor, pleasant or offensive. In clinical medicine, the smell arising from the patient's body, feces, breath, urine, vagina, and clothing may provide valuable information concerning the diagnosis. The smell on clothing may be due to a toxic chemical that spilled on the clothes. Also, a patient may attempt to alter or mask the smell of alcohol on his or her breath by use of a medicated or flavored lozenge, mouthwash, spray, or mint. **3.** A chemical sense dependent upon end organs on the surface of the upper part of the nasal septum and the superior nasal concha. These sensory cells live for an average of 30 days and are affected by a variety of factors including age, nutritional and hormonal states, drugs, and therapeutic radiation. **4.** The property of a thing affecting the olfactory organs; it may be pleasant or unpleasant. SYN: *odor.*

The sense of smell may be affected by many conditions, including the following:

*Anosmia:* A loss of the sense of smell. It may be a local and temporary condition resulting from acute and chronic rhinitis, mouth breathing, nasal polyps, dryness of the nasal mucous membrane, pollens, or very offensive odors. It may also result from disease or injury of the olfactory tract, bone disease near the olfactory nerve, disease of the nasal accessory sinuses, meningitis, or tumors or syphilis affecting the olfactory nerve. It may accompany hysteria. Disease of one cranial hemisphere or of one nasal chamber may account for anosmia. SYN: *anodmia; anosphrasia.*

*Hyperosmia:* An increased sensitivity to odors.

*Kakosmia:* The perception of bad odors where none exist; it may be due to head injuries or occur in hallucinations in certain psychoses. SYN: *cacosmia.*

*Parosmia:* A perverted sense of smell. Odors that are considered agreeable are assumed to be offensive, and disagreeable odors may be found pleasant to those suffering from certain functional derangements and in some catarrhs. SYN: *parosphresia.*

**smile** A facial expression that may represent pleasure, amusement, derision, or scorn. The corners of the mouth are turned up in expressions of pleasure or amusement, and the eyes usually appear to be warm and friendly.

**Smith's fracture** [Robert W. Smith, Irish physician, 1807–1873] A fracture of the lower end of the radius, with forward displacement of the lower fragment.

**Smith-Magenis syndrome** [Ann C. M.

Smith, contemporary U.S. genetics counselor; Ellen Magenis, contemporary U.S. physician] A rare form of genetic mental retardation characterized by chronic ear infections, erratic sleep patterns, head banging, picking at skin, and pulling off fingernails and toenails. There is abnormality of chromosome 17. Treatment is symptomatic.

**Smith-Petersen nail** [Marius N. Smith-Petersen, U.S. orthopedic surgeon, 1886–1953] A special nail that on cross-section has three flanges, used for stabilizing fractures of the neck of the femur.

**Smith-Strang disease** [Allan J. Smith, contemporary Brit. physician; Leonard B. Strang, Brit. physician, b. 1925] Methionine malabsorption syndrome, an inherited disease, which is associated with mental retardation, diarrhea, convulsions, phenylketonuria, and a characteristic odor of the urine. The odor is due to the absorption from the intestinal tract of fermentation products of methionine. SYN: *oasthouse urine disease.*

**smog** [blend of *smoke* and *fog*] Dense fog combined with smoke and other forms of air pollution.

**smoke inhalation injury** Damage to the respiratory tract as a result of inhaling hot gases that may contain toxic substances. Persons exposed to gases produced by burning materials are at risk of developing acute injury to their lungs; and, depending upon the composition of the smoke and the duration of the exposure, the combination of heat and gases may be lethal. Firefighters are esp. at risk from this kind of exposure. Modern construction and decorating materials produce a variety of volatile and irritating substances when burned. Repeated exposure to some of these gases may lead to chronic irritation of the respiratory tract. Firefighters should be aware that the "blackness" of smoke produced by a fire may not be a true indicator of the amount of toxic substances, including carbon monoxide, in the smoke. The normal half-life of carbon monoxide in the body is 4 hr. This can be reduced to 50 min by immediately inhaling 100% oxygen after exposure. Even more effective is the use of hyperbaric oxygen therapy. SEE: *smoke poisoning.*

**smokeless tobacco** Tobacco used in the form of snuff, tobacco powder, or chewing tobacco. These products irritate the oral mucosa and gingiva, and their continued use results in an increased risk of cancer of the mouth, larynx, throat, and esophagus. Use of smokeless tobacco leads to addiction in the same manner as smoked tobacco products. SEE: *tobacco.*

**smoke poisoning** Toxicity produced by inhalation of gases and smoke produced by burning materials. The usual gas is carbon monoxide, but many combustion products will form corrosive acids or alkalies when they reach the moisture present in the upper respiratory tract. This will cause varying degrees of injury to the mucosa, depending on the extent of exposure. This may lead to acute pulmonary edema, shock, and death.

TREATMENT: Corticosteroids and oxygen should be given. Therapy for pulmonary edema should be provided. SEE: *smoke inhalation.*

**smoker's cancer** Cancer of the lip, throat, or lung caused by irritation from excessive smoking. SEE: *tobacco.*

**smoking, passive** The exposure of persons not smoking tobacco products to the smoke produced by other smokers; also called involuntary smoking. The extent and importance of such exposure in the workplace, the home, or in any other circumstance is directly related to the number of cigarettes and other tobacco products used by the smokers. It can lead to injury of the respiratory tract of the nonsmoker and to an increased incidence of all the other pathologic conditions caused by smoking. Prevention of this type of exposure in a home in which smoking is allowed and where children have no alternative but to breathe the tobacco smoke is particularly important. SEE: *tobacco.*

**SMON** *subacute myelo-optic neuropathy.*

**smudging** (smŭj′ĭng) A speech defect in which difficult consonants are omitted.

**Sn** [L. *stannun*] Symbol for the element tin.

**snail** [ME.] A small mollusk having a spiral shell and belonging to the class Gastropoda. Snails are important as intermediate hosts of many species of parasitic flukes.

***s. fever*** Schistosomiasis.

**snake** [ME.] A reptile possessing scales and lacking limbs, external ears, and functional eyelids. In poisonous snakes, venom is produced in a poison gland, which is connected by a tube or groove to a poison fang, one of two sharp elongated teeth present in the upper jaw. In the U.S., the coral snake, copperhead, water moccasin (cottonmouth), and rattlesnake, of which there are 15 species, are poisonous. All except the coral snake belong to a group known as *pit vipers* because of the presence of a distinct pit between the eye and nostril. SEE: illus.

***s. bite*** A puncture wound made by the fangs of a snake. All snakes should be considered poisonous, although only a few secrete enough venom to inoculate poison deeply into the tissues.

FIRST AID: The patient should be transported immediately to a medical facility equipped and staffed to handle snake bites. The absorption of venom should be retarded by placing the victim at rest and splinting the extremity if that was the site of the bite. If possible, a wide constriction band should be placed above the bite. This should be just firm enough to allow a finger to be placed between the band and the skin. The goal is to impede lymph flow,

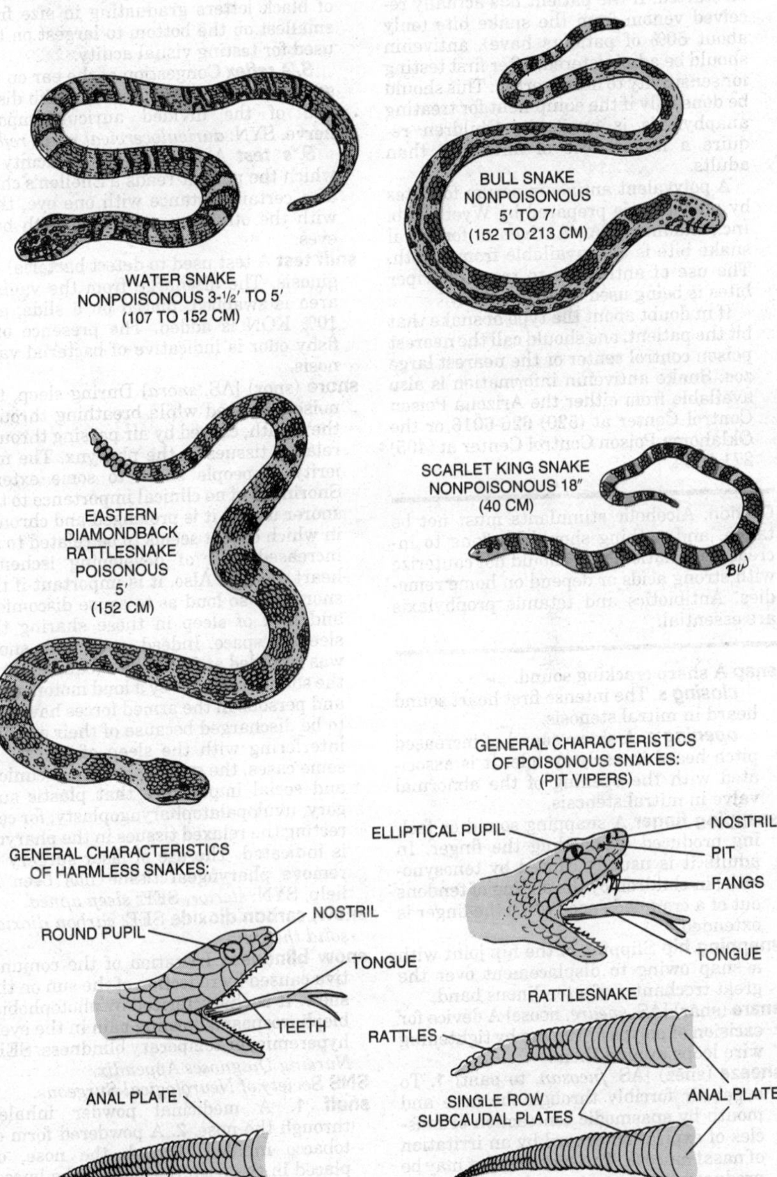
SNAKES
WATER SNAKE
NONPOISONOUS 3-½′ TO 5′
(107 TO 152 CM)
BULL SNAKE
NONPOISONOUS
5′ TO 7′
(152 TO 213 CM)
EASTERN
DIAMONDBACK
RATTLESNAKE
POISONOUS
5′
(152 CM)
SCARLET KING SNAKE
NONPOISONOUS 18″
(40 CM)
GENERAL CHARACTERISTICS
OF POISONOUS SNAKES:
(PIT VIPERS)
ELLIPTICAL PUPIL
NOSTRIL
PIT
FANGS
TONGUE
GENERAL CHARACTERISTICS
OF HARMLESS SNAKES:
ROUND PUPIL
NOSTRIL
TONGUE
TEETH
RATTLESNAKE
RATTLES
ANAL PLATE
SINGLE ROW
SUBCAUDAL PLATES
NO RATTLES
COPPERHEADS AND COTTONMOUTHS
ANAL PLATE
DOUBLE ROW SUBCAUDAL
PLATES

not venous return. As the area begins to swell, the band should be loosened and reapplied away from the swelling.

In the hospital, an intravenous infusion of Ringer's lactate or normal saline should be started. If the patient has actually received venom from the snake bite (only about 50% of patients have), antivenin should be administered, after first testing for sensitivity to horse serum. This should be done only if the equipment for treating anaphylaxis is available. Children require a larger dose of antivenin than adults.

A polyvalent antivenin serum for bites by pit vipers is prepared by Wyeth Lab. Inc., Radnor, PA. Antivenin for coral snake bite is also available from Wyeth. The use of antibodies to treat pit viper bites is being used experimentally.

If in doubt about the type of snake that bit the patient, one should call the nearest poison control center or the nearest large zoo. Snake antivenin information is also available from either the Arizona Poison Control Center at (520) 626-6016 or the Oklahoma Poison Control Center at (405) 271-5854.

---

Caution: Alcoholic stimulants must not be taken, and nothing should be done to increase circulation. One should not cauterize with strong acids or depend on home remedies. Antibiotics and tetanus prophylaxis are essential.

---

**snap** A sharp cracking sound.

***closing s.*** The intense first heart sound heard in mitral stenosis.

***opening s.*** A sharp sound of increased pitch heard in early systole. It is associated with the opening of the abnormal valve in mitral stenosis.

**snapping finger** A snapping sound or feeling produced by bending the finger. In adults it is usually caused by tenosynovitis; in children by the sliding of tendons out of a cramped space when the finger is extended.

**snapping hip** Slipping of the hip joint with a snap owing to displacement over the great trochanter of a tendinous band.

**snare** (snār) [AS. *sneare,* noose] A device for excision of polyps or tumors by tightening wire loops around them.

**sneeze** (snēz) [AS. *fneosan,* to pant] **1.** To expel air forcibly through the nose and mouth by spasmodic contraction of muscles of expiration caused by an irritation of nasal mucosa. The sneeze reflex may be produced by a great number of stimuli. Placing a foot on a cold surface will provoke a sneeze in some people, whereas looking at a bright light or sunlight will cause it in others. Firm pressure applied to the middle of the upper lip and just under the nose will sometimes prevent a sneeze that is about to occur. SEE: *photic sneezing; ptarmus.* **2.** The act of sneezing. SEE: *sternutation; sternutatory.*

**Snellen, Herman** (sněl'ěn) Dutch ophthalmologist, 1834–1908.

***S.'s chart*** A chart imprinted with lines of black letters graduating in size from smallest on the bottom to largest on top; used for testing visual acuity.

***S.'s reflex*** Congestion of the ear on the same side upon stimulation of the distal end of the divided auriculotemporal nerve. SYN: *auriculocervical nerve reflex.*

***S.'s test*** A test for visual acuity in which the patient reads a Snellen's chart at a certain distance with one eye, then with the other eye, and then with both eyes.

**sniff test** A test used to detect bacterial vaginosis. The discharge from the vaginal area is swabbed, placed on a slide, and 10% KON is added. The presence of a fishy odor is indicative of bacterial vaginosis.

**snore** (snor) [AS. *snora*] During sleep, the noise produced while breathing through the mouth, caused by air passing through relaxed tissues in the pharynx. The majority of people snore to some extent. Snoring is of no clinical importance to the snorer unless it is prolonged and chronic, in which case it seems to be related to an increased risk of developing ischemic heart disease. Also, it is important if the snoring is so loud as to cause discomfort and lack of sleep in those sharing the sleeping space. Indeed, one man's snore was recorded at 88 decibels (equivalent to the sound produced by a loud motorcycle), and persons in the armed forces have had to be discharged because of their snoring interfering with the sleep of others. In some cases, the snoring is of such clinical and social importance that plastic surgery, uvulopalatopharyngoplasty, for correcting the relaxed tissues in the pharynx is indicated. The use of laser surgery to remove pharyngeal tissue has been of help. SYN: *stertor.* SEE: *sleep apnea.*

**snow, carbon dioxide** SEE: *carbon dioxide solid therapy.*

**snow blindness** Irritation of the conjunctiva caused by reflection of the sun on the snow. It is characterized by photophobia, blepharospasm, burning pain in the eyes, hyperemia, or temporary blindness. SEE: *Nursing Diagnoses Appendix.*

**SNS** *Society of Neurological Surgeons.*

**snuff** **1.** A medicinal powder inhaled through the nose. **2.** A powdered form of tobacco inhaled through the nose, or placed in the posterior part of the buccal cavity on one side.

**snuffles** (snŭf'ls) [D. *snuffelen,* to snuff] Obstructed nasal breathing with discharge from the nasal mucosa, esp. in infants, chiefly in congenital syphilis.

**SOAP** Acronym for an organized structure for keeping progress notes in the chart. Each entry contains the date, number, and title of the patient's particular problem, followed by the SOAP headings: Subjective findings; Objective findings; Assessment, the documented analysis and conclusions concerning the findings; and Plan for further diagnostic or therapeutic action. If the patient has multiple problems, a SOAP entry on the chart is made for each problem.

**soap** (sōp) [AS. *sape*] A cleansing chemical compound formed by an alkali acting on a fatty acid, such as sodium stearate, $NaC_{18}H_{35}O_2$. Castile soap is made by saponifying olive oil with sodium hydroxide and contains mainly sodium oleate, $NaC_{18}H_{33}O_2$. SEE: *detergent; saponification.*

***green s.*** Soft medicinal s.

***s. liniment*** A solution of soap and camphor in alcohol and water; used as a stimulant and rubefacient.

***soft medicinal s.*** A liquid soap made by saponification of vegetable oils excluding coconut oil and palm kernel oil and without removal of glycerin; used in the treatment of skin diseases. SYN: *green s.*

**SOB** *short of breath.*

**sob** [ME. *sobben,* to catch breath] **1.** To weep with convulsive movements of the chest. **2.** A cry or wail resulting from a sudden convulsive inspiration accompanied by spasmodic closure of the glottis. SEE: *sigh.*

**social interaction, impaired** The state in which an individual participates in an insufficient or excessive quantity or ineffective quality of social exchange. SEE: *Nursing Diagnoses Appendix.*

**social isolation** Aloneness experienced by the individual and perceived as imposed by others and as a negative or threatened state. SEE: *Nursing Diagnoses Appendix.*

**socialization** (sō″shă-lĭ-zā′shŭn) The process of adapting an individual to the social customs of society; in the process he or she becomes a useful member of the society.

**Social and Occupational Functioning Assessment Scale** ABBR: SOFAS. An assessment tool that maps the effects of psychological or medical conditions on a person's level of social and occupational functioning.

**social phobia** Persistent irrational fears and the need to avoid any situation in which one might be exposed to scrutiny by others and potentially embarrassed or humiliated. Even anticipating a phobia-producing situation, such as speaking in public, urinating in a restroom with others present, or eating in public, may cause extreme anxiety. Relaxation therapy, desensitization, or use of beta blockers, such as propranolol, alprazolam, or atenolol, may be of benefit.

**socioacusis** (sō″sē-ō-ă-kū′sĭs) [L. *socius,* companion, + Gr. *akoustikos,* hearing] The long-range ill effects of environmental noise on auditory acuity.

**sociobiology** (sō″sē-ō-bī-ŏl′ō-jē) [″ + Gr. *bios,* life, + *logos,* word, reason] Analysis of social behavior in terms of modern evolutionary theory. It is the study of the social life of animals or humans on the assumption that populations evolve and adapt to their environments in different ways, through individual learning, cultural tradition, or genetic inheritance.

**socioeconomic status** The combined social and economic level of individuals or groups. Such classification is useful in studying the relationship of income and living conditions to the prevalence and incidence of various diseases. Although socioeconomic status is related to income, education, profession, or some combination of these, it is difficult to determine the relative importance of each in influencing mortality and morbidity; and to explain why socioeconomic status operates to influence health.

**sociogram** A diagram used in group analysis and group therapy that shows the pattern of relationships. The origin of the idea is attributed to Jacob L. Moreno, the founder of psychodrama.

**sociology** (sō-sē-ŏl′ō-jē) [″ + *logos,* word, reason] The study of human social behavior and the origins, institutions, and functions of human groups and societies.

**sociomedical** Pert. to sociology and medicine, esp. the interrelationships between the two.

**sociometry** (sō″sē-ŏm′ĕ-trē) [″ + Gr. *metron,* measure] The science concerned with measuring social behavior.

**sociopath** (sō′sē-ō-păth) [″ + Gr. *pathos,* disease, suffering] An individual with antisocial personality disorder. SEE: *personality disorder, antisocial.*

**sociopathy** (sō″sē-ŏp′ă-thē) [″ + Gr. *pathos,* disease, suffering] The condition of being antisocial.

**socket** (sŏk′ĕt) [ME. *soket,* a spearhead] **1.** A hollow in a joint or part for another corresponding organ, as a bone socket or an eye socket. SEE: *acetabulum.* **2.** The proximal portion of a prosthesis, into which the stump of an amputated extremity is fitted.

***alveolar s.*** The bony space occupied by the tooth and periodontal ligament.

***dry s.*** SEE: *osteitis, localized alveolar.*

***tooth s.*** A dental alveolus of the maxilla or mandible; a cavity that contains the root of a tooth.

**soda** (sō′dă) [Med. L., *barilla,* from which soda is made] **1.** A term loosely applied to various salts of sodium, esp. to caustic soda (sodium hydroxide) and baking soda (sodium bicarbonate). SEE: *sodium.* **2.** Short for soda water, which is water charged with carbon dioxide.

***baking s.*** Sodium bicarbonate.

***caustic s.*** Sodium hydroxide.

***s. lime*** A white granular substance consisting of a mixture of calcium hydroxide and sodium hydroxide or potassium hydroxide, or both; used to absorb carbon dioxide.

***s. water*** A solution of carbon dioxide under pressure; carbonic acid.

**sodic** (sō′dĭk) Relating to or containing soda or sodium.

**sodio-** Combining form denoting a compound containing sodium.

**sodium** (sō′dē-ŭm) [LL.] SYMB: Na. A soft metallic element with a strong affinity for oxygen and other nonmetallic elements. Atomic weight 22.9898; atomic number 11; specific gravity 0.971. Sodium constitutes approx. 0.15% of elements of the body. Sodium ($Na^+$), $K^+$, $Ca^{++}$, and $Mg^{++}$ constitute the principal cations of the body, their relative concentration determining the integrity of cell membranes and the bioelectric potentials of tissues. $Na^+$ is the principal cation found in extracellular fluids. Deficiency symptoms include weakness, nerve disorders, loss of weight, "salt hunger," and disturbed digestion. The normal serum sodium level is 135 to 145 mEq/L.

EXCESS: Hypernatremia leads to a decreased level of consciousness, decreased urinary output, muscle twitching followed by muscle paralysis, and decreased cardiac output. Treatment may include diuretics, fluid replacement, and dietary restriction of sodium.

FUNCTION: Sodium is the most abundant cation in extracellular fluids. It contributes to osmotic pressure and osmosis in all water compartments and is part of some buffer systems; its presence in body fluids helps retain water and prevent dehydration. It is essential for nerve impulse transmission and muscle contraction, including that of the heart, both directly and because it influences the levels of potassium and calcium ions.

***s. acetate*** A chemical compound that is used to alkalize the urine, and is used in kidney dialysis solutions.

***s. alginate*** A purified carbohydrate product extracted from certain species of seaweed. It is used as a food additive and as a pharmaceutical aid.

***amobarbital s.*** The monosodium salt of isoamylethylbarbituric acid. It is used as a sedative and hypnotic in control of insomnia, preliminary to surgical anesthesia, and in labor.

***s. ascorbate*** The sodium salt of ascorbic acid, vitamin C. It may be used in a sterile solution when parenteral administration of vitamin C is required.

***s. benzoate*** A white, odorless powder with sweet taste; used as a food preservative.

***s. bicarbonate*** $NaHCO_3$. A white odorless powder with saline taste. It is incompatible with acids, acid salts, ammonium chloride, lime water, ephedrine hydrochloride, and iron chloride. It is used intravenously to treat acidosis, as in diabetic ketoacidosis or cardiopulmonary arrest. Orally it is used as an antacid, although its effectiveness for this purpose is questionable. Externally, it is used as a mild alkaline wash.

***s. carbonate*** $Na_2CO_3$. A white crystalline powder (washing soda); used as an alkali employed chiefly in alkaline baths.

***carboxymethylcellulose s.*** The sodium salt of carboxymethylcellulose.

***s. chloride*** NaCl. Common table salt; used in preparation of normal saline solution, as an emetic, and to add flavor to foods. It is incompatible with silver nitrate. In aqueous solution, sodium chloride, a neutral salt, is a strong electrolyte, being almost completely ionized. The sodium and chlorine ions are important in maintaining the proper electrolyte balance in body fluids. The kidneys regulate retention or excretion of sodium chloride in urine; aldosterone directly increases the renal reabsorption of sodium ions.

***s. citrate*** A white granular powder, saline in taste and soluble in water. Used as an anticoagulant for blood used for transfusion.

***s. fluoride*** NaF. A white crystalline powder, saline in taste, soluble in 25 parts of water. It is added to drinking water and used in solution for local application to teeth for prevention of dental caries. Commercially, it is used in etching glassware and in eradication of rats, insects, ants, and other pests. SEE: *fluoridation; sodium fluoride poisoning.*

***s. hydroxide*** NaOH. A whitish solid; soluble in water, making a clear solution. It is an antacid and a caustic. It is used in laundry detergent and in commercial compounds used to clean sink traps, toilets, and so forth, and in the preparation of soap. SYN: *caustic soda.*

Caution: Great care must be taken in handling it, as it rapidly destroys organic tissues. Protective glasses should be worn while working with this chemical. If splashed in the eye, it may cause blindness.

***s. hypochlorite [solution]*** An antiseptic used in root canal therapy.

Caution: This solution is not suitable for application to wounds.

***s. iodide*** NaI. A colorless crystalline solid that is used as an expectorant.

***s. lactate [injection]*** Sodium salt of inactive lactic acid. In one-sixth or one-fourth molar solution, it is used intravenously to control electrolyte disturbances, esp. acidosis.

***s. lauryl sulfate*** An anionic surface-active agent that is used as a pharmaceutical acid.

***s. monofluorophosphate*** An agent suitable for topical application to teeth to prevent dental caries.

***morrhuate [injection] s.*** The sodium salt of the fatty acids, found in cod liver oil; used as a sclerosing agent for the obliteration of varicose veins.

***s. nitrite*** $NaNO_2$. A white crystalline powder used as an antidote for cyanide poisoning.

***s. nitroprusside*** ABBR: SNP. An antihypertensive and powerful vasodilator used when rapid reduction in blood pressure is required.

---

Caution: Infusion of SNP at the maximum dose rate of 10 μg/kg/min should never last for more than 10 min. For treatment of overdose, SEE: *cyanide poisoning.*

---

***s. phosphate, dibasic*** A chemical that is used as a cathartic.

***s. phosphate P 32 [solution]*** A standardized preparation of radioactive phosphorus ($^{32}P$).

***s. polystyrene sulfonate*** A cation-exchange resin used to lower the potassium level in the body.

***s. propionate*** A pharmaceutical aid that also has antifungal action.

***s. salicylate*** $C_7H_5NaO_3$. A white powder or scales with a sweet saline taste; used as an analgesic and antipyretic. It is incompatible with caffeine citrate and caffeine sodium benzoate.

***s. sulfate*** A salt used as a saline cathartic and diuretic; it also has some uses in veterinary medicine. SYN: *Glauber's salt.*

***s. thiosulfate*** A white crystalline substance, having a cooling taste; it is used externally to remove stains of iodine and intravenously as an antidote for cyanide poisoning.

**sodium fluoride poisoning** A reaction to exposure to a toxic dose of sodium fluoride, a material that is normally used in dentistry or in fluoridating water supplies. Symptoms include conjunctivitis, retching, vomiting, nausea, eventual cardiac weakness, kidney disturbances, and interference with coagulation of blood.

FIRST AID: The affected areas of the skin should be washed and the compound precipitated by addition to the wash solution of soluble calcium salts such as lime water, calcium gluconate, or calcium lactate. Emetics and soothing drinks such as milk, cream, or egg whites should be given. SEE: *Poisons and Poisoning Appendix.*

**sodokosis** (sŏd-ō-kō'sĭs) [Jap. *sodoku,* rat poison, + Gr. *osis,* condition] Rat-bite fever.

**sodoku** (sŏ-dō'koo) Rat-bite fever.

**sodomist, sodomite** (sŏd'ō-mĭst, -mīt) [LL. *Sodoma,* Sodom] A person who practices sodomy.

**sodomy** (sŏd'ō-mē) [LL. *Sodoma,* Sodom] Anal intercourse, usually between men.

**Soemmering, Samuel T. von** (sĕm'ĕr-ĭngz) German anatomist, 1755–1830.

***S.'s bone*** Marginal process of the malar (zygomatic) bone.

***S.'s foramen*** The fovea centralis retinae.

***S.'s ring*** An annular swelling of the periphery of the lens capsule.

***S.'s spot*** The macula lutea of the retina.

**SOFAS** *Social and Occupational Functioning Assessment Scale.*

**soft** (sŏft) [AS. *softe*] Not hard, firm, or solid.

**soft diet** A diet consisting of nothing but soft or semisolid foods or liquids, including fish, egg, and cheese dishes; chicken; cereals; bread; toast; and butter. Excluded are red meats, vegetables or fruits having seeds or thick skins, cellulose, raw fruits, and salads. SYN: *convalescent diet.*

**softening** (sŏf'ĕn-ĭng) [AS.] The process of becoming soft. SYN: *malacia; mollities.*

***s. of bones*** Osteomalacia.

***s. of brain*** Paresis with progressive dementia. SYN: *encephalomalacia.*

***red s.*** Softening of the brain with bleeding into necrosed portions.

**soft palate** The posterior portion of the roof of the mouth, partly separating the mouth and the pharynx. SYN: *velum palatinum.*

**"soft sign"** Any of a number of signs that, when considered collectively, are felt to indicate the presence of damage to the central nervous system. These signs include incoordination, visual motor difficulties, nystagmus, the presence of associated movements, and difficulties with motor control.

**soft sore** Chancroid.

**sol** (sŏl, sōl) [Gr. *sole,* salt water] **1.** State of a colloid system in which the dispersion medium or solvent forms a continuous phase in which the particles of the solute are dispersed, forming a fluid mass. It is called a hydrosol if the dispersion medium is a liquid and an aerosol if a gas. SEE: *gel.* **2.** Solution.

**solace** An object or resource that does or seems to soothe pain or mental stress. In children a teddy bear or a "security" blanket may provide solace. In later life, one's spouse, a friend, or a hobby may be a source of comfort and security.

**Solanaceae** (sōl"ă-nā'sē-ē) A family of herbs, shrubs, and trees from which several important drugs such as scopolamine and belladonna are derived. The potato is one of the species.

**solanaceous** (sŏl"ă-nā'shŭs) Concerning the family Solanaceae.

**solanine** (sō'lă-nēn) A poisonous narcotic alkaloid obtained from potato sprouts and tomatoes. SEE: *poisoning, potato.*

**solar** (sō'lăr) [L. *solaris*] Pert. to the sun or its rays.

**solarium** (sō-lā'rē-ŭm) [L. *solarium,* terrace] **1.** A room or porch exposed to the sun. **2.** A room designed for heliotherapy or for the application of artificial light. **3.** A day or recreational room for patients;

often used as a waiting area for family or visitors.

**solar plexus** The celiac plexus, located behind the stomach and between the suprarenal glands and consisting of two large ganglia, the celiac and superior mesenteric ganglia, from which sympathetic fibers pass to visceral organs.

**solar therapy** Treatment with the sun's rays. SYN: *heliotherapy.*

**solation** (sō-lā′shŭn) In colloidal chemistry, the transformation of a gel into a sol.

**solder** (sŏd′ĕr) Any fusible alloy usually made of tin and lead but may be mostly silver or gold for use in dentistry. The alloy is applied in a melted state to build up or join metal parts.

***building s.*** An alloy of silver with large amounts of copper used to increase the height or bulk of contact areas of dental inlays or crowns; also called *sticky solder.*

***gold s.*** A solder alloy containing a high proportion of gold.

***hard s.*** A solder that is used in dentistry, has a high fusion point, and is stronger and more tarnish-resistant than softer, low-melting-point solders.

***soft s.*** A low-melting-point solder with less strength or tarnishing resistance than hard solder.

**soldering** The joining of two pieces of metal by use of a lower-melting-point alloy. When the melted solder cools and solidifies, it joins the parts together. Soldering is used to join many components of dental appliances or orthodontic bands and to add bulk or contours to crowns or inlays.

**sole** (sōl) [AS. *sole*] **1.** The underpart of the foot. SYN: *planta.* **2.** The portion of a motor endplate at the termination of a motor nerve fiber that is directly adjacent to the contractile substance of a muscle fiber. A large number of muscle nuclei are usually aggregated here. SEE: *antithenar; thenar.*

**soleal line of tibia** A line on the posterior surface of the tibia extending diagonally from below the tibial condyle to the medial border of the tibia. The soleus muscle and fascia are attached to that line.

**solenoid** (sōl′lĕ-noyd) A coil of insulated wire in which a magnetic force is created in the long axis of the coil when an electric current flows through the wire. It may be used to activate switches.

**soleus** (sō′lē-ŭs) [L. *solea,* sole of foot] A flat, broad muscle of the calf of the leg. SEE: *Muscles Appendix.*

**solid** (sŏl′ĭd) [L. *solidus*] **1.** Not gaseous, hollow, or liquid. **2.** A substance not gaseous, liquid, or hollow.

**solipsism** (sōl′ĭp-sĭzm) [L. *solus,* alone, + *ipse,* self] The theory that the self may know only its feelings and changes and there is then only subjective reality.

**solitary** (sŏl′ĭ-tăr-ē) [L. *solitarius,* aloneness] Alone; single or existing separately.

**solitary lymph nodule** One of the small spherical lymphatic nodules found in the lamina propria of the small and large intestine.

**solitude** Being alone. In medicine the voluntary removal of oneself to a place free from stress, noise pollution, and people. This may be accomplished in a variety of settings including walking alone, enjoying sunrises or sunsets, or simply looking at clouds. Some individuals find this capacity to be alone therapeutic, that is, tranquilizing and refreshing. SEE: *relaxation response.*

**solo practitioner** A physician, dentist, or other practitioner who practices alone rather than with a group or partner.

**solubility** (sŏl″ū-bĭl′ĭ-tē) [LL. *solubilis,* to loosen, dissolve] The capability of being dissolved.

**soluble** (sōl′ū-bl) Able to be dissolved.

**soluble immune response suppressor** ABBR: SIRS. A lymphokine that suppresses antibody production.

**solum tympani** (sō′ŭm tĭm′pă-nē) [L.] The floor of the tympanic cavity.

**solute** (sŏl′ūt) [L. *solutus,* to loosen, dissolve] The substance that is dissolved in a solution.

**solutio** (sō-lū′shē-ō) [L. *solutus,* to loosen, dissolve] Solution.

**solution** (sō-lū′shŭn) [L. *solutus,* to loosen, dissolve] **1.** A liquid containing a dissolved substance. **2.** The process by which a solid is homogeneously mixed with a fluid, solid, or gas so that the dissolved substances cannot be distinguished from the resultant fluid. **3.** A mixture formed by dissolution of substances.

The liquid in which the substances are dissolved is called the *solvent* and the substance dissolved, the *solute.*

***aqueous s.*** A solution containing water as the solvent.

***buffer s.*** A solution of a weak acid and its salt (e.g., carbonic acid, sodium bicarbonate) of importance in maintaining a constant pH, esp. of the blood.

***colloidal s.*** A solution in which the solute is suspended and not dissolved, such as gelatin or albumin.

***contrast s.*** A solution containing a radiopaque substance. These solutions are used to facilitate x-ray examination of body cavities.

***hyperbaric s.*** A solution with a specific gravity greater than one, or greater than the solution to which it is being compared. This is important in injecting medicines or anesthetic agents into the spinal fluid in the spinal canal.

***hypertonic s.*** A solution having a greater osmotic pressure than that of cells or body fluids; a solution that draws water out of cells, thus inducing plasmolysis.

***hypotonic s.*** A solution having an osmotic pressure less than that of cells or body fluids; a solution that will cause water to enter cells, thus inducing swelling and possibly lysis.

***iodine s.*** A solution of iodine or potassium iodine used as a source of iodine.

***isobaric s.*** A solution with a specific gravity equal to one or equal to the solution with which it is being compared. SEE: *hyperbaric s.*

***isohydric s.*** A solution having the same hydrogen ion concentration or pH as another.

***isosmotic s.*** A solution with the same osmotic pressure as the solution with which it is being compared.

***isotonic s.*** A solution that has a concentration of electrolytes, nonelectrolytes, or both that will exert osmotic pressure equivalent to that of the solution with which it is being compared. Either 0.16 molar sodium chloride solution (approx. 0.95% salt in water) or 0.3 molar nonelectrolyte solution is approx. isotonic with human red blood cells.

***Locke-Ringer's s.*** A buffered isotonic solution containing 9.0 g sodium chloride, 0.42 g potassium chloride, 0.24 g calcium chloride, 0.5 g sodium bicarbonate, 0.2 g magnesium chloride, 0.5 g dextrose, and distilled water to make 1000 ml.

***molar s.*** A solution containing a gram molecular weight or mole of the reagent dissolved in 1 L (1000 ml) of solution; designated 1M.

***normal s.*** A solution containing 1 g equivalent weight of reagent in 1 L (1000 ml) of solution; designated 1N.

***normal saline s.*** An isotonic saline solution. SEE: *isotonic s.*

***ophthalmic s.*** A sterile preparation suitable for instillation in the eye.

***oral rehydration s.*** A solution used in oral rehydration therapy. The World Health Organization recommends that the solution contain 3.5 g sodium chloride; 2.9 g potassium chloride; 2.9 g trisodium citrate; and 1.5 g glucose dissolved in each liter (approx. 1 qt) of drinking water.

***physiological saline s.*** An isotonic solution of sodium chloride. It is used in irrigating mucous membranes and raw surfaces, in replenishing body water in dehydration, and in restoring circulating blood volume during shock or hemorrhage. SEE: *isotonic s.*

***repair s.*** Any solution given intravenously to treat an electrolyte or metabolic disturbance.

***Ringer's s.*** A solution containing chlorides of sodium, calcium, and potassium. It contains 8.6 g sodium chloride, 0.3 g calcium chloride, 0.3 g potassium chloride, and sufficient distilled water to make 1 L (1000 ml).

***saline s.*** A solution of a salt, usually sodium chloride.

***saturated s.*** A solution containing all the solute it can dissolve. This limit is called the *saturation point*.

***sclerosing s.*** An irritating substance that produces sclerosis when applied to tissues or injected into a vein.

***seminormal s.*** ABBR: 05N or N/2. A solution containing one-half of a gram equivalent weight of reagent in 1 L (1000 ml) of solution.

***standard s.*** A solution containing a definite amount of a substance as a normal solution; used for comparison or analysis.

***supersaturation s.*** A solution in which the saturation point is reached, but when heated, it is possible to dissolve more of the solute.

***test s.*** A reagent solution, one used in performing a particular test.

***Tyrode's s.*** A modified Ringer's solution containing, in addition, a small amount of magnesium chloride and acid and sodium phosphates.

***volumetric s.*** A standard solution containing a definite amount of a substance in 1 L (1000 ml) of solution; used in volumetric analysis.

**solv** [L., *solve*] Dissolve.

**solvate** (sŏl′vāt) A compound formed by reaction between solvent and solute.

**solvent** (sŏl′vĕnt) [L. *solvens*] **1.** Producing a solution, dissolving. **2.** A liquid holding another substance in solution. **3.** A liquid that reacts with a solvent bringing it into solution.

**solvent abuse** SEE: *glue-sniffing.*

**solvolysis** (sŏl-vŏl′ĭ-sĭs) A general term for reactions involving decomposition by hydrolysis, ammonolysis, and sulfolysis.

**soma** (sō′mă) [Gr. *soma,* body] **1.** The body as distinct from the mind. **2.** All of the body cells except the germ cells.

**soman** Pinacolyl methylphosphonofluoridate; an extremely toxic "nerve gas."

**somato-, somat-** (sō′mă-tō) Combining form meaning *body.*

**somatesthesia** (sō″măt-ĕs-thē′zē-ă) [″ + *aisthesis,* sensation] The consciousness of the body; bodily sensation.

**somatic** (sō-măt′ĭk) [Gr. *soma,* body] **1.** Pert. to nonreproductive cells or tissues. **2.** Pert. to the body. **3.** Pert. to structures of the body wall, such as skeletal muscles (somatic musculature) in contrast to structures associated with the viscera, such as visceral muscles (splanchnic musculature).

**somaticosplanchnic** (sō-măt″ĭ-kō-splănk′nĭk) [″ + *splanchnikos,* pert. to the viscera] Somaticovisceral.

**somaticovisceral** (sō-măt″ĭ-kō-vĭs′ĕr-ăl) [″ + L. *viscera,* body organs] Concerning the body and the viscera.

**somatization** (sō″mă-tī-zā′shŭn) The process of expressing a mental condition as a disturbed bodily function.

**somatization disorder** A condition of recurrent and multiple somatic complaints of several years' duration for which medical attention has been sought but no physical basis for the disorder has been found. The age of onset is usually prior to 30. The somatic complaints may be related to virtually any organ system. The essential feature required to establish a diagnosis is a pattern of recurring, multiple, clinically significant complaints resulting in medical treatment or which causes impairment in social, occupational, or other important areas of functioning. If these occur in association with a general medical condition, the physical complaints must be in excess of what would be expected from the medical illness. There must be a history of pain related to at least four different sites or functions such as menstruation, sexual intercourse, or urination. There also must be a history of at least two gastrointestinal symptoms other than pain. There must be a history of at least one sexual or reproductive symptom other than pain (e.g., nausea, vomiting, bloating). In women, this may consist of irregular menses, menorrhagia, or vomiting throughout pregnancy. In men, there may be symptoms such as erectile or ejaculatory dysfunction. Both sexes may be subject to sexual indifference. And there must also be a history of at least one symptom, other than pain, that suggests a neurological condition such as impaired coordination or balance, paralysis or localized weakness, difficulty in swallowing or speaking, urinary retention, hallucinations, loss of touch or pain sensation, double vision, blindness, deafness, seizures, amnesia, and loss of consciousness other than fainting. The unexplained symptoms are not intentionally feigned or produced. SEE: *somatoform disorder.*

**somatoceptors** (sō-măt″ō-sĕp′tors) A term applied to proprioceptors and exteroceptors collectively.

**somatochrome** (sō-măt′ō-krōm) [″ + *chroma,* color] A nerve cell in which the nucleus is completely surrounded by cytoplasm.

**somatocrinin** Growth hormone-releasing factor.

**somatoform disorder** A mental disorder in which the physical symptoms suggest a general medical condition and are not explained by another condition such as a medication or another mental disorder. The symptoms must be clinically significant enough to impair function. A variety of conditions are included in this classification including somatization disorder, conversion disorder, pain disorder, and hypochondriasis. SEE: *Nursing Diagnoses Appendix.*

TREATMENT: The patient should be repeatedly reassured that the disorder is benign. The patient should be seen by as few health care professionals as possible in order to prevent needless repetition of tests and prescriptions for drugs.

**somatogenic** (sō″mă-tō-jĕn′ĭk) [″+ *gennan,* to produce] Originating in the body. SEE: *psychogenic.*

**somatology** (sō″mă-tŏl′ō-jē) [″ + *logos,* word, reason] Comparative study of structure, functions, and development of the human body.

**somatome** (sō′mă-tōm) [″ + *tome,* incision] **1.** A device for cutting the body of the fetus. **2.** A somite.

**somatomedin** Any of a group of insulin-like growth factors (somatomedin C and somatomedin A) that require growth hormone in order to exert their function of stimulating growth. These proteins are produced in the liver and other tissues.

**somatometry** (sō″mă-tŏm′ĕ-trē) [″ + *metron,* measure] Measurement of the body.

**somatopagus** (sō″mă-tŏp′ă-gŭs) [″ + *pagos,* thing fixed] A deformed twin fetus with the trunks merged.

**somatopathic** (sō″mă-tō-păth′ĭk) [″ + *pathos,* disease, suffering] Pert. to organic illness, as distinguished from mental illness.

**somatoplasm** (sō-măt′ō-plăzm) [Gr. *soma,* body, + LL. *plasma,* form, mold] The protoplasm of all the body cells as distinguished from that of the germ plasm.

**somatopleural** (sō″mă-tō-ploor′ăl) Concerning somatopleure.

**somatopleure** (sō-măt′ō-ploor) [″ + *pleura,* side] The lateral and ventral body wall of an embryo, consisting of the outer ectoderm and a layer of somatic mesoderm underlying it. It continues beyond the embryo as the amnion and chorion.

**somatopsychic** (sō″măt-ō-sī′kĭk) [″ + *psyche,* mind] Pert. to both body and mind.

**somatopsychosis** (sō″mă-tō-sī-kō′sĭs) [″ + ″ + *osis,* condition] Any mental disorder that is a symptom of a bodily disease.

**somatoschisis** (sō″mă-tŏs′kĭ-sĭs) [″ + *schistos,* a splitting] A deformed fetus with a cleft in the trunk.

**somatosensory evoked response** ABBR: SER. Response produced by small, painless electrical stimulus administered to large sensory fibers in mixed nerves of the hand or leg. The electroencephalographical record of the character of the subsequent waves produced help to determine the functional state of the nerves involved. SEE: *brainstem auditory evoked responses; evoked response; visual evoked response.*

**somatosexual** (sō″mă-tō-sĕks′ū-ăl) [″ + L. *sexus,* sex] Concerning the body and sexual characteristics.

**somatostatin** (sō-măt′ō-stăt″ĭn) A hormone that inhibits the release of somatotropin; it is produced by the hypothalamus and the delta cells of the pancreas. It also inhibits the secretion of insulin and gastrin. This hormone also inhibits the target tissues of the hormones it inhibits. It has been used experimentally to inhibit hormone production by tumors.

**somatotonia** (sō″mă-tō-tō′nē-ă) [″+ L. *tonus,* a stretching] A personality type, described by the anthropologist Sheldon, in which there is a predominance of physical assertiveness and activity.

**somatotopic** (sō″mă-tō-tŏp′ĭk) [″+ *topos,* place] Concerning the correspondence between a particular part of the body and a particular area of the brain.

**somatotrophic** (sō″mă-tō-trŏf′ĭk) [″ + *tropos,* a turning] **1.** Having selective attraction for or influence on body cells. **2.** Stimulating growth.

**somatotrophin** (sō″mă-tō-trō′fĭn) [″ + *trophe,* nourishment] Growth hormone; somatotropin.

**somatotropic** (sō″mă-tō-trŏp′ĭk) [″ + *trope,* a turn] Influencing the body or body cells.

**somatotropin** (sō″măt-ō-trō′pĭn) [″ + *tropos,* a turning] The anterior pituitary lobe's growth-stimulating principle. In the human, this is called human growth hormone, which increases the rate of cell division and protein synthesis in growing tissues.

***bovine recombinant s.*** A growth hormone made by recombinant methods. It is used in dairy cattle to increase milk production.

**somatotype** (sō-măt′ō-tīp) A particular build or type of body, based on physical characteristics. SEE: *ectomorph; endomorph; mesomorph.*

**somesthetic** (sō-mĕs-thĕt′ĭk) Pert. to sensations and sensory structures of the body.

**somesthetic area** The region in the parietal lobe of the cerebral cortex in which lie the terminations of the axons of general sensory conduction pathways. This area feels and interprets the cutaneous senses and conscious proprioceptive sense.

**somesthetic path** General sensory conduction path leading to the cortex.

**somite** (sō′mīt) [Gr. *soma,* body] Embryonic blocklike segment formed on either side of the neural tube and its underlying notochord. Each somite gives rise to a muscle mass supplied by a spinal nerve and each pair gives rise to a vertebra.

**somnambulism** (sŏm-năm′bū-lĭzm) [L. *somnus,* sleep, + *ambulare,* to walk] Sleepwalking.

**somnambulist** (sŏm-năm′bū-lĭst) One who is subject to sleepwalking.

**somnifacient** (sŏm-nĭ-fā′shĕnt) [″ + *facere,* to make] **1.** Producing sleep. SYN: *hypnotic.* **2.** A drug producing sleep. SYN: *soporific.*

**somniferous** (sŏm-nĭf′ĕr-ŭs) [″ + *ferre,* to bear] Sleep-producing; pert. to that which promotes sleep.

**somniloquism** (sŏm-nĭl′ō-kwĭzm) [″ + ″ + *-ismos,* condition] Talking in one's sleep.

**somnolence** (sŏm′nō-lĕns) [L. *somnolentia,* sleepiness] Prolonged drowsiness or a condition resembling a trance that may continue for a number of days; sleepiness.

**somnolent** (sŏm″nō-lĕnt) [L. *somnolentus*] Sleepy; drowsy.

**somnolentia** (sŏm″nō-lĕn′shē-ă) [L.] **1.** Drowsiness. **2.** The sleep of drunkenness in which the faculties are only partially depressed.

**somnolism** (sŏm′nō-lĭzm) [″ + *-ismos,* condition] The condition of being in a hypnotic trance.

**Somogyi phenomenon** [Michael Somogyi, U.S. biochemist, 1883–1971] In diabetes mellitus, rebound hyperglycemia following an episode of hypoglycemia caused by counter regulatory hormone release. Reduction of insulin dose will help control this condition. SEE: *dawn phenomenon; diabetes mellitus.*

**sone** (sōn) [L. *sonus,* sound] A unit of loudness; the loudness of a pure tone of 1000 cycles per second, 40 decibels above the listener's threshold of hearing.

**sonic** [L. *sonus,* sound] Pert. to sound.

**sonicate** (sŏn′ĭ-kāt) [L. *sonus,* sound] To expose to sound waves.

**sonication** (sŏn″ĭ-kā′shŭn) Exposure to high-frequency sound waves. Used to destroy bacteria.

**sonic boom** (sŏn′ĭk) [L. *sonus,* sound] A noise caused by shock waves from an airborne object traveling faster than the speed of sound. When the waves hit the ground, they may break windows and also affect the hearing.

**Sonoclat coagulation analyzer** An experimental device for measuring blood coagulation function. SEE: *thromboelastogram.*

**sonogram** (sō′nō-grăm) [L. *sonus,* sound, + Gr. *gramma,* something written] The record obtained by use of ultrasonography.

**sonographer** A technologist trained in the application of ultrasound for diagnostic and therapeutic purposes.

***diagnostic medical s.*** One who provides patient services for those using diagnostic ultrasound under the supervision of a doctor of medicine or osteopathy.

**sonography** (sō-nŏg′ră-fē) [″ + Gr. *graphein,* to write] Ultrasonography.

**sonolucent** (sō″nō-loo′sĕnt) In ultrasonography, the condition of not reflecting the ultrasound waves back to their source.

**sonometer** (sō-nŏm′ĕ-tĕr) [″ + Gr. *metron,* a measure] A device used by dentists to cause sound for production of anesthesia.

**sonorous** (sō-nō′rŭs) [L.] Giving forth a loud and rounded sound.

**sophomania** (sŏf″ō-mā′nē-ă) [Gr. *sophos,* wise, + *mania,* madness] An unrealistic belief in one's own wisdom.

**sopor** (sō′por) [L.] Stupor.

**soporiferous** (sō″pō-rĭf′ĕr-ŭs) [″ + *ferre,* to bring] Promoting sleep.

**soporific** (sō-pō-rĭf′ĭk) [″ + *facere,* to make] **1.** Inducing sleep. **2.** Narcotic; a drug producing sleep. SYN: *somnifacient.*

**soporose, soporous** (sō′por-ōs, -ŭs) [L.] Marked by or resembling sound sleep or coma.

**sorbefacient** (sor″bē-fā′shĕnt) [L. *sorbere,* to suck up, + *facere,* to make] Causing or that which causes or promotes absorption.

**sorbitol** $C_6H_{14}O_6$. A crystalline alcohol present in some berries and fruits, used as a sweetening agent and as an excipient in formulating tablets.

**sordes** (sor′dēz) [L. *sordere,* to be dirty] Foul

brown crusts or accumulations on the teeth and about the lips from a foul stomach or secretions of the mouth in mild fever.

NURSING IMPLICATIONS: The nurse prevents this condition by providing frequent oral hygiene for mouth breathers, patients who cannot drink or are not permitted oral fluids, and debilitated patients. A hydrogen peroxide mouthwash (one part hydrogen peroxide to three parts water) or glycerin applied with a soft brush or sponge-stick may be used to remove crusts. Either treatment should always be followed by rinsing with clear water (mouthwashes are astringent, and glycerin dries the mucous membranes). The nurse encourages oral intake if permitted and positions the patient to discourage mouth breathing. If fluids are restricted, the patient should use a water mist or spray to moisten membranes.

**sore** (sor) [AS. *sar,* sore] **1.** Tender; painful. **2.** Any type of tender or painful ulcer or lesion of the skin or mucous membrane.

***bed s.*** SEE: *bedsore.*

***canker s.*** A small lesion of the mucous membrane of the mouth; often accompanying a number of systemic conditions. The cause is unknown. SEE: *stomatitis, aphthous.*

***cold s.*** SEE: *fever blister; herpes simplex.*

***Delhi s.*** Cutaneous leishmaniasis.

***desert s.*** An ulcer of the skin associated with being in the desert.

***hard s.*** A syphilitic chancre; primary lesion of syphilis.

***Oriental s.*** Cutaneous leishmaniasis.

***pressure s.*** A bedsore.

***soft venereal s.*** A soft nonsyphilitic venereal sore occurring on the genitalia. SYN: *venereal s.; chancroid.*

***tropical s.*** Cutaneous leishmaniasis.

***venereal s.*** Soft venereal s.

**sore throat** Inflammation of the tonsils, pharynx, or larynx.

***quinsy s.t.*** Peritonsillar abscess. SEE: *quinsy.*

***septic s.t.*** Severe, epidemic, pseudomembranous inflammation of the fauces and tonsils caused by the hemolytic streptococcus.

***streptococcal s.t.*** SEE: *scarlet fever.*

**soroche** SEE: *mountain sickness, chronic.*

**sorption** (sorp'shŭn) [L. *sorbere,* to suck in] The condition of being absorbed.

**s.o.s.** [L., *si opus sit*] If necessary or required.

**sotalol hydrochloride** (sō'tă-lōl) A beta-adrenergic blocking agent.

**soterenol hydrochloride** (sō'tĕr'ĕ-nōl) An adrenergic medicine used as a bronchodilator.

**souffle** (soof'fl) [Fr. *souffler,* to puff] A soft blowing sound heard in auscultation; a bruit; an auscultatory murmur.

***cardiac s.*** Cardiac murmur.

***fetal s.*** The soft blowing sound heard over the location of the umbilical cord of the fetus in utero and synchronous with the fetal heartbeat during late pregnancy. SYN: *funic s.*

***funic s.*** Fetal s.

***placental s.*** The sound caused by blood entering dilated arteries of the uterus in the last months of pregnancy; synchronous with the maternal pulse rate. It is more frequent than the fetal souffle and is heard as a loud blowing murmur along the side of the uterus and frequently all over it. SYN: *uterine s.*

***splenic s.*** The sound heard over the spleen in malaria.

***uterine s.*** Placental s.

**sound** (sownd) [L. *sonus,* sound] **1.** Auditory sensations produced by vibrations; noise. It is measured in decibels, which is the logarithm of the intensity of sound; thus 20 d. represents not twice 10 d., but 10 times as much. Repeated exposure to excessively loud noises, esp. in certain frequencies, will cause permanent injury to the hearing. SEE: *decibel; noise; sonic boom.* **2.** A form of vibrational energy that gives rise to auditory sensations. SEE: *cochlea; ear; organ of Corti; sonic boom.* **3.** Healthy, not diseased. **4.** Heart sounds. SEE: *diastole; systole.* **5.** [Fr. *sonder,* to probe] An instrument for introduction into a cavity or canal for exploration. SYN: *searcher.*

***adventitious lung s.'s*** Crackles and wheezes superimposed on the normal breath sounds; indicative of respiratory disease. Most adventitious lung sounds can be divided into continuous (wheezing) and discontinuous (crackles) according to acoustical characteristics.

***anasarcous s.*** A moist sound heard on auscultation when the skin is edematous.

***blowing s.*** An organic murmur as of air from an aperture expelled with moderate force.

***bottle s.*** A noise as of fluid in a bottle. SEE: *amphoric.*

***breath s.'s*** Respiratory sounds heard on auscultation of the chest. In a normal chest, they are classified as vesicular, tracheal, and bronchovesicular.

***bronchial s.'s*** Sounds not heard in the normal lung but occurring in pulmonary disease, indicating infiltration and solidification of the lung.

***bronchovesicular s.'s*** A mixture of bronchial and vesicular sounds.

***cracked-pot s.*** A tympanic resonance heard over air cavities. This percussion sound resembles that made by striking a cracked pot.

***ejection s.*** A high-pitched clicking sound heard just after the first heart sound.

***fetal heart s.*** The sound made by the fetal heart.

***friction s.*** A sound produced by rubbing together two inflamed mucous surfaces.

***heart s.'s*** The two sounds "lubb" and

"dupp" resulting from closure of atrial, pulmonic, mitral, and tricuspid valves. Third and fourth heart sounds may be present in some conditions. SEE: *heart*.

***percussion s.*** SEE: *percussion*.

***physiological s.*** A sound perceived when the auditory canals are closed. The sound is produced by the blood flowing through adjacent vessels.

***respiratory s.*** Any sound heard over the lungs, bronchi, or trachea.

***succussion s.*** A splashing sound heard over a cavity with fluid in it.

***to-and-fro s.*** Rasping friction sounds of pericarditis.

***tracheal s.*** A sound normally heard over the trachea or larynx.

***tubular s.*** A sound heard over the trachea or large bronchi.

***urethral s.*** A device suitable for use in exploring the urethra.

***vesicular s.*** A normal sound heard over the entire lung during inspiration resulting from distention of alveoli with air.

***white s.*** A sound made up of all audible frequencies.

**Souques' phenomenon** [A. A. Souques, Fr. neurologist, 1860–1944] Finger extension on the involved side of a hemiplegic patient when the extremity is raised to a position above 90° of shoulder flexion or abduction.

**source-skin distance** In radiation therapy, the distance from the radiation source to the patient's skin.

**source-to-image receptor distance** ABBR: SID. In radiography, the distance from the x-ray tube to the radiographical film or the image digitizer.

**Southern Blot** An analytical method traditionally used in DNA analysis. After a sample of DNA fragments is separated by agarose gel electrophoresis, the fragments are transferred to a solid cellulose support by blotting. The gel is placed between a concentrated salt solution and absorbent paper. Capillary action draws the fragments onto the solid support. The support is then treated with radiolabeled DNA probes.

**soybean oil** The refined oil obtained from seeds of the soya plant.

**sp** [L., *spiritus*] **1.** Spirit. **2.** *Species*.

**spa** (spă) [Spa, a Belgium resort town] A mineral spring, esp. one allegedly having healing properties.

**space** (spās) [L. *spatium*, space] **1.** An area, region, or segment. **2.** A cavity of the body. SYN: *spatium*. **3.** The expanse in which the solar system, stars, and galaxies exist; outside the Earth's atmosphere.

***anatomical dead s.*** The area in the trachea, bronchi, and air passages containing air that does not reach the alveoli during inspiration and is not involved in gas exchange. SYN: *dead s.; deadspace*. SEE: *physiological dead s.*

***axillary s.*** The axilla or space beneath the arm.

***circumlental s.*** The space between the equator of the lens and the ciliary body.

***closest speaking s.*** The space between the teeth during casual repetition of the sound "s." This is considered the closest relationship of the occlusal surfaces and incisal edges of the mandibular teeth to the maxillary teeth during function and rapid speech.

***dead s.*** **1.** Anatomical dead s. SEE: *deadspace*. **2.** The unobliterated space remaining after closure of a surgical wound. This space favors the accumulation of blood, and eventually infection.

***epidural s.*** The space between the dura mater and vertebral periosteum, or between the bones of the cranium and the dura mater, assumed to be lymph spaces.

***extracellular s.*** The space between cells. It contains fluid derived from plasma in the adjacent capillaries. The fluid flows back and forth from capillaries to cells. SEE: *extracellular fluid*.

***s.'s of Fontana*** Spaces in scleral meshwork in angle of the iris through which the aqueous humor passes from the anterior chamber to the canal of Schlemm.

***intercostal s.*** The interval between ribs.

***interfascial s.*** Tenon's s.

***interglobular s.'s*** Czermak's spaces.

***interpleural s.*** The mediastinum.

***interproximal s.*** The space between the surfaces of adjacent teeth in the dental arch. It is divided into the septal space, gingival to the contact point of the teeth and occupied normally by the interdental papilla of the gingiva, and the embrasure, the space occlusal to the contact point of the teeth.

***interradicular s.*** The area between the roots of a multirooted tooth, which contains an alveolar bony septum and the periodontal ligament.

***intervillous s.*** Any area of the maternal side of the placenta where transfer of maternal oxygen, nutrients, and fetal wastes occurs.

***loose s.*** A distensible lung interstitial tissue surrounding the acinus and terminal bronchioles.

***lymph s.*** Any space occupied by lymph tissue.

***Meckel's s.*** Cavum trigeminale.

***mediastinal s.*** The mediastinum.

***medullary s.*** The marrow-containing area of cancellous bone.

***palmar s.*** The midpalmar and thenar spaces of the hand.

***parasinoidal s.'s*** Lateral spaces in the dura mater adjacent to the superior sagittal sinus that receive meningeal and diploic veins.

***perforated s.*** The space pierced by blood vessels at the base of the brain. SYN: *substantia perforata*.

***periodontal ligament s.*** ABBR: PDL space. A radiolucent space that appears on a dental radiograph between the tooth and the adjacent lamina dura. The space is occupied by the periodontal ligament, which lacks the density to be radiopaque.

***perivascular s.'s*** The spaces within adventitia of larger blood vessels of the brain. They communicate with the subarachnoid space.

***personal s.*** In psychiatry, an individual's personal area and the surrounding space. This space is important in interpersonal relations.

***physiological dead s.*** In the respiratory tract, any nonfunctional alveoli that do not receive air that participates in gas exchange. Possible causes include emphysema, pneumothorax, pneumonia, pulmonary edema, and constriction of bronchioles. SEE: *anatomical dead s.*

***plantar s.*** One of four spaces between the fascial layers of the foot. When the foot is infected, pus may be found there.

***pneumatic s.*** Air-containing spaces in bone, esp. those in the paranasal sinuses.

***popliteal s.*** The space in back of the knee joint, containing the popliteal artery and vein and small sciatic and popliteal nerves.

***prezonular s.*** The anterior portion of the posterior chamber of the eye.

***Prussak's s.*** The space in the tympanum behind Shrapnell's membrane.

***retroperitoneal s.*** The potential space outside the parietal peritoneum of the abdominal cavity.

***retropharyngeal s.*** The space behind the pharynx separating prevertebral from visceral fascia. Important in dentistry as a possible path for the spread of infection from oral cavity trauma downward to visceral organs of the mediastinum. SYN: *retropharyngeal fascial cleft.*

***subarachnoid s.*** One of the spaces between the pia mater and arachnoid, containing the cerebrospinal fluid. The spaces, esp. in the cranium, are traversed by numerous trabeculae.

***subdural s.*** Narrow space between the dura and the arachnoid.

***subphrenic s.*** Space between the diaphragm and the abdominal organs.

***suprasternal s.*** Triangular space immediately above the sternum between layers of deep cervical fascia.

***Tenon's s.*** Lymph space between the sclera and Tenon's capsule. SYN: *interfascial s.*

***thenar s.*** A deep fascial space in the hand lying anterior to the adductor pollicis muscle.

***tissue s.*** Any space within tissues not lined with epithelium and containing tissue fluid.

***zonular s.'s*** Spaces within the zonule (suspensory ligament of lens).

**space maintainer** An appliance placed within the dental arch to prevent adjacent teeth from moving into the space left by a missing tooth; it is a temporary placement until the permanent tooth erupts into the space, or until a bridge is placed to replace the missing permanent tooth.

**space medicine** The branch of medical science concerned with the physiological and pathological problems encountered by humans who enter the area beyond the Earth's atmosphere. Included in space medicine are investigation of effects of weightlessness (zero gravity), sensory deprivation, motion sickness, enforced inactivity during lengthy travels in space, and the heat and decelerative forces encountered at the time of reentry into the Earth's atmosphere. With prolonged flights into space, a number of medical problems have arisen, including anemia and loss of blood volume, and loss of bone and muscle mass. These changes also make adjustment to gravity after returning to earth difficult. Medical problems such as these will need to be dealt with when humans are in a weightless environment for several years.

**space sickness** A transient form of physiological vertigo encountered when the head is actively moved in a weightless environment. It may be accompanied by general malaise and nausea, with or without vomiting. The condition resembles seasickness but may or may not occur in individuals who normally experience that disorder while on earth and, conversely, may occur in persons known to be resistant to seasickness.

**spallation** (spawl-lā′shŭn) **1.** The process of breaking into very small parts. The term may be applied to gross structures or to atomic particles. **2.** The release of inert particles into the bloodstream. An example would be the splintering of bits of plastic from the pump used in hemodialysis.

**span** The distance from one fixed point to another, as the distance, when the hand is fully expanded, from the tip of the thumb to the tip of the little finger. Each individual should know that measurement of his or her own hand so that it may be used in estimating the length or size of objects.

**Spanish fly** Cantharides.

**sparer** (spăr′ĕr) [AS. *sparian,* to refrain] A substance destroyed by catabolism but that, nevertheless, decreases catabolic action on other substances.

***protein s.'s*** Carbohydrates and fats, so designated because their presence in diet prevents tissue proteins from being used as a source of energy.

**sparganosis** (spăr″gă-nō′sĭs) Infestation with a variety of Sparganum.

**Sparganum** (spăr′gă-nŭm) *pl.* **spargana** [Gr. *sparganon,* swathing band] The plerocercoid larva of tapeworms, esp. those of the genus *Diphyllobothrium.*

***S. mansoni*** An elongated plerocercoid species, 3 to 14 in. (7.6 to 35 cm) in length, found in muscles and connective tissue, esp. that around the eye; common in the Far East.

***S. mansonoides*** Species occasionally found in the U.S. in larval form.

***S. proliferum*** Minute species infesting humans and producing acne-like nodules. It is thought to proliferate by means of budlike outgrowths.

**spargosis** (spăr-gō′sĭs) [Gr. *spargosis,* swelling] **1.** Distention of the female breasts with milk. **2.** Swelling or thickening of the skin. SYN: *elephantiasis.*

**spasm** (spăzm) [Gr. *spasmos,* convulsion] An involuntary sudden movement or muscular contraction that occurs as a result of some irritant or trauma. Spasms may be clonic (characterized by alternate contraction and relaxation) or tonic (sustained). They may involve either visceral (smooth) muscle or skeletal (striated) muscle. When contractions are strong and painful, they are called cramps. The effect depends on the part affected. Asthma is assumed to be associated with spasm of the muscular coats of smaller bronchi; renal colic to spasm of the muscular coat of the ureter.

TREATMENT: General measures to reduce tension, induce muscle relaxation, and improve circulation are needed. Specific measures include analgesics, massage, relaxation exercises, therapeutic modalities such as heat, cold, or electrotherapy, and, in some cases, gentle therapeutic exercises. Special orthopedic supports or braces are sometimes effective. For vascular spasm, chemical sympathectomy may give relief.

***Bell's s.*** Convulsive tic of the face.

***bronchial s.*** Contraction of the muscle fibers around the bronchial tubes, which occurs in asthma.

***carpopedal s.*** Involuntary muscular contraction of the hands and feet, sometimes seen in hyperventilation syndrome. It is caused by hypocalcemia and commonly encountered during hyperventilation because the lowered carbon dioxide alters the level of ionized calcium. SEE: *hyperventilation, tetany.*

***choreiform s.*** Spasmodic movements resembling chorea.

***clonic s.*** Intermittent contractions and relaxation of muscles.

***diffuse s.*** An esophageal motor disorder characterized by dysphagia, odynophagia, and chest pain.

***s. of the esophagus*** Paroxysmal dysphagia (inability to swallow), often associated with a sense of constriction in the chest. It is characterized by intense dyspnea and occurs in croup, ulceration of the larynx, whooping cough, tetany, hysteria, hydrophobia, and laryngeal crises of locomotor ataxia; when foreign bodies have lodged in the larynx; and when aneurysms or mediastinal tumors press on the recurrent laryngeal nerve and irritate it. The prognosis is indefinite with respect to duration, but the condition is not life-threatening.

TREATMENT: The cause should be discovered and removed. The treatment is largely dietetic, hygienic, and psychological. Dilation by passage of a bougie may be of great value.

***habit s.*** A habitual movement that some people develop. It may persist unchanged throughout life. Included are sniffing, clearing the throat, moving the neck as if relieving collar tension, scratching or rubbing the skin in one place, or eye blinking. Young children are esp. prone to these movements, which may be more prominent during periods of stress or tension. These movements are voluntary but difficult for the individual to suppress. In some cases, they persist for such a long period that they are not noticed by the individual and cannot be controlled. SYN: *tic.* SEE: *jaw-winking; Marcus Gunn syndrome; peotillomania; trichotillomania; Tourette's syndrome.*

***infantile s.*** Seizure activity marked by momentary flexion or extension of the neck, trunk, extremities, or any combination, with onset occurring in the first year of life. Although infantile spasms subside in late infancy, many affected children develop other types of seizure activity and may be severely retarded.

***nodding s.*** A psychogenic condition in adults, causing nodding of the head from clonic spasms of the sternomastoid muscles. A similar nodding occurs in babies, with the head turning from side to side. SYN: *salaam convulsion.*

***saltatory s.*** A tic of the muscles of the lower extremity, causing convulsive leaping upon attempting to stand. SEE: *Jumping Frenchmen of Maine; miryachit; palmus* (2); *Tourette's syndrome.*

***tetanic s.*** A spasm in which contractions continue for a time without interruption.

***tonic s.*** Continued involuntary contractions.

***torsion s.*** A spasm characterized by a turning of a part, esp. the turning of the body at the pelvis.

***toxic s.*** Convulsions due to poison.

***winking s.*** Blepharospasm.

**spasmogen** (spăz′mō-jĕn) [″ + *gennan,* to produce] Something that causes spasms or constrictions as in the bronchospasm associated with asthma.

**spasmolygmus** (spăz-mō-lĭg′mŭs) [″ + *lygmos,* a sob] **1.** A spasmodic hiccup. **2.** Spasmodic sobbing.

**spasmolytic** (spăz-mō-lĭt′ĭk) [″ + *lysis,* dissolution] Arresting spasms or that which acts as an antispasmodic.

**spasmophemia** (spăz-mō-fē′mē-ă) [″ + *pheme,* speech] Stuttering.

**spasmophilia** (spăz-mō-fĭl′ē-ă) [″ + *philein,* to love] A tendency to tetany and convulsions; almost always associated with rickets.

**spasmous** (spăz′mŭs) [Gr. *spasmos,* convulsion] Of the nature of a spasm.

**spasmus** (spăz′mŭs) [Gr. *spasmos,* convulsion] A spasm.

***s. agitans*** Paralysis agitans.

***s. bronchialis*** Bronchial asthma.

***s. caninus*** Risus sardonicus.

***s. coordinatus*** Imitative or compulsive movements, as mimic tics or festination.

***s. cynicus*** A spasmodic contraction of the muscles on both sides of the mouth.

***s. Dubini*** Rhythmic contractions, in rapid succession, of a group or groups of muscles, starting at an extremity or half of the face, and covering a large part or all of the body. It is usually fatal.

***s. glottidis*** Laryngismus.

***s. nictitans*** Blepharospasm.

***s. nutans*** A nodding spasm in infants and young children. The eyes are also involved as manifested by rapid, pendular nystagmoid movements that may be observed in one eye. Spontaneous improvement always occurs.

**spastic** (spăs′tĭk) [Gr. *spastikos,* convulsive] **1.** Resembling or of the nature of spasms or convulsions. **2.** Produced by spasms. **3.** One afflicted with spasms.

**spastic colon** SEE: *colon, irritable.*

**spastic gait** A stiff movement of the legs while walking, usually the result of an upper motor neuron lesion and spasticity in the muscles of the lower extremity. There are several variations. Spasticity in the ankle plantar flexors results in the toes dragging or walking on the toes; spasticity in the hip adductors results in a scissoring or crossing of the legs; spasticity in the quadriceps femoris results in the knee being held rigid. If the upper extremities are involved, the arms do not swing rhythmically but are usually held still with the elbows and wrists flexed.

**spastic hemiplegia** Spasticity occurring in one half of the body, usually owing to a cardiovascular accident or cerebral palsy affecting only half of the brain.

**spasticity** (spăs-tĭs′ĭ-tē) Increased tone or contractions of muscles causing stiff and awkward movements; the result of an upper motor neuron lesion.

**spatial** (spā′shăl) Pert. to space.

**spatial discrimination** The ability to perceive as separate points of contact the two blunt points of a compass when applied to the skin.

**spatial localization disorder** An inability to describe or to find the way even though in familiar surroundings. This neurological condition is usually due to bilateral occipitoparietal lesions of the brain.

**spatial resolution** In radiology, the ability to distinguish two adjacent points of similar density as being separate.

**spatium** (spā′shē-ŭm) *pl.* **spatia** [L.] Space.

**spatula** (spăch′ū-lă) [L. *spatula,* blade] An instrument for spreading or mixing semisolids. It is usually flat, thin, somewhat flexible, and shaped like a knife but without a cutting edge.

***eye s.*** A blade for separating lips of corneal wounds, arresting hemorrhage, or for making pressure; made of sheet metal or rubber.

***nasal s.*** A device for holding mucous flaps in place or to guard against burning from cautery.

**spatulate** (spăch′ŭ-lāt) To mix something by use of a spatula. In dentistry, to mix or manipulate certain dental materials with a spatula to achieve a uniform, homogenous mass.

**spay, spaying** (spā, spā′ĭng) [Gael. *spoth,* castrate] Surgical removal of ovaries, usually said of animals. SEE: *castration.*

**SPCA** *Society for the Prevention of Cruelty to Animals.*

**specialist** (spĕsh′ăl-ĭst) [L. *specialis*] A dentist, nurse, physician, or other health professional who has advanced education and training in one clinical area of practice such as internal medicine, pediatrics, surgery, ophthalmology, neurology, maternal and child health, or cardiology. In most specialized areas of health care, there are organizations offering qualifying examinations. When an individual meets all of the criteria of such a board, he or she is called "board certified" in that area.

**specialization** (spĕsh″ăl-ī-zā′shŭn) The limitation of one's practice to a particular branch of medicine, surgery, dentistry, or nursing. This is customarily done after having received postgraduate training in the area of specialization.

**specialty** (spĕsh′ăl-tē) The branch of medicine, surgery, dentistry, or nursing in which a specialist practices.

**speciation** (spē″sē-ā′shŭn) [L. *species,* a kind] The evolutionary process by which new species of living organisms are formed.

**species** (spē′shēz) [L. *species,* a kind] In biology, a category of classification for living organisms. This group is just below genus and is usually capable of interbreeding.

**species-specific** The characteristics of a species, esp. the immunological nature that differentiates that species from another.

**species type** The original species that served as the basis for identifying a new genus or subgenus.

**specific** (spĕ-sĭf′ĭk) [L. *specificus,* pert. to a kind] **1.** Referring to a remedy having a curative effect on a particular disease or symptom. **2.** Pert. to a species. **3.** Referring to a disease always caused by the same organism. **4.** Restricted, explicit; not generalized.

**specific gravity** ABBR: sp. gr. The weight of a substance compared with the weight of an equal volume of water. For solid and liquid materials, water is used as a standard and considered to have a specific gravity of 1.000. For gases, the weight per unit volume is compared with that of dry air at a specified temperature and usually at atmospheric pressure.

**specificity** (spĕ-sĭ-fĭs′ĭ-tē) The state of being specific; having a relation to a definite result or to a particular cause.

***diagnostic s.*** For a diagnostic or screening test, the proportion of people who are truly free of a specific disease and are so identified by the test. SEE: *sensitivity*.

***s. of exercise*** The design of exercises to stress muscles in a manner similar to the way in which they are to perform. This technique helps the muscle to meet specific demands, including speed and type of contraction, strength and endurance requirements, stabilization, and mobility activities.

**specillum** (spē-sĭl′lŭm) *pl.* **specilla** [L. *specere,* to look] **1.** Lens. **2.** A button-shaped silver probe.

**specimen** (spĕs′ĭ-mĕn) [L. *specere,* to look] A part of a thing intended to show kind and quality of the whole, as a specimen of urine.

---

Caution: Persons handling specimens should wear rubber gloves to protect themselves from accidental exposure to the hepatitis B and AIDS viruses.

---

The following information is important in obtaining, containing, and handling biological and forensic samples.

*Sterilization of glassware:* This is accomplished by the use of hot air or dry heat, boiling water, flowing steam, steam under pressure, certain gases, and germicidal chemicals.

*Labels:* All containers should be labeled with the names of the patient and attending physician and the room number. Labels should be placed on the container, not on the lid. Request forms, sometimes used as labels, are made up to suit the individual laboratory or hospital. Provision is made for recording necessary data as indicated, including the date the specimen was taken, the circumstances, the substances for which the examination is being performed, and any other information desired. SEE: *chain of custody*.

*Time:* If the required specimen cannot be furnished at once, one should note what is needed and inform the patient, supervisor, and any other nurse who may attend the patient in one's absence.

*Charting:* The chart should record all specimens sent to the laboratory, when they were sent, and any other data that seem pertinent such as the appearance of the specimen or unusual occurrences while it was being obtained.

*Care of specimen:* The specimen should be covered immediately after it is deposited in the container. The label or request form should be checked. One should make sure that the container is intact and in no danger of spilling while in transit. Some types of specimens (e.g., blood, urine, tissues) will need special care with respect to the temperature to be maintained while they are stored or transported and the time allowed before being analyzed. SEE: *Universal Precautions Appendix*.

**spectacles** (spĕk′tăk-lz) [L. *spectare,* to see] Glasses.

**spectinomycin hydrochloride, sterile** A sterile preparation of the antibiotic spectinomycin hydrochloride. When diluted with the appropriate amount of sterile water for injection, the medicine may be used intramuscularly.

**spectral** (spĕk′trăl) [L. *spectrum,* image] Concerning a spectrum.

**spectro-** Combining form meaning *appearance, image, form,* or *spectrum*.

**spectrocolorimeter** (spĕk-trō-kŭl-or-ĭm′ĕ-tĕr) [L. *spectrum,* image, + *color,* color, + Gr. *metron,* measure] A device for detecting color blindness by isolating a single spectral color.

**spectrofluorometer** (spĕk″trō-floo″or-ŏm′ĕ-tĕr) An instrument for measuring the degree of fluorescence.

**spectrograph** (spĕk′trō-grăf) [″ + Gr. *graphein,* to write] An instrument designed to photograph spectra on a sensitive photographic plate.

***mass s.*** A device that separates ions of different masses by employing a magnetic field to deflect them as they travel along a given path.

**spectrometer** (spĕk-trŏm′ĕt-ĕr) [″ + Gr. *metron,* measure] A spectroscope so constructed that angular deviation of a ray of light produced by a prism or by a diffraction grating thus indicates the wavelength.

**spectrometry** (spĕk-trŏm′ĕ-trē) [″ + Gr. *metron,* measure] The process of determining the wavelength of light rays by use of a spectrometer.

**spectrophotometer** (spĕk″trō-fō-tŏm′ĕt-ĕr) [″ + Gr. *photos,* light, + *metron,* measure] A device for measuring the amount of color in a solution by comparison with the spectrum.

**spectrophotometry** (spĕk″trō-fō-tŏm′ĕt-rē) An estimation of coloring matter in a solution by use of the spectroscope or spectrophotometer.

**spectropolarimeter** (spĕk″trō-pō″lăr-ĭm′ĕ-tĕr) [″ + *polaris,* pole, + *metron,* measure] A device for measuring the rotation of light rays of a specific wavelength by passage through a translucent solid.

**spectroscope** (spĕk′trō-skōp) [″ + Gr. *skopein,* to examine] An instrument for separating radiant energy into its component frequencies or wavelengths by means of a prism or grating to form a spectrum for inspection.

**spectroscopic** (spĕk″trō-skŏp′ĭk) Concerning a spectroscope.

**spectroscopy** (spĕk-trŏs′kō-pē) **1.** The branch of physical science that treats the phenomena observed with the spectroscope, or those principles on which the action is based. **2.** The art of using the spectroscope.

***nuclear magnetic resonance s.*** ABBR: NMR spectroscopy. A technique that uses the characteristic absorption of nuclei inside a strong magnetic field to identify and characterize molecules.

**spectrum** (spĕk′trŭm) *pl.* **spectra** [L., image] The charted band of wavelengths of electromagnetic vibrations obtained by refraction and diffraction of rays of white light.

***absorption s.*** Spectrum recorded after light rays have passed through a substance that is capable of absorbing some of the wavelengths passing through. This spectrum is specific for various chemicals.

***broad s.*** Refering to antibiotics effective against a variety of microorganisms.

***chromatic s.*** The portion of the spectrum that produces visible light. Wavelengths of about 3900 Å to 7700 Å are visible.

***invisible s.*** The portion of the spectrum either below the red (infrared) or above the violet (ultraviolet), which is invisible to the eye, the waves being too long or too short to affect the retina. The invisible spectrum includes rays less than 3900 Å in length (ultraviolet, roentgen or x, gamma, and cosmic rays) and those exceeding 7700 Å in length (infrared, high-frequency oscillations used in short- and long-wave diathermy, radio, hertzian, and very long waves). These range in length from 7700 Å to 5,000,000 m.

***narrow s.*** A term that refers to an antibiotic effective against only a few microorganisms.

***visible s.*** The portion of the spectrum that is visible. The visible spectrum consists of the colors from red to violet with wavelengths of 3900 Å to 7700 Å. When white light is passed through a prism, the various colors, because of different wavelengths, are refracted to various degrees, giving rise to the diverse colors of the rainbow. These are in order from the shortest wavelength to the longest violet, indigo, blue, green, yellow, orange, and red.

***visible electromagnetic s.*** The complete range of wavelengths of electromagnetic radiation.

**spectrum emission 1.** In spectroscopy and fluorometry, the range of wavelengths emitted by a substance. **2.** In the case of atoms, the lines of emission.

**speculum** (spĕk′ū-lŭm) *pl.* **specula** [L., a mirror] **1.** An instrument for examination of canals. **2.** The membrane separating the anterior cornua of lateral ventricles of the brain. SYN: *septum pellucidum.*

***bivalve s.*** A speculum with two opposed blades that can be separated or closed. SEE: *vaginal s.*

***duck-bill s.*** A bivalve speculum with wide blades.

***ear s.*** A short, funnel-shaped tube, tubular or bivalve (the former being preferable).

***eye s.*** A device for separating the eyelids. Plated steel wire, plain, Luer's, Von Graefe's, and Steven's are the most common types.

***Pedersen s.*** A small vaginal speculum for examining prepubertal patients or others with small vaginal orifices.

***vaginal s.*** A speculum, usually with two opposing portions that, after being inserted, can be pushed apart, for examining the vagina and cervix.

NOTE: A vaginal speculum should be warmed before use.

**speech** [AS. *spaec*] **1.** The verbal expression of one's thoughts. **2.** The act of uttering articulate words or sounds. **3.** Words that are spoken for the purpose of communication.

Historically, certain crude sounds are believed to have served as warnings or threats in much the same way as did facial and bodily expressions. As sounds became highly differentiated, each became associated and gradually identified with a certain idea. These word-symbols are a valuable tool in ideation, and thinking largely depends on this internal speech. Further identifications have made possible visual symbols (written language), although primitive written language was entirely unrelated to speech. The symbols were crude representations of objects.

External speech requires the coordination of the larynx, mouth, lips, chest, and abdominal muscles. These have no special innervation for speech, but the upper neurons respond to complex motor pattern fields that convert the idea into suitable motor stimuli.

***aphonic s.*** Whispering.

***ataxic s.*** Defective speech resulting from muscular incoordination usually the result of cerebellar disorder.

***clipped s.*** Scamping s.

***cued s.*** A language for the deaf that combines lip reading with cues provided by the hands. The use of this technique permits the deaf person to understand a greater variety of words and the mechanics of language than either sign language or lip reading alone.

***echo s.*** Echolalia.

***esophageal s.*** In persons who have had laryngectomies, the modulation of air expelled from the esophagus to produce sound that can be used in speech. The mouth, tongue, and pharynx participate in this.

***explosive s.*** Sudden loud sounds produced by persons with organic brain disease or mental disorders.

***helium s.*** The altered voice produced by inhaling helium and then speaking as the helium is exhaled. The very low density of the helium causes the alteration.

***interjectional s.*** Speech characterized by inarticulate sounds.

***mirror s.*** Speech characterized by reversing the order of syllables of a word.

***paraphasic s.*** Speech that is fluent but may be incomprehensible. Words may have inappropriate syllables inserted, or one word may be substituted for another.

***scamping s.*** Speech characterized by omission of consonants or syllables when unable to pronounce them. SYN: *clipped s.*

***scanning s.*** The pronunciation of words in syllables, or slowly and hesitatingly; pauses between the syllables result in a staccato-like speech. This type of speech is a symptom of certain diseases of the cerebellum and advanced multiple sclerosis. SYN: *staccato s.*

***slurring s.*** Slovenly articulation of letters difficult to pronounce.

***staccato s.*** Scanning s.

**speech abnormality** Any disorder, dysfunction, or impairment of speech as compared with what is considered to be normal. *Speech failure* results in motor aphasia, in which the patient is speechless but there is no paralysis of the muscles of articulation. Although unable to express thoughts in words, the patient can still understand what he or she hears and reads. *Labialism* is the excessive use of labial sounds. *Absence of speech* or *hoarseness* may be part of a hysteria. *Word deafness* is the condition in which a word is heard but the patient has no idea of its meaning. Similarly, *word blindness* means that the written symbol might as well be a foreign word. This is sometimes called *alexia*. *Aphasia* in right-handed patients is classically referable to left-sided brain lesions, but the concept of centers for internal speech esp. is rather misleading. It is probably a diffuse cortical activity, and countless minor distortions occur in addition to those mentioned. Chief of those not enumerated is the slurring speech of *paresis,* in which letters and syllables are omitted without recognition of defect, and this further identifies the abnormality. *Dysarthria* describes any defect of articulation; muscular tone disturbances as seen in cerebellar disease, chorea, paralysis agitans, lenticular degeneration, or multiple sclerosis, producing jerky, monotonous, or scanning speech. Paralysis due to bilateral medullary pathology of the brain results in indistinct enunciation (mouthful speech), which is often entirely unintelligible. Pseudobulbar palsy (as in cases of double hemiplegia) adds a slow spastic characteristic. Peripheral nerve lesions, cleft palate, adenoids, and myasthenia gravis are the source of many possible speech abnormalities.

*Stammering* and *stuttering* are usually psychogenic. Emotional values may be added to speech quality; tremulousness and tension may render the voice high-pitched, irritating, or unsustained and broken. Emotional flattening may occur in the neuroses and psychoses. In the latter, diagnostic changes may occur in the stream of talk.

*Amentia* invariably delays speech appearance, and its faulty development is of diagnostic value. Childish indistinctness (e.g., "r's" replaced by "w's") may persist in mentally handicapped adults.

The delay or nonappearance of speech may be referable to *deafness* (deaf-mutism). Deaf persons may "speak" by using sign language at a slower rate if the normal speech is slow in their geographical area.

**speech and language pathologist** ABBR: SLP. An individual educated and trained to plan, direct, and conduct programs to improve communicative skills of children and adults with language and speech impairments arising from physiological disturbances, defective articulation, or dialect. This individual can evaluate programs and may perform research related to speech and language problems.

**speech synthesizer** An electronic device for producing speech. Activated by a keyboard, it permits persons lacking the ability to speak to communicate.

**speech therapy** The study, diagnosis, and treatment of defects and disorders of the voice and of spoken and written communication.

**"speedballing"** Among abusers of drugs, a combination of cocaine and heroin taken intravenously.

**sperm** (spĕrm) [Gr. *sperma,* seed] **1.** Semen. **2.** Spermatozoa. SEE: illus.

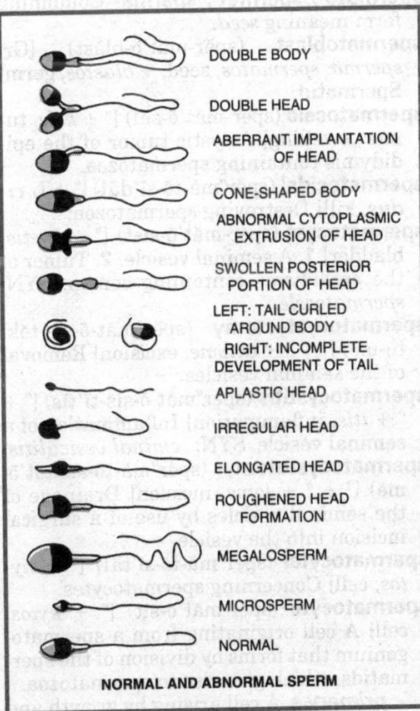

NORMAL AND ABNORMAL SPERM

**sperma-** SEE: *spermato-*.

**sperma** (spĕr′mă) [Gr.] **1.** Semen. **2.** Spermatozoa.

**spermacrasia** (spĕr″măk-rā′zē-ă) [Gr. *sperma,* seed, + *akrasia,* bad mixture] A lack of spermatozoa in the semen. SYN: *aspermia.*

**spermagglutination** Agglutination of spermatozoa.

**spermat-** SEE: *spermato-*.

**spermatemphraxis** (spĕr″măt-ĕm-frăk′sĭs) [″ + *emphraxis,* stoppage] An obstruction to the emission of semen.

**spermatic** (spĕr-măt′ĭk) [Gr. *sperma,* seed] Pert. to semen or sperm.

**spermatic artery** One of two long slender vessels, branches of the abdominal aorta, following each spermatic cord to the testes.

**spermaticide, spermatocide** (spĕrm′ăt-ĭ-sīd, spĕrm′ăt-ō-sīd) [Gr. *sperma,* seed, + L. *cidus,* kill] Spermicide. **spermaticidal** (-sīd″ăl), *adj.*

**spermatic vein** One of two veins draining the testes. The right one empties into the inferior vena cava, the left into the left renal vein. In the spermatic cord, each forms a dilated pampiniform plexus.

**spermatid** (spĕr′mă-tĭd) A cell arising by division of the secondary spermatocyte to become a spermatozoon. SYN: *spermatoblast; spermoblast.*

**spermatin** (spĕr′mă-tĭn) A mucilaginous substance in the semen.

**spermatitis** (spĕr″mă-tī′tĭs) [″ + *itis,* inflammation] Inflammation of the spermatic cord or of the ductus deferens. SYN: *deferentitis; funiculitis.*

**spermato-, spermat-, sperma-** Combining form meaning *seed.*

**spermatoblast** (spĕr-măt′ō-blăst) [Gr. *sperma, spermatos,* seed, + *blastos,* germ] Spermatid.

**spermatocele** (spĕr-măt′ō-sēl) [″ + *kele,* tumor, swelling] A cystic tumor of the epididymis containing spermatozoa.

**spermatocidal** (spĕr″mă-tō-sī′dăl) [″ + L. *cidus,* kill] Destroying spermatozoa.

**spermatocyst** (spĕr-măt′ō-sĭst) [″ + *kystis,* bladder] **1.** A seminal vesicle. **2.** Tumor of the epididymis containing semen. SYN: *spermatocele.*

**spermatocystectomy** (spĕr″măt-ō-sĭs-tĕk′tō-mē) [″ + ″ + *ektome,* excision] Removal of the seminal vesicles.

**spermatocystitis** (spĕr″măt-ō-sĭs-tī′tĭs) [″ + ″ + *itis,* inflammation] Inflammation of a seminal vesicle. SYN: *seminal vesiculitis.*

**spermatocystotomy** (spĕr″mă-tō-sĭs-tŏt′ō-mē) [″ + ″ + *tome,* incision] Drainage of the seminal vesicles by use of a surgical incision into the vesicle.

**spermatocytal** (spĕr″mă-tō-sī′tăl) [″ + *kytos,* cell] Concerning spermatocytes.

**spermatocyte** (spĕr-măt′ō-sīt) [″ + *kytos,* cell] A cell originating from a spermatogonium that forms by division of the spermatids, which give rise to spermatozoa.

***primary s.*** A cell arising by growth and development from a spermatogonium.

***secondary s.*** A cell arising from a primary spermatocyte by a meiotic division. It undergoes a second meiotic division, giving rise to two spermatids with the haploid number of chromosomes.

**spermatogenesis** (spĕr″măt-ō-jĕn′ĕ-sĭs) [″ + *genesis,* generation, birth] The formation of mature functional spermatozoa. In the process, undifferentiated spermatogonia become primary spermatocytes, each of which divides to form two secondary spermatocytes. Each of these divides to form two spermatids, which transform into functional motile spermatozoa. In the process, the chromosome number is reduced from the diploid to the haploid number. SEE: illus.; *gametogenesis; maturation; meiosis.*

**spermatogenic, spermatogenous** (spĕr″mă-tō-jĕn′ĭk, spĕr″mă-tŏj′ĕ-nŭs) Producing sperm.

**spermatogonium** (spĕr″măt-ō-gō′nē-ŭm) *pl.* **spermatogonia** [″ + *gone,* generation] A large unspecialized germ cell that in spermatogenesis gives rise to a primary spermatocyte. SYN: *spermatospore.* SEE: *spermatogenesis.*

**spermatoid** (spĕr′mă-toyd) [″ + *eidos,* form, shape] Resembling a spermatozoon.

**spermatology** (spĕr″mă-tŏl′ō-jē) [″ + *logos,* word, reason] The study of the seminal fluid.

**spermatolysin** (spĕr″măt-ŏl′ĭ-sĭn) [″ + *lysis,* dissolution] A lysin destroying spermatozoa.

**spermatolysis** (spĕr″măt-ŏl′ĭ-sĭs) [″ + *lysis,* dissolution] The dissolution or destruction of spermatozoa.

**spermatolytic** (spĕr″măt-ō-lĭt′ĭk) Destroying spermatozoa.

**spermatopathia, spermatopathy** (spĕr″mă-tō-păth′ē-ă, spĕr-mă-tŏp′ă-thē) [Gr. *spermatos,* seed, + *pathos,* disease] A disease of sperm cells or their secreting glands or ducts.

**spermatophobia** (spĕr″mă-tō-fō′bē-ă) [″ + *phobos,* fear] An abnormal fear of being afflicted with spermatorrhea, involuntary loss of semen.

**spermatopoietic** (spĕr″măt-ō-poy-ĕt′ĭk) [″ + *poiein,* to make] Promoting the formation and secretion of semen.

**spermatorrhea** (spĕr″mă-tō-rē′ă) [″ + *rhoia,* flow] An abnormally frequent involuntary loss of semen without orgasm.

**spermatoschesis** (spĕr″măt-ŏs′kĕ-sĭs) [″ + *schesis,* checking] Suppression of the semen.

**spermatospore** (spĕr-măt′ō-spor) [″ + *sporos,* a seed] Spermatogonium.

**spermatotoxin** (spĕr′mă-tō-tŏk′sĭn) [″ + *toxikon,* poison] Spermatoxin.

**spermatoxin** (spĕr″mă-tŏks′ĭn) [″ + *toxikon,* poison] A toxin that destroys spermatozoa. SYN: *spermatotoxin.*

**spermatozoa** (spĕr″măt-ō-zō′ă) Pl. of spermatozoon.

**spermatozoal** (spĕr″mă-tō-zō′ăl) [″ + *zoon,*

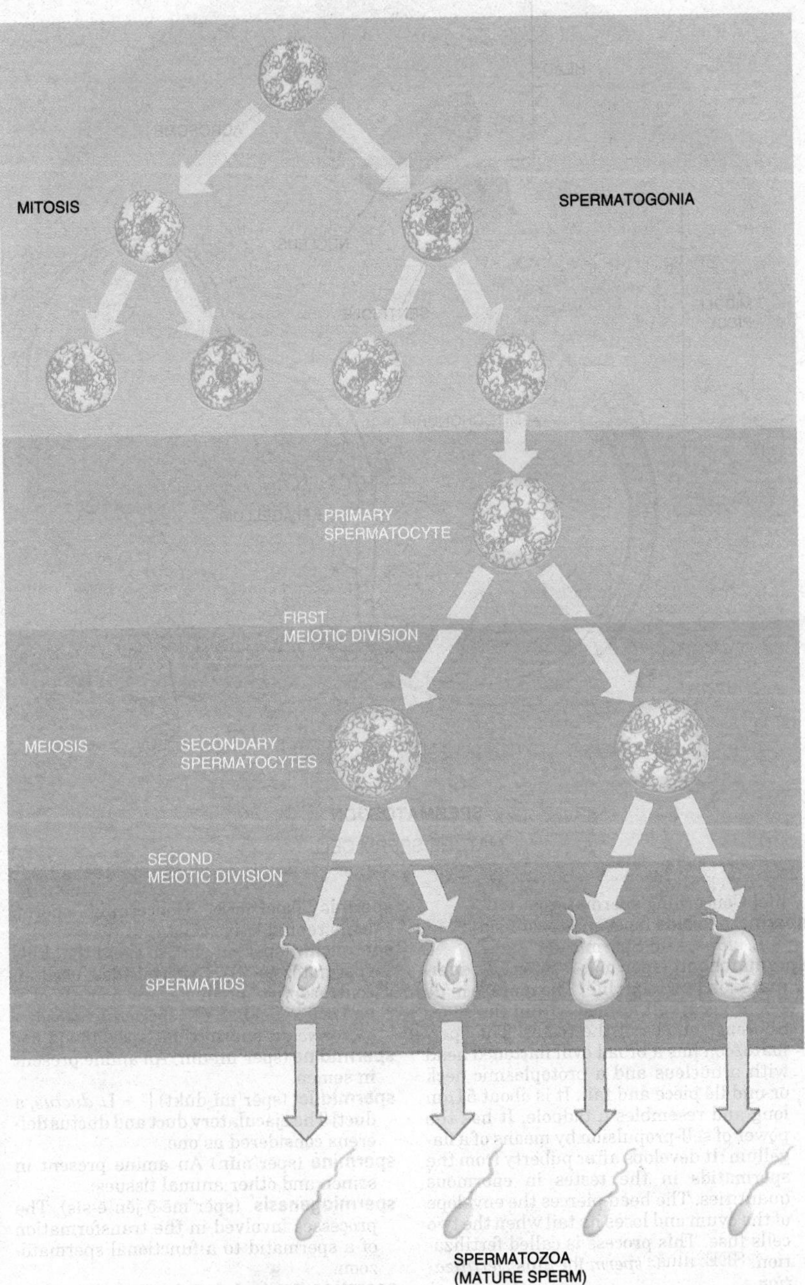


SPERMATOGENESIS

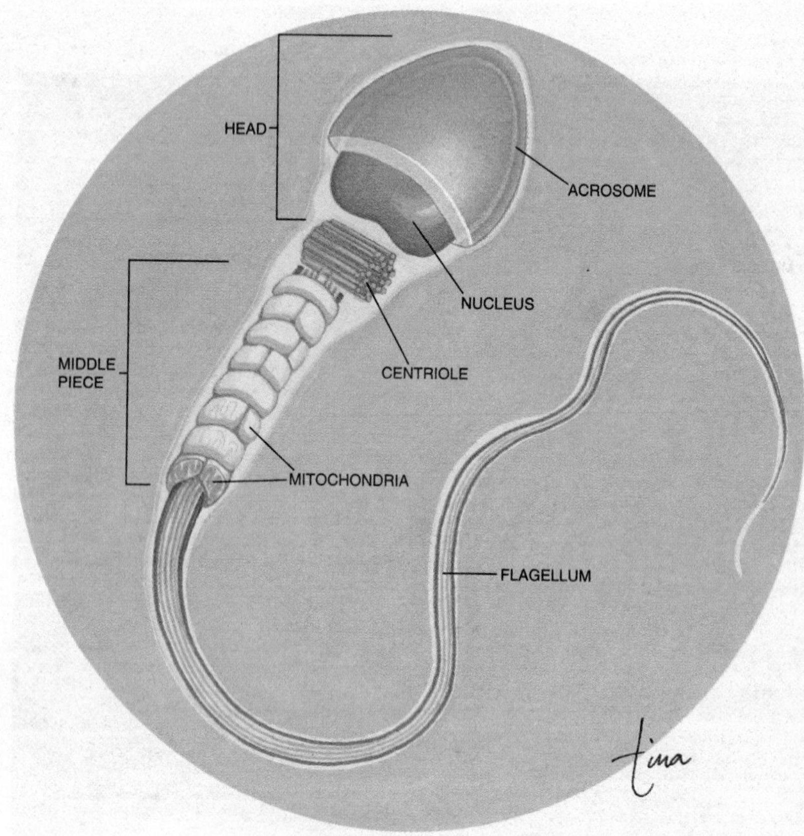


**SPERMATOZOON**

MATURE SPERM CELL

life] Concerning spermatozoa.

**spermatozoicide** (spĕr″mă-tō-zō′ĭ-sīd) [″ + ″ + L. *cidus,* kill] Spermicide.

**spermatozoon** (spĕr″măt-ō-zō′ŏn) *pl.* **spermatozoa** [″ + *zoon,* life] The mature male sex or germ cell formed within the seminiferous tubules of the testes. The spermatozoon has a broad oval flattened head with a nucleus and a protoplasmic neck or middle piece and tail. It is about 51$\mu$m long and resembles a tadpole. It has the power of self-propulsion by means of a flagellum. It develops after puberty from the spermatids in the testes in enormous quantities. The head pierces the envelope of the ovum and loses its tail when the two cells fuse. This process is called fertilization. SEE: illus.; *sperm* for illus.; *fertilization.*

**spermaturia** (spĕr″mă-tū′rē-ă) [″ + *ouron,* urine] Semen discharged with the urine.

**spermectomy** (spĕr-mĕk′tō-mē) [″ + *ektome,* excision] Resection of a portion of the spermatic cord and duct.

**spermic** (spĕr′mĭk) Concerning sperm, male reproductive cells.

**spermicide** (spĕr′mĭ-sīd) An agent that kills spermatozoa. Two spermicides used in contraceptive products are nonoxynol 9 and octoxynol 9. SYN: *spermaticide; spermatozoicide.* **spermicidal** (spĕr″mĭ-sīd′ăl).

**spermidine** (spĕr′mĭ-dĭn) An amine present in semen.

**spermiduct** (spĕr′mĭ-dŭkt) [″ + L. *ductus,* a duct] The ejaculatory duct and ductus deferens considered as one.

**spermine** (spĕr′mĭn) An amine present in semen and other animal tissues.

**spermiogenesis** (spĕr″mē-ō-jĕn′ĕ-sĭs) The processes involved in the transformation of a spermatid to a functional spermatozoon.

**spermiogram** (spĕr′mē-ō-grăm) [″ + *gramma,* something written] A record of examining and classifying sperm in a semen sample.

**spermoblast** (spĕr′mō-blăst) [″ + *blastos,* a germ] Spermatid.

**spermolith** (spĕr′mō-lĭth) [″ + *lithos,* stone] A calculus in the seminal vesicle or spermatic duct.
**spermolysin** (spĕr-mŏl′ĭ-sĭn) A cytolysin formed following the inoculation of spermatozoa.
**spermolytic** (spĕr-mō-lĭt′ĭk) [″ + *lysis,* dissolution] Causing spermatozoa destruction.
**spermoneuralgia** (spĕr″mō-nū-răl′jē-ă) [″ + *neuron,* nerve, + *algos,* pain] Neuralgic pain in the testicles and spermatic cord.
**spermophlebectasia** (spĕr″mō-flē″bĕk-tā′zē-ă) [″ + *phlebos,* vein, + *ektasis,* dilatation] Varicosity of the spermatic veins.
**spermoplasm** (spĕr′mō-plăzm) [″ + LL. *plasma,* form, mold] The protoplasm of a male germ cell.
**spermosphere** (spĕr′mō-sfēr) [″ + *sphaira,* a circle] A mass of spermatoblasts derived from spermatogonia.
**spermospore** (spĕr′mō-spor) [″ + *sporos,* seed] Spermatogonium.
**spermotoxin** (spĕr″mō-tŏk′sĭn) [″ + *toxikon,* poison] Spermatoxin.
**sp. gr.** *specific gravity.*
**sph** *spherical.*
**sphacelate** (sfăs′ĕl-āt) [Gr. *sphakelos,* gangrene] **1.** To develop gangrene. **2.** Gangrenous. SYN: *mortification; necrosis.*
**sphacelation** (sfăs″ĕl-ā′shŭn) Mortification; formation of a mass of gangrenous tissue. SYN: *gangrene; necrosis.*
**sphacelism** (sfăs′ĕl-ĭzm) [″ + *-ismos,* condition] Condition of being affected with sphacelus or gangrene. SYN: *necrosis.*
**sphaceloderma** (sfăs″ĕl-ō-dĕr′mă) [″ + *derma,* skin] Gangrene of the skin. SEE: *Raynaud's disease.*
**sphacelotoxin** (sfăs″ĕl-ō-tŏk′sĭn) [″ + *toxikon,* poison] Poisonous principle obtained from ergot, used to produce abortion.
**sphacelous** (sfăs′ĕl-ŭs) [Gr. *sphakelos,* gangrene] Pert. to a slough or patch of gangrene. SYN: *gangrenous; necrosis; necrotic.*
**sphacelus** (sfăs′ĕl-ŭs) A necrosed mass of tissue. SYN: *gangrene; mortification; necrosis; slough.*
**sphenethmoid** (sfĕn-ĕth′moyd) [Gr. *sphen,* wedge, + *ethmos,* sieve] Sphenoethmoid.
**sphenion** (sfē′nē-ŏn) *pl.* **sphenia** [Gr. *sphen,* wedge] The point at the apex of the sphenoidal angle of the parietal bone.
**spheno-** Combining form meaning *wedge,* or indicating a relationship to the sphenoid bone.
**sphenobasilar** (sfē″nō-băs′ĭ-lăr) [Gr. *sphen,* wedge, + L. *basilaris,* basal] Concerning the sphenoid bone and basilar portion of the occipital bone.
**sphenoccipital** (sfē″nŏk-sĭp′ĭ-tăl) [″ + L. *occipitalis,* occipital] Concerning the sphenoid and occipital bones.
**sphenocephalus** (sfē″nō-sĕf′ă-lŭs) [″ + *kephale,* head] A deformed fetus in which the head is wedge-shaped.
**sphenoethmoid** (sfē″nō-ĕth′moyd) [″ + *ethmos,* sieve, + *eidos,* form, shape] Pert. to the sphenoid and ethmoid bones. SYN: *sphenethmoid.*
**sphenoethmoid recess** Groove back and above the superior concha, or turbinate bone.
**sphenofrontal** (sfē″nō-frŭn′tăl) [″ + L. *frontalis,* frontal] Concerning the sphenoid and frontal bones.
**sphenoid** (sfē′noyd) [″ + *eidos,* form] Cuneiform or wedge-shaped.
**sphenoidal** (sfē-noy′dăl) Concerning the sphenoid bone.
**sphenoid bone** The large bone at the base of the skull between the occipital and ethmoid in front, and the parietal and temporal bones at the side.
**sphenoid fissure** A fissure in sphenoid and frontal bones for nerves and blood vessels.
**sphenoiditis** (sfē″noy-dī′tĭs) [″ + ″ + *itis,* inflammation] **1.** Inflammation of the sphenoidal sinus. **2.** Necrosis of the sphenoid bone.
**sphenoidostomy** (sfē″noy-dŏs′tō-mē) [″ + ″ + *stoma,* mouth] Surgically producing an opening into the sphenoid sinus.
**sphenoidotomy** (sfē″noyd-ŏt′ō-mē) [″ + ″ + *tome,* incision] Incision into the sphenoid bone.
**sphenomalar** (sfē″nō-mā′lăr) [″ + L. *mala,* cheek] Concerning the sphenoid and malar bones.
**sphenomaxillary** (sfē″nō-măk′sĭ-lā-rē) [″ + L. *maxilla,* jawbone] Concerning the sphenoid bone and the maxilla.
**spheno-occipital** (sfē″nō-ŏk-sĭp′ĭ-tăl) [″ + L. *occipitalis,* occipital] Concerning the sphenoid and occipital bones.
**sphenopalatine** (sfē″nō-păl′ă-tēn) [″ + L. *palatum,* palate] Concerning the sphenoid and palatine bones.
**sphenoparietal** (sfē″nō-pă-rī′ĕ-tăl) [″ + L. *paries,* a wall] Concerning the sphenoid and parietal bones.
**sphenorbital** (sfē″nor′bĭ-tăl) [″ + L. *orbita,* track] Concerning the sphenoid bone and the orbits.
**sphenosis** [Gr., wedging] A condition in which fetus becomes wedged in the pelvis.
**sphenosquamosal** (sfē″nō-skwā-mō′săl) [Gr. *sphen,* wedge, + L. *squamosa,* scaly] Concerning the sphenoid bone and the squamous portion of the temporal bone.
**sphenotemporal** (sfē″nō-tĕm′pō-răl) [″ + L. *temporalis,* temporal] Concerning the sphenoid and temporal bones.
**sphenotic** (sfē-nŏt′ĭk) [Gr. *sphen,* wedge, + *eidos,* form, shape] A fetal bone that becomes part of the sphenoid bone.
**sphenotribe** (sfē′nō-trīb) [″ + *tribein,* to crush] An instrument for breaking up the basal part of the fetal cranium.
**sphenoturbinal** (sfē″nō-tŭr′bĭ-năl) [″ + *turbo,* whirl] A thin curved bone anterior to each of the lesser wings of the sphenoid bone.
**sphenovomerine** (sfē″nō-vō′mĕr-ĭn) [″ + L. *vomer,* plowshare] Concerning the sphenoid and vomer bones.
**sphenozygomatic** (sfē″nō-zī″gō-măt′ĭk) [″ +

*zygoma,* cheekbone] Concerning the sphenoid and zygomatic bones.

**sphere** (sfēr) [Gr. *sphaira,* a globe] A ball or globelike structure.

***attraction s.*** A clear region in the cytoplasm close to the nucleus and usually containing a centriole or diplosome (a divided centriole).

***segmentation s.*** The segmented ovum or morula.

**spheresthesia** (sfēr″ĕs-thē′zē-ă) [″ + *aisthesis,* sensation] A morbid sensation, as of a ball or lump ascending from the stomach to the throat; seen in hysteria and other neuroses. SYN: *globus hystericus.*

**spherical** (sfĕr′ĭ-kăl) [Gr. *sphairikos*] Having the form of or pert. to a sphere. SYN: *globular.*

**spherocylinder** (sfē″rō-sĭl′ĭn-dĕr) [Gr. *sphaira,* globe, + *kylindros,* cylinder] A lens with a spherical surface and a cylindrical surface.

**spherocyte** (sfē′rō-sīt) [″ + *kytos,* cell] An erythrocyte that assumes a spheroid shape, and has no central pallor. SEE: illus.

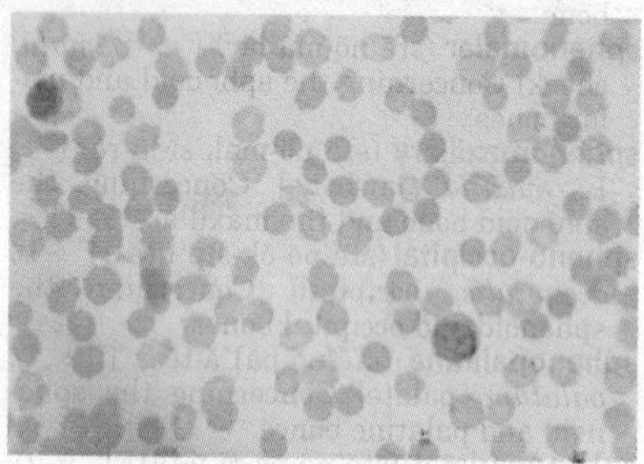

SPHEROCYTES IN PERIPHERAL BLOOD (ORIG. MAG. ×400)

**spherocytosis** (sfē″rō-sī-tō′sĭs) [″ + ″ + *osis,* condition] A condition in which erythrocytes assume a spheroid shape. It occurs in certain hemolytic anemias.

***hereditary s.*** An inherited chronic disease characterized by hemolysis, anemia, spherocytosis, jaundice, and splenomegaly. The only effective treatment is splenectomy but this should be delayed until after the first decade of life. If done prior to age 10, post-splenectomy septicemia may be fatal.

**spheroid** (sfē′royd) [″+ *eidos,* form, shape] **1.** A body shaped like a sphere. **2.** Sphere-shaped.

**spheroidal** (sfē-roy′dăl) Sphere-shaped.

**spherolith** (sfē′rō-lĭth) [″ + *lithos,* stone] A minute concretion in the kidney of the newborn.

**spheroma** (sfē-rō′mă) [″ + *oma,* tumor] A tumor of spherical form.

**spherometer** (sfē-rŏm′ĕt-ĕr) [″ + *metron,* measure] A device to ascertain the curvature of a surface.

**spheroplast** (sfĕr′ō-plăst) In bacteriology, the cell wall remaining after gram-negative organisms have been lysed. Spheroplasts may be formed when synthesis of the cell wall is prevented by the action of certain chemicals while cells are growing. SEE: *protoplast.*

**spherospermia** (sfē″rō-spĕr′mē-ă) [″ + *sperma,* seed] Round spermatozoa without tails.

**spherule** (sfĕr′ūl) [LL. *sphaerula,* little globe] **1.** A very small sphere. **2.** A minute granule found in the center of a centromere of a chromosome. **3.** The structures present in tissues infected with *Coccidioides immitis.* These spherules contain up to hundreds of endospores.

**sphincter** (sfĭngk′tĕr) [Gr. *sphinkter,* band] A circular muscle constricting an orifice. In normal tonic condition, it closes the orifice, that is, the muscle must relax to allow the orifice to open.

***s. ampullae*** A delicate network of fibers about the papilla of Vater, occasionally present in adults, a part of the sphincter of Oddi.

***s. ani*** A sphincter that closes the anus, the external one being of striated muscle, the internal one, of smooth muscle.

***bladder s.*** The smooth muscle about the opening of the bladder into the urethra.

***cardiac s.*** The smooth muscle around the opening of the esophagus into the stomach. SYN: *lower esophageal s.*

***s. choledochus*** The smooth muscle investing the common bile duct just before its junction with the pancreatic duct; a part of the sphincter of Oddi.

***ileocecal s.*** A projection of the ileum into the cecum that acts as a sphincter. SEE: *valve, ileocecal.*

***lower esophageal s.*** Cardiac s.

***s. of Oddi*** A contracted region at the opening of the common bile duct into the duodenum at the papilla of Vater.

***s. pancreaticus*** The smooth muscle encircling the pancreatic duct just before it joins the ampulla.

***precapillary s.*** A smooth muscle cell found at the beginning of a capillary network. It regulates capillary blood flow according to the needs of the tissue. SEE: *artery* for illus.

***pyloric s.*** The smooth muscle around the opening of the stomach into the duodenum.

**sphincteral** (sfĭngk′tĕr-ăl) Concerning a sphincter.

**sphincteralgia** (sfĭngk″tĕr-ăl′jē-ă) [Gr. *sphinkter,* band, + *algos,* pain] Pain in the sphincter ani muscles.

**sphincterectomy** (sfĭngk″tĕr-ĕk′tō-mē) [″+ *ektome,* excision] **1.** Excision of any sphincter muscle. **2.** Excision of part of the iris' pupillary border.

**sphincteric** (sfĭngk-tĕr′ĭk) Concerning a sphincter.

**sphincterismus** (sfĭngk″tĕr-ĭz′mŭs) [″ + *-ismos,* condition] A spasm of the sphincter ani muscles.

**sphincteritis** (sfĭngk″tĕr-ī′tĭs) [″ + *itis,* inflammation] Inflammation of any sphincter muscle.

**sphincterolysis** (sfĭngk″tĕr-ŏl′ĭ-sĭs) [″ + *lysis,* dissolution] Freeing of the iris from the cornea in anterior synechia affecting only the pupillary border.

**sphincteroplasty** (sfĭngk′tĕr-ō-plăs″tē) [″ + *plassein,* to form] A plastic operation on any sphincter muscle.

**sphincteroscope** (sfĭngk′tĕr-ō-skōp″) [″ + *skopein,* to examine] An instrument for inspection of the anal sphincter.

**sphincteroscopy** (sfĭngk″tĕr-ŏs′kō-pē) Inspection of the internal anal sphincter.

**sphincterotome** (sfĭngk′tĕr-ō-tōm″) [″ + *tome,* incision] A surgical instrument for cutting a sphincter.

**sphincterotomy** (sfĭngk″tĕr-ŏt′ō-mē) [″ + *tome,* incision] The cutting of a sphincter muscle.

**sphingolipid** (sfĭng″gō-lĭp′ĭd) [Gr. *sphingein,* to bind, + *lipos,* fat] A lipid containing one of several long-chain bases such as sphingosine or dihydrosphingosine or bases of similar chemical structure but containing longer chains.

**sphingolipidosis** [″ + ″ + *osis,* condition] Any disease marked by a defective metabolism of sphingolipids. These genetically determined errors of metabolism include Sandhoff's disease, Fabry's disease, Tay-Sachs disease, Kufs' disease, Gaucher's disease, Krabbe's leukodystrophy, Niemann-Pick disease, Batten disease, and Spielmeyer-Vogt disease. They are marked by neurological deterioration, usually beginning a few months after birth and eventually leading to death except in the adult form of Gaucher's disease. These diseases can be detected by examining fluid obtained by amniocentesis.

**sphingolipodystrophy** (sfĭng″gō-lĭp″ō-dĭs′trō-fē) [″ + *dys,* bad, + *trophe,* nutrition] A group of diseases caused by defective sphingolipid metabolism.

**sphingomyelins** (sfĭng″gō-mī′ĕl-ĭns) A major group of phosphorus-containing sphingolipids. They are found primarily in nervous tissue and in lipids in the blood. They are derived from choline phosphate and a ceramide.

**sphingosine** (sfĭng′gō-sĭn) A long-chain base, $C_{18}H_{37}O_2N$, present in sphingolipids. SEE: *dihydrosphingosine; sphingolipid.*

**sphygmic** (sfĭg′mĭk) [Gr. *sphygmikos*] Rel. to the pulse.

**sphygmo-** Combining form meaning *pulse.*

**sphygmobolometer** (sfĭg″mō-bō-lŏm′ĕ-tĕr) [Gr. *sphygmos,* pulse, + *bolos,* mass, + *metron,* a measure] A device used to measure the force of the pulse rather than the blood pressure.

**sphygmocardiogram** (sfĭg″mō-kăr′dē-ō-grăm) [″ + *kardia,* heart, + *gramma,* something written] A tracing made by a sphygmocardiograph of the heartbeat and radial pulse.

**sphygmocardiograph** (sfĭg″mō-kăr′dē-ō-grăf) [″ + ″ + *graphein,* to write] A device used for the simultaneous recording of the radial pulse and the heartbeat. SYN: *sphygmocardioscope.*

**sphygmocardioscope** (sfĭg″mō-kăr′dē-ō-skōp) [″ + ″ + *skopein,* to examine] Sphygmocardiograph.

**sphygmochronograph** (sfĭg″mō-krō′nō-grăf) [″ + *chronos,* time, + *graphein,* to write] A sphygmograph recording of the time interval between the heartbeat and the pulse.

**sphygmogram** (sfĭg′mō-grăm) [″ + *gramma,* something written] A tracing of the pulse made by using the sphygmograph.

**sphygmograph** (sfĭg′mō-grăf) [″ + *graphein,* to write] Polygraph.

**sphygmography** (sfĭg-mŏg′ră-fē) Recording the arterial pulse by use of a polygraph.

**sphygmoid** (sfĭg′moyd) [Gr. *sphygmos,* pulse, + *eidos,* form, shape] Resembling the pulse.

**sphygmology** (sfĭg-mŏl′ō-jē) [″ + *logos,* word, reason] The scientific study of the pulse.

**sphygmomanometer** (sfĭg″mō-măn-ŏm′ĕt-ĕr) [″ + *manos,* thin, + *metron,* measure] An instrument for determining arterial blood pressure indirectly. The two types are aneroid and mercury. SEE: *blood pressure.*

***random-zero s.*** A special type of sphygmomanometer that allows the blood pressure to be taken without the observer's knowing where zero pressure is on the device. After the pressure is obtained, the mercury comes to rest at a point. The observed pressure is then corrected by subtracting the at-rest value on the device from the pressure obtained. Although this device was developed to prevent subjective bias in determining blood pressure, it is not necessarily effective in achieving this goal.

**sphygmometer** (sfĭg-mŏm′ĕt-ĕr) [″ + *metron,* measure] An instrument for measuring the pulse. SYN: *polygraph.*

**sphygmopalpation** (sfĭg″mō-păl-pā′shŭn) [″ + L. *palpatio,* palpation] Palpating the pulse.

**sphygmophone** (sfĭg′mō-fōn) [Gr. *sphygmos,* pulse, + *phone,* voice] Instrument for hearing the pulse beat.

**sphygmoplethysmograph** (sfĭg″mō-plĕth-ĭz′mō-grăf) [″ + *plethysmos,* to increase, + *graphein,* to write] A device that traces the pulse with its curve of fluctuation in volume.

**sphygmoscope** (sfĭg′mō-skōp) [″ + *skopein,* to examine] An instrument for showing the heart's movements or pulsations of arteries and veins.

**sphygmosystole** (sfĭg″mō-sĭs′tō-lē) [Gr. *sphygmos,* pulse, + *systole,* contraction]

The segment of the sphygmogram that corresponds to the heart's systole.

**sphygmotonograph** (sfĭg″mō-tō′nō-grăf) [″ + *tonos,* tension, + *graphein,* to write] An instrument for the simultaneous recording and timing of arterial blood pressure, the jugular or carotid pulse, and the brachial pulse.

**sphygmotonometer** (sfĭg″mō-tō-nŏm′ĕt-ĕr) [″ + ″ + *metron,* measure] An instrument for ascertaining the elasticity of walls of an artery.

**sphygmus** (sfĭg′mŭs) [Gr. *sphygmos,* pulse] A pulse or pulsation.

**sphyrectomy** (sfī-rĕk′tō-mē) [Gr. *sphyra,* malleus, + *ektome,* excision] Surgical excision of the malleolus of the ankle.

**sphyrotomy** (sfī-rŏt′ō-mē) [″ + *tome,* incision] Surgical excision of a portion of the malleolus of the ankle.

**spica** (spī′kă) [L., ear of grain] SEE: *bandage, spica.*

**spica hip cast** A cast containing the lower torso and extending to one or both lower extremities. If only one lower extremity is included, it is called a single hip spica; if two are included, it is called a double hip spica. These are used for treating pelvic and femoral fractures.

**spicular** (spĭk′ū-lar) [L. *spiculum,* a dart] Pert. to or resembling a spicule; dartlike.

**spicule** (spĭk′ūl) A small, needle-shaped body. SYN: *spiculum.*

***bony s.*** A needle-shaped fragment of bone.

***cemental s.*** An excementosis or pointed protuberance extending from the surface cementum of a tooth root.

**spiculed red cell** Crenated red blood cells with surface projections. In most instances, this is a normal variation in red cell equilibrium, and is reversible. SEE: *acanthocyte.*

**spiculum** (spĭk′ū-lŭm) *pl.* **spicula** [L., a dart] Spicule.

**spider** (spī′dĕr) **1.** An arachnid, belonging to the order Araneae, class Arachnida, phylum Arthropoda. The body is divided into cephalothorax and abdomen joined by a narrow waist. A spider usually possesses four pairs of legs as well as poison fangs. It often possesses spinnerets. **2.** Anything resembling a spider in appearance.

***arterial s.*** SEE: *spider nevus.*

***s. bite*** SEE: *black widow s.; brown recluse s.*

***black widow s.*** The female of *Latrodectus mactans.* It is glossy black with a brilliant red or yellow spot, usually shaped like an hourglass or two triangles, on the undersurface of the abdomen. Its bite causes excruciating pain and may prove fatal. The bite of a black widow spider initially produces a sensation resembling the prick of a pin. Pain usually lasts for a short period of time and then subsides; later the abdominal muscles become rigid. Within ½ hr, severe abdominal cramps begin. The venom, which is neurotoxic, causes an ascending motor paralysis. Because of the extreme abdominal pain, the patient may be suspected of having an acute condition requiring abdominal surgery. If bitten, all stimulants should be avoided. Suction is of little value as the toxin is rapidly absorbed. Intravenous morphine or benzodiazepine, given slowly and repeated when necessary, controls the pain.

Caution: Respiratory status must be carefully monitored when morphine or benzodiazepine are used.

Heat should be applied either locally or by using a hot tub bath. Forcing fluids is also recommended. Tetanus prophylaxis should be administered. A specific antivenin, *Latrodectus mactans,* is available. This horse serum–containing preparation should be given intramuscularly as soon as the diagnosis is made if respiratory arrest, seizures, or uncontrolled hypotension is present or if the patient is pregnant.

Caution: There is risk of acute hypersensitivity and delayed serum sickness when this antivenin is used.

***brown recluse s.*** *Loxosceles reclusa,* a small, ⅜ in. (10 mm) long spider native to North America. Its venom is quite toxic and is capable of causing death. The venom produces a large area of necrosis at the site of the bite. The venom of the brown recluse spider may produce a large area of necrosis at the site of the bite. Dapsone, if used within the first few days following the bite, may decrease or prevent wound necrosis; however, prior to its use the patient should be tested for G-6-PD deficiency. Ulcers should be cleansed with a solution of hydrogen peroxide suitable for topical applications. Debridement is done if eschar develops. Tetanus prophylaxis should be administered. An antivenin is being investigated experimentally.

**spider-burst** An area on the leg in which capillaries radiate from a central point. The veins, though dilated, are not varicosities.

**spider fingers** Arachnodactyly.

**spider nevus** A branched growth of dilated capillaries on the skin, resembling a spider. This abnormality may be associated with cirrhosis of the liver. SYN: *nevus araneus.* SEE: illus.

**Spielmeyer-Vogt disease** [Walter Spielmeyer, Ger. neurologist, 1879–1935; Oskar Vogt, Ger. neurologist, 1870–1959] Batten disease.

**spigelian line** (spī-jē′lē-ăn) [Adriaan van den Spieghel, Flemish anatomist, 1578–1625] A line on the abdomen lying paral-

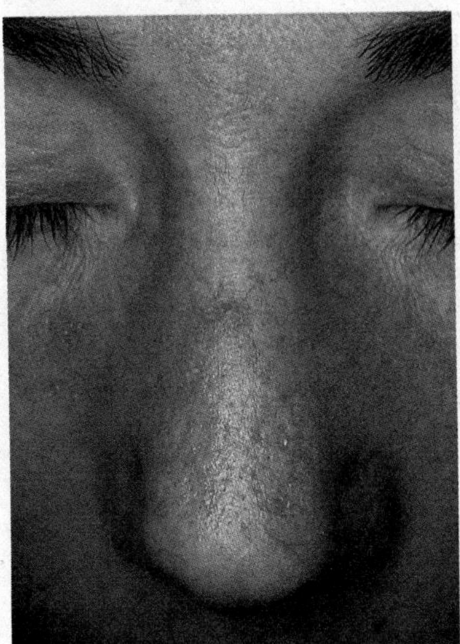

SPIDER NEVUS

lel to the median line and marking the edge of the rectus abdominis muscle. SYN: *linea semilunaris; semilunar line.*

**spigelian lobe** A small lobe behind the right lobe of the liver.

**spike** The main peak in an oscillographical record of the action potential.

**spikeboard** An adapted device for persons with limited upper extremity or one-handed function that allows food to be held in place while it is being prepared.

**spill** (spĭl) [AS. *spillan,* to squander] An overflow.

***cellular s.*** A dissemination of cells through the lymph or the blood resulting in metastasis.

***radioactive s.*** A massive leak of radioactive materials from any source of those materials. SEE: *radiation accidents, emergency handling of.*

**spillway** (spĭl′way) The contour of the teeth that allows food to escape from the cusps during mastication.

**spiloma, spilus** (spī-lō′mă, spī′lŭs) [Gr. *spiloma, spilos,* spot] Nevus.

**spina** (spī′nă) *pl.* **spinae** [L., thorn] **1.** Any spinelike protuberance. **2.** The spine.

***s. bifida cystica*** A congenital defect in the walls of the spinal canal caused by a lack of union between the laminae of the vertebrae. The lumbar portion is the section chiefly affected. As result of this defect, the membranes of the cord are pushed through the opening, forming a tumor known as spina bifida cystic and hydrorrhachis, a condition caused by the fluid contained in the tumor. SYN: *rachischisis.*

***s. bifida occulta*** A failure of the vertebrae to close, without hernial protrusion.

**spinal** (spī′năl) [L. *spinalis*] Pert. to the spine or spinal cord. SYN: *rachial; rachidial.*

**spinal accessory nerve** Accessory nerve.

**spinal anesthesia** Anesthesia produced by an anesthetic injected into the spinal canal. SYN: *narcosis, medullary.*

**spinal canal** A canal of the vertebral column that contains the spinal cord.

**spinal column** The vertebral column enclosing the spinal cord and consisting of 33 vertebrae: seven cervical, 12 dorsal or thoracic, five lumbar, five sacral fused to form one bone, and four in the coccyx fused to form one bone. The number is sometimes increased by an additional vertebra in one region, and sometimes one may be absent in another. SEE: illus.

**spinal cord** An ovoid column of nerve tissue averaging about 44 cm in length, flattened anteroposteriorly, extending from the medulla to the second lumbar vertebra in the spinal canal. Most nerves to the trunk and limbs emerge from the spinal cord, a reflex center for spinal cord reflexes that conducts impulses to and from the brain. In cross section, it does not fill the vertebral space, being surrounded by the pia mater, the cerebrospinal fluid, the arachnoid, and the dura mater, which fuses with the periosteum of the inner surfaces of the vertebrae. The gray matter approximates the shape of an “H,” there being a posterior and an anterior horn in either half. The anterior horn is composed of motor cells from which the fibers making up the motor portions of the peripheral nerves arise. Sensory neurons enter posteriorly. The “H” also divides the surrounding white matter into posterior, lateral, and anterior bundles. These connect the brain and spinal cord in both directions (i.e., with descending and ascending neurons) as well as various portions of the cord itself. SEE: illus.

**spinal cord injury, acute** Acute traumatic injury of the spinal cord. Therapy for this condition includes immobilization, airway maintenance, cardiovascular resuscitation, and insertion of an indwelling catheter. The use of intravenous methylprednisolone given as a bolus dose of 30 mg/kg and then a maintenance dose of 5.4 mg/kg/hr during the acute phase improves neurological recovery.

**spinal curvature** Abnormal curvature of the spine, frequently constitutional in children. It may be angular, lateral (scoliosis), or anteroposterior (kyphosis, lordosis).

**spinal curvature, angular** Pott’s disease.

**spinal curvature, lateral** A deviation of the spine to one side or the other causing a twist of the spine.

**spinal fluid** Cerebrospinal fluid. When normal, it contains 50 to 75 mg of glucose per 100 ml. Its glucose content is lower than that of the blood.

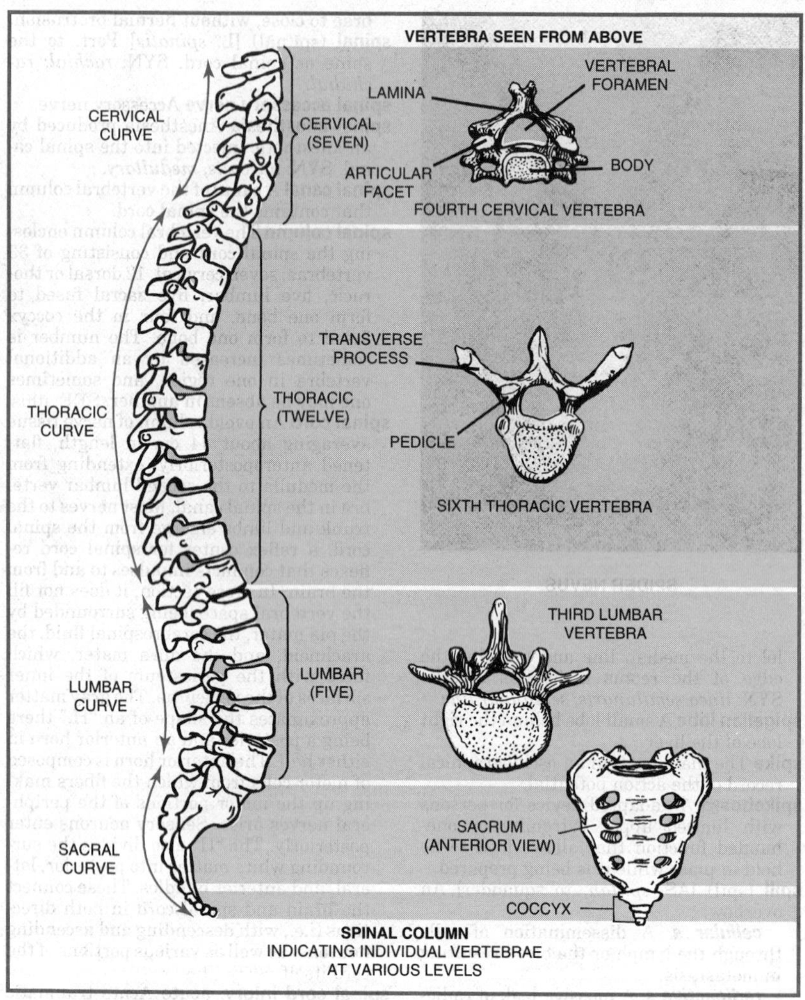

SPINAL COLUMN
INDICATING INDIVIDUAL VERTEBRAE AT VARIOUS LEVELS

DIAGNOSIS: If normal, the cell count is 0 to 5 mononuclear cells per milliliter. This is increased in all diseased states, to hundreds or thousands in meningitis, when fluid becomes opaque. Lymphocytes are found in encephalitis and tuberculous meningitis; polymorphonuclears predominate in septic meningitis and epidemic meningitis. Brain hemorrhages due to arteriosclerosis, high blood pressure, tumors, and other causes lead to bloody fluid. Spinal fluid may contain blood also as a result of a needle having punctured a small blood vessel. In encephalitis, sugar content is increased, the fluid is clear, and the cell count is 100 plus. The presence of globulin in the fluid is abnormal.

*Microorganisms:* Meningococci, streptococci, pneumococci, tubercle bacilli, and influenza bacilli may be present, any of which may be indicative of meningitis. Epidemic meningitis is indicated by gram-negative, intracellular diplococcus, biscuit-shaped microorganisms. Typhoid bacilli may produce meningeal symptoms in typhoid fever. Streptococci may enter the meninges through the ear; the invading point of pneumococci, influenza bacilli, and pneumobacilli is usually the lungs. All these may be found in smears or in culture of the spinal fluid. In meningitis, the spinal fluid glucose level is usually 40% lower than that of blood measured at the same time. In suppurative meningitis, the spinal fluid is puslike and turbid, but it is clear in tuberculous meningitis, encephalitis, and poliomyelitis. In poliomyelitis, the spinal fluid is the same as in encephalitis.

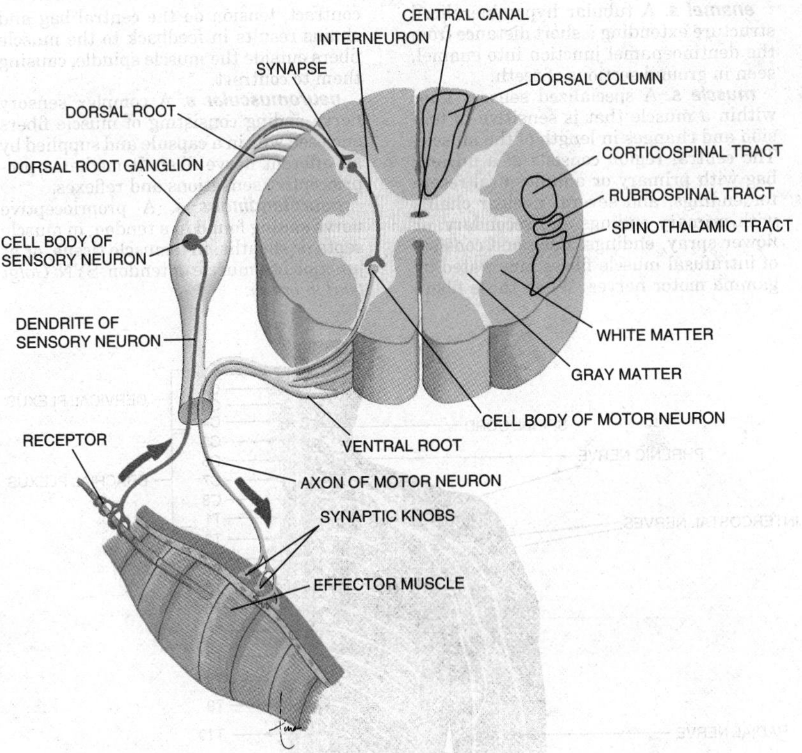


SPINAL CORD

CROSS-SECTION WITH NERVE ROOTS ON LEFT SIDE AND EXAMPLES OF TRACTS ON RIGHT SIDE

**spinal fusion** Surgical immobilization of adjacent vertebrae. This procedure may be done for several conditions, including herniated disk.

**spinal ganglion** An enlargement on the dorsal or posterior root of a spinal nerve, composed principally of cell bodies of somatic and visceral afferent neurons. Also called *dorsal root ganglion*.

**spinalgia** (spī-năl′jē-ă) [L. *spina*, thorn, + Gr. *algos*, pain] Pain in a vertebra under pressure.

**spinalis** (spī-nā′lĭs) [L.] A muscle attached to the spinal process of a vertebra. SEE: *Muscles Appendix*.

**spinal nerve** One of the nerves arising from the spinal cord: 31 pairs, consisting of eight cervical, 12 thoracic, five lumbar, five sacral, and one coccygeal, corresponding with the spinal vertebrae. Each spinal nerve is attached to the spinal cord by two roots: a dorsal or posterior sensory root and a ventral or anterior root. The former consists of afferent fibers conveying impulses to the cord; the latter of efferent fibers conveying impulses from the cord. A typical spinal nerve, on passing through the intervertebral foramen, divides into four branches, a recurrent branch, a dorsal ramus or posterior primary division, a ventral ramus or anterior primary division, and two rami communicantes (white and gray), which pass to ganglia of the sympathethic trunk. SEE: illus.

**spinal puncture** Lumbar puncture.

**spinal stenosis** Narrowing of the spinal canal due to degenerative or traumatic changes in the lumbar spine. It may cause claudication and intractable buttock and leg pain. If physical therapy, back braces, and corticosteroid injections do not provide relief, surgical decompression is indicated.

**spinate** (spī′nāt) Having spines or shaped like a thorn.

**spindle** (spĭn′dl) [AS. *spinel*] **1.** A fusiform-shaped body. **2.** The portion of the achromatic apparatus seen in mitosis consisting of a bundle of delicate fibrils that connect the two centrosomes or asters. The chromosomes arrange themselves on the spindle in an equatorial plate.

***aortic s.*** A dilatation of the aorta following the aortic isthmus.

***enamel s.*** A tubular hypomineralized structure extending a short distance from the dentinoenamel junction into enamel, seen in ground sections of teeth.

***muscle s.*** A specialized sensory fiber within a muscle that is sensitive to tension and changes in length of the muscle. The central region consists of a nuclear bag with primary or annulospiral receptor endings, and several nuclear chains with primary endings and secondary, or flower spray, endings. Each end consists of intrafusal muscle fibers innervated by gamma motor nerves. When these fibers contract, tension on the central bag and chains results in feedback to the muscle fibers outside the muscle spindle, causing them to contract.

***neuromuscular s.*** A complex sensory nerve ending consisting of muscle fibers enclosed within a capsule and supplied by an afferent nerve fiber. It mediates proprioceptive sensations and reflexes.

***neurotendinous s.*** A proprioceptive nerve ending found in a tendon, in muscle septa or sheaths, in a muscle tissue, or at junction of a muscle or tendon. SYN: *Golgi tendon organ.*

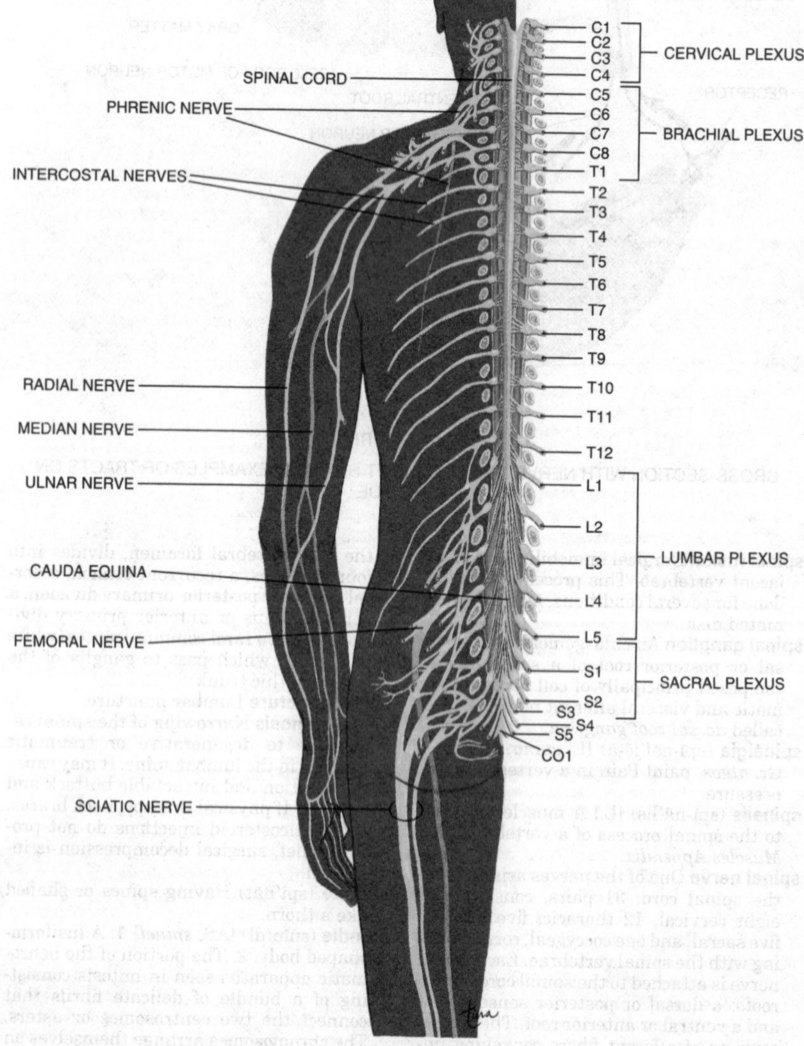


SPINAL NERVES
(LEFT SIDE)

***sleep s.*** Specific waves that appear in the electroencephalogram during light or early sleep.

**spine** (spīn) **1.** A sharp process of bone. **2.** The spinal column, consisting of 33 vertebrae: seven cervical, 12 thoracic, five lumbar, five sacral, and four coccygeal. The bones of the sacrum and coccyx are ankylosed in adult life and counted as one each. SYN: *backbone.*

***alar s.*** The spinous process of the sphenoid bone.

***anterior nasal s.*** The projection formed by the anterior prolongation of the inferior border of the nasal notch of the maxilla.

***bifid s.*** SEE: *spina bifida cystica; spina bifida occulta.*

***fracture of the s.*** A fractured spine often is treated in a plaster jacket with the spine hyperextended to reduce the fracture after essential treatment with skeletal traction. A window is cut in the cast over the abdomen. If the fracture is high, the neck is included. The jacket must be short enough to allow flexion of the thighs. The patient is allowed to walk in the jacket, which is left on for 3 or 4 months. A vest is put on under this plaster, and the prominences are padded with felt.

Traction and Balkan and Stryker frames are used if the fracture involves the cord with paralysis below the injury. Bedsores and urinary tract infections must be prevented. An enema is given when needed.

***frontal s.*** A sharp-pointed medial process extending downward from the nasal process of the frontal bone. SYN: *nasal s.*

***hemal s.*** That part of the hemal arch of a typical vertebra that closes it in.

***Henle's s.*** Suprameatal s.

***iliac s.*** One of four spines of the ilium; namely, the anterior and posterior inferior spines and the anterior and posterior superior spines.

***ischial s.*** The spine of the ischium, a pointed eminence on its posterior border.

***mandibular s.*** The small, tongue-shaped protuberance on the medial aspect of the mandibular ramus near the mandibular foramen, to which the sphenomandibular ligament is attached.

***mental s.*** A small process on the inner surface of the mandible at the back of the symphysis formed of one or more small projections (genial tubercles).

***nasal s.*** Frontal s.

***neural s.*** The spinous process of a vertebra; the posterior projection of the neural arch.

***pharyngeal s.*** The ridge under the basilar process of the occipital bone.

***posterior nasal s.*** The spine formed by medial ends of the horizontal processes of the palatine bones.

***s. of pubis*** A prominent tubercle on the upper border of the pubis.

***s. of scapula*** An osseous plate projecting from the posterior surface of the scapula.

***s. of sphenoid*** The spinous process of the greater sphenoid wing.

***suprameatal s.*** A small spine at the junction of the superior and posterior walls of the external auditory meatus. SYN: *Henle's s.*

***typhoid s.*** An acute arthritis due to infection causing spinal ankylosis during or following typhoid fever.

**spinifugal** (spī-nĭf′ū-găl) [L. *spina,* thorn, + *fugare,* to flee] Moving away from the spinal cord.

**spinipetal** (spī-nĭp′ĕ-tăl) [″ + *petere,* to seek] Conducting nerve impulses toward the spinal cord.

**spinnbarkeit** (spĭn′băr-kīt) [Ger.] ABBR: SBK. Evaluation of the elasticity of cervical mucus used to determine time of ovulation. The cervical secretion is aspirated and placed on a slide. SBK is measured by pulling upward on the secretion with a forceps. Before ovulation, there is no elasticity. On the day of ovulation, elasticity is good, measuring 12 to 24 cm or more. The day after ovulation, elasticity diminishes. Not all women have clear-cut SBK changes. Therefore, this test is used in conjunction with other signs of ovulation. SEE: *basal temperature chart; fern pattern; mittelschmerz; mucorrhea.*

**spinobulbar** (spī″nō-bŭl′băr) [″ + Gr. *bulbos,* a bulb] Concerning the spinal cord and medulla oblongata.

**spinocellular** (spī″nō-sĕl′ū-lăr) [″ + *cellula,* little cell] Pert. to or like prickle cells.

**spinocerebellar** (spī″nō-sĕr-ĕ-bĕl′ăr) [″ + *cerebellum,* little brain] Concerning the spinal cord and cerebellum.

**spinocortical** (spī″nō-kor′tĭ-kăl) [″ + *cortex,* rind] Corticospinal.

**spinocostalis** (spī″nō-kŏs-tā′lĭs) [″ + *costa,* rib] The combination of the superior and inferior serratus muscles.

**spinoglenoid** (spī″nō-glĕn′oyd) [″ + Gr. *glene,* socket, + *eidos,* form, shape] Rel. to the spine of the scapula and the glenoid cavity.

**spinoglenoid ligament** The ligament joining the spine of the scapula to the border of the glenoid cavity.

**spinose** (spī′nōs) [L. *spina,* thorn] Spinous.

**spinotectal** (spī″nō-tĕk′tăl) [″ + *tectum,* roof] Pert. to the spinal cord and the tectum, the dorsal portion (corpora quadrigemina) of the midbrain.

**spinous** (spī′nŭs) [L. *spina,* thorn] Pert. to or resembling a spine. SYN: *spinose.*

**spinous point** A spot over a spinous process very sensitive to pressure.

**spinous process** The prominence at the posterior part of each vertebra.

**spintheropia** (spĭn″thĕr-ō′pē-ă) [Gr. *spinther,* spark, + *ops,* eye] A sensation of sparks before the eyes. SEE: *Moore's lightning streaks.*

**spiradenitis** (spī″răd-ĕn-ī′tĭs) [Gr. *speira,*

coil, + *aden,* gland, + *itis,* inflammation] A funiculus beginning in the coil of a sweat gland. SEE: *hidrosadenitis.*

**spiradenoma** (spī″răd-ĕn-ō′mă) [″ + ″ + *oma,* tumor] A benign tumor of the sweat glands. SYN: *spiroma.*

**spiral** (spī′răl) [L. *spiralis*] Coiling around a center like the thread of a screw.

***Curschmann's s.*** SEE: *Curschmann's spirals.*

**spiral bandage** A roller bandage to be applied spirally.

**spiral lamina** A thin, bony plate projecting from the modiolus into the cochlear canal, dividing it into two portions, the upper scala vestibuli and lower scala tympani. Also called *lamina spiralis.*

**spirilla** (spī-rĭl′ă) [L.] Pl. of spirillum.

**spirillicidal** (spī-rĭl″ĭ-sīd′ăl) [L. *spirillum,* coil, + *cidus,* kill] Destructive to spirochetes or spirilla.

**spirillicide** (spī-rĭl″ĭ-sīd) An agent that is destructive to spirilla.

**spirillolysis** (spī″rĭ-lŏl′ĭ-sĭs) [″ + Gr. *lysis,* dissolution] The destruction of spirilla.

**spirillosis** (spī-rĭl-ō′sĭs) [″ + Gr. *osis,* condition] A disease caused by the presence of spirilla in the blood.

**spirillotropic** (spī″rĭ-lō-trŏp′ĭk) [″ + Gr. *trope,* a turning] Having an attraction to spirilla.

**spirillotropism** (spī″rĭ-lŏt′rō-pĭzm) [″ + ″ + *-ismos,* condition] The ability to attract spirilla.

**Spirillum** (spī-rĭl′ŭm) *pl.* **Spirilla** [L., coil] A genus of spiral-shaped motile microorganisms belonging to the family Pseudomonadaceae, tribe Spirilleae. They are found in fresh water and salt water.

***S. minus*** A species found in the blood of rats and mice; the causative agent of one form of rat-bite fever.

**spirillum** *pl.* **spirilla** A flagellated aerobic bacterium with an elongated spiral shape, of the genus *Spirillum.* SEE: *bacteria* for illus.

**spirit** (spĭr′ĭt) [L. *spiritus,* breath] **1.** A solution of essential or volatile liquid. **2.** Any distilled or volatile liquid. **3.** An alcoholic beverage.

***s. of ammonia*** A pungent solution of approx. 4% ammonium carbonate in 70% alcohol flavored with lemon, lavender, and myristica oil. It is used to elicit reflex stimulation of respiration and as smelling salts to stimulate patients who have fainted.

***s. of bitter almond*** A mixture of oil of bitter almond, almond, and distilled water, used as a flavoring agent.

***s. of camphor*** A mixture of camphor and alcohol, employed locally as a counterirritant.

***s. of juniper*** A mixture of oil of juniper and alcohol.

***s. of lavender*** A mixture of oil of lavender flowers and alcohol, used as a flavoring agent.

***s. of mustard*** A solution of volatile oil of mustard in alcohol, used as a counterirritant.

***s. of peppermint*** A mixture of oil of peppermint, peppermint, and alcohol, used as a carminative.

**spiritual distress** Disruption in the life principle that pervades a person's entire being and that integrates and transcends one's biological and psychosocial nature. SEE: *Nursing Diagnoses Appendix.*

**spiritual therapy** [L. *spiritus,* breath,+ Gr. *therapeia,* treatment] The application of spiritual knowledge in the treatment of mental and physical disorders. It is based on the assumption that humans are spiritual beings living in a spiritual universe, that in proportion to their acceptance of this idea and in proportion to their success in using it, they may control their bodies and maintain the material elements in harmony with a divine plan.

**spiritual well-being, enhanced, potential for** The process of an individual's developing/unfolding or mystery through harmonious interconnectedness that springs from inner strengths. SEE: *Nursing Diagnoses Appendix.*

**spirituous** (spĭr′ĭt-ū-ŭs″) [L., *spiritus,* breath] Containing alcohol.

**spiritus** (spĭr′ĭ-tŭs) [L., breath] An alcoholic solution of a volatile substance. SYN: *spirit.* SEE: *elixir.*

***s. frumenti*** Whiskey.

***s. juniperi*** Gin.

***s. myrciae*** Bay rum.

***s. vini gallici*** Brandy.

**Spirochaeta** (spī″rō-kē′tă) [Gr. *speira,* coil, + *chaite,* hair] A genus of slender, spiral, motile microorganisms belonging to the family Spirochaetaceae, order Spirochaetales.

***S. icterohaemorrhagiae*** A species found in patients with Weil's disease or acute febrile jaundice. SYN: *Leptospira interrogans icterohaemorrhagiae.*

***S. pallida*** The microorganism that causes syphilis. SYN: *Treponema pallidum.*

**Spirochaetales** (spī″rō-kē-tā′lēs) An order of slender spiral organisms belonging to the class Schizomycetes. It includes the families Spirochaetaceae and Treponemataceae.

**spirochetal** (spī″rō-kē′tăl) [″ + *chaite,* hair] Pert. to spirochetes, esp. infections caused by them.

**spirochetalytic** (spī″rō-kē″tă-lĭt′ĭk) [″ + ″ + *lysis,* dissolution] Destructive to spirochetes.

**spirochete** (spī′rō-kēt) Any member of the order Spirochaetales.

**spirochetemia** (spī″rō-kē-tē′mē-ă) [″ + *chaite,* hair, + *haima,* blood] Spirochetes in the blood.

**spirocheticidal** (spī″rō-kē″tĭ-sī′dăl) [″ + ″ + L. *cidus,* kill] Destructive to spirochetes.

**spirocheticide** (spī″rō-kē′tĭ-sīd) Anything that destroys spirochetes.

**spirochetolysis** (spī″rō-kē-tŏl′ĭ-sĭs) [″ +

*chaite,* hair, + *lysis,* dissolution] The destruction of spirochetes by specific antibodies, chemotherapy, or lysins.

**spirochetosis** (spī″rō-kē-tō′sĭs) [″ + ″ + *osis,* condition] Any infection caused by spirochetes.

**spirochetotic** (spī″rō-kē-tŏt′ĭk) Pert. to or marked by spirochetosis.

**spirocheturia** (spī″rō-kē-tū′rē-ă) [Gr. *speira,* coil, + *chaite,* hair, + *ouron,* urine] Spirochetes in the urine.

**spirogram** (spī′rō-grăm″) [L. *spirare,* to breathe, + Gr. *gramma,* something written] A record made by a spirograph indicating respiratory movements.

**spirograph** (spī′rō-grăf) [″ + Gr. *graphein,* to write] A graphic record of respiratory movements.

**spiroid** (spī′royd) [Gr. *speira,* coil, + *eidos,* form, shape] Resembling a spiral.

**spiroma** (spī-rō′mă) [″ + *oma,* tumor] Multiple, benign, cystic epithelioma of the sweat glands. SYN: *spiradenoma.*

**spirometer** (spī-rŏm′ĕt-ĕr) [L. *spirare,* to breathe, + Gr. *metron,* measure] An apparatus, one form of which consists of a cylindrical bell immersed in water and so equipped with outlets that gases can be exhaled into it or inhaled out of it while measurements of volume are made. Less cumbersome forms are also available. The following are typical measurements made on normal men by using the spirometer:

*Complemental air (inspiratory reserve volume):* 1600 cc, the amount that a subject can still inhale by special effort after a normal inspiration.

*Dead space air:* 150 cc, the air inhaled through the nose that gets only as far as nasopharynx, bronchi, bronchioles, and trachea and does not reach the lungs.

*Functional residual air (functional residual capacity):* About 2600 cc, the sum of the supplemental and residual air.

*Minimal air:* Less than 1000 cc, that which remains in the lungs after complete collapse, as in pneumothorax.

*Reserve air:* Supplemental air.

*Residual air (residual volume):* 1000 cc, the amount left in the lungs after a complete expiration.

*Supplemental air (expiratory reserve volume):* 1600 cc that can still be exhaled after a normal exhalation.

*Tidal volume:* 500 cc, the amount exhaled or inhaled during normal respiration.

**spirometry** (spī-rŏm′ĕ-trē) [L. *spirare,* to breathe, + Gr. *metron,* measure] Measurement of the air capacity of the lungs.

***incentive s.*** Spirometry in which visual and vocal stimuli are given to the subject in an attempt to stimulate the maximum effort in performing the test.

**spironolactone** (spī-rō″nō-lăk′tōn) A diuretic drug that blocks the action of aldosterone on the renal tubules. It acts to decrease potassium loss in the urine.

**spissated** (spĭs′āt-ĕd) [L. *spissatus*] Inspissated.

**spissitude** (spĭs′ĭ-tūd) [L. *spissitudo*] The condition of being inspissated, as a fluid thickened by evaporation almost to a solid; thickness.

**spit** (spĭt) [AS. *spittan*] **1.** Saliva. **2.** To expectorate spittle.

**spittle** [AS. *spatl*] Saliva.

**splanchna** (splăngk′nă) [Gr.] The viscera.

**splanchnapophysis** (splăngk″nă-pŏf′ĭ-sĭs) [Gr. *splanchnos,* viscus, + *apophysis,* offshoot] Any skeletal element involved with the function of the alimentary canal, as the lower jaw.

**splanchnectopia** (splăngk″nĕk-tō′pē-ă) [″ + *ektopos,* out of place] Dislocation of a viscus or of the viscera.

**splanchnemphraxis** (splăngk″nĕm-frăk′sĭs) [″ + *emphraxis,* stoppage] Obstruction of any internal organ, particularly the intestine.

**splanchnesthesia** (splăngk″nĕs-thē′zē-ă) [″ + *aisthesis,* sensation] Visceral sensation.

**splanchnesthetic** (splăngk″nĕs-thĕt′ĭk) Rel. to visceral consciousness or sensation.

**splanchnic** (splăngk′nĭk) [Gr. *splanchnikos*] Pert. to the viscera.

**splanchnicectomy** (splăngk″nē-sĕk′tō-mē) [Gr. *splanchnos,* viscus, + *ektome,* excision] Resection of the splanchnic nerves.

**splanchnic nerve** One of three nerves from the thoracic sympathetic ganglia distributed to the viscera.

**splanchnicotomy** (splăngk″nĭ-kŏt′ō-mē) [″ + *tome,* incision] Section of a splanchnic nerve.

**splanchnoblast** (splăngk′nō-blăst) [″ + *blastos,* germ] Incipient rudiment of a viscus. SEE: *anlage; proton.*

**splanchnocele** (splăngk′nō-sēl) **1.** [″ + *koilos,* a cavity] That part of the coelom persisting in the adult, giving rise to the visceral cavities. SYN: *splanchnocoele.* **2.** [″ + *kele,* tumor, swelling] Protrusion of any abdominal viscus.

**splanchnocoele** (splăngk′nō-sēl) [″ + *koilos,* a cavity] Rudimentary embryonic cavity from which the visceral cavities arise. SYN: *splanchnocele* (1).

**splanchnocranium** (splăngk″nō-krā′nē-ŭm) [″ + *kranion,* skull] Viscerocranium.

**splanchnodiastasis** (splăngk″nō-dī-ăs′tă-sĭs) [″ + *diastasis,* a separation] Displacement or separation of any viscus.

**splanchnodynia** (splăngk-nō-dĭn′ē-ă) [Gr. *splanchnos,* viscus, + *odyne,* pain] Pain in the abdominal region.

**splanchnography** (splăngk-nŏg′ră-fē) [″ + *graphein,* to write] Examination of the viscera using fluoroscopy or transillumination.

**splanchnolith** (splăngk′nō-lĭth) [″ + *lithos,* stone] An intestinal calculus.

**splanchnology** (splăngk-nŏl′ō-jē) [″ + *logos,* word, reason] The study of the viscera.

**splanchnomegaly** (splăngk″nō-mĕg′ă-lē) [″ + *megas,* large] Visceromegaly.

**splanchnomicria** (splăngk″nō-mĭk′rē-ă) [″ + *mikros,* small] The condition of having small splanchnic organs.

**splanchnopathia** (splăngk″nō-păth′ē-ă) [″+ *pathos,* disease, suffering] Pathological conditions of the viscera.

**splanchnopleural** (splăngk″nō-ploor′ăl) [″ + *pleura,* side] Concerning the splanchnopleure.

**splanchnopleure** (splăngk′nō-plūr) [″ + *pleura,* side] The embryonic layer formed by the union of the visceral layer of the mesoderm with the entoderm. SEE: *somatopleure.*

**splanchnoptosia, splanchnoptosis** (splăngk″nō-tō′sē-ă, -sĭs) [″ + *ptosis,* a dropping] Prolapse of the viscera. SYN: *enteroptosis; ptosis, abdominal; visceroptosis.*

**splanchnosclerosis** (splăngk″nō-sklĕr-ō′sĭs) [″ + *sklerosis,* to harden] A hardening of any of the viscera through overgrowth or infiltration of connective tissue.

**splanchnoscopy** (splăngk-nŏs′kō-pē) [″ + *skopein,* to examine] Examination of the viscera with the aid of roentgen rays or transillumination.

**splanchnoskeleton** (splăngk″nō-skĕl′ĕ-tŏn) [″ + *skeleton,* a dried-up body] **1.** In primitive vertebrates such as fishes, the cartilaginous or bony arches (branchial) that encircle the pharyngeal portion of digestive tract. **2.** In higher vertebrates, the bones derived from the branchial arches, which include the maxilla, mandible, malleus, incus, stapes, hyoid bone, and cartilages of the larynx.

**splanchnosomatic** (splăngk″nō-sō-măt′ĭk) [″ + *soma,* body] Viscerosomatic.

**splanchnotomy** (splăngk-nŏt′ō-mē) [″+ *tome,* incision] Dissection of the viscera.

**splanchnotribe** (splăngk′nō-trīb) [″ + *tribein,* to rub] A crushing instrument for temporarily closing the lumen of the intestine prior to resection.

**splayfoot** [ME. *splayen,* to spread out, + AS. *fot,* foot] Flatfoot.

**spleen** (splēn) [Gr. *splen*] A dark red, oval organ in the upper left abdominal quadrant posterior and slightly inferior to the stomach. The outer capsule is dense connective tissue and smooth muscle fibers from which trabeculae extend into the pulp (functional tissue) of the spleen. White pulp is mostly lymphocytes and red pulp is a network of venous sinuses. On the inferior side is the hilus, an indentation at which the splenic vessels and nerves enter or exit. Disorders of the spleen include acute and chronic infections and certain infection-like states, hypersplenism, primary splenic thrombocytopenia, primary splenic neutropenia, Felty's syndrome, Banti's disease, congestive splenomegaly, and tumors. SYN: *lien.* SEE: *lymphatic system* for illus; *asplenia syndrome; thrombosis.*

FUNCTION: In the embryo, the spleen forms both red and white blood cells, but after birth, only lymphocytes and monocytes are produced. The macrophages of the spleen remove pathogens of all kinds from circulating blood; they also remove old red blood cells from circulation and form bilirubin (from the heme of the hemoglobin) that will circulate to the liver to be excreted in bile. Because it is so vascular, the spleen may be a reservoir of blood in times of emergency such as hemorrhage. Contraction of the capsule and trabeculae compress the venous sinuses and force the blood in the spleen out into general circulation.

***accessory s.*** Splenic tissue nodules near the spleen.

***floating s.*** An enlarged movable spleen that is not protected by the ribs. SYN: *splenectopia; splenectopy.*

***lardaceous s.*** An enlarged spleen resulting from fatty tissue. SEE: *degeneration, amyloid.*

***sago s.*** A spleen having the appearance of grains of sago.

**splenadenoma** (splēn″ăd-ĕ-nō′mă) [Gr. *splen,* spleen, + *aden,* gland, + *oma,* tumor] An enlarged spleen caused by hyperplasia of its pulp.

**splenalgia** (splē-năl′jē-ă) [″ + *algos,* pain] Neuralgic pain in the spleen. SYN: *splenodynia.*

**splenceratosis** (splēn″sĕr-ă-tō′sĭs) [″ + *keras,* horn, + *osis,* condition] Induration of the spleen.

**splenectasia, splenectasis** (splē″nĕk-tā′zē-ă, splē-nĕk′tă-sĭs) [″ + *ektasis,* dilatation] Enlargement of the spleen.

**splenectomy** (splē-nĕk′tō-mē) [″ + *ektome,* excision] Surgical excision of the spleen. Because of the importance of the spleen in the control of bacteria in the bloodstream, its removal in children less than 10 years of age has resulted in an abnormal risk of the development of fatal septicemia; therefore, unless the condition dictating removal of the spleen is life threatening, the procedure should be delayed. Removal of the spleen in otherwise healthy adults causes only a slight alteration in their ability to resist infections.

**splenectopia, splenectopy** (splē″nĕk-tō′pē-ă, -nĕk′tō-pē) [″ + *ektopos,* out of place] Floating spleen.

**splenelcosis** (splē″nĕl-kō′sĭs) [″ + *helkosis,* ulceration] Ulceration or abscess of the spleen.

**splenemia** (splē-nē′mē-ă) [Gr. *splen,* spleen, + *haima,* blood] **1.** Splenic congestion with blood. **2.** Leukemia with splenic hypertrophy.

**splenemphraxis** (splē″nĕm-frăk′sĭs) [″ + *emphraxis,* an obstruction] Congested condition of the spleen.

**spleneolus** (splē-nē′ō-lŭs) Accessory spleen.

**splenetic** (splē-nĕt′ĭk) **1.** Pert. to the spleen. **2.** Suffering with chronic disease of the spleen. **3.** Surly, fretful, impatient. SYN: *splenic.*

**splenetic cord** One of the poorly defined cords of red pulp of the spleen.

**splenetic nodule** A concentrated mass of white pulp in the spleen. SYN: *malpighi-*

*an body* (2).

**splenetic sinus** One of a series of wide channels with thin walls forming an anastomosing plexus throughout red pulp of spleen. SYN: *terminal vein.*

**splenetic vein** The vein carrying blood from spleen to the portal vein.

**splenial** (splē′nē-ăl) [Gr. *splen,* spleen] Concerning the spleen.

**splenic** (splĕn′ĭk) [Gr. *splenikos*] Splenetic.

**splenic flexure** Junction of transverse and descending colon, making a bend on the left side near the spleen.

**splenicterus** (splē-nĭk′tĕr-ŭs) [Gr. *splen,* spleen, + *ikteros,* jaundice] Inflammation of the spleen associated with jaundice.

**splenification** (splē″nĭ-fĭ-kā′shŭn) [″ + L. *facere,* to make] Splenization.

**spleniform** (splĕn′ĭ-form) [″ + L. *forma,* form] Resembling the spleen.

**splenitis** (splē-nī′tĭs) [″ + *itis,* inflammation] Inflammation of the spleen. This condition comprises acute and chronic hypertrophy, proliferative splenitis, and suppurative inflammation, the result of acute infectious disease. Prognosis depends on the systemic condition underlying the splenitis.

SYMPTOMS: The symptoms may be indefinite or absent; usually there is little pain or tenderness unless perisplenitis exists. Considerable enlargement may be attended by sense of weight, tension, or distress in the left hypochondrium, accompanied perhaps by slight dyspnea, sudden pain appearing in the gastric region followed by vomiting of pus and blood in the course of infectious disease, which may be due to abscess of spleen.

**splenium** (splē′nē-ŭm) [Gr. *splenion,* bandage] **1.** A compress or bandage. **2.** A structure resembling a bandaged part.

***s. corporis callosi*** The thickened posterior end of the corpus callosum.

**splenius** (splē′nē-ŭs) A flat muscle on either side of back of neck and upper thoracic area. SEE: *muscle* for illus.; *Muscles Appendix.*

**splenization** (splē″nī-zā′shŭn) The change in a tissue, as of the lung, when it resembles splenic tissue. SYN: *splenification.*

**spleno-** Combining form meaning *spleen.*

**splenocele** (splē′nō-sēl) [Gr. *splen,* spleen, + *kele,* tumor, swelling] **1.** A hernia of the spleen. **2.** Splenoma.

**splenoceratosis** (splē″nō-sĕr″ă-tō′sĭs) [″ + *keras,* horn, + *osis,* condition] Induration of the spleen.

**splenocleisis** (splē″nō-klī′sĭs) [″ + *kleisis,* closure] Friction on the surface of the spleen or application of gauze in order to induce the formation of fibrous tissue.

**splenocolic** (splē″nō-kŏl′ĭk) [″ + *kolon,* colon] Pert. to the spleen and colon or reference to a fold of peritoneum between the two viscera.

**splenodynia** (splē″nō-dĭn′ē-ă) [″ + *odyne,* pain] Pain in the spleen. SYN: *splenalgia.*

**splenogenic, splenogenous** (splē″nō-jĕn′ĭk, splē-nŏj′ĕn-ŭs) [″ + *gennan,* to produce] Originating in the spleen.

**splenography** (splē-nŏg′ră-fē) [″ + *graphein,* to write] A treatise on, or a description of, the spleen.

**splenohepatomegaly** (splē″nō-hĕp″ă-tō-mĕg′ă-lē) [Gr. *splen,* spleen, + *hepar,* liver, + *megas,* large] Enlargement of the spleen and liver.

**splenoid** (splē′noyd) [″ + *eidos,* form, shape] Resembling the spleen.

**splenokeratosis** (splē″nō-kĕr″ă-tō′sĭs) [″ + *keras,* horn, + *osis,* condition] Induration of the spleen.

**splenolaparotomy** (splē″nō-lăp″ă-rŏt′ō-mē) [″ + *lapara,* flank, + *tome,* incision] Incision through the abdominal wall into the spleen.

**splenology** (splē-nŏl′ō-jē) [″ + *logos,* word, reason] The study of functions and diseases of the spleen.

**splenolymphatic** (splē″nō-lĭm-făt′ĭk) [″ + L. *lympha,* lymph] Concerning the spleen and lymph nodes.

**splenolysin** (splē-nŏl′ĭ-sĭn) [″ + *lysis,* dissolution] An antibody that destroys splenic tissue.

**splenolysis** (splē-nŏl′ĭ-sĭs) Destruction of splenic tissue.

**splenoma** (splē-nō′mă) *pl.* **splenomas, -mata** [″ + *oma,* tumor] A tumor of the spleen. SYN: *splenocele* (2); *splenoncus.*

**splenomalacia** (splē″nō-mă-lā′shē-ă) [″ + *malakia,* softening] Softening of the spleen.

**splenomedullary** (splē″nō-mĕd′ū-lĕr″ē) [″ + L. *medulla,* marrow] Concerning the spleen and bone marrow, or originating in the spleen and bone marrow.

**splenomegalia, splenomegaly** (splē″nō-mē-gā′lē-ă, -mĕg′ă-lē) [″ + *megas,* large] Enlargement of the spleen.

***congestive s.*** A syndrome consisting of anemia, splenic enlargement, hemorrhages, and ultimately cirrhosis of the liver. SYN: *Banti's syndrome.*

***hemolytic s.*** Enlargement of the spleen in association with hemolytic disease of the blood.

**splenometry** (splē-nŏm′ĕ-trē) [″ + *metron,* measure] Determining the size of the spleen.

**splenomyelogenous** (splē-nō-mī″ĕ-lŏj′ĕ-nŭs) [″ + *myelos,* marrow, + *gennan,* to produce] Splenomedullary.

**splenomyelomalacia** (splē″nō-mī″ĕl-ō-mă-lā′shē-ă) [″ + ″ + *malakia,* softening] Abnormal softening of the spleen and bone marrow.

**splenoncus** (splē-nŏng′kŭs) [Gr. *splen,* spleen, + *onkos,* tumor] Splenoma.

**splenonephric** (splē″nō-nĕf′rĭk) [″ + *nephros,* kidney] Rel. to the spleen and kidney. SYN: *lienorenal.*

**splenonephroptosis** (splē″nō-nĕf″rŏp-tō′sĭs) [″ + ″ + *ptosis,* a dropping] Downward displacement of the spleen and kidney.

**splenopancreatic** (splē″nō-păn″krē-ăt′ĭk) [″ + *pankreas,* pancreas] Rel. to the spleen and pancreas.

**splenopathy** (splē-nŏp′ă-thē) [″ + *pathos,* disease, suffering] Any disorder of the spleen.

**splenopexy** (splē′nō-pĕk″sē) [″ + *pexis,* fixation] Artificial fixation of a movable spleen.

**splenophrenic** (splĕn-ō-frĕn′ĭk) [″ + *phren,* diaphragm] Concerning the spleen and diaphragm.

**splenopneumonia** (splē″nō-nū-mō′nē-ă) [″ + *pneumonia,* inflammation of lung] Pneumonia with splenization of the lung.

**splenoportography** (splē″nō-por-tŏg′ră-fē) [″ + L. *porta,* gate, + Gr. *graphein,* to write] Radiography of the spleen and portal vein after injection of a radiopaque contrast medium into the spleen.

**splenoptosis** (splē″nŏp-tō′sĭs) [″ + *ptosis,* a dropping] Downward displacement of the spleen.

**splenorenal** (splē″nō-rē′năl) Pert. to the spleen and kidney.

**splenorenal shunt** Anastomosis of the splenic vein to the renal vein to enable blood from the portal system to enter the general venous circulation; performed in cases of portal hypertension.

**splenorrhagia** (splē″nō-rā′jē-ă) [″ + *rhegnynai,* to burst forth] Hemorrhage from a ruptured spleen.

**splenorrhaphy** (splē-nor′ă-fē) [″ + *rhaphe,* seam, ridge] Suture of a wound of the spleen.

**splenotomy** (splē-nŏt′ō-mē) [″ + *tome,* incision] Incision of the spleen.

**splenotoxin** (splē″nō-tŏks′ĭn) [″ + *toxikon,* poison] Cytotoxin having specific action on splenic cells.

**splenulus** (splĕn′ū-lŭs) [L., a little spleen] A rudimentary or accessory spleen.

**splenunculus** (splē-nŭng′kū-lŭs) An accessory spleen.

**splint** (splĭnt) [MD. *splinte,* a wedge] An appliance made of bone, wood, metal, or plaster of paris, used for the fixation, union, or protection of an injured part of the body. It may be movable or immovable.

***acrylic resin bite-guard s.*** A device fashioned to cover the incisal and occlusal surfaces of a dental arch to stabilize the teeth, treating bruxism, or facilitating proper occlusal positioning.

***Agnew's s.*** A splint used in fractures of the patella and metacarpus.

***air s.*** Inflatable s.

***airplane s.*** An appliance usually used on ambulatory patients in the treatment of fractures of the humerus. It takes its name from the elevated (abducted) position in which it holds the arm suspended away from the body.

***anchor s.*** A splint for fracture of the jaw, with metal loops fitting over the teeth and held together by a rod.

***Ashhurst's s.*** A bracketed splint of wire with a footpiece to cover the thigh and leg after excision of the knee joint.

***Balkan s.*** A splint used for continuous extension in fracture of the femur.

***banjo traction s.*** A splint made out of a steel rod bent to resemble the shape of a banjo. It provides anchor points for attachments to the fingers in the treatment of contractures and fractures of the fingers.

***Bavarian s.*** An immovable dressing in which the plaster is applied between two layers of flannel.

***blow-up s.*** Inflatable s.

***Bond's s.*** A splint used for fracture of the lower end of the radius.

***Bowlby's s.*** A splint used for fracture of the shaft of the humerus.

***box s.*** A splint used for fracture below the knee.

***bracketed s.*** A splint composed of two pieces of metal or wood united by brackets.

***Cabot's s.*** A splint composed of a metal structure placed posterior to the thigh and leg.

***Carter's intranasal s.*** A steel bridge with wings connected by a hinge; used for operation of a depressed nasal bridge.

***coaptation s.*** A small splint adjusted about a fractured part to prevent overriding of the fragments of bones; usually covered by a longer splint for fixation of entire section.

***Denis Browne s.*** A splint used to treat talipes equinovarus (clubfoot), consisting of a curved bar attached to the soles of a pair of high-topped shoes. It is often used in late infancy and applied at bedtime. Its use generally follows casting and manipulation to reduce the deformity.

***dental s.*** A rigid or flexible device or compound used to support, protect, or immobilize teeth that have been loosened, replanted, fractured, or subjected to surgical procedures.

***Dupuytren's s.*** A splint used to prevent eversion in Pott's fracture.

***dynamic s.*** A splint that assists in movements initiated by the patient. SYN: *functional s.*

***flail arm s.*** SEE: *flail arm splint.*

***Fox's s.*** A splint used for fractured clavicle.

***functional s.*** Dynamic s.

***Gibson walking s.*** A splint that is a modification of a Thomas splint.

***Gordon's s.*** A side splint used for the arm and hand in Colles' fracture.

***inflatable s.*** Inflatable device for immobilizing part or all of an extremity. The hollow tubular device is placed around the part and then inflated. SYN: *air s.; blow-up s.*

---

Caution: The splint should not be inflated tightly enough to prevent the flow of blood to and from the extremity. If the patient is to be transported by air, an inflatable splint should not be used without carefully monitoring and adjusting the pressure during flight and at the time of descent.

---

***Jones' nasal s.*** A splint used for the fracture of nasal bones.

***Levis' s.*** A splint of perforated metal extending from below the elbow to the end of the palm; shaped to fit the arm and hand.

***McIntire's s.*** A splint shaped like a double inclined plane, used as a posterior splint for leg and thigh.

***opponens s.*** A splint designed to maintain the thumb in a position to oppose the other fingers.

***padded board s.*** A slat of wood, typically padded on one side and covered with plastic or cloth, to which an injured extremity can be fastened to immobilize it.

***permanent fixed s.*** A nonremovable prosthesis firmly attached to an abutment used to stabilize or immobilize teeth. A fixed bridge may serve as a permanent fixed splint for such support.

***Stromeyer's s.*** A splint with two hinged sections that can be set at any angle, used esp. for the knee.

***temporary removable s.*** One of a variety of splints used for temporary or intermittent support and stabilization of the teeth.

***Thomas s.*** A long wire splint with a proximal ring. The ring fits over the lower extremity and is placed as far as it will go toward the hip. It is used in emergency treatment of femoral fracture.

***Thomas' knee s.*** A rigid metal splint used to remove pressure of body weight from a weak knee joint by transferring weight to the ischium and perineum.

***Thomas' posterior s.*** SEE: *Thomas s.*

***traction s.*** A splint that provides continual traction to a midshaft lower extremity fracture.

***Volkmann's s.*** A splint used for fracture of the lower extremity, consisting of a footpiece and two lateral supports.

**splinter** (splĭn'tĕr) [MD. *splinte,* a wedge] **1.** A fragment from a fractured bone. **2.** A slender, sharp piece of material piercing or imbedded in the skin.

**splinter hemorrhage** A small linear hemorrhage under the fingernails or toenails. It may be due to subacute bacterial endocarditis.

**splinting** Fixation of a dislocation or fracture with a splint. Splints are also used to help support weak joints, to assist actively with functional movement, to immobilize to promote healing, and to protect from injury and deformity.

***abdominal s.*** Involuntary tensing of abdominal muscles to protect underlying inflamed structures. Also called *rigid abdomen.*

**split** (splĭt) [D. *splitten,* to divide] **1.** A longitudinal fissure. **2.** Characterized by a deep fissure.

**split foot** Cleft foot.

**split hand** Cleft hand.

**split pelvis** Congenital failure of pubic bones to form a union at the symphysis.

**splitting** (splĭt'ĭng) [D. *splitten,* to divide] In chemistry, the breaking up of complex molecules into two or more simpler compounds.

**split tongue** A cleft or bifid tongue resulting from developmental arrest.

**$SpO_2$** The saturation of arterial blood with oxygen as measured by pulse oximetry, expressed as a percentage.

**spodogenous** (spō-dŏj'ĕn-ŭs) [Gr. *spodos,* ashes, + *gennan,* to produce] Caused by waste material.

**spodophagous** (spō-dŏf'ă-gŭs) [" + *phagein,* to eat] Destroying the waste matters in the body; said of scavenger cells.

**spondee** (spŏn-dē) Two-syllable words that receive equal stress on each syllable.

**spondee threshold** [Fr., a two-syllable word with equal stress on each syllable] In audiometry, the intensity at which speech is recognized as a meaningful symbol. This is tested by presenting, through an audiometer, two-syllable words in which each symbol is accented equally. SEE: *audiometry.*

**spondyl-** (spŏn'dĭl) SEE: *spondylo-.*

**spondylalgia** (spŏn"dĭl-ăl'jē-ă) [Gr. *spondylos,* vertebra, + *algos,* pain] Painful condition of a vertebra.

**spondylarthritis** (spŏn"dĭl-ăr-thrī'tĭs) [" + *arthron,* joint, + *itis,* inflammation] Inflammation of the joints of the vertebrae; arthritis of the spine. SEE: *spondylitis.*

**spondylarthrocace** (splon"dĭl-ăr-thrŏk'ă-sē) [" + " + *kake,* badness] Tuberculosis of the vertebrae. SYN: *spondylocace.*

**spondylexarthrosis** (spŏn"dĭl-ĕks"ăr-thrō'sĭs) [" + *exarthrosis,* dislocation] Dislocation of a vertebra.

**spondylitic** (spŏn"dĭ-lĭt'ĭk) [" + *itis,* inflammation] **1.** A person with spondylitis. **2.** Concerning spondylitis.

**spondylitis** (spŏn-dĭl-ī'tĭs) [" + *itis,* inflammation] Inflammation of one or more vertebrae, esp. tuberculous disease of the vertebrae (i.e., Pott's disease).

***ankylosing s.*** Rheumatoid s.

***s. deformans*** Inflammation of the vertebral joints resulting in the outgrowth of bone-like deposits on the vertebrae, which may fuse and cause rigid and distorted spine.

***hypertrophic s.*** A condition in which bodies of vertebrae hypertrophy; it occurs in most people over 50. Bony changes such as slipping at bases and the development of bony outgrowths on articular processes occur.

***Kümmell's s.*** A traumatic spondylitis in which symptoms do not appear until some time after the injury.

***Marie-Strümpell s.*** Rheumatoid s.

***rheumatoid s.*** A chronic progressive disease involving the joints between articular processes, costovertebral joints, and sacroiliac joints. Bilateral sclerosis of sacroiliac joints is a diagnostic sign. Changes occurring in joints are similar to those seen in rheumatoid arthritis. Ankylosis may occur, giving rise to stiff back (poker spine). SYN: *ankylosing s.; Marie-Strümpell s.*

***tuberculous s.*** Pott's disease.

**spondylizema** (spŏn″dĭl-ĭ-zē′mă) [Gr. *spondylos,* vertebra, + *izema,* depression] Downward displacement of a vertebra caused by the disintegration of the one below it.

**spondylo-, spondyl-** Combining form meaning *vertebra.*

**spondylocace** (spŏn″dĭ-lŏk′ă-sē) [Gr. *spondylos,* vertebra, + *kake,* badness] Spondylarthrocace.

**spondylodiagnosis** (spŏn″dĭ-lō-dī″ăg-nō′sĭs) [″ + *dia,* through, + *gnosis,* knowledge] Diagnosis by means of visceral reflexes obtained by percussion of the vertebrae.

**spondylodymus** (spŏn″dĭ-lŏd′ĭ-mŭs) [″ + *didymos,* twin] Twin fetuses joined at the vertebrae.

**spondylodynia** (spŏn″dĭ-lō-dĭn′ē-ă) [″ + *odyne,* pain] Pain in a vertebra.

**spondylolisthesis** (spŏn″dĭ-lō-lĭs″thē′sĭs) [″ + *oblisthesis,* a slipping] Any forward slipping of one vertebrae on the one below it. Predisposing factors include spondylolysis, degeneration, elongated pars, elongated pedicles, and birth defects in the spine such as spina bifida. SEE: *retrospondylolisthesis.*

**spondylolisthetic** (spŏn″dĭ-lō-lĭs-thĕt′ĭk) Concerning spondylolisthesis.

**spondylolysis** (spŏn″dĭ-lŏl′ĭ-sĭs) [″ + *lysis,* dissolution] The breaking down of a vertebral structure.

**spondylomalacia** (spŏn″dĭ-lō-mă-lā′shē-ă) [″ + *malakia,* softening] Softening of the vertebrae.

**spondylopathy** (spŏn″dĭl-ŏp′ă-thē) [″ + *pathos,* disease, suffering] Any disorder of the vertebrae.

**spondyloptosis** (spŏn″dĭ-lō-tō′sĭs) [″ + *ptosis,* a dropping] Spondylolisthesis.

**spondylopyosis** (spŏn″dĭ-lō″pī-ō′sĭs) [″ + *pyosis,* suppuration] Suppuration with inflammation of a vertebra.

**spondyloschisis** (spŏn″dĭ-lŏs′kĭ-sĭs) [″ + *schisis,* a splitting] A congenital fissure of one or more of the vertebral arches. SYN: *rhachischisis.*

**spondylosis** (spŏn″dĭ-lō′sĭs) [Gr. *spondylos,* vertebra, + *osis,* condition] Vertebral ankylosis.

***cervical s., lumbar s.*** Degenerative arthritis, osteoarthritis, of the cervical or lumbar vertebrae and related tissues. It may cause pressure on nerve roots with subsequent pain or paresthesia in the extremities.

***rhizomelic s.*** Ankylosis interfering with movements of the hips and shoulders.

**spondylosyndesis** (spŏn″dĭ-lō-sĭn′dĕ-sĭs) [″ + *syndesis,* a binding together] Surgical formation of an ankylosis between vertebrae.

**spondylotherapy** (spŏn″dĭl-ō-thĕr′ă-pē) [″ + *therapeia,* treatment] Spinal therapeutics; spinal manipulation in the treatment of disease.

**spondylotomy** (spŏn″dĭl-ŏt′ō-mē) [″ + *tome,* incision] Removal of part of the vertebral column to correct a deformity. SYN: *rachitomy.*

**spondylous** (spŏn′dĭ-lŭs) [Gr. *spondylos,* vertebra] Concerning a vertebra.

**sponge** (spŭnj) [Gr. *sphongos,* sponge] **1.** Elastic, porous mass forming the internal skeleton of certain marine animals; or rubber or synthetic substance that resembles a sponge in properties and appearance. SYN: *spongia.* **2.** An absorbent pad made of gauze and cotton used to absorb fluids and blood in surgery or to dress wounds. **3.** Short term for sponge bath. **4.** To moisten, clean, cool, or wipe with a sponge.

***abdominal s.*** A flat sponge from ½ to 1 in. (1.27 to 2.54 cm) thick, 3 to 6 in. (7.62 to 15.24 cm) in diameter, used as packing, to prevent closing or obstruction by intrusion of viscera, as covering to prevent tissue injury, and as absorbents.

***contraceptive s.*** A sponge impregnated with a spermicide. It is used intravaginally during sexual intercourse as a method of contraception. SYN: *spermicidal s.* SEE: *contraceptive.*

***gauze s.*** A sterile pad made of absorbent material. It is used during surgery.

***gelatin s.*** A spongy substance prepared from gelatin. This nonantigenic, readily absorbable material is used esp. to stop internal bleeding. It is sold under the trade name of Gelfoam.

Caution: This material may seem effective if used when blood pressure is decreased, as could be the condition during surgery, but may fail as the patient becomes normotensive.

***spermicidal s.*** Contraceptive s.

**sponge diver's disease** Sea anemone sting.

**sponge graft** A sponge placed in an ulcer to cause granulation.

**spongia** (spŏn′jē-ă) [Gr. *sphongos,* sponge] Sponge.

**spongiform** (spŭn′jĭ-form) [Gr. *sphongos,* sponge, + L. *forma,* shape] Having the appearance or quality of a sponge. SYN: *spongioid.*

**spongio-** Combining form meaning *sponge.*

**spongioblast** (spŭn′jē-ō-blăst) [″ + *blastos,* germ] A cell that develops from an embryonic neural tube and serves as forerunner of ependymal cells and astrocytes.

**spongioblastoma** (spŭn″jē-ō-blăs-tō′mă) [″ + ″ + *oma,* tumor] A glioma of the brain derived from spongioblasts.

**spongiocyte** (spŭn′jē-ō-sīt″) [″ + *kytos,* cell] A neuroglial cell.

**spongioid** (spŭn′jē-oyd) [″ + *eidos,* form, shape] Spongiform.

**spongiositis** (spŭn″jē-ō-sī′tĭs) [″ + *itis,* inflammation] Inflammation of the corpus spongiosum of the urethra.

**spongy** (spŭn′jē) Resembling a sponge in texture.

**spontaneous** (spŏn-tā′nē-ŭs) [L.] Occurring unaided or without apparent cause; voluntary.

**spontaneous fracture** Fracture of a demineralized bone as in osteoporosis. This type of fracture may be painless.

ETIOLOGY: Fragilitas ossium; nerve conditions such as tabes; secondary malignant growths; osteoporosis of bones of the aged.

**spontaneous ventilation, inability to sustain** A state in which a patient is unable to maintain adequate breathing to support life. This is measured by deterioration of arterial blood gases, increased work of breathing, and decreasing energy. SEE: *Nursing Diagnoses Appendix.*

**spoon** [AS. *spon,* a chip] Instrument consisting of a small bowl on a handle, used in scooping out tissues or tumors, or in measuring quantities.

**sporadic** (spō-răd′ĭk) [Gr. *sporadikos*] Occurring occasionally or in scattered instances, as a disease. SEE: *endemic; epidemic; pandemic.*

**sporangiophore** (spō-răn′jē-ō-for) [Gr. *sporos,* seed, + *angeion,* vessel, + *phoros,* a bearer] In microbiology, the supporting stalk for a spore sac of certain fungi.

**sporangium** (spō-răn′jē-ŭm) A sac enclosing spores, seen in certain fungi.

**spore** (spor) [Gr. *sporos,* seed] A resistant cell produced by fungi for reproduction or by certain bacteria to withstand harsh environments. Usually spores are asexual, but certain fungi form sexual spores (oospores, zygospores, or ascospores). Spores usually possess a thick wall enabling the cell to withstand unfavorable environmental conditions.

Certain bacteria also form spores; this is not a method of reproduction, but rather a defense when the environment becomes unfavorable. The spores of bacteria are difficult to destroy because they are very resistant to heat and require prolonged exposure to high temperatures to destroy them.

**sporicide** (spor′ĭ-sīd) An agent that destroys bacterial and mold spores. Because spores are more difficult to kill than vegetative cells, a sporicide also acts as a sterilizing agent. **sporicidal,** *adj.* (-ăl).

**sporiferous** (spor-ĭf′ĕr-ŭs) [″ + L. *ferre,* to bear] Producing spores.

**spork** An adapted utensil for persons with limited upper extremity function. The distal end may swivel to allow food to remain level as a result of gravitational force. The bowl end is shaped like a spoon but has modified tines, like a fork.

**sporoblast** (spor′ō-blăst) [″ + *blastos,* germ] The structure within the oocyst of certain parasitic protozoa (*Eimeria* and *Isospora*) that gives rise to a sporocyst and eventually a spore.

**sporocyst** (spor′ō-sĭst) [″ + *kystis,* sac] **1.** Any sac containing spores or reproductive cells. **2.** A sac secreted around a sporoblast by certain protozoa before spore production. **3.** A stage in the life cycle of a trematode worm usually found in the tissues of the first intermediate host, a mollusk. It develops from a miracidium and is essentially a germinal sac containing germ cells. It gives rise to daughter sporocysts or rediae.

**sporogenesis** (spor″ō-jĕn′ĕ-sĭs) [Gr. *sporos,* seed, + *genesis,* generation, birth] The production or formation of spores. SYN: *sporogeny; sporogony.*

**sporogenic** (spor″ō-jĕn′ĭk) [″ + *gennan,* to produce] Having the ability of developing into spores.

**sporogenous** (spor-ŏj′ĕ-nŭs) [″ + *gennan,* to produce] Concerning sporogenesis.

**sporogeny** (spor-ŏj′ĕ-nē) Sporogenesis.

**sporogony** (spor-ŏg′ō-nē) [″ + *goneia,* generation] Sporogenesis.

**sporophore** (spor′ō-for) [″ + *phoros,* bearing] The spore-bearing portion of an organism.

**sporophyte** (spor′ō-fīt) [″ + *phyton,* plant] The spore-bearing stage of a plant exhibiting alternation of generation.

**sporoplasm** (spor′ō-plăzm) [″ + LL. *plasma,* form, mold] The cell protoplasm of spores.

**Sporothrix** (spor′ō-thrĭks) A genus of fungi of the family Moniliaceae; formerly called *Sporotrichum.*

***S. schenckii*** The causative agent of sporotrichosis.

**sporotrichin** (spor-ŏ′trĭ-kĭn) An antigenic substance derived from *Sporothrix* organisms and used for diagnostic purposes.

**sporotrichosis** (spor″ō-trī-kō′sĭs) [″ + *thrix,* hair, + *osis,* condition] A chronic granulomatous infection usually of the skin and superficial lymph node, marked by the formation of abscesses, nodules, and ulcers and caused by the fungus *Sporothrix schenckii.*

**Sporotrichum** (spō-rŏt′rĭ-kŭm) Former name for *Sporothrix.*

***S. schenckii*** SEE: *Sporothrix schenckii.*

**Sporozoa** (spor″ō-zō′ă) [″ + *zoon,* animal] A class of parasitic protozoa of the phylum Apicomplexa (apical microlobule complex), kingdom Protista. The mature forms lack a means of self-locomotion. Important genera are *Plasmodium, Toxoplasma, Cryptosporidium, Microsporidia,* and *Isospora.*

**sporozoan** A protozoon belonging to the group formerly called Sporozoa.

**sporozoite** (spor″ō-zō′īt) [″ + *zoon,* animal] **1.** An animal spore. **2.** An elongated sickle-shaped cell that develops from a sporoblast within the oocyst in the life cycle of the malaria organism. Upon bursting of the oocyst, sporozoites are released into the body cavity and make their way to the salivary gland. They are introduced into human blood by a mosquito and almost immediately enter tissue cells, where they go through two schizogonic divisions and then reenter the bloodstream and infect erythrocytes.

**sport** [ME. *sporten,* to divert] Mutation.

**sports medicine** The application of medical knowledge and science to the physiological and pathological aspects of all persons who indulge in sports and athletics. This includes not only prevention and treatment of injuries but also scientific investigation of training methods and practices.

**sporular** (spor′ū-lăr) [L. *sporula,* little spore] Concerning a spore.

**sporulation** (spor-ū-lā′shŭn) [L. *sporula,* little spore] The production of spores, a method of reproduction of unicellular organisms.

**spot** (spŏt) [MD. *spotte*] A small surface area differing in appearance from its surroundings. SYN: *macula.*

***blind s.*** The optic disk where the optic nerve enters the retina. SEE: *scotoma.*

***blue s.*** Mongolian s.

***cherry-red s.*** A red spot occurring on the retina in cases of Tay-Sachs disease.

***cold s.*** The area on the surface of the skin that, when stimulated, gives rise to a sensation of coldness.

***corneal s.*** Leukoma.

***Fordyce's s.'s*** Ectopic sebaceous glands seen frequently as yellow spots in the oral mucosa of the cheek or lip.

***genital s.*** The area on the nasal mucosa that tends to bleed during menstruation. SEE: *menstruation, vicarious.*

***hot s.*** Warm s.

***hypnogenic s.*** A point on the body that, when pressed, will throw a susceptible person into hypnosis or sleep.

***Koplik's s.'s*** Minute white or bluish-white spots on mucous membrane of mouth before the appearance of the rash of measles.

***liver s.'s*** A popular term for pigmentary skin discolorations, usually in yellow-brown patches. SEE: *chloasma; lentigo.*

***milk s.*** **1.** A thickened and opaque area seen on epicardium at autopsy. **2.** A dense area of macrophages in the omentum.

***mongolian s.*** One of the blue or mulberry-colored spots usually located in the sacral region. It may be present at birth in Asian, American Indian, black, and Southern European infants, and usually disappears during childhood. SYN: *blue s.*

***rose s.'s*** Rose-colored maculae occurring on abdomen or loins in eruption of typhoid fever.

***ruby s.*** Senile angioma.

***temperature s.*** A cutaneous spot that responds to temperature changes. SEE: *cold s.; warm s.*

***warm s.*** An area on the surface of the skin that, when stimulated, causes a sensation of warmth. SYN: *hot s.*

***white s.'s*** Light-colored, elevated areas of various sizes occurring on ventricular surface of the anterior leaflet of the mitral valve.

***yellow s.*** Macula lutea retinae.

**spotted fever** General and imprecise name for various eruptive fevers including typhus, tick fever, and rickettsial fevers. SEE: *Rocky Mountain spotted fever.*

**spotting** The appearance of blood-tinged discharge from the vagina, usually between menstrual periods or at the onset of labor.

**spp** *species* (plural).

**sprain** (sprān) [O. Fr. *espraindre,* to wring] Trauma to a joint that causes pain and disability depending on the degree of injury to the ligaments. In severe sprain, ligaments may be completely torn. The ankle joint is the most often sprained. SEE: *fracture; strain.*

SYMPTOMS: The signs of a sprain are rapid swelling, heat, and disability; these are often accompanied by discoloration and limitation of function. It is important to understand that the intensity of the symptoms and signs may not be accurate indicators of the difference between a sprain and a fracture.

TREATMENT: During the first 24 to 48 hr, cold compresses and a bandage should be applied, and the joint elevated. After initial treatment with cold, heat should be applied. If recovery proves slow, immobilization of the joint is indicated, followed by careful massage.

***s. of ankle, s. of foot*** Trauma to the ankle or foot or both, with soft tissue and possibly ligament and tendon injury, but without fracture. This sprain is marked by pain, tenderness, swelling, ecchymosis of the area, and limitation of motion. SEE: *Nursing Diagnoses Appendix.*

TREATMENT: This should be treated as a fracture until the results of radiological studies of the ankle and foot are available. If there is no fracture, the lower extremity is elevated and immobilized, and cold is applied for 24 hr (ice should not be applied directly to the foot and ankle). Analgesics and nonsteroidal anti-inflammatory agents may be required. If a ligament is partially or completely torn, it may be necessary to immobilize the lower extremity by applying a cast.

***s. of back*** Overstretching of the muscles, ligaments, or other spinal structures, often associated with small fractures. Symptoms include pain, esp. on extreme movements; tenderness; and muscle spasm.

TREATMENT: If the patient is supine, he or she should be kept in that position; if not, the patient should lie down on rigid support. The patient should not be allowed to sit up or walk until fracture is ruled out. Treatment includes intermittent heat; rest, with adhesive strapping, and brace. After the acute symptoms have subsided, physical therapy is prescribed.

***riders' s.*** Sprain of the adductor longus muscles of the thigh, resulting from strain in riding horseback.

**sprain fracture** The separation of a tendon or ligament from its insertion, taking with it a piece of the bone.

**spray** (sprā) [MD. *spraeyen,* to sprinkle] **1.** A jet of fine medicated vapor applied to a diseased part or discharged into the air. **2.** A pressurized container. SYN: *atomizer.* **3.** To discharge fluid in a fine stream.

**spreader** (sprĕd'ĕr) **1.** An instrument for distributing something evenly over a tissue or culture plate. **2.** A bacterial culture that, as it grows, spreads over the surface of the culture medium.

***bladder-neck s.*** An instrument used to expose the bladder neck and prostatic cavity while doing a retropubic prostatectomy.

***root canal s.*** In dentistry, an instrument that is pointed and of variable diameter and taper. It is used to apply force to the material used in filling a root canal.

**spreading** (sprĕd'ĭng) [AS. *spraedan,* to strew] The term indicating a growth on a bacterial culture, extending much (several millimeters or more) beyond the site of inoculation.

**spring** [AS. *springan,* to jump] **1.** The season of the year that comes after winter and before summer. SYN: *vernal.* **2.** The quick movement of a body to its original position through its elasticity.

**spring conjunctivitis** Vernal conjunctivitis.

**spring fever** A feeling of lassitude, rejuvenation, or increased sex drive that affects some people in the spring.

**spring finger** Arrested movement of a finger in flexion or extension followed by a jerk. SYN: *trigger finger.*

**spring ligament** The interior calcaneoscaphoid ligament of the sole of the foot. It joins the os calcis to the scaphoid bone.

**sprue** (sproo) [D. *sprouwe*] In dentistry, the wax, metal, or plastic used to form the aperture(s) through which molten gold or resin will pass to make a casting; also, the part of the casting that later fills the sprue hole.

***celiac s.*** A disease of the intestinal tract characterized by malabsorption, weight loss, abdominal distention, bloating, diarrhea, and steatorrhea. The patients are intolerant to the proteins present in wheat: gluten and gliadin. The microscopic structure of the mucosa of the jejunal portion of the small intestine is abnormal. Diagnosis is difficult because patients may present with only one of the complications such as anemia, bleeding tendency, or unexplained weight loss, which may be attributed to anxiety and depression. There is no specific diagnostic test; however, patients who exhibit virtually complete reversal of symptoms and signs (including changes in bowel mucosa) after beginning a gluten-free diet are considered to have this disease. Treatment is with a gluten-free diet. SYN: *gluten-induced enteropathy; nontropical s.*

***nontropical s.*** Celiac s.

***tropical s.*** A disease endemic in many tropical regions, marked by weakness, anemia, loss of weight, steatorrhea, and malabsorption of essential nutrients. Its cause is unknown but is thought to be a bacterial infection of the intestine. Treatment for tropical sprue is administration of folic acid and tetracyclines for about a month. A longer period of therapy may be required if the disease has been present for years. SEE: *celiac s.*

**spud** (spŭd) [ME. *spudde,* short knife] Short, flattened, spadelike blade to dislodge a foreign substance.

**spur** [AS. *spura,* a pointed instrument] **1.** A sharp or pointed projection. **2.** A sharp horny outgrowth of the skin.

***calcaneal s.*** An exostosis of the heel, often painful and resulting in disability.

***s. cell*** An erythrocyte with spikes caused by a membrane deformity, perhaps the result of excess cholesterol. Spur cells are often seen in alcoholic cirrhosis. SEE: illus.

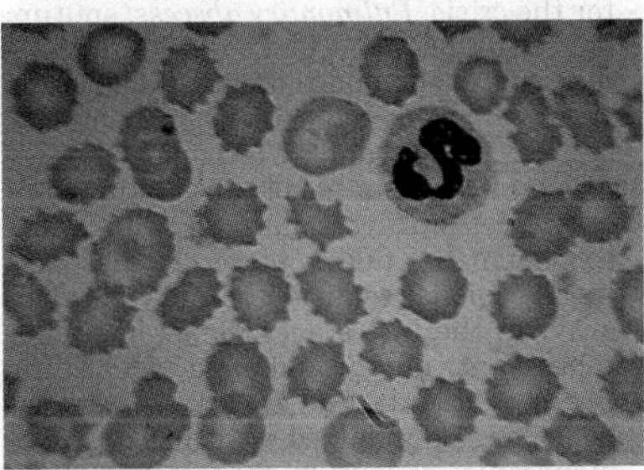

**SPUR CELLS** IN SEVERE LIVER DISEASE (ORIG. MAG. ×640)

***femoral s.*** A spur sometimes present on medial and underside of the neck of the femur.

***scleral s.*** A pointed portion of sclera that projects into the deeper part of the cornea immediately behind the canal of Schlemm at the angle of the iris.

**spurious** (spū'rē-ŭs) [L. *spurius*] Not true or genuine; adulterated; false.

**sputum** (spū'tŭm) *pl.* **sputa** [L.] A substance expelled by coughing or clearing the throat. It may contain a variety of material from the respiratory tract including one or more of the following: cellular debris, mucus, blood, pus, caseous material, and microorganisms. SEE: *Charcot-Leyden crystals.*

DIFFERENTIAL DIAGNOSIS: Copious amounts of sputum are seen in chronic inflammations of the lower respiratory tract. Scanty sputum occurs in all pulmonary bronchial acute inflammations and the early stages of lobar pneumonia and beginning bronchopneumonia. The color of the sputum varies with the origin, cause, and amount of its decomposition.

*Conditions: Anthracosis* (coal dust): sputum is black. *Bronchiectasis:* sputum is mucopurulent and foul if expectoration is infrequent. *Bronchial asthma:* sputum is scanty and frothy, later becoming purulent and grayish, containing eosinophils. *Bronchitis:* sputum is mucous, later purulent, and in chronic cases, greenish-yellow and thick. *Bronchopneumonia:* sputum is frothy, mucoid, thin, mucopurulent, copious, often containing blood. *Calcinosis:* sputum contains particles of lime or chalky deposits such as plaster of paris. *Empyema:* if accompanied by perforations, the sputum resembles that of pulmonary abscess. *Gangrene of the lung and putrid bronchitis:* sputum has an obnoxious odor and is purulent, separates on standing into three layers containing pus cells, hematoidin crystals, and leukocytes. *Lobar pneumonia:* sputum is scanty and viscid, yellowish, and somewhat mucopurulent during the early stages; in later stages, it is rusty, bloody, tenacious and viscid, esp. near or soon after the crisis. *Pulmonary abscess:* sputum is usually purulent and fetid, containing many pus cells and pieces of lung tissue. *Pulmonary tuberculosis:* in early stages, the sputum is scanty, whitish, or grayish-yellow, frothy, and expectorated in small quantities during coughing; later when consolidation takes place, it becomes more copious, tenacious, and yellowish-gray. In the late stages, it becomes mucopurulent, musty and fetid, containing fibers and tubercle bacilli, sometimes blood-tinged or mixed with blood. *Pneumoconiosis:* sputum characteristics depend on the type of inhaled dust that produced the disease. *Siderosis:* sputum contains particles of iron or other metals and resembles that of chronic bronchitis. It also contains alveolar cells. *Silicosis:* sputum contains particles of silica or other stone dusts.

NURSING IMPLICATIONS: Sputum is inspected for color, consistency, and odor. The patient is questioned about times when sputum is raised; about changes in volume, color, consistency, and odor; and about the presence of any blood and whether this increases on coughing. Proper disposal equipment and hygienic instructions for use of this equipment are provided to prevent contamination. The nurse should turn the patient's head away when the patient coughs, wash hands after handling items with sputum, and wear a face mask if the patient has a contagious disease that can be spread through air. The postural drainage technique and its use to promote sputum production are explained.

The patient is kept clean and comfortable. Frequent mouth and nose care are performed to minimize mouth odors and to eliminate unpleasant taste. The patient may suck hard candy to freshen mouth between meals. Prescribed medications are administered to loosen sputum and to alleviate irritation. Those patients who smoke should quit to increase ciliary action and to decrease inflammation. Physical examination of the chest is conducted to assess skin color and general appearance; respiratory rate, depth, and rhythm; and symmetry of chest wall movements. Palpation is performed to detect thoracic excursions, areas of tenderness, and tactile fremitus; percussion to detect dullness owing to fluid or consolidation of lung fields; and auscultation to detect normal and adventitial sounds, their timing, and their location. Adequate hydration is promoted to help liquefy secretions. Disposable equipment is used whenever possible. SEE: *Universal Precautions Appendix.*

***bloody s.*** Hemoptysis.

***nummular s.*** Round, coin-shaped, flat forms that sink in water; seen in bronchiectasis and advanced pulmonary tuberculosis.

***prune juice s.*** The thin, reddish, bloody sputum seen in gangrene, cancer of the lung, and certain pneumonias.

***rusty s.*** Blood-tinged sputum seen in lobar pneumonia.

**sputum specimen** A specimen of material expectorated from the mouth. If produced after a cough, it may contain, in addition to saliva, material from the throat and bronchi. The physical and bacterial characteristics of the sputum depend on the disease process involved and the ability of the patient to cough up material. Some bronchial secretions are quite tenacious and difficult to cough up. SEE: *postural drainage.*

NURSING IMPLICATIONS: The procedure is explained to the patient. The patient should rinse the mouth to remove food particles. Deep breathing is encouraged. Using the collection container provided, the patient collects the specimen in the early morning before ingesting food or drink if possible. The nurse examines the specimen to differentiate between sputum and saliva, documents the characteristics (color, viscosity, odor) and volume, and records the date and time the specimen went to the laboratory and the reason for the specimen. If the patient cannot produce a specimen, heated aerosol may be prescribed to induce expectoration, or the airway may be suctioned with a sputum trap attached to a suction catheter. Postural drainage may also help to produce a specimen. To ensure an uncontaminated specimen, the nurse should give the patient explicit instructions on use of the container. The specimen should be sent to the laboratory immediately or refrigerated. All sputum specimens should be treated as infective until proved otherwise. Appropriate isolation procedures are used for handling specimens.

**sq** *subcutaneous.*

**squalene** (skwăl′ēn) An unsaturated carbohydrate present in shark-liver oil and some vegetable oils. It is an intermediate in the biosynthesis of cholesterol.

**squama** (skwā′mă) *pl.* **squamae** [L.] **1.** A thin plate of bone. **2.** A scale from the epidermis. SYN: *squame.*

**squamate** (skwā′māt) [L. *squama,* scale] Scaly; squamous.

**squamatization** (skwā″mă-tī-zā′shŭn) [L. *squama,* scale] The changing of cells into squamous cells.

**squame** (skwām) [L. *squama,* scale] Squama (2).

**squamocellular** (skwā″mō-sĕl′ū-lăr) [L. *squama,* scale, + *cellula,* little cell] Rel. to or having squamous cells.

**squamofrontal** (skwā″mō-frŏn′tăl) [″ + *frontalis,* frontal] Concerning or belonging to the orbital palate.

**squamomastoid** (skwā″mō-măs′toyd) [″ + Gr. *mastos,* breast, + *eidos,* form, shape] Concerning the squamous and mastoid portions of the temporal bone.

**squamo-occipital** (skwā″mō-ŏk-sĭp′ĭ-tăl) [″ + *occipitalis,* occipital] Concerning the squamous portion of the occipital bone.

**squamoparietal** (skwā″mō-pă-rī′ĕ-tăl) [″ + *paries,* a wall] Rel. to the squamous and parietal bones.

**squamopetrosal** (skwā″mō-pē-trō′săl) [″ + *petrosus,* stony] Concerning the squamous and petrosal portions of the temporal bone.

**squamosa** (skwā-mō′săl) *pl.* **squamosae** [L. scaly] **1.** The squamous part of the temporal bone. **2.** Scaly or platelike.

**squamosal** (skwā-mō″săl) [L. *squama,* scale] Squamous.

**squamosphenoid** (skwā″mō-sfē′noyd) [″ + Gr. *sphen,* wedge, + *eidos,* form, shape] Concerning the squamous portion of the temporal bone and the sphenoid bone.

**squamous** (skwā′mŭs) [L. *squamosus*] Scalelike.

**squamous bone** The upper anterior portion of temporal bone.

**squamous cell** A flat, scaly, epithelial cell.

**squamous epithelium** The flat form of epithelial cells.

**squamous suture** The junction of the temporal and parietal bones.

**squamozygomatic** (sqwā″mō-zī″gō-măt′ĭk) [″ + *zygoma,* cheekbone] Concerning the squamous and zygomatic parts of the temporal bone.

**square knot** Double knot in which ends and standing parts are together and parallel to each other. This knot is used universally because it holds well. It is quite easy to tie but may be very difficult to untie. One should hold one end in each hand, carry the right end over the left end, and make a simple knot. Now this is reversed by carrying the left end over the right end and again tying, thus forming a simple symmetrical knot. If this is not done correctly, a false or granny knot results, a type of knot that usually slips. To untie, the knot is steadied, and one end is taken and drawn until it begins to slip out of the knot. One continues pulling in this direction until the knot slips or jumps and forms two half hitches that may be slipped off. SEE: *knot* for illus.

**square lobe 1.** The quadrate lobe of the liver. **2.** A lobe on upper surface of the cerebellum.

**squarrose, squarrous** (skwăr′ōs, -ŭs) [L. *squarrosus*] Scurfy or scaly; full of scabs or scales.

**squatting position** A position in which person crouches with legs drawn up closely in front of, or beneath, the body; sitting on one's haunches and heels.

**squeeze-bottle** A bottle made of a flexible, semirigid material that can be deformed by applying hand pressure to it. It is used to contain irrigating solutions, esp. those required in ophthalmology.

**squill** (skwĭl) [Gr. *skilla,* a sea onion] A drug derived from a liliaceous plant. It was once popular as an expectorant and diuretic. A form known as red squill has been used as a rat poison.

**squint** (skwĭnt) [ME. *asquint,* sidelong glance] **1.** Abnormality in which the right and left visual axes do not bear toward an objective point simultaneously. SYN: *strabismus.* **2.** To close the eyes partly as in excess light. **3.** To be unable to direct both eyes simultaneously toward a point.

***convergent s.*** Esotropia.

***divergent s.*** Exotropia.

***external s.*** Exotropia.

***internal s.*** Esotropia.

**SR** *sedimentation rate.*

**Sr** Symbol for the element strontium.

**SRF** *somatotropin releasing factor.*

**sRNA** *soluble ribonucleic acid.*

**SRS, SRS-A** *slow-reacting substance; slow-reacting substance of anaphylaxis.*

**SS** *saliva sample; soapsuds; sterile solution.*

**ss** [L. *semis,* half] One-half; *subjects,* as in ss of an experiment or clinical study.

**SSD** *source-skin distance.*

**SSE** *soapsuds enema.*

**SSS** *sterile saline soak.*

**ST** *sedimentation time.*

**S.T. 37** Hexylresorcinol.

**stab** (stăb) [ME. *stob,* stick] **1.** To pierce with a knife. **2.** A wound produced by piercing with a knife or pointed instrument. **3.** A stab culture.

**stab culture** A bacterial culture in which the organism is introduced into a solid gelatin medium with a wire or needle.

**stabile** (stā′bĭl) [L. *stabilis,* stable] Not moving; fixed.

**stability 1.** The condition of remaining unchanged, even in the presence of forces that would normally change the state or condition (e.g., a chemical compound that remains unchanged, or a mature mental state that resists change). **2.** A measure of the ability of an aerosol to remain in suspension. This is determined by the size, type, and concentration of particles, the humidity, and the mobility of the gas in which the particles are transported.

**stabilization** (stā″bĭl-ī-ză′shŭn) [L. *stabilis,* stable] **1.** The act of making something, such as a structure or chemical reaction, stable. **2.** The fixation or seating of a fixed or partial denture so that it will not be displaced in function.

***dynamic s.*** An integrated function of the neuromuscular systems requiring muscles to contract and fixate the body against fluctuating outside forces, providing postural support with fine adjustments in muscle tension. The term usually pertains to a function of the trunk, shoulder, and hip muscles and includes the lower-extremity muscles when they are functioning in a closed chain.

**stable** (stā′bl) **1.** Firm; steady. **2.** The structure of an atom that prevents spontaneous disintegration.

**stable condition** A term used in describing a patient's condition. It indicates that the patient's disease process has not changed precipitously or significantly.

**stachyose** A nonabsorbable carbohydrate present in beans. Because the substance is not absorbed or metabolized in the small intestine, it passes into the colon where it is acted on by bacteria to form gas. This may be related to the flatus produced by eating beans.

**stactometer** (stăk-tŏm′ĕt-ĕr) [Gr. *staktos,* dropping, + *metron,* measure] An instrument for measuring fluid in drops.

**stadium** (stā′dē-ŭm) [Gr. *stadion,* alteration] A stage or period in the progress of a disease. SYN: *stage* (1). SEE: *fastigium.*

***s. fluorescentiae*** The stage of eruption in an exanthematous disease.

***s. sudoris*** The sweating stage of a paroxysm of malaria.

**staff** (stăf) [AS. *staef,* a stick] **1.** An instrument to be introduced into the urethra and bladder as a guide to a surgical knife. **2.** The medical, nursing, and other personnel attached to a hospital.

***attending s.*** The group of physicians and surgeons who are in regular attendance at a hospital.

***consulting s.*** The physicians and surgeons attached to a hospital who may be consulted by members of the attending staff.

***house s.*** SEE: *house staff.*

***s. of Wrisberg*** Prominence of the cuneiform cartilage seen in the normal larynx during examination.

**stage** (stāj) [O. Fr. *estage*] **1.** Period in the course of a disease or in the life history of an organism. SYN: *stadium.* **2.** The platform of a microscope on which the slide is placed.

***algid s.*** The period of chilliness at the beginning of a fever.

***amphibolic s.*** The stage that intervenes between the acme of a disease and its outcome, at a time when the outcome is unknown.

***asphyxial s.*** The preliminary stage of Asiatic cholera.

***cold s.*** The chill or rigor of a malarial paroxysm.

***defervescent s.*** The period in which the temperature is declining.

***eruptive s.*** **1.** The period in which an exanthem appears. **2.** The middle stage in the pre-eruptive, eruptive, or posteruptive categorization of tooth eruption. It is characterized by root elongation and movement of the tooth mesially and toward the occlusal plane.

***expulsive s. of labor*** The stage of dilatation of the cervix uteri during which the child is expelled from uterus. SYN: *second s. of labor.*

***first s. of labor*** The period when the fetal head is molded and the cervix is dilated.

***fourth s. of labor*** The postpartum period beginning immediately after delivery of the placenta.

***hot s.*** Febrile stage in a malarial paroxysm.

***s. of invasion*** The period in which the causative agent is present in the body before the onset of a disease.

***s. of latency*** The incubation period of an infectious disorder.

***placental s. of labor*** The period of labor during which placenta and fetal membranes are discharged. SYN: *third s. of labor.*

***pre-eruptive s.*** The stage following infection and before appearance of eruption.

***pyrogenetic s.*** The stage of onset in a febrile disease.

***resting s.*** Term sometimes used for a cell that is between mitotic divisions. It is not accurate because the cell is metabolically active and is producing a new set of chromosomes for the next division.

***second s. of labor*** The expulsive s. of labor.

***sweating s.*** The third or terminal stage of malaria during which sweating occurs.

***third s. of labor*** The placental s. of labor.

**staggers** (stăg′ĕrz) Vertigo and confusion that occur in decompression illness.

**staging** The process of classifying tumors, esp. malignant tumors, with respect to their degree of differentiation, to their potential for responding to therapy, and to the patient's prognosis.

**stagnation** (stăg-nā′shŭn) [L. *stagnans,* stagnant] **1.** Cessation of motion. **2.** Stasis.

**stain** (stān) [O. Fr. *desteindre,* deprive of color] **1.** Any discoloration. SEE: *antistain formulary.* **2.** A pigment or dye used in coloring microscopic objects and tissues.

**3.** To apply pigment to a tissue or microscopic object.

***acid s.*** A stain in which the color-bearing ion (chromatophore) is the anion (e.g., eosin, commonly used to stain the cytoplasmic or basic elements of cells).

***acid-fast s.*** A stain used in bacteriology, esp. for staining *Mycobacterium tuberculosis.* A special solution of carbolfuchsin is used, which the organism retains in spite of washing with the decolorizing agent acid alcohol. SEE: *Ziehl-Neelsen method.*

***basic s.*** A stain in which the color-bearing ion is the cation (e.g., methylene blue, commonly used to stain the nucleic or acidic elements of cells).

***Commission Certified s.*** A stain that has been certified by the Biological Stain Commission.

***contrast s.*** A stain used to color one part of a tissue or cell, unaffected when another part is stained by another color.

***counter s.*** A stain, usually a contrast stain, used after the staining of specific elements of a tissue.

***dental s.*** A discoloration accumulating on the surface of teeth, denture, or denture base material, most often attributed to the use of tea, coffee, or tobacco. Many stains are due to ingestion of metal-containing dust or drugs. Copper and nickel produce a green stain; manganese and silver a black stain. Mercury produces a green-black stain; and iron a brown stain. A green or green-yellow stain, often present on the gingival third of the maxillary teeth of children, is thought to be caused by bacteria or fungi such as those of the genera *Penicillium* and *Aspergillus.* Both the metallic and stains from microorganisms are thought to be localized in the enamel cuticle remnants on the crown. Yellow, brown, or green fluorescent lines may be incorporated into the calcified structure of teeth as a result of tetracyclines taken while the teeth are forming during infancy and early childhood. Some orange dental stains seen on both labial and lingual surfaces of teeth are thought to be caused by chromogenic bacteria (e.g., *Serratia marcescens*).

***differential s.*** In bacteriology, a stain such as Gram's stain that enables one to differentiate among different types of bacteria.

***double s.*** A mixture of two contrasting dyes, usually an acid and a basic stain.

***Giemsa s.*** A stain that contains azure II–eosin and azure II. It is used in staining tissues including blood cells, Negri bodies, and chromosomes.

***hematoxylin-eosin s.*** A widely used method of staining tissues for microscopic examination. It stains the nuclei a deep blue-black and the cytoplasm pink.

***intravital s.*** A nontoxic dye that, when introduced into an organism, selectively stains certain cells or tissues. SYN: *vital s.*

***inversion s.*** A basic stain that, when under the influence of a mordant, acts as an acid stain.

***metachromatic s.*** A stain with which the constituents of cells or tissues develop a color different from the stain itself.

***neutral s.*** A combination of an acid and a basic stain.

***nuclear s.*** A basic stain affecting nuclei.

***port-wine s.*** Nevus flammeus.

***substantive s.*** A stain that is directly absorbed by the tissues when they are immersed in the staining solution.

***supravital s.*** Stain that will color living cells or tissues that have been removed from the body.

***tumor s.*** In arteriography, an abnormally dense area in a radiographic image caused by the collection of contrast medium in the vessels. This may be a sign of neoplastic growth.

***vital s.*** Intravital s.

***Wright's s.*** A polychrome stain used for staining blood smears. SEE: *Wright's technique.*

**staining** (stān'ĭng) [O. Fr. *desteindre*] The process of impregnating a substance, esp. a tissue, with pigments so that its component parts may be visible under a microscope. SEE: *Wright's technique.*

**staircase breaths** In basic life support, the serial application of several small breaths rather than a single large-volume breath. SEE: *cardiopulmonary resuscitation.*

**staircase phenomenon** The effect exhibited by skeletal and heart muscle when subjected to rapidly repeated maximal stimuli following a period of rest. In the resulting series of contractions, each is greater than the preceding one until a state of maximum contraction is reached. SYN: *treppe.* SEE: *stress test.*

**stalagmometer** (stăl-ăg-mŏm'ĕ-tĕr) [Gr. *stalagmos,* dropping, + *metron,* a measure] An instrument for measuring the number of drops in a given amount of fluid.

**stalk** (stawk) [ME] An elongated structure usually serving to attach or support an organ or structure.

***belly s.*** The structure in an embryo that develops into the umbilical cord.

***body s.*** A bridge of mesoderm that connects the caudal end of the embryo with the chorion. Into it grow the allantois and embryonic blood vessels, the latter forming the umbilical arteries and vein, which connect the embryo with the placenta.

***cerebellar s.*** One of the cerebellar peduncles that connect the cerebellum with the brainstem.

***infundibular s.*** Infundibulum (3).

***optic s.*** The structure that connects the optic vesicle or cup to the forebrain.

***yolk s.*** Vitelline duct.

**stamina** (stăm'ĭ-nă) [L., thread of the warp, thread of human life] Inherent force, constitutional energy; strength; endurance.

**stammering** (stăm'ĕr-ĭng) [AS. *stamerian*]

Stuttering.

***s. of bladder*** An interrupted and irregular flow of urine, with the muscles that control micturition acting spasmodically. SYN: *urinary stuttering.*

**standard** [O. Fr. *estandard,* marking rallying place] That which is established by custom or authority as a model, criterion, or rule for comparison of measurement.

***biological s.*** The standardization of drugs or biological products (vitamins, hormones, antibiotics) by testing their effects on animals. It is used when chemical analysis is impossible or impracticable.

**standard of care** **1.** A statement of actions consistent with minimum safe professional conduct under specific conditions, as determined by professional peer organizations. **2.** In forensic medicine, a measure with which the defendant's conduct is compared to determine negligence or malpractice. **3.** The acts of omission or commission that an ordinary prudent person would have done or not done if in the defendant's position.

**standard deviation** ABBR: S.D. SYMB: $\sigma$. In statistics, the commonly used measure of dispersion or variability in a distribution; the square root of the variance.

**standard error** ABBR: S.E. A measure of variability that could be expected of a statistical constant following the taking of random samples of a given size in a particular set of observations. An important standard error is that of the difference between the means of two samples.

**standard precautions** Guidelines recommended by the Centers for Disease Control and Prevention to reduce the risk of the spread of infection in hospitals. These precautions (e.g., handwashing, gloves, mask, eye protection, gown) apply to blood, all body fluids, secretions, excretions (except sweat), nonintact skin, and mucous membranes of all patients and are the primary strategy for successful nosocomial infection control. SEE: *Universal Precautions Appendix.*

**standard temperature and pressure, dry** ABBR: STPD. Gas volume at 0°C 760 mm Hg total pressure and partial pressure of water of zero (i.e., dry).

**standing orders** Orders, rules, regulations, or procedures prepared by the professional staff of a hospital or clinic and used as guidelines in the preparation and carrying out of medical and surgical procedures.

**standstill** A cessation of activity.

***atrial s.*** Cessation of atrial contractions.

***cardiac s.*** Cessation of contractions of the heart.

***inspiratory s.*** The temporary cessation of inspiration normally following each inspiration, resulting from stimulation of proprioceptors in the alveoli of the lungs. SEE: *Hering-Breuer reflex.*

***respiratory s.*** Cessation of respiratory movements.

***ventricular s.*** Cessation of ventricular contractions.

**stannic** (stăn′ĭk) [L. *stannum,* tin] **1.** Resembling or containing tin. **2.** In chemistry, containing tetravalent tin.

**stannosis** A condition caused by exposure to an inorganic dust produced when tin oxide is used in various manufacturing processes. Signs and symptoms include irritation of the eyes, nasal passages, and other mucous membranes. Because the exposure does not cause pulmonary disease and the clinical symptoms are reversible, the dust is classed as a nuisance dust.

**stannous** (stăn′ŭs) [L. *stannum,* tin] **1.** Resembling or containing tin. **2.** In chemistry, containing divalent tin.

**stannous fluoride** A fluoride compound used in toothpaste to prevent dental caries.

**stannum** (stăn′ŭm) [L.] Tin.

**stanozolol** (stăn′ō-zō-lōl″) An anabolic steroid. Trade name is Winstrol.

**Stanton's disease** Melioidosis.

**stapedectomy** (stā″pē-dĕk′tō-mē) [L. *stapes,* stirrup, + Gr. *ektome,* excision] Excision of the stapes in order to improve hearing, esp. in cases of otosclerosis. The stapes is replaced by a prosthesis.

During the first 24 hr following surgery, the patient remains flat in bed, head movements are kept to a minimum, and the patient is instructed to refrain from blowing his or her nose or sneezing (if possible). In the second 24 hr, the patient moves or arises only if assisted. The patient should not allow the ear to get wet for at least 10 days postoperatively. For 30 days following surgery, the patient should not fly, climb to high altitudes, or be exposed to loud sounds such as those produced by a jet aircraft. Sudden movements, even in elevators, should be avoided. SEE: *Nursing Diagnoses Appendix.*

**stapedial** (stā-pē′dē-ăl) Rel. to the stapes.

**stapediotenotomy** (stā-pē″dē-ō-tĕn-ŏt′ō-mē) [″ + Gr. *tenon,* tendon, + *tome,* incision] Division of the tendon of the stapedius muscle.

**stapediovestibular** (stā-pē″dē-ō-vĕs-tĭb′ū-lar) [″ + *vestibulum,* an antechamber] Rel. to the stapes and vestibule of the ear.

**stapedius** (stā-pē′dē-ŭs) [L. *stapes,* stirrup] A small muscle of the middle ear inserted in the stapes. SEE: *Muscles Appendix.*

**stapes** (stā′pēz) [L., stirrup] The ossicle in the middle ear that articulates with the incus; commonly called the *stirrup.* The footplate of the stapes fits into the oval window. SEE: *ear.*

**staphylectomy** (stăf″ĭ-lĕk′tō-mē) [Gr. *staphyle,* a bunch of grapes + *ektome,* excision] Staphylotomy (1).

**staphyledema** (stăf″ĭl-ē-dē′mă) [″ + *oidema,* swelling] Swelling of the uvula.

**staphyline** (stăf′ĭ-līn) [Gr. *staphyle,* a bunch of grapes] **1.** Resembling a bunch of grapes. SYN: *botryoid.* **2.** Rel. to the uvula. SYN: *uvular.*

**staphylion** (stăf-ĭl′ē-ŏn) [Gr., little grape] **1.** The craniometric point at the median line of the posterior border of the hard palate. **2.** Uvula.

**staphylitis** (stăf″ĭl-ī′tĭs) [Gr. *staphyle,* a bunch of grapes, + *itis,* inflammation] Inflammation of the uvula.

**staphylo-** [Gr. *staphyle,* a bunch of grapes] Combining form indicating the uvula, pert. to or resembling a bunch of grapes, or pert. to *Staphylococcus.*

**staphyloangina** (stăf″ĭl-ō-ăn′jĭ-nă) [″ + L. *angina,* sore throat] Sore throat due to staphylococcus.

**staphylococcal** (stăf″ĭl-ō-kŏk′ăl) [″ + *kokkos,* berry] Pert. to or caused by staphylococci.

**staphylococcal food poisoning** Poisoning by food containing any one of several heat-stable enterotoxins produced by certain strains of staphylococci. When ingested, the toxin causes nausea, vomiting, diarrhea, intestinal cramps, and, in severe cases, prostration and shock. The attack usually lasts 3 to 6 hr. Fatalities are rare. Hygienic preparation techniques can prevent this form of food poisoning. Persons preparing foods should cook all foods thoroughly, refrigerate foods during storage, and wash hands before and after handling foods. Certain foods, such as meat, poultry, fish, and those containing mayonnaise, eggs, or cream, should be refrigerated and used as soon as possible.

NURSING IMPLICATIONS: Patients who contract food poisoning should ingest clear fluids until abdominal pain subsides and return to a normal diet gradually. Fluid and electrolyte balance is monitored, and supportive therapy is maintained as indicated. Enteric precautions are used until evidence of infection subsides.

**staphylococcemia** (stăf″ĭl-ō-kŏk-sē′mē-ă) [″ + ″ + *haima,* blood] The presence of staphylococci in the blood. SYN: *staphylohemia.*

**staphylococci** (stăf″ĭl-ō-kŏk′sē) Pl. of staphylococcus.

**Staphylococcus** (stăf″ĭl-ō-kŏk′ŭs) [Gr. *staphyle,* a bunch of grapes, + *kokkos,* berry] A genus of micrococci belonging to the family Micrococcaceae, order Eubacteriales. They are gram-positive and when cultured on agar produce white, yellow, or orange colonies. Some species are pathogenic, causing suppurative conditions and elaborating endotoxins destructive to tissue cells. Some produce enterotoxins and are the cause of a common type of food poisoning.

***S. aureus*** A species of gram-positive, coagulase-positive anaerobes commonly present on the skin and mucous membranes, esp. those of the nose and mouth, characterized by the production of a golden-yellow pigment. It causes suppurative conditions such as boils, carbuncles, and internal abscesses in humans. Various strains of this species produce toxins including those that cause food poisoning, staphylococcal scalded skin syndrome, and toxic shock syndrome. Some strains also produce hemolysins and staphylokinase.

***S. aureus, methicillin-resistant*** ABBR: MRSA. A strain of *Staphylococcus aureus* resistant to anti-infective agents whose action is based on blocking penicillinase, an enzyme that inactivates penicillin. Patients with MRSA infections should be isolated and appropriate mask-gown-glove precautions used, depending on the site of the infection. SEE: *isolation; resistance, antibiotic.*

***S. aureus, vancomycin-resistant*** A strain of *Staphylococcus aureus* resistant to vancomycin that may become a serious nosocomial pathogen. SEE: *Universal Precautions Appendix.*

***S. epidermidis*** A coagulase-negative species characterized by the formation of white colonies; previously termed *S. albus.* It is the most persistent species of coagulase-negative staphylococci on skin.

***S. hominis*** A coagulase-negative species frequently recovered from skin. It is not consistently pathogenic for humans.

***S. saprophyticus*** A newly classified species that can cause urinary tract infections.

**staphylococcus** (stăf″ĭl-ō-kŏk′ŭs) *pl.* **staphylococci** Term applied loosely to any pathogenic micrococci. SEE: *bacteria* for illus.; *Staphylococcus.*

**staphyloderma** (stăf″ĭ-lō-dĕr′mă) [″ + *derma,* skin] Cutaneous infection with staphylococci.

**staphylodermatitis** (stăf″ĭl-ō-derm″ă-tī′tĭs) [″ + ″ + *itis,* inflammation] A dermatitis caused by staphylococci.

**staphylodialysis** (stăf″ĭ-lō-dī-ăl′ĭ-sĭs) [″ + *dia,* through, + *lysis,* dissolution] Relaxation or elongation of the uvula. SYN: *staphyloptosia; staphyloptosis.*

**staphylohemia** (stăf″ĭ-lō-hē′mē-ă) [″ + *haima,* blood] Staphylococcemia.

**staphylokinase** (stăf″ĭ-lō-kī′nās) A material produced by some strains of *Staphylococcus aureus* that can convert plasminogen to plasmin.

**staphylolysin** (stăf″ĭ-lŏl′ĭ-sĭn) [″ + *lysis,* dissolution] A hemolysin produced by staphylococci.

**staphyloma** (stăf″ĭl-ō′mă) [Gr.] A protrusion of the cornea or sclera of the eye.

***anterior s.*** Globular enlargement of the anterior part of the eye. SYN: *keratoglobus.*

***ciliary s.*** Staphyloma in the region of the ciliary body.

***s. corneae*** Thinning and bulging of the cornea.

***equatorial s.*** Staphyloma in the equatorial region of the eye.

***intercalary s.*** Staphyloma in the region

of the union of the sclera with the periphery of the iris.

***partial s.*** Staphyloma that extends in one direction, displacing the pupil. The remainder of the cornea is clear.

***posterior s.*** A bulging of the sclera backward.

***total s.*** An opaque, protuberant cicatrix found in place of the cornea. It is caused by a perforation of the cornea resulting in poor vision, increased tension, and rupture of thin scar. Treatment involves incision, excision, and ablation.

***uveal s.*** The protrusion of any portion of the uvea through the sclera.

**staphylomatous** (stăf″ĭ-lŏm′ă-tŭs) Concerning or similar to a staphyloma.

**staphyloncus** (stăf″ĭ-lŏng′kŭs) [Gr. *staphyle,* a bunch of grapes, + *onkos,* bulk, mass] A tumor or enlargement of the uvula.

**staphylopharyngeus** (stăf″ĭ-lō-făr-ĭn′jē-ŭs) [″ + *pharynx,* throat] Palatopharyngeus.

**staphylopharyngorrhaphy** (stăf″ĭ-lō-făr″ĭn-gor′ă-fē) [″ + ″ + *rhaphe,* seam, ridge] Any of several different operations on the soft palate and uvula.

**staphyloplasty** (stăf′ĭ-lō-plăs″tē) [″ + *plassein,* to form] Plastic surgery of the uvula or soft palate.

**staphyloptosia, staphyloptosis** (stăf″ĭ-lŏp-tō′sē-ă, -sĭs) [″ + *ptosis,* a dropping] Relaxation or elongation of the uvula. SYN: *staphylodialysis.*

**staphylorrhaphy** (stăf″ĭl-or′ă-fē) [″ + *rhaphe,* seam, ridge] Suture of a cleft palate.

**staphyloschisis** (stăf″ĭ-lŏs′kĭ-sĭs) [″ + *schisis,* a splitting] Cleft palate.

**staphylotome** (stăf′ĭ-lō-tōm) [″ + *tome,* incision] An instrument for cutting the uvula.

**staphylotomy** (stăf″ĭ-lŏt′ō-mē) **1.** [″ + *tome,* incision] Amputation or incision of the uvula. SYN: *staphylectomy.* **2.** [Gr. *staphyloma,* corneal protrusion, + *tome,* incision] Excision of a staphyloma.

**staphylotoxin** (stăf″ĭ-lō-tŏk′sĭn) [Gr. *staphyle,* a bunch of grapes, + *toxikon,* poison] A toxin elaborated by one of the staphylococci, esp. *S. aureus.* Among some of the toxins produced are an enterotoxin, a cause of food poisoning, and exotoxins, including a hemotoxin that lyses red blood cells, a dermonecrotic toxin, toxic shock syndrome toxin-1, and leukocidins.

**staple food** Any food that supplies a substantial part, at least 25% to 35%, of the caloric requirement and is regularly consumed by a certain population.

**stapling** In surgery, a means of fastening tissues together by using special staples compatible with tissues. Staples are made of either titanium or an absorbable polymeric material. The staples are applied in a manner similar to that used in stapling sheets of paper together.

**star** [AS. *steorra*] Any structure resembling a star. SYN: *aster.*

***lens s.*** A starlike structure developing in the lens of the eye as a result of unequal growth of lens fibers.

***s.'s of Verheyen*** Star-shaped masses of veins on the surface of the kidney. SYN: *stellate veins.*

**starch** [AS. *stercan*] Noncrystalline carbohydrate of the polysaccharide group found in plants. Included are vegetable starches, pectins, dextrins, and gums. All are rather easily decomposed, have high molecular weights, and yield monosaccharides on complete hydrolysis. Those that the body can hydrolyze into hexoses are useful as concentrated energy-giving foods. All are reduced to simple sugars before they are absorbed. When some fruits ripen, the starch is changed to sugar, while some vegetables (peas and corn) change sugar into starch as their seeds develop.

The amylases of saliva and pancreatic juice hydrolyze starches to dextrins and maltose. These in turn are hydrolyzed to glucose, which is absorbed into the bloodstream. Glucose not immediately needed for energy is converted into glycogen, a form of starch that is stored in the liver or in muscle tissue. Pure starches, having the formula $(C_6H_{10}O_5)_n$, if normally metabolized, leave no residue and give rise only to carbon dioxide and water.

***animal s.*** Glycogen.

***corn s.*** Starch obtained from ordinary corn or maize (*Zea mays*). It is used as a dusting powder and an absorbent and is a constituent in many pastes and ointments. It is widely used in industry and as a food.

**starch glycerite** A combination of starch, benzoic acid, purified water, and glycerin; used as an emollient in formulations for external use.

**stare** (stār) [AS. *starian*] To gaze fixedly at anyone or anything.

**Star of Life symbol** The symbol approved by the Department of Transportation to represent the emergency medical services, displayed on ambulances and outside of emergency departments. SEE: illus.

**Starling's law of heart** [Ernest Henry Starling, Brit. physiologist, 1866–1927] A law that states that the force of the heartbeat is determined primarily by the length of the fibers constituting its muscular wall (i.e., an increase in diastolic filling increases the force of the heartbeat).

**Starling's law of intestine** A law stating that a stimulus within the intestine (i.e., the presence of food) initiates a band of constriction on the proximal side and relaxation on the distal side. This results in a peristaltic wave.

**starter 1.** A pure culture of bacteria or other microorganism used to initiate a particular fermentation, as in the making of cheese. **2.** Fluid containing bromine ions added to new developer fluid in a processor to decrease overactivity.

**star test pattern** In radiography, a test to

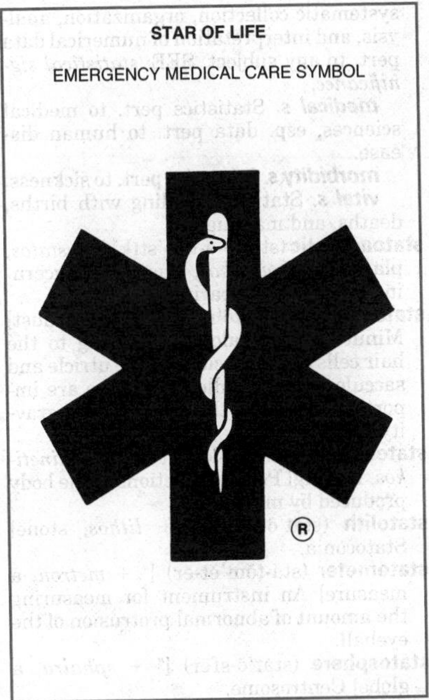


evaluate the resolution of the focal spot of the x-ray tube.

**startle syndrome** The uncontrollable excessive startle reaction that follows any stimulus for which there is usually no adaptation, such as a sudden noise, flash of light, or touching of a person. This causes a stiffening of the body, flexion of the arms, and sometimes a shout and fall to the ground. The verbal portion of the response may be related to what the individual is thinking or viewing at the time and may be a source of embarrassment. This syndrome was originally described as the Jumping Frenchmen of Maine, but it exists in other areas of the world. Treatment with clonazepam is beneficial. SYN: *hyperexplexias.*

**starvation** [AS. *steorfan,* to die] **1.** The condition of being without food for a long period of time. When everything but air and water is withheld, the sequence of events is as follows: (1) hunger, beginning about 4 hr after the last meal, accompanied by gastric contraction and general restlessness, becoming more acute periodically, esp. at times when meals were customarily taken; (2) loss of weight; (3) utilization of glycogen stored in the liver and muscles; (4) utilization of stored fat; (5) spells of nausea and diminishing acuteness of the sensation of hunger; (6) destruction of body protein. The greatest loss of weight is in the fatty tissues, spleen, and liver. **2.** The condition in which the supply of a specific food is below minimum bodily requirements, such as protein starvation. SEE: *kwashiorkor.* **3.** The condition resulting from failure of the body to digest and absorb essential foodstuffs. SEE: *deficiency disease; diet; dietetics.*

**stasibasiphobia** (stă″sĭ-bā″sĭ-fō′bē-ă) [Gr. *stasis,* a standing, + *basis,* step, + *phobos,* fear] The delusion of one's inability to stand or walk, or fear to make the attempt.

**stasimorphia, stasimorphy** (stă″sĭ-mor′fē-ă, -fē) [″ + *morphe,* form] A deformity caused by the failure to develop and grow.

**stasiphobia** (stă″sĭ-fō′bē-ă) [″ + *phobos,* fear] The delusion of one's inability to stand erect or hesitation to make the attempt.

**stasis** (stā′sĭs) [Gr. *stasis,* a standing] Stoppage of the normal flow of fluids, as of the blood or urine, or of the intestinal mechanism. SYN: *stagnation* (2).

***diffusion s.*** Stasis with diffusion of lymph or serum.

***intestinal s.*** Condition in which peristaltic movements fail to move food along the intestine.

***venous s.*** Stasis of blood caused by venous congestion.

**stat** [L., *statim*] Immediately.

**state** [L. *status,* condition] **1.** A condition. **2.** A mode or condition of being.

***anxiety s.*** A condition marked by more or less continuous anxiety and apprehension. SEE: *neurosis, anxiety.*

***central excitatory s.*** ABBR: CES. A condition of increased excitability in the central nervous system, esp. in the spinal cord, following an excitatory stimulus.

***central inhibitory s.*** ABBR: CIS. A condition of decreased excitability in the central nervous system, esp. in the spinal cord, resulting from an inhibitory stimulus.

***dream s.*** The state of diminished consciousness in which the surroundings are perceived as if in a dream.

***excited s.*** The new state produced when energy is added to a nucleus, atom, or molecule. The energy is added by the absorption of photons or by collisions with other particles.

***fatigue s.*** Neurasthenia.

***ground s.*** The state of the lowest energy of a system such as an atom or molecule.

***persistent vegetative s.*** A continuing and unremitting clinical condition of complete unawaremess of the self and the environment accompanied by sleep-wake cycles with either complete or partial preservation of hypothalamic and brainstem autonomic functions. The diagnosis is established if the condition is present for 1 month after acute or nontraumatic brain injury or has lasted for 1 month in patients with degenerative or metabolic disorders or developmental malformations.

***refractory s.*** The condition of reduced

ability to be excited just after a muscle and nerve have been stimulated.

***steady s.*** In physiology, the condition of the metabolic needs of a system such as the muscles being supplied with nutrients at the same rate the energy is expended; dynamic equilibrium.

**static** (stăt'ĭk) [Gr. *statikos,* causing to stand] At rest; in equilibrium; not in motion.

**static balance** Static equilibrium.

**static equilibrium** The ability to maintain a steady position of the head and body in relation to gravity; the opposite of dynamic equilibrium or dynamic balance. SYN: *static balance.*

**static pressure** The pressure existing in all points in the circulation when the heart is stopped. It provides a measure of how well the circulatory bed is filled with blood.

**static reaction** One of the postural reflex responses important to standing and walking. Included are local static reactions acting on individual limbs, segmental static reactions linking the extremities together, and general static reactions to the position of the head in space.

**statics** (stăt'ĭks) The study of matter at rest and of the forces bringing about equilibrium. SEE: *dynamics.*

**static splint** Any orthosis that lacks movable parts and is used for positioning, stability, protection, or support.

**statim** (stăt'ĭm) [L.] ABBR: stat. Immediately; at once.

**station** (stā'shŭn) [L. *statio,* standing] **1.** The manner of standing. **2.** A stopping place. **3.** In obstetrics, the relationship in centimeters between the leading bony portion of the fetal head and the level of the ischial spines. This is useful in judging the level of application of forceps to aid in delivery. SEE: *forceps.*

***aid s.*** A site in the army for collecting the wounded in battle.

***dressing s.*** A temporary station for soldiers wounded during combat.

***rest s.*** A temporary relief station for the sick on a military road or railway.

**stationary** (stā'shŭn-ĕr-ē) [L. *stationarius,* belonging to a station] Remaining in a fixed condition.

**statistical** (stă-tĭs'tĭ-kăl) Pert. to statistics.

**statistical significance** In statistics, after appropriate analysis of the data, the conclusion that the event being investigated had a certain probability of being due to chance, but the probability was so slight that it is presumed that the event was not caused by mere chance. Probability is referred to as the *p value;* and, if the analysis indicated that there was only a one in 20 chance or less (i.e., *p* equal to or less than 0.05) that the observed results occurred due to chance, then the study results are arbitrarily considered to be statistically significant.

**statistics** (stă-tĭs'tĭks) [LL. *statisticus*] The systematic collection, organization, analysis, and interpretation of numerical data pert. to any subject. SEE: *statistical significance.*

***medical s.*** Statistics pert. to medical sciences, esp. data pert. to human disease.

***morbidity s.*** Statistics pert. to sickness.

***vital s.*** Statistics dealing with births, deaths, and marriages.

**statoacoustic** (stăt"ō-ă-koo'stĭk) [Gr. *statos,* placed, + *akoustikos,* acoustic] Concerning balance and hearing.

**statoconia** (stăt"ō-kō'nē-ă) [" + *konos,* dust] Minute bits of calcium adhering to the hair cells of the maculae of the utricle and saccule of the middle ear. These are important in sensing the orientation to gravity. SYN: *statolith.*

**statokinetic** (stăt"kō-kĭn-ĕt'ĭk) [" + *kinetikos,* moving] Pert. to reactions of the body produced by movement.

**statolith** (stăt'ō-lĭth) [" + *lithos,* stone] Statoconia.

**statometer** (stă-tŏm'ĕt-ĕr) [" + *metron,* a measure] An instrument for measuring the amount of abnormal protrusion of the eyeball.

**statosphere** (stăt'ō-sfēr) [" + *sphaira,* a globe] Centrosome.

**stature** (stăt'ūr) [L. *statura*] The height of the body in a standing position.

***short s.*** Body height at a specified age below the level obtained at that age by 70% of the population. A number of disease states, including hormonal, nutritional, and intrauterine growth retardation, may cause this condition. It is important to determine the cause and initiate appropriate therapy as soon as possible.

**status** (stā'tŭs) *pl.* **statuses** [L.] A state or condition.

***s. asthmaticus*** Persistent and intractable asthma.

***s. dysraphicus*** A condition resulting from imperfect closure of neural tube of embryo.

***s. epilepticus*** SEE: *epilepsy.*

***mental s.*** The functional state of the mind as judged by the individual's behavior, appearance, responsiveness to stimuli of all kinds, speech, memory, and judgment.

***s. parathyreoprivus*** A condition resulting from loss of parathyroid tissue.

***s. raptus*** A state of ecstasy.

***s. sternuens*** Continual sneezing that may be caused by transient irritation of the nasal mucosa. Treatment involves application of a topical anesthetic to the nasal mucosa.

***s. verrucosus*** The defective development of the cerebral gyri with many small gyri. This gives a warty appearance to the surface of the brain.

**statute** Laws enacted by a state legislature.

**statutes of limitations** Federal and state laws that set maximum time limits in which lawsuits can be brought and actions, claims, or rights can be enforced. No legal action can be brought outside the time allowed by law even if the person or entity has a claim or cause of action. In medical negligence claims, the statute usually is in effect from the time the wrong occurred or from the time it was or should have been discovered. Time limitations vary from state to state.

**staunch** (stŏnch) [O. Fr. *estanche,* firm] To stop the flow of blood from a wound.

**staurion** (staw′rē-ŏn) [Gr. *stauros,* little cross] The craniometric point where the transverse palatine suture crosses the median one.

**stauroplegia** (staw″rō-plē′jē-ă) [″ + *plege,* stroke] Alternate hemiplegia.

**S.T.D.** **1.** *sexually transmitted disease.* **2.** *skin test dose.* SEE: *Dick test.*

**steal** (stēl) The deviation of blood flow from its normal course or rate of flow.

***subclavian s.*** SEE: *subclavian steal syndrome.*

**steam** (stēm) [AS. *steam,* vapor] **1.** The invisible vapor into which water is converted at the boiling point. **2.** The mist formed by condensation of water vapor. **3.** Any vaporous exhalation.

**steam tent** A device that permits the inhalation of vapors. If no tent is available, a makeshift tent may be improvised. It is important that the method used does not burn the patient.

SOLUTIONS: Approx. 1 qt (or 1 L) of boiling water to which is added 1 tsp (5 ml) of compound tincture of benzoin or 1 tsp (5 ml) of tincture of benzoin (this does not contain aloe), a few crystals of menthol or camphor, or a few drops of methyl salicylate. These ingredients are pleasant to smell but have relatively little therapeutic effect. Most of the value is in the water vapor.

**steapsin** (stē-ăp′sĭn) [Gr. *stear,* fat, + *pepsis,* digestion] A lipolytic enzyme present in pancreatic juice that hydrolyzes fats to fatty acid and glycerine. The bile salts prepare the fats for the action of steapsin by emulsifying them. SYN: *pancreatic lipase.* SEE: *enzyme; pancreas.*

**stearate** (stē′ă-rāt) An ester or salt of stearic acid.

**stearic acid** (stē-ăr′ĭk) [Gr. *stear,* fat] A white, fatty acid found in solid animal fats and a few vegetable fats.

**steariform** (stē-ăr′ĭ-form) [″ + *forma,* shape] Resembling fat.

**stearin** (stē′ă-rĭn) [Gr. *stear,* fat] A white crystalline solid in animal and vegetable fats; $C_3H_5(C_{18}H_{35}O_2)_3$; any of the esters of glycerol and stearic acid, specifically glyceryl tristearate. One of the commonest fats in the body, esp. the solid ones. It breaks down into stearic acid and glycerol.

**stearodermia** (stē″ă-rō-dĕr′mē-ă) [″ + *derma,* skin] A disease of the sebaceous glands of the skin.

**stearopten(e)** (stē″ă-rŏp′tēn) [″ + *ptenos,* volatile] The more solid portion of a volatile oil as distinguished from the more fluid portion or eleoptene. Menthol and thymol are examples.

**stearrhea** (stē″ă-rē′ă) [Gr. *stear,* fat, + *rhoia,* flow] The excessive secretion of sebum or fat from the sebaceous glands of the skin. SYN: *seborrhea oleosa.*

**steatadenoma** (stē-ăt″ăd-ĕ-nō′mă) [Gr. *steatos,* fat, + *aden,* gland, + *oma,* tumor] A tumor of the sebaceous glands.

**steatitis** (stē″ă-tī′tĭs) [″ + *itis,* inflammation] Inflammation of adipose tissue.

**steato-** [Gr. *steatos,* fat] Combining form meaning *fat.* SEE: *adipo-; lipo-.*

**steatocele** (stē-ăt′ō-sēl, stē′ăt-ō-sēl) [″ + *kele,* tumor, swelling] Fatty tumor within the scrotum.

**steatocryptosis** (stē″ă-tō-krĭp-tō′sĭs) [″ + *krypte,* a sac, + *osis,* condition] Any disease of the sebaceous glands. SEE: *stearodermia.*

**steatocystoma multiplex** A skin disorder marked by the development of many sebaceous cysts.

**steatogenous** (stē″ă-tŏj′ĕn-ŭs) [Gr. *steatos,* fat, + *gennan,* to produce] **1.** Causing fatty degeneration. **2.** Producing any sebaceous gland disease.

**steatolysis** (stē″ă-tŏl′ĭ-sĭs) [″ + *lysis,* dissolution] **1.** The process by which fats are first emulsified and then hydrolyzed to fatty acids and glycerine preparatory to absorption. **2.** The decomposition of fat. SYN: *lipolysis.*

**steatolytic** (stē″ă-tō-lĭt′ĭk) Concerning steatolysis.

**steatoma** (stē″ă-tō′mă) [″ + *oma,* tumor] **1.** Sebaceous cyst. **2.** Lipoma.

This smooth, shiny, globular, cutaneous or subcutaneous tumor ranges from a few mm to 10 cm in size. It arises from the sebaceous glands and may occur singly or multiply, usually on the neck, scalp, back, or scrotum. Prolonged irritation may cause suppuration. The tumor should be surgically excised by dissection, without perforating the sac.

**steatomatous** (stē″ă-tō′mă-tŭs) The presence of multiple sebaceous cysts.

**steatonecrosis** (stē″ă-tō-nē-krō′sĭs) [″ + *nekros,* corpse, + *osis,* condition] Necrosis of the fatty tissue in small patches.

**steatopathy** (stē-ă-tŏp′ă-thē) [″ + *pathos,* disease, suffering] Disease of the sebaceous glands of the skin.

**steatopygia** (stē″ă-tō-pĭj′ē-ă) [″ + *pyge,* buttock] Abnormal fatness of the buttocks, occurring more frequently in women than in men. It is seen in some tropical areas of Africa. The location of this excess fat accumulation in the buttocks may represent an adaptation to a very hot climate. It is thought that if this fat were evenly spread throughout the subcutaneous tissue, normal cooling of the skin would be severely limited.

**steatorrhea** (stē″ă-tō-rē′ă) [Gr. *steatos,* fat,

+ *rhoia,* flow] **1.** Increased secretion of fat from the sebaceous glands of the skin. SYN: *seborrhea.* **2.** Fatty stools, as seen in pancreatic diseases.

***idiopathic s.*** Sprue.

***s. simplex*** Excessive secretion of the sebaceous glands of the face.

**steatosis** (stē″ă-tō′sĭs) [″ + *osis,* condition] **1.** Fatty degeneration. **2.** Disease of the sebaceous glands.

**stegnosis** (stĕg-nō′sĭs) [Gr. *stegnosis,* obstruction] **1.** Checking of a secretion or discharge. **2.** Stenosis. **3.** Constipation.

**stegnotic** (stĕg-nŏt′ĭk) Bringing about stegnosis. SYN: *astringent.*

**Stegomyia** (stĕg″ō-mī′ē-ă) A subgenus of mosquito of the genus *Aedes,* family Culicidae, suspected of transmitting the virus of yellow fever.

**Steinert's disease** (stīn′ĕrts) [Hans Steinert, Ger. physician, b. 1875] A hereditary disease characterized by muscular wasting, myotonia, and cataract. SYN: *myotonia dystrophica.*

**Stein-Leventhal syndrome** (stīn-lĕv′ĕn-thăl) [Irving F. Stein, Sr., U.S. gynecologist, b. 1887; Michael L. Leventhal, U.S. obstetrician and gynecologist, 1901–1971] Hyperandrogenism with chronic anovulation in women without specific underlying adrenal or pituitary gland disease. Menses may be regular but later oligomenorrhea develops and then amenorrhea, but infrequently ovulation will occur. Infertility is usually persistent but may be treated with clomiphene, gonadotropins, or wedge resection of the ovary. SYN: *polycystic ovary syndrome.*

**Steinmann's extension** (stīn′mănz) [Fritz Steinmann, Swiss surgeon, 1872–1932] Traction applied to a limb by applying weight to a pin placed through the bone at right angles to the direction of pull of the traction force.

**Steinmann pin** A metal rod used for internal fixation of the adjacent sections of a fractured bone.

**stella** [L.] Star.

***s. lentis hyaloidea*** Posterior pole of the crystalline lens of the eye.

***s. lentis iridica*** Anterior pole of the crystalline lens of the eye.

**stellate** [L. *stellatus*] Star-shaped; arranged with parts radiating from a center.

**stellate bandage** A bandage that is wrapped on the back, crossways.

**stellate cell** Any cell that appears star-shaped (e.g., astrocytes and Kupffer's cells).

**stellate fracture** A fracture with numerous fissures radiating from the central point of injury.

**stellate ganglion** A sympathetic ganglion formed by the fusion of the inferior cervical and first thoracic ganglions.

**stellate ligament** One of the anterior costovertebral ligaments.

**stellate reticulum** The central cellular portion of the enamel organ, considered to be a nutritive store or protective covering of the developing enamel crown. SYN: *enamel pulp.*

**stellate veins** Stars of Verheyen.

**stellectomy** (stĕl-lĕk′tō-mē) [″ + *ektome,* excision] The surgical removal of the stellate ganglion.

**Stellwag's sign** (stĕl′văgs) [Carl Stellwag von Carion, Austrian oculist, 1823–1904] Widening of the palpebral aperture with absence or lessened frequency of winking, seen in Graves' disease.

**stem 1.** [AS. *stemn,* tree trunk] Any stalk-like structure. **2.** To derive from or originate in. **3.** [ME. *stemmen*] To check, stop, or hold back.

**stem cell** Hemocytoblast.

**stenion** (stĕn′ē-ŏn) [Gr. *stenos,* narrow] The craniometric point at the extremities of the smallest transverse diameter in the temporal region.

**steno-** [Gr. *stenos,* narrow] Combining form meaning *narrow* or *short.*

**stenobregmatic** (stĕn″ō-brĕg-măt′ĭk) [″ + *bregma,* front of head] A term applied to a skull with narrowing of the upper and frontal portions.

**stenocephaly** (stĕn″ō-sĕf′ă-lē) [″ + *kephale,* head] Narrowness of the cranium in one or more diameters.

**stenocompressor** (stĕn″ō-kŏm-prĕs′or) [″ + L. *compressor,* that which presses together] An instrument for compressing Stensen's ducts to stop the flow of saliva.

**stenopaic, stenopeic** (stĕn-ŏ-pā′ĭk, -pē′ĭk) [Gr. *stenos,* narrow, + *ope,* opening] Provided with a narrow opening or slit, esp. denoting optical devices to protect against snow blindness.

**stenosal** (stē-nō′săl) [Gr. *stenos,* narrow] Stenotic.

**stenosed** (stē-nōst′, stĕn′ōzd) Marked by stenosis; constricted.

**stenosis** (stĕ-nō′sĭs) [Gr., act of narrowing] The constriction or narrowing of a passage or orifice. SYN: *stricture.*

ETIOLOGY: This may result from embryonic maldevelopment, hypertrophy and thickening of a sphincter muscle, inflammatory disorders, or excessive development of fibrous tissue. It may involve almost any tube or duct.

***aortic s.*** SEE: under *aortic.*

***cardiac s.*** A narrowing or constriction of any of the orifices leading into or from the heart or between the chambers of the heart.

***cicatricial s.*** Stenosis resulting from any contracted cicatrix.

***lumbar s.*** An overgrowth of the laminae of the vertebrae so that the spinal canal is narrowed. This may cause back and leg pain, esp. when walking. SEE: *back pain.*

***mitral s.*** Narrowing of the mitral orifice, obstructing free flow from the atrium to the ventricle. SEE: *Nursing Diagnoses Appendix.*

***pulmonary s.*** Narrowing of the opening into the pulmonary artery from the right cardiac ventricle.

***pyloric s.*** An obstruction caused by hypertrophy of the walls of the pyloric orifice.

***subaortic s.*** A congenital constriction of the aortic tract below the aortic valves.

***tricuspid s.*** Narrowing of the opening to the tricuspid valve.

**stenostomia** (stĕn″ō-stō′mē-ă) [Gr. *stenos,* narrow, + *stoma,* mouth] Narrowing of the mouth.

**stenothorax** (stĕn″ō-thō′răks) [″ + *thorax,* chest] An unusually narrow thorax.

**stenotic** [Gr. *stenosis,* act of narrowing] Produced by or marked by stenosis.

**Stensen's duct** (stĕn′sĕns) [Niels Stensen, Danish anatomist, 1638–1686] The duct leading from the parotid gland to the oral cavity.

**Stensen's foramina** Incisive foramina of the hard palate, transmitting anterior branches of the descending palatine vessels.

**stent** [Charles R. Stent, Brit. dentist, 1845–1901] **1.** Originally a compound used in making dental molds. **2.** Any material or device used to hold tissue in place or to provide a support for a graft or anastomosis while healing is taking place.

***intraluminal coronary artery s.*** A stent made of an inert material, usually stainless steel, with a self-expanding mesh introduced into the coronary artery. It is used to prevent lumen closure (restenosis) following bypass surgery and to treat acute vessel closure after angioplasty.

***urologic s.*** A cylindrical device made of mesh that is inserted into the ureter or urethra during cystoscopy. The stent is kept collapsed while being inserted. After insertion, it opens up and presses against the wall. Eventually the normal tissue grows through the mesh, and within several months this forms a smooth unobstructed lumen. Stents are used in ureters to relieve urinary obstruction due to edema, trauma, or pressure from kidney stones or from a tumor outside the ureter. They are used in the urethra to relieve obstruction from benign prostatic hypertrophy or strictures of the urethra. They are of particular benefit to patients whose physical condition prevents them from undergoing surgery.

**step** A series of rests for the foot used for ascending or descending.

***Rönne's s.*** A steplike defect in the visual field.

**stephanion** (stĕ-fā′nē-ŏn) [Gr. *stephanos,* crown] The point at the intersection of the superior temporal ridge and coronal suture.

**steppage gait** A high-stepping gait seen with paralysis of the dorsiflexors of the ankle; seen in diabetic neuropathy of the peroneal nerve. The patient lifts the foot very high in walking, to raise the drooping toes from the ground or floor.

**steradian** (stē-rā′dē-ăn) The unit of measurement of solid angles. It encloses an area on the surface of a sphere equal to the square of the radius of the sphere.

**sterco-** [L. *stercus,* dung] Combining form meaning *feces.* SEE: *scato-.*

**stercobilin** (stĕr″kō-bī′lĭn) [″ + *bilis,* bile] A brown pigment derived from the bile, giving the characteristic color to feces. SEE: *urobilin.*

**stercobilinogen** (stĕr″kō-bī-lĭn′ō-jĕn) A colorless substance derived from urobilinogen. It is present in the feces and turns brown on oxidation.

**stercolith** (stĕr′kō-lĭth) [″ + Gr. *lithos,* stone] A fecal calculus.

**stercoraceous** (stĕr″kō-rā′shŭs) [L. *stercoraceus*] Having the nature of, pert. to, or containing feces.

**stercorolith** (stĕr′kō-rō-lĭth) [″ + Gr. *lithos,* stone] A fecal concretion. SYN: *coprolith; fecalith.*

**stereo-, stere-** Combining form meaning *solid, having three dimensions,* or *firmly established.*

**stereoagnosis** (stĕr″ē-ō-ăg-nō′sĭs) [Gr. *stereos,* solid, + *a-,* not, + *gnosis,* knowledge] Astereognosis.

**stereoanesthesia** (stĕr″ē-ō-ăn″ĕs-thē′zē-ă) [″ + *an-,* not, + *aisthesis,* sensation] The inability to recognize objects by feeling their form.

**stereoarthrolysis** (stĕr″ē-ō-ăr-thrŏl′ĭ-sĭs) [″ + *arthron,* joint, + *lysis,* dissolution] The surgical formation of a movable new joint in bony ankylosis.

**stereoauscultation** (stĕr″ē-ō-aws″kŭl-tā′shŭn) [″ + L. *auscultare,* listen to] Auscultation by use of a stethoscope with two ends on it so each may be placed on different parts of the chest. One tube of each instrument is inserted into an ear while the other is squeezed shut by the fingers.

**stereocampimeter** (stĕr″ē-ō-kăm-pĭm′ĕ-tĕr) [″ + L. *campus,* field, + Gr. *metron,* measure] A device for measuring the visual field of both eyes simultaneously.

**stereochemical** (stĕr″ē-ō-kĕm′ĭ-kăl) [″ + *chemeia,* chemistry] Concerning stereochemistry.

**stereochemistry** (stĕr″ē-ō-kĕm′ĭs-trē) That branch of chemistry dealing with atoms in their space relationship, and the effect of such a relationship on the action and effects of the molecule.

**stereocilia** (stĕr″ē-ō-sĭl′ē-ă) *sing.* **stereocilium** Nonmotile protoplasmic projections from free surfaces of cells of the ductus epididymis and ductus deferens and on the hair cells of the receptors of the inner ear.

**stereocinefluorography** (stĕr″ē-ō-sĭn″ĕ-flū″or-ŏg′ră-fē) Motion picture photography of the images produced by stereofluorography. This provides a three-dimensional visualization.

**stereoencephalotomy** (stĕr″ē-ō-ĕn-sĕf″ă-lŏt′ō-mē) [″ + *enkephalos,* brain, + *tome,* incision] Surgical incision by use of stereotaxis.

**stereognosis** (stĕr″ē-ŏg-nō′sĭs) [″ + *gnosis,* knowledge] The ability to recognize the form of solid objects by touch.

**stereogram** (stĕr′ē-ō-grăm) [″ + *gramma,* something written] Stereoscopic roentgenogram.

**stereoisomerism** (stĕr″ē-ō-ī-sō′mĕr-ĭzm) A condition in which two or more substances may have the same empirical formula but mirror-image structural formulas.

**stereology** (stĕr″ē-ŏl′ō-jē) [Gr. *stereos,* solid, + *logos,* word, reason] The study of three-dimensional aspects of objects.

**stereometry** (stĕr″ē-ŏm′ĕ-trē) [″ + *metron,* a measure] The measurement of a solid body or the cubic contents of a hollow body.

**stereo-ophthalmoscope** (stĕr″ē-ō-ŏf-thăl′mō-skōp) [″ + *ophthalmos,* eye, + *skopein,* to examine] An ophthalmoscope that is designed to permit the fundus to be seen simultaneously by both eyes of the examiner.

**stereo-orthopter** (stĕr″ē-ō-or-thŏp′tĕr) [″ + *orthos,* straight, + *opsis,* vision] A mirror-reflecting device for the treatment of strabismus.

**stereophantoscope** (stĕr″ē-ō-făn′tō-skōp) [″ + *phantos,* visible, + *skopein,* to examine] A stereoscopic device with rotating disks for testing vision.

**stereophorometer** (stĕr″ē-ō-for-ŏm′ĕ-tĕr) [″ + *phoros,* a bearer, + *metron,* measure] A prism-refracting device for use in correcting extraocular eye muscle imbalance.

**stereophotography** (stĕr″ē-ō-fō-tŏg′ră-fē) [″ + *phos,* light, + *graphein,* to write] Photography that produces the effect of solidity or depth in the pictures.

**stereophotomicrograph** (stĕr″ē-ō-fō″tō-mī′krō-grăf) [″ + ″ + *mikros,* tiny, + *graphein,* to write] A photograph showing the solidity or depth of a microscopic subject.

**stereopsis** (stĕr″ē-ŏp′sĭs) [″ + *opsis,* vision] Stereoscopic vision.

**stereoradiography** (stĕr″ē-ō-rā″dē-ŏg′ră-fē) [″ + L. *radius,* ray, + Gr. *graphein,* to write] Radiography from two slightly different angles so that a stereoscopic effect is produced when the radiographs are viewed through a stereoscope.

**stereoscope** (stĕr′ē-ō-skōp) [″ + *skopein,* to examine] An instrument that creates an impression of solidity or depth of objects seen by combining images of two pictures.

**stereoscopic, stereoscopical** Pert. to the stereoscope or its use.

**stereospecific** (stĕr″ē-ō-spĕ-sĭf′ĭk) Specific for only one of the possible receptors on a cell.

**stereotropism** (stĕr″ē-ŏt′rō-pĭzm) [″ + *tropos,* a turning, + *-ismos,* condition] A response toward (positive stereotropism) or away from (negative stereotropism) a solid object. SYN: *thigmotropism.*

**stereotypic movement disorder** Motor behavior, persisting for at least 4 weeks, that is repetitive, often seemingly driven and nonfunctional to the extent that it interferes with normal activities or results in self-inflicted bodily injury sufficient to require medical treatment. The disorder cannot be accounted for by a compulsion, a tic, or hair pulling, and is not due to the effects of a substance or a general medical condition.

**stereotypy** (stĕr-ē-ō-tī′pē) [″ + *typos,* type] The persistent repetition of words, posture, or movement without meaning; seen in catatonic partial stupors.

**steric** (stē′rĭk) Concerning the spatial arrangement of atoms in a chemical compound.

**sterile** (stĕr′ĭl) [L. *sterilis,* barren] **1.** Free from living microorganisms. Solutions that have passed through certain filters are called sterile solutions because bacteria, fungi, and their spores have been removed. However, viruses can pass through some filters, and the term sterile is incorrectly used in this context. **2.** Not fertile; unable to reproduce young. SYN: *barren.* SEE: *sterility.*

**sterility** (stĕr-ĭl′ĭ-tē) [L. *sterilitas,* barrenness] **1.** The condition of being free from living microorganisms. **2.** The inability of the female to become pregnant or for the male to impregnate a female.

When investigating sterility, both partners should be examined. A routine examination for the female includes a study of the vaginal secretions, a bimanual pelvic examination, visualization of the cervix, in some cases a test for patency of the fallopian tubes, and a record of basal body temperature. A history of pelvic disease in the female is of great importance. The male should have the seminal fluid examined for the number, motility, viability, and normality of the spermatozoa.

TREATMENT: Treatment of sterility depends on the finding and correction of any or all causes of the condition. A high percentage of couples who have an infertility problem during the first year in which they are trying to have a child will, without treatment, produce offspring within 2 to 3 years. SEE: *embryo transfer; gamete intrafallopian transfer; fertilization, in vitro.*

***absolute s.*** The inability to produce offspring as a result of anatomical or physiological factors that prevent production of functional germ cells, conception, or the normal development of a zygote; this type of sterility is incurable.

***female s.*** The inability of a female to conceive.

ETIOLOGY: *Congenital abnormalities:* Absence or maldevelopment of the uterus, tubes, or ovaries; infantile uterus. *Acquired local conditions: Vagina:* Inflammation. *Cervix:* Narrowing of the internal os; acute and chronic endocervicitis; polyps occluding the cervical canal; cervical mucus that, because of either its chemical or physical qualities, is hostile to sperm. *Body of the uterus:* Fibroids of the uterus that block the canal; diseased endometrium, particularly endometritis. *Fallopian tube:* Chronic salpingo-oophoritis with closure of the tubal ostium and where the ovary is embedded in adhesions. *Ovarian dysfunction:* Congenital conditions, or secondary to endocrine disorders, infections, trauma, neoplasms, surgical removal of the ovaries (castration), inactivation of the ovaries by irradiation, or effects of toxic agents. Psychological and emotional disturbances, coital difficulties, and dietary deficiencies may also result in sterility. SEE: *embryo transfer; gamete intrafallopian transfer; fertilization, in vitro.*

***male s.*** The inability of a male either to produce sperm or to produce viable sperm, thereby prohibiting fertilization of the ovum. This may result from congenital factors such as cryptorchidism or maldevelopment of the testicular ducts or testis; acquired factors; and lack of libido, or impotence.

***primary s.*** Sterility resulting from failure of the testis or ovary to produce functional germ cells.

***relative s.*** Sterility due to causes other than a defect of the sex organs.

**sterilization** (stĕr″ĭl-ĭ-zā′shŭn) [L. *sterilis,* barren] **1.** The process of completely removing or destroying all microorganisms on a substance by exposure to chemical or physical agents, exposure to ionizing radiation, or by filtering gas or liquids through porous materials that remove microorganisms. A substance cannot be properly described as being partially sterile. SEE: *sterile.* **2.** The process of rendering barren. This can be accomplished by the surgical removal of the testes or ovaries (castration) or inactivation by irradiation, or by tying off or removing a portion of the reproductive ducts (ductus deferens or uterine tubes). SEE: *salpingectomy; tubal ligation; vasectomy.*

***dry heat s.*** Sterilization of microorganisms by subjection to high temperatures (165°C to 170°C) for 2 to 3 hr in sterilization chambers.

***fractional s.*** Sterilization of microorganisms in which heating is done at separated intervals, so that spores can develop into bacteria and be destroyed. This is usually accomplished by subjecting organisms to free-flowing steam for 15 min for 3 or 4 successive days. SYN: *intermittent s.*

***gas s.*** Exposure to gases such as formaldehyde or ethylene oxide that destroy microorganisms.

***intermittent s.*** Fractional s.

***laparoscopic s.*** Sterilization by use of a laparoscope to gain access to the fallopian tubes so band or clips can be applied to them. In addition, the cut end of the tubes may be electrocoagulated.

***steam s.*** Sterilization by exposure of microorganisms at 212°F (100°C) to flowing steam in an unsealed receptacle or by exposure of microorganisms to steam under pressure in an autoclave.

**sterilize** (stĕr′ĭ-līz) [L. *sterilis,* barren] **1.** To free from microorganisms. **2.** To make incapable of reproduction.

**sterilizer** (stĕr′ĭ-lī″zĕr) An oven or appliance for sterilizing.

***steam s.*** An autoclave that sterilizes by steam under pressure at temperatures above 100°C.

**sternad** (stĕr′năd) [Gr. *sternon,* chest] Toward the sternum.

**sternal** (stĕr′năl) [Gr. *sternalis*] Rel. to the sternum or breastbone.

**sternalgia** (stĕr-năl′jē-ă) [Gr. *sternon,* chest, + *algos,* pain] Pain in the sternum. SYN: *sternodynia.*

**sternal puncture** Use of a large-bore needle to obtain a specimen of marrow from the sternum.

**Sternberg-Reed cell** SEE: *Reed-Sternberg cell.*

**sternebra** (stĕr′nē-bră) [″ + L. *vertebra,* vertebra] Parts of the sternum during development of the fetus.

**sternen** (stĕr′nĕn) [Gr. *sternon,* chest] Concerning the sternum and no other structures.

**sterno-** [Gr. *sternon,* chest] Combining form meaning *sternum.*

**sternoclavicular** (stĕr″nō-klă-vĭk′ū-lăr) [″ + L. *clavicula,* little key] Concerning the sternum and clavicle.

**sternocleidal** (stĕr″nō-klī″dăl) [″ + *clavis,* key] Sternoclavicular.

**sternocleidomastoid** (stĕr″nō-klī″dō-măs′toyd) [″ + *clavis,* key, + *mastos,* breast, + *eidos,* form, shape] One of two muscles arising from the sternum and inner part of the clavicle. SEE: *Muscles Appendix.*

**sternocostal** (stĕr″nō-kŏs′tăl) [″+ L. *costa,* rib] Rel. to sternum and ribs.

**sternodymia** (stĕr″nō-dĭm′ē-ă) [″ + *didymos,* twin] A condition in which deformed twin fetuses are joined at the sternum. SYN: *sternopagia.*

**sternodynia** (stĕr″nō-dĭn′ē-ă) [″ + *odyne,* pain] Pain in the sternum. SYN: *sternalgia.*

**sternohyoid** (stĕr″nō-hī′oyd) [″ + *hyoeides,* U-shaped] The muscle from the medial end of the clavicle and sternum to the hyoid bone. SEE: *Muscles Appendix.*

**sternoid** (stĕr′noyd) [″ + *eidos,* form, shape] Resembling the breastbone.

**sternomastoid** (stĕr″nō-măs′toyd) [″ + *mastos,* breast, + *eidos,* form, shape] Pert. to the sternum and mastoid process of the temporal bone.

**sternomastoid region** The wide area on the lateral region of the neck covered by sternocleidomastoid muscle.

**sternopagia** (stĕr″nō-pā′jē-ă) [″ + *pagos,* thing fixed] Sternodymia.

**sternopericardial** (stĕr″nō-pĕr″ĭ-kăr′dē-ăl) [″ + *peri,* around, + *kardia,* heart] Concerning the sternum and pericardium.

**sternoschisis** (stĕr-nŏs′kĭ-sĭs) [″ + *schisis,* a splitting] A cleft or fissured sternum.

**sternothyroid** (stĕr″nō-thī′royd) [″ + *thyreos,* shield, + *eidos,* form, shape] The muscle extending beneath the sternohyoid that depresses the thyroid cartilage. SEE: *Muscles Appendix.*

**sternotomy** (stĕr-nŏt′ō-mē) [″ + *tome,* incision] The operation of cutting through the sternum.

**sternotracheal** (stĕr″nō-trā′kē-ăl) [″ + *tracheia,* trachea] Concerning the sternum and trachea.

**sternotrypesis** (stĕr″nō-trī-pē′sĭs) [″ + *trypesis,* a boring] Surgical perforation of the sternum.

**sternovertebral** (stĕr″nō-vĕr′tĕ-brăl) [″ + L. *vertebra,* vertebra] Concerning the sternum and vertebrae.

**sternum** (stĕr′nŭm) [L.] The narrow, flat bone in the median line of the thorax in front. It consists of three portions: the manubrium, the body or gladiolus, and the ensiform or xiphoid process. SEE: illus.

***cleft s.*** A congenital fissure of the sternum.

**sternutament** (stĕr-nū′tăm-ĕnt) [L. *sternutare,* to sneeze] A substance causing sneezing.

**sternutatio** (stĕr-nū-tā′shē-ō) [L.] Sneezing.

***s. convulsiva*** Paroxysmal sneezing, as in hay fever.

**sternutation** (stĕr-nū-tā′shŭn) The act of sneezing.

**sternutator** (stĕr′nū-tā″tor) [L. *sternutatorius,* causing sneezing] An agent, such as a war gas, that induces sneezing.

**sternutatory** (stĕr-nū′tă-tō″rē) Causing sneezing.

**steroid** (stĕr′oyd) **1.** An organic compound containing in its chemical nucleus the perhydrocyclopentanophenanthrene ring. SEE: *steroid hormones* for illus.; *perhydrocyclopentanophenanthrene.* **2.** A term applied to any one of a large group of substances chemically related to sterols, including sterols, D vitamins, bile acids, certain hormones, saponins, glucosides of digitalis, and certain carcinogenic substances.

**steroidal withdrawal syndrome** The appearance of symptoms of adrenal insufficiency in persons who discontinue the use of corticosteroids after having been treated with them for a prolonged period. In those patients, adrenal function has been suppressed to such an extent that the adrenal glands do not provide an appropriate response when the patient has a serious infection, surgery, or an accident. This failure to respond to stress may be present for as long as a year after discontinuation of corticosteroid therapy. The syndrome may be prevented by gradual rather than abrupt withdrawal of corticosteroid therapy.

**steroid hormone** One of the sex hormones and hormones of the adrenal cortex. SEE:

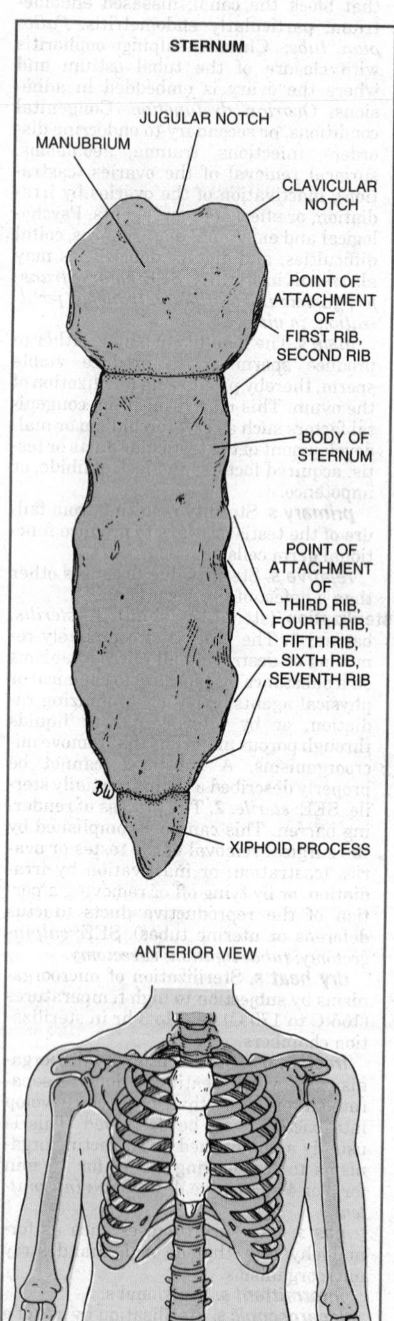

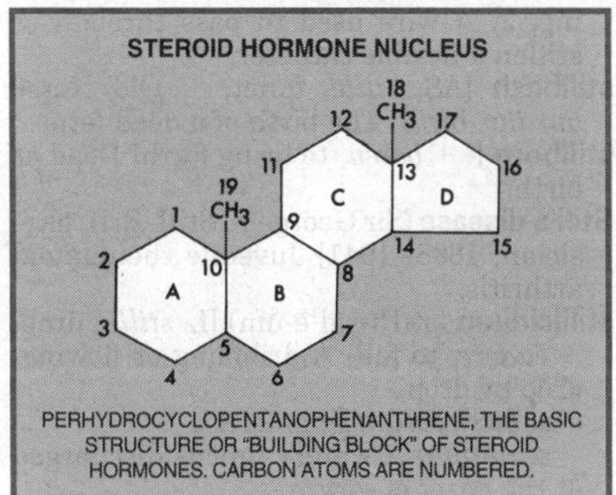

PERHYDROCYCLOPENTANOPHENANTHRENE, THE BASIC STRUCTURE OR "BUILDING BLOCK" OF STEROID HORMONES. CARBON ATOMS ARE NUMBERED.

illus.

**steroid hormone therapy** Treatment with various steroid hormones, esp. those from the adrenal cortex. If therapy is continued for more than a few days, the following general precautions should be observed: low-salt diet; high-protein diet; control of gastric acidity; adequate potassium intake; determination of the need for a prophylactic antibiotic; nitrogen balance (androgen or estrogen therapy may be needed); observation for osteoporosis, particularly in postmenopausal women.

**steroidogenesis** (stē-roy″dō-jĕn′ē-sĭs) Production of steroids.

**sterol** (stĕr′ŏl, stēr′ŏl) [Gr. *stereos,* solid, + L. *oleum,* oil] One of a group of substances (such as cholesterol) related to fats and belonging to the lipids. They are alcohols with a cyclic nucleus (cyclopentanoperhydrophenanthrene) and are found free or esterified with fatty acids (cholesterides). They are found in animals (zoosterols) or in plants (phytosterols). They are generally colorless, crystalline compounds, nonsaponifiable and soluble in certain organic solvents.

**stertor** (stĕr′tor) [NL. *stertor,* to snore] Snoring or laborious breathing owing to obstruction of air passages in the head, seen in certain diseases such as apoplexy.

**stertorous** (stĕr′tō-rŭs) Pert. to laborious breathing provoking a snoring sound.

**stetho-** [Gr. *stethos,* chest] Combining form meaning *chest.*

**stethogram** (stĕth′ō-grăm) [″ + *gramma,* something written] A record of heart sounds. The record may be stored for later comparison with subsequent heart sounds. SYN: *phonocardiogram.*

**stethomyitis, stethomyositis** (stĕth″ō-mī-ī′tĭs, -mī″ō-sī′tĭs) [″ + *mys,* muscle, + *itis,* inflammation] Inflammation of the muscles of the chest.

**stethoparalysis** (stĕth″ō-pă-răl′ĭ-sĭs) [″ + *paralyein,* to disable] Paralysis of the muscles of the chest.

**stethoscope** (stĕth′ō-skōp) [″ + *skopein,* to examine] An instrument used to transmit sounds produced in the body to the examiner's ears. It ordinarily consists of rubber tubing in a Y shape.

***binaural s.*** A stethoscope designed for use with both ears.

***compound s.*** A stethoscope in which more than one set is attached to the same fork and chest piece.

***double s.*** A stethoscope with two earpieces and tubes.

***electronic s.*** A stethoscope equipped to amplify electronically sounds from the body.

***single s.*** A rigid or flexible stethoscope designed for one ear only.

**stethoscopic** (stĕth″ō-skŏp′ĭk) Concerning or done by use of a stethoscope.

**stethospasm** (stĕth′ō-spăzm) [″ + *spasmos,* convulsion] A spasm of the pectoral or chest muscles.

**Stevens-Johnson syndrome** (stē′vĕnz-jŏn′sŏn) [Albert M. Stevens, 1884–1945, Frank C. Johnson, 1894–1934, U.S. pediatricians] A systemic form of erythema multiforme involving fever and lesions of the oral, conjunctival, and vaginal mucous membranes, and marked by a cutaneous rash that is often widespread and severe. Skin loss may lead to dehydration and infection. SEE: illus.; *erythema multiforme.*

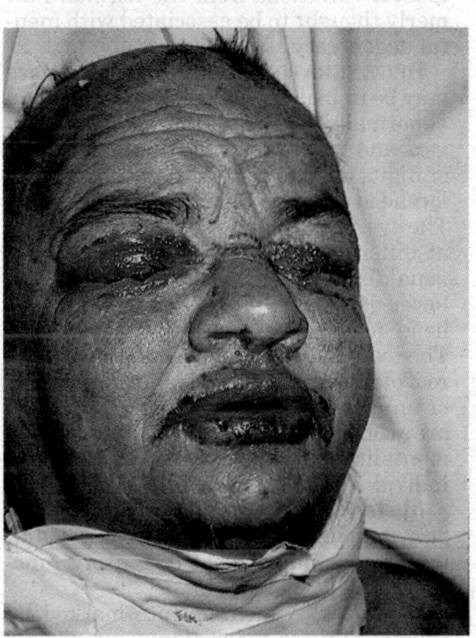
STEVENS-JOHNSON SYNDROME

**STH** *somatotropic hormone.*

**sthenia** (sthē′nē-ă) [Gr. *sthenos,* strength] Normal or unusual strength. Opposite of asthenia.

**sthenic** (sthĕn′ĭk) Active; strong.

**stibialism** (stĭb′ē-ăl-ĭzm) [L. *stibium,* antimony, + Gr. *-ismos,* condition] Antimony poisoning.

**stibiated** (stĭb′ē-āt″ĕd) [L. *stibium,* antimony] Containing antimony.

**stibium** (stĭb′ē-ŭm) [L.] Antimony.

**stibophen** (stĭb′ō-fĕn) A trivalent antimony

compound, used in treating schistosomiasis and granuloma inguinale.

**stiff** [AS. *stif*] Rigid, firm, inflexible.

**stiff joint** A joint with reduced mobility.

**stiff man syndrome** A rare disorder of the central nervous system characterized by fluctuating but progressive muscle rigidity and spasms. The etiology is unknown but is most probably of autoimmune origin. Some cases are associated with carcinoma. Treatment with diazepam or clonazepam may be of benefit. Plasmapharesis has helped some patients.

**stiff neck** Rigidity of neck resulting from spasm of neck muscles. It is a symptom of many disorders. SYN: *torticollis; wryneck.*

**stigma** (stĭg′mă) *pl.* **stigmata, -mas** [Gr., mark] **1.** A mark or spot on the skin; lesions or sores of the hands and feet that resemble crucifixion wounds. **2.** The spot on the ovarian surface where rupture of a graafian follicle occurs. **3.** A social condition marked by attitudinal devaluing or demeaning of persons who, because of disfigurement or disability, are not viewed as being capable of fulfilling valued social roles.

***s. of degeneration*** Any of the developmental variations from the normal. Formerly thought to be associated with mental degeneracy.

DEGENERATION CHANGES: The face may be unusually hairy in the female and abnormally smooth in the male. The fingers and toes may include an extra digit, or digits may be adherent or webbed. The forehead may be sloping and very low. The eyes may be two different colors or set at different levels. The ears may be unusual in many ways. Either the upper or lower jaw may project unusually. The head may be unusually large or small. The teeth may be irregular or project. The roof of the mouth may be high and pointed or unusually narrow. These irregularities are considered indicative of defective mentality only when several occur in one individual.

***hysterical s.*** Any of the peculiar marks or symptoms of hysteria, such as spots on the skin or impairment of sensory functions.

***psychic s.*** A mental state marked by susceptibility to suggestion.

**stigmata** Marks on the body at the same locations as those on Christ's body caused by having been nailed to the cross. Allegedly, these are evidence of divine action, esp. on priests, nuns, and other members of religious orders.

**stigmatic** (stĭg-măt′ĭk) [Gr. *stigma,* mark] Pert. to or marked with a stigma.

**stigmatism 1.** A condition marked by possession of stigmata. **2.** A condition in which light rays are accurately focused on the retina. SEE: *astigmatism.*

**stilbestrol** (stĭl-bĕs′trŏl) Diethylstilbestrol.

**stilet, stilette** (stī-lĕt′) [Fr. *stilette*] **1.** A small, sharp-pointed instrument for probing. **2.** A wire used to pass through or stiffen a flexible catheter.

**stillbirth** [AS. *stille,* quiet, + Old Norse *burdhr,* birth] The birth of a dead fetus.

**stillborn** [″ + *boren,* to bring forth] Dead at birth.

**Still's disease** [Sir George F. Still, Brit. physician, 1868–1941] Juvenile rheumatoid arthritis.

**stillicidium** (stĭl″ĭ-sĭd′ē-ŭm) [L. *stilla,* drop, + *cadere,* to fall] A dribbling or flowing, drop by drop.

***s. lacrimarum*** Epiphora.

***s. narium*** A watery mucus discharged at the onset of coryza.

***s. urinae*** Strangury.

**stimulant** (stĭm′ū-lănt) [L. *stimulans,* goading] Any agent temporarily increasing functional activity. Stimulants may be classified according to the organ upon which they act, as follows: cardiac, bronchial, gastric, cerebral, intestinal, nervous, motor, vasomotor, respiratory, and secretory.

**stimulate** (stĭm′ū-lāt) [L. *stimulare,* to goad on] To increase functional activity of an organ or structure.

**stimulation** (stĭm″ū-lā′shŭn) **1.** The process of being stimulated. **2.** Irritating action of agents on muscles, nerves, or sensory end organs by which activity in a part is evoked.

**stimulator** (stĭm″ū-lā′tor) Something that stimulates.

***long-acting thyroid s.*** A substance present in the blood of persons with hyperthyroidism that stimulates the thyroid. It is an immune gamma globulin.

**stimulus** (stĭm′ū-lŭs) *pl.* **stimuli** [L., a goad] **1.** Any agent or factor able to influence living protoplasm directly, as one capable of causing muscular contraction or secretion in a gland, or of initiating an impulse in a nerve. **2.** A change of environment of sufficient intensity to evoke a response in an organism. **3.** An excitant or irritant.

***adequate s.*** **1.** Any stimulus capable of evoking a response, that is, an environmental change possessing a certain intensity, acting for a certain length of time, and occurring at a certain rate. **2.** A stimulus capable of initiating a nerve impulse in a specific type of receptor.

***chemical s.*** A chemical substance (liquid, gaseous, or solid) that is capable of evoking a response.

***conditioned s.*** A stimulus that gives rise to a conditioned response. SEE: *reflex, conditioned.*

***electric s.*** A stimulus resulting from initiation of or cessation of a flow of electrons as from a battery, induction coil, or generator.

***homologous s.*** A stimulus that acts only on specific sensory end organs.

***iatrotropic s.*** A stimulus or event that makes a person seek or receive medical attention. However, medical care is voluntarily sought by apparently healthy people for many reasons (e.g., an Armed Forces draft examination, pre-employment or premarital examination, or health screening survey). Thus it is possible for disease to be discovered before it would ordinarily make itself known to the individual. Also called the *sick person's chief complaint.*

**liminal s.** Threshold s.

**mechanical s.** A stimulus produced by a physical change such as contact with objects or changes in pressure.

**minimal s.** Threshold s.

**nociceptive s.** A painful and usually injurious stimulus.

**subliminal s.** A stimulus that is weaker than a threshold stimulus.

**thermal s.** A stimulus produced by a change in skin temperature, a rise giving sensations of warmth, a fall giving sensations of coldness.

**threshold s.** The least or weakest stimulus that is capable of initiating a response or giving rise to a sensation. SYN: *liminal s.; miminal s.*

**unconditioned s.** Any stimulus that elicits an unconditioned response (i.e., a response that was inherently present rather than one that was learned).

**sting** [AS. *stingan*] **1.** A sharp, smarting sensation, as of a wound or astringent. **2.** A puncture wound made by an insect. In some cases, the venom of a stinging insect may be more toxic than that of a poisonous snake. Fortunately the insect injects a very small amount of venom into the body. SEE: *bite.*

SYMPTOMS: The reaction of a previously sensitized person is a potentially life-threatening medical emergency that requires prompt, effective therapy. Symptoms may include hives, itching and swelling in areas other than the site of the sting, tightness in the chest and difficulty in breathing, hoarse voice, swelling of the tongue, dizziness or hypotension, unconsciousness, and cardiac arrest.

TREATMENT: Some insect stings contain a substance resembling formic acid and consequently are relieved by topically applied alkalies, as ammonia water or baking soda paste. For intense local pain, injection of local anesthetic may be required. Systemic medication may be needed for generalized pain.

Individuals who have had an allergic reaction to an insect sting may benefit from venom immunotherapy. This treatment involves administration of very small amounts of the insect venom over several weeks until immunity develops. Immunity is then maintained by periodic venom boosters.

Persons who have a history of an anaphylactic reaction to insect stings should avoid exposure to insects by wearing protective clothing, gloves, and shoes. Cosmetics, perfumes, and hair sprays should be avoided because they attract some insects, as do brightly colored and white clothing. Because foods and odor attract insects, particularly yellow jackets, care should be taken when cooking and eating outdoors.

Obviously the reaction of a previously sensitized person is a potentially life-threatening medical emergency that requires prompt, effective therapy. Insect stings cause more deaths than do snake bites. An estimated four persons in 1000 are severely sensitive to insect stings.

**bee s.** SEE: under *bee.*

**caterpillar s.** Irritating contact with the hairs of a butterfly or moth larva. More than 50 species of larvae possess urticating hairs that contain a toxin. Contact can cause numbness and swelling of the infected area, severe radiating pain, localized swelling, enlarged regional lymph nodes, nausea, and vomiting. Although shock and convulsions may occur, no deaths have been reported. The disease is self-limiting. The larva of the flannel moth, *Megalopyge opercularis,* known as the puss caterpillar or woolly worm, is frequently the cause of this sting, particularly in the southern U.S. The fuzz from these larvae can be transported by wind. Treatment involves local application of moist soaks and administration of antihistamines.

**catfish s.** A toxic and allergic reaction caused by exposure to the venom contained in venomous glands at the base of catfish fins. The stung part should be immediately immersed in water as hot as the patient can stand for 1 hr or until the pain is controlled. Tetanus prophylaxis should be administered if needed.

**hornet s.** A sting from a wasp of the family Vespidae, which may cause a general urticaria. In persons who have been previously sensitized to the venom, a severe anaphylactic reaction may develop.

TREATMENT: The stinger should be removed and cold compresses applied. Household ammonia in 10% solution applied to the area is beneficial, and subsequent soothing lotions such as calamine lotion may be used. If pain is intense, a local anesthetic may be injected. If the systemic reaction is intense, 1 ml of epinephrine of 1 : 1000 concentration may be given subcutaneously to adults. An injectable antihistamine may be administered subcutaneously or intravenously if given slowly. If muscle spasms occur, an intravenous infusion of calcium lactate or calcium gluconate is given. In some cases, however, curare (dimethyl tubocurarine chloride) will be required to relieve muscle spasms. SEE: *wasp sting.*

**scorpion s.** SEE: under *scorpion.*

**sea anemone s.** Contact with the nematocysts or stinging cells of certain species of the flowerlike marine coelenterates causing severe dermatitis with chronic ulceration. In some cases, signs and symptoms of a systemic reaction develop, including headache, nausea, vomiting, sneezing, chills, fever, paralysis, delirium, seizures, anaphylaxis, cardiac arrythmias, heart failure, pulmonary edema, and collapse. In rare cases, it is fatal. SYN: *sponge diver's disease.*

TREATMENT: When systemic changes are present, vigorous therapy is indicated for hypotension. Diazepam is administered for convulsions. An electrocardiogram should be monitored for arrhythmias. Treatment for mild stings is symptomatic; application of vinegar to the sting area may inactivate the irritating secretion. All victims should be observed for 6 to 8 hr after initial therapy for rebound phenomenon.

***wasp s.*** SEE: under *wasp.*

**stinger** Burner.

**stingray** Any of the rays of the family Dasyatidae with wide pectoral fins that resemble wings. Soft venom glands are located in the spine running along the top of its whiplike tail; severe injuries can be inflicted if this spine penetrates the skin.

***s. injury*** Penetration of the skin by the spine of a stingray and injection of venom.

TREATMENT: This type of injury should be treated by washing the wound with copious amounts of water; seawater should be used if sterile water is unavailable. The wound should be cleansed thoroughly, and all foreign material should be removed. The wound site should be soaked in water as hot as the patient can tolerate (113°F or 45°C), for 30 to 60 min to inactivate venom. Narcotics may be necessary for pain. Surgical debridement may be necessary. The wound is either packed open or loosely sutured to provide adequate drainage.

**S-T interval** The interval in an electrocardiogram that represents the initial and final ventricular complexes. SEE: *electrocardiogram* for illus.; *QRST complex.*

**stippling** (stĭp′lĭng) [Dutch *stippelen,* to spot] A spotted condition, as in the retina in certain ocular diseases or in basophilic red corpuscles.

***gingival s.*** An orange-peel appearance of healthy gingiva, believed to be due to the enlargement of the underlying connective tissue papillae in response to massage and toothbrushing; the indent lies between the bulging papillae where the epithelia grow downward as rete ridges.

**stirrup, stirrup bone** (stĭr′ŭp) [AS. *stigrap,* a stirrup] A common name for the stapes, the third of the three bones in the middle ear. SEE: *ear.*

**stitch** (stĭch) [AS. *stice,* a pricking] **1.** A local sharp, lancinating, or spasmodic pain. This occurs most often in runners. The following maneuvers may offer relief: bending forward while tightening the abdomen; breathing deeply and exhaling slowly through pursed lips; tightening the belt or pushing one's fingers into the painful area. It is advisable not to eat for 30 to 90 min before exercising, to warm up before exercising, and to work out at a lower intensity for longer periods. **2.** A single loop of suture material passed through skin or flesh by a needle, to facilitate healing of a wound. **3.** Suture.

**St. John's sling** A sling made by applying a triangular bandage with the point downward under the elbow, the upper end over the sound shoulder. The arm is flexed acutely on the chest. The lower end is brought under the affected arm and around the back to knot with the upper end on the sound shoulder. The point is brought up over the elbow and fastened to the base. Support is wholly for the injured shoulder.

**stochastic model** (stō-kăs′tĭk) [Gr. *stokastikos,* skillful in guessing] A statistical model that attempts to reproduce the sequence of events that would be expected to occur in a real-life situation. This technique has some usefulness in predicting the importance and extent of disease in a specified population.

**stock** (stŏk) [AS. *stocc,* tree trunk] The original individual, race, or tribe from which others have descended.

**Stockholm syndrome** The emotional involvement between a hostage and the person holding him or her captive. The hostage's action may be due to sympathy for the terrorist's "cause," to stress, or to the need to cooperate in order to survive. This syndrome is named after the romantic involvement of a terrorist and a bank employee held hostage during a 1973 bank robbery in Stockholm.

**stockinet** A tubular woven material of uniform size that is open at both ends. It is used to hold bandages in place or to place uniform pressure on a leg, finger, arm, or other part of an extremity.

**stocking** A snug covering for the foot and leg. A stocking made of elastic material will place firm, even pressure on the extremity, which is useful in preventing thrombophlebitis of the leg in bedfast patients and in treating varicose veins.

**stocking aid** A device for assisting persons with limited function to put on socks or stockings.

**stoichiometry** (stoy″kē-ŏm′ĕ-trē) [Gr. *stoicheion,* element, + *metron,* measure] The study of the mathematics of chemistry and chemical reactions; chemical calculations.

**stoke** (stōk) [Sir George Stokes, Brit. physicist, 1819–1903] A unit of viscosity equal to $10^{-4}$ m²/sec.

**Stokes-Adams syndrome** (stōks-ăd′ăms) [William Stokes, Irish physician, 1804–1878; Robert Adams, Irish physician, 1791–1875] An altered state of consciousness caused by a decreased flow of blood to the brain. It may be caused by any transient interference with cardiac output such as incomplete or complete heart block. The patient may be lightheaded or become completely unconscious and have convulsions. Treatment includes the administration of intracardiac epinephrine, a sharp blow to the precordium, or use of an external electric pacemaker. SYN: *Adams-Stokes syndrome.*

NURSING IMPLICATIONS: Apical and radial pulses, blood pressure, and cardiac rhythm are monitored and any symptoms and their duration documented. Emergency treatment (atropine sulfate, external pacing) is provided as necessary according to prescribed protocols. The patient is prepared for cardiac pacemaker implantation; the nurse provides reassurance and support to patient and family, teaches pacemaker maintenance, and assists the patient to return to usual activities.

**Stokes' law** (stōks) [William Stokes] A law stating that a muscle lying above an inflamed serous or mucous membrane may be paralyzed.

**Stokes' lens** [George Stokes] Device used to diagnose astigmatism.

**stoma** (stō′mă) *pl.* **stomata, -mas** [Gr., mouth] **1.** A mouth, small opening, or pore. **2.** An artificially created opening between two passages or body cavities or between a cavity or passage and the body's surface. **3.** A minute opening between cells of certain epithelial membranes, esp. peritoneum and pleura.

**stomach** (stŭm′ăk) [Gr. *stomachos,* mouth] A muscular, distensible saclike portion of the alimentary tube between the esophagus and duodenum. SEE: illus.

ANATOMY: It is below the diaphragm to the right of the spleen, partly under the liver. It is composed of an upper fundus, a central body, and a distal pylorus. It has two openings: the upper cardiac orifice opens from the esophagus and is surrounded by the lower esophageal (cardiac) sphincter. The lower pyloric orifice opens into the duodenum and is surrounded by the pyloric sphincter. The wall of the stomach has four layers. The outer serous layer (visceral peritoneum) covers almost all of the organ. The muscular layer just beneath is has three layers of smooth muscle: an outer longitudinal layer, a medial circular layer, and an inner oblique layer. The submucosa is made of connective tissue that contains blood vessels. The mucosa is the lining that contains the gastric glands, simple tubular glands of columnar epithelium that secrete gastric juice. Chief cells secrete pepsinogen; parietal cells secrete hydrochloric acid and the intrinsic factor; mucus cells secrete mucus.

FUNCTION: Gastric juice is secreted at the sight or smell of food, and in larger amounts when food enters the stomach. The presence of food stimulates the production of the hormone gastrin, which increases the secretion of gastric juice. Protein digestion begins in the stomach; pepsin digests proteins to peptones. Hydrochloric acid converts pepsinogen to active pepsin and has little effect on unemulsified fats except those of cream. The

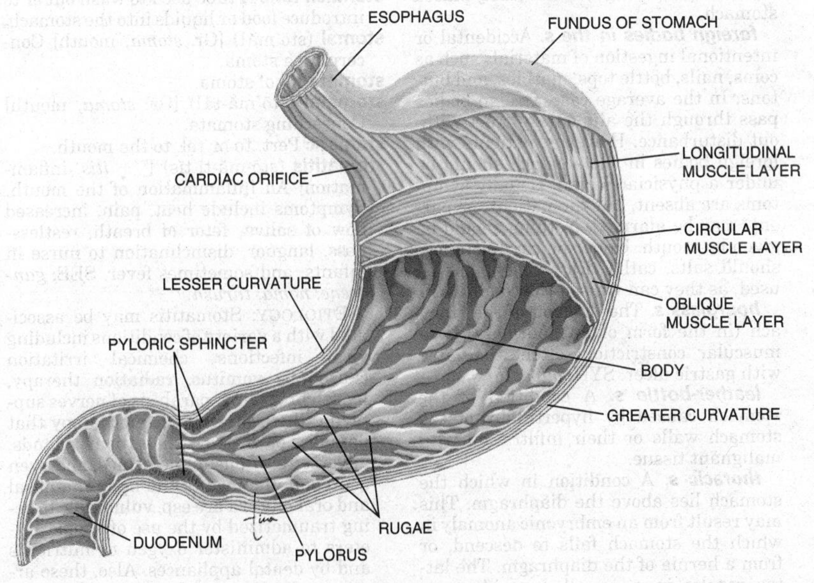


STOMACH
(ANTERIOR VIEW, SECTIONED)

stomach is a reservoir that permits digestion to take place gradually; emptying of the stomach is under both hormonal and nervous control. Secretions and motility are increased by parasympathetic impulses (vagus nerves) and decreased by sympathetic impulses. The intrinsic factor in gastric juice combines with vitamin $B_{12}$ (extrinsic factor) to prevent its digestion and promote its absorption in the small intestine. Little absorption takes place in the stomach because digestion has hardly begun, but water and alcohol are absorbed.

DIET IN SOME DISORDERS: *Atony and hypomotility:* Food is retained longer than normal and decomposition may occur if hydrochloric acid is deficient. Liquids are retained longer than solids. Therefore, diet should consist of quickly and easily digested foods—soft-cooked vegetables, chicken, fish, strained beef, and a moderate amount of skim milk. Liquids, pastries, and rich gravies should be avoided. *Hypermotility:* The stomach empties too rapidly; therefore, the diet should be liquid and soft, given in small frequent feedings. Fats delay the emptying of the stomach. *Hyperacidity:* Protein should be given to combine with acid. Frequent small feedings are advisable.

***bilocular s.*** Hourglass s.

***cardiac s.*** The fundus of the stomach.

***cascade s.*** A form of hourglass stomach in which there is a constriction between the cardiac and pyloric portions. The cardiac portion fills first, and then the contents cascade into the pyloric portion.

***cow horn s.*** A high, transversely placed stomach.

***foreign bodies in the s.*** Accidental or intentional ingestion of materials such as coins, nails, bottle tops, marbles, and buttons. In the average case, foreign bodies pass through the alimentary tract without disturbance. However, patients with foreign bodies in the stomach should be under a physician's care. Usually symptoms are absent, but the patient (or parent) may be alarmed. Nothing should be given by mouth. Under no circumstances should salts, cathartics, and enemas be used, as they can worsen the condition.

***hourglass s.*** The division of the stomach (in the form of an hourglass) by a muscular constriction; often associated with gastric ulcer. SYN: *bilocular s.*

***leather-bottle s.*** A condition of the stomach caused by hypertrophy of the stomach walls or their infiltration with malignant tissue.

***thoracic s.*** A condition in which the stomach lies above the diaphragm. This may result from an embryonic anomaly in which the stomach fails to descend, or from a hernia of the diaphragm. The latter results in a so-called upside-down stomach.

***water-trap s.*** A stomach with the pylorus situated unusually high, causing slow emptying.

**stomach ache** Pain in the stomach. SYN: *gastralgia.*

**stomachal** (stŭm′ă-kăl) [Gr. *stomachos,* mouth] Rel. to the stomach.

**stomach cancer** Cancer of the stomach that may be a carcinoma, lymphoma, or sarcoma.

SYMPTOMS: The general symptoms are those of dyspepsia, with the following characteristic symptoms: continued pain, often tenderness; vomiting of partially digested food; the absence of free hydrochloric acid in gastric juice; hematemesis or blood in stools, slight in amount and blood-altered so it has a coffee-grounds appearance; the presence of tumor; loss of weight and strength; extreme anemia; involvement of the superficial lymph glands. When the pylorus is involved, symptoms of gastric dilatation are present due to blockage of the pyloric outlet.

TREATMENT: The disease should be treated early by surgery and a liquid or semiliquid diet. The prognosis is very poor.

**stomachic** (stō-măk′ĭk) **1.** Concerning the stomach. **2.** A medicine that stimulates the action of the stomach.

**stomach intubation** Passage of a tube into the stomach to obtain gastric contents for examination, for prophylaxis and treatment of ileus, or to remove ingested poisons.

**stomach pump** A device for removing stomach contents through a tube inserted into the stomach through the mouth or nose.

**stomach tube** A tube used to wash out or to introduce food or liquids into the stomach.

**stomal** (stō′măl) [Gr. *stoma,* mouth] Concerning a stoma.

**stomata** Pl. of stoma.

**stomatal** (stō′mă-tăl) [Gr. *stoma,* mouth] Concerning stomata.

**stomatic** Pert. to or rel. to the mouth.

**stomatitis** (stō-mă-tī′tĭs) [″ + *itis,* inflammation] An inflammation of the mouth. Symptoms include heat, pain, increased flow of saliva, fetor of breath, restlessness, languor, disinclination to nurse in infants, and sometimes fever. SEE: *gangrene; noma; thrush.*

ETIOLOGY: Stomatitis may be associated with a variety of conditions including viral infections, chemical irritation caused by vomitus, radiation therapy, mouth breathing, paralysis of nerves supplying the oral area, chemotherapy that damages or destroys the salivary glands, adverse reactions to medicines, and even acute sun damage to the lips. The nasal and oral mucosa are esp. vulnerable to being traumatized by the use of nasal catheters to administer oxygen or nutrients and by dental appliances. Also, these areas may be damaged during surgery when an endotracheal tube is in place.

TREATMENT: Treatment is symptomatic with emphasis on keeping the mucosal surfaces moist and clear of tenacious mucus secretions. Care of the teeth and gingival tissues should be comprehensive and include flossing. The pain of stomatitis may be alleviated by systemic analgesics or application of anesthetic preparations to painful lesions. It is important for patients with dentures to clean the dentures thoroughly. Dentures should be removed from patients who are unconscious or mentally dulled. SEE: *toothbrushing*.

***aphthous s.*** SEE: *aphthous ulcer*.

***catarrhal s.*** Simple stomatitis. General symptoms include those of stomatitis with diffuse red swelling of the mucous membrane. Good hygienic conditions should be maintained, cleansing the mouth with a weak solution of boric acid as a wash.

***corrosive s.*** Stomatitis resulting from intentional or accidental exposure to corrosive substances.

***diphtheritic s.*** Diphtheria of mucous membranes of the gums or cheeks.

***herpetic s.*** Stomatitis marked by cold sores (fever blisters).

***membranous s.*** Stomatitis accompanied by the formation of a false or adventitious membrane.

***mercurial s.*** A form of stomatitis seen in those exposed to elemental mercury or mercury vapors after the administration of very large doses of mercurials.

SYMPTOMS: Early symptoms are tenderness of the gums, redness near insertion of the teeth, metallic taste, and an increase of saliva. Later symptoms include profuse salivation and fetor of breath as well as redness, swelling, and tenderness of the gums. The tongue may be similarly affected and protrude from the mouth. In severe cases, ulceration of the mucous membrane, loss of teeth, and necrosis of the jaw result.

TREATMENT: If the condition is due to acute poisoning, early administration of dimercaprol (British antilewisite) is helpful. If the condition is chronic, dimercaprol is ineffective; the patient should be removed from the source of poison and treated with *N*-acetyl-DL-penicillamine.

***mycotic s.*** Thrush.

***simple s.*** Erythematous inflammation of the mouth occurring in patches on the mucous membranes.

***traumatic s.*** Stomatitis resulting from mechanical injury as from ill-fitting dentures, sharp jagged teeth, or biting the cheek.

***ulcerative s.*** A type of stomatitis thought by some to be an infectious disease, as it often occurs in epidemics and attacks both children and adults when congregated and unable to practice good oral hygiene. The prognosis is guardedly favorable. SYN: *Vincent's s.; trench mouth; Vincent's angina.*

SYMPTOMS: Gums of the lower jaw are chiefly affected, becoming swollen, red, and spongy. Linear ulcers soon form and may extend to the cheek; the gland under the jaw becomes swollen. In severe cases, loosening of teeth and necrosis of the jaw may follow.

TREATMENT: The treatment involves debridement of ulceration, proper dental hygiene, and rinsing of the mouth with saline or a suitable hydrogen peroxide solution. Chemical or physical trauma to the mucosa should be avoided. One should force fluids and provide proper nutrition. Systemic antibiotics are usually not required.

***vesicular s.*** SEE: *aphthous ulcer*.

***Vincent's s.*** Ulcerative s.

**stomato-** Combining form meaning *mouth*.

**stomatocyte** A swollen erythrocyte with a slit-like area of central pallor that is found in hereditary stomatocytosis. SEE: illus.

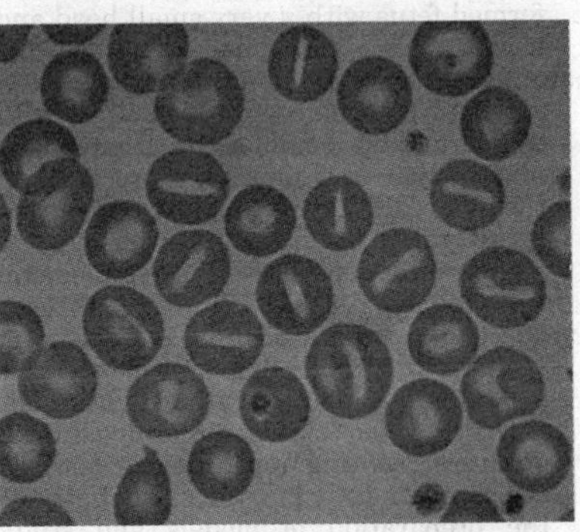

STOMATOCYTES (ORIG. MAG. ×640)

**stomatocytosis, hereditary** A disorder of erythrocytes usually inherited as an autosomal dominant. A membrane defect in the red blood cells permits the entry of excess sodium ions and water, causing the cells to swell. Hemolysis and anemia range from mild to severe. SYN: *hydrocytosis, hereditary*. SEE: *stomatocyte* for illus.

**stomatodynia** (stō″mă-tō-dĭn′ē-ă) [Gr. *stoma*, mouth, + *odyne*, pain] Pain in the mouth.

**stomatogastric** (stō″mă-tō-găs′trĭk) [″ + *gaster*, belly] Concerning the stomach and mouth.

**stomatognathic** (stō″mă-tŏg-năth′ĭk) [″ + *gnathos*, jaw] Indicating the mouth and jaws together.

**stomatologist** (stō″mă-tŏl′ō-jĭst) [″ + *logos*, word, reason] A specialist in the treatment of diseases of the mouth.

**stomatology** (stō″mă-tŏl′ō-jē) The science of the mouth and teeth and their diseases.

**stomatomalacia** (stō″mă-tō-mă-lā′shē-ă) [″ + *malakia*, softening] Pathological softening of any structures of the mouth.

**stomatomenia** (stō″mă-tō-mē′nē-ă) [″ + *meniaia,* menses] Bleeding from the mouth at the time of menstruation.

**stomatomycosis** (stō″mă-tō-mī-kō′sĭs) [″ + *mykes,* fungus, + *osis,* condition] Any disease of the mouth caused by fungi.

**stomatopathy** (stō″mă-tŏp′ă-thē) [″ + *pathos,* disease, suffering] Any mouth disease.

**stomatoplasty** (stō′mă-tō-plăs″tē) [″ + *plassein,* to form] Plastic surgery or repair of the mouth.

**stomatorrhagia** (stō″mă-tō-rā′jē-ă) [″ + *rhegnynai,* to burst forth] Hemorrhage from the mouth or gums.

**stomatosis** (stō″mă-tō′sĭs) [″ + *osis,* condition] Any disease of the mouth.

**stomion** (stō′mē-ŏn) [Gr., dim. of *stoma,* mouth] A landmark used in physical anthropology. It is the central point in the oral fissure when the lips are together.

**stomocephalus** (stō″mō-sĕf′ă-lŭs) [Gr. *stoma,* mouth, + *kephale,* head] A deformed fetus with a very small head and neck.

**stomodeum** (stō″mō-dē′ŭm) [″ + *hodaios,* a way] An external depression lined with ectoderm and bounded by frontonasal, mandibular, and maxillary processes of the embryo. It forms the anterior portion of the oral cavity. Its floor, the pharyngeal membrane, separates the stomodeum from the foregut.

**stone** [AS. *stan*] **1.** Calculus. **2.** In Britain, a unit of weight, 14 lb avoirdupois.

***dental s.*** A hemihydrate of gypsum divided into four classes according to the qualities resulting from differing methods of preparation. It is used in dentistry in the preparation of models and study casts.

***gray s.*** A synthetic stone composed of carborundum and rubber used to polish dental restorations.

***pulp s.*** A calcified structure present in the pulp chamber of a tooth. SYN: *denticle* (2).

***red s.*** An abrasive stone with a garnet as its main component, for polishing dental restorations.

***salivary s.*** A calcified stone present in the ducts of salivary glands; also called *sialolith.*

**stool** (stool) [AS. *stol,* a seat] **1.** Evacuation of the bowels. **2.** Feces.

COLOR: Iron and bismuth turn the stool black, and certain vegetables and berries darken it or produce a distinct color. Pathological stools are usually grayish or whitish and glistening; in hemorrhage, they may be tarry or show fresh blood.

CHARACTERISTICS: *Fatty stools:* These are observed in obstructive jaundice, cancer of the pancreas, pancreatic calculi, and in indigestion or overfeeding in infants.

*Frothy, poorly formed stools:* They may indicate a spastic colon, the presence of gas, or intestinal inflammation.

*Lienteric stools:* These contain much undigested food and are noted in inflammatory conditions of the stomach and upper bowel.

*Tarry stools:* They may indicate gastric hemorrhage, swallowed blood from the nose or lungs, bleeding ulcers of the gastrointestinal tract, hepatic cirrhosis, or cancer. If intestinal transport time is rapid, blood entering the upper gastrointestinal tract may not appear as tarry in the stool but may be bright red.

*Membranous shreds:* They may exist in cancer of the colon, dysentery, relapsing fever, acute proctitis, and in sloughing of intestinal mucosa.

*Mucous stools:* Exist in catarrhal or inflammations of the intestines or rectum, in dysentery, enterocolitis, proctitis, impaction, and ulcerative colitis.

SHAPE: *Cylindrical:* Stools of small caliber may indicate prolapsus ani or annular rectal stricture.

*Ribbon-shaped:* This may indicate stricture or cancer of the rectum; possibly enlargement of the prostate in males, hemorrhoids, spasm of the lower bowel and anus, prostatic abscess, and prolapse of the uterus.

*Scybala:* Rounded masses or balls of fecal matter or hardened feces, these are the result of habitual constipation, atony or sacculation (diverticulum) of the colon, gastric ulcer, dilation, rectal cancer, or dysentery.

***bilious s.*** Yellow or yellow-brown discharges in diarrhea, becoming darker on exposure to air.

***fatty s.*** Fat in the feces, as in pancreatic disease.

***lienteric s.*** Stool containing undigested food.

***pea soup s.*** Liquid stools characteristic of typhoid.

***rice water s.*** Watery serum stools with detached epithelium, as in cholera.

**stool softener** A substance that acts as a wetting agent and thus promotes soft malleable bowel movements. They are not laxatives and therefore are not indicated for constipation caused by decreased or absent peristaltic activity. Docusate sodium or docusate calcium may be used to soften stools.

**stopcock** (stŏp′kŏk) A valve, usually made of glass if used in chemistry, that regulates the flow of fluid from a container.

**stop needle** A needle with an eye at the tip and a disk on the shaft to prevent penetration deeper than desired.

**stoppage** (stŏp′ăj) [AS. *stoppian*] Obstruction of an organ. SEE: *cholestasia.*

**storax** (stō′răks) A balsam obtained from the scarred trunk of *Liquidambar orientalis.* It has been used as an expectorant. It is a component of tincture of benzoin.

**storm** [AS.] A sudden outburst or exacerbation of the symptoms of a disease.

***renal s.*** A sudden attack of renal symptoms accompanying a neurosis, sometimes occurring in patients suffering from aortic regurgitation.

***thyroid s.*** A complication of thyrotoxicosis that, if untreated, is almost always fatal. It consists of the abrupt onset of fever, sweating, tachycardia, pulmonary edema or congestive heart failure, tremulousness, and restlessness. It occurs in patients with untreated or poorly treated thyrotoxicosis. It is usually precipitated by infection, trauma, or a surgical emergency.

**stout** (stowt) [O. Fr. *estout,* bold] **1.** Having a bulky body. SYN: *corpulent.* **2.** Strong, dark beer.

**STP** *standard temperature and pressure.*

**STPD** *standard temperature and pressure, dry.*

**Str** *Streptococcus.*

**strabismal** (stră-bĭz′măl) [Gr. *strabismos,* a squinting] Strabismic.

**strabismic** (stră-bĭz′mĭk) [Gr. *strabismos,* a squinting] Pert. to or afflicted with strabismus.

**strabismometer** (stră-bĭz-mŏm′ĕt-ĕr) [″ + *metron,* a measure] An instrument for determining the amount of strabismus.

**strabismus** (stră-bĭz′mŭs) [Gr. *strabismos,* a squinting] A disorder of the eye in which optic axes cannot be directed to the same object. The squinting eye always deviates to the same extent when the eyes are carried in different directions: *unilateral* when the same eye always deviates; *alternating* when either deviates, the other being fixed; *constant* when the squint remains permanent; *periodic* when the eyes are occasionally free from it. Strabismus can result from reduced visual acuity, unequal ocular muscle tone, or an oculomotor nerve lesion. SYN: *heterotropia; squint.* SEE: *microstrabismus.*

***accommodative s.*** Strabismus due to disorder of ocular accommodation. SYN: *bilateral s.*

***alternating s.*** Strabismus affecting either eye alternately.

***bilateral s.*** Accommodative s.

***concomitant s.*** Strabismus in which both eyes move freely but retain an unnatural relationship to each other.

***convergent s.*** Strabismus in which the deviating eye turns inward.

***divergent s.*** Strabismus in which the deviating eye turns outward.

***horizontal s.*** Strabismus in which the deviation of the visual axis is in the horizontal plane.

***intermittent s.*** Strabismus recurring at intervals.

***monocular s.*** Strabismus in which the same eye habitually deviates.

***monolateral s.*** Strabismus with the squinting eye always the same.

***nonconcomitant s.*** Strabismus of an eye that varies in degree with the change in direction in which the eye moves.

***paralytic s.*** Strabismus due to paralysis of a muscle. The deviation is present only in the sphere of action of the paralyzed muscle. In paralytic squint, the secondary deviation is greater than the primary. This condition results from paralysis of one or more ocular muscles and may point to grave cerebral disease or to some constitutional disease. This form of strabismus is recognized by the fact that if a light or the finger of the examiner is carried from right to left before the face of the patient, the deviating eye fails to follow to its proper limit. This response leads the physician to look for lesions of the sixth nerve in failure of external rectus, of the third nerve in failure of internal rectus of either side, and of the fourth nerve in impairment of superior oblique muscles. In adults, this usually is caused by syphilis involving the nerve centers or trunks. In general, the prognosis is guarded.

TREATMENT: The treatment is directed at the cause. It may involve eyeglasses or contact lenses, miotics, and corrective surgery.

***spastic s.*** Strabismus due to contraction of an ocular muscle.

***vertical s.*** Strabismus in which the eye turns upward. The vision is double (diplopia) unless there is an unconscious suppression of the image in the squinting eye. The expression of the face is bizarre. Vertical strabismus usually is the result of ametropia in childhood or of central nervous system disease in adulthood.

**Strachan syndrome** [William H. W. Strachan, Brit. physician, 1857–1921] The neurological syndrome of amblyopia, painful neuropathy, and orogenital dermatitis that occurs in undernourished persons in many tropical countries. In the U.S., the syndrome occasionally is seen in alcoholic patients. Although it is considered to be due to a nutritional deficiency, it does not seem to be either beriberi or pellagra. Treatment is symptomatic and includes adequate nutrition. Formerly called Jamaican neuritis.

**strain** (strān) **1.** [AS. *streon,* offspring] A stock, said of bacteria or protozoa from a specific source and maintained in successive cultures or animal inoculation. **2.** A hereditary streak or tendency. **3.** [O. Fr. *estreindere,* to draw tight] To pass through, as a filter. **4.** To injure by making too strong an effort or by excessive use. **5.** Excessive use of a part of the body so that it is injured. **6.** Trauma to the muscle or the musculotendinous unit from violent contraction or excessive forcible stretch. It may be associated with failure of the synergistic action of muscles. SEE: *sprain.* **7.** To make a great effort, as in straining to have a bowel movement. This is done by means of the Valsalva maneuver, which increases intra-abdominal pressure and helps to expel feces. **8.** Force applied per unit area. Tension, compression, or shear stress placed on a tissue leads to distortion of the structure and the release of energy.

**strainer** (strān′ĕr) Device used for retaining solid pieces while liquid passes through. SYN: *filter*.

**strain radiography** A radiographical picture taken with the involved region, usually a bone or joint, under static force or tension; used to determine if a partial tear or rupture of the ligaments has occurred. Greater than normal gaping of the joint surfaces indicates a tear. Strain radiography reveals pathological changes that might be inapparent without use of this technique. SYN: *stress radiography*.

**strait** (strāt) [O. Fr. *estreit,* narrow] A constricted or narrow passage.

***inferior s.*** The lower outlet of the pelvic canal.

***s.'s of pelvis*** The inferior and superior openings of the true pelvis.

***superior s.*** The upper opening or inlet of the pelvic canal.

**straitjacket** A shirt with long sleeves laced on a patient and fastened to restrain the arms.

**stramonium** (stră-mō′nē-ŭm) [L.] The dried leaves of *Datura stramonium.* It is used as an ingredient in asthma powder used for its antispasmodic effect. Also called *Jamestown weed*. SYN: *jimson weed*.

**stramonium poisoning** Poisoning in children caused by accidental ingestion of medicine containing stramonium or by a self-administered overdose. The symptoms resemble those of atropine overdose. SEE: *atropine sulfate poisoning*.

**strand** A single thread or fiber.

**strangalesthesia** (străng″găl-ĕs-thē′zē-ă) [L. *strangulare,* halter, + *aisthesis,* sensation] A girdle-like sensation of constriction. SYN: *zonesthesia*.

**strangle** (străng′gl) [L. *strangulare,* halter] **1.** To choke or suffocate. **2.** To be choked from compression of the trachea.

**strangulated** (străng′gū-lā″tĕd) Constricted so that air or blood supply is cut off, as a strangulated hernia.

**strangulation** (străng″gū-lā′shŭn) [L. *strangulare,* halter] The compression or constriction of a part, as the bowel or throat, causing suspension of breathing or of the passage of contents. Congestion accompanies this condition.

***internal s.*** The slipping of a coil of the intestine through the diaphragm or an abnormal opening.

**strangury** (străng′gū-rē) [Gr. *stranx,* drop, squeezed out, + *ouron,* urine] Painful and interrupted urination in drops produced by spasmodic muscular contraction of the urethra and bladder.

**strap** (străp) [Gr. *strophos,* a cord] **1.** A band, as one of adhesive plaster, used to hold dressings in place or to approximate surfaces of a wound. **2.** To bind with strips of adhesive plaster.

**strapping** (străp′ĭng) **1.** An adhesive plaster or other substance used to bind surfaces together or to hold dressings in place. **2.** Application of adhesive plaster strips on a part to give it support or to compress it.

**stratification** (străt″ĭ-fĭ-kā′shŭn) [L. *stratificare,* to arrange in layers] The act or process of arranging in layers.

**stratified** (străt′ĭ-fīd) [L. *stratificare,* to arrange in layers] Arranged in the form of layers.

**stratified epithelium** Epithelium in superimposed layers with differently shaped cells in the various layers.

**stratiform** (străt′ĭ-form) [L. *stratum,* layer, + *forma,* shape] Arranged in layers.

**stratum** (strā′tŭm, străt′ŭm) *pl.* **strata** [L.] A layer.

***s. basale*** **1.** The innermost or deepest layer of the endometrium. **2.** S. germinativum.

***s. compactum*** The superficial or outermost layer of the endometrium.

***s. corneum*** The outermost horny layer of the epidermis.

***s. disjunction*** The outermost layer of the stratum corneum, which is being shed constantly.

***s. germinativum*** The innermost layer of the epidermis; a row of cuboidal cells that divide to replace the rest of the epidermis as it wears away. It is part of the stratum malpighii. SYN: *s. basale* (2). SEE: *s. malpighii*.

***s. granulosum*** A layer of cells containing deeply staining granules of keratohyalin found in the epidermis of the skin lying between the stratum germinativum and the stratum lucidum. It is part of the stratum malpighii. SEE: *s. malpighii*.

***s. lucidum*** The translucent layer of the epidermis lying between the stratum corneum and the stratum granulosum in the palms and soles.

***s. malpighii*** The inner layer of the epidermis. It was first seen with low magnification and described in the 1600s by Marcello Malpighi. It includes both the stratum germinativum and stratum spinosum of today's nomenclature.

***s. papillare*** The papillary layer of the corium lying adjacent to the epidermis.

***s. reticulare*** The recticular layer of the corium lying just beneath the papillary layer.

***s. spinosum*** The prickle cell layer, so called because of its prominent intercellular attachments. It is part of the stratum malpighii. SEE: *s. malpighii*.

***s. spongiosum*** The middle layer of decidua of the endometrium.

***s. submucosum*** The layer of smooth muscle fibers of the myometrium lying contiguous with the endometrium.

***s. subserosum*** The layer of smooth muscle fibers of myometrium that lies immediately under the serous coat.

***s. supravasculare*** The layer of circular and longitudinal muscle fibers lying between the stratum subserosum and the stratum vasculare of the endometrium.

***s. vasculare*** The layer of smooth muscles in myometrium lying between the stratum submucosum and the stratum supravasculare of the endometrium.

**strawberry mark** A soft, modular, vascular nevus usually present on the face or neck, occurring at birth or shortly afterward. SEE: *nevus flammeus.*

**straw itch** A self-limiting skin condition accompanied by itching owing to working in straw or sleeping on a straw mattress. The straw contains a mite that causes the pruritic eruption.

**streak** (strēk) [AS. *strica*] A line or stripe. SYN: *stria.*

***angioid s.*** A dark streak seen in the retinae of individuals with pseudoxanthoma elasticum and sickle cell anemia.

***medullary s.*** A deep longitudinal groove on the dorsal surface of the embryo that becomes the medullary tube.

***meningitic s.*** A red line across the skin formed by drawing a pointed article across it; seen in meningitis and nerve center disorders. SYN: *tache cérébrale.*

***Moore's lightning s.*** The subjective visual sensation of lightning-like flashes at the time of eye movements, esp. noticeable in dim or absent light. They are usually vertical and on the lateral part of the visual field. The flashes are accompanied by or followed by dark spots before the eyes. This condition is not related to significant eye disease.

***primitive s.*** SEE: *primitive streak.*

**stream** (strēm) A steady flow of a liquid.

***cathode s.*** Negatively charged electrons emitted from a cathode and accelerated in a straight line to interact with an anode. X-ray photons are then produced. SEE: *radiation, Bremmstrahlung; ray, cathode.*

**strength 1.** The quality of being strong or powerful as it relates to muscular activity. **2.** The concentration of a solution or substance. **3.** The intensity of light, color, or sound. **4.** The ability to resist deformation, fracture, or abrasion.

***breaking s.*** The point at which an amount of applied force breaks a material. SYN: *tensile strength.*

***compression s.*** The point at which a material loses its shape when force is applied. SYN: *crushing strength.*

***ego s.*** SEE: *ego strength.*

***impact s.*** The force required to fracture a material.

***shear s.*** The resistance of a material to force applied parallel to the plane of the material.

**strephosymbolia** (strĕf″ō-sĭm-bō′lē-ă) [Gr. *strephein,* to twist, + *symbolon,* symbol] **1.** Difficulty in distinguishing between letters that are similar but face in opposite directions (e.g., p-q, b-d). **2.** The perception of objects as reversed, as in a mirror.

**strepitus** (strĕp′ĭ-tŭs) [L.] A sound or noise, as that heard on auscultation.

**strepticemia** (strĕp″tĭ-sē′mē-ă) [Gr. *streptos,* twisted, + *haima,* blood] Streptococcemia.

**strepto-** [Gr. *streptos,* twisted] Combining form meaning *twisted.*

**streptoangina** (strĕp″tō-ăn′jĭ-nă) [″ + L. *angina,* quinsy] A sore throat with membranous formation caused by streptococci.

**streptobacillus moniliformis** A gram-negative bacillus present in the mouths of rats, mice, and cats. It is transmitted to humans through bites or by ingestion of milk contaminated by rats. It causes one form of rat-bite fever, marked by prolonged fever, skin rash, and generalized arthritis. Administration of penicillin is the treatment. SYN: *Haverhill fever.* SEE: *Spirillum minus.*

**streptococcal** (strĕp″tō-kŏk′ăl) [″ + *kokkos,* berry] Caused by or pert. to streptococci.

**streptococcemia** (strĕp″tō-kŏk-sē′mē-ă) [″ + ″ + *haima,* blood] Presence of streptococci in the blood, causing infection. SYN: *strepticemia.*

**streptococci** (strĕp″tō-kŏk′sī) Pl. of streptococcus. SEE: *Streptococcus.*

**streptococcic** (strĕp″tō-kŏk′sĭk) [″ + *kokkos,* berry] Resembling, produced by, or pert. to streptococci.

**streptococcicosis** (strĕp″tō-kŏk″sĭ-kō′sĭs) [″ + ″ + *osis,* condition] Any streptococcal infection.

**streptococcolysin** (strĕp″tō-kŏk-kŏl′ĭ-sĭn) [″ + ″ + *lysis,* dissolution] A hemolysin produced by streptococci. SYN: *streptocolysin; streptolysin.*

**Streptococcus** (strĕp″tō-kŏk′ŭs) [″ + *kokkos,* berry] A genus of bacteria belonging to the family Lactobacillaceae, tribe Streptococceae. They are gram-positive cocci occurring in chains. Most species are harmless saprophytes, but some are among the most common and dangerous pathogens of humans. They are differentiated on the basis of their reactions on blood-agar plates into three types: alpha ($\alpha$), beta ($\beta$), and gamma ($\gamma$). Those of the alpha type form a greenish coloration about colonies and partially hemolyze blood; those of the beta or hemolytic type form clear zones about colonies and completely hemolyze blood; those of the gamma type are nonhemolytic and produce a grayish coloration about colonies. Streptococci were also classified into several immunological groups (Lancefield groups) designated by the letters A through H, and K through O. Most human infections are caused by groups A, B, D, F, G, H, K, and O. More than 55 types of group A beta-hemolytic streptococci have been identified. SEE: *rheumatic fever; scarlet fever.*

***S. agalactiae*** A group B $\beta$-hemolytic species found in raw milk that is the leading cause of bacterial sepsis and meningitis in newborns and a major cause of endometritis and fever in postpartum women.

Infected infants develop early-onset symptoms in the first 5 days of life, including lethargy, jaundice, respiratory distress, shock, pneumonia, and anorexia. The fatality rate is 50% for very low birth weight neonates and 2% to 8% in term infants.

Infected postpartum women develop late-onset symptoms 7 days to several months after giving birth. Symptoms include sepsis, meningitis, seizures, and psychomotor retardation.

**S. bovis** A species found in the alimentary tract of cattle. It may cause endocarditis in humans.

**S. equisimilis** An organism that has been isolated from the upper respiratory tract. It may be associated with erysipelas, puerperal sepsis, pneumonia, osteomyelitis, bacteremia, and endocarditis.

**S. faecalis** A group D enterococcus that may or may not be hemolytic. It may be part of the normal flora of the intestinal tract, and it may be the cause of urinary tract infections.

**S. mutans** A species of streptococci that has been implicated in dental caries and endocarditis.

**S. pneumoniae** A species of bacteria that are oval or spherical, gram-positive, nonmotile, and possess a capsule. The species is made up of a number of distinct strains of which more than 80 serological types have been isolated. It is the causative agent of certain types of pneumonia, esp. lobar pneumonia, and is associated with other infectious diseases such as meningitis, conjunctivitis, endocarditis, periodontitis, septic arthritis, osteomyelitis, otitis media, septicemia, and, rarely, urinary tract infections.

**S. pyogenes** Any of the group A $\beta$-hemolytic streptococci causing suppurative processes. These streptococci are the causative agents of scarlet fever, erysipelas, septic sore throat, puerperal sepsis, and various pyogenic infections.

**S. viridans** A group of $\alpha$-hemolytic streptococci that are normally present in the upper respiratory tract. This is not the name of a particular species. Minor trauma such as vigorous chewing may result in their being admitted to the bloodstream. Thus when heart valves are damaged, these organisms are the ones that most frequently colonize on them. When this occurs, subacute bacterial endocarditis has an excellent chance of developing. *S. mitis* and *S. salivarius* are members of the viridans group. These may be normal inhabitants of the respiratory tract or be pathogenic.

**streptococcus** (strĕp″tō-kŏk′ŭs) *pl.* **streptococci** An organism of the genus *Streptococcus.* SEE: *bacteria* for illus.

**$\alpha$-hemolytic s.** Streptococci that, when grown on blood-agar, produce a zone of partial hemolysis around each colony and often impart a greenish appearance to the agar. Included are *S. pneumoniae* and *S. viridans.*

**$\beta$-hemolytic s.** Streptococci that, when grown on blood-agar, produce hemolysis around each colony. The hemolysis is complete, and a clear zone is present at the site. Included are *S. pyogenes* and *S. agalactiae.*

**group A s.** Beta-hemolytic streptococci that consist of a number of organisms that differ in their ability to cause disease. The clinical features of these diseases include pharyngitis, tonsillitis, otitis media, sinusitis, scarlet fever, erysipelas, cellulitis, impetigo, pneumonia, endometritis, and septicemia. In addition, group A streptococci may cause nonsuppurative sequelae, such as acute rheumatic fever and acute glomerulonephritis.

**group B s.** Beta-hemolytic streptococci that are a leading cause of early-onset neonatal infections and late-onset postpartal infections. In women, this is marked by urinary tract infection, chorioamnionitis, postpartum endometritis, bacteremia, and wound infections complicating cesarean section.

**streptocolysin** (strĕp″tō-kŏl′ĭ-sĭn) [″ + *lysis,* dissolution] A hemolysin produced by streptococci. SYN: *streptococcolysin; streptolysin.*

**streptodermatitis** (strĕp″tō-dĕr″mă-tī′tĭs) [″ + *derma,* skin, + *itis,* inflammation] Inflammation of the skin caused by streptococci.

**streptodornase** (strĕp″tō-dor′nās) One of the enzymes produced by certain strains of hemolytic streptococci. It is capable of liquefying fibrinous and purulent exudates. SEE: *streptokinase.*

**streptokinase** (strĕp″tō-kī′nās) An enzyme produced by certain strains of streptococci that is capable of converting plasminogen to plasmin. It is used as a fibrinolytic agent to help remove fibrin thrombi from arteries. SEE: *reperfusion* (1).

**streptokinase-streptodornase** A mixture of the enzymes streptokinase and streptodornase, which are produced by hemolytic streptococci. This mixture is used topically and in body cavities to remove clotted blood and purulent material.

**streptolysin** (strĕp-tŏl′ĭ-sĭn) A hemolysin produced by streptococci. SYN: *streptococcolysin; streptocolysin.*

**s. O** Streptolysin that is inactivated by oxygen.

**s. S** Streptolysin that is inactivated by heat or acid, but not by oxygen.

**streptomycin sulfate (sterile)** (strĕp″tō-mī′sĭn) An antibiotic derived from a soil microbe, *Streptomyces griseus.*

**streptomycosis** (strĕp″tō-mī-kō′sĭs) [″ + *mykes,* fungus, + *osis,* condition] An infection caused by microorganisms of the genus *Streptomyces.* SYN: *streptococcemia; streptosepticemia.*

**streptosepticemia** (strĕp″tō-sĕp″tĭ-sē′mē-ă) [″ + *septikos,* putrid, + *haima,* blood] Septicemia resulting from streptococcus infection. SYN: *streptococcemia; streptomycosis.*

**stress** (strĕs) [O. Fr. *estresse,* narrowness] In medicine, the result produced when a structure, system, or organism is acted on by forces that disrupt equilibrium or produce strain. In health care, the term denotes the physical (gravity, mechanical force, pathogen, injury) and psychological (fear, anxiety, crisis, joy) forces that are experienced by individuals. It is generally believed that biological organisms require a certain amount of stress in order to maintain their well-being. However, when stress occurs in quantities that the system cannot handle, it produces pathological changes. This biological concept of stress was developed by Hans Selye, who intended originally for stress to indicate cause rather than effect. Through a linguistic error, however, he gave the term stress to effect and later had to use the word stressor for the cause.

The amount of stress humans can withstand without having a pathological reaction to it varies from individual to individual and from situation to situation. Based on data obtained in World War II, individuals exposed to combat stress became nonfunctional at different stress levels, but there was a level of combat stress of such intensity and duration that no one could experience it and remain functional.

In physical sciences, stress may be equated to certain types of forces (e.g., impact, shear, torsion, compression, and tension) that result in deformation or fracture of the material being stressed or tested. In dentistry, the pressure of the upper teeth on the lower teeth in mastication produces stress. Mechanical forces of tension, compression, shear, or torsion may all be applied to teeth or dental prostheses during the movements of mastication and represent stress. SEE: *general adaptation syndrome.*

***oxidative s.*** The cellular damage caused by oxygen-derived free radical formation. The three most important are superoxide ($O_2^-$), hydrogen peroxide ($H_2O_2$), and hydroxyl ions; these are produced during normal metabolic processes as well as in reaction to cell injury. The extent of their damaging potential can be decreased by antioxidants. SEE: *antioxidant; free radical; superoxide; superoxide dismutase.*

**stress-breaker** A device incorporated into a removable denture. It is designed to relieve abutting teeth from excessive stress during chewing.

**stress fracture** A fine hairline fracture that appears without evidence of soft tissue injury. This type of fracture is difficult to diagnose by roentgenographical examination and may not become visible until 3 to 4 weeks after the onset of symptoms. It occurs from repetitive microtraumas, as with running, aerobic dancing, or marching; with use of improper shoes on hard surfaces; or with inadequate healing time after stress.

**stress incontinence** SEE: under *incontinence.*

**stressor** An agent or condition capable of producing stress.

***systemic s.*** A stressor that produces generalized systemic responses.

***topical s.*** Stress that causes mild inflammation or local damage.

**stress radiography** Strain radiography.

**stress test** A method of evaluating cardiovascular fitness. While exercising, usually on a treadmill or a bicycle ergometer, the individual is subjected to steadily increasing levels of work. At the same time, the amount of oxygen consumed is being determined, and an electrocardiogram (ECG) is being monitored. If certain abnormalities are noted in the ECG or chest pain develops, the test is terminated.

***adenosine s.t.*** A test for the diagnosis and evaluation of coronary heart disease. It is used when standard exercise stress testing cannot be done or has been done and yielded unsatisfactory results. The adenosine is administered intravenously and the electrocardiogram is recorded during and after the infusion. It is important that the optimum infusion dose be used.

**stretch** (strĕch) [AS. *streccan,* extend] To draw out or extend to full length.

***static s.*** A sustained, long-duration lengthening of soft tissue such as muscle or tendon applied to increase range of motion. The stretch force is usually applied at a low intensity and continuously for as little as 12 to 15 sec or as long as several minutes.

**stretcher** (strĕch′er) A litter for carrying the sick, injured, or dead.

***basket s.*** A stretcher made of metal or strong synthetic material in which a patient is placed for removal from an accident site. The stretcher may also be lifted by ropes. Also called *Stokes stretcher.*

***orthopedic s.*** A metal stretcher that is hinged along its long axis and designed to be split so that it can be placed on both sides of the patient and then reassembled to lift the patient. SYN: *scoop s.*

***pole s.*** A type of stretcher, also known as the Army type, composed of folding cloth or canvas supported by poles.

***scoop s.*** Orthopedic s.

***spineboard s.*** A wooden board used to secure patients with spinal trauma to prevent movement.

***split-frame (scoop) s.*** A metal stretcher that can be split down the middle, slid under a patient, and reconnected.

**stretching of contractures** The process performed to loosen contracted ligaments, muscles, and adhesions in stiff joints. Force is applied to the part in a direction parallel to the extremity or digit. There should be a slow, steady, and gradually increasing force.

**stretch mark** Stria atrophica.

**stretch receptor** A proprioceptor located in a muscle or tendon that is stimulated by a stretch or pull.

**stria** (strī'ă) *pl.* **striae** [L., a channel] A line or band elevated above or depressed below surrounding tissue, or differing in color and texture. SYN: *streak.*

***striae acusticae*** Horizontal white stripes on the floor of the fourth ventricle of the brain.

***striae atrophica*** A fine pinkish-white or gray line, usually 14 cm long, seen in parts of body where skin has been stretched; commonly seen on thighs, abdomen, and breasts of women who are or have been pregnant; in persons whose skin has been stretched by obesity, tumor, or edema; or in persons who have taken adrenocortical hormones for a prolonged period. Also called a *stretch mark.* SYN: *s. gravidarum.*

***striae gravidarum*** S. atrophica.

***striae longitudinalis lateralis*** One of the longitudinal bands of gray matter, slightly elevated on the upper part of the corpus callosum.

***olfactory striae*** Three bands of fibers (lateral, intermediate, and medial) that form the roots of the olfactory tract.

***striae of Retzius*** The benign incremental lines seen periodically in the calcified enamel of teeth.

***striae terminalis*** A band of fibers in the roof of the inferior horn running to the floor of the body of the lateral ventricle.

**striatal** (strī-ā'tăl) [L. *striatus,* striped] Concerning the corpus striatum.

**striate, striated** (strī'āt, strī'ā-tĕd) [L. *striatus*] Striped; marked by streaks or striae.

**striated artery** One of the branches of the middle cerebral artery that supply the basal nuclei of the brain.

**striated body** Corpus striatum.

**striated vein, inferior** One of the branches of the basal vein that drain the corpus striatum.

**striation** (strī-ā'shŭn) [L. *striatus,* striped] **1.** State of being striped or streaked. **2.** Stria.

**striatum** (strī-ā'tŭm) [L., grooved] Corpus striatum.

**stricture** (strĭk'chŭr) [LL. *strictura,* contraction] A narrowing or constriction of the lumen of a tube, duct, or hollow organ such as the esophagus, ureter, or urethra. Strictures may be congenital or acquired. Acquired strictures may result from infection, trauma, fibrosis resulting from mechanical or chemical irritation, muscular spasm, or pressure from adjacent structures or tumors. They may be temporary or permanent, depending on the cause.

***annular s.*** Ringlike obstruction of an organ involving the entire circumference of a structure.

***anorectal s.*** A fibrotic narrowing of the anorectal canal.

***bridle s.*** A stricture caused by a band of membrane stretched across a tube, partially occluding it.

***cicatricial s.*** A stricture resulting from a scar or wound.

***functional s.*** A stricture caused by muscular spasm.

***impermeable s.*** A stricture closing the lumen of a tube or canal so that an instrument cannot pass through it.

***irritable s.*** A stricture causing pain when an instrument is passed.

***s. of the urethra*** Partial or complete narrowing of the urethra, occuring most commonly in men. The condition is marked by straining to pass urine, esp. at the commencement of urination. It is caused by spasm of the urethral muscle, congestion of the urethra, and fibrous formation.

**stricturotomy** (strĭk"chūr-ŏt'ō-mē) The operation of cutting strictures of the urethra.

**stride length** The length of the stride; useful in measuring the right and left leg stride lengths to determine a neuromuscular disease that affects only one leg.

**strident** (strī'dĕnt) Stridulous.

**stridor** (strī'dor) [L., a harsh sound] A high-pitched, harsh sound heard during respiration. It resembles the blowing of wind due to obstruction of the upper airway.

***congenital laryngeal s.*** Stridor present at birth or occurring during the first weeks or months of life.

***s. dentium*** The noise from grinding of the teeth. SEE: *bruxism.*

***s. serraticus*** A sound of respiration similar to that of sawing, produced by the patient's tracheostomy tube.

**stridulous** (strĭd'ū-lŭs) [L. *stridulus*] Making a shrill, grating sound. SYN: *strident.*

**string-of-pearls deformity** Fusiform enlargement of the proximal and middle phalanges, seen in rickets.

**string sign** A greatly narrowed terminal ileum seen in roentgenological examination of the abdomen in regional enteritis.

**string test** SEE: *Giardia lamblia.*

**striocerebellar** (strī"ō-sĕr"ĕ-bĕl'ăr) [L. *striatus,* striped, + *cerebellum,* little brain] Concerning or affecting the corpus striatum and the cerebellum.

**strip** (strĭp) [AS. *striepan,* to plunder] To remove all contents from a hollow organ or tube, esp. by gentle pressure, as to strip the seminal vesicles.

**stripper** A surgical instrument used to remove a vein.

**strobila** (strō-bī'lă) [Gr. *strobilos,* anything twisted up] The adult form of a tapeworm.

**strobiloid** (strō'bĭ-loyd) [" + *eidos,* form] Resembling a twisted chain. Tapeworm segments have this appearance.

**stroboscope** (strō'bō-skōp) [Gr. *strobos,*

whirl, + *skopein,* to examine] A device that produces an interrupted light. The light is shown on moving or vibrating objects. This makes the object appear to be stationary. A photograph taken at the precise time the light is flashed on the object will not be blurred.

**stroke** (strōk) [ME.] **1.** A sharp blow. **2.** To rub gently in one direction, as in massage. **3.** A gentle movement of the hand across a surface. **4.** In dentistry, a complete simple movement that is often repeated with modifications of position, strength, or speed, perhaps as a part of a continuing activity; for example, the closing stroke in mastication when the jaw closes and the teeth come together. In scaling or planing the roots of teeth, the scaling instrument is introduced carefully into the subgingival area in what is called an exploratory stroke, perhaps followed by a power stroke designed to break or dislodge encrusted calculus. This is followed by a shaving stroke, intended to smooth or plane the root surface. **5.** A sudden loss of consciousness followed by paralysis, caused by one of several different mechanisms including hemorrhage into the brain; formation of an embolus or thrombus that occludes an artery; or rupture of an extracerebral artery causing subarachnoid hemorrhage. Each year about 12 in each 10,000 Americans have a stroke. This illness is the third leading cause of death in the U.S. SYN: *apoplexy; cerebrovascular accident.* SEE: *excitotoxin; transient ischemic attack.*

ETIOLOGY: Stroke may be caused by hemorrhage into the brain, and this accounts for 20% of cases. It is more likely to occur in younger patients. The mechanism is rupture of a vessel or aneurysm, or leakage from a blood vessel. This is usually associated with hypertension. Ischemic stroke, the formation of a blood clot in a vessel supplying blood to the brain, accounts for the other 80%. This is usually related to atherosclerotic changes in a vessel. Another cause is a clot that travels from the heart to the brain and thus occludes an artery.

RISK FACTORS: The risk factors that can be controlled include hypertension, sedentary lifestyle, use of tobacco in any form, elevated blood cholesterol, high salt intake, high alcohol intake, and diabetes.

SYMPTOMS: The onset is usually acute, but may be more gradual if the stroke is caused by thrombosis. The patient becomes unconscious. There is stertorous breathing due to paralysis of a portion of the soft palate; expiration puffs out the cheeks and mouth. The pupils are sometimes unequal, the one on the side of the hemorrhage being larger. Paralysis usually involves one side of the face, and the arm and leg of the opposite side. The eyeballs are turned away from the side of the body that is paralyzed. Skin is covered with clammy sweat; the surface temperature of the skin is often subnormal. Speech may be abnormal or absent.

TREATMENT: The patient should be kept quiet and sitting up or lying down with the head and shoulders elevated. Stimulants should not be given. Cool cloths should be applied to the head and neck. The patient should not be transported unless absolutely imperative, and then it should be done very carefully. Administration of intravenous tissue plasminogen activator results in significant improvement in neurological outcome, although there is an increased risk of symptomatic intracerebral hemorrhage. Use of the experimental drug citicoline within 24 hours of the onset of the stroke has helped injured tissues resist cell death.

PROGNOSIS: This prognosis depends on the symptoms and is often grave. The prognosis is directly related to the degree and length of time blood flow to the affected area of the brain is deficient or completely blocked. A regional cerebral blood flow of at least 15 to 18 ml/100 g of brain tissue is necessary to maintain electrical activity in that part of the brain, but certain functions may remain viable until the flow rate falls to below 10 ml/100 g of tissue. From animal studies, recovery of the function of neuronal tissue is unlikely if occlusion continues longer than 4 to 6 hr. A treatment time beginning within 2 hr of the stroke is probably necessary to avoid or mitigate alterations in function. Thus, the immediate initiation of therapeutic measures is of the utmost importance if the extent of damaged cerebral tissue is to be kept to a minimum. Seventy percent of people who have a stroke remain independent and 10% recover completely. Until the age of 55, men are more likely than women to have a stroke; however, estrogen levels fall in women during menopause, at which time the risk of stroke becomes equal to that of men. SEE: *risk factors.*

NURSING IMPLICATIONS: A patent airway is maintained, and adequate ventilation and oxygenation are provided. As necessary, the trachea or pharynx is suctioned gently to remove secretions. The patient is positioned in the lateral or semiprone position with the head elevated 15 to 30 degrees to decrease cerebral venous pressure. Neurological status (Glasgow Coma Scale; vital signs; pupillary responses; respiratory patterns; and sensory and motor responses to verbal, tactile, and painful stimulation) are monitored for signs of deterioration or improvement, and findings are documented on a neurological flow sheet. A history of the incident is obtained, including time frame, related past medical history (hypertension, use of anticoagulant drugs, cardiac dysrhythmias), and associated injuries. The nurse prepares the patient for prescribed diagnostic studies, including computed tomography scan; nuclear magnetic resonance imaging; x-rays of skull, cervical spine, and soft tissues of neck; arteriography; and lumbar puncture.

The patient is oriented frequently and reassured with verbal and tactile contacts. Aphasia type is assessed, if present, and the patient is supported appropriately. Normal body temperature is maintained, and excessive environmental heat or cold is avoided. Bladder function is assessed; noninvasive measures are used to encourage voiding in the presence of urinary retention, voiding pattern is determined, and the incontinent patient is kept clean and dry. Use of indwelling catheters is avoided because these promote urinary tract infection. Bowel function is assessed, and dietary intervention and stool softeners or laxatives as necessary are used to prevent constipation. Straining at stool or use of enemas is avoided. Fluid and electrolyte balance (intake, output, daily weight, laboratory values) is monitored and maintained. Adequate enteral or parenteral nutrition is provided as appropriate. Nursing measures are instituted to prevent complications of immobility: repositioning at least every 2 hr, maintaining correct body alignment, supporting joints to prevent flexion and rotation contractures, and providing range-of-motion exercises (passive to involved joints, active-assisted or active to uninvolved joints). Irrigation and lubrication prevent oral mucous membranes and eyes (cornea) from drying. Prescribed therapy is administered to decrease cerebral edema, and antihypertensives or anticoagulants are given as appropriate for etiology. The patient is observed for seizure activity, and drug therapy and safety precautions are initiated.

Rehabilitation begins after the acute phase has subsided. The nurse collaborates with speech, physical, and occupational therapist and the patient and family to develop a comprehensive care plan based on realistic goals. All patient efforts should receive positive reinforcement. Patient communication should be a priority. Exercises, proper positioning, and supportive devices help to prevent deformities. Use of foot boards is controversial because they may increase spasticity. Quiet rest periods are provided based on the patient's response to activity. The patient should either assist with or perform own personal hygiene and establish independence in other activities of daily living. The nurse evaluates the patient's ability to feed self and continues to provide enteral feeding as necessary. A bowel and bladder retraining program is initiated, and both patient and family receive instruction in its management. Both patient and family are taught about the therapeutic regimen (activity and rest, diet, and medications), including desired effects and adverse reactions to report. Emotional lability is recognized and explained, and assistance is provided to help the patient deal with outbursts or inappropriate affect. The nurse assists the patient to accept deficits and disabilities, maintaining hope while establishing realistic goals. Both patient and family should participate in available social and financial support groups and services. The patients needs help to accept residual deficits present after 6 months, because these may be permanent. Recovery and survival expectations may be influenced by the patient's age and presence of other chronic illnesses, in addition to early and later responses to stroke damage and therapies.

***heat s.*** An acute and dangerous reaction to heat exposure. The basic defect is failure of the heat-regulating mechanisms of the body. SEE: *heat; hyperpyrexia.*

***ischemic s.*** A stroke due to diminished blood supply to the brain or a particular area of the brain (e.g., the lodging of an embolus from the heart in an artery of the brain).

***little s.*** A pathological change in the brain caused by diminished or lack of blood flow to a very small area of the brain. When this occurs, there may be no clinically detectable changes in the patient, or the changes may be subtle and unnoticed by the patient, but apparent to others. An example would include a person whose habits concerning personal neatness were well known but after the little stroke the person no longer noticed that his or her clothes and appearance were no longer neat and clean. A group of little strokes may cause progressive dementia.

***mini-s.*** SEE: *transient ischemic attack.*

***paralytic s.*** Sudden onset of paralysis resulting from injury to the brain or spinal cord. SEE: *stroke* (5).

**stroke volume** The amount of blood ejected by the left ventricle at each heartbeat. The amount varies with age, sex, and exercise. SYN: *systolic discharge.*

**stroking** A technique of slow tactile stimulation over the posterior primary rami used to inhibit muscle responses and promote relaxation during neuromotor rehabilitation.

**stroma** (strō′mă) *pl.* **stromata** [Gr., bed covering] **1.** Foundation-supporting tissues of an organ. The opposite of parenchyma. **2.** The membranous lipid-protein framework within a red blood cell to which hemoglobin molecules are attached.

**stromal, stromatic** (strō′măl, strō-măt′ĭk) Concerning or resembling the stroma of an organ.

**stromatolysis** (strō″mă-tŏl′ĭ-sĭs) [″ + *lysis,* dissolution] Destruction of the stroma of a cell.

**stromatosis** (strō″mă-tō′sĭs) [″ + *osis,* condition] Presence of mesenchyma-like tissue throughout the endometrium of the uterus.

**Stromeyer's splint** (strō′mī-ĕrz) [Georg F. L. Stromeyer, Ger. surgeon, 1804–1876] A hinged splint for a joint, which can be fixed at an angle.

**Strong Interest Inventory** ABBR: SII. A psychological test that traditionally measures vocational interests but also identifies personality traits. Previous versions (the original was developed in 1927) were known as the Strong Vocational Interest Bank.

**Strongyloides** (strŏn″jĭ-loy′dēz) A genus of roundworms that infect humans.

***S. stercoralis*** A roundworm that infrequently causes infection in humans, which may be fatal. In the U.S., *S. stercoralis* is found mainly in the rural South. The ova hatch in the intestines of the host, and rod-shaped larvae are passed in the stool. In the soil, these may develop into adults and continue their life cycle or may metamorphose into filiform larvae that can infect humans. The filiform larvae enter the skin, pass through the venous system to the lungs, where they migrate upward and are swallowed. A rash or pneumonia may accompany their migration. The rod-shaped larvae have the ability to metamorphose into the filiform larvae in the human intestine. This form then enters the circulation, migrates to the lungs, and begins the cycle again.

This life cycle allows for a massive infection sufficient to cause overwhelming systemic infection with fever, severe abdominal pain, shock, and possibly death. Severe reactions are more likely to occur in immunosuppressed patients or in patients with diseases that alter their immune status. Thiabendazole or mebendazole are the drugs of choice. Repeated courses of treatment may be required.

**strongyloidosis** (strŏn″jĭ-loy-dō′sĭs) [Gr. *strongylos,* compact, + *osis,* condition] Infestation with organisms of the genus *Strongyloides*.

**strongylosis** (strŏn″jĭ-lō′sĭs) Infestation with organisms of the genus *Strongylus*.

**Strongylus** (strŏn′jĭ-lŭs) A genus of parasitic nematodes.

**strontium** (strŏn′shē-ŭm) [Strontian, mining village in Scotland] SYMB: Sr. A dark yellow metal; atomic weight, 87.62; atomic number, 38; specific gravity, 2.6. Medically it is of interest because its radioactive isotope $^{90}$Sr constitutes a radioactive hazard in fallout from atom bombs. The isotope has a half-life of 28 years and is stored in bone when ingested.

**Strophanthus** (strō-făn′thŭs) [Gr. *strophos,* twisted cord, + *anthos,* flower] A genus of plants yielding a poisonous, white, crystalline glucoside, previously used as a heart stimulant.

**strophocephaly** (strŏf″ō-sĕf′ă-lē) [″ + *kephale,* head] Distortion of the head and face resulting from a developmental anomaly.

**structural** (strŭk′tū-răl) [L. *structura,* structure] Pert. to organic structure.

**structure** (strŭk′shŭr) The arrangement of the component parts of an organism.

***denture-supporting s.*** The tissues that support a partial or complete denture.

**struma** (stroo′mă) [L. *struma,* a mass] Goiter.

***s. aberranta*** A struma of the accessory thyroid glands.

***cast iron s.*** Riedel's s.

***s. lymphomatosa*** A rare condition involving a diffuse and extensive infiltration of the entire thyroid gland.

***s. maligna*** Carcinoma of the thyroid gland.

***s. ovarii*** A form of ovarian teratoma in which the mass is composed of typical thyroid follicles filled with colloid.

***Riedel's s.*** A form of chronic thyroiditis in which the gland becomes enlarged, hard, and adherent to adjacent tissues. The follicles become atrophic and fibrosis occurs. SYN: *cast iron s.*

**strumectomy** (stroo-mĕk′tō-mē) [″ + *ektome,* excision] The removal of a goiter.

**strumitis** (stroo-mī′tĭs) [″ + Gr. *itis,* inflammation] Thyroiditis.

**Strümpell's disease** (strĭm′pĕlz) Strümpell-Marie disease.

**Strümpell-Marie disease** [Adolf G. G. von Strümpell, Ger. physician, 1853–1925; Pierre Marie, Fr. neurologist, 1853–1940] Rheumatoid spondylitis.

**Strümpell's sign** (strĭm′pĕls) Dorsiflexion of the foot when the thigh is flexed on the abdomen. This sign may be associated with spastic paralysis of the leg.

**struvite** Crystals of magnesium ammonium phosphate, sometimes found as a harmless ingredient of canned food, where they may be mistaken for glass. Struvite crystals dissolve in vinegar. This simple test will distinguish struvite from glass. Struvite crystals are also present in some renal calculi. They are formed by the action of the bacterial enzyme urease.

**strychnine** (strĭk′nīn, -nēn, -nĭn) [Gr. *strychnos,* nightshade] A poisonous alkaloid obtained from plants, as nux vomica. It has no therapeutic usefulness but has been used as an experimental tool in neuropharmacology.

***s. poisoning*** Toxicity produced by ingestion of strychnine. SEE: *Poisons and Poisoning Appendix.*

**strychninism** (strĭk′nĭn-ĭzm) [″ + *-ismos,* condition] Chronic strychnine poisoning.

**Stryker frame** A device that supports two rectangular pieces of lightweight but strong material so that one side is on the anterior surface of the patient and the other is on the posterior surface. The patient is sandwiched firmly between the pieces of material. The device may be rotated around the patient's long axis. This permits turning the patient without his or her assistance. After a turn is completed,

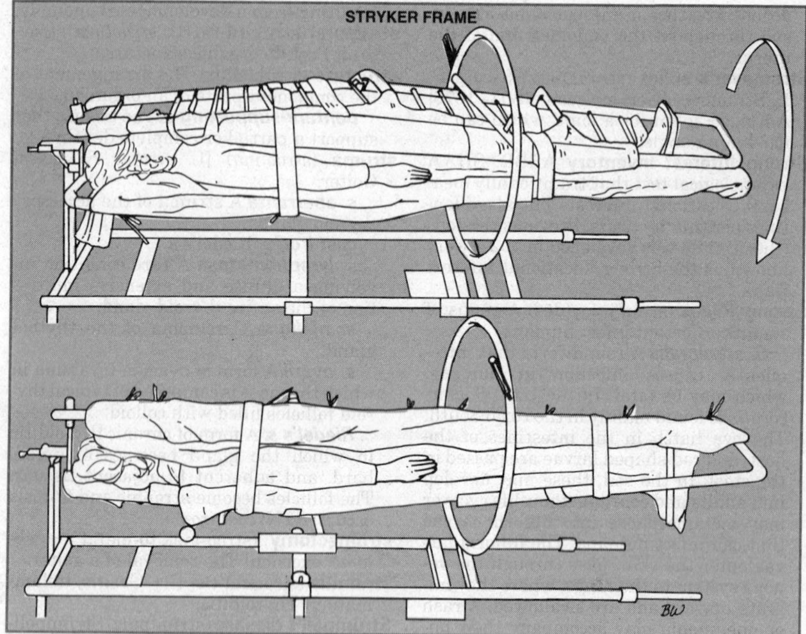


the uppermost portion of the frame can be moved away from the patient. SEE: illus.

**Stryker's saw** An electric-powered oscillating saw that cuts through bone or dense tissue with minimal damage to the underlying soft tissues.

**STS** *serological test for syphilis.*

**STU** *skin test unit.*

**study, case-control** An investigative technique used in epidemiology. Cases are occurrences of the disease or illness in the individuals being investigated. Controls are the individuals being studied who do not have the disease. The frequency of occurrence of possible causes for the disease in the two groups is then obtained and the data analyzed for possible differences. For example, a study might involve a group of patients with cancer and a group from the same population that did not have the disease. The first such study involved an investigation of chimney sweeps in England who developed cancer of the scrotum. The hypothesis was that something peculiar to their occupation led to a higher incidence of cancer than was prevalent in the general population.

**stump** The distal portion of an amputated extremity.

**stump hallucination** Phantom limb.

**stun** (stŭn) [O. Fr. *estoner,* a blow] To render unconscious or stupefied by a blow.

**stupe** (stūp) [L. *stupa,* tow] A counterirritant for topical use, prepared by adding a small amount of an irritant such as turpentine to a hot liquid.

**stupor** (stū′por) [L., numbness] **1.** A condition of unconsciousness, torpor, or lethargy with suppression of sense or feeling. **2.** In psychiatry, a state of lessened responsiveness. Stupor occurs in visceral and infectious diseases, melancholia, catatonia, epilepsy, paresis, poisonings, and hysteria. A benign form is seen in manic-depressive psychosis.

***anergic s.*** Stupor accompanied by immobility; it is seen in certain psychoses.

***epileptic s.*** Stupor that sometimes follows an attack of epilepsy.

***lethargic s.*** Stupor accompanied by lethargy. SEE: *trance.*

**stuporous** Affected with stupor.

**stuporous depression** An extremely depressed phase of manic-depressive psychosis typified by extreme psychomotor retardation and unresponsiveness to surrounding conditions.

**Sturge-Weber syndrome** [William Sturge, Brit. physician, 1850–1919; Frederick Parkes Weber, Brit. physician, 1863–1962] A congenital syndrome marked by port-wine nevi along the distribution of the trigeminal nerve, angiomas of leptomeninges and choroid, intracranial calcifications, mental retardation, epileptic seizures, and glaucoma. SYN: *nevoid amentia.*

**sturine** (stū′rĭn) [NL. *sturio,* sturgeon] Protamine obtained from sperm of sturgeon. SEE: *protamine; salmin(e).*

**stuttering** (stŭt′ĕr-ĭng) [ME. *stutten,* to stutter] A genetically transmitted nervous disorder that probably causes spasmodic disruptions of the auditory feedback loop, which enables the automatic and unconscious monitoring and control of speech. The individual hesitates, repeats, or stumbles spasmodically while attempting to speak. SYN: *stammering.*

This condition occurs in approx. 1% to 2% of the school population. Males are affected four times as often as females. The onset is in two periods: between the ages of 2 and 4 years when speech begins and between 6 and 8 years of age when the need for language increases.

Therapy has been of limited help. Relaxation techniques, hypnosis, delayed auditory feedback, and tranquilizers may help temporarily.

Educational materials are available by calling the Stuttering Foundation of America, Memphis, Tennessee at 800-992-9392; and from American Speech-Language-Hearing Association, Rockville, Maryland by calling 800-638-8255.

***acquired s.*** The appearance of stuttering in patients recovering from aphasic disorders who have never previously stuttered.

***urinary s.*** Irregular, spasmodic urination. SYN: *stammering of bladder.*

**sty(e)** (stī) *pl.* **styes, sties** [AS. *stigan,* to rise] A localized circumscribed inflammatory swelling of one or more of the sebaceous glands of the eyelid. It is caused by a bacterial infection. External styes are superficial and affect Zeis' glands or glands of Moll at the edge of the lid. Internal styes concern the meibomian or tarsal glands under the eyelid and are more severe. SEE: *chalazion.*

SYMPTOMS: General edema of the lid, pain, and localized conjunctivitis mark the condition. As the internal sty progresses, an abscess will form that can be seen through the conjunctiva.

TREATMENT: Frequent application of hot packs usually brings about drainage and resolution. If this fails to do so, incision and drainage are necessary. Topical antibiotics will prevent the spread of infection. SYN: *hordeolum.*

***meibomian s.*** An inflammation of a meibomian gland.

***zeisian s.*** An inflammation of one of the Zeis' glands.

**style, stylet** (stīl, stī'lĕt) [Gr. *stylos,* pillar] **1.** A slender, solid or hollow, plug of metal for making a canal permanent after operation or for stiffening or clearing a cannula or catheter. **2.** A thin probe.

**styliform** (stī'lĭ-form) [" + L. *forma,* form] Long and pointed.

**styliscus** (stī-lĭs'kŭs) [Gr. *styliskos,* a pillar] A slender, cylindrical plug for dilating a channel or for keeping a wound open.

**styloglossus** (stī-lō-glŏs'ŭs) [Gr. *stylos,* pillar, + *glossa,* tongue] A muscle connecting the tongue and styloid process that raises and retracts the tongue. SEE: *Muscles Appendix.*

**stylohyal** (stī"lō-hī'ăl) [" + *hyoeides,* hyoid] Stylohyoid.

**stylohyoid** (stī-lō-hī'oyd) [" + *hyoeides,* hyoid] Pert. to the styloid process of the temporal and hyoid bones. SYN: *stylohyal.*

**stylohyoideus** (stī"lō-hī-oyd'ē-ŭs) A muscle having its origin on the styloid process and its insertion on the hyoid bone. It draws the hyoid bone upward and backward. SEE: *Muscles Appendix.*

**styloid** (stī'loyd) [" + *eidos,* form, shape] Resembling a stylus or pointed instrument.

**styloiditis** (stī"loyd-ī'tĭs) [" + " + *itis,* inflammation] Inflammation of a styloid process.

**styloid process 1.** A pointed process of the temporal bone, projecting downward, and to which some of the muscles of the tongue are attached. **2.** A pointed projection behind the head of the fibula. **3.** A protuberance on the outer portion of the distal end of the radius. **4.** An ulnar projection on the inner side of the distal end.

**stylomandibular** (stī"lō-măn-dĭb'ū-lar) [" + L. *mandibula,* lower jawbone] Concerning the styloid process of the temporal bone and mandible.

**stylomastoid** (stī"lō-măs'toyd) [" + *mastos,* breast, + *eidos,* form, shape] Concerning the styloid and mastoid processes of the temporal bone.

**stylopharyngeus** (stī"lō-făr-ĭn'jē-ŭs) [" + *pharynx,* throat] The muscle connecting the styloid process and the pharynx that elevates and dilates the pharynx. SEE: *Muscles Appendix.*

**stylostaphyline** (stī"lō-stăf'ĭ-līn) [" + *staphyle,* bunch of grapes] Concerning the styloid process of the temporal bone and uvula.

**stylosteophyte** (stī-lŏs'tē-ō-fīt) A peg-shaped outgrowth from bone.

**stylus** (stī'lŭs) [Gr. *stylos,* a pillar] **1.** A probe or slender wire for stiffening or clearing a canal or catheter. **2.** A pointed medicinal preparation in stick form for external application.

**stypsis** (stĭp'sĭs) [Gr., *styphein,* to contract] Astringency or the use of an astringent.

**styptic** (stĭp'tĭk) [Gr. *styptikos,* contracting] **1.** Contracting a blood vessel; stopping a hemorrhage by astringent action. **2.** Anything that stops a hemorrhage such as alum, ferrous sulfate, or tannic acid. SYN: *astringent; hemostat.*

**sub-** [L. *sub,* under, below] Prefix meaning *under, beneath, in small quantity, less than normal.* SEE: *hypo-.*

**subabdominal** (sŭb"ăb-dŏm'ĭ-năl) [L. *sub,* under, below, + *abdomen,* abdomen] Below the abdomen.

**subabdominoperitoneal** (sŭb"ăb-dŏm"ĭ-nō-pĕr"ĭ-tō-nē'ăl) [" + " + Gr. *peritonaion,* peritoneum] Deep to the abdominal peritoneum.

**subacetate** (sŭb-ăs'ĕ-tāt) [" + *acetum,* vinegar] A basic acetate.

**subacid** (sŭb-ăs'ĭd) [" + *acidus,* sour] Moderately acid.

**subacromial** (sŭb-ă-krō'mē-ăl) [" + Gr. *akron,* point, + *osmos,* shoulder] Under the acromial process.

**subacute** (sŭb″ă-kūt′) [″ + *acutus,* sharp] Between acute and chronic, but with some acute features, said of the course of a disease or of the healing process following tissue injury.

**subacute myelo-optic neuropathy** ABBR: SMON. A neurological disease that usually begins with abdominal pain or diarrhea, followed by sensory and motor disturbances in the lower limbs, ataxia, impaired vision, and convulsions or coma. It is reported mostly in Japan and Australia. Most patients survive, but neurological disability remains. Many of those who have the disease have a history of taking drugs of the halogenated oxyquinoline group such as clioquinol (previously called iodochlorhydroxyquin).

**subanconeus** (sŭb″ăn-kō′nē-ŭs) [″ + Gr. *ankon,* elbow] **1.** Below the elbow. **2.** The muscle beneath the elbow that contracts its posterior ligament. SEE: *Muscles Appendix.*

**subapical** (sŭb-ăp′ĭ-kăl) [″ + *apex,* tip] Below the apex.

**subaponeurotic** (sŭb″ăp-ō-nū-rŏt′ĭk) [″ + Gr. *apo,* from, + *neuron,* sinew] Below an aponeurosis.

**subarachnoid** (sŭb″ă-răk′noyd) [″ + Gr. *arachne,* spider, + *eidos,* form, shape] Below or under the arachnoid membrane and the pia mater of the covering of the brain and spinal cord.

**subarachnoid cisternae** Spaces at the base of the brain where the arachnoid becomes widely separated from the pia, giving rise to large cavities.

**subarachnoid space** The space between the pia proper and the arachnoid, containing the cerebrospinal fluid.

**subarcuate** (sŭb-ăr′kū-āt) [L. *sub,* under, below, + *arcuatus,* bowed] Slightly arched.

**subarcuate fossa** A depression that extends backward as a blind tunnel under the superior semicircular canal of the temporal bone.

**subareolar** (sŭb″ă-rē′ō-lăr) [″ + *areola,* a small space] Below the areola.

**subastragalar** (sŭb-ăs-trăg′ă-lăr) [″ + Gr. *astragalos,* ball of the ankle joint] Beneath the astragalus.

**subastringent** (sŭb″ăs-trĭn′jĕnt) [″ + *astringere,* to bind fast] Mildly astringent.

**subatomic** (sŭb″ă-tŏm′ĭk) [″ + Gr. *atomos,* indivisible] Less than the size of an atom.

**subaural** (sŭb-aw′răl) [″ + *auris,* ear] Below the ear.

**subauricular** (sŭb″aw-rĭk′ū-lăr) [″ + *auricula,* little ear] Below an auricle, esp. of the ear.

**subaxial** (sŭb-ăk′sē-ăl) [″ + *axis,* axis] Below an axis.

**subaxillary** (sŭb-ăk′sĭ-lĕr″ē) [″ + *axilla,* armpit] Below the axilla, or armpit.

**subbrachycephalic** (sŭb″brā-kē-sĕ-făl′ĭk) [″ + Gr. *brachys,* short, + *kephale,* head] Having a cephalic index of 78 to 79.

**subcalcarine** (sŭb-kăl′kăr-īn) [″ + *calcar,* spur] Below the calcarine sulcus of the brain.

**subcapsular** (sŭb-kăp′sū-lăr) [″ + *capsula,* little box] Below any capsule, esp. the capsule of the brain, or a capsular ligament.

**subcarbonate** (sŭb-kăr′bō-nāt) [″+ *carbo,* carbon] A basic carbonate; one having a proportion of carbonic acid radical less than the normal carbonate.

**subcartilaginous** (sŭb″kăr-tĭ-lăj′ĭn-ŭs) [″ + *cartilago,* gristle] **1.** Located beneath a cartilage. **2.** Cartilaginous in part.

**subchondral** (sŭb″kŏn′drăl) [″ + Gr. *chondros,* cartilage] Below or under a cartilage.

**subchoroidal** (sŭb″kō-roy′dăl) [″ + Gr. *chorioeides,* skinlike] Below the choroid.

**subclass** (sŭb′klăs) In taxonomy, a category between a class and an order.

**subclavian** (sŭb-klā′vē-ăn) [″ + *clavis,* key] Under the clavicle or collarbone. SYN: *subclavicular.*

**subclavian artery** The large artery at the base of the neck that supplies blood to the arm. The right subclavian artery branches from the innominate artery; the left subclavian artery branches from the aortic arch.

**subclavian steal syndrome** The shunting of blood, which was destined for the brain, away from the cerebral circulation. This occurs when the subclavian artery is occluded. Blood then flows from the opposite vertebral artery across to and down the vertebral artery on the side of the occlusion.

SYMPTOMS: Signs of insufficient blood flow to the brain mark this condition. Symptoms are transient and are aggravated by exercise. Usually the blood pressure in the arm on the affected side will be significantly lower than in the other arm.

**subclavian triangle** The triangle-shaped part of the neck, formed by the clavicle and the omohyoid and sternomastoid muscles.

**subclavian vein** A large vein draining the arm. It unites with the internal jugular vein to form the brachiocephalic (innominate) vein.

**subclavicular** (sŭb″klă-vĭk′ū-lăr) [L. *sub,* under, below, + *clavicula,* little key] Subclavian.

**subclavius** (sŭb-klā′vē-ŭs) [″ + *clavis,* key] A tiny muscle from the first rib to the undersurface of the clavicle. SEE: *Muscles Appendix.*

**subclinical** (sŭb-klĭn′ĭ-kăl) [″ + Gr. *klinikos,* pert. to a bed] Pert. to a period before the appearance of typical symptoms of a disease or to a disease or condition that does not present clinical symptoms. Some infections may not produce characteristic symptoms but can be demonstrated by antigenic reactions.

**subcollateral** (sŭb-kō-lăt′ĕr-ăl) [″ + *con,* together, + *lateralis,* pert. to a side] Below the collateral fissure, indicating a cerebral convolution.

**subconjunctival** (sŭb″kŏn-jŭnk-tī′văl) [″ + *conjungere,* to join together] Beneath the conjunctiva.

**subconsciousness** (sŭb-kŏn′shŭs-nĕs) [″ + *conscius,* aware] **1.** The state of being partially unconscious. **2.** The condition in which mental processes take place without the individual's being aware of their occurrence. SEE: *subliminal.*

**subcontinuous** (sŭb″kŏn-tĭn′ū-ŭs) [″ + *continere,* to hold together] Almost continuous; with periods of abatement.

**subcoracoid** (sŭb-kor′ă-koyd) [″ + Gr. *korakoeides,* like a crow's beak] Beneath the coracoid process.

**subcortex** (sŭb-kor′tĕks) [″ + *cortex,* rind] The white substance of the brain underlying the cortex.

**subcortical** (sŭb-kor′tĭ-kăl) Pert. to the region beneath the cerebral cortex.

**subcostal** (sŭb-kŏs′tăl) [″ + *costa,* rib] Beneath the ribs.

**subcostalgia** (sŭb″kŏs-tăl′jē-ă) [″ + ″ + Gr. *algos,* pain] Pain in the region over the subcostal nerve.

**subcranial** (sŭb-krā′nē-ăl) [″ + Gr. *kranion,* skull] Beneath or below the cranium.

**subcrepitant** (sŭb-krĕp′ĭ-tănt) [″ + *crepitare,* to rattle] Partially crepitant or crackling in character; noting a rale.

**subcrureus** (sŭb-kroo-rē′ŭs) [″ + *crus,* leg] A small muscle between the anterior surface of the femoral shaft and the synovial membrane of the knee joint. SEE: *Muscles Appendix.*

**subculture** (sŭb-kŭl′chūr) [″ + *cultura,* tillage] To make a culture of bacteria with material derived from another culture.

**subcutaneous** (sŭb″kū-tā′nē-ŭs) [″ + *cutis,* skin] Beneath the skin. SYN: *hypodermic.*

**subcutaneous surgery** An operation performed through a small opening in the skin.

**subcutaneous wound** A wound with only a small opening through the skin.

**subcuticular** (sŭb″kū-tĭk′ū-lăr) [L. *sub,* under, below, + *cuticula,* little skin] Subepidermal.

**subcutis** (sŭb-kū′tĭs) The layer of connective tissue beneath the skin.

**subdeltoid** (sŭb-dĕl′toyd) [″ + Gr. *delta,* letter d, + *eidos,* form, shape] Beneath the deltoid muscle.

**subdental** (sŭb-dĕn′tăl) [″ + *dens,* tooth] Beneath the teeth or a tooth.

**subdermal** [″ + Gr. *derma,* skin] Below the skin.

**subdiaphragmatic** (sŭb″dī-ă-frăg-măt′ĭk) [″ + Gr. *diaphragma,* a partition] Beneath the diaphragm. SYN: *subphrenic.*

**subdorsal** (sŭb-dor′săl) [″ + *dorsum,* back] Below the dorsal area.

**subduct** (sŭb-dŭkt′) [″ + *ducere,* to lead] To draw down.

**subdural** (sŭb-dū′răl) [″ + *durus,* hard] Beneath the dura mater.

**subdural space** The space between the arachnoid and the dura mater.

**subendocardial** (sŭb″ĕn-dō-kăr′dē-ăl) [″ + Gr. *endon,* within, + *kardia,* heart] Below the endocardium.

**subendothelial, subendothelium** (sŭb″ĕn-dō-thē′lē-ăl, sŭb″ĕn-dō-thē′lē-ŭm) [″ + Gr. *endon,* within, + *thele,* nipple] Beneath the endothelium.

**subependymal** (sŭb″ĕp-ĕn′dĭ-măl) [″ + Gr. *ependyma,* an upper garment, wrap] Beneath the ependyma.

**subepidermal** (sŭb″ĕp-ĭ-dĕr′măl) [″ + Gr. *epi,* upon, + *derma,* skin] Beneath the epidermis. SYN: *subcuticular.*

**subepithelial** (sŭb″ĕp-ĭ-thē′lē-ăl) [″ + ″ + *thele,* nipple] Beneath the epithelium.

**suberosis** (sū″bĕr-ō′sĭs) [L. *suber,* cork, + Gr. *osis,* condition] Pulmonary hypersensitivity reaction in workers exposed to cork. The antigen is present in a mold in the cork.

**subfamily** (sŭb-făm′ĭ-lē) In taxonomy, the category between a family and a tribe.

**subfascial** (sŭb-făsh′ē-ăl) [L. *sub,* under, below, + *fascia,* a band] Beneath a fascia.

**subfebrile** (sŭb-fē′brĭl) [″ + *febris,* fever] Having a mild fever, usually considered to be less than 101°F (38.3°C).

**subfertility** (sŭb″fĕr-tĭl′ĭ-tē) [″ + *fertilis,* fertile] Fertility considered to be less than normal.

**subflavous** (sŭb-flā′vŭs) [″ + *flavus,* yellow] Yellowish.

**subflavous ligament** The yellowish ligament connecting the laminae of the vertebrae.

**subfolium** (sŭb-fō′lē-ŭm) [″ + *folium,* leaf] A leaflike division of the cerebellar folia.

**subfrontal** (sŭb-frŏn′tăl) [″ + *frontalis,* brow] Below a frontal convolution or lobe of the brain.

**subgenus** (sŭb-jē′nŭs) In taxonomy, the category between a genus and a species.

**subgingival** (sŭb-jĭn′jĭ-văl) [″ + *gingiva,* gum] Beneath the gingiva; rel. to a point or area apical to the margin of the free gingiva, usually within the confines of the gingival sulcus (e.g., subgingival calculus, or the subgingival margin of a restoration).

**subglenoid** (sŭb-glē′noyd) [″ + Gr. *glene,* socket, + *eidos,* form, shape] Below the glenoid fossa or glenoid cavity. SYN: *infraglenoid.*

**subglossal** (sŭb-glŏs′ăl) [″ + Gr. *glossa,* tongue] Sublingual.

**subglossitis** (sŭb-glŏs-sī′tĭs) [″ + ″ + *itis,* inflammation] An inflammation of the undersurface or tissues of the tongue.

**subglottic** (sŭb-glŏt′ĭk) [″ + Gr. *glottis,* back of tongue] Beneath the glottis.

**subgranular** (sŭb-grăn′ū-lăr) [″ + *granulum,* little grain] Not completely granular.

**subgrondation, subgrundation** (sŭb-grŏn-dā′shŭn, -grŭn-dā′shŭn) [Fr.] The depression of one fragment of a broken bone beneath the other, as of the cranium.

**subhepatic** (sŭb″hĕ-păt′ĭk) [L. *sub,* under,

below, + Gr. *hepatikos,* pert. to the liver] Beneath the liver.

**subhyaloid** (sŭb-hī′ă-loyd) [″ + Gr. *hyalos,* glass, + *eidos,* form, shape] Located beneath the hyaloid membrane.

**subhyoid** (sŭb-hī′oyd) [″ + Gr. *hyoeides,* U-shaped] Beneath the hyoid bone.

**subicular** (sŭ-bĭk′ū-lăr) Concerning the uncinate gyrus.

**subiliac** (sŭb-ĭl′ē-ăk) [″ + *iliacus,* pert. to the ilium] **1.** Below the ilium. **2.** Pert. to the subilium.

**subilium** (sŭb-ĭl′ē-ŭm) The lowest part of the ilium.

**subincision** The production of a fistula of the penile urethra, which may interfere with conception. It is used for contraception by some primitive groups, esp. Australian aborigines.

**subintimal** (sŭb-ĭn′tĭ-măl) [″ + *intima,* innermost] Beneath the intima.

**subinvolution** (sŭb″ĭn-vō-lū′shŭn) [L. *sub,* under, below, + *involutio,* a turning into] Imperfect involution; incomplete return of a part to normal dimensions after physiological hypertrophy, as when the uterus fails to reduce to normal size following childbirth. SEE: *uterus.*

**subjacent** (sŭb-jā′sĕnt) [″ + *jacere,* to lie] Lying underneath.

**subject** (sŭb′jĕkt) [L. *subjectus,* brought under] **1.** A patient undergoing treatment, observation, or investigation; this includes a well person participating in a medical or scientific study. **2.** A body used for dissection. **3.** To have a liability to develop attacks of a particular disease. **4.** To submit to a procedure or to the action of another.

**subjective** [L. *subjectivus*] Arising from or concerned with the individual; not perceptible to an observer; the opposite of objective.

**subjective sensation** A sensation occurring when stimuli from internal causes excite the nervous system; one not of objective origin.

**subjective symptoms** A symptom of internal origin, evident only to the patient.

**subjugal** (sŭb-jū′găl) [L. *sub,* under, below, + *jugum,* yoke] Below the malar bone or os zygomaticum.

**sublatio** (sŭb-lā′shē-ō) [L.] Sublation.

***s. retinae*** Detachment of the retina.

**sublation** (sŭb-lā′shŭn) [L. *sublatio,* elevation] The displacement, elevation, or removal of a part. SYN: *sublatio.*

**sublesional** (sŭb-lē′shŭn-ăl) [L. *sub,* under, below, + *laesio,* wound] Beneath a lesion.

**sublethal** (sŭb-lē′thăl) [″ + Gr. *lethe,* oblivion] Less than lethal; almost fatal.

**sublethal dose** A dose containing not quite enough of a toxin or noxious substance to cause death.

**sublimate** (sŭb′lĭ-māt) [L. *sublimare,* to elevate] **1.** A substance obtained or prepared by sublimation. **2.** To cause a solid or gas to change state without becoming a liquid during transition. For example, ice may evaporate without first becoming a liquid. **3.** An ego defense mechanism by which one converts unwanted aggressive or sexual drives into socially acceptable activities.

**sublimation** (sŭb″lĭ-mā′shŭn) [L. *sublimatio*] **1.** The altering of the state of a gas or solid without first changing it into a liquid. **2.** A freudian term pert. to the unconscious mental processes of ego defense whereby unwanted aggressive or sexual drives find an outlet through creative mental work.

**sublime** (sŭb-līm′) [L. *sublimis,* to the limit] To evaporate a substance directly from the solid into the vapor state and condense it again. For example, metallic iodine on heating does not liquefy but forms directly a violet gas.

**subliminal** (sŭb-lĭm′ĭn-ăl) [L. *sub,* under, below, + *limen,* threshold] **1.** Below the threshold of sensation; too weak to arouse sensation or muscular contraction. **2.** Below the normal consciousness.

**subliminal self** In psychiatry, part of the normal individual's personality in which mental processes function without consciousness, under normal waking conditions.

**sublimis** (sŭb-lī′mĭs) [L.] Near the surface.

**sublingual** (sŭb-lĭng′gwăl) [L. *sub,* under, below, + *lingua,* tongue] Beneath or concerning the area beneath the tongue. SYN: *subglossal.*

**sublingual gland** The smallest of the major salivary glands, located in the tissue in the floor of the mouth between the tongue and mandible on each side. It is a mixed seromucous gland. Its main duct opens into or near the submandibular duct, but several smaller ducts may open to the oral cavity independently along the sublingual fold. Numerous minor sublingual glands are scattered throughout the mucosa under the tongue, each with its own duct to the oral surface.

**sublinguitis** (sŭb″lĭng-gwī′tĭs) [″ + ″ + Gr. *itis,* inflammation] An inflammation of the sublingual gland.

**sublobular** (sŭb-lŏb′ū-lăr) [″ + *lobulus,* small lobe] Beneath a lobule.

**sublumbar** (sŭb-lŭm′băr) [″ + *lumbus,* loin] Below the lumbar region.

**subluxation** (sŭb″lŭks-ā′shŭn) [″ + *luxatio,* dislocation] **1.** A partial or incomplete dislocation. **2.** In dentistry, injury to supporting tissues that results in abnormal loosening of teeth without displacement or rotation. When loosely applied to the temporomandibular joint, subluxation refers to the relaxation or stretching of the capsule and ligaments that results in popping noises during movement or partial dislocation of the mandible forward.

**submammary** (sŭb-măm′ă-rē) [″ + *mamma,* breast] Below the mammary gland.

**submandibular** [″ + *mandibula,* lower jawbone] Beneath the mandible or lower jaw.

**submandibular gland** One of the salivary

glands, a mixed tubuloalveolar gland about the size of a walnut that lies in the digastric triangle beneath the mandible. Its main duct (Wharton's duct) opens at the side of the frenulum linguae.

**submandibularitis** An inflammation of or mumps affecting the submandibular gland.

**submarginal** (sŭb-măr′jĭn-ăl) [″ + *marginalis,* border] Close to or next to a margin or border of a part. In dentistry, pert. to a deficiency in material or contour at the margin of a restoration in a tooth.

**submaxillary** Below the maxilla or upper jaw.

**submedial, submedian** (sŭb-mē′dē-ăl, -ăn) [″ + *medianus,* middle] Below or close to the middle.

**submembranous** (sŭb-mĕm′bră-nŭs) [″ + *membrana,* membrane] Containing partly membranous material.

**submental** [″ + *mentum,* chin] Under the chin.

**submerge** (sŭb-mĕrj′) [″ + *mergere,* to immerse] To place under water.

**submerged tooth** A tooth that is below the plane of occlusion; usually a deciduous tooth retained as a result of ankylosis.

**submetacentric** (sŭb″mĕt-ă-sĕn′trĭk) [″ + Gr. *meta,* beyond, + *kentron,* center] Concerning a chromosome in which the centromere is within the two central quarters but away from the middle.

**submicron** [″ + Gr. *mikros,* tiny] A particle smaller than $10^{-5}$ cm in diameter, visible only with an ultramicroscope. SEE: *micron.*

**submicroscopic** [″ + ″ + *skopein,* to examine] Too minute to be seen through a microscope.

**submucosa** (sŭb″mū-kō′să) [L. *sub,* under, below, + *mucosus,* mucus] The layer of connective tissue below the mucosa. It may vary from areolar to quite dense irregular connective tissue and, in addition to the distributing vessels and nerves, may contain extensive deposits of fat, mucous glands, or muscle.

**submucous** (sŭb-mū′kŭs) [″ + *mucus,* mucus] Beneath a mucous membrane.

**submucous resection** Removal of tissue below the mucosa, esp. excision of cartilaginous tissue beneath the mucosal tissue of the nose.

**subnasal** [″ + *nasus,* nose] Under the nose. SYN: *subnasion.*

**subnasale** (sŭb″nā-să′lē) [″ + *nasus,* nose] The base of the anterior nasal spine.

**subnasal point** The craniometric point at the base of the nasal spine.

**subnasion** (sŭb-nā′zē-ŏn) [″ + *nasus,* nose] Subnasal.

**subneural** (sŭb-nū′răl) [″ + Gr. *neuron,* nerve] Beneath the neural axis or the central nervous system.

**subnormal** (sŭb-nor′măl) [″+ *normalis,* acc. to pattern] Less than normal or average.

**subnucleus** (sŭb-nū′klē-ŭs) [″ + *nucleus,* kernel] One of the secondary nuclei into which a nucleus of the central nervous system may be divided.

**suboccipital** (sŭb″ŏk-sĭp′ĭ-tăl) [″ + *occiput,* back of head] Situated below the occiput or occipital bone.

**suboperculum** (sŭb″ō-pĕr′kū-lŭm) [″ + *operculum,* a covering] The portion of the occipital convolution overlapping the insula. SEE: *operculum.*

**suboptimal** (sŭb-ŏp′tĭ-măl) [″ + *optimus,* best] Less than optimum.

**suborbital** (sŭb-or′bĭ-tăl) [″ + *orbita,* track] Beneath the orbit.

**suborder** (sŭb-or′dĕr) In taxonomy, a category below the grouping in the order.

**suboxide** (sŭb-ŏk′sīdz) In a series of oxides, one that contains the smallest amount of oxygen.

**subpapular** (sŭb-păp′ū-lăr) [″ + *papula,* pimple] Very slightly papular, such as papules elevated scarcely more than macules.

**subparietal** (sŭb″pă-rī′ĕ-tăl) [″ + *paries,* a wall] Below the parietal bone or lobe.

**subpatellar** (sŭb″pă-tĕl′ăr) [″ + *patella,* a small pan] Beneath the patella.

**subpectoral** (sŭb-pĕk′tor-ăl) [″ + *pectus,* chest] Below the pectoral area; beneath the pectoral muscles.

**subpeduncular** (sŭb″pē-dŭn′kū-lăr) [″ + *pedunculus,* a little foot] Below a peduncle.

**subpeduncular lobe** A tiny lobe on the undersurface of either cerebellar hemisphere. SYN: *flocculus.*

**subpelviperitoneal** (sŭb-pĕl″vē-pĕr″ĭ-tō-nē′ăl) [L. *sub,* under, below, + *pelvis,* basin, + Gr. *peritonaion,* peritoneum] Beneath the pelvic peritoneum.

**subpericardial** (sŭb″pĕr-ĭ-kăr′dē-ăl) [″+ Gr. *peri,* around, + *kardia,* heart] Beneath the pericardium.

**subperiosteal** (sŭb″pĕr-ē-ŏs′tē-ăl) [″ + ″ + *osteon,* bone] Beneath the periosteum.

**subperitoneal** (sŭb″pĕr-ĭ-tō-nē′ăl) [″ + Gr. *peritonaion,* peritoneum] Beneath the peritoneum. SYN: *subperitoneoabdominal.*

**subperitoneoabdominal** (sŭb″pĕr-ĭ-tō-nē″ō-ăb-dŏm′ĭ-năl) [″ + ″ + L. *abdomen,* belly] Subperitoneal.

**subpharyngeal** (sŭb″făr-ĭn′jē-ăl) [″ + Gr. *pharynx,* throat] Beneath the pharynx.

**subphrenic** (sŭb-frĕn′ĭk) [″ + Gr. *phren,* diaphragm] Subdiaphragmatic.

**subphrenic abscess** A collection of pus beneath the diaphragm.

**subphylum** (sŭb-fī′lŭm) In taxonomy, the category between a phylum and a class.

**subpial** (sŭb-pī′ăl) [″ + *pia,* soft] Beneath the pia.

**subplacenta** (sŭb″plă-sĕn′tă) [″ + *placenta,* a flat cake] During pregnancy, the endometrium that lines the entire uterine cavity except at the site of the implanted blastocyst. SYN: *decidua parietalis.*

**subpleural** (sŭb-plū′răl) [″ + Gr. *pleura,* side] Beneath the pleura.

**subpoena** A court order that requires a person to come to court or appear at a specific time and place to give testimony. Failure to appear can result in punishment by the court.

**subpoena duces tecum** A process used in litigation that compels the party having control of documents, items, and materials relevant to issues in a lawsuit to produce them at a designated time and place.

**subpontine** (sŭb-pŏn′tĭn, -tīn) [″ + *pons,* bridge] Below the pons.

**subpreputial** (sŭb″prē-pū′shăl) [″ + *praeputium,* prepuce] Under the prepuce.

**subpubic** (sŭb-pū′bĭk) [″ + *pubes,* pubic region] Beneath the pubic arch, as a ligament, or performed beneath the pubic arch.

**subpulmonary** (sŭb-pŭl′mō-nā-rē) [″ + *pulmon,* lung] Below the lung.

**subpyramidal** (sŭb″pī-răm′ĭ-dăl) [″ + Gr. *pyramis,* a pyramid] Beneath a pyramid of the kidney.

**subretinal** (sŭb-rĕt′ĭ-năl) [″ + *rete,* a net] Beneath the retina.

**subscapular** (sŭb-skăp′ū-lăr) [″ + *scapula,* shoulder blade] Below the scapula.

**subscleral** (sŭb-sklē′răl) [″ + Gr. *skleros,* hard] Beneath the sclera of the eye. SYN: *subsclerotic* (1).

**subsclerotic** (sŭb-sklē′rŏt-ĭk) [″ + Gr. *skleros,* hard] **1.** Subscleral. **2.** Not completely sclerosed.

**subscription** (sŭb-skrĭp′shŭn) [L. *subscriptas,* written under] The part of a prescription that contains directions for compounding ingredients.

**subserous** (sŭb-sē′rŭs) [L. *sub,* under, below, + *serum,* whey] Beneath a serous membrane.

**subsibilant** (sŭb-sĭb′ĭ-lănt) [″ + *sibilans,* hissing] Having the sound of a muffled whistle.

**subsidence** (sŭb-sīd′ĕns) [L. *subsidere,* to sink down] The gradual disappearance of symptoms or manifestations of a disease.

**subsistence** The minimum amount of something essential for life (e.g., a subsistence diet).

**subspecies** (sŭb′spē-sēz) [L. *sub,* under, below, + *species,* a kind] In taxonomy, subordinate to a species.

**subspinale** (sŭb″spī-nā′lē) [″ + *spina,* thorn] The deepest point between the nasal spine and the crest of the maxilla.

**subspinous** (sŭb-spī′nŭs) [″ + *spina,* thorn] **1.** Beneath any spinous process. **2.** Anterior to or beneath the spinal column.

**subspinous dislocation** A dislocation with the head of the humerus resting below the spine of the scapula.

**substage** (sŭb′stāj) [″ + O. Fr. *estage,* position] The part of the microscope below the stage by which attachments are held in place.

**substance** (sŭb′stăns) [L. *substantia*] **1.** When used in a medicolegal context, a chemical with potential for abuse. A great variety of entities are included such as alcohol, nicotine, caffeine, sedatives, hypnotics, anxiolytics, illicit drugs such as cannabis, heroin, and an array of "street" drugs. Almost any substance may be abused even though its clinical use is approved when used as prescribed. **2.** Material of which any organ or tissue is composed; matter. SYN: *substantia.*

***anterior perforated s.*** The portion of the rhinencephalon lying immediately anterior to the optic chiasm. It is perforated by numerous small arteries.

***anterior pituitary-like s.*** Chorionic gonadotropin.

***black s.*** Substantia nigra.

***chromophilic s.*** A substance found in the cytoplasm of certain cells that stains similar to chromatin with basic dyes. It includes Nissl bodies of neurons and granules in serozymogenic cells.

***colloid s.*** Jelly-like substance in colloid degeneration.

***gray s.*** Gray matter of the brain and spinal cord.

***ground s.*** The matrix or intercellular substance in which the cells of an organ or tissue are embedded.

***high threshold s.*** A substance such as glucose or sodium chloride present in the blood and excreted by the kidney only when its concentration exceeds a certain level.

***ketogenic s.*** A substance that, in its metabolism, gives rise to ketone bodies.

***low threshold s.*** A substance such as urea or uric acid that is excreted by the kidney from the blood almost in its entirety. It occurs in the urine in high concentrations.

***medullary s.*** The soft inner material of any part such as a bone or organ.

***Nissl s.*** The chromatophilic substance of nerve cells. SEE: *Nissl bodies.*

***posterior perforated s.*** A triangular area forming the floor of the interpeduncular fossa. It lies immediately behind the corpora mammillaria and contains numerous openings for blood vessels.

***pressor s.*** A substance that elevates arterial blood pressure.

***reticular s.*** The skein of threads present in some red blood cells. These are visible only when the cells are appropriately stained.

***slow-reacting s.*** SEE: *slow-reacting substance of anaphylaxis.*

***specific soluble s.*** ABBR: SSS. A polysaccharide hapten obtained from the capsules of pneumococci.

***transmitter s.*** Neurotransmitter.

***white s.*** White matter of the brain and spinal cord.

***white s. of Schwann*** A nerve fiber's medullary sheath.

**substance abuse** A maladaptive pattern of behavior in regard to the use of chemically active agents that leads to clinically significant impairment or distress. Commonly abused substances include alcohol; psychoactive chemicals; and therapeutic medications such as sedatives, hypnotics, and anxiolytics. One or more of the following occur within a 12-month period: continued substance use resulting in a failure to fulfill major obligations at work, school, or home (e.g., repeated absences from work or poor work performance; expulsion from school; neglect of children or household); recurrent substance use in hazardous situations such as driving an automobile, flying an airplane, or using a machine; recurrent substance-related legal problems; continued substance use despite having persistent or recurrent social or interpersonal problems caused or exacerbated by the effects of the substance. Substance abuse and induced mental disorders include delirium, dementia, psychosis, mood disorder, anxiety, sexual dysfunction, sleep disorder, and persistent hallucination disorder characterized by "flashbacks." SEE: *alcoholism; substance dependence; Nursing Diagnoses Appendix.*

**substance dependence** A cluster of cognitive, behavioral, and physiological symptoms indicating that the individual continues use of the substance despite the presence of significant substance-related problems. Patients develop a tolerance for the substance and require progressively greater amounts to elicit the effects desired. In addition, patients experience physical and psychological signs and symptoms of withdrawal if the agent is not used. SEE: *alcoholism; substance abuse.*

**substance P** An 11-amino acid peptide that is believed to be important as a neurotransmitter in the pain fiber system. This substance may also be important in eliciting local tissue reactions resembling inflammation. SEE: *neurotransmitter; pain.*

**substandard** Failing to meet the usual or accepted standard.

**substantia** (sŭb-stăn′shē-ă) [L.] The material of which any organ or tissue is composed; matter. SYN: *substance.*

***s. alba*** The white substance of the brain and spinal cord. SYN: *white matter.*

***s. cinerea*** The gray substance of the brain and spinal cord.

***s. ferruginea*** The elongated mass of pigmented cells in the locus ceruleus.

***s. gelatinosa*** The gray matter of the cord surrounding the central canal and capping the head of the posterior horns of the spinal cord.

***s. grisea*** The gray matter of the spinal cord. SYN: *gray matter.*

***s. nigra*** The black substance in a section of the crus cerebri. SYN: *black substance; locus niger.*

***s. propria membranae tympani*** The fibrous middle layer of the drum membrane.

**substantivity** The ability of tissue to absorb an active ingredient and release it slowly over a period of time.

**substernal** (sŭb-stĕr′năl) [L. *sub,* under, below, + Gr. *sternon,* chest] Situated beneath the sternum.

**substernal thrust** In children, a thrusting of the substernal area of the chest. This indicates right ventricular hypertrophy. SEE: *apical heave.*

**substernomastoid** (sŭb-stĕr-nō-măs′toyd) [″ + ″ + Gr. *mastos,* breast, + *eidos,* form, shape] Beneath the sternomastoid muscle.

**substituent** One part of a molecule substituted with another atom or group.

**substitute** (sŭb′stĭ-tūt) Something that may be used in place of another.

***blood s.*** A fluid used to expand the plasma volume, but not a true substitute for the blood. Artificial substances capable of functioning as blood are being investigated, but no completely satisfactory ones are available.

**substitution** (sŭb-stĭ-tū′shŭn) [L. *substitutio,* replacing] **1.** Displacing an atom (or more than one) of an element in a compound by atoms of another element of equal valence. **2.** In psychiatry, the ego defense mechanism of turning from an obstructed desire to one whose gratification is socially acceptable. **3.** The turning from an obstructed form of behavior to a more primitive one, as a substitution neurosis. **4.** The replacement of one substance by another. **5.** In pharmacy, the replacement of one drug by another drug in dispensing. Usually a generic drug is substituted for a proprietary one. SEE: *interchange.*

**substitution product** A compound formed by an element or a radical replacing another element or radical in a compound.

**substitution therapy** In treatment, the use of a substance such as a product of glandular secretion (hormone or enzyme) to replace a natural substance in the body. This method is used when glands fail to secrete properly or the substance secreted is unavailable to tissues.

**substitutive** (sŭb′stĭ-tū″tĭv) [L. *substitutivus*] Causing a change or substitution of characteristics.

**substitutive therapy** Treatment to overcome an inflammation of a specific character by exciting an acute nonspecific inflammation.

**substrate, substratum** (sŭb′strāt, sŭb-strā′tŭm) [L. *substratum,* to lie under] **1.** An underlying layer or foundation. **2.** A base, as of a pigment. **3.** The substance acted upon, as by an enzyme. SYN: *zymolyte.* SEE: *enzyme.*

**substructure** (sŭb′strŭk-chŭr) The underlying structure of supporting material.

**subsultus** (sŭb-sŭl′tŭs) [L., to leap up] Any tremor, twitching, or spasmodic movement.

***s. tendinum*** An involuntary twitching of the muscles, esp. of those of the arms and feet, causing movement of the tendons. It is observed in certain febrile conditions.

**subsylvian** (sŭb-sĭl'vē-ăn) Below the fissure of Sylvius.
**subtarsal** (sŭb-tăr'săl) [L. *sub,* under, below, + Gr. *tarsos,* a broad, flat surface] Below the tarsus.
**subtentorial** Located beneath the tentorium.
**subterminal** (sŭb-tĕr'mĭ-năl) [" + *terminus,* a boundary] Close to the end of an extremity.
**subtetanic** (sŭb"tē-tăn'ĭk) [" + Gr. *tetanikos,* suffering from tetanus] Moderately tetanic.
**subthalamic** (sŭb"thă-lăm'ĭk) [" + Gr. *thalamos,* inner chamber] Located below the thalamus.
**subthalamic nucleus** An elliptical mass of gray matter lying in the ventral thalamus above the cerebral peduncle and rostral to the substantia nigra. It receives fibers from the globus pallidus.
**subthalamus** The portion of the diencephalon lying below the thalamus and above the hypothalamus. SEE: *thalamus.*
**subtile, subtle** (sŭb'tĭl, sŭt'l) [L. *subtilis,* fine] **1.** Very fine or delicate. **2.** Very acute. **3.** Mentally acute or crafty. **4.** Causing injury without attracting attention, as subtle poisons or early symptoms of a disease.
**subtilin** (sŭb'tĭl-ĭn) An antibiotic biosynthesized by *Bacillus subtilis.* It is of low toxicity and effective against gram-positive organisms.
**subtotal** (sŭb-tō'tăl) [L. *sub,* under, below, + *totus,* all] Less than total, as partial removal of a gland.
**subtraction** The process by which undesired, overlying structures can be removed from a radiographical image.
**subtrapezial** (sŭb"tră-pē'zē-ăl) [" + Gr. *trapezion,* a little table] Beneath the trapezius muscle.
**subtribe** (sŭb'trīb) In taxonomy, the category between a genus and a tribe.
**subtrochanteric** (sŭb"trō-kăn-tĕr'ĭk) [" + Gr. *trochanter,* to run] Below a trochanter.
**subtrochlear** (sŭb-trŏk'lē-ăr) [" + Gr. *trokhileia,* system of pulleys] Beneath the trochlea.
**subtuberal** (sŭb-tū'bĕr-ăl) [" + *tuber,* a swelling] Located under a tuber.
**subtympanic** (sŭb-tĭm-păn'ĭk) [" + Gr. *tympanon,* drum] Below the tympanum.
**subumbilical** (sŭb"ŭm-bĭl'ĭ-kăl) [" + *umbilicus,* navel] Below the umbilicus.
**subumbilical space** The triangular space within the body cavity below the navel.
**subungual, subunguial** (sŭb-ŭng'gwăl, -gwē-ăl) [" + *unguis,* nail] Situated beneath the nail of a finger or toe.
**subungual hematoma** A collection of blood under the nail as a result of trauma. This condition may be treated by heating the end of a paper clip and then placing its point against the nail, which permits a small hole to be melted painlessly in the nail and allows the trapped blood to escape.
**subunit** In chemistry, a portion of a compound that represents a smaller part of the molecule than the remainder of the substance. SEE: *beta subunit.*
**suburethral** (sŭb"ū-rē'thrăl) [" + Gr. *ourethra,* urethra] Below the urethra.
**subvaginal** (sŭb-văj'ĭn-ăl) [" + *vagina,* sheath] **1.** Below the vagina. **2.** On the inner side of any tubular sheathing membrane.
**subvertebral** (sŭb-vĕr'tĕ-brăl) [" + *vertebra,* vertebra] Beneath, or on the ventral side of, the vertebral column or a vertebra.
**subvitrinal** (sŭb-vĭt'rĭn-ăl) [" + *vitrina,* vitreous body] Located beneath the vitreous body.
**subvolution** (sŭb"vō-lū'shŭn) [" + *volutus,* turning] A method of turning over a flap surgically to prevent adhesions.
**subzonal** (sŭb-zō'năl) Beneath a zone.
**subzygomatic** (sŭb"zī-gō-măt'ĭk) [" + Gr. *zygoma,* cheekbone] Beneath the zygomatic bone.
**succedaneous** (sŭk"sē-dā'nē-ŭs) [L. *succedaneus,* substituting] **1.** Acting as a substitute or relating to one. **2.** In dentistry, referring to the secondary or permanent set of teeth, which follow an earlier deciduous set.
**succedaneum** (sŭk"sĕ-dā'nē-ŭm) [L. *succedaneus,* substituting] Something that may be used as a substitute.
**succimer** A drug used in treating children with acute lead poisoning when the blood lead level exceeds 45 μg/dl. The chemical name is 2,3-dimercaptosuccinic acid (DMSA). SEE: *lead, acute encephalopathy; lead poisoning, acute.*

Caution: Use of this drug should always be accompanied by identification and removal of the source of the lead exposure.

**succinate** (sŭk'sĭ-nāt) Any salt of succinic acid.
**succinic acid** SEE: *acid, succinic.*
**succinylcholine chloride** (sŭk"sĭ-nĭl-kō'lēn) A drug used for its neuromuscular blocking effect. It is used as an adjuvant in surgical anesthesia, and to prevent trauma in electroconvulsive shock therapy.

Caution: This drug should be used only by physicians who have had extensive training in its use and in a setting where facilities for respiratory and cardiovascular resuscitation are immediately available.

**succinylsulfathiazole** (sŭk"sĭ-nĭl-sŭl"fă-thī'ă-zōl) 2-($N^4$-succinylsulfanilamido)thiazole. Because of lack of evidence of its clinical efficacy, the drug is no longer used.
**succorrhea** (sŭk-kō-rē'ă) [L. *succus,* juice, + Gr. *rhoia,* flow] An unnatural increase in the secretion of any juice, esp. of a digestive fluid.
**succus** (sŭk'kŭs) *pl.* **succi** [L. *succus,* juice]

A juice or fluid secretion.

*s. enterius* The intestinal juice; an alkaline secretion by the minute glands lining the small intestine.

*s. gastricus* The gastric juice.

**succussion** (sŭ-kŭsh′ŭn) [L. *succussio,* a shaking] The shaking of a person to detect the presence of fluid in the body cavity by listening for a splashing sound, esp. in the thorax.

**suck** [AS. *sucan,* to suck] **1.** To draw fluid into the mouth, as from the breast. **2.** To exhaust air from a tube and thus draw fluid from a container. **3.** That which is drawn into the mouth by sucking.

**sucking pad** A mass of fat in the cheeks, esp. well developed in an infant, aiding sucking. SEE: *buccal fat pad.*

**suckle** To nurse at the breast.

**sucralfate** A medicine consisting of a complex formed from sucrose octasulfate and polyaluminum hydroxide. It is effective in treating peptic ulcer by forming a coating over the ulcer crater. The coating will stay in place for over 8 hr. The dose is 1 g 1 hr before each meal and at bedtime. Trade name is Carafate. SEE: *peptic ulcer.*

**sucrase** (sū′krās) [Fr. *sucre,* sugar] An enzyme in the intestinal juice that splits cane sugar into glucose and fructose, the two being absorbed into the portal circulation. SYN: *invertase.*

**sucrose** (sū′krōs) [Fr. *sucre,* sugar] A dissacharide, $C_{12}H_{22}O_{11}$, obtained from sugar cane, sugar beet, and other sources. In the intestine, it is hydrolyzed to glucose and fructose by sucrase present in the intestinal juice.

ACTION/USES: The monosaccharides resulting from the digestion of sucrose are absorbed by the small intestine and carried to the liver, where they may be converted to glycogen and stored if they are not needed immediately for energy.

**sucrosuria** (sū″krō-sū′rē-ă) [″ + Gr. *ouron,* urine] Sucrose in the urine.

**suction** [LL. *suctio,* sucking] The act of, or capacity for, sucking up by reduction of air pressure over the surface of a substance. SEE: *aspiration.*

*nasogastric s.* The suction of gas, fluid, and solid material from the gastrointestinal tract by use of a tube extending from the suction device to the stomach or intestines via the nasal passage. SEE: *Wangensteen tube.*

*post-tussive s.* The suction sound over a lung cavity heard on auscultation after a cough.

**suction abortion** The removal of the products of conception from the uterus using a device that sucks the tissues away from the lining of the uterus.

**suction biopsy** A technique for obtaining tissue by use of a device that applies suction to the area from which the tissue is desired. It is used in obtaining tissue from the mucosa of the stomach and intestines.

**suctorial** (sŭk-tō′rē-ăl) [LL. *suctio,* sucking] **1.** Concerning sucking. **2.** Equipped for sucking.

**sudamen** (sū-dā′mĕn) *pl.* **sudamina** [L., sweat] A noninflammatory eruption from sweat glands marked by whitish vesicles caused by the retention of sweat in the cornified layer of the skin, appearing after profuse sweating or in certain febrile diseases.

**Sudan** (sū-dăn′) One of a number of related biological stains for which fats have a special affinity, including Sudan II, Sudan III (G), Sudan IV, and Sudan R.

**sudanophil** (sū-dăn′ō-fĭl) [*sudan* + Gr. *philein,* to love] A leukocyte that stains readily with Sudan III, indicative of fatty degeneration.

**sudanophilia** (sū-dăn″ō-fĭl′ē-ă) An affinity for Sudan stains.

**sudanophilic** (sū-dăn″ō-fĭl′ĭk) Staining easily with Sudan stain.

**sudden death** Death occurring unexpectedly and instantaneously or within 1 hr of the onset of symptoms in a patient with or without known preexisting heart disease. Sudden death due to cardiac conditions occurs in the U.S. at the rate of one each minute. It may be caused by a number of cardiovascular conditions, including ischemic heart disease, aortic stenosis, coronary embolism, myocarditis, ruptured or dissecting aortic aneurysm, Stokes-Adams syndrome, cerebrovascular accident, pulmonary thromboembolism, and other noncardiovascular-related disorders, such as disturbances of electrolyte balance, drug toxicity, or idiosyncrasy.

**sudden infant death syndrome** ABBR: SIDS. The sudden death of an infant younger than 1 year of age that remains unexplained after a thorough investigation, including a complete autopsy, examination of the death scene, and review of the clinical history. The diagnosis should not be made if the death scene has not been investigated by a trained, competent professional. It is a diagnosis of exclusion in that there are no specific autopsy findings to account for the death. SYN: *crib death.*

SIDS is the most common single cause of death of infants between the ages of 7 days and 1 year. Annually, in the U.S. about 5500 infants die of SIDS. The cause of SIDS is unknown, and attempts to predict which infants will develop the syndrome have been unsuccessful.

RISK FACTORS: Several demographic and environmental factors are associated with a higher incidence of SIDS. Maternal variables include adolescence; unwed marital status; African-American or Native American ethnicity; smoking or substance abuse during pregnancy; severe anemia during pregnancy; and third-trimester bleeding. Infant variables include winter birth, male sex, and low Apgar score. Socioeconomic factors include low income and inadequate housing. Although SIDS infants are apparently normal, healthy, and well-developed, low birth weight and being small for gestational or chronological age have also been noted as risk factors.

PREVENTION: Parents should attempt to remedy those risk factors listed that can be altered or prevented. The prone position for sleep should be avoided. The slogan "Back to Sleep" was devised to remind parents that infants should be positioned on the side or back. A firm sleeping surface is recommended. Soft, plush, or bulky items, such as pillows, rolls of bedding, or cushions should not be placed in the infant's sleeping environment. These items could come into close contact with the infant's face, thereby interfering with ventilation or entrapping the infant's head and causing suffocation. Home monitoring of the infant's cardiorespiratory status is indicated for infants suspected to be at risk of developing SIDS; this is esp. important for subsequent siblings in a family with a SIDS case. SEE: *apnea; apnea alarm mattress.*

NOTE: Loss of an infant because of SIDS may produce a severe grief and guilt reaction. Thus, the family needs expert counseling in the several months after the death.

**Sudeck's disease, Sudeck's atrophy** (soo'dĕks) [Paul Herman Martin Sudeck, Ger. surgeon, 1866–1938] Traumatic osteoporosis.

**sudokeratosis** (sū″dō-kĕr″ă-tō'sĭs) [L. *sudor,* sweat, + Gr. *keras,* horn, + *osis,* condition] Circumscribed horny overgrowths that obstruct the sweat ducts.

**sudomotor** (sū″dō-mō'tor) [″ + *motor,* a mover] Pert. to stimulating the secretion of sweat; noting certain nerves.

**sudor** (sū'dor) [L.] Perspiration; sweat.

***s. cruentus*** Blood-tinged sweat. SYN: *hematidrosis.*

**sudoral** (sū'dor-ăl) Pert. to, caused by, or marked by perspiration.

**sudoresis** (sū″dō-rē'sĭs) [L.] Diaphoresis.

**sudoriferous** (sū-dor-ĭf'ĕr-ŭs) [″ + *ferre,* to bear] Conveying or producing sweat. SYN: *sudoriparous.*

**sudoriferous glands** Sweat-secreting glands of the skin.

**sudorific** (sū″dor-ĭf'ĭk) [L. *sudorificus*] **1.** Secreting or promoting the secretion of sweat. **2.** An agent that produces sweating. SYN: *diaphoretic.*

**sudoriparous** (sū″dor-ĭp'ă-rŭs) [L. *sudor,* sweat, + *parere,* to produce] Sudoriferous.

**suet** (sū'ĕt) [Fr. *sewet,* suet] A hard fat from cattle or sheep kidneys and loins, used as the base of certain ointments and as an emollient.

**suffocate** (sŭf'ō-kāt) [L. *suffocare*] To impair respiration; to smother, asphyxiate.

**suffocation** (sŭf″ō-kā'shŭn) **1.** The state of being choked by obstruction of air passages by drowning, smothering, throttling, or inhalation of noxious gases. SYN: *asphyxiation.* SEE: *asphyxia; resuscitation; unconsciousness.* **2.** The act of obstructing the air passages.

SYMPTOMS: Although insensibility, slight breathing, purple swollen face, and livid lips mark this condition, symptoms are not always present.

TREATMENT: One should splash cold water in the face and slap the chest of the patient. Aromatic spirits of ammonia should be applied to the nostrils. Artificial respiration should be performed. A tracheotomy may be required.

***s., risk for*** Accentuated risk of accidental suffocation (inadequate air available for inhalation). SEE: *Nursing Diagnoses Appendix.*

**suffusion** (sŭ-fū'zhŭn) [L. *suffusio,* a pouring over] **1.** Extravasation. **2.** Pouring of a fluid over the body as treatment.

**sugar** [O. Fr. *zuchre*] A sweet-tasting carbohydrate belonging to the monosaccharide or dissacharide groups. Sugars are crystalline carbohydrates of comparatively low molecular weight that generally have a sweet taste. Sugar has been used topically as a thin paste to treat infected wounds and ulcers, such as decubitus ulcers. Also, sugar taken orally or in appropriate intravenous solution is quite beneficial in preventing the hypoglycemia caused by a dose of excess insulin. SEE: *bedsore; carbohydrates.*

CLASSIFICATION: Sugars are classified in two ways: the number of atoms of simple sugars yielded on hydrolysis by a molecule of the given sugar and the number of carbon atoms in the molecules of the simple sugars so obtained. Therefore, glucose is a monosaccharide because it cannot be hydrolyzed to a simpler sugar; it is a hexose because it contains six carbon atoms per molecule. Sucrose is a disaccharide because on hydrolysis it yields two molecules, one of glucose and one of fructose.

***beet s.*** Sucrose obtained from sugar beets.

***blood s.*** The carbohydrate present in the blood, principally glucose.

***cane s.*** Sucrose obtained from sugar cane.

***diabetic s.*** Glucose in the urine of diabetics.

***fruit s.*** Fructose.

***invert s.*** Mixture consisting of one molecule of glucose and one of fructose resulting from the hydrolysis of sucrose.

***malt s.*** Maltose.

***milk s.*** Lactose.

***muscle s.*** Inositol; not a true sugar.

***wood s.*** Xylose.

**suggestibility** (sŭg-jĕs″tĭ-bĭl'ĭ-tē) [L. *suggestus,* suggested] A condition in which a person responds readily to suggestions or opinions of another.

**suggestible** (sŭg-jĕs'tĭ-bl) Very susceptible to the opinions or suggestions of others.

**suggestion** (sŭg-jĕs′chŭn) [L. *suggestio*] **1.** The imparting of an idea indirectly; the act of implying. **2.** The idea so conveyed. **3.** The psychological process of having an individual adopt or accept an idea without argument or persuasion.

***posthypnotic s.*** A suggestion made to a subject while under hypnosis. After emerging from the hypnotic state, the person usually performs the suggested act.

**suggestive** (sŭg-jĕs′tĭv) Stimulating or pert. to suggestion.

**suggestive therapeutics** The practice of treating disease by hypnotic suggestions.

**suicide** (sū′ĭ-sīd) [L. *sui,* of oneself, + *caedere,* to kill] The intentional and voluntarily taking of one's own life. In the U.S., approx. 30,000 people commit suicide each year, which is equivalent to one suicide every 20 min. Most of these persons have consulted with a physician in the 6 months prior to death, and 10% have seen a physician during the week preceding suicide. These statistics indicate that physicians and other health care workers have great potential for recognizing and treating individuals at risk of suicide.

During the past 30 years, the rate of suicide in persons 15 to 24 years of age, particularly in males, has tripled. Other persons at high risk of suicide include older white men who are without a spouse, unemployed, and in poor health; depressed patients; alcoholics; drug addicts; and those with clinical conditions, including spinal cord injuries, cancer (particularly in men shortly after diagnosis), schizophrenia, or seizure disorders. Suicide occurs in hospitalized patients at 3½ times the rate of the general population. Patients admitted for accidents are believed to be at high risk when the "accident" was in fact a suicide attempt.

Health care professionals should be alert to the warning signs of suicide, such as statements indicating a desire to die or a prediction that suicide will occur. Persons contemplating suicide may be depressed, act to get their lives in order, give away possessions, have failing grades or poor work performance, adopt risk-taking behavior, or have a history of alcoholism or drug abuse.

Management of persons who are contemplating or have attempted suicide includes removal of lethal means from them and the provision of professional, social, and family support. If the patient is being treated as an outpatient, then he or she should be scheduled for specific future appointments and informed of a telephone number where help or assistance will be immediately available on a 24-hr basis. During a crisis, the patient should not be left alone even for a few minutes. For medicolegal reasons, careful and complete medical records should be kept concerning the plans and actions for management of the patient.

**suicide, assisted** SEE: *assisted suicide.*

**suicide cluster** A cluster, of suicides within a defined location and time.

**suicidology** (soo″ĭ-sīd-ŏl′ō-jē) [″ + ″ + Gr. *logos,* word, reason] The science of suicide, including its cause, prediction of those susceptible, and prevention.

**suit 1.** A lawsuit, legal action, or court proceeding by one party against another for damages or other legal remedies. **2.** An outer garment.

***anti-G s.*** SEE: *anti-G suit.*

**sulcal** (sŭl′kăl) [L.] Pert. to a sulcus.

**sulcal artery** A tiny branch of the anterior spinal artery.

**sulcate, sulcated** (sŭl′kāt, -ĕd) [L. *sulcatus*] Furrowed or grooved.

**sulciform** (sŭl′sĭ-form) [L. *sulcus,* groove, + *forma,* form] Resembling a sulcus.

**sulculus** (sŭl′kū-lŭs) [L.] A small sulcus.

**sulcus** (sŭl′kŭs) *pl.* **sulci** [L., groove] A furrow, groove, slight depression, or fissure, esp. of the brain.

***alveololingual s.*** The space in the floor of the mouth between the base of the tongue and the alveolar ridge, on each side extending from the frenum of the tongue back to the retromolar wall.

***calcarine s.*** A deep horizontal fissure on the medial surface of the occipital lobe of the brain.

***s. centralis*** A fissure dividing the frontal and parietal lobes of each cerebral hemisphere. SYN: *Rolando's fissure.*

***collateral s.*** A sulcus on the tentorial surface of the brain. It bounds the inferior lingual gyrus and is parallel to the calcarine and postcalcarine sulci.

***s. cutis*** The ridges on the skin of the palmar surface of the fingers and toes, which comprise the fingerprints.

***gingival s.*** The space or crevice between the free gingiva and the tooth surface. When enlarged by disease, it becomes a periodontal pocket. Also called *gingival crevice* or *pocket.*

***hippocampal s.*** The sulcus on the medial side of the hippocampal gyrus.

***intraparietal s.*** The groove that separates the inferior from the superior parietal bones and lobes.

***nymphocaruncular s.*** The depression between the caruncula of the hymen and the labium minus.

***nymphohymenal s.*** Trench between the labium minus and the hymen on either side.

***s. precentralis*** An interrupted sulcus generally parallel with the fissure of Rolando and anterior to it.

***s. pulmonalis*** A depression on either side of the vertebral column.

***s. spiralis cochleae*** A groove between the labium tympanicum and labium vestibulare.

**sulfacetamide** (sŭl″fă-sĕt′ă-mīd) An antibacterial sulfonamide that is highly soluble. It is particularly useful for topical application to the eye.

***sodium s.*** A very soluble sulfonamide used in solution to treat infections of the cornea and conjunctiva.

**sulfadiazine** (sŭl″fă-dī′ă-zēn) One of a group of diazine derivatives of sulfanilamide. Because it readily penetrates the blood-brain barrier, it has been used extensively in treating meningococcal meningitis. Some strains of meningococci have become resistant to sulfadiazine.

***silver s.*** SEE: *silver sulfadiazine.*

**sulfa drugs** Drugs of the sulfonamide group possessing bacteriostatic properties. SEE: *sulfonamides.*

**sulfamethizole** (sŭl″fă-mĕth′ĭ-zōl) A sulfonamide used in treating urinary tract infections. Trade names are Proklar and Thiosulfil.

**sulfamethoxazole** (sŭl″fă-mĕth-ŏks′ă-zōl) A sulfonamide used in treating urinary tract infections; usually used in combination with trimethoprim. SEE: *trimethoprim.*

**sulfanilamide** (sŭl″făn-ĭl′ă-mīd) Para-aminobenzenesulfonamide. It is a white, slightly bitter crystalline substance from coal tar, the parent of the azo dyes. Formerly it was widely used in the treatment of a number of infections, but because of its toxic reactions it has been superseded by more effective and less toxic sulfonamides.

**sulfapyridine** (sŭl″fă-pĭr′ĭ-dēn) A sulfonamide that is used only in treating dermatitis herpetiformis.

***sodium monohydrate s.*** A soluble salt of sulfapyridine for intravenous use only.

**sulfasalazine** (sŭl″fă-săl′ă-zēn) A sulfonamide that is poorly absorbed from the gastrointestinal tract. It is used in treating ulcerative colitis.

**sulfatase** (sŭl′fă-tās) An enzyme that hydrolyzes sulfuric acid esters.

**sulfate** (sŭl′fāt) [L. *sulphas*] A salt or ester of sulfuric acid.

***cupric s.*** The penta hydrate salt of copper, $CuSO_4 \cdot 5H_2O$, used as an antidote in treating phosphorus poisoning.

***ferrous s.*** An iron compound used in treating iron-deficiency anemia.

***iron s.*** Copperas. It is fatal in large dosages. SEE: *ferrous sulfate; copper salts in Poisons and Poisoning Appendix.*

***magnesium s.*** SEE: *magnesium sulfate.*

**sulfatide** (sŭl′fă-tīd) Any cerebroside with a sulfate radical esterified to the galactose.

**sulfhemoglobin** (sŭlf″hēm-ō-glō′bĭn) Sulfmethemoglobin.

**sulfhemoglobinemia** (sŭlf″hēm-ō-glō″bĭn-ē′mē-ă) A persistent cyanotic condition caused by sulfhemoglobin in blood.

**sulfhydryl** (sŭlf-hī′drĭl) The univalent radical, SH, of sulfur and hydrogen.

**sulfide** (sŭl′fīd) Any compound of sulfur with an element or base.

**sulfinpyrazone** (sŭl″fĭn-pī′ră-zōn) A drug used to promote excretion of uric acid in the urine. Trade name is Anturane.

**sulfisoxazole** (sŭl″fĭ-sŏk′să-zōl) A sulfonamide used for treating certain bacterial infections, esp. certain urinary tract infections.

**sulfmethemoglobin** (sŭlf″mĕt-hē″mō-glō′bĭn) The greenish hemoglobin compound formed when hemoglobin and hydrogen sulfide are combined. SYN: *sulfhemoglobin.*

**sulfobromophthalein** (sŭl″fō-brō″mō-thăl′ē-ĭn) A drug administered intravenously in testing liver function.

**sulfonamide** Any of a group of compounds consisting of amides of sulfanilic acid derived from their parent compound sulfanilamide. They are bacteriostatic. Their action on bacteria results from interference with the functioning of enzyme systems necessary for normal metabolism, growth, and multiplication.

**sulfone** (sŭl′fōn) An oxidation product of sulfur compound in which the $=SO_2$ is united to two hydrocarbon radicals.

**sulfourea** (sŭl″fō-ū-rē′ă) Thiourea.

**sulfoxide** (sŭl-fŏk′sīd) The divalent radical $=SO$.

**sulfoxone sodium** (sŭl-fŏks′ŏn) A drug used in treating leprosy and dermatitis herpetiformis. The leprosy bacillus has, in some areas, become resistant to this drug.

**sulfur** (sŭl′fŭr) [L.] SYMB: S. A pale yellow, crystalline element; atomic weight, 32.06; atomic number, 16; specific gravity, 2.07. It burns with a blue flame, producing sulfur dioxide.

The amount of sulfur excreted in urine varies with the amount of protein in the diet but more or less parallels the amount of nitrogen excreted, as both are derived from protein catabolism. The S:N ratio is approx. 1:14 (i.e., for each gram of sulfur excreted, 14 g of nitrogen are excreted). The amount of sulfur excreted daily is about 1 g. It is oxidized to sulfate and required for the synthesis of body proteins as cystine, cysteine, or their combination.

DEFICIENCY SYMPTOMS: Sulfur deficiency produces dermatitis and imperfect development of hair and nails. A deficiency of cystine or cysteine proteins in the diet inhibits growth and may be fatal. Tissue oxidation of cystine forms inorganic sulfate if the protein intake is sufficient.

***s. dioxide*** An irritating gas used in industry to manufacture acids and as a bactericide and important disinfectant.

***precipitated s.*** A form of sulfur used in various skin diseases, including scabies. Its keratolytic effect helps to make it effective in those disorders.

***sublimed s.*** A form of sulfur used in various skin diseases. Its keratolytic effect helps to make it effective in those disorders. It is a scabicide.

**sulfurated, sulfureted** (sŭl′fū-rā″tĕd, -rĕt″ĕd) Combined or impregnated with sulfur.

**sulfurated hydrogen** $H_2S$. Hydrogen sulfide.

**sulfuric acid poisoning** Injury sustained from contact with sulfuric acid. It is sometimes accidentally taken by mouth, as it resembles syrup or glycerin.

SYMPTOMS: The local effects include burning, with destruction of the skin. If it strikes the eye, it may result in blindness. If taken by mouth, it causes intense injury to the mucosa extending from the mouth to the esophagus and down to the stomach, which results in marked, excruciating pain; swelling of the affected tissues; possibly excessive salivation; painful swallowing; often gasping for breath, and a hoarse voice. The mucous membrane has a grayish-white coating. There is persistent, painful vomiting. The patient quickly goes into shock.

TREATMENT: The acid should be diluted with large volumes of water and neutralized with milk of magnesia, baking soda, or other well-diluted alkalies. This should be followed by soothing substances, such as raw eggs. SEE: *acids in Poisons and Poisoning Appendix.*

---

Caution: Gastric lavage by using a stomach tube should not be attempted if poisoning has occurred more than an hour previously.

---

**sumac** (soo′măk) General term applied to several species of *Rhus.*

***poison s.*** A type of sumac that causes a contact dermatitis. SEE: *poison sumac.*

**summation** (sŭm-ā′shŭn) [L. *summatio,* adding] A cumulative action or effect, as of stimuli; thus, an organ reacts to two or more weak stimuli as if they were a single strong one.

**sunburn** [AS. *sunne,* sun, + *bernan,* to burn] Dermatitis due to excessive exposure to the actinic rays of the sun. The rays that produce the characteristic changes in the skin are ultraviolet, between 290 and 320 nm (sunburn rays). Some people are more resistant to these rays than others, but the skin will be damaged in anyone who has sufficient exposure.

PREVENTION: Direct exposure of the skin to sunlight between 10 AM and 3 PM, when sunburn rays are generally present, should be avoided. Clothing should be worn to cover the skin or a sun-blocking agent with a sun protective factor (SPF) of 15 should be used (to be reapplied each hour if the person is sweating heavily).

TREATMENT: Cool, wet dressings may be applied to the burned area if the reaction is moderate. For severe sunburn, lukewarm baths with oatmeal or cornstarch and baking soda should be given. Aspirin or other nonsteroidal anti-inflammatory agents may reduce inflammation and pain.

**Sunday morning paralysis** Radial nerve palsy, sometimes the indirect result of acute alcoholism resulting from the stuporous patient lying immobile with his or her arm pressed over a projecting surface. SYN: *musculospiral paralysis; Saturday night paralysis.*

**sunflower eyes** Slang term for the appearance of the eyes of patients with Wilson's disease. Deposits of copper around the edge of the cornea (Kayser-Fleischer rings) cause this condition.

**sunglasses** Eyeglasses that protect the eyes from exposure to visible as well as ultraviolet rays. Because of the great variability of sunglasses to perform this function, it is advisable for the potential user to consult an ophthalmologist or optometrist concerning the need for sunglasses and the type needed.

**sunscreen** A substance used to protect the skin from ultraviolet radiation of the sun. It is usually applied as an ointment or cream. SEE: *photosensitivity; ultraviolet radiation.*

**sunscreen protective factor index** In preparations (sunscreens) for protecting the skin from the sun, the ratio of the amount of exposure needed to produce a minimal erythema response with the sunscreen in place divided by the amount of exposure required to produce the same reaction without the sunscreen. SEE: *erythema dose.*

**sunstroke** (sŭn′strōk) [AS. *sunne,* sun, + *strake,* a blow] Heatstroke.

**suntan** Darkening of the skin caused by exposure to the sun. SEE: *tanning salon; sunburn; sunscreen.*

**super-** [L., over, above] Combining form meaning *above, beyond, superior.*

**superabduction** (soo″pĕr-ăb-dŭk′shŭn) [L. *super,* over, above, + *abducens,* drawing away] Pronounced or extreme abduction.

**superacromial** (soo″pĕr-ă-krō′mē-ăl) Supra-acromial.

**superantigen** An antigen that simultaneously activates large numbers of T cells. Exotoxins from bacteria such as staphylococci and group A streptococci act as superantigens.

**superciliary** (soo″pĕr-sĭl′ē-ă-rē) [L. *supercilium,* eyebrow] Pert. to or in the region of an eyebrow. SYN: *supraciliary.*

**supercilium** (soo″pĕr-sĭl′ē-ŭm) *pl.* **supercilia** [L.] **1.** Eyebrow. **2.** A hair of the eyebrow.

**superclass** (soo′pĕr-klăs) In taxonomy, the category between a phylum and a class.

**superego** (soo″pĕr-ē′gō) [″ + *ego,* I; later translators of Freud's writings feel the word *uber-ich* should have been translated to over-I or upper-I and not to superego] In freudian psychoanalytical theory, the portion of the personality associated with ethics, self-criticism, and the moral standard of the community. It is formed in infancy by the individual's adopting as his or her personal standards the values of the significant persons with whom he or she identifies. This helps to form the conscience. The superego functions to protect and to reward when the ego-ideal of behavior or thought is satisfied; and to criticize, punish, and evoke a sense of guilt when the reverse is true. In neuroses, symptoms develop when instinctual drives conflict with those dictated by the superego. SEE: *ego*.

**superexcitation** (soo″pĕr-ĕk″sī-tā′shŭn) [″ + *excitatio,* excitation] Excess excitement.

**superextension** (soo″pĕr-ĕks-tĕn′shŭn) [″ + *extensio,* extension] Excess extension.

**superfamily** (soo″pĕr-făm′ĭ-lē) In taxonomy, the category between an order and a family.

**superfecundation** (soo″pĕr-fē″kŭn-dā′shŭn) [″ + *fecundare,* to fertilize] Successive fertilization by two or more separate instances of sexual intercourse of two or more ova formed during the same menstrual cycle. Fertilization may be by the same male or by two different males.

**superfemale** A female having three X chromosomes.

**superfetation** (soo″pĕr-fē-tā′shŭn) [″ + *fetus,* fetus] The fertilization of two ova in the same uterus at different menstrual periods within a short interval.

**superficial** (soo″pĕr-fĭsh′ăl) [L. *superficialis*] **1.** Pert. to or situated near the surface. **2.** Not thorough; cursory.

**superficialis** (soo″pĕr-fĭsh-ē-ā′lĭs) [L.] Noting a structure such as an artery, vein, or nerve that is near the surface. SYN: *superficial* (1).

**superficies** (soo″pĕr-fĭsh′ē-ēz) [L.] An outer surface.

**superflexion** (soo″pĕr-flĕk′shŭn) [L. *super,* over, above, + *flexio,* flexion] Excess flexion.

**supergenual** (soo″pĕr-jĕn′ū-ăl) [″ + *genu,* knee] Above the knee.

**superglue** An extremely strong adhesive made of cyanoacrylate.

---

Caution: This glue is quite effective in gluing skin to skin. Thus, one should avoid contact with it, esp. on the eyelids.

---

**superinduce** (soo″pĕr-ĭn-dūs′) [″ + *in,* into, + *ducere,* to lead] To bring on, over, or above an already existing condition or situation.

**superinfection** (soo″pĕr-ĭn-fĕk′shŭn) [″ + *infectio,* a putting into] A new infection caused by an organism different from that which caused the initial infection. The microbe responsible is usually resistant to the treatment given for the initial infection.

**superinvolution** (soo″pĕr-ĭn-vō-lū′shŭn) [″ + *involutus,* a turning] Hyperinvolution.

**superior** (soo-pē′rē-or) [L. *superus,* upper] **1.** Higher than; situated above something else. **2.** Better than. **3.** One in charge of others.

**superiority complex** An exaggerated conviction of one's own superiority; a pretense of superiority in order to compensate for one's feeling of inferiority.

**superior vena cava syndrome** A partial occlusion of the superior vena cava with resulting interference of venous blood flow from the head and neck to the heart. This is usually due to some form of cancer. It is marked by venous engorgement and edema of the head and neck.

**superjacent** (soo″pĕr-jā′sĕnt) Immediately above.

**supermedial** (soo″pĕr-mē′dē-ăl) [″ + *medium,* middle] Above the middle.

**supermotility** (soo″pĕr-mō-tĭl′ĭ-tē) [″ + *motilis,* moving] Excessive motility in any part. SYN: *hyperkinesia.*

**supernatant** (soo″pĕr-nā′tănt) [″ + *natare,* to float] **1.** Floating on a surface, as oil on water. **2.** The clear liquid remaining at the top after a precipitate settles. **3.** The cell-derived fluids containing chemical mediators that develop in a laboratory culture of leukocytes mixed with an antigen or mitogen stimulus. Supernatants can be assessed for the presence of monokines or lymphokines by adding them to other white blood cell cultures and measuring cell proliferation and activity.

**supernate** (soo′pĕr-nāt) A supernatant fluid.

**supernumerary** (soo″pĕr-nū′mĕr-ăr″ē) [L. *supernumerarius*] Exceeding the regular number.

**supernumerary teeth** More than the usual number of teeth. Extra teeth develop in approx. 2% of the population, with almost all of them being maxillary incisors or mesiodens. A cleft palate or other developmental disturbances disrupt the dental lamina and often result in palatal supernumerary teeth.

**superolateral** (soo″pĕr-ō-lăt′ĕr-ăl) [″ + *latus,* side] Above and to the side.

**superovulation** (soo″pĕr-ŏv″ū-lā′shŭn) [″ + *ovulum,* little egg] An increased frequency of ovulation or production of a greater number of ova at one time. This is usually caused by the administration of gonadotropins.

**superoxide** A highly reactive form of oxygen. Superoxide is produced during the normal catalytic function of certain enzymes, by the oxidation of hemoglobin to methemoglobin, and when ionizing radiation passes through water. It is also produced when granulocytes phagocytize bacteria. Superoxide is destroyed by the enzyme superoxide dismutase, which catalyzes the conversion of two molecules of superoxide anion to one molecule of oxygen and one of hydrogen peroxide.

**superoxide dismutase** An enzyme that destroys superoxide. One form of the enzyme contains manganese and another contains copper and zinc.

**superparasite** (soo″pĕr-păr′ă-sīt) [″ + Gr. *para,* beside, + *sitos,* food] **1.** A parasite that lives upon another parasite. **2.** A parasite involved in superparasitism.

**superparasitism** (soo″pĕr-păr′ă-sī″tĭzm) [″ + ″ + *-ismos,* condition] A condition in which the host is infested or infected with a greater number of parasites than can be supported.

**superphosphate** (soo″pĕr-fŏs′fāt) Acid phosphate.

**supersaturate** To add more of a substance to a solution than can be dissolved permanently.

**superscription** (soo″pĕr-skrĭp′shŭn) [L. *super,* over, above, + *scriptio,* a writing] The beginning of a prescription noted by the sign ℞, signifying (L.) *recipe,* take.

**supersensitive** (soo″pĕr-sĕn′sĭ-tĭv) [″+ *sensitivus,* feeling] Hypersensitive.

**supersoft** (soo″pĕr-sŏft′) [″ + AS. *softe,* soft] Exceptionally soft; noting roentgen rays of extremely long wavelength and low penetrating power.

**supersonic** (soo″pĕr-sŏn′ĭk) [″ + *sonus,* sound] **1.** Ultrasonic. **2.** Used to describe speeds greater than that of sound. At sea level, in air at 0°C, the speed of sound is about 331 m, or 1087 ft per second (741 mph).

**superstructure** (soo″pĕr-strŭk′chŭr) The visible portion of a structure, esp. those parts external to the main structure.

**supervenosity** (soo″pĕr-vē-nŏs′ĭ-tē) Abnormally decreased oxygen in the venous blood.

**supervention** (soo″pĕr-vĕn′shŭn) [L. *superventio,* a coming over] The development of an additional condition as a complication to an existing disease.

**supervirulent** (soo″pĕr-vĭr′ū-lĕnt) [L. *super,* over, above, + *virulentus,* full of poison] More virulent than usual.

**supervisor** (soo′pĕr-vīz″ĕr) [L. *supervisus,* having looked over] One who directs and evaluates the performance of others. In a health care setting, the supervisor has the knowledge and skills to provide the same service as those being directed (e.g., the supervisor of the pharmacy, physical therapy, or maternity nursing).

**supervitaminosis** Hypervitaminosis.

**supervoltage** (soo′pĕr-vŏl″tĭj) A term applied to x-rays produced by very high voltage.

**supinate** (sū′pĭ-nāt) [L. *supinatus,* bent backward] **1.** To turn the forearm or hand so that the palm faces upward. **2.** To rotate the foot and leg outward.

**supination** (sū″pĭn-ā′shŭn) [L. *supinatio*] **1.** The turning of the palm or the hand anteriorly or the foot inward and upward. **2.** The act of lying flat upon the back. **3.** The condition of being on the back or having the palm of the hand facing upward or the foot turned inward and upward.

**supinator** (sū″pĭn-ā′tor) [L.] A muscle producing the motion of supination of the forearm. SEE: *Muscles Appendix.*

**supine** (sū-pīn′) [L. *supinus,* lying on the back] **1.** Lying on the back with the face upward. **2.** A position of the hand or foot with the palm or foot facing upward; the opposite of prone.

**supplemental** (sŭp″lĕ-mĕn′tăl) [L. *supplementum,* an addition] Referring to something added to supply a need or to reinforce.

**supplemental air** The air that by the most forcible effort can be expelled after an ordinary expiration that has followed a normal inspiration. In men, it averages about 1500 cc. SYN: *reserve air.*

**support** (sŭp-port′) **1.** That which assists in maintaining something in place. **2.** In dentistry, the abutting teeth, alveolar ridge, and mucosal tissues upon which the denture rests.

***s. groups*** Groups of persons with similar concerns who meet to discuss what is known about their problems or disease. The composition and focus of support groups varies. Some groups may be comprised of patients who are experiencing or have experienced the same disorder; such groups may include family members. Discussions often center on current treatments, resources available for assistance, and what individuals can do to improve and maintain their health or adjust to their illness, handicap, or life situation. Other groups may involve those who have experienced the same psychological and emotional trauma, such as rape victims or persons who have lost a loved one. Benefits expressed by members include the knowledge that they are not alone but that others have experienced the same or similar problems and that they have learned to cope effectively.

***s. hose*** Elastic stockings that may extend from the toes to the knee or above. These are worn by bedridden patients to provide sufficient pressure on the tissues to facilitate venous return and to help to prevent the formation of thrombi in the veins of the legs.

***social s.*** Help given by others to provide feedback, satisfy needs, and validate one's experience. A large body of research suggests that the loss of social support is a factor in the etiology of both physical and psychological disease. Nursing practice uses social supports such as tangible materials, teaching, and intimate interactions to restore, promote, and care for patients.

**suppository** (sŭ-pŏz′ĭ-tō-rē) *pl.* **suppositories** [L. *suppositorium,* something placed underneath] A semisolid substance for introduction into the rectum, vagina, or urethra, where it dissolves. It often serves as a vehicle for medicines to be absorbed. It is commonly shaped like a cylinder or cone and may be made of soap, glycerinated gelatin, or cocoa butter (oil of theobroma).

NURSING IMPLICATIONS: Privacy is provided. The nurse instructs the patient to retain the suppository for about 20 min for effectiveness and positions the patient appropriately. The suppository is lubricated and inserted into the appropriate orifice. For neurological rehabilitation, a rectal suppository may be used by the patient after instruction in bowel management. The nurse checks with the patient about effectiveness and notes in chart.

**suppression** (sŭ-prĕsh′ŭn) [L. *suppressio,* a pressing under] **1.** The repression of the external manifestation of a morbid condition. **2.** The complete failure of the natural production of a secretion or excretion, as distinguished from retention, in which normal secretion occurs but the discharge is retained within the organ or body. **3.** In psychoanalysis, the freudian ego defense mechanism of conscious inhibition of an idea or desire, as distinguished from repression, which is considered an unconscious process.

***active immune s.*** The use of agents to block an antigen-specific immune response. An example is the administration of anti-Rh antibodies ($Rh_o$ immune globulin) to Rh-negative mothers during the 28th week of pregnancy to prevent the formation of maternal antibodies that cause erythroblastosis fetalis in the Rh-positive newborn.

**suppression of menses** **1.** Amenorrhea in which menstruation ceases after once being established and from some cause other than hysterectomy, pregnancy, or menopause. **2.** Any suppression of the menses.

**suppressor T cells** A subpopulation of T lymphocytes that slows and stops the specific immune response.

**suppurant** (sŭp′ū-rănt) [L. *suppurans*] **1.** Producing, tending to produce, or marked by pus formation. **2.** An agent causing pus formation. SYN: *suppurative.*

**suppurate** (sŭp′ū-rāt) [L. *suppurare*] To form or generate pus.

**suppuration** (sŭp-ū-rā′shŭn) [L. *suppuratio*] **1.** The process of pus formation. SYN: *pyogenesis.* **2.** The discharge produced by suppuration. SYN: *purulence; pus.*

Inflammation can be caused by the presence of certain microorganisms called pyogenic (pus-forming) bacteria. Suppuration does not always develop even though microorganisms are present in the affected part, as may be the case in erysipelas and acute joint affections where exudate is serous. Liquefaction of tissues and formation of pus will continue while the microorganisms are alive. They cause the death of the leukocytes (white cells) and the cells of the part, liquefying the tissue so that the area becomes filled with a liquid containing the dead and dying cells, which is called pus. An abscess may form because of the accumulation of this liquid. The abscess is indicated by redness, swelling, heat, and pain. It will show fluctuation, which may be felt by palpating it with two fingers. When the abscess reaches the surface, it will burst and discharge its contents. In most cases, it is advisable to incise the abscess surgically rather than to wait for it to burst spontaneously.

**suppurative** (sŭp′ū-rā″tĭv, -ră-tĭv) [L. *suppuratus*] **1.** Producing or associated with generation of pus. **2.** An agent producing pus formation. SYN: *suppurant.*

**supra-** [L.] Combining form meaning *above, beyond, or on the top side.*

**supra-acromial** (soo″pră-ă-krō′mē-ăl) [L. *supra,* above, on top, beyond, + Gr. *akron,* extremity, + *omos,* shoulder] Located above the acromion.

**supra-anal** (soo-pră-ā′năl) [″ + *analis,* anal] Located above the anus.

**supra-auricular** (soo″pră-ŏ-rĭk′ū-lăr) [″ + *auricula,* little ear] Located above the auricle.

**supra-axillary** (soo″pră-ăk′sĭ-lĕr″ē) [″ + *axilla,* underarm] Located above the axilla.

**suprabuccal** (soo″pră-bŭk′ăl) [″ + *bucca,* cheek] Located above the buccal area.

**suprabulge** (soo′pră-bŭlj) The part of the crown of a tooth that curves toward the occlusal surface.

**supracerebellar** (soo″pră-sĕr″ĕ-bĕl′ăr) [″ + *cerebellum,* little brain] Located on or above the upper surface of the cerebellum.

**suprachoroid** (soo″pră-kō′royd) [″ + Gr. *chorioeides,* skinlike] Situated on or above the choroid layer of the eyeball.

**suprachoroidea** (soo″pră-kō-roy′dē-ă) Suprachoroid lamina.

**suprachoroid lamina** The superficial layer of the choroid consisting of thin transparent layers, the outermost adhering to the sclera. SYN: *lamina suprachoroidea; suprachoroidea.*

**supraciliary** (soo″pră-sĭl′ē-ĕr″ē) [L. *supra,* above, on top, beyond, + *cilia,* eyelid] Superciliary.

**supraclavicular** (soo″pră-klă-vĭk′ū-lar) [″ + *clavicula,* little key] Located above the clavicle.

**supraclavicular fossa** A depression on either side of the neck extending down behind the clavicle.

**supraclavicular point** A stimulation point over the clavicle at which contraction of the arm muscles may be produced.

**supracondylar** (soo″pră-kŏn′dĭ-lăr) [″ + Gr. *kondylos,* knuckle] Above a condyle.

**supracostal** (soo″pră-kŏs′tăl) [″ + *costa,* rib] Above the ribs.

**supracotyloid** (soo″pră-kŏt′ĭ-loyd) [″ + Gr. *kotyloeides,* cup-shaped] Above the acetabulum.

**supradiaphragmatic** (soo″pră-dī″ă-frăg-măt′ĭk) [″ + Gr. *dia,* across, + *phragma,* wall] Above the diaphragm.

**supraduction** (soo″pră-dŭk′shŭn) [″ + *ducere,* to lead] Turning upward of the eye.

**supraepicondylar** (soo″pră-ĕp″ĭ-kŏn′dĭ-lăr) [″ + Gr. *epi,* upon, + *kondylos,* condyle] Located above an epicondyle.

**supragingival** Above the gingiva; used in reference to the location of dental restorations, bacterial plaque, or calculus on the tooth. It is often contrasted with subgingival, the gingival margin being the reference point.

**supraglenoid** (soo″pră-glē′noyd) [″ + Gr. *glene,* socket, + *eidos,* form, shape] Above the glenoid cavity or fossa.

**supraglenoid tuberosity** A rough surface of the scapula above the glenoid cavity to which is attached the long head of the biceps muscle.

**supraglottic** (soo″pră-glŏt′ĭk) Located above the glottis.

**supraglottitis** An inflammation of the epiglottis.

**suprahepatic** (soo″pră-hē-păt′ĭk) [″ + Gr. *hepar,* liver] Located above the liver.

**suprahyoid** (soo″pră-hī′oyd) [″ + *hyoeides,* U-shaped] Located above the hyoid bone; denoting accessory thyroid glands within the geniohyoid muscle.

**suprahyoid muscles** The digastric, geniohyoid, mylohyoid, and stylohyoid muscles.

**suprainguinal** (soo″pră-ĭn′gwĭn-ăl) [″ + *inguinalis,* pert. to the groin] Above the groin.

**supraintestinal** (soo″pră-ĭn-tĕs′tĭ-năl) [″ + *intestinum,* intestine] Overlying the intestine.

**supraliminal** (soo″pră-lĭm′ĭ-năl) [L. *supra,* above, on top, beyond, + *limen,* threshold] **1.** Above the threshold of consciousness; conscious. **2.** Exceeding the stimulus threshold. SEE: *subliminal.*

**supralumbar** (soo″pră-lŭm′băr) [″ + *lumbus,* loin] Located above the lumbar region.

**supramalleolar** (soo″pră-mă-lē′ō-lăr) [″ + *malleolus,* little hammer] Located above either malleolus.

**supramammary** (soo″pră-măm′ă-rē) [″ + *mamma,* breast] Located above the breast.

**supramandibular** (soo″pră-măn-dĭb′ū-lăr) [″ + *mandibula,* lower jawbone] Located above the mandible.

**supramarginal** (soo″pră-măr′jĭn-ăl) [″ + *marginalis,* border] Located bove any border.

**supramarginal convolution** A cerebral convolution on the lateral surface of the parietal lobe above the posterior part of the sylvian fissure.

**supramastoid** (soo″pră-măs′toyd) [″ + *mastos,* breast, + *eidos,* form, shape] Located above the mastoid process of the temporal bone.

**supramastoid crest** A ridge on the superior edge of the posterior root of the zygomatic bone. SYN: *temporal line.*

**supramaxillary** (soo″pră-măk′sĭ-lĕr-ē) **1.** Rel. to the upper jaw. **2.** Located above the upper jaw.

**suprameatal** (soo″pră-mē-ā′tăl) [″ + *meatus,* passage] Above a meatus, esp. the exterior auditory meatus, noting the spine of Henle, a small bony projection at the posterosuperior margin of the external auditory meatus.

**suprameatal triangle** The triangular space bordered by the posterior wall of the external auditory meatus and the posterior root of the zygomatic process of the temporal bone.

**supramental** (soo″pră-mĕn′tăl) [L. *supra,* above, on top, beyond, + *mentum,* chin] Located above the chin.

**supranasal** (soo″pră-nā′zăl) [″ + *nasus,* nose] Located above the nose.

**supranuclear** (soo″pră-nū′klē-lăr) [″ + *nucleus,* little kernel] Concerning nerve fibers located above a nucleus in the brain.

**supraoccipital** (soo″pră-ŏk-sĭp′ĭ-tăl) [″ + *occiput,* back of head] Lying above or in the upper portion of the occiput.

**supraocclusion** (soo″pră-ŏ-kloo′zhŭn) [″ + *occlusio,* occlusion] The condition of teeth that are beyond the occlusal plane.

**supraorbital** (soo″pră-or′bĭ-tăl) [″ + *orbita,* track] Located above the orbit.

**supraorbital neuralgia** Neuralgia of the supraorbital nerve. SYN: *hemicrania* (1).

**supraorbital notch** A notch in the superior margin of the orbital arch for transmitting supraorbital vessels and nerve.

**suprapatellar** (soo″pră-pă-tĕl′ăr) [″ + *patella,* a small pan] Located above the patella.

**suprapelvic** (soo″pră-pĕl′vĭk) [″ + *pelvis,* basin] Located above the pelvis.

**suprapontine** (soo″pră-pŏn′tīn) [″ + *pons,* bridge] Located above the pons varolii.

**suprapubic** (soo″pră-pū′bĭk) [″ + NL. *(os) pubis,* bone of the groin] Located above the pubic arch.

**suprapubic aspiration of urine** A procedure for draining the bladder when it is not possible to use a urethral catheter. The skin over the lower abdominal area is cleansed. An incision in the abdominal wall is made with a needle or trocar to gain access to the bladder. To prevent complications during the procedure, it is important to observe the following guidelines: The patient should be positioned in the marked Trendelenburg position. The bladder should be distended with 400 ml of fluid. Any previous abdominal wall incisions that may have left the bladder or bowel adherent to the scar tissue should be noted. The incision should be no more than 3 cm above the pubic symphysis. The trocar should be inserted 30 degrees toward the bladder, that is, away from the pubic symphysis (if in doubt, a small gauge needle should be inserted for orientation); the trocar should not be placed in a vertical direction. The depth of trocar insertion should be monitored, using gentle pressure on the trocar to prevent damage to the bladder base.

Caution: The needle may pierce a loop of bowel that is lying over the anterior surface of the bladder.

**suprapubic catheter** A catheter inserted through a suprapubic incision into the bladder to drain urine; generally used when unable to insert through the urethra due to obstruction or there is a need to allow the urethra and bladder sphincter to heal. SEE: *suprapubic aspiration of urine.*

NURSING IMPLICATIONS: The nurse observes for hemorrhage or prolonged hematuria and signs of local or systemic infection. Aseptic technique is used during dressing or equipment changes. Bladder irrigation is performed as prescribed. Medications such as analgesics, antispasmodics, and bowel stimulants are administered as prescribed. The patient's ability to micturate is evaluated. Intake and output are monitored and recorded. Fluids are forced unless otherwise restricted to ensure passage of dilute urine.

**suprarenal** (soo″pră-rē′năl) [L. *supra,* above, on top, beyond, + *ren,* kidney] **1.** Located above the kidney. **2.** Pert. to the gland above each kidney. SEE: *adrenal gland.*

**suprarenalectomy** (soo″pră-rē″năl-ĕk′tō-mē) [″ + ″ + Gr. *ektome,* excision] Adrenalectomy.

**suprarenal gland** An endocrine gland lying adjacent to and in a superior and medial position to the kidney. SYN: *adrenal gland.* SEE: *ACTH; adrenalin; corticosterone; cortisone; endocrine gland; epinephrine; norepinephrine.*

**suprarenalopathy** (soo″pră-rē-năl-ŏp′ă-thē) [″ + ″ + Gr. *pathos,* disease, suffering] A disorder caused by abnormal functioning of the adrenal glands.

**suprascapular** (soo″pră-skăp′ū-lăr) [″ + *scapula,* shoulder blade] Located above the scapula.

**suprascleral** (soo″pră-sklē′răl) [″ + Gr. *skleros,* hard] Located on the surface of the sclera.

**suprasegmental** [″ + *segmentum,* segment] Located above the segmented portion.

**suprasegmental brain** The cerebrum, midbrain, and cerebellum as distinguished from the segmental portion (pons and medulla oblongata).

**suprasellar** (soo″pră-sĕl′ăr) [″ + *sella,* saddle] Located above or over the sella turcica.

**suprasonic, supersonic** (soo″pră-sŏn′ĭk) [″ + *sonus,* sound] Noting sound with frequencies of vibration above 20,000 cycles per second. SEE: *supersonic.*

**supraspinal** (soo″pră-spī′năl) [″ + *spina,* thorn] Located above a spine.

**supraspinous** Located above any spinous process.

**supraspinous fossa** A groove above the spine of the scapula.

**suprastapedial** (soo″pră-stă-pē′dē-ăl) [″ + *stapes,* stirrup] Located above the stapes of the inner ear.

**suprasternal** (soo″pră-stĕr′năl) [L. *supra,* above, on top, beyond, + Gr. *sternon,* chest] Located above the sternum. SYN: *episternal.*

**suprasylvian** (soo″pră-sĭl′vē-ăn) Located above the sylvian fissure of the brain.

**supratemporal** (soo″pră-tĕm′pō-răl) [″ + *temporalis,* temporal] Located above the temporal bone or fossa.

**supratentorial** (soo″pră-tĕn-tō′rē-ăl) Located above the tentorium.

**suprathoracic** (soo″pră-thō-răs′ĭk) [″ + Gr. *thorax,* chest] Located above the thorax.

**supratonsillar** (soo″pră-tŏn′sĭ-lăr) [″ + *tonsilla,* almond] Located above the tonsil.

**supratrochlear** (soo″pră-trŏk′lē-ăr) [″ + *trochlea,* pulley] Located above a trochlea, esp. that of the humerus.

**supratympanic** (soo″pră-tĭm-păn′ĭk) [″ + *tympanon,* drum] Located above the tympanic membrane of the ear.

**supravaginal** (soo″pră-văj′ĭ-năl) [″ + *vagina,* sheath] Located above the vagina or any sheathing membrane.

**supraventricular** (soo″pră-vĕn-trĭk′ū-lăr) [″ + *ventriculus,* a little belly] Located above the ventricle, esp. the heart ventricles.

**supravergence** (soo″pră-vĕr′jĕns) [″ + *vergere,* to be inclined] A condition in which one eye moves upward in the vertical plane while the other does not.

**supraversion** (soo″pră-vĕr′zhŭn) [″ + *versio,* a turning] **1.** A turning upward. **2.** In dentistry, a tooth out of occlusal line.

**sura** (sū′ră) [L.] The calf of the leg; the muscular posterior portion of the lower leg.

**sural** (sū′răl) Rel. to the calf of the leg.

**suramin sodium** (soo′ră-mĭn) A urea derivative used in treating African trypanosomiasis (sleeping sickness). It is available only from the Parasitic Disease Division of the Centers for Disease Control (CDC), Atlanta, Georgia 30333.

**surefooted** Being able to walk or run without stumbling or falling.

**surface** (sŭr′fĕs) [Fr. *sur,* above, + L. *facies,* face] **1.** The exterior boundary of an object. **2.** The external or internal exposed portions of a hollow structure, as the outer or inner surfaces of the cranium or stomach. **3.** The face or faces of a body such as a bone. **4.** The side of a tooth or the dental arch; usually named for the adjacent tissue or space. The outer or facial surface is called the labial surface of the incisors or canines, and the buccal surface of the premolars and molars. The facial surface may also be called the vestibular surface. The inner surface of each tooth is called the lingual or oral surface. Within the arch, each tooth is said to have a mesial surface, the side toward the midpoint in the front of the dental arch, and a distal surface, the side of the tooth farthest from the midpoint in the front of the dental arch. SEE: illus.

***body s.*** SEE: *body surface area.*

**surface tension** A condition at the surface of a liquid in contact with a gas or another liquid that causes its surface to act as a stretched rubber membrane. It results from the mutual attraction of the molecules to each other, thus producing a cohesive state that causes liquids to assume

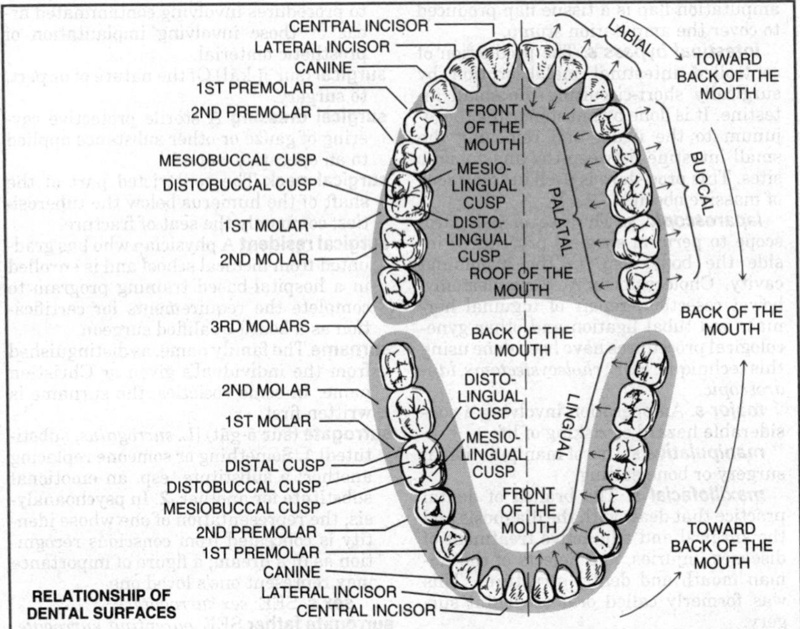

RELATIONSHIP OF DENTAL SURFACES

a shape presenting the smallest surface area to the surrounding medium. This accounts for the spherical shape assumed by fluids, such as drops of oil or water.

**surfactant** (sŭr-făk′tănt) A surface-active agent that lowers surface tension (e.g., oils and various forms of detergents). Artificial surfactants may be given endotracheally to relieve respiratory distress.

***modified natural s.*** A replacement phospholipid from a natural source with some components removed. Trade name is Survanta.

***pulmonary s.*** A substance in the lung that regulates the amount of surface tension of the fluid lining the alveoli. Synthetic lung surfactant is available for treating patients with respiratory distress syndrome. SYN: *lung surfactant.* SEE: *lecithin-sphingomyelin ratio.*

**surfer's ear** The growth of a bony area in the subcutaneous area of the ear owing to prolonged exposure to cold, as may occur in persons who participate in surfing.

**surfer's knots** A nodular swelling and possibly bone changes of the area of the lower leg and foot exposed to pressure and trauma while on a surfboard. Such nodules may be painful.

**surgeon** (sŭr′jŭn) [L. *chirurgia*] A medical practitioner who specializes in surgery.

**surgeon general** The chief medical officer in one of the armed forces of the U.S. or the U.S. Public Health Service.

**surgery** (sŭr′jĕr-ē) [L. *chirurgia*] **1.** The branch of medicine dealing with manual and operative procedures for correction of deformities and defects, repair of injuries, and diagnosis and cure of certain diseases. **2.** A surgeon's operating room. **3.** Treatment or work performed by a surgeon. SYN: *operation.* SEE: *Nursing Diagnoses Appendix.*

***ablative s.*** Operation in which a part is removed.

***ambulatory s.*** Surgery done between the time the patient is admitted in the morning and the time the patient is discharged the same day. Also called *day surgery.*

***aseptic s.*** An operative procedure carried on under aseptic conditions or in the absence of pathogenic organisms.

***aural s.*** Surgery of the ear.

***conservative s.*** Surgery in which as much as possible of a part or structure is retained. The opposite of radical surgery.

***cosmetic s.*** Surgery done to revise or change the texture, configuration, or relationship of contiguous structures of any feature of the human body that would be considered by the average observer to be within the broad range of normal and acceptable variation for age and ethnic origin. In addition, the procedure is performed for a condition that is judged by competent medical opinion to be without potential for jeopardy to physical or mental health. (Adapted from the official A.M.A. definition, 1974.) SEE: *plastic s.*

***exploratory s.*** An operation performed for diagnostic purposes.

***flap s.*** A surgical procedure in which a flap of tissue or periosteum is raised. An amputation flap is a tissue flap produced to cover the amputation stump.

***intestinal bypass s.*** The production of controlled intestinal malabsorption by surgically short-circuiting the small intestine. It is done by anastomosing the jejunum to the ileum and removing the small intestine between the anastomotic sites. This procedure is used in treatment of massive obesity.

***laparoscopic s.*** The use of a laparoscope to perform surgical procedures inside the body, esp. in the abdominal cavity. Cholecystectomy, appendectomy, bowel resection, repair of inguinal hernias, and tubal ligation and other gynecological procedures have been done using this technique. SEE: *cholecystectomy, laparoscopic.*

***major s.*** An operation involving a considerable hazard or risking of life.

***manipulative s.*** Use of manipulation in surgery or bone-setting.

***maxillofacial s.*** The branch of dental practice that deals with the diagnosis and the surgical and adjunctive treatment of diseases, injuries, and defects of the human mouth and dental structures. This was formerly called oral or dental surgery.

***minor s.*** A simple operation not considered to involve a risk to life.

***mucogingival s.*** A plastic surgical method for correcting disease conditions relating to the gingiva and adjacent mucosa of the mouth.

***open heart s.*** Surgery involving direct visualization of the exposed heart.

***oral s.*** Maxillofacial s.

***orthopedic s.*** Surgical prevention and correction of musculoskeletal deformities.

***plastic s.*** Surgery concerned with the repair or restoration of defective or missing structures, frequently involving the transference of tissue from a part or person to another part or person. SEE: *cosmetic s.; tissue expansion, soft.*

***radical s.*** An operation performed to remove a large amount of damaged or neoplastic tissue or adjoining areas of lymphatic drainage in an attempt to obtain complete cure. This is the opposite of conservative surgery.

***reconstructive s.*** An operation to repair a loss or defect.

***second-look s.*** Surgery some months or as much as a year after the original operation for cancer. The second look is to detect possible recurrences.

***subtotal s.*** An operation in which only a portion of the organ is removed, as subtotal removal of the thyroid gland.

**surgery, antimicrobial prophylaxis in** The use of antibiotics prior to and during a surgical procedure. Even though this may decrease the incidence of infection in certain procedures the benefit must be considered with respect to the potential side effects. This practice is more nearly suited to procedures involving contaminated areas or those involving implantation of prosthetic material.

**surgical** (sŭr'jĭ-kăl) Of the nature of or pert. to surgery.

**surgical dressing** A sterile protective covering of gauze or other substance applied to an operative wound.

**surgical neck** The constricted part of the shaft of the humerus below the tuberosities; commonly the seat of fracture.

**surgical resident** A physician who has graduated from medical school and is enrolled in a hospital-based training program to complete the requirements for certification as a board-qualified surgeon.

**surname** The family name, as distinguished from the individual's given or Christian name. In some societies, the surname is written first.

**surrogate** (sŭr'ō-gāt) [L. *surrogatus,* substituted] **1.** Something or someone replacing another; a substitute, esp. an emotional substitute for another. **2.** In psychoanalysis, the representation of one whose identity is concealed from conscious recognition as in a dream; a figure of importance may represent one's loved one.

***sex s.*** SEE: *sex surrogate.*

**surrogate father** SEE: *parenting, surrogate.*

**surrogate mother** SEE: under *mother.*

**sursumduction** (sŭr"sŭm-dŭk'shŭn) [L. *sursum,* upward, + *ducere,* to lead] Elevation, as the power or act of turning an eye upward independently of the other one.

**sursumvergence** (sŭr"sŭm-vĕr'jĕns) [" + *vergere,* to turn] An upward turning, as of the eyeballs.

**sursumversion** (sŭr"sŭm-vĕr'zhŭn) [" + *versio,* turning] The process of turning upward; simultaneous movement of both eyes upward.

**surveillance** (sŭr-vāl'ăns) The monitoring or controlling of something.

***immunological s.*** The idea that the body defenses recognize alien materials or malignant cells and destroy them when they appear.

**survey** The study of a particular disease or condition, esp. its epidemiological aspects.

**survival** Continuing to live, esp. under conditions in which death would be the expected outcome.

**survivor guilt** The feeling of guilt present in some persons who have survived an event in which others have lost their lives (e.g., a war, ship sinking, holocaust, or prison camp).

**susceptibility** (sŭs-sĕp"tĭ-bĭl'ĭ-tē) The state of being susceptible.

**susceptible** (sŭ-sĕp'tĭ-bl) [L. *susceptibilis,* capable of receiving] **1.** Having little resistance to a disease or foreign protein. **2.** Easily impressed or influenced.

**sushi** (soo'shē) A general term for a food made of raw fish, usually wrapped in a soft rice shell. Some raw fish contain adults or larvae of the nematodes of the family Anisakidae. In order to prevent these organisms from infecting persons who eat raw fish, the U.S. Food and Drug Administration has directed that prior to serving, the fish must be suddenly frozen to −31°F (−34.4°C) or below for 15 hr, or held in a commercial freezer at −4°F (−20°C) for 24 hr. After that period, the fish may be thawed and served. SEE: *anisakiasis*.

**suspended** (sŭs-pĕnd′ĕd) [L. *suspendere*, to hang up] **1.** Hanging. **2.** Temporarily inactive.

**suspension** (sŭs-pĕn′shŭn) [L. *suspensio*, a hanging] **1.** A condition of temporary cessation, as of any vital process. **2.** Treatment using a hanging support to immobilize a body part in a desired position. **3.** The state of a solid when its particles are mixed with, but not dissolved in, a fluid or another solid; also a substance in this state.

***cephalic s.*** The supported suspension of a patient by the head to extend the vertebral column.

***colloid s.*** A colloidal solution in which particles of the dispersed phase are relatively large. SYN: *suspensoid*.

***tendon s.*** Fixation of a tendon. SYN: *tenodesis*.

**suspensoid** (sŭs-pĕn′soyd) [″ + Gr. *eidos*, form, shape] Colloid suspension.

**suspensory** (sŭs-pĕn′sō-rē) [L. *suspensorius*, hanging] **1.** Supporting a part, as a muscle, ligament, or bone. **2.** A structure of the body that supports a part. **3.** A bandage or sac for supporting or compressing a part, esp. the scrotum.

**suspiration** (sŭs″pĭr-ā′shŭn) [L. *suspiratio*] A sigh or the act of sighing.

**suspirious** (sŭs-pī′rē-ŭs) [L. *suspirare*, to sigh] Breathing with apparent effort; sighing.

**sustentacular** (sŭs″tĕn-tăk′ū-lăr) [L. *sustentaculum*, support] Supporting; upholding.

**sustentacular cell** A supporting cell such as those found in the acoustic macula, organ of Corti, olfactory epithelium, taste buds, or testes. Those in the testes secrete the hormone inhibin and are also called *Sertoli cells*. SEE: *Sertoli cell*.

**sustentacular fibers of Müller** [Friedrich von Müller, Ger. physician, 1858–1941] Fibers forming the supporting framework of the retina.

**sustentaculum** (sŭs″tĕn-tăk′ū-lŭm) *pl.* **sustentacula** [L.] A supporting structure.

***s. hepatis*** A fold of peritoneum upon which rests the right margin of the liver.

***s. lienis*** The phrenocolic ligament that apparently supports the spleen.

***s. tali*** A process of the calcaneum that supports part of the astragalus or talus.

**sutilains** (soo′tĭ-lāns) Proteolytic enzymes derived from the bacterium *Bacillus subtilis*. Calculated on the dry basis, it contains not less than 2,500,000 USP casein units. It is used in ointment form to debride necrotic lesions.

Caution: This product should be kept away from the eyes.

**Sutton's disease** (sŭt′ŏnz) **1.** [Richard L. Sutton, Sr., U.S. dermatologist, 1878–1952] A halo nevus. **2.** [Richard L. Sutton, Jr., U.S. dermatologist, b. 1908] Granuloma fissuratum.

**Sutton's law** A law that indicates one should look for diseases where they are most likely to be (e.g., malaria in tropical areas that harbor *Anopheles* mosquitoes; atherosclerosis in patients who are middle-aged or older). Originally, it meant that a bank robber robs banks because "that is where the money is." A reporter coined the phrase "Sutton's law" and attributed it to Willie Sutton, a U.S. bank robber.

**sutura** (sū-tū′ră) *pl.* **suturae** [L., a seam] **1.** Suture (1). SEE: *synarthrosis*. **2.** Any kind of suture.

***s. dentata*** A sutura with interlocking of bony processes resembling the teeth of a saw.

***s. harmonia*** A simple apposition of two contiguous bones.

***s. limbosa*** A beveled suture in which opposing margins fit in parallel ridges as between the parietal and frontal bones.

***s. notha*** A false suture with ill-defined projections.

***s. serrata*** A suture with deeper and more irregular indentations than a dental suture.

***s. squamosa*** A suture formed by the overlapping of contiguous bones by broad beveled edges as in the suture between the squamous portion of the temporal and parietal bones.

***s. vera*** A true suture in which no movement of united bones can occur.

**sutural** (sū′tū-răl) [L. *sutura*, a seam] Rel. to a suture.

**sutural joint** An articulation between two bones.

**sutural ligament** Fibers that unite opposed bones forming a cranial suture.

**suturation** (sū″tū-rā′shŭn) The application of sutures; stitching.

**suture** (sū′chūr) [L. *sutura*, a seam] **1.** The line of union in an immovable articulation, as those between the skull bones; also such an articulation itself. SYN: *sutura*. SEE: *raphe; synarthrosis*. **2.** An operation in which soft tissues of the body are united by stitching them together. **3.** The thread, wire, or other material used to stitch parts of the body together. **4.** The seam or line of union formed by surgical stitches. **5.** To unite by stitching.

***absorbable surgical s.*** A sterile strand prepared from collagen derived from healthy mammals or from a synthetic polymer. This type of suture is absorbed and thus does not need to be removed.

***apposition s.*** The suture in the superficial layers of the skin in order to produce precise apposition of the edges.

***approximation s.*** A deep suture for joining the deep tissues of a wound.

***basilar s.*** The suture between the occipital bone and sphenoid bone that persists until the 16th to 18th year as the anteroposterior growth center of the base of the skull; also called *spheno-occipital synchondrosis*.

***bifrontal s.*** The suture between the frontal and parietal bones.

***biparietal s.*** The suture between the two parietal bones.

***buried s.*** A suture placed so that it is completely covered by skin.

***button s.*** A suture in which the threads are passed through buttons on the surface and tied to prevent the suture material from cutting into the skin. SEE: *quilled s.*

***catgut s.*** A suture material made from a portion of the small intestine of sheep. It can be sterilized. Eventually it is absorbed by body fluids.

***coaptation s.*** A superficial suture for cutaneous wounds.

***cobbler's s.*** A suture in which the thread has a needle at each end.

***continuous s.*** The closure of a wound by means of one continuous thread, usually by transfixing one edge of the wound and then the other alternately from within outward. SYN: *uninterrupted s.*

***coronal s.*** A suture between the frontal and parietal bones. SYN: *frontoparietal s.*

***cranial s.*** One of the sutures between the bones of the skull.

***dentate s.*** A suture consisting of long and toothlike processes.

***ethmoidofrontal s.*** A suture between the ethmoid and frontal bones.

***ethmoidolacrimal s.*** A suture between the ethmoid and lacrimal bones.

***ethmosphenoid s.*** A suture between the ethmoid and sphenoid bones.

***false s.*** Any form of suture in which one surface is smooth.

***figure-of-eight s.*** A suture shaped like the figure eight.

***frontal s.*** An occasional suture in the frontal bone from the sagittal suture to the root of the nose. SYN: *mediofrontal s.; metopic s.*

***frontolacrimal s.*** A suture between the frontal and lacrimal bones.

***frontomalar s.*** A suture between the frontal and malar bones.

***frontomaxillary s.*** Suture between the frontal bone and superior maxilla.

***frontonasal s.*** A suture between the frontal bone and the alae of the sphenoid bone.

***frontoparietal s.*** Coronal s.

***frontotemporal s.*** A suture between the frontal and temporal bones.

***glover's s.*** A continuous suture in which the needle is passed through the loop of the preceding stitch.

***harmonic s.*** A suture in which there is simple apposition of bone.

***implanted s.*** A suture formed by placing pins opposite each other on the two sides of a wound, and approximating the lips of the wound by winding thread or other similar material about the pins.

***intermaxillary s.*** A suture between the superior maxillae.

***internasal s.*** A suture between the nasal bones.

***interparietal s.*** Sagittal s.

***interrupted s.*** A suture formed by single stitches inserted separately, the needle usually being passed through one lip of the wound from without inward and through the other from within outward.

***lambdoid s.*** A suture between the parietal bones and the two superior borders of the occipital bone. SYN: *occipital s.; occipitoparietal s.*

***longitudinal s.*** Sagittal s.

***maxillolacrimal s.*** A suture between the maxilla and lacrimal bone.

***mediofrontal s.*** Frontal s.

***metopic s.*** Frontal s.

***nasomaxillary s.*** A suture between the nasal bone and superior maxilla.

***nonabsorbable s.*** A suture made from a material that is not absorbed by the body, such as silk, silkworm gut, horsehair, certain synthetic materials, or wire.

***nonabsorbable surgical s.*** A sterile or nonsterile strand of material that is suitably resistant to the action of living mammalian fluids and tissue. This suture should be used only in those applications in which it may eventually be removed or its staying in the tissues will cause no harm.

***occipital s.*** Lambdoid s.

***occipitomastoid s.*** A suture between the occipital bone and the mastoid portion of the temporal bone. SYN: *temporo-occipital s.*

***occipitoparietal s.*** Lambdoid s.

***palatine s.*** A suture between the palatine bones.

***palatine transverse s.*** A suture between the palatine processes and superior maxilla.

***parietal s.*** Sagittal s.

***parietomastoid s.*** A suture between the parietal bone and the mastoid portion of the temporal bone.

***petro-occipital s.*** A suture between the petrous portion of the temporal bone and the occipital bone.

***petrosphenoidal s.*** A suture between the petrous portion of the temporal bone and the ala magna of the sphenoid bone.

***purse-string s.*** A suture entering and exiting around the periphery of a circular opening. Drawing the suture taut closes the opening.

***quilled s.*** An interrupted suture in which a double thread is passed deep into the tissues below the bottom of the wound, the needle being so withdrawn as to leave a loop hanging from one lip of the wound and the two free ends of the thread from the other. A quill, or more commonly a piece of bougie, is passed through the loops, which are tightened upon it, and the free ends of each separate thread are tied together over a second quill. The purpose of a quilled suture is prevention of tearing when tension becomes greater. SEE: *button s.*

***relaxation s.*** A suture that may be loosened to relieve excessive tension.

***relief s.*** A row of supplementary sutures including the tissues to the extent of 1 to 1½ in. (2.5 to 3.8 cm) on each side of a fistula or a deep wound, for the purpose of lessening the strain on the coaptation sutures.

***right-angled s.*** A suture used in sewing intestine. The needle is passed in the same direction as the long axis of the incision, and the process is repeated on the opposite side of the incision, the suture being continuous.

***sagittal s.*** A suture between the two parietal bones. SYN: *interparietal s.; longitudinal s.; parietal s.*

***serrated s.*** An articulation by suture in which there is an interlocking of bones by small, fine, and delicate projections and indentations.

***shotted s.*** A suture in which both ends of a wire or silkworm gut are passed through a perforated shot that is then compressed tightly over them.

***silk s.*** A suture made of silk. It may be twisted, braided, or floss.

***silkworm gut s.*** A suture that causes little friction, is pliable, does not curl or twist, and is less liable to produce irritation.

***sphenoparietal s.*** The suture between the parietal bone and the ala magna of the sphenoid bone.

***sphenosquamous s.*** An articulation of the great wing of the sphenoid with the squamous portion of the temporal bone.

***sphenotemporal s.*** A suture between the sphenoid and temporal bones.

***squamoparietal s.*** A suture between the parietal and squamous portions of the temporal bone.

***squamosphenoidal s.*** A suture between the squamous portion of the temporal bone and great wing of the sphenoid bone.

***squamous s.*** A suture between flat overlapping bones.

***subcuticular s.*** A buried continuous suture in which the needle is passed horizontally under the epidermis into the cutis vera, emerging at the edge of the wound but beneath the skin, then in a similar manner passed through the cutis vera of the opposite side of the wound, and so on until the other angle of the wound is reached.

***temporo-occipital s.*** Occipitomastoid s.

***temporoparietal s.*** The suture between the temporal and parietal bones.

***twisted s.*** A suture in which pins are passed through the opposite lips of a wound and material is wound about the pins, crossing them first at one end and then at the other in a figure-of-eight fashion, thus holding the lips of the wound firmly together.

***uninterrupted s.*** Continuous s.

***vertical mattress s.*** An interrupted suture in which a deep stitch is taken and the needle inserted upon the same side as that from which it emerged, and passed back through both lips of the wound. The suture is then tied to the free end on the side the needle originally entered. This suture is particularly useful in holding together thick fragile tissues.

***wire s.*** A suture adapted for cases in which there is tension or resection, or for uniting ends of bones. Usually stainless steel or silver wire is used.

**suxamethonium chloride** (sŭk″să-mĕ-thō′nē-ŭm) Succinylcholine chloride.

**Sv** *sievert.*

**SvO$_2$** *venous oxygen saturation.*

**SV 40 virus** Simian virus 40, which is a member of the papovavirus family. The virus produces sarcomas after subcutaneous inoculation into newborn hamsters.

**swab** (swăb) [Dutch *swabbe,* mop] **1.** Cotton or gauze on the end of a slender stick, used for cleansing cavities, applying remedies, or for obtaining a piece of tissue or secretion for bacteriological examination. **2.** To wipe with a swab.

***test tube s.*** A swab for cleansing tubes.

***urethral s.*** A slender rod for holding cotton used in examinations with the speculum, in treating ulcers, or removing secretions. The male urethral swab is a rod about 7 in. (17.8 cm) long.

***uterine s.*** A slender flattened wire, or a plain rod or one with coarse thread on the distal end for absorbing or wiping away discharges.

**swage** (swāj) **1.** To shape metal, esp. around something in order to make a close fit. **2.** Fusing a suture to a needle.

**swager** A dental tool or device used to shape silver amalgam or gold by applying pressure from different directions simultaneously.

**swallow** (swăl′ō) [AS. *swelgan*] To cause or enable the passage of something from the mouth through the throat and esophagus into the stomach by muscular action. SYN: *deglutition.*

**swallowed blood syndrome** SEE: *APT test.*

**swallowing** (swăl′ō-ĭng) A complicated act, usually initiated voluntarily but always completed reflexively, whereby food is moved from the mouth through the pharynx and esophagus to the stomach. It occurs in the following three stages. SYN: *deglutition.*

In the *first stage,* food is placed on the surface of the tongue. The tip of the tongue is placed against the hard palate; then elevation of the larynx and backward movement of the tongue forces food through the isthmus of the fauces in the pharynx.

In the *second stage,* the food passes through the pharynx. This involves constriction of the walls of the pharynx, backward bending of the epiglottis, and an upward and forward movement of the larynx and trachea. This may be observed externally with the bobbing of the Adam's apple. Food is kept from entering the nasal cavity by elevation of the soft palate and from entering the larynx by closure of the glottis and backward inclination of the epiglottis. During this stage, respiratory movements are inhibited by reflex.

In the *third stage,* food moves down the esophagus and into the stomach. This movement is accomplished by momentum from the second stage, peristaltic contractions, and gravity. With the body in upright position, liquids pass rapidly and do not require assistance from the esophagus. However, second-stage momentum and peristaltic contractions are sufficient to allow liquids to be drunk even when the head is lower than the stomach.

Difficulty in swallowing is called dysphagia. It may be caused by congenital defects such as cleft palate or esophageal obstruction; neural and psychogenic disturbances; muscular dysfunction; or local conditions such as presence of tumors, abscesses, and inflammation.

***air s.*** Introduction of air into the stomach or intestines while eating, drinking, chewing gum, or smoking. May be habitual on the part of the patient or brought on by hysteria. SYN: *aerophagia.*

***impaired s.*** The state in which an individual has decreased ability to voluntarily pass fluids and/or solids from the mouth to the stomach. SEE: *Nursing Diagnoses Appendix.*

***tongue s.*** A condition in which the tongue tends to fall backward and obstruct the openings to the larynx and esophagus. The tongue is not swallowed and the term is inaccurate; nevertheless, it is commonly used. The condition is due to excessive flaccidity of the tongue during unconsciousness. Control of this requires forceful elevation of the chin and extension of the head during artificial respiration in order to help provide an airway. The tongue may also be pulled forward to clear the airway.

**swallow's nest** Cerebral depression between the uvula and the posterior velum. SYN: *nidus hirundinis.*

**Swan-Ganz catheter** [Harold James Swan, U.S. physician, b. 1922; Willian Ganz, U.S. physician, b. 1919] A soft, flexible catheter that contains a balloon near its tip. The sterile catheter is passed through the vein to the right heart, being carried along by the blood returning to the heart. The balloon then helps, without the use of fluoroscopy, to guide the catheter to the pulmonary artery. Once in the pulmonary artery, the balloon is inflated sufficiently to block the flow of blood from the right heart to the lung. This allows the back pressure in the pulmonary artery distal to the balloon to be recorded. This pressure reflects the pressure transmitted back from the left atrial chamber of the heart.

A catheter similar to the Swan-Ganz was originally developed in 1953 and used in dogs by the U.S. physiologists Michael Lategola and Hermann Rahn.

**swan-neck deformity** A finger deformity frequently seen in rheumatoid arthritis marked by flexion of the distal interphalangeal joints and hyperextension of the proximal interphalangeal joints owing to hypermobility in the proximal interphalangeal joint and slipping of the link ligament posteriorly. The interossei muscles may become tight as a result of the position.

**swarming** (sworm'ĭng) The spread of bacteria over a culture medium.

**sway-back** (swā'băk) A faulty, slouched posture in which the pelvis is shifted forward and the thorax posteriorly. Lordosis occurs in the lower lumbar spinal region; a compensating reversal to kyphosis occurs in the upper lumbar and thoracic regions.

**sway, postural** Forward and backward movement of the body with motion occurring around the ankle joints when the feet are fixed on the floor. Backward sway is controlled by the anterior tibialis, quadriceps, and abdominal muscles; forward sway is controlled by the gastrocnemius, hamstring, and paraspinal muscles.

**sweat** (swĕt) [AS. *sweatan*] **1.** The secretion of the sudoriferous glands of the skin. SYN: *perspiration; sudor.* SEE: *glands, Moll's.* **2.** The condition of perspiring or of being made to perspire freely, as to order a sweat for a patient. **3.** To emit moisture through the skin's pores. SYN: *perspire.* **4.** To cause to emit moisture through the pores.

Perspiration is a colorless, slightly turbid, salty, aqueous fluid, although that from the sweat glands in the axillae, around the anus, and of the ceruminous glands has an oily consistency. It contains urea, fatty substances, and sodium chloride. This salty, watery fluid is difficult to collect without contamination with sebum. Perspiration is controlled by the sympathetic nervous system through true secretory fibers supplying sweat glands.

Ingestion of spicy foods such as those flavored with chili peppers may cause sweating. Capsaicin, a chemical in chili that activates nerve endings in the mouth and tongue, causes sweating of the face. SEE: *perspiration, insensible; perspiration, sensible.*

FUNCTION: Sweat cools the body by evaporation and rids it of what waste may be expressed through the pores of the skin. The daily amount is about a liter;

this figure is subject to extreme variation according to physical activity and atmospheric conditions, and in hot conditions may be as much as 10 to 15 L in 24 hr.

***bloody s.*** Hemathidrosis.

***colliquative s.*** Profuse, clammy sweat.

***colored s.*** Chromidrosis.

***fetid s.*** Bromidrosis.

***night s.*** Sweating during the night; it may be a symptom of pulmonary tuberculosis or sleep apnea.

***profuse s.*** Hyperhidrosis.

***scanty s.*** Anhidrosis.

**sweat center** One of the principal centers controlling perspiration located in the hypothalamus; secondary centers are present in the spinal cord.

**sweat gland** A simple, coiled, tubular gland found on all body surfaces except the margin of the lips, glans penis, and inner surface of the prepuce. The coiled secreting portion lies in the corium or subcutaneous portion of skin; the secretory duct follows a straight or oblique course through the dermis but becomes spiral in passing through the epidermis to its opening, a sweat pore. Most sweat glands are merocrine; those of the axilla, areola, mammary gland, labia majora, and circumanal region are apocrine. Sweat glands are most numerous on the palms of the hands and soles of the feet. SEE: illus.; *gland, apocrine; gland, eccrine.*

**sweating** (swĕt′ĭng) [AS. *swat,* sweat] **1.** The act of exuding sweat. **2.** Emitting sweat. **3.** Causing profuse sweat.

***deficiency of s.*** Anhidrosis.

***excessive s.*** Hyperhidrosis.

***gustatory s.*** Sweating and flushing over the distribution of the auriculotemporal nerve in response to chewing.

***insensible s.*** The evaporation of water from the skin without the production of visible sweat. This is done by the water vapor diffusing through the skin rather than being secreted by the sweat glands.

***sensible s.*** The production of moisture on the skin by means of the secretions of the sweat glands.

***urinous s.*** Uridrosis.

**Swedish gymnastics** A system of active and passive exercise of the various muscles and joints of the body without using apparatus.

**Swedish massage** Massage combined with Swedish gymnastics.

**sweet** [AS. *swete,* sweet] **1.** Pleasing to the taste or smell. SEE: *taste.* **2.** Containing or derived from sugar. **3.** Free from excess of acid, sulfur, or corrosive salts.

**Sweet's procedure** A radiographical procedure used to locate foreign objects in the eye.

**Sweet's syndrome** [R. D. Sweet, contemporary Brit. physician] A condition marked by fever; raised painful plaques on the limbs, face, and neck; neutrophil leukocytosis; and dense dermal infiltration with mature neutrophil polymorphs. The cause is unknown, but treatment with adrenal cortical hormone is usually effective.

**swelling** (swĕl′ĭng) [AS. *swellan,* swollen] An abnormal transient enlargement, esp.

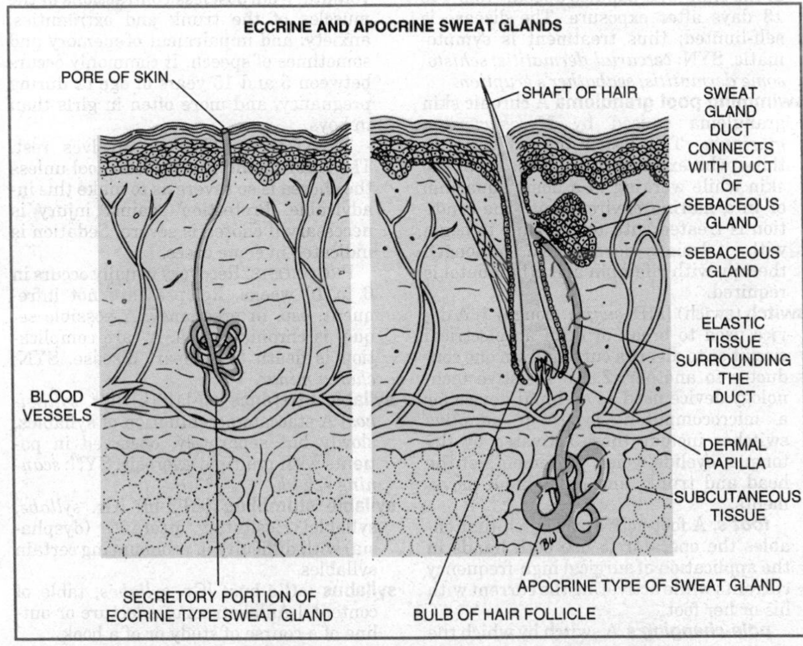

one appearing on the surface of the body. Ice water applied to the area helps to reduce swelling. SEE: *edema.*

***albuminous s.*** Cloudy s.

***Calabar s.*** A swelling occurring in infestations by the nematode *Loa loa.* Temporary and painless, the swelling is thought to be the result of temporary sensitization.

***cloudy s.*** A degeneration of tissues marked by a cloudy appearance, swelling, and the appearance of tiny albuminoid granules in the cells as observed with the microscope. SYN: *albuminous s.*

***fugitive s.*** A temporary swelling such as those occurring in infestations of *Loa loa,* which appear at one place, persist for 2 or 3 days, then disappear, possibly to recur at another position.

***glassy s.*** A swelling occurring in amyloid degeneration of tissues. SEE: *amyloid degeneration; erythredema.*

***white s.*** A swelling seen in tuberculous arthritis, esp. of the knee.

**Swift's disease** Acrodynia.

**swimmer's ear** A type of external otitis seen in persons who swim for a considerable period of time or fail to completely dry their ear canals after swimming. If excess cerumen is not present, the condition can be prevented by placing a few drops of 70% alcohol in the ear canals at the end of each swimming session.

**swimmer's itch** The appearance of papules resembling insect bites on the skin of persons who swim in water containing the cercariae of certain schistosomes. It is usually present only on exposed surfaces of the skin. The papules appear from 4 to 13 days after exposure. The disease is self-limited; thus treatment is symptomatic. SYN: *cercarial dermatitis; schistosome dermatitis; seabather's eruption.*

**swimming pool granuloma** A chronic skin granuloma caused by *Mycobacterium marinum.* The lesion may develop in those who experience an abrasion of the skin while working in a home aquarium or in a marine environment. The condition is treated with tetracycline to begin with; if lesions do not heal, prolonged therapy with rifampin and ethambutol is required.

**switch** (swĭch) [MD. *swijch,* bough] **1.** A device used to break or open an electrical circuit or to divert a current from one conductor to another. **2.** An assistive technology device used as an input device for a microcomputer. Types of adaptive switches include those activated by the tongue, eyelids, voice, movements of the head and trunk, and gross hand movements.

***foot s.*** A foot-activated switch that enables the operator to use both hands in the application of surgical high-frequency currents while activating the current with his or her foot.

***pole-changing s.*** A switch by which the polarity of a circuit may be reversed.

**swoon** [AS. *swogan,* to suffocate] **1.** Syncope. **2.** To faint.

**sycoma** (sī-kō'mă) [Gr. *sykoma*] Condyloma.

**sycosiform** (sī-kō'sĭ-form) [Gr. *sykosis,* figlike disease, + L. *forma,* shape] Resembling sycosis.

**sycosis** (sī-kō'sĭs) [Gr. *sykosos,* figlike disease] A chronic inflammation of the hair follicles.

SYMPTOMS: The patient has inflammation of hairy areas of the body marked by an aggregation of papules and pustules, each of which is pierced by a hair. The pustules show no disposition to rupture but dry to form yellow-brown crusts. There is itching and burning. If the disease persists, it may lead to extreme destruction of hair follicles and permanent alopecia. The organism should be cultured and tested to determine the systemic and topical antibiotic of choice. The disease is curable with prolonged treatment and relapses do occur. *Staphylococcus aureus* and *epidermidis* entering through hair follicles cause the disease. Trauma and disability are predisposing factors.

***s. barbae*** Sycosis of the beard marked by papules and pustules perforated by hairs and surrounded by infiltrated skin.

***lupoid s.*** A pustular lesion of the hair follicles of the beard.

**Sydenham's chorea** (sĭd'ĕn-hămz) [Thomas Sydenham, Brit. physician, 1624–1689] A disease of childhood usually associated with rheumatic fever and marked by involuntary purposeless contractions of the muscles of the trunk and extremities; anxiety; and impairment of memory and sometimes of speech. It commonly occurs between 5 and 15 years of age or during pregnancy, and more often in girls than in boys.

TREATMENT: Therapy involves rest. The child should remain in school unless the chorea is so severe as to make this inadvisable. Protection against injury is necessary if chorea is severe. Sedation is indicated in some cases.

PROGNOSIS: Recovery usually occurs in 6 to 10 weeks. Relapses are not infrequent, esp. in pregnancy. A possible sequel is chronic chorea. A rare complication is death from heart disease. SYN: *chorea minor.*

**syllabic utterance** (sĭ-lăb'ĭk) [Gr. *syllabikos*] A staccato accentuation of syllables, slowly but separately, observed in patients with multiple sclerosis. SYN: *scanning speech.*

**syllable stumbling** (sĭl'ă-bl) [Gr. *syllabe,* syllable] Hesitating utterance (dysphasia) with difficulty in pronouncing certain syllables.

**syllabus** (sĭl'ă-bŭs) [Gr. *syllabos,* table of contents] An abstract of a lecture or outline of a course of study or of a book.

**sylvatic plague** Bubonic plague that is endemic among wild rodents. The causative organism is transmitted by fleas. SEE: *plague.*

**sylvian aqueduct** (sĭl′vē-ăn) [François (Franciscus del la Boë) Sylvius, Dutch anatomist, 1614–1672] A narrow canal from the third to the fourth ventricle.

**sylvian artery** [François Sylvius] The middle cerebral artery in the fissure of Sylvius.

**sylvian fissure** [François Sylvius] SEE: *fissure of Sylvius.*

**sylvian line** [François Sylvius] Line on exterior of the cranium, marking direction of the sylvian fissure.

**sym-** [Gr. *syn,* together] Combining form meaning *with, along, together with, beside.*

**symballophone** (sĭm-băl′ō-fōn) [″ + *ballein,* to throw, + *phone,* sound] A special stethoscope with two chest pieces. Its use assists in locating a lesion in the chest by comparing the different sounds detected by the two chest pieces.

**symbion, symbiont** (sĭm′bē-ŏn, -bē-ŏnt) [Gr. *syn,* together, + *bios,* life] An organism that lives with another in a state of symbiosis.

**symbiosis** (sĭm″bē-ō′sĭs) [Gr.] **1.** The living together in close association of two organisms of different species. If neither organism is harmed, this is called *commensalism*; if the association is beneficial to both, *mutualism*; if one is harmed and the other benefits, *parasitism*. **2.** In psychiatry, a dependent, mutually reinforcing relationship between two persons. In a healthy context, it is characteristic of the infant-mother relationship. In an unhealthy context, it may reinforce the psychopathology present in close associates.

**symbiote** (sĭm′bī-ōt) [Gr. *syn,* together, + *bios,* life] An organism symbiotic with another.

**symbiotic** (sĭm″bī-ŏt′ĭk) Concerning symbiosis.

**symblepharon** (sĭm-blĕf′ă-rŏn) [″ + *blepharon,* eyelid] An adhesion between the conjunctivae of the lid and eyeball resulting from injuries, esp. burns from lime or acids. It is seen also in trachoma, in pemphigus, and following operations. Interference with movement of the eyeball and conjunctival irritation mark this condition. This condition requires division of the cicatricial bands, maintaining the separation of the raw surfaces, and mucous membrane grafts.

**symblepharopterygium** (sĭm-blĕf″ă-rō-tĕr-ĭj′ē-ŭm) [″ + ″ + *pterygion,* wing] The abnormal joining of the eyelid to the eyeball.

**symbol** (sĭm′bŏl) [Gr. *symbolon,* a sign] **1.** An object or sign that represents an idea or quality by association, resemblance, or convention. SEE: Prescription Writing and Symbols in *Abbreviations Appendix.* **2.** In psychology, an object used as an unconscious substitute that is not connected consciously with the libido, but into which the libido is concentrated. **3.** A mark or letter representing an atom or an element in chemistry.

***phallic s.*** An object that bears some resemblance to the penis.

**symbolia** (sĭm-bō′lē-ă) The ability to identify or recognize an object by the sense of touch.

**symbolism** (sĭm′bŏl-ĭzm) [″ + *-ismos,* condition] **1.** The unconscious substitutive expression of subconscious thoughts of sexual significance in terms recognized by the objective consciousness. **2.** An abnormal condition in which everything that occurs is interpreted as a symbol of the patient's own thoughts.

**symbolization** An unconscious process by which an object or idea comes to represent another object or idea on the basis of similarity or association.

**symbolophobia** (sĭm″bŏl-ō-fō′bē-ă) [″ + *phobos,* fear] A hesitancy in expressing oneself in words or action for fear that it may be interpreted as possessing a symbolic meaning.

**symbrachydactyly** (sĭm-brăk″ē-dăk′tĭ-lē) [″ + *brachys,* short, + *daktylos,* finger] The webbing of abnormally short fingers.

**Syme's operation** (sīmz) [James Syme, Scottish surgeon, 1799–1870] **1.** Amputation of the foot at the ankle joint with removal of the malleoli. **2.** Excision of the tongue. **3.** External urethrotomy.

**symmelia** (sĭm-mē′lē-ă) [Gr. *syn,* together, + *melos,* limb] Fusion of limbs.

**symmelus, symelus** (sĭm′ĕ-lŭs, -ē-lŭs) [″ + *melos,* limb] Sirenomelia.

**symmetromania** (sĭm″ĕ-trō-mā′nē-ă) [Gr. *symmetria,* symmetry, + *mania,* madness] A compulsive impulse to make symmetrical motions such as moving both arms instead of one.

**symmetry** (sĭm′ĕt-rē) Correspondence in shape, size, and relative position of parts on opposite sides of a body.

***bilateral s.*** Symmetry of an organism or body whose right and left halves are mirror images of each other or in which a median longitudinal section divides the organism or body into equivalent right and left halves.

***radial s.*** Symmetry of an organism whose parts radiate from a central axis.

**sympathectomize** (sĭm″pă-thĕk′tō-mīz) To perform a sympathectomy.

**sympathectomy** (sĭm″pă-thĕk′tō-mē) [Gr. *sympathetikos,* sympathy, + *ektome,* excision] Excision of a portion of the sympathetic division of the autonomic nervous system. It may include a nerve, plexus, ganglion, or a series of ganglia of the sympathetic trunk. SYN: *sympathicectomy.*

***chemical s.*** The use of drugs to destroy or temporarily inactivate part of the sympathetic nervous system.

***periarterial s.*** Removal of the sheath of an artery in which sympathetic nerve fibers are located; used in trophic disturbances.

**sympatheoneuritis** (sĭm-păth″ē-ō-nū-rī′tĭs) [″ + *neuron,* nerve, + *itis,* inflammation] An inflammation of the sympathetic nerve.

**sympathetic** (sĭm″pă-thĕt′ĭk) **1.** Pert. to the sympathetic nervous system. **2.** Caused by or pert. to sympathy.

**sympatheticalgia** (sĭm″pă-thĕt″ĭ-kăl′jē-ă) [″ + *algos,* pain] Pain in the cervical sympathetic ganglion.

**sympathetic irritation** The irritation of one structure caused by irritation of a related one.

**sympathetic nervous system** SEE: *system, sympathetic nervous.*

**sympatheticoparalytic** (sĭm″pă-thĕt″ĭ-kō-păr″ă-lĭt′ĭk) [″ + *paralysis,* a loosening at the sides] Resulting from paralysis of the sympathetic nervous system.

**sympatheticopathy** (sĭm″pă-thĕt″ĭ-kŏp′ă-thē) [″ + *pathos,* disease, suffering] Any condition resulting from a disorder of the sympathetic nervous system.

**sympathetic ophthalmia** Inflammation of the uveal tract in one eye caused by a similar inflammation in the other eye.

**sympatheticotonia** (sĭm″pă-thĕt″ĭ-kō-tō′nē-ă) [″ + *tonos,* act of stretching, tension] A condition marked by excessive tone of the sympathetic nervous system with unusually high blood pressure, fine tremor of the hands, and insomnia; the opposite of vagotonia. It may be present in thyrotoxic patients.

**sympathetic plexus** One of the plexuses formed at intervals by the sympathetic nerves and ganglia.

**sympathicectomy** (sĭm-păth″ĭ-sĕk′tō-mē) [″ + *ektome,* excision] Sympathectomy.

**sympathicolytic** (sĭm-păth″ĭ-kō-lĭt′ĭk) [″ + *lytikos,* dissolving] Interfering with, opposing, inhibiting, or destroying impulses from the sympathetic nervous system. SYN: *sympatholytic.*

**sympathiconeuritis** (sĭm-păth″ĭ-kō-nū-rī′tĭs) [″ + *neuron,* nerve, + *itis,* inflammation] An inflammation of the sympathetic nerves.

**sympathicopathy** (sĭm-păth″ĭ-kŏp′ă-thē) [″ + *pathos,* disease, suffering] A disease or disordered function caused by a malfunction of the autonomic nervous system.

**sympathicotripsy** (sĭm-păth″ĭ-kō-trĭp′sē) [″ + *tripsis,* a crushing] The crushing of a sympathetic ganglion.

**sympathicotropic** (sĭm-păth″ĭ-kō-trŏp′ĭk) [″ + *tropos,* a turning] Having a special affinity for the sympathetic nerve.

**sympathicus** (sĭm-păth′ĭ-kŭs) The sympathetic nervous system.

**sympathoadrenal** (sĭm″păth-ō-ă-drē′năl) [″ + L. *ad,* to, + *ren,* kidney] Concerning the sympathetic part of the autonomic nervous system and the adrenal medulla.

**sympathoblastoma** (sĭm″păth-ō-blăs-tō′mă) [″ + ″ + *oma,* tumor] A malignant tumor made up of sympathetic nerve cells.

**sympathoglioblastoma** (sĭm″păth-ō-glī″ō-blăs-tō′mă) [Gr. *sympathetikos,* sympathy, + *glia,* glue, + *blastos,* germ, + *oma,* tumor] A tumor made up primarily of sympathoblasts with scattered neuroblasts and spongioblasts.

**sympathogonia** (sĭm″pă-thō-gō′nē-ă) [″ + *gone,* seed] Primitive cells from which sympathetic nervous system cells are derived.

**sympathogonioma** (sĭm″pă-thō-gō″nē-ō′mă) [″ + ″ + *oma,* tumor] A tumor containing sympathogonia.

**sympatholytic** Sympathicolytic.

**sympathomimetic** (sĭm″pă-thō-mĭm-ĕt′ĭk) [″ + *mimetikos,* imitating] Adrenergic; producing effects resembling those resulting from stimulation of the sympathetic nervous system, such as effects following the injection of epinephrine.

**sympathy** (sĭm′pă-thē) [Gr. *sympatheia*] **1.** An association or feeling of closeness between individuals such that something that affects one affects the other. SEE: *empathy.* **2.** In biology, something that affects one of a paired organ influencing the other. The mechanism of this interaction is not always clearly understood.

**sympexion** (sĭm-pĕks′ē-ŏn) [Gr. *sympexis,* concretion] A concretion in certain sites such as the prostate or seminal vesicles.

**symphalangism** (sĭm-făl′ăn-jĭzm) [Gr. *syn,* together, + *phalanx,* closely knit row] **1.** An ankylosis of the joints of the fingers or toes. **2.** A web-fingered or web-toed condition.

**symphyogenetic** (sĭm″fē-ō-jĕ-nĕt′ĭk) [Gr. *syn,* together, + *phyein,* to grow, + *gennan,* to produce] Concerning the combined effect of heredity and environment upon the development and function of an organism.

**symphyseal** (sĭm-fĭz′ē-ăl) [Gr. *symphysis,* growing together] Pert. to symphysis.

**symphyseotomy** (sĭm-fĭz″ē-ŏt′ō-mē) [″ + *tome,* incision] A section of the symphysis pubis to enlarge the pelvic diameters during delivery. SYN: *pubiotomy; symphysiotomy.*

**symphysiectomy** (sĭm-fĭz″ē-ĕk′tō-mē) [″ + *ektome,* excision] Resection of the symphysis pubis to facilitate delivery.

**symphysion** (sĭm-fĭz′ē-ŏn) [Gr. *symphysis,* growing together] The most anterior point of the alveolar process of the lower jaw.

**symphysiorrhaphy** (sĭm-fĭz″ē-or′ă-fē) [″ + *rhaphe,* seam, ridge] The surgical repair of a divided symphysis.

**symphysiotome** (sĭm-fĭz′ē-ō-tōm) [″ + *tome,* incision] An instrument for dividing a symphysis.

**symphysiotomy** (sĭm-fĭz″ē-ŏt′ō-mē) [″ + *tome,* incision] Symphyseotomy.

**symphysis** (sĭm′fĭ-sĭs) *pl.* **symphyses** [Gr., growing together] **1.** A line of fusion between two bones that are separate in early development, as symphysis of the mandible. **2.** A form of synchondrosis in which the bones are separated by a disk of fibrocartilage, as in joints between bodies of vertebrae or between pubic bones. SEE: *intervertebral disk.*

***s. cartilaginosa*** Synchondroses.

***s. of jaw*** An anterior, median, vertical ridge on the outer surface of the lower jaw representing a line of union of its halves.

***s. ligamentosa*** Syndesmoses.

***s. mandibulae*** S. menti.

***s. menti*** The symphysis of the chin or the ridge marking the line of union of the two halves of the mandible. SYN: *s. mandibulae.*

***s. pubis*** The junction of the pubic bones on the midline in front; the bony eminence under the pubic hair.

**symphysodactyly** (sĭm″fĭ-sō-dăk′tĭ-lē) [″ + *daktylos,* finger] Syndactylism.

**sympodia** (sĭm-pō′dē-ă) [″ + *pous,* foot] A condition in which the lower extremities are united.

**symporter** (sĭm-por′tĕr) A mechanism for carrying two different molecules or ions in the same direction through a membrane.

**symptom** (sĭm′tŭm, sĭmp-) [Gr. *symptoma,* occurrence] Any perceptible change in the body or its functions that indicates disease or the kind or phases of disease. Symptoms may be classified as objective, subjective, cardinal, and, sometimes, constitutional. However, another classification considers all symptoms as being subjective, with objective indications being called signs.

Aspects of general symptom analysis include the following: *onset:* date, manner (gradual or sudden), and precipitating factors; *characteristics:* character, location, radiation, severity, timing, aggravating or relieving factors, and associated symptoms; *course since onset:* incidence, progress, and effects of therapy.

ABDOMEN: The abdominal area may be distended, rigid, flat, flabby, adipose, tympanitic, shiny, enlarged, or bulging in certain areas with certain discolorations, stripings, or markings. The muscles may be tensed and little affected by pressure. Cold or hot areas may be noted. Various sounds may be heard such as splashings, roarings, and rumblings (borborygmi, also known as intestinal flatus).

*Pain* is closely associated with abdominal symptoms. The exact area affected should be located and the nature, duration, time when it arises, and any causes that might be responsible noted. Also the effect of movement or pressure on the pain, and the alteration in the pain if the pressure applied to the area is suddenly released, should be noted. SEE: *rebound tenderness.*

*Emesis* is another condition associated with symptoms pert. to the abdominal region. It may consist of simple regurgitation of the stomach contents or may be extremely forcible. In the latter case, it is called projectile vomiting. Emesis may be watery, clear, or contain mucus or undigested food; it may be stertorous, bilious, frothy, profuse, purulent, colored from food or medication, or contain blood (hematemesis). If blood is present in large quantity and has been acted on by gastric juices, it may resemble coffee grounds. Emesis may be sour, may have the odor of feces or garlic, may be ammoniacal, or may have an odor characteristic of some food or drug.

The patient may complain of abdominal distention, gas, pain caused by gas, and interference with respiration. Heartburn may be present, as may gastritis and regurgitation. Pain may be felt when food enters the stomach or may be relieved by eating or shortly after eating or by changing body position. Distention after eating and the desire to eructate or expel flatus should be noted. Colicky pains in the abdomen may be accompanied by pain in the shoulder. Pain at the pit of the stomach and in the lower right quadrant may indicate appendicitis. When pains are over the lower right ribs or a little below, disease of the gallbladder may be suspected. SEE: *abdomen; emesis.*

BACK: The dorsal side of the body may reveal edema, deformities, irregularities of the spine, discolorations, eruptions, impaired motion, decubitus, or any condition affecting the skin. SEE: *back pain.*

BREATH: The breath may have a fecal, sweet (acetone), wet hay, fishy, ammonia, urine, blood, or pus odor. Respiration may be abdominal or thoracic and show dyspnea, orthopnea, apnea, or it may be normal (eupnea). SEE: *apnea; breath; dyspnea; orthopnea.*

CHEST: The chest may show abnormalities and deformities. It may move asymmetrically with one lung being inflated much less than the other. Coughing may be whooping, hacking, crowing, hoarse, dry, rasping, or hysterical. There may or may not be expectoration. A cough may be spasmodic or occur on awakening. During sleep, it may awaken the patient. It may or may not produce sputum. It may occur when swallowing food, when the patient is in a horizontal position, or when the patient is subjected to temperature changes. Hiccupping should be noted if and when it occurs. Sputum may be mucoid, yellowish, thick, tenacious, ropy, gelatinous, dark green, offensive in odor, copious, streaked with bright (brick red) or dark blood (hemoptysis), or it may resemble cheesy lumps. It may be clear and watery, scanty, or profuse.

Frequency of coughing and clearing the throat should be noted. The patient's respirations may be shallow. Dyspnea, an inability to expand the lungs, complaints of irritation, sticking pains, or catchy pains on inspiration may be present. There may be an accumulation of phlegm in the air passages or a tickling in the throat. The patient may not be able to take deep inspirations or may yawn constantly. There may be migrating knifelike pains in the region of the heart or throughout the chest. Heart-consciousness, a fluttering feeling about the heart, or cardiac pain may be present. Queer sensations, the loud beating of the heart, and heaviness in the cardiac region are other symptoms. SEE: *apnea; chest; cough; dyspnea; hiccough; sputum.*

DEFECATION: Symptoms to observe are the frequency of defecation; the presence of constipation; hemorrhoids; the nature of the feces such as formation (ribbon-shaped, soft, semiformed, hard or scybalous, cylindrical) and whether watery, liquid, or semiliquid; the color, whether dark brown, light brown, clay-colored, green, yellowish, black, bloody; and whether lienteric, serous, mucous, purulent, tarry, or containing membranous shreds, calculi, or foreign substances. The amount should be noted, as small, medium, large, or copious. The odor may be characteristic of various conditions: sour, putrid, offensive, or fetid. The nature of the evacuation should be noted, as natural, difficult, involuntary, or painful. SEE: *feces; stool.*

DENTITION: Teeth may be discolored, irregular, missing, misshapen, or affected by caries. There may be a partial or complete denture. Dental hygiene may be good or poor. There may be a loosening of teeth, a film over them, or they may show the presence of sordes.

EARS: Tinnitus aurium (ringing in the ears) occurs in certain diseases. Pain in or about the ears, or swelling under either or both, should be noted. Impacted cerumen, foreign bodies, or insects may be present in the auditory canals. SEE: *ear.*

EYES: The eyes may stare, look excited, or be expressionless. Nystagmus, strabismus, and coma vigil may be present. Pupils may be contracted or dilated, or one pupil may be affected. The patient may keep the eyes closed constantly, or keep one open and the other closed. Eyes may be sunken or protruding. Lacrimation may be present. Eyelids may be edematous. The eyeball may be soft to the touch or extremely hard. Accommodation may be faulty. Nictitation, squinting, or tremor of the eyelids should always be recorded. Blurring of vision usually is associated with other symptoms. The patient may complain of colorless or colored specks dancing before the eyes (muscae volitantes). SEE: *eye.*

GAIT: The gait may be faltering, scissors, festinating, unsteady, staggering, weakened, or swaying; or movements may be stiff, awkward, or unusual. There may be total disability or immobility. SEE: *gait.*

GENERAL APPEARANCE: The face may show an expression of anxiety or have a pinched look or a drawn expression. The patient may have an air of apathy, a distorted or a blank look, an emotional expression, a risus sardonicus, or lack of all expression (masklike).

GENERAL SYMPTOMS: Burning sensations may be complained of in various parts of the body, as in the head, throat, arms, chest, or abdomen. They may or may not be accompanied by tenderness. The complaint may be of feeling too hot or too cold without apparent cause, or of having a general feeling of distress.

Anorexia and nausea upon taking food, at the thought of food, or with no reference to food are significant and should be noted. When the nausea occurs should also be noted: on awakening, when taking fluids, after eating, when changing a position, when taking medication, or in the presence of odors. There always should be an explanation for nausea, either somatic or psychiatric.

Fear of death (angor animi), anxiety, agitation, or panic may be present.

LIMBS: The symptoms pert. to the skin, of course, also apply to the skin of the limbs. Deformities, abnormalities, impaired motion, discolorations, sensitivity, and varicosities should be noted.

LIPS: These may be pale, dry, cyanotic, edematous, drawn, deformed, out of proportion, motionless and expressionless, flushed, or fissured; or they may show other lesions or growths. SEE: *lip.*

MOUTH AND GUMS: The patient's mouth and gums may be pale or ulcerated, highly inflamed and red, infected, discolored, edematous, or abnormally shaped. Pyorrhea or edema may be present. The patient may complain of bitter, sweet, salty, sour, fishy, or flat tastes, or an absence of taste. Medication may have much to do with temporary disorders of taste. SEE: *gum; mouth.*

NOSE: The nose may appear deformed, discolored, edematous, or enlarged. The nostrils may discharge or show obstruction. There may be an inability to breathe through one or both nostrils. The patient may complain of odors not usually manifested as objective symptoms or for which there is no known cause. SEE: *nose.*

PAIN: One should determine if the patient's perception of pain is local or referred so that the exact area affected can be ascertained. The wording of the patient's complaint of pain must be charted or reported. One should note if the pain is in the nature of a cramp or spasm; if it is dull, superficial, deep, remittent, shifting, shooting, lancinating, gnawing, fixed, or sharp; or if there is an absence of pain, esp. in conditions in which pain usually occurs. Whether pain is relieved or increased by pressure, heat, cold, change of body position or environment, or other conditions should be noted, as should when the pain is experienced, how often the same type of pain recurs, and whether it awakens the patient from sleep, esp. at night. The patient's facial expression during an attack of pain should be observed and the patient's description listened to carefully.

The patient may locate a *headache* around the eyes and nose, in the center of the forehead, above the nose, in one or both temples accompanied by throbbing, at the top of the head, or at the base of the skull. It may be felt as a tight, bandlike sensation around the head above the eyes. It may be in the center of the forehead above the eyebrow line, in the upper region of the center forehead, all over the top of the head, over one or both ears, or the back of both ears. The pain may be sharp, dull, or shifting. It may accompany head noises, or a roaring in the head may be experienced without pain. Vertigo or a sensation of fainting may be present. Pulsations may be felt in the occiput or in the temporal region. A patient may be very sensitive to light and sound, and headaches may be accompanied by nausea, vomiting, the sensation of flashing lights, and chills. Tenderness or soreness may be associated with rigidity. SEE: *headache; pain.*

POSITIONS AND POSTURES: An inability to lie down; to arise; or to lie on one side, on the back, or in any special position reveals much to the physician. Whether the patient lies on the affected or the unaffected side is also important to observe. Left or right legs, or both, may be flexed, or there may be an inclination to lie with the arms above the head. The legs may be restless. SEE: *posture.*

SKIN: The skin may appear pale, flushed all over or in spots; may be cyanotic, jaundiced, shiny, erupted, burned, blistered, sunburned, wrinkled, lacerated, nodular, bruised; may exhibit dermographia, lesions, growth, or deformities; or may be puffy and edematous, ashy, gray, wet with perspiration, or discolored. SEE: *skin.*

THROAT: The throat may show abnormalities, discoloration, swelling, inflammation, diseased tonsils, and presence of adenoids. Dysphagia and hoarseness or aphonia and other conditions affecting the voice may be present. A lump in the throat (globus hystericus) or a dry, scratchy irritation or fullness or pulsations may be present.

TONGUE: The tongue may be coated, clean, smooth, atrophic, shiny, dry on top and moist on the sides or dry all over. It may look like raw beef or appear furry, glossy, tremulous, or sharp-pointed. It may be edematous or abnormal in size. Fissures may be present. The papillae may have disappeared. The patient may have a strawberry tongue, or the tongue may have various colors. The tongue may deviate from the midline. SEE: *tongue.*

URINE: The urine may be blue, milky, pale, lemon, smoky, brick-colored, clear, amber, straw-colored, orange, or almost any other color. Hematuria may be present. Polyuria, oliguria, or frequent urination of small amounts may occur. The odors may be ammoniacal, aromatic, stercorous, or like that of new-mown hay, ripe apples, or violets. There may be retention, suppression, or dribbling, and urination may be painful. SEE: *urine.*

***accessory s.*** A minor symptom, or a nonpathognomonic one. SYN: *assident s.*

***accidental s.*** A symptom occurring incidentally during the course of a disease but having no relationship to the disease.

***assident s.*** Accessory s.

***cardinal s.*** A principal symptom in the diagnosis of a disease.

***concomitant s.*** A symptom occurring along with the essential symptoms of a disease.

***constitutional s.*** A symptom caused by or indicating systemic disease. SYN: *general s.*

***delayed s.*** A symptom appearing sometime after the precipitating cause.

***direct s.*** A symptom resulting from direct effects of the disease.

***dissociation s.*** Anesthesia to heat, cold, and pain without loss of tactile sensibility; seen in syringomyelia.

***equivocal s.*** A symptom that may occur in several diseases.

***focal s.*** A symptom at a specific location.

***general s.*** Constitutional s.

***indirect s.*** A symptom occurring secondarily as a result of a disease.

***labyrinthine s.*** A group of symptoms, such as tinnitus, vertigo, or nausea, indicating a disease or lesion of the inner ear.

***local s.*** A symptom indicating the specific location of the pathological process.

***negative pathognomonic s.*** A symptom that never occurs in a certain disease or condition; hence, its occurrence rules out the existence of that disease.

***objective s.*** A symptom apparent to the observer. SEE: *sign.*

***passive s.*** Static s.

***pathognomonic s.*** A symptom that is unmistakably associated with a particular disease.

***presenting s.*** The symptom that led the patient to seek medical care.

***prodromal s.*** Prodrome.

***rational s.*** Subjective s.

***signal s.*** A symptom that is premonitory of an impending condition such as the aura that precedes an attack of epilepsy or migraine.

***static s.*** A symptom pert. to the condition of a single organ or structure without reference to the remainder of the body. SYN: *passive s.*

***subjective s.*** A symptom apparent only to the patient. SYN: *rational s.*

***sympathetic s.*** A symptom for which there is no specific inciting cause and usually occurring at a point more or less remote from the point of disturbance. SEE: *sympathy* (1).

***withdrawal s.*** One of the symptoms following sudden withdrawal of a substance to which a person has become addicted.

**symptomatic** (sĭmp″tō-măt′ĭk) [Gr. *symptomatikos*] Of the nature of or concerning a symptom.

**symptomatology** (sĭmp″tō-mă-tŏl′ō-jē) [Gr. *symptoma,* symptom, + *logos,* word, reason] **1.** The science of symptoms and indications. **2.** All of the symptoms of a given disease as a whole.

**symptom complex** Syndrome.

**symptom magnification syndrome** A term relating to the rehabilitation of persons with work-related injuries, used in reference to behaviors that exaggerate the pain or functional limitation.

**sympus** (sĭm′pŭs) [″ + *pous,* foot] A deformed fetus fused at the lower limbs.

**syn-** [Gr., together] Prefix meaning *joined, together*. SEE: *con-*.

**synactosis** (sĭn″ăk-tō′sĭs) [Gr. *syn,* together, + L. *actio,* function, + Gr. *osis,* condition] A malformation resulting from the abnormal fusion of parts.

**synadelphus** (sĭn″ă-dĕl′fŭs) [″ + *adelphos,* brother] A deformed fetus with eight limbs.

**synalgic** (sĭn-ăl′jĭk) Pert. to or marked by referred pain.

**synapse** (sĭn′ăps) [Gr. *synapsis,* point of contact] The space between the junction of two neurons in a neural pathway, where the termination of the axon of one neuron comes into close proximity with the cell body or dendrites of another. The electrical impulse traveling along a presynaptic neuron to the end of its axon releases a chemical neurotransmitter that stimulates or inhibits an electrical impulse in the postsynaptic neuron; synaptic transmission is in one direction only. Synapses are susceptible to fatigue, offer a resistance to the passage of impulses, and are markedly susceptible to the effects of oxygen deficiency, anesthetics, and other agents, including therapeutic drugs and toxic chemicals. SYN: *synapsis* (1). SEE: illus.

***axodendritic s.*** The synapse between an axon of one neuron and the dendrites of another.

***axodendrosomatic s.*** The synapse between the axon of one neuron and the dendrites and cell body of another.

***axosomatic s.*** The synapse between the axon of one neuron and the cell body of another.

**synapsis** (sĭn-ăp′sĭs) [Gr., point of contact] **1.** Synapse. **2.** The process of first maturation division in gametogenesis, in which there is conjugation of pairs of homologous chromosomes forming double or bivalent chromosomes. In the resulting meiotic division, the chromosome number is reduced from the diploid to the haploid number. It is at this stage that crossing

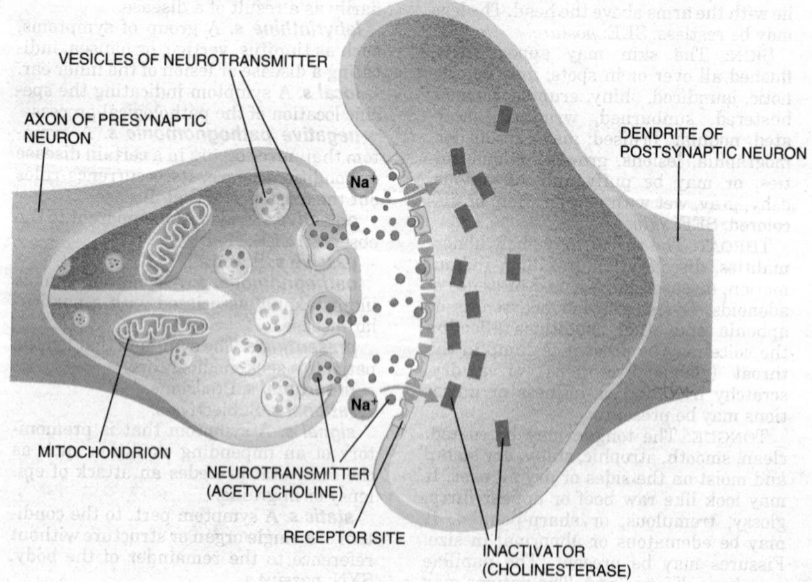


**SYNAPSE**

TRANSMISSION AT AN EXCITATORY SYNAPSE (ARROW INDICATES DIRECTION OF IMPULSE)

over occurs.

**synaptic** Pert. to a synapse or synapsis.

**synaptic field** A field in the cerebral cortex, cerebellar cortex, and retina where large numbers of contacts between neurons can take place.

**synaptolemma** (sĭn-ăp″tō-lĕm′ă) The membrane at a synapse separating two neurons.

**synaptology** (sĭn″ăp-tŏl′ō-jē) [″ + *logos,* word, reason] The study of synapses.

**synarthrodia** (sĭn″ăr-thrō′dē-ă) [Gr. *syn,* together, + *arthron,* joint, + *eidos,* form, shape] Synarthrosis.

**synarthrodial** Pert. to a synarthrosis.

**synarthrophysis** (sĭn″ăr-thrō-fī′sĭs) [″ + *arthron,* joint, + *physis,* growth] A progressive ankylosis of joints.

**synarthrosis** [″ + *arthron,* joint, + *osis,* condition] A type of joint in which the skeletal elements are united by a continuous intervening substance (cartilage, fibrous tissue, or bone). Movement is absent or limited, and a joint cavity is lacking. It includes the synchondrosis, suture, and syndesmosis types of joints. SYN: *synarthrodia.*

**syncanthus** (sĭn-kăn′thŭs) [″ + *kanthos,* angle] An adhesion of the eyeball to the structures of the orbit.

**syncephalus** (sĭn-sĕf′ă-lŭs) [″ + *kephale,* head] A deformed fetus with one head, one face, and four ears.

**synchilia** (sĭn-kī′lē-ă) [″+ *cheilos,* lip] The congenital adhesion of the lips or atresia of the mouth.

**synchiria** (sĭn-kī′rē-ă) [″+ *cheir,* hand] A disorder of sensibility in which a stimulus applied to one side of the body is felt on both sides. SEE: *achiria; allochiria; dyschiria.*

**synchondroseotomy** (sĭn″kŏn-drō″sē-ŏt′ō-mē) [″+ *chondros,* cartilage, + *tome,* incision] An operation of cutting through the sacroiliac ligaments and closing the arch of the pubes in the congenital absence of the anterior wall of the bladder (exstrophy).

**synchondrosis** (sĭn″kŏn-drō′sĭs) [″ + ″ + *osis,* condition] An immovable joint having surfaces between the bones connected by cartilages. This may be temporary, in which case the cartilage eventually becomes ossified, or permanent. SYN: *symphysis cartilaginosa.*

**synchondrotomy** (sĭn-kŏn-drŏt′ō-mē) [″ + ″ + *tome,* incision] **1.** The division of articulating cartilage of a synchondrosis. **2.** A section of the symphysis pubis to facilitate childbirth. SYN: *symphyseotomy.*

**synchorial** (sĭn-kō′rē-ăl) [″ + *chorion,* chorion] Pert. to multiple fetuses that share a single placenta.

**synchronism** (sĭn′krō-nĭzm) [″+ *chronos,* time, + *-ismos,* condition] The simultaneous occurrence of acts or events.

**synchronous** (sĭn′krō-nŭs) Occurring simultaneously.

**synchrony** The simultaneous occurrence of separate events.

**synchysis** (sĭn′kĭs-ĭs) [Gr., confound] The fluid state of the vitreous of the eye.

***s. scintillans*** Bright flashes of light resulting from the presence of crystals of cholesterol or fat substances in the vitreous body.

**syncinesis** (sĭn″sĭn-ē′sĭs) [″ + *kinesis,* movement] An involuntary movement produced in association with a voluntary one. SYN: *synkinesis.*

***imitative s.*** An involuntary movement occurring on the sound side when a movement is attempted on the paralyzed side.

***spasmodic s.*** Syncinesis occurring on the paralyzed side when muscles of the opposite side are voluntarily moved.

**synciput** (sĭn′sĭ-pŭt) The anterior upper half of the cranium. SYN: *sinciput.*

**synclinal** (sĭn-klī′năl) [Gr. *synklinein,* to lean together] Inclined in the same direction toward a point.

**synclitism** (sĭn′klĭt-ĭzm) [Gr. *synklinein,* to lean together, + *-ismos,* condition] Parallelism between the planes of the fetal head and those of the maternal pelvis.

**synclonus** (sĭn′klō-nŭs) [″ + *klonos,* turmoil] **1.** Clonic contraction of several muscles together. **2.** A disease marked by muscular spasms.

***s. ballismus*** Paralysis agitans.

***s. tremens*** Generalized tremor.

**syncopal** (sĭn′kō-păl) [Gr. *synkope,* fainting] Rel. to or marked by syncope.

**syncope** (sĭn′kō-pē) [Gr. *synkope,* fainting] A transient loss of consciousness resulting from an inadequate blood flow to the brain. The patient experiences a generalized weakness of muscles, loss of postural tone, inability to continue standing, and loss of consciousness. At onset, the person is usually upright. The patient may not have sufficient warning to drop to the floor or stop driving to prevent harm to himself or herself or others. The condition may last for a few seconds or as long as half an hour. SYN: *fainting; swoon.* SEE: *coma; transient ischemic attack; unconsciousness.*

ETIOLOGY: Syncope or fainting may be due to deficient blood flow resulting from peripheral circulatory failure, cerebral vascular accident (stroke), cardiac arrhythmia or transient cardiac standstill in Stokes-Adams syndrome, or altered blood chemistry as in hyperventilation or hypoglycemia. Predisposing factors include fatigue, prolonged standing, nausea, pain, emotional disturbances, anemia, dehydration, and poor ventilation.

FIRST AID: The person should be placed in a horizontal position, preferably with the head low in order to facilitate blood flow to the brain. At the same time, a clear airway should be ensured. The clothing must be loose, esp. if a tight collar was being worn. Fainting usually is of short duration and is counteracted by the individual's being in a supine position. Nevertheless it is important to attempt to establish the cause of the faint before dismissing the episode as being of no consequence. If recovery from fainting is not prompt, the person should be moved to a hospital.

***s. anginosa*** Syncope occurring with anginal pain.

***cardiac s.*** Syncope of cardiac origin as in Stokes-Adams syndrome, aortic stenosis, tachycardia, bradycardia, or myocardial infarction.

***carotid sinus s.*** Syncope resulting from pressure on, or hypersensitivity of, the carotid sinus. It may result from turning the head to one side or from wearing too tight a collar.

***cough s.*** Syncope occurring during a coughing spell.

***defecation s.*** SEE: *defecation syncope*.

***hysterical s.*** Syncope resulting from anxiety.

***laryngeal s.*** Brief unconsciousness following coughing and tickling in the throat.

***local s.*** Numbness of a part with sudden blanching, as of the fingers; a symptom of Raynaud's disease or of local asphyxia.

***micturition s.*** The abrupt loss of consciousness during urination. It usually occurs in men who get up at night to urinate. The pathophysiology of this is not understood. Recovery is uneventful.

***neurocardiogenic s.*** SEE: *vasodepressor s.*

***swallow s.*** Fainting that occurs in relation to swallowing. This may be related to an abnormality of the esophagus or heart but may also occur in normal persons.

***tussive s.*** Fainting following a paroxysm of coughing. This is a rare condition in patients with chronic bronchitis. SYN: *laryngeal vertigo*.

***vasodepressor s.*** Syncope resulting from a fall in blood pressure owing to failure of peripheral resistance with concomitant reduced venous return, or due to slowing of the heart. It may be caused by emotional stress, pain, acute loss of blood, fear, or by assuming an upright position after having been in bed for a prolonged period. Either drug therapy or the use of an artificial pacemaker may be helpful when this condition is associated with recurrent bradycardia or asystole. SYN: *vasovagal s.*

***vasovagal s.*** Vasodepressor s.

**syncretio** (sĭn-krē′shē-ō) [L.] The development of adhesions between opposing inflamed surfaces.

**syncytial** (sĭn-sĭ′shăl) Of the nature of a syncytium.

**syncytioma** (sĭn″sĭt-ē-ō′mă) [″ + ″ + *oma,* tumor] A tumor of the chorion. SYN: *chorioma; deciduoma.*

***s. benignum*** A mole.

***s. malignum*** A tumor formed of cells from the syncytium and chorion, occurring frequently after abortion or during puerperium at the site of the placenta.

**syncytiotrophoblast** (sĭn-sĭt″ē-ō-trō′fō-blăst) [″ + ″ + *trophe,* nourishment, + *blastos,* germ] The outer layer of cells covering the chorionic villi of the placenta. These cells are in contact with the maternal blood or decidua. SYN: *syntrophoblast.*

**syncytium** (sĭn-sĭt′ē-ŭm) [″ + *kytos,* cell] **1.** A multinucleated mass of protoplasm such as a striated muscle fiber. **2.** A group of cells in which the protoplasm of one cell is continuous with that of adjoining cells such as the mesenchyme cells of the embryo. SYN: *coenocyte.*

**syndactylism** (sĭn-dăk′tĭl-ĭzm) [″ + *daktylos,* finger, + *-ismos,* condition] A fusion of two or more toes or fingers.

**syndactylous** (sĭn-dăk′tĭ-lŭs) [″ + *daktylos,* finger] Concerning syndactylism.

**syndectomy** (sĭn-dĕk′tō-mē) [″ + *dein,* to bind, + *ektome,* excision] The excision of a circular strip of the conjunctiva around the cornea to relieve pannus. SYN: *peritomy* (1).

**syndesis** (sĭn-dē′sĭs) [″ + *desis,* binding] **1.** The condition of being bound together. **2.** Surgical fixation or ankylosis of a joint.

**syndesmectomy** (sĭn″dĕs-mĕk′tō-mē) [Gr. *syndesmos,* ligament, + *ektome,* excision] The excision of a section of a ligament.

**syndesmectopia** (sĭn″dĕs-mĕk-tō′pē-ă) [″ + *ektopos,* out of place] An abnormal position of a ligament.

**syndesmitis** (sĭn″dĕs-mī′tĭs) [″ + *itis,* inflammation] **1.** An inflammation of a ligament or ligaments. **2.** An inflammation of the conjunctiva.

**syndesmochorial** (sĭn″dĕs″mō-kor′ē-ăl) Pert. to a type of placenta found in ungulates (e.g., sheep and goats) in which there is destruction of the surface layer of the uterine mucosa, thus allowing chorionic villi to come into direct contact with maternal blood vessels.

**syndesmography** (sĭn-dĕs-mŏg′ră-fē) [Gr. *syndesmos,* ligament, + *graphein,* to write] A treatise on the ligaments.

**syndesmologia** (sĭn″dĕs-mō-lō′jē-ă) [″ + *logos,* word, reason] A term concerned with the articulations of joints and their related ligaments.

**syndesmology** (sĭn″dĕs-mŏl′ō-jē) [″ + *logos,* word, reason] The study of the ligaments, joints, their movements, and their disorders.

**syndesmoma** (sĭn″dĕs-mō′mă) [″ + *oma,* tumor] A connective tissue tumor.

**syndesmopexy** (sĭn-dĕs′mō-pĕk″sē) [″ + *pexis,* fixation] Joining of two ligaments or fixation of a ligament in a new place, used in correction of a dislocation.

**syndesmophyte** (sĭn-dĕs′mō-fīt) [″ + *phyton,* plant] **1.** A bony bridge formed between adjacent vertebrae. **2.** A bony outgrowth from a ligament.

**syndesmoplasty** (sĭn-dĕs′mō-plăs″tē) [″ + *plassein,* to form] Plastic surgery on a ligament.

**syndesmorrhaphy** (sĭn″dĕs-mor′ă-fē) [″ + *rhaphe,* seam, ridge] The repair or suture of a ligament.

**syndesmosis** (sĭn″dĕs-mō′sĭs) *pl.* **syndesmoses** [Gr. *syndesmos,* ligament, + *osis,* condition] An articulation in which the bones are united by ligaments. SYN: *symphysis ligamentosa.*

**syndesmotomy** (sĭn″dĕs-mŏt′ō-mē) [″ + *tome,* incision] The surgical section of ligaments.

**syndrome** (sĭn′drōm) [Gr., a running together] A group of symptoms and signs of disordered function related to one another by means of some anatomical, physiological, or biochemical peculiarity. This definition does not include a precise cause of an illness but does provide a framework of reference for investigating it. **syndromic** (sĭn-drŏm′ĭk), *adj.*

***acute chest s.*** A complication of sickle cell disease resulting from occlusion in the pulmonary vasculature and marked by chest pain, tachypnea, fever, rales and rhonchi, leukocytosis, and lobar consolidation.

***Adair-Dighton s.*** A familial condition marked by fragility of bones, deafness, and blue sclerae. SEE: *osteogenesis imperfecta.*

***adiposogenital s.*** Fröhlich's s.

***adrenogenital s.*** A syndrome marked by abnormally early puberty in children, overmasculinization in adults, virilism, and hirsutism, caused by the excessive production of adrenocortical hormones. SEE: *Cushing's syndrome.*

***Angelman s.*** A rare genetic condition marked by severe mental retardation, microcephaly, and paroxysms of laughter. It is due to an abnormal chromosome 15 of maternal origin. SEE: *Prader-Willi s.*

***Angelucci's s.*** Palpitation, excitable temperament, and vasomotor disturbance in some individuals who experience spring conjunctivitis.

***antiphospholipid antibody s.*** An inherited hypercoagulable condition that frequently causes recurrent vascular thrombotic events. The diagnosis is established by one or more major criteria: venous thrombosis, arterial thrombosis or vasculopathy, recurrent pregnancy loss, and thrombocytopenia. Additionally, patients test positive for lupus anticoagulant and have a moderate-to-high anticardiolipin antibody level.

***cleft lip–cleft palate s.*** SEE: *Van der Woude's syndrome.*

***chronic pain s.*** Long-standing low back pain in patients who have developed illness behavior and hopelessness where there is no longer a direct relationship between the pain and the apparent disability. Treatment of the painful symptoms usually does not change the condition; the patient may require psychological and sociological intervention and behavior modification techniques. SEE: *back pain.*

***congenital rubella s.*** Infection of the fetus from maternal rubella. The newborn may have severe central nervous system impairment, including deafness and mental retardation. SEE: *vaccine, rubella.*

***cri du chat s.*** A hereditary congenital anomaly so named because the infant's cry resembles the cry of a cat. Characterized by mental retardation, microcephaly, dwarfism, epicanthal folds, and laryngeal defect. Due to a deletion of the short arm of chromosome 4 or 5 of the B group.

***cubital tunnel s.*** Medial elbow pain, hand fatigue, and sensations in the fourth and fifth fingers resulting from ulnar nerve damage in the cubital tunnel. This condition is frequently seen in athletes who throw objects.

***culture bound s.*** A recurrent, locality-specific pattern of behavior that is not recognized by traditional psychiatry.

***cumulative trauma s.*** Overuse syndrome.

***dumping s.*** A symptom complex that may follow partial or complete gastrectomy. It appears to be related to the rapid emptying of the gastric pouch and occurs immediately after eating. This syndrome consists of weakness, varying degrees of syncope, nausea, sweating, and palpitation, and sometimes diarrhea and a sensation of warmth. Lying down usually affords some relief.

***Fröhlich's s.*** A syndrome in adolescent boys marked by an increase in fat, atrophy of the genitals, a transition to feminine type owing to lesions of the pituitary and hypothalamus. SYN: *adiposogenital s.*

***Gerstmann-Sträussler-Scheinker s.*** ABBR: GSS syndrome. A rare hereditary spinocerebellar degenerative disease caused by prions. Clinically, the onset of symptoms and signs in midlife are related to progressive cerebellar dysfunction with ataxia, unsteadiness, incoordination, and progressive gait difficulty. The prognosis is poor and there is no specific therapy. SEE: *prion disease.*

***Gradenigo's s.*** Paralysis of the external rectus muscle with severe temporoparietal pain and suppurative otitis media on the affected side. It is caused by an infection in the petrous portion of the temporal bone involving the sixth nerve.

***hantavirus pulmonary s.*** An acute infectious disease caused by hantavirus, an agent not known to cause human disease prior to the spring of 1993. It is thought to be caused by inhalation of aerosols from the droppings of rodents such as mice. Clinically, the onset is sudden with generalized malaise and fever followed within 4 to 5 days by cough and dyspnea. Severe respiratory distress and a shock-like state may then develop within hours. If the shock and hypoxemia are not fatal, the leakage of fluid into the lungs resolves within a few days. The fatality rate is approx. 50%.

Measuring the rising antibody titers to hantavirus antigens is a useful diagnostic tool as is immunohistochemical staining of lung and kidney tissues. Treatment includes avoidance of excess administration of fluids. Pressor drugs should be given to maintain blood pressure.

***hepatopulmonary s.*** A combination of liver disease, decreased arterial oxygen concentration, and dilatation of the blood vessels of the lung. Clinically the patient may have signs and symptoms of liver disease including gastrointestinal bleeding, esophageal varices, ascites, palmar erythema, and splenomegaly. Pulmonary signs include clubbing of the fingers, cyanosis, dyspnea, and decreased arterial oxygen concentration while in an upright position (orthodeoxia). With the exception of liver transplantation, therapy has been ineffective.

***hepatorenal s.*** Renal failure that occurs in patients with liver disease in the absence of clinical, laboratory, or anatomical evidence of other known causes. The disease usually occurs in patients with alcoholic cirrhosis, but cirrhosis is not necessary for its development. Most patients with this syndrome die.

***Horner's s.*** A condition marked by contracted pupils and ptosis, enophthalmos, and a dry, cool face on the affected side produced by paralysis of sympathetic nerves. It is caused by tumors in the neck, trauma, apical tuberculosis, tabes, syringomyelia, and neuritis of the cervical plexus.

***HTLV-1 induced lymphoproliferative s.*** A disease seen in persons infected with human T-cell leukemia-lymphoma virus (HTLV-1). The clinical signs are lymphadenopathy, hepatomegaly, splenomegaly, cutaneous infiltration with neoplastic T cells, hypercalcemia, lymphocytosis, and skeletal changes. Most of these patients develop T-cell leukemia.

TREATMENT: Patients are treated with combination chemotherapy. The median duration of remission is 12 months.

***idiopathic hyperkinetic heart s.*** Hyperactivity of the heart not due to a disease process. Its cause is unknown and it is benign. No treatment is required.

***iliotibial band s.*** ABBR: ITB or IT band. An inflammatory overuse syndrome caused by mechanical friction between the iliotibial band and the lateral femoral condyle. It is commonly seen in distance runners and cyclists. Pain is manifested over the lateral aspect of the knee along the iliotibial band with no effusion of the knee.

***impingement s.*** The compromise of soft tissues in the subacromial space, causing pain with overhead motions or rotational motions with an abducted arm (e.g., throwing). This syndrome is seen in repetitive overhead activities. It is treated with rotator cuff strengthening exercises, anti-inflammatory medications, and subacromial steroid injection. If conservative management fails, subacromial decompression (acromioplasty) is used.

***incompetent palatal s.*** Incomplete or ineffective separation by the soft palate of the nasopharynx from the oropharynx, characterized by hypernasality and distortion of speech called whinolalia. This syndrome may be due to congenital or acquired defects of the palate or to psychiatric disorders.

***irritable bowel s.*** ABBR: IBS. A syndrome that is probably a group of disorders that manifest themselves in various ways so that some symptoms present in some patients but not in others. The cause of these variations in symptomatology is thought to be related to the different causes of IBS. The diagnostic criteria for IBS are (1) abdominal pain or discomfort relieved with defecation or associated with a change in frequency or consistency of stools and (2) an irregular pattern of defecation at least 25% of the time, consisting of three or more of the following: altered stool frequency, altered stool form (hard or loose and watery), altered stool passage (straining or urgency, feeling of incomplete evacuation), passage of mucus, and bloating or feeling of abdominal distention. Although these criteria may not be perfect, they were developed as a consensus and do provide a useful definition. Abdominal pain and altered bowel habits are nonspecific symptoms present in many illnesses. SEE: *disease, inflammatory bowel.*

Epidemiological data are not firmly established because it is estimated that only 14% to 50% of adults with symptoms of IBS seek medical attention. Nevertheless, IBS is reported in 10% to 20% of adults, with a slight predominance in women. Patients with IBS who seek medical attention have an increased prevalence of psychiatric diagnoses, including anxiety, depression, and somatization. Though psychosocial factors are not thought to cause the symptoms of IBS, they influence how the illness is experienced and acted upon by the patient. A cause and effect link between stress and IBS has not been proved.

TREATMENT: Management of IBS should begin with establishing a therapeutic physician-patient relationship and educating the patient about the benign nature of the illness and the excellent long-term prognosis. Initial recommendations are concerned with dietary modifications that may lessen the symptoms. Foods that the patient has found to cause difficulties are eliminated (dairy foods and gas-forming foods often cause symptoms). A number of medications are used in treating IBS, but evidence that any therapy is effective is lacking. Even so an individual patient may benefit from a particular medicine because of the placebo effect. In addition, though drugs do not offer a cure, specific symptoms can be alleviated with antidiarrheal agents or antispasmodics. Alternative therapy, including psychotherapy, hypnotherapy, imagery, and biofeedback alone or in combination may be effective in some patients. SEE: *Crohn's disease.*

***Korsakoff's s.*** A psychosis, ordinarily due to chronic alcoholism, with polyneuritis, disorientation, insomnia, muttering delirium, hallucinations, and a bilateral wrist drop or footdrop.

***lactase deficiency s.*** An absence of the lactase enzyme in intestinal mucosa, leading to abdominal cramps, bloating, and diarrhea in persons who ingest lactase. This enzyme deficiency may be hereditary but can be present in almost any digestive tract disease that damages the intestinal mucosa. The treatment for this syndrome is avoidance of milk. SEE: *breath test for lactase deficiency; yogurt.*

***lip-pit s.*** SEE: *Van der Woude's syndrome.*

***locked-in s.*** Pseudocoma in patients who are awake but have no means of communication. They cannot talk or move limbs or face muscles. The syndrome is due to infarction or hemorrhage into the brain in the central pons area. The ability to move the eyes vertically and to blink are generally normal, and those movements may be used to give signals and respond to questions.

***long QT s.*** QT s.

***maxillofacial s.*** Maxillofacial dysostosis.

***multiple chemical sensitivity s.*** ABBR: MCSS. A condition in which some persons experience physical symptoms allegedly related to prolonged exposure to low levels of environmental pollutants. Current evidence to support this concept is insufficient to establish MCSS as an accepted clinical diagnosis.

***myeloplastic s.*** ABBR: MDS. Any of a group of disorders of the blood termed refractory anemias because they do not respond to any known treatment. Even though these disorders are acquired, the cause is unknown. Some of the patients will eventually develop leukemia. Many cases require no treatment. Those who do are treated symptomatically.

***nursing-bottle s.*** Tooth decay that results when an infant is allowed to drink from a nursing bottle for a prolonged period. The sugar in the bottle contents promotes bacterial growth on the tooth surface.

***ovarian hyperstimulation s.*** ABBR: OHSS. A potentially life-threatening complication that occurs in some women having induced ovulation for in vitro fertilization. The acute onset occurs within the first week ovulation is induced and is characterized by marked cystic ovarian enlargement, ascites, hydrothorax, arterial hypotension, tachycardia, hemoconcentration, oliguria, sodium retention, hypernatremia, and in severe cases renal failure. Treatment includes symptomatic therapy to maintain circulatory function, bed rest, low sodium diet, and diuretic therapy.

***Persian Gulf s.*** ABBR: PGS. A general term used to describe a variety of symptoms experienced by veterans of the Persian Gulf war. Many of the almost 700,000 persons involved in the Persian Gulf war, 1990–1991, have reported fatigue, loss of memory, muscle and joint pains, shortness of breath, and symptoms of respiratory and gastrointestinal complaints. The cause of these complaints remains obscure. The conclusion is that there is no single disease or syndrome apparent but rather multiple illnesses with overlapping symptoms and causes. It has been recommended that the veterans' reports of ill health not be lumped into one syndrome.

***POEMS s.*** A rare multisystem disease characterized by the presence of polyneuropathy, organomegaly, endocrinopathy, monoclonal gammopathy, and skin changes. It often presents with osteosclerotic bone lesions associated with plasma cell dyscrasia. Whether or not POEMS is a distinct disease is controversial. The cause in unknown.

***postcardiotomy s.*** Postpericardiotomy s.

***postconcussion s.*** The persistence of fatigue, dizziness, headache, and difficulty in concentrating after mild head injury.

***postfall s.*** The inability to stand or walk without support for fear of repeating a fall. It is not associated with any physical disability and usually occurs in the elderly.

***postmaturity s.*** A condition occurring in infants born after 42 weeks' gestation who exhibit signs of perinatal compromise related to diminished intrauterine oxygenation and nutrition secondary to placental insufficiency. During labor the fetal monitor may display late decelerations, and fetal hypoxia may result in meconium expulsion and aspiration. Characteristic assessment findings include skin desquamation and an absence of lanugo and vernix caseosa. Laboratory findings may include polycythemia and hypoglycemia. Postmature infants may also be at increased risk of cold stress due to diminished subcutaneous fat.

***postpericardiotomy s.*** Fever, pericardial friction rub, and chest pain occurring several days or weeks after cardiac surgery. The syndrome appears to be an autoimmune response to damaged cardiac cells. Congestive heart failure may ensue.

SYN: *postcardiotomy s.*

***posttachycardia s.*** Secondary ST and T wave changes associated with decreased filling of the coronary arteries and subsequent ischemia during tachycardia.

***Prader-Willi s.*** A rare congenital condition marked by genetic obesity, mental retardation, short stature, sexual infantilism, and hypotonia. The cause is an abnormal chromosome 15 of maternal origin. SEE: *Angelman s.*

***QT s.*** A syndrome marked by a prolonged Q-T interval combined with torsades de pointes. This condition may be congenital or may be acquired as a result of drug administration. Also called *prolonged QT interval syndrome* or *long QT syndrome.*

***refeeding s.*** The potentially fatal metabolic response of a starved individual to feeding, either enteral or parenteral. The correction of electrolyte imbalances is imperative before gradual refeeding to prevent cardiac and respiratory failure.

***Rendu-Osler-Weber s.*** Hereditary hemorrhagic telangiectasia.

***sepsis s.*** The signs and symptoms caused by significant hypotension and inadequate blood and oxygen flow to organs as the result of serious systemic infection. Chemical mediators of inflammation and the cell-mediated immune response, particularly tumor necrosis factors and interleukins, cause the physiological changes that produce clinical signs. Initially there is vasodilation, increased vascular perfusion, and movement of plasma out of blood vessels, producing hypovolemia and hypotension. Compensatory vasoconstriction occurs in an effort to maintain blood flow to vital organs; as sepsis progresses, the vasoconstriction produces tissue hypoxia and organ dysfunction. Tissue hypoxia is increased by abnormal stimulation of the coagulation cascade and by neutrophil aggregation in the capillaries, which produce microthrombi. Within the lung, damage to the capillary endothelium may cause adult respiratory distress syndrome. The classic clinical signs include fever, hypotension, hypoxemia, tachycardia, respiratory distress, oliguria, coagulopathy, decreased level of consciousness, petechiae, and multiple organ failure.

TREATMENT: A third-generation cephalosporin (e.g., ceftriaxone) or extended-spectrum penicillin (e.g., ticarcillin) plus an aminoglycoside (e.g., amikacin) provides antibiotic coverage until an organism is positively identified. Fluid and electrolyte balance must be maintained; vasopressors such as dopamine or dobutamine are used to stabilize blood pressure. Use of corticosteroids is not supported by research.

***shoulder-hand s.*** Reflex sympathetic dystrophy.

***sick sinus s.*** SEE: *sick sinus syndrome.*

***skin-eye s.*** A syndrome consisting of deposits on the anterior surface of the lens and posterior cornea, and skin pigmentation. It is due to extensive medication with some of the phenothiazine-type tranquilizers. SEE: *iatrogenic disorder.*

***Stokes-Adams s.*** A syndrome of bradycardia with loss of consciousness caused by decreased blood flow to the brain. It is caused by partial or complete heart block.

***supine hypotensive s.*** A profound fall in blood pressure in a pregnant woman who is lying flat on her back, caused by impaired venous return due to compression of the inferior vena cava by the enlarged gravid uterus. This condition occurs most commonly in late pregnancy. SYN: *vena caval s.*

***s. of inappropriate antidiuretic hormone*** ABBR: SIADH. A syndrome of increased ADH activity in spite of reduced plasma osmolarity. Often first recognized by a relative hyponatremia, it is most commonly associated with disorders of the central nervous system, various tumors, and drugs.

***systemic inflammatory response s.*** An acute illness marked by generalized activation of the endothelial cells in response to infectious and noninfectious conditions such as trauma, burns, pancreatitis, adrenal insufficiency, pulmonary embolism, dissecting or ruptured aortic aneurysm, myocardial infarction, anaphylaxis, or drug overdose. The condition is seen in a severe form when shock is the result of gram-negative bacteremia. In this syndrome, the cytokines interleukin-1 and tumor necrosis factor stimulate the endothelial cells to act as coagulants rather than anticoagulants. Response to infectious and noninfectious conditions such as trauma, burns, pancreatitis, adrenal insufficiency, pulmonary embolism, dissecting or ruptured aortic aneurysm, myocardial infarction, anaphylaxis, or drug overdose. Therapy directed at blockage of these cytokines has been tried.

***toxic shock s.*** SEE: *toxic shock syndrome.*

***vena caval s.*** Supine hypotensive s.

***Weber's s.*** Paralysis of the hypoglossal nerve on one side and of the oculomotor nerve on the other, with paralysis of the limbs owing to a lesion of a cerebral peduncle.

**synechia** (sĭn-ĕk′ē-ă) *pl.* **synechiae** [Gr. *synecheia,* continuity] An adhesion of parts, esp. adhesion of the iris to the lens and cornea.

***annular s.*** An adhesion of the iris to the lens throughout its entire pupillary margin.

***anterior s.*** An adhesion of the iris to the cornea.

***posterior s.*** An adhesion of the iris to the capsule of the lens.

***total s.*** An adhesion of the entire surface of the iris to the lens.

***s. vulvae*** Fusion of the vulvae, usually congenital.

**synechotomy** (sĭn″ĕk-ŏt′ō-mē) [″ + *tome,* incision] The division of a synechia or adhesion.

**synechtenterotomy** (sĭn″ĕk-tĕn″tĕr-ŏt′ō-mē) [″ + *enteron,* intestine, + *tome,* incision] The division of an intestinal adhesion.

**synecology** (sĭn″ē-kŏl′ō-jē) [Gr. *syn,* together, + *oikos,* house, + *logos,* word, reason] The study of organisms in relationship to their environment in group form.

**synencephalocele** (sĭn″ĕn-sĕf′ă-lō-sēl″) [″ + *enkephalos,* brain, + *kele,* tumor, swelling] An encephalocele with adhesions to adjacent structures.

**syneresis** (sĭn-ĕr′ĕ-sĭs) [Gr. *synairesis,* drawing together] The contraction of a gel resulting in its separation from the liquid, as a shrinkage of fibrin when blood clots.

**synergetic** (sĭn″ĕr-jĕt′ĭk) [Gr. *syn,* together, + *ergon,* work] Exhibiting cooperative action, said of certain muscles; working together. SYN: *synergic.*

**synergia** (sĭn-ĕr′jē-ă) The association and correlation of the activity of synergetic muscle groups.

**synergic** (sĭn-ĕr′jĭk) [″ + *ergon,* work] Rel. to or exhibiting cooperation, as certain muscles. SYN: *synergetic.*

**synergism** (sĭn′ĕr-jĭzm) [″ + ″ + *-ismos,* condition] The harmonious action of two agents, such as drugs or organs, producing an effect that neither could produce alone or one that is greater than the total effects of each agent operating by itself.

**synergist** (sĭn′ĕr-jĭst) **1.** A remedy that acts to enhance the action of another. SYN: *adjuvant.* **2.** A muscle or organ functioning in cooperation with another, as the flexor muscles; the opposite of antagonist.

**synergistic** (sĭn″ĕr-jĭs′tĭk) **1.** Concerning synergy. **2.** Acting together.

**synergy** (sĭn′ĕr-jē) [Gr. *synergia*] An action of two or more agents or organs working with each other, cooperating. Their action is combined and coordinated. SEE: *synergism.*

**synesthesia** (sĭn″ĕs-thē′zē-ă) [Gr. *syn,* together, + *aisthesis,* sensation] **1.** A sensation in one area from a stimulus applied to another part. **2.** A subjective sensation of a sense other than the one being stimulated. Hearing a sound may also produce the sensation of smell. SEE: *phonism.*

***s. algica*** Painful synesthesia.

**synesthesialgia** (sĭn″ĕs-thē-zē-ăl′jē-ă) [″ + ″ + *algos,* pain] A painful sensation giving rise to a subjective one of different character. SEE: *synesthesia.*

**Syngamus** (sĭn′gă-mŭs) A genus of nematode worms parasitic in the respiratory tract of birds and mammals.

***S. laryngeus*** A species normally parasitic in ruminants but sometimes accidentally infesting humans.

**syngamy** (sĭn′gă-mē) [Gr. *syn,* together, + *gamos,* marriage] **1.** Sexual reproduction. **2.** The final stage of fertilization in which the haploid chromosome sets from the male and female gametes come together following breakdown of the pronuclear membranes to form the zygote. SYN: *sexual reproduction.*

**syngeneic** Descriptive of individuals or cells without detectable tissue incompatibility. Strains of mice that are inbred for a great number of generations become syngeneic. Identical twins may be syngeneic.

**syngenesis** (sĭn-jĕn′ĕ-sĭs) [″ + *genesis,* generation, birth] Arising from the germ cells derived from both parents, rather than from a single cell from one parent.

**syngnathia** (sĭn-nā′thē-ă) [″ + *gnathos,* jaw] Congenital adhesions between the jaws.

**synizesis** (sĭn″ĭ-zē′sĭs) [Gr. *synizesis*] **1.** An occlusion or shutting. **2.** A clumping of nuclear chromatin during the prophase of mitosis.

***s. pupillae*** Closure of the pupil of the eye with loss of vision.

**synkaryon** (sĭn-kăr′ē-ŏn) [Gr. *syn,* together, + *karyon,* kernel] A nucleus resulting from fusion of two pronuclei.

**synkinesis** (sĭn″kĭ-nē′sĭs) [″ + *kinesis,* movement] An involuntary movement of one part occurring simultaneously with reflex or voluntary movement of another part.

***imitative s.*** An involuntary movement in a healthy or normal muscle accompanying an attempted movement of a paralyzed muscle on the opposite side.

**synnecrosis** (sĭn″nĕ-krō′sĭs) [″ + *nekrosis,* state of death] The condition of association between groups or individuals that causes mutual inhibition or death.

**synonym** (sĭn′ō-nĭm) [Gr. *synonymon*] ABBR: syn. One of two words that have the same or very similar meaning; an additional or substitute name for the same disease, sign, symptom, or anatomical structure.

**synophrys** (sĭn-ŏf′rĭs) [Gr. *syn,* together, + *ophrys,* eyebrow] A condition in which the eyebrows grow across the midline.

**synophthalmus** (sĭn″ŏf-thăl′mŭs) [″ + *ophthalmos,* eye] Cyclops.

**synopsia** (sĭn′ŏp-sē-ă) [″ + *opsis,* vision] A condition in which there is a congenital fusion of the eyes.

**synopsis** (sĭn-ŏp′sĭs) [Gr.] A summary; a general review of the whole.

**synoptophore** (sĭn-ŏp′tō-for) [″ + *ops,* sight, + *phoros,* bearing] An apparatus for diagnosis and treatment of strabismus. SYN: *synoptoscope.*

**synoptoscope** (sĭn-ŏp′tō-skōp) [″ + ″ + *skopein,* to examine] Synoptophore.

**synorchidism, synorchism** (sĭn-or′kĭd-ĭzm, -kĭzm) [″ + *orchis,* testicle, + *-ismos,* condition] The union or partial fusion of the testicles.

**synoscheos** (sĭn-ŏs′kē-ŏs) [″ + *oscheon,* scrotum] An adhesion between the penis and scrotum.

**synosteology** (sĭn″ŏs-tē-ŏl′ō-jē) [″ + ″ + *logos,* word, reason] The branch of medical science concerned with joints and articulations.

**synosteosis** (sĭn″ŏs-tē-ō′sĭs) Synostosis.

**synosteotomy** (sĭn″ŏs-tē-ŏt′ō-mē) [″ + *osteon,* bone, + *tome,* incision] Dissection of joints.

**synostosis** (sĭn″ŏs-tō′sĭs) *pl.* **synostoses** [″ + ″ + *osis,* condition] **1.** Articulation by osseous tissue of adjacent bones. **2.** Union of separate bones by osseous tissue.

**synostotic** (sĭn″ŏs-tŏt′ĭk) [″ + ″ + *osis,* condition] Concerning synostosis.

**synotia** (sĭn-ō′shē-ă) [″ + *ous,* ear] The union of, or approximation of, the ears occurring in embryonic development, usually associated with absence of, or incomplete development of, the lower jaw.

**synotus** (sī-nō′tŭs) [″ + *ous,* ear] A fetus with synotia.

**synovectomy** (sĭn″ō-vĕk′tō-mē) [L. *synovia,* joint fluid, + Gr. *ektome,* excision] Excision of the synovial membrane.

**synovia** (sĭn-ō′vē-ă) [L.] Synovial fluid.

**synovial** (sĭn-ō′vē-ăl) Pert. to synovia, the lubricating fluid of the joints.

**synovial bursa** Bursa.

**synovial crypt** Diverticulum of a synovial membrane of a joint.

**synovial cyst** Accumulation of synovia in a bursa, synovial crypt, or sac of a synovial hernia, causing a tumor.

**synovial fluid** Clear viscid lubricating fluid of the joint, bursae, and tendon sheaths, secreted by the synovial membrane of a joint. It contains mucin, albumin, fat, and electrolytes. SYN: *synovia.* SEE: *joint, synovial* for illus.

**synovial fold** One of the smooth folds of synovial membrane on the inner surface of the joint capsule. SYN: *plica, synovial.*

**synovial hernia** Protrusion of a portion of synovial membrane through a tear in the stratum fibrosum of a joint capsule.

**synovial tendon sheath** One of the sheaths that develop in osteofibrous canals through which tendons pass. Each is a double-layered tube, the space between the two layers being occupied by synovial fluid. SYN: *vagina mucosa tendinis.*

**synovial villi** Slender avascular processes on the free surface of a synovial membrane projecting into the joint cavity.

**synovioma** (sĭn″ō-vē-ō′mă) [L. *synovia,* joint fluid, + Gr. *oma,* tumor] A tumor arising from a synovial membrane.

**synoviparous** (sĭn″ō-vĭp′ă-rŭs) [″ + *parere,* to produce] Forming synovia.

**synovitis** (sĭn″ō-vī′tĭs) [″ + Gr. *itis,* inflammation] Inflammation of a synovial membrane. Simple inflammation may be the result of an aseptic wound, a subcutaneous injury (contusion or sprain), irritation produced by damaged cartilage, or exposure to cold and dampness. SEE: *Nursing Diagnoses Appendix.*

SYMPTOMS: The joint is painful, much more so on motion, esp. at night. It is swollen and tense. The condition may fluctuate. In synovitis of the knee, the patella is floated up from the condyles, and it can be readily depressed, to rise again when pressure is taken off. The part is never in full extension, as this increases the pain. Skin, which is very sensitive to pressure only at certain points, is neither thickened nor reddened. After a few days, when pain lessens and swelling diminishes as the effusion and extravasated blood are absorbed, the limb returns to its natural position, and recovery follows.

***chronic s.*** Synovitis in which an undue amount of fluid remains in the cavity and the membrane itself is edematous. Later, if the disease does not subside, membrane and articular structures become irregularly thickened by plastic exudation and formation of fibrous tissue. The joint is weak but not esp. painful, except on pressure and sometimes not even then. Movements, esp. in extension, are restricted, and generally attended by some grating or creaking. Symptoms are well marked when there is great accumulation of liquid. Fluid, which is straw-colored, somewhat viscid, sometimes flocculent, and may or may not be bloodstained, can be drawn off with a hypodermic needle.

***dendritic s.*** Synovitis with villous growths developing in the sac.

***dry s.*** Synovitis with little or no effusion. SYN: *s. sicca.*

***purulent s.*** Synovitis with purulent effusion within the sac. SYN: *suppurative arthritis.*

***serous s.*** Synovitis with nonpurulent, copious effusion.

***s. sicca*** Dry s.

***simple s.*** Synovitis with only slightly turbid, if not clear, effusion.

***tendinous s.*** Inflammation of a tendon sheath. SYN: *vaginal s.*

***vaginal s.*** Tendinous s.

***vibration s.*** Synovitis resulting from a wound near a joint.

**synovium** (sĭn-ō′vē-ŭm) [L. *synovia,* joint fluid] A synovial membrane.

**syntactic** (sĭn-tăk′tĭk) Concerning or affecting syntax.

**syntaxis** (sĭn-tăk′sĭs) [″ + *taxis,* arrangement] A junction between two bones. SYN: *articulation.*

**synthase** Synthetase.

**synthermal** (sĭn-thĕr′măl) [″ + *therme,* heat] Having the same temperature.

**synthesis** (sĭn′thĕs-ĭs) [Gr.] In chemistry, the union of elements to produce compounds; the process of building up. In general, the process or processes involved in the formation of a complex substance from simpler elements or compounds, as the synthesis of proteins from amino acids. Synthesis is the opposite of decomposition.

**synthesize** (sĭn″thĕ-sīz′) To produce by synthesis.

**synthetase** (sĭn′thĕ-tās) An enzyme that acts as a catalyst for joining two molecules with the loss or splitting off of a high-energy phosphate group. SYN: *ligase; synthase.*

**synthetic** (sĭn-thĕt′ĭk) [Gr. *synthetikos*] Rel. to or made by synthesis; artificially prepared.

**synthorax** (sĭn-thō′răks) [Gr. *syn,* together, + *thorax,* chest] Thoracopagus.

**syntone** (sĭn′tōn) [″ + *tonos,* act of stretching, tension] An individual whose personality indicates a stable responsiveness to the environment and its social demands. SEE: *syntonic.*

**syntonic** (sĭn-tŏn′ĭk) Pert. to a personality characterized by an even temperament, a normal emotional responsiveness to life situations; the opposite of schizoid. SEE: *syntone.*

**syntonin** (sĭn′tō-nĭn) An acid albumin formed by the action of dilute hydrochloric acid on muscle during gastric digestion.

**syntoxoid** (sĭn-tŏk′soyd) [Gr. *syn,* together, + *toxikon,* poison, + *eidos,* form, shape] A toxoid having the same degree of affinity for an antitoxin as that possessed by the toxin.

**syntrophism** (sĭn′trōf-ĭzm) [″ + *trophe,* nourishment, + *-ismos,* condition] Stimulation of an organism to grow by mixing with or through the closeness of another strain.

**syntrophoblast** (sĭn-trŏf′ō-blăst) [″ + ″ + *blastos,* germ] The outer syncytial layer of the trophoblast. SEE: *trophoblast.*

**syntropic** (sĭn-trŏp′ĭk) [″ + *trope,* a turn] Concerning syntropy.

**syntropy** (sĭn′trō-pē) [″ + *trope,* a turn] Turning or pointing in the same direction.

**synulosis** (sĭn″ū-lō′sĭs) [Gr. *synoulosis*] The formulation of scar tissue.

**synulotic** (sĭn″ū-lŏt′ĭk) **1.** Promoting cicatrization. **2.** An agent stimulating cicatrization.

**syphilid(e)** (sĭf″ĭl-ĭd) *pl.* **syphilides** [Fr.] A skin eruption caused by secondary syphilis.

**syphiliphobia** (sĭf″ĭl-ĭ-fō′bē-ă) [″ + Gr. *phobos,* fear] Syphilophobia (1).

**syphilis** (sĭf′ĭ-lĭs) [*Syphilis,* shepherd having the disease in a Latin poem] An infectious, chronic venereal disease marked by lesions that may involve any organ or tissue. Cutaneous manifestions usually occur, relapses are frequent, and the disease may exist without symptoms for years. SYN: *lues.* SEE: illus.; *Universal Precautions Appendix.*

SYMPTOMS: *Primary stage:* Initial lesion appears 2 to 4 weeks after inoculation, changing from a small red papule to a small ulcer to a hard chancre. The lesion is found usually on the prepuce or vulva but may be on any skin or mucous membrane site. Lymph nodes enlarge about 2 weeks after the appearance of the lesion.

*Secondary stage:* Symptoms appear about 6 weeks after the primary lesion occurs, principally in the form of lesions of the skin and mucous membranes. The character of the skin lesions is protean; syphilis is often called the "great imitator." Systemic symptoms such as head-

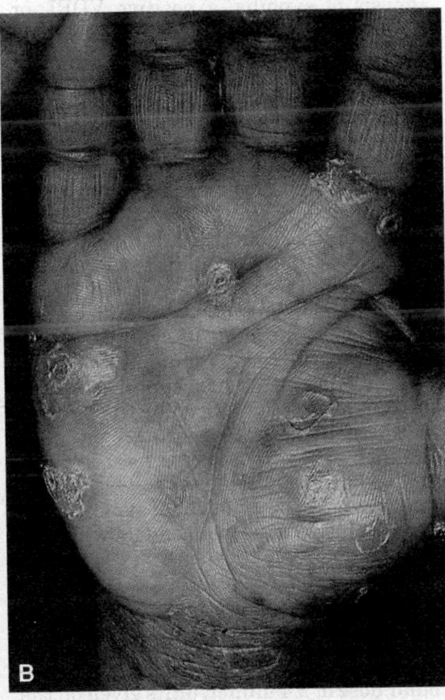


**SYPHILIS**

SECONDARY SYPHILITIC RASH ON **(A)** BACK AND **(B)** PALM

ache, fever, and malaise are common but may be absent. Enlargement and induration of regional lymph nodes occur. Eruptions of skin, maculae (roseola), syphilides, and reddish-brown coppery spots continue for a week or two and may recur later.

*Tertiary stage:* The heart and blood vessels (cardiovascular syphilis) and the central nervous system (neurosyphilis) are frequently involved. Tabes dorsalis, paresis (dementia paralytica), and various types of psychoses may result.

ETIOLOGY: The causative organism is *Treponema pallidum,* a spirochete that is usually transmitted by sexual contact, or in utero by the passage of the spirochete from mother to fetus, and rarely by contact of broken skin with contaminated objects. The bacteria may enter through broken skin or any mucous membrane.

DIAGNOSIS: Laboratory tests for syphilis are based on three procedures: *microscopic,* dark-field demonstration of spirochetes in material taken from a chancre or other early lesion; *biopsy,* examination of cerebrospinal fluid; *serologic tests for syphilis* (S.T.S.), done on blood and spinal fluid. The VDRL (Venereal Disease Research Laboratory), microhemagglutination assay for antibody to *T. pallidum* immobilization (MAA-TP), fluorescent treponemal antibody absorbed (FTA-Abs), and rapid plasma reagin (RPR) tests also are useful in diagnosing syphilis and distinguishing it from biological false-positive serologic reactions. To establish a diagnosis of syphilis, a positive VDRL or RPR test must be confirmed by an FTA-Abs test. Serological tests for syphilis yield negative results during the primary and early secondary stages of the disease.

---

Caution: A person who contracts gonorrhea also may have been exposed to syphilis at the same time. Because the clinical signs and symptoms of gonorrhea develop several weeks before those of syphilis, the patient may be treated for that disease. The treatment for gonorrhea may be sufficient to mask or delay the signs of syphilis but insufficient to rid the patient of the spirochetes. When this occurs, syphilis will develop and may be unnoticed by the patient. It is therefore of vital importance either to treat each case of gonorrhea as if syphilis had also been contracted, or to test the patient for serological evidence of syphilis each month for at least 4 months following the treatment for gonorrhea.

---

TREATMENT: The treatment of choice for all types and stages of syphilis is long-acting penicillin G in a single intramuscular dose of 2.4 million units given on the day of diagnosis. Should allergic reactions occur, other antibiotics (doxycycline or tetracycline) may be substituted.

NURSING IMPLICATIONS: The nurse teaches the patient about the illness and the importance of locating all contacts, treatment, and follow-up care. Penicillin is administered as prescribed or an alternative antibiotic if the patient is allergic to penicillin. The patient is referred to a public health agency to assist in identifying contacts. Preventive methods are taught, and supportive counseling is provided. The nurse should use caution when handling laboratory specimens. The patient should avoid sexual contact with anyone until the full course of therapy has been completed, including previous partners who have not received adequate evaluation and treatment, if indicated, for syphilis. Secretory precautions are instituted from the time the disease is suspected until 24 hr after initiation of proper antibiotic therapy. SEE: *Universal Precautions Appendix.*

***cardiovascular s.*** Syphilis involving the heart and great blood vessels, esp. the aorta. Saccular aneurysms of the aorta and aortic insufficiency frequently result.

***congenital s.*** Syphilis transmitted from the mother to the fetus in utero. Transplacental fetal infection may occur if a pregnant woman is not treated by the 18th week of gestation or contracts the disease later in pregnancy. SYN: *prenatal s.* SEE: *Nursing Diagnoses Appendix.*

***endemic s.*** Chronic, nonvenereal syphilis infection of childhood. It is characterized in its early stages by mucocutaneous or membrane lesions. Later, gummas of bone and skin occur. The causative organism is *T. pallidum.* Penicillin is the treatment of choice.

***extragenital s.*** Syphilis in which the primary chancre is located elsewhere than on genital organs.

***latent s.*** The phase of syphilis during which symptoms are absent and the disease can be diagnosed only by serological tests.

***meningovascular s.*** A form of neurosyphilis in which the meninges and vascular structures of the brain and spinal cord are involved. It may be localized or general.

***neuro-s.*** Involvement of the nervous system by syphilis.

***prenatal s.*** Congenital s.

***visceral s.*** Syphilis in which visceral organs are involved.

**syphilitic** (sĭf″ĭ-lĭt′ĭk) [L. *syphiliticus*] Rel. to, caused by, or affected with syphilis.

**syphilitic macule** One of the small red eruptions manifested in secondary syphilis, often covering the entire body. These eruptions are associated with chancre or scar, alopecia, pain in bones, swollen glands, and sore throat.

**syphiloderm, syphiloderma** (sĭf′ĭl-ō-dĕrm″, sĭf″ĭl-ō-dĕr′mă) [″ + Gr. *derma,* skin] A syphilitic cutaneous disorder.

**syphiloid** (sĭf′ĭ-loyd) [″ + Gr. *eidos,* form,

shape] Resembling syphilis.

**syphilology** (sĭf″ĭl-ŏl′ō-jē) The study of syphilis and its treatment.

**syphiloma** (sĭf″ĭl-ō′mă) [″ + Gr. *oma,* tumor] A syphilitic tumor; a gumma.

**syphilomania** (sĭf″ĭl-ō-mā′nē-ă) [″ + Gr. *mania,* madness] Syphilophobia (1).

**syphilophobia** (sĭf″ĭl-ō-fō′bē-ă) [″ + Gr. *phobos,* fear] **1.** A morbid fear of syphilis. **2.** A delusion of having syphilis.

**syphilophobic** (sĭf″ĭl-ō-fō′bĭk) Pert. to or affected with syphilophobia.

**syphilotherapy** (sĭf″ĭl-ō-thĕr′ă-pē) [″ + Gr. *therapeia,* treatment] The treatment of syphilis.

**syr** [L., *syrupus*] Syrup.

**syrigmophonia** (sĭr″ĭg-mō-fō′nē-ă) [Gr. *syrigmos,* a whistle, + *phone,* voice] **1.** A sibilant rale. **2.** A whistling sound in pronunciation of "s" due to a denture peculiarity.

**syrigmus** (sĭr-ĭg′mŭs) [Gr. *syrigmos,* a whistle] A subjective sound such as a hissing or ringing heard in the ears.

**syringadenoma** (sĭr-ĭng″ă-dē-nō′mă) [Gr. *syrinx,* pipe, + *aden,* gland, + *oma,* tumor] Tumor of a sweat gland.

**syringe** (sĭr-ĭnj′, sĭr′ĭng) [Gr. *syrinx,* pipe] **1.** An instrument for injecting fluids into cavities or vessels. **2.** To wash out or introduce fluid with a syringe.

***hand s.*** A hollow rubber bulb that is fitted to a nozzle and delivers air when squeezed.

***hypodermic s.*** A syringe, fitted with a needle, used to administer drugs by injecting them into the subcutaneous tissue.

***oral s.*** A syringe made of plastic or glass. It is not fitted with a needle but is graduated and is used to dispense liquid medication to children. The tip is constructed to prevent its breaking in the child's mouth.

**syringectomy** (sĭr″ĭn-jĕk′tō-mē) [″ + *ektome,* excision] Removal of the walls of a fistula.

**syringocarcinoma** (sĭ-rĭng″gō-kăr″sĭ-nō′mă) [″ + *karkinos,* crab, + *oma,* tumor] Carcinoma of a sweat gland.

**syringocele** (sĭr-ĭn′gō-sēl) [″ + *koilia,* cavity] **1.** The central canal of the myelon or spinal cord. **2.** A form of meningomyelocele that contains a cavity in the ectopic spinal cord.

**syringocystadenoma** (sĭr-ĭn″gō-sĭs″tă-dĕ-nō′mă) [″ + *kystis,* bladder, sac, + *aden,* gland, + *oma,* tumor] Adenoma of the sweat glands, characterized by tiny, hard, papular formations.

**syringocystoma** (sĭr-ĭn″gō-sĭs-tō′mă) [″+ ″ + *oma,* tumor] A cystic tumor having its origin in ducts of the sweat gland.

**syringoencephalomyelia** (sĭ-rĭng″gō-ĕn-sĕf″ă-lō-mī-ē′lē-ă) [″ + *enkephalos,* brain, + *myelos,* marrow] A condition of cavities in the brain and spinal cord.

**syringoid** (sĭr-ĭn′goyd) [Gr. *syrinx,* pipe, + *eidos,* form, shape] Resembling a tube; fistulous.

**syringoma** (sĭr″ĭn-gō′mă) [″ + *oma,* tumor] A tumor of the sweat glands.

**syringomeningocele** (sĭr-ĭn″gō-mĕn-ĭn′gō-sēl) [″ + *meninx,* membrane, + *kele,* tumor, swelling] A meningocele that is similar to a syringomyelocele.

**syringomyelia** (sĭr-ĭn″gō-mī-ē′lē-ă) [″ + *myelos,* marrow] A chronic progressive disease of the spinal cord characterized by the development of cavities and gliosis of surrounding tissue. It usually begins before age 30 and is more common among men than among women. Its cause is unknown. SEE: *Nursing Diagnoses Appendix.*

SYMPTOMS: Cavitation occurs in cervical and lumbar regions and soon involves pathways of the cord that carry impulses of pain and temperature sensations, resulting in dissociated sensory loss. Destruction of lateral and anterior gray matter causes muscular atrophy and weakness.

TREATMENT: There is no satisfactory treatment. Sudden enlargement of a cavity may warrant surgical intervention with decompression of the cavity. Persistent pain may necessitate chordotomy or medullary tractotomy for relief.

**syringomyelitis** (sĭr-ĭn″gō-mī″ĕ-lī′tĭs) [″ + *myelos,* marrow, + *itis,* inflammation] Inflammation coincident with abnormal dilation of the central canal of the spinal cord.

**syringomyelocele** (sĭr-ĭn″gō-mī″ĕl-ō-sēl) [″ + ″ + *kele,* tumor, swelling] A form of spina bifida in which the cavity of the projecting portion communicates with the central canal of the spinal cord.

**syringomyelus** (sĭr-ĭn″gō-mī′ĕl-ŭs) An abnormal dilatation of the central canal of the spinal cord.

**syringopontia** (sĭr-ĭn″gō-pŏn′shē-ă) [″ + L. *pons,* bridge] Cavity formation in the pons varolii similar to syringomyelia.

**syringosystrophy** (sĭr-ĭn″gō-sĭs′trō-fē) [″ + *systrophe,* a twist] Twisting of the oviduct.

**syringotomy** (sĭr″ĭn-gŏt′ō-mē) An operation for incision of a fistula.

**syrinx** (sĭr′ĭnks) [Gr., pipe] **1.** A tube or pipe. **2.** A pathological cavity in the spinal cord or brain. **3.** A fistula.

**syrup** (sĭr′ŭp) [L. *syrupus*] ABBR: syr. A concentrated solution of sugar in water to which specific medicinal substances are usually added. Syrups usually do not represent a very high percentage of the active drug. Some syrups are used principally to give a pleasant odor and taste to solutions.

***simple s.*** A combination of purified water and sucrose.

**syssarcosis** (sĭs″ăr-kō′sĭs) [Gr. *syn,* together, + *sarkosis,* fleshy growth] The union of bones by muscles; a muscular articulation such as the hyoid and patella.

**systaltic** (sĭs-tăl′tĭk) [Gr. *systaltikos,* contracting] Pulsating.

**system** (sĭs′tĕm) [Gr. *systema,* a composite whole] **1.** An organized grouping of related structures or parts. **2.** A group of structures or organs related to each other and performing certain functions together (e.g., the digestive system). **3.** A group of cells or aggregations of cells that perform a particular function (e.g., the mononuclear phagocyte, and the cardiovascular, respiratory, and central nervous systems).

***alimentary s.*** Digestive s.

***autonomic nervous s.*** That portion of the peripheral nervous system that innervates all smooth muscle, cardiac muscle, and glands, the activities of which are involuntary. It includes the craniosacral (parasympathetic) and thoracolumbar (sympathetic) divisions, each of which provides fibers for most of the visceral structures or organs. SYN: *vegetative nervous s.; visceral efferent s.*

***cardiovascular s.*** The heart and blood vessels (aorta, arteries, arterioles, capillaries, venules, veins, venae cavae).

***centimeter-gram-second s.*** ABBR: CGS. Metric s.

***central nervous s.*** That portion of the nervous system consisting of the brain and spinal cord.

***chromaffin s.*** The mass of tissue forming paraganglia and medulla of suprarenal glands, which secretes epinephrine and stains readily with chromium salts. Similar tissue is found in the organs of Zuckerkandl and in the liver, testes, ovary, and heart.

***circulatory s.*** A system concerned with circulation of body fluids. It includes the cardiovascular and lymphatic systems.

***conduction s. of the heart*** SEE: *heart, conduction system of.*

***cytochrome s.*** SEE: *cytochrome transport system.*

***digestive s.*** The alimentary canal (oral cavity, pharynx, esophagus, stomach, small and large intestines) and the accessory organs (teeth, tongue, salivary glands, liver, and pancreas). SEE: *digestive system* for illus.; *digestion.*

***endocrine s.*** The ductless glands or the glands of internal secretion, which include the pineal body, pancreas, and paraganglia and the pituitary, thyroid, parathyroid, and adrenal glands as well as the ovaries and testes. SEE: *endocrine gland.*

***extrapyramidal motor s.*** The functional system that includes all descending fibers arising in cortical and subcortical motor centers that reach the medulla and spinal cord by pathways other than recognized corticospinal tracts. The system is important in maintenance of equilibrium and muscle tone.

***genital s.*** Reproductive s.

***genitourinary s.*** The reproductive organs combined with the urinary organs. SEE: *genitalia* for illus.

***haversian s.*** Architectural unit of bone consisting of a central tube (haversian canal) with alternate layers of intercellular material (matrix) surrounding it in concentric cylinders. Alternating layers of matrix and cells are called haversian lamellae.

***health care s.*** An organized system of the various components relating to the provision of health care. Elements include physicians and their assistants, dentists and their associates, nurses and their surrogates, the various levels of diagnostic and care facilities, voluntary organizations, medical administrators including those in hospitals and government agencies, the medical insurance industry, and the pharmaceutical and medical device manufacturers. An ideal health care system would emphasize preventive medicine and encourage preventive self-care; enable access to primary care for assessment of and assistance with health problems; provide secondary or acute care involving emergency medical services and complex medical and surgical services; facilitate tertiary care for patients who need referral to facilities that provide rehabilitative services; offer respite care to allow families temporary relief from the daily tasks of caring for individuals for whom they are responsible; provide continuing supportive services for those whose mental or physical illness or disability is such that they need assistance with everyday tasks of living (e.g., home health and nursing home care); and provide hospice care for those with terminal illnesses.

***hematopoietic s.*** The blood-forming tissues and organs of the body. It includes the bone marrow, spleen, and lymphatic tissue.

***heterogeneous s.*** Any system whose components may be separated mechanically.

***homogeneous s.*** Any system whose components cannot be separated mechanically.

***hypophyseoportal s.*** The series of vessels that lead from the hypothalamus to the anterior lobe of the pituitary. The releasing factors are carried to the pituitary through this system.

***impulse-conducting s.*** A system of atypical muscle fibers (Purkinje fibers) within the heart that conduct impulses regulating contractions of the atria and ventricles. It includes the SA and AV nodes and the bundle of His.

***integumentary s.*** The skin and its derivatives (hair, nails) and the subcutaneous tissue. It is the largest system in the body.

***International s. of Units*** ABBR: SI. The modern version of the metric system. SEE: *SI Units Appendix.*

***lymphatic s.*** The system concerned with lymph circulation, the protection of the body against pathogens, and the establishment of immunity to certain diseases. It includes lymph vessels and ducts and lymphatic organs (lymph nodes, tonsils, thymus, spleen). SEE: *lymph; lymphatic.*

***lymphoreticular s.*** In general, the lymphatic tissue and the reticuloendothelial system. Specifically the system includes fixed and mobile cellular tissue involved in body defense by macrophage activity and immunological mechanisms but does not include the granulocytic cells of the blood (i.e., neutrophils, eosinophils, and basophils.)

***metric s.*** A system of weights and measures based on the meter (39.37 in.) as the unit of linear measure; the gram (15.432 gr) as the unit of weight; and the liter (1.057 qt) as the unit of volume. SYN: *centimeter-gram-second s.* SEE: Metric System and SI Units in *Weights and Measures Appendix.*

***microsomal ethanol oxidizing s.*** ABBR: MEOS. A hepatic enzyme system that catabolizes drugs and other potentially toxic substances. Ethanol ingested in relatively small amounts is catabolized by the hepatic enzyme alcohol dehydrogenase. Whenever ingested amounts of ethanol are large enough to overcome or deplete the alcohol dehydrogenase system, the microsomal ethanol oxidizing system (MEOS) becomes the major route for ethanol catabolism. Ethanol breakdown by the MEOS is not thought to produce as much energy as alcohol dehydrogenase breakdown, resulting in less weight gain than would be expected from the ethanol calories consumed.

***muscular s.*** The system that includes the skeletal muscles and their tendons. SEE: *muscle.*

***needleless intravenous infusion s.*** A device for administering intravenous solutions that permits intravascular access without the necessity of handling a needle. These systems were developed to reduce the number of needle-stick injuries related to traditional intravenous administration of fluids. The possiblity that their use increases the patient's chance of infection is being investigated. SEE: *needle-stick injury.*

***nervous s.*** The system that includes the brain, spinal cord, ganglia, and nerves.

***osseous s.*** The bony structures of the body; the skeleton. SEE: *skeleton.*

***oxygen delivery s.*** An apparatus that provides a concentration of inhaled oxygen greater than that of room air. A *fixed-performance* oxygen delivery system provides a consistent oxygen concentration. A *variable-performance* oxygen delivery system provides an oxygen concentration that may vary with changes in the patient's breathing pattern.

***parasympathetic nervous s.*** SEE: *parasympathetic nervous system.*

***peripheral nervous s.*** That part of the nervous system outside the central nervous system.

***portal s.*** A system of vessels in which blood passes through a capillary network, a large vessel, and then another capillary network before returning to the systemic circulation (e.g., the circulation of blood through the liver).

***prosthetic control s.*** A mechanical system of cables and attachments that, used with a harness, permits the wearer of a prosthetic device to perform desired movements, such as grasping objects.

***reproductive s.*** The gonads and their associated structures and ducts. In the female, this system includes the ovaries, uterine tubes (oviducts), uterus, vagina, and vulva. In the male, it includes the testes, efferent ducts, epididymis, ductus deferens, ejaculatory duct, urethra and accessory glands (bulbourethral, prostate, seminal vesicles), and penis. SYN: *genital s.* SEE: *genitalia* for illus.

***respiratory s.*** The organs involved in the interchange of gases between an organism and the atmosphere. In humans, this system consists of the air passageways and organs (nasal cavities, oral cavity, pharynx, larynx, trachea, and lungs, including bronchi, bronchioles, alveolar ducts, and alveoli) and the respiratory muscles. SEE: illus.; *lung* for illus.

***reticuloendothelial s.*** ABBR: RES. Collectively, all the phagocytic cells of the body, except the leukocytes. This system includes macrophages, histiocytes, Kupffer cells of the liver, reticular cells of the lymphatic organs, the microglia of the brain, and many others. These cells are responsible for phagocytosis of damaged or old cells, cellular debris, foreign substances, and pathogens, removing them from the circulation. They play an important role in the nonspecific immune response. Also called the *mononuclear phagocyte system.*

***seated s.*** Adapted seating device.

***skeletal s.*** The bony framework of the body. SEE: *skeleton.*

***sympathetic nervous s.*** The thoracolumbar division of the autonomic nervous system. Preganglionic fibers originate in the thoracic and lumbar segments of the spinal cord and synapse with postganglionic neurons in the sympathetic ganglia. Most of these ganglia are in two chains lateral to the backbone, and others are within the trunk; postganglionic fibers extend to the organs innervated. Some effects of sympathetic stimulation are increased heart rate, dilation of the bronchioles, dilation of the pupils, vasoconstriction in the skin and viscera, vasodilation in the skeletal muscles, slowing of peristalsis, conversion of glycogen to glucose by the liver, and secretion of epinephrine and norephinephrine by the adrenal medulla. Sympathetic effects are general rather than specific and prepare the body to cope with stressful situations. SEE: *autonomic nervous system* for illus.;

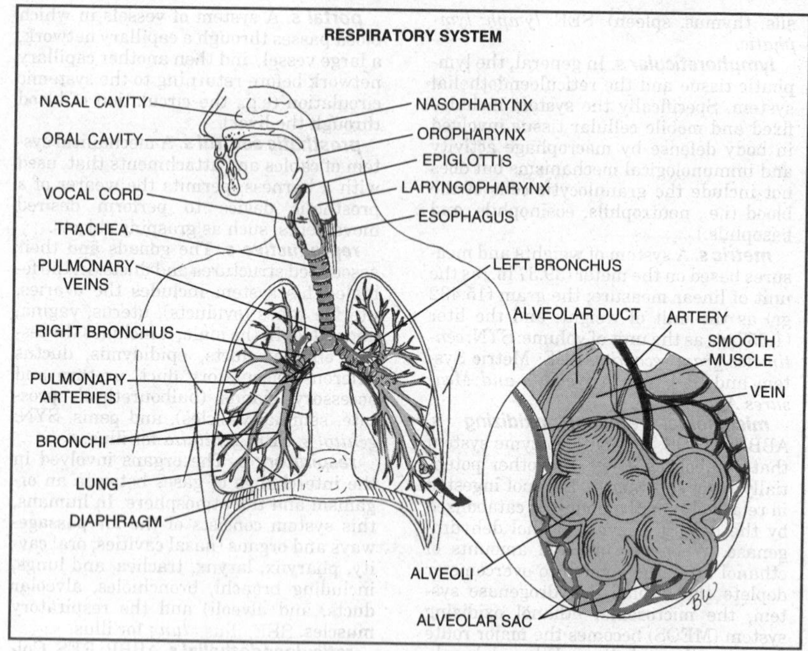


RESPIRATORY SYSTEM

(A) ANTERIOR VIEW, (B) ALVEOLI AND PULMONARY CAPILLARIES

*parasympathetic nervous system.*

***token economy s.*** Any program using positive reinforcement (operant conditioning) to teach or train desired skills or behaviors.

***urinary s.*** The kidneys, ureters, bladder, and urethra.

***urogenital s.*** The urinary and reproductive systems combined. SEE: *genitalia* for illus.

***vascular s.*** The system of all the blood vessels (arteries, capillaries, and veins).

***vasomotor s.*** The part of the nervous system that controls the size of the vascular system vessels.

***vegetative nervous s.*** Autonomic nervous s.

***visceral efferent s.*** Autonomic nervous s.

**systema** (sĭs-tē′mă) [Gr., a composite whole] System.

**systematic** (sĭs″tĕ-măt′ĭk) Concerning a system or organized according to a system.

**systematization** (sĭs-tĕm″ă-tī-zā′shŭn) The process of organizing something according to a plan.

**systemic** (sĭs-tĕm′ĭk) Pert. to a whole body rather than to one of its parts; somatic.

**systemic circulation** The blood flow from the left ventricle through the aorta and all its branches (arteries) to the capillaries of the tissues and its return to the heart through veins and the venae cavae, which empty into the right atrium.

**systemic lupus erythematosus** SEE: under *lupus.*

**systemic remedy** A remedy that acts on the body as a whole.

**systemoid** (sĭs′tĕ-moyd) [″ + *eidos,* form, shape] **1.** Resembling a system. **2.** Pert. to tumors made up of several types of tissues.

**Systems Model** SEE: *Nursing Theory Appendix.*

**systems theory** As used in clinical medicine, an approach that considers the human being as a whole as opposed to his or her parts. Human beings are considered open systems constantly exchanging information, matter, and energy with the environment. There are three levels of reference for systems: the system level on which one is focusing, such as a person; the suprasystems level above the focal system, such as the person's family, community, and culture; and the subsystem, that below the focal system, such as the bodily systems and the cell. Those involved in health care must view persons as being affected constantly by suprasystems and subsystems. Health care, in the systems approach, transcends the idea of treating illness and addresses the larger issue of attaining and maintaining health through assessment and treatment of the total person. SEE: *holism; holistic medicine.*

**systole** (sĭs′tō-lē) [Gr., contraction] Contraction of the chambers of the heart. The myocardial fibers shorten, making the chamber smaller and forcing blood out. In the cardiac cycle, atrial systole precedes ventricular systole, which pumps blood into the aorta and pulmonary artery. SEE: *diastole; murmur; presystole.*

***aborted s.*** A premature cardiac systole in which arterial pressure is increased little if at all because of inadequate filling of ventricles resulting from shortening of the preceding diastole.

***anticipated s.*** A systole that is aborted because it occurs before the ventricle is filled.

***arterial s.*** The rebound or recoil of the stretched elastic walls of the arteries following ventricular systole.

***atrial s.*** The contraction of the atria; it precedes the ventricular systole.

***electrical s.*** The total duration of the QRST complex in an electrocardiogram; it is approx. the same as that of the mechanical systole.

***premature s.*** Extrasystole.

***ventricular s.*** Ventricular contraction.

**systolic** (sĭs-tŏl′ĭk) [Gr. *systole,* contraction] Pert. to the systole.

**systolic discharge** The amount of blood ejected by the heart at each systole.

**systolic murmur** A cardiac murmur during systole.

**systolic pressure** Maximum blood pressure. This occurs during contraction of the ventricle. SEE: *blood pressure; diastolic pressure; pulse; pulse pressure.*

**systremma** (sĭs-trĕm′ă) [Gr. *systremma,* anything twisted together] A cramp in the calf of the leg, the muscles forming a hard knot.

**syzygial** (sĭ-zĭj′ē-ăl) [Gr. *syzygia,* conjunction] Pert. to a syzygium.

**syzygiology** (sĭ-zĭj″ē-ŏl′ō-jē) [″ + *logos,* word, reason] The study of interdependence or interrelationship of the whole as opposed to that of isolated functions or separate parts. SEE: *holism.*

**syzygium** (sĭ-zĭj′ē-ŭm) [Gr. *syzygia,* conjunction] Fusion of two parts or structures without loss of identity of the parts.

**syzygy** (sĭz′ĭ-jē) Fusion of organs, each remaining distinct.

# T

**T** *temperature; time; intraocular tension.*
**t** *temporal;* L. *ter,* three times.
**T1, T2, etc.** *first thoracic nerve, second thoracic nerve,* and so forth.
**$T_{1/2}$, $t_{1/2}$** In nuclear medicine, the symbol of half-life of a radioactive substance.
**$T_3$** *Triiodothyronine.*
**$T_4$** *Thyroxine.*
**T-1824** Evans blue.
**T.A.** *toxin-antitoxin.*
**Ta** Symbol for the element tantalum.
**tabacosis** (tăb″ă-kō′sĭs) [″ + Gr. *osis,* condition] Chronic tobacco poisoning or pneumoconiosis from inhaling tobacco dust.
**tabanid** (tăb′ă-nĭd) [L. *tabanus,* horsefly] A member of the dipterous family Tabanidae.
**Tabanidae** (tă-băn′ĭ-dē) [L. *tabanus,* horsefly] A family of insects belonging to the order Diptera. It includes horseflies, gadflies, deer flies, and mango flies, all bloodsucking insects that attack humans and other warm-blooded animals. Tabanidae is of medical importance because flies serve in the transmission of the filaria worm, *Loa loa,* tularemia, anthrax, and other diseases. Their bites are extremely painful and heal with difficulty.
**Tabanus** (tă-bā′nŭs) [L., horsefly] A genus of flies of the family Tabanidae.
**tabardillo** (tăb″ăr-dē′lyō) [Sp.] An epidemic louse-borne typhus fever occurring in parts of Mexico. SEE: *typhus.*
**tabatière anatomique** (tă-bă″tē-ār′ ă-nă″tō-mēk′) [Fr., anatomical snuffbox] The triangular area of the dorsum of the hand at the base of the thumb. When the thumb is extended, the tendons of the long and short extensor muscles of the thumb bound this area, which appears as a depression. When snuff was used, a small pinch could be placed in this "box" and snuffed up into the nose from that site. Tenderness in this area may be present when the navicular bone is fractured. SYN: *anatomical snuffbox.*
**tabella** (tă-bĕl′ă) *pl.* **tabellae** [L., tablet] A medicated mass of material formed into a small disk. SEE: *lozenge; tablet; troche.*
**tabes** (tā′bēz) [L., wasting disease] A gradual, progressive wasting in any chronic disease.

***diabetic t.*** Peripheral neuritis affecting diabetics; may affect the spinal cord and simulate tabes caused by syphilis.

***t. dorsalis*** Sclerosis of the posterior columns of the spinal cord, caused by infection of the central nervous system with *Treponema pallidum,* the causative agent of syphilis. SYN: *locomotor ataxia.* SEE: *syphilis.*

SYMPTOMS: Postural instability, esp. when the eyes are closed, and a staggering wide-base gait are characteristic of this disease; hence the name locomotor ataxia. Pain and paresthesias are common, esp. lightning pains, described as sharp, stabbing, and paroxysmal. Ankle and knee reflexes are diminished or lost. Many symptoms characteristic of syphilis such as pupillary changes, optic atrophy, bladder disturbances, and development of trophic ulcers, esp. on the feet, make diagnosis certain.

TREATMENT: The patient should be treated for syphilis. Special measures should be taken to relieve severe pains. Rehabilitation measures are often essential for those with disturbed gait.

***t. ergotica*** Tabes resulting from the use of ergot.

***t. mesenterica*** Emaciation and general disorder of the functions of nutrition caused by engorgement and tubercular degeneration of the mesenteric glands.

**tabetic** (tă-bĕt′ĭk) [L. *tabes,* wasting disease] Pert. to or afflicted with tabes.

***t. foot*** Twisted foot in locomotor ataxia.

**tabetiform** (tă-bĕt′ĭ-form) [″ + *forma,* shape] Resembling or characteristic of tabes.
**tablature** (tăb′lă-chūr) The formation of the cranial bones into two outer hard layers and a spongy center, the diploë.
**table** (tā′bl) [L. *tabula,* board] **1.** A flat-topped structure, as an operating table. **2.** A thin flat plate, as of bone.

***periodic t.*** SEE: *periodic table.*

***t.'s of the skull*** The inner and outer condensed layers of the cranial bone separated by diploë (cancellous bony tissue).

***tilt t.*** A table that may be tilted. A person is secured to it, and the circulatory response to various angles of tilt from flat to perpendicular is observed and recorded. It is useful in studying postural hypotension.

***vitreous t.*** The inner cranial table.

***water t.*** The level at which rock or any underground stratum is saturated with water. This overlies an impervious stratum.

**tablespoon** (tā′bl-spoon) ABBR: Tbs. A rough measure using a household spoon. To administer a tablespoon of medicine, 15 ml of the substance should be given.
**tablet** (tăb′lĕt) [O. Fr. *tablete,* a small table] A small, disklike mass of medicinal powder.

***buccal t.*** A tablet designed to be placed in the mouth and held between the cheek and gum until dissolved and absorbed through the buccal mucosa.

***coated t.*** A type of tablet usually made

by coating a compressed substance with sugar or chocolate.

***compressed t.*** A tablet made by forcibly compressing the powdered substances into the desired shape. These tablets may be very hard and not readily soluble.

***dispensing t.*** A tablet that contains a comparatively large amount of the active drug. It is used by pharmacists and dispensing physicians to avoid the necessity of weighing small amounts of a potent drug in filling prescriptions.

***enteric-coated t.*** A tablet with an outer layer that is resistant to dissolution by gastric juices.

***fluoride t.*** A tablet of sodium fluoride for prevention of dental caries.

***hypodermic t.*** A tablet that frequently contains, in addition to the active drug, some agents that produce chemical action when water is added, thus causing a rapid disintegration of the mass. It is used to form injectable solutions.

***sublingual t.*** A small, flat, oval tablet placed beneath the tongue to permit direct absorption of the active substance.

***t. triturate*** A tablet made by moistening the medication mixed with a powdered lactose or sucrose, and then molding it into shape and allowing the liquid to evaporate. They usually disintegrate readily and are a very desirable form for administering certain drugs.

**tablier** (tă-blyā′) [Fr., apron] Pudendal apron; enlarged vulvae. SEE: *Hottentot apron.*

**taboo** [Polynesian *tabu, tapu,* inviolable] An act, object, or social custom separated or set aside as being sacred or profane, thus forbidden for general use.

**taboparalysis** (tā″bō-păr-ăl′ĭ-sĭs) [L. *tabes,* wasting disease, + Gr. *paralyein,* to disable] Tabes associated concurrently with general paralysis. SYN: *taboparesis.*

**taboparesis** (tā″bō-păr-ē′sĭs, -păr′ĕ-sĭs) [″ + Gr. *paresis,* relaxation] Taboparalysis.

**tabophobia** (tā″bō-fō′bē-ă) [″ + Gr. *phobos,* fear] A morbid fear of being afflicted with tabes, a common symptom of neurasthenia.

**tabular** (tăb′ū-lăr) [L. *tabula,* board] **1.** Resembling a table. **2.** Set up in columns, as a tabulation.

***t. bone*** A flat bone, or one with two compact bonelike parts with cancellous tissue between them.

**tabun** Ethyl *N*-dimethylphosphoramidocyanidate; an extremely toxic nerve gas.

**tache** (tŏsh) [Fr., spot] A colored spot or macule on the skin, as a freckle.

***t. bleuâtre*** Macula caerulea.

***t. cérébrale*** The red line that occurs in meningitis and other nervous disorders when a fingernail is drawn across the skin.

***t. motrice*** The motor endplate of a striated muscle fiber.

***t. noire*** A small round or oval ulcer covered by a black scab; the primary lesion of boutonneuse fever and rickettsialpox.

**tachetic** (tăk-ĕt′ĭk) [Fr. *tache,* spot] Marked by purple or reddish blue patches (taches).

**tachistoscope** (tă-kĭs′tō-skōp) [Gr. *tachistos,* swiftest, + *skopein,* to view] A device used to determine the speed of visual perception. The time of exposure can be adjusted so that the length of time needed for detection of the viewed object can be measured.

**tachy-** Combining form meaning *swift, rapid.*

**tachyarrhythmia** (tăk″ē-ă-rĭth′mē-ă) [Gr. *tachys,* swift, + *a,* not, + *rhythmos,* rhythm] Irregularity of heartbeat combined with rapid rate.

**tachycardia** (tăk″ē-kăr′dē-ă) [″ + *kardia,* heart] An abnormal rapidity of heart action, usually defined as a heart rate greater than 100 beats per minute in adults.

***atrial t.*** Rapid heart rate, usually less than 200 beats per minute. The beats arise from an atrial focus.

***atrioventricular reentrant t.*** ABBR: AVNRT. Tachycardia due to the presence of two conduction pathways involving the AV node: the normal (fast) one and the abnormal (slow) one. During normal sinus rhythm, conduction of a stimulus to the atrial myocardium is via the fast pathway. In AVNRT, premature atrial depolarization occurs when the normal fast pathway may be blocked. In that case, the slow pathway transmits the stimulus, reenters the fast pathway and atrial tachycardia is the result. The condition can be treated by radiofrequency ablation of the slow pathway. SEE: *ablation; atrial fibrillation.*

***ectopic t.*** A rapid heartbeat caused by stimuli arising from outside the sinoatrial node.

***essential t.*** Rapid persistent heart action caused by functional disturbance.

***fetal t.*** A fetal heart rate faster than 160 beats per minute that persists throughout one 10-min period.

***nodal t.*** Tachycardia resulting from an increase in rhythmicity of the AV node over the SA node. It may be the result of digitalis therapy.

***pacemaker-mediated t.*** A problem of dual-chamber cardiac pacemakers in which tachycardia develops due to improper functioning of the pacemaker. This can be treated by reprogramming the electronic signals to the atrium.

***paroxysmal atrial t.*** Atrial tachycardia beginning and ending suddenly. The rate is usually from 150 to 240 beats per minute. Short episodes occurring infrequently do not usually require treatment. Longer episodes characterized by significant tachycardia, however, may signify underlying disease.

NURSING IMPLICATIONS: The nurse advises the patient to seek medical assessment if episodes occur frequently and are accompanied by palpitations and anxiety. Valsalva's maneuver can be taught to reduce heart rate during mild episodes.

***paroxysmal nodal t.*** Tachycardia due to increased activity of the AV junctional focus. The rate is usually from 120 to 180 beats per minute.

***paroxysmal supraventricular t.*** Rapid ectopic atrial arrhythmia originating proximal to the His bundle bifurcation. A reentry impulse occurs in the atria, AV node, or His bundle.

***paroxysmal ventricular t.*** Ventricular tachycardia beginning and ending suddenly.

***polymorphic ventricular t.*** Very rapid ventricular tachycardia characterized by a gradually changing QRS complex in the electrocardiogram. It is usually self-limiting but may change into ventricular fibrillation. SYN: *torsade de pointes.*

***reflex t.*** Tachycardia resulting from stimuli outside the heart, reflexly accelerating the heart rate or depressing vagal tone.

***sinus t.*** Uncomplicated tachycardia when the sinus rhythm is faster than 100 beats per minute, as that caused by exercise. Causes other than exercise include hyperthermia, thyrotoxicosis, hemorrhage, anoxia, infections, cardiac failure, and certain drugs such as atropine, epinephrine, and nicotine.

TREATMENT: Tachycardia sometimes ceases following procedures that cause vagal stimulation. Among these are pressure on one or both carotid sinuses, pressure on the eyeballs, induction of gagging or vomiting, attempted expiration with glottis closed, lying down with the feet in the air, and bending over. If these procedures when employed singly are unsuccessful, two or more combined may produce desirable results. If these general measures are ineffective, specific therapy based on etiological factors will be required.

***t. strumosa exophthalmica*** Tachycardia occurring as a symptom of exophthalmic goiter.

***ventricular t.*** A series of beats arising from a ventricular focus at a rate greater than 100 beats per minute. The beats usually arise from a single focus and are at a rate of 150 to 200 beats per minute.

**tachycardia-bradycardia syndrome** A form of sick sinus syndrome; a group of arrhythmias produced by a defect in the sinus node impulse generation or conduction. Arrhythmias associated may include supraventricular tachycardias, atrial fibrillation, atrial flutter that alternates with sinus arrest, and sinus bradycardia.

**tachycardiac** (tăk″ē-kăr′dē-ăk) [Gr. *tachys,* swift, + *kardia,* heart] Pert. to or afflicted with tachycardia.

**tachygastria** Increased rate of contractions of the stomach.

**tachylalia** (tăk″ē-lā′lē-ă) [″ + *lalein,* to speak] Rapid speech.

**tachyphasia** (tăk″ē-fā′zē-ă) [″ + *phasis,* speech] Tachyphrasia.

**tachyphrasia** (tăk″ē-frā′zē-ă) [″ + *phrasis,* speech] Excessive volubility or rapidity of speech, as seen in mental disorders. SYN: *tachyphasia.*

**tachyphrenia** (tăk″ē-frē′nē-ă) [″ + *phren,* mind] Abnormally rapid mental activity.

**tachyphylaxis** (tăk″ē-fī-lăk′sĭs) [″ + *phylaxis,* protection] Rapid immunization to a toxic dose of a substance by previously injecting tiny doses of the same substance.

**tachypnea** (tăk″ĭp-nē′ă) [″ + *pnoia,* breath] Abnormal rapidity of respiration.

***nervous t.*** Respiratory rate of 40 or more per minute. It occurs in hysteria and neurasthenia. If prolonged, it will cause excess loss of $CO_2$ and the hyperventilation syndrome will develop. SEE: *alkalosis, respiratory; hyperventilation.*

***transient t. of the newborn*** ABBR: TTN. A self-limited condition of newborns marked by early onset of respiratory rate greater than 60/min and other signs of respiratory distress. It is thought to be caused by delayed clearance of fetal lung liquid. Recovery usually occurs within 3 days.

**tachyrhythmia** (tăk″ē-rĭth′mē-ă) [″ + *rhythmos,* rhythm] **1.** Tachycardia. **2.** Increase in the frequency of brain waves in electroencephalography up to 12 to 50 per second.

**tachysterol** (tă-kĭs′tĕ-rŏl) One of the isomers of ergosterol obtained by irradiation.

**tacrine** The first medication approved by the U.S. Food and Drug Administration for the treatment of Alzheimer's disease. It is recommended for use in the early stages and does not cure the disease, but helps to reduce the symptoms.

**tactile** (tăk′tĭl) [L. *tactilis*] Perceptible to the touch. SYN: *tactual.*

***t. defensiveness*** A defense reaction owing to sensitivity to being touched.

***t. discrimination*** The ability to localize two points of pressure on the surface of the skin and to identify them as discrete sensations.

***t. disk*** The tiny expanded end of a sensory nerve fiber found in the epidermis and in the epithelial root sheath of a hair.

***t. localization*** An individual's ability to accurately identify the site of tactile stimulation (touch, pressure, or pain). Tactile localization is often tested in sensory evaluations following disease or trauma of the nervous system.

***t. system*** That portion of the nervous system concerned with the sensation of touch. It includes sensory nerve endings (Meissner's corpuscles, Merkel's tactile disks, hair-root endings), afferent nerve fibers, conducting pathways in the cord and brain, and the sensory (somesthetic) area of the cerebral cortex.

**taction** (tăk'shŭn) [L. *tactio*] **1.** The sense of touch. **2.** Touching.

**tactometer** (tăk-tŏm'ĕt-ĕr) [L. *tactus,* touch, + Gr. *metron,* measure] An instrument for determining the acuity of tactile sensitiveness.

**tactual** (tăk'tū-ăl) [L. *tactus,* touch] Tactile.

**tactus** (tăk'tŭs) [L.] Touch (1).

***t. eruditus*** A sensitivity of touch acquired by long practice.

**taedium vitae** (tē'dē-ŭm vē"tī) [L.] Weariness of life, with suicidal inclination.

**taen-, taeni-** Combining form meaning *tapeworm.* SEE: *ten-.*

**Taenia** (tē'nē-ă) [L., tape] A genus of parasitic flatworms belonging to the class Cestoda, phylum Platyhelminthes. They are elongated ribbon-like worms consisting of a scolex, usually with suckers and perhaps hooks, and a chain of segments (proglottids). Adults live as intestinal parasites of vertebrates; larvae parasitize both vertebrates and invertebrates, which serve as intermediate hosts. SEE: *taeniasis; tapeworm.*

***T. echinococcus*** *Echinococcus granulosus.*

***T. lata*** *Diphyllobothrium latum.*

***T. saginata*** A tapeworm whose larvae live in cattle. The adult worm lives in the intestines of humans, who acquire it by eating insufficiently cooked beef infested with the encysted larval form (cysticercus or bladderworm). Adult worms may reach a length of 15 to 20 ft (4.6 to 6.1 m) or longer. SYN: *beef tapeworm.* SEE: illus.

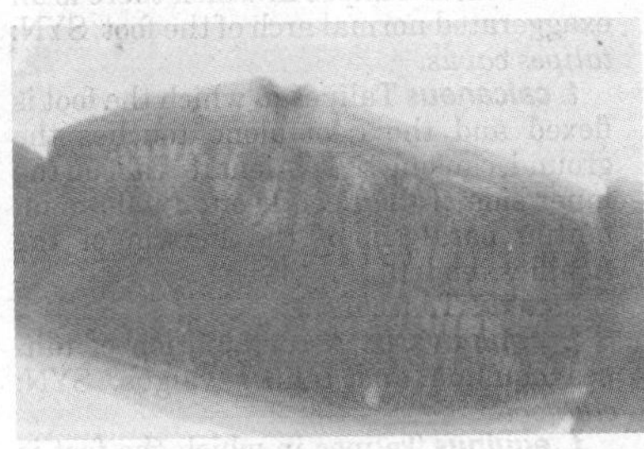

**TAENIA SAGINATA**

GRAVID PROGLOTTID (ORIG. MAG. ×5)

***T. solium*** A tapeworm whose larvae live in hogs; its scolex possesses a row of hooks about the rostellum. The adult worm lives in the intestines of humans, who acquire it by eating insufficiently cooked pork infested with the larval form. Infected pork containing the bladderworm *(Cysticercus cellulosae)* is called measly pork. The cysticerci may also develop in humans; infection occurs from self-infection with eggs from contaminated hands or by hatching of eggs liberated in the intestine. The condition is treated with niclosamide or praziquantel.

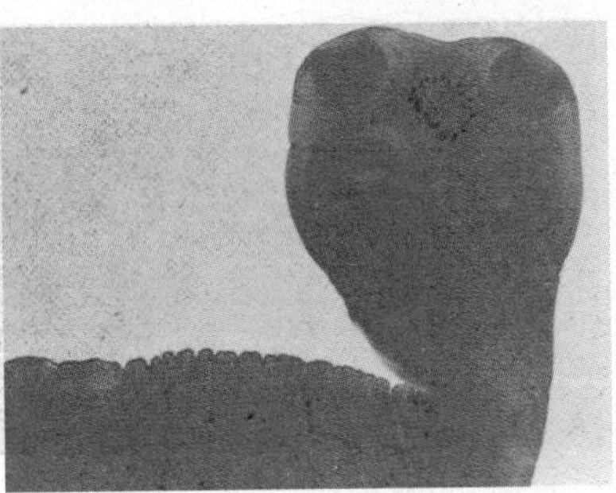

**TAENIA SOLIUM** (ORIG. MAG. ×100)

SYN: *armed tapeworm; pork tapeworm.* SEE: illus.

**taenia** (tē'nē-ă) [L., tape] **1.** A flat band or strip of soft tissue. **2.** A tapeworm of the genus *Taenia.* SYN: *tenia.*

***t. coli*** One of three bands of the large intestines into which muscular fibers are collected. They are taenia mesocolica (mesenteric insertion), taenia libera (opposite mesocolic band), and taenia omentalis (at place of attachment of omentum to transverse colon).

***t. fimbriae*** The folded or recurved lateral edge of the fimbria to which the epithelium covering the choroid plexus of the inferior horn of the lateral ventricle is attached.

***t. pontis*** One or two small transverse bands of fiber at the rostral border of the pons.

***t. semicircularis*** Stria terminalis.

***t. thalami*** A structure separating the superior surface from the lateral surface of the thalamus, its lateral portion containing the stria medullaris.

***t. ventriculi tertii*** The taenia of the third ventricle.

**taeniacide** (tē'nē-ă-sīd) [L. *taenia,* tapeworm, + *cidus,* kill] An agent that kills tapeworms.

**taeniafuge** (tē'nē-ă-fūj") [" + *fugere,* to put to flight] Tenifuge.

**taeniasis** (tē-nī'ă-sĭs) [" + Gr. *-iasis,* condition] The condition of being infested with tapeworms of the genus *Taenia.* SEE: *tapeworm.*

**taeniform** (tē'nĭ-form) [" + *forma,* shape] Having the structure of, or resembling, a tapeworm.

**taenifuge** (tē'nĭ-fūj) [" + *fuga,* flight] Tenifuge.

**taeniophobia** (tē"nē-ō-fō'bē-ă) [" + Gr. *phobos,* fear] The morbid fear of becoming infested with tapeworms.

**tag 1.** A small polyp or growth. **2.** A label or tracer; or the application of a label or tracer.

***hemorrhoidal t.*** The remaining anal skin tag from an old external hemorrhoid.

***radioactive t.*** A radioactive isotope that is incorporated into a chemical or organic

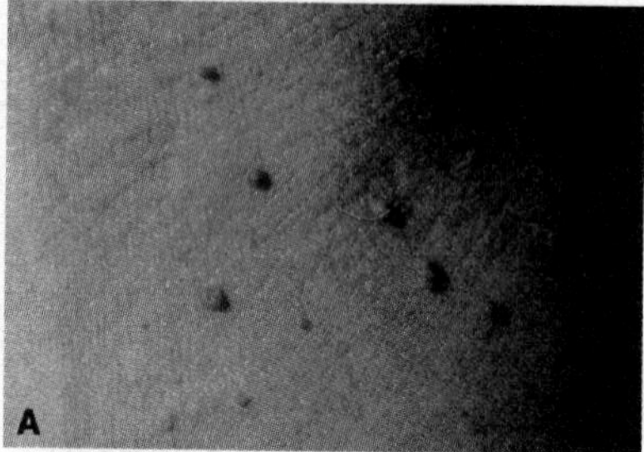


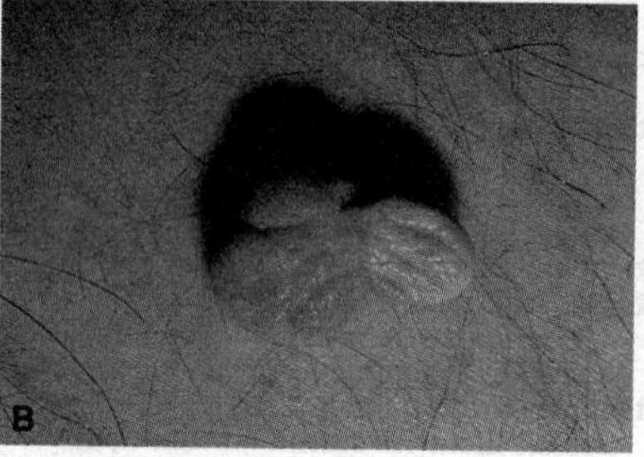


**SKIN TAGS**

**(A)** MULTIPLE TAGS ON NECK, **(B)** PEDUNCULATED TAG

material to allow its detection in metabolic or chemical processes.

***skin t.*** A small outgrowth of skin, usually occurring on the neck, axilla, and groin. SEE: illus.; *acrochordon.*

**tagging** Introduction of a radioactive isotope into a molecule in order to distinguish the molecule from others without that "tag." SYN: *labeling.*

**tagliacotian operation** (tă-lē-ă-kō'shē-ăn) [Gasparo Tagliacozzi, It. surgeon, 1546–1599] A plastic operation on the nose in which skin is used from another part of the body.

**tail** (tāl) [AS. *taegel*] **1.** A posterior, long, flexible terminus, as the extremity of the spinal column. SEE: *cauda.* **2.** An uninterrupted extension of the insurance policy period; also called the *extended reporting endorsement*. SEE: *professional liability insurance.*

**tailgut** (tāl'gŭt) A transient diverticulum of the entodermal cloaca of the embryo. It extends into the tail.

**tailor's cramp** An occupational syndrome marked by spasm of the muscles of the arms and hands.

**taint** (tānt) [O. Fr. *teint,* color, tint] To spoil or cause putrefaction, as in tainted meat.

**Takayasu's arteritis** [Michishige Takayasu, Japanese physician, 1872–1938] An inflammatory disease of the aorta that occludes one or more of the large branches of the aortic arch. This decreases the flow of blood to the areas supplied by these branches, which in turn leads to a lack of pulse in those areas. The etiology is unknown and the only effective treatment is to implant vascular grafts to bypass the occluded vessels. SYN: *pulseless disease.*

**take** To be effective, as in administering a vaccine; or to be successful in grafting skin or transplanting an organ.

**talalgia** (tăl-ăl'jē-ă) [L. *talus,* heel, + Gr. *algos,* pain] Pain in the heel or ankle.

**talar** (tā'lăr) [L. *talaris,* of the ankle] Pert. to the talus, the ankle.

**talc** (tălk) [Persian *talk*] Powdered soapstone; a soft, soapy powder; native hydrous magnesium silicate, $Mg_3Si_4O_{10}(OH)_2$, used as a dusting powder. SYN: *talcum.*

---

Caution: Talc used for industrial, cosmetic, or health products should not contain asbestos fibers.

---

**talcosis** (tăl-kō'sĭs) [Persian *talk,* talc, + Gr. *osis,* condition] A disease caused by the inhalation or implantation of talc in the body.

**talcum** (tălk'ŭm) [L.] Talc.

**tali** (tā'lī) Pl. of talus.

**talipes** (tăl'ĭ-pēz) [L. *talus,* ankle, + *pes,* foot] Any of several deformities of the foot, esp. those occurring congenitally; a nontraumatic deviation of the foot in the direction of one or two of the four lines of movement.

***t. arcuatus*** Talipes in which there is an exaggerated normal arch of the foot. SYN: *talipes cavus.*

***t. calcaneus*** Talipes in which the foot is flexed and the heel alone touches the ground, causing the patient to walk on the inner side of the heel. It often follows infantile paralysis of the muscle of the Achilles tendon.

***t. cavus*** T. arcuatus.

***t. equinovarus*** A combination of talipes equinus and talipes valgus. SYN: *clubfoot.*

***t. equinus*** Talipes in which the foot is extended and the person walks on the toes.

***t. percavus*** Talipes in which there is excessive plantar curvature.

***t. valgus*** Talipes in which the heel and foot are turned outward.

***t. varus*** Talipes in which the heel is turned inward from the midline of the leg.

**talipomanus** (tăl"ĭp-ŏm'ăn-ŭs) [L. *talus,* ankle, + *pes,* foot, + *manus,* hand] A deformity of the hand in which it is twisted out of position. SYN: *clubhand.*

**tallow** (tăl'ō) Fat obtained from suet, the solid fat of certain ruminants.

**talocalcaneal** (tā"lō-kăl-kā'nē-ăl) [" + *calcaneus,* heel bone] Pert. to the talus and calcaneus, bones of the tarsus.

**talocrural** (tā"lō-kroo'răl) [" + *crus,* leg]

Pert. to the talus and leg bones.

**talocrural articulation** **1.** The ankle joint. **2.** A ginglymoid joint or hinge joint.

**talofibular** (tā″lō-fĭb′ū-lăr) [″ + *fibula,* pin] Concerning the talus and fibula.

**talon** (tăl′ōn) [L.] The portion of the claw of a bird, esp. a bird of prey, that projects posteriorly.

***t. noir*** Minute intracutaneous black areas of the heels, toes, or hands. They are thought to be areas of hemorrhage caused by trauma.

**talonavicular** (tā″lō-nă-vĭk′ū-lăr) [L. *talus,* ankle, + *navicula,* boat] Concerning the talus and navicular bones. SYN: *taloscaphoid.*

**talonid** (tăl′ō-nĭd) [ME. *talon,* heel] The crushing region, the posterior or heel part, of a lower molar tooth.

**taloscaphoid** (tā″lō-skăf′oyd) [L. *talus,* ankle, + Gr. *skaphe,* skiff, + *eidos,* form, shape] Talonavicular.

**talotibial** (tā″lō-tĭb′ē-ăl) [″ + *tibia,* shinbone] Concerning the talus and tibial bones.

**talus** (tā′lŭs) *pl.* **tali** [L., ankle] The ankle bone articulating with the tibia, fibula, calcaneus, and navicular bone; formerly called astragalus.

**tambour** (tăm-boor′) [Fr., drum] A shallow, drum-shaped appliance used in transmitting and registering arterial pulsations, blood pressure, and respiratory movements.

**Tamm-Horsfall mucoprotein** [Igor Tamm, Russian-born U.S. virologist, 1922–1971; Frank L. Horsfall, Jr., U.S. physician, 1906–1971] A normal mucoprotein in the urine. It is not derived from plasma but is produced by the ascending limb of the loop of Henle. When this protein is concentrated at low pH, it forms gel. These conditions may be met when the urine is exposed to myoglobin, hemoglobin, albumin, Bence-Jones protein, and pyelographical contrast media. This protein is contained in most urinary casts and is identical to human uromedulin.

**tamoxifen citrate** (tă-mŏks′ĭ-fĕn) An antiestrogen drug used in treating carcinoma of the breast.

**tampon** (tăm′pŏn) [Fr., plug] A roll or pack made of various absorbent substances, such as cotton, rayon, wool, and gauze, used to arrest hemorrhage or absorb secretions from a wound or body cavity.

***menstrual t.*** An absorbent material suitably shaped and prepared to provide a hygienic means of absorbing menstrual fluid in the vagina. A cord is attached and remains outside the vagina to facilitate removal. These tampons are made for self-insertion. SEE: *menstruation; sanitary napkin.*

***Mikulicz's t.*** Mikulicz's drain.

***nasal t.*** A soft rubber bulb dilated with compressed air, used in plugging nostrils to stop hemorrhage from the nose.

**tamponade** (tăm″pŏn-ād′) [Fr., plug] **1.** The act of using a tampon. SYN: *tamponage; tamponing; tamponment.* **2.** The pathological compression of a part.

***balloon t.*** Producing pressure against some object by the use of a catheter surrounded by an elongated balloon; often used in the esophagus to arrest bleeding from varices. The Sengstaken-Blakemore tube, which is most frequently used, is a three-lumen tube: one lumen to administer fluids to the patient or to provide gastric suction, another going to a balloon inserted in the stomach to hold the tube in place, and the third attached to the balloon for application of pressure to the esophageal walls. SEE: *epistaxis; varicose veins.*

NURSING IMPLICATIONS: After balloon insertion, vital signs, electrolyte status, and changes in hematocrit are monitored. Because the balloon prevents swallowing, fluids and tube feedings are administered as prescribed. The nurse instructs the patient to expectorate saliva and provides an emesis basin for oral secretions. Aspiration of secretions is necessary. Comatose patients require continuous drainage of the esophagus above the balloon.

***cardiac t.*** A pathological condition resulting from the accumulation of excess fluid in the pericardium; it may result from pericarditis or injuries to the heart or great blood vessels, with accumulation of blood.

A rapid rise in intrapericardial pressure impairs diastolic filling of the heart in cardiac tamponade. The rise in pressure usually results from blood or fluid accumulating in the pericardial sac. If fluid accumulates rapidly, as little as 250 ml can create an emergency situation. Slow accumulation and a rise in pressure, as in pericardial effusion associated with cancer, may not produce immediate signs and symptoms because the fibrous wall of the pericardial sac can gradually stretch to accommodate as much as 1 to 2 L of fluid.

ETIOLOGY: Cardiac tamponade may be idiopathic (Dressler's syndrome) or may result from any of the following causes: effusion (in cancer, bacterial infections, tuberculosis, and, rarely, acute rheumatic fever); hemorrhage from trauma (such as gunshot or stab wounds of the chest, perforation by catheter during cardiac or central venous catheterization, or after cardiac surgery); hemorrhage from nontraumatic causes (such as rupture of the heart or great vessels, or anticoagulant therapy in a patient with pericarditis); viral, postirradiation, or idiopathic pericarditis; acute myocardial infarction; chronic renal failure during dialysis; drug reaction (procainamide, hydralazine, minoxidil, isoniazid, penicillin, methysergide, and daunorubicin); or connective tissue disorders (such as rheumatoid arthritis, systemic lupus erythematosus, rheumatic fever, vasculitis, and scleroderma). Pressure resulting from fluid accumulation in the pericardium decreases ventricular filling and cardiac output, resulting in cardiogenic shock and death if untreated (esp. in acute situations).

DIAGNOSIS: Cardiac tamponade is diagnosed by chest radiograph (slightly widened mediastinum and enlargement of the cardiac silhouette), ECG (reduced QRS amplitude, electrical alternans of the P wave, QRS complex, and T wave and generalized ST-segment elevation), pulmonary artery pressure monitoring (increased right atrial pressure, right ventricular diastolic pressure, and central venous pressure), and echocardiography (pericardial effusion with signs of right ventricular and atrial compression).

TREATMENT: Treatment is directed to relieving intrapericardial pressure and cardiac compression by removing accumulated blood or fluid. Pericardiocentesis (needle aspiration of the pericardial cavity) or surgical creation of a pericardial opening or window dramatically improves systemic arterial pressure and cardiac output. A drain may be inserted in the pericardial sac to relieve effusion and left in place until the effusion stops or windowing is performed. In cases of infection, antibiotics can be instilled through the drain. Supportive therapies (fluid replacement and vasopressors or inotropics) are used as necessary for the hypotensive patient, and known causes are treated.

NURSING IMPLICATIONS: The patient is assessed for a history of disorders that can cause tamponade and for symptoms such as acute pain and dyspnea. Other symptoms include orthopnea, diaphoresis, anxiety, restlessness, and pallor or cyanosis. The neck vein is inspected for distention; peripheral pulses are palpated for rapidity and weakness; the liver is palpated and percussed for hepatomegaly; the anterior chest wall percussed for a widening area of flatness; and the blood pressure auscultated for decreased arterial pressure, pulsus paradoxus (an abnormal inspiratory drop of greater than 15 mm Hg in systemic blood pressure), and narrow pulse pressure. Heart sounds may be muffled. A quiet heart with faint sounds usually accompanies only severe tamponade and occurs within minutes of the tamponade (as in cardiac rupture or trauma). The lungs are clear.

When these symptoms are apparent, the patient is transferred to intensive care immediately for hemodynamic monitoring. The patient is monitored for signs of increasing tamponade, increasing dyspnea, and arrhythmias and for signs of respiratory distress such as increasing tachypnea and changes in the level of consciousness. Prescribed inotropic drugs, intravenous solutions to maintain the patient's blood pressure, and oxygen are administered as necessary and prescribed. Supportive care is provided as indicated by the patient's condition and the underlying cause of the tamponade.

The patient is prepared for central line insertion, pericardiocentesis, thoracotomy, or other therapeutic measures as indicated; brief explanations of procedures and expected sensations are provided, and the patient is reassured to decrease anxiety. The patient is observed for a decrease in central venous pressure and a concomitant rise in blood pressure after treatment, which indicate relief of cardiac compression.

If the patient is not acutely ill, the patient is educated about the condition, including its cause and its treatment. The importance of reporting any worsening of symptoms immediately is stressed.

***nasal t.*** SEE: *epistaxis; nosebleed* for illus.

**tamponage** (tăm′pŏn-ŏj) [Fr., plug] Tamponade.

**tamponing, tamponment** (tăm′pŏn-ĭng, tăm-pŏn′mĕnt) Tamponade.

**tandem** A curved stainless steel tube inserted into the uterine canal during brachytherapy to hold radioactive sources.

**tang 1.** A strong taste or flavor. **2.** A long slender projection or prong forming a part of a chisel, file, or knife. **3.** In dentistry, an apparatus for joining the rests and retainers to palatal or lingual bars of a denture.

**Tangier disease** (tăn-jēr′) [Tangier Island, in Chesapeake Bay, where the disease was first discovered] A rare disease caused by familial high-density lipoprotein deficiency. Symptoms and signs include polyneuropathy, lymphadenopathy, orange-yellow discoloration of enlarged tonsillar tissue, hepatosplenomegaly, and a marked decrease in high-density lipoproteins. Cholesterol esters accumulate in various organs. There is no specific therapy.

**tannin** (tăn′ĭn) [Fr. *tanin*] **1.** An acid substance found in the bark of certain plants and trees or their products, usually from nutgall. It is found in coffee and to a greater extent in tea. **2.** Any of several substances containing tannin.

ACTION/USES: Tannin is used as an astringent, an antidote for various poisons, and a topical hemostatic. It is constipating. It is partly eliminated in the urine as gallic acid.

**tanning salon** A place equipped to provide exposure to artificial light in order to produce a "suntan." The ultraviolet radiation emitted by the units is different from that in natural sunlight. If this type of tan is obtained and the individual is then exposed to sunlight, the skin damage may be greater than that induced by sunlight alone. SEE: *photosensitivity*.

**tantalum** (tăn′tă-lŭm) SYMB: Ta. A rare metallic element derived from tantalite;

atomic weight, 180.947; atomic number, 73. Because it is noncorrosive and malleable, it has been used to repair cranial defects, as a wire suture, and in prostheses.

**tantrum** (tăn'trŭm) A display of great anger, which may or may not include violent action.

***temper t.*** A stage of anger and reaction in which the individuals, esp. children, are no longer in control of themselves and are unaware of how their condition appears to others. The parents or associates need to realize that it is not possible to talk the child out of this behavior or reaction. The child needs to be separated, at that time, from the person or situation the child thinks caused the incident. The parents or those involved should not demean or make fun of the child during the episode. The child will eventually learn that control of anger is important and that, at times, controlled anger is an appropriate response to certain situations.

**Tanyoz's sign** **1.** In ascites, the downward displacement of the umbilicus. **2.** In pregnancy, the upward displacement of the umbilicus.

**tap** (tăp) **1.** [AS. *taeppa*] To puncture or to empty a cavity of fluid. SEE: *lumbar puncture; paracentesis; thoracentesis.* **2.** [O. Fr. *taper*] A light blow.

***spinal t.*** SEE: *spinal puncture.*

**tape** (tāp) [AS. *taeppe*] **1.** A long, flexible, narrow strip of linen, cotton, paper, or plastic such as adhesive tape. **2.** To wrap a part with a long bandage made of adhesive or other type of material.

***adhesive t.*** A fabric, film, or paper, one side of which is coated with an adhesive substance, that adheres to the skin. SYN: *adhesive plaster.*

**tapeinocephalic** (tăp"ĭ-nō-sĕ-făl'ĭk) [Gr. *tapeinos,* low-lying, + *kephale,* head] Pert. to tapeinocephaly.

**tapeinocephaly** (tăp"ĭ-nō-sĕf'ă-lē) A flattened head in which the vertical index of the skull is less than 72.

**tapetum** (tă-pē'tŭm) [NL., a carpet] A layer of fibers from the corpus callosum forming the roof and lateral walls of the inferior and posterior horns of the lateral ventricles of the brain. The fibers pass to the temporal and occipital lobes.

***t. choroideae*** tapetum lucidum.

***t. lucidum*** A layer of tissue in the choroid of the eye between the vascular and capillary layers in some animals, but not in humans. This membrane reflects light shined into the animal's eyes. It produces a green reflection, readily seen in cats. SYN: *tapetum choroideae.*

**tapeworm** [AS. *taeppe,* a narrow band, + *wyrm,* worm] Any of the species of parasitic worms belonging to the class Cestoda, phylum Platyhelminthes. A typical tapeworm consists of a scolex with hooks and suckers for attachment and a series of segments or proglottids that vary in number from a few to several thousand. New proglottids are budded off of the scolex, so that a worm is actually a linear colony consisting of immature, mature, and ripe or gravid proglottids. Adults live as endoparasites in the intestine. The terminal ripe proglottids containing the ova break off and pass out with the feces. The eggs develop into minute six-hooked oncospheres, which, when ingested by the proper intermediate host (usually another vertebrate), develop in muscle tissues into an encysted larva known as a cysticercus. Infestation occurs when uncooked meat containing encysted larvae is eaten. These larvae develop into the mature adult in the primary host.

Species of medical importance are *Diphyllobothrium latum, Echinococcus granulosus, Hymenolepis nana, H. diminuta, Taenia saginata,* and *T. solium.* SEE: *cysticercosis; cysticercus; hydatid; taeniasis.*

SYMPTOMS: Often symptoms are absent. If tapeworms are numerous, they may cause intestinal obstruction. Occasionally mild systemic symptoms may occur from absorption of metabolic wastes, and sometimes there are dyspeptic symptoms.

***armed t.*** *Taenia solium.*

***beef t.*** *Taenia saginata.*

***broad t.*** *Diphyllobothrium latum.*

***dog t.*** *Dipylidium caninum.*

***dwarf t.*** *Hymenolepis nana.*

***fish t.*** *Diphyllobothrium latum.*

***hydatid t.*** *Echinococcus granulosus.*

***mouse t.*** *Hymenolepis nana.*

***pork t.*** *Taenia solium.*

***rat t.*** *Hymenolepis nana.*

***unarmed t.*** *Taenia saginata.*

**taphephobia** (tăf"ĕ-fō'bē-ă) [Gr. *taphos,* grave, + *phobos,* fear] An abnormal fear of being buried alive.

**taphophilia** (tăf"ō-fĭl'ē-ă) [" + *philos,* love] An abnormal attraction for graves.

**Tapia syndrome** (tā'pē-ă) [Antonio García Tapia, Sp. physician, 1875–1950] Paralysis of the pharynx and larynx on one side and atrophy of the tongue on the opposite side, caused by a lesion affecting the vagus (10th) and hypoglossal (12th) cranial nerves on the side in which the pharynx is affected.

**tapinocephalic** (tăp"ĭn-ō-sĕf-ăl'ĭk) [Gr. *tapeinos,* lying low, + *kephale,* head] Pert. to flatness of the top of the cranium.

**tapinocephaly** (tăp"ĭn-ō-sĕf'ă-lē) Flatness of the top of the cranium.

**tapotement** (tă-pōt-mŏn') [Fr.] Percussion in massage. Techniques include beating with the clinched hand, clapping performed with the palm of the hand, hacking with the ulnar border of the hand, and punctuation with the tips of the fingers. The strength of the manipulations is an essential factor in the massage treatment, and care must be taken not to bruise the patient. As a rule, one should begin with moderate pressure, and then ascertain from the patient the sensation.

A lubricating lotion or cream should be used to avoid abrading the skin. SYN: *tapping* (1). SEE: *massage.*

**tapping** (tăp′ĭng) **1.** [O.Fr. *taper,* of imitative origin] Tapotement. **2.** [AS. *taeppa,* tap] Paracentesis.

**tar** A dark, viscid mass of complex chemicals obtained by destructive distillation of coal, shale, and organic matter, esp. wood from pine and juniper trees.

***coal t.*** A tar produced in the destructive distillation of bituminous coal. It is used as an ingredient in ointments for treating eczema and other skin diseases.

***juniper t.*** A material obtained from the destructive distillation of oil of the wood of the juniper tree, *Juniperus oxycedrus.* It is used in certain medicines applied topically in treating certain skin diseases.

***pine t.*** A product obtained from the distillation of pine wood.

**tarantism** (tăr′ăn-tĭzm) [*Taranto,* seaport in southern Italy, + Gr. *-ismos,* condition] A nervous disorder marked by stupor, melancholy, and uncontrollable dancing mania; popularly attributed to the bite of the tarantula. SYN: *tarentism.*

**tarantula** (tă-răn′tū-lă) A large venomous spider feared by many people; however, its bite is comparable in severity to a bee sting. SEE: *spider bite.*

**Tardieu's spot** (tăr-dyūz′) [Auguste A. Tardieu, Fr. physician, 1818–1879] One of the subpleural spots of ecchymosis following death by strangulation.

**tardive** (tăr′dĭv) [Fr., tardy] Characterized by lateness, esp. pert. to a disease in which the characteristic sign or symptom appears late in the course of the disease. SEE: *dyskinesia, tardive.*

**tare** (tăr) The weight of an empty container. That weight is subtracted from the total weight of the vessel and substance added to it in order to determine the precise weight of the material added to the container.

**tared** A container of known and predetermined tare.

**tarentism** (tăr′ĕn-tĭzm) Tarantism.

**target** (tăr′gĕt) [O. Fr. *targette,* light shield] **1.** A structure or organ to which something is directed. **2.** The portion of the anode of an x-ray or therapeutic tube in which electrons from the filament or electron gun are focused and x-ray photons are produced; usually made of a heavy metal such as tungsten or molybdenum.

**target cell** An erythrocyte with a rounded central area surrounded by a lightly stained clear ring, which in turn is surrounded by a dense ring of peripheral protoplasm. It is present in certain blood disorders. SEE: illus.

**tarichatoxin** (tăr″ĭk-ă-tŏk′sĭn) A neurotoxin from the *Taricha* newt.

**Tarnier's sign** (tăr-nē-āz′) [Etienne Stéphene Tarnier, Fr. obstetrician, 1828–1897] A sign of impending miscarriage; the disappearance of the angle between the upper and lower uterine segments in pregnancy.

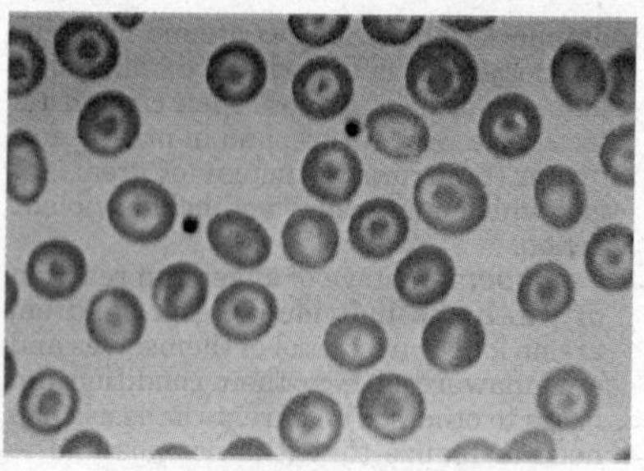

**TARGET CELLS** IN HEMOGLOBIN C DISEASE (ORIG. MAG. ×600)

**tarnish** Surface discoloration or reduced luster of metals owing to the effect of corrosive substances or galvanic action. In dental restorations, such action may be enhanced by accumulation of bacterial plaque.

**tarsadenitis** (tăr″săd-ĕn-ī′tĭs) [Gr. *tarsos,* a broad, flat surface, + *aden,* gland, + *itis,* inflammation] An inflammation of the tarsal or meibomian glands of the eyelid.

**tarsal** (tăr′săl) [Gr. *tarsalis*] **1.** Pert. to the tarsus or supporting plate of the eyelid. **2.** Pert. to the ankle or tarsus.

**tarsal bone** One of the seven bones of the ankle, hind foot, and midfoot, consisting of the talus, calcaneus, navicular, cuboid, and three cuneiform bones. SYN: *tarsale.*

**tarsal cartilage** SEE: *plate, tarsal.*

**tarsale** (tăr-sā′lē) *pl.* **tarsalia** [L.] A tarsal bone.

**tarsalgia** (tăr-săl′jē-ă) [Gr. *tarsos,* a broad, flat surface, + *algos,* pain] Pain in the tarsus or ankle; it may be due to flatfoot, shortening of the Achilles tendon, or other causes.

**tarsalis** (tăr-sā′lĭs) [L.] One of the tarsal muscles. SEE: *Muscles Appendix.*

**tarsal tunnel syndrome** Neuropathy of the distal portion of the tibial nerve at the ankle caused by chronic pressure on the nerve at the point it passes through the tarsal tunnel. It causes pain in and numbness of the sole of the foot and weakness of the plantar flexion of the toes.

**tarsectomy** (tar-sĕk′tō-mē) [″ + *ektome,* excision] **1.** An excision of the tarsus or a tarsal bone. **2.** The removal of the tarsal plate of an eyelid.

**tarsectopia** (tăr″sĕk-tō′pē-ă) A dislocation of the tarsus.

**tarsitis** (tăr-sī′tĭs) [″ + *itis,* inflammation] **1.** An inflammation of the tarsus of the foot. **2.** Blepharitis.

**tarso-** [Gr. *tarsos,* a broad, flat surface] Combining form indicating *the flat of the foot* or *the edge of the eyelid.*

**tarsocheiloplasty** (tăr″sō-kī′lō-plăs″tē) [″ + *cheilos,* lip, + *plassein,* to form] The plastic repair of the borders of the eyelid.

**tarsoclasia, tarsoclasis** (tăr″sō-klā′sē-ă, tăr-sŏk′lăs-ĭs) [″ + *klasis,* a breaking] A surgical fracture of the tarsus for the correction of clubfoot.

**tarsomalacia** (tăr″sō-mă-lā′sē-ă) [″ + *malakia,* a softening] The softening of the tarsal cartilages of the eyes.

**tarsomegaly** (tăr″sō-mĕg′ă-lē) [″ + *megas,* large] An enlargement of the heel bone, calcaneus.

**tarsometatarsal** (tăr″sō-mĕt″ă-tăr′săl) [″ + *meta,* between, + *tarsos,* a broad, flat surface] Pert. to the tarsus and the metatarsus.

**tarso-orbital** (tăr″sō-or′bĭ-tăl) [″ + L. *orbita,* track] Concerning the tarsus of the eyelid and the orbit.

**tarsophalangeal** (tăr″sō-fă-lăn′jē-ăl) [″ + *phalanx,* closely knit row] Concerning the tarsus of the foot and the phalanges of the toes.

**tarsophyma** (tăr″sō-fī′mă) [″ + *phyma,* a growth] Sty.

**tarsoplasia, tarsoplasty** (tăr″sō-plā′zē-ă, tăr′sō-plăs″tē) [″ + *plassein,* to form] Blepharoplasty.

**tarsoptosis** (tăr″sŏp-tō′sĭs) [″ + *ptosis,* falling] Flatfoot; fallen arch of the foot.

**tarsorrhaphy** (tăr-sor′ă-fē) [″ + *rhaphe,* seam, ridge] Blepharorrhaphy.

**tarsotarsal** (tăr″sō-tăr′săl) [″ + *tarsos,* a broad, flat surface] Concerning the articulation between two rows of tarsal bones.

**tarsotibial** (tăr″sō-tĭb′ē-ăl) [″ + L. *tibia,* shinbone] Concerning the tarsus and the tibia of the foot.

**tarsotomy** (tăr-sŏt′ō-mē) [″ + *tome,* incision] **1.** An incision of the tarsal cartilage of an eyelid. **2.** Any surgical incision of the tarsus of the foot.

**tarsus** (tăr′sŭs) *pl.* **tarsi** [Gr. *tarsos,* a broad, flat surface] **1.** The ankle with its seven bones located between the bones of the lower leg and the metatarsus and forming the proximal portion of the foot. It consists of the calcaneus (os calcis), talus (astragalus), cuboid (os cuboideum), navicular (scaphoid), and first, second, and third cuneiform bones. The talus articulates with the tibia and fibula, the cuboid and cuneiform bones with the metatarsals. SEE: *foot; skeleton;* names of individual bones. **2.** A curved plate of dense white fibrous tissue forming the supporting structure of the eyelid; also called the *tarsal plate.*

***t. inferior palpebrae*** The firm layer of connective tissue that provides internal support for the lower eyelid.

***t. superior palpebrae*** The firm layer of connective tissue that provides internal support for the upper eyelid.

**tartar** [Gr. *tartaron,* dregs] **1.** An acid compound found in the juice of grapes and deposited on the sides of casks during winemaking. **2.** Dental plaque.

***cream of t.*** Potassium bitartrate.

***t. emetic*** Antimony potassium tartrate; used as an emetic.

**tartrate** A salt of tartaric acid.

**tartrazine** A pyrazole aniline dye widely used to color foods, cosmetics, drugs, and textiles.

**task, cancellation** A type of cognitive test that measures attention by determining an individual's ability to select and mark a line through selected target letters or symbols within a larger field of many letters or symbols.

**taste** (tāst) [O. Fr. *taster,* to feel, to taste] **1.** To attempt to determine the flavor of a substance by touching it with the tongue. **2.** A chemical sense dependent on the sense organs on the surface of the tongue. These organs, called *taste buds*, when appropriately stimulated, produce one or a combination of the four fundamental taste sensations: sweet, bitter, sour, and salty. The nervous impulses are carried to the brain by the facial nerve (from the anterior two thirds of the surface of the tongue) and the glossopharyngeal nerve (from the posterior third). Loss of taste may be due to bilateral disease of the facial nerve and of gustatory fibers of the glossopharyngeal nerve or to cytotoxic drugs used therapeutically.

The cells of the taste buds have an average life span of 10 to 10½ days; thus, they are constantly being renewed. If a cytotoxic agent used in cancer therapy destroys the cells, taste will return in a minimum of 10 days but usually over a much longer period.

***t. area*** An area in the cerebral cortex at the lower end of the somesthetic area in the parietal lobe.

***t. blindness*** An inability to taste certain substances such as phenylthiocarbamide (PTC). This inability is due to a hereditary factor that is transmitted as an autosomal recessive trait.

***t. bud*** One of the sensory end organs that mediate the sensation of taste. They are oval structures located on the surface of the tongue, esp. the sides of the circumvallate papillae, on the soft palate, epiglottis, and portions of the pharynx. Each contains sensory and gustatory (taste) cells and supporting (sustentacular) cells. When stimulated by chemical stimuli, they give rise to the sense of taste. SEE: *chemoreceptor*.

***t. cell*** One of the neuroepithelial cells within a taste bud that serve as receptors for the sense of taste. Each possesses on the free surface a short taste hair that projects through the inner taste pore. SYN: *gustatory cell.*

**taster** (tās′tĕr) A person capable of detecting a particular substance by using the taste sense. SEE: *phenylthiocarbamide.*

**TAT** *thematic apperception test.*

**T.A.T.** *tetanus antitoxin; toxin-antitoxin.*

**tattooing** (tă-too′ĭng) [Tahitian *tatau*] **1.** Indelible marking of the skin produced by introducing minute amounts of pigments into the skin. Tattooing is usually done to produce a certain design, picture, or name. When it is done commercially, sterile procedures are rarely used and hepatitis B or C or AIDS virus may be transmitted to the customer. The technique may also be used to conceal a corneal leukoma, to mask pigmented areas of skin, or to color skin to look like the areola in mammoplasty. **2.** In radiation therapy, the induction of a small amount of indelible pigment under the skin for a permanent marker of an area treated with radiation.

***removal of t.*** Use of a ruby laser to "erase" the pigment in an unwanted tattoo. This usually causes no permanent skin changes.

***traumatic t.*** Following abrasion of the skin, embedding of fine dirt particles under the superficial layers of the skin; or as a result of forceful deposit of gunpowder granules. This can be prevented by immediate removal of the particles.

**taurine** (taw'rĭn) A derivative of cysteine. It is present in bile, as taurocholic acid, in combination with bile acid.

**taurocholate** (taw"rō-kō'lāt) A salt of taurocholic acid.

**taurocholemia** (taw"rō-kō-lē'mē-ă) [Gr. *tauros,* a bull, + *chole,* bile, + *haima,* blood] Taurocholic acid in the blood.

**taurodontism** (taw"rō-dŏn'tĭzm) [" + *odous,* tooth, + *-ismos,* condition] A condition in which the teeth have greatly enlarged pulp chambers that are deepened. In that shape, the pulp chamber encroaches on the roots of the teeth.

**Taussig-Bing syndrome** (tau'sĭg-bĭng) [Helen B. Taussig, U.S. pediatrician, 1898–1986; Richard J. Bing, U.S. surgeon, 1909–1986] A congenital deformity of the heart in which the aorta arises from the right ventricle and the pulmonary artery arises from both ventricles. An intraventricular septal defect is present.

**tauto-** Prefix meaning *identical.*

**tautomer** (taw'tō-mĕr) [" + *meros,* a part] A chemical that is capable of tautomerism.

**tautomeral, tautomeric** (taw-tŏm'ĕr-ăl, -tō-mĕr'ĭk) [" + *meros,* a part] Pert. to certain neurons that send processes to the white matter on the same side of the spinal cord.

**tautomerase** (taw-tŏm'ĕr-ās) [" + " + *-ase,* enzyme] An enzyme that catalyzes tautomeric reactions.

**tautomerism** (taw-tŏm'ĕr-ĭzm) [" + " + *-ismos,* condition] A phenomenon in which two formulas are possible and exist in dynamic equilibrium so that as the amount of one substance is altered, the second is changed into the other form in order to maintain the equilibrium. SEE: *isomerism.*

**tautorotation** (taw"tō-rō-tā'shŭn) [" + L. *rotare,* to turn round] A change in specific rotation that occurs when a solution of certain sugars stands for a while.

**taxis** (tăk'sĭs) [Gr., arrangement] **1.** The manual replacement or reduction of a hernia or dislocation. **2.** The response of an organism to its environment; a turning toward (positive taxis) or away from (negative taxis) a particular stimulus. SEE: *chemotaxis.*

**taxol** A chemical obtained from the bark of the yew tree, *Taxus brevifolia.* In clinical trials, taxol has shown great promise in treating certain advanced cancers of the ovary and the breast. Like all drugs, taxol can cause undesired side effects.

**taxon** (tăk'sŏn) [Gr. *taxis,* arrangement] A taxonomic group.

**taxonomic** (tăk"sō-nŏm'ĭk) Concerning taxonomy.

**taxonomy** (tăks-ŏn'ō-mē) [" + *nomos,* law] The laws and principles of classification of living organisms; also used for classification of learning objectives.

**Taylor brace** (tā'lĕr) [Charles Fayette Taylor, U.S. surgeon, 1827–1899] A brace with two rigid posterior oblique portions and soft straps crossed anteriorly over the chest.

**Taylor, Euphemia Jane** [U.S. nurse, 1878–1957.] A pioneer of psychiatric nursing. She graduated from the Johns Hopkins Hospital School of Nursing in 1907 and became Director of Nursing Services at the Henry Phipps Clinic at Johns Hopkins from 1913–1919. Due to her efforts, Johns Hopkins was the first general hospital school of nursing to offer a course in psychiatric nursing. She became the Dean of the Yale School of Nursing in 1934 and served in this position until 1944. She was also a leader in the International Council of Nurses until her death.

**Tay-Sachs disease** [Warren Tay, Brit. physician, 1843–1927; Bernard Sachs, U.S. neurologist, 1858–1944] An inherited disease transmitted as an autosomal recessive trait. The rate of occurrence in Ashkenazi Jews in the U.S. is estimated to be 400 per 1 million births. Because of the lack of the enzyme hexosaminidase A, which is important in sphingolipid metabolism, sphingolipids accumulate in the cells, esp. those of the nerves and the brain. Death usually occurs before the age of 4. There is no specific therapy. SEE: *Nursing Diagnoses Appendix.*

SYMPTOMS: This disease is marked by neurological deterioration characterized by mental and physical retardation, blindness, cherry-red spots on the macula, an exaggerated startle response, spasticity, convulsions, and enlargement of the head. Carriers of the trait can be accurately detected by assay of hexosaminidase A. Affected embryos may be detected by measurement of hexosaminidase A in the amniotic fluid.

**Tay's spot** Cherry-red spot.

**TB** Colloquialism for *tuberculosis.*

**Tb** Symbol for the element terbium.

**t.b.** *tubercle bacillus; tuberculosis.*

**T bandage** A bandage resembling the letter T, used for the head and the perineum.

**T-bar** T-shaped tubing connected to an endotracheal tube in situ; used to deliver oxygen therapy to an intubated patient who does not require mechanical ventilation.

**TBI** *total body irradiation.*

**TBP** *thyroxine-binding protein.*

**Tbs** *tablespoon.*

**TBSA** *total body surface area.*

**Tc** Symbol for the element technetium.

**T cell growth factor** Interleukin-2.

**T-cell–mediated immunity** SEE: *immunity, cell-mediated.*

**T-cell receptor** ABBR: TCR. One of the molecules on the surface of T cells that are specific for an antigen. Thus, for each of the great number of antigens to which the human may be exposed, there is a specific TCR for each one. As T cells mature, a mechanism deletes those carrying receptors that would react with self-antigens. This process, called negative selection, promotes self-tolerance and reduces the risk of autoimmune diseases. SEE: *autoimmunity; immune response; cell, T.*

**$TCID_{50}$** *Tissue culture infective dose.*

**t.d.s.** L. *ter die sumendum,* to be taken three times a day.

**Te** Symbol for the element tellurium.

**tea** (tē) **1.** An infusion of a medicinal plant. **2.** The leaves of the plant *Thea chinensis* or *Camellia sinensis,* from which a beverage is made by steeping the leaves in boiling hot water.

COMPOSITION: The principal ingredients are caffeine, tannin, and a volatile oil that gives the beverage prepared from tea leaves its characteristic taste and aroma. Caffeine, which constitutes 1% to 4% of tea leaves, is one of the medically important ingredients in tea. Fluoride is present in green tea at about twice the amount in black tea, but in both teas the concentration is sufficient to help prevent tooth decay. The caloric content is negligible until sugar and milk are added to the beverage. SEE: *caffeine; caffeine withdrawal.*

***black t.*** Tea made from leaves that have been fermented before they are dried.

***green t.*** Tea prepared by heating leaves in open trays.

***herb t.*** Tea made of a variety of plants, including leaves of certain flowers, herbs, barks, and grasses. Some herbs used in these teas are known to be harmful.

***Paraguay copper t.*** Tea made from the leaves and stems of *Ilex paraguayensis*. It is a stimulating drink and contains volatile oil, tannin, and caffeine.

**TEAB** *tetraethylammonium bromide.*

**TEAC** *tetraethylammonium chloride.*

**tear** (tār) [AS. *taer*] To separate or pull apart by force.

***bucket handle t.*** A longitudinal tear, usually beginning in the middle of a meniscus (cartilage) of the knee.

**tears** (tērs) [AS. *tear*] The watery saline solution secreted continuously by the lacrimal glands. They lubricate the surfaces between the eyeball and eyelids (i.e., the conjunctiva). These are called continuous tears. Irritant tears are produced when a foreign object or substance is in the eye. SEE: *Schirmer's test.*

***artificial t.'s*** A solution of materials used to lubricate the conjunctivae.

***crocodile t.'s*** Excess tear production that occurs when salivary glands are stimulated during eating. This condition may be present in patients with incomplete recovery from facial paralysis.

**tease** (tēz) [AS. *taesan,* to pluck] To separate a tissue into minute parts with a needle to prepare it for microscopy.

**teaspoon** (tē′spoon) ABBR: tsp. A household measure equal to approx. 5 ml. Teaspoons used in the home vary from 3 to 6 ml. Because household measures are not accurate, when a teaspoon dose is prescribed or ordered, 5 ml of the substance should be given.

**teat** (tēt) [ME. *tete,* from AS. *tit,* teat] **1.** The nipple of the mammary gland. SYN: *papilla, mammae.* SEE: *nipple; breast.* **2.** Any protuberance resembling a nipple.

**teatulation** (tēt″ū-lā′shŭn) [AS. *tit,* teat] The development of a nipple-like elevation.

**technetium** (tĕk-nē′shē-ŭm) SYMB: Tc. A synthetic metallic chemical element; atomic weight, 98.9062; atomic number, 43.

**technetium-99m** SYMB: $^{99m}$Tc. An isomer of technetium that emits gamma rays. It has a half-life of 6 hr.

**technetium Tc 99m albumin aggregated injection** A radioactive isotope of technetium-99m. It is used intravenously for scanning the lung.

**technical** (tĕk′nĭ-kăl) [Gr. *tekhnikos,* skilled] Requiring technique or special skill.

**technician** (tĕk-nĭsh′ăn) An individual who has the knowledge and skill required to carry out specific technical procedures. This individual usually has a diploma from a specialized school or an associate degree from college or has received training through preceptorship.

***biomedical engineering t.*** A technician who assembles, repairs, and adapts medical equipment used for the delivery of health care and assists in the development and maintenance of these systems.

***certified pulmonary function t.*** An individual trained to evaluate respiratory function who has passed the examination offered by the National Board for Respiratory Care.

***certified respiratory therapy t.*** An entry-level respiratory care practitioner who has passed the examination offered by the National Board for Respiratory Care.

***dental t.*** A technician who constructs complete and partial dentures, makes orthodontic appliances, and fixes bridgework, crowns, and other dental restorations as authorized by dentists.

***dialysis t.*** A technician who operates and maintains an artificial kidney machine following approved methods to provide dialysis treatment for patients with kidney disorders.

***dietetic t.*** A technician who assists the food service manager and dietitian in a health care facility with planning, implementing, and evaluating food programs, and may train and supervise dietary aides.

***electrocardiographical t.*** A technician who operates and maintains electrocardiographic machines, records the heart's electrical activity, and provides data for diagnosis and treatment of heart ailments by physicians.

***electromyographical t.*** A technician who assists the physician in recording and analyzing bioelectric potentials that originate in muscle tissue. This includes the operation of various electronic devices, maintenance of electronic equipment, assisting with patient care during testing, and record keeping.

***emergency medical t.—paramedic*** A technician who responds to medical emergency calls, evaluates the nature of the emergency, and carries out specific diagnostic measures and emergency treatment procedures under the standing orders or specific directions of a physician.

***environmental health t.*** A technician who assists in the survey of environmental hazards and performs technical duties under professional supervision in areas such as pollution control, radiation protection, and sanitation.

***histological t.*** A technician who works under the supervision of a pathologist in sectioning, staining, and mounting human and animal tissue and fluid for microscopic study.

***medical laboratory t.*** A technician who performs biological and chemical tests requiring limited independent judgment or correlation competency under the supervision of a medical technologist, pathologist, or physician.

***medical record t.*** A technician who assists the medical record administrator by coding, analyzing, and preserving patients' medical records and compiling reports, disease indices, and statistics in health care institutions.

***orthopedic t.*** A technician who is trained in maintaining traction devices, applies all types of traction, makes casts, and applies splints.

***pharmacy t.*** A technician who assists the pharmacist in certain activities such as medication profile reviews for drug incompatibilities, typing of prescription labels, prescription packaging, handling of purchase records, inventory control, and may, where state law and hospital policy permit, dispense drugs to patients under the supervision of a registered pharmacist.

***psychiatric t.*** A technician who works under the supervision of a professional in the care of mentally ill patients in a psychiatric care facility. This person assists in carrying out the prescribed treatment plan and assigned individual and group activities with patients.

***respiratory therapy t.*** A technician who routinely treats patients requiring noncritical respiratory care and who recognizes and responds to specified respiratory emergencies.

**technique** (tĕk-nēk′) [Fr., Gr. *technikos*] **1.** A systematic procedure or method by which an involved or scientific task is completed. **2.** The skill in performing details of a procedure or operation. **3.** In radiology, the various technical factors that must be determined in order to produce a diagnostic radiograph, such as kilovoltage, milliamperage, time of exposure, and focal-film distance.

***bisecting angle t.*** A dental radiographic technique that requires (1) placement of the film as close as possible to the teeth, causing the film to rest against the crown; (2) visualization of a bisector, which bisects the angle formed by the long axis of the teeth and the film; and (3) positioning of the central ray perpendicular to the bisector. The image produced is distorted in a buccolingual direction. Also called *short-cone technique*. SEE: *Cieszynski's rule*.

***compensatory t.*** The use of modified procedures or assistive devices to enable the successful performance of tasks by persons with a disability.

***enzyme-multiplied immunoassay technique*** ABBR: EMIT. A widely used clinical chemistry procedure.

***forced expiration t.*** A type of cough that facilitates clearance of bronchial secretions while reducing the risk of bronchiolar collapse. One or two expirations are forced from average to low lung volume with an open glottis. A period of diaphragmatic breathing and relaxation follows.

***minimal leak t.*** ABBR: MLT. A method of determining cuff inflation volume on endotracheal tubes.

***paralleling t.*** A dental radiographic technique that requires placement of the film parallel to the teeth and positioning of the central ray perpendicular to the teeth. The orientation of the film, teeth, and central ray produce a radiograph with minimal geometric distortion. Also called *right-angle* or *long-cone technique*.

**techno-** Combining form meaning *art, skill.*

**technologist** (tĕk″nŏl′ō-jĭst) [Gr. *techne,* art, + *logos,* word, reason] An individual specializing in the application of scientific knowledge in solving practical or theoretical problems. The knowledge and skills required for performing these functions are achieved through formal education and a period of supervised clinical practice.

***blood bank t.*** A technologist trained to assist in all of the routine and special functions and tasks concerned with blood bank and transfusion services.

***cardiovascular t.*** A technologist who performs a wide range of tests related to the functions and therapeutic care of the heart and lung system. These include operating and maintaining a heart-lung machine, assisting in cardiac catheterization, cardiac resuscitation, postoperative monitoring, and the care and treatment of patients who have undergone heart or lung surgery.

***electroencephalographic t.*** A technologist who operates and maintains electroencephalographic machines.

***histologic t.*** A technologist who performs all the functions of the histological technician, as well as more complex procedures for processing tissues, such as identifying tissue structures, cell components, and their staining characteristics, and relates them to physiological functions. He or she may also implement and test new techniques and procedures.

***medical t.*** A technologist who works in conjunction with pathologists, physicians, and scientists in all general areas of the clinical laboratory. Independent and correlational judgments are made in a wide range of complex procedures. A medical technologist may teach and supervise laboratory personnel.

***nuclear medicine t.*** Radiation therapy t.

***radiation therapy t.*** ABBR: RT(T). A technologist trained to assist the radiation oncologist in the safe application of radiation for therapeutic purposes. Also called *radiation therapist*. SYN: *nuclear medicine t.*

***radiological t.*** A technologist trained in the safe application of ionizing radiation to portions of the body to assist the physician in the diagnosis of injuries and disease. This individual may also supervise or teach others. Technology programs approved by the Joint Review Commission on Education in the Radiologic Sciences are conducted in hospitals, medical schools, and colleges with hospital affiliations.

***registered pulmonary function t.*** An individual who has completed the pulmonary function registry examination administered by the National Board for Respiratory Care.

***surgical t.*** A technologist who assists in providing a safe environment for surgical care and assists surgeon, nurses, and other operating room staff.

**technology** (těk-nŏl′ō-jē) [″ + *logos,* word, reason] **1.** The application of scientific knowledge. **2.** The entire scientific knowledge used in solving or approaching problems and situations. **3.** The entire body of knowledge available to a civilization.

***adaptive t.*** Assistive t.

***assistive t.*** A device or adaptation that enables or assists persons with disability to perform everyday tasks of living. Assistive technologies are categorized by rehabilitation personnel as high technology or low technology, with the former including devices that use microprocessors. An example of a high-technology device would be an environmental control unit or robotic aid. An example of a low technology device would be a reacher or a tool with a built-up handle. SYN: *adaptive t.; adaptive device.*

**tectocephalic** (tĕk″tō-sĕ-făl′ĭk) [L. *tectum,* roof, + Gr. *kephale,* head] Concerning tectocephaly.

**tectocephaly** (tĕk-tō-sĕf′ăl-ē) Scaphocephalism.

**tectorial** (tĕk-tō′rē-ăl) [L. *tectum,* roof] Pert. to tectorium.

**tectorium** (tĕk-tō′rē-ŭm) *pl.* **tectoria** [L. *tectorium,* a covering] **1.** Any rooflike structure. SYN: *tectum; tegmentum; tegument.* **2.** The membrane that overhangs the receptors for hearing (hair cells) in the organ of Corti.

**tectospinal** (tĕk″tō-spī′năl) [L. *tectum,* roof, + *spina,* thorn] From the tectum mesencephali to the spinal cord.

**tectospinal tract** A tract of white fibers of the spinal cord passing from the tectum of the midbrain and going down through the medulla to the spinal cord. It begins on one side and crosses to the other.

**tectum** (tĕk′tŭm) [L., roof] **1.** Any structure serving as, or resembling, a roof. SYN: *tectorium; tegmentum; tegument.* **2.** The dorsal portion of the midbrain consisting of the superior and inferior colliculi (corpora quadrigemina). SYN: *tegmentum.*

***t. mesencephali*** The roof of the midbrain, including the corpora quadrigemina.

**T.E.D.** *threshold erythema dose.*

**teenage** Adolescent.

**teeth** (tēth) *sing.,* **tooth** [AS. *toth,* tooth] Hard bony projections in the jaws serving as organs of mastication, there being 32 permanent teeth, 16 in each jaw. They include the following types: incisors, canines (cuspids), premolars (bicuspids), and molars. An average child should have 6 teeth at 1 year, 12 at 18 months, 16 at 2 years, and 20 at 2½ years. A child may be born with teeth, and in other cases the teeth may not appear until 16 months. SEE: *dentition* for illus.; *tooth; plaque, dental; periodontal disease.*

***anterior t.*** Teeth located close to the midline of the dental arch on either side of the jaw, including the incisors and canines.

***auditory t.*** Minute toothlike projections along the free margin of the labium vestibulare of the cochlea. SYN: *Huschke's auditory teeth.*

***charting and numbering of t.*** The var-

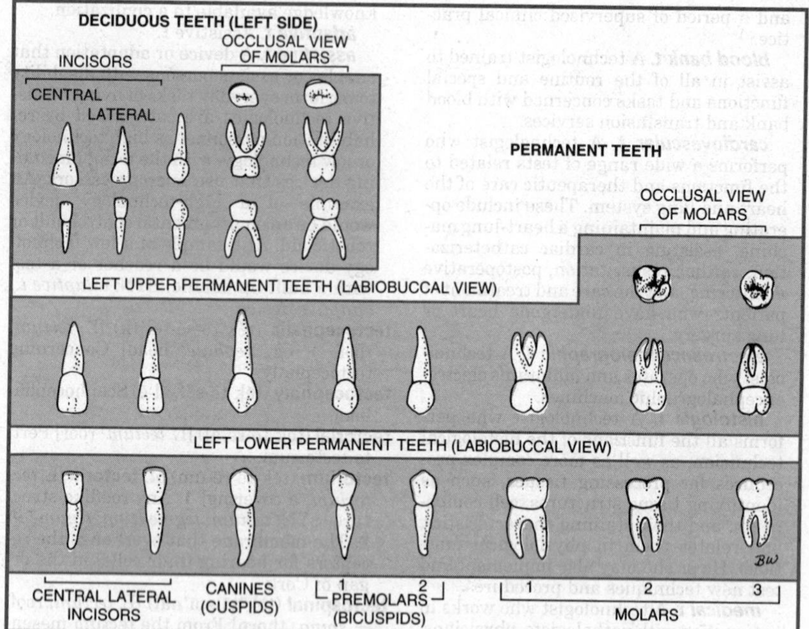


ious systems developed for designating teeth in a chart system including numbers, letters, or symbols. They are not uniformly accepted. Widely used are the two-digit system of Federation Dentaire Internationale (FDI system) and the American system, which numbers the permanent teeth consecutively from the upper right third molar as #1 through the maxillary teeth to #16, and then to the left mandibular third molar as #17 and through the mandibular teeth to the right third molar as #32.

***deciduous t.*** Teeth making up the first dentition, which are shed and replaced by the permanent teeth. SYN: *milk t.; temporary t.* SEE: illus.

***malacotic t.*** Teeth that are esp. prone to decay, soft in structure and white in color.

***milk t.*** Deciduous t.

***permanent t.*** Teeth that develop as the second dentition, replacing the deciduous teeth. SYN: *secondary t.* SEE: *deciduous t.* for illus.

***reimplantation or repair of t.*** The preservation and restoration of teeth dislodged or broken by trauma.

First Aid: If a tooth is completely knocked out of its socket by trauma or fracture, the tooth or fragment should be gently cleaned (not scrubbed), placed in clean water, and taken with the patient without delay to a dentist. For an adult who is conscious, the tooth may be replaced in the socket during transport to the dentist. The dentist may be able to save the tooth by gluing the fragments to the remaining part of the tooth.

***sclerotic t.*** Yellowish teeth that are naturally hard and not subject to ready decay.

***secondary t.*** Permanent t.

***stained t.*** Deep or superficial discoloration of teeth. A number of conditions cause this (e.g., exposure of the fetus to tetracycline the mother took during pregnancy or mottling caused by exposure to high levels of fluoride in drinking water). No matter what the cause, the stains may be covered up by applying a plastic resin or porcelain laminate coating over them, a process called bonding. This same technique may be used to rebuild or repair chipped or cracked teeth.

***temporary t.*** Deciduous t.

***twinning of t.*** A dental anomaly in which two teeth are joined together.

***wisdom t.*** The third molar teeth of the permanent dentition, which are the last to erupt.

**teething** (tēth′ĭng) [AS. *toth,* tooth] Eruption of the teeth. SEE: *dentition.*

**Teflon** Trade name for polytetrafluorethylene.

**tegmen** (tĕg′mĕn) *pl.* **tegmina** [L. *tegmen,* covering] A structure that covers a part.

***t. mastoideum*** The bony roof of mastoid cells.

***t. tympani*** The roof of the tympanum separating the middle ear from the cranial cavity.

***t. ventriculi quarti*** The roof of the fourth ventricle.

**tegmental** (tĕg-mĕn′tăl) [L. *tegmentum,* covering] Relating to a tegmentum.

**tegmental nucleus** One of several masses of gray matter lying in the tegmentum of the midbrain and upper portion of the pons; it includes the dorsal, pedunculopontile, reticular, and ventral nuclei.

**tegmentum** (tĕg-mĕn′tŭm) [L. *tegmentum,* covering] **1.** A roof or covering. SYN: *tectorium; tegument.* **2.** The dorsal portion of the cruri cerebri of the midbrain. It contains the red nucleus and nuclei and roots of the oculomotor nerve. SYN: *tectum.*

**tegument** (tĕg′ū-mĕnt) **1.** Integument. **2.** A covering structure.

**tegumental, tegumentary** (tĕg″ū-mĕn′tăl, -tă-rē) Concerning the skin or tegument; covering.

**teichoic acid** A polymer found in the wall of certain bacteria.

**teichopsia** (tī-kŏp′sē-ă) [Gr. *teichos,* wall, + *opsis,* vision] Zigzag lines bounding a luminous area appearing in the visual field. It causes temporary blindness in that portion of the field of vision. This condition is sometimes associated with migraine headaches or mental or physical strain. SYN: *scintillating scotoma.*

**teinodynia** (tī″nō-dĭn′ē-ă) [Gr. *tenon,* tendon, + *odyne,* pain] Tenodynia.

**tel-, tele- 1.** Combining form meaning *end.* **2.** Combining form meaning *distant.*

**tela** (tē′lă) *pl.* **telae** [L. *tela,* web] Any weblike structure.

***t. choroidea*** Part of the pia mater covering the roof of the third and fourth cerebral ventricles.

***t. conjunctiva*** Connective tissue.

***t. elastica*** Elastic tissue.

***t. subcutanea*** Subcutaneous connective tissue; superficial fascia.

***t. submucosa*** The submucosa of the intestine.

**telalgia** (tĕl-ăl′jē-ă) [Gr. *tele,* distant, + *algos,* pain] Pain felt at a distance from its stimulus. SYN: *pain, referred.*

**telangiectasia, telangiectasis** (tĕl-ăn″jē-ĕk-tā′zē-ă, -ĕk′tă-sĭs) [Gr. *telos,* end, + *angeion,* vessel, + *ektasis,* dilatation] A vascular lesion formed by dilatation of a group of small blood vessels. It may appear as a birthmark or become apparent in young children. It may also be caused by long-term sun exposure. Although the lesion may occur anywhere on the skin, it is seen most frequently on the face and thighs. SEE: illus.

***hereditary hemorrhagic t.*** A hereditary disease marked by thinness of the walls of the blood vessels of the nose, skin, and digestive tract as well as a tendency to hemorrhage. SYN: *Rendu-Osler-Weber syndrome.*

***t. lymphatica*** A tumor composed of dilated lymph vessels.

***spider t.*** A stellate angioma

**telangiectatic** (tĕl-ăn″jē-ĕk-tăt′ĭk) Concerning telangiectasia.

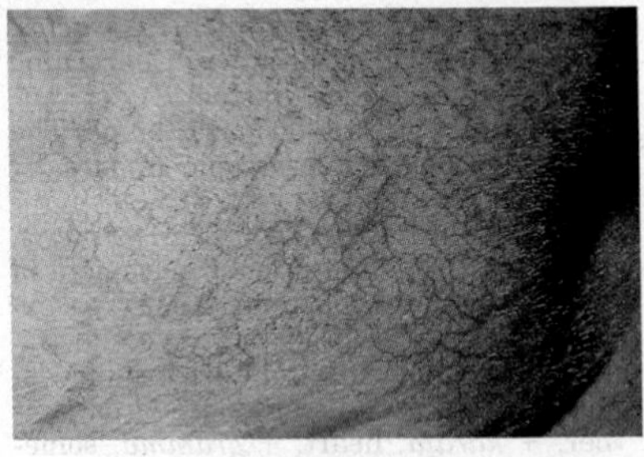

TELANGIECTASIA
(FROM SUN EXPOSURE)

**telangiectodes** (tĕl-ăn″jē-ĕk-tō′dēz) Tumors that have telangiectasia.

**telangiitis** (tĕl-ăn″jē-ī′tĭs) [″ + ″ + *itis,* inflammation] An inflammation of the capillaries.

**telangioma** (tĕl-ăn″jē-ō′mă) [Gr. *telos,* end, + *angeion,* vessel, + *oma,* tumor] A tumor made up of dilated capillaries or arterioles.

**telangion** (tĕl-ăn′jē-ŏn) [″ + *angeion,* vessel] A capillary or terminal arteriole.

**telangiosis** (tĕl″ăn-jē-ō′sĭs) [″ + ″ + *osis,* condition] A disease of capillary vessels.

**telecanthus** (tĕl″ĕ-kăn′thŭs) [Gr. *tele,* distant, + *kanthos,* corner of the eye] Increased distance between the inner canthi of the eyelids.

**telecardiogram** (tĕl″ĕ-kăr′dē-ō-grăm) [″ + *kardia,* heart, + *gramma,* something written] A cardiogram that records at a distance from the patient. The signal is transmitted electronically to the recording device. SYN: *telelectrocardiogram.*

**telecardiography** (tĕl″ĕ-kăr″dē-ŏg′ră-fē) [″ + ″ + *graphein,* to write] The process of taking telecardiograms.

**telecardiophone** (tĕl″ĕ-kăr′dē-ō-fōn) [″ + ″ + *phone,* voice] A stethoscope that will magnify heart sounds so they may be heard at a distance from the patient.

**teleceptive** (tĕl-ĕ-sĕp′tĭv) [″ + L. *ceptivus,* take] Relating to a teleceptor.

**teleceptor** (tĕl′ĕ-sĕp″tor) [″ + L. *ceptor,* a receiver] A distance receptor; a sense organ that responds to stimuli arising some distance from the body, such as the eye, ear, and nose. SYN: *teloceptor.*

**telecurietherapy** (tĕl-ĕ-kū″rē-thĕr′ă-pē) [″ + *curie,* + Gr. *therapeia,* treatment] The application of radiation therapy from a source distant from the lesion or patient.

**teledendrite, teledendron** (tĕl-ĕ-dĕn′drīt, -dĕn′drŏn) [Gr. *telos,* end, + *dendron,* a tree] One of the terminal processes of an axon. SYN: *telodendron.*

**telediagnosis** (tĕl″ĕ-dī″ăg-nō′sĭs) [Gr. *tele,* distant, + *diagignoskein,* to discern] Diagnosis made on the basis of data transmitted electronically to the physician's location.

**telediastolic** (těl″ĕ-dī-ă-stŏl′ĭk) [Gr. *telos,* end, + *diastole,* a dilatation] Concerning the last phase of the diastole.

**telefluoroscopy** (těl″ĕ-floo″or-ŏs′kō-pē) The transmission of fluoroscopic images by electronic means.

**telekinesis** (těl″ĕ-kĭ-nē′sĭs) [″ + *kinesis,* movement] The intentional movement of articles without touching them. The existence of this ability is controversial.

**telelectrocardiogram** (těl″ē-lĕk″trō-kăr′dē-ō-grăm) [Gr. *tele,* distant, + *elektron,* amber, + *kardia,* heart, + *gramma,* something written] Telecardiogram.

**telemedicine** The use of telecommunications equipment to transmit the image of and general information about a patient at a distant site. This technique has proven to be of great value in providing comprehensive medical and surgical consultation for those caring for patients in remote areas or battlefields with limited hospital facilities.

**telemeter** (těl′ĕ-mē″tĕr) [″ + *metron,* measure] An electronic device used to transmit information to a distant point.

**telemetry** (tĕ-lĕm′ĕ-trē) The transmission of data electronically to a distant location.

**telencephalic** (těl″ĕn-sĕf-ăl′ĭk) [Gr. *telos,* end, + *enkephalos,* brain] Pert. to the endbrain (telencephalon).

**telencephalization** (těl″ĕn-sĕf″ăl-ī-zā′shŭn) The evolutionary degree of control over functions previously mediated by lower nerve centers.

**telencephalon** (těl-ĕn-sĕf′ă-lŏn) [″ + *enkephalos,* brain] The embryonic endbrain or posterior division of the prosencephalon from which the cerebral hemispheres, corpora striata, and rhinencephalon develop.

**teleneurite** (těl″ĕ-nū′rīt) [″ + *neuron,* nerve] The branching end of an axon.

**teleneuron** (těl″ĕ-nū′rŏn) [″ + *neuron,* nerve] A nerve ending.

**teleo-** Combining form meaning *perfect, complete.*

**teleological** (tē″lē-ō-lŏj′ĭ-kăl) Concerning teleology.

**teleology** (těl-ē-ŏl′ō-jē) [Gr. *teleos,* complete, + *logos,* word, reason] **1.** The belief that everything is directed toward some final purpose. **2.** The doctrine of final causes.

**teleomitosis** (těl″ē-ō-mī-tō′sĭs) [″ + *mitos,* thread, + *osis,* condition] Completed mitosis.

**teleonomy** (těl″ē-ŏn′ō-mē) [″ + *nomos,* law] The concept that, in an organism or animal, the existence of a structure, capability, or function indicates that it had a survival function. **teleonomic** (těl″ē-ō-nŏm′ĭk), *adj.*

**teleoperator** A machine or device operated by a person at a distance. Such a machine allows tasks to be done deep in the ocean or on orbiting satellites, and allows radioactive materials to be manipulated without danger of exposure to the radioactivity.

**teleopsia** (těl-ē-ŏp′sē-ă) [Gr. *tele,* distant, + *ops,* eye] A visual disorder in which objects perceived in space have excessive depth or in which close objects appear far away.

**teleotherapeutics** (těl″ē-ō-thĕr-ă-pū′tĭks) [Gr. *tele,* distant, + *therapeutikos,* treating] The use of hypnotic suggestion in the treatment of disease. SYN: *suggestive therapeutics.*

**telepathy** (tĕ-lĕp′ă-thē) Communication of one mind with another at a distance without any physical or psychological explanation. SYN: *telesthesia* (1).

**teleradiogram** (těl″ĕ-rā′dē-ō-grăm) [Gr. *tele,* distant, + L. *radius,* ray, + Gr. *gramma,* something written] An x-ray picture obtained by teleradiography.

**teleradiography** (těl″ĕ-rā-dē-ŏg′ră-fē) [″] Radiography with the radiation source about 2 m (6½ ft) from the body. Because the rays are virtually parallel at that distance, distortion is minimized. SYN: *teleroentgenography.*

**teleradiology** The transmission of an x-ray image to a distant center where it may be interpreted by a radiologist.

**teleradium** (těl″ĕ-rā′dē-ŭm) A radium source distant from the area being treated.

**teleroentgenogram** (těl″ĕ-rĕnt-gĕn′ō-grăm) Teleradiogram.

**teleroentgenography** (těl″ĕ-rĕnt″gĕn-ŏg′ră-fē) [″ + ″ + Gr. *graphein,* to write] Teleradiography.

**telesthesia** (těl-ĕs-thē′zē-ă) [″ + *aisthesis,* sensation] **1.** Telepathy. SEE: *paranormal.* **2.** Distance perception.

**telesystolic** (těl″ĕ-sĭs-tŏl′ĭk) [Gr. *telos,* end, + *systole,* contraction] Pert. to the termination of the cardiac systole.

**teletactor** (těl″ĕ-tăk′tor) [″ + L. *tactus,* touch] A device used by the deaf to receive vibrations through the skin.

**teletherapy** (těl-ĕ-thĕr′ă-pē) [Gr. *tele,* distant, + *therapeia,* treatment] **1.** Treatment of disease by telepathy. **2.** Cancer treatment in which the radiation source is placed outside the body.

**teletypewriter** ABBR: TTY. A typewriter that may be connected to a telephone. This device permits deaf persons to communicate by sending and receiving typewritten messages.

**telluric** (tĕ-lūr′ĭk) [L. *tellus,* earth] Of or rel. to the earth.

**tellurism** (těl′ū-rĭzm) [″ + Gr. *-ismos,* condition] The concept that emanations from the earth cause disease.

**tellurium** (těl-ū′rē-ŭm) [L. *tellus,* earth] SYMB: Te. A nonmetallic element used as an electric rectifier and in coloring glass; atomic weight, 127.60; atomic number, 52; specific gravity, 6.24.

**tellurium poisoning** Toxicity resulting from the ingestion of tellurium. It is marked by a garlic odor of all secretions and excretions and a disagreeable breath odor. Perspiration and saliva are suppressed, resulting in dry skin and mouth. Anorexia, nausea, drowsiness, and weakness may be present. Treatment includes administration of saline cathartics and an increase in fluid intake. In addition, perspiration should be induced; otherwise, treatment is symptomatic.

**telocentric** (tĕl″ō-sĕn′trĭk) [Gr. *telos,* end, + *kentron,* center] Location of the centromere in the extreme end of the replicating chromosome so that there is only one arm on the chromosome.

**teloceptor** Teleceptor.

**telodendron** (tĕl-ō-dĕn′drŏn) [Gr. *telos,* end, + *dendron,* tree] Teledendrite.

**telogen** (tĕl′ō-jĕn) [″ + *genesis,* generation, birth] The resting stage of the hair growth cycle. SEE: *anagen; catagen.*

**teloglia** (tĕl-ŏg′lē-ă) The Schwann cells at the end of a motor nerve fiber near the neuromuscular junction.

**telolecithal** Concerning an egg in which the large yolk mass is concentrated at one pole.

**telolemma** (tĕl″ō-lĕm′mă) [″ + *lemma,* rind] The membrane of the axon terminal at a neuromuscular junction.

**telomerase** An enzyme present in cancer cells that enables them to divide indefinitely.

**telomere** (tĕl′ō-mēr) [″ + *meros,* part] The end of an arm of a chromosome.

**telophase** (tĕl′ō-fāz) [″ + *phasis,* an appearance] The final phase or stage of mitosis (karyokinesis) during which reconstruction of the daughter nuclei takes place and the cytoplasm of the cell divides, giving rise to two daughter cells.

**telophragma** (tĕl″ō-frăg′mă) [″ + *phragmos,* a fencing in] The Z line or disk in striated muscle. SEE: *Z disk.*

**telosynapsis** (tĕl″ō-sĭ-năp′sĭs) [″ + *synapsis,* point of contact] End-to-end union of pairs of homologous chromosomes during gametogenesis.

**TEM** *triethylenemelamine.*

**tempeh** A wheat-soybean food developed as an excellent inexpensive source of protein for children. It is used in economically depressed countries. The quality of protein in tempeh is almost equal to casein.

**temper** [AS. *temprian,* to mingle] The state of an individual's mood, disposition, or mind (e.g., even-tempered or foul-tempered).

**temperament** (tĕm′pĕr-ă-mĕnt) [L. *temperamentum,* mixture] The combination of intellectual, emotional, ethical, and physical characteristics of a specific individual.

**temperance** Moderation in one's thoughts and actions, esp. with respect to use of alcoholic beverages.

**temperate** (tĕm′pĕr-ĭt) Moderate; not excessive.

**temperature** (tĕm′pĕr-ă-tūr) [L. *temperatura,* proportion] **1.** The degree of heat of a living body. **2.** The degree of hotness or coldness of a substance.

Body temperature varies with the time of day and the site of measurement. Oral temperature is usually 97.5° to 99.5°F (36° to 38°C), and the temperature in the liver may be 105°F (40.6°C). Daily fluctuations in an individual may be 1° or 2°F. Body temperature may be measured by a clinical thermometer placed in the mouth, in the rectum, or under the arm. Rectal temperature is usually from 0.5° to 1.0°F (0.28° to 0.56°C) higher than by mouth; axillary temperature is about 0.5°F (0.28°C) lower than by mouth. Oral temperature may be inaccurate if taken just after the patient has ingested cold substances or has been breathing with the mouth open.

Body temperature is regulated by thermoregulatory centers in the hypothalamus that balance heat production and heat loss. Eighty-five percent of body heat is lost through the skin (radiation, conduction, sweating) and the remainder through the lungs and fecal and urinary excretions. Muscular work (including shivering) is a mechanism for raising body temperature. Elevation of temperature above normal is called fever (pyrexia), and subnormal temperature is hypothermia. SEE: illus.; *ear thermometry.*

***absolute t.*** The temperature measured from absolute zero, which is −273.15°C.

***ambient t.*** The surrounding temperature or that present in the place, site, or location indicated.

***axillary t.*** The temperature obtained by placing a thermometer in the apex of the axilla with the arm pressed closely to the side of the body. The temperature obtained by this method is usually 0.5° to 1.0°F (0.28° to 0.56°C) lower than oral.

***basal t. chart*** SEE: *basal temperature chart.*

***body t.*** The temperature of the body. SEE: *temperature.*

***core t.*** SEE: *core temperature.*

***critical t.*** The temperature below which a gas may be converted to liquid form by pressure.

***inverse t.*** A condition in which the body temperature is higher in the morning than in the evening.

***maximum t.*** The temperature above which bacterial growth will not take place.

***mean t.*** The average temperature for a stated period in a given locality.

***minimum t.*** In bacteriology, the temperature below which bacterial growth will not take place.

***normal t.*** The temperature of the body, taken orally, in a healthy individual: 97.5° to 99.5°F (36° to 38°C) in humans.

***optimum t.*** The temperature at which a procedure is best carried out, such as the culture of a given organism or the action of an enzyme.

***oral t.*** The temperature obtained by placing a thermometer under the pa-

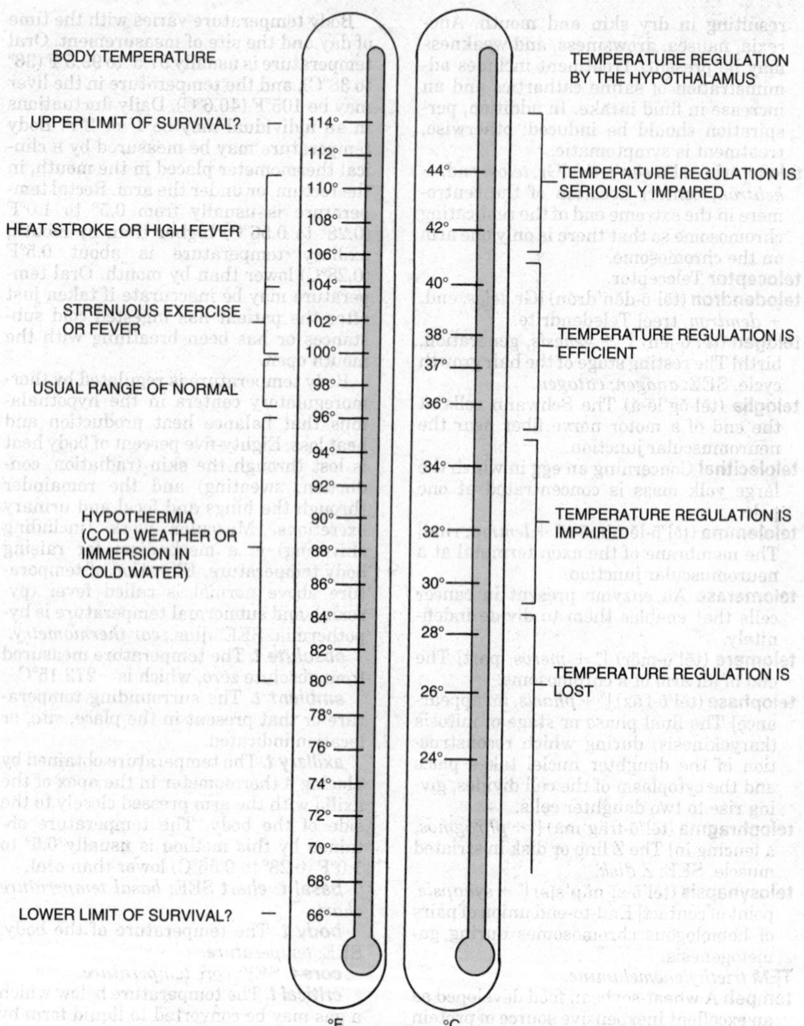

**TEMPERATURE REGULATION**
EFFECTS OF CHANGES IN BODY TEMPERATURE

tient's tongue with lips closed for 3 min. It should not be taken for at least 10 min after ingestion of hot or cold liquids. It is not advisable for infants, individuals who breathe through the mouth, comatose patients, or those extremely ill.

***rectal t.*** The temperature obtained by inserting a thermometer into the anal canal to a depth of at least 1½ in. (3.8 cm) and allowing it to remain there for 3 to 5 min. This method should not be used following a rectal operation or if the rectum is diseased. A rectal temperature is more accurate than either oral or axillary temperatures. It averages about 1°F (0.56°C) higher than the oral temperature and approx. 1.5°F (0.84°C) higher than axillary temperature.

***room t.*** The temperature between 65° and 80°F (18.3° and 26.7°C).

***subnormal t.*** A body temperature below the normal range of 97.5° to 99.5°F (36° to 38°C).

***tympanic t.*** The temperature obtained by placing an electronic probe in the ear canal. SEE: *ear thermometry; thermometer, tympanic.*

**temperature senses** The sensations of warmth resulting from raising the temperature of the skin and that of cold aroused by lowering it. The sensation of warmth is mediated by Ruffini's corpuscles; that of cold, by the end-bulbs of Krause. These receptors are distributed so as to form cold and warm sensing spots on the skin. Afferent impulses from receptors, on reaching the thalamus, may give rise to crude uncritical temperature sensations; on being relayed to the somesthetic area of the cortex, they result in discrete and fairly well localized sensations of heat and cold. Adaptation is rapid.

**template** (tĕm′plāt) A pattern, mold, or form used as a guide in duplicating a shape, structure, or device.

***occlusal t.*** A stone or metal base made from a wax occlusal registration against which artificial teeth are set in the preparation of a denture.

***wax t.*** A wax impression of the occlusion of teeth made by closing the jaw until the teeth are embedded in the wax plate.

**temple** (tĕm′pl) [O. Fr. from L. *tempora,* pl. of *tempus,* temple] The region of the head in front of the ear and over the zygomatic arch.

**tempolabile** (tĕm″pō-lā′bl) [L. *tempus,* period of time, + *labi,* to slip] Becoming altered spontaneously within a definite time.

**tempora** (tĕm′pō-ră) [L. pl. of *tempus,* period of time] The temples.

**temporal** (tĕm′por-ăl) [L. *temporalis,* period of time] **1.** Pert. to or limited in time. **2.** Rel. to the temples.

**temporal bone** A bone on both sides of the skull at its base. It is composed of squamous, mastoid, and petrous portions, the latter enclosing the receptors for hearing and equilibrium. SYN: *os temporale.* SEE: *Arnold's canal; mastoid; petrosa; styloid process.*

**temporalis** (tĕm″pō-ră′lĭs) [L.] The muscle in the temporal fossa that elevates the mandible. SEE: *Muscles Appendix.*

**temporal line** One of two lines on the lateral surface of the frontal and parietal bones that mark the upper limit of the temporal fossa.

**temporal lobe** The lobe of the cerebrum located laterally and below the frontal and occipital lobes. It contains auditory receptive areas.

**temporal-sequential organization** The ability of a child to develop concepts of time and sequence. This function is localized in the left hemisphere of the brain. This ability is essential to the function of a child in daily activities concerned with routines such as telling time or following multistep directions. Skill in this function increases with age. SEE: *digit span test.*

**temporo-** [L.] Combining form meaning *temple* of the head.

**temporoauricular** (tĕm″pō-rō-aw-rĭk′ū-lăr) [″ + *auricula,* little ear] Concerning the temples and auricular areas.

**temporohyoid** (tĕm″pō-rō-hī′oyd) [″ + Gr. *hyoeides,* U-shaped] Concerning the temporal and hyoid bones.

**temporomalar** (tĕm″pō-rō-mā′lăr) [″ + *mala,* cheek] Temporozygomatic.

**temporomandibular** (tĕm″pō-rō-măn-dĭb′ū-lăr) [″ + *mandibula,* lower jawbone] Pert. to the temporal and mandible bones; esp. important in dentistry because of the articulation of the bones of the temporomandibular joint.

**temporomandibular joints** The encapsulated, double, synovial joints between the condyles of the mandible and the temporal bones of the skull. SYN: *craniomandibular joints.*

**temporomandibular joint syndrome** ABBR: TMJ syndrome. Severe aching pain in and about the temporomandibular joint, made worse by chewing. The syndrome is marked by limited movement of the joint and clicking sounds during chewing. Tinnitus, pain, and deafness may be present. Causes include lesions of the temporomandibular joint tissues, malocclusion, overbite, poorly fitting dentures, and tissue changes resulting in pressure on nerves. Treatment consists of definitive therapy for the primary disease or condition. SYN: *Costen's syndrome.*

**temporomaxillary** (tĕm″pō-rō-măk′sĭ-lĕr-ē) [″ + *maxilla,* jawbone] Pert. to the temporal and maxillary bones.

**temporo-occipital** (tĕm″pō-rō-ŏk-sĭp′ĭ-tăl) [″ + *occipitalis,* pert. to the occiput] Pert. to the temporal and occipital bones or their regions.

**temporoparietal** (tĕm″pō-rō-pă-rī′ĕ-tăl) [″ + *paries,* wall] Concerning the temporal and parietal bones.

**temporopontine** [″ + *pons,* bridge] Concerning or situated between the temporal lobe of the brain and the pons.

**temporosphenoid** (tĕm″pō-rō-sfē′noyd) [″ + Gr. *sphen,* wedge, + *eidos,* form, shape] Pert. to the temporal and sphenoid bones.

**temporozygomatic** (tĕm″pō-rō-zī″gō-măt′ĭk) [″ + Gr. *zygoma,* cheekbone] Concerning the temporal and zygomatic bones. SYN: *temporomalar.*

**tempostabile** (tĕm″pō-stā′bĭl) [L. *tempus,* time, + *stabilis,* stable] Descriptive of something, esp. a chemical compound, that remains stable with the passage of time.

**ten-** SEE: *taen-.*

**tenacious** (tĕ-nā′shŭs) [L. *tenax*] Adhering to; adhesive; retentive.

**tenacity** (tĕ-năs′ĭ-tē) Condition of being tough, stubborn, or obstinate.

**tenaculum** (tĕn-ăk′ū-lŭm) [L., a holder] Sharp, hooklike, pointed instrument with a slender shank for grasping and holding an anatomical part.

**tenalgia** (tĕn-ăl′jē-ă) [Gr. *tenon,* tendon, + *algos,* pain] Tenodynia.

***t. crepitans*** An inflammation of a tendon sheath that on movement results in a crackling sound. SYN: *tendosynovitis crepitans; tenosynovitis crepitans.*

**Tenckhoff peritoneal catheter** A catheter placed into the peritoneal cavity through the anterior abdominal wall. It is left in for an extended period and is used for peritoneal dialysis. SEE: *dialysis, continuous ambulatory peritoneal.*

**tender loving care** ABBR: TLC. The concept of administering medical and nursing care and attention to a patient in a kindly, compassionate, and humane manner as distinguished from a cold technical approach. This is particularly important in intensive care units, where patients are connected to electronic monitors and devices.

**tenderness** (tĕn′dĕr-nĕs) Sensitivity to pain upon pressure.

***rebound t.*** Production of or intensification of pain when pressure is released. SEE: *Blumberg's sign.*

**tendinitis, tendonitis** (tĕn″dĭn-ī′tĭs) [L. *tendo,* tendon, + Gr. *itis,* inflammation] An inflammation of a tendon. SYN: *tenonitis; tenontitis.*

***rotator cuff t.*** A frequent cause of shoulder pain thought to be due to pressure on the tendons of the shoulder, esp. that of the supraspinatus. The onset usually follows injury or overuse during activities involving repeated elevation of the arm such as in certain occupations and sports (e.g., baseball, basketball, tennis, or swimming). Persons older than age 40 are particularly susceptible. Treatment consists of conservative therapy; if that is not of benefit and functional loss is present, then surgery is indicated.

**tendinoplasty** (tĕn′dĭ-nō-plăs″tē) [″ + Gr. *plassein,* to form] Plastic surgery of tendons. SYN: *tendoplasty; tenontoplasty; tenoplasty.*

**tendinosis 1.** Degeneration of a tendon from repetitive microtrauma. **2.** Tendinitis without inflammation. **3.** Collagen degeneration.

**tendinosuture** (tĕn″dĭn-ō-sū′tūr) [″ + *sutura,* a seam] The suturing of a divided tendon. SYN: *tenorrhaphy.*

**tendinous** (tĕn′dĭ-nŭs) [L. *tendinosus*] Pert. to, composed of, or resembling tendons.

**tendinous synovitis** An inflammation of a tendon's synovial sheath.

**tendo-** SEE: *teno-.*

**tendo** [L.] A tendon.

**tendolysis** (tĕn-dŏl′ĭ-sĭs) [″ + Gr. *lysis,* dissolution] The process of freeing a tendon from adhesions. SYN: *tenolysis.*

**tendon** (tĕn′dŭn) [L. *tendo,* tendon] Fibrous connective tissue serving for the attachment of muscles to bones and other parts. SYN: *sinew; tendo.*

***Achilles t.*** The large tendon at the lower end of the gastrocnemius muscle, inserted into the os calcis. It is the strongest and thickest tendon in the body. SYN: *calcaneal t.*

***calcaneal t.*** Achilles t.

***central t.*** The central portion of the diaphragm, consisting of a flat aponeurosis into which the muscle fibers of the diaphragm are inserted.

***superior t. of Lockwood*** The portion of the fibrous ring from which the superior oblique muscle of the eye originates.

***t. of Zinn*** The portion of the fibrous ring (annulus tendineus communis) from which the inferior rectus muscle of the eye originates.

**tendon action** Passive movement of a joint when a two-joint or multi-joint muscle is stretched across it.

**tendon cell** One of the fibroblasts of white fibrous connective tissue of tendons that are arranged in parallel rows.

**tendonitis, tendinitis** [″ + Gr. *itis,* inflammation] An inflammation of a tendon.

**tendon reflex** A reflex act in which a muscle contracts when its tendon is percussed.

***patellar t.r.*** Slight extension of the leg when the tendon of the quadriceps muscle is tapped immediately below the patella. When the patient is lying in bed, the leg should be slightly bent at the knee in order to test this reflex. When the patient is sitting on the edge of the bed, this reflex may be tested while the leg hangs free. SYN: *knee jerk; patellar reflex.* SEE: *Jendrassik's maneuver.*

**tendon spindle** A fusiform nerve ending in a tendon.

**tendoplasty** (tĕn′dō-plăs″tē) [″ + Gr. *plassein,* to mold] Reparative surgery of an injured tendon. SYN: *tendinoplasty; tenontoplasty; tenoplasty.*

**tendosynovitis** (tĕn″dō-sĭn″ō-vī′tĭs) [″ + *synovia,* joint fluid, + Gr. *itis,* inflammation] Tenosynovitis.

**tendotome** (tĕn′dō-tōm) [″ + Gr. *tome,* incision] Tenotome.

**tendotomy** (tĕn-dŏt′ō-mē) Tenotomy.

**tendovaginal** (tĕn″dō-văj′ĭ-năl) [L. *tendo,* tendon, + *vagina,* sheath] Rel. to a tendon and its sheath.

**tendovaginitis** (tĕn″dō-văj″ĭn-ī′tĭs) [″ + ″ + Gr. *itis,* inflammation] Tenosynovitis. SYN: *tendosynovitis.*

**Tenebrio** (tĕ-nĕb′rē-ō) A genus of beetles including the species of *T. molitor,* which serves as an intermediate host of helminth parasites of vertebrates.

**tenectomy** [″ + *ektome,* excision] Excision of a lesion of a tendon or tendon sheath.

***graduated t.*** Partial division of a tendon.

**tenesmus** (tĕ-nĕz′mŭs) [Gr. *teinesmos,* a stretching] Spasmodic contraction of anal or bladder sphincter with pain and persistent desire to empty the bowel or bladder, with involuntary ineffectual straining efforts. **tenesmic** (tĕn-ĕz′mĭk), *adj.*

**teni-** SEE: *taen-.*

**tenia** (tē′nē-ă) [L. *taenia,* tape] Taenia.

**teniasis** (tē-nī′ă-sĭs) [L. *taenia,* tapeworm, + Gr. *-iasis,* a condition] Presence of tapeworms in the body.

**tenicide** (tĕn′ĭ-sīd) [″ + *cidus,* killing] Taeniacide.

**tenifuge** (tĕn′ĭ-fūj) [″ + *fuga,* flight] Causing

or that which causes expulsion of tapeworms.

**tennis elbow** A condition marked by pain over the lateral epicondyle of the humerus or the head of the radius. The pain radiates to the outer side of the arm and forearm due to injury or overuse of the extensor carpi radialis brevis or longus muscle, as may occur in playing tennis. The condition is aggravated by resisted wrist extension or forearm supination, or by a stretch force with the wrist flexed, forearm pronated, and elbow extended. Present are weakness of the wrist and difficulty in grasping objects. A reliable diagnostic sign is increased pain when the middle finger is extended against resistance. SYN: *epicondylitis, lateral humeral.*

TREATMENT: In mild cases, treatment includes immobilization by a splint or adhesive strapping, supplemented by application of cold, as well as use of nonsteroidal anti-inflammatory agents and muscle relaxants. Also, it may be possible to decrease the pain and inflammation by applying a wide strap just below the elbow. This will alter the action of the stressed muscles in the forearm and splint the area. This strap should be worn during exercise. Injection of cortisone and local anesthetic into the painful area may be of assistance in cases that have not been helped by conservative therapy. In persistent cases, surgical intervention may be indicated.

**teno-, tendo-** Combining form meaning *tendon.*

**tenodesis** (tĕn-ŏd′ĕ-sĭs) [Gr. *tenon,* tendon, + *desis,* a binding] **1.** Surgical fixation of a tendon. Usually a tendon is transferred from its initial point of origin to a new origin in order to restore muscle balance to a joint, to restore lost function, or to increase active power of joint motion. **2.** Closing of the fingers through tendon action of the extrinsic finger flexor muscles when they are stretched across the wrist joint during wrist extension. This mechanism is used for functional grip in the quadriplegic individual when paralysis is due to loss below the sixth cervical vertebra. SEE: *tendon action.*

**tenodesis splint** Orthosis fabricated to allow pinch and grasp movements through use of wrist extensors. Also called *wrist-driven flexor hinge hand splint.*

**tenodynia** (tĕn″ō-dĭn′ē-ă) [″ + *odyne,* pain] Pain in a tendon. SYN: *teinodynia; tenalgia; tenontodynia.*

**tenofibril** (tĕn′ō-fī″brĭl) [″ + *fibrilla,* little fiber] A fine thread present in the cytoplasm of epithelial cells.

**tenolysis** (tĕn-ŏl′ĭ-sĭs) [″ + *lysis,* dissolution] Tendolysis.

**tenometer** Tenonometer.

**tenomyoplasty** (tĕn″ō-mī′ō-plăs″tē) [″ + *mys,* muscle, + *plassein,* to form] Reparative operation upon a tendon and muscle. SYN: *tenontomyoplasty.*

**tenomyotomy** (tĕn″ō-mī-ŏt′ō-mē) [″ + ″ + *tome,* incision] Excision of lateral portion of a tendon or muscle.

**Tenon's capsule** (tē′nŏns) [Jacques R. Tenon, Fr. surgeon, 1724–1816] A thin connective tissue envelope of the eyeball behind the conjunctiva.

**tenonectomy** (tĕn″ō-nĕk′tō-mē) [″ + *ektome,* excision] Excision of a portion of a tendon.

**tenonitis** (tĕn″ō-nī′tĭs) [″ + *itis,* inflammation] **1.** Inflammation of a tendon. SYN: *tenontitis.* **2.** Inflammation of Tenon's capsule.

**tenonometer** (tĕn″ō-nŏm′ĕ-tĕr) [Gr. *teinein,* to stretch, + *metron,* measure] A device for measuring degree of intraocular tension. SYN: *tonometer.*

**Tenon's space** Space between the posterior surface of the eyeball and Tenon's capsule.

**tenontitis** (tĕn″ŏn-tī′tĭs) [Gr. *tenontos,* tendon, + *itis,* inflammation] Inflammation of a tendon. SYN: *tendinitis; tenositis.*

**tenontodynia** (tĕn″ŏn-tō-dĭn′ē-ă) [″ + *odyne,* pain] Tenodynia.

**tenontography** (tĕn″ŏn-tŏg′ră-fē) [″ + *graphein,* to write] A treatise on tendons.

**tenontolemmitis** (tĕn-ŏn″tō-lĕm-mī′tĭs) [″ + *lemma,* rind, + *itis,* inflammation] Tenosynovitis.

**tenontology** (tĕn″ŏn-tŏl′ō-jē) [″ + *logos,* word, reason] The study of tendons.

**tenontomyoplasty** (tĕn-ŏn″tō-mī′ō-plăs″tē) [″ + *mys,* muscle, + *plassein,* to form] Plastic surgery, including muscle and tendon repair in treatment of hernia. SYN: *myotenontoplasty; tenomyoplasty.*

**tenontomyotomy** (tĕn-ŏn″tō-mī-ŏt′ō-mē) [″ + ″ + *tome,* incision] Cutting of the principal tendon of a muscle with excision of the muscle in part or in whole. SYN: *myotenotomy.*

**tenontoplasty** (tĕn-ŏn′tō-plăs″tē) [″ + *plassein,* to form] Plastic surgery of defective or injured tendons. SYN: *tenoplasty.*

**tenontothecitis** (tĕn-ŏn″tō-thē-sī′tĭs) [″ + *theke,* sheath, + *itis,* inflammation] An inflammation of a tendon and its sheath. SYN: *tendosynovitis; tendovaginitis; tenosynovitis.*

***t. stenosans*** A chronic form of tenontothecitis with narrowing of the sheath.

**tenophyte** (tĕn′ō-fīt) [″ + *phyton,* a growth] A cartilaginous or osseous growth on a tendon.

**tenoplastic** (tĕn″ō-plăs′tĭk) Concerning tenoplasty.

**tenoplasty** (tĕn′ō-plăs″tē) [″ + *plassein,* to form] Reparative surgery of tendons. SYN: *tendinoplasty; tenontoplasty.*

**tenoreceptor** (tĕn″ō-rē-sĕp′tor) [″ + L. *receptor,* receiver] Proprioceptive nerve ending in a tendon.

**tenorrhaphy** (tĕn-or′ă-fē) [″ + *rhaphe,* seam, ridge] Suturing of a tendon.

**tenositis** (tĕn″ō-sī′tĭs) [″ + *itis,* inflammation] An inflammation of a tendon. SYN: *tenontitis.*

**tenostosis** (tĕn″ŏs-tō′sĭs) [Gr. *tenon,* tendon, + *osteon,* bone, + *osis,* condition] Calcification of a tendon.

**tenosuspension** (tĕn″ō-sŭs-pĕn′shŭn) [″ + L. *suspensio,* a hanging under] In surgery, use of a tendon to support a structure.

**tenosuture** (tĕn″ō-sū′chūr) [″ + L. *sutura,* a seam] Suture of a partially or completely divided tendon. SYN: *tenorrhaphy.*

**tenosynovectomy** (tĕn″ō-sĭn″ō-vĕk′tō-mē) [″ + *synovia,* joint fluid, + Gr. *ektome,* excision] Excision of a tendon sheath.

**tenosynovitis** (tĕn″ō-sĭn″ō-vī′tĭs) [″ + ″ + Gr. *itis,* inflammation] An inflammation of a tendon sheath. SYN: *tendosynovitis; tendovaginitis.*

***t. crepitans*** An inflammation of a tendon sheath in which a crackling sound is heard on motion. It most commonly affects flexor tendons. Symptoms include pain and excessive tenderness. This condition may follow puncture wounds, contusions, and lacerations or be caused by lymphatic extension of inflammation. Treatment includes early drainage, rest, heat, and appropriate antibiotics.

***t. hyperplastica*** Painless swelling of extensor tendons over the wrist joint.

**tenotome** (tĕn′ō-tōm) [″ + *tome,* incision] An instrument used for dividing a tendon. SYN: *tendotome.*

**tenotomist** (tĕ-nŏt′ō-mĭst) Specialist in tenotomy.

**tenotomy** (tĕ-nŏt′ō-mē) Surgical section of a tendon.

**tenovaginitis** (tĕn″ō-văj″ĭn-ī′tĭs) [″ + L. *vagina,* sheath, + Gr. *itis,* inflammation] Inflammation of a tendon sheath. SYN: *tendosynovitis; tenontothecitis; tenosynovitis.*

**TENS** *transcutaneous electrical nerve stimulation.*

**tense** (tĕns) Tight, rigid, anxious, under mental stress.

**Tensilon test** Diagnostic test for juvenile myasthenia gravis. Tensilon (edrophonium chloride) is injected intravascularly with an improvement of muscle strength that lasts for 5 min.

**tensiometer** (tĕn″sē-ŏm′ĕ-tĕr) [L. *tensio,* a stretching, + Gr. *metron,* measure] **1.** A device for determining the surface tension of liquids. **2.** A device used to measure the amount of force a muscle can produce. Also called *cable tensiometer.*

**tension** (tĕn′shŭn) [L. *tensio,* a stretching] **1.** Process or act of stretching; state of being strained or stretched. **2.** Pressure, as arterial tension. **3.** Expansive force of a gas or vapor. **4.** Mental, emotional, or nervous strain.

***arterial t.*** Tension resulting from the force exerted by the blood pressure on the walls of arteries.

***intraocular t.*** The pressure of the fluid within the eyeball. SEE: *tonometry.*

***intravenous t.*** Force exerted by the blood pressure on the walls of a vein.

***muscular t.*** Condition of a muscle in which fibers tend to shorten and thus perform work or liberate heat.

***premenstrual t.*** Condition occurring periodically in some individuals a few days before menstruation; marked by varying degrees of nervousness and irritability, rapidly changing emotions, headaches, and sometimes depression. Usually disappears a short time after onset of menstrual flow. SEE: *premenstrual syndrome.*

***surface t.*** Molecular property of film on surface of a liquid to resist rupture. The molecules are mutally attracted and their cohesive state presents the smallest surface area to the surrounding medium.

***tissue t.*** The theoretical state of equilibrium between the cells of a tissue.

**tension headache** Headache caused by sustained tension of muscles of the face, neck, and scalp.

**tension myalgia** SEE: *fibromyalgia.*

**tension of gases** Gas pressure usually measured in millimeters of mercury (mm Hg).

**tension pneumothorax** Valvular pneumothorax.

**tension suture** A suture used to reduce the pull on the edges of a wound.

**tensometer** (tĕn-sŏm′ĕ-tĕr) [L. *tensio,* a stretching, + Gr. *metron,* measure] A device for testing the tensile strength of materials.

**tensor** (tĕn′sor) [L., a stretcher] Any muscle that makes a part tense. SEE: *Muscles Appendix.*

**tent** (tĕnt) [O. Fr. *tente,* from L. *tenta,* stretched out] **1.** A plug of soft material used to maintain or dilate the opening to a sinus, canal, or body cavity. A variety of cylindrically shaped materials may be used. **2.** A portable covering or shelter composed of fabric.

***cool mist t.*** An aerosolized enclosure with cooling by ice or refrigeration, used in treating croup (laryngobracheobronchitis) in children.

***laminaria t.*** A plug made of *Laminaria digitata,* that is placed in the cervical canal of the uterus to dilate it.

***oxygen t.*** A tent that can be placed over a bed for the continuous administration of oxygen.

***sponge t.*** A plug made of compressed sponge that is placed in the cervical canal to dilate it.

**tentacle** (tĕn′tă-k′l) A slender projection of invertebrates. It is used for prehension, tactile purposes, or feeding.

**tentative** (tĕn′tă-tĭv) [L. *tentativus,* feel, try] **1.** Rel. to a diagnosis subject to change because of insufficient data. **2.** Indecisive.

**tenth cranial nerve** Nerve supplying most of the abdominal viscera, the heart, lungs, and esophagus. SYN: *vagus nerve.* SEE: *cranial nerves.*

**tentorial** (tĕn-tō′rē-ăl) Pert. to a tentorium.

**tentorial notch** SEE: under *notch.*

**tentorial pressure cone** Projection of a portion of the temporal lobe of the cerebrum through the incisure of the tentorium due to increased intracranial pressure.

**tentorium** (tĕn-tō′rē-ŭm) *pl.* **tentoria** [L., tent] A tentlike structure or part.

***t. cerebelli*** The process of the dura mater between the cerebrum and cerebellum supporting the occipital lobes.

**tephromyelitis** (tĕf″rō-mī″ĕl-ī′tĭs) [″ + *myelos,* marrow, + *itis,* inflammation] Inflammation of the gray matter of the spinal cord.

**tephrylometer** (tĕf″rĭ-lŏm′ĕ-tĕr) [″ + *hyle,* matter, + *metron,* measure] A device for measuring the thickness of the cerebral cortex, the gray matter of the brain.

**tepid** (tĕp′ĭd) [L. *tepidus,* lukewarm] Slightly warm; lukewarm.

**TEPP** *tetraethylpyrophosphate.*

**ter-** [L., thrice] Combining form meaning *three times.*

**teracurie** (tĕr″ă-kū′rē) A unit of radioactivity, $10^{12}$ curies.

**teramorphous** (tĕr-ă-mor′fŭs) [Gr. *teras,* monster, + *morphe,* form] Similar to, or of the nature of, a congenitally deformed fetus, infant, or child.

**teras** (tĕr′ăs) *pl.* **terata** [Gr.] A severely deformed fetus.

**teratic** (tĕr-ăt′ĭk) [Gr. *teratikos,* monstrous] Pert. to a severely malformed fetus.

**teratism** (tĕr′ă-tĭzm) [Gr. *teratisma*] An anomaly or structural abnormality either inherited or acquired.

***acquired t.*** Abnormality resulting from a prenatal environmental influence.

***atresic t.*** Teratism in which natural openings such as the mouth or anus fail to form.

***ceasmic t.*** Teratism in which a normal union of parts fails to occur (e.g., as in spina bifida or cleft palate).

***ectogenic t.*** Condition in which parts are absent or defective.

***ectopic t.*** Abnormality in which a part becomes displaced.

***hypergenic t.*** Teratism in which a part is duplicated (e.g., polydactylism).

***symphysic t.*** Teratism in which parts that are normally separate are fused.

**terato-** Combining form meaning *monster.*

**teratoblastoma** (tĕr″ă-tō-blăs-tō′mă) [Gr. *teratos,* monster, + *blastos,* germ, + *oma,* tumor] A tumor that contains embryonic material but that is not representative of all three germinal layers. SEE: *teratoma.*

**teratocarcinoma** (tĕr″ă-tō-kăr″sĭ-nō′mă) [″ + *karkinos,* cancer, + *oma,* tumor] A carcinoma that has developed from the epithelial cells of a teratoma.

**teratogen** (tĕr-ăt′ō-jĕn) [″ + *gennan,* to produce] Anything that adversely affects normal cellular development in the embryo or fetus. Known teratogens include certain chemicals, some therapeutic and illicit drugs, radiation, and intrauterine viral infections. SEE: table; *mutagen.*

**teratogenesis** (tĕr″ă-tō-gĕn′ĕ-sĭs) [″ + *genesis,* generation, birth] The development of abnormal structures in an embryo.

**teratogenetic** (tĕr″ă-tō-jĕ-nĕt′ĭk) [″ + *gene-*

## Common Teratogenic or Fetotoxic Drugs

| | |
|---|---|
| Alcohol | Antidiabetics<br>Oral hypoglycemics |
| Amebicides | Antihypertensives<br>Diazoxide, thiazide diuretics, reserpine |
| Analgesics and antipyretics<br>Aspirin and other salicylates (in third trimester); narcotics (prolonged use) | Antineoplastics<br>All agents |
| Antibiotics<br>Aminoglycosides, chloramphenicol, tetracycline, trimethoprim, sulfonamides (in third trimester) | Antithyroid drugs<br>Radioiodine, propylthiouracil, methimazole |
| Antifungal drugs<br>Griseofulvin, ketoconazole | Disulfiram (Antabuse) |
| | Ergotamine |
| Antiparasitic drugs<br>Lindane, mebendazole, Fansidar (sulfadoxine and pyrimethamine), and others | Hormones<br>Estrogens, diethylstilbestrol, progestins, androgens |
| Antiviral drugs<br>Amantadine, ribavirin, and others | Isotretinoin (Accutane) |
| | Nonsteroidal anti-inflammatory drugs (in third trimester) |
| Anticoagulants<br>Warfarin, dicumarol and other coumarin derivatives | Psychoactive drugs<br>Lithium, benzodiazepines, amitriptyline |
| Anticonvulsants<br>Aminoglutethimide, ethotoin, phenytoin, paramethadione, trimethadione, valproic acid | Tobacco |

SOURCE: Tierney, L. M. et al., eds., Current Medical Diagnosis and Treatment. Appleton and Lange, Norwalk, CT, 1993.

*sis,* generation, birth] Concerning teratogenesis.

**teratogenic** (tĕr″ă-tō-gĕn′ĭk) Causing abnormal development of the embryo.

**teratoid** (tĕr′ă-toyd) [Gr. *teratos,* monster, + *eidos,* form, shape] Resembling a severely malformed fetus.

**teratoid tumor** Tumor of embryonic remains from all germinal layers. SYN: *teratoma.*

**teratologic** (tĕr″ă-tō-lŏj′ĭk) Concerning teratology.

**teratology** (tĕr-ă-tŏl′ō-jē) [″ + *logos,* word, reason] Branch of science dealing with the study of congenitally deformed fetuses.

**teratoma** (tĕr-ă-tō′mă) [″ + *oma,* tumor] A congenital tumor containing one or more of the three primary embryonic germ layers. Thus, hair and teeth as well as endodermal elements may be present. SYN: *dermoid cyst.* SEE: *fetus in fetu.*

**teratomatous** (tĕr″ă-tō′mă-tŭs) Pert. to or resembling a teratoma.

**teratophobia** (tĕr″ă-tō-fō′bē-ă) [″ + *phobos,* fear] An abnormal fear of giving birth to a malformed fetus or being in contact with one.

**teratosis** (tĕr″ă-tō′sĭs) [″ + *osis,* condition] A deformed fetus.

**teratospermia** (tĕr″ă-tō-spĕr′mē-ă) [″ + *sperma,* seed] Malformed sperm in semen.

**terazosin hydrochloride** A hypertensive agent.

**terbium** (tĕr′bē-ŭm) SYMB: Tb. Atomic weight, 158.9254; atomic number, 65; specific gravity, 8.272. A metal of the rare earths.

**terbutaline sulfate** A synthetic sympathomimetic amine used in treating asthma. It is an effective bronchodilator.

**terchloride** (tĕr-klō′rīd) Trichloride.

**terebrant** (tĕr′ĕ-brănt) Piercingly painful.

**terebration** (tĕr″ĕ-brā′shŭn) [L. *terebratio*] **1.** Boring; trephination. **2.** A boring pain.

**teres** (tĕ′rēz) [L., round] Round and smooth; cylindrical; used to describe certain muscles and ligaments.

**tergal** (tĕr′găl) [L. *tergum,* back] Concerning the back or dorsal surface.

**tergum** (tĕr′gŭm) [L.] The back.

**ter in die** (tĕr ĭn dē′ă) [L.] ABBR: t.i.d. Three times a day.

**term** [L. *terminus,* a boundary] **1.** A limit or boundary. **2.** A definite or limited period of duration such as the normal period of pregnancy, approx. nine calendar months or 38 to 42 weeks' gestation.

**terminal** (tĕr′mĭ-năl) [L. *terminalis*] Pert. to or placed at the end.

**terminal arteriole** An arteriole that has no branches but splits into capillaries.

**terminal bars** Minute bars of dense intercellular cement that occupy and close spaces between epithelial cells and bind them together.

**terminal cancer** Term used to describe the condition of having advanced cancer.

**terminal device** ABBR: TD. Component of an upper extremity prosthesis that substitutes for the functions of the hand. There are many types of terminal devices, some of which are designed for use with specific tools and implements. These devices are classified basically by whether or not the action of the prosthesis wearer results in opening the device (voluntary opening) or closing it (voluntary closing). SYN: *hook.*

**terminal ganglia** Ganglia of the parasympathetic division of the autonomic nervous system that are located in or close to walls or visceral structures such as the heart or intestines.

**terminal illness** An illness that, because of its nature, can be expected to cause the patient to die. Usually a chronic disease for which there is no known cure.

NURSING IMPLICATIONS: The nurse supports the patient and family by anticipating their loss and grief and helps the patient to deal with major concerns: pain, fear, hopelessness, dependency, disability, loss of self-esteem, and loss of pleasure. Hospice care is provided if desired and available. The patient receives caring comfort and help in adjusting to decreased quality of life to ensure that death is with dignity.

**terminal infection** Infection appearing in the late stage of another disease; often fatal.

**terminal vein** One of two veins (anterior and posterior) draining portions of the brain and emptying into the interior cerebral veins.

**terminatio** (tĕr″mĭ-nā′shē-ō) [L.] The termination or ending.

**termination** [L. *terminatio,* limiting] **1.** The distal end of a part. **2.** The cessation of anything.

**terminology** (tĕr-mĭ-nŏl′ō-jē) [L. *terminus,* a boundary, + Gr. *logos,* word] The vocabulary of scientific and technical terms used in specific arts, trades, or professions. SYN: *nomenclature.*

**terminus** (tĕr′mĭ-nŭs) [L.] An ending; a boundary.

**terpene** (tĕr′pēn) Any member of the family of hydrocarbons of the formula $C_{10}H_{16}$.

**terpin hydrate** (tĕr′pĭn hī′drāt) A white crystalline substance with a turpentine taste; made by the interaction of rectified spirits of turpentine, alcohol, and nitric acid. It is in the form of an elixir and is used as an expectorant.

**terra** (tĕr′ă) [L.] Earth; soil.

***t. alba*** White clay.

***t. fullonica*** Fuller's earth.

**terracing** (tĕr′ăs-ĭng) [O. Fr. *terrasse*] Suturing in several rows through thick tissues in closing a wound.

**territoriality** (tĕr″ĭ-tor″ē-ăl′ĭ-tē) The tendency of animals and humans to defend a particular area or region.

**terror** [L. *terrere,* to frighten] Very great fear.

***night t.'s*** SEE: *night terrors.*

**tertian** (tĕr′shŭn) [L. *tertianus,* the third] Occurring every third day; usually pert. to a form of malarial fever.

**tertiary** (tĕr′shē-ār-ē) [L. *tertiarius*] Third in order or stage.

**tertiary alcohol** Alcohol containing the trivalent group ≡COH.

**tertiary care** A level of medical care that would be available only in large medical care institutions. Included would be techniques and methods of therapy and diagnosis involving equipment and personnel that would not be economically feasible to have in a smaller institution because of the lack of utilization. SEE: *primary care; secondary care.*

**tertiary syphilis** The third and most advanced stage of syphilis.

**tertigravida** (tĕr″shē-grăv′ĭ-dă) [″ + *gravida,* pregnant] A woman pregnant for the third time.

**tertipara** (tĕr-shĭp′ă-ră) [L. *tertius,* third, + *parere,* to bring forth] A woman who has had three pregnancies terminating after the 20th week of gestation or has produced three infants weighing at least 500 g, regardless of their viability.

**tesla** [Nikola Tesla, U.S. physicist, 1856–1943] ABBR: T. In the SI system, a measure of magnetic strength; 1 tesla equals 1 weber per square meter.

**tessellated** (tĕs′ĕ-lā″tĕd) [L. *tessella,* a square] Composed of little squares.

**test** [L. *testum,* earthen vessel] **1.** An examination. **2.** A method to determine the presence or nature of a substance or the presence of a disease. **3.** A chemical reaction. **4.** A reagent or substance used in making a test.

***acetic acid t.*** A test for albumin in urine. Adding a few drops of acetic acid to urine that has been boiled causes a white precipitate if albumin is present.

***acetone t.*** A test for the presence of acetone in the urine; made by adding a few drops of sodium nitroprusside to the urine along with strong ammonia water. The presence of acetone causes the formation of a magenta ring at outline of contacts.

***agglutination t.*** A widely used test in which adding an antiserum containing antibodies to cells or bacteria causes them to agglutinate.

***alkali denaturation t.*** A test for hemoglobin F (fetal hemoglobin) in the blood. Spectrophotometry is used in this test.

***Allen-Doisy t.*** A test to determine the amount of estrogen content in female blood serum by its reaction on secretions of mice.

***apprehension t.*** A test of chronic joint instability. If this is present, the patient displays apprehension or discomfort when a joint is put in a position of risk for dislocation. There is an obvious facial display of discomfort; the patient may try to resist the maneuver by muscle contraction.

*Patella:* The patient lies supine with a relaxed quadriceps, and the examiner places digital pressure on the patella, attempting to locate it laterally.

*Shoulder:* The arm is abducted to 90° and rotated externally. With continued external rotation, the patient with an unstable shoulder complains of pain and expresses fear of dislocation.

***aptitude t.*** A test used to determine an individual's capability in various areas, esp. specific occupations.

***Aschheim-Zondek t.*** A test for pregnancy performed by injecting the patient's urine subcutaneously into immature female mice. If the patient is pregnant, the ovaries of the mouse begin to mature prematurely.

***association t.*** A test used to determine an individual's response to word stimuli. The nature of the response and time required may provide insight into the subject's personality and previous experiences.

***autohemolysis t.*** A test of the rate of hemolysis of sterile defibrinated whole blood incubated at 37°C. Normal cells hemolyze at a certain rate and blood cells from persons with certain types of disease hemolyze at a faster rate.

***biuret t.*** A test to determine the presence of proteins or urea.

***block design t.*** A neuropsychological test involving the placement of wooden blocks according to three-dimensional drawings. The test assesses the presence of constructional apraxia, often exhibited in patients with brain lesions.

***box and block t.*** A standardized, timed test of manual dexterity and endurance, used in rehabilitation, in which the subject transfers small blocks from one side of a box to another.

***caries activity t.*** Any laboratory test that measures the degree of caries activity in a dental patient. The tests may identify the number of cariogenic bacteria or the acid production from saliva samples.

***challenge t.*** Administering a substance in order to determine its ability to cause a response, esp. the giving of an antigen and observing or testing for the antibody response.

***chromatin t.*** A test for genetic sex in which blood or tissue cells are examined for the presence or absence of Barr bodies.

***coin t.*** A test for pneumothorax. A metal coin is placed flat on the chest and struck with another coin. The chest is auscultated at the same time. If a pneumothorax is present, a sharp, metallic ringing sound is heard.

***complement-fixation t.*** SEE: *complement fixation.*

***concentration t.*** A kidney function test based on the ability of the person to produce concentrated urine under conditions that would normally cause such production, as in intentional dehydration.

***conjunctival t.*** An allergy test in which the suspected antigen is placed in the conjunctival sac; if it is allergenic for that patient, the conjunctiva becomes red and itchy and tears are produced.

***cover t.*** A test for strabismus. The eyes are observed and the patient is asked to focus on an object. A cover is placed first over one eye and then the other. If either eye moves, strabismus is present.

***creatinine clearance t.*** A laboratory test to determine the ability of the kidneys to remove creatinine from the blood for excretion into the urine. It is the best indicator of renal function and is therefore useful for a physician prescribing medications that are excreted by the kidneys. The normal creatinine clearance for men ranges from 95 to 135 ml/min. For women, the value is slightly less. As a person ages, the creatinine clearance decreases.

***Developmental T. of Visual Motor Integration*** A test of visual perception and motor planning requiring the copying of shapes and forms.

***double-blind t.*** SEE: *double-blind technique.*

***effort-independent t.*** A test whose accuracy or success does not depend on patient compliance.

***finger-to-finger t.*** A test for coordination of the movements of the upper extremities. The patient is asked to touch the tips of the fingers of one hand to the opposite fingertips.

***finger-nose t.*** A test of cerebellar function wherein the patient is asked to, while keeping the eyes open, touch the nose with the finger and remove the finger, and repeat this rapidly. The test is done by using a finger of each hand successively or in concert. How fast and well this is done is recorded.

***Friedman t.*** One of the first tests for pregnancy in which the patient's urine was injected into unmated mature female rabbits; a positive reaction was indicated by formation of corpora lutea and corpora haemorrhagica. This test is no longer used.

***foam stability t.*** Shake t.

***galactose tolerance t.*** A test of the ability of the liver to metabolize galactose. A standard dose of galactose is administered to the fasting patient, and the amount of galactose excreted in the urine in the next 5 hr is determined. If the liver is damaged, the galactose is not metabolized to glycogen but is instead excreted in the urine.

***glucose tolerance t.*** SEE: *glucose tolerance test.*

***guaiac t.*** A test for occult blood in the feces. An alcoholic solution of guaiac resin and hydrogen peroxide is mixed with the specimen. The appearance of a blue color indicates a positive test. This test is effective in detecting tumors of the colon. The feces should be tested twice daily for 3 days to enhance detection of occult blood.

***hardness t.*** A test designed to determine the relative hardness of materials by correlating the size or depth of an indent produced by a particular instrument with a known amount of compressive force. SEE: *hardness number.*

***histamine t.*** **1.** Injection of histamine subcutaneously to stimulate gastric secretion of hydrochloric acid. **2.** A test for vasomotor headache; a histamine injection precipitates the onset of a headache in persons with this disease.

***human repeated patch insult t.*** The serial application of substances to the skin to test for reaction. The material is applied fresh to the same skin site every other day for 10 applications. Each application remains on for 48 hr. After a rest period of about 2 weeks, the test material is applied again for 48 hr to a different skin site than that originally used. This area is examined daily for the next 4 days for evidence of irritation. The test measures the ability of the test substance to cause sensitization or irritation reactions or both.

***in-home t.*** A test done in the home to provide information about an individual's health status. Examples include tests to measure blood sugar (glucose), cholesterol, occult blood in feces, and blood pressure, as well as ovulation predictors and pregnancy tests. The materials and devices needed for in-home tests are available over the counter (i.e., a prescription from a health care professional is not needed).

***intelligence t.*** A test designed to assess the intelligence of an individual, used as a basis for determining intelligence quotient (IQ). It is now believed that some of the standardized tests of intelligence were more nearly achievement tests. SEE: *intelligence; quotient, intelligence.*

***intracutaneous t.*** A test done by injecting an antigen intracutaneously and observing the response.

***limulus amebocyte lysate t.*** ABBR: LAL test. A test used to detect minute quantities of bacterial endotoxins and to test for pyrogens in various materials; it is also used to detect septicemia due to gram-negative bacteria. Limulus amebocyte lysate is formed from the lysed circulating amebocytes of the horseshoe crab *(Limulus polyphemus).*

***liver function t.*** A blood test for a specific aspect of liver metabolism. Because of the diversity of liver functions and the disorders that may affect those functions, no single test provides a reliable measure of overall liver function. The ability to excrete bile pigments is measured by determining the serum bilirubin level; the levels of serum enzymes such as the aminotransferases aspartate (AST) and alanine (ALT) may be used to assess damage to the liver cells and biliary tract obstruction or dysfunction. Levels of the serum proteins albumin and globulin and their ratio are used to judge the extent of liver damage. Certain blood clotting factors are synthesized in the liver, and abnormalities can be determined by measuring the rate of conversion of prothrombin to thrombin by the one-stage prothrombin time test. Blood ammonia levels are elevated in some patients with either acute or chronic liver disease; marked elevations usually indicate severe necrosis of the liver cells. SEE: *liver*.

***loading t.*** The administration of a substance to determine individual's ability to metabolize or excrete it. Thus, a glucose tolerance test is one form of this test.

***McMurray t.*** A test for a torn meniscus of the knee. The examiner flexes the patient's knee completely, rotates the tibia outward, and applies a valgus force against the knee while slowly extending it. A painful click indicates a torn medial meniscus. If a click is felt when the tibia is rotated inward and a varus force is applied against the knee during extension, the lateral meniscus is torn.

***Motor-Free Visual Perception T.*** A standardized test of visual perception that does not require motor performance.

***multiple-puncture t.*** Any skin test, but esp. a tuberculin test, in which the material is placed on the skin and multiple superficial punctures are produced under the material, thus allowing the material to enter the skin.

***neutralization t.*** A test of the ability of an antibody to neutralize the toxic effects of an antigen.

***ninhydrin t.*** A neurological test of sensation following peripheral nerve injury; used to detect a sympathetic response as indicated by sweat.

***nonstress t.*** ABBR: NST. An external electronic monitoring procedure to assess fetal well-being. An acceleration in fetal heart rate should be evident in response to fetal movement. *Reactive test:* Two criteria indicate satisfactory fetal status. The monitor records a minimum of two episodes of heart rate acceleration accompanying fetal movement within one 20-min period, and accelerations of 15 beats per minute persist for a minimum of 15 sec per episode. *Nonreactive test:* The monitor record does not meet either criterion for reactivity. This indicates the need for a second test within the nest several hours, contraction stress testing, a fetal biophysical profile, or all three. *Inconclusive test:* The monitor records less than one acceleration in 20 min or an acceleration less than 15 bpm lasting less than 15 sec.

***patch t.*** A skin test in which a low concentration of a substance is applied to the skin under an occlusive dressing for 48 hr to assess for hypersensitivity to a suspected allergen. If the concentration of the agent is too high or an allergy exists to the material used in the dressing, false-positive reactions can occur because of local irritation. False-negative reactions may result if the concentration of the suspected allergen is too low. Intradermal injection may be used instead of patch testing as another form of delayed hypersensitivity skin testing.

***pinprick t.*** A test for cutaneous pain receptors. A small, clean, sharp object such as a pin or needle is gently applied to the skin and the patient is asked to describe the sensation. One must be certain the patient is reporting the sensation of pain rather than that of pressure. Usually, application of the sharp object is interspersed with application of a dull object, and the patient is asked to state each time whether a sharp or dull sensation was felt. The patient is not, of course, allowed to observe the test procedure.

---

Caution: The sharp object should not penetrate the dermis, and to prevent passage of infectious material from one patient to another, the test objects should be either discarded after use or sterilized before their use on another patient.

---

***precipitin t.*** An antigen-antibody test in which a specific antigen is added to a solution. If the solution contains the antibody to that antigen, a precipitate is formed.

***pregnancy t.*** SEE: *pregnancy test*.

***prothrombin consumption t.*** A test for the amount of thromboplastin present in the plasma that reacts with prothrombin. This is determined by quantitating the prothrombin that remains in the serum after coagulation is complete.

***psychometric t.*** A measurement technique used to assist in diagnosing cognitive and behavioral difficulties in infants and children. Several different tests are available.

***pulp vitality t.*** A determination of the vitality of a tooth pulp by the application of hot, cold, or electrical stimuli. Also called *vitalometry*.

***radioimmunosorbent t.*** ABBR: RIST. Use of radioimmunoassay to measure the immune globulin E (IgE) antibody in serum.

***rapid surfactant t.*** Shake t.

***Rubin t.*** The original test for patency of the fallopian tubes by insufflation with carbon dioxide; used in investigating the cause of sterility. SYN: *tubal insufflation*.

***Schiller's t.*** A test for detection of cancer of the cervix by painting the tissue with iodine solution; areas that contain glycogen are stained by the iodine. Those sites that do not stain, but become white or yellow, are assumed to be abnormal. Tissue is taken from those areas for microscopic examination.

***scratch t.*** An allergy test in which the antigen is applied to skin that has been lightly scratched.

***secretin injection t.*** A test performed by injecting secretin intravenously and then measuring changes in gastrin in the serum when attempting to diagnose gastrinoma, or measuring changes in the duodenal fluid when investigating pancreatic insufficiency and malabsorption.

***Sensory Integration and Praxis T.'s*** ABBR: SIPT. A standardized battery of assessment tests to identify motor planning and sensory processing deficits in children 4 through 8 years of age. It includes 17 subtests.

***serial sevens t.*** SEE: *serial sevens test.*

***serologic t.*** Any test done on serum.

***shake t.*** A quick test to estimate fetal lung maturity. A sample of amniotic fluid is diluted with normal saline, mixed with 95% ethyl alcohol, and shaken for 30 sec. The continued presence of small foamy bubbles in the solution after 15 min confirms the presence of pulmonary surfactant. SYN: *foam stability t.; rapid surfactant t.*

***sickling t.*** A test for the ability of red cells to sickle. The red cells are placed in an atmosphere of reduced oxygen tension. If they contain hemoglobin S, they will sickle.

***standardized t.*** A test that has been developed empirically, has adequate norms, definite instructions for administration, and evidence of reliability and validity.

***starch-iodine t.*** A test for the presence of starch. When an iodine solution is applied to a substance or material that contains starch, a dark blue color appears.

***sulfosalicylic acid t.*** A test for protein in the urine.

***thematic apperception t.*** A projective test in which the subject is shown life situations in pictures that could be interpreted in several ways. The subject is asked to provide a story of what the picture represents. The results may provide insights into the subject's personality.

***three-glass t.*** A test to identify the site of a urinary tract infection. On awakening, the patient empties the bladder by passing urine sequentially into three test tubes (glasses). The amount of cellular debris visible to the naked eye in the glasses helps to determine whether the infection is located in the anterior urethra, posterior urethra, or prostate. If the first glass is turbid and the other two are clear, the anterior urethra is inflamed but the rest of the urinary tract is clear. If the initial specimen is clear and the second and third ones are turbid, the posterior urethra or prostate is inflamed. If only the third specimen is turbid, then only the prostate is inflamed.

***tine t.*** SEE: *tine test.*

***tolerance t.*** A test of the ability of the patient or subject to endure the medicine given or exercise taken.

***tourniquet t.*** A test for capillary fragility. A blood pressure cuff is inflated sufficiently to occlude venous return from the arm. It is kept in place for a set time. After the cuff is removed, the skin distal to the cuff is examined for petechiae.

***tuberculin t.*** SEE: *tuberculin test.*

***up and go t.*** A timed test of lower-extremity mobility. It measures the time required to rise from a chair, walk 10 ft, turn, and return to the sitting position. Performance on this test is affected by abnormal gaits that increase the risk of falling.

***urea balance t.*** A test of kidney function by measuring intake and output of urea.

***wrinkle t.*** A test of sensibility following complete transection of or damage to peripheral nerves based on the characteristic sympathetic response of skin following extended immersion in water. SEE: *nerve.*

**testa** (tĕs′tă) [L.] A shell.

**testalgia** (tĕs-tăl′jē-ă) [L. *testis,* testicle, + Gr. *algos,* pain] Pain in the testicle.

**testectomy** (tĕs-tĕk′tō-mē) [″ + Gr. *ektome,* excision] **1.** Removal of a testicle. SYN: *castration.* **2.** Removal of a corpus quadrigeminum.

**testes** (tĕs′tēs) [L.] Pl. of testis.

**testicle** (tĕs′tĭ-kl) [L. *testiculus,* a little testis] A testis.

***self-examination of t.*** A technique that enables a man to detect changes in the size and shape of his testicles and evaluate any tenderness. Each testicle is examined separately and in comparison with the other. The best time to perform the test is just after a warm bath or shower, when the scrotal tissue is more nearly relaxed. The man places his thumbs on the anterior surface of the testicle, supporting it with the index and middle fingers of both hands. Each testicle is gently rolled between the fingers and thumbs and carefully felt for lumps, hardness, or thickening, esp. as compared with the other testicle. The epididymis is a soft, slightly tender, tubelike body behind the testicle. Abnormal findings should be reported immediately to a health care professional.

**testicond** (tĕs′tĭ-kŏnd) [L. *testis,* testicle, + *condere,* to hide] The condition of having the testicles remain undescended. It is abnormal in man and in many animals.

**testicular** (tĕs-tĭk′ū-lăr) Rel. to a testicle.

**testicular cancer, germ-cell** A particular type of testicular cancer. Metastatic cancer of this type is treated with ifosfamide and mesna.

**testis** (tĕs′tĭs) *pl.* **testes** [L.] The male gonad or testicle. It is one of two reproductive glands located in the scrotum that produces the male reproductive cells (spermatozoa) and the male hormones testos-

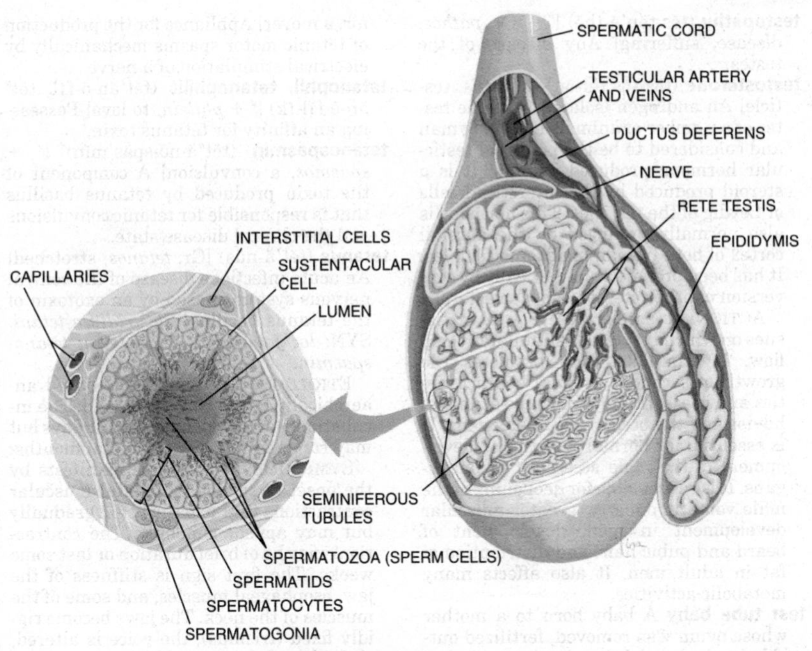


**TESTIS**

MIDSAGITTAL SECTION OF TESTIS AND EPIDIDYMIS (RIGHT), CROSS-SECTION THROUGH A SEMINIFEROUS TUBULE (LEFT)

terone and inhibin. SEE: illus.

ANATOMY: Each is an ovoid body about 4 cm long and 2 to 2.5 cm in width and thickness, enclosed within a dense inelastic fibrous tunica albuginea. The testis is divided into numerous lobules separated by septa, each lobule containing one to three seminiferous tubules within which the spermatozoa arise. The lobules lead to straight ducts that join a plexus, the rete testis, from which 15 to 20 efferent ducts lead to the epididymis. The epididymis leads to the ductus deferens, through which sperm are conveyed to the urethra. Between the seminiferous tubules are the interstitial cells (cells of Leydig), which secrete testosterone, and the sustentacular cells, which secrete inhibin. The testes are suspended from the body by the spermatic cord, a structure that extends from the inguinal ring to the testis and contains the ductus deferens, testicular vessels (spermatic artery, vein, lymph vessels), and nerves.

DISORDERS: Hyperfunction (hypergonadism) may cause early maturity such as dentition, large sexual organs with early functional activity, and increased growth of hair. Hypofunction (hypogonadism) is indicated by undeveloped testes, absence of body hair, high-pitched voice, sterility, smooth skin, loss of sexual desire, low metabolism, and eunuchoid or eunuch body type.

***descent of t.*** Change in position of the testis from the abdominal cavity to the scrotum during gestation of the fetus.

***displaced t.*** A testis located abnormally within the inguinal canal or pelvis.

***femoral t.*** An inguinal testis near or over the femoral ring.

***inverted t.*** A testis reversed in the scrotum so that the epididymis attaches to the anterior instead of the posterior part of the gland.

***perineal t.*** A testis located in the perineal region outside the scrotum.

***undescended t.*** A testis remaining in the inguinal canal or abdominal cavity. This may be present at birth or develop later.

**testis compression reflex** Contraction of abdominal muscles following moderate compression of a testis.

**testitis** (tĕs-tī′tĭs) [L. *testis*, testicle, + Gr. *itis*, inflammation] Inflammation of a testis. SEE: *orchitis*.

**test meal** A meal usually small and of definite quality and composition, given to aid in chemical analysis of the stomach contents or radiographical examination of the stomach.

**testoid** (tĕs′toyd) Resembling a testis.

**testolactone** (tĕs-tō-lăk′tōn) An antineoplastic agent used in treating carcinoma of the breast in postmenopausal women.

**testopathy** (tĕs-tŏp′ă-thē) [″ + Gr. *pathos,* disease, suffering] Any disease of the testes.

**testosterone** (tĕs-tŏs′tĕr-ōn) [L. *testis,* testicle] An androgen isolated from the testes of a number of animals including man and considered to be the principal testicular hormone produced in man. It is a steroid produced by the interstitial cells of Leydig of the testicles. This hormone is also normally produced by the adrenal cortex of both human males and females. It has been prepared synthetically by conversion of other sterols, esp. cholesterol.

ACTION: It accelerates growth in tissues on which it acts and stimulates blood flow. It stimulates and promotes the growth of secondary sexual characteristics and is essential for normal sexual behavior and the occurrence of erections. It is essential for normal growth and development of the male accessory sexual organs. It is responsible for deepening of the male voice at puberty, greater muscular development in men, development of beard and pubic hair, and distribution of fat in adult men. It also affects many metabolic activities.

**test tube baby** A baby born to a mother whose ovum was removed, fertilized outside her body, and then implanted in her uterus. SEE: *gamete intrafallopian transfer; in vitro fertilization.*

**test type** Letters or figures of various size printed on paper. These are used in testing visual acuity.

**tetanic** (tĕ-tăn′ĭk) [Gr. *tetanikos*] **1.** Pert. to or producing tetanus. **2.** Any agent producing tetanic spasms.

**tetanic convulsion** A tonic convulsion with constant muscular contraction.

**tetaniform** (tĕ-tăn′ĭ-form) [Gr. *tetanos,* stretched, + L. *forma,* shape] Resembling tetanus.

**tetanigenous** (tĕt″ă-nĭj′ĕ-nŭs) [″ + *gennan,* to produce] Causing tetanus or tetanic spasms.

**tetanism** (tĕt′ă-nĭzm) [″ + *-ismos,* condition] Persistent muscular hypertonicity resembling tetanus, esp. in infants.

**tetanization** (tĕt″ă-nī-zā′shŭn) [Gr. *tetanos,* stretched] **1.** Production of tetanus or tetanic spasms by induction of the disease. **2.** Induction of tetanic contractions in a muscle by electrical stimuli.

**tetanize** (tĕt′ă-nīz) To induce tonic muscular spasms.

**tetanode** (tĕt′ă-nōd) [″ + *eidos,* form, shape] In tetany, the quiet period between spasms.

**tetanoid paraplegia** Paralysis of lower extremities due to lateral sclerosis of the spinal cord. SYN: *paraplegia, spastic.*

**tetanolysin** (tĕt″ă-nŏl′ĭ-sĭn) A hemolytic component of the toxin produced by *Clostridium tetani,* causative organism of tetanus. It does not cause the clinical signs and symptoms of this disease.

**tetanomotor** (tĕt″ăn-ō-mō′tor) [″ + L. *motor,* a mover] Appliance for the production of tetanic motor spasms mechanically by electrical stimulation of a nerve.

**tetanophil, tetanophilic** (tĕt′ăn-ō-fĭl, tĕt″ăn-ō-fĭl′ĭk) [″ + *philein,* to love] Possessing an affinity for tetanus toxin.

**tetanospasmin** (tĕt″ă-nō-spăs′mĭn) [″ + *spasmos,* a convulsion] A component of the toxin produced by tetanus bacillus that is responsible for tetanic convulsions and the clinical disease state.

**tetanus** (tĕt′ă-nŭs) [Gr. *tetanos,* stretched] An acute infectious disease of the central nervous system caused by an exotoxin of the tetanus bacillus, *Clostridium tetani.* SYN: *lockjaw.* SEE: *tetanolysin; tetanospasmin.*

ETIOLOGY: The toxin is produced anaerobically at the site of a wound. The incubation period is usually 3 to 21 days but may range from 1 day to several months.

SYMPTOMS: The disease manifests by the onset of extremely painful muscular contractions that usually begin gradually but may appear suddenly. The contractions may be of brief duration or last some weeks. The first sign is stiffness of the jaw, esophageal muscles, and some of the muscles of the neck. The jaws become rigidly fixed (trismus), the voice is altered, and the muscles of the face contract, producing a wild excited expression and a combination of bitter laughter and crying. The muscles of the back and extremities become tetanic. The paroxysms are reflex and are excited by noises, currents of air, and irritation of bedclothes. The temperature usually rises and may become extremely high. The patient also suffers from hunger, thirst, and lack of sleep. The mind is clear. This disease is usually fatal, with the patient expiring from asphyxia or exhaustion.

TREATMENT: The patient is treated in an intensive care unit. The wound should be debrided, and the patient should be given penicillin if the wound is infected. Tetanus immune globulin should be given intramuscularly. If this is unavailable, 10,000 units of tetanus antitoxin are given intravenously after testing for horse serum sensitivity. Antiserum does not neutralize toxin fixed to central nervous system cells and is of little use in patients with symptoms present at the time of hospitalization. It is esp. beneficial if administered early in mild to moderately severe cases. Patients should receive antibiotics to treat infection and to stop toxin production. The muscle spasms are treated with sedatives, muscle relaxants, or neuromuscular blocking agents. Airway management is of utmost importance, esp. in patients with diffuse rigidity. Tracheostomy is an important treatment and reduces the risk of aspiration when laryngospasm prevents respiration. Intravenous access should be established. A Foley catheter should be inserted to prevent urinary retention.

NOTE: Recovery from tetanus does not guarantee natural immunity. Therefore, the patient should begin an immunization series before leaving the hospital.

PREVENTION: Initial immunization should begin in infancy. The toxoid should be given in three doses at 4- to 8-week intervals when the infant is 6 to 8 weeks old, and a fourth dose 6 to 12 months thereafter. A fifth dose is usually administered at 4 to 6 years of age before school entry. The tetanus toxoid is commonly given in combination with diphtheria toxoid and pertussis vaccine (DPT). Active immunization with adsorbed tetanus toxoid provides protection for at least 10 years. Although it has been the practice to give a tetanus booster every 10 years, current advice is to give a single booster dose at age 50 if the individual received all 5 doses as a child.

***t. anticus*** Form of tetanus in which the body is bowed forward.

***artificial t.*** Tetanus produced by a drug such as strychnine.

***ascending t.*** Tetanus in which muscle spasms occur first in the lower part of the body and then spread upward, finally involving muscles of the head and neck.

***cephalic t.*** A form of tetanus due to a wound of the head, esp. one near the eyebrow. It is marked by trismus, facial paralysis on one side, and pronounced dysphagia. It resembles rabies and is often fatal. SYN: *hydrophobic t.*

***cerebral t.*** A form of tetanus produced by inoculating the brain of animals with tetanus antitoxin; it is marked by epileptiform convulsions and excitement.

***chronic t.*** **1.** A latent infection in a healed wound, reactivated on opening the wound. **2.** A form of tetanus in which the onset and progress of the disease are slower and more prolonged and the symptoms are less severe.

***cryptogenic t.*** Tetanus in which the site of entry of the organism is not known.

***descending t.*** Tetanus in which muscle spasms occur first in the head and neck and later are manifested in other muscles of the body.

***t. dorsalis*** Tetanus in which the body is bent backward.

***extensor t.*** Tetanus that affects the extensor muscles.

***hydrophobic t.*** Cephalic t.

***idiopathic t.*** Tetanus that occurs without any visible lesion.

***imitative t.*** Hysteria that simulates tetanus.

***t. infantum*** T. neonatorum.

***t. lateralis*** A form of tetanus in which the body is bent sideways.

***local t.*** Tetanus marked by spasticity of a group of muscles near the wound. Trismus, tonic contraction of jaw muscles, is usually absent.

***t. neonatorum*** Tetanus of very young infants, usually due to infection of the navel caused by using nonsterile technique in ligating the umbilical cord.

***t. paradoxus*** Cephalic tetanus combined with paralysis of the facial or other cranial nerve.

***postoperative t.*** Tetanus that follows an operation.

***puerperal t.*** Tetanus that occurs following childbirth.

***toxic t.*** Tetanus produced by overdose of strychnine.

**tetanus antitoxin** **1.** An antibody that develops in the blood of humans or other animals (horses) as a result of infection by the tetanus organism *(Clostridium tetani)* or inoculation with tetanus toxin or toxoid. **2.** An antitoxin derived from the blood of horses or cattle immunized against tetanus toxin. It is used to produce passive immunity to prevent the development of tetanus and in the treatment of active tetanus. The prophylactic dose is 1500 units injected subcutaneously; the dose for active tetanus is 5000 to 20,000 units injected intravenously or subcutaneously.

**tetanus immune globulin** Immune globulin from human blood for use in persons not previously immunized against tetanus whose wound would indicate the need for tetanus prophylaxis. Tetanus immune globulin (human) produces fewer side effects than does tetanus antitoxin produced from horse serum.

**tetanus toxoid** Tetanus toxin modified so that its toxicity is greatly reduced, while retaining its capacity to promote active immunity.

**tetany** (tĕt′ă-nē) [Gr. *tetanos,* stretched] A nervous disorder marked by intermittent tonic spasms that are usually paroxysmal and involve the extremities. It may occur in infants, esp. newborns in intensive care units. High risk infants include premature newborns of diabetic mothers and those who have had perinatal asphyxia.

SYMPTOMS: The condition is marked by nervousness, irritability, and apprehension; numbness and tingling of the extremities; cramps of the various muscles (particularly those of the hands, producing a typical accoucheur type of hand, such as carpopedal spasm); and extreme extension of the feet. Bilateral tonic spasms occur in the arms and legs, with the jaws involved rarely. Contractions are usually paroxysmal and are attended with pain. There may be slight edema. Sensation is not disturbed, the mind is clear, and fever is slight or absent.

SIGNS: Characteristic diagnostic signs are Trousseau's sign, Chvostek's sign, and the peroneal sign. Prolongation of the isoelectric phase of the S-T segment of the electrocardiogram usually indicates low calcium. SEE: *Chvostek's sign; hyperventilation; Trousseau's sign.*

ETIOLOGY: Tetany is induced by changes in pH and by a deficiency of extracellular calcium that increase nervous and muscular excitability. Causative factors are parathyroid deficiency or inadvertent operative removal of parathyroids during thyroidectomy, alkalosis, vitamin D deficiency, or hyperventilation.

PROGNOSIS: The outcome is usually favorable. Attacks following thyroidectomy are sometimes fatal, however.

***alkalotic t.*** Tetany resulting from respiratory alkalosis, as in hyperventilation, or from metabolic alkalosis induced by excessive intake of sodium bicarbonate or excessive loss of chlorides by vomiting, gastric lavage, or suction.

***duration t.*** Continuous contraction, esp. in degenerated muscles, in response to a continuous electric current.

***epidemic t.*** A form of tetany occurring in Europe, esp. in the winter season. It is of short duration and is seldom fatal.

***gastric t.*** A severe form of tetany from stomach disorders accompanied by tonic, painful spasms of the extremities.

***hyperventilation t.*** Tetany caused by continued hyperventilation.

***hypocalcemic t.*** Tetany due to low serum calcium and high serum phosphate levels. This may be due to lack of vitamin D, factors that interfere with calcium absorption such as steatorrhea or infantile diarrhea, or defective renal excretion of phosphorus.

***latent t.*** Tetany that requires mechanical or electrical stimulation of nerves to show characteristic signs of excitability; the opposition of manifest tetany.

***manifest t.*** Tetany in which the characteristic symptoms such as carpopedal spasm, laryngospasm, and convulsions are present; the opposite of latent tetany.

***parathyroid t.*** Tetany resulting from excision of the parathyroid glands or from hyposecretion of the parathyroid glands as a result of disease or disorders of the glands. SEE: *hypoparathyroidism.*

***rachitic t.*** Tetany due to hypocalcemia accompanying vitamin D deficiency.

***thyreoprival t.*** Tetany resulting from removal of the thyroid gland accompanied by removal of the parathyroid glands.

**tetarcone** (tĕt′ăr-kōn) [Gr. *tetartos,* fourth, + *konos,* cone] The fourth or distolingual cusp of an upper premolar tooth. SYN: *tetartocone.*

**tetartanopia, tetartanopsia** (tĕt″ăr-tăn-ō′pē-ă, -ŏp′sē-ă) [″ + *opsis,* vision] Symmetrical blindness in the same quadrant of each visual field. SYN: *quadrantanopsia.*

**tetartocone** (tĕt-ăr′tō-kōn) [″ + *konos,* cone] Tetarcone.

**tetra-, tetr-** Combining form meaning *four.*

**tetrabasic** (tĕt″ră-bā′sĭk) [Gr. *tetras,* four, + *basis,* base] Having four replaceable hydrogen atoms, said of an acid or acid salt.

**tetrablastic** (tĕt″ră-blăs′tĭk) [″ + *blastos,* germ] Having four germinal layers: the ectoderm, endoderm, and two mesodermic layers.

**tetrabrachius** (tĕt″ră-brā′kē-ŭs) [″ + *brachion,* arm] A deformed fetus with four arms.

**tetrabromofluorescein** (tĕt″ră-brōm″ō-flū-or-ĕs′ĭn, -ē-ĭn) A dye, $C_{20}H_8Br_4O_5$, obtained from action of bromine on fluorescein, used as a stain in microscopy. SYN: *eosin.*

**tetracaine hydrochloride** A local anesthetic agent used topically and by infiltration. Trade name is Pontocaine Hydrochloride.

**tetrachirus** (tĕt″ră-kī′rŭs) [″ + *cheir,* hand] A deformed fetus with four hands.

**tetrachlorethylene** (tĕt″ră-klor-ĕth′ĭ-lēn) A clear, colorless liquid with a characteristic odor, used as a solvent.

**tetrachloride** (tĕt″ră-klō′rīd) A radical with four atoms of chlorine.

**tetracid** (tĕ-trăs′ĭd) [″ + L. *acidus,* sour] **1.** Able to react with four molecules of a monoacid or two of a diacid to form a salt or ester, said of a base or alcohol. This term is disapproved by some authorities. **2.** Having four hydrogen atoms replaceable by basic atoms or radicals, said of acids.

**Tetracoccus** (tĕt″ră-kŏk′ŭs) [″ + *kokkos,* berry] A genus of micrococcus arranged in groups of four by division into two planes.

**tetracrotic** (tĕt″ră-krŏt′ĭk) [″ + *krotos,* beat] Noting a pulse or pulse tracing with four upward strokes in the descending limb of the wave.

**tetracycline** (tĕt″ră-sī′klēn) A member of the tetracycline group of broad-spectrum antibiotics having similar pharmacological activity (i.e., tetracycline, chlortetracycline, oxytetracycline). Adverse effects may include hypersensitivity, burning of the eyes, glossitis, gastrointestinal disorders, various leukocyte changes, liver and kidney disorders, and staining of the teeth of a child whose mother took tetracycline during pregnancy. There are a great number of trade names for this antibiotic.

**tetrad** (tĕt′răd) [Gr. *tetras,* four] **1.** A group of four things with something in common. **2.** An element having a valence or combining power of four. **3.** A group of four similar bodies. **4.** A group of four parts, said of cells produced by division in two planes, or of a chromosome in four parts in preparation for two mitotic divisions in maturation.

**tetradactyly** (tĕt″ră-dăk′tĭ-lē) [″ + *daktylos,* finger] Having four digits on a hand or foot.

**tetraethylpyrophosphate** (tĕt-ră-ĕth″ĭl-pī-rō-fŏs′fāt) ABBR: TEPP. A powerful cholinesterase inhibitor used as an insecticide. It is poisonous to humans; the antidote is atropine.

**tetrahydrocannabinol** (tĕt″ră-hī″drō-kă-năb′ĭ-nŏl) A chemical, $C_{21}H_{30}O_2$, that is the principal active component in cannabis, or marijuana.

**tetrahydrozoline hydrochloride** (tĕt″ră-hī-drō′zō-lēn) A vasoconstrictor agent used as a nasal decongestant and ophthalmic vasoconstrictor.

**tetraiodothyronine** (tĕt″ră-ī″ō-dō-thī′rō-nēn) Thyroxine.

**tetralogy** The combination of four symptoms or elements.

***t. of Fallot*** An anomaly of the heart consisting of pulmonary stenosis, interventricular septal defect, dextroposed aorta that receives blood from both ventricles, and hypertrophy of the right ventricle.

**tetramastia, tetramazia** (tĕt″ră-măs′tē-ă, tĕt″ră-mā′zē-ă) [″ + *mastos, mazos,* breast] A condition characterized by the presence of four breasts.

**tetramastigote** (tĕt″ră-măs′tĭ-gōt) [″ + *mastix,* lash] Having four flagella.

**tetrameric, tetramerous** (tĕt″ră-mĕr′ĭk, tĕt-răm′ĕr-ŭs) [″ + *meros,* a part] Having four parts.

**tetranopsia** (tĕt″ră-nŏp′sē-ă) [″ + *an-,* not, + *opsis,* vision] Obliteration of one quarter of the visual field.

**tetraotus** (tĕt″ră-ō′tŭs) [Gr. *tetras,* four, + *otos,* ear] Tetrotus.

**tetraparesis** (tĕt″ră-păr′ĕ-sĭs) [″ + *parienai,* to let fall] Muscular weakness of all four extremities.

**tetrapeptide** (tĕt″ră-pĕp′tīd) A peptide that yields four amino acids when it is hydrolyzed.

**tetraplegia** (tĕt″ră-plē′jē-ă) [″ + *plege,* a stroke] Quadriplegia.

**tetraploid** (tĕt′ră-ployd) [″ + *ploos,* a fold, + *eidos,* form, shape] **1.** Concerning tetraploidy. **2.** Having four sets of chromosomes.

**tetrapus** (tĕt′ră-pŭs) [″ + *pous,* foot] A deformed fetus having four feet.

**tetrasaccharide** (tĕt″ră-săk′ă-rīd) A carbohydrate composed of four monosaccharides.

**tetrascelus** (tĕt-răs′ē-lŭs) [″ + *skelos,* leg] A deformed fetus having four legs.

**tetrasomic** (tĕt-ră-sō′mĭk) [″ + *soma,* body] Possessing four instead of the usual pair of chromosomes in an otherwise diploid cell; that is, having a chromosome number of 2n+2.

**tetraster** (tĕt-răs′tĕr) [″ + *aster,* star] A mitotic figure in which there are four asters instead of the usual two; occurring abnormally in mitosis.

**tetrastichiasis** (tĕt″ră-stĭ-kī′ă-sĭs) [″ + *stichos,* row, + *-iasis,* condition] A deformed fetus having four rows of eyelashes.

**tetratomic** (tĕt″ră-tŏm′ĭk) [″ + *atomos,* indivisible] Having four atoms.

**tetravalent** (tĕt″ră-vā′lĕnt) Having a valence or combining power of four. SYN: *quadrivalent.*

**tetrodotoxin** (tĕt″rō-dō-tŏks′ĭn) A powerful nerve poison found in the eggs of the California newt and in certain puffer fish in Japan. In concentrated form, it is more toxic than cyanide.

**tetrotus** (tĕt-rō′tŭs) [″ + *otos,* ear] A deformed fetus with two faces, four eyes, and four ears.

**tetroxide** (tĕ-trŏk′sīd) A chemical compound containing four oxygen atoms.

**textiform** (tĕks′tĭ-form) [L. *textum,* something woven, + *forma,* shape] Resembling a network, web, or mesh.

**textoblastic** (tĕks″tō-blăs′tĭk) [L. *textus,* tissue, + Gr. *blastos,* germ] Forming adult tissue; regenerative.

**textural** (tĕks′tū-răl) [L. *textura,* weaving] Concerning the texture or constitution of a tissue.

**texture** (tĕks′tūr) [L. *textura*] The organization of a tissue or structure.

**textus** (tĕks′tŭs) [L.] Tissue.

**T fracture** Fracture in which bone splits both longitudinally and transversely.

**T-group** A group of individuals who meet in training sessions to become more sensitive to themselves and others.

**Th** Symbol for the element thorium.

**thalamencephalon** (thăl″ă-mĕn-sĕf′ă-lŏn) [Gr. *thalamos,* inner chamber, + *enkephalos,* brain] The part of the diencephalon that includes the thalamus, pineal body, and geniculate bodies.

**thalamic** (thăl-ăm′ĭk) [Gr. *thalamos,* inner chamber] Pert. to the thalamus.

**thalamic syndrome** A syndrome caused by an optic thalamic lesion, with vascular lesions of the thalamus, causing disturbances of sensation and partial or complete paralysis of one side of the body. An extremely severe, sharp, boring-type pain may occur spontaneously. There also is a tendency to overrespond to a sensory stimulus and to be aware of the stimulus long after it has ceased.

**thalamo-** **1.** Combining form meaning *chamber.* **2.** Combining form meaning *thalamus.*

**thalamocele, thalamocoele** (thăl′ăm-ō-sēl) [Gr. *thalamos,* inner chamber, + *koilia,* a hollow] The third ventricle of the brain.

**thalamocortical** (thăl″ăm-ō-kor′tĭ-kăl) [″ + L. *cortex,* rind] Pert. to the optic thalamus and the cerebral cortex.

**thalamolenticular** (thăl′ăm-ō-lĕn-tĭk′ū-lăr) [″ + L. *lenticula,* lentil] Concerning the optic thalamus and the lenticular nucleus.

**thalamotomy** (thăl-ă-mŏt′ō-mē) [″ + *tome,* incision] Destruction by one of several methods of a portion of the thalamus to treat psychosis or intractable pain.

**thalamus** (thăl′ă-mŭs) *pl.* **thalami** [L.] The largest subdivision of the diencephalon on either side, consisting chiefly of an ovoid gray nuclear mass in the lateral wall of the third ventricle. Each consists of a number of nuclei (anterior, medial, lateral, and ventral), the medial and lateral geniculate bodies, and the pulvinar.

FUNCTION: All sensory stimuli, with the exception of olfactory, are received by the thalamus. These are associated, integrated, and then relayed through thalamocortical radiations to specific cortical areas. Impulses are also received from the cortex, hypothalamus, and corpus striatum and relayed to visceral and somatic effectors. The thalamus is also the center for appreciation of primitive uncritical sensations of pain, crude touch, and temperature.

**thalassemia** (thăl-ă-sē'mē-ă) [Gr. *thalassa,* sea, + *haima,* blood] A group of hereditary anemias occurring in populations bordering the Mediterranean and in Southeast Asia. Anemia is produced by either a defective production rate of the alpha or beta hemoglobin polypeptide chain or a decreased synthesis of the beta chain. Heterozygotes are usually asymptomatic. The severity in homozygotes varies according to the complexity of the inheritance pattern, but thalassemia may be fatal. SEE: *anemia, sickle cell.*

***t. intermedia*** A chronic hemolytic anemia caused by deficient alpha chain synthesis. It is also called *hemoglobin H disease.*

***t. major*** The homozygous form of deficient beta chain synthesis, which is very severe and presents during childhood. It is characterized by fatigue, splenomegaly, severe anemia, enlargement of the heart, slight jaundice, leg ulcers, and cholelithiasis. Increased bone marrow activity causes thickening of the cranial bones and increased malar eminences. Prognosis varies; however, the younger the child when the disease appears, the more unfavorable the outcome. SYN: *Cooley's anemia.* SEE: illus.

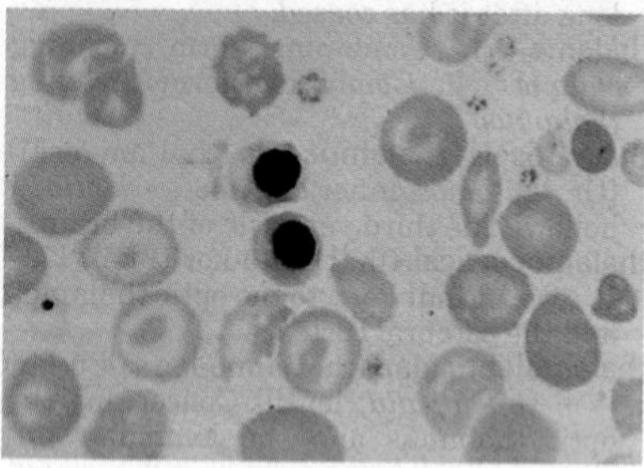

THALASSEMIA MAJOR

PERIPHERAL BLOOD WITH NORMOBLASTS AND TARGET CELLS (ORIG. MAG. ×600)

***t. minor*** A mild disease produced by heterozygosity for either beta or alpha chain. It may be completely asymptomatic. It is usually revealed by chance or as a result of study of the family of an individual having thalassemia major. The prognosis is excellent.

**thalassophobia** (thăl-ăs"ō-fō'bē-ă) [Gr. *thalassa,* sea, + *phobos,* fear] An abnormal fear of the sea.

**thalassotherapy** (thăl-ăs"sō-thĕr'ă-pē) [" + *therapeia,* treatment] Treatment of disease by living at the seaside, by sea bathing, or by sea voyages.

**thalidomide** (thă-lĭd'ō-mīd) A hypnotic drug that, if taken in early pregnancy, may cause severe malformation in limbs of developing fetuses. It is used in treating erythema nodosum leprosum and is being investigated as an immunosuppresive agent. SEE: *phocomelia.*

Caution: This drug should not be administered to women of childbearing age.

**thallitoxicosis** (thăl"ĭ-tŏk"sĭ-kō'sĭs) Poisoning by accidental ingestion of thallium sulfate–containing pesticides. SYN: *thallotoxicosis.* SEE: *thallium* in *Poisons and Poisoning Appendix.*

**thallium** (thăl'ē-ŭm) [Gr. *thallos,* a young shoot] SYMB: Tl. A metallic element. Atomic weight, 204.37; atomic number, 81; specific gravity, 11.85. Its salts are poisonous.

***t. sulfate*** A chemical used as a rodenticide. It is also quite toxic to humans.

**thallium poisoning** Poisoning characterized by severe abdominal pain, vomiting, diarrhea, tremors, delirium, convulsions, paralysis, coma, and death. SEE: *Poisons and Poisoning Appendix.*

**thallotoxicosis** (thăl"ō-tŏk"sĭ-kō'sĭs) Thallitoxicosis.

**thanato-** Combining form meaning *death.*

**thanatobiological** (thăn"ă-tō-bī-ō-lŏj'ĭ-kăl) [Gr. *thanatos,* death, + *bios,* life, + *logos,* word, reason] Rel. to the processes of life and death.

**thanatognomonic** (thăn"ăt-ŏg-nō-mŏn'ĭk) [" + *gnomonikos,* knowing] Indicative of the approach of death.

**thanatology** (thăn"ă-tŏl'ō-jē) [Gr. *thanatos,* death, + *logos,* word, reason] The study of death.

**thanatomania** (thăn"ă-tō-mā'nē-ă) [" + *mania,* madness] The condition of homicidal or suicidal mania.

**thanatophidia** (thăn"ă-tō-fĭd'ē-ă) [" + *ophis,* snake] Venomous snakes.

**thanatophobia** (thăn"ă-tō-fō'bē-ă) [" + *phobos,* fear] A morbid fear of death. SYN: *necrophobia.*

**thanatophoric dwarfism** Dwarfism caused by generalized failure of endochondral bone formation. It is characterized by a large head, a prominent forehead, hypertelorism, a saddle nose, and short limbs extending straight out from the trunk. Most of these infants die soon after birth. SEE: *dwarf, micromelic.*

**Thayer-Martin medium** A special medium used for growing the causative organism of gonorrhea, *Neisseria gonorrhoeae.*

**theaism** (thē'ă-ĭzm) [L. *thea,* tea, + Gr. *-ismos,* condition] Chronic caffeine poisoning from excessive tea drinking.

**thebaine** (thē-bā'ĭn) An alkaloid present in opium.

**thebesian foramen** (thē-bē'zē-ăn) [Adam Christian Thebesius, Ger. physician, 1686–1732] The orifice of a thebesian vein, opening into the right atrium of the heart.

**thebesian valve** An endocardial fold at the entrance of the coronary sinus into the right atrium.

**thebesian veins** Venules conveying blood from the myocardium to the atria or ventricles.

**theca** (thē′kă) *pl.* **thecae** [Gr. *theke,* sheath] A sheath of investing membrane.

***t. cordis*** Pericardium that sheaths the heart.

***t. folliculi*** The outer wall of a graafian follicle, consisting of an inner vascular layer (theca interna) and outer fibrous layer (theca externa).

**thecal** (thē′kăl) [Gr. *theke,* sheath] Pert. to a sheath.

**thecitis** (thē-sī′tĭs) [″ + *itis,* inflammation] Inflammation of the sheath of a tendon.

**theco-** Combining form meaning *sheath, case, receptacle.*

**thecodont** (thē′kō-dŏnt) [Gr. *theke,* sheath, + *odous,* tooth] Having teeth that are inserted in sockets.

**thecoma** (thē-kō′mă) [″ + *oma,* tumor] A tumor of the ovary usually occurring during or after menopause. It is usually benign.

**thecomatosis** (thē″kō-mă-tō′sĭs) [″ + ″ + *osis,* condition] Increased connective tissue in the ovary.

**thecostegnosia, thecostegnosis** (thē″kō-stĕg-nō′sē-ă, -nō′sĭs) [″ + *stegnosis,* a narrowing] Constriction of a tendon sheath.

**thelalgia** (thē-lăl′jē-ă) [Gr. *thele,* nipple, + *algos,* pain] Pain in the nipples.

**thelarche** (thē-lăr′kē) [″ + *arche,* beginning] The beginning of breast development at puberty. SEE: *pubarche; semenarche.*

**Thelazia** (thē-lā′zē-ă) [Gr. *thelazo,* to suck] A genus of nematodes that inhabit the conjunctival sac and lacrimal ducts of various species of vertebrates. Occasionally species of *Thelazia* are found in humans.

**thelaziasis** (thē″lā-zī′ă-sĭs) [″ + *-iasis,* condition] The condition of being infested by worms of the genus *Thelazia.*

**theleplasty** (thē′lĕ-plăs″tē) [Gr. *thele,* nipple, + *plassein,* to form] Plastic surgery of the nipple. SYN: *mammilliplasty.*

**thelerethism** (thēl-ĕr′ĕ-thĭzm) [″ + *erethisma,* stimulation] Erection of the nipple.

**thelitis** (thē-lī′tĭs) [″ + *itis,* inflammation] Inflammation of the nipples. SYN: *acromastitis.*

**thelium** (thē′lē-ŭm) *pl.* **thelia** [L.] **1.** A papilla. **2.** A nipple. **3.** A cellular layer.

**theloncus** (thē-lŏn′kŭs) [″ + *onkus,* bulk, mass] A tumor of a nipple.

**thelophlebostemma** (thē″lō-flĕb″ō-stĕm′mă) [″ + *phelps,* vein, + *stemma,* wreath] A dark or venous circle of veins about the nipple.

**thelorrhagia** (thē″lō-rā′jē-ă) [″ + *rhegnynai,* to burst forth] Hemorrhage from a nipple.

**thelygenic** (thē″lē-jĕn′ĭk) [Gr. *thelys,* female, + *gennan,* to produce] Producing only female children.

**thenad** (thē′năd) [Gr. *thenar,* palm, + L. *ad,* toward] Toward the palm or thenar eminence.

**thenal** (thē′năl) [Gr. *thenar,* palm] Pert. to the palm or thenar eminence.

**thenal aspect** The outer side of the palm.

**thenar** (thē′năr) [Gr. *thenar,* palm] **1.** The palm of the hand or sole of the foot. **2.** A fleshy eminence at the base of the thumb. **3.** Concerning the palm.

**thenar cleft** A fascial cleft of the palm overlying the volar surface of the adductor pollicis muscle.

**thenar eminence** A prominence at the base of the thumb.

**thenar fascia** A thin membrane covering the short muscles of the thumb.

**thenar muscle** The abductor or flexor muscle of the thumb.

**theobromine** (thē-ō-brō′mēn) [Gr. *theos,* god, + *broma,* food] A white powder obtained from *Theobroma cacao,* the plant from which chocolate is obtained. It dilates blood vessels in the heart and peripherally. It is used as a mild stimulant and as a diuretic.

**theomania** (thē-ō-mā′nē-ă) [Gr. *theos,* god, + *mania,* madness] Religious insanity; esp. that in which the patient thinks he or she is a deity or has divine inspiration.

**theophobia** (thē″ō-fō′bē-ă) [″ + *phobos,* fear] An abnormal fear of the wrath of God.

**theophylline** (thē″ō-fĭl′ēn, -ĭn) [L. *thea,* tea, + Gr. *phyllon,* plant] A white crystalline powder with action resembling caffeine and theobromine. SEE: *aminophylline.*

***t. ethylenediamine*** Previously used name for aminophylline.

**theorem** (thē′ō-rĕm) [Gr. *theorema,* principle arrived at by speculation] A proposition that can be proved by use of logic, or by argument, from information previously accepted as being valid.

**theory** (thē′ō-rē) [Gr. *theoria,* speculation as opposed to practice] A statement that best explains all the available evidence on a given topic. It is not a guess. If evidence that contradicts the theory becomes available, the theory must be abandoned, modified or changed to incorporate it. When a theory becomes generally accepted and firmly established, it may be called a doctrine or principle, although the term "theory" is often used, as in "cell theory."

***t. of aging*** A compilation of theories that deal with aging at cellular and biological levels.

***cell t.*** The proposition that living things are composed of cells capable of life.

***clonal selection t. of immunity*** The theory formulated by the Australian Nobel prize winner F. M. Burnett, in 1959, that mesenchymal cells, precursors of the cells that form antibodies, are made up of innumerable clones. The clones capable of reacting with "self" components (i.e., the individual's own cells) are eliminated or suppressed in the prenatal period. Those clones not eliminated or suppressed that are specific for foreign substances react with the antigen fitting to the receptor, and this leads to the proliferation of that clone.

***germ t.*** The proposition that infectious diseases are caused by microorganisms.

***learning t.*** An approach to understanding how learning comes about by applying certain laws of learning; learning represents a change in behavior that has come about as a result of practice, education, and experience.

***nursing t.*** A theory that explores, describes, and analyzes the epistemological origins of nursing knowledge.

***quantum t.*** The proposition that energy can be emitted in discrete quantities (quanta) and that atomic particles can exist only in certain energy states. Quanta are measured by multiplying the frequency of the radiation, *v*, by Planck's constant, *h*.

***recapitulation t.*** The theory that during development an individual organism goes through the same progressive stages as did the species in developing from the lower to the higher forms of life. The theory that ontogeny recapitulates phylogeny.

***target t.*** A model used in radiobiology to describe cell survival from radiation. Each cell has a certain number of critical structures (targets) that must be inactivated for the cell to die. If all are inactivated, the cell will recover.

**Theory of Clinical Nursing** A nursing theory developed by Reva Rubin that focuses on patients' experiences of tension or stress in health problem situations. The goal of nursing is to help patients adjust to, endure through, and usefully integrate health problem situations. SEE: *Nursing Theory Appendix.*

**Theory of Cultural Care Diversity and Universality** A nursing theory developed by Madeleine Leininger that focuses on diversities and universalities in human care. The goal of nursing is to provide culturally congruent care to people. SEE: *Nursing Theory Appendix.*

**Theory of Health as Expanding Consciousness** A nursing theory developed by Margaret Newman that proposes that all people in every situation, no matter how disordered and hopeless the situation may seem, are part of the universal process of expanding consciousness. The goal of nursing is the authentic involvement of nurse and patient in a mutual relationship of pattern recognition and augmentation. SEE: *Nursing Theory Appendix.*

**Theory of Human Becoming** A nursing theory developed by Rosemarie Parse that focuses on the individual's experiences of health. The goal of nursing is to respect and facilitate the quality of life as perceived by the individual and the family. SEE: *Nursing Theory Appendix.*

**Theory of Human Caring** A nursing theory developed by Jean Watson that focuses on the transpersonal caring relationship between nurse and patient and the caring actions or interventions used by nurses. The goal of nursing is to help individuals to gain a higher degree of harmony within the mind, body, and soul through the use of 10 nursing interventions. SEE: *Nursing Theory Appendix.*

**Theory of Interpersonal Relations** A nursing theory developed by Hildegard Peplau that identifies the four phases of the interpersonal process between the nurse and the patient: orientation, identification, exploitation, and resolution. The goal of nursing is to promote favorable changes in patients. SEE: *Nursing Theory Appendix.*

**Theory of the Nursing Process Discipline** A nursing theory developed by Ida Jean Orlando Pelletier that focuses on how the nurse identifies patients' immediate needs for help. The goal of nursing is to identify and meet patients' immediate needs for help through use of the deliberative nursing process. SEE: *Nursing Theory Appendix.*

**theotherapy** (thē″ō-thĕr′ă-pē) [Gr. *theos*, god, + *therapeia*, treatment] The treatment of disease by spiritual and religious methods.

**thèque** (tĕk) [Fr., a box] A nest of nevus cells or other cells close to the basal layer of the epidermis.

**therapeutic** (thĕr-ă-pū′tĭk) [Gr. *therapeutikos*, treating] **1.** Pert. to results obtained from treatment. **2.** Having medicinal or healing properties. **3.** A healing agent.

**therapeutic exercise** Scientific supervision of exercise for the purpose of preventing muscular atrophy, restoring joint and muscle function, increasing muscular strength, and improving efficiency of cardiovascular and pulmonary function.

**therapeutic recreation** A specialized field within recreation whose specialists plan and direct recreational activities for patients recovering from physical or mental illness or who are attempting to cope with a permanent or temporary disability.

**therapeutic regimen (community), ineffective management of** A pattern of regulating and integrating into community processes programs for treatment of illness and the sequelae of illness that is unsatisfactory for meeting health-related goals. SEE: *Nursing Diagnoses Appendix.*

**therapeutic regimen (families), ineffective management of** A pattern of regulating and integrating into family processes a program for treatment of illness and the sequelae of illness that is unsatisfactory for meeting specific health needs. SEE: *Nursing Diagnoses Appendix.*

**therapeutic regimen (individual), effective management of** A pattern of regulating and integrating into daily living a program for treatment of illness and its sequelae that is satisfactory for meeting specific health goals. SEE: *Nursing Di-*

*agnoses Appendix.*

**therapeutic regimen (individual), ineffective management of** A pattern of regulating and integrating into daily living a program for treatment of illness and the sequelae of illness that is unsatisfactory for meeting specific health goals. SEE: *Nursing Diagnoses Appendix.*

**therapeutics** (thĕr″ă-pū′tĭks) [Gr. *therapeutike,* treatment] That branch of medicine concerned with the application of remedies and the treatment of disease. SYN: *therapy.*

**therapia sterilisans magna** (thĕr″ă-pē′ă stē-rĭl′ĭ-săns măg′nă) [L.] Ehrlich's method of administering a chemical agent that would destroy in one large dose all the parasites in a patient without causing serious injury to the patient.

**therapist** (thĕr′ă-pĭst) [Gr. *therapeia,* treatment] A person skilled in giving therapy, usually in a specific field of health care.

***licensed occupational t.*** ABBR: LOTR; OTR/L. An occupational therapist who has been certified by the American Occupational Therapy Certification Board as a registered occupational therapist (OTR). Some state governments, as part of their licensure statutes, permit use of the OTR/L or LOTR designations.

***occupational t.*** ABBR: OT. One who provides assessment and intervention to ameliorate physical and psychological deficits that interfere with the performance of activities and tasks of living.

***physical t.*** Registered physical t.

***radiation t.*** Radiation therapy technologist.

***registered physical t.*** ABBR: RPT. An individual who has successfully completed an accredited physical therapy education program and has passed a licensing examination, and who is then legally responsible for evaluating, planning, conducting, and supervising a physical therapy program using rehabilitative and therapeutic exercise techniques and physical modalities.

***respiratory t.*** A person skilled in managing the techniques and equipment used in treating those with acute and chronic respiratory diseases.

***speech t.*** A person skilled in assisting patients who have speech and language difficulties.

**therapy** (thĕr′ă-pē) [Gr. *therapeia,* treatment] Treatment of a disease or pathological condition. SYN: *therapeutics.* SEE: *treatment.*

***adjuvant t.*** SEE: *adjuvant therapy.*

***anticoagulant t.*** The use of anticoagulants to decrease the tendency of the blood to coagulate and cause thrombosis.

***aversion t.*** SEE: *aversion therapy.*

***behavior t.*** In psychiatry, the use of conditioning techniques to directly modify behavior. Even though the technique may be of benefit, the basic cause of the difficulty is not abolished.

***biological t.*** SEE: *immunotherapy.*

***collapse t.*** The production of a pneumothorax on one side to treat pulmonary tuberculosis. It allows the lung on that side to be at rest.

***electroconvulsive t.*** SEE: *electroconvulsive therapy.*

***estrogen replacement t.*** SEE: under *estrogen.*

***fever t.*** Therapy involving artificially produced fever. This is accomplished by exposure to high environmental temperature or by the injection of foreign proteins.

***group t.*** SEE: *group therapy.*

***home drug infusion t.*** Out-of-hospital management of diseases or disorders that require intravenous administration of therapeutic agents. Patients who receive this form of therapy will need to be carefully selected and trained. Their home care providers also will need to be experienced in the procedures. When these qualifications are not met, the patients are at high risk for adverse events including severe infection, shock, and even death.

***hormone replacement t.*** ABBR: HRT. The use of synthetic hormones to replace hormones that are absent or deficient. It is typically used for menopausal and postmenopausal women when estrogen is replaced orally, transdermally, or vaginally. It is believed that the concurrent use of estrogen and progesterone provides all the benefits ascribed to estrogen replacement therapy and reduces the risk of estrogen-stimulated malignancies. SEE: *estrogen replacement therapy.*

***immunological t.*** SEE: *immunological therapy.*

***immunosuppressive t.*** SEE: *immunosuppressive agent.*

***inhalation t.*** The administration of medicines, water vapor, gases (e.g., oxygen, carbon dioxide, or helium), or anesthetics by inhalation. The medicines usually are nebulized by using an aerosol or spray apparatus. SEE: *intermittent positive-pressure breathing.*

***insulin shock t.*** SEE: *shock, insulin.*

***light t.*** Treatment with radiation from the visible spectrum.

***liquid air t.*** The therapeutic application of air that is so cold as to be liquefied. SEE: *$CO_2$ therapy; cryotherapy; hypothermia.*

***milieu t.*** A method of psychotherapy that controls the environment of the patient to provide interpersonal contacts that will develop trust, assurance, and personal autonomy.

***neoadjuvant t.*** SEE: *neoadjuvant therapy.*

***nonspecific t.*** The use of injections of foreign proteins or bacterial vaccines in the treatment of infection to stimulate general cellular activity. SEE: *specific t.*

***occupational t.*** Therapeutic use of

work, self-care, and play activities to increase independent function, enhance development, and prevent disability; it may include adaptation of task or environment to achieve maximum independence and to enhance quality of life.

***opsonic t.*** The use of bacterial vaccines to elevate the opsonic index of the blood. SYN: *vaccine t.*

***parenteral t.*** A medicine or solution administered via a route other than ingestion.

***photodynamic t.*** A method of treating cancer by using light-absorbing chemicals that are selectively retained by malignant cells. When these cells are exposed to light in the visible range, the cancer cells are killed.

***physical t.*** ABBR: PT. The appropriate use of therapeutic exercise, rehabilitative programs, and physical agents such as massage, heat, hydrotherapy, radiation, and electricity, under the direction of a licensed physical therapist.

***play t.*** The use of play, esp. with dolls and toys, to allow children to express their feelings. This may permit insight into their thought processes that could not be obtained through verbal communication.

***radiation t.*** SEE: *radiation therapy.*

***replacement t.*** The therapeutic use of a medicine to substitute for a natural substance that is either absent or diminished (e.g., insulin or thyroid hormone).

***serum t.*** The use of injections of blood serum from immunized animals or persons in the treatment of disease. SYN: *serotherapy.*

***shock t.*** SEE: *shock therapy.*

***specific t.*** Administration of a remedy acting directly against the cause of a disease, as penicillin for syphilis or acyclovir for the herpes simplex virus. SEE: *nonspecific t.*

***speech t.*** SEE: *speech therapy.*

***spiritual t.*** SEE: *spiritual therapy.*

***substitution t.*** Administration of a substance that the body normally produces, such as a hormone.

***transgenerational t.*** A type of psychotherapy that addresses longstanding patterns from at least three generations of the patient's family. This method focuses on functional and nonfunctional family processes by using theoretical concepts from Murry Bowen, Ivan Boszormenyi-Nagy, Carl Whitaker, and Nathan Ackerman.

***vaccine t.*** Injection of bacteria or their products to produce active immunization against a disease. SYN: *opsonic t.*

***validation t.*** A technique used for patients with moderate-to-late dementia in which the caregiver agrees with the patient's statement or beliefs. This method helps prevent argumentative and agitated behavior. It is used when reality orientation is not successful.

**therapy putty** The generic name for a malleable plastic material used as a therapeutic modality to provide resistance in various hand exercises. One brand is available under the trade name Theraplast.

**therm** [Gr. *therme,* heat] Term used to indicate a variety of quantities of heat. SEE: *MET.*

**thermacogenesis** (thĕr″mă-kō-jĕn′ĕs-ĭs) [Gr. *therme,* heat, + *genesis,* generation, birth] Production of an increase of body temperature by drug therapy or biological methods, such as injection of malarial parasites.

**thermal** (thĕr′măl) [Gr. *therme,* heat] Pert. to heat.

**thermal death point** In bacteriology, the degree of heat that will kill organisms in a fluid culture in 10 min.

**thermalgesia** (thĕr″măl-jē′zē-ă) [″ + *algesis,* sense of pain] Pain caused by heat. SYN: *thermoalgesia.*

**thermalgia** (thĕr-măl′jē-ă) [″ + *algos,* pain] Neuralgia accompanied by an intense burning sensation, pain, redness, and sweating of the area involved. SYN: *causalgia.*

**thermal radiation** Heat radiation.

**thermal sense** Thermesthesia.

**thermanesthesia** (thĕrm″ăn-ĕs-thē′zē-ă) [″ + ″ + *aisthesis,* sensation] Thermoanesthesia.

**thermatology** (thĕr-mă-tŏl′ō-jē) [Gr. *therme,* heat, + *logos,* word, reason] The study of heat in the treatment of disease.

**thermelometer** (thĕr″mĕl-ŏm′ĕ-tĕr) [″ + *elektron,* amber, + Gr. *metron,* a measure] An electric thermometer used to indicate temperature changes too slight to be measured on an ordinary thermometer.

**thermesthesia** (thĕr″mĕs-thē′zē-ă) [″ + *aisthesis,* sensation] The capability of perceiving heat and cold; temperature sense. SYN: *thermal sense; thermoesthesia.*

**thermesthesiometer** (thĕrm″ĕs-thē-zē-ŏm′ĕt-ĕr) [″ + *aisthesis,* sensation, + *metron,* a measure] A device for determining sensibility to heat.

**thermic** (thĕr′mĭk) [Gr. *therme,* heat] Pert. to heat.

**thermic sense** The temperature sense; ability to react to heat stimuli.

**thermistor** (thĕr-mĭs′tọr) An apparatus for quickly determining very small changes in temperature. Materials that alter their resistance to the flow of electricity as the temperature changes are used in these devices.

**thermo-** Combining form indicating *hot, heat.*

**thermoalgesia** (thĕr″mō-ăl-jē′zē-ă) [Gr. *therme,* heat, + *algesis,* sense of pain] Thermalgesia.

**thermoanesthesia** (thĕr″mō-ăn″ĕs-thē′zē-ă) [″ + ″ + *aisthesis,* sensation] **1.** Inability to distinguish between heat and cold. **2.** Insensibility to heat or temperature changes. SYN: *thermanesthesia.*

**thermobiosis** (thĕr″mō-bī-ō′sĭs) [″ + *biosis,* way of life] The ability to withstand high temperature.

**thermobiotic** (thĕr″mō-bī-ŏt′ĭk) [″ + *bios,* life] Able to exist at high temperature.

**thermocauterectomy** (thĕr″mō-kaw-tĕr-ĕk′tō-mē) [″ + *kauterion,* branding iron, + *ektome,* excision] Excision by thermocautery.

**thermocautery** (thĕr″mō-kaw′tĕr-ē) **1.** Cautery by application of heat. **2.** Cauterizing iron.

**thermochemistry** (thĕr″mō-kĕm′ĭs-trē) The branch of science concerned with the interrelationship of heat and chemical reactions.

**thermochroic** (thĕr″mō-krō′ĭk) [″ + *chroa,* color] Concerning thermochroism.

**thermochroism** (thĕr-mŏk′rō-ĭzm) [″ + *chroa,* color] Property of a substance reflecting or transmitting portions of thermal radiation and absorbing or altering others.

**thermocoagulation** (thĕr″mō-kō-ăg-ū-lā′shŭn) [″ + L. *coagulatio,* clotting] The use of high-frequency currents to produce coagulation to destroy tissue.

**thermocouple** (thĕr′mō-kŭ″pl) [″ + L. *copula,* a bond] Thermopile.

**thermocurrent** (thĕr″mō-kŭr′ĕnt) An electric current produced by thermoelectric means.

**thermode** A device for heating or cooling a part of the body. Thermodes have been used in studying the effect on body function when the temperature of some organ or tissue is changed.

**thermodiffusion** (thĕr″mō-dĭ-fū′zhŭn) Increased diffusion of a substance as a result of increased heat.

**thermodilution** (thĕr″mō-dī-lū′shŭn) The use of an injected cold liquid such as sterile saline into the bloodstream and measurement of the temperature change downstream. This technique has been used to determine cardiac output.

**thermoduric** (thĕr″mō-dū′rĭk) [″ + L. *durus,* resistant] Thermophilic.

**thermodynamics** (thĕr″mō-dī-năm′ĭks) [″ + *dynamis,* power] The branch of physics concerned with laws that govern heat production, changes, and conversion into other forms of energy.

**thermoelectric** (thĕr″mō-ē-lĕk′trĭk) Concerning thermoelectricity.

**thermoelectricity** (thĕr″mō-ē-lĕk-trĭs′ĭ-tē) Electricity generated by heat.

**thermoesthesia** (thĕr″mō-ĕs-thē′zē-ă) [Gr. *therme,* heat, + *aisthesis,* sensation] Thermesthesia.

**thermoexcitatory** (thĕr″mō-ĕk-sī′tă-tor-ē) [″ + L. *excitare,* to irritate] Stimulating the production of heat in the body.

**thermogenesis** (thĕr″mō-jĕn′ĕ-sĭs) [″ + *genesis,* generation, birth] The production of heat, esp. in the body.

***dietary t.*** The heat-producing response to ingesting food. For several hours after eating, the metabolic rate increases. Heat is a byproduct of the energy required for digesting, absorbing, and metabolizing food components, and synthesizing and storing protein and fat. The calories used in the thermic response are expended and thus are not stored in the form of fat. Because the caloric requirement for this thermic response is greater for ingested fat than it is for carbohydrate and protein, it might be assumed that a mixed meal containing a preponderance of fat would contribute less to storage of excess calories than meals high in protein or carbohydrate. The practical importance of this concept is being investigated.

***nonshivering t.*** A limited physiological response of the newborn infant to chilling. Hypothermia increases the metabolic rate, generating heat and catabolizing glycogen stored in brown fat to liberate glucose to meet the increased energy needs. Brown fat catabolism also liberates fatty acids, which lower blood pH, increase the risk of metabolic acidosis, and interfere with bilirubin transport. SEE: *hypothermia.*

**thermograph** (thĕr′mō-grăf) [″ + *graphein,* to write] A device for registering variations of heat.

**thermography** In medicine, the use of a device that detects and records the heat present in very small areas of the part being studied. When these multiple readings are accumulated, the relatively hot and cold spots on the body surface are revealed. The technique has been used to study blood flow to limbs and to detect cancer of the breast.

**thermohyperalgesia** (thĕr″mō-hī″pĕr-ăl-jē′zē-ă) [″ + *hyper,* excessive, + *algesis,* sense of pain] Unbearable pain on the application of heat.

**thermohyperesthesia** (thĕr″mō-hī″pĕr-ĕs-thē′zē-ă) [″ + *hyper,* excessive, + *aisthesis,* sensation] Exceptional sensitivity to heat.

**thermohypesthesia** (thĕr″mō-hī″pĕs-thē′zē-ă) [″ + *hypo,* below, + *aisthesis,* sensation] Diminished perception of heat.

**thermoinhibitory** (thĕr″mō-ĭn-hĭb′ĭ-tor″ē) [″ + L. *inhibere,* to restrain] Arresting or impeding the generation of body heat.

**thermolamp** (thĕr′mō-lămp) [″ + *lampe,* torch] A lamp used for providing heat.

**thermology** (thĕr-mŏl′ō-jē) [″ + *logos,* word, reason] The science of heat.

**thermoluminescent dosimeter** A monitoring device consisting of a small crystal in a container that can be attached to a patient or to a health care worker. It stores energy when struck by ionizing radiation. When heated, it will emit light proportional to the amount of radiation to which it has been exposed.

**thermolysis** (thĕr-mŏl′ĭ-sĭs) [″ + *lysis,* dissolution] **1.** Loss of body heat, as by evaporation. **2.** Chemical decomposition by heat.

**thermolytic** (thĕr″mō-lĭt′ĭk) [″ + *lytikos,* dissolving] Promoting thermolysis.

**thermomassage** (thĕr″mō-mă-săzh′) Massage by use of heat.

**thermometer** (thĕr-mŏm′ĕ-tĕr) [″ + *metron*, measure] An instrument for indicating the degree of heat or cold. First mention of the use of a thermometer in diagnosis of disease was given by Italian physician Sanctorius in 1626. The glass clinical thermometer used today differs little from the one he used. **thermometric** (thĕr″mō-mĕt′rĭk), *adj.*

***alcohol t.*** A thermometer containing alcohol.

***Celsius t.*** A thermometric scale generally used in scientific notation. Temperature of boiling water at sea level is 100°C and the freezing point is 0°C. SYN: *centigrade t.* SEE: tables.

***centigrade t.*** Celsius t.

***clinical t.*** A thermometer for measuring the body temperature; one in which the mercury remains stationary at the registration point until shaken down.

***differential t.*** A thermometer recording slight variations of temperature.

***Fahrenheit t.*** A thermometric scale used in English-speaking countries, in which the boiling point is 212°F and the freezing point is 32°F. SEE: tables at *Celsius t.*

***gas t.*** A thermometer filled with gas, such as air, helium, or oxygen.

***Kelvin t.*** A thermometric scale in which absolute zero is 0°K; the freezing point of water is 273.15°K; and the boiling point of water is 373.15°K. Thus 1°K on the Kelvin scale is exactly equivalent to 1°C.

***mercury t.*** A thermometer containing mercury for measurement of temperature.

***recording t.*** A device with a suitable sensor that continuously monitors and records temperature.

**Comparative Thermometric Scale**

| | Celsius* | Fahrenheit |
|---|---|---|
| Boiling point of water | 100° | 212° |
| | 90 | 194 |
| | 80 | 176 |
| | 70 | 158 |
| | 60 | 140 |
| | 50 | 122 |
| | 40 | 104 |
| Body temperature | 37° | 98.6° |
| | 30 | 86 |
| | 20 | 68 |
| | 10 | 50 |
| Freezing point of water | 0° | 32° |
| | −10 | 14 |
| | −20 | −4 |

CONVERSION: *Fahrenheit to Celsius*: Subtract 32 and multiply by 5/9. *Celsius to Fahrenheit*: Multiply by 9/5 and add 32.

* Also called *Centigrade*.

***rectal t.*** A thermometer that is inserted into the rectum for determining body temperature.

***self-registering t.*** A thermometer recording variations of temperature.

***spirit t.*** A thermometer filled with alcohol instead of mercury for registering low temperatures.

***surface t.*** A thermometer for indicating the temperature of the body's surface.

***tympanic t.*** A thermometer that determines the temperature electronically by measuring it from the tympanic membrane of the ear. SEE: *ear thermometry; temperature, tympanic.*

***wet-and-dry-bulb t.*** A device for determining relative humidity consisting of two thermometers, the bulb of one being kept saturated with water vapor. The difference in temperatures between the two depends on relative humidity.

**thermometer, disinfection of** Disinfection of a thermometer with a substance that is able to kill ordinary bacteria and *Mycobacterium tuberculosis* as well as viruses. A variety of chemical solutions are used, but the effectiveness of these agents can be greatly diminished if the thermometer is not washed thoroughly before being disinfected.

**thermometry** (thĕr-mŏm′ĕ-trē) Measurement of temperature.

***clinical t.*** Measurement of the temperature of warm-blooded organisms, esp. humans. The oral temperature of the healthy human body ranges between 96.6° and 100°F (35.9° and 37.8°C). During a 24-hr period, a person's body temperature may vary from 0.5° to 2.0°F (0.28° to 1.1°C). It is highest in late afternoon and lowest during sleep in the early hours of the morning. It is slightly increased by eating, exercising, and external heat, and is reduced about 1.5°F (0.8°C) during sleep. In disease, the temperature of the body deviates several degrees above or below that considered the average in healthy persons.

In acute infections such as meningitis, pneumonia, scarlatina, typhoid, typhus, and intermittent fever, body temperature sometimes rises as high as 106° to 107°F (41.1° to 41.7°C). In other febrile diseases, it rarely reaches 104°F (40°C). However, the temperature may reach as high as 110°F (43.3°C) in sunstroke. The lowest extreme of temperature is found sometimes in the cold stage of cholera, when temperature may be very low (85° to 90°F or 29.4° to 32.2°C) for several days.

Subnormal temperatures, below 98°F (36.7°C), are observed during convalescence from certain febrile conditions; after pneumonia and typhoid fever; in collapse resulting from shock, hemorrhage, or rupture of a viscus, as the bowel in typhoid or the stomach in perforating ulcer.

In general, for every degree of fever the pulse rises 10 beats per minute, but ele-

## Thermometric Equivalents (Celsius and Fahrenheit)

| C° | F° | C° | F° | C° | F° | C° | F° |
|---|---|---|---|---|---|---|---|
| 0 | 32 | 27 | 80.6 | 54 | 129.2 | 81 | 177.8 |
| 1 | 33.8 | 28 | 82.4 | 55 | 131 | 82 | 179.6 |
| 2 | 35.6 | 29 | 84.2 | 56 | 132.8 | 83 | 181.4 |
| 3 | 37.4 | 30 | 86.0 | 57 | 134.6 | 84 | 183.2 |
| 4 | 39.2 | 31 | 87.8 | 58 | 136.4 | 85 | 185 |
| 5 | 41 | 32 | 89.6 | 59 | 138.2 | 86 | 186.8 |
| 6 | 42.8 | 33 | 91.4 | 60 | 140 | 87 | 188.6 |
| 7 | 44.6 | 34 | 93.2 | 61 | 141.8 | 88 | 190.4 |
| 8 | 46.4 | 35 | 95 | 62 | 143.6 | 89 | 192.2 |
| 9 | 48.2 | 36 | 96.8 | 63 | 145.4 | 90 | 194 |
| 10 | 50 | 37 | 98.6 | 64 | 147.2 | 91 | 195.8 |
| 11 | 51.8 | 38 | 100.4 | 65 | 149 | 92 | 197.6 |
| 12 | 53.6 | 39 | 102.2 | 66 | 150.8 | 93 | 199.4 |
| 13 | 55.4 | 40 | 104 | 67 | 152.6 | 94 | 201.2 |
| 14 | 57.2 | 41 | 105.8 | 68 | 154.4 | 95 | 203 |
| 15 | 59 | 42 | 107.6 | 69 | 156.2 | 96 | 204.8 |
| 16 | 60.8 | 43 | 109.4 | 70 | 158 | 97 | 206.6 |
| 17 | 62.6 | 44 | 111.2 | 71 | 159.8 | 98 | 208.4 |
| 18 | 64.4 | 45 | 113 | 72 | 161.6 | 99 | 210.2 |
| 19 | 66.2 | 46 | 114.8 | 73 | 163.4 | 100 | 212 |
| 20 | 68 | 47 | 116.6 | 74 | 165.2 | | |
| 21 | 69.8 | 48 | 118.4 | 75 | 167 | | |
| 22 | 71.6 | 49 | 120.2 | 76 | 168.8 | | |
| 23 | 73.4 | 50 | 122 | 77 | 170.6 | | |
| 24 | 75.2 | 51 | 123.8 | 78 | 172.4 | | |
| 25 | 77 | 52 | 125.6 | 79 | 174.2 | | |
| 26 | 78.8 | 53 | 127.4 | 80 | 176 | | |

vation of temperature to 99.5°F (37.5°C) provides greater evidence of disease than a pulse rate increase from 70 to 90 beats per minute. If the temperature remains above normal after general symptoms subside during convalescence, the patient is in danger of a relapse or the occurrence of some other disease. The range of the increase of heat in different febrile diseases extends to 110°F (43.3°C) or more and, as a rule, the amount of increase is a criterion of the intensity of the disease.

Artificial fever induced through diathermy, continuous hot bath, or injection of malarial organisms was formerly used in treating some diseases but is seldom used in modern medicine.

**thermoneurosis** (thĕr″mō-nū-rō′sĭs) [Gr. *therme,* heat, + *neuron,* nerve, + *osis,* condition] Elevation of body temperature in hysteria and other nervous conditions.

**thermonuclear** (thĕr″mō-nū′klē-ăr) Concerning thermonuclear reactions.

**thermopenetration** (thĕr″mō-pĕn-ĕ-trā′shŭn) [″ + L. *penetrare,* to go within] Application of heat to the deeper tissues of the body by diathermy. SYN: *thermoradiotherapy.*

**thermophilic** (thĕr″mō-fĭl′ĭk) [″ + *philein,* to love] Preferring or thriving best at high temperatures, said of bacteria that thrive best at temperatures between 40° and 70°C (104° and 158°F). SYN: *thermoduric.*

**thermophils** (thĕr′mō-fĭlz) Organisms that grow best at elevated temperatures (i.e., 40° to 70°C).

**thermophobia** (thĕr″mō-fō′bē-ă) [″ + *phobos,* fear] An abnormal dread of heat.

**thermophore** (thĕr′mō-for) [″ + *phoros,* a bearer] An apparatus for applying heat to a part, consisting of a water heater and tubes conveying water to a coil and returning to the heater or salts that produce heat when moistened.

**thermophylic** (thĕr″mō-fī′lĭk) [″ + *phylake,* guard] Resistant to destruction by heat, characteristic of certain bacteria.

**thermopile** (thĕr′mō-pīl) [″ + L. *pila,* pile] In physical therapy, a thermoelectric battery used in measuring small variations in the degree of heat. It consists of a number of connected dissimilar metallic plates. Under the influence of heat, these plates produce an electric current. SYN: *thermocouple.*

**thermoplastic** (thĕr″mō-plăs′tĭk) Concerning or being softened or made malleable by heat.

**thermopolypnea** (thĕr″mō-pŏl-ĭp-nē′ă) [″ + *polys,* many, + *pnoia,* breath] Quickened breathing caused by high fever or increased ambient temperature.

**thermoradiotherapy** (thĕr″mō-rā″dē-ō-thĕr′ă-pē) [″ + L. *radius,* ray, + Gr. *therapeia,* treatment] Application of heat to the deep tissues by diathermy. SYN: *thermopenetration.*

**thermoreceptor** (thĕr″mō-rē-sĕp′tor) [″ + L. *receptor,* a receiver] A sensory receptor that is stimulated by a rise of body temperature.

**thermoregulation** (thĕr″mō-rĕg″ū-lā′shŭn) Heat regulation.

***ineffective t.*** The state in which the individual's temperature fluctuates between hypothermia and hyperthermia. SEE: *Nursing Diagnoses Appendix.*

**thermoregulatory** (thĕr″mō-rĕg′ū-lă-tor″ē) Pert. to the regulation of temperature, esp. body temperature.

**thermoregulatory center** A center in the hypothalamus that regulates heat production and heat loss, esp. the latter, so that a normal body temperature is maintained. It is influenced by nervous impulses from cutaneous receptors and by the temperature of the blood flowing through it.

**thermoresistant** (thĕr″mō-rē-zĭs′tănt) [″ + L. *resistentia,* resistance] An ability to survive in relatively high temperature; characteristic of some types of bacteria.

**thermostabile** (thĕr″mō-stā′bĭl) [″ + L. *stabilis,* stable] Not changed or destroyed by heat.

**thermostat** (thĕr′mō-stăt) [″ + *statikos,* standing] An automatic device for regulating the temperature.

**thermosterilization** Bacterial sterilization by use of heat.

**thermotaxis** (thĕr″mō-tăks′ĭs) [″ + *taxis,* arrangement] **1.** Regulation of bodily temperature. **2.** Reaction of organisms or of protoplasm in the living body to heat. **3.** The movement of certain organisms or cells toward (positive thermotaxis) or away from (negative thermotaxis) heat.

**thermotherapy** (thĕr″mō-thĕr′ă-pē) [″ + *therapeia,* treatment] The therapeutic application of heat. Heat may be applied locally by radiant heating devices that give off infrared rays and by conductive heating that uses hot water bottles, paraffin baths, or moist hot packs. The temperature of the body may be increased by artificial fever, by raising environmental temperature, or by preventing heat loss from the body. SEE: *heat; hyperthermia.*

**thermotolerant** (thĕr″mō-tŏl′ĕr-ănt) [″ + L. *tolerare,* to tolerate] Able to live normally in high temperature.

**thermotonometer** (thĕr″mō-tō-nŏm′ĕ-tĕr) [″ + *tonos,* tension, + *metron,* measure] A device for measuring muscle contraction caused by heat stimuli.

**theroid** (thē′royd) [Gr. *theriodes,* beastlike] Having animal instincts and characteristics.

**thiabendazole** (thī″ă-bĕn′dă-zŏl) An antihelmintic drug used in treating cutaneous larva migrans and strongyloidiasis.

**thiaminase** (thī-ăm′ĭ-nās) An enzyme that hydrolyzes thiamine.

**thiamine hydrochloride** $C_{12}H_{17}ClN_4OS \cdot HCl$. A white crystalline compound occurring naturally and produced synthetically. It is widely distributed in various animal and plant foods. Dry yeast and wheat germ are the richest natural sources. It is present in the outer layers of seeds and in nuts, legumes, most vegetables, and in some meats (pork, liver, heart, and kidneys). The daily requirement for children and adults is 0.5 mg per 1000 kcal of food intake. SYN: *vitamin* $B_1$.

FUNCTION: It is essential for the normal metabolism of carbohydrates and fats. Because it acts as a coenzyme of carboxylases in the decarboxylation of pyruvic acid, thiamine hydrochloride is essential for the liberation of energy and the transfer of pyruvic acid into the Krebs cycle.

DEFICIENCY SYMPTOMS: Moderate deficiency results in impaired functioning of nervous, circulatory, digestive, and endocrine systems. Neurasthenia, neurological disorders, and cardiac and gastrointestinal symptoms may result. Loss of appetite, fatigue, muscle tenderness, and increased irritability are symptoms. Severe prolonged deficiency results in beriberi.

**thiamine pyrophosphate** An enzyme important in carbohydrate metabolism. It is the active form of thiamine. SYN: *cocarboxylase.*

**Thiersch's graft** (tērsh′ĕz) [Karl Thiersch, Ger. surgeon, 1822–1895] A method of skin grafting using the epidermis and a portion of the dermis.

**thiethylperazine malate** (thī-ĕth″ĭl-pĕr′ă-zēn) An antiemetic drug.

**thigh** (thī) [AS. *theoh*] The proximal portion of the lower extremity; the portion lying between the hip joint and the knee. SEE: *femur; hip; pectineus; sartorius.*

**thigmesthesia** (thĭg″mĕs-thē′zē-ă) [Gr. *thigma,* touch, + *aisthesis,* sensation] Sensitivity to touch.

**thigmotaxis** (thĭg″mō-tăks′ĭs) [″ + *taxis,* arrangement] The negative or positive response of certain motile cells to touch.

**thigmotropism** (thĭg-mŏt′rō-pĭzm) [″ + *tropos,* a turning, + *-ismos,* condition] The response of certain motile cells to move toward something that touches them.

**thimerosal** (thī-mĕr′ō-săl) An organic mercurial antiseptic used topically and as a preservative in pharmaceutical preparations.

**thinking** The highest order of intellectual activity, which is difficult to describe and analyze. Involved in thinking are the interpretation and ordering of symbols for learning, for organizing information, and for problem solving. The logical progression of this process would be to have and develop the capacity to reason and make sound judgments.

**thin-layer chromatography** ABBR: TLC. Chromatography involving the adsorption and partitioning of compounds on a thin porous solid applied as a thin layer on a glass plate.

**thiocyanate** (thī″ō-sī′ă-nāt) Any compound containing the radical —SCN.

**thiogenic** (thī″ō-jĕn′ĭk) [Gr. *theion,* sulfur, + *gennan,* to produce] Able to convert hydrogen sulfide into higher sulfur compounds, said of bacteria in the water of some mineral springs.

**thioglucosidase** (thī″ō-glū-kō′sĭ-dās) An enzyme that catalyzes the hydrolysis of thioglycoside to a thiol and a sugar.

**thioguanine** (thī″ō-gwă′nēn) An antimetabolite used in treating certain types of leukemia. It also acts as an immunosuppressant.

**thiopectic, thiopexic** (thī-ō-pĕk′tĭk, -pĕks′ĭk) [″ + *pexis,* fixation] Pert. to the fixation of sulfur.

**thiopental sodium** (thī″ō-pĕn′tăl) An ultra–short-acting barbiturate used as an adjuvant in surgical anesthesia.

**thiophil, thiophilic** (thī′ō-fĭl, thī″ō-fĭl′ĭk) [Gr. *theion,* sulfur, + *philein,* to love] Thriving in the presence of sulfur or its compounds, which is true of some bacteria.

**thioridazine hydrochloride** (thī″ō-rĭd′ă-zēn) An antipsychotic drug.

**thiosulfate** (thī″ō-sŭl′fāt) Any salt of thiosulfuric acid.

**thiotepa** (thī″ō-tē′pă) An alkylating agent that is cytotoxic. It is used in treating certain types of neoplasms.

---

Caution: Great care should be taken to prevent inhaling particles of thiotepa or exposing the skin to it.

---

**thiothixene** (thī″ō-thĭks′ēn) An antipsychotic drug.

**thiourea** (thī″ō-ūr-ē′ă) [Gr. *theion,* sulfur, + *ouron,* urine] A colorless crystalline compound of urea in which sulfur replaces the oxygen. SYN: *sulfourea.*

**thiram poisoning** Toxic exposure to thiram. This may occur in those engaged either in manufacturing or applying this compound in agricultural work.

**third cranial nerve** Oculomotor nerve. SEE: *cranial nerves.*

**third intention** Healing of a wound by filling with granulation tissue. SEE: *healing.*

**third ventricle** The third ventricle of the brain, a narrow cavity between the two optic thalami. It communicates anteriorly with the lateral ventricles and posteriorly, via the cerebral aqueduct of Sylvius, with the fourth ventricle. SYN: *ventriculus tertius.*

**thirst** [AS. *thurst*] The bodily sensation resulting from the lack of or desire for liquids. Thirst may result from drying of mucous membranes, esp. those of the pharynx, or from reduced salivary secretion. It also results from general dehydration, as may occur following hemorrhage, profuse sweating, vomiting, or excessive loss of urine as in diabetes mellitus or insipidus.

**Thiry's fistula** (tē′rēz) [Ludwig Thiry, Austrian physiologist, 1817–1897] An artificial fistula placed in a dog's intestines for obtaining intestinal juices for experimental purposes.

**thixolabile** (thĭk″sō-lā′bĭl) Esp. susceptible to being changed by shaking.

**thixotropy** (thĭks-ŏt′rō-pē) [Gr. *thixis,* a touching, + *trope,* turning] The property of certain gels in which they liquefy when agitated and revert to a gel on standing.

**thlipsencephalus** (thlĭp″sĕn-sĕf′ă-lŭs) [Gr. *thlipsis,* pressure, + *enkephalos,* brain] A deformed fetus with a malformed or absent skull.

**Thomas splint** [Hugh Owen Thomas, Brit. orthopedic surgeon, 1834–1891] A splint originally developed to treat hip-joint disease. It is now used mainly to place traction on the leg in its long axis, in treating fractures of the upper leg. It consists of a proximal ring that fits around the upper leg and to which two long rigid slender steel rods are attached. These extend down to another smaller ring distal to the foot.

**Thomas-White hypothesis** [Clayton Thomas, b. 1921, U.S. physician; Arthur White, b. 1925, U.S. physician] The hypothesis that there will eventually be reported a congenital abnormality in which a fetus has two umbilici.

**Thompson test** A test to evaluate the integrity of the Achilles tendon. The patient kneels on the examination table with the feet hanging off; the examiner squeezes the calf while observing for plantar flexion. The result is positive if there is no movement of the foot; this indicates an Achilles tendon rupture.

**Thomsen's disease** (tŏm′sĕnz) [Asmus Julius Thomsen, Danish physician, 1815–1896] Myotonia congenita.

**thorac-** SEE: *thoraco-.*

**thoracalgia** (thō″răk-ăl′jē-ă) [Gr. *thorakos,* chest, + *algos,* pain] Pain in the chest wall. SYN: *pleurodynia.*

**thoracectomy** (thō″ră-sĕk′tō-mē) [″ + *ektome,* excision] Incision of the chest wall with resection of a portion of rib.

**thoracentesis** (thō″ră-sĕn-tē′sĭs) [″ + *kentesis,* a puncture] Surgical puncture of the chest wall for removal of fluids; usually done by using a large-bore needle. SYN: *pleurocentesis; thoracocentesis.*

Nursing Implications: Before the procedure, the chest x-ray report should be obtained if available. The procedure should be explained to the patient and the signed consent verified. The nurse should prepare the patient for sensations that may be experienced and emphasize the importance of the patient's remaining still during the procedure. Baseline vital signs should be obtained. Allergies should be identified and a sedative, if prescribed, should be administered. The patient should be positioned comfortably. The nurse should assist the physician and support the patient throughout the procedure. The patient's vital signs should be checked frequently throughout the procedure. The nurse should assess for dizziness, faintness, tachycardia, dyspnea, chest pain, nausea, pallor or cyanosis, weakness, diaphoresis, and cough or expectoration of blood. An occlusive dressing should be applied to the puncture wound as the needle or cannula is removed. The specimen should be sent for diagnostic testing as ordered, and the procedure and patient response documented. The nurse should arrange for a postprocedure chest radiograph to detect pneumothorax and evaluate the results. Vital signs and dressing status should continue to be monitored, and the patient assessed for coughing or expectoration of blood.

**thoraci-** SEE: *thoraco-*.

**thoracic** (thō-răs′ĭk) [Gr. *thorax,* chest] Pert. to the chest or thorax.

**thoracic cage** The bony structure surrounding the thorax, consisting of the 12 paired ribs, the thoracic vertebrae, and the sternum.

**thoracic duct** The main lymph duct of the body, having its origin at the cisterna chyli on the abdomen. It passes upward through the diaphragm into the thorax, continuing upward alongside the aorta and esophagus to the neck, where it turns to the left and enters the left subclavian vein near its junction with the left internal jugular vein. It receives lymph from all parts of the body except the right side of the head, neck, and thorax and right upper extremity. SEE: *lymphatic system* for illus.

**thoracic limb** One of the upper extremities.

**thoracicoabdominal** (thō-răs″ĭ-kō-ăb-dŏm′ĭ-năl) Concerning the thorax and abdomen.

**thoracicohumeral** (thō-răs″ĭ-kō-hū′mĕr-ăl) Concerning the thorax and humerus bone.

**thoracic outlet compression syndrome** A symptom complex caused by conditions in which nerves or vessels are compressed in the neck or axilla. Anatomically, the cause is compression by structures, such as the first rib pressing against the clavicle. Also, the condition may be associated with a cervical rib or scalenus anticus syndrome. It is characterized by brachial neuritis with or without vascular or vasomotor disturbance in the upper extremities. The condition may be confused with cervical disk lesions, osteoarthritis affecting cervical vertebrae, bursitis, brachial plexus injury, angina, and lung cancer.

**thoracic squeeze** A rare occurrence in divers who are skilled enough to go approx. 80 to 100 ft (24.4 to 30.5 m) deep while holding their breath. The lungs become compressed sufficiently to cause rupture of alveolar capillaries. Treatment involves immediately removing the patient from the water and giving artificial respiration, preferably with an apparatus that will deliver increased oxygen concentration rather than just air.

**thoracic surgery** Surgery involving the rib cage and structures contained within the thoracic cage.

NURSING IMPLICATIONS: *Preoperative:* Preparation involves the usual preoperative teaching, with special emphasis on breathing and coughing, incisional splinting, pain evaluation, invasive and noninvasive relief measures that will be available, and basic information about the chest drainage tube and system that will be required in most such surgeries. The nurse should encourage the patient to voice fears and concerns, allay misapprehensions, and correct misconceptions. *Postoperative:* Vital signs and breath sounds should be monitored. Water-seal chest drainage should be maintained as prescribed, and the volume and characteristics of drainage should be monitored. The nurse should maintain sterile impervious wound dressings; provide analgesia and comfort measures to ensure patient cooperation with respiratory toilet, exercises, and rest and activity; provide emotional support and encouragement; and provide instructions to be followed by the patient and family after discharge and follow-up care.

**thoraco-** Combining form meaning *chest, chest wall.*

**thoracoacromial** (thō″ră-kō-ă-krō′mē-ăl) Concerning the thorax and acromion.

**thoracobronchotomy** (thō″răk-ō-brŏn-kŏt′ō-mē) [Gr. *thorakos,* chest, + *bronchos,* windpipe, + *tome,* incision] Incision through the thoracic wall into the bronchus.

**thoracocautery** (thō″răk-ō-kaw′tĕr-ē) [″ + *kauterion,* branding iron] The use of cautery in breaking up pulmonary adhesions to collapse the lung.

**thoracoceloschisis** (thō″răk-ō-sē-lŏs′kĭ-sĭs) [Gr. *thorakos,* chest, + *koilia,* belly, + *schisis,* a splitting] A congenital fissure of the thoracic and abdominal cavities.

**thoracocentesis** (thō″răk-ō-sĕn-tē′sĭs) [″ + *kentesis,* a puncture] Thoracentesis.

**thoracodelphus** (thō″ră-kō-dĕl′fŭs) [″ + *adelphos,* brother] A deformed fetus with a single head and thorax, but four legs.

**thoracodidymus** (thō″ră-kō-dĭd′ĭ-mŭs) [″ + *didymos,* twin] Conjoined twins united at the thorax.

**thoracodynia** (thō″răk-ō-dĭn′ē-ă) [″ + *odyne,* pain] Pain in the thorax.

**thoracogastroschisis** (thō″răk-ō-găs-trŏs′kĭ-sĭs) [″ + *gaster,* belly, + *schisis,* a splitting] A congenital fissure of the abdomen and thorax.

**thoracograph** (thō-răk′ō-grăf) [″ + *graphein,* to write] A device for plotting and recording the contour of the thorax and its change during inspiration and expiration.

**thoracolaparotomy** (thō″ră-kō-lăp″ă-rŏt′ō-mē) [″ + *lapara,* loin, + *tome,* incision] A surgical incision of the thoracic wall and the diaphragm to gain access to adjacent areas.

**thoracolumbar** (thō″răk-ō-lŭm′bar) [″ + L.

*lumbus,* loin] Pert. to the thoracic and lumbar parts of the spine; denoting their ganglia and the fibers of the sympathetic nervous system.

**thoracolysis** (thō″răk-ŏl′ĭ-sĭs) [″ + *lysis,* dissolution] The freeing of a lung that is attached to the chest wall. SYN: *pneumonolysis.*

**thoracomelus** (thō″ră-kŏm′ē-lŭs) [″ + *melos,* limb] A deformed fetus with an extra leg attached to the thorax.

**thoracometer** (thō″ră-kŏm′ĕ-tĕr) [Gr. *thorakos,* chest, + *metron,* measure] A device for measuring the expansion of the chest.

**thoracometry** (thō″ră-kŏm′ĕt-rē) [″ + *metron,* measure] The measurement of the thorax.

**thoracomyodynia** (thō″ră-kō-mī″ō-dĭn′ē-ă) [″ + *mys,* muscle, + *odyne,* pain] Pain in the chest muscles.

**thoracopagus** (thō″ră-kŏp′ă-gŭs) [″ + *pagos,* fixed] Two malformed fetuses joined at the thorax.

**thoracoparacephalus** (thō″ră-kō-păr″ă-sĕf′ă-lŭs) [″ + *para,* beside, + *kephale,* head] Thoracopagus twins in which a rudimentary head is attached to the smaller twin.

**thoracopathy** (thō″răk-ŏp′ă-thē) [″ + *pathos,* disease, suffering] Any disease of the thorax, thoracic organs, or tissues.

**thoracoplasty** (thō′ră-kō-plăs″tē, thō-ră′kō-plăs″tē) [″ + *plassein,* to form] A plastic operation on the thorax; removal of portions of the ribs in stages to collapse diseased areas of the lung. SEE: *empyema.*

**thoracopneumoplasty** (thō″ră-kō-nū′mō-plăs-tē) [″ + *pneumon,* lung, + *plassein,* to form] Plastic surgery involving the chest and lung.

**thoracoschisis** (thō″ră-kŏs′kĭ-sĭs) [″ + *schisis,* a splitting] A congenital fissure of the chest wall.

**thoracoscope** (thō-rā′kō-skōp, -răk′ō-skōp) [″ + *skopein,* to examine] An instrument for inspection of the thoracic cavity. It has an electric light and is inserted through an intercostal space.

**thoracoscopy** (thō″ră-kŏs′kō-pē) A diagnostic examination of the pleural cavity with an endoscope.

**thoracostenosis** (thō″ră-kō-stĕn-ō′sĭs) [″ + *stenosis,* act of narrowing] Narrowness of the thorax due to atrophy of trunk muscles.

**thoracostomy** (thō″răk-ŏs′tō-mē) [″ + *stoma,* mouth] Resection of the chest wall to allow drainage of the chest cavity.

**thoracotomy** (thō″răk-ŏt′ō-mē) [″ + *tome,* incision] Surgical incision of the chest wall.

**thorax** (thō′răks) *pl.* **thoraces, thoraxes** [Gr., chest] That part of the body between the base of the neck superiorly and the diaphragm inferiorly. SYN: *chest.* SEE: illus.

The surface of the thorax is divided into regions as follows: *Anterior surface:* supraclavicular, above the clavicles; suprasternal, above the sternum; clavicular, over the clavicles; sternal, over the sternum; mammary, the space between the third and sixth ribs on either side; inframammary, below the mammae and above the lower border of the 12th rib on either

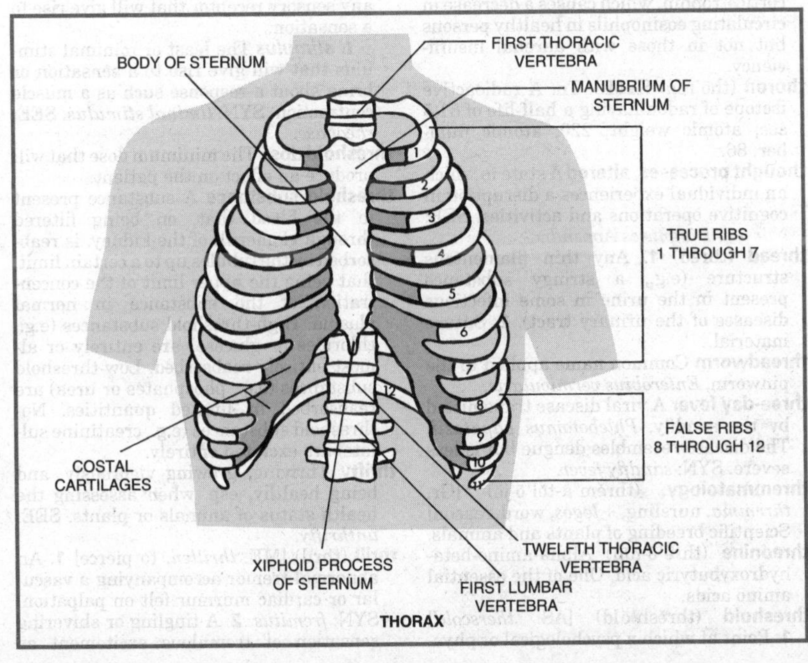

THORAX

side. *Posterior surface:* scapular, over the scapulae; interscapular, between the scapulae; infrascapular, below the scapulae. *On sides:* axillary, above the sixth rib.

***barrel-shaped t.*** A malformed chest rounded like a barrel, seen in advanced pulmonary emphysema.

***bony t.*** The part of the skeleton that is made up of the thoracic vertebrae, 12 pairs of ribs, and the sternum.

***t. paralyticus*** The long, flat chest of patients with constitutional visceroptosis.

***Peyrot's t.*** A chest that has an obliquely oval deformed shape, seen with large pleural effusions.

**Thorazine** Trade name for chlorpromazine hydrochloride. It is an antipsychotic agent useful in controlling excited psychotic behavior. It is also valuable as an antiemetic. It must be used with caution when given concomitantly with sedatives and general anesthetics, as it potentiates their actions.

**Thorel's bundle** (tō'rĕlz) [Christen Thorel, Ger. physician, 1880–1935] A muscle bundle in the heart that connects the sinoatrial and atrioventricular nodes and passes medial to the orifice of the inferior vena cava.

**thorium** (thō'rē-ŭm) SYMB: Th. A radioactive metallic element. Atomic weight, 232.038; atomic number, 90. At one time, it was used to outline blood vessels in radiography.

**Thorn test** [George W. Thorn, U.S. physician, b. 1906] A test for adrenal insufficiency involving the administration of corticotrophin, which causes a decrease in circulating eosinophils in healthy persons but not in those with adrenal insufficiency.

**thoron** (thō'rŏn) SYMB: Tn. A radioactive isotope of radon having a half-life of 51.5 sec; atomic weight, 220; atomic number, 86.

**thought processes, altered** A state in which an individual experiences a disruption in cognitive operations and activities. SEE: *Nursing Diagnoses Appendix.*

**thread** (thrĕd) **1.** Any thin filamentous structure (e.g., a stringy substance present in the urine in some infectious diseases of the urinary tract). **2.** Suture material.

**threadworm** Common name applied to the pinworm, *Enterobius vermicularis.*

**three-day fever** A viral disease transmitted by the sandfly, *Phlebotomus papatasii.* The disease resembles dengue but is less severe. SYN: *sandfly fever.*

**thremmatology** (thrĕm"ă-tŏl'ō-jē) [Gr. *thremma,* nursling, + *logos,* word, reason] Scientific breeding of plants and animals.

**threonine** (thrē'ō-nīn) Alpha-amino-beta-hydroxybutyric acid. One of the essential amino acids.

**threshold** (thrĕsh'ōld) [AS. *therscold*] **1.** Point at which a psychological or physiological effect begins to be produced. **2.** A measure of the sensitivity of an organ or function that is obtained by finding the lowest value of the appropriate stimulus that will give the response.

***absolute t.*** The lowest amount or intensity of a stimulus that will give rise to a sensation or a response.

***acoustic reflex t.*** SEE: *acoustic reflex threshold.*

***anaerobic t.*** The point at which increased carbon dioxide production and minute ventilation result from increased levels of lactic acid during exercise.

***auditory t.*** Minimum audible sound perceived.

***t. of consciousness*** In psychoanalysis, the point at which a stimulus is just barely perceived.

***differential t.*** The lowest limit at which two stimuli can be differentiated from each other.

***erythema t.*** The stage in which erythema of the skin due to radiation just begins.

***ketosis t.*** The lower limit at which ketone bodies (acetoacetic acid, hydroxybutyric acid, and acetone), on their accumulation in the blood, are excreted by the kidney. At that point, ketone bodies are being produced faster by the liver than the body can oxidize them.

***renal t.*** The concentration at which a substance in the blood normally not excreted by the kidney begins to appear in the urine. The renal threshold for glucose is 160 to 180 mg/dl.

***sensory t.*** The minimal stimulus for any sensory receptor that will give rise to a sensation.

***t. stimulus*** The least or minimal stimulus that will give rise to a sensation or bring about a response such as a muscle contraction. SYN: *liminal stimulus.* SEE: *rheobase.*

**threshold dose** The minimum dose that will produce an effect on the patient.

**threshold substance** A substance present in the blood that, on being filtered through glomeruli of the kidney, is reabsorbed by the tubules up to a certain limit, that being the upper limit of the concentration of the substance in normal plasma. High-threshold substances (e.g., chlorides or glucose) are entirely or almost entirely reabsorbed. Low-threshold substances (e.g., phosphates or urea) are reabsorbed in limited quantities. No-threshold substances (e.g., creatinine sulfate) are excreted entirely.

**thrifty** Thriving, growing vigorously, and being healthy, esp. when assessing the health status of animals or plants. SEE: *unthrifty.*

**thrill** (thrĭl) [ME. *thrillen,* to pierce] **1.** An abnormal tremor accompanying a vascular or cardiac murmur felt on palpation. SYN: *fremitus.* **2.** A tingling or shivering sensation of tremulous excitement as from pain, pleasure, or horror.

***aneurysmal t.*** A thrill felt on palpation of an aneurysm.

***aortic t.*** A thrill heard over an aortic aperture on lesions of valves.

***arterial t.*** A thrill heard over an artery.

***diastolic t.*** A thrill felt over the heart during diastole of the ventricle.

***hydatid t.*** A peculiar tremor felt on palpation of a hydatid cyst.

***presystolic t.*** A thrill sometimes felt over the apex of the heart preceding ventricular contraction.

***systolic t.*** A thrill felt during systole over the precordium. It may be associated with aortic or pulmonary stenosis, or an interventricular septal defect.

**thrix** Hair.

***t. annulata*** Hair with light and dark segments alternating along the shaft.

**-thrix** [Gr. *thrix,* hair] A word ending indicating hair.

**throat** (thrōt) [AS. *throte*] **1.** The pharynx and fauces. **2.** The cavity from the arch of the palate to the glottis and superior opening of the esophagus. **3.** The anterior portion of the neck. **4.** Any narrow orifice.

**throat, foreign bodies in** The presence of foreign objects in the pharynx or throat. Symptoms depend somewhat on the location and size of the foreign body, and vary from simple discomfort to distressing coughing, difficulty in breathing, retching, and cyanosis. If not relieved, suffocation results in unconsciousness.

If the symptoms are relieved but it is not known whether the foreign body has been removed, it is important to seek medical attention in case the object has moved farther down the respiratory tract.

FIRST AID: If complete airway obstruction is present as evidenced by an inability to speak or absence of intake of air, the Heimlich maneuver should be performed. This consists of (1) wrapping one's arms around the victim's waist from behind; (2) making a fist with one hand and placing it against the victim's abdomen between the navel and rib cage; and (3) clasping the fist with the free hand and pressing in with a quick, forceful upward thrust. This may be repeated several times if necessary. If the airway remains obstructed, tracheostomy will be required to save the patient's life. SEE: *Heimlich maneuver* for illus.

---

Caution: The Heimlich maneuver should not be performed unless complete airway obstruction is present. If the patient can cough, this maneuver should not be performed. Children and infants should be placed head down to facilitate removal of the obstruction.

---

**throb** (thrŏb) [ME. *throbben,* of imitative origin] **1.** A beat or pulsation, as of the heart. **2.** To pulsate.

**throbbing** (thrŏb'ĭng) Pulsation.

**Throckmorton's reflex** (thrŏk'mor"tŭnz) [Thomas Bentley Throckmorton, U.S. neurologist, 1885–1961] The extension of the great toe and flexion of the other toes when the dorsum of the foot is percussed in the metatarsophalangeal region.

**thrombase** (thrŏm'bās) Thrombin.

**thrombasthenia** (thrŏm"băs-thē'nē-ă) [Gr. *thrombos,* clot, + *astheneia,* weakness] A hemorrhagic disorder caused by abnormal platelet function characterized by abnormal clot retraction, prolonged bleeding time, and lack of aggregation of the platelets on a blood smear.

**thrombectomy** (thrŏm-bĕk'tō-mē) [" + *ektome,* excision] Excision of a thrombus.

**thrombi** (thrŏm'bī) Pl. of thrombus.

**thrombin** (thrŏm'bĭn) [Gr. *thrombos,* clot] **1.** An enzyme formed in shed blood from prothrombin, which reacts with soluble fibrinogen converting it to fibrin, which forms the basis of a blood clot. SEE: *coagulation, blood.* **2.** A sterile plasma protein substance prepared from prothrombin of bovine origin. It is used topically to control capillary oozing during surgical procedures. When used alone, it is not capable of controlling arterial bleeding.

**thrombinogen** (thrŏm-bĭn'ō-jĕn) An obsolete term for prothrombin.

**thrombo-** Combining form meaning *clot.*

**thromboangiitis** (thrŏm"bō-ăn"jē-ī'tĭs) [Gr. *thrombos,* clot, + *angeion,* vessel, + *itis,* inflammation] Inflammation of the inner coat of a blood vessel with clot formation. SEE: *thrombosis.*

***t. obliterans*** A chronic, recurring, inflammatory, vascular occlusive disease, chiefly of the peripheral arteries and veins of the extremities. The disease is seen most commonly in men 20 to 40 years of age who smoke cigarettes. SYN: *Buerger's disease.*

SYMPTOMS: The patient experiences occlusion; thrombosis; excruciating pain in the leg or foot that is worse at night; cyanotic, clammy, cold extremities; and a diminished sense of heat and cold. Gangrene of the toes or foot may develop.

**thromboarteritis** (thrŏm"bō-ăr-tē-rī'tĭs) [" + *arteria,* artery, + *itis,* inflammation] Inflammation of an artery in connection with thrombosis. SYN: *thromboendarteritis.*

**thromboclasis** (thrŏm-bŏk'lă-sĭs) [" + *klasis,* a breaking] Thrombolysis.

**thromboclastic** (thrŏm"bō-klăs'tĭk) Thrombolytic.

**thrombocyst** (thrŏm'bō-sĭst) [Gr. *thrombos,* clot, + *kystis,* a sac] A membranous sac enveloping a thrombus. SYN: *thrombocystis.*

**thrombocystis** Thrombocyst.

**thrombocyte** (thrŏm'bō-sīt) [" + *kytos,* cell] Platelet.

**thrombocythemia** (thrŏm"bō-sī-thē'mē-ă) [" + " + *haima,* blood] An absolute increase in the number of platelets in the blood.

**thrombocytocrit** (thrŏm″bō-sī′tō-krĭt) [″ + ″ + *krinein,* to separate] A device for estimating the platelet content of the blood.

**thrombocytolysis** (thrŏm″bō-sī-tŏl′ĭ-sĭs) [″ + ″ + *lysis,* dissolution] Dissolution of thrombocytes.

**thrombocytopathy** (thrŏm″bō-sī-tŏp′ă-thē) [″ + ″ + *pathos,* disease, suffering] Deficient function of platelets.

**thrombocytopenia** (thrŏm″bō-sī″tō-pē′nē-ă) [″ + ″ + *penia,* lack] An abnormal decrease in number of the blood platelets. SYN: *thrombopenia.*

NURSING IMPLICATIONS: The patient is watched for signs of internal hemorrhage, esp. intracranial pressure, as well as hematuria, hematemesis, bleeding gums, abdominal distention, melena, prolonged menstruation, epistaxis, ecchymosis, petechiae, or purpura, and is handled gently to prevent trauma and hemorrhage. Emesis, urine, and stools are evaluated for evidence of occult bleeding. Bleeding is controlled by applying pressure to bleeding sites. Bedrest is encouraged to prevent excessive activity and exhaustion. The patient should avoid constipation and straining as well as exposure to upper respiratory infections, which may cause sneezing and coughing. Use of a soft toothbrush helps to prevent injury. An electric razor should be used for shaving. Platelet transfusions are administered as prescribed, and the patient is observed for chills, fever, or allergic reactions. Aspirin and other nonsteroidal anti-inflammatory agents should be avoided, because these drugs may inhibit platelet function. If splenectomy is performed, preoperative and postoperative nursing care is provided as required. The nurse should encourage the patient to express feelings and concerns.

**thrombocytopoiesis** (thrŏm″bō-sī″tō-poy-ē′sĭs) [″ + ″ + *poiesis,* production] The formation of blood platelets.

**thrombocytosis** (thrŏm″bō-sī-tō′sĭs) [″ + *kytos,* cell] An increase in the number of blood platelets.

**thromboelastogram** ABBR: TEG. A device used to determine the presence of intravascular fibrinolysis and for monitoring the effect of antifibrinolytic therapy on the formation and dissolution of clots. SEE: *Sonoclat coagulation analyzer.*

**thromboembolism** (thrŏm″bō-ĕm′bō-lĭzm) [″ + *embolos,* thrown in, + *-ismos,* condition] An embolism; the blocking of a blood vessel by a thrombus that has become detached from its site of formation.

**thromboendarterectomy** (thrŏm″bō-ĕnd″ăr-tĕr-ĕk′tō-mē) [″ + *endon,* within, + *arteria,* artery, + *ektome,* excision] Surgical removal of a thrombus from an artery, and removal of the diseased intima of the artery.

**thromboendarteritis** (thrŏm″bō-ĕnd-ăr″tĕr-ī′tĭs) [″ + ″ + ″ + *itis,* inflammation] Thromboarteritis.

**thromboendocarditis** (thrŏm″bō-ĕn″dō-kăr-dī′tĭs) [″ + *endon,* within, + *kardia,* heart, + *itis,* inflammation] Formation of a clot on an inflamed surface of a heart valve.

**thrombogenesis** (thrŏm″bō-jĕn′ĕ-sĭs) [″ + *genesis,* generation, birth] The formation of a blood clot.

**thrombogenic** (thrŏm″bō-jĕn′ĭk) [″ + *gennan,* to produce] Producing or tending to produce a clot.

**thromboid** (thrŏm′boyd) [″ + *eidos,* form, shape] Resembling a thrombus or clot.

**thrombokinase** (thrŏm″bō-kĭn′ās) [″ + *kinesis,* movement] Obsolete term for the 10th blood coagulation factor (factor X) or Stuart factor.

**thrombokinesis** (thrŏm″bō-kĭ-nē′sĭs) [″ + *kinesis,* movement] The coagulation of the blood.

**thrombolymphangitis** (thrŏm″bō-lĭm″făn-jī′tĭs) [″ + L. *lympha,* lymph, + Gr. *angeion,* vessel, + *itis,* inflammation] Inflammation of a lymphatic vessel due to obstruction by thrombus formation.

**thrombolysis** (thrŏm-bŏl′ĭ-sĭs) [″ + *lysis,* dissolution] The breaking up of a thrombus. SYN: *thromboclasis.*

***reperfusion t.*** Use of thrombolytic agents to remove a thrombus that is blocking one or more arteries, esp. coronary arteries of the heart. When the blockage is removed, the tissues normally supplied with blood by the artery are reperfused. The quicker this is accomplished following a heart attack, the greater the chances for survival. SEE: *myocardial infarction.*

**thrombolytic** (thrŏm-bō-lĭt′ĭk) Pert. to or causing the breaking up of a thrombus.

**thrombomodulin** A protein released by the vascular endothelium. Acting in concert with other factors, it helps to prevent formation of intravascular thrombi. SEE: *endothelium.*

**thrombon** (thrŏm′bŏn) [Gr. *thrombos,* clot] The portion of the hematopoietic system concerned with platelet formation.

**thrombopathy** (thrŏm-bŏp′ă-thē) [″ + *pathos,* disease, suffering] A defect in the coagulation apparatus of the blood.

**thrombopenia** (thrŏm-bō-pē′nē-ă) [″ + *penia,* lack] An abnormal decrease in the number of blood platelets.

**thrombophilia** (thrŏm-bō-fĭl′ē-ă) [″ + *philein,* to love] A tendency to form blood clots.

**thrombophlebitis** (thrŏm″bō-flē-bī′tĭs) [″ + *phleps,* vein, + *itis,* inflammation] Inflammation of a vein in conjunction with the formation of a thrombus. It usually occurs in an extremity, most frequently a leg. SEE: *phlebitis; phlegmasia alba dolens; Nursing Diagnoses Appendix.*

TREATMENT: The therapeutic goal is to prevent a thrombus from becoming an embolus that may reach the lung. The anticoagulant heparin is used but requires careful monitoring of the patient's response. Therapy may also include ligation of the vein proximal to the thrombus to prevent pulmonary embolism.

NURSING IMPLICATIONS: Prevention includes identifying patients at risk and encouraging leg exercises, use of antiembolic stockings, and early ambulation to prevent venous stasis. Prolonged pressure on the popliteal areas should be avoided. The patient should be assessed at regular intervals for signs of inflammation, tenderness, aching, and differences in calf circumference measurements. The physician's prescribed regimen should be followed regarding elevation of the leg or keeping it flat and intermittent or continuous application of warm, moist heat. The nurse should administer anticoagulants as prescribed, evaluating the patient for signs of bleeding, and monitor coagulation results; instruct the patient to avoid rubbing or massaging the extremities; assess the patient every 2 hr for signs of pulmonary emboli, dyspnea, tachypnea, hypotension, chest pain, changes of level of consciousness, arterial blood gas abnormalities, or electrocardiogram changes; and prepare the patient for the diagnostic procedures and medical or surgical interventions prescribed.

***t. migrans*** Recurring attacks of thrombophlebitis in various sites.

***postpartum iliofemoral t.*** Thrombophlebitis of the iliofemoral artery that occurs during the postpartum period.

**thromboplastic** (thrŏm″bō-plăs′tĭk) [″ + *plassein,* to form] Pert. to or causing acceleration of clot formation in the blood.

**thromboplastid** (thrŏm″bō-plăs′tĭd) A blood platelet.

**thromboplastin** (thrŏm″bō-plăs′tĭn) [″+ *plassein,* to form] The third blood coagulation factor (factor III), a substance found in both blood and tissues. Tissue thromboplastin is found in most parts of the body as an intracellular substance. A substance with thromboplastic activity is also present in red blood cells. Even though these two substances are separate and act in different manners, both are able to accelerate the clotting of blood.

**thromboplastinogen** (thrŏm″bō-plăs-tĭn′ō-jĕn) Blood clotting factor VIII. SEE: *coagulation factors.*

**thrombopoiesis** (thrŏm″bō-poy-ē′sĭs) [″ + *poiesis,* production] The formation of blood platelets.

**thrombopoietin** A chemical substance that acts on the bone marrow to stimulate platelet production.

**thrombosed** (thrŏm′bōzd) [Gr. *thrombos,* a clot] **1.** Coagulated; clotted. **2.** Denoting a vessel containing a thrombus.

**thrombosinusitis** (thrŏm″bō-sī-nŭs-ī′tĭs) [″ + L. *sinus,* a curve, hollow, + Gr. *itis,* inflammation] Thrombus formation of a dural sinus in the brain.

**thrombosis** (thrŏm-bō′sĭs) [″ + *osis,* condition] The formation, development, or existence of a blood clot or thrombus within the vascular system. This is a life-saving process when it occurs during hemorrhage. It is a life-threatening event when it occurs at any other time because the clot can occlude a vessel and stop the blood supply to an organ or a part. The thrombus, if detached, becomes an embolus and occludes a vessel at a distance from the original site; for example, a clot in the leg may break off and cause a pulmonary embolus.

ETIOLOGY: Trauma (esp. following an operation and parturition), cardiac and vascular disorders, obesity, heredity, increasing age, an excess of erythrocytes and of platelets, an overproduction of fibrinogen, and sepsis are predisposing causes.

SYMPTOMS: *Lungs:* Obstruction of the smaller vessels in the lungs causes an infarct that may be accompanied by sudden pain in the side of the chest, similar to pleurisy; also present are the spitting of blood, a pleural friction rub, and signs of consolidation. *Kidneys:* Blood appears in the urine. *Skin:* Small hemorrhagic spots may appear in the skin. *Spleen:* Pain is felt in the left upper abdomen. *Extremities:* If a large artery in one of the extremities, such as the arm, is suddenly obstructed, the part becomes cold, pale, bluish, and the pulse disappears below the obstructed site. Gangrene of the digits or of the whole limb may ensue. The same symptoms may be present with an embolism.

If the limb is swollen, one should watch for pressure sores. Burning with a hot water bottle or electric pad should be guarded against. Prolonged bedrest may be necessary, depending on the patient's condition.

TREATMENT: Anticoagulant therapy is necessary. When a thrombus or embolus is large, surgical removal may be necessary.

***cardiac t.*** Thrombosis of an artery supplying the heart muscle (myocardium).

***coagulation t.*** Thrombosis due to coagulation of fibrin in a blood vessel.

***coronary t.*** Thrombosis of a coronary artery; a common cause of myocardial infarction.

SYMPTOMS: Symptoms include the sudden onset of severe and prolonged substernal oppression and pain, the pain arising over the precordium and being referred to the upper and middle sternum and often radiating to the left and sometimes right arm and into the neck or back. Blood pressure usually falls, pulse becomes rapid, and fever and leukocytosis are usually observed within 24 hr. Erythrocyte sedimentation rate becomes elevated and electrocardiographic changes occur.

Certain enzyme tests are very helpful

in diagnosing myocardial infarction. The serum level of creatine phosphokinase (CPK) is elevated in the first 24 hr following the infarction; the degree of elevation is proportional to the amount of cardiac muscle damaged. The CPK level may also be elevated if skeletal muscle damage is present. In that case, other enzyme tests such as aspartate aminotransferase (AST) or lactic dehydrogenase (LDH) will be helpful in diagnosis.

TREATMENT: The patient requires complete physical and mental rest for a variable length of time depending on severity. This is sometimes best accomplished by allowing the patient to rest in a reclining chair rather than a bed and to use a bedside toilet instead of having to strain to use a bedpan. Special nursing care is desirable. Prompt and complete relief from pain is achieved by use of intravenous morphine sulfate; oxygen administration is sometimes necessary. Vasopressor drugs are used to elevate blood pressure. Digitalis is given when there is evidence of congestive heart failure. Cardiac arrhythmias, esp. tachycardia, must be treated. Anticoagulants are given. Treatment in the coronary care unit is usually mandatory.

If given within the first several hours after the acute thrombosis, medicines such as streptokinase or tissue plasminogen activator given to lyse the thrombus have greatly improved the prognosis in these patients. SEE: *streptokinase; tissue plasminogen activator.*

DIET: Diet is as requested by the patient, but caloric intake is restricted to 1000 to 1500 kcal. Salt intake is restricted, and fluid intake and output are recorded.

COMPLICATIONS: Complications include shock, acute pulmonary edema, pulmonary embolism, paroxysmal ventricular tachycardia, congestive heart failure, and aneurysm of the ventricle.

Most patients develop some form of cardiac arrhythmia. This can be simple sinus tachycardia, bradycardia, atrial fibrillation, ventricular tachycardia, ventricular fibrillation, or cardiac arrest. The latter two are life threatening and require prompt and diligent therapeutic intervention. Depending on the cause, the arrhythmia will be treated with one or more of the following: atropine, lidocaine, digitalis, defibrillation, or a pacemaker.

NURSING IMPLICATIONS: Cardiovascular monitoring is maintained during the acute phase to detect complications such as shock, pulmonary edema or embolism, or an abnormal heart rate or rhythm. Medications are administered as prescribed to relieve pain, and treatment effectiveness is observed. Support and reassurance and opportunities to ask questions and to discuss concerns are provided to the patient and family. The nurse teaches the patient about medications, lifestyle modification, and return to normal activities before discharge.

***deep venous t.*** ABBR: DVT. Thrombosis of one or more veins in the deep venous system of the upper or lower extremities. This may occur without obvious cause but is more likely to result from any condition that involves venous stasis or damage to the endothelial area of a vein, or as a result of conditions associated with certain surgical procedures and the accompanying inactivity of the patient. In many cases, the result of this is that the thrombus will form and a portion of it will travel to the lung and create pulmonary embolism. To prevent this, anticoagulants, antithrombosis stockings, operative thrombectomy, or vena caval interruption may be used. Also, a vena caval filter may be inserted to prevent emboli from entering the lung. DVT may be detected by ultrasound when traditional methods fail to provide evidence of the thrombosis. SEE: *embolism, pulmonary.*

***embolic t.*** Thrombosis caused by an embolus obstructing a vessel.

***hepatic vein t.*** A usually fatal thrombotic occlusion of the hepatic veins, marked clinically by hepatomegaly, weight gain, ascites, and abdominal pain. SYN: *Budd-Chiari syndrome.*

***infective t.*** Thrombosis in which there is bacterial infection.

***marasmic t.*** Thrombosis due to wasting diseases of infancy and old age.

***placental t.*** Thrombi in the placenta and veins of the uterus.

***plate t.*** Thrombus formed from an accumulation of blood platelets.

***puerperal t.*** Coagulation in veins following labor.

***sinus t.*** Formation of a blood clot in a venous sinus.

***traumatic t.*** Thrombosis due to a wound or injury of a part.

***venous t.*** Thrombosis of a vein. SEE: *Nursing Diagnoses Appendix.*

**thrombostasis** (thrŏm-bŏs′tă-sĭs) [″ + *stasis,* standing still] Stasis of blood in a part, causing or caused by formation of a thrombus.

**thrombosthenin** (thrŏm″bō-sthē′nĭn) [″ + *sthenos,* strength] A contractile protein present in the platelets. This protein is active in clot retraction.

**thrombotic** (thrŏm-bŏt′ĭk) [Gr. *thrombos,* clot] Related to, caused by, or of the nature of a thrombus.

**thromboxane $A_2$** ABBR: $TXA_2$. An unstable compound synthesized in platelets and other cells from a prostaglandin, $PGH_2$. It acts to aggregate platelets. In addition, it is a potent vasoconstrictor. SEE: *eicosanoid; prostaglandins; prostanoids.*

**thrombus** (thrŏm′bŭs) [Gr. *thrombos*] A blood clot that obstructs a blood vessel or a cavity of the heart. Anticoagulants are used in prevention and treatment of this condition.

***agonal t.*** A blood clot formed in the heart just at the time of death.

***annular t.*** A thrombus whose circumference is attached to the walls of a vessel, while an opening still remains in the center.

***antemortem t.*** A clot formed in the heart or large vessels before death.

***ball t.*** A round clot in the heart, esp. in the atria.

***hyaline t.*** A thrombus having a glassy appearance, usually occurring in smaller blood vessels.

***lateral t.*** Mural t.

***milk t.*** A curdled milk tumor in the female breast caused by obstruction in a lactiferous duct.

***mural t.*** A thrombus attached to the wall of a vessel or the heart. SYN: *lateral t.; parietal t.*

***obstructing t.*** A thrombus completely occluding the lumen of a vessel.

***occluding t.*** A thrombus that completely closes the vessel.

***parietal t.*** Mural t.

***postmortem t.*** Blood clot formed in the heart or a large blood vessel after death.

***progressive t.*** Propagated t.

***propagated t.*** A thrombus that increases in size. SYN: *progressive t.*

***stratified t.*** A thrombus composed of layers.

***white t.*** A pale thrombus in any site; made up principally of platelets.

**through-and-through drainage** Irrigation and drainage of a cavity or an organ such as the bladder by placing two perforated tubes, drains, or catheters in the area. A solution is instilled through one tube, usually by continuous drip, and the other tube is attached to either straight or gravity drainage or to a suction machine.

**through illumination** Passage of light through the walls of an organ or cavity for medical examination. SYN: *transillumination.*

**throwback** SEE: *atavism.*

**thrush** (thrŭsh) [D. *troske,* rotten wood] An infection of the mouth or throat, esp. in infants and young children, caused by *Candida albicans.* It is characterized by formation of white patches and ulcers and frequently by fever and gastrointestinal inflammation. Thrush is a specific form of oral candidiasis characterized by creamy white, curdlike patches on the tongue and other oral mucosal surfaces. The easily scraped off patches consist of *Candida,* epithelial cells, leukocytes, bacteria, keratin, necrotic tissue, and food debris. The use of inhaled corticosteroids in treating asthma, esp. in children, is frequently associated with the development of thrush. Cancer patients and persons with AIDS have a high incidence of thrush. SEE: *aphtha; candidiasis; sprue; stomatitis.*

**thrust 1.** To move forward suddenly and forcibly, as in tongue thrust when the tongue is pushed against the teeth or alveolar ridge at the beginning of deglutition. This may cause open bite or malformed jaws. **2.** In physical therapy, a manipulative technique in which the therapist applies a rapid movement to tear adhesions and increase flexibility of restricted joint capsules.

**thrypsis** (thrĭp′sĭs) [Gr., breaking in pieces] A fracture in which the bone is splintered or crushed.

**thulium** (thū′lē-ŭm) SYMB: Tm. A rare metallic element found in combination with minerals; atomic weight, 168.934; atomic number, 69.

**thumb** (thŭm) [AS. *thuma,* thumb] The short thick first finger on the radial side of the hand, having two phalanges and being opposable to the other four digits. SYN: *pollex.* SEE: *hand* for illus.

***skier's t.*** Chronic radial subluxation of the metacarpophalangeal joint of the thumb. Also called *gamekeeper's thumb.*

***tennis t.*** Calcification and inflammation of the tendon of the flexor pollicis longus muscle owing to repeated irritation and stress while playing tennis.

**thumb sign** Protrusion of the thumb across the palm and beyond the clenched fist; seen in children with Marfan's syndrome.

**thumb sucking** The habit of sucking one's thumb. Intermittent thumb sucking is not abnormal, but prolonged and intensive thumb sucking past the time the first permanent teeth erupt at 5 or 6 years of age can lead to a misshapen mouth and displaced teeth. If the habit persists, combined dental and psychological therapy should be instituted.

**thymectomize** (thī-mĕk′tō-mīz) To surgically remove the thymus gland.

**thymectomy** (thī-mĕk′tō-mē) [Gr. *thymos,* mind, + *ektome,* excision] Surgical removal of the thymus gland.

**thymelcosis** (thī″mĕl-kō′sĭs) [″ + *helkosis,* ulceration] Ulceration of the thymus gland.

**-thymia** [Gr. *thymos,* mind] A word ending indicating *a state of the mind.*

**thymic** (thī′mĭk) [L. *thymicus*] Rel. to the thymus gland.

**thymicolymphatic** (thī″mĭ-kō-lĭm-făt′ĭk) Rel. to the thymus and lymph glands.

**thymidine** (thī′mĭ-dēn) A nucleoside present in deoxyribonucleotide. It is formed from the condensation product of thymine and deoxyribase.

**thymine** (thī′mĭn) $C_5N_2H_6O_2$. A pyrimidine base present in DNA (not RNA) where it is paired with adenine.

**thymitis** (thī-mī′tĭs) [Gr. *thymos,* mind, + *itis,* inflammation] Inflammation of the thymus gland.

**thymo- 1.** Combining form meaning *thymus.* **2.** Combining form meaning *mind.*

**thymocyte** (thī′mō-sīt) [Gr. *thymos,* mind, + *kytos,* cell] A cell in the thymus that migrated there as a prothymocyte from the bone marrow. Thymocytes mature as they develop, and some of them leave the thymus to become various types of T lymphocytes.

**thymokesis** (thī″mō-kē′sĭs) An abnormal enlargement of the thymus in the adult.

**thymokinetic** (thī″mō-kĭ-nĕt′ĭk) [″ + *kinesis,* movement] Stimulating the thymus gland.

**thymol** (thī′mōl) [Gr. *thumon,* thyme, + L. *oleum,* oil] White crystals obtained from oil of thyme; formerly used in treatment of hookworm.

***t. iodide*** An antifungal and antibacterial agent.

**thymolytic** (thī-mō-lĭt′ĭk) Destructive to thymus tissue.

**thymoma** (thī-mō′mă) [″ + *oma,* tumor] A tumor originating in the epithelial tissues of the thymus gland.

**thymopathy** (thī-mŏp′ă-thē) A disease of the thymus.

**thymopexy** (thī″mō-pĕks′ē) [″ + *pexis,* fixation] Fixation of an enlarged thymus in a new position.

**thymopoietin** (thī″mō-poy′ĕ-tĭn) A substance produced by the thymus that stimulates differentiation of thymocytes.

**thymoprivic** (thī″mō-prĭv′ĭk) [″ + L. *privus,* deprived of] Concerning or caused by removal of the thymus.

**thymotoxic** (thī″mō-tŏks′ĭk) [″ + *toxikon,* poison] Poisonous to thymic tissue.

**thymus** (thī′mŭs) [Gr. *thymos*] An unpaired organ located in the mediastinal cavity anterior to and above the heart. It consists of two flattened symmetrical lobes, each enclosed in a capsule, from which trabeculae extend into the gland and divide each lobe into many lobules. These contain a cortex and medulla. The cortex is composed of dense lymphoid tissue containing many cells (thymocytes) closely packed together. The medulla also contains thymocytes but they are less numerous. It also contains characteristic thymic (Hassall's) corpuscles. SEE: illus.

At birth, the average weight of the thymus is 10 to 15 g. Growth is rapid during the first 2 years, then slows. The thymus attains a weight of about 40 g at puberty, after which it begins to undergo involution and the thymic tissue is replaced with adipose and connective tissue.

FUNCTION: The organ is important in the development of the immune response in the newborn. Its removal during early childhood has been associated with an increased susceptibility to acute infectious diseases at a later time.

The thymus is essential to the maturation of the thymic lymphoid cells, called T cells. When the T cells enter the circulation, they are the small- and medium-sized lymphocytes; they may survive for up to 5 years. These cells are important in the body's cellular immune response.

PATHOLOGY: Sometimes it is much larger than it should be and is then known as an enlarged thymus. Children

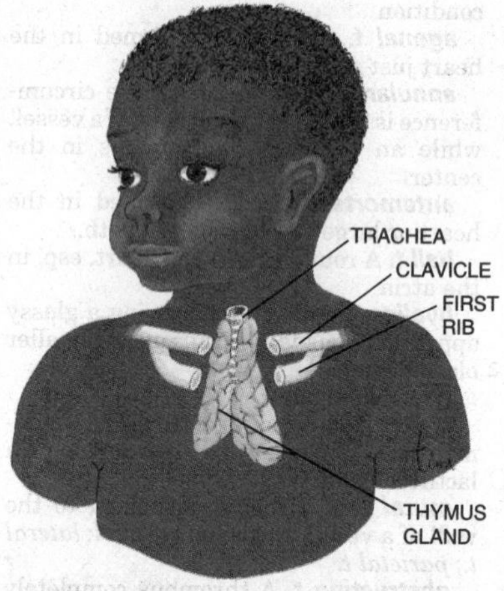


**THYMUS** IN A YOUNG CHILD

having these enlarged structures were routinely irradiated in the past. This practice has been discontinued because of the high incidence of cancer of the thyroid in these individuals when they reached adulthood. It is recommended that anyone who has undergone thymus irradiation be examined for possible thyroid cancer.

***accessory t.*** A lobule isolated from the mass of the thymus gland.

***t. persistens hyperplastica*** Thymus persisting into adulthood, sometimes hypertrophying.

**thymus dependent antigen** One of the foreign antigens that require B lymphocyte stimulation by T cells before production of antibodies and memory cells can occur.

**thymus independent antigen** One of the foreign antigens that are capable of stimulating B cell activation and the production of antibodies without T cell interaction. Most of these antibodies fall into the IgM class. A few memory cells are created.

**thymusectomy** (thī″mŭs-ĕk′tō-mē) [Gr. *thymos,* mind, + *ektome,* excision] Surgical excision of the thymus.

**thyreo-, thyro-** [Gr. *thyreos,* shield] Combining form indicating *thyroid.*

**thyreoplasia** Defective functioning of the thyroid gland owing to abnormal development.

**thyroadenitis** (thī″rō-ăd-ĕ-nī′tĭs) [″ + *aden,* gland, + *itis,* inflammation] Inflammation of the thyroid gland.

**thyroaplasia** (thī″rō-ă-plā′zē-ă) [″ + *a-,* not, + *plasis,* a molding] Imperfect development of the thyroid gland.

**thyroarytenoid** (thī″rō-ă-rĭt′ĕn-oyd) [″ + *arytaina,* ladle, + *eidos,* form, shape] Rel. to the thyroid and arytenoid cartilages.

**thyrocalcitonin** (thī″rō-kăl″sĭ-tō′nĭn) Calcitonin.

**thyrocardiac** (thī″rō-kăr′dē-ăk) [″ + *kardia,* heart] **1.** Pert. to the heart and thyroid gland. **2.** A person suffering from thyroid disease complicated by a heart disorder.

**thyrocele** (thī′rō-sēl) [″ + *kele,* tumor, swelling] Goiter.

**thyrochondrotomy** (thī″rō-kŏn-drŏt′ō-mē) [″ + *chondros,* cartilage, + *tome,* incision] Surgical incision of thyroid cartilage.

**thyrocolloid** (thī″rō-kŏl′oyd) Colloid contained in the thyroid gland.

**thyrocricotomy** (thī″rō-krī-kŏt′ō-mē) [″ + *krikos,* ring, + *tome,* incision] A division of the cricothyroid membrane.

**thyroepiglottic** (thī″rō-ĕp″ĭ-glŏt′ĭk) [″ + *epi,* upon, + *glottis,* back of tongue] Rel. to the thyroid and epiglottis.

**thyroepiglottic muscle** A muscle arising on the inner surface of the thyroid cartilage. It extends upward and backward and is inserted on the epiglottis. It depresses the epiglottis.

**thyroepiglottideus** (thī″rō-ĕp″ĭ-glŏt-ĭd′ē-ŭs) A muscle in the thyroid cartilage that depresses the epiglottis.

**thyrofissure** (thī″rō-fĭsh′ŭr) Surgical creation of an opening through the thyroid cartilage to expose the inside of the larynx.

**thyrogenic, thyrogenous** (thī-rō-jĕn′ĭk, thī-rŏj′ĕ-nŭs) [″ + *gennan,* to produce] Having its origin in the thyroid.

**thyroglobulin** (thī″rō-glŏb′ū-lĭn) [″ + L. *globulus,* globule] **1.** An iodine-containing protein secreted by the thyroid gland and stored within its colloid substance, from which thyroxine and triiodothyronine are derived. **2.** A substance obtained by the fractionation of thyroid glands from the hog, *Sus scrofa.*

**thyroglossal** (thī″rō-glŏs′săl) [″ + *glossa,* tongue] Pert. to the thyroid gland and the tongue.

**thyroglossal duct** A duct that in the embryo connects the thyroid diverticulum with the tongue. It eventually disappears, its point of origin being indicated as a pit, the foramen cecum. It sometimes persists as an anomaly.

**thyrohyal** (thī″rō-hī′ăl) Concerning the thyroid cartilage and the hyoid bone.

**thyrohyoid** (thī″rō-hī′oyd) [″ + *hyoeides,* U-shaped] Rel. to thyroid cartilage and hyoid bone.

**thyroid** (thī′royd) [″ + *eidos,* form, shape] **1.** An endocrine gland in the neck, anterior to and partially surrounding the thyroid cartilage and upper rings of the trachea. SEE: *thyroid gland.* **2.** The cleaned, dried, and powdered thyroid gland of animals, usually pigs, slaughtered for food. The preparation is free of fat and connective tissue.

ACTION/USES: It is used in cases of deficient action of the gland (hypothyroidism) or following thyroidectomy.

ADMINISTRATION: It is given orally in tablet form. The maximum effect will not be obtained for at least 7 to 10 days. It is advisable to start with a small dose and increase it gradually until the proper dose is determined.

**thyroid cachexia** Exophthalmic goiter. SEE: *hyperthyroidism.*

**thyroid cartilage** The principal cartilage of the larynx, consisting of two broad laminae united anteriorly to form a V-shaped structure. It forms a subcutaneous projection called the laryngeal prominence or Adam's apple. SEE: *thyroid gland* for illus.

**thyroid crisis** Thyroid storm.

**thyroidea accessoria, thyroidea ima** (thī-roy′dē-ă) Accessory thyroid.

**thyroidectomized** (thī″roy-dĕk′tō-mīzd) [″ + *eidos,* form, shape, + *ektome,* excision] With the thyroid gland removed.

**thyroidectomy** (thī″royd-ĕk′tō-mē) Excision of the thyroid gland. SEE: *Nursing Diagnoses Appendix.*

NURSING IMPLICATIONS: *Preoperative:* A calm atmosphere is provided. A diet high in carbohydrates, protein, and supplemental vitamins restores a positive nitrogen balance. Prescribed antithyroid drugs are administered to establish a euthyroid state, and the patient's response and side effects are reported. Usual preoperative teaching is carried out in addition to special considerations pert. to movement of the head and voice rest.

*Postoperative:* Vital signs and intake and output are assessed, emotional support is provided, and prescribed analgesics are administered. The nurse assesses the patient frequently during the initial 48 hr for signs of tracheal compression with acute airway obstruction (choking, irregular respirations, or stridor). Oxygen, suction, and tracheostomy equipment should be readily available at bedside. The incision is observed for signs of swelling or bleeding; dressings at the back of the neck where blood would accumulate also are assessed. The patient is maintained in a semi-Fowler position as tolerated, and the head is immobilized with sandbags or pillows and supported during moving or turning. The patient is assessed for signs of damage to the recurrent laryngeal nerve (hoarseness or weak whispery voice persisting for more than 4 days). Answering questions with hand signals or a "magic slate" or other written communication tool gives the voice a rest. The patient is assessed for signs of tetany (tingling of toes, fingers, and circumoral area; positive Chvostek's and Trousseau's signs) leading to seizure activity. Calcium chloride is available for emergency IV administration. The patient is also evaluated for signs of thyroid storm (hyperpyrexia, tachydysrhythmias, profuse diaphoresis, hypotension, and diarrhea), which can progress to delirium, coma, cardiovascular collapse, and death.

*Discharge planning:* The nurse teaches the patient to observe for and report signs

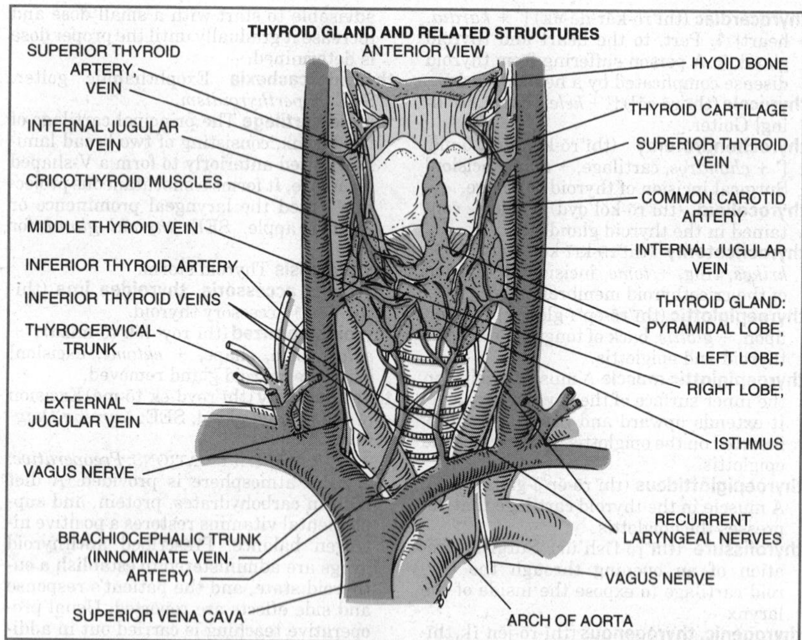


of hypothyroid or hyperthyroid function. Neck exercises are encouraged for optimal range of motion after suture removal. The nurse also teaches the patient about prescribed medications and about the importance of rest, relaxation, and good nutrition.

***subtotal t.*** Surgical excision of most of the thyroid to relieve hyperthyroidism.

**thyroid function test** A test for evidence of increased or decreased thyroid function, including a clinical physical examination, which is usually reliable, and a variety of reliable laboratory tests. Some of the more common tests are based on direct or indirect determination of the two thyroid hormones, triiodothyronine ($T_3$) and tetraiodothyronine ($T_4$). Also frequently used are tests on radioactive iodine uptake by the thyroid.

Thyroid function tests may be unreliable in certain circumstances. They may be influenced by the patient's having been exposed to organic or inorganic iodides or to drugs that interfere with the binding capacity of serum proteins.

Hypothyroidism is confirmed by finding a subnormal level of free serum thyroxine ($T_4$) in the serum.

In 95% of patients with hyperthyroidism, the level of free serum thyroxine ($T_4$) is increased. It is also helpful to obtain the serum thyroid stimulating hormone level, which is decreased in hyperthyroidism. SEE: *goiter, exophthalmic; hyperthyroidism.*

**thyroid gland** An endocrine gland located in the base of the neck on both sides of the lower part of the larynx and upper part of the trachea. It consists of two lateral lobes connected by an isthmus. Sometimes a third medial or pyramidal lobe extends upward from the isthmus. Histologically, it consists of a large number of closed vesicles called follicles that contain a homogeneous substance called colloid, which contains the thyroglobulin. It in turn contains various active substances such as thyroxine and triiodothyronine. Parafollicular cells secrete the hormone calcitonin. The thyroid gland is enlarged in goiter and it may pulsate due to its increased blood supply. SEE: illus.

**thyroidism** (thī′royd-ĭzm) A disease caused by hyperactivity of the thyroid gland.

**thyroiditis** (thī″royd-ī′tĭs) [″ + *eidos,* form, shape, + *itis,* inflammation] Inflammation of the thyroid gland. SEE: *struma, Riedel's.*

***giant cell t.*** Thyroiditis characterized by the presence of giant cells, round-cell infiltration, fibrosis, and destruction of follicles.

***Hashimoto's t.*** SEE: *Hashimoto's thyroiditis.*

***Reidel's t.*** A rare form of thyroiditis characterized by fibrotic destruction of the thyroid gland. The fibrotic tissue extends beyond the capsule of the gland into the surrounding structures of the neck and may develop sufficiently to compress the trachea. The etiology is unknown.

**thyroidomania** (thī″royd-ō-mā′nē-ă) [″ + ″ + *mania,* frenzy] A mental disorder associated with hyperthyroidism.

**thyroidotomy** (thī″royd-ŏt′ō-mē) [″ + ″ + *tome,* incision] Incision of the thyroid gland.

**thyroidotoxin** (thī″royd-ō-tŏk′sĭn) A substance that is specifically toxic for cells of the thyroid gland.

**thyroid-stimulating hormone** ABBR: TSH. A hormone secreted by the anterior lobe of the pituitary that stimulates the thyroid gland to secrete thyroxine and triiodothyronine. SYN: *thyrotropic hormone; thyrotropin.*

**thyroid storm** A complication of thyrotoxicosis that if untreated is almost uniformly fatal. It consists of an abrupt onset of fever, sweating, tachycardia, pulmonary edema or congestive heart failure, tremulousness, and restlessness. It occurs in a patient in whom existing thyrotoxicosis has been treated poorly or not at all. It usually is precipitated by infection, trauma, or a surgical emergency. SYN: *thyroid crisis; thyrotoxic crisis.*

TREATMENT: The condition is treated with catecholamine inhibitors. Both guanethidine and propranolol have been reported to be quite effective.

**thyrolysin** (thī-rŏl′ĭ-sĭn) Anything that destroys thyroid tissue.

**thyrolytic** (thī″rō-lĭt′ĭk) [Gr. *thyreos,* shield, + *lysis,* dissolution] Causing destruction of thyroid tissue.

**thyromegaly** (thī″rō-mĕg′ă-lē) [″ + *megas,* large] Enlargement of the thyroid gland.

**thyroparathyroidectomy** (thī″rō-păr″ă-thī″royd-ĕk′tō-mē) [″ + *para,* beside, + *thyreos,* shield, + *eidos,* form, shape, + *ektome,* excision] Surgical removal of the thyroid and parathyroid glands.

**thyropathy** (thī-rŏp′ă-thē) [″ + *pathos,* disease, suffering] Any disease of the thyroid.

**thyroplasty** A surgical procedure for altering the configuration of the thyroid cartilage adjacent to the vocal cords. This is done to treat certain types of dysphonia.

**thyroprival** (thī″rō-prī′văl) [″ + L. *privus,* single, set apart] Pert. to a condition resulting from loss of function or removal of the thyroid gland.

**thyroprivia** (thī″rō-prĭv′ē-ă) [″ + L. *privus,* single, set apart] Hypothyroidism due to deficient action of or removal of the thyroid.

**thyroptosis** (thī″rŏp-tō′sĭs) [″ + *ptosis,* a dropping] Downward displacement of the thyroid into the thorax.

**thyrotherapy** (thī″rō-thĕr′ă-pē) [″ + *therapeia,* treatment] Treatment with thyroid gland extracts.

**thyrotome** (thī′rō-tōm) [″ + *tome,* incision] A knife for cutting the thyroid cartilage.

**thyrotomy** (thī-rŏt′ō-mē) **1.** The splitting of the thyroid cartilage anteriorly in midline to expose laryngeal structures. **2.** Surgery on the thyroid gland.

**thyrotoxic** (thī″rō-tŏks′ĭk) [″ + *toxikon,* poison] Pert. to, affected by, or marked by toxic activity of the thyroid gland.

**thyrotoxic crisis** Thyroid storm.

**thyrotoxicosis** (thī″rō-tŏks″ĭ-kō′sĭs) [″ + ″ + *osis,* condition] A toxic condition caused by hyperactivity of the thyroid gland. Symptoms include rapid heart action, tremors, elevated basal metabolism, enlarged gland, exophthalmos, nervous symptoms, and weight loss. SYN: *goiter, exophthalmic.* SEE: *Nursing Diagnoses Appendix.*

NURSING IMPLICATIONS: The nurse provides a restful environment, encouraging expression of feelings, and promoting avoidance of stressors and stimulants to assist the patient in coping with the anxiety and irritability associated with this condition. Nutritional intake should consist of foods high in carbohydrates, proteins, and vitamins to maintain an anabolic state and to prevent muscle weakness and wasting. Comfort measures are provided to reduce effects of pyrexia, diaphoresis, abdominal cramping, and diarrhea. Fluids and electrolytes lost by diaphoresis or diarrhea are replaced as ordered. Use of methylcellulose eye drops, moist compresses, protective shields or glasses, and proper position protect the patient's eyes from injuries due to exophthalmia. Prescribed antithyroid drugs and iodides are administered and evaluated for desired effects and adverse reactions. The nurse prepares the patient for surgical treatment if scheduled.

**thyrotropic** (thī″rō-trŏp′ĭk) [″ + *trope,* a turning] That which has an affinity for or stimulates the thyroid gland.

**thyrotropic hormone** Thyrotropin.

**thyrotropin** (thī-rŏt′rō-pĭn) A hormone secreted by the anterior lobe of the pituitary that stimulates the thyroid gland. SYN: *thyroid-stimulating hormone; thyrotropic hormone.*

**thyrotropin-releasing hormone** ABBR: TRH. The major hypothalamic mediator of thyroid-stimulating hormone (TSH).

**thyrotropism** (thī-rŏt′rō-pĭzm) Affinity for the thyroid.

**thyroxine** (thī-rŏks′ĭn) [Gr. *thyreos,* shield] ABBR: $T_4$. One of the principal hormones secreted by the thyroid gland that increases the use of all food types for energy production and increases the rate of protein synthesis in most tissues. It is used to treat hypothyroidism. Chemically, it is 3,5,3′,5′-tetraiodothyronine. SYN: *tetraiodothyronine.* SEE: *thyroid; thyroid function tests; triiodothyronine.*

**Ti** Symbol for the element titanium.

**TIA** *transient ischemic attack.*

**tibia** (tĭb′ē-ă) [L., *tibia,* shinbone] The inner and larger bone of the leg between the knee and the ankle; it articulates with the femur above and with the talus below.

***saber-shaped t.*** A deformity of the tibia caused by gummatous periostitis (syphilitic) in which it curves outward.

***t. valga*** A bulging of the lower legs in

which the convexity is inward. SYN: *genu valgum.*

***t. vara*** A bowing of the lower legs in which the convexity is outward. SYN: *genu varum.*

**tibiad** (tĭb′ē-ăd) [″ + *ad,* to] Toward the tibia.

**tibial** (tĭb′ē-ăl) [L. *tibialis*] Concerning the tibia.

**tibialgia** (tĭb″ē-ăl′jē-ă) [″ + Gr. *algos,* pain] Pain in the tibia.

**tibialis** (tĭb″ē-ā′lĭs) [L.] Pert. to the tibia.

**tibioadductor reflex** (tĭb″ē-ō-ăd-dŭk′tor) [L. *tibia,* shinbone, + *adducere,* to lead to] Adduction of either the stimulated leg or the opposite one when the tibia is percussed on the inner side.

**tibiocalcanean** (tĭb″ē-ō-kăl-kā′nē-ăn) Concerning the tibia and calcaneus bones.

**tibiofemoral** (tĭb″ē-ō-fĕm′or-ăl) [″ + L. *femur,* thigh] Rel. to the tibia and femur.

**tibiofibular** (tĭb″ē-ō-fĭb′ū-lăr) [″ + L. *fibula,* pin] Rel. to the tibia and fibula. SYN: *tibioperoneal.*

**tibionavicular** (tĭb″ē-ō-nă-vĭk′ū-lăr) Concerning the tibia and navicular bones. SYN: *tibioscaphoid.*

**tibioperoneal** (tĭb″ē-ō-pĕr″ō-nē′ăl) Tibiofibular.

**tibioscaphoid** (tĭb″ē-ō-skăf′oyd) Tibionavicular.

**tibiotarsal** (tĭb″ē-ō-tăr′săl) [″ + Gr. *tarsos,* broad, flat surface] Rel. to the tibia and tarsus.

**tic** (tĭk) [Fr.] A spasmodic muscular contraction, most commonly involving the face, mouth, eyes, head, neck, or shoulder muscles. The spasms may be tonic or clonic. The movement appears purposeful, is often repeated, is involuntary, and can be inhibited for a short time only to burst forth with increased severity.

Children between the ages of 5 and 10 years are esp. likely to develop tics or habit spasms. These tend to cease in a few weeks if they are ignored. SYN: *habit spasm.* SEE: *neuralgia; Tourette's syndrome.*

ETIOLOGY: In most cases, the cause is unknown. In some individuals, the tic is related to anxiety and nervous tension.

***convulsive t.*** Spasm of the facial muscles supplied by the seventh cranial nerve.

***t. douloureux*** Degeneration of or pressure on the trigeminal nerve, resulting in neuralgia of that nerve. The pain comes on in severe lightning-like stabs and radiates from the angle of the jaw along one of the involved branches. If it is the first branch, a shocklike pain is felt along the eye and back over the forehead. If it is the middle fiber, the upper lip, nose, and cheek under the eye are affected. If it is the third branch, pain is in the lower lip and outer border of the tongue on the affected side. Pain is momentary but may occur repetitively for as long as 20 sec. Paroxysms may last for hours and then subside for weeks or months. SYN: *trigeminal neuralgia.* SEE: *Nursing Diagnoses Appendix.*

TREATMENT: The condition is treated with carbamazepine, phenytoin, or baclofen. Surgical therapy may be required to relieve pressure from arteries pressing on the root of the trigeminal nerve.

NURSING IMPLICATIONS: The characteristics of each attack are observed and recorded. The patient should maintain independence and participate in social activities. Analeptic drugs are administered as prescribed and observed for side effects. In the patient receiving alcohol injections, pain will return with nerve regeneration, and the physician should be notified of pain recurrence. Before surgery, causative factors such as extreme temperatures of foods and jarring of the bed should be eliminated. The patient should use a cotton pad to cleanse the face and a blunt-toothed comb to comb the hair.

After surgery, sensory deficits are assessed to prevent trauma to the face and affected areas. The patient who has had an ophthalmic branch resection should examine the eye for foreign substances with a hand mirror every hour. The patient who has had a mandibular or maxillary branch resection should take care when eating: the patient should chew food on the unaffected side to prevent inner cheek injury. Frequent dental examinations detect abnormalities that the patient cannot feel. The nurse provides emotional support.

***facial t.*** Tic of the facial muscles.

***habit t.*** Habitual repetition of a grimace or muscular action.

***t. rotatoire*** Spasmodic torticollis in which the head and neck are forcibly rotated or turned from one side to the other.

***spasmodic t.*** Tonic contractions and paralysis of the muscles of one or both sides of the face.

***vocal t.'s*** Grunts and barking sounds that may be made by persons with Tourette's syndrome.

**ticarcillin disodium, sterile** (tī″kăr-sĭl′ĭn) A semisynthetic penicillin esp. effective against *Pseudomonas aeruginosa.*

**tick** (tĭk) [ME. *tyke*] Any of the numerous bloodsucking acarids of the order Acarida. Ixodidae is the hard tick family and Argasidae the soft. Ticks transmit specific diseases to humans and lower animals. SEE: illus.

***t. bite*** A puncture wound caused by a tick. Ticks can be vectors for several diseases, including Rocky Mountain spotted fever, Q fever, tularemia, borreliosis, human babesiosis, human ehrlichiosis, and Lyme disease, but the bite itself usually produces a mildly itching papule. If the tick is incompletely removed, the retained mouth parts may cause a pruritic nodule. The nodule should be surgically excised.

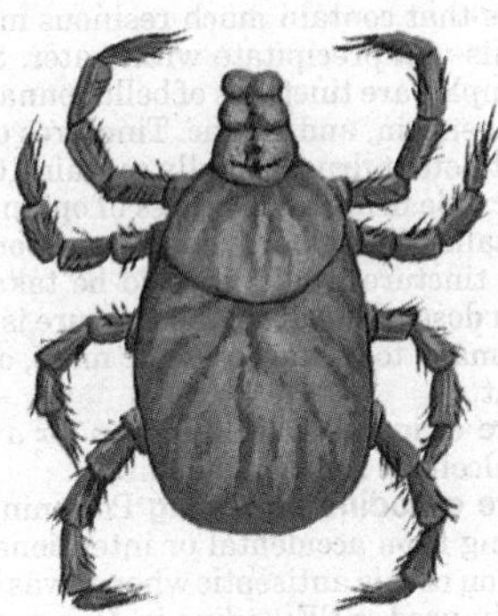

TICK

WOOD TICK (DERMACENTOR) (ORIG. MAG. ×4)

Removal of a tick should not be done by crushing but by either gentle traction or application of petroleum jelly, oil, or nail polish to the tick, which will facilitate removal. SEE: *paralysis, tick-bite.*

***wood t.*** *Dermacentor andersoni,* an important North American species of tick, which causes tick paralysis and transmits causative organisms of Rocky Mountain spotted fever and tularemia. SEE: *tick* for illus.

**tick-borne rickettsiosis** The spotted-fever group (SFG) of tick-borne rickettsioses. Included are infections caused by the pathogenic organism *Rickettsia rickettsii,* which causes Rocky Mountain spotted fever. There are six other pathogenic SFG rickettsial species, five of which (*R. conorii, R. sibirica, R. japonica, R. australis,* and *R. africae*) are most likely to be transmitted by a tick bite. *R. akari,* which causes rickettsialpox, is transmitted to humans by mouse mites.

**tickle** (tĭk′l) [ME. *tikelen*] **1.** Peculiar sensation caused by titillation or touching, esp. in certain areas of the body, resulting in reflex muscular movements, laughter, or hysteria. **2.** To arouse such a sensation by touching a surface lightly.

**tickling** (tĭk′lĭng) Gentle stimulation of a sensitive surface and its reflex effect, such as involuntary laughter. SYN: *titillation.*

**t.i.d.** L. *ter in die,* three times a day.

**tidal** (tī′dăl) Periodically rising and falling, increasing and decreasing.

**tidal air** SEE: *volume, tidal.*

**tidal drainage** The drainage of a paralyzed bladder by use of an automatic irrigation apparatus.

**tide** [AS. *tid,* time] Alternate rise and fall; a space of time.

***acid t.*** Temporary increase in acidity of urine caused by increased secretion of alkaline substances into the duodenum or by fasting.

***alkaline t.*** Temporary decrease in acidity of urine following awakening and after meals. The former results from an increased rate of breathing, in which excess carbon dioxide is eliminated; the latter results from an increase of base in the blood following the secretion of HCl into gastric juice.

***fat t.*** Increased fat in the lymph and blood after a fatty meal.

**Tietze's syndrome** (tĕt′sĕz) [Alexander Tietze, Ger. surgeon, 1864–1927] Inflammation of the costochondral cartilages. This self-limiting disease is of unknown etiology. The pain may be confused with that of myocardial infarction. There is no specific therapy, but some relief is provided by injecting the area with procaine and corticosteroids.

**tigering** [Gr. *tigris,* tiger] Tigerlike striped appearance of the heart muscle owing to irregular areas of fatty degeneration. This is seen in conditions that cause severe anoxemia, such as anemia.

**tigretier** (tē-grĕt″ē-ā′) [Fr.] A dancing mania or form of tarantism caused by the bite of a poisonous spider, occurring in Tigré, Abyssinia.

**tigroid** (tī′groyd) [Gr. *tigroeides,* tiger-spotted] Striped, spotted, or marked like a tiger.

**tigroid bodies** Masses of chromophil substance present in the cell bodies of neurons. SYN: *Nissl bodies.*

**tigrolysis** (tĭg″rŏl′ĭ-sĭs) Chromatolysis.

**tilmus** (tĭl′mŭs) [Gr. *tilmos,* a plucking] Carphology.

**tiltometer** (tĭl-tŏm′ĕ-tĕr) A device for measuring the degree of tilt of a bed or operating table; used to determine which end of the spinal canal is lower when spinal anesthesia has been given.

**timbre** (tĭm′bĕr, tăm′br) [Fr., a bell to be struck with a hammer] The resonance quality of a sound by which it is distinguished, other than pitch or intensity, depending on the number and character of the vibrating body's overtones.

**time** (tīm) [AS. *tima,* time] The interval between beginning and ending; measured duration.

***bleeding t.*** The time required for bleeding from a small wound to cease; usually tested by puncturing the earlobe. The normal time is 1 to 3 min. SEE: *bleeding time.*

***clot retraction t.*** The time required following withdrawal of blood for a clot to completely contract and express the serum entrapped within the fibrin net. The normal time is about 1 hr. Clot retraction depends on the number of platelets in the specimen.

***coagulation t.*** The time required for clotting to occur in whole blood that has been placed in tubes coated with silicone. The time required is somewhat different for each laboratory but will usually be from 20 to 60 min.

***doubling t.*** The length of time needed for a malignant tumor cell population to double in size.

***median lethal t.*** The time required for the death of 50% of the individuals of an organism group that were exposed to ionizing radiation.

***partial thromboplastin t.*** The time needed for plasma to clot after the addition of partial thromboplastin; used to test for defects of the clotting system.

***prothrombin t.*** The time required for plasma coagulation in the formation of thrombin from prothrombin. Normal levels of calcium, thromboplastin, and other essential tissue coagulation factors are required. Normal values range from 11 to 12.5 sec.

***reaction t.*** The period between application of a stimulus and the response.

***setting t.*** The time required for a material to polymerize or harden, as in dental amalgam, cement, plaster, resin, or stone.

***thermal death t.*** The time required to kill a bacterium at a certain temperature.

**time frame** The limits of time for any event or occurrence.

**time inventory** An assessment approach used by occupational therapists to determine a patient's perception of the value of time and its organization.

**time-out** An alternative method of discipline that involves removing the child from social interaction and placing him or her in a nonstimulating location (i.e., in a chair facing a corner) for a few minutes after an unacceptable behavior has occurred.

**timer** (tĭm′ĕr) A device for measuring, signaling, recording, or otherwise indicating elapsed time. Various forms of timers are used in radiographic, surgical, and laboratory work.

**tin** (tĭn) [AS.] SYMB: Sn. A metallic element used in various industries and in making certain tissue stains; atomic weight, 118.69; atomic number, 50. SEE: *tin poisoning*.

**tinct** *tincture*.

**tinctable** (tĭnk′tă-bl) Stainable.

**tinction** (tĭnk′shŭn) [L. *tingere*, to dye] **1.** The process of staining. **2.** A stain.

**tinctorial** (tĭnk-tō′rē-ăl) [L. *tinctorius*, dyeing] Rel. to staining or color.

**tinctura** (tĭnk-tū′ră) *pl.* **tincturae** [L., a dyeing] Tincture.

**tincturation** (tĭnk″tū-rā′shŭn) Making a tincture from an appropriate drug.

**tincture** (tĭnk′chūr) [L. *tincture*, a dyeing] An alcoholic extract of vegetable or animal substances. Simple alcoholic solutions of pure substances such as iodine and quinine are no longer called tinctures. The name of the material contained in the tincture other than alcohol is added to the name of the tincture. SYN: *tinctura*.

This class of preparations usually contains tannic acid, so, in most instances, cannot be used with agents that are incompatible with that drug. Those tinctures that contain much resinous matter or oils will precipitate with water. Some examples are tinctures of belladonna, ginger, benzoin, and guaiac. Tinctures of the most potent drugs usually contain 10% of the crude drug, as tinctures of opium and digitalis. When more than a teaspoon of a 10% tincture would have to be taken to get a dose of the drug, the tincture is usually made to contain 20%, or more, of the agent.

**tincture of iodine** Obsolete term for a simple alcoholic solution of iodine.

**tincture of iodine poisoning** Poisoning resulting from accidental or intentional ingestion of this antiseptic when it was commonly used. SEE: *iodine* in *Poisons and Poisoning Appendix*.

SYMPTOMS: The patient experiences a very strong irritation of the mouth, esophagus, and stomach. Membranes are stained dark brown or black. Pain is intense and leads to early vomiting and purging, extreme thirst, and often collapse.

TREATMENT: The patient must be given large amounts of water, milk, and starchy paste; and gruels, such as boiled rice or cream of wheat. Gastric lavage should be performed with either 1% to 10% starch solution, or sodium thiosulfite or protein solution such as egg white or milk. Pain, circulatory collapse, and fluid and electrolyte balance should be controlled with appropriate therapy. Tracheotomy may be required.

**tine** A sharp, pointed prong.

**tinea** (tĭn′ē-ă) [L., worm] Any fungus skin disease occurring on various parts of the body. It is commonly called ringworm. SEE: *dermatomycosis*.

SYMPTOMS: There are two types of symptoms. Superficial symptoms are marking by scaling; slight itching; reddish or grayish patches; and dry, brittle hair that is easily extracted with the hair shaft. The deep type is characterized by flat, reddish, kerion-like tumors, the surface studded with dead or broken hairs or by gaping follicular orifices. Nodules may be broken down in the center, discharging pus through dilated follicular openings.

TREATMENT: Griseofulvin, terbinafine, or ketoconazole is given orally for all types of true trichophyton infections. Local treatment alone is of little benefit in ringworm of the scalp, nails, and in most cases the feet. Topical preparations containing fungicidal agents are useful in the treatment of tinea cruris and tinea pedis.

Personal hygiene is important in controlling these two common diseases. The use of antiseptic foot baths to control tinea pedis does not prevent spread of the infection from one person to another. Persons affected should not let others use their personal items such as clothes, towels, and sports equipment.

Tinea of the scalp, tinea capitis, is particularly resistant if due to *Microsporum audouinii*. It should not be treated topically. Systemic griseofulvin is quite effective.

**t. amiantacea** Sticky scaling of the scalp following infection or trauma.

**t. barbae** A fungus skin disease of the bearded portions of the neck and face. SYN: *barber's itch*.

**t. capitis** A fungal infection of the scalp. It may be due to one of several types of *Microsporum* or *Trichophyton tonsurans*. SEE: illus.; *kerion*.

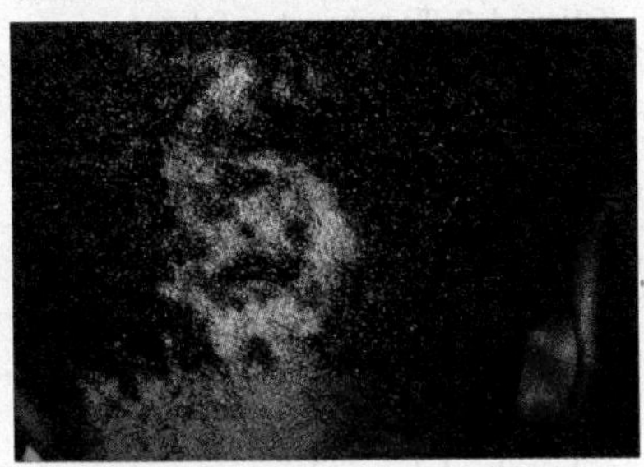

**TINEA CAPITIS** WITH HAIR LOSS

**t. corporis** Tinea of the body. It begins with red, slightly elevated scaly patches that on examination reveal minute vesicles or papules. New patches spring from the periphery while the central portion clears up. There is often considerable itching. SEE: illus.

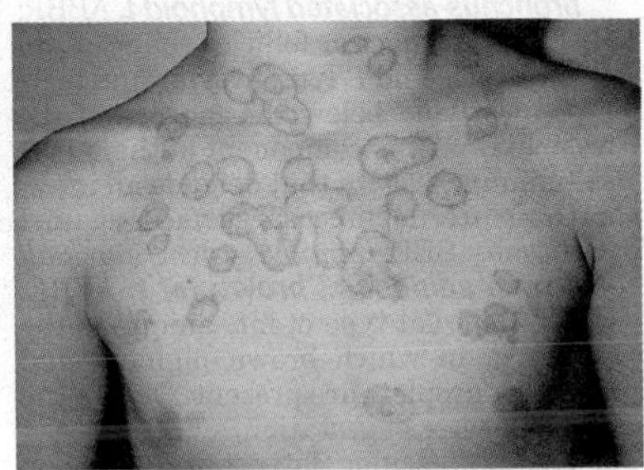

**TINEA CORPORIS**

**t. cruris** A fungus skin disease of surfaces of contact in the scrotal, crural, anal, and genital areas. Also called "jock itch." SYN: *dhobie itch*. SEE: illus.

**t. imbricata** Chronic tinea caused by *Trichophyton concentricum*. It is present in tropical regions. The annular lesions have scales at their periphery.

**t. kerion** Kerion.

**t. nigra** An asymptomatic superficial fungal infection that affects the skin of the palms. Caused by *Cladosporium werneckii* or *C. mansonii,* it is characterized by deeply pigmented, macular, nonscaly

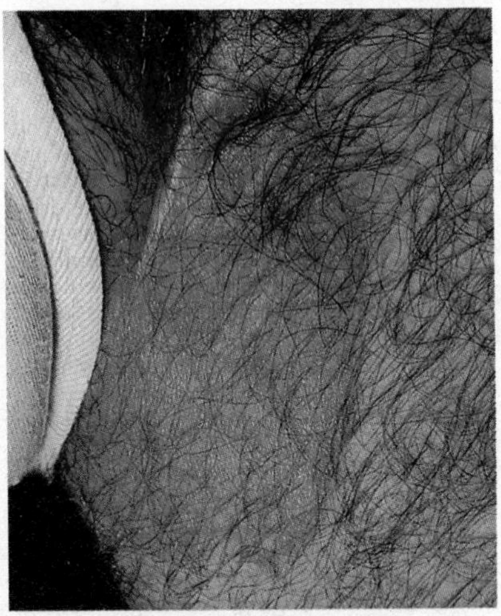

**TINEA CRURIS** ON INNER THIGH

patches. SYN: *pityriasis nigra*.

**t. nodosa** Sheathlike nodular masses in the hair of the beard and mustache from growth of either *Piedraia hortae,* which causes black piedra, or *Trichosporon beigelii,* which causes white piedra. The masses surround the hairs, which become brittle; hairs may be penetrated by fungus and thus split. SYN: *piedra*.

**t. pedis** Athlete's foot.

**t. profunda** A rare type of tinea characterized by indolent nodules and plaques, which may ulcerate.

**t. sycosis** T. barbae.

**t. tonsurans** T. capitis.

**t. unguium** Onychomycosis.

**t. versicolor** A fungus infection of the skin producing yellow or fawn-colored branny patches. A topically applied azole antifungal cream or 2% selenium sulfide lotion is effective in treating the causative agent, the fungus *Malassezia furfur*. SYN: *pityriasis versicolor*. SEE: illus.

**TINEA VERSICOLOR** ON BACK

**Tinel's sign** (tĭn-ĕlz′) [Jules Tinel, Fr. neurologist, 1879–1952] A cutaneous tingling sensation produced by pressing on or tapping the nerve trunk that has been damaged or is regenerating following trauma.

**tine test** A skin test for tuberculosis. The tuberculin is on metal tines that are barely pressed into the skin. The test is read in 48 and 72 hr. The unit is sterile and disposable and therefore is very useful in mass surveys. Several multiple puncture tests are available including Mantoux, Aplitest, and Heaf tests. SEE: *tuberculin test.*

**tingibility** (tĭn″jĭ-bĭl′ĭ-tē) The property of being stainable.

**tingible** (tĭn′jĭ-bl) [L. *tingere,* to stain] Capable of being stained by a dye.

**tingle** (tĭng′gl) A prickling or stinging sensation that may be caused by cold or nerve injury.

**tinnitus** (tĭn-ī′tŭs) [L., a jingling] A subjective ringing or tinkling sound in the ear.

***t. aurium*** Ringing, tinkling, buzzing, or other sounds in the ear, found in certain diseases of the exterior, middle, or inner ear.

ETIOLOGY: It may be caused by impacted cerumen, myringitis, otitis media, labyrinthitis, Ménière's symptom complex, otosclerosis, or hysteria. It also may follow prolonged therapy with drugs such as quinine and salicylates, including aspirin.

**tin poisoning** Poisoning from tin in soldered containers. This is exceedingly rare. Symptoms include a metallic taste in the mouth, gastrointestinal irritation, nausea, vomiting, cramping, and diarrhea. The stomach should be washed out and bland or soothing drinks administered.

**tintometer** (tĭn-tŏm′ĕ-ter) [L. *tinctus,* a dyeing, + Gr. *metron,* a measure] A scale of different shades of color to determine by comparison the intensity of color of the blood or other fluid.

**tintometric** (tĭn″tō-mĕt′rĭk) Rel. to tintometry.

**tintometry** (tĭn-tŏm′ĕ-trē) Estimation of color by comparison with a scale of colors.

**tip** (tĭp) [ME] A point or apex of a part.

**tipped uterus** Malposition of the uterus. In the past, this has been invoked as the cause of numerous conditions, including pelvic pain, back pain, abnormal uterine bleeding, infertility, and emotional difficulties. Simple malposition of the uterus without evidence of a specific disease condition that accounts for the malposition is felt to be harmless and virtually symptomless. It is essential therefore that individuals who have been told that a tipped uterus is the cause of their symptoms be carefully examined to attempt to find a specific organic cause for the symptoms. If in the absence of other findings a vaginal pessary relieves symptoms associated with a retrodisplaced uterus and these symptoms return when the pessary is removed, then surgical suspension of the uterus is indicated. If surgery is not acceptable to the patient, the pessary may be worn intermittently. Evidence is lacking that a tipped uterus is an important cause of pelvic pain and discomfort.

**tipping** (tĭp′ĭng) Angulation of a structure, such as a tooth about its long axis, the patella when it moves away from the frontal plane of the femur, or the scapula when the inferior angle moves away from the ribcage.

**tiqueur** (tĭ-kĕr′) [Fr.] One afflicted with a tic.

**tire** (tīr) [AS. *teorian,* to tire] **1.** To become fatigued. **2.** To exhaust or fatigue.

**tirefond** (tēr-fŏn′) [Fr.] An appliance like a corkscrew for raising depressed portions of bone or for removing foreign bodies.

**tires** (tīrz) Trembles.

**tiring** (tīr′ĭng) Fastening wire around the fragments of a bone.

**tissue** (tĭsh′ū) [O. Fr. *tissu,* from L. *texere,* to weave] A group or collection of similar cells and their intercellular substance that act together in the performance of a particular function. The primary tissues are epithelial, connective, skeletal, muscular, glandular, and nervous.

***adenoid t.*** Lymphoid t.

***adipose t.*** Fat.

***areolar t.*** A form of loose connective tissue consisting of fibroblasts in a matrix of tissue fluid and collagen and elastin fibers. Many white blood cells are present. It is found subcutaneously and beneath the epithelium of all mucous membranes. SEE: *connective t.* for illus.

***bony t., bone t.*** Osseous t.

***bronchus-associated lymphoid t.*** ABBR: BALT. Small sacs or follicles that contain clusters of T and B lymphocytes and macrophages lying below the mucosa of the bronchial wall; a component of the mucosal immune system that defends all internal and external mucosal surfaces against pathogens. SEE: *immune system, mucosal.*

***brown adipose t., brown fat t.*** ABBR: BAT. A special type of fat, unique to the newborn, in which brown pigment and small fat droplets are present. During the last trimester of gestation, small deposits of highly vascular fatty tissue develop around the fetal neck, between the scapulae, behind the sternum, around the kidneys and adrenal glands, and in the axillae. In response to cold stress, these deposits are catabolized to produce heat and energy.

***cancellous t.*** Spongy bone with many marrow cavities. It is present at the ends of long articular bones and in the interior of most flat bones.

***cartilage t.*** The dense connective tissue of cartilage consisting of cells embedded in a matrix.

***chondroid t.*** Embryonic cartilage.

***chordal t.*** Tissue of the notochord or derived from it. The nucleus pulposus is derived from the notochord.

***chromaffin t.*** Tissue containing cells that give the chromaffin reaction. It is found in the adrenal medulla and near the sympathetic ganglia. SEE: *chromaffin system.*

***cicatricial t.*** The thick fibrous tissue formed as part of the healing process in soft tissue wounds. SYN: *scar t.*

***connective t.*** Tissue that supports and connects other tissues and parts of the body. Connective tissue has comparatively few cells. Its bulk consists of intercellular substance or matrix, whose nature gives each type of connective tissue its particular properties. Connective tissue, with the exception of cartilage, is highly vascular. Connective tissue proper includes the following types: mucous, fibrous (areolar, white fibrous, yellow fibrous, or elastic), reticular, and adipose. Dense connective tissue includes cartilage and bone (osseous tissue). Blood is sometimes considered a connective tissue. SEE: illus.

***elastic t.*** A form of connective tissue in which yellow elastic fibers predominate. It is found in certain ligaments and the walls of blood vessels, esp. the larger arteries.

***embryonic t.*** Mucous t.

***endothelial t.*** Endothelium.

***epithelial t.*** Epithelium.

***erectile t.*** Spongy tissue, the spaces of which fill with blood, causing it to harden and expand. It is found in the penis, clitoris, and nipples.

***extracellular t.*** All of the tissue and fluids outside of the cells of the body, including plasma, serum, lymph, aqueous and vitreous humors, and connective tissue such as collagen, cartilage, and some bone.

***fatty t.*** Fat.

***fibrous t.*** Connective tissue consisting principally of fibers. The three types are areolar or loose connective, white fibrous, and yellow fibrous or elastic.

***gelatiginous t.*** Tissue from which gelatin may be obtained by treating it with hot water.

***glandular t.*** A group of epithelial cells capable of producing secretions.

***granulation t.*** The newly formed vascular and cellular tissue produced in the early stages of wound healing.

***hard t.*** In dentistry, the term used to denote any of the three calcified tissue components of the tooth: enamel, dentin, and cementum.

***homologous t.'s*** Tissues that are identical in structure.

***indifferent t.*** Tissue composed of undifferentiated cells as in embryonic tissue.

***interstitial t.*** Connective tissue that forms a network with the cellular elements of an organ.

***lymphadenoid t.*** Lymphoid tissue present in various sites, including the spleen and bone marrow.

***lymphoid t.*** A collection of developing and mature lymphocytes mingled with a supporting lattice of connective tissue. Such collections are present in the adenoids, in the tonsils, and in Peyer's patches in the intestines. SYN: *adenoid t.*

***mesenchymal t.*** The embryonic mesenchyme.

***mucous t.*** Jelly-like tissue from which connective tissue is derived. SYN: *embryonic t.*

***muscular t.*** The cells composing the muscles. *Voluntary:* Striated or skeletal muscle attached to bones or the skin. The cells are long cylinders with apparent striations and several nuclei each. *Involuntary:* Smooth or visceral muscle not under voluntary control, found mainly in the walls of hollow organs such as the stomach, intestines, arteries, veins, and uterus. The cells are small and tapered with no striations and one nucleus each. *Cardiac:* Found only in the walls of the chambers of the heart; not under voluntary control. The cells are branched, with striations and one nucleus each. SEE: *muscle.*

***myeloid t.*** The red bone marrow in which most blood cells are formed.

***nerve t., nervous t.*** All of the tissue of the central and peripheral nervous systems.

***osseous t.*** Connective tissue with intercellular substance impregnated with phosphate and carbonate of calcium, the mineral substances being two thirds of the bone's dry weight. It may be in its usual or abnormal site (i.e., in calcified tissue). SYN: *bony t.*

***reticular t.*** A type of connective tissue consisting of delicate fibers forming interlacing networks. Fibers stain selectively with silver stains and are called argyrophil fibers. Reticular tissue supports lymph nodes and is found in muscular tissue and bone marrow, the spleen, liver, lungs, kidneys, and mucous membranes of the gastrointestinal tract, and the walls of blood vessels.

***scar t.*** Cicatricial t.

***sclerous t.*** Firm connective tissue such as bone and cartilage.

***skeletal t.*** Bone.

***splenic t.*** The highly vascular splenic pulp.

***subcutaneous t.*** Areolar tissue under and becoming part of the corium.

***subcutaneous adipose t.*** Adipose tissue within subcutaneous tissue.

***white fibrous t.*** Connective tissue made primarily of collagen fibers. Strong and inelastic, it forms tendons, ligaments, deep fascia, and the dermis.

***white nervous t.*** Nervous tissue made of myelinated nerve fibers. SYN: *white matter.*

**tissue bank** A facility for collecting, processing, and storing tissue for later transplan-

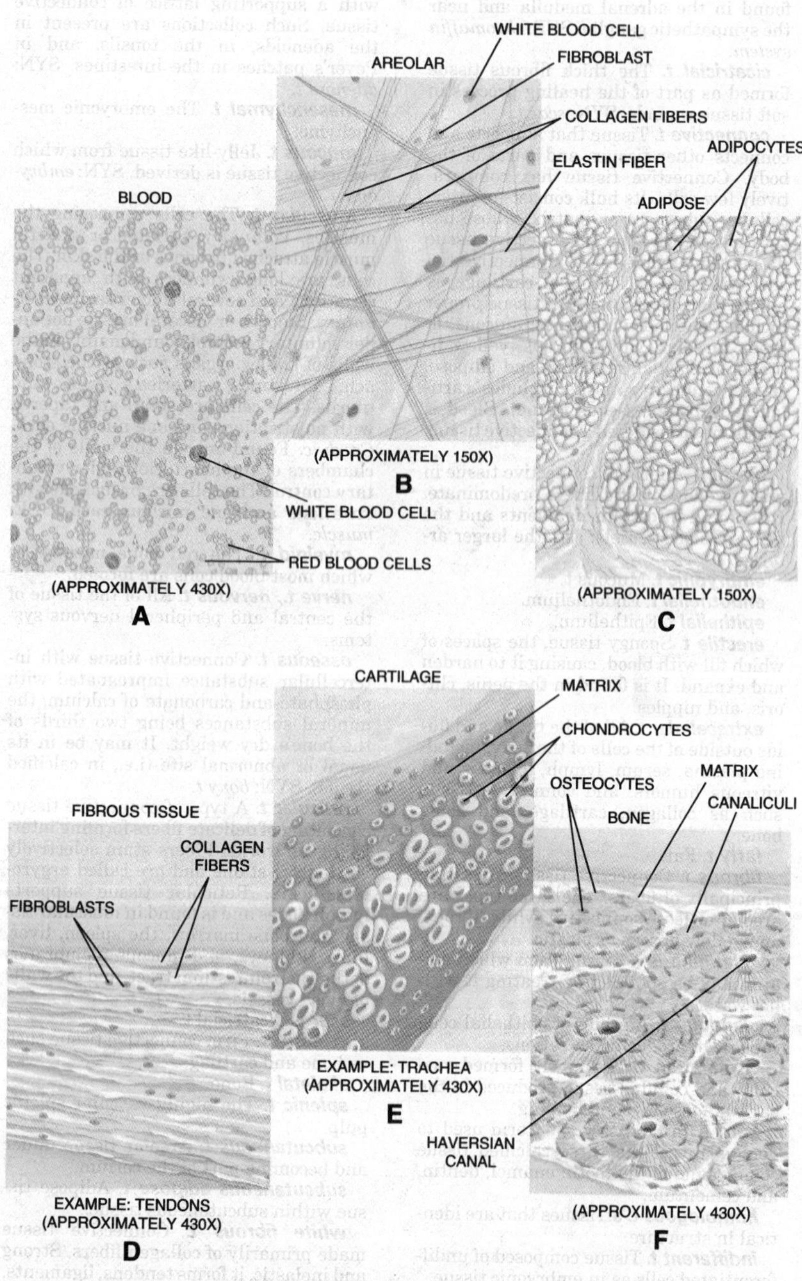


**CONNECTIVE TISSUES**

**(A)** BLOOD, **(B)** AREOLAR, **(C)** ADIPOSE, **(D)** FIBROUS, **(E)** CARTILAGE, **(F)** BONE

tation. Tissue stored includes bone, skin, nerve, fascial, tendon, heart valve, dura mater, cornea, and bone marrow. These are tested for microbial pathogens and stored either in a freeze-dried or frozen state.

**tissue culture** Growth of tissue in vitro on artificial media for experimental research.

**tissue culture ineffective dose** ABBR: $TCID_{50}$. Dose that will produce a cytopathic effect in 50% of the cultures inoculated.

**tissue expansion, soft** A technique used in plastic surgery to expand skin to remove an area for cosmetic reasons. One or more expander balloons are inserted under the skin. The balloons are then expanded by progressively increasing the amount of saline solution in them. This is done on a weekly basis for whatever time is required to sufficiently stretch the overlying skin. Once the expansion is completed, the plastic surgical procedure is done. This permits removal of skin without having to cover the area by a skin graft. SEE: *surgery, plastic; W-plasty; Z-plasty.*

**tissue factor** ABBR: TF. Coagulation factor III.

**tissue integrity, impaired** A state in which an individual experiences damage to mucous membrane or corneal, integumentary, or subcutaneous tissue. SEE: *Nursing Diagnoses Appendix.*

**tissue perfusion, altered** The state in which an individual experiences a decrease in nutrition and oxygenation at the cellular level due to a deficit in capillary blood supply. Tissue perfusion problems (cerebral, cardiopulmonary, renal, gastrointestinal, peripheral) can exist without decreased cardiac output; however, there may be a relationship between cardiac output and tissue perfusion. SEE: *Nursing Diagnoses Appendix.*

**tissue plasminogen activator** ABBR: TPA. A drug used to dissolve the blood clots (thrombolysis) that cause occlusion of the arteries in myocardial infarction. It is administered within the first 6 hr of the attack. It has been shown to reduce the chances of dying following a heart attack by more than 50%. The undesired side effect of causing intracranial bleeding as a result of the therapy has not been a problem when the correct dose is given; and the drug may have a place in the treatment of stroke caused by intravascular clots in the arteries of the central nervous system. Patients over 75 years of age or any patient with a history of stroke or history of potential bleeding sites should not be given the drug. In addition, it should be used cautiously in pregnant women. This drug has a half-life of about 5 min. It is metabolized in the liver and excreted in the urine. Within 10 min of its administration, about 80% of a dose has been cleared from the blood. SYN: *recombinant TPA.* SEE: *reperfusion; streptokinase.*

NURSING IMPLICATIONS: The patient maintains strict bedrest throughout infusion. Additional IV access sites are initiated for adjuvant therapies or required blood studies before administering TPA. No further needle sticks should occur during therapy. The IV access site is inspected for bleeding throughout therapy, and the patient is assessed for indications of intracerebral or gastric bleeding. Heparin is administered with or after therapy as prescribed to maintain activated partial thromboplastin time at two times the patient's normal baseline. The nurse evaluates for indications of reperfusion: sudden cessation of chest pain, early peak of creatine phosphokinase-MB enzyme (at 12 hr after injury), resolution of electrocardiographic injury current patterns, and "reperfusion dysrhythmias," including accelerated idioventricular rhythm, ventricular tachycardia, sinus bradycardia, and atrioventricular block with hypotension. Mild allergic reactions to therapy (pruritus, urticaria, flushing, fever, headache, nausea, and malaise) are assessed, documented, and treated, as well as more acute reactions (bronchospasm, angioedema). In the case of acute reactions, emergency treatment is initiated promptly to protect the airway and to prevent circulatory collapse.

**tissue reaction** The response of living tissues to altered conditions or types of restorative materials, metals, cements.

**tissue typing** Technique for determining the histocompatibility of tissues to be used in grafts and transplants with the recipient's tissues and cells. SEE: *transplantation.*

**tissular** (tĭsh′ū-lăr) Concerning living tissues.

**titanium** (tī-tā′nē-ŭm) [L. *titan,* the sun] SYMB: Ti. A metallic element found in combination with minerals; atomic weight, 47.90; atomic number, 22; specific gravity, 4.54. In dentistry, it is used as an alloy chiefly for appliances and implants because of its biological acceptance and resistance to corrosion.

***t. dioxide*** A chemical used to protect the skin from the sun. It is also used in industrial applications to produce white in paints and plastics.

**titer** (tī′tĕr) [F. *titre,* standard] Standard of strength per volume of a volumetric test solution.

***agglutination t.*** The highest dilution of a serum that will cause clumping or agglutination of the bacteria being tested.

***antibody t.*** A measure of the amount of antibody against a particular antigen present in the blood. One use is in detection of antibodies against herpes simplex and Epstein-Barr viruses. Researchers believe that any elevated antibody titers may indicate a decrease in lymphocyte activity as the result of the stress response or other condition, as these viruses are generally controlled by T lymphocytes. This titer is also useful in following the course of many acute infectious diseases. A rising titer usually indicates the disease is present and the body is reacting to the specific antigen.

**titillation** (tĭt″ĭl-ā′shŭn) [L. *titillatio,* a tickling] **1.** The act of tickling. **2.** The state of being tickled. **3.** The sensation produced by tickling.

**titin** An elastic protein in sarcomeres that anchors myosin filaments to the Z disks.

**titrate** (tī′trāt) To determine or estimate by titration.

**titration** (tī-trā′shŭn) [Fr. *titre,* a standard] **1.** Estimation of the concentration of a chemical solution by adding known amounts of standard reagents until alteration in color or electrical state occurs. **2.** Determination of the quantity of antibody in an antiserum.

**titre** Titer.

**titrimetric** (tī″trĭ-mĕt′rĭk) [″ + Gr. *metron,* measure] Employing the process of titration.

**titrimetry** (tī-trĭm′ĕ-trē) [*titration* + Gr. *metron,* measure] Analysis by titration.

**titubation** (tĭt″ū-bā′shŭn) [L. *titubatio,* a staggering] A coarse and backward tremor of the trunk. In patients with cerebellar disease, standing sometimes provokes this tremor.

***lingual t.*** Stuttering.

**Tl** Symbol for the element thallium.

**TLC** **1.** *tender loving care.* **2.** *total lung capacity.* **3.** *thin-layer chromatography.* SEE: *chromatography, thin-layer.*

**TLD** *Thermoluminescent dosimeter.*

**T.L.R.** *tonic labyrinthine reflex.*

**Tm** **1.** Symbol for the element thulium. **2.** Symbol for maximal tubular excretory capacity of the kidneys.

**TMJ** *temporomandibular joint.*

**TMP** *trimethoprim.*

**Tn** Symbol for normal intraocular tension.

**TNF** *tumor necrosis factor.*

**TNM classification** Method of classifying malignant tumors with respect to primary *t*umor, involvement of regional lymph *n*odes, and presence or absence of *m*etastases. SEE: *cancer.*

**TNT** *trinitrotoluene.*

**TO** *old tuberculin* (also abbr. OT).

**toadskin** (tōd′skĭn) A condition characterized by excessive dryness, wrinkling, and scaling of skin sometimes seen in vitamin deficiencies.

**toadstool** (tōd′stool) Any of various fungi with an umbrella-shaped cap, esp. a poisonous mushroom.

**toadstool poisoning** The toxicity experienced from ingestion of a poisonous mushroom.

SYMPTOMS: Symptoms appear from a few minutes to 15 hr after ingestion and are characterized by marked abdominal pain, vomiting, and intense diarrhea. Profound weakness comes early and remains. Sometimes perspiration and lacrimation and occasionally convulsions or coma are present.

FIRST AID: The patient should be kept on absolute bedrest. Stomach and bowels should be emptied promptly and completely with gastric lavage and quick-acting cathartic and enemas. Atropine is esp. helpful and may be given by any route. Fluid, sodium chloride, and high carbohydrate intake should be maintained intravenously if required. Excitement, hypotension, convulsions, pain, and fever are treated symptomatically. Dialysis has been used in treating poisoning caused by *Amanita phalloides.* SEE: *Amanita* in *Poisons and Poisoning Appendix.*

**tobacco** (tō-băk′ō) [Sp. *tabaco*] Dried leaves of *Nicotiana tabacum* and other species. It contains nicotine, pyridine, picoline, and collidin, and is widely used in forms of cigars, cigarettes, pipe tobacco, snuff, and chewing tobacco. During its combustion, various products are given off, the most important being nicotine and certain compounds that have an adverse effect on the lungs. For this reason, the use of tobacco products has proved injurious to health. Although chewing tobacco and snuff are not smoked, they, too, are harmful. SEE: *risk factors; smokeless tobacco; smoking, passive.*

**tobramycin** (tō″brā-mī′sĭn) An antibiotic drug.

**tocainide** (tō-kāy′nīd) A lidocaine analogue used in treating ventricular arrhythmias. Trade name is Tonocard.

**toco-** Combining form indicating relationship to *labor* or *childbirth.*

**tocodynagraph** (tō″kō-dī′nă-grăf) [Gr. *tokos,* birth, + *dynamis,* power, + *graphein,* to write] A device for measuring the intensity of uterine contractions.

**tocodynamometer** (tō″kō-dī″năm-ŏm′ĕ-tĕr) [″ + *dynamis,* power, + *metron,* a measure] A device for estimating the force of uterine contractions in labor.

**tocograph** (tŏk′ō-grăf) [″ + *graphein,* to write] A device for estimating and recording the force of uterine contractions.

**tocography** (tō″kŏg′ră-fē) Recording the intensity of uterine contractions.

**tocology** (tō-kŏl′ō-jē) [″ + *logos,* word, reason] Science of parturition and obstetrics.

**tocolysis** (tō″kō-lī′sĭs) [″ + *lysis,* dissolution] Inhibition of uterine contractions. Drugs used for this include adrenergic agonists, magnesium sulfate, and ethanol.

**tocopherol** (tō-kŏf′ĕr-ŏl) [″ + *pherein,* to carry, + L. *oleum,* oil] Generic term for vitamin E (alpha-tocopherol) and a number of chemically related compounds, most of which have the biological activity of vitamin E.

**tocophobia** (tō″kō-fō′bē-ă) [″ + *phobos,* fear] An abnormal fear of childbirth.

**tocus** (tō′kŭs) [L.] Parturition; childbirth.

**toe** (tō) [AS. *ta*] A digit of the foot. SYN: *digit.* SEE: *foot* for illus.

***claw t.*** Hammertoe.

***dislocation of the t.*** Traumatic displacement of bones of a toe. This condition is treated essentially the same as dislocation of the finger. SEE: *finger, dislocation of.*

***fanning of t.'s*** Spreading of toes, esp. when the sole is stroked.

***Morton's t.*** Metatarsalgia.

***pigeon t.*** Walking with the toes turned inward.

***turf t.*** A hyperextension injury of the first metatarsophalangeal (MTP) joint. Severe hyperextension also injures the plantar sesamoids and flexor tendons. The injury commonly occurs on artificial surfaces such as astroturf, where the competitors wear light, flexible-soled shoes that allow MTP hyperextension on the firm surface.

***webbed t.'s*** Toes joined by webs of skin.

**toe clonus** Contraction of the big toe caused by sudden extension of the first phalanx.

**toe drop** Inability to lift the toes.

**toenail** (tō′nāl) Unguis. SEE: *nail.*

**toe reflex** A reflex in which strong flexion of the great toe flexes all the muscles below the knee.

**Togaviridae** [L. *toga,* coat, + *virus,* poison] A family of viruses that include the genus *Alphavirus*. They cause Western and Eastern equine encephalitis. Other Togaviridae include the rubiviruses (e.g., rubella virus).

**toilet** (toy′lĕt) [Fr. *toilette,* a little cloth] **1.** Cleansing of a wound after operation or of an obstetrical patient. **2.** An apparatus for use during defecation and urination to collect and dispose of these waste products. The disposal may be immediate by flushing with water, by chemical digestion, or by incineration.

**toilet training** Teaching a child to control urination and defecation until placed on a toilet. The bowel movements of an infant may habitually occur at the same time each day very early in life, but it is not advisable to begin to train the child until the end of the second year. Close to that time, placing the child on a small potty chair for a short period at regular intervals may allow the child to stay dry. First the diapers are removed while the child is awake. Later they are removed during naps and the child is told he or she should be able to stay dry. This schedule may need to be interrupted for a period if the child does not remain dry. Later on there will be no need for diapers during the day or night. To protect the bed, a rubber sheet should be used during the training period. Children who are unsuccessful in remaining dry or training their bowel habits should not be punished. To do so may promote the later development of enuresis or constipation.

**toko-** Toco-.

**tolazamide** (tŏl-ăz′ă-mīd) An oral hypoglycemia agent of the sulfonylurea class.

Caution: This drug should be used only in patients with non–insulin-dependent diabetes who cannot be treated with diet alone and who are unwilling or unable to take insulin if weight reduction and dietary control fail.

**tolazoline hydrochloride** (tŏl-ăz′ō-lēn) An alpha-adrenergic blocking agent used to produce peripheral vasodilation.

**tolbutamide** (tŏl-bū′tă-mīd) An oral hypoglycemic agent of the sulfonylurea class.

Caution: This drug should be used only in patients with non–insulin-dependent diabetes who cannot be treated with diet alone and who are unwilling or unable to take insulin if weight reduction and dietary control fail.

**tolerance** (tŏl′ĕr-ăns) [L. *tolerantia,* tolerance] Capacity for enduring a large amount of a substance (food, drug, or poison) without an adverse effect and showing a decreased sensitivity to subsequent doses of the same substance.

***drug t.*** The progressive decrease in the effectiveness of a drug.

***exercise t.*** The amount of physical activity that can be done under supervision before exhaustion.

***glucose t.*** The ability of the body to absorb and use glucose. SEE: *glucose tolerance test.*

***immunological t.*** A state of immunological inactivity or diminution so that an antigen that would ordinarily induce an immune response does not.

***pain t.*** The degree of pain an individual can withstand.

***radiation t.*** The level below which tissue radiation exposure will be least harmful. Some organs are less tolerant to radiation than others.

***tissue t.*** The ability of specific tissues to withstand the effects of ionizing radiation.

**tolerant** Capable of enduring or withstanding drugs without experiencing ill effects.

**tolerogen** (tŏl′ĕr-ō-jĕn) That which causes immunological tolerance or failure of the body to react to an antigen by forming an antibody. The mechanism of formation of this specific unresponsive state is poorly understood.

**tolerogenic** (tŏl″ĕr-ō-jĕn′ĭk) Producing immunological tolerance.

**tollwut** (tŏl-voot′) [Ger.] Rabies.

**tolnaftate** (tŏl-năf′tāt) A synthetic antifungal agent used topically in treating various forms of tinea.

**tolu balsam** A balsam obtained from *Myroxylon balsamum,* used as an expectorant.

**toluene** A hydrocarbon derived from coal tar.

**toluene poisoning** SEE: *benzene* in *Poisons*

*and Poisoning Appendix.*

**toluidine** (tŏl-ū′ĭ-dĭn) $C_7H_9N$. Aminotoluene, a derivative of toluene.

**tomaculous neuropathy** (tō-mā′cū-lŭs) [L. *tomaculum,* a kind of sausage] The presence of sausage-shaped areas of thickened myelin with secondary axon constriction in some cases of familial recurrent brachial neuropathy.

**tomatine** (tō′mă-tēn) A substance derived from tomato plants affected by wilt. It has antifungal action.

**-tome** Combining form meaning *cutting, cutting instrument.*

**tomo-** Combining form indicating *section, layer.*

**tomogram** (tō′mō-grăm) [Gr. *tome,* incision, + *gramma,* something written] The radiograph obtained during tomography.

**tomograph** (tō′mō-grăf) [″ + *graphein,* to write] An x-ray tube attached to a Bucky diaphragm by a rigid rod allowing rotation around a fixed point (fulcrum) during the radiographical exposure for tomography.

**tomography** (tō-mŏg′ră-fē) A radiographic technique that selects a level in the body and blurs out structures above and below that plane, leaving a clear image of the selected anatomy. This is accomplished by moving the x-ray tube in the opposite direction from the imaging device around a stationary fulcrum defining the plane of interest. Tube movements can be linear, curvilinear, circular, elliptical, figure eight, hypocycloidal, or trispiral. SYN: *body section radiography.*

***computed t.*** ABBR: CT. Tomography in which transverse planes of tissue are swept by a pinpoint radiographic beam and a computerized analysis of the variance in absorption produces a precise reconstructed image of that area. This technique has a greater sensitivity in showing the relationship of structures than conventional radiography.

***computerized axial t.*** ABBR: CAT. SEE: *magnetic resonance imaging; tomography, computed.*

***positron emission t.*** ABBR: PET. Reconstruction of brain sections by using positron-emitting radionuclides. By using several different radionuclides, researchers can measure regional cerebral blood flow, blood volume, oxygen uptake, and glucose transport and metabolism, and can locate neurotransmitter receptors. PET has been used with fludeoxyglucose F 18 to identify and localize regional lymph node metastases and to help assess response to therapy.

The images produced by PET are in colors that indicate the degree of metabolism or blood flow. The highest rates appear red, those lower appear yellow, then green, and the lowest rates appear blue. The images in various disease states may then be compared to those of normal subjects. SEE: illus.; *Alzheimer's disease, Parkinson's disease, and cerebrovascular accident* for illus.

***single photon emission computed t.*** ABBR: SPECT. A medical imaging method for reconstructing cross-sectional images of radiotracer distributions. It is used in diagnosing and treating stroke, dementia, and epilepsy, and in diagnosing heart and liver disease. SEE: *nuclear medicine scanning tests; positron emission t.*

**-tomy** Combining form meaning *cutting, incision.*

**tonaphasia** (tō″nă-fā′sē-ă) [L. *tonus,* a stretching, + *a-,* not, + *phasis,* speech] Inability to remember a tune owing to cerebral lesion.

**tone** (tōn) [L. *tonus,* a stretching] **1.** That state of a body or any of its organs or parts

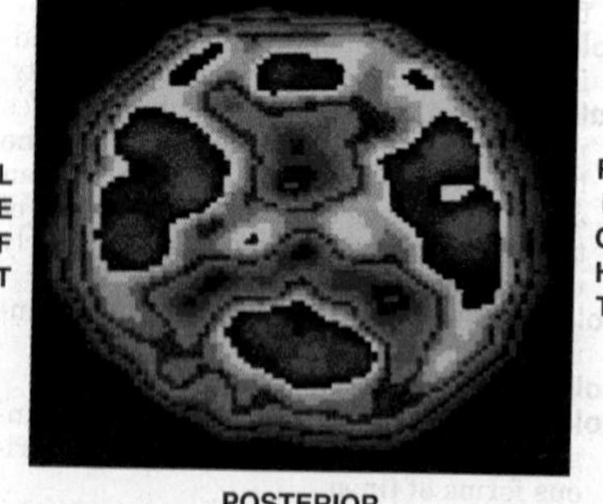


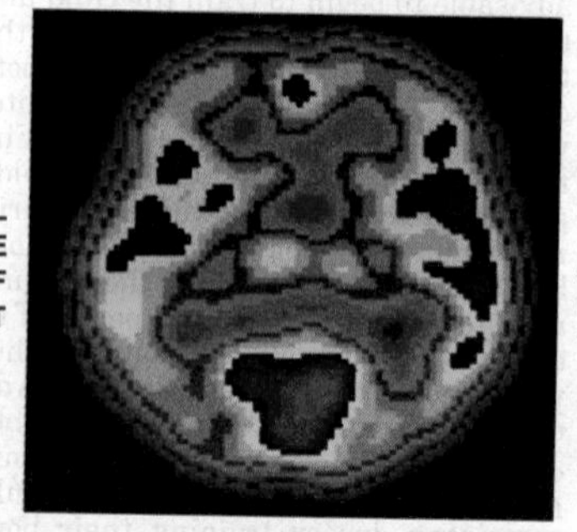


**PET SCAN OF BRAIN**

TRANSVERSE SECTION IN **(A)** NORMAL YOUNG PATIENT, **(B)** NORMAL AGING PATIENT

in which the functions are healthy and normal. In a more restricted sense, the resistance of muscles to passive elongation or stretch. **2.** Normal tension or responsiveness to stimuli, as of arteries or muscles, seen particularly in involuntary muscle (such as the sphincter of the urinary bladder). SYN: *tonicity* (2); *tonus*. **3.** A musical or vocal sound.

***muscular t.*** The state of slight contraction usually present in muscles that contributes to posture and coordination; the ability of a muscle to resist a force for a considerable period without change in length.

**tone deafness** The inability to detect differences in musical sounds. SYN: *amusia*.

**tongs, Crutchfield** SEE: *Crutchfield tongs*.

**tongue** (tŭng) [AS. *tunge*] A freely movable muscular organ lying partly in the floor of the mouth and partly in the pharynx. Its function is manipulation of food in mastication and deglutition, speech production, and taste. Its surface is covered with mucous membrane. SYN: *lingua*. SEE: illus.

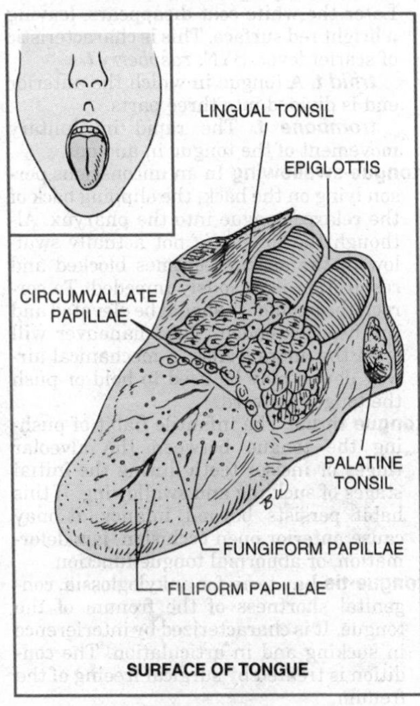


SURFACE OF TONGUE

ANATOMY: The tongue consists of a body and root and is attached by muscles to the hyoid bone below, the mandible in front, the styloid process behind, and the palate above, and by mucous membrane to the floor of the mouth, the lateral walls of the pharynx, and the epiglottis. A median fold, the frenulum linguae, connects the tongue to the floor of the mouth. The surface of the tongue bears numerous papillae of three types: filiform, fungiform, and vallate. Taste buds are present on the surfaces of many of the papillae, esp. the vallate papillae. Mucous and serous glands (lingual glands) are present, their ducts opening on the surface. Lymphoid tissue composing the lingual tonsils is present in the posterior third of the tongue. A median fibrous septum extends the entire length of the tongue.

*Arteries:* Lingual, exterior maxillary, and ascending pharyngeal. *Muscles:* Extrinsic muscles include genioglossus, hyoglossus, and styloglossus. Intrinsic muscles consist of four groups: superior, inferior, transverse, and vertical lingualis muscles. *Nerves:* Lingual nerve (containing fibers from trigeminal and facial nerves), glossopharyngeal, vagus, and hypoglossal.

DIFFERENTIAL DIAGNOSIS: Pain occurs in local lesions, fissures, glossitis, malignancies, and pernicious anemia. Protrusion and movement occur with very sick patients, as in advanced typhoid fever and toxemia. The tongue is tremulous in early typhoid and in meningitis. In chorea, it is thrust out suddenly and at once withdrawn. If it protrudes very slowly or is left exposed after being shown, it is a sign of great exhaustion, vascular congestion, or disorder of the nerve supply. If the tongue when protruded points to the right or left involuntarily, a central or peripheral lesion of the nerve supply is present. Some persons have the ability to curl the tongue along its long axis. This ability is genetically determined. When the tongue is thrust to one side and continually held in this position, hemiplegia is indicated. In hemiplegia, the tongue is turned toward the paralyzed side if the face is affected. If turned toward the unaffected side, it denotes a lesion of the medulla. Scars may be the result of injury or bulbar palsy causing ulceration. Spasm occurs in multiple sclerosis, general paresis, melancholia, and stuttering. Tremors are noted in asthenia, alcoholism, bulbar palsy, and Graves' disease. Tremulousness occurs in all acute diseases but is of no particular significance in chronic nervous disorders.

*Color:* The tongue may be temporarily discolored by a variety of colored medicines, foods, and liquids. *Black coating:* Glossophytia; this may be due to stain or presence of microphytes. In dysentery, this indicates impending death. The onset of jaundice is usually first detectable in the yellowish discoloration of the area under the tongue visualized when its tip is placed against the roof of the mouth. *Black hairy:* SEE: *hairy tongue*. *Bluish:* This denotes impaired circulation, interference with respiration, heart disease, asthma, or cyanosis. *Pale:* This indicates severe anemia. The tongue appears smaller than normal. *Red:* This is an early sign in typhoid fever. *Bright red:* This indicates glossitis or stomatitis. *Clean red:* With papillae prominent, or a white-coated tongue with papillae projecting through the fur, this indicates scarlatina. A red tip and edges, or having a red dry streak in the center, is typical of typhoid. *Strawberry:* White fur through which project bright red and prominent papillae is seen in the early stage of scarlet fever. *Yellow:* With thick fur covering the tongue, this indicates jaundice.

*Macroglossia:* A large tongue is generally congenital or may result from inflammation, Ludwig's angina, glossitis, actinomycosis, acromegaly, or myxedema. If localized, it may be due to gumma, carcinoma, or local trauma. *Microglossia:* A small tongue is observed in anemia, emaciation, and convalescence from typhoid. These conditions are temporary.

***bifid t.*** A tongue with a cleft at its anterior end. SYN: *cleft t.; forked t.*

***burning t.*** Burning sensation of the tongue. SYN: *glossopyrosis.*

***cleft t.*** Bifid t.

***coated t.*** A tongue covered with a layer of whitish or yellowish material consisting of desquamated epithelium, bacteria, or food debris. The significance of this is difficult to interpret. It may mean only that the patient slept with the mouth open or has not eaten because of loss of appetite. If darkly coated, it may indicate a fungus infection.

***deviation of t.*** Marked turning of the tongue from the midline when protruded, indicative of lesions of the hypoglossal nerve.

***dry t.*** A tongue that is dry and shriveled, usually indicative of dehydration. It may also be the result of mouth breathing.

***fern-leaf t.*** A tongue possessing a prominent central furrow and lateral branches.

***filmy t.*** A tongue possessing symmetrical whitish patches.

***fissured t.*** A tongue bearing deep furrows in its epithelium, which may be normal. Causes are obscure. If deep and inflamed, it may be due to syphilitic infection, dissecting glossitis, a broken tooth, chronic dysentery, hepatic disease, or diabetes mellitus.

***forked t.*** Bifid t.

***furred t.*** A coated tongue on which the surface epithelium appears as a coat of white fur. It is seen in nearly all fevers. Unilateral furring may result from disturbed innervation, as in conditions affecting the second and third branches of the fifth nerve. It has been noted in neuralgia of those branches and in fractures of the skull involving the foramen rotundum. Yellow fur indicates jaundice.

***geographic t.*** A tongue with white raised areas resembling mountain ranges on a relief map. Areas consist of heaped-up epithelium surrounding areas of atrophy.

***hairy t.*** A tongue covered with hairlike papillae entangled with threads produced by the fungus *Aspergillus niger* or *Candida albicans.* This condition is usually seen as the result of antibiotic therapy that inhibits growth of bacteria normally present in the mouth, permitting overgrowth of fungi. SYN: *glossotrichia; lingua nigra.*

***magenta t.*** A magenta-colored tongue seen in cases of riboflavin deficiency.

***parrot t.*** A dry shriveled tongue seen in typhus.

***raspberry t.*** Strawberry t.

***scrotal t.*** A furrowed and fissured tongue, resembling the skin of the scrotum. SEE: *fissured t.*

***smoker's t.*** Leukoplakia.

***smooth t.*** A condition of the tongue resulting from atrophy of papillae. It is characteristic of many conditions, such as anemia and malnutrition.

***strawberry t.*** A tongue that first has a white coat except at the tip and along the edges, with enlarged papillae standing out distinctly against the white surface. Later the white coat disappears, leaving a bright red surface. This is characteristic of scarlet fever. SYN: *raspberry t.*

***trifid t.*** A tongue in which the anterior end is divided into three parts.

***trombone t.*** The rapid involuntary movement of the tongue in and out.

**tongue-swallowing** In an unconscious person lying on the back, the slipping back of the relaxed tongue into the pharynx. Although the tongue is not actually swallowed, the airway becomes blocked and respiration is seriously impeded. To correct, the shoulders should be elevated and the head extended. This maneuver will open the airway. Also, a mechanical airway device may be used to hold or push the tongue forward.

**tongue thrust** The infantile habit of pushing the tongue between the alveolar ridges or incisor teeth during the initial stages of suckling and swallowing. If this habit persists beyond infancy, it may cause anterior open occlusion, jaw deformation, or abnormal tongue function.

**tongue-tie** Lay term for ankyloglossia, congenital shortness of the frenum of the tongue. It is characterized by interference in sucking and in articulation. The condition is treated by surgical freeing of the frenum.

**tonic** (tŏn′ĭk) [Gr. *tonikos,* from *tonos,* tone] **1.** Pert. to or characterized by tension or contraction, esp. muscular tension. **2.** Restoring tone. **3.** A medicine that increases strength and tone. Tonics are subdivided according to action, such as cardiac or general.

**tonicity** (tō-nĭs′ĭ-tē) [Gr. *tonos,* act of stretching] **1.** Property of possessing tone, esp. muscular tone. **2.** Tone (2).

**tonic labyrinthine reflex** In animals, the

postural reflex. In decerebrate humans, this reflex manifests as extension of the four extremities when the person is in a supine position with the head in midline.

**tonicoclonic** (tŏn″ĭ-kō-klŏn′ĭk) Tonoclonic.

**tonic spasm** A persistent, involuntary, firm or violent muscular contraction. SEE: *clonic spasm.*

**tonoclonic** (tŏn″ō-klŏn′ĭk) [″ + *klonos,* tumult] Both tonic and clonic, said of muscular spasms. SYN: *tonicoclonic.*

**tonofibril** (tŏn′ō-fī″brĭl) Tenofibril.

**tonofilament** (tŏn″ō-fĭl′ă-mĕnt) A filament of a tonofibril.

**tonogram** (tō′nō-grăm) [″ + *gramma,* something written] The record produced by a tonograph.

**tonograph** (tō′nō-grăf) [″ + *graphein,* to write] A recording tonometer.

**tonography** (tō-nŏg′ră-fē) The recording of changes in intraocular pressure.

**tonometer** (tōn-ŏm′ĕ-tĕr) [″ + *metron,* measure] An instrument for measuring tension or pressure, esp. intraocular pressure.

***Schiötz t.*** An instrument for measuring intraocular pressure by the degree of indentation produced by pressure on the cornea.

**tonometry** (tōn-ŏm′ĕ-trē) The measurement of tension of a part, as intraocular tension. This test is extremely useful in detecting glaucoma.

***analytical t.*** A technique used in blood gas analysis in which the liquid blood sample and its gas are held at equilibrium and the partial pressures of oxygen and carbon dioxide are measured.

***digital t.*** Determining intraocular pressure by use of the fingers.

***noncontact t.*** Determining intraocular pressure by measuring the degree of indentation of the cornea produced by a puff of air.

**tonoplast** (tŏn′ō-plăst) [″ + *plassein,* to form] The membrane surrounding an intracellular vacuole.

**tonsil** (tŏn′sĭl) [L. *tonsilla,* almond] **1.** A mass of lymphatic tissue located in depressions of the mucous membrane of the fauces and pharynx. **2.** A rounded mass on the inferior surface of the cerebellum lying lateral to the uvula.

FUNCTION: The tonsil produces lymphocytes and monocytes, and contains macrophages that phagocytize pathogens that get through the epithelium.

***cerebellar t.*** One of a pair of cerebellar lobules on either side of the uvula, projecting from the inferior surface of the cerebellum.

***faucial t.*** Palatine t.

***lingual t.*** A mass of lymphoid tissue located in the root of the tongue.

***Luschka's t.*** Pharyngeal t.

***nasal t.*** Lymphoid tissue on the nasal septum.

***palatine t.*** A mass of lymphoid tissue that lies in tonsillar fossa on each side of the oral pharynx between the glossopalatine and pharyngopalatine arches. The free surface of each tonsil is covered with stratified squamous epithelium that forms deep indentations or crypts extending into the substance of the tonsil. The lateral surface of each tonsil is covered with a firm fibrous capsule. Efferent lymph vessels convey lymph from the tonsil. SYN: *faucial t.*

***pharyngeal t.*** Lymphoid tissue on the roof of the posterior superior wall of the nasopharynx. SYN: *Luschka's t.* SEE: *adenoid.*

***tubal t.*** Lymphatic tissue present in the mucous membrane of the auditory tube near its opening into the pharynx.

**tonsilla** (tŏn-sĭl′ă) [L.] A general anatomical term for a small, discrete, rounded mass of tissue.

**tonsillar** (tŏn′sĭ-lăr) Pert. to a tonsil, esp. the faucial or palatine tonsil.

**tonsillar area** An area composed of the palatine arch, tonsillar fossa, glossopalatine sulcus, and posterior faucial pillar.

**tonsillar crypt** A deep indentation into the pharyngeal surface of a tonsil. It is lined with stratified epithelium.

**tonsillar fossa** A depression, located between the glossopalatine and pharyngopalatine arches, in which the palatine tonsil is situated.

**tonsillar ring** The almost complete ring of tonsillar tissue encircling the pharynx. It includes the palatine, lingual, and pharyngeal tonsils. SEE: *Waldeyer's ring.*

**tonsillar sinus** The space lying between the plica triangularis and the anterior surface of the palatine tonsil.

**tonsillectomy** (tŏn-sĭl-ĕk′tō-mē) [L. *tonsilla,* almond + Gr. *ektome,* excision] Surgical removal of the tonsils. SEE: *Nursing Diagnoses Appendix.*

NURSING IMPLICATIONS: *Preoperative:* The nurse explains the anesthetic methods and expected sensations to the adult patient. For children, the nurse explains the anesthetic methods and hospital routines in simple, nonthreatening language; permits the child to try on hospital garb; and shows the child the operating and recovery room areas as appropriate to age. Parents are encouraged to remain with the child.

*Postoperative:* A patent airway is maintained, and the patient is placed in a semiprone or sidelying position until he or she has fully recovered from anesthesia. Vital signs are monitored, and the patient is assessed for bleeding (excessive swallowing in a semiconscious child), restlessness, tachycardia, and pallor. After the patient's gag reflex has returned, water and nonirritating fluids are permitted by mouth. Deep breathing and turning help to prevent pulmonary complications. Ice packs are applied and analgesics administered as prescribed. The nurse encourages voice rest and instructs the patient not to clear the throat or cough, because this may precipitate bleeding. Written discharge instructions covering use of fluids and soft diet and avoidance of overactivity are provided to the patient and family. Within 5 to 10 days postoperatively, a white scab will form in the patient's throat; the patient or family should report any bleeding, ear discomfort, or persistent fever.

**tonsillitis** (tŏn-sĭl-ī'tĭs) [" + Gr. *itis,* inflammation] Inflammation of a tonsil, esp. the faucial tonsil. SEE: *Nursing Diagnoses Appendix.*

***acute parenchymatous t.*** Tonsillitis in which the entire tonsil is affected.

***acute t.*** Inflammation of the lymphatic tissue of the pharynx, esp. the palatine or faucial tonsils. It may occur sporadically or in epidemic form. Acute tonsillitis is usually self-limited, but serious complications such as sinusitis, otitis media, mastoiditis, or peritonsillar abscess may occur. SEE: *rheumatic fever.*

SYMPTOMS: The onset is sudden, usually accompanied by chills. The temperature may reach 105°F (40.6°C). Malaise, headache, pains and aches in the back and extremities, and pain in the tonsils, esp. when swallowing, may be present. The tonsils appear enlarged and red with yellowish exudate projecting from the crypts.

ETIOLOGY: This may be caused by a variety of organisms. If due to group A beta-hemolytic streptococci, sequelae such as rheumatic fever, carditis, and nephritis must be considered.

TREATMENT: General treatment includes bedrest, liquid diet, antipyretics, and hot saline or 30% glucose gargles or throat irrigations. The specific therapy involves the use of procaine penicillin or tetracycline drugs.

If the disease is thought to be due to group A beta-hemolytic streptococci, the throat should be cultured and then penicillin therapy instituted for a full 10-day course. If therapy was instituted before the report of the culture and the result is negative for these organisms, the penicillin therapy may be discontinued when clinical signs of infection have subsided.

If throat culture technique is not available and infection with group A beta-hemolytic streptococci is suspected, then a full 10-day course of penicillin should be given. This regimen may prevent rheumatic fever, rheumatic heart disease, or glomerulonephritis, which are rare but often serious immunological reactions following such infections. Administration of penicillin for fewer than 10 days when tonsillitis is due to group A beta-hemolytic streptococci is not advisable, even though clinical signs of infection may disappear within the first several days of treatment.

***follicular t.*** Tonsillitis in which the crypts are affected.

**tonsillolith** (tŏn'sĭl-ō-lĭth) [" + Gr. *lithos,* stone] A concretion within a tonsil. SYN: *amygdalolith.*

**tonsillopathy** (tŏn"sĭ-lŏp'ă-thē) Any disease of the tonsil.

**tonsilloscopy** (tŏn"sĭl-lŏs'kō-pē) [" + Gr. *skopein,* to examine] Inspection of the tonsils.

**tonsillotome** (tŏn-sĭl'ō-tōm) A surgical instrument used in tonsillectomy.

**tonsillotomy** (tŏn"sĭl-ŏt'ō-mē) [" + Gr. *tome,* incision] Incision of the tonsils.

**tonus** (tō'nŭs) [L., tension] The partial steady contraction of muscle that determines tonicity or firmness; the opposite of clonus. SYN: *tone; tonicity.*

**tooth** [AS. *toth*] One of the conical hard structures of the upper and lower jaws used for mastication. A tooth consists of a crown portion above the gum, a root portion embedded in a socket (alveolus) of the jaw bone, and a neck or cervical constricted region between the crown and root. The soft tissue gingiva covers the neck and root to a variable extent, depending on age and oral hygiene. The major portion of a tooth consists of dentin, which surrounds the pulp chamber in the crown and root of the tooth. Dentin is harder than bone. Enamel, the hardest tissue of the body, covers the crown. Cementum is similar to bone and covers the root, attaching the tooth to the surrounding bony socket by the periodontal ligament fibers embedded in both bone and cementum. The pulp cavity contains the dental pulp, a loose connective tissue containing many cells, nerves, and blood or lymph vessels. Each tooth has five surfaces: occlusal, medial, distal, lingual, and facial or buccal. SEE: illus.; *dentition; periodontal disease; plaque, dental; teeth; teeth, reimplantation or repair of; teeth, stained.*

***accessional t.*** The permanent molar tooth that arises without deciduous predecessors in the dental arch.

***anatomic t.*** An artificial tooth that duplicates the anatomical form of a natural tooth.

***baby t.'s*** Deciduous teeth.

***hypersensitive t.*** A tooth that is sensitive to temperature changes, sweets, or percussion. It may exhibit gingival recession, exposed root dentin, caries, or periodontal disease.

***impacted t.*** A tooth that is unable to erupt due to adjacent teeth or malposition of the tooth.

***implanted t.*** An artificial tooth implanted permanently into the jaw.

***t. surface*** The external aspect of a tooth. Each tooth has five surfaces, usually named for the adjacent tissue or space. The outer (facial) surface is called the *labial* surface for the incisors or canines, and the *buccal* surface for the premolars and molars. The inner surface of

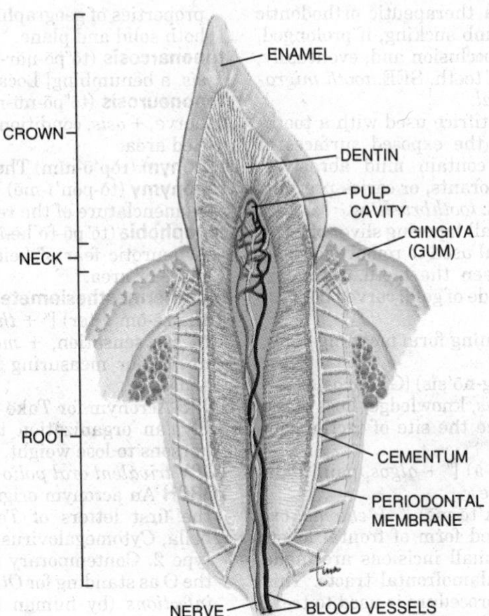


TOOTH STRUCTURE
(LONGITUDINAL SECTION)

each tooth is called the *lingual* (oral) surface. Within the arch, each tooth has a *mesial* surface, the side toward the midpoint in the front of the dental arch, and a *distal* surface, the side farthest from the midpoint in the front of the dental arch. The *occlusal* surface comes in contact with a tooth in the opposing jaw.

**toothache** Pain in a tooth or the region about a tooth. SYN: *dentalgia; odontalgia; odontodynia*.

**tooth bleaching** The application of chemical bleaching agents to teeth to make them whiter.

**toothbrushing** The act of cleaning the teeth by using a soft brush specifically designed for this purpose. The toothbrush consists of tufts of soft, synthetic fibers or natural bristles mounted in a handle that may be straight or angled for better access or brushing action. It is usually used with fluoride toothpaste (a mildly abrasive, flavored dentifrice) in a manner suggested by dentists and dental hygienists as being a suitable method for cleaning. The proper use of a toothbrush stimulates periodontal tissue. SEE: *hygiene, oral; periodontal disease; plaque, dental; teeth; tooth*.

Good oral hygiene, consisting of proper brushing of the teeth with a soft bristle brush, use of a fluoride-containing toothpaste, and daily use of dental floss, will help to prevent dental plaque. If brushing or flossing causes bleeding, pain, or irritation, a dentist should be seen without delay.

Some people with conditions that limit motion of their hands may have difficulty holding and using a toothbrush. This may be overcome by attaching the brush handle to the hand with a wide elastic band, or the handle may be enlarged by attaching a rubber or foam ball to it. Those with limited shoulder or elbow movement may find that lengthening the handle by attaching it to a long piece of wood or plastic is beneficial. In addition, an electric toothbrush may be of benefit.

Caution: If the toothbrush used has hard bristles or if any toothbrush is used too forcibly, gingival tissue may be eroded and damaged.

**tooth migration, pathological** Drifting or movement of teeth due to the pathological changes in areas adjacent to the moving teeth. SEE: *drift, mesial; tooth movement*.

**tooth migration, physiological** The natural and expected movement of teeth as growth and development occur. SEE: *drift, mesial; tooth migration, pathological; tooth movement*.

**tooth movement** The change in position of a tooth or teeth in the dental arch. This may be due to abnormal pressure from the tongue, pathological changes in tooth-supporting structures, malocclusion, missing teeth, or a therapeutic orthodontic procedure. Thumb sucking, if prolonged, may cause malocclusion and, eventually, displacement of teeth. SEE: *tooth migration, pathological.*

**toothpaste** A dentifrice used with a toothbrush to clean the exposed surfaces of teeth. It may contain mild abrasives, whiteners, deodorants, or caries-preventing agents. SEE: *toothbrushing.*

**toothpick** Any small tapering sliver of wood or other material used to remove food debris from between the teeth. Early examples were made of gold, carved bone, or ivory.

**top-, topo-** Combining form meaning *place, locale.*

**topagnosis** (tŏp″ăg-nō′sĭs) [Gr. *topos,* place, + *a,* not, + *gnosis,* knowledge] Loss of the ability to localize the site of tactile sensations.

**topalgia** (tō-păl′jē-ă) [″ + *algos,* pain] Pain in a localized site.

**topectomy** (tō-pĕk′tō-mē) [″ + *ektome,* excision] A modified form of frontal lobotomy in which small incisions are made through the thalamofrontal tracts. This psychosurgical procedure is used to treat certain mental diseases.

**topesthesia** (tŏp″ĕs-thē′zē-ă) [″ + *aisthesis,* sensation] The ability through tactile sense to determine that skin is touched. SYN: *topognosia.*

**tophaceous** (tō-fā′shŭs) [L. *tophaceus,* sandy] **1.** Relating to a tophus. **2.** Sandy or gritty.

**tophus** (tō′fŭs) *pl.* **tophi** [L., porous stone] **1.** A deposit of sodium biurate in tissues near a joint, in the ear, or in bone in gout. **2.** A salivary calculus. **3.** Tartar on the teeth.

**tophyperidrosis** (tŏf″ĭ-pĕr″ĭ-drō′sĭs) [Gr. *topos,* place, + *hyper,* above, + *hidros,* sweat] Excessive sweating in local areas.

**topical** [Gr. *topos,* place] Pert. to a definite surface area; local.

**topoalgia** (tō″pō-ăl′jē-ă) [″ + *algos,* pain] Localized pain, common in neurasthenia following emotional upsets.

**topoanesthesia** (tō″pō-ăn″ĕs-thē′zē-ă) [″ + *an-,* not, + *aisthesis,* sensation] Loss of the ability to recognize the location of a tactile sensation.

**topognosia, topognosis** (tō″pŏg-nō′sē-ă, -sĭs) [″ + *gnosis,* knowledge] Recognition of the location of a tactile sensation. SYN: *topesthesia.*

**topographical** (tŏp″ō-grăf′ĭk) [″ + *graphein,* to write] Pert. to description of special regions.

**topographical anatomy** A study of all the structures and their relationships in a given region (e.g., the axilla).

**topography** (tō-pŏg′ră-fē) Description of a part of the body.

**topology** (tō-pŏl′ō-jē) **1.** Topographical anatomy. **2.** In obstetrics, the relationship of the presenting fetal part to the pelvic outlet. **3.** In mathematics, the study of the properties of geographical configurations, both solid and plane.

**toponarcosis** (tō″pō-năr-kō′sĭs) [″ + *narkosis,* a benumbing] Local anesthesia.

**toponeurosis** (tō″pō-nū-rō′sĭs) [″ + *neuron,* nerve, + *osis,* condition] Neurosis of a limited area.

**toponym** (tŏp′ō-nĭm) The name of a region.

**toponymy** (tō-pŏn′ĭ-mē) [″ + *onoma,* name] Nomenclature of the regions of the body.

**topophobia** (tō″pō-fō′bē-ă) [″ + *phobos,* fear] A neurotic fear of being in a particular place or area.

**topothermesthesiometer** (tŏp″ō-thĕr″mĕs-thē-zē-ŏm′ĕ-ter) [″ + *therme,* heat, + *aisthesis,* sensation, + *metron,* measure] A device for measuring local temperature sense.

**TOPS** Acronym for *T*ake *O*ff *P*ounds *S*ensibly, an organization that assists obese persons to lose weight.

**TOPV** *trivalent oral polio vaccine.*

**TORCH** An acronym originally coined from the first letters of *T*oxoplasmosis, *R*ubella, *C*ytomegalovirus, and *H*erpesvirus type 2. Contemporary revisions describe the O as standing for *Other transplacental infections* (by human immunodeficiency virus, hepatitis B, human parvovirus, and syphilis). TORCH infections can attack a growing embryo or fetus and cause abortion, abnormal fetal development, severe congenital anomalies, mental retardation, and fetal or neonatal death.

**torcular herophili** (tor′kū-lăr) The confluence of sinuses at the internal occipital protuberance of the skull.

**toric** (tō′rĭk) Concerning a torus.

**tormina** (tor′mĭn-ă) *sing.,* **tormen** [L., twistings] Intestinal colic with griping pains.

**torose, torous** (tō′rōs, -rŭs) [L. *torosus,* full of muscle] Knobby or bulging; tubercular.

**torpent** (tor′pĕnt) [L. *torpens,* numbing] **1.** Medicine that modifies irritation. **2.** Not capable of functioning; dormant, apathetic, torpid.

**torpid** (tor′pĭd) [L. *torpidus,* numb] Not acting vigorously; sluggish.

**torpidity** (tor-pĭd′ĭ-tē) Sluggishness; inactivity.

**torpor** [L. *torpor,* numbness] Abnormal inactivity; dormancy; numbness; apathy.

***t. retinae*** Reduced sensitivity of retina to light stimuli.

**torque** (tork) [L. *torquere,* to twist] **1.** A force producing rotary motion. **2.** In dentistry, the application of force to rotate a tooth around its long axis.

**torr** (tor) The pressure of 1/760 of the standard atmospheric pressure. This is virtually equivalent to the pressure of 1 mm Hg.

**torrefaction** (tor″ĕ-făk′shŭn) [L. *torrefactio*] Roasting or parching something, esp. a drug, to dry it.

**torsade de pointes** Very rapid ventricular tachycardia characterized by a gradually changing QRS complex in the ECG. It is usually self-limiting but may change into ventricular fibrillation. SYN: *polymorphic ventricular tachycardia.*

**torsiometer** (tor″sē-ŏm′ĕ-tĕr) A device for measuring the rotation of the eyeball around the visual axis (i.e., its anterior-posterior axis).

**torsion** (tor′shŭn) [L. *torsio,* a twisting] **1.** The act of twisting or the condition of being twisted. **2.** In dentistry, the state of a tooth when rotated around its long axis. **3.** Rotation of the vertical meridians of the eye.

**torsionometer** (tor″shŭn-ŏm′ĕ-tĕr) [″ + Gr. *metron,* measure] A device for measuring the rotation of the vertebral column around the long axis.

**torsive** (tor′sĭv) Twisted, as in a spiral.

**torsiversion** (tor″sĭ-vĕr′zhŭn) Rotation of a tooth around its long axis.

**torso** (tor′sō) [It.] The trunk of the body.

**torsoclusion** (tor″sō-kloo′zhŭn) [″ + L. *occlusio,* to occlude] **1.** Acupressure in combination with torsion to stop a bleeding vessel. **2.** Malocclusion characterized by rotation of a tooth on its long axis.

**tort** A wrongful act or injury, committed by one person against another person or another person's property, that may be pursued in civil court by the injured party. The purpose of tort law is to make amends to the injured party, primarily through monetary compensation or damages.

***intentional t.*** An intentional wrongful act by a person who means to cause harm, or who knows or is reasonably certain that harm will result from the act.

***unintentional t.*** An unintended wrongful act against another person that produces injury or harm.

**torticollar** (tor″tĭ-kŏl′ăr) Concerning torticollis.

**torticollis** (tor″tĭ-kŏl′ĭs) [L. *tortus,* twisted, + *collum,* neck] A deformity of the neck secondary to shortening of neck muscles, which tilts the head to the affected side with the chin pointing to the other side. It may be congenital or acquired. The muscles affected are principally those supplied by the spinal accessory nerve. SYN: *wryneck.*

ETIOLOGY: The condition may be caused by scars, disease of cervical vertebrae, adenitis, tonsillitis, rheumatism, enlarged cervical glands, retropharyngeal abscess, or cerebellar tumors. It may be spasmodic (clonic) or permanent (tonic). The latter type may be due to Pott's disease (tuberculosis of the spine).

***fixed t.*** An abnormal position of the head owing to organic shortening of the muscles.

***intermittent t.*** Spasmodic t.

***ocular t.*** Torticollis from inequality in sight of the two eyes.

***rheumatic t.*** Symptomatic t.

***spasmodic t.*** Torticollis with recurrent but transient contractions of the muscles of the neck and esp. of the sternocleidomastoid. SYN: *intermittent t.*

TREATMENT: Botulinus toxin has been used experimentally with good results. The toxin inhibits the spastic contractions of the affected muscles. SEE: *toxin, botulinus.*

***spurious t.*** Torticollis from caries of the cervical vertebrae.

***symptomatic t.*** Rheumatic stiff neck. SYN: *rheumatic t.*

**tortipelvis** (tor″tĭ-pĕl′vĭs) [″ + *pelvis,* basin] Muscular spasms that distort the spine and hip. SYN: *dystonia musculorum deformans.*

**tortuous** (tor′choo-ŭs) [L. *tortuosus,* fr. *torqueo,* to twist] Having many twists or turns.

**torture** (tor′chūr) [LL. *tortura,* a twisting] Infliction of severe mental or physical pain by various methods, usually for the purpose of coercion.

**Torula** (tor′ū-lă) Former name of a genus of yeastlike organisms, now called *Cryptococcus.*

**toruloid** (tor′ū-loyd) [L. *torulus,* a little bulge, + Gr. *eidos,* form, shape] Beaded; noting an aggregate of colonies like those seen in the budding of yeast.

**toruloma** (tor-ū-lō′mă) [*Torula,* old name for Cryptococcus, + *oma,* tumor] The nodular lesion of cryptococcosis (torulosis).

**Torulopsis glabrata** A yeast of the family Cryptococcaceae, closely related to the *Candida* species. It is usually nonpathogenic for humans but may cause serious illness in immunocompromised patients no matter what the cause and in patients receiving immunosuppressive drugs, antibiotics, or corticosteroids.

**torulosis** (tor-ū-lō′sĭs) Cryptococcosis.

**torulus** (tor′ū-lŭs) [L. *torulus,* a little elevation] Papilla.

***t. tactiles*** A tactile cutaneous elevation on the palms and soles.

**torus** (tō′rŭs) *pl.* **tori** [L., swelling] A rounded elevation or swelling.

***t. mandibularis*** An exostosis that develops on the lingual aspect of the body of the mandible, perhaps transmitted as a genetic trait.

***t. palatinus*** A benign exostosis located in the midline of the hard palate. SYN: *palatine protuberance.*

**total allergy syndrome** The mistaken belief of some patients, and occasionally their medical advisers, that they are allergic to everything in their environment. Even though their symptoms resemble an allergic condition, the difficulty is most probably caused by acute or chronic emotional stress. These individuals may go to great lengths to isolate themselves from environmental materials. Treatment is difficult, but psychotherapy should be tried. This condition has also been termed "20th century syndrome."

**total hip replacement** Surgical procedure used in treating severe arthritis of the hip. Both the head of the femur and the acetabulum are replaced with synthetic components. SEE: *arthroplasty*.

NURSING IMPLICATIONS: *Preoperative:* The nurse determines the patient's knowledge of the procedure, postoperative care, and expected outcome and provides necessary information and corrects misconceptions. The nurse also teaches the patient about postoperative limitations, hip abduction methods, use of a trapeze, mobility regimen, gluteal and quadriceps setting, and triceps exercises. The importance of respiratory toilet is explained, and the proper technique taught. Prescribed antibiotics and other drugs are administered. Reports of laboratory and radiological studies are reviewed, and the physician is notified of any abnormal findings. The nurse teaches the patient pain evaluation and explains the availability of analgesics. Preoperative preparations are carried out (skin, gastrointestinal tract, urinary bladder, and premedication), and their significance is explained to the patient. The nurse encourages the patient to verbalize feelings and concerns.

*Postoperative:* Dressings and drainage devices are monitored for excessive bleeding, and the area beneath the buttocks is inspected for gravity pooling of drainage. Dressings are replaced or reinforced according to the surgeon's protocol and aseptic technique. Vital signs are monitored, and neurovascular status of the affected extremity is checked frequently. Analgesics are administered as prescribed and required, and the patient is evaluated for response. The patient is repositioned frequently in prescribed positions, and the integrity of all supportive equipment (splints, pillows, traction devices) is maintained during repositioning. The patient should avoid leg crossing and internal rotation, which enhance the potential for prosthesis dislocation and interfere with venous return. Respiratory status is assessed, and deep breathing and coughing are encouraged to prevent pulmonary complications. An exercise program and ambulation should begin as prescribed by the surgeon (type and extent of weight bearing on affected limb) and in collaboration with the physical therapist. Raised toilet seats and semireclining chairs are used to prevent hip flexion. A diet high in protein and vitamin C is provided, wound healing assessed, and skin breakdown prevented. Antiembolic devices are applied to the legs if prescribed, and the patient is assessed for such complications as thrombophlebitis, embolism, and dislocation. Discharge teaching focuses on the exercise regimen and activity limitations, stressing the importance of swimming and walking programs. Outpatient orthopedic follow-up and physical therapy are arranged as required. The patient should participate in a weight reduction program if necessary.

**total joint replacement** SEE: *knee, replacement of; total hip replacement; Nursing Diagnoses Appendix*.

**total parenteral nutrition** ABBR: TPN. The intravenous provision of total nutritional needs for a patient who is unable to take appropriate amounts of food enterally. For short-term support (7 to 10 days), peripheral total parenteral nutrition (TPN) using the smaller peripheral veins is the method of choice because there are fewer complications and there is a lower incidence of infection than with a central line. The disadvantage is that fewer calories can be delivered, although the use of lipid emulsions allows for 2000 to 2500 kcal per 24-hr delivery. The maximum concentration tolerated is less than 900 mOsm/kg.

With central TPN, patients have been maintained in a healthy state for prolonged periods with nutrients given through a catheter extending through the subclavian vein to the superior vena cava. Feedings of 1800 mOsm/kg are usually tolerated with the addition of calorie-rich lipid emulsions. The daily feeding of 2500 to 3000 kcal for an adult includes 2500 to 3000 ml of water; 100 to 130 g protein hydrolysate (amino acids) containing 12 to 18 g nitrogen; 525 to 625 g dextrose; 125 to 150 mEq sodium; 75 to 120 mEq potassium; 4 to 8 mEq magnesium; and vitamins A, D, E, and C, as well as thiamine, riboflavin, niacin, and pantothenic acid. Calcium, phosphorus, and iron are given as required; vitamins $B_{12}$ and K and folic acid are given intramuscularly as needed. Trace elements are required after 1 month of continuous TPN.

NURSING IMPLICATIONS: The procedure is explained to the patient, and a nutritional assessment is obtained. Intake and output are monitored and recorded. The nurse assists with catheter insertion and observes for adverse effects, documents procedure and initial fluid administration, and continues to monitor fluid intake. The catheter insertion site is inspected and redressed every 25 to 48 hr; a strict aseptic technique is used for this procedure. The condition of the site and position of the catheter are documented, and the catheter is evaluated for leakage; if present, this should be reported to the physician. Electrolytes are monitored. Vitamin supplements are administered as prescribed. The patient is observed for edema and dehydration. If diarrhea or nausea occurs, the infusion rate is slowed. Urine sugar and acetone tests are performed every 6 hr, and blood sugar levels are monitored as prescribed. Daily weights are obtained. The solution should never be discontinued abruptly but tapered off with isotonic glucose administered for several hours. In the event of catheter blockage or removal, the physician should be notified immediately. The nurse provides home-care instructions for the patient and family.

**totipotency** (tō″tē-pō′tĕn-sē) The ability of a cell to develop into any of the various types of cell, tissue, or complex structure present in the body.

**totipotent** (tō-tĭp′ō-tĕnt) [L. *totus*, all, + *potentia*, power] In embryology, the ability of a cell or group of cells to produce all of the tissues required for human development (i.e., the embryonic membranes, the embryo, and finally the fetus).

**touch** (tŭch) [O. Fr. *tochier*] **1.** To perceive by the tactile sense; to feel with the hands, to palpate. **2.** The sense by which pressure on the skin or mucosa is perceived; the tactile sense. **3.** Examination with the hand. SYN: *palpation*.

Various disorders may disturb or impair the tactile sense or the ability to feel normally. There are a number of words and suffixes pert. to sensation and its modifications. A few of the more important ones are as follows: algesia, -algia, anesthesia, dysesthesia, -dynia, esthesia, esthesioneurosis, hyperesthesia, paresthesia, and synesthesia.

***abdominal t.*** Palpation of the abdomen.

***after-t.*** Persistence of the sensation of touch after contact with stimulus has ceased.

***double t.*** Vaginal and rectal examination made at the same time.

***rectal t.*** Digital examination of the rectum.

***vaginal t.*** Digital examination of the vagina.

***vesical t.*** Digital examination of the bladder.

**tour de maître** (toor″ dĕ mā-tr′) [Fr., the master's turn] A method of introducing a catheter or sound into the male bladder or into the uterus. This involves very carefully turning and angulating the device so as to follow the curvature of the passageway.

**Tourette's syndrome** [Georges Gilles de la Tourette, Fr. neurologist, 1857–1904] A rare condition of unknown etiology that begins in childhood and may continue throughout life. It is thought to be a neurological rather than a psychiatric disease. The syndrome, which occurs three times more frequently in boys than in girls, is estimated to affect 0.1 to 0.5 per thousand in the U.S. Symptoms include lack of muscle coordination, involuntary purposeless movements, tics, and incoherent grunts and barks that may represent stifled obscenities. At puberty, some victims begin to experience attacks of coprolalia and involuntary swearing. This aspect of the condition complicates social adjustment. Certain drugs, including haloperidol and clonidine, have produced dramatic improvement in some patients. SYN: *Gilles de la Tourette's syndrome*. SEE: *tic*.

**Tournay's sign** (tūr-nāz′) [Auguste Tournay, Fr. ophthalmologist, 1878–1969] Dilatation of the pupil of the eye on unusually strong lateral fixation.

**tourniquet** (toor′nĭ-kĕt) [Fr., a turning instrument] Any constrictor used on an extremity to apply pressure over an artery and thereby control bleeding; also used to distend veins to facilitate venipuncture or intravenous injections.

*Arterial hemorrhage:* The tourniquet is applied between the wound and the heart, close to the wound, placing a hard pad over the point of pressure. This should be discontinued as soon as possible and a tight bandage substituted under the loosened tourniquet. SEE: *bleeding, arterial* for table.

Caution: A tourniquet should never be left in place too long. Ordinarily, it should be released from 12 to 18 min after application to determine whether bleeding has ceased. If it has, the tourniquet is left loosely in place so that it may be retightened if necessary. If bleeding has not ceased, it should be retightened at once. In general, a tourniquet should not be used if steady firm pressure over the bleeding site will stop the flow.

***rotating t.*** The application of blood pressure cuffs to three extremities; used in certain types of medical emergencies, such as acute pulmonary edema, to reduce the return of blood to the heart. The patient is placed in a head-high position (Fowler's). The pressure is kept midway between systolic and diastolic. Every 10 min, the cuffs are deflated and when inflated, the previously free extremity is now used. This allows each extremity to be free of a tourniquet for 10 min out of each 40-min cycle. Obviously, a cuff would not be applied to an extremity into which an intravenous infusion is running.

**tourniquet paralysis** Nerve injury caused by leaving a tourniquet on too long or too tightly.

**tourniquet test** A test for determining the ability of capillaries to withstand increased pressure. SEE: illus.

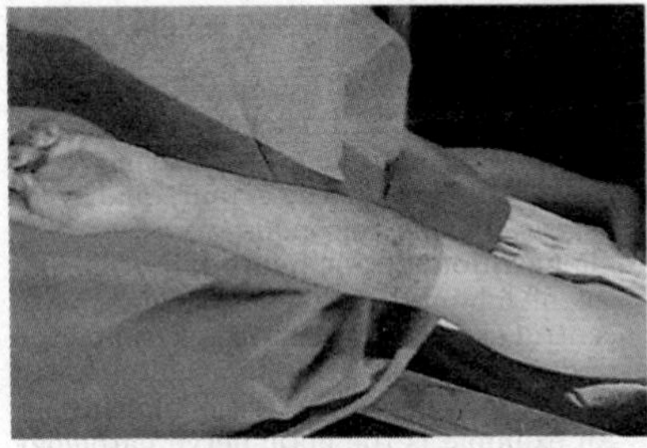

TOURNIQUET TEST
POSITIVE TEST FOR IDIOPATHIC THROMBOCYTOPENIC PURPURA

**Touton cell** (toot′ŏn) [Karl Touton, Ger. dermatologist, 1858–1934] A giant multinucleated cell found in lesions of xanthomatosis.

**towelette** (tow″ĕl-ĕt′) [ME. *towelle,* towel] A small towel for surgical or obstetrical use.

**tox-** SEE: *toxi-*

**toxanemia** (tŏks″ă-nē′mē-ă) [Gr. *toxikon,* poison, + *an-,* not, + *haima,* blood] Anemia due to a hemolytic toxin.

**toxemia** (tŏk-sē′mē-ă) [″ + Gr. *haima,* blood] Distribution throughout the body of poisonous products of bacteria growing in a focal or local site, thus producing generalized symptoms.

SYMPTOMS: The condition is marked by fever, diarrhea, vomiting, quickened or depressed pulse and respiration, and shock. In tetanus, the nervous system is esp. affected; in diphtheria, nerves and muscles are affected. **toxemic** (-mĭk), *adj.*

***alimentary t.*** Illness due to absorption of bacterial or other toxins from the gastrointestinal tract.

***eclamptogenic t.*** T. of pregnancy.

***t. of pregnancy*** Previously used term for pregnancy-induced hypertension. SEE: *eclampsia; pre-eclampsia; Nursing Diagnoses Appendix.*

**toxenzyme** (tŏks-ĕn′zīm) [″ + Gr. *en,* in, + *zyme,* leaven] A poisonous enzyme.

**toxi-, tox-, toxo-** Combining form meaning *poison.*

**toxic-** SEE: *toxico-.*

**toxic** (tŏks′ĭk) [Gr. *toxikon,* poison] Pert. to, resembling, or caused by poison. SYN: *poisonous.*

**toxic-allergic syndrome** A disease characterized by toxic-allergic pneumonopathy, with respiratory distress, fever, headache, nausea, myalgia, abdominal pains, rash, hepatosplenomegaly, and eosinophilia. This syndrome is caused by ingestion of rapeseed oil adulterated with aniline and containing acetanilide. There is no specific therapy, but mechanically assisted respiratory therapy and corticosteroids are helpful.

**toxicant** (tŏks′ĭ-kănt) [L. *toxicans,* poisoning] **1.** Poisonous; toxic. **2.** Any poison.

**toxicemic** Toxemic.

**toxic erythema** Redness of the skin or a rash resulting from toxic agents such as drugs.

**toxicide** (tŏks′ĭ-sīd) [Gr. *toxikon,* poison, + L. *cidus,* kill] **1.** Destructive to toxins. **2.** A chemical antidote for poisons.

**toxicity** (tŏks-ĭs′ĭ-tē) The extent, quality, or degree of being poisonous.

**toxic-nutritional optic neuropathy** The onset of bilateral visual impairment with central scotomas, occurring over a period of days or weeks. This is usually associated with a toxic or nutritional disorder. An example is the optic nerve pathology caused by ingestion of methyl alcohol.

**toxico-, toxic-** [Gr. *toxikon,* poison] Combining form meaning *poisonous.*

**Toxicodendron** (tŏk″sĭ-kō-dĕn′drŏn) A genus of plants that includes poison ivy and poison oak.

**toxicoderma** (tŏks″ĭ-kō-dĕr′mă) [″ + *derma,* skin] Any skin disease resulting from a poison. SYN: *toxicodermatosis; toxidermitis.*

**toxicodermatitis** (tŏks″ĭ-kō-dĕrm-ă-tī′tĭs) [″ + ″ + *itis,* inflammation] Inflammation of the skin caused by a poison.

**toxicodermatosis** (tŏks″ĭ-kō-dĕrm-ă-tō′sĭs) [″ + ″ + *osis,* condition] Toxicoderma.

**toxicogenic** (tŏks″ĭ-kō-jĕn′ĭk) [″ + *gennan,* to produce] Caused by, or producing, a poison.

**toxicoid** (tŏks′ĭ-koyd) [″ + *eidos,* form, shape] Of the nature of a poison.

**toxicologist** (tŏks″ĭ-kŏl′ō-jĭst) [″ + *logos,* word, reason] A specialist in the field of poisons or toxins.

**toxicology** (tŏks″ĭ-kŏl′ō-jē) Division of medical and biological science concerned with toxic substances, detecting them, studying their chemistry and pharmacological actions, and establishing antidotes and treatment of toxic manifestations, prevention of poisoning, and methods for controlling exposure to harmful substances.

**toxicopathy** (tŏks″ĭ-kŏp′ă-thē) [″ + *pathos,* disease, suffering] Any disease caused by a poison.

**toxicophidia** (tŏk″sĭ-kō-fĭd′ē-ă) [″ + Gr. *ophis,* snake] Poisonous snakes. SYN: *thanatophidia.*

**toxicophobia** (tŏks″ĭ-kō-fō′bē-ă) [″ + *phobos,* fear] An abnormal fear of being poisoned by any medium: food, gas, water, or drugs.

**toxicosis** (tŏks″ĭ-kō′sĭs) [″ + *osis,* condition] A disease resulting from poisoning.

***endogenic t.*** A disease due to poisons generated within the body. SYN: *autointoxication.*

***exogenic t.*** Any toxic condition resulting from a poison not generated in the body.

***retention t.*** Toxicosis from retained products that normally are excreted shortly after formation.

**toxic shock-like syndrome** ABBR: TSLS. An infection in which the initial site is skin or soft tissue. This may occur in adults or children and it is readily transmitted from person to person. Typically there is a history of a minor usually nonpenetrating local trauma that within the next 1 to 3 days develops into the usual toxic shock syndrome (TSS) caused by a toxin elaborated by certain strains of *Staphylococcus aureus.* SEE: *toxic shock syndrome.*

**toxic shock syndrome** ABBR: TSS. A rare and sometimes fatal disease caused by a toxin or toxins produced by certain strains of the bacterium *Staphylococcus aureus.* SEE: *Nursing Diagnoses Appendix.*

INCIDENCE: The disease has occurred in young menstruating women, most of whom were using vaginal tampons for menstrual protection. About one half of the total cases reported occur in men, menstruating women who are not using tampons, and women who do not menstruate. Toxic shock syndrome has also occurred in patients with streptococcal infections. SEE: *streptococcal t.s.s.*

DIAGNOSIS: The diagnosis is made when the following criteria are met: fever of 102°F (38.9°C) or greater; diffuse macular erythematous rash followed in 1 or 2 weeks by desquamation, particularly of the palms and soles; hypotension or orthostatic syncope; and involvement of three or more of the following organ systems: gastrointestinal (vomiting or diarrhea at the onset of illness), muscular (severe myalgia), mucous membrane (vaginal, oropharyngeal, or conjunctival hyperemia), renal, hepatic, hematological (platelets less than 100,000/cu mm), and central nervous system (disorientation or alteration in consciousness without focal neurological signs when fever and hypotension are absent). In addition, the following are helpful in diagnosis: negative results on blood, throat, or cerebrospinal fluid culture; possible positive result on blood culture for *Staphylococcus aureus;* and no rise in titer to tests for Rocky Mountain spotted fever, leptospirosis, or rubeola.

Caution: Anyone who develops these symptoms and signs should seek medical attention immediately. If a tampon is being used, it should be removed at once.

TREATMENT: Beta-lactamase–resistant antimicrobials should be given, as well as immediate therapy for shock and renal failure, if present.

***streptococcal t.s.s.*** A syndrome similar to toxic shock syndrome but caused by group A streptococcus. Procedures such as suction lipectomy, hysterectomy, vaginal delivery, bunionectomy, and bone pinning may provide a portal of entry, but this is undetermined in approx. half the cases. SEE: *toxic shock syndrome.*

**toxic substance** Any substance that can cause acute or chronic injury to the human body or that is suspected of being able to cause disease or injury under some conditions. In the U.S., the National Institute of Occupational Safety and Health (NIOSH) publishes a registry of toxic chemicals. SEE: *hazardous material; health hazard; permissible exposure limits; right-to-know law.*

**toxidermitis** (tŏks″ĭ-dĕr-mī′tĭs) [″ + *derma,* skin, + *itis,* inflammation] Toxicoderma.

**toxigenic** (tŏks″ĭ-jĕn′ĭk) [″ + *gennan,* to produce] Producing toxins or poisons.

**toxigenicity** (tŏks″ĭ-jĕn-ĭs′ĭ-tē) The virulence of a toxin-producing pathogenic organism.

**toxin** (tŏks′ĭn) [Gr. *toxikon,* poison] A poisonous substance of animal or plant origin. SEE: *antitoxin; phytotoxin; toxoid.*

***bacterial t.*** A toxin produced by bacteria, including exotoxins, which diffuse from bacterial cells into the surrounding medium, and endotoxins, the cell walls of gram-negative bacteria, which remain toxic after the bacteria have been destroyed. SEE: *bacteria.*

***botulinus t.*** A neurotoxin that blocks acetylcholine release, produced by *Clostridium botulinum,* the causative organism for botulism. Seven types of the toxin have been identified.

***dermonecrotic t.*** Any one of a group of different toxins that can cause necrosis of the skin. Coagulase-positive *Staphylococcus aureus* produce several such toxins. SEE: *Kawasaki disease; scalded skin syndrome, staphylococcal; toxic shock syndrome.*

***Dick t.*** An erythrogenic toxin produced by some streptococci. SYN: *erythrogenic t.*

***diphtheria t.*** The specific toxin produced by *Corynebacterium diphtheriae.*

***dysentery t.*** The exotoxin of various species of *Shigella.*

***erythrogenic t.*** Dick t.

***extracellular t.*** Exotoxin.

***intracellular t.*** Endotoxin.

***plant t.*** Any toxin produced by a plant; a phytotoxin.

**toxin-antitoxin** (tŏks′ĭn-ăn″tĭ-tŏks′ĭn) [Gr. *toxikon,* poison, + *anti,* against, + *toxikon,* poison] ABBR: T.A.T. Diphtheria toxin with its antitoxin in a nearly neutral mixture, the diphtheria toxin being about 85% neutralized; used for immunization against diphtheria.

**toxinicide** (tŏks-ĭn′ĭs-īd) [″ + *cidus,* kill] That which is destructive to toxins.

**toxinosis** (tŏk″sĭ-nō′sĭs) [″ + Gr. *osis,* condition] Any disease or condition caused by a toxin.

**toxipathy** (tŏks-ĭp′ă-thē) [″ + Gr. *pathos,* disease, suffering] Any disease caused by poison.

**toxiphobia** (tŏks″ĭ-fō′bē-ă) [″ + Gr. *phobos,* fear] An abnormal fear of being poisoned.

**toxisterol** (tŏk-sĭs′tĕr-ŏl) A toxic derivative obtained by radiating ergosterol.

**toxitherapy** (tŏks″ĭ-thĕr′ă-pē) [″ + Gr. *therapeia,* treatment] The use of toxins in treatment of disease (e.g., the use of botulinum toxin injected locally to treat certain eye muscle imbalance conditions and to treat spasmodic torticollis).

**toxituberculid** (tŏks″ĭ-tū-bĕr′kū-lĭd) A skin lesion resulting from the action of a toxin produced by *Mycobacterium tuberculosis.*

**toxo-** SEE: *toxi-.*

**toxocariasis** (tŏks″ō-kăr-ī′ă-sĭs) [″ + *kara,* head, + *-iasis,* condition] A self-limiting disease due to infection with nematode worms *Toxocara canis* or *T. cati.* In humans, the eggs penetrate the bowel wall and enter the circulation. Larvae may be carried to any part of the body where the blood vessel is large enough to accommodate them. They may end up in the brain, retinal vessels, liver, lung, or heart. The larvae cause hemorrhage, inflammation, and necrosis in these tissues. Thus the patient may have myocarditis, endophthalmitis, epilepsy, or encephalitis. Diagnosis is made by immunological tests and by the presence of larvae in tissue obtained by liver biopsy. It is important that toxocariasis be considered in cases diagnosed as retinoblastoma. SYN: *visceral larva migrans.*

**toxogenin** (tŏks-ŏj'ĕn-ĭn) [Gr. *toxikon,* poison, + *gennan,* to produce] Hypothetical substance in the blood caused by injection of antigens, innocuous in itself, but causing anaphylaxis on addition of fresh antigen.

**toxoid** (tŏks'oyd) [" + *eidos,* form, shape] A toxin that has been treated to destroy its toxicity but is still capable of inducing formation of antibodies on injection. SYN: *anatoxin.*

***alum-precipitated t.*** Toxoid of diphtheria or tetanus precipitated with alum.

***diphtheria t.*** Diphtheria toxin detoxified by formaldehyde treatment.

***tetanus t.*** SEE: *tetanus toxoid.*

**toxolecithin** (tŏks"ō-lĕs'ĭ-thĭn) [" + *lekithos,* egg yolk] A compound of lecithin with a toxin such as certain snake venoms.

**toxolysin** (tŏks-ŏl'ĭ-sĭn) [" + *lysis,* dissolution] A substance that destroys toxins. SYN: *antitoxin; toxicide.*

**toxomucin** (tŏks"ō-mū'sĭn) [" + L. *mucus,* mucus] Specific toxic albuminoid from cultures of tubercle bacilli.

**toxonosis** (tŏks"ō-nō'sĭs) [" + *osis,* condition] Toxicosis.

**toxopeptone** (tŏks"ō-pĕp'tōn) [" + *pepton,* digesting] A protein derivative produced by action of a toxin on peptones.

**toxophil(e)** (tŏks'ō-fĭl, -fīl) [" + *philein,* to love] Having a special affinity for toxins.

**toxophilic** (tŏk"sō-fĭl'ĭk) [" + *philein,* to love] Concerning a toxophile.

**toxophore** (tŏks'ō-for) [" + *phoros,* a bearer] The portion of a toxin that gives the toxin its poisonous qualities.

**toxophorous** (tŏk-sŏf'ō-rŭs) Concerning a toxophore.

**toxophylaxin** (tŏks"ō-fī-lăks'ĭn) [" + *phylax,* guard] A substance that neutralizes bacterial toxins.

**Toxoplasma** (tŏks"ō-plăs'mă) A genus of protozoa.

***T. gondii*** The causative agent of toxoplasmosis.

**toxoplasmin** (tŏk"sō-plăs'mĭn) An antigen obtained from mouse peritoneal fluid infected with *Toxoplasma gondii.*

**toxoplasmosis** (tŏks-ō-plăs-mō'sĭs) A disease caused by infection with the protozoan *Toxoplasma gondii.* The organism is found in many mammals and birds. Symptoms may be so mild as to be barely noticeable or may be more severe with lymphadenopathy, malaise, muscle pain, and little if any fever. The severe disseminated form produces pneumonitis, hepatitis, and encephalitis. In the congenital form, destructive lesions of the central nervous system, jaundice, anemia, and generalized lymphadenopathy usually are present. In AIDS patients, dormant protozoa may become active and contribute to brain deterioration. Diagnosis is by identification of culture of the organism and by serological test.

TREATMENT: Although treatment is not entirely satisfactory, trisulfapyrimidines or pyrimethamine and sulfadiazine are indicated. The latter combination is less toxic if folinic acid is given with each dose. This therapy helps prevent bone marrow depression. Pregnant women may be treated with spiramycin to prevent placental infections.

**Toynbee maneuver** [Joseph Toynbee, Brit. physician, 1815–1866] Changing the pressure within the middle ear by swallowing or blowing while the nose is pinched closed and the mouth is tightly shut. This maneuver is used to "clear the ears" when quickly changing altitude, as in an airplane flight.

In some cases, the effect of this maneuver may be enhanced by tilting the head backward while it is done. This places tension on the tensor tympani muscle and helps to open the eustachian tubes. SEE: *Valsalva's maneuver.*

**TPA** *total parenteral alimentation; tissue plasminogen activator.*

**T.P.I. test** *Treponema pallidum immobilizing test* (for syphilis).

**TPN** *triphosphopyridine nucleotide; total parenteral nutrition.*

**TPR** *temperature, pulse, respiration.*

**tr** L. *tinctura,* tincture.

**trabecula** (tră-bĕk'ū-lă) *pl.* **trabeculae** [L., a little beam] **1.** The fibrous cord of connective tissue that serves as supporting fiber by forming a septum that extends into an organ from its wall or capsule. **2.** The network of osseous tissue that makes up the cancellous structure of a bone.

***t. carnea cordis*** Any of the thick muscular tissue bands attached to the inner walls of the ventricles of the heart. SYN: *columna carnea.*

**trabecular** (tră-bĕk'ū-lăr) Concerning a trabecula.

**trabecularism** (tră-bĕk'ū-lăr-ĭzm) The condition of having a trabecular structure.

**trabeculate** (tră-bĕk'ū-lāt) Having trabeculae.

**trabeculoplasty** Surgical procedure on the trabecular meshwork of the eye. This procedure is used to allow the escape of aqueous humor in the treatment of glaucoma. SEE: *glaucoma.*

**trabs** (trăbz) *pl.* **trabes** [L., a beam] A supporting band.

***t. cerebri*** An arched band of white fibers connecting the cerebral hemispheres. SYN: *corpus callosum.*

**trace** (trās) [O. Fr. *tracier*] **1.** A very small

quantity. **2.** A visible mark or sign.

***primitive t.*** A pale white streak in the germinal area indicating the beginning of the development of the blastoderm. SYN: *primitive streak.*

**trace element** An organic element normally found in minute quantities in foods and tissues (e.g., aluminum, bromine, chromium, cobalt, copper, fluorine, iron, iodine, manganese, nickel, silicon, zinc, and other rare minerals).

**tracer** A radioactive isotope, capable of being incorporated into compounds, that when introduced into the body "tags" a specific portion of the molecule so that its course may be traced. This is used in absorption and excretion studies, in identification of intermediary products of metabolism, and in determination of distribution of various substances in the body. Radioactive carbon ($^{14}C$), calcium ($^{42}Ca$), and iodine ($^{131}I$) are examples of tracers commonly used. SEE: *label.*

**trachea** (trā'kē-ă) *pl.* **tracheae** [Gr. *tracheia,* rough] A cylindrical cartilaginous tube, 4½ in. (11.3 cm) long, from the larynx to the primary bronchi. It extends from the sixth cervical to the fifth dorsal vertebra, where it divides at a point called the carina into two bronchi, one leading to each lung. The mucosa is made of ciliated epithelium that sweeps mucus, trapped dust, and pathogens upward. SYN: *windpipe.* SEE: *bronchi.*

**tracheaectasy** (trā"kē-ă-ĕk'tă-sē) [Gr. *tracheia,* rough, + *ektasis,* dilatation] Dilatation of the trachea.

**tracheal** (trā'kē-ăl) Pert. to the trachea.

**trachealgia** (trā"kē-ăl'jē-ă) [" + *algos,* pain] Pain in the trachea.

**trachealis** (trā"kē-ā'lĭs) [L.] A muscle composed of smooth muscle fibers that extends between the ends of the tracheal rings. Its contraction reduces the size of the lumen.

**tracheal tickle** A maneuver designed to elicit a reflex cough.

**tracheal tugging** A slight downward movement of the trachea with each inspiratory effort due to descent of the diaphragm in a person with a low, flat diaphragm.

**tracheitis** (trā"kē-ī'tĭs) [Gr. *tracheia,* rough, + *itis,* inflammation] An inflammation of the trachea. It may be acute or chronic and may be associated with bronchitis and laryngitis. SYN: *trachitis.*

NURSING IMPLICATIONS: Vital signs are monitored, and the patient is assessed for fever and acute airway obstruction (croupy cough, stridor) due to the presence of copious, thick, and purulent secretions. Humidified oxygen is administered as prescribed, and suctioning is performed as necessary to remove secretions. Antibiotics are administered as prescribed. If airway obstruction persists, emergency endotracheal intubation or tracheostomy is performed. The nurse provides comfort to the patient to reduce anxiety.

**trachelectomopexy** (trā"kĕ-lĕk'tŏm-ō-pĕk"sē) [" + *ektome,* excision, + *pexis,* fixation] Fixation of the uterine neck with partial excision.

**trachelectomy** (trā"kĕl-ĕk'tō-mē) [" + *ektome,* excision] Amputation of the cervix uteri.

**trachelematoma** (trā"kĕl-ĕm"ă-tō'mă) [" + *haima,* blood, + *oma,* tumor] A hematoma situated on the neck.

**trachelism, trachelismus** (trā'kĕ-lĭzm, trā-kĕ-lĭz'mŭs) [" + *-ismos,* condition] Backward spasm of the neck, sometimes preceding an epileptic attack.

**trachelitis** (trā-kĕ-lī'tĭs) [" + *itis,* inflammation] Inflammation of the mucous membrane of the cervix uteri. SYN: *cervicitis.*

**trachelo-** Combining form meaning *neck.*

**trachelobregmatic** (trā"kĕ-lō-brĕg-măt'ĭk) [Gr. *trachelos,* neck, + *bregma,* front of the head] Pert. to the neck and the bregma.

**trachelocele** (trăk'ĕ-lō-sēl) [" + *kele,* tumor, swelling] Tracheocele.

**trachelocyrtosis** (trā"kĕ-lō-sĭr-tō'sĭs) [" + *kyrtos,* curved, + *osis,* condition] Trachelokyphosis.

**trachelocystitis** (trā"kĕl-ō-sĭs-tī'tĭs) [" + *kystis,* bladder, + *itis,* inflammation] Inflammation of the neck of the bladder.

**trachelodynia** (trā"kĕ-lō-dĭn'ē-ă) [" + *odyne,* pain] Pain in the neck.

**trachelokyphosis** (trā"kĕl-ō-kī-fō'sĭs) [" + *kyphosis,* humpback] Excessive anterior curvature of cervical portion of spine. SYN: *trachelocyrtosis.*

**trachelology** (trā"kĕ-lŏl'ō-jē) [" + *logos,* word, reason] Scientific study of the neck, its diseases, and its injuries.

**trachelomastoid** (trā"kĕ-lō-măs'toyd) [" + *mastos,* breast, + *eidos,* form, shape] A muscle of the neck. SEE: *Muscles Appendix.*

**trachelomyitis** (trā"kĕ-lō-mī-ī'tĭs) [" + *mys,* muscle, + *itis,* inflammation] Inflammation of the muscles of the neck.

**trachelopexy** (trā'kĕl-ō-pĕks"ē) [" + *pexis,* fixation] Surgical fixation of the cervix uteri to an adjacent part.

**tracheloplasty** (trā'kĕl-ō-plăs"tē) [" + *plassein,* to form] Surgical repair or plastic surgery of the neck of the uterus.

**trachelorrhaphy** (trā"kĕl-or'ă-fē) [" + *rhaphe,* seam, ridge] Suturing of a torn cervix uteri.

**tracheloschisis** (trā"kĕ-lŏs'kĭ-sĭs) [" + *schisis,* a splitting] Congenital opening or fissure in the neck.

**trachelotomy** (trā"kĕl-ŏt'ō-mē) [" + *tome,* incision] Incision of the cervix of the uterus.

**tracheo-** Combining form meaning *trachea, windpipe.*

**tracheoaerocele** (trā"kē-ō-ĕr'-ō-sēl) [Gr. *tracheia,* rough, + *aer,* air, + *kele,* tumor, swelling] Hernia or cyst of trachea containing air.

**tracheobronchial** (trā″kē-ō-brŏng′kē-ăl) Concerning the trachea and bronchus.

**tracheobronchomegaly** (trā″kē-ō-brŏng″kō-mĕg′ă-lē) Congenitally enlarged size of the trachea and bronchi.

**tracheobronchoscopy** (trā″kē-ō-brŏng-kŏs′kō-pē) [″ + *bronchos,* windpipe, + *skopein,* to examine] Inspection of the trachea and bronchi through a bronchoscope.

**tracheocele** (trā′kē-ō-sēl) [″ + *kele,* hernia] Protrusion of mucous membrane through the wall of the trachea. SYN: *trachelocele.*

**tracheoesophageal** (trā″kē-ō-ē-sŏf″ă-jē′ăl) [″ + *oisophagos,* esophagus] Pert. to the trachea and esophagus.

**tracheolaryngeal** (trā″kē-ō-lăr-rĭn′jē-ăl) Concerning the trachea and larynx.

**tracheolaryngotomy** (trā″kē-ō-lăr″ĭn-gŏt′ō-mē) [″ + *larynx,* larynx, + *tome,* incision] Incision into the larynx and trachea.

**tracheomalacia** (trā″kē-ō-mă-lā′shē-ă) Softening of the tracheal cartilage. It may be caused by pressure of the left pulmonary artery on the trachea.

**tracheopathia, tracheopathy** (trā″kē-ō-păth′ē-ă, -ŏp′ă-thē) [″ + *pathos,* disease, suffering] A disease of the trachea.

**tracheopharyngeal** (trā″kē-ō-făr-ĭn′jē-ăl) [″ + *pharynx,* throat] Pert. to both the trachea and the pharynx.

**tracheophony** (trā″kē-ŏf′ō-nē) [″ + *phone,* a sound] The sound heard over the trachea in auscultation.

**tracheoplasty** (trā′kē-ō-plăs″tē) [″ + *plassein,* to form] Plastic operation on the trachea.

**tracheopyosis** (trā″kē-ō-pī-ō′sĭs) [″ + *pyon,* pus, + *osis,* condition] Tracheitis with suppuration.

**tracheorrhagia** (trā″kē-ō-rā′jē-ă) [Gr. *tracheia,* rough, + *rhegnynai,* to burst forth] Tracheal hemorrhage.

**tracheoschisis** (trā″kē-ŏs′kĭs-ĭs) [″ + *schisis,* a splitting] A fissure of the trachea.

**tracheoscopy** (trā″kē-ŏs′kō-pē) [″ + *skopein,* to examine] Inspection of the interior of the trachea by means of reflected light.

**tracheostenosis** (trā″kē-ō-stĕn-ō′sĭs) [″ + *stenosis,* act of narrowing] Contraction or narrowing of the lumen of the trachea.

**tracheostoma** (trā″kē-ŏs′tō-mă) Opening into the trachea, via the neck.

**tracheostomize** (trā″kē-ŏs′tō-mīz) To perform a tracheostomy.

**tracheostomy** (trā″kē-ŏs′tō-mē) [″ + *stoma,* mouth] The operation of incising the skin over the trachea and making a surgical wound in the trachea to permit an airway during tracheal obstruction. This technique is used to provide an airway in emergency situations and to replace the airway provided by an endotracheal tube that has been in place for more than several weeks. The latter indication is necessary to prevent permanent damage of the larynx. SEE: *tube, endotracheal.*

---

Caution: Tracheostomy should be done by someone who is thoroughly trained in performing this surgical procedure.

---

NURSING IMPLICATIONS: Vital signs are monitored frequently after surgery. Warm, humidified oxygen is administered. The patient is placed in the semi-Fowler position to enhance drainage and to promote ease of breathing. A restful environment is provided. Communication is established by questions with simple yes and no answers, hand signals, and simple sign language and with use of a “magic slate” or an alphabet board for writing. (Written communication requires vision, hand strength, and dexterity and is often difficult or impossible for acutely ill patients.) Later, the patient is taught how to cover the tracheostomy to permit vocalization. The nurse should be alert to the patient’s unmet needs and assist with these to prevent increased anxiety. Establishment of range-of-motion exercises and chest physiotherapy promotes aeration of the lung. Analgesics, antibiotics, and other prescribed medications are administered. Intake and output are monitored and recorded, and adequate fluids and nutrition are provided. Suctioning of secretions and tracheostomy care are provided as necessary. Dressing is changed frequently during the first 24 hr postoperatively, and the surgical site is observed for excessive bleeding. Coughing and deep breathing are encouraged at regular intervals. A teaching plan should cover stoma care, which includes cleansing, removing crusts, and filtering air with a suitable filter. The nurse should be alert for signs of infection. The patient should avoid crowds, continue coughing and deep-breathing exercises, maintain adequate fluids and nutrition, and avoid smoking. Activities may be gradually increased to include noncontact sports but should not include swimming. Showering may be permitted if the patient wears a protective plastic bib or uses the hand to cover the stoma. The nurse should reassure the patient that secretions will decrease and that taste and smell will gradually return and should stress the importance of follow-up care.

***mini-t.*** Placement of a 4 mm (about 1/6th of an inch) cannula through an incision made through the cricothyroid membrane into the trachea. This is done using local anesthesia. This type of tracheostomy is esp. useful in removing sputum retained in the tracheobronchial tree.

**tracheostomy care** Management of the tracheostomy wound and the airway device. The patient should be suctioned as often as necessary to remove secretions. Before suctioning, the patient should be aerated well, which can be accomplished by using an Ambu bag attached to a source of oxygen. Sterile technique is maintained throughout the procedure. Before suctioning, the patency of the suction catheter is tested by aspirating sterile normal saline through it. The catheter is inserted without applying suction until the patient coughs. Suction is applied intermittently and the catheter withdrawn in a rotating motion. The airway is assessed by auscultating the lungs, and the suctioning procedure is repeated until the airway is clear. Each suctioning episode should take no longer than 15 sec, and the patient should be allowed to rest and breathe between suctioning episodes. The suction catheter is cleansed with sterile normal saline solution, as is the oral cavity if necessary. The inner cannula should be cleansed or replaced after each aspiration. Metal cannulas should be cleansed with sterile water.

An emergency tracheotomy kit is kept at the bedside at all times. A Kelly clamp is also kept at the bedside to hold open the tracheostomy site in an emergency. Cuffed tracheostomy tubes must be inflated if the patient is on positive-pressure ventilation unless ordered otherwise. In other cases, the cuff is kept deflated if the patient has problems with aspiration. The dressing and tape are changed every 8 hr using aseptic technique. Tracheostomies should always be covered with an oval dressing between the airway device and the skin to prevent skin breakdown. To apply neck tapes, two lengths of twill tape approx. 10 in. (25 cm) long are obtained; the end of each is folded and a slit is made ½ in. (1.3 cm) long about 1 in. (2.5 cm) from the fold. The slit end is slipped under the neck plate and the other end of the tape pulled through the slit. This is repeated for the other side. The tape is wrapped around the neck and secured with a square knot on the side. Neck tapes should be left in place until new tapes are attached. Tracheal secretions are cultured as ordered; their color, viscosity, amount, and abnormal odor, if any, are observed. The site is inspected daily for bleeding, hematoma formation, subcutaneous emphysema, and signs of infection. Appropriate skin care is provided. One should help to alleviate the patient's anxiety and apprehension, and provide a communication process. The patient's response is documented.

**tracheotome** (trā′kē-ō-tōm) [″ + *tome,* incision] An instrument used to open the trachea.

**tracheotomy** (trā″kē-ŏt′ō-mē) Incision of the trachea through the skin and muscles of the neck overlying the trachea. SEE: *tracheostomy.*

**trachitis** (trā-kī′tĭs) [″ + *itis,* inflammation] Tracheitis.

**trachoma** (trā-kō′mă) [Gr., roughness] A chronic contagious form of conjunctivitis, noted by hypertrophy of the conjunctiva and formation of follicles with subsequent cicatricial changes. Complications include pannus, ptosis, and corneal ulcers. The disease may result in blindness, corneal opacities, ectropion, entropion, staphyloma, symblepharon, and trichiasis. The disease affects 400,000,000 people, mostly in Asia and Africa, but is also seen in the southwestern part of the U.S. Approx. 20,000,000 persons have been blinded by this disease. Children with ocular infections are the primary reservoir of the infection, and the spread is by hand-to-eye contact between children or on the feet of flies who feed on the exudate from the children with active infection. The important treatment procedures are facial cleanlinesss and reduction of household fly density. SYN: *Egyptian ophthalmia; granular conjunctivitis.*

ETIOLOGY: The causative agent is a strain of *Chlamydia trachomatis.* Chlamydial organisms are responsible for psittacosis, inclusion conjunctivitis, lymphogranuloma venereum, genital tract infections, neonatal infections, and pneumonia. The disease is readily transmitted, esp. in its early stages. Transmission occurs by direct contact with trachomatous material or indirectly through contaminated articles such as towels or handkerchiefs. SEE: *Universal Precautions Appendix.*

TREATMENT: Topical tetracycline or erythromycin and systemic tetracycline, sulfonamides, erythromycin, or azithromycin are effective. Surgery may be necessary when lid deformities occur.

***brawny t.*** Trachoma with general lymphoid infiltration without granulation of the conjunctiva.

***t. deformans*** Trachoma with cicatricial contractions.

***diffuse t.*** Trachoma with large granulations.

**trachomatous** (tră-kō′mă-tŭs) Concerning trachoma.

**trachychromatic** (trā″kĭ-krō-măt′ĭk) [Gr. *trachys,* rough, + *chroma,* color] Pert. to a nucleus with very deeply staining chromatin.

**trachyphonia** (trā″kĭ-fō′nē-ă) [″ + *phone,* voice] Roughness or hoarseness of the voice.

**tracing** (trā′sĭng) **1.** A graphic record of some event that changes with time such as respiratory movements or electrical activity of the heart or brain. **2.** In dentistry, a graphic display of movements of the mandible.

**tract** (trăkt) [L. *tractus,* extent] **1.** A course or pathway. **2.** A group or bundle of nerve fibers within the spinal cord or brain that constitutes an anatomical and functional unit. SEE: *fasciculus.* **3.** A group of organs or parts forming a continuous pathway.

***afferent t.*** Ascending t.

***alimentary t.*** The canal or passage from the mouth to the anus. SYN: *digestive t.*

***ascending t.*** White fibers in the spinal cord that carry nerve impulses toward the brain. SYN: *afferent t.*

***biliary t.*** SEE: *biliary tract.*

***corticospinal t.*** Pyramidal t.

***descending t.*** Fibers in the spinal cord that carry nerve impulses from the brain.

***digestive t.*** Alimentary t.

***dorsolateral t.*** A spinal cord tract superficial to the tip of the dorsal horn. It is made up of short pain and temperature fibers that are processes of neurons having their cell bodies in the dorsal root ganglion.

***extrapyramidal t.*** SEE: *system, extrapyramidal.*

***gastrointestinal t.*** The stomach and intestines.

***genitourinary t.*** The genital and urinary pathways.

***iliotibial t.*** A thickened area of fascia lata extending from the lateral condyle of the tibia to the iliac crest.

***intestinal t.*** The small and large intestines.

***motor t.*** A descending pathway that conveys motor impulses from the brain to the lower portions of the spinal cord.

***olfactory t.*** A narrow white band that extends from the olfactory bulb to the anterior perforated substance of the brain.

***optic t.*** Fibers of the optic nerve that continue beyond the optic chiasma, most of which terminate in the lateral geniculate body of the thalamus. Some continue to the superior colliculus of the midbrain; others enter the hypothalamus and terminate in the supraoptic and medial nuclei.

***pyramidal t.*** One of three descending tracts (lateral, ventral, ventrolateral) of the spinal cord. The tract consists of fibers arising from the giant pyramidal cells of Betz present in the motor area of the cerebral cortex. SYN: *corticospinal tract.*

***respiratory t.*** The respiratory organs in continuity.

***rubrospinal t.*** A descending tract of fibers arising from cell bodies located in the red nucleus of the midbrain. Fibers terminate in the gray matter of the spinal cord.

***supraopticohypophyseal t.*** A tract consisting of fibers arising from cell bodies located in supraoptic and paraventricular nuclei of the hypothalamus and terminating in the posterior lobe of the hypophysis.

***urinary t.*** The urinary passageway from the kidney to the outside of the body, including the pelvis of the kidney, ureter, bladder, and urethra.

***uveal t.*** The vascular and pigmented tissues that constitute the middle coat of the eye, including the iris, ciliary body, and choroid.

**tractellum** (trăk-tĕl′ŭm) [L.] An anterior flagellum of a protozoan. It propels the body by traction.

**traction** (trăk′shŭn) [L. *tractio*] The process of drawing or pulling. SEE: *Nursing Diagnoses Appendix.*

***axis t.*** Traction in line with the long axis of a course through which a body (fetus) is to be drawn.

***cervical t.*** Traction applied to the cervical spine by applying a force to lift the head or a mobilization technique to distract individual joints of the vertebrae. SEE: *Crutchfield tongs.*

***elastic t.*** Traction exerted by elastic devices such as rubber bands.

***external t.*** Traction applied to any fracture (e.g., compression fractures of the face using metal or plaster headgear for anchorage).

***head t.*** Traction applied to the head as in the treatment of injuries to cervical vertebrae.

***intermittent t.*** The force of traction alternately applied and released at specified intervals.

***lumbar t.*** Traction applied to the lumbar spine usually by applying a force to pull on the pelvis or by using a mobilization technique to distract individual joints of the lumbar vertebrae.

***manual t.*** The application of traction to the joints of the spine or extremities by a therapist trained to know appropriate positions and intensities for the force.

***maxillomandibular t.*** Traction applied to the maxilla and mandible by means of elastic or wire ligatures and interdental wiring or splints.

***mechanical t.*** The use of a device or mechanical linkage (i.e., pulleys and weights) to apply a traction force.

***sustained t.*** The application of a constant traction force up to ½ hr.

***weight t.*** Traction exerted by means of weights.

**tractor** (trăk′tor) [L., drawer] Any device or instrument for applying traction.

**tractotomy** (trăk-tŏt′ō-mē) Surgical section of a fiber tract of the central nervous system. It is sometimes resorted to for relief of intractable pain.

**tractus** (trăk′tŭs) *pl.* **tractus** [L.] A tract or path.

**tragacanth** (trăg′ă-kănth) [Gr. *tragakantha,* a goat thorn] The dried gummy exudation from the plant *Astragalus gummifer* and related species, grown in Asia. It is used in the form of mucilage as a greaseless lubricant and as an application for chapped skin.

**tragal** (trā′găl) [Gr. *tragos,* goat] Relating to the tragus.

**tragi** (trā′jī) Pl. of tragus.

**tragicus** (trăj′ĭk-ŭs) [L.] The muscle on the outer surface of the tragus. SEE: *Muscles Appendix.*

**tragion** (trăj′ē-ŏn) An anthropometric point at the upper margin of the tragus of the ear.

**tragomaschalia** (trăg″ō-măs-kāl′ē-ă) [Gr. *tragos,* goat, + *maschale,* the armpit] Odorous perspiration (bromidrosis) of the axilla.

**tragophonia, tragophony** (trăg″ō-fō′nē-ă, -ŏf′ō-nē) [″ + *phone,* voice] A bleating sound heard in auscultation at the level of fluid in hydrothorax. SYN: *egophony.*

**tragopodia** (trăg″ō-pō′dē-ă) [″ + *pous,* foot] Knock-knee.

**tragus** (trā′gŭs) *pl.* **tragi** [Gr. *tragos,* goat] A cartilaginous projection in front of the exterior meatus of the ear.

**train** (trān) To participate in a special program of instruction to attain competence in a certain occupation or profession.

**trainable** (trān′ă-bl) Having the ability to be instructed and to learn from being taught. In classifying severity of mental retardation or brain damage, it is important to know to what extent individuals may be trainable in various areas such as safety, personal care, or self-feeding.

**training** An organized system of instruction.

***assertiveness t.*** A type of behavior therapy in which the patient is taught to respond in a more positive and assertive manner to the normal stimuli encountered in daily activities. The goal is to be able to express one's true feelings, positive or negative. Role playing in group therapy may be used to teach this to patients.

***athletic t.*** **1.** The physical and mental conditioning program used by athletes to increase their proficiency in sports endeavors. **2.** Performing the tasks that an athletic trainer is prepared to do.

***aversive t.*** SEE: *aversion therapy.*

***habit t.*** The development in young children of specific behavior patterns for performing basic activities such as eating, dressing, using the toilet, and sleeping.

***social skills t.*** The components of rehabilitation programs that focus on the skills necessary for effective interaction in social situations.

**trait** (trāt) A distinguishing feature; a characteristic or property of an individual.

***acquired t.*** A trait that is not inherited; one resulting from the effects of the environment.

***inherited t.*** A trait due to genes transmitted through germ cells.

***personality t.*** An enduring pattern of perceiving, communicating, and thinking about oneself, others, and the environment that is exhibited in multiple contexts. When personality traits become maladaptive, a personality disorder ensues.

**trajector** (tră-jĕk′tor) [L. *trajectus,* thrown across] A device for determining the approximate location of a bullet in a wound.

**trance** (trăns) [L. *transitus,* a passing over] A sleeplike state, as in deep hypnosis, appearing also in hysteria and in some spiritualistic mediums, with limited sensory and motor contact with the ordinary surroundings, and with subsequent amnesia of what has occurred during the state.

***death t.*** A trance simulating death.

***induced t.*** A trance caused by some external event such as hypnosis.

**tranexamic acid** An antifibrinolytic drug that is approximately 10 times as potent and with more sustained activity than aminocaproic acid. It is used to decrease bleeding time during surgical procedures. Loss of blood is decreased when this drug is used.

**tranquilizer** (trăn″kwĭ-līz′ĕr) [L. *tranquillus,* calm] A drug that acts to reduce mental tension and anxiety without interfering with normal mental activity. This ideal state of tranquilization is difficult to attain. Thus, patients taking these medicines may find that their reactions are slowed. The use of tranquilizers has facilitated the treatment of severely disturbed psychiatric patients. Among the drugs in use are chlordiazepoxide (Librium), chlorpromazine (Thorazine), diazepam (Valium), meprobamate (Miltown, Equanil), alprazolam (Xanax), and reserpine (Serpasil).

Side effects, particularly from chlorpromazine and reserpine, have included jaundice, nausea, rashes, and in some instances severe mental depression. The U.S. Public Health Service has warned of "a significant incidence of severe depression, with suicidal tendencies in some instances," in persons receiving a heavy reserpine dosage.

Persons taking tranquilizers regularly should not discontinue their use suddenly. To prevent withdrawal signs, which include convulsions, muscle cramps, sweating, and vomiting, the dose is reduced gradually.

---

Caution: Some tranquilizers may injure the developing embryo. Therefore, before prescribing one, one should know whether it is approved for use during pregnancy, esp. early pregnancy.

---

**trans-** [L.] Prefix meaning *across, over, beyond, through.*

**transabdominal** (trăns″ăb-dŏm′ĭ-năl) Through or across the abdomen or abdominal wall.

**transacetylation** (trăns-ăs″ē-tĭl-ā′shŭn) Transfer of an acetyl group ($CH_3CO$—) in a chemical reaction.

**transaction** The interaction of a person with others.

**transactional analysis** Psychotherapy involving role playing in an attempt to understand the relationship between the patient and the therapist and eventually that between the patient and reality.

**transamidination** (trăns-ăm″ĭ-dĭn-ā′shŭn) The transfer of an amidine group from one amino acid to another.

**transaminase** (trăns-ăm′ĭn-ās) An enzyme that catalyzes transamination.

***glutamic-oxaloacetic t.*** Aspartate aminotransferase.

***glutamic-pyruvic t.*** Alanine aminotransferase.

**transamination** (trăns″ăm-ĭ-nā′shŭn) The transfer of an amino group from one compound to another or the transposition of an amino group within a single compound.

**transaortic** (trăns″ā-or′tĭk) Done through the aorta (e.g., a surgical procedure).

**transatrial** (trăns-ā′trē-ăl) Done through the atrium (e.g., a surgical procedure).

**transaudient** (trăns-aw′dē-ĕnt) [″ + *audire,* to hear] Permeable to sound waves.

**transaxial** (trăns-ăk′sē-ăl) Across the long axis of a structure or part.

**transbronchial** Across the bronchi or the bronchial wall.

**transcalent** (trăns-kā′lĕnt) [″ + *calere,* to be hot] Permeable by heat rays. SYN: *diathermal.*

**transcapillary** (trăns″kăp′ĭl-lă-rē) [″ + *capillaris,* relating to hair] Across the endothelial wall of a capillary.

**transcapillary exchange** The passage of substances between blood and tissue (interstitial) fluid.

**transcervical** (trăns-sĕr′vĭ-kăl) Done through the cervical os of the uterus.

**transcortical** (trăns-kor′tĭ-kăl) Joining two parts of the cerebral cortex.

**transcortin** (trăns-kor′tĭn) A corticosteroid-binding globulin.

**transcriptase** (trăns-krĭp′tās) A polymerase that performs transcription by converting a DNA base sequence into its complementary RNA base sequence. SYN: *RNA polymerase.*

**transcription** (trăn-skrĭp′shŭn) In protein synthesis, the process of copying the genetic information from the DNA in the chromosomes to the ribosomes, cell organelles in the cytoplasm that are the site of protein synthesis. This is done by a molecule of messenger RNA (mRNA), which carries this information.

**transcutaneous** Percutaneous.

**transcutaneous electrical nerve stimulation** ABBR: TENS. The application of mild electrical stimulation to skin electrodes placed over a painful area. It causes interference with transmission of painful stimuli.

**transcutaneous oxygen monitoring** The use of a modified Clark electrode, warmed and applied to the skin of an infant, to measure oxygen tension continuously.

**transdermal infusion system** A method of delivering medicine by placing it in a special gel-like matrix that is applied to the skin. The medicine is absorbed through the skin at a fixed rate. Each application will provide medicine for from one to several days. Nitroglycerin and scopolamine are examples of medicines that have been prepared for use in this type of system. SYN: *transdermal drug-delivery system.*

**transducer** (trăns-dū′sĕr) [L. *trans,* across, + *ducere,* to lead] A device that converts one form of energy to another. The telephone is an example. It is used in medical electronics to receive the energy produced by sound or pressure and relay it as an electrical impulse to another transducer, which can either convert the energy back into its original form or produce a record of it on a recording device.

***ultrasonic t.*** A device used in ultrasound that sends and receives the sound wave signal.

**transduction** (trăns-dŭk′shŭn) A phenomenon causing genetic recombination in bacteria in which DNA is carried from one bacterium to another by a bacteriophage. SEE: *transformation.*

**transection, transsection** (trăn-sĕk′shŭn, trăns-sĕk′shŭn) [″ + *sectio,* cutting] A cutting made across a long axis; a cross section.

**trans fatty acid** SEE: under *fatty acid.*

**transfection** (trans-fĕk′shŭn) The infection of bacteria by purified phage DNA after pretreatment with calcium ions or conversion to spheroplasts.

**transfer, transference** (trăns′fer, trăns-fĕr′ĕns) [″ + *ferre,* to bear] **1.** The mental process whereby a person transfers patterns of feelings and behavior that had previously been experienced with important figures such as parents or siblings to another person. Quite often these feelings are shifted to the caregiver. **2.** The state in which the symptoms of one area are transmitted to a similar area.

***zygote intrafallopian t.*** ABBR: ZIFT. An in vitro fertilization technique in which a woman's ova are surgically removed and mixed with her partner's sperm. The resulting zygotes are placed in her fallopian tube. SEE: *embryo transfer; fertilization, in vitro; GIFT.*

**transferase** (trăns′fĕr-ās) An enzyme that catalyzes the transfer of atoms or groups of atoms from one chemical compound to another.

**transfer board** A device used to bridge the space between a wheelchair and a bed, toilet, or carseat; used to facilitate independent or assisted transferring of the patient from one of these sites to another. It is also called a *sliding board.*

**transfer factor** In immunology, a factor present in lymphocytes that have been sensitized to antigens, which can, in humans, be transferred to a nonsensitized recipient. Thus, the recipient will react to the same antigen that was originally used to sensitize the lymphocytes of the donor. In humans, the factor can be transferred by injecting the recipient with either intact lymphocytes or extracts of disrupted cells.

**transferrin** (trăns-fĕr′rĭn) A globulin in the blood that binds and transports iron.

***carbohydrate-deficient t.*** A globulin used as a marker for alcohol abuse. The compound is elevated in those who are chronic heavy drinkers, but is not present in nondrinkers. SEE: *alcoholism.*

**transferring** The act of moving a person with limited function from one location to another. This may be accomplished by the patient or with assistance.

**transfix** (trăns-fĭks′) [″ + *figere,* to fix] To pierce through or impale with a sharp instrument.

**transfixion** (trăns-fĭk′shŭn) A maneuver in performing an amputation in which a knife is passed into the soft parts and cutting is from within outward.

**transforation** (trăns″for-ā′shŭn) [″ + *forare,* to pierce] The perforation of the fetal skull at the base in craniotomy.

**transforator** (trăns′for-ā″tor) An instrument for perforating the fetal skull.

**transformation** (trăns″for-mā′shŭn) [″ + *formatio,* a forming] **1.** Change of shape or form. SYN: *metamorphosis.* **2.** In oncology, the change of one tissue into another. SEE: *metastasis.* **3.** A type of mutation occurring in bacteria. It results from DNA of a bacterial cell penetrating the host cell and becoming incorporated into the genotype of the host.

**transformer** (trăns-form′er) [″ + *formare,* to form] A stationary induction apparatus to change electrical energy at one voltage and current to electrical energy at another voltage and current through the medium of magnetic energy, without mechanical motion.

***step-down t.*** A transformer that changes electricity to a lower voltage.

***step-up t.*** A transformer that changes electricity to a higher voltage.

**transfuse** The act of transfusion.

**transfusion** (trăns-fū′zhŭn) [″ + *fusio,* a pouring] **1.** The injection of blood or a blood component into the bloodstream. SEE: *blood transfusion; interosseous infusion.* **2.** The injection of saline or other solutions into a vein for a therapeutic purpose.

***autologous t.*** A procedure for collecting and storing a patient's own blood several weeks before its anticipated need by the patient. Alternatively, blood lost during a surgical procedure can be recovered from the operation site and processed for transfusion. This method of providing blood for an individual is used to prevent the transmission of disease that can occur with the use of donor blood. SEE: *blood doping.*

***cadaver blood t.*** A transfusion using blood obtained from a cadaver within a short time after death.

***direct t.*** The transfer of blood directly from one person to another.

***exchange t.*** The transfusion and withdrawal of small amounts of blood repeated until blood volume is almost entirely exchanged. This method is used in infants born with hemolytic disease and in patients with uremia. SYN: *replacement t.*

***indirect t.*** A transfusion of blood from a donor to a suitable storage container and then to the patient.

***replacement t.*** Exchange t.

***single unit t.*** SEE: *blood, transfusion of a single unit.*

**transfusion reaction** One of a variety of reactions that can occur as a result of blood transfusions. The most serious is the response of the recipient when incompatible blood is administered, in which case massive intravascular clumping and lysis of red blood cells occur. Other causes of hemolytic reactions are administering hemolyzed or fragile red blood cells due to the age of the blood or to its having been stored at an inappropriate temperature or having come in contact with incompatible intravenous solutions. If the reaction is severe, the patient will experience a bursting feeling in the head, face flushing, pain in the neck and lumbar area, vomiting, and shock. If the blood contains something to which the patient is allergic, the symptoms of urticaria, edema, wheezing, and headache will be present. Infrequently, anaphylactic shock will occur. Some patients with compromised cardiovascular systems will experience heart failure, shock, pulmonary edema, and cyanosis if too much blood is administered. The transfusion must be stopped when these symptoms and signs appear. Such patients should not receive whole blood.

Prevention of these types of reactions depends on meticulous attention to detail and accuracy in labeling the patient's blood sample for typing and cross-matching, double-checking this at the time of transfusion, and starting the blood flow very slowly during the first 15 min and observing carefully for reactions. To prevent allergic reactions in persons with a history of allergies, an antihistamine may be administered orally or intramuscularly just before the transfusion is started.

**transfusion syndrome, multiple** The development of hemorrhagic tendency caused by multiple transfusions with blood low in platelets and by increased fibrinolytic activity in the blood. In treating these patients, one should transfuse with blood that is only a few hours old and give fibrinogen. SEE: *post-transfusion syndrome.*

**transgenic** An organism into which hereditary (i.e., genetic) material from another organism has been introduced.

**Transgrow** Proprietary name of a special medium for culturing *Neisseria gonorrhoeae.* The specimen may be placed in the medium and then shipped to the laboratory. The bacteria will remain viable although they were not incubated while being transported.

**transient** [L. *transi,* to go by] Not lasting; of brief duration.

**transient ischemic attack** ABBR: TIA. Temporary interference with blood supply to the brain. The symptoms of neurological deficit may last for only a few moments or for several hours. After the attack, no evidence of residual brain damage or neurological damage remains. It is not necessarily true that individuals who have experienced TIAs will within the predictable future develop a full vascular occlusion and have a stroke. SEE: *bruit, carotid; stroke*.

SYMPTOMS: Usually there is an abrupt onset of giddiness or a light-headed sensation. The specific signs and symptoms depend on the portion of the brain affected. Thus, any one or a combination of several of the following may be present: fleeting monocular blindness, hemiparesis, hemiplegia, aphasia, astereognosis, dizziness, staggering, numbness, difficulty in swallowing, or paresthesias.

ETIOLOGY: This condition is caused by insufficient blood flow to the brain as a result of decreased cardiac output, hypotension, overmedication with antihypertensive agents, or cerebrovascular spasm. Intravascular microembolization is suspected of causing some cases.

NURSING IMPLICATIONS: The nurse supports the patient and family during diagnostic procedures by explaining the procedures and expected sensations and by encouraging verbalization of feelings and concerns. Therapeutic interventions are provided, and the patient is instructed about desired effects and adverse reactions of prescribed drugs. Safety measures are instituted to prevent injury associated with uncoordinated gait or weakness in subsequent attacks.

**transiliac** (trăns-ĭl′ē-ăk) [L. *trans*, across, + *iliacus*, pert. to ilium] Extending between the two ilia.

**transilient** (trăns-sĭl′ē-ĕnt) Jumping across or passing over as occurs when nerve fibers in the brain link nonadjacent convolutions.

**transillumination** (trăns″ĭl-lū″mĭ-nā′shŭn) [″ + *illuminare*, to light up] Inspection of a cavity or organ by passing a light through its walls. When pus or a lesion is present, the transmission of light is diminished or absent.

**transinsular** (trăns-ĭn′sū-lăr) Across the insula of the brain.

**transischiac** (trăns-ĭs′kē-ăk) Across or between the ischia of the pelvis.

**transisthmian** (trăns-ĭs′mē-ăn) Across an isthmus.

**transition** (trăn-zĭ′shŭn) [L. *transitio*, a going across] **1.** Passage from one state or position to another, or from one part to another part; a change in health status, roles, family, abilities, and other important areas. Transitions often require adaptations within the person, the group, or the environment and define the need for and context of nursing care. **2.** In obstetrics, the final phase of the first stage of labor. Cervical dilation is 8 to 10 cm and strong uterine contractions occur every 1.5 to 2 min and persist for 60 to 90 sec. Accompanying behavioral changes include increasing irritability and anxiety, declining coping abilities, and expressions of a strong desire for the labor to be ended immediately.

**transitional** (trăn-zĭsh′ŭn-ăl) Marked by or relating to change.

**translation** (trăns-lā′shŭn) [L. *trans*, across, + *latus*, borne] **1.** The synthesis of proteins under the direction of ribonucleic acid. **2.** To change to another place or to convert into another form.

**translocation** (trăns″lō-kā′shŭn) [″ + *locus*, place] **1.** The alteration of a chromosome by transfer of a portion of it either to another chromosome or to another portion of the same chromosome. The latter is called shift or intrachange. When two chromosomes interchange material, it is called reciprocal translocation. **2.** Movement of bacteria across the intestinal wall to invade the body. **3.** The linear motion of one structure across the parallel surface of another.

**translucent** (trăns-lū′sĕnt) [″ + *lucens*, shining] Not transparent but permitting passage of light.

**transmethylase** (trăns-mĕth′ĭ-lās) Methyltransferase.

**transmethylation** (trăns″mĕth-ĭ-lā′shŭn) The process in the metabolism of amino acids in which a methyl group is transferred from one compound to another; for example, the conversion in the body of homocysteine to methionine. In this case, the methyl group is furnished by choline or betaine.

**transmigration** (trănz″mī-grā′shŭn) [″ + *migrare*, to move from place to place] Wandering across or through, esp. the passage of white blood cells through capillary membranes into the tissues.

***external t.*** Transfer of an ovum from an ovary to an opposite tube through the pelvic cavity.

***internal t.*** Transfer of an ovum through the uterus to the opposite oviduct.

**transmissible** (trăns-mĭs′ă-bl) [L. *transmissio*, a sending across] Capable of being carried from one person to another, as an infectious disease.

**transmission** (trăns-mĭsh′ŭn) Transfer of anything, as a disease or hereditary characteristics.

***airborne t.*** The spread of infectious organisms by aerosol or dust particles.

***biological t.*** A condition in which the organism that transmits the causative agent of a disease plays an essential role in the life history of a parasite or germ.

***duplex t.*** The passage of impulses through a nerve trunk in both directions.

***mechanical t.*** The passive transfer of causative agents of disease, esp. by arthropods. This may be indirect, as when flies pick up organisms from excreta of humans or animals and deposit them on food, or direct, as when they pick up organisms from the body of a diseased individual and directly inoculate them into the body of another individual by bites or through open sores. SEE: *vector*.

***neuromyal t.*** The transmission of excitation from a motor neuron to a muscle fiber at a neuromyal (myoneural) junction.

***placental t.*** The transmission of substances in the mother's blood to the blood of the fetus by way of the placenta.

***synaptic t.*** The release of a neurotransmitter by a neuron that initiates or inhibits an electrical impulse in the next neuron in the pathway.

***transovarial t.*** The transmission of causative agents of disease to offspring following invasion of the ovary and infection of eggs; occurs in ticks and mites.

***vertical t.*** **1.** In certain insects, transovarial passage of infection from one generation to the next. **2.** In mammals, passage of infection from the mother's body fluids to the infant either in utero, during delivery, or during the neonatal period (via breast milk).

**transmission-based precautions** Measures suggested by the Centers for Disease Control and Prevention to reduce the risk of airborne, droplet, and direct-contact transmission of infection in hospitals. SEE: *Universal Precautions Appendix*.

**transmural** (trăns-mū′răl) [L. *trans,* across, + *murus,* a wall] Across the wall of an organ or structure, as in transmural myocardial thrombosis, in which the tissue in the entire thickness of a portion of the cardiac wall is affected.

**transmutation** (trăns″mū-tā′shŭn) [L. *transmutatio,* a changing across] A transformation or change, as the evolutionary change of one species into another.

**transocular** (trăns-ŏk′ū-lăr) [″ + *oculus,* eye] Across the eye.

**transonance** (trăns′ō-năns) [L. *trans,* across + *sonans,* sounding] The transmission of sounds through an organ, as heart sounds through the lungs and chest wall.

**transorbital** (trăns-or′bĭ-tăl) [″ + *orbita,* track] Passing through the orbit of the eye.

**transovarial passage** (trăns-ō-vā′rē-ăl) The passage of infectious or toxic agents into the ovary, a process that might invade and infect the oocytes.

**transparent** (trăns-păr′ĕnt) [″ + *parere,* to appear] **1.** Transmitting light rays so that objects are visible through the substance. **2.** Pervious to radiant energy.

**transparietal** (trăns″pă-rī′ĕ-tăl) [″ + *paries,* a wall] Through a parietal region or wall.

**transpeptidase** (trăns-pĕp′tĭ-dās) An enzyme that catalyzes the transfer of a peptide from one compound to another.

**transperitoneal** (trăns″pĕr-ĭ-tō-nē′ăl) Across or through the peritoneum.

**transphosphorylase** (trăns-fŏs-for′ĭ-lās) An enzyme that catalyzes the transfer of a phosphate group from one compound to another.

**transphosphorylation** (trăns-fŏs″for-ĭ-lā′shŭn) The exchange of phosphate groups from one compound to another.

**transpirable** (trăns-pī′ră-bl) [″ + *spirare,* to breathe] Permitting secretion through the skin or membranes, as perspiration.

**transpiration** (trăns″pī-rā′shŭn) [″ + *spirare,* to breathe] **1.** The passage of water, gas, or vapor through the skin or a membrane. SEE: *perspiration*. **2.** The substance exhaled.

***cutaneous t.*** Perspiration.

***pulmonary t.*** The escape of watery vapor from the blood to the air in the lungs.

**transpire** To emit vapor through the skin or other tissues. SEE: *perspire*.

**transplacental** (trăns″plă-sĕn′tăl) Through the placenta, esp. penetration of the placenta by a toxin, chemical, or organism that would affect the fetus.

**transplant** [″ + *plantare,* to plant] **1.** (trăns-plănt′) To transfer tissue or an organ from one part to another as in grafting or plastic surgery. **2.** (trăns′plănt) A piece of tissue or organ used in transplantation.

**transplantar** (trăns-plăn′tăr) [″ + *planta,* sole] Across the sole of the foot.

**transplantation** (trăns″plăn-tā′shŭn) **1.** The grafting of living tissue from its normal position to another site or the transplantation of an organ or tissue from one person to another. Organs and tissues that have been successfully transplanted include the heart, lung, kidney, liver, pancreas, cornea, large blood vessels, tendon, cartilage, skin, bone, and bone marrow. Brain tissue has been implanted experimentally in treating parkinsonism. The most important factor in successful transplantation is the matching of histocompatibility antigens that differentiate one individual's cells from another's. Cyclosporine has been used to attempt to prevent rejection of the transplant. SEE: *autotransplantation; graft; heart transplantation; organ donation; renal transplantation; replantation*. **2.** In dentistry, the transfer of a tooth from one alveolus to another.

***allogeneic t.*** Transplantation of material from a donor to another person.

***autologous t.*** Transplantation of material from one location in the body to another site.

***autoplastic t.*** Transplantation of tissue from one part to another part of the same body. SYN: *homoplastic t*.

***bone marrow t.*** SEE: *bone marrow transplantation*.

***combined liver-small intestine t.*** An experimental procedure in which both the liver and small intestine have been replaced. The procedure has been done successfully.

***hair t.*** A surgical procedure for placing plugs of skin containing hair follicles from one body site to another. This technique is very time consuming but has some success in treatment of alopecia of the scalp.

***heart t.*** Surgical transplantation of the heart from a patient who died of trauma or a disease that left the heart intact and capable of functioning in the recipient. This procedure was performed frequently in the 1970s, after which very few were done. As techniques for matching the donor and recipient have improved, the procedure is now done in many hospitals but is limited by the availability of donor hearts.

***heteroplastic t.*** Transplantation of a part from one individual to another individual of the same or a closely related species.

***heterotopic t.*** Transplantation in which the transplant is placed in a different location in the host than it had been in the donor.

***homoplastic t.*** Autoplastic t.

***homotopic t.*** Transplantation in which the transplant occupies the same location in the host as it had in the donor.

***small intestine t.*** An experimental procedure in which the small intestine is replaced. The procedure has been done successfully.

***syngeneic t.*** A specific type of allogeneic transplantation of material between identical twins.

**transplantation antigen** The commonly used term for one of the histocompatibility antigens that cause the immune system of one individual to reject transplanted tissue.

**transpleural** (trăns-ploor′răl) Through the pleura.

**transport** Movement or transfer of substances in a biological system, esp. movement of electrolytes, nutrients, and liquids across cell membranes. Transport may occur actively, passively, or with the assistance of a carrier.

***active t.*** Transfer of a substance across a membrane even though its concentration may be higher on the side toward which the movement is taking place.

**transportation of the injured** The process of moving an injured person to a hospital or other treatment center.

*Carrying in arms:* The patient is picked up in both arms, as the carrying of a child.

*One-arm assist:* The patient's arm is placed about the neck of the bearer, and the bearer's arm is placed about the patient's waist, thus assisting the patient to walk.

*Chair carry, chair stretcher:* Any ordinary firm chair may be used. The patient is seated on the tilted-back chair. One bearer grasps the back of the chair and the other the legs of the chair (either the front or rear, depending on the construction of the chair). Both bearers face in the same direction.

*Fireman's drag:* The patient's wrists are crossed and tied with a belt or rope. The bearer kneels astride the patient, with his or her head under the patient's wrists, and walks on all fours, dragging the patient underneath.

*Fireman's lift:* The bearer grasps the patient's left wrist with the right hand. The bearer's head is placed under the patient's left armpit, drawing the patient's body over the bearer's left shoulder. The bearer's left arm should encircle both thighs, then lift the patient. The patient's wrist is transferred to the bearer's left hand, thus leaving one hand free to remove obstacles or to open doors.

*Four-handed basket seat:* Each of two bearers grasps own wrist and then grasps the partner's free wrist. The patient sits on this support.

*Pack-strap carry:* The patient is supported along the bearer's back. The patient's right arm is brought over the bearer's right shoulder and held by the bearer's left hand. The patient's left arm is brought over the left shoulder and held by the bearer's right hand. The patient is thus carried on the back, with the arms resembling pack straps.

*Piggyback carry:* The patient is supported along the bearer's back with the knees raised to the sides of the bearer's torso. This leaves the patient practically in a sitting position astride the bearer's back, with arms around the bearer's neck or trunk.

*Six- or eight-person carry:* This is done as the three-person carry, except three or four bearers are on each side of the patient, thus dividing the patient's weight more uniformly.

*Three-handed basket seat:* The bearer grasps his or her own wrist; the partner grasps the bearer's wrist and leaves one arm free for supporting the patient.

*Three- or four-person carry:* This is the litter-type carry used by emergency squads. Three persons kneel on one side of the patient, place their hands under the patient and lift up. The head bearer supports the patient's head and shoulders, the center bearer lifts the waist and hips, and the third bearer lifts both the lower extremities. A fourth person, if available, should help steady the patient while he or she is being lifted.

*Two-handed seat:* The bearers kneel on either side of the patient. Each passes one arm around the patient's back (under the armpits) and the other arm under the knees and lifts the patient carefully in a sitting position.

*Wheelchair, improvised:* To make this, the legs of a chair, preferably one with arms, are fastened to parallel boards and skates or casters are attached to the bottom of the boards. A footrest can be made by attaching a broom handle or stick across the parallel boards in front of the chair.

*Vehicles:* If an ambulance is not available, stretchers can be improvised with ropes and chairs, ladders, or poles. The patient should always be tied to the stretcher during transportation. Several bearers will be necessary to assist entering and leaving the vehicle.

**transport protein** One of the proteins important to transporting materials such as hormones from their site of origin to the site of cellular action and metabolism.

**transpose** To change places (e.g., moving the insertion of a muscle or ligament to another site).

**transposition** (trănz″pō-zĭ′shŭn) [L. *trans,* across, + *positio,* a placing] **1.** A transfer of position from one spot to another. SYN: *metathesis.* **2.** Displacement of an organ, esp. a viscus, to the opposite side. **3.** Transplantation of a flap of tissue without severing it entirely from its original position until it has united in the new position.

**transposition of great vessels** A fetal deformity of the heart in which the aorta arises from the right ventricle and the pulmonary artery arises from the left ventricle.

**transposon** (trănz-pō′zŏn) A genetic unit such as a DNA sequence that is transferred from one cell's genetic material to another.

**trans-retinal** The form of retinal created when light strikes the retina. It separates from the opsin of the photopigment (rhodopsin in rods), which is then said to be bleached. The enzyme retinal isomerase converts it back to cis-retinal, and the photopigment is again able to respond to light.

**transsegmental** (trăns″sĕg-mĕn′tăl) [″ + *segmentum,* a cutting] Extending across or beyond a segment, as of a limb.

**transseptal** (trăns-sĕp′tăl) [″ + *saeptum,* partition] Across a septum.

**transsexual** (trăns-sĕks′ū-ăl) [″ + *sexus,* sex] **1.** An individual who has an overwhelming desire to be of the opposite sex. **2.** An individual who has had his or her external sex changed by surgery.

**transsexualism** (trăns-sĕks′ū-ă-lĭzm) The condition of being of a certain definite sex (i.e., male or female) but feeling and acting as if a member of the opposite sex. In some instances, the desire to alter this situation leads individuals to seek medical and surgical assistance to alter anatomical characteristics so that their anatomy would more nearly match their feelings about their true sexuality. The success of this therapy is controversial.

**transsexual surgery** Surgical therapy for alteration of the anatomical sex of an individual whose psychological gender is not consistent with the anatomical sexual characteristics.

**transsphenoidal** (trăns″sfē-noy′dăl) Through or across the sphenoid bone.

**transtemporal** (trăns-tĕm′pō-răl) [″ + *temporalis,* pert. to a temple] Crossing the temporal lobe of the cerebrum.

**transthalamic** (trăns″thăl-ăm′ĭk) [″ + Gr. *thalamos,* chamber] Passing across the optic thalamus.

**transthoracic** (trăns″thō-răs′ĭk) [″ + Gr. *thorax,* chest] Across the thorax.

**transthoracotomy** (trăns″thō-ră-kŏt′ō-mē) [″ + Gr. *thorax,* chest, + *tome,* incision] The operation of incising across the thorax.

**transthyretin** ABBR: TTR. A normal serum prealbumin protein that binds and transports thyroxine ($T_4$).

**transtracheal** Across or through the trachea.

**transtracheal jet insufflation** The life-saving technique of ventilating a patient with a complete airway obstruction. A small catheter is placed via a cricothyroid puncture and attached to a pressure-controlled oxygen outlet via a one-way valve.

**transtympanic neurectomy** Surgical interruption of the parasympathetic nerve supply to the parotid and submandibular glands by bilateral sectioning of the tympanic and chorda tympani nerves. The technique is used in treating sialorrhea in mentally retarded children.

**transubstantiation** (trăn″sŭb-stăn″shē-ā′shŭn) [″ + *substantia,* substance] The process of replacing one tissue for another.

**transudate** (trăns′ū-dāt) [″ + *sudare,* to sweat] The fluid that passes through a membrane, esp. that which passes through capillary walls. Compared to an exudate, a transudate has fewer cellular elements and is of a lower specific gravity.

**transudation** (trăns-ū-dā′shŭn) Oozing of a fluid through pores or interstices, as of a membrane.

**transureteroureterostomy** (trăns″ū-rē″tĕr-ō-ū-rē″tĕr-ŏs′tō-mē) Section of one ureter and joining both ends to the opposite ureter.

**transurethral** (trăns″ū-rē′thrăl) [″ + Gr. *ourethra,* urethra] Pert. to an operation performed through the urethra.

**transurethral resection of the prostate** ABBR: TUR, TURP. The removal of prostatic tissue using a device inserted through the urethra. SEE: *prostate.*

**transvaginal** (trăns-văj′ĭn-ăl) [″ + *vagina,* sheath] Through the vagina or across its wall as in a surgical procedure.

**transvector** (trăns-vĕk′tor) An animal that transmits a toxin that it does not produce and by which it is itself unaffected, as when a bivalve mollusc, such as the oyster, filters viruses out of the water and transmits them to those who ingest the mollusc.

**transvenous** Through a vein.

**transversalis** (trăns″vĕr-să′lĭs) [″ + *vertere,* to turn] A structure occurring at right angles to the long axis of the body.

**transversalis fascia** A thin membrane forming the peritoneal surface of the transversus muscle and its aponeurosis.

**transverse** (trăns-vĕrs′) [L. *transversus*] Lying at right angles to the long axis of the body; crosswise.

**transversectomy** (trăns″vĕr-sĕk′tō-mē) [″ +

Gr. *ektome,* excision] Excision of a transverse vertebral process.

**transverse foramen** A canal through the transverse processes of the cervical vertebrae for passage of the vertebral arteries.

**transverse plane** A plane that divides the body into a top and bottom portion.

**transversion** (trăns-vĕr′zhŭn) The eruption of a tooth at an abnormal site.

**transversocostal** (trăns-vĕr″sō-kŏs′tăl) Costotransverse.

**transversospinalis** (trăns-vĕr″sō-spī-nā′lĭs) [L. *transversus,* turned across, + *spina,* thorn] Semispinalis capitis, semispinalis cervicis. SEE: *Muscles Appendix.*

**transversourethralis** (trăns-vĕr″sō-ū″rē-thrā′lĭs) The transverse fibers of the sphincter urethrae muscle.

**transversus** (trăns-vĕr′sŭs) [L.] **1.** Any of several small muscles. SEE: *Muscles Appendix.* **2.** Lying across the long axis of a part or organ.

**transvesical** (trăns-vĕs′ĭ-kăl) Across or through the bladder.

**transvestism, transvestitism** (trăns-vĕst′ĭzm, -ĭ-tĭzm) [L. *trans,* across, + *vestitus,* clothed, + Gr. *-ismos,* condition] The desire to dress in the clothes of and be accepted as a member of the opposite sex.

**transvestite** (trăns-vĕs′tīt) An individual who practices transvestism.

**Trantas' dots** (trăn′tăs) [Alexios Trantas, Gr. ophthalmologist, 1867–1960] Chalky concretions of the conjunctiva around the limbus. These are associated with vernal conjunctivitis.

**tranylcypromine** (trăn″ĭl-sī′prō-mēn) An antidepressant drug. Trade name is Parnate.

**trap, food** A space or area in or between teeth where particles of food may become lodged.

**trapeze bar** Triangular device suspended above a bed to facilitate transferring and positioning the patient; also called a *swivel trapeze bar.*

**trapezial** (tră-pē′zē-ăl) Concerning the trapezium.

**trapeziform** (tră-pē′zĭ-form) Shaped like a trapezoid.

**trapezii** The trapezium and trapezoid carpal bones once they have fused. They function as one bone in the mechanics of the wrist.

**trapeziometacarpal** (tră-pē″zē-ō-mĕt″ă-kăr′păl) Concerning or connecting the trapezium and the metacarpus of the thumb.

**trapezium** (tră-pē′zē-ŭm) [Gr. *trapezion,* a little table] **1.** A four-sided, single-plane geometric figure in which none of the sides are parallel. **2.** The os trapezium, the first bone on the radial side of the distal row of the bones of the wrist. It articulates with the base of the metacarpal bone of the thumb. SYN: *greater multangular bone.*

**trapezius** (tră-pē′zē-ŭs) A flat, triangular muscle covering the posterior surface of the neck and shoulder. SEE: *Muscles Appendix.*

**trapezoid** (trăp′ĕ-zoyd) [Gr. *trapezoeides,* table-shaped] A four-sided figure having two parallel sides and two divergent sides.

**trapezoid body** A bundle of transverse fibers in the ventral portion of the tegmentum of pons. SYN: *corpus trapezoideum.*

**trapezoid bone** The second bone in the distal row of carpal bones. It lies between the trapezium and capitate bones. SYN: *lesser multangular bone.*

**trapezoid ligament** The lateral portion of the coracoclavicular ligament.

**trauma** (traw′mă) *pl.* **traumata, traumas** [Gr. *trauma,* wound] **1.** A physical injury or wound caused by external force or violence. It may be self-inflicted. In the U.S., trauma is the principal cause of death between the ages of 1 and 44 years. In addition to each death from trauma, there are at least two cases of permanent disability caused by trauma. The principal types of trauma involved include motor vehicle accidents, falls, burns, gunshot wounds, and drowning. The majority of deaths occur in the first several hours after the event. **2.** An emotional or psychological shock that may produce disordered feelings or behavior.

***birth t.*** Injury to the fetus during the birthing process.

***high risk for t.*** Accentuated risk of accidental tissue injury (e.g., wound, burn, fracture). SEE: *Nursing Diagnoses Appendix.*

***occlusal t.*** Any injury to part of the masticatory system as a result of malocclusion or occlusal dysfunction. It may be abrupt in its development in response to a restoration or ill-fitting prosthetic device, or result from years of tooth wear, drift, or faulty oral habits. It may produce adverse periodontal changes, tooth mobility, or excessive wear, pain in the temporomandibular joints, or spasms and pain in the muscles of mastication.

***psychic t.*** A painful emotional experience that may cause anxiety.

***toothbrush t.*** Abrasion or grooving of teeth and gingival injury or recession as a result of improper brushing with a stiff-textured brush.

**trauma center** A regional hospital capable of providing care for critically injured patients. Available on a 24-hr basis are a surgical team, operating suite, surgical subspecialties, intensive care unit, and specialized nursing team.

**Trauma Score** Numerical grading system that combines the Glasgow Coma Scale and measurements of cardiopulmonary function as a gauge of severity of injury and predictor of survival after blunt trauma to the head. Each parameter is given a number (high for normal and low for impaired or absent function). Severity of injury is estimated by summing the

**Trauma Score**

| Cardiopulmonary* | | |
|---|---|---|
| Respiratory rate | 10–24/min | 4 |
| | 24–35/min | 3 |
| | 36/min or greater | 2 |
| | 1–9/min | 1 |
| | None | 0 |
| Respiratory expansion | Normal | 1 |
| | Retractive | 0 |
| Systolic blood pressure | 90 mm Hg or greater | 4 |
| | 70–89 mm Hg | 3 |
| | 50–69 mm Hg | 2 |
| | 0–49 mm Hg | 1 |
| Pulse | None | 0 |
| Capillary refill | Normal | 2 |
| | Delayed | 1 |
| | None | 0 |
| Cardiopulmonary assessment | | |

| Neurological† (Glasgow Coma Scale) | | |
|---|---|---|
| Eye opening | Spontaneous | 4 |
| | To voice | 3 |
| | To pain | 2 |
| | None | 1 |
| Verbal response | Oriented | 5 |
| | Confused | 4 |
| | Inappropriate speech | 3 |
| | Incomprehensible sounds | 2 |
| | None | 1 |
| Motor response | Obeys command | 6 |
| | Localizes pain | 5 |
| | Withdraws (pain) | 4 |
| | Flexion (pain) | 3 |
| | Extension (pain) | 2 |
| | None | 1 |
| Glasgow Coma Score Total | | |
| **Total Glasgow Coma Scale Points**<br>14 – 15 = 5<br>11 – 13 = 4<br>8 – 10 = 3<br>5 – 7 = 2<br>3 – 4 = 1 | Conversion = Approximately one third total value | |
| Neurological assessment | | |

Total trauma score = Cardiopulmonary + Neurological

* Adapted from Champion, HR, Sacco, WJ, Carnazzo, AJ, et al: Trauma score. Crit Care Med 9(9):672–676, 1981.

† Adapted from Teasdale, G, and Jennett, B: Lancet II, 1974, p. 81, and Teasdale, G, et al: Acta Neurochirurgica Suppl. 28, 1979, pp 13–16.

numbers. The lowest score is 1, the highest 16. SEE: table.

**traumatic** (traw-măt′ĭk) [Gr. *traumatikos*] Caused by or relating to an injury.

**traumatic psychosis** Psychosis resulting from physical injuries or emotional shock.

**traumatism** (traw′mă-tĭzm) [Gr. *traumatismos*] Morbid condition of a system owing to an injury or a wound.

**traumato-** Combining form meaning *trauma.*

**traumatology** (traw-mă-tŏl′ō-jē) [Gr. *trauma,* wound, + *logos,* word, reason] The branch of surgery dealing with wounds and their care.

**traumatopathy** (traw″mă-tŏp′ă-thē) [″ + *pathos,* disease, suffering] Pathological state caused by trauma.

**traumatophilia** (traw″mă-tō-fĭl′ē-ă) [″ + *philein,* to love] The enjoyment of or unconscious desire to be traumatized, either mentally or physically. SEE: *masochism.*

**traumatopnea** (traw″mă-tŏp-nē′ă) [″ + *pnoia,* breath] The passage of air in and out of a wound in the chest wall.

**traumatopyra** (traw″mă-tō-pī′ră) [″ + *pyr,* fever] Fever caused by trauma.

**traumatotherapy** (traw″mă-tō-thĕr′ă-pē) Treatment of injury.

**travel, medical preparation for** The process of advance consideration and planning for the environmental, physical, and social changes that may be encountered during travel.

For travel in the U.S., no particular medical provisions need be made other than the usual ones concerning a spare pair of glasses, provisions for any medicines taken regularly, and suitable clothing. International travel requires more planning with respect to required immunizations, knowledge of climatic conditions that will be encountered, and the availability of medical care in the places that will be visited. Knowledge of the altitude of the area to be visited is particularly important if the traveler has chronic diseases of the heart or lungs. Persons who use wheelchairs will need to know how well suited the places to be visited are for wheelchair access. It is also important to know whether or not one's medical insurance will cover medical expenses incurred abroad. SEE: *diarrhea, travelers'*.

**tray** (trā) A flat surface with raised edges.

***impression t.*** In dentistry, a U-shaped receptacle with raised edges made of metal or acrylic resin used to carry impression material and support it in contact with the surfaces to be recorded until the impression material is set or firm.

**Treacher Collins syndrome** [Edward Treacher Collins, Brit. ophthalmologist, 1862–1919] Mandibulofacial dysostosis.

**treatment** (trēt'mĕnt) [ME. *treten,* to handle] **1.** Medical, surgical, dental, or psychiatric management of a patient. **2.** Any specific procedure used for the cure or the amelioration of a disease or pathological condition. SEE: *therapy.*

***active t.*** Treatment directed specifically toward cure of a disease.

***causal t.*** Treatment directed toward removal of the cause of the disease.

***conservative t.*** **1.** The withholding of administration of medicine or use of operative procedures until such procedures are clearly indicated. **2.** In surgical cases, the preservation of the organ or part if at all possible with the least possible mutilation.

***dental t.*** Any of a variety of treatments of the teeth and adjacent tissues to restore or maintain normal oral health and function.

***dietetic t.*** Treatment of disease based on regulation of diet.

***electric shock t.*** Electroshock therapy; shock therapy.

***empiric t.*** Treatment based on observation and experience rather than having a scientific basis.

***expectant t.*** Relief of symptoms as they arise (i.e., not directed at the specific cause).

***palliative t.*** Treatment designed for the relief of symptoms of the disease rather than curing the disease.

***preventive t.*** Treatment directed at the prevention of disease.

***radiation t.*** The administration of high-energy x-ray photons, electrons, or nuclear emissions for the cure of cancer or palliation of symptoms.

***rational t.*** Treatment based on scientific principles.

***shock t.*** Electroshock therapy; shock therapy.

***specific t.*** Treatment directed at the cause of a disease.

***supportive t.*** Special measures employed to supplement specific therapy.

***surgical t.*** Treatment by performance of an operation.

***symptomatic t.*** Treatment directed toward constitutional symptoms, such as pyrexia, shock, and pain.

**treatment plan** The projected series and sequence of treatment procedures based on an individualized evaluation of what is needed to restore or improve the health and function of a patient.

**tree** A structure that resembles a tree.

***bronchial t.*** The right or left bronchus with its branches and their terminal arborizations.

***tracheobronchial t.*** The trachea, bronchi, and their branches.

**trehala** (trē-hā'lă) A sweet substance secreted by the insect *Larinus maculatus.*

**trehalase** (trē-hā'lās) An enzyme that hydrolyzes trehalose to form two molecules; D-glucose.

**trehalose** (trē-hā'lōs) A disaccharide of trehala. It is also present in certain fungi.

**Trematoda** (trĕm"ă-tō'dă) [Gr. *trematodes,* pierced] A class of flatworms commonly called flukes belonging to the phylum Platyhelminthes. It includes two orders: Monogenea, which are external or semi-external parasites having direct development with no asexual multiplication, and Digenea, internal parasites with asexual generation in their life cycle. The Digenea usually require two or more hosts, the hosts alternating. SEE: *fluke.*

**trematode** (trĕm'ă-tōd) A parasitic flatworm belonging to the class Trematoda. SEE: *cercaria; fluke.*

**trematodiasis** (trĕm"ă-tō-dī'ă-sĭs) Infestation with a trematode.

**tremble** (trĕm'bl) [O. Fr. *trembler*] **1.** An involuntary quivering or shaking. **2.** To shiver, quiver, or shake.

**trembles** (trĕm'blz) A condition resulting from ingestion of plants such as snakeroot *(Eupatorium urticaefolium)* or jimmyweed *(Haplopappus heterophyllus).* The condition is common in domestic animals and may occur in humans as a result of ingesting the plants or more commonly from drinking milk or eating the meat of poisoned animals. Symptoms are weakness, anorexia, nausea and vomiting, and prostration, possibly resulting in death. In humans, the illness is called milk sickness.

**tremelloid, tremellose** (trĕm'ĕ-loyd, -lōs) Jelly-like.

**tremetol** (trĕm'ĕ-tŏl) A poisonous substance occurring in snakeroot, rayless goldenrod, and other plants that may cause trembles in animals or humans. SEE: *trembles.*

**tremograph** (trĕm'ō-grăf) [" + Gr. *graphein,* to write] A device for recording tremors.

**tremolabile** (trē"mō-lā'bl) [" + *labi,* to slip]

Easily destroyed or inactivated by shaking; said of a ferment.

**tremophobia** (trē″mō-fō′bē-ă) [″ + Gr. *phobos*, fear] An abnormal fear of trembling.

**tremor** (trĕm′or, trē′mor) [L. *tremor*, a shaking] **1.** A quivering, esp. a continuous quivering of a convulsive nature. **2.** An involuntary movement of a part or parts of the body resulting from alternate contractions of opposing muscles. SEE: *subsultus.*

Tremors may be classified as involuntary, static, dynamic, kinetic, hereditary, and hysteric. Pathological tremors are independent of the will. The trembling may be fine or coarse, rapid or slow, and may appear on movement (intention tremor) or improve when the part is voluntarily exercised. It is often caused by organic disease; trembling may also express an emotion (e.g., fear). All abnormal tremors except palatal and ocular myoclonus disappear during sleep.

***action t.*** Intention t.

***alcoholic t.*** The visible tremor exhibited by alcoholics.

***cerebellar t.*** An intention tremor of 3 to 5 Hz frequency, associated with cerebellar disease.

***coarse t.*** A tremor in which oscillations are relatively slow.

***continuous t.*** A tremor that resembles tremors of paralysis agitans.

***enhanced physiological t.*** An action tremor associated with catecholamine excess (e.g., in association with anxiety, thyrotoxicosis, hypoglycemia, or alcohol withdrawal). It may occur as a side effect of drugs, such as epinephrine, caffeine, theophylline, amphetamines, levodopa, tricyclic antidepressants, lithium, and corticosteroids.

***essential t.*** A benign tremor, usually of the head, chin, outstretched hands, and occasionally the voice, that needs to be differentiated from the tremor of parkinsonism. Essential tremor, which is made worse by anxiety or action, is usually 8 to 10 cycles per second and that of parkinsonism 4 to 5. In essential tremor, there is usually a family history but not in parkinsonism. The medicines that are effective in treating parkinsonism have no effect on essential tremor.

***familial t.*** A tremor indistinguishable from essential tremor in its clinical manifestation. The difference is this tremor occurs in several members of a family. It is inherited as an autosomal dominant trait.

***fibrillary t.*** A tremor caused by consecutive contractions of separate muscular fibrillae rather than of a muscle or muscles.

***fine t.*** A rapid tremor.

***flapping t.*** Asterixis.

***forced t.*** A tremor continuing after voluntary motion has ceased.

***Hunt's t.*** A tremor associated with all voluntary movements. It is present in certain cerebellar lesions.

***hysterical t.*** A fine tremor occurring in hysteria. It may be limited to one extremity or generalized.

***intention t.*** A tremor exhibited or intensified when attempting coordinated movements. SYN: *action t.*

***intermittent t.*** A tremor common to paralyzed muscles in hemoplegia when attempting voluntary movement.

***muscular t.*** Slight oscillating muscular contractions in rhythmical order.

***parkinsonian t.*** A rest tremor that is suppressed briefly during voluntary activity. Parkinson's disease can occur without tremor. The tremor disappears during all but the lightest phases of sleep.

***physiological t.*** A tremor occurring in normal individuals. It may be transient and occur in association with excessive physical exertion, excitement, hunger, fatigue, or other causes. SEE: *enhanced physiological t.*

***rest t.*** A tremor present when the involved part is at rest but absent or diminished when active movements are attempted. SYN: *static t.*

***senile t.*** A tremor indistinguishable from essential tremor in its clinical manifestation. The difference is this type of tremor has its onset in late adult life.

***static t.*** Rest t.

***volitional t.*** Trembling of the limbs or of the body when making a voluntary effort; seen in multiple sclerosis and other nervous diseases.

**tremorgram** (trĕm′or-grăm) Graphic representation of a tremor recorded on a tremograph.

**tremulor** (trĕm′ū-lor) A device for administering vibratory massage.

**tremulous** (trĕm′ū-lŭs) [L. *tremulus*] Trembling or shaking.

**trench fever** A nonfatal, febrile disease of diverse signs, symptoms, and severity. Usually present are headache; malaise; pain; tenderness, esp. in the shins; splenomegaly; and sometimes a transient macular rash. The causative rickettsial organism, *Rochalimaea quintana,* may be cultured from the blood. Even though humans are the hosts for the organism, the disease is not directly transmitted from person to person. The body louse, *Pediculus humanus humanus,* is the intermediate host. It begins to excrete infectious feces 5 to 12 days after ingesting blood from an infected human. The causative organism is sensitive *in vitro* to antibiotics such as tetracyclines and chloramphenicol, but there is no evidence that these are clinically effective.

**trench foot** A condition resembling frostbite affecting the feet of soldiers who are obliged to keep their feet in wet socks and shoes for long periods.

**trench mouth** Acute necrotizing ulcerative gingivitis.

**trend** [ME. *trenden,* to revolve] The inclination to proceed in a certain direction or at a certain rate; used to describe the prognosis or course of a symptom or disease.

**Trendelenburg gait** A side lurching of the trunk over the stance leg due to weakness in the gluteus medius muscle.

**Trendelenburg position** (trĕn-dĕl′ĕn-bŭrg) [Friedrich Trendelenburg, Ger. surgeon, 1844–1924] A position in which the patient's head is low and the body and legs are on an elevated and inclined plane. This may be accomplished by having the patient flat on a bed and elevating the foot of the bed. In this position, the abdominal organs are pushed up toward the chest by gravity. The foot of the bed may be elevated by resting it on blocks. This position is used in abdominal surgery. In treating shock, this position is usually used, but if there is an associated head injury, the head should not be kept lower than the trunk. SEE: *position* for illus.

**Trendelenburg sign** A pelvic drop on the side of the elevated leg when the patient stands on one leg and lifts the other. It indicates weakness or instability of the gluteus medius muscle on the stance side.

**Trendelenburg test** A test to evaluate the strength of the gluteus medius muscle. The examiner stands behind the patient and observes the pelvis as the patient stands on one leg and then the other. A positive result determines muscle weakness on the standing leg side when the pelvis tilts down on the opposite side.

**trepan** (trē-păn′) [Gr. *trypanon,* a borer] **1.** To perforate the skull with a trepan to relieve the brain from pressure. **2.** An instrument resembling a carpenter's bit for incision of the skull. SYN: *trephine.*

**trepanation** (trĕp″ă-nā′shŭn) [L. *trepanatio*] Surgery using a trepan.

***corneal t.*** Keratoplasty.

**trephination** (trĕf″ĭn-ā′shŭn) [Fr. *trephine,* a bore] The process of cutting out a piece of bone with the trephine.

**trephine** (trē-fīn′) **1.** To perforate with a trephine. **2.** A cylindrical saw for cutting a circular piece of bone out of the skull. SYN: *trepan.*

**trephining** The process of cutting bone with a trephine.

**trephocyte** (trĕf′ō-sīt) [Gr. *trephein,* to feed, + *kytos,* cell] Trophocyte.

**trepidant** (trĕp′ĭ-dănt) [L. *trepidans,* trembling] Marked by tremor.

**trepidatio** (trĕp″ĭ-dā′shē-ō) [L.] Trepidation.

**trepidation** (trĕp″ĭ-dā′shŭn) [L. *trepidatio,* a trembling] **1.** Fear, anxiety. **2.** Trembling movement, esp. when involuntary.

**Treponema** (trĕp″ō-nē′mă) [Gr. *trepein,* to turn, + *nema,* thread] A genus of spirochetes, parasitic in humans, which belongs to the family Treponemataceae. They move by flexing, snapping, and bending. SEE: *bacteria* for illus.

***T. carateum*** The causative agent of pinta, an infectious disease of the skin.

***T. pallidum*** The causative organism of syphilis. SYN: *Spirochaeta pallida.*

***T. pertenue*** The causative organism of yaws (frambesia).

**Treponemataceae** (trĕp″ō-nē″mă-tā′sē-ē) A family of spiral organisms belonging to the order Spirochaetales; includes the genera *Borrelia, Leptospira,* and *Treponema.*

**treponematosis** (trĕp″ō-nē-mă-tō′sĭs) Infection with *Treponema.*

**treponeme** (trĕp′ō-nēm) Any organism of the genus *Treponema.*

**treponemiasis** (trĕp″ō-nē-mī′ă-sĭs) [″ + *nema,* thread, + *-iasis,* condition] Infestation with *Treponema.*

**treponemicidal** (trĕp″ō-nē″mĭ-sī′dăl) [″ +″ + L. *cidus,* to kill] Destructive to *Treponema.*

**trepopnea** (trĕp-ŏp′nē-ă) [″ + *pnoia,* breath] The condition of being able to breathe with less difficulty when in a certain position.

**treppe** Staircase phenomenon.

**tretinoin** (trĕt′ĭ-noyn) All-transretinoic acid. It is a keratolytic agent used topically in treating acne. Trade name is Retin-A.

**TRH** *thyrotropin-releasing hormone.*

**tri-** [Gr.] Prefix meaning *three.*

**triacetate** (trī-ăs′ĕ-tāt) Any acetate that contains three acetic acid groups.

**triacetin** (trī-ăs′ĕ-tĭn) An antifungal agent used topically, whose previously used name was glyceryl triacetate.

**triacidic** (trī″ă-sĭd′ĭk) Containing three acidic hydrogen ions.

**triacylglycerols** Combination of glycerol and three fatty acids. The fatty acids may be all the same or each different. They are the major components of the storage (or deposit) of fat in plant and animal cells. These substances are referred to as fats, neutral fats, or triglycerides. These fats provide the major source of stored energy in the body. SEE: *fat.*

**triad** (trī′ăd) [Gr. *trias,* group of three] **1.** Any three things having something in common. **2.** A trivalent element. **3.** Trivalent.

***Hutchinson's t.*** A syndrome characteristic of prenatal syphilis consisting of notched teeth, interstitial keratitis, and eighth-nerve deafness due to meningeal involvement.

**triage** (trē-ăzh′) [Fr., sorting] The screening and classification of sick, wounded, or injured persons during war or other disasters to determine priority needs for the efficient use of medical and nursing personnel, equipment, and facilities. It is also done in emergency rooms and in acute care clinics to determine priority of treatment. The use of triage is essential if the maximum number of lives is to be saved during an emergency situation that produces many more sick and wounded individuals than the available medical care facilities and personnel can handle.

It is important to provide a quick, convenient method of noting the condition of each casualty. This task may be accomplished by attaching a color-coded tag to the body of the patient or labeling untraumatized skin with a marking pen. The classification is then upgraded or downgraded as indicated by the improvement or deterioration of the patient.

NURSING IMPLICATIONS: For each patient, the emergency room staff must obtain a brief history, perform a rapid physical assessment including vital signs, perform first aid if necessary, assist in determining the severity of illness, and transfer the patient to the appropriate place of care. In order of diagnosis and treatment, bleeding with subsequent shock is the second priority after establishment of an airway and basic life-support measures. Arterial bleeding, whether internal or external, needs immediate care. Next, neurological status and traumatized bones and tissues receive attention. After diagnosis and treatment of emergency conditions, the staff should perform an orderly and complete physical examination to ensure that no life-threatening condition has been neglected. The patient is reassessed frequently, and prescribed care is altered as necessary.

**triakaidekaphobia** (trī″ă-kī″dĕk-ă-fō′bē-ă) [Gr. *treis,* three, + *kai,* and, + *deka,* ten, + *phobos,* fear] Superstition regarding the number 13. SYN: *triskaidekaphobia.*

**triamcinolone** (trī″ăm-sĭn′ō-lōn) A synthetic glucosteroid drug.

**triamterene** (trī-ăm′tĕr-ēn) A potassium-sparing diuretic drug.

**triangle** (trī′ăng-gl) [L. *triangulum*] A figure or area formed by three angles and three sides.

***anal t.*** The triangle with its base between the two ischial tuberosities and its apex at the coccyx.

***anterior t. of neck*** The space bounded by the middle line of the neck, the anterior border of the sternocleidomastoid muscle, and a line running along the lower border of the mandible and continued to the mastoid process of the temporal bone.

***cephalic t.*** The triangle on the anteroposterior plane of the skull formed by lines joining the occiput and forehead and chin, and a line uniting the occiput and the chin.

***digastric t.*** The triangular region of the neck. Its borders are the mandible, stylohyoid muscle, and the anterior belly of the digastric muscle.

***t. of elbow*** The area in front of the elbow bounded by the brachioradialis and the pronator teres muscles on the sides, and with the base toward the humerus.

***facial t.*** The triangle bounded by the lines uniting the basion and the alveolar and nasal points, and one uniting the nasal and basion.

***femoral t.*** The triangle on the inner part of the thigh, bounded by the sartorius and adductor longus muscles and above by the inguinal ligament. SYN: *Scarpa's t.*

***frontal t.*** The triangle bounded by the maximum frontal diameter and the lines joining its extremities and the glabella.

***Hesselbach's t.*** The interval in the groin bounded by Poupart's ligament, the edge of the rectus muscle, and the deep epigastric artery.

***inferior carotid t.*** The space bounded by the middle line of the neck, the sternomastoid muscle, and the anterior belly of the omohyoid muscle. SYN: *muscular t.; t. of necessity.*

***inferior occipital t.*** The area having the bimastoid diameter for its base and the inion for its apex.

***Lesser's t.*** The triangle bounded below by the anterior and posterior bellies of the digastric muscle and above by the hypogastric nerve.

***lumbocostoabdominal t.*** The triangle bounded in front by the obliquus abdominis externus, above by the lower border of the serratus posticus inferior and the point of the 12th rib, behind by the outer edge of the erector spinae, and below by the obliquus abdominis internus.

***muscular t.*** Inferior carotid t.

***mylohyoid t.*** The triangular space formed by the mylohyoid muscle and the two bellies of the digastric muscle.

***t. of necessity*** Inferior carotid t.

***occipital t. of the neck*** The triangle bounded by the sternocleidomastoid, the trapezius, and the omohyoid muscles.

***omoclavicular t.*** Subclavian t.

***omohyoid t.*** Superior carotid t.

***t. of Petit*** The space above the hip bone between the exterior oblique muscle, the latissimus dorsi, and the interior oblique muscle.

***posterior cervical t.*** The triangle bounded by the upper border of the clavicle, the posterior border of the sternocleidomastoid muscle, and the anterior border of the trapezius muscle.

***pubourethral t.*** A triangular space in the perineum bounded externally by the ischiocavernous muscle, internally by the bulbocavernous muscle, and posteriorly by the transversus perinei muscle.

***Scarpa's t.*** Femoral t.

***subclavian t.*** A triangular space bounded by the posterior belly of the omohyoid, the upper border of the clavicle, and the posterior margin of the sternocleidomastoid. SYN: *omoclavicular t.; supraclavicular t.*

***submandibular t.*** The triangular region of the neck, bounded by the inferior border of the mandible, the stylohyoid muscle and the posterior belly of the digastric muscle, and the anterior belly of the digastric muscle; it is one of three triangles included in the anterior triangle of the neck. This was formerly called submaxillary triangle.

***suboccipital t.*** The triangle bounded by the obliquus inferior and superior muscles on two sides and the rectus capitis posterior major muscle on the third side. The floor contains the posterior arch of the atlas bone and the vertebral artery. It is covered by the semispinalis capitis muscle.

***superior carotid t.*** The space bounded by the anterior belly of the omohyoid muscle, the posterior belly of the digastricus muscle, and the sternomastoid muscle. SYN: *omohyoid t.*

***supraclavicular t.*** Subclavian t.

***suprameatal t.*** The triangle slightly above and behind the exterior auditory meatus. It is bounded above by the root of the zygoma and anteriorly by the posterior wall of the exterior auditory meatus.

***urogenital t.*** The triangle with its base formed by a line between the two ischial tuberosities and its apex just below the symphysis pubis.

***vesical t.*** Trigone.

**triangular** Having three sides; shaped like a triangle. SYN: *triquetral; triquetrous.*

**triangular bandage** A square bandage folded diagonally. When folded, the several thicknesses can be applied to afford support. SEE: illus.; *bandage.*

**triangularis** (trī-ăng″gū-lā′rĭs) [L.] A muscle of the chin. SEE: *Muscles Appendix.*

**triangular ligament** One of two ligaments, right and left, connecting posterior portions of the right and left lobes of the liver with corresponding portions of the diaphragm.

**triangular nucleus of Schwalbe** The chief or dorsal nucleus of the vestibular division of the eighth cranial nerve. It is located in the pons and occupies most of the acoustic area of the rhomboid fossa.

**triangulation** In qualitative research, a technique for enhancing validity by comparing information gathered from several sources. Qualitative research, and thus triangulation, is being used increasingly in the rehabilitation sciences and in behavioral medicine.

**Triatoma** (trī-ăt′ō-mă) A genus of blood-sucking insects belonging to the order Hemiptera, family Reduviidae; commonly called cone-nosed bugs or assassin bugs. It includes the species *T. braziliensis, T. dimidiata, T. infestans, T. protracta, T. recuva, T. rubida,* and others. They are house-infesting pests and some species, esp. *T. infestans,* transmit *Trypanosoma cruzi,* the causative agent of Chagas' disease.

**triatomic** (trī″ă-tŏm′ĭk) Composed of three atoms.

**tribade** A lesbian.

**tribadism** (trĭb′ăd-ĭzm) [Gr. *tribein,* to rub, + *-ismos,* condition] A relationship in which women attempt to imitate heterosexual intercourse with each other.

**tribasic** (trī-bā′sĭk) [Gr. *treis,* three, + L. *basis,* base] Capable of neutralizing or accepting three hydrogen ions.

**tribasilar** (trī-băs′ĭl-ăr) [″ + L. *basilaris,*

TRIANGULAR BANDAGE

STEPS IN MAKING SLING FOR ARM

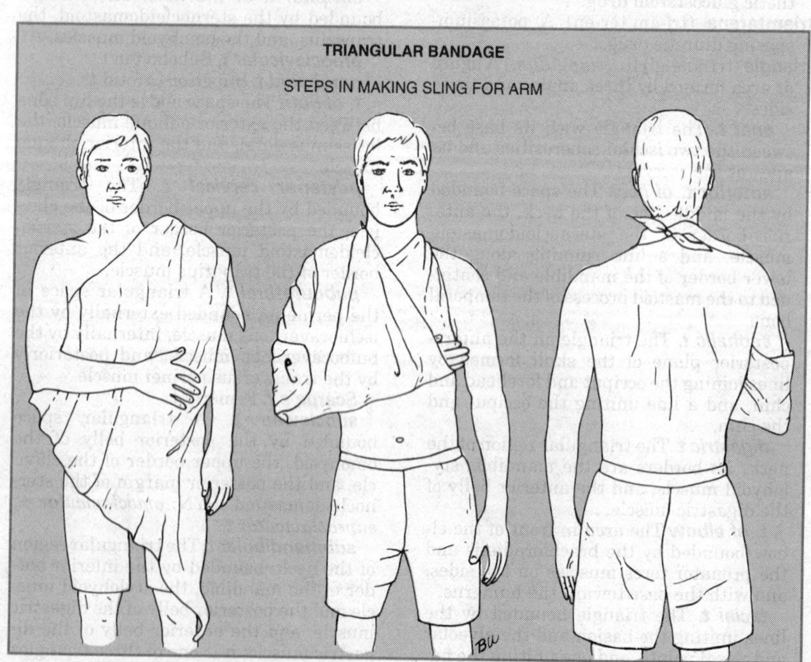

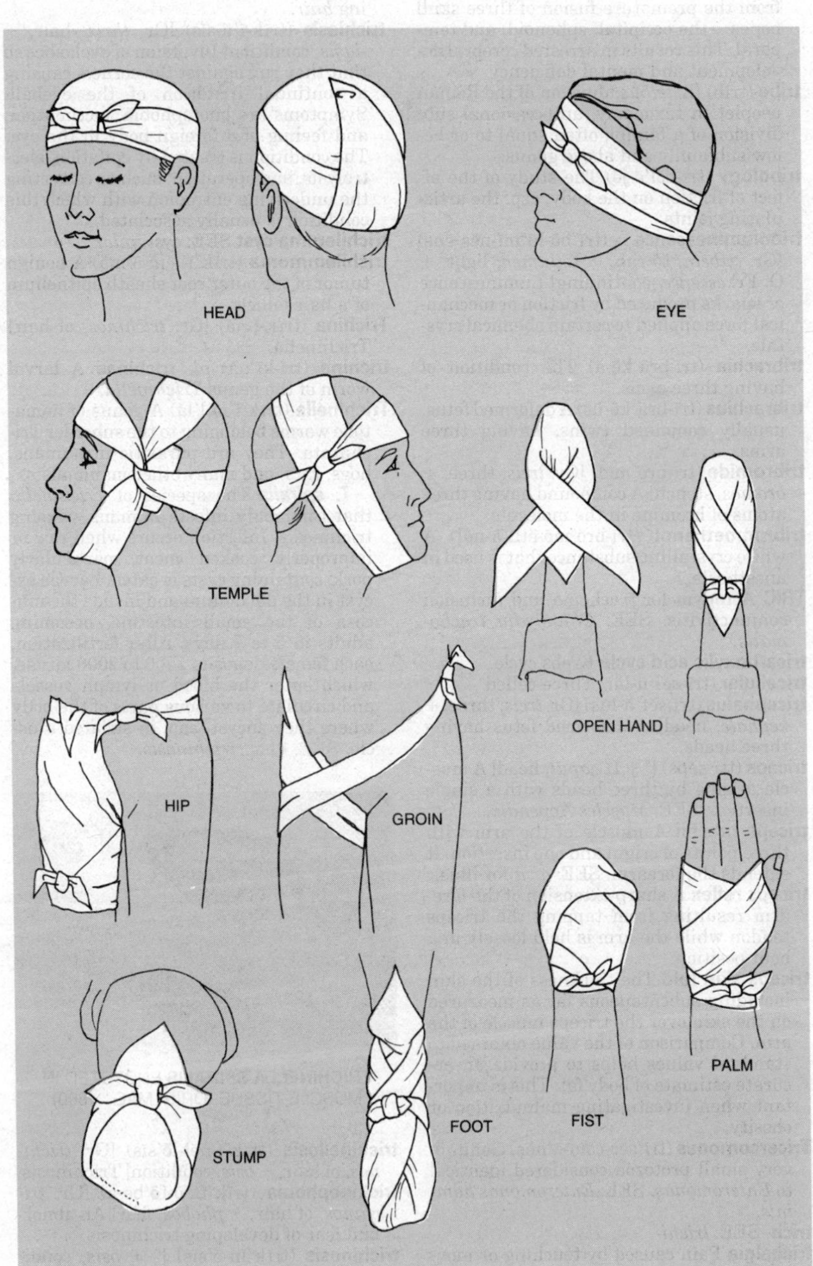


TRIANGULAR BANDAGES

base] Having three bases.

**tribasilar synostosis** A condition resulting from the premature fusion of three skull bones—the occipital, sphenoid, and temporal. This results in arrested cerebral development and mental deficiency.

**tribe** (trīb) [L. *tribus,* division of the Roman people] In taxonomy, an occasional subdivision of a family; often equal to or below subfamily and above genus.

**tribology** (trĭ-bŏl′ō-jē) The study of the effect of friction on the body, esp. the articulating joints.

**triboluminescence** (trī″bō-lū″mĭ-nĕs′ĕns) [Gr. *tribein,* to rub, + L. *lumen,* light, + O. Fr. *escence,* continuing] Luminescence or sparks produced by friction or mechanical force applied to certain chemical crystals.

**tribrachia** (trī-brā′kē-ă) The condition of having three arms.

**tribrachius** (trī-brā′kē-ŭs) A deformed fetus, usually conjoined twins, having three arms.

**tribromide** (trī-brō′mīd) [Gr. *treis,* three, + *bromos,* stench] A compound having three atoms of bromine in the molecule.

**tribromoethanol** (trī-brō″mō-ĕth′ă-nŏl) A white crystalline substance that is used in anesthesia.

**TRIC** Acronym for *tr*achoma and *i*nclusion *c*onjunctivitis. SEE: *Chlamydia trachomatis.*

**tricarboxylic acid cycle** Krebs cycle.

**tricellular** (trī-sĕl′ū-lăr) Three-celled.

**tricephalus** (trī-sĕf′ă-lŭs) [Gr. *treis,* three, + *kephale,* head] A deformed fetus having three heads.

**triceps** (trī′sĕps) [″ + L. *caput,* head] A muscle arising by three heads with a single insertion. SEE: *Muscles Appendix.*

**triceps brachii** A muscle of the arm with three points of origin and one insertion. It extends the forearm. SEE: *arm* for illus.

**triceps reflex** A sharp extension of the forearm resulting from tapping the triceps tendon while the arm is held loosely in a bent position.

**triceps skin fold** The thickness of the skin including subcutaneous fat as measured on the skin over the triceps muscle of the arm. Comparison of the value obtained to standard values helps to provide an accurate estimate of body fat. This is important when investigating malnutrition or obesity.

**Tricercomonas** (trī″sĕr-cŏm-ō′năs) Genus of very small protozoa considered identical to *Enteromonas.* SEE: *Enteromonas hominis.*

**trich-** SEE: *trichi-.*

**trichalgia** Pain caused by touching or moving the hair.

**trichangiectasia, trichangiectasis** (trĭk″ăn-jē-ĕk-tā′zē-ă, -ĕk′tă-sĭs) [Gr. *thrix,* hair, + *angeion,* vessel, + *ektasis,* dilatation] Telangiectasia.

**trichatrophia** (trĭk″ă-trō′fē-ă) [″ + *atrophia,* atrophy] Brittleness of hair resulting from atrophy of the root.

**trichi-, trich, tricho-** Combining form meaning *hair.*

**trichiasis** (trĭk-ī′ă-sĭs) [Gr. *thrix,* hair, + *-iasis,* condition] Inversion of eyelashes so that they rub against the cornea, causing a continual irritation of the eyeball. Symptoms are photophobia, lacrimation, and feeling of a foreign body in the eye. The condition is treated by epilation, electrolysis, and operation, such as correcting the underlying entropion with which this condition is usually associated.

**trichilemma cyst** SEE: *cyst, pilar.*

**trichilemmoma** (trĭk″ĭ-lĕm-ō′mă) A benign tumor of the outer root sheath epithelium of a hair follicle.

**Trichina** (trĭk-ī′nă) [Gr. *trichinos,* of hair] Trichinella.

**trichina** (trĭ-kī′nă) *pl.* **trichinae** A larval worm of the genus *Trichinella.*

**Trichinella** (trĭk″ĭ-nĕl′lă) A genus of nematode worms belonging to the suborder Trichurata. They are parasitic in humans, hogs, rats, and many other mammals.

***T. spiralis*** The species of *Trichinella* that commonly infests humans, causing trichinosis. Infection occurs when raw or improperly cooked meat, particularly pork, containing cysts is eaten. Larvae excyst in the duodenum and invade the mucosa of the small intestine, becoming adults in 5 to 7 days. After fertilization, each female deposits 1000 to 2000 larvae, which enter the blood or lymph vessels and circulate to various parts of the body where they encyst, esp. in striated muscle. SEE: illus.; *trichinosis.*

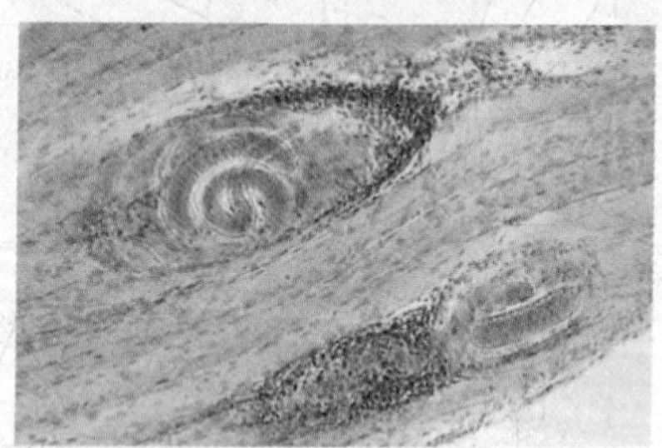

**TRICHINELLA SPIRALIS** ENCYSTED IN MUSCLE TISSUE (ORIG. MAG. ×800)

**trichinellosis** (trĭk″ĭ-nĕl-lō′sĭs) [Gr. *trichinos,* of hair, + *osis,* condition] Trichinosis.

**trichinophobia** (trĭk″ĭn-ō-fō′bē-ă) [Gr. *trichinos,* of hair, + *phobos,* fear] An abnormal fear of developing trichinosis.

**trichinosis** (trĭk″ĭn-ō′sĭs) [″ + *osis,* condition] A disease caused by the ingestion of *Trichinella spiralis* when raw or insufficiently cooked infected pork or wild game (e.g., bear, seals, or moose) is eaten. SYN: *trichinellosis.* SEE: *Nursing Diagnoses Appendix.*

SYMPTOMS: Sometimes symptoms are

lacking. When large numbers of the organism have been ingested, gastrointestinal symptoms, such as pain, nausea, vomiting, and serous diarrhea, develop in a few days. In 1 to 2 weeks, muscular symptoms develop. Muscles become swollen, firm, and extremely painful. Movement is inhibited and dyspnea results from involvement of respiratory muscles. Edema, esp. of the face, is a prominent symptom. Profuse sweating is observed sometimes, and high fever and eosinophilia are usually present.

In the third to sixth week of the disease, signs and symptoms of encephalitis and meningitis with visual and auditory symptoms may develop.

TREATMENT: For the acute stage, thiabendazole may be helpful. In later stages, after the worms have involved the muscles, muscle pains should be relieved by analgesics. Corticosteroids are indicated for allergic reaction or central nervous system involvement. Treatment is in general symptomatic and supportive to enable the patient to survive the acute toxemia following invasion of the muscles. After encystment, the only symptom is vague muscular pains, which may persist for weeks.

PROGNOSIS: The prognosis depends on the number of worms ingested. The majority of patients recover.

PREVENTION: Proper cooking of food, esp. pork and wild animal meat, can prevent this disease. Meat should be heated long enough for all parts to reach at least 160°F (71°C). Freezing for a certain time can also prevent the disease, but other methods, such as smoking or pickling, are ineffective in destroying this roundworm. Low-level gamma irradiation effectively sterilizes pork; at high levels, it kills trichina encysted larvae.

NURSING IMPLICATIONS: The nurse provides support and encourages the patient to report adverse symptoms, because treatment is primarily directed at their relief. The patient should also obtain sufficient rest.

**trichinous** (trĭk′ĭn-ŭs) [Gr. *trichinos,* of hair] Infested with trichinae.

**trichinous myositis** Myositis trichinosa.

**trichion** (trĭk′ē-ŏn) [Gr.] The anthropometric point at which the midsagittal plane of the head intersects the hairline.

**trichitis** (trĭk-ī′tĭs) [Gr. *thrix,* hair, + *itis,* inflammation] Inflammation of hair bulbs.

**trichloride** (trī-klō′rīd) A compound containing three atoms of chlorine.

**trichlormethiazide** (trī-klor″mĕ-thī′ă-zīd) A diuretic drug of the thiazide type.

**trichloroacetic acid** A drug used as a caustic to destroy certain types of warts, condylomata, keratoses, and hyperplastic tissue.

**trichloroethylene** (trī″klor-ō-ĕth′ĭl-ēn) A colorless clear volatile liquid with a specific gravity of 1.47 at 59°F (15°C). It is used as an analgesic and anesthetic agent to supplement the action of nitrous oxide. It should not be used with epinephrine.

---

Caution: This substance should not be used in a system that requires soda lime. The heat generated in this type of system by the action of carbon dioxide and the lime will break down trichloroethylene to form the toxic gas phosgene and hydrochloric acid. Also, in the presence of alkali the toxic and flammable substance dichloroacetylene is formed.

---

**2,4,5-trichlorophenoxyacetic acid** ABBR: 2,4,5-T. A widely used herbicide that contains dioxin, a toxic and undesirable contaminant.

**tricho-** [Gr. *thrix, trichos,* hair] SEE: *trichi-*.

**trichoanesthesia** (trĭk″ō-ăn″ĕs-thē′zē-ă) Loss of sensibility of the hair.

**trichobacteria** (trĭk″ō-băk-tē′rē-ă) [Gr. *thrix, trichos,* hair, + *bakterion,* rod] **1.** Filamentous bacteria. **2.** Bacteria possessing flagella.

**trichobezoar** (trĭk″ō-bē′zor) [″ + Arabic *bazahr,* protecting against poison] Hairball.

**trichocardia** (trĭk-ō-kăr′dē-ă) [″ + *kardia,* heart] Pericardial inflammation with elevations resembling hair. SYN: *shaggy pericardium.*

**trichoclasia, trichoclasis** (trĭk″ō-klā′zē-ă, -ŏk′lăs-ĭs) [″ + *klasis,* a breaking] Brittleness of the hair.

**trichocryptosis** (trĭk″ō-krĭp-tō′sĭs) [″ + *kryptos,* concealed] Any disease of the hair follicles.

**trichocyst** (trĭk′ō-sĭst) [″ + *kystis,* bladder] **1.** A cell structure derived from cytoplasm. **2.** In some single-celled organisms, a vesicle equipped with a thread that can be thrust out for the purposes of defense or attack.

**Trichodectes** (trĭk″ō-dĕk′tēz) [″ + *dektes,* biter] A genus of lice of the suborder Mallophaga. These lice do not bite humans.

**trichoepithelioma** (trĭk″ō-ĕp″ĭ-thē-lē-ō″mă) [″ + *epi,* upon, + *thele,* nipple, + *oma,* tumor] A benign skin tumor originating in the hair follicles.

**trichoesthesia** (trĭk″ō-ĕs-thē′zē-ă) [″ + *aisthesis,* sensation] **1.** The sensation felt when a hair is touched. **2.** A paresthesia causing a sensation of the presence of a hair on a mucous membrane or on the skin.

**trichogen** (trĭk′ō-jĕn) [″ + *gennan,* to produce] An agent stimulating hair growth.

**trichogenous** (trĭk-ŏj′ĕn-ŭs) Promoting hair growth.

**trichoglossia** (trĭk″ō-glŏs′ē-ă) [″ + *glossa,* tongue] Hairy condition of the tongue.

**trichohyalin** (trĭk″ō-hī′ă-lĭn) [″ + *hyalos,* glass] The hyaline of the hair.

**trichoid** (trĭk′oyd) [″ + *eidos,* form, shape] Hairlike.

**trichokryptomania** (trĭk″ō-krĭp″tō-mā′nēă) [″ + *kryptos,* hidden, + *mania,* madness]

An abnormal desire to break off the hair or beard with the fingernail.

**tricholith** (trĭk′ō-lĭth) [″ + *lithos,* stone] **1.** A hairy nodule on the hair; seen in piedra. **2.** A calcified intestinal bezoar that contains hair.

**trichology** (trĭk-ŏl′ō-jē) [″ + *logos,* word, reason] The study of the hair and its care and treatment.

**trichoma** (trĭk-ō′mă) [Gr., hairiness] **1.** Inversion of one or more eyelashes. SYN: *entropion.* **2.** Matted, verminous, encrusted state of the hair.

**trichomatosis** (trĭk″ō-mă-tō′sĭs) [″ + *osis,* condition] Entangled matted hair caused by fungus disease of the scalp and lack of cleanliness.

**trichomatous** (trĭ-kŏm′ă-tŭs) Of the nature of or affected with trichoma.

**trichome** (trī′kōm) [Gr. *trichoma,* a growth of hair] **1.** A hair or other appendage of the skin. **2.** A colony of blue-green algae that grows end-to-end in a chainlike fashion.

**trichomegaly** (trĭk″ō-mĕg′ă-lē) [Gr. *trichos,* hair, + *megas,* large] Long, coarse eyebrows.

**trichomonacide** (trĭk″ō-mō′nă-sīd) Anything that is lethal to trichomonads.

**trichomonad** (trĭk″ō-mō′năd) Related to or resembling the genus of flagellate *Trichomonas.*

**Trichomonas** (trĭk″ō′mō′năs) [″ + *monas,* unit] Genus of flagellate parasitic protozoa.

***T. hominis*** A benign trichomonas found in the large intestine.

***T. tenax*** A benign trichomonas that may be present in the mouth.

***T. vaginalis*** A species found in the vagina that produces discharge. *T. vaginalis* is fairly common in women, esp. during pregnancy or following vaginal surgery. It is sometimes found in the male urethra and may be transmitted through sexual intercourse. SEE: illus.; *colpitis macularis.*

SYMPTOMS: *T. vaginalis* causes persistent burning, redness, and itching of the vulvar tissue associated with a profuse vaginal discharge that may be frothy or malodorous or both. Occasionally, infection with *T. vaginalis* is asymptomatic.

TREATMENT: Metronidazole (Flagyl) is taken orally by the woman and her sexual partner. Alcohol should not be consumed during metronidazole therapy.

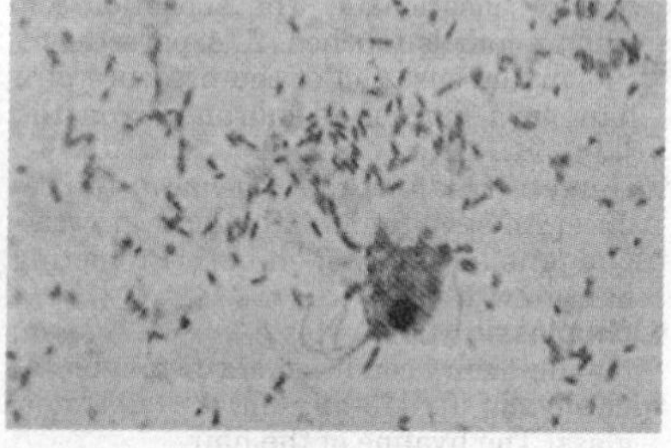


TRICHOMONAS VAGINALIS AND BACTERIA IN VAGINAL SMEAR (ORIG. MAG. ×1000)

**trichomoniasis** (trĭk″ō-mō-nī′ă-sĭs) [″ + ″ + *-iasis,* infection] Infestation with a parasite of the genus *Trichomonas.*

**trichomycosis** (trĭk″ō-mī-kō′sĭs) [″ + *mykes,* fungus, + *osis,* condition] Any disease of the hair caused by a fungus.

***t. axillaris*** An affection of the axillary region and sometimes pubic hairs caused by *Nocardia tenuis.*

***t. nodosa*** Piedra.

**trichonosis, trichonosus** (trĭk-ō-nō′sĭs, -ŏn′ō-sŭs) [Gr. *trichos,* hair, + *nosos,* disease] Any disease of the hair. SYN: *trichopathy.*

**trichopathophobia** (trĭk″ō-păth″ō-fō′bē-ă) [″ + *pathos,* disease, suffering, + *phobos,* fear] A morbid fear of hair on the face experienced by women, or any abnormal anxiety regarding hair.

**trichopathy** (trĭk-ŏp′ă-thē) [″ + *pathos,* disease, suffering] Trichonosis.

**trichophagia, trichophagy** (trĭk-ō-fā′jē-ă, -ŏf′ă-jē) [″ + *phagein,* to eat] The habit of eating hair.

**trichophobia** (trĭk″ō-fō′bē-ă) [″ + *phobos,* fear] An abnormal dread of hair or of touching it.

**trichophytic** (trĭk″ō-fĭt′ĭk) [″ + *phyton,* plant] **1.** Relating to *Trichophyton.* **2.** Promoting hair growth.

**trichophytic granulosa** (trĭk″ō-fĭt′ĭk) Tinea profunda.

**trichophytid** (trĭ-kŏf′ĭ-tĭd) A skin disorder considered to be an allergic reaction to fungi of the genus *Trichophyton.*

**trichophytin** (trĭ-kŏf′ĭ-tĭn) An extract prepared from cultures of the fungi of the genus *Trichophyton;* used as an antigen for skin tests and for the treatment of certain trichophytid infections.

**trichophytobezoar** (trĭk-ō-fī″tō-bē′zor) [″ + *phyton,* plant, + Arabic *bazahr,* protecting against poison] A hairball found in the stomach or intestine composed of hair, vegetable fibers, and miscellaneous debris.

**Trichophyton** (trĭ-kŏf′ĭt-ŏn) A genus of parasitic fungi that lives in or on the skin or its appendages (hair and nails) and is the cause of various dermatomycoses and ringworm infections. Species that produce spores arranged in rows on the outside of the hair are designated ectothrix; if spores are within the hair, endothrix.

***T. mentagrophytes*** A species, one form of which, called *granulare,* is parasitic on several mammals including horses, dogs, and rodents and can also affect humans. Another variety, called interdigitale, is associated with tinea pedis.

***T. schoenleinii*** The causative agent of favus of the scalp. SEE: *favus.*

***T. tonsurans*** The most frequent cause of ringworm of the scalp. SEE: *tinea capitis.*

***T. violaceum*** The causative agent of some forms of ringworm of the scalp, beard, or nails.

**trichophytosis** (trĭk″ō-fī-tō′sĭs) [″ + *phyton,* plant, + *osis,* condition] Infestation with *Trichophyton* fungi.

**trichoptilosis** (trĭk″ŏp-tĭl-ō′sĭs) [″ + *ptilon,* feather, + *osis,* condition] **1.** The splitting of hairs at their ends, giving them a featherlike appearance. **2.** A disease of hair marked by development of nodules along the hair shaft, at which point it splits off.

**trichoscopy** (trĭk-ŏs′kō-pē) [″ + *skopein,* to examine] Inspection of the hair.

**trichosiderin** (trĭk″ō-sĭd′ĕr-ĭn) [″ + *sideros,* iron] An iron-containing pigment normally present in red hair.

**trichosis** (trī-kō′sĭs) [″ + *osis,* condition] Any disease of the hair or its abnormal growth or development in an abnormal place.

***t. decolor*** Any abnormal coloring or lack of coloring of the hair. SYN: *canities.*

***t. setosa*** Coarse hair.

**Trichosporon** (trĭ-kŏs′pō-rŏn) [″ + *sporos,* a seed] A genus of fungi that grows on hair and causes piedra.

***T. beigelii*** The causative agent of white piedra. SEE: *piedra.*

**trichosporosis** (trĭk″ō-spō-rō′sĭs) [″ + ″ + *osis,* condition] Infestation of the hair with *Trichosporon.*

**trichostasis spinulosa** (trĭ-kŏs′tă-sĭs spĭn″ū-lō′să) [″ + *stasis,* a standing] A congenital condition in which the hair follicle is plugged with keratin and fine, lanugo hairs.

**trichostrongyliasis** (trĭk″ō-strŏn-jĭ-lī′ă-sĭs) Infestation with the intestinal parasite *Trichostrongylus;* a rare disease in the U.S.

**trichostrongylosis** (trĭk″ō-strŏn″jĭ-lō′sĭs) Infestation with *Trichostrongylus.*

**Trichostrongylus** (trĭk″ō-strŏn′jĭ-lŭs) A genus of nematode worms of the family Trichostrongylidae. These worms are of economic importance because of the damage they cause to domestic animals and birds.

**Trichothecium** (trĭk″ō-thē′sē-ŭm) [″ + *theke,* a box] A genus of mold fungi causing disease of the hair.

***T. roseum*** A species of mold fungus found in certain cases of inflammation of the eardrum (mycomyringitis).

**trichotillomania** (trĭk″ō-tĭl″ō-mā′nē-ă) [″ + *tillein,* to pull, + *mania,* madness] The unnatural and irresistible urge to pull out one's own hair. It is estimated that 8 million Americans are affected by this compulsive action. Clomipramine has been effective in treating this condition.

**trichotomous** (trī-kŏt′ō-mŭs) [Gr. *tricha,* threefold, + *tome,* incision] Divided into three.

**trichotomy** (trī-kŏt′ō-mē) Division into three parts.

**trichotoxin** (trĭk″ō-tŏks′ĭn) [Gr. *trichos,* hair, + *toxikon,* poison] An antibody or cytotoxin that destroys ciliated epithelial cells.

**trichotrophy** (trĭ-kŏt′rō-fē) [″ + *trophe,* nourishment] Nutrition of the hair.

**trichroic** (trī-krō′ĭk) [Gr. *treis,* three, + *chroa,* color] Presenting three different colors when viewed along each of three different axes.

**trichroism** (trī′krō-ĭzm) [″ + ″ + *-ismos,* condition] Quality of showing a different color when viewed along each of three axes. SYN: *trichromatism.*

**trichromatic** (trī″krō-măt′ĭk) [″ + *chroma,* color] Rel. to or able to see the three primary colors; denoting normal color vision. SYN: *trichromic.*

**trichromatism** (trī-krō′mă-tĭzm) Trichroism.

**trichromatopsia** (trī″krō-mă-tŏp′sē-ă) Normal color vision.

**trichromic** (trī-krō′mĭk) Pert. to normal color vision or the ability to see the three primary colors. SYN: *trichromatic.*

**trichterbrust** (trĭch′tĕr-broost) [Ger.] Funnel chest.

**trichuriasis** (trĭk″ū-rī′ă-sĭs) [Gr. *trichos,* hair, + *oura,* tail + *-iasis,* condition] The presence of worms of the genus *Trichuris* in the colon or in the ileum.

**Trichuris** (trĭ-kū′rĭs) Parasitic nematode worms that belong to the class Nematoda.

***T. trichiura*** A species of *Trichuris* that infects humans when the ova that have undergone incubation in the soil are ingested. The larvae develop into adults, which inhabit the large intestine. If the infection is heavy, the patient will develop diarrhea and abdominal pain. Rectal prolapse may occur if a great number of worms are present. It is not definitely known that infection with *Trichuris* causes intestinal blood loss. Mebendazole is the drug of choice; albendazole or ivermectin may be of benefit. SYN: *whipworm.* SEE: illus.

**tricipital** (trī-sĭp′ĭ-tăl) [Gr. *treis,* three, + L. *caput,* head] Three-headed, as the triceps muscle.

**tricitrates oral solution** A solution of sodium citrate, potassium citrate, and citric acid in a suitable aqueous medium. The sodium and potassium ion contents of the solution are approx. 1 mEq/ml.

**triclofos sodium** (trī′klō-fōs) A sedative-hypnotic drug.

**tricornic** (trī-kor′nĭk) [″ + L. *cornu,* horn] Having three horns or cornua. SYN: *tricornute.*

**tricornute** (trī-kor′nūt) [″ + L. *cornutus,* horned] Having three horns or cornua. SYN: *tricornic.*

**tricrotic** (trī-krŏt′ĭk) [Gr. *trikrotos,* rowed with a triple stroke] A condition in which three accentuated waves or notches occur on a sphygmograph tracing from one beat of the pulse.

**tricrotism** (trī′krŏt-ĭzm) [″ + *-ismos,* condition] The condition of being tricrotic.

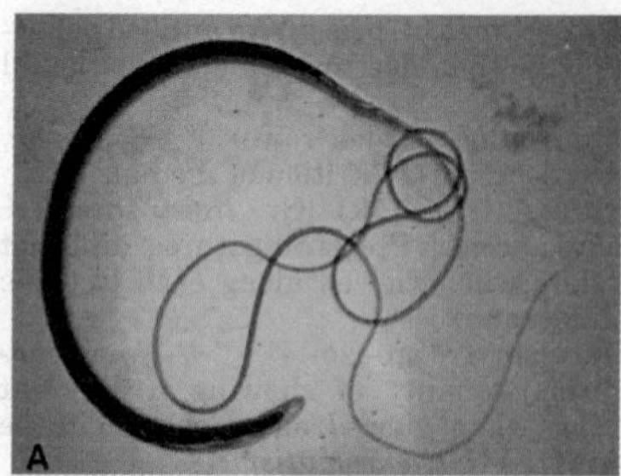

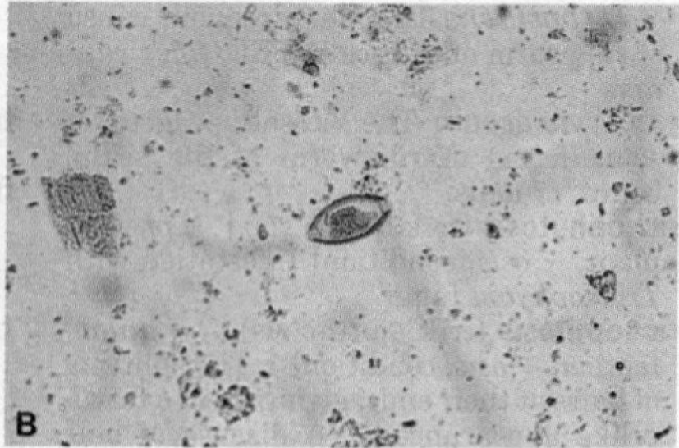



**TRICHURIS TRICHIURA**

**(A)** ADULT FEMALE (ORIG. MAG. ×4), **(B)** EGGS IN FECES (ORIG. MAG. ×100)

**tricuspid** (trī-kŭs′pĭd) [Gr. *treis,* three, + L. *cuspis,* point] **1.** Pert. to the tricuspid valve. **2.** Having three points or cusps.

**tricuspid area** The lower portion of the body of the sternum where sounds of the right atrioventricular orifice are best heard.

**tricuspid atresia** Stenosis of the tricuspid valve. A fairly uncommon congenital malformation that causes cyanosis and clubbing. Symptoms include paroxysmal dyspnea and difficulty in feeding.

**tricuspid murmur** A murmur caused by stenosis of the tricuspid valve or by its incompetency.

**tricuspid orifice** Right atrioventricular cardiac aperture.

**tricuspid tooth** A tooth with a crown that has three cusps.

**tricuspid valve** SEE: under *valve.*

**trident, tridentate** (trī′dĕnt, trī-dĕn′tāt) [L. *tres, tria,* three, + *dens,* tooth] Having three prongs.

**tridermic** (trī-dĕr′mĭk) [Gr. *treis,* three, + *derma,* skin] Developed from the ectoderm, endoderm, and mesoderm.

**tridermoma** (trī″dĕr-mō′mă) [″ + ″ + *oma,* tumor] A teratoid growth containing all three germ layers.

**tridihexethyl chloride** (trī″dī-hĕks-ĕth′ĭl) An anticholinergic drug that acts similarly to belladonna.

**trielcon** (trī-ĕl′kŏn) [″ + *helkein,* to draw] An instrument with three branches for removing bullets or other foreign bodies from wounds.

**triencephalus** (trī″ĕn-sĕf′ă-lŭs) [″ + *enkephalos,* brain] A deformed fetus lacking the organs of sight, hearing, and smell.

**triethylenemelamine** (trī-ĕth″ĭ-lēn-mĕl′ă-mēn) ABBR: TEM. One of the nitrogen mustard compounds. SEE: *nitrogen mustards.*

**triethylenethiophosphoramide** (trī-ĕth″ĭ-lēn-thī″ō-fŏs-for′ă-mīd) Thiotepa.

**trifacial** (trī-fā′shăl) [L. *trifacialis*] Trigeminal.

**trifacial neuralgia** Tic douloureux.

**trifid** (trī-fĭd) [L. *trifidus,* split thrice] Split into three; having three clefts.

**trifluoperazine hydrochloride** (trī″floo-ō-păr′ă-zēn) An antipsychotic drug.

**triflupromazine** (trī″floo-prō′mă-zēn) An antipsychotic drug that is also used in treating nausea and vomiting.

**trifurcation** (trī″fŭr-kā′shŭn) [Gr. *treis,* three, + L. *furca,* fork] **1.** Division into three branches. **2.** In dentistry, the area of root division in a tooth with three or more roots.

**trifurcation involvement** The extension of periodontitis or a periodontal pocket into an area where the tooth roots divide.

**trigastric** (trī-găs′trĭk) [Gr. *treis,* three, + *gaster,* belly] Having three bellies, as certain muscles.

**trigeminal** (trī-jĕm′ĭn-ăl) [L. *tres, tria,* three, + *geminus,* twin] Pert. to the trigeminus or fifth cranial nerve. SYN: *trifocal.*

**trigeminal cough** A reflex cough from irritation of the trigeminal terminations in respiratory upper passages.

**trigeminal nerve** A large mixed nerve arising superficially from the side of the pons near its superior border. It is attached to the brainstem by two roots: a large sensory root and a small motor root. The sensory root bears an enlargement, the semilunar gasserian ganglion, from which three large branches arise. These are *ophthalmic,* purely sensory, from the skin of the upper part of the head, mucous membranes of the nasal cavity and sinuses, cornea, and conjunctiva; *maxillary,* purely sensory, from the dura mater, gums and teeth of the upper jaw, upper lip, and orbit; and *mandibular,* the largest division, containing sensory fibers from the tongue, gums, and teeth of the lower jaw, skin of the cheek, lower jaw, and lip, and motor fibers supplying principally the muscles of mastication. SYN: *fifth cranial nerve.* SEE: *Cranial Nerves Appendix.*

**trigeminal neuralgia** Tic douloureux.

**trigeminal pulse** A pulse with a longer or shorter interval after each three beats because the third beat is an extrasystole.

**trigeminus** (trī-jĕm′ĭ-nŭs) Trigeminal nerve.

**trigeminy** (trī-jĕm′ĭ-nē) Occurring in threes, esp. three pulse beats in rapid succession.

**trigenic** (trī-jĕn′ĭk) [Gr. *treis,* three, + *gennan,* to produce] In genetics, a condition in which three alleles are present at any particular locus on the chromosome.

**trigger** (trĭg′ĕr) [D. *trekker,* something pulled] **1.** Stimulus. **2.** To initiate or start with suddenness.

**trigger action** A physiological process or a pathological change initiated by a sudden stimulus.

**trigger finger** A state in which flexion or extension of a digit is arrested temporarily but is finally completed with a jerk. Any finger may be involved, but the ring or middle finger is most often affected.

TREATMENT: A finger splint or cortisone injection may be used to treat this condition. Surgery may be required.

**trigger point, trigger zone 1.** An area that when stimulated will initiate an attack of neuralgia. **2.** An area of the cerebral cortex that, when stimulated, produces abnormal reactions similar to those in acquired epilepsy. SEE: *epileptogenic zone.*

**trigger substance** A chemical substance that initiates a function or action.

**triglycerides** (trī-glĭs′ĕr-īds) Combinations of glycerol with three of five different fatty acids. These substances, triacylglycerols, are also called neutral fats. A large portion of the fatty substances (i.e., lipids) in the blood is triglycerides. Because these lipids are insoluble in water, they are transported in combination with proteins (lipoproteins). About 1 or 2 g of triglycerides per kilogram of body weight are ingested daily in the usual diet in the U.S. In addition, they are produced in the liver. SEE: *hyperlipoproteinemia.*

***medium-chain t.*** Triglycerides with 8 to 10 carbon atoms. They are digested and absorbed differently than the usual dietary fats and, for that reason, have been useful in treating malabsorption.

**trigonal** (trĭg′ō-năl) [Gr. *trigonon,* a three-cornered figure] Triangular; pert. to a trigone.

**trigone** (trī′gōn) A triangular space, esp. one at the base of the bladder, between the two openings of the ureters and the urethra. SYN: *t. of bladder; trigonum; vesical t.*

***t. of bladder*** Trigone.

***carotid t.*** The triangular area in the neck bounded by the posterior belly of the digastric muscle, the sternocleidomastoid muscle, and the midline of the neck.

***olfactory t.*** A small triangular eminence at the root of the olfactory peduncle and anterior to the anterior perforated space of the base of the brain.

***vesical t.*** Trigone.

**trigonectomy** (trī″gōn-ĕk′tō-mē) [″ + *ektome,* excision] Excision of the base of the bladder.

**trigonid** (trī-gō′nĭd) The first three cusps of a lower molar tooth.

**trigonitis** (trĭg″ō-nī′tĭs) [″ + *itis,* inflammation] Inflammation of the mucous membrane of the trigone of the bladder.

**trigonocephalic** (trī″gō-nō-sĕ-făl′ĭk) [″ + *kephale,* head] Having a head shaped like a triangle.

**trigonocephalus** (trĭg″ō-nō-sĕf′ă-lŭs) A fetus exhibiting trigonocephaly.

**trigonocephaly** (trī-gō″nō-sĕf′ă-lē) The condition of the head of the fetus being shaped like a triangle.

**trigonum** (trī-gō′nŭm) *pl.* **trigona** [L.] Trigone.

***t. lumbale*** Triangle of Petit.

**trihexyphenidyl hydrochloride** (trī-hĕk″sē-fĕn′ĭ-dĭl) An anticholinergic drug used in treating parkinsonism. Trade names are Antitrem, Artane, Pipanol, and Tremin.

**trihybrid** (trī-hī′brĭd) [Gr. *treis,* three, + L. *hybrida,* mongrel] In genetics, the offspring of a cross between two individuals differing in three unit characters.

**triiniodymus** (trī″ĭn-ē-ŏd′ĭ-mŭs) [″ + *inion,* nape of the neck, + *didymos,* twin] A deformed fetus with a single body and three heads joined at the occiput.

**triiodothyronine** (trī″ī-ō″dō-thī′rō-nēn) ABBR: $T_3$. One of two forms of the principal hormone secreted by the thyroid gland. Chemically it is 3,5,3′-triiodothyronine (liothyronine). SEE: *tetraiodothyronine; thyroid-function test.*

**trikates** A solution of potassium acetate, potassium bicarbonate, and potassium citrate; used in treating electrolyte deficiencies.

**trilabe** (trī′lāb) [Gr. *treis,* three, + *labe,* a handle] Three-pronged forceps for removing foreign substances from the bladder.

**trilaminar** (trī-lăm′ĭ-năr) Composed of three layers.

**trilateral** (trī-lăt′ĕr-ăl) [″ + L. *latus,* side] Concerning three sides.

**trill** (trĭl) [It. *trillare,* probably imitative] A tremulous sound, esp. in vocal music.

**trilobate** (trī-lō′bāt) [″ + *lobos,* lobe] Having three lobes.

**trilocular** (trī-lŏk′ū-lăr) [″ + L. *loculus,* cell] Having three compartments.

**trilogy** (trĭl′ō-jē) A series of three events.

**trimanual** (trī-măn′ū-ăl) [″ + *manualis,* by hand] Performed with three hands, as an obstetrical maneuver.

**trimensual** (trī-mĕn′shū-ăl) [″ + *mensualis,* monthly] Occurring every 3 months.

**trimeprazine tartrate** (trī-mĕp′ră-zēn) A drug used for its antipruritic action.

**trimester** (trī-mĕs′tĕr) A 3-month period.

***first t.*** The first 3 months of pregnancy.

***second t.*** The middle 3 months of pregnancy.

***third t.*** The third and final 3 months of pregnancy.

**trimethadione** (trī″mĕth-ă-dī′ōn) An anticonvulsive agent used in treating certain forms of epilepsy.

**trimethaphan camsylate** (trī-mĕth′ă-făn) A ganglionic blocking agent used to diminish blood pressure in acute hypertensive crisis.

**trimethidinium methosulfate** (trī-mĕth″ĭ-dĭn′ē-ŭm) An antihypertensive drug.

**trimethobenzamide hydrochloride** (trī-mĕth″ō-bĕn′ză-mīd) An antiemetic drug.

**trimethoprim** (trī-mĕth′ō-prĭm) An antibacterial drug usually used in combination with sulfamethoxazole because they interfere with two sequential steps in the metabolism of certain bacteria. The combination is useful in treating various bacterial infections, esp. urinary tract pathogens such as *Pseudomonas aeruginosa, Proteus mirabilis, Escherichia coli,* and *Klebsiella* species. Also, the combination is used in treating *Pneumocystis carinii* pneumonia and travelers' diarrhea caused by susceptible strains of enterotoxigenic *E. coli*. SEE: *sulfamethoxazole.*

**trimethylene** (trī-mĕth′ĭ-lēn) Cyclopropane.

**trimmer** A device or instrument used to shape something by cutting off the material along its margin.

***gingival margin t.*** A cutting instrument for shaping gingival contours. It has a curved and angled shaft for use either on the right or left sides and on the mesial or distal surfaces.

***model t.*** A rotary flat grinder used to trim dental plaster or stone casts. Water keeps the cutting surface clean and obviates any dust problem as the casts are squared into proper study models.

**trimorphous** (trī-mor′fŭs) [″ + *morphe,* form] **1.** Having three different forms as the larva, pupa, and adult of certain insects. **2.** Having three different forms of crystals.

**trinitrophenol** (trī″nī-trō-fē′nōl) A yellow crystalline powder that precipitates proteins. It is used as a dye and as a reagent. SYN: *picric acid.*

**trinitrotoluene** (trī″nī-trō-tŏl′ū-ēn) ABBR: TNT. An explosive compound.

**triocephalus** (trī″ō-sĕf′ă-lŭs) [″ + *kephale,* head] A deformed fetus with a rudimentary head without eyes, nose, or mouth.

**triolein** Olein.

**triolism** (trī′ō-lĭzm) Sexual activity involving two persons of one sex and one person of the opposite sex.

**triophthalmos** (trī″ŏf-thăl′mōs) [″ + *ophthalmos,* eye] A deformed fetus with three eyes.

**triopodymus** (trī″ō-pŏd′ĭ-mŭs) [″ + *ops,* face, + *didymos,* twin] A deformed fetus with three fused heads and three faces.

**triorchid, triorchis** (trī-or′kĭd, -kĭs) [″ + *orchis,* testicle] A person who has three testicles.

**triorchidism** (trī-or′kĭd-ĭzm) [″ + ″ + *-ismos,* condition] The condition of having three testicles.

**triose** (trī′ōs) A monosaccharide having three carbon atoms in its molecule.

**triotus** (trī-ō′tŭs) [″ + *ous,* ear] A person with a third ear.

**trioxsalen** (trī-ŏk′să-lĕn) An agent used to promote repigmentation in vitiligo. Trade name is Trisoralen. SEE: *psoralen; vitiligo.*

**trip** (trĭp) A slang term used to refer to hallucinations produced by various drugs, including LSD, mescaline, and some narcotics.

**tripara** (trĭp′ă-ră) [L. *tres, tria,* three, + *parere,* to bear] A woman who has had three pregnancies that have lasted beyond 20 weeks or that have produced an infant of at least 500 g; also designated Para III. SYN: *tertipara.*

**tripelennamine citrate** (trī″pĕ-lĕn′ă-mĭn) An antihistamine drug.

**tripeptide** (trī-pĕp′tīd) [Gr. *treis,* three, + *pepton,* digested] The product of a combination of three amino acids formed during proteolytic digestion.

**triphalangia** (trī″fă-lăn′jē-ă) [″ + *phalanx,* closely knit row] A deformity marked by the presence of three phalanges in a thumb or great toe.

**triphasic** (trī-fā′sĭk) [″ + *phasis,* phase] Consisting of three phases or stages, said of electric currents.

**triphenylmethane** (trī-fĕn″ĭl-mĕth′ān) A coal tar–derived chemical that serves as the basis of some dyes and stains.

**Tripier's amputation** (trĭp-ē-āz′) [Léon Tripier, Fr. surgeon, 1842–1891] Amputation of a foot with part of the calcaneus removed.

**triple** (trĭp′l) [L. *triplus,* threefold] Consisting of three; threefold; treble.

**triplegia** (trī-plē′jē-ă) [″ + *plege,* stroke] Hemiplegia with paralysis of one limb on the other side of the body.

**triple response** The three reactions of the skin to injury: a red reaction along the line of injury; a red area (flare or erythema) about the injury; and an elevated area (welt or wheal) resulting from localized edema.

**triplet** (trĭp′lĕt) [L. *triplus,* threefold] **1.** One of three children produced in one gestation and one birth. SEE: *Hellin's law.* **2.** A combination of three of a kind.

**triplex** (trī′plĕks, trĭp′lĕks) [Gr. *triploos,* triple] Triple; threefold.

**triploblastic** (trĭp″lō-blăst′ĭk) [″ + *blastos,* germ] Consisting of three germ layers: ectoderm, entoderm, and mesoderm.

**triploid** (trĭp′loyd) Concerning triploidy.

**triploidy** (trĭp′loy-dē) In the human, having three sets of chromosomes.

**triplokoria** (trĭp″lō-kor′ē-ă) [″ + *kore,* pupil] Possessing three pupillary openings in one eye.

**triplopia** (trĭp-lō′pē-ă) [″ + *ope,* vision] A condition in which three images of the same object are seen.

**tripod** (trī′pŏd) [Gr. *treis,* three, + *pous,* foot] A stand having three supports, usually legs.

**tripodia** (trī-pō′dē-ă) Having three feet.

**tripoding** (trī′pŏd-ĭng) The use of three bases for support (e.g., two legs and a cane, or one leg and two crutches).

**triprolidine hydrochloride** (trī-prō′lĭ-dēn)

An antihistamine drug.
**triprosopus** (trī″prō-sō′pŭs) [″ + *prosopon,* face] A deformed fetus with three faces.
**tripsis** (trĭp′sĭs) [Gr. *tripsis,* friction] **1.** The process of trituration. **2.** Massage.
**-tripsy** (trĭp′sē) [Gr. *tripsis,* friction] A word ending indicating intentional crushing of something.
**triquetral** (trī-kwē′trăl) [L. *triquetrus*] Triangular.
**triquetral bone 1.** The third carpal bone in the proximal row, enumerated from the radial side. **2.** Any wormian bone. SYN: *cuneiform bone.*
**triquetrous** (trī-kwē′trŭs) [L. *triquetrus,* triangular] Triangular.
**triquetrum** (trī-kwē′trŭm) [L.] Three-cornered.
**triradial, triradiate** (trī-rā′dē-ăl, -āt) [Gr. *treis,* three, + L. *radiatus,* rayed] Having three rays; radiating in three directions.
**triradius** (trī-rā′dē-ŭs) In classifying fingerprints, the point of convergence of dermal ridges coming from three directions.
**trisaccharide** (trī-săk′ă-rīd) A carbohydrate that on hydrolysis yields three molecules of simple sugars (monosaccharides).
**triskaidekaphobia** (trĭ-skī-dĕk-ă-fō′bē-ă) [Gr. *triskaideka,* thirteen, + *phobos,* fear] Superstition concerning the number 13. SYN: *triakaidekaphobia.*
**trismic** (trĭz′mĭk) Concerning trismus.
**trismoid** (trĭz′moyd) [Gr. *trismos,* grating, + *eidos,* form, shape] **1.** Of the nature of trismus. **2.** A form of trismus nascentium; once thought to be due to pressure on the occiput during delivery.
**trismus** (trĭz′mŭs) [Gr. *trismos,* grating] Tonic contraction of the muscles of mastication; may occur in mouth infections, encephalitis, inflammation of salivary glands, and tetanus. SYN: *ankylostoma; lockjaw.*
**trisomic** (trī-sōm′ĭk) In genetics, an individual possessing 2n+1 chromosomes, that is, one set of chromosomes contains an extra (third) chromosome. SEE: *chromosome; karyotype.*
**trisomy** (trī′sō-mē) In genetics, having three homologous chromosomes per cell instead of two.

***t. 13*** Trisomy of chromosome 13, which causes severe congenital deformation and mental retardation. Children with trisomy 13 usually do not survive past the first year of life. They have a large broad nose, widely spaced small eyes (hypertelorism), low-set ears, and a poorly formed lower jaw.

***t. 18*** Trisomy of chromosome 18, which causes severe deformity and mental retardation. Children with trisomy 18 usually do not survive beyond the first year of life. The condition is characterized by a prominent occiput, overlapping of the index finger over the third finger, frequent facial abnormalities, a straight nose coming off sharply from the forehead, low-set ears, and a cleft palate and lip.

***t. 21*** Down syndrome.
**trisplanchnic** (trī-splănk′nĭk) [Gr. *treis,* three, + *splanchna,* viscera] Pert. to the three large body cavities: the skull, thorax, and abdomen.
**tristichia** (trī-stĭk′ē-ă) [″ + *stichos,* row] The presence of three rows of eyelashes.
**tristimania** (trĭs″tĭ-mā′nē-ă) [L. *tristis,* sad, + Gr. *mania,* madness] Melancholia.
**trisulcate** (trī-sŭl′kāt) [L. *tres, tria,* three, + *sulcus,* groove] Having three grooves or furrows.
**trisulfapyrimidines oral suspension** (trī-sŭl″fă-pī-rĭm′ĭ-dēnz) A combination of sulfadiazene, sulfamerazine, and sulfamethazine. This antimicrobial combination was developed to reduce the precipitation of crystals of the sulfonamides in the urinary tract.
**trisulfate** (trī-sŭl′f āt) A chemical compound containing three sulfate, $SO_4$, groups.
**trisulfide** (trī-sŭl′fīd) A chemical compound containing three sulfur atoms.
**tritanomalopia** (trī″tă-nŏm′ă-lō-pē-ă) [Gr. *tritos,* third, + *anomalos,* irregular, + *ope,* sight] A color vision defect similar to tritanopia but less pronounced. SYN: *tritanomaly.*
**tritanomaly** (trī″tă-nŏm′ă-lē) Tritanomalopia.
**tritanopia** (trī″tă-nō′pē-ă) [Gr. *tritos,* third, + *an-,* not, + *ope,* vision] Blue blindness; color blindness in which there is a defect in the perception of blue. SEE: *color blindness.*
**tritiate** (trĭt′ē-āt) To treat with tritium.
**tritiated thymidine** $^3$H-Tdr. A radioactively labeled nucleoside used to measure T lymphocyte proliferation in vitro. Thymidine is essential for DNA synthesis, thus the amount of $^3$H-Tdr taken up is a general measure of the number of new lymphocytes produced.
**triticeous** (trĭt-ĭsh′ŭs) [L. *triticeus,* of wheat] Shaped like a grain of wheat.

***t. cartilage*** A cartilaginous nodule in the thyrohyoid ligament.
**tritium** (trĭt′ē-ŭm, trĭsh′ē-ŭm) [Gr. *tritos,* third] The mass three isotope of hydrogen; triple-weight hydrogen.
**triturable** (trĭt′ū-ră-bl) [L. *triturare,* to pulverize] Capable of being powdered.
**triturate** (trĭt′ū-rāt) **1.** To reduce to a fine powder by rubbing. **2.** A finely divided substance made by rubbing.
**trituration** (trĭt-ū-rā′shŭn) [LL. *triturare,* to pulverize] **1.** The act of reducing to a powder. **2.** A finely ground and easily mixed powder. **3.** The creation of a homogenous mixture of metal alloy particles and mercury to form dental amalgam. SYN: *amalgamation.*
**trivalence** (trĭv′ă-lĕns) Condition of being trivalent.
**trivalent** (trī-vā′lĕnt, trĭv′ăl-ĕnt) [Gr. *treis,* three, + L. *valens,* powerful] Combining with or replacing three hydrogen atoms.
**trivalve** (trī′vălv) Having three valves.
**trivial name** A nonsystematic or semisyste-

matic name and qualifying term used to name drugs. These names do not provide assistance in determining biological action or function of the drug. Examples are aspirin, caffeine, and belladonna.

**trizonal** (trī-zō′năl) Having three zones or layers.

**tRNA** *transfer RNA.*

**trocar** (trō′kăr) [Fr. *trois quarts,* three quarters] A sharply pointed surgical instrument contained in a cannula; used for aspiration or removal of fluids from cavities.

**trochanter** (trō-kăn′tĕr) [Gr. *trokhanter,* to run] Either of the two bony processes below the neck of the femur.

***greater t.*** T. major.

***lesser t.*** T. minor.

***t. major*** A thick process at the upper end of the femur projecting upward externally to the union of the neck and shaft. SYN: *greater t.*

***t. minor*** A conical tuberosity on the inner and posterior surface of the upper end of the femur, at the junction of the shaft and neck. SYN: *lesser t.; trochantin.*

***t. tertius*** The gluteal ridge of the femur when it is unusually prominent. SYN: *third t.*

***third t.*** T. tertius.

**trochanterian, trochanteric** (trō″kăn-tē′rē-ăn, trō-kăn-tĕr′ĭk) Rel. to a trochanter.

**trochanterplasty** (trō-kăn′tĕr-plăs″tē) Plastic surgery of the neck of the femur.

**trochantin** (trō-kăn′tĭn) Trochanter minor.

**trochantinian** (trō″kăn-tĭn′ē-ăn) Concerning the lesser trochanter of the femur.

**troche, troch** (trō′kē, trōk′) [Gr. *trokhiskos,* a small wheel] A solid, discoid, or cylindrical mass consisting chiefly of medicinal powder, sugar, and mucilage. Troches are used by placing them in the mouth and allowing them to remain until, through slow solution or disintegration, their mild medication is released. SYN: *lozenge.*

**trochiscus** (trō-kĭs′kŭs) [L., Gr. *trochiskos,* a small disk] A medicated tablet or troche.

**trochlea** (trŏk′lē-ă) *pl.* **trochleae** [Gr. *trokhileia,* system of pulleys] **1.** A structure having the function of a pulley; a ring or hook through which a tendon or muscle projects. **2.** The articular smooth surface of a bone on which glides another bone.

**trochlea of the elbow** A surface on the distal humerus that articulates with the ulna.

**trochlear** (trŏk′lē-ăr) **1.** Of the nature of a pulley. **2.** Pert. to a trochlea.

**trochlear fovea** A depression on the orbital plate of the frontal bone for attachment of the cartilaginous pulley of the superior oblique muscle.

**trochleariform** (trŏk″lē-ăr′ĭ-form) Pulley-shaped.

**trochlearis** (trŏk″lē-ā′rĭs) [L.] The superior oblique muscle of the eye. SEE: *Muscles Appendix.*

**trochlear nerve** A small mixed nerve exiting from the dorsal surface of the midbrain. It contains efferent motor fibers to the superior oblique muscle of the eye and afferent sensory fibers conveying proprioceptive impulses from the same muscle. SYN: *fourth cranial nerve.* SEE: *Cranial Nerves Appendix.*

**trochocardia** (trō″kō-kăr′dē-ă) [Gr. *trokhos,* a wheel, + *kardia,* heart] Rotary displacement of the heart on its axis.

**trochocephalia, trochocephaly** (trō″kō-sē-fā′lē-ă, -sĕf′ă-lē) [″ + *kephale,* head] Roundheadedness, a deformity due to premature union of the frontal and parietal bones.

**trochoid** (trō′koyd) [Gr. *trokhos,* a wheel, + *eidos,* form, shape] Rotating or revolving, noting an articulation resembling a pivot or pulley. SEE: *joint, pivot.*

**trochoides** (trō-koy′dēz) A pivot or rotary joint.

**Troglotrematidae** (trŏg″lō-trē-măt′ĭ-dē) A family of flukes that includes *Paragonimus* (human lung fluke).

**Troisier's node** (trwă-zē-āz′) [Charles E. Troisier, Fr. physician, 1844–1919] Sentinel node.

**trolamine** (trō′lă-mēn) An alkalizing agent.

**troland** (trō′lănd) A unit of visual stimulation to the retina of the eye. It is equal to the illumination received per square millimeter of the pupil from a source of 1 lux brightness.

**troleandomycin** (trō″lē-ăn-dō-mī′sĭn) An antibacterial drug.

**trolnitrate phosphate** (trŏl-nī′trāt) A vasodilator drug. Trade name is Metamine.

**Trombicula** (trŏm-bĭk′ū-lă) A genus of mites belonging to the Trombiculidae. The larvae, called redbugs or chiggers, cause an irritating dermatitis and rash. They may serve as vectors of various diseases.

***T. akamushi*** A species of mites that transmits the causative agent of scrub typhus.

**trombiculiasis** (trŏm-bĭk″ū-lī′ă-sĭs) Infestation with Trombiculidae.

**Trombiculidae** (trŏm-bĭk′ū-lī″dē) A family of mites; only the genus *Trombicula* is of medical significance.

**tromethamine** (trō-mĕth′ă-mēn) A drug used intravenously to correct acidosis. It should not be used longer than 1 day except in life-threatening emergencies.

**troph-** SEE: *tropho-.*

**trophectoderm** (trŏf-ĕk′tō-dĕrm) [Gr. *trophe,* nourishment, + *ectoderm*] In embryology, the peripheral cells of the blastocyst that form the chorion surrounding the embryo, and eventually the placenta.

**trophedema** (trŏf″ĕ-dē′mă) [Gr. *trophe,* nourishment, + *oidema,* a swelling] Localized edema caused by congenital hypoplasia of lymphatic vessels or resulting secondarily from obstruction to lymph flow by external pressure. Repeated low-grade infection may also obstruct the flow of lymph.

**trophic** (trŏf′ĭk) [Gr. *trophikos*] Concerned with nourishment; applied particularly to a type of efferent nerves believed to control the growth and nourishment of the parts they innervate. SEE: *autotrophic.*

**trophism** (trŏf'ĭzm) Nutrition.

**tropho-, troph-** Combining form meaning *nourishment.*

**trophoblast** (trŏf'ō-blăst) [Gr. *trophe,* nourishment, + *blastos,* germ] The outermost layer of the developing blastocyst (blastodermic vesicle) of a mammal. It differentiates into two layers, the cytotrophoblast and syntrophoblast, the latter coming into intimate relationship with the uterine endometrium, with which it establishes nutrient relationships. SEE: *fertilization* for illus.

**trophoblastic** (trŏf"ō-blăs'tĭk) Concerning trophoblasts.

**trophoblastoma** (trŏf"ō-blăs-tō'mă) [" + " + *oma,* tumor] A neoplasm due to excessive proliferation of chorionic epithelium. SYN: *chorioepithelioma.*

**trophocyte** (trŏf'ō-sīt) A cell that nourishes (e.g., Sertoli cells of the testicle, which support developing spermatozoa). SYN: *trephocyte.*

**trophoneurosis** (trŏf"ō-nū-rō'sĭs) [" + *neuron,* nerve, + *osis,* condition] Any trophic disorder caused by defective function of the nerves concerned with nutrition of the part.

***disseminated t.*** Thickening and hardening of the skin. SYN: *sclerema; scleroderma.*

***facial t.*** Progressive facial atrophy.

***muscular t.*** Muscular changes in connection with nervous disorders.

**trophonucleus** (trŏf"ō-nū'klē-ŭs) [" + *nucleus,* kernel] Protozoan nucleus concerned with vegetative functions in metabolism and not reproduction.

**trophopathia** (trŏf"ō-păth'ē-ă) [" + *pathos,* disease, suffering] **1.** Any disorder of nutrition. **2.** A trophic disease.

**trophozoite** (trŏf"ō-zō'īt) [" + *zoon,* animal] A sporozoan nourished by its hosts during its growth stage.

**tropia** (trō'pē-ă) [Gr. *trope,* turn] Deviation of the eye or eyes away from the visual axis; observed with the eyes open and uncovered. Esotropia indicates inward or nasal deviation; exotropia, outward; hypertropia, upward; hypotropia, downward. SYN: *manifest squint; strabismus.* SEE: *-phoria.*

**tropical** (trŏp'ĭ-kal) [Gr. *tropikos,* turning] Pert. to the tropics.

**tropical immersion foot** A syndrome with severe wrinkling and maceration of the soles of the feet and marked lowering of the threshold of pain. The condition is due to prolonged exposure of the feet to warm water, as would occur in the tropics. It may be prevented by allowing the feet to dry thoroughly each night, using dry socks and shoes the next day, and protecting the feet with silicone grease.

**tropical lichen** Acute inflammation of the sweat glands. SYN: *prickly heat.*

**tropical sprue** Sprue.

**tropicamide** (trō-pĭk'ă-mīd) An anticholinergic drug used to produce mydriasis and cycloplegia in treating eye conditions.

**-tropin** [Gr. *tropos,* a turn] Combining form, used as a suffix, indicating the stimulating effect of a substance, esp. a hormone, on its target organ.

**tropine** (trō'pĭn) An alkaloid, $C_8H_{15}NO$, that smells like tobacco. It is present in certain plants.

**tropism** (trō'pĭzm) [Gr. *trope,* turn, + *-ismos,* condition] **1.** Reaction of living organisms involuntarily toward or away from light, darkness, heat, cold, or other stimuli. **2.** The involuntary response of an organism as a bending, turning, or movement toward (positive tropism) or away from (negative tropism) an external stimulus. SYN: *taxis.* SEE: *chemotropism; phototropism.*

**tropocollagen** (trō"pō-kŏl'ă-jĕn) [" + *collagen*] The basic molecular unit of collagen fibrils, composed of three polypeptide chains.

**tropometer** (trŏp-ŏm'ĕ-ter) [" + *metron,* measure] **1.** A device for measuring the rotation of the eyeballs. **2.** An instrument for measuring torsion in long bones.

**tropomyosin** (trō"pō-mī'ō-sĭn) An inhibitory protein in muscle fibers; it blocks myosin from forming cross-bridges with actin until shifted by troponin-calcium ion interaction.

**troponin** (trō'pō-nĭn) An inhibitory protein in muscle fibers. The action potential at the sarcolemma causes the sarcoplasmic reticulum to release calcium ions, which bond to troponin and shift tropomyosin away from the myosin-binding sites of actin, permitting contraction.

**Trotter's syndrome** A unilateral neuralgia in the mandible, tongue, and ear. The causes are mandibular nerve lesions, deafness on the same side due to eustachian tube lesions, and damage to the levator palatini muscle resulting in kinesthesia of the soft palate.

**trough** (trŏf) A groove or channel.

***focal t.*** A three-dimensional area within which structures are accurately reproduced on a panoramic radiograph. Positioning the patient within the focal trough is critical to producing a panoramic radiograph that clearly reproduces oral structures.

***gingival t.*** Gingival sulcus.

***synaptic t.*** The depression in a muscle fiber that is occupied by the axon termination in a motor endplate.

**Trousseau's sign** (troo-sōz') [Armand Trousseau, Fr. physician, 1801–1867] A muscular spasm resulting from pressure applied to nerves and vessels of the upper arm. It is indicative of latent tetany and also occurs in osteomalacia. SEE: *tetany.*

**Trousseau's spots** Streaking of the skin with the fingernail, seen in meningitis and other cerebral diseases.

**Trousseau's symptom** Spasmodic muscular contractions produced by pressing the principal vessel and nerve of the limb. Presence of this symptom is a sign of tetany.

**troy weight** A system of weighing gold, silver, precious metals, and jewels in which 5760 gr equal 1 lb; 1 gr equals 0.0648 g. SEE: *Weights and Measures Appendix.*

**true** (troo) [AS. *treowe,* faithful] Not false; real; genuine.

**true conjugate diameter of pelvic inlet** The distance from the posterior surface of the symphysis pubis to the promontory of the sacrum (about 11 cm in the female).

**true pelvis** The portion of the pelvis that falls below the iliopectineal line.

**true ribs** The seven upper ribs on each side with cartilages articulating directly with the sternum. SYN: *costa vera.* SEE: *rib.*

**truncal** (trŭng′kăl) [L. *truncus,* trunk] Rel. to the trunk.

**truncate** (trŭng′kāt) [L. *truncare,* to cut off] **1.** Having a square end as if it were cut off; lacking an apex. **2.** To shorten by amputation of a part of the entity.

**truncus** (trŭng′kŭs) Trunk (2).

***t. arteriosus*** The arterial trunk from the embryonic heart.

***t. brachiocephalicus*** The initial branch of the arch of the aorta.

***t. celiacus*** Celiac trunk.

***t. pulmonalis*** Pulmonary trunk.

**trunk** (trŭnk) [L. *truncus,* trunk] **1.** The body exclusive of the head and limbs. SYN: *torso.* **2.** The main stem of a lymphatic vessel, nerve, or blood vessel.

***celiac t.*** The trunk arising from the abdominal aorta. Most of the blood supply for the liver, stomach, spleen, gallbladder, pancreas, and duodenum comes from this trunk. SYN: *truncus celiacus.*

***lumbosacral t.*** Part of the fourth and all of the fifth lumbar spinal nerves. These nerves accompany part of the first, second, and third sacral nerves to form the sciatic nerve.

***pulmonary t.*** The great vessel that arises from the right ventricle of the heart and gives rise to the right and left pulmonary arteries to the lungs. SYN: *truncus pulmonalis.*

***sympathetic t.*** The two long chains of ganglia, connected by sympathetic nerve fibers, that extend along the vertebral column from the skull to the coccyx.

**trusion** (troo′zhŭn) [L. *trudere,* to show] Malposition of a tooth or teeth.

**truss** (trŭs) [ME. *trusse,* a bundle] **1.** A restraining device for pushing a hernia, esp. an inguinal or abdominal wall hernia, back in place. **2.** To tie or bind as with a cord or string.

**trust** In the relations between health care providers and patients, reliance by both parties on the integrity and sincerity of each other, and the patient's confidence in the ability of the care provider or confidence that the provider would be willing to seek assistance when his or her ability is lacking. Trust is essential in the relationship between patients and those who provide medical care for them.

**truth serum** One of several hypnotic drugs supposedly having the effect of causing a person on questioning to talk freely and without inhibition. In actual practice, serum is not given, but a short-acting barbiturate or Pentothal Sodium is given intravenously. The reliability of the information obtained is questionable.

**trybutyrase** An enzyme present in the stomach that digests the short-chain diglycerides of butter. SEE: *digestion.*

**try-in** The temporary placement of a dental restoration or device to determine its fit and comfortableness.

**trypanocide** (trĭp-ăn′ō-sīd) [Gr. *trypanon,* a borer, + L. *cide,* kill] **1.** Destructive to trypanosomes. **2.** An agent that kills trypanosomes. SYN: *trypanosomicide.* **trypanocidal** (trĭp″ăn-ō-sī′dăl), *adj.*

**trypanolysis** (trĭp-ăn-ŏl′ĭ-sĭs) [″ + *lysis,* dissolution] The dissolution of trypanosomes.

**Trypanoplasma** (trī″păn-ō-plăz′mă) [″ + LL. *plasma,* form, mold] A genus of protozoan parasites resembling trypanosomes.

**Trypanosoma** (trī″păn-ō-sō′mă) [″ + *soma,* a body] A genus of parasitic, flagellate protozoa found in the blood of many vertebrates, including humans. The protozoa are transmitted by insect vectors. SEE: illus.

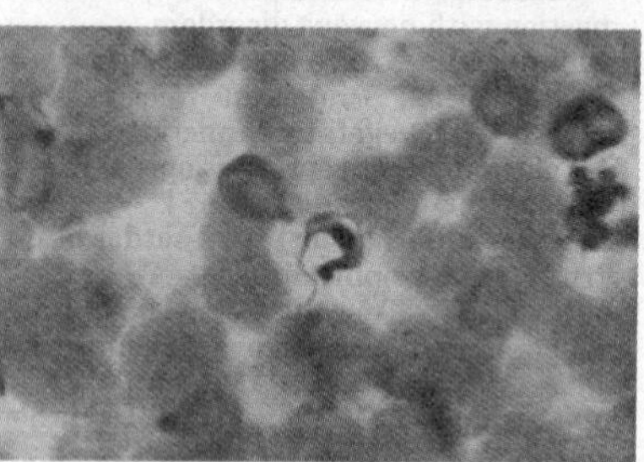
20μm

TRYPANOSOMA (CENTER) IN BLOOD (ORIG. MAG. ×1000)

***T. brucei*** The causative agent of trypanosomiasis in horses and other domestic animals. This organism is nonpathogenic in humans.

***T. cruzi*** The causative agent of American trypanosomiasis in many animals and specifically Chagas' disease in humans. It is transmitted by blood-sucking insects (triatomids) belonging to the family Reduviidae.

***T. gambiense*** The causative agent of African sleeping sickness. It is transmitted by the tsetse fly.

***T. rhodesiense*** An organism parasitic in wild game and domestic animals of portions of Africa. It may cause East African sleeping sickness in humans.

**trypanosomal** (trī-păn-ō-sō′măl) Pert. to trypanosomata.

**trypanosome** (trī′păn-ō-sōm) Any protozoan belonging to the genus Trypanosoma.

**trypanosomiasis** (trī-păn″ō-sō-mī′ă-sĭs) [″ + *soma,* body, + *-iasis,* infection] Any of the several diseases occurring in humans and domestic animals caused by a species of *Trypanosoma*. SEE: *sleeping sickness.*

***African t.*** African sleeping sickness, caused by *Trypanosoma gambiense.* SEE: *eflornithine.*

***South American t., American t.*** A disease caused by *Trypanosoma cruzi* and transmitted by the biting reduviid bug. It is characterized by fever, lymphadenopathy, hepatosplenomegaly, and facial edema. Chronic cases may be mild or asymptomatic, or may be accompanied by myocardiopathy, megaesophagus, and megacolon, with fatal outcome. SYN: *Chagas' disease.*

TREATMENT: The only drug available in the U.S. for treatment is nifurtimox, available from the Centers for Disease Control and Prevention. Outside of this, patients who tolerate nifurtimox poorly can use benzinazole.

**trypanosomic** (trī-păn″ō-sō′mĭk) Concerning trypanosomes.

**trypanosomicide** Trypanocide.

**trypanosomid** (trī-păn′ō-sō-mĭd) A skin eruption in any disease caused by a trypanosome.

**tryparsamide** (trĭp-ărs′ă-mĭd, -mīd) An arsenic compound containing about 25% arsenic; used chiefly in treating sleeping sickness.

**trypsin** (trĭp′sĭn) [Gr. *tripsis,* friction] **1.** A proteolytic enzyme formed in the intestine from the action of enterokinase of the intestinal juice (succus entericus) on trypsinogen secreted by the pancreas and present in pancreatic juice. It catalyzes the hydrolysis of peptide bonds in partly digested proteins and some native proteins, the final products being amino acids and various polypeptides. **2.** A proteolytic enzyme crystallized from an extract of the pancreas gland of an ox. SEE: *chymotrypsin; digestion; enzyme; pancreas.*

***crystallized t.*** A standardized preparation of the proteolytic enzyme trypsin. It is extracted from the pancreas of the ox, *Bos taurus.*

**trypsinized** (trĭp′sĭ-nīzd) Subjected to the action of trypsin, thus having antitryptic power abolished.

**trypsinogen** (trĭp-sĭn′ō-jĕn) [″ + *gennan,* to produce] The proenzyme or inactive form of trypsin found in pancreatic juice. It is activated when mixed in the intestine with the enterokinase of the succus entericus.

**tryptic** (trĭp′tĭk) Rel. to trypsin.

**tryptolysis** (trĭp-tŏl′ĭ-sĭs) [″ + *lysis,* dissolution] The hydrolysis of proteins or their derivatives by trypsin.

**tryptone** (trĭp′tōn) A peptide produced by the action of trypsin on a protein.

**tryptophan** (trĭp′tō-făn) An essential amino acid present in high concentrations in animal and fish protein. It is necessary for normal growth and development. Tryptophan is a precursor of serotonin, a neurotransmitter in the central nervous system. In high doses, it may cause nausea and vomiting.

**tryptophanase** (trĭp′tō-f ān-ās) An enzyme that catalyzes the splitting of tryptophan into indole, pyruvic acid, and ammonia.

**tryptophanuria** (trĭp″tō-fă-nū′rē-ă) [*tryptophan* + Gr. *ouron,* urine] The presence of excessive levels of tryptophan in the urine.

**T/S** *thyroid:serum* (thyroid to serum iodine ratio).

**T.S.** *test solution; triple strength.*

**TSD** *target skin distance.*

**tsetse fly** (tsĕt′sē) [S. African] One of several species of blood-sucking flies belonging to the genus *Glossina,* order Diptera, confined to Africa south of the Sahara Desert. It is an important transmitter of trypanosomes, the causative agents of African sleeping sicknesses in humans and nagana and other diseases of cattle and game animals. SEE: *Trypanosoma; trypanosomiasis.*

**TSH** *thyroid-stimulating hormone.*

**TSH-RF** *thyroid-stimulating hormone releasing factor.*

**tsp** *teaspoon.*

**TSTA** *tumor-specific transplantation antigen.*

**tsutsugamushi disease** (soot″soo-gă-moo′shĭ) [Japanese, dangerous bug] Scrub typhus.

**TT** *transit time* of blood through heart and lungs.

**T-tube** A device inserted into the biliary duct after removal of the gallbladder. It allows for drainage of the gallbladder and introduction of contrast medium for postoperative radiographical study of the bile duct.

**T.U.** *toxic unit; toxin unit.*

**tuaminoheptane sulfate** (too-ăm″ĭ-nō-hĕp′tān) A sympathomimetic drug used to produce vasoconstriction of the nasal mucosa or the conjunctiva.

**tub** (tŭb) [ME. *tubbe*] **1.** A receptacle for bathing. **2.** The use of a cold bath. **3.** To treat by using a cold bath.

**tuba** (too′bă) [L. *tubus,* tube] Tube.

**tubal** (tū′băl) [L. *tubus,* tube] Pert. to a tube, esp. the fallopian tube.

**tubal nephritis** Inflammation of kidney tubules.

**tubal pregnancy** SEE: *pregnancy, tubal.*

**tubatorsion** (tū″bă-tor′shŭn) [″ + *torsio,* a twisting] The twisting of an oviduct.

**tubba, tubboe** (tŭb′ă, -ō) Yaws that attacks the palms and soles.

**tube** (tūb) [L. *tubus,* a tube] A long, hollow,

cylindrical structure.

***auditory t.*** Eustachian t.

***Cantor t.*** Intestinal decompression t.

***cathode ray t.*** A vacuum tube with a thin window at the end opposite the cathode to allow the cathode rays to pass outside. More generally, any discharge tube in which the vacuum is fairly high.

***Coolidge t.*** A kind of hot-cathode tube that is so highly exhausted that the residual gas plays no part in the production of the cathode stream, and that is regulated by variable heating of the cathode filament.

***Crookes' t.*** A vacuum tube used in producing roentgen rays.

***cuffed endotracheal t.*** An airway catheter used to provide an airway through the trachea and at the same time to prevent aspiration of foreign material into the bronchus. This is accomplished by an inflatable cuff that surrounds the tube. The cuff is inflated after the tube is placed in the trachea.

***drainage t.*** A glass or rubber tube that, when inserted into a cavity, drains away its fluid contents.

***endobronchial t.*** A double-lumen tube used in anesthesia. One tube may be used to aerate a portion of the lung, while the other is occluded to deflate the other lung or a portion of it.

***endotracheal t.*** A catheter inserted into the trachea to provide an airway.

***esophageal t.*** Stomach t.

***eustachian t.*** The tube passing from the nasopharynx to the middle ear. SYN: *auditory t.; otopharyngeal t.*

***fallopian t.*** One of two oviducts leading from the ovary into the uterine cavity. SYN: *uterine t.*

***fermentation t.*** A U-shaped tube open at one end. If gas is produced by the bacteria cultured, the level of fluid decreases in the side of the tube with the closed end.

***gastrostomy t.*** A tube placed directly into the stomach for long-term enteral feeding. This may be done laparoscopically, with a percutaneous endoscopic gastrostomy (PEG) tube, or surgically. SEE: *percutaneous endoscopic gastrostomy.*

***hot-cathode t.*** A vacuum tube in which the cathode is electrically heated to incandescence and in which the supply of electrons depends on the temperature of the cathode.

***hot-cathode roentgen-ray t.*** An evacuated glass envelope, containing a positive anode and negative cathode separated by a gap, that produces x-ray photons. Electrons are supplied from a heated cathode in the form of a stream that interacts with the anode when a potential difference is placed between the anode and cathode.

***intestinal t.*** A flexible tube, usually made of plastic or rubber, placed in the intestinal tract to suck gas, fluid, or solids from the stomach or intestines; or to administer fluids, electrolytes, or nutrients to the patient. The tube may be passed through the nose, mouth, or anus, or through a colostomy opening.

NURSING IMPLICATIONS: When an intestinal tube is inserted, the nurse must aid its movement into the intestinal tract. The patient is usually placed on the right side for ½ hr, then the left side for ½ hr, and then on the back. These position changes, as well as ambulation, will facilitate movement of the tube into the intestinal tract.

Because the tube may drain feces, drainage should be kept from the patient's view. Frequent oral hygiene is needed to prevent oral ulceration because the patient will not be taking fluids by mouth. When the tube is removed, the patient's emotional reaction must be considered. Immediate oral hygiene is performed, particularly since drainage from the tube can easily cause the patient to become nauseated.

While the tube is in, the patient should be taught not to mouth breathe or swallow air. This enhances entry of air into the gastrointestinal tract and works counter to the principle of intestinal tubes and drainage.

***intestinal decompression t.*** A tube placed in the intestinal tract, usually via the nose and esophagus, to relieve gas pressure produced when paralytic ileus or intestinal obstruction is present. Tubes may be plain; made of rubber, plastic, or silicone; or equipped with a mercury-filled tip to facilitate passage into the intestinal tract. The latter type is called a Cantor tube. The tubes are impregnated with a radiopaque substance to allow radiographic visualization of their location.

***intubation t.*** A tube for passing into the larynx to facilitate breathing. SEE: *intubation.*

***jejunostomy t.*** A tube placed directly into the jejunum for long-term enteral feeding. This may be done laporoscopically, with a percutaneous endoscopic jejunostomy tube, or surgically. It is not as commonly used as the gastrostomy tube.

***Levin t.*** A tube passed via the nose into the gastrointestinal tract.

***Miller-Abbott t.*** A double-channel intestinal tube used to relieve intestinal distention. Inserted through a nostril, the tube is passed through the stomach into the small intestine.

***nasoduodenal t.*** A flexible tube of silicone or a similar synthetic material, inserted through the nose into the duodenum for short-term enteral feeding. The small weight on the distal end of the tube moves the tube into place through the stomach into the duodenum. Aspiration is less likely than with a nasogastric tube. SEE: *Miller-Abbott t.*

***nasogastric t.*** A tube inserted through

the nose and extending into the stomach. It may be used for emptying the stomach of gas and liquids or for administering liquids to the patient.

***nasointestinal t.*** A long tube inserted through the nose into the stomach for decompression. The weight at the end promotes its advancement into the small intestine. The most common use is to relieve the abdominal distention associated with intestinal obstruction.

***nasojejunal t.*** A tube passed through the nose into the jejunum for formula feeding.

***neural t.*** SEE: *neural tube.*

***otopharyngeal t.*** Eustachian t.

***photomultiplier t.*** ABBR: PMT. A very high sensitivity photosensor used in many clinical laboratory instruments.

***Sengstaken-Blakemore t.*** A three-element nasogastric tube used in treating esophageal bleeding. One tube is for aspiration, another is for feeding, and the third is attached to an elongated balloon that surrounds the tubes. The balloon is inflated after the tube is inserted. The goal is to compress the bleeding areas.

***Southey's t.*** A very small tube pushed into tissue to help drain edema fluid; used in severe congestive heart failure to relieve edema of the legs.

***stomach t.*** A rubber tube for introducing food into the stomach or for washing out the stomach. SYN: *esophageal t.*

***test t.*** A glass tube closed at one end. It is used in chemistry to hold chemicals and materials being tested.

***thoracostomy t.*** A tube inserted into the pleural space via the chest wall to remove air or fluid present in the space.

***tracheotomy t.*** A tube for insertion into the trachea.

***transnasal t.*** A tube passed through the nose into the gastrointestinal tract for feeding.

***uterine t.*** Fallopian t.

***ventilation t.*** SEE: *grommet.*

***Wangensteen t.*** A tube used in the Wangensteen method.

**tubectomy** (too-běk'tō-mē) Surgical removal of all or part of a tube, esp. the fallopian tube.

**tube feeding** Providing the patient's fluids and nutritional requirements by instilling foods into the stomach via a nasogastric tube. An alternative method uses a gastrostomy tube inserted into the stomach via the abdominal wall. This can be done under local anesthesia. This method of providing food for comatose patients who have no hope of recovery is controversial.

**tuber** (tū'běr) *pl.* **tubera** [L., a swelling] A swelling or enlargement.

***t. cinereum*** A part of the base of the hypothalamus bordered by the mammillary bodies, the optic chiasma, and on either side by the optic tract. It is connected by the infundibulum with the posterior lobe of the pituitary.

**tubercle** (tū'běr-kl) [L. *tuberculum,* a little swelling] **1.** A small rounded elevation or eminence on a bone. **2.** A small nodule, esp. a circumscribed solid elevation of the skin or mucous membrane. **3.** The characteristic lesion resulting from infection by tubercle bacilli. It consists typically of three parts: a central giant cell, a midzone of epithelioid cells, and a peripheral zone of nonspecific structure. SYN: *tuberculum.* SEE: *tuberculosis.*

***adductor t.*** The tubercle of the femur to which is attached the tendon of the adductor magnus.

***articular t.*** The tubercle at the base of the zygomatic arch to which is attached the temporomandibular ligament; it is lateral to the articular eminence of the glenoid fossa, with which it is often confused. SYN: *zygomatic t.*

***condyloid t.*** An eminence on the mandibular condyle for the attachment of the lateral ligament of the temporomandibular joint.

***deltoid t.*** The tubercle on the clavicle or humerus for attachment of the deltoid muscle.

***dental t.*** A small elevation of variable size on the crown of a tooth representing a thickened area of enamel or an accessory cusp.

***fibrous t.*** A fibrous tissue that has replaced a previously inflamed area.

***genial t.*** The tubercle on either side of the lower jawbone.

***genital t.*** The embryonic structure that becomes the clitoris or the penis.

***lacrimal t.*** A small tubercle between the lacrimal crest and the frontal process of the maxilla.

***laminated t.*** The cerebellar nodule.

***Lisfranc's t.*** A tubercle on the first rib for attachment of the scalenus anticus muscle.

***mental t.*** A small tubercle on either side of the midline of the chin.

***miliary t.*** A small tubercle resembling a millet seed, caused by tuberculosis. SEE: *tuberculosis, miliary.*

***olfactory t.*** An elevation at the rostral end of the anterior perforated substance of the brain. It is well developed in lower mammals but rudimentary in humans.

***pharyngeal t.*** The point of attachment of the superior pharyngeal constrictor and its fibrous raphe on the inferior surface of the basilar part of the occipital bone.

***pubic t.*** A small projection at the lateral end of the crest of the pubic bone. The inguinal ligament attaches to it.

***supraglenoid t.*** A rough, elevated area just above the glenoid cavity of the scapula. The long head of the biceps muscle of the arm attaches to this tubercle.

***t. of the upper lip*** The prominence of the upper part of the vermilion border that represents the distal termination of the philtrum of the upper lip.

***zygomatic t.*** Articular t.

**tubercula** (tū-bĕr′kū-lă) Pl. of tuberculum.

**tubercular** (tū-bĕr′kū-lăr) [L. *tuberculum,* a little swelling] Relating to or marked by nodules. SYN: *torose; tuberculate; tuberculated.*

**tuberculate, tuberculated** (tū-bĕr′kū-lāt, -lāt″ĕd) [L. *tuberculum,* a small swelling] Tubercular.

**tuberculation** (tū-bĕr″kū-lā′shŭn) The formation of tubercles.

**tuberculid, tuberculide** (tū-bĕr′kū-lĭd, -līd) [L. *tuberculum,* a little swelling] A tuberculous cutaneous eruption caused by toxins of tuberculosis. SYN: *tuberculoderma.*

***follicular t.*** A cutaneous eruption characterized by the presence of groups of follicular lesions, esp. on the trunk.

***papulonecrotic t.*** A form of tuberculid characterized by symmetrically distributed bluish papules, esp. on the extremities. These undergo central necrosis and, on healing, leave deep scars.

**tuberculin** (tū-bĕr′kū-lĭn) [L. *tuberculum,* a little swelling] **1.** A soluble cell substance prepared from the tubercle bacillus (usually the human type), which is used to determine the presence of a tuberculosis infection. Among the types of tuberculin used are Koch's original or old tuberculin (OT) and tuberculin purified protein derivative (PPD). **2.** The tuberculin used for diagnostic tests of the ability of the skin to react to the intradermal injection of tuberculin.

***new t.*** A suspension of tubercle bacilli fragments from which the soluble materials have been removed and to which glycerin has been added.

***old t.*** ABBR: OT. Tuberculin originally prepared by (H.H.) Robert Koch from cultures of *Mycobacterium tuberculosis.*

***purified protein derivative t.*** ABBR: PPD. A purified tuberculin obtained by the same technique as that used for old tuberculin except a synthetic broth is used to culture the *Mycobacterium tuberculosis.*

**tuberculin test** A test to determine the presence of a tuberculosis infection based on a positive reaction of the subject to tuberculin. Tests commonly used are Mantoux test, involving intradermal injection of tuberculin, and other multiple-puncture tests. In all tests, a local inflammatory reaction is observed in infected persons after 48 to 96 hr. Tests do not reveal whether infection is active or inactive. It is important to record the date and site of the test and the lot number of the PPD solution. The results of the test are positive when the area around the injection site is indurated. The diameter of the area of induration is recorded in millimeters. SEE: *tine test.*

**tuberculin tine test** A tuberculin test performed by using a special disposable instrument that contains multiple sharp points or prongs for piercing the skin. These tines penetrate the skin and introduce the tuberculin that has been applied to them. The test is read in 48 to 72 hr.

**tuberculitis** (tū″bĕr-kū-lī′tĭs) Inflammation of a tubercle.

**tuberculocele** (tū-bĕr′kū-lō-sēl″) [″ + *kele,* tumor] Tuberculosis of the testis.

**tuberculocidal** (tū-bĕr″kū-lō-sī′dăl) Anything that destroys *Mycobacterium tuberculosis.*

**tuberculoderma** (tū-bĕr″kū-lō-dĕr′mă) [″ + Gr. *derma,* skin] Tuberculid.

**tuberculofibroid** (tū-bĕr″kū-lō-fī′broyd) [″ + *fibra,* fiber, + Gr. *eidos,* form, shape] Denoting fibroid degeneration of tubercles.

**tuberculofibrosis** (tū-bĕr″kū-lō-fī-brō′sĭs) [″ + ″ + Gr. *osis,* condition] **1.** Chronic pulmonary inflammation with formation of fibrous tissue. **2.** Interstitial pneumonia.

**tuberculoid** (tū-bĕr′kū-loyd) [L. *tuberculum,* a little swelling, + Gr. *eidos,* form, shape] Resembling tuberculosis or a tubercle.

**tuberculoma** (tū-bĕr″kū-lō′mă) [″ + Gr. *oma,* tumor] **1.** A tuberculous abscess. **2.** Any tuberculous neoplasm.

**tuberculophobia** (tū-bĕr″kū-lō-fō′bē-ă) [″ + Gr. *phobos,* fear] An abnormal fear of being infected with tuberculosis.

**tuberculoprotein** (tū-bĕr″kū-lō-prō′tē-ĭn) A protein derived from tubercle bacilli.

**tuberculosilicosis** (tū-bĕr″kū-lō-sĭl″ĭ-kō′sĭs) Silicosis and pulmonary tuberculosis at the same time.

**tuberculosis** (tū-bĕr″kū-lō′sĭs) [″ + Gr. *osis,* condition] ABBR: TB. An infectious disease caused by the tubercle bacillus, *Mycobacterium tuberculosis,* and characterized pathologically by inflammatory infiltrations, formation of tubercles, caseation, necrosis, abscesses, fibrosis, and calcification. It most commonly affects the respiratory system, but other parts of the body such as the gastrointestinal and genitourinary tracts, bones, joints, nervous system, lymph nodes, and skin may also become infected. Fish, amphibians, birds, and mammals (esp. cattle) are subject to the disease. Three types of the tubercle bacillus exist: human, bovine, and avian. Humans may become infected by any of the three types, but in the U.S. the human type predominates. Infection usually is acquired from contact with an infected person or an infected cow or through drinking contaminated milk.

Tuberculosis may occur in an acute generalized form (miliary tuberculosis) or in a chronic localized form. In humans, the primary infection usually consists of localized lesions in the lung with enlarged lymph nodes in the surrounding area. Macrophages surround the bacilli in an attempt to engulf them but cannot, producing granulomas with a soft, cheesy (caseous) core. From this state, lesions may heal by fibrosis and calcification and the disease may exist in an arrested or inactive stage. Reactivation or exacerbation of the disease or reinfection gives rise to the chronic progressive form.

The incidence of tuberculosis decreased significantly until around 1990, when multidrug-resistant strains began appearing. Tuberculosis is most commonly seen in homeless people, refugees from Asia, those in prisons and long-term psychiatric facilities, the elderly, particularly those in residential facilities, and people infected with HIV. All patients on immunosuppressive drug therapy, and those with chronic respiratory disorders, diabetes, renal failure, or poor nutritional status, are also at risk. Any patient in one of these categories who is diagnosed with pneumonia should be tested for tuberculosis; all health care workers should be tested annually. SEE: illus.; *immunological therapy; tine test; tuberculin test; Nursing Diagnoses Appendix.*

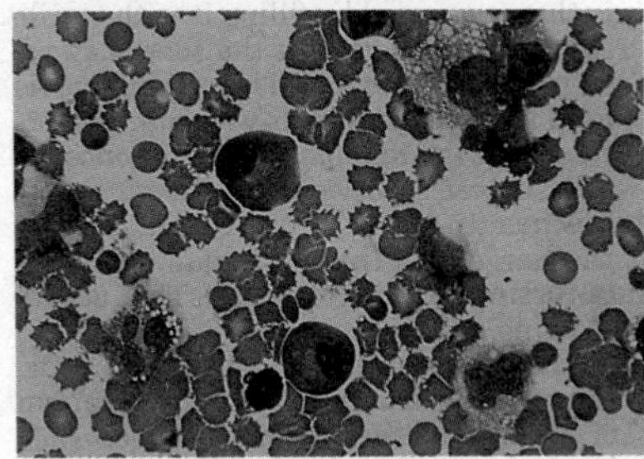

**TUBERCULOSIS**

PLEURAL FLUID WITH PLASMA CELLS (ORIG. MAG. ×1000)

INCUBATION PERIOD: Approx. 4 to 12 weeks will elapse between the time of infection and the time a demonstrable primary lesion or positive tuberculin skin test occurs.

DIAGNOSIS: A positive tuberculin skin test indicates the patient has had a tuberculous infection; however, unless repeated tests indicate a recent change from negative, it is impossible to tell how recently the infection occurred. A presumptive diagnosis of active disease is made by finding acid-fast bacilli in stained smears from sputum or other body fluids. The diagnosis is confirmed by isolating *Mycobacterium tuberculosis* on culture. The culture will take at least 3 weeks and usually 4 to 6 weeks. Recently a nucleic acid probe test has become available that can detect *Mycobacterium tuberculosis* in sputum specimens in 4 to 5 hr.

NOTE: Many varieties of *Mycobacterium* that previously were thought to be nonpathogenic for humans have been found to cause chronic progressive pulmonary disease closely resembling pulmonary tuberculosis. These organisms have been termed anonymous or atypical *Mycobacterium*. They have been classified into four groups: photochromogens, scotochromogens, nonphotochromogens, and rapid growers.

TREATMENT: For treating uncomplicated tuberculosis, daily isoniazid (INH), pyrazinamide (PZA), and rifampin (RMP) for 2 months followed by 4 months of daily RMP and INH is effective. In this regimen, the medicines are self-administered. To ensure compliance and to help prevent the development of drug-resistant strains of the tubercle bacillus, directly observed preventive therapy (DOPT) should be used. Preventive therapy is recommended for patients infected with HIV and household members of patients with tuberculosis. Multidrug-resistant tuberculosis is extremely difficult to treat; mortality may be as high as 80%. Recommended therapies include ethambutol plus RMP for 6 months followed by PZA plus RMP for 9 months, or PZA plus ciprofloxacin for 6 to 12 months; the effectiveness of these treatment plans is still being investigated. SEE: *multidrug-resistant t.*

**avian t.** Tuberculosis of birds caused by *Mycobacterium avium.*

**bovine t.** Tuberculosis of cattle caused by *Mycobacterium bovis.*

**endogenous t.** Tuberculosis originating in a tubercle in another body site.

**exogenous t.** Tuberculosis originating from a source outside the body.

**hematogenous t.** The spread of tuberculosis from a primary site to another site via the bloodstream.

**miliary t.** Tuberculosis that spreads throughout the body via the bloodstream. It may be fatal.

**multidrug resistant t.** ABBR: MDR-TB. *Mycobacterium tuberculosis* bacilli that are resistant to therapy with a variety of drugs that had been effective in treating tuberculosis in the past. The development of MDR-TB may be related to failure to test the causative organism for drug sensitivity, failure to initiate adequate therapy, failure to modify the treatment regimen when susceptibility testing indicates the need for change, or failure to identify and remedy patient noncompliance by directly observed preventive therapy (DOPT).

**open t.** Tuberculosis in which the tubercle bacilli are present in bodily secretions that leave the body.

**tuberculostatic** (tū-bĕr″kū-lō-stăt′ĭk) Arresting the growth of the tubercle bacillus.

**tuberculotic** (tū-bĕr″kū-lŏt′ĭk) Concerning tuberculosis.

**tuberculous** (tū-bĕr′kū-lŭs) [L. *tuberculum*, a little swelling] Relating to or affected with tuberculosis, or conditions marked by infiltration of a specific tubercle, as opposed to the term tubercular, referring to a nonspecific tubercle.

**tuberculum** (tū-bĕr′kū-lŭm) *pl.* **tubercula**

[L. *tuberculum,* a little swelling] A small knot or nodule; a tubercle.

*t. acusticum* The dorsal nucleus of the cochlear nerve.

*t. impar* A small median eminence on the floor of the embryonic oral cavity that plays a minor role in tongue development.

*t. majus humeri* The larger tuberosity of the humerus at the upper end of its lateral surface, giving attachment to the infraspinatus, supraspinatus, and teres minor muscles.

*t. minus humeri* The projection at the proximal end of the anterior humerus, providing attachment to the subscapularis muscle.

**tuberosis** (tū″bĕr-ō′sĭs) A condition in which nodules develop; a nonspecific term that indicates no specific disease process.

**tuberositas** (tū-bĕr-ŏs′ĭt-ăs) *pl.* **tuberositates** [L.] A projection, nodule, or prominence.

**tuberosity** (tū-bĕr-ŏs′ĭ-tē) [L. *tuberositas,* tuberosity] **1.** An elevated round process of a bone. **2.** A tubercle or nodule.

*ischial t.* A palpable prominence on the inferior margin of the ischium that supports a person's weight when sitting.

*maxillary t.* A rounded eminence on the posteroinferior surface of the maxilla that enlarges with the development and eruption of the third molar. It articulates medially with the palatine bone and laterally with the lateral pterygoid process of the sphenoid. It forms the anterior surface of the pterygopalatine fossa, including a groove for the passage of the maxillary nerve which is anesthetized in this region for a maxillary or second-division block.

**tuberous** (tū′bĕr-ŭs) Pert. to tubers.

**tubo-** Combining form meaning *tube.*

**tuboabdominal** (tū″bō-ăb-dŏm′ĭn-ăl) [L. *tubus,* tube, + *abdominalis,* pert. to the abdomen] Pert. to the fallopian tubes and the abdomen.

**tuboabdominal pregnancy** Ectopic gestation with the embryo partly in the tube and partly in the abdominal cavity.

**tubocurarine chloride** (tū″bō-kū-ră′rĭn klō′rīd) A drug used to produce skeletal muscle relaxation during anesthesia and convulsive states and to treat poisoning caused by black widow spider bites. Tubocurarine was originally obtained from the Indian arrow poison, curare.

---

Caution: Tubocurarine should be administered only by those who have the proper equipment and are fully capable of providing artificial ventilation, tracheal intubation, appropriate antidotes, and additional therapy in case of overdose.

---

**tuboligamentous** (tū″bō-lĭg-ă-mĕn′tŭs) [″ + *ligamentum,* a band] Pert. to the fallopian tube and broad ligament of the uterus.

**tubo-ovarian** (tū″bō-ō-vā′rē-ăn) [″ + LL. *ovarium,* ovary] Pert. to the fallopian tube and the ovary.

**tubo-ovariotomy** (tū″bō-ō-vā-rē-ŏt′ō-mē) [″ + LL. *ovarium,* ovary, + Gr. *tome,* incision] Excision of ovaries and oviducts.

**tubo-ovaritis** (tū″bō-ō″vă-rī′tĭs) [″ + ″ + Gr. *itis,* inflammation] Inflammation of the ovary and fallopian tube.

**tuboperitoneal** (tū″bō-pĕr-ĭ-tō-nē′ăl) [″ + Gr. *peritonaion,* peritoneum] Rel. to the oviduct and peritoneum.

**tuboplasty** (tū′bō-plăs″tē) **1.** Plastic repair of any tube. **2.** Plastic repair of a fallopian tube or tubes in an attempt to restore patency so that fertilization of the ovum may occur. SYN: *salpingoplasty.*

**tuboplasty, transcervical balloon** An experimental procedure for treating occlusion of the fallopian tubes. The procedure does not involve surgery. A balloon catheter is inserted through the cervical os of the uterus and into the fallopian tube to the point of occlusion in the tube. The balloon is then expanded by filling it with sterile saline. This dilation of the tube may restore tubal patency. This technique is used to help individuals with bilateral occlusion of the fallopian tubes to conceive. SEE: *catheter, balloon; infertility.*

**tuborrhea** (tū-bor-rē′ă) [″ + Gr. *rhoia,* flow] Discharge from the eustachian tube.

**tubotorsion** (tū″bō-tor′shŭn) The act of twisting a tube.

**tubotympanal** (tū″bō-tĭm′pă-năl) [″ + Gr. *tympanon,* a drum] Rel. to the tympanum of the ear and the eustachian tube.

**tubouterine** (tū″bō-ū′tĕr-ĭn) [″ + *uterinus,* pert. to the uterus] Rel. to the oviduct and the uterus.

**tubovaginal** (tū″bō-văj′ĭ-năl) Concerning the fallopian tube and vagina.

**tubular** (tū′bū-lăr) [L. *tubularis,* like a tube] Rel. to or having the form of a tube or tubule.

**tubule** (tū′būl) [L. *tubulus,* a tubule] A small tube or canal.

*collecting t.* The tubule in the renal medulla that is the last part of a nephron.

*convoluted t.'s of the kidney* The proximal and distal convoluted tubules of the nephron that, with the loop of Henle and collecting tubule, form the renal tubule through which the glomerular filtrate passes before entering the renal pelvis. SEE: *kidney* for illus.; *nephron.*

*convoluted seminiferous t.* One of the tubules present in each lobe of the testes.

*dentinal t.* One of the very small canals in the dentin. These extend from the pulp cavity of the tooth to the enamel and are occupied by odontoblastic processes and occasional nerve filaments.

*excretory t.* Renal t.

*galactophorous t.* One of the lactiferous ducts of the breast. It provides a channel for the milk formed in the lobes of the breast to pass to the nipple. SYN: *lactiferous t.*

*Henle's t.* Henle's loop.

*junctional t.* The short segment of a renal tubule that connects the distal convoluted tubule with the collecting tubule.

***lactiferous t.*** Galactophorous t.

***mesonephric t.*** One of the embryonic tubules consisting of two groups, cranial and caudal. The cranial group gives rise in the male to the efferent ductules of the testes and appendix epididymis; in the female, it gives rise to the epoophoron and vesicular appendices. The caudal group gives rise in the male to the paradidymis and aberrant ductules; in the female, it gives rise to the paroophoron. All structures except the efferent ductules of the testes are vestigial. SYN: *wolffian tubules.*

***metanephritic t.*** One of the tubes that make up the permanent kidneys of amniotes.

***renal t.*** The part of a nephron through which renal filtrate from the renal corpuscle flows and is changed to urine by absorption and secretion. The parts, in order, are the proximal convoluted tubule, the loop of Henle, the distal convoluted tubule, and collecting tubule. SYN: *excretory t.* SEE: *kidney* for illus; *nephron.*

***seminiferous t.*** One of the very small channels of the testes in which spermatozoa develop and through which they leave the testes.

***transverse t.*** ABBR: T-tubule. An invagination of the cell membrane of a muscle fiber that carries the action potential to the interior of the cell and the innermost sarcomeres.

***uriniferous t.*** SEE: *renal t.*

**tubulin** (tū′bū-lĭn) A protein present in the microtubules of cells.

**tubulization** (too″bū-lī-zā′shŭn) A method of repairing severed nerves in which the nerve ends are placed in a tube of absorbable material.

**tubuloalveolar** Consisting of tubes and alveoli, as in a tubuloalveolar salivary gland.

**tubulocyst** (too′bū-lō-sĭst) The cystic dilatation of a functionless duct or canal.

**tubulodermoid** (tū″bū-lō-dĕr′moyd) [″ + Gr. *derma,* skin, + *eidos,* form, shape] A dermoid tumor caused by the persistent embryonic tubular structure.

**tubuloracemose** (too″bū-lō-răs′ĕ-mōs) Pert. to a gland that has tubular and racemose characteristics.

**tubulorrhexis** (too″bū-lō-rĕk′sĭs) [″ + *rhexis,* a breaking] Focal ruptures of renal tubules.

**tubulus** (tū′bū-lŭs) *pl.* **tubuli** [L.] A tubule.

**tubus** (too′bŭs) [L.] Tube.

***t. digestorius*** The alimentary canal.

**tuft** A small clump, cluster, or coiled mass.

***enamel t.*** An abnormal structure formed in the development of enamel, consisting of poorly calcified twisted rods.

***malpighian t.*** The renal glomerulus.

**tugging** A dragging or pulling.

***tracheal t.*** An indication of a thoracic aneurysm. There is a sense of downward pulling of the larynx with cardiac systole when the thyroid cartilage is gently raised between the finger and thumb.

**tularemia** (tū-lăr-ē′mē-ă) [*Tulare,* part of California where disease was first discovered] An acute plaguelike infectious disease caused by *Francisella tularensis* (formerly classed as *Pasteurella tularensis*). It is transmitted to humans by the bite of an infected tick or other bloodsucking insect, by direct contact with infected animals, by eating inadequately cooked meat, or by drinking water that contains the organism. Streptomycin or gentamicin is effective in treating the disease. SYN: *deer fly fever; rabbit fever.*

SYMPTOMS: The symptoms may appear from 1 to 10 days, but averaging 3 days, after infection and include headache, chilliness, vomiting, aching pains, and fever. An ulcer develops at the entry site of the bacteria, and regional lymph nodes enlarge, become painful, and may develop into abscesses. Serious cases involve pneumonia, debilitation, and an extended recovery period.

**tumbu fly** A species of fly belonging to the genus *Cordylobia* in Africa and the genus *Dermatobia* in tropical America. Their larvae develop in the skin of wild domesticated animals, and humans are frequently attacked.

**tumefacient** (tū-mĕ-fā′shĕnt) [L. *tumefaciens,* producing swelling] Producing or tending to produce swelling; swollen.

**tumefaction** (tū″mĕ-făk′shŭn) [L. *tumefactio,* a swelling] Intumescence.

**tumentia** (tū-mĕn′shē-ă) [L.] Swelling.

***vasomotor t.*** Irregular swellings in the lower extremities associated with vasomotor disturbances.

**tumescence** (tū-mĕs′ĕns) **1.** A condition of being swollen or tumid. **2.** A swelling.

**tumor** (tū′mor) [L. *tumor,* a swelling] **1.** A swelling or enlargement. **2.** Swelling, one of the four classical signs of inflammation. The others are calor (heat), dolor (pain), and rubor (redness). **3.** A spontaneous new growth of tissue forming an abnormal mass. It is, with few exceptions of unknown cause, noninflammatory, and develops independent of and unrestrained by normal laws of growth and morphogenesis. SYN: *neoplasm.* SEE: *cancer.*

TYPES: *Myeloid sarcoma* or *giant-celled sarcoma:* This consists of elements formed chiefly of protoplasm containing two or more nuclei, up to 20 or even 50, with a varying number of round, spindle, or mixed cells. Consistency varies from that of jelly to that of muscle. The tumors more frequently occur on the lower jaw, femur, and tibia. *Round-celled sarcoma:* This is usually soft, vascular, and rapidly growing, becoming large, and it gives rise to metastatic deposits in distant parts and in viscera. Tumors occur in periosteum, bone, lymphatic glands, subcutaneous tissue, testicle, eye, ovary, uterus, lung, and kidneys, although they may occur wherever fibrous tissue exists. *Glioma:* This grows from the connective tissue of nerve centers and its basic substance resembles that structure. It occurs in retina and brain. *Melanotic sarcoma:* Cells may be of either the round or the spindle variety. This type of tumor is extremely malignant. *Spindle-cell sarcoma:* Cells vary greatly in size, from small oat-shaped cells to greatly elongated bodies with long, fine, tapering extremities. These occur chiefly in bones. *Endothelioma:* This may occur, in different forms, in the testicle, pia mater, pleura, and peritoneum.

*Acinous or spheroidal-celled carcinoma:* This occurs in two forms: 1) hard, spheroidal-celled (scirrhus or chronic carcinoma) and 2) soft, spheroidal-celled (encephaloid or acute carcinoma). It resembles brain tissue in appearance and consistency. It may occur in the testicle, liver, bladder, kidney, ovary, fundus oculi, and more rarely breast. SEE: *scirrhus*. *Colloid carcinoma:* This is one of the preceding varieties that has undergone mucoid degeneration and so distended the alveoli that they may be seen by the naked eye. It occurs in the stomach, intestine, omentum, and ovary. *Epithelial carcinoma:* The squamous-celled epitheliomata always develop from the skin or mucous membranes or their glands, esp. at junctions of mucous and cutaneous surfaces. They are not encapsulated and commence as a wartlike growth, flattened tubercle, or fissure; ulceration in all these forms sets in early. Cylindrical or columnar-celled epitheliomata are a less common form of carcinoma. They originate from either the cylindrical surface epithelium of a mucous membrane or its glands, closely imitating these structures in microscopic appearance. These growths form indurated infiltrating masses in the walls of the organs attacked, producing considerable stenosis of lumina of hollow viscera such as rectal and small intestinal obstruction. These occur in the uterus and intestinal tract.

*Warty or villous growth (papillomata):* These resemble in their structure hypertrophied papillae of the skin or mucous membrane. These include condylomata and mucous tubercles and occur about the anus and genitals or in the mouth and throat. Warts and warty growths arise on the skin of the hands and genitalia and on the mucous surface of the larynx, and villous growths of the bladder, rectum, and larynx may occur. *Teratoma:* These tumors contain bone, hair, or teeth and are usually situated in the ovaries or testicles but may also be present in other tissues.

***carotid body t.*** A benign tumor of the carotid body.

***connective tissue t.*** Any tumor of connective tissue such as fibroma, lipoma, chondroma, or sarcoma.

***desmoid t.*** A tumor of the fibrous connective tissue.

***erectile t.*** A tumor composed of erectile tissue.

***Ewing's t.*** A malignant tumor of bone.

***false t.*** An enlargement due to hemorrhage into tissue or extravasation of fluid into a space but not due to a neoplastic growth.

***fibroid t.*** A benign fibrous tissue tumor of the myometrium.

***giant cell t. of bone*** A benign or malignant tumor of bone in which the cells are multinucleated and surrounded by cellular spindle cell stroma.

***giant cell t. of tendon sheath*** A localized nodular tenosynovitis.

***granulosa t., granulosa cell t.*** An estrin-secreting tumor of the granulosa cells of the ovary.

***granulosa-theca cell t.*** An estrogen-secreting tumor of the ovary made up of either granulosa or theca cells.

***heterologous t.*** A tumor in which the tissue differs from that in which it is growing.

***homoiotypic t., homologous t.*** A tumor in which the tissue resembles that in which it is growing.

***Hürthle cell t.*** A benign or malignant tumor of the thyroid gland. The cells are large and acidophilic.

***islet cell t.*** A tumor of the islets of Langerhans of the pancreas.

***Krukenberg's t.*** A tumor of the ovary caused by metastases from a tumor in the gastrointestinal tract.

***lipoid cell t. of the ovary*** A masculinizing tumor of the ovary. It may be malignant.

***mast cell t.*** A benign nodular accumulation of mast cells.

***melanotic neuroectodermal t.*** A benign tumor of the jaw, occurring mostly during the first year of life.

***mesenchymal mixed t.*** A tumor composed of tissue that resembles mesenchymal cells.

***t. of pregnancy*** The abdominal swelling produced by the growing conceptus of pregnancy.

***phantom t.*** An apparent tumor due to muscular contractions or flatus seen in hysteria.

***sand t.*** Psammoma.

***turban t.*** Multiple cutaneous cylindromata that cover the scalp like a turban.

**tumoraffin** (tū′mor-ăf-ĭn) [L. *tumor*, a swelling, + *affinis*, related] Having an affinity for tumor cells.

**tumor angiogenesis factor** ABBR: TAF. A protein present in animal and human cancer tissue that in experimental studies appears to be essential to growth of the cancer. The substance is thought to act by stimulating the growth of new blood capillaries for supplying the tumor with nutrients and removing waste products.

**tumor burden** The sum of cancer cells present in the body.
**tumoricidal** (too″mor-ĭ-sī′dăl) Lethal to neoplastic cells.
**tumorigenesis** (too″mor-ĭ-jĕn′ĕ-sĭs) The production of tumors.
**tumorigenic** (tū″mor-ĭ-jĕn′ĭk) [″ + Gr. *genesis,* generation, birth] Oncogenic.
**tumor marker** A substance whose presence in blood serum serves as a biochemical indicator for the possible presence of a malignancy. Examples of markers and the malignancies they may indicate are carcinoembryonic antigen for cancers of the colon, lung, breast, and ovary; beta subunit of chorionic gonadotropin for trophoblastic and testicular tumors; alpha-fetoprotein for testicular teratocarcinoma and primary hepatocellular carcinoma; and prostatic acid phosphatase and prostate-specific antigen for malignancy of the prostate.
**tumor necrosis factor** ABBR: TNF. A protein mediator or cytokine released primarily by macrophages and T lymphocytes that helps regulate the immune response and some hematopoietic functions. There are two factors: alpha (TNF$\alpha$), also called cachectin, produced by macrophages, and beta (TNF$\beta$) called lymphotoxin, which is produced by activated CD4+ T cells. The functions of TNFs are very similar to those of interleukin-1. SEE: *cytokine; interleukin-1.*
**tumorous** (too′mor-ŭs) Tumor-like.
**tumultus** (tū-mŭl′tŭs) [L.] Excessive or agitated activity.
***t. cordis*** Irregular heart action with palpitation.
***t. sermonis*** Extreme stuttering due to a pathological cause.
**Tunga** (tŭng′ă) A genus of fleas of the family Hectopsyllidae.
***T. penetrans*** A small flea common in tropical regions. It infests humans, cats, dogs, rats, pigs, and other animals and produces a severe local inflammation frequently liable to secondary infection.
**tungiasis** (tŭng-gī′ă-sĭs) Infestation of the skin with *Tunga penetrans.*
**tungsten** (tŭng′stĕn) SYMB: W (for wolfram). A metallic element; atomic weight, 183.85; atomic number, 74.
**tunic** (tū′nĭk) [L. *tunica,* a sheath] An investing membrane.
***Bichat's t.*** Tunica intima.
**tunica** (tū′nĭ-kă) *pl.* **tunicae** [L. *tunica,* a sheath] A coat or covering; in anatomy, the term defines a covering or lining layer of connective tissue or epithelium, respectively.
***t. adventitia*** The outermost fibroelastic layer of a blood vessel or other tubular structure. SYN: *t. externa.*
***t. albuginea*** The white fibrous coat of the eye, testicle, ovary, or spleen.
***t. conjunctiva*** Conjunctiva.
***t. dartos*** The muscular, contractile tissue beneath the skin of the scrotum.
***t. externa*** T. adventitia.
***t. interna*** SEE: *t. intima.*
***t. intima*** The lining of a blood vessel composed of an epithelial (endothelium) layer and the basement membrane, a subendothelial connective tissue layer, and usually an internal elastic lamina. SYN: *Bichat's tunic.*
***t. media*** The middle layer in the wall of a blood vessel composed of circular or spiraling smooth muscle and some elastic fibers.
***t. mucosa*** The mucous membrane lining of various structures.
***t. muscularis*** The smooth muscule layer in the walls of organs such as the bronchi, intestines, and blood vessels.
***t. serosa*** The membrane lining the walls of the closed body cavities and folded over the organs in those cavities, forming the outermost layer of the wall of these organs. The body cavities are the thoracic, abdominal, and pericardial cavities.
***t. vaginalis*** The serous membrane surrounding the front and sides of the testicle.
***t. vasculosa*** Any vascular layer.
**tuning fork** A device that, when struck at the forked end, vibrates and thus can be heard and felt. It is used in testing the sensations of hearing, including bone conduction and vibration. A fork that vibrates at 256 cycles/sec is suitable for use in these tests.
**tunnel** (tŭn′ĕl) A narrow channel or passageway.
***carpal t.*** The canal in the wrist bounded by osteofibrous material through which the flexor tendons and the median nerve pass. SYN: *flexor t.*
***flexor t.*** Carpal t.
***inner t.*** The triangular canal lying between the inner and outer pillars of Corti in the organ of Corti of the inner ear.
***tarsal t.*** The osteofibrous canal in the tarsal area bounded by the flexor retinaculum and tarsal bones. The posterior tibial vessels, tibial nerve, and flexor tendons pass through this tunnel.
**TUR** *transurethral resection* (of the prostate).
**turbid** (tŭr′bĭd) [L. *turba,* a tumult] Cloudy; not clear. SEE: *turbidity.*
**turbidimeter** (tŭr-bĭ-dĭm′ĕ-ter) [L. *turbidus,* disturbed, + Gr. *metron,* measure] A device for estimating the degree of turbidity of a fluid.
**turbidimetry** (tŭr-bĭ-dĭm′ĕ-trē) [″ + Gr. *metron,* measure] Estimation of the turbidity of a liquid.
**turbidity** (tŭr-bĭd′ĭ-tē) [L. *turbiditas,* turbidity] Opacity due to the suspension of flaky or granular particles in a normally clear liquid.
**turbinal, turbinate** (tŭr′bĭ-năl, -nāt) [L. *turbinalis,* fr. *turbo,* a child's top] Shaped like an inverted cone.
**turbinated** (tŭr′bĭ-nā″tĕd) [L. *turbo,* whirl]

Top-shaped or cone-shaped. SEE: *concha*.

**turbinectomy** (tŭr-bĭn-ĕk′tō-mē) [″ + Gr. *ektome,* excision.] Excision of a turbinated bone.

**turbinotome** (tŭr-bĭn′ō-tōm) [″ + Gr. *tome,* incision] An instrument for excision of a turbinated bone.

**turbinotomy** (tŭr-bĭn-ŏt′ō-mē) [″ + Gr. *tome,* incision] Surgical incision of a turbinated bone.

**turgescence** (tŭr-jĕs′ĕns) [L. *turgescens,* swelling] Swelling or enlargement of a part.

**turgescent** (tŭr-jĕs′ĕnt) [L. *turgescens,* swelling] Swollen; inflated.

**turgid** (tŭr′jĭd) [L. *turgidus,* swollen] Swollen; bloated.

**turgometer** (tŭr-gŏm′ĕ-tĕr) [L. *turgor,* swelling, + Gr. *metron,* measure] A device for measuring turgescence.

**turgor** [L., a swelling] **1.** Normal tension in a cell. **2.** Distention, swelling.

***skin t.*** The resistance of the skin to deformation, esp. to being grasped between the fingers. In a healthy person, when the skin on the back of the hand is grasped between the fingers and released, it returns to its normal appearance either immediately or relatively slowly. The state of hydration of the skin can determine which of these reactions occurs, but age is the most important factor. As a person ages, the skin returns much more slowly to its normal position after having been pinched between the fingers. The skin over the forehead or sternum may be used when assessing turgor in elderly persons.

***t. vitalis*** Normal fullness of the capillaries and blood vessels.

**turista** (tū-rēs′tă) [Sp.] One of the many names applied to travelers' diarrhea, esp. that which occurs in tourists in Mexico.

**Türk's irritation cell** A cell resembling a plasma cell, found in cases of severe anemia or chronic infection.

**Turner's syndrome** [Henry Hubert Turner, U.S. physician, 1892–1970] A congenital endocrine disorder caused by failure of the ovaries to respond to pituitary hormone stimulation. Clinically, there is amenorrhea, failure of sexual maturation, and usually short stature. About one third of these patients have webbing of the neck and may have marked cubitus valgus. Intelligence may be impaired. These patients usually have only 45 chromosomes, the second X chromosome being absent. SYN: *gonadal dysgenesis*. SEE: *karyotype*.

**turning** [AS. *turnian,* to turn] Version.

**turpentine** (tŭr′pĕn-tīn) [Gr. *terebinthos,* turpentine tree] Oleoresin obtained from various species of pine trees. It is a mixture of terpenes and other hydrocarbons obtained from pine trees. It was previously used in liniments and counterirritants, applied topically, and is the source of oil of turpentine or spirits of turpentine.

**turpentine poisoning** Toxicity resulting usually from inhalation of turpentine. SEE: *Poisons and Poisoning Appendix*.

SYMPTOMS: Symptoms include a warm or burning sensation in the esophagus and stomach, followed by cramping, vomiting, and diarrhea. Pulse and respiration become weak, slow, and irregular. Irritation of the urinary tract and central nervous system resembles alcoholic intoxication.

FIRST AID: Gastric lavage should be performed, soothing drinks and stimulants should be given, and fluid intake should be increased.

**turunda** (tū-rŭn′dă) [L.] **1.** A surgical tent, drain, or tampon. **2.** A suppository.

**tussal** (tŭs′ăl) [L. *tussis,* cough] Tussive.

**tussicular** (tŭ-sĭk′ū-lăr) [L. *tussis,* cough] Pert. to a cough.

**tussiculation** (tŭ-sĭk″ū-lā′shŭn) A short, dry cough.

**tussis** (tŭs′ĭs) [L.] A cough.

**tussive** (tŭs′ĭv) [L. *tussis,* cough] Relating to a cough. SYN: *tussal*.

**tussive syncope** SEE: *laryngeal vertigo*.

**tutamen** (tū-tā′mĕn) *pl.* **tutamina** [L.] Any tissue that has a protective action.

***tutamina oculi*** The structures around the eye that protect it: the eyebrows, eyelids, and eyelashes.

**T wave** The portion of the electrocardiogram that is due to repolarization of the ventricles. The wave may be positive or negative depending on the lead involved in recording the ECG and whether or not the electrical activity of the heart is within normal limits. SEE: *electrocardiogram; QRST complex*.

**twelfth cranial nerve** One of a pair of cranial nerves distributing to the base of the tongue. SEE: *cranial nerve; hypoglossal nerve; Nerves Appendix*.

**twig** The final branch of a structure such as a nerve or vessel.

**twilight sleep** A state of partial anesthesia and hypoconsciousness in which pain sense has been greatly reduced by the injection of morphine and scopolamine. The patient responds to pain, but afterward the memory of the pain is dulled or effaced. SEE: *labor*.

**twilight state** A state in which consciousness is disordered, making possible actions subsequently forgotten. This may occur in hysteria and epilepsy.

**twin** (twĭn) [AS. *twinn*] One of two children developed within the uterus at the same time from the same impregnation. Identical and fraternal twins provide a unique resource for investigating the origin and natural history of various diseases and in attempts to discover the differential importance of environmental and hereditary factors in causing physical and mental disorders. The latter type of investigation is esp. important in following the course of identical twins who were separated shortly after birth and grew up in differ-

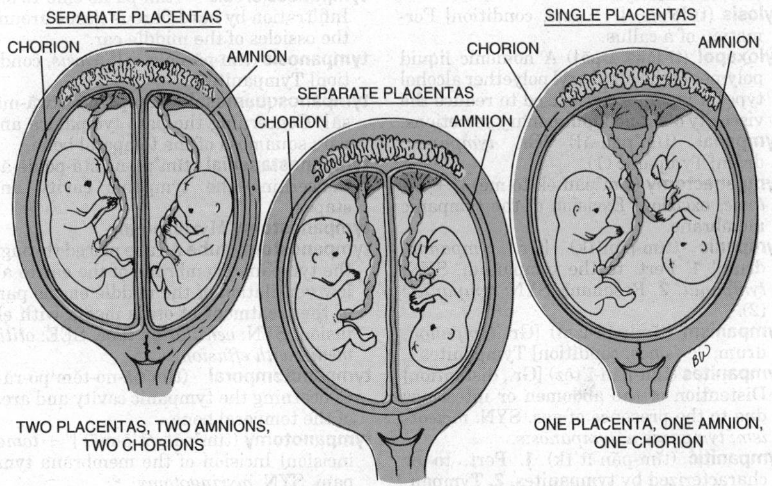


ent social, economic, educational, and environmental conditions. In one study, the second twin to emerge was reputed to be at increased risk of an unfavorable outcome (e.g., need for intubation and resuscitation, lower 5-min Apgar score), even when delivered by cesarean section. SEE: illus.; *fetus papyraceus; Hellin's law.*

***biovular t.'s*** Dizygotic t.'s.

***conjoined t.'s*** Twins that are united. SEE: *Siamese twins.*

***dizygotic t.'s*** Twins from two separate ova fertilized at the same time. SYN: *biovular t.'s; fraternal t.'s.* SEE: *monozygotic t.'s.*

***enzygotic t.'s*** Monozygotic t.'s.

***fraternal t.'s*** Dizygotic t.'s.

***growth discordant t.*** The unequal growth of twins while in utero. The smaller twin is at greater risk of having congenital anomalies than is the normal birth-weight twin. SYN: *unequal t.'s.*

***identical t.'s*** Monozygotic t.'s.

***impacted t.'s*** Twins so entwined in utero as to prevent normal delivery.

***interlocked t.'s*** Twins in which the neck of one becomes interlocked with the head of the other, making vaginal delivery impossible.

***monozygotic t.'s*** Twins that develop from a single fertilized ovum. Monozygotic twins have the same genetic makeup and, consequently, are of the same sex and resemble each other strikingly physically, physiologically, and mentally. They develop within a common chorionic sac and have a common placenta. Each usually develops its own amnion and umbilical cord. Such twins may result from development of two inner cell masses within a blastocyst, development of two embryonic axes on a single blastoderm, or the division of a single embryonic axis into two centers. SYN: *enzygotic t.'s; identical t.'s; true t.'s; uniovular t.'s.*

***parasitic t.*** The smaller of a pair of conjoined twins, when there is a marked disparity in size.

***Siamese t.'s*** SEE: *Siamese twins.*

***true t.'s*** Monozygotic t.'s.

***unequal t.'s*** Growth discordant t.'s.

***uniovular t.'s*** Monozygotic t.'s.

***vanishing t.*** SEE: *gestation, multiple.*

**twinge** (twĭnj) [AS. *twengan,* to pinch] A sudden keen pain.

**twinning** (twĭn′ĭng) Delivery of or producing twins.

**twitch** (twĭch) [ME. *twicchen*] **1.** A single contraction of one muscle fiber in response to one nerve impulse. SEE: *myokymia.* **2.** To jerk convulsively.

**twitching** (twĭtch′ĭng) Repeated contractions of portions of muscles.

**two-point discrimination test** A test of cutaneous sensation involving determination of the ability of the patient to detect that the skin is being touched by two pointed objects at once. It is used to determine the degree of sensory loss following disease or trauma affecting the nervous system.

**$TXA_2$** *thromboxane $A_2$.*

**tybamate** (tī′bă-māt) A minor tranquilizer.

**tylectomy** (tī-lĕk′tō-mē) [Gr. *tylos,* knot, + *ektome,* excision] Lumpectomy.

**tylion** (tĭl′ē-ŏn) [Gr. *tyleion,* knot] The point at the middle of the anterior edge of the optic groove.

**tyloma** (tī-lō′mă) [Gr. *tylos,* knot, + *oma,* tumor] A callosity.

**tylosis** (tī-lō′sĭs) [″ + *osis,* condition] Formation of a callus.

**tyloxapol** (tī-lŏks′ă-pōl) A nonionic liquid polymer of the alkyl aryl polyether alcohol type. It is a mucolytic used to reduce the viscosity of bronchopulmonary secretions.

**tympanal** (tĭm′păn-ăl) [Gr. *tympanon,* drum] Tympanic (1).

**tympanectomy** (tĭm″păn-ĕk′tō-mē) [″ + *ektome,* excision] Excision of the tympanic membrane.

**tympanic** (tĭm-păn′ĭk) [Gr. *tympanon,* drum] **1.** Pert. to the tympanum. SYN: *tympanal.* **2.** Resonant. SYN: *tympanitic* (2).

**tympanism** (tĭm′păn-ĭzm) [Gr. *tympanon,* drum, + *-ismos,* condition] Tympanites.

**tympanites** (tĭm-păn-ī′tēz) [Gr., distention] Distention of the abdomen or intestines due to the presence of gas. SYN: *meteorism; tympanism; tympanosis.*

**tympanitic** (tĭm-păn-ĭt′ĭk) **1.** Pert. to or characterized by tympanites. **2.** Tympanic (2).

**tympanitic resonance** A sound produced by percussion over an air-filled or gas-filled cavity.

**tympanitis** (tĭm-păn-ī′tĭs) [Gr. *tympanon,* drum, + *itis,* inflammation] Otitis media.

**tympano-** [Gr. *tympanon,* drum] Combining form indicating *eardrum, tympanum of the ear.*

**tympanocentesis** Drainage of fluid from the middle ear by using a small gauge needle to puncture the tympanic membrane. The fluid is cultured to determine the identity of any bacteria that are present.

**tympanoeustachian** (tĭm″pă-nō-ū-stā′kē-ăn) Concerning the tympanic cavity and eustachian tube.

**tympanography** Radiographic examination of the eustachian tubes and middle ear after introduction of a contrast medium.

**tympanohyal** (tĭm″pă-nō-hī′ăl) Concerning the tympanic cavity and hyoid arch.

**tympanomalleal** (tĭm″pă-nō-măl′ē-ăl) Concerning the tympanic membrane and malleus.

**tympanomandibular** (tĭm″pă-nō-măn-dĭb′ū-lăr) Concerning the middle ear and mandible.

**tympanomastoiditis** (tĭm″păn-ō-măs″toy-dī′tĭs) [″ + *mastos,* breast, + *eidos,* form, shape, + *itis,* inflammation] Inflammation of the tympanum and mastoid cells.

**tympanometry** (tĭm″pă-nŏm′ĕ-trē) A procedure for objective evaluation of the mobility and patency of the eardrum and for detection of middle-ear disorders and patency of the eustachian tubes. SEE: *audiometry.*

**tympanoplasty** (tĭm″păn-ō-plăs′tē) [″ + *plassein,* to form] Any one of several surgical procedures designed either to cure a chronic inflammatory process in the middle ear or to restore function to the sound-transmitting mechanism of the middle ear. SEE: *Nursing Diagnoses Appendix.*

**tympanosclerosis** (tĭm″pă-nō-sklĕ-rō′sĭs) Infiltration by hard fibrous tissue around the ossicles of the middle ear.

**tympanosis** (tĭm-pă-nō′sĭs) [″ + *osis,* condition] Tympanites.

**tympanosquamosal** (tĭm″pă-nō-skwă-mō′săl) Concerning the pars tympanica and pars squamosa of the temporal bone.

**tympanostapedial** (tĭm″pă-nō-stă-pē′dē-ăl) Concerning the tympanic cavity and stapes.

**tympanostomy** Myringotomy.

**tympanostomy tube** A tube placed through the tympanic membrane of the ear to allow ventilation of the middle ear as part of the treatment of otitis media with effusion. SYN: *ventilation tube.* SEE: *otitis media with effusion.*

**tympanotemporal** (tĭm″pă-nō-tĕm′pō-răl) Concerning the tympanic cavity and area of the temporal bone.

**tympanotomy** (tĭm″păn-ŏt′ō-mē) [″ + *tome,* incision] Incision of the membrana tympani. SYN: *myringotomy.*

**tympanous** (tĭm′păn-ŭs) [Gr. *tympanon,* a drum] Marked by abdominal distention with gas.

**tympanum** (tĭm′păn-ŭm) [L.; Gr. *tympanon*] The middle ear or tympanic cavity. SYN: *cavum tympani; eardrum.* SEE: *ear, middle.*

**tympany** (tĭm′pă-nē) **1.** Abdominal distention with gas. **2.** Tympanic resonance on percussion. It is a clear hollow note like that of a drum. It indicates a pathological condition of the lung or of a cavity.

**type** (tīp) [Gr. *typos,* mark] The general character of a person, disease, or substance.

***asthenic t.*** Having a thin, flat, long-chested body build with poor muscular development.

***athletic t.*** Having broad shoulders, a deep chest, flat abdomen, thick neck, and excellent muscular development.

***blood t.*** SEE: *blood groups.*

***phage t.*** Distinguishing subgroups of bacteria by the type of bacteriophage associated with that specific bacterium.

***pyknic t.*** Having a rounded body, large chest, thick shoulders, broad head, thick neck, and usually short stature.

**type A personality** SEE: *behavior pattern, type A.*

**type B personality** SEE: *behavior, type B.*

**typhlectasis** (tĭf-lĕk′tă-sĭs) [Gr. *typhlon,* cecum, + *ektasis,* dilatation] Cecal distention.

**typhlectomy** (tĭf-lĕk′tō-mē) [″ + *ektome,* excision] Excision of the cecum. SYN: *cecectomy.*

**typhlenteritis** (tĭf″lĕn-tĕr-ī′tĭs) [″ + *enteron,* intestine, + *itis,* inflammation] Inflammation of the cecum. SYN: *typhlitis; typhloenteritis.*

**typhlitis** (tĭf-lī′tĭs) [″ + *itis,* inflammation] Inflammation of the cecum. SYN: *typhlenteritis; typhloenteritis.*

**typhlo-** 1. Combining form meaning *cecum.* 2. Combining form meaning *blindness.*

**typhlodicliditis** (tĭf″lō-dĭk-lĭ-dī′tĭs) [″ + *diklis,* door, + *itis,* inflammation] Inflammation of the ileocecal valve.

**typhloempyema** (tĭf″lō-ĕm-pī-ē′mă) [″ + *en,* in, + *pyon,* pus, + *haima,* blood] An abdominal abscess following appendicitis.

**typhloenteritis** (tĭf″lō-ĕn-tĕr-ī′tĭs) [″ + *enteron,* intestine, + *itis,* inflammation] Inflammation of the cecum. SYN: *typhlenteritis; typhlitis.*

**typhlolithiasis** (tĭf″lō-lĭ-thī′ă-sĭs) [Gr. *typhlon,* cecum, + *lithos,* stone, + *-iasis,* condition] Formation of a concretion in the cecum.

**typhlomegaly** (tĭf″lō-mĕg′ă-lē) [Gr. *typhlon,* cecum, + *megas,* large] An abnormally large cecum.

**typhlon** (tĭf′lŏn) [Gr.] The cecum.

**typhlopexy** (tĭf′lō-pĕks″ē) [Gr. *typhlon,* cecum, + *pexis,* fixation] Suturing of a movable cecum to the abdominal wall.

**typhlorrhaphy** (tĭf-lor′ă-fē) Surgical repair of the cecum.

**typhlospasm** (tĭf′lō-spăsm) Spasm of the cecum.

**typhlostenosis** (tĭf″lō-stĕn-ō′sĭs) [Gr. *typhlon,* cecum, + *stenosis,* act of narrowing] Stenosis or stricture of the cecum.

**typhlostomy** (tĭf-lŏs′tō-mē) [″ + *stoma,* mouth] Establishment of a permanent cecal fistula.

**typhlotomy** (tĭf-lŏt′ō-mē) [Gr. *typhlon,* cecum, + *tome,* incision] Incision of the cecum.

**typhloureterostomy** (tĭf″lō-ū-rē″tĕr-ŏs′tō-mē) [″ + *oureter,* ureter, + *stoma,* mouth] Implantation of a ureter in the cecum.

**typho-** [Gr. *typhos,* fever] Combining form meaning *fever, typhoid.*

**typhoid** (tī′foyd) [Gr. *typhos,* fever, + *eidos,* form, shape] Resembling typhus.

**typhoidal** (tī-foy′dăl) Resembling typhoid.

**typhoid carrier** An individual who has recovered from typhoid fever but who harbors the bacteria, usually in the gallbladder, and who excretes it in the urine and feces.

**typhoid fever** An acute infectious disease characterized by definite lesions in Peyer's patches, mesenteric glands, and the spleen accompanied by fever, headache, and abdominal pain. The incubation period generally varies from 1 to 3 weeks; however, this period may be as short as 3 days or as long as 3 months. Immunity can ordinarily be established by administering one of several types of vaccine available. SYN: *enteric fever.* SEE: *typhoid vaccine.*

SYMPTOMS: Early symptoms are headache, general weakness, indefinite pains, and nosebleed. Constipation may occur. Within a few days to a week, the temperature may reach a maximum of 104° to 105°F (40° to 40.6°C) and during this time, or up to the 10th day, rose spots can usually be seen, particularly on the abdomen, though they may be observed on the chest and back. They usually occur in crops during a period of several days and will blanch on pressure. Abdominal tenderness develops and with it, generally, distention. Splenomegaly is found in more than half of the cases by the end of the first week.

During the following weeks, fever is characterized by marked daily remissions, evening temperature being from 1° to 3°F (0.56° to 1.7°C) higher than that in the morning. In the young, the temperature often rises very abruptly. When the diurnal remissions are slight, a protracted case is forecast. As defervescence advances, the temperature becomes more irregular. Remissions are more decided, and not infrequently a higher temperature is recorded in the morning. Rapid respiratory rate, slight cough, and bronchial crackles are common. The pulse is usually slow in comparison with the temperature rise and is dicrotic. Heart sounds are often feeble, expression is dull and heavy, cheeks are somewhat flushed, conjunctivae are clear, and pupils are dilated.

The tongue is tremulous. It is red at the tip and edges and covered posteriorly with a whitish furlike material. In severe cases, the tongue becomes dry, brown, and fissured and sordes collect on the teeth. Gastric symptoms are not common but, when present, they are obstinate. Vomiting sometimes develops and becomes a serious complication. The abdomen is tympanitic and tender on palpation, esp. in the iliac fossa. Diarrhea is usually present but is not constant. Bowel movements vary from three to six or more a day and are thin and yellowish, with an offensive smell. Stupor, muttering, delirium, twitching of the muscles, carphologia, and coma vigil may be present. Proteinuria and urinary retention are common. White blood count demonstrates a leukopenia. Convalescence is marked by anemia, loss of hair, and often desquamation. The patient shows evidence of having suffered from a protracted illness that has produced general mental and physical debilitation.

ETIOLOGY: The causative organism is *Salmonella typhi,* a gram-negative, motile bacillus. It may be transmitted by infected water or milk supplies. Human carriers, particularly food handlers, may be responsible for spread of infection. Body discharges from active or convalescent cases may be the means of infecting others.

DIFFERENTIAL DIAGNOSIS: Paratyphoid, pneumonia, dysentery, meningitis, smallpox, and appendicitis are among the differential diagnoses. Diagnostic points of value are the presence of rose spots, splenomegaly, leukopenia, the Widal serological test result, blood culture, and examination of feces for the presence of the causative organism. The best means of providing bacterial confirmation is through bone marrow culture. This method is successful even after patients have received antibiotics. SEE: *paratyphoid fever.*

TREATMENT: Antibiotics such as chloramphenicol, amoxicillin, trimethoprim, and sulfamethoxazole are effective in treating typhoid fever, as are ofloxacin and third-generation cephalosporins such as ceftriaxone. Quinolones should not be used in children or pregnant women.

General care, isolation of the patient, and disinfection of all discharges are of primary importance. Those caring for the typhoid patient should be immunized against the disease. All precautions applicable to such infections must be adopted. Articles in contact with the patient must be sterilized or disinfected before being handled by persons other than the immediate attendant. SEE: *Universal Precautions Appendix.*

It is necessary to guard against the development of bedsores. Because delirium is not infrequent, the patient may require constant watching to prevent his or her leaving the bed. The mouth should be kept as clean as possible to prevent the development of sordes.

Ice bags and cold sponging are little used at present. On the other hand, sponging with tepid water, or with alcohol, is sometimes used when the temperature has reached unusual heights. Surgical intervention is necessary if antibiotics and bowel decompression fail to control severe hemorrhage or if intestinal perforation occurs.

COMPLICATIONS: These occur in approx. 25% of untreated cases and account for the majority of deaths. The most frequent and dangerous complications are intestinal hemorrhage and intestinal perforation. An abrupt fall of several degrees in temperature suggests intestinal hemorrhage or perforation. This usually occurs during the third or fourth week.

PROGNOSIS: The prognosis should always be guarded, no matter how mild the case appears to be. The fatality rate varies in different epidemics. Hemorrhages in any form, together with excessive diarrhea, are unfavorable signs.

NURSING IMPLICATIONS: Enteric precautions (handwashing, patient handwashing, glove and gown for disposal of feces or fecally contaminated objects) are followed until three consecutive stool cultures at 24-hr intervals are negative. Drugs are administered as prescribed, and the patient is observed for signs and symptoms of complications, such as bacteremia, intestinal bleeding, and bowel perforation. During the acute phase, the temperature is monitored, and prescribed antipyretics are administered; tepid sponge baths are also provided to promote vasodilation without shivering. The incontinent patient is cleansed, and high fluid intake by mouth or IV is encouraged to maintain adequate hydration. Frequent oral hygiene and skin care are provided. The patient is repositioned, and passive to active range-of-motion exercises are carried out. Bladder distention is noted, and intake and output are monitored. Adequate nutrition is maintained. The nurse explains the importance of follow-up care and examination to ensure that the patient is not a carrier.

*Charting:* A 4-hr chart should be kept of temperature, pulse, and respiration, although pulse should be monitored much more frequently. In the third week, the temperature should be taken every 2 hr. A sudden drop in temperature indicates hemorrhage.

*Disinfection:* The usual methods of disinfection should be observed in handling all excreta and secretions, linens, and utensils. Disinfection for the nurse is also very important. SEE: *Universal Precautions Appendix.*

**typhoid vaccine** A vaccine containing killed *Salmonella typhi.* Although its effectiveness in preventing typhoid fever is limited to protecting only those who have experienced a small infecting dose of *S. typhi,* its use is advisable in persons who will be exposed to typhoid bacilli. An oral live vaccine using *S. typhi* strain Ty21a and a parenteral vaccine containing polysaccharide Vi antigen are currently available. The former should not be given to patients receiving antibiotics or the antimalarial drug mefloquine. SEE: *typhoid fever.*

**typholysin** (tī-fŏl′ĭ-sĭn) [″ + *lysis,* dissolution] A lysin destructive to typhoid bacilli.

**typhomalarial** (tī″fō-mă-lā′rē-ăl) [″ + It. *malaria,* bad air] Having symptoms of both typhoid and malarial fevers.

**typhomania** (tī-fō-mā′nē-ă) [″ + *mania,* madness] Muttering delirium characteristic of typhoid fever and typhus.

**typhopneumonia** (tī″fō-nū-mō′nē-ă) [″ + *pneumon,* lung, + *-ia,* condition, abnormal state] **1.** Pneumonia occurring in typhoid fever. **2.** Pneumonia with typhoid symptoms.

**typhous** (tī′fŭs) [Gr. *typhos,* fever] Pert. to typhus fever.

**typhus** (tī′fŭs) [Gr. *typhos,* fever] Any of a group of acute infectious diseases characterized by great prostration, severe headache, generalized maculopapular rash, sustained high fever, and usually progressive neurological involvement, ending in a crisis in 10 to 14 days.

Several diseases are included in the group: epidemic (louse-borne) typhus, caused by *Rickettsia prowazekii;* Brill-Zinsser disease (recrudescent typhus), caused by *Rickettsia prowazekii;* scrub typhus (Tsutsugamushi disease or mite-borne typus fever), caused by *Rickettsia tsutsugamushi;* and murine (flea-borne) typhus, caused by *Rickettsia typhi.* Although clinically and pathologically similar, they differ in intensity of symptoms, severity, and mortality rate.

Epidemic typhus is particularly prevalent amid unsanitary conditions. It often develops on shipboard, in army camps, and where living conditions are unfavorable and congestion is marked. The disease is rare in the U.S. Typhoid fever, Henoch's purpura, epidemic meningitis of fulminating type, and ulcerative endocarditis may have to be considered in the differential diagnosis. The incubation period is generally 1 to 2 weeks, except in Brill-Zinsser disease, which may recur years after the initial attack. SEE: *Nursing Diagnoses Appendix.*

SYMPTOMS: The onset of symptoms is sudden. Severe headache, pain in the back and limbs, and extreme prostration occur. The fever rises rapidly, often reaching 104° to 105°F (40° to 40.6°C) in 2 to 3 days; remains high for about 10 days; and then falls by the time of crisis. The pulse is rapid, weak, and often dicrotic. The tongue is tremulous and may be covered with whitish fur; in severe cases, it becomes black and rolled up like a ball in the back of the mouth. The face is dusky, the conjunctivae are injected, and the pupils are contracted. The patient demonstrates stupor, delirium, muscle twitching, and picking at the bedclothes (carphologia).

On the fourth to fifth day, bluish petechial spots appear over the body, esp. on the abdomen, which do not disappear on pressure. The extent of eruption indicates the severity of the attack. Sometimes there is a diffuse, dark red, subcuticular mottling. The bowels are constipated and the urine is scanty, pigmented, and often albuminous.

TREATMENT: *Preventive:* Absolute cleanliness, sterilization of clothing, and the use of protective apparel prevent infestation by the body louse. The patient must be isolated. Absolute rest and a liquid diet are necessary. *Specific:* Broad-spectrum antibiotics, such as the tetracyclines and chloramphenicol, give excellent results. SEE: *Universal Precautions Appendix.*

COMPLICATIONS: Bronchopneumonia occurs more frequently than lobar pneumonia. Hypostatic congestion of the lungs, nephritis, and parotid abscess also may occur.

PROGNOSIS: The prognosis is variable. Mortality may be quite high in epidemic typhus and almost nonexistent in murine typhus. Broad-spectrum antibiotics are life saving if given early enough.

***endemic t.*** Murine t.

***epidemic t.*** An infectious disease caused by *Rickettsia prowazekii* and transmitted by human body louse *(Pediculus humanus corporis).*

***flea-borne t.*** Murine t.

***Mexican t.*** A louse-borne epidemic typhus present in certain portions of Mexico. SYN: *tabardillo.*

***mite-borne t.*** Scrub t.

***murine t.*** A disease caused by *Rickettsia typhi* and occurring in nature as a mild infection of rats and transmitted from rat to rat by the rat-louse or flea. Humans may acquire it by being bitten by infected rat fleas or ingesting food contaminated by rat urine or flea feces. SYN: *endemic t.; flea-borne t.*

***recrudescent t.*** The recurrence of epidemic typhus after the initial attack.

***scrub t.*** A self-limited febrile disease of 2 weeks' duration caused by *Rickettsia tsutsugamushi* and transmitted by two species of mites (chiggers) of the genus *Thrombicula.* It occurs principally in the Pacific-Asiatic area. SYN: *mite-borne t.; tsutsugamushi disease.*

**typhus vaccine** A sterile suspension of the killed rickettsial organism of a strain or strains of epidemic typhus rickettsiae.

**typical** (tĭp′ĭ-kăl) [Gr. *typikos,* pert. to type] Having the characteristics of, pert. to, or conforming to a type, condition, or group.

**typing** (tīp′ĭng) Identification of type.

***bacteriophage t.*** Determination of the subdivision of a bacterial species using a type-specific bacteriophage.

***blood t.*** Determination of the specific blood group of an individual. SEE: *blood transfusion.*

***tissue t.*** Determination of the histocompatibility of tissues to be used in grafts and transplants. SEE: *transplantation.*

**typo-** Combining form meaning *type.*

**typodont** A replica of the natural dentition and alveolar mucosa used in training dental students.

**typoscope** (tī′pō-skōp) [Gr. *typos,* type, + *skopein,* to examine] A reading aid device for patients with amblyopia or cataract.

**typus** (tī′pŭs) [L.] Type.

**tyramine** (tī′ră-mēn) An intermediate product in the conversion of tyrosine to epinephrine. Tyramine is found in most cheeses and in beer, broad bean pods, yeast, wine, and chicken liver. When persons taking certain types of antidepressant monoamine oxidase inhibitors also eat these foods, they may experience severe hypertension, headache, palpitation, neck pain, and perhaps intracranial hemorrhage. This is due to the tyramine's not being inactivated by monoamine oxidation. This has been called the "cheese reaction."

**tyrannism** (tĭr′ăn-ĭzm) [Gr. *tyrannos,* tyrant, + *-ismos,* condition] Sadism.

**tyrogenous** (tī-rŏj′ĕn-ŭs) [Gr. *tyros,* cheese, + *gennan,* to produce] Having origin in or produced by cheese.

**Tyroglyphus** (tī-rŏg′lĭ-fŭs) [Gr. *tyros,* cheese, + *glyphein,* to carve] A genus of sarcoptoid mites commonly known as cheese mites. They infest cheese and dried vegetable food products and occasionally infest humans, causing pruritus. This genus includes species that cause grocer's itch, vanillism, and copra itch.

**tyroid** (tī'royd) [″ + *eidos,* form, shape] Caseous; cheesy.

**tyroma** (tī-rō'mă) A tumor that contains cheeselike material.

**tyromatosis** (tī″rō-mă-tō'sĭs) [″ + *oma,* tumor, + *osis,* condition] Caseation (1).

**tyrosinase** (tī-rō'sĭn-ās) [Gr. *tyros,* cheese] An enzyme that acts on tyrosine to produce melanin.

**tyrosine** (tī'rō-sĭn) An amino acid present in many proteins, esp. casein. It serves as a precursor of epinephrine, thyroxine, and melanin. Two vitamins, ascorbic acid and folic acid, are essential for its metabolism.

**tyrosinemia** (tī″rō-sĭ-nē'mē-ă) A disease of tyrosine metabolism caused by a deficiency of the enzyme tyrosine aminotransferase. In addition to an accumulation of tyrosine in the blood, mental retardation, keratitis, and dermatitis are present. Treatment consists of controlling phenylalanine and tyrosine intake.

**tyrosinosis** (tī″rō-sĭn-ō'sĭs) [″ + *osis,* condition] A condition resulting from faulty metabolism of tyrosine, whereby its oxidation products appear in the urine.

**tyrosinuria** (tī″rō-sĭn-ū'rē-ă) [″ + *ouron,* urine] Tyrosine in the urine.

**tyrosis** (tī-rō'sĭs) [″ + *osis,* condition] **1.** Curdling of milk. **2.** Vomiting of cheesy substance by infants. **3.** Caseation (1).

**tyrosyluria** (tī″rō-sĭl-ū'rē-ă) Increased tyrosine-derived products in the urine.

**tyrothricin** (tī″rō-thrī'sĭn) An antibacterial drug.

**tyrotoxism** (tī″rō-tŏks'ĭzm) [″ + *toxikon,* a poison, + *-ismos,* condition] Poisoning produced by a milk product or by cheese.

**Tyrrell's fascia** (tĭr'rĕlz) [Frederick Tyrrell, Brit. anatomist, 1797–1843] An ill-defined fibromuscular layer from the middle aponeurosis of the perineum, behind the prostate gland.

**Tyson's gland** (tī'sŭnz) [Edward Tyson, Brit. physician and anatomist, 1650–1708] One of the modified sebaceous glands located on the neck of the penis and the inner surface of the prepuce. The secretion of these glands is one of the components of smegma. SYN: *preputial gland.*

**tysonitis** (tī″sŏn-ī'tĭs) Inflammation of Tyson's glands.

**tyvelose** (tī'vĕl-ōs) A carbohydrate, 3-6-dideoxy-D-mannose, derived from certain strains of *Salmonella.* It is a somatic antigen.

**Tzanck cell** A degenerated cell from the keratin layer of the skin, disconnected from adjacent cells. It is seen in pemphigus.

**Tzanck test** (tsănk) [Arnault Tzanck, Russ. dermatologist in Paris, 1886–1954] The examination of tissue from the lower surface of a lesion in vesicular disease to determine the cell type.

**tzetze** (sĕt'sē) Tsetse fly.

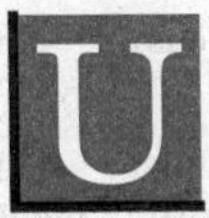

**U** **1.** *unit.* **2.** Symbol for the element uranium.

**$^{235}$U** Isotope of uranium with mass number 235.

**UAO** *upper airway obstruction.*

**ubiquinol** (ū-bĭk′wĭ-nŏl) Coenzyme $QH_2$, the reduced form of ubiquinone.

**ubiquinone** (ū-bĭk′wĭ-nōn) [*ubi*quitous + coenzyme *quinone*] Coenzyme Q, a lipid-soluble quinone present in virtually all cells. It collects reducing equivalents during intracellular respiration and is converted to its reduced form, ubiquinol, while involved in this process.

**ubiquitin** A small protein present in eukaryotic cells that combines with other proteins and makes these proteins susceptible to destruction. It is also important in promoting the functions of proteins that make up ribosomes.

**UDP** *uridine diphosphate.*

**Uffelmann's test** (oof′ĕl-mănz) [Jules Uffelmann, Ger. physician, 1837–1894] A test for the determination of lactic acid in gastric juice.

**Uhthoff's sign** (oot′hŏfs) [Wilhelm Uhthoff, Ger. ophthalmologist, 1853–1927] The nystagmus that occurs in multiple disseminated sclerosis.

**ulcer** (ŭl′sĕr) [L. *ulcus,* ulcer] An open sore or lesion of the skin or mucous membrane accompanied by sloughing of inflamed necrotic tissue. If the sore becomes infected, pus is formed. Simple ulcers may result from trauma, caustics, intense heat or cold, or arterial or venous stasis. They may occur as a complication of varicose veins due to stasis of blood leading to inflammation, necrosis, and sloughing of tissue. Ulcers of the mucous membrane of the stomach or duodenum are usually caused by gastric acid and pepsin. The secretion from cutaneous sores caused by early syphilis (chancre) contains the causative agent *Treponema pallidum.*

***amputating u.*** An ulcer that destroys tissue to the bone by encircling the part.

***aphthous u.*** SEE: *aphthous ulcer.*

***atonic u.*** A chronic ulcer with scant tendency to heal.

***callous u.*** A chronic ulcer with indurated, elevated edges and no granulations. It heals very slowly.

***chronic leg u.*** Any long-standing, slow-to-heal ulcer of a lower extremity, esp. one caused by occlusive disease of the arteries or veins or by varicose veins.

***Curling's u.*** A peptic ulcer that sometimes occurs following severe burns to the body; a form of stress ulcer.

***decubitus u.*** SEE: *decubitus ulcer.*

***denture u.*** An ulcer of the oral mucosa caused by irritation from wearing dentures.

***duodenal u.*** An ulcer on the mucosa of the duodenum caused by the action of the gastric juice. SEE: *peptic ulcer.*

***follicular u.*** A tiny ulcer originating in a lymph follicle and affecting a mucous membrane.

***fungus u.*** An ulcer in which the granulations protrude above the edges of the wound and bleed easily.

***gastric u.*** An ulcer of the gastric mucosa. SEE: *peptic ulcer.*

***Hunner's u.*** A painful, slow-to-heal ulcer of the urinary bladder.

***indolent u.*** A nearly painless ulcer usually found on the leg, characterized by an indurated and elevated edge and a nongranulating base.

***peptic u.*** SEE: *peptic ulcer.*

***perforating u.*** An ulcer that permeates the entire thickness of the part, such as the foot or intestine.

***phagedenic u.*** An ulcer that spreads rapidly and disintegrates the tissues, producing a slough and discharge.

***pressure u.*** SEE: *pressure sore.*

***rodent u.*** SEE: *rodent ulcer.*

***serpiginous u.*** A creeping ulcer that heals in one part and extends to another.

***simple u.*** A local ulcer with no severe inflammation or pain.

***specific u.*** An ulcer caused by a specific disease, as syphilis or lupus.

***stercoral u.*** **1.** An ulcer caused by pressure from impacted feces. **2.** A perforating ulcer through which feces escape.

***stress u.*** A peptic ulcer caused by acute or chronic physical or mental stress such as may accompany cerebral trauma, burns, surgery, acute infection, prolonged adrenal corticosteroid therapy, or central nervous system disease.

***traumatic u.*** An ulcer due to injury of the oral mucosa. Causes include biting, denture irritation, toothbrush injury, and sharp edges of teeth or restorations.

***trophic u.*** An ulcer caused by the failure to supply nutrients to a part.

***tropical u.*** **1.** An indolent ulcer, usually of a lower extremity, that occurs in persons living in hot, humid areas. The etiology may or may not be known, and it may be caused by a combination of bacterial, environmental, and nutritional factors. **2.** The tropical sore caused by leishmaniasis.

***varicose u.*** An ulcer, esp. of the lower extremity, associated with varicose veins.

***venereal u.*** An ulcer caused by a venereal disease (i.e., chancre or chancroid).

***venous stasis u.*** A poorly healing ulcer

that results from inadequate venous drainage.

**ulcera** Pl. of ulcus.

**ulcerate** (ŭl′sĕr-āt) [L. *ulcerare,* to form ulcers] To produce or become affected with an ulcer.

**ulcerated** (ŭl′sĕr-ā″tĕd) Of the nature of an ulcer or affected with one.

**ulcerated tooth** Suppuration of the alveolar periosteum with ulceration of the gum surrounding the decaying root of a tooth.

**ulceration** (ŭl″sĕr-ā′shŭn) Suppuration occurring on a free surface, as on the skin or on a mucous membrane, to form an ulcer. SEE: *eye, trophic ulceration of.*

**ulcerative** (ŭl′sĕr-ā-tĭv) [L. *ulcerare,* to form ulcers] Pert. to or causing ulceration.

**ulcerative colitis** SEE: *disease, inflammatory bowel.*

**ulcerogangrenous** (ŭl″sĕr-ō-găng′grĕ-nŭs) Rel. to an ulcer that contains gangrenous tissue.

**ulcerogenic drug** A medicine that, because of its systemic rather than local effects, may cause peptic ulcers.

**ulceromembranous** (ŭl″sĕr-ō-mĕm′brăn-ŭs) [″ + *membrana,* membrane] Pert. to ulceration and formation of a fibrous pseudomembrane.

**ulceromembranous tonsillitis** Tonsillitis that ulcerates and develops a membranous film.

**ulcerous** (ŭl′sĕr-ŭs) Pert. to or affected with an ulcer.

**ulcus** (ŭl′kŭs) *pl.* **ulcera** [L.] Ulcer.

**ulegyria** (ū″lē-jī′rē-ă) [Gr. *oule,* scar, + *gyros,* ring] A condition in which gyri of the cerebral cortex are abnormal due to scar tissue from injuries, usually occurring in early development.

**ulerythema** (ū-lĕr-ĭ-thē′mă) [″ + *erythema,* redness] An erythematous disorder with atrophic scar formation.

***u. ophryogenes*** Folliculitis of the eyebrows, characterized by falling out of hair and scarring.

***u. sycosiforme*** Inflammation of the hair follicles of the beard with alopecia in the affected area.

**uletomy** (ū-lĕt′ō-mē) [″ + *tome,* incision] Incision of a scar to relieve tension. SYN: *cicatricotomy.*

**uliginous** (ū-lĭj′ĭ-nŭs) [L. *uliginosus,* wet] Muddy; slimy.

**ulitis** Gingivitis.

**ulna** (ŭl′nă) [L., elbow] The inner and larger bone of the forearm, between the wrist and the elbow, on the side opposite that of the thumb. It articulates with the head of the radius and humerus proximally, and with the radius and carpals distally.

**ulnad** (ŭl′năd) [″ + *ad,* to] In the direction of the ulna.

**ulnar** (ŭl′năr) [L. *ulna,* elbow] Rel. to the ulna, or to the nerve or artery named from it.

**ulnar drift** A joint change at the metacarpophalangeal joints frequently seen in rheumatoid arthritis, resulting from chronic synovitis. In this condition, the long axis of the fingers deviates in an ulnar direction with respect to the metacarpals.

**ulnaris** (ŭl-nā′rĭs) **1.** Ulnar. **2.** Concerning the ulna.

**ulnocarpal** (ŭl″nō-kăr′păl) [″ + Gr. *karpos,* wrist] Relating to the carpus and ulna, or to the ulnar side of the wrist.

**ulnoradial** (ŭl″nō-rā′dē-ăl) [″ + *radius,* spoke of a wheel] Rel. to the ulna and radius, as their ligaments and articulations.

**ulo-** Combining form meaning *scar, scarring.*

**ulodermatitis** (ū″lō-dĕrm-ă-tī′tĭs) [Gr. *oule,* scar, + *derma,* skin, + *itis,* inflammation] Dermatitis with scar tissue formation.

**uloid** (ū′loyd) [″ + *eidos,* form, shape] **1.** Scarlike. **2.** A scarlike lesion caused by subcutaneous degeneration.

**ulosis** (ū-lō′sĭs) [″ + *osis,* condition] Cicatrization.

**ulotic** (ū-lŏt′ĭk) [″] Cicatricial.

**ulotrichous** (ū-lŏt′rĭk-ŭs) [Gr. *oulos,* woolly, + *thrix,* hair] Having short woolly hair, characteristic of some races.

**ultimate** (ŭl′tĭm-ĭt) [L. *ultimus,* last] Final or last.

**ultimobranchial body** (ŭl″tĭ-mō-brăng′kē-ăl) One of two embryonic pharyngeal pouches usually considered as rudimentary fifth pouches. They become separated from the pharynx and incorporated into the substance of the thyroid gland, where they give rise to parafollicular cells that secrete calcitonin, a hormone used to regulate the blood calcium level.

**ultra-** [L.] Prefix meaning *beyond, excess.*

**ultrabrachycephalic** (ŭl″tră-brăk″ĭ-sē-făl′ĭk) [L. *ultra,* beyond, + Gr. *brachys,* short, + *kephale,* head] Having a cephalic index of 90 or more.

**ultracentrifugation** (ŭl″tră-sĕn-trĭf″ū-gā′shŭn) Treatment or preparation of substances by use of the ultracentrifuge.

**ultracentrifuge** (ŭl-tră-sĕn′trĭ-fūj) [″ + *centrum,* center, + *fugere,* to flee] A high-speed centrifuge capable of producing centrifugal forces more than 100,000 times gravity; used in the study of proteins, viruses, and other substances present in blood.

**ultradian** (ŭl-tră′dē-ăn) [″ + *dies,* day] Concerning biological rhythms that occur less frequently than every 24 hr.

**ultrafilter** (ŭl-tră-fĭl′tĕr) A filter by which colloidal particles may be separated from their dispersion medium or from crystalloids.

**ultrafiltration** (ŭl″tră-fĭl-trā′shŭn) [″ + *filtrum,* a filter] Filtration of a colloidal substance in which the dispersed particles, but not the liquid, are held back.

**ultraligation** (ŭl″tră-lī-gā′shŭn) [″ + *ligare,* to bind] Ligation of a blood vessel beyond the origin of a branch.

**ultramicrobe** (ŭl″tră-mī′krōb) [″ + Gr. *mikros,* small, + *bios,* life] A microorganism too small to be visible by an ordinary microscope.

**ultramicroscope** (ŭl″tră-mī′krō-skōp) [″ + ″ + *skopein,* to examine] A microscope by which objects invisible through an ordinary microscope may be seen by means of powerful side illumination. SYN: *darkfield microscope.*

**ultramicroscopy** (ŭl″tră-mī-krŏs′kō-pē) The use of the ultramicroscope.

**ultramicrotome** (ŭl″tră-mī′krō-tōm) A microtome that makes extremely thin slices of tissue.

**ultrasonic** (ŭl-tră-sŏn′ĭk) [″ + *sonus,* sound] Pert. to sounds of frequencies above approx. 20,000 cycles/sec, which are inaudible to the human ear. SEE: *supersonic; ultrasonography; ultrasound.*

**ultrasonic cleaning** The use of ultrasonic energy to clean objects, including medical and surgical instruments.

**ultrasonics** (ŭl-tră-sŏn′ĭks) The division of acoustics that studies inaudible sounds (i.e., those with frequencies greater than 20,000 cycles/sec). Biological effects may result, depending on the intensity of the beams. Heating effects are produced by beams of low intensity, paralytic effects by those of moderate intensity, and lethal effects by those of high intensity. The lethal action of ultrasonics is primarily the result, either directly or indirectly, of cavitation of tissues. Ultrasonics is used clinically for therapeutic and diagnostic purposes. In dentistry, instruments producing 29,000 cycles/sec are used in periodontal surgery, curettage, and root planing. SEE: *ultrasound.*

**ultrasonogram** (ŭl″tră-sŏn′ō-grăm) The image produced by use of ultrasonography.

**ultrasonography** (ŭl-tră-sŏn-ŏg′ră-fē) The use of ultrasound to produce an image or photograph of an organ or tissue. Ultrasonic echoes are recorded as they strike tissues of different densities.

***Doppler u.*** The shift in frequency produced when an ultrasound wave is echoed from something in motion. The use of the Doppler effect permits measuring the velocity of that which is being studied (e.g., blood flow in a vessel).

***gray-scale u.*** Use of a television scan technique to process the strength of ultrasound echoes with the strongest being registered as white and the weakest as different shades of gray.

**ultrasound** Inaudible sound in the frequency range of approx. 20,000 to 10 billion ($10^9$) cycles/sec. Ultrasound has different velocities in tissues that differ in density and elasticity from others. This property permits the use of ultrasound in outlining the shape of various tissues and organs in the body. The diagnostic and therapeutic use of ultrasound requires special equipment. In physical therapy, the thermal effects of ultrasound are used to treat musculoskeletal injuries, weaken scar tissue, stretch tendons, and warm tissue. Ultrasound may be used with phonophoresis to facilitate movement of ions into tissue and with electric current for muscular stimulation. SEE: *phonophoresis; ultrasonography.*

***A-mode u.*** Sonographic information presented as a single line representing the time it takes for the ultrasound wave to reach the interface of a structure and reflect back to the transducer.

***real-time u.*** A sonographic procedure that provides rapid, multiple images of an anatomical structure in the form of motion.

**ultrastructure** (ŭl′tră-strŭk″chŭr) The fine structure of tissues. It is visible only by use of electron microscopy.

**ultraviolet** (ŭl″tră-vī′ō-lĕt) [″ + *viola,* violet] Beyond the visible spectrum at its violet end, said of rays between the violet rays and x-rays. SEE: *infrared rays.*

**ultraviolet radiation** ABBR: UVR. Rays emitted by natural and artificial sources, including very hot bodies, the sun, and ionized gases with wavelengths between 290 and 400 nm. From a therapeutic standpoint, physiological effects include erythema production, skin pigmentation, antirachitic effect through production of vitamin D, bactericidal effects, and various effects on metabolism. In clinical practice, dosage is measured in terms of minimum erythema dose.

In addition to erythema, UVR can cause degenerative and neoplastic changes in the skin, retinal damage, cataracts, and modification of the immunological system of the skin.

The UVR spectrum has been described and categorized as follows:

UV-A, which includes wavelengths of 320 to 400 nm, can produce skin erythema, but the required dose is 1000 times that of UV-B.

UV-B, with the included wavelength of 290 to 320 nm, is the principal portion of the UVR spectrum that causes sunburn. A large portion of the UV-B emitted by the sun is absorbed by the ozone layer in the earth's atmosphere.

UV-C includes those wavelengths below 290 nm. These rays are completely absorbed by the ozone layer and have no role in causing pathological changes caused by exposure to sunlight.

UVR in combination with various chemical compounds may cause phototoxic or photoallergic reactions. SEE: *erythema dose; sunscreen; tanning salon.*

**ultraviolet therapy** Treatment with ultraviolet radiation. SEE: *heliotherapy; light therapy.*

**ululation** (ŭl″ū-lā′shŭn) [L. *ululare,* to howl] The crying and screaming of mentally ill persons.

**umbilical** (ŭm-bĭl′ĭ-kăl) [L. *umbilicus,* navel] Pert. to the umbilicus.

**umbilical cord** The attachment connecting the fetus with the placenta. It contains two arteries and one vein surrounded by

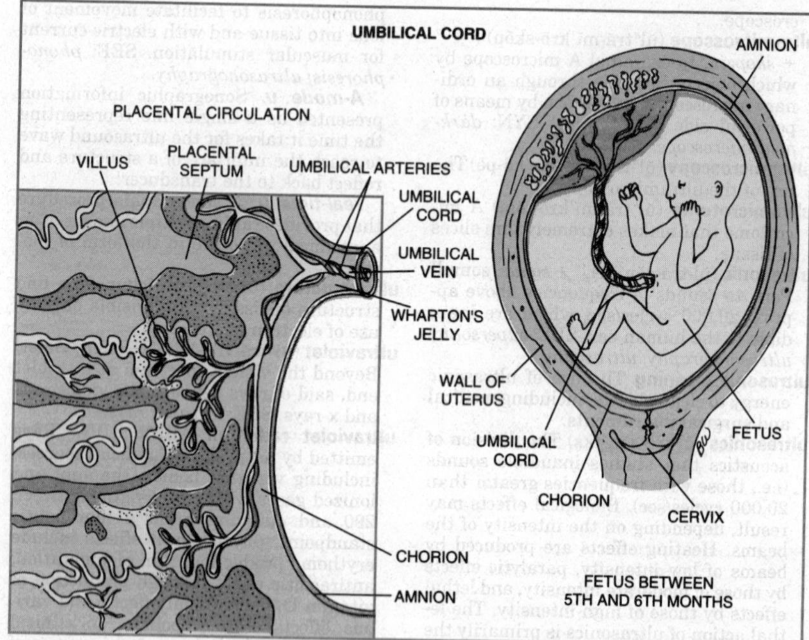


a gelatinous substance, Wharton's jelly. The umbilical arteries carry blood from the fetus to the placenta, where nutrients are obtained and carbon dioxide and oxygen are exchanged; this oxygenated blood returns to the fetus through the umbilical vein. SEE: illus.

The umbilical cord is surgically severed after the birth of the child. To give the infant a better blood supply, the cord should not be cut or tied until the umbilical vessels have ceased pulsating. However, in preterm infants, the cord should be clamped and cut before pulsation ceases to avoid maternal-newborn transfusion and reduce the risk of hypovolemia, polycythemia, and hyperbilirubinemia.

The stump of the severed cord atrophies and leaves a depression on the abdomen of the child, called a navel or umbilicus.

**umbilical fissure** In the fetus, the portion of the hepatic longitudinal fissure in which the umbilical vein is lodged.

**umbilical hernia** A hernia in the region of the umbilicus.

**umbilical souffle** A hissing sound said to arise from the umbilical cord.

**umbilical vein catheter** A catheter placed in the umbilical vein of an infant to facilitate administration of medicines parenterally or to do an exchange transfusion.

**umbilical vesicle** That part of the embryonic yolk sac leading from the umbilicus.

**umbilicate** (ŭm-bĭl′ĭ-kāt) [L. *umbilicatus,* dimpled] Pert. to or shaped like the navel, denoting a bacterial colony with a central depression resembling an umbilicus.

**umbilication** (ŭm-bĭl-ĭ-kā′shŭn) [L. *umbilicatus,* dimpled] **1.** A depression resembling a navel. **2.** Formation at the apex of a pustule or vesicle of a pit or depression.

**umbilicus** (ŭm-bĭ-lī′kŭs, -bĭl′ĭ-kŭs) *pl.* **umbilici** [L., a pit] A depressed point in the middle of the abdomen; the scar that marks the former attachment of the umbilical cord to the fetus. SEE: *Cullen's sign; nodule, Sister Mary Joseph; Tanyoz's sign.*

**umbo** (ŭm′bō) [L., boss of a shield] The projecting center of a round surface.

***u. of tympanic membrane*** The central depressed portion of the concavity on the lateral surface of the tympanic membrane. It marks the point where the handle (manubrium of malleus) is attached to the inner surface.

**umbra** (ŭm′bră) [L., shade, shadow] The edge of the radiographic image proper.

**umbrella filter** A filter placed in a blood vessel to prevent emboli from passing that point. It has been used in the vena cava to prevent emboli in the veins from reaching the lungs.

**UMP** *uridine monophosphate.*

**un-** [AS.] Prefix meaning *back, reversal, annulment, not.*

**uncal** (ŭng′kăl) Concerning the uncus of the brain.

**uncal herniation** Transtentorial herniation.

**unciform, unciforme** (ŭn′sĭ-form) [L. *uncus,* hook, + *forma,* shape] Uncinate.

**unciform bone** The hook-shaped bone on the ulnar side of the distal row of the carpus. SYN: *os hamatum.*

**unciform fasciculus** A bundle of fibers connecting the frontal cerebral lobes with the temporosphenoid lobes.

**unciform process** **1.** Long thin lamina of bone from the orbital plate of the ethmoid articulating with the inferior turbinate. **2.** The hook at the anterior end of the hippocampal gyrus. **3.** The hooked end of the unciform bone.

**uncinariasis** (ŭn″sĭn-ă-rī′ă-sĭs) The condition of being infested with hookworms (i.e., worms of the genus *Uncinaria).*

**uncinate** (ŭn′sĭn-āt) [L. *uncinatus,* hooked] Hook-shaped; hooked. SYN: *unciform.*

**uncinate bundle of Russell** [James S. Risien Russell, Brit. physician, 1863–1939] Fibers that arise in the fastigial superior cerebellar peduncle and pass inferiorly to the vestibular nuclei and reticular formation by which impulses are carried to muscles, esp. those of the neck and body.

**uncinate convolution** Uncinate gyrus.

**uncinate epilepsy** A form of epilepsy occurring in disease of the uncinate area of the temporal lobe of the brain.

**uncinate fasciculus** The bundle of fibers connecting the orbital gyri of the frontal lobe with the rostral portion of the temporal lobe. They curve sharply as they pass over the lateral cerebral fissure.

**uncinate fit** An episodic attack characterized by olfactory and gustatory hallucinations, usually disagreeable; a sense of unreality; and sometimes convulsions and temporary loss of senses of taste and smell. This is associated with lesions of the uncinate gyrus of the brain.

**uncinate gyrus** A gyrus of the temporal lobe of the brain consisting of the recurved rostral portion of the hippocampal gyrus. SYN: *uncinate convolution; uncus* (2).

**uncinatum** (ŭn″sĭ-nā′tŭm) [L.] Hooked.

**uncipressure** (ŭn′sĭ-prĕsh″ŭr) [L. *uncus,* hook, + *pressura,* pressure] Pressure applied with the use of a blunt hook to arrest bleeding.

**uncomplemented** (ŭn-kŏm′plē-mĕnt″ĕd) Not joined or associated with complement and thus inactive.

**unconditioned reflex** An inborn or natural reflex, not dependent on previous experience or training.

**unconscious** (ŭn-kŏn′shŭs) [AS. *un,* not, + L. *conscius,* aware] **1.** Insensible; lacking in awareness of the environment. In this state, a person experiences no sensory impressions and has no subjective experiences. SEE: *unconsciousness.* **2.** In freudian psychiatry, that part of our personality consisting of a complex of feelings and drives of which we are unaware and that are not available to our consciousness.

***collective u.*** One of two divisions of the unconscious, according to Carl Jung, the other category being personal unconscious. The personal unconscious includes all of the material stored in the unconscious that was acquired through personal experience. The collective unconscious comprises material that the species inherits. Thus, the collective unconscious would be common to all members of a society, a people, or to humankind in general. Instinct is included in the collective unconscious. SEE: *sociobiology.*

**unconsciousness** (ŭn-kŏn′shŭs-nĕs) [AS. *un,* not, + L. *conscius,* aware] The state of being insensible or without conscious experiences. Unconsciousness physiologically occurs in sleep; pathologically, it may occur temporarily as in syncope (fainting) or be prolonged and vary in depth from stupor (semiconsciousness) to coma (profound unconsciousness). The patient whose unconsciousness is due to a pathological process is unable to swallow, the eyes do not react, and he or she is unaware of surroundings. Unconsciousness can be caused by alcohol, barbiturate and bromide intoxication; anoxia; brain tumor; carbon monoxide poisoning; cardiac decompensation; cerebral accident (hemorrhage, thrombosis, embolism); concussion; diabetes; eclampsia; epilepsy; fear; fracture of skull; fright; heatstroke; hemorrhage (esp. subarachnoid); hypertensive encephalopathy; meningitis; neurosyphilis; opium poisoning; overdose of insulin; pneumonia; severe infections; subdural hematoma; or uremia. SEE: *coma; Glasgow Coma Scale; Nursing Diagnoses Appendix.*

TREATMENT: If the face is flushed or if hemorrhage is present or suspected, the patient's head should not be lowered, and he or she should not be given stimulants. In other instances, however, it is desirable to lower the patient's head and shoulders, loosen clothing, and keep him or her comfortably warm but not hot. Dentures should be removed. The head should be turned to one side to prevent aspiration of vomitus. Artificial respiration should be given as needed. One should observe for evidence of blows to the head, fractures, and paralysis. Pulse, respiration, breath odor, skin color and condition, and pupils should be tested. It is important to diagnose the cause of unconsciousness before instituting specific therapy.

---

Caution: The patient should be examined for a Medic Alert bracelet or pendant or a medical record card indicating chronic illness, critical medications, or drug allergies.

---

NURSING IMPLICATIONS: In the initial approach, the ABCs of emergency care are followed, with evaluation of airway, bleeding, and consciousness. Examination is made for fractures, esp. of the head. Adequate circulation and ventilation are established. Dentures are removed. The nurse assesses the patient for other health problems and treats those of immediate concern. Safety measures are implemented to prevent further trauma. The nurse re-examines the patient and, if the patient is conscious, obtains a history. Fluid and electrolyte balance is monitored, level of consciousness assessed frequently, and a neurological flow sheet started. As ordered, blood is drawn for the following laboratory studies: arterial blood gases, blood glucose, blood ammonia, electrolytes, blood urea nitrogen, and depressant drugs of abuse (alcohol, barbiturates, narcotics). The patient is turned and positioned often to allow drainage of secretions; aspiration is performed if needed. Oxygen is administered as prescribed. Eye care is performed. A Foley catheter is inserted if the patient is incontinent. Intake and output are monitored. Oral hygiene is provided frequently. Temperature is monitored, and antipyretic measures are instituted.

Moving an Unconscious Patient, Stretcher to Bed: *Method I:* The draw sheet is folded in half lengthwise and placed across the center of the stretcher; the excess is pleated and the ends tucked under for about 6 in. before the patient is put on the stretcher. (This sheet should be under the buttocks when the patient is on the stretcher.) The stretcher is placed parallel with the bed and as close as possible to it. Three other people are needed to assist—one person is positioned at the patient's head, one at the feet, one at the side, and one at the far side of the bed. The people at the sides take firm hold of the ends of the draw sheet and all four lift together, with the person at the far side pulling the draw sheet toward the bed.

*Method II:* This movement requires three people. The stretcher is placed at right angles to the foot of the bed with the patient's head at the end of bed nearest the stretcher. Standing side by side, the three people put their arms under the patient and lift and swing the patient around onto the bed.

**unco-ossified** (ŭn″kō-ŏs′ĭ-fīd) Not ossified into one bone.

**uncovertebral** (ŭn″kō-vĕr′tĕ-brăl) Concerning the uncinate process of a vertebra.

**unction** (ŭnk′shŭn) [L. *unctio,* ointment] **1.** The application of an ointment. **2.** Ointment.

**uncus** (ŭn′kŭs) [L. *uncus,* hook] **1.** Any structure that is hook-shaped. **2.** Uncinate gyrus.

**undecylenic acid** An antifungal drug used topically to treat tinea pedis.

**underachiever** A person whose achievements are less than what is predicted to be possible.

**underbite** A condition in which the lower incisors pass in front of the upper incisors when the mouth is closed.

**undercut** (ŭn′dĕr-kŭt) A condition of having overhanging tissue as could be the case in preparing a dental cavity for restoration. Undercutting helps to keep the filling material in place.

**undernutrition** (ŭn″dĕr-nū-trĭsh′ŭn) [AS. *under,* beneath, + LL. *nutritio,* nourish] Inadequate nutrition from any cause.

Symptoms: This condition is marked by loss of body weight representing at first mostly loss of body fat and then loss of protein, manifested by atrophy of muscles, weakness, and edema.

**undertoe** (ŭn′dĕr-tō) [″ + *ta,* toe] The condition of displacement of the great toe underneath the others.

**underweight** (ŭn′dĕr-wāt″) An imprecise term to describe a condition in which the body weight is at least 10% less than what would be considered normal for a particular individual.

**undifferentiation** (ŭn-dĭf″ĕr-ĕn-shē-ā′shŭn) [AS. *un,* not, + L. *differens,* bearing apart] An alteration in cell character to a more embryonic type or toward a malignant state. SYN: *anaplasia.*

**undinism** (ŭn′dĭn-ĭzm) An awakening of the libido by running water, as by urination or at the sight of urine. SEE: *urolagnia.*

**undulant** (ŭn′dū-lănt) [L. *undulatio,* wavy] Rising and falling like waves, or moving like them.

**undulant fever** (ŭn′dū-lănt) Brucellosis.

**undulate** (ŭn′dū-lāt) [L. *undulatio,* wavy] Wavy; having a wavy border with shallow sinuses, said of bacterial colonies.

**undulation** (ŭn-dū-lā′shŭn) A continuous wavelike motion or pulsation.

**ung** [L.] *unguentum,* ointment.

**ungual** (ŭng′gwăl) [L. *unguis,* nail] Pert. to or resembling the nails.

**ungual phalanx** The terminal phalanx of each finger and toe.

**ungual tuberosity** The spatula-shaped extremity of the terminal phalanx that supports the nails of fingers and toes.

**unguent** (ŭng′gwĕnt) [L. *unguentum,* ointment] Ointment.

**unguentum** (ŭn-gwĕn′tŭm) [L., ointment] Ointment.

**unguis** (ŭng′gwĭs) *pl.* **ungues** [L., nail] **1.** A fingernail or toenail. SYN: *onyx.* **2.** The lacrimal bone. **3.** A white prominence on the floor of the posterior horn of the lateral ventricle. SYN: *hippocampus minor.*

***u. incarnatus*** An ingrowing nail, esp. a toenail.

**uni-** Combining form meaning *one.* SEE: *mono-.*

**uniarticular** (ū″nē-ăr-tĭk′ū-lăr) [L. *unus,* one, + *articulus,* joint] Pert. to a single joint.

**uniaxial** (ū″nē-ăk′sē-ăl) [″ + *axis,* axis] Having a single axis.

**unibasal** (ū″nē-bā′săl) [″ + *basis,* base] Having a single base.

**unicameral** (ū″nĭ-kăm′ĕr-ăl) [″ + *camera,* vault] Having a single cavity.

**unicellular** (ū″nĭ-sĕl′ū-lăr) [″ + *cellula,* a little box] Having only one cell.

**unicentral** (ū″nĭ-sĕn′trăl) [″ + *centrum,* center] Having a single center.

**uniceps** (ū′nĭ-sĕps) [″ + *caput,* head] Having

a single head or origin, as in muscles.

**unicorn, unicornous** (ū′nĭ-korn, ū-nĭ-kor′nŭs) [″ + *cornu,* horn] Having a single cornu or horn.

**unicuspid** (ū″nĭ-kŭs′pĭd) Having a single cusp.

**uniform** Having the identical shape or form of other objects of the same class.

**unigerminal** (ū″nĭ-jĕr′mĭ-năl) Concerning a single ovum or germ.

**uniglandular** (ū″nĭ-glăn′dū-lăr) Concerning one gland.

**unigravida** (ū″nĭ-grăv′ĭ-dă) [″ + *gravida,* pregnant] A woman who is pregnant for the first time. SEE: *primigravida.*

**unilaminar** (ū″nĭ-lăm′ĭ-năr) Having a single layer.

**unilateral** (ū″nĭ-lăt′ĕr-ăl) [″ + *latus,* side] Affecting or occurring on only one side. SEE: *contralateral; homolateral; ipsilateral.*

**unilateral neglect** The state in which an individual is perceptually unaware of and inattentive to one side of the body and the immediate unilateral area that the patient visualizes. SEE: *Nursing Diagnoses Appendix.*

**unilobar** (ū″nĭ-lō′băr) Having a single lobe.

**unilocular** (ū″nĭ-lŏk′ū-lăr) [″ + *loculus,* a small space] Having only one cavity.

**uninuclear** (ū″nĭ-nū′klē-ăr) [″ + *nucleus,* a kernel] Having only one nucleus.

**uninucleated** (ū″nĭ-nū′klē-āt″ĕd) Having a single nucleus.

**uniocular** (ū″nē-ŏk′ū-lăr) [″ + *oculus,* eye] Pert. to or having only one eye.

**union** (ūn′yŭn) [L. *unio*] **1.** The act of joining two or more things into one part, or the state of being so united. **2.** Growing together of severed or broken parts, as of bones or lips of a wound. SEE: *healing.*

***secondary u.*** A healing by second intention with adhesion of granulating surfaces. SEE: *healing.*

***vicious u.*** The union of the ends of a broken bone in such a way as to cause deformity.

**unioval** (ū″nē-ō′văl) [L. *unus,* one, + *ovum,* egg] Developed from one ovum, as identical twins.

**uniovular** (ū″nē-ŏv′ū-lăr) [″ + *ovum,* egg] Monozygotic, as in the case of twins that develop from a single ovum.

**unipara** (ū-nĭp′ă-ră) [″ + *parere,* to bring forth, to bear] A woman who has had one pregnancy of more than 20 weeks' duration or has produced a fetus weighing at least 500 g, regardless of the fetus's viability. SEE: *primipara.*

**uniparous** (ū-nĭp′ă-rŭs) [″ + *parere,* to bring forth, to bear] **1.** Giving birth to one offspring at a time. **2.** Having produced one child weighing at least 500 g or having a pregnancy lasting 20 weeks, regardless of the fetus' viability.

**unipolar** (ū″nĭ-pō′lăr) [″ + *polus,* pole] **1.** Having or pert. to one pole. **2.** Having a single process, as a unipolar neuron.

**unipotent, unipotential** (ū-nĭp′ō-tĕnt, ū″nĭ-pō-tĕn′shăl) Concerning a cell that can only develop in a specific way to produce a certain end result.

**uniseptate** (ū″nē-sĕp′tāt) Having only one septum.

**unisex 1.** Lack of gender distinction by external appearance, esp. with respect to hairstyle or clothing. **2.** Suitable for use by either sex.

**unit** (ū′nĭt) [L. *unus,* one] ABBR: u. **1.** One of anything. **2.** A determined amount adopted as a standard of measurement.

***amboceptor u.*** The smallest amount of amboceptor required in the presence of which a given quantity of red blood corpuscles will be hemolyzed by an excess of complement.

***angström u.*** ABBR: Å; A.U. An internationally adopted unit of measurement of wavelength, 1/10,000,000 mm, or 1/254,000,000 in.

***antigen u.*** The smallest quantity of antigen required to fix one unit of complement.

***antitoxin u.*** A unit for expressing the strength of an antitoxin. Originally, the various units were defined biologically but now are compared with a weighed standard specified by the U.S. Public Health Service and the World Health Organization.

***atomic mass u.*** ABBR: AMU. One-twelfth of the mass of a neutral carbon atom; equal to $1.657 \times 10^{-24}$ g.

***Bodansky u.*** In clinical chemistry, a unit of alkaline phosphatase equal to that which will liberate 1 mg of phosphorus as inorganic phosphate after 1 hr of incubation with a buffered substrate containing sodium β-glycerophosphate. SEE: *phosphatase, alkaline.*

***British thermal u.*** ABBR: BTU. The amount of heat necessary to raise the temperature of 1 lb of water from 39°F to 40°F.

***u. of capacity*** The capacity of a condenser that gives a difference of potential of 1 volt when charged with 1 coulomb. SYN: *curie; farad.*

***cat u.*** The amount of drug per kilogram of body weight just sufficient to kill a cat when injected intravenously slowly and continuously.

***complement u.*** The smallest quantity of complement required for hemolysis of a given amount of red blood corpuscles with one amboceptor (hemolysin) unit present.

***dental u.*** **1.** A masticatory unit consisting of a single tooth and its adjacent tissues. **2.** A mobile or fixed piece of equipment, usually complete with chair, light, engine, and other accessories or utilities necessary for dental examinations or operations.

***electrostatic u.*** ABBR: ESU or ESE (from the German *elektrostatische Einheit*). Any static electricity unit based on the unit electrostatic charge expressed in the centimeter-gram-second system of measurement.

***hemolytic u.*** The amount of inactivated immune serum that causes complete hemolysis of 1 ml of a 5% emulsion of washed red blood corpuscles in the presence of complement.

***international u.*** ABBR: I.U. An internationally accepted amount of a substance. Usually this form of expressing quantity is used for fat-soluble vitamins and some hormones, enzymes, and biologicals such as vaccines. These units are defined by the International Conference for Unification of Formulae.

***light u.*** A foot-candle, or the amount of light 1 ft from a standard candle. The ideal amount of light required for work varies with the specific type of work being done. The term *foot-candle* took the place of *candle power*, but light intensity in the International System of Units is indicated by lumen. SEE: *candela; lumen.*

***Mache u.*** ABBR: M.u. A unit of measurement of radium emanation.

***motor u.*** A somatic motor neuron and all the muscle cells it innervates.

***mouse u.*** SEE: *Allen-Doisy unit.*

***rat u.*** The greatest dilution of estrogen that will cause desquamation and cornification of the vaginal epithelium if given to a mature spayed rat in three injections, one every 4 hr. This must occur in the first day of treatment.

***SI u.*** Any of the units specified by the International System of Units adopted by an International Conference of Weights and Measures in 1960. SEE: *SI Units* for tables; SEE: *SI Units Appendix.*

***terminal duct lobular u.*** ABBR: TDLU. The blind ending of the lactiferous duct that contains the lobule and its duct. Most benign and malignant breast lesions arise here.

***Todd u.*** In a test of inhibition hemolysis by enzymes such as antistreptolysin O, the reciprocal of the highest dilution that inhibits hemolysis.

***USP u.*** Any unit specified in the U.S. Pharmacopeia.

**unitarian** (ū-nĭ-tār′ē-ăn) [L. *unitarius*] Composed of a single unit.

**unitary** (ū′nĭ-tĕr-ē) Rel. to a single unit.

**unit dose** A dose form in which individual doses of medicine are prepared in each packet. This saves time in dispensing medicines, esp. to hospitalized patients.

**United Network for Organ Sharing** ABBR: UNOS. An organization established in 1984 to facilitate donation of organs for possible transplantation. All hospitals are required by law to inform relatives of potential donors about UNOS. SEE: *death; dying; do not resuscitate; organ donation; transplantation.*

**United States Adopted Names** ABBR: USAN. Dictionary of nonproprietary names, brand names, code designations, and Chemical Abstracts Service registry numbers for drugs published by the U.S. Pharmacopeial Convention, Inc. The purpose is to have nonproprietary names assigned to new drugs in accordance with established principles. SEE: *USAN and the USP Dictionary of Drug Names.*

**United States Pharmacopeia** SEE: *Pharmacopeia, United States.*

**United States Public Health Service** ABBR: USPHS. An agency of the U.S. Department of Health and Human Services (HHS). Broadly, its function is to assess needs and promote national and international health. Included in the organization are the Centers for Disease Control and Prevention (CDC); Food and Drug Administration (FDA); Alcohol, Drug Abuse and Mental Health Administration; Agency for Toxic Substances and Disease Registry; and various USPHS Regional Offices.

**uniterminal** (ū″nĭ-tĕr′mĭn-ăl) [L. *unus,* one, + *terminus,* end] Having only one terminal.

**univalence** (ū″nĭ-vā′lĕns) The condition of having only one valence.

**univalent** (ū″nĭ-vā′lĕnt, ū-nĭv′ă-lĕnt) [″ + *valens,* to be powerful] Possessing the power of combining or replacing one atom of hydrogen. SYN: *monovalent.*

**universal** (ū″nĭ-vĕr′săl) [L. *universalis,* combined into one whole] General or applicable or common to all situations or conditions.

**universal antidote** An antidote used in poisoning where the specific antidote is unknown or not available; consisting of two parts activated charcoal, one part tannic acid, and one part magnesium oxide. A paste of five heaping teaspoons of the mixture dissolved in a glass of water is given orally. After the patient has swallowed the antidote, the stomach contents should be removed by gastric lavage. In general, there is no "universal" antidote; however, the preferred general antidote is activated charcoal alone.

---

Caution: Gastric lavage should not be used in patients who have ingested caustics. The stomach or esophagus may be ruptured during introduction of the tube.

---

**universal cuff** An adapted device fitted around the palm of the hand to permit attachment of self-care tools when normal grasp is absent. SYN: *palmar cuff.*

**universal donor** A person whose blood type is O, Rh negative. As a rule, blood from a universal donor may be transfused without danger of untoward reactions into persons belonging to any of the other ABO blood groups.

NOTE: Because there are multiple blood type factors in addition to those of ABO, it would be dangerous to assume that type O, Rh-negative blood could, without further compatibility testing, be given to persons of a different blood type.

**universal dressing** A large flat bandage that

may be folded several times to make a relatively large dressing or folded several more times to make a smaller and thicker bandage. This process can be continued until the unit is suitable for use as a cervical collar. SEE: *dressing, universal* for illus.

**universal precautions** Guidelines designed to protect workers with occupational exposure to bloodborne pathogens (such as HIV and hepatitis B virus). These "universal blood and body fluid precautions" (e.g., gloves, masks, and gowns), originally recommended by the Centers for Disease Control and Prevention in 1985, were mandated by the OSHA Bloodborne Pathogens Standard in 1991 for workers in all U.S. health care settings. SEE: *Universal Precautions Appendix.*

**universal recipient** A person belonging to blood type AB, Rh positive, whose serum will not agglutinate the cells of the other ABO blood. Nevertheless, the recipient's blood must be tested by cross-matching before the transfusion.

**unlicensed assistive personnel** Persons who assist the licensed nurse in providing care to patients (formerly called nurse's aides or nursing attendants).

**unmedullated** (ŭn-mĕd′ū-lāt″ĕd) Unmyelinated.

**unmyelinated** (ŭn-mī′ĕ-lĭ-nāt″ĕd) Lacking a myelin sheath; used of neurons. SYN: *unmedullated.*

**Unna's paste** (oo′năz) [Paul G. Unna, Ger. dermatologist, 1850–1929] A mixture of 15% zinc oxide in a glycogelatin base.

**Unna's (paste) boot** A bootlike dressing of the lower extremity made of layers of gauze and Unna's paste. It is used in treating chronic ulcers of the leg, usually caused by varicosities.

**UNOS** *United Network for Organ Sharing.*

**unsaturated** (ŭn-săt′ū-rāt″ĕd) [AS. *un,* not + L. *saturare,* to fill] **1.** Capable of dissolving or absorbing to a greater degree. **2.** Not combined to the greatest possible extent.

**unsaturated compound** An organic compound having double or triple bonds between the carbon atoms.

**unsex** (ŭn-sĕks′) [″ + L. *sexus,* sex] **1.** To castrate; to spay or excise the ovaries. **2.** To deprive of sexual character.

**unstriated** (ŭn-strī′āt-ĕd) [″ + *striatus,* striped] Unstriped, as smooth muscle fiber.

**unthrifty** Not healthy or robust, esp. when describing plants or animals.

**Unverricht's disease, Unverricht's syndrome** (oon′fĕr-ĭkts) [Heinrich Unverricht, Ger. physician, 1853–1912] A rare, fatal disease inherited as an autosomal recessive trait. It is characterized by the onset in later childhood of progressive myoclonic epilepsy, tetraplegia, and dementia. Also called *Unverricht-Lafora disease.*

**upper airway obstruction** ABBR: UAO. A condition of the respiratory system in which it has the capability of functioning but is prevented from doing so by an obstruction in the upper portion of the airway, such as the main bronchus, larynx, mouth, or nose. SEE: *cardiopulmonary resuscitation; tracheostomy.*

**upper GI** *upper gastrointestinal.*

**upper motor neuron lesion** A neurological condition caused by damage to the corticospinal or pyramidal tract in the brain or spinal cord. This lesion results in hemiplegia, paraplegia, or quadriplegia, depending on its location and extent. Clinical signs include loss of voluntary movement, spasticity, sensory loss, and pathological reflexes.

**upper respiratory infection** ABBR: URI. An imprecise term for almost any kind of infectious disease process involving the nasal passages, pharynx, and bronchi. The etiological agent may be bacterial or viral.

**upsiloid** (ŭp′sĭ-loyd) [Gr. *upsilon,* letter U, + *eidos,* form, shape] Shaped like the letter U or V.

**uptake** (ŭp′tāk) The absorption of nutrients, chemicals (including radioactive materials), and medicines by tissues or by an entire organism.

**urachal** (ū′ră-kăl) [Gr. *ourachos,* fetal urinary canal] Rel. to the urachus.

**urachus** (ū′ră-kŭs) [Gr. *ourachos,* fetal urinary canal] An epithelioid cord surrounded by fibrous tissue extending from the apex of the bladder to the umbilicus. In the embryo, it is continuous with the allantoic stalk; postnatally it forms the middle umbilical ligament of the bladder.

***patent u.*** A condition in which the urachus remains as a hollow tube that connects the vertex of the bladder with the umbilicus, resulting in an umbilical urinary fistula.

**uracil** (ū′ră-sĭl) $C_4H_4N_2O_2$. A pyrimidine base found in RNA (not DNA) which, if paired, pairs with adenine.

**uracil mustard** An alkylating type of cytotoxic drug used in treating certain types of malignant tumors.

---

Caution: This drug must be handled with exceptional care, in a well-ventilated hood, and using a protective mask, protective glasses, and gloves. The work area should be thoroughly cleaned afterward. The hands should be rinsed in water for several minutes, then washed with soap and water.

---

**uraniscoñitis** (ū-răn-ĭs″kōn-ī′tĭs) [Gr. *ouraniskos,* palate, + *itis,* inflammation] Inflammation of the palate.

**uraniscoplasty** (ū-răn-ĭs′kō-plăs″tē) [″ + *plassein,* to form] Operation for repair of a cleft palate.

**uraniscorrhaphy** (ū″răn-ĭs-kor′ră-fē) [″ + *rhaphe,* seam, ridge] Operation for suturing of a cleft palate. SYN: *uraniscoplasty.*

**uraniscus** (ū-răn-ĭs′kŭs) [Gr. *ouraniskos,* palate] The palate, or the roof of the mouth.

**uranium** (ū-rā′nē-ŭm) [LL., planet Uranus] SYMB: U. A radioactive element, the parent of radium and other radioelements; atomic weight, 238.029; atomic number, 92. Uranium ore contains the isotopes $^{238}U$, $^{235}U$, and $^{234}U$.

**uranoplegia** (ū″ră-nō-plē′jē-ă) [″ + *plege,* stroke] Paralysis of muscles of the soft palate.

**uranoschisis** (ū-răn-ŏs′kĭs-ĭs) [″ + *schisis,* a splitting] Cleft palate.

**uranostaphyloschisis** (ū″ră-nō-stăf″ĭ-lŏs′kĭ-sĭs) Cleft of the hard and soft palates.

**uranyl** (ū′ră-nĭl) The bivalent uranium radical $UO^{2+}$. It forms salts with many acids. An example is uranyl nitrate, $UO_2(NO_3)_2$.

**urapostema** (ū″ră-pŏs-tē′mă) [Gr. *ouron,* urine, + *apostema,* abscess] An abscess containing urine.

**uraroma** (ū-ră-rō′mă) [″ + *aroma,* spice] Aromatic spicy odor of freshly voided urine.

**urarthritis** (ū″răr-thrī′tĭs) Arthritis due to gout.

**urase** (ū′rās) Urease.

**urate** (ū′rāt) [Gr. *ouron,* urine] The combination of uric acid with a base; a salt of uric acid. Urates are normally present in urine.

**uratemia** (ū″ră-tē′mē-ă) [″ + *haima,* blood] Urates, esp. sodium urate, in the blood.

**uratosis** (ū″ră-tō′sĭs) Any condition leading to deposition of urates in tissues.

**uraturia** (ū″ră-tū′rē-ă) [Gr. *ouron,* urine] Excess of urates in the urine. SYN: *lithuria.*

**urceiform** (ŭr-sē′ĭ-form) [L. *urceus,* pitcher, + *forma,* shape] Pitcher-shaped.

**ur-defense(s)** (ŭr″dē-fĕns′) [Ger. *ur,* ultimate, + *defense*] Basic beliefs, such as religious or scientific ones, that are thought by the individual to be essential to people's emotional well-being. These beliefs may include faith in a personal or universal God or the fundamental goodness of humankind.

**urea** (ū-rē′ă) [Gr. *ouron,* urine] **1.** The diamide of carbonic acid, a crystalline solid having the formula $CH_4N_2O$; found in blood, lymph, and urine. It is formed in the liver from ammonia derived from amino acids by deamination. It may also be formed directly from arginine.

Urea is the chief nitrogenous constituent of urine and, along with carbon dioxide, the final product of protein metabolism in the body. In normal conditions, urea represents 80% to 90% of the total urinary nitrogen. It is odorless and colorless, appears as white prismatic crystals, and forms salts with acids. Its excess is one of the signs of uremia. The amount of urea excreted varies directly with the amount of protein in the diet. Its excretion is increased in fever, diabetes, or increased activity of the adrenal gland. **2.** A standardized preparation of urea used as a diuretic.

**urea cycle** The complex cyclic chemical reactions in some (ureotelic) animals, including humans, that produce urea from the metabolism of nitrogen-containing foods. This cycle provides a method of excreting the nitrogen produced by the metabolism of amino acids as urea. The cycle was first described by Sir Hans Krebs [1900–1981].

**urea frost** White flaky deposits of urea seen on the skin in patients with advanced uremia.

**ureagenetic** (ū-rē″ă-jĕn-ĕt′ĭk) [″ + *genesis,* generation, birth] Pert. to or producing urea.

**ureametry** (ū-rē-ăm′ĕt-rē) Determination of the amount of urea in urine.

**urea nitrogen** The nitrogen of urea as distinguished from nitrogen in blood proteins.

**Ureaplasma urealyticum** A microorganism of the genus *Mycoplasma,* usually sexually transmitted. It may cause inflammation of the urogenital tract in males and females.

**urease** (ū′rē-ās) [Gr. *ouron,* urine] An enzyme that accelerates the hydrolysis of urea into carbon dioxide and ammonia. It is used in determining the amount of urea in blood or in urine.

**urelcosis** (ū-rĕl-kō′sĭs) [″ + *helkosis,* ulceration] Ulceration of the urinary tract.

**uremia** (ū-rē′mē-ă) [″ + *haima,* blood] A toxic condition associated with renal insufficiency produced by the retention in the blood of nitrogenous substances normally excreted by the kidney. SEE: *azotemia; coma, uremic.*

SYMPTOMS: Symptoms include nausea, vomiting, headache, dizziness, dimness of vision, coma or convulsions, and urinous odor of breath and perspiration. Stupor and stertorous respiration also are associated with this condition. There is no change in pupillary reaction. Dry skin, hard rapid pulse, elevated blood pressure, and scanty urine containing casts and albumin further characterize uremia. There is a reduction of urea in the urine, and tube casts are present. Urea retention is at least 150 to 500 mg/dl of blood.

ETIOLOGY: Uremia may result from the disturbed kidney function seen in nephritis or from suppression or deficient urinary secretion of any cause.

TREATMENT: Dialysis is the treatment for this condition.

***extrarenal u.*** Prerenal u.

***prerenal u.*** Uremia resulting not from primary renal disease but from other conditions such as disturbances in circulation, fluid balance, or metabolism arising in other parts of the body. SYN: *extrarenal u.*

**uremic** (ū-rē′mĭk) Pert. to or caused by uremia.

**uremigenic** (ū-rē″mĭ-jĕn′ĭk) [Gr. *ouron,* urine, + *haima,* blood, + *gennan,* to produce] Caused by or producing uremia.

**ureogenesis** (ūr″ē-ō-jĕn′ĕ-sĭs) [″ + *genesis,* generation, birth] Formation of urea.

**ureotelic** (ū″rē-ō-tĕl′ĭk) [*urea* + Gr. *telikos,* belonging to the completion] Concerning animals that excrete amino nitrogen in the form of urea. Included in this group are mammals, including most terrestrial vertebrates. SEE: *urea cycle; uricotelic.*

**uresis** (ū-rē′sĭs) [Gr. *ouresis*] Urination.

**ureter** (ū′rĕ-ter, ū-rē′tĕr) [Gr. *oureter*] The tube that carries urine from the kidney to the bladder. It originates in the pelvis of the kidney and terminates in the base of the bladder. Each kidney has one ureter measuring from 28 to 34 cm long, the right being slightly shorter than the left. The diameter varies from 1 mm to 1 cm. The wall consists of three layers: the mucosal, muscular, and fibrous layers. SEE: *kidney; urethra.*

**ureteral** (ū-rē′tĕr-ăl) Concerning the ureter. SYN: *ureteric.*

**ureteralgia** (ū″rē-tĕr-ăl′jē-ă) [″ + *algos,* pain] Pain in the ureter.

**uretercystoscope** (ū-rē″tĕr-sĭs′tō-skōp) [″ + *kystis,* bladder, + *skopein,* to examine] A cystoscope combined with a ureteral catheter. SYN: *ureterocystoscope.*

**ureterectasis** (ū-rē″tĕr-ĕk′tă-sĭs) [″ + *ektasis,* dilatation] Dilatation of the ureter.

**ureterectomy** (ū-rē″tĕr-ĕk′tō-mē) [″ + *ektome,* excision] Excision of a ureter.

**ureteric** (ū″rĕ-tĕr′ĭk) Ureteral.

**ureteritis** (ū-rē″tĕr-ī′tĭs) [″ + *itis,* inflammation] Inflammation of the ureters.

**uretero-** Combining form indicating *ureter.*

**ureterocele** (ū-rē′tĕr-ō-sēl) [″ + *kele,* tumor, swelling] Cystlike dilatation of the ureter near its opening into the bladder; usually a result of congenital stenosis of the ureteral orifice.

**ureterocelectomy** (ū-rē″tĕr-ō-sē-lĕk′tō-mē) [″ + ″ + *ektome,* excision] Surgical removal of a ureterocele.

**ureterocervical** (ū-rē″tĕr-ō-sĕr′vĭ-kăl) [″ + L. *cervicalis,* pert. to cervix] Concerning the ureter and the cervix uteri.

**ureterocolostomy** (ū-rē″tĕr-ō-kō-lŏs′tō-mē) [″ + *kolon,* colon, + *stoma,* mouth] The implantation of the ureter into the colon.

**ureterocystoscope** (ū-rē″tĕr-ō-sĭs′tō-skōp) [″ + ″ + *skopein,* to view] Uretercystoscope.

**ureteroenterostomy** (ū-rē″tĕr-ō-ĕn-tĕr-ŏs′tō-mē) [″ + *enteron,* intestine, + *stoma,* mouth] Formation of a passage between a ureter and the intestine.

**ureterography** (ū-rē″tĕr-ŏg′ră-fē) [″ + *graphein,* to write] Radiography of the ureter after injection of a radiopaque substance into it.

**ureteroheminephrectomy** (ū-rē″tĕr-ō-hĕm″ĭ-nĕ-frĕk′tō-mē) [″ + *hemi-,* half, + *nephros,* kidney, + *ektome,* excision] In cases of reduplication of the upper urinary tract on one side, surgical removal of the reduplicated portion.

**ureterohydronephrosis** (ū-rē″tĕr-ō-hī″drō-nĕ-frō′sĭs) [″ + *hydor,* water, + *nephros,* kidney, + *osis,* condition] Dilatation of the ureter and the pelvis of the kidney resulting from a mechanical or inflammatory obstruction in the urinary tract.

**ureteroileostomy** (ū-rē″tĕr-ō-ĭl″ē-ŏs′tō-mē) [″ + *ileum,* ileum, + *stoma,* mouth] Surgical anastomosis of a ureter to an isolated segment of the ileum. The ileum is connected to an abdominal stoma so that urine leaves the body via that opening.

**ureterolith** (ū-rē′tĕr-ō-lĭth) [″ + *lithos,* stone] A stone or calculus in the ureter.

**ureterolithiasis** (ū-rē″tĕr-ō-lĭth-ī′ăs-ĭs) [″ + ″ + *iasis,* condition] Development of a calculus in the ureter.

**ureterolithotomy** (ū-rē″tĕr-ō-lĭth-ŏt′ō-mē) [″ + ″ + *tome,* incision] Surgical incision for removal of a calculus from the ureter.

**ureterolysis** (ū-rē″tĕr-ŏl′ĭ-sĭs) [″ + *lysis,* dissolution] **1.** Rupture of a ureter. **2.** Paralysis of the ureter. **3.** The process of loosening adhesions around the ureter.

**ureteroneocystostomy** (ū-rē″tĕr-ō-nē″ō-sĭs-tŏs′tō-mē) [″ + *neos,* new, + *kystis,* bladder, + *stoma,* mouth] Surgical formation of a new passage between a ureter and the bladder.

**ureteroneopyelostomy** (ū-rē″tĕr-ō-nē″ō-pī-ĕ-lŏs′tō-mē) [″ + ″ + *pyelos,* pelvis, + *stoma,* mouth] Excision of a portion of the ureter with attachment of the severed end of the lower portion to a new aperture in the renal pelvis. SYN: *ureteropyelostomy.*

**ureteronephrectomy** (ū-rē″tĕr-ō-nĕf-rĕk′tō-mē) [″ + *nephros,* kidney, + *ektome,* excision] Removal of a kidney and its ureter.

**ureteropelvioplasty** (ū-rē″tĕr-ō-pĕl′vē-ō-plăs″tē) [Gr. *oureter,* ureter, + L. *pelvis,* basin, + Gr. *plassein,* to mold] Plastic surgery of the junction of the ureter and the pelvis of the kidney.

**ureteroplasty** (ū-rē′tĕr-ō-plăs″tē) [″ + *plassein,* to form] Plastic surgery of the ureter.

**ureteroproctostomy** (ū-rē″tĕr-ō-prŏk-tŏs′tō-mē) [″ + *proktos,* anus, + *stoma,* mouth] The formation of a passage from the ureter to the lower rectum.

**ureteropyelitis** (ū-rē″tĕr-ō-pī-ĕl-ī′tĭs) [″ + *pyelos,* pelvis, + *itis,* inflammation] Inflammation of the pelvis of the kidney and a ureter.

**ureteropyelonephritis** (ū-rē″tĕr-ō-pī″ĕl-ō-nĕf-rī′tĭs) [″ + ″ + *nephros,* kidney, + *itis,* inflammation] Inflammation of the renal pelvis and the ureter.

**ureteropyeloplasty** (ū-rē″tĕr-ō-pī′ĕl-ō-plăs″tē) [″ + ″ + *plassein,* to mold] Plastic surgery of the ureter and renal pelvis.

**ureteropyelostomy** (ū-rē″tĕr-ō-pī″ĕ-lŏs′tō-mē) [″ + ″ + *stoma,* mouth] Ureteroneopyelostomy.

**ureteropyosis** (ū-rē″tĕr-ō-pī-ō′sĭs) [″ + *pyon,* pus, + *osis,* condition] Suppurative inflammation within a ureter.

**ureterorrhagia** (ū-rē″tĕr-or-rā′jē-ă) [″ + *rhegnynai,* to burst forth] Hemorrhage from the ureter.

**ureterorrhaphy** (ū-rē″tĕr-or′ră-fē) [″ + *rha-*

*phe,* seam, ridge] Suture of the ureter, as for fistula.

**ureterosigmoidostomy** (ū-rē″tĕr-ō-sĭg-moyd-ŏs′tō-mē) [″ + *sigma,* letter S, + *eidos,* shape, + *stoma,* mouth] Surgical implantation of the ureter into the sigmoid flexure.

**ureterostegnosis** (ū-rē″tĕr-ō-stĕg-nō′sĭs) Stricture of a ureter.

**ureterostoma** (ū″rē-tĕr-ŏs′tō-mă) [Gr. *oureter,* ureter, + *stoma,* mouth] The orifice through which the ureter enters the urinary bladder.

**ureterostomy** (ū-rē″tĕr-ŏs′tō-mē) [″ + *stoma,* mouth] The formation of a permanent fistula for drainage of a ureter.

***cutaneous u.*** Surgical implantation of the ureter into the skin. This allows urine to drain via the ureter to the outside of the body by going through the stoma.

**ureterotomy** (ū-rē″tĕr-ŏt′ō-mē) [″ + *tome,* incision] Incision or surgery of the ureter.

**ureterotrigonoenterostomy** (ū-rē″tĕr-ō-trī-gō″nō-ĕn″tĕr-ŏs′tō-mē) [″ + *trigonon,* three-sided figure, + *enteron,* intestine, + *stoma,* mouth] Surgical removal of the trigone of the bladder with one or both of the ureteral openings and implantation of it into the intestine.

**ureteroureterostomy** (ū-rē″tĕr-ō-ū-rē″tĕr-ŏs′tō-mē) [″ + ″ + *stoma,* mouth] **1.** The formation of a connection from one ureter to the other. **2.** The re-establishment of a passage between the ends of a divided ureter.

**ureterouterine** (ū-rē″tĕr-ō-ū′tĕr-ĭn) [″ + L. *uterus,* womb] Concerning the ureter and uterus or a fistula between them.

**ureterovaginal** (ū-rē″tĕr-ō-văj′ĭ-năl) [″ + L. *vagina,* sheath] Relating to a ureter and the vagina, denoting a fistula connecting them.

**ureterovesicostomy** (ū-rē″tĕr-ō-vĕs″ĭ-kŏs′tō-mē) [″ + ″ + Gr. *stoma,* mouth] Reimplantation of a ureter into the bladder.

**urethra** (ū-rē′thră) [Gr. *ourethra*] A canal for the discharge of urine extending from the bladder to the outside. In females, its orifice lies in the vestibule between the vagina and clitoris; in males, the urethra passes through the prostate gland and the penis, opening at the tip of the glans penis. In males, it serves as the passage for semen as well as urine. Its lining, the mucosa, is thrown into folds and contains openings of lacunae into which the glands of Littre open. Surrounding the mucosa is a lamina propria containing many elastic fibers and blood vessels, outside of which is an indefinite muscular layer. SEE: *penis.*

***u. muliebris*** The female urethra.

***u. virilis*** The male urethra.

**urethral** (ū-rē′thrăl) [Gr. *ourethra,* urethra] Relating to the urethra.

**urethralgia** (ū-rē-thrăl′jē-ă) [″ + *algos,* pain] Pain in the urethra.

**urethral syndrome** SEE: *acute urethral syndrome.*

**urethratresia** (ū-rē″thră-trē′zē-ă) [″ + *a-,* not, + *tresis,* a perforation] Occlusion or imperforation of the urethra.

**urethrectomy** (ū-rē-thrĕk′tō-mē) [″ + *ektome,* excision] Surgical excision of the urethra or part of it.

**urethreurynter** (ū-rēth″rūr-ĭn′tĕr) [″ + *eurynein,* to dilate] An appliance for dilating the urethra.

**urethrism, urethrismus** (ū′rē-thrĭzm, ū″rē-thrĭz′mŭs) [″ + *-ismos,* condition] Irritability or spasm of the urethra.

**urethritis** (ū″rē-thrī′tĭs) [″ + *itis,* inflammation] Inflammation of the urethra.

***anterior u.*** Inflammation of that portion of the urethra anterior to the anterior layer of the triangular ligament.

***gonococcal u.*** Urethritis caused by gonococcus.

***nongonococcal u.*** ABBR: NGU. A urethral inflammation caused by organisms other than *Neisseria gonorrhoeae.* NGU is the most common sexually transmitted disease in men. It accounts for 4 to 6 million physician visits annually. Clinically the symptoms usually develop within about 7 to 14 days but may range from 2 to 35 days. The symptoms usually include painful urination and a urethral discharge. Because of the similarity of NGU to gonococcal urethritis, the disease is diagnosed from bacteriological culture of the discharge. The two organisms most frequently associated with NGU are *Chlamydia trachomatis* and *Ureaplasma urealyticum.* Other causes include herpes simplex virus, *Trichomonas vaginalis, Haemophilus influenzae, Gardnerella vaginalis,* and *Clostridium difficile.*

TREATMENT: NGU due to *C. trachomatis* or *U. urealyticum* is treated with doxycycline or azithromycin. Appropriate antibiotics are used for other causative organisms.

***nonspecific u.*** ABBR: NSU. Nongonococcal u.

***posterior u.*** Inflammation of membranous and prostatic portions of the urethra.

***specific u.*** Urethritis due to a specific organism, usually gonococcus.

**urethro-** [Gr. *ourethra*] Combining form meaning *urethra.*

**urethrobulbar** (ū-rē″thrō-bŭl′băr) Concerning the urethra and the bulbar penis.

**urethrocele** (ū-rē′thrō-sēl) [″ + *kele,* tumor, swelling] **1.** Pouchlike protrusion of the urethral wall in the female. **2.** Thickening of connective tissue around the urethra in the female.

**urethrocystitis** (ū-rē″thrō-sĭs-tī′tĭs) [″ + *kystis,* bladder, + *itis,* inflammation] Inflammation of the urethra and bladder.

**urethrocystopexy** (ū-rē″thrō-sĭs′tō-pĕk″sē) [″ + *kystis,* bladder, + *pexis,* fixation] Plastic surgery of the urethral-bladder junction to relieve urinary stress incontinence.

**urethrograph** (ū-rē′thrō-grăf) A device for

recording the caliber of the urethra.

**urethrography** (ū-rē-thrŏg′ră-fē) [″ + *graphein,* to write] Radiography of the urethra after it has been filled with contrast medium.

***voiding u.*** Radiographic examination of the urethra during micturition after the introduction of a contrast medium.

**urethrometer** (ū-rē-thrŏm′ĕt-ĕr) [Gr. *ourethra,* urethra, + *metron,* measure] An instrument for measuring the diameter of the urethra or the lumen of a stricture.

**urethropenile** (ū-rē″thrō-pē′nīl) [″ + L. *penis,* penis] Relating to the urethra and penis.

**urethroperineal** (ū-rē″thrō-pĕr-ĭ-nē′ăl) [″ + *perinaion,* perineum] Rel. to the urethra and perineum.

**urethroperineoscrotal** (ū-rē″thrō-pĕr-ĭ-nē″ō-skrō′tăl) [″ + ″ + L. *scrotum,* a bag] Relating to the urethra, perineum, and scrotum.

**urethropexy** (ū-rē′thrō-pĕks-ē) [″ + Gr. *pexis,* fixation] Surgical fixation of the urethra.

**urethrophraxis** (ū-rē-thrō-frăks′ĭs) [″ + *phrassein,* to obstruct] Urethral obstruction.

**urethroplasty** (ū-rē′thrō-plăs″tē) [″ + *plassein,* to mold] Reparative surgery of the urethra.

**urethroprostatic** (ū-rē″thrō-prŏs-tăt′ĭk) Concerning the urethra and prostate.

**urethrorectal** (ū-rē″thrō-rĕk′tăl) [Gr. *ourethra,* urethra, + L. *rectus,* straight] Rel. to the urethra and rectum.

**urethrorrhagia** (ū-rē″thror-ā′jē-ă) [″ + *rhegnynai,* to burst forth] Hemorrhage from the urethra.

**urethrorrhaphy** (ū-rē-thror′ăf-ē) [″ + *rhaphe,* seam, ridge] Suture of the urethra or of a urethral fistula.

**urethrorrhea** (ū-rē″thror-ē′ă) [″ + *rhoia,* flow] An abnormal discharge from the urethra.

***u. ex libidine*** The discharge of normal glandular secretions resulting from sexual stimulation, esp. that preceding sexual intercourse. SEE: *Cowper's glands.*

**urethroscopy** (ū-rē-thrŏs′kō-pē) An examination of the mucous membrane of the urethra with a urethroscope.

**urethrospasm** (ū-rē′thrō-spăzm) [″ + *spasmos,* a convulsion] Spasmodic stricture of the urethra.

**urethrostenosis** (ū-rē″thrō-stĕn-ō′sĭs) [″ + *stenosis,* act of narrowing] Stricture of the urethra.

**urethrostomy** (ū-rē-thrŏs′tō-mē) [″ + *stoma,* mouth] The formation of a permanent fistula opening into the urethra by perineal section and fixation of the membranous urethra in the perineum.

**urethrotome** (ū-rē′thrō-tōm) [″ + *tome,* incision] An instrument for incision of a urethral stricture.

**urethrotomy** (ū-rē-thrŏt′ō-mē) Incision of a urethral stricture.

**urethrotrigonitis** (ū-rē″thrō-trī″gō-nī′tĭs) [″ + *trigonon,* three-sided figure, + *itis,* inflammation] Inflammation of the urethra and the trigone of the bladder.

**urethrovaginal** (ū-rē″thrō-văj′ĭ-năl) [″ + L. *vagina,* sheath] Pert. to the urethra and vagina.

**urethrovesical** (ū-rē″thrō-vĕs′ĭ-kăl) [″ + L. *vesicula,* little bladder] Concerning the urethra and the bladder.

**urgency** A sudden, almost uncontrollable need to urinate.

**urhydrosis** (ūr″hī-drō′sĭs) [Gr. *ouron,* urine, + *hidros,* sweat] Excretion of urea in sweat.

**URI** *upper respiratory infection.*

**uric** (ū′rĭk) [Gr. *ourikos,* urine] Of or pert. to urine.

**uric acid** $C_5H_4N_4O_3$. A crystalline acid occurring as an end product of purine metabolism. It is formed from purine bases derived from nucleic acids (DNA and RNA). It is a common constituent of urinary and renal calculi and of gouty concretions. SEE: illus.

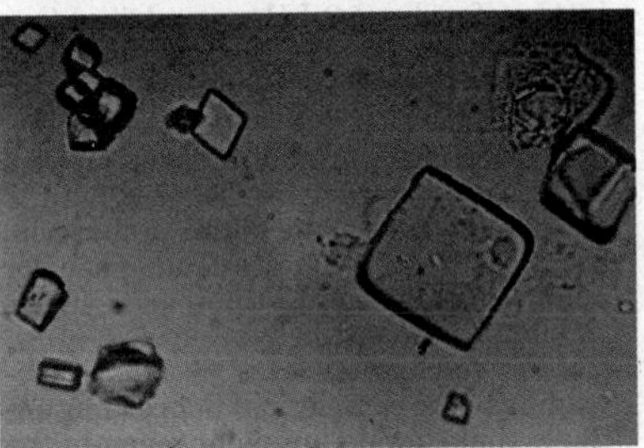

URIC ACID CRYSTALS (ORIG. MAG. ×400)

OUTPUT: The uric acid output should be between 0.8 and 1 g/day if the patient is on an ordinary mixed diet. Uric acid must be excreted because it cannot be metabolized.

Increased elimination is observed in ingestion of proteins and nitrogenous foods, after exercise, after administration of cytotoxic agents, and in gout, leukemia, and acute articular rheumatism. Decreased elimination is observed in nephritis, chlorosis, and lead poisoning, and in those following a protein-free diet.

***endogenous u.a.*** Uric acid derived from purines undergoing metabolism from the nucleic acid of body tissues.

***exogenous u.a.*** Uric acid derived from purines from food made up of free purines and nucleic acids. SEE: *urate; uraturia.*

**uricacidemia** (ū″rĭk-ăs-ĭd-ē′mē-ă) [Gr. *ourikos,* urine, + L. *acidus,* sour, + Gr. *haima,* blood] Excessive uric acid in the blood.

**uricaciduria** (ū″rĭk-ăs-ĭd-ū′rē-ă) [″ + ″ + Gr. *ouron,* urine] Uricemia.

**uricase** (ū′rĭ-kāz) [″ + *-ase,* enzyme] An enzyme present in the liver and kidneys of most mammals, but not humans. This enzyme is capable of oxidizing uric acid into allantoin and carbon dioxide.

**uricemia** (ū-rĭ-sē′mē-ă) [″ + *haima,* blood] Excessive uric acid in the blood. SYN: *uricacidemia.*

**uricocholia** (ū″rĭ-kō-kō′lē-ă) [″ + *chole,* bile] Uric acid in the bile.

**uricopoiesis** (ū″rĭ-kō-poy-ē′sĭs) [″ + *poiesis,* formation] Producing uric acid.

**uricosuria** (ū″rĭ-kō-sū′rē-ă) [″ + *ouron,* urine] The excessive excretion of uric acid in the urine.

**uricosuric** (ū″rĭ-kō-sū′rĭk) Potentiating the excretion of uric acid in the urine.

**uricosuric agent** A drug (such as probenecid) that increases the urinary excretion of uric acid, thereby reducing the concentration of uric acid in the blood. It is used to treat gout.

NURSING IMPLICATIONS: The nurse assesses the patient for a history of gastrointestinal complaints or ulceration and for drug sensitivities and drug regimens to prevent interactions. The patient should take drugs with milk or food. Fluid intake of at least 3 L/day is advised (unless contraindicated), and alkalinization of urine with sodium bicarbonate and alkaline-ash diet to prevent uric acid crystallization until serum urate levels return to normal. The patient should avoid the use of salicylates while taking probenecid; the patient may use acetaminophen for analgesia. Gastrointestinal side effects should be reported.

**uricotelic** (ū″rĭ-kō-tĕl′ĭk) [″ + *telikos,* belonging to the completion] Concerning animals that excrete amino nitrogen in the form of uric acid. Included in this group are birds, snakes, and lizards. SEE: *urea cycle; ureotelic.*

**uricoxidase** (ū″rĭk-ŏks′ĭ-dās) [″ + *oxys,* sharp, + *-ase,* enzyme] An enzyme capable of oxidizing uric acid.

**uridine** (ūr′ĭ-dĭn) A nucleoside that is one of the four main riboside components of ribonucleic acid. It consists of uracil and D-ribose.

***u. diphosphate*** A uridine-containing nucleotide important in certain metabolic reactions, in which it transports sugars such as glucose and galactose.

**uridrosis** (ū-rĭ-drō′sĭs) [″ + *hidrosis,* a sweating] The presence of urea in the sweat. Evaporation may show white scales, the crystals of urea.

***u. crystallina*** Urea frost.

**urin-** SEE: *urino-.*

**urinaccelerator** (ū″rĭn-ăk-sĕl′ĕr-ā″tor) Musculus bulbospongiosus.

**urinal** (ū′rĭn-ăl) [L. *urina,* urine] **1.** A container into which one urinates. **2.** A toilet or bathroom fixture for receiving urine and flushing it away.

***condom u.*** Condom catheter.

**urinalysis** (ū″rĭ-năl′ĭ-sĭs) [″ + Gr. *ana,* apart, + *lysis,* a loosening] Analysis of the urine. SEE: *urine.*

**urinary** (ū′rĭ-nār″ē) [L. *urina,* urine] Pert. to, secreting, or containing urine.

**urinary bladder** A receptacle for urine excreted by the kidneys. SEE: *bladder.*

**urinary calculus** A concretion formed in the urinary passages. These vary in composition but may contain urates, calcium, oxalate, calcium carbonate, phosphates, and cystine. SEE: *calculus, renal; lithotriptor.*

NURSING IMPLICATIONS: The patient is encouraged to verbalize anxieties and concerns regarding severe pain. Pain relief measures are instituted as prescribed; they include analgesics, antispasmodics, and warm, moist heat. All urine is strained for stones, and any calculus is sent for laboratory analysis. If a lithotriptor is to be used, the duration of the procedure and follow-up care are explained. The nurse explains all diagnostic studies and encourages the patient to verbalize fears and concerns. Urine is observed for hematuria, and voided specimens are tested for specific gravity. Vital signs are monitored; if temperature is elevated, antipyretic measures are instituted as ordered. Fluids are forced to enhance dilution of urine, and intake and output are monitored. The nurse stays alert for complications such as infection, stasis, and retention. A catheter is inserted as ordered. Dietary management is based on the composition of the stone. If calcium stones are present, patients should reduce their intake of dietary calcium and increase their intake of foods that acidify the urine, such as cereals and cranberry and grape juices. If phosphate stones are present, patients should increase their intake of acid-ash foods such as cereals, eggs, meat, and cranberry and grape juices. Persons prone to uric acid stones should consume an alkaline-ash diet of green vegetables and fruits. To minimize urinary tract infections, esp. for female patients, the nurse teaches the patient proper perineal hygiene and emphasizes the need for increased fluid intake.

**urinary cast** A cast of the kidney tubules passed in the urine.

**urinary director appliance** A hand-held, hollow, plastic device that fits over the vulva, enabling a woman to urinate while standing. The device collects urine and allows it to be directed away from the user through an outlet spout. Intended use is for women who are active outdoors and need to urinate without partially disrobing. Medically, the appliance has been found to be useful in patients who have had a radical vulvectomy. Trade name is Sani-Fem Urinary Director and it is available from Sani-Fem, Downey, California.

Other devices for use by women in collecting urine are available. Some of these have the capacity to contain the specimen for later disposal rather than merely redirecting the flow.

**urinary diversion** The surgical redirection of

urine flow. SEE: *Nursing Diagnoses Appendix.*

**urinary elimination, altered patterns of** The state in which an individual experiences a disturbance in urine elimination. SEE: *Nursing Diagnoses Appendix*.

**urinary incontinence** SEE: *incontinence; incontinence, stress urinary*.

**urinary pigments** Urochrome, urobilin, uroerythrin, and hematoporphyrin.

**urinary retention** The state in which the individual experiences incomplete emptying of the bladder. High urethral pressure inhibits voiding until increased abdominal pressure causes urine to be involuntarily lost, or high urethral pressure inhibits complete emptying of the bladder. SEE: *Nursing Diagnoses Appendix*.

**urinary stammering** Temporary interruptions in voiding urine.

**urinary system** Kidneys, ureters, bladder, and urethra. SEE: illus.

**urinary tract** Urinary system.

**urinary tract infection** ABBR: UTI. Infection of the urinary tract with microorganisms. This condition may be asymptomatic, esp. during pregnancy. Asymptomatic UTI during pregnancy is a contributing factor to maternal and fetal morbidity. SYN: *cystitis*. SEE: *clean-catch method*.

ETIOLOGY: The most common cause (80%) of symptomatic UTI is *Escherichia coli;* an additional 5% to 15% are due to *Staphylococcus saprophyticus*. The small remaining percentage of infection may be caused by enterococci, *Klebsiella, Proteus mirabilis,* or other organisms. Symptomatic urethritis may be due to *Chlamydia trachomatis*.

SYMPTOMS: The most common symptoms include dysuria, urinary frequency,

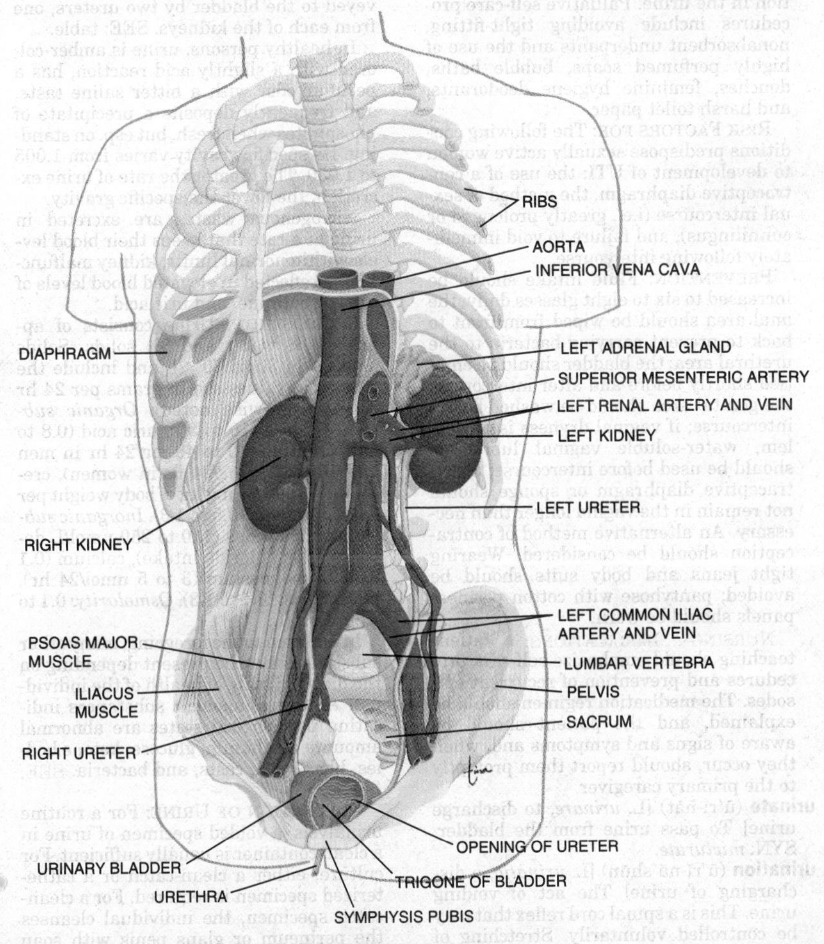


URINARY SYSTEM

and urgency. On occasion, women also complain of a feeling of not emptying the bladder and "heaviness" in the lower abdomen.

DIAGNOSIS: Microscopic examination of the urine reveals bacteria and an abnormal number of leukocytes. A variety of methods have been used to detect asymptomatic UTI, but the current belief is that the most effective method is by microscopic examination of Gram-stained urinary sediment.

TREATMENT: The antibiotic used will depend on the causative organism and the susceptibility of those bacteria to antibiotics available. The duration of therapy may be as short as several days for UTI in men and women who are not pregnant. In pregnant patients, asymptomatic UTI may need to be treated throughout the entire pregnancy. Daily fluid intake should be increased to 3 L; drinking water is important to dilute the bacterial concentration in the urine. Palliative self-care procedures include avoiding tight-fitting, nonabsorbent underpants and the use of highly perfumed soaps, bubble baths, douches, feminine hygiene deodorants, and harsh toilet paper.

RISK FACTORS FOR: The following conditions predispose sexually active women to development of UTI: the use of a contraceptive diaphragm, the method of sexual intercourse (i.e., greatly prolonged or cunnilingus), and failure to void immediately following intercourse.

PREVENTION: Fluid intake should be increased to six to eight glasses daily; the anal area should be wiped from front to back to prevent carrying bacteria to the urethral area; the bladder should be emptied shortly before and after intercourse; the genital area should be washed before intercourse; if vaginal dryness is a problem, water-soluble vaginal lubricants should be used before intercourse; a contraceptive diaphragm or sponge should not remain in the vagina longer than necessary. An alternative method of contraception should be considered. Wearing tight jeans and body suits should be avoided; pantyhose with cotton perineal panels should be worn.

NURSING IMPLICATIONS: Patient teaching should emphasize self-care procedures and prevention of recurrent episodes. The medication regimen should be explained, and the patient should be aware of signs and symptoms and, when they occur, should report them promptly to the primary caregiver.

**urinate** (ū′rĭ-nāt) [L. *urinare,* to discharge urine] To pass urine from the bladder. SYN: *micturate.*

**urination** (ū″rĭ-nā′shŭn) [L. *urinatio,* a discharging of urine] The act of voiding urine. This is a spinal cord reflex that may be controlled voluntarily. Stretching of the bladder initiates nerve impulses to the spinal cord; returning motor impulses cause contraction of the detrusor muscle of the bladder and relaxation of the bladder sphincter. Contraction of the external urethral sphincter may temporarily prevent urination. SYN: *micturition; uresis.*

DIFFERENTIAL DIAGNOSIS: Increased frequency is seen in polyuria; nervous excitement; irritation of the bladder, urethra, or urinary meatus; disease of the spinal cord; enlarged prostate in males; pregnancy in females; beer drinking; interstitial nephritis; diabetes; and phimosis. Decreased frequency occurs after dehydration, sweating, diarrhea, or bleeding; and in anuria, oliguria, uremia, brain disease, increased salt intake, drug poisoning, coma, and parenchymatous nephritis. SEE: *urine.*

**urine** (ū′rĭn) [L. *urina;* Gr. *ouron,* urine] The fluid excreted by the kidneys, stored in the bladder, and discharged, usually voluntarily, through the urethra. It is conveyed to the bladder by two ureters, one from each of the kidneys. SEE: table.

In healthy persons, urine is amber-colored with a slightly acid reaction, has a peculiar odor with a bitter saline taste, and frequently deposits a precipitate of phosphates when fresh, but esp. on standing. Its specific gravity varies from 1.005 to 1.030. The greater the rate of urine excretion, the lower the specific gravity.

Nitrogenous wastes are excreted in urine at a rate that keeps their blood levels within normal limits; kidney malfunction is reflected in elevated blood levels of urea, creatinine, and uric acid.

COMPOSITION: Urine consists of approx. 95% water and 5% solids. Solids amount to 30 to 70 g/L and include the following (values are in grams per 24 hr unless otherwise noted): *Organic substances:* urea (10 to 30), uric acid (0.8 to 1.0), creatine (10 to 40 mg/24 hr in men and 10 to 270 mg/24 hr in women), creatinine (15 to 25 mg/kg of body weight per day), ammonia (0.5 to 1.3). *Inorganic substances:* chlorides (110 to 250 nmol/L depending on chloride intake), calcium (0.1 to 0.2), magnesium (3 to 5 nmol/24 hr), phosphorus (0.4 to 1.3). *Osmolarity:* 0.1 to 2.5 mOsm/L.

In addition to the foregoing, many other substances may be present depending on the diet and state of health of the individual. Among component substances indicating pathological states are abnormal amounts of albumin, glucose, ketone bodies, blood, pus, casts, and bacteria. SEE: illus.

COLLECTION OF URINE: For a routine urinalysis, a voided specimen of urine in a clean container is usually sufficient. For culture, either a clean-catch or a catheterized specimen is required. For a clean-catch specimen, the individual cleanses the perineum or glans penis with soap and water or an antiseptic solution such

## Significance of Changes in Urine

| Normal | Abnormal | Significance |
|---|---|---|
| ***Quantity*** | | |
| 1000–1500 ml (approx. 95% $H_2O$) | | Depends on water and fluid, foods consumed, exercise, temperature, kidney function |
| | High (polyuria) | Diabetes mellitus, diabetes insipidus, nervous diseases, certain types of chronic nephritis (kidney disorder), diuretics (e.g., caffeine, digitalis) causing increased urinary excretion |
| | Low (oliguria) | Acute nephritis, heart disease, fevers, eclampsia, diarrhea, vomiting, inadequate fluid intake |
| | None (anuria) | Uremia (nitrogenous wastes in blood), acute nephritis, metal poisoning (e.g., due to bichloride of mercury), complete obstruction of urinary tract |
| ***Color*** | | |
| Yellow to amber | | Depends on concentration of pigment (urochrome) |
| | Pale | Diabetes insipidus; due to a very dilute urine |
| | Milky | Fat globules, pus in genitourinary infections |
| | Reddish | Blood pigments, drugs, or food pigments |
| | Greenish | Bile pigment, associated with jaundice |
| | Brown-black | Poisoning (mercury, lead, phenol), hemorrhage |
| ***Transparency*** | | |
| Clear | | Normal |
| Cloudy on standing | | Precipitation of mucin from urinary tract; not pathological |
| Turbid | | Precipitation of calcium phosphate; not pathological |
| | Milky | Presence of fat globules; pathological |
| | Turbid | Presence of pus due to inflammation of urinary tract; pathological |
| ***Odor*** | | |
| Faintly aromatic | | Normal |
| | Pleasant (sweet) | Acetone, associated with diabetes mellitus |
| | Unpleasant | Decomposition or ingestion of certain drugs or foods |
| Peppermint | | Menthol ingestion |
| Acrid | | Asparagus in diet |
| Spicy | | Ingestion of sandalwood oil or saffron |

*Table continued on following page*

**Significance of Changes in Urine** (Continued)

| *Proteinuria* | | |
|---|---|---|
| **Normal** | **Abnormal** | **Significance** |
| Albumin and globulin | | Excretion of 10–100 mg each 24 hr is normal but this amount is not detected by usual tests |
| | Albumin | Evidence of altered renal function; may be due to renal pathology or a systemic disease such as diabetes mellitus |
| | Globulin | Bence Jones proteins associated with multiple myeloma and diseases of globulin metabolism. Other types of globulins may be present in acute and chronic pyelonephritis |

| *Specific Gravity* | | |
|---|---|---|
| **Normal** | **Abnormal** | **Significance** |
| 1.010–1.025 specific gravity; can vary in the absence of pathology | | Ordinary; specific gravity inversely proportional to volume |
| | Low (chronic) | Dilution if volume is large; otherwise nephritis |
| | High (chronic) | Acute nephritis; concentrated if volume is small; otherwise, if light colored and volume is large, diabetes mellitus |

| *Acidity* | | |
|---|---|---|
| **Normal** | **Abnormal** | **Significance** |
| Acid (slight) | | Diet of acid-forming foods (meats, eggs, prunes, wheat) overbalances the base-forming foods (vegetables and fruits) |
| | High acidity | Acidosis, diabetes mellitus, many pathological disorders (fevers, starvation) |
| | Alkaline | Vegetarian diet changes urea into ammonium carbonate; infection or ingestion of alkaline compounds |

as benzalkonium chloride before voiding. A midstream specimen of urine is then collected in a sterilized container. A catheterized specimen is obtained by passing a catheter into the bladder, using sterile technique. SEE: *suprapubic catheter*.

NOTE: A urine specimen may be obtained to test for excretion of drugs of abuse. In such cases, care must be taken to ensure that the specimen was produced by the individual and that there was no opportunity for the specimen to be diluted with water or someone else's urine.

DIAGNOSIS: *Color:* Normal urine is amber colored, resulting from the presence of urobilin, a pigment mainly derived from bilirubin, in the bile. This pigment is found in excessive quantities in fever and may indicate excess destruction of red blood cells. The effect of food and medication must be considered before concluding that the color of the urine is abnormal. *Black:* This may indicate melanuria, malignant pigmented tumor, melanotic cancer, or carbolic acid poisoning. *Bile-colored:* This is seen in jaundice. *Blue:* Urine that is blue may result from methylene blue or the presence of indigo. *Colorless:* This is known as achromaturia and is usually due to the urine's being extremely dilute. *Lime green:* The presence of a blue substance such as methylene blue or indican and yellow urochrome produces this color. *Milky:* Urine that is milky may be due to chyluria, lipuria, or pus. *Orange-red:* This may indicate the presence of pyridine dyes. *Pale:* Pale urine indicates an excess of fluid intake; it is found in conditions causing polyuria. *Red or reddish:* This may be due to the presence of blood in the urine, hematuria, phenolsulfonphthalein, or to senna or rhubarb, which may color the urine either brown or orange. Psychopathic or malingering patients have added ketchup or tomato juice to their urine specimen to make it appear to be blood stained.

*Odor: Ammoniacal:* This odor may re-

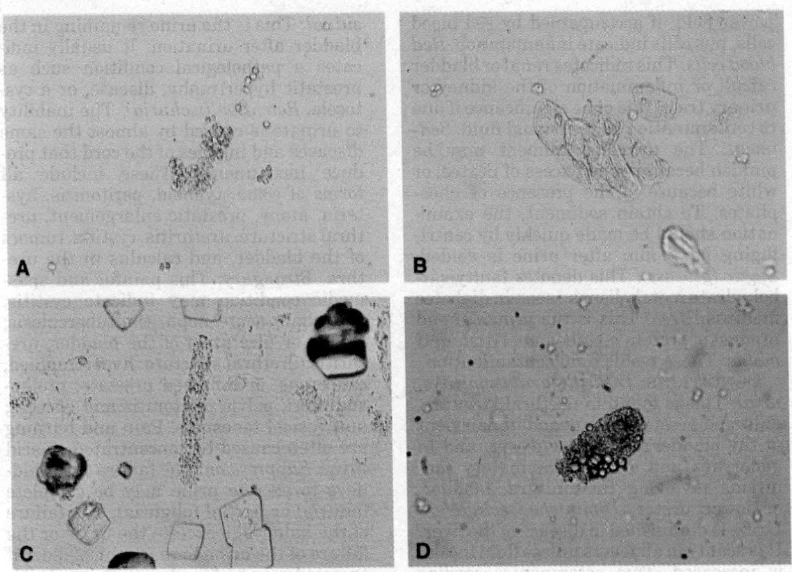


URINE

(A) WHITE BLOOD CELLS, (B) SQUAMOUS EPITHELIAL CELLS, (C) GRANULAR CAST AND URIC ACID CRYSTALS, (D) FAT BODY (ORIG. MAG. ×400)

sult from decomposition products. *Aromatic:* This is the odor of normal urine. *Fecal:* This may be due to fistulous communications between the intestinal and urinary tracts. *Fishy:* A fishy odor indicates cystitis. *New-mown hay:* This indicates diabetes. *Overripe apple:* An odor such as this may indicate acetonuria or the presence of acetone bodies in the urine. *Violet:* This odor may be caused by turpentine.

NOTE: Some foods, esp. asparagus, may cause the urine to have a characteristic odor. This is a transient phenomenon.

PRODUCTS IN DISEASE: *Acidic:* Urine that is acidic may be found in acidosis and pyelonephritis. *Alkaline:* A white sediment characterizes alkaline urine. *Albumin:* This is due to nephritis and inflammation of the mucous membrane of any portion of the urinary apparatus. *Acetone:* The presence of acetone represents the byproducts of excessive fat metabolism excreted by the kidneys and known as ketonuria. *Animal parasites:* These are rare, found as a result of contamination. *Bacteria:* Bacteria in the urine are usually regarded as being of little importance if fewer than 100,000 can be cultured from each milliliter of urine. The urine appears cloudy. *Bile:* Bile in the urine indicates abnormal retention of bile. *Blood:* Urine containing blood shows a smoky sediment and is reddish-brown. It may indicate hemorrhagic nephritis, calculi, congestion of a kidney, renal carcinoma, tuberculosis of the kidney, chronic infections, or trauma. *Casts:* These indicate renal disease. A few hyaline casts in the aged denote slight damage to the kidneys. Casts are found in large numbers in nephritis. The less acute the disease, the finer are the granular casts. *Crystals:* Calcium oxalate and uric acid crystals are present in acid urine, and crystals of ammonium biurate and phosphates in alkaline urine. The only crystals having significance are leucine and tyrosine crystals, which may indicate liver disease. *Cylindroids:* This has no special significance. *Acetoacetic acid:* This is due to deficient carbohydrate metabolism of an advanced stage and is preceded by the presence of acetone. *Epithelial cells (squamous):* If in large numbers from the urinary bladder and ureters, they indicate inflammation of these parts; epithelial cells of the kidney indicate serious kidney damage. *Fat droplets:* These indicate fatty degeneration of the kidneys and lipemia. *Froth:* This indicates the presence of bile. *Indican:* This is of little significance but is seen in intestinal putrefaction. *Mucus:* If mucus is visible and in quantity, urethritis is indicated. It is of no special significance in women if the quantity is small. *Mucous threads:* These mucoid ribbon-like structures are of no great significance. *Pus:* This is mucoid and shows a white sediment. It is found in bacterial infections of the urinary tract. The presence of the occasional pus cell may be normal per high-power field; if accompanied by red blood cells, pus cells indicate inflammation. *Red blood cells:* This indicates renal or bladder calculi or inflammation of the kidney or urinary tract. It is of no significance if due to contamination by menstrual fluid. *Sediment:* The urinary sediment may be pinkish because of an excess of urates, or white because of the presence of phosphates. To obtain sediment, the examination should be made quickly by centrifuging for 3 min after urine is voided. *Sugar (glucose):* This denotes faulty carbohydrate metabolism as seen in diabetes mellitus. *Urea:* This is the principal end product of protein metabolism. *Yeasts and molds:* These result from contamination.

CONDITIONS: *Difficult urination (dysuria):* This is found in urethral stricture, enlarged prostate, atony and impairment of the bladder's muscular power, and in gonorrhea and other inflammatory conditions involving the urethra, bladder, or lower ureter. *Diminished (oliguria):* Urine is diminished in disease of the liver. It is scanty in all fevers unless fluid intake is increased. This accompanies cardiac failure; acute, chronic, and parenchymatous nephritis; obstruction of return venous circulation of the kidney; thrombosis of the renal vein or inferior vena cava; loss of fluids through hemorrhages, vomiting, or diarrhea; inadequate fluid intake; obstruction or pressure on the ureter; and lead poisoning.

*Incontinence (enuresis):* An inability to retain urine because of paralysis or relaxation of sphincters or contraction of the longitudinal muscular layer of the bladder results in incontinence and dribbling. This can occur in all forms of coma, during an epileptic seizure, shock, typhoid, and typhus. It may also occur in conjunction with injuries to or tumors of the spinal cord, transverse myelitis, spinal meningitis, locomotor ataxia, paralysis, and reflex excitability of the nervous system. Other causes include local irritation of the bladder, cystitis, phimosis, vesical calculus, contracted meatus, ascarides, and very concentrated urine. SEE: *incontinence, urinary stress.*

*Increased (polyuria):* This occurs in fevers, esp. if weight is lost; after pregnancy; during parturition; and after the intake of large quantities of liquid. It may indicate chronic interstitial nephritis; diabetes mellitus or insipidus; amyloid disease of the kidney; reabsorption of effusions; and functional disease of the nervous system, as in hysteria and neurasthenia. It is persistent in bulbar, cerebellar, and spinal tumors; locomotor ataxia; and meningitis. *Obstructive:* This is the result of occlusion of one or both ureters or occlusion of the urethra. *Painful:* This is from dysuria or irritation of the bladder with spasmodic contractions. There is a persistent desire to urinate. *Residual:* This is the urine remaining in the bladder after urination. It usually indicates a pathological condition such as prostatic hypertrophy, disease, or a cystocele. *Retention (ischuria):* The inability to urinate is caused by almost the same diseases and injuries of the cord that produce incontinence. These include all forms of coma, typhoid, peritonitis, hysteria, atony, prostatic enlargement, urethral stricture, urethritis, cystitis, tumors of the bladder, and calculus in the urethra. *Strangury:* This painful and spasmodic condition may indicate cystitis; neuralgia; acute nephritis; tuberculosis; cancer or ulceration of the bladder; urethritis; urethral stricture; hypertrophied, cancerous, or inflamed prostate; prolapsus uteri; pelvic peritonitis and abscess; and vesical tenesmus. Pain and burning are often caused by concentrated or acid urine. *Suppression:* The failure of the kidneys to excrete urine may be complete (anuria) or partial (oliguria). The failure of the kidneys to excrete the urine or the failure of the urine to reach the bladder if excreted may be found in acute nephritis or congestion, renal abscess, and the last stages of chronic nephritis. Renal damage may be caused by the patient's having received a blood transfusion with incompatible blood.

**double-voided u.** A urine sample voided 30 min after the patient has emptied the bladder.

**midstream specimen of u.** A specimen collected after the initial flow of urine has begun. This permits obtaining a sample free of urethral debris. SEE: *clean-catch method.*

**residual u.** SEE: *residual urine.*

**urino-, urin-** Combining form meaning *urine.* SEE: *uro-.*

**urinogenital** (ū″rĭ-nō-jĕn′ĭ-tăl) [″ + *genitalia,* genitals] Urogenital.

**urinology** (ū″rĭ-nŏl′ō-jē) Urology.

**urinoma** (ū″rĭ-nō′mă) [″ + Gr. *oma,* mass] A cyst containing urine.

**urinometer** (ū″rĭ-nŏm′ĕ-tĕr) [″ + Gr. *metron,* measure] A device, a form of hydrometer, for determining the specific gravity of urine. A weighted float is placed in the urine and the depth to which it sinks is noted on a scale suitable for urine specific gravity. The calibration temperature of the urinometer is 60°F (15.6°C). If the urine is not at that temperature, the specific gravity reading will need to be adjusted for the actual temperature of the urine. For every 5.4°F (3°C) that the urine is above 60°F, 0.001 is added to the reading; for every 5.4°F (3°C) that the temperature of the urine is below the calibration temperature, 0.001 is subtracted from the reading. Example: The urinometer reading is 1.015 and the temperature of the urine is 82°F, a difference of 22°F from the calibration temperature of 60°F. Thus 22 divided by 5.4 equals 4.07. This times

0.001 is approximately 1.004. This added to the 1.015 reading indicates the specific gravity is 1.019. SEE: *hydrometer*.

**urinophil** (ū′rĭ-nō-fĭl) [″ + Gr. *philein*, to love] Capable of existing in the urine, such as bacteria that grow best in urine.

**urinose, urinous** (ū′rĭ-nōs, ū′rĭ-nŭs) [L. *urina*, urine] Having the characteristics of or containing urine.

**uriposia** (ū″rĭ-pō′zē-ă) [″ + *posis*, drinking] Drinking of urine.

**uro-** [Gr. *ouron*, urine] Combining form meaning *urine*. SEE: *urino-*.

**uroammoniac** (ū″rō-ă-mō′nē-ăk) Containing urine and ammonia.

**urobilin** (ū″rō-bī′lĭn) [″ + L. *bilis*, bile] A brown pigment formed by the oxidation of urobilinogen, a decomposition product of bilirubin. Urobilin may be formed from the urobilinogen in stools or in urine after exposure to air.

**urobilinemia** (ū″rō-bī″lĭn-ē′mē-ă) [″ + ″ + Gr. *haima*, blood] Urobilin in the blood.

**urobilinicterus** (ū″rō-bī-lĭn-ĭk′tĕr-ŭs) [″ + L. *bilis*, bile, + Gr. *ikteros*, jaundice] Jaundice resulting from urobilinemia.

**urobilinogen** (ū″rō-bī-lĭn′ō-jĕn) [″ + ″ + Gr. *gennan*, to produce] A colorless derivative of bilirubin, from which it is formed by the action of intestinal bacteria.

**urobilinogenemia** (ū″rō-bī″lĭn-ō-jĕn-ē′mē-ă) [″ + ″ + ″ + *haima*, blood] Urobilinogen in the blood.

**urobilinuria** (ū″rō-bī″lĭn-ū′rē-ă) [″ + ″ + Gr. *ouron*, urine] Excess of urobilin in the urine.

**urocele** (ū′rō-sēl) [″ + *kele*, tumor, swelling] Escape of urine into the scrotum. SYN: *uroscheocele*.

**urochesia** (ū-rō-kē′zē-ă) [″ + *chezein*, to defecate] A discharge of urine in the feces.

**urochrome** (ū′rō-krōm) [″ + *chroma*, color] The pigment that gives urine its characteristic color. It is derived from urobilin.

**urocyanin** (ū-rō-sī′ă-nĭn) [″ + *kyanos*, blue] A blue pigment present in the urine in certain diseases, esp. scarlet fever.

**urocyanogen** (ū″rō-sī-ăn′ō-jĕn) [″ + ″ + *gennan*, to produce] A blue pigment in urine, esp. in cholera patients.

**urocyanosis** (ū″rō-sī-ăn-ō′sĭs) [″ + ″ + *osis*, condition] Blue discoloration of the urine; possibly due to the presence of indigo blue from oxidation of indican or to ingestion of drugs such as methylene blue. SEE: *indicanuria*.

**urodynamics** (ū″rō-dī-năm′ĭks) The study of the holding or storage of urine in the bladder, the facility with which it empties, and the rate of movement of urine out of the bladder during micturition.

**urodynia** (ū″rō-dĭn′ē-ă) [″ + *odyne*, pain] Pain associated with urination.

**uroerythrin** (ū″rō-ĕr′ĭth-rĭn) [″ + *erythros*, red] Purpurin (2).

**uroflavin** (ū″rō-flā′vĭn) A fluorescent compound present in the urine of persons taking riboflavin.

**uroflowmeter** A device for recording urine flow; used to quantitate obstruction to urine flowing from the bladder.

**urofuscin** (ū″rō-fūs′ĭn) [″ + L. *fuscus*, dark brown] A red-brown pigment sometimes found in samples of urine, esp. in cases of porphyrinuria.

**urofuscohematin** (ū″rō-fūs″kō-hĕm′ăt-ĭn) [″ + ″ + Gr. *haima*, blood] A reddish-brown pigment in urine in some diseases.

**urogastrone** (ū″rō-găs′trōn) [″ + *gaster*, belly] A polypeptide present in urine that has an inhibitory effect on gastric secretion.

**urogenital** (ū″rō-jĕn′ĭ-tăl) [″ + L. *genitalia*, genitals] Pert. to the urinary and reproductive organs. SYN: *urinogenital*.

**urogenous** (ū-rŏj′ĕn-ŭs) [″ + *gennan*, to produce] **1.** Producing urine. **2.** Originating in urine.

**urogram** (ū′rō-grăm) [″ + *gramma*, something written] A radiograph of the urinary tract.

**urography** (ū′rŏg′ră-fē) [Gr. *ouron*, urine, + *graphein*, to write] Radiography of the urinary tract after the introduction of a contrast medium.

***ascending u.*** Urography in which the radiopaque dye is injected into the bladder during cystoscopy. SYN: *cystoscopic u.; retrograde u.*

***cystoscopic u.*** Ascending u.

***descending u.*** Urography in which an injected dye is excreted by the kidney and studied by x-ray examination during excretion. SYN: *excretion u.; intravenous u.*

***excretion u., excretory u.*** Descending u.

***intravenous u.*** Descending u.

***retrograde u.*** Ascending u.

**urohematin** (ū″rō-hĕm′ăt-ĭn) [″ + *haima*, blood] Pigment in urine, considered as identical with hematin, that alters the color of urine in proportion to the degree of oxidation.

**urohematonephrosis** (ū″rō-hĕm″ă-tō-nē-frō′sĭs) [″ + ″ + *nephros*, kidney] A pathological condition of the kidney in which the pelvis is distended with blood and urine.

**urohematoporphyrin** (ū″rō-hĕm″ă-tō-por′fĭr-ĭn) [″ + ″ + *porphyra*, purple] Iron-free hematin in urine when intravascular hemolysis occurs.

**urokinase** (ū-rō-kī′nās) An enzyme obtained from human urine; used experimentally for dissolving venous thrombi and pulmonary emboli. It is administered intravenously.

**urokinetic** (ū″rō-kĭ-nĕt′ĭk) [″ + *kinesis*, movement] Resulting reflexly from stimulation of the urinary organs.

**urolagnia** (ū-rō-lăg′nē-ă) [″ + *lagneia*, lust] Sexual excitation associated with urine or urination (e.g., watching another person urinate or having another person urinate on one's own body). SEE: *undinism*.

**urolith** (ū′rō-lĭth) [″ + *lithos*, stone] A concretion in the urine.

**urolithiasis** (ū″rō-lĭ-thī′ă-sĭs) [″ + ″ + *-iasis*,

condition] The formation of urinary calculi and the illness associated with the presence of calculi in the urinary tract. SEE: *calculus, renal; Nursing Diagnoses Appendix.*

**urolithic** (ū″rō-lĭth′ĭk) Concerning urinary calculi.

**urological** (ū-rō-lŏj′ĭk-ăl) [″ + *logos,* word, reason] Pert. to urology.

**urologist** (ū-rŏl′ō-jĭst) A physician who specializes in the practice of urology.

**urology** (ū-rŏl′ō-jē) [″+ *logos,* word, reason] The branch of medicine concerned with the urinary tract in both sexes and the male genital tract.

**urolutein** (ū-rō-lū′tē-ĭn) [″ + L. *luteus,* yellow] A yellow pigment seen in the urine.

**uromedulin, human** The most abundant protein of renal origin in normal urine. This glycoprotein is the same protein termed Tamm-Horsfall mucoprotein. SEE: *mucoprotein, Tamm-Horsfall.*

**uromelanin** (ū-rō-mĕl′ăn-ĭn) [″ + *melas,* black] A black pigment occurring in urine resulting from the decomposition of urochrome.

**uromelus** (ū-rŏm′ē-lŭs) [Gr. *oura,* tail, + *melos,* limb] A congenitally deformed fetus in which the lower extremities are fused. SYN: *sirenomelia.*

**uronephrosis** (ū″rō-nĕf-rō′sĭs) [″ + *nephros,* kidney, + *osis,* condition] Dilatation of the renal structures from obstruction of the urinary flow; distention of the renal pelvis and tubules with urine. SYN: *hydronephrosis.*

**uronophile** (ū-rŏn′ō-fĭl) [″ + *philein,* to love] A microorganism that grows best in a culture containing urine.

**uropathogen** (ū″rō-păth′ō-jĕn) [″+ *pathos,* disease, suffering, + *gennan,* to produce] A microorganism capable of causing disease of the urinary tract.

**uropathy** (ū-rŏp′ă-thē) Any disease affecting the urinary tract.

***obstructive u.*** Any disease resulting from obstruction of the urinary tract.

**uropepsin** (ū″rō-pĕp′sĭn) The end product of pepsin metabolism. It is excreted in the urine.

**urophein, urophaein** (ū″rō-fē′ĭn) [″ + *phaios,* gray] Gray pigment sometimes found in urine.

**urophosphometer** (ū″rō-fŏs-fŏm′ĕ-tĕr) [″ + L. *phosphas,* phosphorus] A device for estimating the amount of phosphorus in the urine.

**uroplania** (ū″rō-plā′nē-ă) [″ + *plane,* a wandering] A condition in which urine is present in or discharged from parts other than the urinary organs.

**uropoiesis** (ū″rō-poy-ē′sĭs) [Gr. *ouron,* urine, + *poiesis,* production] The formation of urine by the kidneys.

**uropoietic** (ū″rō-poy-ĕt′ĭk) [″+ *poiein,* to form] Pert. to the formation of urine.

**uroporphyria** (ū″rō-por-fĭr′ē-ă) Porphyria in which an excess amount of uroporphyrin is excreted in the urine.

**uroporphyrin** (ū″rō-por′fĭ-rĭn) A red pigment present in the urine and feces in cases of porphyria; may also be present in the urine of persons taking certain drugs.

**uroporphyrinogen** (ū″rō-por″fĭ-rĭn′ō-jĕn) Any one of several porphyrins that are the precursors of uroporphyrins.

***u. I*** An abnormal isomer of a precursor of protoporphyrin, which accumulates in one form of porphyria. It causes the urine to be red, the teeth to fluoresce brightly in ultraviolet light, and the skin to be abnormally sensitive to sunlight. This is observed in congenital erythropoietic porphyria.

**uropsammus** (ū″rō-săm′ŭs) [″+ *psammos,* sand] Gravel or calcareous sediment in the urine.

**uropyoureter** (ū″rō-pī″ō-ū-rē′tĕr) [″+ ″ + *oureter,* ureter] Accumulation of urine and pus in the ureter.

**urorrhodin** (ū-rō-rō′dĭn) [″ + *rhodon,* rose] A rose-colored pigment in the urine in certain infectious diseases such as typhoid fever and tuberculosis.

**uroscheocele** (ū-rŏs′kē-ō-sēl) [″ + *oscheon,* scrotum, + *kele,* tumor, swelling] Urocele.

**uroschesis** (ū-rŏs′kĕs-ĭs) [″ + *schesis,* a holding] **1.** Suppression of urine. **2.** Retention of urine.

**uroscopy** (ū-rŏs′kō-pē) [″+ *skopein,* to examine] **1.** Examination of the urine. **2.** Diagnosis by examination of the urine.

**urotoxin** (ū″rō-tŏk′sĭn) Toxic substances in the urine.

**uroureter** (ū″rō-ū′rē-tĕr, ū″rō-ū-rē′tĕr) [″ + *oureter,* ureter] Distention of the ureter with urine caused by stricture or obstruction.

**uroxanthin** (ū″rō-zăn′thĭn) [″ + *xanthos,* yellow] Yellow pigment of the urine; an indigo-forming substance.

**uroxin** (ū-rŏk′sĭn) [″ + *oxys,* sharp] Alloxantin, a derivative of alloxan.

**ursodiol** A drug used to treat cholesterol gallstones. SEE: *gallstone.*

**urtica** (ŭr-tī′kă) *pl.* **urticae** [L., nettle] A wheal.

**urticant** (ŭr′tĭ-kănt) That which causes an urticarial reaction in the skin.

**urticaria** (ŭr-tĭ-kā′rē-ă) [L. *urtica,* nettle] A vascular reaction of the skin characterized by a sudden general eruption of pale evanescent wheals or papules, which are associated with severe itching. This condition may be caused by contact with an external irritant such as the nettle, physical agents, foods, insect bites, serum sickness, pollens, drugs, or neurogenic factors. SYN: *hives; nettle rash.* SEE: illus.; *allergy; angioneurotic edema.*

TREATMENT: Unless a preventable cause can be identified, the treatment is symptomatic. Antihistamines are effective in most cases. In severe cases that do not respond to antihistamines, corticosteroids are used.

***aquagenic u.*** Urticaria caused by exposure of the skin to ordinary water.

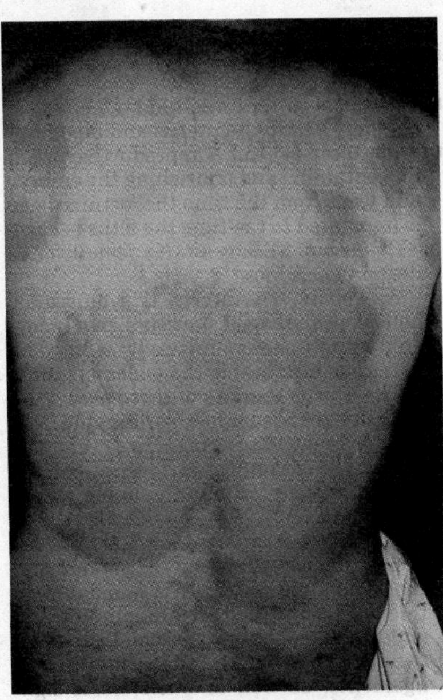

URTICARIA

LARGE WHEALS IN PATIENT ALLERGIC TO PENICILLIN

***u. bullosa*** Eruption of temporary vesicles with infusion of fluid under the epidermis.

***cold u.*** Cold-induced urticarial eruption that may progress to angioedema.

***u. factitia*** Urticaria following slight irritation of the skin. SYN: *dermatographia*.

***u. gigantea*** Angioneurotic edema.

***u. haemorrhagica*** Urticaria with lesions infiltrated with blood.

***u. maculosa*** A chronic form of urticaria with red-colored lesions.

***u. medicamentosa*** Urticaria due to certain drugs.

***u. papulosa*** A form of urticaria in which the wheal is followed by a lingering papule that is attended by considerable itching; most commonly observed in debilitated children. SYN: *lichen urticatus; prurigo simplex*.

***u. pigmentosa*** A form of urticaria characterized by persistent, pigmented maculopapular lesions that urticate when stroked (Darier's sign). It typically occurs in childhood. Biopsy reveals infiltration by mast cells.

***pressure u.*** Urticaria that is produced by pressure perpendicular to the surface of the skin. The persistent red swelling appears after a delay of 1 to 4 hr.

***solar u.*** Urticaria occurring in certain individuals following exposure to sunlight.

**urticarial** (ŭr″tĭ-kā′rē-ăl) [L. *urtica,* nettle] Pert. to urticaria.

**urticate** (ŭr′tĭ-kāt) **1.** To produce urticaria. **2.** Marked by the appearance of wheals.

**urushiol** (ū-roo′shē-ŏl″) [Japanese *urushi,* lac, + L. *oleum,* oil] The principal toxic irritant substance of plants such as poison ivy, which produces characteristic severe dermatitis on contact.

**U.S. AEC** *U.S. Atomic Energy Commission.*

**USAN** *United States Adopted Names* (for drugs).

**USAN and the USP Dictionary of Drug Names** A dictionary of nonproprietary names, brand names, code designations, and Chemical Abstracts Service registry numbers for drugs. The 1995 edition is cumulative for U.S. adopted names (USAN) from June 15, 1961, through June 15, 1994.

**USDA** *United States Department of Agriculture.*

**Usher's syndrome** [Charles Howard Usher, Brit. ophthalmologist, 1865–1942] A hereditary disorder characterized by a combination of congenital deafness and retinitis pigmentosa that results in a gradual loss of vision.

**USP, U.S. Phar.** *United States Pharmacopeia.*

**U.S.P.H.S.** *United States Public Health Service.*

**USP-PRN** *United States Pharmacopeia–Practitioners' Reporting Network.*

**ustilaginism** (ŭs-tĭl-ăj′ĭn-ĭzm) [L. *ustulatus,* scorched, + Gr. *-ismos,* condition] Poisoning resulting from eating corn infected with smut fungus, *Ustilago maydis.*

**Ustilago** (ŭs-tĭl-ā′gō) A moldlike fungus, *Ustilago maydis,* commonly called smut.

**uta** (ū′tă) American leishmaniasis.

**Utah Elbow** A myoelectric prosthesis that uses an electrode and microprocessors to control both the elbow and the terminal device. The system is also designed to permit a natural elbow swing during walking.

**ut dict** L. *ut dictum,* as directed.

**utend** L. *utendus,* to be used.

**uter-** SEE: *utero-.*

**uteralgia** (ū″tĕr-ăl′jē-ă) [L. *uterus,* womb, + Gr. *algos,* pain] Uterine pain.

**uterectomy** (ū″tĕr-ĕk′tō-mē) [″ + Gr. *ektome,* excision] Hysterectomy.

**uterine** (ū′tĕr-ĭn, -īn) [L. *uterinus*] Pert. to the uterus.

**uterine artery Doppler velocimetry** SEE: *Doppler echocardiography.*

**uterine bleeding** Bleeding from the uterus. Physiological bleeding via the vagina occurs in normal menstruation. Abnormal forms include excessive menstrual flow (hypermenorrhea, menorrhagia) or too frequent menstruation (polymenorrhea). Nonmenstrual bleeding is called metrorrhagia. Pseudomenstrual or withdrawal bleeding may occur following estrogen therapy. Breakthrough bleeding is the term used for intermenstrual bleeding that sometimes occurs in women who take progestational agents such as birth control pills or receive estrogen-progesterone replacement therapy. SEE: *amenorrhea; menstruation; tampon, menstrual; Nursing Diagnoses Appendix.*

**uterine gland** One of the tubular glands in the endometrium.

**uterine souffle** A vascular sound that may be heard in the pregnant uterus by using a stethoscope.

**uterine subinvolution** Failure of the uterus to return to its normal size after childbirth. A uterus that weighs more than 100 g is considered to be enlarged.

**uterine tube** Fallopian tube.

**utero-, uter-** Combining form meaning *uterus.* SEE: *hystero-; metro-.*

**uteroabdominal** (ū″tĕr-ō-ăb-dŏm′ĭ-năl) [L. *uterus,* womb, + *abdomen,* belly] Pert. to both the uterus and abdomen.

**uterocele** (ū-tĕr′ō-sēl) [″ + Gr. *kele,* tumor, swelling] Hernia containing the uterus.

**uterocervical** (ū″tĕr-ō-sĕr′vĭ-kăl) [″ + *cervix,* neck] Rel. to the uterus and cervix.

**uterocystostomy** (ū″tĕr-ō-sĭs-tŏs′tō-mē) [″ + Gr. *kystis,* bladder, + *stoma,* mouth] The formation of a passage between the uterine cervix and the bladder.

**uterofixation** (ū″tĕr-ō-fĭks-ā′shŭn) [″ + *fixatio,* a fixing] Fixation of a displaced uterus.

**uterography** (ū″tĕr-ŏg′ră-fē) [″ + Gr. *graphein,* to write] Radiography of the uterus.

**uterolith** (ū′tĕr-ō-lĭth) [″ + Gr. *lithos,* stone] A uterine concretion.

**uterometer** (ū″tĕr-ŏm′ĕt-er) [″ + Gr. *metron,* measure] A device for measuring the uterus and determining its position.

**uteroovarian** (ū″tĕr-ō-ō-vā′rē-ăn) [″ + LL. *ovarium,* ovary] Rel. to the uterus and ovary.

**uteropexia, uteropexy** (ū″tĕr-ō-pĕks′ē-ă, ū′tĕr-ō-pĕks″ē) [″ + Gr. *pexis,* fixation] Fixation of the uterus to the abdominal wall.

**uteroplacental** (ū″tĕr-ō-plă-sĕn′tăl) [″ + *placenta,* a flat cake] Rel. to the placenta and uterus.

**uteroplasty** (ū″tĕr-ō-plăs′tē) [″ + Gr. *plassein,* to form] Plastic surgery of the uterus. SYN: *metroplasty.*

**uterorectal** (ū″tĕr-ō-rĕk′tăl) Concerning the uterus and rectum.

**uterosacral** (ū″tĕr-ō-sā′krăl) [″ + *sacralis,* pert. to the sacrum] Rel. to the uterus and sacrum.

**uterosalpingography** (ū″tĕr-ō-săl-pĭng-ŏg′ră-fē) [″ + Gr. *salpinx,* tube, + *graphein,* to write] Radiography of the uterus and fallopian tubes after the introduction of a contrast medium.

**uterotomy** (ū-tĕr-ŏt′ō-mē) Incision of the uterus.

**uterotractor** (ū″tĕr-ō-trăk′tor) [″ + *tractor,* drawer] An instrument for applying traction to the cervix uteri.

**uterotubal** (ū″tĕr-ō-tū′băl) [″ + *tuba,* tube] Relating to the uterus and oviducts.

**uterovaginal** (ū″tĕr-ō-văj′ĭ-năl) [″ + *vagina,* sheath] Rel. to the uterus and vagina.

**uteroventral** (ū″tĕr-ō-vĕn′trăl) Uteroabdominal.

**uterovesical** (ū″tĕr-ō-vĕs′ĭ-kăl) [″ + *vesica,* bladder] Rel. to the uterus and bladder.

**uterus** (ū′tĕr-ŭs) [L.] A reproductive organ for containing and nourishing the embryo and fetus from the time the fertilized egg is implanted to the time the fetus is born. SYN: *womb.* SEE: *genitalia, female* for illus.; *pregnancy test.*

ANATOMY: The uterus is a muscular, hollow, pear-shaped structure, partly covered by peritoneum; the cavity is lined by a mucous membrane, the endometrium.

The uterus consists of three areas: the body or expanded upper portion, the isthmus or constricted central area, and the cervix, the lowermost cylindrical portion that joins the uterus to the upper end of the vagina.

The uterus is situated in the midpelvis, approx. halfway between the sacrum and the symphysis pubis. It is supported in this position by the pelvic diaphragm and supplemented by two broad ligaments, two round ligaments, and two uterosacral ligaments, as well as other lesser ligaments. The rounded portion of the body lying above the openings of the two uterine tubes is the fundus. The lateral borders of the fundus to which the tubes are attached are called the cornual ends. The fallopian tubes communicate with the peritoneal cavity and provide the pathway for the ova to go from the ovary to the uterine cavity. The cavity of the uterus, a potential space, is triangular, with the base of the triangle in the fundal portion. The canal of the cervix is long and narrow and is constricted at the upper end by the internal os and at the lower end by the external os.

The largest portion of the uterus is made up of smooth muscle that is longitudinal and circular. The outer covering of the uterus is the peritoneum, with the exception of that part on which the bladder rests and the vaginal portion of the cervix. The lining of the body of the uterus varies in form and histological structure with the period of life in which it is studied, the prepuberty stage, the actively menstruating stage, and the menopausal stage, each having its own characteristics. The uterus is normally anteflexed. Its blood supply is derived from the uterine and ovarian arteries.

POSITIONS: *Anteflexion:* The uterus bends forward. *Anteversion:* The fundus is displaced forward toward the pubis, while the cervix is tilted up toward the sacrum. *Retroflexion:* The uterus bends backward at the junction of the body and the cervix. *Retroversion:* The uterus inclines backward with retention of the normal curve; this position is the opposite of anteversion.

AUSCULTATION: After the fourth

month of gestation, if the uterus contains a living fetus, three distinct sounds may be heard. *Fetal heart sounds:* These consist of a succession of short, rapid, double pulsations varying in frequency from 120 to 140 per minute. The first sound is short, feeble, and obscure, whereas the second, the one usually heard, is loud and distinct; it sounds like the ticking of a watch wrapped in a napkin. The sound is usually transmitted over a space on the abdominal wall of 3 or 4 in. (7.6 to 10.2 cm) square. Location is determined by the position of the fetus. Generally, when maximum intensity is on the level of or above the umbilicus, it is a breech presentation. During labor, examinations should be made between uterine contractions. In protracted labor, the fetal heart sound is of value in indicating the time for manual or instrumental interference to save the child's life. Irregularity and feebleness of sound indicate a life-threatening situation for the fetus.

*Funic souffle:* This is the soft blowing sound heard over the location of the umbilical cord of the fetus in utero and synchronous with the fetal heartbeat during late pregnancy.

*Uterine bruit:* This sound is single, intermittent in character, and a combination of blowing and hissing sounds. It increases in intensity up to the period of labor. This bruit is believed to depend on the rapid passage of blood from the arteries into the distended venous sinuses of the uterus. Synchronous with the maternal pulse, and subject to the same variations, it is always heard before the pulsations of the fetal heart. The area over which it is audible varies, with the greatest point of intensity in a median line a little above the pubes.

PALPATION: During the third month of pregnancy, if the abdominal walls are not too thick, the examiner may palpate by placing the patient on her back with her head raised and thighs flexed, and pressing the points of the fingers gently downward and backward above the pubes. A hard round mass will be found beneath the median line, rising out of the pelvis. Between 2 and 4 weeks later, the increase is marked. As pregnancy advances, the mass loses its hardness and becomes more elastic, like a cyst filled with water. In doubtful cases in which decided abdominal enlargement is present, a standard hormonal test for pregnancy should be done.

By vaginal examination, one may be able to diagnose the stage of gestation, stage of parturition, or, if the woman is near term, the progress of labor, the presentation and position of the fetus, and the position of the uterus. The tip of the cervix of an unimpregnated uterus feels firm and cartilaginous (e.g., like touching the tip of the nose). The impregnated uterus feels soft like velvet (e.g., like touching the lips), but deeper, beyond the softness, is a hardness (e.g., like touching a board).

PERCUSSION: The nonpregnant uterus is inaccessible to touch externally or to percussion. At the end of the second month of pregnancy, a dull sound on percussion just above the pubes indicates the enlarging uterus. Later, as the uterus increases in volume and rises into the abdomen, strong presumptive evidence of pregnancy may be established, by the oval tumor felt in the hypogastrium and by the circumscribed area of dullness corresponding to the situation of the tumor. This presumption becomes strengthened if the area of dullness increases as gestation progresses. Palpation and percussion, however, are not sufficient to determine whether the enlargement is due to pregnancy or to some other form of new growth. After the fifth month, both of these methods are inferior to auscultation.

***u. acollis*** A uterus without a cervix.

***u. arcuatus*** A uterus with a depressed arched fundus.

***u. bicornis*** A uterus in which the fundus is divided into two parts.

***u. biforis*** A uterus in which the external os is divided into two parts by a septum.

***u. bilocularis*** A uterus in which the cavity is divided into two parts by a partition.

***bipartite u.*** A uterus in which the body is partially divided by a median septum.

***cancer of u.*** A malignant neoplasm of the uterus, detected by size, intermittent bleeding, purulent discharge, vaginal or Papanicolaou smear, or cervical or endometrial biopsy. Cancer may produce sterility, abortion, hemorrhage, or sepsis. Uterine cancer is extremely rare in pregnancy; however, if present, a tumor will usually increase in size during pregnancy.

***u. cordiformis*** A heart-shaped uterus.

***u. didelphys*** A double uterus.

***u. duplex*** A double uterus resulting from failure of union of müllerian ducts.

***fetal u.*** A uterus that is retarded in development and possesses an extremely long cervical canal.

***fibroids of u.*** SEE: *fibroma, uterine.*

***gravid u.*** A pregnant uterus.

***u. masculinus*** The prostatic utricle.

***u. parvicollis*** A normal uterus with a disproportionately small vaginal portion.

***prolapse of u.*** A condition in which a defective pelvic floor allows the uterus or part of it to protrude out of the vagina. In first-degree uterine prolapse, the cervix uteri reaches down to the vaginal introitus. In second-degree uterine prolapse, it protrudes out from the vagina. In third-degree uterine prolapse, the entire uterus lies outside of the vagina. SYN: *descensus uteri*. SEE: *procidentia*.

SYMPTOMS: The condition is most often

seen following instrumental deliveries or when the patient has been allowed to bear down during labor before the cervix is fully dilated. Frequently associated with this is a prolapse of the anterior and posterior vaginal walls, as seen in cystocele and rectocele. In the early stages, there are dragging sensations in the lower abdomen, back pain while standing and on exertion, a sensation of weight and bearing down in the perineum, and frequency of urination and incontinence of urine in cases associated with cystocele. In the later stages, a protrusion or swelling at the vulva is noticed on standing or straining, and leukorrhea is present. In procidentia, there is frequently pain on walking, an inability to urinate unless the mass is reduced, and cystitis.

ETIOLOGY: This condition may be congenital or acquired; most often, however, it is acquired. The etiological factors are congenital weakness of the uterine supports and injury to the pelvic floor or uterine supports during childbirth.

TREATMENT: The treatment depends on the age of the patient, the degree of prolapse, and the associated pathology. Abdominal surgery with fixation of the uterus is required if the prolapse is complete.

***pubescent u.*** An adult uterus that resembles that of a prepubertal female.

***rupture of u. in pregnancy*** Loss of continuity of the wall of the uterus. This rare but serious event may be spontaneous or traumatic. The fetus and amniotic sac may be expelled into the peritoneal cavity. SEE: *Nursing Diagnoses Appendix.*

SYMPTOMS: Obstruction usually precedes symptoms. Abdominal pains, shock, and hemorrhage may characterize the occurrence. The fetus is easily palpated. However, spontaneous rupture may occur without warning.

ETIOLOGY: The event may be caused by obstruction or by weakness of the uterine wall. Scars may cause such a weakness.

TREATMENT: The condition must be treated by combating the shock and hemorrhage, and surgically removing the products of conception from the peritoneal cavity.

***subinvolution of u.*** The lack of involution of the uterus following childbirth, manifested by a large uterus (greater than 100 g) and a continuation of lochia rubra beyond the usual time. It is caused usually by puerperal infection, overdistention of the uterus by multiple pregnancy or polyhydramnios, lack of lactation, malposition of the uterus, and retained secundines. Involution is aided by the certainty that the placenta is intact at the time of delivery and the use of ecbolics to cause uterine contraction.

***tipped u.*** SEE: *tipped uterus.*

***tumors of u.*** Uterine tumors, which may cause sterility or abortion or obstruct labor; they may become infected or twisted on their attachments. Myomata (fibroids) are possible but not common in young women; fibroids are more common in women beyond age 30 and in black women. Subserous tumors do not affect pregnancy, may impede labor, or may disappear after labor. Interstitial and submucous types may interfere with pregnancy and produce abortion.

EFFECTS ON LABOR: Tumors usually have no effect on labor. If low, they may cause malpresentation or impossible labor; labor pains may be weak and inefficient. Often there will be severe pains and rupture of the uterus. Submucous tumors may protrude before or after birth. The placenta may be retained. The tumor may be infected postpartum. The knee-chest position helps the patient if the tumor is in the pelvis. If in the fundus, delivery is through the vagina; if not, cesarean section may be needed.

***u. unicornis*** A uterus possessing only one lateral half and usually having only one uterine tube.

**utilization review** Evaluation of the necessity, quality, effectiveness, or efficiency of medical services, procedures, and facilities. In regard to a hospital, the review includes appropriateness of admission, services ordered and provided, length of stay, and discharge practices.

**utricle** (ū′trĭk′l) [L. *utriculus,* a little bag] **1.** One of two sacs of the membranous labyrinth in the bony vestibule of the inner ear. It communicates with the semicircular ducts by five openings on the posterior wall and with the sacculus and endolymphatic duct by an opening on the anterior wall. On its inner surface is an area of sensory epithelium, the macula utriculi, containing cells that respond to movement of otoliths caused by changes in position. **2.** Any small sac. SYN: *utriculus.*

***prostatic u.*** A small blind pouch of the urethra extending into the substance of the prostate gland. It is a remnant of the embryonic mullerian duct. SYN: *utriculus, masculinus; utriculus, prostaticus; uterus masculinus.*

***u. of urethra*** The prostatic vesicle of the male.

***u. of vestibule*** The vestibular cavity connecting with the semicircular canals.

**utricular** (ū-trĭk′ū-lăr) [L. *utriculus,* a little bag] **1.** Pert. to the utricle. **2.** Like a bladder.

**utriculitis** (ū-trĭk-ū-lī′tĭs) [″ + Gr. *itis,* inflammation] Inflammation of the utricle, that of either the vestibule or the prostate.

**utriculoplasty** (ū-trĭk′ū-lō-plăs″tē) [″ + Gr. *plassein,* to form] Surgical reduction of the size of the uterus by excision of a longitudinal wedge-shaped section.

**utriculosaccular** (ū-trĭk″ū-lō-săk′ū-lăr) [″ + *sacculus,* a small bag] Pert. to the utricle and saccule of the labyrinth.

**utriculosaccular duct** A duct uniting the utricle and saccule.

**utriculus** (ū-trĭk′ū-lŭs) [L., a little bag] A utricle.

***u. masculinus*** Prostatic utricle.

***u. prostaticus*** Prostatic utricle.

**uvea** (ū′vē-ă) [L. *uva,* grape] The highly vascular middle layer of the eyeball, immediately beneath the sclera. It consists of the iris, ciliary body, and choroid, and forms the pigmented layer.

**uveal** (ū′vē-ăl) Pert. to the middle layer of the eye, or uvea.

**uveitic** (ū-vē-ĭt′ĭk) [″ + Gr. *itis,* inflammation] Marked by or pert. to uveitis.

**uveitis** (ū-vē-ī′tĭs) A nonspecific term for any intraocular inflammatory disorder. The uveal tract structures—iris, ciliary body, and choroid—are usually involved, but other nonuveal parts of the eye, including the retina and cornea, may be involved.

Uveitis that is not associated with known infections or that is associated with diseases of unknown cause is termed endogenous uveitis. This is thought to be due to an autoimmune phenomenon.

TREATMENT: Corticosteroids and other immunosuppressive agents, including cyclosporine, are used in treating some causes of uveitis, but their use may make some types of uveitus worse.

Short-acting cycloplegic agents such as hematropine, scopolamine, or cyclopentolate are used during therapy to prevent inflammatory adhesions (posterior synechiae) between the iris and lens.

***sympathetic u.*** Severe, bilateral uveitis that starts as inflammation of the uveal tract of one eye resulting from a puncture wound. The injured eye is termed the "exciting eye." If the affected eye is not removed within 10 days of the accident that caused the wound, blindness will occur. SEE: *ophthalmia, sympathetic.*

**uveoparotitis** (ū″vē-ō-păr-ō-tī′tĭs) [″ + Gr. *para,* beside, + *ous,* ear, + *itis,* inflammation] Inflammation of the parotid gland and uveitis.

**uveoplasty** (ū′vē-ō-plăs″tē) [″ + Gr. *plassein,* to form] Reparative operation of the uvea.

**uveoscleritis** (ū″vē-ō-sklĕr-ī′tĭs) Inflammation of the sclera in which the infection has spread from the uvea.

**uviform** (ū′vĭ-form) [″ + *forma,* form] Shaped like a grape.

**uviofast** (ū′vē-ō-făst) Uvioresistant.

**uviol** (ū′vē-ŏl) Glass that is unusually transparent to ultraviolet rays.

**uvioresistant** (ū″vē-ō-rē-zĭs′tănt) Resistant to the effects of ultraviolet radiation. SYN: *uviofast.*

**uviosensitive** (ū″vē-ō-sĕn′sĭ-tĭv) Sensitive to the effects of ultraviolet radiation.

**uvula** (ū′vū-lă) [L. *uvula,* a little grape] A small, soft structure hanging from the free edge of the soft palate in the midline above the root of the tongue. It is composed of muscle, connective tissue, and mucous membrane. SYN: *staphyle.*

***u. of cerebellum*** A small lobule of the cerebellum lying on the inferior surface of the inferior vermis, anterior to the pyramis.

***u. fissa*** A cleft uvula.

***u. vermis*** A small, triangular elevation on the vermis of the cerebellum of the brain.

***u. vesicae*** A median projection of mucous membrane of the urinary bladder located immediately anterior to the orifice of the urethra.

**uvulaptosis** (ū″vū-lăp-tō′sĭs) [″ + Gr. *ptosis,* a dropping] Uvuloptosis.

**uvular** (ū′vū-lăr) [L. *uvula,* little grape] Pert. to the uvula.

**uvularis** (ū-vū-lā′rĭs) [L.] The azygos uvulae muscle. SEE: *Muscles Appendix.*

**uvulectomy** (ū″vū-lĕk′tō-mē) [″ + Gr. *ektome,* excision] Surgical removal of the uvula.

**uvulitis** (ū″vū-lī′tĭs) [″ + Gr. *itis,* inflammation] Inflammation of the uvula.

**uvulopalatopharyngoplasty** ABBR: UPPP. Plastic surgery of the oropharynx in which redundant soft palate, uvula, pillars, fauces, and sometimes posterior pharyngeal wall mucosa are removed. The procedure may be done by using laser therapy. It is usually done to correct intractable snoring or sleep apnea. SEE: *sleep disorders; snore.*

**uvuloptosis** (ū″vū-lŏp-tō′sĭs) [″ + Gr. *ptosis,* a dropping] A relaxed and pendulous condition of the palate. SYN: *uvulaptosis.*

**U wave** In the electrocardiogram, a low-amplitude deflection that follows the T wave. Its significance is unknown, and its absence does not indicate abnormality. SEE: *QRST complex; electrocardiogram.*

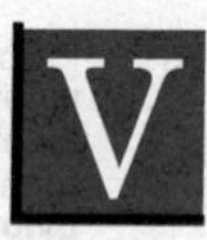

**V** **1.** *Vibrio; vision; visual acuity.* **2.** Symbol for the element vanadium.

**V̇** **1.** Symbol for gas flow. **2.** Symbol for ventilation.

**v** L. *vena,* vein; *volt.*

**vaccina** (văk-sī′nă) Vaccinia.

**vaccinable** (văk-sĭn′ă-b′l) Capable of being successfully vaccinated.

**vaccinal** (văk′sĭn-ăl) Rel. to vaccine or to vaccination.

**vaccinate** (văk′sĭn-āt) [L. *vaccinus,* pert. to cows] To inoculate with vaccine to produce immunity against disease.

**vaccination** (văk″sĭ-nā′shŭn) [L. *vaccinus,* pert. to cows] **1.** Inoculation with any vaccine or toxoid to establish resistance to a specific infectious disease. SEE: *immunization.* **2.** A scar left on the skin by inoculation of a vaccine.

**vaccine** (văk′sēn, văk-sēn′) [L. *vaccinus,* pert. to cows] A suspension of infectious agents, or some part of them, given for the purpose of establishing resistance to an infectious disease. SEE: table.

Vaccines comprise four general classes:

1. Those containing living attenuated infectious organisms, such as vaccine for poliomyelitis.
2. Those containing infectious agents killed by physical or chemical means, such as vaccines used to protect human beings against typhoid fever, rabies, and whooping cough.
3. Those containing soluble toxins of microorganisms, sometimes used as such, but generally forming toxoids, such as the one used in the prevention of diphtheria and tetanus.
4. Those containing substances extracted from infectious agents, such as capsular polysaccharides extracted from pneumococci.

FUNCTION: Vaccines are used to stimulate an immune response in the body by creating antibodies or activated T lymphocytes capable of controlling the organism. The result is protection against a disease; the duration depends on the particular vaccine. Recovery from measles or diphtheria, for example, usually provides lifelong immunity. The immune system has produced antibodies and memory cells for these pathogens so that subsequent exposure does not result in disease. A successful vaccine does the same thing, usually without risk of illness. The measles vaccine is believed to provide lifelong immunity, but the diphtheria vaccine requires periodic booster doses. More than one type of vaccine may be available for immunization against a specific infectious agent. SEE: *diphtheria; immune response; immunity; immunization; immunobiologics.*

***autogenous v.*** Bacterial vaccine prepared from lesions of the individual to be inoculated. SYN: *homologous v.*

***bacterial v.*** A suspension of killed or attenuated bacteria; used for injection into the body to induce development of active immunity to the same organism.

***BCG v.*** Bacille Calmette-Guérin, a preparation of a dried, living culture of *Mycobacterium tuberculosis.* In areas with a high incidence of tuberculosis, it is used in prophylactic vaccination of infants against tuberculosis. It is also used in adults who are at high and unavoidable risk of becoming infected with tuberculosis. A disadvantage of use of this vaccine is that it produces hypersensitivity to tuberculin. As a result, the skin test for tuberculin sensitivity becomes positive and may persist for 5 years. There is no way to distinguish a positive skin test due to BCG from one caused by infection with *Mycobacterium tuberculosis.*

***cholera v.*** A vaccine prepared from killed *Vibrio cholerae.* It is effective for only a few months.

***diphtheria v.*** SEE: *DPT v.*

***DPT v.*** A combination of diphtheria and tetanus toxoids and killed pertussis bacilli that is administered intramuscularly to immunize children against diphtheria, tetanus, and pertussis.

***DTaP v.*** A preparation of diphtheria and tetanus toxoids and acellular pertussis proteins. It may be used for the fourth and fifth injections in the series.

***Haemophilus influenzae type b v.*** A vaccine prepared from the bacterial polysaccharide (HbPV) or polysaccharide converted to protein (HbCV).

***hepatitis B v.*** A vaccine prepared from hepatitis B protein antigen produced by genetically engineered yeast.

***heterologous v.*** A vaccine derived from an organism different from the organism against which the vaccine is used.

***homologous v.*** Autogenous v.

***human diploid cell rabies v.*** ABBR: HDCV. An inactivated virus vaccine prepared from fixed rabies virus grown in human diploid cell tissue culture.

***inactivated poliovirus v.*** An injectable vaccine made from three types of inactivated polioviruses. Previously used name: poliomyelitis vaccine. SYN: *Salk v.*

***influenza virus v.*** A polyvalent vaccine containing inactivated antigenic variants of the influenza virus (types A and B either individually or combined) for use in areas expected to have epidemics. Its use

**Vaccines**

| Name | Age Administered | Booster Schedule | Comments |
|---|---|---|---|
| BCG (bacillus of Calmette and Guérin) | In epidemic conditions, administered to infants as soon as possible after birth. | None | The only contra-indications are symptomatic human immunodeficiency virus (HIV) infection or other illnesses known to suppress immunity. |
| Cholera | See Comments | Every 3 to 6 mo for those who remain in epidemic areas. | Only those traveling to countries where cholera is present need to be vaccinated. Whole cell vaccines provide partial protection for 3 to 6 mo. |
| DPT (diphtheria, pertussis, tetanus) | At 2 mo, 4 mo, 6 mo, and 15–18 mo. A fifth dose may be given at 4–6 yr. | Tetanus and diphtheria immunization every 10 yr, esp. for people over 50. Persons who have received five doses of tetanus toxoid in childhood may not need a booster until age 50. | Tetanus booster may be required following a wound even though all routine and booster immunizations have been received. Booster of diphtheria toxoid should be given if child under 6 is exposed to diphtheria. Vaccine is contraindicated in cases of acute infection, previous central nervous system damage, or convulsions. |
| *Haemophilus influenzae* b (polysaccharide or conjugate) | At 2 mo, 4 mo, discretionally at 6 mo, and at 12–15 mo. | None | SEE: *Haemophilus influenzae type b infection.* |
| Hepatitis B | At birth, 2 mo, and 6–18 mo, or at 1–2 mo, 4 mo, and 6–18 mo. All ages if risk is present. | None | Recommended as a routine childhood vaccine. All health care workers should receive it. Immune globulin or hepatitis B globulin may be given to produce passive immunity in exposed contacts. They are contraindicated for those allergic to yeast products. |
| Influenza (flu) | All ages. | Annually, given prior to time influenza is expected. | Recommended for the elderly, health care professionals, residents of long-term care facilities, and those of any age who have chronic disease of the heart or lungs, metabolic diseases such as diabetes, or immunosuppression. |

*continued on following page*

**Vaccines** (Continued)

| Name | Age Administered | Booster Schedule | Comments |
|---|---|---|---|
| MMR (measles [live attenuated rubeola], mumps, rubella) | 12–15 mo. | 4–6 yr or 11–12 yr. | Vaccine will usually prevent measles if given within 2 days after a child has been exposed to the disease. Not given to adults. Contraindicated for those with allergy to egg or neomycin, active infection, or severe immunosuppression. |
| Plague | See Comments | See Comments | Recommended for those traveling to Southeast Asia, persons who work closely with wild rodents in plague areas, and laboratory personnel working with *Yersinia pestis* organisms. |
| Pneumococcal vaccine, polyvalent | Should not be given to children under age 2 or to pregnant women. | None | Vaccine is effective against the 23 most prevalent types of pneumococci. Administered to those who have an increased risk of developing pneumococcal pneumonia. Included are those who have chronic diseases, have had a splenectomy, are in chronic care facilities, or are 65 years of age or older. |
| Polio (live oral trivalent vaccine) | At 2 mo, 4 mo, and 6–18 mo. | At 4–6 mo or 11–12 yr. | Administration is postponed in those with persistent vomiting, diarrhea, acute illness, or immunosuppression and in those who live in the same household as an immunosuppressed person. An alternate polio vaccine is available for immunosuppressed children. |
| Rabies | See Comments | See Comments | Each exposure to rabies needs to be evaluated on an individual basis by the physician. Postexposure prophylaxis includes the human diploid cell vaccine and rabies immune globulin. |

**Vaccines** (Continued)

| Name | Age Administered | Booster Schedule | Comments |
|---|---|---|---|
| Typhoid | See Comments | See Comments | Immunization is indicated when a person has come into contact with a known typhoid carrier, if there is an outbreak of typhoid fever, or prior to traveling to an area where typhoid is endemic. |
| *Varicella zoster* (chickenpox) | 12–18 mo. | None | Immunizes against chickenpox in adulthood as well as childhood. The illness is much more serious in adults than in children. |
| Yellow fever | See Comments | Every 10 years. | Vaccine should be given to all persons traveling or living in areas where yellow fever is present. |

is particularly helpful to the aged and chronically ill.

***killed v.*** A vaccine prepared from dead microorganisms. This type of vaccine is used for strains that have a high virulence.

***live attenuated measles (rubeola) virus v.*** A vaccine prepared from live strains of the measles virus. It is the preferred form except in patients who have one of the following: lymphoma, leukemia, or other generalized malignancy; radiation therapy; pregnancy; active tuberculosis; egg sensitivity; prolonged treatment with drugs that suppress the immune response (i.e., corticosteroids or antimetabolites); or administration of gamma globulin, blood, or plasma. Those persons should be given immune globulin immediately following exposure.

***live measles and mumps virus v.*** A standardized vaccine containing attenuated measles and mumps viruses.

***live measles and rubella virus v.*** A standardized vaccine containing attenuated measles and rubella viruses.

***live measles, mumps, and rubella virus v.*** ABBR: MMR vaccine. A standardized vaccine containing attenuated measles, mumps, and rubella viruses.

***live measles virus v.*** A standardized attenuated virus vaccine for use in immunizing against measles.

***live oral poliovirus v.*** A vaccine prepared from three types of live attenuated poliovirus. SYN: *Sabin v.*

***live rubella virus v.*** An attenuated virus vaccine used to prevent rubella (German measles). All nonpregnant susceptible women of childbearing age should be provided with this vaccine to prevent fetal infection and the congenital rubella syndrome (i.e., possible fetal death, prematurity, impaired hearing, cataract, mental retardation, and other serious conditions). SEE: *rubella.*

***meningococcal v.*** A vaccine prepared from bacterial polysaccharides from certain types of meningococci. Meningococcal polysaccharide vaccines A, C, Y, and W135 are available for preventing diseases caused by those serogroups. A vaccine for meningococcal serogroup B is not available. SEE: *meningitis, acute meningococcal.*

***mumps v.*** A live attenuated vaccine used to prevent mumps. Its use should be governed by the same restrictions listed for live attenuated measles virus vaccine.

***pertussis v.*** SEE: *DPT v.*

***plague v.*** A vaccine made from a crude fraction of killed plague bacilli for immunizing against plague.

***polyvalent v.*** A vaccine produced from cultures of a number of strains of the same species.

***polyvalent pneumococcal v.*** A vaccine that contains 23 of the known 83 pneumococcal capsular polysaccharides, and induces immunity for 3 to 5 years. This vaccine is estimated to protect against 90% of the pneumococcal types that produce serious disease in patients over 2 years of age. Children at high risk can be vaccinated at age 6 months and reinoculated at age 2 years. The vaccine is particularly indicated in high-risk groups such as persons with sickle cell diseases, chronic debilitating disease, immunological defects, and the elderly.

***rabies* v.** A vaccine prepared from killed, fixed virus of rabies, used prophylactically following a bite by a rabid animal. SEE: *human diploid cell rabies v.; rabies.*

***Sabin* v.** Live oral poliovirus v. SEE: *poliomyelitis.*

***Salk* v.** Inactivated poliovirus v.

***sensitized* v.** A vaccine prepared from bacteria treated with their specific immune serum.

***smallpox* v.** A vaccine made from the lymph of cowpox vesicles obtained from healthy vaccinated bovine animals. NOTE: This vaccine is no longer used because smallpox has been eradicated worldwide.

***tetanus* v.** SEE: *DPT v.*

***typhoid* v.** A vaccine made of killed *Salmonella typhi* organisms for immunizing against typhoid. It may not be effective if the person receives unusually large doses of the live organism at the time of exposure.

***varicella (chickenpox)* v.** A chickenpox vaccine prepared from attenuated virus. SEE: *chickenpox; herpes zoster.*

***yellow fever* v.** A vaccine made from a live attenuated strain of yellow fever virus.

**vaccinia** (văk-sĭn′ē-ă) [L. *vaccinus,* pert. to cows] A contagious disease of cattle, produced in humans by inoculation with cowpox virus to confer immunity against smallpox. Papules form about the third day after vaccination, changing to umbilicated vesicles about the fifth day, and at the end of the first week becoming umbilicated pustules surrounded by red areolae. They dry and form scabs, which fall off about the second week, leaving a white pitted depression. SYN: *cowpox; vaccina.* SEE: *vaccination; varicella; variola.*

**v. *necrosum*** Spreading necrosis at the site of a smallpox vaccination; may be accompanied by similar necrotic areas elsewhere on the body.

**vaccinia immune globulin** Hyperimmune gamma globulin; the therapeutic agent of choice for dermal complications of vaccination for smallpox (i.e., eczema vaccinatum and progressive vaccinia).

NOTE: There is no longer a need for this material because smallpox has been eradicated worldwide.

**vacciniform** (văk-sĭn′ĭ-form) [L. *vaccinus,* pert. to cows, + *forma,* shape] Of the nature of vaccinia or cowpox.

**vaccinogenous** (văk″sĭn-ŏj′ĕn-ŭs) [L. *vaccinus,* pert. to cows, + Gr. *gennan,* to produce] Producing vaccine or pert. to its production.

**vaccinostyle** (văk-sĭn′ō-stīl) A pointed stylus used in vaccination.

**vaccinotherapeutics** (văk″sĭn-ō-thĕr″ă-pū′tĭks) Treatment by injection of bacterial vaccines.

**vacuolar** (văk′ū-ō-lăr) [L. *vacuum,* empty] Pert. to or possessing vacuoles.

**vacuolar degeneration** Swelling of cells with an increase in the number and size of vacuoles. SYN: *cloudy swelling.*

**vacuolated** (văk′ū-ō-lāt″ĕd) Possessing or containing vacuoles.

**vacuolation** (văk″ū-ō-lā′shŭn) Formation of vacuoles. SYN: *vacuolization.*

**vacuole** (văk′ū-ōl) [L. *vacuum,* empty] A clear space in cell protoplasm filled with fluid or air.

***autophagic* v.** A vacuole that contains recognizable fragments of the ribosomes or mitochondria.

***contractile* v.** A cavity filled with fluid in the cytoplasm of a protozoan. The cavity is emptied by sudden contraction of its walls.

***heterophagous* v.** A vacuole that contains substances that come from outside the cell.

***plasmocrine* v.** A vacuole present in the cytoplasm of a secretory cell that is filled with crystalloid material.

***rhagiocrine* v.** A vacuole present in the cytoplasm of a secretory cell that is filled with colloid material.

**vacuolization** (văk″ū-ō-lĭ-zā′shŭn) [L. *vacuum,* empty] Vacuolation.

**vacuum** (văk′ū-ŭm) [L., empty] A space exhausted of its air content.

**vacuum aspiration** Removal of uterine contents by using a hollow curet or catheter to which a suction apparatus is attached. It is used before the 12th week of pregnancy.

**vacuum extractor** A device for applying traction to the fetus during delivery by using a suction cup attached to the fetal head. Its use may be hazardous except in the hands of experts.

**vacuum tube** A vessel of insulating material (usually glass) that is sealed and has a vacuum sufficiently high to permit the free flow of electrons between the electrodes that extend into the tube from the outside. In England, it is called a vacuum valve.

**vagabond's disease** Discoloration of the skin caused by exposure and scratching owing to the presence of lice. SEE: *pediculosis corporis.*

**vagal** (vā′găl) [L. *vagus,* wandering] Pert. to the vagus nerve.

**vagal attack** A condition of dyspnea with cardiac distress and a fear of impending death. The sinking sensation associated with the attack is assumed to be the result of vasomotor spasm.

**vagal escape** A condition in which one or more beats of the heart occur even though the vagus nerve is being continuously stimulated. Stimulation of the vagus normally inhibits heartbeat.

**vagi** (vā′gī) Pl. of vagus.

**vagina** (vă-jī′nă) *pl.* **vaginae, vaginas** [L.,

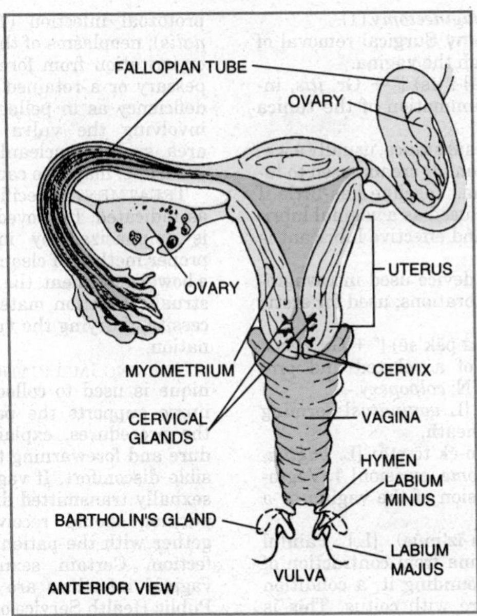


VAGINA AND OTHER FEMALE ORGANS

sheath] **1.** A sheathlike part. **2.** A musculomembranous tube that forms the passageway between the cervix uteri and the vulva. SEE: illus.

ANATOMY: In the uppermost part, the cervix divides the vagina into four fornices: the two lateral, the anterior, and the posterior. The bladder is situated adjacent to the anterior wall of the vagina, and the rectum is behind the posterior wall. The vagina represents a potential space, the walls of which are in contact with each other. Close to the cervix uteri the walls form a horizontal crescent shape, at the midpoint an H shape, and close to the vulva the shape of a vertical slit. The vagina is lined by a mucous membrane made up of squamous epithelium. It is surrounded by fasciae that allow for easy distensibility. The blood supply of the vagina is furnished from the inferior vesical, inferior hemorrhoidal, and uterine arteries. Except for the area close to the entrance, the vaginal tissue and mucosa contain few, if any, sensory nerve endings. The vagina is a passage for the intromission of the penis, for the reception of semen, and for the discharge of the menstrual flow. It also serves as a passageway through which the fetus is delivered.

***artificial* v.** A vagina constructed by plastic surgery for a patient whose vagina was removed for treatment of carcinoma or one who has congenital absence of the vagina.

***bulb of* v.** The small erectile body on each side of the vestibule. SYN: *Bartholin's glands; vestibuli of vagina.*

***v. fibrosa tendinis*** A fibrous sheath surrounding a tendon that usually confines it to an osseous groove.

***foreign bodies in* v.** SEE: *foreign bodies.*

***v. masculina*** The prostatic utricle.

***v. mucosa tendinis*** A synovial sheath that develops about a tendon.

***septate* v.** A congenital condition in which the vagina is divided longitudinally into two parts. This division may be partial or complete.

**vaginal** (văj′ĭn-ăl) [L. *vagina,* sheath] Pert. to the vagina or to any enveloping sheath.

**vaginal atrophy, postmenopausal** Atrophy of the vagina and vaginal mucosa that may occur following menopause. Hormonal changes occur following menopause. These changes are believed to influence the onset of vaginal atrophy. Menopausal women who continue to engage in sexual intercourse during menopause and following have less vaginal atrophy than do those women who become sexually inactive.

**vaginal birth after previous cesarean** ABBR: VBAC. Normal childbirth subsequent to cesarean delivery of a previous pregnancy. It was once erroneously believed that, in pregnancies subsequent to cesarean delivery, normal labor and vaginal birth were contraindicated by the risk of uterine rupture.

**vaginalectomy** (văj″ĭn-ăl-ĕk′tō-mē) [″ + Gr. *ektome,* excision] Excision of the tunica vaginalis. SYN: *vaginectomy* (1).

**vaginal hysterectomy** Surgical removal of the uterus through the vagina.

**vaginalitis** (văj-ĭn-ăl-ī'tĭs) [" + Gr. *itis,* inflammation] Inflammation of the tunica vaginalis testis.

**vaginal lubricant** A substance, usually a water-soluble ointment or cream, used to lubricate the vagina. Vaseline has little if any benefit when used as a vaginal lubricant. A natural and effective lubricant is human saliva.

**vaginal vibrator** A device used intravaginally to produce vibrations; used for erotic stimulation.

**vaginapexy** (văj"ĭn-ă-pĕk'sē) [" + Gr. *pexis,* fixation] Repair of a relaxed and prolapsed vagina. SYN: *colpopexy.*

**vaginate** (văj'ĭn-āt) [L. *vaginatus*] Forming or enclosed in a sheath.

**vaginectomy** (văj-ĭn-ĕk'tō-mē) [L. *vagina,* sheath, + Gr. *ektome,* excision] **1.** Vaginalectomy. **2.** Excision of the vagina or a part of it.

**vaginismus** (văj"ĭn-ĭz'mŭs) [L.] Painful spasm of the vagina from contraction of the muscles surrounding it, a condition that may interfere with coitus. This is usually the result of real, imagined, or anticipated attempts at vaginal penetration. A physical condition (i.e., an anatomical abnormality) may account for the condition, but this is not usually the case. The patient and her sex partner should be seen together by the physician. If there are no anatomical causes, the following therapy may help: The patient is desensitized through learning relaxation techniques. This is followed by self-insertion of a small vaginal dilator. Over time, the dilator size is increased and, eventually, when both the patient and her sex partner are agreeable, female-superior intercourse may be tried with the man being passive. Later, male-superior intercourse is prescribed. SEE: *Nursing Diagnoses Appendix.*

**vaginitis** (văj-ĭn-ī'tĭs) [L. *vagina,* sheath, + Gr. *itis,* inflammation] **1.** Inflammation of a sheath. **2.** Inflammation of the vagina. SYN: *colpitis.* SEE: *sexually transmitted disease; Nursing Diagnoses Appendix.*

SYMPTOMS: The patient experiences free purulent vaginal discharge, sometimes malodorous and occasionally stained with blood. There is irritation and itching of the vulvae and perineum, increased frequency of micturition, and smarting pain on the passage of urine. The vaginal mucous membrane is reddened and there may be superficial ulceration.

ETIOLOGY: This condition may be caused by microorganisms such as gonococci, chlamydiae, *Gardnerella vaginalis,* staphylococci, streptococci, spirochetes; viruses; irritation from use of strong chemicals in douching; fungus infection (candidiasis) caused by *Candida albicans;* protozoal infection (*Trichomonas vaginalis*); neoplasms of the cervix or vagina; or irritation from foreign bodies (e.g., a pessary or a retained tampon). Vitamin deficiency as in pellagra and conditions involving the vulva and surrounding area, such as uncleanliness or intestinal parasites, may also cause this condition.

TREATMENT: Specific therapy is given as indicated. Improved perineal hygiene is emphasized by instructing in the proper method of cleaning the anus after a bowel movement, the proper use of menstrual protection materials, and the necessity of drying the vulva following urination.

NURSING IMPLICATIONS: Aseptic technique is used to collect specimens. The nurse supports the patient throughout the procedures, explaining each procedure and forewarning the patient of possible discomfort. If vaginitis is due to a sexually transmitted disease, the sexual partner should receive treatment together with the patient to prevent reinfection. Certain sexually transmitted vaginal infections are reported to local Public Health Service officials along with the patient's known sexual contacts.

***v. adhaesiva*** Inflammation of the vagina causing adhesions between its walls.

***atrophic v.*** Vaginitis following menopause. SYN: *postmenopausal v.; senile v.*

***candidal v.*** Vaginitis due to infection with *Candida albicans.*

TREATMENT: Specific therapy with intravaginal miconazole cream, clotrimazole, or butoconazole is effective, as is ketaconazole administered orally. The ingestion of yogurt containing *Lactobacillus acidophilus* is also effective in decreasing colonization of the vagina by *Candida.*

NOTE: Some manufacturers may claim their yogurt contains lactobacilli even when this is not true.

***chlamydial v.*** Vaginitis caused by infection with *Chlamydia trachomatis.*

***diphtheritic v.*** Vaginitis with membranous exudate caused by infection with *Corynebacterium diphtheriae.*

***emphysematous v.*** Vaginitis with gas-bubble formation in connective tissues.

***Gardnerella vaginalis v.*** SEE: *Gardnerella vaginalis vaginitis; vaginosis, bacterial.*

***granular v.*** Vaginitis with cellular infiltration and enlargement of papillae.

***nonspecific v.*** In the past, a term used to describe virtually all cases of vaginitis in which no specific etiological agent could be identified. It is now known that the majority of such cases are caused by either *Gardnerella vaginalis* or *Trichomonas vaginalis* organisms. SEE: *vaginosis, bacterial.*

DIAGNOSIS: A fresh specimen diluted with normal saline will on microscopic examination reveal *Trichomonas* organisms. If short motile rods are seen to cover vaginal epithelial cells ("clue" cells), then *Gardnerella* organisms are the cause. In the latter, the vaginal aspirate is usually acid and, when mixed with a 10% potassium hydroxide solution, emits a characteristic offensive (fishy) odor. Metronidazole is used to treat *Trichomonas* or *Gardnerella* infection.

***postmenopausal v.*** Atrophic v.

***senile v.*** Atrophic v.

***v. testis*** Inflammation of the tunica vaginalis of the testis.

***Trichomonas vaginalis v.*** Vaginitis associated with or caused by infection by *Trichomonas vaginalis,* a flagellate protozoon. *T. vaginalis* may be present in the vagina without causing disease in the host. Because the causative organism may be spread by direct contact during sexual intercourse, *T. vaginalis* vaginitis is classified as a sexually transmitted disease.

**vaginoabdominal** (văj″ĭn-ō-ăb-dŏm′ĭn-ăl) [L. *vagina,* sheath, + *abdominalis,* abdominal] Rel. to the vagina and abdomen.

**vaginocele** (văj′ĭn-ō-sēl) [″ + Gr. *kele,* tumor, swelling] Vaginal hernia. SYN: *colpocele.*

**vaginodynia** (văj″ĭn-ō-dĭn′ē-ă) [″ + Gr. *odyne,* pain] Pain in the vagina.

**vaginogenic** (văj″ĭn-ō-jĕn′ĭk) [″ + Gr. *gennan,* to produce] Developed from or originating in the vagina.

**vaginogram** (văj′ĭn-ō-grăm) [″ + gramma, something written] A radiograph of the vagina.

**vaginography** (văj-ĭn-ŏg′ră-fē) [″ + Gr. *graphein,* to write] Radiography of the vagina. This technique is useful in diagnosing ureterovaginal fistula.

**vaginolabial** (văj″ĭn-ō-lā′bē-ăl) [″ + *labium,* lip] Rel. to the vagina and labia.

**vaginometer** (văj-ĭn-ŏm′ĕ-tĕr) [″ + Gr. *metron,* measure] A device for measuring the length and expansion of the vagina.

**vaginomycosis** (văj″ĭn-ō-mī-kō′sĭs) [″ + Gr. *mykes,* fungus, + *osis,* condition] A fungus infection (mycosis) of the vagina.

**vaginopathy** (văj″ĭ-nŏp′ă-thē) [″ + Gr. *pathos,* disease, suffering] Any disease of the vagina.

**vaginoperineal** (văj″ĭn-ō-pĕr-ĭ-nē′ăl) [″ + Gr. *perinaion,* perineum] Rel. to the vagina and perineum.

**vaginoperineoplasty** Plastic surgery involving the vagina and perineum.

**vaginoperineorrhaphy** (văj″ĭn-ō-pĕr″ĭ-nē-or′ăf-ē) [″ + ″ + *rhaphe,* seam, ridge] Repair of a laceration involving both the perineum and vagina. SYN: *colpoperineorrhaphy.*

**vaginoperineotomy** (văj″ĭn-ō-pĕr″ĭn-ē-ŏt′ō-mē) [″ + ″ + *tome,* incision] Surgical incision of the vagina and perineum; usually done to facilitate childbirth. SEE: *episiotomy.*

**vaginoperitoneal** (văj″ĭn-ō-pĕr″ĭ-tō-nē′ăl) Rel. to the vagina and peritoneum.

**vaginoplasty** (vă-jī′nō-plăs″tē) [″ + Gr. *plassein,* to form] Plastic surgery on the vagina.

**vaginoscope** (văj′ĭn-ō-skōp) [″ + Gr. *skopein,* to examine] An instrument for inspection of the vagina. This may be a speculum or an optical instrument.

**vaginoscopy** (văj″ĭn-ŏs′kō-pē) Visual examination of the vagina.

**vaginosis, bacterial** Inflammation of the vagina caused by *Gardnerella vaginalis.* Before this organism was identified, this condition was classed as nonspecific vaginitis. The diagnosis is confirmed when *Candida* and trichomonal vaginitis are excluded, the characteristic "clue" cells are found in vaginal secretions, and the characteristic fishy odor is produced when the vaginal discharge is mixed with 10% potassium hydroxide. SEE: *Gardnerella vaginalis vaginitis.*

**vaginotome** (vă-jī′nō-tōm) [″ + Gr. *tome,* incision] An instrument for making an incision in the vaginal walls.

**vaginotomy** (văj″ĭ-nŏt′ō-mē) [″ + Gr. *tome,* incision] Incision of the vagina.

**vaginovesical** (văj″ĭ-nō-vĕs′ĭ-kăl) [″ + *vesica,* bladder] Rel. to the vagina and bladder. SYN: *vesicovaginal.*

**vaginovulvar** (văj″ĭn-ō-vŭl′văr) [″ + *vulva,* covering] Vulvovaginal.

**vagitis** (vă-jī′tĭs) [L. *vagus,* wandering, + Gr. *itis,* inflammation] Inflammation of the vagal nerve.

**vagitus** (vă-jī′tŭs) [L. *vagire,* to squall] The first cry of a newborn.

***v. uterinus*** The crying of a fetus while still in the uterus.

***v. vaginalis*** The cry of an infant with its head still in the vagina.

**vagolysis** (vā-gŏl′ĭ-sĭs) [L. *vagus,* wandering, + Gr. *lysis,* dissolution] Surgical destruction of the vagus nerve.

**vagolytic** (vā″gō-lĭt′ĭk) **1.** Concerning vagolysis. **2.** An agent, surgical or chemical, that prevents function of the vagus nerve.

**vagomimetic** (vā″gō-mĭ-mĕt′ĭk) [″ + Gr. *mimetikos,* imitating] Resembling action caused by stimulation of the vagus nerve.

**vagosympathetic** (vā″gō-sĭm-pă-thĕt′ĭk) [″ + Gr. *sympathetikos,* suffering with] The cervical sympathetic and vagus nerves considered together.

**vagotomy** (vā-gŏt′ō-mē) [″ + Gr. *tome,* incision] Section of the vagus nerve.

***medical v.*** Administration of drugs to prevent function of the vagus nerve.

**vagotonia** (vā″gō-tō′nē-ă) [″ + Gr. *tonos,* tension] Hyperirritability of the parasympathetic nervous system. SEE: *sympatheticotonia.*

**vagotonic** (vā″gō-tŏn′ĭk) Pert. to vagotonia.

**vagotropic** (vā″gō-trŏp′ĭk) [″ + Gr. *tropos,* a turning] Acting on the vagus nerve.

**vagotropism** (vā-gŏt′rō-pĭzm) [″ + ″ + *-ismos,* condition] Affinity for the vagus nerve, as a drug.

**vagovagal** (vā″gō-vā′găl) Concerning reflex activity mediated entirely through the vagus nerve (i.e., via efferent and afferent impulses transmitted through the vagus nerve).

**vagrant** (vā′grănt) [L. *vagrans*] **1.** Wandering from place to place without a fixed home. **2.** A homeless person who wanders from place to place.

**vagus** (vā′gŭs) *pl.* **vagi** [L., wandering] The pneumogastric or 10th cranial nerve. It is a mixed nerve, having motor and sensory functions and a wider distribution than any of the other cranial nerves. SEE: illus.; *cranial nerves*.

**vagus pulse** Decreased heart rate caused by the slowing action of stimuli from the vagus nerve. SEE: *vagotomy; vagotonia*.

**vagusstoff** (vā′gŭs-stŏf) [″ + Ger. *Stoff*, substance] Acetylcholine.

**valence, valency** (vā′lĕns, -lĕn-sē) [L. *valens*, powerful] **1.** The property of an atom or group of atoms causing them to combine in definite proportion with other atoms or groups of atoms. Valency may be as high as 8 and is determined by the number of electrons in the outer orbit of the atom. **2.** The degree of the combining power or replacing power of an atom or group of atoms, the hydrogen atom being the unit of comparison. The number indicates how many atoms of hydrogen can unite with one atom of another element.

**Valentin's ganglion** (văl′ĕn-tēnz) [Gabriel Gustav Valentin, Ger. physician, 1810–1883] A small ganglion at the junction of the middle and posterior branches of the superior dental plexus.

**valethamate bromide** (văl-ĕth′ă-māt) An anticonvulsant drug.

**valgus** (văl′gŭs) [L., bowlegged] Bent outward or twisted, used esp. of deformities

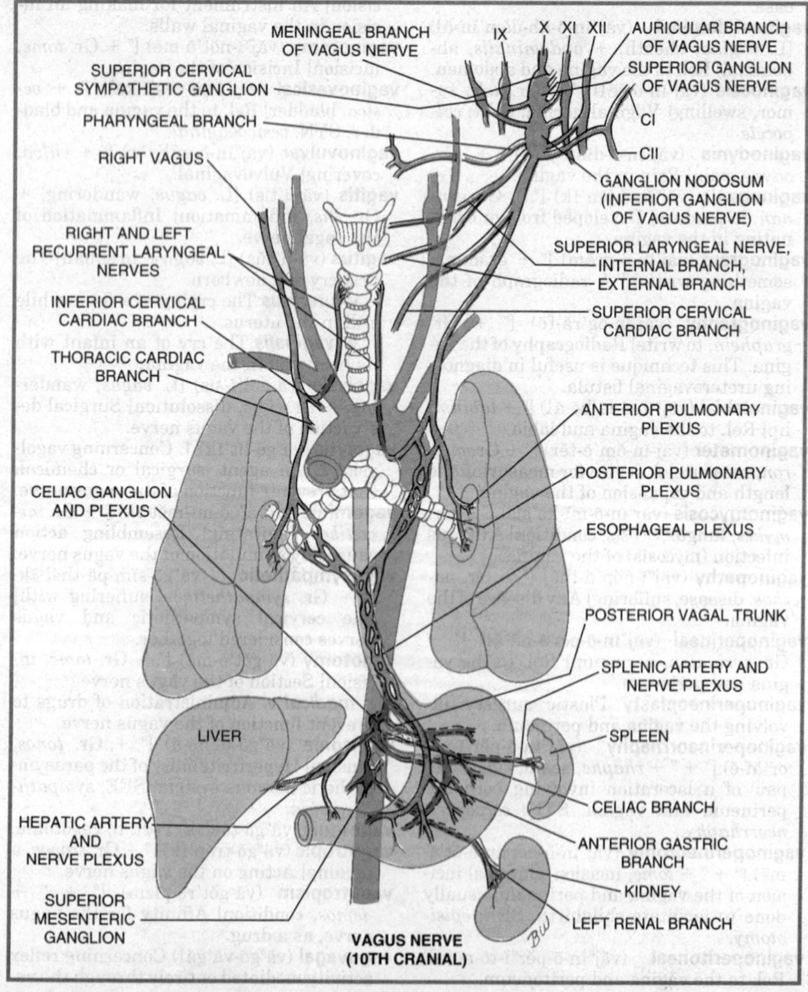

in which the most distal anatomical part is bent outward and away from the midline of the body, as talipes valgus or hallux valgus. SEE: *knock-knee; varus.*

**valid** [L. *validus,* strong] Producing the desired effect; correct.

**validate** To ensure that the item in question is valid and correct.

**validity** (vă-lĭd′ĭ-tē) **1.** The degree to which data or results of a study are correct or true. **2.** The extent to which a situation as observed reflects the true situation.

**valine** (văl′ēn, vā′lēn) $C_5H_{11}NO_2$. An amino acid derived from digestion of proteins. It is essential in the diet, esp. for normal growth in infants.

**valinemia** (văl″ĭ-nē′mē-ă) Increased valine in the blood.

**vallate** (văl′āt) [L. *vallatus,* walled] Having a rim around a depression.

**vallate papilla** A circumvallate papilla; one of a group of papillae forming a V-shaped row on the posterior dorsal surface of the tongue.

**vallecula** (văl-lĕk′ū-lă) [L., a depression] A depression or crevice.

***v. cerebelli*** A deep fissure on the inferior surface of the cerebellum. SYN: *valley of cerebellum.*

***v. epiglottica*** A depression lying lateral to the median epiglottic fold and separating it from the pharyngoepiglottic fold.

***v. ovata*** A depression in the liver in which rests the gallbladder.

***v. sylvii*** A depression marking the beginning of the fissure of Sylvius in the brain.

***v. unguis*** A fold of skin in which the proximal and lateral edges of the nails are embedded.

**Valleix's points** (văl-lāz′) [François L. I. Valleix, Fr. physician, 1807–1855] In neuralgia, distinct painful points along the course of the affected nerve.

**valley of cerebellum** Vallecula cerebelli.

**valley fever** Coccidioidomycosis.

**vallum unguis** (văl′ŭm ŭng′gwĭs) The fold of skin overlapping the nail.

**VALPAR component work samples** ABBR: VCWS. Trade name for standardized assessment modules used to determine the vocation-related rehabilitation needs of persons with various limitations and disabilities. The modules assess abilities and skills, including tool use, dexterity, problem solving, strength, and movement as applied to specific work tasks. It is widely used by occupational therapists in work-related rehabilitation settings.

**Valsalva's maneuver** (văl-săl′văz) [Antonio Maria Valsalva, It. anatomist, 1666–1723] An attempt to forcibly exhale with the glottis, nose, and mouth closed. This maneuver causes increased intrathoracic pressure, slowing of the pulse, decreased return of blood to the heart, and increased venous pressure. If the eustachian tubes are not obstructed, the pressure on the tympanic membranes also will be increased. When this maneuver is done with just the glottis closed, only intrathoracic pressure will increase. This maneuver is helpful in "clearing" ears that have become blocked during a descent from high altitude. SEE: *Müller maneuver; Toynbee maneuver.*

**Valsalva's sinuses** Three dilatations in the wall of the aorta behind the three flaps of the aortic semilunar valve.

**value** (văl′ū) [ME. from L. *valere,* to be of value] **1.** The amount of a specific substance or the magnitude of an entity. **2.** Something that is cherished or held dear.

**valvate** (văl′vāt) [L. *valva,* leaf of a folding door] Valvular.

**valve** (vălv) [L. *valva,* leaf of a folding door] Any one of various membranous structures in a hollow organ or passage that temporarily close to permit the flow of fluid in one direction only.

***aortic v.*** The valve at the junction of the left ventricle and the ascending aorta; composed of three segments (semilunar cusps). The aortic valve prevents regurgitation at the entrance of the aorta to the heart. SEE: *cardiac v.* for illus.

***bicuspid v.*** The valve that closes the orifice between the left cardiac atrium and the left ventricle. SYN: *left atrioventricular v.; mitral v.* SEE: *cardiac v.* for illus.

***Bjork-Shiley concavoconvex heart v.*** A synthetic artificial heart valve that is no longer commercially available but remains implanted in thousands of patients. The valve has been known to fracture during use, which results in death in the majority of cases.

***cardiac v.*** One of the four valves that control the flow of blood into, through, and out of the heart. In order of the entry of the venous blood into the right atrium, they are right atrioventricular, pulmonary, left atrioventricular, and aortic. SEE: illus.

***coronary v.*** The coronary sinus valve at the entrance of the coronary sinus into the right atrium. SYN: *thebesian v.*

***Houston's v.*** One of the mucosal folds of the rectum. SYN: *plicae transversales recti.*

***ileocecal v.*** A projection of the ileum of the small intestine into the cecum of the colon. It prevents backup of fecal material into the small intestine. It is composed of two membranous folds. SYN: *v. of Varolius; valvula coli.*

***left atrioventricular v.*** Bicuspid v.

***mitral v.*** Bicuspid v.

***prosthetic heart v.*** A substitute valve used to replace a diseased valve. Most valves are artificial and not made of biological tissues.

***pulmonary v.*** The valve at the junction of the right ventricle and pulmonary artery. It is composed of three cusps and prevents regurgitation of blood from the pulmonary artery to the right ventricle.

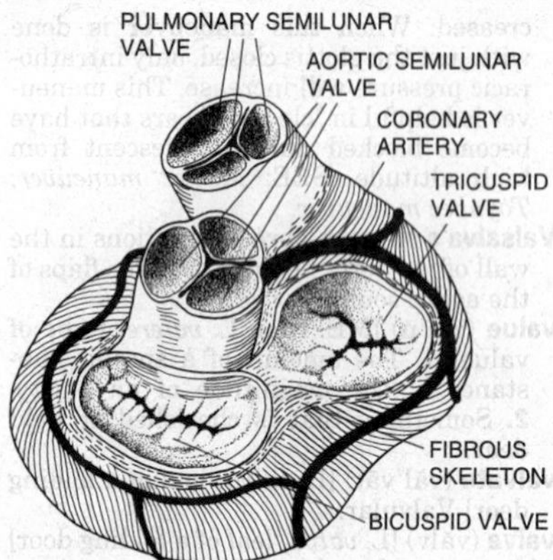


CARDIAC VALVES
(SUPERIOR VIEW WITH ATRIA REMOVED)

SEE: *cardiac v.* for illus.

***pyloric v.*** The prominent circular membranous fold at the pyloric orifice of the stomach. SYN: *valvula pylori.*

***reducing v.*** A device used to reduce the pressure of gas that has been compressed in a cylinder.

***right atrioventricular v.*** Tricuspid v.

***semilunar v.*** The type of valve separating the heart and aorta and the heart and pulmonary artery. SYN: *valvula semilunaris.* SEE: *cardiac v.* for illus.

***thebesian v.*** Coronary v.

***tricuspid v.*** The valve between the right atrium and right ventricle of the heart. SYN: *right atrioventricular v.; valvula tricuspidalis.* SEE: *cardiac v.* for illus.

***v. of Varolius*** Ileocecal v.

**valvectomy** Surgical excision of a valve, esp. a heart valve. SEE: *valvuloplasty.*

**valvotomy** (văl-vŏt′ō-mē) [″ + Gr. *tome,* incision] Valvulotomy.

***mitral balloon v.*** Expansion of a balloon placed in the orifice of a stenotic mitral valve. This method of treating mitral stenosis is believed to be as effective as surgical repair of a stenotic valve. SYN: *valvuloplasty.*

**valvula** (văl′vū-lă) *pl.* **valvulae** [L., a small fold] A valve, specifically a small valve.

***v. bicuspidalis*** Bicuspid valve.

***v. coli*** Ileocecal valve.

***v. pylori*** Pyloric valve.

***v. semilunaris*** Semilunar valve.

***v. tricuspidalis*** Tricuspid valve.

**valvulae** (văl′vū-lē) Pl. of valvula.

***v. conniventes*** Plicae circulares.

**valvular** (văl′vū-lăr) [L. *valvula,* a small fold] Rel. to or having one or more valves. SYN: *valvate.*

**valvulitis** (văl″vū-lī′tĭs) [″ + Gr. *itis,* inflammation] Inflammation of a valve, esp. a cardiac valve.

**valvuloplasty** (văl′vū-lō-plăs″tē) Plastic or restorative surgery on a valve, esp. a cardiac valve.

***percutaneous balloon v.*** The percutaneous insertion of one or more balloons across a stenotic heart valve. Inflating the balloons decreases the constriction. This technique has been esp. helpful in treating pulmonic stenosis.

**valvulotome** (văl′vū-lō-tōm) [″ + Gr. *tome,* incision] An instrument for incising a valve.

**valvulotomy** (văl″vū-lŏt′ō-mē) The process of cutting through a valve, as a rectal fold that is rigid and causing constriction. SYN: *valvotomy.*

**vanadium** (vă-nā′dē-ŭm) [*Vanadis,* a Scandinavian goddess] SYMB: V. A light gray metallic element; atomic weight, 50.941; atomic number, 23.

**vanadiumism** (vă-nā′dē-ŭm-ĭzm) Toxicity due to chronic exposure to vanadium. The symptoms include bronchitis, pneumonitis, conjunctivitis, and anemia.

**van Buren's disease** (văn bū′rĕnz) [William Holme van Buren, U.S. surgeon, 1819–1883] Induration of the corpora cavernosa of the penis. SYN: *Peyronie's disease.*

**vancomycin hydrochloride** (văn′kō-mī″sĭn) An antibacterial drug.

**van den Bergh's test** (văn″dĕnbŭrgz′) [A. A. Hijmans van den Bergh, Dutch physician, 1869–1943] A test to detect the presence of bilirubin in blood serum or plasma.

**van der Hoeve's syndrome** [Jan van der Hoeve, Dutch ophthalmologist, 1878–1952] Conductive deafness caused by otosclerosis-like changes in the temporal bone. Blue sclerae and osteogenesis imperfecta are also present.

**van der Waals forces** [Johannes D. van der Waals, Dutch physicist, 1837–1923] The definite but weak forces of attraction between the nuclei of atoms of compounds. These forces do not exist on the basis of ionic attraction, hydrogen bonding, or sharing of electrons.

**Van der Woude's syndrome** An autosomal dominant syndrome marked by cleft lip, palate, or both, paramedian pits of the lower lip, hypodontia, and missing second premolar teeth. SYN: *cleft lip–cleft palate syndrome; lip-pit syndrome.*

**vanilla** (vă-nĭl′ă) [Sp. *vainilla,* little sheath] Any one of a group of tropical orchids. The cured seed pods of *Vanilla planifolia* contain an aromatic substance, also called vanilla, that is used for flavoring.

**vanillin** A crystalline compound found in vanilla pods or produced synthetically; used for flavoring foods and in pharmaceuticals.

**vanillism** (vă-nĭl′ĭzm) Irritation of the skin, mucous membranes, and conjunctiva sometimes experienced by workers handling raw vanilla. It is caused by a mite.

**vanillylmandelic acid** ABBR: VMA. 3-methoxy-4-hydroxymandelic acid. Approx. 90% of the catecholamines epinephrine and norepinephrine are metabolized to VMA and are secreted in the urine. Persons with pheochromocytoma produce excess amounts of catecholamines; thus, increased amounts of VMA are present in their urine.

**vanishing twin** SEE: *gestation, multiple.*

**van't Hoff's rule** [Jacobus Henricus van't Hoff, Dutch chemist, 1852–1911] The rule that the speed of chemical reactions is doubled, at least, for each 10°C rise in temperature.

**vapor** (vā′por) [L., steam] **1.** The gaseous state of any substance. **2.** A medicinal substance for administration by inhalation.

**vaporization** (vā″por-ī-zā′shŭn) [L. *vapor,* steam] **1.** The conversion of a liquid or solid into vapor. **2.** Therapeutic use of a vapor.

**vaporize** (vā′por-īz) To change a material to a vapor form.

**vaporizer** (vā′por-ī″zer) A device for converting liquids into a vapor spray.

**vaporous** (vā′por-ŭs) [L. *vapor,* steam] Consisting of, pert. to, or producing vapors.

**vapor-permeable membrane** A membrane, usually transparent, that is permeable to oxygen and water vapor. It may be prepared with an adhesive backing that will stick only to dry skin. This type of membrane has been used in treating wounds. The membrane must be applied properly without wrinkles and changed as often as necessary to prevent excess accumulation of fluid and bacteria under it.

**Vaquez's disease** (vă-kāz′) [Louis Henri Vaquez, Fr. physician, 1860–1936] Polycythemia vera.

**variability** (văr″ē-ă-bĭl′ĭ-tē) The ability and tendency to change.

***baseline v.*** Fluctations in the fetal heart rate, recorded by the electronic monitor, that reflect the status of the fetal autonomic nervous system. Absence of short-term variability (beat-to-beat changes) is a sign of fetal compromise. Long-term variability (wavelike undulations) occurs normally three to five times per minute. Increased long-term variability is common during fetal sleep but may reflect prematurity, congenital abnormalities such as anencephaly, or fetal response to drugs.

**variable** (vā′rē-ă-b′l) [L. *variare,* to vary] **1.** Anything that is not constant but can and does change in different circumstances. In statistics, it is often possible to graph the relationship of one variable to another (e.g., the increase in height and weight in the growing child). **2.** Changing form, or structure, behavior, or physiology.

***dependent v.*** In research studies, a variable influenced by the independent variable.

***independent v.*** In research studies, a variable controlled by the investigator.

**variance** (văr′ē-ăns) [L. *variare,* to vary] A statistical index of the degree to which measurements in a data set are different from each other or deviate from the mean; the square of the standard deviation.

**variant** (văr′ē-ănt) That which is different from the characteristics of the other organisms or entities in a particular classification, esp. a disease, species, or physical appearance.

**variate** (vā′rē-āt) Variable (2).

**variation** (vā″rē-ā′shŭn) Differences between individuals of a certain species or class.

***continuous v.*** Variation in which the difference between successive groups or individuals is quite small.

***meristic v.*** Variation in number as opposed to kind.

**varication** (văr″ĭ-kā′shŭn) **1.** Formation of a varix. **2.** The condition of a varicosity.

**variced** Concerning a varix.

**varicella** (văr″ĭ-sĕl′ă) [L., a tiny spot] An acute, highly contagious viral disease characterized by an eruption that makes its appearance in successive crops, and passes through stages of macules, papules, vesicles, and crusts. Incubation time is from 2 to 3 weeks; usually 13 to 17 days. The prognosis is always favorable except in a very severe type, called varicella gangrenosa, in which gangrene may develop about the site of the lesions. SYN: *chickenpox.* SEE: *varicella-zoster immune globulin.*

SYMPTOMS: There may be a slight elevation of temperature at onset, followed within 24 hr by appearance of the eruption, after which time the temperature usually rises still further. Eruption first appears on the back and chest, crops continuing to make their appearance for an average of 2 to 3 days. Each crop requires about 36 hr to pass through the several stages. Because of this, macules, papules, vesicles, and crusts may be found side by side in the same general locality. Lesions are superficial and rupture very easily. They tend to be ovoid. On the chest, their distribution is often particularly marked along the course of the intercostal nerves. Some, although possibly few, scars nearly always remain as evidence of a varicella attack. The extremities are relatively free, as compared with the trunk.

ETIOLOGY: This virus is caused by varicella-zoster, which also causes herpes zoster. It may occur at any age, but is far less common in adults than in children. Epidemics are most frequent in winter and spring and in temperate zones. Approx. 75% of all children will contract varicella by age 15.

DIFFERENTIAL DIAGNOSIS: Confusion between this disease and smallpox is responsible for the chief importance given varicella. Impetigo, dermatitis herpetiformis, herpes zoster, and furunculosis may also require consideration.

COMPLICATIONS: Secondary infections may occur, caused by scratching, which may result in abscess formation; at times, development of erysipelas or even septicemia may result. Occasionally, lesions in the vicinity of the larynx may cause edema of the glottis and threaten the life of the patient. Encephalitis is a rare complication. Varicella may be fatal in children with leukemia or children who are taking adrenocorticosteroids.

PREVENTION: Administration of varicella-zoster immune globulin (VZIg) within 72 hr of exposure will prevent clinical varicella in susceptible, healthy children. The following conditions should alert one to the possible need for use of VZIg: immunocompromised children; newborns of mothers who develop varicella in the period 5 days before to 48 hr after delivery; postnatal exposure of newborns (esp. those who are premature) to varicella; healthy adults who are susceptible to varicella and who have been exposed; pregnant women who have no history of having had varicella and who have had significant exposure. The use of VZIg in pregnant women will not prevent fetal infection or congenital varicella syndrome. Live attenuated vaccine is now available for general use.

Caution: Because severe illness and death have resulted from varicella in children being treated with corticosteroids, these children should avoid exposure to varicella.

TREATMENT: Acyclovir should be given to adolescents and adults and to high-risk patients (e.g., premature infants) within 24 hr of onset of the disease. The use of calamine lotion locally may alleviate irritation. The skin, bedclothes, and sheets should be kept clean to help prevent skin infections. The fingernails should be cropped to prevent a secondary infection from pruritic skin lesions. Aspirin should be avoided because of the risk of Reye's syndrome. The usual duration of the disease is from 2 to 3 weeks. Patients are usually contagious from 5 days before skin eruption until not more than 6 days after the first crop of vesicles. SEE: *Universal Precautions Appendix.*

***v. gangrenosa*** Varicella in which necrosis occurs around the vesicles, resulting in gangrenous ulceration.

**varicella-zoster immune globulin** ABBR: VZIg. An immune globulin obtained from the blood of healthy persons found to have high antibody titers to varicella-zoster. SEE: *varicella.*

**varicelliform** (vär″ĭ-sĕl′ĭ-form) Resembling varicella. SYN: *varicelloid.*

**varicelloid** (vär″ĭ-sĕl′oyd) [″ + Gr. *eidos,* form, shape] Varicelliform.

**varices** (văr′ĭ-sēz) [L.] Pl. of varix.

**variciform** (văr-ĭs′ĭ-form) [L. *varix,* twisted vein, + *forma,* shape] Varicose.

**varicoblepharon** (văr″ĭ-kō-blĕf′ă-rŏn) [″ + Gr. *blepharon,* eyelid] Varicose tumor of the eyelid.

**varicocele** (văr′ĭ-kō-sēl) [″ + Gr. *kele,* tumor, swelling] Enlargement of the veins of the spermatic cord (pampiniform plexus), commonly occurring on the left side in adolescent males; these seldom require treatment. SYN: *varicole.*

SYMPTOMS: The vessels on the affected side of the scrotum are full, feel like a bundle of worms, and are sometimes purplish. There is a dull ache along the cord and a slight dragging sensation in the groin.

TREATMENT: The dragging sensation from an exceptionally large varicocele may be relieved by reducing the weight applied to the scrotum through use of a suspensory. Surgery is required for persistent symptomatic varicocele.

***ovarian v.*** Varicosity of the veins of the ovarian or pampiniform plexus of the broad ligament.

***utero-ovarian v.*** Varicosity of the veins of the ovarian (pampiniform) plexus and the uterine plexus of the broad ligament.

**varicocelectomy** (văr″ĭ-kō-sē-lĕk′tō-mē) [L. *varix,* twisted vein, + Gr. *kele,* tumor, swelling, + *ektome,* excision] Excision of a portion of the scrotal sac with ligation of the dilated veins to relieve varicocele.

**varicography** (văr″ĭ-kŏg′ră-fē) [″ + Gr. *graphein,* to write] Radiography of varicose veins after the injection of a contrast medium.

**varicoid** (văr′ĭ-koyd) [″ + Gr. *eidos,* form, shape] Resembling a varix.

**varicole** (văr′ĭ-kōl) Varicocele.

**varicomphalus** (văr″ĭ-kŏm′fă-lŭs) [″ + Gr. *omphalos,* navel] Varicose tumor of the navel.

**varicophlebitis** (văr″ĭ-kō-flē-bī′tĭs) [″ + Gr. *phleps,* vein, + *itis,* inflammation] Phlebitis combined with varicose veins.

**varicose** (văr′ĭ-kōs) [L. *varicosus,* full of dilated veins] Pert. to varices; distended, swollen, knotted veins. SYN: *variciform.*

**varicose ulcer** An ulcer that forms as a result of varicose veins. When thrombophlebitis develops in varicose veins, this leads to venous stasis and eventually edema and ulcer formation.

NURSING IMPLICATIONS: The patient maintains bedrest. Warm, moist compresses are continuously applied to relieve discomfort and infection. Aseptic technique is used in applying dressings and therapeutic agents.

**varicose vein** An enlarged, twisted superficial vein. This condition may occur in almost any part of the body but is most common in the lower extremities and in the esophagus. SEE: *Nursing Diagnoses Appendix.*

SYMPTOMS: Pain in the feet and ankles, swelling, and ulcers on the skin characterize this condition. Severe bleeding occurs if a vein is injured. SEE: illus.

ETIOLOGY: The condition is caused by incompetent venous valves that may be

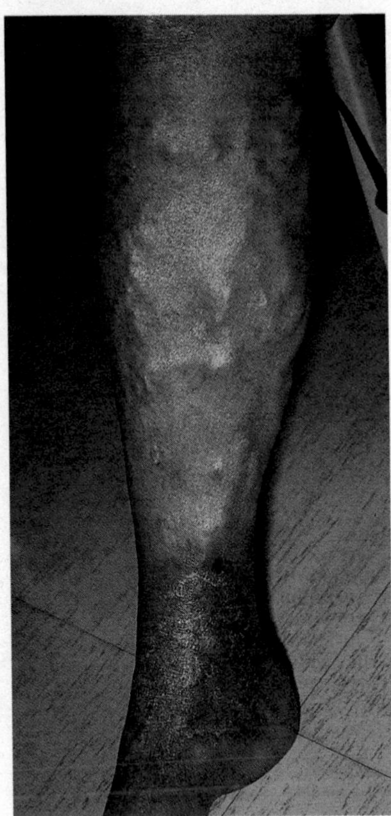

**VARICOSE VEINS** AND STASIS DERMATITIS OF THE ANKLE

acquired or congenital. The development of varicose veins is promoted and aggravated by pregnancy, obesity, and occupations that require prolonged standing. Esophageal varices are caused by portal hypertension that accompanies cirrhosis of the liver.

FIRST AID: In hemorrhage, elevation of the extremity and gentle but firm pressure over the wound will stop the bleeding. The pressure may be applied by holding a medium-sized coin firmly against the bleeding site. The use of a tourniquet is undesirable. A sterile dressing should be held in place with a firm bandage. The patient should not be permitted to walk until the acute condition is controlled. The Sengstaken-Blakemore tube may be used to control bleeding caused by hemorrhage from esophageal varices. SEE: *tamponade, balloon.*

TREATMENT: In general, treatment consists of rest, elevation of the extremity, and use of an external support. The use of elastic stockings is much preferred to elastic bandages. Unna's paste boots are recommended for elderly or debilitated persons with cutaneous ulcers. Injection of sclerosing solutions may be used for small varicosities. High ligation and removal of the vein by stripping may be necessary for major varicosities.

NURSING IMPLICATIONS: The nurse teaches the patient to avoid anything that impedes venous return, such as wearing garters and tight girdles, crossing the legs at the knees, and prolonged sitting. After the legs have been elevated for 10 to 15 min, support hose are applied. The patient should not sit in a chair for longer than 1 hr at a time. Ambulation is encouraged for at least 5 min every hour. The patient should elevate the legs whenever possible, but no less than twice a day for 30 min each time, and should avoid prolonged standing. Signs of thrombophlebitis, a complication of varicose veins, include heat and local pain. If surgery is performed, elastic stockings or antithrombus devices are applied postoperatively and the foot of the bed is elevated above the level of the heart. Overweight patients need to lose weight.

**varicosis** (văr″ĭ-kō′sĭs) [L.] Varicose condition of veins.

**varicosity** (văr″ĭ-kŏs′ĭ-tē) [L. *varix,* twisted vein] **1.** Condition of being varicose. **2.** Varix (1).

**varicotomy** (văr″ĭ-kŏt′ō-mē) [″ + Gr. *tome,* incision] Excision of a varicose vein.

**varicula** (văr-ĭk′ū-lă) [L., a tiny dilated vein] A small varix, esp. of the conjunctiva.

**variety** (vă-rī′ĕ-tē) [L., *varietas,* variety] A term used in classifying individuals in a subpopulation of a species.

**variola** (vă-rī′ō-lă) [L., pustule] An acute, contagious, systemic viral disease characterized by a prodromal stage during which the constitutional symptoms usually are severe, followed by an eruption that passes through the successive stages of macules, papules, vesicles, pustules, and crusts. SYN: *smallpox.* **variolar** (-lăr), *adj.*

NOTE: This disease is considered to have been completely eradicated worldwide. Cultures of the virus are kept in only one or two research laboratories.

***v. minor*** A mild form of smallpox with sparse rash and low-grade fever.

**varix** (vā′rĭks) *pl.* **varices** [L., twisted vein] **1.** A tortuous dilatation of a vein. SEE: *varicose vein.* **2.** Less commonly, dilatation of an artery or lymph vessel.

***aneurysmal v.*** A direct communication between an artery and a varicose vein without an intervening sac.

***arterial v.*** A varicosity or dilation of an artery.

***chyle v.*** A varix of a lymphatic vessel that conveys chyle.

***esophageal v.*** SEE: *esophageal varix; Nursing Diagnoses Appendix.*

***lymphaticus v.*** Dilatation of a lymphatic vessel.

***turbinal v.*** Permanent dilatation of veins of turbinate bodies.

**varnish** (văr′nĭsh) A solution of gums and resins in a solvent. When these are applied to a surface, the solvent evaporates and leaves a hard, more or less flexible film. In dentistry, varnishes are used to protect sensitive tooth areas such as the pulp.

***cavity v.*** The material applied to the walls and floor of a tooth cavity preparation to protect against acidic cements or metallic restorations. It reduces microleakage and seals the dentinal tubules, thereby reducing pulp irritation.

***periodontal v.*** A protective coating applied to the outer tooth surface to alleviate pain and promote healing after deep scaling or curettage.

**varolian** (vă-rō′lē-ăn) [Costanzo Varolio (Varolius), It. anatomist, 1543–1575] Rel. to the pons varolii.

**varolian bend** The anterior extension of the hindgut on its ventral surface in the fetus.

**varus** (vā′rŭs) [L.] Bent inward or twisted, used esp. of deformities in which the most distal part of the anatomy is turned inward. There are many varus conditions. In *coxa varus*, the shaft of the femur turns inward with respect to the neck of the femur. In *genu varus*, either the femur or tibia turns inward at the knee, causing a bowlegged deformity. *Talipes varus* is a clubfooted condition in which the foot turns inward and the person walks on the outer border of the foot. SEE: *valgus*.

**vas** (văs) *pl.* **vasa** [L., vessel] A vessel or duct.

***v. aberrans*** **1.** A narrow tube varying in length from 1½ to 14 in. (3.8 to 35.6 cm), occasionally found connected with the lower part of the canal of the epididymis or with the commencement of the vas deferens. **2.** A vestige of the biliary ducts sometimes found in the liver.

***v. afferens*** An afferent vessel of a lymph node.

***v. afferens glomeruli*** The afferent arteriole that conveys blood to the glomerulus of a renal corpuscle.

***v. capillare*** A capillary blood vessel.

***v. deferens*** The secretory duct of the testis, a continuation of the epididymis. This slim, muscular tube, approx. 18 in. (45.7 cm) long, transports the sperm from each testis to the ejaculatory duct, which empties into the prostatic urethra. SYN: *ductus deferens*. SEE: illus.; *genitalia* for illus.

***v. lymphaticum*** One of the vessels carrying the lymph.

***v. prominens*** Blood vessel on the cochlea's accessory spiral ligament.

***v. spirale*** A large blood vessel beneath the tunnel of Corti in the basilar membrane.

**vasa** (vā′să) [L. *vas*, vessel] Pl. of vas.

***v. afferentia*** The lymphatic vessels en-

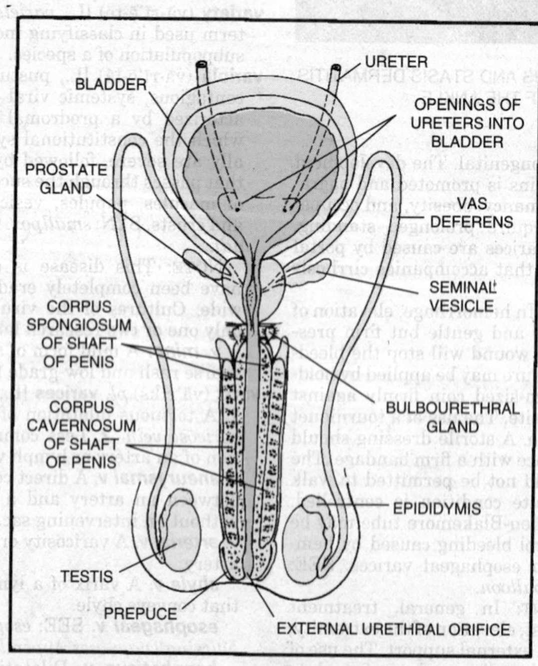


**VAS DEFERENS AND OTHER MALE ORGANS**

tering a lymph node.

***v. brevia*** Branches of the splenic artery going to the greater curvature of the stomach.

***v. efferentia*** **1.** Lymphatics that leave a lymph node. **2.** The secretory ducts of the testis to the head of the epididymis.

***v. praevia*** The blood vessels of the umbilical cord presenting before the fetus.

***v. recta*** **1.** Tubules that become straight before entering the mediastinum testis. **2.** Straight collecting tubules of the kidney.

***v. vasorum*** Minute blood vessels that are distributed to the walls of the larger veins and arteries.

***v. vorticosa*** Stellate veins of the choroid, carrying blood to the superior ophthalmic vein.

**vasal** (vā′săl) [L. *vas,* vessel] Rel. to a vas or vessel.

**vasalgia** (vă-săl′jē-ă) Pain in a vessel of any kind.

**vascular** (văs′kū-lăr) [L. *vasculum,* a small vessel] Pert. to or composed of blood vessels.

**vascular endothelium** The cellular tissue lining the blood vessels. In addition to serving as a semipermeable barrier between the blood and the vascular smooth muscle, the endothelium is highly active as a metabolic and endocrine organ. The cells may function to inactivate vasoactive substances and, in turn, produce vasodilator substances. Damage to the endothelium leads to increased production of prostaglandins.

**vascularity** (văs″kū-lăr′ĭ-tē) The state of being vascular.

**vascularization** (văs″kū-lăr-ī-zā′shŭn) [L. *vasculum,* a small vessel] The development of new blood vessels in a structure.

**vascularize** (văs′kū-lăr″īz) [L. *vasculum,* a small vessel] To become vascular by development of new blood vessels.

**vascular ring** A congenital abnormality in which an arterial ring encircles the trachea and esophagus. This causes signs of compression of their structures. Surgery may be required to relieve the symptoms.

**vascular system** The blood vessels: the arteries, capillaries, and veins. Pulmonary and systemic circulation are included.

**vascular tuft** One of the vascular processes on the chorion in the fetus at an early stage of development. SYN: *chorionic villi.*

**vascular tumor** Hemangioma; telangioma.

**vasculature** (văs′kū-lă-tūr″) The arrangement of blood vessels in the body or any part of it, including their relationship and functions.

**vasculitis** (văs″kū-lī′tĭs) [″ + *itis,* inflammation] Inflammation of a blood or lymph vessel. SYN: *angiitis.*

***livedoid v.*** Vascular inflammation combined with intravascular thrombosis. These purpuric lesions are slow to heal. The cause in most cases in unknown, but they may be associated with diseases such as systemic lupus or scleroderma.

**vasculogenesis** (văs″kū-lō-jĕn′ĕ-sĭs) [″ + Gr. *genesis,* generation, birth] Development of the vascular system.

**vasculomotor** (văs″kū-lō-mō′tor) Vasomotor.

**vasectomy** (vă-sĕk′tō-mē) [L. *vas,* vessel, + Gr. *ektome,* excision] Removal of all or a segment of the vas deferens. Bilateral vasectomy is the most successful method of male contraception. The question of the possible increased risk of prostate cancer in individuals who have had a vasectomy has been investigated, but the findings are inconclusive. SEE: illus.

NOTE: Persons who have had this surgical procedure ejaculate in a normal manner but the ejaculate does not contain sperm. There are no anatomical or physiological reasons for sterilization by this method to alter the sex drive or libido. Nevertheless, hematomas may occur postoperatively, and granulomas in response to leakage of sperm may occur.

---

Caution: The patient should have about two dozen ejaculations to help ensure that sterility has been accomplished. Sterility is not considered to have been achieved until two ejaculates have been found to be free of sperm. Spontaneous reanastomosis has been reported.

---

NURSING IMPLICATIONS: Ice bags are applied after surgery to reduce swelling and to promote comfort. Sitz baths may promote comfort in the days immediately after the surgery. Surgery does not prevent sexually transmitted diseases.

**vasectomy reversal** Surgical procedure for the rejoining of the previously severed vas deferens. Although this procedure may be successful, the chance of success varies in published reports.

**vasiform** (văs′ĭ-form) [″ + *forma,* shape] Resembling a tubular structure or vas.

**vasitis** (vă-sī′tĭs) Inflammation of the ductus deferens of the testicle.

**vaso-** [L. *vas,* vessel] Combining form meaning *vessel,* as a blood vessel.

**vasoactive** (văs″ō-ăk′tĭv) Affecting blood vessels.

**vasoactive intestinal polypeptide** ABBR: VIP. A peptide present in the mucosa of the gastrointestinal tract. One of its principal actions is to inhibit gastric function including gastric acid secretion. Vasoactive intestinal polypeptide is also present in nerve fibers of the female genital tract.

**vasoconstriction** (văs″ō-kŏn-strĭk′shŭn) A decrease in the caliber of blood vessels.

***hypoxic pulmonary v.*** Narrowing of the small arterioles in the alveoli in response to hypoxia.

**vasoconstrictive** (văs″ō-kŏn-strĭk′tĭv) [″ + *constrictus,* bound] Causing constriction of the blood vessels.

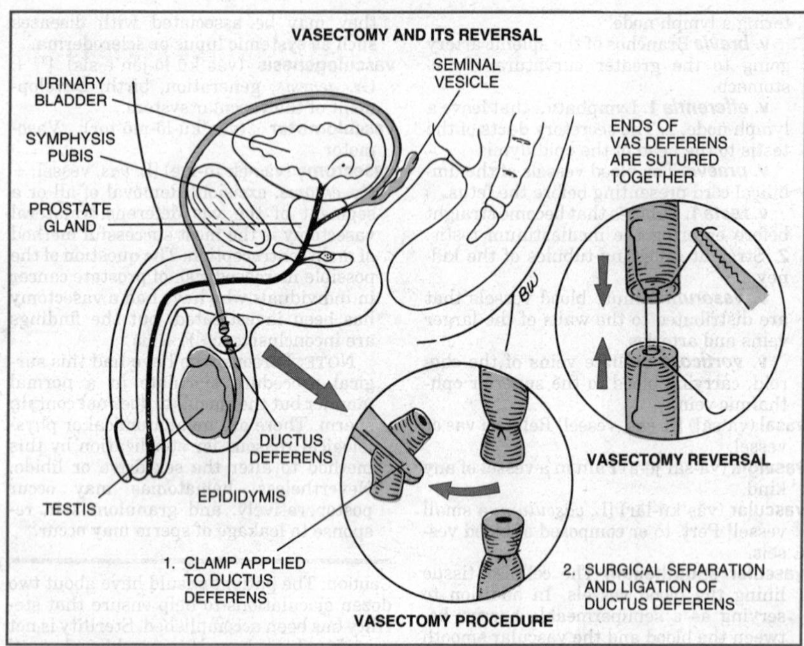


**vasoconstrictor** (văs″ō-kŏn-strĭk′tor) [″ + *constrictor,* a binder] **1.** Causing constriction of the blood vessels. **2.** That which constricts or narrows the caliber of blood vessels, as a drug or a nerve.

**vasodentin** (văs″ō-dĕn′tĭn) [″ + *dens,* tooth] Modified dentin provided with blood capillaries. This is present in fish but seldom seen in other animals.

**vasodepression** (văs″ō-dē-prĕsh′ŭn) [″ + *depressio,* a pressing down] Vasomotor depression or collapse.

**vasodepressor** (văs″ō-dē-prĕs′or) [″ + *depressor,* that which presses down] **1.** Having a depressing influence on the circulation, lowering blood pressure by dilatation of blood vessels. **2.** An agent that decreases circulation.

**vasodilatation** (văs″ō-dīl-ă-tā′shŭn) [″ + *dilatare,* to enlarge] Dilatation of blood vessels, esp. small arteries and arterioles.

***antidromic v.*** Vasodilatation resulting from stimulation of the dorsal root of a spinal nerve.

***reflex v.*** Blood vessel dilation caused by stimulation of its dilator nerves or inhibition of its constrictor substance or nerves. This can be done by stimulating the sensory reflex arc.

**vasodilation** (văs″ō-dī-lā′shŭn) An increase in the caliber of blood vessels.

**vasodilative** (văs″ō-dī′lā-tĭv) Causing dilation of blood vessels.

**vasodilator** (văs″ō-dī-lā′tor) [″ + *dilatare,* to enlarge] **1.** Causing relaxation of blood vessels. **2.** A nerve or drug that dilates blood vessels.

**vasoepididymostomy** (văs″ō-ĕp″ĭ-dĭd-ĭ-mŏs′tō-mē) [″ + Gr. *epi,* upon, + *didymos,* testicle, + *stoma,* mouth] The formation of a passage between the vas deferens and the epididymis.

**vasofactive** (văs″ō-făk′tĭv) [″ + *facere,* to make] Forming new blood vessels.

**vasoganglion** (văs″ō-găng′glē-ŏn) Any mass of blood vessels.

**vasography** (văs-ŏg′ră-fē) [″ + Gr. *graphein,* to write] Radiography of the blood vessels, usually after the injection of a contrast medium.

**vasohypertonic** (văs″ō-hī″pĕr-tŏn′ĭk) [″ + Gr. *hyper,* over, above, excessive, + *tonikos,* pert. to tension] Vasoconstrictor.

**vasohypotonic** (văs″ō-hī″pō-tŏn′ĭk) [″ + Gr. *hypo,* under, beneath, below, + *tonikos,* pert. to tension] Vasodilator.

**vasoinhibitor** (văs″ō-ĭn-hĭb′ĭ-tor) [″ + *inhibere,* to restrain] An agent that decreases the action of vasomotor nerves.

**vasoinhibitory** (văs″ō-ĭn-hĭb′ĭ-tor-ē) Restricting vasomotor activity.

**vasoligation** (văs″ō-lī-gā′shŭn) [″ + *ligare,* to bind] Ligation of a vessel, specifically the vas deferens.

**vasomotion** (văs″ō-mō′shŭn) [″ + *motio,* movement] Change in caliber of a blood vessel.

**vasomotor** (văs″ō-mō′tor) [″ + *motor,* a mover] Pert. to the nerves having muscular control of the blood vessel walls. The circularly arranged fibers of the muscles of arteries and veins can contract or relax; the affected region is accordingly either blanched or flushed. The former effect can commonly be produced by stimulating sympathetic fibers and is consequently called vasoconstrictor. Certain other nerves, on stimulation, cause vasodilation, examples being the nervus chorda tympani and the nervi erigentes. A vasomotor reflex is one in which the stimulus, such as a horrifying sight, results in a change in vasomotor tone (e.g., pallor). SEE: *vasoconstrictor; vasodilator.*

**vasomotor epilepsy** Epilepsy with vasomotor changes in the skin.

**vasomotor reflex** Constriction of cutaneous blood vessels in response to a stimulus to the skin.

**vasomotor spasm** Spasm of smaller arteries.

**vasoneuropathy** (văs″ō-nū-rŏp′ă-thē) Disease due to the combined effect of the vascular and nervous systems.

**vasoneurosis** (văs″ō-nū-rō′sĭs) [L. *vas,* vessel, + Gr. *neuron,* nerve, + *osis,* condition] A neurosis affecting blood vessels; a disorder of the vasomotor system.

**vaso-orchidostomy** (văs″ō-or″kĭd-ŏs′tō-mē) [″ + Gr. *orchis,* testicle, + *stoma,* mouth] Surgical connection of the epididymis to the severed end of the vas deferens.

**vasoparesis** (văs″ō-păr-ē′sĭs) [″ + Gr. *parienai,* to let fall] Partial paralysis or weakness of the vasomotor nerves.

**vasopressin** (văs″ō-prĕs′ĭn) A hormone formed in the supraoptic and paraventricular nuclei of the hypothalamus and transported to the posterior lobe of the hypophysis through the hypothalamohypophyseal tract. It has an antidiuretic effect and a pressor effect that elevates blood pressure. This drug should not be used as an agent to increase blood pressure because of its effect of reducing coronary artery blood flow. SYN: *antidiuretic hormone.* SEE: *oxytocin.*

**vasopressin injection** A sterile solution, in a suitable diluent, of material containing the polypeptide hormone having the properties of causing the contraction of vascular and other smooth muscle, and of diuresis.

**vasopressor** (văs″ō-prĕs′or) **1.** Causing contraction of the smooth muscle of arteries and arterioles. This increases resistance to the flow of blood and thus elevates blood pressure. **2.** An agent that stimulates contraction of smooth muscle of arteries and arterioles.

**vasopuncture** (văs′ō-pŭnk″chūr) [″ + *punctura,* prick] Puncture of the vas deferens.

**vasoreflex** (văs″ō-rē′flĕx) A reflex that alters the caliber of blood vessels.

**vasorrhaphy** (văs-or′ă-fē) [″ + Gr. *rhaphe,* seam, ridge] Surgical suture of the vas deferens.

**vasosection** (văs″ō-sĕk′shŭn) [″ + *sectio,* a cutting] Surgical division of the vasa deferentia.

**vasosensory** (văs″ō-sĕn′sō-rē) [″ + *sensorius,* pert. to sensation] Rel. to sensation in the blood vessels.

**vasospasm** (văs′ō-spăzm) [″ + Gr. *spasmos,* a convulsion] Spasm of a blood vessel. SYN: *angiohypotonia; angiospasm; vasoconstriction.*

**vasospastic** (văs″ō-spăs′tĭk) Concerning or characterized by vasospasm.

**vasostimulant** (văs″ō-stĭm′ū-lănt) [L. *vas,* vessel, + *stimulans,* goading] Exciting vasomotor action.

**vasostomy** (vă-sŏs′tō-mē) [″ + Gr. *stoma,* mouth] Surgical procedure of making an opening into the vas deferens.

**vasotomy** (văs-ŏt′ō-mē) [″ + Gr. *tome,* incision] Incision of the vas deferens.

**vasotonia** (văs″ō-tō′nē-ă) [″ + Gr. *tonos,* act of stretching, tension] The tone of blood vessels.

**vasotonic** (văs″ō-tŏn′ĭk) [″ + Gr. *tonikos,* pert. to tone] **1.** Pert. to the tone of a vessel. **2.** Causing vasotonia.

**vasotrophic** (văs″ō-trŏf′ĭk) [″ + Gr. *trophe,* nourishment] Concerned with the nutrition of blood vessels.

**vasotropic** (văs″ō-trŏp′ĭk) Affecting blood vessels.

**vasovagal** (văs″ō-vā′găl) Concerning the action of stimuli from the vagus nerve on blood vessels.

**vasovagal syncope** Sudden faint due to hypotension induced by the response of the nervous system to abrupt emotional stress, pain, or trauma. This is accompanied by pallor, sweating, hyperventilation, and bradycardia. Vagal stimulation causes this reaction. Treatment consists of having the patient lie flat and being certain that there is a clear airway; the underlying condition is treated if indicated. Anticholinergic agents, such as propantheline bromide, may be helpful. Vomiting does not usually occur, but if it does, the patient should be positioned to prevent aspiration of vomitus.

**vasovasostomy** (văs″ō-vă-sŏs′tō-mē) [″ + *vas,* vessel, + *stoma,* mouth] Rejoining of the previously severed ductus deferens of the testicle.

**vasovesiculectomy** (văs″o-vĕ-sĭk″ū-lĕk′tō-mē) [″ + *vesicula,* tiny sac, + Gr. *ektome,* excision] Excision of the vas deferens and seminal vesicles.

**vasovesiculitis** (văs″ō-vĕ-sĭk″ū-lī′tĭs) [″ + *vesicula,* a tiny bladder, + Gr. *itis,* inflammation] Inflammation of the vas deferens and seminal vesicles.

**vastus** (văs′tŭs) [L., vast] **1.** Great, large, extensive. **2.** One of three muscles of the thigh. SEE: *Muscles Appendix.*

**Vater's ampulla** (fă′tĕrz) [Abraham Vater, Ger. anatomist, 1684–1751] Former name for Vater's papilla.

**Vater's corpuscles** Ovoid end organs of nerves supplying the skin. SYN: *pacinian corpuscles.*

**Vater's papilla** The duodenal end of the drainage systems of the pancreatic and common bile ducts. Formerly called Vater's ampulla.

**vault** (vawlt) A part or structure resembling

a dome or arched roof.

**VBAC** *vaginal birth after previous cesarean.*

**VC** *vital capacity.*

**VD** *venereal disease.*

**VDH** *valvular disease of the heart.*

**VDRL** *Venereal Disease Research Laboratories.*

**vection** (vĕk′shŭn) [L. *vectio,* a carrying] **1.** Transfer of disease agents by a vector from the sick to the well. **2.** Illusion of self-motion. This may be produced experimentally by having the subject seated within a drum that rotates while the subject remains stationary.

**vectis** (vĕk′tĭs) [L., pole] A curved lever for making traction on the presenting part of the fetus.

**vector** (vĕk′tor) [L., a carrier] **1.** Any force or influence that is a quantity completely specified by magnitude, direction, and sense, which can be represented by a straight line of appropriate length and direction. **2.** A carrier, usually an insect or other arthropod, that transmits the causative organisms of disease from infected to noninfected individuals, esp. one in which the organism goes through one or more stages in its life cycle.

***biological v.*** An animal vector in which the disease-causing organism multiplies or develops prior to becoming infective for a susceptible individual.

***mechanical v.*** A vector in or upon which growth and development of the infective agent do not occur.

**vectorcardiogram** (vĕk″tor-kăr′dē-ō-grăm) [″ + Gr. *kardia,* heart, + *gramma,* something written] A graphic record of the direction and magnitude of the electrical forces of the heart's action by means of a continuous series of vector loops. Analysis of the configuration of these loops permits certain statements to be made about the state of health or diseased condition of the heart. At any moment the electrical activity of the heart can be represented as an electrical vector with a specific direction and magnitude. This is called the instantaneous cardiac vector. A series of these vectors may be established for the entire cardiac cycle. By joining the tips of these vectors with a continuous line, the vectorcardiogram loop is formed. The configuration so obtained may be projected on the frontal plane or viewed as a three-dimensional loop. Three vectorcardiogram loops are formed during each cardiac cycle—one for the electrical activity of the atrium; one for ventricular depolarization; one for ventricular repolarization.

***spatial v.*** Depiction of the vectorcardiogram in three planes—frontal, sagittal, and horizontal.

**vectorcardiography** Analysis of the direction and magnitude of the electrical forces of the heart's action by a continuous series of loops (vectors) that represent the cardiac cycle.

**vectorial** (vĕk-tō′rē-ăl) [L. *vector,* a carrier] Rel. to a vector.

**VEE** *Venezuelan equine encephalitis.*

**vegan** (vĕj′ăn) A vegetarian who omits all animal protein from the diet.

**veganism** (vĕj′ă-nĭzm) Strict vegetarianism in which one eats no food, including milk or cheese products, from an animal source.

**vegetable** (vĕj′ĕ-tă-bl) **1.** Pert. to, of the nature of, or derived from plants. **2.** A herbaceous plant, esp. one cultivated for food. **3.** The edible part or parts of plants that are used as food, including the leaves, stems, seeds and seed pods, flowers, roots, tubers, and fruits.

Vegetables are important sources of minerals and vitamins; provide bulk, which stimulates intestinal motility; and are sources of energy. Caloric value is indirectly proportional to water content. Vegetables in general are valuable for their mineral content and for their fiber content. Copper is estimated at 1.2 mg/kg for leafy vegetables, and 0.7 mg/kg for nonleafy ones.

Plant and vegetable proteins are nutritionally inferior to those from animal sources, but by combining certain vegetables in the diet, a completely adequate and balanced mixture of essential amino acids can be provided. Corn is low in lysine but has adequate amounts of tryptophan; beans are adequate in lysine but low in tryptophan. While neither of these two foods contains adequate amounts of essential amino acids, they are adequate when eaten in combination. Similarly, rice and soybeans eaten together provide adequate essential amino acids even though each is lacking in essential amino acids. SEE: *incaparina.*

All starches in vegetables must be changed to sugars before they can be absorbed. Dry heat changes starch to dextrin; heat and acid or an enzyme change dextrin to dextrose. In germinating grain, starch is changed to dextrin and dextrose. Fermented dextrose produces alcohol and carbon dioxide.

***cruciferous v.*** One of a group of vegetables, named for their crosslike flowers, including broccoli, brussels sprouts, cabbage, and cauliflower. These vegetables contain chemicals such as indoles that are thought to be protective against cancer.

**vegetal** (vĕj′ĕ-tăl) **1.** Pert. to plants. **2.** Tropic or nutritional, esp. with reference to that part of an ovum which contains the yolk. SEE: *pole, vegetal.*

**vegetarian** (vĕj-ĕ-tā′rē-ăn) [from *vegetable,* coined 1847 by the Vegetarian Society] One whose diet consists mainly of vegetables, sometimes also excluding dairy products. A carefully planned vegetarian diet, even if devoid of dairy products, may provide adequate nutrition; but if the diet is limited to fats, oils, refined carbohydrates, starches, or alcohol, it may not be nutritionally adequate.

**vegetarianism** (věj-ĕ-tā'rē-ăn-ĭzm) [" + Gr. *-ismos,* condition] The belief and practice of eating vegetables and fruits only; may or may not exclude dairy products.

**vegetate** (věj'ĕ-tāt) [LL. *vegetare,* to grow] **1.** To grow luxuriantly with the production of fleshy or warty outgrowths such as a polyp. **2.** To lead a passive existence mentally or physically, or both; to do little more than eat and maintain autonomic body functions.

**vegetation** (věj-ĕ-tā'shŭn) A morbid luxurious outgrowth on any part, esp. wartlike projections made up of collections of fibrin in which are enmeshed white and red blood cells; sometimes seen on denuded areas of the endocardium covering the valves of the heart.

***adenoid v.*** Funguslike masses of lymphoid tissue in the nasopharynx.

**vegetative** (věj'ĕ-tā"tĭv) **1.** Having the power to grow, as plants. **2.** Functioning involuntarily. **3.** Quiescent, passive, denoting a stage of development.

**vegetative state** SEE: under *state.*

**vegetoanimal** (věj"ĕ-tō-ăn'ĭ-măl) Concerning plants and animals.

**vehicle** (vē'ĭ-kl) [L. *vehiculum,* that which carries] An inert agent that carries the active ingredient in a medicine (e.g., a syrup in liquid preparations).

**veil** (vāl) [L. *velum,* a covering] **1.** Any veil-like structure. **2.** A piece of the amniotic sac occasionally covering the face of a newborn infant. SYN: *caul.* **3.** Slight alteration in the voice in order to disguise it.

**vein** (vān) [L. *vena,* vein] A vessel carrying deoxygenated (dark red) blood to the heart, except for the pulmonary veins, which carry oxygenated blood. Veins have three coats: inner, middle, and outer. They differ from arteries in their larger capacity and greater number; also in their thinner walls, larger and more frequent anastomoses, and presence of valves that prevent backward circulation. They consist of two sets, superficial or subcutaneous, and the deep veins, with frequent communications between the two. The former do not usually accompany an artery, as do the latter. The systemic veins consist of three groups—those entering the heart through the superior vena cava, those through the inferior vena cava, and those through the coronary sinus. Blood from the capillary plexuses enters the right atrium of the heart. SEE: illus.; *circulation; vena; Veins Appendix.*

***brachiocephalic v.'s*** The right and left veins, each formed by the union of the internal jugular with the subclavian vein.

***innominate v.'s*** Brachiocephalic v.'s.

**velamen** (vē-lā'mĕn) *pl.* **velamina** [L., veil] Any covering membrane.

***v. nativum*** The skin covering the body.

***v. vulvae*** Hottentot apron.

**velamentous** (věl"ă-mĕn'tŭs) Expanding like a veil, or sheet.

**velamentum** (věl"ă-mĕn'tŭm) *pl.* **velamenta** [L., a cover] A membranous covering.

**velar** (vē'lăr) [L. *velum,* a veil] Pert. to a velum or veil-like structure.

**Velcro** Trade name for fabric tape closures frequently used in orthotic fabrication and in adapting garments and devices for use by disabled persons with limited upper extremity function. The material contains a hooked side that adheres to the opposite (looped) side when the two are pressed together. The material may be applied and removed many times without losing its ability to adhere.

**veliform** (věl'ĭ-form) Velamentous.

**vellus** (věl'ŭs) [L., fleece] The fine hair present on the body after the lanugo hair of the newborn is gone.

**velopharyngeal** (věl"ō-fă-rĭn'jē-ăl) [L. *velum,* veil, + Gr. *pharynx,* throat] Concerning the soft palate and the pharynx.

**Velpeau's bandage** (věl-pōz') [Alfred Velpeau, Fr. surgeon, 1795–1867] A special immobilizing roller bandage that incorporates the shoulder, forearm, and arm. SEE: *bandage* for illus.

**Velpeau's deformity** Deformity seen in Colles' fracture, in which the lower fragment is displaced backward.

**velum** (vē'lŭm) [L., veil] Any veil-like structure.

***v. palatinum*** The soft palate.

**vena** (vē'nă) *pl.* **venae** [L.] A vein. SEE: *Veins Appendix.*

***v. cava inferior*** The principal vein draining blood from the lower portion of the body. It is formed by junction of the two common iliac veins and terminates in the right atrium of the heart. SEE: *heart.*

***v. cava superior*** The principal vein draining blood from the upper portion of the body. It is formed by the junction of the right and left brachiocephalic veins and empties into the right atrium of the heart. SEE: *heart.*

**venacavography** (vē"nă-kā-vŏg'ră-fē) Radiography of the vena cava during the injection of a contrast medium.

**venae comitantes** [L.] Two or more veins accompanying an artery. They are usually present with the deep arteries of the extremities.

**venation** The distribution of veins to an organ or structure.

**venectasia** (vē"nĕk-tā'zē-ă) [L. *vena,* a vein, + Gr. *ektasis,* dilation] Dilation of a vein. SYN: *phlebectasia.*

**venectomy** (vē-nĕk'tō-mē) [" + Gr. *ektome,* excision] Phlebectomy.

**veneer** In dentistry, a manmade material, such as an acrylic resin, that can be bonded to the surface of a tooth. It is sometimes used for cosmetic reasons.

**venene** (vē-nēn') A mixture of venoms from poisonous snakes.

**venenosalivary** (vĕn"ĕ-nō-săl'ĭ-vĕr"ē) Venomosalivary.

**venenosity** (vĕn"ĕ-nŏs'ĭ-tē) State of being

venomous.

**venenous** (věn′ĕn-ŭs) [L. *venenum*, poison] Poisonous.

**venepuncture** (věn′ē-pŭnk″chūr) [L. *vena*, vein, + *punctura*, a point] Venipuncture.

**venereal** (vē-nē′rē-ăl) [L. *venereus*] Pert. to or resulting from intercourse.

**venereal bubo** Enlarged lymph node in the groin, the result of a venereal disease.

**venereal collar** SEE: *leukoderma, syphilitic.*

**venereal disease** Disease acquired ordinarily as a result of heterosexual or homosexual intercourse with an individual who is afflicted. The diseases so classified in-

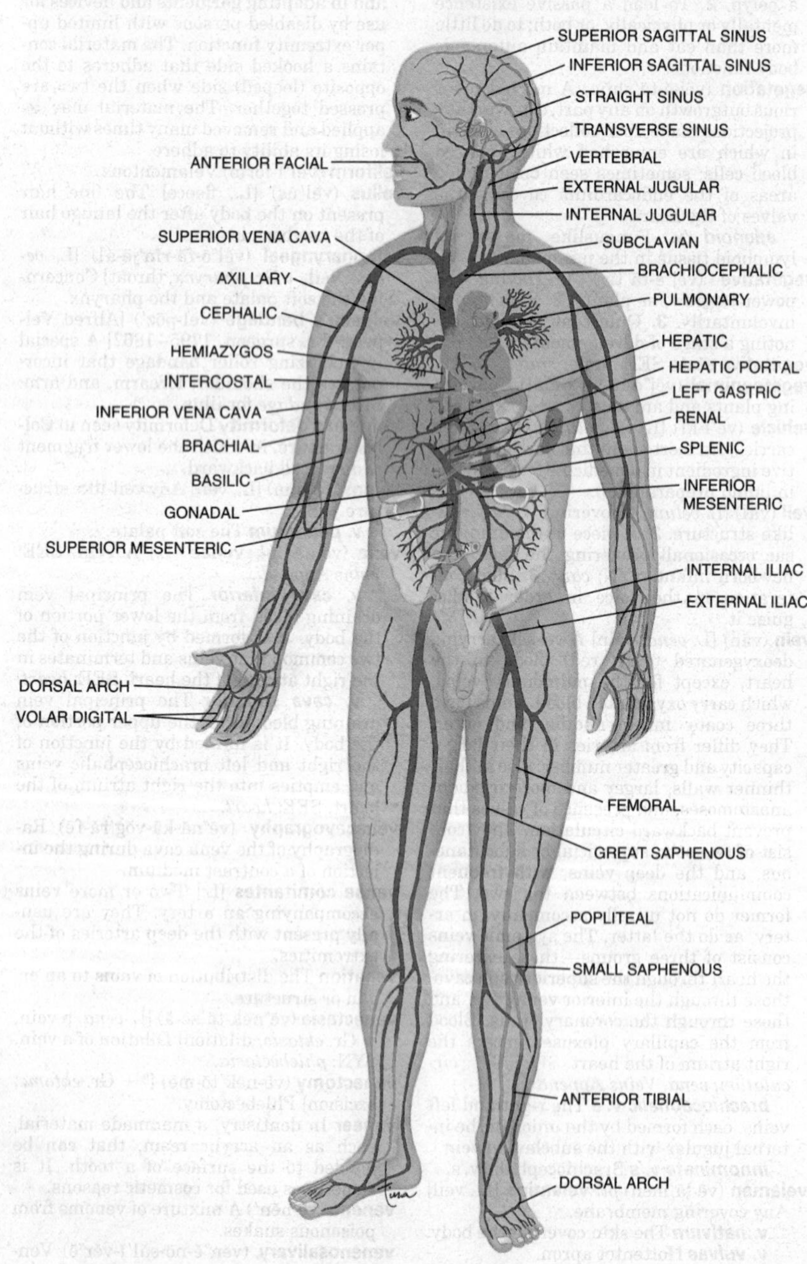

SYSTEMIC VEINS

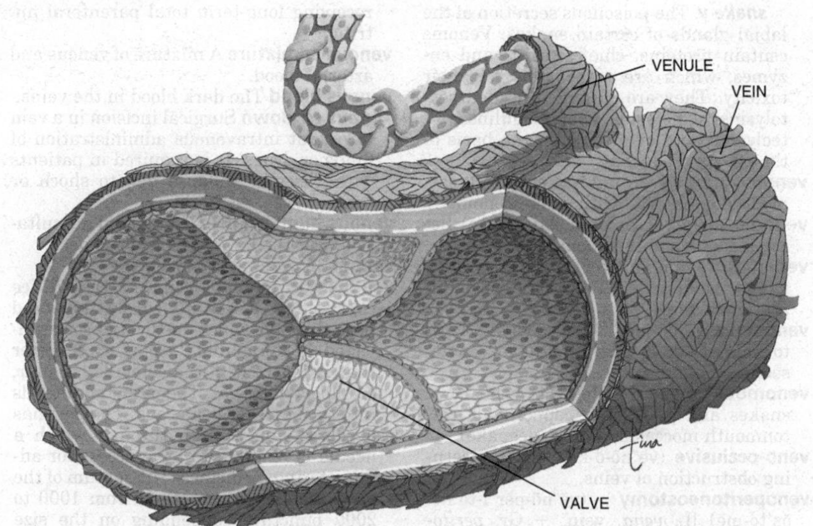


STRUCTURE OF A VEIN AND VENULE

clude gonorrhea, nonspecific urethritis, chlamydiosis, syphilis, AIDS, and chancroid. *Trichomonas vaginalis* vaginitis can be, but is not always, contracted through sexual intercourse. Genital candidiasis, lymphogranuloma venereum, granuloma inguinale, genital herpes, genital warts, balanoposthitis, and proctitis are also included in this classification. Bacterial pathogens, such as those of the genera *Salmonella, Shigella, Campylobacter,* and parasitic organisms including those of the genera *Giardia* and *Amoeba* may be transmitted by sexual activity involving anal-oral contact. Scabies may also be a venereal disease. SYN: *sexually transmitted disease.* SEE: *AIDS; Nursing Diagnoses Appendix.*

**venereal sore** Chancroid.

**venereal urethritis** Urethritis occurring in gonorrhea.

**venereal wart** Moist reddish elevation on the genitals and anus. SYN: *condyloma; verruca acuminata.*

**venereologist** (vē-nĕr″ē-ŏl′ō-jĭst) [″ + Gr. *logos,* word, reason] A doctor who specializes in the treatment of venereal diseases.

**venereology** (vē-nĕr″ē-ŏl′ō-jē) The scientific study and treatment of venereal diseases.

**venereophobia** (vē-nĕr″ē-ŏ-fō′bē-ă) [L. *venereus,* pert. to sexual intercourse, + Gr. *phobos,* fear] Abnormal fear of venereal disease. SYN: *cypridophobia.*

**venesection** (vĕn″ĕ-sĕk′shŭn) [L. *vena,* vein, + *sectio,* a cutting] Surgical opening of a vein for withdrawal of blood. SYN: *phlebotomy.*

**venin(e)** (vĕn′ĭn) [L. *venenum,* poison] Toxic substance in snake venom. SYN: *venene.*

**venipuncture** (vĕn′ĭ-pŭnk″chūr) [L. *vena,* vein, + *punctura,* a point] Puncture of a vein for any purpose. The pain of venipuncture may be diminished by several methods, including application of cold to the area just prior to the puncture; injection of sterile, normal saline intracutaneously to produce blanching of the site; and use of a local anesthetic to produce a wheal at the site. SEE: *intravenous infusion* for illus.

**venisuture** (vĕn′ĭ-sū″chūr) [″ + *sutura,* a seam] Suture of a vein. SYN: *phleborrhaphy.*

**veno-** Combining form meaning *vein.*

**venoatrial** (vē″nō-āt′rē-ăl) [″ + *atrium,* corridor] Rel. to the vena cava and the atrium. SYN: *venoauricular.*

**venoauricular** (vē″nō-aw-rĭk′ū-lăr) [″ + *auricula,* little ear] Venoatrial.

**venoclysis** (vē-nŏk′lĭ-sĭs) [″ + Gr. *klysis,* a washing] The continuous injection of medicinal or nutrient fluid intravenously.

**venofibrosis** (vē″nō-fī-brō′sĭs) Phlebosclerosis.

**venogram** (vē′nō-grăm) [″ + Gr. *gramma,* something written] **1.** A radiograph of the veins. SYN: *phlebogram.* **2.** A tracing of the venous pulse.

**venography** (vē-nŏg′ră-fē) [″ + Gr. *graphein,* to write] **1.** A radiographic procedure to visualize veins filled with a contrast medium; most commonly used to detect thrombophlebitis. **2.** The making of a tracing of the venous pulse.

**venom** (vĕn′ŏm) [L. *venenum,* poison] A poison secreted by some animals, such as insects, spiders, or snakes, and transmitted by bites or stings.

***Russell's viper v.*** SEE: *Russell's viper venom.*

***snake v.*** The poisonous secretion of the labial glands of certain snakes. Venoms contain proteins, chiefly toxins and enzymes, which are responsible for their toxicity. They are classified as neurocytolysins, hemolysins, hemocoagulins, proteolysins, and cytolysins on the basis of the effects produced.

**venomization** (vĕn″ŭm-ī-zā′shŭn) Treatment of a material with snake venom.

**venomosalivary** (vĕn″ō-mō-săl′ĭ-vĕr″ē) Secreting saliva with venom in it.

**venomotor** (vē″nō-mō′tor) [L. *vena,* vein, + *motus,* moving] Pert. to constriction or dilatation of veins.

**venomous** (vĕn′ō-mŭs) **1.** Poisonous. **2.** Pert. to animals or insects that have venom-secreting glands.

**venomous snake** In the U.S., the coral snakes and pit vipers (copperhead, cottonmouth moccasin, and rattlesnake).

**veno-occlusive** (vē″nō-ŏ-kloo′sĭv) Concerning obstruction of veins.

**venoperitoneostomy** (vē″nō-pĕr″ĭ-tō″nē-ŏs′tō-mē) [L. *vena,* vein, + Gr. *peritonaion,* peritoneum, + *stoma,* mouth] Surgical insertion of the cut end of the saphenous vein into the cavity of the peritoneum. This is done to allow ascitic fluid from the peritoneal cavity to drain into the vein.

**venosclerosis** (vē″nō-sklĕ-rō′sĭs) [″ + Gr. *sklerosis,* to harden] Sclerosis of veins. SYN: *phlebosclerosis.*

**venosinal** (vē″nō-sī′năl) Concerning the vena cava and the right atrium of the heart.

**venosity** (vē-nŏs′ĭ-tē) [L. *vena,* vein] **1.** A condition in which there is an excess of venous blood in a part, causing venous congestion. **2.** Deficient aeration of venous blood.

**venospasm** (vē′nō-spăzm) [″ + Gr. *spasmos,* a convulsion] Contraction of a vein, which may follow infusion of a cold or irritating substance into the vein.

**venostasis** (vē″nō-stā′sĭs) [″ + Gr. *stasis,* standing still] The trapping of blood in an extremity by compression of veins, a method sometimes employed for reducing the amount of blood being returned to the heart.

**venostat** (vē′nō-stăt) [″ + Gr. *statikos,* standing] An appliance for performing venous compression.

**venothrombotic** (vē″nō-thrŏm-bŏt′ĭk) Having the property of inducing the formation of thrombi in veins.

**venotomy** (vē-nŏt′ō-mē) [″ + Gr. *tome,* incision] Incision of a vein.

**venous** (vē′nŭs) [L. *vena,* vein] Pert. to the veins or blood passing through them.

**venous access device** A specially designed catheter for use in gaining and maintaining access to the venous system. This device provides access for patients who require intravenous fluids or medications for several days or more (e.g., those having a bone marrow transplant or who are receiving long-term total parenteral nutrition).

**venous admixture** A mixture of venous and arterial blood.

**venous blood** The dark blood in the veins.

**venous cutdown** Surgical incision in a vein to permit intravenous administration of fluids or drugs. It is required in patients with vascular collapse due to shock or other causes. SEE: illus.

**venous hum** A murmur heard on auscultation over the larger veins of the neck.

**venous hyperemia** Venosity (1).

**venous port** Part of a venous access device consisting of a subcutaneously implanted port through which medications are injected. Leading from the port is a catheter that is inserted in the cephalic, jugular, or subclavian vein. The catheter extends into the superior vena cava. The port has a self-sealing septum through which a needle is inserted to have access for administering medicines. The septum of the port is made to withstand from 1000 to 2000 punctures depending on the size needle used. Sterile technique is used each time a needle enters the port. The port permits unrestricted patient activity. Each time it is used care must be taken to be certain the line is open and that the catheter in the vein has remained in the proper position.

**venous return** The amount of blood returning to the atria of the heart.

**venous sinus** A channel that carries venous blood. Important venous sinuses are those of the dura mater draining the brain and those of the spleen.

**venous sinus of sclera** Schlemm's canal.

**venovenostomy** (vē″nō-vē-nŏs′tō-mē) [″ + ″ + Gr. *stoma,* mouth] The formation of an anastomosis of a vein joined to a vein.

**vent** (vĕnt) [O. Fr. *fente,* slit] An opening in any cavity, esp. one for excretion.

***alveolar v.*** An opening between adjacent alveoli of the lung.

**venter** (vĕn′tĕr) [L., belly] **1.** A belly-shaped part. **2.** The cavity of the abdomen. **3.** The wide swelling part or belly of a muscle.

**ventilation** (vĕn″tĭ-lā′shŭn) [L. *ventilare,* to air] **1.** Circulation of fresh air in a room and withdrawal of foul air. **2.** In physiology, the amount of air inhaled per day. This can be estimated by spirometry, multiplying the tidal air by the number of respirations per day. An average figure is 10,000 L. This must not be confused with the total amount of oxygen consumed, which is on the average only 360 L/day. These volumes are more than doubled during hard physical labor.

***abdominal displacement v.*** A noninvasive type of artificial ventilation that relies on displacement of the abdominal contents to move the patient's diaphragm.

***airway pressure release v.*** A type of mechanical ventilation in which continuous airway pressure is intermittently released to a lower pressure.

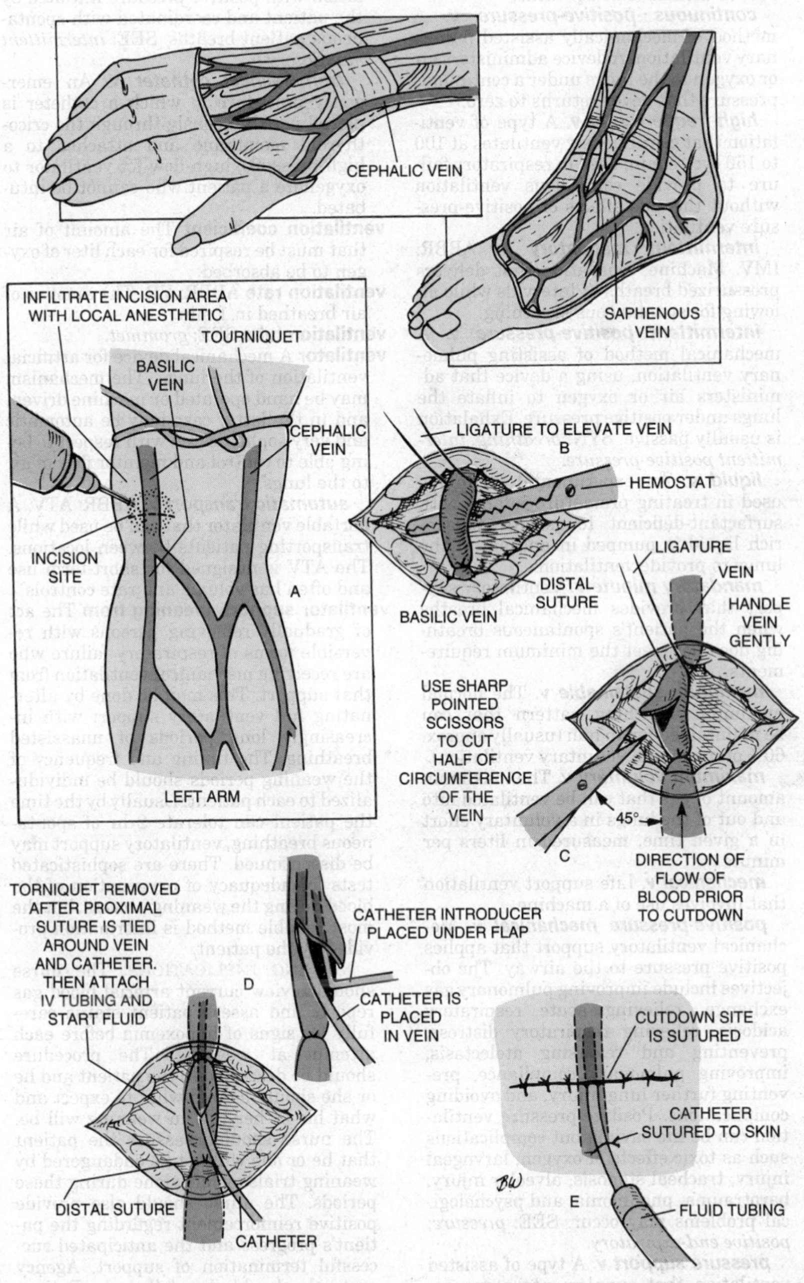
VENOUS CUTDOWN
CEPHALIC VEIN
SAPHENOUS VEIN
INFILTRATE INCISION AREA WITH LOCAL ANESTHETIC
TOURNIQUET
BASILIC VEIN
CEPHALIC VEIN
INCISION SITE
A
LEFT ARM
LIGATURE TO ELEVATE VEIN
B
HEMOSTAT
LIGATURE
DISTAL SUTURE
BASILIC VEIN
VEIN
HANDLE VEIN GENTLY
USE SHARP POINTED SCISSORS TO CUT HALF OF CIRCUMFERENCE OF THE VEIN
45°
C
DIRECTION OF FLOW OF BLOOD PRIOR TO CUTDOWN
TORNIQUET REMOVED AFTER PROXIMAL SUTURE IS TIED AROUND VEIN AND CATHETER. THEN ATTACH IV TUBING AND START FLUID
CATHETER INTRODUCER PLACED UNDER FLAP
D
CATHETER IS PLACED IN VEIN
DISTAL SUTURE
CATHETER
CUTDOWN SITE IS SUTURED
CATHETER SUTURED TO SKIN
E
FLUID TUBING
BW

***alveolar v.*** The movement of gas into and out of the alveoli. Its measure is corrected for anatomical deadspace and reflected in the arterial partial pressure of carbon dioxide ($PaCO_2$) value.

***continuous positive-pressure v.*** A method of mechanically assisted pulmonary ventilation. A device administers air or oxygen to the lungs under a continuous pressure that never returns to zero.

***high-frequency jet v.*** A type of ventilation that continuously ventilates at 100 to 150 cycles/min; used in respiratory failure to provide continuous ventilation without the side effects of positive-pressure ventilation.

***intermittent mandatory v.*** ABBR: IMV. Machine ventilation that delivers pressurized breaths at intervals while allowing for spontaneous breathing.

***intermittent positive-pressure v.*** A mechanical method of assisting pulmonary ventilation, using a device that administers air or oxygen to inflate the lungs under positive pressure. Exhalation is usually passive. SYN: *breathing, intermittent positive-pressure.*

***liquid v.*** An experimental technique used in treating premature infants with surfactant-deficient lungs. An oxygen-rich liquid is pumped in and out of the lungs to provide ventilation.

***mandatory minute v.*** Ventilatory support that provides mechanical breaths when the patient's spontaneous breathing does not meet the minimum requirements.

***maximum sustainable v.*** The normal maximum breathing pattern that can be maintained for 15 min (usually approx. 60% of maximum voluntary ventilation).

***maximum voluntary v.*** The maximum amount of gas that can be ventilated into and out of the lungs in a voluntary effort in a given time, measured in liters per minute.

***mechanical v.*** Life support ventilation that involves use of a machine.

***positive-pressure mechanical v.*** Mechanical ventilatory support that applies positive pressure to the airway. The objectives include improving pulmonary gas exchange, relieving acute respiratory acidosis, relieving respiratory distress, preventing and reversing atelectasis, improving pulmonary compliance, preventing further lung injury, and avoiding complications. Positive-pressure ventilation can be life saving, but complications such as toxic effects of oxygen, laryngeal injury, tracheal stenosis, alveolar injury, barotrauma, pneumonia, and psychological problems may occur. SEE: *pressure, positive end-expiratory.*

***pressure support v.*** A type of assisted ventilation that supplements a spontaneous breath. The patient controls the frequency and the duration and flow of inspiration.

***pulmonary v.*** The inspiration and expiration of air from the lungs.

***synchronized intermittent mandatory v.*** ABBR: SIMV. Periodic assisted ventilation with positive pressure initiated by the patient and coordinated with spontaneous patient breaths. SEE: *intermittent mandatory v.*

***transtracheal catheter v.*** An emergency procedure in which a catheter is placed percutaneously through the cricothyroid membrane and attached to a high-pressure, high-flow jet ventilator to oxygenate a patient who cannot be intubated.

**ventilation coefficient** The amount of air that must be respired for each liter of oxygen to be absorbed.

**ventilation rate** ABBR: VR. The amount of air breathed in 1 min.

**ventilation tube** SEE: *grommet.*

**ventilator** A mechanical device for artificial ventilation of the lungs. The mechanism may be hand operated or machine driven, and in the latter case may be automatic and very sophisticated with respect to being able to control and monitor flow of air to the lungs.

***automatic transport v.*** ABBR: ATV. A portable ventilator that can be used while transporting patients between locations. The ATV is designed for short-term use and often has volume and rate controls.

**ventilator support, weaning from** The act of gradually removing persons with reversible forms of respiratory failure who are receiving mechanical ventilation from that support. This may be done by alternating full ventilatory support with increasingly long periods of unassisted breathing. The timing and frequency of the weaning periods should be individualized to each patient. Usually by the time the patient can tolerate 2 hr of spontaneous breathing, ventilatory support may be discontinued. There are sophisticated tests for adequacy of oxygenation of the blood during the weaning process, but the most reliable method is information provided by the patient.

NURSING IMPLICATIONS: The nurse should review current arterial blood gas reports and assess patient status carefully for signs of hypoxemia before each attempt at weaning. The procedure should be described to the patient and he or she should be told what to expect and what his or her role in weaning will be. The nurse should reassure the patient that he or she will not be endangered by weaning trials or left alone during these periods. The nurse should also provide positive reinforcement regarding the patient's progress and the anticipated successful termination of support. Agency protocol should be followed. Patient status and response to the procedure should be continuously evaluated. Nursing actions, patient response, and status should be recorded and reported.

**ventilatory weaning response, dysfunctional** ABBR: DVWR. A state in which a patient cannot adjust to lowered levels of mechanical ventilator support, which interrupts and prolongs the weaning process. SEE: *Nursing Diagnoses Appendix.*

**ventouse** (vĕn-toos′) [Fr.] A glass or glass-shaped vessel used in cupping.

**ventrad** (vĕn′trăd) [L. *venter,* belly, + *ad,* to] Toward the ventral aspect; the opposite of dorsad.

**ventral** (vĕn′trăl) [L. *ventralis,* pert. to the belly] Pert. to the belly; the opposite of dorsal. Hence, in quadrupeds, pert. to the lower or underneath side of the body; in humans, pert. to the anterior portion or the front side of the body.

**ventral hernia** A hernia through the abdominal wall, esp. at points other than the umbilicus and groin.

**ventralis** (vĕn-trā′lĭs) [L.] Anterior, or closer to the front.

**ventricle** (vĕn′trĭk-l) [L. *ventriculus,* a little belly] **1.** A small cavity. **2.** Either of two lower chambers of the heart that, when filled with blood, contract to propel it into the arteries. The right ventricle forces blood into the pulmonary artery and thence into the lungs; the left pumps blood into the aorta to the rest of the body. **3.** One of the fluid-filled cavities of the brain. SEE: illus.; *Arantius' body.*

***aortic v.*** The left ventricle of the heart.

***v. of Arantius*** The terminal depression of the median sulcus of the fourth ventricle of the brain.

***fifth v.*** The cavity of the septum lucidum of the brain. It is between the two laminae of the septum lucidum.

***fourth v.*** The cavity posterior to the pons and medulla and anterior to the cerebellum of the brain. It extends from the central canal of the upper end of the spinal cord to the aqueduct of the midbrain. Its roof is the cerebellum and the superior and inferior medullary vela. Its floor is the rhomboid fossa.

***v. of larynx*** The space between the true and false vocal cords.

***lateral v.*** The cavity in each cerebral hemisphere that communicates with the third ventricle through the interventricular foramen. It consists of a triangular central body and four horns, two inferior and two posterior.

***left v.*** The cavity of the heart that receives blood from the left atrium and pumps it into the system circulation via the aorta.

***Morgagni's v.*** The recess in the lateral wall on each side of the larynx between the vestibular and vocal folds.

***pineal v.*** The pineal recess of the third ventricle of the brain.

***right v.*** The cavity of the heart that re-

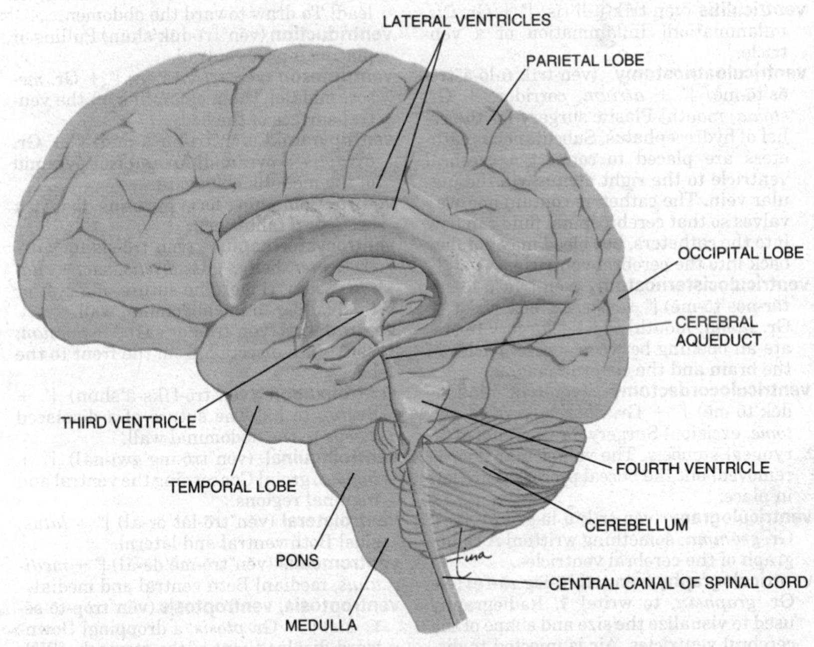


VENTRICLES OF THE BRAIN
(LEFT LATERAL VIEW)

ceives blood from the right atrium and pumps it into the lungs via the pulmonary artery.

***third v.*** The median cavity in the brain bounded by the thalamus and hypothalamus on either side, anteriorly by the optic chiasm; the floor is made up of the tuber cinereum, mammillary body, the posterior perforated substance and tegmentum of the cerebral peduncle; the roof is the ependyma. Anteriorly, it communicates with the lateral ventricles, and posteriorly, with the aqueduct of the midbrain.

**ventricornu** (vĕn″trĭ-kor′nū) [L. *venter,* belly, + *cornu,* horn] The anterior ventral horn of gray matter of the spinal cord.

**ventricular** (vĕn-trĭk′ū-lăr) [L. *ventriculus,* a little belly] Pert. to a ventricle.

**ventricular assist pumping** Use of a device to temporarily replace the pumping action of a diseased or nonfunctioning heart.

**ventricular compliance** Distensibility or stiffness of the relaxed ventricle of the heart.

**ventricular fold** One of the false vocal cords or folds of mucous membrane parallel to or above the true vocal cords.

**ventricular ligament** A narrow band of fibrous tissue lying within each ventricular fold.

**ventricular septal defect** A defect in the septum between the left and right ventricles of the heart. This permits blood to be shunted between the ventricles.

**ventriculitis** (vĕn-trĭk″ū-lī′tĭs) [″ + Gr. *itis,* inflammation] Inflammation of a ventricle.

**ventriculoatriostomy** (vĕn-trĭk″ū-lō-ā″trē-ŏs′tō-mē) [″ + *atrium,* corridor, + Gr. *stoma,* mouth] Plastic surgery for the relief of hydrocephalus. Subcutaneous catheters are placed to connect a cerebral ventricle to the right atrium via the jugular vein. The catheters contain one-way valves so that cerebrospinal fluid can flow into the catheters, but blood may not flow back into the cerebral ventricle.

**ventriculocisternostomy** (vĕn-trĭk″ū-lō-sĭs″tĕr-nŏs′tō-mē) [″ + *cisterna,* box, chest, + Gr. *stoma,* mouth] Plastic surgery to create an opening between the ventricles of the brain and the cisterna magna.

**ventriculocordectomy** (vĕn-trĭk″ū-lō-kor-dĕk′tō-mē) [″ + Gr. *khorde,* cord, + *ektome,* excision] Surgery for the relief of laryngeal stenosis. The ventricular floor is removed, but the buccal processes are left in place.

**ventriculogram** (vĕn-trĭk′ū-lō-grăm) [″ + Gr. *gramma,* something written] A radiograph of the cerebral ventricles.

**ventriculography** (vĕn-trĭk″ū-lŏg′ră-fē) [″ + Gr. *graphein,* to write] **1.** Radiography used to visualize the size and shape of the cerebral ventricles. Air is injected to display the cerebrospinal fluid that normally fills these cavities. This technique has been replaced by computed tomography and magnetic resonance imaging. **2.** Visualization of ventricles of the heart by radiograph after injection of a contrast material.

**ventriculometry** (vĕn-trĭk″ū-lŏm′ĕ-trē) [″ + Gr. *metron,* measure] The measurement of the intraventricular cerebral pressure.

**ventriculonector** (vĕn-trĭk″ū-lō-nĕk′tor) [L. *ventriculus,* a little belly, + *nector,* a joiner] The atrioventricular bundle.

**ventriculopuncture** (vĕn-trĭk′ū-lō-pŭnk″tūr) [″ + *punctura,* a point] The use of a needle to puncture a lateral ventricle of the brain.

**ventriculoscopy** (vĕn-trĭk″ū-lŏs′kō-pē) [″ + Gr. *skopein,* to examine] Examination of the ventricles of the brain with an endoscope.

**ventriculostomy** (vĕn-trĭk″ū-lŏs′tō-mē) [″ + Gr. *stoma,* mouth] Plastic surgery to establish communication between the floor of the third ventricle of the brain and the cisterna interpeduncularis. This is done to treat hydrocephalus.

**ventriculosubarachnoid** (vĕn-trĭk″ū-lō-sŭb″ă-răk′noyd) Concerning the cerebral ventricles and the subarachnoid spaces.

**ventriculotomy** (vĕn-trĭk″ū-lŏt′ō-mē) [″ + Gr. *tome,* incision] Surgical incision of a ventricle.

**ventriculus** (vĕn-trĭk′ū-lŭs) [L., a little belly] **1.** Ventricle. **2.** The stomach. **3.** A ventricle of the brain or heart.

***v. tertius*** Third ventricle.

**ventriduct** (vĕn′trĭ-dŭkt) [″ + *ducere,* to lead] To draw toward the abdomen.

**ventriduction** (vĕn″trĭ-dŭk′shŭn) Pulling or placing a part ventrad.

**ventrimeson** (vĕn″trĭ-mĕs′ŏn) [″ + Gr. *mesos,* middle] The median line on the ventral surface of the body.

**ventripyramid** (vĕn″trĭ-pĭr′ă-mĭd) [″ + Gr. *pyramis,* a pyramid] An anterior pyramid of the medulla oblongata.

**ventro-** Combining form meaning *abdomen* or *ventral* (anterior).

**ventrocystorrhaphy** (vĕn″trō-sĭs-tor′ă-fē) [L. *venter,* belly, + Gr. *kystis,* sac, + *rhaphe,* seam, ridge] The suture of a cyst or the bladder to the abdominal wall.

**ventrodorsal** (vĕn″trō-dor′săl) [″ + *dorsum,* back] In a direction from the front to the back.

**ventrofixation** (vĕn″trō-fĭks-ā′shŭn) [″ + *fixatio,* to fix] The suture of a displaced viscus to the abdominal wall.

**ventroinguinal** (vĕn″trō-ĭng′gwĭ-năl) [″ + *inguen,* groin] Concerning the ventral and inguinal regions.

**ventrolateral** (vĕn″trō-lăt′ĕr-ăl) [″ + *latus,* side] Both ventral and lateral.

**ventromedial** (vĕn″trō-mē′dē-ăl) [″ + *medianus,* median] Both ventral and medial.

**ventroptosia, ventroptosis** (vĕn″trŏp-tō′sē-ă, -sĭs) [″ + Gr. *ptosis,* a dropping] Downward displacement of the stomach. SYN: *gastroptosis.*

**ventroscopy** (vĕn-trŏs′kō-pē) [L. *venter,* belly, + Gr. *skopein,* to examine] Examination of the abdominal cavity by illumination. SYN: *celioscopy.*

**ventrose** (vĕn′trōs) Having a swelling like a belly.

**ventrosity** (vĕn-trŏs′ĭ-tē) Having an enlarged belly; corpulence.

**ventrosuspension** (vĕn″trō-sŭs-pĕn′shŭn) [″ + *suspensio,* a hanging] The fixation of a displaced uterus to the abdominal wall.

**ventrotomy** (vĕn-trŏt′ō-mē) [″ + Gr. *tome,* incision] Incision into the abdominal cavity. SYN: *celiotomy; laparotomy.*

**ventrovesicofixation** (vĕn″trō-vĕs″ĭ-kō-fĭks-ā′shŭn) [″ + L. *vesica,* bladder, + *fixare,* to fix] The suture of the uterus to the abdominal wall and bladder. SYN: *hysterocystopexy.*

**Venturi mask** [Giovanni Battista Venturi, It. scientist, 1746–1822] A special mask for administering a controlled concentration of oxygen to a patient.

**venturimeter** (vĕn″tūr-ĭm′ĕ-tĕr) A device for measuring the flow of fluids through vessels.

**venula** (vĕn′ū-lă) [L., little vein] Venule.

**venule** (vĕn′ūl) [L., *venula,* little vein] A tiny vein continuous with a capillary. SYN: *venula.*

**Venus, crown of** A papular eruption around the hairline on the forehead caused by secondary syphilis.

**Venus, mount of** The mons pubis.

**Venus's collar** (vē′nŭs) [L., the Roman goddess of love] Pigmentation around the neck; an eruption due to syphilis.

**verbigeration** (vĕr-bĭj″ĕr-ā′shŭn) [L. *verbigerare,* to chatter] Repetition of words that are either meaningless or have no significance.

**verbomania** (vĕr″bō-mā′nē-ă) [L. *verba,* word, + Gr. *mania,* madness] The flow of talk in some forms of psychosis.

**verdigris** (vĕr″dĭ-grĭs) [O. Fr. *vert de Grece,* green of Greece] **1.** Mixture of basic copper acetates. **2.** The green-gray deposit of copper carbonate on copper and bronze vessels.

**verdigris poisoning** Poisoning due to ingestion of verdigris, which contains copper salts. Symptoms are identical to those caused by ingesting copper sulfate. SEE: *copper salts* in *Poisons and Poisoning Appendix.*

**verdohemoglobin** (vĕr″dō-hēm′ō-glōb″ĭn) A greenish pigment occurring as an intermediate product in the formation of bilirubin from hemoglobin.

**Verga's ventricle** (vĕr′găz) [Andrea Verga, It. neurologist, 1811–1895] A cleftlike space between the corpus callosum and the body of the fornix of the brain.

**verge** (vĕrj) An edge or margin.

***anal v.*** The transitional area between the smooth perianal area and the hairy skin.

**vergence** (vĕr′jĕns) [L. *vergere,* to bend] A turning of one eye with reference to the other; may be horizontal (convergence or divergence) or vertical (intravergence or supravergence). SEE: *-phoria.*

**Verheyen's stars** (fĕr-hī′ĕns) [Philippe Verheyen, Flemish anatomist, 1648–1710] Starlike venous plexuses on the surface of the kidney below its capsule.

**vermicidal** (vĕr″mĭ-sī′dăl) [L. *vermis,* worm, + *cidus,* kill] Destroying worms parasitic in the intestines.

**vermicide** (vĕr′mĭ-sīd) **1.** Destroying worms. **2.** An agent that will kill intestinal worms.

**vermicular** (vĕr-mĭk′ū-lăr) [L. *vermicularis*] Resembling a worm.

**vermicular pulse** A small rapid pulse resulting in wormlike feeling in the fingers.

**vermiculation** (vĕr-mĭk″ū-lā′shŭn) [L. *vermiculare,* to wriggle] A wormlike motion, as in the intestines. SEE: *peristalsis.*

**vermicule** (vĕr′mĭ-kūl) [L. *vermiculus,* a small worm] **1.** A small worm. **2.** Having a wormlike shape.

**vermiculose, vermiculous** (vĕr-mĭk′ŭ-lōs, vĕr-mĭk′ū-lŭs) [L. *vermicularis,* wormlike] **1.** Infested with worms or larvae. **2.** Wormlike.

**vermiform** (vĕr′mĭ-form) [L. *vermis,* worm, + *forma,* shape] Shaped like a worm.

**vermiform appendix** A long, narrow, worm-shaped tube connected to the cecum. It varies in length from less than 1 in. to more than 8 in. (2.5 to 20.3 cm) with an average of about 3 in. (7.6 cm). Its distal end is closed. It is lined with mucosa similar to that of the large intestine. Its inflammation is called appendicitis. SEE: illus.

VERMIFORM APPENDIX

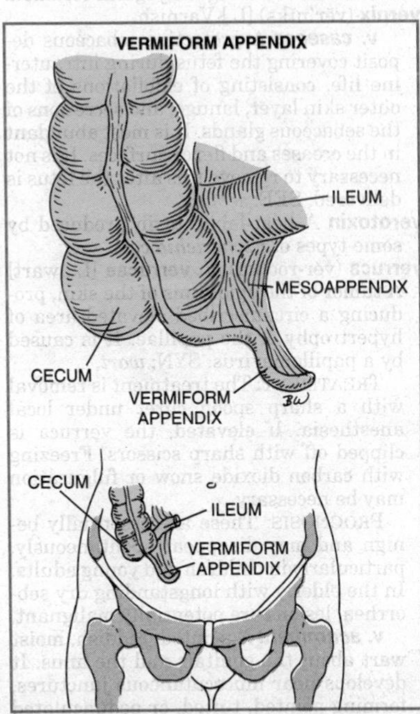

**vermifugal** (vĕr-mĭf′ū-găl) [″ + *fugare,* to put to flight] Expelling worms from the intestines.
**vermifuge** (vĕr′mĭ-fūj) Anthelmintic.
**vermilionectomy** (vĕr-mĭl″yŏn-ĕk′tō-mē) [″ + Gr. *ektome,* excision] Surgical removal of the vermilion border of the lip.
**vermin** (vĕr′mĭn) [L. *vermis,* worm] Small insects and animals such as mice, lice, or bedbugs that are annoying or cause destruction or disease.
**verminal** (vĕr′mĭ-năl) Concerning or caused by worms.
**vermination** (vĕr″mĭn-ā′shŭn) Vermin or worm infestation.
**verminosis** (vĕr″mĭn-ō′sĭs) [″ + Gr. *osis,* condition] Infestation with vermin.
**vermiphobia** (vĕr″mĭ-fō′bē-ă) [″ + Gr. *phobos,* fear] An abnormal fear of being infested with worms.
**vermis** (vĕr′mĭs) [L. worm] **1.** A worm. **2.** Vermis cerebelli.

***v. cerebelli*** Median connecting lobe of the cerebellum.

***inferior v.*** The anteroinferior portion of the vermis of the cerebellum, which includes the nodule, uvula, pyramis, and tuber.

***superior v.*** The posterior dorsal portion of the vermis, which includes the folium, declive, culmen, and central lobule.

**vernal** (vĕr′năl) [L. *vernalis,* pert. to spring] Occurring in or pert. to the spring.
**Vernet's syndrome** (vĕr-nāz′) [Maurice Vernet, Fr. physician, b. 1887] Paralysis of the glossopharyngeal, vagus, and spinal accessory nerves on the opposite side of a lesion involving the jugular foramen.
**vernix** (vĕr′nĭks) [L.] Varnish.

***v. caseosa*** A protective sebaceous deposit covering the fetus during intrauterine life, consisting of exfoliations of the outer skin layer, lanugo, and secretions of the sebaceous glands. It is most abundant in the creases and flexor surfaces. It is not necessary to remove this after the fetus is delivered. SEE: *sebum.*

**verotoxin** A heat-labile toxin produced by some types of *Escherichia coli.*
**verruca** (vĕr-roo′kă) *pl.* **verrucae** [L., wart] A tumor of the epidermis of the skin, producing a circumscribed elevated area of hypertrophy of the papillae. It is caused by a papillomavirus. SYN: *wart.*

TREATMENT: The treatment is removal with a sharp spoon curet under local anesthesia. If elevated, the verruca is clipped off with sharp scissors. Freezing with carbon dioxide snow or fulguration may be necessary.

PROGNOSIS: These are essentially benign and may disappear spontaneously, particularly in children and young adults. In the elderly with longstanding dry seborrhea, lesions are potentially malignant.

***v. acuminata*** A pointed, reddish, moist wart about the genitals and the anus. It develops near mucocutaneous junctures, forming pointed, tufted, or pedunculated pinkish or purplish projections of varying lengths and consistency. Venereal warts should be treated with topically applied podophyllum resin. SYN: *condyloma; genital wart; venereal wart.*

***v. digitata*** A form of verruca seen on the face and scalp, possibly serving as a starting point of cutaneous horns. Several filiform projections with horny caps are formed, closely grouped on a comparatively narrow base that in turn may be separated from the skin surface by a slightly contracted neck.

***v. filiformis*** A small threadlike growth on the neck and eyelids covered with smooth and apparently normal epidermis.

***v. gyri hippocampi*** One of the small wartlike protuberances on the convex surface of the gyrus hippocampi.

***v. plana*** A flat or slightly raised wart.

***v. plantaris*** Plantar wart.

***v. vulgaris*** The common wart, usually found on the backs of the hands and fingers; however, it may occur on any area of the skin.

**verruciform** (vĕ-roo′sĭ-form) [L. *verruca,* wart, + *forma,* shape] Wartlike.
**verrucose, verrucous** (vĕr′roo-kōs, vĕr-roo′kŭs) [L. *verrucosus,* wartlike] Wartlike, with raised portions.
**verrucosis** (vĕr″oo-kō′sĭs) [L. *verruca,* wart, + Gr. *osis,* condition] The condition of having multiple warts.
**verruga peruana** (vĕ-roo′gă pĕr-wăn′ă) [Sp., Peruvian wart] The eruptive second clinical stage of bartonellosis. Oroya fever is the first or febrile stage.
**versicolor** (vĕr′sĭ-kŏl″or) [L., of changing colors] **1.** Having many shades or colors. **2.** Changeable in color. SEE: *tinea versicolor.*
**version** (vĕr′zhŭn) [L. *versio,* a turning] **1.** Altering of the position of the fetus in the uterus. It may occur naturally or may be done mechanically by the physician to facilitate delivery. SEE: *conversion.* **2.** Deflection of an organ such as the uterus from its normal position.

***bipolar v.*** Changing of the position of the fetus by combined internal and external manipulation.

***cephalic v.*** Turning of the fetus so that the head presents.

***combined v.*** Mechanical version by combined internal and external manipulation.

***external v.*** Version of the fetus through the abdominal wall.

***internal v.*** Podalic v.

***pelvic v.*** Version of a cross-presentation until it is changed to a pelvic presentation.

***podalic v.*** Version of the fetus by the feet so that the breech presents; done with one hand inserted in the vagina. SYN: *internal v.*

***spontaneous v.*** Version of the fetus by uterine muscular contraction without artificial assistance.

**vertebra** (věr′tĕ-bră) *pl.* **vertebrae** [L.] Any of the 33 bony segments of the spinal column: 7 cervical, 12 thoracic, 5 lumbar, 5 sacral, and 4 coccygeal vertebrae. In adults, the five sacral vertebrae fuse to form a single bone, the sacrum, and the four rudimentary coccygeal vertebrae fuse to form the coccyx.

A typical vertebra consists of a ventral body and a dorsal or neural arch. In the thoracic region, the body bears on each side two costal pits for reception of the head of the rib. The arch that encloses the vertebral foramen is formed of two roots or pedicles and two laminae. The arch bears seven processes: a dorsal spinous process, two lateral transverse processes, and four articular processes (two superior and two inferior). A deep concavity, the inferior vertebral notch, on the inferior border of the arch provides a passageway for a spinal nerve. The successive vertebral foramina surround the spinal cord.

The bodies of successive vertebrae articulate with one another and are separated by intervertebral disks, disks of fibrous cartilage enclosing a central mass, the nucleus pulposus. The inferior articular processes articulate with the superior articular processes of the next succeeding vertebra in the caudal direction. Several ligaments (supraspinous, interspinous, anterior and posterior longitudinal, and the ligamenta flava) hold the vertebrae in position, yet permit a limited degree of movement. Motions of the vertebral column include forward bending (flexion), backward bending (extension), side bending (lateral flexion), and rotation. Lateral flexion and rotation motions are coupled so that whenever the vertebrae bend to the side, they also rotate and vice versa. SEE: *sacrum* for illus.

***basilar v.*** The lowest of the lumbar vertebrae.

***cervical v.*** One of the seven vertebrae of the neck.

***coccygeal v.*** One of the rudimentary vertebrae of the coccyx.

***v. dentata*** The second cervical vertebra. SYN: *odontoid v.; axis.*

***false v.*** The sacral and coccygeal vertebrae that fuse. SYN: *fixed v.*

***fixed v.*** False v.

***lumbar v.*** One of the five vertebrae between the thoracic vertebrae and the sacrum.

***v. magnum*** The sacrum.

***odontoid v.*** V. dentata.

***v. prominens*** The seventh cervical vertebra.

***sacral v.*** One of the five fused vertebrae forming the sacrum. SEE: *sacrum* for illus.

***sternal v.*** One of the segments of the sternum.

***thoracic v.*** One of the 12 vertebrae that connect the ribs and form part of the posterior wall of the thorax. SEE: *spinal column* for illus.

***true v.*** One of the vertebrae that remain unfused through life: the cervical, thoracic, and lumbar.

**vertebral** (věr′tĕ-brăl) [L. *vertebra,* vertebra] Pert. to a vertebra or the vertebral column.

**vertebral arch** The thoracic portion of a vertebra that encloses a vertebral foramen.

**vertebral canal** Spinal canal.

**vertebral column** Spinal column.

**vertebral foramen** The hollow space enclosed by a vertebral arch.

**vertebral groove** The groove lying on either side of the spinous processes of the vertebrae.

**vertebral notch** SEE: under *notch.*

**vertebral rib** One of the lower two, or floating, ribs.

**vertebrarium** (věr″tĕ-brā′rē-ŭm) [L.] The vertebral column.

**Vertebrata** (věr″tĕ-brā′tă) A subphylum of the phylum Chordata characterized by possession of a segmented backbone or spinal column. It includes the following classes: Agnatha (cyclostomes), Chondrichthyes (cartilaginous fishes), Osteichthyes (bony fishes), Amphibia, Reptilia, Aves, and Mammalia. Members of this subphylum possess an axial notochord at some period of their existence.

**vertebrate** (věr′tĕ-brāt) [L. *vertebra,* vertebra] Having or resembling a vertebral column.

**vertebrated** (věr′tĕ-brāt″ĕd) Composed of jointed segments.

**vertebrectomy** (věr″tĕ-brĕk′tō-mē) [″ + Gr. *ektome,* excision] Excision of a vertebra or part of one.

**vertebro-** Combining form indicating *vertebra.*

**vertebroarterial** (věr″tĕ-brō-ăr-tē′rē-ăl) [″ + Gr. *arteria,* artery] Concerning the vertebral artery.

**vertebrobasilar** (věr″tĕ-brō-băs′ĭ-lăr) [″ + *basilaris,* basilar] Concerning the vertebral and basilar arteries.

**vertebrochondral** (věr″tĕ-brō-kŏn′drăl) [″ + Gr. *chondros,* cartilage] Pert. to the vertebra and the costal cartilages.

**vertebrocostal** (věr″tĕ-brō-kŏs′tăl) [″ + *costa,* rib] Costovertebral.

**vertebrofemoral** (věr″tĕ-brō-fĕm′or-ăl) [″ + *femur,* thigh] Concerning the vertebrae and femur.

**vertebroiliac** (věr″tĕ-brō-ĭl′ē-ăk) [″ + *iliacus,* pert. to ilium] Concerning the vertebrae and ilium.

**vertebromammary** (věr″tĕ-brō-măm′mă-rē) [″ + *mamma,* breast] Pert. to the vertebral and mammary areas.

**vertebrosacral** (věr″tĕ-brō-sā′krăl) [″ + *sacrum,* sacred] Concerning the vertebrae and sacrum.

**vertebrosternal** (věr″tĕ-brō-stĕr′năl) [″ + Gr. *sternon,* chest] Pert. to a vertebra and the sternum.

**vertex** (vĕr′tĕks) [L., summit] The top of the head. SYN: *corona capitis; crown.*

***v. cordis*** The apex of the heart.

**vertical** (vĕr′tĭ-kăl) [L. *verticalis,* summit] **1.** Pert. to or situated at the vertex. **2.** Perpendicular to the plane of the horizon of the earth; upright.

**verticalis** (vĕr″tĭ-kā′lĭs) [L.] Vertical, indicating any plane that passes through the body parallel to the long axis of the body.

**verticality** The ability to perceive accurately the vertical position in the absence of environmental cues.

**verticillate** (vĕr-tĭs′ĭl-āt, -tĭs-ĭl′āt) [L. *verticillus,* a little whirl] Arranged like the spokes of a wheel or a whorl.

**verticomental** (vĕr″tĭ-kō-mĕn′tăl) [L. *vertex,* summit, + *mentum,* chin] Concerning the crown of the head and the chin.

**vertiginous** (vĕr-tĭj′ĭ-nŭs) [L. *vertiginosus,* one suffering from dizziness] Pert. to or afflicted with vertigo.

**vertigo** (vĕr′tĭ-gō, vĕr-tī′gō) [L. *vertigo,* a turning round] The sensation of moving around in space (subjective vertigo) or of having objects move about the person (objective vertigo). This is true vertigo and is a result of a disturbance of the equilibrium. Vertigo is sometimes used as a synonym for dizziness, lightheadedness, or giddiness. It may be caused by a variety of entities, including middle ear disease; toxic conditions such as those caused by salicylates, alcohol, or streptomycin; sunstroke; postural hypotension; or toxemia due to food poisoning or infectious diseases. SEE: *vection* (2).

NURSING IMPLICATIONS: Assessment should include whether the patient experiences a sense of turning or whirling and its direction; whether it is intermittent and the time of day it occurs; whether it is associated with drugs, occupation, or menses; whether it is associated with nausea and vomiting or with nystagmus and migraine. Safety measures, such as the use of siderails in bed, are instituted. The patient should ambulate gradually after a slow, assisted move from a sitting position. The call bell should be available at all times; tissues, water, and other supplies should be within easy reach; and furniture and other obstacles should be removed from the path of ambulation. The patient who received a fenestration operation on the ear and experiences severe vertigo should be confined to bed for several days and then begin to gradually increase activity.

***alternobaric v.*** Vertigo associated with a sudden decrease in the pressure to which the inner ear is exposed. This could occur when a scuba diver ascends quickly or when an aircraft ascends quickly. SEE: *bends.*

***auditory v.*** Vertigo due to disease of the ear.

***benign positional v.*** A disorder of the labyrinth of the inner ear characterized by paroxysmal vertigo and nystagmus only when the head is in a certain position or moves in a certain direction. The diagnosis is made at the bedside by moving the patient from the sitting position to recumbency with the head tilted down 30° over the end of the table and 30° to one side. This causes a paroxysm of vertigo. This test is called the Hallpike maneuver. The episodes may last less than a minute but may recur for months. SYN: *positional vertigo of Bárány.*

***central v.*** Vertigo caused by disease of the central nervous system.

***cerebral v.*** Vertigo due to brain disease.

***epidemic v.*** Vertigo that may occur in epidemic form. It is believed to be due to vestibular neuronitis.

***epileptic v.*** Vertigo accompanying or following an epileptic attack.

***essential v.*** Vertigo from an unknown cause.

***gastric v.*** Vertigo associated with a gastric disturbance.

***horizontal v.*** Vertigo that occurs while the patient is supine.

***hysterical v.*** Vertigo accompanying hysteria.

***labyrinthine v.*** SEE: *Ménière's disease.*

***laryngeal v.*** Vertigo and fainting during a coughing spell in patients with chronic bronchitis. SYN: *laryngeal syncope.*

***objective v.*** Vertigo in which stationary objects appear to be moving.

***ocular v.*** Vertigo caused by disease of the eye.

***organic v.*** Vertigo due to a brain lesion.

***peripheral v.*** Vertigo due to disturbances in the peripheral areas of the central nervous system.

***positional v., postural v.*** Vertigo that occurs when the head is in a specific position.

***rotary v.*** Subjective v.

***subjective v.*** Vertigo in which the patient has the sensation of turning or rotating. SYN: *rotary v.*

***toxic v.*** Vertigo caused by the presence of a toxin in the body.

***vertical v.*** Vertigo produced by standing or by looking up or down.

***vestibular v.*** Vertigo due to disease or malfunction of the vestibular apparatus.

**verumontanitis** (vĕr″ū-mŏn″tăn-ī′tĭs) [L. *veru,* spit, dart, + *montanus,* mountainous, + Gr. *itis,* inflammation] Inflammation of the verumontanum. SYN: *colliculitis.*

**verumontanum** (vĕr″ū-mŏn-tā′nŭm) [L. *veru,* spit, dart, + *montanus,* mountainous] An elevation on the floor of the prostatic portion of the urethra where the seminal ducts enter.

**very low–density lipoprotein** ABBR: VLDL. A plasma lipid that is bound to albumin consisting of chylomicrons and prelipoproteins. These lipoproteins contain a greater ratio of lipid than low-density lipoproteins and are the least dense. SEE: *lipoprotein.*

**vesalianum** (vĕs-ā″lē-ā′nŭm) [Andreas Vesalius, Flemish anatomist and physician, 1514–1564] One of the sesamoid bones in the tendon of origin of the gastrocnemius muscle, and another on the outer border of the foot in the angle between the cuboid and fifth metatarsal.

**Vesalius, foramen of** (vĕs-ā′lē-ŭs) [Andreas Vesalius] The opening in the base of the skull transmitting an emissary vein.

**Vesalius, vein of** The small emissary vein from the cavernous sinus passing through the foramen of Vesalius and conveying blood to the pterygoid plexus.

**vesica** (vĕ-sī′kă) [L.] A bladder.

***v. fellea*** The gallbladder.

***v. prostatica*** A minute pouch in the prostatic urethra, remnant of the müllerian duct. SYN: *utriculus prostaticus.*

***v. urinaria*** The urinary bladder.

**vesical** (vĕs′ĭ-kăl) Pert. to or shaped like a bladder.

**vesical reflex** An inclination to urinate caused by moderate bladder distention.

**vesicant** (vĕs′ĭ-kănt) [L. *vesicare,* to blister] **1.** Blistering; causing or forming blisters. **2.** An agent used to produce blisters. It is much less severe in its effects than are escharotics. **3.** A blistering gas used in chemical warfare. SYN: *vesicatory.* SEE: *gas, vesicant.*

**vesication** (vĕs″ĭ-kā′shŭn) **1.** The process of blistering. **2.** A blister.

**vesicatory** (vĕs′ĭ-kă-tor″ē) Vesicant.

**vesicle** (vĕs′ĭ-kl) [L. *vesicula,* a little bladder] **1.** A small sac or bladder containing fluid. **2.** A blisterlike small elevation on the skin containing serous fluid. Vesicles may vary in diameter from a few millimeters to a centimeter. They may be round, transparent, opaque, or dark elevations of the skin, sometimes containing seropurulent or bloody fluid. In sudamina, they result from sweat that cannot escape from the skin; in herpes, they are mounted on an inflammatory base, having no tendency to rupture but associated with burning pain. In herpes zoster, they follow the line of the nerve trunks. In dermatitis venenata, they result from contact with poison ivy or oak and are accompanied by great itching. They are also seen in dermatitis herpetiformis or multiformis. In impetigo contagiosa, they occur, esp. in children, in discrete form, flat and umbilicated, filled with straw-colored fluid, with no tendency to break. They dry up, forming yellow crusts with little itching. They are also seen in vesicular eczema, molluscum contagiosum, miliaria (prickly heat or heat rash), chickenpox, smallpox, and scabies. SEE: illus.; *herpes; miliaria.*

***allantoic v.*** The hollow, enlarged part of the allantois, esp. in birds and reptiles.

***auditory v.*** That portion of the cerebral vesicle from which the exterior ear is formed. SYN: *otic v.*

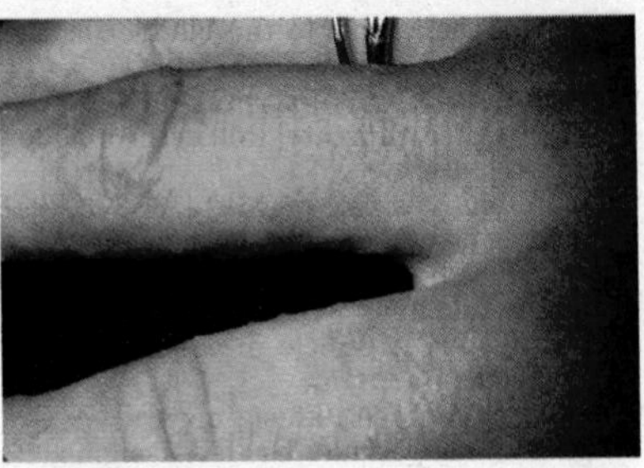

VESICLES OF POMPHOLYX ON FINGERS

***blastodermic v.*** The sac developed from the blastoderm.

***brain v.*** One of the five embryonic subdivisions of the brain. SYN: *encephalic v.*

***cerebral v.*** Brain v.

***chorionic v.*** The outer villus-covered layer of the early embryo. It encloses the embryo, amnion, umbilical cord, and yolk stalk.

***compound v.*** Multilocular v.

***encephalic v.*** Brain v.

***lens v.*** The embryonic vesicle formed from the lens pit. It develops into the lens of the eye.

***multilocular v.*** A vesicle that contains multiple chambers.

***optic v.*** A hollow outgrowth from the lateral aspects of the embryonic brain. The retinae and optic nerves develop from these paired vesicles.

***otic v.*** Auditory v.

***primary brain v.*** One of the three earliest subdivisions of the embryonic neural tube.

***seminal v.*** One of the two membranous sacculated tubes situated at the base of the bladder, between it and the rectum, serving as a reservoir for semen and having a secretion of its own.

***umbilical v.*** The portion of the embryonic yolk sac outside the body cavity.

**vesico-** (vĕs′ĭ-kō) Combining form meaning *bladder, vesicle.*

**vesicoabdominal** (vĕs″ĭ-kō-ăb-dŏm′ĭ-năl) [L. *vesica,* bladder, + *abdomen,* belly] Concerning the urinary bladder and the abdomen.

**vesicocele** (vĕs′ĭ-kō-sēl″) [L. *vesica,* bladder, + Gr. *kele,* tumor, swelling] Hernia of the bladder into the vagina. SYN: *cystocele.*

**vesicocervical** (vĕs″ĭ-kō-sĕr′vĭ-kăl) [″ + *cervix,* neck] Rel. to the urinary bladder and cervix uteri.

**vesicoclysis** (vĕs″ĭ-kŏk′lĭ-sĭs) [″ + Gr. *klysis,* a washing] Injection of fluid into the bladder.

**vesicoenteric** (vĕs″ĭ-kō-ĕn-tĕr′ĭk) [″ + Gr. *enteron,* intestine] Concerning the urinary bladder and intestine.

**vesicofixation** (vĕs″ĭ-kō-fĭks-ā′shŭn) [L. *vesica,* bladder, + *fixatio,* a fixing] Attachment of the uterus to the bladder or the bladder to the abdominal wall.

**vesicoprostatic** (vĕs″ĭ-kō-prŏs-tăt′ĭk) [″ + Gr. *prostates,* prostate] Rel. to the bladder and prostate.

**vesicopubic** (vĕs″ĭ-kō-pū′bĭk) [″ + NL. *(os) pubis,* bone of the groin] Pert. to the bladder and os pubis.

**vesicopustule** (vĕs″ĭ-kō-pŭs′tūl) [″ + *pustula,* blister] A vesicle in which pus has developed.

**vesicosigmoid** (vĕs″ĭ-kō-sĭg′moyd) [″ + Gr. *sigmoid,* shaped like Gr. letter sigma, σ] Concerning the urinary bladder and sigmoid colon.

**vesicosigmoidostomy** (vĕs″ĭ-kō-sĭg″moy-dŏs′tō-mē) [″ + ″ + *stoma,* mouth] Surgical creation of an anastomosis between the urinary bladder and sigmoid colon.

**vesicospinal** (vĕs″ĭ-kō-spī′năl) [″ + *spina,* thorn] Rel. to the urinary bladder and spinal cord.

**vesicostomy** (vĕs″ĭ-kŏs′tō-mē) [″ + Gr. *stoma,* mouth] Surgical production of an opening into the bladder.

**vesicotomy** (vĕs″ĭ-kŏt′ō-mē) [″ + Gr. *tome,* incision] Incision of the bladder.

**vesicoumbilical** (vĕs″ĭ-kō-ŭm-bĭl′ĭ-kăl) [″ + *umbilicus,* navel] Concerning the urinary bladder and umbilicus.

**vesicoureteral** (vĕs″ĭ-kō-ū-rē′tĕr-ăl) [″ + Gr. *oureter,* ureter] Concerning the urinary bladder and a ureter.

**vesicouterine** (vĕs″ĭ-kō-ū′tĕr-ĭn) [″ + *uterinus,* pert. to the womb] Pert. to the urinary bladder and uterus.

**vesicouterine pouch** Downward extension of the peritoneal cavity located between the bladder and uterus.

**vesicouterovaginal** (vĕs″ĭ-kō-ū″tĕr-ō-văj′ĭ-năl) [″ + *uterus,* womb, + *vagina,* sheath] Concerning the urinary bladder, the uterus, and the vagina.

**vesicovaginal** (vĕs″ĭ-kō-văj′ĭ-năl) [″ + *vagina,* sheath] Vaginovesical.

**vesicovaginorectal** (vĕs″ĭ-kō-văj″ĭ-nō-rĕk′tăl) [″ + *vagina,* sheath, + *rectum,* straight] Concerning the urinary bladder, vagina, and rectum.

**vesicula** (vĕ-sĭk′ū-lă) *pl.* **vesiculae** [L.] A small bladder or vesicle.

***v. seminalis*** Seminal vesicle.

**vesicular** (vĕ-sĭk′ū-lăr) Pert. to vesicles or small blisters.

**vesicular eczema** Eczema accompanied by the formation of vesicles.

**vesicular murmur** The normal sound of respiration heard on auscultation.

**vesicular resonance** Percussion sound heard over the normal lung.

**vesiculated** (vĕ-sĭk′ū-lāt″ĕd) Having vesicles present.

**vesiculation** (vĕ-sĭk″ū-lā′shŭn) [L. *vesicula,* a tiny bladder] The formation of vesicles or the state of having or forming them.

**vesiculectomy** (vĕ-sĭk″ū-lĕk′tō-mē) [″ + Gr. *ektome,* excision] Partial or complete excision of a vesicle, particularly a seminal vesicle.

**vesiculiform** (vĕ-sĭk′ū-lĭ-form) [″ + *forma,* shape] Having the shape of a vesicle.

**vesiculitis** (vĕ-sĭk″ū-lī′tĭs) [″ + Gr. *itis,* inflammation] Inflammation of a vesicle, particularly the seminal vesicle.

**vesiculobronchial** (vĕ-sĭk″ū-lō-brŏng′kē-ăl) [″ + Gr. *bronchos,* windpipe] Both vesicular and bronchial.

**vesiculocavernous** (vĕ-sĭk″ū-lō-kăv′ĕr-nŭs) [″ + *caverna,* a hollow] Vesicular and cavernous.

**vesiculogram** (vĕ-sĭk′ū-lō-grăm) [″ + Gr. *gramma,* something written] A radiograph of the seminal vesicles.

**vesiculography** (vĕ-sĭk″ū-lŏg′ră-fē) [″ + Gr. *graphein,* to write] Radiography of the seminal vesicles after the injection of a contrast medium. This procedure has been replaced by ultrasound imaging.

**vesiculopapular** (vĕ-sĭk″ū-lō-păp′ū-lăr) [″ + *papula,* pimple] Composed of vesicles and papules.

**vesiculopustular** (vĕ-sĭk″ū-lō-pŭs′tū-lăr) [″ + *pustula,* blister] Having both vesicles and pustules.

**vesiculotomy** (vĕ-sĭk″ū-lŏt′ō-mē) [″ + Gr. *tome,* incision] Surgical incision into a vesicle, as a seminal vesicle.

**vesiculotubular** (vĕ-sĭk″ū-lō-tū′bū-lăr) [″ + *tubularis,* like a tube] Sounds from auscultation of the chest that have both vesicular and tubular qualities.

**vesiculotympanic** (vĕ-sĭk″ū-lō-tĭm-păn′ĭk) [″ + Gr. *tympanon,* drum] Having both vesicular and tympanic qualities.

**Vespidae** [L. *vespa,* wasp] Family of wasps, including paper wasps, hornets, and yellow jackets.

**vessel** (vĕs′ĕl) [O. Fr. from L. *vascellum,* a little vessel] A tube, duct, or canal to convey the fluids of the body. SYN: *vas.*

***absorbent v.'s*** The lacteals, lymphatics, and capillaries of the intestines.

***blood v.*** Any of the vessels carrying blood (i.e., arteries, veins, and capillaries).

***chyliferous v.*** One of the vessels arising in the villi of the intestinal walls carrying chyle and terminating in the thoracic duct.

***collateral v.*** A vessel parallel to the vessel from which it arose.

***great v.*** One of the large blood vessels entering and leaving the heart.

***lacteal v.*** A lymph vessel that collects chyle from the intestinal villi.

***lymphatic v.*** A thin-walled vessel that conveys lymph from the tissues. These vessels resemble veins in structure, possessing three layers (intima, media, and adventitia) and paired valves.

***nutrient v.*** One of the vessels supplying specific areas such as the interior of bones.

***radicular v.*** A branch of a vertebral artery supplying the cerebral nerve root.

**vestibular** (vĕs-tĭb′ū-lăr) [L. *vestibulum,* vestibule] Pert. to a vestibule.

**vestibular bulb** One of the two sacculated

collections of veins, lying on either side of the vagina beneath the bulbocavernosus muscle, connected anteriorly by the pars intermedia, and through this strip of cavernous tissue communicating with the erectile tissue of the clitoris. The vestibular bulbs are the homologues of the male corpus spongiosum. Injury during labor may give rise to troublesome bleeding. SEE: *Bartholin's glands; vagina; vestibule of vagina.*

**vestibular nerve** A main division of the auditory nerve; arises in the vestibular ganglion and is concerned with equilibrium.

**vestibule** (vĕs′tĭ-būl) A small space or cavity at the beginning of a canal, such as the aortic vestibule.

***aortic v.*** The part of the left ventricle of the heart just below the aortic valve.

***buccal v.*** The part of the oral cavity bounded by the teeth, gingiva, and alveolar processes and laterally by the cheek.

***v. of ear*** The middle part of the inner ear, behind the cochlea, and in front of the semicircular canals; it contains the utriculus and sacculus.

***v. of larynx*** The portion of the larynx above the vocal cords.

***v. of mouth*** The part of the oral cavity between the lips and the cheeks and between the teeth and the gums.

***v. of nose*** The anterior part of the nostrils, containing the vibrissae.

***v. of pharynx*** The space surrounded by the soft palate, base of the tongue, and the palatoglossal and palatopharyngeal arches.

***v. of vagina*** An almond-shaped space between the lines of attachment of the labia minora. The clitoris is situated at the superior angle; the inferior boundary is the fourchette. The vestibule is approx. 4 to 5 cm long and 2 cm in greatest width when the labia minora are separated. Four major structures open into the vestibule: the urethra anteriorly, the vagina into the midportion, and the two secretory ducts of the glands of Bartholin laterally. The covering membranes are pink and constructed of delicate stratified squamous epithelium. SEE: *Bartholin's glands; vagina; vestibular bulb.*

**vestibulocochlear nerve** (vĕs-tĭb″ū-lō-kŏk′lē-ăr) [L. *vestibulum,* vestibule, + Gr. *kokhlos,* land snail] The eighth cranial nerve, which emerges from the brain behind the facial nerve between the pons and medulla oblongata. SYN: *acoustic nerve.* SEE: illus.

**vestibuloplasty** (vĕs-tĭb′ū-lō-plăs″tē) [″ + Gr. *plassein,* to mold] Plastic surgery of the vestibule of the mouth.

**vestibulotomy** (vĕs-tĭb″ū-lŏt′ō-mē) [″ + Gr. *tome,* incision] Surgical incision into the vestibule of the inner ear.

**vestibulourethral** (vĕs-tĭb″ū-lō-ū-rē′thrăl) [″ + Gr. *ourethra,* urethra] Rel. to the vestibule of the vagina and urethra.

**vestibulum** (vĕs-tĭb′ū-lŭm) *pl.* **vestibula** [L.] Vestibule.

**vestige** (vĕs′tĭj) [L. *vestigium,* footstep] A small degenerate or incompletely developed structure that has been more fully developed in the embryo or in a previous

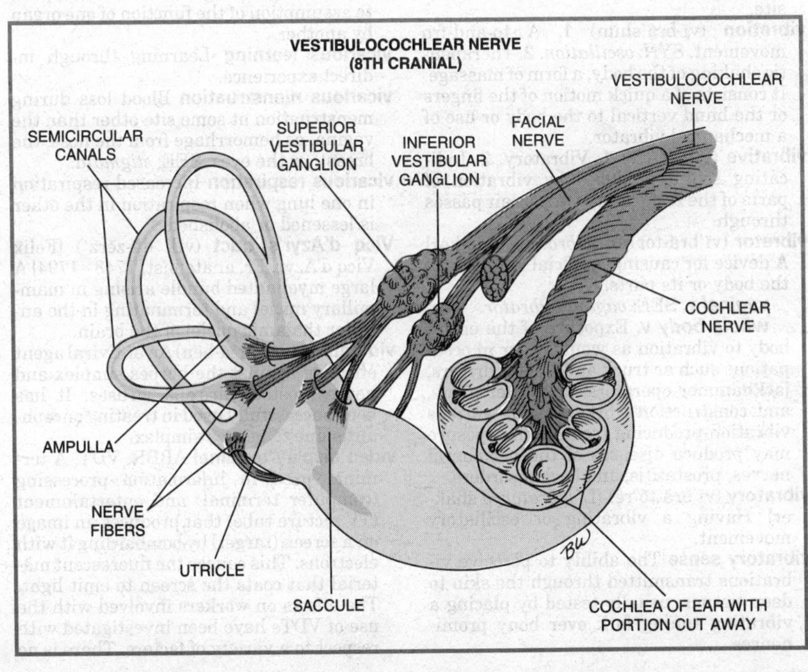

stage of the species.

**vestigial** (vĕs-tĭj'ē-ăl) Of the nature of a vestige. SYN: *rudimentary*.

**vestigium** (vĕs-tĭj'ē-ŭm) *pl.* **vestigia** [L., a footstep] Vestige.

**veterinarian** (vĕt″ĕr-ĭ-nār'ē-ăn) One who is trained and licensed to practice veterinary medicine and surgery.

**veterinary** (vĕt'ĕr-ĭ-nār″ē) **1.** Pert. to animals, their diseases, and their treatment. **2.** A veterinarian.

**veterinary medicine** The branch of medicine that deals with diseases of animals and their treatment.

**VF** *ventricular fibrillation; vocal fremitus.*

**V.H.** *viral hepatitis.*

**via** (vē'ă, vī'ă) *pl.* **viae** [L.] Any passage in the body such as nasal, intestinal, or vaginal.

**viability** (vī″ă-bĭl'ĭ-tē) [L. *vita,* life, + *habilis,* fit] Ability to live, grow, and develop.

**viable** (vī'ă-bl) [L. *vita,* life, + *habilis,* fit] Capable of living, as a newborn or a fetus that has reached a stage, usually 24 weeks or greater than 500 g, that will permit it to live outside the uterus.

**vial** (vī'ăl) [Gr. *phiale,* a drinking cup] A small glass bottle for medicines or chemicals.

**vibex** (vī'bĕks) *pl.* **vibices** [L. *vibix,* mark of a blow] A narrow linear mark of hemorrhage into the skin.

**vibrapuncture** (vī″bră-pŭnk'tūr) The medical use of a tattoo technique to introduce medicine into skin lesions. Multiple punctures are made into the skin by a needle that has passed through a small amount of the solution of medicine placed on the site.

**vibration** (vī-brā'shŭn) **1.** A to-and-fro movement. SYN: *oscillation.* **2.** Therapeutic shaking of the body, a form of massage. It consists of a quick motion of the fingers or the hand vertical to the body or use of a mechanical vibrator.

**vibrative** (vĭb'ră-tĭv) **1.** Vibratory. **2.** Indicating sound produced by vibration of parts of the respiratory tract as air passes through.

**vibrator** (vī'brā-tor) [L. *vibrator,* a shaker] A device for causing artificial vibration of the body or its parts.

***vaginal v.*** SEE: *vaginal vibrator.*

***whole body v.*** Exposure of the entire body to vibration as would occur in occupations such as truck and tractor drivers, jackhammer operators, helicopter pilots, and construction workers using various vibration-producing tools. Such exposure may produce diseases of the peripheral nerves, prostatitis, and back disorders.

**vibratory** (vī'bră-tō″rē) [L. *vibrator,* a shaker] Having a vibrating or oscillatory movement.

**vibratory sense** The ability to perceive vibrations transmitted through the skin to deep tissues; usually tested by placing a vibrating tuning fork over bony prominences.

**Vibrio** (vĭb'rē-ō) A genus of curved, motile, gram-negative bacilli, several of which may be pathogenic for humans.

***V. cholerae*** The causative agent of cholera.

***V. vulnificus*** A gram-negative bacillus commonly found in seawater. It may cause a fulminant gangrene if it contaminates wounds or may cause a fatal septicemia if ingested by those with impaired gastric, liver, kidney, or immune function. The usual source in such cases is raw shellfish.

**vibrio** (vĭb'rē-ō) *pl.* **vibriones** An organism of the genus *Vibrio.* SEE: *bacteria* for illus.

**vibriocidal** (vĭb″rē-ō-sī'dăl) Destructive to vibrio organisms.

**vibrion** (vē″brē-ŏn') [Fr.] A vibrio organism.

**vibriosis** (vĭb″rē-ō'sĭs) The condition of being infected with organisms of the genus *Vibrio.*

**vibrissae** (vī-brĭs'ē) *sing.,* **vibrissa** [L. *vibrissa,* that which shakes] Stiff hairs within the nostrils at the anterior nares.

**vibromassage** (vī″brō-mă-săj') A massage given by a mechanical vibrator.

**vibrometer** (vī-brŏm'ĕt-ĕr) [L. *vibrare,* to shake, + Gr. *metron,* measure] A device used to measure the vibratory sensation threshold. It is particularly useful in judging the progression or remission of peripheral neuropathy.

**vibrotherapeutics** (vī″brō-thĕr″ă-pū'tĭks) [″ + Gr. *therapeutikos,* treating] The therapeutic application of vibration.

**vicarious** (vī-kā'rē-ŭs) [L. *vicarius,* change, alternation] Acting as a substitute; pert. to assumption of the function of one organ by another.

**vicarious learning** Learning through indirect experience.

**vicarious menstruation** Blood loss during menstruation at some site other than the vagina, as hemorrhage from the nose, the breast, or the eyes. SEE: *stigmata.*

**vicarious respiration** Increased respiration in one lung when respiration in the other is lessened or abolished.

**Vicq d'Azyr's tract** (vĭk dă-zērz') [Felix Vicq d'Azyr, Fr. anatomist, 1748–1794] A large myelinated bundle arising in mammillary nuclei and terminating in the anterior thalamic nuclei of the brain.

**vidarabine** (vī-dăr'ă-bēn) An antiviral agent effective against the herpes simplex and herpes zoster–varicella viruses. It has been successfully used in treating encephalitis due to herpes simplex.

**video display terminal** ABBR: VDT. A terminal used in information processing (computer terminal) and entertainment (TV picture tube) that produces an image on a screen (target) by bombarding it with electrons. This causes the fluorescent material that coats the screen to emit light. The effects on workers involved with the use of VDTs have been investigated with respect to a variety of factors. There is no evidence that reproductive or visual health is impaired by working with VDTs. Those who work with VDTs may experience musculoskeletal difficulties if the workplaces are poorly designed. This may be due to the screen being positioned in a way that promotes poor posture, or the chair being of improper design. These conditions may be avoided by adapting simple commonsense remedies. SEE: *radiation, low-level.*

**videognosis** (vĭd″ē-ŏg-nō′sĭs) [L. *videre,* to see, + Gr. *gnosis,* knowledge] Diagnosis using data and radiographic images transmitted by the use of television.

**video-stroboscope** A closed-circuit television recording technique used to obtain images while the field is illuminated by use of a stroboscope. Using this method provides precise, sequential views of the organ being photographed as it moves.

**vidian artery** (vĭd′ē-ăn) [Guido Guidi (L. *Vidius*), It. physician, 1500–1569] The artery passing through the pterygoid canal.

**vidian canal** A canal in the medial pterygoid plate of the sphenoid bone for transmission of pterygoid (vidian) vessels and nerve. SYN: *pterygoid canal.*

**vidian nerve** A branch from the sphenopalatine ganglion. SEE: *Nerves Appendix.*

**view box** In radiology, a uniform light source used to view a radiograph.

**vigil** (vĭj′ĭl) [L., awake] Insomnia, wakefulness.

***coma v.*** A condition of muttering delirium in which the patient is partially conscious and not completely comatose. SEE: *vigilambulism.*

**vigilambulism** (vĭj″ĭl-ăm′bū-lĭzm) [″ + *ambulare,* to walk, + Gr. *-ismos,* condition] Automatism that occurs while the person is awake; resembles somnambulism.

**vigilance** (vĭj′ĭ-lăns) [L. *vigilantia,* wastefulness] The condition of being attentive, alert, and watchful.

**vigintinormal** (vī-jĭn″tĭ-nor′măl) [L. *viginti,* twenty, + *normal,* rule] Consisting of one twentieth of what is normal, as a solution.

**vignetting** In radiology, a loss in brightness and focus toward the periphery of the output phosphor during image intensification.

**vigor** (vĭg′or) [L.] Active force or strength of body or mind.

**Villaret's syndrome** (vē-lăr-āz′) [Maurice Villaret, Fr. neurologist, 1877–1946] Ipsilateral paralysis of the 9th, 10th, 11th, 12th, and sometimes the 7th cranial nerves and the cervical sympathetic fibers. It is caused by a lesion in the posterior retroparotid space. The signs and symptoms include paralysis and anesthesia of the pharyngeal area with difficulty swallowing; loss of taste sensation in the posterior third of the tongue; paralysis of the vocal cords, and the sternocleidomastoid and trapezius muscles; and Horner's syndrome.

**villi** (vĭl′ī) [L.] Pl. of villus.

**villiferous** (vĭl-ĭf′ĕr-ŭs) [″ + *ferre,* to bear] Having villi or tufts of hair.

**villoma** (vĭ-lō′mă) [L. *villus,* tuft of hair, + Gr. *oma,* tumor] A villous tumor.

**villose, villous** (vĭl′ōs, vĭl′ŭs) [L. *villus,* tuft of hair] Pert. to or furnished with villi or with fine hairlike extensions.

**villositis** (vĭl″ōs-ī′tĭs) [″ + Gr. *itis,* inflammation] Inflammation of the placental villi.

**villosity** (vĭ-lŏs′ĭ-tē) The condition of being covered with villi.

**villus** (vĭl′ŭs) *pl.* **villi** [L., tuft of hair] A small fold or projection of some mucous membranes.

***arachnoid v.*** A protrusion of the cerebral arachnoid into the dural wall of a venous sinus or its lacuna; a pathway for reabsorption of cerebrospinal fluid.

***chorionic villi*** One of the tiny vascular projections of the chorionic surface that become vascular and help to form the placenta. SEE: *embryo* for illus.; *chorion.*

***intestinal v.*** One of the multiple, minute projections of the intestinal mucosa into the lumen of the small intestines. These projections increase the surface area for absorption of water and nutrients; each contains a capillary network and a lacteal. SEE: illus.

***synovial v.*** One of the thin projections of the synovial membrane into the joint cavity.

**villusectomy** (vĭl″ŭs-ĕk′tō-mē) [″ + Gr. *ektome,* excision] Surgical removal of a synovial villus.

**vinblastine sulfate** (vĭn-blăs′tēn) A fraction of an extract obtained from the periwinkle plant, *Vinca rosea,* a species of myrtle. It is a cytotoxic agent used in treating certain types of malignant tumors.

---

Caution: Vinblastine sulfate must be handled with great care because it is a potent cytotoxic agent.

---

**Vinca** (vĭn′kă) A genus of herbs including periwinkles, from which vincristine and vinblastine are obtained.

**Vincent's angina** Acute necrotizing ulcerative gingivitis.

**vincristine sulfate** (vĭn-krĭs′tēn) A fraction of an extract obtained from the periwinkle plant, *Vinca rosea,* a species of myrtle. It is a cytotoxic agent used in treating certain types of malignant tumors.

---

Caution: Vincristine sulfate must be handled with great care because it is a potent cytotoxic agent.

---

**vinculum** (vĭn′kū-lŭm) *pl.* **vincula** [L., to bind, tie] A uniting band or bundle. SYN: *frenulum; frenum; ligament.*

***v. tendinum*** **1.** Slender tendinous filaments connecting the phalanges with the flexor tendons. **2.** The ringlike ligament of

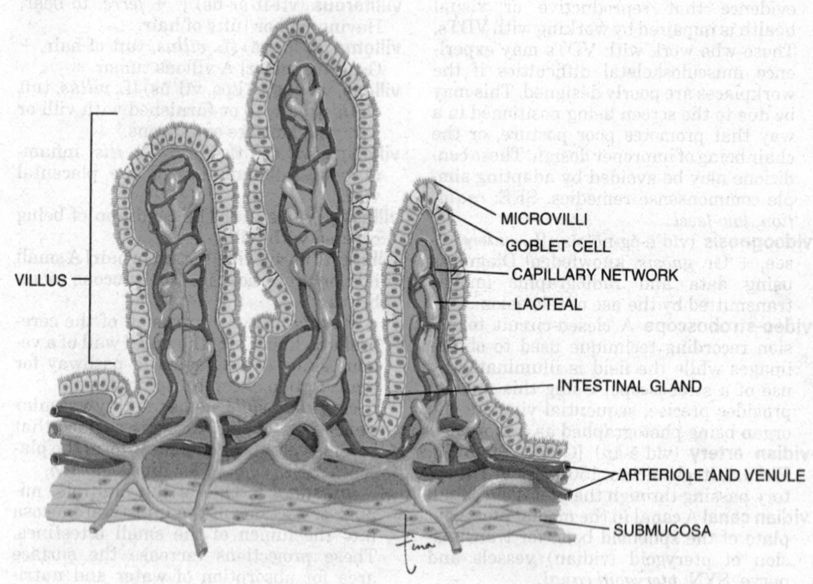


VILLI OF SMALL INTESTINE

the ankle or wrist.

**vinegar** (vĭn′ĕ-găr) [ME. *vinegre,* from Fr. *vin,* wine, + *aigre,* sour] The product of fermentation of weak alcoholic solutions such as apple cider. It is a weak, impure solution of acetic acid, usually containing between 4% and 6%. SEE: *condiment.*

**vinyl** (vī′nĭl) The univalent ethenyl hydrocarbon molecule, $CH_2{=}CH{-}$.

***v. chloride*** A vinyl radical attached to a chlorine atom, $CH_2{=}CHCl$. Some individuals exposed to vinyl chloride have developed malignant lung tumors.

***v. cyanide*** A toxic liquid compound, $CH_2{=}CHCN$, used in making plastics. SYN: *acrylonitrile.*

***v. ether*** An anesthetic agent that is virtually obsolete because it is explosive or flammable in the concentration required to produce anesthesia.

**violaceous** (vī″ĕ-lā′shŭs) [L. *violaceus,* violet] Having a purple discoloration, esp. of the skin.

**violate** (vī′ĕ-lāt″) [L. *violare,* to injure] To harm or injure a person, esp. to rape a female.

**violence** (vī′ō-lĕnts) [L. *violentia*] **1.** The use of force or physical compulsion to abuse or damage. **2.** The act of violent behavior.

***risk for v., directed at self/others*** *Self-directed:* Behaviors in which an individual demonstrates that he or she can be physically, emotionally, or sexually harmful to the self. *Directed at others:* Behaviors in which an individual demonstrates that he or she can be physically, emotionally, or sexually harmful to others. SEE: *Nursing Diagnoses Appendix.*

**violet** (vī′ō-lĕt) [ME. *violett,* from L. *viola,* violet] One of the colors of the spectrum; similar to purple.

***gentian v.*** SEE: *gentian violet.*

**violet blindness** Inability to see violet tints.

**viomycin** (vī-ō-mī′sĭn) An antibiotic produced by strains of *Streptomyces griseus.*

**viosterol** (vī-ŏs′tĕr-ōl) A solution of irradiated ergosterol in vegetable oil. SYN: *calciferol.*

**viper** (vī′pĕr) Any venomous snake of the family Viperidae.

**vipoma** [*v*asoactive *i*ntestinal *p*olypeptide + *oma,* tumor] A rare form of islet cell tumor of the pancreas that is characterized by watery diarrhea, hypokalemia, and achlorhydria. This is caused by the release of vasoactive intestinal peptide from the tumor.

**viraginity** (vĭr″ă-jĭn′ĭ-tē) [L. *virago,* an amazon or manlike woman] A condition in which a woman believes that she should be a male even though she is aware that her body is female. SEE: *transsexual.*

**viral** Pert. to or caused by a virus.

**viral gastroenteritis** SEE: *epidemic viral gastroenteropathy.*

**viral interference** The inhibition of the multiplication of one type of virus by the presence of another virus in the same cell. SEE: *interferon.*

**Virchow's node** SEE: *node, signal.*

**viremia** (vī″rēm′ē-ă) The presence of viruses in the blood.

**vires** (vī′rēs) Pl. of vis.

**virga** [L., a rod] Penis.

**virgin** (vĕr′jĭn) [L. *virgo,* a maiden] **1.** A woman or man who has not had sexual intercourse. **2.** Uncontaminated; fresh; new.

**virginal** (vĕr′jĭn-ăl) [L. *virgo,* a maiden] Rel. to a virgin or to virginity.

**virginity** (vĕr-jĭn′ĭt-ē) [L. *virginitas,* maidenhood] The state of being a virgin; not having experienced sexual intercourse.

**virile** (vĭr′ĭl) [L. *virilis,* masculine] Masculine.

**virile reflex 1.** The sudden downward movement of a completely relaxed penis when the prepuce or glans is pulled upward. SYN: *bulbocavernosus reflex.* **2.** The contraction of the bulbocavernous muscle on percussing the dorsum of the penis. **3.** The contraction of the bulbocavernous muscle resulting from compression of the glans penis.

**virilescence** (vĭr-ĭl-ĕs′ĕns) [L. *virilis,* masculine] The acquisition of secondary masculine characteristics in the female.

**virilia** (vĭr-ĭl′ē-ă) [L.] The male sexual organs.

**virilism** (vĭr′ĭl-ĭzm) [″ + Gr. *-ismos,* condition] The presence or development of male secondary characteristics in a woman.

**virility** (vĭr-ĭl′ĭ-tē) [L. *virilitas,* masculinity] **1.** The state of possessing masculine qualities. **2.** Sexual potency in the male.

**virilization** (vĭr″ĭ-lī-zā′shŭn) The production of masculine secondary sex changes in a woman. Included would be voice change, development of male-type baldness, clitoral enlargement, and increased growth of facial and body hair. Virilization may be caused by one of several endocrine diseases that lead to excess production of testosterone, or by the woman's taking anabolic steroids. In the latter case, this is often done to attempt to enhance muscular development.

**virion** (vī′rē-ŏn, vĭ′rē-ŏn) A complete virus particle; a unit of genetic material, the genome, surrounded by a protective protein coat, the capsid. Sometimes the capsid is surrounded by a lipid envelope. SEE: *capsid.*

**viripotent** (vī-rĭp′ō-tĕnt) [L. *viripotens*] Sexually mature, as applied to a man.

**viroid** A small, naked, infectious molecule of RNA. Viroids differ from viruses by the absence of a dormant phase and by genomes that are much smaller than those of known viruses.

**virology** (vī-rŏl′ō-jē) [L. *virus,* poison, + Gr. *logos,* word, reason] The study of viruses and viral diseases.

**viropexis** (vī″rō-pĕk′sĭs) [″ + Gr. *pexis,* fixation] The fixation of a virus particle to a cell. This leads to the inclusion of the virus inside the cell.

**virtual** (vĕr′tū-ăl) [L. *virtus,* capacity] Appearing to exist but not existing in actual fact or form.

**virucidal** (vĭr-ū-sī′dăl) [L. *virus,* poison, + *cidus,* to kill] Destructive of a virus.

**virucide** An agent that destroys or inactivates a virus, esp. a chemical substance used on living tissue.

**virulence** (vĭr′ū-lĕns) [LL. *virulentia,* stench] **1.** The relative power and degree of pathogenicity possessed by organisms. Properties that influence the virulence of an organism include (1) the strength of its adhesion molecules, which link it to the target cell; (2) its ability to secrete enzymes or exotoxins that damage target cells, or endotoxins that interfere with the body's normal regulatory systems; and (3) its ability to inhibit or evade the actions of white blood cells and their chemical mediators. SEE: *immunocompetent; immunocompromised.* **2.** The property of being virulent; venomousness, as of a disease. SEE: *attenuation.*

**virulent** (vĭr′ū-lĕnt) [L. *virulentus,* poison] **1.** Very poisonous. **2.** Infectious; able to overcome the host's defensive mechanism.

**viruria** (vīr-ūr′ē-ă) [″ + Gr. *ouron,* urine] The presence of viruses in the urine.

**virus** (vī′rŭs) [L., poison] The smallest organism identified by use of electron microscopy. Viruses can live only inside cells. Because they cannot obtain food or reproduce outside cells, they are called obligate intracellular parasites. Viruses comprise a central core of either deoxyribonucleic acid (DNA) or ribonucleic acid (RNA), surrounded by a protein coating, or capsid; some viruses create an additional covering called an envelope from the cytoplasm of the cell.

Viruses with envelopes have a greater ability to adhere to cell membranes and to avoid destruction by the immune system. Both the capsid and envelope have antigens (protein markers recognizable to white blood cells). Many of these antigens change frequently, so that the body is unable to create one immunoglobulin (antibody) that can neutralize both the original antigen and its replacement. The common influenza viruses have antigens that mutate or combine readily, requiring new vaccines with each mutation. The body's primary immune defenses against viruses are cytotoxic T lymphocytes, interferons, and to some extent immunoglobulins (antibodies); destruction of the virus often requires destruction of the host cell.

When viruses enter a cell, they may immediately trigger a disease process or remain quiescent for many years. They damage the host cell by blocking its normal protein synthesis and using its metabolic machinery for their own reproduction. New virus particles are then released either by destroying their host cell or by forming small buds that break off and infect other cells. One virus may produce different symptoms according to the immune defenses of the individual infected; in contrast, several viruses cause

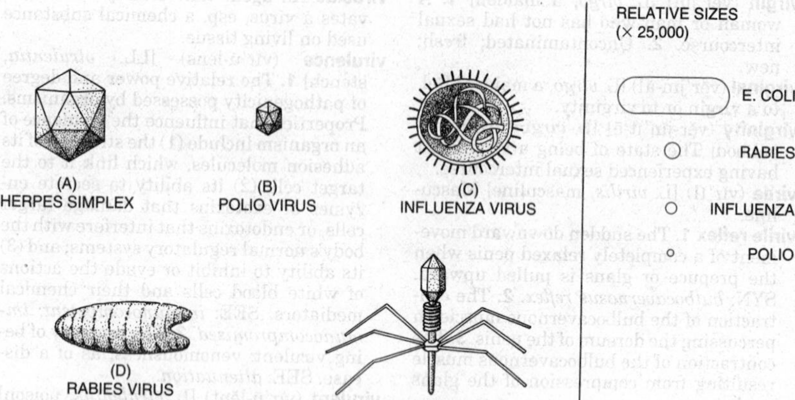


**VIRUSES**

the same signs in many people (e.g., viruses that infect the upper respiratory tract).

Some viruses are called oncogenic because data indicate that they may alter a cell's DNA and induce cells to become malignant. Viruses that remain quiescent inside the cell are called latent viruses, waiting for a time when the body's immune defenses are decreased to begin replication and produce symptoms. For example, all of the herpesvirus family are latent; adults may develop shingles after childhood exposure to the varicella zoster virus, which causes chickenpox. SEE: illus.; table.

CLASSIFICATION: The 400 known viruses are classified in several ways: by genome core (RNA or DNA), host (animals, plants, or bacteria), method of reproduction (e.g., retrovirus), mode of transmission (e.g., enterovirus), and disease pro-

**Common Viral Infections**

| Virus | Type of Infection and/or Site |
|---|---|
| Adenovirus | Respiratory tract |
| Herpes virus group | |
| HSV-1 | Cold sores/fever blisters; keratitis |
| HSV-2 | Genital herpes |
| Cytomegalovirus | Central nervous system damage and hemolysis in newborn |
| | Opportunistic: retinitis, gastrointestinal tract, lungs |
| Epstein-Barr | Infectious mononucleosis |
| | Opportunistic: lymphoma, hairy leukoplakia |
| Varicella zoster | Skin (chickenpox); Neurons (shingles) |
| Hepatitis (A, B, C, D, E) | Liver |
| Human papillomavirus | Genital warts, cervical neoplasia |
| Human immunodeficiency virus (HIV I and II) | AIDS |
| Influenza (A, B, C) | "Flu," bronchiolitis, pneumonia |
| Poliovirus | Poliomyelitis |
| Respiratory syncytial virus | Bronchiolitis, pneumonia |
| Rhinovirus | Upper respiratory tract (common cold) |
| Rubella | German measles |
| Rubeola | Measles |

duced (e.g., hepatitis virus).

***arbor v.*** Former name for arbovirus.

***attenuated v.*** A virus with reduced pathogenicity due to treatment or repeated passage through hosts.

***bacterial v.*** A bacteriophage.

***chikungunya v.*** A mosquito-borne virus that causes a denguelike disease with hemorrhagic complications.

***coxsackie v.*** SEE: *coxsackievirus.*

***cytomegalic v.*** ABBR: CMV. Cytomegalovirus.

***defective v.*** A virus particle that, because of a lack of certain essential factors, is unable to replicate. Sometimes this can be overcome by the presence of a helper virus that provides the missing factor or factors.

***EB v.*** Epstein-Barr virus.

***enteric v.*** Enterovirus.

***enteric cytopathogenic human orphan v.*** ABBR: ECHO virus. A virus that was accidentally discovered in human feces and not known to be associated with a disease, thus the name "orphan." Initially 33 ECHO virus serotypes were designated, but numbers 10 and 28 have been reclassified. Various serotypes have been associated with aseptic meningitis, encephalitis, acute upper respiratory infection, enteritis, pleurodynia, and myocarditis.

***enteric orphan v.*** SEE: *enteric cytopathogenic human orphan v.*

***filtrable v.*** A virus causing infectious disease, the essential elements of which are so tiny that they retain infectivity after passing through a filter of the Berkefeld type. SEE: *filter, Berkefeld.*

***fixé v., fixed v.*** A rabies virus that was stabilized and modified but only partially attenuated by serial passage through rabbits.

***helper v.*** A virus that permits a defective virus present in the same cell to replicate. SEE: *defective v.*

***herpes v.*** Herpesvirus.

***human immunodeficiency v.*** ABBR: HIV. SEE: *human immunodeficiency virus.*

***latent v.*** A virus that has the ability to infect the host, initially causing little or no signs of illness but persisting for the lifetime of the infected individual; later on, a specific triggering mechanism may cause the virus to produce a clinically apparent disease. This occurs with herpes simplex virus that remains latent in sensory ganglia and is reactivated by trauma to the skin supplied by the distal sensory nerves associated with these ganglia. After reactivation, the virus may cause localized or generalized lesions in the affected area and the central nervous system.

***lytic v.*** Any virus that, after infecting a cell, lyses it.

***masked v.*** A virus that ordinarily occurs in the host in a noninfective state but is activated and demonstrated by indirect methods.

***neurotropic v.*** A virus that reproduces in nerve tissue.

***oncogenic v.*** A virus that produces tumors. Although there is a relationship between viruses and human cancer, their exact role is not fully understood.

***orphan v.*** One of several viruses that initially were not thought to be associated with pathogenicity. However, since then, a number of them have been shown to be associated with disease. This group includes the enteroviruses and rhinoviruses.

***parainfluenza v.*** One of a group of viruses that affect infants and young children. It causes respiratory infections that may be mild or may progress to pneumonia. Most infections are so mild as to be clinically inapparent.

***plant v.*** Any virus that is pathogenic for plants.

***pox v.*** Poxvirus.

***respiratory syncytial v.*** A virus that is a major cause of lower respiratory tract disease during infancy and early childhood. It induces the formation of cell masses in which the cellular protoplasms are connected (syncytium) in cell cultures. Attempts to develop an effective and safe vaccine have been in vain. Because it is difficult to recognize the disease early and inapparent cases are frequent, isolation and public health measures are not adequate to control the spread of the disease. Ribavirin is the primary drug used in its treatment. The administration of high doses of respiratory syncytial virus immune globulin is an effective means of preventing lower respiratory tract infection in infants and young children at high risk for contracting this disease.

***slow v.*** SEE: *slow virus infection.*

***street v.*** A rabies virus obtained from an infected animal rather than from a laboratory strain.

***tumor v.*** A virus that causes malignant neoplasms. This is known to occur in a variety of species, including some primates, but proof that any human tumor is virus-induced is inconclusive. Viruses suspected of being oncogenic (i.e., tumor-inducing) in humans are Epstein-Barr virus linked with African Burkitt's lymphoma, hepatitis B virus with primary hepatocellular carcinoma, herpes simplex type 2 with carcinoma of the cervix, and cytomegalovirus with Kaposi's sarcoma.

**virusemia** (vī″rŭs-ēm′ē-ă) [″ + Gr. *haima,* blood] Viremia.

**virus shedding** The release of a virus from the host.

**virustatic** (vīr″ū-stăt′ĭk) [″ + Gr. *statikos,* bringing to a standstill] Stopping the growth of viruses.

**vis** (vĭs) *pl.* **vires** [L., strength] Force, strength, energy, power.

**viscera** (vĭs′ĕr-ă) *sing.,* **viscus** [L.] Internal organs enclosed within a cavity, esp. the abdominal organs. SEE: *celosomia; evisceration; splanchnic.*

**viscerad** (vĭs′ĕr-ăd) [″ + *ad,* toward] Toward the viscera.

**visceral** (vĭs′ĕr-ăl) [L. *viscera,* body organs] **1.** Pert. to viscera. **2.** Pert. to or derived from the gill arches of vertebrates.

**visceral cavity** The body cavity containing the viscera.

**visceral cleft** One of the fissures separating the visceral arches.

**visceral skeleton** The pelvis, ribs, and sternum enclosing the viscera.

**viscerimotor** (vĭs″ĕr-ĭ-mō′tor) [″ + *motor,* mover] Visceromotor.

**viscero-** (vĭs′ĕr-ō) [L. *viscera,* body organs] Combining form meaning *viscera.*

**viscerocranium** (vĭs″ĕr-ō-krā′nē-ŭm) That portion of the skull derived from the pharyngeal arches.

**viscerogenic** (vĭs″ĕr-ō-jĕn′ĭk) [″ + Gr. *gennan,* to produce] Originating in the viscera.

**visceroinhibitory** (vĭs″ĕr-ō-ĭn-hĭb′ĭ-tō-rē) [″ + *inhibere,* to restrain] Checking the action of the viscera.

**visceromegaly** (vĭs″ĕr-ō-mĕg′ă-lē) [″ + Gr. *megalos,* great] Generalized enlargement of the abdominal visceral organs.

**visceromotor** (vĭs″ĕr-ō-mō′tor) [L. *viscera,* body organs, + *motor,* a mover] Rel. to a nerve conveying motor impulses to the viscera. SYN: *viscerimotor.*

**visceromotor reflex** An increase in tonus of the abdominal muscles resulting from painful stimuli originating in a viscus.

**visceroparietal** (vĭs″ĕr-ō-pă-rī′ĕ-tăl) [″ + *paries,* wall] Rel. to the viscera and abdominal wall.

**visceroperitoneal** (vĭs″ĕr-ō-pĕr″ĭ-tō-nē′ăl) [″+ Gr. *peritonaion,* peritoneum] Rel. to the abdominal viscera and peritoneum.

**visceropleural** (vĭs″ĕr-ō-ploo′răl) [″+ Gr. *pleura,* a side] Rel. to the thoracic viscera and pleura. SYN: *pleurovisceral.*

**visceroptosis** (vĭs″ĕr-ŏp-tō′sĭs) [″ + Gr. *ptosis,* a dropping] Downward displacement of a viscus.

**visceroreceptors** (vĭs″ĕr-ō-rē-sĕp′torz) A group of receptors that includes those located in visceral organs. Their stimulation gives rise to poorly localized and ill-defined sensations. In hollow visceral organs, they are stimulated principally by excessive contraction or by distention.

**viscerosensory** (vĭs″ĕr-ō-sĕn′sō-rē) [″ + *sensorius,* sensory] Pert. to sensations aroused by stimulation of visceroreceptors.

**viscerosensory reflex** Pain or tenderness elicited in somatic structures (skin and muscle) caused by visceral disorder. SEE: *pain, referred.*

**visceroskeletal** (vĭs″ĕr-ō-skĕl′ĕt-ăl) [″ + Gr. *skeleton,* a dried-up body] Rel. to the visceral skeleton.

**viscerosomatic** (vĭs″ĕr-ō-sō-măt′ĭk) [″ + Gr. *soma,* body] Rel. to the viscera and the body.

**viscerosomatic reaction** A reaction occurring in muscles of the body wall as a result of stimulation of visceroreceptors.

**viscerotome** (vĭs′ĕr-ō-tōm) [″ + Gr. *tome,* incision] The part of an abdominal organ that is supplied with afferent nerves from a single posterior root.

**viscerotonia** (vĭs″ĕr-ō-tōn′ē-ă) [″ + Gr. *tonos,* tension] Personality traits characterized by predominance of social over intellectual and physical traits. The individual is sociable and convivial, exhibits unusual appreciation of food, and loves company, affection, social support, and approval.

**viscerotrophic** (vĭs″ĕr-ō-trŏf′ĭk) [″ + Gr. *trophe,* nourishment] Pert. to trophic changes rel. to or associated with visceral conditions.

**viscerotropic** (vĭs″ĕr-ō-trŏp′ĭk) [″ + Gr. *tropos,* a turn] Primarily affecting the viscera.

**viscerovisceral reaction** (vĭs″ĕr-ō-vĭs′ĕr-ăl) A reaction taking place in the viscera as a result of stimulation of visceral receptors. Such reactions are usually below the level of consciousness.

**viscid** (vĭs′ĭd) [L. *viscum,* mistletoe, birdlime] Adhering, glutinous, sticky. In bacteriology, said of a colony that strings out by clinging to a needle when it is touched to the culture and withdrawn. The sediment rises in a coherent whirl when the liquid culture is shaken.

**viscoelasticity** The property of being viscous and elastic.

**viscosimeter** (vĭs″kŏs-ĭm′ĕ-tĕr) [LL. *viscosus,* viscous, + Gr. *metron,* measure] A device for estimating the viscosity of a fluid, esp. of blood.

**viscosimetry** (vĭs″kō-sĭm′ĕ-trē) Measurement of the viscosity of a substance.

**viscosity** (vĭs″kŏs′ĭ-tē) [LL. *viscosus,* viscous] **1.** The state of being sticky or gummy. **2.** Resistance offered by a fluid to change of form or relative position of its particles due to attraction of molecules to each other.

***specific v.*** The internal friction of a fluid, measured by comparing the rate of flow of the liquid through a tube with that of some standard liquid, or by measuring the resistance to rotating paddles.

**viscous** (vĭs′kŭs) Sticky, gummy, gelatinous, with high viscosity.

**viscus** (vĭs′kŭs) *pl.* **viscera** [L., body organ] Any internal organ enclosed within a cavity, such as the thorax or abdomen.

**visibility** (vĭz″ĭ-bĭl′ĭ-tē) [L. *visibilitas*] The quality of being visible.

**visible** (vĭz′ĭ-bl) [L. *visibilis*] Capable of being seen.

**visile** (vĭz′ĭl) [L. *visum,* seeing] **1.** Pert. to vision. **2.** Readily recalling what is seen, more than that which is audible or motile.

**vision** (vĭzh′ŭn) [L. *visio,* a seeing] **1.** Act of viewing external objects. SYN: *sight.* SEE: *reading machine for the blind.* **2.** Sense by which light and color are apprehended. **3.** An imaginary sight.

***achromatic v.*** Complete color blindness.

***artificial v.*** A technique, still in the experimental stage, designed to make it possible for some persons who are blind to see. SEE: *Optacon.*

***binocular v.*** The visual sensation that is produced when the images perceived by each eye are fused to appear as one.

***central v.*** Vision resulting from rays falling on the fovea centralis.

***day v.*** A condition in which one sees better during the day than at night, found in peripheral lesions of the retina such as retinitis pigmentosa. SYN: *photopic v.*

***dichromatic v.*** A form of defective color vision in which only two of the primary colors are perceived.

***double v.*** Diplopia.

***field of v.*** The space within which an object can be seen while the eye remains fixed on one point.

***half v.*** Hemianopia.

***indirect v.*** Peripheral v.

***low v.*** A significant loss of vision that cannot be corrected medically, surgically, or with eyeglasses.

***monocular v.*** Vision using only one eye.

***multiple v.*** Polyopia.

***night v.*** Ability to see when illumination is reduced. SYN: *scotopic v.*

***oscillating v.*** Oscillopsia.

***peripheral v.*** Vision resulting from rays falling on the retina outside of the macular field. SYN: *indirect v.*

***phantom v.*** An experience of visual sensations following surgical removal of an eye; usually a transient condition.

***photopic v.*** Day v.

***scotopic v.*** Night v.

***stereoscopic v.*** Vision in which things have the appearance of solidity and relief, as though seen in three dimensions. Binocular vision produces this effect. SYN: *stereopsis.*

***tunnel v.* 1.** A condition seen in hysteria in which the field of vision is the same regardless of distance from the visual screen. **2.** Severe constriction of the visual field caused by advanced chronic glaucoma.

***v. without sight*** The ability of individuals who are blind and unable to perceive visual stimuli including bright light, to respond to light. This has been investigated by determining melatonin secretion in blind persons. In sighted individuals, the hormone is secreted during sleep. Some completely blind individuals also secrete melatonin during sleep as if their sense of sight were intact. In others, melatonin is not secreted during sleep. This investigation concluded that the central nervous system in some blind persons responds to light even though they are without sight.

**visit** An encounter between a patient and a health professional that requires either the patient to travel from his or her home to the professional's usual place of practice (office visit) or vice versa (home visit).

**Visiting Nurse Association** A voluntary health agency that provides nursing services in the home, including health supervision, education and counseling, and maintenance of the medical regimen. Nurses and other personnel such as home health aides who are specifically trained for tasks of personal bedside care provide the services offered by the agency. These agencies originated in the visiting or district nurse service provided to the poor in their homes by voluntary agencies such as the New York City Mission, which existed in the 1870s. The first visiting nurse associations were established in Buffalo, Boston, and Philadelphia between 1886 and 1887.

**visual** (vĭzh′ū-ăl) [L. *visio,* a seeing] **1.** Pert. to vision. **2.** One whose learning and memorizing processes are largely of a visual nature.

**visual acuity** A measure of the resolving power of the eye; usually determined by one's ability to read letters of various sizes at a standard distance from the test chart. The result is expressed as a fraction. For example, 20/20 is normal vision, meaning the subject's eye has the ability to see from a distance of 20 ft (6.1 m) what the normal eye would see at that distance. Visual acuity of 20/40 means that a person sees at 20 ft (6.1 m) what the normal eye could see at 40 ft (12.2 m).

**visual angle** The angle between the line of sight and the extremities of the object seen.

**visual axis** The line of vision from the object seen through the pupil's center to the macula lutea.

**visual cone** The cone whose vertex is at the eye and whose generating lines touch the boundary of a visible object.

**visual evoked response** ABBR: VER. A reaction produced in response to visual stimuli. While the patient is watching a pattern projected on a screen, the electroencephalogram is recorded. The characteristics of the wave form, its latency, and the amplitude of the wave can be compared with the normal, and important information concerning the function of the visual apparatus in transmitting stimuli to the brain can be obtained. SEE: *brainstem auditory evoked responses; evoked responses; somatosensory evoked responses.*

**visual field** The area within which objects may be seen when the eye is fixed. SEE: *perimetry.*

**visual function** The process of receiving stimuli transmitted to the eye and then to the brain and translating those stimuli into images. There are three aspects of visual function: form sense, color sense, and light sense. Form sense is tested by determining visual acuity; color sense by having the patient distinguish colors depicted in standard charts; and light sense by testing peripheral vision.

There is evidence that the human eye must see an object twice to form an image of the object in the brain. This is done when the eye fixes on an object and then almost instantaneously and imperceptibly shifts to look at the object from a slightly different angle.

**visualization** (vĭzh″ū-ăl-ī-zā′shŭn) The act of viewing or sensing a picture of an object, esp. the picture of a body structure as obtained by radiographic study.

**visualize** (vĭzh′ū-ăl-īz) **1.** To make visible. **2.** To imagine or picture something in one's mind.

**visual object agnosia** Loss of the ability to visually recognize objects presented, even though some degree of ability to see is intact.

**visual plane** The plane in which both optic axes lie.

**visual point** The center of vision.

**visuoauditory** (vĭzh″ū-ō-aw′dĭ-tor″ē) [L. *visio,* a seeing, + *auditorius,* pert. to hearing] Rel. to sight and hearing, as connecting nerve fibers between auditory and visual centers.

**visuognosis** (vĭzh″ū-ŏg-nō′sĭs) [″ + Gr. *gnosis,* knowledge] The recognition and appreciation of what is seen.

**visuopsychic** (vĭzh″ū-ō-sī′kĭk) [″ + Gr. *psyche,* soul, mind] Both visual and psychic, applied to the cerebral area involved in perception of visual sensations.

**visuosensory** (vĭzh″ū-ō-sĕn′sō-rē) [L. *visio,* a seeing, + *sensorius,* sensory] Rel. to the recognition of visual impressions.

**visuospatial** Concerning the ability to discern spatial relationships from visual presentations.

**vita glass** (vī′tă-glăs) [L. *vita,* life, + AS. *glaes,* glass] Window glass containing quartz for transmitting the ultraviolet rays of sunlight.

**vital** (vī′tăl) [L. *vitalis,* pert. to life] **1.** Pert. to or characteristic of life. **2.** Contributing to or essential for life.

**vital center** The respiratory center in the medulla.

**vitalism** (vī′tăl-ĭzm) [″ + Gr. *-ismos,* condition] The opinion that a force neither chemical nor mechanical is responsible for some phenomena.

**vitalist** (vī′tăl-ĭst) [L. *vitalis,* pert. to life] One who believes in vitalism.

**vitalistic** (vī-tăl-ĭs′tĭk) Relating to vitalism.

**vitality** (vī-tăl′ĭ-tē) **1.** That which distinguishes living things from the nonliving. **2.** Animation, action. **3.** The state of being alive.

**vitalize** (vī′tăl-īz) To instill life or force in anything.

**vitalometer** A diagnostic device that measures the response of a nerve in the pulp of a tooth to an electrical stimulus.

**vital signs** The traditional signs of life (i.e., heartbeat, body temperature, respiration, and blood pressure).

**vital statistics** Statistics relating to births (natality), deaths (mortality), marriages, health, and disease (morbidity). Vital statistics for the U.S. are published annually by the National Center for Health Statistics of the Department of Health and Human Services.

**vitamer** (vī′tă-mĕr) Any one of a number of compounds that have specific vitamin activity.

**vitamin** (vī′tă-mĭn) [L. *vita,* life, + *amine*] Any of a group of organic substances other than proteins, carbohydrates, fats, and organic salts that are essential for normal metabolism, growth, and development of the body. Vitamins are required in very small quantities. They are not energy sources, but some are essential for the release of energy from food. Others are part of enzymes (coenzymes) necessary for the synthesis of DNA, clotting factors, collagen, and hemoglobin.

The chemical structure of the known vitamins has been determined, and some may be synthesized. In general, none of the vitamins can be formed in the body but must be obtained preformed from animal or plant sources. Exceptions are the formation of vitamin A from its precursor, carotene, the formation of vitamin D by the action of ultraviolet light on the skin, and the formation of vitamin K by symbiotic bacteria of the intestines. Some vitamins are unstable, being readily destroyed by oxidation, heat, esp. in an alkaline medium, strong acids, light, and aging. SEE: *Vitamins Appendix.*

There are several broad classifications of vitamins, such as the fat-soluble (A, D, E, and K) and the water-soluble (B and C) vitamins. This distinction is of clinical importance in patients with diseases that interfere with digestion of fat because they will eventually develop deficiencies of the fat-soluble vitamins, which are essential to body growth, development, and function. Certain vitamins cannot be manufactured by certain species. Humans belong to one of the few species that cannot manufacture vitamin C.

A variety of conditions increase the need for vitamins above the usual recommended dose. These include lactation, pregnancy, use of certain drugs, excessive use of alcohol or tobacco, and certain illnesses.

***antiberiberi v.*** Vitamin $B_1$.

***antineuritic v.*** Vitamin $B_1$.

***antipellagra v.*** Nicotinamide.

***antirachitic v.*** The vitamin D group.

***antiscorbutic v.*** Vitamin C.

***antixerophthalmic v.*** Vitamin A.

**vitamin A** A fat-soluble vitamin formed in the body from precursors, yellow pigments of plants (alpha, beta, and gamma carotene). It is essential for normal growth and development, the normal function and integrity of epithelial tissues, formation of visual purple, and normal tooth and bone development. It is stored in the liver. The recommended daily requirement for women is 800 $\mu g$ and for men 1000 $\mu g$. Retinol is the form of vitamin A found in mammals. One retinol equivalent is equal to 6 $\mu g$ of beta-carotene. The use of beta-carotene instead of vitamin A as a dietary supplement has the advantage that the latter in large doses may be toxic, while beta-carotene is virtually nontoxic. Excessive intake of vitamin A may cause acute or chronic effects. SYN: *retinol*. SEE: *hypervitaminosis; Vitamins Appendix.*

SOURCES: Butter, butterfat in milk, egg yolks, and cod liver oil are rich sources. The vitamin is found also in liver, green leafy and yellow vegetables, prunes, pineapples, oranges, limes, and cantaloupes.

STABILITY: This vitamin resists boiling for some time if not exposed to oxidation. It is quite stable with brief exposure to heat but not with continued high temperatures (above 100°C or 212°F).

DEFICIENCY DISORDERS: A deficiency of vitamin A causes interference with growth, reduced resistance to infections, and interference with nutrition of the cornea, conjunctiva, trachea, hair follicles, and renal pelvis. Thus these tissues have an increased susceptibility to infections. Vitamin A deficiency also interferes with the ability of the eyes to adapt to darkness (night blindness) and impairs visual acuity. Children with vitamin A deficiency will experience impaired growth and development. SEE: *Bitot's spots.*

**vitamin $A_1$** A form of vitamin A found in fish liver oils.

**vitamin $A_2$** A compound found in the livers of freshwater fish; similar in properties to vitamin A but with different ultraviolet absorption spectra.

**vitamin B complex** A group of water-soluble vitamins isolated from liver, yeast, and other sources. Only grain-made yeast preserves its potency if dried. Among vitamins included are thiamine ($B_1$), riboflavin ($B_2$), niacin (nicotinic acid), pyridoxine ($B_6$), biotin, folic acid, and cyanocobalamin ($B_{12}$).

SOURCES: *Thiamine:* Whole grains, wheat embryo, brewer's yeast, legumes, nuts, egg yolk, fruits, and vegetables. *Riboflavin:* Brewer's yeast, liver, meat, esp. pork and fish, poultry, eggs, milk, and green vegetables. *Nicotinic acid:* Brewer's yeast, liver, meat, poultry, and green vegetables. *Pyridoxine:* Rice, bran, and yeast. *Folic acid:* Leafy green vegetables, organ meats, lean beef and veal, and wheat cereals.

ACTION/USES: Vitamin B affects growth, appetite, lactation, and the gastrointestinal, nervous, and endocrine systems; aids in marasmus; stimulates appetite; is important in metabolism of carbohydrates, including sugar; stimulates biliary action; and is used as an adjunct when some antituberculosis drugs are used.

Vitamin $B_1$, thiamine, affects growth and nutrition and carbohydrate metabolism. $B_2$, riboflavin, affects growth and cellular metabolism. Nicotinic acid prevents pellagra.

Although not destroyed by ordinary cooking, B complex vitamins may be destroyed by excessive heating for 2 to 4 hr. Bicarbonate of soda used in cooking aids destruction. Riboflavin and nicotinic acid, more stable than thiamine, are not destroyed by heat or oxidation.

NOTE: Prolonged use of antibiotics may destroy the intestinal bacteria that normally produce some of the B vitamins. In those cases, supplemental vitamins will be required.

STABILITY: Long-continued cooking or high-temperature cooking destroys vitamin B; bicarbonate of soda used in cooking aids its destruction. Ordinary cooking or heat does not destroy it.

DEFICIENCY DISORDERS: Deficiency causes beriberi, pellagra, digestive disturbances, enlargement of the liver, disturbance of the thyroid, degeneration of sex glands, and disturbance of the nervous system. It also induces edema; affects the heart, liver, spleen, and kidneys; enlarges the adrenals; and causes dysfunction of the pituitary and salivary glands.

**vitamin $B_1$** Thiamine, or thiamine hydrochloride. The recommended daily allowance is approx. 1.5 mg for men and 1.1 mg for women. SEE: *Vitamins Appendix.*

**vitamin $B_2$** Riboflavin. SEE: *Vitamins Appendix.*

**vitamin $B_6$** Pyridoxine; found in rice, bran, and yeast. Excess doses (2 to 5 g/day for months) have caused impairment of central nervous system function. SEE: *Vitamins Appendix.*

**vitamin $B_{12}$** A red crystalline substance, a cobamide, extracted from the liver, that is essential for the formation of red blood cells. Its deficiency results in pernicious anemia. It is used for prophylaxis and treatment of these and other diseases in which there is defective red cell formation. The recommended adult daily requirement is 2 $\mu g$/day. The terms vitamin $B_{12}$ and cyanocobalamin are used interchangeably as the generic term for all of the cobamides active in humans. SYN: *cyanocobalamin*. SEE: *Vitamins Appendix.*

**vitamin C** Ascorbic acid, a factor necessary for formation of collagen in connective tissues and essential in maintenance of integrity of intercellular cement in many tissues, esp. capillary walls. Vitamin C deficiency leads to scurvy. SEE: *Vitamins Appendix.*

NOTE: The recommended adult daily allowance is 60 mg. Large daily doses of vitamin C have been recommended for prevention and treatment of the common cold. Although the effectiveness of vitamin C for this purpose has not been established, it is felt that the vitamin may at least decrease the severity of cold symptoms. Excess doses of vitamin C for an extended period can interfere with absorption of vitamin $B_{12}$, cause uricosuria, and promote formation of oxalate kidney stones.

SOURCES: Vitamin C is found in raw cabbage, young carrots, orange juice, lettuce, celery, onions, tomatoes, radishes, and green peppers. Citrus fruits and rutabagas are esp. rich in this vitamin. Strawberries are about as rich a source as tomatoes. Apples, pears, apricots, plums, peaches, and pineapples also contain vitamin C.

STABILITY: The vitamin is destroyed easily by heat in the presence of oxygen, as in open-kettle boiling. It is less affected by heat in an acid medium; otherwise, it is stable.

DEFICIENCY DISORDERS: Vitamin C deficiency causes scurvy, imperfect prenatal skeletal formation, defective teeth, pyorrhea, anorexia, and anemia. It also leads to undernutrition injury to bone, cells, and blood vessels.

**vitamin D** One of several vitamins having antirachitic activity. The vitamin D group, which is fat-soluble, includes $D_2$ (calciferol), $D_3$ (irradiated 7-dehydrocholesterol), $D_4$ (irradiated 22-dihydroergosterol), and $D_5$ (irradiated dehydrositosterol). It is essential in calcium and phosphorus metabolism; consequently, it is required for normal development of bones and teeth. The recommended daily allowance is 10 $\mu$g. The stability of this vitamin is not affected by oxidation; heat, unless over 100°C (212°F); or long-continued cooking. A deficiency of vitamin D causes imperfect skeletal formation, bone diseases, rickets, and caries. SEE: *Vitamins Appendix*.

SOURCES: Milk, cod liver oil, salmon and cod livers, egg yolk, and butter fat contain vitamin D. Ergosterol in the skin activated by sunlight or ultraviolet radiation possesses vitamin D potency.

ACTION/USES: Vitamin D is necessary for the absorption of calcium and phosphorus from food in the small intestine. It is called the antirachitic vitamin because its deficiency interferes with calcium and phosphorus use, which in turn causes rickets. Sun or ultraviolet radiation exposure synthesizes this vitamin in the body. Its presence is necessary for the most efficient absorption of calcium and phosphorus. It is used to treat and prevent infantile rickets, spasmophilia (infantile tetany), and softening of bone. Vitamin D is also important in normal growth and mineralization of skeleton and teeth.

Prolonged excessive doses of vitamin D (100,000 IU daily) cause hypercalcemia with anorexia, nausea, vomiting, polyuria, polydipsia, weakness, anxiety, pruritus, and altered renal function.

**vitamin E** Alpha-tocopherol, an essential nutrient for humans, although the exact biochemical mechanism whereby it functions in the body is unknown. Because of the amount of vitamin E present in foods, its deficiency is absent in the general population. Excessive doses (100 mg/kg/day) in low-birth-weight neonates have been implicated in the development of necrotizing enterocolitis and sepsis. The recommended adult daily allowance is 10 mg for men and 8 mg for women. SEE: *Vitamins Appendix*.

**vitamin K** An antihemorrhagic factor whose activity is associated with compounds derived from naphthoquinone. Vitamin K, which is fat soluble, is present in alfalfa, fats, oats, wheats, and rye; vitamin $K_2$, in fishmeal. Vitamin $K_3$ is synthesized as menadione sodium bisulfite. Vitamin K is necessary for synthesis of clotting factors VII, IX, X, and prothrombin by the liver. Its deficiency prolongs blood-clotting time and causes hemorrhages. In the newborn, the colon is sterile until food is ingested and bacteria colonize the site. Because this bacterial source of vitamin K is not immediately available, an intramuscular injection of 1 mg of water-soluble vitamin $K_1$ (phytonadione) is recommended for all newborns.

Large doses may cause hemolysis in persons with G6PD deficiency and in some healthy individuals. Large doses in the newborn may lead to anemia and kernicterus. The recommended adult daily allowance is 65 $\mu$g for women and 80 $\mu$g for men. SEE: *Vitamins Appendix*.

ACTION/USES: Vitamin K helps to eliminate prolonged bleeding in operations and in the biliary tract of jaundiced patients. Bile salts are necessary for its absorption.

**vitamin loss** Loss of vitamin content in food products because of vitamin instability, esp. in oxidation and during heating. Methods of preserving foods add to the loss of vitamins. Pickling, salting, curing, or fermenting processes usually cause complete loss of vitamin C. Commercial canning destroys from 50% to 85% of vitamin C contained in peas, lima beans, spinach, and asparagus. Pasteurization, unless special precautions are observed, causes a loss of from 30% to 60% of vitamin C. Apple pie and freshly prepared applesauce retain only from 20% to 30% of the vitamin C value of the apple. Vitamin $B_1$ in wheat is lost through milling because the wheat embryo, rich in vitamin $B_1$, is removed during this process.

**vitamin supplement** Any vitamin tablet or capsule containing one or more vitamins. Thus, a tablet or capsule may contain a single vitamin or many, and in some instances, a preparation will contain more than a dozen vitamins and an even greater number of minerals. The rationale for daily use of this latter type of vitamin and mineral supplement has not been established. In general, healthy adult men and healthy nonpregnant, nonlactating women consuming a normal, varied diet do not need vitamin supplements.

The difficulty of individuals choosing to treat themselves with vitamin supplements are: (1) People who take the supplements are usually already consuming an adequate diet. (2) The vitamins chosen are often not the ones inadequate in their diet. (3) The dose may be many times greater than the daily needs.

Some cardiologists, epidemiologists, and nutritionists feel that the combination of antioxidants and vitamin supplements such as vitamin C and vitamin E decreases the risk of developing heart disease. Others disagree and feel that essential nutrients should be and can be obtained from a healthy diet.

Also, excessive doses of pyridoxine (vitamin $B_6$) or vitamins A and D can cause toxic symptoms. SEE: *Food Guide Pyramid; vitamin C.*

**vitellary** (vĭt′ĕl-ā-rē) [L. *vitellus,* yolk of an egg] Vitelline.

**vitellin** (vī-tĕl′ĭn) A protein that can be extracted from egg yolk and contains lecithin. SEE: *nucleoprotein; ovovitellin.*

**vitelline** (vī-tĕl′ēn) Pert. to the yolk of an egg or the ovum.

**vitelline circulation** The embryonic circulation of blood to the yolk sac via the vitelline arteries and its return to general circulation through the vitelline veins.

**vitelline duct** The narrow duct connecting the yolk sac with the embryonic gut.

**vitelline vein** One of two veins conveying blood from the yolk sac.

**vitellogenesis** (vī″tĕl-ō-jĕn′ĕ-sĭs) The production of yolk.

**vitellointestinal** (vī″tĕl-ō-ĭn-tĕs′tĭn-ăl) Concerning the embryonic yolk sac and the intestinal tract.

**vitellolutein** (vī″tĕl-ō-lū′tē-ĭn) [L. *vitellus,* yolk, + *luteus,* yellow] A yellow pigment present in lutein.

**vitellorubin** (vī″tĕl-ō-rū′bĭn) [″ + *ruber,* red] A red pigment present in lutein.

**vitellose** (vī-tĕl′ōs) A proteose present in vitellin.

**vitellus** (vī-tĕl′ŭs) [L.] The yolk of an ovum, esp. the yolk of a hen's egg.

**vitiation** (vĭsh″ē-ā′shŭn) [L. *vitiare,* to corrupt] Injury, contamination, impairment of use or efficiency.

**vitiligines** (vĭt″ĭ-lĭj′ĭ-nēz) Depigmented areas of skin. SEE: *vitiligo.*

**vitiliginous** (vĭt″ĭ-lĭj′ĭ-nŭs) Concerning vitiligo.

**vitiligo** (vĭt-ĭl-ī′gō) [L.] An acquired cutaneous disorder characterized by white patches, surrounded by areas of normal pigmentation. It is more common in the tropics and in blacks. Although the cause is unknown, the condition may be associated with systemic diseases such as

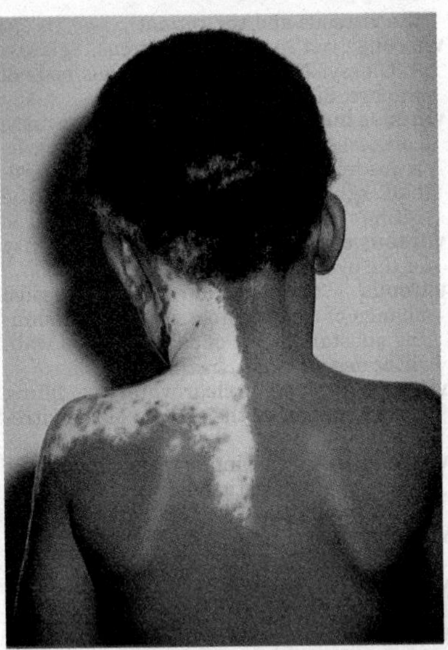

**VITILIGO**

hypothyroidism or hyperthyroidism, diabetes mellitus, Addison's disease, pernicious anemia, leprosy, or chronic mucocutaneous candidiasis syndrome. SYN: *leukoderma; skin, piebald.* SEE: illus.

TREATMENT: Oral and topical synthetic trioxsalen and a natural psoralen, methoxsalen, are used with exposure to long-wave ultraviolet light, but the efficacy is doubtful. The lesions may be masked by use of cosmetic preparations. Vitiliginous areas should be protected from sunburn by applying a 5% aminobenzoic acid solution or gel to the affected areas. The use of 5% fluorouracil cream applied under an occlusive dressing to the depigmented areas may cause erosion of the dermis and, after re-epithelialization, pigment may reappear.

***v. capitis*** Vitiligo of the scalp with depigmentation of the hairs of the affected area.

***perinevic v.*** Vitiligo surrounding a nevus.

**vitium** (vĭsh′ē-ŭm) *pl.* **vitia** [L., fault] A fault, defect, or vice.

**vitrectomy** (vĭ-trĕk′tō-mē) [L. *vitreus,* glassy, + Gr. *ektome,* excision] The use of a special instrument to remove the contents of the vitreous chamber and replace them with a sterile physiological saline solution.

**vitreocapsulitis** (vĭt″rē-ō-kăp″sū-lī′tĭs) [L. *vitreus,* glassy, + *capsula,* capsule, + Gr. *itis,* inflammation] Inflammation of the vitreous humor. SYN: *hyalitis.*

**vitreodentin** (vĭt″rē-ō-dĕn′tĭn) A particularly hard and brittle form of dentin.

**vitreoretinal** (vĭt″rē-ō-rĕt′ĭ-năl) Concerning

the vitreous and the retina.

**vitreous** (vĭt'rē-ŭs) [L. *vitreus*, glassy] **1.** Glassy. **2.** Pert. to the vitreous body of the eye. **3.** The vitreous body.

**vitreous body** A transparent jelly-like mass composed of collagen fibrils and a gel (vitreous humor). It fills the cavity of the eyeball, behind the lens and in front of the retina.

**vitreous chamber** The portion of the cavity of the eyeball behind the lens.

**vitreous degeneration** Retrogressive change of a part into a translucent shining substance, esp. of a blood vessel wall. SEE: *degeneration, hyaline*.

**vitreous humor** The clear watery gel filling the interstices of the stroma of the vitreous body.

**vitreous table** The inner layer of compact tissue characteristic of most of the bones of the cranium.

**vitrescence** (vĭ-trĕs'ĕns) Becoming hard and transparent like glass.

**vitreum** (vĭt'rē-ŭm) The vitreous body of the eye.

**vitrification** The process of converting a silicate material into a smooth, viscous substance by heat. The silicate material hardens on cooling and possesses a smooth, glossy surface. In dentistry, it is related to the extensive use of ceramics, cements, and porcelains. These vary by the additive components that determine their density and refractive qualities.

**vitriol** (vĭt'rē-ōl) [L. *vitriolum*] A sulfate of any of various metals.

**vitropression** (vĭt"rō-prĕsh'ŭn) [L. *vitrum*, glass, + *pressio*, a squeezing] A method of temporarily eliminating redness of the skin caused by hyperemia by pressure with a glass slide on the skin for the purpose of studying any lesions or discolorations.

**vivi-** (vĭv'ĭ) [L. *vivus*] Combining form meaning *alive*.

**vividiffusion** (vĭv"ĭ-dĭf-ū'zhŭn) [L. *vivus*, alive, + *dis*, apart, + *fundere*, to pour] The process of removing diffusible substances from the blood of a living animal by allowing it to flow through dialyzing membranes immersed in saline solution.

**vivification** (vĭv"ĭ-fĭ-kā'shŭn) [" + *facere*, to make] **1.** Trimming of the surface layer of a wound to aid the union of tissues. **2.** Transformation of protein through assimilation into the living matter of cellular organisms.

**viviparity** (vĭv"ĭ-păr'ĭ-tē) The ability to produce living young rather than producing young by laying an egg and then having it hatch.

**viviparous** (vĭv-ĭp'ăr-ŭs) [" + *parere*, to bring forth, to bear] Developing young within the body, the young being expelled and born alive; the opposite of oviparous.

**vivisect** (vĭv'ĭ-sĕkt) [L. *vivus*, alive, + *sectio*, a cutting] To dissect a living animal for experimental purposes.

**vivisection** (vĭv"ĭ-sĕk'shŭn) [" + *sectio*, a cutting] Cutting of or operation on a living animal for physiological investigation and the study of disease. The operations are usually performed on an anesthetized animal under conditions similar to those encountered in an operating room of a hospital.

**vivisectionist** (vĭv"ĭ-sĕk'shŭn-ĭst) One who practices or believes in vivisection. SEE: *antivivisection*.

**vivisector** (vĭv-ĭs-ĕk'tor) [" + *sector*, a cutting] One who practices vivisection.

**VLDL** *very low–density lipoprotein.*

**Vleminckx's solution** (flĕm'ĭnks) [Jean François Vleminckx, Belgian physician, 1800–1876] A solution of sulfurated lime used in various skin diseases.

**VMA** *vanillylmandelic acid.*

**$V_{max}$** *maximum velocity.*

**V.N.A.** *Visiting Nurse Association.*

**vocal** (vō'kăl) [L. *vocalis*, talking] Pert. to the voice.

**vocal cord** Either of two thin, reedlike folds of tissue within the larynx that vibrate as air passes between them, producing sounds that are the basis of speech.

**vocal cords, false** The ventricular folds of the larynx.

**vocal cords, true** Vocal folds.

**vocal folds** The thin edges of the vocal lips of the larynx, each of which encloses the vocal ligament. They form the edges of the rima glottidis and are involved in the production of sound. SYN: *true vocal cords*.

**vocal fremitus** Chest-wall vibration felt on palpation while the patient is speaking.

**vocal ligament** A strong band of elastic tissue lying within the vocal fold.

**vocal lips** Two shelflike projections of the lateral walls of the larynx. Their edges bear the vocal folds.

**vocal muscle** The inner portion of the thyroarytenoid muscle, which lies in the vocal lip lateral to and in contact with the vocal ligament.

**vocal process** The area of the arytenoid cartilage to which are attached the vocal cords.

**vocal resonance** The sound heard during auscultation of the lung while the patient is speaking.

**vocal signs** The indication of disease by changes in the voice.

**voces** (vō'sēz) [L.] Pl. of vox.

**voice** (voys) [L. *vox*] A sound, uttered by human beings, produced by vibration of the vocal cords.

***amphoric v.*** Cavernous v.

***cavernous v.*** A hollow voice sound heard during auscultation of the chest, indicating a pulmonary cavity. SEE: *amphoric v.*

***eunuchoid v.*** The characteristic high-pitched voice of a male in whom the normal sexual development has not occurred or in a male who was castrated before puberty.

**voiceprint** A technique for depicting graphically the characteristics of an individual's speech pattern. Because voiceprints, like fingerprints, can be used to distinguish one person from another, the technique is useful in medicine and in identifying the voices of criminal suspects.

**voices** (voys'ĕz) In psychiatry, verbal-auditory hallucinations expressed as being heard by the patient.

**void** (voyd) [O. Fr. *voider,* to empty] To evacuate the bowels or bladder.

**vol** *volume.*

**vol%** *volume percent.*

**vola, volar** (vō'lă, vō'lăr) [L.] Terms originally used to refer to the palm of the hand or sole of the foot. The preferred terms for reference to the palm of the hand are palmar and palmaris.

**vola manus** (vō'lă) Palm.

**vola pedis** The sole of the foot.

**volaris** (vō-lā'rĭs) Volar.

**volatile** (vŏl'ă-tĭl) [L. *volatilis,* flying] Easily vaporized or evaporated. Examples of volatile liquids are ether (boiling point, 34.5°C) and ethyl chloride (boiling point, 12.2°C).

**volatilization** (vŏl"ă-tĭl-ī-zā'shŭn) Conversion of a solid or liquid into a vapor.

**volatilize** (vŏl'ă-tĭl-īz) To vaporize a liquid or solid.

**volition** (vō-lĭsh'ŭn) [L. *volitio,* will] The act or power of willing or choosing.

**volitional** (vō-lĭsh'ŭn-ăl) Performed by volition.

**Volkmann's canals** (fōlk'mănz) [Alfred Wilhelm Volkmann, Ger. physiologist, 1800–1877] Vascular channels in compact bone. They are not surrounded by concentric lamellae as are the haversian canals.

**Volkmann's contracture** (fōlk'mănz) [Richard von Volkmann, Ger. surgeon, 1830–1889] Degeneration, contracture, fibrosis, and atrophy of a muscle resulting from injury to its blood supply; usually seen in the hand. SYN: *ischemic paralysis.*

**volley** (vŏl'ē) [L. *volare,* to fly] The simultaneous or nearly simultaneous discharge of a number of nerve impulses from a center within the brain or spinal cord.

**volt** (vōlt) [Count Alessandro Volta, It. physicist, 1745–1827] An electrical unit of pressure, the electromotive force required to produce 1 ampere of current through a resistance of 1 ohm.

**voltage** (vōl'tĭj) Electromotive force or difference in potential expressed in volts.

**voltaic** (vŏl-tā'ĭk) Concerning electricity produced by a battery.

**voltaism** (vŏl'tă-ĭzm) Galvanism.

**voltammeter** (vōlt-ăm'mē-tĕr) A device for measuring both volts and amperes.

**voltampere** (vōlt-ăm'pēr) The value obtained by multiplying volts times amperes.

**voltmeter** A device for measuring voltage, esp. for determining the voltage between two points of an electrical circuit.

**volubility** (vŏl"ū-bĭl'ĭ-tē) [L. *volubilitas,* flow of discourse] Excessive speech.

**volume** (vŏl'ūm) The space occupied by a substance, usually a gas or liquid. Liquid volume is expressed in liters or milliliters; gas volume in cubic centimeters.

***closing v.*** The amount of gas remaining in the lung when the small airways close during a maximum expiratory effort. It is increased in patients with small airway disease.

***compressed v.*** The volume lost to the patient as pressurized deadspace in ventilation circuits.

***expiratory reserve v.*** The maximal amount of air that can be forced from the lungs after normal expiration.

***inspiratory reserve v.*** The maximal amount of air that can be inhaled after a normal inspiration.

***mean corpuscular v.*** ABBR: MCV. The mean volume of an average erythrocyte. Normal values range from 82 to 92 cubic microns.

***minute v.*** The volume of gas expired or inspired per minute in quiet breathing, usually measured as expired ventilation.

***packed cell v.*** Hematocrit.

***residual v.*** ABBR: RV. The volume of air remaining in the lungs after maximal expiration. This amount of air is essential for continuous gas exchange.

***stroke v.*** The amount of blood discharged by a ventricle in one contraction. It is determined by dividing the minute volume by the number of heartbeats occurring in 1 min.

***tidal v.*** The volume of air inspired and expired in a normal breath.

**volumenometer** (vŏl"ūm-nŏm'ĕ-tĕr) Volumometer.

**volume percent** ABBR: vol%. The number of cubic centimeters (milliliters) of a substance (usually oxygen or carbon dioxide) contained in 100 ml of another substance (e.g., blood).

**volumetric** (vŏl"ū-mĕt'rĭk) [L. *volumen,* a volume, + Gr. *metron,* measure] Pert. to measurement of volume.

**volumometer** (vŏl"ū-mŏm'ĕ-tĕr) A device for measuring volume. SYN: *volumenometer.*

**voluntary** (vŏl'ŭn-tĕr"ē) [L. *voluntas,* will] Pert. to or under control of the will.

**voluntary health agency** Any nonprofit, nongovernmental agency, governed by lay or professional individuals and organized on a national, state, or local level, whose primary purpose is health related. This term applies to agencies supported mainly by voluntary public contributions. These agencies are usually engaged in programs of service, education, and research related to a particular disability or group of diseases and disabilities; for example, the American Heart Association, American Cancer Society, National Lung Institute, and their state and local affiliates. The term can also be applied to such agencies as nonprofit hospitals, visiting nurse associations, and other local service organizations that have both lay and professional governing boards and are supported by both voluntary contributions and charges and fees for service provided.

**voluntary muscle** Any muscle that is normally controlled by the will. These muscles are generally attached to the skeleton and are innervated by myelinated nerves coming directly from the brain or spinal cord. Microscopically, they consist of long cylindrical fibers bearing crosswise striations. The terms voluntary, striped, striated, cross-striated, and skeletal are practically synonymous when applied to muscle.

**voluptuous** (vō-lŭp′tū-ŭs) [L. *voluptas,* pleasure] **1.** Pert. to, arising from, or provoking, consciously or otherwise, sensual desire, usually applied to the female sex. **2.** Given to sensualism.

**volute** (vō-lūt′) [L. *volutus,* rolled] Convoluted.

**volvulosis** (vŏl″vū-lō′sĭs) Onchocerciasis.

**volvulus** (vŏl′vū-lŭs) [L. *volvere,* to roll] A twisting of the bowel on itself, causing obstruction. A prolapsed mesentery is the predisposing cause. This usually occurs at the sigmoid and ileocecal areas of the intestines.

**vomer** (vō′mĕr) [L., plowshare] The plowshaped bone that forms the lower and posterior portion of the nasal septum, articulating with the ethmoid, the sphenoid, the two palate bones, and the two superior maxillary bones.

**vomerine** (vō′mĕr-ĭn) Pert. to the vomer.

**vomerobasilar** (vō″mĕr-ō-băs′ĭ-lăr) Concerning the vomer and base of the skull.

**vomeronasal** (vō″mĕr-ō-nā′săl) Pert. to the vomer and nasal bones.

**vomeronasal cartilage** One of two narrow strips of cartilage lying along the anterior portion of the inferior border of the septal cartilage of the nose.

**vomeronasal organ** A small tubular epithelial sac lying on the anteroinferior surface of the nasal septum; rudimentary in humans. SYN: *Jacobson's organ.*

**vomica** (vŏm′ĭ-kă) *pl.* **vomicae** [L., ulcer] **1.** A cavity in the lungs, as from suppuration. **2.** Sudden and profuse expectoration of putrid purulent matter.

**vomicose** (vŏm′ĭ-kōs) Marked by many ulcers; ulcerous; purulent.

**vomit** (vŏm′ĭt) [L. *vomere,* to vomit] **1.** Material that is ejected from the stomach through the mouth. **2.** To eject stomach contents through the mouth. SEE: *melena; nausea; vomitus.*

PHYSIOLOGY: The act is usually a reflex involving the coordinated activity of both voluntary and involuntary muscles. A certain position is assumed, the glottis is closed, the diaphragm and abdominal muscles contract, and the cardiac sphincter of the stomach relaxes while antiperistaltic waves course over the duodenum, stomach, and esophagus.

***bilious v.*** Bile forced back into the stomach and ejected with vomited matter.

***black v.*** Vomit containing blood acted on by the gastric juice; seen in the worst form of yellow fever.

***coffee-ground v.*** Vomit having the appearance and consistency of coffee grounds because of blood mixed with gastric contents. It occurs in any condition associated with hemorrhage into the stomach.

**vomiting** (vŏm′ĭt-ĭng) [L. *vomere,* to vomit] Ejection through the mouth of the gastric contents, and, in cases of bowel obstruction, intestinal contents. It may result from toxins from ptomaines, drugs, uremia, and specific fevers; cerebral tumors and meningitis (often unaccompanied by nausea and failing to relieve associated headache); diseases of the stomach such as ulcer, cancer, dilatation, dyspepsia; reflex from pregnancy, uterine or ovarian disease, irritation of the fauces, intestinal parasites, biliary colic; intestinal obstruction; motion sickness; and nervous disorders such as hysteria and migraine. Vomiting may result from taking toxic doses of drugs or poisons such as arsenic, aconite, antimony, barium, colchicum, cantharides, copper, corrosive alkalis, acids, digitalis, iodine, mercury, phenol, phosphorus, veratrum, wood alcohol (methanol), food toxins or poisons, and zinc. Periodic vomiting may be in itself a neurosis or associated with the gastric crises of locomotor ataxia. Esophageal vomiting results from obstruction, and the vomitus is alkaline in reaction. SYN: *emesis.* SEE: *anorexia nervosa; bulimia.*

TREATMENT: Antinausea medicines should be taken by mouth if possible, otherwise intramuscularly or intravenously. Fluids may be given by mouth if the patient will accept them. If vomiting continues, intravenous fluids and electrolytes will be required to replace those lost in the vomitus.

*In pregnancy (hyperemesis gravidarum):* If severe, fluid intake by mouth should be restricted but maintained by intravenous route. In less severe cases, frequent small feedings of more or less dry foods are advisable.

Caution: It is of utmost importance not to use medicines during pregnancy unless there is evidence that the drug being prescribed has been investigated and found to be harmless to the embryo and its development.

NURSING IMPLICATIONS: Causative factors such as drugs, food, disease entities, and psychological factors are assessed and removed if possible. Frequency, amount, time, and characteristics of vomitus are assessed. The patient is positioned to prevent aspiration, and suction equipment is available. Antiemetics are administered as prescribed. Food and fluids are withheld for several hours, and frequent mouth care is offered. If surgery during pregnancy is required, restriction of foods and fluids for approximately 8 hr before surgery helps to prevent vomiting. Comfort measures, such as a cool cloth applied to the face, are instituted. Serum electrolytes are monitored, and accurate intake and output records are kept to ensure proper fluid replacement. Vital signs are monitored, and if the temperature is elevated, antipyretic measures are instituted. To help prevent vomiting, the patient should take deep breaths and swallow. The nurse promotes a calm environment and provides distraction.

***cyclic* v.** Periodic and recurring attacks of vomiting occurring in patients with a nervous temperament. Continued vomiting causes metabolic alkalosis as a result of chloride loss.

SYMPTOMS: Dizziness, loss of appetite, headache, and nausea may occur. The patient then vomits about every half hour for 1 to 2 days. Great thirst, slight rise of temperature, rapid pulse, and prostration are present.

NURSING IMPLICATIONS: The patient's symptoms are assessed and documented, vital signs monitored, fluid and electrolyte balance maintained, and prescribed medications administered to relieve headache, nausea, and vomiting. A calm, stress-free environment is provided.

***dry* v.** Nausea and retching without vomitus.

***epidemic* v.** Sudden unexplained attacks of gastroenteritis characterized by nausea, vomiting, and sometimes diarrhea. Although not proven, the symptoms are believed to be due to a virus. Treatment is symptomatic.

***induced* v.** The production of vomiting by administering certain types of emetics (e.g., syrup of ipecac or amorphine) or by physical stimulation of the posterior pharynx.

---

Caution: In the past, salt solutions were used to induce vomiting. Because sodium chloride in high doses is toxic and may be lethal, it should not be used.

---

***pernicious* v.** Severe vomiting of pregnancy.

***v. of pregnancy*** The vomiting, esp. morning sickness, that some women experience during pregnancy.

***projectile* v.** Ejection of vomitus with great force.

***psychogenic* v.** Occasional or persistent vomiting associated with severe emotional stress. Each person has the potential for this reaction to emotional stress, but the threshold varies from one person to another.

***stercoraceous* v.** Vomiting of fecal matter.

**vomitus** (vŏm′ĭ-tŭs) Material ejected from the stomach by vomiting.

CHARACTERISTICS: *Ammoniacal odor:* This indicates uremia. *Bilious:* Green or greenish-yellow vomitus, containing bile, appears after frequent and violent vomiting. *Fecal:* This may indicate intestinal obstruction, general peritonitis, or an abnormal communication between the intestines and stomach. *Garlic odor:* This may denote phosphorus poisoning.

*Hematemesis:* If bright and fluid, the blood has not been long in the stomach; otherwise, it has the appearance of coffee grounds and is reddish-brown, or it forms in clots. This may indicate rupture of an aneurysm into the stomach or esophagus or rupture of esophageal varicose veins; gastric ulcer; cirrhosis of the liver; an enlarged spleen; or carcinoma of the stomach. It is not necessarily fatal. Hematemesis may result from swallowed blood. It may occur in vicarious menstruation, gastritis, or corrosive poisoning; it may follow ingestion of strong alkalies or acids; or it may result from anemia, leukemia, or Hodgkin's disease. Sometimes it is present in chronic nephritis, scurvy, purpura hemorrhagica, acute yellow atrophy of the liver, or malaria.

*Profuse:* The ejection of large quantities of frothy fermented material is highly significant of gastric dilatation. *Purulent:* This may result from the rupture of an abscess into the esophagus or stomach. *Without nausea, distress, or other phenomena:* This may occur in certain neuroses, in hysteria, uremia, central nervous system disease as from a tumor, or as a precursor of apoplexy. The vomitus may be colored by certain fruits, by wine, coffee, cocoa, soups, or bile.

***coffee-ground* v.** Vomitus of dark red or black granular material (resembling coffee grounds), which is blood. The blood has been in the stomach or intestinal tract long enough to be changed from red to black by the action of gastric and intestinal juices. It occurs in conditions associated with hemorrhage into the stomach.

**von Gierke disease** (fŏn gēr′kĕz) [Edgar von Gierke, Ger. pathologist, 1877–1945] Glycogen storage disease type 1a. SYN: *glycogenosis; glycogen storage disease.*

**von Graefe's sign** (fŏn grā′fēz) [Albrecht von Graefe, Ger. ophthalmologist, 1828–1870] The failure of the eyelid to move downward promptly with the eyeball; the lid moves tardily and jerkily. This sign is seen in exophthalmic goiter.

**von Hippel's disease** Hippel's disease.

**von Jaksch's disease** [Rudolf von Jaksch-Wartenhorst, Austrian physician, 1855–1947] A symptom complex consisting of anemia, hepatosplenomegaly, and infections that are associated with a number of chronic diseases such as tuberculosis and malnutrition.

**von Pirquet's test** (fŏn pēr'kāz) [Clemens Peter Johann von Pirquet, Austrian pediatrician, 1874–1929] A diagnostic test for tuberculosis in which a small amount of tuberculin is applied to a scarified area of the skin of the arm. A positive reaction is seen if a red papillar eruption appears several days later at the site of inoculation.

**von Recklinghausen's canals** Recklinghausen's canals.

**von Recklinghausen's disease** Type 1 neurofibromatosis.

**von Recklinghausen's tumor** Recklinghausen's tumor.

**von Willebrand's disease** [Erik Adolph von Willebrand, Finnish physician, 1870–1949] A congenital bleeding disorder caused by a deficiency of coagulation factor VIII. This disease is inherited as an autosomal dominant trait. The bleeding tendency manifests at an early age, usually as epistaxis and easy bruising and, rarely, petechiae. Bleeding in the intestinal tract during surgery and excess loss of blood during menstruation are common. The symptoms decrease in severity with age and during pregnancy. The disorder is diagnosed by prolonged bleeding time and factor VIII deficiency. Treatment involves administering factor VIII 24 to 48 hr before surgery or during attacks of bleeding.

**Voorhees' bag** (voor'ēz) [James Ditmors Voorhees, U.S. obstetrician, 1869–1929] An inflatable rubber bag for dilating the cervix uteri to induce and facilitate labor.

**voracious** (vō-rā'shŭs) [L. *vorare,* to devour] Having an insatiable or ravenous appetite.

**vortex** (vor'tĕks) *pl.* **vortices** [L., a whirlpool] A structure having a spiral or whorled appearance.

***coccygeal v.*** The region over the coccyx where lanugo hairs of the embryo come to a point.

***v. of heart*** The region at the apex of the heart where muscle fibers of the ventricles make a tight spiral and turn inward.

***v. lentis*** Spiral patterns on the surface of the lens owing to a concentric pattern of fiber growth.

**vortices** (vor'tĭ-sēz) [L.] Pl. of vortex.

***v. pilorum*** Hair whorls as in arrangement of hairs on the scalp.

**vorticose** (vor'tĭk-ōs) [L. *vortices,* whirlpools] Whirling or having a whorled arrangement.

**vorticose vein** One of four veins (two superior and two inferior) that receive blood from all parts of the choroid of the eye. They empty into posterior ciliary and superior ophthalmic veins.

**vox** (vŏks) *pl.* **voces** [L.] Voice.

**voyeur** (voy-yĕr') [Fr., one who sees] One who derives sexual pleasure from observing nude persons or the sexual activity of others.

**voyeurism** (voy'yĕr-ĭzm) The experiencing of sexual gratification by observing nude persons or the sexual activity of others.

**V.R.** *right vision; ventilation rate; vocal resonance.*

**VRE** *vancomycin-resistant enterococcus.*

**V.S.** *vesicular sound; vital signs; volumetric solution.*

**VSD** *ventricular septal defect.*

**vuerometer** (vū"ĕr-ŏm'ĕ-tĕr) [Fr. *vue,* sight, + Gr. *metron,* measure] An apparatus for measuring the interpupillary distance of the eyes.

**vulgaris** (vŭl-gā'rĭs) [L.] Ordinary, common.

**vulnerable** (vŭl'nĕr-ă-bl) [L. *vulnerare,* to wound] Easily injured or wounded.

**vulnerant** (vŭl'nĕr-ănt) **1.** Something that wounds or injures. **2.** To inflict injury.

**vulnerary** (vŭl'nĕr-ăr"ē) **1.** Pert. to wounds. **2.** An agent, esp. a folk remedy or herb, used to promote wound healing.

**Vulpian-Heidenhain-Sherrington phenomenon** [Edme-Felix Alfred Vulpian, French physician, 1826–1887; Rudolph Peter Heinrich Heidenhain, Ger. physiologist, 1834–1897; Sir Charles Scott Sherrington, Brit. physiologist, 1857–1952] Contraction of denervated skeletal muscle by stimulating autonomic cholinergic fibers innervating its blood vessels.

**vulsella, vulsellum** (vŭl-sĕl'ă, vŭl-sĕl'ŭm) [L. *vulsella,* tweezers] A forceps with a hook on each blade.

**vulva** (vŭl'vă) *pl.* **vulvae** [L., covering] That portion of the female external genitalia lying posterior to the mons veneris, consisting of the labia majora, labia minora, clitoris, vestibule of the vagina, vaginal opening, and bulbs of the vestibule. SYN: *pudendum femininum.* SEE: illus.

***v. connivens*** Vulva in which the labia majora are in apposition.

***v. hians*** Vulva in which the labia majora are gaping.

***velamen v.*** An abnormally elongated clitoris.

**vulval, vulvar** [L. *vulva,* covering] Relating to the vulva.

**vulvar dystrophy** One of the nonneoplastic epithelial disorders of the vulvar skin and mucosa. These conditions may be associated with squamous cell hyperplasia, lichen sclerosus, or other dermatoses.

**vulvar leukoplakia** A condition characterized by diffuse or focal translucent thickening of the vulva; often gives rise to carcinoma.

**vulvar vestibulitis syndrome** The presence of severe pain on pressing or touching the vestibule of the vagina or on attempted vaginal entry. Physical findings of a mild degree of localized erythema are limited to the mucosa of the vestibule. The etiology of this distressing syndrome is unknown, and therapy, including vestibulectomy, has not been 100% effective.

**vulvectomy** (vŭl-vĕk'tō-mē) [" + Gr. *ektome,* excision] Excision of the vulva.

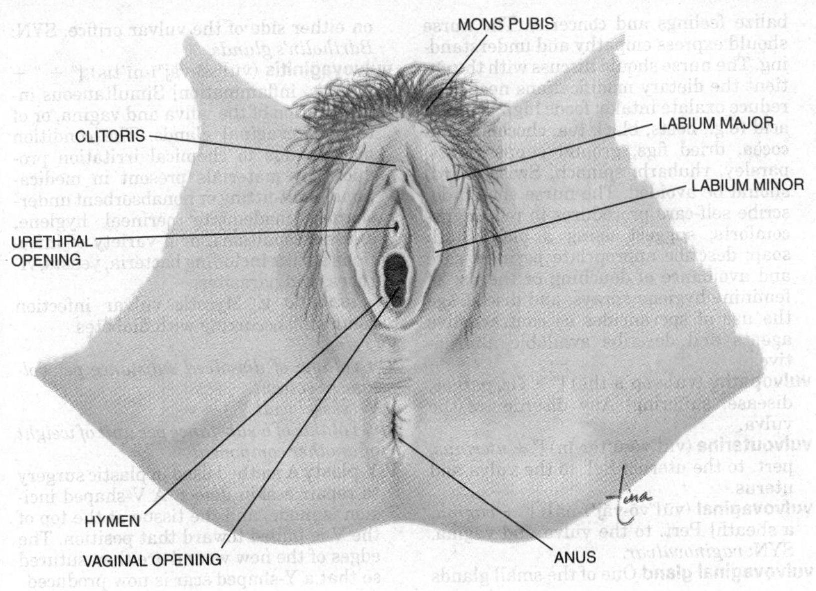


VULVA
(INFERIOR VIEW OF THE PERINEUM)

NURSING IMPLICATIONS: In preparing the patient for surgery, the nurse attempts to allay fear and anxiety and provides information about the procedure and expected sensations and opportunities for the patient to ask questions. The patient having a simple vulvectomy may resume sexual intercourse after the wound has healed. Skin cleansing is performed as indicated, and prophylactic medications are administered to prevent infection after surgery. Wound care is carried out postoperatively as indicated; usually the wound is cleansed daily and exposed to air at frequent intervals to decrease the possibility of tissue breakdown. Comfort measures are instituted; positioning pillows to support the legs helps to relieve tension on the wound. Medications are administered to relieve pain during the healing process, which is usually slow. Aseptic technique is used for uretheral and catheter care, and sitz baths are discouraged because infections are easily acquired. The patient should participate in wound care before discharge, with the assistance of a family member if necessary. The nurse should allow opportunities for the patient to discuss anxieties and encourage gradual resumption of normal activities on the patient's return home.

**vulvitis** (vŭl-vī′tĭs) [L. *vulva,* covering, + Gr. *itis,* inflammation] Inflammation of the vulva.

***acute nongonorrheal v.*** Vulvitis resulting from chafing of the opposed lips of the vulva or from accumulated sebaceous material around the clitoris.

***follicular v.*** Inflammation of the hair follicles of the vulva.

***gangrenous v.*** Necrosis and sloughing of areas of the vulva, often a complication of infectious diseases such as diphtheria, scarlatina, herpes genitalis, or typhoid fever.

***leukoplakic v.*** A chronic atrophic vulvitis. SEE: *kraurosis vulvae.*

***mycotic v.*** Vulvitis caused by various fungi, most commonly *Candida albicans.*

**vulvo-** Combining form meaning *covering, vulva.*

**vulvocrural** (vŭl″vō-kroo′răl) [L. *vulva,* covering, + *cruralis,* pert. to the leg] Rel. to the vulva and thigh.

**vulvodynia** [″ + *dynia,* pain] A nonspecific syndrome that has no known cause. Although no specific cause is known, in some patients the symptoms have been relieved by excluding oxalate-containing foods from the diet to reduce the oxalate in the urine. It is characterized by pain, esp. during sexual intercourse; itching; and discomfort. SEE: *pruritus, vulvar.*

The Vulvar Pain Foundation provides information and support for women with vulvodynia. Their address is P.O. Box 4177, Graham, NC 27253. Phone 910-226-0704.

NURSING IMPLICATIONS: The patient's history should be carefully reviewed for coexisting disorders and factors or events that preceded or increased symptoms. The patient should be encouraged to verbalize feelings and concerns. The nurse should express empathy and understanding. The nurse should discuss with the patient the dietary modifications needed to reduce oxalate intake: foods high in oxalic acid (e.g., beets, black tea, chocolate and cocoa, dried figs, ground pepper, nuts, parsley, rhubarb, spinach, Swiss chard) should be avoided. The nurse should describe self-care procedures to reduce discomforts; suggest using a bland bath soap; describe appropriate perineal care and avoidance of douching or the use of feminine hygiene sprays; and discourage the use of spermicides as contraceptive agents and describe available alternatives.

**vulvopathy** (vŭl-vŏp′ă-thē) [″ + Gr. *pathos,* disease, suffering] Any disorder of the vulva.

**vulvouterine** (vŭl″vō-ū′tĕr-ĭn) [″ + *uterinus,* pert. to the uterus] Rel. to the vulva and uterus.

**vulvovaginal** (vŭl″vō-văj′ĭ-năl) [″ + *vagina,* a sheath] Pert. to the vulva and vagina. SYN: *vaginovulvar.*

**vulvovaginal gland** One of the small glands on either side of the vulvar orifice. SYN: *Bartholin's glands.*

**vulvovaginitis** (vŭl″vō-văj″ĭ-nī′tĭs) [″ + ″ + Gr. *itis,* inflammation] Simultaneous inflammation of the vulva and vagina, or of the vulvovaginal glands. The condition may be due to chemical irritation produced by materials present in medications, tight-fitting or nonabsorbent underclothes, inadequate perineal hygiene, allergic conditions, or a variety of infectious agents including bacteria, yeasts, viruses, and parasites.

***diabetic v.*** Mycotic vulvar infection commonly occurring with diabetes.

**vv** *veins.*

**v/v** *volume of dissolved substance per volume of solvent.*

**V.W.** *vessel wall.*

**v/w** *volume of a substance per unit of weight of another component.*

**V-Y-plasty** A method used in plastic surgery to repair a skin defect. A V-shaped incision is made, and the tissue at the top of the V is pulled toward that position. The edges of the new wound are then sutured so that a Y-shaped scar is now produced.

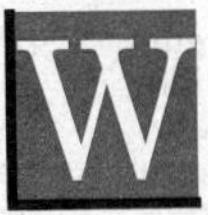

**W** Symbol for the element tungsten (wolfram).

**w** *watt; week; wife; with.*

**Waardenburg syndrome** [Petrus Johannes Waardenburg, Dutch ophthalmologist, 1886–1979] A congenital defect involving pigmentation. It consists of a white forelock, vitiligo, heterochromic irides, broad nasal root, dystopia canthorum (lateral displacement of the inner canthi), deficient pigmentation of the fundus, synophrys (growing together of the two eyebrows), and cutaneous hypopigmentation. Congenital deafness may or may not be present. The condition is inherited as an autosomal dominant trait.

**Wachendorf's membrane** (vŏk'ĕn-dorfs) [Eberhard J. Wachendorf, Dutch physician, 1703–1758] **1.** A thin membrane occluding the pupil of the embryo. **2.** The outer membrane ensheathing a cell.

**wafer** (wā'fĕr) [Ger. *wafel*] **1.** A thin sheet of flour paste used to enclose a medicinal dose of powder. **2.** A flat vaginal suppository.

**Wagstaffe's fracture** (wăg'stăfs) [William Warwick Wagstaffe, Brit. surgeon, 1843–1910] A fracture with separation of the medial malleolus of the ankle.

**waist** (wāst) [ME. *wast,* growth] The small part of the human trunk between the thorax and hips. SEE: *sensation, cincture.*

**wakeful** (wāk'fŭl) [AS. *wacian,* to be awake, + *full,* complete] Not able to sleep; sleepless.

**Walcher's position** (vŏl'kĕrz) [Gustav Adolf Walcher, Ger. gynecologist, 1856–1935] A position in which the patient assumes a dorsal recumbent posture with the hips at the edge of the bed and the legs hanging down.

**Wald, Lillian** (wăld) U.S. nurse, 1867–1940, who founded the Henry Street Settlement in New York City, one of the world's first visiting nurse associations.

**Wald cycle** The transformations involved in the breakdown of resynthesis of rhodopsin.

**Waldenström's disease** (văl'dĕn-strĕmz) [Johann Henning Waldenström, Swedish surgeon, b. 1877] Osteochondritis deformans juvenilis.

**Waldeyer's gland** (vŏl'dī-ĕrz) [Wilhelm von Waldeyer, Ger. anatomist, 1836–1921] A sweat gland of the eyelids; usually found most prominently in the lower lid margin.

**Waldeyer's neuron** The nerve cell and its processes.

**Waldeyer's ring** SEE: *ring, lymphoid.*

**walk 1.** A method of locomotion of upright bipeds such as humans. **2.** The particular way an individual moves. SEE: *gait.*

**walker** A device used to assist a person in walking. It consists of a stable platform made of light-weight metal tubing that is at a height that permits it to be grasped by the hands and used as support while taking a step. The walker is then moved forward and another step is taken. SEE: *crutch.*

**walking** [AS. *wealcan,* to roll] The act of moving on foot; advancing by steps.

**walking cast** A cast that allows the patient to be ambulatory.

**walking system** A complex device that enables patients with spinal injuries resulting in paralysis of the legs to walk. The device uses computer-controlled electrical stimulation to muscles so that walking may be accomplished. Each of these devices is made esp. for each patient, and their use is experimental.

**walking well** Persons who are indeed ill but still able to walk.

**walking wounded** In military medicine, an ambulatory case.

**wall** [AS. *weall*] The limiting or surrounding substance or material of a cell, vessel, or cavity such as an artery, vein, chest, or bladder. In dentistry, it may refer to specific boundaries of a cavity preparation or its location within the tooth, for example, cavity walls: buccal, lingual, mesial, distal, pulpal, coronal, axial, cervical, facial, incisal, gingival, or enamel.

**Wallenberg's syndrome** (vŏl'ĕn-bĕrgz) [Adolf Wallenberg, Ger. physician, 1862–1949] A complex of symptoms resulting from occlusion of the posteroinferior cerebellar artery or one of its branches supplying the lower portion of the brainstem. Dysphagia, muscular weakness or paralysis, impairment of pain and temperature senses, and cerebellar dysfunction are characteristic.

**wallerian degeneration** (wŏl-ē'rē-ăn) [Augustus Volney Waller, Brit. physician, 1816–1870] The degeneration of a nerve fiber (axon) that has been severed from its cell body. The myelin sheath also degenerates and is transformed into a chain of lipoid droplets that stains by the Marchi method, which is used in tracing the course of injured nerve fibers. The neurilemma does not degenerate but forms a tube that directs the growth of the regenerating axon.

**walleye** [ME. *wawil-eghed*] **1.** An eye in which the iris is light-colored or white. **2.** Leukoma or dense opacity of the cornea. **3.** A squint in which both visual axes diverge. SYN: *strabismus, divergent.*

**Walthard's islets, Walthard's inclusions** [Max Walthard, Swiss gynecologist,

1867–1933] Nests or small cysts of embryological squamous epithelium-like cells in the superficial parts of the ovary, tubes, and uterine ligaments. They are thought to represent the beginning Brenner tumor.

**wand, dressing** Dressing stick.

**wandering** (wăn′dĕr-ĭng) [AS. *wandrian*] Moving about; not fixed.

**wandering abscess** An abscess that burrows and comes to the surface at a point distant from its origin.

**wandering kidney** A dislocated floating kidney.

**wandering spleen** A dislocated floating spleen.

**Wangensteen tube** (wăn′gĕn-stēn) [Owen H. Wangensteen, U.S. surgeon, 1898–1981] A double-lumen tube used for relieving postoperative abdominal distention, nausea, vomiting, and certain cases of mechanical bowel obstruction. It is used as an intranasal catheter in combination with a suction siphonage apparatus. SEE: *decompression.*

**Warburg apparatus** [Otto H. Warburg, Ger. biochemist, 1883–1970] A capillary manometer used for determining oxygen consumption and carbon dioxide production of small bits of cellular tissue. It is widely used in metabolism studies.

**ward** [AS. *weard,* watching over] A large room in a hospital for the care of several patients.

***accident w.*** A ward reserved for accident cases.

***psychiatric w.*** A ward in a general hospital for mentally ill patients.

**Wardrop's disease** (wăr′drŏps) [James Wardrop, Brit. surgeon, 1782–1869] An acute inflammation of the nailbed with fetid ulceration and loss of the nail.

**Wardrop's operation** Ligation of an artery for aneurysm at a distance beyond the sac.

**warehousemen's itch** Eczema of the hands resulting from touching irritating substances.

**warfarin poisoning** Poisoning caused by accidental administration of an overdose of warfarin or by the cumulative effect of repeated administration of the drug. Warfarin is also used as a rodenticide. Repeated ingestion of this material by children may cause poisoning. SEE: *Poisons and Poisoning Appendix.*

NURSING IMPLICATIONS: The nurse instructs the patient to observe for signs of bleeding such as epistaxis, bleeding gums, hematuria, melena, and skin trauma (ecchymosis, purpura, or petechia). Preventive measures should include gentle blowing of the nose, use of an electric razor and a soft-bristled toothbrush, gentle cleaning of the anal area, and avoidance of constrictive clothing. The importance of regular blood studies and medical follow-up is stressed. The patient should wear or carry a medical identification tag listing the prescribed drug, dosage, frequency of administration, and physician's name and telephone number. Because many drugs interact with anticoagulants to interfere with their action, the patient should consult with the physician before taking over-the-counter medication.

**warfarin potassium** An anticoagulant drug. Trade name is Athrombin-K.

**warfarin sodium** [name derived from initials of *W*isconsin *A*lumni *R*esearch *F*oundation] An anticoagulant drug. Coumadin and Panwarfin are trade names.

**war gases** Any chemical substances, whether solid, liquid, or vapor, used to produce poisonous or irritant effects. SEE: *gas, war.*

**wart** (wort) [AS. *wearte*] A circumscribed cutaneous elevation resulting from hypertrophy of the papillae and epidermis. It is caused by a papillomavirus. This term is applied also to benign conditions, such as verruca, that resemble warts. SEE: illus.

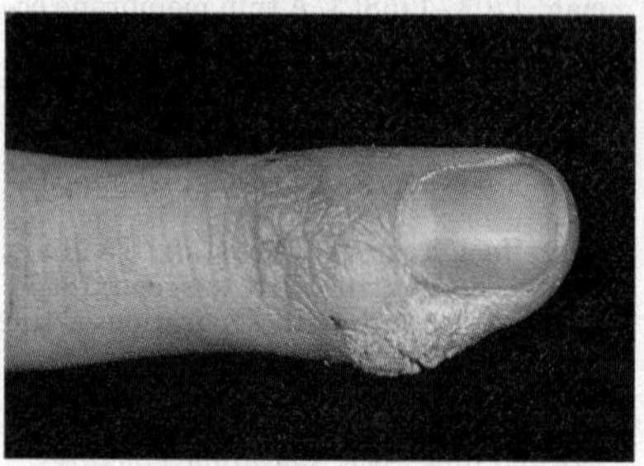

PERIUNGUAL WART

***common w.*** SEE: *verucca vulgaris.*

***genital w.*** A wart of the genitalia, caused by human papillomavirus (HPV). In women, these warts may be associated with cancer of the cervix. An estimated 1 million new cases of genital warts occur each year in the U.S. SEE: illus.

TREATMENT: A variety of therapies, including topically applied chemicals such as podophyllin, laser therapy, surgery, and recombinant interferon alfa-2a, have been used with varying degrees of success. Nevertheless, there is no completely safe and effective therapy available for genital warts.

NURSING IMPLICATIONS: A history is obtained for unprotected sexual contact with a partner with known infection, a new partner, or multiple partners. Universal precautions are used to examine the patient, to collect a specimen, or to perform associated procedures. The nurse inspects the genitalia for warts growing on the moist genital surfaces, such as the subpreputial sac; the urethral meatus; and less commonly, the penile shaft or scrotum in male patients and the vulva

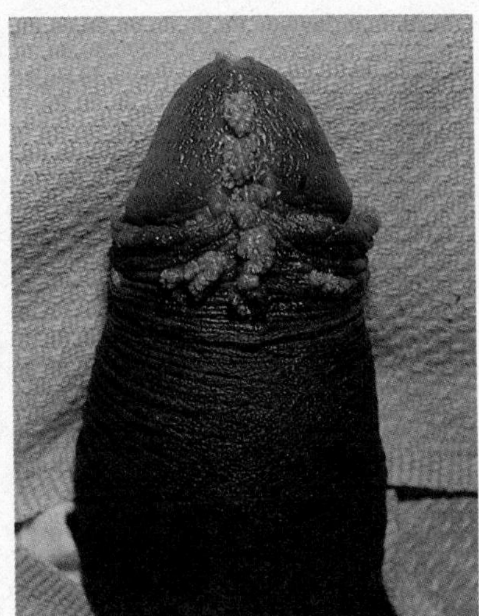

GENITAL WARTS ON PENIS

and vaginal and cervical wall in female patients. In both sexes, the papillomas spread to the perineum and perianal area. These warts begin as tiny pink or red swellings and may grow as large as 4 in. (10 cm) and become pedunculated. Multiple warts have a cauliflower-like appearance. The patient usually reports no other symptoms, but a few complain of itching and pain. Infected lesions become malodorous. The patient is monitored for signs of genital cancer and for infection. A nonthreatening, nonjudgmental atmosphere is provided to encourage the patient to verbalize feelings about perceived changes in sexual behavior and body image. Sexual abstinence or condom use during intercourse is recommended until healing is complete. The patient must inform sexual partners about the risk for genital warts and the need for evaluation. The patient should be tested for human immunodeficiency virus and for other sexually transmitted diseases. Genital warts can recur and the virus can mutate, causing warts of a different strain. The patient should report for weekly treatment until all warts are removed and then schedule a checkup for 3 months after all warts have disappeared. Female patients should have a Papanicolaou test every 6 months.

***plantar w.*** A wart on a pressure-bearing area, esp. the sole of the foot. SYN: *verruca plantaris*. SEE: illus.

***seborrheic w.*** Seborrheic keratosis.

***venereal w.*** A vegetating growth on the skin, esp. on the mucocutaneous juncture of the genitals, having an offensive discharge. SYN: *verruca acuminata*.

**wash** (wăsh) [AS. *wacsan*] **1.** The act of cleaning, esp. a part or all of the body.

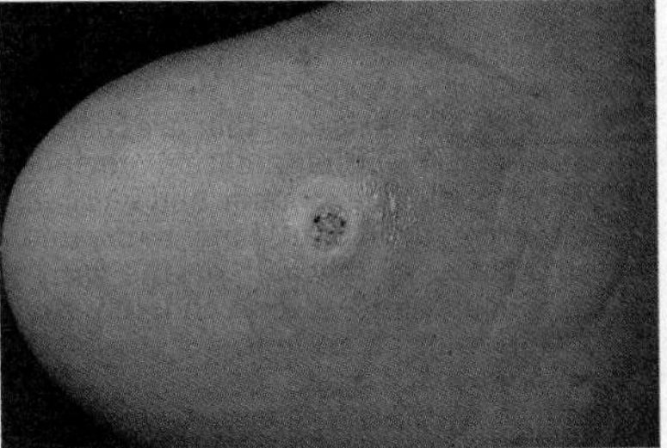

PLANTAR WART

**2.** A medicinal preparation used in washing or coating.

***eye w.*** A lotion for the eyes. SYN: *collyrium*.

**washerwoman's itch** Eczema of the hands of laundry workers who are repeatedly exposed to harsh soaps.

**washout, nitrogen** The removal of nitrogen from the body by breathing either 100% oxygen or a combination of oxygen and helium. Although complete removal of nitrogen requires 12 hr of breathing nitrogen-free air, 2 hr may be sufficient to prevent the development of bends in aviators preparing to ascend to high altitudes.

**wasp** [AS. *waesp*] Term sometimes applied to all insects belonging to the suborder Apocrita, order Hymenoptera (except the Formicidae or ants), but more generally restricted to the superfamilies Scolioidea, Vespoidea, and Specoidea. Members have the base of the abdomen constricted, and females have a piercing ovipositor, which in many species is modified into a sting. Many are social, living in large colonies. Common representatives are yellow jackets and hornets.

**wasp sting** The injection of wasp venom into the skin, resulting in a painful wound and sometimes a mild systemic reaction. Multiple stings may be dangerous, esp. to sensitized individuals.

TREATMENT: The area should be cooled as quickly and efficiently as possible to prevent the venom from gaining access to the general circulation. Bicarbonate of soda paste, strong epsom salt, or household ammonia solution should be applied locally. If pain is severe, the area should be infiltrated with 2% procaine solution. Severe allergic reaction may require injection of 0.2 to 0.5 ml of epinephrine subcutaneously. An antihistamine suitable for intravenous injection should be given slowly. If shock and collapse seem imminent, hydrocortisone should be given. If muscle spasms occur, an intravenous infusion of calcium lactate or calcium gluconate is given. In some cases, however, curare (dimethyl tubocurarine chloride) will be required to relieve muscle spasms.

**waste** (wāst) [L. *vastus*, empty] **1.** Cachexia. **2.** Loss by breaking down of bodily tissue.

3. Excreted material no longer useful to an organism.

**waste products** Products of metabolism or wear and tear of tissues that are removed from the body by elimination. Included are carbon dioxide, organic and inorganic salts, urine, dead skin, hair, nails, undigested foods, soluble salts in the form of nitrogenous salts (urea) and inorganic salts (sodium chloride), and gas in the form of carbon dioxide.

**wasting** (wāst'ĭng) [L. *vastare,* to devastate] Enfeebling; causing loss of strength or size; emaciating. SEE: *marasmus.*

**water** (wă'tĕr) [AS. *waeter*] $H_2O$, hydrogen combined with oxygen, forming a tasteless, clear, odorless fluid.

Water freezes at 32°F (0°C) and boils at 212°F (100°C). It is the principal chemical constituent of the body, composing approx. 65% of the body weight of an adult male and 55% of the adult female. It is distributed within the intracellular fluid and outside of the cells in the extracellular fluid. Water is indispensable for metabolic activities within cells, as it is the medium in which chemical reactions usually take place. Outside of cells, it is the principal transporting agent of the body. The following properties of water are important to living organisms: it is almost a universal solvent; it is a medium in which acids, bases, and salts ionize, and the concentrations of these substances (electrolytes) must be and are normally regulated quite precisely by the body; it possesses a high specific heat and has a high latent heat of vaporization, important in regulation and maintenance of a constant body temperature; it possesses a high surface tension; and it is an important reacting agent and essential in all hydrolytic reactions.

Water is the principal constituent of all body fluids (blood, lymph, tissue fluid), secretions (salivary juice, gastric juice, bile, sweat), and excretory fluid (urine). Intake of water is determined principally by the sense of thirst. Excessive intake may lead to water intoxication; excessive loss to dehydration. Humans can survive for only a short time without water intake. The exact length of survival time varies with ambient temperature, moisture in available food, and amount of physical activity.

***bound w.*** Water that in protoplasm is attached to organic substances. It is not available for metabolic processes.

***deionized w.*** Water that has been passed through a substance that removes cations and anions present as contaminants.

***distilled w.*** Water that has been purified by distillation. It is used in preparing pharmaceuticals.

***emergency preparation of safe drinking w.*** The purification of water when only unclean water is available or when the available drinking water is believed to be contaminated. One of the following methods may be used: (1) Water is strained through a clean cloth and boiled vigorously for 30 min. (2) Three drops of alcoholic solution of iodine are added to each quart (approx. 1 L) of water. The water is then mixed well and left to stand for 30 min before using. (3) Ten drops of 1% chlorine bleach, 2 drops of 4% to 6% chlorine bleach, or 1 drop of 7% to 10% chlorine bleach is added to each quart (liter) of water. The water is then mixed well and left to stand for 30 min. If the water is cloudy to begin with, double the amount of chlorine is used.

When the water is contaminated by *Giardia* organisms, heating to 55°C (131°F) kills the protozoa (method 1). Methods 2 and 3 also kill the cysts, but more time is required. Vegetative bacteria and viruses are killed by water kept at 60°C (140°F) for 30 min.

NOTE: When traveling in an area where the potability of water is questionable and no easy method of purification is available, using water from the hot water tap may decrease the possibility of ingesting live pathogenic microorganisms. The water is allowed to cool to drinking temperature.

***hard w.*** Water that contains dissolved salts of magnesium or calcium.

***heavy w.*** $D_2O$. An isotopic variety of water, esp. deuterium oxide, in which hydrogen has been displaced by its isotope, deuterium. Its properties differ from ordinary water in that heavy water has a higher freezing and boiling point and is incapable of supporting life.

***w. for injection*** Water for parenteral use that has been distilled and sterilized. Distilled, sterilized water that is stored in sealed containers remains free of pyrogens and may be used after longer periods of storage.

***lime w.*** Aqueous calcium hydroxide solution.

***potable w.*** Water suitable for drinking, in that it is hygienic and free of odor, pathogenic microorganisms, and objectionable minerals.

***purified w.*** Water that is mineral free; obtained by distillation, or deionization.

***pyrogen-free w.*** Water that has been rendered free of fever-producing proteins (bacteria and their metabolic products). SEE: *w. for injection.*

***soft w.*** Water that contains very little, if any, dissolved salts of magnesium or calcium.

**water bed** A rubber mattress partially filled with warm water (100°F or 37.8°C). When too full, the mattress is hard. It is used to prevent and treat bedsores.

**water cure** Hydrotherapy.

**waterhammer pulse** A pulse marked by a quick, powerful beat, collapsing suddenly; associated with aortic insufficiency. SYN: *Corrigan's pulse.*

**Waterhouse-Friderichsen syndrome** [Rupert Waterhouse, Brit. physician, 1873–1958; Carl Friderichsen, Danish physician, b. 1886] An acute adrenal insufficiency due to hemorrhage into the adrenal gland caused by meningococcal infection. SEE: *adrenal gland; meningitis, acute meningococcal.*

**waters** The common term for the amniotic fluid surrounding the fetus.

**water syringe** In dentistry, a syringe for delivering water spray to a localized area. The flow, pressure, and temperature are controlled.

**Watson-Crick helix** [James Dewey Watson, U.S. biochemist, b. 1928; Francis Harry Compton Crick, Brit. biochemist, b. 1916] The double helix of DNA, named after the two scientists who established its structure. Each strand consists of nucleotides of phosphate, deoxyribose, and nitrogenous bases. The sequence of bases is the genetic code for the organism and is transmitted to new cells in mitosis or to offspring in egg and sperm. SEE: *code, triplet; deoxyribonucleic acid.*

**Watson, Margaret Jean Harman** A nursing educator, born 1940, who developed the Theory of Human Caring. SEE: *Nursing Theory Appendix.*

**Watson-Schwartz test** (wŏt′sŏn-shwărts) [Cecil J. Watson, U.S. physician, 1901–1983; Samuel Schwartz, U.S. physician, b. 1916] A test used in acute porphyria to differentiate porphobilinogen from urobilinogen.

**watt** [James Watt, Scottish engineer, 1736–1819] ABBR: w. A unit of electrical power. One watt is the power produced by 1 ampere of current flowing with a force or pressure (i.e., electromotive force) of 1 volt. In SI units, 1 w equals 1 J/sec. In other units, 1 w equals 1 newton m/sec. This is also equal to 0.7376 ft-lb/sec. SEE: *electromotive force.*

**wattage** (wŏt′ĭj) The electrical energy produced or consumed by an electrical device, expressed in watts.

**wave** (wāv) [ME. *wave*] **1.** A disturbance, usually orderly and predictable, observed as a moving ridge on the surface of a liquid. **2.** An undulating or vibrating motion. **3.** An oscillation seen in the recording of an electrocardiogram, electroencephalogram, or other graphic record of physiological activity. SEE: illus.

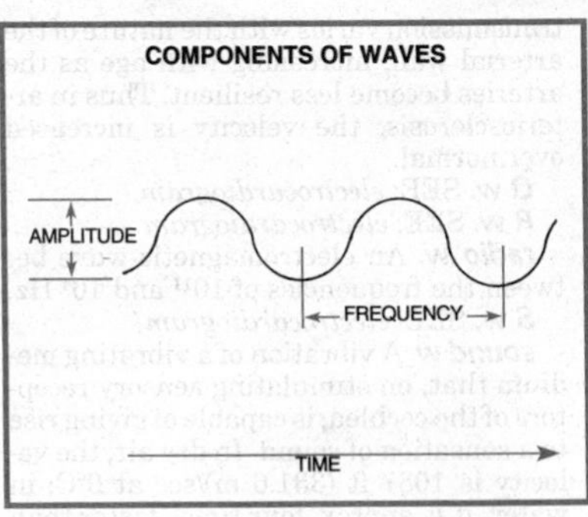


***a* w. 1.** A venous neck wave produced by atrial contraction. **2.** A component of right atrial and pulmonary artery wedge pressure tracings produced by atrial contraction. The a wave just precedes the first heart sound. It is absent in atrial fibrillation and is larger in atrioventricular dissociation and in conditions causing dilation of the right atrium.

***alpha* w.** SEE: *rhythm, alpha.*

***beta* w.** SEE: *rhythm, beta.*

***brain* w.** The fluctuation, usually rhythmic, of electrical impulses produced by the brain. SEE: *electroencephalography.*

***c* w.** A component of right atrial and pulmonary capillary wedge pressure waves. It reflects the closing of the tricuspid valve at the beginning of ventricular systole. An abnormal configuration is seen in increased right heart pressure and with abnormalities of the tricuspid valve.

***delta* w.** SEE: *rhythm, delta.*

***electromagnetic* w.** A wave-form produced by simultaneous oscillation of electric and magnetic fields perpendicular to each other. The direction of propagation of the wave is perpendicular to the oscillations. The following waves, in order of increasing frequency and decreasing wavelength, are electromagnetic: radio, television, microwave, infrared, visible light, ultraviolet, x-rays, and gamma rays. SEE: *electromagnetic spectrum* for table.

***excitation* w.** The excitatory impulse(s) that originate in the sinoatrial node of the heart and sweep through the musculature of the atria, stimulating the atrioventricular node and then continuing through the conductile tissue of the ventricles. They bring about contractions of the chambers of the heart.

***F* w.** A flutter wave seen as a "sawtooth" or "picket fence" base line on the electrocardiogram tracing of atrial flutter. F waves are caused by a re-entry electrophysiological mechanism.

***f* w.** A fibrillatory wave seen as the wavy base line on the electrocardiogram tracing of atrial fibrillation. These waves are caused by multiple ectopic foci in the atria.

***light* w.** An electromagnetic wave that produces the sensation of visible light on the retina.

***P* w.** SEE: *electrocardiogram.*

***pulse* w.** The pressure wave originated by the systolic discharge of blood into the aorta. It is not due to the passage of the ejected blood but is the result of the impact being transmitted through the arterial walls. The velocity in the aorta may be as high as 500 cm/sec and as low as 0.07 cm/sec in capillaries. The speed of transmission varies with the nature of the arterial wall, increasing with age as the arteries become less resilient. Thus in arteriosclerosis, the velocity is increased over normal.

***Q* w.** SEE: *electrocardiogram.*

***R* w.** SEE: *electrocardiogram.*

***radio* w.** An electromagnetic wave between the frequencies of $10^{11}$ and $10^4$ Hz.

***S* w.** SEE: *electrocardiogram.*

***sound* w.** A vibration of a vibrating medium that, on stimulating sensory receptors of the cochlea, is capable of giving rise to a sensation of sound. In dry air, the velocity is 1087 ft (331.6 m)/sec at 0°C; in water, it is approx. four times faster than in air.

***T* w.** SEE: *electrocardiogram.*

***theta* w.** A brain wave present in the electroencephalogram. It has a frequency of about 4 to 7 Hz.

***ultrashort* w.** An arbitrary designation of radio waves of a wavelength of less than 1 m.

***ultrasonic* w.** A sound wave of greater frequency than 20 kHz. These waves do not produce sound audible to the human ear.

**wavelength** (wāv′lĕngth) The distance between the beginning and end of a single wave cycle, usually measured from the top of one wave to the top of the next one.

**wax** [AS. *weax*] **1.** A substance obtained from bees (beeswax), plants, or petroleum (paraffin). It is solid at room temperature. In medicine, a purified form, white wax, is used in making ointments and to stop bleeding from bones during surgery. **2.** Any substance with the consistency of beeswax. **3.** Earwax. SYN: *cerumen.*

***bone* w.** A nontoxic, biocompatible wax used during surgery to plug cavities in cranial bones and other bones to control bleeding.

***casting* w.** A mixture of several waxes that can be carved or formed into shapes to be cast in metal.

***dental* w.** A variety of waxes compounded for their specific properties desired for dental procedures (e.g., baseplate wax, bone wax, boxing wax, burnout wax, casting wax, inlay wax, and pattern wax).

**waxing-up** In dentistry, the shaping of wax around the contours of a trial denture.

**waxy** (wăks′ē) [AS. *weax,* wax] Resembling or pert. to wax.

**waxy cast** A dense, highly refractile urinary cast. Such casts have clean-cut contours, sometimes irregular curves and notches. These casts occurs in severe chronic renal disease.

**waxy degeneration** Amyloid degeneration seen in wasting diseases.

**WBC** *white blood cells; white blood count.*

**weak** (wēk) [Old Norse *veikr,* flexible] **1.** Lacking physical strength or vigor; infirm, esp. as compared with what would be the normal or usual for that individual. **2.** Dilute, as in a weak solution, or weak tea.

**weakness** A precise but subjective term used by a patient to indicate a lack of strength as compared with what he or she feels is normal. The cause may be organic disease or a combination of an organic disease and a mental state. In either event, the symptom, if it is unremitting, requires careful investigation with special attention being given to determining potentially lethal causes that may be curable (e.g., cancer, anemia, certain parasitic or infectious diseases, or neurological conditions).

**wean** (wēn) [AS. *wenian*] **1.** To accustom an infant to discontinuation of breast milk by substitution of other nourishment. **2.** The slow discontinuation of ventilatory support therapy. SEE: *ventilator support, weaning from.*

**weanling** A young child or infant recently changed from breast to formula feeding.

**weanling diarrhea** Severe gastroenteritis that sometimes occurs in infants who recently have been weaned.

**web** A tissue or membrane extending across a space.

***esophageal* w.** A tissue in the form of a web that extends across the esophageal lumen and thus interferes with the swallowing of food.

***terminal* w.** A microscopic weblike network that is beneath the microvilli of intestinal absorption cells and beneath the hair cells of the inner ear.

**webbed** (wĕbd) [AS. *webb,* a fabric] Having a membrane or tissue connecting adjacent structures, as the toes of a duck's feet.

**Weber-Christian disease** (wĕb′ĕr-krĭs′chĕn) [Fredrick Parkes Weber, Brit. physician, 1863–1962; Henry A. Christian, U.S. physician, 1876–1951] Relapsing, febrile, nodular, nonsuppurative panniculitis, a generalized disorder of fat metabolism characterized by recurring episodes of fever and the development of crops of subcutaneous fatty nodules.

**Weber's gland** (vā′bĕrz) [Moritz I. Weber, Ger. anatomist, 1795–1875] One of the mucous glands of the tongue.

**Weber's paralysis** (wĕb′ĕrz) [Sir Hermann David Weber, Brit. physician, 1823–1918] Paralysis of the oculomotor nerve on one side with contralateral spastic hemiplegia. It is caused by a lesion of the crus cerebri.

**Weber test** [Friedrich Eugen Weber, Ger. otologist, 1823–1891] A test for unilateral deafness. A vibrating tuning fork held against the midline of the top of the head is perceived as being so located by those with equal hearing ability in the ears; to persons with unilateral conductive-type deafness, the sound will be perceived as being more pronounced on the diseased side; in persons with unilateral nerve-type deafness, the sound will be perceived as being louder in the good ear. SEE:

*hearing.*

**Wechsler Intelligence Scale for Children** ABBR: WISC. A widely used intelligence test for children aged 5 to 16.

**wedge 1.** A solid object with a broad base and two sides arising from the base to intersect each other and to form an acute angle opposite the base. **2.** In radiography, a filter placed in the primary x-ray beam to vary the intensity.

***step w.*** A device consisting of increasing thicknesses of absorber through which radiographs are taken to determine the amounts of radiation reaching the film.

**wedge pressure** Pulmonary artery wedge pressure.

**WEE** *western equine encephalomyelitis.*

**WeeFIM** The Functional Independence Measure adapted for children aged 6 months to 7 years. SEE: *Functional Independence Measure.*

**weeping** [AS. *wepan,* to lament] **1.** Shedding tears. **2.** Moist, dripping.

**weeping eczema** Dermatitis with eruption of vesicles exuding serum.

**weeping sinew** A circumscribed cystic swelling of a tendon sheath.

**Wegener's granulomatosis, Wegener's syndrome** [Frederich Wegener, Ger. pathologist, 1843–1917] A rare condition characterized by vasculitis, granulomatous lesions of the entire respiratory tract, and glomerulonephritis. The symptoms are fever, weakness, malaise, weight loss, purulent rhinitis, sinusitis, polyarthralgia, ulcerations of the nasal septum, and signs of severe progressive renal disease. The prognosis is very good if it is diagnosed early and treated initially with cyclophosphamide and corticosteroids and then with cyclophosphamide alone. If cyclophosphamide causes undesired side effects, azathioprine may be used in its place. If the condition is not treated early, death results, usually within 1 year.

**Weidel reaction** (vī'dĕl) [Hugo Weidel, Austrian chemist, 1849–1899] **1.** A test for the presence of xanthine bodies. **2.** A test for the presence of uric acid.

**Weigert's law** (vī'gĕrts) [Carl Weigert, Ger. pathologist, 1845–1904] An observation stating that loss or destruction of tissue results in an excess of new tissue during repair.

**weighing, underwater** SEE: *hydrodensitometry.*

**weight** (wāt) [AS. *gewiht*] The gravitational force exerted on an object, usually by the earth. The unit of weight is the newton; 1 newton equals 0.225 lb. The difference between weight and mass is that the weight of an object varies with the force of gravity, but the mass remains the same. For example, an object weighs less on the moon than on earth because the force of gravity is less on the moon; but the object's mass is the same in both places. SEE: *mass* (3).

The weight of the body increases in pathological obesity and decreases in Addison's disease, AIDS, cancer, chronic diarrhea, chronic suppurations, untreated type I diabetes mellitus, hysteria, anorexia, fevers, lactation when prolonged, marasmus, obstruction of the pylorus or thoracic duct, starvation, tuberculosis, and ulcer of the stomach.

Normal weight depends on the frame of the individual. SEE: table.

***apothecaries' w.*** SEE: *apothecaries' weights and measures.*

***atomic w.*** ABBR: at. wt. The weight of an atom of an element compared with that of 1/12 the weight of carbon-12.

***avoirdupois w.*** SEE: *avoirdupois measure.*

***w. cycling*** Yo-yo diet.

***equivalent w.*** The weight of a chemical element that is equivalent to and will replace a hydrogen atom (1.008 g) in a chemical reaction.

***molecular w.*** ABBR: mol. wt. The weight of a molecule attained by totaling the atomic weight of its constituent atoms. SEE: *atomic w.*

***set point w.*** The concept that body weight is controlled by the central nervous system and set at a certain value; the value is more or less stable until something occurs to alter it. An example of resetting of the set point occurs in persons with a disturbance of hypothalamic function that interferes with the satiety and feeding centers.

***w. in volume*** ABBR: w/v. The amount by weight of a solid substance dissolved in a measured quantity of liquid. Percent w/v expresses the number of grams of an ingredient in 100 ml of solution.

***w. in weight*** ABBR: w/w. The amount by weight of a solid substance dissolved in a known amount (by weight) of liquid. Percent w/w expresses the number of grams of one ingredient in 100 g of solution.

**weighting** In radiation therapy using two opposing fields, the use of a higher dose for one of the fields.

**weightlessness** The condition of not being acted on by the force of gravity. It is present when astronauts travel in areas so distant from the earth, moon, or planets that the force of gravity is virtually absent.

**weights and measures** SEE: *Weights and Measures Appendix.*

**Weil's disease** (vīlz) [Adolf Weil, Ger. physician, 1848–1916] Severe leptospirosis caused by any one of several serotypes of *Leptospira interrogans* such as *L. icterohemorrhagica* in rats, *L. pomona* in swine, or *L. canicola* in dogs. All of these may be pathogenic for humans.

ETIOLOGY: The infection is caused by an organism found in rat urine and feces, and acquired by humans through contaminated food or water or by contact of bro-

### 1983 Metropolitan Height and Weight Tables for Men and Women According to Frame, Ages 25 to 59

| Men | | | | | Women | | | | |
|---|---|---|---|---|---|---|---|---|---|
| Height (in shoes)* | | Weight in Pounds (in indoor clothing)† | | | Height (in shoes)* | | Weight in Pounds (in indoor clothing)† | | |
| *Ft.* | *In.* | *Small Frame* | *Medium Frame* | *Large Frame* | *Ft.* | *In.* | *Small Frame* | *Medium Frame* | *Large Frame* |
| 5 | 2 | 128–134 | 131–141 | 138–150 | 4 | 10 | 102–111 | 109–121 | 118–131 |
| 5 | 3 | 130–136 | 133–143 | 140–153 | 4 | 11 | 103–113 | 111–123 | 120–134 |
| 5 | 4 | 132–138 | 135–145 | 142–156 | 5 | 0 | 104–115 | 113–126 | 122–137 |
| 5 | 5 | 134–140 | 137–148 | 144–160 | 5 | 1 | 106–118 | 115–129 | 125–140 |
| 5 | 6 | 136–142 | 139–151 | 146–164 | 5 | 2 | 108–121 | 118–132 | 128–143 |
| 5 | 7 | 138–145 | 142–154 | 149–168 | 5 | 3 | 111–124 | 121–135 | 131–147 |
| 5 | 8 | 140–148 | 145–157 | 152–172 | 5 | 4 | 114–127 | 124–138 | 134–151 |
| 5 | 9 | 142–151 | 148–160 | 155–176 | 5 | 5 | 117–130 | 127–141 | 137–155 |
| 5 | 10 | 144–154 | 151–163 | 158–180 | 5 | 6 | 120–133 | 130–144 | 140–159 |
| 5 | 11 | 146–157 | 154–166 | 161–184 | 5 | 7 | 123–136 | 133–147 | 143–163 |
| 6 | 0 | 149–160 | 157–170 | 164–188 | 5 | 8 | 126–139 | 136–150 | 146–167 |
| 6 | 1 | 152–164 | 160–174 | 168–192 | 5 | 9 | 129–142 | 139–153 | 149–170 |
| 6 | 2 | 155–168 | 164–178 | 172–197 | 5 | 10 | 132–145 | 142–156 | 152–173 |
| 6 | 3 | 158–172 | 167–182 | 176–202 | 5 | 11 | 135–148 | 145–159 | 155–176 |
| 6 | 4 | 162–176 | 171–187 | 181–207 | 6 | 0 | 138–151 | 148–162 | 158–179 |

SOURCE OF BASIC DATA: Build Study, 1979, Society of Actuaries and Association of Life Insurance Medical Directors of America, 1980.
Copyright 1983 Metropolitan Life Insurance Company.
* Shoes with 1-in. heels.
† Indoor clothing weighing 5 lb for men and 3 lb for women.

ken skin with an infected rat or its feces or urine. It is a specific infection accompanied by muscular pains, fever, jaundice, and enlargement of the liver and spleen.

TREATMENT: Treatment is symptomatic. In severely ill patients who are unable to take medicine, penicillin G is given orally or ampicillin intravenously. In less severe cases when oral medication can be tolerated, doxycycline, an oral form of penicillin G, or amoxicillin is given.

PREVENTION: Doxycycline may be used to prevent infection in those exposed to the spirochetes.

**Weil-Felix reaction, Weil-Felix test** (vīl-fā′lĭks) [Edmund Weil, Austrian bacteriologist, 1880–1922; Arthur Felix, Ger. bacteriologist, 1887–1956] The agglutination of certain *Proteus* organisms caused by the development of *Proteus* antibodies in certain rickettsial diseases.

**Weir Mitchell's treatment** (wēr mĭt′chĕlz) [Silas Weir Mitchell, U.S. neurologist, 1829–1914] The treatment for hysteria and neurasthenia that consists of bedrest, massage, nourishing diet, and a change of environment.

**weismannism** (wīs′măn-ĭzm) [August F. L. Weismann, Ger. biologist, 1834–1914] The theory that acquired characteristics are not inherited.

**Weitbrecht's foramen** (vīt′brĕkts) [Josias Weitbrecht, Ger.-born Russian anatomist, 1702–1747] An opening in the articular cartilage of the shoulder joint.

**Weitbrecht's ligament** The oblique cord connecting the ulna and radius.

**Welch's bacillus** (wĕlsh′ĕz) [William Henry Welch, U.S. pathologist, 1850–1934] *Clostridium perfringens,* the causative organism of gas gangrene. SEE: *gangrene, gas.*

**Wellens' syndrome** The signs of occlusion of the left anterior descending coronary artery. Electrocardiography shows an inverted symmetrical T wave with little or no associated change of the ST segment or R wave. Inversion appears principally, but not exclusively, in the $V_2$ and $V_3$ leads. The finding is a noninvasive means of identifying patients with this type of occlusion who are at risk for an extensive myocardial infarction.

**wellness** The condition of being in good health, including the appreciation and enjoyment of health. Wellness is more than a lack of disease symptoms; it is a state of mental and physical balance and fitness.

**welt** [ME. *welte*] An elevation on the skin produced by a lash, blow, or allergic stimulus. The skin is unbroken and the mark is reversible.

**wen** (wĕn) [AS.] A cyst resulting from the retention of secretion in a sebaceous gland. One or more rounded or oval elevations, varying in size from a few millimeters to about 10 cm, appear slowly on the scalp, face, or back. They are painless, rather soft, and contain a yellow-white caseous mass. The sac and contents should be carefully dissected to prevent its recurrence. SYN: *sebaceous cyst; steatoma.* SEE: *Fordyce's disease.*

**Wenckebach's period, Wenckebach's phenomenon** (věn'kĕ-băks) [Karel F. Wenckebach, Dutch-born Aust. internist, 1864–1940] A form of incomplete heart block in which, as detected by electrocardiography, there is progressive lengthening of the P-R interval until there is no ventricular response; and then the cycle of increasing P-R intervals begins again.

**Werdnig-Hoffmann disease** (věrd'nĭg-hŏf'măn) [Guido Werdnig, Austrian neurologist, 1844–1919; Johann Hoffmann, Ger. neurologist, 1857–1919] A hereditary, progressive, infantile form of muscular atrophy resulting from degeneration of the anterior horn cells of the spinal cord. It is characterized by early onset, hypotonia and wasting of muscles, complete flaccid paralysis, and death.

**Werdnig-Hoffmann paralysis** Infantile muscular atrophy, considered by some to be identical with amyotonia congenita.

**Werdnig-Hoffmann syndrome** SEE: *Werdnig-Hoffmann paralysis.*

**Werlhof's disease** (věrl'hŏfs) [Paul G. Werlhof, Ger. physician, 1699–1767] Idiopathic thrombocytopenic purpura.

**Wermer's syndrome** [Paul Wermer, U.S. physician, d. 1975] Multiple endocrine neoplasia.

**Wernicke's aphasia** (věr'nĭ-kēz) [Karl Wernicke, Ger. neurologist, 1848–1905] An injury to the Wernicke's area in the temporal lobe of the dominant hemisphere of the brain, resulting in an inability to comprehend the spoken or written word. Visual and auditory pathways are unaffected; however, patients are unable to differentiate between words or interpret their meaning. Although patients speak fluently, they are unable to function socially because their ability to communicate effectively is impaired by a disordered speech pattern called paraphasia (i.e., inserting inappropriate syllables into words or substituting one word for another). They also may be unable to repeat spoken words. If the condition is due to a stroke, the aphasia usually improves with time. In some cases, there are no associated neurological changes and the aphasic patient may be incorrectly diagnosed as being psychotic. The disorder is caused by impairment of blood flow through the lower division of the left middle cerebral artery. SEE: *speech, paraphasic.*

**Wernicke's center** An area in the dominant hemisphere of the brain that recalls, recognizes, and interprets words and other sounds in the process of using language.

**Wernicke's encephalopathy** Encephalopathy associated with thiamine deficiency; usually associated with chronic alcoholism, gastric carcinoma, or hyperemesis gravidarum.

**Wernicke's syndrome** A frequent condition of old age marked by loss of memory and disorientation with confabulation. SEE: *polioencephalitis, anterior superior.*

**western blotting** A technique for analyzing protein antigens. Initially, the antigens are separated by electrophoresis and transferred to a solid membrane by blotting. The membrane is incubated with antibodies, and then the bound antibodies are detected by enzymatic or radioactive methods. This method is used to detect small amounts of antibodies.

**Westphal-Edinger nucleus** [Karl Westphal, Ger. neurologist, 1833–1890; Ludwig Edinger, Ger. neurologist, 1855–1918] A small group of nerve cells in the rostral portion of the nucleus of the oculomotor nerve. Efferent fibers pass to the ciliary ganglion conveying impulses destined for the intrinsic muscles of the eye.

**Westphal-Strümpell pseudosclerosis** (věst'făl-strĭm'p'l) [K. Westphal; Adolf G. G. von Strümpell, Ger. physician, 1853–1925] Wilson's disease.

**West Tool Sort** Trade name for a commercial assessment device used in industrial rehabilitation to measure perceived abilities. The test consists of 80 cards, depicting various tools, that the individual sorts into piles according to the perceived ability to perform work-related tasks.

**wet** (wĕt) [AS. *waet*] Soaked with moisture, usually water.

**wet brain** An increased amount of cerebrospinal fluid with edema of the meninges; may be associated with alcoholism.

**wet cup** A cupping glass used after scarification.

**wet dream** Nocturnal emission.

**wet nurse** A woman who breastfeeds another's child.

**wet nurse phenomenon** The production of milk in response to repeated stimulation of the nipples in unpregnant women who have previously been pregnant.

**wet pack** A form of bath given by wrapping a patient in hot or cold wet sheets, covered with a blanket, used esp. to reduce fever.

**Wetzel grid** (wĕt'sĕl) [Norman C. Wetzel, U.S. pediatrician, b. 1897] A graph for use in evaluating growth and development in children aged 5 to 18 years.

**Wharton's duct** (hwăr'tŏnz) [Thomas Wharton, Brit. anatomist, 1614–1673] The duct of the submandibular salivary gland opening into the mouth at the side of the frenulum linguae.

**Wharton's jelly** A gelatinous intercellular substance consisting of primitive connective tissue of the umbilical cord. It is rich in hyaluronic acid.

**wheal** (hwēl) **1.** [AS. *hwele*] A more or less round and evanescent elevation of the skin, white in the center with a pale-red periphery, accompanied by itching. It is seen in urticaria, insect bites, anaphylaxis, and angioneurotic edema. SYN:

*pomphus*. **2.** [ME. *wale,* a stripe] An elongated mark or ridge. Such a ridge is produced by intradermal injection.

**wheat** (hwēt) [AS. *hwaete*] Any of various cereal grasses, widely cultivated for its important edible grain used in making flour. Boiled whole wheat is an excellent food. Wheat preparations and pastas include macaroni, vermicelli, and noodles, which are made from flour and water, molded, dried, and slightly baked. They are easy to digest. SEE: *bread*.

STRUCTURE: Wheat is composed of the husk or outer coat, which is removed before grinding; bran coats, which are removed in making white flour and contain the mineral substances; gluten, which contains the fat and protein; and starch, the center of the kernel. Refined wheat products do not include the bran and germ, which contain B complex vitamins, phosphorus, and iron.

**wheat germ** The embryo portion of wheat. It is an excellent source of B vitamins and vitamin E.

**wheat germ oil** The oil expressed from the germ of the wheat seed.

**wheatstone bridge** An electric circuit with two branches, each containing two resistors. These branches are joined to complete the circuit. If the resistance in three resistors is known, the resistance of the fourth and unknown one can be calculated.

**wheel** A disk attached through its middle to an axle that rotates. In dentistry, small wheels are attached to a handpiece and used for polishing and shaping teeth and restorations.

***carborundum w.*** A cutting wheel containing silicon carbide, in variable grit sizes.

***diamond w.*** In dentistry, a wheel that contains diamond powder or chips.

***polishing w.*** In dentistry, a wheel made of soft material suitable for polishing teeth or restorations.

***wire w.*** A wheel containing pieces of wire. It is used for cleaning metal surfaces.

**wheelchair** A type of mobility device for personal transport. Traditional wheelchairs have a seating area positioned between two large wheels, with two smaller wheels at the front. These can be self-propelled through handrims or pushed by another person. Advances in wheelchair design have provided alternatives that better accommodate obstacles and rough terrain. Lightweight, collapsible modes exist, as well as models designed for racing and sports. Powered wheelchairs and scooters, driven by electric motors, can be controlled through electronic switches and enable mobility by persons with muscle weakness or even paralysis.

**wheeze** (hwēz) [ME. *whesen*] A continuous musical sound caused by narrowing of the lumen of a respiratory passageway. Often noted only by the use of a stethoscope, it occurs in asthma, croup, hay fever, mitral stenosis, and pleural effusion. It may result from the presence of tumors, foreign obstructions, bronchial spasm, tuberculosis, obstructive emphysema, or edema.

**wheezing** The production of whistling sounds during difficult breathing such as occurs in asthma, coryza, croup, and other respiratory disorders. SEE: *wheeze*.

**whey** The watery material separated from the curd of milk that has coagulated.

**whinolalia** (wĭn″ō-lā′lē-ă) [AS. *whinan,* whine, + Gr. *lalein,* to talk] Hypernasality and distortion of speech, which occurs in incompetent palate syndrome.

**whiplash injury** An imprecise term for injury to the cervical vertebrae and adjacent soft tissues. It is produced by a sudden jerking or relative backward or forward acceleration of the head with respect to the vertebral column. This type of injury may occur in a vehicle that is suddenly and forcibly struck from the rear.

**Whipple's disease** (hwĭp′ĕlz) [George Hoyt Whipple, U.S. pathologist, 1878–1976] Intestinal lipodystrophy, characterized by abnormal skin pigmentation, fatty stools, loss of weight and strength, chronic arthritis, a distinctive lesion of the mucosa of the jejunum and ileum, and other signs of a malabsorption syndrome. This rare disease resembles idiopathic steatorrhea. SYN: *intestinal lipodystrophy*.

ETIOLOGY: It is believed that the causative organism is a gram-positive bacillus, *Tropheryma whippelii*.

TREATMENT: Intensive antibiotic therapy with procaine penicillin followed by maintenance therapy with tetracycline yields good results.

**whipworm** Trichuris trichiura.

**whirlbone 1.** The patella. **2.** The head of the femur.

**whiskey, whisky** (hwĭs′kē) A distilled alcoholic liquor made from grain. The alcohol present is ethyl alcohol.

Caution: Wood or methyl alcohol should never be used in alcoholic beverages intended for human consumption. It is extremely toxic and may cause death. In those who survive, blindness is a common occurrence.

**whisper** (hwĭs′pĕr) [AS. *hwisprian*] **1.** Speech with a low, soft voice; a low, sibilant sound. **2.** To utter in a low sound.

***cavernous w.*** Direct transmission of a whisper through a cavity in auscultation.

**whistle** (hwĭs′ĕl) **1.** A sound produced by pursing one's lips and blowing. **2.** A tubular device driven by wind that produces a loud and usually shrill sound.

**whistling face syndrome** A congenital malformation with muscle dysfunction that produces a masklike "whistling face," hypoplastic nasal bones, and clubfeet. The genetic transmission may be autosomal recessive.

**white** (hwīt) [AS. *hwit*] **1.** The achromatic color of maximum lightness that reflects all rays of the spectrum. **2.** The color of milk or fresh snow; opposite of black.

**white cell** The leukocyte.

**white-damp** Carbon monoxide formed in a mine following an explosion.

**white of egg** The albumin of an egg.

**white of eye** The part of the sclera visible around the iris.

**white fingers** Decreased blood flow to the hand and fingers as a result of working with tools that produce vibration, such as chain saws, impact wrenches, and jackhammers. The fingers become pale and then red after the exposure to the vibration is stopped.

**white gangrene** Gangrene caused by local anemia.

**whitehead** (hwīt'hĕd) A closed comedo containing pale, dried sebum. SEE: *blackhead; comedo.*

**white leg** SEE: *phlegmasia alba dolens.*

**white line** Linea alba.

**white lotion** A combination of zinc sulfate and sulfurated potassium diluted in purified water, used in treating certain skin diseases.

**white ointment** An ointment containing white wax and white petroleum.

**whitepox** (hwīt'pŏks) Variola minor.

**white precipitate** Ammoniated mercury.

**whites** Slang for leukorrhea.

**white softening** The stage of softening of any substance in which the affected area has become white and anemic.

**whitlow** (hwĭt'lō) [ME. *whitflawe,* white flow] Suppurative inflammation at the end of a finger or toe. It may be deep seated, involving the bone and its periosteum, or superficial, affecting parts of the nail. SYN: *felon; panaris; paronychia; runaround.*

***herpetic w.*** Whitlow due to herpes simplex virus. It is painful and accompanied by lymphadenopathy.

**Whitmore's disease** [Alfred Whitmore, Brit. surgeon, 1876–1946] Melioidosis.

**WHO** *World Health Organization.*

**whole body counter** An instrument that detects the radiation present in the entire body.

**whole bowel irrigation** A decontamination technique to cleanse mechanically the entire gastrointestinal tract in cases of poisoning in which emesis is dangerous because aspiration may occur, or in which ingested pills are too big to be evacuated via gastric lavage. It involves oral administration of several liters of an isotonic solution.

**wholism** Holism.

**wholistic health** SEE: *holistic medicine.*

**whoop** (hoop) [AS. *hwopan,* to threaten] The sonorous and convulsive inspiratory crow following a paroxysm of whooping cough.

**whooping cough** Pertussis.

**whorl** (hwŭrl) [ME. *whorle*] **1.** A spiral arrangement of cardiac muscular fibers. SYN: *vortex.* **2.** A type of fingerprint in which the central papillary ridges turn through at least one complete circle. SEE: *fingerprint* for illus.

**WIC** *Special Supplementary Food Program for Women, Infants, and Children.*

**Widal's reaction, Widal's test** (vē-dălz') [Georges Fernand Isidore Widal, Fr. physician, 1862–1929] An agglutination test for typhoid fever.

**wig** A covering for the head to simulate hair if the individual is bald or partially bald. Wigs may be made of hair or synthetic fibers such as acrylic. Wigs are esp. beneficial for use by patients who have lost their hair due to exposure to certain types of cytotoxic agents used in cancer chemotherapy.

**wild cherry** The dried bark of *Prunus serotina,* used principally in the form of syrup as a flavored vehicle for cough medicine.

**will** [AS.] **1.** The mental faculty used in choosing or deciding on an act or thought. **2.** The power of controlling one's actions or emotions.

**Willis, Thomas** (wĭl'ĭs) British anatomist, 1621–1675.

***circle of W.*** An arterial anastomosis that encircles the optic chiasm and hypophysis, from which the principal arteries supplying the brain are derived. It receives blood from the two internal carotid arteries and the basilar artery formed by union of the two vertebral arteries. SEE: illus.

**Willis' cord** One of the cords crossing the superior longitudinal sinus transversely.

**Wilms' tumor** (vĭlmz) [Max Wilms, Ger. surgeon, 1867–1918] A rapidly developing tumor of the kidney that usually occurs in children. In the past, the mortality from this type of cancer was extremely high; however, newer approaches to therapy have been very effective in controlling the tumor. SYN: *embryonal carcinosarcoma; nephroblastoma.* SEE: *Nursing Diagnoses Appendix.*

**Wilson's disease** (wĭl'sŭnz) [Samuel Alexander Kinnier Wilson, Brit. internist, 1877–1937] A hereditary syndrome transmitted as an autosomal recessive trait in which a decrease of ceruloplasmin permits accumulation of copper in various organs (brain, liver, kidney, and cornea) associated with increased intestinal absorption of copper. A pigmented ring (Kayser-Fleischer ring) at the outer margin of the cornea is pathognomonic. This syndrome is characterized by degenerative changes in the brain, cirrhosis of the liver, splenomegaly, tremor, muscular rigidity, involuntary movements, spastic contractures, psychic disturbances, dysphagia, and progressive weakness and emaciation. SYN: *hepatolenticular de-*

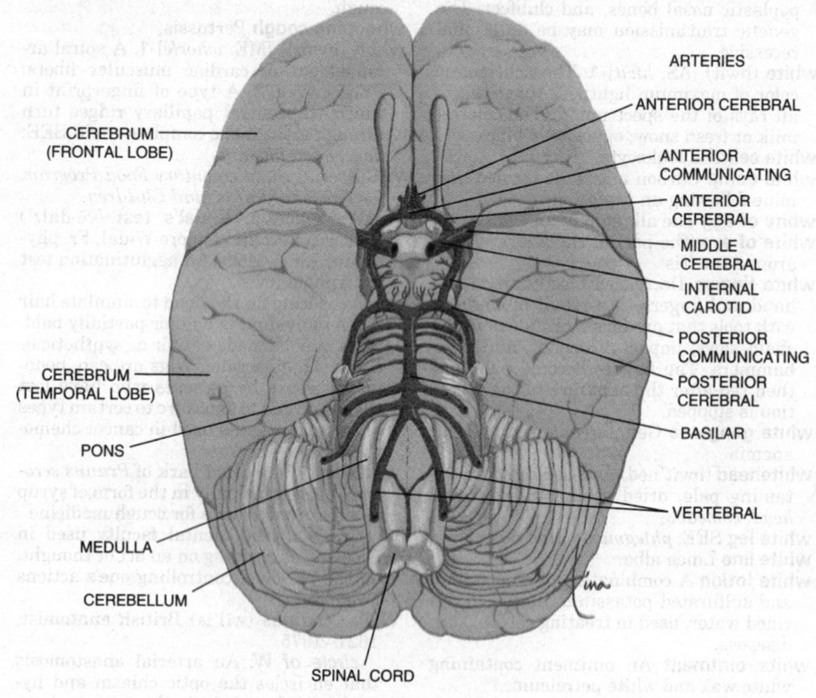


CIRCLE OF WILLIS

(INFERIOR VIEW OF BRAIN)

*generation; Westphal-Strümpell pseudosclerosis.*

TREATMENT: The untreated disease is fatal. The goal is to prevent further copper accumulation in tissues by avoiding foods high in copper such as organ meats, shellfish, nuts, dried legumes, chocolate, and whole cereals. Reduction of the copper in the tissues is achieved by giving the copper binder, D-penicillamine, orally until the serum copper level returns to normal. Carefully controlled doses of this therapy will probably be required for the patient's entire lifetime. Blood cell counts and hemoglobin should be monitored every 2 weeks during the first 6 weeks of treatment. Nonsteroidal anti-inflammatory drugs or systemic corticosteroids may help to relieve symptoms.

Caution: The copper binder, D-penicillamine, may cause pyridoxine and iron deficiency.

**Wilson-Mikity syndrome** [Miriam G. Wilson, U.S. pediatrician, b. 1922; Victor G. Mikity, U.S. radiologist, b. 1919] A so-called pulmonary dysmaturity syndrome seen in premature infants. The symptoms are insidious onset of dyspnea, tachypnea, and cyanosis in the first month of life. Radiographs of the lungs reveal evidence of emphysema that develops into multicysts. Therapy is directed at the pulmonary insufficiency and cardiac failure. The death rate is about 25%.

**Winckel's disease** (vĭng'kĕlz) [Franz von Winckel, Ger. gynecologist, 1837–1911] A fatal disease of the newborn characterized by profuse hemorrhages, hematuria, jaundice, enlarged spleen, collapse, and convulsions.

**windburn** Erythema and irritation of the skin caused by exposure to wind. Simultaneous exposure to the sun, moisture, wind, and cold may cause a severe dermatitis.

**windchill** The cooling effect wind has on exposed human skin. The effect is intensified if the skin is moist or wet.

**windchill factor** Loss of heat from exposure of skin to wind. Heat loss is proportional to the speed of the wind. Thus, skin exposed to a wind velocity of 20 mph (32 km/hr) when the temperature is 0°F (−17.8°C) is cooled at the same rate as in still air at −46°F (−43.3°C). Similarly, when the temperature is 20°F (−6.7°C) and the wind is 10, 20, or 35 mph (16.1, 32.2, or 56.3 km/hr), the equivalent skin temperature is −4°, −18°, or −28°F

(−20°, −27.8°, or −33.3°C), respectively. The windchill factor is calculated for dry skin; skin that is wet from any cause and exposed to wind loses heat at a much higher rate. Wind blowing over wet skin can cause frostbite, even on a comfortably warm day as judged by the thermometer.

**windchill index** A table listing the windchill factor for various combinations of temperature and wind velocity.

**window** [Old Norse *vindauga*] **1.** An aperture for the admission of light or air or both. **2.** A small aperture into a cavity, esp. that of the inner ear. SYN: *fenestra.*

***aortic w.*** In radiology, in a left anterior oblique or lateral view of the chest, a clear area bounded by the aortic arch, the bifurcation of the trachea, and the pericardial border.

***beryllium w.*** The part of a radiographic tube through which the x-ray photons pass to the outside.

***cochlear w.*** The fenestra cochleae.

***w. level*** ABBR: WL. In computed tomography, the center of the range of gray scale in the image.

***oval w.*** The fenestra vestibuli.

***radiation w.*** A translucent lead glass window in a radiographic control booth.

***radiographic w.*** A thinner area on the glass envelope of an x-ray tube from which x-rays are emitted toward the patient.

***round w.*** The fenestra cochleae.

***vestibular w.*** The fenestra vestibuli.

***window w.*** ABBR: WW. In computed tomography, the number of shades of gray in an image.

**windowing** Cutting a hole in anything, esp. a plaster cast, to relieve pressure on the skin or a bony area.

**windpipe** Trachea.

**wine** (wīn) [L. *vinum,* wine] **1.** Fermented juice of any fruit, usually made from grapes and containing 10% to 15% alcohol. **2.** The solution of a medicinal substance in wine. SYN: *vinum.*

**wineglass** A fluid measure of approx. 2 fl oz (60 ml).

**wine sore** Slang term for a superficial infected area of the skin seen in alcoholics with poor personal hygiene; erroneously thought to be due to specific action of the wine.

**wing** [Old Norse *vaengi*] A structure resembling the wing of a bird, esp. the great and small wings of the sphenoid bone. SEE: *ala.*

**wink** [AS. *wincian*] The brief, voluntary closure of one eye. In hemiplegia, the patient may not be able to blink or close the eye on the paralyzed side without simultaneously closing the other eye. This is called *Revilliod sign* or *orbicularis sign.* SEE: *blink; Marcus Gunn syndrome.*

**winking** SEE: *wink.*

***jaw w.*** The involuntary simultaneous closing of the eyelid as the jaw is moved.

***jaw w. syndrome*** The unilateral ptosis of the eye at rest, and the rapid exaggerating elevation of the lid when the mandible is either depressed or moved to the opposite side of the ptosed lid. SYN: *Marcus Gunn syndrome.*

**Winslow, foramen of** (wĭnz′lō) [Jacob Benignus Winslow, Danish-born Fr. anatomist, 1669–1760] The epiploic foramen.

**Winslow, ligament of** The oblique popliteal ligament located at the back of the knee.

**Winslow, pancreas of** The processus uncinatus of the pancreas.

**wintergreen oil** Methyl salicylate. This colorless, yellowish, or reddish liquid has a characteristic taste and odor. It is used as a flavoring substance and as a counterirritant applied topically in the form of salves, lotions, and ointments.

**winter itch** A mild form of eczematous dermatitis of the lower legs of elderly persons during dry periods of the year. The skin contains fine cracks and there is no erythema. Excessive skin dryness should be avoided. The skin should be rehydrated with a cream or emulsion of water in oil. SYN: *asteatotic eczema; pruritus hiemalis.*

**wire** (wīr) **1.** Metal drawn out into threads of varying thickness. **2.** To join fracture fragments together by use of wire.

***arch w.*** In dentistry, application of wire around the dental arch to correct irregularities of position of the teeth.

***Kirschner w.*** SEE: *Kirschner wire.*

***ligature w.*** A soft, thin wire used in orthodontics to anchor other dental devices to an arch wire.

***separating w.*** A soft wire used in dentistry to separate teeth before banding them.

**wired** Slang for tense and anxious, esp. when the condition is caused by the effect of a psychoactive drug.

**wiring** (wīr′ĭng) Fastening bone fragments together with wire.

***circumferential w.*** A method of treating a fractured mandible by passing wires around the bone and a splint in the oral cavity.

***continuous loop w.*** The forming of wire loops on both mandibular and maxillary teeth to provide attachment sites for rubber bands. These are used in treating fractures of the mandible. SYN: *Stout's w.*

***craniofacial suspension w.*** Wiring using bones not contiguous with the oral cavity for attachment of wires that lead from those bones to the fractured jaw segments.

***Gilmer w.*** Wiring of single opposed teeth by use of wire passed circumferentially around the two teeth and the ends twisted together. The twisted ends are placed where they will not irritate adjacent soft tissues. This procedure is used to produce intermaxillary fixation.

***Ivy loop w.*** The placement of wire around adjacent teeth to provide an attachment site for rubber bands.

***perialveolar w.*** The use of wires to fix a splint to the mandible. The wires are passed through the alveolar process from the buccal plate to the palate.

***pyriform w.*** Wiring using the nasal bones to stabilize a fracture of the jaw. The wires are passed through the pyriform aperture of the nasal bone and then to the segment.

***Stout's w.*** Continuous loop w.

**Wirsung, duct of** (vēr′soong) [Johann Georg Wirsung, Ger. physician, 1600–1643] The main secretory duct of the pancreas. SYN: *pancreatic duct.*

**wisdom tooth** (wĭz′dŏm) The last molar tooth on each side of the jaw. These four molars may appear as late as the 25th year or may never erupt.

**Wiskott-Aldrich syndrome** [Alfred Wiskott, Ger. pediatrician, 1898–1978; Robert A. Aldrich, U.S. pediatrician, b. 1917] An immunodeficiency disorder occurring in boys, marked by defects in both T and B cell function. Patients have eczema, recurring bloody diarrhea, thrombocytopenia with bleeding tendency, and infections, esp. of the ears. Treatment consists of bone marrow transplantation. In patients for whom a suitable bone marrow donor is unavailable, splenectomy is helpful. Prophylactic antibiotics or intravenous immune globulin is regularly used to prevent sepsis. The prognosis has improved and some patients treated with splenectomy have reached adulthood. Patients who have been successfully treated by bone marrow transplantation should have a normal life expectancy.

**withdrawal** Cessation of administration of a drug, esp. a narcotic, or alcohol to which the individual has become either physiologically or psychologically addicted. Withdrawal symptoms vary with the type of drug used. Neonates may exhibit withdrawal symptoms from drugs or alcohol ingested by the mother during pregnancy. SEE: *drug addiction.*

**withdrawal syndrome** Partial collapse resulting from the withdrawal of alcohol, stimulants, or some opiates.

**witkop** (wĭt′kŏp) [Afrikaans, white scalp] Matted crusts in the hair producing a scalplike structure; seen in South African natives.

**witness** A person having knowledge or information about a particular subject or event.

***expert w.*** A qualified person who assists a judge and jury in understanding technical aspects of a lawsuit, such as breaches of the standard of care and damages or injuries sustained.

***fact w.*** A person who has knowledge of circumstances surrounding the events of the alleged incident in a complaint or petition for damages. SYN: *material w.*

***material w.*** Fact w.

**Witzel jejunostomy** [Friedrich O. Witzel, Ger. surgeon, 1865–1925] A jejunostomy created by inserting a rubber catheter into the jejunum and bringing it to the skin surface. Medication and feedings can be administered on a long-term basis. SEE: *jejunostomy.*

**witzelsucht** (vĭt′sĕl-zookt) [M. Jastrowitz, Ger. physician, b. 1839] A condition produced by frontal lobe lesions characterized by self-amusement from poor jokes and puns. SEE: *moria.*

***primary affective w.*** A peculiar variety of witzelsucht characterized by teutonization of nomenclature.

**Wohlfahrtia** (vōl-făr′tē-ă) [Peter Wohlfahrtia, Ger. author, 1675–1726] A genus of flies parasitic in animal tissue, belonging to the family Sarcophagidae, order Diptera.

***W. magnifica*** A species found in southeast Europe. The larvae may occur in human and animal wounds.

***W. opaca*** A species occurring in Canada. This species commonly infests wild animals; human infants also may become infested.

***W. vigil*** A species found in Canada and the northern United States.

**wolffian body** (wool′fē-ăn) [Kaspar Friedrich Wolff, Ger. anatomist, 1733–1794] Mesonephros. SEE: *embryo; paroophoron; parovarium.*

**wolffian cyst** A cyst lying in one of the broad ligaments of the uterus.

**wolffian duct** The duct in the embryo leading from the mesonephros to the cloaca. From it develop the ductus epididymis, ductus deferens, seminal vesicle, ejaculatory duct, ureter, and pelvis of the kidney. SYN: *mesonephric duct.*

**wolffian tubule** One of 30 to 34 tubules that develop within the mesonephros and empty into the mesonephric duct. Most are transitional, persisting for only a short time. Some persist in men as the efferent ductules of the testis; others persist only as vestigial structures. SYN: *mesonephric tubule.* SEE: *epoophoron; paradidymis; paroophoron.*

**Wolff-Parkinson-White syndrome** [Louis Wolff, U.S. cardiologist, 1898–1972; Sir John Parkinson, Brit. physician 1885–1976; Paul Dudley White, U.S. cardiologist, 1886–1973] ABBR: WPW. An abnormality of cardiac rhythm that manifests as supraventricular tachycardia. The diagnosis is made by use of electrocardiography. The P-R interval is less than 0.12 sec and the QRS complex contains an initial slur, called the delta wave, that broadens the complex. SEE: *pre-excitation, ventricular.*

**wolfram** (wool′frăm) Tungsten.

**wolfsbane** (wŏlfs′bān) Old name for aconite root.

**Wolhynia fever** Trench fever.

**Wolman's disease** [Moshe Wolman, Israeli physician, b. 1914] An inherited metabolic disorder in which infants develop hepatosplenomegaly, calcification of the adrenal glands, and foam cells in the bone marrow and other tissues.

**woman** An adult human female. SEE: *man.*

**womb** (woom) [AS. *wamb*] A uterus.

**wood alcohol** SEE: *alcohol, methyl.*

**Wood's rays** [Robert Williams Wood, U.S. physicist, 1868–1955] Ultraviolet rays; used to detect fluorescent materials in the skin and hair in certain disease states such as tinea capitis. The terms Wood's light and Wood's lamp have become synonymous with Wood's rays, even though these are misnomers.

**wool** The curly hair that composes the fleece of sheep and other animals. Lanolin is obtained from sheep wool.

**wool fat** Anhydrous lanolin, a fatty substance obtained from sheep's wool; used as a base for ointments.

**woolsorter's disease** A pulmonary form of anthrax that develops in those who handle wool contaminated with *Bacillus anthracis.*

**word blindness** Alexia.

**word salad** The use of words with no apparent meaning attached to them or to their relationship with one another; usually found in schizophrenia.

**work** [Ger. *wirken*] **1.** A force moving a resistance. The amount of work done is the product of the force in the direction of movement times the distance the resisting object is moved. Regardless of the force applied, if the resisting object is not moved, then no work has been done. This is not to say that energy has not been expended. Work is measured in units of force times distance, or newton meters. SEE: *calorie; erg.* **2.** The job, occupation, or task one performs as a means of providing a livelihood.

**work of breathing** ABBR: WOB. The amount of effort used to expand and contract the lungs. It is determined by lung and thorax compliance, airway resistance, and the use of accessory muscles for inspiration or forced expiration.

**work hardening** A series of conditioning exercises that an injured worker performs in a rehabilitation program. These are designed to simulate the functional tasks encountered on the job to which the individual will return.

**working through** In psychiatry, the combined endeavor of the patient and the therapist to understand the unconscious genesis of a symptom or mental illness.

**workout** In athletics, a practice or training session.

**work-up** The process of obtaining all of the necessary data for diagnosing and treating a patient. It should be done in an orderly manner so that essential elements will not be overlooked. Included are retrieval of all previous medical and dental records, the patient's family and personal medical history, social and occupational history, physical examination, laboratory studies, x-ray examinations, and indicated diagnostic surgical procedures. The patient's work-up is an ongoing process wherein all hospital personnel involved cooperate in attempting to determine the correct diagnosis and effective therapy. SEE: *nursing histories* for table; *medical record, problem-oriented.*

**World Health Organization** ABBR: WHO. The United Nations agency concerned with health. Its definition of health is as follows:

"Health is a state of complete physical and social well being, and not merely the absence of disease or infirmity. The enjoyment of the highest attainable standards of health is one of the fundamental rights of every human being without distinction of race, religion, political belief, economic or social condition. The health of all peoples is fundamental to the attainment of peace and security and is dependent upon the fullest cooperation of individuals and States. The achievement of any State in the promotion and protection of health is of value to all."

**worm** (wŭrm) [AS. *wyrm*] **1.** An elongated invertebrate belonging to one of the following phyla: Platyhelminthes (flatworms); Nemathelminthes or Aschelminthes (roundworms or threadworms); Acanthocephala (spinyheaded worms); and Annelida (Annulata) (segmented worms). SYN: *helminth.* **2.** Any small, limbless, creeping animal. **3.** The median portion of the cerebellum. **4.** Any wormlike structure.

**wormian bone** (wŭr′mē-ăn) [Ole Worm, Danish physician, 1588–1654] One of the small, irregular bones found along the cranial sutures.

**wormwood** (wĕrm′wood) A toxic substance, absinthium, obtained from *Artemisia absinthium.* It was used in certain alcoholic beverages (absinthe), but because of its toxicity such use is prohibited in most countries.

**worried well** Persons who are indeed well, but who, because of their anxiety or an imagined illness, frequent medical care facilities seeking reassurance concerning their health.

**wound** (woond) [AS. *wund*] A break in the continuity of soft parts of body structures caused by violence or trauma to tissues. In treating any wound, the previously immunized patient should be given a tetanus toxoid booster injection. If not previously immunized, the patient should be given tetanus immune globulin. If tetanus immune globulin is not available, the equine form may be used, but the patient must be tested for hypersensitivity before the full dose is administered.

***abdominal w.*** A common wound involving damage to the structure of the abdominal wall. The wound is debrided and sutured only after a careful examination had been made to determine whether tissues and organs in the abdominal cavity have been damaged. When a cavity has been opened, and esp. if viscera have been exposed, the area must be kept sterile and moist to help prevent infection. When viscera have been damaged, measures are taken to repair the damage. If the intestines have been penetrated, prophylactic antibodies and intestinal drainage are needed.

***bullet w.*** A puncture wound from a bullet. Usually there is a small point of entrance, and, if the bullet left the body, a larger point of exit. Bullet wounds are associated with injuries of bone, tendon, adjacent vital organs, or blood vessels. The symptoms depend on the wound site and the speed and character of the bullet. SEE: *Nursing Diagnoses Appendix.*

TREATMENT: Tetanus booster injection or tetanus immune globulin and antibiotics, if indicated, should be given. An appropriate bandage should be applied. Complications, including hemorrhage and shock, should be treated.

***cellulitis of w.*** The local inflammation of a wound, occurring when the wound has been closed without drainage, esp. in appendicitis. Symptoms are elevated temperature from the fourth to the seventh day, with an accompanying tenderness. The dressing should be inspected and findings charted. The abscess should be evacuated and hot, wet dressings applied. Antibiotics may be required.

***contused w.*** A bruise in which the skin is not broken. It may be caused by a blunt instrument. Injury of the tissues under the skin, leaving the skin unbroken, traumatizes the soft tissue. Ruptured blood vessels underneath the skin cause discoloration. If extravasated blood becomes encapsulated, it is termed hematoma; if it is diffuse, ecchymosis. SEE: *ecchymosis; hematoma.*

TREATMENT: Cold compresses, pressure, and rest, along with elevation of the injured area, will help prevent or reduce swelling. When the acute stage is over (within 24 to 48 hr), continued rest, heat, and elevation are prescribed. Aseptic drainage may be indicated.

***crushing w.*** Trauma due to force applied to tissues so they are mashed or compressed, but with minimal or no lacerations. If there is no bleeding, cold should be applied; if the wound is bleeding, application of the dressing should be followed by cold packs until the patient can be given definitive surgical treatment. If the bone is fractured, a splint should be applied.

***fishhook w.*** An injury caused by a fishhook becoming embedded in soft tissue. Deeply embedded fishhooks are difficult to remove. One should push the hook through, then cut off the barb with an instrument, and pull the remainder of the fishhook out by the route of entry. Antitetanus treatment should be given as indicated. Because these injuries often become infected, prophylactic use of a broad-spectrum antibiotic is indicated.

***incised w.*** Any sharp cut in which the tissues are not severed; a clean cut caused by a keen cutting instrument. The wound may be either aseptic or infected, depending on the circumstances that caused it.

An aseptic wound, one occurring under surgical conditions, should heal if conditions are favorable and no contaminations caused by pathogenic organisms or foreign material enter into it. During the healing process, the area of the wound must be kept aseptic. The skin must be cleansed with mild soap and normal saline solution, rinsed thoroughly, and covered securely with sterile dressings to keep the wound clean. A clean wound should be left alone. The dressings should be changed only often enough to keep the wound clean. There should be no squeezing or pulling of its edges.

***lacerated w.*** An unclean wound with torn ragged edges, the type of wound that provides many avenues for infection. It can be caused by implements that may be covered with any kind of pathogenic bacteria; thus, a wide variety of types of wound infections may be expected. Antitetanus and gas gangrene prophylaxis may be needed.

TREATMENT: The wound should be cleansed with mild soap and water and rinsed thoroughly. Ragged wound edges need to be trimmed and dead tissue removed. The patient should be given tetanus antitoxin or tetanus booster, depending on previous history. The wound should never be sealed. It is best to hold the wound open with some form of drain.

***nonpenetrating w.*** A wound in which the surface of the skin remains intact.

***open w.*** A contusion in which the skin is also broken, such as a gunshot, incised, or lacerated wound.

***penetrating w.*** A wound in which the skin is broken and the agent causing the wound enters subcutaneous tissue or a deeplying structure or cavity.

***perforating w.*** A wound in which the object that caused it, such as a bullet, projectile, or knife, entered and emerged from the body.

***puncture w.*** A wound made by a sharp-pointed instrument such as a dagger, ice pick, or needle. The chief danger is from thrombosis and possible release of emboli. A puncture wound usually is collapsed, which provides ideal conditions for infection. The placement of a drain, antitetanus therapy or prophylaxis, and gas gangrene prophylaxis may be required. This will depend on the nature of the instrument that caused the injury.

***subcutaneous w.*** A wound, such as contusion, that is unaccompanied by a break in the skin.

***tunnel w.*** A wound having a small entrance and exit of uniform diameter.

**wound ballistics** The study of the effects on the body produced by penetrating projectiles.

**wound healing** SEE: *inflammation.*

**W-plasty** A technique used in plastic surgery to prevent contractures in straight-line scars. Each side of the edges of a wound is cut in the form of connected W's, and the edges are sutured together in a zig-zag fashion. SEE: *tissue expansion; Z-plasty.*

**wrap, Coban** Coban.

**wreath** (rēth) A structure that encircles something so that it resembles a circlet of leaves and branches worn around the head.

**Wright's stain** [James H. Wright, U.S. pathologist, 1871–1928] A combination of eosin and methylene blue used in staining blood cells to reveal malarial parasites and to differentiate the kinds of white blood cells. SEE: *Wright's technique.*

**Wright's technique** A method of staining blood smears. The following procedures are used: (1) The dried blood smear is covered with 5 to 10 drops of Wright's stain and left to stand for 1 min. (2) An equal amount of neutral distilled water is added to the stain. The diluted stain is left to stand for 3 to 10 min. A metallic sheen should appear. (3) The stain is removed by gently washing with distilled water. (4) The slide is stood on end and allowed to dry. (5) The slide is mounted in balsam or methacrylate. If staining results are good, red cells will be pink or copper, white cells will have densely stained blue nuclei, and the cytoplasmic granules will stain variously in the different types of leukocytes. SEE: *leukocyte.*

**wrinkle** (rĭng'kl) [AS. *gewrinclian,* to wind] **1.** A crevice, furrow, or ridge in the skin. **2.** To make creases or furrows, as in the skin by habitual frowning.

**Wrisberg's cardiac ganglion** (rĭs'bŭrgz) [Heinrich August Wrisberg, Ger. anatomist, 1739–1808] Wrisberg's ganglion.

**Wrisberg's cartilages** The cuneiform cartilages of the larynx.

**Wrisberg's ganglion** A ganglion of the superficial cardiac plexus, between the aortic arch and the pulmonary artery. SYN: *Wrisberg's cardiac ganglion.* SEE: *ganglion, cardiac.*

**Wrisberg's nerve 1.** The medial brachial cutaneous nerve, a branch of the medial cord of the brachial plexus. **2.** The nervus intermedius (pars intermedia), a branch of the facial nerve lying between the motor root and the acoustic nerve.

**wrist** (rĭst) [AS] The joint or region lying between the hand and the forearm.

**wrist bone** One of the eight bones composing the carpus. SEE: *hand* for illus.; *skeleton.*

**wrist drop** A condition in which the hand is flexed at the wrist and cannot be extended; may be due to injury of the radial nerve or paralysis of the extensor muscles of the wrist and hand.

**wrist unit** A component of an upper-extremity prosthesis that attaches the terminal device to the forearm section and provides for pronation or supination.

**writing** The act of placing characters, letters, or words on a surface, usually paper, for the purpose of communicating ideas.

***dextrad w.*** Writing that progresses from left to right.

***mirror w.*** Writing so that letters and words are reversed and appear as in a mirror.

**writing hand** The position of the hand seen in paralysis agitans, marked by contraction of the hand muscles. The fingers assume a position similar to that used in holding a pen.

**wrongful birth, wrongful life** The idea that conception would have been prevented or pregnancy would have been interrupted if the parents had been adequately informed of the possibility that the mother would give birth to a physically or mentally defective child.

**wryneck** (rī'nĕk) A contracted state of one or more muscles of the neck, producing an abnormal position of the head. Occasionally, it is acute, caused by cold or trauma. In this case, it generally passes away under the influence of rest, heat, and time. More commonly, it is chronic, spastic in character, and dependent on nerve irritation. Wryneck has been produced by habitual malposition of the head assumed because of an existing ocular defect. It may be congenital. Chronic wryneck may require surgical therapy. SYN: *loxia; torticollis.*

**w.s.** *water-soluble.*

**wt** *weight.*

**Wuchereria** (voo"kĕr-ē'rē-ă) [Otto Wucherer, Ger. physician, 1820–1873] A genus of filarial worms belonging to the superfamily Filarioidea, class Nematoda; common in warm regions of the world.

***W. bancrofti*** The causative agent of elephantiasis. Adults of the species live in human lymph nodes and ducts. Females

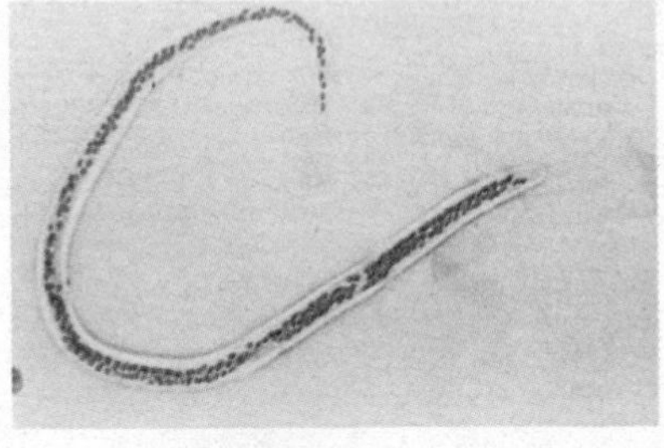


**WUCHERERIA BANCROFTI**

MICROFILARIA (ORIG. MAG. ×400)

give birth to sheathed microfilariae, which remain in internal organs during the day but at night are in circulating blood, where they are sucked up by night-biting mosquitoes, in which they continue their development, becoming infective larvae in about 2 weeks. They are then passed on to humans when the mosquito bites. There is no satisfactory treatment but diethylcarbamazine citrate has been used to reduce the number of microfilariae in the peripheral blood. It is less effective against adult worms. Ivermectin is similar in its effectiveness. SYN: *Filaria bancrofti*. SEE: illus.

***W. malayi*** A species occurring in Southeast Asia and largely responsible for lymphangitis and elephantiasis in that region. It closely resembles *W. bancrofti*.

**wuchereriasis** (voo″kĕr-ē-rī′ă-sĭs) Elephantiasis.

**w/v** *weight in volume.*

**w/w** *weight in weight.*

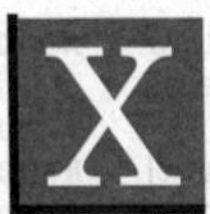

**X** Symbol for Kienböck's unit of x-ray dose; symbol for xanthine.

**Xanax** Trade name for alprazolam, a triazolo-benzodiazepine antianxiety agent.

**xanchromatic** (zăn″krō-măt′ĭk) Xanthochromic.

**xanthelasma** (zăn″thĕl-ăz′mă) [Gr. *xanthos,* yellow, + *elasma,* plate] Xanthoma.

**xanthematin** (zăn-thĕm′ă-tĭn) A yellow substance produced by the action of nitric acid on hematin.

**xanthemia** (zăn-thē′mē-ă) [″ + *haima,* blood] Carotenemia.

**xanthene** (zăn′thēn) A crystalline compound, $O{=}(C_6H_4)_2{=}CH_2$, from which various dyes are formed, including rhodamine and fluorescein.

**xanthic** (zăn′thĭk) [Gr. *xanthos,* yellow] **1.** Yellow. **2.** Pert. to xanthine.

**xanthine** (zăn′thĭn, -thēn) A nitrogenous compound present in muscle tissue, liver, spleen, pancreas, and other organs, and in the urine. It is formed during the degradation of adenosine monophosphate to uric acid.

***dimethyl-x.*** Theobromine.

**xanthine base** A group of chemical compounds including xanthine, hypoxanthine, uric acid, and theobromine, which have a purine as their base. SYN: *purine base.*

**xanthiuria** (zăn″thē-ū′rē-ă) The excretion of large amounts of xanthine in the urine. SYN: *xanthuria.*

**xanthochromia** (zăn″thō-krō′mē-ă) [″ + *chroma,* color] Yellow discoloration, as of the skin in patches or of the cerebrospinal fluid, resembling jaundice.

**xanthochromic** (zăn″thō-krō′mĭk) **1.** Pert. to anything yellow. **2.** Pert. to xanthochromia.

**xanthocyanopia, xanthocyanopsia** (zăn″thō-sī-ăn-ŏ′pē-ă, -ŏp′sē-ă) [Gr. *xanthos,* yellow, + *kyanos,* blue, + *opsis,* sight] A form of color blindness in which yellow and blue are distinguishable, but not red and green. SYN: *xanthokyanopy.*

**xanthocyte** (zăn′thō-sīt) [″ + *kytos,* cell] A cell containing yellow pigment.

**xanthoderma** (zăn″thō-dĕr′mă) [″ + *derma,* skin] Yellowness of the skin.

**xanthodont** (zăn′thō-dŏnt) [″ + *odous,* tooth] An individual who has yellow teeth.

**xanthogranuloma** (zăn″thō-grăn″ū-lō′mă) [″ + L. *granulum,* grain, + *oma,* tumor] A tumor having characteristics of both an infectious granuloma and a xanthoma.

***juvenile x.*** A skin disease that may be present at birth or develop in the first months of life. The firm dome-shaped yellow, pink, or orange papules, ranging from a few millimeters to 4 cm in diameter, are usually present on the scalp, face, and upper trunk. Biopsy of these lesions reveals lipid-filled histiocytes, inflammatory cells, and Touton giant cells (multinucleated vacuolated cells with a wreath of nuclei and peripheral rim of foamy cytoplasm). Although this illness is distressing, there is no need to attempt to treat the lesions because they regress spontaneously during the first years of life.

**xanthokyanopy** (zăn″thō-kī-ăn′ō-pē) [″ + *kyanos,* blue, + *opsis,* sight] Xanthocyanopia.

**xanthoma** (zăn-thō′mă) [Gr. *xanthos,* yellow, + *oma,* tumor] A flat or slightly elevated, soft rounded plaque or nodule, usually on the eyelids, esp. near the inner canthus. It may occur in patches of yellowish macule on the orbital regions in middle or later life. It consists of a degenerative process involving fibers of the orbicularis muscle.

***diabetic x.*** A cutaneous disease associated with uncontrolled diabetes mellitus.

***x. disseminatum*** A condition characterized by the presence of xanthomata throughout the body, esp. on the face, in tendon sheaths, and in mucous membranes. SYN: *Hand-Schüller-Christian disease.*

***x. multiplex*** Xanthomata all over the body.

***x. palpebrarum*** Xanthoma affecting the eyelids.

***x. tuberosum*** A form of xanthoma that may appear on the neck, shoulders, trunk, or extremities, consisting of small elastic and yellowish nodules.

**xanthomatosis** (zăn″thō-mă-tō′sĭs) [″ + ″ + *osis,* condition] A condition in which there is a deposition of lipid in tissues, usually accompanied by hyperlipemia. Cholesterol may accumulate in tumor nodules (xanthoma) or in individual cells, esp. histiocytes and reticuloendothelial cells.

**xanthomatous** (zăn-thō′mă-tŭs) Concerning xanthoma.

**Xanthomonas maltophilia** Gram-negative, motile, strictly aerobic bacteria of the genus *Pseudomonas* that frequently cause infections related to the use of central venous catheters and in wounds, pneumonia, meningitis, endocarditis, and conjunctivitis. Infections are treated with ticarcillin, clavulanate, trimethoprim, or sulfamethoxazole.

**xanthophose** (zăn′thō-fōz) [″ + *phos,* light] Any yellow phose. SEE: *phose.*

**xanthophyll** (zăn′thō-fĭl) [″ + *phyllon,* leaf] A yellow pigment derived from carotene. It is present in some plants and egg yolk.

**xanthoprotein** (zăn″thō-prō′tē-ĭn) A yellow substance produced by heating proteins with nitric acid.

**xanthopsia** (zăn-thŏp′sē-ă) [″ + *opsis*, sight] A condition in which objects appear to be yellow.

**xanthopsis** (zăn-thŏp′sĭs) A yellow pigmentation seen in certain cancers and degenerating tissue.

**xanthosis** (zăn-thō′sĭs) [″ + *osis*, condition] A yellowing of the skin seen in carotenemia resulting from ingestion of excessive quantities of carrots, squash, egg yolk, and other foods containing carotenoids. The condition is usually harmless, but it may indicate an increase of lipochromes in the blood caused by other conditions such as hypothyroidism, diabetes, or a malignancy.

**xanthous** (zăn′thŭs) [Gr. *xanthos*, yellow] Yellow.

**xanthurenic acid** $C_{10}H_7NO_4$. 4,8-dihydroxyquinaldic acid. An acid excreted in the urine of pyridoxine-deficient animals after they are fed tryptophan.

**xanthuria** (zăn-thū′rē-ă) [″ + *ouron*, urine] Xanthiuria.

**X chromosome** The chromosome that determines female sex characteristics. In the normal female, there are two X chromosomes, and in the normal male, one X chromosome and one Y chromosome. SEE: *chromosome*.

**x-disease** Poisoning caused by ingestion of peanuts or peanut products contaminated with *Aspergillus flavus* or other *Aspergillus* strains that produce aflatoxin. Farm animals and humans are susceptible to this toxicosis. SYN: *aflatoxicosis*.

**Xe** Symbol for the element xenon.

**xeno-** [Gr. *xenos*, stranger] Combining form indicating *strange, foreign*.

**xenobiotic** (zĕn″ō-bī-ŏt′ĭk) An antibiotic chemical substance not produced by the body, and thus foreign to it.

**xenogeneic** (zĕn″ō-jĕn-ā′ĭk) [″ + *gennan*, to produce] Tissues used for transplantation that are obtained from a species different from that of the recipient. SEE: *heterologous*.

**xenogenous** (zĕn-ŏj′ĕn-ŭs) [Gr. *xenos*, stranger, + *gennan*, to produce] **1.** Caused by a foreign body. **2.** Originating in the host, as a toxin resulting from stimuli applied to cells of the host.

**xenograft** (zĕn′ō-grăft) [″ + L. *graphium*, stylus] A surgical graft of tissue from an individual of one species to an individual of a different species. SYN: *heterograft*.

**xenomenia** (zĕn-ō-mē′nē-ă) [″ + *meniaia*, menses] Menstruation from a part of the body other than the uterus. SYN: *stigmata; vicarious menstruation*.

**xenon** (zē′nŏn) [Gr. *xenos*, stranger] SYMB: Xe. A gaseous element in the atmosphere; atomic weight, 131.29; atomic number, 54.

**xenon-133** A radioactive isotope of xenon used in photoscanning studies of the lung.

**xenoparasite** (zĕn″ō-păr′ă-sīt) An ectoparasite of a weakened animal, one that would not normally serve as a host.

**xenophobia** (zĕn″ō-fō′bē-ă) [″ + *phobos*, fear] Abnormal dread of strangers.

**xenophonia** (zĕn″ō-fō′nē-ă) [″ + *phone*, voice] Alteration in accent and intonation of a person's voice resulting from a speech defect.

**xenophthalmia** (zĕn″ŏf-thăl′mē-ă) [″ + *ophthalmia*, eye inflammation] Inflammation of the eye caused by a foreign body.

**Xenopsylla** (zĕn″ŏp-sĭl′ă) [″ + *psylla*, flea] A genus of fleas belonging to the family Pulicidae, order Siphonaptera.

***X. cheopis*** The rat flea; other hosts include humans and various animals. This species is a vector for a number of pathogens including *Hymenolepis nana*, the dwarf tapeworm; *Salmonella* organisms; and causative organisms of bubonic and sylvatic plague and endemic typhus.

**xenorexia** (zĕn″ō-rĕk′sē-ă) [″ + *orexis*, appetite] An abnormality of appetite marked by persistent swallowing of foreign objects. SEE: *pica*.

**xenotransplantation** Transplantation of animal tissues or organs into humans.

**xerantic** (zē-răn′tĭk) [Gr. *xeros*, dry] Causing dryness. SYN: *siccant; siccative*.

**xerasia** (zē-rā′sē-ă) [Gr. *xeros*, dry] A disease of the hair in which there is abnormal dryness and brittleness, and eventually hair loss.

**xero-** Combining form meaning *dry*.

**xerocheilia** (zē″rō-kī′lē-ă) [″ + *cheilos*, lip] Dryness of the lips; a type of cheilitis.

**xerocyte** An erythrocyte that is dehydrated and appears to have "puddled" at one end, seeming half dark and half light. This type of cell is found in hereditary xerocytosis. SEE: illus.; *xerocytosis, hereditary*.

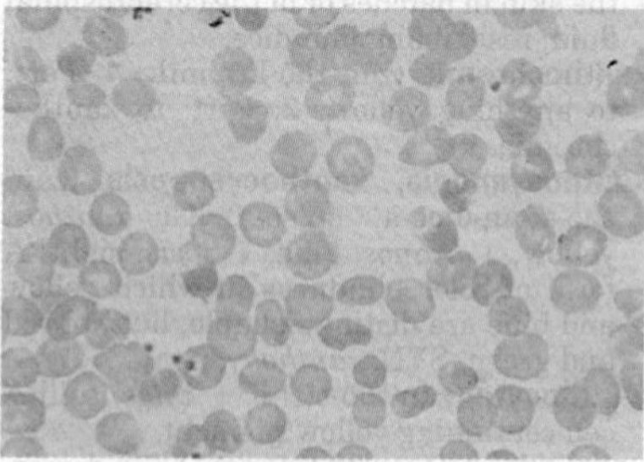

XEROCYTES

**xerocytosis, hereditary** A disorder of erythrocytes usually inherited as an autosomal dominant trait. A membrane defect in the red blood cells permits the loss of excess potassium ions and water, causing dehydration of the cells. Hemolysis and anemia range from mild to severe. SEE: *xerocyte* for illus.

**xeroderma** (zē″rō-dĕr′mă) [″ + *derma*, skin]

Roughness and dryness of the skin; mild ichthyosis.

***x. pigmentosum*** A rare, progressive, autosomal recessive, degenerative disease characterized by severe photosensitivity developing in the first years of life. There is rapid onset of erythema, bullae, pigmented macules, hypochromic spots, and telangiectasia. The skin becomes atrophic, dry, and wrinkled. A variety of benign and malignant growth appear early in life. The condition is treated symptomatically and sunlight is avoided. SYN: *Kaposi's disease; melanosis lenticularis.*

**xerography** (zē-rŏg′ră-fē) Xeroradiography.

**xeroma** (zē-rō′mă) [″ + *oma,* tumor] Xerophthalmia.

**xeromammography** (zē″rō-măm-mŏg′ră-fē) Xeroradiography of the breast.

**xeromycteria** (zē″rō-mĭk-tē′rē-ă) [″ + *mykter,* nose] Dryness of the nasal passages.

**xerophthalmia** (zē-rŏf-thăl′mē-ă) [″ + *ophthalmos,* eye] Conjunctival dryness with keratinization of the epithelium following chronic conjunctivitis and in disease caused by vitamin A deficiency. SYN: *xeroma; xerophthalmus.* SEE: *Schirmer's test.*

**xerophthalmus** (zē″rŏf-thăl′mŭs) Xerophthalmia.

**xeroradiography** (zē″rō-rā″dē-ŏg′ră-fē) A method of photoreproduction used in radiography. It is a dry process involving the use of metal plates covered with a powdered substance, such as selenium, electrically and evenly charged. The x-rays alter the charge of the substance to varying degrees, depending on the tissues they have traversed. This produces the image. This procedure has been replaced by film and screen mammography because of its high radiation dose.

**xerosis** (zē-rō′sĭs) [Gr.] Abnormal dryness of the skin, mucous membranes, or conjunctiva. SEE: illus.

**xerostomia** (zē″rō-stō′mē-ă) [″ + *stoma,* mouth] Dryness of the mouth caused by abnormal reduction in the amount of salivary secretion. It may occur in diabetes, hysteria, paralysis of the facial nerve involving the chorda tympani, acute infections, and some types of neuroses. It is induced by certain drugs such as nicotine and atropine. SEE: *ptyalism; Sjögren's syndrome.*

**xerotic** (zē-rŏt′ĭk) [Gr. *xeros,* dry] Dry; characterized by dryness.

**xerotocia** (zē″rō-tō′sē-ă) [″ + *tokos,* birth] Dry labor caused by a diminished amount of amniotic fluid.

**xiphi-, xipho-, xiph-** Combining form meaning *sword-shaped, xiphoid.*

**xiphisternum** (zĭf″ĭ-stĕr′nŭm) [Gr. *xiphos,* sword, + *sternon,* chest] Xiphoid process.

**xiphocostal** (zĭf″ō-kŏs′tăl) [″ + L. *costa,* rib] Rel. to the xiphoid cartilage and ribs.

**xiphocostal ligament** The ligament connecting the xiphoid cartilage to the cartilage of the eighth rib.

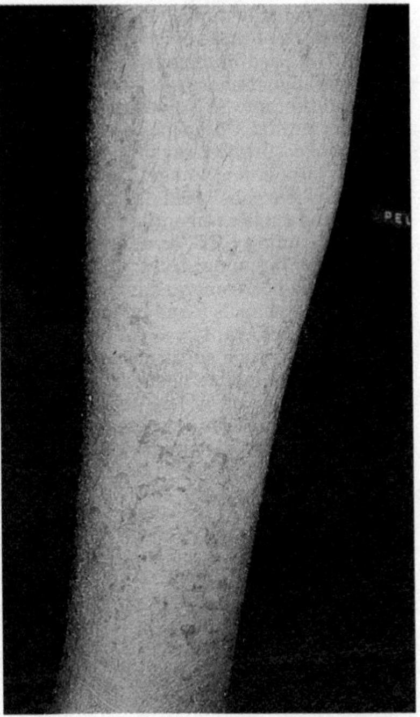

XEROSIS OF LEG

**xiphodynia** (zĭf″ō-dĭn′ē-ă) [″ + *odyne,* pain] Pain in the ensiform cartilage.

**xiphoid** (zĭf′oyd) [Gr. *xiphos,* sword, + *eidos,* form, shape] Sword-shaped. SYN: *ensiform; gladiate.*

**xiphoiditis** (zĭf″oyd-ī′tĭs) [″ + ″ + *itis,* inflammation] Inflammation of the ensiform or xiphoid cartilage.

**xiphoid process** The lowest portion of the sternum; a sword-shaped cartilaginous process supported by bone. No ribs attach to the xiphoid process; however, some abdominal muscles are attached. The xiphoid process ossifies in the aged. SYN: *xiphisternum.* SEE: *sternum* for illus.

**xiphopagotomy** (zī-fŏp″ă-gŏt′ō-mē) Surgical separation of twins joined at the xiphoid process.

**xiphopagus** (zī-fŏp′ă-gŭs) [″ + *pagos,* thing fixed] Symmetrical twins joined at the xiphoid process.

**X-linked** Denoting characteristics that are transmitted by genes on the X chromosome.

**X-linked disorder** A disease caused by genes located on the X chromosome. SEE: *choroideremia; hemophilia.*

**x radiation 1.** Electromagnetic waves or energy composed of x-rays. **2.** Treatment with or exposure to x-rays.

**x-ray photon** An uncharged particle of energy, moving in waves produced by the interaction of high-speed electrons with a target (comonly tungsten). These particles vary from those of lower energy (1 to 0.1 A.U.), used in diagnostic imaging, to those of higher energy (0.1 to $10^{-4}$ A.U.), used in therapy. SYN: *roentgen ray.*

**x-ray dermatitis** Cutaneous inflammation due to exposure to x-ray photons.

**xylene** (zī′lēn, zī-lēn′) A mixture of isomeric dimethylbenzenes used in making lacquers and rubber cement. SYN: *xylol.*

**xylene poisoning** SEE: *benzene* in *Poisons and Poisoning Appendix.*

**xylenol** (zī′lĕ-nŏl) General name for a series of dimethylphenols found in the pine-type coal tar disinfectants.

**xylitol** A five-carbon sugar alcohol that has a sweet taste and has chemical properties similar to those of sucrose. It may be used in place of sucrose as a sweetener. The use of xylitol in the diet might reduce tooth decay in children.

**xylol** (zī′lŏl) Xylene.

**xylometazoline hydrochloride** (zī″lō-mĕt″ă-zō′lēn) A vasoconstrictor used as a nasal decongestant. Trade name is Otrivin Hydrochloride.

**xylose** (zī′lōs) [Gr. *xylon,* wood] Wood sugar, a crystalline, nonfermentable pentose.

**xylulose** (zī′lū-lōs) A pentose sugar present in nature as L-xylulose. It appears in the urine in essential pentosuria and in the form of D-xylulose.

**xylyl** (zī′lĭl) A radical, $CH_3C_6H_4CH_2$—, formed by the removal of a hydrogen atom from xylene.

**xyrospasm** (zī′rō-spăzm) [Gr. *xyron,* razor, + *spasmos,* a convulsion] An occupational spasm or neurosis involving the fingers and arms; seen in barbers.

**xyster** (zĭs′tĕr) [Gr., scraper] Raspatory.

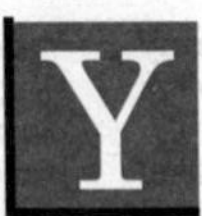

**Y** Symbol for the element yttrium.

**Yale brace** A type of head-cervical-thoracic orthosis designed to control flexion, extension and rotation of the head, and moderate restriction of lateral bending.

**Yankauer suction catheter** A rigid suction tip used to aspirate secretions from the oropharynx.

**yard** [AS. *gerd,* a rod] A measure of 3 ft or 36 in.; equal to 0.9144 m. SEE: *Weights and Measures Appendix.*

**yaw** (yaw) The primary lesion of yaws.

***mother y.*** A papilloma that is the initial lesion of yaws, occurring at the site of inoculation 3 to 4 weeks after infection. This lesion persists for several weeks or months and is painless unless there is a secondary infection. SYN: *frambesioma.*

**yawn** (yawn) [AS. *geonian*] **1.** To open the mouth involuntarily and usually take a deep breath as in drowsiness or fatigue; yawning may also be an expression of boredom. Yawning may stimulate observers to yawn. **2.** The involuntary act of gaping, accompanied by attempts at inspiration, excited by drowsiness.

**yawning** (yawn′ĭng) Deep inspiration with the mouth wide open; induced by drowsiness, boredom, or fatigue. SEE: *pandiculation.*

**yaws** (yawz) An infectious nonvenereal disease caused by a spirochete, *Treponema pertenue,* and mainly found in humid, equatorial regions. The disease is marked by febrile disturbances, rheumatism, and eruption of tubercles with a caseous crust on the hands, feet, face, and external genitals. The infection is rarely, if ever, fatal but can be disfiguring and disabling. The treatment is administration of penicillin. SYN: *frambesia; pian.*

**Yb** Symbol for the element ytterbium.

**Y cartilage** The cartilage that connects the pubis, ilium, and ischium and extends into the acetabulum.

**Y chromosome** The chromosome that determines the male sex. Normal males possess one Y chromosome and one X chromosome; normal females possess two X chromosomes. SEE: *chromosome; Lyon hypothesis.*

**Y-connector** A glass or plastic connector that divides one incoming line into two outgoing ones.

**years of life lost** The number of years a person is estimated to have remained alive if the disease experienced had not intervened.

**yeast** (yēst) [AS. *gist*] **1.** Any of several unicellular fungi of the genus *Saccharomyces,* which reproduce by budding. They are capable of fermenting carbohydrates. Yeasts, esp. *Candida albicans,* may cause systemic infections as well as vaginitis. Yeast infections are frequently present in patients with malignant lymphomas, severe diabetes mellitus, AIDS, or other conditions causing immunocompromise. SEE: illus.; *candida; candidiasis; fungi.*

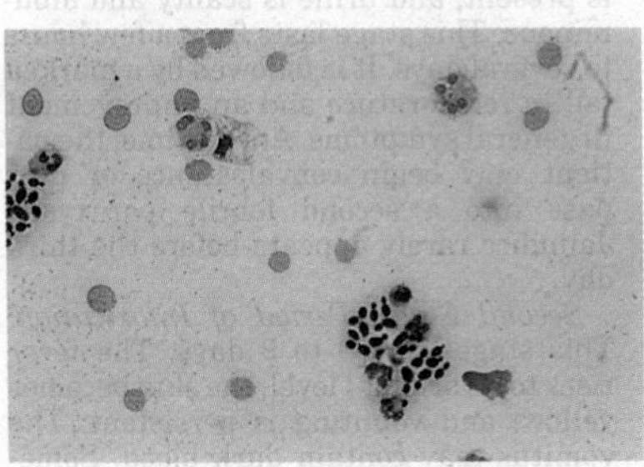

BUDDING **YEAST** IN PERITONEAL FLUID (ORIG. MAG. ×400)

**2.** A commercial product composed of meal impregnated with living yeast.

***brewer's y.*** Yeast obtained during the brewing of beer. It may be used in the dried form as a good source of vitamin B.

***dried y.*** Dried yeast cells from strains of *Saccharomyces cerevisiae.* It is used as a source of proteins and vitamins, esp. B complex.

**yellow** (yĕl′ō) [AS. *geolu*] **1.** One of the primary colors resembling that of a ripe lemon. **2.** Colored yellow, as the skin in disease.

***visual y.*** SEE: *visual yellow.*

**yellow body** The corpus luteum.

**yellow fever** An acute infectious viral disease characterized by jaundice, epigastric tenderness, vomiting, hemorrhages, and a febrile course consisting of two paroxysms.

There are two forms of yellow fever: urban, in which the transmission cycle is mosquito to human to mosquito; and sylvan, in which the reservoir is wild primates. Also, in sylvan yellow fever, the mosquito will remain infected for life.

Except for a few cases in Trinidad in 1954, urban yellow fever has not been reported in North or South America since 1942. Outbreaks do occur in parts of Africa near rain forests. Yellow fever has not been reported in Asia or the eastern coast of Africa. Sylvan yellow fever is enzootic in South America and parts of Africa.

In general, the disease is erroneously thought to be minor with respect to the number of annual cases. Further study has revealed that the true incidence is usually underestimated.

SYMPTOMS: *First Stage:* The disease, which has an incubation period of 3 to 6 days, begins with the sudden onset of fever, sometimes accompanied by a chill, followed by head, back, and limb pain, nausea, and vomiting. The temperature rises rapidly until it reaches its maximum 103° to 105°F (39.4° to 40.6°C). The pulse may be slow and weak (Faget's sign). The face is flushed, conjunctivae are injected, and the pupils are small. Gastroenteritis is present, and urine is scanty and albuminous. This stage lasts from a few hours to several days. It is followed by a marked fall in temperature and an improvement in general symptoms. At this time, the patient may begin convalescence or may pass into a second febrile paroxysm. Jaundice rarely appears before the third day.

*Second Stage, Period of Intoxication:* This stage lasts 3 to 9 days. The fever rises to its original level, the skin becomes yellow, and vomiting is persistent. The vomitus may contain dark blood. Sometimes hemorrhages occur from other mucous membranes. The pulse is rapid but not in proportion to the fever. Urine becomes very scanty and contains albumin and casts. Death frequently results from exhaustion or uremia, although recovery may follow the gravest symptoms.

ETIOLOGY: The virus of yellow fever, genus *Flavivirus,* Flaviviridae family, is usually transmitted by the bite of a female mosquito, *Aedes aegypti.* However, in Africa, other species of *Aedes* are responsible for the spread of this virus between monkeys and humans.

DIAGNOSIS: Diagnosis on clinical grounds alone is almost impossible during the period of infection or in atypical mild forms. Yellow fever viral antigen or antibodies may be detected during the acute phase of the illness.

PROPHYLAXIS: Preventive measures include mosquito control by screening, spraying with nontoxic insecticides, and destruction of breeding areas. Yellow fever vaccine prepared from the 17D strain is available for those who plan to travel or live in areas where the disease is endemic. The vaccine is contraindicated in the first 4 months of life and the first trimester of pregnancy.

TREATMENT: Although there is no specific therapy, absolute rest in a cool, well-ventilated room; a liquid diet; and vitamin K and calcium gluconate for hemorrhagic tendency are recommended. Dehydration and electrolyte balance must be controlled by appropriate intravenous fluid replacement therapy. Parenteral fluids containing 10% to 20% glucose should be given to prevent fluid overload. Transfusion may be required. Heparin may be required if disseminated intravascular coagulation occurs. Dopamine may be required to maintain blood pressure in cases that do not respond to fluid administration. Fever is controlled by cool applications. Analgesics are given for pain.

PROGNOSIS: The prognosis is always grave. Mortality is 5% for natives of an area where the disease is endemic.

**yellow ointment** An ointment containing yellow wax and petrolatum.

**yellow spot 1.** The yellow nodule of the anterior end of the vocal cord. SYN: *macula flava laryngis.* **2.** The center of the retina, the point of clearest vision. SYN: *macula lutea retinae.*

**yellow vision** A condition in which objects seem yellow in color. SYN: *xanthopsia.*

**Yersinia** (yĕr-sĭn′ē-ă) [Alexandre Emil Jean Yersin, Swiss bacteriologist who worked in Paris, 1863–1943] A genus of gram-negative bacteria.

***Y. enterocolitica*** A species of large coccobacilli that are pathogenic for humans. Clinical infections may be characterized by acute mesenteric lymphadenitis or enterocolitis. The disease may progress to a septicemic form in children, and mortality may be as high as 50%. Therapy with trimethoprim-sulfamethoxazole, aminoglycosides, tetracycline, third-generation cephalosporin, or quinolones is effective.

***Y. pestis*** The causative organism of plague; formerly termed *Pasteurella pestis.*

***Y. pseudotuberculosis*** A gram-negative coccoid or ovoid organism that produces pseudotuberculosis in humans.

**yersiniosis** (yĕr-sĭn″ē-ō′sĭs) Infection with *Yersinia* organisms.

**yin-yang** The Chinese symbol of opposing but complementary entities or concepts such as light-dark, male-female, and sun-moon. In Chinese philosophy and medicine, the goal is to have a proper balance of such biological forces. Applied to contemporary biology, this would embody a feedback type of control of physiological phenomena. SEE: illus.

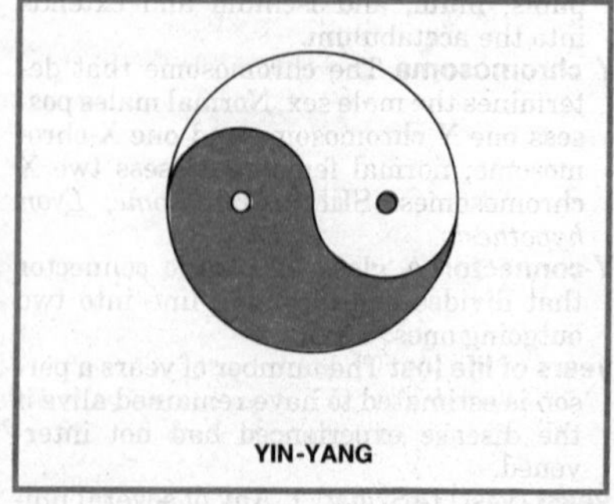

YIN-YANG

**-yl** [Gr. *hyle,* matter, substance] Suffix signifying a radical in chemistry.

**-ylene** Suffix denoting a bivalent hydrocarbon radical in chemistry.

**Y ligament** A Y-shaped band covering the upper and anterior portions of the hip joint. Also called *iliofemoral ligament*.

**yoga** [Sanskrit, union] A system of beliefs and practices, the goal of which is to attain a union of the individual self with Supreme Reality or the Universal Self. The term yoga, as used in the Western world, has been associated almost exclusively with physical postures and regulation of breathing. These are yoga exercises but not yoga in the spiritual sense.

**yogurt, yoghurt** (yōg′hŭrt) [Turkish] A form of curdled milk; the curdling is caused by action of *Lactobacillus bulgaricus*. Extensive but unsubstantiated claims have been made concerning the therapeutic value of yogurt for various ailments. Yogurt may be of benefit in persons with lactase deficiency. SEE: *milk*.

**yohimbine** (yō-hĭm′bēn) A poisonous alkaloid derived from the bark of the tree *Corynanthe yohimbi*. It is an alpha-adrenergic blocking agent that causes antidiuresis, increased blood pressure, tachycardia, irritability, tremor, sweating, dizziness, nausea, and vomiting.

**yoke** (yōk) A tissue connecting two structures.

**yolk** (yōk) [AS. *geolca*] The contents of the ovum; sometimes only the nutritive portion. SYN: *vitellus*. SEE: *zona pellucida*.

***y. sac*** In mammals, the embryonic membrane that is the site of formation of the first red blood cells and the cells that will become oogonia or spermatogonia. SEE: *embryo* for illus.

***y. stalk*** The umbilical duct connecting the yolk sac with the embryo.

**Young-Helmholtz theory** (yŭng-hĕlm′hōlts) [Thomas Young, Brit. physician, 1773–1829; Hermann Ludwig Ferdinand von Helmholtz, Ger. physician, 1821–1894] The theory that color vision depends on three different sets of retinal fibers responsible for perception of red, green, and violet. The loss of red, green, or violet as color perceptive elements in the retina causes an inability to perceive a primary color or any color of which it forms a part.

**Young's rule** (yŭngz) [Thomas Young] A method previously used for calculating the dose of a drug appropriate for administration to a child. No such rule is adequate to guarantee the efficacy and safety of a dose of a drug used for pediatric patients, esp. newborns. The dose used should be based on pharmacokinetic data for a given age group and adjusted in accordance with each individual's ability to handle the drug.

**youth** (yooth) [AS. *geoguth*] The period between childhood and maturity.

In some modern societies, there is a fascination with being young or with avoiding becoming old. Thus, a large industry has developed to provide potions, pills, and devices promoted to prevent aging.

**ypsiliform** (ĭp-sĭl′ĭ-form) Y-shaped.

**y.s.** *yellow spot* of the retina.

**ytterbium** (ĭ-tŭr′bē-ŭm) SYMB: Yb. A rare metallic earth element used in screens in radiography; atomic weight, 173.04; atomic number, 70.

**yttrium** (ĭt′rē-ŭm) SYMB: Y. A metallic element; atomic weight, 88.905; atomic number, 39.

**yushi** Minamata disease.

# Z

**Z 1.** Ger. *Zuckung,* contraction. **2.** Symbol for atomic number.

**z** *zero; zone.*

**Z-79 Committee of the American National Standards Institute** A committee that develops standards for anesthetic and ventilatory equipment. The label "Z-79" signifies that a device meets the established standard.

**Zaglas' ligament** (ză′glŭs) The part of the posterior sacroiliac ligament from the posterosuperior spinous process of the ilium to the side of the sacrum.

**Zahn's line** (zŏnz) [Frederick W. Zahn, Ger. pathologist, 1845–1904] One of the transverse whitish marks on the free surface of a thrombus made by the edges of the lamellae of blood platelets.

**Zang's space** (zăngz) [Christoph B. Zang, Ger. surgeon, 1772–1835] The space between the two lower tendons of the sternomastoid muscle in the supraclavicular fossa.

**Zaroxolyn** Trade name for metolazone.

**Zavanelli maneuver** In obstetrics, the manual return of the head of a partially born fetus with intractable shoulder dystocia to the vagina. This is followed by cesarean section.

**Z disk** A thin, dark disk that transversely bisects the I band (isotropic band) of a striated muscle fiber. The thin filaments, made primarily of actin, are attached to the Z disk; the area between the two Z disks is a sarcomere, the unit of contraction. SYN: *Krause's membrane.*

**zea** Maize or corn.

**zeatin** (zē′ă-tĭn) A cytotoxin that can be isolated from sweet corn.

**zeaxanthin** (zē″ă-zăn′thĭn) A carotenoid that is an isomer of xanthophyll. It is present in a great number of plants and animals.

**zein** (zē′ĭn) [Gr. *zeia,* a kind of grain] A protein obtained from maize. It is deficient in tryptophan and lysine.

**Zeis' gland** [Eduard Zeis, Ger. ophthalmologist, 1807–1868] One of the sebaceous glands of the eyelid, close to the free edge of the lid. Each gland is associated with an eyelash. SEE: *Moll's glands.*

**zeisian** (zī′sē-ăn) Pert. to something originally described by Eduard Zeis.

**zeitgeber** [German *zeitgeber,* timekeeper] Any of the mechanisms in nature that keep internal biological clocks synchronized (entrained) with the environment. Zeitgebers can be physical, involving light or temperature (e.g., sunrise, sunset), or social, involving regular activities (e.g., consistent mealtimes).

**zeitgeist** [German] The spirit of the people, or trend of thought at a particular time.

**zelotypia** (zē″lō-tĭp′ē-ă) [Gr. *zelos,* zeal, + *typtein,* to strike] **1.** Morbid or monomaniacal zeal in the interest of any project or cause. **2.** Insane jealousy.

**Zenker, Friedrich Albert von** (zĕng′kĕr) German pathologist, 1825–1898.

***Z.'s degeneration*** A glassy or waxy hyaline degeneration of skeletal muscles in acute infectious diseases, esp. in typhoid. SYN: *zenkerism.*

***Z.'s diverticulum*** Herniation of the mucous membrane of the esophagus through a defect in the wall of the esophagus. The location is usually in the posterior hypopharyngeal wall. Small diverticuli are asymptomatic. Large ones trap food and cause halitosis. Also they may cause esophageal obstruction and dysphagia. Treatment is surgical. SYN: *hypopharyngeal diverticulum.*

**zenkerism** (zĕng′kĕr-ĭzm) Zenker's degeneration.

**Zenker's fluid** [Konrad Zenker, 19th-century Ger. histologist] A tissue fixative consisting of mercuric chloride, potassium dichromate, glacial acetic acid, and water. It is used to examine cells, and particularly nuclei, in detail.

**zero** (zē′rō) [It.] **1.** Corresponding to nothing. SYMB: 0. **2.** The point from which the graduation figures of a scale commence.

On the Celsius scale, zero (0°) is the temperature of melting ice, equivalent to 32° on the Fahrenheit scale. To obtain this fixed point, the thermometer is immersed in melting ice, and when the mercury column ceases to fall, the level at which it remains is fixed as 0° on the C and as 32° on the F scale. SEE: *thermometer.*

***absolute z.*** The temperature at which all atoms and molecules cease movement or at which all gases liquefy: −273.15°C or −459.67°F.

***limes z.*** SYMB: L0. The greatest amount of toxin that, when mixed with one unit of antitoxin and injected into a guinea pig weighing 250 g, will cause no local edema.

**zero population growth** ABBR: ZPG. The demographic condition when in a given period of time the population neither increases nor decreases.

**zero-sum game** A game in which the sum of the wins is equal to the sum of the losses.

**zestocausis** (zĕs″tō-kŏw′sĭs) [Gr. *zestos,* boiling hot, + *kausis,* burning] Cauterization with a tube containing heated steam.

**zidovudine** An antiviral medicine used in treating AIDS. It was formerly called azidothymidine.

**Ziehl-Neelsen method** (zēl-nēl′sĕn) [Franz Ziehl, Ger. bacteriologist, 1857–1926; Friedrich Karl Adolf Neelsen, Ger. pathologist, 1854–1894] A method for staining *Mycobacterium tuberculosis*. A solution of carbolfuchsin is applied, which the organism retains after rinsing with acid alcohol.

**Zieve's syndrome** [L. Zieve, U.S. physician, b. 1915] Hyperlipidemia, jaundice, hemolytic anemia, and abdominal pain following the intake of a large amount of alcoholic beverages.

**ZIFT** *zygote intrafallopian transfer*.

**Zim jar opener** Trademarked name for a variety of devices allowing one-handed opening of bottles and jars for persons with disability.

**zinc** (zĭnk) [L. *zincum*] SYMB: Zn. A bluish-white, crystalline metallic element that boils at 906°C; atomic weight, 65.37; atomic number, 30; specific gravity, 7.13. It is found as a carbonate and silicate, known as calamine, and as a sulfide (blende). Sources are meat, including liver; eggs; seafood; and, to a lesser extent, grain products.

FUNCTION: Zinc is an essential dietary element for animals, including humans. It is involved in most metabolic pathways. The recommended dietary allowance is 10 to 15 mg of zinc daily for adults, 19 mg daily during the first 6 months of pregnancy, and 5 mg daily for infants.

DEFICIENCY SYMPTOMS: Loss of appetite, growth retardation, hypogonadism and dwarfism, skin changes, immunological abnormalities, altered rate of wound healing, and impaired taste characterize this condition. Zinc deficiency during pregnancy may lead to developmental disorders in the child.

***z. acetate*** White, pearly crystals; used as an astringent and antiseptic, chiefly in eye solutions, in a 0.1% to 0.5% solution.

***z. bacitracin*** SEE: *bacitracin, zinc*.

***z. cadmium sulfide*** A fluorescent material used in radiographic screens.

***z. carbonate*** A mild astringent used topically in dusting powders.

***z. chloride*** A white granular powder used as an antiseptic.

***z. gelatin*** A combination of zinc oxide, glycerin, and purified water. This smooth jelly is placed between layers of gauze dressing to serve as a protective dressing and to support varicosities. It is removed by soaking in warm water.

***z. oxide*** A very fine white powder of zinc. It is slightly antiseptic and astringent and is used chiefly in the form of ointment containing 20% zinc oxide. SYN: *white z.*

***z. oxide and eugenol*** Two substances that react together to produce a relatively hard mass, used in dentistry for impression material, cavity liners, temporary restorations, and cementing layers.

***z. salts*** A bluish-white metal used to make various containers and also to galvanize iron to prevent rust. The most commonly used compounds are zinc oxide as a pigment for paints and ointments. The salts also are used as a wood preservative, in soldering, in medicine to neutralize tissue, and in dilute solutions as an astringent and emetic. SEE: *zinc salts poisoning*.

***z. stearate*** A very fine smooth powder used as a nonirritating antiseptic and astringent for burns, scalds, and abrasions.

***z. sulfate*** An astringent agent used as a 0.25% solution for temporary relief of minor eye irritation.

***z. undecylenate*** An antifungal agent used in treating fungal infection of the feet.

***white z.*** Z. oxide.

**zinc-eugenol cement** A cement and protectant used in dentistry. SEE: *zinc oxide and eugenol*.

**zinciferous** (zĭng-kĭf′ĕr-ŭs) Containing zinc.

**zinc salts poisoning** A poisoning caused by zinc ingestion, characterized by metallic taste with prompt burning of the mouth, throat, esophagus, and stomach. There is violent vomiting, often bloody; increased salivation; painful diarrhea; and coma. If the patient recovers, neurologic complications are frequent. First aid treatment involves washing out the stomach and treating the patient as for sulfuric acid ingestion. SEE: *Poisons and Poisoning Appendix*.

**Zinn's ligament** (zĭnz) [Johann G. Zinn, Ger. anatomist, 1727–1759] Connective tissue giving attachment to the rectus muscles of the eyeball. SEE: *zonule of Zinn*.

**zipper pull** An adaptive device allowing persons with limited function to fasten zippers on clothing, esp. those in back.

**zirconium** (zĭr-kō′nē-ŭm) SYMB: Zr. A metallic element found only in combination; atomic weight, 91.22; atomic number, 40. It is used in corrosion-resistant alloys and as a white pigment in dental porcelain and other ceramics.

**Zn** Symbol for the element zinc.

**zoacanthosis** (zō″ăk-ăn-thō′sĭs) Dermatitis due to foreign bodies such as bristles, hairs, or stingers from animals.

**zoanthropy** (zō-ăn′thrō-pē) [Gr. *zoon*, animal, + *anthropos*, man] The delusion that one is an animal.

**Zollinger-Ellison syndrome** [Robert M. Zollinger, 1903–1992; Edwin H. Ellison, 1918–1970, U.S. surgeons] A condition caused by non–insulin-secreting pancreatic tumors, which secrete excess amounts of gastrin. This stimulates the stomach to secrete great amounts of hydrochloric acid and pepsin, which in turn leads to peptic ulceration of the stomach and small intestine. About 60% of the tumors are malignant. Total gastrectomy and local excision of the pancreatic tumor should be performed if metastases have not appeared.

**zona** (zō′nă) *pl.* **zonae** [L., a girdle] **1.** A band or girdle. **2.** Herpes zoster.

***z. ciliaris*** Ciliary zone.

***z. facialis*** Herpes zoster of the face.

***z. fasciculata*** The adrenal cortex.

***z. glomerulosa*** The outer layer of the adrenal cortex just inside the capsule.

***z. ophthalmica*** Old name for herpes zoster of the area supplied by the ophthalmic nerve.

***z. pellucida*** The inner, solid, thick, membranous envelope of the ovum. It is pierced by many radiating canals, giving it a striated appearance. SYN: *z. radiata; z. striata; membrane, vitelline.*

***z. radiata*** Z. pellucida.

***z. reticularis*** The inner layer of the cortex of the adrenal gland.

***z. striata*** Z. pellucida.

**zonae** Pl. of zona.

**zonal** (zō′năl) [L. *zonalis*] Pert. to a zone.

**zonary** (zō′năr-ē) [L. *zona,* a girdle] Pert. to or shaped like a zone.

**zonary placenta** Placenta arranged in the form of a broad ring around the chorion.

**Zondek-Aschheim test** (zŏn′dĕk-ăsh′hīm) [Bernhardt Zondek, Ger.-born Israeli obstetrician-gynecologist, 1891–1966; Selmar Aschheim, Ger. gynecologist, 1878–1965] A test for pregnancy by injecting the patient's urine subcutaneously into immature female mice.

**zone** (zōn) [L. *zona,* a girdle] An area or belt.

***cell-free z.*** In dentistry, an area below the odontoblastic layer of the dental pulp that has relatively few cells; also called the *zone of Weil.*

***cell-rich z.*** The area of increased cell frequency between the cell-free zone and the central pulp of the tooth.

***chemoreceptor trigger z.*** ABBR: CTZ. A zone in the medulla that is sensitive to certain chemical stimuli. Stimulation of this zone may produce nausea.

***ciliary z.*** The peripheral part of the anterior surface of the iris of the eye.

***comfort z.*** The range of temperature, humidity, and, when applicable, solar radiation and wind in which an individual doing work at a specified rate and in a certain specified garment is comfortable.

***epileptogenic z.*** Any area of the brain that after stimulation produces an epileptic seizure.

***erogenous z.*** An area of the body that may produce erotic desires when stimulated. These areas include, but are not limited to, the breasts, lips, genital and anal regions, buttocks, and sometimes the special senses that cause sexual excitation, such as the sense of smell or taste.

***H z.*** H band.

***hypnogenic z., hypnogenous z.*** Any area of the body that, when pressed on, induces hypnosis.

***lung z.*** Any of four regions of the lung, differentiated by the hemodynamic conditions acting on blood flow. They include the middle, intermediate, and lowest regions, and all areas where alveolar pressure equals or exceeds pulmonary arterial pressure.

***transitional z.*** The area of the lens of the eye where the epithelial capsule cells change into lens fibers.

**zonesthesia** (zōn″ĕs-thē′zē-ă) [″ + *aisthesis,* sensation] A sensation, as a cord constricting the body. SYN: *sensation, cincture; girdle pain.*

**zonifugal** (zō-nĭf′ū-găl) [″ + *fugere,* to flee] Passing outward from within any zone or area.

**zoning** The occurrence of a stronger fixation of complement in a lesser amount of suspected serum; a phenomenon occasionally observed in diagnosing syphilis by the complement-fixation method.

**zonipetal** (zō-nĭp′ĕt-ăl) [″ + *petere,* to seek] Passing from outside into a zone or area of the body.

**zonography** A type of tomography, using a tomographic angle less than 10°, that produces an image of a larger thickness of tissue. This technique is used for kidneys or structures lacking inherent contrast.

**zonoskeleton** (zōn″ō-skĕl′ĕ-tŏn) The proximal bones to which limbs attach, such as the hip bone, scapula, and clavicle.

**zonula** (zōn′ū-lă) [L.] A small zone. SYN: *zonule.*

***z. adherens*** The portion of the junctional complex between columnar epithelial cells below the zonula occludens where there is an intercellular space of about 200 A.U. and the cellular membranes are supported by filamentous material.

***z. ciliaris*** The suspensory ligament of the crystalline lens. SYN: *zonule of Zinn.*

***z. occludens*** The portion of the junctional complex between columnar epithelial cells just below the free surface where the intercellular space is obliterated. Also called *tight junction.*

**zonular** (zōn′ū-lăr) Pert. to a zonula.

**zonular cataract** A cataract with opacity limited to certain layers of the lens.

**zonular fiber** One of the interlacing fibers of the zonula ciliaris.

**zonular space** A space between the fibers of the ligaments of the lens.

**zonule** (zōn′ūl) [L. *zonula,* small zone] A small band or area. SYN: *zonula.*

***z. of Zinn*** Zonula ciliaris.

**zonulitis** (zōn-ū-lī′tĭs) [″ + Gr. *itis,* inflammation] Inflammation of the zonule of Zinn.

**zonulolysis** (zŏn″ū-lŏl′ĭ-sĭs) [″ + Gr. *lysis,* dissolution] The use of enzymes to dissolve the zonula ciliaris of the eye. SYN: *zonulysis.*

**zonulotomy** (zŏn″ū-lŏt′ō-mē) [″ + Gr. *tome,* incision] Surgical incision of the ciliary zonule.

**zonulysis** (zŏn″ū-lī′sĭs) Zonulolysis.

**zoo-** Combining form meaning *animal, animal life.*

**zoobiology** (zō″ō-bī-ŏl′ō-jē) [Gr. *zoon,* animal, + *bios,* life, + *logos,* word, reason] The biology of animals.

**zoochemistry** (zō″ō-kĕm′ĭs-trē) Biochemistry of animals.

**zooerasty** (zō″ō-ē′răs-tē) Bestiality.

**zoofulvin** (zō″ō-fŭl′vĭn) A yellow pigment derived from certain animal feathers.

**zoogenous** (zō-ŏj′ĕn-ŭs) [″ + *gennan,* to produce] Derived or acquired from animals.

**zoogeny** (zō″ŏj′ĕ-nē) [″ + *gennan,* to produce] The development and evolution of animals.

**zoogeography** (zō″ō-jē-ŏg′ră-fē) The study of the distribution of animals on the earth.

**zooglea** (zō″ō-glē′ă) [″ + *gloios,* sticky] A stage in development of certain organisms in which colonies of microbes are embedded in a gelatinous matrix.

**zoograft** (zō′ō-grăft) [″ + L. *graphium,* stylus] A graft of tissue obtained from an animal.

**zoografting** (zō″ō-grăft′ĭng) The use of animal tissue in grafting on a human body.

**zooid** (zō′oyd) [″ + *eidos,* form, shape] **1.** Resembling an animal. **2.** A form resembling an animal; an organism produced by fission. **3.** An animal cell that can move or exist independently.

**zoolagnia** (zō″ō-lăg′nē-ă) [″ + *lagneia,* lust] Sexual desire for animals.

**zoologist** (zō-ŏl′ō-jĭst) [″ + *logos,* word, reason] A biologist who specializes in the study of animal life.

**zoology** (zō-ŏl′ō-jē) The science of animal life.

**zoom lens** A type of lens that can be adjusted to focus on near or distant objects.

**zoomania** (zō″ō-mā′nē-ă) [Gr. *zoon,* animal, + *mania,* madness] A morbid and excessive affection for animals.

**Zoomastigophora** A class of unicellular organisms within the phylum Sarcomastigophora. These organisms usually have one or more flagella but these may be absent in certain amoebae. It includes free-living and parasitic species such as *Giardia lamblia.*

**zoonosis** (zō-ō-nō′sĭs) *pl.* **zoonoses** [″ + *nosos,* disease] A disease communicable from animals to humans. Over 250 organisms are known to cause zoonotic infections, of which 30 to 40 spread from pets and animals used by the blind and deaf. Patients with AIDS are esp. at risk of developing zoonoses.

**zoonotic** (zō″ō-nŏt′ĭk) Concerning zoonoses.

**zooparasite** (zō″ō-păr′ă-sīt) [″ + *para,* beside, + *sitos,* food] An animal parasite.

**zoopathology** (zō″ō-păth-ŏl′ō-jē) [″ + *pathos,* disease, + *logos,* word, reason] The science of the diseases of animals.

**zoophilia** The preference for obtaining sexual gratification by having intercourse or other sexual activity with animals.

**zoophile** (zō′ō-fīl) [″ + *philein,* to love] **1.** One who likes animals. **2.** An antivivisectionist.

**zoophilism** (zō-ŏf′ĭl-ĭzm) [″ + ″ + *-ismos,* condition] An abnormal love of animals.

**zoophobia** (zō″ō-fō′bē-ă) [″ + *phobos,* fear] An abnormal fear of animals.

**zoophyte** (zō′ō-fīt) [″ + *phyton,* plant] A plantlike animal; any of numerous invertebrate animals resembling plants in appearance or mode of growth.

**zooplankton** (zō″ō-plănk′tŏn) [″ + *planktos,* wandering] A small animal organism present in natural waters. SEE: *phytoplankton.*

**zoopsia** (zō-ŏp′sē-ă) [″ + *opsis,* vision] Hallucinations involving animals. SYN: *zooscopy* (1).

**zoopsychology** (zō″ō-sī-kŏl′ō-jē) Animal psychology.

**zoosadism** (zō″ō-sā′dĭzm) The act of being sadistic to animals.

**zooscopy** (zō-ŏs′kō-pē) [″ + *skopein,* to examine] **1.** Zoopsia. **2.** The scientific observation of animals.

**zoosmosis** (zō″ŏs-mō′sĭs) [Gr. *zoe,* life, + *osmos,* impulsion] The process of living protoplasm passing into the tissues from blood vessels.

**zoospore** (zō′ō-spor) [″ + *sporos,* seed] A motile asexual spore that moves by means of one or more flagella.

**zoosterol** (zō″ō-stē′rŏl) Any sterol derived from animals.

**zootechnics** (zō″ō-tĕk′nĭks) [Gr. *zoon,* animal, + *techne,* art] The complete care, management, and breeding of domestic animals.

**zootic** (zō-ŏt′ĭk) Concerning animals.

**zootomy** (zō-ŏt′ō-mē) [″ + *tome,* incision] Dissection of animals.

**zootoxin** (zō″ō-tŏks′ĭn) [″ + *toxikon,* poison] Any toxin or poison produced by an animal (e.g., snake venom).

**zootrophic** (zō″ō-trŏf′ĭk) [″ + *trophe,* nutrition] Concerning animal nutrition.

**zoster** (zŏs′tĕr) [Gr. *zoster,* girdle] Herpes zoster.

***z. auricularis*** Herpes zoster of the ear.

***z. ophthalmicus*** Herpes zoster affecting the ophthalmic nerve.

**zosteroid** (zŏs′tĕr-oyd) [″ + *eidos,* form, shape] Resembling herpes zoster.

**ZPG** *zero population growth.*

**Z-plasty** A technique with a Z-shaped incision used in plastic surgery to relieve tension in scar tissue. The area under tension is lengthened at the expense of the surrounding elastic tissue. SEE: illus.; *tissue expansion; W-plasty.*

**Zr** Symbol for the element zirconium.

**Z-track** An injection technique in which the surface (skin and subcutaneous) tissues are pulled and held to one side before insertion of the needle deep into the muscle in the identified site. The medication is injected slowly, followed by a 10-sec delay; then the needle is removed, and the tissues are quickly permitted to resume their normal position. This provides a Z-shaped track, which makes it difficult for the injected irritating drug to seep back

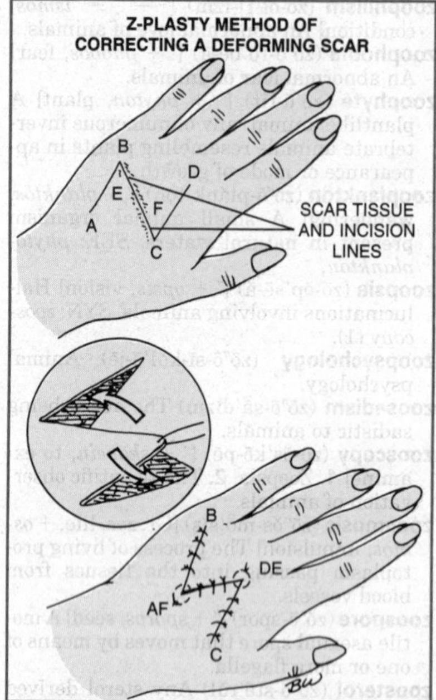


into subcutaneous tissues.

**zwitterion** (tsvĭt′ĕr-ī″ŏn) A dipolar ion that contains positive and negative charges of equal strength. This ion is therefore not attracted to either an anode or cathode. In a neutral solution, amino acids function as zwitterions.

**zygal** (zī′găl) [Gr. *zygon,* yoke] Concerning or shaped like a yoke.

**zygapophyseal** (zī″gă-pō-fĭz′ē-ăl) Concerning a zygapophysis.

**zygapophysis** (zī″gă-pŏf′ĭ-sĭs) [″ + *apo,* from, + *physis,* growth] One of the articular processes of the neural arch of a vertebra.

**zygion** (zĭj′ē-ŏn) *pl.* **zygia** [Gr. *zygon,* yoke] The craniometrical point on the zygoma at either end of the bizygomatic diameter.

**zygocyte** Zygote.

**zygodactyly** (zī″gō-dăk′tĭl-ē) [″ + *daktylos,* digit] Syndactylism.

**zygoma** (zī-gō′mă) [Gr., cheekbone] **1.** The long arch that joins the zygomatic processes of the temporal and malar bones on the sides of the skull. **2.** The malar bone.

**zygomatic** (zī″gō-măt′ĭk) Pert. to the zygoma.

**zygomatic arch** The formation, on each side of the cheeks, of the zygomatic process of each malar bone articulating with the zygomatic process of the temporal bone.

**zygomatic bone** The bone on either side of the face below the eye. SYN: *malar bone.*

**zygomaticoauricularis** (zī″gō-măt″ĭ-kō-ăw-rĭk″ū-lā′rĭs) [L.] The muscle that draws the pinna of the ear forward. SEE: *Muscles Appendix.*

**zygomaticofacial** (zī″gō-măt″ĭ-kō-fā′shăl) Concerning the zygoma and face.

**zygomaticofrontal** (zī″gō-măt″ĭ-kō-frŏn′tăl) Concerning the zygoma and frontal bone of the face.

**zygomaticomaxillary** (zī″gō-măt″ĭ-kō-măk′sĭ-lĕr″ē) Concerning the zygoma and maxilla.

**zygomatico-orbital** (zī″gō-măt″ĭ-kō-or′bĭ-tăl) Concerning the zygoma and orbit of the eye.

**zygomaticosphenoid** (zī″gō-măt″ĭ-kō-sfē′noyd) Concerning the zygoma and sphenoid bone.

**zygomaticotemporal** (zī″gō-măt″ĭ-kō-tĕm′por-ăl) Concerning the zygoma and temporal bone.

**zygomatic process 1.** A thin projection from the temporal bone bounding its squamous portion. **2.** A part of the malar bone helping to form the zygoma.

**zygomatic reflex** The movement of the lower jaw toward the percussed side when the zygoma is percussed.

**zygomaticum** (zī″gō-măt′ĭ-kŭm) [L.] The zygomatic bone.

**zygomaticus** (zī″gō-măt′ĭk-ŭs) [L.] A muscle that draws the upper lip upward and outward. SEE: *Muscles Appendix.*

**zygomaxillary** (zī″gō-măks′ĭl-ār-ē) [Gr. *zygoma,* cheekbone, + L. *maxilla,* jawbone] Pert. to the cheekbone and upper jaw.

**zygomaxillary point** A craniometrical point marked at the lower end of the zygomatic suture.

**Zygomycetes** A class of fungi that includes those which cause mucormycosis and entomophthoramycosis.

**zygomycosis** Fungal infections caused by various species including those involved in mucormycosis and entomophthoramycosis.

**zygon** (zī′gŏn) [Gr.] The short crossbar connecting the parallel limbs of a cerebral fissure.

**zygopodium** (zī″gō-pō′dē-ŭm) The intermediate-distal portion of a limb, such as the ulna and radius, and the tibia and fibula.

**zygosis** (zī-gō′sĭs) [Gr. *zygosis,* a balancing] The sexual union of two unicellular animals.

**zygosity** (zī-gŏs′ĭ-tē) [Gr. *zygon,* yoke] Concerning zygosis.

**zygosperm** (zī′gō-spĕrm) Zygospore.

**zygospore** (zī′gō-spor) A spore formed by fusion of morphologically identical structures. SYN: *zygosperm.*

**zygote** (zī′gōt) [Gr. *zygotos,* yoked] The cell produced by the union of two gametes; the fertilized ovum. SYN: *oosperm; zygocyte.*

**zygote intrafallopian transfer** SEE: under *transfer.*

**zygotene** (zī′gō-tēn) [Gr. *zygotos,* yoked] The second stage of the prophase of the first meiotic division. During this stage, the homologous chromosomes pair side by side. SEE: *cell division.*

**zygotic** (zī-gŏt′ĭk) Concerning a zygote.

**zygotoblast** (zī-gō′tō-blăst) [″ + *blastos,*

germ] Sporozoite.

**zygotomere** (zī-gō'tō-mēr) [" + *meros,* part] Sporoblast.

**zymase** (zī'mās) [Gr. *zyme,* leaven, + *-ase,* enzyme] Any of a group of enzymes that, in the presence of oxygen, convert certain carbohydrates into carbon dioxide and water or, in the absence of oxygen, into alcohol and carbon dioxide or lactic acid. It is found in yeast, bacteria, and higher plants and animals. SEE: *enzyme, fermenting.*

**zymic** (zī'mĭk) Concerning enzymes.

**zymogen** (zī'mō-jĕn) [" + *gennan,* to produce] A substance that develops into a chemical ferment or enzyme. It exists in an inactive form antecedent to the active enzyme. SYN: *proenzyme.* SEE: *pepsinogen; trypsinogen.*

**zymogene** (zī'mō-jēn) A microbe causing fermentation.

**zymogen granule** A secretory granule of a pre-enzyme substance seen in cells of synthetic organs such as salivary glands or the pancreas.

**zymogenic** (zī"mō-jĕn'ĭk) **1.** Causing a fermentation. **2.** Pert. to or producing a zymogen. SYN: *zymogenous.*

**zymogenous** (zī-mŏj'ĕ-nŭs) Zymogenic.

**zymogram** (zī'mō-grăm) An electrophoretic graph of the separation of the enzymes in a solution.

**zymohexase** (zī"mō-hĕk'sās) The enzyme involved in splitting fructose 1,6-diphosphate into dihydroxyacetone phosphate and phosphoglyceric aldehyde.

**zymologist** (zī-mŏl'ō-jĭst) One who specializes in the study of ferments.

**zymology** (zī-mŏl'ō-jē) The science of fermentation.

**zymolysis** (zī-mŏl'ĭ-sĭs) [Gr. *zyme,* leaven, + *lysis,* dissolution] The changes produced by an enzyme; the action of enzymes. SYN: *fermentation.*

**zymolyte** (zī'mō-līt") Substrate.

**zymolytic** (zī"mō-lĭt'ĭk) [" + *lytikos,* dissolved] Causing fermentation; fermentative.

**zymometer** (zī-mŏm'ĕ-tĕr) [" + *metron,* measure] A device for measuring fermentation.

**Zymonema** (zī"mō-nē'mă) [" + *nema,* thread] A genus of fungi.

**zymoprotein** (zī"mō-prō'tē-ĭn) Any protein that also functions as an enzyme.

**zymosan** (zī'mō-săn) An anticomplement obtained from the walls of yeast cells.

**zymose** (zī'mōs) Invertase.

**zymosterol** (zī-mŏs'tĕr-ŏl) A sterol obtained from yeast.

**zymotic** (zī-mŏt'ĭk) Rel. to or produced by fermentation.

**Z.Z.'Z."** Symbol for increasing strengths of contraction.

# Appendices

## Table of Contents

# Index to Appendices

# APPENDIX 1
# Universal Precautions

## Appendix 1–1 OSHA Bloodborne Pathogens Standard

### WHO IS COVERED?

The Occupational Safety and Health Administration (OSHA) standard protects employees who may be occupationally exposed to blood and other potential infectious materials, which includes but is not limited to physicians, nurses, phlebotomists, emergency medical personnel, operating room personnel, therapists, orderlies, laundry workers, and other health care workers.

Blood means human blood, blood products, or blood components. Other potentially infectious materials include human body fluids such as saliva in dental procedures, semen, vaginal secretions; cerebrospinal, synovial, pleural, pericardial, peritoneal, and amniotic fluids; body fluids visibly contaminated with blood; unfixed human tissues or organs; HIV-containing cell or tissue cultures; and HIV- or HBV-containing culture mediums or other solutions.

Occupational exposure means a "reasonably anticipated skin, eye, mucous membrane, or parenteral contact with blood or other potentially infectious materials that may result from the performance of the employee's duties."

Federal OSHA authority extends to all private sector employers with one or more employees, as well as federal civilian employees. In addition, many states administer their own occupational safety and health programs through plans approved under section 18(b) of the OSH Act. These plans must adopt standards and enforce requirements that are at least as effective as federal requirements. Of the current 25 state plan states and territories, 23 cover the private and public (state and local governments) sectors and 2 cover the public sector only.

Determining occupational exposure and instituting control methods and work practices appropriate for specific job assignments are key requirements of the standard. The required written exposure control plan and methods of compliance show how employee exposure can be minimized or eliminated.

### THE EXPOSURE CONTROL PLAN

A written exposure control plan is necessary for the safety and health of workers. At a minimum, the plan must include the following:

- Identify job classifications where there is exposure to blood or other potentially infectious materials.
- Explain the protective measures currently in effect in the acute care facility and/or a schedule and methods of compliance to be implemented, including hepatitis B vaccination and post-exposure follow-up procedures; how hazards are communicated to employees; personal protective equipment; housekeeping; and recordkeeping.
- Establish procedures for evaluating the circumstances of an exposure incident.

The schedule of how and when the provisions of the standard will be implemented may be a simple calendar with brief notations describing the compliance methods, an annotated copy of the standard, or a part of another document, such as the infection control plan.

The written exposure control plan must be available to workers and OSHA representatives and updated at least annually or whenever changes in procedures create new occupational exposures.

### WHO HAS OCCUPATIONAL EXPOSURE?

The exposure determination must be based on the definition of occupational exposure **without regard to personal protective clothing and equipment.** Exposure determination begins by reviewing job classifications of employees within the work environment and then making a list divided into two groups: job classifications in which **all** of the employees have occupational exposure, and those classifications in which **some** of the employees have occupational exposure.

Where **all** employees are occupationally exposed, it is not necessary to list specific work tasks. Some examples include phlebotomists, lab technicians, physicians, nurses, nurse's aides, surgical technicians, and emergency room personnel.

Where only **some** of the employees have exposure, specific tasks and procedures causing exposure must be listed. Examples include ward clerks or secretaries who occasionally handle blood or infectious specimens, and housekeeping staff who may be exposed to contaminated objects and/or environments some of the time.

When employees with occupational exposure have been identified, the next step is to communicate the hazards of the exposure to the employees.

## COMMUNICATING HAZARDS TO EMPLOYEES

The initial training for current employees must be scheduled within 90 days of the effective date of the bloodborne pathogens standard, at no cost to the employee, and during working hours.[1] Training also is required for new workers at the time of their initial assignment to tasks with occupational exposure or when job tasks change, causing occupational exposure, and annually thereafter.

Training sessions must be comprehensive in nature, including information on bloodborne pathogens as well as on OSHA regulations and the employer's exposure control plan. The person conducting the training must be knowledgeable in the subject matter as it relates to acute care facilities.

Specifically, the training program must do the following:

1. Explain the regulatory text and make a copy of the regulatory text accessible.
2. Explain the epidemiology and symptoms of bloodborne diseases.
3. Explain the modes of transmission of bloodborne pathogens.
4. Explain the employer's written exposure control plan.
5. Describe the methods to control transmission of HBV and HIV.
6. Explain how to recognize occupational exposure.
7. Inform workers about the availability of free hepatitis B vaccinations, vaccine efficacy, safety, benefits, and administration.
8. Explain the emergency procedures for and reporting of exposure incidents.
9. Inform workers of the post-exposure evaluation and follow-up available from health care professionals.
10. Describe how to select, use, remove, handle, decontaminate, and dispose of personal protective clothing and equipment.
11. Explain the use and limitations of safe work practices, engineering controls, and personal protective equipment.
12. Explain the use of labels, signs, and color coding required by the standard.
13. Provide a question-and-answer session on training.

In addition to communicating hazards to employees and providing training to identify and control hazards, other preventive measures also must be taken to ensure employee protection.

## PREVENTIVE MEASURES

Preventive measures such as hepatitis B vaccination, universal precautions, engineering controls, safe work practices, personal protective equipment, and housekeeping measures help reduce the risks of occupational exposure.

### Hepatitis B Vaccination

The hepatitis B vaccination series must be made available within 10 working days of initial assignment to every employee who has occupational exposure. The hepatitis B vaccination must be made available without cost to the employee, at a reasonable time and place for the employee, by a licensed health care professional,[2] and according to recommendations of the U.S. Public Health Service, including routine booster doses.[3]

The health care professional designated by the employer to implement this part of the standard must be provided with a copy of the bloodborne pathogens standard. The health care professional must provide the employer with a written opinion stating whether the hepatitis B vaccination is indicated for the employee and whether the employee has received such vaccination.

Employers are not required to offer hepatitis B vaccination (a) to employees who have previously completed the hepatitis B vaccination series, (b) when immunity is confirmed through antibody testing, or (c) if vaccine is contraindicated for medical reasons. Participation in a prescreening program is not a prerequisite for receiving hepatitis B vaccination. Employees who decline the vaccination may request and obtain it at a later date, if they continue to be exposed. Employees who decline to accept the hepatitis B vaccination must sign a declination form, indicating that they were offered the vaccination but refused it.

### Universal Precautions

The single most important measure to control transmission of HBV and HIV is to treat all human blood and other potentially infectious materials AS IF THEY WERE infectious for HBV and HIV. Application of this approach is referred to as "universal precautions." *Blood and certain body fluids from all acute care patients should be considered as potentially infectious materials.*[4] These fluids cause *contamination,* defined in the standard as "the presence or the reasonably anticipated presence of blood or other potentially infectious materials on an item or surface."

## METHODS OF CONTROL

### Engineering and Work Practice Controls

Engineering and work practice controls are the primary methods used to control the transmission of HBV and HIV in acute care facilities. Engineering controls isolate or remove the hazard from employees and are used in conjunction with work practices. Personal protective equipment also shall be used when occupational exposure to bloodborne pathogens remains even after instituting these controls. Engineering controls must be examined and maintained, or replaced, on a scheduled basis. Some engineering controls that apply to acute care facilities and are required by the standard include the following:

1. Use puncture-resistant, leak-proof containers, color-coded red or labeled, according to the standard (see table) to discard contaminated items like needles, broken glass, scalpels, or other items that could cause a cut or puncture wound.
2. Use puncture-resistant, leak-proof containers, color-coded red or labeled to store contaminated reusable sharps until they are properly reprocessed.
3. Store and process reusable contaminated sharps in a way that ensures safe handling. For example, use a mechanical device to retrieve used instruments from soaking pans in decontamination areas.
4. Use puncture-resistant, leak-proof containers to collect, handle, process, store, transport, or ship blood specimens and potentially infectious materials. Label these specimens if shipped outside the facility. Labeling is not required when specimens are handled by employees trained to use universal precautions with all specimens and when these specimens are kept within the facility.

Similarly, work practice controls reduce the likelihood of exposure by altering the manner in which the task is performed. All procedures shall minimize splashing, spraying, splattering, and generation of droplets. Work practice requirements include the following:

1. Wash hands when gloves are removed and as soon as possible after contact with blood or other potentially infectious materials.
2. Provide and make available a mechanism for immediate eye irrigation, in the event of an exposure incident.
3. Do not bend, recap, or remove contaminated needles unless required to do so by specific medical procedures or the employer can demonstrate that no alternative is feasible. In these instances, use mechanical means such as forceps, or a one-handed technique to recap or remove contaminated needles.
4. Do not shear or break contaminated needles.
5. Discard contaminated needles and sharp instruments in puncture-resistant, leak-proof, red or biohazard-labeled containers[5] that are accessible, maintained upright, and not allowed to be overfilled.
6. Do not eat, drink, smoke, apply cosmetics, or handle contact lenses in areas of potential occupational exposure. (Note: use of hand lotions is acceptable.)
7. Do not store food or drink in refrigerators or on shelves where blood or potentially infectious materials are present.
8. Use red, or affix biohazard labels to, containers to store, transport, or ship blood or other potentially infectious materials, such as lab specimens. (See figure below.)
9. Do not use mouth pipetting to suction blood or other potentially infectious materials; **it is prohibited.**

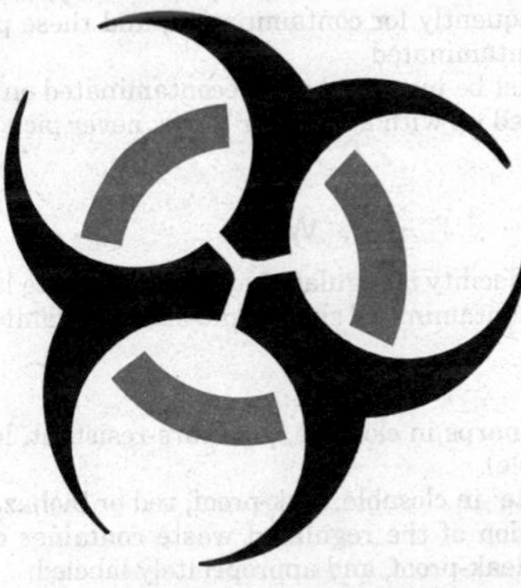

BIOHAZARD SYMBOL

## Personal Protective Equipment

In addition to instituting engineering and work practice controls, the standard requires that appropriate personal protective equipment be used to reduce worker risk of exposure. Personal protective equipment is specialized clothing or equipment used by employees to protect against direct exposure to blood or other potentially infectious materials. Protective equipment must not allow blood or other potentially infectious materials to pass through to workers' clothing, skin, or mucous membranes. Such equipment includes, but is not limited to, gloves, gowns, laboratory coats, face shields or masks, and eye protection.

The employer is responsible for providing, maintaining, laundering, disposing, replacing, and assuring the proper use of personal protective equipment. The employer is responsible for ensuring that workers have access to the protective equipment, at no cost, including proper sizes and types that take allergic conditions into consideration.

An employee may temporarily and briefly decline to wear personal protective equipment **under rare and extraordinary circumstances** and when, in the employee's professional judgment, it prevents the delivery of health care or public safety services or poses an increased or life-threatening hazard to employees. In general, **appropriate personal protective equipment is expected to be used whenever occupational exposure may occur.**

The employer also must ensure that employees observe the following precautions for safely handling and using personal protective equipment:

1. Remove all personal protective equipment immediately following contamination and upon leaving the work area, and place in an appropriately designated area or container for storing, washing, decontaminating, or discarding.
2. Wear appropriate gloves when contact with blood, mucous membranes, non-intact skin, or potentially infectious materials is anticipated; when performing vascular access procedures;[6] and when handling or touching contaminated items or surfaces.
3. Provide hypoallergenic gloves, liners, or powderless gloves or other alternatives to employees who need them.
4. Replace disposable, single-use gloves as soon as possible when contaminated, or if torn, punctured, or barrier function is compromised.
5. Do not reuse disposable (single-use) gloves.
6. Decontaminate reusable (utility) gloves after each use and discard if they show signs of cracking, peeling, tearing, puncturing, deteriorating, or failing to provide a protective barrier.
7. Use full face shields or face masks with eye protection, goggles, or eyeglasses with side shields when splashes of blood and other bodily fluids may occur and when contamination of the eyes, nose, or mouth can be anticipated (e.g., during invasive and surgical procedures).
8. Also wear surgical caps or hoods and/or shoe covers or boots when gross contamination may occur, such as during surgery and autopsy procedures.

**Remember: The selection of appropriate personal protective equipment depends on the quantity and type of exposure expected.**

## Housekeeping Procedures

### Equipment

The employer must ensure a clean and sanitary workplace. Contaminated work surfaces must be decontaminated with a disinfectant upon completion of procedures or when contaminated by splashes, spills, or contact with blood, other potentially infectious materials, and at the end of the work shift. Surfaces and equipment protected with plastic wrap, foil, or other nonabsorbent materials must be inspected frequently for contamination; and these protective coverings must be changed when found to be contaminated.

Waste cans and pails must be inspected and decontaminated on a regularly scheduled basis. Broken glass should be cleaned up with a brush or tongs; never pick up broken glass with hands, even when wearing gloves.

### Waste

Waste removed from the facility is regulated by local and state laws. Special precautions are necessary when disposing of contaminated sharps and other contaminated waste, and include the following:

1. Dispose of contaminated sharps in closable, puncture-resistant, leak-proof, red or biohazard-labeled containers (see table).
2. Place other regulated waste[7] in closable, leak-proof, red or biohazard-labeled bags or containers. If outside contamination of the regulated waste container occurs, place it in a second container that is closable, leak-proof, and appropriately labeled.

## LABELING REQUIREMENTS

| *Item* | *No Label Needed If Universal Precautions Are Used and Specific Use of Container Is Known to All Employees* | | *Biohazard Label* | | *Red Container* |
|---|---|---|---|---|---|
| Regulated waste container (e.g., contaminated sharps containers) | | | X | or | X |
| Reusable contaminated sharps container (e.g., surgical instruments soaking in a tray) | | | X | or | X |
| Refrigerator/freezer holding blood or other potentially infectious material | | | X | | |
| Containers used for storage, transport, or shipping of blood | | | X | or | X |
| Blood/blood products for clinical use | X | | | | |
| Individual specimen containers of blood or other potentially infectious materials remaining in facility | X | or | X | or | X |
| Contaminated equipment needing service (e.g., dialysis equipment, suction apparatus) | | | X Plus a label specifying where the contamination exists | | |
| Specimens and regulated waste shipped from the primary facility to another facility for service or disposal | | | X | or | X |
| Contaminated laundry | * | or | X | or | X |
| Contaminated laundry sent to another facility that does not use universal precautions | | | X | or | X |

* Alternative labeling or color coding is sufficient if it permits all employees to recognize the containers as requiring compliance with universal precautions.

### Laundry

Laundering contaminated articles, including employee lab coats and uniforms meant to function as personal protective equipment, is the responsibility of the employer. Contaminated laundry shall be handled as little as possible with minimum agitation. This can be accomplished through the use of a washer and dryer in a designated area on-site, or the contaminated items can be sent to a commercial laundry. The following requirements should be met with respect to contaminated laundry:

1. Bag contaminated laundry as soon as it is removed and store in a designated area or container.
2. Use red laundry bags or those marked with the biohazard symbol unless universal precautions are in effect in the facility and all employees recognize the bags as contaminated and have been trained in handling the bags.
3. Clearly mark laundry sent off-site for cleaning, by placing it in red bags or bags clearly marked with the orange biohazard symbol; and use leak-proof bags to prevent soak-through.
4. Wear gloves or other protective equipment when handling contaminated laundry.

## WHAT TO DO IF AN EXPOSURE INCIDENT OCCURS

An exposure incident is the specific eye, mouth or other mucous membrane, non-intact skin, parenteral contact with blood or other potentially infectious materials that results from the performance of an employee's duties. An example of an exposure incident would be a puncture from a contaminated sharp.

The employer is responsible for establishing the procedure for evaluating exposure incidents.

When evaluating an exposure incident, immediate assessment and confidentiality are critical issues. Employees should immediately report exposure incidents to enable timely medical evaluation and follow-up by a health care professional as well as a prompt request by the employer for testing of the source individual's blood for HIV and HBV. The "source individual" is any patient whose blood or body fluids are the source of an exposure incident to the employee.

At the time of the exposure incident, the exposed employee must be directed to a health care professional. The employer must provide the health care professional with a copy of the bloodborne pathogens standard; a description of the employee's job duties as they relate to the incident; a report of the specific exposure, including route of exposure; relevant employee medical records, including hepatitis B vaccination status; and results of the source individual's blood tests, if available. At that time, a baseline blood sample should be drawn from the employee, if he/she consents. If the employee elects to delay HIV testing of the sample, the health care professional must preserve the employee's blood sample for at least 90 days.[8]

Testing the source individual's blood does not need to be repeated if the source individual is known to be infectious for HIV or HBV; and testing cannot be done in most states without written consent.[9] The results of the source individual's blood tests are confidential. As soon as possible, however, the test results of the source individual's blood must be made available to the exposed employee through consultation with the health care professional.

Following post-exposure evaluation, the health care professional will provide a written opinion to the employer. This opinion is limited to a statement that the employee has been informed of the results of the evaluation and told of the need, if any, for any further evaluation or treatment. The employer must provide a copy of the written opinion to the employee within 15 days. This is the only information shared with the employer following an exposure incident; all other employee medical records are confidential.

All evaluations and follow-up must be available at no cost to the employee and at a reasonable time and place, performed by or under the supervision of a licensed physician or another licensed health care professional, such as a nurse practitioner, and according to recommendations of the U.S. Public Health Service guidelines current at the time of the evaluation and procedure. In addition, all laboratory tests must be conducted by an accredited laboratory and at no cost to the employee.

## RECORDKEEPING

There are two types of records required by the bloodborne pathogens standard: medical and training.

A medical record must be established for each employee with occupational exposure. **This record is confidential and separate from other personnel records.** This record may be kept on-site or may be retained by the health care professional who provides services to employees. The medical record contains the employee's name, social security number, hepatitis B vaccination status, including the dates of vaccination and the written opinion of the health care professional regarding the hepatitis B vaccination. If an occupational exposure occurs, reports are added to the medical record to document the incident and the results of testing following the incident. The post-evaluation written opinion of the health care professional is also part of the medical record. The medical record also must document what information has been provided to the health care provider. Medical records must be maintained 30 years past the last date of employment of the employee.

Emphasis is on confidentiality of medical records. No medical record or part of a medical record should be disclosed without direct, written consent of the employee or as required by law.

Training records document each training session and are to be kept for 3 years. Training records must include the date, content outline, trainer's name and qualifications, and names and job titles of all persons attending the training sessions.

If the employer ceases to do business, medical and training records are transferred to the successor employer. If there is no successor employer, the employer must notify the Director of the National Institute for Occupational Safety and Health, U.S. Department of Health and Human Services, for specific directions regarding disposition of the records at least 3 months prior to disposal.

Upon request, both medical and training records must be made available to the Assistant Secretary of Labor of Occupational Safety and Health. Training records must be available to employees upon request. Medical records can be obtained by the employee or anyone having the employee's written consent.

Additional recordkeeping is required for employers with 11 or more employees (see OSHA's "Recordkeeping Guidelines for Occupational Injuries and Illnesses" for more information).

## OTHER SOURCES OF OSHA ASSISTANCE

### Consultation Programs

Consultation assistance is available to employers who want help in establishing and maintaining a safe and healthful workplace. Largely funded by OSHA, the service is provided at no cost to the employer. Primarily developed for smaller employers with more hazardous operations, the consultation service is delivered by state government agencies or universities employing professional safety consultants and health consultants. Comprehensive assistance includes an appraisal of all mechanical, physical work practice, and environmental hazards of the workplace and all aspects of the employer's present job safety and health program. No penalties are proposed or citations issued for hazards identified by the consultant.

### Voluntary Protection Programs

Voluntary protection programs (VPPs) and on-site consultation services, when coupled with an effective enforcement program, expand worker protection to help meet the goals of the OSH Act. The three VPPs—Star, Merit, and Demonstration—are designed to recognize outstanding achievement by companies that have successfully incorporated comprehensive safety and health programs into their total management system. They motivate others to achieve excellent safety and health results in the same outstanding way, and they establish a cooperative relationship between employers, employees, and OSHA.

### Training and Education

OSHA's area offices offer a variety of informational services, such as publications, audiovisual aids, technical advice, and speakers for special engagements. Each regional office has a bloodborne pathogens coordinator to assist employers.

OSHA's Training Institute in Des Plaines, IL, provides basic and advanced courses in safety and health for federal and state compliance officers, state consultants, federal agency personnel, and private sector employers, employees, and their representatives.

OSHA also provides funds to nonprofit organizations, through grants, to conduct workplace training and education in subjects where OSHA believes there is a lack of workplace training. Current grant subjects include agricultural safety and health, hazard communication programs, and HIV and HBV. Grants are awarded annually, with a 1-year renewal possible. Grant recipients are expected to contribute 20 percent of the total grant cost.

For more information on grants, and training and education, contact the OSHA Training Institute, Office of Training and Education, 1555 Time Drive, Des Plaines, IL 60018, (708) 297-4810.

For more information on AIDS, contact the Centers for Disease Control National AIDS Clearinghouse, (800) 458-5231.

---

[1] Employees who received training in the year preceding the effective date of the standard need only receive training pertaining to any provisions not already included.

[2] Licensed health care professional is a person whose legally permitted scope of practice allows him or her to perform independently the activities required under paragraph (f) of the standard regarding hepatitis B vaccination and post-exposure and follow-up.

[3] Health care professionals can call the Centers for Disease Control disease information hotline (404) 332-4555, extension 234, for updated information on hepatitis B vaccination.

[4] SEE ALSO: "Recommendations for Prevention of HIV Transmission in Health-Care Settings," *MMWR* (36) 2S: August 21, 1987.

[5] Biohazard labeling requires a fluorescent orange or orange-red label with the biological hazard symbol as well as the word **Biohazard** in contrasting color affixed to the bag or container.

[6] Phlebotomists in volunteer blood donation centers are exempt in certain circumstances. See section (d)(3)(ix)(D) of the standard for specific details.

[7] Liquid or semiliquid blood or other potentially infectious materials; items contaminated with these fluids and materials, which could release these substances in a liquid or semiliquid state, if compressed; items caked with dried blood or other potentially infectious materials that are capable of releasing these materials during handling; contaminated sharps; and pathological and microbiological wastes containing blood or other potentially infectious materials.

[8] If, during this time, the employee elects to have the baseline sample tested, testing shall be performed as soon as feasible.

[9] If consent is not obtained, the employer must show that legally required consent could not be obtained. Where consent is not required by law, the source individual's blood, if available, should be tested and the results documented.

SOURCE: Bloodborne Pathogens and Acute Care Facilities (OSHA 3128), Occupational Safety and Health Administration, Washington, DC, 1992.

# Appendix 1–2 CDC Isolation Precautions

## BACKGROUND AND SUMMARY

In January 1996, the Centers for Disease Control and Prevention (CDC) issued new guidelines for isolation precautions in hospitals. The guidelines, based on the latest epidemiologic information on transmission of infection in hospitals, are intended primarily for use in acute-care hospitals, although some of the recommendations may be applicable to subacute-care or extended-care facilities. The recommendations are not intended for use in day care, well care, or domiciliary care programs.

The revised guidelines contain two tiers of precautions. In the first, and most important, tier are those precautions designed for the care of all patients in hospitals regardless of their diagnosis or presumed infection status. Implementation of these "Standard Precautions" is the primary strategy for successful nosocomial infection control. In the second tier are precautions designed only for the care of specified patients. These additional "Transmission-Based Precautions" are used for patients known or suspected to be infected or colonized with epidemiologically important pathogens that can be transmitted by airborne or droplet transmission or by contact with dry skin or contaminated surfaces.

**Standard Precautions** synthesize the major features of Universal (Blood and Body Fluid) Precautions (designed to reduce the risk of transmission of bloodborne pathogens) and Body Substance Isolation (designed to reduce the risk of transmission of pathogens from moist body substances). Standard Precautions apply to (1) blood; (2) all body fluids, secretions, and excretions *except sweat,* regardless of whether they contain visible blood; (3) nonintact skin; and (4) mucous membranes. Standard Precautions are designed to reduce the risk of transmission of both recognized and unrecognized sources of infection in hospitals.

**Transmission-Based Precautions** are designed for patients documented or suspected to be infected or colonized with highly transmissible or epidemiologically important pathogens for which additional precautions beyond Standard Precautions are needed to interrupt transmission in hospitals. There are three types of Transmission-Based Precautions: *Airborne Precautions, Droplet Precautions,* and *Contact Precautions.* They may be combined for diseases that have multiple routes of transmission. When used either singly or in combination, they are to be used in addition to Standard Precautions.

**Airborne Precautions** are designed to reduce the risk of airborne transmission of infectious agents. Airborne transmission occurs by dissemination of either airborne droplet nuclei (small-particle residue [5 microns or smaller in size] of evaporated droplets that may remain suspended in the air for long periods of time) or dust particles containing the infectious agent. Microorganisms carried in this manner can be dispersed widely by air currents and may become inhaled by or deposited on a susceptible host within the same room or over a longer distance from the source patient, depending on environmental factors; therefore, special air handling and ventilation are required to prevent airborne transmission. Examples of diseases spread by airborne droplet nuclei include measles, varicella (including disseminated zoster), and tuberculosis.

**Droplet Precautions** are designed to reduce the risk of droplet transmission of infectious agents. Droplet transmission involves contact of the conjunctivae or the mucous membranes of the nose or mouth of a susceptible person with large-particle droplets (larger than 5 microns in size) containing microorganisms generated from a person who has a clinical disease or who is a carrier of the microorganism. Droplets are generated from the source person primarily during coughing, sneezing, or talking and during the performance of certain procedures such as suctioning and bronchoscopy. Transmission via large-particle droplets requires close contact between source and recipient persons, because droplets do not remain suspended in the air and generally travel only short distances, usually 3 ft or less, through the air. Because droplets do not remain suspended in the air, special air handling and ventilation are not required to prevent droplet transmission.

Examples of illnesses spread by large-particle droplets include invasive *Haemophilus influenzae* type B disease (including meningitis, pneumonia, epiglottitis, and sepsis); invasive *Neisseria meningitidis* disease (including meningitis, pneumonia, and sepsis); diphtheria (pharyngeal); mycoplasma pneumonia; pertussis; pneumonic plague; streptococcal pharyngitis, pneumonia, or scarlet fever in infants and young children; adenovirus, influenza; mumps; parvovirus B19; and rubella.

**Contact Precautions** are designed to reduce the risk of transmission of epidemiologically important microorganisms by direct or indirect contact. Direct-contact transmission involves skin-to-skin contact and physical transfer of microorganisms to a susceptible host from an infected or colonized person, such as occurs when personnel turn patients, bathe patients, or perform other patient-care activities that require physical contact. Direct-contact transmission can also occur between two patients (e.g., by hand contact), with one serving as the source of infectious microorganisms and the other as a susceptible host. Indirect-contact transmission involves contact of a susceptible host with a contaminated intermediate object, usually inanimate, in the patient's environment.

Examples of illnesses spread by direct contact include gastrointestinal, respiratory, skin, or wound infections or colonization with multidrug-resistant bacteria judged by the infection control program (based on current state, regional, or national recommendations) to be of special clinical and epidemiologic significance; enteric infections with a low infectious dose or prolonged environmental survival, including *Clostridium difficile;* for diapered or incontinent patients: enterohemorrhagic *Escherichia coli* O157:H7, *Shigella,* hepatitis A, or rotavirus; respiratory syncytial virus, parainfluenza virus, or enteroviral infections in infants and young children; viral/hemorrhagic conjunctivitis; viral hemorrhagic infections (Ebola, Lassa, or Marburg); and skin infections that are highly contagious or that may occur on dry skin, including:

Diphtheria (cutaneous)
Herpes simplex virus (neonatal or mucocutaneous)
Impetigo
Major (noncontained) abscesses, cellulitis, or decubiti
Pediculosis
Scabies
Staphylococcal furunculosis in infants and young children
Zoster (disseminated or in the immunocompromised host)

## STANDARD PRECAUTIONS

Use the following Standard Precautions, or the equivalent, for the care of all patients.

- **Handwashing:**
  1. Wash hands after touching blood, body fluids, secretions, excretions, and contaminated items, whether or not gloves are worn. Wash hands immediately after gloves are removed, between patient contacts, and when otherwise indicated to avoid transfer of microorganisms to other patients or environments. It may be necessary to wash hands between tasks and procedures on the same patient to prevent cross-contamination of different body sites.
  2. Use a plain (nonantimicrobial) soap for routine handwashing.
  3. Use an antimicrobial agent or a waterless antiseptic agent for specific circumstances (e.g., control of outbreaks or hyperendemic infections), as defined by the infection control program. (See Contact Precautions for additional recommendations on using antimicrobial and antiseptic agents.)
- **Gloves:** Wear gloves (clean, nonsterile gloves are adequate) when touching blood, body fluids, secretions, excretions, and contaminated items. Put on clean gloves just before touching mucous membranes and nonintact skin. Change gloves between tasks and procedures on the same patient after contact with material that may contain a high concentration of microorganisms. Remove gloves promptly after use, before touching noncontaminated items and environmental surfaces, and before going to another patient, and wash hands immediately to avoid transfer of microorganisms to other patients or environments.
- **Mask, Eye Protection, Face Shield:** Wear a mask and eye protection or a face shield to protect mucous membranes of the eyes, nose, and mouth during procedures and patient-care activities that are likely to generate splashes or sprays of blood, body fluids, secretions, and excretions.
- **Gown:** Wear a gown (a clean, nonsterile gown is adequate) to protect skin and to prevent soiling of clothing during procedures and patient-care activities that are likely to generate splashes or sprays of blood, body fluids, secretions, or excretions. Select a gown that is appropriate for the activity and amount of fluid likely to be encountered. Remove a soiled gown as promptly as possible, and wash hands to avoid transfer of microorganisms to other patients or environments.
- **Patient-Care Equipment:** Handle used patient-care equipment soiled with blood, body fluids, secretions, and excretions in a manner that prevents skin and mucous membrane exposures, contamination of clothing, and transfer of microorganisms to other patients and environments. Ensure that reusable equipment is not used for the care of another patient until it has been cleaned and reprocessed appropriately. Ensure that single-use items are discarded properly.
- **Environmental Control:** Ensure that the hospital has adequate procedures for the routine care, cleaning, and disinfection of environmental surfaces, beds, bedrails, bedside equipment, and other frequently touched surfaces, and ensure that these procedures are being followed.
- **Linen:** Handle, transport and process used linen soiled with blood, body fluids, secretions, and excretions in a manner that prevents skin and mucous membrane exposures and contamination of clothing, and that avoids transfer of microorganisms to other patients and environments.
- **Occupational Health and Bloodborne Pathogens:**
  1. Take care to prevent injuries when using needles, scalpels, and other sharp instruments or devices; when handling sharp instruments after procedures; when cleaning used instruments; and when disposing of used needles. Never recap used needles, or otherwise manipulate them using both hands, or use any other technique that involves directing the point of a needle toward any part of the body; rather, use either a one-handed "scoop" technique or a mechanical device designed for holding the needle sheath. Do not remove used needles from disposable syringes by hand, and do not bend, break, or otherwise manipulate used needle by hand. Place used disposable syringes and needles, scalpel blades, and other sharp items in appropriate puncture-resistant containers, which are located as close as practical to the area in which the items were used, and place reusable syringes and needles in a puncture-resistant container for transport to the reprocessing area.

2. Use mouthpieces, resuscitation bags, or other ventilation devices as an alternative to mouth-to-mouth resuscitation methods in areas where the need for resuscitation is predictable.

- **Patient Placement:** Place a patient who contaminates the environment or who does not (or cannot be expected to) assist in maintaining appropriate hygiene or environmental control in a private room. If a private room is not available, consult with infection control professionals regarding patient placement or other alternatives.

## TRANSMISSION-BASED PRECAUTIONS

### Airborne Precautions

In addition to Standard Precautions, use Airborne Precautions, or the equivalent, for patients known or suspected to be infected with microorganisms transmitted by airborne droplet nuclei (small-particle residue [5 microns or smaller in size] of evaporated droplets containing microorganisms that remain suspended in the air and that can be dispersed widely by air currents within a room or over a long distance).

- **Patient Placement:** Place the patient in a private room that has (1) monitored negative air pressure in relation to the surrounding areas, (2) 6–12 air changes per hour, and (3) appropriate discharge of air outdoors or monitored high-efficiency filtration of room air before the air is circulated to other areas in the hospital. Keep the room door closed and the patient in the room. When a private room is not available, place the patient in a room with a patient who has active infection with the same microorganism unless otherwise recommended, but with no other infection. When a private room is not available and cohorting is not desirable, consultation with infection control professionals is advised before patient placement.
- **Respiratory Protection:** Wear respiratory protection when entering the room of a patient with known or suspected infectious pulmonary tuberculosis. Susceptible persons should not enter the room of patients known or suspected to have measles (rubeola) or varicella (chickenpox) if other immune caregivers are available. If susceptible persons must enter the room of a patient known or suspected to have measles or varicella, they should wear respiratory protection. Persons immune to measles or varicella need not wear respiratory protection.
- **Patient Transport:** Limit the movement and transport of the patient from the room to essential purposes only. If transport or movement is necessary, minimize patient dispersal of droplet nuclei by placing a surgical mask on the patient, if possible.

#### Additional Precautions for Preventing Transmission of Tuberculosis

Consult CDC "Guidelines for Preventing the Transmission of Tuberculosis in Health-Care Facilities"[1] for additional prevention strategies.

### Droplet Precautions

In addition to Standard Precautions, use Droplet Precautions, or the equivalent, for a patient known or suspected to be infected with microorganisms transmitted by droplets (large-particle droplets [larger than 5 microns in size] that can be generated during coughing, sneezing, talking, or the performance of procedures).

- **Patient Placement:** Place the patient in a private room. When a private room is not available, place the patient in a room with a patient(s) who has active infection with the same microorganism but with no other infection (cohorting). When a private room is not available and cohorting is not achievable, maintain spatial separation of at least 3 ft between the infected patient and other patients and visitors. Special air handling and ventilation are not necessary, and the door may remain open.
- **Mask:** In addition to standard precautions, wear a mask when working within 3 ft of the patient. (Logistically, some hospitals may want to implement the wearing of a mask to enter the room.)
- **Patient Transport:** Limit the movement and transport of the patient from the room to essential purposes only. If transport or movement is necessary, minimize patient dispersal of droplets by masking the patient, if possible.

### Contact Precautions

In addition to Standard Precautions, use Contact Precautions, or the equivalent, for specified patients known or suspected to be infected or colonized with epidemiologically important microorganisms that can be transmitted by direct contact with the patient (hand or skin-to-skin contact that occurs when performing patient-care activities that require touching the patient's dry skin) or indirect contact (touching) with environmental surfaces or patient-care items in the patient's environment.

- **Patient Placement:** Place the patient in a private room. When a private room is not available, place the patient in a room with a patient(s) who has active infection with the same microorganism but with no other infection (cohorting). When a private room is not available and cohorting is not achievable, consider the epidemiology of the microorganism and the patient population when determining patient placement. Consultation with infection control professionals is advised before patient placement.

- **Gloves and Handwashing:** In addition to wearing gloves as outlined under Standard Precautions, wear gloves (clean, nonsterile gloves are adequate) when entering the room. During the course of providing care for a patient, change gloves after having contact with infective material that may contain high concentrations of microorganisms (fecal material and wound drainage). Remove gloves before leaving the patient's environment and wash hands immediately with an antimicrobial agent or a waterless antiseptic agent. After glove removal and handwashing, ensure that hands do not touch potentially contaminated environmental surfaces or items in the patient's room to avoid transfer of microorganisms to other patients or environments.
- **Gown:** In addition to wearing a gown as outlined under Standard Precautions, wear a gown (a clean, nonsterile gown is adequate) when entering the room if you anticipate that your clothing will have substantial contact with the patient, environmental surfaces, or items in the patient's room, or if the patient is incontinent or has diarrhea, an ileostomy, a colostomy, or wound drainage not contained by a dressing. Remove the gown before leaving the patient's environment. After gown removal, ensure that clothing does not contact potentially contaminated environmental surfaces to avoid transfer of microorganisms to other patients or environments.
- **Patient Transport:** Limit the movement and transport of the patient from the room to essential purposes only. If the patient is transported out of the room, ensure that precautions are maintained to minimize the risk of transmission of microorganisms to other patients and contamination of environmental surfaces or equipment.
- **Patient-Care Equipment:** When possible, dedicate the use of noncritical patient-care equipment to a single patient (or cohort of patients infected or colonized with the pathogen requiring precautions) to avoid sharing between patients. If use of common equipment or items is unavoidable, then adequately clean and disinfect them before use for another patient.

## Additional Precautions for Preventing the Spread of Vancomycin Resistance

Consult the Hospital Infection Control Practices Advisory Committee report on preventing the spread of vancomycin resistance for additional prevention strategies.[2]

---

[1] Centers for Disease Control and Prevention. Guidelines for preventing the transmission of tuberculosis in health-care facilities, 1994. *MMWR* 1994; 43 (RR-13):1–132, and *Federal Register* 1994; 59 (208):54242–54303.

[2] Hospital Infection Control Practices Advisory Committee. Recommendations for preventing the spread of vancomycin resistance. *Amer J Infect Control* 1995; 23:87–94, *Infect Control Hosp Epidemiol* 1995; 16:105–113, and *MMWR* 1995; 44 (RR-12):1–13.

SOURCE: Adapted from Garner, JS, Hospital Infection Control Practices Advisory Committee. Guidelines for isolation precautions in hospitals. *Infect Control Hosp Epidemiol* 1996; 17:53–80.

# APPENDIX 2
# Anatomy

## Appendix 2–1 Muscles

The muscles in the body number over 650, the total varying according to the authority, as some list as separate muscles what others regard as portions of adjacent muscles. Most of the muscles occur in pairs; five are single muscles.

### HEAD AND FACE

**auricularis anterior** (aw-rĭk″ū-lă′rĭs ăn-tē′rĭ-or). ACTION: Draws pinna of ear forward and upward. ORIGIN: Superficial temporal fascia. INSERTION: Helix of ear anteriorly. INNERVATION: Facial.

**auricularis posterior** (aw-rĭk″ū-lă′rĭs pŏs-tē′rē-or). ACTION: Draws pinna of ear backward. ORIGIN: Mastoid process. INSERTION: Root of auricle. INNERVATION: Facial.

**auricularis superior** (aw-rĭk″ū-lă′rĭs sū-pē′rē-or). ACTION: Elevates pinna of ear. ORIGIN: Galea aponeurotica. INSERTION: Upper portion of pinna of ear. INNERVATION: Facial.

**buccinator** (bŭk″sĭn-ā′tor). ACTION: Compresses cheek, retracts angle of mouth. ORIGIN: Alveolar process of maxilla, pterygomandibular ligament, buccinator ridge of mandible. INSERTION: Orbicularis oris. INNERVATION: Facial.

**ciliaris** (sĭl-ĭ-ā′rĭs). ACTION: Alters shape of crystalline lens in accommodation. ORIGIN: (1) Meridional: Junctions of cornea and sclera. (2) Circular: Fibers forming a circle close to iris. INSERTION: (1) External layers of choroid. (2) Ciliary process. INNERVATION: Short ciliary.

**corrugator supercilii** (kōr′ū-gā′tōr sū-pĕr-sĭl′ĭ-ī). ACTION: Draws eyebrows down and in. ORIGIN: Inner end of superciliary arch. INSERTION: Skin above orbital arch. INNERVATION: Facial.

**depressor anguli oris** (dē-prĕs′or ăng′ū-lī ō′rĭs). ACTION: Depresses angle of mouth. ORIGIN: External oblique line of mandible. INSERTION: Angle of mouth. INNERVATION: Facial.

**depressor labii inferioris** (dē-prĕs′or lā′bĭ-ī ĭn-fē″rĭ-ō′rĭs). ACTION: Draws lower lip down. ORIGIN: External oblique line of the mandible. INSERTION: Lower lip and orbicularis oris. INNERVATION: Facial.

**depressor septi nasi** (dē-prĕs′or sĕp′tī nā′sī). ACTION: Draws outer wall of nostril downward. ORIGIN: Incisive fossa of superior maxillary bone. INSERTION: Septum and ala of nose. INNERVATION: Facial.

**dilator naris anterior** (dĭl′ă-tor nā′rĭs ăn-tē′rĭ-or). ACTION: Dilates apertures of nostril. ORIGIN: Cartilage of ala of nose. INSERTION: Border of ala. INNERVATION: Facial.

**dilator naris posterior** (dĭl′ă-tor nā′rĭs pŏs-tē′rē-or). ACTION: Dilates apertures of nostril. ORIGIN: Nasal notch of superior maxilla and the sesamoid cartilages. INSERTION: Integument of margin of nostril. INNERVATION: Facial.

**levator anguli oris** (lē-vā′tor ăng′ū-lī ō′rĭs). ACTION: Elevates angle of mouth. ORIGIN: Canine fossa of maxilla. INSERTION: Angle of mouth and orbicularis oris. INNERVATION: Facial.

**levator labii superioris** (lē-vā′tor lā′bĭ-ī sū-pē″rē-ŏ′rĭs). ACTION: Elevates and extends upper lip. ORIGIN: Lower margin of orbit, malar bone. INSERTION: Upper lip. INNERVATION: Infraorbital branch of facial.

**levator labii superioris alaeque nasi** (lē-vā′tor lā′bĭ-ī sū-pē″rē-ō′rĭs ā-lē′kwĕ nā′sī). ACTION: Elevates upper lip, dilates nostril. ORIGIN: Nasal process of maxilla. INSERTION: Cartilage of ala of nose and upper lip. INNERVATION: Infraorbital branch of facial.

**levator palpebrae superioris** (lē-vā′tor păl′pē-brē sū-pē″rē-ō′rĭs). ACTION: Raises upper eyelid. ORIGIN: Lesser wing of the sphenoid bone. INSERTION: Upper tarsal cartilage. INNERVATION: Oculomotor.

**masseter** (mă-sē′tĕr). ACTION: Raises mandible. ORIGIN: Zygomatic arch and malar process of superior maxilla. INSERTION: Angle of ramus and coronoid process of mandible. INNERVATION: Mandibular division of trigeminal.

**mentalis** (mĕn-tā′lĭs). ACTION: Elevates and protrudes lower lip, wrinkles skin of chin. ORIGIN: Incisive fossa of mandible. INSERTION: Integument of chin. INNERVATION: Facial.

**nasalis** (nā-sā′lĭs). Consists of transverse and alar parts. ACTION: Depresses cartilaginous part of nose and draws the alae medially. ORIGIN: Maxilla. INSERTION: Bridge of nose. INNERVATION: Buccal branches of facial.

**obliquus inferior oculi** (ŏb-lī′kwŭs ĭn-fē′rĭ-or ŏk′ū-lī). ACTION: Rotates eyeball up and out. ORIGIN: Orbital plate of superior maxillary bone. INSERTION: Sclerotic coat at right angles to insertion of rectus externus just below it. INNERVATION: Oculomotor.

**obliquus superior oculi** (ŏb-lī′kwŭs sū-pē′rē-or ŏk′ū-lī). ACTION: Rotates eyeball down and out. ORIGIN: Above optic foramen. INSERTION: By a tendon through trochlea to the sclerotic coat. INNERVATION: Trochlear.

**occipitofrontalis** (ŏk-sĭp′ĭ-tō-frŏn-tā′lĭs).

Consists of (1) occipitalis and (2) frontalis bellies. ACTION: (1) Draws scalp back. (2) Draws scalp forward, raises eyebrows. ORIGIN: (1) Occipital and temporal bones. (2) Procerus, corrugator, and orbicularis oris muscles. INSERTION: Galea aponeurotica. INNERVATION: Facial.

**orbicularis oculi** (or-bĭk″ū-lā′rĭs ŏk′ū-lī). ACTION: Closes eyelid, wrinkles forehead vertically, compresses lacrimal sac. ORIGIN: (1) *(Pars lacrimalis)* Lacrimal bone. (2) *(Pars orbitalis)* Frontal processes of maxilla and frontal bone. (3) *(Pars palpebralis)* Inner canthus. INSERTION: (1) Joins palpebral portion. (2) Encircles orbit to orbit. (3) Outer canthus. INNERVATION: Facial.

**orbicularis oris** (or-bĭk″ū-lā′rĭs ō′rĭs). ACTION: Closes lips. ORIGIN: Nasal septum and canine fossa of mandible by accessory fibers. INSERTION: Buccinator and adjacent muscles surrounding mouth. INNERVATION: Facial.

**procerus** (prō-sē′rŭs). ACTION: Draws skin of forehead down. ORIGIN: Bridge of nose. INSERTION: Skin over root of nose. INNERVATION: Facial.

**pterygoideus lateralis** (tĕr-ĭ-goyd′ē-ŭs lăt″ĕr-ā′lĭs). ACTION: Brings jaw forward, moves jaw from side to side, opens jaws. ORIGIN: (1) Outer plate of pterygoid process. (2) Great wing of sphenoid and infratemporal ridge. INSERTION: Neck of condyle of mandible. INNERVATION: Lateral pterygoid from trigeminal nerve.

**pterygoideus medialis** (tĕr-ĭ-goyd′ē-ŭs mē-dĭ-ā′lĭs). ACTION: Closes jaw by raising and advancing it. ORIGIN: Pterygoid fossa of sphenoid bone. INSERTION: Inner surface of angle of mandible. INNERVATION: Medial pterygoid from trigeminal nerve.

**rectus externus or lateralis** (rĕk′tŭs ĕks-tĕr′nŭs, lăt″ĕr-ā′lĭs). ACTION: Rotates eyeball outward. ORIGIN: Margin of sphenoidal fissure and outer margin of optic foramen. INSERTION: Sclerotic coat. INNERVATION: Abducent.

**rectus inferior** (rĕk′tŭs ĭn-fē′rĭ-or). ACTION: Rotates eyeball downward. ORIGIN: Lower margin of optic foramen. INSERTION: Sclerotic coat. INNERVATION: Oculomotor.

**rectus internus or medialis** (rĕk′tŭs ĭn-tĕr′nŭs, mē-dĭ-ā′lĭs). ACTION: Rotates eyeball inward. ORIGIN: Lower margin of optic foramen. INSERTION: Sclerotic coat. INNERVATION: Oculomotor.

**rectus superior** (rĕk′tŭs sū-pē′rē-or). ACTION: Rotates eyeball upward. ORIGIN: Upper margin of optic foramen. INSERTION: Sclerotic coat. INNERVATION: Oculomotor.

**risorius** (rĭ-sō′rĭ-ŭs). ACTION: Draws angle of mouth outward ("laughing muscle"). ORIGIN: Fascia over masseter muscle. INSERTION: Angle of mouth. INNERVATION: Facial, buccal branch.

**temporalis** (tĕm-pō-rā′lĭs). ACTION: Closes jaws. ORIGIN: Temporal fossa and temporal fascia. INSERTION: Coronoid process of lower jaw. INNERVATION: Trigeminal, mandibular division.

**zygomaticus major** (zī-gō-măt′ĭ-kŭs mā′jor). ACTION: Draws upper lip backward, upward, and outward. ORIGIN: Zygomatic bone, zygomatic arch. INSERTION: Angle of mouth. INNERVATION: Facial.

**zygomaticus minor** (zī-gō-măt′ĭ-kŭs mī′nor). ACTION: Draws the upper lip up and out. ORIGIN: Zygomatic bone behind the maxillary arch. INSERTION: Angle of mouth, orbicularis oris. INNERVATION: Facial.

## EAR

**antitragicus** (an-tī-tră′jĭ-kŭs). ORIGIN: Anterior part of antitragus. INSERTION: Opposite side at larger auricular fissure. INNERVATION: Posterior auricular branch of facial.

**helicis major and minor** (hĕl′ĭ-sĭs mā′jor, mī′nor). ACTION: Tighten the skin of auditory canal. ORIGIN: Tuberosity on helix. INSERTION: Rim of helix. INNERVATION: Auriculotemporal and posterior auricular.

**obliquus auriculae** (ŏb-lī′kwŭs aw-rĭk′ū-lē). ORIGIN: Concha of the ear. INSERTION: Fossa of antihelix. INNERVATION: Posterior auricular branch of facial.

**stapedius** (stă-pē′dĭ-ŭs). ACTION: Depresses base of the stapes. ORIGIN: Interior of pyramid. INSERTION: Neck of stapes. INNERVATION: Tympanic branch of facial.

**tensor tympani** (tĕn′sor tĭm′păn-ī). ACTION: Draws the membrana tympani tense. ORIGIN: Temporal tube, eustachian tube and canal. INSERTION: Handle of malleus. INNERVATION: Branch of mandibular through otic ganglion.

**tragicus** (tră′jĭ-kŭs). ORIGIN and INSERTION: Outer part of tragus. INNERVATION: Temporal branch of facial.

**transversus auriculae** (trăns-vĕr′sŭs aw-rĭk′ū-lē). ACTION: Retracts helix. ORIGIN: Cranial surface of pinna. INSERTION: Circumference of pinna. INNERVATION: Posterior auricular branch of facial.

## NECK

**constrictor pharyngis inferior** (kŏn-strĭk′tor făr-ĭn′jĭs ĭn-fē′rĭ-or). ACTION: Narrows pharynx, as in swallowing. ORIGIN: Sides of cricoid and thyroid cartilage. INSERTION: Posterior raphe of pharyngeal wall. INNERVATION: Pharyngeal plexus.

**constrictor pharyngis medius** (kŏn-strĭk′tor făr-ĭn′jĭs mē′dē-ŭs). ACTION: Narrows pharynx, as in swallowing. ORIGIN: Both cornua of hyoid bone and stylohyoid ligament. INSERTION: Middle of posterior pharyngeal wall. INNERVATION: Pharyngeal plexus.

**constrictor pharyngis superior** (kŏn-strĭk'tor făr-ĭn'jĭs sū-pē'rē-or). ACTION: Narrows pharynx, as in swallowing. ORIGIN: Internal pterygoid plate, pterygomandibular ligament, jaw, side of tongue. INSERTION: Posterior pharyngeal wall. INNERVATION: Pharyngeal plexus.

**digastricus** (dī-găs'trĭ-kŭs). Consists of (1) anterior and (2) posterior bellies. ACTION: (1) Draws hyoid bone forward. (2) Draws hyoid bone backward. ORIGIN: (1) Lower border of lower jaw. (2) Mastoid groove of temporal bone. INSERTION: Intermediate tendon between both bellies. INNERVATION: (1) Mylohyoid. (2) Facial.

**genioglossus** (jē-nē"ō-glŏs'ŭs). ACTION: Protrudes and retracts tongue, elevates hyoid. ORIGIN: Inner surface of symphysis of mandible. INSERTION: Hyoid and bottom of tongue. INNERVATION: Hypoglossal.

**geniohyoideus** (jē-nē"ō-hī-oyd'ē-ŭs). ACTION: Elevates and advances hyoid and helps to depress jaw. ORIGIN: Mental spine of inferior maxilla. INSERTION: Hyoid. INNERVATION: Hypoglossal.

**glossopalatinus** (glŏs"ō-păl-ă-tī'nŭs). ACTION: Elevates back of tongue and constricts fauces. ORIGIN: Undersurface of soft palate. INSERTION: Side of tongue. INNERVATION: Pharyngeal plexus.

**hyoglossus** (hī"ō-glŏs'ŭs). ACTION: Depresses side of tongue and retracts tongue. ORIGIN: Cornua and body of hyoid. INSERTION: Side of tongue. INNERVATION: Hypoglossal.

**levator veli palatini** (lē-vā'tor vē'lī păl"ă-tī'nī). ACTION: Elevates soft palate. ORIGIN: Petrous portion of temporal bone and cartilaginous eustacian tube. INSERTION: Aponeurosis of soft palate. INNERVATION: Pharyngeal plexus.

**linguae** (lĭng-gwē). ACTION: Elevates sides and center of tongue. ORIGIN: Undersurface of tongue. INSERTION: Edge of tongue. INNERVATION: Hypoglossal.

**longus capitis** (lŏng'ŭs kăp'ĭ-tĭs). ACTION: Flexes head. ORIGIN: Transverse processes of 3rd to 6th cervical vertebrae. INSERTION: Occipital bone, basilar process. INNERVATION: Branches of 1st to 3rd cervical nerves.

**longus colli** (lŏng'ŭs kōl'ī). Consists of three parts: (1) superior oblique, (2) inferior oblique, and (3) vertical. ACTION: Twists and bends neck forward. ORIGIN: (1) Transverse processes of 3rd to 5th cervical vertebrae. (2) Bodies of 1st to 3rd thoracic vertebrae. (3) Bodies of three upper thoracic and three lower cervical vertebrae. INSERTION: (1) Anterior tubercle of atlas. (2) Transverse processes of 5th and 6th cervical vertebrae. (3) Bodies of 2nd to 4th cervical vertebrae. INNERVATION: Branches of 2nd to 7th cervical.

**mylohyoideus** (mī"lō-hī-oyd'ē-ŭs). ACTION: Elevates floor of mouth and hyoid, depresses jaw. ORIGIN: Mylohyoid line of mandible. INSERTION: Body of hyoid and median raphe. INNERVATION: Mylohyoid.

**omohyoideus** (ō"mō-hī-oyd'ē-ŭs). ACTION: Depresses hyoid. ORIGIN: Upper border of scapula. INSERTION: Hyoid bone. INNERVATION: Upper cervical through ansa hypoglossi.

**pharyngopalatinus** (făr-ĭn"gō-păl-ă-tī'nŭs). ACTION: Narrows fauces and shuts off nasopharynx. ORIGIN: Soft palate. INSERTION: Thyroid cartilage and aponeurosis of the pharynx. INNERVATION: Pharyngeal plexus.

**platysma** (plă-tĭz'mă). ACTION: Wrinkles skin of neck and chest, depresses jaw and lower lip. ORIGIN: Clavicle, acromion and fascia over deltoid, and pectoralis major. INSERTION: Lower border of mandible, risorius, and opposite platysma. INNERVATION: Cervical branch of facial.

**rectus capitis anterior** (rĕk'tŭs kăp'ĭ-tĭs ăn-tē'rĭ-or). ACTION: Turns and inclines the head. ORIGIN: Base of atlas. INSERTION: Occipital bone, basilar process. INNERVATION: Between 1st and 2nd cervical.

**rectus capitis lateralis** (rĕk'tŭs kăp'ĭ-tĭs lăt"ĕr-ā'lĭs). ACTION: Inclines head laterally and supports it. ORIGIN: Transverse process of atlas. INSERTION: Jugular process of occipital bone. INNERVATION: Between 1st and 2nd cervical nerves.

**salpingopharyngeus** (săl-pĭn"gō-făr-ĭn'jē-ŭs). ACTION: Elevates nasopharynx. ORIGIN: Eustachian tube close to nasopharynx. INSERTION: Posterior portion of the pharyngopalatinus. INNERVATION: Pharyngeal plexus.

**scalenus anterior** (skā-lē'nŭs ăn-tē'rĭ-or). ACTION: Elevates 1st rib and flexes neck. ORIGIN: Transverse processes of 3rd to 6th cervical vertebrae. INSERTION: Tubercle of 1st rib. INNERVATION: Cervical plexus.

**scalenus medius** (skā-lē'nŭs mē'dē-ŭs). ACTION: Elevates 1st rib and flexes neck. ORIGIN: Transverse processes of 2nd to 6th cervical vertebrae. INSERTION: First rib. INNERVATION: Cervical plexus.

**scalenus posterior** (skā-lē'nŭs pŏs-tē'rē-or). ACTION: Elevates 2nd rib and flexes neck. ORIGIN: Transverse processes of 4th to 6th cervical vertebrae. INSERTION: Second rib. INNERVATION: Cervical and brachial plexus.

**sternocleidomastoideus** (stĕr"nō-klī-dō-măs-toyd'ē-ŭs). ACTION: Rotates and laterally flexes neck. ORIGIN: By two heads, from sternum and clavicle. INSERTION: Mastoid process and outer part of superior curved line of occipital bone. INNERVATION: Spinal accessory.

**sternohyoideus** (stĕr"nō-hī-oyd'ē-ŭs). ACTION: Depresses hyoid bone. ORIGIN: Manubrium sterni and 1st costal cartilage. INSERTION: Body of hyoid bone. INNERVATION: Upper cervical through ansa hypoglossi.

**sternothyroideus** (stĕr"nō-thī-rē-oyd'ē-ŭs). ACTION: Depresses thyroid cartilage. ORIGIN: Sternum and 1st costal cartilage. INSERTION: Side of thyroid cartilage. INNERVATION: Upper cervical through ansa hypoglossi.

**styloglossus** (stī"lō-glŏs'ŭs). ACTION: Retracts and elevates tongue. ORIGIN: Styloid process. INSERTION: Side of tongue. INNERVATION: Hypoglossal.

**stylohyoideus** (stī″lō-hī-oyd′ē-ŭs). ACTION: Elevates hyoid, drawing it up and back. ORIGIN: Styloid process. INSERTION: Body of hyoid bone. INNERVATION: Facial.

**stylopharyngeus** (stī″lō-făr-ĭn′jē-ŭs). ACTION: Elevates and dilates pharynx. ORIGIN: Styloid process. INSERTION: Thyroid cartilage and side of pharynx. INNERVATION: Glossopharyngeal.

**tensor veli palatini** (tĕn′sōr vē′lī păl″ă-tī′nī). ACTION: Stretches soft palate. ORIGIN: Spine of sphenoid, scaphoid fossa of internal pterygoid process and eustachian tube. INSERTION: Posterior border of hard palate and aponeurosis of soft palate. INNERVATION: Otic ganglion, trigeminal nerve.

**thyrohyoideus** (thī-rō-hī-oyd′ē-ŭs). ACTION: Depresses hyoid bone; elevates thyroid cartilage if hyoid bone is fixed. ORIGIN: Side of thyroid cartilage. INSERTION: Cornu and body of hyoid bone. INNERVATION: Hypoglossal.

**uvulae** (ū′vū-lē). ACTION: Elevates the uvula. ORIGIN: Posterior nasal spine. INSERTION: Forms large part of uvula. INNERVATION: Pharyngeal plexus.

## LARYNX AND EPIGLOTTIS

**aryepiglotticus** (ăr″ē-ĕp″ĭ-glŏt′ĭk-ŭs). ACTION: Closes glottic opening. ORIGIN: Arytenoid cartilage. INSERTION: Epiglottis. INNERVATION: Laryngeal, recurrent.

**arytenoideus** (ăr″ē-tē-noyd′ē-ŭs). Consists of (1) arytenoideus obliquus and (2) arytenoideus transversus. ACTION: Closes glottic opening. ORIGIN: Arytenoid cartilage. INSERTION: (1) Aryepiglottic fold. (2) Crosses between the two cartilages of the obliquus portion. INNERVATION: Laryngeal, recurrent.

**cricoarytenoideus lateralis** (krī″kō-ăr″ē-tē-noyd′ē-ŭs lăt″ĕr-ā′lĭs). ACTION: Narrows glottis. ORIGIN: Upper border of arch of cricoid cartilage. INSERTION: Muscular process of arytenoid cartilage. INNERVATION: Laryngeal, recurrent.

**cricoarytenoideus posterior** (krī″kō-ăr″ē-tē-noyd′ē-ŭs pŏs-tē′rē-or). ACTION: Opens glottis. ORIGIN: Back of cricoid cartilage. INSERTION: Muscular process of arytenoid cartilage. INNERVATION: Laryngeal, recurrent.

**cricothyroideus** (krī″kō-thī-royd′ē-ŭs). ACTION: Tightens vocal cords. ORIGIN: Anterior surface of cricoid cartilage. INSERTION: Thyroid cartilage. INNERVATION: Laryngeal, superior.

**thyroarytenoideus** (thī″rō-ăr″ē-tē-noyd′ē-ŭs). ACTION: Relaxes vocal cords. ORIGIN: Thyroid cartilage. INSERTION: Arytenoid cartilage. INNERVATION: Laryngeal, recurrent.

**thyroepiglotticus** (thī″rō-ĕp″ĭ-glŏt′ĭk-ŭs). ACTION: Depresses epiglottis. ORIGIN: Thyroid cartilage. INSERTION: Epiglottis and sacculus laryngis. INNERVATION: Laryngeal, recurrent.

## BACK

**iliocostalis cervicis** (ĭl″ē-ō-kŏs-tă′lĭs sĕr′vĭ-sĭs). ACTION: Extends cervical spine. ORIGIN: Angles of 3rd to 6th ribs. INSERTION: Transverse processes of 4th to 6th cervical vertebrae. INNERVATION: Cervical plexus.

**iliocostalis lumborum** (ĭl″ē-ō-kŏs-tă′lĭs lŭm-bō′rŭm). ACTION: Extends lumbar spine. ORIGIN: With sacrospinalis. INSERTION: In angles of 5th to 12th ribs. INNERVATION: Branches of thoracic and lumbar nerves.

**iliocostalis thoracis** (ĭl″ē-ō-kŏs-tă′lĭs thō-ră′sĭs). ACTION: Keeps dorsal spine erect. ORIGIN: Angles of 12th to 7th ribs. INSERTION: Sixth to 1st ribs and 7th cervical vertebra. INNERVATION: Branches of thoracic nerves.

**interspinales** (ĭn-tĕr-spī-nă′lēz). A series. ACTION: Supports and extends vertebral column. ORIGIN: Undersurface of spine of one vertebra. INSERTION: Spine of vertebra above. INNERVATION: Branches of cervical, thoracic, and lumbar nerve.

**intertransversarii** (ĭn-tĕr-trăns-vĕr-să′rĭ-ī). ACTION: Flexes vertebral column. ORIGIN: Between transverse processes of contiguous vertebrae. INNERVATION: Branches of cervical, thoracic, and lumbar nerves.

**latissimus dorsi** (lă-tĭs′ĭ-mŭs dŏr′sī). ACTION: Adducts, extends, and rotates arm. ORIGIN: Lower thoracic and lumbar vertebrae, sacrum, and tip of iliac crest. INSERTION: Intertubercular groove of humerus. INNERVATION: Brachial plexus.

**levator scapulae** (lē-vā′tor skăp′ū-lē). ACTION: Elevates posterior angle of scapula. ORIGIN: Transverse process of four upper cervical vertebrae. INSERTION: Superior edge of scapula. INNERVATION: Dorsal scapular from 5th cervical and branches of 3rd and 4th cervical.

**longissimus capitis** (lŏn-jĭs′ĭ-mŭs kăp′ĭ-tĭs). ACTION: Keeps head erect, draws it backward or to one side. ORIGIN: Upper thoracic and lower and middle cervical vertebrae. INSERTION: Mastoid process. INNERVATION: Cervical plexus.

**longissimus cervicis** (lŏn-jĭs′ĭ-mŭs sĕr′vĭ-sĭs). ACTION: Extends cervical spine. ORIGIN: Upper thoracic vertebrae. INSERTION: Ribs and upper lumbar and thoracic vertebrae. INNERVATION: Cervical plexus and upper thoracic nerves.

**longissimus thoracis** (lŏn-jĭs′ĭ-mŭs thō-ră′sĭs). ACTION: Extends spinal column. ORIGIN: Transverse processes of lumbar and dorsal vertebrae. INSERTION: Lowest ribs and lumbar and dorsal vertebrae. INNERVATION: Lumbar and thoracic nerves.

**multifidus** (mŭl-tĭf'ĭ-dŭs). ACTION: Rotates spinal column. ORIGIN: Sacrum, iliac spine, lumbar, cervical, and dorsal vertebrae. INSERTION: Laminae and spinous processes of next four vertebrae above. INNERVATION: Thoracic and lumbar nerves.

**obliquus capitis inferior** (ŏb-lī'kwŭs kăp'ĭ-tĭs ĭn-fē'rĭ-or). ACTION: Rotates head. ORIGIN: Spine of axis. INSERTION: Transverse process of atlas. INNERVATION: Suboccipital.

**obliquus capitis superior** (ŏb-lī'kwŭs kăp'ĭ-tĭs sū-pē'rē-or). ACTION: Rotates head. ORIGIN: Transverse process of axis. INSERTION: Occipital bone. INNERVATION: Suboccipital.

**rectus capitis posterior major** (rĕk'tŭs kăp'ĭ-tĭs pŏs-tē'rē-or mā'jor). ACTION: Rotates and draws head backward. ORIGIN: Spine of axis. INSERTION: Inferior curved line of occipital bone. INNERVATION: Suboccipital.

**rectus capitis posterior minor** (rĕk'tŭs kăp'ĭ-tĭs pŏs-tē'rē-or mī'nor). ACTION: Rotates and draws head backward. ORIGIN: Posterior tubercle of atlas. INSERTION: Inferior curved line of occipital bone. INNERVATION: Suboccipital.

**rhomboideus major** (rŏm-boy'dē-ŭs mā'jor). ACTION: Retracts, elevates, and downwardly rotates scapula. ORIGIN: Spinous processes of 2nd to 5th thoracic vertebrae. INSERTION: Vertebral border of scapula below spine. INNERVATION: Dorsal scapular from brachial plexus.

**rhomboideus minor** (rŏm-boy'dē-ŭs mī'nor). ACTION: Retracts and elevates scapula. ORIGIN: Spinous processes of 7th cervical vertebra and 1st thoracic vertebra. INSERTION: Border of scapula above spine. INNERVATION: Dorsal scapular from brachial plexus.

**rotatores** (rō-tā-tō'rēz). ACTION: Extends and rotates the vertebral column. ORIGIN: Transverse processes of 2nd to 12th dorsal vertebrae. INSERTION: Lamina of next vertebra above. INNERVATION: Branches of cervical, thoracic, and lumbar nerves.

**sacrospinalis** (să"krō-spī-nā'lĭs). ACTION: Extends vertebral column. ORIGIN: Sacrum, lumbar vertebrae, iliac crest. INSERTION: Iliocostalis and longissimus thoracis. INNERVATION: Branches of thoracic and lumbar nerves.

**semispinalis capitis** (sĕm"ē-spī-nā'lĭs kăp'ĭ-tĭs). ACTION: Rotates and draws head backward. ORIGIN: Transverse processes of upper six or seven thoracic and lower four cervical vertebrae. INSERTION: Occipital bone, between inferior and superior curved line. INNERVATION: Branches of cervical nerves.

**semispinalis cervicis** (sĕm"ē-spī-nā'lĭs sĕr'vĭ-sĭs). ACTION: Extends the vertebral column and rotates it toward the opposite side. ORIGIN: Transverse processes of upper five or six thoracic vertebrae. INSERTION: Spines from axis to 5th cervical vertebra. INNERVATION: Branches of cervical nerves.

**semispinalis thoracis** (sĕm"ē-spī-nā'lĭs thō-ră'sĭs). ACTION: Extends the vertebral column and rotates it toward the opposite side. ORIGIN: Transverse processes of 6th to 10th thoracic vertebrae. INSERTION: Spines of upper four thoracic and lower two cervical vertebrae. INNERVATION: Branches of thoracic nerves.

**serratus posterior inferior** (sĕr-ā'tŭs pŏs-tē'rē-or ĭn-fē'rĭ-or). ACTION: Draws ribs back and downward. ORIGIN: Spines of lower two thoracic and upper two lumbar vertebrae. INSERTION: Lower four ribs. INNERVATION: Branches of 9th to 12th thoracic nerves.

**serratus posterior superior** (sĕr-ā'tŭs pŏs-tē'rē-or sū-pē'rē-or). ACTION: Elevates the ribs. ORIGIN: Spines of 7th cervical and two upper thoracic vertebrae. INSERTION: Angles of 2nd to 5th ribs. INNERVATION: Branches of thoracic nerves.

**spinalis capitis** (spī-nā'lĭs kăp'ĭ-tĭs). ORIGIN: Inconstant; from spines of upper dorsal and lower cervical vertebrae. INSERTION: Blends with the semispinalis capitis.

**spinalis cervicis** (spī-nā'lĭs sĕr'vĭ-sĭs). ACTION: Extends cervical spine. ORIGIN: Spines of 5th, 6th, and 7th cervical vertebrae. INSERTION: Axis and, occasionally, the two vertebrae below. INNERVATION: Branches of cervical nerves.

**spinalis thoracis** (spī-nā'lĭs thō-ră'sĭs). ACTION: Erects spinal column. ORIGIN: Spines of first two lumbar and last two thoracic vertebrae. INSERTION: Spines of middle and upper thoracic vertebrae. INNERVATION: Branches of thoracic and lumbar nerves.

**splenius capitis** (splē'nē-ŭs kăp'ĭ-tĭs). ACTION: Rotates and extends head. ORIGIN: Ligamentum nuchae, 7th cervical and first three thoracic vertebrae. INSERTION: Mastoid process and superior curved line of occiput. INNERVATION: Branches of cervical nerves.

**splenius cervicis** (splē'nē-ŭs sĕr'vĭ-sĭs). ACTION: Rotates and flexes head and neck. ORIGIN: Spines of 3rd to 6th thoracic vertebrae. INSERTION: Transverse processes of 1st and 2nd cervical vertebrae. INNERVATION: Branches of cervical nerves.

**suspensorius duodeni** (sŭs-pĕn-sō'rē-ŭs doo"ō-dē'nē). ACTION: Acts as a suspensory ligament. Wide, flat band of smooth muscle attached to the left crus of diaphragm and continuous with the muscular layer of the duodenum at its junction with the jejunum. INNERVATION: Celiac plexus.

**trapezius** (tră-pē'zē-ŭs). ACTION: Extends head, raises and rotates scapula. ORIGIN: Superior curved line of occipital, spinous processes of 7th cervical and all thoracic vertebrae. INSERTION: Clavicle, acromion, base of spine of scapula. INNERVATION: Spinal accessory and cervical plexus.

## ABDOMEN

**cremaster** (krē-măs'tĕr). ACTION: Raises testicle. ORIGIN: Midportion of inguinal ligament. INSERTION: Cremasteric fascia and pubic bone. INNERVATION: Genitofemoral.

**obliquus externus abdominis** (ŏb-lī'kwŭs ĕks-tĕr'nŭs ăb-dŏm'ĭ-nĭs). ACTION: Contracts abdomen and viscera. ORIGIN: Lower eight ribs. INSERTION: Iliac crest, Poupart's ligament, linea alba, pubic crest. INNERVATION: Iliohypogastric, ilioinguinal, and branches of intercostal.

**obliquus internus abdominis** (ŏb-lī'kwŭs ĭn-tĕr'nŭs ăb-dŏm'ĭ-nĭs). ACTION: Compresses viscera, flexes thorax forward. ORIGIN: Iliac crest, inguinal ligament, lumbar fascia. INSERTION: Few lowest ribs, linea alba, pubic crest. INNERVATION: Iliohypogastric, ilioinguinal, and branches of intercostal.

**pyramidalis** (pĭ-răm"ĭ-dă'lĭs). ACTION: Tightens linea alba. ORIGIN: Pubic crest. INSERTION: Linea alba. INNERVATION: Branch of 12th thoracic.

**quadratus lumborum** (kwăd-rā'tŭs lŭm-bō'rŭm). ACTION: Flexes trunk laterally and assists lumbar vertebral extension. ORIGIN: Iliac crest, iliolumbar ligament, lower lumbar vertebrae. INSERTION: Twelfth rib and the upper lumbar vertebrae. INNERVATION: Branches of 1st lumbar and 12th thoracic.

**rectus abdominis** (rĕk'tŭs ăb-dŏm'ĭ-nĭs). ACTION: Compresses or flattens abdomen. ORIGIN: Pubis. INSERTION: Cartilage of 5th to 7th ribs. INNERVATION: Branches of 7th to 12th intercostal.

**transversus abdominis** (trăns-vĕr'sŭs ăb-dŏm'ĭ-nĭs). ACTION: Compresses abdomen, flexes thorax. ORIGIN: Lumbar fascia, 7th to 12th costal cartilages, inguinal ligament, iliac crest. INSERTION: Xiphoid cartilage, linea alba, pubic crest, and iliopectineal line. INNERVATION: Iliohypogastric, ilioinguinal, branches of intercostal.

## PERINEUM

**bulbospongiosus** (bŭl"bō-spŏn"jē-ō'sŭs). ACTION: Constricts bulbous urethra in male; constricts urethra in female. ORIGIN: Central point of perineum and medial raphe. INSERTION: Undersurface of bulb, spongy and cavernous part of penis; root of clitoris. INNERVATION: Perineal branch of pudendal.

**coccygeus** (kŏk-sĭj'ē-ŭs). ACTION: Supports coccyx, closes pelvic outlet. ORIGIN: Ischial spine and sacrospinous ligament. INSERTION: Coccyx and lowest portion of sacrum. INNERVATION: Third and 4th sacral.

**corrugator cutis ani** (kōr'ū-gā'tōr kū'tĭs ā'nī). ACTION: Wrinkles skin of anus. ORIGIN: Submucous tissue, interior of anus. INSERTION: Subcutaneous tissue on opposite side of anus. INNERVATION: Sympathetic.

**depressor urethrae** (dē-prĕs'or ū-rē'thrē). ACTION: Depresses urethra. ORIGIN: Ramus of ischium near the transversus perinei profundus. INSERTION: Fibers of constrictor vaginae.

**ischiocavernosus** (ĭs"kē-ō-kă"vĕr-nō'sŭs). ACTION: Maintains erection of penis or clitoris. ORIGIN: Tuberosity of ischium and great sacrosciatic ligament. INSERTION: Corpora cavernosa of clitoris or penis. INNERVATION: Perineal branch of pudendal.

**levator ani** (lē-vā'tor ā'nī). ACTION: Supports rectum and pelvic floor, aids in defecation. ORIGIN: Pubis, pelvic fascia, ischial spine. INSERTION: Rectum, coccyx, and fibrous raphe of perineum. INNERVATION: Sacral and perineal.

**sphincter ani externus** (sfĭngk'tĕr ā'nī ĕks-tĕr'nŭs). ACTION: Closes anus. ORIGIN: Ring of fibers surrounding anus. INSERTION: Coccyx and central point of perineum. INNERVATION: Hemorrhoidal branch of pudendal.

**sphincter ani internus** (sfĭngk'tĕr ā'nī ĭn-tĕr'nŭs). ACTION: Contracts rectum and anus, but not voluntarily. ORIGIN: Muscular ring of rectal fibers above canal.

**sphincter urethrae membranaceae** (sfĭngk'tĕr ū-rē'thrē mĕm-bră-nā'sē-ē). ACTION: Constricts membranous urethra. ORIGIN: Ramus of pubis. INSERTION: Behind and in front of urethra. INNERVATION: Perineal branch of pudendal.

**sphincter vesicae** (sfĭngk'tĕr vĕs'ĭ-kē). ACTION: Shuts off internal orifice of urethra. ORIGIN: Near urethral orifice of bladder. INNERVATION: Sacral and hypogastric.

**transversus perinei profundus** (trăns-vĕr'sŭs pĕr-ĭ-nē'ī prō-fŭn'dŭs). ACTION: Assists compressor urethrae. ORIGIN: Ramus of ischium. INSERTION: Central tendon. INNERVATION: Perineal branch of pudendal.

**transversus perinei superficialis** (trăns-vĕr'sŭs pĕr-ĭ-nē'ī soo"pĕr-fĭsh-ē-ā'lĭs). ACTION: Tenses central tendon. ORIGIN: Ramus of ischium. INSERTION: Central point of perineum. INNERVATION: Perineal branch of pudendal.

## THORAX

**diaphragma** (dī"ă-frăg'mă). ACTION: Increases chest capacity and decreases pressure within the thoracic cavity. ORIGIN: Ensiform cartilage, 7th to 12th ribs, arcuate ligaments, and lumbar vertebrae. INSERTION: Central tendon. INNERVATION: Phrenic.

**intercostalis externus** (ĭn"tĕr-kŏs-tă'lĭs ĕks-tĕr'nŭs). ACTION: Draws ribs together and raises ribs. ORIGIN: Lower border of rib. INSERTION: Upper border of rib below. INNERVATION: Intercostal.

**intercostalis internus** (ĭn"tĕr-kŏs-tă'lĭs ĭn-tĕr'nŭs). ACTION: Draws ribs together and lowers ribs. ORIGIN: Lower border of rib. INSERTION: Upper border of rib below. INNERVATION: Intercostal.

**levatores costarum** (lē-vā-tō'rez kŏs-tā'rŭm). ACTION: Raises ribs, flexes vertebral column. ORIGIN: Transverse process of 7th cervical and upper 11 thoracic vertebrae. INSERTION: Rib next below. INNERVATION: Branches of intercostal.

**subcostales** (sŭb-kŏs-tā'lēz). ACTION: Draws ribs together and lowers ribs. ORIGIN: Inconstant; inner surface of the ribs. INSERTION: Inner surface of one of the ribs just below. INNERVATION: Intercostal.

**transversus thoracis** (trăns-vĕr'sŭs thō-ră'sĭs). ACTION: Narrows the chest. ORIGIN: Xiphoid cartilage and sternum. INSERTION: Costal cartilages, 2nd to 6th ribs. INNERVATION: Branches of intercostal.

## SHOULDER

**deltoideus** (dĕl-toy'dē-ŭs). ACTION: Raises and rotates arm. ORIGIN: Clavicle, acromion process, and spine of scapula. INSERTION: Shaft of humerus. INNERVATION: Axillary (circumflex) from brachial plexus.

**infraspinatus** (ĭn"fră-spī-nā'tŭs). ACTION: Rotates arm back and out. ORIGIN: Infraspinous fossa of scapula. INSERTION: Great tuberosity of humerus. INNERVATION: Suprascapular from brachial plexus.

**pectoralis major** (pĕk"tō-ră'lĭs mā'jor). ACTION: Flexes, adducts, and rotates arm. ORIGIN: Sternum, clavicle, and cartilages of 1st to 6th ribs. INSERTION: Bicipital ridge of humerus. INNERVATION: Pectoral from brachial plexus.

**pectoralis minor** (pĕk"tō-ră'lĭs mī'nor). ACTION: Draws down scapula and point to shoulder, raises ribs. ORIGIN: Third to 5th ribs. INSERTION: Coracoid process of scapula. INNERVATION: Pectoral from brachial plexus.

**serratus anterior** (sĕr-ā'tŭs ăn-tē'rĭ-or). ACTION: Elevates ribs, rotates scapula. ORIGIN: Upper eight or nine ribs. INSERTION: Angles and vertebral border of scapula. INNERVATION: Long thoracic from brachial plexus.

**subclavius** (sŭb-klā'vē-ŭs). ACTION: Draws clavicle down and forward or elevates the 1st rib. ORIGIN: First rib and cartilage. INSERTION: Undersurface of clavicle. INNERVATION: Branches of 5th and 6th cervical.

**subscapularis** (sŭb-skăp-ū-lă'rĭs). ACTION: Rotates humerus inward and lowers it. ORIGIN: Subscapular fossa. INSERTION: Lesser tubercle of humerus. INNERVATION: Subscapular.

**supraspinatus** (soo"pră-spī-nā'tŭs). ACTION: Abducts and raises arm. ORIGIN: Supraspinous fossa of scapula. INSERTION: Greater tubercle of humerus. INNERVATION: Branches of suprascapular.

**teres major** (tĕ'rēz mā'jor). ACTION: Inwardly rotates, adducts, and extends arm. ORIGIN: Axillary border of scapula. INSERTION: Lesser tubercle of humerus. INNERVATION: Branch of lower subscapular.

**teres minor** (tĕ'rēz mī'nor). ACTION: Rotates arm outward. ORIGIN: Axillary border of scapula. INSERTION: Greater tubercle of humerus. INNERVATION: Branch of axillary (circumflex).

## ARM AND FOREARM

**anconeus** (ăn-kō'nē-ŭs). ACTION: Extends forearm. ORIGIN: Lateral epicondyle of humerus. INSERTION: Olecranon and posterior surface of ulna. INNERVATION: Branch of radial.

**biceps brachii** (bī'sĕps brā'kē-ī). ACTION: Flexes arm and forearm and supinates forearm. ORIGIN: (1) Short head from coracoid process. (2) Long head from the supraglenoid tuberosity at the margin of the glenoid cavity. INSERTION: Bicipital tuberosity of radius. INNERVATION: Musculocutaneous.

**brachialis** (brā"kē-ăl'ĭs). ACTION: Flexes forearm. ORIGIN: Lower half of anterior surface of humerus. INSERTION: Coronoid process of ulna. INNERVATION: Musculocutaneous and radial.

**brachioradialis** (brā"kē-ō-rā"dē-ă'lĭs). ACTION: Flexes and supinates forearm. ORIGIN: Supracondylar ridge of humerus. INSERTION: Styloid process of radius. INNERVATION: Branch of radial. SYN: *supinator longus*.

**coracobrachialis** (kor"ă-kō-brā"kē-ăl'ĭs). ACTION: Raises and adducts arm. ORIGIN: Coracoid process of scapula. INSERTION: Middle of inner border of humerus. INNERVATION: Musculocutaneous.

**extensor carpi radialis brevis** (ĕks-tĕn'sōr kar'pī rā"dē-ā'lĭs brĕ'vĭs). ACTION: Extends and abducts wrist. ORIGIN: External condyloid ridge of humerus. INSERTION: Base of 3rd metacarpal. INNERVATION: Branch of radial.

**extensor carpi radialis longus** (ĕks-tĕn'sōr kar'pī rā"dē-ā'lĭs lŏng'ŭs). ACTION: Extends and abducts wrist. ORIGIN: External condyloid ridge of humerus. INSERTION: Base of 2nd metacarpal. INNERVATION: Branch of radial.

**extensor carpi ulnaris** (ĕks-tĕn'sōr kar'pī ŭl-nā'rĭs). ACTION: Extends and adducts hand and wrist. ORIGIN: Lateral epicondyle of humerus. INSERTION: Base of 5th metacarpal. INNERVATION: Branch of radial.

**extensor digiti minimi** (ĕks-tĕn'sōr dĭj'ĭ-tī mĭn'ĭm-ī). ACTION: Extends little finger. ORIGIN: External epicondyle of humerus. INSERTION: Dorsum of 1st phalanx of little finger. INNERVATION: Branch of radial.

**extensor digitorum communis** (ĕks-tĕn'sōr dĭj-ĭ-tō'rŭm kŏm-mū'nĭs). ACTION: Extends fingers and wrist. ORIGIN: External epicondyle of humerus. INSERTION: Second and 3rd phalanges. INNERVATION: Branch of radial.

**extensor indicis proprius** (ĕks-tĕn'sōr ĭn'dĭ-sĭs prō'prē-ŭs). ACTION: Extends index finger. ORIGIN: Dorsal surface of ulna and interosseous membrane. INSERTION: First tendon of extensor digitorum communis. IN-

NERVATION: Branch of radial.

**extensor pollicis brevis** (ĕks-tĕn′sŏr pŏl′ĭ-sĭs brĕ′vĭs). ACTION: Extends thumb and abducts 1st metacarpal. ORIGIN: Dorsal surface of radius. INSERTION: Base of 1st phalanx of thumb. INNERVATION: Branch of radial.

**extensor pollicis longus** (ĕks-tĕn′sŏr pŏl′ĭ-sĭs lŏng′ŭs). ACTION: Extends terminal phalanx of thumb and abducts hand. ORIGIN: Dorsal surface of ulna. INSERTION: Base of 2nd phalanx of thumb. INNERVATION: Branch of radial.

**flexor carpi radialis** (flĕks′or kar′pī rā″dē-ā′lĭs). ACTION: Flexes and abducts wrist. ORIGIN: Medial epicondyle of humerus. INSERTION: Base of 2nd metacarpal. INNERVATION: Branch of median.

**flexor carpi ulnaris** (flĕks′or kar′pī ŭl-nā′rĭs). Consists of (1) humeral head and (2) ulnar head. ACTION: Flexes and adducts wrist. ORIGIN: (1) Medial epicondyle of humerus. (2) Olecranon process and posterior border of ulna. INSERTION: Pisiform bone and 5th metacarpal. INNERVATION: Branch of ulnar.

**flexor digitorum profundus** (flĕks′or dĭj-ĭ-tō′rŭm prō-fŭn′dŭs). ACTION: Flexes the distal interphalangeal joints of the fingers. ORIGIN: Upper three fourths of shaft of ulna. INSERTION: Terminal phalanges of fingers. INNERVATION: Branch of ulnar and branch of median.

**flexor digitorum sublimis** (flĕks′or dĭj-ĭ-tō′rŭm sŭb-lī′mĭs). SYN: *flexor digitorum superficialis.*

**flexor digitorum superficialis** (flĕks′or dĭj-ĭ-tō′rŭm soo″pĕr-fĭsh-ē-ā′lĭs). Consists of three heads: (1) humeral, (2) ulnar, and (3) radial. ACTION: Flexes the middle and proximal phalanges, carpal flexion of hand. ORIGIN: (1) Medial epicondyle of humerus. (2) Medial side of coronoid process. (3) Outer border of radius. INSERTION: Second phalanx of each finger. INNERVATION: Branches of median. SYN: *flexor digitorum sublimis.*

**flexor pollicis longus** (flĕks′or pŏl′ĭ-sĭs lŏng′ŭs). ACTION: Flexes thumb. ORIGIN: Anterior surface of middle third of radius. INSERTION: Terminal phalanx of thumb. INNERVATION: Branch of median.

**palmaris longus** (păl-mā′rĭs lŏng′ŭs). ACTION: Tightens palmar fascia, flexes wrist. ORIGIN: Medial epicondyle of humerus. INSERTION: Transverse carpal ligament and palmar fascia. INNERVATION: Branch of median.

**pronator quadratus** (prō-nā′tor kwăd-rā′tŭs). ACTION: Pronates forearm. ORIGIN: Lower fourth of ulna. INSERTION: Lower fourth of radius. INNERVATION: Volar interosseous.

**pronator teres** (prō-nā′tor tĕ′rēz). Consists of (1) humeral head and (2) ulnar head. ACTION: Pronates hand. ORIGIN: (1) Medial epicondyle of humerus. (2) Coronoid process of ulna. INSERTION: Lateral surface of shaft of radius. INNERVATION: Branch of median.

**supinator** (soo″pĭ-nā′tor). ACTION: Supinates forearm. ORIGIN: Lateral epicondyle of humerus, oblique line of ulna, elbow joint. INSERTION: Outer surface of radius. INNERVATION: Branch of radial.

**supinator longus** (soo″pĭ-nā′tor lŏng′ŭs). SYN: *brachioradialis.*

**triceps brachii** (trī′sĕps brā′kē-ī). Consists of three heads: (1) long, (2) lateral, and (3) medial. ACTION: Extends forearm and arm. ORIGIN: (1) Infraglenoid tubercle of scapula. (2) Posterior surface of humerus below great tubercle. (3) Humerus below radial groove. INSERTION: Olecranon process of ulna. INNERVATION: Branches of radial.

## HAND

**abductor digiti minimi manus** (ăb-dŭk′tor dĭj-ĭ-tī mĭn′ĭ-mī mă′nŭs). ACTION: Abducts little finger. ORIGIN: Pisiform bone and ligaments. INSERTION: Inner side of 1st phalanx of little finger. INNERVATION: Ulnar, palmar branch.

**abductor pollicis brevis** (ăb-dŭk′tor pŏl′ĭ-sĭs brĕ′vĭs). ACTION: Abducts thumb. ORIGIN: Ridge of trapezius and transverse carpal ligament. INSERTION: Outer side of 1st phalanx of thumb. INNERVATION: Branch of median.

**abductor pollicis longus** (ăb-dŭk′tor pŏl′ĭ-sĭs lŏng′ŭs). ACTION: Abducts and assists in extending thumb. ORIGIN: Posterior surface of radius and ulna. INSERTION: Outer side of base of 1st metacarpal. INNERVATION: Branch of radial.

**adductor pollicis** (ăd-dŭk′tor pŏl′ĭ-sĭs). ACTION: Adducts thumb. ORIGIN: Third metacarpal bone. INSERTION: Inner side of base of 1st phalanx of thumb. INNERVATION: Ulnar.

**flexor digiti quinti brevis manus** (flĕks′or dĭj-ĭ-tī kwĭn′tī brĕ′vĭs mă′nŭs). ACTION: Flexes 1st phalanx of little finger. ORIGIN: Unciform bone. INSERTION: First phalanx of little finger. INNERVATION: Branch of ulnar.

**flexor pollicis brevis** (flĕks′or pŏl′ĭ-sĭs brĕ′vĭs). ACTION: Flexes 1st phalanx of thumb. ORIGIN: Transverse carpal ligament, metacarpal bone. INSERTION: Base of 1st phalanx of thumb. INNERVATION: Branch of median and ulnar.

**interossei dorsales manus** (ĭn″tĕr-ŏs′ē-ī dŏr-sā′lēz mă′nŭs). Four. ACTION: Abducts and adducts fingers. ORIGIN: Sides of metacarpal bones. INSERTION: First phalanges. INNERVATION: Branch of ulnar.

**interossei volares** (ĭn″tĕr-ŏs′ē-ī vō-lā′rēz). Three. ACTION: Adducts index finger, abducts ring and little fingers. ORIGIN: Metacarpal bones laterally. INSERTION: Ulnar side of index finger, and radial sides of ring and little fingers. INNERVATION: Branch of ulnar.

**lumbricales manus** (lŭm-brĭ-kā′lēz mă′nŭs). Four. ACTION: Flexes 1st and extends 2nd and 3rd phalanges. ORIGIN: Tendon of flexor digitorum profundus. INSERTION: First phalanx and extensor tendon. INNERVATION: Median and ulnar.

**opponens digiti quinti** (ŏp-pō'nĕns dĭj-ĭ-tī kwĭn'tī). ACTION: Flexes and adducts little finger. ORIGIN: Unciform bone, transverse carpal ligament. INSERTION: Fifth metacarpal bone. INNERVATION: Branch of ulnar.

**opponens pollicis** (ŏp-pō'nĕns pŏl'ĭ-sĭs). ACTION: Flexes and adducts thumb. ORIGIN: Trapezium and transverse carpal ligament. INSERTION: First metacarpal bone. INNERVATION: Median.

**palmaris brevis** (păl-mā'rĭs brĕ'vĭs). ACTION: Wrinkles skin on inner side of hand. ORIGIN: Central portion of palmar aponeurosis and transverse carpal ligament. INSERTION: Skin of ulnar side of hand. INNERVATION: Branch of ulnar.

## HIP, THIGH, LOWER EXTREMITY

**adductor brevis** (ăd-dŭk'tor brĕ'vĭs). ACTION: Flexes, adducts, and tends to rotate thigh medially. ORIGIN: Ramus of pubis. INSERTION: Upper portion of linea aspera of femur. INNERVATION: Branch of obturator.

**adductor longus** (ăd-dŭk'tor lŏng'ŭs). ACTION: Adducts, flexes, and tends to rotate thigh medially. ORIGIN: Pubic crest and symphysis. INSERTION: Middle of linea aspera of femur. INNERVATION: Branch of obturator.

**adductor magnus** (ăd-dŭk'tor măg'nŭs). ACTION: Adducts thigh and rotates it outward. ORIGIN: Ramus of ischium and pubis. INSERTION: Linea aspera of femur and medial condyle. INNERVATION: Branch of sciatic and obturator.

**articularis genus** (ăr-tĭk"ū-lā'rĭs jē'nŭs). ACTION: Elevates capsule of knee joint. ORIGIN: Lower quarter of anterior surface of femoral shaft. INSERTION: Synovial membrane of knee joint. INNERVATION: Branch of femoral.

**biceps femoris** (bī'sĕps fĕm'ō-rĭs). ACTION: Flexes knee and rotates it outward. ORIGIN: (1) Short head from linea aspera. (2) Long head from ischial tuberosity. INSERTION: Head of fibula; lateral condyle of tibia. INNERVATION: (1) Peroneal and (2) tibial portions of sciatic.

**gemellus inferior** (jĕ-mĕl'ŭs ĭn-fē'rĭ-or). ACTION: Rotates thigh outward. ORIGIN: Ischial tuberosity. INSERTION: Medial surface of greater trochanter. INNERVATION: Sacral.

**gemellus superior** (jĕ-mĕl'ŭs sū-pē'rē-or). ACTION: Rotates thigh outward. ORIGIN: Spine of ischium. INSERTION: Medial surface of greater trochanter. INNERVATION: Sacral plexus.

**gluteus maximus** (gloo'tē-ŭs măk'sē-mŭs). ACTION: Extends and rotates thigh. ORIGIN: Superior curved iliac line and crest, coccyx, and sacrum. INSERTION: Fascia lata and femur below greater trochanter. INNERVATION: Inferior gluteal.

**gluteus medius** (gloo'tē-ŭs mē'dē-ŭs). ACTION: Abducts and rotates thigh. ORIGIN: Lateral surface of ilium. INSERTION: Greater trochanter. INNERVATION: Branches of superior gluteal.

**gluteus minimus** (gloo'tē-ŭs mĭn'ĭ-mŭs). ACTION: Abducts and extends thigh. ORIGIN: Lateral surface of ilium. INSERTION: Greater trochanter. INNERVATION: Branch of superior gluteal.

**gracilis** (grăs'ĭ-lĭs). ACTION: Flexes and adducts leg, adducts thigh. ORIGIN: Symphysis pubis and pubic arch. INSERTION: Medial surface of shaft of tibia. INNERVATION: Branch of obturator.

**iliacus** (ĭ-lī'ă-kŭs). ACTION: Flexes and rotates thigh. ORIGIN: Margin of iliac fossa. INSERTION: Lesser trochanter. INNERVATION: Branches of femoral.

**obturator internus** (ŏb'tū-rā"tor ĭn-tĕr'nŭs). ACTION: Rotates thigh outward. ORIGIN: Pubes, ischium, obturator foramen. INSERTION: Inner surface of greater trochanter. INNERVATION: Branch of obturator.

**pectineus** (pĕk-tĭn'ē-ŭs). ACTION: Flexes and adducts thigh. ORIGIN: Pubic spine, iliopectineal line. INSERTION: Pectineal line of femur. INNERVATION: Branch of obturator and femoral.

**piriformis** (pĭ-rĭ-for'mĭs). ACTION: Abducts and rotates thigh outward. ORIGIN: Margins of anterior sacral foramina and sacrosciatic notch of ilium. INSERTION: Upper margin of greater trochanter. INNERVATION: Branch of sacral.

**psoas major** (sō'ăs mā'jor). ACTION: Flexes thigh, adducts and rotates it medially. ORIGIN: Last thoracic and all of the lumbar vertebrae. INSERTION: Lesser trochanter of femur. INNERVATION: Lumbar plexus.

**psoas minor** (sō'ăs mī'nor). ACTION: Tenses iliac fascia. ORIGIN: Twelfth thoracic and 1st lumbar vertebrae. INSERTION: Iliac fascia and iliopectineal tuberosity. INNERVATION: Branch of lumbar.

**quadratus femoris** (kwăd-rā'tŭs fĕm'ō-rĭs). ACTION: Rotates thigh outward. ORIGIN: Ischial tuberosity. INSERTION: Intertrochanteric ridge. INNERVATION: Sciatic.

**quadriceps femoris** (kwăd'rĭ-sĕps fĕm'ō-rĭs). ACTION: Extends leg. ORIGIN: By four heads: rectus femoris, vastus medialis, vastus lateralis, and vastus intermedius. INSERTION: Patella and tibial tuberosity. INNERVATION: Branches of femoral.

**rectus femoris** (rĕk'tŭs fĕm'ō-rĭs). ACTION: Extends leg and assists flexion of thigh. ORIGIN: Iliac spine, upper margin of acetabulum. INSERTION: Base of patella. INNERVATION: Femoral.

**sartorius** (săr-tō'rē-ŭs). ACTION: Flexes and rotates thigh and leg. ORIGIN: Anterior superior iliac spine. INSERTION: Tibial tuberosity. INNERVATION: Branches of femoral.

**semimembranosus** (sĕm"ē-mĕm"brăn-ō'sŭs). ACTION: Flexes and rotates leg, extends thigh. ORIGIN: Ischial tuberosity. INSERTION: Medial condyle of tibia. INNERVATION: Tibial portion of sciatic.

**semitendinosus** (sĕm″ē-tĕn″dĭn-ō′sŭs). ACTION: Flexes and rotates leg, extends thigh. ORIGIN: Ischial tuberosity. INSERTION: Shaft of tibia below internal tuberosity. INNERVATION: Tibial portion of sciatic.

**tensor fasciae latae** (tĕn′sōr făsh′ē-ē lā′tē). ACTION: Flexes and rotates thigh. ORIGIN: Iliac crest, iliac spine, fascia lata. INSERTION: Iliotibial band of fascia lata. INNERVATION: Branch of superior gluteal.

**vastus intermedius** (văs′tŭs ĭn″tĕr-mē′dē-ŭs). ORIGIN: Upper part of anterior surface of shaft of femur. INSERTION: Common tendon of quadriceps femoris. INNERVATION: Branches of femoral.

**vastus lateralis** (văs′tŭs lăt″ĕr-ā′lĭs). ACTION: Extends knee. ORIGIN: Linea aspera to greater trochanter. INSERTION: Common tendon of quadriceps femoris. INNERVATION: Branches of femoral.

**vastus medialis** (văs′tŭs mē-dĭ-ā′lĭs). ACTION: Extends leg, draws patella in. ORIGIN: Linea aspera of femur. INSERTION: Common tendon of quadriceps femoris. INNERVATION: Branches of femoral.

## LEG

**extensor digitorum longus** (ĕks-tĕn′sōr dĭj-ĭ-tō′rŭm lŏng′ŭs). ACTION: Extends toes, dorsiflexes foot. ORIGIN: External tuberosity of tibia; body of fibula. INSERTION: Second and 3rd phalanges of toes. INNERVATION: Branches of peroneal.

**extensor hallucis longus** (ĕks-tĕn′sōr hăl-oo′sĭs lŏng′ŭs). ACTION: Extends great toe, flexes foot. ORIGIN: Front of fibula and interosseous membrane. INSERTION: Terminal phalanx of great toe. INNERVATION: Branch of peroneal.

**flexor digitorum longus** (flĕks′or dĭj-ĭ-tō′rŭm lŏng′ŭs). ACTION: Flexes the toes. ORIGIN: Posterior surface of tibia. INSERTION: Terminal phalanges of lesser toes. INNERVATION: Branch of tibial.

**flexor hallucis longus** (flĕks′or hăl-oo′sĭs lŏng′ŭs). ACTION: Flexes phalanges, primarily the distal phalanges, and plantar flexes the foot. ORIGIN: Lower portion of shaft of fibula. INSERTION: Distal phalanx of great toe. INNERVATION: Posterior tibial.

**gastrocnemius** (găs″trŏk-nē′mē-ŭs). ACTION: Plantar flexes foot and flexes knee. ORIGIN: External and internal femoral condyles. INSERTION: By tendo calcaneus into os calcis. INNERVATION: Branches of tibial.

**peroneus brevis** (pĕr-ō-nē′ŭs brĕ′vĭs). ACTION: Extends and abducts foot. ORIGIN: Midportion of shaft of fibula. INSERTION: Base of 5th metatarsal bone. INNERVATION: Branch of peroneal.

**peroneus longus** (pĕr-ō-nē′ŭs lŏng′ŭs). ACTION: Extends, abducts, and everts foot. ORIGIN: Upper fibula and external condyle of tibia. INSERTION: By tendon to internal cuneiform and 1st metatarsal bone. INNERVATION: Branch of peroneal.

**peroneus tertius** (pĕr-ō-nē′ŭs tĕr′shē-ŭs). ACTION: Flexes foot. ORIGIN: Lower part of fibula. INSERTION: Fifth metatarsal bone. INNERVATION: Branch of peroneal.

**plantaris** (plăn-tăr′ĭs). ACTION: Extends foot. ORIGIN: External supracondyloid ridge of femur. INSERTION: Inner border of tendo calcaneus. INNERVATION: Branch of tibial.

**popliteus** (pŏp-lĭt′ē-ŭs). ACTION: Flexes leg and rotates it inward. ORIGIN: External condyle of femur. INSERTION: Posterior surface of tibia. INNERVATION: Branch of tibial.

**soleus** (sō′lē-ŭs). ACTION: Plantar flexes foot. ORIGIN: Upper shaft of fibula, oblique line of tibia. INSERTION: By tendo calcaneus to os calcis. INNERVATION: Tibial.

**tibialis anterior** (tĭb″ē-ā′lĭs ăn-tē′rĭ-or). ACTION: Dorsiflexes foot and increases the arch in the takeoff of walking. ORIGIN: Upper tibia, interosseus membrane, and intermuscular septum. INSERTION: Internal cuneiform and 1st metatarsal. INNERVATION: Branch of peroneal.

**tibialis posterior** (tĭb″ē-ā′lĭs pŏs-tē′rē-or). ACTION: Plantar flexes foot. ORIGIN: Shaft of fibula and tibia. INSERTION: Tuberosity of scaphoid, 2nd to 4th metatarsal, internal cuneiform. INNERVATION: Branch of tibial.

## FOOT

**abductor digiti minimi pedis** (ăb-dŭk′tor dĭj-ĭ-tī mĭn′ĭ-mī pē′dĭs). ACTION: Abducts little toe. ORIGIN: Outer tuberosity of calcaneus, plantar fascia, and intermuscular septum. INSERTION: External side of 1st phalanx of little toe. INNERVATION: Lateral plantar.

**abductor hallucis** (ăb-dŭk′tor hăl-oo′sĭs). ACTION: Abducts great toe. ORIGIN: Inner tuberosity of os calcis, plantar fascia. INSERTION: Inner side, 1st phalanx of great toe. INNERVATION: Medial plantar.

**adductor hallucis** (ăd-dŭk′tor hăl-oo′sĭs). ACTION: Adducts great toe. ORIGIN: Tarsal terminations of the three middle metatarsal bones. INSERTION: Lateral side of base of 1st phalanx of great toe. INNERVATION: Branch of lateral plantar.

**extensor digitorum brevis** (ĕks-tĕn′sōr dĭj-ĭ-tō′rŭm brĕ′vĭs). ACTION: Extends toes. ORIGIN: Dorsal surface of os calcis. INSERTION: To 1st phalanx of great toe and the tendons of extensor digitorum longus. INNERVATION: Branch of peroneal.

**flexor accessorius** (flĕks′or ăk-sĕ-sō′rē-ŭs). SYN: *quadratus plantae*.

**flexor digiti quinti brevis pedis** (flĕks′or dĭj-ĭ-tī kwĭn′tī brĕ′vĭs pē′dĭs). ACTION: Flexes the little toe. ORIGIN: Base of metatarsal of little toe and sheath of peroneus longus. IN-

SERTION: Outer side of base of 1st phalanx of little toe. INNERVATION: External plantar.

**flexor digitorum brevis** (flĕks′or dĭj-ĭ-tō′rŭm brĕ′vĭs). ACTION: Flexes toe. ORIGIN: Os calcis and plantar fascia. INSERTION: Second phalanges of lesser toes. INNERVATION: Internal plantar.

**flexor hallucis brevis** (flĕks′or hăl-oo′sĭs brĕ′vĭs). ACTION: Flexes great toe. ORIGIN: Internal surface of cuboid and middle and external cuneiform bones. INSERTION: Sides of base of 1st phalanx of great toe. INNERVATION: Internal and external plantar.

**interossei dorsales pedis** (ĭn″tĕr-ŏs′ē-ī dōr-sā′lēz pē′dĭs). Four. ACTION: Adducts 2nd toe, abducts 2nd, 3rd, and 4th toes. ORIGIN: Shafts of adjacent metatarsal bones. INSERTION: First phalanges of lesser toes. INNERVATION: External plantar.

**interossei plantares** (ĭn″tĕr-ŏs′ē-ī plăn-tăr′ĭs). Three. ACTION: Adducts three outer toes. ORIGIN: Third, 4th, and 5th metatarsal bones. INSERTION: First phalanx of corresponding toe. INNERVATION: External plantar.

**lumbricales pedis** (lŭm-brĭ-kā′lēz pē′dĭs). Four. ACTION: Flexes the 1st and extends the 2nd and 3rd phalanges. ORIGIN: Tendons of flexor digitorum longus. INSERTION: First phalanx and extensor tendon. INNERVATION: External and internal plantar.

**quadratus plantae** (kwăd-rā′tŭs plăn′tē). ACTION: Assists flexion of toes. ORIGIN: Inferior surface of os calcis by two heads from outer and inner borders. INSERTION: Tendons of flexor digitorum longus. INNERVATION: Branch of lateral plantar. SYN: *flexor accessorius.*

## GENERAL

**arrectores pilorum** (ă″rĕk-tō′rēz pĭl-ō′rŭm). ACTION: Elevates hairs of skin. ORIGIN: Papillary layer of skin. INSERTION: Hair follicles. INNERVATION: Sympathetic.

# Appendix 2–2 Principal Joints

| Name | Type | Ligaments |
|---|---|---|
| Acromioclavicular | Gliding | Capsular; superior and inferior acromioclavicular; articular disk; coracoclavicular (trapezoid and conoid) |
| Atlas and axis | Pivot (trochoid) | Capsular; anterior and posterior atlantoaxial; transverse |
| Atlas and occipital | Condyloid | Capsular; anterior and posterior atlanto-occipital membrane; lateral; tectorial membrane; alar; apical odontoid |
| Calcaneocuboid | Gliding | Capsular; dorsal calcaneocuboid; bifurcated; long plantar; plantar calcaneocuboid |
| Carpometacarpal | Gliding | Dorsal; volar; interosseous |
| Femur and tibia | Hinge (ginglymus) | Capsular; patellar; oblique and arcuate popliteal; tibial and fibular collateral; anterior and posterior cruciate; medial and lateral menisci; transverse; coronary |
| Hip bone and femur | Ball and socket (enarthrosis) | Capsular; iliofemoral; pubocapsular; ischiofemoral; round ligament of femur; transverse acetabular |
| Humerus and ulna | Hinge (ginglymus) | Capsular; ulnar and radial collateral |
| Intercarpal | | |
| Carpal, proximal | Gliding | Dorsal; volar; interosseous |
| Carpal, distal | Gliding | Dorsal; volar; interosseous |
| Carpal bones, two rows with each other | | Volar; dorsal; collateral |
| Interphalangeal | Hinge (ginglymus) | Collateral; volar in fingers and plantar in toes |

**Principal Joints** (Continued)

| *Name* | *Type* | *Ligaments* |
|---|---|---|
| Mandible and temporal | Condyloid | Capsular; temporomandibular; sphenomandibular; articular disk; stylomandibular |
| Metacarpophalangeal | Condyloid | Volar; collateral |
| Metatarsophalangeal | Condyloid | Plantar; collateral |
| Pubic bones | Symphysis | Superior and arcuate pubic; interpubic fibrocartilaginous layer |
| Radioulnar, distal | Pivot (trochoid) | Ulnar collateral; articular disk |
| Radioulnar, proximal | Pivot (trochoid) | Annular |
| Ribs, heads of | Gliding | Capsular; radiate; intra-articular |
| Ribs, tubercles and necks of | Gliding | Capsular; anterior and posterior costotransverse; neck of rib; tubercle of rib |
| Sacrococcygeal | Symphysis | Anterior, posterior, and lateral sacrococcygeal; interposed fibrocartilaginous; interarticular |
| Sacroiliac | Gliding (slight) | Anterior and posterior sacroiliac; interosseous |
| Scapula and humerus | Ball and socket (enarthrosis) | Capsular; coracohumeral; glenohumeral; transverse humeral; glenoid of humerus |
| Sternoclavicular | Double gliding | Capsular; anterior and posterior sternoclavicular; inter- and costoclavicular; articular disk |
| Sternocostal | Gliding | Capsular; radiate and intra-articular sternocostal; costoxiphoid |
| Talus and calcaneus | Gliding | Capsular; anterior, posterior, lateral, medial, and interosseous; talocalcaneal |
| Talus and navicular | Gliding | Capsular; dorsal talonavicular |
| Tarsometatarsal | Gliding | Dorsal; plantar; interosseous |
| Tibia-fibula and talus (ankle) | Hinge (ginglymus) | Capsular; deltoid; anterior and posterior talofibular; calcaneofibular |
| Tibiofibular, proximal | Gliding | Capsular; anterior; posterior |
| Tibiofibular, distal | Syndesmosis | Anterior and posterior tibiofibular; inferior transverse; interosseous |
| Vertebral arches | Gliding | Capsular; flaval; supraspinal; nuchal; interspinal; intertransverse |
| Vertebral bodies | Symphysis | Anterior and posterior longitudinal; intervertebral fibrocartilaginous |
| Radius-ulna and carpals (wrist) | Condyloid | Volar and dorsal radiocarpal; ulnar and radial collateral |

# Appendix 2–3 Nerves

| *Name* | *Nomina Anatomica Term* | *Origin* | *Function* | *Distribution* |
|---|---|---|---|---|
| Abducent (6th cranial n.) | N. abducens | Pons | Motor | Lateral rectus muscle of eye |
| Accessory (11th cranial n.) | N. accessorius | Medulla oblongata and spinal cord | Motor | Sternomastoid and trapezius |
| Alveolar, inferior | N. alveolaris inferior | Mandibular div. of trigeminal | Sensory and motor | Teeth of lower jaw, mylohyoid muscle, and skin of chin |
| Alveolar, superior | Nn. alveolares superiores | Maxillary div. of trigeminal | Sensory | Upper teeth and gums |
| Auditory (8th cranial n.) SEE: *Vestibulocochlear* | | | | |
| Auricular, great | N. auricularis magnus | Second and third cervical through cervical plexus | Sensory | Side of neck; skin of ear and cheek |
| Auricular, posterior | N. auricularis posterior | Facial | Motor | Posterior auricular muscle |
| Auriculotemporal | N. auriculotemporalis | Mandibular div. of trigeminal | Sensory | Side of scalp |
| Buccal | N. buccalis | Mandibular div. of trigeminal | Sensory | Skin and mucous membrane of cheek |
| Cervical n., superficial (Cutaneous cervical n.; transverse n. of neck) | N. transversus colli | Second and third cervical through cervical plexus | Sensory | Skin of front of neck |
| Chorda tympani | | Facial | Motor and sensory | Sublingual and submaxillary glands; sense of taste |
| Ciliary, long | Nn. ciliares longi | Nasal | Sensory and motor | Cornea, iris, and ciliary body |
| Ciliary, short | Nn. ciliares breves | Ciliary ganglion | Sensory and motor | Cornea, iris, and ciliary body |
| Circumflex (Axillary) | N. axillaris | Posterior cord of brachial plexus | Motor and sensory | Deltoid, teres minor, shoulder joint, and overlying skin |

| | | | | |
|---|---|---|---|---|
| Coccygeal | N. coccygeus | Spinal cord | Motor and sensory | Coccygeus muscle and skin over coccyx |
| Cochlear | N. cochlearis | Auditory | Sense of hearing | Cochlea |
| Cutaneous, lateral, of forearm | N. cutaneus antebrachii medialis | Musculocutaneous nerve | General sensory | Side of forearm |
| Cutaneous, medial, of forearm | N. cutaneus antebrachii medialis | Brachial plexus | General sensory | Front and medial forearm |
| Cutaneous, posterior, of forearm | N. cutaneus antebrachii posterior | Radial nerve | General sensory | Back of forearm |
| Cutaneous, lateral inferior, of arm | N. cutaneus brachii lateralis inferior | Radial nerve | General sensory | Lateral side of arm |
| Cutaneous, lateral superior, of arm | N. cutaneus brachii lateralis superior | Axillary nerve | General sensory | Back of arm |
| Cutaneous, medial, of arm | N. cutaneus brachii medialis | Brachial plexus | General sensory | Middle and back of arm |
| Cutaneous, posterior, of arm | N. cutaneus brachii posterior | Radial nerve in axilla | General sensory | Back of arm |
| Cutaneous, intermediate dorsal | N. cutaneus dorsalis intermedius | Superficial peroneal nerve | General sensory | Front of lower leg; dorsum of foot; toes |
| Cutaneous, lateral dorsal | N. cutaneus dorsalis lateralis | Sural nerve | General sensory | Lateral side of foot |
| Cutaneous, medial dorsal | N. cutaneus dorsalis medialis | Superficial peroneal nerve | General sensory | Medial side of foot; big toe; second and third toes |
| Cutaneous, lateral femoral | N. cutaneus femoralis lateralis | Lumbar plexus | General sensory | Lateral and front thigh |
| Cutaneous, posterior femoral | N. cutaneus femoralis posterior | Sacral plexus | General sensory | Buttocks; external genitals; back of thigh and calf |
| Cutaneous, lateral, of calf | N. cutaneus surae lateralis | Common fibular nerve | General sensory | Lateral side of back of leg |
| Cutaneous, medial, of calf | N. cutaneus surae medialis | Tibial nerve | General sensory | Back of leg |
| Digastric | | Facial | Motor | Stylohyoid and posterior belly of digastric muscle |
| Facial (7th cranial n.) | N. facialis | Pons | Motor | Muscles of expression; sense of taste |

**Nerves** (Continued)

| *Name* | *Nomina Anatomica Term* | *Origin* | *Function* | *Distribution* |
|---|---|---|---|---|
| Femoral (Anterior crural n.) | N. femoralis | 2nd, 3rd, and 4th lumbar | Motor and sensory | Muscles and skin of thigh |
| Frontal | N. frontalis | Ophthalmic div. of trigeminal | Sensory | Skin of forehead |
| Genitofemoral (Genitocrural n.) | N. genitofemoralis | 1st and 2nd lumbar | Sensory and motor | Cremaster muscle and skin of groin and upper part of thigh |
| Glossopharyngeal (9th cranial n.) | N. glossopharyngeus | Medulla oblongata | Motor and sensory | Muscles and mucous membrane of pharynx, fauces, and posterior third of tongue; sense of taste |
| Gluteal, inferior | N. gluteus inferior | 5th lumbar and 1st and 2nd sacral | Motor | Gluteus maximus |
| Gluteal, superior | N. gluteus superior | 4th and 5th lumbar and 1st sacral | Motor | Gluteus medius and minimus, tensor fasciae femoris |
| Hypogastric | N. hypogastricus | Iliohypogastric | Motor and sensory | Muscles and skin of abdominal wall |
| Hypoglossal (12th cranial n.) | N. hypoglossus | Hypoglossal nucleus in medulla oblongata | Motor | Intrinsic and extrinsic muscles of tongue |
| Iliohypogastric | N. iliohypogastricus | 1st lumbar | Sensory and motor | Muscles and skin of hypogastrium |
| Ilioinguinal | N. ilioinguinalis | 1st lumbar | Sensory and motor | Muscles of abdominal wall, skin of upper thigh, skin of root of penis and scrotum (in male), and skin of mons pubis and labium majus (in female) |
| Infraorbital | N. infraorbitalis | Maxillary div. of trigeminal | Sensory | Skin of cheek and all upper teeth except molars |
| Infratrochlear | N. infratrochlearis | Nasociliary | Sensory | Skin of lower eyelid and root of nose, conjunctiva, and lacrimal sac and caruncle |

| | | | | |
|---|---|---|---|---|
| Intercostal | Nn. intercostales | Thoracic | Sensory and motor | Muscles and skin of back, thorax, and upper abdomen |
| Intercostobrachial | Nn. intercostobrachiales | 2nd intercostal | Sensory | Skin of axilla and medial side of arm |
| Interosseous, anterior (Volar interosseous n.) | N. interosseus anterior | Median | Motor | Deep flexor and pronator muscles of forearm |
| Interosseous, posterior | N. interosseus posterior | Musculospiral (Radial) | Motor and sensory | Muscles and skin of back of forearm and wrist |
| Lacrimal | N. lacrimalis | Ophthalmic div. of trigeminal | Sensory | Lacrimal gland, conjunctiva, and skin of upper eyelid |
| Laryngeal, inferior | N. laryngeus inferior | Branch of recurrent laryngeal | Motor | Muscles of larynx except cricothyroid |
| Laryngeal, recurrent | N. laryngeus recurrens | Vagus | Motor | Muscles of larynx except cricothyroid |
| Laryngeal, superior | N. laryngeus superior | Vagus | Motor and sensory | Mucous membrane of larynx; arytenoid and cricothyroid muscles |
| Lingual | N. lingualis | Mandibular div. of trigeminal | Sensory | Mucous membrane of anterior two thirds of tongue and floor and outer wall of mouth |
| Lumbar | Nn. lumbales | Spinal cord | Motor and sensory | Loins and front of lower abdomen and thigh to help in forming lumbar and sacral plexuses |
| Mandibular | N. mandibularis | Trigeminal | Motor and sensory | Teeth, gums, and skin of lower jaw and cheek; muscles of mastication; mucous membrane of anterior two thirds of tongue |
| Masseteric | N. massetericus | Mandibular div. of trigeminal | Motor | Masseter muscle |
| Maxillary | N. maxillaris | Trigeminal | Sensory | Nasal pharynx, palate, teeth of upper jaw and skin of cheek |

**Nerves** (Continued)

| *Name* | *Nomina Anatomica Term* | *Origin* | *Function* | *Distribution* |
|---|---|---|---|---|
| Median | N. medianus | Internal and external cords of brachial plexus | Motor and sensory | Pronators and flexors of forearm, two external lumbricales, thenar muscles, skin of palm and first four fingers |
| Mental | N. mentalis | Inferior alveolar | Sensory | Skin and mucous membrane of lower lip and chin |
| Musculocutaneous | N. musculocutaneous | External cord of brachial plexus | Motor and sensory | Flexors of upper arm and skin of external aspect of forearm |
| Mylohyoid | N. mylohyoideus | Inferior alveolar | Motor | Mylohyoid muscle and anterior belly of digastric muscle |
| Nasal (Nasociliary n.) | N. nasociliaris | Ophthalmic div. of trigeminal | Sensory | Ciliary ganglion, iris, conjunctiva, ethmoid cells, mucous membrane and skin of nose |
| Nasopalatine | N. nasopalatinus | Meckel's ganglion (Sphenopalatine ganglion) | Sensory | Mucous membrane of nose and palate |
| Obturator | N. obturatorius | 2nd, 3rd, and 4th lumbar through lumbar plexus | Motor and sensory | Adductors of thigh, hip, and knee joints; skin of inner aspect of thigh |
| Occipital, greater | N. occipitalis major | 2nd cervical | Motor and sensory | Muscles of back of neck; skin over occiput |
| Occipital, lesser | N. occipitalis minor | 2nd and 3rd cervical | Sensory | Skin behind ear and on back of scalp |
| Occipital, third | N. occipitalis tertius | 3rd cervical | Sensory | Skin of back of head and nape of neck |
| Oculomotor (3rd cranial n.) | N. oculomotorius | Floor of aqueduct of Sylvius | Motor | All ocular muscles except lateral rectus and superior oblique |
| Olfactory (1st cranial n.) | Nn. olfactorii | Olfactory lobe | Special sense of smell | Olfactory receptors |

| | | | | |
|---|---|---|---|---|
| Ophthalmic | N. ophthalmicus | 1st div. of trigeminal | Sensory | Lacrimal gland, conjunctiva, skin of forehead, skin and mucous membrane of nose |
| Optic (2nd cranial n.) | N. opticus | Corpora quadrigemina | Special sense of sight | Retina |
| Palatine, anterior, middle, and posterior | Nn. palatini | Meckel's ganglion | Sensory and motor | Mucous membrane of palate; autonomic to glands |
| Pectoralis | N. pectoralis lateralis<br>N. pectoralis medialis | Brachial plexus | Motor | Pectoralis minor and major muscles |
| Perineal | N. perineales | Pudendal | Motor and sensory | Muscles and skin of perineum |
| Peroneal, common | N. peroneus communis | Sciatic | Motor and sensory | Extensor muscles of lower leg and foot and overlying skin |
| Phrenic | N. phrenicus | 3rd, 4th, and 5th cervical | Motor and sensory | Diaphragm |
| Pneumogastric. SEE: *Vagus n.* | | | | |
| Pterygoid | N. pterygoideus lateralis medialis | Mandibular div. of trigeminal | Motor | Lateral and medial pterygoid muscles |
| Pterygoid canal, n. of (Vidian n.) | N. canalis pterygoidei | Facial | Sensory | Meckel's ganglion (sphenopalatine ganglion) |
| Pterygopalatine | N. pterygopalatini | Maxillary div. of trigeminal | Sensory | Meckel's ganglion |
| Pudendal | N. pudendus | 2nd, 3rd, and 4th sacral | Sensory | Skin and muscles of perineum and genitalia |
| Radial (musculospiral n.) | N. radialis | Brachial plexus | Motor and sensory | Skin of back of entire arm and hand; extensor muscles of entire arm and hand |
| Sacral | Nn. sacrales | Spinal cord | Motor and sensory | Muscles and skin of loins and lower extremities |
| Saphenous, external or short. SEE: *Sural n.* | | | | |

**Nerves** (Continued)

| *Name* | *Nomina Anatomica Term* | *Origin* | *Function* | *Distribution* |
|---|---|---|---|---|
| Saphenous, internal or long | N. saphenus | Femoral | Sensory | Skin of inner aspect of knee, leg, ankle, and dorsum of foot |
| Sciatic (Great sciatic n.) | N. ischiadicus | Sacral plexus | Motor and sensory | Muscles of calf and back of thigh; skin of lower calf and upper surface of foot |
| Spinal accessory. SEE: *Accessory n. (11th cranial n.)* | | | | |
| Stapedial | N. stapedius | Facial | Motor | Stapedius muscle |
| Stylohyoid | | Facial | Motor | Stylohyoid muscle |
| Suboccipital | N. suboccipitalis | Posterior div. of 1st cervical | Motor | Complexus oblique and rectus muscles of back of neck |
| Subscapular | N. subscapularis | Posterior cord of brachial plexus | Motor | Teres major and subscapularis muscles |
| Supraclavicular, intermediate (Supraclavicular n., middle; supraclavicular n.) | Nn. supraclaviculares intermedii | 3rd and 4th cervical | Sensory | Skin of fossa below collarbone |
| Supraclavicular, lateral (Supraclavicular n., posterior; supra-acromial n.) | Nn. supraclaviculares laterales | 3rd and 4th cervical | Sensory | Skin of shoulder |
| Supraclavicular, medial (Supraclavicular n., anterior; suprasternal n.) | Nn. supraclaviculares mediales | 3rd and 4th cervical | Sensory | Skin over upper part of thorax |
| Supraorbital | N. supraorbitalis | Frontal | Sensory | Forehead, upper eyelid, scalp, and frontal sinus |
| Suprascapular | N. suprascapularis | 5th and 6th cervical | Motor | Supraspinatus and infraspinatus muscles and the shoulder joint |
| Supratrochlear | N. supratrochlearis | Frontal | Sensory | Skin of upper eyelid and root of nose |

| Sural | N. suralis | Common peroneal and tibial n.s | Sensory | Skin of calf and medial side of foot to great toe |
|---|---|---|---|---|
| Temporal, deep | Nn. temporales profundi | Mandibular div. of trigeminal | Motor | Temporal muscle |
| Thoracic | Nn. thoracici | Spinal cord | Motor and sensory | Muscles and skin of thorax |
| Thoracic, long (Posterior thoracic n.; external respiratory n. of Bell). | N. thoracicus longus | 5th, 6th, and 7th cervical | Motor | Serratus anterior muscle |
| Tibial | N. tibialis | Sciatic | Motor and sensory | Flexor muscles of back of knee joint and calf; skin of lower leg |
| Trigeminal (5th cranial n.; trifacial n.) | N. trigeminus | Midbrain and pons | Motor and sensory | Skin of face, tongue, teeth; muscles of mastication |
| Trochlear (4th cranial n.; pathetic n.) | N. trochlearis | Floor of aqueduct of Sylvius | Motor | Superior oblique muscle of eye |
| Typanic (Jacobson's n.) | N. tympanicus | Glossopharyngeal | Sensory | Tympanum, eustachian tube, and structures of middle ear |
| Ulnar | N. ulnaris | Medial cord of brachial plexus | Motor and sensory | Muscles and skin of forearm and hand |
| Vagus (10th cranial n.; pneumogastric n.) | N. vagus | Medulla oblongata | Motor and sensory | Pharynx, larynx, heart, lungs, stomach and other abdominal viscera |
| Vestibulocochlear (8th cranial n.; acoustic n.; auditory n.) | N. vestibulocochlearis | Ganglion of Scarpa and ganglion of Corti | Sense of hearing and equilibrium | Cochlea, semicircular canals, utricle, and saccule |
| Zygomatic | N. zygomaticus | Maxillary div. of trigeminal | Sensory | Skin of temple and cheekbone |

## Appendix 2–4 Nerve Plexuses

**aortic** (ā-or′tĭk). *(Abdominal.)* ORIGIN: Semilunar, lumbar ganglia, renal and solar plexuses. LOCATION: Sides and front of aorta. DISTRIBUTION: Inferior mesenteric, spermatic and hypogastric plexus. Filaments to inferior vena cava. *(Thoracic.)* ORIGIN: Thoracic ganglia of sympathetic nerve, cardiac plexus. LOCATION: Surrounding the thoracic aorta. DISTRIBUTION: Solar plexus, aorta.

**brachial** (brā′kē-ăl). ORIGIN: Anterior branches of 5th, 6th, 7th, 8th cervical, and greater part of 1st thoracic nerves. LOCATION: Lower part of neck to axilla. DISTRIBUTION: Sixteen branches of suprascapular, subscapular, rhomboid, median, ulnar, musculospiral, posterior thoracic, musculothoracic, circumflex, musculocutaneous nerves.

**cardiac** (kăr′dē-ăk). *(Great or Deep.)* ORIGIN: Cardiac nerves of cervical ganglion of sympathetic and vagus. LOCATION: In front of bifurcation of trachea. DISTRIBUTION: Pulmonary, coronary and cardiac plexuses. *(Superficial or Anterior.)* ORIGIN: Left superior cardiac nerve, branch of vagus, and filaments of deep cardiac plexus. LOCATION: Beneath arch of aorta. Front of right pulmonary artery. DISTRIBUTION: Coronary and pulmonary plexuses.

**carotid** (kă-rŏt′ĭd). *(External.)* ORIGIN: Pharyngeal plexus, superior cardiac nerve, and superior cervical ganglion. LOCATION: Around external carotid artery. DISTRIBUTION: External carotid artery and its branches. *(Internal.)* ORIGIN: Postganglionic sympathetic fibers. LOCATION: Surrounding internal carotid artery. DISTRIBUTION: Tympanic plexus, sphenopalatine ganglion, abducens and oculomotor nerves, the cerebral vessels, and the ciliary ganglion.

**cavernous** (kăv′ĕr-nŭs). ORIGIN: 3rd to 6th cranial nerves and ophthalmic ganglion. LOCATION: Cavernous sinus. DISTRIBUTION: Wall of internal carotid artery.

**celiac** (sē′lē-ăk). ORIGIN: Solar plexus, branches from lesser splanchnic and vagus nerves. LOCATION: Behind stomach, in front of aorta at level of origin of celiac artery. DISTRIBUTION: Coronary, hepatic, pyloric, gastroduodenal, gastroepiploic, and splenic plexuses. SYN: *solar plexus.*

**cervical** (ser′vĭ-kăl). ORIGIN: Anterior branches of first four cervical nerves. LOCATION: Beneath sternocleidomastoid muscle opposite first four cervical vertebrae. DISTRIBUTION: Skin and muscles of neck; phrenic nerve to diaphragm.

**coccygeal** (kŏk-sĭj′ē-ăl). ORIGIN: Fourth and 5th sacral and the coccygeal nerves. LOCATION: Dorsal surface of coccyx and caudal end of sacrum. DISTRIBUTION: Anococcygeal nerves.

**cystic** (sĭs′tĭk). ORIGIN: Hepatic plexus. LOCATION: At gallbladder. DISTRIBUTION: Gallbladder.

**esophageal** (ē-sŏf″ă-jē′ăl). ORIGIN: Vagus nerve, thoracic sympathetic ganglia. LOCATION: Around the esophagus. DISTRIBUTION: Esophagus.

**gastric** (găs′trĭk). ORIGIN: Celiac plexus and continuations of esophageal plexuses. LOCATION: Gastric artery. DISTRIBUTION: Stomach.

**hemorrhoidal** (hĕm-ō-roy′dăl). ORIGIN: Pelvic and inferior mesenteric plexuses. LOCATION: Rectum and sides of rectum. DISTRIBUTION: Rectum.

**hepatic** (hē-păt′ĭk). ORIGIN: Celiac plexus, left vagus, right phrenic. LOCATION: Accompanies hepatic artery. DISTRIBUTION: Liver.

**hypogastric** (hī″pō-găs′trĭk). ORIGIN: Aortic plexus and lumbar ganglia. LOCATION: Promontory of sacrum. DISTRIBUTION: Pelvic plexus.

**lumbar** (lŭm′băr). ORIGIN: Anterior branches of first four lumbar nerves. LOCATION: Psoas muscle. DISTRIBUTION: Iliohypogastric, ilioinguinal, genitocrural, external cutaneous, obturator, accessory, and anterior crural nerves.

**Meissner's** (mīs′nĕrz). ORIGIN: Superior mesenteric plexus (controls secretions of the bowels). LOCATION: Submucosa of alimentary tube. DISTRIBUTION: Mucosal glands and smooth muscle. SYN: *submucosal plexus.*

**mesenteric** (mĕs″ĕn-tĕr′ĭk). ORIGIN: Celiac plexus and left side of aortic plexus. LOCATION: Surrounding the inferior and superior mesenteric arteries. DISTRIBUTION: Descending colon, sigmoid, rectum, intestines.

**myenteric** (mī″ĕn-tĕr′ĭk). ORIGIN: Sympathetic and parasympathetic nerves. LOCATION: Between circular and longitudinal smooth muscle layers of alimentary tube. DISTRIBUTION: Smooth muscle of alimentary tube; controls peristalsis. SYN: *Auerbach's plexus.*

**ophthalmic** (ŏf-thăl′mĭk). ORIGIN: Internal carotid plexus. LOCATION: Around ophthalmic artery and optic nerve. DISTRIBUTION: Optic region.

**pancreatic** (păn″krē-ăt′ĭk). ORIGIN: Splenic plexus. LOCATION: Near pancreas. DISTRIBUTION: Filaments to pancreas.

**pancreaticoduodenal** (păn″krē-ăt″ĭ-kō-dū-ō-dē′năl). ORIGIN: Hepatic plexus. LOCATION: Near head of pancreas. DISTRIBUTION: Filaments to pancreas and duodenum.

**pelvic** (pĕl′vĭk). ORIGIN: Hypogastric plexus, 2nd to 4th sacral nerves, 1st and 2nd sacral ganglia (pelvic brain). LOCATION: Side of rectum and bladder. DISTRIBUTION: Viscera of pelvis, pelvic plexus.

**phrenic** (frĕn′ĭk). ORIGIN: Cervical plexus, semilunar ganglia. LOCATION: Accompanies phrenic artery to diaphragm. DISTRIBUTION: Diaphragm and suprarenal capsules.

**prostatic** (prŏs-tăt′ĭk). ORIGIN: Hypogastric

plexus. LOCATION: Vesical arteries. DISTRIBUTION: Bladder.

**pulmonary** (pŭl′mō-nĕ-rē). ORIGIN: Anterior and posterior pulmonary branches of vagus and sympathetic nerves. LOCATION: Root of lungs, front and back. DISTRIBUTION: Root of lungs.

**pyloric** (pī-lor′ĭk). ORIGIN: Hepatic plexus. LOCATION: Near pylorus. DISTRIBUTION: Filaments to pylorus.

**renal** (rē′năl). ORIGIN: Solar and aortic plexuses and semilunar ganglia. LOCATION: Renal artery. DISTRIBUTION: Kidneys, posterior vena cava, spermatic plexus.

**sacral** (sā′krăl). ORIGIN: Anterior branch of 4th and 5th lumbar and 1st, 2nd, 3rd, and 4th sacral nerves. LOCATION: Front of sacrum on piriformis muscle. DISTRIBUTION: Muscular, pudic, superior gluteal, great and small sciatic nerves.

**solar** (sō′lăr). *(Epigastric.)* ORIGIN: Splanchnics and right vagus. LOCATION: Back of stomach. DISTRIBUTION: Semilunar ganglia, suprarenal, renal, spermatic, celiac, superior mesenteric, and aortic plexuses. Called *abdominal brain.* SYN: *celiac plexus.*

**spermatic** (spĕr-măt′ĭk). *(Ovarian.)* ORIGIN: Aortic plexus. LOCATION: Accompanies spermatic vessels to testes or ovaries. DISTRIBUTION: Testes or ovaries.

**splenic** (splĕn′ĭk). ORIGIN: Celiac plexus, left semilunar ganglion, right vagus nerve. LOCATION: Accompanies splenic artery. DISTRIBUTION: Spleen, pancreatic plexus, left gastroepiploic plexus.

**suprarenal** (soo″pră-rē′năl). ORIGIN: Diaphragmatic, solar, and renal plexuses. LOCATION: Around suprarenal capsules. DISTRIBUTION: Filaments to medulla of suprarenal capsules.

**thyroid** (thī′royd). *(Inferior.)* ORIGIN: Middle cervical ganglion. LOCATION: Around external carotid and inferior thyroid arteries. DISTRIBUTION: Larynx, pharynx, thyroid gland. *(Superior.)* ORIGIN: Superior laryngeal and cardiac nerves. LOCATION: Around the thyroid gland. DISTRIBUTION: Thyroid region.

**uterine** (ū′tĕriĭn). ORIGIN: Pelvic plexus. LOCATION: Accompanies uterine arteries. DISTRIBUTION: Cervix and lower part of uterus.

**vaginal** (văj′ĭn-ăl). ORIGIN: Pelvic plexus. LOCATION: Vaginal walls. DISTRIBUTION: Vagina.

**vertebral** (vĕr′tĕ-brăl). ORIGIN: First part thoracic ganglion, upper cervical nerves. LOCATION: Surrounding basilar and vertebral arteries. DISTRIBUTION: Vertebral and cerebellar regions.

**vesical** (vĕs′ĭ-kăl). ORIGIN: Pelvic plexus. LOCATION: Accompanies vesical arteries. DISTRIBUTION: Vesicula seminalis, vas deferens.

## Appendix 2–5 Cranial Nerves

| No. | Name | Nomina Anatomica Term | Origin | Function | Distribution |
|---|---|---|---|---|---|
| 1st | Olfactory | Nn. olfactorii | Olfactory lobe | Smell | Olfactory receptors |
| 2nd | Optic | N. opticus | Retina | Sight | Retina |
| 3rd | Oculomotor | N. oculomotorius | Floor of aqueduct of Sylvius | Motor | All ocular muscles except lateral rectus and superior oblique; iris |
| 4th | Trochlear | N. trochlearis | Floor of aqueduct of Sylvius | Motor | Superior oblique muscle of eye |
| 5th | Trigeminal | N. trigeminus | Midbrain and pons | Motor and chief sensory n. of face | Skin of face; tongue; teeth; muscles of mastication |
| 6th | Abducent | N. abducens | Pons | Motor | Lateral rectus muscle of eye |
| 7th | Facial | N. facialis | Pons | Motor and sensory | Muscles of expression; salivary glands; sense of taste |
| 8th | Auditory | N. vestibulocochlearis | Brain | Hearing and equilibrium | Cochlea, semicircular canals, utricle and saccule |
| 9th | Glossopharyngeal | N. glossopharyngeus | Medulla oblongata | Motor and sensory | Sensation of pharynx and posterior third of tongue; parotid gland; sense of taste; carotid sinus |
| 10th | Vagus | N. vagus | Medulla oblongata | Motor and sensory | Pharynx; larynx; heart; lungs; esophagus; aortic sinus; stomach and other abdominal viscera |
| 11th | Accessory | N. accessorius | Medulla oblongata and spinal cord | Motor | Sternomastoid and trapezius muscles |
| 12th | Hypoglossal | N. hypoglossus | Medulla oblongata | Motor | Intrinsic and extrinsic muscles of tongue |

# Appendix 2–6 Arteries

| *Name* | *Nomina Anatomica Term* | *Origin* | *Distribution* | *Branches* |
|---|---|---|---|---|
| Alveolar, inferior | A. alveolaris inferior | Maxillary | Lower anterior skull | Dental; mylohyoid; mental |
| Angular | A. angularis | Terminal branch of external maxillary | Neck and face | |
| Aorta. SEE: *aorta* in vocabulary | | | | |
| Arcuate (Metatarsal a.) | A. arcuata pedis | Dorsal a. of foot | Foot and toes | Deep plantar; dorsal metatarsal; dorsal digital |
| A. of the pterygoid canal | A. canalis pterygoidei | Maxillary | Roof of pharynx; auditory (eustachian) tube | |
| Auditory, internal | A. labyrinthi | Middle of basilar or anterior inferior cerebellar | Internal ear | |
| Auricular, deep | A. auricularis profunda | Maxillary | Skin of auditory canal, tympanic membrane, and temporomandibular joint | |
| Auricular, posterior | A. auricularis posterior | External carotid | Middle ear; mastoid cells; auricle; parotid gland | Stylomastoid; auricular; occipital |
| Axillary | A. axillaris | Subclavian | Forms brachial artery and seven branches | Superior; thoracic; thoracoacromial; lateral thoracic; subscapular; anterior and posterior humeral; thoracodorsal; brachial |
| Basilar | A. basilaris | Vertebral | Pons | Posterior cerebral; pontine; internal auditory; anterior inferior cerebellar; superior cerebellar |

**Arteries** (Continued)

| *Name* | *Nomina Anatomica Term* | *Origin* | *Distribution* | *Branches* |
|---|---|---|---|---|
| Brachial | A. brachialis | Axillary | Upper arm | Deep brachial; nutrient; superior and inferior collateral; muscular |
| Brachial, deep | A. profunda brachii | Brachial | Accompanies radial nerve | |
| Brachiocephalic trunk (Innominate a.) | Truncus brachiocephalicus | Arch of aorta | Right side of head, neck, and arm | Right subclavian; right common carotid |
| Bronchial | Rr. bronchiales | Thoracic aorta | Bronchi; lower trachea; pulmonary vessels; pericardium; part of esophagus | Left and right bronchial |
| Buccal (Buccinator a.) | A. buccalis | Maxillary | Buccinator muscle; mucous membrane of mouth | |
| Capsular, middle. SEE: *Suprarenal a., middle.* | | | | |
| Carotid, common | A. carotis communis | Brachiocephalic trunk (right); aortic arch (left) | Neck and thyroid | External and internal carotid |
| Carotid, external | A. carotis externa | Common carotid | Neck; face; skull | Superior thyroid; ascending pharyngeal; lingual; facial; occipital; posterior auricular; superficial temporal; maxillary |
| Carotid, internal | A. carotis interna | Common carotid | Anterior brain; eyes; forehead; nose | Caroticotympanic; vidian; cavernous; hypophyseal; semilunar; anterior meningeal; ophthalmic; anterior and middle cerebral; posterior communicating; choroidal |

| | | | | |
|---|---|---|---|---|
| Celiac | Truncus celiacus | Abdominal aorta | Stomach; liver; pancreas; duodenum; spleen | Left gastric; common hepatic; splenic |
| Cerebellar, anterior inferior | A. cerebelli inferior anterior | Basilar | Anterior undersurface of cerebellum | |
| Cerebellar, posterior inferior | A. cerebelli inferior posterior | Vertebral | Cerebellum | |
| Cerebellar, superior | A. cerebelli superior | Near termination of basilar | Upper cerebellum; midbrain; pineal body | |
| Cerebral, anterior | A. cerebri anterior | Internal carotid | Cerebrum | Cortical; central; anterior communicating |
| Cerebral, posterior | A. cerebri posterior | Basilar | Cerebrum | Central; posterior choroidal; cortical temporal; calcarine; parieto-occipital |
| Cervical, ascending | A. cervicalis ascendens | Inferior thyroid | Muscles of neck and spinal cord | |
| Cervical, superficial | | Thyroid axis | Muscles of shoulder | |
| Cervical, transverse | A. transversa colli | Thyroid axis | Muscles and glands of neck | Deep and superficial rami |
| Choroidal, anterior (Choroid) | A. choroides anterior | Internal carotid | Internal capsule | |
| Ciliary, anterior | Aa. ciliares anteriores | Ophthalmic and lacrimal | Iris; conjunctiva | |
| Ciliary, long posterior | Aa. ciliares posteriores longae | Ophthalmic | Iris and ciliary process | |
| Ciliary, short posterior | Aa. ciliares posteriores breves | Ophthalmic | Choroid coat of eye | |
| Circumflex, anterior humeral | A. circumflexa humeri anterior | Lateral side of axillary | Shoulder joint and upper arm | |
| Circumflex iliac a., deep | A. circumflexa ilium profunda | External iliac | Muscles of skin and lower abdomen | |
| Circumflex, posterior humeral | A. circumflexa humeri posterior | Axillary | Deltoid and shoulder joint; upper arm | |
| Colic, left | A. colica sinistra | Inferior mesenteric | Descending and transverse colon | Ascending and descending colic |
| Colic, middle | A. colica media | Superior mesenteric | Transverse colon | Right and left colic |

**Arteries** (Continued)

| *Name* | *Nomina Anatomica Term* | *Origin* | *Distribution* | *Branches* |
|---|---|---|---|---|
| Colic, right | A. colica dextra | Superior mesenteric | Ascending colon | Ascending and descending colic |
| Collateral, inferior ulnar | A. collateralis ulnaris inferior | Brachial | Muscles at back of elbow | |
| Collateral, superior ulnar | A. collateralis ulnaris superior | Brachial | Elbow joint and triceps muscles | |
| Communicating, posterior | A. communicans posterior cerebri | Internal carotid | Hippocampus; thalamus | |
| Coronary, left | A. coronaria sinistra | Ascending aorta | Left ventricle and atrium | Anterior descending coronary; circumflex |
| Coronary, right | A. coronaria dextra | Ascending aorta | Right ventricle and atrium | Posterior descending; marginal |
| Cystic | A. cystica | Proper hepatic | Gallbladder; liver | |
| Digital, common palmar | Aa. digitales palmares communes | Palmar arch | Fingers | Proper palmar digital |
| Digital, proper palmar (Collateral digital a.) | Aa. digitales palmares propriae | Common palmar digital | Fingers | |
| Dorsal, of foot | A. dorsalis pedis | Continuation of anterior tibial | Foot | Lateral and medial tarsal; deep plantar; arcuate; first dorsal metatarsal |
| Epigastric, inferior | A. epigastrica inferior | External iliac | Abdominal muscles; peritoneum | Cremasteric |
| Epigastric, superficial | A. epigastrica superficialis | Femoral | Skin of abdomen; superficial fascia; inguinal lymph nodes | |
| Epigastric, superior | A. epigastric superior | Internal thoracic | Abdominal muscles and skin; diaphragm | |
| Esophageal | | In front of aorta | Esophagus | |
| Ethmoidal, anterior | A. ethmoidalis anterior | Ophthalmic | Ethmoidal cells and frontal sinus; dura mater; nasal cavity | Anterior meningeal |

| | | | | |
|---|---|---|---|---|
| Ethmoidal, posterior | A. ethmoidalis posterior | Ophthalmic | Ethmoidal cells; dura mater; nasal cavity | Posterior meningeal |
| Facial (External maxillary a.) | A. facialis | Carotid triangle | Face; tonsil; palate; submandibular gland | Ascending palatine; tonsillar; submental; inferior and superior labial; angular; glandular; lateral nasal; muscular |
| Facial, transverse | A. transversa faciei | Superficial temporal | Parotid gland; skin of face; masseter muscle | |
| Femoral | A. femoralis | Continuation of external iliac | Lower abdominal wall; external genitalia; lower extremity | Superficial epigastric; superficial circumflex iliac; external pudendal; deep femoral; descending genicular |
| Femoral, deep | A. profunda femoris | Femoral | Thigh muscles; hip joint; gluteal muscles; femur | Perforating; medial and lateral circumflex |
| Femoral, lateral circumflex | A. circumflexa femoris lateralis | Deep femoral a. | Hip joint; thigh muscles | Ascending; descending; transverse |
| Femoral, medial circumflex | A. circumflexa femoris medialis | Medial aspect of deep femoral a. | Hip joint; thigh muscles | Deep; acetabular; transverse; superficial |
| Fibula. SEE: *Peroneal a.* | | | | |
| Frontal | A. supratrochlearis | Ophthalmic | Forehead muscles; cranium | |
| Gastric, left | A. gastrica sinistra | Celiac trunk | Abdominal section of esophagus; stomach; left lobe of liver | Anterior and posterior gastric; cardioesophageal |
| Gastric, right | A. gastrica dextra | Common hepatic | Lesser curvature of stomach | |
| Gastric, short | Aa. gastricae breves | End of splenic | Greater curvature of stomach | |
| Gastroduodenal | A. gastroduodenalis | Common hepatic trunk | Stomach; duodenum; pancreas; greater omentum | Superior pancreaticoduodenal; right gastroepiploic; retroduodenal |

**Arteries** (Continued)

| *Name* | *Nomina Anatomica Term* | *Origin* | *Distribution* | *Branches* |
|---|---|---|---|---|
| Gastro-omental, left | A. gastro-omentalis sinistra | Splenic | Stomach; greater omentum | |
| Gastro-omental, right | A. gastro-omentalis dextra | Gastroduodenal | Stomach; greater omentum | Ascending pyloric and ascending branches to stomach |
| Genicular, descending | A. genus descendens | Femoral | Knee joint; skin of upper and medial section of leg | Saphenous; musculo-articular |
| Genicular, inferior | A. genus inferior lateralis | Popliteal | Knee joint; skin of upper and middle leg | |
| Genicular, middle | A. genus media | Popliteal | Knee joint, ligaments and synovial membrane of knee | |
| Genicular, superior | A. genus superior lateralis | On either side of popliteal | Knee joint; femur; patella | |
| Gluteal, inferior | A. glutea inferior | Internal iliac | Buttocks and back of thigh | Sciatic |
| Gluteal, superior | A. glutea superior | Internal iliac | Gluteal region | Superficial and deep gluteal |
| Hemorrhoidal, middle | A. rectalis media | Internal iliac | Rectum; prostate; seminal vesicles | |
| Hemorrhoidal, superior | A. rectalis superior | Inferior mesenteric | Rectum | |
| Hepatic, common | A. hepatica communis | Celiac trunk | Stomach; pancreas; duodenum; liver; gallbladder; greater omentum | Right gastric; gastroduodenal; proper hepatic |
| Hepatic, proper | A. hepatica propria | Common hepatic | Liver and gallbladder | Cystic |
| Ileocolic | A. ileocolica | Superior mesenteric | Ileum; cecum; appendix; ascending colon | Superior and inferior ileocolic; appendicular |
| Iliac, common | A. iliaca communis | End of abdominal aorta | Pelvis; abdominal wall; lower limbs | External and internal iliac |

| | | | | |
|---|---|---|---|---|
| Iliac, external | A. iliaca externa | Common iliac | Abdominal wall; external genitalia; lower limb | Inferior epigastric; deep circumflex iliac |
| Iliac, internal | A. iliaca interna | Common iliac | Walls and viscera of pelvis, buttocks, reproductive organs; medial side of thighs | Superior, middle, and inferior vesical; middle hemorrhoidal; obturator; internal pudendal; inferior gluteal; uterine; vaginal; iliolumbar; lateral sacral; superior gluteal |
| Iliac, superficial circumflex | A. circumflexa ilium superficialis | Femoral | Inguinal glands; skin of thigh and abdomen | |
| Infraorbital | A. infraorbitalis | Maxillary | Maxillary sinus; center of face | Anterior superior alveolar; orbital |
| Intercostal | Aa. intercostales posteriores | Thoracic aorta | Intercostal spaces; back muscles; vertebral column; thoracic wall | Anterior and posterior rami |
| Interosseous, anterior (Volar interosseous a.) | A. interossea anterior | Common interosseous | Deep structures of anterior forearm | Median; nutrient; muscular |
| Interosseous, common | A. interossea communis | Ulnar | Deep structure of forearm | Anterior and posterior interosseous |
| Interosseous, posterior | A. interossea posterior | Common interosseous | Muscles of posterior forearm | Recurrent interosseous |
| Intestinal | | Superior mesenteric | Jejunum and ileum | |
| Labial, inferior | A. labialis inferior | Near angle of mouth | Lower lip | |
| Labial, superior | A. labialis superior | Near angle of mouth | Upper lip | |
| Lacrimal | A. lacrimalis | Ophthalmic | Lacrimal gland; eyelid; conjunctiva | Lateral palpebral; zygomatic; recurrent |
| Laryngeal, inferior | A. laryngea inferior | Inferior thyroid | Muscles and mucous membrane of trachea and larynx | |

**Arteries** (Continued)

| *Name* | *Nomina Anatomica Term* | *Origin* | *Distribution* | *Branches* |
|---|---|---|---|---|
| Laryngeal, superior | A. laryngea superior | Superior thyroid | Muscles, mucous membrane, and glands of larynx | |
| Lingual | A. lingualis | External carotid | Undersurface of tongue; tonsil; epiglottis | Suprahyoid; dorsal and deep lingual; sublingual |
| Lingual, deep | A. profunda linguae | End of lingual | Undersurface of tongue | |
| Lingual, dorsal | Rr. dorsales linguae | Lingual | Mucous membrane on dorsum of tongue; glossopalatine arch; tonsil; soft palate; epiglottis | |
| Lumbar | Aa. lumbales | Abdominal aorta | Abdominal wall; vertebrae; lumbar muscles; renal capsule | Posterior lumbar; muscular |
| Malleolar, lateral anterior | A. malleolaris anterior lateralis | Anterior tibial | Ankle joint | |
| Malleolar, medial anterior | A. malleolaris anterior medialis | Anterior tibial | Ankle joint | |
| Malleolar, medial posterior | Rr. malleolares mediales arteriae tibialis posterioris | Peroneal | Tibial malleolus | |
| Masseteric | A. masseterica | Maxillary | Masseter muscle | |
| Maxillary (Internal maxillary a.) | A. maxillaris | External carotid | Jaws and teeth; muscles of mastication; ear; meninges; nose; nasal sinus; palate | Anterior tympanic; deep auricular; middle and accessory meningeal; inferior and posterior superior alveolar; deep temporal; pterygoid; masseteric; buccal; infraorbital; greater palatine; pharyngeal; sphenopalatine |
| Maxillary, external. SEE: *Facial a.* | | | | |

| | | | | |
|---|---|---|---|---|
| Mediastinal, anterior | Rr. mediastinales arteriae thoracicae internae | Internal thoracic | Anterior mediastinal cavity; portion of thymus | |
| Medullary (Bulbar a.) | | Vertebral | Medulla oblongata | |
| Meningeal, middle | A. meningea media | Maxillary | Dura mater; cranial bones | Superficial; petrosal; superior tympanic; orbital; temporal; and numerous small vessels |
| Mesenteric, inferior | A. mesenterica inferior | Abdominal aorta | Left half of transverse colon; descending, iliac, and sigmoid colon; part of rectum | Left colic; sigmoid; superior hemorrhoidal |
| Mesenteric, superior | A. mesenterica superior | Abdominal aorta | Small intestine; cecum; ascending colon; part of transverse colon | Inferior pancreaticoduodenal; jejunal; ileal; ileocolic; right and middle colon |
| Metacarpal, palmar | Aa. metacarpales palmares | Deep palmar arch | Interosseous muscles and bones | |
| Metatarsal, first dorsal | | Dorsal a. of foot | Medial border of foot | |
| Musculophrenic | A. musculophrenica | Internal thoracic | Diaphragm; abdominal and thoracic walls | |
| Nasal, dorsal | A. dorsalis nasi | Ophthalmic | Lacrimal sac; integuments of nose | Lacrimal |
| Obturator | A. obturatoria | Internal iliac | Pelvis and thigh | Iliac; vesical; pubic; anterior and posterior obturator |
| Occipital | A. occipitalis | Posterior part of external carotid | Muscles of neck and scalp; meninges; mastoid | Muscular; meningeal; sternomastoid; descending occipital; auricular |
| Ophthalmic | A. ophthalmica | Internal carotid | Eye and adjacent structures of face | Lacrimal; supraorbital; posterior and anterior ethmoidal; medial palpebral; frontal; dorsal nasal; central a. of retina; short posterior, long posterior, and anterior ciliary; muscular |
| Ovarian | A. ovarica | Abdominal aorta | Ovaries; uterine tubes; ureter | Ureteral |

**Arteries** (Continued)

| *Name* | *Nomina Anatomica Term* | *Origin* | *Distribution* | *Branches* |
|---|---|---|---|---|
| Palatine, ascending | A. palatina ascendens | Facial | Base of skull; palate; auditory tube | |
| Palatine, greater | A. palatina major | Maxillary | Palate and tonsils | Greater and lesser palatine |
| Palpebral, medial (Internal Palpebral a.) | Aa. palpebrales mediales | Ophthalmic | Upper and lower eyelids | Superior and inferior palpebral |
| Pancreaticoduodenal, inferior | Aa. pancreaticoduodenales inferiores | Superior mesenteric | Pancreas; duodenum | |
| Pancreaticoduodenal, superior | Aa. supraduodenales superiores | Gastroduodenal | Pancreas; duodenum | |
| Perforating | Aa. perforantes | Deep femoral | Back of thigh | |
| Pericardiacophrenic | A. pericardiacophrenica | Internal thoracic | Diaphragm; pericardium; pleura | |
| Peroneal (Fibular) | A. peronea (A. fibularis) | Posterior tibial | Ankle; deep calf muscles | Perforating; communicating; calcaneal; tibial and fibular nutrient; lateral and medial malleolar |
| Pharyngeal, ascending | A. pharyngea ascendens | Posterior part of external carotid | Pharynx; soft palate; ear; meninges; cranial nerves; capitis muscles | Pharyngeal; palatine; posterior meningeal; prevertebral; inferior tympanic |
| Phrenic | Aa. phrenicae inferiores and Aa. phrenicae superiores | Aorta, abdominal Aorta, thoracic | Diaphragm; adrenal glands Diaphragm | Medial, lateral, and superior adrenal |
| Plantar, deep | R. plantaris profunda | Dorsal a. of foot | Sole of foot | First plantar metatarsal |
| Plantar, lateral | A. plantaris lateralis | Posterior tibial | Toes and sole of foot | Plantar arch and plantar metatarsal |
| Plantar, medial | A. plantaris medialis | Posterior tibial | Muscles and skin of sole of foot and toes | Superficial digital |

| | | | | |
|---|---|---|---|---|
| Popliteal | A. poplitea | Continuation of femoral | Knee and calf | Anterior and posterior tibial; lateral and medial superior genicular; middle, sural, lateral, and medial inferior genicular; genicular articular |
| Pudendal, external | Aa. pudendae externae | Femoral | External genitalia; medial thigh | |
| Pudendal, internal | A. pudenda interna | Internal iliac | External genitalia | Posterior scrotal or posterior labial; inferior hemorrhoidal; perineal; urethral; a. of bulb of penis or vestibule; deep a. of penis or clitoris; dorsal a. of penis or clitoris |
| Pulmonary | Truncus pulmonalis | Right ventricle | Lungs | Right and left pulmonary |
| Pulmonary, left | A. pulmonalis sinistra | Pulmonary trunk | Left lung | Numerous branches |
| Pulmonary, right | A. pulmonalis dextra | Pulmonary trunk | Right lung | Numerous branches |
| Radial | A. radialis | Brachial | Forearm; wrist; hand | Recurrent radial; muscular; palmar and dorsal carpal; superficial palmar; first dorsal metacarpal; principal a. of thumb; perforating; recurrent; palmar |
| Radial, of index finger | A. radialis indicis | Principal a. of thumb | Index finger | |
| Recurrent, anterior tibial | A. recurrens tibialis anterior | Anterior tibial | Knee joint | |
| Recurrent, posterior tibial | A. recurrens tibialis posterior | Anterior tibial | Knee joint | |
| Recurrent, radial | A. recurrens radialis | Below elbow from radial | Elbow joint; muscles of forearm | |
| Recurrent, ulnar | A. recurrens ulnaris | Ulnar | Elbow joint; skin and muscles of elbow | Anterior and posterior recurrent |
| Renal | A. renalis | Abdominal aorta | Kidney; suprarenal gland; ureter | Inferior suprarenal |

**Arteries** (Continued)

| *Name* | *Nomina Anatomica Term* | *Origin* | *Distribution* | *Branches* |
|---|---|---|---|---|
| Retroduodenal | | Gastroduodenal | Head of pancreas; duodenum; bile duct | |
| Sacral, lateral | Aa. sacrales laterales | Internal iliac | Coccyx and sacrum | |
| Sacral, middle | A. sacralis mediana | Abdominal aorta | Sacrum; coccyx; rectum | Lowest lumbar |
| Scapula, circumflex a. of | A. circumflexa scapulae | Subscapular | Lateral border of scapula; infraspinous fossa | |
| Scapular, descending (Dorsal scapular a.) | A. scapularis descendens | Subclavian | Medial border of scapula | |
| Sigmoid | Aa. sigmoideae | Inferior mesenteric | Iliac, sigmoid, and pelvic colon | |
| Spermatic, internal. SEE: *Testicular a.* | | | | |
| Sphenopalatine (Nasopalatine a.) | A. sphenopalatina | Maxillary | Nose | Posterior lateral nasal; posterior septal |
| Spinal, anterior (Ventral spinal a.) | A. spinalis anterior | Vertebral | Anterior spinal cord | |
| Spinal, posterior (Dorsal spinal a.) | A. spinalis posterior | Vertebral | Posterior spinal cord | |
| Splenic | A. splenica | Celiac trunk | Pancreas; spleen; stomach; greater omentum | Pancreatic; left gastroepiploic; short gastric; splenic |
| Sternomastoid | Rr. sternocleidomastoidei arteriae occipitalis | Occipital or external carotid | Sternocleidomastoid muscles | |
| Stylomastoid | A. stylomastoidea | Posterior auricular | Mastoid; tympanic cavity; stapedius muscle | |
| Subclavian | A. subclavia | Brachiocephalic trunk (right); arch of aorta (left) | Brain; meninges; spinal cord; neck; thoracic walls; upper limbs | Vertebral; internal thoracic; thyrocervical; costocervical; transverse cervical |

| | | | | |
|---|---|---|---|---|
| Subcostal | A. subcostalis | Thoracic aorta | Upper abdominal wall | Dorsal and spinal |
| Sublingual | A. sublingualis | Anterior margin of hypoglossus | Sublingual gland and mucous membrane of mouth and gums | |
| Submental | A. submentalis | Facial | Mylohyoid muscle; submandibular and sublingual glands; lower lip | |
| Subscapular | A. subscapularis | Axillary | Shoulder | Scapular circumflex and thoracodorsal |
| Supraorbital | A. supraorbitalis | Ophthalmic | Forehead; frontal sinus; upper eyelid; upper muscles of orbit | |
| Suprarenal, middle (Middle capsular a.) | A. suprarenalis media | Abdominal aorta | Suprarenal gland | |
| Suprascapular (Transverse scapular a.) | A. suprascapularis | Thyroid axis | Scapular; clavicle; shoulder joint | Acromial; suprasternal |
| Sural | Aa. surales | Popliteal opposite knee joint | Calf | |
| Tarsal, lateral | A. tarsalis lateralis | Dorsal a. of foot | Muscles and joints of tarsus | |
| Tarsal, medial | Aa. mediales | Dorsal a. of foot | Middle portion of foot | |
| Temporal, middle | A. temporalis media | Above zygomatic arch | Temporal muscle | |
| Temporal, superficial | A. temporalis superficialis | End of external carotid | Parotid gland; auricle; scalp; skin of face; masseter muscle | Transverse facial; middle temporal; anterior auricular; frontal; parietal |
| Testicular (Internal spermatic a.) | A. testicularis | Abdominal aorta | Ureter; epididymis; testes | Ureteral |
| Thoracic, internal (Internal mammary a.) | A. thoracica interna | Subclavian | Anterior thoracic wall; mediastinal structures; diaphragm | Pericardiacophrenic; anterior mediastinal; pericardial; sternal; intercostal; perforating; musculophrenic; superior epigastric |

## Arteries (Continued)

| *Name* | *Nomina Anatomica Term* | *Origin* | *Distribution* | *Branches* |
|---|---|---|---|---|
| Thoracic, lateral | A. thoracica lateralis | Axillary | Shoulder muscles and axillary glands | In the female, external mammary |
| Thoracic, superior | A. thoracica suprema | Thoracoacromial | Muscles of chest | |
| Thoracoacromial | A. thoracoacromialis | Axillary | Muscles and skin of upper arm, shoulder, and chest | Pectoral; acromial; clavicular; deltoid |
| Thoracodorsal | A. thoracodorsalis | Subscapular | Posterior portion of axillary | |
| Thumb, principal a. of | A. princeps pollicis | Radial | Sides and palmar aspect of thumb | Radial a. of index finger |
| Thyroid, inferior | A. thyroidea inferior | Thyroid axis | Thyroid gland; esophagus | Inferior laryngeal; tracheal; muscular; esophageal; ascending cervical |
| Thyroid, superior | A. thyroidea superior | External carotid | Hyoid muscles; larynx; thyroid gland; pharynx | Hyoid; sternomastoid; superior laryngeal; cricothyroid |
| Tibial, anterior | A. tibialis anterior | Popliteal | Leg; ankle; foot | Anterior and posterior tibial recurrent; fibular; lateral and medial anterior malleolar |
| Tibial, posterior | A. tibialis posterior | Lower end of popliteal | Leg; foot; heel | Peroneal; lateral and medial posterior malleolar; communicating; plantar; tibial and fibular nutrient |
| Tympanic, anterior | A. tympanica anterior | Maxillary | Lining of tympanic arch | |
| Tympanic, inferior | A. tympanica inferior | Ascending pharyngeal | Tympanic cavity | |

| | | | | |
|---|---|---|---|---|
| Ulnar | A. ulnaris | Brachial | Forearm; wrist and hand | Anterior and posterior recurrent; common interosseous; muscular; palmar and dorsal carpal; deep palmar; superficial palmar arch |
| Uterine | A. uterina | Internal iliac | Uterus; uterine tubes; ovary; vagina | Vaginal; ovarian; tubal |
| Vaginal | A. vaginalis | Uterine | Vagina; bladder | |
| Vertebral | A. vertebralis | Subclavian | Muscles of neck; vertebrae; spinal cord; cerebellum; interior of cerebrum | Spinal; muscular; anterior and posterior spinal; posterior inferior cerebellar; medullary |
| Vesical, inferior | A. vesicalis inferior | Internal iliac | Bladder; prostate; seminal vesicles | |
| Vesical, superior | Aa. vesicales superiores | Internal iliac | Upper part of bladder | A. to the ductus deferens |

## Appendix 2–7 Veins

| *Name* | *Nomina Anatomica Term* | *Origin* | *Distribution* | *Description* |
|---|---|---|---|---|
| Angular | V. angularis | Union of supratrochlear and supraorbital veins | Continues inferiorly as facial v. | Short superficial v. in nasal region |
| Antebrachial, median | V. mediana antebrachii | Base of dorsum of thumb | Ascends forearm between cephalic and basilic veins to elbow where it joins these veins | Superficial v. in forearm |
| Auricular, posterior | V. auricularis posterior | Plexus on side of head | From side of head it descends behind the pinna where it unites with retromandibular v. to form the external jugular v. | Superficial v. that drains parietal and posterior part of temporal region |

**Veins** (Continued)

| *Name* | *Nomina Anatomica Term* | *Origin* | *Distribution* | *Description* |
|---|---|---|---|---|
| Axillary | V. axillaris | Junction of basilic and brachial veins | Lower border of teres major muscles to lateral border of first rib where it becomes the subclavian v. | Portion of venous trunk of upper extremity |
| Azygos | V. azygos | Arises from ascending lumbar v. | From level of diaphragm up posterior thoracic wall on right of vertebral bodies to superior vena cava | Trunk that connects superior and inferior venae cavae |
| Basilic | V. basilica | Ulnar side of dorsal rete of hand | Ascends posteriorly on the forearm. Below the elbow it moves to exterior surface where it joins axillary v. | Superficial v. of hand and forearm |
| Brachial | Vv. brachiales | Tributaries from structures in upper arm | Follows course of brachial artery and joins axillary v. | Each v. drains an arm |
| Brachiocephalic (Innominate v.) | Vv. brachiocephalicae (dextra et sinistra) | Union of internal jugular and subclavian veins | From sternal end of clavicle it descends below the cartilage of first rib to form superior vena cava | Paired veins that drain blood from head, neck, and upper extremities and unite to form superior vena cava |
| Bronchial | Vv. bronchiales | Capillaries of bronchi and roots of lungs | Empties into azygos v. on the right and into hemiazygos or superior intercostal veins on left | Several veins that return blood from larger bronchi and roots of lungs |
| Cardiac | Vv. cordis<br>Vv. cardiaca (4) | Capillaries of myocardium | Usually empty into coronary sinus | Drain blood from myocardium |
| Cardinal | | Each v. receives a v. from caudal and cephalic portions of embryo | Include precardinal and postcardinal veins | First veins to appear in body of embryo |
| Cephalic | V. cephalica | Radial border of dorsal rete of hand | Winds anteriorly up arm and empties into axillary v. | Superficial v. of arm and forearm |

| | | | | |
|---|---|---|---|---|
| Cerebellar, inferior | Vv. cerebelli inferiores | Undersurface of cerebellum | Empty into transverse, superior, petrosal, and occipital sinuses | Large veins of undersurface of cerebellum |
| Cerebellar, superior | Vv. cerebelli superiores | Upper surface of cerebellum | Empty into straight sinus or transverse sinus | Veins from upper surface of cerebellum |
| Cerebral, great | V. cerebri magna | Formed by union of two internal cerebral veins | Curves backward and upward around the splenium of the corpus callosum and continues as a straight sinus | Short median trunk |
| Cerebral, inferior | Vv. cerebri inferiores | Tributaries in lobes of cerebrum | From various lobes they empty into cavernous and transverse sinuses | Small-sized veins that drain undersurfaces of hemispheres |
| Cerebral, internal | Vv. cerebri internae | Formed near interventricular foramen by union of terminal and choroid veins | Run backward parallel to one another and unite at the splenium of the corpus callosum to form great cerebral v. | Two veins that drain deep parts of hemispheres |
| Cerebral, superficial middle | V. cerebri media superficialis | Lateral surface of cerebral hemisphere | Follows lateral cerebral fissure and empties into cavernous sinus | Drains lateral surface of cerebral hemisphere |
| Cerebral, superior | Vv. cerebri superiores | Capillaries of cerebrum | From cerebrum to longitudinal cerebral fissure, opening into superior sagittal sinus | Eight to twelve veins that drain the surface of the cerebral hemisphere |
| Cervical, deep | V. cervicalis profunda | Plexus in suboccipital triangle | Follows deep cervical artery down neck and empties into vertebral or brachiocephalic v. | Deep v. of neck |
| Cervical, transverse | Vv. transversae cervicis | Capillaries of supraspinous region of scapula and neck | From supraspinous region of scapula diagonally across shoulder to subclavian or external jugular v. | Drain blood from supraspinous region of scapula and neck |
| Cutaneous | V. cutanea | Capillaries of superficial tissues of body wall | Throughout subcutaneous tissue of body wall | One of the veins located beneath layers of superficial fascia immediately under the skin |

**Veins** (Continued)

| *Name* | *Nomina Anatomica Term* | *Origin* | *Distribution* | *Description* |
|---|---|---|---|---|
| Cystic | V. cystica | Capillaries of gallbladder | From gallbladder along cystic duct to enter right branch of portal v. just below liver | Drains gallbladder |
| Deep | | Extremities | Throughout the body | Accompany homonymous arteries and usually enclosed in sheaths with those vessels |
| Digital, palmar | Vv. digitales palmares | Capillaries of superficial tissues of palmar surface of fingers | Along proper and common digital arteries | Superficial veins of palmar surface of fingers |
| Digital, plantar | Vv. digitales plantares | Capillaries of toes | Along plantar surface of toes to foot to form four metatarsal veins | Veins of plantar surface of toes |
| Diploic | Vv. diploicae | Spongy bone between internal and external skull surfaces | Connect with meningeal veins, sinuses of the dura mater, and veins of the pericranium | Large veins of the skull. Main veins are frontal, anterior and posterior temporal, and occipital. |
| Emissary | Vv. emissariae | Cerebral sinuses | Pass through foramina of skull | Small valveless veins that connect sinuses inside the skull and veins external to it |
| Epigastric, inferior | V. epigastrica inferior | Capillaries of internal surface of lower anterior abdominal walls | Internal surface of abdominal wall diagonally across wall to flow into external iliac v. | V. of lower anterior abdominal wall |
| Epigastric, superficial | V. epigastrica superficialis | Superficial tissues of lower portion of anterior abdominal wall | Follows superficial epigastric artery and opens into great saphenous v. | Drains lower and medial portion of abdominal wall |
| Esophageal | Vv. esophageae | Capillaries of esophagus | From esophagus empty into inferior thyroid, hemiazygos, azygos, or left brachiocephalic v. | Several small trunks that drain esophagus |

| | | | | |
|---|---|---|---|---|
| Facial | V. facialis | Continuation of angular v. | From inner angle of orbit it passes diagonally downward and outward to lower jaw | Deep v. of face. Branches drain deep structures of face. |
| Femoral | V. femoralis | Continuation of popliteal v. | From posterior region of knee it follows course of femoral artery, becoming external iliac v. at inguinal ligament | Large v. of thigh |
| Femoral, deep | V. profunda femoris | Tributaries from posterior region of thigh | Accompanies deep femoral artery to femoral triangle where it joins femoral v. | Deep v. of thigh |
| Gastric, left | V. gastrica sinistra | Gastrohepatic omentum | Right to left along lesser curvature of stomach to enter portal v. | Drains both surfaces of stomach |
| Gastric, right (Pyloric) | V. gastrica dextra | Small v. from upper portion of stomach | From upper stomach runs left to right along pyloric portion of lesser curvature of stomach to end in portal v. | Drains upper portion of stomach |
| Gastric, short | Vv. gastricae breves | Capillaries of fundus of stomach | From wall of stomach empty into splenic v. | Drain wall of stomach |
| Gastro-omental, left | V. gastro-omentalis sinistra | Branches from stomach and greater omentum | Right to left on greater curvature of stomach to empty into splenic v. | V. of upper stomach |
| Gastro-omental, right | V. gastro-omentalis dextra | Branches from greater omentum and lower surfaces of stomach | Left to right on greater curvature of stomach to empty into superior mesenteric v. | V. of lower stomach |
| Gluteal, inferior (Sciatic v.) | Vv. gluteae inferiores | Capillaries of upper part of back of thigh | Upper back thigh through lower sciatic foramen where they unite into a single v. and empty into internal iliac v. | V. of lower region of hip |
| Gluteal, superior | Vv. gluteae superiores | Capillaries of gluteal and adjacent muscles | From tissues of hip they pass through sciatic foramen to empty into internal iliac v. | Drain muscles of buttocks |

**Veins** (Continued)

| *Name* | *Nomina Anatomica Term* | *Origin* | *Distribution* | *Description* |
|---|---|---|---|---|
| Hemiazygos | V. hemiazygos | Left ascending lumbar v. | Lumbar region through diaphragm, crossing in front of spine and emptying into azygos v. | Single v. of lower left thoracic wall |
| Hemiazygos, accessory | V. hemiazygos accessoria | Capillaries of upper intercostal spaces | From left side of vertebra crosses over spine to enter azygos v. | Drains blood from intercostal spaces above level of sixth to seventh |
| Hepatic | Vv. hepaticae | Tissues of liver | From liver empty into inferior vena cava | Drain the liver |
| Ileocolic | V. ileocolica | Capillaries of organs in area of ileum and colon | From lower portion of ascending colon runs parallel with ileocolic artery and empties into superior mesenteric v. | Large tributary of mesenteric v. that drains the ileum, appendix, cecum, and lower part of ascending colon |
| Iliac, common | V. iliaca communis | Union of internal and external iliac veins | Diagonally across pelvis | Large v. that drains blood from pelvis and leg. One on each side meets to form inferior vena cava |
| Iliac, deep circumflex | V. circumflexa ilium profunda | Capillaries of deep muscles of upper portion of thigh and lower portion of abdomen | Deep tissues of anterior superior spine along inner surface of pelvic brim to external iliac v. | V. of deep structures of iliac region |
| Iliac, external | V. iliaca externa | Begins behind inguinal ligament as continuation of external iliac v. | Behind inguinal ligament to sacroiliac articulation where it unites with internal iliac v. to form common iliac v. | Upward continuation of external iliac v. |
| Iliac, internal (Hypogastric v.) | V. iliaca interna | Near upper part of greater sciatic foramen | Upper part of greater sciatic foramen | Short v. that draws blood from pelvis |

| | | | | |
|---|---|---|---|---|
| Intercostal | | Tributaries of other veins of intercostal spaces | Intercostal spaces to region of lower ribs | One of a number of veins (anterior, posterior, right, left, superior, and highest) that drain blood from intercostal spaces |
| Intervertebral | V. intervertebralis | Vertebral plexuses | Vertebral plexuses through intervertebral foramina where they empty into regional veins | One of numerous veins that drain vertebral plexuses and accompany spinal nerves |
| Jugular, anterior | V. jugularis anterior | From veins of region of lower lip | From lower jaw descends neck anteriorly and enters external jugular v. | Superficial v. of anterior region of neck |
| Jugular, external | V. jugularis externa | Formed at parotid gland by union of posterior auricular and retromandibular veins | From parotid gland descends perpendicularly in neck to empty into subclavian, internal jugular, or brachiocephalic v. | A large superficial v. that receives greater part of blood from exterior of cranium and deep parts of face |
| Jugular, internal | V. jugularis interna | Continuous from transverse sinus at base of skull | Runs vertically in neck and unites with subclavian v. at root of neck to form the brachiocephalic v. | Largest v. of head and neck. Collects blood from brain, superficial parts of face, and neck |
| Lingual | V. lingualis | Capillaries of tongue and sublingual areas | Follows distribution of lingual artery | Deep v. of tongue |
| Lumbar | Vv. lumbales | Capillaries of abdominal walls | Abdominal walls to ascending lumbar v., inferior vena cava, and iliolumbar v. | Four or five veins of abdominal walls |
| Lumbar, ascending | V. lumbalis ascendens | Lateral sacral veins | Lateral sacral v. along lateral border of spinal column to first lumbar vertebra where it becomes azygos v. on right side and hemiazygos v. on left side | Longitudinal v. that connects lumbar veins |
| Meningeal | Vv. meningeae | Meninges of brain | Accompany meningeal arteries from meninges and empty into regional sinuses and veins | Multiple veins of dura mater of brain |

## Veins (Continued)

| *Name* | *Nomina Anatomica Term* | *Origin* | *Distribution* | *Description* |
|---|---|---|---|---|
| Mesenteric, superior | V. mesenterica superior | Capillaries of small intestine | From ileum in right iliac fossa it follows distribution of its artery and unites with splenic v. behind pancreas to form portal v. | Large v. from small intestine |
| Mesenteric, inferior | V. mesenterica inferior | Capillaries of colon and rectum | As a continuation of superior rectal v. ascends behind peritoneum and enters splenic v. | Drains blood from rectum and sigmoid and descending parts of colon |
| Metacarpal, dorsal | Vv. metacarpeae dorsales | Capillaries of hand | From digital venous arches join to form dorsal venous rete of hand | Superficial veins of back of hand |
| Metacarpal, palmar | Vv. metacarpeae palmares | Capillaries of palm | Deep tissues of palm along metacarpal bone to deep venous arches | Deep veins on both sides of hand |
| Metatarsal, dorsal | Vv. metatarsales dorsales | Dorsal digital veins of toes | Through metatarsal spaces to unite to form dorsal venous arch | Deep veins of back of foot |
| Metatarsal, plantar | Vv. metatarsales plantares | Plantar digital veins | From toes to ankles and open into plantar venous arch | Deep veins of solar aspect of foot |
| Musculophrenic | Vv. musculophrenicae | Capillaries of upper abdominal wall, lower intercostal spaces, and diaphragm | Along thoracic surface of diaphragm upward lateral to sternum to unite with superior epigastric v. to form internal thoracic v. | Drains blood from thoracic surface of diaphragm and from walls of thorax and abdomen |
| Obturator | Vv. obturatoriae | Union of tributaries of hip and muscle of upper posterior thigh | From upper portion of adductor region of thigh run through upper part of obturator foramen and run back to empty into internal iliac v. | Drain blood from obturator foramen |

| | | | | |
|---|---|---|---|---|
| Occipital | Vv. occipitales | Plexus at back part of vertex of skull | From plexus of occipital region, occasionally following course of occipital artery, extends to internal or external jugular v. | Superficial veins that drain occipital region |
| Ophthalmic, inferior | V. ophthalmica inferior | Venous network at forepart of orbit | Runs backward in lower orbit and divides into two branches. One passes through inferior orbital fissure and joins pterygoid venous plexus; the second enters cranium through superior orbital fissure and ends in cavernous sinus | Ophthalmic v. that divides into two terminal branches |
| Ophthalmic, superior | V. ophthalmica superior | Inner angle of orbit | Follows course of ophthalmic artery into cavernous sinus | Paired veins of orbital cavity |
| Ovarian, right and left | V. ovarica dextra and V. ovarica sinistra | Capillaries of ovaries, uterine tubes, and adjacent structures | Pampiniform plexus of broad ligament into inferior vena cava on right and left renal v. on left | Drains ovaries |
| Palatine, external | V. palatina externa | Capillaries of deep tissues of neck | Palatine regions into facial v. | Drains blood from tonsils and soft palate |
| Pancreatic | Vv. pancreaticae | Capillaries of pancreas | From pancreas into splenic and superior mesenteric veins | V. of pancreas |
| Parietal emissary | V. emissaria parietalis | Upper skull | Connects superior sagittal sinus with extracranial veins | Small v. that passes through the parietal foramen of the skull |
| Parumbilical | Vv. parumbilicales | Cutaneous veins in region of umbilicus | From region of umbilicus run backward and upward to left portal v. | Small important veins that establish communication between portal v. and superior and inferior epigastric veins |
| Penis, dorsal v. of | V. dorsalis profunda penis | Capillaries of skin or tissue of penis | Runs length of penis between two dorsal arteries | Two (deep and superficial) veins of penis |
| Peroneal (Fibular veins) | Vv. peroneae (fibulares) | Veins of ankle and capillaries of tissues of leg | From venous plexus in region of heel upward along lateral region of deep tissue to flow into posterior tibial v. | Deep veins of leg |

**Veins** (Continued)

| *Name* | *Nomina Anatomica Term* | *Origin* | *Distribution* | *Description* |
|---|---|---|---|---|
| Pharyngeal | Vv. pharyngeae | Pharyngeal plexus | Empty from pharyngeal plexus into internal jugular v. | Drain pharyngeal plexus |
| Phrenic, inferior | Vv. phrenicae inferiores | Tissues of diaphragm | From diaphragm flow to inferior vena cava on right side and left suprarenal v. on left side | Drain abdominal surface of diaphragm |
| Popliteal | V. poplitea | Union of tibial veins at lower border of popliteus muscle | From tibial veins upward to adductor hiatus to become femoral v. | Large v. in posterior region of knee |
| Portal | V. portae hepatis | Union of superior mesenteric and splenic veins | Abdominal cavity | Subdivision of systemic venous system. Collects blood from digestive tract and conveys it to the liver. |
| Pudendal, external | Vv. pudendae externae | Capillaries of superficial tissues of lower abdomen, scrotum, or labia | From lower abdomen transversely across upper region of thigh to great saphenous or femoral v. | Drain blood from superficial regions of medial aspect of upper thigh and receive subcutaneous dorsal veins of external genitals |
| Pudendal, internal | V. pudenda interna | Deep vein of penis or clitoris | Follows course of internal pudendal artery and opens into internal iliac v. | Drains the perineum and external genitals |
| Pulmonary | Vv. pulmonales | Capillaries around air sacs of lungs | Lungs to left atrium | Four veins that return oxygenated blood from lungs to left atrium of heart |
| Radial | Vv. radiales | Palmar arches of hand | From palmar arches of hand accompany radial artery along lateral side of forearm in deep tissues to unite with ulnar v. to form brachial v. | Large deep veins on radial side of forearm |
| Rectal, inferior | Vv. rectales inferiores | Venous plexus of anal canal | Anal canal to internal pudendal v. | Drain the rectal plexus |

| | | | | |
|---|---|---|---|---|
| Rectal, middle | Vv. rectales mediae | Rectal plexus with tributaries from bladder, prostate, and seminal vesicles | Run laterally from rectal plexus to internal iliac v. | Drain the rectal plexus |
| Rectal, superior | V. rectalis superior | Capillaries of rectum | Ascends from rectal plexus to brim of pelvis into inferior mesenteric v. | Drains upper part of rectal plexus |
| Renal | Vv. renales | Capillaries of kidneys. The left v. receives the left suprarenal v. and left gonadal v. | From kidneys transversely across posterior abdominal wall to inferior vena cava | Short thick trunks that drain the kidneys. The left is longer than the right |
| Sacral, lateral | Vv. sacrales laterales | Tissues of posterior pelvic wall | Posterior pelvic wall upward along sacrum to empty into internal iliac v. | Large v. of posterior pelvic wall veins |
| Sacral, middle | V. sacralis mediana | Capillaries of tissues of posterior pelvic wall | From pelvic wall in sacral region follows middle sacral artery to empty into common iliac v. | Large v. of posterior pelvic wall |
| Saphenous, great | V. saphena magna | Medial marginal v. of dorsum of foot | Dorsum of foot to femoral v. just below the inguinal ligament | Longest v. in body |
| Saphenous, small | V. saphena parva | Continuation of marginal v. | From behind malleolus ascends back of leg to knee joint where it opens into popliteal v. | Large superficial v. of back of leg |
| Sciatic. SEE: *Gluteal v., inferior.* | | | | |
| Spinal, anterior and posterior | Vv. spinales anteriores and Vv. superiores | Spinal cord and its pia mater | Spinal cord through roots to internal vertebral venous plexuses | Network of veins draining blood from spinal cord |
| Splenic | V. splenica | Union of several small veins at the hilus of the spleen | From spleen transversely across abdomen to head of pancreas; forms portal v. by joining the superior mesenteric v. | Large v. that drains blood from spleen and part of stomach |

**Veins** (Continued)

| *Name* | *Nomina Anatomica Term* | *Origin* | *Distribution* | *Description* |
|---|---|---|---|---|
| Subcardinal | | | | Paired vessels in embryo that replace postcardinal veins. SEE: *Cardinal v.* |
| Subclavian | V. subclavia | Continuation of axillary v. | Outer border of first rib to sternal end of clavicle where it joins the internal jugular v. to form the brachiocephalic v. | Main venous trunk of upper extremity |
| Supraorbital | V. supraorbitalis | Capillaries and superficial tissues of region of eye | From region of eye along lateral wall of orbital cavity to root of nose where it unites with supratrochlear v. to form angular v. | Drains upper portion of orbital cavity |
| Suprarenal, left | V. suprarenalis sinistra | Capillaries of left adrenal gland | Hilum of left suprarenal gland, ascending to left renal v. | V. of left adrenal gland |
| Suprarenal, right | V. suprarenalis dextra | Capillaries of right adrenal gland | Hilum of right adrenal gland to inferior vena cava | V. of right adrenal gland |
| Supratrochlear (Frontal v.) (2) | Vv. supratrochleares | Capillaries of anterior region of scalp | From venous plexuses in forehead diagonally to left of root of nose where they unite with supra-orbital v. to form angular v. | Drain the anterior scalp |
| Temporal, middle | V. temporalis media | Substance of temporal muscle | From lateral superficial plexus of skull it passes to zygoma where it joins superficial temporal v. to form retromandibular v. | Superficial v. of lateral portion of stomach |
| Temporal, superficial | Vv. temporales superficiales | Lateral scalp in parietal and frontal region | Temporal region of scalp diagonally to ear and downward to mandible where they unite with maxillary v. to form retromandibular v. | Veins of superficial tissues of skull |

| | | | | |
|---|---|---|---|---|
| Testicular | V. testicularis dextra and sinistra | Capillaries of testes | From brim of pelvis upward along posterior abdominal wall to inferior vena cava on right and renal v. on left | Receives blood from testis and epididymis |
| Thoracic, internal | Vv. thoracicae internae | Tributaries from tissues of intercostal spaces | Tributaries form a single trunk that runs up medial side of internal thoracic artery and ends in brachiocephalic v. | Deep v. of chest draining intercostal spaces |
| Thoracic, lateral (Long thoracic v.) | V. thoracica lateralis | Capillaries of muscles and glands of anterior chest | Tissues of anterior chest muscles to axillary v. | A large tributary v. of the axillary v. that drains the lateral thoracic wall |
| Thoracoepigastric | Vv. thoracoepigastricae | Region of superficial epigastric v. | Run laterally along trunk from superficial epigastric v. to lateral thoracic v. | Superficial v. of trunk that establishes an important communication between the femoral and axillary veins |
| Thyroid, inferior | V. thyroidea inferior | Veins from thyroid glands | Downward to brachiocephalic v. | Two or more veins that arise in venous plexuses on thyroid gland |
| Thyroid, superior | V. thyroidea superior | Substance and surface of thyroid gland | Accompanies superior thyroid artery and empties into internal jugular v. | One v. from either side of thyroid |
| Tibial, anterior | Vv. tibiales anteriores | Capillaries of leg tissue and dorsal metatarsal v. | Accompany anterior tibial artery, ascending between tibia and fibula and uniting with posterior tibial v. to form popliteal v. | Deep veins of anterior aspect of leg |
| Tibial, posterior | Vv. tibiales posteriores | Capillaries of deep tissues of leg | From ankle up posterior aspect of leg to unite with anterior tibial v. to form popliteal v. just below knee | Deep veins of back of leg |

**Veins** (Continued)

| *Name* | *Nomina Anatomica Term* | *Origin* | *Distribution* | *Description* |
|---|---|---|---|---|
| Ulnar | Vv. ulnares | Palmar arches of hand | Palmar arches of hand upward in deep tissues along ulnar side of forearm to form brachial v. with radial v. at elbow | Large deep veins of medial aspect of forearm |
| Umbilical | V. umbilicalis sinistra | Placental tissues | Along umbilical cord through umbilicus to liver upward through inferior vena cava to heart | V. that carries blood from placenta to fetus |
| Uterine | Vv. uterinae | Tissues of uterus | Uterine plexus through part of the broad ligament to empty into internal iliac v. | Veins carrying blood from uterus |
| Vena cava inferior | V. cava inferior | Right and left iliac veins | From union of iliac veins at level of fifth lumbar vertebra to right atrium of heart | Returns blood from lower half of body |
| Vena cava superior | V. cava superior | Two brachiocephalic veins | From below right costal cartilage to right atrium of heart | Drains blood from upper half of body |
| Vertebral | V. vertebralis | Numerous small tributaries in the suboccipital triangle | Base of skull down neck, opening into brachiocephalic v. | Drains blood from internal vertebral venous plexuses |
| Vertebral, anterior | V. vertebralis anterior | Plexus around transverse process of upper cervical vertebrae | Descends from region of upper cervical vertebrae with ascending cervical artery and opens into terminal part of vertebral v. | Small v. |

# APPENDIX 3

# Normal Reference Laboratory Values

## BLOOD, PLASMA, OR SERUM VALUES

| *Determination* | Reference Range | | *Minimal ml Required** | *Note* |
|---|---|---|---|---|
| | *Conventional* | *SI* | | |
| Acetoacetate plus acetone | Negative | | 1-B | |
| Aldolase | 1.3–8.2 U/L | 22–137 nmol · $sec^{-1}$/L | 2-S | Use unhemolyzed serum |
| Ammonia | 12–55 μmol/L | 12–55 μmol/L | 2-B | Collect in heparinized tube; deliver *immediately* packed in ice |
| Amylase | 4–25 units/ml | 4–25 arb. unit | 1-S | |
| Ascorbic acid | 0.4–1.5 mg/100 ml | 23–85 μmol/L | 7-B | Collect in heparinized tube before any food is given |
| Bilirubin | Direct: up to 0.4 mg/100 ml<br>Total: up to 1.0 mg/100 ml | Up to 7 μmol/L<br>Up to 17 μmol/L | 1-S | |
| Blood volume | 8.5–9.0% of body weight in kg | 80–85 ml/kg | | |
| Calcium | 8.5–10.5 mg/100 ml (slightly higher in children) | 2.1–2.6 mmol/L | 1-S | |
| Carbamazepine | 4.0–12.0 μg/ml | 17–51 μmol/L | | |
| Carbon dioxide content | 24–30 mEq/L | 24–30 mmol/L | 1-S | Fill tube to top |
| Carbon monoxide | Less than 5% of total hemoglobin | | 3-B | Fill tube to top |
| Carotenoids | 0.8–4.0 μg/ml | 1.5–7.4 μmol/L | 3-S | Vitamin A may be done on same specimen |
| Ceruloplasmin | 27–37 mg/100 ml | 1.8–2.5 μmol/L | 2-S | |
| Chloramphenicol | 10–20 μg/ml | 31–62 μmol/L | .0.2-S | |
| Chloride | 100–106 mEq/L | 100–106 mmol/L | 1-S | |
| CK isoenzymes | 5% MB or less | | 0.2-S | |
| Copper | Total: 100–200 μg/100 ml | 16–31 μmol/L | 1-S | |
| Creatine kinase (CK) | Female: 10–79 U/L<br>Male: 17–148 U/L | 167–1317 nmol · $sec^{-1}$/L<br>283–2467 nmol. · $sec^{-1}$/L | 1-S | |
| Creatinine | 0.6–1.5 mg/100 ml | 53–133 μmol/L | 1-S | |
| Ethanol | 0 mg/100 ml | 0 mmol/L | 2-B | Collect in oxalate and refrigerate |
| Glucose | Fasting: 70–110 mg/100 ml | 3.9–5.6 mmol/L | 1-P | Collect with oxalate–fluoride mixture |
| Iron | 50–150 μg/100 ml (higher in males) | 9.0–26.9 μmol/L | 1-S | |

## BLOOD, PLASMA, OR SERUM VALUES (Continued)

| Determination | Reference Range: Conventional | Reference Range: SI | Minimal ml Required* | Note |
|---|---|---|---|---|
| Iron-binding capacity | 250–410 μg/100 ml | 44.8–73.4 μmol/L | 1-S | |
| Lactic acid | 0.6–1.8 mEq/L | 0.6–1.8 mmol/L | 2-B | Collect with oxalate–fluoride; deliver immediately packed in ice |
| Lactic dehydrogenase | 45–90 U/L | 750–1500 nmol · $sec^{-1}$/L | 1-S | Unsuitable if hemolyzed |
| Lead | 50 μg/100 ml or less | Up to 2.4 μmol/L | 2-B | Collect with oxalate–fluoride mixture |
| Lipase | 2 units/ml or less | Up to 2 arb. unit | 1-S | |
| Lipids | | | | |
| Cholesterol | 120–220 mg/100 ml | 3.10–5.69 mmol/L | 1-S | Fasting |
| Triglycerides | 40–150 mg/100 ml | 0.4–1.5 g/L | 1-S | Fasting |
| Lipoprotein electrophoresis (LEP) | | | 2-S | Fasting, do not freeze serum |
| Lithium | 0.5–1.5 mEq/L | 0.5–1.5 mmol/L | 1-S | |
| Magnesium | 1.5–2.0 mEq/L | 0.8–1.3 mmol/L | 1-S | |
| 5′ Nucleotidase | 1–11 U/L | 17–183 nmol · $sec^{-1}$/L | 1-S | |
| Osmolality | 280–296 mOsm/kg water | 280–296 mmol/kg | 1-S | |
| Oxygen saturation (arterial) | 96–100% | 0.96–1.00 | 3-B | Deliver in sealed heparinized syringe packed in ice |
| $PCO_2$ | 35–45 mm Hg | 4.7–6.0 kPa | 2-B | Collect and deliver in sealed heparinized syringe |
| pH | 7.35–7.45 | Same | 2-B | Collect without stasis in sealed heparinized syringe; deliver packed in ice |
| $PO_2$ | 75–100 mm Hg (dependent on age) while breathing room air<br>Above 500 mm Hg while on 100% $O_2$ | 10.0–13.3 kPa | 2-B | |
| Phenobarbital | 15–50 μg/ml | 65–215 μmol/L | 1-S | |
| Phenytoin (Dilantin) | 5–20 μg/ml | 20–80 μmol/L | 1-S | |
| Phosphatase (acid) | Male—Total: 0.13–0.63 sigma U/ml<br>Female—Total: 0.01–0.56 sigma U/ml | 36–175 nmol · $sec^{-1}$/L<br>2.8–156 nmol · $sec^{-1}$/L | 1-S | Must always be drawn just before analysis or stored as frozen serum; avoid hemolysis |

| | | | | |
|---|---|---|---|---|
| | Prostatic: 0–0.5 Fishman–Lerner U/100 ml | | | |
| Phosphatase (alkaline) | 13–39 U/L, infants and adolescents up to 104 U/L | 217–650 nmol · $sec^{-1}$/L, up to 1.26 $\mu$mol · $sec^{-1}$/L | 1-S | |
| Phosphorus (inorganic) | 3.0–4.5 mg/100 ml (infants in first year up to 6.0 mg/100 ml) | 1.0–1.5 mmol/L | 1-S | |
| Potassium | 3.5–5.0 mEq/L | 3.5–5.0 mmol/L | 1-S | Serum must be separated promptly from cells |
| Primidone (Mysoline) | 4–12 $\mu$g/ml | 18–55 $\mu$mol/L | 1-S | |
| Procainamide | 4–10 $\mu$g/ml | 17–42 $\mu$mol/L | 1-S | |
| Protein: Total | 6.0–8.4 g/100 ml | 60–84 g/L | 1-S | |
| Albumin | 3.5–5.0 g/100 ml | 35–50 g/L | 1-S | |
| Globulin | 2.3–3.5 g/100 ml | 23–35 g/L | | Globulin equals total protein minus albumin |
| Electrophoresis | (% of total protein) | | 1-S | Quantitation by densitometry |
| Albumin | 52–68 | | | |
| Globulin: | | | | |
| $Alpha_1$ | 4.2–7.2 | | | |
| $Alpha_2$ | 6.8–12 | | | |
| Beta | 9.3–15 | | | |
| Gamma | 13–23 | | | |
| Pyruvic acid | 0–0.11 mEq/L | 0–0.11 mmol/L | 2-B | Collect with oxalate fluoride. Deliver immediately packed in ice |
| Quinidine | 1.2–4.0 $\mu$g/ml | 3.7–12.3 $\mu$mol/L | 1-S | |
| Salicylate: | 0 | | 2-P | |
| Therapeutic | 20–25 mg/100 ml; 25–30 mg/100 ml to age 10 yr 3 hr post dose | 1.4–1.8 mmol/L<br>1.8–2.2 mmol/L | | |
| Sodium | 135–145 mEq/L | 135–145 mmol/L | 1-S | |
| Sulfonamide | 5–15 mg/100 ml | | 2-P | |
| Transaminase, aspartate aminotransferase | 7–27 U/L | 117–450 nmol · $sec^{-1}$/L | 1-S | |
| Transaminase, alanine aminotransferase | 1–21 U/L | 17–350 nmol · $sec^{-1}$/L | 1-S | |
| Urea nitrogen (BUN) | 8–25 mg/100 ml | 2.9–8.9 mmol/L | 1-S | |
| Uric acid | 3.0–7.0 mg/100 ml | 0.18–0.42 mmol/L | 1-S | |
| Vitamin A | 0.15–0.6 $\mu$g/ml | 0.5–2.1 $\mu$mol/L | 3-S | |

## URINE VALUES

| Determination | Reference Range: Conventional | Reference Range: SI | Minimal Quantity Required* | Note |
|---|---|---|---|---|
| Acetone plus acetoacetate (quantitative) | 0 | 0 mg/L | 2 ml | |
| Amylase | 24–76 units/ml | 24–76 arb. unit | | |
| Calcium | 300 mg/day or less | 7.5 mmol/day or less | 24-hr specimen | Collect in special bottle with 10 ml of concentrated HCl |
| Catecholamines | Epinephrine: under 20 $\mu$g/day<br>Norepinephrine: under 100 $\mu$g/day | <109 nmol/day<br><590 nmol/day | 24-hr specimen | Should be collected with 10 ml of concentrated HCl (pH should be between 2.0 and 3.0) |
| Chorionic gonadotropin | 0 | 0 arb. unit | 1st morning void | |
| Copper | 0–100 $\mu$g/day | 0–1.6 $\mu$mol/day | 24-hr specimen | |
| Coproporphyrin | 50–250 $\mu$g/day<br>Children under 80 lb (36 kg): 0–75 $\mu$g/day | 80–380 nmol/day<br>0–115 nmol/day | 24-hr specimen | Collect with 5 g of sodium carbonate |
| Creatine | Under 100 mg/day or less than 6% of creatinine. In pregnancy: up to 12%. In children under 1 yr: may equal creatinine. In older children: up to 30% of creatinine. | <0.75 mmol/day | 24-hr specimen | Also order creatinine |
| Creatinine | 15–25 mg/kg of body weight/day | 0.13–0.22 mmol · $kg^{-1}$/day | 24-hr specimen | |
| Cystine or cysteine | 0 | 0 | 10 ml | Qualitative |
| Hemoglobin and myoglobin | 0 | | Freshly voided sample | Chemical examination with benzidine |
| 5-Hydroxyindoleacetic acid | 2–9 mg/day (women lower than men) | 10–45 $\mu$mol/day | 24-hr specimen | Collect with 10 ml of concentrated HCl |
| Lead | 0.08 $\mu$g/ml or 120 $\mu$g/day or less | 0.39 $\mu$mol/L or less | 24-hr specimen | |
| Phosphorus (inorganic) | Varies with intake; average, 1 g/day | 32 mmol/day | 24-hr specimen | Collect with 10 ml of concentrated HCl |
| Porphobilinogen | 0 | 0 | 10 ml | Use freshly voided urine |
| Protein: | | | | |
| Quantitative | <150 mg/24 hr | <0.15 g/day | 24-hr specimen | |

| | | | | |
|---|---|---|---|---|
| Steroids: | | | | |
| 17-Ketosteroids (per day) | Age / Male / Female<br>10 / 1–4 mg / 1–4 mg<br>20 / 6–21 / 4–16<br>30 / 8–26 / 4–14<br>50 / 5–18 / 3–9<br>70 / 2–10 / 1–7 | 3–14 μmol / 3–14 μmol<br>21–73 / 14–56<br>28–90 / 14–49<br>17–62 / 10–31<br>7–35 / 3–24 | 24-hr specimen | Not valid if patient is receiving meprobamate |
| 17-Hydroxysteroids | 3–8 mg/day (women lower than men) | 8–22 μmol/day as tetrahydrocortisol | 24-hr specimen | Keep cold; chlorpromazine and related drugs interfere with assay |
| Sugar: | | | | |
| Quantitative glucose | 0 | 0 mmol/L | 24-hr or other timed specimen | |
| Urobilinogen | Up to 1.0 Ehrlich U | To 1.0 arb. unit | 2-hr sample (1–3 p.m.) | |
| Uroporphyrin | 0–30 μg/day | <36 nmol/day | See *Coproporphyrin* | |
| Vanillylmandelic acid (VMA) | Up to 9 mg/24 hr | Up to 45 μmol/day | 24-hr specimen | Collect as for catecholamines |

## SPECIAL ENDOCRINE TESTS

### Steroid Hormones

| | Reference Range | | | |
|---|---|---|---|---|
| ***Determination*** | ***Conventional*** | ***SI*** | ***Minimal ml Required**** | ***Note*** |
| Aldosterone | Excretion: 5–19 μg/24 hr | 14–53 nmol/day | 5/day | Keep specimen cold |
| | Supine: 48 ± 29 pg/ml | 133 ± 80 pmol/L | 3-S, P | Fasting, at rest, 210-mEq sodium diet |
| | Upright (2 hr): 65 ± 23 pg/ml | 180 ± 64 pmol/L | | Upright, 2 hr, 210-mEq sodium diet |
| | Supine: 107 ± 45 pg/ml | 279 ± 125 pmol/L | | Fasting, at rest, 110-mEq sodium diet |
| | Upright (2 hr): 239 ± 123 pg/ml | 663 ± 341 pmol/L | | Upright, 2 hr, 110-mEq sodium diet |
| | Supine: 175 ± 75 pg/ml | 485 ± 208 pmol/L | | Fasting, at rest, 10-mEq sodium diet |

## SPECIAL ENDOCRINE TESTS (Continued)

### Steroid Hormones

| Determination | Reference Range: Conventional | Reference Range: SI | Minimal ml Required* | Note |
|---|---|---|---|---|
| Cortisol | Upright (2 hr): 532 ± 228 pg/ml | 1476 ± 632 pmol/L | | Upright, 2 hr, 10-mEq sodium diet |
| | 8 a.m.: 5–25 μg/100 ml | 0.14–0.69 μmol/L | 1-P | Fasting |
| | 8 p.m.: Below 10 μg/100 ml | 0–0.28 μmol/L | 1-P | At rest |
| | 4-hr ACTH test: 30–45 μg/100 ml | 0.83–1.24 μmol/L | 1-P | 20 U ACTH, IV per 4 hr |
| | Overnight suppression test: Below 5 μg/100 ml | 0.14 nmol/L | 1-P | 8 a.m. sample after 0.5 mg dexamethasone by mouth at midnight |
| | Excretion: 20–70 μg/24 hr | 55–193 nmol/day | 2/day | Keep specimen cold |
| Dehydroepiandrosterone (DHEA) | Male: 0.5–5.5 ng/ml | 1.7–19 nmol/L | 2-S, P | |
| | Female: 1.4–8.0 ng/ml | 4.9–28 nmol/L | | Adult |
| | 0.3–4.5 ng/ml | 1.0–15.6 nmol/L | | Postmenopausal |
| Dehydroepiandrosterone sulfate (DHEA-S) | Male: 151–446 μg/100 ml | 3.9–11.4 μgmol/L | 2-S, P | |
| | Female: 84–433 μg/100 ml | 2.2–11.1 μmol/L | | Adult |
| | 1.7–177 μg/100 ml | 0.04–4.5 μmol/L | | Postmenopausal |
| 11-Deoxycortisol | Responsive: Over 7.5 μg/100 ml | >0.22 μmol/L | 1-P | 8 a.m. sample, preceded by 4.5 g of metyrapone by mouth per 24 hr or by single dose of 2.5 g by mouth at midnight |
| Estradiol | Male: <50 pg/ml | <184 pmol/L | 5-S, P | |
| | Female: 23–361 pg/ml | 84–1325 pmol/L | | Adult |
| | <30 pg/ml | <110 pmol/L | | Postmenopausal |
| | <20 pg/ml | <73 pmol/L | | Prepubertal |
| Progesterone | Male: <1.0 ng/ml | <3.2 nmol/L | 5-S, P | |
| | Female: 0.2–0.6 ng/ml | 0.6–1.9 nmol/L | | Follicular phase |

| Determination | Conventional | SI | Minimal ml Required* | Note |
|---|---|---|---|---|
| | 0.3–3.5 ng/ml | 0.95–11 nmol/L | | Midcycle peak |
| | 6.5–32.2 ng/ml | 21–102 nmol/L | | Postovulatory |
| Testosterone | Adult male: | | 1-P | a.m. sample |
| | 300–1100 ng/100 ml | 10.4–38.1 nmol/L | | |
| | Adolescent male: | | | |
| | Over 100 ng/100 ml | >3.5 nmol/L | | |
| | Female: | | | |
| | 25–90 ng/100 ml | 0.87–3.12 nmol/L | | |
| Unbound testosterone | Adult male: | | 2-P | a.m. sample |
| | 3.06–24.0 ng/100 ml | 106–832 pmol/L | | |
| | Adult female: | | | |
| | 0.09–1.28 ng/100 ml | 3.1–44.4 pmol/L | | |

## Polypeptide Hormones

| Determination | Reference Range | | Minimal ml Required* | Note |
|---|---|---|---|---|
| | Conventional | SI | | |
| Adrenocorticotropin (ACTH) | 15–70 pg/ml | 3.3–15.4 pmol/L | 5-P | Place specimen on ice and send promptly to laboratory. Use EDTA tube only. |
| Alpha subunit | <0.5–2.5 ng/ml | <0.4–2.0 nmol/L | 2-S | Adult male or female |
| | <0.5–5.0 ng/ml | <0.4–4.0 nmol/L | | Postmenopausal female |
| Calcitonin | Male: 0–14 pg/ml | 0–4.1 pmol/L | 5-S | Test done only on known or suspected cases of medullary carcinoma of the thyroid |
| | Female: 0–28 pg/ml | 0–8.2 pmol/L | | |
| | >100 pg/ml in medullary carcinoma | >29.3 pmol/L | | |
| Follicle-stimulating hormone (FSH) | Male: 3–18 mU/ml | 3–18 arb. unit | 5-S, P | Same sample may be used for LH |
| | Female: 4.6–22.4 mU/ml | 4.6–22.4 arb. unit | | Pre- or postovulatory |
| | 13–41 mU/ml | 13–41 arb. unit | | Midcycle peak |
| | 30–170 mU/ml | 30–170 arb. unit | | Postmenopausal |
| Growth hormone | Below 5 ng/ml | <233 pmol/L | 1-S | Fasting, at rest |
| | Children: Over 10 ng/ml | >465 pmol/L | | After exercise |
| | Male: Below 5 ng/ml | <233 pmol/L | | |
| | Female: Up to 30 ng/ml | 0–1395 pmol/L | | |
| | Male: Below 5 ng/ml | <233 pmol/L | | After glucose load |
| | Female: Below 5 ng/ml | <233 pmol/L | | |

## Polypeptide Hormones (Continued)

| Determination | Reference Range: Conventional | Reference Range: SI | Minimal ml Required* | Note |
|---|---|---|---|---|
| Insulin | 6–26 μU/ml | 43–187 pmol/L | 1-S | Fasting |
| | Below 20 μU/ml | <144 pmol/L | | During hypoglycemia |
| | Up to 150 μU/ml | 0–1078 pmol/L | | After glucose load |
| Luteinizing hormone (LH) | Male: 3–18 mU/ml | 3–18 arb. unit | 5-S, P | Same sample may be used for FSH |
| | Female: | | | |
| | 2.4–34.5 mU/ml | 2.4–34.5 arb. unit | | Pre- or postovulatory |
| | 43–187 mU/ml | 43–187 arb. unit | | Midcycle peak |
| | 30–150 mU/ml | 30–150 arb. unit | | Postmenopausal |
| Parathyroid hormone | <25 pg/ml | <2.94 pmol/L | 5-P | Keep blood on ice, or plasma must be frozen if it is to be sent any distance; a.m. sample |
| Prolactin | 2–15 ng/ml | 0.08–6.0 nmol/L | 2-S | |
| Renin activity | Supine: | | 4-P | EDTA tubes, on ice, normal diet |
| | 1.1 ± 0.8 ng/ml/hr | 0.9 ± 0.6 nmol/L/hr | | |
| | Upright: | | | |
| | 1.9 ± 1.7 ng/ml/hr | 1.5 ± 1.3 nmol/L/hr | | |
| | Supine: | | | Low-sodium diet |
| | 2.7 ± 1.8 ng/ml/hr | 2.1 ± 1.4 nmol/L/hr | | |
| | Upright: | | | |
| | 6.6 ± 2.5 ng/ml/hr | 5.1 ± 1.9 nmol/L/hr | | |
| | Diuretics: | | | Low-sodium diet |
| | 10.0 ± 3.7 ng/ml/hr | 7.7 ± 2.9 nmol/L/hr | | |
| Somatomedin C (Sm-C, IGF-1) | 0.08–2.8 U/ml | 0.08–2.8 arb. unit | 2-P | EDTA plasma |
| | | | | Prepubertal |
| | 0.9–5.9 U/ml | 0.9–5.9 arb. unit | | During puberty |
| | 0.34–1.9 U/ml | 0.34–1.9 arb. unit | | Adult males |
| | 0.45–2.2 U/ml | 0.45–2.2 arb. unit | | Adult females |

## Thyroid Hormones

| Determination | Reference Range: Conventional | Reference Range: SI | Minimal ml Required* | Note |
|---|---|---|---|---|
| Thyroid-stimulating hormone (TSH) | 0.5–5.0 μUlml | 0.5–5.0 arb. unit | 2-S | |
| Thyroxine-binding globulin capacity | 15–25 μg $T_4$/100 ml | 193–322 nmol/L | 2-S | |
| Total triiodothyronine ($T_3$) | 75–195 ng/100 ml | 1.16–3.00 nmol/L | 2-S | |
| Reverse triiodothyronine (rT3) | 13–53 ng/ml | 0.2–0.8 nmol/L | 2-S | |
| Total thyroxine by RIA ($T_4$) | 4–12 μg/100 ml | 52–154 nmol/L | 1-S | |
| $T_3$ resin uptake | 25–35% | 0.25–0.35 | 2-S | |
| Free thyroxine index ($FT_4I$) | 1–4 | | 2-S | |

## VITAMIN D DERIVATIVES

| Determination | Reference Range: Conventional | Reference Range: SI | Minimal ml Required* | Note |
|---|---|---|---|---|
| 1,25-Dihydroxy-vitamin D | 26–65 pg/ml | 62–155 pmol/L | 1-S | |
| 25-Hydroxy-vitamin D | 8–55 ng/ml | 19.4–137 nmol/L | 1-S | |

## HEMATOLOGIC VALUES

| Determination | Reference Range: Conventional | Reference Range: SI | Minimal ml Required* | Note |
|---|---|---|---|---|
| Coagulation factors: | | | | |
| Factor I (fibrinogen) | 0.15–0.35 g/100 ml | 4.0–10.0 μmol/L | 4.5-P | Collect in Vacutainer containing sodium citrate |
| Factor II (prothrombin) | 60–140% | 0.60–1.40 | 4.5-P | Collect in plastic tubes with 3.8% sodium citrate |
| Factor V (accelerator globulin) | 60–140% | 0.60–1.40 | 4.5-P | Collect as in factor II determination |
| Factor VII-X (proconvertin-Stuart) | 70–130% | 0.70–1.30 | 4.5-P | Collect as in factor II determination |

## HEMATOLOGIC VALUES (Continued)

| Determination | Reference Range: Conventional | Reference Range: SI | Minimal ml Required* | Note |
|---|---|---|---|---|
| Factor X (Stuart factor) | 70–130% | 0.70–1.30 | 4.5-P | Collect as in factor II determination |
| Factor VIII (antihemophilic globulin) | 50–200% | 0.50–2.0 | 4.5-P | Collect as in factor II determination |
| Factor IX (plasma thromboplastic cofactor) | 60–140% | 0.60–1.40 | 4.5-P | Collect as in factor II determination |
| Factor XI (plasma thromboplastic antecedent) | 60–140% | 0.60–1.40 | 4.5-P | Collect as in factor II determination |
| Factor XII (Hageman factor) | 60–140% | 0.60–1.40 | 4.5-P | Collect as in factor II determination |
| Coagulation screening tests: | | | | |
| Bleeding time (Simplate) | 3–9.5 min | 180–570 sec | | |
| Prothrombin time | Less than 2-sec deviation from control | Less than 2-sec deviation from control | 4.5-P | Collect in Vacutainer containing 3.8% sodium citrate |
| Partial thromboplastin time (activated) | 25–38 sec | 25–38 sec | 4.5-P | Collect in Vacutainer containing 3.8% sodium citrate |
| Whole-blood clot lysis | No clot lysis in 24 hr | 0/day | 2.0-whole blood | Collect in sterile tube and incubate at 37°C |
| Fibrinolytic studies: | | | | |
| Euglobin lysis | No lysis in 2 hr | 0/2 hr | 4.5-P | Collect as in factor II determination |
| Fibrinogen split products | Negative reaction at >1:4 dilution | 0 (at 1:4 dilution) | 4.5-S | Collect in special tube containing thrombin and epsilon aminocaproic acid |
| Thrombin time | Control ±5 sec | Control ±5 sec | 4.5-P | Collect as in factor II determination |
| "Complete" blood count: | | | | |
| Hematocrit | Male: 45–52%<br>Female: 37–48% | Male: 0.45–0.52<br>Female: 0.37–0.48 | 1-B | Use EDTA as anticoagulant; the seven listed tests are performed automatically on the Ortho ELT 800, which directly determines cell counts, hemoglobin (as the cyanmethemoglobin derivative), and MCV and computes hematocrit, MCH, and MCHC |
| Hemoglobin | Male: 13–18 g/100 ml<br>Female: 12–16 g/100 ml | Male: 8.1–11.2 mmol/L<br>Female: 7.4–9.9 mmol/L | | |
| Leukocyte count | 4300–10,800/mm$^3$ | 4.3–10.8 × $10^9$/L | | |
| Erythrocyte count | 4.2–5.9 million/mm$^3$ | 4.2–5.9 × $10^{12}$/L | | |
| Mean corpuscular volume (MCV) | 86–98 $\mu m^3$/cell | 86–98 fl | | |
| Mean corpuscular hemoglobin (MCH) | 27–32 pg/RBC | 1.7–2.0 pg/cell | | |
| Mean corpuscular hemoglobin concentration (MCHC) | 32–36% | 0.32–0.36 | | |

| | | | | |
|---|---|---|---|---|
| Erythrocyte sedimentation rate | Male: 1–13 mm/hr<br>Female: 1–20 mm/hr | Male: 1–13 mm/hr<br>Female: 1–20 mm/hr | 5-B | Use EDTA as anticoagulant |
| Erythrocyte enzymes: | | | | |
| Glucose-6-phosphate dehydrogenase | 5–15 U/g Hb | 5–15 U/g | 9-B | Use special anticoagulant (ACD solution) |
| Pyruvate kinase | 13–17 U/g Hb | 13–17 U/g | 8-B | Use special anticoagulant (ACD solution) |
| Ferritin (serum) | | | | |
| Iron deficiency | 0–12 ng/ml<br>13–20 Borderline | 0–4.8 nmol/L<br>5.2–8 nmol/L Borderline | | |
| Iron excess | >400 ng/L | >160 nmol/L | | |
| Folic acid | | | | |
| Normal | >3.3 ng/ml | >7.3 nmol/L | 1-S | |
| Borderline | 2.5–3.2 ng/ml | 5.75–7.39 nmol/L | 1-S | |
| Haptoglobin | 40–336 mg/100 ml | 0.4–3.36 g/L | 1-S | |
| Hemoglobin studies: | | | | |
| Electrophoresis for abnormal hemoglobin | | | 5-B | Collect with anticoagulant |
| Electrophoresis for | | | 5-B | Use oxalate as anticoagulant |
| $A_2$ hemoglobin | 3.0% | 0.015–0.035 | | |
| Borderline | 0.3–3.5% | 0.03–0.035 | | |
| Hemoglobin F (fetal hemoglobin) | Less than 2% | <0.02 | 5-B | Collect with anticoagulant |
| Hemoglobin, met- and sulf- | 0 | 0 | 5-B | Use heparin as anticoagulant |
| Serum hemoglobin | 2–3 mg/100 ml | 1.2–1.9 $\mu$mol/L | 2-S | |
| Thermolabile hemoglobin | 0 | 0 | 1-B | Any anticoagulant |
| Lupus anticoagulant | 0 | 0 | 4.5-P | Collect as in factor II determination |
| LE (lupus erythematosus) preparation: | | | | |
| Method I | 0 | 0 | 5-B | Use heparin as anticoagulant |
| Method II | 0 | 0 | 5-B | Use defibrinated blood |
| Leukocyte alkaline phosphatase: | | | 20-Isolated blood leukocytes | Special handling of blood necessary |
| Qualitative method | Males: 33–188 U<br>Females (off contraceptive pill): 30–160 U | 33–188 U<br>30–160 U | Smear-B | |
| Muramidase | Serum, 3–7 $\mu$g/ml<br>Urine, 0–2 $\mu$g/ml | 3–7 mg/L<br>0–2 $\mu$g/L | 1-S<br>1-U | |

## HEMATOLOGIC VALUES (Continued)

| *Determination* | Reference Range: *Conventional* | Reference Range: *SI* | *Minimal ml Required** | *Note* |
|---|---|---|---|---|
| Osmotic fragility of erythrocytes | Increased if hemolysis occurs in over 0.5% NaCl; decreased if hemolysis is incomplete in 0.3% NaCl | | 5-B | Use heparin as anticoagulant |
| Peroxide hemolysis | Less than 10% | 0.10 | 6-B | Use EDTA as anticoagulant |
| Platelet count | 150,000–350,000/mm$^3$ | 150–350 × $10^9$/L | 0.5-B | Use EDTA as anticoagulant; counts are performed on Clay Adams Ultraflow; when counts are low, results are confirmed by hand counting |
| Platelet function tests: | | | | |
| Clot retraction | 50–100%/2 hr | 0.50–1.00/2 hr | 4.5-P | Collect as in factor II determination |
| Platelet aggregation | Full response to ADP, epinephrine, and collagen | 1.0 | 18-P | Collect as in factor II determination |
| Platelet factor 3 | 33–57 sec | 33–57 sec | 4.5-P | Collect as in factor II determination |
| Reticulocyte count | 0.5–2.5% red cells | 0.005–0.025 | 0.1-B | |
| Vitamin $B_{12}$ | 205–876 pg/ml | 150–674 pmol/L | 12-S | |
| Borderline | 140–204 pg/ml | 102.6–149 pmol/L | | |

## CEREBROSPINAL FLUID VALUES

| *Determination* | Reference Range: *Conventional* | Reference Range: *SI* | *Minimal ml Required** | *Note* |
|---|---|---|---|---|
| Bilirubin | 0 | 0 | 2 | |
| Cell count | 0–5 mononuclear cells | | 0.5 | |
| Chloride | 120–130 mEq/L | 120–130 mmol/L | 0.5 | |
| Colloidal gold | 0000000000–0001222111 | Same | 0.1 | |
| Albumin | Mean: 29.5 mg/100 ml<br>±2 SD: 11–48 mg/100 ml | 0.295 g/L<br>±2 SD: 0.11–0.48 | 2.5 | |
| IgG | Mean: 4.3 mg/100 ml<br>±2 SD: 0–8.6 mg/100 ml | 0.043 g/L<br>±2 SD: 0–0.086 | | |

| | | | | |
|---|---|---|---|---|
| Glucose | 50–75 mg/100 ml | 2.8–4.2 mmol/L | 0.5 | |
| Pressure (initial) | 70–180 mm of water | 70–180 arb. unit | | |
| Protein: | | | | |
| Lumbar | 15–45 mg/100 ml | 0.15–0.45 g/L | 1 | |
| Cisternal | 15–25 mg/100 ml | 0.15–0.25 g/L | 1 | |
| Ventricular | 5–15 mg/100 ml | 0.05–0.15 g/L | 1 | |

## MISCELLANEOUS VALUES

| Determination | Reference Range: Conventional | Reference Range: SI | Minimal ml Required* | Note |
|---|---|---|---|---|
| Carcinoembryonic antigen (CEA) | 0–2.5 ng/ml | 0–2.5 μg/L | 20-P | Must be sent on ice |
| Chylous fluid | | | | Use fresh specimen |
| Digitoxin | 17 ± 6 ng/ml | 22 ± 7.8 nmol/L | 1-S | Medication with digitoxin or digitalis |
| Digoxin | 1.2 ± 0.4 ng/ml | 1.54 ± 0.5 nmol/L | 1-S | Medication with digoxin 0.25 mg per day |
| | 1.5 ± 0.4 ng/ml | 1.92 ± 0.5 nmol/L | 1-S | Medication with digoxin 0.5 mg per day |
| Duodenal drainage | | | | pH should be in proper range with minimal amount of gastric juice |
| pH (urine) | 5–7 | 5–7 | | |
| Gastric analysis | Basal: | | | |
| | Females: 2.0 ± 1.8 mEq/hr | 0.6 ± 0.5 μmol/sec | | |
| | Males: 3.0 ± 2.0 mEq/hr | 0.8 ± 0.6 μmol/sec | | |
| | Maximal (after histalog or gastrin): | | | |
| | Females: 16 ± 5 mEq/hr | 4.4 ± 1.4 μmol/sec | | |
| | Males: 23 ± 5 mEq/hr | 6.4 ± 1.4 μmol/sec | | |
| Gastrin-I | 0–200 pg/ml | 0–95 pmol/L | 4-P | Heparinized sample |
| Immunologic tests: | | | | |
| Alpha-fetoprotein | Undetectable in normal adults | | 2-S | |
| Alpha-1-antitrypsin | 85–213 mg/100 ml | 0.85–2.13 g/L | 10-B | |
| Rheumatoid factor | <60 IU/ml | | 10 ml clotted blood | Fasting sample preferred |
| Antinuclear antibodies | Negative at a 1:8 dilution of serum | | 2-S | Send to laboratory promptly |

## MISCELLANEOUS VALUES (Continued)

| Determination | Reference Range: Conventional | Reference Range: SI | Minimal ml Required* | Note |
|---|---|---|---|---|
| Anti-DNA antibodies | Negative at a 1:10 dilution of serum | | 2-S | |
| Antibodies to Sm and RNP (ENA) | None detected | | 10 ml clotted blood | |
| Antibodies to SS-A (Ro) and SS-B (La) | None detected | | 10 ml clotted blood | |
| Autoantibodies to: | | | | |
| Thyroid colloid and microsomal antigens | Negative at a 1:10 dilution of serum | | 2-S | Low titers in some elderly normal women |
| Gastric parietal cells | Negative at a 1:20 dilution of serum | | 2-S | |
| Smooth muscle | Negative at a 1:20 dilution of serum | | 2-S | |
| Mitochondria | Negative at a 1:20 dilution of serum | | 2-S | |
| Interstitial cells of the testes | Negative at a 1:10 dilution of serum | | 2-S | |
| Skeletal muscle | Negative at a 1:60 dilution of serum | | 2-S | |
| Adrenal gland | Negative at a 1:10 dilution of serum | | 2-S | |
| Bence Jones protein | No Bence Jones protein detected in a 50-fold concentrate of urine | | 50-U | |
| Complement, total hemolytic | 150–250 U/ml | | 10-B | Must be sent on ice |
| Cryoprecipitable proteins | None detected | 0 arb. unit | 10-S | Collect and transport at 37°C |
| C3 | Range, 83–177 mg/100 ml | 0.83–1.77 g/L | 2-S | |
| C4 | Range, 15–45 mg/100 ml | 0.15–0.45 g/L | 2-S | |
| Factor B | 12–30 mg/100 ml | | 5 ml clotted blood | |
| C1 esterase inhibitor | 13.2–24 mg/100 ml | | 5 ml clotted blood | |
| Hemoglobin $A_{1e}$ | 3.8–6.4% | 0.038–0.064 | 5-P | Send EDTA tube on ice promptly to laboratory |

| | | | | |
|---|---|---|---|---|
| Hypersensitivity pneumonitis screen | No antibodies to those antigens assayed | | 5 ml clotted blood | |
| Immunoglobulins: | | | | |
| IgG | 639–1349 mg/100 ml | 6.39–13.49 g/L | 2-S | |
| IgA | 70–312 mg/100 ml | 0.7–3.12 g/L | 2-S | |
| IgM | 86–352 mg/100 ml | 0.86–3.52 g/L | 2-S | |
| Viscosity | 1.4–1.8 relative viscosity units | | 10-B | Expressed as the relative viscosity of serum compared with water |
| Iontophoresis | Children: 0–40 mEq sodium/L<br>Adults: 0–60 mEq sodium/L | 0–40 mmol/L<br>0–60 mmol/L | | Value given in terms of sodium |
| Propranolol (includes bioactive 4-OH metabolite) | 100–300 ng/ml | 386–1158 nmol/L | 1-S | Obtain blood sample 4 hr after last dose of beta-blocking agent |
| Stool fat | Less than 5 g in 24 hr or less than 4% of measured fat intake in 3-day period | <5 g/day | 24-hr or 3-day specimen | |
| Stool nitrogen | Less than 2 g/day or 10% of urinary nitrogen | <2 g/day | 24-hr or 3-day specimen | |
| Synovial fluid: | | | | |
| Glucose | Not less than 20 mg/100 ml lower than simultaneously drawn blood sugar | See Blood Glucose | ml of fresh fluid | Collect with oxalate–fluoride mixture |
| D-Xylose absorption | 5–8 g/5 hr in urine; 40 mg per 100 ml in blood 2 hr after ingestion of 25 g of D-xylose | 33–53 mmol/day<br>2.7 mmol/L | 5-U<br>5-B | For directions see Benson et al.: N Engl J Med 256:335, 1957 |

* Abbreviations used: SI, Système International d'Unités; P, plasma; S, serum; B, blood; and U, urine.

SOURCE: From Scully, Robert E. (ed): Case Records of the Massachusetts General Hospital, New England Journal of Medicine, vol. 314, pp. 39–49, January 2, 1986. Used with permission.

APPENDIX 4

# Prefixes, Suffixes, and Combining Forms

**a-, an-.** Without; away from; not.
**ab-, abs-.** From; away from; absent.
**abdomin-, abdomino-.** Abdomen.
**abs-.** SEE: *ab-*.
**acantho-.** Thorn; spine.
**acro-.** Extremity; top; extreme point.
**actino-.** Ray; some form of radiation.
**ad-.** Adherence; increase; toward.
**-ad.** Toward; in the direction of.
**aden-, adeno-.** Gland.
**adip-, adipo-.** Fat.
**-aemia.** Blood.
**aer-, aero-.** Air.
**-aesthesia, aesthesio-.** SEE: *-esthesia.*
**-agogue.** Producer; leader.
**-agra.** Sudden severe pain.
**-al.** Relating to (e.g., abdominal, intestinal). In chemistry, an aldehyde.
**-algesia, -algia.** Suffering; pain.
**algi-.** Pain.
**all-.** SEE: *allo-*.
**allo-, all-.** Other.
**amb-, ambi-.** Both; on both sides; around; about.
**amph-, amphi-, ampho-.** Both; on both sides; on all sides; double; around; about.
**an-.** SEE: *a-*.
**ana-, an-.** Up; against; back.
**andro-.** Man; male; masculine.
**angi-, angio-.** Blood or lymph vessels.
**aniso-.** Unequal; asymmetrical; dissimilar.
**ankyl-, ankylo-.** Crooked; bent; fusion or growing together of parts.
**ante-.** Before.
**antero-.** Anterior; front; before.
**anthropo-.** Human beings; human life.
**ant-, anti-.** Against.
**antr-, antro-.** Antrum.
**apo-.** From; derived from; separated from; opposed.
**arch-, arche-, archi-.** First; principal; beginning; original.
**arteri-, arterio-.** Artery.
**arthr-, arthro-.** Joint.
**-ase.** Enzyme.
**-asis, -esis, -iasis, -isis, -sis.** Condition; pathological state.
**astro-.** Star; star-shaped.
**atelo-.** Imperfect; incomplete.
**atmo-.** Steam; vapor.
**atreto-.** Absence of an opening.
**aut-, auto-.** Self.
**axio-.** Axis; the long axis of a tooth.
**axo-.** Axis; axon.
**bacteri-, bacterio-.** Bacteria; bacterium.
**balan-, balano-.** Glans clitoridis; glans penis.
**baro-.** Weight; pressure.
**basi-, basio-.** Base; foundation.
**bi-, bis-.** Two; double; twice.
**bili-.** Bile.
**bio-.** Life.
**bis-.** SEE: *bi-*.
**blast-, -blast.** Germ; bud; embryonic state of development.
**blenn-, blenno-.** Mucus.
**blephar-, blepharo-.** Eyelid.
**brachy-.** Short.
**brady-.** Slow.
**brom-, bromo-.** Bromine.
**bronch-, bronchi-, broncho-.** Airway.
**cac-, caci-, caco-.** Bad; ill.
**cardi-, cardio-.** Heart.
**carpo-.** Carpus.
**cary-, caryo-.** SEE: *kary-*.
**cat-, cata-, cath-, kat-, kata-.** Down; downward; destructive; against; according to.
**cath-.** SEE: *cat-*.
**cel-, celo-. 1.** Tumor; hernia. **2.** Cavity.
**-cele.** Tumor; swelling; hernia.
**cent-.** Hundred.
**cephal-, cephalo-.** Head.
**cervic-, cervico-.** Neck; the neck of an organ.
**cheil-, cheilo-.** SEE: *chil-*.
**chil-, chilo-,** Lip; lips.
**chrom-, chromo-.** Color.
**-cide.** Causing death.
**cine-.** Movement.
**circum-.** Around.
**-cle, -cule.** Little (e.g., molecule, corpuscle).
**cleid-, cleido-.** Clavicle.
**co-, com-, con-.** Together.
**colp-, colpo-.** SEE: *kolp-*.
**contra-.** Against; opposite.
**crani-, cranio-.** Skull; cranium.
**cry-, cryo-.** Cold.
**cyan-, cyano-.** Blue.
**cycl-, cyclo-.** Circular; cyclical; ciliary body of the eye.
**cyst-, cysto-, -cyst.** Cyst; urinary bladder.
**cyt-, cyto-, -cyte.** Cell.
**dacry-.** Tears.
**dactyl-.** Fingers.
**de-.** From; down; not.
**dec-, deca-.** Ten.
**deci-.** One tenth.
**demi-.** Half.
**dent-, denti-, dento-.** Teeth.
**derm-, derma-, dermato-, dermo-.** Skin.
**deuter-, deutero-, deuto-.** Second; secondary.
**dextro-.** Right.
**di-.** Double; twice; two; apart from.
**dia-.** Through; between; asunder.
**dipla-, diplo-.** Double; twin.
**dis-.** Negative; double; twice; apart; absence of.
**dors-, dorsi-, dorso-.** Back.
**-dynia.** Pain.
**dys-.** Difficult; bad; painful.
**ec-, ecto-.** Out; on the outside.
**-ectomy.** Excision.
**ectro-.** Congenital absence of a part.
**ef-, es-, ex-, exo-.** Out.

**electr-, electro-.** Electricity.
**-emesis.** Vomiting.
**-emia.** Blood.
**en-.** In; into.
**enantio-.** Opposite.
**end-, endo-.** Within.
**ent-, ento-.** Within; inside.
**enter-, entero-.** Intestine.
**ep-, epi-.** Upon; over; at; in addition to; after.
**erythr-, erythro-.** Red.
**-esis.** SEE: *-asis*.
**-esthesia.** Sensation.
**etio-.** Causation.
**eu-.** Well; good; healthy; normal.
**eury-.** Broad.
**ex-.** Out; away from; completely.
**exo-.** Out; outside of; without.
**extra-.** Outside of; in addition; beyond.
**-facient.** Causing; making happen.
**-ferous.** Producing.
**ferri-, ferro-.** Iron.
**fibro-.** Fibers; fibrous tissues.
**fluo-.** Flow.
**fore-.** Before; in front of.
**-form.** Form.
**-fuge.** To expel; to drive away; fleeing.
**galact-, galacto-.** Milk.
**gam-, gamo-.** Marriage; sexual union.
**gaster-, gastero-, gastr-, gastro-.** Stomach.
**gen-.** Producing; forming.
**-gen, -gene, -genesis, -genetic, -genic.** Producing; forming.
**genito-.** Organs of reproduction.
**gero-.** Old age.
**giga-.** Billion.
**glosso-.** Tongue.
**gluc-, gluco-, glyc-, glyco-.** Sugar; glycerol or similar substance.
**gnath-, gnatho-.** Jaw; cheek.
**-gog, -gogue.** To make flow.
**gon-, gono-.** Semen; seed; genitals; offspring.
**-gram.** A tracing; a mark.
**-graph.** Instrument used to make a drawing or record.
**-graphy.** Writing; record.
**gyn-, gyne-, gyneco-, gyno-.** Woman; female.
**gyro-.** Circle; spiral; ring.
**hem-, hema-, hemato-, hemo-.** Blood.
**hemi-.** Half.
**hepat-, hepato-.** Liver.
**heredo-.** Heredity.
**heter-, hetero-.** Other; different.
**hex-, hexa-.** Six.
**histo-.** Tissue.
**hol-, holo-.** Complete; entire; homogenous.
**homeo-.** Likeness; resemblance; constant unchanging state.
**homo-.** Same; likeness.
**hydra-, hydro-, hydr-.** Water.
**hyo-.** Hyoid bone.
**hyp-, hyph-, hypo-.** Less than; below; under.
**hyper-.** Above; excessive; beyond.
**hypno-.** Sleep; hypnosis.
**hyster-, hystero-.** Uterus.
**-ia.** Condition, esp. an abnormal state.
**-iasis.** SEE: *-asis*.
**-iatric.** Medicine; medical profession; physicians.
**-ic.** Pertaining to; relating to.
**ichthyo-.** Fish.
**-id.** Secondary skin eruption distant from primary infection site.
**ideo-.** Mental images.
**idio-.** Individual; distinct.
**ileo-.** Ileum.
**ilio-.** Ilium; flank.
**im-.** SEE: *in-*. Used before b, m, or p.
**in-.** In; inside; within; intensive action; negative.
**infra-.** Below; under; beneath; inferior to; after.
**inter-.** Between; in the midst.
**intra-, intro-.** Within; in; into.
**ipsi-.** Same.
**irid-, irido-.** Iris.
**ischio-.** Ischium.
**-isis.** SEE: *-asis*.
**-ism.** Condition; theory.
**iso-.** Equal.
**-ite. 1.** Of the nature of. **2.** In chemistry, a salt of an acid with the termination *-ous*.
**-itis.** Inflammation of.
**-ize.** To treat by special method.
**jejuno-.** Jejunum.
**juxta-.** Close proximity.
**kary-, karyo-, cary-, caryo-.** Nucleus; nut.
**kat-, kata-.** SEE: *cat-*.
**kera-, kerato-.** Horny substance; cornea.
**kilo-.** Thousand.
**kinesi-, kino-, -kinesis.** Movement.
**klepto-.** To steal.
**kolp-, kolpo-, colp-, colpo-.** Vagina.
**kypho-.** Humped.
**lact-.** Milk.
**laparo-.** Flank; abdominal wall.
**laryng-, laryngo-.** Larynx.
**latero-.** Side.
**leio-.** Smooth.
**lepido-.** Flakes; scales.
**lepto-.** Thin; fine; slight; delicate.
**leuk-, leuko-.** White; colorless; rel. to a leukocyte.
**linguo-.** Tongue.
**lip-, lipo-.** Fat.
**-lite, -lith, lith-, litho-.** Stone; calculus.
**-logia, -logy.** Science of; study of.
**lumbo-.** Loins.
**lyo-.** Dissolution; decomposition.
**-lysis. 1.** Setting free; disintegration. **2.** In medicine, reduction of; relief from.
**macr-, macro-.** Large; long.
**mal-.** Ill; bad; poor.
**-mania.** Frenzy; madness.
**med-, medi-, medio-.** Middle.
**mega-, megal-, megalo-.** Large; of great size.
**-megalia, -megaly.** Enlargement of a body part.
**meio-, mio-.** Less; smaller.
**melan-, melano-.** Black.
**mening-, meningo-.** Meninges.
**mes-, meso-. 1.** Middle. **2.** In anatomy, the mesentery. **3.** In medicine, secondary; partial.
**mesio-.** Toward the middle.
**meta-. 1.** Change; transformation; next in a series. **2.** In chemistry, the 1,3 position of benzene derivatives.

**-meter.** Measure.
**metr-, metra-, metro-.** Uterus.
**micr-, micro-.** Small.
**mio-.** SEE: *meio-*.
**mon-, mono-.** Single; one.
**muc-, muci-, muco-, myxa-, myxo-.** Mucus.
**multi-.** Many; much.
**musculo-, my-, myo-.** Muscle.
**my-, myo-.** SEE: *musculo-*.
**myc-, myco-.** Fungus.
**myel-, myelo-.** Spinal cord; bone marrow.
**myx-, myxo-.** SEE: *muc-*.
**nano-. 1.** One billionth. **2.** Dwarfism (nanism).
**narco-.** Numbness; stupor.
**naso-.** Nose.
**necr-, necro-.** Death; necrosis.
**neo-.** New; recent.
**nephr-, nephra-, nephro-.** Kidney.
**neur-, neuri, neuro-.** Nerve; nervous system.
**nitr-, nitro-.** Nitrogen.
**non-.** No.
**normo-.** Normal; usual.
**noso-.** Disease.
**noto-.** The back.
**nucleo-.** Nucleus.
**nyct-, nycto-.** Night; darkness.
**ob-.** Against.
**occipito-.** Occiput.
**octa-, octo-.** Eight.
**oculo-.** Eye.
**-ode, -oid.** Form; shape; resemblance.
**odont-, odonto-.** Tooth; teeth.
**-odynia, odyno-.** Pain.
**-oid.** SEE: *-ode.*
**oleo-.** Oil.
**olig-, oligo-.** Few; small.
**-ology.** Science of; study of.
**-oma.** Tumor.
**omo-.** Shoulder.
**omphal-, omphalo-.** Navel.
**onco-.** Tumor; swelling; mass.
**onych-, onycho-.** Fingernails; toenails.
**oo-, ovi-, ovo-.** Egg; ovum.
**oophor-, oophoro-, oophoron-.** Ovary.
**ophthalm-, ophthalmo-.** Eye.
**-opia.** Vision.
**opisth-, opistho-.** Backward.
**optico-, opto-.** Eye; vision.
**orchi-, orchid-, orchido-.** Testicle.
**oro-.** Mouth.
**orth-, ortho-.** Straight; correct; normal; in proper order.
**os-.** Mouth; bone.
**oscheo-.** Scrotum.
**-ose. 1.** Carbohydrate. **2.** Primary alteration of a protein.
**-osis.** Condition; status, process; abnormal increase.
**osmo-. 1.** Odor; smell. **2.** Impulse. **3.** Osmosis.
**oste-, osteo-.** Bone.
**-ostomosis, -ostomy, -stomosis, -stomy.** A created mouth or outlet.
**ot-, oto-.** Ear.
**-otomy.** Cutting.
**-ous. 1.** Possessing; full of. **2.** Pertaining to.
**ovi-, ovo-.** SEE: *oo-*.
**ox-.** Oxygen.
**oxy-. 1.** Sharp; keen; acute; acid; pungent. **2.** Oxygen in a compound. **3.** Hydroxyl group.
**pach-, pachy-.** Thick.
**-pagus.** Twins joined at a specific site (e.g., craniopagus).
**pali-, palin-.** Recurrence; repetition.
**pan-.** All; entire.
**pant-, panto-.** All or the whole of something.
**papulo-.** Pimple; papule.
**para-, -para. 1.** Prefix: near; alongside of; departure from normal. **2.** Suffix: Bearing offspring.
**path-, patho-, -path, -pathic, -pathy.** Disease; suffering.
**ped-, pedi-, pedo-.** Foot.
**pedia-.** Child.
**-penia.** Decrease from normal; deficiency.
**pent-, penta-.** Five.
**per-.** Throughout; through; utterly; intense.
**peri-.** Around; about.
**perineo-.** Perineum.
**peritoneo-.** Peritoneum.
**pero-.** Deformed.
**petro-.** Stone; the petrous portion of the temporal bone.
**-pexy.** Fixation, usually surgical.
**phaco-.** Lens of the eye.
**phag-, phago-.** Eating; ingestion; devouring.
**phall-.** Penis.
**pharmaco-.** Drug; medicine.
**pharyng-, pharyngo-.** Pharynx.
**-phil, -philia, -philic.** Love for; tendency toward; craving for.
**phlebo-.** Vein.
**-phobia.** Abnormal fear or aversion.
**phono-.** Sound; voice.
**-phoresis.** Transmission.
**-phoria.** In ophthalmology, a turning with reference to the visual axis.
**photo-.** Light.
**phren-, phreno-, -phrenia.** Mind; diaphragm.
**-phylaxis.** Protection.
**physico-.** Physical; natural.
**physio-.** Rel. to nature.
**physo-.** Air; gas.
**phyt-, phyto-.** Plant; something that grows.
**pico-.** One trillionth.
**picr-, picro-.** Bitter.
**-piesis.** Pressure.
**pimel-, pimelo-.** Fat.
**plagio-.** Slanting; oblique.
**-plasia.** Growth; cellular proliferation.
**plasm-, -plasm. 1.** Prefix: Living substance or tissue. **2.** Suffix: To mold.
**-plastic.** Molded; indicates restoration of lost or badly formed features.
**platy-.** Broad.
**-plegia.** Paralysis; stroke.
**pleur-, pleuro-.** Pleura; side; rib.
**-ploid.** Chromosome pairs of a specific number.
**plur-, pluri-.** Several; more.
**pneo-.** Breath; breathing.
**pneum-, pneuma-, pneumato-.** Air; gas; respiration.
**pneumo-, pneumono-.** Air; lung.
**pod-, podo-.** Foot.
**-poiesis, -poietic.** Production; formation.

**polio-.** Gray matter of the nervous system.
**poly-.** Much; many.
**post-.** After.
**postero-.** Posterior; behind; toward the back.
**-praxis. 1.** Act; activity. **2.** Practice; use.
**pre-.** Before; in front of.
**presby-.** Old age.
**pro-.** Before; in behalf of.
**proct-, procto-.** Anus; rectum.
**proso-.** Forward, anterior.
**proto-. 1.** First. **2.** In chemistry, the lowest of a series of compounds with the same elements.
**pseud-, pseudo-.** False.
**psych-, psycho-.** Mind; mental processes.
**psychro-.** Cold.
**pubio-, pubo-.** Pubic bone or region.
**pulmo-.** Lung.
**py-, pyo-.** Pus.
**pycn-, pycno-, pykn-, pykno-.** Dense; thick; compact; frequent.
**pyelo-.** Pelvis.
**pyg-, pygo-.** Buttocks.
**pykn-, pykno-.** SEE: *pycn-.*
**pyle-.** Orifice, esp. of the portal vein.
**pyloro-.** Gatekeeper; applied to the pylorus.
**pyreto-.** Fever.
**pyro-.** Heat; fire.
**quadr-, quadri-.** Four.
**quinqu-.** Five.
**rachi-, rachio-.** Spine.
**radio-. 1.** Radiant energy; a radioactive substance. **2.** In chemistry, a radioactive isotope.
**re-.** Back; again.
**recto-.** Straight; rectum.
**ren-, reno-.** Kidney.
**reticulo-.** Reticulum.
**retro-.** Backward; back; behind.
**rhabdo-.** Rod.
**rheo-, -(r)rhea.** Current; stream; to flow; to discharge.
**rhino-.** Nose.
**rhizo-.** Root.
**rhodo-.** Red.
**roseo-.** Rose-colored.
**-(r)rhage, -(r)rhagia.** Rupture; profuse fluid discharge.
**-(r)rhaphy.** A suturing or stitching.
**-(r)rhexis.** Rupture of a specific body part.
**sacchar-, saccharo-.** Sugar.
**sacro-.** Sacrum.
**salping-, salpingo-.** Auditory tube; fallopian tube.
**sapro-.** Putrid; rotten.
**sarco-.** Flesh.
**scapho-.** Boat-shaped; scaphoid.
**scapulo-.** Shoulder.
**scato-.** Dung; fecal matter.
**schisto-.** Split; cleft.
**schizo-.** Division.
**scirrho-.** Hard; hard tumor or scirrhus.
**sclero-.** Hard; relating to the sclera.
**-sclerosis.** Dryness; hardness.
**-scope.** Instrument for viewing or examining (includes other methods of examination).
**-scopy.** Examination.
**scoto-.** Darkness.
**sebo-.** Fatty substance.
**semi-.** Half.
**septi-.** Seven.
**sero-.** Serum.
**sesqui-.** One and one half.
**sial-, sialo-.** Saliva.
**sidero-.** Iron; steel.
**-sis.** SEE: *-asis.*
**sitio-, sito-.** Bread; made from grain; food.
**skeleto-.** Skeleton.
**skia-.** Shadow.
**sodio-.** Sodium.
**somat-, somato-.** Body.
**spectro-.** Appearance; image; form; spectrum.
**sperma-, spermat-, spermato-.** Sperm; spermatozoa.
**spheno-.** Wedge; sphenoid bone.
**sphygmo-.** Pulse.
**spleno-.** Spleen.
**spondyl-, spondylo-.** Vertebra.
**spongio-.** Spongelike.
**staphylo-.** Uvula; bunch of grapes; *Staphylococcus.*
**steato-.** Fat.
**steno-.** Narrow; short.
**sterco-.** Feces.
**stere-, stereo-.** Three dimensions.
**sterno-.** Sternum.
**stetho-.** Chest.
**stomato-.** Mouth.
**-stomosis, -stomy.** SEE: *-ostomosis.*
**strepto-.** Twisted.
**sub-.** Under; beneath; in small quantity; less than normal.
**super-.** Above; beyond; superior.
**supra-.** Above; beyond; on top.
**sym-.** With; together with; along; beside.
**syn-.** Joined; together.
**tachy-.** Swift; rapid.
**taen-, taeni-, ten-, teni-.** Tapeworm.
**tarso-.** Flat of the foot; edge of the eyelid.
**tauto-.** Same.
**techno-.** Art; skill.
**tel-, tele-. 1.** End. **2.** Distant; far.
**teleo-.** Perfect; complete.
**temporo-.** Temples of the head.
**ten-, teni-.** SEE: *taen-.*
**tendo-, teno-.** Tendon.
**ter-.** Three.
**tera-.** One trillionth.
**terato-.** Severely malformed fetus.
**tetra-.** Four.
**thalamo-.** Chamber; part of the brain where a nerve originates; thalamus.
**thanato-.** Death.
**theco-.** Sheath; case; receptacle.
**thermo-.** Hot; heat.
**thio-.** Sulfur.
**thorac-, thoraci-, thoraco-.** Chest; chest wall.
**thrombo-.** Blood clot; thrombus.
**thymo-. 1.** Thymus. **2.** Soul; emotions.
**thyro-.** Thyroid gland; oblong; shield.
**toco-.** Childbirth.
**-tome.** Cutting instrument.
**tomo-.** Section; layer.
**-tomy.** Cutting operation; excision.
**top-, topo-.** Place; locale.
**tox-, toxi-, toxico-, toxo-, -toxic.** Toxin; poison; toxic.

**trachelo-.** Neck.
**tracheo-.** Trachea; windpipe.
**trans-.** Across; over; beyond; through.
**traumato-.** Trauma.
**tri-.** Three.
**trich-, trichi-, tricho-.** Hair.
**troph-, tropho-, -trophic.** Nourishment.
**-tropin.** Stimulation of a target organ by a substance, esp. a hormone.
**tubo-.** Tube.
**tympano-.** Eardrum; tympanum.
**typhlo-. 1.** Cecum. **2.** Blindness.
**typho-.** Fever; typhoid.
**ulo-.** Scar; scarring.
**ultra-.** Beyond; excess.
**uni-.** One.
**uretero-.** Ureter.
**urethro-.** Urethra.
**-uria.** Urine.
**urin-, urino, uro-.** Urine.
**uter-, utero-.** Uterus.
**vaso-.** Vessel (e.g., blood vessel).
**veno-.** Vein.
**ventro-, ventr-, ventri-.** Abdomen; anterior surface of the body.
**vertebro-.** Vertebra; vertebrae.
**vesico-.** Bladder; vesicle.
**viscero-.** Viscera.
**vulvo-.** Covering; vulva.
**xanth-.** Yellow.
**xeno-.** Strange; foreign.
**xero-.** Dry.
**xiph-, xiphi-, xipho-.** Xiphoid cartilage.
**zoo-.** Animal; animal life.

# APPENDIX 5
# Latin and Greek Nomenclature

## Appendix 5–1 English with Latin and Greek Equivalents

**acid.** Acidum.
**ague.** Febris.
**and.** Et.
**arm.** Brachium. Gr., brachion.
**artery.** Arteria.
**attachment.** Adhesio.
**back.** Tergum; dorsum.
**backbone.** Spina.
**backward.** Retro.
**bath.** Balneum.
**beef.** Bubula.
**belly.** Venter; abdomen.
**bend.** Flexus.
**bile.** Bilis. Gr., chole.
**bladder.** Vesica.
**bleed.** Fluere.
**blind.** Caecus.
**blister.** Pustula vesicatorium.
**bloat.** Tumere.
**blood.** Sanguis. Gr., haima.
**blood vessel.** Vena.
**body.** Corpus. Gr., soma.
**boiling up.** Effervescens.
**bone.** Os. Gr., osteon.
**bony.** Osseus.
**bowels.** Intestina; viscera.
**bowlegged.** Valgus.
**brain.** Cerebrum. Gr., enkephalos.
**breach.** Ruptura.
**breast.** Mamma. Gr., mastos.
**breath.** Halitus.
**bubble.** Pustula.
**bulb.** Bulbus.
**buttock.** Clunis. Gr., gloutos.
**calcareous.** Calci similis.
**canal.** Canalis.
**cartilage.** Cartilago. Gr., chondros.
**catarrh.** Coryza.
**cavity.** Caverna.
**change.** Mutatio.
**chest.** Thorax. Gr., thorax.
**chin.** Mentum. Gr., geneion.
**choke.** Strangulare.
**clavicle.** Clavicula.
**congestion.** Conglobatio.
**consumption.** Phthisis, pulmonaria.
**convulsion.** Convulsio.
**cord.** Corda.
**corn.** Callus-clavus.
**cornea.** Cornu. Gr., keras.
**costive.** Astrictus.
**cough.** Tussio.
**countenance.** Vultus.
**cramp.** Spasmus.
**crisis.** Dies crisimus.
**cup.** Poculum.
**cure.** Sanare.
**curvature.** Curvatura.
**cuticle.** Cuticula.
**daily.** Diurnus.
**dandruff.** Furfures capitis.
**day.** Dies.
**dead.** Mortuus; defunctus.
**deadly.** Lethalis.
**deafness.** Surditas.
**decompose.** Desolvere.
**dental.** Dentalis.
**depression.** Depressio.
**digestive.** Digestorius; pepticus.
**dilute.** Diluere.
**discharge.** Eluvies; effluens.
**disease.** Morbus.
**dorsal.** Dorsalis.
**dose.** Potio.
**dram.** Drachma.
**drink.** Bibere; potis.
**dropsy.** Hydrops; opis.
**drug.** Medicamentum.
**duct.** Ductus.
**dysentery.** Dysenteria.
**ear.** Auris. Gr., ous.
**eat.** Edere. Gr., phagos.
**egg.** Ovum.
**elbow.** Cubitum. Gr., ankon.
**embryo.** Partus immaturus.
**emission.** Emissio.
**entrails.** Viscera.
**epidemic.** Epidemus.
**epilepsy.** Morbus comitalis; epilepsia.
**epileptic.** Epilepticus.
**erection.** Erectio.
**erotic.** Amatorius.
**eunuch.** Eunuchus.
**every.** Omnis.
**excrement.** Excrementum.
**excretion.** Excrementum; excretio.
**exhalation.** Exhalatio.
**exhale.** Exhalare.
**expel.** Expellere.
**expire.** Expirare.
**external.** Externus.
**extract.** Extractum.
**eye.** Oculus. Gr., ophthalmos.
**eyeball.** Pupula.
**eyebrow.** Supercilium.
**eyelid.** Palpebra.
**eyetooth.** Dens caninus.
**face.** Facies.
**faculty.** Facultas.
**faint.** Collabi.
**fat.** Adeps. Gr., lipos.
**feature.** Lineomentum.
**febrile.** Febriculosus.
**fecundity.** Fecunditas.
**feel.** Tactus.
**fever.** Febris.

**film.** Membranula.
**filter.** Percolare.
**finger.** Digitus. Gr., daktylos.
**fistula.** Fistula putris.
**fit.** Accessus.
**flesh.** Carnis. Gr., sarx.
**fluid.** Fluidus.
**food.** Cibus.
**foot.** Pes, pedis. Gr., pous.
**forearm.** Brachium.
**forehead.** Frons.
**freckle.** Lentigo.
**gall.** Bilis.
**gangrene.** Gangraena.
**gargle.** Gargarizein.
**gland.** Glandula.
**gleet.** Ichor.
**gout.** Morbus articularis; (in feet) podagra.
**grain.** Granum.
**gravel.** Calculus.
**grinder tooth.** Dens maxillaris.
**gullet.** Gula.
**gum.** Gingiva.
**gut.** Intestinum.
**hair.** Capillus. Gr., thrix.
**half.** Dimidius.
**hand.** Manus. Gr., cheir.
**harelip.** Labrum fissum.
**haunch.** Clunis.
**head.** Caput. Gr., kephale.
**heal.** Sanare.
**healer.** Medicus.
**healing.** Salutaris.
**health.** Sanitas.
**healthful.** Salutaris; saluber.
**healthy.** Sanus.
**hear.** Audire.
**hearing.** Auditio; (sense of) auditus.
**heart.** Cor. Gr., kardia.
**heartburn.** Redundatio stomachi.
**heat.** Calor.
**hectic.** Hecticus.
**heel.** Calx, talus.
**hirsute.** Hirsutus.
**homeopathic.** Homeopathicus.
**hysterics.** Hysteria.
**illness.** Morbus.
**incisor.** Dens acutus.
**infant.** Infans; puerilis.
**infect.** Inficere.
**infectious.** Contagiosus.
**infirm.** Infirmus; debilis.
**inflammation.** Inflammatio; (of lungs) inflammatio pulmonaria.
**injection.** Injectio.
**insane.** Insanus.
**intellect.** Intellectus.
**intercourse.** Congressus.
**internal.** Intestinus.
**intestine.** Intestinum. Gr., enteron.
**itch.** Scabies.
**itching.** Pruritus.
**jaw.** Maxilla.
**joint.** Artus. Gr., arthron.
**jugular vein.** Vena jugularis.
**kidney.** Ren. Gr., nephros.
**knee.** Genu. Gr., gonu.
**kneepan.** Patella.
**knuckle.** Condylus.
**labor.** Partus.
**labyrinth.** Labyrinthus.
**lacerate.** Lacerare.
**larynx.** Guttur.
**lateral.** Lateralis.
**leech.** Sanguisuga.
**leg.** Tibia.
**leprosy.** Lepra.
**ligament.** Ligamentum. Gr., syndesmos.
**ligature.** Ligatura.
**limb.** Membrum.
**lime.** Calx.
**listen.** Auscultare.
**liver.** Jecur. Gr., hepar.
**livid.** Lividus.
**loin.** Lumbus. Gr., lapara.
**looseness.** Laxitas.
**lotion.** Lotio.
**lukewarm.** Tepidus.
**lung.** Pulmo. Gr., pneumon.
**lymph.** Lympha.
**mad.** Insanus.
**malady.** Morbus.
**male.** Masculinus.
**malignant.** Malignus.
**maternity.** Conditio matris.
**medicated.** Medicatus.
**medicine.** (Remedy) Medicamentum.
**milk.** Lac.
**mind.** Animus.
**mix.** Miscere.
**mixture.** Mistura.
**moist.** Humidus.
**molar.** Dens molaris.
**month.** Mensis.
**monthly.** Menstruus.
**morbid.** Morbidus.
**mouth.** Os. Gr., stoma.
**mucous.** Mucosus.
**muscle.** Musculus. Gr., mys.
**mustard.** Sinapis.
**nail.** Unguis.
**navel.** Umbilicus. Gr., omphalos.
**neck.** Cervix; collum. Gr., trachelos.
**nerve.** Nervus. Gr., neuron.
**nipple.** Papilla.
**no, none.** Nullus.
**normal.** Normalis.
**nose.** Nasus. Gr., rhis.
**nostril.** Naris.
**not.** Non.
**nourish.** Nutrire.
**nourishment.** Alimentus.
**now.** Nunc.
**nudity.** Nudatio.
**nurse.** Nutrix.
**obesity.** Obesitas.
**ocular.** Ocularis.
**oculist.** Ocularis medicus.
**oil.** Oleum.
**ointment.** Unguentum.
**operator.** Manus curatio.
**opiate.** Medicamemtum somnificum.
**optics.** Optica.
**orifice.** Foramen.
**pain.** Dolor.
**palate.** Palatum.
**palm.** Palma.
**parasite.** Parasitus.

**part.** Pars.
**patient.** Patiens.
**pectoral.** Pectoralis.
**pedal.** Pedale.
**phlegm.** Pituita.
**pill.** Pilus.
**pimple.** Pustula.
**plaster.** Emplastrum.
**poison.** Venenum.
**poultice.** Cataplasma.
**powder.** Pulvis.
**pregnant.** Gravida.
**prepare.** Parare.
**prescribe.** Praescribere.
**prescription.** Praescriptum.
**puberty.** Pubertas.
**pubic bone.** Os pubis. Gr., pecten.
**pulverize.** Pulverare.
**pupil.** Pupilla.
**purgative.** Purgativus.
**putrid.** Putridus.
**quinsy.** Cynanche; angina.
**rash.** Exanthema.
**recover.** Convalescere.
**recumbent.** Recumbens.
**recur.** Recurrere.
**redness.** Rubor.
**remedy.** Remedium.
**respiration.** Respiratio.
**rheum.** Fluxio.
**rib.** Costa.
**rigid.** Rigidus.
**ringing.** Tinnitus.
**rupture.** Hernia.
**saliva.** Sputum.
**sallow.** Salix.
**salt.** Sal.
**salve.** Unguentum.
**sane.** Sanus.
**scab.** Scabies.
**scalp.** Pericranium.
**scaly.** Squamosus.
**scar.** Cicatrix.
**sciatica.** Ischias.
**scruple.** Scrupulum.
**seed.** Semen.
**senile.** Senilis.
**serum.** Sanguinis pars equosa.
**sheath.** Vagina.
**shin.** Tibia.
**shock.** Concussio; (of electricity) ictus electricus.
**short.** Brevis.
**shoulder.** Humerus. Gr., omos.
**shoulder blade.** Scapula.
**shudder.** Tremor.
**sick.** Aegrotus.
**side.** Latus.
**sinew.** Nervus.
**skeleton.** Gr., skeleton.
**skin.** Cutis. Gr., derma.
**skull.** Cranium. Gr., kranion.
**sleep.** Somnus.
**smallpox.** Variola.
**smell.** Odoratus.
**soap.** Sapo.
**socket.** Cavum.
**soft.** Mollis.
**solid.** Solidus.
**solution.** Dilutum.
**soporific.** Soporus.
**sore.** Ulcus.
**spasm.** Spasmus.
**spinal.** Dorsalis; spinalis.
**spine.** Spina.
**spirit.** Spiritus.
**spittle.** Sputum.
**spleen.** Lien.
**spoon.** Cochleare.
**sprain.** Luxatio.
**stomach.** Stomachus. Gr., gaster.
**stone.** Calculus.
**stricture.** Strictura.
**sugar.** Saccharum.
**suture.** Sutura.
**swallow.** Glutire.
**sweat.** Sudor. Gr., hidros.
**symptom.** Symptoma.
**system.** Systema.
**tail.** Cauda.
**take.** Sumere.
**tapeworm.** Taenia.
**taste.** Gustatus.
**tear.** Lacrima.
**teeth.** Dentes.
**tendon.** Tendo. Gr., tenon.
**testicle.** Testis. Gr., orchis.
**thigh.** Femur.
**throat.** Fauces. Gr., pharynx.
**throb.** Palpitare.
**thumb.** Pollex.
**tongue.** Lingua. Gr., glossa.
**tonsil.** Tonsilla.
**tooth.** Dens. Gr., odous.
**troche.** Trochiscus.
**tube.** Tuba.
**twin.** Geminus.
**twitching.** Subsultus.
**ulcer.** Ulcus.
**unless.** Nisi.
**urine.** Urina.
**uterine.** Uterinus.
**vaccine.** Vaccinum.
**vagina.** Vagina. Gr., kolpos.
**valve.** Valvula.
**vein.** Vena. Gr., phleps.
**vertebra.** Vertebra. Gr., spondylos.
**vessel.** Vas.
**wash.** Lavare.
**water.** Aqua.
**wax.** Cera.
**waxed dressing.** Ceratum.
**weary.** Lassus.
**wet.** Humidus.
**windpipe.** Arteria aspera.
**wine.** Vinum.
**woman.** Femina.
**womb.** Uterus. Gr., hystera.
**worm.** Vermis.
**wound.** Vulnus.
**wrist.** Carpus. Gr., karpos.
**yolk.** Luteum.

## COLORS

**black.** Niger; nigra; nigrum.
**blue.** Caeruleus; cyaneus; lividus.

**brown.** Fulvus.
**crimson.** Coccum; coccineus.
**gray.** Cinereus.
**green.** Viridis.
**lemon.** Citreus.
**pink.** Rosaceus.
**purple.** Purpura; purpureus.
**red.** Ruber.
**scarlet.** Coccineus.
**violet.** Violaceus.
**white.** Albus.
**yellow.** Flavus; luteus; croceus.

## QUALITIES

**bitter.** Acerbus.
**chill.** Friguscolum.
**cold.** Frigidus.
**dry.** Aridus.
**dull.** Stupidus; hebes.
**faintness.** Languor.
**fat.** Obesus; pinguis.
**heat.** Calor; ardor; fervor.
**heavy.** Gravis; ponderosus.
**hot.** Calidus; fervens; candens.
**light.** Levis.
**liquid.** Liquidus.
**moist.** Humidus; uvidus.
**sharp.** Acutus.
**short.** Brevis.
**sour.** Acidus.
**sweet.** Dulcis.
**tall.** Longus; celsus; procerus.
**thick.** Densus.
**thin.** Tenuis; macer.
**warm.** Calidus.
**warmth.** Calor.
**weary.** Lassus; languidus; fatigatus.
**wet.** Humidus.

## METALS

**copper.** Cuprum; cuprinus.
**gold.** Aurum; aureus.
**iron.** Ferrum; ferreus.
**silver.** Argentum; argenteus.
**tin.** Stannum; plumbum album.

## TIME

**afternoon.** Post meridiem.
**age.** Aetas; maturus; adultus; impubis.
**autumn.** Autumnus.
**birth.** Partus; natales.
**breakfast.** Prandium.
**child.** Infans; puer; filius.
**daily.** Diurnus.
**date.** Status diei.
**dawn.** Prima lux.
**day.** Dies.
**death.** Mors.
**dinner.** Cena.
**evening.** Vesper.
**hour.** Hora.
**infant.** Infans.
**maturity.** Maturitas; aetas matura.
**meal.** Epulae.
**midnight.** Media nox.
**midsummer.** Media aestas.
**moment.** Punctum.
**month.** Mens.
**monthly.** Menstruus.
**morning.** Matutinum.
**night.** Nox, noctis.
**noon.** Meridies.
**old.** Antiquus.
**puberty.** Pubertas.
**second.** Secundum.
**spring.** Ver; veris.
**summer.** Aestas.
**sunrise.** Solis ortus.
**sunset.** Solis occasus.
**supper.** Cena.
**time.** Tempus.
**winter.** Hiems, hiemis.
**year.** Annus.
**young.** Parvus; infans.
**youth.** Adolescentia.

## NUMERALS (ROMAN)

**SEE:** *Roman Numerals Appendix.*

# Appendix 5–2 Greek Alphabet

| *Name of Letter* | *Capital* | *Lowercase* | *Transliteration* | *Name of Letter* | *Capital* | *Lowercase* | *Transliteration* |
|---|---|---|---|---|---|---|---|
| alpha | Α | α | a | xi | Ξ | ξ | x |
| beta | Β | ϐ or β | b | omicron | Ο | ο | o short |
| gamma | Γ | γ | g | pi | Π | π | p |
| delta | Δ | δ | d | rho | Ρ | ρ | r |
| epsilon | Ε | ϵ | e short | sigma | Σ | σ or s | s |
| zeta | Ζ | ζ | z | tau | Τ | τ | t |
| eta | Η | η | e long | upsilon | Υ | υ | y |
| theta | Θ | θ | th | phi | Φ | ϕ or φ | f |
| iota | Ι | ι | i | chi | Χ | χ | ch as in German "echt" |
| kappa | Κ | κ | k, c | | | | |
| lambda | Λ | λ | l | | | | |
| mu | Μ | μ | m | psi | Ψ | ψ | ps |
| nu | Ν | ν | n | omega | Ω | ω | o long |

# Appendix 5–3 Roman Numerals

A line placed over a letter increases its value one thousand times.

| | | | | | | |
|---|---|---|---|---|---|---|
| 1 I | 6 VI | 11 XI | 40 XL | 90 XC | 5,000 $\overline{V}$ | |
| 2 II | 7 VII | 12 XII | 50 L | 100 C | 10,000 $\overline{X}$ | |
| 3 III | 8 VIII | 15 XV | 60 LX | 500 D | 100,000 $\overline{C}$ | |
| 4 IV | 9 IX | 20 XX | 70 LXX | 1000 M | 1,000,000 $\overline{M}$ | |
| 5 V | 10 X | 30 XXX | 80 LXXX | 2000 MM | | |

# APPENDIX 6
# Medical Abbreviations

| | |
|---|---|
| a | artery |
| ā | of each |
| aa | of each; arteries |
| ABG | arterial blood gas |
| a.c. | before a meal |
| AD | advance directive |
| ad | to; up to |
| add. | add |
| ad lib. | freely; as desired |
| admov. | apply |
| ad sat. | to saturation |
| AF | atrial fibrillation |
| AI | aortic incompetence |
| ALT | alanine aminotransferase |
| alt. dieb. | every other day |
| alt. hor. | every other hour |
| alt. noc. | every other night |
| AM | morning |
| ant. | anterior |
| A-P | anterior-posterior |
| ap | before dinner |
| AQ, aq | water |
| aq. dest. | distilled water |
| aq. frig. | cold water |
| ARMD | age-related macular degeneration |
| AST | aspartate aminotransferase |
| at. wt. | atomic weight |
| AV | atrioventricular |
| av. | avoirdupois |
| bib. | drink |
| b.i.d. | twice a day |
| b.i.n. | twice a night |
| BM | bowel movement |
| bol. | pill |
| BP | blood pressure |
| B.P. | British Pharmacopeia |
| BUN | blood urea nitrogen |
| C | Calorie (kilocalorie); Celsius |
| c | calorie (small calorie) |
| c̄ | with |
| ca. | about; approximately |
| cap. | a capsule |
| CBC | complete blood count |
| CC | chief complaint |
| cc | cubic centimeter |
| cg | centigram |
| Ci | curie |
| CIS | carcinoma in situ |
| cm | centimeter |
| c.m.s. | to be taken tomorrow morning |
| c.n. | tomorrow night |
| CNS | central nervous system |
| comp. | compound; compounded of |
| CSF | cerebrospinal fluid |
| CV | cardiovascular |
| D | diopter; dose |
| d | density; right |
| /d | per day |
| D and C | dilatation and curettage |
| dB | decibel |

| | |
|---|---|
| dc | discontinue |
| det. | let it be given |
| dieb. alt. | every other day |
| dieb. tert. | every third day |
| dil. | dilute; diluted |
| dim. | halved |
| DNA | deoxyribonucleic acid |
| DNR | do not resuscitate |
| DOA | dead on arrival |
| DPT | diphtheria-pertussis-tetanus (vaccine) |
| dr. | dram |
| dur. dolor | while pain lasts |
| Dx | diagnosis |
| ECF | extracellular fluid |
| ECG | electrocardiogram |
| ECT | electroconvulsive therapy |
| ED | Emergency Department |
| EDC | estimated date of confinement |
| EEG | electroencephalogram |
| elix. | elixir |
| EMG | electromyogram |
| EMS | emergency medical service |
| ENT | ear, nose, and throat |
| EOM | extraocular muscles |
| ER | Emergency Room |
| ESR | erythrocyte sedimentation rate |
| F | Fahrenheit |
| f | female |
| FEV | forced expiratory volume |
| Fld | fluid |
| fl. dr. | fluidram |
| fl. oz. | fluidounce |
| FP | family practice |
| FSH | follicle-stimulating hormone |
| g, gm | gram |
| garg | a gargle |
| GERD | gastroesophageal reflux disease |
| GI | gastrointestinal |
| gr | grain |
| grad | by degrees |
| GRAS | generally recognized as safe |
| Gtt, gtt | drops |
| guttat. | drop by drop |
| GYN | gynecology |
| h, hr | hour |
| Hg | mercury |
| hgb | hemoglobin |
| hor. decub. | bedtime |
| hor. som., h.s. | bedtime |
| Hz | hertz (cycles per second) |
| ICSH | interstitial cell–stimulating hormone |
| IM | intramuscular |
| in d. | daily |
| INF | interferon |
| inj. | injection |
| instill. | instillation |
| IOP | intraocular pressure |

IQ intelligence quotient
I.U. international unit
IUCD intrauterine contraceptive device
IUD intrauterine device
IUFD intrauterine fetal death
IV intravenous
IVP intravenous pyelogram
J joule
kg kilogram
KUB kidney, ureter, and bladder
L liter
lab. laboratory
lb pound
$LD_{50}$ lethal dose, median
LE lupus erythematosus
LH luteinizing hormone
liq. liquid; fluid
lmp last menstrual period
LTD lowest tolerated dose
M molar; thousand; muscle
m male; meter; minim
man. prim. first thing in the morning
MED minimum effective dose
mEq milliequivalent
mg milligram
mist. a mixture
ml milliliter
MLD minimum lethal dose
mm millimeter
mMol millimole
MMR measles-mumps-rubella (vaccine)
mol. wt. molecular weight
mor. dict. as directed
mor. sol. as accustomed
MPC maximum permitted concentration
MPN most probable number
mr milliroentgen
MRI magnetic resonance imaging
MS mitral stenosis; multiple sclerosis
mV millivolt
$\mu$Eq microequivalent
$\mu$g microgram
n nerve
n.b. note well
nCi nanocurie
NMR nuclear magnetic resonance
nn nerves
noct. maneq. night and morning
non rep., n.r. do not repeat
NPN nonprotein nitrogen
n.p.o. nothing by mouth
NSAID nonsteroidal anti-inflammatory drug
NSR normal sinus rhythm
O pint
OB obstetrics
OC oral contraceptive
O.D. right eye
om. mane vel noc. every morning or night
omn. hor. every hour
omn. noct. every night
O.S. left eye
oz ounce
P, p melting point

p̄ after
part. vic. in divided doses
PBI protein-bound iodine
p.c. after meals
$PCO_2$ carbon dioxide pressure
PERRLA pupils equal, regular, react to light and accommodation
pH hydrogen ion concentration
PI present illness; previous illness
pil. pill
PM afternoon/evening
PMI point of maximal impulse
post. posterior
ppm parts per million
p.r. through the rectum
p.r.n. as needed
pt pint
p.v. through the vagina
q.h. every hour
q.2h. every 2 hours
q.3h. every 3 hours
q.i.d. four times a day
q.l. as much as wanted
q.p. as much as desired
q.s. as much as is needed
qt quart
quotid. daily
rad radiation absorbed dose
RBC red blood cell; red blood count
REM rapid eye movements
RNA ribonucleic acid
RPM revolutions per minute
RQ respiratory quotient
S mark
s̄ without
SA sinoatrial
SC, sc, s.c. subcutaneous(ly)
S.D. standard deviation
S.E. standard error
semih. half an hour
SOB shortness of breath
s.o.s. if necessary
S/P no change after
sp. gr. specific gravity
spt. spirit
s.q. subcutaneous(ly)
st. let it (them) stand
stat. immediately
STD sexually transmitted disease
syr. syrup
T temperature
tab. medicated tablet
temp. temperature
t.i.d. three times a day
t.i.n. three times a night
tinct., tr. tincture
TLC, tlc tender loving care; thin-layer chromatography; total lung capacity
top. topically
trit. triturate or grind
TSD time since death
TSH thyroid-stimulating hormone
UHF ultrahigh frequency
ult. praes. the last ordered
ung. ointment

| | |
|---|---|
| URI | upper respiratory infection |
| USAN | United States Adopted Name |
| USP | United States Pharmacopeia |
| UTI | urinary tract infection |
| UV | ultraviolet |
| v | vein |
| vol. | volume |
| vol. % | volume percent |
| vv | veins |
| WBC | white blood cell; white blood count |
| WDWN | well developed, well nourished |
| WF/BF | white female/black female |
| WM/BM | white male/black male |
| wt. | weight |
| w/v. | weight in volume |
| x | multiplied by |
| yr | year |
| Z | atomic number |

# APPENDIX 7
# Symbols

| | |
|---|---|
| ♏ | Minim. |
| ℈ | Scruple. |
| ʒ | Dram. |
| fʒ | Fluidram. |
| ℥ | Ounce. |
| f℥ | Fluidounce. |
| O | Pint. |
| ℔ | Pound. |
| ℞ | Recipe (L. take). |
| M | Misce (L. mix). |
| $\overline{aa}$ | Of each. |
| A, Å, AU | angström unit. |
| C-1, C-2, etc. | Complement. |
| c, $\bar{c}$ | cum (L. with). |
| Δ | Change; heat. |
| $E_0$ | Electroaffinity. |
| $F_1$ | First filial generation. |
| $F_2$ | Second filial generation. |
| mμ | Millimicron, nanometer. |
| μg | Microgram. |
| mEq | Milliequivalent. |
| mg | Milligram. |
| mg% | Milligrams percent; milligrams per 100 ml. |
| $QO_2$ | Oxygen consumption. |
| *m*- | Meta-. |
| *o*- | Ortho-. |
| *p*- | Para-. |
| $\bar{p}$ | After. |
| $PO_2$ | Partial pressure of oxygen. |
| $PCO_2$ | Partial pressure of carbon dioxide. |
| $\bar{s}$ | Without. |
| $\overline{ss}$, ss | [L. semis]. One half. |
| μm | Micrometer. |
| μ | Micron (former term for micrometer). |
| μμ | Micromicron. |
| + | Plus; excess; acid reaction; positive. |
| − | Minus; deficiency; alkaline reaction; negative. |
| ± | Plus or minus; either positive or negative; indefinite. |
| # | Number; following a number, pounds. |
| ÷ | Divided by. |
| × | Multiplied by; magnification. |
| / | Divided by. |
| = | Equals. |
| ≈ | Approximately equal. |
| > | Greater than; from which is derived. |
| < | Less than; derived from. |
| ≮ | Not less than. |
| ≯ | Not greater than. |
| ≦ | Equal to or less than. |
| ≧ | Equal to or greater than. |
| ≠ | Not equal to. |
| $\sqrt{\ }$ | Root; square root; radical. |
| $\sqrt[2]{\ }$ | Square root. |
| $\sqrt[3]{\ }$ | Cube root. |
| ∞ | Infinity. |
| : | Ratio; "is to." |
| :: | Equality between ratios, "as." |
| ∴ | Therefore. |
| ° | Degree. |
| % | Percent. |
| π | 3.1416—ratio of circumference of a circle to its diameter. |
| □, ♂ | Male. |
| ○, ♀ | Female. |
| ⇌ | Denotes a reversible reaction. |
| n | Subscripted n indicates the number of the molecules can vary from two to greater. |
| ↑ | Increase. |
| ↓ | Decrease. |

# APPENDIX 8
# Units of Measurement (Including SI Units)

## Appendix 8–1 Scientific Notation

Sometimes it is necessary to use very large and very small numbers. These can best be indicated and handled in calculations by use of scientific notation, which is to say by use of exponents. Use of scientific notation requires writing the number so that it is the result of multiplying some whole number power of 10 by a number between 1 and 10. Examples are:

$$1234 = 1.234 \times 10^{3}$$

$$0.01234 = 1.234 \times \frac{1}{100} = 1.234 \times 10^{-2}$$

$$0.001234 = 1.234 \times \frac{1}{1000} = 1.234 \times 10^{-3}$$

To convert a number to its equivalent in scientific notation:

Place the decimal point to the right of the first non-zero digit. This will now be a number between 1 and 9.

Multiply this number by a power of 10, the exponent of which is equal to the number of places the decimal point was moved. The exponent is positive if the decimal point was moved to the left, and negative if it was moved to the right. For example:

$$\frac{1{,}234{,}000.0 \times 0.000072}{6000.0} = \frac{1.234 \times 10^{6} \times 7.2 \times 10^{-5}}{6.0 \times 10^{3}}$$

Now, by simply adding or subtracting the exponents of ten, and remembering that moving an exponent from the denominator of the fraction to the numerator changes its sign,

$$= \frac{1.234 \times 10^{6} \times 10^{-5} \times 10^{-3} \times 7.2}{6} = \frac{1.234 \times 10^{-2} \times 7.2}{6}$$

Now, dividing by 6,

$$= 1.234 \times 10^{-2} \times 1.2 = 1.4808 \times 10^{-2} = \frac{1.4808}{100} = 0.014808$$

The last operation changed $1.4808 \times 10^{-2}$ into the final value, 0.014808, which is not expressed in scientific notation.

## Appendix 8–2 SI Units (Système International d'Unités or International System of Units)

This system includes two types of units important in clinical medicine. The *base units* are shown in the first table, derived units in the second table, and derived units with special names in the third table.

### SI BASE UNITS

| *Quantity* | *Name* | *Symbol* |
|---|---|---|
| Length | meter | m |
| Mass | kilogram | kg |
| Time | second | s |
| Electric current | ampere | A |
| Temperature | kelvin | K |
| Luminous intensity | candela | cd |
| Amount of a substance | mole | mol |

## SOME SI DERIVED UNITS

| Quantity | Name of Derived Unit | Symbol |
|---|---|---|
| Area | square meter | $m^2$ |
| Volume | cubic meter | $m^3$ |
| Speed, velocity | meter per second | m/s |
| Acceleration | meter per second squared | $m/s^2$ |
| Mass density | kilogram per cubic meter | $kg/m^3$ |
| Concentration of a substance | mole per cubic meter | $mol/m^3$ |
| Specific volume | cubic meter per kilogram | $m^3/kg$ |
| Luminescence | candela per square meter | $cd/m^2$ |

## SI DERIVED UNITS WITH SPECIAL NAMES

| Quantity | Name | Symbol | Expressed in Terms of Other Units |
|---|---|---|---|
| Frequency | hertz | Hz | $s^{-1}$ |
| Force | newton | N | $kg \cdot m \cdot s^{-2}$ or $kg \cdot m/s^2$ |
| Pressure | pascal | Pa | $N \cdot m^{-2}$ or $N/m^2$ |
| Energy, work, amount of heat | joule | J | $kg \cdot m^2 \cdot s^{-2}$ or $N \cdot m$ |
| Power | watt | W | $J \cdot s$ or J/s |
| Quantity of electricity | coulomb | C | $A \cdot s$ |
| Electromotive force | volt | V | W/A |
| Capacitance | farad | F | C/V |
| Electrical resistance | ohm | Ω | V/a |
| Conductance | siemens | S | A/V |
| Inductance | henry | H | W$\phi$/A |
| Illuminance | lux | lx | $ln/m^2$ |
| Absorbed (radiation) dose | gray | Gy | J/kg |
| Dose equivalent (radiation) | sievert | Sv | J/kg |
| Activity (radiation) | becquerel | Bq | $s^{-1}$ |

## PREFIXES AND MULTIPLES USED IN SI

| Prefix | Symbol | Power | Multiple or Portion of a Multiple |
|---|---|---|---|
| tera | T | $10^{12}$ | 1,000,000,000,000 |
| giga | G | $10^9$ | 1,000,000,000 |
| mega | M | $10^6$ | 1,000,000 |
| kilo | k | $10^3$ | 1,000 |
| hecto | h | $10^2$ | 100 |
| deca | da | $10^1$ | 10 |
| unity | | | 1 |
| deci | d | $10^{-1}$ | 0.1 |
| centi | c | $10^{-2}$ | 0.01 |
| milli | m | $10^{-3}$ | 0.001 |
| micro | $\mu$ | $10^{-6}$ | 0.000001 |
| nano | n | $10^{-9}$ | 0.000000001 |
| pico | p | $10^{-12}$ | 0.000000000001 |
| femto | f | $10^{-15}$ | 0.000000000000001 |
| atto | a | $10^{-18}$ | 0.000000000000000001 |

# Appendix 8–3 Metric System

## MASSES

| Table | | Grams | | Grains |
|---|---|---|---|---|
| 1 Kilogram | = | 1000.0 | = | 15,432.35 |
| 1 Hectogram | = | 100.0 | = | 1,543.23 |
| 1 Decagram | = | 10.0 | = | 154.323 |
| 1 Gram | = | 1.0 | = | 15.432 |

### MASSES (Continued)

| Table | | Grams | | Grains |
|---|---|---|---|---|
| 1 Decigram | = | 0.1 | = | 1.5432 |
| 1 Centigram | = | 0.01 | = | 0.15432 |
| 1 Milligram | = | 0.001 | = | 0.01543 |
| 1 Microgram | = | $10^{-6}$ | = | $15.432 \times 10^{-6}$ |
| 1 Nanogram | = | $10^{-9}$ | = | $15.432 \times 10^{-9}$ |
| 1 Picogram | = | $10^{-12}$ | = | $15.432 \times 10^{-12}$ |
| 1 Femtogram | = | $10^{-15}$ | = | $15.432 \times 10^{-15}$ |
| 1 Attogram | = | $10^{-18}$ | = | $15.432 \times 10^{-18}$ |

Arabic numbers are used with masses and measures, as 10 g, or 3 ml, etc. Portions of masses and measures are usually expressed decimally. $10^{-1}$ indicates 0.1; $10^{-6} = 0.000001$; etc. SEE: *Scientific Notation Appendix.*

# Appendix 8–4 Weights and Measures

Arabic numerals are used with masses and measures, as 10 g, or 3 ml, etc. Portions of masses and measures are usually expressed decimally. For practical purposes, 1 cm³ (cubic centimeter) is equivalent to 1 ml (milliliter) and 1 drop (gtt.) of water is equivalent to a minim (m).

### LENGTH

| *Millimeters (mm)* | *Centimeters (cm)* | *Inches (in.)* | *Feet (ft)* | *Yards (yd)* | *Meters (m)* |
|---|---|---|---|---|---|
| 1.0 | 0.1 | 0.03937 | 0.00328 | 0.0011 | 0.001 |
| 10.0 | 1.0 | 0.3937 | 0.03281 | 0.0109 | 0.01 |
| 25.4 | 2.54 | 1.0 | 0.0833 | 0.0278 | 0.0254 |
| 304.8 | 30.48 | 12.0 | 1.0 | 0.333 | 0.3048 |
| 914.40 | 91.44 | 36.0 | 3.0 | 1.0 | 0.9144 |
| 1000.0 | 100.0 | 39.37 | 3.2808 | 1.0936 | 1.0 |

1 $\mu$m = 1 micrometer = 0.001 millimeter. 1 mm = 100 $\mu$m.
1 km = 1 kilometer = 1000 meters = 0.62137 statute mile.
1 statute mile = 5280 feet = 1.609 kilometers.
1 nautical mile= 6076.042 feet= 1852.276 meters.

### VOLUME (FLUID)

| *Milliliters (ml)* | *U.S. Fluidrams (f℥)* | *Cubic Inches (in.³)* | *U.S. Fluidounces (f℥)* | *U.S. Fluid Quarts (qt)* | *Liters (L)* |
|---|---|---|---|---|---|
| 1.0 | 0.2705 | 0.061 | 0.03381 | 0.00106 | 0.001 |
| 3.697 | 1.0 | 0.226 | 0.125 | 0.00391 | 0.00369 |
| 16.3866 | 4.4329 | 1.0 | 0.5541 | 0.0173 | 0.01639 |
| 29.573 | 8.0 | 1.8047 | 1.0 | 0.03125 | 0.02957 |
| 946.332 | 256.0 | 57.75 | 32.0 | 1.0 | 0.9463 |
| 1000.0 | 270.52 | 61.025 | 33.815 | 1.0567 | 1.0 |

1 gallon = 4 quarts = 8 pints = 3.785 liters.
1 pint = 473.16 ml.

### WEIGHT

| *Grains (gr)* | *Grams (g)* | *Apothecaries' Ounces (℥)* | *Avoirdupois Pounds (lb)* | *Kilograms (kg)* |
|---|---|---|---|---|
| 1.0 | 0.0648 | 0.00208 | 0.0001429 | 0.000065 |
| 15.432 | 1.0 | 0.03215 | 0.002205 | 0.001 |
| 480.0 | 31.1 | 1.0 | 0.06855 | 0.0311 |
| 7000.0 | 453.5924 | 14.583 | 1.0 | 0.45354 |
| 15432.358 | 1000.0 | 32.15 | 2.2046 | 1.0 |

1 microgram ($\mu$g) = 0.001 milligram.
1 mg = 1 milligram = 0.001 g; 1000 mg = 1 g.

## APOTHECARIES' WEIGHT

20 grains = 1 scruple
8 drams = 1 ounce
3 scruples = 1 dram
12 ounces = 1 pound

## AVOIRDUPOIS WEIGHT

27.343 grains = 1 dram
16 ounces = 1 pound
2000 pounds = 1 short ton
1 oz troy = 480 grains
1 lb troy = 5760 grains
16 drams = 1 ounce
100 pounds = 1 hundredweight
2240 pounds = 1 long ton
1 oz avoirdupois = 437.5 grains
1 lb avoirdupois = 7000 grains

## CIRCULAR MEASURE

60 seconds = 1 minute
90 degrees = 1 quadrant
60 minutes = 1 degree
4 quadrants = 360 degrees = circle

## CUBIC MEASURE

1728 cubic inches = 1 cubic foot
2150.42 cubic inches = 1 standard bushel
1 cubic foot = about four fifths of a bushel
27 cubic feet = 1 cubic yard
268.8 cubic inches = 1 dry (U.S.) gallon
128 cubic feet = 1 cord (wood)

## DRY MEASURE

2 pints = 1 quart
8 quarts = 1 peck
4 pecks = 1 bushel

## LIQUID MEASURE

16 ounces = 1 pint
1000 milliliters = 1 liter
4 gills = 1 pint
4 quarts = 1 gallon
31.5 gallons = 1 barrel (U.S.)
2 pints = 1 quart
2 barrels = 1 hogshead (U.S.)
1 quart = 946.35 milliliters
1 liter = 1.0566 quart

Barrels and hogsheads vary in size. A U.S. gallon is equal to 0.8327 British gallon; therefore, a British gallon is equal to 1.201 U.S. gallons. 1 liter is equal to 1.0567 quarts.

## LINEAR MEASURE

1 inch = 2.54 centimeters
12 inches = 1 foot
1 statute mile = 5280 feet
40 rods = 1 furlong
3 feet = 1 yard
3 statute miles = 1 statute league
8 furlongs = 1 statute mile
5.5 yards = 1 rod
1 nautical mile = 6076.042 feet

## TROY WEIGHT

24 grains = 1 pennyweight
20 pennyweights = 1 ounce
12 ounces = 1 pound

Used for weighing gold, silver, and jewels.

## HOUSEHOLD MEASURES* AND WEIGHTS

Approximate Equivalents: 60 gtt. = 1 teaspoonful = 5 ml = 60 minims
= 60 grains = 1 dram = ⅛ ounce

1 teaspoon = ⅛ fl. oz; 1 dram
3 teaspoons = 1 tablespoon
1 tablespoon = ½ fl. oz; 4 drams
16 teaspoons (liquid) = 1 cup
12 tablespoons (dry) = 1 cup
1 cup = 8 fl. oz
1 tumbler or glass = 8 fl. oz; ½ pint

* Household measures are not precise. For instance, a household tsp will hold from 3 to 5 ml of liquid. Therefore, household equivalents should not be substituted for medication prescribed by the physician.

Note: Traditionally, the word "weights" is used in these tables, but "masses" is the correct term.

# Appendix 8–5 Conversion Rules and Factors

To convert units of one system into the other, multiply the number of units in column I by the equivalent factor opposite that unit in column II.

## WEIGHT

| | | |
|---|---|---|
| 1 attogram | = | $15.432 \times 10^{-18}$ grains |
| 1 femtogram | = | $15.432 \times 10^{-15}$ grains |
| 1 picogram | = | $15.432 \times 10^{-12}$ grains |
| 1 nanogram | = | $15.432 \times 10^{-9}$ grains |
| 1 microgram | = | $15.432 \times 10^{-6}$ grains |
| 1 milligram | = | 0.015432 grain |
| 1 centigram | = | 0.15432 grain |
| 1 decigram | = | 1.5432 grains |
| 1 decagram | = | 154.323 grains |
| 1 hectogram | = | 1543.23 grains |
| 1 gram | = | 15.432 grains |
| 1 gram | = | 0.25720 apothecaries' dram |
| 1 gram | = | 0.03527 avoirdupois ounce |
| 1 gram | = | 0.03215 apothecaries' or troy ounce |
| 1 kilogram | = | 35.274 avoirdupois ounces |
| 1 kilogram | = | 32.151 apothecaries' or troy ounces |
| 1 kilogram | = | 2.2046 avoirdupois pounds |
| 1 grain | = | 64.7989 milligrams |
| 1 grain | = | 0.0648 gram |
| 1 apothecaries' dram | = | 3.8879 gram |
| 1 avoirdupois ounce | = | 28.3495 grams |
| 1 apothecaries' or troy ounce | = | 31.1035 grams |
| 1 avoirdupois pound | = | 453.5924 grams |

## VOLUME (AIR OR GAS)

| | | |
|---|---|---|
| 1 cubic centimeter ($cm^3$) | = | 0.06102 cubic inch |
| 1 cubic meter ($m^3$) | = | 35.314 cubic feet |
| 1 cubic meter | = | 1.3079 cubic yard |
| 1 cubic inch ($in^3$) | = | 16.3872 cubic centimeters |
| 1 cubic foot ($ft^3$) | = | 0.02832 cubic meter |

## CAPACITY (FLUID OR LIQUID)

| | | |
|---|---|---|
| 1 milliliter | = | 16.23 minims |
| 1 milliliter | = | 0.2705 fluidram |
| 1 milliliter | = | 0.0338 fluidounce |
| 1 liter | = | 33.8148 fluidounces |
| 1 liter | = | 2.1134 pints |
| 1 liter | = | 1.0567 quart |
| 1 liter | = | 0.2642 gallon |
| 1 fluidram | = | 3.697 milliliters |
| 1 fluidounce | = | 29.573 milliliters |
| 1 pint | = | 473.1765 milliliters |
| 1 quart | = | 946.353 milliliters |
| 1 gallon | = | 3.785 liters |

## TIME

1 millisecond = one thousandth (0.001) of a second
1 second = 1⁄60 of a minute
1 minute = 1⁄60 of an hour
1 hour = 1⁄24 of a day

## TEMPERATURE*

Given a temperature on the Fahrenheit scale; to convert it to degrees Celsius, subtract 32 and multiply by 5/9. Given a temperature on the Celsius scale; to convert it to degrees Fahrenheit, multiply by 9/5 and add 32. Degrees celsius are equivalent to degrees Centigrade.

* SEE: *thermometer, Celsius* for table.

## PRESSURE

| TO OBTAIN | MULTIPLY | BY |
|---|---|---|
| lb/sq in. | atmospheres | 14.696 |
| lb/sq in. | in. of water | 0.03609 |
| lb/sq in. | ft of water | 0.4335 |
| lb/sq in. | in. of mercury | 0.4912 |
| lb/sq in. | kg/sq meter | 0.00142 |
| lb/sq in. | kg/sq cm | 14.22 |
| lb/sq in. | cm of mercury | 0.1934 |
| lb/sq ft | atmospheres | 2116.8 |
| lb/sq ft | in. of water | 5.204 |
| lb/sq ft | ft of water | 62.48 |
| lb/sq ft | in. of mercury | 70.727 |
| lb/sq ft | cm of mercury | 27.845 |
| lb/sq ft | kg/sq meter | 0.20482 |
| lb/cu in. | gm/ml | 0.03613 |
| lb/cu ft | lb/cu in. | 1728.0 |
| lb/cu ft | gm/ml | 62.428 |
| lb/U.S. gal | gm/L | 8.345 |
| in. of water | in. of mercury | 13.60 |
| in. of water | cm of mercury | 5.3543 |
| ft of water | atmospheres | 33.95 |
| ft of water | lb/sq in. | 2.307 |
| ft of water | kg/sq meter | 0.00328 |
| ft of water | in. of mercury | 1.133 |
| ft of water | cm of mercury | 0.4461 |
| atmospheres | ft of water | 0.02947 |
| atmospheres | in. of mercury | 0.03342 |
| atmospheres | kg/sq cm | 0.9678 |
| bars | atmospheres | 1.0133 |
| in. of mercury | atmospheres | 29.921 |
| in. of mercury | lb/sq in. | 2.036 |
| mm of mercury | atmospheres | 760.0 |
| g/ml | lb/cu in. | 27.68 |
| g/sq cm | kg/sq meter | 0.1 |
| kg/sq meter | lb/sq in. | 703.1 |
| kg/sq meter | in. of water | 25.40 |
| kg/sq meter | in. of mercury | 345.32 |
| kg/sq meter | cm of mercury | 135.95 |
| kg/sq meter | atmospheres | 10332.0 |
| kg/sq cm | atmospheres | 1.0332 |

## FLOW RATE

| TO OBTAIN | MULTIPLY | BY |
|---|---|---|
| cu ft/hr | cc/min | 0.00212 |
| cu ft/hr | L/min | 2.12 |
| L/min | cu ft/hr | 0.472 |

## PARTS PER MILLION

Conversion of parts per million (ppm) to percent:
1 ppm = 0.0001%, 10 ppm = 0.001%, 100 ppm = 0.01% 1000 ppm = 0.1%, 10,000 ppm = 1%, etc.

## ENERGY

1 foot pound = 1.35582 joule
1 joule = 0.2389 Calorie (kilocalorie)
1 Calorie (kilocalorie) = 1000 calories = 4184 joules
A large Calorie, or kilocalorie, is always written with a capital C.

## pH

The pH scale is simply a series of numbers stating where a given solution would stand in a series of solutions arranged according to acidity or alkalinity. At one extreme (high pH) lies a highly alkaline solution, which may be made by dissolving 4 g of sodium hydroxide in water to make a liter of solution; at the other extreme (low pH) is an acid solution containing 3.65 g of hydrogen chloride per liter of water. Halfway between lies purified water, which is neutral. All other solutions can be arranged on this scale, and their acidity or alkalinity can be stated by giving the numbers that indicate their relative positions. If the pH of a certain solution is 5.3, it falls between gastric juice and urine on the above scale, is moderately acid, and will turn litmus red.

| | | |
|---|---|---|
| Tenth-normal HCl | − 1.00 | Litmus is red in this acid range. |
| Gastric juice | *1.4 | |
| Urine | *6.0 | |
| Water | 7.00—Neutral | |
| Blood | 7.35–7.45 | Litmus is blue in this alkaline range. |
| Bile | *7.5 | |
| Pancreatic juice | 8.5 | |
| Tenth-normal NaOH | 13.00 | |

* These body fluids vary rather widely in pH; typical figures have been used for simplicity. Urine samples obtained from healthy individuals may have pH anywhere between 4.7 and 8.0.

# APPENDIX 9
# Nutrition

## Appendix 9–1 Recommended Daily Dietary Allowances[a] (Revised 1989)

| Category | Age (yr) or Condition | Weight[b] (kg) | Weight[b] (lb) | Height[b] (cm) | Height[b] (in.) | Protein (g) | Vitamin A (μg RE)[c] | Vitamin D (μg)[d] | Vitamin E (mg α-TE)[e] | Vitamin K (μg) | Vitamin C (mg) | Thiamin (mg) | Riboflavin (mg) | Niacin (mg NE)[f] | Vitamin $B_6$ (mg) | Folate (μg) | Vitamin $B_{12}$ (μg) | Calcium (mg) | Phosphorus (mg) | Magnesium (mg) | Iron (mg) | Zinc (mg) | Iodine (μg) | Selenium (μg) |
|---|---|---|---|---|---|---|---|---|---|---|---|---|---|---|---|---|---|---|---|---|---|---|---|---|
| | | | | | | | Fat-Soluble Vitamins | | | | Water-Soluble Vitamins | | | | | | | Minerals | | | | | | |
| Infants | 0.0–0.5 | 6 | 13 | 60 | 24 | 13 | 375 | 7.5 | 3 | 5 | 30 | 0.3 | 0.4 | 5 | 0.3 | 25 | 0.3 | 400 | 300 | 40 | 6 | 5 | 40 | 10 |
| | 0.5–1.0 | 9 | 20 | 71 | 28 | 14 | 375 | 10 | 4 | 10 | 35 | 0.4 | 0.5 | 6 | 0.6 | 35 | 0.5 | 600 | 500 | 60 | 10 | 5 | 50 | 15 |
| Children | 1–3 | 13 | 29 | 90 | 35 | 16 | 400 | 10 | 6 | 15 | 40 | 0.7 | 0.8 | 9 | 1.0 | 50 | 0.7 | 800 | 800 | 80 | 10 | 10 | 70 | 20 |
| | 4–6 | 20 | 44 | 112 | 44 | 24 | 500 | 10 | 7 | 20 | 45 | 0.9 | 1.1 | 12 | 1.1 | 75 | 1.0 | 800 | 800 | 120 | 10 | 10 | 90 | 20 |
| | 7–10 | 28 | 62 | 132 | 52 | 28 | 700 | 10 | 7 | 30 | 45 | 1.0 | 1.2 | 13 | 1.4 | 100 | 1.4 | 800 | 800 | 170 | 10 | 10 | 120 | 30 |
| Males | 11–14 | 45 | 99 | 157 | 62 | 45 | 1000 | 10 | 10 | 45 | 50 | 1.3 | 1.5 | 17 | 1.7 | 150 | 2.0 | 1200 | 1200 | 270 | 12 | 15 | 150 | 40 |
| | 15–18 | 66 | 145 | 176 | 69 | 59 | 1000 | 10 | 10 | 65 | 60 | 1.5 | 1.3 | 20 | 2.0 | 200 | 2.0 | 1200 | 1200 | 400 | 12 | 15 | 150 | 50 |
| | 19–24 | 72 | 160 | 177 | 70 | 58 | 1000 | 10 | 10 | 70 | 60 | 1.5 | 1.7 | 19 | 2.0 | 200 | 2.0 | 1200 | 1200 | 350 | 10 | 15 | 150 | 70 |
| | 25–50 | 79 | 174 | 176 | 70 | 63 | 1000 | 5 | 10 | 80 | 60 | 1.5 | 1.7 | 19 | 2.0 | 200 | 2.0 | 800 | 800 | 350 | 10 | 15 | 150 | 70 |
| | 51 + | 77 | 170 | 173 | 68 | 63 | 1000 | 5 | 10 | 80 | 60 | 1.2 | 1.4 | 15 | 2.0 | 200 | 2.0 | 800 | 800 | 350 | 10 | 15 | 150 | 70 |
| Females | 11–14 | 46 | 101 | 157 | 62 | 46 | 800 | 10 | 8 | 45 | 50 | 1.1 | 1.3 | 15 | 1.4 | 150 | 2.0 | 1200 | 1200 | 280 | 15 | 12 | 150 | 45 |
| | 15–18 | 55 | 120 | 163 | 64 | 44 | 800 | 10 | 8 | 55 | 60 | 1.1 | 1.3 | 15 | 1.5 | 180 | 2.0 | 1200 | 1200 | 300 | 15 | 12 | 150 | 50 |
| | 19–24 | 58 | 128 | 164 | 65 | 46 | 800 | 10 | 8 | 60 | 60 | 1.1 | 1.3 | 15 | 1.6 | 180 | 2.0 | 1200 | 1200 | 280 | 15 | 12 | 150 | 55 |
| | 25–50 | 63 | 138 | 163 | 64 | 50 | 800 | 5 | 8 | 65 | 60 | 1.1 | 1.3 | 15 | 1.6 | 180 | 2.0 | 800 | 800 | 280 | 15 | 12 | 150 | 55 |
| | 51 + | 65 | 143 | 160 | 63 | 50 | 800 | 5 | 8 | 65 | 60 | 1.0 | 1.2 | 13 | 1.6 | 180 | 2.0 | 800 | 800 | 280 | 10 | 12 | 150 | 55 |
| Pregnant | | | | | | 60 | 800 | 10 | 10 | 65 | 70 | 1.5 | 1.6 | 17 | 2.2 | 400 | 2.2 | 1200 | 1200 | 300 | 30 | 15 | 175 | 65 |
| Lactating | 1st 6 months | | | | | 65 | 1300 | 10 | 12 | 65 | 95 | 1.6 | 1.8 | 20 | 2.1 | 280 | 2.6 | 1200 | 1200 | 355 | 15 | 19 | 200 | 75 |
| | 2nd 6 months | | | | | 62 | 1200 | 10 | 11 | 65 | 90 | 1.6 | 1.7 | 20 | 2.1 | 260 | 2.6 | 1200 | 1200 | 340 | 15 | 16 | 200 | 75 |

[a] The allowances, expressed as average daily intakes over time, are intended to provide for individual variations among most normal persons as they live in the United States under usual environmental stresses. Diets should be based on a variety of common foods in order to provide other nutrients for which human requirements have been less well defined.

[b] Weights and heights of reference adults are actual medians for the U.S. population of the designated age, as reported by NHANES II [second National Health and Nutrition Examination Survey]. The median weights and heights of those under 19 years of age were taken from Hamill et al. [Physical Growth: National Center for Health Statistics percentiles. Am J Clin Nutr 32:607, 1979]. The use of these figures does not imply that the height-to-weight ratios are ideal.

[c] Retinol equivalents. 1 RE = 1 μg retinol or 6 μg beta-carotene.

[d] As cholecalciferol. 10 μg cholecalciferol = 400 IU (International Units) of vitamin D.

[e] Alpha-tocopherol equivalents. 1 mg d-alpha tocopherol = 1 alpha-TE.

[f] 1 NE (niacin equivalent) = 1 mg of niacin or 60 mg of dietary tryptophan.

SOURCE: National Research Council (Food and Nutrition Board): Recommended Dietary Allowances, ed 10. National Academy Press, Washington, DC, 1989.

# Appendix 9–2 Estimated Safe and Adequate Daily Dietary Intakes of Selected Vitamins and Minerals[a]

| | | Vitamins | | Trace Elements[b] | | | | |
|---|---|---|---|---|---|---|---|---|
| *Category* | *Age (yr)* | *Biotin (μg)* | *Pantothenic Acid (mg)* | *Copper (mg)* | *Manganese (mg)* | *Fluoride (mg)* | *Chromium (μg)* | *Molybdenum (μg)* |
| Infants | 0.0–0.5 | 10 | 2 | 0.4–0.6 | 0.3–0.6 | 0.1–0.5 | 10–40 | 15–30 |
| | 0.5–1.0 | 15 | 3 | 0.6–0.7 | 0.6–1.0 | 0.2–1.0 | 20–60 | 20–40 |
| Children and Adolescents | 1–3 | 20 | 3 | 0.7–1.0 | 1.0–1.5 | 0.5–1.5 | 20–80 | 25–50 |
| | 4–6 | 25 | 3–4 | 1.0–1.5 | 1.5–2.0 | 1.0–2.5 | 30–120 | 30–75 |
| | 7–10 | 30 | 4–5 | 1.0–2.0 | 2.0–3.0 | 1.5–2.5 | 50–200 | 50–150 |
| | 11+ | 30–100 | 4–7 | 1.5–2.5 | 2.0–5.0 | 1.5–2.5 | 50–200 | 75–250 |
| Adults | | 30–100 | 4–7 | 1.5–3.0 | 2.0–5.0 | 1.5–4.0 | 50–200 | 75–250 |

[a] Because there is less information on which to base allowances, these figures are not given in the main table of RDA and are provided here in the form of ranges of recommended intakes.

[b] Because the toxic levels for many trace elements may be only several times usual intakes, the upper levels for the trace elements given in this table should not be habitually exceeded.

SOURCE: National Research Council (Food and Nutrition Board): Recommended Dietary Allowances, ed 10. National Academy Press, Washington, DC, 1989, p 284.

# Appendix 9–3 **Vitamins***

| *Vitamin* | *Chief Functions* | *Results of Deficiency* | *Characteristics* | *Good Sources* |
|---|---|---|---|---|
| VITAMIN A<br>Retinol (animal source)<br>Carotene<br>Beta-carotene | Essential for maintaining the integrity of epithelial membranes<br>Helps maintain resistance to infections<br>Necessary for the formation of rhodopsin and prevention of night blindness<br>Necessary for proper bone growth<br>Facilitates RNA formation from DNA<br>Thought to be cancer preventive because of antioxidative properties associated with control of free radical damage to DNA and cell membranes | *Mild:*<br>Retarded growth<br>Increased susceptibility to infection<br>Abnormal function of gastrointestinal, genitourinary and respiratory tracts due to altered epithelial membranes<br>Skin dries, shrivels, thickens; sometimes pustule formation<br>Night blindness<br>*Severe:*<br>Xerophthalmia, a characteristic eye disease, and other local infections | Fat soluble<br>Not destroyed by ordinary cooking temperatures<br>Is destroyed by high temperatures when oxygen is present<br>Marked capacity for storage in the liver<br>NOTE: Excessive intake of carotene, from which vitamin A is formed, may produce yellow discoloration of the skin (carotenemia). Excessive vitamin A intake causes symptoms similar to those of deficiency conditions | Liver<br>Animal fats<br>Butter<br>Cheese<br>Cream<br>Egg yolk<br>Whole milk<br>Fish liver oil<br>Liver<br>Vegetables<br>Green leafy, esp. escarole, kale, parsley<br>Yellow, esp. carrots<br>*Artificial:*<br>Concentrates in several forms<br>Irradiated fish oils |
| VITAMIN D<br>Calciferol<br>Ergocalciferol<br>Cholecalciferol<br>Calcitriol<br>Antirachitic factor | Hormone-like regulation of calcium and phosphorus metabolism by promotion of<br>Gastrointestinal absorption<br>Bone and tooth mineralization<br>Renal reabsorption<br>Skeletal reserves<br>Antirachitic | *Mild:*<br>Interferes with utilization of calcium and phosphorus in bone and tooth formation<br>Irritability<br>Weakness<br>*Severe:*<br>Rickets in young children<br>Osteomalacia in adults | Soluble in fats and organic solvents<br>Relatively stable under refrigeration<br>Stored in liver<br>Often associated with vitamin A | Formed in the skin by exposure to sunlight<br>Fortified milk and dairy products<br>Egg yolk<br>Fish liver oils<br>Fish having fat distributed through the flesh, salmon, tuna, herring, sardines<br>Liver<br>Oysters<br>Artificially prepared forms |

* See App. 9–1 for recommended daily allowances.

| | | | | |
|---|---|---|---|---|
| VITAMIN E<br>Alpha-tocopherol<br>Beta-tocopherol<br>Gamma-tocopherol | Important antioxidant that<br>Prevents red blood cell hemolysis<br>Protects vitamin A and unsaturated fatty acids from oxidation<br>Promotes cell membrane integrity<br>Improves immune response<br>May protect against cancer | Red blood cell resistance to rupture is decreased, but deficiency seldom occurs except in premature infants and people with chronic fat malabsorption. | Soluble in fat<br>Stable to heat in absence of oxygen and ultraviolet light<br>Unstable under freezing and processing | Vegetable oils<br>Margarine<br>Whole grain or fortified cereals<br>Wheat germ<br>Green leafy vegetables |
| VITAMIN K<br>Menadione<br>Phylloquinone<br>Menaquinone | Promotes synthesis of clotting factors | Prolonged clotting time, resulting in bleeding<br>NOTE: Seldom occurs in the absence of anticoagulant drugs. In addition to food sources, intestinal bacteria manufacture approx. half the body's requirement.<br>Fat malabsorption can cause deficiency<br>Synthetic form (menadione) does not depend on fat absorption | Soluble in fat<br>Stable to heat | Green leafy vegetables<br>Meats<br>Dairy products<br>Intestinal bacteria |
| VITAMIN C<br>Ascorbic acid | Essential to formation of intracellular cement substances in a variety of tissues including skin, dentin, cartilage, and bone matrix<br>Important in healing of wounds and bone fractures<br>Prevents scurvy<br>Facilitates absorption of iron | *Mild:*<br>Lowered resistance to infections<br>Joint tenderness<br>Susceptibility to dental caries, pyorrhea, and bleeding gums<br>Delayed wound healing<br>Bruising<br>*Severe:*<br>Hemorrhage<br>Anemia | Soluble in water<br>Easily destroyed by oxidation; heat hastens the process<br>Lost in cooking, particularly if water in which food was cooked is discarded. Also loss is greater if cooked in iron or copper utensils.<br>Quick-frozen foods lose little of their vitamin C. | Abundant in most fresh fruits and vegetables, esp. citrus fruit and juices, tomato and orange<br>*Artificial:*<br>Ascorbic acid<br>Cevitamic acid |

**Vitamins** (Continued)

| *Vitamin* | *Chief Functions* | *Results of Deficiency* | *Characteristics* | *Good Sources* |
|---|---|---|---|---|
| | Protects folate<br>Antioxidant<br>Promotes capillary permeability | Scurvy<br>NOTE: Many drugs affect availability. | Stored in the body to a limited extent | |
| THIAMINE<br>Vitamin $B_1$ | Important role in carbohydrate metabolism<br>Essential for maintenance of normal appetite<br>Essential for normal functioning of nervous tissue<br>Coenzyme for cellular energy production | *Mild:*<br>Loss of appetite<br>Impaired metabolism of starches and sugars<br>Emaciation<br>Irritability<br>*Severe:*<br>Various nervous disorders<br>Loss of coordinating power of muscles<br>Beriberi<br>Paralysis in humans | Soluble in water<br>Not readily destroyed by ordinary cooking temperature<br>Destroyed by exposure to heat, alkali, or sulfites<br>Is not stored in body<br>NOTE: Deficiency is often associated with alcoholism. | Widely distributed in plant and animal tissues but seldom occurs in high concentration, except in brewer's yeast<br>Enriched or whole grain cereals<br>Pork<br>Peas, beans<br>Nuts<br>*Artificial:*<br>Concentrates from yeast<br>Rice polishings<br>Wheat germ |
| RIBOFLAVIN<br>Vitamin $B_2$ | Important as coenzyme in cellular oxidation<br>Essential to normal growth<br>Participates in light adaptation<br>Vital to protein metabolism<br>Associated with niacin and vitamin $B_6$ functions | Impaired growth<br>Lassitude and weakness<br>Cheilosis<br>Glossitis<br>Dermatitis<br>Anemia<br>Photophobia<br>Cataracts | Water soluble<br>Alcohol soluble<br>Not destroyed by heat in cooking unless with alkali<br>Unstable in light, esp. in presence of alkali | Milk and milk products<br>Enriched foods<br>Whole grain breads and cereals<br>Liver<br>Meats<br>Eggs |
| NIACIN<br>Nicotinic acid<br>Nicotinamide<br>Antipellagra vitamin | As the component of two important enzymes, it is important in glycolysis, tissue respiration, fat synthesis, and cellular energy production | Pellagra<br>Gastrointestinal disturbances<br>Mental disturbances<br>NOTE: Associated with alcoholism | Soluble in hot water and alcohol<br>Not destroyed by heat, light, air, or alkali<br>Not destroyed in ordinary cooking | Milk<br>Eggs<br>Meats<br>Legumes<br>Enriched foods<br>Whole grain cereals |

| | | | | |
|---|---|---|---|---|
| | Nicotinic acid, but not nicotinamide, causes vasodilation and flushing<br>Prevents pellagra | | | Nuts<br>NOTE: Also formed in the body from dietary tryptophan (amino acid) |
| VITAMIN $B_6$<br>Pyridoxine<br>Pyridoxal<br>Pyridoxamine | Used in hemoglobin synthesis<br>Essential for metabolism of tryptophan to niacin<br>Needed for utilization of certain other amino acids | Anemias<br>Depressed immunity<br>Dermatitis around eyes and mouth<br>Neuritis<br>Anorexia, nausea, and vomiting | Soluble in water and alcohol<br>Rapidly inactivated in presence of heat, sunlight, or air | Meats<br>Cereal grains<br>Some fruits<br>Nuts |
| FOLATE<br>Folacin<br>Folic acid | Essential for normal functioning of hematopoietic system<br>Important coenzyme for RNA and DNA synthesis<br>Important in fetal development<br>Functions interrelated with those of vitamin $B_{12}$ | Anemia<br>NOTE: Neural tube defects (e.g., spina bifida) are associated with maternal deficiency. Alcohol and contraceptives interfere with absorption. | Slightly soluble in water<br>Easily destroyed by heat in presence of acid<br>Decreases when food is stored at room temperature<br>NOTE: A large dose may prevent appearance of anemia in a case of pernicious anemia but still permit neurological symptoms to develop. | Liver<br>Green leafy vegetables<br>Peas, beans<br>Some fruits |
| VITAMIN $B_{12}$<br>Cyanocobalamin<br>Hydroxycobalamin | Necessary for myelin synthesis<br>Essential for normal development of red blood cells<br>Associated with folate metabolism | Pernicious anemia<br>Neurological disorders | Soluble in water or alcohol<br>Unstable in hot alkaline or acid solutions | Found only in animal products (e.g., meats, eggs, dairy products)<br>Most of vitamin $B_{12}$ required by humans is synthesized by intestinal bacteria. Can also be recycled. |

# APPENDIX 10
# Phobias

| *Fear of* | *Condition* |
|---|---|
| Air | Aerophobia |
| Animals | Zoophobia |
| Anything new | Neophobia |
| Bacilli | Bacillophobia |
| Bearing a deformed child | Teratophobia |
| Bees | Apiphobia, melissophobia |
| Being buried alive | Taphephobia |
| Birds | Ornithophobia |
| Blood | Hematophobia, hemophobia |
| Blushing | Ereuthrophobia |
| Brain disease | Meningitophobia |
| Bridges (crossing of) | Gephyrophobia |
| Cats | Ailurophobia, galeophobia |
| Change or novelty | Kainophobia |
| Childbirth | Tocophobia |
| Choking | Pnigophobia |
| Cold or something cold | Psychrophobia |
| Color(s) | Chromatophobia, chromophobia |
| Confinement | Claustrophobia |
| Contamination or infection | Molysmophobia |
| Corpses | Necrophobia |
| Crowds | Ochlophobia |
| Dampness | Hygrophobia |
| Darkness | Nyctophobia, scotophobia |
| Dawn | Eosophobia |
| Daylight | Phengophobia |
| Death | Thanatophobia |
| Definite, specific disease | Monopathophobia |
| Deformity | Dysmorphophobia |
| Depth | Bathophobia |
| Developing a phobia | Phobophobia |
| Dirt | Mysophobia, rupophobia |
| Disease | Nosophobia, pathophobia |
| Dogs | Cynophobia |
| Dolls | Pediophobia |
| Drafts | Anemophobia |
| Dust | Amathophobia |
| Eating | Phagophobia |
| Electricity | Electrophobia |
| Emptiness | Kenophobia, cenophobia |
| Error | Hamartophobia |
| Everything | Panphobia, panophobia, pantophobia |
| Excrement | Coprophobia |
| Eyes | Ommatophobia |
| Failure | Kakorrhaphiophobia |
| Fatigue | Kopophobia |
| Feathers | Pteronophobia |
| Fever | Pyrexeophobia |
| Filth | Mysophobia |
| Filth or odor, personal | Automysophobia |
| Fire | Pyrophobia |
| Fish | Ichthyophobia |
| Floods | Antlophobia |
| Fog | Homichlophobia |
| Food | Cibophobia, sitophobia |
| Forest | Hylophobia |
| Frogs | Batrachophobia |
| Ghosts | Phasmophobia |
| Girls | Parthenophobia |
| Glare of light | Photaugiaphobia |
| Glass | Crystallophobia, hyalophobia |
| God | Theophobia |
| Gravity | Barophobia |
| Hair | Trichopathophobia |
| Heat | Thermophobia |
| Height | Acrophobia |
| Hell | Hadephobia, stygiophobia |
| Heredity and hereditary disease | Patroiophobia |
| High objects or being on tall buildings | Batophobia |
| House, being in a | Domatophobia, oikophobia |
| Ideas | Ideophobia |
| Injury | Traumatophobia |
| Innovation | Neophobia |
| Insane, becoming | Maniaphobia |
| Insects | Acarophobia, entomophobia |
| Jealousy | Zelophobia |
| Justice | Dikephobia |
| Knife or pointed objects | Aichmophobia |
| Large objects | Megalophobia |
| Left | Levophobia |
| Light | Photophobia |
| Lightning | Astraphobia, astrapophobia, keraunophobia |
| Locked in, being | Clithrophobia |
| Looked at, being | Scopophobia |
| Machinery | Mechanophobia |
| Men | Androphobia |
| Many things | Polyphobia |
| Marriage | Gamophobia |
| Medicine | Pharmacophobia |
| Metals | Metallophobia |
| Mice | Musophobia |
| Mirror and seeing oneself in | Eisoptrophobia, spectrophobia |
| Missiles | Ballistophobia |
| Moisture | Hygrophobia |
| Money | Chrematophobia |
| Motion | Kinesophobia |

**Phobias** (Continued)

| *Fear of* | *Condition* | *Fear of* | *Condition* |
|---|---|---|---|
| Myths | Mythophobia | Sitting down | Kathisophobia |
| Naked body | Gymnophobia | Skin of animals | Doraphobia |
| Name, hearing a certain | Onomatophobia | Skin disease | Dermatosiophobia |
| | | Skin lesion | Dermatophobia |
| Needles | Belonephobia | Sleep | Hypnophobia |
| Neglect or omission of duty | Paralipophobia | Small objects | Microphobia, microbiophobia |
| Night | Noctiphobia, nyctophobia | Smothering | Pnigerophobia |
| | | Snake | Ophidiophobia |
| Northern lights | Auroraphobia | Snow | Chionophobia |
| Novelty | Kainophobia | Solitude or being alone | Eremophobia |
| Odor | Olfactophobia, osmophobia, osphresiophobia | | |
| | | Sounds | Acousticophobia |
| | | Sourness | Acerophobia |
| Odor, personal | Bromidrosiphobia | Speaking, talking | Lalophobia |
| Open space | Agoraphobia | Spider | Arachnophobia |
| Overwork | Ponophobia | Stairs | Climacophobia |
| Pain | Algophobia, odynophobia | Standing up | Stasiphobia |
| | | Standing or walking | Stasibasiphobia |
| Parasites | Parasitophobia | Stars | Siderophobia |
| People | Anthropophobia | Stealing | Kleptophobia |
| Place | Topophobia | Stories | Mythophobia |
| Pleasure | Hedonophobia | Strangers | Xenophobia |
| Pointed objects | Aichmophobia | Street | Agyiophobia |
| Poison | Iophobia, toxicophobia | String | Linonophobia |
| | | Sunlight | Heliophobia |
| Poverty | Peniaphobia | Symbolism | Symbolophobia |
| Precipices | Cremnophobia | Syphilis | Syphilophobia |
| Punishment | Poinephobia | Tapeworms | Taeniophobia |
| Rabies | Cynophobia, lyssophobia | Taste | Geumaphobia |
| | | Teeth | Odontophobia |
| Railroad or train | Siderodromophobia | Thinking | Phronemophobia |
| Rain or rain storm | Ombrophobia | Thunder | Astraphobia, brontophobia |
| Rectum | Proctophobia | | |
| Red | Erythrophobia | Time | Chronophobia |
| Responsibility | Hypengyophobia | Touched, being | Haphephobia, haptephobia |
| Returning home | Nostophobia | | |
| Right | Dextrophobia | Travel | Hodophobia |
| River | Potamophobia | Trembling | Tremophobia |
| Robbers | Harpaxophobia | Trichinosis | Trichinophobia |
| Rod or instrument of punishment | Rhabdophobia | Tuberculosis | Phthisiophobia, tuberculophobia |
| Ruin | Atephobia | Vaccination | Vaccinophobia |
| Sacred things | Hierophobia | Vehicle, being in | Amaxophobia |
| Scabies | Scabiphobia | Venereal disease | Cypridophobia |
| School | School phobia | Voice, one's own | Phonophobia |
| Scratches or being scratched | Amychophobia | Void | Kenophobia |
| | | Vomiting | Emetophobia |
| Sea | Thalassophobia | Walking | Basiphobia |
| Self | Autophobia | Water | Hydrophobia |
| Semen, loss of | Spermatophobia | Weakness | Asthenophobia |
| Sex | Genophobia | Wind | Anemophobia |
| Sexual intercourse | Coitophobia | Women | Gynephobia |
| Shock | Hormephobia | Words, hearing certain | Onomatophobia |
| Sin | Hamartophobia | | |
| Sinning | Peccatiphobia | Work | Ergasiophobia |
| Sitting | Thaasophobia | Writing | Graphophobia |

Adapted from Campbell, R.J.: Psychiatric Dictionary, ed 5. Oxford University Press, N.Y., 1981.

# APPENDIX 11
# Manual Alphabet

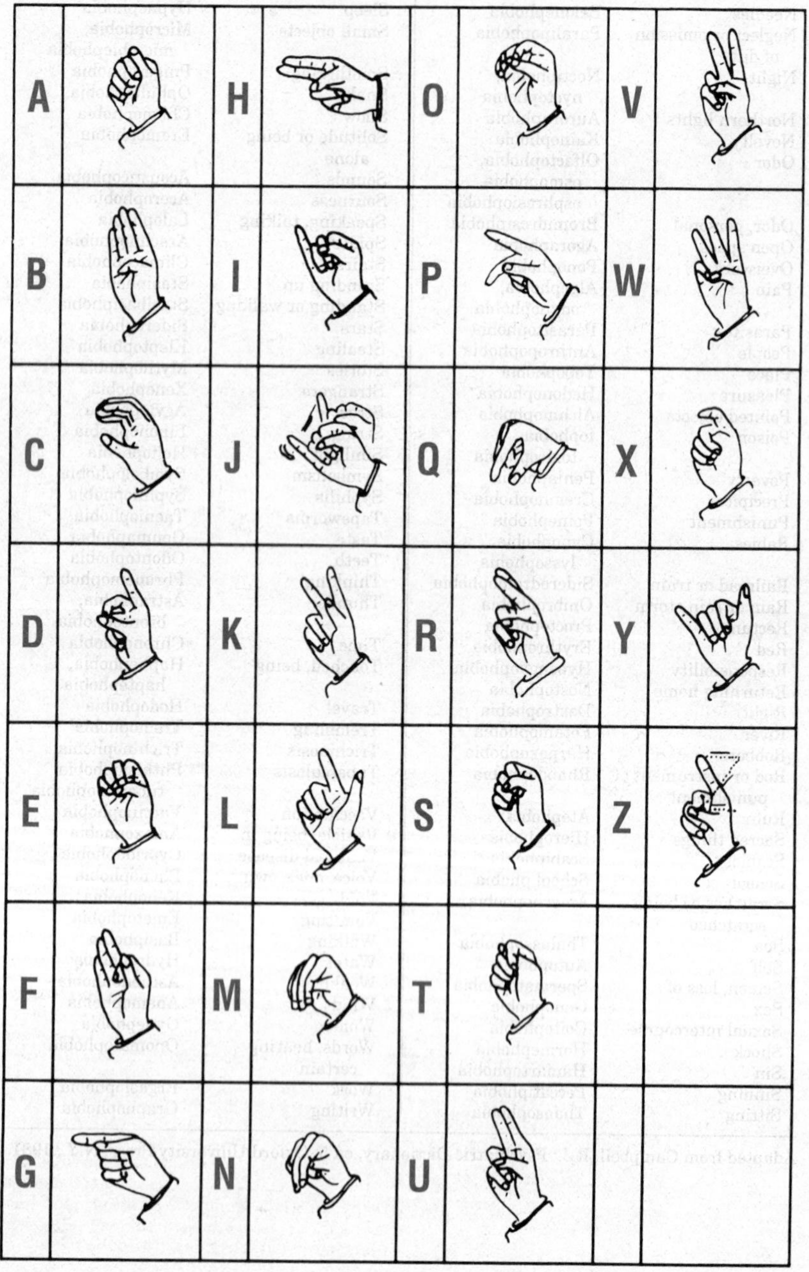

| | | | |
|---|---|---|---|
| A | H | O | V |
| B | I | P | W |
| C | J | Q | X |
| D | K | R | Y |
| E | L | S | Z |
| F | M | T | |
| G | N | U | |

APPENDIX 12

# The Interpreter in Three Languages

## Basic Medical Diagnosis and Treatment in English, Spanish, and French

TABLE OF CONTENTS



## INTRODUCTION

**When attempting to communicate with a patient whose language is foreign to you, it is important to establish that while you may be able to say a few words in his or her language you will not be able to understand the patient's replies. The patient may need to use signs in replying. The following paragraphs are given for your convenience in explaining your language difficulty to the patient.**

### English

**Hello. I want to help you. I do not speak (English) but will use this book to ask you some questions. I will not be able to understand your spoken answers. Please respond by shaking your head or raising one finger to indicate "no"; nod your head or raise two fingers to indicate "yes."**

### Spanish

**Translation**

**Saludos. Quiero ayudarlo. Yo no hablo español, pero voy a usar este libro para hacerle algunas preguntas. No voy a poder entender sus respuestas; por eso haga el favor de contestar, engando con la cabeza o levantando un dedo para indicar "no" y afirmando con la cabeza o levantando dos dedos para indicar "sí."**

**Phonetic**

**Sah-loo'dohs. Ki-air'oh ah-joo-dar'loh. Joh noh ah'bloh es'panyohl, pair'oh voy ah oo-sawr' es'tay lee'broh pahr'ah ah-sair'lay ahl-goo'nahs pray-goon'tahs. Noh voy ah poh-dair' en-ten-dair' soos res-poo-es'tahs; pore es-soh ah'gah el fah-vohr' day kohn-tes-tahr', nay-gahn'doh kohn lah kah-bay'thah oh lay-vahn-tahn'doh oon day'doh pahr'ah een-dee-kahr' noh ee ah-feer-mahn'doh kohn lah kah-bay'thah oh lay-vahn-tahn'doh dohs day'dohs pahr'a een-dee-kahr' see.**

## French

**Translation**
Bonjour. Je veux bien vous aider. Je ne parle pas français mais tout en me servant de ce livre je vais vous poser des questions. Je ne comprendrai pas ce que vous dites en français. Je vous en prie, pour répondre: pour indiquer "non", secouez la tête ou levez un seul doigt; pour indiquer "oui", faites un signe de tête ou levez deux doigts.

**Phonetic**
Bon-zhoor′. Zheh veh bih-ehn′ vooz ay-day′. Zheh neh parl pah frahn-say′ may toot ahn meh sehr-vahn′ d′ seh lee′vrah zheh vay voo poh-say′ day kehs-tih-on′. Zheh neh kahm-prahn′dry pah seh keh voo deet ahn frahn-say′. Zheh vooz ahn pree, por ray-pahn′drah; por ahn-dee-kay nohn, seh-kway′ lah teht oo leh-vay′ oon sool dwoit; por ahn-dee-kay wee′, fayt oon seen deh teht oo leh-vay′ duh dwoit.

## GENERAL

### Basic Questions and Replies

| *English* | *Spanish* | *French* |
|---|---|---|
| Good morning. | Buenos días. | Bonjour. |
| My name is . . . I am a (nurse, physician, social worker, psychologist, etc.). | Me llamo . . . soy (enfermera, médico, trabador social, psicólogo, etc.) | Je m'appelle . . . Je suis (infirmière, médecin, assistante sociale, psychologue, etc.) |
| What is your name? | ¿Cómo se llama? | Quel est votre nom? |
| How old are you? | ¿Cuántos años tiene? | Quel âge avez-vous? |
| Do you understand me? | ¿Me entiende? | Me comprenez-vous? |
| Answer only . . . | Conteste solamente . . . | Répondez seulement . . . |
| Yes No | Sí No | Oui Non |
| What do you say? | ¿Qué dice? | Que dites-vous? |
| Speak slower. | Hable más despacio. | Parlez plus lentement. |
| Say it once again. | Repítalo, por favor. | Répétez ça. |
| Don't be afraid. | No tenga miedo. | N'ayez pas peur. |
| Try to recollect. | Trate de recordar. | Cherchez à vous rappeler. |
| You cannot remember? | ¿No recuerda? | Vous ne vous en souvenez pas? |
| Come to my office. | Venga a mi oficina. | Venez à mon bureau. |
| Please remove all your clothes and put on this gown. | Por favor, quítese la ropa y póngase esta bata. | S'il vous plaît, déshabillez-vous et mettez cette robe. |
| You will? | ¿Ud. quiere?* | Vous voulez bien? |
| You will not? | ¿No quiere Ud.? | Vous ne voulez pas? |
| You don't know? | ¿No sabe? | Vous ne savez pas? |
| Is it impossible? | ¿Es imposible? | C'est impossible? |
| It is necessary. | Es necesario. | C'est necéssaire. |
| That is right. | Está bien. | C'est bien. |
| Show me . . . | Enseñeme . . . | Montrez-moi . . . |
| Here There | Aquí Allí | Ici Là |
| Which side? | ¿En qué lado? | Quel côté? |
| Since when? | ¿Desde cuándo? | Depuis quand? |
| Right | Derecha | A droite |
| Left | Izquierda | A gauche |
| More or less | Más o menos | Plus ou moins |
| How long? | ¿Cuánto tiempo? | Combien de temps? |
| Not much | No mucho | Pas beaucoup |
| Try again. | Trate otra vez. | Essayez encore une fois. |
| Never | Nunca | Jamais |
| Never mind. | Olvídelo. | Ça ne fait rien. |
| That will do. | Suficiente. | Ça suffit. |
| About how much daily? | ¿Más o menos qué cantidad diaramente? | A peu près combien par jour? |

### Seasons

| | | |
|---|---|---|
| Spring | Primavera | Printemps |
| Summer | Verano | Été |
| Autumn | Otoño | Automne |
| Winter | Invierno | Hiver |

* Ud.—Usted.

| English | Spanish | French |
|---|---|---|
| **Months** | | |
| January | Enero | Janvier |
| February | Febrero | Février |
| March | Marzo | Mars |
| April | Abril | Avril |
| May | Mayo | Mai |
| June | Junio | Juin |
| July | Julio | Juillet |
| August | Agosto | Août |
| September | Septiembre | Septembre |
| October | Octubre | Octobre |
| November | Noviembre | Novembre |
| December | Diciembre | Décembre |
| **Days of the Week** | | |
| Sunday | Domingo | Dimanche |
| Monday | Lunes | Lundi |
| Tuesday | Martes | Mardi |
| Wednesday | Miércoles | Mercredi |
| Thursday | Jueves | Jeudi |
| Friday | Viernes | Vendredi |
| Saturday | Sábado | Samedi |
| **Numbers and Time** | | |
| One | Uno | Un |
| Two | Dos | Deux |
| Three | Tres | Trois |
| Four | Cuatro | Quatre |
| Five | Cinco | Cinq |
| Six | Seis | Six |
| Seven | Siete | Sept |
| Eight | Ocho | Huit |
| Nine | Nueve | Neuf |
| Ten | Diez | Dix |
| Twenty | Veinte | Vingt |
| Thirty | Treinta | Trente |
| Forty | Cuarenta | Quarante |
| Fifty | Cincuenta | Cinquante |
| Sixty | Sesenta | Soixante |
| Seventy | Setenta | Soixante-dix |
| At 10:00 | A las diez | A dix heures |
| At 2:30 | A las dos y media | A deux heures et demie |
| Early in the morning | Temprano por la mañana | De bon matin |
| In the daytime | En el día | Pendant la journée |
| At noon | Al mediodía | A midi |
| At bedtime | Al acostarse | A l'heure de se coucher |
| At night | Por la noche | Le soir |
| With meals | Con las comidas | Avec les repas |
| Before meals | Antes de las comidas | Avant les repas |
| After meals | Después de las comidas | Après les repas |
| Today | Hoy | Aujourd'hui |
| Tomorrow | Mañana | Demain |
| Every day | Todos los días | Chaque jour |
| Every other day | Cada dos días | Tous les deux jours |
| Every hour | Cada hora | Chaque heure |
| How long have you felt this way? | ¿Desde cuándo se siente así? | Depuis quand vous sentez-vous comme ça? |
| It came all of a sudden? | ¿Vino de repente? | Ça vous est arrivé tout à coup? |
| For how many days or weeks? | ¿Cuántos días o semanas? | Depuis combien de jours ou semaines? |
| Do they come every day? | ¿Los tiene todos los días? | Ça vous gêne tous les jours? |
| At the same hour? | ¿A la misma hora? | A la même heure? |
| At intervals? | ¿De vez en cuando? | De temps à autre? |
| It will be too late. | Será demasiado tarde. | Çe sera trop tard. |

| English | Spanish | French |
|---|---|---|
| **Colors** | | |
| Black | Negro | Noir |
| Blue | Azul | Bleu |
| Green | Verde | Vert |
| Pink | Rosado | Rose |
| Red | Rojo | Rouge |
| White | Blanco | Blanc |
| Yellow | Amarillo | Jaune |
| **Parts of Body** | | |
| In the abdomen | En el vientre | Dans l'abdomen |
| The ankle | El tobillo | La cheville |
| The arm | El brazo | Le bras |
| The back | La espalda | Le dos |
| The bones | Los huesos | Les os |
| The chest | El pecho | La poitrine |
| The ears | Los oídos | Les oreilles |
| The elbow | El codo | Le coude |
| The eye | El ojo | L'oeil |
| The foot | El pie | Le pied |
| The gums | Las encías | Les gencives |
| The hand | La mano | La main |
| The head | La cabeza | La tête |
| The heart | El corazón | Le coeur |
| The leg | La pierna | La jambe |
| The liver | El hígado | Le foie |
| The lungs | Los pulmones | Les poumons |
| The mouth | La boca | La bouche |
| The muscles | Los músculos | Les muscles |
| The neck | El cuello | Le cou |
| The nerves | Los nervios | Les nerfs |
| The nose | La nariz | Le nez |
| The penis | El pene | Le pénis |
| The perineum | El perineo | Le périnée |
| The rectal area | La parte rectal | La partie rectale |
| The ribs | Las costillas | Les côtes |
| The shoulder blades | Las paletillas | Les omoplates |
| The side | El flanco | Le côté |
| The skin | La piel | La peau |
| The skull | El cráneo | Le crâne |
| The stomach | El estómago | L'estomac |
| The teeth | Los dientes | Les dents |
| The temples | Las sienes | Les tempes |
| The thigh | El muslo | La cuisse |
| The throat | La garganta | La gorge |
| The thumb | El dedo pulgar | Le pouce |
| The tongue | La lengua | La langue |
| The wrist | La muñeca | Le poignet |
| The vagina | La vagina | Le vagin |

## HISTORY

### Family

| English | Spanish | French |
|---|---|---|
| Are you married? | ¿Es Ud. casado? | Etes-vous marié? |
| A widower? | ¿Viudo? | Veuf? |
| A widow? | ¿Viuda? | Veuve? |
| Do you have children? | ¿Tiene Ud. hijos? | Avez-vous des enfants? |
| Are they still living? | ¿Viven todavía? | Sont-ils encore vivants? |
| Do you have any sisters? | ¿Tiene hermanas? | Avez-vous des soeurs? |
| Do you have any brothers? | ¿Tiene hermanos? | Avez-vous des frères? |
| Of what did your mother die? | ¿De qué murió su madre? | De quoi est morte votre mère? |
| And your father? | ¿Y su padre? | Et votre père? |
| Your grandfather? | ¿Su abuelo? | Votre grand-père? |
| Your grandmother? | ¿Su abuela? | Votre grand-mère? |

| *English* | *Spanish* | *French* |
|---|---|---|
| **General** | | |
| Do you have . . . ? | ¿Tiene . . . ? | Avez-vous . . . ? |
| Have you ever had . . . ? | ¿Ha tenido . . . ? | Avez-vous jamais eu . . . ? |
| Chills | Escalofríos | Les frissons |
| Dizziness | El vértigo | Le vertige |
| Shortness of breath | Corto de aliento | Essoufflement |
| Night sweats | Sudores de noche | Transpiration dans la nuit |
| An attack of fever | Un ataque de calentura | Une attaque de fièvre |
| Toothache | Dolor de muelas | Mal aux dents |
| Hemorrhage | Hemorragia | Hémorragie |
| Hoarseness | Ronquera | Enrouement |
| Nosebleeds | Hemorragia por la nariz | Saignements de nez |
| Unusual vaginal bleeding | Hemorragia vaginal fuera de los períodos | Du saignement vaginal anormal |
| When did you last have a period? | ¿Cuándo tuvo Ud. su última menstruación? | Quand avez-vous eu vos règles pour la dernière fois? |
| Are you menopausal? | ¿Padece de la menopausia? | Passez-vous par la ménopause? |
| Are you on hormone therapy? | ¿Sigue un tratamiento hormonal? | Faites-vous un traitment hormonal? |
| Do you take birth control pills? | ¿Toma. Ud. píldoras anticonceptivas? | Est-ce que vous prenez des médicaments anti-conceptionnels? |
| How many pregnancies (abortions or miscarriages) have you had? | ¿Cuántos embarazos (abortos, abortos involuntarios) ha tenido Ud.? | Combien de grossesses (avortements, fausses couches) avez-vous eu? |
| How many living children do you have? What are their ages? | ¿Cuántos hijos vivos tiene Ud.? ¿Cuántos años de edad tienen? | Combien d'enfants vivants avez-vous? Quel âge ont-ils? |
| Any difficulties in pregnancies? Deliveries? | ¿Dificultades con el embarazo? ¿En el parto? | Des difficultés avec la grossesse? Avec l'accouchement? |
| Do you have any sexual difficulties? | ¿Tiene problemas sexuales? | Avez-vous des problèmes sexuels? |
| **Work History** | | |
| What work do you do? | ¿Cuál es su ocupación? | Quelle est votre profession? |
| Is it heavy physical work? | ¿Es un trabajo corporal pesado? | Est-ce que c'est un travail physiquement fatigant? |
| What work have you done? | ¿Qué trabajo ha hecho? | A quoi avez-vous travaillé? |
| **Diseases** | | |
| What diseases have you had? | ¿Qué enfermedades ha tenido? | Quelles maladies avez-vous eu? |
| What type of allergy (types of allergies) do you have? | ¿Qué clase de alergia tiene Ud.? | Quelle sorte d'allergie avez-vous? |
| What is the reaction? | ¿Cuál es la reacción? | Quelle est la réaction? |
| What is the treatment? | ¿Cuál es el tratamiento? | Quel est le traitement? |
| Anemia | Anemia | L'anémie |
| Bleeding tendency | Tendencia a sangrar | Une tendance à saigner |
| Bowel problems | Problemas de vientre (evacuación) | Problèmes au ventre (évacuation) |
| Broken bones | Huesos partidos | Des os cassés |
| Cancer | Cáncer | Le cancer |
| Chicken pox | Varicela | La varicelle |
| Diabetes | Diabetes | Le diabète |
| Diphtheria | Difteria | La diphthérie |
| German measles | Rubéola | Rubéole |
| Gonorrhea | Gonorrea | La gonorrhée |
| Heart disease | Enfermedad del corazón | Une maladie de coeur |
| High blood pressure | Presíon sanguínea elevada | La tension artérielle trop élevée |
| HIV (AIDS) | HIV (SIDA) | HIV (SIDA) |
| Influenza | Gripe (influenza) | La grippe |
| Injuries | Daños | Blessures |

| English | Spanish | French |
|---|---|---|
| Lead poisoning | Envenenamiento con plomo | Empoisonnement causé par le plomb |
| Liver disease | Enfermedad del hígado | Une maladie de foie |
| Malaria | Malaria (paludismo) | La malaria |
| Measles | Sarampión | La rougeole |
| Mental disease | Enfermedades mentales | Une maladie mentale |
| Mumps | Paperas | Les oreillons |
| Nervous disease | Enfermedades nerviosas | Une maladie nerveuse |
| Pleurisy | Pleuresía | Une pleurésie |
| Pneumonia | Pulmonía | Pneumonie |
| Rheumatic fever | Reumatismo (fiebre reumática) | La fièvre rhumatismale |
| Rheumatism | Reumatismo | Le rhumatisme |
| Scarlet fever | Escarlatina | La fièvre scarlatine |
| Seizures | Ataques | Des crises |
| Skin rashes | Erupciones de la piel | Eruptions de la peau |
| Smallpox | Viruela | La variole |
| Syphilis | Sífilis | La syphilis |
| Tuberculosis | Tuberculosis | Tuberculose |
| Typhoid fever | Tifoidea | La fièvre typhoide |
| What immunizations have you had? | ¿Qué inmunizaciones ha tenido Ud.? | Quelles immunisations avez-vous eu? |

## EXAMINATION

### General

| English | Spanish | French |
|---|---|---|
| How do you feel? | ¿Cómo se siente? | Comment vous sentez-vous? |
| Good | Bien | Bien |
| Bad | Mal | Mal |
| Let me look at . . . ; listen to your heart/lungs. | Déjeme reconocerle el corazón/los pulmones. | Permettez-moi de vous examiner le coeur/les poumons. |
| Let me feel your pulse. | Déjeme tomarle el pulso. | Permettez-moi de vous tâter le pouls. |
| Let me check your temperature. | Déjeme tomarle la temperatura. | Permettez-moi de vous prendre la température. |
| Whisper: one, two, three. | Repita en voz baja: uno, dos, tres. | Dites tout bas: un, deux, trois. |
| Say it out loud. | Dígalo en voz alta. | Dites-le à voix haute. |
| Sit down. | Siéntese. | Asseyez-vous. |
| Stand up. | Levántese. | Levez-vous. |
| Walk a little way. | Ande algunos pasos. | Faites quelques pas. |
| Turn back and come this way. | Dé la vuelta y regrese por aquí. | Faites demi-tour et revenez par ici. |
| Do you feel like falling? | ¿Le parece que se va a caer? | Vous sentez-vous comme si vous allez tomber? |
| Do you feel dizzy? | ¿Tiene Ud. vértigo? | Avez-vous le vertige? |
| Are you tired? | ¿Está Ud. cansado? | Êtes vous fatigué? |
| Do you exercise? What type? How often? How long? | ¿Hace ejercicio? ¿De qué tipo? ¿Con qué frecuencia? ¿Por cuánto tiempo? | Prenez-vous de l'exercice? De quelle sorte? Combien de fois? Pour combien de temps? |
| Do you sleep well? | ¿Duerme Ud. bien? | Dormez-vous bien? |
| Do you wake up feeling rested? | ¿Se despierta Ud. descansado(a)? | Vous réveillez-vous bien reposé(e)? |
| Do you have any difficulty in breathing? | ¿Tiene dificultad para respirar? | Avez-vous du mal à respirer? |
| Have you lost weight? | ¿Ha perdido Ud. peso? | Avez-vous maigri? |
| How long have you had this skin rash? | ¿Desde cuándo tiene Ud. esta erupción en la piel? | Depuis quand avez-vous cette éruption sur la peau? |
| Are you usually (now) cold? | ¿Tiene Ud. frío usualmente (ahora)? | Avez-vous froid d'habitude (maintenant)? |
| Are you usually (now) warm? | ¿Tiene Ud. calor usualmente (ahora)? | Avez-vous chaud d'habitude (maintenant)? |
| Can you swallow easily? | ¿Puede Ud. tragar facilmente? | Pouvez-vous avaler facilement? |

| English | Spanish | French |
|---|---|---|
| Have you a good appetite? | ¿Tiene Ud. buen apetito? | Avez-vous bon appétit? |
| Are you thirsty? | ¿Tiene sed? | Avez-vous soif? |
| Do you feel weak? | ¿Se siente Ud. débil? | Vous sentez-vous faible? |
| Had you been drinking alcohol? Have you been drinking alcohol? | ¿Había tomado Ud. alcohol? ¿Ha tomado Ud. alcohol? | Aviez-vous bu de l'alcool? Avez-vous bu de l'alcool? |
| Do you drink wine? Beer? Whisky? Gin? Rum? Vodka? Something else? | ¿Toma Ud. vino? ¿Cerveza, whisky, gin, ron, vodka? ¿Otra cosa? | Buvez-vous du vin? Bière, whisky, gin, rhum, vodka? Quelque chose d'autre? |
| Are you a drinking person? | ¿Toma Ud. bebidas alcohólicas normalmente? | Buvez-vous de l'alcool d'habitude? |
| How much do you drink at one time? | ¿Cuánto toma Ud. cada vez? | Combien buvez-vous chaque fois? |
| How often do you drink? Every day? On weekends? | ¿Con qué frecuencia toma Ud.? ¿Cada día? ¿El fin de semana? | Combien de fois buvez-vous? Tous les jours? Le weekend? |
| Do you smoke tobacco? Cigarettes? Pipe? Cigars? | ¿Fuma Ud. tobaco? ¿Cigarrilos? ¿Pipa? ¿Cigarros? | Fumez-vous le tabac? Cigarettes? Pipe? Cigares? |
| How many do you smoke per day? | ¿Cuántos fuma Ud. al día? | Combien fumez-vous par jour? |
| For how many years? | ¿Por cuántos años? | Depuis combien d'années? |
| Do you inhale? | ¿Traga Ud. el humo? | Avalez-vous la fumée? |
| Do you use caffeine? What beverages? | ¿Usa Ud. la cafeína? ¿Qué bebidas? | Prenez-vous de la caféine? Quelles boissons? |
| How much/how frequently? | ¿Cuántas/con qué frecuencia? | Combien/combien de fois? |
| What drugs do you take (prescriptions, over-the-counter, street)? | ¿Qué medicinas/drogas toma Ud. (recetas, sin-recetas, droga de la calle)? | Quels médicaments/drogues prenez-vous (ordonnances, sans-ordonnance, drogues de la rue)? |
| Are you nervous? | ¿Está Ud. nervioso? | Etes-vous nerveux? |
| When were you first taken sick? | ¿Cuándo le empezó esta enfermedad? | Quand êtes-vous tombé malade d'abord? |
| How did this illness begin? | ¿Cómo empezó esta enfermedad? | Comment cette maladie a-t-elle commencé? |
| Did you take anything for it? | ¿Tomó algo para mejorarla? | Avez-vous pris quelque chose pour cela? |
| Have you taken the (any) medicine? | ¿Ha tomado Ud. la (alguna) medicina? | Avez-vous pris du (quelque) médicament? |
| Did it (the medicine) help? | ¿Le ayudó (la medicina)? | Il vous a fait du bien (le médicament)? |
| Did a dog bite you? | ¿Le mordió un perro? | Est-ce qu'un chien vous a mordu? |
| Did an insect sting you? | ¿Le picó un insecto? | Un insecte vous a piqué? |
| Did you prick yourself with a pin? | ¿Se ha pinchado con un alfiler? | Vous êtes-vous piqué avec une épingle? |
| Did you burn yourself? | ¿Se quemó? | Vous êtes-vous brûlé? |
| Did you twist your ankle? | ¿Se torció Ud. el tobillo? | Vous êtes-vous tordu la cheville? |

## Pain

| English | Spanish | French |
|---|---|---|
| Have you any pain? | ¿Tiene dolor? | Avez-vous mal quelque part? |
| Show me where it hurts. | Enséñeme donde le duele. | Montrez-moi où vous avez mal. |
| Does it move to another area? | ¿Se mueve para otra parte? | Cela se déplace à un autre endroit? |
| What did you feel in the beginning? | ¿Qué sentía cuando empezó? | Qu'avez-vous senti au commencement? |
| Sharp pain | Dolor agudo | Elancement |
| Shooting pains | Dolores agudos | Des élancements |
| Dull pain | Dolor sordo | Douleur sourde |
| Heavy aching pain | Dolor continuo fuerte | Grosse et vive douleur |
| Is the pain always there? | ¿Le duele constantemente? | Ça vous fait mal continuellement? |
| Does it come and go? | ¿Se va y vuelve? | Ça s'en va et revient? |
| How bad is the pain now? usually? | ¿Cuánto le duele ahora? ¿Usualmente? | Combien de mal avez-vous maintenant? D'habitude? |

| English | Spanish | French |
|---|---|---|
| Small/little | Un poco/muy poco | Un peu/très peu |
| Very bad | Muchísimo | Beaucoup |
| In between | Así, así | Entre les deux |
| Does anything make it worse? | ¿Hay algo que lo hace peor? | Quelque chose le rend pire? |
| Does anything make it better/easier? | ¿Hay algo que lo hace mejor/más fácil? | Quelque chose le rend mieux/plus facile? |
| Is the pain better since the medicine I gave you? | ¿El dolor está mejor con la medicina que le di? | La douleur va mieux depuis le médicament que je vous ai donné? |
| A little better? A lot? | ¿Un poco mejor? ¿Mucho mejor? | Un peu mieux? Beaucoup mieux? |
| **Head** | | |
| How does your head feel? | ¿Cómo siente la cabeza? | Comment va votre tête? |
| Can you remember things that happened? | ¿Puede Ud. recordar lo que le ha pasado? | Pouvez-vous vous souvenir de ce qui s'est passé? |
| Can you remember what you did today? Yesterday? Last month/year? Many years ago? | ¿Puede Ud. recordar lo que hizo hoy? ¿Ayer? ¿El mes/año pasado? ¿Muchos años atrás? | Pouvez-vous vous souvenir de ce que vous avez fait aujourd'hui? Hier? Le mois dernier? L'année dernière? Il y a beaucoup d'années? |
| Have you any pain in the head? | ¿Le duele la cabeza? | Avez-vous mal à la tête? |
| Did you fall? | ¿Se cayó? | Etes-vous tombé? |
| How did you fall? | ¿Cómo se cayó? | Comment êtes-vous tombé? |
| Did you faint? | ¿Se desmayó? | Vous êtes-vous évanoui? |
| Have you ever had fainting spells? | ¿Ha tenido desmayos alguna vez? | Avez-vous jamais eu des évanouissements? |
| Do you feel dizzy? | ¿Tiene Ud. vértigo? | Avez-vous le vertige? |
| **Ears** | | |
| Do you have ringing in the ears? | ¿Le pitan los oídos? | Avez-vous des bourdonnements d'oreilles? |
| Can you hear me speaking? [Examiner then repeats more loudly and more softly.] | ¿Puede Ud. oírme cuando hablo? | Pouvez-vous m'entendre quand je parle? |
| [Examiner should look for discharge from ears rather than ask about it.] | | |
| **Eyes** | | |
| Do you wear eyeglasses? Contact lenses? What type? | ¿Usa Ud. anteojos? ¿Lentes de contacto? ¿Qué tipo? | Portez-vous des lunettes? Des verres de contact? Quelle sorte? |
| When did you last have your eyes examined? | ¿Cuándo fue la última vez que le examinaron los ojos? | Quand est-ce que vous vous êtes fait examiner les yeux la dernière fois? |
| Look up. | Mire para arriba. | Regardez en haut. |
| Look down. | Mire para abajo. | Regardez en bas. |
| Look toward your nose. | Mire la nariz. | Regardez le nez. |
| Look at me. | Míreme. | Regardez-moi. |
| Can you see what is on the wall? | ¿Puede ver lo que está en la pared? | Pouvez-vous voir ce qu'il y a contre le mur? |
| Can you see it now? | ¿Puede verlo ahora? | Le voyez-vous maintenant? |
| And now? | ¿Y ahora? | Et maintenant? |
| What is it? | ¿Qué es esto? | Qu'est-ce que c'est? |
| Tell me what number it is. | Dígame qué número es éste. | Dites-moi quel est le numéro. |
| Tell me what letter it is. | Dígame qué letra es ésta. | Dites-moi quelle est la lettre. |
| Can you see clearly? | ¿Puede ver claramente? | Pouvez-vous voir clairement? |
| Better at a distance? | ¿Mejor a cierta distancia? | Mieux à distance? |
| (Can you see) better at close range? | ¿Puede Ud. ver mejor de cerca? | Pouvez-vous voir mieux de près? |

| *English* | *Spanish* | *French* |
|---|---|---|
| Is your vision cloudy? Blurred? Double? | ¿Tiene Ud. la vista velada? ¿Borrosa? ¿Doble? | Avez-vous la vue trouble? Voilée? Double? |
| Do you see haloes/rings around things? | ¿Ve Ud. halos/anillos alrededor de las cosas? | Voyez-vous des halos/ronds autour des choses? |
| Do you see flashing lights? | ¿Ve Ud. destellos? | Voyez-vous des lumières à éclats? |
| Does light (sun) bother your eyes? | ¿La luz (el sol) le molesta los ojos? | La lumière (le soleil) vous gêne les yeux? |
| Do(es) your eye(s) hurt? Sting? Burn? Itch? | ¿Le duele(n) el ojo (los ojos)? ¿Le pica(n)? ¿Está(n) irritado(s)? ¿Le arde(n)? | Avez-vous mal à l'oeil (aux yeux)? Cela pique, brûle, démange? |
| Can you read? | ¿Puede Ud. leer? | Pouvez-vous lire? |
| Can you read a newspaper/ newsprint? | ¿Puede Ud. leer el periódico? | Pouvez-vous lire le journal? |
| Do your eyes water a good deal? | ¿Le lagrimean mucho los ojos? | Est-ce que les yeux vous coulent beaucoup? |
| Can't you open your eye? | ¿No puede abrir el ojo? | Ne pouvez-vous pas ouvrir l'oeil? |
| Did anything get into your eye? | ¿Le entró algo en el ojo? | Est-ce que quelque chose est entré dans l'oeil? |
| Does the eyeball feel as if it were swollen? | ¿Le parece que el ojo está hinchado? | L'oeil vous semble-t-il gonflé? |
| Wear this patch (shield) on your eye [give time frame]. | Use Ud. este parche en el ojo. | Mettez-vous ce couvre-oeil. |
| It would harm your eyes. | Le haría daño a los ojos. | Cela vous abîmerait les yeux. |
| How long has your eyesight been failing? | ¿Desde cuando ha bajado su vista? | Depuis quand diminue votre vue? |

## Nose, Throat, and Mouth

| *English* | *Spanish* | *French* |
|---|---|---|
| How long have you been hoarse? | ¿Desde cuando está Ud. ronco(a)? | Depuis quand êtes-vous enroué(e)? |
| Can you breathe through your nose? | ¿Puede Ud. respirar por la nariz? | Pouvez-vous respirer par le nez? |
| Can you breathe through each nostril? | ¿Puede Ud. respirar por cada ventana de la nariz? | Pouvez-vous respirer par chaque narine? |
| Open your mouth. | Abra la boca. | Ouvrez la bouche. |
| Can you swallow easily? | ¿Puede Ud. tragar facilmente? | Pouvez-vous avaler facilement? |
| Does it hurt you to open your mouth? | ¿Le duele al abrir la boca? | Ouvrir la bouche vous fait-il mal? |
| Do you go to (have you been to) a dentist? | ¿Consulta Ud. (ha consultado) a un dentista? | Consultez-vous (avez-vous consulté) un dentiste? |
| Do you go regularly? When was the last time? | ¿Lo consulta regularmente? ¿Cuándo fue la última vez? | Vous le consultez regulièrement? Quand a été la dernière fois? |
| Do you brush your teeth? | ¿Se lava Ud. los dientes? | Vous lavez-vous les dents? |
| Do you floss? | ¿Usa Ud. hilo dental? | Utilizez-vous le fil dentaire? |
| Do you wear dentures? | ¿Usa Ud. dentadura postiza? | Portez-vous des dentiers? |
| Please remove your denture(s). | Por favor, quítese la(s) dentadura(s). | S'il vous plaît, enlevez le(s) dentier(s). |
| Take a deep breath. | Respire profundamente. | Respirez profondément. |
| Cough. | Tosa. | Toussez. |
| Cough again. | Tosa otra vez. | Toussez encore une fois. |
| How long have you had this cough? | ¿Desde cuándo tiene la tos? | Depuis quand avez-vous la toux? |
| Is it worse at night? In the morning? | ¿Está peor por la noche? ¿Por la mañana? | C'est pire dans la nuit? Pendant le matin? |
| Do you expectorate much? | ¿Escupe mucho? | Crachez-vous beaucoup? |
| What is the color of your expectorations? | ¿De qué color es el esputo? | De quelle couleur sont vos crachats? |
| Does your tongue feel swollen? | ¿Siente Ud. la lengua hinchada? | Est-ce que la langue vous paraît gonflée? |
| Do you have a sore throat? | ¿Le duele la garganta? | Avez-vous mal à la gorge? |
| Does it hurt to swallow? | ¿Le duele al tragar? | Ça vous fait mal quand vous avaler? |

| English | Spanish | French |
|---|---|---|
| | **Upper Extremities** | |
| Let me see your hand. | Enséñeme la mano. | Montrez-moi la main. |
| Grasp my hand. | Apriete mi mano. | Serrez-moi la main. |
| Squeeze (my hand) harder. | Apriete Ud. (mi mano) más fuerte. | Serrez-moi (la main) plus fort. |
| Can you not do it better than that? | ¿No puede hacerlo más fuerte? | Vous ne pouvez pas serrer plus fort que cela? |
| Your arm feels paralyzed? | ¿Parece que el brazo está paralizado? | Est-ce que le bras vous paraît paralysé? |
| Raise your arm. | Levante el brazo. | Levez le bras. |
| Raise it more. | Más alto. | Plus haut. |
| Now the other. | Ahora el otro. | Maintenant l'autre. |
| Hold both arms out in front of you and push against my hand. | Extienda los brazos delante de Ud. y empuje contra mi mano. | Tendez vos bras devant vous et poussez contre ma main. |
| Your arm feels weak? | ¿El brazo le parece débil? | Le bras vous semble faible? |
| How long have you had no strength in your arm? | ¿Desde cuándo no tiene fuerza en el brazo? | Depuis quand vous n'avez pas de force dans le bras? |
| Had you been sleeping on your arm? | ¿Ha dormido encima del brazo? | Vous êtes-vous endormi sur le bras? |
| | **Cardiopulmonary** | |
| Do you experience a rapid (irregular) heartbeat? | ¿Siente el latido del corazón rápido (irregular)? | Eprouvez-vous le battement du coeur rapide (irrégulier)? |
| Do you have pain in your chest? Your jaw? Your arm? | ¿Le duele el pecho? ¿La mandíbula? ¿El brazo? | Avez-vous mal à la poitrine? A la mâchoire? Au bras? |
| Do you get short of breath? With exertion? | ¿Se le corta la respiración? ¿Después de un esfuerzo? | Vous vous essoufflez? Après de l'effort? |
| Do you breathe more easily sitting upright? | ¿Respira mejor cuando está sentado? | Respirez-vous mieux quand vous êtes assis? |
| How many pillows do you need to sleep? | ¿Cuántas almohadas necesita Ud. para dormir? | Vous avez besoin de combien d'oreillers pour dormir? |
| Does it hurt you to breathe? | ¿Le duele cuando respira? | Vous avez mal quand vous respirez? |
| Do you breathe in dust or chemicals at home? At work? | ¿Respira Ud. polvos o productos químicos en casa? ¿En el trabajo? | Respirez-vous des poussières ou des produits chimiques chez vous? Au travail? |
| Do you cough up mucus (phlegm/sputum)? | ¿Tose mocos (flema/esputo)? | Toussez-vous gras (flegme/crachats)? |
| What is the color of your sputum? | ¿De qué color es el esputo? | De quelle couleur sont les crachats? |
| [Examiner should demonstrate any desired motion for patient.] | | |
| | **Gastrointestinal** | |
| Do you have stomach cramps? | ¿Tiene calambres en el estómago? | Avez-vous des crampes de l'estomac? |
| How long has your tongue been that color? | ¿Desde cuándo tiene la lengua de ese color? | Depuis quand votre langue a-t-elle cette couleur? |
| Have you a pain in the pit of your stomach? | ¿Tiene dolor en la boca del estómago? | Est-ce que ça vous fait mal dans le creux de l'estomac? |
| Does eating make you vomit? | ¿El comer le hace vomitar? | Rendez-vous ce que vous mangez? |
| Are you constipated? | ¿Está estreñido? | Etes-vous constipé? |
| Do you have diarrhea? | ¿Tiene diarrea? | Avez-vous la diarrhée? |
| Do you pass any blood? | ¿Con sangre? | Y-a-t-il du sang? |
| Do you belch gas? | ¿Eructa Ud. (gases)? | Eructez-vous (des gaz)? |
| Do you have burning pain (indigestion)? | ¿Padece Ud. de la rescoldera (indigestión)? | Avez-vous des brûlures d'estomac (indigestions)? |

| English | Spanish | French |
|---|---|---|
| What have you been eating? How much? How often? | ¿Qué come? ¿Cuánto? ¿Con qué frecuencia? | Qu'est-ce que vous mangez? Combien? Combien de fois? |
| Are your stools formed? Soft? Hard? Liquid? | ¿Cómo son sus evacuaciones de vientre? ¿Sueltas? ¿Duras? ¿Líquidas? | Comment sont vos évacuations de ventre? Molles? Dures? Liquides? |
| When do you usually have a bowel movement? | ¿Cuándo evacúa el vientre usualmente? | Quand évacuez-vous le ventre d'habitude? |
| Do you pass gas? | ¿Suelta gases del vientre? | Lâchez-vous des gaz du ventre? |
| Do you pass stools involuntarily? | ¿Evacúa el vientre sin querer? | Evacuez-vous le ventre involontairement? |
| Do you feel nauseated (sick to your stomach)? | ¿Tiene náuseas (asco grande)? | Avez-vous la nausée (mal au coeur)? |
| Have you been vomiting? How long? How many times? | ¿Ha vomitado? ¿Desde cuándo? ¿Cuántas veces? | Avez-vous vomi? Depuis quand? Combien de fois? |
| What does the vomitus look like? | ¿A qué se parece el vómito? | A quoi ressemble le vomissement? |
| Is the vomitus (or stool) brown? Black? | ¿Es de color café el vómito (o la evacuación)? ¿Negro? | Le vomissement est brun (ou la selle)? Noir? |

### Genitourinary

| English | Spanish | French |
|---|---|---|
| Have you any difficulty passing water? | ¿Tiene dificultad en orinar? | Avez-vous de la difficulté à uriner? |
| Do you pass water involuntarily? | ¿Orina sin querer? | Urinez-vous involontairement? |
| Are any of your limbs swollen? | ¿Están hinchados algunos de sus miembros? | Avez-vous des membres gonflés? |
| How long have they been swollen like this? | ¿Desde cuándo estan hinchados así? | Depuis quand sont-ils gonflés comme ça? |
| Were they ever swollen before? | ¿Han estado hinchados alguna vez antes? | Ont-ils jamais été gonflés autrefois? |
| What color is your urine? Is it clear? | ¿De qué color es su orina? ¿Clara? | De quelle couleur est votre urine? Claire? |
| Do you have any burning when you urinate? | ¿Le arde al orinar? | Cela brûle quand vous urinez? |
| Do you have vaginal itching? Burning? Discharge? | ¿Tiene irritación vaginal? ¿Sensaciones ardientes? ¿Derrames? | Avez-vous de l'irritation vaginale? Sensations de chaleur? Ecoulements? |
| What does the discharge look like? | ¿A qué se parece el derrame? | A quoi ressemblent les écoulements? |
| Do your breasts hurt? | ¿Le duelen los senos? | Avez-vous mal aux seins? |
| Are there any lumps? | ¿Hay alguna masa? | Il y a des grosseurs? |
| Is there any discharge from the nipples? | ¿Hay derrame de los pezones? | Les bouts des seins écoulent? |
| Were they ever swollen before? | ¿Han estado hinchados antes? | Ils ont été gonflés avant? |
| Have you ever breastfed? Are you breastfeeding? | ¿Ha criado al pecho alguna vez? ¿Cría al pecho ahora? | Avez-vous allaité un enfant? Vous allaitez maintenant? |

### Back and Lower Extremities

| English | Spanish | French |
|---|---|---|
| Is your movement limited in any way? | ¿Está Ud. limitado para moverse de alguna forma? | Etes-vous limité pour vous déplacer de quelque manière? |
| Do your legs/feet hurt? Feel cold? Numb? | ¿Le duelen las piernas/los pies? ¿Sensación de frío? ¿Entumecidas/entumecidos? | Avez-vous mal aux jambes/aux pieds? Sensation de froid? Engourdies/engourdis? |
| Do you have pins and needles? | ¿Tiene sensaciones de pinchazos? | Eprouvez-vous des fourmillements? |
| Is the pain/symptom worse when you walk? | ¿El dolor/síntoma está peor cuando Ud. anda? | La douleur/le symptôme est pire quand vous marchez? |
| Is it eased when you stop walking? | ¿Se alivia cuando deja de andar? | Ça se calme quand vous arrêtez de marcher? |

| *English* | *Spanish* | *French* |
|---|---|---|
| Raise your right leg (your left leg) (both legs). | Levante su pierna derecha (su pierna izquierda) (las dos piernas). | Levez la jambe droite (la jambe gauche) (les deux jambes). |
| Bend your knees. | Doble las rodillas. | Pliez les genoux. |
| Wiggle your toes. | Mueva los dedos (de pie). | Remuez les doigts (de pied). |
| Do you have back pain? Where? | ¿Le duele la espalda? ¿Dónde? | Avez-vous mal au dos? Où? |
| Bend forward at the waist. | Inclínese hacia adelante. | Penchez-vous en avant. |
| Bend from side to side. | Inclínese de lado en lado. | Penchez-vous d'un côté à l'autre. |
| [Examiner should demonstrate desired motion for patient.] | | |
| I need to check other pulses in your legs. | Necesito tomarle otros pulsos en sus piernas. | J'ai besoin de vous tâter d'autres pouls dans vos jambes. |

## TREATMENT

### General

| | | |
|---|---|---|
| It is nothing serious. | No es nada grave. | Ce n'est rien de grave. |
| You will get better. | Ud. se mejorará. | Vous vous remettrez. |
| You will need to follow these directions. | Tiene Ud. que seguir estas instrucciones. | Vous devez suivre ces indications. |
| You will need to take this medicine until it is finished. | Tiene Ud. que tomar esta medicina hasta que se le acabe. | Il faut prendre ce médicament jusqu'à le terminer. |
| You will need to take this treatment until your doctor (nurse) tells you to stop. | Tiene Ud. que seguir este tratamiento hasta que el médico (la enfermera) diga que lo deje. | Vous devez suivre ce traitement jusqu'à ce que le médecin (l'infirmière) vous dise de l'arrêter. |
| Take a bath. | Tome un baño. | Prenez un bain. |
| A sponge bath. | Un baño de esponja. | Un bain à l'éponge. |
| An oatmeal bath. | Un baño de harina de avena. | Un bain de farine d'avoine. |
| A cornmeal bath. | Un baño de harina de maíz. | Un bain de farine de maïs. |
| Soak in warm water (for 20 minutes three times a day for the next week). | Báñese en agua caliente (por 20 minutos tres veces al día durante la semana que viene). | Baignez-vous dans de l'eau chaude (pour 20 minutes trois fois par jour pendant la semaine prochaine). |
| [Length and duration of treatment are specified.] | | |
| Apply ice (for 20 minutes of every hour for the next 2 days). | Ponga hielo (por 20 minutos de cada hora durante los 2 próximos días). | Mettez de la glace (pour 20 minutes de chaque heure pendant les 2 jours suivants). |
| [Length and duration of treatment are specified.] | | |
| Wash the wound with . . . | Lave la herida con . . . | Lavez la blessure avec . . . |
| Apply a bandage to . . . | Ponga un vendaje a . . . | Mettez un bandage à . . . |
| Keep the bandage dry and clean. | Mantenga el vendaje limpio y seco. | Gardez le bandage propre et sec. |
| Wash your hands thoroughly before and after treatment (caring for the wound/ applying drops). | Lávese las manos completamente antes y después del tratamiento (cuidando la herida/aplicando gotas). | Lavez-vous les mains complètement avant et après le traitement (soignant la blessure/ applicant les gouttes). |
| Apply ointment (lotion/ cream/powder). | Aplíquese ungüento (loción, crema, polvos). | Appliquez un onguent, lotion, crème, poudre). |
| Keep very quiet. | Estése muy quieto. | Restez tranquille. |
| You must not speak. | No debe hablar. | Vous ne devez pas parler. |
| Swallow small pieces of ice. | Trague pedacitos de hielo. | Avalez de petits morceaux de glace. |

| *English* | *Spanish* | *French* |
|---|---|---|

## Diet

| *English* | *Spanish* | *French* |
|---|---|---|
| In a few days you may eat food. | Dentro de algunos días podrá comer. | Après quelques jours vous pouvez prendre de la nourriture. |
| You will need to eat a special (high-protein/low-fat/ diabetic) diet. | Tiene que estar a una dieta de (alta proteína/baja grasa/diabética). | Vous devez suivre un régime de (haute protéine/basses graisses/diabétique). |
| You may eat . . . | Puede comer . . . | Vous pouvez manger . . . |
| Soft foods only. | Solamente comida blanda. | Seulement de la nourriture molle. |
| Your regular diet when your symptoms are gone. | Su dieta normal cuando terminados sus síntomas. | Votre régime normal quand vos symptômes seront terminés. |
| You may drink . . . | Puede tomar . . . | Vous pouvez boire . . . |
| Water | Agua | De l'eau |
| Clear liquids (tea, bouillon, Jell-O) | Líquidos claros (té, caldo, Jell-O) | Liquides claires (thé, bouillon, Jell-O) |
| All liquids including milk and juices | Todo líquido, inclusive leche y jugo | Toute liquide, lait et jus y compris |
| No caffeine (coffee, tea, chocolate, cola) | Ninguna cafeína (café, té, chocolate, cola) | Pas de caféine (café, thé, chocolat, cola) |
| Only decaffeinated drinks | Unicamente bebidas descafeínadas | Seulement les boissons décaféinées |

## Surgery

| *English* | *Spanish* | *French* |
|---|---|---|
| You will need an operation on your . . . (to remove . . . ) | Tendrá Ud. que operarse en su . . . (para quitarle . . . ) | Il faut que l'on vous fasse une opération (pour enlever votre . . . ) |
| You will need tests before the operation (blood tests, chest radiograph, electrocardiogram). | Tendrá que hacerse análisis antes de la operación (análisis de sangre, radiografía del pecho, electrocardiograma). | Il faut que l'on vous fasse des analyses avant l'opération (analyse du sang, radiographie de la poitrine, electrocardiogramme). |
| [Examiner explains nature of tests and tells patient when and where they will be given.] | | |
| You will be in the hospital for [length of time]. | Ud. estará en el hospital por [cuanto tiempo]. | Vous resterez à l'hôpital pour [combien de temps]. |
| [Examiner tells patient when and where the surgery will take place.] | | |

## Medication (use with Numbers and Time)

| *English* | *Spanish* | *French* |
|---|---|---|
| I will give you something for that. | Le daré algo para eso. | Je vous donnerai quelque chose pour cela. |
| I will leave a prescription. | Le dejaré una receta. | Je laisserai une ordonnance. |
| Use it as directed [give dosing intervals] until it is gone (until you are told to stop). | Tómelo según indicado [intervalo de dósis] hasta terminarlo (hasta que se le diga dejarlo). | Prenez-le [intervalle de dose] jusqu'au bout (jusqu'à ce que l'on vous dise d'arrêter). |
| Take 1 teaspoonful three times daily (in water). | Tome 1 cucharadita tres veces al día, con agua. | Prenez-en une cuillerée à café trois fois par jour (avec de l'eau). |
| Take 1 tablespoonful. | Tome una cucharada. | Prenez-en une cuillerée à soupe. |
| Mix in [amount] of water (juice) and drink the entire amount. | Mescle en [cantidad] de agua (jugo) y beba lo todo. | Mélangez avec [quantité] d'eau (de jus) et buvez le tout. |
| Gargle. | Haga gárgaras. | Gargarissez-vous. |

| English | Spanish | French |
|---|---|---|
| Inject the drug into your abdomen (arm, leg, buttock, muscle tissue). | Inyéctese la medicina en el abdomen (el brazo, la pierna, la nalga, el tejido muscular). | Faites-vous une piqûre du médicament dans l'abdomen (le bras, la jambe, la fesse, le tissu musculaire). |
| Insert the suppository into your rectum (vagina). | Métase el supositorio en el recto (la vagina). | Mettez le suppositoire dans votre rectum (votre vagin). |
| A pill | Una píldora | Une pilule |
| Do not crush the tablet (open the capsule). | No aplaste el comprimido (no abra la cápsula). | N'écrasez pas le comprimé (n'ouvrez pas la capsule). |
| Drop [number of drops] into the right (left) eye. | Vierta [número de gotas] en el ojo derecho (izquierdo). | Versez [nombre de gouttes] dans l'oeil droit (gauche). |
| Drop [number of drops] into each eye. | Vierta [número de gotas] en cada ojo. | Versez [nombre de gouttes] dans chaque oeil. |
| Who is available to assist you at home? With medications? With diet? | ¿Quién está disponible en su casa para atenderle a Ud.? ¿Con las medicinas? ¿Con la dieta? | Qui est disponible chez vous pour vous aider? Avec les médicaments? Avec le régime? |
| Who is available to transport you to the doctor (hospital) (home)? | ¿Quién está disponible para llevarle al médico (hospital) (a casa)? | Qui est disponible pour vous conduire au médecin (à l'hôpital) (chez vous)? |

## NURSING CARE CONCERNS

| English | Spanish | French |
|---|---|---|
| Do you need to pass water? | ¿Necesita Ud. orinar? | Avez-vous besoin d'uriner? |
| Do you need to have a bowel movement? | ¿Necesita Ud. evacuar el vientre? | Avez-vous besoin d'évacuer le ventre? |
| Do you need a drink of water? | ¿Necesita Ud. tomar agua? | Avez-vous besoin de prendre de l'eau? |
| Do you need your mouth rinsed? | ¿Necesita que le limpien la boca? | Avez-vous besoin de vous faire rincer la bouche? |
| Do you need something to eat? | ¿Necesita Ud. algo de comer? | Avez-vous besoin de manger quelque chose? |
| Do you need your position changed? | ¿Necesita que le cambien de posición? | Avez-vous besoin de vous faire changer de position? |
| Do you need medicine for pain? | ¿Necesita medicina contra el dolor? | Avez-vous besoin d'un médicament pour la douleur? |
| You will be getting oxygen. | Le van a poner oxígeno. | On va vous donner de l'oxigène. |
| You will be getting a breathing treatment. | Le van a dar un tratamiento de respiración. | On va vous donner un traitement de respiration. |
| You will be getting intravenous fluid. | Le van a dar un flúido intravenoso. | On va vous donner un fluide intraveineux. |
| You will be getting a bland diet. | Le van a poner una dieta blanda. | On va vous mettre au régime simple. |
| You will be getting an injection. | Le van a dar una inyección. | On va vous faire une piqûre. |

# APPENDIX 13
# Medical Emergencies

## Appendix 13–1 Poisons and Poisoning

| *Substances* | *Pathology* | *Symptoms* | *Emergency Measures* | *Comments* |
|---|---|---|---|---|
| Acetaminophen | Production of toxic intermediate metabolite that cannot be detoxified due to glutathione depletion. | Phase 1 (0–24 hr): Sometimes asymptomatic—anorexia, nausea, vomiting.<br>Phase 2 (24–48 hr): GI symptoms resolve; hepatotoxicity is subclinical, but liver function tests and coagulation tests are abnormal. If liver damage is significant, patient may progress to phase 3.<br>Phase 3: (48–96 hr): Problems due to severe hepatic compromise—bleeding disorders, hypoglycemia, hepatic encephalopathy.<br>Phase 4 (>96 hr): Recovery period. Laboratory values return to normal and symptoms resolve. | Gastric lavage or emesis. Toxicity is unlikely at a dose <140 mg/kg. For significant serum levels of acetaminophen, acetylcysteine can be administered orally in a loading dose followed by a maintenance regimen. | In general, patients require hospitalization for observation and supportive treatment. Hepatic failure can occur, and renal complications or failure can develop. Most recover fully without further sequelae. In some instances, hepatic failure may require transplantation. |
| Acids<br>Acetic<br>Hydrochloric<br>Nitric<br>Phosphoric<br>Sulfuric<br>Any other strong acid | Immediate destruction and necrosis with eschar formation of mucous membranes and tissues on contact. | Burning pain on contact with mucous membranes of the mouth and throat, dysphagia, abdominal pain, nausea, hematemesis, thirst, esophageal or gastric perforation, shock, death. | Establishment of airway patency, aggressive volume resuscitation, radiographic evaluation of damage, water or milk for minute or dilute ingestion. Surgical intervention may be required. | Permanent damage to the esophagus and stomach can result in chronic dysphagia and stricture formation. |

**Poisons and Poisoning** (Continued)

| *Substances* | *Pathology* | *Symptoms* | *Emergency Measures* | *Comments* |
|---|---|---|---|---|
| Alkalis | Irreversible destruction and liquefactive tissue necrosis that penetrates beyond surface contact with alkali. | Immediate burning and blistering of tissue on contact; severe pain of mouth, esophagus, and chest; esophageal or gastric perforation; pancreatitis; hematemesis; shock; death. | Establishment of airway patency, aggressive volume resuscitation, radiographic evaluation of damage, water or milk for minute or dilute ingestion. Surgical intervention may be required. | Permanent damage to the esophagus and stomach can result in chronic dysphagia, stricture formation, and necrosis of tissue. |
| Ammonia and ammonium hydroxide | Tissue destruction due to alkaline injury on contact with mucous membranes. Degree of destruction depends on alkalinity of product and amount and length of exposure. | Burning of mouth and throat, chest pain, esophageal and gastric damage, hematemesis. Inhalation of gas can cause coughing, bronchospasm, and pulmonary edema. | Airway protection if there are signs of involvement, supplemental humidified oxygen and bronchodilators for inhalation exposures, moderate amounts of water or milk to dilute ingestion, analgesics for pain. Additional procedures may be required to assess extent of tissue injury. | Most significant damage is seen with intentional massive ingestions or occupational exposures to concentrated strengths of ammonia. Most accidental exposures to household strength products resolve without residual damage. |
| Amphetamines and amphetamine-like agents | Excessive stimulation of the CNS and of peripheral alpha and beta receptor sites. | Excitement, restlessness, tremors, hyperactive reflexes, nausea, vomiting, diarrhea, palpitations, arrhythmias, hypertension, hyperthermia, dehydration, mydriasis, agitation, seizures, coma, death. | Supportive care including airway maintenance and cardiac monitoring; gastric lavage; administration of activated charcoal and cathartic; cooling measures for hyperthermia; benzodiazepines for seizures; vasodilators and beta-adrenergic blocking agents. | Toxicity can occur with slightly higher than therapeutic doses. Tolerance can readily develop with repeated use. |

| | | | | |
|---|---|---|---|---|
| Antidepressants: selective serotonin reuptake inhibitors (SSRI)<br>Fluoxetine<br>Paroxetine<br>Sertraline | CNS depression, excessive stimulation of serotonin receptors. | Serotonin syndrome: hypomania, confusion, myoclonus, diaphoresis, hyperreflexia, tremor, hyperthermia, agitation, restlessness, insomnia, nausea, vomiting, drowsiness, ataxia, coma. | Maintenance of airway, breathing, circulation; gastric decontamination by emesis or lavage for large ingestions; administration of activated charcoal and cathartic. The serotonin antagonists cyproheptadine and methysergide have reportedly been used with success. | These agents are considered relatively safe, even in overdoses. As a class, the SSRIs do cause the anticholinergic effects seen with cyclic antidepressants. However, they are less toxic in excessive doses. |
| Antidepressants: cyclic<br>Amitriptyline<br>Amoxapine<br>Desipramine<br>Doxepin<br>Imipramine<br>Nortriptyline | Toxic cardiovascular and CNS effects secondary to anticholinergic activity, inhibited reuptake of neurotransmitters, peripheral alpha-adrenergic blockade, alteration of cardiac cells resulting in conduction disturbances. | Confusion, dizziness, altered mental status (lethargy to coma), hypotension, tachycardia, hyperthermia, mydriasis, dry mucous membranes, prolonged QRS complex, cardiac dysrhythmias, seizures. | Cardiac monitoring, gastric decontamination with activated charcoal and cathartic, gastric lavage for large ingestions, benzodiazepines for seizures, sodium bicarbonate for conduction disturbances. | Death can ocur within a few hours of an overdose. |
| Antihistamines: sedating (major classes)<br>Alkylamines<br>Ethanolamines<br>Ethylenediamines<br>Phenothiazines<br>Piperazines | Excessive central and peripheral anticholinergic effects. | Lethargy, agitation, confusion, miosis, tachycardia, hyperthermia, decreased GI motility, hypotension, respiratory depression, ataxia, stupor, seizures, dysrhythmias, coma, circulatory collapse, death. | Maintenance of airway, breathing, circulation, and fluids for hypotension; gastric decontamination by emesis if ingestion was recent; activated charcoal and cathartic. For massive ingestion or if patient is sedated, intubation and gastric lavage followed by activated charcoal and cathartic; IV physostigmine for anticholinergic toxicity; benzodiazepines for seizures. | Most ingestions are complex to manage because many antihistamines are commercially available in combination with various analgesics and decongestants. With early intervention, most overdoses have excellent outcomes without sequelae. Some newer antihistamines have a minimal CNS effect. |

**Poisons and Poisoning** (Continued)

| *Substances* | *Pathology* | *Symptoms* | *Emergency Measures* | *Comments* |
|---|---|---|---|---|
| Arsenic and arsenic salts | Disruption of enzymatic reactions that are essential for cellular metabolism; possible phosphate replacement or interaction with sulfhydryl groups. | Nausea, vomiting, hemorrhagic gastritis, severe watery diarrhea, dehydration, pulmonary edema, hypotension, delirium, encephalopathy, arrhythmias, convulsions, shock, death. Symptoms may have delayed onset. | Aggressive fluid replacement, activated charcoal or gastric lavage for larger ingestions, dimercaprol (BAL) 3–5 mg/kg IM every 4–6 hr for symptomatic patients. | Toxicity depends on the type of arsenic, amount involved, and route of exposure. Systemic toxicity can result from percutaneous absorption. Arsenic is a carcinogen. |
| Aspirin—SEE: *salicylates* | | | | |
| Atropine and anticholinergic agents | Acetylcholine blockage at muscarinic receptor sites; affects exocrine glands and cardiac tissue. | Dry mouth and burning pain in throat, thirst, blurred vision, mydriasis, dry, hot, flushed skin, hyperpyrexia, tachycardia, palpitations, restlessness, excitement, confusion, convulsions, delirium; rarely, death. | Airway maintenance and ventilation assistance, emesis or gastric lavage, activated charcoal and cathartic, diazepam for sedation and control of convulsions, physostigmine 0.5–1 mg IV for severe atropine toxicity, cooling measures for hyperthermia. | Classes of drugs that possess anticholinergic activity include antihistamines, antipsychotics, antispasmodics, cyclic antidepressants, and skeletal muscle relaxants. Atropine in ophthalmic preparations may be toxic to infants and young children. |
| Barbiturates<br>Amobarbital<br>Aprobarbital<br>Butabarbital<br>Mephobarbital<br>Methohexital<br>Pentobarbital<br>Phenobarbital<br>Secobarbital | Depressed neuronal activity of brain, hypotension caused by depression of central sympathetic tone, inhibition of cardiac contractility. | Drowsiness, confusion, ataxia, vertigo, slurred speech, shallow respiration and pulse, headache, stupor, hypotension, areflexia, cyanosis, hypothermia, cardiovascular collapse, respiratory arrest, death. | Airway maintenance and ventilation assistance, treatment of hypotension, gastric lavage, activated charcoal and cathartic, alkalinization of urine to enhance phenobarbital elimination, hemoperfusion for severe toxicity. | Severity of toxicity depends on the agent ingested. |

| | | | | |
|---|---|---|---|---|
| Benzene<br>Xylene<br>Toluene | Irritation of mucous membranes and airway caused by agents and their metabolites, CNS depression, myocardial effects resulting in conduction disturbances. | Burning sensation of mouth and stomach, nausea, vomiting, chest pain, cough, headache, pneumonitis (if inhaled), vertigo, ataxia, confusion, stupor, ventricular dysrhythmias, convulsions, coma, respiratory failure, death. | Airway maintenance and ventilation assistance, activated charcoal and cathartic, therapy for arrhythmias and seizures. Gastric lavage within 30 min is useful for larger ingestions. | Chronic exposure can result in permanent renal damage, bone marrow suppression, and neuropsychological damage. |
| Benzodiazepines<br>Alprazolam<br>Chlordiazepoxide<br>Clorazepate<br>Diazepam<br>Estazolam<br>Flurazepam<br>Lorazepam<br>Midazolam<br>Oxazepam<br>Prazepam<br>Temazepam<br>Triazolam | Generalized CNS depressant effects caused by enhanced activity of gamma-aminobutyric acid, an inhibitory neurotransmitter. | Confusion, dizziness, somnolence, ataxia, hypotension, coma, respiratory depression, cardiovascular depression. | Airway maintenance and ventilation assistance, gastric lavage, activated charcoal and cathartic, flumazenil IV administered and repeated to reverse unconsciousness or respiratory depression, fluids and vasopressors for hypotension. | Generally considered safe, even in high doses. Fatalities are rare and usually due to coingestions with other CNS depressants. |
| Boric acid and borate salts | Exact mechanism of toxicity unknown. | Headache, nausea, vomiting (vomitus may be blue green), fever, oliguria or anuria, diarrhea, stomach pain, lethargy, restlessness, distinctive erythroderma, tremor, convulsions, renal and hepatic injury or failure, cyanosis, coma, shock with vascular collapse, death. | Airway maintenance and ventilation assistance, emesis or gastric lavage for large ingestions, activated charcoal (may not offer much benefit), hemodialysis for large ingestions. | Reports of toxicity from boric acid ingestions and exposures has declined in recent years due to decreased use as an irrigant and antiseptic agent. |

**Poisons and Poisoning** (Continued)

| *Substances* | *Pathology* | *Symptoms* | *Emergency Measures* | *Comments* |
|---|---|---|---|---|
| Botulinum toxin | Potent neurotoxicity produced by *Clostridium botulinum;* prevents release of acetylcholine by irreversibly binding to cholinergic nerve terminals. | Nausea, vomiting, occasional diarrhea, dysphagia, diplopia, loss of visual acuity and pupillary reflexes, profuse sweating, rapid and weak pulse, death usually caused by respiratory failure. Symptoms may present up to a week after ingestion. | Emesis or gastric lavage for recent ingestion, activated charcoal and cathartic, aggressive supportive care for symptomatic patients. Guanidine may enhance acetylcholine release. Botulism antitoxin can be administered to bind circulating free toxin. Sensitivity to horse serum should be determined before antitoxin administration. | Even with excellent supportive care, recovery may take months to years. Common long-term sequelae include dysgeusia, dry mouth, dyspepsia, constipation, tachycardia, arthralgias, and fatigue. Botulinum toxin is available from the local health department or the Centers for Disease Control and Prevention [(404) 329-2888]. |
| Cadmium salts or fumes | Diverse multisystemic toxicities that are not clearly understood. | Nausea, vomiting, diarrhea, abdominal cramps, salivation, gastritis, headache, vertigo, exhaustion, collapse, acute renal failure, chemical pneumonitis with pulmonary edema on inhalation, death. | No specific treatment is available. Gastric lavage and catharsis may be useful for acute noncaustic ingestions. Inhalation requires aggressive respiratory support. | Long-term effects vary with duration and severity of exposure. Renal function may be affected. Chronic exposures have resulted in osteomalacia, emphysema, and increased risk of lung or prostate cancer. |
| Calcium channel blockers<br>Myocardial and vascular effects<br>Bepridil<br>Diltiazem<br>Verapamil<br>Primarily vascular effects<br>Amlodipine<br>Isradipine<br>Nicardipine<br>Nifedipine | Prevention of calcium entry into cells, resulting in decreased myocardium contractility, blockade of AV and SA nodes, and peripheral vasodilation. | Nausea, vomiting, dizziness, headache, confusion, stupor, hyperglycemia, hypotension, bradycardia, metabolic acidosis, cardiac conduction disturbances, seizures, coma, death. | Maintenance of airway, breathing, and circulation; fluids and vasopressors for hypotension; gastric lavage and cathartic; multiple-dose activated charcoal; whole bowel irrigation; calcium chloride or calcium gluconate for hypotension and bradydysrhythmias, atropine or isoproterenol for bradycardia. | Intentional overdoses of calcium channel blockers are life threatening and often fatal despite aggressive management. |

| | | | | |
|---|---|---|---|---|
| Camphor | CNS stimulant with toxic effects; underlying mechanism is not known. | Burning of mouth and throat, nausea, vomiting, headache, CNS hyperactivity followed by CNS depression, vertigo, liver function abnormalities, delirium, tremor, convulsions, apnea, coma, death from respiratory arrest secondary to status epilepticus. | Airway maintenance, gastric lavage with copious amounts of fluid, activated charcoal and cathartic, benzodiazepines for seizures. | Fatalities have been reported with 1- or 2-g doses; however, most exposures can be effectively managed and resolved without residual complications. |
| Carbon monoxide | Hemoglobin binding preventing delivery of oxygen to cells; has significantly greater affinity for hemoglobin than oxygen. | Mild headache, dyspnea with moderate exertion, irritability, fatigue, nausea, vomiting, confusion, ataxia, syncope, convulsions, death from respiratory arrest. | 100% oxygen by face mask or endotracheal tube, IV fluids, cardiac monitoring, hyperbaric oxygen for significant exposures. | Residual effects can include dementia, psychosis, paralysis, peripheral neuropathy, and parkinsonism. |
| Carbon tetrachloride | Metabolites cause renal and hepatic toxicity; potent CNS depressant effects. | Nausea, vomiting, abdominal pain, headache, confusion, drowsiness, coma, renal and hepatic failure. Death is caused by respiratory arrest, circulatory collapse, or ventricular fibrillation. | Airway maintenance and ventilation asistance, gastric lavage, activated charcoal and cathartic, acetylcysteine to decrease effects of intermediate metabolite. | Toxicity from inhalation can be severe; small ingestions (<10 ml) can be fatal. |
| Chlorate salts | Potent oxidative properties that destroy red blood cells; toxicity to kidneys due to direct effects and hemolysis. | Abdominal pain, nausea, vomiting, diarrhea, methemoglobinemia, intravascular hemolysis, delirium, coagulopathy, coma, convulsions, cyanosis, renal failure, death. | Gastric lavage and activated charcoal, methylene blue for mild toxicities, hemodialysis to remove toxin. Sodium thiosulfate IV has been used to inactivate the chlorate ion, with inconsistent results. | In some instance, exchange transfusions have been advocated to reverse effects of poisoning. |
| Chlorinated compounds<br>Chlorine<br>Chlorine gas<br>Sodium hypochlorite | Corrosive effect on contact with mucous membranes. | Immediate burning of mouth and throat, coughing, choking, bronchospasm, chest and abdominal pain, stridor, pulmonary edema, esophageal burns. | For inhalation, humidified supplemental oxygen and bronchodilators; for dilute ingestions, water or milk; for concentrated ingestions, gastric lavage and endoscopic evaluation. | Esophageal damage can result in stricture formation. |

**Poisons and Poisoning** (Continued)

| *Substances* | *Pathology* | *Symptoms* | *Emergency Measures* | *Comments* |
|---|---|---|---|---|
| Chlorinated hydrocarbon pesticides<br>Aldrin<br>Chlordane<br>DDT (chlorophenothane)<br>Dieldrin<br>Heptachlor<br>Lindane<br>Thiodan<br>Toxaphene | Direct toxicity to neuronal axons, interfering with transmission; affects myocardium stability resulting in arrhythmias. | Vomiting, headache, fatigue, tremors, ataxia, weakness, confusion, seizures, respiratory depression, arrhythmias, coma. In agents other than DDT, seizure may be first sign of toxicity. | Maintenance of airway, breathing, circulation; activated charcoal and cathartic; lavage for large ingestions; multiple-dose activated charcoal and cholestyramine to enhance removal; appropriate therapy for seizures and arrhythmias. | These agents can be absorbed transdermally and by inhalation. Toxicity and outcomes vary. |
| Cocaine | CNS stimulation and inhibition of neuronal uptake of catecholamines, depressed conduction and myocardial contractility. | Anxiety, agitation, delirium, hypertension, tachycardia, hyperthermia, diaphoresis, tremor, mydriasis, flushing, seizures, ECG abnormalities, areflexia, coma, death. | Airway maintenance and ventilation assistance, cardiac monitoring, activated charcoal or whole-bowel irrigation for ingestion, beta blockers and vasodilators, benzodiazepines, cooling measures. | Cocaine continues to be a popular drug of abuse and a high number of fatalities continue to be reported each year. |
| Copper salts | Mucous membrane irritation, multisystemic toxicities with salts. Elemental copper is poorly absorbed and causes little toxicity. | Pain in mouth, esophagus, and stomach; abdominal pain; vomiting; gastroenteritis; shock; hepatic and renal injury; hemolysis; seizures; coma; death. | Fluid replacement and pressors, gastric lavage; dimercaprol and penicillamine for large ingestions. | Long-term copper exposures have resulted in liver fibrosis, cirrhosis, and renal dysfunction. |
| Cyanide | Nonspecific inhibition of enzyme systems; binds to cytochrome oxidase of cells, blocking oxygen use. | Nausea, vomiting, abdominal pain, almond odor of breath, headache, dyspnea, agitation, confusion, syncope, convulsions, lethargy, coma, cardiovascular collapse, death. Onset of symptoms is abrupt. | Oxygen and assisted ventilation if needed, gastric lavage, activated charcoal and cathartic, inhalation of amyl nitrite pearls until antidote is available. Antidote kit contains amyl and sodium nitrites and sodium thiosulfate. | Delayed neurological sequelae including dystonias and parkinsonism have been reported following acute cyanide poisoning. |

| | | | | |
|---|---|---|---|---|
| Digoxin and digitalis | Excessive excitability and automaticity of myocardium resulting in conduction disturbances and dysrhythmias; AV blockade. | In minutes to hours, anorexia, nausea, vomiting, diarrhea, headache, fatigue, weakness, drowsiness, electrolyte disturbances, confusion, delirium, visual disturbances, dysrhythmias, bradycardia, AV block, death from ventricular fibrillation. | Cardiac monitoring, emesis or gastric lavage, activated charcoal, digoxin-specific antibody fragments (Fab) for severe toxicity, lidocaine or phenytoin for ventricular irritability. | Most poisonings result from ingestion of prescribed digoxin. Digitalis is also found in plants including foxglove, lily of the valley, dogbane, and oleander. |
| Dinitrophenol and pentachlorophenol | Uncoupling of oxidative phosphorylation in mitochondria, hypermetabolic state and lactic acid production. Dinitrophenol oxidizes hemoglobin to methemoglobin. | Fatigue, thirst, nausea, vomiting, abdominal pain, sweating, flushing, restlessness, excitement, hyperthermia, tachycardia, hyperpnea, metabolic acidosis, cyanosis, seizures, coma, death from respiratory or circulatory failure. | Maintenance of airway, breathing, circulation; activated charcoal and cathartic; gastric lavage for large ingestions; methylene blue IV; fluid replacement; benzodiazepines; cooling measures. | Ingestion of 1–3 g of these agents can be lethal. Many accidental transdermal poisonings have been reported. |
| Ergotamines or ergot alkaloids | Central sympatholytic effects: serotonin release and interference with neuronal uptake. Peripherally, may act as a partial alpha-adrenergic agonist or an antagonist at adrenergic, dopaminergic, and tryptaminergic receptors. | Nausea, vomiting, dizziness, diarrhea, headache, thirst, weak pulse, tingling and numbness of extremities, dyspnea, hallucinations, blood pressure changes, hemorrhagic vesiculations, paresthesias, peripheral ischemia, convulsions, loss of conciousness, gangrene. | Emesis and multiple-dose activated charcoal and cathartic; for peripheral symptoms, nitroprusside/nitroglycerine IV to maintain perfusion. Other agents including captopril, prazosin, and nifedipine have been used successfully. | Outcome is based on route and amount of ingestion. |
| Ethanol | CNS depression; effects can be additive when combined with other CNS depressants. | Impaired motor coordination, slurred speech, inebriation, ataxia, peripheral vasodilation, rapid pulse, nausea, vomiting, drowsiness, stupor, coma, peripheral vascular collapse, hypotension, tachycardia, hypothermia, death from respiratory or circulatory failure. | Emesis or gastric lavage for substantial, recent ingestions, warming measures for hypothermia, hemodialysis in deteriorating conditions. | Ethanol is often coingested with other toxic substances in suicide attempts; emergency treatment may vary depending on other substances ingested. |

**Poisons and Poisoning** (Continued)

| *Substances* | *Pathology* | *Symptoms* | *Emergency Measures* | *Comments* |
|---|---|---|---|---|
| Ethylene glycol | Metabolism to oxalic, glyoxylic, and glycolic acids; conversion to lactate, increasing the lactic acid level; calcium oxalate crystal formation and deposition in tissues; metabolite toxicity to kidneys, CNS, and lungs. | Nausea, vomiting, excitability, hypotension, abdominal cramps, weakness, metabolic acidosis, ataxia, vertigo, arrhythmias, stupor, coma, death from respiratory failure or renal failure with uremia. | Maintenance of airway, breathing, circulation; sodium bicarbonate and IV calcium; emesis or gastric lavage; ethanol to prevent toxic metabolite formation; folic acid, thiamine, and pyridoxine; therapy for seizures and arrhythmias; hemodialysis for severe toxicity. | Outcomes vary; in general, comatose patients have a poor prognosis. |
| Fluoride salts | Direct metabolic and cytotoxic effects; multiple adverse effects from calcium and magnesium binding. | Salivation, thirst, nausea, abdominal pain, vomiting, diarrhea, muscle weakness, hypocalcemia, hyperkalemia, tetanic contractions, death due to vascular collapse and shock. | Maintenance of airway, breathing, circulation; cardiac monitoring; emesis or gastric lavage; calcium salts; for severe toxicity, IV calcium chloride; therapy for electrolyte disturbances. | Degree of toxicity depends on salt solubility and the amount of elemental fluoride ingested. Pediatric toxicities are often caused by fluorinated toothpaste ingestions. |
| Hydrogen sulfide gas | Inhibition of oxidative phosphorylation enzymes, potent inhibition of cytochrome oxidase. Exposure results in cellular hypoxia. | Irritated mucous membranes, conjunctivitis, headache, nausea, vomiting, weakness, bradycardia, hypotension, dyspnea, rapid loss of consciousness with larger exposures, pulmonary edema, cyanosis, convulsions, coma, death due to cardiac or respiratory arrest. | High-flow oxygen, advanced cardiac life support as indicated, sodium nitrite, blood pressure monitoring, hyperbaric oxygen if available. Methemoglobin level should be recorded 30 min after infusion. | If patient is immediately removed from the exposure, recovery may be rapid and complete. More severe exposures have resulted in permanent neurological changes and myocardial ischemia. |
| Ipecac syrup or fluid extract | Cardiac and neuromuscular toxicity with systemic absorption; toxicities are seen with chronic and prolonged use. | Vomiting, diarrhea, lethargy, irritability, hypothermia, hypotonia, dehydration, gastritis, seizures, cardiac toxicity, neuromuscular toxicity, shock, death. | Activated charcoal or gastric lavage for large ingestions, fluid replacement, correction of electrolyte abnormalities, cardiac monitoring, therapy for arrhythmias. | Chronic exposures are reported in patients with eating disorders; cases of toxicity secondary to Munchausen's syndrome by proxy have also been documented. |

| | | | | |
|---|---|---|---|---|
| Iron salts | Several mechanisms: direct corrosive effects on GI mucosa, hepatocellular toxicity, cardiovascular compromise, metabolic acidosis. Neurological manifestations are caused by hypoperfusion, metabolic acidosis, and hepatic compromise. | Nausea, vomiting, severe gastroenteritis, hematemesis, diarrhea, tachypnea, tachycardia, hypotension, lethargy, cyanosis, convulsions, coma, shock leading to death. | Emesis or gastric lavage with normal saline; if tablets are found on radiograph, whole bowel irrigation; deferoxamine to chelate iron 4–6 hours postingestion for high serum levels or signs of systemic toxicity. | Patients with systemic complications require hospital admission, constant monitoring, and supportive care until resolution. Late complications (2–8 wk) include GI stricture and obstruction. Toxicity is unlikely at a dose <20 mg/kg. |
| Isopropanol<br>Isopropyl alcohol<br>Rubbing alcohol | Potent CNS depressant metabolized to acetone; may contribute to CNS depression. | Nausea, vomiting, abdominal pain, hypotension, ataxia, areflexia, inebriation, muscle weakness, ketonemia, ketonuria, respiratory depression, hemorrhagic tracheobronchitis, myocardial depression, coma, death. | Emesis, gastric lavage, and activated charcoal soon after exposure; hemodialysis for severe clinical problems. | A majority of cases resolve without sequelae. |
| Lead and lead salts | Heavy metal interaction with sulfhydryl groups and interference with action of numerous enzymes, interference with heme production and survival of red blood cells. Chronic exposure can cause irreversible CNS and developmental effects. | Abdominal pain, vomiting, lethargy, behavioral changes, ataxia, arthralgias, abdominal or renal colic, anemia, acute encephalopathy, seizures, coma, death. | Emesis or gastric lavage, activated charcoal and cathartic (charcoal may not offer much benefit), dimercaprol or EDTA for symptoms or significant serum levels of lead, supportive care as needed. | Chronic exposure to lead can result in developmental and neuropsychiatric defects. |
| Lithium | At therapeutic doses, possible alteration of cAMP activity, efefect on norepinephrine availability, and displacement of other cations intracellularly. These effects may be disrupted or exaggerated at high doses; electrolyte imbalance may occur. | Nausea, vomiting, diarrhea, fine resting tremor, lethargy, confusion, tremors, ataxia, ECG abnormalities, profound weakness, muscle fasciculations, hyperreflexia, clonus, stupor, seizures, acute renal failure, coma, death. | Maintenance of airway, breathing, circulation, hydration; for acute ingestions, emesis or gastric lavage; whole bowel irrigation if a sustained-release product was ingested; activated charcoal for coingestions; hemodialysis for severe cases or renal insufficiency or failure. | Chronic or acute-on-chronic overdoses are more life threatening than acute poisonings. Chronic exposure permits intracellular accumulation. In acute poisonings, most lithium remains in the extracellular fluid for many hours, causing toxicity. |

## Poisons and Poisoning (Continued)

| *Substances* | *Pathology* | *Symptoms* | *Emergency Measures* | *Comments* |
|---|---|---|---|---|
| Mercuric salts | Reaction with carboxyl, sulfhydryl, phosphoryl, and amide groups; interference with enzyme and cellular functions; toxicity involving multiple organ systems. | Burning of mouth and throat, thirst, abdominal pain, nausea, corrosive gastroenteritis, hematemesis, diarrhea, dehydration, shock, acute tubular necrosis. | Gastric lavage, activated charcoal (does not adsorb mercuric salts effectively), dimercaprol, aggressive fluid replacement. Hemodialysis may be required for acute renal failure. | Doses of 1–4 g of mercuric chloride can be fatal. Chronic poisonings have resulted in neurological abnormalities, renal dysfunction, and gastrointestinal symptoms. |
| Methanol | Metabolism to formaldehyde and formic acid. | Latent period (24–72 hr) before development of symptoms, dizziness, inebriation, blurred vision, headache, nausea, vomiting, abdominal pain, delirium, visual disturbances that may progress to blindness, weak and rapid pulse, shallow respirations, cyanosis, coma, metabolic acidosis, respiratory failure, death. | Activated charcoal for recent ingestion, ethanol IV or orally to inhibit toxic metabolites, hemodialysis in severe cases, aggressive management of metabolic acidosis. | Visual impairment, optic atrophy, and blindness are due to effects of formic acid on the optic nerve. |
| Mushrooms–containing muscarine<br>*Amanita muscaria* (fly agaric)<br>*Amanita panterina* (panther)<br>*Clitocybe dealbata* (sweater)<br>*Clitocybe dilatata*<br>*Clitocybe illudens*<br>Most *Inocybe* species | Peripheral cholinergic effect due to muscarine; stimulation of autonomic nervous system. | Lacrimation, diaphoresis, salivation, abdominal cramps, vomiting, loss of bowel and bladder control. | Atropine 1–2 mg IV, repeated and titrated depending on clinical presentation; supportive care including fluid replacement. | Patients typically recover without residual effects. |

| | | | | |
|---|---|---|---|---|
| Mushrooms–containing cyclopeptides<br>*Amanita phalloides* (death cap)<br>*Amanita tennifolia*<br>*Amanita virosa* (destroying angel)<br>*Galerina autumnalis*<br>*Galerina marginata*<br>*Galarina venenata*<br>*Lepiota helveola*<br>*Lepiota josserandii* | Cytotoxicity of cyclopeptides (phallotoxins, amatoxins, virotoxins), cellular insult causing hepatic, renal, GI, and CNS damage. | Phase 1 (6–12 hr): Nausea, abdominal pain, vomiting, watery diarrhea, thirst.<br>Phase 2 (12–24 hr): Symptomatic improvement, elevated hepatic enzymes.<br>Phase 3 (1–6 days): Restlessness, delirium, hallucinations, hematuria, gastroenteritis, pancreatitis, hypoglycemia, shock, acute renal failure, jaundice, hepatic coma, death. | Gastric lavage and multiple-dose activated charcoal every 2–4 hr, activated charcoal hemoperfusion, fluid and electrolyte resuscitation, hepatic transplantation in fulminant hepatic failure. | Cyclopeptide-containing mushrooms are responsible for most mushroom fatalities in North America. Toxic cyclopeptides are heat stable, insoluble in water, and not affected by drying. |
| Naphthalene | Metabolism to numerous byproducts including alpha-napthol, a potent hemolytic agent. | Fever, nausea, vomiting, abdominal pain, diarrhea, lethargy, seizures, hemolysis, pallor, jaundice, cyanosis. | Emesis, gastric lavage for larger ingestions, activated charcoal and cathartic, IV hydration and urinary alkalinization, transfusions for hemolysis. | Hemolysis is acute and severe in patients with glucose-6-phosphate dehydrogenase deficiency. Naphthalene was used in mothballs and toilet bowl cleaners, but less toxic agents have been used recently. |
| Nicotine | Binding to cholinergic nicotine receptors; toxicity due to sympathetic and parasympathetic stimulation followed by ganglionic and neuromuscular blockade. | Nausea, vomiting, abdominal pain, headache, salivation, diarrhea, hyperpnea, diaphoresis, tachycardia, hypertension, pallor, agitation, tremor, ataxia, confusion, dysrhythmias, hypotension, shock, muscle paralysis, coma, death. | Maintenance of airway, breathing, circulation; multiple-dose activated charcoal and cathartic for large oral ingestions; lavage for large, recent liquid ingestion; thorough washing of exposed skin; therapy for seizures, hypertension, hypotension, and arrhythmias. | Because most commercial sources of nicotine are not concentrated, a majority of exposures cause mild toxicity and resolve without complications. |
| Nitroglycerines, nitrates, nitrites | Vasodilation causing hypotension. Nitrites are potent oxidizing agents that cause methemoglobinemia. | Headache, hypotension, skin flushing, nausea, methemoglobinemia, cyanosis, symptoms of cardiac ischemia or cerebrovascular disease, seizures secondary to hypotension. | Maintenance of airway, breathing, circulation; emesis for recent ingestion; activated charcoal and cathartic; lavage for large ingestions; fluids and vasopressors for hypotension; antidote methylene blue IV for symptomatic methemoglobinemia; exchange transfusion for severe toxicity. | Most cases can be managed successfully with early, aggressive interventions; life-threatening complications are due to hypotension and methemoglobinemia. |

## Poisons and Poisoning (Continued)

| *Substances* | *Pathology* | *Symptoms* | *Emergency Measures* | *Comments* |
|---|---|---|---|---|
| Nonsteroidal anti-inflammatory agents | Inhibition of prostacyclin and prostaglandin $E_2$ production resulting in acute renal failure. | Nausea, vomiting, gastrointestinal distress and bleeding, tinnitus, metabolic acidosis, CNS depression, respiratory depression, mild hepatic toxicity, acute renal failure, seizures. | Gastric decontamination with activated charcoal, gastric lavage and activated charcoal for patients requiring intubation; multiple-dose activated charcoal for severe toxicity or ingestion of agents with long half-lives; therapy for seizures. | Baseline renal and hepatic function should be assessed. Most toxic exposures to this class of agents are successfully treated and resolve fully without residual sequelae. |
| Opioids and Opiates<br>Codeine<br>Fentanyl<br>Heroin<br>Morphine<br>Methadone and other synthetic opioids | Excessive stimulation of CNS opiate receptors causing sedation and respiratory failure. | Drowsiness, nausea, dysphoria, bradypnea, miosis, hypothermia, respiratory depression, hypotension, bradycardia, weak pulse, coma, apnea, death. | Maintenance of airway, breathing, circulation if necessary; emesis for initial treatment in alert patient, or intubation and gastric lavage; activated charcoal and cathartic; single or multiple doses of naloxone, naltrexone, or nalmefene parenterally. | Antidotes are useful in reversing effects of the opiates, but administration may precipitate severe withdrawal symptoms. |
| Oxalic acid and oxalate salts | Corrosion of tissues on contact; precipitation with calcium to form insoluble deposits throughout organs, causing systemic damage. | Irritation of mouth and esophagus, vomiting, weakness, shock, tetany, convulsions, cardiac arrest, death. Inhalation can cause pneumonitis and pulmonary edema. | Calcium chloride, calcium gluconate, or calcium carbonate to precipitate oxalate; flushing and lavage with copious amounts of water; IV calcium chloride or calcium gluconate for symptomatic hypocalcemia; maintenance of high urine output, therapy for seizures and arrhythmias. | Ingestions of 5–15 g of oxalic acid have resulted in death. |

| | | | | |
|---|---|---|---|---|
| Parathion and other organophosphates | Acetylcholinesterase inhibition, resulting in excessive acetylcholine stimulation of muscarinic and nicotinic receptors. | Nausea, vomiting, diarrhea, abdominal pain, tremor, muscle fasciculations, excessive salivation and sweating, dehydration, bradycardia, weakness, shock, death usually caused by respiratory paralysis. | Maintenance of airway, breathing, circulation; activated charcoal and cathartic; gastric lavage for large, recent ingestions; repeated atropine IV depending on signs and symptoms of toxicity; pralidoxime IV bolus followed by continuous infusion to restore acetylcholinesterase activity and detoxify organophosphates; diazepam for convulsions. | Toxicity depends on the relative toxicity of the organophosphate and the quantity involved. |
| Phenol | Corrosive injury to skin, eyes, and respiratory tract; protein denaturation and coagulation necrosis. | Vomiting, diarrhea, gastrointestinal injury, agitation, confusion, seizures, hypotension, shock, coma, respiratory failure, death. | Multiple-dose activated charcoal and cathartic; washing of exposed areas; benzodiazepines for seizures. Low molecular weight polyethylene glycol has been used for gastric decontamination and topical exposures. If corrosion has occurred, tube passage may cause rupture. | Corrosive burns of the skin and mucous membranes and GI perforation can occur. Esophageal stricture and renal failure rarely occur. |
| Phenothiazines and neuroleptics | Prominent cardiovascular and CNS effects; toxicity due to inhibitory effects of dopaminergic, cholinergic, alpha-adrenergic, histaminic, and seritonergic receptors. | Sedation, somnolence, stupor, dry mouth, tachycardia, labile blood pressure, hypothermia or hyperthermia, dysrhythmias, extrapyramidal symptoms, acathisias, coma, NMS, seizures, cardiac arrest, death. | Maintenance of airway, breathing, circulation; emesis for recent ingestion; activated charcoal and cathartic; lavage for large ingestions; diphenhydramine or benztropine IV for dystonias; sodium bicarbonate for dysrhythmias; vasopressors; rapid cooling and benzodiazepines for NMS. | Death from neuroleptic agent overdose is rare; many intentional ingestions are taken with other agents that complicate care and outcome. |

**Poisons and Poisoning** (Continued)

| *Substances* | *Pathology* | *Symptoms* | *Emergency Measures* | *Comments* |
|---|---|---|---|---|
| Phosphorus and phosphides | Local irritation and tissue burns; direct toxic effect to myocardium and vessels; hepatic, renal, and GI damage due to latent systemic toxicity. | Painful burns to mucous membranes and skin on contact, nausea, vomitus and diarrhea with garlicky odor, jaundice, metabolic derangements, dysrhythmias, coma, shock, seizures, hepatic or renal failure, cardiac arrest. Inhalation can cause pneumonitis and pulmonary edema. | Maintenance of airway, breathing, circulation; endoscopy to assess GI burns; cautious gastric lavage with hydrogen peroxide or potassium permanganate, followed by activated charcoal and mineral oil cathartic; fluid replacement and correction of electrolyte imbalance. | After acute effects from ingestion, a symptom-free period of a few weeks may be followed by a stage of systemic toxicity involving the liver, kidneys, heart, CNS, and GI tract. |
| Salicylates<br>Aspirin<br>Salicylate salts | Effect on multiple organ systems, metabolic derangement. Effects are due to stimulation of respiratory center, intracellular uncoupling of oxidative phosphorylation, and alteration of platelet function. | Nausea, vomiting, agitation, hyperthermia, lethargy, hyperglycemia or hypoglycemia, hyperpnea, tachypnea, tinnitus, hemorrhagic gastritis, delirium, stupor, acid-base disturbances, electrolyte imbalance, cerebral edema, convulsions, cardiovascular collapse. | Maintenance of airway, breathing, circulation; emesis for recent ingestion; lavage for several hours (may be needed to eliminate bezoars); multiple-dose activated charcoal; urinary alkalinization; correction of acid-base and fluid-electrolyte abnormalities; hemodialysis for severe toxicity or deteriorating condition. | The prognosis of patients suffering from an acute toxic ingestion can be assessed on the basis of serum levels obtained within 6 hr of ingestion. |
| Strychnine | Competitive antagonism of glycine at postsynaptic spinal cord motor neuron. | Muscle twitching, extensor spasm, opisthotonos, trismus or facial grimacing, seizures, medullary paralysis, death. Symptoms occur within 20 min. | Gastric lavage and activated charcoal, dark and quiet environment, benzodiazepines or neuromuscular blockade, mechanical ventilation. | Poisonings are rare since commercial use in rodenticides has decreased. Most exposures result in death. The approximate fatal dose for a child is 15 mg; for an adult, 5–10 mg/kg. |

| | | | | |
|---|---|---|---|---|
| Thallium salts | Combination with mitrochondrial sulfhydryl groups, interference with oxidative phosphorylation. | Nausea, vomiting, abdominal pain, hematemesis, bloody diarrhea, headache, alopecia, hematuria, proteinuria, elevated hepatic enzymes, lethargy, tremors, ataxia, delirium, seizures, coma, death. | Syrup of ipecac or gastric lavage; activated charcoal with sorbitol; fluid, electrolyte, and glucose treatment to prevent shock; benzodiazepines for seizures. Hemoperfusion and hemodialysis may be moderately successful. | Alopecia and Mee's sign, single white transverse lines on the nails 2–3 weeks postexposure, are common diagnostic features. Long-term neurological impairment can occur. |
| Theophylline—SEE: *xanthine derivatives* | | | | |
| Xanthine derivatives<br>Aminophylline<br>Caffeine<br>Theophylline | Antagonism of adenosine activity and release of catecholamines; in high doses, phosphodiesterase inhibition. Toxic effects are secondary to smooth muscle relaxation, peripheral vasodilation, myocardial stimulation, and CNS excitation. | Nausea, protracted vomiting, hypotension, respiratory alkalosis, metabolic acidosis, hypokalemia, tachycardia, hypercalcemia, ventricular dysrhythmias, seizures, death due to cardiovascular collapse. | Emesis or gastric lavage, activated charcoal and cathartic, multiple-dose activated charcoal if levels continue to rise. Whole bowel irrigation may decrease effectiveness of activated charcoal. For larger ingestions or deteriorating condition, charcoal hemoperfusion can enhance removal. Patient should be monitored for toxicity (cardiac, electrolyte, acid-base, and theophylline levels); fluid replacement and vasopressors may be required. | Most theophylline preparations are sustained release and can form bezoars. A theophylline level should be determined every 2 hr until a decline is demonstrated with two successive levels. |
| Warfarin and related anticoagulant compounds | Inhibition of vitamin K 2,3-epoxide reductase and quinone reductase activity (these are necessary to activate vitamin K, which is essential in coagulation). | Fatigue, hematuria, nosebleeds, ecchymoses, GI hemorrhage, hypotension, intracranial hemorrhage, hemorrhagic shock, death (rare). Onset of symptoms occurs after 2–5 days. | Emesis or gastric lavage; for large ingestions, serial PTs every 12–24 hr until patient is stabilized; vitamin $K_1$ (phytonadione) to correct coagulopathy. | Most accidental ingestions resolve without further sequelae. Intentional ingestions or delay in seeking treatment may re sult in severe coagulopathy. Symptomatic patients require hospitalization and aggressive therapy to prevent further complications. |

AV = atrioventricular; BAL = British anti-lewisite; CNS = central nervous system; ECG = electrocardiogram; EDTA = ethylenediamenetetra-acetic acid; GI = gastrointestinal; NMS = neuroleptic malignant syndrome; PT = prothrombin time; SA = sinoatrial.

SOURCE: Goldfrank, LR, et al.: Goldfrank's Toxicologic Emergencies, ed. 5. Appleton and Lange, East Norwalk, CT, 1994.

## Appendix 13–2 Toxicity Rating Chart

| *Toxicity Rating or Class* | Probable Oral LETHAL Dose (Human) *Dose* | | *For 70-kg (150-lb) Person* |
|---|---|---|---|
| 6 Super toxic | less than 5 | mg/kg | A taste (less than 7 drops) |
| 5 Extremely toxic | 5–50 | mg/kg | Between 7 drops and 1 teaspoonful |
| 4 Very toxic | 50–500 | mg/kg | Between 1 tsp and 1 ounce |
| 3 Moderately toxic | 0.5–5 | g/kg | Between 1 oz and 1 pint (or 1 lb) |
| 2 Slightly toxic | 5–15 | g/kg | Between 1 pt and 1 quart |
| 1 Practically nontoxic | above 15 | g/kg | More than 1 qt (2.2 lb) |

SOURCE: Gosselin, RE, Smith, RP, and Hodge, HC: Clinical Toxicology of Commercial Products, ed. 5. The Williams & Wilkins Co., Baltimore, 1984, with permission.

## Appendix 13–3 Substances Generally Nontoxic When Ingested*

Ball-point inks (amt. in 1 pen)
Barium sulfate
Bathtub toys (floating)
Blackboard chalk (calcium carbonate)
Candles (insect-repellent type may be toxic)
Carbowax (polyethylene glycol)
Carboxymethylcellulose (dehydrating material packed with drugs, film, etc.)
Castor oil
Cetyl alcohol
Crayons (children's: marked A.P., C.P., or C.S. 130–46)
Detergents, anionic and nonionic
Dichloral (herbicide)
Dry cell battery
Glycerol
Glyceryl monostearate
Graphite
Gums (acacia, agar, ghatti, etc.)
Hormones
Kaolin
Lanolin
Lauric acid
Linoleic acid
Linseed oil (not boiled)
Lipstick
Magnesium silicate (antacid)
Matches
Methylcellulose
Modeling clay
Paraffin, chlorinated
Pencil lead (graphite)
Pepper, black (except inhaled in mass)
Petrolatum
Polyethylene glycols
Polyethylene glycol stearate
Polysorbate (Tweens®)
Putty
Red oil (turkey-red oil, sulfated castor oil)
Silica (silicon dioxide)
Spermaceti
Stearic acid
Sweetening agents
Talc (except when inhaled)
Tallow
Thermometer fluid or mercury
Titanium oxide
Triacetin (glyceryl triacetate)
Vitamins, children's multiple (with or without iron)
Vitamins, multiple without iron

* Substances listed here may, however, be present in combination with phenol, petroleum distillate vehicles, or other toxic chemicals. Because manufactured products may be changed in their composition, this table is intended only as a guide, and prudence requires that a poison center be consulted for up-to-date information.

SOURCE: The Merck Manual, Ed. 16, Merck Sharp and Dohme, 1992, with permission.

# Appendix 13–4 Emergency Situations

| *Medical Emergency* | *Pathophysiology* | *History and Physical Examination* | *Treatment* |
|---|---|---|---|
| Acute Myocardial Infarction (MI, AMI) | Acute blockage of coronary arteries resulting in death of myocardial tissue. Risk factors often present include tobacco use, hypertension, hypercholesterolemia, diabetes mellitus, or family history of heart disease. Men are at greater risk than premenopausal women. Modification of risk factors lowers the risk for disease. | Usually, tightness, pressure, heaviness, or burning in the chest. Pain may radiate to the neck, jaw, back, or arms. Often the patient feels short of breath. Palpitations, nausea, and vomiting may occur. The physical examination is often normal. Breath sounds may have crackles, indicating congestive heart failure. A new heart murmur may be present. Pulses may become thready. Skin may be pale and clammy. A 12-lead ECG may show evidence of an MI (up to 40% of patients may have a nondiagnostic ECG initially). Cardiac enzymes demonstrate a characteristic pattern. | Oxygen, nitroglycerin, and aspirin are the initial therapies. Heparin is used to prevent further blood clot formation when there are no contraindications. Thrombolytic agents or angioplasty may be used to open the blocked vessel. Morphine is given for pain and anxiety. |
| Airway Obstruction | Complete or partial obstruction caused by foreign bodies, anatomical abnormalities, allergic reactions, infection, or trauma. | Probable agitation in the early phases of airway obstruction. Loss of consciousness if the obstruction is not relieved. Signs of respiratory distress (labored, ineffective breaths) until patient becomes unconscious and apneic. | Foreign body airway obstruction is treated using the Heimlich maneuver in adults and back blows and chest thrusts in infants and children. Treatment of other causes may be more advanced and specialized. |
| Angina Pectoris | Inadequate supply of oxygen to the myocardium caused by arteriosclerosis when oxygen demand exceeds supply. Unstable angina, marked by more frequent attacks, pain with less exertion or at rest, reduced response to nitroglycerin, or more severe episodes may indicate a progression in the patient's coronary artery disease and a higher risk for MI. Stable | Similar to MI. Chest discomfort is short lasting—usually less than 5 min, but may last up to 30 min. Nitroglycerin and rest usually reduce or eliminate symptoms. There may be evidence of ischemia on a 12-lead ECG. Cardiac enzymes will not demonstrate the characteristic pattern of an MI. | Oxygen, nitroglycerin, and aspirin are the initial therapies. Heparin is used in unstable angina when there are no contraindications. Generally the patient with unstable or new onset angina will require risk assessment, either in the hospital or as an outpatient. Several options include stress testing and cardiac catheterization. |

**Emergency Situations** (Continued)

| *Medical Emergency* | *Pathophysiology* | *History and Physical Examination* | *Treatment* |
|---|---|---|---|
| | angina is discomfort typical of the patient's usual pattern. | | |
| Asthma | Episodic reversible bronchospasm. Immunoglobulins released in response to various stimuli cause bronchiolar constriction, resulting in difficulty in exhalation. | Difficulty breathing, wheezing, and chest tightness. Patients are often able to identify the triggering event. They may report that their inhalers are not providing adequate relief. Physical findings include tachycardia and labored breathing. Patient may be frightened, agitated, or, in the final stages of a severe attack, sleepy. Lung sounds have a prolonged expiratory phase. The most common sound will be wheezes. In severe cases there may be no lung sounds. | Emergency treatment includes administration of nebulized bronchodilators (e.g., albuterol and oxygen). Epinephrine may be injected subcutaneously in severe cases. Oral or intravenous steroids are helpful in reducing the return of symptoms once the acute attack has been aborted. Severe cases may require intubation. |
| Cerebrovascular Accident (CVA, stroke) | Inadequate blood flow to an area of the brain causing tissue death. In thrombotic CVAs, blood vessels narrowed by atherosclerosis limit delivery of oxygenated blood to the brain or a portion of it. In embolic CVAs, clots travel from other areas of the body to block cerebral vessels. Hemorrhagic CVAs result from bleeding caused by hypertension or rupture of cerebral aneurysms. | Commonly, paresthesias, slurred speech, facial droops, hemiparesis, paralysis, and confusion. Onset may be sudden or gradual. | Emergency treatment involves oxygen administration and blood pressure control. A computed tomography (CT) scan of the brain is indicated to rule out hemorrhage as a cause of neurological deficits. Anticoagulation may be indicated if a hemorrhagic CVA is not suspected. |
| Chronic Obstructive Pulmonary Disease (COPD) | Progressive chronic emphysema and bronchitis marked by cough, dyspnea, poor gas exchange, and airway obstruction. Most cases are caused by cigarette smoking. In emphysema there is destruction of the lung parenchyma and loss of alveoli (anatomic unit where gas | Shortness of breath, labored breathing, difficulty in breathing with exertion that progresses to rest dyspnea. Often a concurrent pulmonary infection exacerbates the COPD. Tachycardia and tachypnea are present. Patient may have cyanosis. Breath sounds | Treatment generally involves supplying supplemental oxygen and attempting to relieve bronchoconstriction using inhaled bronchodilators. Antibiotics may be necessary if the patient has a respiratory infection. |

| | | | |
|---|---|---|---|
| | exchange occurs). Chronic bronchitis is caused by airway inflammation and excessive bronchial mucus production. | may be distant, with wheezes or congestion. A COPD exacerbation may be difficult to distinguish from congestive heart failure. | |
| Cold-induced soft tissue injury (frostnip, chilblain, frostbite) | *Frostnip:* superficial, reversible injury caused by ice crystal formation on the surface of the skin. *Chilblain:* superficial injury caused by exposure to cold humid air. Tissue does not freeze. *Frostbite:* destruction of tissue by freezing. The extent of tissue loss reflects the duration of cold exposure and the magnitude of temperature depression. | *Frostnip:* usually, paresthesias, pain, and numbness. *Chilblain:* redness, itching, numbness, burning, and pain. *Frostbite:* similar to chilblain. Frostbitten skin may be waxy and white or mottled and cyanotic. The frozen part will have no sensation. Surrounding tissue may be painful and tender. As the tissue thaws its appearance changes. In partial-thickness frostbite the skin becomes red and warm. Blisters containing clear fluid may appear. In full-thickness frostbite the blisters contain a bloody fluid. There is no sensation in full-thickness frostbite. | Initial treatment involves removing the patient from the cold environment. Concomitant hypothermia is a hazard. The frozen parts should not be rewarmed if there is danger of refreezing. Rapid rewarming should be performed by soaking the injured part in warm water (42°C). Rubbing or other manipulation of frozen tissue may worsen the injury. Further treatment may be needed for more serious injuries. |
| Congestive Heart Failure (CHF) | Ventricular failure resulting from cardiac ischemia, previous heart attacks, or diseased heart valves. In right-sided heart failure, fluid accumulates in dependent areas. In left-sided heart failure, fluid accumulates in the lungs. Often the patient experiences both right and left failure. | Reduced exercise tolerance, ankle edema, shortness of breath, and possible chest tightness, with either gradual or acute onset. Findings can include tachycardia, hyper- or hypotension, tachypnea, and labored breathing. Signs of right-sided heart failure include distended neck veins, ankle edema, and hepatic congestion. Wheezes or crackles may be heard in left-sided heart failure. | Emergency treatment often includes a diuretic. In left-sided heart failure, oxygen, nitroglycerin, and possibly morphine are used. Angiotensin-converting enzyme inhibitors also reduce the workload of the heart. Patients with new onset or worsening CHF may have an echocardiogram to estimate the functional capacity of the heart. |
| Gastrointestinal Bleeding | Peptic ulcers, gastritis, esophagitis, diverticular disease, hemorrhoids, or cancer. Bleeding may be mild or severe. | Digested blood resembling coffee grounds in the patient's vomitus or as black tarry stools. Red blood may appear in either stool or vomitus. Patient may or may not have pain. Significant blood loss, whether gradual | Significant blood loss will require intravenous fluids and possibly blood transfusions. A cause of the bleeding must be sought. |

**Emergency Situations** (Continued)

| *Medical Emergency* | *Pathophysiology* | *History and Physical Examination* | *Treatment* |
|---|---|---|---|
| | | or sudden, causes pallor and lightheadedness or faintness. Patient may be tachycardic with weak pulse. Hypotension may be present. | |
| Hyperglycemia | High blood glucose, caused most often by impaired glucose metabolism. It may result from inadequate insulin secretion, insulin resistance, steroid use, pregnancy, infection and, in diabetic patients, overeating. | Gradual onset of symptoms. Sick or run down feeling, frequent urination, excessive thirst or hunger. A serious infection may have caused the hyperglycemia. Patients may be significantly dehydrated due to excessive urination caused by the body's attempt to eliminate glucose via the urine. | Efforts are directed at lowering the blood glucose level. Insulin may be required. Intravenous hydration may also be useful. |
| Hyperthermia (Heat cramps, heat exhaustion, heatstroke) | Inability of the body to cope with heat stress resulting from excessive heat production or decreased heat loss. *Heat cramps:* muscle cramps and fatigue accompanied by water and mild salt depletion. *Heat exhaustion:* serious dehydration with water and electrolyte depletion. Patients maintain thermoregulatory control. Heat exhaustion may progress to *heatstroke,* characterized by thermoregulatory failure and profound dehydration. | The person with heat cramps complains of painful muscle spasms. There is a history of recent exertion in a hot environment. The patient has been sweating profusely with inadequate or hypotonic fluid replacement. The patient with heat exhaustion has also been sweating in a hot environment. Symptoms include thirst, weakness, fatigue, vomiting, and anorexia. The skin is cool and clammy. Body temperature may be normal or subnormal. The heatstroke victim will have an altered mental status and will be tachycardic, hypotensive, hyperthermic, and tachypneic. Signs of dehydration will be present. | First aid begins with removal of the patient from the hot environment. Heat cramp victims are treated with an oral or intravenous fluid and electrolyte solution. Heat exhaustion is treated by intravenous fluids. Patients with severe dehydration may require more than 4 L of IV fluid. Patients with heatstroke require rapid cooling. Many techniques are available, but evaporation with water is practical and effective. The patient may be sprayed with water and fanned until the core temperature is about 38.5°C. Cooling beyond this may cause overshoot hypothermia. IV fluid resuscitation as for heat exhaustion is also needed. |

| | | | |
|---|---|---|---|
| Hypoglycemia | Low blood glucose, typically found in diabetic patients. It generally results from excessive insulin administration or inadequate food intake. | Weakness or faintness; pale, moist skin. Mental status may vary from confused and agitated to unconscious. Onset of symptoms is sudden and progressive if untreated. Hypoglycemia may mimic CVAs or seizures. | Sugar should be given if hypoglycemia is suspected. This may be done by mouth if the patient is able to safely eat or drink. Intravenous glucose is used when the patient is unable to take sugar by mouth. Hospitalization may be necessary if the patient has taken an overdose of long-acting insulin or an oral antihyperglycemic agent. |
| Hypothermia | Core temperature less than 35°C (95°F), caused by decreased heat production, increased heat loss, or impaired temperature regulation. Central nervous system, cardiovascular, and respiratory systems are impaired when the temperature is below 35°C. | Lethargy, confusion, and fatigue in mild cases. Heart rate and respiratory rate may be increased. As hypothermia worsens the patient stops shivering. Heart rate, blood pressure, and respirations slow. The patient eventually loses consciousness. Respirations and pulses may be difficult to detect. | Treatment generally involves warming the patient. First aid includes removing the patient from exposure to cold. Wet clothing should be removed. Warm blankets, warm oxygen, and warm IV fluids may be used. An accurate core temperature must be recorded, if possible. Temperatures less than 32°C may require more aggressive rewarming techniques, such as gastric lavage, peritoneal lavage, hemodialysis, or cardiopulmonary bypass. If pulses are absent, cardiopulmonary resuscitation is indicated. |
| Seizure | Disorderly neuronal discharges from the cerebral cortex of the brain. The nature of the seizure depends on the location of the origin of abnormal activity and on its propagation through the brain. Seizures vary from behavioral or emotional changes to staring episodes or vigorous muscle contractions. Prolonged seizures can result in acidosis, hypoxia, and neuronal damage. | Most often, a previous history of a seizure disorder. During a generalized motor seizure, altered mental status and vigorous muscle activity. Patient may bite the tongue and lose control of bladder or bowel function. Trauma may occur when the patient falls to the ground. Tachycardia and irregular breathing are present. Eyes may deviate to one side or the other, or may "roll back into the head." After the seizure the patient may be unconscious initially. There is usually a gradual return to normal wakeful- | During the seizure, the patient should be guarded against injury. This may involve helping the patient to the floor and moving furniture out of the way. Supplemental oxygen should be given. Objects should not be inserted into the patient's mouth—an obstructed airway may result. The patient cannot swallow the tongue. Medications such as diazepam or phenytoin may be used. Most seizure patients will require some investigation into the cause of the seizure. This may include checking blood levels of antiseizure medications. Patients |

Emergency Situations (Continued)

| *Medical Emergency* | *Pathophysiology* | *History and Physical Examination* | *Treatment* |
|---|---|---|---|
| | | ness. The patient may not recall that a seizure has occurred. | with first-time seizures may need a more extensive evaluation, including a CT scan, an EEG, blood work, and a spinal tap. |
| Thermal burns | *First- and second-degree burns:* partial-thickness injuries involving only the epidermis or the epidermis and dermis. Third-degree burns: full-thickness injuries involving the deeper tissues. Burns impair the skin's ability to prevent heat and water loss. Burned skin is not an effective barrier to infection. Severity depends on the character and temperature of the agent, the duration of exposure, and the type of skin injured. | *First-degree burns:* red and painful. *Second-degree burns:* red, painful, and weeping. These burns heat without scarring. *Third-degree burns:* may be white or charred. The subcutaneous nerves have been destroyed; thus there is no pain. Surrounding areas are painful. Full-thickness burns heal poorly, leaving a scar. | The first step is to stop the burning process. Oxygen should be administered if there has been smoke inhalation. Jewelry and clothing should be removed in anticipation of swelling. Sterile sheets or dressings should be applied to the burned areas. The use of moist dressings is controversial; they may promote hypothermia if a large percentage of the body surface is burned. |
| Transient Ischemic Attack (TIA) | Duration <24 hr; otherwise similar to CVAs. May indicate increased risk for CVA. | Signs and symptoms similar to those of CVA, but shorter in duration. | Typical treatment is aspirin as a blood thinner and a search for the cause of TIA. A CT scan, electrocardiogram, echocardigram, and carotid artery Doppler ultrasound may be done. |

# APPENDIX 14
# Computer Glossary

**-86-xx** A designation used by the computer industry for models of the central processing unit in a microcomputer (e.g., 486-66). Newer and faster chips carry higher number designations. SEE: *central processing unit.*

**AI** *artificial intelligence.*

**ALT** *alternate.*

**alternate** ABBR: ALT. A board key that, when depressed in conjunction with other keys, sends a code to the computer instructing it to perform an operation.

**American Standard Code for Information Interchange** SEE: *ASCII.*

**application** A software package or program that performs a set of tasks (e.g., word processing, graphics, spreadsheet).

**artificial intelligence** ABBR: AI. A high-level series of computer-based processes that allows the computer to perform certain tasks "learned" from previous instructions. Complex AI systems are capable of similarly complex tasks. Medical field use is being developed in areas such as orthopedic surgery, physical therapy, and so forth.

**ASCII** *American Standard Code for Information Interchange.* A basic format for storing and transferring text-based materials from one computer or software package to another.

**attribute** A characteristic of a file (e.g., read only, system, hidden). DOS help instructions explain the use of these codes.

**autoexec.bat** A file used by an IBM-type computer on start-up to discover any instructions that should be automatically executed. Installation programs of many software packages modify this file to facilitate the operation of the computer.

**axis** Either of the two lines on a bar or line graph that act as the scale. The horizontal line is the X axis; the vertical line is the Y axis. Line graph format is often used to record the length of hospital stays.

**backup** A copy of a file, program, or disk made to prevent loss of data.

***battery b.*** A copy of a file, disk, or program created automatically when power is lost, permitting an organized shutdown of the computer. Loss of power during computer use can lead to serious data loss, which is potentially damaging to the hard disk. SEE: *universal power supply.*

**basic input/output system** ABBR: BIOS. A chip that determines how data are channeled into and out of the computer through the central processing unit chip. SEE: *central processing unit.*

**bat** *batch file.*

**batch file** SEE: under *file.*

**battery** A chip that maintains information relating to the configuration of the computer. It contains essential origination and setup information and is maintained by a battery.

**battery backup** SEE: under *backup.*

**baud** One pulse per second.

***b. rate*** A measure used to indicate speed of data transmission via a modem. Higher baud rates indicate faster transmission (e.g., 28,000 baud is faster than 14,400 baud).

**BBS** *Bulletin Board Service.*

**benchmark** A standard against which machine-operating parameters are compared. It is used to test the speed of a computer and its processor.

**binary system** A number system to "base" the system used by all microcomputers. All of the information placed into a computer is in binary form, that is, numbers made up of zeros and ones (0 and 1). In this system each "place" in a binary number represents a power of 2 (i.e., the number of times 2 is to be multiplied by itself).

**BIOS** *basic input/output system.*

**bit** Abbreviation for binary digit. Computers work with binary numbers (bytes) made up of zeros and ones (0 and 1). A bit is one such digit in a binary number. SEE: *binary system; byte.*

**bitmap** A graphic image stored as a pattern of dots. Some graphic image files are referred to as bitmap images; such files are identified by the extension *.bmp.*

**bits per second** ABBR: bps. The number of bits transmitted in a second. SEE: *bit.*

**board** SEE: *bulletin board; circuit board; clipboard; motherboard.*

**boilerplate** Text that has been prepared in one document and stored for use in others. Boilerplating is convenient for forms, headings, contract language, and paragraphs of standard text used frequently in various documents.

**boot** To start or restart a computer. All information stored in random access memory is erased, and the machine executes all initiation instructions.

***cold b.*** Initiation of a machine system by turning the computer off and then on again.

***hot b.*** Reinitiation of a program or machine system without turning off the main power switch. This is done most often by the concurrent pressing of the control, alternate, and delete (CTRL-ALT-DEL) keys. Also called *warm boot.*

**bps** *bits per second.*

**browser** A program that allows free travel through the Internet resources. Several software development services provide web browsers, which are relatively easy to install on a personal computer. The fastest modem possible should be used to facilitate the accessing and transfer of Internet data.

***web b.*** A program that provides an interface to the World Wide Web.

**buffer** A temporary storage area of computer memory that holds data until it can be processed (e.g., by a printer).

**bug** A fault in a program instruction that causes malfunction of the computer or program.

**bulletin board** A message system usually accessible by modem. It allows users a wide range of informational services. Users may advertise; receive and store electronic mail; or contact other users interested in various subjects.

**Bulletin Board Service** ABBR: BBS. A system of telephonically interconnecting computers. SEE: *bulletin board.*

**byte** A unit of data usually composed of eight bits. It takes one byte to represent an ASCII character. SEE: *binary system; bit.*

**cache** A method of storing data in a section of temporary random access memory. This method is used for storing instructions to a hard disk or video card to facilitate processing speed.

**CAD** *computer-assisted design.*

**card** A hard plastic, sometimes glass-reinforced board on which all circuit components are mounted and electrically "wired" to each other by printed copper paths. Numerous types of boards provide graphics representation, color capability, boost of storage capacity, and other features to a computer. SYN: *circuit board.*

***graphics c.*** A circuit board enabling display of graphic images.

***sound c.*** A circuit board that permits the computer to produce sound effects or text recognition in a multimedia package.

***video c.*** A plug-in board that determines proper operation of the monitor.

**carriage return** ABBR: CR. The key that indicates the decision to accept and perform a command or enter recently typed information. Until CR is used, entered data can be altered or the entire command canceled. Also called *ENTER.*

**cartridge 1.** An insertable device containing data or program information; often used with central processing units or laser printers to extend memory capacity. **2.** An insert for a laser printer or office copier containing toner.

**cathode ray tube** ABBR: CRT. Technical term for a monitor or screen.

**CD-ROM** *compact disk, read-only memory.*

**central processing unit** ABBR: CPU. The basic box or cabinet containing all of a computer's circuit boards. Sometimes only the single main chip on a circuit board (e.g., the 486 chip) is known as the CPU.

**Check Disk** ABBR: CHKDSK. A program built into MS-DOS, permitting a quick examination of the hard disk drive to make sure files are stored properly and ready to use.

**chip** An integrated circuit. Complete electronic subsystems or operating systems can be included in a single chip.

**CHKDSK** *Check Disk.*

**circuit board** Card. SEE: *motherboard.*

**click** Use of the left, middle, or right button of a mouse to initiate an action. This is equivalent to hitting the ENTER or ESCAPE key or initiating other functions of the keyboard. "Double click" is the rapid succession of two clicks on a mouse button at a specified location.

**client** In a local area network hookup, any computer that draws its information from a server. Any client may have access to all or only some programs or data stored on the server, depending on the decisions made by the systems operator. SEE: *server.*

**clipboard** A temporary storage file that holds recently cut or deleted information for subsequent retrieval. The data may be restored in either a different location or the original source. Clipboards are widely used in Windows applications for transfer to another location in the same or another application package.

**cold boot** SEE: under *boot.*

**command** An instruction issued to the computer for execution of a specific task.

**communications port** SEE: under *port.*

**communications protocol** A standard way in which one computer communicates with others or with other terminals. Protocols are usually established and selected by system managers. Names include XMODEM and KERMIT. All such protocols are software driven and mostly unseen to the casual modem user.

**compact disk, read-only memory** ABBR: CD-ROM. A storage medium that uses a laser beam to retrieve data for use by the computer. It is widely used for large data sets such as encyclopedias and full volumes of text. A full multimedia package often contains sound and video files. Writable CD-ROMs can be assembled by an author and subsequently edited.

**compatibility** The ability of one computer to run a program generated on or written for another.

**COM port** SEE: under *port.*

**compressed file** SEE: under *file.*

**computer** An electronic device for storing and retrieving numerical or textual data and for processing and analyzing numerical or mathematical data. In medicine and the biological sciences, the use of computers has made it possible to store and retrieve from quantities of data that would require an inordinate amount of space if stored in conventional files.

***laptop c.*** A small, portable computer.

***mainframe c.*** A major computer installation requiring one or more large cabinets. Mainframe computers are fixed in place.

***personal c.*** ABBR: PC. Microcomputer.

**computer-assisted design** ABBR: CAD. The use of computer systems to assist in designing two- or three-dimensional objects. Application may occur in plastic surgery or in orthopedics to design replacement parts, such as an artificial hip.

**CONFIG.SYS** A file prepared by the user to tell the machine what devices to use. It is loaded automatically on start-up.

**configuration** The manner in which hardware and software are programmed and arranged to operate a system or network.

**console** ABBR: CON. A monitor or screen.

**control** ABBR: CTRL. One of the special keys on an IBM-type computer. Depressing it in conjunction with another key or keys generates a different set of commands or characters.

**control-alternate-delete** ABBR: CTRL-ALT-DEL. Three keys that, if struck simultaneously, will reboot the computer. SEE: *boot, hot*.

**controller** A special card or a part of a hard drive. It translates the signals coming from the central processing unit into physical motion of the read-write head, as well as its read-write functions.

**conventional memory** SEE: *memory*.

**conversion** The changing of data or a file into a format different from the one in which it was generated.

**CPU** *central processing unit*.

**crash** A sudden and unexpected program termination that may cause a computer to cease operating or "hang up" and require a reboot. SEE: *hangup*.

**CRT** *cathode ray tube*.

**CTRL** *control* (key).

**CTRL-ALT-DEL** *control-alternate-delete* (keys).

**cursor** A flashing line, square, or rectangle on the monitor that moves each time a key is struck and indicates where the next keystroke will appear.

**data** (Pl. of datum) Information. Data units in order of increasing size are bit, byte, word, line, paragraph, and page. Data may be alphabetical, numerical, or graphic, and may be manipulated with all conventional mathematical functions.

***d. security*** **1.** The automatic prevention of updates to the same file by more than one operator at one time. **2.** The automatic prevention of unauthorized use or theft of information in a computer.

***d. transfer*** The moving of information from one machine to another. It is accomplished through a hard-wire direct connection, a local area network, or an intermediate telephone link.

**database** A collection of data, either numerical or textual, that has been keyed in and stored on disk or another storage medium. A database is usually created in a specific format, allowing easy insertion of future additions and sorting of information according to identified categories or sequences.

**default** A value automatically used in calculations and operations unless changed by the user. Rebooting always restores default values.

**default drive** SEE: under *drive*.

**defragment** To rearrange information using a special program that stores all files in contiguous sectors. With continual storage changes (removal of old and addition of new material), segments of one file can be scattered over the disk, which is then said to be "fragmented." This slows retrieval and causes extra wear on the drive.

**desktop publishing** ABBR: DTP. The computerized production of documents ready for duplication. The necessary equipment includes a scanner, a word processing and typesetting program, a graphics and layout program, and a laser printer.

**destination drive** SEE: under *drive*.

**device name** The names and conventional abbreviations assigned to computer system components. Major components are central processing unit (CPU), keyboard (KBD), monitor/console (CON), printer (PRN) or line printer (LPT), and communications port (COM port).

**diagnostics** The use of a special program to check the inner workings of a computer. The technician can find every bit stored and its location, as well as critical machine parameters, peripherals, and procedures.

**dialogue box** In Windows and similar programs, a menu of choices offered in a graphic area indicating that a specific response is required for the program to proceed.

**digital radiography** Radiography using computerized imaging instead of conventional film or screen imaging.

**DIR** *directory*.

**directory** ABBR: DIR. A listing of all the filenames presently in working order in a specified location or sublocation of a disk.

***root d.*** The top-level directory of a formatted disk; most often C:\. SEE: *subdirectory*.

**disk** A round plastic or metal platter coated with a magnetic medium and used for data storage.

***backup d.*** **1.** A precautionary or safety disk used to duplicate information from a master disk. Backup disks are usually used for archiving or storage and to preserve data in case the master disk is lost or damaged. **2.** A set of disks to which all of the information on a hard disk drive or floppy disks will be copied for safe storage and retrieval in case the original data are no longer usable.

***d. capacity*** The number of bytes that can be stored on a disk.

***destination d.*** The disk to which information is transferred from the source disk. SEE: *source d.*

***d. drive*** SEE: *drive*.

***floppy d.*** A thin, flexible plastic platter inside a protective covering. SYN: *diskette*.

***hard d.*** A nonremovable set of platters sealed in an airtight metal case within the central processing unit. A hard disk rotates and reacts much faster than a floppy disk drive.

***source d.*** The disk from which data are copied to the destination disk. SEE: *destination d.*

***virtual d.*** A section of the computer's random access memory that is designated to function like a hard disk drive. The advantage is that data transfer is much faster than with a mechanical drive. The disadvantage is that the data exist in the virtual memory only while the computer is turned on and must be saved to a permanent storage medium before it is turned off. Also called *virtual memory*.

**diskette** SEE: *disk, floppy*.

**disk operating system** ABBR: DOS. A basic set of files and commands that controls the computer's operation, such as input/output control or data management.

**display** A visual image of numbers, letters, and graphic characters on the monitor screen.

**document** Any body of text that is typed and stored in a file.

**documentation** Manuals, instruction books, and programs or help menus that provide guidance to a user.

**DOS** *disk operating system*.

**download** To transfer and save a program or data from a computer at a remote location. SEE: *upload*.

**drag** To move an item from one location to another by holding down the mouse button until the desired location has been reached.

**drive** The mechanism that rotates the floppy disk, or the platters in a hard disk drive, and lowers the read-write heads when data are to be transferred. Also called *disk drive*.

***default d.*** The disk drive automatically used by the computer for data storage and retrieval unless the user specifies otherwise. Usually the default drive is designated by the letter "C."

***destination d.*** The drive to which data to be stored are sent.

***disk d.*** SEE: *drive*.

***logical d.*** Partition.

***removable hard d.*** ABBR: removable HD. A hard disk drive with interchangeable modules that can be moved from one computer to another.

***tape d.*** A high-speed storage medium to receive and hold data from a computer. It is used primarily as a backup device so that data lost or damaged on the machine's hard disk drive can be restored if needed.

***zip d.*** A device that allows safe, relatively easy backup of hard drive data. The data are transferred onto 3.5-in. disk cartridges that can hold up to 100 MB. Zip drives are attached to the LPT1 (parallel) printer port and can be transported easily from one computer to another.

**driver** A set of instructions (a miniature program) that permits the central processing unit to interact with a peripheral device. The most commonly required is a printer driver, specific to the make and model of the device. Drivers are most often supplied by the equipment vendor or are included within a larger software package.

**DTP** *desktop publishing*.

**electronic mail** ABBR: e-mail. Messages created on a computer, then sent to another computer and stored there until the recipient responds. E-mail packages are used widely for rapid communication. They are usually mounted within total communications packages that allow a wide use of e-mail through the Internet. SEE: *Internet*.

**e-mail** *electronic mail*.

**EMM** *expanded memory management*.

**ENTER** A key that is the official "do it" command. Before this key is pressed, issued instructions can usually be changed or canceled. Also called *carriage return*.

**error message** A message appearing on the screen that indicates a problem with either the hardware or a software application. Most error messages may be interpreted by consulting the appropriate manual. Some error messages require interpretation by a technician.

**ESC** *escape* (key).

**escape** The key marked "ESC" on the top row of the keyboard. It is usually used to exit a specific activity within a program or to return to a menu.

**Ethernet** A major protocol and hardware for a local area network.

**.EXE** An extension used to indicate an executable file.

**executable file** SEE: under *file*.

**expanded memory** SEE: *memory*.

**expanded memory management** ABBR: EMM. A program that allocates and manages an area of expanded memory in which several programs are contending for the same locations. SEE: *memory, random access*.

**extended memory** SEE: *memory*.

**extended memory specification** ABBR: XMS memory. Extended memory accessible by using the eXtended Memory Specification. SEE: *memory*.

**extension** The three letters following the period at the end of a filename (e.g., autoexec.bat).

**external** A peripheral item, such as a modem or CD-ROM drive, that is outside the computer cabinet. It has its own power supply and must be connected by cables.

**eye-gaze communicator** An electronic (assistive) device that allows a person to control a computer by eye movement directed toward the screen or other connected device.

**fax modem** SEE: under *modem*.

**file** A collection of data, computer instructions, or text that is stored as a single unit.

***batch f.*** ABBR: bat. A file that completes more than one task (e.g., autoexec.bat).

***compressed f.*** A file that has been processed by a software routine to take up less space on a disk. Special software must be used for compressing and decompressing such files. Also called *zipped file*. SEE: *PKZIP/PKUNZIP*.

***executable f.*** A type of file that can be run from the prompt without typing in the extension. It is usually the file that makes a program operate.

***hidden f.*** A file that is not normally listed in a directory. It is not meant to be modified by a user.

**filename 1.** An assigned name given to a collection of data that enables the user to retrieve that file by name. **2.** A program that can be initiated by typing the name..

**font** The typeface, type size, and type style of a document. Fonts are easily changed in most word processing packages.

**footer** In desktop publishing, text repeated at the bottom of each page. SEE: *header*.

**format** **1.** To install the primary divisions and structure required for storage and retrieval on a new disk. All new disks must be formatted by the user unless preformatted by the manufacturer. **2.** The structural arrangement (sectors and tracks) of a disk.

**freeze** SEE: *hangup*.

**function key** Any of several keys whose designation begins with the letter "F." Alone or in conjunction with the ALT or SHIFT key, it executes many different, often programmable, routines. On most keyboards, function keys are found on the top row.

**GANTT chart** A graphic, annotated representation of a project, used for scheduling. It shows when tasks are to be started and finished, and the crews assigned to each component of the work.

**garbage in, garbage out** ABBR: GIGO. An expression indicating that flawed input will surely lead to flawed or useless output.

**GIF** *Graphical Interface Format*.

**gigabyte** A storage capacity of 1,000,000,000 bytes, used in hard-drive data storage.

**GIGO** *garbage in, garbage out*.

**gopher** A network resource client-server feature within the Internet. It is designed like a menu so that users can select areas of interest and eliminates the need for complex searching. Once the selection has been made, the gopher facilitates connection to the selected topic.

**Graphical Interface Format** ABBR: GIF. Copyright of Compuserve (pronounced "jif"). A bit-mapped file that sends instructions to the computer about what to do with each pixel of the picture (e.g., on, off, highlighted, color).

**graphics card** SEE: under *card*.

**graphic user interface** ABBR: GUI (pronounced "gooey"). A representation of icons that, when "clicked on" with a mouse, initiate specific programs or actions. Examples include Windows and OS/2.

**groupware** Software designed for use by more than one individual. It is used by groups of people working on a single project and sharing the same or similar data.

**GUI** *graphic user interface*.

**hangup** A nonoperational condition, in which the computer does not respond to any keystroke. When the computer "hangs up" (i.e., crashes or freezes), it is necessary to reboot the computer. SEE: *boot*.

**hardware** The central processing unit, monitor, keyboard, printer, and any add-on circuit boards or other devices installed in or connected to the computer.

**hard-wire** Connection by wire rather than by radio waves to interrelate two or more computers in a network.

**header** In desktop publishing, text repeated at the top of each page. SEE: *footer*.

**hertz** ABBR: Hz. A unit of frequency equal to 1 cycle/sec; in computer terminology, usually used to judge the relative speed of a machine.

**hidden file** SEE: under *file*.

**high memory** SEE: under *memory*.

**home page** On the Internet World Wide Web, an initial location related to the selected or searched topic. It may relate to a person, a corporation or institution, a subject, or combination of any of these. The content may be linked to several other locations or to similar pages. Home pages are accessed by uniform resource locators. SEE: *browser; Hypertext Markup Language; Internet; uniform resource locator*.

**hot boot** SEE: under *boot*.

**hot key** A designated key or keys, used in conjunction with a memory-resident program, that brings up the program on the screen. Using the ESCAPE key usually closes the program.

**HTML** *Hypertext Markup Language*.

**hypertext** A system of help screens interconnected in layers. Each lower or higher layer is accessible by clicking on a key word or icon. Hypertext is used in developing teaching-learning packages, home pages for the Internet, and other applications. SEE: *Hypertext Markup Language*.

**Hypertext Markup Language** ABBR: HTML. A software language used by developers to construct home pages for use on the Internet. It allows linkages with other pages, graphic files, compressed video or sound files, or simply additional text. SEE: *hypertext*.

**Hz** *hertz*.

**icon** A small symbol on the screen that corresponds to a program and is interactive with the user. Clicking on the icon will start the program or execute a specific function using the program.

**import** To bring material from a different source into a working program; most often done with text, spreadsheets, pictures, and symbols.

**input and output** ABBR: I/O. The transfer of data between the central processing unit and its peripherals.

**insert** To place a letter, number, or graphics character between two others. Text is usually typed in Insert mode. Pressing the INSERT toggle key changes the mode to Strikeover or Typeover, in which the new text replaces the existing text as it is typed in. Pressing INSERT again changes the mode back to Insert.

**INTEL** A major developer and supplier of computer chips such as (in order of increasing speed of operation) the 8088, 80286, 80386, 80486, and Pentium.

**interactive** Term used for a computer application that waits for user input and performs tasks responsively.

**interface** A connection among devices or software packages that allows compatibility or performance of a desired function. Modems are telephone interfaces, for example.

**internal** Term applied to equipment enclosed within the main computer.

**Internet** A worldwide linkage of computers designed to facilitate communication and information exchange. Features include worldwide electronic mail, home pages of information, bulletin boards, special interest groups, and file downloads to personal computers. Participation includes universities, corporations, governments, agencies, and individuals. SEE: *home page; uniform resource locator*.

**I/O** *input and output*.

**keypad** A secondary grouping of keys to the right of the typewriter keyboard similar to that of an adding machine. It contains numbers and several special keys, such as directional arrows. SYN: *numberpad*.

**joystick** A controller for video computer games. It moves the onscreen pointer left and right or up and down.

**justification** Text alignment at the left or right margin or both. Many word processing programs have automatic justification capability that may be selected through a dialogue box.

**label** In a spreadsheet, text made up of alphabetical characters, as opposed to *value*, which is numerical.

**LAN** *local area network*.

**landscape** A page orientation in which the long dimension is horizontal. SEE: *orientation; portrait*.

**laptop** A lightweight, portable computer that is usually battery operated. SEE: *notebook*.

**laser printer** SEE: under *printer*.

**LCD panel** *liquid crystal display panel*.

**liquid crystal display panel** ABBR: LCD panel. A screen that accepts output directly from a computer adapter and projects the image from the computer via an overhead projector. The panel fits over the projector like a transparency, allowing the computer screen to be greatly enlarged. This technology is effective for presentations.

**local area network** ABBR: LAN. A system of two or more computers, hard-wired to each other, in the same office or building. Special cables are required, but no telephone is involved.

**logical drive** Partition.

**login** The process of attaching an outlying computer (the client) to the server electronically. To obtain access to the local area network, the user must provide a name and password. SEE: *client; logout; server*.

**logout** The process of ending a local area network session. SEE: *login*.

**low-radiation monitor** SEE: under *monitor*.

**LPT1, LPT2, LPT3, PRN** Parallel ports through which signals flow to line printers. LPT1 and PRN are synonyms. In most cases, printers are connected to the LPT1 port of a personal computer. SEE: *port*.

**M, MB** *megabyte*.

**manual** Printed instructions that provide procedural and operational information and guidance. SEE: *documentation*.

**Massachusetts General Hospital Utility Multi-Programming System** ABBR: MUMPS. A programming language designed to handle complex data, such as patient records.

**MEDLINE** A series of databases accessible by modem through the 24-hr retrieval system provided by the National Library of Medicine. MEDLINE resources include information on the history of medicine and related sciences, toxic effects of chemical substances, cancer research projects, and the entire spectrum of patient care.

**megabyte** ABBR: M, MB. 1,048,576 bytes.

**memory** The basic volatile memory space, or random access memory area. In this area, unsaved data are processed by programs before being committed to hard storage. The first 640K are called conventional memory. The remaining 360K are expanded memory and are used for special purposes. Beyond the first 1000 K, special memory chips (usually in multiple megabytes) can be added, called extended memory. It is not unusual to recommend that a personal computer be equipped with 16 MB of random access memory (RAM). All changes made to RAM and not saved to a disk are lost when the machine is turned off.

***high m.*** The area above the first 640K of conventional random access memory. Special techniques are required to access this area.

***random access m.*** ABBR: RAM. The segment of central processing unit internal memory that is available to the user for programs, data manipulation, and storage. RAM can be changed as often as desired. All changes made to RAM are lost when the machine is turned off. SEE: *memory*.

***read-only m.*** ABBR: ROM. The portion of a computer's memory that contains permanent instructions as opposed to random access memory. ROM cannot be changed and is not lost when power is turned off. ROM information is programmed into an on-board chip.

***m. upgrade*** The addition of memory chips to provide more space for data.

***XMS m.*** *extended memory specification*.

**menu-driven** Term applied to a programming technique that permits the user to make all required choices from a list shown on the monitor. Selecting appropriate numbers or letters from the menu will help lead the user through necessary commands.

**microcomputer** A computer in which all equipment fits on a desk and is readily transportable to another location. SYN: *personal computer*.

**MIDI** *musical instrument digital interface*.

**MIDI sequencer** A program that plays or records songs in the form of musical instrument digital interface (MIDI) files.

**minicomputer** A computer with size and computing capacity between those of a mainframe computer and a microcomputer. The central processing unit is usually a floor model cabinet with hard disk drives of gigabyte capacity. A minicomputer may be moved if necessary.

**modem** An internal or external device that

allows data to be transmitted over conventional telephone lines. SEE: *fax m.; baud rate.*

***fax m.*** An external device or internal board that plugs into a personal computer, permitting the receipt and transmission of data across telephone lines. It may connect to a facsimile (fax) machine or another fax modem.

**monitor** A viewing screen, similar to a television screen, connected to a computer to enable entering and reading of text, graphics, and data.

***low-radiation m.*** A monitor designed for minimum emission of electromagnetic energy into the atmosphere.

**Mosaic** A World Wide Web client server developed by the National Center for Supercomputing Applications at the University of Illinois. A graphic user interface, it allows users to navigate easily through the Internet and to access hypertext documents relating to the designated search area. SEE: *browser.*

**motherboard** The primary circuit board containing the main central processing unit chip. All other boards, controllers, and peripherals are plugged into the motherboard, from which they derive their power and instructions.

**mouse** A hand-manipulated device that generates electrical signals in relation to its motion and position. Signals interpreted by the central processing unit reflect corresponding motion of a cursor, arrow, or other indicator on the monitor screen. Clicking a mouse button sends a specific instruction to an application.

**MS-DOS** *Microsoft disk operating system.* SEE: *disk operating system.*

**multimedia** The production of sound, animation, full-motion video, or a combination of these for learning or entertainment. CD-ROM encyclopedias, game packages, and other applications make full use of multimedia. The personal computer requires a sound card, a CD-ROM, and speakers.

**multi-task** To perform several tasks at the same time. In Windows, printing from one package and entering data into another is a use of multi-tasking capabilities.

**MUMPS** *Massachusetts General Hospital Utility Multi-Programming System* (language).

**Musical Instrument Digital Interface** ABBR: MIDI. A board that causes the computer to play music by converting computer information into analog signals that are processed by audio circuits. Information needed to play a song is stored in a MIDI file. Keyboards attached to computers use a MIDI interface.

**network** SEE: *local area network; wide area network.*

**notebook** A lightweight computer very similar to a laptop but smaller and lighter (about 4 lb).

**Novell** A major vendor of local area networks. It uses its own operating system, distinct from DOS.

**numberpad** Keypad.

**NUM LOCK** A board toggle key that forces all the calculator keys into numerical mode, so that arrows and other motion keys are no longer operational. Pressing NUM LOCK again switches back to arrow key functions.

**OCR** *optical character reader.*

**optical character reader** ABBR: OCR. A device that reads printed or handwritten characters and transforms the information into data adaptable to computer processing. It is always used with a scanner and scanning software.

**orientation** The position of the long dimension of a page—vertical (portrait) or horizontal (landscape).

**OS/2** A graphic user interface developed by IBM Corporation to run on personal computers. It is a multiprocessing operating system that can run native programs as well as programs designed for Windows and DOS.

**palette** The collection of colors available in a graphics package.

**parameter** A value that can be added to customize a command to perform a specific task. If a parameter is not specified by the user, a predetermined parameter (default) is used.

**partition** Any of several divisions of a large hard disk drive. Although physically part of the actual drive (e.g., C:), it is assigned a different letter (D:, E:) and functions as a separate unit. Modern drives, coupled with better controllers and newer versions of DOS, can handle all available disk storage space as a single drive, C:. Earlier versions of DOS could manage no more than 32 MB at a time, so that a higher-capacity drive had to be split into two or more partitions. SYN: *logical drive.*

**password** An identification code or name that allows a user access to a network, a computer, a computer program, or a computer-related service such as a bulletin board. Passwords are effective in protecting word processing files.

**PC** *personal computer.*

**Pentium** The newest computer chip; faster than the 486.

**peripheral** Any piece of equipment added to the basic computer (central processing unit, monitor, keyboard). Major peripherals include the printer, external modem, joystick, mouse, sound speakers, and external CD-ROM.

**pixel** Abbreviation for picture element; the smallest area on the screen that can be turned on or off. The greater the number of pixels, the sharper the definition of alphanumeric characters or graphic representations. Hundreds of thousands of pixels are often necessary to create a useful graphic image.

**PKZIP/PKUNZIP** A form of file compression (PKZIP) and uncompression (PKUNZIP). SEE: *file, compressed.*

**plotter** Equipment that uses one or more drawing pens to generate a graphic or pictorial image on paper.

**pocket LAN** A connector between a computer and a telephone that makes it possible to hook a remote portable or laptop computer to the server at home base. SEE: *local area network*.

**port** An input-output connection through which data flow can be directed. The mouse is connected to one of the COM ports; the printer is most often connected to LPT1, a parallel port.

***COM p.*** *communications port.*

***communications p.*** ABBR: COM port. A device used for output to any device that responds to data. Typical devices connected to COM ports are the modem and mouse.

***printer p.*** The port designated to receive the data output and route it to a printer. Possibilities are LPT1, LPT2, LPT3, and PRN (equivalent to LPT1). Most printers are connected to LPT1.

**portrait** A page orientation in which the short dimension is horizontal. SEE: *landscape; orientation.*

**printer** An keyless device that physically prints output data from a computer. Also called a *line printer*.

***inkjet p.*** A printer that generates characters by using ink cartridges and directing minute sprays of ink onto the paper. This type of printer produces high-quality color and black and white output.

***laser p.*** A printer capable of very high quality type and photographic resolution. It uses toner and a laser beam to fabricate the image on plain paper.

***line p.*** SEE: *printer.*

**printer port** SEE: under *port.*

**print-screen** A keyboard command that causes the image on the screen to be printed out on paper. The key is often marked PRT SCRN.

**prompt** A standard symbol that appears onscreen, indicating that the computer is ready to receive commands. The most common is the C:> prompt, which indicates that a command may be executed directly to the C: drive.

**RAM** *random access memory.*

**random access memory** SEE: under *memory.*

**read-only memory** SEE: under *memory.*

**remote access** A mode in which a user can control unattended terminals in another location.

**removable hard drive** SEE: under *drive.*

**removable HD** *removable hard drive.*

**resolution** The degree of detail, measured in dots per inch, that a monitor, scanner, printer, or fax machine can create in an image. Typical values range from 75 × 75 (very coarse) to 1280 × 1024 (fine).

**restore** To retrieve data from a backup source (e.g., tape, disk) and replace it on the computer's hard drive. SEE: *backup.*

**ROM** *read-only memory.*

**root directory** SEE: under *directory.*

**save** To send information to a permanent storage medium such as a disk.

**scanner** Equipment that reads characters or graphic material on a page and converts them into a computer file.

**screen-print** SEE: *print-screen.*

**screen saver** Any moving pattern that prevents burning of the screen phosphor by keeping the same material from remaining onscreen too long. It is usually activated by a timer after a few minutes of screen inactivity and is released by any keystroke.

**server** The source of data and programs for all the computers in a local area network. Any information required can be retrieved, updated, and restored. A server should not be used as an active terminal.

**setup** **1.** Preparation of the computer system for operation. **2.** The command used to install many applications in the Windows environment.

**shareware** Software that a user can obtain on a trial basis. Programs are available on disks from commercial sources for $3 to $5 or may be downloaded free from a bulletin board service. Payment of $20 to $40 is usually required if use of the program continues beyond 30 days.

**SHIFT** A board key that capitalizes all letters or accesses the characters above the numbers. It also provides alternate responses for the function keys (F1 to F12) and some other keys.

**SIG** *special-interest group.*

**software** Programs written for the computer (e.g., word processing, data processing, graphics, utilities, spreadsheets, games).

**sound card** SEE: under *card.*

**special-interest group** ABBR: SIG. Computer users who share a common focus. Segments of bulletin board service networks, Internet chat groups, and other such facilities are devoted to the use of SIGs.

**spreadsheet** A program that presents columns of numerical data; used in accounting and other administrative settings. It allows sorting of entered data and, through formulas, the modification of related cells.

**SQL** *Structured Query Language.*

**storage** A method of retaining data, text, or graphics by preserving the information on larger disk drives (hard drives) within the computer or on removable (floppy) disks. Information may be transferred from one computer to another by using data stored on removable disks.

***primary s.*** The location where data and programs are kept during processing.

***secondary s.*** The location of space not being used to store data and programs during processing.

**Structured Query Language** ABBR: SQL. A high-level language that permits almost ordinary, sentence-like expressions by the user.

**subdirectory** A directory that branches off from the root directory (e.g., C:\subdir).

**tape drive** SEE: under *drive.*

**telecommunication** The transmission of data over telephone lines. SEE: *modem.*

**terminal** A work station, usually consisting of a keyboard and monitor, with no storage device (i.e., hard disk). The terminal relies on a network server for its files and program.

*dumb t.* A work station that does not have storage facilities. It relies on a remote server for input and storage.

**Terminate and Stay Resident** ABBR: TSR. Term usually applied to a program that is not apparently accessible but can be instantly called up with one or two "hot keys." A TSR does not need to be reloaded each time it is to be used. Typical TSRs are calendars, clocks, telephone dialers, alarms, and so forth. SEE: *hot key*.

**trackball** A point-and-click device, similar to a mouse. The ball, placed at the top, is the only moving part. It is rotated by hand in any direction to achieve the desired motion on-screen.

**TSR** *Terminate and Stay Resident*.

**typeface** The design of type. Two broad categories are serif and sans serif. Serif faces vary in stroke thickness and include a thin line (finial) at the end of each stroke. A typical example is Times Roman, the typeface used in most newspapers. Sans serif (without serif) type has no thickness variation and no finials. Helvetica, most often seen in headings, is typical. SEE: *font*.

**type size** The height and width of type, expressed in points. There are 12 points per pica and 72 points per in. Newspaper type size is generally nine points. SEE: *font*.

**type style** Any variation within the same typeface family. There are four variations: normal (roman), italic, bold, and bold italic. Normal type is generally straight up and down, italic type is slanted, and bold type has a heavier body. SEE: *font*.

**uniform resource locator** ABBR: URL. An address uniquely identifying a home page within the World Wide Web Internet resource. When entered in the proper field carefully (they are case sensitive), URLs take the user directly to the identified page or area of interest. Web browsers automatically select the appropriate URLs when a search path has been executed. Also called *web page address*.

**universal power supply** ABBR: UPS. An electronically controlled emergency power source that is activated almost instantly when utility electricity is lost. The UPS keeps batteries on a trickle charge during normal operation, but during a power failure converts their stored energy into output that is usually enough for 15 min of emergency operation.

**upload** To transfer data from one computer to another at a remote site. Files that the user has prepared may be uploaded to a bulletin board or other appropriate site. SEE: *download*.

**upper memory area** From 640K to 1024K of conventional memory.

**UPS** *universal power supply*.

**URL** *uniform resource locator*.

**utility program** A program that facilitates and speeds the operation of a computer.

**value** A number or numerical symbol in a spreadsheet. SEE: *label*.

**vaporware** A denigrating nickname for computer software that is always on the verge of "coming to market" but never does.

**video** The computer monitor display, or the output to it.

**virtual disk** SEE: under *disk*.

**virus** A flaw deliberately introduced into a program to cause humorous, annoying, or destructive results. The most severe result is a disk crash, in which all data and programs are lost. Most viruses are transmitted by programs downloaded from a bulletin board service. Programs and devices are available to spot viruses and eliminate them before they activate, multiply across the system, and cause major damage. Computers should have antivirus programs installed as soon as they are purchased.

**voice recognition** The capacity of a computer to transform spoken input into electronic signals that it can process and interpret as an instruction.

**WAN** *wide area network*.

**warm boot** SEE: *boot, hot*.

**web page** SEE: *home page*.

**wide area network** ABBR: WAN. A system in which computers are linked by telephone lines. This system, spread among several buildings, may extend over several cities or even countries. SEE: *local area network*.

**Windows** A graphic user interface that depends on icons and a mouse for program manipulation selection and startup, rather than using conventional, keyed-in DOS commands.

**word wrap** The automatic movement of text to the next line when the end of a line is reached. Use of the return key is not necessary.

**World Wide Web** An extremely large set of hypertext resources (pages) found within the Internet. Web pages can be located by conducting a search on the Internet or by directly entering the universal resource locator (web page address). This resource is growing rapidly each year and can provide a wealth of information to researchers. SEE: *Internet*.

**write protect** To safeguard information on a diskette and prevent the overwriting of old material with new material. The square notch on the floppy disk is blocked, thereby preventing writing to the disk. Data on a protected disk can be read and used but not altered.

**WYSIWYG** Acronym for "What You See Is What You Get"; a program in which the printed product mimics exactly what is shown on screen.

**XMS memory** *extended memory specification*. SEE: under *memory*.

**zip drive** SEE: under *drive*.

**zipped file** SEE: *file, compressed*.

# APPENDIX 15
# Health Care Resource Organizations

## Appendix 15–1 Resource Organizations in the United States

AIDS

**American Red Cross**
National Headquarters
AIDS Education Program
Jefferson Park
8111 Gatehouse Road
Falls Church, VA 22042
(703) 206-7130

**CDC National AIDS Clearinghouse**
P.O. Box 6003
Rockville, MD 20840-6003
(800) 458-5231
(800) 243-7012 (Deaf access)

**CDC National AIDS Hot Line**
P.O. Box 13827
Research Triangle Park, NC 27709
(800) 342-AIDS
(800) 344-7432 (Spanish)
(800) 243-7889 (Deaf access)

**National Association of People with AIDS**
1413 K Street NW
Washington, DC 20005
(202) 898-0414

**National Hospice Organization**
1901 N. Moore Street, Suite 901
Arlington, VA 22209
(800) 658-8898

ALCOHOLISM
SEE: *Substance Abuse*

ALZHEIMER'S DISEASE

**Alzheimer's Association**
919 N. Michigan Avenue, Ste. 1000
Chicago, IL 60611
(312) 335-8700
(800) 272-3900

ASTHMA
SEE: *Respiratory Disorders*

BLINDNESS
SEE: *Visual Impairment*

BURNS

**American Burn Association**
c/o Secretary of Jeffrey R. Saffle, M.D.
University of Utah Medical Center
Department of Surgery
50 N. Medical Drive
Salt Lake City, UT 84132
(800) 548-2876

**National Burn Victim Foundation**
32-34 Scotland Road
Orange, NJ 07050
(201) 676-7700

CANCER

**American Cancer Society**
1599 Clifton Road NE
Atlanta, GA 30329-4251
(800) ACS-2345

**Leukemia Society of America**
600 3rd Avenue
New York, NY 10016
(212) 573-8484
(800) 955-4LSA

**National Cancer Institute**
Cancer Information Service
9000 Rockville Pike
Bethesda, MD 20892
(800) 4-CANCER

**R.A. Bloch Cancer Foundation**
4400 Main
Kansas City, MO 64111
(816) 932-8453

CEREBRAL PALSY

**United Cerebral Palsy Associations**
1660 L Street NW, Ste. 700
Washington, DC 20036
(800) USA-5UCP

DEAFNESS
SEE: *Hearing Impairment*

DEPRESSION
SEE: *Mental Health*

DIABETES

**American Diabetes Association**
1660 Duke Street
Alexandria, VA 22314
(800) ADA-DISC

**Juvenile Diabetes Foundation International**
120 Wall Street
New York, NY 10005
(800) JDF-CURE

DISABILITY

**Job Accommodation Network**
918 Chestnut Ridge Road, Ste. 1
P.O. Box 6080
Morgantown, WV 26506
(800) 526-7234

**National Rehabilitation Information Center**
8455 Colesville Road., Ste. 935
Silver Spring, MD 20919-3319
(301) 588-9284
(800) 346-2742

DIVING ACCIDENTS

**Divers Alert Network**
3100 Tower Blvd., Ste. 1300
Durham, NC 27707
(919) 684-8111

DOWN SYNDROME

**National Down Syndrome Society**
666 Broadway
New York, NY 10012
(800) 221-4602

DRUG ABUSE
SEE: *Substance Abuse*

DYSLEXIA

**Orton Dyslexia Society**
Chester Bldg., Ste. 382
860 LaSalle Road
Baltimore, MD 21286-2044
(800) ABCD-123

EATING DISORDERS

**National Association of Anorexia Nervosa and Associated Disorders**
Box 7
Highland Park, IL 60035
(708) 831-3438

ELDERLY

**American Association of Retired Persons**
601 E Street NW
Washington, DC 20049
(202) 434-2277

**American Geriatric Society**
770 Lexington Avenue, Ste. 300
New York, NY 10015
(212) 308-1414

**Gerontological Society of America**
1275 K Street NW, Ste. 350
Washington, DC 20005
(202) 842-1275

EMERGENCY RESPONSE SYSTEM

**Lifeline Systems, Inc.**
640 Memorial Drive
Cambridge, MA 01239
(800) 321-2042

EPILEPSY

**Epilepsy Foundation of America**
4351 Garden City Drive
Landover, MD 20785
(800) EFA-1000

GASTROINTESTINAL

**Crohn's and Colitis Foundation of America**
386 Park Avenue S.
New York, NY 10016-8804
(800) 932-2423

HEARING IMPAIRMENT

**Alexander Graham Bell Association for the Deaf**
3417 Volta Place NW
Washington, DC 20007
(202) 337-5220

**Better Hearing Institute**
P.O. Box 1840
Washington, DC 20013
(800) EAR WELL
(703) 642-6050

**International Hearing Society**
20361 Middlebelt Road
Livonia, MI 48512
(800) 521-5247

**National Association of the Deaf**
814 Thayer Avenue
Silver Spring, MD 20910
(301) 587-1788

HEART DISEASE

**American Heart Association**
7272 Greenville Avenue
Dallas, TX 75231-4596
(800) 242-8715

**Mended Hearts**
7272 Greenville Avenue
Dallas, TX 75231-4596
(214) 706-1442

**National Heart Savers Association**
9140 W. Dodge Road
Omaha, NE 68114
(402) 398-1993

HEMOPHILIA

**National Hemophilia Foundation**
110 Greene Street, Ste. 303
New York, NY 10012
(800) 424-2634

KIDNEY DISEASE

**American Kidney Fund**
6110 Executive Blvd., Ste. 1010
Rockville, MD 20852
(800) 638-8299

**National Kidney Foundation**
30 E. 33 Street, Suite 1100
New York, NY 10016
(800) 622-9010

LIVER DISEASE

**American Liver Foundation**
1425 Pompton Avenue
Cedar Grove, NJ 07009
(800) 223-0179

LUNG DISEASES
SEE: *Respiratory Disorders*

LUPUS ERYTHEMATOSUS

**Lupus Foundation of America**
4 Research Place, Ste. 180
Rockville, MD 20850-3226
(301) 670-9292
(800) 558-0121

MENTAL HEALTH

**Anxiety Disorders Association of America**
6000 Executive Blvd., Ste. 513
Rockville, MD 20852
(301) 231-9350

**Depression and Related Affective Disorders**
600 N. Wolfe Street
Baltimore, MD 21287-7381
(410) 955-4647

**National Depressive and Manic-Depressive Association**
730 N. Franklin Street, Ste. 501
Chicago, IL 60610
(312) 642-0049

**National Mental Health Association**
1015 Prince Street
Alexandria, VA 22314-2971
(703) 684-7722
(800) 969-NMHA

NEUROLOGICAL DISORDERS

**Amyotrophic Lateral Sclerosis Association**
21021 Ventura Blvd., Ste. 321
Woodland Hills, CA 91364
(800) 782-4747

**Multiple Sclerosis Foundation**
6350 N. Andrews Avenue
Fort Lauderdale, FL 33309
(800) 441-7055

**Muscular Dystrophy Association**
3300 E. Sunrise Drive
Tucson, AZ 85718
(602) 529-2000

**National Multiple Sclerosis Society**
733 3rd Avenue, 6th Fl.
New York, NY 10017
(212) 986-3240
(800) FIGHT-MS

**Norris MDA/ALS Center**
California Pacific Medical Center
P.O. Box 7999
San Francisco, CA 94120
(415) 923-3604

ORGAN DONATION

**Living Bank**
4545 Post Oak Place, Ste. 315
Houston, TX 77027
(800) 528-2971

**United Network for Organ Sharing**
P.O. Box 13770
Richmond, VA 23225
(800) 24-DONOR

PAIN

**American Chronic Pain Association**
PO Box 850
Rocklin, CA 95677
(916) 632-0922

**International Association for the Study of Pain**
909 NE 43rd Street, Ste. 306
Seattle, WA 98105-6020
(206) 547-6409

PARKINSON'S DISEASE

**National Parkinson Foundation**
1501 N.W. 9th Avenue
Bob Hope Road
Miami, FL 33136
(800) 433-7022

**Parkinson's Disease Foundation, Inc.**
710 W. 168th Street
New York, NY 10032
(212) 923-4700
(800) 457-6676

PESTICIDES

**National Pesticide Telecommunication Network**
Ag Chem Extension, Oregon State University
333 Weniger
Corvallis, OR 97331-6502
(800) 858-7378

RARE DISORDERS

**National Organization for Rare Disorders**
P.O. Box 9823
New Fairfield, CT 16812
(800) 999-6673

RESPIRATORY DISORDERS

**American Lung Association**
1740 Broadway
New York, NY 10019
(212) 315-8700
(800) LUNG-USA

**Asthma and Allergy Foundation of America**
11225 15th Street, NW, Ste. 502
Washington, DC 20005
(202) 466-7643
(800) 7ASTHMA

**Cystic Fibrosis Foundation**
6931 Arlington Road, No. 200
Bethesda, MD 20814
(800) 344-4823

REYE'S SYNDROME

**National Reye's Syndrome Foundation**
426 N. Lewis Street
Bryan, OH 433506
(800) 233-7393

SICKLE CELL ANEMIA

**Sickle Cell Disease Association of America, Inc.**
200 Corporate Pointe, Ste. 495
Culver City, CA 90230-7633
(800) 421-8453

SPINA BIFIDA

**Spina Bifida Association of America**
4590 MacArthur Blvd. NW, Ste. 250
Washington, DC 20007
(202) 944-3285
(800) 621-3141

SPINAL CORD INJURY

**National Spinal Cord Injury Association**
545 Concord Avenue, Ste. 29
Cambridge, MA 02138
(800) 962-9629

SUBSTANCE ABUSE

**Cottage Program International**
57 W. South Temple, Ste. 420
Salt Lake City, UT 84101-1511
(800) 752-6100

**National Families in Action**
2296 Henderson Mill Road, Ste. 300
Atlanta, GA 30345
(404) 934-6364

TAY-SACHS DISEASE

**National Foundation for Jewish Genetic Diseases**
250 Park Avenue, Ste. 1000
New York, NY 10177
(212) 371-1030

VISUAL IMPAIRMENT

**American Foundation for the Blind**
11 Penn Plaza, Ste. 300
New York, NY 10001
(212) 502-7600

**Lighthouse National Center for Education**
111 E. 59th Street
New York, NY 10022
(800) 334-5497

**National Association for Visually Handicapped**
22 W. 21st Street
New York, NY 10010
(212) 889-3141

**Recording for the Blind and Dyslexic**
20 Roszel Road
Princeton, NJ 08540
(800) 221-4792

SOURCES: Margolis, S and Moses, H, eds: The Johns Hopkins Medical Handbook, Random House, New York, 1992; and Schwartz, CA and Turner, RL: Encyclopedia of Associations: National Organizations of the U.S., ed 29, Gale Research, Detroit, 1995.

# Appendix 15–2 Resource Organizations in Canada

AIDS

**AIDS Committee of Ottawa**
207 Queens Street, 4th Fl.
Ottawa, Ontario K1P 6E5
(613) 238-5014

**Canadian Public Health Association**
National AIDS Information Clearing House
1565 Carling Avenue, Ste. 400
Ottawa, Ontario K1Z 8R1
(613) 725-3769

ALZHEIMER'S DISEASE

**Alzheimer Society of Canada**
1320 Yonge Street, Ste. 201
Toronto, Ontario M4T 1X2
(416) 925-3552

ARTHRITIS

**Arthritis Society**
250 Bloor Street E, Ste. 901
Toronto, Ontario M4W 3P2
(416) 967-1414

BIRTH DEFECTS

**AboutFace**
99 Crowns Lane, 4th Fl.
Toronto, Ontario M5R 3P4
(800) 665-3223

CANCER

**Canadian Cancer Society**
National Office
10 Alcorn Avenue, Ste. 200
Toronto, Ontario M4V 3B1
(416) 961-7223

DIABETES

**Canadian Diabetes Association**
15 Toronto Street, Ste. 800
Toronto, Ontario M5C 2E3
(416) 363-3373

EATING DISORDERS

**National Eating Disorders Information Centre**
College Wing, 1-211
200 Elizabeth Street
Toronto, Ontario M5G-2C4
(416) 340-4156
(416) 340-3440

HEARING IMPAIRMENT

**Canadian Association of the Deaf**
205-2435 Holly Lane
Ottawa, Ontario K1V 7P2
(613) 526-4785
(613) VOICE/TTY

HEART DISEASE

**Canadian Adult Congenital Heart Network**
The Toronto Hospital
200 Elizabeth Street, Rm. 12NU-119
Toronto, Ontario M5G 2C4
(416) 340-3872
(416) 340-5014

**Canadian Cardiovascular Society**
360 Victoria Avenue, Rm. 401
Westmont, Quebec H3Z 2N4
(514) 482-3407
(514) 482-6574

HEMOPHILIA

**World Federation of Hemophilia**
1310 Greene Avenue, Ste. 500
Montreal, Quebec H3Z 2B2
(514) 933-7944

KIDNEY

**Kidney Foundation of Canada**
2300 René LeVesque Blvd.
Montreal, Quebec H3Z 2Z3
(514) 938-4515

LIVER

**Canadian Liver Foundation**
365 Bloor Street E, Ste. 200
Toronto, Ontario M4W 3L4
(416) 964-1953

MENTAL HEALTH

**Canadian Mental Health Association**
1560 Yonge Street
Toronto, Ontario M4S 2Z3
(416) 484-7750

NEUROLOGICAL DISORDERS

**ALS Society of Canada**
220 - 6 Adelaide Street E
Toronto, Ontario M5C 1H6
(416) 362-0269
(800) 267-4ALS

**Canadian Association of Friedreich's Ataxia**
5620, rue C.A. Jobin
Montreal, Quebec H1P 1H8
(514) 321-8684

ORGAN DONATION

**M.O.R.E. of Ontario**
984 Bay Street, Ste. 503
Toronto, Ontario M5S 2A5
(416) 921-1130
(800) 263-2833

REPRODUCTIVE DISORDERS

**Canadian Pelvic Inflammatory Disease Society**
P.O. Box 33804, Sta. D
Vancouver, British Columbia V6J 4L6

**Infertility Awareness Association of Canada**
774 Echo Drive, Ste. 523
Ottawa, Ontario K7S 5N8
(613) 730-1322

RESPIRATORY DISORDERS

**International Cystic Fibrosis (Mucoviscidosis) Association**
323 Lippens Avenue
Montreal, Quebec H2M 1H7
(514) 381-0922

**Lung Association**
Three Raymond Street
Ottawa, Ontario K1R 1A3
(613) 230-4200

VISUAL IMPAIRMENT

**Canadian Council of the Blind**
405-396 Cooper Street
Ottawa, Ontario K2P 2H7
(613) 567-0311

SOURCE: Thurn, L, ed: Encyclopedia of Associations: International Organizations, ed 30. Gale Research, New York, 1996.

# APPENDIX 16
# Documentation System Definitions

**ALERT.** A charting system used primarily in long-term care in which the patient's chart is tagged to indicate that special charting procedures/precautions need to be initiated and followed for a specified time.

**CBE.** Acronym for *C*harting *B*y *E*xception, a system for documentation that eliminates the need to chart repetitious findings and tasks. The health care provider uses specially designed admission history and flow sheets that highlight important findings and trends. Only significant findings or exceptions to established standards of care and protocols are documented in the progress notes.

**CLINICAL PROGRESSION.** A critical path that has been enhanced by the addition of (1) nursing diagnosis, (2) intermediate and discharge goals, and (3) variance tracking. This type of plan is usually used for longer hospital stays not requiring critical care.

**CORE.** A documentation system designed to support the nursing process. Key elements include database, care plans, flow sheets, progress notes, and discharge summaries. Progress notes use a three-column format and are organized using patient *D*atabase; *A*ction of the health care provider; and *E*valuation of patient outcome.

**CRITICAL PATH.** A cause-and-effect grid that outlines usual interventions by health care providers against a timeline for a case type (diagnosis-related group; see App. 17) or otherwise defined homogeneous patient population. This type of plan is usually used in cases requiring critical care.

**DAR.** Acronym for the organizing structure for writing progress notes using Focus Charting©. Each Focus entry includes *D*atabase describing the current patient condition; *A*ction taken by the health care provider; and patient *R*esponse or outcome to the intervention.

**FACT.** Acronym for a documentation system including these key elements: *F*lowsheets for specific patient populations; standardized *A*ssessment parameters printed on the chart form; *C*oncise integrated progress notes; and *T*imely entries by health care providers at the time care is given.

**FOCUS CHARTING©.** Trademark title for a three-column format for organizing the progress notes in the patient record. The FOCUS column serves as an index. The body of the note is organized by identifying the DATAbase describing the current patient condition; ACTION taken by the health care provider; and patient RESPONSE to or outcome of the intervention.

**PIE.** Acronym for a process-oriented documentation system. The progress notes in the patient record use (P) to define the particular *P*roblem; (I) to document *I*ntervention; and (E) to *E*valuate the patient outcome. PIE charting integrates care planning with progress notes.

**POMR.** Acronym for *P*roblem-*O*riented *M*edical *R*ecord, a method of establishing and maintaining the patient's medical record so that problems are clearly stated. These data are kept in the front of the chart and are evaluated as frequently as indicated with respect to recording changes in the patient's problems as well as progress made in solving the problems. Use of this system may bring a degree of comprehensiveness to total patient care that might not be possible with conventional medical records.

**SOAP.** Acronym for an organized structure for keeping progress notes in the chart. Each entry contains the date, number, and title of the patient's particular problem, followed by the SOAP headings: *S*ubjective findings; *O*bjective findings; *A*ssessment, the documented analysis and conclusions concerning the findings; and *P*lan for further diagnostic or therapeutic action. If the patient has multiple problems, a SOAP entry on the chart is made for each problem.

**SOAPIER.** Adds to the SOAP headings listed above: documentation of *I*ntervention implemented to solve the identified problem; *E*valuation of the effectiveness of the intervention; and care plan *R*evisions indicated.

**VARIANCE.** A task or outcome that does not occur as described or within the time frame identified on a critical path or clinical progression.

APPENDIX 17

# Diagnosis-Related Groups (DRG)

| *DRG* | *Description* |
|---|---|
| 1 | Craniotomy, age >17 except for trauma |
| 2 | Craniotomy for trauma, age >17 |
| 3 | Craniotomy, age 0 to 17 |
| 4 | Spinal procedures |
| 5 | Extracranial vascular procedures |
| 6 | Carpal tunnel release |
| 7 | Peripheral and cranial nerve and other nervous system procedures with CC |
| 8 | Peripheral and cranial nerve and other nervous system procedures without CC |
| 9 | Spinal disorders and injuries |
| 10 | Nervous system neoplasms with CC |
| 11 | Nervous system neoplasms without CC |
| 12 | Degenerative nervous system disorders |
| 13 | Multiple sclerosis and cerebellar ataxia |
| 14 | Specific cerebrovascular disorders except transient ischemic attack |
| 15 | Transient ischemic attack and precerebral occlusions |
| 16 | Nonspecific cerebrovascular disorders with CC |
| 17 | Nonspecific cerebrovascular disorders without CC |
| 18 | Cranial and peripheral nerve disorders with CC |
| 19 | Cranial and peripheral nerve disorders without CC |
| 20 | Nervous system infection except viral meningitis |
| 21 | Viral meningitis |
| 22 | Hypertensive encephalopathy |
| 23 | Nontraumatic stupor and coma |
| 24 | Seizure and headache, age >17 with CC |
| 25 | Seizure and headache, age >17 without CC |
| 26 | Seizure and headache, age 0 to 17 |
| 27 | Traumatic stupor and coma, coma >1 hour |
| 28 | Traumatic stupor and coma, coma <1 hour, age >17 with CC |
| 29 | Traumatic stupor and coma, coma <1 hour, age >17 without CC |
| 30 | Traumatic stupor and coma, coma <1 hour, age 0 to 17 |
| 31 | Concussion, age >17 with CC |
| 32 | Concussion, age >17 without CC |
| 33 | Concussion, age 0 to 17 |
| 34 | Other disorders of nervous system with CC |
| 35 | Other disorders of nervous system without CC |
| 36 | Retinal procedures |
| 37 | Orbital procedures |
| 38 | Primary iris procedures |
| 39 | Lens procedures with or without vitrectomy |
| 40 | Extraocular procedures except orbit, age >17 |
| 41 | Extraocular procedures except orbit, age 0 to 17 |
| 42 | Intraocular procedures except retina, iris, and lens |
| 43 | Hyphema |
| 44 | Acute major eye infections |
| 45 | Neurological eye disorders |
| 46 | Other disorders of the eye, age >17 with CC |
| 47 | Other disorders of the eye, age >17 without CC |
| 48 | Other disorders of the eye, age 0 to 17 |
| 49 | Major head and neck procedures |
| 50 | Sialoadenectomy |
| 51 | Salivary gland procedures except sialoadenectomy |
| 52 | Cleft lip and palate repair |
| 53 | Sinus and mastoid procedures, age >17 |
| 54 | Sinus and mastoid procedures, age 0 to 17 |
| 55 | Miscellaneous ear, nose, mouth, and throat procedures |
| 56 | Rhinoplasty |
| 57 | Tonsillectomy and adenoidectomy procedures except tonsillectomy and/or adenoidectomy only, age >17 |
| 58 | Tonsillectomy and adenoidectomy procedures except tonsillectomy and/or adenoidectomy only, age 0 to 17 |
| 59 | Tonsillectomy and/or adenoidectomy only, age >17 |

**Diagnosis-Related Groups (DRG)** (Continued)

| *DRG* | *Description* |
|---|---|
| 60 | Tonsillectomy and/or adenoidectomy only, age 0 to 17 |
| 61 | Myringotomy with tube insertion, age >17 |
| 62 | Myringotomy with tube insertion, age 0 to 17 |
| 63 | Other ear, nose, mouth, and throat OR procedures |
| 64 | Ear, nose, mouth, and throat malignancy |
| 65 | Dysequilibrium |
| 66 | Epistaxis |
| 67 | Epiglottitis |
| 68 | Otitis media and URI, age >17 with CC |
| 69 | Otitis media and URI, age >17 without CC |
| 70 | Otitis media and URI, age 0 to 17 |
| 71 | Laryngotracheitis |
| 72 | Nasal trauma and deformity |
| 73 | Other ear, nose, mouth, and throat diagnoses, age >17 |
| 74 | Other ear, nose, mouth, and throat diagnoses, age 0 to 17 |
| 75 | Major chest procedures |
| 76 | Other respiratory system OR procedures with CC |
| 77 | Other respiratory system OR procedures without CC |
| 78 | Pulmonary embolism |
| 79 | Respiratory infections and inflammations, age >17 with CC |
| 80 | Respiratory infections and inflammations, age >17 without CC |
| 81 | Respiratory infections and inflammations, age 0 to 17 |
| 82 | Respiratory neoplasms |
| 83 | Major chest trauma with CC |
| 84 | Major chest trauma without CC |
| 85 | Pleural effusion with CC |
| 86 | Pleural effusion without CC |
| 87 | Pulmonary edema and respiratory failure |
| 88 | Chronic obstructive pulmonary disease |
| 89 | Simple pneumonia and pleurisy, age >17 with CC |
| 90 | Simple pneumonia and pleurisy, age >17 without CC |
| 91 | Simple pneumonia and pleurisy, age 0 to 17 |
| 92 | Interstitial lung disease with CC |
| 93 | Interstitial lung disease without CC |
| 94 | Pneumothorax with CC |
| 95 | Pneumothorax without CC |
| 96 | Bronchitis and asthma, age >17 with CC |
| 97 | Bronchitis and asthma, age >17 without CC |
| 98 | Bronchitis and asthma, age 0 to 17 |
| 99 | Respiratory signs and symptoms with CC |
| 100 | Respiratory signs and symptoms without CC |
| 101 | Other respiratory system diagnoses with CC |
| 102 | Other respiratory system diagnoses without CC |
| 103 | Heart transplant |
| 104 | Cardiac valve procedures with cardiac catheterization |
| 105 | Cardiac valve procedures without cardiac catheterization |
| 106 | Coronary bypass with cardiac catheterization |
| 107 | Coronary bypass without cardiac catheterization |
| 108 | Other cardiothoracic procedures |
| 109 | No longer valid |
| 110 | Major cardiovascular procedures with CC |
| 111 | Major cardiovascular procedures without CC |
| 112 | Percutaneous cardiovascular procedures |
| 113 | Amputation for circulatory system disorders except upper limb and toe |
| 114 | Upper limb and toe amputation for circulatory system disorders |
| 115 | Permanent cardiac pacemaker implant with AMI, heart failure, or shock |
| 116 | Other permanent cardiac pacemaker implant or AICD lead or generator procedure |
| 117 | Cardiac pacemaker revision except device replacement |
| 118 | Cardiac pacemaker device replacement |
| 119 | Vein ligation and stripping |
| 120 | Other circulatory system OR procedures |
| 121 | Circulatory disorders with AMI and cardiovascular complication, discharged alive |
| 122 | Circulatory disorders with AMI without cardiovascular complication, discharged alive |
| 123 | Circulatory disorders with AMI, expired |
| 124 | Circulatory disorders except AMI with cardiac catheterization and complex diagnosis |

**Diagnosis-Related Groups (DRG)** (Continued)

| *DRG* | *Description* |
|---|---|
| 125 | Circulatory disorders except AMI with cardiac catheterization without complex diagnosis |
| 126 | Acute and subacute endocarditis |
| 127 | Heart failure and shock |
| 128 | Deep vein thrombophlebitis |
| 129 | Cardiac arrest, unexplained |
| 130 | Peripheral vascular disorders with CC |
| 131 | Peripheral vascular disorders without CC |
| 132 | Atherosclerosis with CC |
| 133 | Atherosclerosis without CC |
| 134 | Hypertension |
| 135 | Cardiac congenital and valvular disorders, age >17 with CC |
| 136 | Cardiac congenital and valvular disorders, age >17 without CC |
| 137 | Cardiac congenital and valvular disorders, age 0 to 17 |
| 138 | Cardiac arrhythmia and conduction disorders with CC |
| 139 | Cardiac arrhythmia and conduction disorders without CC |
| 140 | Angina pectoris |
| 141 | Syncope and collapse with CC |
| 142 | Syncope and collapse without CC |
| 143 | Chest pain |
| 144 | Other circulatory system diagnoses with CC |
| 145 | Other circulatory system diagnoses without CC |
| 146 | Rectal resection with CC |
| 147 | Rectal resection without CC |
| 148 | Major small and large bowel procedures with CC |
| 149 | Major small and large bowel procedures without CC |
| 150 | Peritoneal adhesiolysis with CC |
| 151 | Peritoneal adhesiolysis without CC |
| 152 | Minor small and large bowel procedures with CC |
| 153 | Minor small and large bowel procedures without CC |
| 154 | Stomach, esophageal, and duodenal procedures, age >17 with CC |
| 155 | Stomach, esophageal, and duodenal procedures, age >17 without CC |
| 156 | Stomach, esophageal, and duodenal procedures, age 0 to 17 |
| 157 | Anal and stomal procedures with CC |
| 158 | Anal and stomal procedures without CC |
| 159 | Hernia procedures except inguinal and femoral, age >17 with CC |
| 160 | Hernia procedures except inguinal and femoral, age >17 without CC |
| 161 | Inguinal and femoral hernia procedures, age >17 with CC |
| 162 | Inguinal and femoral hernia procedures, age >17 without CC |
| 163 | Hernia procedures, age 0 to 17 |
| 164 | Appendectomy with complicated principal diagnosis with CC |
| 165 | Appendectomy with complicated principal diagnosis without CC |
| 166 | Appendectomy without complicated principal diagnosis with CC |
| 167 | Appendectomy without complicated principal diagnosis without CC |
| 168 | Mouth procedures with CC |
| 169 | Mouth procedures without CC |
| 170 | Other digestive system OR procedures with CC |
| 171 | Other digestive system OR procedures without CC |
| 172 | Digestive malignancy with CC |
| 173 | Digestive malignancy without CC |
| 174 | GI hemorrhage with CC |
| 175 | GI hemorrhage without CC |
| 176 | Complicated peptic ulcer |
| 177 | Uncomplicated peptic ulcer with CC |
| 178 | Uncomplicated peptic ulcer without CC |
| 179 | Inflammatory bowel disease |
| 180 | GI obstruction with CC |
| 181 | GI obstruction without CC |
| 182 | Esophagitis, gastroenteritis, and miscellaneous digestive disorders, age >17 with CC |
| 183 | Esophagitis, gastroenteritis, and miscellaneous digestive disorders, age >17 without CC |
| 184 | Esophagitis, gastroenteritis, and miscellaneous digestive disorders, age 0 to 17 |
| 185 | Dental and oral diseases except extractions and restorations, age >17 |
| 186 | Dental and oral diseases except extractions and restorations, age 0 to 17 |
| 187 | Dental extractions and restorations |
| 188 | Other digestive system diagnoses, age >17 with CC |

Diagnosis-Related Groups (DRG) (Continued)

| DRG | Description |
|---|---|
| 189 | Other digestive system diagnoses, age >17 without CC |
| 190 | Other digestive system diagnoses, age 0 to 17 |
| 191 | Pancreas, liver, and shunt procedures with CC |
| 192 | Pancreas, liver, and shunt procedures without CC |
| 193 | Biliary tract procedures except only cholecystectomy with or without common duct exploration with CC |
| 194 | Biliary tract procedures except only cholecystectomy with or without common duct exploration without CC |
| 195 | Cholecystectomy with common duct exploration with CC |
| 196 | Cholecystectomy with common duct exploration without CC |
| 197 | Cholecystectomy except by laparoscope without common duct exploration with CC |
| 198 | Cholecystectomy except by laparoscope without common duct exploration without CC |
| 199 | Hepatobiliary diagnostic procedure for malignancy |
| 200 | Hepatobiliary diagnostic procedure for nonmalignancy |
| 201 | Other hepatobiliary or pancreas OR procedures |
| 202 | Cirrhosis and alcoholic hepatitis |
| 203 | Malignancy of hepatobiliary system or pancreas |
| 204 | Disorders of pancreas except malignancy |
| 205 | Disorders of liver except malignancy, cirrhosis, and alcoholic hepatitis with CC |
| 206 | Disorders of liver except malignancy, cirrhosis, and alcoholic hepatitis without CC |
| 207 | Disorders of the biliary tract with CC |
| 208 | Disorders of the biliary tract without CC |
| 209 | Major joint and limb reattachment procedures of lower extremity |
| 210 | Hip and femur procedures except major joint procedures, age >17 with CC |
| 211 | Hip and femur procedures except major joint procedures, age >17 without CC |
| 212 | Hip and femur procedures except major joint procedures, age 0 to 17 |
| 213 | Amputation for musculoskeletal system and connective tissue disorders |
| 214 | Back and neck procedures with CC |
| 215 | Back and neck procedures without CC |
| 216 | Biopsies of musculoskeletal system and connective tissue |
| 217 | Wound debridement and skin graft except hand for musculoskeletal and connective tissue disorders |
| 218 | Lower extremity and humerus procedures except hip, foot, and femur, age >17 with CC |
| 219 | Lower extremity and humerus procedures except hip, foot, and femur, age >17 without CC |
| 220 | Lower extremity and humerus procedures except hip, foot, and femur, age 0 to 17 |
| 221 | Knee procedures with CC |
| 222 | Knee procedures without CC |
| 223 | Major shoulder/elbow procedures or other upper extremity procedures with CC |
| 224 | Shoulder, elbow, or forearm procedures except major joint procedures without CC |
| 225 | Foot procedures |
| 226 | Soft tissue procedures with CC |
| 227 | Soft tissue procedures without CC |
| 228 | Major thumb or joint procedures or other hand or wrist procedures with CC |
| 229 | Hand or wrist procedures except major joint procedures without CC |
| 230 | Local excision and removal of internal fixation devices of hip and femur |
| 231 | Local excision and removal of internal fixation devices except hip and femur |
| 232 | Arthroscopy |
| 233 | Other musculoskeletal system and connective tissue OR procedures with CC |
| 234 | Other musculoskeletal system and connective tissue OR procedures without CC |
| 235 | Fractures of femur |
| 236 | Fractures of hip and pelvis |
| 237 | Sprains, strains, and dislocations of hip, pelvis, and thigh |
| 238 | Osteomyelitis |
| 239 | Pathological fractures and musculoskeletal and connective tissue malignancy |
| 240 | Connective tissue disorders with CC |
| 241 | Connective tissue disorders without CC |
| 242 | Septic arthritis |
| 243 | Medical back problems |
| 244 | Bone diseases and specific arthropathies with CC |
| 245 | Bone diseases and specific arthropathies without CC |
| 246 | Nonspecific arthropathies |
| 247 | Signs and symptoms of musculoskeletal system and connective tissue |
| 248 | Tendonitis, myositis, and bursitis |
| 249 | Aftercare, musculoskeletal system and connective tissue |

**Diagnosis-Related Groups (DRG)** (Continued)

| *DRG* | *Description* |
|---|---|
| 250 | Fractures, sprains, strains, and dislocations of forearm, hand, and foot, age >17 with CC |
| 251 | Fractures, sprains, strains, and dislocations of forearm, hand, and foot, age >17 without CC |
| 252 | Fractures, sprains, strains, and dislocations of forearm, hand, and foot, age 0 to 17 |
| 253 | Fractures, sprains, strains, and dislocations of upper arm and lower leg except foot, age >17 with CC |
| 254 | Fractures, sprains, strains, and dislocations of upper arm and lower leg except foot, age >17 without CC |
| 255 | Fractures, sprains, strains, and dislocations of upper arm and lower leg except foot, age 0 to 17 |
| 256 | Other musculoskeletal system and connective tissue diagnoses |
| 257 | Total mastectomy for malignancy with CC |
| 258 | Total mastectomy for malignancy without CC |
| 259 | Subtotal mastectomy for malignancy with CC |
| 260 | Subtotal mastectomy for malignancy without CC |
| 261 | Breast procedure for nonmalignancy except biopsy and local excision |
| 262 | Breast biopsy and local excision for nonmalignancy |
| 263 | Skin graft and/or debridement for skin ulcer or cellulitis with CC |
| 264 | Skin graft and/or debridement for skin ulcer or cellulitis without CC |
| 265 | Skin graft and/or debridement except for skin ulcer or cellulitis with CC |
| 266 | Skin graft and/or debridement except for skin ulcer or cellulitis without CC |
| 267 | Perianal and pilonidal procedures |
| 268 | Skin, subcutaneous tissue, and breast plastic procedures |
| 269 | Other skin, subcutaneous tissue, and breast procedures with CC |
| 270 | Other skin, subcutaneous tissue, and breast procedures without CC |
| 271 | Skin ulcers |
| 272 | Major skin disorders with CC |
| 273 | Major skin disorders without CC |
| 274 | Malignant breast disorders with CC |
| 275 | Malignant breast disorders without CC |
| 276 | Nonmalignant breast disorders |
| 277 | Cellulitis, age >17 with CC |
| 278 | Cellulitis, age >17 without CC |
| 279 | Cellulitis, age 0 to 17 |
| 280 | Trauma to skin, subcutaneous tissue, and breast, age >17 with CC |
| 281 | Trauma to skin, subcutaneous tissue, and breast, age >17 without CC |
| 282 | Trauma to skin, subcutaneous tissue, and breast, age 0 to 17 |
| 283 | Minor skin disorders with CC |
| 284 | Minor skin disorders without CC |
| 285 | Amputation of lower limb for endocrine, nutritional, and metabolic disorders |
| 286 | Adrenal and pituitary procedures |
| 287 | Skin grafts and wound debridement for endocrine, nutritional, and metabolic disorders |
| 288 | OR procedures for obesity |
| 289 | Parathyroid procedures |
| 290 | Thyroid procedures |
| 291 | Thyroglossal procedures |
| 292 | Other endocrine, nutritional, and metabolic OR procedures with CC |
| 293 | Other endocrine, nutritional, and metabolic OR procedures without CC |
| 294 | Diabetes, age >35 |
| 295 | Diabetes, age 0 to 35 |
| 296 | Nutritional and miscellaneous metabolic disorders, age >17 with CC |
| 297 | Nutritional and miscellaneous metabolic disorders, age >17 without CC |
| 298 | Nutritional and miscellaneous metabolic disorders, age 0 to 17 |
| 299 | Inborn errors of metabolism |
| 300 | Endocrine disorders with CC |
| 301 | Endocrine disorders without CC |
| 302 | Kidney transplant |
| 303 | Kidney, ureter, and major bladder procedures for neoplasm |
| 304 | Kidney, ureter, and major bladder procedures for nonneoplasms with CC |
| 305 | Kidney, ureter, and major bladder procedures for nonneoplasms without CC |
| 306 | Prostatectomy with CC |
| 307 | Prostatectomy without CC |
| 308 | Minor bladder procedures with CC |
| 309 | Minor bladder procedures without CC |
| 310 | Transurethral procedures with CC |

**Diagnosis-Related Groups (DRG)** (Continued)

| *DRG* | *Description* |
|---|---|
| 311 | Transurethral procedures without CC |
| 312 | Urethral procedures, age >17 with CC |
| 313 | Urethral procedures, age >17 without CC |
| 314 | Urethral procedures, age 0 to 17 |
| 315 | Other kidney and urinary tract OR procedures |
| 316 | Renal failure |
| 317 | Admission for renal dialysis |
| 318 | Kidney and urinary tract neoplasms with CC |
| 319 | Kidney and urinary tract neoplasms without CC |
| 320 | Kidney and urinary tract infections, age >17 with CC |
| 321 | Kidney and urinary tract infections, age >17 without CC |
| 322 | Kidney and urinary tract infections, age 0 to 17 |
| 323 | Urinary stones with CC and/or ESW lithotripsy |
| 324 | Urinary stones without CC |
| 325 | Kidney and urinary tract signs and symptoms, age >17 with CC |
| 326 | Kidney and urinary tract signs and symptoms, age >17 without CC |
| 327 | Kidney and urinary tract signs and symptoms, age 0 to 17 |
| 328 | Urethral stricture, age >17 with CC |
| 329 | Urethral stricture, age >17 without CC |
| 330 | Urethral stricture, age 0 to 17 |
| 331 | Other kidney and urinary tract diagnoses, age >17 with CC |
| 332 | Other kidney and urinary tract diagnoses, age >17 without CC |
| 333 | Other kidney and urinary tract diagnoses, age 0 to 17 |
| 334 | Major male pelvic procedures with CC |
| 335 | Major male pelvic procedures without CC |
| 336 | Transurethral prostatectomy with CC |
| 337 | Transurethral prostatectomy without CC |
| 338 | Testes procedures for malignancy |
| 339 | Testes procedures for nonmalignancy, age >17 |
| 340 | Testes procedures for nonmalignancy, age 0 to 17 |
| 341 | Penis procedures |
| 342 | Circumcision, age >17 |
| 343 | Circumcision, age 0 to 17 |
| 344 | Other male reproductive system OR procedures for malignancy |
| 345 | Other male reproductive system OR procedures except for malignancy |
| 346 | Malignancy of male reproductive system with CC |
| 347 | Malignancy of male reproductive system without CC |
| 348 | Benign prostatic hypertrophy with CC |
| 349 | Benign prostatic hypertrophy without CC |
| 350 | Inflammation of the male reproductive system |
| 351 | Sterilization, male |
| 352 | Other male reproductive system diagnoses |
| 353 | Pelvic evisceration, radical hysterectomy, and radical vulvectomy |
| 354 | Uterine and adnexa procedures for nonovarian/adnexal malignancy with CC |
| 355 | Uterine and adnexa procedures for nonovarian/adnexal malignancy without CC |
| 356 | Female reproductive system reconstructive procedures |
| 357 | Uterine and adnexa procedures for ovarian or adnexal malignancy |
| 358 | Uterine and adnexa procedures for nonmalignancy with CC |
| 359 | Uterine and adnexa procedures for nonmalignancy without CC |
| 360 | Vagina, cervix, and vulva procedures |
| 361 | Laparoscopy and incisional tubal interruption |
| 362 | Endoscopic tubal interruption |
| 363 | D and C, conization, and radioimplant for malignancy |
| 364 | D and C, conization except for malignancy |
| 365 | Other female reproductive system OR procedures |
| 366 | Malignancy of female reproductive system with CC |
| 367 | Malignancy of female reproductive system without CC |
| 368 | Infections of female reproductive system |
| 369 | Menstrual and other female reproductive system disorders |
| 370 | Cesarean section with CC |
| 371 | Cesarean section without CC |
| 372 | Vaginal delivery with complicating diagnoses |
| 373 | Vaginal delivery without complicating diagnoses |
| 374 | Vaginal delivery with sterilization and/or D and C |
| 375 | Vaginal delivery with OR procedure except sterilization and/or D and C |
| 376 | Postpartum and postabortion diagnoses without OR procedure |

**Diagnosis-Related Groups (DRG)** (Continued)

| *DRG* | *Description* |
|---|---|
| 377 | Postpartum and postabortion diagnoses with OR procedure |
| 378 | Ectopic pregnancy |
| 379 | Threatened abortion |
| 380 | Abortion without D and C |
| 381 | Abortion with D and C, aspiration curettage, or hysterotomy |
| 382 | False labor |
| 383 | Other antepartum diagnoses with medical complications |
| 384 | Other antepartum diagnoses without medical complications |
| 385 | Neonates, died or transferred to another acute care facility |
| 386 | Extreme immaturity or respiratory distress syndrome of neonate |
| 387 | Prematurity with major problems |
| 388 | Prematurity without major problems |
| 389 | Full-term neonate with major problems |
| 390 | Neonate with other significant problems |
| 391 | Normal newborn |
| 392 | Splenectomy, age >17 |
| 393 | Splenectomy, age 0 to 17 |
| 394 | Other OR procedures of the blood and blood-forming organs |
| 395 | Red blood cell disorders, age >17 |
| 396 | Red blood cell disorders, age 0 to 17 |
| 397 | Coagulation disorders |
| 398 | Reticuloendothelial and immunity disorders with CC |
| 399 | Reticuloendothelial and immunity disorders without CC |
| 400 | Lymphoma and leukemia with major OR procedures |
| 401 | Lymphoma and nonacute leukemia with other OR procedure with CC |
| 402 | Lymphoma and nonacute leukemia with other OR procedure without CC |
| 403 | Lymphoma and nonacute leukemia with CC |
| 404 | Lymphoma and nonacute leukemia without CC |
| 405 | Acute leukemia without major OR procedure, age 0 to 17 |
| 406 | Myeloproliferative disorders or poorly differentiated neoplasms with major OR procedures with CC |
| 407 | Myeloproliferative disorders or poorly differentiated neoplasms with major OR procedures without CC |
| 408 | Myeloproliferative disorders or poorly differentiated neoplasms with other OR procedures |
| 409 | Radiotherapy |
| 410 | Chemotherapy without acute leukemia as secondary diagnosis |
| 411 | History of malignancy without endoscopy |
| 412 | History of malignancy with endoscopy |
| 413 | Other myeloproliferative disorders or poorly differentiated neoplasm diagnoses with CC |
| 414 | Other myeloproliferative disorders or poorly differentiated neoplasm diagnoses without CC |
| 415 | OR procedure for infectious and parasitic diseases |
| 416 | Septicemia, age >17 |
| 417 | Septicemia, age 0 to 17 |
| 418 | Postoperative and posttraumatic infections |
| 419 | Fever of unknown origin, age >17 with CC |
| 420 | Fever of unknown origin, age >17 without CC |
| 421 | Viral illness, age >17 |
| 422 | Viral illness and fever of unknown origin, age 0 to 17 |
| 423 | Other infectious and parasitic diseases diagnoses |
| 424 | OR procedures with principal diagnosis of mental illness |
| 425 | Acute adjustment reactions and disturbances of psychosocial dysfunction |
| 426 | Depressive neuroses |
| 427 | Neuroses except depressive |
| 428 | Disorders of personality and impulse control |
| 429 | Organic disturbances and mental retardation |
| 430 | Psychoses |
| 431 | Childhood mental disorders |
| 432 | Other mental disorder diagnoses |
| 433 | Alcohol/drug abuse or dependence, left against medical advice |
| 434 | Alcohol/drug abuse or dependence, detoxification, or other symptomatic treatment with CC |
| 435 | Alcohol/drug abuse or dependence, detoxification, or other symptomatic treatment without CC |

**Diagnosis-Related Groups (DRG)** (Continued)

| *DRG* | *Description* |
|---|---|
| 436 | Alcohol/drug dependence with rehabilitation therapy |
| 437 | Alcohol/drug dependence with combined rehabilitation and detoxification therapy |
| 438 | No longer valid |
| 439 | Skin grafts for injuries |
| 440 | Wound debridements for injuries |
| 441 | Hand procedures for injuries |
| 442 | Other OR procedures for injuries with CC |
| 443 | Other OR procedures for injuries without CC |
| 444 | Traumatic injury, age >17 with CC |
| 445 | Traumatic injury, age >17 without CC |
| 446 | Traumatic injury, age 0 to 17 |
| 447 | Allergic reactions, age >17 |
| 448 | Allergic reactions, age 0 to 17 |
| 449 | Poisoning and toxic effects of drugs, age >17 with CC |
| 450 | Poisoning and toxic effects of drugs, age >17 without CC |
| 451 | Poisoning and toxic effects of drugs, age 0 to 17 |
| 452 | Complications of treatment with CC |
| 453 | Complications of treatment without CC |
| 454 | Other injury, poisoning and toxic effect diagnoses with CC |
| 455 | Other injury, poisoning, and toxic effect diagnoses without CC |
| 456 | Burns, transferred to another acute care facility |
| 457 | Extensive burns without OR procedure |
| 458 | Nonextensive burns with skin graft |
| 459 | Nonextensive burns with wound debridement or other OR procedure |
| 460 | Nonextensive burns without OR procedure |
| 461 | OR procedures with diagnoses of other contact with health services |
| 462 | Rehabilitation |
| 463 | Signs and symptoms with CC |
| 464 | Signs and symptoms without CC |
| 465 | Aftercare with history of malignancy as secondary diagnosis |
| 466 | Aftercare without history of malignancy as secondary diagnosis |
| 467 | Other factors influencing health status |
| 468 | Extensive OR procedure unrelated to principal diagnosis |
| 469 | Principal diagnosis invalid as discharge diagnosis |
| 470 | Ungroupable |
| 471 | Bilateral or multiple major joint procedures of lower extremity |
| 472 | Extensive burns with OR procedure |
| 473 | Acute leukemia without major OR procedure, age >17 |
| 474 | No longer valid |
| 475 | Respiratory system diagnosis with ventilator support |
| 476 | Prostatic OR procedure unrelated to principal diagnosis |
| 477 | Nonextensive OR procedure unrelated to principal diagnosis |
| 478 | Other vascular procedures with CC |
| 479 | Other vascular procedures without CC |
| 480 | Liver transplant |
| 481 | Bone marrow transplant |
| 482 | Tracheostomy for face, mouth, and neck diagnoses |
| 483 | Tracheostomy except for face, mouth, and neck diagnoses |
| 484 | Craniotomy for multiple significant trauma |
| 485 | Limb reattachment, hip, and femur procedures for multiple significant trauma |
| 486 | Other OR procedures for multiple significant trauma |
| 487 | Other multiple significant trauma |
| 488 | HIV with extensive OR procedure |
| 489 | HIV with major related condition |
| 490 | HIV with or without other related condition |
| 491 | Major joint and limb reattachment procedures of upper extremity |
| 492 | Chemotherapy with acute leukemia as secondary diagnosis |
| 493 | Laparoscopic cholecystectomy without common duct exploration with CC |
| 494 | Laparoscopic cholecystectomy without common duct exploration without CC |
| 495 | Lung transplant |

AICD = automatic implantable cardioverter-defibrillator; AMI = acute myocardial infarction; CC = comorbidity or complication; D and C = dilation and curettage; ESW = extracorporeal shock wave; GI = gastrointestinal; HIV = human immunodeficiency virus; OR = operating room
SOURCE: DRG Guidebook, St. Anthony Publishing, Reston, VA, 1995, with permission.

# APPENDIX 18
# Professional Designations and Titles in the Health Sciences

ACCE ASPO (American Society for Psychoprophylaxis in Obstetrics) Certified Childbirth Educator
AOCN American Oncology Certified Nurse
ARRT American Registry of Radiologic Technologists
ART Accredited Record Technologist
ATC Athletic Trainer, Certified
BS Bachelor of Science; Bachelor of Surgery
BSN Bachelor of Science in Nursing
CAPA Certified Ambulatory Post-Anesthesia Nurse
CARN Certified Addiction Registered Nurse
CB Bachelor of Surgery
CCCN Certified Continence Care Nurse
CCM Certified Case Manager
CCP Certified Clinical Perfusionist
CCRN Certified Critical Care Registered Nurse
CDE Certified Diabetes Educator
CEN Certified Emergency Nurse
CETN Certified Enterostomal Therapy Nurse
CFNP Certified Family Nurse Practitioner
CFRN Certified Flight Registered Nurse
CGN Certified Gastroenterology Nurse
CGRN Certified Gastroenterology Registered Nurse
CGT Certified Gastroenterology Technician
ChB Bachelor of Surgery
ChD Doctor of Surgery
CHN Certified Hemodialysis Nurse
CIC Certified Infection Control Nurse
CLPNI Certified Licensed Practitioner Nursing, Intravenous
CLS Clinical Laboratory Scientist
CMA-A Certified Medical Assistant, Administrative
CMA-C Certified Medical Assistant, Clinical
CNA Certified Nursing Assistant; Certified in Nursing Administration
CNAA Certified in Nursing Administration, Advanced
CNDLTC Certified Nursing Director of Long-Term Care
CNM Certified Nurse Midwife
CNMT Certified Nuclear Medical Technologist
CNN Certified Nephrology Nurse
CNOR Certified Nurse, Operating Room
CNRN Certified Neuroscience Registered Nurse
CNSN Certified Nutrition Support Nurse
COCN Certified Ostomy Care Nurse
COHN Certified Occupational Health Nurse
COHN-S Certified Occupational Health Nurse—Specialty
CORLN Certified Otorhinolaryngology Nurse
CPAN Certified Post-Anesthesia Nurse
CPDN Certified Peritoneal Dialysis Nurse
CPN Certified Pediatric Nurse
CPNP Certified Pediatric Nurse Practitioner
CPON Certified Pediatric Oncology Nurse
CPSN Certified Plastic Surgical Nurse
CRNA Certified Registered Nurse Anesthetist
CRNFA Certified Registered Nurse, First Assistant
CRNH Certified Registered Hospice Nurse
CRNI Certified Registered Nurse, Intravenous
CRNO Certified Registered Nurse, Ophthalmology
CRRN Certified Rehabilitation Registered Nurse
CRTT Certified Respiratory Therapy Technician
CSN Certified School Nurse
CURN Certified Urology Registered Nurse
CWCN Certified Wound Care Nurse
DC Doctor of Chiropractic
DCh Doctor of Surgery
DDS Doctor of Dental Surgery
DMD Doctor of Dental Medicine
DME Doctor of Medical Education
DMSc Doctor of Medical Science
DO Doctor of Osteopathy; Doctor of Optometry
DP Doctor of Pharmacy
DPH Doctor of Public Health
DPhil Doctor of Philosophy
DPM Doctor of Podiatric Medicine
DrPH Doctor of Public Health
DS Doctor of Science

| | |
|---|---|
| **DSc** | Doctor of Science |
| **DSW** | Doctor of Social Work |
| **EdD** | Doctor of Education |
| **EMT-B** | Emergency Medical Technician—Basic |
| **EMT-D** | Emergency Medical Technician—Defibrillation |
| **EMT-I** | Emergency Medical Technician—Intermediate |
| **EMT-P** | Emergency Medical Technician—Paramedic |
| **FAAFP** | Fellow of the American Academy of Family Physicians |
| **FAAN** | Fellow of the American Academy of Nursing |
| **FACC** | Fellow of the American College of Cardiology |
| **FACP** | Fellow of the American College of Physicians |
| **FACS** | Fellow of the American College of Surgeons |
| **FACSM** | Fellow of the American College of Sports Medicine |
| **FAOTA** | Fellow of the American Occupational Therapy Association |
| **FAPHA** | Fellow of the American Public Health Association |
| **FCPS** | Fellow of the College of Physicians and Surgeons |
| **FFA** | Fellow of the Faculty of Anaesthetists |
| **FFARCS** | Fellow of the Faculty of Anaesthetists of the Royal College of Surgeons |
| **FNP** | Family Nurse Practitioner |
| **FP** | Family Practitioner |
| **FRCGP** | Fellow of the Royal College of General Practitioners |
| **FRCOG** | Fellow of the Royal College of Obstetricians and Gynaecologists |
| **FRCP** | Fellow of the Royal College of Physicians |
| **FRCPC** | Fellow of the Royal College of Physicians of Canada |
| **FRCR** | Fellow of the Royal College of Radiologists |
| **FRCS** | Fellow of the Royal College of Surgeons |
| **FRCSC** | Fellow of the Royal College of Surgeons of Canada |
| **FRS** | Fellow of the Royal Society |
| **GPN** | General Pediatric Nurse |
| **HT** | Histologic Technician/Histologic Technologist |
| **LAT** | Licensed Athletic Trainer |
| **LATC** | Licensed Athletic Trainer, Certified |
| **LPN** | Licensed Practical Nurse |
| **LVN** | Licensed Visiting Nurse; Licensed Vocational Nurse |
| **MCh** | Master of Surgery |
| **MD** | Doctor of Medicine |
| **ME** | Medical Examiner |
| **MEd** | Master of Education |
| **MLT** | Medical Laboratory Technician |
| **MPH** | Master of Public Health |
| **MPharm** | Master in Pharmacy |
| **MRCP** | Member of the Royal College of Physicians |
| **MRCS** | Member of the Royal College of Surgeons |
| **MS** | Master of Science; Master of Surgery |
| **MSc** | Master of Surgery |
| **MSN** | Master of Science in Nursing |
| **MSurg** | Master of Surgery |
| **MT** | Medical Technologist |
| **MTA** | Medical Technologist Assistant |
| **MT(ASCP)** | Medical Technologist (American Society of Clinical Pathologists) |
| **ND** | Doctor of Nursing |
| **NMP** | Nurse Massage Therapist; Nursing Massage Therapist |
| **NP** | Nurse Practitioner |
| **NREMT-P** | National Registry of Emergency Medical Technician–Paramedics |
| **OCN** | Oncology Certified Nurse |
| **OD** | Doctor of Optometry |
| **ONC** | Orthopedic Nurse Certified |
| **OT-C** | Occupational Therapist (Canada) |
| **OTR** | Registered Occupational Therapist |
| **PA** | Physician's Assistant |
| **PA-C** | Physician's Assistant Certified |
| **PD** | Doctor of Pharmacy |
| **PharmD** | Doctor of Pharmacy |
| **PharmG** | Graduate in Pharmacy |
| **PhD** | Doctor of Philosophy |
| **PNP** | Pediatric Nurse Practitioner |
| **PT** | Physical Therapist |
| **RD** | Registered Dietician |
| **RDH** | Registered Dental Hygienist |
| **RDMS** | Registered Diagnostic Medical Sonographer |
| **R EEG T** | Radiologic Electroencephalography Technologist |
| **R EP T** | Registered Evoked Potentials Technologist |
| **RN** | Registered Nurse |
| **RNC** | Registered Nurse Certified (OB/GYN and Neonatal) |
| **RPh** | Registered Pharmacist |
| **RPT** | Registered Physical Therapist |
| **RRA** | Registered Record Administrator |
| **RRT** | Registered Respiratory Therapist |
| **RTR** | Registered Recreational Therapist |
| **RVT** | Registered Vascular Technologist |
| **ScD** | Doctor of Science |
| **SCT** | Specialist in Cytotechnology |
| **SM** | Master of Surgery |

# APPENDIX 19
# Nursing Organizations

## Appendix 19–1 Nursing Organizations in the United States

**Academy of Medical-Surgical Nurses**
E. Holly Ave., Box 56, Pitman, NJ 08071; (609) 256-2323

**American Academy of Ambulatory Nursing Administration**
E. Holly Ave., Box 56, Pitman, NJ 08071; (609) 582-9617

**American Academy of Nurse Practitioners**
Box 12846, Austin, TX 78711; (512) 442-4262

**American Academy of Nursing**
2420 Pershing Rd., Kansas City, MO 64108; (816) 474-5720

**American Assembly for Men in Nursing**
Box 31753, Independence, OH 44131; (216) 524-3504

**American Association of Critical-Care Nurses**
101 Columbia, Aliso Viejo, CA 92656; (800) 899-2226

**American Association of Diabetes Educators**
500 N. Michigan Ave., Ste. 1400, Chicago, IL 60611; (312) 661-1700

**American Association of Neuroscience Nurses**
222 S. Prospect, Park Ridge, IL 60068-4001; (708) 692-7050

**American Association of Nurse Anesthetists**
216 W. Higgins Rd., Park Ridge, IL 60068-5790; (708) 692-7050

**American Association of Occcupational Health Nurses**
50 Lenox Pointe, Atlanta, GA 30324; (404) 262-1162

**American Association of Spinal Cord Injury Nurses**
75–20 Astoria Blvd., Jackson Heights, NY 11370-1178; (718) 803-3782

**American Board of Neuroscience Nursing**
224 N. DesPlaines, Ste. 601, Chicago, IL 60661

**American Board for Occupational Health Nurses**
10503 N. Cedarburg Rd., Mequon, WI 53092-4403; (414) 242-0704

**American Board of Post Anesthesia Nursing Certification**
11512 Allecingie Pky., Richmond, VA 23235; (804) 378-4936

**American College of Nurse-Midwives**
1522 K St. NW, Suite 1000, Washington, DC 20005; (202) 728-9860

**American Licensed Practical Nurses Association**
1090 Vermont Ave. NW, Suite 1200, Washington, DC 20005; (202) 682-5800

**American Nephrology Nurses' Association**
E. Holly Ave., Box 56, Pitman, NJ 08071; (609) 256-2320

**American Nurses Association**
600 Maryland Ave. SW, Suite 100 West, Washington, DC 20024-2571; (202) 651-7000

**American Nurses' Foundation**
600 Maryland Ave SW, Ste. 100 West, Washington, DC 20024; (202) 651-7227

**American Organization of Nurse Executives**
One N. Franklin, 34th Fl., Chicago, IL 60606; (312) 422-4503

**American Psychiatric Nurses Association**
1200 19th St. NW, Ste. 300, Washington, DC 20036; (202) 857-1133

**American Society of Ophthalmic Registered Nurses, Inc.**
Box 193030, San Francisco, CA 94119; (415) 561-8513

**American Society of Plastic and Reconstructive Surgical Nurses**
E. Holly Ave., Box 56, Pitman, NJ 08071; (609) 256-2340

**American Society of Post Anesthesia Nurses**
6900 Grove Rd., Thorofare, NJ 08086; (609) 845-5557

**American Thoracic Society, Section on Nursing**
1749 Broadway, New York, NY 10019; (212) 315-8700

**American Urological Association Allied**
11512 Allecingie Pky., Richmond, VA 23235; (804) 379-1306

**Assembly of Hospital Schools of Nursing**
American Hospital Association, Center for Nursing, 840 N. Lake Shore Dr., Chicago, IL 60611; (312) 280-6432

**Association of Operating Room Nurses**
2170 S. Parker Rd., Ste. 300, Denver, CO 80231; (303) 755-6300

**Association of Pediatric Oncology Nurses**
5700 Old Orchard Rd., Skokie, IL 60077; (708) 966-3723

**Association of Rehabilitation Nurses**
4700 W. Lake Ave., Glenview, IL 60025-1485; (847) 375-4710

**Association of Women's Health, Obstetric, and Neonatal Nurses**
700 14th St. NW, Ste. 600, Washington, DC 20005-2019; (202) 662-1600

**Baromedical Nurses Association**
Box 2727, Palm Desert, CA 92261; (619) 770-3676

**Cassandra: Radical Feminist Nurses Network**
Box 181039, Cleveland Heights, OH 44118

**Commission on Graduates of Foreign Nursing Schools**
3600 Market St., Ste. 400, Philadelphia, PA 19104; (215) 222-8454

**Council on Certification of Nurse Anesthetists**
222 S. Prospect Ave., Park Ridge, IL 60068; (708) 692-7050

**Dermatology Nurses Association**
E. Holly Ave., Box 56, Pitman, NJ 08071; (609) 582-1915

**Emergency Nurses Association**
216 Higgins Rd., Park Ridge, IL 60068; (708) 698-9400

**Federation for Accessible Nursing Education and Licensure**
Box 1418, Lewisburg, WV 24901; (304) 645-4357

**Frontier Nursing Service**
100 Wendover Rd., Wendover, KY 41775; (606) 672-2317

**International Flying Nurses Association**
c/o Terri A. Sinkowski, R.N., Box 561218, Harwood Heights, IL 60656

**Intravenous Nurses Society**
Fresh Pond Sq., 10 Fawcett St., Cambridge, MA 02138; (617) 441-3008

**National Association of Hispanic Nurses**
1501 16th St. NW, Washington, DC 20036; (202) 387-2477

**National Association of Orthopaedic Nurses**
E. Holly Ave., Box 56, Pitman, NJ 08071; (609) 256-2310

**National Association of Pediatric Nurse Associates and Practitioners**
1101 Kings Hwy. N., 206, Cherry Hill, NJ 08034; (609) 667-1773

**National Association of Physician Nurses**
900 S. Washington St., G-13, Falls Church, VA 22046; (703) 237-8616

**National Association of Registered Nurses**
11508 Allecingie Pky., Ste. C, Richmond, VA 23235; (804) 794-6513

**National Association of School Nurses**
Lamplighter Lane, Box 1300, Scarborough, ME 04070; (207) 883-2117

**National Black Nurses Association, Inc.**
1511 K St. NW, Washington, DC 20005; (202) 347-3808

**National Certification Corporation for the Obstetric, Gynecologic, and Neonatal Specialties**
645 N. Michigan Ave., Ste. 900, Chicago, IL 60611; (312) 951-0207

**National Council of State Boards of Nursing, Inc.**
676 N. St. Clair St., Ste. 550, Chicago, IL 60611; (312) 787-6555

**National Federation of Licensed Practical Nurses, Inc.**
1418 Aversboro Rd., Garner, NC 27529-4547; (919) 779-0046

**National Federation for Specialty Nursing Organizations**
E. Holly Ave., Box 56, Pitman, NJ 08071; (609) 256-2333

**National Flight Nurses Association**
c/o Christine Dorsen, 6900 Grove Rd., Thorofare, NJ 08086; (609) 384-6725

**National Geronotological Nurses Association**
7520 Parkway Dr., Ste. 510, Hanover, MD 21076

**National League for Nursing**
350 Hudson St., New York, NY 10014; (212) 989-9393

**National Nurses Society on Addictions**
4101 Lake Boone Trl., Ste. 201, Raleigh, NC 27607

**National Organization for Associate Degree Nursing**
11250 Roger Bacon Dr., Ste. 8, Reston, VA 22090-5202; (703) 525-5202

**National Student Nurses' Association**
555 W. 57th St., Ste. 1327, New York, NY 10019; (212) 581-2211

**North American Nursing Diagnosis Association**
1211 Locust St., Philadelphia, PA 19107; (215) 545-8105

**Nurse Consultants Association, Inc.**
414 Plaza Dr., Suite 209, Westmont, IL 60559; (708) 655-0087

**Nurses Educational Funds**
555 W. 57th St., 13th fl., New York, NY 10019; (212) 582-8820

**Nurses' House**
350 Hudson St., New York, NY 10014; (212) 989-9393

**Nurses Organization of Veterans Affairs**
6728 Old McLean Village Dr., McLean, VA 22101

**Oncology Nursing Society**
501 Holiday Dr., Pittsburgh, PA 15220; (412) 921-7373

**Respiratory Nursing Society**
4700 W. Lake Ave., Glenview, IL 60025; (708) 375-4700

**Society of Gastrointestinal Nurses and Associates**
401 N. Michigan Ave., Chicago, IL 60611-4267; (800) 245-7462

**Society of Otorhinolaryngology and Head/Neck Nurses**
116 Canal St., Ste. A, New Smyrna Beach, FL 32168; (904) 428-1695

**Society for Vascular Nursing**
309 Winter St., Norwood, MA 02062; (617) 762-3630

**Visiting Nurse Associations of America**
3801 E. Florida Ave., Ste. 900, Denver, CO 80210; (303) 753-0218

**Wound, Ostomy, and Incontinence Nurses**
2755 Bristol St., Ste. 100, Costa Mesa, CA 92626; (714) 476-0268

# Appendix 19–2 Nursing Organizations in Canada

## NATIONAL ORGANIZATIONS

**Academy of Chief Executive Nurses of Teaching Hospitals**
Director of Nursing, Saint John Regional Hospital, Box 2100, Saint John, New Brunswick E2L 4L2; (506) 648-6369

**Canadian Association of Burn Nurses**
Wellesley Hospital, 160 Wellesley St. E., Toronto, Ontario M4Y 1J3; (416) 926-7693

**Canadian Association of Critical Care Nurses**
Box 22006, London, Ontario N6C 4N0; (519) 649-5284

**Canadian Association for Enterostomal Therapy**
Victorian Order of Nurses, Winnipeg Branch, 311-167 Lombard Ave., Winnipeg, Manitoba R3B 0T6; (204) 957-0650, ext. 37

**Canadian Association for the History of Nursing**
430 Hendon Dr. NW, Calgary, Alberta T2K 1Z7; (403) 289-3194

**Canadian Association of Nephrology Nurses and Technicians**
6431 Seaforth St., Halifax, Nova Scotia B3L 1R4; (902) 428-5517

**Canadian Association of Neuroscience Nurses**
416 Preston Ave., Saskatoon, Saskatchewan S7H 2V2; (306) 966-1889

**Canadian Association of Nurse Administrators**
c/o Medicine Hat Regional Hospital, Office of AEO-Patient Services, 666 Fifth St. SW, Medicine Hat, Alberta T1A 4H6; (403) 529-8018

**Canadian Association of Nurses in AIDS Care**
Montreal General Hospital, 1650 Cedar Ave., Room 7112, Montreal, Quebec H3E 1A4; (514) 934-8070

**Canadian Association of Nurses in Independent Practice**
55 McCaul St., Box 155, Toronto, Ontario M5T 2N7; (416) 683-3754

**Canadian Association of Nurses in Oncology**
c/o Manitoba Cancer Treatment and Research Foundation, 100 Olivia St., Winnipeg, Manitoba R3E 0V9; (204) 787-2233

**Canadian Association for Nursing Law**
1 Evergreen Place, Winnipeg, Manitoba R3C 0E9

**Canadian Association of Pediatric Nurses**
44 Dayfoot Dr., Georgetown, Ontario L7G 2L1; (416) 840-1440
151 Bloor St. W., Suite 480, Toronto, Ontario M5S 1T3

**Canadian Association of Rehabilitation Nurses**
1 Place Ville-Marie, Suite 3725, Montreal, Quebec H3B 3P4; (514) 937-3661, ext. 119

**Canadian Correctional Nurses Association**
c/o New Brunswick Training School, R.R. #6, Fredericton, New Brunswick E3B 4X7; (506) 453-7800

**Canadian Council of Cardiovascular Nurses**
160 George St., Suite 200, Ottawa, Ontario K1N 9M2; (613) 237-4361

**Canadian Diabetes Association, Professional Health Workers Section**
902-2060 Bellwood, Burnaby, British Columbia V5B 4V2; (416) 789-9551

**Canadian Federation of Mental Health Nurses**
331 Montgomery Ave., Winnipeg, Manitoba R3L 1T6; (204) 787-3345

**Canadian Gerontological Nursing Association**
Dean, Faculty of Nursing, University of New Brunswick, Box 4400, Fredericton, New Brunswick E3B 5A3; (506) 453-4642

**Canadian Holistic Nurses Association**
Box 1752, Kingston, Ontario K7L 5J6; (613) 549-6646

**Canadian Intravenous Nurses Association**
200-4433 Sheppard Ave. E., Agincourt, Ontario M1S 1V3; (416) 292-0687

**Canadian Nurse Educators Association**
2280–15th Sideroad, R.R. #4, Thunder Bay, Ontario P7C 4Z2; (807) 475-6306

**Canadian Nurses Respiratory Society**
c/o Canadian Lung Association, 908-75 Albert St., Ottawa, Ontario K1P 5E7; (613) 237-1208

**Canadian Nursing Research Group**
CSB-5-123, Faculty of Nursing, University of Alberta, Edmonton, Alberta T6G 2G3; (403) 492-2996

**Canadian Obstetric Gynecologic and Neonatal Nurses**
4375 Royal Ave., Montreal, Quebec H4A 2M7; (514) 934-4400, ext. 2389

**Canadian Orthopaedic Nurses Association**
410-9890 Manchester Dr., Burnaby, British Columbia V3N 4R4; (604) 875-4053

**Canadian Society of Gastroenterology Nurses and Associates**
GI Investigations Unit 4W1, Chedoke-McMaster Hospital, McMaster Div., 1200 Main St. W., Hamilton, Ontario L8N 3Z5

**Community Health Nurses Association of Canada**
1049 Flintlock Court, London, Ontario N6H 4M3; (519) 613-9900

**Community and Hospital Infection Control Association – Canada**
Senior Infection Control Nurse, Vancouver General Hospital, 855 12th Ave., Vancouver, British Columbia V5Z 1M9

**Indian and Inuit Nurses of Canada**
55 Murray St., 4th fl., Ottawa, Ontario K1N 5M3; (613) 230-1864

**National Association of Occupational Health Nurses**
B. F. Goodrich Canada Inc., Scotford Chemical Group, Box 3418, Fort Saskatchewan, Alberta T8L 2T3; (403) 998-8780

**National Emergency Nurses' Affiliation**
55 Highfield Park Dr., Apt. 101, Dartmouth, Nova Scotia B3A 4S4; (902) 463-6061

**Nursing Sisters Association of Canada**
52 Thorncliffe Dr., Suite 301, Toronto, Ontario M4N 1K5; (416) 424-1440

**Operating Room Nurses Association of Canada**
2864 W. 3rd Ave., Vancouver, British Columbia V6K 1M7; (604) 682-2344, ext. 2330

## PROVINCIAL AND TERRITORIAL ASSOCIATIONS

**Alberta Association of Registered Nurses**
11620–168 St., Edmonton, Alberta T5M 4A6; (403) 451-0043

**Registered Nurses Association of British Columbia**
2855 Arbutus St., Vancouver, British Columbia V6J 3Y8; (604) 736-7331

**Manitoba Association of Registered Nurses**
647 Broadway, Winnipeg, Manitoba R3C 0X2; (204) 774-3477

**Nurses Association of New Brunswick**
165 Regent St., Fredericton, New Brunswick E3B 3W5; (506) 458-8731

**Association of Registered Nurses of Newfoundland**
55 Military Rd., Box 6116, St. John's, Newfoundland A1C 5X8; (709) 753-6040

**Northwest Territories Registered Nurses Association**
Box 2757, Yellowknife, Northwest Territories X1A 2R1; (403) 873-2745

**Nurses Association of Nova Scotia**
120 Eileen Stubbs Ave., Suite 104, Dartmouth, Nova Scotia B3H 1Y1; (902) 468-9744

**Registered Nurses Association of Ontario**
33 Price St., Toronto, Ontario M4W 1Z2; (800) 268-7199; (416) 923-3523
For information on registration/licensure in Ontario, contact College of Nurses of Ontario, 101 Davenport Rd., Toronto, Ontario M5R 3P1; (800) 387-5526; (416) 928-0900.

**Association of Registered Nurses of Prince Edward Island**
Box 1838, Charlottetown, Prince Edward Island C1A 7N5; (902) 368-3764
For information on registration/licensure in Quebec, contact l'Ordre des infirmières et infirmiers du Quebec, 4200 ouest, boul. Dorchester, Montreal, Quebec H3Z 1V4; (800) 363-6048; (514) 935-2501

**Saskatchewan Registered Nurses Association**
2066 Retallack St., Regina, Saskatchewan S4T 2K2; (306) 757-4643

**Yukon Registered Nurses Association**
Box 5371, Whitehorse, Yukon Y1A 4Z2; (403) 667-4062

SOURCES: Encyclopedia of Associations, ed 30 (Gale Research Co., Detroit, 1996); Canadian Nurses Association, Ottawa, Ontario.

# APPENDIX 20
# Conceptual Models and Theories of Nursing*

Jacqueline Fawcett, PhD, FAAN

## Appendix 20–1 The Forerunners

### FLORENCE NIGHTINGALE'S NOTES ON NURSING

#### Overview

Nightingale maintained that *every* woman is a nurse because every woman, at one time or another in her life, has charge of the personal health of someone. Nightingale equated knowledge of nursing with knowledge of sanitation. The focus of nursing knowledge was how to keep the body free from disease or in such a condition that it could recover from disease. According to Nightingale, nursing ought to signify the proper use of fresh air, light, warmth, cleanliness, quiet, and the proper selection and administration of diet — all at the least expense of vital power to the patient. That is, she maintained that the purpose of nursing was to put patients in the best condition for nature to act upon them.

#### Implications for Nursing Practice

Nursing practice encompasses care of both well and sick people. Nursing actions focus on both patients and their environments. Thirteen "hints" provided the boundaries of nursing practice:

1. **Ventilation and warming**–the nurse must be concerned first with keeping the air that patients breathe as pure as the external air, without chilling them.
2. **Health of houses**–attention to pure air, pure water, efficient drainage, cleanliness, and light will secure the health of houses.
3. **Petty management**–all the results of good nursing may be negated by one defect: not knowing how to manage what you do when you are there and what shall be done when you are not there.
4. **Noise**–unnecessary noise, or noise that creates an expectation in the mind, is that which hurts patients. Anything that wakes patients suddenly out of their sleep will invariably put them into a state of greater excitement and do them more serious and lasting mischief than any continuous noise, however loud.
5. **Variety**–the nerves of the sick suffer from seeing the same walls, the same ceiling, the same surroundings during a long confinement to one or two rooms. The majority of cheerful cases is to be found among those patients who are not confined to one room, whatever their suffering, and the majority of depressed cases will be seen among those subjected to a long monotony of objects about them.
6. **Taking food**–the nurse should be conscious of patients' diets and remember how much food each patient has had and ought to have each day.
7. **What food?**–to watch for the opinions the patient's stomach gives, rather than to read "analyses of foods," is the business of all those who have to decide what the patient should eat.
8. **Bed and bedding**–the patient should have a clean bed every 12 hours. The bed should be narrow, so that the patient does not feel "out of humanity's reach." The bed should not be so high that the patient cannot easily get in and out of it. The bed should be in the lightest spot in the room, preferably near a window. Pillows should be used to support the back below the breathing apparatus, to allow shoulders room to fall back, and to support the head without throwing it forward.
9. **Light**–with the sick, second only to their need of fresh air is their need of light. Light, especially direct sunlight, has a purifying effect upon the air of a room.
10. **Cleanliness of rooms and walls**–the greater part of nursing consists in preserving cleanliness. The inside air can be kept clean only by excessive care to rid rooms and their furnishings of the organic matter and dust with which they become saturated. Without cleanliness, you cannot have all the effects of ventilation; without ventilation, you can have no thorough cleanliness.

---

* SOURCE: Adapted from overviews written by Jacqueline Fawcett for the videotape series, *The Nurse Theorists: Portraits of Excellence*, produced by Studio Three, Samuel Merritt College of Nursing, Oakland, CA and funded by the Helene Fuld Health Trust (1987–1990); from Fawcett, J. (1993). *Analysis and evaluation of nursing theories*. Philadelphia: F. A. Davis; and from Fawcett, J. (1995). *Analysis and evaluation of conceptual models of nursing* (3rd ed.). Philadelphia: F. A. Davis.

11. **Personal cleanliness**–nurses should always remember that if they allow patients to remain unwashed or to remain in clothing saturated with perspiration or other excretion, they are interfering injuriously with the natural processes of health just as much as if they were to give their patients a dose of slow poison.
12. **Chattering hopes and advices**–there is scarcely a greater worry which invalids have to endure than the incurable hopes of their friends. All friends, visitors, and attendants of the sick should avoid the practice of attempting to cheer the sick by making light of their danger and by exaggerating their probabilities of recovery.
13. **Observation of the sick**–the most important practical lesson nurses can learn is what to observe, how to observe, which symptoms indicate improvement, which indicate the reverse, which are important, which are not, and which are the evidence of neglect and what kind of neglect.

### Implications for Nursing Education

Nightingale's primary contribution to nursing education was her belief that nursing schools should be administratively and economically independent from hospitals, even though the training could take place in the hospital. The purpose of nursing education was to teach the theoretical and practical knowledge underlying physician's orders. Knowledge of the 13 "hints" for nursing practice was considered an essential part of the training of every nurse.

### Reference

Nightingale, F. (1859). *Notes on nursing: What it is, and what it is not.* London: Harrison and Sons. [Commemorative edition printed by J. B. Lippincott Company, Philadelphia, 1992]

## VIRGINIA HENDERSON'S DEFINITION OF NURSING

### Overview

The unique function of the nurse is to help individuals, sick or well, to perform those activities contributing to health or its recovery (or to peaceful death) that they would perform unaided if they had the necessary strength, will, or knowledge, and to do this in such a way as to help them gain independence as soon as possible.

### Implications for Nursing Practice

The practice of nursing requires nurses to know and understand patients by putting themselves in the place of the patients. Nurses should not take at face value everything that patients say, but rather should interact with patients to ascertain their true feelings. *Basic nursing care* involves helping the patient perform the following activities unaided:

1. Breathe normally.
2. Eat and drink adequately.
3. Eliminate body wastes.
4. Move and maintain desirable postures.
5. Sleep and rest.
6. Select suitable clothes and dress and undress.
7. Maintain body temperature within normal range by adjusting clothing and modifying the environment.
8. Keep the body clean and well groomed and protect the integument.
9. Avoid dangers in the environment and avoid injuring others.
10. Communicate with others in expressing emotions, needs, fears, or opinions.
11. Worship according to one's faith.
12. Work in such a way that there is a sense of accomplishment.
13. Play or participate in various forms of recreation.
14. Learn, discover, or satisfy the curiosity that leads to normal development and health and use the available health facilities.

### Implications for Nursing Education

Henderson's definition of nursing identifies an area of health and human welfare in which the nurse is an expert and independent practitioner. This kind of nursing requires a liberal education within a college or university, with grounding in the physical, biological, and social sciences and ability to use analytic processes. The professional aspects of the curriculum should focus on the nurse's major function of supplementing patients when they need strength, will, or knowledge in performing daily activities or in carrying out prescribed therapy, with emphasis on the individualization of patient care.

### Reference

Henderson, V. (1966). *The nature of nursing. A definition and its implications for practice, research, and education.* New York: Macmillan.

# Appendix 20–2 Conceptual Models

A conceptual model is defined as a set of abstract and general concepts and the propositions that describe and link those concepts. Conceptual models of nursing, which also are referred to as conceptual frameworks, conceptual systems, and paradigms, provide distinctive frames of reference for thinking about people, their environments, their health, and nursing.

## DOROTHY JOHNSON'S BEHAVIORAL SYSTEM MODEL

### Overview

Focus is on the person as a behavioral system, made up of all the patterned, repetitive, and purposeful ways of behavior that characterize life. Seven subsystems carry out specialized tasks or functions needed to maintain the integrity of the whole behavioral system and to manage its relationship to the environment:

1. **Attachment or affiliative**–function is the security needed for survival as well as social inclusion, intimacy, and formation and maintenance of social bonds.
2. **Dependency**–function is the succoring behavior that calls for a response of nurturance as well as approval, attention or recognition, and physical assistance.
3. **Ingestive subsystem**–function is appetite satisfaction in terms of when, how, what, how much, and under what conditions the individual eats, all of which is governed by social and psychological considerations as well as biological requirements for food and fluids.
4. **Eliminative**–function is elimination in terms of when, how, and under what conditions the individual eliminates wastes.
5. **Sexual**–functions are procreation and gratification, with regard to behaviors dependent upon the individual's biological sex and gender role identity, including but not limited to courting and mating.
6. **Aggressive**–function is protection and preservation of self and society.
7. **Achievement**–function is mastery or control of some aspect of self or environment, with regard to intellectual, physical, creative, mechanical, social, and care-taking (of children, partner, home) skills.

The *structure* of each subsystem includes four elements:

1. **Drive or goal**–the motivation for behavior.
2. **Set**–the individual's predisposition to act in certain ways to fulfill the function of the subsystem.
3. **Choice**–the individual's total behavioral repertoire for fulfilling subsystem functions, which encompasses the scope of action alternatives from which the person can choose.
4. **Action**–the individual's actual behavior in a situation. Action is the only structural element that can be observed directly; all other elements must be inferred from the individual's actual behavior and from the consequences of that behavior.

Three *functional requirements* are needed by each subsystem to fulfill its functions:

1. **Protection** from noxious influences with which the system cannot cope.
2. **Nurturance** through the input of appropriate supplies from the environment.
3. **Stimulation** to enhance growth and prevent stagnation.

### Implications for Nursing Practice

Nursing practice is directed toward restoration, maintenance, or attainment of behavioral system balance and dynamic stability at the highest possible level for the individual. The nursing diagnostic and treatment process has four steps:

1. **Determination of the existence of a problem** in behavioral subsystem functions or structural elements.
2. **Diagnostic classification of problems** as internal subsystem problems or intersystem problems.
3. **Management of nursing problems** through three types of treatments:
   *Fulfill subsystem functional requirements* by protecting the patient from overwhelming noxious influences, supplying adequate nurturance, and providing stimulation.
   *Impose external regulatory or control mechanisms on behavior,* such as setting limits for behavior, inhibiting ineffective behavioral responses, and assisting patients to acquire new behavioral responses.
   *Change the structural elements of the subsystems* by altering set through instruction or counseling and adding choices through teaching new skills.
4. **Evaluate the efficacy of nursing treatments** by comparing extent of behavior system stability and balance before and after the treatments.

### Implications for Nursing Education

Education for nursing practice requires a thorough grounding in the natural and social sciences, with emphasis on the genetic, neurological, and endocrine bases of behavior; psychological and social mechanisms for the regulation and control of behavior; social learning theories; and motivational structures and processes. The professional aspects of the curriculum focus on study of the behavioral system as a whole and as a composite of subsystems; pathophysiology; the clinical sciences of nursing and medicine; and the health care system.

## References

Johnson, D. E. (1980). The behavioral system model for nursing. In J. P. Riehl & C. Roy, *Conceptual models for nursing practice* (2nd ed., pp. 207–216). New York: Appleton-Century-Crofts.

Johnson, D. E. (1990). The behavioral system model for nursing. In M. E. Parker (Ed.), *Nursing theories in practice* (pp. 23–32). New York: National League for Nursing.

# IMOGENE KING'S GENERAL SYSTEMS FRAMEWORK

## Overview

Focus is on the continuing ability of individuals to meet their basic needs so that they may function in their socially defined roles, and on individuals' interactions within three open, dynamic, interacting systems.

1. **Personal systems** are individuals, who are regarded as rational, sentient, social beings. Concepts related to the personal system are:
   **Perception**–a process of organizing, interpreting, and transforming information from sense data and memory that gives meaning to one's experience, represents one's image of reality, and influences one's behavior.
   **Self**–a composite of thoughts and feelings that constitute a person's awareness of individual existence, of who and what he or she is.
   **Growth and development**–cellular, molecular, and behavioral changes in human beings that are a function of genetic endowment, meaningful and satisfying experiences, and an environment conducive to helping individuals move toward maturity.
   *Body image*–a person's perceptions of his or her body.
   *Time*–the duration between the occurrence of one event and the occurrence of another event.
   *Space*–the physical area called territory that exists in all directions.
   *Learning*–gaining knowledge.
2. **Interpersonal systems** are composed of two, three, or more individuals interacting in a given situation. The concepts associated with this system are:
   *Interactions*–the acts of two or more persons in mutual presence; a sequence of verbal and nonverbal behaviors that are goal directed.
   *Communication*–the vehicle by which human relations are developed and maintained; encompasses intrapersonal, interpersonal, verbal, and nonverbal communication.
   *Transaction*–a process of interaction in which human beings communicate with the environment to achieve goals that are valued; goal-directed human behaviors.
   *Role*–a set of behaviors expected of a person occupying a position in a social system.
   *Stress*–a dynamic state whereby a human being interacts with the environment to maintain balance for growth, development, and performance, involving an exchange of energy and information between the person and the environment for regulation and control of stressors.
   *Coping*–a way of dealing with stress.
3. **Social systems** are organized boundary systems of social roles, behaviors, and practices developed to maintain values and the mechanisms to regulate the practices and roles. The concepts related to social systems are:
   *Organization*–composed of human beings with prescribed roles and positions who use resources to accomplish personal and organizational goals.
   *Authority*–a transactional process characterized by active, reciprocal relations in which members' values, backgrounds, and perceptions play a role in defining, validating, and accepting the authority of individuals within an organization.
   *Power*–the process whereby one or more persons influence other persons in a situation.
   *Status*–the position of an individual in a group or a group in relation to other groups in an organization.
   *Decision making*–a dynamic and systematic process by which goal-directed choice of perceived alternatives is made and acted upon by individuals or groups to answer a question and attain a goal.
   *Control*–being in charge.

## Implications for Nursing Practice

Nursing practice is directed toward helping individuals maintain their health so they can function in their roles. The *theory of goal attainment* describes an interaction-transaction nursing process that depicts a sequence in which the nurse and the client meet in a situation.

1. **Assessment phase**–the nurse and the client perceive each other, make mental judgments about each other, take some mental action, react to each other's perceptions of the other, communicate, and begin to interact.
2. **Planning phase**–interactions between the nurse and the client continue and can be observed directly. The specific data of interaction, which can be recorded, are the concerns, problems, or disturbances identified by the client and the nurse, their mutual goal setting, their exploration of means to achieve the goal, and their agreement on the means required to achieve the goal.
3. **Implementation phase**–transactions are made and can be observed in the form of goal attainment measures.
4. **Evaluation phase**–a decision is made with regard to whether the goal was attained and, if necessary, the determination of why the goal was not attained.

### Implications for Nursing Education

The General Systems Framework and the theory of goal attainment lead to a focus on the dynamic interaction of the nurse-client dyad. This focus, in turn, leads to emphasis on nursing student behavior as well as client behavior. The concepts related to the personal, interpersonal, and social systems serve as the theoretical content for nursing courses in associate degree, baccalaureate, and master's nursing programs. The theoretical knowledge is used by students in learning experiences involving concrete nursing situations.

### References

King, I. M. (1981). *A theory for nursing. Systems, concepts, process.* New York: Wiley.
King, I. M. (1986). *Curriculum and instruction in nursing.* Norwalk, CT: Appleton-Century-Crofts.
King, I.M. (1992). King's theory of goal attainment. *Nursing Science Quarterly*, 5, 19–26.

## MYRA LEVINE'S CONSERVATION MODEL

### Overview

Focus is on conservation of the person's wholeness. Adaptation is the process by which people maintain their wholeness or integrity as they respond to environmental challenges and become congruent with the environment. Sources of challenges are:

1. **Perceptual environment**–encompasses that part of the environment to which individuals respond with their sense organs.
2. **Operational environment**–includes those aspects of the environment that are not directly perceived, such as radiation, odorless and colorless pollutants, and microorganisms.
3. **Conceptual environment**–the environment of language, ideas, symbols, concepts, and invention.

Individuals respond to the environment by means of four integrated processes:

1. *Fight-or-flight mechanism*
2. *Inflammatory-immune* response
3. *Stress* response
4. *Perceptual awareness*–includes the basic orienting, haptic, auditory, visual, and taste-smell systems.

### Implications for Nursing Practice

Nursing practice is directed toward promoting wholeness for all people, well or sick. Patients are partners or participants in nursing care and are temporarily dependent on the nurse. The nurse's goal is to end the dependence as quickly as possible. The nursing process of this conceptual model is conservation, which is defined as "keeping together," and consists of three steps:

1. **Trophicognosis**–a nursing care judgment arrived at by the scientific method. Involves observation, awareness of provocative facts, and construction of a testable hypothesis, which is the trophicognosis.
2. **Intervention**–two types of nursing interventions:

   *Therapeutic*–when nursing intervention influences adaptation favorably or toward renewed social well-being.

   *Supportive*–when nursing intervention cannot alter the course of the adaptation and can only maintain the status quo or fail to halt a downward course.

   Intervention is structured according to four conservation principles:

   *Principle of conservation of energy*–balancing the patient's energy output and energy input to avoid excessive fatigue.

   *Principle of conservation of structural integrity*–focusing attention on healing by maintaining or restoring the structure of the body through prevention of physical breakdown and promotion of healing.

   *Principle of conservation of personal integrity*–maintaining or restoring the individual patient's sense of identity, self-worth, and acknowledgment of uniqueness.

*Principle of conservation of social integrity*–acknowledging patients as social beings and helping them to preserve their places in family, community, and society.

### Implications for Nursing Education

Education focuses on understanding both the person and the environment, with emphasis placed on processes by which the person adapts to environmental challenges. Theoretical and clinical knowledge related to the four conservation principles provides the structure for nursing courses. Students are prepared for the practice of holistic nursing and for lifelong learning.

### References

Levine, M. E. (1973). *Introduction to clinical nursing* (2nd ed.). Philadelphia: F. A. Davis.

Schaefer, K. M., & Pond, J. B. (Eds.). (1991). *Levine's conservation model: A framework for nursing practice*. Philadelphia: F. A. Davis.

## BETTY NEUMAN'S SYSTEMS MODEL

### Overview

Focus is on the wellness of the client system in relation to environmental stress and reactions to stress. The client system, which can be an individual, a family or other group, or a community, is a composite of five interrelated variables:

1. **Physiological variables**–bodily structure and function.
2. **Psychological variables**–mental processes and relationships.
3. **Sociocultural variables**–social and cultural functions.
4. **Developmental variables**–developmental processes of life.
5. **Spiritual variables**–aspects of spirituality on a continuum from complete unawareness or denial to a consciously developed high level of spiritual understanding.

The client system is depicted as a central core, which is a basic structure of survival factors common to the species, surrounded by three types of concentric rings:

1. **Flexible line of defense**–the outermost ring; a protective buffer for the client's normal or stable state that prevents invasion of stressors and keeps the client system free from stressor reactions or symptomatology.
2. **Normal line of defense**–lies between the flexible line of defense and the lines of resistance; represents the client system's normal or usual wellness state.
3. **Lines of resistance**–the innermost concentric rings; involuntarily activated when a stressor invades the normal line of defense. They attempt to stabilize the client system and foster a return to the normal line of defense. If they are effective, the system can reconstitute; if ineffective, death may ensue.

Environment is defined as "all internal and external factors or influences surrounding the client system":

1. **Internal environment**–"all forces or interactive influences internal to or contained solely within the boundaries of the defined client system"; the source of *intrapersonal stressors*.
2. **External environment**–all forces or interaction influences external to or existing outside the defined client system; the source of *interpersonal and extrapersonal stressors*.
3. **Created environment**–subconsciously developed by the client as a symbolic expression of system wholeness. It supersedes and encompasses the internal and external environments, and functions as a subjective safety mechanism that may block the true reality of the environment and the health experience.

### Implications for Nursing Practice

Nursing practice is directed toward facilitating optimal wellness through retention, attainment, or maintenance of client system stability. The three steps of the nursing process are:

1. **Nursing diagnosis**–formulated on the basis of assessment of the variables and lines of defense and resistance making up the client system.
2. **Nursing goals**–negotiated with the client for desired prescriptive changes to correct variances from wellness.
3. **Nursing outcomes**–determined by evaluation of the results of three types of prevention-as-intervention modalities:

   *Primary prevention*–action required to *retain* client system stability; selected when the risk of or hazard from a stressor is known but a reaction has not yet occurred. Interventions attempt to reduce the possibility of the client's encounter with the stressor or strengthen the flexible line of defense to decrease the possibility of a reaction when the stressor is encountered.

   *Secondary prevention*–action required to *attain* system stability; selected when a reaction to a stressor has already occurred. Interventions deal with existing symptoms and attempt to strengthen the lines of resistance through use of the client's internal and external resources.

*Tertiary prevention*–action required to *maintain* system stability; selected when some degree of client system stability has occurred following secondary prevention interventions.

### Implications for Nursing Education

The model is an appropriate curriculum guide for all levels of nursing education. The components of the model serve as curriculum content, including the five variable areas (physiological, psychological, sociocultural, developmental, spiritual), the three categories of stressors (intrapersonal, interpersonal, extrapersonal) and the three prevention-as-intervention modalities (primary, secondary, tertiary).

### Reference

Neuman, B. (1995). *The Neuman Systems Model* (3rd ed.). Norwalk, CT: Appleton and Lange.

## DOROTHEA OREM'S SELF-CARE FRAMEWORK

### Overview

Focus is on the nurse's deliberate action related to systems of therapeutic self-care for individuals who have limitations in their abilities to provide continuing self-care or care of dependent others. The six central concepts are:

1. **Self-care**–behavior directed by individuals to themselves or their environments to regulate factors that affect their own development and functioning in the interests of life, health, or well-being.
2. **Self-care agency**–a complex capability of maturing and mature individuals to determine the presence and characteristics of specific requirements for regulating their own functioning and development, make judgments and decisions about what to do, and perform care measures to meet specific self-care requisites. The person's ability to perform self-care is influenced by 10 *power components:*
   - Ability to maintain attention and exercise requisite vigilance with respect to self as self-care agent and internal and external conditions and factors significant for self-care.
   - Controlled use of available physical energy that is sufficient for the initiation and continuation of self-care operations.
   - Ability to control the position of the body and its parts in the execution of the movements required for the initiation and completion of self-care operations.
   - Ability to reason within a self-care frame of reference.
   - Motivation (i.e., goal orientations for self-care that are in accord with its characteristics and its meaning for life, health, and well-being).
   - Ability to make decisions about care of self and to operationalize these decisions.
   - Ability to acquire technical knowledge about self-care from authoritative sources, to retain it, and to operationalize it.
   - A repertoire of cognitive, perceptual, manipulative, communication, and interpersonal skills adapted to the performance of self-care operations.
   - Ability to order discrete self-care actions or action systems into relationships with prior and subsequent actions toward the final achievement of regulatory goals of self-care.
   - Ability to consistently perform self-care operations, integrating them with relevant aspects of personal, family, and community living.

   The person's ability to perform self-care as well as the kind and amount of self-care that is required are influenced by 10 internal and external factors called *basic conditioning factors:*
   - Age
   - Gender
   - Developmental state
   - Health state
   - Sociocultural orientation
   - Health care system factors; for example, medical diagnostic and treatment modalities
   - Family system factors
   - Patterns of living including activities regularly engaged in
   - Environmental factors
   - Resource availability and adequacy
3. **Therapeutic self-care demand**–the action demand on individuals to meet three types of self-care requisites:
   - *Universal self-care requisites*–actions that need to be performed to maintain life processes, the integrity of human structure and function, and general well-being.
   - *Developmental self-care requisites*–actions that need to be performed in relation to human developmental processes, conditions, and events and in relation to events that may adversely affect development.
   - *Health deviation self-care requisites*–actions that need to be performed in relation to genetic and constitutional defects, human structural and functional deviations and their

effects, and medical diagnostic and treatment measures prescribed or performed by physicians.

4. **Self-care deficit**–the relationship of inadequacy between self-care agency and the therapeutic self-care demand.
5. **Nursing agency**–a complex property or attribute that enables nurses to know and help others to know their therapeutic self-care demands, meet their therapeutic self-care demands, and regulate the exercise or development of their self-care agency.
6. **Nursing system**–a series of coordinated deliberate practical actions performed by nurses and patients directed toward meeting the patient's therapeutic self-care demand and protecting and regulating the exercise or development of the patient's self-care agency.

### Implications for Nursing Practice

Nursing practice is directed toward helping people to meet their own and their dependent others' therapeutic self-care demands. The six operations that describe and give direction to nursing practice are:

1. **Nursing diagnosis**–a professional operation focusing on determining why the person needs nursing care. This requires calculation of the person's therapeutic self-care demand through assessment of the self-care requisites, assessment of self-care agency, including determination of the influence of the power components and the basic conditioning factors, and identification of the self-care deficit.
2. **Nursing prescription**–a professional operation that specifies the means to be used to meet particular self-care requisites, all care measures needed to meet the entire therapeutic self-care demand, and the roles to be played by the nurse and the self-care agent in meeting the patient's therapeutic self-care demand and in regulating the patient's exercise or development of self-care agency.
3. **Nursing system design**–a professional operation that involves selection of a nursing system and one or more methods of helping. The three types of regulatory nursing system designs are:

   *Wholly compensatory nursing system*–selected when the patient cannot or should not perform self-care actions.

   *Partly compensatory nursing system*–selected when the patient can perform some, but not all, self-care actions.

   *Supportive-educative nursing system*–selected when the patient can and should perform all self-care actions.

   The five methods of helping are:

   Acting for or doing for another
   Guiding and directing
   Providing physical or psychological support
   Providing and maintaining an environment that supports personal development
   Teaching
4. **Planning**–a case management operation that requires specification of the time, place, environmental conditions, equipment and supplies, the organization and timing of tasks to be performed, and the number and the qualifications of nurses or others necessary to produce a designed nursing system, to evaluate effects, and to make needed adjustments.
5. **Regulatory care**–a professional operation that involves the actual production and management of the designated nursing system and methods of helping.
6. **Controlling**–a case management operation that encompasses observation and evaluation of the efficacy of the nursing system.

### Implications for Nursing Education

The Self-Care Framework provides a body of knowledge that can be used for curriculum development. The focus of both undergraduate and graduate nursing curricula is on components of self-care, self-care agency, self-care deficits, nursing agency, and nursing systems. Education for clinical skills emphasizes the methods of helping.

### Reference

Orem, D. E. (1995). *Nursing: Concepts of practice* (5th ed.). St. Louis: Mosby.

## MARTHA ROGERS' SCIENCE OF UNITARY HUMAN BEINGS

### Overview

Focus is on unitary, irreducible human beings and their environments. The four basic concepts are:

1. **Energy fields**–irreducible, indivisible, pandimensional unitary human beings and environments that are identified by pattern and manifesting characteristics that are specific to the whole and cannot be predicted from knowledge of the parts. Human and environmental energy fields are integral with each other.

2. **Openness**–a characteristic of human and environmental energy fields; energy fields are continuously and completely open.
3. **Pattern**–the distinguishing characteristic of an energy field. Pattern is perceived as a single wave that gives identity to the field. Each human field pattern is unique and is integral with its own unique environmental field pattern. Pattern is an abstraction that cannot be seen; what is seen or experienced are manifestations of field pattern.
4. **Pandimensionality**–a nonlinear domain without spatial or temporal attributes.

The three principles of homeodynamics, which describe the nature of human and environmental energy fields, are:

1. **Resonancy**–asserts that human and environmental fields are identified by wave patterns that manifest continuous change from lower to higher frequencies.
2. **Helicy**–asserts that human and environmental field patterns are continuous, innovative, and unpredictable, and are characterized by increasing diversity.
3. **Integrality**–emphasizes the continuous mutual human field and environmental field process.

### Implications for Nursing Practice

Nursing practice is directed toward promoting the health and well-being of all persons, wherever they are. The Rogerian practice methodology encompasses two phases:

1. **Pattern manifestation appraisal**–the continuous process of identifying manifestations of the human and environmental fields that relate to current health events. Human field pattern is appraised through manifestations of the pattern in the form of experience, perception, and expressions. Experiences of pattern manifestation are accompanied by perception and are expressed in such diverse forms as verbal responses, responses to questionnaires, and personal ways of living and relating. Relevant pattern information includes sensations, thoughts, feelings, awareness, imagination, memory, introspective insights, intuitive apprehensions, recurring themes and issues that pervade one's life, metaphors, visualizations, images, nutrition, work and play, exercise, substance use, sleep/wake cycles, safety, decelerated/accelerated field rhythms, space-time shifts, interpersonal networks, and professional health care access and use.
2. **Deliberative mutual patterning**–the continuous process whereby the nurse with the client patterns the environmental field to promote harmony related to the health events. The nurse helps to create an environment where healing conditions are optimal and invites clients to heal themselves as they participate in various modalities used in deliberative mutual patterning, including noninvasive modalities such as therapeutic touch, imagery, meditation, relaxation, unconditional love, attitudes of hope, humor, and upbeat moods, and the use of sound, color, and motion.

### Implications for Nursing Education

Education for nursing practice requires a commitment to lifelong learning. Education for professional nursing occurs at the baccalaureate, masters, and doctoral levels in college and university settings. The purpose of professional nursing educational programs is to provide the knowledge and tools necessary for nursing practice. The liberal arts and sciences are a predominant component of the curriculum. The principles of resonancy, helicy, and integrality represent the major integrating concepts of the nursing courses.

### References

Madrid, M., & Barrett, E. A. M. (Eds.). (1994). *Rogers' scientific art of nursing practice*. New York: National League for Nursing.

Rogers, M. E. (1990). Nursing: Science of unitary, irreducible, human beings: Update 1990. In E. A. M. Barrett (Ed.), *Visions of Rogers' science-based nursing* (pp. 5–11). New York: National League for Nursing.

Rogers, M. E. (1992). Nursing science and the space age. *Nursing Science Quarterly*, 5, 27–34.

## CALLISTA ROY'S ADAPTATION MODEL

### Overview

Focuses on the responses of the human adaptive system to a constantly changing environment. Adaptation is the central feature of the model. Problems in adaptation arise when the adaptive system is unable to cope with or respond to constantly changing stimuli from the internal and external environments in a manner that maintains the integrity of the system. Environmental stimuli are categorized as:

1. **Focal**–the stimuli most immediately confronting the person.
2. **Contextual**–the contributing factors in the situation.
3. **Residual**–other unknown factors that may influence the situation. When the factors making up residual stimuli become known, they are considered focal or contextual stimuli.

Adaptation occurs through two types of innate or acquired coping mechanisms used to respond to changing environmental stimuli:

1. **Regulator subsystem**–receives input from the external environment and from changes in the person's internal state and processes the changes through neural-chemical-endocrine channels to produce responses.
2. **Cognator subsystem**–also receives input from external and internal stimuli that involve psychological, social, physical, and physiological factors, including regulator subsystem outputs. These stimuli then are processed through cognitive/emotive pathways, including perceptual/information processing, learning, judgment, and emotion.

Responses take place in four modes:

1. **Physiological mode**–concerned with basic needs requisite to maintaining the physical and physiological integrity of the human system; encompasses oxygenation, nutrition, elimination, activity and rest, protection, the senses, fluids and electrolytes, neurological functions, and endocrine functions.
2. **Self-concept mode**–deals with people's conceptions of the
   *Physical self*–body sensation and body image.
   *Personal self*–self-consistency, self-ideal, and the moral-ethical-spiritual self.
3. **Role function mode**–concerned with people's performance of roles on the basis of their positions within society.
4. **Interdependence mode**–involves the willingness and ability to love, respect, and value others, and to accept and respond to love, respect, and value given by others; concerned primarily with relationships with significant others and social support systems.

The four modes are interrelated. Responses in any one mode may have an effect on or act as a stimulus in one or all of the other modes.

Responses in each mode:

1. **Adaptive**–those that promote the integrity of the person in terms of the goals of the human adaptive system, including survival, growth, reproduction, and mastery.
2. **Ineffective**–those that do not contribute to the goals of the human adaptive system.

## Implications for Nursing Practice

Nursing practice is directed toward promoting adaptation in each of the four response modes, thereby contributing to the person's health, quality of life, and dying with dignity. The nursing process encompasses six steps:

1. **Assessment of behavior**–collection of data regarding adaptive system behaviors; determination of adaptive and ineffective responses; setting priorities for further assessment.
2. **Assessment of stimuli**–identification of the focal and contextual stimuli that influence adaptive system behaviors.
3. **Nursing diagnosis**–judgments regarding adaptation status.
4. **Goal setting**–statement of behavioral outcomes of nursing intervention.
5. **Nursing intervention**–management of environmental stimuli by increasing, decreasing, maintaining, removing, or otherwise altering or changing relevant focal and/or contextual stimuli.
6. **Evaluation**–judgments regarding the effectiveness of nursing intervention.

## Implications for Nursing Education

The model is an appropriate curriculum guide for diploma, associate degree, baccalaureate degree, and master's degree nursing education programs. Curriculum content is based on the components of the conceptual model. The vertical strands of the curriculum focus on theory and practice. The theory strand encompasses content on the adapting person, health/illness, and stress/disruption. The practice strand emphasizes nursing management of environmental stimuli. The horizontal strands include the nursing process and student adaptation and leadership.

## Reference

Roy, C., & Andrews, H. A. (1991). *The Roy Adaptation Model: The definitive statement*. Norwalk, CT: Appleton and Lange.

# Appendix 20–3 Nursing Theory

A theory is defined as a set of relatively specific and concrete concepts and the statements that describe or link those concepts. Nursing theories are derived from more abstract and general conceptual models and describe, explain, or predict phenomena of interest to nursing. A grand theory is more abstract than a middle-range theory.

## MADELEINE LEININGER'S THEORY OF CULTURAL CARE DIVERSITY AND UNIVERSALITY

### Overview

A grand theory focusing on the discovery of human care diversities and universalities and ways to provide culturally congruent care to people. The concepts of the theory are:

1. **Care**–abstract and concrete phenomena related to assisting, supporting, or enabling experiences or behaviors toward or for others with evident or anticipated needs to ameliorate or improve a human condition or lifeway.
2. **Caring**–the actions and activities directed toward assisting, supporting, or enabling another individual or group with evident or anticipated needs to ameliorate or improve a human condition or lifeway or to face death.
3. **Culture**–the learned, shared, and transmitted values, beliefs, norms, and lifeways of a particular group that guides thinking, decisions, and actions in patterned ways; encompasses several cultural and social structure dimensions: technological factors, religious and philosophical factors, kinship and social factors, political and legal factors, economic factors, educational factors, and cultural values and lifeways.
4. **Language**–word usages, symbols, and meanings about care.
5. **Ethnohistory**–past facts, events, instances, experiences of individuals, groups, cultures, and institutions that are primarily people centered (ethno) and which describe, explain, and interpret human lifeways within particular cultural contexts and over short or long periods of time.
6. **Environmental context**–the totality of an event, situation, or particular experiences that give meaning to human expressions, interpretations, and social interactions in particular physical, ecological, sociopolitical, and/or cultural settings.
7. **Health**–a state of well-being that is culturally defined, valued, and practiced, and which reflects the ability of individuals (or groups) to perform their daily role activities in culturally expressed, beneficial, and patterned lifeways.
8. **Worldview**–the way people tend to look out on the world or their universe to form a picture of or a value stance about their life or the world around them.
9. **Cultural care**–the subjectively and objectively transmitted values, beliefs, and patterned lifeways that assist, support, or enable another individual or group to maintain well-being and health, to improve his or her human condition and lifeway, to deal with illness, handicaps, or death. The two dimensions are:

    *Cultural care diversity*–the variabilities and/or differences in meanings, patterns, values, lifeways, or symbols of care within or between collectivities that are related to assistive, supportive, or enabling human care expressions.

    *Cultural care universality*–the common, similar, or dominant uniform care meanings, patterns, values, lifeways, or symbols that are manifest among many cultures and reflect assistive, supportive, facilitative, or enabling ways to help people.
10. **Care systems**–the values, norms, and structural features of an organization designed for serving people's health needs, concerns, or conditions. The two types of care systems are:

    *Generic lay care system*–traditional or local indigenous health care or cure practices that have special meanings and uses to heal or assist people, which are generally offered in familiar home or community environmental contexts with their local practitioners.

    *Professional health care system*–professional care or cure services offered by diverse health personnel who have been prepared through formal professional programs of study in special educational institutions.
11. **Cultural-congruent nursing care**–cognitively based assistive, supportive, facilitative, or enabling acts or decisions that are tailored to fit with individual, group, or institutional cultural values, beliefs, and lifeways in order to provide or support meaningful, beneficial, and satisfying health care or well-being services. The three modes of cultural-congruent nursing care are:

    *Cultural care preservation or maintenance*–assistive, supportive, facilitative, or enabling professional actions and decisions that help people of a particular culture to retain and/or preserve relevant care values so that they can maintain their well-being, recover from illness, or face handicaps and/or death.

    *Cultural care accommodation or negotiation*–assistive, supportive, facilitative, or enabling creative professional actions and decisions that help people of a designated culture to adapt to, or to negotiate with, others for a beneficial or satisfying health outcome with professional care providers.

    *Cultural care repatterning or restructuring*–assistive, supportive, facilitative, or enabling professional actions and decisions that help clients reorder, change, or greatly modify their lifeways for a new, different and beneficial health care pattern while respecting the clients' cultural values and beliefs and still providing a beneficial or healthier lifeway than before the changes were coestablished with the clients.

### Implications for Nursing Practice

Nursing practice is directed toward improving and providing culturally congruent care to people. The three modes of cultural-congruent nursing care are used as the basis for nursing interventions.

### Implications for Nursing Education

Professional nursing care, learned in formal educational programs, builds upon the generic care given by naturalistic lay and folk care givers. The curriculum emphasizes transcultural nursing knowledge, with formal study about different cultures in the world, as well as culture-universal and culture-specific health care needs of people and nursing care practices. Transcultural nurse generalists are prepared at the baccalaureate level for the general use of transcultural nursing concepts, principles, and practices. Transcultural nurse specialists, who are prepared at the doctoral level, have in-depth understanding of a few cultures and can function as field practitioners, teachers, researchers, or consultants. Certification is awarded by the Transcultural Nursing Society to nurses who have educational preparation in transcultural nursing or the equivalent and who demonstrate basic clinical competence in transcultural nursing.

### Reference

Leininger, M. M. (Ed.). (1991). *Culture care diversity and universality: A theory of nursing.* New York: National League for Nursing.

## NEWMAN'S THEORY OF HEALTH AS EXPANDING CONSCIOUSNESS

### Overview

A grand theory focusing on health as the expansion of consciousness, with emphasis on the idea that every person in every situation, no matter how disordered and hopeless the situation may seem, is part of the universal process of expanding consciousness. The concepts of the theory are:

1. **Time**–the amount of time perceived to be passing (subjective time); clock time (objective time).
2. **Space**–encompasses personal space, inner space, and life space as dimensions of space relevant to the individual, and territoriality, shared space, and distancing as dimensions relevant to the family.
3. **Movement**–an essential property of matter; a means of communicating; the means whereby one perceives reality and becomes aware of self; the natural condition of life.
4. **Consciousness**–the informational capacity of human beings, that is, the ability of humans to interact with their environments. Consciousness encompasses interconnected cognitive and affective awareness, physiochemical maintenance including the nervous and endocrine systems, growth processes, the immune system, and the genetic code. Consciousness can be seen in the quantity and quality of the interaction between human beings and their environments. The process of life is toward higher levels of consciousness; sometimes this process is smooth, pleasant, harmonious; other times it is difficult and disharmonious, as in disease.
5. **Pattern**–a fundamental attribute that gives unity in diversity; information that depicts the whole; relatedness. People are identified by their pattern. The evolution of expanding consciousness is seen in the pattern of movement-space-time.

### Implications for Nursing Practice

Nursing practice is directed toward facilitating pattern recognition by connecting with the client in an authentic way, and assisting the client to discover new rules for a higher level of organization or consciousness. The nurse-client relationship is a rhythmic coming together and moving apart that occurs in three ongoing steps:

1. **Meeting**–occurs when there is a mutual attraction of nurse and client via congruent patterns.
2. **Forming shared consciousness**–sharing of the whole between the nurse and the client to form a connection; when the connection is formed, pattern recognition is facilitated by means of the application of the four components of Newman's research methodology:
   *Establishing the mutuality of the process of inquiry.*
   *Focusing on the most meaningful persons and events in the person's life.*
   *Organizing the data in narrative form and displaying it as sequential patterns over time.*
   *Sharing the person's perception of the pattern with him or her and seeking revision or confirmation.*
3. **Moving apart**–occurs when the client is able to center without being connected to the nurse.

### Implications for Nursing Education

Education for nursing should be the professional doctoral degree, the Doctor of Nursing (ND), which requires a strong arts and sciences background as pre-professional education. Students and practicing nurses who plan to use the Theory of Health as Expanding Consciousness have to be prepared for personal transformation in the way that they view the world and nursing.

### Reference

Newman, M. A. (1994). *Health as expanding consciousness* (2nd ed.). New York: National League for Nursing.

## IDA JEAN ORLANDO'S THEORY OF THE NURSING PROCESS DISCIPLINE

### Overview

A middle-range predictive theory focusing on an interpersonal process that is directed toward facilitating identification of the nature of the patient's distress and his or her immediate needs for help. The concepts of the theory are:

1. **Patient's behavior**–behavior observed by the nurse in an immediate nurse-patient situation. The two dimensions are:

   *Need for help*–a requirement of the patient which, if supplied, relieves or diminishes immediate distress or improves immediate sense of adequacy or well-being.

   *Improvement*–an increase in patients' mental and physical health, their well-being, and their sense of adequacy. The need for help and improvement can be expressed in both nonverbal and verbal forms. Visual manifestations of nonverbal behavior include such motor activities as eating, walking, twitching, and trembling, as well as such physiological forms as urinating, defecating, temperature and blood pressure readings, respiratory rate, and skin color. Vocal forms of nonverbal behavior—nonverbal behavior that is heard—include crying, moaning, laughing, coughing, sneezing, sighing, yelling, screaming, groaning, and singing. Verbal behavior refers to what a patient says, including complaints, requests, questions, refusals, demands, and comments or statements.

2. **Nurse's reaction**–the nurse's nonobservable response to the patient's behavior. The three dimensions are:

   *Perception*–physical stimulation of any one of the five senses by the patient's behavior.

   *Thought*–an idea which occurs in the nurse's mind.

   *Feeling*–a state of mind inclining the nurse toward or against a perception, thought, or action; occurs in response to the nurse's perceptions and thoughts.

3. **Nurse's activity**–the observable actions taken by nurses in response to their reactions, including instructions, suggestions, directions, explanations, information, requests, and questions directed toward the patient; making decisions for the patient; handling the patient's body; administering medications or treatments; and changing the patient's immediate environment. The two dimensions of nurse's activity are:

   *Automatic nursing process*–actions decided on by the nurse for reasons other than the patient's immediate need.

   *Deliberative nursing process* (process discipline)—a specific set of nurse behaviors or actions directed toward the patient's behavior that ascertain or meet the patient's immediate needs for help.

### Implications for Nursing Practice

Nursing practice is directed toward identifying and meeting the patient's immediate needs for help through use of the deliberative nursing process, which occurs when three requirements are met:

1. What the nurse says to the patient must match the nurse's reaction, what the nurse does nonverbally must be verbally expressed, and the expression must match the nurse's reaction.
2. The nurse must clearly communicate to the patient that what is expressed belongs to himself or herself. (*I* think that . . . )
3. The nurse must ask the patient about the item expressed in order to obtain correction or verification. (Is that so?)

### Implications for Nursing Education

Students should be trained in the use of the deliberative nursing process for all person-to-person contacts. The purpose of training is to change the nurse's activity from personal and automatic to disciplined and professional. Training is facilitated by use of process recordings that include perceptions of or about the patient, thoughts and/or feelings about the perception, and what was said and/or done to, with, or for the patient. The process discipline can be successfully taught in 6 to 12 weeks.

### References

Orlando, I. J. (1961). *The dynamic nurse-patient relationship: Function, process and principles.* New York: G. P. Putnam's Sons. [Reprinted 1990, New York: National League for Nursing]

Orlando, I. J. (1972). *The discipline and teaching of nursing process: An evaluative study.* New York: G. P. Putnam's Sons.

## ROSEMARIE PARSE'S THEORY OF HUMAN BECOMING

### Overview

A grand theory focusing on human experiences of participation with the universe in the cocreation of health. The concepts of the theory are:

1. **Meaning**–encompasses three subconcepts:
   *Imaging*–symbolizing or picturing; making concrete the meaning of multidimensional experiences.
   *Valuing*–choosing to confirm a cherished belief; the process of confirming cherished beliefs.
   *Languaging*–expressing valued images; sharing valued images through symbols of words, gesture, gaze, touch, and posture.
2. **Rhythmicity**–referring to cadence or order; the subconcepts are:
   *Revealing-concealing*–the simultaneous disclosing of some aspects of self and hiding of others; a paradoxical rhythm in the pattern of relating with others.
   *Enabling-limiting*–a rhythmical pattern of relating; in choosing, there are an infinite number of opportunities and an infinite number of limitations: thus one is enabled-limited by all choices.
   *Connecting-separating*–a rhythmical process of moving together and moving apart.
3. **Cotranscendence**–referring to going beyond the actual in interrelationships with others; the subconcepts are:
   *Powering*–struggling with the tension of pushing-resisting.
   *Originating*–springing from; emerging; creating anew, generating unique ways of living which surface through interconnections with people and projects.
   *Transforming*–the changing of change, coconstituting anew in a deliberate way; the shifting of views of the familiar as different light is shed on what is known.

The three major principles of the theory of human becoming are:

1. **Structuring meaning multidimensionally is cocreating reality through the languaging of valuing and imaging**–means that humans construct what is real for them from choices made at many realms of the universe.
2. **Cocreating rhythmical patterns of relating is living the paradoxical unity of revealing-concealing and enabling-limiting while connecting-separating**–means that humans live in rhythm with the universe coconstituting patterns of relating.
3. **Cotranscending with the possibles is powering unique ways of originating in the process of transforming**–means that humans forge unique paths with shifting perspectives as a different light is cast on the familiar.

### Implications for Nursing Practice

Nursing practice is directed toward respecting the quality of life as perceived by the person and the family. The practice methodology encompasses three dimensions and three processes:

1. The dimension, *illuminating meaning,* is shedding light through uncovering what was, is, and will be, as it is appearing now. It happens in explicating what is. The process of *explicating* is making clear what is appearing now through languaging.
2. The dimension, *synchronizing rhythms,* happens in dwelling with the pitch, yaw, and roll of the interhuman cadence. The process of *dwelling with* is giving self over to the flow of the struggle in connecting-separating.
3. The dimension, *mobilizing transcendence,* happens in moving beyond the meaning moment to what is not-yet. The process of *moving beyond* is propelling toward an imaged possible in transforming.

### Implications for Nursing Education

Course content flows from the three principles of the theory. Clinical courses emphasize the knowledge and skills requisite to the application of the practice methodology. Graduate education builds on baccalaureate education and prepares specialists who concentrate on creating and testing concepts of the theory of human becoming.

### References

Parse, R. R. (1992). Human becoming: Parse's theory of nursing. *Nursing Science Quarterly,* 5, 35–42.

Parse, R. R. (Ed.). (1995). *Illuminations: The human becoming theory in practice and research.* New York: National League for Nursing.

## HILDEGARD PEPLAU'S THEORY OF INTERPERSONAL RELATIONS

### Overview

A middle-range descriptive theory focusing on the phases of the interpersonal process that occurs when an ill person and a nurse come together to resolve a difficulty felt in relation to health. The one concept of the theory is nurse-patient relationship, which has four discernible phases:

1. **Orientation**–occurs as the patient has a felt need signifying a health problem and seeks assistance to clarify the problem. The patient participates by asking questions, by trying to find out what needs to be known in order to feel secure, and by observing ways in which professional people respond. The nurse participates by helping the patient to recognize and understand the health problem and the extent of need for assistance, to understand what professional services can offer, to plan the use of professional services, and to harness energy from tension and anxiety connected with felt needs.
2. **Identification**–occurs as the patient learns how to make use of the nurse-patient relationship as both come to know and to respect one another, as persons who have likes and differences of opinions, in ways of looking at a situation, in responding to events. The nurse makes use of professional education and skill in aiding the patient to arrive at a point where full use can be made of the relationship in order to solve the health problem.
3. **Exploitation**–occurs as the patient makes full use of available professional services.
4. **Resolution**–occurs as the nurse helps the patient to organize actions so that the patient will want to be free for more productive social activities and relationships.

### Implications for Nursing Practice

Nursing practice is directed toward promoting favorable changes in patients, which is accomplished through the nurse-patient relationship. Within that relationship, the nurse's major function is to study the interpersonal relations between the patient/client and others. The five characteristics of professional nursing practice are:

1. The focus of professional nursing is the patient.
2. The nurse uses participant observation rather than spectator observation.
3. The nurse is aware of the various roles she assumes in the nurse-patient relationship.
4. Professional nursing is primarily investigative, with emphasis on observation and collection of data that are made available to the patient, rather than task-oriented.
5. Professional nursing is grounded in the use of theory.

Three interlocking performances in interpersonal relations make it possible for nurses to study what is happening in their contacts with patients:

1. Nurses *observe* the ways in which patients transform energy into patterns of action that bring satisfaction or security in the face of a recurring problem.
2. Nurses and patients *communicate* with one another in terms of their views of themselves and their expectations of others.
3. Nurses *record* the verbatim difficulties of patients and desymbolize the recordings to reveal hidden wishes and longings that may be the root of the problem.

### Implications for Nursing Education

Nursing is an educative instrument, a maturing force, that aims to promote forward movement of personality in the direction of creative, constructive, productive, personal, and community living. The task of each school of nursing is the fullest development of the nurse as a person who is aware of how he or she functions in a situation and as a person who wants to nurse patients in a helpful way.

### References

Peplau, H. E. (1952). *Interpersonal relations in nursing.* New York: G. P. Putnam's Sons. [Reprinted 1991. New York: Springer]

Peplau, H. E. (1992). Interpersonal relations: A theoretical framework for application in nursing practice. *Nursing Science Quarterly, 5,* 13–18.

## REVA RUBIN'S THEORY OF CLINICAL NURSING

### Overview

A grand theory focusing on patients as persons undergoing subjectively involved experiences of varying degrees of tension or stress in a health problem situation. The major concepts are the situation of the patient and nursing care. Statements related to the patient situation and nursing care are:

1. Nursing care is dependent on the best estimate available of the situation of the patient.
2. Nursing care exists in a one-to-one relationship with the patient.
3. The relationship of nursing care to the situation of the patient is an ever-changing process of interaction.
4. The situation of the patient is expressed as a fraction or ratio that reflects the level or intensity of nursing care required.

If the situation for the patient is relatively insignificant, one that the patient can cope with quite well, then nursing care probably need not go beyond careful assessment.

If the situation for the patient is overwhelming, nursing care may have to encompass a whole series of activities to reduce the effects of the situation or reinforce the capacities of the patient in coping with the situation.

5. Situations within the sphere of proper nursing concern are fluid.

## Implications for Nursing Practice

Nursing practice is directed toward helping the patient adjust to, endure through, and usefully integrate the health problem situation in its many ramifications through the phenomenon of *situational fluidity,* which characterizes nursing care in terms of:

1. **Time**–nursing operates within the immediate present; patient needs and behavior have an immediacy if not an urgency.
2. **Definition or diagnostic sets**–nursing diagnoses are based on the definition of capacities and limitations of the persons who are patients in relation to the situations in which they find themselves.
3. **Actions**–nursing actions are primarily directed toward helping the patient realign observations and expectations into a better "fit" with each other; nursing conveys a message to patients about themselves in their immediate situations.

## Implications for Nursing Education

Education for nursing practice and nursing research emphasizes learning the naturalistic method of observation of patients in action, involved in a natural situation and setting. The learners typically are graduate students in nursing. The nurse-observer is viewed as an identifiable and functional part of the setting, as well as a helpful adjunct in the situation. The student is trained to observe while providing nursing care for the patient in a particular situation and to then record the entire nurse-patient interaction. The recorded observation serves as a database for evaluation of the quality and adequacy of nursing care as well as for generation of new theories.

## References

Rubin, R. (1968). A theory of clinical nursing. *Nursing Research, 17,* 210–212.

Rubin, R. (1984). *Maternal identity and the maternal experience.* New York: Springer.

# JEAN WATSON'S THEORY OF HUMAN CARING

## Overview

A middle-range descriptive theory focusing on the caring actions taken by nurses as they interact with others. The concepts of the theory are:

1. **Transpersonal caring**–human-to-human connectedness whereby each person is touched by the human center of the other; the four components are:
   *Self*–the organized consistent conceptual gestalt composed of perceptions of the characteristics of the "I" or "me" and the perceptions of the relationships of the "I" or "me" to others and to various aspects of life, together with the values attached to those perceptions.
   *Phenomenal field*–made up of the totality of human experience; the individual's frame of reference that can be known only to the person; the person's subjective reality.
   *Actual caring occasion of the patient and the nurse*–the event when the giver and the recipient of care come together, which involves action and choice by both the nurse and the individual.
   *Intersubjectivity*–refers to an intersubjective human-to-human relationship in which the person of the nurse affects and is affected by the person of the other. Both are fully present in the moment and feel a union with the other. They share a phenomenal field which becomes part of the life history of both and are coparticipants in becoming in the now and the future.
2. **Carative factors**–nursing interventions or caring processes; the 10 carative factors are:
   *Formation of a humanistic-altruistic system of values.*
   *Instillation of faith-hope.*
   *Cultivation of sensitivity to one's self and to others.*
   *Development of a helping-trusting, human care relationship.*
   *Promotion and acceptance of the expression of positive and negative feelings.*
   *Systematic use of a creative problem-solving caring process.*
   *Promotion of transpersonal teaching-learning.*
   *Provision for a supportive, protective, and/or corrective mental, physical, societal, and spiritual environment.*
   *Assistance with gratification of human needs.*
   *Allowance for existential-phenomenological-spiritual forces.*

## Implications for Nursing Practice

Nursing practice is directed toward helping persons gain a higher degree of harmony within the mind, body, and soul which generates self-knowledge, self-reverence, self-healing, and self-care processes while increasing diversity, which is pursued through use of the 10 carative factors.

## Implications for Nursing Education

Professional nursing education should be at the postbaccalaureate level of the Doctorate of Nursing (N.D.). The nature of human life is the subject matter of nursing. The curriculum acknowledges caring as a moral ideal and incorporates philosophical theories of human caring, health, and healing. Core areas of content are the humanities, social-biomedical science, and human caring content and process. Courses should use art, music, literature, poetry, drama, and movement to facilitate understanding of responses to health and illness as well as to new caring-healing modalities.

## References

Watson, J. (1985). *Nursing: Human science and human care. A theory of nursing*. Norwalk, CT: Appleton-Century-Crofts. [Reprinted 1988. New York: National League for Nursing]

Watson, J. (1990). Transpersonal caring: A transcendent view of person, health, and nursing. In M. E. Parker (Ed.), *Nursing theories in practice* (pp. 277–288). New York: National League for Nursing.

# APPENDIX 21
# Nursing Diagnoses*

## Quick View of Contents



Appendices 21–1 and 21–2 **Organize all approved NANDA nursing diagnoses by two nursing models: Gordon's Functional Health Patterns and Doenges & Moorhouse's Diagnostic Divisions. The use of a nursing model as a framework helps to organize the data needed to identify and validate nursing diagnoses.**

Appendix 21–3 **Lists the most recently approved NANDA nursing diagnoses for quick reference.**

Appendix 21–4 **Provides a guide to choosing appropriate nursing diagnoses by alphabetically listing almost 300 diseases/disorders with their commonly associated nursing diagnoses. Each of the listed diseases/disorders has been cross-referenced from its position in the body of the dictionary. The nursing diagnoses are written in the form of patient problem statements, also known as PES format (Problem, Etiology, Signs/ Symptoms). The phrases "may be related to" and "possibly evidenced by" in the patient problem statements serve to help one individualize the care for the specific patient situations. A "risk for" diagnosis is not evidenced by signs and symptoms, as the problem has not occurred and nursing interventions are directed at prevention. Because the patient's health status is perpetual and ongoing, other nursing diagnoses may be appropriate based on changing patient situations. To identify other applicable nursing diagnoses check Appendix 21–1, then turn to Appendix 21–5 to test and validate your choices.**

Appendix 21–5 **Details the NANDA-approved diagnoses through the 12th Conference in alphabetical order with their associated etiology [Related/Risk Factors] and signs and symptoms [Defining Characteristics]. This specific focus on assessment data/evaluation criteria helps you complete the validation process.**

---

* **Adapted from North American Nursing Diagnosis Association (1994). NANDA Nursing Diagnoses: Definitions and Classification 1995–1996. Philadelphia: NANDA.**

# Appendix 21–1 Gordon's Functional Health Patterns

HEALTH PERCEPTION – HEALTH MANAGEMENT PATTERN

Energy Field Disturbance
Health Maintenance, altered
Health-Seeking Behaviors (specify)
Infection, risk for
Injury, risk for
Noncompliance (specify) [compliance, altered]
Perioperative Positioning Injury, risk for
Poisoning, risk for
Protection, altered
Suffocation, risk for
Therapeutic Regimen (Community), ineffective management of
Therapeutic Regimen (Families), ineffective management of
Therapeutic Regimen (Individual), effective management of
Therapuetic Regimen (Individual), ineffective management of
Trauma, risk for

NUTRITIONAL – METABOLIC PATTERN

Aspiration, risk for
Body Temperature, altered, risk for
Breastfeeding, effective
Breastfeeding, ineffective
Breastfeeding, interrupted
Fluid Volume Deficit [active loss]
Fluid Volume Deficit [regulatory failure]
Fluid Volume Deficit, risk for
Fluid Volume Excess
Hyperthermia
Hypothermia
Infant Feeding Pattern, ineffective
Nutrition: altered, less than body requirements
Nutrition: altered, more than body requirements
Nutrition: altered, risk for more than body requirements
Oral Mucous Membrane, altered
Skin Integrity, impaired
Skin Integrity, impaired, risk for
Swallowing, impaired
Thermoregulation, ineffective
Tissue Integrity, impaired

ELIMINATION PATTERN

Bowel Incontinence
Constipation
Constipation, colonic
Constipation, perceived
Diarrhea
Incontinence, functional
Incontinence, reflex
Incontinence, stress
Incontinence, total
Incontinence, urge
Urinary Elimination, altered patterns of
Urinary Retention [acute/chronic]

ACTIVITY – EXERCISE PATTERN

Activity Intolerance [specify level]
Activity Intolerance, risk for
Airway Clearance, ineffective
Breathing Pattern, ineffective
Cardiac Output, decreased
Disorganized Infant Behavior
Disorganized Infant Behavior, risk for
Disuse Syndrome, risk for
Diversional Activity Deficit
Dysreflexia
Enhanced Organized Infant Behavior, potential for
Fatigue
Gas Exchange, impaired
Growth and Development, altered
Home Maintenance Management, impaired
Peripheral Neurovascular Dysfunction, risk for
Physical Mobility, impaired
Self-Care Deficit [specify level]: feeding, bathing/hygiene, dressing/grooming, toileting
Spontaneous Ventilation, inability to sustain
Tissue Perfusion, altered (specify): cerebral, cardiopulmonary, renal, gastrointestinal, peripheral
Ventilatory Weaning Response, dysfunctional (DVWR)

SLEEP – REST PATTERN

Sleep Pattern Disturbance

COGNITIVE – PERCEPTUAL PATTERN

Adaptive Capacity: intracranial, decreased
Confusion, Acute
Confusion, Chronic
Decisional Conflict
Environmental Interpretation Syndrome, impaired
Knowledge Deficit [learning need] (specify)
Memory, impaired
Pain
Pain, acute
Pain, chronic
Sensory/Perceptual Alterations (specify): visual, auditory, kinesthetic, gustatory, tactile, olfactory
Thought Processes, altered
Unilateral Neglect

SELF-PERCEPTION – SELF-CONCEPT PATTERN

Anxiety [Mild, Moderate, Severe, Panic]

Body Image Disturbance
Fear
Hopelessness
Loneliness, risk for
Personal Identity Disturbance
Powerlessness
Self-Esteem, chronic low
Self-Esteem Disturbance
Self-Esteem, situational low
Self-Mutilation, risk for

ROLE – RELATIONSHIP PATTERN
Caregiver Role Strain
Caregiver Role Strain, risk for
Communication, impaired, verbal
Family process, altered: alcoholism [substance abuse]
Family processes, altered
Grieving, anticipatory
Grieving, dysfunctional
Parental Role Conflict
Parent/Infant/Child Attachment, altered, risk for
Parenting, altered
Parenting, altered, risk for
Relocation Stress Syndrome
Role Performance, altered
Social Interaction, impaired
Social Isolation
Violence, [actual]/risk for, directed at self/ others

SEXUALITY – REPRODUCTIVE PATTERN
Rape-Trauma Syndrome [specify]
Rape-Trauma Syndrome: compound reaction
Rape-Trauma Syndrome: silent reaction
Sexual Dysfunction
Sexuality Patterns, altered

COPING – STRESS TOLERANCE PATTERN
Adjustment, impaired
Community Coping, Enhanced, potential for
Community Coping, ineffective
Coping, defensive
Coping, individual, ineffective
Denial, ineffective
Family Coping, ineffective: compromised
Family Coping, ineffective: disabling
Family Coping: potential for growth
Post-Trauma Response [specify stage]

VALUE – BELIEF PATTERN
Spiritual Distress (distress of the human spirit)
Spiritual Well-being, enhanced, potential for

NOTE: Information appearing in brackets has been added to clarify and facilitate the use of nursing diagnoses.
SOURCE: Adapted from Gordon, M: Manual of Nursing Diagnosis, 1995–1996. St. Louis, Mosby–Year Book, Inc., 1995.

# Appendix 21–2 Doenges & Moorhouse's Diagnostic Divisions

ACTIVITY/REST
Activity Intolerance [specify level]
Activity Intolerance, risk for
Disuse Syndrome, risk for
Diversional Activity Deficit
Fatigue
Sleep Pattern Disturbance

CIRCULATION
Adaptive Capacity: intracranial, decreased
Cardiac Output, decreased
Dysreflexia
Tissue Perfusion, altered (specify): cerebral, cardiopulmonary, renal, gastrointestinal, peripheral

EGO INTEGRITY
Adjustment, impaired
Anxiety [Mild, Moderate, Severe, Panic]
Body Image Disturbance
Coping, defensive
Coping, individual, ineffective
Decisional Conflict
Denial, ineffective
Energy Field Disturbance
Fear
Grieving, anticipatory
Grieving, dysfunctional
Hopelessness
Personal Identity Disturbance
Post-Trauma Response [specify stage]
Powerlessness
Rape-Trauma Syndrome [specify]
Rape-Trauma Syndrome: compound reaction
Rape-Trauma Syndrome: silent reaction
Relocation Stress Syndrome
Self-Esteem, chronic low
Self-Esteem Disturbance
Self-Esteem, situational low
Spiritual Distress (distress of the human spirit)
Spiritual Well-being, enhanced, potential for

ELIMINATION
Bowel Incontinence
Constipation
Constipation, colonic
Constipation, perceived

Diarrhea
Incontinence, functional
Incontinence, reflex
Incontinence, stress
Incontinence, total
Incontinence, urge
Urinary Elimination, altered patterns of
Urinary Retention [acute/chronic]

FOOD/FLUID
Breastfeeding, effective
Breastfeeding, ineffective
Breastfeeding, interrupted
Fluid Volume Deficit [active loss]
Fluid Volume Deficit [regulatory failure]
Fluid Volume Deficit, risk for
Fluid Volume Excess
Infant Feeding Pattern, ineffective
Nutrition: altered, less than body requirements
Nutrition: altered, more than body requirements
Nutrition: altered, risk for more than body requirements
Oral Mucous Membrane, altered
Swallowing, impaired

HYGIENE
Self-Care Deficit [specify level]: feeding, bathing/hygiene, dressing/grooming, toileting

NEUROSENSORY
Confusion, acute
Confusion, chronic
Disorganized Infant Behavior
Disorganized Infant Behavior, risk for
Enhanced Organized Infant Behavior, potential for
Memory, impaired
Peripheral Neurovascular Dysfunction, risk for
Sensory/Perceptual Alterations (specify): visual, auditory, kinesthetic, gustatory, tactile, olfactory
Thought Processes, altered
Unilateral Neglect

PAIN/DISCOMFORT
Pain
Pain, acute
Pain, chronic

RESPIRATION
Airway Clearance, ineffective
Aspiration, risk for
Breathing Pattern, ineffective
Gas Exchange, impaired
Spontaneous Ventilation, inability to sustain
Ventilatory Weaning Response, dysfunctional (DVWR)

SAFETY
Body Temperature, altered, risk for
Environmental Interpretation Syndrome, impaired
Health Maintenance, altered
Home Maintenance Management, impaired
Hyperthermia
Hypothermia
Infection, risk for
Injury, risk for
Perioperative Positioning Injury, risk for
Physical Mobility, impaired
Poisoning, risk for
Protection, altered
Self-Mutilation, risk for
Skin Integrity, impaired
Skin Integrity, impaired, risk for
Suffocation, risk for
Thermoregulation, ineffective
Tissue Integrity, impaired
Trauma, risk for
Violence, [actual]/risk for, directed at self/others

SEXUALITY [Component of Ego Integrity and Social Interaction]
Sexual Dysfunction
Sexuality Patterns, altered

SOCIAL INTERACTION
Caregiver Role Strain
Caregiver Role Strain, risk for
Communication, impaired, verbal
Community Coping, enhanced, potential for
Community Coping, ineffective
Family Coping, ineffective: compromised
Family Coping, ineffective: disabling
Family Coping: potential for growth
Family Process, altered: alcoholism [substance abuse]
Family Processes, altered
Loneliness, risk for
Parental Role Conflict
Parent/Infant/Child Attachment, altered, risk for
Parenting, altered
Parenting, altered, risk for
Role Performance, altered
Social Interaction, impaired
Social Isolation

TEACHING/LEARNING
Growth and Development, altered
Health-Seeking Behaviors (specify)
Knowledge Deficit [learning need] (specify)
Noncompliance (specify) [compliance, altered]
Therapeutic Regimen (Community), ineffective management of
Therapeutic Regimen (Families), ineffective management of
Therapeutic Regimen (Individual), effective management of
Therapeutic Regimen (Individual), ineffective management of

SOURCE: Adapted from Doenges, ME and Moorhouse, MF: Nurse's Pocket Guide: Nursing Diagnoses with Interventions, ed. 5, F.A. Davis, Philadelphia, 1995, with permission.

# Appendix 21–3 Nursing Diagnoses Approved at the 11th and 12th NANDA Conferences

## NANDA 11th Conference, 1994 (Approved)

Adaptive Capacity: intracranial, decreased
Community Coping, enhanced, potential for
Community Coping, ineffective
Confusion, acute
Confusion, chronic
Disorganized Infant Behavior
Disorganized Infant Behavior, risk for
Energy Field Disturbance
Enhanced Organized Infant Behavior, potential for
Environmental Interpretation Syndrome, impaired
Family Process, altered: alcoholism [substance abuse]
Loneliness, risk for
Memory, impaired
Parent/Infant/Child Attachment, altered, risk for
Perioperative Positioning Injury, risk for
Spiritual Well-Being, enhanced, potential for
Therapeutic Regimen (Community), ineffective management of
Therapeutic Regimen (Families), ineffective management of
Therapeutic Regimen (Individual), effective management of

# Appendix 21–4 Nursing Diagnoses Grouped by Diseases/Disorders

**abortion, spontaneous**

Fluid volume deficit [active loss] may be related to excessive blood loss, possibly evidenced by decreased pulse volume and pressure, delayed capillary refill, or changes in sensorium.

Anxiety [specify level] may be related to changes in health status of fetus/self, threat of death, possibly evidenced by restlessness, tremors, facial tension, focus on self, or feeling of uncertainty.

Knowledge deficit [learning need] regarding cause of abortion, self-care, contraception/future pregnancy may be related to lack of familiarity with new self/health-care needs, sources for support, possibly evidenced by requests for information and statement of concern/misconceptions.

Grieving [expected] related to perinatal loss, possibly evidenced by crying, expressions of sorrow, or changes in eating habits/sleep patterns.

Sexuality patterns, altered, risk for: risk factors may include increasing fear of pregnancy and/or repeat loss, impaired relationship with significant other(s), self-doubt regarding own femininity.

**abruptio placentae**

Fluid volume deficit [active loss] may be related to excessive blood loss, possibly evidenced by hypotension, increased heart rate, decreased pulse volume and pressure, delayed capillary refill, or changes in sensorium.

Fear related to threat of death (perceived or actual) to fetus/self, possibly evidenced by verbalization of specific concerns, increased tension, sympathetic stimulation.

Pain [acute] may be related to collection of blood between uterine wall and placenta, possibly evidenced by verbal reports, abdominal guarding, muscle tension, or alterations in vital signs.

Gas exchange, impaired, fetal may be related to altered uteroplacental oxygen transfer, possibly evidenced by alterations in fetal heart rate and movement.

**abscess, brain** (acute)

Pain [acute] may be related to inflammation, edema of tissues, possibly evidenced by reports of headache, restlessness, irritability, and moaning.

Hyperthermia, risk for: risk factors may include inflammatory process/hypermetabolic state and dehydration.

Confusion, acute may be related to physiologic changes (e.g., cerebral edema/altered perfusion, fever), possibly evidenced by fluctuation in cognition/level of consciousness, increased agitation/restlessness, hallucinations.

Suffocation/Trauma, risk for: risk factors may include development of clonic/tonic muscle activity and changes in consciousness (seizure activity).

**achalasia**

Swallowing, impaired may be related to neuromuscular impairment, possibly evidenced by observed difficulty in swallowing or regurgitation.

Nutrition, altered, less than body requirements may be related to inability and/or reluctance to ingest adequate nutrients to meet metabolic demands/nutritional needs, possibly evidenced by reported/observed inadequate intake, weight loss, and pale conjunctiva and mucous membranes.

Pain, [acute] may be related to spasm of the lower esophageal sphincter, possibly evidenced by reports of substernal pressure, recurrent heartburn, or gastric fullness (gas pains).

Anxiety [specify level]/Fear may be related to recurrent pain, choking sensation, altered health status, possibly evidenced by verbalizations of distress, apprehension, restlessness, or insomnia.

Aspiration, risk for: risk factors may include regurgitation/spillover of esophageal contents.

Knowledge deficit [learning need] regarding condition, prognosis, and treatment needs may be related to lack of familiarity with pathology and treatment of condition, possibly evidenced by requests for information, statement of concern, or development of preventable complications.

**acidosis, metabolic**

Refer to *diabetic ketoacidosis*.

**acute respiratory distress syndrome** (ARDS)

Airway clearance, ineffective may be related to loss of ciliary action, increased amount and viscosity of secretions, and increased airway resistance, possibly evidenced by presence of dyspnea, changes in depth/rate of respiration, use of accessory muscles for breathing, wheezes/crackles, cough with or without sputum production.

Gas exchange, impaired may be related to changes in pulmonary capillary permeability with edema formation, alveolar hypoventilation and collapse, with intrapulmonary shunting; possibly evidenced by tachypnea, use of accessory muscles, cyanosis, hypoxia per ABGs/oximetry, anxiety, and changes in mentation.

Fluid volume deficit, risk for: risk factors may include active loss from diuretic use and restricted intake.

Cardiac output, decreased, risk for: risk factors may include alteration in preload (hypovolemia, vascular pooling, diuretic therapy, and increased intrathoracic pressure/use of ventilator/PEEP).

Anxiety [specify level]/Fear may be related to physiologic factors (effects of hypoxemia); situational crisis; change in health status/threat of death, possibly evidenced by increased tension, apprehension, restlessness, focus on self, and sympathetic stimulation.

**Addison's disease**

Fluid volume deficit [regulatory failure] may be related to vomiting, diarrhea, increased renal losses, possibly evidenced by delayed capillary refill, poor skin turgor, dry mucous membranes, report of thirst.

Cardiac output, decreased may be related to hypovolemia and altered electrical conduction (dysrhythmias) and/or diminished cardiac muscle mass, possibly evidenced by alterations in vital signs, changes in mentation, and irregular pulse or pulse deficit.

Fatigue may be related to decreased metabolic energy production, altered body chemistry (fluid, electrolyte, and glucose imbalance), possibly evidenced by unremitting/overwhelming lack of energy, inability to maintain usual routines, decreased performance, impaired ability to concentrate, lethargy, and disinterest in surroundings.

Body image disturbance may be related to changes in skin pigmentation and mucous membranes, loss of axillary/pubic hair, possibly evidenced by verbalization of negative feelings about body and decreased social involvement.

Physical mobility, impaired, risk for: risk factors may include neuromuscular impairment (muscle wasting/weakness) and dizziness/syncope.

Nutrition, altered, less than body requirements may be related to glucocorticoid deficiency; abnormal fat, protein, and carbohydrate metabolism, nausea, vomiting, anorexia, possibly evidenced by weight loss, muscle wasting, abdominal cramps, diarrhea, and severe hypoglycemia.

Home maintenance management, impaired, risk for: risk factors may include effects of disease process, impaired cognitive functioning, and inadequate support systems.

**adenoidectomy**

Anxiety [specify level]/Fear may be related to separation from supportive others, unfamiliar surroundings, and perceived threat of injury/abandonment, possibly evidenced by crying, apprehension, trembling, and sympathetic stimulation (pupil dilation, increased heart rate).

Airway clearance, ineffective, risk for: risk factors may include sedation, collection of secretions/blood in oropharynx, and vomiting.

Fluid volume deficit, risk for: risk factors may include operative trauma to highly vascular site/hemorrhage.

Pain, [acute] may be related to physical trauma to oronasopharynx, presence of packing, possibly evidenced by restlessness, crying, and facial mask of pain.

**adrenalectomy**

Tissue perfusion, altered (specify) may be related to hypovolemia and vascular pooling (vasodilation), possibly evidenced by diminished pulse, pallor/cyanosis, hypotension, and changes in mentation.

Infection, risk for: risk factors may include inadequate primary defenses (incision, traumatized tissues), suppressed inflammatory response, invasive procedures.

Knowledge deficit [learning need] regarding condition, prognosis, and treatment needs may be related to unfamiliarity with long-term therapy requirements, possibly evidenced by request for information and statement of concern/misconceptions.

**affective disorder**

Refer to *bipolar disorder* and *depressive disorders, major depression, dysthymia.*

**AIDS** (acquired immunodeficiency syndrome)

Infection, risk for progression to sepsis/onset of new opportunistic infection: risk factors may include depressed immune system, use of antimicrobial agents, inadequate primary defenses, broken skin, traumatized tissue, malnutrition, and chronic disease processes.

Fluid volume deficit, risk for: risk factors may include excessive losses: copious diarrhea, profuse sweating, vomiting, hypermetabolic state, and fever; impaired intake (nausea, anorexia, lethargy).

Pain [acute/chronic] may be related to tissue inflammation/destruction: infections, internal/external cutaneous lesions, rectal excoriation, malignancies, necrosis, peripheral neuropathies, myalgias, and arthralgias, possibly evidenced by verbal reports, self-focusing/narrowed focus, alteration in muscle tone, paresthesias, paralysis, guarding behaviors, changes in vital signs (acute), autonomic responses, and restlessness.

Nutrition, altered, less than body requirements may by related to altered ability to ingest, digest, and/or absorb nutrients (nausea/vomiting, hyperactive gag reflex, intestinal disturbances), increased metabolic activity/nutritional needs (fever, infection), possibly evidenced by weight loss, decreased subcutaneous fat/muscle mass, lack of interest in food/aversion to eating, altered taste sensation, abdominal cramping, hyperactive bowel sounds, diarrhea, sore and inflamed buccal cavity.

Fatigue may be related to decreased metabolic energy production, increased energy requirements (hypermetabolic state), overwhelming psychologic/emotional demands, altered body chemistry (side effects of medication, chemotherapy), possibly evidenced by unremitting/overwhelming lack of energy, inability to maintain usual routines, decreased performance, impaired ability to concentrate, lethargy/restlessness, and disinterest in surroundings.

Social isolation may be related to changes in physical appearance/mental status, state of wellness, perceptions of unacceptable social or sexual behavior/values, physical isolation, phobic fear of others (transmission of disease); possibly evidenced by expressed feelings of rejection, absence of supportive significant others, and withdrawal from usual activities.

Thought processes, altered/Confusion, chronic may be related to physiologic changes (hypoxemia, CNS infection by HIV, brain malignancies, and/or disseminated systemic opportunistic infection); alteration of drug metabolism/excretion; accumulation of toxic elements (renal failure, severe electrolyte imbalance, hepatic insufficiency), possibly evidenced by clinical evidence of organic impairment, altered attention span, distractibility, memory deficit, disorientation, cognitive dissonance, delusional thinking, impaired ability to make decisions/problem solve, inability to follow complex commands/mental tasks, and loss of impulse control and altered personality.

**aldosteronism, primary**

Fluid volume deficit [regulatory failure] may be related to increased urinary losses, possibly evidenced by dry mucous membranes, poor skin turgor, dilute urine, excessive thirst, weight loss.

Physical mobility, impaired may be related to neuromuscular impairment, weakness, and pain, possibly evidenced by impaired coordination, decreased muscle strength, paralysis, and positive Chvostek's and Trousseau's signs.

Cardiac output, decreased, risk for: risk factors may include hypovolemia and altered electrical conduction/dysrhythmias.

**Alzheimer's disease**

Trauma, risk for: risk factors may include inability to recognize/identify danger in environment, disorientation, confusion, impaired judgment, weakness, and muscular incoordination.

Thought processes, altered/Confusion, chronic may be related to physiologic changes (neuronal degeneration), sleep deprivation, and psychologic conflicts; possibly evidenced by inaccurate interpretation of environment, memory deficit, impaired ability to make decisions/problem solve, distractibility, disorientation, inappropriate/nonreality-based thinking, impaired socialization, and altered personality.

Sensory/Perceptual alterations (specify) may be related to altered sensory reception, transmission, and/or integration (neurologic disease/deficit), socially restricted environment (homebound/institutionalized), possibly evidenced by memory loss, changes in usual response to stimuli, and exaggerated emotional responses (anxiety, paranoia, hallucinations).

Sleep pattern disturbance may be related to sensory impairment, changes in activity patterns, psychological stress (neurologic impairment), possibly evidenced by wakefulness, disorientation (day/night reversal), increased aimless wandering, inability to identify need/time for sleeping, changes in behavior/performance, lethargy; dark circles under eyes and frequent yawning.

Health maintenance, altered may be related to deterioration affecting ability in all areas, cognitive impairment, ineffective individual/family coping, possibly evidenced by reported or observed inability to take responsibility for meeting basic health practices, lack of equipment/financial or other resources, and impairment of personal support system.

Family coping, ineffective: compromised/Caregiver role strain may be related to family disorganization, role changes, family/caregiver isolation, long-term illness/complexity and amount of homecare needs exhausting supportive/financial capabilities of family member(s); possibly evidenced by verbalizations of frustrations in dealing with day-to-day care, reports of conflict, feelings of depression, expressed anger/guilt directed toward patient, and withdrawal from interaction with patient/social contacts.

Relocation stress syndrome, risk for: risk factors may include little or no preparation for transfer to a new setting, changes in daily routine, sensory impairment, physical deterioration, separation from support systems.

**amputation**

Tissue perfusion, altered, peripheral, risk for: risk factors may include reduced arterial/venous blood flow, tissue edema, hematoma formation, hypovolemia.

Pain [acute] may be related to tissue and nerve trauma, psychologic impact of loss of body part, possibly evidenced by reports of incisional/phantom pain, guarding behavior, narrowed/self-focus, and autonomic responses.

Physical mobility, impaired may be related to loss of limb, altered sense of balance, pain/discomfort, possibly evidenced by reluctance to attempt movement, impaired coordination; decreased muscle strength, control, and mass.

Body image disturbance may be related to loss of a body part, possibly evidenced by verbalization of feelings of powerlessness, grief, preoccupation with loss, and unwillingness to look at/touch stump.

**amyotrophic lateral sclerosis**

Physical mobility, impaired may be related to muscle wasting/weakness, possibly evidenced by impaired coordination, limited range of motion, and impaired purposeful movement.

Breathing pattern, ineffective may be related to neuromuscular impairment, decreased energy, fatigue, tracheobronchial obstruction, possibly evidenced by shortness of breath, fremitus, respiratory depth changes, and reduced vital capacity.

Swallowing, impaired may be related to muscle wasting and fatigue, possibly evidenced by recurrent coughing/choking and signs of aspiration.

Powerlessness [specify level] may be related to chronic/debilitating nature of illness, lack of control over outcome, possibly evidenced by expressions of frustration about inability to care for self and depression over physical deterioration.

Grieving, anticipatory may be related to perceived potential loss of self/physiopsychosocial well-being, possibly evidenced by sorrow, choked feelings, expression of distress, changes in eating habits/sleeping patterns, and altered communication patterns/libido.

Communication, impaired verbal may be related to physical barrier (neuromuscular impairment), possibly evidenced by impaired articulation, inability to speak in sentences, and use of nonverbal cues (changes in facial expression).

Caregiver role strain, risk for: risk factors may include illness severity of care receiver, complexity and amount of homecare needs, duration of caregiving required, caregiver is spouse, family/caregiver isolation, lack of respite/recreation for caregiver.

**anemia**

Tissue perfusion, altered (specify) may be related to exchange problems (reduction of cellular components necessary for delivery of oxygen/nutrients to the cells), possibly evidenced by palpitations, angina, pallor, cold extremities, changes in blood pressure, inability to concentrate.

Activity intolerance may be related to imbalance between oxygen supply (delivery) and demand, possibly evidenced by reports of fatigue and weakness, abnormal heart rate or blood pressure response, decreased exercise/activity level, and exertional discomfort or dyspnea.

Knowledge deficit [learning need] regarding condition, prognosis, and treatment needs may be related to inadequate understanding or misinterpretation of dietary/physiologic needs, possibly evidenced by inadequate dietary intake, request for information, and development of preventable complications.

**anemia, sickle cell**

Gas exchange, impaired may be related to decreased oxygen-carrying capacity of blood, reduced red blood cell life span, abnormal red blood cell structure, increased blood viscosity, predisposition to bacterial pneumonia/pulmonary infarcts, possibly evidenced by dyspnea, use of accessory muscles, cyanosis/signs of hypoxia, tachycardia, changes in mentation, and restlessness.

Tissue perfusion, altered (specify) may be related to stasis, vaso-occlusive nature of sickling, inflammatory response, AV shunts in pulmonary and peripheral circulation, myocardial damage (small infarcts, iron deposits, fibrosis), possibly evidenced by signs and symptoms dependent on system involved, for example, renal—decreased specific gravity and pale urine in face of dehydration; cerebral—paralysis and visual disturbances; peripheral—distal ischemia, tissue infarctions, ulcerations, bone pain; cardiopulmonary—angina, palpitations.

Pain [acute/chronic] may be related to intravascular sickling with localized vascular stasis, occlusion, infarction/necrosis, deprivation of oxygen and nutrients, accumulation of noxious metabolites, possibly evidenced by reports of localized, generalized, or migratory joint and/or abdominal/back pain, guarding and distraction behaviors (moaning, crying, restlessness), facial grimacing, narrowed focus, and autonomic responses.

Knowledge deficit [learning need] regarding disease process, genetic factors, prognosis, and treatment needs may be related to lack of exposure/recall, misinterpretation of information, unfamiliarity with resources, possibly evidenced by questions, statement of concern/misconceptions, exacerbation of condition, inadequate follow-through of therapy instructions, and development of preventable complications.

Growth and development, altered may be related to effects of physical condition, possibly evidenced by altered physical growth and delay/difficulty performing skills typical of age group.

Family coping, ineffective: compromised may be related to chronic nature of disease/disability, family disorganization, presence of other crises/situations impacting significant person/parent, lifestyle restrictions, possibly evidenced by significant person/parent expressing preoccupation with own reaction and displaying protective behavior disproportionate to patient's ability or need for autonomy.

**angina pectoris**

Pain [acute] may be related to decreased myocardial blood flow, increased cardiac workload/oxygen consumption, possibly evidenced by verbal reports, narrowed focus, distraction behaviors (restlessness, moaning), and autonomic responses (diaphoresis, changes in vital signs).

Cardiac output, decreased may be related to inotropic changes (transient/prolonged myocardial ischemia, effects of medications), alterations in rate/rhythm and electrical conduction, possibly evidenced by changes in hemodynamic readings, dyspnea, restlessness, decreased tolerance for activity, fatigue, diminished peripheral pulses, cool/pale skin, changes in mental status, and continued chest pain.

Anxiety [specify level] may be related to situational crises, change in health status and/or threat of death, possibly evidenced by verbalized apprehension, facial tension, extraneous movements, and focus on self.

Activity intolerance may be related to imbalance between oxygen supply and demand, possibly evidenced by exertional dyspnea, abnormal pulse/blood pressure response to activity, and ECG changes.

Knowledge deficit [learning need] regarding condition, prognosis, and treatment needs may be related to lack of exposure, inaccurate/misinterpretation of information, possibly evidenced by questions, request for information, statement of concern, and inaccurate follow-through of instructions.

Adjustment, impaired, risk for: risk factors may include condition requiring long-term therapy/change in lifestyle, assault to self-concept, and altered locus of control.

**anorexia nervosa**

Nutrition, altered, less than body requirements may be related to psychologic restrictions of food intake and/or excessive activity, self-induced vomiting, laxative abuse, possibly evidenced by weight loss, poor skin turgor/muscle tone, denial of hunger, unusual hoarding or handling of food, amenorrhea, electrolyte imbalance, cardiac irregularities, hypotension.

Fluid volume deficit, risk for: risk factors may include inadequate intake of food and liquids, consistent self-induced vomiting, chronic/excessive laxative/diuretic use.

Body image disturbance/Self-esteem, chronic low may be related to altered perception of body, perceived loss of control in some aspect of life, unmet dependency needs, personal vulnerability, dysfunctional family system, possibly evidenced by negative feelings, distorted view of body, use of denial, feeling powerless to prevent/make changes, expressions of shame/guilt, overly conforming, dependence on other's opinions.

Coping, individual, ineffective may be related to maturational crisis and attempt to control environment, possibly evidenced by verbalization of inability to cope/ask for help, poor self-esteem and difficulty meeting role expectations/basic needs, poor problem-solving capabilities, verbal manipulation, destructive behavior toward self.

Family coping, ineffective: disabling may be related to ambivalent family relationships and ways of transacting issues of control, possibly evidenced by enmeshed family with lack of separation of individual members who may speak for one another, distortion of reality regarding patient's health problem.

**anxiety disorder, generalized**

Anxiety [specify level]/Powerlessness may be related to real or perceived threat to physical integrity or self-concept (may or may not be able to identify the threat), unconscious conflict about essential values/beliefs and goals of life, unmet needs, negative self-talk, possibly evidenced by sympathetic stimulation, extraneous movements (foot shuffling, hand/arm fidgeting, rocking movements, restlessness), persistent feelings of apprehension and uneasiness, a general anxious feeling that patient has difficulty alleviating, poor eye contact, focus on self, impaired functioning, and free-floating anxiety.

Sleep pattern disturbance may be related to psychologic stress, repetitive thoughts, possibly evidenced by reports of difficulty in falling asleep/awakening earlier or later than desired, reports of not feeling rested, dark circles under eyes, and frequent yawning.

Coping, individual, ineffective may be related to level of anxiety being experienced by the patient, personal vulnerability, unrealistic perceptions and inadequate coping methods, possibly evidenced by verbalization of inability to cope/problem solve, excessive compulsive behaviors (e.g., smoking, drinking), emotional tension, alteration in societal participation, and high rate of accidents.

Family coping, ineffective: compromised, risk for: risk factors may include inadequate/incorrect information or understanding by a primary person, temporary family disorganization and role changes, prolonged disability that exhausts the supportive capacity of significant other(s).

Social interaction, impaired/Social isolation may be related to low self-concept, inadequate personal resources, misinterpretation of internal/external stimuli, possibly evidenced by discomfort in social situations, withdrawal from or reported change in pattern of interactions, dysfunctional interactions, expressed feelings of difference from others, sad, dull affect.

**aortic stenosis**

Cardiac output, decreased may be related to structural changes of heart valve, left ventricular outflow obstruction, alteration of afterload (increased LVEDP and SVR), alteration in electrical conduction, possibly evidenced by fatigue, dyspnea, altered vital signs, and syncope.

Pain, [acute], risk for: risk factors may include ischemia of cardiac muscle.

Activity intolerance may be related to imbalance between oxygen supply and demand, possibly evidenced by exertional dyspnea, reported fatigue/weakness, and ECG changes/dysrhythmias.

**appendicitis**

Pain, [acute] may be related to inflammation, possibly evidenced by verbal reports, guarding behavior, narrowed focus, and autonomic responses (diaphoresis, changes in vital signs).

Fluid volume deficit, risk for: risk factors may include nausea, vomiting, anorexia, and hypermetabolic state.

Infection, risk for: risk factors may include release of pathogenic organisms into peritoneal cavity.

**arrhythmia, cardiac**

Refer to *dysrhythmia, cardiac*.

**arthritis, juvenile rheumatoid** (also refer to *arthritis, rheumatoid*)

Growth and development, altered may be related to effects of physical disability and required therapy, possibly evidenced by lack of/delay in performing skills typical for age, and altered physical growth.

Social isolation, risk for: risk factors may include delay in accomplishing developmental task, altered state of wellness, and changes in physical appearance.

**arthritis, rheumatoid**

Pain, chronic may be related to joint/muscle inflammation, degeneration, deformity, possibly evidenced by verbal reports, narrowed focus, guarded movement, and physical and social withdrawal.

Physical mobility, impaired may be related to musculoskeletal deformity, pain, decreased muscle strength, possibly evidenced by limited range of motion, impaired coordination, reluctance to attempt movement, and decreased muscle strength/control and mass.

Self-care deficit (specify) may be related to musculoskeletal impairment, decreased strength/endurance and range of motion, pain on movement, possibly evidenced by inability to manage activities of daily living.

Body image disturbance may be related to change in body structure/function, impaired mobility/ability to perform usual tasks, focus on past strength/function/appearance, change in lifestyle/physical abilities, dependence on others for assistance, possibly evidenced by negative self-talk, feelings of helplessness, and decreased social involvement.

**arthroplasty**

Infection, risk for: risk factors may include breach of primary defenses (surgical incision), stasis of body fluids at operative site, and altered inflammatory response.

Fluid volume deficit, risk for: risk factors may include surgical procedure/trauma to vascular area.

Physical mobility, impaired may be related to decreased strength, pain, musculoskeletal changes, possibly evidenced by impaired coordination and reluctance to attempt movement.

Pain, [acute] may be related to tissue trauma, local edema, possibly evidenced by verbal reports, narrowed focus, guarded movement, and autonomic responses (diaphoresis, changes in vital signs).

**arthroscopy**

Knowledge deficit [learning need] regarding procedure/outcomes and self-care needs may be related to unfamiliarity with information/resources, misinterpretations, possibly evidenced by questions and requests for information and misconceptions.

**asthma** (also refer to *emphysema*)

Airway clearance, ineffective may be related to increased production/retained pulmonary secretions, bronchospasm, decreased energy/fatigue, possibly evidenced by wheezing, difficulty breathing, changes in depth/rate of respirations, use of accessory muscles, and persistent ineffective cough with or without sputum production.

Gas exchange, impaired may be related to altered delivery of inspired oxygen/air trapping, alveolar destruction, possibly evidenced by dyspnea, confusion, restlessness, reduced tolerance for activity, cyanosis, and changes in ABGs and vital signs.

Anxiety [specify level] may be related to perceived threat of death, possibly evidenced by apprehension, fearful expression, and extraneous movements.

Activity intolerance may be related to imbalance between oxygen supply and demand, possibly evidenced by fatigue and exertional dyspnea.

**athlete's foot**

Skin integrity, impaired may be related to fungal invasion, humidity, secretions, possibly evidenced by disruption of skin surface, reports of painful itching.

Infection, risk for spread: risk factors may include multiple breaks in skin, exposure to moist/warm environment.

**autistic disorder**

Social interaction, impaired may be related to disturbance in self-concept; lack of bonding and development of trust; inadequate sensory stimulation or abnormal response to sensory input; organic brain dysfunction; possibly evidenced by lack of responsiveness to others; lack of eye contact or facial responsiveness; treating persons as objects; lack of awareness of feelings in others; indifference/aversion to comfort, affection, or physical contact; failure to develop cooperative social play and peer friendships in childhood.

Communication, impaired verbal may be related to inability to trust others, withdrawal into self, organic brain dysfunction, inadequate sensory stimulation, maternal deprivation, possibly evidenced by lack of interactive communication mode, does not use gestures or spoken language, absent or abnormal nonverbal communication, lack of eye contact or facial expression, peculiar patterns of speech (form, content, or speech production), and impaired ability to initiate or sustain conversation despite adequate speech.

Self-mutilation, risk for: risk factors may include organic brain dysfunction; inability to trust others; disturbance in self-concept; inadequate sensory stimulation or abnormal response to sensory input; history of physical, emotional, or sexual abuse; and response to demands of therapy, realization of severity of condition.

Personal identity disturbance may be related to organic brain dysfunction, lack of development of trust, maternal deprivation, fixation at presymbiotic phase of development, possibly evidenced by lack of awareness of the feelings or existence of others, increased anxiety resulting from physical contact with others, absent or impaired imitation of others, repeats what others say, persistent preoccupation with parts of objects, obsessive attachment to objects, marked distress over changes in environment, autocratic/ritualistic behaviors, self-touching, rocking, swaying.

Family coping, ineffective: compromised/disabling may be related to family members unable to express feelings; excessive guilt, anger, or blaming among family members regarding child's condition; ambivalent or dissonant family relationships, prolonged coping with problem exhausting supportive ability of family members, possibly evidenced by denial of existence or severity of disturbed behaviors, preoccupation with personal emotional reaction to situation, rationalization that problem will be outgrown, attempts to intervene with child are achieving increasingly ineffective results, family withdraws from or becomes overly protective of child.

**battered child syndrome**

Self-esteem disturbance may be related to deprivation and negative feedback of family members, possibly evidenced by lack of eye contact, withdrawal from social contacts, and discounting own needs.

Post-trauma response may be related to sustained/recurrent physical or emotional abuse, possibly evidenced by acting-out behavior, development of phobias, poor impulse control, and emotional numbness.

Parenting, altered may be related to poor role model/identity, unrealistic expectations, presence of stressors, and lack of support, possibly evidenced by verbalization of negative feelings, inappropriate caretaking behaviors, and evidence of physical/psychologic trauma to child.

Family coping, ineffective: compromised/disabling may be related to situational or developmental crisis and family disorganization, possibly evidenced by verbalized concern about ability to deal with current situation, and displaying protective behaviors disproportionate to child's ability or need for autonomy.

**benign prostatic hypertrophy**

Urinary retention [acute/chronic] may be related to mechanical obstruction (enlarged prostate), decompensation of detrusor musculature, inability of bladder to contract adequately, possibly evidenced by frequency, hesitancy, inability to empty bladder completely, incontinence/dribbling, bladder distention, residual urine.

Pain [acute] may be related to mucosal irritation, bladder distension, colic, urinary infection, and radiation therapy, possibly evidenced by reports (bladder/rectal spasm), narrowed focus, altered muscle tone, grimacing, distraction behaviors, restlessness, and autonomic responses.

Fluid volume deficit, risk for: risk factors may include postobstructive diuresis, endocrine/electrolyte imbalances.

Fear/Anxiety [specify level] may be related to change in health status (possibility of surgical procedure/malignancy); embarrassment/loss of dignity associated with genital exposure before, during, and after treatment, and concern about sexual ability, possibly evidenced by increased tension, apprehension, worry, expressed concerns regarding perceived changes, and fear of unspecified consequences.

**bipolar disorder**

Violence, risk for, directed at others/self: risk factors may include irritability; impulsive behavior; delusional thinking; angry response when ideas are refuted or wishes denied; manic excitement, with possible indicators of threatening body language/verbalizations; increased motor activity; overt and aggressive acts; and hostility.

Nutrition, altered, less than body requirements may be related to inadequate intake in relation to metabolic expenditures, possibly evidenced by body weight 20% or more below ideal weight, observed inadequate intake, inattention to mealtimes, and distraction from task of eating.

Poisoning, risk for lithium toxicity: risk factors may include narrow therapeutic range of drug, patient's ability (or lack of) to follow through with medication regimen and monitoring, and denial of need for information/therapy.

Sleep pattern disturbance may be related to psychologic stress, lack of recognition of fatigue/need to sleep, hyperactivity, possibly evidenced by denial of need to sleep, interrupted nighttime sleep, one or more nights without sleep, changes in behavior and performance, increasing irritability/restlessness, and dark circles under eyes.

Sensory/Perceptual alterations (specify and/or overload) may be related to decrease in sensory threshold, endogenous chemical alteration, psychologic stress, sleep deprivation, possibly evidenced by increased distractibility and agitation, anxiety, disorientation, poor concentration, auditory/visual hallucination, bizarre thinking, and motor incoordination.

Family processes, altered may be related to situational crises (illness, economics, change in roles), euphoric mood and grandiose ideas/actions of patient, manipulative behavior and limit-testing, patient's refusal to accept responsibility for own actions, possibly evidenced by statements of difficulty coping with situation, lack of adaptation to change or not dealing constructively with illness, ineffective family decision-making process, failure to send and to receive clear messages, and inappropriate boundary maintenance.

**borderline personality disorder**

Self-mutilation/Violence, risk for, directed at self/others: risk factors may include use of projection as a major defense mechanism, pervasive problems with negative transference, feelings of guilt/need to "punish" self, distorted sense of self, inability to cope with increased psychologic/physiologic tension in a healthy manner.

Thought processes, altered may be related to psychologic conflicts and brief psychotic episodes, delusional thinking, cognitive distortions, increasing anxiety/fear, and poor reality base, possibly evidenced by persecutory thoughts of "I am a victim," perception of events as either grossly distorted or "did not happen at all," and interference with ability to think clearly and logically.

Anxiety [severe to panic] may be related to unconscious conflicts, perceived threat to self-concept, unmet needs, possibly evidenced by transient psychotic symptoms, abuse of alcohol/other drugs, easy frustration and feelings of hurt, and performance of self-mutilating acts.

Self-Esteem/Personal Identity disturbance may be related to lack of positive feedback, unmet dependency needs, retarded ego development/fixation at an earlier level of development, possibly evidenced by difficulty identifying self or defining self-boundaries, feelings of depersonalization, extreme mood changes, lack of tolerance of rejection or being alone, unhappiness with self, striking out at others, performance of ritualistic self-damaging acts, and belief that punishing self is necessary.

Social isolation may be related to immature interests, unaccepted social behavior, inadequate personal resources, and inability to engage in satisfying personal relationships, possibly evidenced by alternating clinging and distancing behaviors, difficulty meeting expectations of others, experiencing feelings of difference from others, expressing interests inappropriate to developmental age, and showing behavior unaccepted by dominant cultural group.

**brain tumor**

Pain, [acute] may be related to pressure on brain tissues, possibly evidenced by reports of headache, facial mask of pain, narrowed focus, and autonomic responses (changes in vital signs).

Thought processes, altered may be related to altered circulation to and/or destruction of brain tissue, possibly evidenced by memory loss, personality changes, impaired ability to make decisions/conceptualize, and altered level of consciousness.

Sensory/Perceptual alterations (specify) may be related to compression/displacement of brain tissue, disruption of neuronal conduction, possibly evidenced by changes in visual acuity, alterations in sense of balance/gait disturbance, and paresthesia.

Fluid volume deficit, risk for: risk factors may include recurrent vomiting from irritation of vagal center in medulla, and decreased intake.

Self-care deficit (specify) may be related to sensory/neuromuscular impairment interfering with ability to perform tasks, possibly evidenced by unkempt/disheveled appearance, body odor, and verbalization/observation of inability to perform activities of daily living.

**bronchitis**

Airway clearance, ineffective may be related to excessive, thickened mucous secretions, possibly evidenced by presence of rhonchi, tachypnea, and ineffective cough.

Activity intolerance may be related to imbalance between oxygen supply and demand, possibly evidenced by reports of fatigue, dyspnea, and abnormal vital sign response to activity.

Pain, [acute] may be related to localized inflammation, persistent cough, aching associated with fever, possibly evidenced by reports of discomfort, distraction behavior, and facial mask of pain.

**bronchopneumonia** (also refer to *bronchitis*)

Airway clearance, ineffective may be related to tracheal bronchial inflammation, edema formation, increased sputum production, pleuritic pain, decreased energy, fatigue, possibly evidenced by changes in rate/depth of respirations, abnormal breath sounds, use of accessory muscles, dyspnea, cyanosis, effective/ineffective cough (with or without sputum production).

Gas exchange, impaired may be related to inflammatory process, collection of secretions affecting exchange across alveolar membrane, and hypoventilation, possibly evidenced by restlessness/changes in mentation, dyspnea, tachycardia, pallor, cyanosis, and ABGs/oximetry evidence of hypoxia.

Infection, risk for spread: risk factors may include decreased ciliary action, stasis of secretions, presence of existing infection.

**burn** (dependent on type, degree, and severity of the injury)

Fluid volume deficit, risk for: risk factors may include loss of fluids through wounds, capillary damage and evaporation, hypermetabolic state, insufficient intake, and hemorrhagic losses.

Infection, risk for: risk factors may include loss of protective dermal barrier, traumatized/necrotic tissue, decreased hemoglobin, suppressed inflammatory response, environmental exposure/invasive procedures.

Pain [acute] may be related to destruction of/trauma to tissue and nerves, edema formation, and manipulation of impaired tissues, possibly evidenced by verbal reports, narrowed focus, distraction and guarding behaviors, facial mask of pain, and autonomic responses (changes in vital signs).

Nutrition, altered, less than body requirements, risk for: risk factors may include hypermetabolic state in response to burn injury/stress, inadequate intake, protein catabolism.

Post-trauma response may be related to life-threatening event, possibly evidenced by re-experiencing the event, repetitive dreams/nightmares, psychic/emotional numbness, and sleep disturbance.

Diversional activity deficit may be related to long-term hospitalization, frequent lengthy treatments, and physical limitations, possibly evidenced by boredom, restlessness, withdrawal, and requests for something to do.

Growth and development, altered may be related to effects of physical disability, separation from significant others, and environmental deficiencies, possibly evidenced by loss of previously acquired skills and inability/reluctance to perform self-care.

**bursitis**

Pain, [acute/chronic] may be related to inflammation of affected joint, possibly evidenced by verbal reports, guarding behavior, and narrowed focus.

Physical mobility, impaired may be related to inflammation and swelling of joint and pain, possibly evidenced by diminished range of motion, reluctance to attempt movement, and imposed restriction of movement by medical treatment.

**calculus, urinary**

Pain, [acute] may be related to tissue trauma and edema formation, possibly evidenced by reports of sudden, severe, colicky pains, guarding, and distraction behaviors.

Urinary retention, risk for: risk factors may include obstruction of urinary flow.

Infection, risk for: risk factors may include stasis of urine.

Knowledge deficit [learning need] regarding condition, prognosis, and treatment needs may be related to lack of exposure/recall and information misinterpretation, possibly evidenced by requests for information, statements of concern, and recurrence/development of preventable complications.

**cancer** (also refer to *chemotherapy*)

Fear/Anxiety [specify level] may be related to situational crises, threat to/change in health/socioeconomic status, role functioning, interaction patterns; threat of death, separation from family, interpersonal transmission of feelings, possibly evidenced by expressed concerns, feelings of inadequacy/helplessness, insomnia, increased tension, restlessness, focus on self, sympathetic stimulation.

Grieving, anticipatory may be related to potential loss of physiologic well-being (body part/function), perceived separation from significant others/lifestyle (death), possibly evidenced by anger, sadness, withdrawal, choked feelings, changes in eating/sleep patterns, activity level, libido, and communication patterns.

Pain, [acute] may be related to the disease process (compression of nerve tissue, infiltration of nerves or their vascular supply, obstruction of a nerve pathway, inflammation), or side effects of therapeutic agents, possibly evidenced by verbal reports, self-focusing/narrowed focus, alteration in muscle tone, facial mask of pain, distraction/guarding behaviors, autonomic responses, and restlessness.

Fatigue may be related to decreased metabolic energy production, increased energy requirements (hypermetabolic state), overwhelming psychologic/emotional demands, and altered body chemistry (side effects of medications, chemotherapy), possibly evidenced by unremitting/overwhelming lack of energy, inability to maintain usual routines, decreased performance, impaired ability to concentrate, lethargy/listlessness, and disinterest in surroundings.

Home maintenance management, impaired may be related to debilitation, lack of resources, and/or inadequate support systems, possibly evidenced by verbalization of problem, request for assistance, and lack of necessary equipment or aids.

Family coping, ineffective: compromised/disabling may be related to chronic nature of disease and disability, ongoing treatment needs, parental supervision, and lifestyle restrictions, possibly evidenced by expression of denial/despair, depression, and protective behavior disproportionate to patient's abilities or need for autonomy.

Family coping: potential for growth may be related to the fact that the individual's needs are being sufficiently gratified and adaptive tasks effectively addressed, enabling goals of self-actualization to surface, possibly evidenced by verbalizations of impact of crisis on own values, priorities, goals, or relationships.

**cardiac surgery**

Anxiety (specify level)/Fear may be related to change in health status and threat to self-concept/of death, possibly evidenced by sympathetic stimulation, increased tension, and apprehension.

Cardiac output, decreased, risk for: risk factors may include decreased preload (hypovolemia), depressed myocardial contractility, changes in systemic vascular resistance (afterload), and alterations in electrical conduction (dysrhythmias).

Fluid volume deficit [active loss] may be related to intraoperative bleeding with inadequate blood replacement; bleeding related to insufficient heparin reversal, fibrinolysis, or platelet destruction; or volume depletion effects of intraoperative/postoperative diuretic therapy, possibly evidenced by increased pulse rate, decreased pulse volume/pressure, decreased urine output, hemoconcentration.

Gas exchange, impaired, risk for: risk factors may include alveolar-capillary membrane changes (atelectasis), intestinal edema, inadequate function or premature discontinuation of chest tubes, and diminished oxygen-carrying capacity of the blood.

Pain, [acute] may be related to tissue inflammation/trauma, edema formation, intraoperative nerve trauma, and myocardial ischemia, possibly evidenced by reports of incisional discomfort/pain in chest and donor site, paresthesia/pain in hand, arm, shoulder; anxiety; restlessness; irritability; distraction behaviors; and autonomic responses.

Skin/Tissue integrity, impaired related to mechanical trauma (surgical incisions, puncture wounds) and edema evidenced by disruption of skin surface/tissues.

**care, long-term** (also refer to condition requiring/contributing to need for facility placement)

Anxiety [specify level]/Fear may be related to change in health status, role functioning, interaction patterns, socioeconomic status, environment; unmet needs, recent life changes, and loss of friends/significant other(s), possibly evidenced by apprehension, restlessness, insomnia, repetitive questioning, pacing, purposeless activity, expressed concern regarding changes in life events, and focus on self.

Grieving, anticipatory may be related to perceived/actual or potential loss of physiopsychosocial well-being, personal possessions, and significant other(s), as well as cultural beliefs about aging, possibly evidenced by denial of feelings, depression, sorrow, guilt; alterations in activity level, sleep patterns, eating habits, and libido.

Poisoning, risk for drug toxicity: risk factors may include effects of aging (reduced metabolism, impaired circulation, precarious physiologic balance, presence of multiple diseases/organ involvement), and use of multiple prescribed/over-the-counter drugs.

Thought processes, altered may be related to physiologic changes of aging (loss of cells and brain atrophy, decreased blood supply), altered sensory input, pain, effects of medications, and psychologic conflicts (disrupted life pattern), possibly evidenced by slower reaction times, memory loss, altered attention span, disorientation, inability to follow, altered sleep patterns, and personality changes.

Sleep pattern disturbance may be related to internal factors (illness, psychologic stress, inactivity) and external factors (environmental changes, facility routines), possibly evidenced by reports of difficulty in falling asleep/not feeling rested, interrupted sleep/awakening earlier than desired, change in behavior/performance, increasing irritability, and listlessness.

Sexuality Patterns, altered, risk for: risk factors may include biopsychosocial alteration of sexuality, interference in psychologic/physical well-being, self-image, and lack of privacy/significant other(s).

Relocation stress syndrome, risk for: risk factors may include multiple losses, feeling of powerlessness, lack of/inappropriate use of support system, and changes in psychosocial/physical health status.

**carpal tunnel syndrome**

Pain, [acute]/chronic may be related to pressure on median nerve, possibly evidenced by verbal reports, reluctance to use affected extremity, guarding behaviors, expressed fear of reinjury, altered ability to continue previous activities.

Physical mobility, impaired may be related to neuromuscular impairment and pain, possibly evidenced by decreased hand strength, weakness, limited range of motion, and reluctance to attempt movement.

Peripheral neurovascular dysfunction, risk for: risks include mechanical compression (e.g., brace, repetitive tasks/motions), immobilization.

Knowledge deficit [learning need] regarding condition, prognosis, and treatment/safety needs may be related to lack of exposure/recall, information misinterpretation, possibly evidenced by questions, statements of concern, request for information, and inaccurate follow-through of instructions/development of preventable complications.

**cast** (also refer to *fracture*)

Peripheral neurovascular dysfunction, risk for: risk factors may include presence of fracture(s), mechanical compression (cast), tissue trauma, immobilization, vascular obstruction.

Skin integrity, impaired, risk for: risk factors may include pressure of cast, moisture/debris under cast, objects inserted under cast to relieve itching, and/or altered sensation/circulation.

Self-care deficit (specify) may be related to impaired ability to perform self-care tasks, possibly evidenced by statements of need for assistance and observed difficulty in performing activities of daily living.

**cataract**

Sensory/Perceptual alteration, visual may be related to altered sensory reception/status of sense organs and therapeutically restricted environment (surgical procedure, patching), possibly evidenced by diminished acuity, visual distortions, and change in usual response to stimuli.

Trauma, risk for: risk factors may include poor vision and reduced hand/eye coordination.

Anxiety [specify level]/Fear may be related to alteration in visual acuity and threat of permanent loss of vision/independence, possibly evidenced by expressed concerns, apprehension, and feelings of uncertainty.

Knowledge deficit [learning need] regarding ways of coping with altered abilities, therapy choices, lifestyle changes may be related to lack of exposure/recall, misinterpretation, or cognitive limitations, possibly evidenced by requests for information, statement of concern, inaccurate follow-through of instructions/development of preventable complications.

**cat scratch disease**

Pain, [acute] may be related to effects of circulating toxins (fever, headache, and lymphadenitis), possibly evidenced by verbal reports, guarding behavior, and autonomic response (changes in vital signs).

Hyperthermia may be related to inflammatory process, possibly evidenced by increased body temperature, flushed warm skin, tachypnea, and tachycardia.

**cerebrovascular accident**

Tissue perfusion, altered, cerebral may be related to interruption of blood flow (occlusive disorder, hemorrhage, cerebral vasospasm/edema), possibly evidenced by altered level of consciousness, changes in vital signs, changes in motor/sensory responses, restlessness, memory loss, sensory, language, and intellectual and emotional deficits.

Physical mobility, impaired may be related to neuromuscular involvement (weakness, paresthesia, flaccid/hypotonic or spastic paralysis), perceptual/cognitive impairment, possibly evidenced by inability to purposefully move involved body parts, limited range of motion, impaired coordination, or decreased muscle strength/control.

Communication, impaired verbal [and/or written] may be related to impaired cerebral circulation, neuromuscular impairment, loss of facial/oral muscle tone and control; generalized weakness/fatigue possibly evidenced by impaired articulation, does not/cannot speak (dysarthria), inability to modulate speech, find and/or name words, identify objects and/or inability to comprehend written/spoken language, inability to produce written communication.

Self-care deficit (specify) may be related to neuromuscular impairment, decreased strength/endurance, loss of muscle control/coordination, perceptual/cognitive impairment, pain/discomfort, and depression, possibly evidenced by stated/observed inability to perform activities of daily living, requests for assistance, disheveled appearance, and incontinence.

Swallowing, impaired, risk for: risk factors may include muscle paralysis and perceptual impairment.

Unilateral neglect, risk for: risk factors may include sensory loss of part of visual field with perceptual loss of corresponding body segment.

Home maintenance management, impaired may be related to condition of individual family member, insufficient finances/family organization or planning, unfamiliarity with resources, and inadequate support systems, possibly evidenced by members expressing difficulty in managing home in a comfortable manner/requesting assistance with home maintenance, disorderly surroundings, and overtaxed family members.

Self-esteem/Body image disturbance/Role performance, altered may be related to biophysical, psychosocial, and cognitive/perceptual changes, possibly evidenced by actual change in structure and/or function, change in usual patterns of responsibility/physical capacity to resume role; and verbal/nonverbal response to actual or perceived change.

**cesarean birth, unplanned**

Knowledge deficit [learning need] regarding underlying procedure, pathophysiology, and self-care needs may be related to incomplete/inadequate information, possibly evidenced by request for information, verbalization of concerns/misconceptions and inappropriate/exaggerated behavior.

Anxiety [specify level] may be related to actual/perceived threat to mother/fetus, emotional threat to self-esteem, unmet needs/expectations, and interpersonal transmission, possibly evidenced by increased tension, apprehension, feelings of inadequacy, sympathetic stimulation, restlessness, and narrowed focus.

Self-esteem, situational low, risk for: risk factors may include perceived "failure" at life event.

Pain [acute], risk for: risk factors may include increased/prolonged contractions, psychologic reaction.

Infection, risk for: risk factors may include invasive procedures, rupture of amniotic membranes, break in skin, decreased hemoglobin, exposure to pathogens.

**chemotherapy** (also refer to *cancer*)

Fluid volume deficit, risk for: risk factors may include gastrointestinal losses (vomiting), interference with adequate intake (stomatitis/anorexia), losses through abnormal routes (indwelling tubes, wounds, fistulas), and hypermetabolic state.

Nutrition, altered, less than body requirements may be related to inability to ingest adequate nutrients (nausea, anorexia, stomatitis, and fatigue) or hypermetabolic state, possibly evidenced by weight loss (wasting); aversion to eating; reported altered taste sensation; sore, inflamed buccal cavity; and diarrhea or constipation.

Oral mucous membranes, altered may be related to side effects of therapeutic agents/radiation, dehydration, and malnutrition, possibly evidenced by ulcerations, leukoplakia, decreased salivation, and reports of pain.

Body image disturbance may be related to anatomical/structural changes; loss of hair and weight, possibly evidenced by negative feelings about body, preoccupation with change, feelings of helplessness/hopelessness, and change in social involvement.

**cholecystectomy**

Pain, [acute] may be related to interruption in skin/tissue layers with mechanical closure (sutures/staples) and invasive procedures (including NG tube), possibly evidenced by verbal reports, guarding/distraction behaviors, and autonomic responses (changes in vital signs).

Breathing pattern, ineffective may be related to decreased lung expansion (pain and muscle weakness), decreased energy/fatigue, ineffective cough, possibly evidenced by fremitus, tachypnea, and decreased respiratory depth/vital capacity.

Fluid volume deficit, risk for: risk factors may include vomiting/NG aspiration, medically restricted intake, altered coagulation.

**cholelithiasis**

Pain, [acute] may be related to inflammation and distention of tissues, ductal spasm, possibly evidenced by verbal reports, guarding/distraction behaviors, and autonomic responses (changes in vital signs).

Nutrition: altered, less than body requirements may be related to inability to ingest/absorb adequate nutrients (food intolerance/pain, nausea/vomiting, anorexia), possibly evidenced by aversion to food/decreased intake and weight loss.

Knowledge deficit [learning need] regarding pathophysiology, therapy choices, and self-care needs may be related to lack of information or misinterpretation, possibly evidenced by verbalization of concerns, questions, and recurrence of condition.

**chronic obstructive pulmonary disease**

Gas exchange, impaired may be related to altered oxygen delivery (obstruction of airways by secretions/bronchospasm, air-trapping) and alveoli destruction, possibly evidenced by dyspnea, confusion, restlessness, abnormal ABG values, and reduced tolerance for activity.

Airway clearance, ineffective may be related to bronchospasm, increased production of tenacious secretions, retained secretions, and decreased energy/fatigue, possibly evidenced by presence of wheezes, crackles, tachypnea, dyspnea, pallor or cyanosis, and chest x-ray findings.

Activity intolerance may be related to imbalance between oxygen supply and demand, and generalized weakness, possibly evidenced by verbal reports of fatigue, exertional dyspnea, and abnormal vital sign response.

Nutrition, altered, less than body requirements may be related to inability to ingest adequate nutrients (dyspnea, fatigue, medication side effect, sputum production, anorexia), possibly evidenced by weight loss, decreased muscle mass/subcutaneous fat, poor muscle tone, reported altered taste sensation, aversion to eating, and lack of interest in food.

Infection, risk for: risk factors may include decreased ciliary action, stasis of secretions, and debilitated state/malnutrition.

**cirrhosis**

Nutrition, altered, less than body requirements may be related to inability to ingest/absorb nutrients (anorexia, nausea, indigestion, abnormal bowel function, impaired storage of vitamins), possibly evidenced by aversion to eating, observed lack of intake, muscle wasting, weight loss, and imbalances in nutritional studies.

Fluid volume excess may be related to compromised regulatory mechanism (e.g., decreased plasma proteins/malnutrition) and excess sodium/fluid intake, possibly evidenced by generalized or abdominal edema, weight gain, dyspnea, blood pressure changes, positive hepatojugular reflex, change in mentation, altered electrolytes, changes in urine specific gravity, and pleural effusion.

Skin integrity, impaired, risk for: risk factors may include altered circulation/metabolic state, poor skin turgor, skeletal prominence, and presence of edema/ascites.

Thought processes, altered, risk for: risk factors may include physiologic changes (increased serum ammonia level and inability of liver to detoxify certain enzymes/drugs).

Self-esteem/Body image disturbance may be related to biophysical changes/altered physical appearance, uncertainty of prognosis, changes in role function, personal vulnerability, self-destructive behavior (alcohol-induced disease), possibly evidenced by verbalization of changes in lifestyle, fear of rejection/reaction of others, negative feelings about body/abilities, and feelings of helplessness/hopelessness/powerlessness.

Injury, risk for hemorrhage: risk factors may include abnormal blood profile (altered clotting factors), portal hypertension/development of esophageal varices.

**cocaine hydrochloride poisoning, acute**

Breathing pattern, ineffective may be related to pharmacologic effects on respiratory center of the brain, possibly evidenced by tachypnea, altered depth of respiration, shortness of breath, and abnormal ABGs.

Cardiac output, decreased, risk for: risk factors may include drug effect on myocardium (degree dependent on drug purity/quality used), alterations in electrical rate/rhythm/conduction, preexisting myocardiopathy.

Nutrition, altered: less than body requirements may be related to anorexia, insufficient/inappropriate use of financial resources, possibly evidenced by reported inadequate intake, weight loss/less than normal weight gain, lack of interest in food, poor muscle tone, signs/laboratory evidence of vitamin deficiencies.

Thought processes, altered may be related to pharmacologic stimulation of the nervous system, possibly evidenced by altered attention span, disorientation, and hallucinations.

Coping, individual, ineffective may be related to personal vulnerability, negative role modeling, inadequate support systems, ineffective/inadequate coping skills with substitution of drug, possibly evidenced by use of harmful substance, despite evidence of undesirable consequences.

Sensory/Perceptual alteration (specify) may be related to exogenous chemical, altered sensory reception/transmission/integration (hallucination), altered status of sense organs, possibly evidenced by responding to internal stimuli from hallucinatory experiences, bizarre thinking, changes in sensory acuity (sense of smell/taste).

**coccidioidomycosis** (San Joaquin/Valley Fever)

Pain [acute] may be related to inflammation, possibly evidenced by verbal reports, distraction behaviors, and narrowed focus.

Fatigue may be related to decreased energy production; states of discomfort, possibly evidenced by reports of overwhelming lack of energy, inability to maintain usual routine, emotional lability/irritability, impaired ability to concentrate, and decreased endurance/libido.

Knowledge deficit [learning need] regarding nature/course of disease and therapy needs may be related to lack of information, possibly evidenced by statements of concern and questions.

**colitis, ulcerative**

Diarrhea may be related to inflammation or malabsorption of the bowel, presence of toxins and/or segmental narrowing of the lumen, possibly evidenced by increased bowel sounds/peristalsis, urgency, frequent/watery stools (acute phase), changes in stool color, and abdominal pain/cramping.

Pain, [acute/chronic] may be related to inflammation of the intestines/hyperperistalsis and anal/rectal irritation, possibly evidenced by verbal reports, guarding/distraction behaviors.

Fluid volume deficit, risk for: risk factors may include continued gastrointestinal losses (diarrhea, vomiting, capillary plasma loss), altered intake, hypermetabolic state.

Nutrition, altered, less than body requirements may be related to altered intake/absorption of nutrients (medically restricted intake, fear that eating may cause diarrhea) and hypermetabolic state, possibly evidenced by weight loss, decreased subcutaneous fat/muscle mass, poor muscle tone, hyperactive bowel sounds, steatorrhea, pale conjunctiva and mucous membranes, and aversion to eating.

Coping, individual, ineffective may be related to chronic nature and indefinite outcome of disease, multiple stressors (repeated over time), personal vulnerability, severe pain, inadequate sleep, lack of/ineffective support systems, possibly evidenced by verbalization of inability to cope, discouragement, anxiety, preoccupation with physical self, chronic worry, emotional tension, depression, and recurrent exacerbation of symptoms.

Powerlessness, risk for: risk factors may include unresolved dependency conflicts, feelings of insecurity/resentment, repressing anger and aggressive feelings, lacking a sense of control in stressful situations, sacrificing own wishes for others, and retreat from aggression or frustration.

**colostomy**

Skin integrity, impaired, risk for: risk factors may include absence of sphincter at stoma and chemical irritation from caustic bowel contents, reaction to product/removal of adhesive, and improper fitting of appliance.

Diarrhea/Constipation, risk for: risk factors may include interruption/alteration of normal bowel function, changes in dietary/fluid intake, and effects of medication.

Knowledge deficit [learning need] regarding changes in physiologic function and self-care/treatment needs may be related to lack of exposure/recall, information misinterpretation, possibly evidenced by questions, statement of concern, and inaccurate follow-through of instruction/development of preventable complications.

Body image disturbance may be related to biophysical changes (presence of stoma; loss of control of bowel elimination) and psychosocial factors (altered body structure, disease process/associated treatment regimen, e.g., cancer, colitis), possibly evidenced by verbalization of change in perception of self, negative feelings about body, fear of rejection/reaction of others, not touching/looking at stoma, and refusal to participate in care.

Social interaction, impaired may be related to fear of embarrassing situation secondary to altered bowel control with loss of contents, odor, possibly evidenced by reduced participation and verbalized/observed discomfort in social situations.

Sexual dysfunction, risk for: risk factors may include altered body structure/function, radical resection/treatment procedures, vulnerability/psychologic concern about response of significant other(s), and disruption of sexual response pattern (e.g., erection difficulty).

**coma, diabetic**

Refer to *diabetic ketoacidosis*.

**concussion of the brain**

Pain, [acute] may be related to trauma to/edema of cerebral tissue, possibly evidenced by reports of headache, guarding/distraction behaviors, and narrowed focus.

Fluid volume deficit, risk for: risk factors may include vomiting, decreased intake, and hypermetabolic state (fever).

Knowledge deficit [learning need] regarding condition, treatment/safety needs, and potential complications may be related to lack of recall, misinterpretation, cognitive limitation, possibly evidenced by questions/statement of concerns, development of preventable complications.

**congestive heart failure**

Cardiac output, decreased may be related to altered myocardial contractility/inotropic changes; alterations in rate, rhythm, and electrical conduction; and structural changes (valvular defects, ventricular aneurysm), possibly evidenced by tachycardia/dysrhythmias, changes in blood pressure, extra heart sounds, decreased urine output, diminished peripheral pulses, cool/ashen skin, orthopnea, crackles, dependent/generalized edema, and chest pain.

Fluid volume excess may be related to reduced glomerular filtration rate/increased ADH production, and sodium/water retention, possibly evidenced by orthopnea and abnormal breath sounds, $S_3$ heart sound, jugular vein distention, positive hepatojugular reflex, weight gain, hypertension, oliguria, and generalized edema.

Gas exchange, impaired, risk for: risk factors may include alveolar-capillary membrane changes (fluid collection/shifts into interstitial space/alveoli).

Activity intolerance may be related to imbalance between oxygen supply/demand, generalized weakness, and prolonged bedrest/sedentary lifestyle, possibly evidenced by reported/observed weakness, fatigue, changes in vital signs, presence of dysrhythmias, dyspnea, pallor, and diaphoresis.

Knowledge deficit [learning need] regarding cardiac function/disease process may be related to lack of information/misinterpretation, possibly evidenced by questions, statements of concern/misconceptions, development of preventable complications or exacerbations of condition.

**Conn's syndrome**
Refer to *aldosteronism, primary.*

**constipation**
Constipation may be related to weak abdominal musculature, GI obstructive lesions, pain on defecation, diagnostic procedures, pregnancy, possibly evidenced by change in character/frequency of stools, feeling of abdominal/rectal fullness or pressure, changes in bowel sounds, abdominal distension.

Pain, [acute] may be related to abdominal fullness/pressure, straining to defecate, and trauma to delicate tissues, possibly evidenced by verbal reports, reluctance to defecate, and distraction behaviors.

Knowledge deficit [learning need] regarding dietary needs, bowel function, and medication effect may be related to lack of information/misconceptions, possibly evidenced by development of problem and verbalization of concerns/questions.

**coronary artery bypass surgery**
Cardiac output, decreased may be related to decreased myocardial contractility, diminished circulating volume (preload), alterations in electrical conduction, and increased systemic vascular resistance (afterload), possibly evidenced by changes in blood pressure, presence of ECG changes/dysrhythmias, and diminished peripheral pulses.

Fluid volume deficit [active loss] may be related to intraoperative blood loss or use of diuretics, possibly evidenced by decreased blood pressure, concentrated urine with elevated specific gravity, and decreased pulse volume/pressure.

Pain [acute] may be related to direct chest tissue/bone trauma, invasive tubes/lines, and donor site incision, possibly evidenced by verbal reports, autonomic responses (changes in vital signs), and distraction behaviors/restlessness or irritability.

Sensory/Perceptual alterations (specify) may be related to restricted environment (postoperative/acute), sleep deprivation, effects of medications, continuous environmental sounds/activities, and psychologic stress of procedure, possibly evidenced by disorientation, alterations in behavior, exaggerated emotional responses, and visual/auditory distortions.

**Crohn's disease** (also refer to *colitis, ulcerative*)
Nutrition, altered, less than body requirements may be related to intestinal pain after eating, and decreased transit time through bowel, possibly evidenced by weight loss, aversion to eating, and observed lack of intake.

Diarrhea may be related to inflammation of small intestines, particularly dietary intake, possibly evidenced by hyperactive bowel sounds, cramping, and frequent, loose liquid stools.

Knowledge deficit [learning need] regarding condition, nutritional needs, and prevention of recurrence may be related to insufficient information/misinterpretation, unfamiliarity with resources, possibly evidenced by statements of concern/questions, inaccurate follow-through of instructions, and development of preventable complications/exacerbation of condition.

**croup**
Airway clearance, ineffective may be related to presence of thick, tenacious mucus, and swelling/spasms of the epiglottis, possibly evidenced by harsh/brassy cough, tachypnea, use of accessory breathing muscles, and presence of wheezes.

Fluid volume deficit [active loss] may be related to decreased ability/aversion to swallowing, presence of fever, and increased respiratory losses, possibly evidenced by dry mucous membranes, poor skin turgor, and scanty/concentrated urine.

**croup, membranous** (also refer to *croup*)
Suffocation, risk for: risk factors may include inflammation of larynx with formation of false membrane.

Anxiety [specify level]/Fear may be related to change in environment, perceived threat to self (difficulty breathing), and transmission of anxiety of adults, possibly evidenced by restlessness, facial tension, glancing about, and sympathetic stimulation.

**Cushing's syndrome**
Infection, risk for: risk factors may include immunosuppressed inflammatory response, skin and capillary fragility, and negative nitrogen balance.

Nutrition, altered, less than body requirements may be related to inability to utilize nutrients (disturbance of carbohydrate metabolism), possibly evidenced by decreased muscle mass and increased resistance to insulin.

Self-care deficit (specify) may be related to muscle wasting, generalized weakness, fatigue, and demineralization of bones, possibly evidenced by statements of/observed inability to complete or perform activities of daily living.

Body image disturbance may be related to change in structure/appearance (effects of disease process, drug therapy), possibly evidenced by negative feelings about body, feelings of helplessness, and changes in social involvement.

Sexual dysfunction may be related to loss of libido, impotence, and cessation of menses, possibly evidenced by verbalization of concerns and/or dissatisfaction and alteration in relationship with significant other.

Trauma, risk for fractures: risk factors may include increased protein breakdown, negative protein balance, demineralization of bones.

**cystic fibrosis**

Airway clearance, ineffective may be related to excessive production of thick mucus and decreased ciliary action, possibly evidenced by abnormal breath sounds, ineffective cough, cyanosis, and altered respiratory rate/depth.

Infection, risk for: risk factors may include stasis of respiratory secretions and development of atelectasis.

Nutrition, altered, less than body requirements may be related to impaired digestive process and malabsorption of nutrients, possibly evidenced by failure to gain weight, muscle wasting, and retarded physical growth.

Knowledge deficit [learning need] regarding pathophysiology of condition, medical management, and available community resources may be related to insufficient information/misconceptions, possibly evidenced by statements of concern, questions, inaccurate follow-through of instructions, development of preventable complications.

Family coping, ineffective: compromised may be related to chronic nature of disease and disability and parental supervision and lifestyle restrictions, possibly evidenced by protective behavior disproportionate to patient's abilities or need for autonomy.

**cystitis**

Pain, [acute] may be related to inflammation and bladder spasms, possibly evidenced by verbal reports, distraction behaviors, and narrowed focus.

Urinary elimination, altered may be related to inflammation/irritation of bladder, possibly evidenced by frequency, nocturia, and dysuria.

Knowledge deficit [learning need] regarding condition, treatment, and prevention of recurrence may be related to inadequate information/misconceptions, possibly evidenced by statements of concern and questions or recurrent infections.

**cytomegalic inclusion disease**

Refer to *herpes*.

**dehiscence** (abdominal)

Skin integrity, impaired may be related to altered circulation, altered nutritional state (obesity/malnutrition), and physical stress on incision, possibly evidenced by poor/delayed wound healing and disruption of skin surface/wound closure.

Infection, risk for: risk factors may include inadequate primary defenses (separation of incision, traumatized intestines, environmental exposure).

Tissue integrity, impaired, risk for: risk factors may include exposure of abdominal contents to external environment.

Fear/Anxiety, severe may be related to crises, perceived threat of death, possibly evidenced by fearfulness, restless behaviors, and sympathetic stimulation.

Knowledge deficit [learning need] regarding condition/prognosis and treatment needs may be related to lack of information/recall and misinterpretation of information, possibly evidenced by development of preventable complication, requests for information, and statement of concern.

**dehydration**

Fluid volume deficit (specify) may be related to etiology as defined by specific situation, possibly evidenced by dry mucous membranes, poor skin turgor, decreased pulse volume/pressure, and thirst.

Oral mucous membranes, altered, risk for: risk factors may include dehydration and decreased salivation.

Knowledge deficit [learning need] regarding fluid needs may be related to lack of information/misinterpretation, possibly evidenced by questions, statement of concern, and inadequate follow-through of instructions/development of preventable complications.

**delirium tremens**

Sensory/Perceptual alterations (specify) may be related to exogenous/endogenous chemical alterations, sleep deprivation, and psychologic stress, possibly evidenced by disorientation, restlessness, irritability, exaggerated emotional responses, and visual and auditory distortions/hallucinations.

Fluid volume deficit, risk for: risk factors may include reduced intake, profuse diaphoresis, and agitation.

Trauma, risk for: risk factors may include alterations in balance, reduced muscle coordination, cognitive impairment, and involuntary clonic/tonic muscle activity.

Nutrition, altered, less than body requirements may be related to poor dietary intake, effects of alcohol on organs involved in digestion, interference with absorption/metabolism of nutrients and amino acids, possibly evidenced by reports of inadequate food intake, altered taste sensation, lack of interest in food, debilitated state, decreased subcutaneous fat/muscle mass, signs of mineral/electrolyte deficiency, including abnormal laboratory findings.

**dementia, presenile/senile** (also refer to *Alzheimer's disease*)

Thought processes, altered may be related to irreversible cerebral neuronal degeneration, loss of memory, sleep deprivation, psychologic conflicts, possibly evidenced by memory deficit, decreased ability to grasp ideas/problem solve and make decisions, altered attention span, disorientation, delusions, and inappropriate social behavior/affect.

Memory, impaired may be related to neurological disturbances, possibly evidenced by observed experiences of forgetting, inability to determine if a behavior was performed, inability to perform previously learned skills, inability to recall factual information or recent/past events.

Trauma, risk for: risk factors may include changes in muscle coordination/balance, impaired judgment, seizure activity.

Caregiver role strain, risk for: risk factors may include illness severity of care receiver, duration of caregiving required, care receiver exhibits deviant/bizarre behavior; family/caregiver isolation, lack of respite/recreation, spouse is caregiver.

**depressive disorders, major depression, dysthymia**

Violence, risk for, directed at self/others: risk factors may include depressed mood and feelings of worthlessness and hopelessness.

Anxiety [moderate to severe]/Thought processes, altered may be related to psychological conflicts, unconscious conflict about essential values/goals of life, unmet needs, threat to self-concept, sleep deprivation, interpersonal transmission/contagion, possibly evidenced by reports of nervousness or fearfulness, feelings of inadequacy, agitation, angry/tearful outbursts, rambling/discoordinated speech, restlessness, hand rubbing or wringing, tremulousness, poor memory/concentration, decreased ability to grasp ideas, inability to follow/impaired ability to make decisions, numerous/repetitious physical complaints without organic cause, ideas of reference, hallucinations/delusions.

Sleep pattern disturbance may be related to biochemical alterations (decreased serotonin), unresolved fears and anxieties, and inactivity, possibly evidenced by difficulty in falling/remaining asleep, early morning awakening/awakening later than desired, reports of not feeling rested, and physical signs (e.g., dark circles under eyes, excessive yawning).

Social isolation/Social interaction, impaired may be related to alterations in mental status/thought processes (depressed mood), inadequate personal resources, decreased energy/inertia, difficulty engaging in satisfying personal relationships, feelings of worthlessness/low self-concept, inadequacy in or absence of significant purpose in life, and knowledge/skill deficit about social interactions, possibly evidenced by decreased involvement with others, expressed feelings of difference from others, remaining in home/room/bed, refusing invitations/suggestions of social involvement, and dysfunctional interaction with peers, family, and/or others.

Family processes, altered may be related to situational crises of illness of family member with change in roles/responsibilities, developmental crises (e.g., loss of family member/relationship), possibly evidenced by statements of difficulty coping with situation, family system not meeting needs of its members, difficulty accepting or receiving help appropriately, ineffective family decision-making process, and failure to send and to receive clear messages.

Injury, risk for [adverse effects of electroconvulsive therapy (ECT)]: risk factors may include electroconvulsive effects on the cardiovascular, respiratory, musculoskeletal, and nervous systems, and pharmacologic effects of anesthesia.

**dermatitis seborrheica**

Skin integrity, impaired may be related to chronic inflammatory condition of the skin, possibly evidenced by disruption of skin surface with dry or moist scales, yellowish crusts, erythema, and fissures.

**diabetes mellitus**

Knowledge deficit [learning need] regarding disease process/treatment and individual care needs may be related to unfamiliarity with information/lack of recall, misinterpretation, possibly evidenced by requests for information, statements of concern/misconceptions, inadequate follow-through of instructions, and development of preventable complications.

Nutrition, altered, less than body requirements may be related to inability to utilize nutrients (imbalance between intake and utilization of glucose) to meet metabolic needs, possibly evidenced by change in weight, muscle weakness, increased thirst/urination, and hyperglycemia.

Adjustment, impaired, risk for: risk factors may include all-encompassing change in lifestyle and self-concept requiring lifelong adherence to therapeutic regimen and internal/altered locus of control.

Infection, risk for: risk factors may include decreased leukocytic function, circulatory changes, and delayed healing.

Family coping, ineffective: compromised may be related to inadequate or incorrect information or understanding by primary person(s), other situational/developmental crises or situations the significant person(s) may be facing, lifelong condition requiring behavioral changes impacting family, possibly evidenced by family expression of confusion about what to do, verbalization that they are having difficulty coping with situation, family does not meet physical/emotional needs of its members, significant other(s) preoccupied with personal reaction (e.g., guilt, fear), significant other(s) display protective behavior disproportionate (too little/too much) to patient's abilities or need for autonomy.

**diabetic ketoacidosis**

Fluid volume deficit [regulatory failure] may be related to hyperosmolar urinary losses, gastric losses, and inadequate intake, possibly evidenced by increased urinary output/dilute urine, reports of weakness, thirst, sudden weight loss, hypotension, tachycardia, delayed capillary refill, dry mucous membranes, poor skin turgor.

Nutrition, altered, less than body requirements may be related to inadequate utilization of nutrients (insulin deficiency), decreased oral intake, hypermetabolic state, possibly evidenced by recent weight loss, reports of weakness, lack of interest in food, gastric fullness/abdominal pain, increased ketones, and imbalance between glucose/insulin levels.

Sensory/Perceptual alteration (specify), risk for: risk factors may include endogenous chemical alteration (glucose/insulin and/or electrolyte imbalance).

Infection, risk for: risk factors may include high glucose levels, decreased leukocyte function, stasis of body fluids, invasive procedures, and alteration in circulation/perfusion.

**dialysis, general** (also refer to *dialysis, peritoneal*; *hemodialysis*)

Nutrition, altered: less than body requirements may be related to inadequate ingestion of nutrients (dietary restrictions, anorexia, nausea/vomiting, stomatitis), loss of protein during procedure, possibly evidenced by reported inadequate intake, aversion to eating, altered taste sensation, poor muscle tone/weakness, sore/inflamed buccal cavity, pale conjunctiva/mucous membranes.

Grieving, anticipatory may be related to actual or perceived loss, chronic and/or fatal illness, and thwarted grieving response to a loss, possibly evidenced by verbal expression of distress/unresolved issues, denial of loss, altered eating habits, sleep and dream patterns, activity levels, libido; crying, labile affect, feelings of sorrow, guilt, and anger.

Body image disturbance/Role performance, altered may be related to situational crisis and chronic illness with changes in usual roles, possibly evidenced by verbalization of changes in lifestyle, focus on past function, negative feelings about body, feelings of helplessness/powerlessness, extension of body boundary to incorporate environmental objects (e.g., dialysis setup), change in social involvement, overdependence on others for care, not taking responsibility for self-care/lack of follow-through, and self-destructive behavior.

Coping, individual, ineffective may be related to situational crises/personal vulnerability, multiple life changes, inadequate support systems, and severe pain/overwhelming threat to self, possibly evidenced by verbalization of inability to cope/asking for help, chronic worry, fatigue, insomnia, anxiety/depression, and inappropriate use of defense mechanism.

Powerlessness may be related to illness-related regimen and health-care environment, possibly evidenced by verbal expression of having no control, depression over physical deterioration, nonparticipation in care, anger, and passivity.

Family coping, ineffective: compromised/disabling may be related to inadequate or incorrect information or understanding by a primary person, temporary family disorganization and role changes, patient providing little support in turn for the primary person, and prolonged disease/disability progression that exhausts the supportive capacity of significant persons, possibly evidenced by expressions of concern or reports about significant other's/family's response to patient's health problem, preoccupation of significant other(s) with own personal reactions, display of intolerance/rejection, and protective behavior disproportionate (too little or too much) to patient's abilities or need for autonomy.

**dialysis, peritoneal** (also refer to *dialysis, general*)

Fluid volume excess, risk for: risk factors may include inadequate osmotic gradient of dialysate, fluid retention (dialysate drainage problems/inappropriate osmotic gradient of solution), excessive PO/IV intake.

Pain, [acute] may be related to procedural factors (catheter irritation, improper catheter placement), presence of edema/abdominal distention, inflammation, or infection, rapid infusion/infusion of cold or acidic dialysate, possibly evidenced by verbal reports, guarding/distraction behaviors, and self-focus.

Infection, risk for: risk factors may include contamination of catheter/infusion system, skin contaminants, sterile peritonitis (response to composition of dialysate).

Breathing pattern, ineffective, risk for: risk factors may include increased abdominal pressure with restricted diaphragmatic excursion, rapid infusion of dialysate, pain/discomfort, inflammatory process (e.g., atelectasis/pneumonia).

**diarrhea**

Knowledge deficit [learning need] regarding causative/contributing factors and therapeutic needs may be related to lack of information/misconceptions, possibly evidenced by statements of concern, questions, and development of preventable complications.

Fluid volume deficit, risk for: risk factors may include excessive losses through GI tract, altered intake.

Pain, [acute] may be related to abdominal cramping and irritation/excoriation of skin, possibly evidenced by verbal reports, facial grimacing, and autonomic responses.

Skin integrity, impaired may be related to effects of excretions on delicate tissues, possibly evidenced by reports of discomfort and disruption of skin surface/destruction of skin layers.

**digitalis poisoning**

Cardiac output, decreased may be related to altered myocardial contractility/electrical conduction, properties of digitalis (long half-life and narrow therapeutic range), concurrent medications, age/general health status and electrolyte/acid-base balance possibly evidenced by changes in rate/rhythm/conduction (development/worsening of dysrhythmias), changes in mentation, worsening of congestive heart failure, elevated serum drug levels.

Fluid volume deficit/excess, risk for: risk factors may include excessive losses from vomiting/diarrhea, decreased intake/nausea, decreased plasma proteins, malnutrition, continued use of diuretics; excess sodium/fluid retention.

Knowledge deficit [learning need] regarding condition/therapy needs may be related to information misinterpretation and lack of recall, possibly evidenced by inaccurate follow-through of instructions and development of preventable complications.

Thought processes, altered, risk for: risk factors may include physiologic effects of toxicity/reduced cerebral perfusion.

**dilation and curettage** (also refer to *abortion, spontaneous*)

Knowledge deficit [learning need] regarding surgical procedure, possible postprocedural complications, and therapeutic needs may be related to lack of exposure/unfamiliarity with information, possibly evidenced by requests for information and statements of concern/misconceptions.

**disruptive behavior disorder** (childhood, adolescence), **conduct disorder**

Coping, ineffective, individual may be related to inadequate coping strategies, maturational crisis, multiple life changes, lack of control of impulsive actions, and personal vulnerability, possibly evidenced by inappropriate use of defense mechanisms, inability to meet role expectations, poor self-esteem, failure to assume responsibility for own actions, and excessive smoking/drinking/drug use.

Violence, risk for, directed at self/others: risk factors may include dysfunctional family system and loss of significant relationships.

Adjustment, impaired may be related to nonexistent or unsuccessful ability to be involved in problem solving or goal setting, losses connected with current and/or past occurrences in individual situation (e.g., loss of self-esteem, family member/friends), poor school performance, relocation, lack of movement toward independence, and difficulty limiting expectations of self, possibly evidenced by ambivalence toward parent(s), anxiety, self-blame, anger, and feelings of rejection, assault to self-esteem, and altered locus of control.

Family coping, ineffective: compromised/disabling may be related to excessive guilt, anger, or blaming among family members regarding child's behavior; parental inconsistencies; disagreements regarding discipline, limit-setting, and approaches; and exhaustion of parental resources (prolonged coping with disruptive child), possibly evidenced by unrealistic parental expectations, rejection or overprotection of child; and exaggerated expressions of anger, disappointment, or despair regarding child's behavior or ability to improve or change.

Social interaction, impaired may be related to retarded ego development, low self-esteem, dysfunctional family system, and neurologic impairment, possibly evidenced by difficulty waiting turn in games or group situations, does not seem to listen to what is being said, has difficulty playing quietly and maintaining attention to task or play activity, often shifting from one activity to another and interrupting or intruding on others.

**disseminated intravascular coagulation**

Anxiety [specify level]/Fear may be related to sudden change in health status and threat of death, interpersonal transmission/contagion, possibly evidenced by sympathetic stimulation, restlessness, focus on self, and apprehension.

Fluid volume deficit, risk for: risk factors may include failure of regulatory mechanism (coagulation process) and active loss/hemorrhage.

Tissue perfusion, altered (specify) may be related to alteration of arterial/venous flow (microemboli throughout circulatory system and hypovolemia), possibly evidenced by changes in respiratory rate and depth, changes in mentation, decreased urinary output, and development of acral cyanosis/focal gangrene.

Gas exchange, impaired, risk for: risk factors may include reduced oxygen-carrying capacity, development of acidosis, fibrin deposition in microcirculation, and ischemic damage of lung parenchyma.

Pain, [acute] may be related to bleeding into joints/muscles, hematoma formation, and ischemic tissues with areas of acral cyanosis/focal gangrene, possibly evidenced by verbal reports, narrowed focus, alteration in muscle tone, guarding/distraction behaviors, restlessness, and autonomic responses.

**dissociative disorders** (including multiple personality)

Anxiety [severe/panic]/Fear may be related to maladaption of ineffective coping continuing from early life, unconscious conflict(s), threat to self-concept, unmet needs, or phobic stimulus, possibly evidenced by maladaptive response to stress (e.g., dissociating self/fragmentation of the personality), increased tension, feelings of inadequacy, and focus on self, projection of personal perceptions onto the environment.

Violence, risk for, directed at self/others: risk factors may include depressed mood, dissociative state/conflicting personalities, panic states, and suicidal/homicidal behaviors.

Personal identity disturbance may be related to psychologic conflicts (dissociative state), childhood trauma/abuse, threat to physical integrity/self-concept, and underdeveloped ego, possibly evidenced by alteration in perception or experience of self, loss of one's own sense of reality/the external world, poorly differentiated ego boundaries, confusion about sense of self, purpose or direction in life, memory loss, presence of more than one personality within the individual.

Family coping, ineffective: compromised may be related to multiple stressors repeated over time, prolonged progression of disorder that exhausts the supportive capacity of significant people, family disorganization and role changes, possibly evidenced by family/significant other describing inadequate understanding or knowledge that interferes with effective assistive or supportive behaviors, and relationship/marital conflict.

**diverticulitis**

Pain, [acute] may be related to inflammation of intestinal mucosa, abdominal cramping, and presence of fever/chills, possibly evidenced by reports, guarding/distraction behaviors, autonomic responses, and narrowed focus.

Diarrhea/Constipation may be related to altered structure/function and presence of inflammation, possibly evidenced by signs and symptoms dependent on specific problem (e.g., increase/decrease in frequency of stools and change in consistency).

Knowledge deficit [learning need] regarding disease process, potential complications, and therapeutic needs may be related to lack of information/misconceptions, possibly evidenced by statements of concern, request for information, and development of preventable complications.

Powerlessness, risk for: risk factors may include chronic nature of disease process with recurrent episodes despite cooperation with medical regimen.

**Down syndrome** (also refer to *mental retardation*)

Growth and development, altered may be related to effects of physical/mental disability, possibly evidenced by altered physical growth, delay/inability in performing skills and self-care/self-control activities appropriate for age.

Trauma, risk for: risk factors may include cognitive difficulties and poor muscle tone/coordination and weakness.

Nutrition, altered, less than body requirements may be related to poor muscle tone and protruding tongue, possibly evidenced by weak and ineffective sucking/swallowing and observed lack of adequate intake with weight loss/failure to gain.

Family processes, altered may be related to situational/maturational crisis requiring incorporation of new skills into family dynamics, possibly evidenced by confusion about what to do, verbalized difficulty coping with situation, unexamined family myths.

Grieving, dysfunctional, risk for: risk factors may include loss of "the perfect child," chronic condition requiring long-term care, and unresolved feelings.

Parenting, altered, risk for: risk factors may include interference/delayed development of parenting, and attachment behaviors.

Social isolation, risk for: risk factors may include withdrawal from usual social interactions and activities, assumption of total child care, and becoming overindulgent/overprotective.

**drug overdose, acute** (depressants)

Breathing pattern, ineffective/Gas exchange, impaired may be related to neuromuscular impairment/central nervous system depression, decreased lung expansion, possibly evidenced by changes in respirations, cyanosis, and abnormal ABGs.

Trauma/Suffocation/Poisoning, risk for: risk factors may include CNS depression/agitation, hypersensitivity to the drug(s), or psychological stress.

Violence, risk for, directed at self/others: risk factors may include suicidal behaviors, toxic reactions to drug(s).

Infection, risk for: risk factors may include IV drug injection techniques, impurities in injected drugs, localized trauma, malnutrition, or altered immune state.

**Duchenne's muscular dystrophy**

Physical mobility, impaired may be related to musculoskeletal impairment/weakness, possibly evidenced by decreased muscle strength, control, and mass; limited range of motion; and impaired coordination.

Growth and development, altered may be related to effects of physical disability, possibly evidenced by altered physical growth and altered ability to perform self-care/self-control activities appropriate to age.

Nutrition, altered, risk for more than body requirements: risk factors may include sedentary lifestyle and dysfunctional eating patterns.

Family coping, ineffective: compromised may be related to situational crisis/emotional conflicts around issues about hereditary nature of condition and prolonged disease/disability that exhausts supportive capacity of family members, possibly evidenced by preoccupation with personal reactions regarding disability and displaying protective behavior disproportionate (too little/too much) to patient's abilities/need for autonomy.

**dysmenorrhea**

Pain, [acute] may be related to exaggerated uterine contractility, possibly evidenced by reports, guarding/distraction behaviors, narrowed focus, and autonomic responses (changes in vital signs).

Activity intolerance, risk for: risk factors may include severity of pain and presence of secondary symptoms (nausea, vomiting, syncope, chills), depression.

Coping, individual, ineffective may be related to chronic, recurrent nature of problem, anticipatory anxiety, and inadequate coping methods, possibly evidenced by muscular tension, headaches, general irritability, chronic depression, verbalization of inability to cope, and report of poor self-esteem.

**dysrhythmia, cardiac**

Cardiac output, decreased: may be related to altered electrical conduction and reduced myocardial contractility, possibly evidenced by alterations in hemodynamic readings, ECG changes, fatigue, dyspnea, and syncope.

Anxiety [specify level] may be related to perceived threat of death, possibly evidenced by increased tension, apprehension, and expressed concerns.

Pain, [acute], risk for: risk factors may include ischemia of cardiac muscle.

Knowledge deficit [learning need] regarding medical condition/therapy needs may be related to lack of information/misinterpretation and unfamiliarity with information resources, possibly evidenced by questions, statement of misconception, failure to improve on previous regimen, and development of preventable complications.

Activity intolerance, risk for: risk factors may include imbalance between myocardial oxygen supply and demand, and cardiac depressant effects of certain drugs (beta blockers, antidysrhythmics).

**eclampsia**

Refer to *pregnancy-induced hypertension*.

**ectopic pregnancy** (tubal)

Pain, [acute] may be related to distention/rupture of fallopian tube, possibly evidenced by reports, guarding/distraction behaviors, facial mask of pain, and autonomic responses (diaphoresis, changes in vital signs).

Fluid volume deficit, risk for: risk factors may include hemorrhagic losses and decreased/restricted intake.

Anxiety [specify level] may be related to threat of death and possible loss of ability to conceive, possibly evidenced by increased tension, apprehension, sympathetic stimulation, restlessness, and focus on self.

**eczema** (dermatitis)

Pain [discomfort] may be related to cutaneous inflammation and irritation, possibly evidenced by verbal reports, irritability, and scratching.

Infection, risk for: risk factors may include broken skin and tissue trauma.

Social isolation may be related to alterations in physical appearance, possibly evidenced by expressed feelings of rejection and decreased interaction with peers.

**edema, pulmonary**

Fluid volume excess may be related to decreased cardiac functioning, excessive fluid/sodium intake, possibly evidenced by dyspnea, presence of crackles (rales), pulmonary congestion on x-ray, restlessness, anxiety, and increased CVP.

Gas exchange, impaired may be related to altered blood flow and decreased alveolar-capillary exchange (fluid collection/shifts into interstitial space/alveoli), possibly evidenced by hypoxia, restlessness, and confusion.

Anxiety [specify level]/Fear may be related to perceived threat of death (inability to breathe), possibly evidenced by responses ranging from apprehension to panic state, restlessness, and focus on self.

**emphysema**

Gas exchange, impaired may be related to alveolar capillary membrane changes/destruction, possibly evidenced by dyspnea, restlessness, changes in mentation, abnormal ABG values.

Airway clearance, ineffective may be related to increased production/retained tenacious secretions, decreased energy level, and muscle wasting, possibly evidenced by abnormal breath sounds (rhonchi), ineffective cough, changes in rate/depth of respirations, and dyspnea.

Activity intolerance may be related to imbalance between oxygen supply and demand, possibly evidenced by reports of fatigue/weakness, exertional dyspnea, and abnormal vital sign response to activity.

Nutrition, altered, less than body requirements may be related to inability to ingest food (shortness of breath, anorexia, generalized weakness, and medication side effects), possibly evidenced by lack of interest in food, reported altered taste, loss of muscle mass and tone, fatigue, and weight loss.

Infection, risk for: risk factors may include inadequate primary defenses (stasis of body fluids, decreased ciliary action), chronic disease process, and malnutrition.

Powerlessness may be related to illness-related regimen and health care environment, possibly evidenced by verbal expression of having no control, depression over physical deterioration, nonparticipation in care, anger, and passivity.

**encephalitis**

Tissue perfusion, altered, cerebral, risk for: risk factors may include cerebral edema altering/interrupting cerebral arterial/venous blood flow, hypovolemia, exchange problems at cellular level (acidosis).

Hyperthermia may be related to increased metabolic rate, illness, and dehydration, possibly evidenced by increased body temperature, flushed/warm skin, and increased pulse and respiratory rates.

Pain, [acute] may be related to inflammation/irritation of the brain and cerebral edema, possibly evidenced by verbal reports of headache, distraction behaviors, restlessness, and autonomic response (changes in vital signs).

Trauma/Suffocation, risk for: risk factors may include restlessness, clonic/tonic activity, altered sensorium, and cognitive impairment.

**endocarditis**

Cardiac output, decreased, risk for: risk factors may include inflammation of heart lining and structural change in valve leaflets.

Anxiety [specify level] may be related to change in health status and threat of death, possibly evidenced by apprehension, expressed concerns, and focus on self.

Pain, [acute] may be related to generalized inflammatory process and effects of embolic phenomena, possibly evidenced by reports, narrowed focus, distraction behaviors, and autonomic responses (changes in vital signs).

Tissue perfusion, altered (specify), risk for: risk factors may include embolic interruption of arterial flow (embolization of thrombi/valvular vegetations).

**endometriosis**

Pain, [acute/chronic] may be related to pressure of concealed bleeding/formation of adhesions, possibly evidenced by verbal reports (pain between/with menstruation), guarding/distraction behaviors, and narrowed focus.

Sexual dysfunction may be related to pain secondary to presence of adhesions, possibly evidenced by verbalization of problem, and altered relationship with partner.

Knowledge deficit [learning need] regarding pathophysiology of condition and therapy needs may be related to lack of information/misinterpretations, possibly evidenced by statements of concern and misconceptions.

**enteritis**
Refer to *colitis, ulcerative*; *Crohn's disease*.

**epididymitis**
Pain, [acute] may be related to inflammation, edema formation, and tension on the spermatic cord, possibly evidenced by verbal reports, guarding/distraction behaviors (restlessness), and autonomic responses (changes in vital signs).
Infection, risk for spread: risk factors may include presence of inflammation/infectious process, insufficient knowledge to avoid spread of infection.
Knowledge deficit [learning need] regarding pathophysiology, outcome, and self-care needs may be related to lack of information/misinterpretations, possibly evidenced by statements of concern, misconceptions, and questions.

**epilepsy**
Knowledge deficit [learning need] regarding condition and medication control may be related to lack of information/misinterpretations, scarce financial resources, possibly evidenced by questions, statements of concern/misconceptions, incorrect use of anticonvulsant medication, or recurrent episodes/uncontrolled seizures.
Self-esteem/Body image disturbance may be related to perceived neurologic functional change/weakness, stigma associated with condition, possibly evidenced by negative feelings about "brain"/self, change in social involvement, feelings of helplessness, and preoccupation with perceived change or loss.
Social interaction, impaired may be related to unpredictable nature of condition and self concept disturbance, possibly evidenced by decreased self-assurance, verbalization of concern, discomfort in social situations, inability to receive/communicate a satisfying sense of belonging/caring, and withdrawal from social contact/activities.
Trauma/Suffocation, risk for: risk factors may include weakness, balancing difficulties, cognitive limitations/altered consciousness, loss of large- or small-muscle coordination (during seizure).

**failure to thrive**
Nutrition, altered, less than body requirements may be related to inability to ingest/digest/absorb nutrients (defects in organ function/metabolism, genetic factors), and physical deprivation/psychosocial factors), possibly evidenced by lack of appropriate weight gain/weight loss, poor muscle tone, pale conjunctiva, and laboratory tests reflecting nutritional deficiency.
Growth and Development, altered may be related to inadequate caretaking (physical/emotional neglect or abuse), indifference, inconsistent responsiveness, multiple caretakers, environmental and stimulation deficiencies, possibly evidenced by altered physical growth, flat affect, listlessness, decreased response, delay or difficulty in performing skills or self-control activities appropriate for age group.
Parenting, altered, risk for: risk factors may include lack of knowledge, inadequate bonding, unrealistic expectations for self/infant, and lack of appropriate response of child to relationship.
Knowledge deficit [learning need] regarding pathophysiology of condition, nutritional needs, growth/development expectations, and parenting skills may be related to lack of information/misinformation or misinterpretation, possibly evidenced by verbalization of concerns, questions, misconceptions; and development of preventable complications.

**fetal alcohol syndrome**
Injury, risk for CNS damage: risk factors may include external chemical factors (alcohol intake by mother), placental insufficiency, fetal drug withdrawal in utero/postpartum, and prematurity.
Infant behavior, disorganized may be related to prematurity, environmental overstimulation, lack of containment/boundaries, possibly evidenced by change from baseline physiological measures, tremors, startles, twitches, hyperextension of arms/legs, deficient self-regulatory behaviors, deficient response to visual/auditory stimuli.

Parenting, altered, risk for: risk factors may include mental and/or physical illness, inability of mother to assume the overwhelming task of unselfish giving and nurturing, presence of stressors (financial/legal problems), lack of available or ineffective role model, interruption of bonding process, lack of appropriate response of child to relationship.

Coping, individual, ineffective (mother) may be related to personal vulnerability, low self-esteem, inadequate coping skills, and multiple stressors (repeated over period of time), possibly evidenced by inability to meet basic needs/role expectations/problem solving, and excessive use of drug(s).

Family coping, ineffective: disabling may be related to lack of/insufficient support from others, mother's drug problem and treatment status, together with poor coping skills, lack of family stability/overinvolvement of parents with children and multigenerational addictive behaviors, possibly evidenced by abandonment, rejection, neglectful relationships with family members, and decisions and actions by family that are detrimental.

**fetal demise**

Grieving, [expected] may be related to death of fetus/infant (wanted/unwanted) possibly evidenced by verbal expression of distress, anger, loss, crying, alteration in eating habits or sleep pattern.

Self-Esteem, situational low may be related to perceived "failure" at a life event, possibly evidenced by negative self-appraisal in response to life event in a person with a previous positive self-evaluation, verbalization of negative feelings about the self (helplessness, uselessness), difficulty making decisions.

Spiritual distress, risk for: risk factors may include challenged belief and value system (birth is supposed to be the beginning of life, not of death) and intense suffering.

**fracture** (also refer to *cast*)

Trauma, risk for additional injury: risk factors may include loss of skeletal integrity/movement of skeletal fragments, use of traction apparatus.

Pain, [acute] may be related to muscle spasms, movement of bone fragments, tissue trauma/edema, traction/immobility device, stress and anxiety, possibly evidenced by verbal reports, distraction behaviors, self-focusing/narrowed focus, facial mask of pain, guarding/protective behavior, alteration in muscle tone, and autonomic responses (changes in vital signs).

Physical mobility, impaired may be related to neuromuscular/skeletal impairment, pain/discomfort, restrictive therapies (bed rest, extremity immobilization), and psychological immobility, possibly evidenced by inability to purposefully move within the physical environment, imposed restrictions, reluctance to attempt movement, limited range of motion, and decreased muscle strength/control.

Gas exchange, impaired, risk for: risk factors may include altered blood flow, blood/fat emboli, alveolar/capillary membrane changes (interstitial/pulmonary edema, congestion).

Knowledge deficit [learning need] regarding healing process, therapy requirements, and potential complications may be related to lack of exposure, misinterpretation of information, possibly evidenced by statements of concern, questions, and misconceptions.

**frostbite**

Tissue integrity, impaired may be related to altered circulation and thermal injury, possibly evidenced by damaged/destroyed tissue.

Pain, [acute] may be related to diminished circulation with tissue ischemia/necrosis and edema formation, possibly evidenced by reports, guarding/distraction behaviors, narrowed focus, and autonomic responses (changes in vital signs).

Infection, risk for: risk factors may include traumatized tissue/tissue destruction and compromised immune response in affected area.

**gallstone**

Refer to *cholelithiasis*.

**gangrene, dry**

Tissue perfusion, altered, peripheral may be related to interruption in arterial flow, possibly evidenced by cool skin temperature, change in color (black), atrophy of affected part, and presence of pain.

Pain, [acute] may be related to tissue hypoxia and necrotic process, possibly evidenced by reports, guarding/distraction behaviors, narrowed focus, and autonomic responses (changes in vital signs).

**gas, lung irritant**

Airway clearance, ineffective may be related to irritation/inflammation of airway, possibly evidenced by marked cough, abnormal breath sounds (wheezes), dyspnea, and tachypnea.

Gas exchange, impaired, risk for: risk factors may include irritation/inflammation of alveolar membrane (dependent on type of agent and length of exposure).

Anxiety [specify level] may be related to change in health status and threat of death, possibly evidenced by verbalizations, increased tension, apprehension, and sympathetic stimulation.

**gastritis, acute**

Pain [acute] may be related to irritation/inflammation of gastric mucosa, possibly evidenced by reports, guarding/distraction behaviors, and autonomic responses (changes in vital signs).

Fluid volume deficit, risk for: risk factors may include excessive losses through vomiting and diarrhea, continued bleeding, or reluctance to ingest/restrictions of oral intake.

**gastritis, chronic**

Nutrition: altered, less than body requirements, risk for: risk factors may include inability to ingest adequate nutrients (prolonged nausea/vomiting, anorexia, epigastric pain).

Knowledge deficit [learning need] regarding pathophysiology, psychologic factors, therapy needs, and potential complications may be related to lack of information/misinterpretation, possibly evidenced by verbalization of concerns, questions, misconceptions, and continuation of problem.

**gastroenteritis**

Refer to *gastritis, chronic*.

**gender identity disorder**

Anxiety [specify level] may be related to unconscious/conscious conflicts about essential values/beliefs (ego-dystonic gender identification), threat to self-concept, and unmet needs, possibly evidenced by increased tension, helplessness, hopelessness, feelings of inadequacy, uncertainty, insomnia, focus on self, and impaired daily functioning.

Role performance, altered/Personal identity disturbance may be related to crisis in development in which person has difficulty knowing to which sex he or she belongs; sense of discomfort and inappropriateness about anatomic sex characteristics, possibly evidenced by confusion about sense of self, purpose or direction in life, sexual identification/preference, verbalization of desire to be/insistence that person is the opposite sex, change in self-perception of role, and conflict in roles.

Sexuality patterns, altered may be related to ineffective or absent role models and conflict with sexual orientation and/or preferences, possibly evidenced by verbalizations of discomfort with sexual orientation and lack of information about human sexuality.

Family coping, ineffective: compromised/disabling, risk for: risk factors may include inadequate/incorrect information or understanding, temporary family disorganization and role changes, and patient providing little support in turn for primary person.

Family coping, potential for growth may be related to fact that individual's basic needs are sufficiently gratified and adaptive tasks effectively addressed to enable goals of self-actualization to surface, possibly evidenced by family member(s) attempt(s) to describe growth/impact of crisis on own values, priorities, goals, or relationships; family member(s) is/are moving in direction of health-promotion and enriching lifestyle that supports patient's search for self; and choosing experiences that optimize wellness.

**glaucoma**

Sensory/perceptual alterations, visual may be related to altered sensory reception and altered status of sense organ (increased intraocular pressure/atrophy of optic nerve head), possibly evidenced by progressive loss of visual field.

Anxiety [specify level] may be related to change in health status, presence of pain, possibility/reality of loss of vision, unmet needs, and negative self-talk, possibly evidenced by apprehension, uncertainty, and expressed concern regarding changes in life event.

**glomerulonephritis**

Fluid volume excess may be related to failure of regulatory mechanism (inflammation of glomerular membrane inhibiting filtration), possibly evidenced by weight gain, edema/anasarca, intake greater than output, and blood pressure changes.

Pain, [acute] may be related to effects of circulating toxins and edema/distension of renal capsule, possibly evidenced by reports, guarding/distraction behaviors, and autonomic responses (changes in vital signs).

Nutrition, altered, less than body requirements may be related to anorexia and dietary restrictions, possibly evidenced by aversion to eating, reported altered taste, weight loss, and decreased intake.

Diversional activity deficit may be related to treatment modality/restrictions, fatigue, and malaise, possibly evidenced by statements of boredom, restlessness, and irritability.

**gonorrhea** (also refer to *sexually transmitted disease*)

Infection, risk for dissemination/bacteremia: risk factors may include presence of infectious process in highly vascular area and lack of recognition of disease process.

Pain, [acute] may be related to irritation/inflammation of mucosa and effects of circulating toxins, possibly evidenced by verbal reports of genital or pharyngeal irritation, perineal/pelvic pain, or guarding/distraction behaviors.

Knowledge deficit [learning need] regarding disease cause/transmission, therapy, and self-care needs may be related to lack of information/misinterpretation, denial of exposure, possibly evidenced by statements of concern, questions, misconceptions, and inaccurate follow-through of instructions/development of preventable complications.

**gout**

Pain, [acute] may be related to inflammation of joint(s), possibly evidenced by verbal reports, guarding/distraction behaviors, and autonomic responses (changes in vital signs).

Physical mobility, impaired may be related to joint pain/edema, possibly evidenced by reluctance to attempt movement, limited range of motion, and therapeutic restriction of movement.

Knowledge deficit [learning need] regarding cause, treatment, and prevention of condition may be related to lack of information/misinterpretation, possibly evidenced by statements of concern, questions, misconceptions, and inaccurate follow-through of instructions.

**Guillain-Barré syndrome** (acute polyneuritis)

Breathing pattern/Airway clearance, ineffective, risk for: risk factors may include weakness/paralysis of respiratory muscles, impaired gag/swallow reflexes, decreased energy/fatigue.

Sensory/Perceptual alterations (specify) may be related to altered sensory reception/transmission/integration (altered status of sense organs, sleep deprivation), therapeutically restricted environment, endogenous chemical alterations (electrolyte imbalance, hypoxia), and psychologic stress, possibly evidenced by reported or observed change in usual response to stimuli, altered communication patterns, and measured change in sensory acuity and motor coordination.

Physical mobility, impaired may be related to neuromuscular impairment, pain/discomfort, possibly evidenced by impaired coordination, partial/complete paralysis, decreased muscle strength/control.

Anxiety [specify level]/Fear may be related to situational crisis, change in health status/threat of death, possibly evidenced by increased tension, restlessness, helplessness, apprehension, uncertainty, fearfulness, focus on self, and sympathetic stimulation.

Disuse syndrome, risk for: risk factors include paralysis and pain.

**hay fever**

Pain, [discomfort] may be related to irritation/inflammation of upper airway mucous membranes and conjunctiva, possibly evidenced by reports, irritability, and restlessness.

Knowledge deficit [learning need] regarding underlying cause, appropriate therapy, and required lifestyle changes may be related to lack of information, possibly evidenced by statements of concern, questions, and misconceptions.

**heatstroke**

Hyperthermia may be related to prolonged exposure to hot environment/vigorous activity with failure of regulating mechanism of the body, possibly evidenced by high body temperature (above 105°F/40.6°C), flushed/hot skin, tachycardia, and seizure activity.

Cardiac output, decreased may be related to functional stress of hypermetabolic state, altered circulating volume/venous return, and direct myocardial damage secondary to hyperthermia, possibly evidenced by decreased peripheral pulses, dysrhythmias/tachycardia, and changes in mentation.

**hemodialysis** (also refer to *dialysis, general*)

Injury, risk for loss of vascular access: risk factors may include clotting/thrombosis, infection, or disconnection/hemorrhage.

Fluid volume deficit, risk for: risk factors may include excessive fluid losses/shifts via ultrafiltration, hemorrhage (altered coagulation/disconnection of shunt), and fluid restrictions.

Fluid volume excess, risk for: risk factors may include excessive fluid intake, rapid IV, blood/plasma expanders/saline to support BP during procedure.

**hemophilia**

Fluid volume deficit, risk for: risk factors may include impaired coagulation/hemorrhagic losses.

Pain, [acute/chronic], risk for: risk factors may include nerve compression from hematomas, nerve damage, or hemorrhage into joint space.

Physical mobility, impaired, risk for: risk factors may include joint hemorrhage, swelling, degenerative changes, and muscle atrophy.

Family coping, ineffective: compromised may be related to prolonged nature of condition that exhausts the supportive capacity of significant people, possibly evidenced by protective behaviors disproportionate to patient's abilities/need for autonomy.

**hemorrhoidectomy**

Pain, [acute] may be related to edema/swelling and tissue trauma, possibly evidenced by verbal reports, guarding/distraction behaviors, focus on self, and autonomic responses (changes in vital signs).

Urinary retention, risk for: risk factors may include perineal trauma, edema/swelling, and pain.

Knowledge deficit [learning need] regarding therapeutic treatment and potential complications may be related to lack of information/misconceptions, possibly evidenced by statements of concern and questions.

**hemorrhoids**

Pain, [acute] may be related to inflammation and edema of prolapsed varices, possibly evidenced by verbal reports, and guarding/distraction behaviors.

Constipation may be related to pain on defecation and reluctance to defecate, possibly evidenced by frequency less than usual pattern and hard, formed stools.

**hemothorax** (also refer to *pneumothorax*)

Trauma/Suffocation, risk for: risk factors may include concurrent disease/injury process, dependence on external device (chest drainage system), and lack of safety education/precautions.

Anxiety [specify level] may be related to change in health status and threat of death, possibly evidenced by increased tension, restlessness, expressed concern, sympathetic stimulation, and focus on self.

**hepatitis, acute viral**

Fatigue may be related to decreased metabolic energy production and altered body chemistry, possibly evidenced by reports of lack of energy/inability to maintain usual routines, decreased performance, and increased physical complaints.

Nutrition, altered, less than body requirements may be related to inability to ingest adequate nutrients (nausea, vomiting, anorexia), hypermetabolic state, altered absorption and metabolism, possibly evidenced by aversion to eating/lack of interest in food, observed lack of intake, and weight loss.

Pain, [acute] may be related to inflammation and swelling of the liver, arthralgias, urticarial eruptions, and pruritus, possibly evidenced by verbal reports, guarding/distraction behavior, focus on self, and autonomic responses (changes in vital signs).

Home maintenance management, impaired, risk for: risk factors may include debilitating effects of disease process and inadequate support systems (family, financial, role model).

Knowledge deficit [learning need] regarding disease process/transmission, treatment needs, and future expectations may be related to lack of information/recall, misinterpretation, unfamiliarity with resources, possibly evidenced by questions, statement of concerns/misconceptions, inaccurate follow-through of instructions, and development of preventable complications.

**hernia, hiatal**

Pain, chronic may be related to regurgitation of acidic gastric contents, possibly evidenced by verbal reports, facial grimacing, and focus on self.

Knowledge deficit [learning need] regarding pathophysiology and prevention of complications may be related to lack of information/misconceptions, possibly evidenced by statements of concern, questions, and recurrence of condition.

**herniation of nucleus pulposus** (ruptured intervertebral disk)

Pain, [acute/chronic] may be related to nerve compression/irritation and muscle spasms, possibly evidenced by verbal reports, guarding/distraction behaviors, preoccupation with pain, self/narrowed focus, and autonomic responses (changes in vital signs when pain is acute), altered muscle tone/function, changes in eating/sleeping patterns and libido, physical/social withdrawal.

Physical mobility, impaired may be related to pain (muscle spasms), therapeutic restrictions (e.g., bedrest, traction/braces), muscular impairment, and depression, possibly evidenced by reports of pain on movement, reluctance to attempt/difficulty with purposeful movement, decreased muscle strength, impaired coordination, and limited range of motion.

Diversional activity deficit may be related to length of recuperation period and therapy restrictions, physical limitations, pain and depression, possibly evidenced by statements of boredom, disinterest, "nothing to do," restlessness, irritability, withdrawal.

**herpes, herpes simplex**

Pain, [acute] may be related to presence of localized inflammation and open lesions, possibly evidenced by verbal reports, distraction behaviors, and restlessness.

Infection, risk for secondary infection: risk factors may include broken/traumatized tissue, altered immune response, and untreated infection/treatment failure.

Sexuality patterns, altered, risk for: risk factors may include lack of knowledge, values conflict, and/or fear of transmitting the disease.

**herpes zoster**

Pain, [acute] may be related to inflammation/local lesions along sensory nerve(s), possibly evidenced by verbal reports, guarding/distraction behaviors, narrowed focus, and autonomic responses (changes in vital signs).

Knowledge deficit [learning need] regarding pathophysiology, therapeutic needs, and potential complications may be related to lack of information/misinterpretation, possibly evidenced by statements of concern, questions, and misconceptions.

**HIV positive** (also refer to *AIDS*)

Adjustment, impaired may be related to life-threatening and stigmatizing condition/disease, assault to self-esteem, altered locus of control, inadequate support systems, incomplete grieving, medication side effects (fatigue/depression), possibly evidenced by verbalization of nonacceptance/denial of diagnosis, nonexistent or unsuccessful involvement in problem solving/goal setting, extended period of shock and disbelief or anger, lack of future-oriented thinking.

Knowledge deficit [learning need] regarding disease, prognosis, and treatment needs may be related to lack of exposure/recall, information misinterpretation, unfamiliarity with information resources, or cognitive limitation, possibly evidenced by statement of misconception/request for information, inappropriate/exaggerated behaviors (hostile, agitated, hysterical, apathetic), inaccurate follow-through of instructions/development of preventable complications.

**Hodgkin's disease** (also refer to *cancer; chemotherapy*)

Anxiety [specify level]/Fear may be related to threat to self-concept and threat of death, possibly evidenced by apprehension, insomnia, focus on self, and increased tension.

Knowledge deficit [learning need] regarding diagnosis, pathophysiology, treatment, and prognosis may be related to lack of information/misinterpretation, possibly evidenced by statements of concern, questions, and misconceptions.

Pain, [acute/discomfort] may be related to manifestations of inflammatory response (fever, chills, night sweats) and pruritus, possibly evidenced by verbal reports, distraction behaviors, and focus on self.

Breathing pattern/Airway clearance, ineffective, risk for: risk factors may include tracheobronchial obstruction (enlarged mediastinal nodes and/or airway edema).

**hydrocephalus**

Tissue perfusion, altered: cerebral may be related to decreased arterial/venous blood flow (compression of brain tissue), possibly evidenced by changes in mentation, restlessness, irritability, reports of headache, pupillary changes, and changes in vital signs.

Sensory-perceptual alterations: visual may be related to pressure on sensory/motor nerves, possibly evidenced by reports of double vision, development of strabismus, nystagmus, pupillary changes, and optic atrophy.

Physical mobility, impaired, risk for: risk factors may include neuromuscular impairment, decreased muscle strength, and impaired coordination.

Infection, risk for: risk factors may include invasive procedure/presence of shunt.

Knowledge deficit [learning need] regarding condition, prognosis, and long-term therapy needs/medical follow-up may be related to lack of information/misperceptions, possibly evidenced by questions, statement of concern, request for information, and inaccurate follow-through of instruction/development of preventable complications.

**hyperbilirubinemia**

Injury, risk for CNS involvement: risk factors may include prematurity, hemolytic disease, asphyxia, acidosis, hyponatremia, and hypoglycemia.

Injury, risk for effects of treatment: risk factors may include physical properties of phototherapy and effects on body regulatory mechanisms, invasive procedure (exchange transfusion), abnormal blood profile, or chemical imbalances.

Knowledge deficit [learning need] regarding condition, prognosis, treatment/safety needs may be related to lack of exposure/recall and information misinterpretation, possibly evidenced by questions, statement of concern, and inaccurate follow-through of instructions/development of preventable complications.

**hyperemesis gravidarum**

Fluid volume deficit [active loss] may be related to excessive gastric losses and reduced intake, possibly evidenced by dry mucous membranes, decreased/concentrated urine, decreased pulse volume and pressure, thirst, and hemoconcentration.

Nutrition: altered, less than body requirements may be related to inability to ingest/digest/absorb nutrients (prolonged vomiting), possibly evidenced by reported inadequate food intake, lack of interest in food/aversion to eating, and weight loss.

Coping, individual, ineffective, risk for: risk factors may include situational/maturational crisis (pregnancy, change in health status, projected role changes, concern about outcome).

**hypertension**

Knowledge deficit [learning need] regarding condition, therapeutic regimen, and potential complications may be related to lack of information/recall, misinterpretation, cognitive limitations, and/or denial of diagnosis, possibly evidenced by statements of concern or questions and misconceptions, inaccurate follow-through of instructions, and lack of blood pressure control.

Adjustment, impaired may be related to condition requiring change in lifestyle, altered locus of control, and absence of feelings/denial of illness, possibly evidenced by verbalization of nonacceptance of health status change and lack of movement toward independence.

Sexual dysfunction, risk for: risk factors may include side effects of medication.

Cardiac output, decreased, risk for: risk factors may include increased afterload (vasoconstriction) myocardial ischemia, ventricular hypertrophy/rigidity.

Pain, [acute] may be related to increased cerebral vascular pressure, possibly evidenced by verbal reports of throbbing pain located in suboccipital region, present on awakening and disappearing spontaneously after being up and about; reluctance to move head; avoidance of bright lights and noise; or increased muscle tension.

**hyperthyroidism** (also refer to *thyrotoxicosis*)

Fatigue may be related to hypermetabolic imbalance with increased energy requirements, irritability of central nervous system, and altered body chemistry, possibly evidenced by verbalization of overwhelming lack of energy to maintain usual routine, decreased performance, emotional lability/irritability, and impaired ability to concentrate.

Anxiety [specify level] may be related to increased stimulation of the central nervous system (hypermetabolic state, pseudocatecholamine effect of thyroid hormones), possibly evidenced by increased feelings of apprehension, overexcited/distressed, irritability/emotional lability, shakiness, restless movements, or tremors.

Nutrition: altered, risk for less than body requirements: risk factors may include inability to ingest adequate nutrients for hypermetabolic rate/constant activity, impaired absorption of nutrients (vomiting/diarrhea), hyperglycemia, or relative insulin insufficiency.

Tissue integrity, impaired, risk for: risk factors may include altered protective mechanisms of eye related to periorbital edema, reduced ability to blink, eye discomfort/dryness and development of corneal abrasion/ulceration.

**hypoglycemia**

Thought processes, altered may be related to inadequate glucose for cellular brain function and effects of endogenous hormone activity, possibly evidenced by irritability, changes in mentation, memory loss, altered attention span, and emotional lability.

Nutrition, altered, risk for less than body requirements: risk factors may include inadequate glucose metabolism and imbalance of glucose/insulin levels.

Knowledge deficit [learning need] regarding pathophysiology of condition and therapy/self-care needs may be related to lack of information/recall, misinterpretations, possibly evidenced by development of hypoglycemia and statements of questions/misconceptions.

**hypoparathyroidism** (acute)

Injury, risk for: risk factors may include neuromuscular excitability/tetany and formation of renal stones.

Pain, [acute] may be related to recurrent muscle spasms and alteration in reflexes, possibly evidenced by verbal reports, distraction behaviors, and narrowed focus.

Airway clearance, ineffective, risk for: risk factors may include spasm of the laryngeal muscles.

**hypothermia** (systemic) (also refer to *frostbite*)

Hypothermia may be related to exposure to cold environment, inadequate clothing, age extremes (very young/elderly), damage to hypothalamus, consumption of alcohol/medications causing vasodilation, possibly evidenced by reduction in body temperature below normal range, shivering, cool skin, or pallor.

Knowledge deficit [learning need] regarding risk factors, treatment needs, and prognosis may be related to lack of information/recall, misinterpretation, possibly evidenced by statement of concerns/misconceptions, occurrence of problem, and development of complications.

**hypothyroidism**

Physical mobility, impaired may be related to weakness, fatigue, muscle aches, altered reflexes, and mucin deposits in joints and interstitial spaces, possibly evidenced by decreased muscle strength/control and impaired coordination.

Fatigue may be related to decreased metabolic energy production, possibly evidenced by verbalization of unremitting/overwhelming lack of energy, inability to maintain usual routines, impaired ability to concentrate, decreased libido, irritability, listlessness, decreased performance, increase in physical complaints.

Sensory-perceptual alterations (specify) may be related to mucin deposits and nerve compression, possibly evidenced by paresthesias of hands and feet or decreased hearing.

Constipation may be related to decreased peristalsis/physical activity, possibly evidenced by frequency less than usual pattern; decreased bowel sounds; hard, dry stool; and development of fecal impaction.

**hysterectomy**

Pain, [acute] may be related to tissue trauma/abdominal incision, edema/hematoma formation, possibly evidenced by verbal reports, guarding/distraction behaviors, and autonomic responses (changes in vital signs).

Urinary elimination, altered/Urinary retention, acute, risk for: risk factors may include mechanical trauma, surgical manipulation, presence of localized edema/hematoma, or nerve trauma with temporary bladder atony.

Sexuality patterns, altered/Sexual dysfunction, risk for: risk factors may include concerns regarding altered body function/structure, changes in hormone levels, loss of libido, and changes in sexual response pattern.

**ileocolitis**

Refer to *colitis, ulcerative*.

**ileostomy**

Refer to *colostomy*.

**ileus**

Pain, [acute] may be related to distension/edema and ischemia of intestinal tissue, possibly evidenced by verbal reports, guarding/distraction behaviors, narrowed focus, and autonomic responses (changes in vital signs).

Diarrhea/Constipation may be related to presence of obstruction/changes in peristalsis, possibly evidenced by changes in frequency and consistency or absence of stool, alterations in bowel sounds, presence of pain, and cramping.

Fluid volume deficit, risk for: risk factors may include increased intestinal losses (vomiting and diarrhea), and decreased intake.

**impetigo**

Skin integrity, impaired may be related to presence of infectious process and pruritus, possibly evidenced by open/crusted lesions.

Pain, [acute] may be related to inflammation and pruritus, possibly evidenced by verbal reports, distraction behaviors, and self-focusing.

Infection, risk for secondary infection: risk factors may include broken skin, traumatized tissue, altered immune response, and virulence/contagious nature of causative organism.

Infection, risk for transmission: risk factors may include virulent nature of causative organism, insufficient knowledge to prevent infection of others.

**influenza**

Pain, [discomfort] may be related to inflammation and effects of circulating toxins, possibly evidenced by verbal reports, distraction behaviors, and narrowed focus.

Fluid volume deficit, risk for: risk factors may include excessive gastric losses, hypermetabolic state, and altered intake.

Hyperthermia may be related to effects of circulating toxins and dehydration, possibly evidenced by increased body temperature, warm/flushed skin, and tachycardia.

**insulin shock**

Refer to *hypoglycemia*.

**intestinal obstruction**

Refer to *ileus*.

**Kawasaki disease**

Hyperthermia may be related to increased metabolic rate and dehydration, possibly evidenced by increased body temperature greater than normal range, flushed skin, increased respiratory rate, and tachycardia.

Pain, [acute] may be related to inflammation and edema/swelling of tissues, possibly evidenced by verbal reports, restlessness, guarding behavior, and narrowed focus.

Skin integrity, impaired may be related to inflammatory process, altered circulation, and edema formation, possibly evidenced by disruption of skin surface including macular rash and desquamation.

Oral mucous membranes, altered may be related to inflammatory process, dehydration, and mouth breathing, possibly evidenced by pain, hyperemia, and fissures of lips.

Cardiac output, decreased, risk for: risk factors may include structural changes/inflammation of coronary arteries and alterations in rate/rhythm or conduction.

**labor, induced/augmented**

Knowledge deficit [learning need] regarding procedure, treatment needs, and possible complications may be related to lack of exposure/recall, information misinterpretation, and unfamiliarity with information resources, possibly evidenced by questions, statement of concern/misconception, and exaggerated behaviors.

Injury, risk for maternal: risk factors may include adverse effects/response to therapeutic interventions.

Gas exchange, impaired, risk for fetal: risk factors may include altered placental perfusion/cord prolapse.

Pain, [acute] may be related to altered characteristics of chemically stimulated contractions, psychologic concerns, possibly evidenced by verbal reports, increased muscle tone, distraction/guarding behaviors, and narrowed focus.

**labor, preterm**

Activity intolerance may be related to muscle/cellular hypersensitivity, possibly evidenced by continued uterine contractions/irritability.

Poisoning, risk for: risk factors may include dose-related toxic/side effects of tocolytics.

Injury, risk for fetal: risk factors may include delivery of premature/immature infant.

Anxiety [specify level] may be related to situational crisis, perceived or actual threats to self/fetus and inadequate time to prepare for labor, possibly evidenced by increased tension, restlessness, expressions of concern, and autonomic responses (changes in vital signs).

Knowledge deficit [learning need] regarding preterm labor treatment needs and prognosis may be related to lack of information and misinterpretation, possibly evidenced by questions, statement of concern, misconceptions, inaccurate follow-through of instruction, and development of preventable complications.

**labor, stage I** (active phase)

Pain, [acute/discomfort] may be related to contraction-related hypoxia, dilation of tissues, and pressure on adjacent structures combined with stimulation of both parasympathetic and sympathetic nerve endings, possibly evidenced by verbal reports, distraction/guarding behaviors (restlessness), muscle tension, and narrowed focus.

Urinary elimination, altered may be related to altered intake/dehydration, hormonal changes, hemorrhage, severe intrapartal hypertension, mechanical compression of bladder, and effects of regional anesthesia, possibly evidenced by changes in amount/frequency of voiding, urinary retention, slowed progression of labor, and reduced sensation.

Coping, individual/couple, ineffective, risk for: risk factors may include stressors accompanying labor, personal vulnerability, use of ineffective coping mechanisms, inadequate support systems, and pain.

Self-esteem disturbance, risk for: risk factors may include use of medications to relieve intense contractions and inability to carry out wish for an unmedicated childbirth.

**labor, stage II** (expulsion)

Pain, [acute] may be related to strong uterine contractions, tissue stretching/dilation and compression of nerves by presenting part of the fetus, and bladder distention, possibly evidenced by verbal reports, facial grimacing, distraction/guarding behaviors (restlessness), narrowed focus, and autonomic responses (diaphoresis).

Cardiac output, altered [fluctuation] may be related to repeated, prolonged Valsalva's maneuvers, effects of anesthesia/medications, dorsal recumbent position occluding the inferior vena cava and partially obstructing the aorta (fluctuations in venous return), changes in systemic vascular resistance, possibly evidenced by decreased venous return, changes in vital signs (blood pressure, pulse), urinary output, or fetal bradycardia.

Gas exchange, impaired fetal, risk for: risk factors may include mechanical compression of head/cord (causing bradycardia and hypoxia), maternal position/prolonged labor affecting placental perfusion, and effects of maternal anesthesia.

Skin/Tissue integrity, impaired, risk for: risk factors may include untoward stretching/lacerations of delicate tissues (precipitous labor, hypertonic contractile pattern, adolescence, large fetus) and application of forceps.

Fatigue, risk for: risk factors may include increased energy requirements, overwhelming psychologic/emotional demands, or presence of pain.

**laminectomy** (lumbar)

Peripheral/[spinal nerve root] neurovascular dysfunction, risk for: risk factors may include orthopedic surgery, tissue trauma, mechanical compression (dressing, edema/hematoma formation).

Trauma, risk for, spinal: risk factors may include temporary weakness of spinal column, balancing difficulties, and changes in muscle tone/coordination.

Pain, [acute] may be related to traumatized tissues, localized inflammation, and edema, possibly evidenced by alteration in muscle tone, verbal reports, and distraction/guarding behaviors.

Physical mobility, impaired may be related to imposed medical restrictions, neuromuscular impairment, and pain, possibly evidenced by limited range of motion, decreased muscle strength/control, impaired coordination, and reluctance to attempt movement.

Urinary retention, risk for: risk factors may include pain and swelling in operative area and reduced mobility/restrictions of position.

**laryngectomy** (also refer to *cancer*; *chemotherapy*)

Airway clearance, ineffective may be related to partial/total removal of the glottis, temporary or permanent change to neck breathing, edema formation, and copious/thick secretions, possibly evidenced by dyspnea/difficulty breathing, changes in rate/depth of respiration, use of accessory respiratory muscles, weak/ineffective cough, abnormal breath sounds, and cyanosis.

Communication, impaired verbal may be related to anatomic deficit (removal of vocal cords), physical barrier (tracheostomy tube), and required voice rest, possibly evidenced by inability to speak, change in vocal characteristics, and impaired articulation.

Skin/Tissue integrity, impaired may be related to surgical removal of tissues/grafting, effects of radiation or chemotherapeutic agents, altered circulation/reduced blood supply, compromised nutritional status, edema formation, and pooling/continuous drainage of secretions, possibly evidenced by disruption of skin/tissue surface and destruction of skin/tissue layers.

Oral mucous membranes, altered may be related to dehydration/absence of oral intake, poor/inadequate oral hygiene, pathologic condition (oral cancer), mechanical trauma (oral surgery), decreased saliva production, difficulty swallowing and pooling/drooling of secretions, and nutritional deficits, possibly evidenced by xerostomia (dry mouth), oral discomfort, thick/mucoid saliva, decreased saliva production, dry and crusted/coated tongue, inflamed lips, absent teeth/gums, poor dental health, and halitosis.

**laryngitis**

Refer to *croup*.

**lead poisoning, acute** (also refer to *lead poisoning, chronic*)

Trauma, risk for: risk factors may include loss of coordination, altered level of consciousness, clonic or tonic muscle activity, neurologic damage.

Fluid volume deficit, risk for: risk factors may include excessive vomiting, diarrhea, or decreased intake.

Knowledge deficit [learning need] regarding sources of lead and prevention of poisoning may be related to lack of information/misinterpretation, possibly evidenced by statements of concern, questions, and misconceptions.

**lead poisoning, chronic (also refer to *lead poisoning, acute*)**

Nutrition, altered, less than body requirements may be related to decreased intake (chemically induced changes in the gastrointestinal tract), possibly evidenced by anorexia, abdominal discomfort, reported metallic taste, and weight loss.

Thought processes, altered may be related to deposition of lead in central nervous system and brain tissue, possibly evidenced by personality changes, learning disabilities, and impaired ability to conceptualize and reason.

Pain, chronic may be related to deposition of lead in soft tissues and bone, possibly evidenced by verbal reports, distraction behaviors, and focus on self.

**leukemia, acute** (also refer to *chemotherapy*)

Infection, risk for: risk factors may include inadequate secondary defenses (alterations in mature white blood cells, increased number of immature lymphocytes, immunosuppression and bone marrow suppression), invasive procedures, and malnutrition.

Anxiety [specify level]/Fear may be related to change in health status, threat of death, and situational crisis, possibly evidenced by sympathetic stimulation, apprehension, feelings of helplessness, focus on self, and insomnia.
Activity intolerance may be related to reduced energy stores, increased metabolic rate, imbalance between oxygen supply and demand, or therapeutic restrictions (bedrest)/effect of drug therapy, possibly evidenced by generalized weakness, reports of fatigue, exertional dyspnea, and abnormal heart rate or blood pressure response.
Pain, [acute] may be related to physical agents (infiltration of tissues/organs/central nervous system, expanding bone marrow) and chemical agents (antileukemic agents), possibly evidenced by verbal reports (abdominal discomfort, arthralgia, bone pain, headache), distraction behaviors, narrowed focus, and autonomic responses (changes in vital signs).
Fluid volume deficit, risk for: risk factors may include excessive losses (vomiting, hemorrhage, diarrhea), decreased intake (nausea, anorexia), increased fluid need (hypermetabolic state/fever).

**long-term care**
Refer to *care, long-term.*

**lupus erythematosus, systemic**
Pain, [acute] may be related to widespread inflammatory process affecting connective tissues, blood vessels, serosal surfaces, and mucous membranes, possibly evidenced by multiple verbal reports, guarding/distraction behaviors, self-focusing, and autonomic responses (changes in vital signs).
Skin/Tissue integrity, impaired may be related to chronic inflammation, edema formation, and altered circulation, possibly evidenced by presence of skin rash/lesions, ulcerations of mucous membranes, and photosensitivity.
Fatigue may be related to increased energy requirements (chronic inflammation) and altered body chemistry (including effects of drug therapy), possibly evidenced by reports of overwhelming lack of energy/inability to maintain usual routines, decreased performance, lethargy, and malaise.
Body image disturbance may be related to presence of chronic condition with rash, lesions, ulcers, purpura, mottled erythema of hands, alopecia, loss of strength, and altered body function, possibly evidenced by hiding body parts, negative feelings about body, feelings of helplessness, and change in social involvement.

**Lyme disease**
Pain, [acute] may be related to systemic effects of toxins, presence of rash, urticaria, and joint swelling/inflammation, possibly evidenced by verbal reports, guarding behavior, autonomic responses, and narrowed focus.
Fatigue may be related to increased energy requirements, altered body chemistry, and states of discomfort, possibly evidenced by reports of overwhelming lack of energy/inability to maintain usual routines, decreased performance, lethargy, and malaise.
Cardiac output, decreased, risk for: risk factors may include alteration in rate/rhythm/conduction.

**Mallory-Weiss syndrome** (also refer to *achalasia*)
Fluid volume deficit, risk for: risk factors may include excessive vascular losses, presence of vomiting, and reduced intake.
Knowledge deficit [learning need] regarding causes, treatment, and prevention of condition may be related to lack of information/misinterpretation, possibly evidenced by statements of concern, questions, and recurrence of problem.

**mastectomy**
Skin/Tissue integrity, impaired may be related to surgical removal of skin/tissue, altered circulation, drainage, presence of edema, changes in skin elasticity/sensation, and tissue destruction (radiation), possibly evidenced by disruption of skin surface and destruction of skin layers/subcutaneous tissues.
Physical mobility, impaired may be related to neuromuscular impairment, pain, and edema formation, possibly evidenced by reluctance to attempt movement, limited range of motion, and decreased muscle mass/strength.

Self-care deficit, bathing/dressing may be related to temporary loss/altered action of one or both arms, possibly evidenced by statements of inability to perform/complete self-care tasks.

Body image disturbance may be related to loss of body part denoting femininity, possibly evidenced by not looking at/touching area, negative feelings about body, preoccupation with loss, and change in social involvement/relationship.

**mastitis**

Pain, [acute] may be related to erythema and edema of breast tissues, possibly evidenced by verbal reports, guarding/distraction behaviors, self-focusing, autonomic responses (changes in vital signs).

Infection, risk for spread/abscess formation: risk factors may include traumatized tissues, stasis of fluids, and insufficient knowledge to prevent complications.

Knowledge deficit [learning need] regarding pathophysiology, treatment, and prevention may be related to lack of information/misinterpretation, possibly evidenced by statements of concern, questions, and misconceptions.

**mastoidectomy**

Infection, risk for spread: risk factors may include pre-existing infection, surgical trauma, and stasis of body fluids in close proximity to brain.

Pain, [acute] may be related to inflammation, tissue trauma, and edema formation, possibly evidenced by verbal reports, distraction behaviors, restlessness, self-focusing, and autonomic responses (changes in vital signs).

Sensory/Perceptual alterations, auditory may be related to presence of surgical packing, edema, and surgical disturbance of middle ear structures, possibly evidenced by reported/tested hearing loss in affected ear.

**measles**

Pain, [acute] may be related to inflammation of mucous membranes, conjunctiva, and presence of extensive skin rash with pruritus, possibly evidenced by verbal reports, distraction behaviors, self-focusing, and autonomic responses (changes in vital signs).

Hyperthermia may be related to presence of viral toxins and inflammatory response, possibly evidenced by increased body temperature, flushed/warm skin, and tachycardia.

Infection, risk for, secondary: risk factors may include altered immune response and traumatized dermal tissues.

Knowledge deficit [learning need] regarding condition, transmission, and possible complications may be related to lack of information/misinterpretation, possibly evidenced by statements of concern, questions, misconceptions, and development of preventable complications.

**meningitis, acute meningococcal**

Infection, risk for spread: risk factors may include hematogenous dissemination of pathogen, stasis of body fluids, suppressed inflammatory response (medication-induced), and exposure of others to pathogens.

Tissue perfusion, altered, cerebral, risk for: risk factors may include cerebral edema altering/interrupting cerebral arterial/venous blood flow, hypovolemia, exchange problems at cellular level (acidosis).

Hyperthermia may be related to infectious process (increased metabolic rate) and dehydration, possibly evidenced by increased body temperature, warm/flushed skin, and tachycardia.

Pain, [acute] may be related to inflammation/irritation of the meninges with spasm of extensor muscles (neck, shoulders, and back), possibly evidenced by verbal reports, guarding/distraction behaviors, narrowed focus, and autonomic responses (changes in vital signs).

Trauma/Suffocation, risk for: risk factors may include alterations in level of consciousness, possible development of clonic/tonic muscle activity (seizures), and generalized weakness/prostration.

**meniscectomy**

Physical mobility, impaired may be related to pain, joint instability, and imposed medical restrictions of movement, possibly evidenced by decreased muscle strength/control, limited range of motion, and reluctance to attempt movement.

Knowledge deficit [learning need] regarding postoperative expectations, prevention of complications, and self-care needs may be related to lack of information, possibly evidenced by statements of concern, questions, and misconceptions.

**mental retardation** (also refer to *Down syndrome*)

Communication, impaired, verbal may be related to developmental delay/impairment of cognitive and motor abilities, possibly evidenced by impaired articulation, difficulty with phonation, and inability to modulate speech/find appropriate words (dependent on degree of retardation).

Self-care deficit (specify), risk for: risk factors may include impaired cognitive ability and motor skills.

Nutrition, altered, risk for more than body requirements: risk factors may include decreased metabolic rate coupled with impaired cognitive development, dysfunctional eating patterns, and sedentary level.

Social interaction, impaired may be related to impaired thought processes, communication barriers, and knowledge/skill deficit about ways to enhance mutuality, possibly evidenced by dysfunctional interactions with peers, family and/or significant other(s), and verbalized/observed discomfort in social situation.

Family coping, ineffective: compromised may be related to chronic nature of condition and degree of disability that exhausts supportive capacity of significant other(s), other situational or developmental crises or situations the significant other may be facing, or unrealistic expectations of significant other, possibly evidenced by preoccupation of significant other with personal reaction, significant other withdraws or enters into limited interaction with individual, protective behavior disproportionate (too much or too little) to patient's abilities or need for autonomy.

Home maintenance management, impaired may be related to impaired cognitive functioning, insufficient finances/family organization or planning, lack of knowledge, and inadequate support systems, possibly evidenced by requests for assistance, expression of difficulty in maintaining home, disorderly surroundings, and overtaxed family members.

Sexual dysfunction, risk for: risk factors may include biopsychosocial alteration of sexuality, ineffectual/absent role models, misinformation/lack of knowledge, lack of significant other(s), and lack of appropriate behavior control.

**mitral stenosis**

Activity intolerance may be related to imbalance between oxygen supply and demand, possibly evidenced by reports of fatigue, weakness, exertional dyspnea, and tachycardia.

Gas exchange, impaired may be related to altered blood flow, possibly evidenced by restlessness, hypoxia, and cyanosis (orthopnea/paroxysmal nocturnal dyspnea).

Knowledge deficit [learning need] regarding pathophysiology, therapeutic needs, and potential complications may be related to lack of information/recall, misinterpretation, possibly evidenced by statements of concern, questions, inaccurate follow-through of instructions, and development of preventable complications.

**mononucleosis, infectious**

Fatigue may be related to decreased energy production, states of discomfort, and increased energy requirements (inflammatory process), possibly evidenced by reports of overwhelming lack of energy, inability to maintain usual routines, lethargy, and malaise.

Pain, [discomfort] may be related to inflammation of lymphoid and organ tissues, irritation of oropharyngeal mucous membranes, and effects of circulating toxins, possibly evidenced by verbal reports, distraction behaviors, and self-focusing.

Hyperthermia may be related to inflammatory process, possibly evidenced by increased body temperature, warm/flushed skin, and tachycardia.

Knowledge deficit [learning need] regarding disease transmission, self-care needs, medical therapy, and potential complications may be related to lack of information/misinterpretation, possibly evidenced by statements of concern, misconceptions, and inaccurate follow-through of instructions.

**mood disorders**

Refer to *depressive disorders*.

**multiple personality**
Refer to *dissociative disorders*.

**multiple sclerosis**
Physical mobility, impaired may be related to neuromuscular and perceptual impairment, decreased strength/endurance, fatigue, pain/discomfort, depression, possibly evidenced by impaired coordination, decreased muscle control/mass, and altered ability to move purposefully or perform routine tasks.
Sensory-perceptual alterations, visual, kinesthetic, tactile may be related to delayed/interrupted neuronal transmission, possibly evidenced by impaired vision, diplopia, disturbance of vibratory or position sense, paresthesias, numbness, and blunting of sensation.
Thought processes, altered may be related to physiologic changes, involvement of pathways of emotional control, and depression, possibly evidenced by impaired judgment, emotional lability, and altered attention span.
Powerlessness/Hopelessness may be related to illness-related regimen and lifestyle of helplessness, possibly evidenced by verbal expressions of having no control or influence over the situation, depression over physical deterioration that occurs despite patient compliance with regimen, nonparticipation in care or decision making when opportunities are provided, passivity, or decreased verbalization/affect.
Home maintenance management, impaired may be related to effects of debilitating disease, impaired cognitive and/or emotional functioning, insufficient finances, and inadequate support systems, possibly evidenced by reported difficulty, observed disorderly surroundings, and poor hygienic conditions.
Family coping, ineffective: compromised/disabling may be related to temporary family disorganization and role changes, patient providing little support in turn for significant other(s), prolonged disease/disability progression that exhausts the supportive capacity of significant other(s), feelings of guilt, anxiety, hostility, despair, and highly ambivalent family relationships, possibly evidenced by patient expressing/confirming concern or report about significant other(s) response to patient's illness, significant other(s) preoccupied with own personal reactions, intolerance, abandonment, neglectful care of the patient, and distortion of reality regarding patient's illness.

**mumps**
Pain, [acute] may be related to presence of inflammation, circulating toxins, and enlargement of salivary glands, possibly evidenced by verbal reports, guarding/distraction behaviors, self-focusing, and autonomic responses (changes in vital signs).
Hyperthermia may be related to inflammatory process (increased metabolic rate), and dehydration, possibly evidenced by increased body temperature, warm/flushed skin, and tachycardia.
Fluid volume deficit, risk for: risk factors may include hypermetabolic state and painful swallowing with decreased intake.

**muscular dystrophy** (Duchenne's)
Refer to *Duchenne's muscular dystrophy*.

**myasthenia gravis**
Breathing pattern/Airway clearance, ineffective may be related to neuromuscular weakness and decreased energy/fatigue, possibly evidenced by dyspnea, changes in rate/depth of respiration, ineffective cough, and adventitious breath sounds.
Communication, impaired verbal may be related to neuromuscular weakness, fatigue, and physical barrier (intubation), possibly evidenced by facial weakness, impaired articulation, hoarseness, and inability to speak.
Swallowing, impaired may be related to neuromuscular impairment of laryngeal/pharyngeal muscles and muscular fatigue, possibly evidenced by reported/observed difficulty swallowing, coughing/choking, and evidence of aspiration.
Anxiety [specify level]/Fear may be related to situational crisis, threat to self-concept, change in health/socioeconomic status or role function, separation from support systems, lack of knowledge, and inability to communicate, possibly evidenced by expressed concerns, increased tension, restlessness, apprehension, sympathetic stimulation, crying, focus on self, uncooperative behavior, withdrawal, anger, and noncommunication.

Knowledge deficit [learning need] regarding drug therapy, potential for crisis (myasthenic or cholinergic) and self-care management may be related to inadequate information/ misinterpretation, possibly evidenced by statements of concern, questions, and misconceptions; development of preventable complications.

Physical mobility, impaired may be related to neuromuscular impairment, possibly evidenced by reports of progressive fatigability with repetitive/prolonged muscle use, impaired coordination, and decreased muscle strength/control.

Sensory-perceptual alterations, visual may be related to neuromuscular impairment, possibly evidenced by visual distortions (diplopia) and motor incoordination.

**myocardial infarction** (also refer to *myocarditis*)

Pain, [acute] may be related to ischemia of myocardial tissue, possibly evidenced by verbal reports, guarding/distraction behaviors (restlessness), facial mask of pain, self-focusing, and autonomic responses (diaphoresis, changes in vital signs).

Anxiety [specify level]/Fear may be related to threat of death, threat of change of health status/ role functioning and lifestyle or interpersonal transmission/contagion, possibly evidenced by increased tension, fearful attitude, apprehension, expressed concerns/ uncertainty, restlessness, sympathetic stimulation, and somatic complaints.

Cardiac output, decreased, risk for: risk factors may include changes in rate and electrical conduction, reduced preload, increased systemic vascular resistance, and altered muscle contractility/depressant effects of some medications.

**myocarditis**

Activity intolerance may be related to imbalance in oxygen supply and demand (myocardial inflammation/damage), cardiac depressant effects of certain drugs, and enforced bedrest, possibly evidenced by reports of fatigue, exertional dyspnea, tachycardia/palpitations in response to activity, ECG changes/dysrhythmias, and generalized weakness.

Cardiac output, decreased, risk for: risk factors may include degeneration of cardiac muscle.

Knowledge deficit [learning need] regarding pathophysiology of condition/outcomes, treatment, and self-care needs/lifestyle changes may be related to lack of information/misinterpretation, possibly evidenced by statements of concern, misconceptions, inaccurate follow-through of instructions, and development of preventable complications.

**myringotomy**

Refer to *mastoidectomy*.

**myxedema** (also refer to *hypothyroidism*)

Body image disturbance may be related to change in structure/function (loss of hair/thickening of skin, masklike facial expression, enlarged tongue, menstrual and reproductive disturbances), possibly evidenced by negative feelings about body, feelings of helplessness, and change in social involvement.

Nutrition, altered, more than body requirements may be related to decreased metabolic rate and activity level, possibly evidenced by weight gain greater than ideal for height and frame.

Cardiac output, decreased, risk for: risk factors may include altered electrical conduction and myocardial contractility.

**neonate, normal newborn**

Gas exchange, impaired, risk for: risk factors may include prenatal or intrapartal stressors, excess production of mucus, or cold stress.

Body temperature, altered, risk for: risk factors may include large body surface in relation to mass, limited amounts of insulating subcutaneous fat, nonrenewable sources of brown fat and few white fat stores, thin epidermis with close proximity of blood vessels to the skin, inability to shiver, and movement from a warm uterine environment to a much cooler environment.

Parent/Infant attachment, altered, risk for: risk factors may include developmental transition (gain of a family member); anxiety associated with the parent role, or lack of privacy.

Nutrition, altered, less than body requirements, risk for: risk factors may include rapid metabolic rate, high caloric requirement, increased insensible water losses through pulmonary and cutaneous routes, fatigue, and a potential for inadequate or depleted glucose stores.

Infection, risk for: risk factors may include inadequate secondary defenses (inadequate acquired immunity, e.g., deficiency of neutrophils and specific immunoglobulins) and inadequate primary defenses (e.g., environmental exposure, broken skin, traumatized tissues, decreased ciliary action).

**neonate, premature newborn**

**Gas exchange, impaired may be related to alveolar-capillary membrane changes (inadequate surfactant levels), altered blood flow (immaturity of pulmonary arteriole musculature), altered oxygen supply (immaturity of central nervous system and neuromuscular system, tracheobronchial obstruction), altered oxygen-carrying capacity of blood (anemia), and cold stress, possibly evidenced by respiratory difficulties, inadequate oxygenation of tissues, and acidemia.**

**Breathing pattern, ineffective may be related to immaturity of the respiratory center, poor positioning, drug-related depression, metabolic imbalances, or decreased energy/fatigue, possibly evidenced by dyspnea, tachypnea, periods of apnea, nasal flaring/use of accessory muscles, cyanosis, abnormal ABGs, or tachycardia.**

**Thermoregulation, ineffective, risk for: risk factors may include immature CNS development (temperature regulation center), decreased ratio of body mass to surface area, decreased subcutaneous fat, limited brown fat stores, inability to shiver or sweat, poor metabolic reserves, muted response to hypothermia, and frequent medical/nursing manipulations and interventions.**

**Fluid volume deficit, risk for: risk factors may include extremes of age and weight or excessive fluid losses (thin skin, lack of insulating fat, increased environmental temperature, immature kidney/failure to concentrate urine).**

**Infant behavior, disorganized, risk for: risk factors may include prematurity, lack of containment/boundaries, pain, or overstimulation.**

**nephrectomy**

**Pain, [acute] may be related to surgical tissue trauma with mechanical closure (suture), possibly evidenced by verbal reports, guarding/distraction behaviors, self-focusing, and autonomic responses (changes in vital signs).**

**Fluid volume deficit, risk for: risk factors may include excessive vascular losses and restricted intake.**

**Breathing pattern, ineffective may be related to incisional pain with decreased lung expansion, possibly evidenced by tachypnea, fremitus, changes in respiratory depth/chest expansion, and changes in ABGs.**

**Constipation may be related to reduced dietary intake, decreased mobility, gastrointestinal obstructions (paralytic ileus), and incisional pain with defecation, possibly evidenced by decreased bowel sounds, reduced frequency/amount of stool, and hard/formed stool.**

**nephrotic syndrome**

**Fluid volume excess may be related to compromised regulatory mechanism with changes in hydrostatic/oncotic vascular pressure and increased activation of the renin-angiotensin-aldosterone system, possibly evidenced by edema/anasarca, effusions/ascites, weight gain, intake greater than output, and blood pressure changes.**

**Nutrition, altered, less than body requirements may be related to excessive protein losses and inability to ingest adequate nutrients (anorexia), possibly evidenced by weight loss/muscle wasting (may be difficult to assess due to edema), lack of interest in food, and observed inadequate intake.**

Infection, risk for: risk factors may include chronic disease and steroidal suppression of inflammatory responses.

Skin integrity, impaired, risk for: risk factors may include presence of edema and activity restrictions.

**neuralgia, trigeminal**

Pain, [acute] may be related to neuromuscular impairment with sudden violent muscle spasm, possibly evidenced by verbal reports, guarding/distraction behaviors, self-focusing, and autonomic responses (changes in vital signs).

Knowledge deficit [learning need] regarding control of recurrent episodes, medical therapies, and self-care needs may be related to lack of information/recall and misinterpretation, possibly evidenced by statements of concern, questions, and exacerbation of condition.

**neuritis**

Pain, [acute]/chronic may be related to nerve damage usually associated with a degenerative process, possibly evidenced by verbal reports, guarding/distraction behaviors, self-focusing, and autonomic responses (changes in vital signs).

Knowledge deficit [learning need] regarding underlying causative factors, treatment, and prevention may be related to lack of information/misinterpretation, possibly evidenced by statements of concern, questions, and misconceptions.

**obesity**

Nutrition, altered, more than body requirements may be related to excessive intake in relation to metabolic needs, possibly evidenced by weight 20 percent greater than ideal for height and frame, sedentary activity level, reported/observed dysfunctional eating patterns, and excess body fat by triceps skinfold/other measurements.

Body image disturbance may be related to view of self in contrast with societal values, family/subculture encouragement of overeating; control, sex, and love issues; possibly evidenced by negative feelings about body, fear of rejection/reaction of others, feelings of hopelessness/powerlessness, and lack of follow-through with treatment plan.

Activity intolerance may be related to imbalance between oxygen supply and demand, and sedentary lifestyle, possibly evidenced by fatigue or weakness, exertional discomfort, and abnormal heart rate/blood pressure response.

Coping, individual, ineffective may be related to personal vulnerability, unmet expectations, and inadequate coping methods, possibly evidenced by verbalization of difficulty dealing with anxiety and tension, overeating, and eating in response to stress.

**osteoarthritis** (degenerative joint disease)

Refer to *arthritis, rheumatoid*.

(Although this is a degenerative process versus the inflammatory process of rheumatoid arthritis, nursing concerns are the same.)

**osteomyelitis**

Pain, [acute] may be related to inflammation and tissue necrosis, possibly evidenced by verbal reports, guarding/distraction behaviors, self-focus, and autonomic responses (changes in vital signs).

Hyperthermia may be related to increased metabolic rate and infectious process, possibly evidenced by increased body temperature and warm/flushed skin.

Tissue perfusion, altered, bone may be related to inflammatory reaction with thrombosis of vessels, destruction of tissue, edema, and abscess formation, possibly evidenced by bone necrosis, continuation of infectious process, and delayed healing.

Knowledge deficit [learning need] regarding pathophysiology of condition, long-term therapy needs, activity restriction, and prevention of complications may be related to lack of information/misinterpretation, possibly evidenced by statements of concern, questions and misconceptions, and inaccurate follow-through of instructions.

**osteoporosis**

Trauma, risk for: risk factors may include loss of bone integrity, increasing risk of fracture with minimal or no stress.

Pain, [acute]/chronic may be related to vertebral compression on spinal nerve/muscles/ligaments, spontaneous fractures, possibly evidenced by verbal reports, guarding/distraction behaviors, self-focus, and changes in sleep pattern.

Physical mobility, impaired may be related to pain and musculoskeletal impairment, possibly evidenced by limited range of motion, reluctance to attempt movement/expressed fear of reinjury, and imposed restrictions/limitations.

**palsy, cerebral** (spastic hemiplegia)

Physical mobility, impaired may be related to muscular weakness/hypertonicity, increased deep tendon reflexes, tendency to contractures, and underdevelopment of affected limbs, possibly evidenced by decreased muscle strength/control/mass, limited range of motion, and impaired coordination.

Family coping, ineffective: compromised may be related to permanent nature of condition, situational crisis, emotional conflicts/temporary family disorganization, and incomplete information/understanding of patient's needs, possibly evidenced by verbalized anxiety/guilt regarding patient's disability, inadequate understanding and knowledge base, and displaying protective behaviors disproportionate (too little/too much) to patient's abilities/need for autonomy.

Growth and development, altered may be related to effects of physical disability, possibly evidenced by altered physical growth, delay, or difficulty in performing skills (motor, social, expressive), and altered ability to perform self-care/self-control activities appropriate to age.

**pancreatitis**

Pain, [acute] may be related to obstruction of pancreatic/biliary ducts, chemical contamination of peritoneal surfaces by pancreatic exudate/autodigestion, extension of inflammation to the retroperitoneal nerve plexus, possibly evidenced by verbal reports, guarding/distraction behaviors, self-focus, grimacing, autonomic responses (changes in vital signs), and alteration in muscle tone.

Fluid volume deficit, risk for: risk factors may include excessive gastric losses (vomiting, nasogastric suctioning), increase in size of vascular bed (vasodilation, effects of kinins), third-space fluid transudation, ascites formation, alteration of clotting process, hemorrhage.

Nutrition, altered, less than body requirements may be related to vomiting, decreased oral intake as well as altered ability to digest nutrients (loss of digestive enzymes/insulin), possibly evidenced by reported inadequate food intake, aversion to eating, reported altered taste sensation, weight loss, and reduced muscle mass.

Infection, risk for: risk factors may include inadequate primary defenses (stasis of body fluids, altered peristalsis, change in pH secretions), immunosuppression, nutritional deficiencies, tissue destruction, and chronic disease.

**paranoid disorders**

Violence, risk for, directed at self/others: risk factors may include perceived threats of danger and increased feelings of anxiety.

Anxiety [severe] may be related to inability to trust (has not mastered tasks of trust versus mistrust), possibly evidenced by rigid delusional system (serves to provide relief from stress that justifies the delusion), frightened of other people and own hostility.

Powerlessness may be related to feelings of inadequacy, lifestyle of helplessness, maladaptive interpersonal interactions (e.g., misuse of power, force, abusive relationships), sense of severely impaired self-esteem, and belief that individual has no control over situation(s), possibly evidenced by use of paranoid delusions, use of aggressive behavior to compensate, and expressions of recognition of damage paranoia has caused self and others.

Thought processes, altered may be related to psychologic conflicts, increased anxiety, and fear, possibly evidenced by difficulties in the process and character of thought, interference with the ability to think clearly and logically, delusions, or fragmentation and autistic thinking.

Family coping, ineffective: compromised may be related to temporary or sustained family disorganization/role changes, prolonged progression of condition that exhausts the supportive capacity of significant other(s), possibly evidenced by family system not meeting physical/emotional/spiritual needs of its members, inability to express or to accept wide range of feelings, inappropriate boundary maintenance; significant other(s) describes preoccupation with personal reactions.

**paraplegia** (also refer to *quadriplegia*)

Physical mobility, impaired may be related to neuromuscular impairment (flaccid/spastic paralysis), possibly evidenced by loss of muscle control and coordination, muscle atrophy/contractures, and inability to move purposefully.

Sensory-perceptual alterations, kinesthetic and tactile may be related to neurologic deficit with loss of sensory reception and transmission, possibly evidenced by reported/measured change in sensory acuity and loss of usual response to stimuli.

Incontinence, reflex may be related to loss of nerve conduction above the level of the reflex arc, possibly evidenced by lack of awareness of bladder filling/fullness, absence of urge to void, and uninhibited bladder contraction.

Body image disturbance/Role performance, altered may be related to loss of body functions, change in physical ability to resume role, perceived loss of self/identity, possibly evidenced by negative feelings about body/self, feelings of helplessness/powerlessness, delay in taking responsibility for self-care/participation in therapy, and change in social involvement.

Sexual dysfunction may be related to loss of sensation, altered function, vulnerability, possibly evidenced by seeking of confirmation of desirability, verbalization of concern, and alteration in relationship with significant other, and change in interest in self/others.

**parathyroidectomy**

Pain, [acute] may be related to presence of surgical incision and effects of calcium imbalance (bone pain, tetany), possibly evidenced by verbal reports, guarding/distraction behaviors, self-focus, and autonomic responses (changes in vital signs).

Fluid volume excess, risk for: risk factors may include preoperative renal involvement, stress-induced release of ADH, and changing calcium/electrolyte levels.

Airway clearance, ineffective, risk for: risk factors may include edema formation and laryngeal nerve damage.

Knowledge deficit [learning need] regarding postoperative care/complications and long-term needs may be related to lack of information/recall, misinterpretation, possibly evidenced by statements of concern, questions, and misconceptions.

**Parkinson's disease**

Physical mobility, impaired may be related to neuromuscular impairment (muscle weakness, tremors, bradykinesia) and musculoskeletal impairment (joint rigidity), possibly evidenced by decreased muscle strength/control, impaired coordination, and limited range of motion.

Swallowing, impaired may be related to neuromuscular impairment/muscle weakness, possibly evidenced by reported/observed difficulty in swallowing, drooling, evidence of aspiration (choking, coughing).

Communication, impaired, verbal may be related to muscle weakness and incoordination, possibly evidenced by impaired articulation, difficulty with phonation, and changes in rhythm and intonation.

**pelvic inflammatory disease**

Infection, risk for spread: risk factors may include presence of infectious process in highly vascular pelvic structures or delay in seeking treatment.

Pain, [acute] may be related to inflammation, edema, and congestion of reproductive/pelvic tissues, possibly evidenced by verbal reports, guarding/distraction behaviors, self-focus, and autonomic responses (changes in vital signs).

Hyperthermia may be related to inflammatory process/hypermetabolic state, possibly evidenced by increased body temperature, warm/flushed skin, and tachycardia.

Knowledge deficit [learning need] regarding cause/complications of condition, therapy needs, and transmission of disease to others may be related to lack of information/misinterpretation, possibly evidenced by statements of concern, questions, misconceptions, and development of preventable complications.

**periarteritis nodosa**

Refer to *polyarteritis (nodosa)*.

**pericarditis**

Pain, [acute] may be related to inflammation and presence of effusion, possibly evidenced by verbal reports, guarding/distraction behaviors, self-focus, and autonomic responses (changes in vital signs).

Activity intolerance may be related to imbalance between oxygen supply and demand (restriction of cardiac filling/ventricular contraction, reduced cardiac output), possibly evidenced by reports of weakness/fatigue, exertional dyspnea, abnormal heart rate or blood pressure response, and signs of congestive heart failure.

Cardiac output, decreased, risk for: risk factors may include accumulation of fluid (effusion) restricting cardiac filling/contractility.

Anxiety [specify level] may be related to change in health status and perceived threat of death, possibly evidenced by increased tension, apprehension, restlessness, and expressed concerns.

**peripheral vascular disease** (atherosclerosis)

Tissue perfusion, altered, peripheral may be related to reductions or interruptions of arterial/venous blood flow, possibly evidenced by changes in skin temperature/color, lack of hair growth, blood pressure/pulse changes in extremity, presence of bruits, and reports of claudication.

Activity intolerance may be related to imbalance between oxygen supply and demand, possibly evidenced by reports of muscle fatigue/weakness and exertional discomfort (claudication).

Tissue integrity, impaired, risk for: risk factors may include altered circulation with decreased sensation and impaired healing.

**peritonitis**

Infection, risk for spread/septicemia: risk factors may include inadequate primary defenses (broken skin, traumatized tissue, altered peristalsis), inadequate secondary defenses (immunosuppression), and invasive procedures.

Fluid volume deficit [active loss] may be related to fluid shifts from extracellular, intravascular, and interstitial compartments into intestines and/or peritoneal space, excessive gastric losses (vomiting, diarrhea, nasogastric tube), hypermetabolic state, and restricted intake, possibly evidenced by dry mucous membranes, poor skin turgor, delayed capillary refill, weak peripheral pulses, diminished urinary output, dark/concentrated urine, hypotension, and tachycardia.

Pain, [acute] may be related to chemical irritation of parietal peritoneum, trauma to tissues, accumulation of fluid in abdominal/peritoneal cavity, possibly evidenced by verbal reports, muscle guarding/rebound tenderness, distraction behaviors, facial mask of pain, self-focus, autonomic responses (changes in vital signs).

Nutrition, altered, less than body requirements, risk for: risk factors may include nausea/vomiting, intestinal dysfunction, metabolic abnormalities, or increased metabolic needs.

**pheochromocytoma**

Anxiety [specify level] may be related to excessive physiologic (hormonal) stimulation of the sympathetic nervous system, situational crises, threat to/change in health status, possibly evidenced by apprehension, shakiness, restlessness, focus on self, fearfulness, diaphoresis, and sense of impending doom.

Fluid volume deficit [active loss/regulatory failure] may be related to excessive gastric losses (vomiting/diarrhea), hypermetabolic state, diaphoresis, and hyperosmolar diuresis, possibly evidenced by hemoconcentration, dry mucous membranes, poor skin turgor, thirst, and weight loss.

Cardiac output, decreased/Tissue perfusion, altered (specify) may be related to altered preload/decreased blood volume, altered systemic vascular resistance, and increased sympathetic activity (excessive secretion of catecholamines), possibly evidenced by cool/clammy skin, change in blood pressure (hypertension/postural hypotension), visual disturbances, severe headache, and angina.

Knowledge deficit [learning need] regarding pathophysiology of condition, outcome, preoperative and postoperative care needs may be related to lack of information/recall, possibly evidenced by statements of concern, questions, and misconceptions.

**phlebitis**

Refer to *thrombophlebitis*.

**phobia** (also refer to *anxiety disorder, generalized*)

Fear may be related to learned irrational response to natural or innate origins (phobic stimulus), or unfounded morbid dread of a seemingly harmless object/situation, possibly evidenced by sympathetic stimulation and reactions ranging from apprehension to panic.

Social interaction, impaired may be related to intense fear of encountering feared object/activity or situation and anticipated loss of control, possibly evidenced by reported change of style/pattern of interaction, discomfort in social situations, and avoidance of phobic stimulus.

**placenta previa**

Fluid volume deficit, risk for: risk factors may include excessive vascular losses (vessel damage and inadequate vasoconstriction).

Gas exchange, impaired, fetal may be related to altered blood flow, altered carrying capacity of blood (maternal anemia), and decreased surface area of gas exchange at site of placental attachment, possibly evidenced by changes in fetal heart rate/activity and release of meconium.

Fear may be related to threat of death (perceived or actual) to self or fetus, possibly evidenced by verbalization of specific concerns, increased tension, sympathetic stimulation.

Diversional activity deficit, risk for: risk factors may include imposed activity restrictions/bedrest.

**pleurisy**

Pain, [acute] may be related to inflammation/irritation of the parietal pleura, possibly evidenced by verbal reports, guarding/distraction behaviors, self-focus, and autonomic responses (changes in vital signs).

Breathing pattern, ineffective may be related to pain on inspiration, possibly evidenced by decreased respiratory depth, tachypnea, and dyspnea.

Infection, risk for pneumonia: risk factors may include stasis of pulmonary secretions, decreased lung expansion, and ineffective cough.

**pneumonia**

Refer to *bronchitis*; *bronchopneumonia*.

**pneumothorax** (also refer to *hemothorax*)

Breathing pattern, ineffective may be related to decreased lung expansion (fluid/air accumulation), pain, inflammatory process, possibly evidenced by dyspnea, tachypnea, altered chest excursion, respiratory depth changes, cough, cyanosis, and abnormal ABGs.

Cardiac output, decreased, risk for: risk factors may include compression/displacement of cardiac structures.

Pain, [acute] may be related to irritation of nerve endings within pleural space by foreign object (chest tube), possibly evidenced by verbal reports, guarding/distraction behaviors, self-focus, and autonomic responses (changes in vital signs).

**polyarteritis** (nodosa)

Tissue perfusion, altered (specify) may be related to reduction/interruption of blood flow, possibly evidenced by organ tissue infarctions, changes in organ function, and development of organic psychosis.

Hyperthermia may be related to widespread inflammatory process, possibly evidenced by increased body temperature and warm/flushed skin.

Pain, [acute] may be related to inflammation, tissue ischemia, and necrosis of affected area, possibly evidenced by verbal reports, guarding/distraction behaviors, self-focus, and autonomic responses (changes in vital signs).

Grieving, anticipatory may be related to perceived loss of self, possibly evidenced by expressions of sorrow and anger, altered sleep and/or eating patterns, and changes in activity level or libido.

**polycythemia vera**

Activity intolerance may be related to imbalance between oxygen supply and demand, possibly evidenced by reports of fatigue/weakness.

Tissue perfusion, altered (specify) may be related to reduction/interruption of arterial/venous blood flow (insufficiency, thrombosis, or hemorrhage), possibly evidenced by pain in affected area, impaired mental ability, visual disturbances, and color changes of skin/mucous membranes.

**polyradiculitis**

Refer to *Guillain-Barré syndrome*.

**postoperative recovery period**

Breathing pattern, ineffective may be related to neuromuscular and perceptual/cognitive impairment, decreased lung expansion/energy, and tracheobronchial obstruction, possibly evidenced by changes in respiratory rate and depth, reduced vital capacity, apnea, cyanosis, and noisy respirations.

Body temperature, altered, risk for: risk factors may include exposure to cool environment, effect of medications/anesthetic agents, extremes of age/weight, and dehydration.

Sensory-perceptual alteration (specify)/Thought processes, altered may be related to chemical alteration (use of pharmaceutical agents, hypoxia), therapeutically restricted environment, excessive sensory stimuli and physiologic stress, possibly evidenced by changes in usual response to stimuli, motor incoordination, impaired ability to concentrate, reason, and make decisions; and disorientation to person, place, and time.

Fluid volume, deficit, risk for: risk factors may include restriction of oral intake, loss of fluid through abnormal routes (indwelling tubes, drains), normal routes (vomiting, loss of vascular integrity, changes in clotting ability), and extremes of age and weight.

Pain, [acute] may be related to disruption of skin, tissue, and muscle integrity, musculoskeletal/bone trauma, and presence of tubes and drains, possibly evidenced by verbal reports, alteration in muscle tone, facial mask of pain, distraction/guarding behaviors, narrowed focus, and autonomic responses.

Skin/Tissue integrity, impaired may be related to mechanical interruption of skin/tissues, altered circulation, effects of medication, accumulation of drainage, and altered metabolic state, possibly evidenced by disruption of skin surface/layers and tissues.

Infection, risk for: risk factors may include broken skin, traumatized tissues, stasis of body fluids, presence of pathogens/contaminants, environmental exposure, and invasive procedures.

**postpartal period**

Family processes, altered, risk for: risk factors may include developmental transition (gain of a family member) and transient period of disequilibrium.

Fluid volume deficit, risk for: risk factors may include excessive blood loss during delivery, reduced intake/inadequate replacement, nausea/vomiting, or increased urine output.

Pain, [acute]/Discomfort may be related to tissue trauma/edema, muscle contractions, bladder fullness, and physical/psychologic exhaustion, possibly evidenced by reports of cramping (afterpains), self-focusing, alteration in muscle tone, distraction behavior, and autonomic responses (changes in vital signs).

Urinary elimination, altered may be related to physiologic return to nonpregnant state (decrease in circulating blood volume, continued elevation in renal plasma flow), mechanical trauma/tissue edema, and effects of medication/anesthesia, possibly evidenced by frequency, dysuria, urgency, incontinence, or retention.

Constipation may be related to decreased muscle tone associated with diastasis recti, prenatal effects of progesterone, dehydration, excess analgesia or anesthesia, pain (hemorrhoids, episiotomy, or perineal tenderness), prelabor diarrhea, and lack of intake, possibly evidenced by frequency less than usual pattern, hard-formed stool, straining at stool, decreased bowel sounds, and abdominal distension.

Sleep pattern disturbance may be related to pain/discomfort, intense exhilaration/excitement, anxiety, exhausting process of labor/delivery, and needs/demands of family members, possibly evidenced by verbal reports of difficulty in falling asleep/not feeling well-rested, interrupted sleep, frequent yawning, irritability, or dark circles under eyes.

**post-traumatic stress disorder**

Post-trauma response related to having experienced a traumatic life event, possibly evidenced by re-experiencing of the event, somatic reactions, psychic/emotional numbness, altered lifestyle, impaired sleep.

Anxiety [severe to panic]/Fear may be related to memory of traumatic life event, threat to self-concept/death, change in environment, and negative self-talk, possibly evidenced by increased tension/wariness, sense of helplessness, apprehension, fearfulness, uncertainty/confusion, restlessness, somatic complaints, sense of impending doom, and sympathetic stimulation with cardiovascular excitement/palpitations.

Violence, risk for, directed at self/others: risk factors may include a startle reaction, an intrusive memory of an event causing a sudden acting-out of a feeling as if the event were occurring, use of alcohol/other drugs to ward off painful effects and produce psychic numbing, breaking through the rage that has been walled off, response to intense anxiety or panic state, and loss of control.

Coping, individual, ineffective may be related to personal vulnerability, inadequate support system, unrealistic perceptions, unmet expectations, overwhelming threat to self, and multiple stressors repeated over period of time, possibly evidenced by verbalization of inability to cope or difficulty asking for help, muscular tension/headaches, chronic worry, and emotional tension.

Grieving, dysfunctional may be related to actual/perceived object loss (loss of self as seen before the traumatic incident occurred as well as other losses incurred in/after the incident), loss of physiopsychosocial well-being, thwarted grieving response to a loss, and lack of resolution of previous grieving responses, possibly evidenced by verbal expression of distress at loss, anger, sadness, labile affect, alterations in eating habits, sleep/dream patterns, libido; reliving of past experiences, expression of guilt, and alterations in concentration.

Family processes, altered may be related to situational crisis, possibly evidenced by expressions of confusion about what to do and expressions of difficulty coping, family system not meeting physical/emotional/spiritual needs of its members, not adapting to change or dealing with traumatic experience constructively, and ineffective family decision-making process.

**pregnancy** (prenatal period)

Nutrition, altered, less than body requirements, risk for: risk factors may include changes in appetite, insufficient intake (nausea/vomiting, inadequate financial resources and nutritional knowledge) to meet increased metabolic demands (increased thyroid activity associated with the growth of fetal and maternal tissues).

[Discomfort]/Pain may be related to hormonal influences, physical changes, possibly evidenced by verbal reports (nausea, breast changes, leg cramps, hemorrhoids, nasal stuffiness), alteration in muscle tone, restlessness, and autonomic responses (changes in vital signs).

Injury, risk for, fetal: risk factors may include environmental/hereditary factors and problems of maternal well-being that directly affect the developing fetus (e.g., malnutrition, substance use).

Cardiac output, [maximally compensated] may be related to increased fluid volume/maximal cardiac effort and hormonal effects of progesterone and relaxin (that place the patient at risk for hypertension and/or circulatory failure), and changes in peripheral resistance (afterload), possibly evidenced by variations in blood pressure and pulse, syncopal episodes, or presence of pathological edema.

Family coping, potential for growth may be related to situational/maturational crisis with anticipated changes in family structure/roles, needs sufficiently met and adaptive tasks effectively addressed to enable goals of self-actualization to surface, as evidenced by movement toward health-promoting and enriching lifestyle, choosing experiences that optimize condition/pregnancy experience.

Constipation, risk for: risk factors may include changes in dietary/fluid intake, smooth muscle relaxation, decreased peristalsis, and effects of medications (e.g., iron).

Fatigue/Sleep pattern disturbance may be related to increased carbohydrate metabolism, altered body chemistry, increased energy requirements to perform activities of daily living, discomfort, anxiety, inactivity, possibly evidenced by reports of overwhelming lack of energy/inability to maintain usual routines, difficulty falling asleep/not feeling well-rested, interrupted sleep, irritability, lethargy, and frequent yawning.

Role performance, altered, risk for: risk factors may include maturational crisis, developmental level, history of maladaptive coping, or absence of support systems.

Knowledge deficit [learning need] regarding normal physiologic/psychologic changes may be related to lack of information/recall and misinterpretation, possibly evidenced by questions, statement of concern, misconceptions, and inaccurate follow-through of instructions/development of preventable complications.

**pregnancy, adolescent** (also refer to *pregnancy, prenatal period*)

Family processes, altered may be related to situational/developmental transition (economic, change in roles/gain of a family member), possibly evidenced by family expressing confusion about what to do, unable to meet physical/emotional/spiritual needs of the members, family inability to adapt to change or to deal with traumatic experience constructively, does not demonstrate respect for individuality and autonomy of its members, ineffective family decision-making process, and inappropriate boundary maintenance.

Social isolation may be related to alterations in physical appearance, perceived unacceptable social behavior, restricted social sphere, stage of adolescence, and interference with accomplishing developmental tasks, possibly evidenced by expressions of feelings of aloneness/rejection/difference from others, uncommunicative, withdrawn, no eye contact, seeking to be alone, unacceptable behavior, and absence of supportive significant other(s).

Body image/Self-esteem disturbance may be related to situational/maturational crisis, biophysical changes in body and fear of failure at life events, absence of support systems, possibly evidenced by self-negating verbalizations, expressions of shame/guilt, fear of rejection/reaction of others, hypersensitivity to criticism, and lack of follow-through/nonparticipation in prenatal care.

Knowledge deficit [learning need] regarding pregnancy, developmental/individual needs, future expectations may be related to lack of exposure, information misinterpretation, unfamiliarity with information resources, lack of interest in learning, possibly evidenced by questions, statement of concern/misconception, sense of vulnerability/denial of reality, inaccurate follow-through of instruction, and development of preventable complications.

Parenting, altered, risk for: may be related to chronological age/developmental stage, unmet social/emotional/maturational needs of parenting figures, unrealistic expectation of self/infant/partner, ineffective role model/social support, lack of role identity, and presence of stressors (e.g., financial).

**pregnancy-induced hypertension** (pre-eclampsia)

Fluid volume deficit [regulatory failure] may be related to a plasma protein loss, decreasing plasma colloid osmotic pressure allowing fluid shifts out of vascular compartment, possibly evidenced by edema formation, sudden weight gain, hemoconcentration, nausea/vomiting, epigastric pain, headaches, visual changes, decreased urine output.

Tissue perfusion, altered, renal may be related to decreased blood flow (vasoconstriction) and relative hypovolemia, possibly evidenced by decreased urine output and abnormal laboratory values for renal function studies.

Gas exchange, impaired/Nutrition, altered, less than body requirements, fetal may be related to vasospasm of spiral arteries and relative hypovolemia, possibly evidenced by changes in fetal heart rate/activity, reduced weight gain, and premature delivery.

Knowledge deficit [learning need] regarding pathophysiology of condition, therapy, self-care/nutritional needs, and potential complications may be related to lack of information/recall, misinterpretation, possibly evidenced by statements of concern, questions, misconceptions, inaccurate follow-through of instructions/development of preventable complications.

**premenstrual tension syndrome** (PMS)

Pain, [acute]/chronic may be related to cyclic changes in female hormones affecting other systems (e.g., vascular congestion/spasms), possibly evidenced by increased tension, apprehension, jitteriness, verbal reports, distraction behaviors, somatic complaints, and self-focusing.

Fluid volume excess may be related to abnormal alterations of hormonal levels, possibly evidenced by edema formation, weight gain, and periodic changes in emotional status/irritability.

Anxiety [specify level] may be related to cyclic changes in female hormones affecting other systems, possibly evidenced by feelings of inability to cope/loss of control, depersonalization, increased tension, apprehension, jitteriness, somatic complaints, and impaired functioning.

Knowledge deficit [learning need] regarding pathophysiology of condition and self-care/treatment needs may be related to lack of information/misinterpretation, possibly evidenced by statements of concern, questions, misconceptions, and continuation of condition.

**pressure ulcer or sore** (also refer to *ulcer, decubitus*)

Tissue perfusion, altered, peripheral may be related to reduced/interrupted blood flow, possibly evidenced by presence of inflamed, necrotic lesion.

Knowledge deficit [learning need] regarding cause/prevention of condition and potential complications may be related to lack of information/misinterpretation, possibly evidenced by statements of concern, questions, misconceptions, and inaccurate follow-through of instructions.

**preterm labor**

Refer to *labor, preterm*.

**prostatectomy**

Urinary elimination, altered may be related to mechanical obstruction (blood clots, edema, trauma, surgical procedure, pressure/irritation of catheter/balloon), and loss of bladder tone, possibly evidenced by dysuria, frequency, dribbling, incontinence, retention, bladder fullness, suprapubic discomfort.

Fluid volume deficit, risk for: risk factors may include trauma to highly vascular area with excessive vascular losses, restricted intake.

Pain, [acute] may be related to irritation of bladder mucosa and tissue trauma/edema, possibly evidenced by verbal reports (bladder spasms), distraction behaviors, self-focus, and autonomic responses (changes in vital signs).

Body image disturbance may be related to perceived threat of altered body/sexual function, possibly evidenced by preoccupation with change/loss, negative feelings about body, and statements of concern regarding functioning.

Sexual dysfunction, risk for: risk factors may include situational crisis (incontinence, leakage of urine after catheter removal, involvement of genital area) and threat to self-concept/change in health status.

**pruritus**

Pain, [acute] may be related to cutaneous hyperesthesia and inflammation, possibly evidenced by verbal reports, distraction behaviors, and self-focus.

Skin integrity, impaired, risk for: risk factors may include mechanical trauma (scratching) and development of vesicles/bullae that may rupture.

**psoriasis**

Skin integrity, impaired may be related to increased epidermal cell proliferation and absence of normal protective skin layers, possibly evidenced by scaling papules and plaques.

Body image disturbance may be related to cosmetically unsightly skin lesions, possibly evidenced by hiding affected body part, negative feelings about body, feelings of helplessness, and change in social involvement.

**pulmonary embolus**

Breathing pattern, ineffective may be related to tracheobronchial obstruction (inflammation, copious secretions or active bleeding), decreased lung expansion, inflammatory process, possibly evidenced by changes in depth and/or rate of respiration, dyspnea/use of accessory muscles, altered chest excursion, abnormal breath sounds (crackles, wheezes), and cough (with or without sputum production).

Gas exchange, impaired may be related to altered blood flow to alveoli or to major portions of the lung, alveolar-capillary membrane changes (atelectasis, airway/alveolar collapse, pulmonary edema/effusion, excessive secretions/active bleeding), possibly evidenced by profound dyspnea, restlessness, apprehension, somnolence, cyanosis, and changes in ABGs/pulse oximetry (hypoxemia and hypercapnia).

Tissue perfusion, altered, cardiopulmonary may be related to interruption of blood flow (arterial/venous), exchange problems at alveolar level or at tissue level (acidotic shifting of the oxyhemoglobin curve), possibly evidenced by radiology/laboratory evidence of ventilation/perfusion mismatch, dyspnea, and central cyanosis.

Fear/Anxiety [specify level] may be related to severe dyspnea/inability to breathe normally, perceived threat of death, threat to or change in health status, physiologic response to hypoxemia/acidosis, and concern regarding unknown outcome of situation, possibly evidenced by restlessness, irritability, withdrawal or attack behavior, sympathetic stimulation (cardiovascular excitation, pupil dilation, sweating, vomiting, diarrhea), crying, voice quivering, and impending sense of doom.

**purpura, idiopathic thrombocytopenic**

Injury, risk for: risk factors may include abnormal blood profile/risk of hemorrhage.

Activity intolerance may be related to decreased oxygen-carrying capacity/imbalance between oxygen supply and demand, possibly evidenced by reports of fatigue/weakness.

Knowledge deficit [learning need] regarding therapy choices, outcomes, and self-care needs may be related to lack of information/misinterpretation, possibly evidenced by statements of concern, questions, and misconceptions.

**pyelonephritis**

Pain, [acute] may be related to acute inflammation of renal tissues, possibly evidenced by verbal reports, guarding/distraction behaviors, self-focus, and autonomic responses (changes in vital signs).

Hyperthermia may be related to inflammatory process/increased metabolic rate, possibly evidenced by increase in body temperature, warm/flushed skin, tachycardia, and chills.

Urinary elimination, altered may be related to inflammation/irritation of bladder mucosa, possibly evidenced by dysuria, urgency, and frequency.

Knowledge deficit [learning need] regarding therapy needs and prevention may be related to lack of information/misinterpretation, possibly evidenced by statements of concern, questions, misconceptions, and recurrence of condition.

**quadriplegia** (also refer to *paraplegia*)

Breathing pattern, ineffective may be related to neuromuscular impairment (diaphragm and intercostal muscle function), reflex abdominal spasms, gastric distention, possibly evidenced by decreased respiratory depth, dyspnea, cyanosis, and abnormal ABGs.

Trauma, risk for additional spinal injury: risk factors may include temporary weakness/instability of spinal column.

Grieving, anticipatory may be related to perceived loss of self, anticipated alterations in lifestyle and expectations, and limitation of future options/choices, possibly evidenced by expressions of distress, anger, sorrow, choked feelings, and changes in eating habits, sleep, and communication patterns.

Self-care deficit, all areas related to neuromuscular impairment, possibly evidenced by inability to perform self-care tasks.

Dysreflexia, risk for: risk factors may include altered nerve function (spinal cord injury at T-6 or above), bladder/bowel/skin stimulation (tactile, pain, thermal).

Home maintenance management, impaired may be related to permanent effects of injury, inadequate/absent support systems and finances, and lack of familiarity with resources, possibly evidenced by expressions of difficulties, requests for information and assistance, outstanding debts/financial crisis, and lack of necessary aides and equipment.

**rape**

Knowledge deficit [learning need] regarding prophylactic treatment for individual concerns (sexually transmitted diseases, pregnancy), required medical/legal procedures, community resources/supports may be related to lack of information, possibly evidenced by statements of concern, questions, misconceptions, and exacerbation of symptoms.

Rape-trauma syndrome (acute phase) related to actual or attempted sexual attack without consent, possibly evidenced by wide range of emotional reactions, including anxiety, fear, anger, embarrassment, and multisystem physical complaints.

Tissue integrity, impaired, risk for: risk factors may include forceful sexual penetration and trauma to fragile tissues.

Coping, individual, ineffective may be related to personal vulnerability, unmet expectations, unrealistic perception, inadequate support systems/coping methods, multiple stressors repeated over time, overwhelming threat to self, possibly evidenced by verbalizations of inability to cope or difficulty asking for help, muscular tension/headaches, emotional tension, chronic worry.

Sexual dysfunction may be related to biopsychosocial alteration of sexuality (stress of post-trauma response), vulnerability, loss of sexual desire, impaired relationship with significant other, possibly evidenced by alteration in achieving sexual satisfaction, change in interest in self/others, preoccupation with self.

**Raynaud's phenomenon**

Pain, [acute]/chronic may be related to vasospasm/altered perfusion of affected tissues and ischemia/destruction of tissues, possibly evidenced by verbal reports, guarding of affected parts, self-focusing, and restlessness.

Tissue perfusion, altered, peripheral may be related to periodic reduction of arterial blood flow to affected areas, possibly evidenced by pallor, cyanosis, coolness, numbness, paresthesia, slow healing of lesions.

Knowledge deficit [learning need] regarding pathophysiology of the condition, potential for complications, therapy/self-care needs may be related to lack of information/misinterpretation, possibly evidenced by statements of concern, questions, and misconceptions; development of preventable complications.

**reflex sympathetic dystrophy** (RSD)

Pain, [acute]/chronic may be related to continued nerve stimulation, possibly evidenced by verbal reports, distraction/guarding behaviors, narrowed focus, changes in sleep patterns, and altered ability to continue previous activities.

Tissue perfusion, altered, peripheral may be related to reduction of arterial blood flow (arteriole vasoconstriction), possibly evidenced by reports of pain, decreased skin temperature and pallor, diminished arterial pulsations, and tissue swelling.

Sensory-perceptual alteration, tactile may be related to altered sensory reception (neurologic deficit, pain), possibly evidenced by change in usual response to stimuli/abnormal sensitivity of touch, physiologic anxiety, and irritability.

Role performance, altered, risk for: risk factors may include situational crisis, chronic disability, and debilitating pain.

Family coping, ineffective: compromised, risk for: risk factors may include temporary family disorganization and role changes and prolonged disability that exhausts the supportive capacity of significant other(s).

**renal failure, acute**

Fluid volume excess may be related to compromised regulatory mechanisms (decreased kidney function), possibly evidenced by weight gain, edema/anasarca, intake greater than output, venous congestion, and altered electrolyte levels.

Nutrition, altered, less than body requirements may be related to inability to ingest/digest adequate nutrients (anorexia, nausea/vomiting, ulcerations of oral mucosa, and increased metabolic needs) in addition to therapeutic dietary restrictions, possibly evidenced by lack of interest in food/aversion to eating, observed inadequate intake, weight loss, or loss of muscle mass.

Infection, risk for: risk factors may include depression of immunologic defenses, invasive procedures/devices, and changes in dietary intake/malnutrition.

Thought processes, altered may be related to accumulation of toxic waste products and altered cerebral perfusion, possibly evidenced by disorientation, changes in recent memory, apathy, and episodic obtundation.

Fatigue may be related to decreased metabolic energy production/dietary restrictions, anemia, increased energy requirements, (e.g., fever/inflammation and tissue regeneration), possibly evidenced by overwhelming lack of energy, inability to maintain usual activities, decreased performance, lethargy, and disinterest in surroundings.

**renal transplantation**

Fluid volume excess, risk for: risk factors may include compromised regulatory mechanism (implantation of new kidney requiring adjustment period for optimal functioning).

Body image disturbance may be related to failure and subsequent replacement of body part and medication-induced changes in appearance, possibly evidenced by preoccupation with loss/change, negative feelings about body, and focus on past strength/function.

Fear may be related to potential for transplant rejection/failure and threat of death, possibly evidenced by increased tension, apprehension, concentration on source and verbalizations of concern.

Infection, risk for: risk factors may include broken skin/traumatized tissue, stasis of body fluids, immunosuppression, invasive procedures, nutritional deficits, and chronic disease.

**respiratory distress syndrome** (premature infant) (also refer to *neonate, premature newborn*)

Gas exchange, impaired may be related to alveolar-capillary membrane changes (inadequate surfactant levels), altered oxygen supply (tracheobronchial obstruction, atelectasis), altered blood flow (immaturity of pulmonary arteriole musculature), and altered oxygen-carrying capacity of blood (anemia), and cold stress, possibly evidenced by tachypnea, use of accessory muscles/retractions, expiratory grunting, pallor or cyanosis, abnormal ABGs, and tachycardia.

Spontaneous ventilation, inability to sustain may be related to respiratory muscle fatigue and metabolic factors, possibly evidenced by dyspnea, increased metabolic rate, restlessness, use of accessory muscles, and abnormal ABGs.

Infection, risk for: risk factors may include inadequate primary defenses (decreased ciliary action, stasis of body fluids, traumatized tissues), inadequate secondary defenses (deficiency of neutrophils and specific immunoglobulins), invasive procedures, and malnutrition (absence of nutrient stores, increased metabolic demands).

Tissue perfusion, altered, gastrointestinal, risk for: risk factors may include persistent fetal circulation and exchange problems.

Parent/Infant/Child attachment, altered, risk for: risk factors may include premature/ill infant who is unable to effectively initiate parental contact due to altered behavioral organization, separation, physical barriers, anxiety associated with the parental role/demands of infant.

**retinal detachment**

Sensory-perceptual alterations, visual related to decreased sensory reception, possibly evidenced by visual distortions, decreased visual field, and changes in visual acuity.

Knowledge deficit [learning need] regarding therapy, prognosis, and self-care needs may be related to lack of information/misconceptions, possibly evidenced by statements of concern and questions.

Home maintenance management, impaired, risk for: risk factors may include postoperative activity restrictions/limitations.

**Reye's syndrome**

Fluid volume deficit [active loss/regulatory failure] may be related to failure of regulatory mechanism (diabetes insipidus), excessive gastric losses (pernicious vomiting), and altered intake, possibly evidenced by increased/dilute urine output, sudden weight loss, decreased venous filling, dry mucous membranes, decreased skin turgor, hypotension, and tachycardia.

Tissue perfusion, decreased, cerebral may be related to diminished arterial/venous blood flow and hypovolemia, possibly evidenced by memory loss, altered consciousness, and restlessness/agitation.

Trauma, risk for: risk factors may include generalized weakness, reduced coordination, and cognitive deficits.

Breathing pattern, ineffective may be related to decreased energy and fatigue, cognitive impairment, tracheobronchial obstruction, and inflammatory process (aspiration pneumonia), possibly evidenced by tachypnea, abnormal ABGs, cough, and use of accessory muscles.

**rheumatic fever**

Pain, [acute] may be related to migratory inflammation of joints, possibly evidenced by verbal reports, guarding/distraction behaviors, self-focus, and autonomic responses (changes in vital signs).

Hyperthermia may be related to inflammatory process/hypermetabolic state, possibly evidenced by increased body temperature, warm/flushed skin, and tachycardia.

Activity intolerance may be related to generalized weakness, joint pain, and medical restrictions/bedrest, possibly evidenced by reports of fatigue, exertional discomfort, and abnormal heart rate in response to activity.

Cardiac output, decreased, risk for: risk factors may include cardiac inflammation/enlargement and altered contractility.

**rickets** (osteomalacia)

Growth and development, altered may be related to dietary deficiencies/indiscretions, malabsorption syndrome, and lack of exposure to sunlight, possibly evidenced by altered physical growth and delay or difficulty in performing motor skills typical for age.

Knowledge deficit [learning need] regarding cause, pathophysiology, and therapy needs/prevention may be related to lack of information, possibly evidenced by statements of concern, questions, misconceptions, and inaccurate follow-through of instructions.

**ringworm, tinea** (also refer to *athlete's foot*)

Skin integrity, impaired may be related to fungal infection of the dermis, possibly evidenced by disruption of skin surfaces/presence of lesions.

Knowledge deficit [learning need] regarding infectious nature, therapy, and self-care needs may be related to lack of information/misinformation, possibly evidenced by statements of concern, questions, and recurrence/spread.

**rubella**

Pain, [acute/Discomfort] may be related to inflammatory effects of viral infection and presence of desquamating rash, possibly evidenced by verbal reports, distraction behaviors/restlessness.

Knowledge deficit [learning need] regarding contagious nature, possible complications, and self-care needs may be related to lack of information/misinterpretation, possibly evidenced by statements of concern, questions, and inaccurate follow-through of instructions.

**scabies**

Skin integrity, impaired may be related to presence of invasive parasite and development of pruritus, possibly evidenced by disruption of skin surface and inflammation.

Knowledge deficit [learning need] regarding communicable nature, possible complications, therapy, and self-care needs may be related to lack of information/misinterpretation, possibly evidenced by questions and statements of concern about spread to others.

**scarlet fever**

Hyperthermia may be related to effects of circulating toxins, possibly evidenced by increased body temperature, warm/flushed skin, and tachycardia.

Pain, [Discomfort] may be related to inflammation of mucous membranes and effects of circulating toxins (malaise, fever), possibly evidenced by verbal reports, distraction behaviors, guarding (decreased swallowing), and self-focus.

Fluid volume deficit, risk for: risk factors may include hypermetabolic state (hyperthermia) and reduced intake.

**schizophrenia** (schizophrenic disorders)

Thought process, altered may be related to disintegration of thinking processes, impaired judgment, presence of psychologic conflicts, disintegrated ego boundaries, sleep disturbance, ambivalence, and concomitant dependence, possibly evidenced by impaired ability to reason/problem solve, inappropriate affect, presence of delusional system, command hallucinations, obsessions, ideas of reference, and cognitive dissonance.

Social isolation may be related to alterations in mental status, mistrust of others/delusional thinking, unacceptable social behaviors, inadequate personal resources, and inability to engage in satisfying personal relationships, possibly evidenced by difficulty in establishing relationships with others, dull affect, uncommunicative/withdrawn behavior, seeking to be alone, and inadequate/absent significant purpose in life.

Health maintenance, altered may be related to altered ability to make deliberate and thoughtful judgments, altered communications, and lack of/inappropriate use of material resources, possibly evidenced by inability to take responsibility for meeting basic health practices in any or all functional areas and demonstrated lack of adaptive behaviors to internal or external environmental changes.

Violence, risk for, directed at self/others: risk factors may include disturbances of thinking/feeling (depression, paranoia, suicidal ideation), catatonic/manic excitement, and toxic reactions to drugs (alcohol).

Coping, individual, ineffective may be related to personal vulnerability, inadequate support system(s), unrealistic perceptions, inadequate coping methods, and disintegration of thought processes, possibly evidenced by impaired judgment/cognition and perception, diminished problem-solving/decision-making capacities, poor self-esteem, chronic anxiety, depression, inability to perform role expectations, and alteration in social participation.

Family coping, ineffective: disabling may be related to ambivalent family system/relationships and difficulty of family members in coping effectively with patient's maladaptive behaviors, possibly evidenced by patient's expressions of despair at family's lack of reaction/involvement, neglectful relationships with patient, extreme distortion regarding patient's health problem including denial about its existence/severity or prolonged overconcern, impaired restructuring of a meaningful life for individual family members, and impaired individuation.

Self-care deficit (specify) may be related to perceptual and cognitive impairment, immobility (withdrawal/isolation and decreased psychomotor activity), and side effects of psychotropic medications, possibly evidenced by inability or difficulty in areas of feeding self, keeping body clean, dressing appropriately, toileting self, or changes in bowel/bladder elimination.

**sciatica**

Pain, [acute]/chronic may be related to peripheral nerve root compression, possibly evidenced by verbal reports, guarding/distraction behaviors, and self-focus.

Physical mobility, impaired may be related to neurologic pain and muscular involvement, possibly evidenced by reluctance to attempt movement and decreased muscle strength/mass.

**scleroderma** (also refer to *lupus erythematosus, systemic*)

Physical mobility, impaired may be related to musculoskeletal impairment and associated pain, possibly evidenced by decreased strength, decreased range of motion, and reluctance to attempt movement.

Tissue perfusion, altered (specify) may be related to reduced arterial blood flow (arteriolar vasoconstriction), possibly evidenced by changes in skin temperature/color, ulcer formation, and changes in organ function (cardiopulmonary, gastrointestinal, renal).

Nutrition, altered, less than body requirements may be related to inability to ingest/digest/absorb adequate nutrients (sclerosis of the tissues rendering mouth immobile, decreased peristalsis of esophagus/small intestines, atrophy of smooth muscle of colon), possibly evidenced by weight loss, decreased intake/food and reported/observed difficulty swallowing.

Adjustment, impaired may be related to disability requiring change in lifestyle, inadequate support systems, assault to self-concept, and altered locus of control, possibly evidenced by verbalization of nonacceptance of health status change and lack of movement toward independence/future-oriented thinking.

Body image disturbance may be related to skin changes with induration, atrophy, and fibrosis, loss of hair, and skin and muscle contractures, possibly evidenced by verbalization of negative feelings about body, focus on past strength/function or appearance, fear of rejection/reaction by others, hiding body part, and change in social involvement.

**scoliosis**

Body image disturbance may be related to altered body structure, use of therapeutic device(s), and activity restrictions, possibly evidenced by negative feelings about body, change in social involvement, and preoccupation with situation or refusal to acknowledge problem.

Knowledge deficit [learning need] regarding pathophysiology of condition and therapy needs and possible outcomes may be related to lack of information/misinterpretation, possibly evidenced by statements of concern, questions, misconceptions, and inaccurate follow-through of instructions.

Adjustment, impaired may be related to lack of comprehension of long-term consequences of behavior, possibly evidenced by failure to adhere to treatment regimen/keep appointments and evidence of failure to improve.

**sepsis, puerperal** (also refer to *septicemia*)

Infection, risk for spread/septic shock: risk factors may include presence of infection, broken skin, traumatized tissues, high vascularity of involved area, stasis of body fluids, invasive procedures, increased environmental exposure, chronic disease (e.g., diabetes, anemia, malnutrition), altered immune response, and untoward effect of medications (e.g., opportunistic/secondary infections).

Hyperthermia may be related to inflammatory process/hypermetabolic state, possibly evidenced by increase in body temperature, warm/flushed skin, and tachycardia.

Parenting, altered may be related to presence of physical illness, medical/therapeutic interruption in bonding process, and threat to own survival, possibly evidenced by incomplete parental attachment behaviors and verbalized concern regarding role inadequacy.

Tissue perfusion, altered, peripheral, risk for: risk factors may include interruption/reduction of blood flow (presence of infectious thrombi).

**septicemia** (also refer to *sepsis, puerperal*)
Tissue perfusion, altered (specify) may be related to changes in arterial/venous blood flow (selective vasoconstriction, presence of microemboli) and hypovolemia, possibly evidenced by changes in skin temperature/color, changes in blood/pulse pressure, changes in sensorium, and decreased urinary output.
Fluid volume deficit, risk for: risk factors may include marked increase in vascular compartment/massive vasodilation, vascular shifts to interstitial space, and reduced intake.
Cardiac output, decreased, risk for: risk factors may include decreased preload (venous return and circulating volume), altered afterload (increased systemic vascular resistance), negative inotropic effects of hypoxia, complement activation, and lysosomal hydrolase.

**serum sickness**
Pain, [acute] may be related to inflammation of the joints and skin eruptions, possibly evidenced by verbal reports, guarding/distraction behaviors, and self-focus.
Knowledge deficit [learning need] regarding nature of condition, treatment needs, potential complications, and need to avoid causative agent may be related to lack of information/misinterpretation, possibly evidenced by statements of concern, questions, misconceptions, and inaccurate follow-through of instructions.

**sexually transmitted disease** (STD)
Infection, risk for transmission: risk factors may include contagious nature of infecting agent and insufficient knowledge to avoid exposure to/transmission of pathogens.
Skin/Tissue integrity, impaired may be related to invasion of/irritation by pathogenic organism(s), possibly evidenced by disruptions of skin/tissue and inflammation of mucous membranes.
Knowledge deficit [learning need] regarding condition, prognosis/complications, therapy needs, and transmission may be related to lack of information/misinterpretation, lack of interest in learning, possibly evidenced by statements of concern, questions, misconceptions, inaccurate follow-through of instructions, and development of preventable complications.

**shock** (also refer to *shock, cardiogenic; shock, hemorrhagic*)
Tissue perfusion, altered (specify) may be related to changes in circulating volume and/or vascular tone, possibly evidenced by changes in skin color/temperature and pulse pressure, reduced blood pressure, changes in mentation, and decreased urinary output.
Anxiety [specify level] may be related to change in health status and threat of death, possibly evidenced by increased tension, apprehension, sympathetic stimulation, restlessness, and expressions of concern.

**shock, cardiogenic**
Cardiac output, decreased may be related to structural damage, decreased myocardial contractility, and presence of dysrhythmias, possibly evidenced by ECG changes, variations in hemodynamic readings, jugular vein distention, cold/clammy skin, diminished peripheral pulses, and decreased urinary output.

**shock, hemorrhagic**
Fluid volume deficit [active loss] may be related to excessive vascular loss, inadequate intake/replacement, possibly evidenced by hypotension, tachycardia, decreased pulse volume and pressure, change in mentation, and decreased/concentrated urine.

**sick sinus syndrome**
Cardiac output, decreased may be related to alterations in rate, rhythm, and electrical conduction, possibly evidenced by ECG evidence of dysrhythmias, reports of palpitations/weakness, changes in mentation/consciousness, and syncope.
Trauma, risk for: risk factors may include changes in cerebral perfusion with altered consciousness/loss of balance.

**snow blindness**
Sensory-perceptual alterations, visual may be related to altered status of sense organ (irritation of the conjunctiva, hyperemia), possibly evidenced by intolerance to light (photophobia) and decreased/loss of visual acuity.
Pain, [acute] may be related to irritation/vascular congestion of the conjunctiva, possibly evidenced by verbal reports, guarding/distraction behaviors, and self-focus.

Anxiety [specify level] may be related to situational crisis and threat to/change in health status, possibly evidenced by increased tension, apprehension, uncertainty, worry, restlessness, and focus on self.

**somatoform disorders**

Coping, individual, ineffective may be related to severe level of anxiety that is repressed, personal vulnerability, unmet dependency needs, fixation in earlier level of development, retarded ego development, and inadequate coping skills, possibly evidenced by verbalized inability to cope/problem solve, high illness rate, multiple somatic complaints of several years' duration, decreased functioning in social/occupational settings, narcissistic tendencies with total focus on self/physical symptoms, demanding behaviors, history of "doctor shopping" and refusal to attend therapeutic activities.

Pain, chronic may be related to severe level of repressed anxiety, low self-concept, unmet dependency needs, history of self or loved one having experienced a serious illness, possibly evidenced by verbal reports of severe/prolonged pain, guarded movement/protective behaviors, facial mask of pain, fear of reinjury, altered ability to continue previous activities, social withdrawal, demands for therapy/medication.

Social Interaction, impaired may be related to inability to engage in satisfying personal relationships, preoccupation with self and physical symptoms, altered state of wellness, chronic pain, and rejection by others, possibly evidenced by preoccupation with own thoughts, sad/dull affect, absence of supportive significant other(s), uncommunicative/withdrawn behavior, lack of eye contact, and seeking to be alone.

Violence, risk for, directed at self: risk factors may include depressed mood, feelings of powerlessness over physical condition, belief that he or she has serious illness, and hysterical response to chronic pain.

**sprain of ankle or foot**

Pain, [acute] may be related to trauma to/swelling in joint, possibly evidenced by verbal reports, guarding/distraction behaviors, self-focusing, and autonomic responses (changes in vital signs).

Physical mobility, impaired may be related to musculoskeletal injury, pain, and therapeutic restrictions, possibly evidenced by reluctance to attempt movement and limited range of motion.

**stapedectomy**

Trauma, risk for: risk factors may include increased middle-ear pressure with displacement of prosthesis and balancing difficulties/dizziness.

Infection, risk for: risk factors may include surgically traumatized tissue, invasive procedures, and environmental exposure to upper respiratory infections.

Pain, [acute] may be related to surgical trauma, edema formation, and presence of packing, possibly evidenced by verbal reports, guarding/distraction behaviors, and self-focus.

**substance dependency/abuse rehabilitation** (also refer to *drug overdose*)

Denial/Coping, individual, ineffective may be related to personal vulnerability, difficulty handling new situations, previous ineffective/inadequate coping skills with substitution of drug(s), and anxiety/fear, possibly evidenced by lack of acceptance that drug use is causing the present situation, use of manipulation to avoid responsibility for self, altered social patterns/participation, impaired adaptive behavior and problem-solving skills, employment difficulties, financial affairs in disarray, and decreased ability to handle stress of illness/hospitalization.

Powerlessness may be related to substance addiction with/without periods of abstinence, episodic compulsive indulgence, attempts at recovery, and lifestyle of helplessness, possibly evidenced by ineffective recovery attempts, statements of inability to stop behavior/requests for help, continuous/constant thinking about drug and/or obtaining drug, alteration in personal/occupational and social life.

Nutrition, altered, less than body requirements may be related to insufficient dietary intake to meet metabolic needs for psychologic/physiologic/economic reasons, possibly evidenced by weight less than normal for height/body build, decreased subcutaneous fat/muscle mass, reported altered taste sensation, poor muscle tone, sore/inflamed buccal cavity, lack of interest in food, and laboratory evidence of protein/vitamin deficiencies.

Family coping, ineffective: compromised or disabling/Caregiver role strain may be related to personal vulnerability of individual family members, codependency issues, situational crises, compromised social systems, family disorganization/role changes, prolonged/progressive condition that exhausts supportive capability of family members, significant other with chronically unexpressed feelings of guilt, anger, hostility, and despair, possibly evidenced by denial, lack of acceptance that drinking/drug use is causing the present situation, or belief that all problems are due to substance use, severely dysfunctional family (e.g., family violence, spouse/child abuse, separation/divorce), financial affairs in disarray, employment difficulties, altered social patterns/participation, significant other(s) demonstrating enabling or codependent behaviors.

Sexual dysfunction may be related to altered body function (neurologic damage and debilitating effects of drug use), changes in appearance, possibly evidenced by progressive interference with sexual functioning; significant degree of testicular atrophy, gynecomastia, or impotence/decreased sperm counts in men; and loss of body hair, thin/soft skin, spider angiomas, and amenorrhea/increase in miscarriages in women.

Family process, altered: alcoholism may be related to abuse/history of alcoholism, inadequate coping skills/lack of problem-solving skills, genetic predisposition/biochemical influences, possibly evidenced by feelings of anger, frustration, responsibility for alcoholic's behavior, guilt, vulnerability, disturbed family dynamics/deterioration in family relationships, family denial, closed communication systems, triangulating family relationships, manipulation, or blaming.

**surgery, general**

Anxiety [specify level]/Fear may be related to situational crisis, unfamiliarity with environment, change in health status, threat of death and separation from usual support systems, possibly evidenced by increased tension, apprehension, decreased self-assurance, fear of unspecific consequences, focus on self, sympathetic stimulation, and restlessness.

Knowledge deficit [learning need] regarding surgical procedure/expectation, postoperative routines/therapy, and self-care needs may be related to lack of information/misinterpretation, possibly evidenced by statements of concern, questions, and misconceptions.

Perioperative positioning injury, risk for: risk factors may include disorientation, immobilization, muscle weakness, obesity/edema.

Breathing pattern, ineffective, risk for: risk factors may include chemically induced muscular relaxation, perception/cognitive impairment, decreased energy, and incisional pain.

Fluid volume deficit, risk for: risk factors may include preoperative/postoperative fluid deprivation, blood loss, and excessive GI losses (vomiting/gastric suction).

Pain, [acute] may be related to intraoperative positioning, muscle retractions, and tissue trauma/presence of incision, tubes or drains, possibly evidenced by verbal reports, guarding/distraction/protective behaviors, self-focus, alteration in muscle tone, facial mask of pain, and autonomic responses (changes in vital signs).

**synovitis** (knee)

Pain, [acute] may be related to inflammation of synovial membrane of the joint with effusion, possibly evidenced by verbal reports, guarding/distraction behaviors, self-focus, and autonomic responses (changes in vital signs).

Physical mobility, impaired may be related to pain and decreased strength of joint, possibly evidenced by limited range of motion and reluctance to attempt movement.

**syphilis, congenital** (also refer to *sexually transmitted disease*)

Pain, [acute] may be related to inflammatory process, edema formation, and development of skin lesions, possibly evidenced by irritability/crying that may be increased with movement of extremities and autonomic responses (changes in vital signs).

Skin/Tissue integrity, impaired may be related to exposure to pathogens during vaginal delivery, possibly evidenced by disruption of skin surfaces and rhinitis.

Growth and development, altered may be related to effects of infectious process, possibly evidenced by altered physical growth and delay or difficulty performing skills typical of age group.

Knowledge deficit [learning need] regarding pathophysiology of condition, transmissibility, therapy needs, expected outcomes, and potential complications may be related to caretaker/parental lack of information/misinterpretation, possibly evidenced by statements of concern, questions, and misconceptions.

**syringomyelia**

Sensory-perceptual alterations (specify) may be related to altered sensory perception (neurologic lesion), possibly evidenced by change in usual response to stimuli and motor incoordination.

Anxiety [specify level]/Fear may be related to change in health status, threat of change in role functioning and socioeconomic status, and threat to self-concept, possibly evidenced by increased tension, apprehension, uncertainty, focus on self, and expressed concerns.

Physical mobility, impaired may be related to neuromuscular and sensory impairment, possibly evidenced by decreased muscle strength, control and mass, and impaired coordination.

Self-care deficit (specify) may be related to neuromuscular and sensory impairments, possibly evidenced by statement of inability to perform care tasks.

**Tay-Sachs disease**

Growth and development, altered may be related to effects of physical condition, possibly evidenced by altered physical growth, loss of/failure to acquire skills typical of age, flat affect, and decreased responses.

Sensory-perceptual alterations, visual may be related to neurologic deterioration of optic nerve, possibly evidenced by loss of visual acuity.

Grieving, anticipatory (family) may be related to expected eventual loss of infant, possibly evidenced by expressions of distress, denial, guilt, anger, and sorrow; choked feelings; changes in sleep/eating habits; and altered libido.

Powerlessness (family) may be related to absence of therapeutic interventions for progressive/fatal disease, possibly evidenced by verbal expressions of having no control over situation/outcome and depression over physical/mental deterioration.

Spiritual distress, risk for: risk factors may include challenged belief and value system by presence of fatal condition with racial/religious connotations and intense suffering.

Family coping, ineffective: compromised may be related to situational crisis, temporary preoccupation with managing emotional conflicts and personal suffering, family disorganization, and prolonged/progressive disease, possibly evidenced by preoccupation with personal reactions, expressed concern about reactions of other family members, inadequate support of one another, and altered communication patterns.

**thrombophlebitis**

Tissue perfusion, altered, peripheral may be related to interruption of venous blood flow, possibly evidenced by changes in skin color/temperature over affected area, development of edema, diminished peripheral pulses, slow capillary refill.

Pain, [acute/Discomfort] may be related to vascular inflammation/irritation and edema formation (accumulation of lactic acid), possibly evidenced by verbal reports, guarding/distraction behaviors, and self-focus.

Physical mobility, impaired, risk for: risk factors may include pain and discomfort and restrictive therapies/safety precautions.

Knowledge deficit [learning need] regarding pathophysiology of condition, therapy/self-care needs, and risk of embolization may be related to lack of information/misinterpretation, possibly evidenced by statements of concern, questions, inaccurate follow-through of instructions, and development of preventable complications.

**thrombosis, venous**

Refer to *thrombophlebitis*.

**thyroidectomy** (also refer to *hyperthyroidism; hypoparathyroidism; hypothyroidism*)

Airway clearance, ineffective, risk for: risk factors may include hematoma/edema formation with tracheal obstruction or laryngeal spasm.

Communication, impaired verbal may be related to tissue edema, pain/discomfort, and vocal cord injury/laryngeal nerve damage, possibly evidenced by impaired articulation, does not/cannot speak, and use of nonverbal cues or gestures.

Injury, risk for, tetany: risk factors may include chemical imbalance/excessive CNS stimulation.

Trauma, risk for, head/neck: risk factors may include loss of muscle control/support and position of suture line.

Pain, [acute] may be related to presence of surgical incision/manipulation of tissues/muscles, postoperative edema, possibly evidenced by verbal reports, guarding/distraction behaviors, narrowed focus, and autonomic responses (changes in vital signs).

**thyrotoxicoxis** (also refer to *hyperthyroidism*)

Cardiac output, decreased, risk for: risk factors may inlcude uncontrolled hypermetabolic state increasing cardiac workload, changes in venous return and systemic vascular resistance, and alteration in rate, rhythm, and electrical conduction.

Anxiety [specify level] may be related to physiologic factors/CNS stimulation (hypermetabolic state and pseudocatecholamine effect of thyroid hormones), possibly evidenced by increased feelings of apprehension, shakiness, loss of control, panic, changes in cognition, distortion of environmental stimuli, extraneous movements, restlessness, and tremors.

Thought processes, altered, risk for: risk factors may include physiologic changes (increased CNS stimulation/accelerated mental activity), and altered sleep patterns.

Knowledge deficit [learning need] regarding condition, treatment needs, and potential for complications/crisis situation may be related to lack of information/recall, misinterpretation, possibly evidenced by statements of concern, questions, misconceptions, and inaccurate follow-through of instructions.

**tic douloureux**

Refer to *neuralgia, trigeminal*.

**tonsillectomy**

Refer to *adenoidectomy*.

**tonsillitis**

Pain, [acute] may be related to inflammation of tonsils and effects of circulating toxins, possibly evidenced by verbal reports, guarding/distraction behaviors, reluctance/refusal to swallow, self-focus, and autonomic responses (changes in vital signs).

Hyperthermia may be related to presence of inflammatory process/hypermetabolic state and dehydration, possibly evidenced by increased body temperature, warm/flushed skin, and tachycardia.

Knowledge deficit [learning need] regarding cause/transmission, treatment needs, and potential complications may be related to lack of information/misinterpretation, possibly evidenced by statements of concern, questions, inaccurate follow-through of instructions, and recurrence of condition.

**total joint replacement**

Infection, risk for: risk factors may include inadequate primary defenses (broken skin, exposure of joint), inadequate secondary defenses/immunosuppression (long-term corticosteroid use), invasive procedures, surgical manipulation, implantation of foreign body, and decreased mobility.

Physical mobility, impaired may be related to pain and discomfort, musculoskeletal impairment, and surgery/restrictive therapies, possibly evidenced by reluctance to attempt movement, difficulty purposefully moving within the physical environment, reports of pain/discomfort on movement, limited range of motion, and decreased muscle strength/control.

Tissue perfusion, altered, peripheral, risk for: risk factors may include reduced arterial/venous blood flow, direct trauma to blood vessels, tissue edema, improper location/dislocation of prosthesis, and hypovolemia.

Pain, [acute] may be related to physical agents (traumatized tissues/surgical intervention, degeneration of joints, muscle spasms) and psychologic factors (anxiety, advanced age), possibly evidenced by verbal reports, distraction/guarding behaviors, self-focus, and autonomic responses (changes in vital signs).

**toxemia of pregnancy**

Refer to *pregnancy-induced hypertension*.

**toxic shock syndrome** (also refer to *septicemia*)

Hyperthermia may be related to inflammatory process/hypermetabolic state and dehydration, possibly evidenced by increased body temperature, warm/flushed skin, and tachycardia.

Fluid volume deficit [active loss] may be related to increased gastric losses (diarrhea, vomiting), fever/hypermetabolic state, and decreased intake, possibly evidenced by dry mucous membranes, increased pulse, hypotension, delayed venous filling, decreased/concentrated urine, and hemoconcentration.

Pain, [acute] may be related to inflammatory process, effects of circulating toxins, and skin disruptions, possibly evidenced by verbal reports, guarding/distraction behaviors, self-focus, and autonomic responses (changes in vital signs).

Skin/Tissue integrity, impaired may be related to effects of circulating toxins and dehydration, possibly evidenced by development of desquamating rash, hyperemia, and inflammation of mucous membranes.

**traction** (also refer to *cast*)

Pain, [acute] may be related to direct trauma to tissue/bone, muscle spasms, movement of bone fragments, edema, injury to soft tissue, traction/immobility device, anxiety, possibly evidenced by verbal reports, guarding/distraction behaviors, self-focus, and autonomic responses (changes in vital signs).

Physical mobility, impaired may be related to neuromuscular/skeletal impairment, pain, psychologic immobility, and therapeutic restrictions of movement, possibly evidenced by limited range of motion, inability to move purposefully in environment, reluctance to attempt movement, and decreased muscle strength/control.

Infection, risk for: risk factors may include invasive procedures (including insertion of foreign body through skin/bone), presence of traumatized tissue, and reduced activity with stasis of body fluids.

Diversional activity deficit may be related to length of hospitalization and environmental lack of usual activity, possibly evidenced by statements of boredom, restlessness, and irritability.

**trichinosis**

Pain, [acute] may be related to parasitic invasion of muscle tissues, edema of upper eyelids, small localized hemorrhages, and development of urticaria, possibly evidenced by verbal reports, guarding/distraction behaviors (restlessness), and autonomic responses (changes in vital signs).

Fluid volume deficit [active loss] may be related to hypermetabolic state (fever, diaphoresis), excessive gastric losses (vomiting, diarrhea), and decreased intake/difficulty swallowing, possibly evidenced by dry mucous membranes, decreased skin turgor, hypotension, decreased venous filling, decreased/concentrated urine, and hemoconcentration.

Breathing pattern, ineffective may be related to myositis of the diaphragm and intercostal muscles, possibly evidenced by resulting changes in respiratory depth, tachypnea, dyspnea, and abnormal ABGs.

Knowledge deficit [learning need] regarding cause/prevention of condition, therapy needs, and possible complications may be related to lack of information/misinterpretation, possibly evidenced by statements of concern, questions, and misconceptions.

**tuberculosis** (pulmonary)

Infection, risk for spread/reactivation: risk factors may include inadequate primary defenses (decreased ciliary action/stasis of secretions, tissue destruction/extension of infection), lowered resistance/suppressed inflammatory response, malnutrition, environmental exposure, and insufficient knowledge to avoid exposure to pathogens, or inadequate therapeutic intervention.

Airway clearance, ineffective may be related to thick, viscous or bloody secretions, fatigue/poor cough effort, and tracheal/pharyngeal edema, possibly evidenced by abnormal respiratory rate, rhythm, and depth; adventitious breath sounds (rhonchi, wheezes); stridor and dyspnea.

Gas exchange, impaired, risk for: risk factors may include decrease in effective lung surface, atelectasis, destruction of alveolar-capillary membrane, bronchial edema, thick, viscous secretions.

Activity intolerance may be related to imbalance between oxygen supply and demand, possibly evidenced by reports of fatigue, weakness, and exertional dyspnea.

Nutrition, altered, less than body requirements may be related to inability to ingest adequate nutrients (anorexia, effects of drug therapy, fatigue, insufficient financial resources), possibly evidenced by weight loss, reported lack of interest in food/altered taste sensation, and poor muscle tone.

Noncompliance (specify) [Compliance, altered], risk for: risk factors may include lengthy therapy requirements even after remission of symptoms as well as side effects of therapy.

**tympanoplasty**
Refer to *stapedectomy*.

**typhus** (tick-borne fever/Rocky Mountain spotted fever)
Hyperthermia may be related to generalized inflammatory process (vasculitis), possibly evidenced by increased body temperature, warm/flushed skin, and tachycardia.
Pain, [acute] may be related to generalized vasculitis and edema formation, possibly evidenced by verbal reports, guarding/distraction behaviors, self-focus, and autonomic responses (changes in vital signs).
Tissue perfusion, altered (specify) may be related to reduction/interruption of blood flow (generalized vasculitis/thrombi formation), possibly evidenced by reports of headache/abdominal pain, changes in mentation, and areas of peripheral ulceration/necrosis.

**ulcer, decubitus**
Skin/Tissue integrity, impaired may be related to altered circulation, nutritional deficit, fluid imbalance, impaired physical mobility, irritation of body excretions/secretions, and sensory impairments, evidenced by tissue damage/destruction.
Pain, [acute] may be related to destruction of protective skin layers and exposure of nerves, possibly evidenced by verbal reports, distraction behaviors, and self-focus.
Infection, risk for: risk factors may include broken/traumatized tissue, increased environmental exposure, and nutritional deficits.

**ulcer, peptic** (acute)
Fluid volume deficit [active loss] may be related to vascular losses (hemorrhage), possibly evidenced by hypotension, tachycardia, delayed capillary refill, changes in mentation, restlessness, concentrated/decreased urine, pallor, diaphoresis, and hemoconcentration.
Tissue perfusion, altered (specify), risk for: risk factors may include hypovolemia.
Fear/Anxiety [specify level] may be related to change in health status and threat of death, possibly evidenced by increased tension, restlessness, irritability, fearfulness, trembling, tachycardia, diaphoresis, lack of eye contact, focus on self, verbalization of concerns, withdrawal, and panic or attack behavior.
Pain, [acute] may be related to caustic irritation/destruction of gastric tissues, possibly evidenced by verbal reports, distraction behaviors, self-focus, and autonomic responses (changes in vital signs).
Knowledge deficit [learning need] regarding condition, therapy/self-care needs, and potential complications may be related to lack of information/recall, misinterpretation, possibly evidenced by statements of concern, questions, misconceptions; inaccurate follow-through of instructions, and development of preventable complications/recurrence of condition.

**unconsciousness** (coma)
Suffocation, risk for: risk factors may include cognitive impairment/loss of protective reflexes and purposeful movement.
Trauma, risk for: risk factors may include cognitive impairment, generalized weakness/reduced coordination, and absence of purposeful movement.
Self-care deficit, total may be related to cognitive impairment and absence of purposeful activity, possibly evidenced by inability to perform activities of daily living.
Tissue perfusion, altered, cerebral, risk for: risk factors may include reduced or interrupted arterial/venous blood flow (direct injury, edema formation).
Infection, risk for: risk factors may include stasis of body fluids (oral, pulmonary, urinary), invasive procedures, and nutritional deficits.

**urinary diversion**
Skin integrity, impaired, risk for: risk factors may include absence of sphincter at stoma, character/flow of urine from stoma, reaction to product/chemicals, and improper fitting of appliance or removal of adhesive.
Body image/Self-esteem disturbance: related factors may include biophysical factors (presence of stoma, loss of control of urine elimination) and psychosocial factors (altered body structure, disease process/associated treatment regimen [cancer]), possibly evidenced by verbalization of change in body image, fear of rejection/reaction of others, negative feelings about body, not touching/looking at stoma, refusal to participate in care.

Pain, [acute] may be related to physical factors (disruption of skin/tissues, presence of incisions/drains), biologic factors (activity of disease process, such as cancer, trauma), and psychologic factors (fear, anxiety), possibly evidenced by verbal reports, self-focusing, guarding/distraction behaviors, restlessness, and autonomic responses (changes in vital signs).

Urinary elimination, altered may be related to surgical diversion, tissue trauma, and post-operative edema, possibly evidenced by loss of continence, changes in amount and character of urine, and urinary retention.

**urolithiasis** (urinary calculi)

Pain, [acute] may be related to distention, trauma, and edema formation in sensitive tissue, cellular ischemia, possibly evidenced by verbal reports, guarding/distraction behaviors, self-focus, and autonomic responses (changes in vital signs).

Urinary elimination, altered may be related to edema formation and irritation/inflammation of ureteral and bladder tissues, possibly evidenced by urgency, frequency, retention, and hematuria.

Fluid volume deficit, risk for: risk factors may include stimulation of renal-intestinal reflexes causing nausea, vomiting, and diarrhea; changes in urinary output, postoperative diuresis, and decreased intake.

**uterine bleeding, abnormal**

Anxiety [specify level] may be related to perceived change in health status and unknown etiology, possibly evidenced by apprehension, uncertainty, fear of unspecified consequences, expressed concerns, and focus on self.

Activity intolerance may be related to imbalance between oxygen supply and demand/decreased oxygen-carrying capacity of blood (anemia), possibly evidenced by reports of fatigue/weakness.

**uterus, rupture of, in pregnancy**

Fluid volume deficit [active loss] may be related to excessive vascular losses, possibly evidenced by hypotension, increased pulse rate, decreased venous filling, and decreased urine output.

Cardiac output, decreased may be related to decreased preload (hypovolemia), possibly evidenced by cold/clammy skin, decreased peripheral pulses, variations in hemodynamic readings, tachycardia, and cyanosis.

Pain, [acute] may be related to tissue trauma and irritation of accumulating blood, possibly evidenced by verbal reports, guarding/distraction behaviors, self-focus, and autonomic responses (changes in vital signs).

Anxiety [specify level] may be related to threat of death of self/fetus, interpersonal contagion, physiological response (release of catecholamines), possibly evidenced by fearful/scared affect, sympathetic stimulation, stated fear of unspecified consequences, and expressed concerns.

**vaginismus**

Pain, [acute] may be related to muscle spasm and hyperesthesia of the nerve supply to vaginal mucous membrane, possibly evidenced by verbal reports, distraction behaviors, and self-focus.

Sexual dysfunction may be related to physical and/or psychologic alteration in function (severe spasms of vaginal muscles), possibly evidenced by verbalization of problem, inability to achieve desired satisfaction, and alteration in relationship with significant other.

**vaginitis**

Tissue integrity, impaired may be related to irritation/inflammation and mechanical trauma (scratching) of sensitive tissues, possibly evidenced by damaged/destroyed tissue, presence of lesions.

Pain, [acute] may be related to localized inflammation and tissue trauma, possibly evidenced by verbal reports, distraction behaviors, and self-focus.

Knowledge deficit [learning need] regarding hygienic/therapy needs and sexual behaviors/transmission of organisms may be related to lack of information/misinterpretation, possibly evidenced by statements of concern, questions, and misconceptions.

**varices, esophageal** (also refer to *ulcer, peptic [acute]*)
Fluid volume deficit [active loss] may be related to excessive vascular loss, reduced intake, and gastric losses (vomiting), possibly evidenced by hypotension, tachycardia, decreased venous filling, and decreased/concentrated urine.
Anxiety [specify level]/Fear may be related to change in health status and threat of death, possibly evidenced by increased tension/apprehension, sympathetic stimulation, restlessness, focus on self, and expressed concerns.

**varicose veins**
Pain, chronic may be related to venous insufficiency and stasis, possibly evidenced by verbal reports.
Body image disturbance may be related to change in structure (presence of enlarged, discolored tortuous superficial leg veins), possibly evidenced by hiding affected parts and negative feelings about body.
Skin/Tissue integrity, impaired, risk for: risk factors may include altered circulation/venous stasis and edema formation.

**venereal disease**
Refer to *sexually transmitted disease*.

**Wilms' tumor** (also refer to *cancer*; *chemotherapy*)
Anxiety [specify level]/Fear may be related to change in environment and interaction patterns with family members and threat of death with family transmission and contagion of concerns, possibly evidenced by fearful/scared affect, distress, crying, insomnia, and sympathetic stimulation.
Injury, risk for: risk factors may include nature of tumor (vascular, mushy with very thin covering) with increased danger of metastasis when manipulated.
Family processes, altered may be related to situational crisis of life-threatening illness, possibly evidenced by a family system that has difficulty meeting physical, emotional, and spiritual needs of its members, and inability to deal with traumatic experience effectively.
Diversional activity deficit may be related to environmental lack of age-appropriate activity (including activity restrictions) and length of hospitalization/treatment, possibly evidenced by restlessness, crying, lethargy, and acting-out behavior.

**wound, bullet** (depends on site and speed/character of bullet)
Fluid volume deficit, risk for: risk factors may include excessive vascular losses, altered intake/restrictions.
Pain, [acute] may be related to destruction of tissue (including organ and musculoskeletal), surgical repair, and therapeutic interventions, possibly evidenced by verbal reports, guarding/distraction behaviors, self-focus, and autonomic responses (changes in vital signs).
Infection, risk for: risk factors may include tissue destruction and increased environmental exposure, invasive procedures, and decreased hemoglobin.
Post-trauma response, risk for: risk factors may include nature of incident (catastrophic accident, assault, suicide attempt) and possibly injury/death of other(s) involved.

# Appendix 21–5 Nursing Diagnoses Through the 12th NANDA Conference in Alphabetical Order

Information appearing in brackets has been added by the authors to clarify and facilitate the use of nursing diagnoses.

A "RISK FOR" diagnosis is *not* evidenced by signs and symptoms, because the problem has not yet occurred, and nursing interventions are directed at prevention. Therefore, *risk* factors that are present are noted instead.

New nursing diagnoses from the NANDA 11th Conference (1994) and 12th Conference (1996) appear on page 2331.

## ACTIVITY INTOLERANCE [SPECIFY LEVEL]

*Diagnostic Division: Activity/Rest*

**Definition:** A state in which an individual has insufficient physiological or psychological energy to endure or complete required or desired daily activities.

### RELATED FACTORS

Generalized weakness; Sedentary lifestyle; Imbalance between oxygen supply and demand; Bedrest or immobility; [Cognitive deficits/emotional status; underlying disease process/depression]

### DEFINING CHARACTERISTICS

**Subjective**

Report of fatigue or weakness; Exertional discomfort or dyspnea; [Pain, weakness, vertigo, extreme stress]; [Verbalizes no desire and/or lack of interest in activity]

**Objective**

Abnormal heart rate or blood pressure response to activity; Electrocardiographic changes reflecting dysrhythmias or ischemia; [Pallor]; [Cyanosis]

## ACTIVITY INTOLERANCE, RISK FOR

*Diagnostic Division: Activity/Rest*

**Definition:** A state in which an individual is at risk of experiencing insufficient physiologic or psychologic energy to endure or complete required or desired daily activities.

### RISK FACTORS

History of previous intolerance; Presence of circulatory/respiratory problems; Deconditioned status; Inexperience with the activity; [Diagnosis of progressive disease state/debilitating condition such as cancer, multiple sclerosis; extensive surgical procedures]; [Verbalized reluctance/inability to perform expected activity]

## ADAPTIVE CAPACITY: INTRACRANIAL, DECREASED

*Diagnostic Division: Circulation*

**Definition:** A clinical state in which intracranial fluid dynamic mechanisms that normally compensate for increases in intracranial volumes are compromised, resulting in repeated, disproportionate increases in intracranial pressure (ICP) in response to a variety of noxious and non-noxious stimuli.

### RELATED FACTORS

Brain injuries; Sustained increase in ICP greater than or equal to 10 to 15 mm Hg; Decreased cerebral perfusion pressure less than or equal to 50 to 60 mm Hg; Systemic hypotension with intracranial hypertension

### DEFINING CHARACTERISTICS

**Objective**

Repeated increases in ICP of greater than 10 mm Hg for more than 5 min following a variety of external stimuli; Disproportionate increases in ICP following single environmental or nursing maneuver stimulus; Elevated P2 ICP waveform; Volume pressure response test variation (volume-pressure ratio greater than 2, pressure equals volume index less than 10); Baseline ICP equal to or greater than 10 mm Hg; Wide-amplitude ICP waveform

## ADJUSTMENT, IMPAIRED

*Diagnostic Division: Ego Integrity*

**Definition:** The state in which the individual is unable to modify his/her lifestyle or behavior in a manner consistent with a change in health status.

### RELATED FACTORS

Disability requiring change in lifestyle; Inadequate support systems; Impaired cognition, sensory overload; Assault to self-esteem, altered locus of control; Incomplete grieving [severe emotional loss] [Physical and/or learning disability] [Life-threatening condition or disease]

### DEFINING CHARACTERISTICS

**Subjective**

Verbalization of nonacceptance of health status change

**Objective**
Nonexistent or unsuccessful ability to be involved in problem-solving or goal setting; Lack of movement toward independence; Extended period of shock, disbelief, or anger regarding health status change; Lack of future-oriented thinking; [Lack of ability to limit expectations of self]

## AIRWAY CLEARANCE, INEFFECTIVE

*Diagnostic Division: Respiration*

**Definition:** A state in which an individual is unable to clear secretions or obstructions from the respiratory tract.

### RELATED FACTORS
Tracheobronchial infection, obstruction, secretion; Sputum, tenacious and copious; Decreased energy and fatigue; Perceptual/cognitive impairment; Trauma

### DEFINING CHARACTERISTICS
**Subjective**
Verbal communication of difficulty with sputum; Communicates chest congestion

**Objective**
Abnormal breath sounds; crackles, gurgles, wheezes; Cough, ineffective or absent

## ANXIETY [MILD, MODERATE, SEVERE, PANIC]

*Diagnostic Division: Ego Integrity*

**Definition:** A vague uneasy feeling, the source of which is often nonspecific or unknown to the individual.

### RELATED FACTORS
Unconscious conflict about essential values, [beliefs], and goals of life; Situational and [or] maturational crises; Interpersonal transmission and contagion; Threat to self-concept [perceived or actual], [unconscious conflict]; Threat of death [perceived or actual]; Threat to or change in health status [progressive/debilitating disease, terminal illness], role functioning, environment [safety], interaction patterns [socioeconomic status]; Unmet needs; [Positive or negative self-talk]; [Physiologic factors, such as hyperthyroidism, pheochromocytoma, use of steroids]

### DEFINING CHARACTERISTICS
**Subjective**
Increased tension; Painful and persistent increased helplessness; Scared; Shakiness; Regretful; Overexcited; Rattled; Distressed; Apprehension; Uncertainty; Fearful; Feelings of inadequacy; Fear of unspecific consequences; Expressed concern regarding changes in life events; Anxious; Worried; Jittery; [Somatic complaints, especially chest, back, and neck pain]; [Sleeplessness]; [Sense of impending doom]; [Hopelessness] [Forgetfulness, inability to concentrate]

**Objective**
Sympathetic stimulation: cardiovascular excitation, superficial vasoconstriction, pupil dilation; Increased wariness; Extraneous movements: foot shuffling; hand/arm movements; Increased perspiration; Restlessness; Insomnia; Glancing about; poor eye contact; Trembling; hand tremors; Facial tension; Voice quivering; Focus on self; [crying, tearfulness]; [Urinary frequency]; [Repetitive questioning]; [Pacing; purposeless activity]; [Impaired functioning; immobility]

## ASPIRATION, RISK FOR

*Diagnostic Division: Respiration*

**Definition:** The state in which an individual is at risk for entry of gastrointestinal secretions, oropharyngeal sections, [or exogenous food] or solids or fluids into tracheobronchial passages [due to dysfunction or absence of normal protective mechanisms].

### RISK FACTORS
Reduced level of consciousness; Depressed cough and gag reflexes; Presence of tracheostomy or endotracheal tube; [Overinflated tracheostomy/endotracheal tube cuff]; [Inadequate tracheostomy/endotracheal tube cuff inflation]; Gastrointestinal tubes; Tube feedings/medication administration; Situation hindering elevation of upper body [weakness, paralysis]; Increased intragastric pressure; Increased gastric residual; Decreased gastrointestinal motility; Delaying gastric emptying; Impaired swallowing [owing to inability of the epiglottis and true vocal cords to move to close off tracheal]; Facial/oral/neck surgery or trauma; Wired jaws; Incomplete

lower esophageal sphincter [hiatal hernia or other esophageal disease affecting stomach valve function]

## BODY IMAGE DISTURBANCE

*Diagnostic Division: Ego Integrity*

**Definition:** Disruption in the way one perceives one's body image.

### RELATED FACTORS

Biophysical [physical trauma/mutilation, pregnancy, physical change caused by biochemical agents (drugs), dependence on machine]; Psychosocial; Cultural or spiritual; [Cognitive/perceptual]; [Significance of body part or functioning with regard to age, sex, developmental level, or basic human needs]; [Maturational changes]

### DEFINING CHARACTERISTICS

A or B must be present to justify the diagnosis of Body Image Disturbance. A = verbal response to actual or perceived change in structure and/or function; B = nonverbal response to actual or perceived change in structure and/or function. The following clinical manifestations may be used to validate the presence of A or B:

**Subjective**

Change in lifestyle; Fear of rejection or of reaction by others; Focus on past strength, function, or appearance; Negative feelings about body; Feelings of helplessness, hopelessness, or powerlessness; Preoccupation with change or loss; [depersonalization/grandiosity]; Refusal to verify actual change; Emphasis on remaining strengths, heightened achievement; Personalization of part or loss by name; Depersonalization of part or loss by impersonal pronouns; Extension of body boundary to incorporate environmental objects

**Objective**

Missing body part; Actual change in structure and/or function; Not looking at/not touching body part; Trauma to nonfunctioning part; Change in ability to estimate spatial relationship of body to environment; Hiding or overexposing body part (intentional or unintentional); Change in social involvement; [Inability to differentiate internal/external stimuli/loss of ego boundaries]; [Inability to accept change in body boundaries (e.g., stroke patient unaware of paralysis)]; [Aggression, low frustration tolerance level]

## BODY TEMPERATURE, ALTERED, RISK FOR

*Diagnostic Division: Safety*

**Definition:** The state in which the individual is at risk for failure to maintain body temperature within normal range.

### RISK FACTORS

Extremes of age; Extremes of weight; Exposure to cold/cool or warm/hot environments; Dehydration; Inactivity or vigorous activity; Medications causing vasoconstriction/vasodilation, altered metabolic rate, sedation, [use or overdose of certain drugs or exposure to anesthesia]; Inappropriate clothing for environmental temperature; Illness or trauma affecting temperature regulation; [Infections, systemic or localized]; [Neoplasms, tumors, collagen vascular disease]

## BOWEL INCONTINENCE

*Diagnostic Division: Elimination*

**Definition:** A state in which an individual experiences a change in normal bowel habits characterized by involuntary passage of stool.

### RELATED FACTORS

Gastrointestinal disorders [fecal impaction]; Neuromuscular disorders; Colostomy; Loss of renal sphincter control; Impaired cognition; [Severe anxiety, depression]

### DEFINING CHARACTERISTICS

**Objective**

Involuntary passage of stool

## BREASTFEEDING, EFFECTIVE

*Diagnostic Division: Food/Fluid*

**Definition:** The state in which a mother-infant dyad/family exhibits adequate proficiency and satisfaction with breastfeeding process.

**RELATED FACTORS**

Basic breastfeeding knowledge; Normal breast structure; Normal infant oral structure; Infant gestational age greater than 34 weeks; Support sources [available]; Maternal confidence

**DEFINING CHARACTERISTICS**

**Subjective**

Maternal verbalization of satisfaction with the breastfeeding process

**Objective**

Mother able to position infant at breast to promote a successful latch-on response; Infant is content after feedings; Regular and sustained sucking at the breast (8 to 10 times/24 hours); Appropriate infant weight patterns for age; Signs and/or symptoms of oxytocin release (let-down or milk ejection reflex); [Infant] Soft stools; over 6 wet diapers per day of unconcentrated urine; Eagerness of infant to nurse

## BREASTFEEDING, INEFFECTIVE

*Diagnostic Division: Food/Fluid*

**Definition:** The state in which a mother, infant, or child experiences dissatisfaction or difficulty with the breastfeeding process.

**RELATED FACTORS**

Prematurity; Infant anomaly; Maternal breast anomaly; Previous breast surgery; Previous history of breastfeeding failure; Infant receiving [numerous or repeated] supplemental feedings with artificial nipple; Poor infant sucking reflex; Nonsupportive partner/family; Knowledge deficit; Interruption in breastfeeding; Maternal anxiety or ambivalence; Painful nipples/breast engorgement

**DEFINING CHARACTERISTICS**

**Subjective**

Unsatisfactory breastfeeding process; Persistence of sore nipples beyond the first week of breastfeeding; Insufficient emptying of each breast per feeding; Actual or perceived inadequate milk supply

**Objective**

Observable signs of inadequate infant intake [decrease in number of wet diapers, inappropriate weight loss or inadequate gain]; Nonsustained or insufficient opportunity for suckling at the breast; Infant inability [failure] to attach on to maternal breast correctly; Infant arching and crying at the breasts; Resisting latching on; Infant exhibiting fussiness and crying within the first hour after breastfeeding; Unresponsive to other comfort measures; No observable signs of oxytocin release

## BREASTFEEDING, INTERRUPTED

*Diagnostic Division: Food/Fluid*

**Definition:** A break in the continuity of the breastfeeding process as a result of inability or inadvisability to put a baby to breast for feeding.

**RELATED FACTORS**

Maternal or infant illness; Prematurity; Maternal employment; Contraindications to breastfeeding (e.g., drugs, true breast milk jaundice); Need to abruptly wean infant

**DEFINING CHARACTERISTICS**

**Subjective**

Infant does not receive nourishment at the breast for some or all of feedings; Maternal desire to maintain lactation and provide (or eventually provide) her breast milk for her infant's nutritional needs; Lack of knowledge regarding expression and storage of breast milk

**Objective**

Separation of mother and infant

## BREATHING PATTERN, INEFFECTIVE

*Diagnostic Division: Respiration*

**Definition:** The state in which the rate, depth, timing, rhythm, or chest/abdominal wall excursion during inspiration, expiration, or both does not maintain optimum ventilation for the individual.

**RELATED FACTORS**

Neuromuscular/musculoskeletal impairment; Anxiety; Pain; Perception or cognitive impairment; Decreased energy and fatigue

**DEFINING CHARACTERISTICS**

**Subjective**

Dyspnea (shortness of breath)

**Objective**

Respiratory rate: adults (14 or older), less than 11 or greater than 24; infants, less than 25 or greater than 60; ages 1 through 4, less than 20 or greater than 30, ages 5 to 14, less than 15 or greater than 25; Depth of breathing: adults, VT less than 200 ml or greater than 500 ml/kg at rest; infants 6–8 ml/kg at rest; Timing ratio of inspiration and expiration (if measured): inspiratory time less than 1:2 or greater than 2:4; fractional inspiratory time less than .36 or greater than .47; inspiration longer than expiration; Irregular breathing rhythm (e.g., apnea, frequent signs, use of accessory breathing muscles inappropriate to level of activity, asynchronous thoracoabdominal motion); Grunting; Nasal flaring; Paradoxical breathing patterns; Use of accessory muscles; Altered chest excursion

## CARDIAC OUTPUT, DECREASED

*Diagnostic Division: Circulation*

**Definition:** A state in which the blood pumped by the heart is inadequate to meet the metabolic demands of the body.

NOTE: In a hypermetabolic state, although cardiac output may be within normal range, it may still be inadequate to meet the needs of the body's tissues. Cardiac output and tissue perfusion are interrelated, although there are differences. When cardiac output is decreased, tissue perfusion problems will develop; however, tissue perfusion problems can exist without decreased cardiac output.

**RELATED FACTORS**

To be developed by NANDA (Mechanical: alteration in preload [e.g., decreased venous return, altered myocardial contractility]; afterload [e.g., alteration in systemic vascular resistance]; inotropic changes in heart. Electrical: alterations in rate, rhythm, conduction. Structural [e.g., ventricular-septal rupture, ventricular aneurysm, papillary muscle rupture, valvular disease.])

NOTE: These factors were identified when this diagnosis was originally accepted and have been retained here to assist the user until NANDA completes its work.

**DEFINING CHARACTERISTICS**

**Subjective**

Fatigue; Dyspnea; Orthopnea/PND; Chest pain

**Objective**

Variations in blood pressure readings; Arrhythmias; Jugular vein distention; Skin color changes; Crackles; Oliguria; Decreased peripheral pulses; Cold, clammy skin; Restlessness; Weight gain; Wheezing; Edema; Elevated PA pressures; Increased respiratory rate; Use of accessory muscules; ECG changes; Ejection factor < 40%; Abnormal chest x-ray (pulmonary vascular congestion); Abnormal cardiac enzymes; Altered mental status

**OTHER POSSIBLE CHARACTERISTICS**

**Subjective**

Syncope; Vertigo; Weakness; Shortness of breath; [Angina]

**Objective**

Edema; Change in mental status; Frothy sputum; Gallop rhythm, abnormal heart sounds; Cough; [Liver engorgement/ascites]

## CAREGIVER ROLE STRAIN

*Diagnostic Division: Social Interaction*

**Definition:** A caregiver's felt difficulty in performing the family caregiver role.

**RELATED FACTORS**

**Pathophysiologic/Physiologic**

Illness severity of the care receiver; Addiction or codependency; Premature birth/Congenital defect; Discharge of family member with significant home care needs; Caregiver health impairment; Unpredictable illness course or instability in the care receiver's health; Caregiver is female

**Developmental**

Caregiver is not developmentally ready for caregiver role (e.g., young adult needing to provide care for a middle-aged parent); Developmental delay or retardation of the care receiver or caregiver

**Psychosocial**

Psychosocial or cognitive problems in care receiver; Marginal family adaptation or dysfunction prior to the caregiving situation; Marginal caregiver's coping patterns; Past history of poor relationship between caregiver and care receiver; Care receiver exhibits deviant, bizarre behavior; Caregiver is spouse

**Situational**

Presence of abuse or violence; Presence of situational stressors that normally affect families, such as significant loss, disaster, or crisis, poverty or economic vulnerability, major life events (e.g., birth, hospitalization, leaving home, returning home, marriage, divorce, [changes in] employment, retirement, death); Duration of caregiving required; Inadequate physical environment for providing care (e.g., housing, transportation, community services, equipment) Family/caregiver isolation; Lack of respite and recreation for caregiver; Inexperience with caregiving; Caregiver's competing role commitments; Complexity/amount of caregiving tasks

NOTE: The presence of this problem may encompass other numerous problems/high-risk concerns such as Diversional Activity deficit; Sleep Pattern disturbance; Fatigue; Anxiety; Coping, Individual, ineffective; Family coping; Decisional Conflict; Denial, ineffective; Grieving, anticipatory/[actual]; Hopelessness; Powerlessness; Spiritual Distress; Health Maintenance, altered; Home Maintenance Management, impaired; Sexuality Patterns, altered; Family Coping: potential for growth; Family Processes, altered; Social Isolation. Careful attention to data gathering will identify and clarify the client's specific needs, which can then be coordinated under this single diagnostic label.]

**DEFINING CHARACTERISTICS**

**Subjective**

80% of caregivers report one or more of these defining characteristics: Do not have enough resources to provide the care needed; Find it hard to do specific caregiving activities; Worry about such things as the care receiver's health and emotional state, having to put the care receiver in an institution, and who will care for the care receiver if something should happen to the caregiver; [Believe] feel that caregiving interferes with other important roles in their lives [such as being a worker, parent, spouse, or friend]; Feel loss because the care receiver is like a different person compared to before caregiving began or, in the case of a child, that the care receiver was never the child the caregiver expected; Feel family conflict around issues of providing care [e.g., believing that other family members do not do their share in providing care to the care receiver or that not enough appreciation is shown for what the caregiver does]; Feel stress or nervousness in their relationship with the care receiver; Feel depressed

**Objective**

[Inability to meet role expectations/basic needs of caregiver and/or care receiver]; [Disorderly surroundings, tasks not done (e.g., bills unpaid)]; [Alteration in social participation]; Authors' note: Although objective characteristics were not included in the NANDA diagnosis, if caregiver is in a state of denial, subjective statements may not be made by caregiver; however, statements of care receiver and observations of family members and/or other healthcare providers may indicate presence of problem.

## CAREGIVER ROLE STRAIN, RISK FOR

*Diagnostic Division: Social Interaction*

**Definition:** A caregiver is vulnerable for felt difficulty in performing the family caregiver role.

**RISK FACTORS**

**Pathophysiologic**

Illness severity of the care receiver; Addiction or codependency; Premature birth/Congenital defect; Discharge of family member with significant home care needs; Caregiver health impairment; Unpredictable illness course or instability in the care receiver's health; Caregiver is female; Psychological or cognitive problems in care receiver

**Developmental**

Caregiver is not developmentally ready for caregiver role (e.g., young adult needing to provide care for a middle-aged parent); Developmental delay or retardation of the care receiver or caregiver

**Psychosocial**

Marginal family adaptation or dysfunction prior to the caregiving situation; Marginal caregiver's coping patterns; Past history of poor relationship between caregiver and care receiver; Care receiver exhibits deviant, bizarre behavior; Caregiver is spouse

**Situational**

Presence of abuse or violence; Presence of situational stressors that normally affect families, such as significant loss, disaster, or crisis, poverty or economic vulnerability, major life events (e.g., birth, hospitalization, leaving home, returning home, marriage, divorce, [change in] employment, retirement, death); Duration of caregiving required; Inadequate physical environment for providing care (e.g., housing, transportation, community services, equipment); Family/caregiver isolation; Lack of respite and recreation for caregiver; Inexperience with caregiving; Caregiver's competing role commitments; Complexity/amount of caregiving tasks

## COMMUNICATION, IMPAIRED, VERBAL

*Diagnostic Division: Social Interaction*

**Definition:** The state in which an individual experiences a decreased or absent ability to use or to understand language in human interaction.

### RELATED FACTORS

Decrease in circulation to brain; Brain tumor; Anatomic deficit, cleft palate; Developmental or age-related; Physical barrier (tracheostomy, intubation); Psychologic barriers, psychosis, lack of stimuli [depression, panic, anger]; Cultural difference; [Drug intake, chemical imbalance]

### DEFINING CHARACTERISTICS

**Subjective**

[Reports of difficulty expressing self]

**Objective**

Unable to speak dominant language; Speaks or verbalizes with difficulty; Does not or cannot speak; Disorientation; Stuttering, slurring; Dyspnea; Difficulty forming words or sentences; Difficulty expressing thought verbally; Inappropriate verbalization [incessant, loose association of ideas, flight of ideas]; [Inability to modulate speech]; [Message inappropriate to content]; [Use of nonverbal cues, (e.g., facial expression, gestures, pleading eyes, turning away)]; [Frustration, anger, hostility]

## COMMUNITY COPING, ENHANCED, POTENTIAL FOR

*Diagnostic Division: Social Interaction*

**Definition:** A pattern of community activities for adaptation and problem solving that is satisfactory for meeting the demands or needs of the community but can be improved for management of current and future problems/stressors.

### RELATED FACTORS

Social supports available; Resources available for problem solving; Community has a sense of power to manage stressors

### DEFINING CHARACTERISTICS

**Objective**

Deficits in one or more characteristics that indicate effective coping; Active planning by community for predicted stressors; Active problem solving by community when faced with issues; Agreement that community is responsible for stress management; Positive communication among community members; Positive communication between community/aggregates and larger community; Programs available for recreation and relaxation; Resources sufficient for managing stressors

## COMMUNITY COPING, INEFFECTIVE

*Diagnostic Division: Social Interaction*

**Definition:** A pattern of community activities for adaptation and problem solving that is unsatisfactory for meeting the demands or needs of the community. [Community is defined as "a group of people with a common identity or perspective, occupying space during a given period of time, and functioning through a social system to meet its needs within a larger social environment."]

### RELATED FACTORS

Deficits in social support; Inadequate resources for problem solving; Powerlessness

### DEFINING CHARACTERISTICS

**Subjective**

Community does not meet its own expectations; Expressed difficulty in meeting demands for change; Expressed vulnerability; Stressors perceived as excessive

**Objective**

Deficits of community participation; Deficits in communication methods; Excessive community conflicts; High illness rates

## CONFUSION, ACUTE

*Diagnostic Division: Neurosensory*

**Definition:** The abrupt onset of a cluster of global, transient changes and disturbances in attention, cognition, psychomotor activity level of consciousness, and/or sleep/wake cycle.

### RELATED FACTORS

Over 60 years of age; Dementia; Alcohol abuse, drug abuse; Delirium [including febrile epilepticum (following or instead of an epileptic attack), toxic and traumatic]; [Medication reaction/interaction; anesthesia/surgery; metabolic imbalances]; [Exacerbation of a chronic illness, hypoxemia]; [Severe pain]; [Sleep deprivation]

NOTE: Although no time frame is presented to aid in differentiating acute from chronic confusion, the definition of chronic confusion identifies an irreversible state. Therefore, our belief is that acute confusion is potentially reversible.

### DEFINING CHARACTERISTICS

**Subjective**

Hallucinations [Visual/auditory]; [Exaggerated emotional responses]

**Objective**

Fluctuation in cognition; Fluctuation in sleep/wake cycle; Fluctuation in level of consciousness; Fluctuation in psychomotor activity [tremors, body movement]; Increased agitation or restlessness; Misperceptions, [inappropriate responses]; Lack of motivation to initiate and/or follow through with goal-directed or purposeful behavior

## CONFUSION, CHRONIC

*Diagnostic Division: Neurosensory*

**Definition:** An irreversible, long-standing, and/or progressive deterioration of intellect and personality characterized by decreased ability to interpret environmental stimuli, decreased capacity for intellectual thought processes, and manifested by disturbances of memory, orientation, and behavior.

### RELATED FACTORS

Alzheimer's disease; Korsakoff's psychosis; Multi-infarct dementia; Cerebrovascular accident; Head injury

### DEFINING CHARACTERISTICS

**Objective**

Clinical evidence of organic impairment; Altered interpretation/response to stimuli; Progressive/long-standing cognitive impairment; No change in level of consciousness; Impaired socialization; Impaired memory (short term, long term); Altered personality

## CONSTIPATION

*Diagnostic Division: Elimination*

**Definition:** A state in which an individual experiences a change in normal bowel habits characterized by a decrease in frequency and/or passage of hard, dry stools.

### RELATED FACTORS

To be developed by NANDA: [Neuromuscular/Musculoskeletal impairment, weak abdominal musculature]; [Gastrointestinal obstructive lesions]; [Megacolon] [Pain on defecation], [Hemorrhoids, back injury]; [Diagnostic procedures], [Treatments, drug side effects/interactions]; [Pregnancy]; [Lack of exercise, inadequate diet and fluid intake, lack of privacy]

NOTE: These factors were identified when this diagnosis was originally accepted and have been retained here to assist the user until NANDA completes its work.

### DEFINING CHARACTERISTICS

**Subjective**

Frequency less than usual pattern; Reported feeling of abdominal or rectal fullness or pressure; [Less than usual amount of stool]; [Nausea]

**Objective**

Hard, formed stools; Straining at stool; Palpable mass; Decreased activity level; [Immobility]; [Decreased bowel sounds]; [Abdominal distention]

### OTHER POSSIBLE CHARACTERISTICS

**Subjective**

Abdominal/back pain; Headache; Interference with daily living; Appetite impairment; Use of laxatives

## CONSTIPATION, COLONIC

*Diagnostic Division: Elimination*

**Definition:** The state in which an individual's pattern of elimination is characterized by hard, dry stool which results from a delay in passage of food residue.

**RELATED FACTORS**

Less than adequate fluid/dietary intake; less than adequate fiber; Less than adequate physical activity; Immobility; Lack of privacy; Emotional disturbances; Stress; Change in daily routine; Chronic use of medication and enemas; Metabolic problems (e.g., hypothyroidism, hypocalcemia, hypokalemia); [Neuromuscular/musculoskeletal impairment; Weak abdominal musculature]; [Gastrointestinal obstructive lesions; Megacolon]; [Pain on defecation: Hemorrhoids, Back injury]; [Diagnostic procedures, medication side effects/interactions]; [Pregnancy]

**DEFINING CHARACTERISTICS**

**Subjective**

Decreased frequency; Painful defecation; Abdominal distention; Abdominal pain; Rectal pressure; Appetite impairment; Headache

**Objective**

Hard, dry stool; Straining at stool; Palpable mass

## CONSTIPATION, PERCEIVED

*Diagnostic Division: Elimination*

**Definition:** The state in which an individual makes a self-diagnosis of constipation and ensures a daily bowel movement through abuse of laxatives, enemas, and suppositories.

**RELATED FACTORS**

Cultural/family health beliefs; Faulty appraisal; Impaired thought processes; [Long-term expectations/habits]

**DEFINING CHARACTERISTICS**

**Subjective**

Expectation of a daily bowel movement with the resulting overuse of laxatives, enemas, and suppositories; Expected passage of stool at same time every day

## COPING, DEFENSIVE

*Diagnostic Division: Ego Integrity*

**Definition:** The state in which an individual repeatedly projects falsely positive self-evaluation based on a self-protective pattern which defends against underlying perceived threats to positive self-regard.

**RELATED FACTORS**

[Refer to Coping, Individual, ineffective]

**DEFINING CHARACTERISTICS**

**Subjective**

Denial of obvious problems/weaknesses; Projection of blame/responsibility; Rationalizes failures; Hypersensitive to slight/criticism; Grandiosity; [Refuses or rejects assistance]

**Objective**

Superior attitude toward others; Difficulty establishing/maintaining relationships, [avoidance of intimacy]; Hostile laughter or ridicule of others, [aggressive behavior]; Difficulty in reality-testing perceptions; Lack of follow-through or participation in treatment or therapy; [Attention-seeking behavior]

## COPING, INDIVIDUAL, INEFFECTIVE

*Diagnostic Division: Ego Integrity*

**Definition:** Impairment of adaptive behaviors and abilities of a person in meeting life's demands and roles.

**RELATED FACTORS**

Situational/maturational crises; Personal vulnerability; [Inadequate support systems]; [Poor nutrition]; [Work overload, no vacations, too many deadlines]; Unrealistic perceptions; [Multiple stressors, repeated over period of time]; [Multiple life changes, conflict]; [Inadequate relaxation, little or no exercise]; [Unmet expectations]; [Inadequate coping method]; [Impairment of nervous system; cognitive/sensory/perceptual impairment]; [Memory loss]; [Severe pain, overwhelming threat to self]

**DEFINING CHARACTERISTICS**

**Subjective**

Verbalization of inability to cope or inability to ask for help; [Reports of chronic worry/anxiety/depression, poor self-esteem]; [Reports of muscular/emotional tension, lack of appetite, chronic fatigue, insomnia, general irritability]

**Objective**

Inability to problem-solve; Inability to meet role expectations/basic needs; Alteration in societal participation; Inappropriate use of defense mechanisms [including excessive use of denial, withdrawal]; Change in usual communication patterns; Verbal manipulation; High illness rate [including high blood pressure, ulcers, irritable bowel, frequent headaches/neckaches]; High rate of accidents; Destructive behavior toward self or others [including overeating, excessive smoking/drinking, overuse of prescribed/OTC medications, alcohol]; [Lack of assertive behaviors]

## DECISIONAL CONFLICT

*Diagnostic Division: Ego Integrity*

**Definition:** The state of uncertainty about course of action to be taken when choice among competing actions involves risk, loss, or challenge to personal life values.

**RELATED FACTORS**

Unclear personal values/beliefs; Perceived threat to value system; Lack of experience or interference with decision making; Lack of relevant information; Support system deficit; Multiple or divergent sources of information; [Age, developmental state]; [Family system, sociocultural factors]; [Cognitive, emotional, behavioral level of functioning]

**DEFINING CHARACTERISTICS**

**Subjective**

Verbalized uncertainty about choices or of undesired consequences of alternative actions being considered; Verbalized feelings of distress or questioning personal values and beliefs while attempting a decision

**Objective**

Vacillation between alternative choices; Delayed decision-making; Self-focusing; Physical signs of distress or tension (increased heart rate, increased muscle tension, restlessness, etc.)

## DENIAL, INEFFECTIVE

*Diagnostic Division: Ego Integrity*

**Definition:** The state of a conscious or unconscious attempt to disavow the knowledge or meaning of an event to reduce anxiety/fear to the detriment of health.

**RELATED FACTORS**

To be developed by NANDA: [Personal vulnerability; unmet self-needs]; [Presence of overwhelming anxiety-producing feelings/situation; reality factors that are consciously intolerable]; [Fear of consequences, negative past experiences]; [Learned response patterns (e.g., avoidance)]; [Cultural factors, personal/family value systems]

**DEFINING CHARACTERISTICS**

**Subjective**

Minimizes symptoms; displaces source of symptoms to other organs; Unable to admit impact of disease on life pattern; Displaces fear of impact of the condition; Does not admit fear of death or invalidism

**Objective**

Delays seeking or refuses health care attention to the detriment of health; Does not perceive personal relevance of symptoms or danger; Makes dismissive gestures or comments when speaking of distressing events; Displays inappropriate affect; Uses home remedies (self-treatment) to relieve symptoms

## DIARRHEA

*Diagnostic Division: Elimination*

**Definition:** A state in which an individual experiences a change in normal bowel habits characterized by the frequent passage of loose, fluid, unformed stools.

**RELATED FACTORS**
Gastrointestinal disorders [e.g., inflammation, irritation, or malabsorption of bowel], fecal impaction; Metabolic/endocrine disorders; Nutritional disorders, changes in dietary intake; Infectious processes; Tube feedings; Adverse effects of medications [radiation, toxins, contaminants]; High stress levels

**DEFINING CHARACTERISTICS**
**Subjective**
Abdominal pain; Urgency; Cramping

**Objective**
Increased frequency; Increased frequency of bowel sounds; Loose, liquid stools

**OTHER POSSIBLE CHARACTERISTICS**
Change in color

## DISORGANIZED INFANT BEHAVIOR

*Diagnostic Division: Neurosensory*

**Definition:** Alteration in integration and modulation of the physiologic and behavioral systems of functioning (i.e., autonomic, motor, state, organizational, self-regulatory, and attentional-interactional systems).

**RELATED FACTORS**
Pain; Oral/motor problems; Feeding intolerance; Lack of containment/boundaries; Prematurity; [immaturity of the central nervous system; genetic problems that alter neurologic and/or physiologic functioning; conditions resulting in hypoxia and/or birth asphyxia]; [Malnutrition; infection; drug addiction]; [Environmental events or conditions such as separation from parents, exposure to loud noise, excessive handling, bright lights]; Environmental overstimulation; Invasive/painful procedures

**DEFINING CHARACTERISTICS**
Change from baseline physiologic measures [e.g., dramatic fluctuations in heart rate, breathing pattern, color; decrease in $TCPO_2$/oxygen saturation]; Tremors, startles, twitches; [flaccidity or hypertonicity] Hyperextension of arms and legs; Diffuse/unclear sleep; Deficient self-regulatory behaviors; Deficient response to visual/auditory stimuli; Yawning; Apnea; [Inability to move smoothly between states]; [averted head/eyes, "locking in"—inability to look away from stimulus]

## DISORGANIZED INFANT BEHAVIOR, RISK FOR

*Diagnostic Division: Neurosensory*

**Definition:** Risk for alteration in integration and modulation of the physiologic and behavioral systems of functioning (i.e., autonomic, motor, state, organizational, self-regulatory, and attentional-interactional systems).

**RISK FACTORS**
Pain; Oral/motor problems; Environmental overstimulation; Lack of containment/boundaries; Prematurity; [immaturity of the central nervous system; genetic problems that alter neurologic and/or physiologic functioning conditions resulting in hypoxia and/or birth asphyxia]; [Malnutrition; infection; drug addiction]; [Environmental events or conditions such as separation from parents, exposure to loud noise, excessive handling, bright lights] Invasive/painful procedures

## DISUSE SYNDROME, RISK FOR

*Diagnostic Division: Activity/Rest*

**Definition:** A state in which an individual is at risk for deterioration of body systems as the result of prescribed or unavoidable musculoskeletal inactivity.

NOTE: NANDA identifies complications from immobility including pressure ulcer, constipation, stasis of pulmonary secretions, thrombosis, urinary tract infection/retention, decreased strength/endurance, orthostatic hypotension, decreased range of joint motion, disorientation, body image disturbance, and powerlessness.

**RISK FACTORS**
**Subjective**
Severe pain, [chronic pain]

**Objective**
Paralysis; Mechanical or prescribed immobilization; Altered level of consciousness

## DIVERSIONAL ACTIVITY DEFICIT

*Diagnostic Division: Activity/Rest*

**Definition:** The state in which an individual experiences a decreased stimulation from or interest or engagement in recreational or leisure activities (because of internal/external factors that may or may not be beyond the individual's control).

**RELATED FACTORS**

Environmental lack of diversional activity; Long-term hospitalization; Frequent, lengthy treatments; [Physical limitations]; [Bedridden]; [Situational, developmental problem, lack of sources]; [Psychologic condition, e.g., depression]; [Fatigue, pain]

**DEFINING CHARACTERISTICS**

**Subjective**

Patient's statement regarding the following: Boredom; Wish there were something to do, to read, etc.; Usual hobbies cannot be undertaken in hospital [or home]; [changes in abilities/physical limitations]

**Objective**

[Flat affect]; [Disinterested, inattentive]; [Restless]; [Crying]; [Lethargy]; [Withdrawn]; [Hostile]; [Overeating or lack of interest in eating; weight loss or gain]

## DYSREFLEXIA

*Diagnostic Division: Circulation*

**Definition:** The state in which an individual with a spinal cord injury at T-7 or above experiences a life-threatening uninhibited sympathetic response of the nervous system to a noxious stimulus.

**RELATED FACTORS**

Bladder or bowel distention [catheter insertion, obstruction, irrigation]; Skin irritation; Lack of patient and caregiver knowledge; [Sexual excitation]; [Environmental temperature extremes]

**DEFINING CHARACTERISTICS**

Individual with spinal cord injury (T-7 or above) with:

**Subjective**

Headache (a diffuse pain in different portions of the head and not confined to any nerve distribution area); Paresthesia; chilling; blurred vision; chest pain; metallic taste in mouth; nasal congestion

**Objective**

Paroxysmal hypertension (sudden periodic elevated blood pressure where systolic pressure is over 140 mm Hg and diastolic is above 90 mm Hg); Bradycardia or tachycardia (pulse rate of less than 60 or over 100 beats per minute); Diaphoresis (above the injury); red splotches on skin (above the injury); pallor (below the injury); Horner's syndrome (contraction of the pupil, partial ptosis of the eyelid, enophthalmos and sometimes loss of sweating over the affected side of the face); conjunctival congestion; Pilomotor reflex (gooseflesh formation when skin is cooled)

## ENERGY FIELD DISTURBANCE

*Diagnostic Division: Ego Integrity*

**Definition:** A disruption of the flow of energy [aura] surrounding a person's being that results in a disharmony of the body, mind, and/or spirit.

**RELATED FACTORS**

To be developed by NANDA: [Block in energy field]; [Depression]; [Increased state of anxiety]; [Impaired immune system]; [Pain]

**DEFINING CHARACTERISTICS**

**Objective**

Temperature change (warmth/coolness); Visual changes (image/color); Disruption of the field (vacant/hole/spike/bulge); Movement (wave/spike/tingling/dense/flowing); Sounds (tone/words)

## ENHANCED ORGANIZED INFANT BEHAVIOR, POTENTIAL FOR

*Diagnostic Division: Neurosensory*

**Definition:** A pattern of modulation of the physiologic and behavioral systems of functioning of an infant (i.e., autonomic, motor, state, organizational, self-regulatory, and attentional-interactional systems) that is satisfactory but that can be improved, resulting in higher levels of integration in response to environmental stimuli.

**RELATED FACTORS**
Prematurity; Pain

**DEFINING CHARACTERISTICS**
**Objective**
Stable physiologic measures; Definite sleep-wake states; Use of some self-regulatory behaviors; Response to visual/auditory stimuli

## ENVIRONMENTAL INTERPRETATION SYNDROME, IMPAIRED

*Diagnostic Division: Safety*

**Definition:** Consistent lack of orientation to person, place, time, or circumstances over more than 3 to 6 months, necessitating a protective environment.

**RELATED FACTORS**
Dementia (Alzheimer's disease, multi-infarct dementia, Pick's disease, AIDS dementia); Parkinson's disease; Huntington's disease; Depression; Alcoholism

**DEFINING CHARACTERISTICS**
**Subjective**
[Loss of occupation or social function from memory decline]

**Objective**
Consistent disorientation in known and unknown environments; Chronic confusional states; Loss of occupation or social function from memory decline; Inability to follow simple directions, instructions; Inability to reason; Inability to concentrate; Slowness in responding to questions

## FAMILY COPING, INEFFECTIVE: COMPROMISED

*Diagnostic Division: Social Interaction*

**Definition:** A usually supportive primary person (family member or close friend [significant other]) is providing insufficient, ineffective, or compromised support, comfort, assistance, or encouragement that may be needed by the client to manage or master adaptive tasks related to his or her health challenge.

**RELATED FACTORS**
Inadequate or incorrect information or understanding by a primary person; Temporary preoccupation by a significant person who is trying to manage emotional conflicts and personal suffering and is unable to perceive or to act effectively in regard to [patient's] needs; Temporary family disorganization and role changes; Other situational or developmental crises or situations the significant person may be facing; [Client] providing little support in turn for the primary person; Prolonged disease or disability progression that exhausts the supportive capacity of significant people; [Unrealistic expectations of patient/significant other(s) or each other]; [Lack of mutual decision-making skills]; [Diverse coalitions of family members]

**DEFINING CHARACTERISTICS**
**Subjective**
Client expresses or confirms a concern or complaint about significant other's response to his or her health problem; Significant person describes preoccupation with personal reaction (e.g., fear, anticipatory grief, guilt, anxiety to illness/disability, or to other situational or developmental crises); Significant person describes or confirms an inadequate understanding or knowledge base that interferes with effective assistive or supportive behaviors

**Objective**
Significant person attempts assistive or supportive behaviors with less than satisfactory results; Significant person withdraws or enters into limited or temporary personal communication with [client] at time of need; Significant person displays protective behavior disproportionate (too little or too much) to [client] abilities or need for autonomy; [Significant person displays sudden outbursts of emotions/shows emotional lability or interferes with necessary nursing/medical interventions]

## FAMILY COPING, INEFFECTIVE: DISABLING

*Diagnostic Division: Social Interaction*

**Definition:** The behavior of a significant person (family member or other primary person) disables his or her own capacities and the capacities to effectively address tasks essential to either person's adaptation to the health challenge.

**RELATED FACTORS**

Significant person with chronically unexpressed feelings of guilt, anxiety, hostility, despair, etc.; Dissonant discrepancy of coping styles being used to deal with the adaptive tasks by the significant person and client or among significant people; Highly ambivalent family relationships; Arbitrary handling of a family's resistance to treatment, which tends to solidify defensiveness because it fails to deal adequately with underlying anxiety; [High-risk family situations, such as single or adolescent parent, abusive relationship, substance abuse, acute/chronic disabilities, member with terminal illness]

**DEFINING CHARACTERISTICS**

**Subjective**

[Expresses despair regarding family reactions/lack of involvement]

**Objective**

Intolerance; Abandonment; Psychosomatic tendency; Agitation, depression, aggression, hostility; Rejection; Desertion; Taking on illness signs of client; Neglectful relationships with other family members; Carrying on usual routines disregarding [client's] needs; Neglectful care of the client in regard to basic human needs and/or illness treatment; Distortion of reality regarding the health problem, including extreme denial about its existence or severity; Decisions and actions by family that are detrimental to economic or social well-being; Impaired restructuring of a meaningful life for self; impaired individualization; prolonged overconcern for client; Client's development of helpless, inactive dependence

## FAMILY COPING: POTENTIAL FOR GROWTH

*Diagnostic Division: Social Interaction*

**Definition:** Effective managing of adaptive tasks by family member involved with the health challenge who now is exhibiting desire and readiness for enhanced health and growth in regard to self and in relation to the client.

**RELATED FACTORS**

Needs sufficiently gratified and adaptive tasks effectively addressed to enable goals of self-actualization to surface; [Developmental stage, situational crises/supports]

**DEFINING CHARACTERISTICS**

**Subjective**

Family member attempting to describe growth impact of crisis on his/her own values, priorities, goals, or relationships; Individual expresses interest in making contact on a one-to-one basis or on a mutual-aid group basis with another person who has experienced a similar situation

**Objective**

Family member is moving in direction of health-promoting and enriching lifestyle that supports and monitors maturational processes, audits and negotiates treatment programs, and generally chooses experiences that optimize wellness

## FAMILY PROCESS, ALTERED: ALCOHOLISM [SUBSTANCE ABUSE]

*Diagnostic Division: Social Interaction*

**Definition:** The state in which the psychosocial, spiritual, and physiologic functions of the family unit are chronically disorganized, leading to conflict, denial of problems, resistance to change, ineffective problem-solving, and a series of self-perpetuating crises.

**RELATED FACTORS**

Abuse of alcohol; Family history of alcoholism; Resistance to treatment; Inadequate coping skills; Genetic predisposition; Addictive personality; Lack of problem-solving skills; Biochemical influences

**DEFINING CHARACTERISTICS**

**Subjective**

**Feelings**

Decreased self-esteem/Worthlessness; Anger/Suppressed rage; Frustration; Powerlessness; Anxiety/Tension/Distress; Insecurity; Repressed emotions; Responsibility for alcoholic's behavior; Lingering resentment; Shame/Embarrassment; Hurt; Unhappiness; Guilt; Emotional isolation/Loneliness; Vulnerability; Mistrust; Hopelessness; Rejection; Depression; hostility; fear; confusion; dissatisfaction; loss; Being different from other people; misunderstood; Emotional control by others; being unloved; lack of identity; Abandonment; confused love and pity; moodiness; failure

**Roles and Relationships**

Deterioration in family relationships/Disturbed family dynamics; Ineffective spouse communication/Marital problems; Altered role function/Disruption of family roles; Inconsistent parenting/Low perception of parental support; Family denial; Intimacy dysfunction; Chronic family problems; Lack of skills necessary for relationships; lack of cohesiveness; disrupted family rituals; Family unable to meet security needs of its members; Pattern of rejection; economic problems; neglected obligations

**Objective**
**Roles and Relationships**
Closed communication systems; Triangulating family relationships; reduced ability of family members to relate to each other for mutual growth and maturation; Family does not demonstrate respect for individuality and autonomy of its members

**Behaviors**
Expression of anger inappropriately; Difficulty with intimate relationships; Loss of control of drinking; Impaired communication; Ineffective problem-solving skills; Enabling to maintain drinking [substance abuse]; Inability to meet emotional needs of its members; Manipulation; Dependency; Criticizing; Alcohol [substance] abuse; Broken promises; Rationalization/Denial of problems; Refusal to get help/Inability to accept and receive help appropriately; Blaming; Inadequate understanding or knowledge of alcoholism [substance abuse]; Inability to meet spiritual needs of its members; Inability to express or accept wide range of feelings; Orientation toward tension relief rather than achievement of goals; Family special occasions are alcohol centered; Escalating conflict; Lying; Contradictory, paradoxical communication; Lack of dealing with conflict; Harsh self-judgment; Isolation; Nicotine [/other substance] addiction; Difficulty having fun; Self-blaming; Unresolved grief; Controlling communication/power struggles; Inability to adapt to change; Immaturity; Stress-related physical illnesses; Inability to deal with traumatic experiences constructively; Seeking approval and affirmation; Lack of reliability; Disturbances in academic performance in children; Disturbances in concentration; Chaos; Substance abuse other than alcohol; Failure to accomplish current or past developmental tasks/Difficulty with life cycle transitions; Verbal abuse of spouse or parent; Agitation; Diminished physical contact

## FAMILY PROCESSES, ALTERED

*Diagnostic Division: Social Interaction*

**Definition:** The state in which a family that normally functions effectively experiences a dysfunction.

### RELATED FACTORS
Situational transition and/or crises [e.g., economic, change in roles, illness, trauma, disabling/expensive treatments]; Development transition and/or crises [e.g., loss or gain of a family member, adolescence, leaving home for college]

### DEFINING CHARACTERISTICS
**Subjective**
Family uninvolved in community activities; Unexamined family myths; [rigidity in functions, rules, roles]; [Family expresses confusion about what to do, verbalizes they are having difficulty coping with situation]

**Objective**
Family system unable to [does not] meet physical/emotional/spiritual needs of its members; Family unable to [does not] meet security needs of its members; Inability to accept or to receive help appropriately; Family inability to [does not] adapt to change or to deal with traumatic experience constructively; Parents do not demonstrate respect for each other's views on child-rearing practices; Inability to express or to accept wide range of feelings/feelings of members; Inability of family members to relate to each other for mutual growth and maturation; Rigidity in function and roles; Family does not demonstrate respect for individuality and autonomy of its members; Family fails to accomplish current or past developmental task; Unhealthy family decision-making process; Failure to send and to receive clear messages; Inappropriate level and direction of energy; Inappropriate boundary maintenance; Inappropriate or poorly communicated family rules, rituals, symbols

## FATIGUE

*Diagnostic Division: Activity/Rest*

**Definition:** An overwhelming sustained sense of exhaustion and decreased capacity for physical and mental work.

### RELATED FACTORS
Decreased/increased metabolic energy production; Overwhelming psychological or emotional demands; Increased energy requirements to perform activities of daily living; Excessive social

and/or role demands; States of discomfort; Altered body chemistry (e.g., medications, drug withdrawal, chemotherapy)

**DEFINING CHARACTERISTICS**

**Subjective**

Verbalization of an unremitting and overwhelming lack of energy; Inability to maintain usual routines; Perceived need for additional energy to accomplish routine tasks; Impaired ability to concentrate; Decreased libido

**Objective**

Increase in physical complaints; Emotionally labile or irritable; Lethargic or listless; Disinterest in surroundings/introspection; Decreased performance; Accident prone

## FEAR [SPECIFY FOCUS]

*Diagnostic Division: Ego Integrity*

**Definition:** Feeling of dread related to an indentifiable source which the individual validates.

**RELATED FACTORS**

To be developed by NANDA: (Natural or innate origins; environmental stimuli (e.g., sudden noise, loss of physical support, heights, pain); (Learned response: conditioning, modeling from, or identification with others); (Separation from support system in a potentially threatening situation such as hospitalization, treatments, etc.); (Knowledge deficit or unfamiliarity); (Phobic stimulus or phobia); (Language barrier) [or inability to communicate]; (Sensory impairment); [Threat of death, perceived or actual]

NOTE: These factors were identified when this diagnosis was originally accepted and have been retained here to assist the user until NANDA completes its work.

**DEFINING CHARACTERISTICS**

**Subjective**

Ability to identify object of fear; Panic; Scared; Jittery; [Increased tension; Apprehension; Frightened; Terrified]; [Impulsiveness]; [Decreased self-assurance]; [Associated physical symptoms: nausea, "heart beating fast," etc.]

**Objective**

[Attack/fight behavior—aggressive; flight behavior—withdrawal]; [Wide-eyed; Increased alertness; Concentration on source]; [Sympathetic stimulation: cardiovascular excitation, superficial vasoconstriction (paleness/loss of color), pupil dilation, vomiting, diarrhea, diaphoresis, etc.]

## FLUID VOLUME DEFICIT [ACTIVE LOSS]

*Diagnostic Division: Food/Fluid*

**Definition:** The state in which an individual experiences vascular, cellular, or intracellular dehydration (in excess of needs or replacement capabilities owing to active loss).

**RELATED FACTORS**

Active loss [e.g., burns, abdominal cancer, hemorrhage, gastric intubation, diarrhea, fistulas, use of hyperosmotic radiopaque contrast agents]

**DEFINING CHARACTERISTICS**

**Objective**

Decreased urine output; Output greater than intake; Decreased venous filling; Increased serum sodium; Concentrated urine; Sudden weight loss; Hemoconcentration

**OTHER DEFINING CHARACTERISTICS:**

**Subjective**

Thirst; Weakness

**Objective**

Hypotension [postural]; Decreased skin turgor; Increased pulse rate; Dry skin; Dry mucous membranes; Increased body temperature; Change in mental state.

## FLUID VOLUME DEFICIT [REGULATORY FAILURE]

*Diagnostic Division: Food/Fluid*

**Definition:** The state in which an individual experiences vascular, cellular, or intracellular dehydration [in excess of needs or replacement capabilities owing to failure of regulatory mechanisms].

### RELATED FACTORS
Failure of regulatory mechanisms [e.g., adrenal disease, recovery phase of acute renal failure, uncontrolled diabetes mellitus/insipidus]

### DEFINING CHARACTERISTICS
**Subjective**
[Reports of fatigue, nervousness, exhaustion]

**Objective**
Increased urine output; Dilute urine; Sudden weight loss; Decreased venous filling; Hemoconcentration; Altered serum sodium

### OTHER DEFINING CHARACTERISTICS:
**Subjective**
Thirst; Weakness

**Objective**
Hypotension [postural]; Increased pulse rate; Decreased skin turgor; Decreased pulse volume and pressure; Change in mental status [e.g., confusion]; Increased body temperature; Dry skin/ mucous membranes; [Edema; possible weight gain]

## FLUID VOLUME DEFICIT, RISK FOR

*Diagnostic Division: Food/Fluid*

**Definition:** The state in which an individual is at risk of experiencing vascular, cellular, or intracellular dehydration.

### RISK FACTORS
Extremes of age and weight; Loss of fluid through abnormal routes, e.g., indwelling tubes; Knowledge deficiency related to fluid volume; Factors influencing fluid needs, e.g., hypermetabolic states; Medications, e.g., diuretics; Excessive losses through normal routes, e.g., diarrhea; Deviations affecting access to, intake of, or absorption of fluids, e.g., physical immobility

## FLUID VOLUME EXCESS

*Diagnostic Division: Food/Fluid*

**Definition:** The state in which an individual experiences increased isotonic fluid retention.

### RELATED FACTORS
Compromised regulatory mechanism [e.g., SIADH or decreased plasma proteins as found in conditions such as malnutrition, draining fistulas, burns, organ failure]; Excess fluid intake; Excess sodium intake; [Drug therapies, e.g., chlorpropamide, tolbutamide, vincristine, tryptyline, carbamazepine]

### DEFINING CHARACTERISTICS
**Subjective**
Shortness of breath

**Objective**
Edema; Effusion; Anasarca; Weight gain; Intake greater than output; Abnormal breath sounds: crackles (rales); Decreased hemoglobin, hematocrit; Increased central venous pressure; Jugular vein distention; Positive hepatojugular reflex

## GAS EXCHANGE, IMPAIRED

*Diagnostic Division: Respiration*

**Definition:** The state in which the individual experiences an excess or deficit in oxygenation and/or carbon dioxide elimination at the alveolar-capillary membrane (specify: hypercapnia or hypoxemia). [This may be an entity of its own, but it also may be an end result of other pathology with an interrelatedness between airway clearance and/or breathing pattern problems.]

### RELATED FACTORS
Ventilation perfusion imbalance [as in the following: Altered blood flow (e.g., pulmonary embolus, increased vascular resistance), vasospasm, heart failure, hypovolemic shock]; [Alveolar-capillary membrane changes (e.g., acute respiratory distress syndrome); chronic conditions such as restrictive/obstructive lung disease, pneumoconiosis, respiratory depressant drugs, brain injury, asbestosis/ silicosis]; [Altered oxygen supply (e.g., altitude sickness)]; [Altered oxygen-carrying capacity of blood (e.g., sickle cell/other anemia, carbon monoxide poisoning)]

**DEFINING CHARACTERISTICS**
**Subjective**
Dyspnea; Headache upon awakening; Vision disturbances

**Objective**
Confusion; [decreased mental acuity]; Abnormal ABGs; Hypoxia; Hypercapnia; Cyanosis (in neonates only); Somnolence, [lethargy]; Restlessness; Irritability, [agitation]; [Tachypnea]; [Changes in heart rate/rhythm]; [Polycythemia]

## GRIEVING, ANTICIPATORY

*Diagnostic Division: Ego Integrity*

**Definition:** Intellectual and emotional responses and behaviors by which individuals (families, communities) work through the process of modifying self-concept based on the perception of potential loss.

NOTE: May be a healthy response requiring interventions of support and information-giving.

**RELATED FACTORS**
To be developed by NANDA: [Perceived potential loss of significant other (body part/function, social role), physiopsychosocial well-being, lifestyle, personal possessions]

**DEFINING CHARACTERISTICS**
**Subjective**
Expression of distress at potential loss; Denial of potential loss; Denial of the significance of the loss; Guilt; Anger; Sorrow; Alteration in: eating habits, sleep patterns, dream patterns, activity level, libido; Difficulty taking on new or different roles

**Objective**
Potential loss of significant object; Altered communication patterns; [Altered affect]; [Crying]; Bargaining; Resolution of grief prior to the reality of loss

## GRIEVING, DYSFUNCTIONAL

*Diagnostic Division: Ego Integrity*

**Definition:** Extended, unsuccessful use of intellectual and emotional responses by which individuals (families, communities) attempt to work through the process of modifying self-concept based on the perception of potential loss.

**RELATED FACTORS**
Actual or perceived object loss (*object loss* is used in the broadest sense). Objects include people, possessions, a job, status, home, ideals, parts and processes of the body [e.g., amputation, paralysis, chronic/fatal illness]; [Thwarted grieving response to a loss]; [Lack of resolution of previous grieving response]; [Absence of anticipatory grieving]

**DEFINING CHARACTERISTICS**
**Subjective**
Expression of distress at loss; Denial of loss; Expression of guilt; Expression of unresolved issues; Anger; Sadness; Alterations in eating habits, sleep and dream patterns, activity level, libido, concentration and/or pursuits of tasks; Idealization of lost object; Reliving of past experiences with little or reduction (diminishment) of intensity of the grief; [Hopelessness]

**Objective**
Repetitive use of ineffectual behaviors associated with attempts to reinvest in relationships; Prolonged interference with life functioning; onset or exacerbation of somatic or psychosomatic responses; Crying; Difficulty in expressing loss; Developmental regression; Labile affect; [Isolation]; [Withdrawal]

## GROWTH AND DEVELOPMENT, ALTERED

*Diagnostic Division: Teaching/Learning*

**Definition:** The state in which an individual demonstrates deviations in norms from his/her age group.

**RELATED FACTORS**
Inadequate caretaking; Indifference, inconsistent responsiveness, multiple caretakers; Separation from significant others; Environmental and stimulation deficiencies; Effects of physical disability [handicapping condition]; Prescribed dependence [insufficient expectations for self-care]; [Physical/emotional neglect/abuse]

### DEFINING CHARACTERISTICS

**Subjective**

Inability to perform self-care or self-control activities appropriate for age; [Loss of previously acquired skills; precocious or accelerated skill attainment]

**Objective**

Delay or difficulty in performing skills (motor, social, or expressive) typical of age group; Altered physical growth; Flat affect, listlessness, decreased responses [Sleep disturbances, negative mood/response]

## HEALTH MAINTENANCE, ALTERED

*Diagnostic Division: Safety*

**Definition:** Inability to identify, manage, and/or seek out help to maintain health. [This diagnosis contains components of other nursing diagnoses. We recommend subsuming health maintenance interventions under the "basic" nursing diagnosis when a single causative factor is identified, e.g., Knowledge Deficit; Communication, impaired verbal; Thought Processes, altered; Individual/Family Coping, ineffective; Growth and Development, altered.]

### RELATED FACTORS

Lack of or significant alteration in communication skills (written, verbal, and/or gestural); Complete or partial lack of gross and/or fine motor skills; Unachieved developmental tasks; Lack of ability to make deliberate and thoughtful judgments; Perceptual or cognitive impairment; Ineffective individual coping; dysfunctional grieving; Lack of material resource; Ineffective family coping: disabling; spiritual distress

### DEFINING CHARACTERISTICS

**Subjective**

Expressed interest in improving health behaviors; Reported lack of equipment, financial and/or other resources; Impairment of personal support system

**Objective**

Demonstrated lack of knowledge regarding basic health practices; Observed inability to take the responsibility for meeting basic health practices in any or all functional pattern areas; Demonstrated lack of adaptive behaviors to internal or external environmental changes; History of lack of health-seeking behavior; Observed impairment of personal support system; lack of equipment, financial and/or other resources; [Observed compulsive behaviors]

## HEALTH-SEEKING BEHAVIORS (SPECIFY)

*Diagnostic Division: Teaching/Learning*

**Definition:** A state in which an individual in stable health is actively seeking ways to alter personal health habits and/or the environment in order to move toward higher level of health.

### RELATED FACTORS

[Situation/maturation occurrence precipitating concern about current health status]

### DEFINING CHARACTERISTICS

**Subjective**

Expressed desire to seek a higher level of wellness; [Expressed desire to modify codependent behavior]; Expressed desire for increased control of health practice; Expression of concern about current environmental conditions on health status; Stated unfamiliarity with wellness community resources

**Objective**

Observed desire to seek a higher level of wellness; Observed desire for increased control of health practice; Demonstrated or observed lack of knowledge in health promotion behaviors, unfamiliarity with wellness community resources

## HOME MAINTENANCE MANAGEMENT, IMPAIRED

*Diagnostic Division: Safety*

**Definition:** Inability to independently maintain a safe, growth-promoting immediate environment.

### RELATED FACTORS

Disease or injury of individual or family member; Insufficient finances; Impaired cognitive or emotional functioning; Lack of role modeling; Insufficient family organization or planning; Unfamiliarity with neighborhood resources; Lack of knowledge; Inadequate support systems.

**DEFINING CHARACTERISTICS**
**Subjective**
Household members express difficulty in maintaining their home in a comfortable [safe] fashion; Household requests assistance with home maintenance; Household members describe outstanding debts or financial crises

**Objective**
Disorderly surroundings; Accumulation of dirt, food or hygienic wastes; Inappropriate household temperature; Lack of necessary equipment or aids; Presence of vermin or rodents; Unwashed or unavailable cooking equipment, clothes, or linen; Offensive odors; Overtaxed family members, e.g., exhausted, anxious; Repeated hygienic disorders, infestations, or infections.

## HOPELESSNESS

*Diagnostic Division: Ego Integrity*

**Definition:** A subjective state in which an individual sees limited or no alternatives or personal choices available and is unable to mobilize energy on own behalf.

**RELATED FACTORS**
Prolonged activity restriction, creating isolation; Failing or deteriorating physiologic condition; Long-term stress; Abandonment; Lost belief in transcendent values/God

**DEFINING CHARACTERISTICS**
**Subjective**
Verbal cues (despondent content, "I can't," sighing); [believes things will not change/problems will always be there]

**Objective**
Passivity, decreased verbalization; Decreased affect; Lack of initiative; Decreased response to stimuli [depressed cognitive functions, problems with decisions, thought processes; regression]; Turning away from speaker; Closing eyes; Shrugging in response to speaker; Decreased appetite, increased/decreased sleep; Lack of involvement in care/passively allowing care; Withdrawal from environs; [Lack of involvement/interest in significant other(s) (children, spouse)] [Angry outbursts]

## HYPERTHERMIA

*Diagnostic Division: Safety*

**Definition:** A state in which an individual's body temperature is elevated above his/her normal range.

**RELATED FACTORS**
Exposure to hot environment; Vigorous activity; Medications/anesthesia; Inappropriate clothing; Increased metabolic rate, illness or trauma; Dehydration; Inability or decreased ability to perspire

**DEFINING CHARACTERISTICS**
**Subjective**
[Headache]

**Objective**
Flushed skin, warm to touch; Increase in body temperature above normal range; Increased respiratory rate, tachycardia; Seizures/convulsions; [Unstable blood pressure]; [Muscle rigidity]; [Muscle fasciculations]; [Confusion]

## HYPOTHERMIA

*Diagnostic Division: Safety*

**Definition:** The state in which an individual's body temperature is reduced below normal range.

**RELATED FACTORS**
Exposure to cool or cold environment [prolonged exposure, e.g., homeless, immersion in cold water/near drowning, induced hypothermia/cardiopulmonary bypass]; Inadequate clothing; Evaporation from skin in cool environment; Inability or decreased ability to shiver; Aging [or very young]; [Debilitating] illness or trauma, damage to hypothalamus; Malnutrition; Decreased metabolic rate; Inactivity; Consumption of alcohol; Medications causing vasodilation; [Vasodilation, e.g., sepsis, drug overdose]

### DEFINING CHARACTERISTICS

**Objective**

Reduction in body temperature below normal range; Shivering (mild); Cool skin; Pallor (moderate); Slow capillary refill; Cyanotic nail beds; Hypertension; Tachycardia; Piloerection; [Core temperature 95°F/35°C: increased respirations, poor judgment, shivering]; [Core temperature 95° to 93.2°F/35° to 34°C: bradycardia or tachycardia, myocardial irritability/dysrhythmias, muscle rigidity, shivering, lethargic/confused, decreased coordination]; [Core temperature 93.2° to 86°F/34° to 30°C: hypoventilation, bradycardia, generalized ridigity, metabolic acidosis, coma] [Core temperature below 86°F/30°C: no apparent vital signs, heart rate unresponsive to drug therapy, comatose, cyanotic, dilated pupils, apneic, areflexic, no shivering (appears dead)]

## INCONTINENCE, FUNCTIONAL

*Diagnostic Division: Elimination*

**Definition:** The state in which an individual experiences an involuntary, unpredictable passage of urine.

### RELATED FACTORS

Altered environment [e.g., poor lighting or inability to locate bathroom]; Sensory, cognitive [e.g., inattentiveness to urge to void, use of sedation], or mobility deficits [including difficulty in removing clothes]; [Increased urine production]; [Reluctance to use call light or bedpan]

### DEFINING CHARACTERISTICS

**Subjective**

Urge to void or bladder contractions sufficiently strong to result in loss of urine before reaching an appropriate receptacle; [Voiding in large amounts]

## INCONTINENCE, REFLEX

*Diagnostic Division: Elimination*

**Definition:** The state in which an individual experiences an involuntary loss of urine, occurring at somewhat predictable intervals when a specific bladder volume is reached.

### RELATED FACTORS

Neurologic impairment (e.g., spinal cord lesion that interferes with conduction of cerebral messages [nerve impulses] above the level of the reflex arc); [Cerebral lesion abolishing voluntary control]

### DEFINING CHARACTERISTICS

**Subjective**

No [or only partial] awareness of bladder filling; No urge to void or feelings of bladder fullness; [Voids in large amounts]; [Unaware of being incontinent]

**Objective**

Uninhibited bladder contraction/spasm at regular intervals; [Interrupted, complete, or involuntary void]; [Normal/increased anal tone]

## INCONTINENCE, STRESS

*Diagnostic Division: Elimination*

**Definition:** The state in which an individual experiences a loss of urine of less than 50 ml occurring with increased abdominal pressure.

### RELATED FACTORS

Degenerative changes in pelvic muscles and structural supports associated with increased age; High intra-abdominal pressure (e.g., obesity, gravid uterus); Incompetent bladder outlet; Overdistention between voidings; Weak pelvic muscles and structural supports [e.g., straining with chronic constipation]

### DEFINING CHARACTERISTICS

**Subjective**

Reported dribbling with increased abdominal pressure [e.g., coughing, sneezing, lifting, impact aerobics, changing position]; Urinary urgency, urinary frequency (more often than every 2 hours)

**Objective**

Observed dribbling with increased abdominal pressure.

## INCONTINENCE, TOTAL

*Diagnostic Division: Elimination*

**Definition:** The state in which an individual experiences a continuous and unpredictable loss of urine.

**RELATED FACTORS**

Neuropathy preventing transmission of reflex [signals to the reflex arc] indicating bladder fullness; Neurologic dysfunction causing triggering of micturition at unpredictable times [cerebral lesions]; Independent contraction of detrusor reflex owing to surgery; Trauma or disease affecting spinal cord nerves [destruction of sensory or motor neurons below the injury level]; Anatomic (fistula)

**DEFINING CHARACTERISTICS**

**Subjective**

Constant flow of urine occurs at unpredictable times without distention or uninhibited bladder contractions/spasm; Nocturia; Lack of perineal or bladder filling awareness; Unawareness of incontinence

**Objective**

Unsuccessful incontinence refractory treatments

## INCONTINENCE, URGE

*Diagnostic Division: Elimination*

**Definition:** The state in which an individual experiences involuntary passage of urine occurring soon after a strong sense of urgency to void.

**RELATED FACTORS**

Decreased bladder capacity (e.g., history of PID, abdominal surgeries, indwelling urinary catheter); Irritation of bladder stretch receptors causing spasm (e.g., bladder infection [atrophic urethritis, vaginitis]); alcohol; caffeine; increased fluids; increased urine concentration; overdistention of bladder; [Medication use, such as diuretics, sedatives, anticholinergic agents]; [Constipation/stool impaction]; [Restricted mobility; psychological disorder such as depression, change in mentation/confusional state]

**DEFINING CHARACTERISTICS**

**Subjective**

Urinary urgency; Frequency (voiding more often than every 2 hours); Bladder contracture/spasm; Nocturia (more than two times per night)

**Objective**

Inability to reach toilet in time; Voiding in small amounts (less than 100 ml) or in large amounts (more than 550 ml)

## INFANT FEEDING PATTERN, INEFFECTIVE

*Diagnostic Division: Food/Fluid*

**Definition:** A state in which an infant demonstrates an impaired ability to suck or coordinate the suck-swallow response.

**RELATED FACTORS**

Prematurity; Neurological impairment/delay; Oral hypersensitivity; Prolonged NPO; Anatomic abnormality

**DEFINING CHARACTERISTICS**

**Subjective**

[Caregiver reports infant is unable to initiate or sustain an effective suck]

**Objective**

Inability to initiate or sustain an effective suck; Inability to coordinate sucking, swallowing, and breathing

## INFECTION, RISK FOR

*Diagnostic Division: Safety*

**Definition:** The state in which an individual is at increased risk for being invaded by pathogenic organisms.

**RISK FACTORS**

Inadequate primary defenses (broken skin, traumatized tissue, decrease of ciliary action, stasis of body fluids, change in pH secretions, altered peristalsis); Inadequate secondary defenses (e.g., decreased hemoglobin, leukopenia, suppressed inflammatory response) and immunosuppression; Inadequate acquired immunity; tissue destruction and increased environmental exposure; Chronic disease; Invasive procedures; Malnutrition; Trauma; Pharmaceutical agents [including antibiotic therapy]; Rupture of amniotic membranes; Insufficient knowledge to avoid exposure to pathogens

## INJURY, RISK FOR

*Diagnostic Division: Safety*

**Definition:** A state in which the individual is at risk of injury as a result of environmental conditions interacting with the individual's adaptive and defensive resources.

NOTE: The potential for injury differs from individual to individual, and situation to situation. It is our belief that the environment is not safe, and there is no way to list everything that might present a danger to someone. Rather, we believe nurses have the responsibility to educate people throughout their life cycles to live safely in their environment.

**RISK FACTORS**

**Internal**

Biochemical, regulatory function: (sensory, integrative, effector dysfunction; tissue hypoxia), immune-autoimmune dysfunction; malnutrition; abnormal blood profile (leukocytosis/leukopenia; altered clotting factors; thrombocytopenia; sickle cell, thalassemia; decreased hemoglobin); Physical: (broken skin, altered mobility); development age; (physiologic, psychosocial); Psychologic (affective, orientation)

**External**

Biologic: (immunization level of community, microorganism); Chemical: (pollutants, poisons, drugs, pharmaceutical agents, alcohol, caffeine, nicotine, preservatives, cosmetics, and dyes), nutrients (vitamins, food types); Physical: (design, structure, and arrangement of community, building and/or equipment); mode of transport/transportation; People/provider (nosocomial agent; staffing patterns; cognitive, affective, and psychomotor factors)

## KNOWLEDGE DEFICIT [LEARNING NEED] (SPECIFY)

*Diagnostic Division: Teaching/Learning*

**Definition:** Absence or deficiency of cognitive information related to specific topic. [Lack of specific information necessary for patient/significant other(s) to make informed choices regarding condition/lifestyle changes.]

NOTE: The 1994 Preconference Workgroup for this diagnosis recommends the use of knowledge deficit as an etiology rather than as a nursing diagnosis.

**RELATED FACTORS**

Lack of exposure; Cognitive limitation; Information misinterpretation; Lack of interest in learning; Unfamiliarity with information resources; [Patient's request for no information]; Lack of recall; [Inaccurate/incomplete information presented]

**DEFINING CHARACTERISTICS**

**Subjective**

Verbalization of the problem; [Statement of misconception]; [Request for information]

**Objective**

Inaccurate follow-through of instruction; Inadequate performance of test; Inappropriate or exaggerated behaviors, e.g., hysterical, hostile, agitated, apathetic; [Development of preventable complication]

## LONELINESS, RISK FOR

*Diagnostic Division: Social Interaction*

**Definition:** A subjective state in which an individual is at risk of experiencing vague dysphoria.

**RISK FACTORS**

Affectional deprivation; Physical isolation; Cathectic deprivation; Social isolation

## MEMORY, IMPAIRED

*Diagnostic Division: Neurosensory*

**Definition:** The state in which an individual experiences the inability to remember or recall bits of information or behavioral skills. Impaired memory may be attributed to pathophysiologic or situational causes that are either temporary or permanent.

**RELATED FACTORS**

Acute or chronic hypoxia; Anemia; Decreased cardiac output; Fluid and electrolyte imbalance; Neurological disturbances [e.g., brain injury/concussion]; Excessive environmental disturbances; [manic state, fugue, traumatic event]; [Substance use/abuse; effects of medications]; [Age]

**DEFINING CHARACTERISTICS**

**Subjective**

Reported experiences of forgetting; Inability to recall recent or past events, factual information, [or familiar persons, places, items]

**Objective**

Observed experiences of forgetting; Inability to determine if a behavior was performed; Inability to learn or retain new skills or information; Inability to perform a previously learned skill; Forget to perform a behavior at a scheduled time

## NONCOMPLIANCE (SPECIFY) [COMPLIANCE, ALTERED]

*Diagnostic Division: Teaching/Learning*

**Definition:** A person's informed decision not to adhere to a therapeutic recommendation.

NOTE: Noncompliance is a term that may create a negative situation for patient and caregiver that may foster difficulties in resolving the causative factors. Because patients have a right to refuse therapy, we see this as a situation in which the professional need is to accept the patient's point of view/behavior/choice(s) and to work together to find alternate means to meet original and/or revised goals.

**RELATED FACTORS**

Patient value system: Health beliefs, cultural influences, spiritual values; Client-provider relationships; [Fear/anxiety]; [Altered thought processes such as depression, paranoia]; [Difficulty changing behavior, as in addictions]; [Inadequate resources, support systems]; [Issues of secondary gain]

**DEFINING CHARACTERISTICS**

**Subjective**

Statements by patient or significant other(s) [e.g., does not perceive illness/risk to be serious, does not believe in efficacy of therapy, unwilling to follow treatment regimen or accept side effects/limitations]

**Objective**

Behavior indicative of failure to adhere (by direct observation); Objective tests (physiologic measures, detection of markers); Evidence of development of complications; Failure to keep appointments; Evidence of exacerbation of symptoms; Failure to progress; [Inability to set or to attain mutual goals] [Denial]

## NUTRITION: ALTERED, LESS THAN BODY REQUIREMENTS

*Diagnostic Division: Food/Fluid*

**Definition:** The state in which an individual experiences an intake of nutrients insufficient to meet metabolic needs.

**RELATED FACTORS**

Inability to ingest or to digest food or to absorb nutrients because of biologic, psychologic, or economic factors; [Increased metabolic demands (e.g., burns)]

**DEFINING CHARACTERISTICS**

**Subjective**

Reported inadequate food intake less than RDA; Lack of interest in food; Reported lack of food; Perceived inability to ingest food; Aversion to eating; Satiety immediately after ingesting food; Reported altered taste sensation; Abdominal cramping; Abdominal pain with or without pathologic conditions; Lack of information; misinformation; misconceptions

**Objective**

Body weight 20% or more under ideal [for height and frame]; Loss of weight with adequate food intake; Evidence of lack of food [available]; Poor muscle tone; Weakness of muscles required for swallowing or mastication; Sore, inflamed buccal cavity; Capillary fragility; Hyperactive bowel sounds; Diarrhea and/or steatorrhea; Pale conjunctiva and mucous membranes; Excessive loss of hair [or increased growth of hair on body (lanugo)]; [Decreased subcutaneous fat/muscle mass]; [Abnormal laboratory studies (e.g., decreased albumin, total proteins; iron deficency; electrolyte imbalances)]

## NUTRITION: ALTERED, MORE THAN BODY REQUIREMENTS

*Diagnostic Division: Food/Fluid*

**Definition:** The state in which an individual is experiencing an intake of nutrients which exceeds metabolic needs.

### RELATED FACTORS

Excessive intake in relationship to metabolic need

NOTE: Underlying cause is often complex and may be difficult to diagnose/treat.

### DEFINING CHARACTERISTICS

**Subjective**

Reported dysfunctional eating patterns: Pairing food with other activities; Eating in response to external cues such as time of day, social situation; Concentrating food intake at end of day; Eating in response to internal cues other than hunger, e.g., anxiety; Sedentary activity level

**Objective**

Weight 20% over ideal for height and frame [obese]; Triceps skinfold greater than 15 mm in men and 25 mm in women; Weight 10% over ideal for height and frame [overweight]; Observed dysfunctional eating patterns [as noted in Subjective]; [Percentage of body fat greater than 22% for trim women and 15% for trim men]

## NUTRITION: ALTERED, RISK FOR MORE THAN BODY REQUIREMENTS

*Diagnostic Division: Food/Fluid*

**Definition:** The state in which an individual is at risk of experiencing an intake of nutrients that exceeds metabolic needs.

### RISK FACTORS

Reported/observed obesity in one or both parents [/spouse; hereditary predisposition]; Rapid transition across growth percentiles in infants or children [adolescents]; Reported use of solid food as major food source before 5 months of age; Reported/observed higher baseline weight at beginning of each pregnancy, [frequent, closely spaced pregnancies]; Dysfunctional eating patterns: pairing food with other activities, eating in response to external cues such as time of day or social situation, concentrating food intake at end of day, eating in response to internal cues other than hunger, e.g., anxiety; Observed use of food as reward or comfort measure; [Frequent/repeated dieting]; [Socially/culturally isolated; lacking other outlets]; [Alteration in usual activity patterns/sedentary lifestyle]; [Alteration in usual coping patterns]; [Majority of foods consumed are concentrated, high-calorie sources/fat]; [Significant/sudden decline in financial resources; lower socioeconomic status]

## ORAL MUCOUS MEMBRANE, ALTERED

*Diagnostic Division: Food/Fluid*

**Definition:** The state in which the individual experiences disruptions in the tissue layers of the oral cavity.

### RELATED FACTORS

Pathologic conditions: oral cavity (radiation to head and/or neck); Trauma: Chemical, e.g., acidic foods, drugs, noxious agents, alcohol; Trauma: Mechanical, e.g., ill-fitting dentures, braces, tubes (endotracheal, nasogastric), surgery in oral cavity; Dehydration; NPO for more than 24 hours; Malnutrition; Lack of or decreased salivation; Ineffective oral hygiene; Mouth breathing; Infection; Medication

### DEFINING CHARACTERISTICS

**Subjective**

Xerostomia (dry mouth); Oral pain or discomfort

**Objective**

Coated tongue; Oral lesions or ulcers; Stomatitis; Lack of or decreased salivation; Leukoplakia; Edema; Hyperemia; Oral plaque; Desquamation; Vesicles; Hemorrhagic gingivitis; Carious teeth; Halitosis

## PAIN

*Diagnostic Division: Pain / Discomfort*

**Definition:** An unpleasant sensory and emotional experience arising from actual or potential tissue damage or described in terms of such damage (International Association for the Study of Pain)

Refer to *pain, acute; pain, chronic.*

## PAIN, ACUTE

*Diagnostic Division: Pain / Discomfort*

**Definition:** Sudden or slow onset of any intensity from mild to severe with an anticipated or predictable end and a duration of less than 6 months.

**RELATED FACTORS**

Injuring agents: biologic, chemical, physical, psychologic

**DEFINING CHARACTERISTICS**

**Subjective**

Verbal or coded report; [Expect fewer complaints from patients under 40, males, some cultural groups]; [Pain unrelieved and/or increased beyond tolerance]

**Objective**

Observed evidence; Antalgic position; Protective behavior; Guarding behavior; Antalgic gestures; Facial mask; Sleep disturbance (eyes lack luster, "beaten look," fixed or scattered movement, grimace); Self-focus; Narrowed focus (altered time perception, impaired thought process, reduced interaction with people and environment); Distraction behavior (pacing, seeking out other people and/or activities, repetitive activities); Autonomic alteration in muscle tone (may span from listless [flaccid] to rigid); Autonomic responses (diaphoresis, blood pressure, respiration and pulse changes, pupillary dilation); Expressive behavior (restlessness, moaning, crying, vigilance, irritability, sighing); Changes in appetitie and eating; [Fear/panic]

## PAIN, CHRONIC

*Diagnostic Division: Pain / Discomfort*

**Definition:** Sudden or slow onset of any intensity from mild to severe, constant or recurring without anticipated or predictable end and a duration of greater than 6 months. [Pain is a signal that something is wrong. Chronic pain can be recurrent and periodically disabling (e.g., migraine headaches) or may be unremitting. While chronic pain syndrome includes various learned behaviors, psychologic factors become the primary contribution to impairment. It is a complex entity, combining elements from other nursing diagnoses (e.g., Powerlessness; Diversional Activity deficit; Family Processes, altered; Self-care deficit).]

**RELATED FACTORS**

Chronic physical/psychosocial disability

**DEFINING CHARACTERISTICS**

**Subjective**

Verbal or coded report of pain experienced for more than 6 months; Changes in sleep patterns; Anorexia; Weight changes; Fatigue; Fear of reinjury; Reduced interaction with people; Altered ability to continue previous activities; [Changes in appetite]; [Preoccupation with pain]; [Desperately seeks alternative solutions/therapies for relief/control of pain]

**Objective**

Observed evidence of: Protective behavior; Guarding behavior; Facial mask; Irritability; Self-focusing; Restlessness; Depression; Atrophy of involved muscle group; Sympathetic mediated responses (temperature, cold, changes of body position, hypersensitivity)

## PARENTAL ROLE CONFLICT

*Diagnostic Division: Social Interaction*

**Definition:** The state in which a parent experiences role confusion and conflict in response to crisis.

**RELATED FACTORS**

Separation from child due to chronic illness [/disability]; Intimidation with invasive or restrictive modalities (e.g., isolation, intubation), specialized care centers, policies; Home care of a child with special needs (e.g., apnea monitoring, postural drainage, hyperalimentation); Change in marital status; Interruptions of family life due to home care regimen (treatments, caregiver's lack of respite)

**DEFINING CHARACTERISTICS**

**Subjective**

Parent(s) express concerns/feelings of inadequacy to provide for child's physical and emotional needs during hospitalization or in the home; Parent(s) express concerns about changes in parental role, family functioning, family communication, family health; Parent(s) express concern about perceived loss of control over decisions relating to their child; Parent(s) verbalize feelings of guilt, anger, fear, anxiety, and/or frustration about effect of child's illness on family process

**Objective**

Demonstrated disruption in caretaking routines; Reluctance to participate in usual caretaking activities, even with encouragement and support; Demonstrated feelings of guilt, anger, fear, anxiety, and/or frustration about effect of child's illness on family process

## PARENT/INFANT/CHILD ATTACHMENT, ALTERED, RISK FOR

*Diagnostic Division: Social Interaction*

**Definition:** Disruption of the interactive process between parent/significant other and infant that fosters the development of a protective and nurturing reciprocal relationship.

**RISK FACTORS**

Inability of parents to meet the personal needs; Anxiety associated with the parent role; Substance abuse; Premature infant, ill infant/child who is unable to effectively initiate parental contact due to altered behavioral organization; Separation; Physical barriers; Lack of privacy; [Parents who themselves experienced altered attachment]; [Uncertainty of paternity; conception as a result of rape/sexual abuse]; [Difficult pregnancy and/or birth (actual or perceived)]

## PARENTING, ALTERED

*Diagnostic Division: Social Interaction*

**Definition:** The state in which a nurturing figure(s) experiences an inability to create an environment which promotes the optimum growth and development of another human being. (It is important to state as a preface to this diagnosis that adjustment to parenting in general is a normal maturational process that elicits nursing behaviors of prevention of potential problems and health promotion.)

**RELATED FACTORS**

Lack of available role model/ineffective role model; Lack of support between/from significant other(s); Interruption in bonding process [e.g., maternal, paternal, other]; Mental and/or physical illness; Lack of knowledge; Limited cognitive functioning; Multiple pregnancies; Unrealistic expectation for self, infant, partner; Physical and psychosocial abuse of nurturing figure; Unmet social/emotional maturation needs of parenting figures; Perceived threat to own survival, physical and emotional; Presence of stress (financial, legal, recent crisis, cultural move [e.g., from another country, nationality]); Lack of role identity; Lack of or inappropriate response of child to relationship

**DEFINING CHARACTERISTICS**

**Subjective**

Verbalization cannot control child; Constant verbalization of disappointment in gender or physical characteristics of the infant/child; Verbalization of resentment toward the infant/child; Verbalization of role inadequacy [inability to care for/promote self-discipline in child]; Verbal disgust at body functions of infant/child; Verbalizes desire to have child call him/her by first name versus traditional cultural tendencies

**Objective**

Abandonment; Runaway; Incidence of physical and psychologic trauma; Inattention to infant/child needs; Inappropriate caretaking behaviors (toilet training, sleep/rest, feeding); History of child abuse or abandonment by primary caretaker; [Current] incidence of physical and psychological trauma; Lack of parental attachment behaviors: inappropriate visual/tactile/auditory stimulation, negative identification of infant/child characteristics, negative attachment of meanings to infant/child characteristics, noncompliance with health appointments for self and/or infant/child; Inappropriate or inconsistent discipline practices; Frequent accidents/illness; Growth and development lag in the child; Child receives care from multiple caretakers without consideration for the needs of the infant/child; Compulsive seeking of role approval from others

## PARENTING, ALTERED, RISK FOR

*Diagnostic Division: Social Interaction*

**Definition:** The state in which a nurturing figure(s) is at risk to experience an inability to create an environment which promotes the optimum growth and development of another human being. (It is important to state as a preface to this diagnosis that adjustment to parenting in general is a normal maturational process that elicits nursing behaviors of prevention of potential problems and health promotion.)

### RISK FACTORS

Lack of available model/ineffective role model; Lack of support between/from significant other(s); Interruption in bonding process, (e.g., maternal, paternal, other); Mental and/or physical illness; Lack of knowledge; Limited cognitive functioning; Multiple pregnancies; Unrealistic expectation for self, infant, partner; Physical and psychosocial abuse of nurturing figure; Unmet social/emotional maturation needs of parenting figures; Perceived threat to own survival, physical and emotional; Presence of stress (financial, legal, recent crisis, culture move [e.g., from another country, nationality]); Lack of role identity; Lack of or inappropriate response of child to relationship

## PERIOPERATIVE POSITIONING INJURY, RISK FOR

*Diagnostic Division: Safety*

**Definition:** A state in which the client is at risk for injury as a result of the environmental conditions found in the perioperative setting.

### RISK FACTORS

Disorientation; Immobilization; Muscle weakness; [pre-existing musculoskeletal conditions]; Sensory/perceptual disturbances due to anesthesia; Obesity; Emaciation; Edema; [Elderly]

## PERIPHERAL NEUROVASCULAR DYSFUNCTION, RISK FOR

*Diagnostic Division: Neurosensory*

**Definition:** A state in which an individual is at risk of experiencing a disruption in circulation, sensation, or motion of an extremity.

### RISK FACTORS

Fractures; Mechanical compression (e.g., tourniquet, cast, brace, dressing, or restraint); Orthopedic surgery; Trauma; Immobilization; Burns; Vascular obstruction

## PERSONAL IDENTITY DISTURBANCE

*Diagnostic Division: Ego Integrity*

**Definition:** Inability to distinguish between self and nonself.

### RELATED FACTORS

To be developed by NANDA: [Organic brain syndrome]; [Poor ego differentiation, as in schizophrenia]; [Panic/dissociative states]; [Biochemical body change]

### DEFINING CHARACTERISTICS

(To be developed by NANDA)

**Subjective**

[Confusion about sense of self, purpose or direction in life, sexual identification/preference]

**Objective**

[Difficulty in making decisions]; [Poorly differentiated ego boundaries]; [Refer to ND *Anxiety [panic]* for additional characteristics]

## PHYSICAL MOBILITY, IMPAIRED

*Diagnostic Division: Safety*

**Definition:** A state in which the individual experiences a limitation of ability for independent physical movement.

### RELATED FACTORS

Intolerance to activity/decreased strength and endurance; Pain/discomfort; Neuromuscular/musculoskeletal impairment; Perceptual/cognitive impairment; Depression/severe anxiety; [Restrictive therapies/safety precautions, e.g., bed rest, limb immobilization]; [Effects of medications (antipsychotics, muscle relaxants)]

### DEFINING CHARACTERISTICS

**Subjective**

Reluctance to attempt movement; [Report of pain/discomfort on movement]

**Objective**

Inability to purposefully move within the physical environment, including bed mobility, transfer, and ambulation; Impaired coordination; Limited range of motion; Decreased muscle strength, control, and/or mass; Imposed restrictions of movement, including mechanical, medical protocol

## POISONING, RISK FOR

*Diagnostic Division: Safety*

**Definition:** Accentuated risk of accidental exposure to or ingestion of drugs or dangerous products in doses sufficient to cause poisoning [/Or the adverse effects of prescribed medication/drug use].

### RISK FACTORS

**Internal (Individual)**

Reduced vision; Lack of safety or drug education; Lack of proper precaution; [unsafe habits, disregard for safety measures, lack of supervision] Insufficient finances; Verbalization of occupational setting without adequate safeguards; Cognitive or emotional difficulties; [behavioral]; [Age, e.g., young child, elderly]; [Chronic disease state, disability]; [Cultural or religious beliefs/practices]

**External (Environmental)**

Large supplies of drugs in house; Dangerous products placed or stored within the reach of children or confused persons; Flaking, peeling paint or plaster in presence of young children; Paint, lacquer, etc., in poorly ventilated areas or without effective protection; Medicines stored in unlocked cabinets accessible to children or confused persons; Availability of illicit drugs potentially contaminated by poisonous additives; Chemical contamination of food and water; Unprotected contact with heavy metals or chemicals; Presence of poisonous vegetation; Presence of atmospheric pollutants; [close proximity to industrial chemicals]; [Therapeutic margin of safety of specific drugs (e.g., therapeutic versus toxic level, half-life, method of uptake and degradation in body, adequacy of organ function)]

## POST-TRAUMA RESPONSE [SPECIFY STAGE]

*Diagnostic Division: Ego Integrity*

**Definition:** The state of an individual's experiencing a sustained painful response to an overwhelming traumatic event(s).

### RELATED FACTORS

Disasters [e.g., floods, earthquakes, tornadoes, airplane crashes], wars, epidemics, rape, assault, torture, catastrophic illness or accident, [being held hostage]

### DEFINING CHARACTERISTICS

**Subjective**

Re-experience of the traumatic event which may be identified in cognitive, affective, and/or sensory motor activities (flashbacks, intrusive thoughts, repetitive dreams or nightmares, excessive verbalization of the traumatic event, verbalization of survival guilt or guilt about behavior required for survival); [Somatic reactions: reports of chronic pains/headaches, nausea, changes in appetite, sensitivity to noise, insomnia, dizziness, unsteadiness, chronic fatigue and easy fatigability, sleep disturbance]

**Objective**

Psychic/emotional numbness (impaired interpretation of reality, confusion, dissociation or amnesia, vagueness about traumatic event, constricted affect); Altered lifestyle (self-destructiveness such as substance abuse, suicide attempt, or other acting-out behavior; difficulty with interpersonal relationships [loss of interest in usual activities, detachment, loss of feeling of intimacy/sexuality]; development of phobia regarding trauma; poor impulse control/irritability and explosiveness); [Disturbance of mood, e.g., depression, anxiety, embarrassment, fear, humiliation, self-blame, low self-esteem, fear of violence toward self or others]; [Cognitive disruption: confusion, loss of memory/concentration, indecisiveness]; [Social reactions: dependence on others, work/school failure, avoidance of close relationships, social isolation]

**Stages**

Acute subtype: begins within 6 months and does not last longer than 6 months; Chronic subtype: lasts more than 6 months; Delayed subtype: period of latency of 6 months or more before onset of symptoms

## POWERLESSNESS [SPECIFY LEVEL]

*Diagnostic Division: Ego Integrity*

**Definition:** Perception that one's own action will not significantly affect an outcome; a perceived lack of control over a current situation or immediate happening.

### RELATED FACTORS

Health care environment [e.g., loss of privacy, personal possessions, control over therapies]; Interpersonal interaction [e.g., misuse of power, force; abusive relationships]; Illness-related regimen [e.g., chronic/debilitating conditions]; Lifestyle of helplessness [e.g., repeated failures, dependency]

### DEFINING CHARACTERISTICS

**Subjective**

**Severe**

Verbal expressions of having no control or influence over situation, outcome, or self-care; Depression over physical deterioration that occurs despite patient compliance with regimens

**Moderate**

Expressions of dissatisfaction and frustration over inability to perform previous tasks and/or activities; Expression of doubt regarding role performance; Reluctance to express true feelings, fearing alienation from caregivers

**Low**

Expressions of uncertainty about fluctuating energy levels

**Objective**

**Severe**

Apathy; [Anger]; [Withdrawn]; [Resigned]; [Crying]

**Moderate**

Does not monitor progress; Nonparticipation in care or decision making when opportunities are provided; Dependence on others that may result in irritability, resentment, anger, and guilt; Inability to seek information regarding care; Does not defend self-care practices when challenged

**Low**

Passivity

## PROTECTION, ALTERED

*Diagnostic Division: Safety*

**Definition:** The state in which an individual experiences a decrease in the ability to guard the self from internal or external threats such as illness or injury.

### RELATED FACTORS

Extremes of age; Inadequate nutrition; Alcohol abuse; Abnormal blood profiles (leukopenia, thrombocytopenia, anemia, coagulation); Drug therapies (antineoplastic, corticosteroid, immune, anticoagulant, thrombolytic); Treatments (surgery, radiation); Diseases (e.g., cancer and immune disorders)

### DEFINING CHARACTERISTICS

**Subjective**

Neurosensory alterations; Chilling; Itching; Insomnia; Fatigue; Weakness; Anorexia

**Objective**

Deficient immunity; Impaired healing; Altered clotting; Maladaptive stress response; Perspiring [inappropriate]; Dyspnea; Cough; Restlessness; Immobility; Disorientation; Pressure sores

NOTE: The purpose of this diagnosis seems to be to combine multiple diagnoses under a single heading for ease of planning care when a number of variables may be present. Outcomes/evaluation criteria and interventions are specifically tied to individual related factors that are present, such as: Extremes of age: Concerns may include body temperature/thermoregulation or thought process/sensory-perceptual alterations, as well as risk for trauma, suffocation, or poisoning; and fluid volume imbalances; Inadequate nutrition: Brings up issues of nutrition, less than body requirements; infection, altered thought processes, trauma, ineffective coping, and altered family processes; Alcohol abuse: May be situational or chronic with problems ranging from ineffective breathing patterns, decreased cardiac output, and fluid volume deficit to nutritional problems, infection, trauma, altered thought processes, and coping/family process difficulties; Abnormal blood profile: Suggests possibility of fluid volume deficit, decreased tissue perfusion, impaired gas exchange, activity intolerance, or risk for infection; Drug therapies, treatments, and disease concerns: Would include risk for infection, fluid volume imbalances, altered skin/tissue integrity, pain, nutritional problems, fatigue, and emotional responses. It is suggested that the user refer to specific nursing diagnoses based on identified related factors and individual concerns for this patient in order to find appropriate outcomes and interventions.

## RAPE-TRAUMA SYNDROME [SPECIFY]

*Diagnostic Division: Ego Integrity*

**Definition:** Rape is forced and violent sexual penetration against the victim's will and without the victim's consent. The trauma syndrome that develops from an attack or attempted attack includes an acute phase of disorganization of the victim's lifestyle and a long-term process of reorganization of lifestyle. This syndrome includes the following three subcomponents: [A] Rape-Trauma, [B] Compound Reaction, and [C] Silent Reaction.

[NOTE: While attacks are most often directed toward women, men also may be victims.]

### DEFINING CHARACTERISTICS

**A: Rape-Trauma**

**Acute Phase**

Emotional reactions: anger, fear of physical violence and death, self-blame, embarrassment, humiliation, thoughts of revenge; Multiple physical symptoms: muscle tension, sleep pattern disturbance, gastrointestinal irritability, genitourinary discomfort

**Long-Term Phase**

Changes in lifestyle (changes in residence; dealing with repetitive nightmares and phobias; seeking family support; seeking social network support)

**B: Compound Reaction**

All defining characteristics listed under A: Rape-Trauma; Reactivated symptoms of previous conditions, e.g., physical illness, psychiatric illness; Reliance on alcohol and/or drugs

**C: Silent Reaction**

Abrupt changes in relationship with men; Increase in nightmares; Increasing anxiety during interview, e.g., blocking of associations, long periods of silence, minor stuttering, physical distress; Marked changes in sexual behavior; No verbalization of the occurrence of rape; Sudden onset of phobic reactions

## RELOCATION STRESS SYNDROME

*Diagnostic Division: Ego Integrity*

**Definition:** Physiologic and/or psychological disturbances as a result of transfer from one environment to another.

### RELATED FACTORS

Past, concurrent, and recent losses; Losses involved with decision to move; Feeling of powerlessness; Lack of adequate support system; Little or no preparation for the impending move; Moderate to high degree of environmental change; History and types of previous transfers; Impaired psychosocial health status; Decreased physical health status

### DEFINING CHARACTERISTICS

**Subjective**

Anxiety; Apprehension; Depression; Loneliness; Verbalization of unwillingness to relocate; Sleep disturbance; Change in eating habits; Gastrointestinal disturbances; Insecurity; Lack of trust; Unfavorable comparison of post-transfer/pre-transfer staff; Verbalization of being concerned/upset [angry] about transfer

**Objective**

Change in environment/location; Increased confusion (elderly population) [/cognitively impaired]; Increased (frequency of) verbalization of needs; Dependency; Sad affect; Vigilance; Weight change; Withdrawal; Hostile behavior/outbursts

## ROLE PERFORMANCE, ALTERED

*Diagnostic Division: Social Interaction*

**Definition:** Disruption in the way one perceives one's role performance.

### RELATED FACTORS

To be developed by NANDA: [Crisis:] [Situational, e.g., male head of household is in a passive, dependent patient role, absence of role model, transitions, conflicts between various roles]; [Developmental (age, values/beliefs)]; and/or [Health-illness, e.g., chronic illness, change in physical capacity, perceptual problems].

**DEFINING CHARACTERISTICS**

**Subjective**

Change in self-perception of role; Denial of role; Lack of knowledge of role

**Objective**

Change in others' perception of role; Change in usual patterns or responsibility; Conflict in roles; Change in physical capacity to resume role; [Failure to assume role]

## SELF-CARE DEFICIT [SPECIFY LEVEL]: FEEDING, BATHING/HYGIENE, DRESSING/GROOMING, TOILETING

*Diagnostic Division: Hygiene*

**Definition:** A state in which the individual experiences an impaired ability to perform or to complete feeding, bathing/hygiene, toileting, dressing, and grooming activities for oneself (on a temporary, permanent, or progressing basis).

[NOTE: Self-care also may be expanded to include the practices used by the client to promote health, the individual responsibility for self, a way of thinking. Refer to Home Maintenance Management, impaired; Health Maintenance, altered.]

**RELATED FACTORS**

Intolerance to activity, decreased strength and endurance; Neuromuscular impairment; Depression; severe anxiety; Pain, discomfort; Perceptual or cognitive impairment; Musculoskeletal impairment; Impaired transfer ability (self-toileting); Impaired mobility status (self-toileting); [Mechanical restrictions such as cast, splint, traction, ventilator]

**DEFINING CHARACTERISTICS**

**A. Self-Feeding Deficit:**

Inability to bring food from a receptacle to the mouth; [Inability to open packages, cook/prepare food]

**B. Self-Bathing/Hygiene Deficit:**

Inability to wash body or body parts; to obtain or to get to water source; to regulate temperature or flow

**C. Self-Dressing/Grooming Deficit:**

Impaired ability to put on or to take off necessary items of clothing; to obtain or to replace articles of clothing; to fasten clothing; to maintain appearance at a satisfactory level

**D. Self-Toileting Deficit:**

Unable to get to toilet or commode; Unable to manipulate clothing for toileting; Unable to sit on or rise from toilet or commode; Unable to carry out proper toilet hygiene; Unable to flush toilet or empty commode

## SELF-ESTEEM, CHRONIC LOW

*Diagnostic Division: Ego Integrity*

**Definition:** Longstanding negative self-evaluation/feelings about self or self-capabilities.

**RELATED FACTORS**

To be developed by NANDA: [Continual negative evaluation of self/capabilities from childhood]; [Personal vulnerability]; [Life choices perpetuating failure; ineffective social/occupational functioning]; [Feelings of abandonment by significant other; willingness to tolerate possibly life-threatening domestic violence]; [Chronic physical/psychiatric conditions; antisocial behaviors]

**DEFINING CHARACTERISTICS**

**Subjective**

[Observations or] self-reports of self-negation; Shame; Guilt; Evaluating self as unable to deal with events

**Objective**

Observations [or self-reports] of Rationalizing away/rejecting positive feedback about self; Exaggerating negative feedback; Hesitant to try new things/situations; Frequent lack of success in work and other life events; Being overly conforming or dependent on others' opinions; Lack of culturally appropriate eye contact; Nonassertion; Passivity; Indecisiveness; Excessively seeking reassurance

## SELF-ESTEEM DISTURBANCE

*Diagnostic Division: Ego Integrity*

**Definition:** Negative self-evaluation/feelings about self or self-capabilities that may be directly or indirectly expressed. [Self-esteem is a human need for survival.]

### RELATED FACTORS

To be developed by NANDA: [Unsatisfactory parent-child relationship]; [Unrealistic expectations (on the part of self and others)]; [Unmet dependency needs]; [Absent, erratic, or inconsistent parental discipline]; [Dysfunctional family system]; [Child/sexual abuse or neglect]; [Underdeveloped ego and punitive superego, retarded ego development]; [Negative role models]; [Disorganized or chaotic environments]; [Extreme poverty]; [Lack of positive feedback, repeated negative feedback resulting in diminished self-worth]; [Perceived/numerous failures (learned helplessness); "Failure" at life events (e.g., loss of job, divorce, relationship problems)]; [Impaired cognition fostering negative view of self]; [Aging]

### DEFINING CHARACTERISTICS

#### Subjective

Self-negating verbalization; Evaluates self as unable to deal with events; Expressions of shame/guilt; [Inability to accept positive reinforcement]

#### Objective

Rationalizes away/rejects positive feedback and exaggerates negative feedback about self; Hesitant to try new things/situations; Hypersensitive to slight or criticism; Denial of problems obvious to others; Projection of blame/responsibility for problems; Rationalizing personal failures; [Not taking responsibility for self-care (self-neglect)]; [Lack of follow-through]; [Nonparticipation in therapy]; [Self-destructive behavior; accident prone]; [Lack of eye contact]

NOTE: Taxonomically this diagnosis is a broad category that has been subdivided into situational low and chronic low. When initial assessment reveals this diagnosis, further evaluation is required to determine the patient's specific needs.

## SELF-ESTEEM, SITUATIONAL LOW

*Diagnostic Division: Ego Integrity*

**Definition:** Episodic feelings about self or capabilities which develop in response to a loss or change.

### RELATED FACTORS

To be developed by NANDA: ["Failure" at life event (e.g., loss of job, relationship problems, divorce)]; [Feelings of abandonment by significant other]; [Maturational transitions, adolescence, aging]; [Perceived loss of control in some aspect of life]; [Loss of health status/body part/independent functioning]; [Memory deficits/cognitive impairment]; [Loss of capability for effective verbal communication]

### DEFINING CHARACTERISTICS

#### Subjective

[Observations or] self-reports of: Self-negation; Shame; Guilt; Inability to handle situations/events; Difficulty making decisions

#### Objective

Self-reports of: Significant recent loss or change; Negative feelings about self

## SELF-MUTILATION, RISK FOR

*Diagnostic Division: Safety*

**Definition:** A state in which the individual is at risk to perform an act upon the self to injure, not kill, which produces tissue damage and tension relief.

### RISK FACTORS

#### Groups at Risk

Clients with borderline personality disorder, especially females 16 to 25 years of age; Clients in psychotic state—frequently males in young adulthood; Emotionally disturbed and/or battered children; [Clients with organic conditions, e.g.,] mental retardation and autism, [encephalitis, Tourette's syndrome, acute intoxication, Addison's disease] Clients with a history of self-injury; Clients with a history of physical, emotional, or sexual abuse

[The following factors originally noted by NANDA as Risk Factors are now classified as Defining Characteristics. Because a risk diagnosis is not evidenced by signs and symptoms, we will continue to list these as Risk Factors.]

Inability to cope with increased psychological-physiologic tension in a healthy manner; Feelings of depression, rejection, self-hatred, separation anxiety, guilt, and depersonalization; Fluctuating emotions; Command hallucinations; Need for sensory stimuli; Parental emotional deprivation; Dysfunctional family

## SENSORY/PERCEPTUAL ALTERATIONS (SPECIFY): VISUAL, AUDITORY, KINESTHETIC, GUSTATORY, TACTILE, OLFACTORY

*Diagnostic Division: Neurosensory*

**Definition:** A state in which an individual experiences a change in the amount or patterning of oncoming stimuli accompanied by a diminished, exaggerated, distorted, or impaired response to such stimuli.

### RELATED FACTORS

Altered environmental stimuli, excessive or insufficient; [Therapeutically restricted environments, e.g., isolation, intensive care, bed rest, traction, confining illnesses, incubator]; [Socially restricted environment (e.g., institutionalization, homebound, aging, chronic/terminal illness, dying, infant deprivation; stigmatized (e.g., mentally ill/retarded/handicapped); bereaved]; [Excessive noise level, e.g., work environment, patient's immediate environment (ICU with support machinery, etc.)]; Altered sensory reception, transmission, and/or integration: [Neurologic disease/trauma/deficit, altered status of sense organs, inability to communicate/understand/speak/respond, sleep deprivation, and/or pain (phantom limb)]; Chemical alterations: endogenous (electrolyte) [elevated BUN, elevated ammonia, hypoxia], exogenous (drugs, etc.) [central nervous system stimulants or depressants, mind-altering drugs]; Psychologic stress [narrowed perceptual fields caused by anxiety]

### DEFINING CHARACTERISTICS

**Subjective**

Anxiety [panic state]; Indication of body image alteration; Reported change in sensory acuity [e.g., photosensitivity, hypoesthesia/hyperesthesia, diminished/altered sense of taste, inability to tell position of body parts (proprioception), visual/auditory distortions]; [Reports of pain]

**Objective**

Measured change in sensory acuity; Change in problem-solving abilities; [Lack of/poor concentration]; Altered abstraction/conceptualization; [Disordered thought sequencing]; Disoriented in time, in place, or with persons; Altered communication patterns; Change in usual response to stimuli; [Rapid mood swings, exaggerated emotional responses]; Change in behavior pattern; Apathy; Restlessness, irritability; [Bizarre thinking]; [Motor incoordination; altered sense of balance/falls, e.g., Ménière's syndrome]

### OTHER POSSIBLE CHARACTERISTICS

**Subjective**

Complaints [reports] of fatigue

**Objective**

Change in muscular tension; Hallucinations; Alteration in posture; Inappropriate responses

## SEXUAL DYSFUNCTION

*Diagnostic Division: Sexuality (Component of Social Interaction)*

**Definition:** The state in which an individual experiences a change in sexual function that is viewed as unsatisfying, unrewarding, or inadequate.

### RELATED FACTORS

Biopsychosocial alteration of sexuality: Ineffectual or absent role models; Vulnerability; Misinformation or lack of knowledge; Physical abuse; Values conflict; Lack of privacy; Altered body structure or function: pregnancy, recent childbirth, drugs, surgery, anomalies, disease process, trauma [paraplegia/quadriplegia], radiation; Psychosocial abuse, e.g., harmful relationships; Lack of significant other; [Loss of sexual desire]; [Disruption of sexual response pattern, e.g., premature ejaculation, dyspareunia, vaginismus]

### DEFINING CHARACTERISTICS

**Subjective**

Verbalization of problem; Actual or perceived limitation imposed by disease and/or therapy; Inability to achieve desired satisfaction; Alterations in achieving perceived sex role; Conflicts involving values; Alterations in achieving sexual satisfaction; Seeking of confirmation of desirability

**Objective**

Alteration in relationship with significant other; Change of interest in self and others

## SEXUALITY PATTERNS, ALTERED

*Diagnostic Division: Sexuality (Component of Social Interaction)*

**Definition:** The state in which an individual expresses concern regarding his/her sexuality.

**RELATED FACTORS**

Knowledge/skill deficit about alternative responses to health-related transitions, altered body function or structure, illness or medical treatment; Lack of privacy; Lack of significant other; Ineffective or absent role models; Conflicts with sexual orientation or variant preferences; Fear of pregnancy or of acquiring a sexually transmitted disease; Impaired relationship with a significant other

**DEFINING CHARACTERISTICS**

**Subjective**

Reported difficulties, limitations, or changes in sexual behaviors or activities; [Expressions of feeling of alienation, loneliness, loss, powerlessness, anger]

## SKIN INTEGRITY, IMPAIRED

*Diagnostic Division: Safety*

**Definition:** A state in which the individual's skin is adversely altered. [An interruption in the integumentary system, the largest multifunctional organ of the body.]

**RELATED FACTORS**

**External (Environmental)**

Hyperthermia or hypothermia; Chemical substance; Radiation; Physical immobilization; Humidity; Mechanical factors (shearing forces, pressure, restraint); [Excretions/secretions]; [Trauma: injury/surgery]

**Internal (Somatic)**

Medication; Altered nutritional state (obesity, emaciation); Metabolic state; Circulation; Sensation; Pigmentation; Skeletal prominence; Developmental factors; Alterations in turgor (change in elasticity); Immunologic deficit; [Psychogenic]; [Presence of edema]

**DEFINING CHARACTERISTICS**

**Subjective**

[Reports of itching/pain/numbness of affected/surrounding area]

**Objective**

Disruption of skin surface; Destruction of skin layers; Invasion of body structures

## SKIN INTEGRITY, IMPAIRED, RISK FOR

*Diagnostic Division: Safety*

**Definition:** A state in which the individual's skin is at risk of being adversely altered.

**RISK FACTORS**

**External (Environmental)**

Chemical substance; Hypothermia or hyperthermia; Radiation; Physical immobilization; Excretions and secretions; Humidity; Mechanical factors (shearing forces, pressure, restraint)

**Internal (Somatic)**

Medication; Alterations in nutrition state (obesity, emaciation); Metabolic state; Circulation; Sensation; Pigmentation; Skeletal prominence; Developmental factors; Alterations in skin turgor (change in elasticity); Psychogenic; Immunologic; [Presence of edema]

## SLEEP PATTERN DISTURBANCE

*Diagnostic Division: Activity/Rest*

**Definition:** Disruption of sleep time, which causes patient discomfort or interferes with desired lifestyle.

**RELATED FACTORS**

Sensory alterations: Internal factors: illness, [pain]; psychologic stress [anxiety, depression]; [inactivity]; External factors: environmental changes [including change of work shift, hospital routine]; social cues [e.g., demands of caring for others]

**DEFINING CHARACTERISTICS**

**Subjective**

Verbal complaints [reports] of difficulty in falling asleep; Verbal complaints [reports] of not feeling well rested; Awakening earlier or later than desired; Interrupted sleep; [Falls asleep during activities]

**Objective**

Changes in behavior and performance: Increasing irritability, Disorientation, Listlessness, Restlessness, Lethargy; Physical signs: Mild, fleeting nystagmus, Ptosis of eyelid, Slight hand tremor, Expressionless face; Thick speech with mispronunciation and incorrect words; Dark circles under eyes; Changes in posture; Frequent yawning

## SOCIAL INTERACTION, IMPAIRED

*Diagnostic Division: Social Interaction*

**Definition:** The state in which an individual participates in an insufficient or excessive quantity or ineffective quality of social exchange.

**RELATED FACTORS**

Knowledge/skill deficit about ways to enhance mutuality; Communication barriers [including head injury, stroke, other neurologic conditions affecting ability to communicate]; Self-concept disturbance; Absence of available significant others or peers; Limited physical mobility [e.g., neuromuscular disease]; Therapeutic isolation; Sociocultural dissonance; Environmental barriers; Altered thought processes

**DEFINING CHARACTERISTICS**

**Subjective**

Verbalized discomfort in social situations; Verbalized inability to receive or communicate a satisfying sense of belonging, caring, interest, or shared history; Family report of change of style or pattern of interaction

**Objective**

Observed discomfort in social situations; Observed inability to receive or communicate a satisfying sense of belonging, caring, interest, or shared history; Observed use of unsuccessful social interaction behaviors; Dysfunctional interaction with peers, family, and/or others

## SOCIAL ISOLATION

*Diagnostic Division: Social Interaction*

**Definition:** Aloneness experienced by the individual and perceived as imposed by others and as a negative or threatened state.

**RISK FACTORS**

Factors contributing to the absence of satisfying personal relationships, such as the following: Delay in accomplishing developmental tasks; Alterations in mental status; Altered state of wellness; Immature interests; Alterations in physical appearance; Unaccepted social behavior; Unaccepted social values; Inadequate personal resources; Inability to engage in satisfying personal relationships; [Traumatic incidents or events causing physical and/or emotional pain]

**DEFINING CHARACTERISTICS**

**Subjective**

Expresses feeling of aloneness imposed by others; Expresses values acceptable to subculture, but unable to accept values of dominant culture; Inability to meet expectations of others; Expresses feelings of rejection; Experiences feelings of difference from others; Inadequacy in or absence of significant purpose in life; Expresses interests inappropriate to developmental age or stage; Insecurity in public

**Objective**

Sad, dull affect; Absence of supportive significant other(s)—family, friends, group; Evidence of physical and/or mental handicap or altered state of wellness; Uncommunicative, withdrawn; no eye contact; Preoccupation with own thoughts; repetitive, meaningless actions; Inappropriate or immature interest and activities for developmental age or stage; Projects hostility in voice, behavior; Seeks to be alone or exists in subculture; Shows behavior unaccepted by dominant cultural group

## SPIRITUAL DISTRESS (DISTRESS OF THE HUMAN SPIRIT)

*Diagnostic Division: Ego Integrity*

**Definition:** Disruption in the life principle that pervades a person's entire being and that integrates and transcends one's biologic and psychosocial nature.

**RELATED FACTORS**

Separation from religious and cultural ties; Challenged belief and value system, e.g., result of moral or ethical implications of therapy or result of intense suffering

**DEFINING CHARACTERISTICS**

**Subjective**

Expresses concern with meaning of life and death and/or belief systems; Verbalizes inner conflict about beliefs; concern about relationship with deity; Questions moral and ethical implications of therapeutic regimen; Description of nightmares or sleep disturbances; [Unable to accept self]; [Engages in self-blame]; [Description of somatic symptoms]; Anger toward God (as defined by the person); Questions meaning of suffering; Questions meaning of own existence; Seeks spiritual assistance; Unable [or chooses not] to participate in usual religious practices; Displacement of anger toward religious representatives; [Regards illness as punishment]; [Does not experience that God is forgiving]; Denies responsibilities for problems

**Objective**

Alteration in behavior or mood evidenced by anger, crying, withdrawal, preoccupation, anxiety, hostility, apathy, etc.; Gallows humor

## SPIRITUAL WELL-BEING, ENHANCED, POTENTIAL FOR

*Diagnostic Division: Ego Integrity*

**Definition:** The process of an individual's developing/unfolding of mystery through harmonious interconnectedness that springs from inner strengths. [The ability to invest meaning, value, and purpose in life that gives harmony, peace, and contentment, providing for life-affirming relationships with deity, self, community, and environment.]

### DEFINING CHARACTERISTICS

**Subjective**

Inner strength: A sense of awareness, self-consciousness, sacred source, unifying force, inner core, and transcendence; Unfolding mystery: One's experience about life's purpose and meaning, mystery, uncertainty, and struggles; Harmonious interconnectedness: Relatedness, connectedness, harmony with self, others, higher power/God, and the environment

## SPONTANEOUS VENTILATION, INABILITY TO SUSTAIN

*Diagnostic Division: Respiration*

**Definition:** A state in which the response pattern of decreased energy reserves results in an individual's inability to maintain breathing adequate to support life.

### RELATED FACTORS

Metabolic factors; [hypermetabolic state (e.g., infection), nutritional deficits/depletion of energy stores]; Respiratory muscle fatigue; [Airway size/resistance; problems with secretion management]

### DEFINING CHARACTERISTICS

**Subjective**

Dyspnea; Apprehension

**Objective**

Increased metabolic rate; Increased restlessness; Increased use of accessory muscles; Decreased tidal volume; Increased heart rate; Decreased $Po_2$; Increased $Pco_2$; Decreased cooperation; Decreased $Sao_2$

## SUFFOCATION, RISK FOR

*Diagnostic Division: Safety*

**Definition:** Accentuated risk of accidental suffocation (inadequate air available for inhalation).

### RISK FACTORS

**Internal (individual)**

Reduced olfactory sensation; Reduced motor abilities; Lack of safety education, precautions; Cognitive or emotional difficulties [altered consciousness/mentation]; Disease or injury process.

**External (environmental)**

Pillow/propped bottle placed in an infant's crib; Vehicle warming in closed garage [faulty exhaust system]; Children playing with plastic bags or inserting small objects into their mouths or noses; Discarded or unused refrigerators or freezers without removed doors; Children left unattended in bathtubs or pools; Household gas leaks; Smoking in bed; Use of fuel-burning heaters not vented to outside; Low-strung clothesline; Pacifier hung around infant's head; Eating of large mouthfuls of food

## SWALLOWING, IMPAIRED

*Diagnostic Division: Food/Fluid*

**Definition:** The state in which an individual has decreased ability to voluntarily pass fluids and/or solids from the mouth to the stomach.

**RELATED FACTORS**

Neuromuscular impairment (e.g., decreased or absent gag reflex, decreased strength or excursion of muscles involved in mastication [and swallowing], perceptual impairment [decreased sensation in oral cavity], facial paralysis); Mechanical obstruction (e.g., edema, tracheostomy tube, tumor); Fatigue; Limited awareness; Reddened, irritated oropharyngeal cavity

**DEFINING CHARACTERISTICS**

**Objective**

Observed evidence of difficulty in swallowing (e.g., stasis of food in oral cavity [pocketing/squirreling of food, food sticking], coughing/choking); [drooling, stranding phlegm, swallowing incoordination—repeated swallows, nasal regurgitation, wet/hoarse voice]; Evidence of aspiration, [foamy phlegm]; [Facial droop, difficulty chewing]

## THERAPEUTIC REGIMEN (COMMUNITY), INEFFECTIVE MANAGEMENT OF

*Diagnostic Division: Teaching/Learning*

**Definition:** A pattern of regulating and integrating into community processes programs for treatment of illness and the sequelae of illness that are unsatisfactory for meeting health-related goals.

**RELATED FACTORS**

To be developed by NANDA: [Lack of safety for community members]; [Economic insecurity]; [Health care not available]; [Unhealthy environment]; [Education not available for all community members]; [Does not possess means to meet human needs for recognition, fellowship, security, and membership]

**DEFINING CHARACTERISTICS**

**Subjective**

[Community members/agencies verbalize inability to meet therapeutic needs of all members]; [Community members/agencies verbalize overburdening of resources for meeting therapeutic needs of all members]

**Objective**

Deficits in persons and programs to be accountable for illness care of aggregates; Deficits in advocates for aggregates; Deficit in community activities for [primary medical care/prevention]/secondary and tertiary prevention; Illness symptoms above the norm expected for the number and type of population; unexpected acceleration of illness(es); Number of healthcare resources insufficient[/unavailable] for the incidence or prevalence of illness(es); [Deficits in community for collaboration and development of coalitions to address programs for treatment of illness and the sequelae of illness]

## THERAPEUTIC REGIMEN (FAMILIES), INEFFECTIVE MANAGEMENT OF

*Diagnostic Division: Teaching/Learning*

**Definition:** A pattern of regulating and integrating into family processes a program for treatment of illness and the sequelae of illness that is unsatisfactory for meeting specific health needs.

**RELATED FACTORS**

Complexity of health care system; Complexity of therapeutic regimen; Decisional conflicts; Economic difficulties; Excessive demands made on individual or family; Family conflict

**DEFINING CHARACTERISTICS**

**Subjective**

Verbalized difficulty with regulation/integration of one or more effects or prevention of complication; [inability to manage treatment regimen]; Verbalized desire to manage the treatment of illness and prevention of the sequelae; Verbalizes that family did not take action to reduce risk factors for progression of illness and sequelae

**Objective**

Inappropriate family activities for meeting the goals of a treatment or prevention program; Acceleration (expected or unexpected) of illness symptoms of a family member; Lack of attention to illness and its sequelae

## THERAPEUTIC REGIMEN (INDIVIDUAL), EFFECTIVE MANAGEMENT OF

*Diagnostic Division: Teaching/Learning*

**Definition:** A pattern of regulating and integrating into daily living a program for treatment of illness and its sequelae that is satisfactory for meeting specific health goals.

**DEFINING CHARACTERISTICS**

**Subjective**

Verbalized desire to manage the treatment of illness and prevention of sequelae; Verbalized intent to reduce risk factors for progression of illness and sequelae

**Objective**

Appropriate choices of daily activities for meeting the goals of a treatment or prevention program; Illness symptoms are within a normal range of expectation

## THERAPEUTIC REGIMEN (INDIVIDUAL), INEFFECTIVE MANAGEMENT OF

*Diagnostic Division: Teaching/Learning*

**Definition:** A pattern of regulating and integrating into daily living a program for treatment of illness and the sequelae of illness that is unsatisfactory for meeting specific health goals.

**RELATED FACTORS**

Complexity of health care system; Complexity of therapeutic regimen; Decisional conflicts; Economic difficulties; Excessive demands made on individual or family; Family conflict; Family patterns of health care; Inadequate number and types of cues to action; Knowledge deficits; Mistrust of regimen and/or health care personnel; Perceived seriousness; Perceived susceptibility; Perceived barriers; Perceived benefits; Powerlessness; Social support deficits

**DEFINING CHARACTERISTICS**

**Subjective**

Verbalized desire to manage the treatment of illness and prevention of sequelae; Verbalized difficulty with regulation/integration of one or more prescribed regimens for treatment of illness and its effects or prevention of complications; Verbalized that did not take action to include treatment regimens in daily routines; Verbalized that did not take action to reduce risk factors for progression of illness and sequelae

**Objective**

Inappropriate choices of daily living for meeting the goals of a treatment or prevention program; Acceleration (expected or unexpected) of illness symptoms

## THERMOREGULATION, INEFFECTIVE

*Diagnostic Division: Safety*

**Definition:** The state in which the individual's temperature fluctuates between hypothermia and hyperthermia.

**RELATED FACTORS**

Trauma or illness [e.g., cerebral edema, cerebrovascular accident, intracranial surgery, or head injury]; Immaturity, aging [e.g., loss/absence of brown adipose tissue]; Fluctuating environmental temperature; [Changes in hypothalamic tissue, causing alterations in emission of thermosensitive cells and regulation of heat loss/production]; [Changes in level/action of thyroxine and catecholamines]; [Changes in metabolic rate/activity]; [Chemical reactions in contracting muscles]

**DEFINING CHARACTERISTICS**

**Objective**

Fluctuations in body temperature above or below the normal range; (Also refer to) defining characteristics present in hypothermia and hyperthermia.

## THOUGHT PROCESSES, ALTERED

*Diagnostic Division: Neurosensory*

**Definition:** A state in which an individual experiences a disruption in cognitive operations and activities.

**RELATED FACTORS**

To be developed by NANDA: [Physiologic changes, aging, hypoxia, head injury, malnutrition, infections]; [Biochemical changes, medications, substance abuse]; [Sleep deprivation]; [Psychological conflicts, emotional changes, mental disorders]

**DEFINING CHARACTERISTICS**

**Subjective**

[Ideas of reference, hallucinations, delusions]

**Objective**

Inaccurate interpretation of environment; Memory deficit/problems [disorientation to time, place, person, circumstances, and events, loss of short-term/remote memory]; Hypervigilance/hypovigilance; Cognitive dissonance, [Decreased ability to grasp ideas, make decisions, problem-solve, reason-abstract or conceptualize, calculate]; Disordered thought sequencing; Distractibility [altered attention span]; Egocentricity; [Confabulation]; [Inappropriate social behavior]

**OTHER POSSIBLE CHARACTERISTICS**
**Objective**
Inappropriate/nonreality-based thinking

## TISSUE INTEGRITY, IMPAIRED

*Diagnostic Division: Safety*

**Definition:** A state in which an individual experiences damage to mucous membrane or corneal, integumentary, or subcutaneous tissue.

**RELATED FACTORS**
Altered circulation; Nutritional deficit/excess; Fluid deficit/excess; [metabolic or endocrine dysfunction]; Knowledge deficit; Impaired physical mobility; Irritants, chemical (including body excretions, secretions, medications); [infections]; Thermal (temperature extremes); Mechanical (pressure, shear, friction), radiation (including therapeutic radiation), [surgery]

**DEFINING CHARACTERISTICS**
**Objective**
Damaged or destroyed tissue (cornea, mucous membrane, integumentary, or subcutaneous)

## TISSUE PERFUSION, ALTERED (SPECIFY TYPE): CEREBRAL, CARDIOPULMONARY, RENAL, GASTROINTESTINAL, PERIPHERAL

*Diagnostic Division: Circulation*

**Definition:** The state in which an individual experiences a decrease in nutrition and oxygenation at the cellular level due to a deficit in capillary blood supply. [Tissue perfusion problems can exist without decreased cardiac output; however, there may be a relationship between cardiac output and tissue perfusion.]

**RELATED FACTORS**
Interruption of flow: arterial, venous; Hypervolemia; Exchange problems; Hypovolemia

**DEFINING CHARACTERISTICS**
**Subjective**
Claudication (M-1/H-2)*; [resting or aching pain]; [Angina]; [Palpitations]

**Objective**
Skin temperature: cold extremities (H-1/L-2); Skin color: dependent, blue or purple (M-1/L-2) [or mottled]; pale on elevation and color does not return on lowering leg (H-1/H-2); Diminished[/absent] arterial pulsations (H-1/H-2) (critical); Skin quality: shining (H-1/L-2); Lack of lanugo (H-1/M-2); Round scars covered with atrophied skin (H-1/M-2); Gangrene (L-1/H-2); Slow-growing, dry thick brittle nails (H-1/M-2); Blood pressure changes in extremities; Bruits (M-1/M-2); Slow healing of lesions (H-1/L-2); [Delayed capillary refill]

Further work and development are required for the subcomponents, specifically cerebral, renal, and gastrointestinal

**Cerebral**
**Objective**
[Restlessness]; [Behavior changes]; [Decreased cognition; memory loss]; [Altered consciousness]

**Renal**
**Objective**
[Decreased urinary output, changes in specific gravity]; [Edema formation]; [Hypertension]; [Changes in laboratory values]

**Gastrointestinal**
**Subjective**
[Pain]; [Nausea/vomiting]

**Objective**
[Changes in bowel sounds]; [Abdominal distention]; [Melena]

*H = high; M = moderate; L = low; 1 = chances that characteristic will be present, given diagnosis; 2 = estimated sensitivities and specificities; chances that characteristic will not be explained by any other diagnosis.

## TRAUMA, RISK FOR

*Diagnostic Division: Safety*

**Definition:** Accentuated risk of accidental tissue injury, e.g., wound, burn, fracture.

### RISK FACTORS

**Internal (individual)**

Weakness; Balancing difficulties; Reduced large, or small, muscle coordination; Lack of safety education/precautions; Cognitive or emotional difficulties; Poor vision; Reduced temperature and/or tactile sensation; Reduced hand/eye coordination; Insufficient finances to purchase safety equipment or to effect repairs; History of previous trauma

**External (environmental) [includes but is not limited to:]**

Slippery floors, (e.g., wet or highly waxed); Bathtub without hand grip or antislip equipment; Unsturdy or absent stair rails; High beds; Children playing without gates at top of stairs; Inappropriate call-for-aid mechanisms for bedresting client; Snow or ice on stairs, walkways; Unanchored rugs; Use of unsteady ladder or chairs; Entering unlighted rooms; Unanchored electric wires; Litter or liquid spills on floors or stairways; Obstructed passageways; Unsafe window protection in homes with young children; Pot handles facing toward front of stove; Potential igniting of gas leaks; Bathing in very hot water (e.g., unsupervised bathing of young children); Experimenting with chemicals or gasoline; Children playing with matches, candles, cigarettes; Highly flammable children's toys or clothing; Overloaded fuse boxes; Sliding on coarse bed linen or struggling within bed [/chair] restraints; Contact with acids or alkalis; Contact with intense cold; Overexposure to sun, sun lamps, radiotherapy; Guns or ammunition stored unlocked; Children playing with sharp-edged toys; Driving a mechanically unsafe vehicle; Driving at excessive speeds; Children riding in the front seat of car; Delayed lighting of gas burner or oven; Unscreened fires or heaters; Wearing of plastic aprons or flowing clothing around open flame; Inadequately stored combustibles or corrosives, (e.g., matches, oily rags, lye); Contact with rapidly moving machinery, industrial belts, or pulleys; Faulty electrical plugs, frayed wires, or defective appliances; Playing with fireworks or gunpowder; Use of cracked dishware or glasses; Knives stored uncovered; Large icicles hanging from roof; Exposure to dangerous machinery; High-crime neighborhood and vulnerable clients; Driving after partaking of alcoholic beverages or [other] drugs; Driving without necessary visual aids; Smoking in bed or near oxygen; Grease waste collected on stoves; Unrestrained infants/children riding in car; Unsafe road or road-crossing conditions; Play or work near vehicle pathways (e.g., driveways, lanes, railroad tracks); Overloaded electrical outlets; Use of thin or worn pot holders [or mitts]; Nonuse or misuse of seat restraints; Nonuse or misuse of necessary headgear for motorized cyclists or young children carried on adult bicycles

## UNILATERAL NEGLECT

*Diagnostic Division: Neurosensory*

**Definition:** The state in which an individual is perceptually unaware of and inattentive to one side of the body [and the immediate unilateral territory/space.]

### RELATED FACTORS

Effects of disturbed perceptual abilities, e.g., [homonymous] hemianopsia [or visual inattention]; One-sided blindness, neurologic illness or trauma; [Impaired cerebral blood flow]

### DEFINING CHARACTERISTICS

**Subjective**

[Reports feeling that part does not belong to own self]

**Objective**

Consistent inattention to stimuli on an affected side; Inadequate self-care [inability to satisfactorily perform activities of daily living]; [Lack of] Positioning and/or safety precautions in regard to the affected side; Does not look toward affected side; Leaves food on plate on the affected side; [Does not touch affected side]; [Failure to use the affected side of the body without being reminded to do so]

## URINARY ELIMINATION, ALTERED PATTERNS OF

*Diagnostic Division: Elimination*

**Definition:** The state in which an individual experiences a disturbance in urine elimination.

### RELATED FACTORS

Multiple causality, including: Sensory motor impairment; Anatomical obstruction; Urinary tract infection; [Mechanical trauma]; [Surgical diversion]; [Fluid/volume states]; [Psychogenic factors]

**DEFINING CHARACTERISTICS**
**Subjective**
Frequency; Hesitancy; Dysuria; Nocturia; [Enuresis]; [Urgency]

**Objective**
Incontinence; Retention

## URINARY RETENTION [ACUTE/CHRONIC]

*Diagnostic Division: Elimination*

**Definition:** The state in which the individual experiences incomplete emptying of the bladder. [High urethral pressure inhibits voiding until increased abdominal pressure causes urine to be involuntarily lost, or high urethral pressure inhibits timely/complete emptying of bladder.]

**RELATED FACTORS**
High urethral pressure caused by weak detrusor [absent detrusor]; Inhibition of reflex arc; Strong sphincter; Blockage [e.g., BPH, perineal swelling]; [Habituation of reflex arc]; [Use of medications with side effect of retention, e.g., atropine, belladonna, psychotropics, antihistamines, opiates]; [Infections]; [Neurologic diseases/trauma]

**DEFINING CHARACTERISTICS**
**Subjective**
Sensation of bladder fullness; Dribbling; Dysuria

**Objective**
Bladder distention; Small, frequent voiding or absence of urine output; Residual urine [150 ml or more]; Overflow incontinence; [Reduced stream]

## VENTILATORY WEANING RESPONSE, DYSFUNCTIONAL (DVWR)

*Diagnostic Division: Respiration*

**Definition:** A state in which a patient cannot adjust to lowered levels of mechanical ventilator support, which interrupts and prolongs the weaning process.

**RELATED FACTORS**
**Physical**
Ineffective airway clearance; Sleep pattern disturbance; Inadequate nutrition; Uncontrolled pain or discomfort; [Muscle weakness/fatigue, inability to control respiratory muscles; immobility]

**Psychological**
Knowledge deficit of the weaning process, patient role; Patient-perceived inefficacy about the ability to wean; Decreased motivation; Decreased self-esteem; Anxiety (moderate, severe); fear; insufficient trust in the nurse; Hopelessness; Powerlessness; [Unprepared for weaning attempt]

**Situational**
Uncontrolled episodic energy demands or problems; Inappropriate pacing of diminished ventilator support; Inadequate social support; Adverse environment (noisy, active environment, negative events in the room, low nurse-patient ratio, extended nurse absence from bedside, unfamiliar nursing staff); History of ventilator dependence >1 week; History of multiple unsuccessful weaning attempts

**DEFINING CHARACTERISTICS**
**Mild DVWR**
**Subjective**
Expressed feelings of increased need for oxygen, breathing discomfort, fatigue, warmth; Queries about possible machine malfunction

**Objective**
Restlessness; Slight increased respiratory rate from baseline; Increased concentration on breathing

**Moderate DVWR**
**Subjective**
Apprehension

**Objective**
Slight increase from baseline blood pressure <20 mm Hg; Slight increase from baseline heart rate <20 beats/min; Baseline increase in respiratory rate <5 breaths/min; Hypervigilance to activities; Inability to respond to coaching; Inability to cooperate; Diaphoresis; Eye widening ("wide-eyed look"); Decreased air entry on ausculation; Color changes: pallor, slight cyanosis; Slight respiratory accessory muscle use